			13/IIIa	14/IVa	15/Va	16/VIa	17/VIIa	0 2 He 4.002602 2
			+3 5 B 10.811 2-3	+2 +4 6 C 12.0107 2-4	±1 ±2 ±3 +4 +5 7 N 14.0067 2-5	−2 8 O 15.9994 2-6	−1 9 F 18.9984032 2-7	0 10 Ne 20.1797 2-8
			+3 13 Al 26.9815386 2-8-3	+2 +4 14 Si 28.0855 2-8-4	±3 +5 15 P 30.973762 2-8-5	+4 +6 −2 16 S 32.065 2-8-6	±1 +5 +7 17 Cl 35.453 2-8-7	0 18 Ar 39.948 2-8-8

10/VIII	11/Ib	12/IIb						
+2 +3 28 Ni 58.6934 -8-16-2	+1 +2 29 Cu 63.546 -8-18-1	+2 30 Zn 65.409 -8-18-2	+3 31 Ga 69.723 -8-18-3	+2 +4 32 Ge 72.64 -8-18-4	±3 +5 33 As 74.92160 -8-18-5	+4 +6 −2 34 Se 78.96 -8-18-6	±1 +5 35 Br 79.904 -8-18-7	0 36 Kr 83.798 -8-18-8
+2 +4 46 Pd 106.42 -18-18-0	+1 47 Ag 107.8682 -18-18-1	+2 48 Cd 112.411 -18-18-2	+3 49 In 114.818 -18-18-3	+2 +4 50 Sn 118.710 -18-18-4	±3 +5 51 Sb 121.760 -18-18-5	+4 +6 −2 52 Te 127.60 -18-18-6	±1 +5 +7 53 I 126.90447 -18-18-7	0 54 Xe 131.293 -18-18-8
+2 +4 78 Pt 195.084 -32-16-2	+1 +3 79 Au 196.966569 -32-18-1	+1 +2 80 Hg 200.59 -32-18-2	+1 +3 81 Tl 204.3833 -32-18-3	+2 +4 82 Pb 207.2 -32-18-4	+3 +5 83 Bi 208.98040 -32-18-5	+2 +4 84 Po (208.9824) -32-18-6	±1 +5 +7 85 At (209.9871) -32-18-7	0 86 Rn (222.0176) -32-18-8
110 Ds	111 Rg (272.1535)	112 *Uub		114 *Uuq		116 *Uuh		

Noble Gases

+2 +3 63 Eu 151.964 -25-8-2	+3 64 Gd 157.25 -25-9-2	+3 65 Tb 158.92535 -27-8-2	+3 66 Dy 162.500 -28-8-2	+3 67 Ho 164.93032 -29-8-2	+3 68 Er 167.259 -30-8-2	+3 69 Tm 168.93421 -31-8-2	+2 +3 70 Yb 173.04 -32-8-2	+3 71 Lu 174.967 -32-9-2
+3 +4 +5 +6 95 Am (243.0614) -25-8-2	+3 96 Cm (247.0704) -25-9-2	+3 +4 97 Bk (247.0703) -27-8-2	+3 98 Cf (251.0796) -28-8-2	+3 99 Es (252.0830) -29-8-2	+3 100 Fm (257.0951) -30-8-2	+2 +3 101 Md (258.0984) -31-8-2	+2 +3 102 No (259.1010) -32-8-2	+3 103 Lr (262.1097) -32-9-2

Note: Elements with atomic numbers 112 and above have been reported but not fully authenticated.

* Symbols based on IUPAC systematic names.

THE MERCK INDEX

FOURTEENTH EDITION

1st Edition—1889
2nd Edition—1896
3rd Edition—1907
4th Edition—1930
5th Edition—1940
6th Edition—1952
7th Edition—1960
8th Edition—1968
9th Edition—1976
10th Edition—1983
11th Edition—1989
12th Edition—1996
13th Edition—2001
14th Edition—2006

OTHER MERCK HANDBOOKS

THE MERCK MANUAL OF DIAGNOSIS AND THERAPY
First Edition, 1899

THE MERCK VETERINARY MANUAL
First Edition, 1955

THE MERCK MANUAL OF GERIATRICS
First Edition, 1990

THE MERCK MANUAL OF MEDICAL INFORMATION—HOME EDITION
First Edition, 1997

THE MERCK MANUAL OF HEALTH & AGING
First Edition, 2004

The Merck Handbooks are published as a not-for-profit service
to the scientific community and the public.

THE

MERCK INDEX

AN ENCYCLOPEDIA OF
CHEMICALS, DRUGS, AND BIOLOGICALS

FOURTEENTH EDITION

Maryadele J. O'Neil, *Editor*
Patricia E. Heckelman, *Senior Associate Editor*
Cherie B. Koch, *Associate Editor*
Kristin J. Roman, *Assistant Editor*

Catherine M. Kenny, *Editorial Assistant*
Maryann R. D'Arecca, *Administrative Associate*

Published by
Merck Research Laboratories
Division of

MERCK & CO., INC.
Whitehouse Station, NJ, USA

2006

Library of Congress Catalog Card Number 89-60001
ISBN Number 0-911910-00-X
ISBN Number 978-0-911910-00-1

Printed in the USA

FOREWORD

For more than a century, *The Merck Index*, Chemistry's Constant Companion™, has provided quick and reliable answers to questions arising in the course of the scientist's work. The Fourteenth Edition continues this tradition to publish an authoritative, multidisciplinary reference handbook committed to scientific excellence.

Each edition is reflective of key scientific discoveries of its time period. Once again, significant new compounds have been carefully selected from biomedicine, agriculture, and various disciplines of chemistry. With the particular needs of the research scientist in mind, every effort has been made to include additional physical property information in the monographs. Coverage of important new tools for pharmacological research and organic synthesis has been expanded and includes more than 140 monographs on Name Reagents. The Organic Name Reactions have again been updated and now include 450 entries.

The Supplemental Tables have been extensively revised. More than 70 pages of hard-to-find information complement the material presented in the other sections. New for this edition is a table describing vaccine preparations for use in the prevention of infectious disease, an area of research never before covered in this reference work. Another new table provides the expanded meanings for acronyms encountered in biomedical and pharmaceutical research.

An important new feature introduced for this edition is the companion CD that accompanies the printed volume. This new multimedia reference set allows the scientist to use whichever format is most useful—hardcopy at the lab bench and CD in the laptop. The text searchable CD uses CambridgeSoft's ChemFinder® software to enable quick retrieval of data and provides access to nearly 1000 monographs retired from the 12th and 13th editions that are no longer available in print.

Merck & Co., Inc. is one of the world's largest pharmaceutical companies. Merck is committed to providing trusted medical and scientific information and continues to publish *The Merck Index* and all of the Merck Handbooks as a not-for-profit service to the scientific community and the public. We hope that this edition of *The Merck Index* will be an indispensable resource to all who use it.

ACKNOWLEDGMENTS

The successful publication of the Fourteenth Edition of *The Merck Index* would not have been possible without the close collaboration of many dedicated people who have generously contributed their expertise and special talents.

The Merck Index Staff wishes to acknowledge our coworkers whose contributions have been particularly significant: *Beverly Grodzinski* for system support and for organizing and tracking the production process; *John Ho* and *Bob Dougherty* for computer expertise, custom programming and technical guidance; *Sharon O'Brien* for designing the CD artwork; *Debra Shelinsky Greene* and *Hilary Wandall* for advice and counsel on intellectual property and contractual issues; *Pamela Barnes-Paul* for coordinating the advertising and marketing effort; *Margaret Hill*, *Ann Smith*, and the entire staff of the MRL Library for their ongoing assistance.

We are especially indebted to the many readers who took the time to contact us with comments, additions and corrections and to the generations of Merck scientists who have contributed to this and previous editions of *The Merck Index*.

Finally, special thanks are due to *Dr. John D. Irvin* of Merck Research Laboratories for his personal interest, encouragement and support; and to *Gary Zelko*, our publisher, for his collaboration and expertise in producing this edition.

TABLE OF CONTENTS

EXPLANATORY NOTES

The Fourteenth edition of *The Merck Index* contains 10,200 monographs describing significant chemicals, drugs, and biological substances. The entries cover a wide range of compounds which have been selected on the basis of present or historic importance and interest. Since the publication of the Thirteenth Edition in 2001, over 5,000 monographs have been significantly revised and updated. More than five hundred monographs have either been combined or deleted from the manuscript to make room for hundreds of new entries. Nearly 450 of these monographs, as well as 540 monographs archived from the Twelfth Edition, are presented in their original form on the companion CD which accompanies this volume.

Entries are generally limited to single substances and related compounds such as isomers or salts. While multi-component drugs are, for the most part, excluded, there are a number of monographs devoted to families of natural products or biological substances. Monographs vary greatly in length. The length of a monograph, however, is not necessarily indicative of the importance of a compound, but rather may simply be an indication of the amount of relevant published information available for the compound.

For the purpose of illustrating the general monograph format, a typical monograph is depicted and the components are identified. While all possible categories of information in a monograph are described below, it must be emphasized that not all categories are present in every monograph.

Monograph Number. Sequential accession numbers are assigned to monographs which are alphabetized by title. Entries in the indices are referenced to these accession numbers, not to page numbers. (*Note:* Monograph numbers in the Fourteenth Edition do not correspond to Thirteenth Edition monograph numbers.)

Monograph Title. Titles are usually simple chemical names or in the case of drugs, the commonly used generic name such as the USAN (United States Adopted Name) or INN (International Nonproprietary Name). Registered trademarks, designated by ®, are used for a small number of entry titles, primarily when nonproprietary terms are not available. Plant monographs are titled using a common name rather than the full botanical name.

Chemical Abstracts Registry Number(s). The Chemical Abstracts Service (CAS) Registry Number appears following the title. These unique identifiers are provided for title substances and for selected derivatives. Where appropriate, numbers for isomeric and unspecified forms of the compound are listed. Descriptors are appended to the entry if more than one registry number has been associated with the compound.

Chemical Abstracts Name(s). The uninverted form of the CAS Index Name appears in native font following the CAS Registry Number. When a specific isomer is being discussed, stereochemical descriptors have been included to more clearly delineate that isomer. CAS Registry Numbers and CAS Index Names are provided as aids for further searching of the compound of interest in *Chemical Abstracts* and elsewhere.

Alternate Name(s). Other chemical names, trivial names, experimental drug codes, and trademarks that identify the entry are listed. Listing of trademarks

Title

Chemical Abstracts Registry Number

Chemical Abstracts Name

Monograph number

1565. ***n*-Butyl Cyanoacrylate.** [6606-65-1] 2-Cyano-2-propenoic acid butyl ester; enbucrilate; NBCA; *n*-butyl 2-cyanoacrylate; Histoacryl; Indermil; Liquiband; Tisuacryl; Vetbond. $C_8H_{11}NO_2$; mol wt 153.18. C 62.73%, H 7.24%, N 9.14%, O 20.89%. Monomer rapidly polymerizes upon contact with fluid or tissue to form a strong, biodegradable adhesive. Preparative methods: A. E. Ardis, **US 2467927** (1949 to B. F. Goodrich); C. H. McKeever, **US 2912454** (1959 to Rohm & Haas). Prepn, polymerization and degradation: F. Leonard *et al., J. Appl. Polym. Sci.* **10**, 259 (1966). Mechanism of polymerization and nanoparticle formation: N. Behan *et al., Biomaterials* **22**, 1335 (2001). Characterization of polymer nanoparticles by particle size analysis: A. Bootz *et al., Eur. J. Pharm. Biopharm.* **57**, 369 (2004); by MS: *idem et al., ibid.* **60**, 391 (2005). Clinical experience in ophthalmic applications: A. B. Leahey *et al., Ophthalmology* **100**, 173 (1993); in closure of surgical incisions: G. E. Amiel *et al., J. Am. Coll. Surg.* **189**, 21 (1999). Clinical evaluation in augmentation rhinoplasty: M. E. Sachs, *Arch. Otolaryngol.* **111**, 389 (1985); in management of bleeding gastric varices: B. D. Greenwald *et al., Am. J. Gastroenterol.* **98**, 1982 (2003). Review of biomedical applications: C. Vauthier *et al., Adv. Drug Delivery Rev.* **55**, 519-548 (2003).

Molecular formula

Percentage composition

Alternate names and/or trademarks (capitalized) of title compound

Molecular weight

Chemical information

Literature references

Biological and pharmacological information

Reviews

Structure

H_3C—O—C(=O)—C(CN)=CH_2

Derivative Compound Chemical Abstracts Registry Number

Derivative of title compound

Non-medical use

Therapeutic category (in humans)

Colorless liquid. $bp_{1.8}$ 68°. d^{20} 0.989. n_D^{20} 1.4424. n_D^{25} 1.4410. Insol in water. Flash pt, closed cup: >176°F (>80°C). Vapor pressure (25°): <0.5 mmHg. Surface tension: 31.11 dynes/cm. *Highly reactive with water and weak bases.*

Polymer. [25154-80-7] Poly(butyl 2-cyanoacrylate).

USE: Adhesive. Polymer nanoparticles as pharmaceutic aid for controlled release drug delivery.

THERAP CAT: Tissue adhesive.

THERAP CAT (VET): Tissue adhesive.

Physical data for title compound

Alternate names and/or trademarks of the derivative compound

Therapeutic category (veterinary)

ix

is for information purposes only and it should not be assumed that the trademarks are in current use. The first letter of each trademark is capitalized; absence of capitalization, however, does not preclude that a name may either currently be a proprietary name, or may once have been the subject of proprietary rights. If known, the company associated with a particular trademark (as a manufacturer, distributor or trademark owner) is listed alongside the trademark in the Name Index.

Molecular Formula, Molecular Weight, % Composition. Elements in the molecular formula are listed according to the Hill convention (C, H, then other elements in alphabetical order). Formula and molecular weight are provided for title compounds having a specific known structure. All molecular weights have been recalculated using the 2005 IUPAC Table of Standard Atomic Weights.

Literature References. A concise reference history of each compound is provided. Frequently, there is a brief description or capsule statement to summarize the significance of the compound. References to isolation, preparation or synthesis, patent information, and structural studies are cited. While reference is made to various methods of synthesis, the intent is to give a representative, but by no means exhaustive list. Patent numbers are provided merely as a source of preparative information; however, whenever possible, the product patent has been cited in monographs. Patents are cited using the two letter international country code followed by the number in boldface print; the year of publication and the assignee are included if known. References to pharmacology or biological activity, clinical trials, and toxicity studies may be included, where appropriate. Review articles are usually cited at the end of the references. Reviews pertaining to a group of closely related compounds or to a family of natural substances are generally listed only in the monograph for the parent element or compound. Literature references are cited in the conventional manner; journal abbreviations generally correspond to those in CASSI (CAS Source Index®) or in the *List of Journals Indexed in Index Medicus*. The number of the first page of the reference is given; first and last page numbers are listed for reviews.

Structure. For this edition, all structures have been drawn according to current conventions using CambridgeSoft's ChemDraw® software package. Structural depictions, including stereochemistry, if relevant, are included in nearly 6,700 monographs. Structures that do not correspond precisely to the monograph title have been labeled to identify the specific form depicted. Standard conventions of heavy wedges and dotted lines to show bonds directed above or below the plane of the paper are used where appropriate. Whenever possible, double bond geometry has been defined within the structure. Amino acid residues are assumed to be L unless specified otherwise. In addition, 1,850 monographs contain line formulae showing molecular arrangements.

Physical Data. Data are cited as found in the literature. When several alternate data values appear in the literature, the data is evaluated and representative selections are made. The values are then reported with the corresponding source. Whenever possible, the color of a substance is stated, but the absence of color (white or colorless) is often omitted. Temperatures are given in degrees Celsius, unless otherwise noted. When solubilities are determined at room temperature (about 25°C), the temperature is generally omitted. When optical rotations are measured in water, the solvent is usually not specified. For ultraviolet absorption measurements, the solvent is given within parentheses.

An effort has been made to provide toxicity data (e.g. LD_{50}, LC_{50}) and to identify the source of this information. *Caution* and/or *Note* statements are also provided in a number of monographs. Specific statements are given for compounds on the U.S. Government's Schedules of Controlled Substances in Title 21 of the Code of Federal Regulations (CFR), for compounds listed as suspected or confirmed carcinogens in the *Eleventh Report on Carcinogens* issued in 2004 by the U.S. Department of Health and Human Services (USDHHS), and for chemicals considered potential occupational hazards as described in sources such as the *NIOSH Pocket Guide to Chemical Hazards (USDHHS)*. *Note:* Absence of toxicity data or specific cautions does not imply that toxic effects do not exist.

Derivatives. When derivatives (isomers, salts, etc.) of the title compound are described in a monograph, the information appears in the paragraph(s) directly following the physical data. These paragraphs may also be used to describe specific members of a large family of natural substances. Derivative data presentation mirrors that of the title compound and may include registry numbers, chemical and alternate names, molecular weights, percentage composition, literature references, and physical properties.

Use. Descriptions of specific uses, which are not medical or veterinary therapeutic applications, are summarized under this heading.

Therapeutic Category and Therapeutic Category (Veterinary). In most cases, therapeutic categories reflect the accepted terminology in the medical literature. When available, mode of action information is included in the literature references section of the monograph. Monographs for human drugs have been indexed by both therapeutic category and biological activity beginning on page THER-1.

The Merck Index is not intended as an official therapeutic guide. Inclusion of a drug or any other compound in this book is not an endorsement, but merely a statement of the fact that such a substance exists. THERAPEUTIC CATEGORY and THERAPEUTIC CATEGORY (VETERINARY) paragraphs are intended only as summary statements of major pharmacological properties or indications for the individual compounds. For additional information on uses, dosage, side effects, and adverse reactions, readers are directed to consult pertinent scientific and professional publications, product circulars, information sheets or material safety data sheets prepared or published by the respective manufacturers.

Indices. Four indices—Name, Formula, CAS Registry Number and Therapeutic Category—are included; each entry directs the reader to the number of the monograph in which the substance of interest is described. More than 60,000 synonyms, including titles, CAS names, alternate names, trademarks, and derivative names are contained in the **Name Index.** If known, trademarks have been matched with an associated company. An abbreviated form of the company name appears in brackets following the trademark. The complete company name and location is listed in an unpdated and expanded Company Register in the TABLES section of the book. Company names are provided as a source of additional information and do not necessarily imply trademark ownership. Due to reorganizations or mergers, some company names may have changed since the original matching process was completed.

More than 7,500 entries appear in the **Formula Index.** This index contains the molecular formula for the title compounds and derivatives other than acid addition salts, hydrates or isomers.

The **CAS Registry Number Index** of more than 12,000 entries arranged in ascending Registry Number order. Descriptors are appended to the entry if more than one registry number may be associated with the compound.

In the **Therapeutic Category and Biological Activity Index,** monographs describing human drugs have been listed by one or more therapeutic indications and/or mechanisms of action. Cross references to closely related categories and mechanisms have been included. Whenever appropriate, subclassifications have been developed by grouping compounds according to chemical or pharmacological similarities.

Organic Name Reactions. This section is comprised of 450 named reactions and an index. A concise reference history and associated reaction schema are provided for each reaction or subreaction.

Tables. A compilation of over 70 pages of tables is provided to supplement the material presented in the monographs. This section has been extensively revised for this edition and now includes tables of Acronyms, Vaccines, and Physical Constants.

Great care has been taken to assure the accuracy of the information contained in *The Merck Index.* However, the Editorial Staff and the Publisher cannot be responsible for errors incurred in publication or for any consequences arising from use of the information published in *The Merck Index.* Accordingly, reference to original sources is strongly encouraged, as is reporting of errors and omissions in order to assure that appropriate changes may be made in the next edition.

Abbreviations

Included are abbreviations commonly used in *The Merck Index*. Please consult the Acronyms and Glossary
(Suppl. Tables Section) for additional definitions.

α_D^{25}	specific optical rotation at 25° C for D (sodium) line; absence of brackets indicates optical rotation of a liquid in a 1 decimeter cell, neat
Å	angstrom
A	absorbance
Ab	antibody
abs	absolute; absorption
abs config	absolute configuration
Ag	antigen
alc	alcohol; ethanol; ethyl alcohol
alk	alkali(ne)
a_M	molar absorptivity
amps	ampules; amperes
anhydr	anhydrous
Ann.	*Justus Liebig's Annalen der Chemie*
approx; ~	approximate(ly)
aq	aqueous
as-; asym-	asymmetrical; unsymmetrical
at.	atomic
at. no.	atomic number
at. wt.	atomic weight
atm	atmosphere(s)
B.P.C.	British Pharmaceutical Codex
Bé	Baumé (a specific gravity scale)
Beilstein	*Beilstein's Handbuch der Organischen Chemie*
Ber.	*Chemische Berichte* (Berichte der Deutschen Chemischen Gesellschaft)
bp	basepair; boiling point
°C	Celsius degrees
c	concentration
ca.	(*circa*) about
cal	calorie(s)
calc(d)	calculate; calculated
cc	cubic centimeter(s) (milliliter)
cf.	(*confer*) compare
Ci	curie
coll. vol.	collective volume
compd	compound
compn	composition
concd	concentrated
concn	concentration
config	configuration
constit	constituent(s)
contd	continued
contg	containing
corr	corrected
corresp	corresponding; corresponds
C_p	heat capacity (constant pressure)
crit press	critical pressure
crit temp	critical temperature
cryst	crystalline; crystals
crystn	crystallization
Δ (delta)	indicates the locant of the double bond

d	density; specific gravity (d_4^{19} specific gravity at 19° referred to water at 4°)
d-	*dextro* (rotatory); the opposite of *l*
D-	*Dextro* configuration; opposite of L
Da	daltons
dec; decomp; decompn	decompose(s); decomposition
deg	degree
deliquesc	deliquescent
deriv	derivative
determn	determination
dil	dilute; diluted; dilution
distln	distillation
dl-	racemic
DL-	optically inactive by external compensation as contrasted with *meso-*
dyn	dynes
ε (epsilon)	molar extinction coefficient; dielectric constant
η (eta)	viscosity
E.C. No.	Enzyme Commission Number
e.g.	(*exempli gratia*) for example
$E_{1cm}^{1\%}$	the absorbance of a solution containing one gram per 100 ml contained in a cell having an absorption path of one cm
Ed(s).	editor(s)
ed.	edition
eidem	the same (authors); plural of *idem*
E_M	molar extinction coefficient (concn in g-moles/l)
equiv	equivalent
et al.	(*et alii*) and others
etc.	(*et cetera*) and so forth
eV	electron volt
evac	evacuated
evapn	evaporation
exptl	experimental(ly)
ext(d)	extract; extracted
extern	externally
°F	Fahrenheit degrees
fp	freezing point
Frdl.	*P. Friedlander Fortschritte der Teer-farbenfabrikation*, a collection of patents
g	gram(s)
Gmelin's	*Gmelin's Handbuch der Anorganischen Chemie*
habit.	habitat
Houben	a German collection of medicinal patents
Houben Weyl	*Houben-Weyl Methoden der Organischen Chemie*
hr	hour
i.e.	(*id est*) that is
i.g.	intragastric
i.m.	intramuscular
i.p.	intraperitoneal
I.U.	international unit
i.v.	intravenous

Abbreviations (Continued)

ibid.	(*ibidem*) at the same place	pK	log of the reciprocal of the dissociation constant
idem	the same (author); plural: *eidem*, the same (authors)	ppm	parts per million
incl	including	ppt; pptd	precipitate; precipitated
incompat	incompatibility	prepd; prepn	prepared; preparation
inorg	inorganic	press.	pressure
insol	insoluble	pt	point
Intl	International	*q.q.v.*	(*quae vide*) which see, plural
isoln	isolation	*q.v.*	(*quod vide*) which see
K	dissociation constant; equilibrium constant; Kelvin temperature	*r-*	racemic
		recryst(n)	recrystallize; recrystallization
λ (lambda)	wavelength; microliter	ref	reference
l	liter	rep [REP]	"roentgen equivalent physical" means a dose of ionizing radiation capable of producing energy absorption of 93 ergs per gram of tissue
l-	*levo*(rotatory); the opposite of *d*		
L-	*Levo* configuration; opposite of D		
LC_{50}	median lethal concentration; the concn of a chemical that is estimated to be fatal to 50% of the organism tested	resp	respectively
		s.c.	subcutaneous
LD_{50}	median lethal dose; the quantity of a chemical that is estimated to be fatal to 50% of the organisms tested	sapon(if)	saponification
		satd	saturated
		sec	second(s)
loc. cit.	(*loco citato*) in the place cited	sepn	separation
log	logarithm (common)	sol	soluble
log *P*	logarithm of the partition coefficient	soly	solubility
M	molar (concentration; moles/liter)	solidif	solidifies; solidification
m-	*meta* chemical locant for ring substituents	soln	solution
Mab; mAb	monoclonal antibody	sp gr	specific gravity
mass spec	mass spectrometry	*sp.*	species
MD	molecular rotation $\dfrac{[\alpha]_{\mathrm{D}} \times \text{mol wt}}{100}$	spec	spectroscopy; spectrum; spectral
		spp.	species (plural)
Mellor's	*Mellor's Comprehensive Treatise on Inorganic and Theoretical Chemistry*	*sqq*	(*sequentia*) and following
		subl	sublimes
Mfg; manuf	manufacturing	suppl	supplement
mfr	manufacturer	*sym-*	symmetrical
misc	miscible	$t_{1/2}$	half-life
mixt	mixture	tabl	tablet(s)
mol wt	molecular weight	tech	technical
Monatsh.	*Monatshefte für Chemie*	temp	temperature
mp	melting point	uncor(r)	uncorrected
M_r	relative molecular mass	*unsym-*	unsymmetrical; asymmetrical
N	normal concentration or nitrogen as a locant	UV; uv	ultraviolet
n	index of refraction (n_{D}^{20} for 20° and sodium light); normal, as *n*-propyl	v	volt(s)
		v-	(*vicinal*) adjacent
o-	*ortho* chemical locant for ring substituents	v/v	percent "volume in volume" expresses the number of milliliters of an active constituent in 100 milliliters of solution
op. cit.	(*opere citato*) in the work cited		
org	organic		
OsM	osmolar; osmole	var	variety
ψ (psi)	pseudo	*viz.*	(*videlicet*) that is to say; namely
P	poise	vol	volume
p-	*para* chemical locant for ring substituents	vs	versus
p; pp	page(s)	w/v	percent "weight in volume" expresses the number of grams of an active constituent in 100 milliliters of solution, and is used regardless of whether water or another liquid is the solvent
Pa	pascal		
passim	here and there; scattered		
pat.	patent		
petr	petroleum	w/w	percent "weight in weight" expresses the number of grams of an active constituent in 100 grams of solution or mixture
pH	acid-base scale; log of reciprocal of hydrogen ion concentration		
pI	isoelectric point	wt	weight

MONOGRAPHS

THE MERCK INDEX

OF CHEMICALS, DRUGS, AND BIOLOGICALS

A

1. Abacavir. [136470-78-5] (1S,4R)-4-[2-Amino-6-(cyclopropylamino)-9H-purin-9-yl]-2-cyclopentene-1-methanol; (−)-cis-4-[2-amino-6-(cyclopropylamino)-9H-purin-9-yl]-2-cyclopentene-1-methanol; 1592U89. $C_{14}H_{18}N_6O$; mol wt 286.33. C 58.73%, H 6.34%, N 29.35%, O 5.59%. Nucleoside reverse transcriptase inhibitor (NRTI). Prepn: S. M. Daluge, **EP 349242** (1990 to Wellcome Found.); idem, **US 5034394** (1991 to Burroughs Wellcome). Asymmetric synthesis: M. T. Crimmins, B. W. King, J. Org. Chem. **61**, 4192 (1996). Pharmacology and biological profile: S. M. Daluge et al., Antimicrob. Agents Chemother. **41**, 1082 (1997). Review of antiviral activity and clinical evaluations: R. H. Foster, D. Faulds, Drugs **55**, 729-736 (1998). Clinical trial of triple nucleoside regimen in HIV patients: S. Staszewski et al., J. Am. Med. Assoc. **285**, 1155 (2001).

White solid foam from acetonitrile, mp 165°. uv max (pH 1): 296, 255 nm (ε 14000, 10700); uv max (pH 7): 284, 259 nm (ε 15900, 9200); uv max (pH 13): 284, 259 nm (ε 15800, 9100). $[\alpha]_D^{20}$ −59.7°; $[\alpha]_{436}^{20}$ −127.8°; $[\alpha]_{365}^{20}$ −218.1° (c = 0.15 in methanol). Log P (1-octanol/0.1M sodium phosphate): 1.22 ±0.03 (pH 7.4). pKa 5.01. Soly in water (25°): >80 mM (pH 7).

Sulfate. [188062-50-2] Ziagen. $(C_{14}H_{18}N_6O)_2 \cdot H_2SO_4$; mol wt 670.74.

THERAP CAT: Antiviral.

2. Abamectin. [71751-41-2] Avermectin B_1; 5-O-demethylavermectin A_{1a} and 5-O-demethyl-25-de(1-methylpropyl)-25-(1-methylethyl)avermectin A_{1a} (4:1); avermectin $B_{1a/b}$; MK-936; Agri-Mek; Avid; Zephyr. Mixture of avermectins, q.v., containing at least 80% of avermectin B_{1a} ($C_{48}H_{72}O_{14}$) and not more than 20% of avermectin B_{1b} ($C_{47}H_{70}O_{14}$). Isoln from Streptomyces avermitilis: G. Albers-Schönberg et al., **DE 2717040**; eidem, **US 4310519** (1977, 1982 both to Merck & Co.). Separation of components: T. W. Miller et al., Antimicrob. Agents Chemother. **15**, 368 (1979); by semi-preparative HPLC: C. C. Ku et al., J. Liq. Chromatogr. **7**, 2905 (1984). Structure determn: G. Albers-Schönberg et al., J. Am. Chem. Soc. **103**, 4216 (1981). Absolute configuration: J. P. Springer et al., ibid. 4221. Partial synthesis of B_{1a}: K. C. Nicolaou et al., ibid. **106**, 4189 (1984). Total synthesis: S. Hanessian et al., ibid. **108**, 2776 (1986). Anthelmintic activity: L. S. Blair, W. C. Campbell, J. Parasitol. **64**, 1032 (1978); J. R. Egerton et al., Antimicrob. Agents Chemother. **15**, 372 (1979); K. S. Todd et al., Am. J. Vet. Res. **45**, 976 (1984). Pesticidal activity: I. Putter et al., Experientia **37**, 963 (1981); R. A. Dybas, A. St. J. Green, Proc. Br. Crop Prot. Conf. - Pests Dis. **1984**, 947. Control of red imported fire ants: J. A. Greenblatt et al., J. Agric. Entomol. **3**, 233 (1986). Interaction with GABA receptors: S. S. Pong et al., J. Neurochem. **34**, 351 (1980); T. N. Mellin et al., Neuropharmacology **22**, 89 (1983). Receptor binding studies: S. S. Pong, C. C. Wang, ibid. **19**, 311 (1980); G. Drexler, W. Sieghart, Eur. J. Pharmacol. **99**, 269 (1984). Fate in soil and plants: D. L. Bull et al., J. Agric. Food Chem. **32**, 94 (1984); H. A. Moye et al., ibid. **35**, 859 (1987); M. S. Maynard et al., ibid. **37**, 178, 184 (1989). Review: J. R. Babu, ACS Symp. Ser. **380**, 91-108 (1988). Reviews of modes of action: C. C. Wang, S. S. Pong, Prog. Clin. Biol. Res. **97**, 373-395 (1982); D. J. Wright, Biochem. Soc. Trans. **15**, 65-67 (1987); of insecticidal activities and use: L. Strong, T. A. Brown, Bull. Entomol. Res. **77**, 357-389 (1987). Book: Ivermectin and Abamectin, W. C. Campbell, Ed. (Springer-Verlag, New York, 1989) 363 pp.

component B_{1a}, R = C_2H_5 component B_{1b}, R = CH_3

Odorless, off-white to yellow crystals from methanol, mp 150-155° (dec). $[\alpha]_D$ +55.7 ±2° (c = 0.87 in $CHCl_3$). uv max (methanol): 237, 245, 253 nm (log ε 4.48, 4.53, 4.34). Vapor pressure: 1.5×10^{-9} torr. Soly at 21° (μg/l): water 10; (mg/ml): acetone 100; n-butanol 10; chloroform 25; cyclohexane 6; ethanol 20; isopropanol 70; kerosene 0.5; methanol 19.5; toluene 350. Hydrolysis does not occur in aq soln at pH 3, 5, 7. LD_{50} (technical grade) orally in sesame oil in mouse, rat: 13.5, 10.0 mg/kg; dermally in rabbit: >2000 mg/kg. LD_{50} in mallard duck, bobwhite quail: 84.6, >2000 mg/kg. LC_{50} (96 hr) in rainbow trout, bluegill: 3.6, 9.6 μg/l; LC_{50} (48 hr) in Daphnia magna: 0.34 μg/l (Merck Technical Data Sheet).

USE: Acaricide; insecticide.

THERAP CAT (VET): Anthelmintic.

3. Abarelix. [183552-38-7] N-Acetyl-3-(2-naphthalenyl)-D-alanyl-4-chloro-D-phenylalanyl-3-(3-pyridinyl)-D-alanyl-L-seryl-N-methyl-L-tyrosyl-D-asparaginyl-L-leucyl-N^6-(1-methylethyl)-L-lysyl-L-prolyl-D-alaninamide; Ac-D-Nal¹-4-Cl-D-Phe²-D-Pal³-N-Me-Tyr⁵-D-Asn⁶-Lys(iPr)⁸-D-Ala¹⁰-LH-RH; PPI-149; Plenaxis. $C_{72}H_{95}ClN_{14}O_{14}$; mol wt 1416.06. C 61.07%, H 6.76%, Cl 2.50%, N 13.85%, O 15.82%. Decapeptide LH-RH antagonist. Prepn: R. W. Roeske, **WO 9640757** (1996 to Indiana Univ. Found.); idem, **US 5843901** (1998 to Adv. Res. Technol. Inst.). Pharmacology and suppression of plasma gonadotropins: C. J. Molineaux et al., Mol. Urol. **2**, 265 (1998). Clinical comparison with leuprolide in prostate cancer: J. Trachtenberg et al., J. Urol. **167**, 1670 (2002). Clinical pharmacology: S. L. Wong et al., Clin.

Pharmacol. Ther. **73**, 304 (2003); of depot formulation: *eidem, J. Clin. Pharmacol.* **44**, 495 (2004). Review of clinical development: P. Mongiat-Artus, P. Teillac, *Expert Opin. Pharmacother.* **5**, 2171-2179 (2004).

White solid. Sol in water.

THERAP CAT: Antineoplastic (hormonal).

4. Abatacept. [332348-12-6] 1-25-Oncostatin M (human precursor) fusion protein with CTLA-4 (antigen)(human) fusion protein with immunoglobulin G1 (human heavy chain fragment); CTLA-4Ig; BMS-188667; Orencia. Selective costimulation modulator that inhibits T cell activation via the CD28/B7 receptor pathway. Recombinant chimeric fusion protein composed of the extracellular domain of human cytotoxic lymphocyte-associated antigen 4 (CTLA-4) fused to the heavy constant region of human IgG. Prepn: P. S. Linsley *et al., J. Exp. Med.* **174**, 561 (1991); *eidem*, **WO 9300431**; *eidem*, **US 5434131** (1993, 1995 both to Bristol-Myers Squibb). CE and HPLC analysis: K. F. Greve *et al., J. Chromatogr. A* **723**, 273 (1996). Pharmacokinetics: N. R. Srinivas *et al., J. Pharm. Sci.* **85**, 1 (1996). Clinical evaluation in psoriasis: J. R. Abrams *et al., J. Clin. Invest.* **103**, 1243 (1999); in rheumatoid arthritis (RA): J. M. Kremer *et al., Arthritis Rheum.* **52**, 2263 (2005); M. C. Genovese *et al., N. Engl. J. Med.* **353**, 1114 (2005). Review of pharmacology: N. Najafian, M. H. Sayegh, *Expert Opin. Invest. Drugs* **9**, 2147-2157 (2000); of mechanism of action and clinical development in RA: G. G. Teng *et al., Expert Opin. Biol. Ther.* **5**, 1245-1254 (2005).

THERAP CAT: Immunosuppressant; antipsoriatic.

5. Abciximab. [143653-53-6] Anti-(human integrin $\alpha_{IIb}\beta_3$) immunoglobulin G1 Fab fragment (human-mouse monoclonal c7E3 clone p7E3V_Hh$C_{\gamma l}$ γ_1-chain) disulfide with human-mouse monoclonal c7E3 clone p7E3V_κhC_κ κ-chain; c7E3 Fab; ReoPro. Platelet aggregation inhibitor. Fab fragment of chimeric human-murine monoclonal antibody c7E3 directed against the human platelet glycoprotein IIb/IIIa (GPIIb/IIIa) receptor. Chimeric fragment consists of the variable regions of murine *7E3* reconstructed with human constant regions of the Fab fragment. Mol wt ~47,600. Prepn: B. S. Coller, D. M. Knight, **WO 9512412** (1995 to Centocor and Res. Found. State Univ. New York); D. M. Knight *et al., Mol. Immunol.* **32**, 1271 (1995). Pharmacology: C. Kohmura *et al., Arterioscler. Thromb.* **13**, 1837 (1993). Clinical pharmacodynamics: J. E. Tcheng *et al., Circulation* **90**, 1757 (1994). Clinical studies as adjunct in prevention of ischemic complications associated with coronary revascularization: EPIC Investigators, *N. Engl. J. Med.* **330**, 956 (1994); EPILOG Investigators, *ibid.* **336**, 1689 (1997). Review of development, binding studies and preclinical testing: R. E. Jordan *et al.* in *Adhesion Receptors as Therapeutic Targets*, M. A. Horton, Ed. (CRC Press, Boca Raton, 1996) p 281-305; of pharmacology and clinical efficacy: R. H. Foster, L. R. Wiseman, *Drugs* **56**, 629-665 (1998).

THERAP CAT: Antithrombotic.

6. Abetimus Sodium. [169147-32-4] d(C-A-C-A-C-A-C-A-C-A-C-A-C-A-C-A-C-A-C-A-C-A)-DNA 5'-ester with 1,2-ethanediylbis(oxy-2,1-ethanediyl) bis[2-(21,21-dihydroxy-21-oxido-4,11-dioxo-20-oxa-13-thia-3,10-diaza-21-phophaheneicos-1-yl)-23,23-dihydroxy-23-oxido-6,13-dioxo-22-oxa-15-thia-2,5,12-triaza-23-phosphatricosanoate] (4:1) complex with d(T-G-T-G-T-G-T-G-T-G-T-G-T-G-T-G-T-G-T-G)-DNA (1:1) hexapentacontahectasodium salt; LJP-394; Riquent. B-cell toleragen which prevents the expression of anti-ds-DNA. Consists of four identical ds-DNA oligonucleotides (20 basepairs) attached through a linker to a non-immunogenic modified triethylene glycol base. Relative mass of 54 kDa. Prepn: S. M. Coutts *et al., EP 642798*; *eidem*, **US 5552391** (1995, 1996 both to La Jolla Pharm.); D. S. Jones *et al., J. Med. Chem.* **38**, 2138 (1995). Clinical evaluation in systemic lupus erythematosus (SLE): R. A. Furie *et al., J. Rheumatol.* **28**, 257 (2001), in prevention of SLE renal flare: D. Alarcon-Segovia *et al., Arthritis Rheum.* **48**, 442 (2003). Review of clinical pharmacology: D. J. Wallace, *Expert Opin. Invest. Drugs* **10**, 111-117 (2001); of clinical experience: M. H. Cardiel, *ibid.* **14**, 77-88 (2005).

Colorless aqueous solution with an osmolality of 255-310 mmol/kg at pH 6.8-7.8.

THERAP CAT: Immunosuppressant in treatment of SLE and associated nephritis.

7. Abietic Acid. [514-10-3] [1R-(1α,4aβ,4bα,10aα)]-1,-2,3,4,4a,4b,5,6,10,10a-Decahydro-1,4a-dimethyl-7-(1-methylethyl)-1-phenanthrenecarboxylic acid; 13-isopropylpodocarpa-7,13-dien-15-oic acid; sylvic acid. $C_{20}H_{30}O_2$; mol wt 302.45. C 79.42%, H 10.00%, O 10.58%. A widely available organic acid, prepared by isomerization of rosin: Harris, Sanderson, *Org. Synth.* **coll. vol. IV**, 1 (1963); Fieser, Fieser, *The Chemistry of Natural Products Related to Phenanthrene* (New York, 3rd ed., 1949). Synthesis from dehydroabietic acid: A. W. Burgstahler, L. W. Worden, *J. Am. Chem. Soc.* **83**, 2587 (1961); E. Wenkert *et al., ibid.* **86**, 2038 (1964). Chromatographic study: A. G. Douglas, T. G. Powell, *J. Chromatogr.* **43**, 241 (1969). Metabolism in rabbits: Y. Asakawa *et al., Xenobiotica* **16**, 753 (1986).

Monoclinic plates from alcohol + water, mp 172-175°. $[\alpha]_D^{24}$ $-106°$ (c = 1 in abs alc). uv max: 235, 241.5, 250 nm (ε 19500, 22000, 14300). Insol in water. Sol in alc, benzene, chloroform, ether, acetone, carbon disulfide, dil NaOH soln. Commercial abietic acid made by heating rosin alone or with acids may be glassy or partly crystalline, usually of yellow color and melting as low as 85°.

Methyl ester *see* Methyl Abietate.

USE: Manufacture of esters (ester gums), e.g., methyl, vinyl and glyceryl esters for use in lacquers and varnishes. Manufacture of "metal resinates", soaps, plastics and paper sizes. Assists growth of lactic and butyric acid bacteria.

8. Abikoviromycin. [31774-33-1] 7-Ethylidene-1a,2,3,-7-tetrahydrocyclopent[*b*]oxireno[*c*]pyridine; 4,4a-epoxy-5-ethylidene-2,3,4,4a-tetrahydro-5*H*-1-pyridine; abicoviromycin; latumcidin. $C_{10}H_{11}NO$; mol wt 161.20. C 74.51%, H 6.88%, N 8.69%, O 9.93%. Antiviral antibiotic produced by *Streptomyces abikoensis* and *Streptomyces rubescens*. Chromatographic isoln from broth cultures: Umezawa *et al., Jpn. Med. J.* **4**, 331 (1951); *C.A.* **46**, 7167 (1952); Umezawa, **JP 54 6200** (1954 to Nippon). Identity with latumcidin: Sakagami *et al., J. Antibiot.* **11A**, 231 (1958). Structure: Gurevich *et al., Tetrahedron Lett.* **1968**, 2209. Stereochemistry: Kono *et al., J. Antibiot.* **23**, 572 (1970); Gurevich *et al., Khim. Prir. Soedin.* **7**, 104 (1971), *C.A.* **75**, 5752e (1971). Crystal and molecular structure of the selenate: Y. Kono *et al., Acta Crystallogr.* **B27**, 2341 (1971). *In vitro* antiviral activity: V. M. Roikhel, N. A. Zeitlenok, *Antibiotiki* **14**, 969 (1969), *C.A.* **72**, 19394q (1969).

Highly unstable and polymerizes promptly on isolation even at −50°; however, it can be handled in dilute solutions and in the form of its salts. uv max (neutral ethanol or 0.1*N* KOH): 218, 244, 289 nm (log ε 3.83, 3.99, 3.94); (0.1*N* HCl) 236, 341 nm (log ε 3.99, 4.05).

9. Abrin. [1393-62-0] Agglutinin; toxalbumin. A toxic lectin and hemagglutinin obtained from seeds of *jequirity, Abrus precatorius* L., *Leguminosae*, a common vine of tropical countries; also found in central and southern Florida. Isoln and purification: J. Y. Lin *et al., J. Formosan Med. Assoc.* **68**, 518 (1969), *C.A.* **72**, 98695 (1970); *eidem, Toxicon* **9**, 97 (1971). The high toxicity of abrin was originally believed to result from its hemagglutinating activity, but subsequent studies have shown that separate proteins are responsible for the toxicity and agglutination: S. Olsnes, A. Pihl, *Eur. J. Biochem.* **35**, 179 (1973). Five glycoproteins have been purified from the seeds of *A. precatorius:* **Abrus agglutinin** and the toxic principles, abrins a-d. *Abrus* agglutinin is a tetramer of 134,900 Da, is non-toxic to animal cells and a potent hemagglutinator. Abrins a through d (mol wt 63,000-67,000 Da) are composed of two disulfide-linked polypeptide chains. The smaller A-chain inhibits protein synthesis and causes cell death; the larger B-chain binds to the cell plasma membrane. Purification of major components: C. H. Wei *et al., J. Biol. Chem.* **249,** 3061 (1974). Crystallographic study: C. H. Wei, J. R. Einstein, *ibid.* 2985. Improved purification, properties, crystallography of *Abrus* agglutinin: C. H. Wei *et al., ibid.* **250,** 4790 (1975). Physical properties of the toxic principles: M. S. Herrmann, W. D. Behnke, *Biochim. Biophys. Acta* **621,** 43 (1980); *eidem, ibid.* **667,** 397 (1981). Isoln and purification of all five proteins: J. Y. Lin *et al., Toxicon* **19,** 41 (1981). Amino acid sequence of the A-chain of abrin-a and comparison with ricin: G. Funatsu *et al., Agric. Biol. Chem.* **52,** 1095 (1988). Antitumor effects in animals: V. V. S. Reddy, M. Sirsi, *Cancer Res.* **29,** 1447 (1969); J. Y. Lin *et al., Nature* **227,** 292 (1970); O. Fodstad *et al., Cancer Res.* **37,** 4559 (1977). Immunoelectron microscopy studies of abrin toxic action on tumor cells: C. T. Lin *et al., J. Ultrastruct. Res.* **73,** 310 (1980). Studies on toxicity and binding kinetics: M. Witten *et al., Exp. Cell Biol.* **49,** 306 (1981); C. E. Bennett *et al., ibid.* 319. Use of A-chain in cell-type-specific cytotoxic agents known as "immunotoxins": A. J. Cumber *et al., Methods Enzymol.* **112,** 207 (1985). Toxicity study: J. Y. Lin *et al., J. Formosan Med. Assoc.* **68,** 322 (1969), *C.A.* **71,** 121926 (1969). *See also* Ricin, Lectins.

Yellowish-white powder. Sol in solns of sodium chloride, usually with turbidity. The toxic portion is heat-stable to incubation at 60° for 30 min; at 80°, most of the toxicity is lost in 30 min. LD_{50} i.p. in mice: 0.020 mg/kg (Lin p. 322).

Caution: Seeds of *A. precatorius* are extremely toxic; one seed, if thoroughly masticated, can cause fatal poisoning, *cf.* J. M. Kingsbury, *Poisonous Plants of the United States and Canada* (Prentice-Hall, New Jersey, 1964) p 303; K. Genest *et al., Arzneim.-Forsch.* **21,** 888 (1971). *Note:* Do not confuse with abrine, *q.v.*

USE: Exptly in cancer research.

10. Abrine. [526-31-8] *N*-Methyl-L-tryptophan; α-methylamino-β-(3-indole)propionic acid. $C_{12}H_{14}N_2O_2$; mol wt 218.25. C 66.04%, H 6.47%, N 12.84%, O 14.66%. Not to be confused with the albuminous substance abrin, *q.v.* Obtained from the seeds of *Abrus precatorius* L., *Leguminosae* (jequirity): Hoshino, *Ann.* **520,** 31 (1935). Synthesis: Miller, Robson, *J. Chem. Soc.* **1938,** 1910. Configuration: Cahill, Jackson, *J. Biol. Chem.* **126,** 29 (1938).

Prisms from water, dec 295°. $[\alpha]_D^{21}$ +44° (0.28 g in 10 ml 0.5*N* HCl). One gram dissolves in about 100 ml methanol, slightly sol in water, insol in ether. Sol in dil acids, alkalies.

Hydrochloride. $C_{12}H_{14}N_2O_2 \cdot$ HCl. Needles, mp 222°, soluble in water.

Nitrate. $C_{12}H_{14}N_2O_2 \cdot$ HNO₃. Needles, dec 143°.

Acetyl derivative. $C_{14}H_{16}N_2O_3$. mp 176°. $[\alpha]_D^{25}$ −148° (43 mg in 5 ml 0.1*N* NaOH).

11. Abscisic Acid. [21293-29-8] (2*Z*,4*E*)-5-[(1*S*)-Hydroxy-2,6,6-trimethyl-4-oxo-2-cyclohexen-1-yl]-3-methyl-2,4-pentadienoic acid; abscisin II; dormin; ABA. $C_{15}H_{20}O_4$; mol wt 264.32. C 68.16%, H 7.63%, O 24.21%. Abscission-accelerating plant hormone; naturally occurring as the (+)-*cis,trans*-form. Regulates seed maturation and germination and mediates the plant response to environmental stress. Isoln from young cotton fruit: K. Ohkuma *et al., Science* **142,** 1592 (1963); from sycamore leaves: J. W. Cornforth *et al., Nature* **205,** 1269 (1965). Identification in sycamore, birch, rose, cabbage, potato, lemon, avocado: *eidem, ibid.* **210,** 627 (1966). Structure and synthesis of (±)-*cis,trans*-form: *eidem, ibid.* **206,** 715 (1965); and enantiomers: F. Kienzle *et al., Helv. Chim. Acta* **61,** 2616 (1978). Absolute configuration of

naturally occurring form: G. Ryback, *Chem. Commun.* **1972,** 1190. Crystal and molecular structure: H. W. Schmalle *et al., Acta Crystallogr.* **B33,** 2218 (1977). *Review:* F. T. Addicott, J. L. Lyon, *Annu. Rev. Plant Physiol.* **20,** 139 (1969). Review of role in root growth regulation: P. E. Pilet, P. W. Barlow, *Plant Growth Regul.* **6,** 217-265 (1987); of metabolism: J. A. D. Zeevaart, R. A. Creelman, *Annu. Rev. Plant Physiol. Plant Mol. Biol.* **39,** 439-473 (1988); of signal transduction: J. Leung, J. Giraudat, *ibid.* **49,** 199-222 (1998).

Crystals from ethyl acetate + hexane, mp 161-163°. Sublimes at 120°. $[\alpha]_D^{20}$ +411.1° (c = 1 in ethanol). $[\alpha]_D^{20}$ +426.5° (c = 1 in 0.005*N* methanolic H_2SO_4). Sol in aq NaHCO₃, chloroform, acetone, ethyl acetate, ether; slightly sol in benzene, water; sparingly sol in petr ether. uv max (methanol): 252 nm (ε 25200).

(−)-cis,trans-Form. [14398-53-9] (*R*)-(−)-Abscisic acid. mp 162-163°. $[\alpha]_D^{20}$ −426.2° (c = 1 in 0.005*N* H_2SO_4).

(±)-cis,trans-Form. [14375-45-2] Crystals, mp 188-190°.

12. Absinthin. [1362-42-1] [3*S*-(3α,3aα,6β,6aα,6bβ,7α,-7aβ,8α,10aβ,11β,13aα,13bα,13cβ,14bβ)]-3,3a,4,5,6,6a,6b,7,7a,8,-9,10,10a,13a,13c,14b-Hexadecahydro-6,8-dihydroxy-3,6,8,11,14,-15-hexamethyl-2*H*-7,13b-ethenopentaleno[1″,2″:6,7;5″,4″:6′,-7′]dicyclohepta[1,2-b:1′,2′-b′]difuran-2,12(11*H*)-dione; absinthiin; absynthin. $C_{30}H_{40}O_6$; mol wt 496.64. C 72.55%, H 8.12%, O 19.33%. Chief bitter principle of wormwood, *Artemisia absinthium* L., *Compositae.* Isoln by chromatography: V. Herout *et al., Collect. Czech. Chem. Commun.* **21,** 1485 (1956); see also *Chem. Ind. (London)* **1955,** 569. Structural studies: L. Novotny *et al., ibid.* **1958,** 465; *Collect. Czech. Chem. Commun.* **25,** 1492 (1960); K. Vokác *et al., Tetrahedron Lett.* **9,** 3855 (1968). Structure: J. Beauhaire *et al., ibid.* **21,** 3191 (1980). Total synthesis: W. Zhang *et al., J. Am. Chem. Soc.* **127,** 18 (2005).

Colorless crystals from benzene, mp 165-166° (dec). $[\alpha]_D^{20}$ +107.0° (c = 1.9 in CHCl₃); $[\alpha]_D^{20}$ +103.5° (c = 1.0 in CHCl₃).

13. Acacetin. [480-44-4] 5,7-Dihydroxy-2-(4-methoxyphenyl)-4*H*-1-benzopyran-4-one; 5,7-dihydroxy-4′-methoxyflavone; apigenin-4′-methyl ether. $C_{16}H_{12}O_5$; mol wt 284.26. C 67.60%, H 4.26%, O 28.14%. The aglycon of linarin, *q.v.,* and of acaciin. Isoln from linarin: Zemplén, Bognar, *Ber.* **74B,** 1818 (1941). From acaciin: Hattori, *Acta Phytochim.* **2,** 105 (1925). Isoln from *Robinia pseudoacacia* L., *Leguminosae:* Nakazawa, Matsuura, *J. Pharm. Soc. Jpn.* **73,** 481 (1953). Structure: Baker *et al., J. Chem. Soc.* **1951,** 691. Synthesis: Robinson, Venkataraman, *ibid.* **1926,** 2348; Zemplén, Bognar, *Ber.* **76B,** 452 (1943); Narasimhachari, Seshadri, *Proc. Indian Acad. Sci.* **30A,** 151 (1949); Simpson, *Sci. Proc. R. Dublin Soc.* **27,** 111 (1956), *C.A.* **51,** 8082a (1957).

Yellow needles from 95% alcohol, mp 263°. Sol in hot alc, practically insol in ether. Sol in alkalies with yellow color.

7-Rhamnoglucoside. Acaciin. $C_{28}H_{32}O_{14}$. From *Robinia pseudacacia* L., *Leguminosae:* Freudenberg, Hartmann, *Ann.* **587**, 207 (1954). Structure: Zemplén, Mester, *Magy. Kem. Foly.* **56**, 2 (1950), *C.A.* **45**, 7977d (1951). Needles from pyridine + water, mp 263°. $[\alpha]$ −85.3° (pyridine); −99.5° (glacial acetic acid). Sparingly soluble in cold, more sol in boiling water; slightly sol in organic solvents.

14. Acacia. [9000-01-5] Gum Arabic. Estimations of mol wt range from about 240,000: Oakley, *Trans. Faraday Soc.* **31**, 136 (1935), to 580,000: Anderson *et al., Carbohyd. Res.* **3**, 308 (1967). According to the U.S.P., acacia is the dried gummy exudation from the stems and branches of *Acacia senegal* (L.) Willd., *Leguminosae*, or other African species of Acacia. According to C. L. Mantell, *The Water-Soluble Gums* (New York, 1947), Kordofan gum (hashab geneina), the gum from *Acacia verek* Guill. & Perr. from plantations in the Kordofan province (Sudan) is considered the best commercial variety. Grades of Kordofan gum which are clear, white (sun bleached) and tasteless are preferred for food prepns and pharmaceuticals. (There is a close relationship between color and flavor due to the presence of tannins.) Acacia was originally thought to be composed only of (−)-arabinose, (+)-galactose, (−)-rhamnose, (+)-glycuronic acid. Revised composition and structural studies: Anderson *et al., J. Chem. Soc. C* **1966**, 1959. *See also* Swenson *et al., J. Polym. Sci. Part A-2* **6**, 1593 (1968). General review: Anderson, Dea, *J. Soc. Cosmet. Chem.* **22**, 61-76 (1971). Review of use as food additive: D. M. W. Anderson, *Food Addit. Contam.* **3**, 225-230 (1986).

Occurs in spheroidal tears up to 32 mm in diameter. Also flakes and powder. Solns of gum from *Acacia verek* are levorotatory; other acacia species are dextrorotatory: Hamy, *Bull. Sci. Pharmacol.* **35**, 421 (1928). Specific gravity: 1.35-1.49 (samples dried at 100° are heavier). Moisture content usually varies from 13-15%. U.S.P. limit 15%. Material containing less than 12% chips easily and produces dust during transportation. Insol in alcohol. Almost completely sol in twice its weight of water. 100 grams of a satd soln contains 37 g at 25°; 38 g at 50°; 40 g at 90°: Taft, Malm, *Trans. Kans. Acad. Sci.* **32**, 49 (1929). Aq soln acid to litmus. Also sol in glycerol and in propylene glycol, but prolonged heating (several days) may be necessary for complete solution (about 5%). *Incompat.* Precipitates or jellies result upon addition of solns of ferric salts, borax, basic lead acetate (lead subacetate, but not neutral lead acetate), alcohol, sodium silicate, gelatin, ammoniated tincture of guaiac.

USE: As mucilage, excipient for tablets, size, emulsifier, thickener, also in candy, other foods; as colloidal stabilizer. In the manufacture of spray-dried "fixed" flavors—stable, powdered flavors used in packaged dry-mix products (puddings, desserts, cake mixes) where flavor stability and long shelf life are important.

15. Acacic Acid. [1962-14-7] $(3\beta,16\alpha,21\beta)$-Trihydroxyolean-12-en-28-oic acid. $C_{30}H_{48}O_5$; mol wt 488.70. C 73.73%, H 9.90%, O 16.37%. Isoln from pods of *Acacia concinna* D.C., *Leguminosae:* Varshney, Shamsuddin, *Tetrahedron Lett.* **1964**, 2055; from bark of *A. concinna* D.C.: R. Banerji, S. K. Nigam, *J. Indian Chem. Soc.* **57**, 1043 (1980). Structure and stereochemistry: Varshney *et al., ibid.* **1965**, 1187. Revised structure: A. K. Barua *et al., Trans. Bose Res. Inst. (Calcutta)* **39**, 61 (1976), *C.A.* **87**, 53460c (1977).

Needles from methanol, mp 280-281°.

Methyl ester. $C_{31}H_{50}O_5$. Needles from methanol, mp 223-224°.

Diacetyl lactone. $C_{34}H_{50}O_6$. Crystals, mp 235-236°.

16. Acadesine. [2627-69-2] 5-Amino-1-β-D-ribofuranosyl-1*H*-imidazole-4-carboxamide; 5-amino-4-imidazolecarboxamide ribonucleoside; AICA-riboside; Arasine; Protara. $C_9H_{14}N_4O_5$; mol wt 258.23. C 41.86%, H 5.46%, N 21.70%, O 30.98%. Purine nucleoside analog. Prototype adenosine regulating agent; enhances endogenous adenosine levels in ischemic tissue. Biosynthesis, isoln, and characterization: G. R. Greenberg, E. L. Spilman, *J. Biol. Chem.* **219**, 411 (1956). Chemical synthesis: J. Baddiley *et al., Proc. Chem. Soc. London* **1957**, 149; J. P. Ferris *et al., J. Org. Chem.* **50**, 747 (1985); T. Saito *et al., Chem. Pharm. Bull.* **42**, 2263 (1994). Pharmacology: Z.-Q. Zhao *et al., Cardiovasc. Res.* **29**, 495 (1995). Antiplatelet activity: D. A. Bullough *et al., J. Clin. Invest.* **94**, 1524 (1994). Disposition and metabolism: R. Dixon *et al., J. Clin. Pharmacol.* **33**, 955 (1993). HPLC determn in plasma: L.-S. Chen *et al., J. Liq. Chromatogr.* **18**, 1451 (1995). Review of pharmacology: K. Mullane, M. Young, *Drug Dev. Res.* **28**, 336-343 (1993); of development: K. Mullane *et al., Trends Cardiovasc. Med.* **3**, 227-234 (1993). Meta-analysis of clinical trials in coronary artery bypass graft surgery: D. T. Mangano *et al., J. Am. Med. Assoc.* **277**, 325-332 (1997).

Crystals from methanol or water, mp 213-214° (dec). Also reported as slightly brownish prisms from 90% aq ethanol, mp 206-208° (dec) (Saito). uv max (pH 7 and 1*N* NaOH): 265 nm (ε 12400). uv max (1*N* HCl): 245, 265 nm (ε 8670, 10320).

THERAP CAT: Cardioprotective.

17. Acamprosate Calcium. [77337-73-6] 3-(Acetylamino)-1-propanesulfonic acid calcium salt (2:1); calcium acetyl homotaurinate; Ca-AOTA; calcium bisacetyl homotaurine; Aotal; Campral. $C_{10}H_{20}CaN_2O_8S_2$; mol wt 400.48. C 29.99%, H 5.03%, Ca 10.01%, N 6.99%, O 31.96%, S 16.01%. GABA (γ-aminobutyric acid, *q.v.*) agonist. Prepn: J. P. Durlach, **DE 3019350**; *idem,* **US 4355043** (1980, 1982 both to Lab. Meram). Physicochemical and pharmacological study: C. Chabenat *et al., Methods Find. Exp. Clin. Pharmacol.* **10**, 311 (1988). Pharmacology: J. Durlach *et al., ibid.* 437; A. Guiet-Bara *et al., Alcohol* **5**, 63 (1988). Suppression of ethanol intake in rats: F. Boismare *et al., Pharmacol. Biochem. Behav.* **21**, 787 (1984); J. Le Magnen *et al., Alcohol* **4**, 97 (1987). Evaluation of abuse potential: K. A. Grant, W. L. Woolverton, *Pharmacol. Biochem. Behav.* **32**, 607 (1989). HPLC determn in plasma: C. Chabenat *et al., J. Chromatogr.* **414**, 417 (1987). Clinical evaluation in relapse prevention in weaned alcoholics: J. P. L'Huintre *et al., Lancet* **1**, 1014 (1985); J. P. L'Huintre *et al., Alcohol Alcohol.* **25**, 613 (1990). Review of clinical efficacy in maintenance of abstinence in alcoholics: L. J. Scott *et al., CNS Drugs* **19**, 445-464 (2005); of mechanism of action: P. De Witte *et al., ibid.* 517-537.

Colorless crystalline powder, mp 270°. uv max (water): 192 nm (ε 7360). Freely sol in water. Practically insol in absolute ethanol, dichloromethane. LD_{50} i.p. in male mice: 1.87 g/kg (Durlach, 1982).

THERAP CAT: In treatment of alcoholism.

18. Acarbose. [56180-94-0] O-4,6-Dideoxy-4-[[[1S-(1α,4α,5β,6α)]-4,5,6-trihydroxy-3-(hydroxymethyl)-2-cyclohexen-1-yl]amino]-α-D-glucopyranosyl-(1 → 4)-O-α-D-glucopyranosyl-(1 → 4)-D-glucose; 4'',6''-dideoxy-4''-[(1S)-(1,4,6/5)-4,5,6-trihydroxy-3-hydroxymethyl-2-cyclohexenylamino]maltotriose; Bay g 5421; Glucobay; Prandase; Precose. $C_{25}H_{43}NO_{18}$; mol wt 645.60. C 46.51%, H 6.71%, N 2.17%, O 44.61%. Pseudotetrasaccharide containing an unsaturated cyclitol moiety. An α-glucosidase inhibitor that reduces sugar absorption in the gastrointestinal tract. Isoln from strains of *Actinoplanes:* W. Frommer *et al., DE 2347782; eidem,* **US 4062950** (1975, 1977 both to Bayer). Total synthesis: S. Ogawa, Y. Shibata, *Chem. Commun.* **1988**, 605; *eidem, Carbohydr. Res.* **189,** 309 (1989). Biosynthetic studies: U. Degwert *et al., J. Antibiot.* **40,** 855 (1987). Glucosidase inhibition studies: D. D. Schmidt *et al., Naturwissenschaften* **64,** 535 (1977); W. Puls *et al., ibid.* 536. Use in treatment of diabetic adults: D. Sailor, G. Roder, *Arzneim.-Forsch.* **30,** 2182 (1980); H. Laube *et al., ibid.* 1154. Long-term study in sulfonylurea-treated diabetics: H. Vierhapper *et al., Diabetologia* **20,** 586 (1981). Potential use in prophylaxis of dental caries: N. E. Fiehn, D. Moe, *Scand. J. Dent. Res.* **90,** 124 (1982). Review of pharmacodynamics, pharmacokinetics and therapeutic potential: S. P. Clissold, C. Edwards, *Drugs* **35,** 214-243 (1988).

Amorphous powder. $[\alpha]_D^{18}$ +165° (c = 0.4 in water).
THERAP CAT: Antidiabetic.

19. Acebutolol. [37517-30-9] N-[3-Acetyl-4-[2-hydroxy-3-[(1-methylethyl)amino]propoxy]phenyl]butanamide; 3'-acetyl-4'-[2-hydroxy-3-(isopropylamino)propoxy]butyranilide; 1-(2-acetyl-4-n-butyramidophenoxy)-2-hydroxy-3-isopropylaminopropane; 5'-butyramido-2'-(2-hydroxy-3-isopropylaminopropoxy)acetophenone. $C_{18}H_{28}N_2O_4$; mol wt 336.43. C 64.26%, H 8.39%, N 8.33%, O 19.02%. Cardioselective β-adrenergic blocker. Prepn: K. R. H. Wooldridge, B. Basil, *ZA 6808345; eidem,* **US 3857952** (1969, 1974 both to May & Baker). Pharmacology: Cuthbert, Owusu-Ankomah, *Br. J. Pharmacol.* **43,** 639 (1971); Basil *et al., ibid.* **48,** 198 (1973); Lewis *et al., Br. Heart J.* **35,** 743 (1973). HPLC determn in plasma and urine: M. Piquette-Miller *et al., J. Chromatogr.* **526,** 129 (1990). Crystal structure: A. Carpy *et al., Acta Crystallogr.* **B35,** 185 (1979). Review of pharmacology and therapeutic efficacy: B. N. Singh *et al., Drugs* **29,** 531-569 (1985); G. DeBono *et al., Am. Heart J.* **109,** 1211-1223 (1985). Comprehensive description: R. T. Foster, R. A. Carr, *Anal. Profiles Drug Subs.* **19,** 1-26 (1990).

Crystals, mp 119-123°.
Hydrochloride. [34381-68-5] M & B 17803A; IL-17803A; Acecor; Acetanol; Neptal; Prent; Sectral. $C_{18}H_{28}N_2O_4$.HCl; mol wt 372.89. Crystals from anhydr methanol-anhydr diethyl ether, mp 141-143°. Freely sol in water. Soly at room temperature (mg/ml): water 200; ethanol 70.

THERAP CAT: Antihypertensive; antianginal; antiarrhythmic (class II).

20. Acecainide. [32795-44-1] 4-(Acetylamino)-N-[2-(diethylamino)ethyl]benzamide; 4'-[[2-(diethylamino)ethyl]carbamoyl]acetanilide; N-acetylprocainamide; NAPA. $C_{15}H_{23}N_3O_2$; mol wt 277.36. C 64.96%, H 8.36%, N 15.15%, O 11.54%. Metabolite of procainamide, q.v. Prepn: E. C. Schreiber, **DE 2062978** (1971 to Squibb), *C.A.* **75,** 76427 (1972). Pharmacokinetics: M. Wierzchowiecki *et al., Int. J. Clin. Pharmacol. Ther. Toxicol.* **18,** 272 (1980). Clinical pharmacology and antiarrhythmic efficacy: J. Kluger *et al., Am. J. Cardiol.* **45,** 1250 (1980); R. A. Winkle *et al., ibid.* **47,** 123 (1981). HPLC determn in plasma: D. Raphanaud *et al., Ther. Drug Monit.* **8,** 365 (1986). Review of pharmacology and therapeutic potential: D. W. G. Harron, R. N. Brogden, *Drugs* **39,** 720-740 (1990).

Hydrochloride. [34118-92-8] ASL-601. $C_{15}H_{23}N_3O_2$.HCl; mol wt 313.82. Crystals, mp 190-193°.
THERAP CAT: Antiarrhythmic.

21. Acecarbromal. [77-66-7] N-[(Acetylamino)carbonyl]-2-bromo-2-ethylbutanamide; N-acetyl-N-bromodiethylacetylurea; acetylbromodiethylacetylcarbamide; N-acetyl-N'-α-bromo-α-ethylbutyrylcarbamide; acetylcarbromal; Abasin; Sedamyl. C_9H_{15}-BrN_2O_3; mol wt 279.13. C 38.73%, H 5.42%, Br 28.63%, N 10.04%, O 17.20%. Prepn: **DE 327129** (1920 to Bayer), *Frdl.* **13,** 809 (1923). HPLC determn in plasma, urine: M. Höbel, G. Bender, *Arch. Toxicol.* **37,** 307 (1977). GC-MS screening procedure in urine: H. H. Maurer, *J. Chromatogr.* **530,** 307 (1990).

Crystals, slightly bitter taste, mp 108-109°. Slightly sol in water; freely sol in alcohol, ethyl acetate.
THERAP CAT: Sedative, hypnotic.

22. Aceclofenac. [89796-99-6] 2-[(2,6-Dichlorophenyl)-amino]benzeneacetic acid carboxymethyl ester; 2-[(2,6-dichlorophenyl)amino]phenylacetoxyacetic acid; glycolic acid [o-(2,6-dichloroanilino)phenyl]acetate ester; PR-82/3; Airtal; Falcol; Gerbin; Preservex. $C_{16}H_{13}Cl_2NO_4$; mol wt 354.18. C 54.26%, H 3.70%, Cl 20.02%, N 3.95%, O 18.07%. Prepn: A. V. Casas, **ES 8404783;** *idem,* **US 4548952** (1984, 1985 both to Prodes). Gastrointestinal tolerance in rats in comparison with diclofenac, q.v.: V. Rimbau *et al., Farmaco Ed. Prat.* **43,** 19 (1988). Clinical trial in comparison with acetaminophen, q.v., in episiotomal pain: A. Yscla, *Drugs Exp. Clin. Res.* **14,** 491 (1988). Clinical evaluation in rheumatoid arthritis: R. Ballesteros *et al., Clin. Trials J.* **27,** 12 (1990).

White crystals from cyclohexane, mp 149-150°. uv max (ethanol): 275 nm (log ε 4.14).
THERAP CAT: Anti-inflammatory; analgesic.

23. Acediasulfone. [80-03-5] N-[4-[(4-Aminophenyl)sulfonyl]phenyl]glycine; N-p-sulfanilylphenylglycine; p-amino-p'-

(carboxymethylamino)diphenyl sulfone; 4-carboxymethylamino-4'-aminodiphenylsulfone; diaminodiphenylsulfone-N-acetic acid. $C_{14}H_{14}N_2O_4S$; mol wt 306.34. C 54.89%, H 4.61%, N 9.14%, O 20.89%, S 10.47%. Prepn: Jackson, *J. Am. Chem. Soc.* **70**, 680 (1948); **CH 254803** and **CH 278482** (1949, 1952, to Cilag Ltd.); Rawlins, **US 2589211** (1952 to Parke, Davis).

Crystals, mp 194°. Sol in methanol, dil sodium hydroxide, acetone.

Sodium salt. [127-60-6] Sulfon-Cilag. $C_{14}H_{13}N_2NaO_4S$; mol wt 328.32.

Morpholine salt. Bentrofene. $C_{18}H_{23}N_3O_5S$; mol wt 393.46. Prepn: Martin, Habicht, **US 2751382** (1956 to Cilag Ltd.). Glittering crystals, mp 133-135° (dec).

THERAP CAT: Antibacterial.

24. Acefylline. [652-37-9] 1,2,3,6-Tetrahydro-1,3-dimethyl-2,6-dioxopurine-7-acetic acid; carboxymethyltheophylline; 7-theophyllineacetic acid. $C_9H_{10}N_4O_4$; mol wt 238.20. C 45.38%, H 4.23%, N 23.52%, O 26.87%. Prepn: **DE 352980** (1922 to E. Merck); *Frdl.* **14**, 1320; S. M. Ride et al., *Pharmazie* **32**, 672 (1977). Prepn of salts: J. Baisse, *Bull. Soc. Chim. Fr.* **1949**, 769; M. Milletti, F. Virgili, *Chimica* **6**, 394 (1951), *C.A.* **46**, 8615h (1952). GC determn in urine: J. Zuidema, H. Hilbers, *J. Chromatogr.* **182**, 445 (1980). HPLC determn in serum and pharmacokinetics: S. Sved et al., *Biopharm. Drug Dispos.* **2**, 177 (1981).

Crystals from water, mp 271°.

Sodium salt. [837-27-4] $C_9H_9N_4NaO_4$. Silky needles, mp >300°.

Compd with piperazine. Acefylline piperazine; acepifylline; Dynaphylline; Etaphylline; Etafillina. Undefined mixture of the 1:1 and 2:1 salts; contains 75-78% theophylline acetic acid and 22-25% anhydrous piperazine.

THERAP CAT: Bronchodilator.

25. Aceglutamide. [2490-97-3] N^2-Acetyl-L-glutamine; α-N-acetyl-L-glutamine; Acutil-S. $C_7H_{12}N_2O_4$; mol wt 188.18. C 44.68%, H 6.43%, N 14.89%, O 34.01%. Prepn: P. Karrer et al., *Helv. Chim. Acta* **9**, 301 (1926); **GB 792576** (1958 to Merck & Co.), *C.A.* **53**, 2109a (1959); I. J. Maschler, N. Lichtenstein, *Biochim. Biophys. Acta* **57**, 252 (1962). Stability study: G. Sekules, G. Guadagnini, *Farmaco Ed. Prat.* **21**, 22 (1966). NMR study: W. Voelter et al., *Z. Naturforsch.* **26B**, 213 (1971). Fermentation study: T. Nakanishi, *J. Ferment. Technol.* **56**, 573 (1978). Prepn of the aluminum complex: T. Kagawa et al., **DE 2127176** corresp to **US 3787466** (1971, 1974 both to Kyowa). Physico-chemical properties: E. Hayakawa et al., *Yakugaku Zasshi* **97**, 731 (1977), *C.A.* **87**, 141198 (1977). Effect on exptl chronic gastric ulcer: H. Tanaka et al., *Oyo Yakuri* **7**, 1035 (1973), *C.A.* **81**, 33283v (1974). Cytoprotective effect: H. Tanaka, *Arzneim.-Forsch.* **36**, 1485 (1986).

Crystals from ethanol, mp 197°. $[\alpha]_D^{20}$ −12.5° (c = 2.9 in water).

Aluminum complex. [12607-92-0] Pentakis (N^2-acetyl-L-glutaminato)tetrahydroxytrialuminum; aceglutamide aluminum; KW-110; Glumal. $C_{35}H_{59}Al_3N_{10}O_{24}$; mol wt 1084.84. White powder, mp 221° (dec). Sol in water. Practically insol in methanol, ethanol, acetone. LD_{50} in male mice, rats (g/kg): 14.3, >14.5 orally; 5.0, 4.2 i.p.; 0.46, 0.40 i.v. (Kagawa).

THERAP CAT: Free acid as nootropic; aluminum complex as antiulcerative.

26. Acemannan. Carrisyn. Long-chain, polydispersed, β-(1,4)-linked acetylated mannan obtained from the mucilage of *Aloe barbadensis,* Miller, *Liliaceae* (aloe vera). Isolation, purification, and characterization: B. H. McAnalley, **WO 8700052**; idem, **US 4735935** (1987, 1988 both to Carrington Labs.). Structural study: S. Manna, B. H. McAnalley, *Carbohydr. Res.* **241**, 317 (1993). Immunostimulant effect *in vitro:* D. Womble, J. H. Helderman, *Int. J. Immunopharmacol.* **10**, 967 (1988). Inhibition of HIV-1 replication *in vitro:* J. B. Kahlon et al., *Mol. Biother.* **3**, 127 (1991). Veterinary trial in feline-leukemia virus infection: M. A. Sheets et al., *ibid.* 41; in canine and feline spontaneous tumors: C. Harris et al., *ibid.* 207. Toxicological evaluation: R. W. Fogleman et al., *Vet. Hum. Toxicol.* **34**, 201 (1992).

THERAP CAT: Antiviral; immunomodulator.

THERAP CAT (VET): Antiviral.

27. Acemetacin. [53164-05-9] 1-(4-Chlorobenzoyl)-5-methoxy-2-methyl-1*H*-indole-3-acetic acid carboxymethyl ester; [[1-(4-chlorobenzoyl)-5-methoxy-2-methylindol-3-yl]acetoxy]acetic acid; TV-1322; Acemix; Emflex; Rantudil; Solart. $C_{21}H_{18}$-ClNO$_6$; mol wt 415.82. C 60.66%, H 4.36%, Cl 8.53%, N 3.37%, O 23.09%. Deriv of indomethacin, q.v. Prepn: K. H. Boltze et al., **DE 2234651**; eidem, **US 3910952** (1972, 1975 both to Troponwerke). Series of articles on chemistry, analysis, pharmacodynamics, toxicology and clinical trials: *Arzneim.-Forsch.* **30**, 1313-1468 (1980). Toxicity data: H. Jacobi, H.-D. Dell, *ibid.* 1398.

Very fine pale yellow crystals from petr ether, mp 150-153°. LD_{50} in male, female mice, male, female rats (mg/kg): 55.5, 18.42, 24.2, 30.1 orally; 34.1, 51.1, 38.1, 28.3 i.v. (Jacobi, Dell).

THERAP CAT: Anti-inflammatory.

28. Acenaphthene. [83-32-9] 1,2-Dihydroacenaphthylene; peri-ethylenenaphthalene; 1,8-ethylenenaphthalene. $C_{12}H_{10}$; mol wt 154.21. C 93.46%, H 6.54%. Occurs in coal tar. Isoln: Ges. f. Teerverwertung, **DE 277110**; *Chem. Zentralbl.* **1914, II**, 597. In petroleum residues: Orloff et al., *C.A.* **31**, 2800⁹ (1937). By passing ethylene and benzene or naphthalene though a red hot tube: Berthelot, *Bull. Soc. Chim.* [2] **7**, 274; **8**, 226, 245 (1867). By heating tetrahydroacenaphthene with sulfur to 180°: Braun et al., *Ber.* **55**, 1694 (1922). From acenaphthenone or acenaphthenequinone by high pressure hydrogenation in decalin with nickel at 180-240°: Braun, Bayer, *Ber.* **59**, 921, 923 (1926). From acenaphthenone oxime: Morgan, Stanley, *J. Soc. Chem. Ind. London* **44**, 494T (1925). Review of toxicology and human exposure: *Toxicological Profile for Polycyclic Aromatic Hydrocarbons* (PB95-264370, 1995) 487 pp.

Orthorhombic bipyramidal needles from alcohol. d 1.189. mp 95°. bp 279°. uv spectrum: Seshan, *Proc. Indian Acad. Sci.* **A3**, 148 (1936). Factors influencing the uv spectrum: Jones, *J. Am. Chem. Soc.* **67**, 2127 (1945). Insol in water. One gram dissolves in 31 ml alcohol, 56 ml methanol, 25 ml propanol, 2.5 ml chloroform, 5 ml benzene or toluene. 3.2 g are sol in 100 ml glacial acetic acid. Forms water-sol, cryst complexes with desoxycholic acid, containing two molecules of the bile acid as a rule. The complexes crystallize when concentrated solns of the proper amount of the components in alcohol or dioxane are allowed to cool slowly.

USE: Dye intermediate; manuf plastics; insecticide; fungicide.

29. Acenocoumarol. [152-72-7] 4-Hydroxy-3-[1-(4-nitrophenyl)-3-oxobutyl]-2H-1-benzopyran-2-one; 3-(α-acetonyl-p-nitrobenzyl)-4-hydroxycoumarin; 3-(α-p-nitrophenyl-β-acetylethyl)-4-hydroxycoumarin; acenocoumarin; nicoumalone; G-23350; Mini-Sintrom; Sinthrome; Sintrom. $C_{19}H_{15}NO_6$; mol wt 353.33. C 64.59%, H 4.28%, N 3.96%, O 27.17%. Vitamin K antagonist; structurally similar to warfarin, q.v. Prepn: W. Stoll, F. Litvan, US 2648682 (1953 to Geigy); I. C. Ivanov et al., Arch. Pharm. 323, 521 (1990). Resolution and abs config of enantiomers: C. R. Wheeler, W. F. Trager, J. Med. Chem. 22, 1122 (1979). Pharmacology and toxicity: M. Leroux, B. Jamain, Therapie 11, 85 (1956). GC-MS determn in plasma: F. Pommier et al., J. Chromatogr. B 654, 35 (1994). Clinical trial: D. P. M. Brandjes et al., N. Engl. J. Med. 327, 1485 (1992).

Crystals, mp 196-199°. Sparingly sol in water and most organic solvents. Forms water-sol salt with alkalies. LD_{50} orally in mice, rats: 1470, 1000 mg/kg (Leroux, Jamain).

THERAP CAT: Anticoagulant.

30. Aceperone. [807-31-8] N-[[1-[4-(4-Fluorophenyl)-4-oxobutyl]-4-phenyl-4-piperidinyl]methyl]acetamide; N-[[1-[1-[3-(p-fluorobenzoyl)propyl]-4-phenyl-4-piperidyl]methyl]acetamide; 1-(p-fluorophenyl)-4-(4-phenyl-4-acetamidomethylpiperidino)-1-butanone; 1-[γ-(4-fluorobenzoyl)propyl]-4-acetamidomethyl-4-phenylpiperidine; N-[1-[3-(p-fluorobenzoyl)propyl]-4-phenylpiperidin-4-ylmethyl]acetamide; 4'-fluoro-4-(4-acetamidomethyl-4-phenylpiperido)butyrophenone; acetabutone; acetobuton; R-3248. $C_{24}H_{29}FN_2O_2$; mol wt 396.50. C 72.70%, H 7.37%, F 4.79%, N 7.07%, O 8.07%. Prepd by reacting γ-chloro-4-fluorobutyrophenone with 4-acetamidomethyl-4-phenylpiperidine: P. A. J. Janssen, BE 606849 (1961), corresp to US 3083205 (1961, 1963 both to Janssen). Crystal structure: N. Van Opdenbosch et al., Acta Crystallogr. 33B, 171 (1977).

Crystals, mp 97-100°.

31. Acephate. [30560-19-1] Acetylphosphoramidothioic acid O,S-dimethyl ester; Ortho 12420; Orthene. $C_4H_{10}NO_3PS$; mol wt 183.17. C 26.23%, H 5.50%, N 7.65%, O 26.20%, P 16.91%, S 17.51%. Prepn and activity: Magee, US 3716600 and US 3845172 (1973, 1974 both to Chevron).

White solid, mp 64-68° (impure). Very sol in water; moderately sol in acetone, alc. Low soly in aromatic solvents. LD_{50} orally in rats: 700 mg/kg (Magee, 1973).

USE: Contact and systemic insecticide.

32. Acepromazine. [61-00-7] 1-[10-[3-(Dimethylamino)propyl]-10H-phenothiazin-2-yl]ethanone; 10-[3-(dimethylamino)propyl]phenothiazin-2-yl methyl ketone; 2-acetyl-10-(3-dimethylaminopropyl)phenothiazine; 3-acetyl-10-(3-dimethylaminopropyl)phenothiazine; 10-(3-dimethylaminopropyl)phenothiazine-3-ethylone; acetazine; acetopromazine; acetylpromazine; 1522-CB. $C_{19}H_{22}N_2OS$; mol wt 326.46. C 69.90%, H 6.79%, N 8.58%, O 4.90%, S 9.82%. Prepn: J. Schmitt et al., Bull. Soc. Chim. Fr. 1957, 938. Pharmacology and toxicology: W. Wirth et al., Arch. Int. Pharmacodyn. 123, 78 (1959). GLC determn in plasma: S. Ballard, T. Tobin, J. Toxicol. Environ. Health 7, 745 (1981). Clinical trial in cats: D. H. Dyson et al., Can. Vet. J. 33, 462 (1992); in horses: A. Hashem, H. Keller, J. Vet. Pharmacol. Ther. 16, 359 (1993). Brief review of clinical experience: N. Brock, Can. Vet. J. 35, 458-459 (1994).

Yellow-colored oil, $bp_{0.5}$ 220-240°.

Maleate. [3598-37-6] Atravet; Calmivet; Plegicil; PromAce; Sedalin; Vetranquil. $C_{19}H_{22}N_2OS \cdot C_4H_4O_4$; mol wt 442.53. Yellow crystals from ethyl acetate, mp 135-136°. pKa 9.3. Sol in water, alcohol, chloroform. pH of aq solns: ~4.0. LD_{50} orally in rats: 400 mg/kg; i.v. in mice: 59 mg/kg (Wirth).

THERAP CAT (VET): Tranquilizer.

33. Acequinocyl. [57960-19-7] 2-(Acetyloxy)-3-dodecyl-1,4-naphthalenedione; AKD-2023; DPX-3792; DPX-T3792; AC-145; Kanemite. $C_{24}H_{32}O_4$; mol wt 384.51. C 74.97%, H 8.39%, O 16.64%. Naphthoquinone miticide which inhibits mitochondrial electron transfer. Prepn: NL 7505470; R. F. Bellina, D. L. Fost, US 4082848 (1975, 1978 both to Du Pont). Field study on mites: D. A. Marsden, W. W. Allen, J. Econ. Entomol. 73, 168 (1980). Acaricidal mechanism: Y. Koura et al., J. Pestic. Sci. 23, 18 (1998). Review of physical properties, mode of action, and biological characteristics: F. Wakasa, S. Watanabe, Agrochem. Jpn. 75, 17 (1999).

Fine yellowish powder, mp 59.6°. Soly in water at 25°: 6.7×10^{-6} g/l. Vapor pressure at 40°: 5.18×10^{-5} Pa. Log P (octanol/water): > 6.2. LD_{50} in rats (mg/kg): > 5000 orally, > 2000 dermally; in mice (mg/kg): > 5000 orally. LC_{50} (96hr) in carp, rainbow trout (mg/l): > 96.5, > 33 (Wakasa).

USE: Acaricide.

34. Acerin. [8001-08-9] An extract from the dried fruit of the Norway maple Acer plantanoides L., Aceraceae. Freshly prepd solutions of acerin destroy E. coli and vaccinia virus in 5 min but are less effective on the Staphylococcus Twort virus. Phagicidal action also exists even in the presence of the host cells. Extraction and properties: G. Fischer, Acta Pathol. Microbiol. Scand. 31, 433 (1952); 34, 482 (1954); Fischer et al., Experientia 10, 329 (1954).

Practically insol in methanol, ethanol, ether, acetone. Does not dialyze through a cellophane membrane at room temp but passes through a Seitz filter. Sodium chloride precipitates the active principle in acerin preparations as does also normal serum with 1:800 solns of acerin. Strong acerin preparations acquire reddish-brown color after treatment with alkali and oxidation in air. In general, the substance behaves similarly to vegetable tannins.

35. Acerola. The ripe fruit of Malpighia punicifolia L., Malpighiaceae, also called West Indian Cherry. Habit. Central

America, Puerto Rico. Probably the richest natural source of ascorbic acid. Analysis of pitted fruit: Water 92.28%; ascorbic acid 1690 mg/100 g; vitamin A 11.0 mg/100 g; niacin 407 γ/100 g; vitamin B_6 8.7 γ/100 g; thiamine-HCl 30.0 γ/100 g; fluorine 10 γ/100 g; carbohydrates 6.4%. pH of juice 3.3. The pits comprise 19.25% of the fruit. *Ref:* Derse, Elvehjem, *J. Am. Med. Assoc.* **156**, 1501 (1954). Commercial aspects: *J. Agric. Food Chem.* **2**, 1155 (1954). *Review:* Moscoso, *Econ. Bot.* **10**, 280 (1956). Method of preparing acerola juice concentrates: Morse, **US 3012942**; **US 3012943** (both 1961 to Nutrilite Products).

THERAP CAT: Nutrient.

36. ACES. [7365-82-4] 2-[(2-Amino-2-oxoethyl)amino]-ethanesulfonic acid; *N*-(carbamoylmethyl)taurine; *N*-(2-acetamido)-2-aminoethanesulfonic acid. $C_4H_{10}N_2O_4S$; mol wt 182.20. C 26.37%, H 5.53%, N 15.38%, O 35.12%, S 17.60%. One of several zwitterionic N-substituted amino acids known as "Good" buffers. Active in pH range 6-8. Prepn: N. E. Good *et al., Biochemistry* **5**, 467 (1966). Thermodynamic parameters: D. C. McGlothlin, J. Jordan, *Anal. Lett.* **9**, 245 (1976). Metal complexation in solns: J. M. Pope *et al., Anal. Biochem.* **36**, 173 (1970). Effect of temperature on pK values: R. N. Roy *et al., J. Chem. Eng. Data* **42**, 41 (1997). Use as buffer in electrophoresis: D. J. Chappell, *Clin. Chem.* **31**, 1384 (1985); Q. Liu *et al., Anal. Biochem.* **270**, 112 (1999); in chromatography: Z. Yu, D. Westerlund, *Chromatographia* **44**, 589 (1997).

Crystals from alcohol and water, dec 293°. pKa at 0.1M (0°): 7.32; (20°): 6.88; (37°): 6.56. ΔpKa/°C: −0.020.

USE: Buffer for biological systems.

37. Acesulfame. [33665-90-6] 6-Methyl-1,2,3-oxathiazin-4(3*H*)-one 2,2-dioxide; 6-methyl-3,4-dihydro-1,2,3-oxathiazin-4-one 2,2-dioxide; acetosulfam. $C_4H_5NO_4S$; mol wt 163.15. C 29.45%, H 3.09%, N 8.59%, O 39.23%, S 19.65%. Non-nutritive artificial sweetener. Prepn: K. Clauss, H. Jensen, **DE 2001017**; *eidem,* **US 3689486** (1971, 1972 to Hoechst); K. Clauss *et al., Z. Lebensm.-Unters. Forsch.* **162**, 37 (1976). Crystal structure: E. F. Paulus, *Acta Crystallogr.* **B31**, 1191 (1975). HPLC analysis: H. Grosspietsch, H. Hachenberg, *Z. Lebensm.-Unters. Forsch.* **171**, 41 (1980). *Book: Acesulfame-K*, D. G. Mayer, F. H. Kemper, Eds. (Marcel Dekker, Inc., New York, 1991) 243 pp.

Needles from benzene or chloroform, mp 123-123.5°.

Potassium salt. [55589-62-3] Acesulfame-K; HOE-095K; Sunette. $C_4H_4KNO_4S$; mol wt 201.24. Colorless, odorless powder. Dec pt ~225°. d (solid) 1.81 g/cm³; d (bulk) 1.1-1.3 kg/dm³. uv max: 227 nm (ε 1.0762×10⁴). Very sol in water, DMF, DMSO. Sol in alc, glycerin-water. Soly in water (g/l): ~150 (0°); ~210 (10°); ~270 (20°); ~360 (30°); ~460 (40°); ~580 (50°); ~830 (70°); ~1300 (100°). Soly at 20° (g/l): methanol ~10; ethanol (anhydrous) ~1; glycerol (anhydrous) ~30; glycerol/water (80:20, v/v) ~82; glycerol/water (50:50, v/v) ~162; acetone ~0.8; glacial acetic acid ~130. Soly at 23° (g/l): ethanol/water (80:20, v/v) ~46; ethanol/water (60:40, v/v) ~100; ethanol/water (40:60, v/v) ~155; ethanol/water (20:80, v/v) ~221. LD_{50} in rats (mg/kg): 7431 orally, 2243 i.p. (Mayer, Kemper).

USE: Potassium salt as sweetener for foods, cosmetics.

38. Acetal. [105-57-7] 1,1-Diethoxyethane; diethylacetal; acetaldehyde diethyl acetal; ethylidene diethyl ether. $C_6H_{14}O_2$; mol wt 118.17. C 60.98%, H 11.94%, O 27.08%. CH_3-$CH(OC_2H_5)_2$. Made from acetaldehyde and alcohol in the presence of anhydrous calcium chloride or of small quantities of mineral acid: H. Adkins, B. H. Nissen, *J. Am. Chem. Soc.* **44**, 2750 (1922);

eidem, Org. Synth. **coll. vol. I,** 1 (2nd ed., 1941). Toxicity study: H. F. Smyth *et al., J. Ind. Hyg. Toxicol.* **31**, 60 (1949).

Volatile liquid. d_4^{20} 0.8254. bp_{760} 102.7°; bp_{200} 66.3°; bp_{60} 39.8°; bp_{40} 31.9°; bp_{20} 19.6°; bp_{10} 8.0°; bp_5 −2.3°; $bp_{1.0}$ −23°. n_D^{20} 1.38193. Flash pt, closed cup: 97°F (36°C). uv spectrum: Purvis, *J. Chem. Soc.* **127**, 9 (1925). 100 g water dissolve 5 g acetal. Misc with alcohol, 60% alcohol, ether. Sol in heptane, methylcyclohexane, propyl-, isopropyl-, butyl-, isobutyl alcohol, and ethyl acetate. Tends to polymerize on standing. Stable to alkalies. LD_{50} orally in rats: 4.57 g/kg (Smyth).

USE: Solvent; in synthetic perfumes such as jasmine; in organic syntheses.

39. Acetaldehyde. [75-07-0] Ethanal; "aldehyde"; acetic aldehyde; ethylaldehyde. C_2H_4O; mol wt 44.05. C 54.53%, H 9.15%, O 36.32%. CH_3CHO. Produced by oxidation of alcohol with $Na_2Cr_2O_7$ and H_2SO_4; usually from acetylene, dil H_2SO_4 and mercuric oxide as catalyst; also by passing alcohol vapor over a heated metallic catalyst. Lab procedure from ethanol: Wertheim, *J. Am. Chem. Soc.* **44**, 2658 (1922); Fricke, Havestadt, *Angew. Chem.* **36**, 546 (1923); Gattermann-Wieland, *Praxis des Organischen Chemikers* (de Gruyter, Berlin, 40th ed., 1961) p 180; from acetylene: Gattermann-Wieland, *op. cit.* 183; from paraldehyde: A. I. Vogel, *Practical Organic Chemistry* (Longmans, London, 3rd ed., 1959) p 324; by catalytic oxidation of ethylene in aq soln: J. Smidt *et al., Angew. Chem.* **71**, 176 (1959); by oxidation of ethylene in fuel cells in the gas phase: K. Otsuka *et al., Chem. Commun.* **1988**, 1272. Manuf: *Faith, Keyes & Clark's Industrial Chemicals*, F. A. Lowenheim, M. K. Moran, Eds. (Wiley-Interscience, New York, 4th ed., 1975) pp 1-7. Toxicity data: Smyth, *Arch. Ind. Hyg. Occup. Med.* **4**, 119 (1951). *Review:* H. J. Hagemeyer in *Kirk-Othmer Encyclopedia of Chemical Technology* **vol. 1** (John Wiley & Sons, New York, 4th ed., 1991) pp 94-109.

Flammable liquid; characteristic, pungent odor. d_4^{16} 0.788. mp −123.5°. bp 21°. n_D^{20} 1.3316. Flash pt, closed cup: −36°F (−38°C). Miscible with water, alcohol. *Keep cold. Chill thoroughly before opening.* LD_{50} orally in rats: 1930 mg/kg (Smyth).

Caution: Potential symptoms of overexposure are eye, nose and throat irritation; conjunctivitis; coughing; CNS depression; eye and skin burns; dermatitis; delayed pulmonary edema. *See NIOSH Pocket Guide to Chemical Hazards* (DHHS/NIOSH 97-140, 1997) p 2. *See also Clinical Toxicology of Commercial Products*, R. E. Gosselin *et al.,* Eds. (Williams & Wilkins, Baltimore, 5th ed., 1984) Section II, p 186. This substance is reasonably anticipated to be a human carcinogen: *Report on Carcinogens, Eleventh Edition* (PB2005-104914, 2004) p III-1.

USE: Manuf paraldehyde, acetic acid, butanol, perfumes, flavors, aniline dyes, plastics, synthetic rubber; silvering mirrors, hardening gelatin fibers. Flavoring agent in foods and beverages. Fumigant for storage of apples and strawberries.

40. Acetaldehyde Ammonia. [75-39-8] 1-Aminoethanol; α-aminoethyl alcohol; aldehyde ammonia. C_2H_7NO; mol wt 61.08. C 39.33%, H 11.55%, N 22.93%, O 26.19%. CH_3-$CH(OH)NH_2$. Prepd from acetaldehyde and ammonia: Aschan, *Ber.* **48**, 874 (1915).

Crystals; gradually turns yellow to brown in air. mp 97°. bp 110°, partly decomposing. Freely sol in water, slightly in ether. *Protect from light and air.*

Caution: Irritates eyes, mucous membranes.

USE: For preparing pure acetaldehyde; in organic syntheses.

41. Acetaldehyde Sodium Bisulfite. [918-04-7] 1-Hydroxyethanesulfonic acid sodium salt. $C_2H_5NaO_4S$; mol wt 148.11. C 16.22%, H 3.40%, Na 15.52%, O 43.21%, S 21.65%. $CH_3CH(OH)SO_3Na$.

Hemihydrate. Crystals, decomposed by acids. Freely sol in water. Insol in alcohol.

Caution: Irritates skin, mucous membranes.

USE: Making pure acetaldehyde; in organic synthesis.

42. Acetaldoxime. [107-29-9] Acetaldehyde oxime; aldoxime; ethylidenehydroxylamine. C_2H_5NO; mol wt 59.07. C 40.67%, H 8.53%, N 23.71%, O 27.09%. $CH_3CH=NOH$. Prepn: Dunstan, Dymond, *J. Chem. Soc.* **61**, 470 (1892). Manuf: Donaruma, **US 2763686** (1956 to du Pont).

Two crystalline modifications, mp 12° (β-form), mp 46.5° (α-form). d 0.966. bp 114.5°. n_D^{20} 1.415. Dec by aq HCl into acetaldehyde and hydroxylamine. Very sol in water, alcohol, ether.

43. Acetamide. [60-35-5] Acetic acid amide. C_2H_5NO; mol wt 59.07. C 40.67%, H 8.53%, N 23.71%, O 27.09%. CH_3-$CONH_2$. Prepd by fractional distillation of ammonium acetate: Coleman, Alvarado, *Org. Synth.* **coll. vol. I,** 3 (2nd ed., 1941); Gattermann-Wieland, *Praxis des Organischen Chemikers* (40th ed., 1961) p 118; Vogel, *Practical Organic Chemistry* (3rd ed., 1959) p 401. Prepn from methyl acetate, W. P. Munro *et al.,* **US 2106697** (1936 to Calco Chem.); from ethyl acetate, Vogel, *op. cit.,* p 403. Studies of acetamide as an ionizing solvent: Jauder, Winkler, *J. Inorg. Nucl. Chem.* **9,** 24, 32, 39 (1959). Toxicological study: Weisburger *et al., Toxicol. Appl. Pharmacol.* **14,** 163 (1969).

Deliquescent hexagonal crystals. Odorless when pure, but frequently has a mousy odor. d_4^{20} 1.159. mp 81°. bp_{760} 222°; bp_{100} 158°; bp_{40} 136°; bp_{20} 120°; bp_{10} 105°; bp_5 92°. n_D^{78} 1.4274. Neutral reaction. pKb (25°): 14.51. One gram dissolves in 0.5 ml water, 2 ml alcohol, 6 ml pyridine. Sol in chloroform, glycerol, hot benzene.

USE: Solvent; molten acetamide is an excellent solvent for many organic and inorganic compounds. Solubilizer; renders sparingly soluble substances more soluble in water by mere addition or by fusion. Plasticizer; stabilizer. Manuf methylamine, denaturing alcohol. In organic syntheses.

44. Acetamidine Hydrochloride. [124-42-5] Ethanimidamide hydrochloride; ethanamidine hydrochloride; α-amino-α-iminoethane hydrochloride; ethenylamidine hydrochloride; acediamine hydrochloride; SN-4455. $C_2H_7ClN_2$; mol wt 94.54. C 25.41%, H 7.46%, Cl 37.50%, N 29.63%. Prepd by passing HCl into a soln of acetonitrile in abs alcohol, then passing NH_3 into the reaction mixture: Pinner, *Ber.* **16,** 1654 (1883); **17,** 178 (1884); Dox, *Org. Synth.* **coll. vol. I,** 5 (New York, 2nd ed., 1941). *See also* Fargher, *J. Chem. Soc.* **117,** 674 (1920). *Review:* Shriner, Neumann, *Chem. Rev.* **35,** 351-425 (1944).

Long prisms from alcohol, somewhat deliquescent, mp 174° (Fargher); mp 164-166° (Dox). Very sol in water. Sol in alcohols. Practically insol in acetone, ether. Should be stored in a closed container and in a cool place. If alkali is added to an aq soln, the free base is liberated.

Free base. $C_2H_6N_2$. uv max: 224 nm (ε 4000). pK$_1$ (25°): 12.1. Has a strong alkaline reaction and on slight warming dissociates into ammonia and acetic acid.

Caution: Irritates mucous membranes, skin. Avoid tasting, swallowing, inhalation of the dust, skin contact.

USE: In the synthesis of imidazoles, pyrimidines, triazines.

45. ε-Acetamidocaproic Acid. [57-08-9] 6-(Acetylamino)hexanoic acid; 6-acetamidohexanoic acid; acetaminocaproic acid; acexamic acid; N-acetyl-6-aminohexanoic acid. $C_8H_{15}NO_3$; mol wt 173.21. C 55.47%, H 8.73%, N 8.09%, O 27.71%. CH_3-$CONH(CH_2)_5COOH$. Prepn: Offe, *Z. Naturforsch.* **2b,** 182 (1947); **FR M2332** (1964 to Rowa), *C.A.* **61,** 577b (1964). Anti-inflammatory activity of salts: O. Guillard *et al., Pharmacology* **34,** 296 (1987). Clinical comparison with ranitidine in gastroduodenal ulcer: M. J. Varas Lorenzo, *Curr. Ther. Res.* **39,** 19 (1986).

Crystals from acetone, mp 104-105.5° (**FR M2332**), mp 112° (Offe).

Sodium salt. [7234-48-5] Plastenan. $C_8H_{14}NNaO_3$; mol wt 195.19.

Zinc salt. [70020-71-2] Zinc acexamate; Copinal. $C_{16}H_{28}N_2$-O_6Zn; mol wt 409.81.

THERAP CAT: Anti-inflammatory; zinc salt as antiulcerative.

46. Acetamidoeugenol. [305-13-5] N,N-Diethyl-2-[2-methoxy-4-(2-propenyl)phenoxy]acetamide; 2-(4-allyl-2-methoxyphenoxy)-N,N-diethylacetamide; N,N-diethyl-2-methoxy-4-allylphenoxyacetamide; 2-methoxy-4-allylphenoxyacetic acid N,N-diethylamide; 2-M-4-A; G-29505; Detrovel; Estil. $C_{16}H_{23}NO_3$;

mol wt 277.36. C 69.29%, H 8.36%, N 5.05%, O 17.31%. Prepn: **GB 792490; GB 837995** (1958, 1960 to Geigy).

Oil. $bp_{0.001}$ 143-146°; n_D^{25} 1.5300. Soluble in water, pH of 5% aq soln 7.3.

THERAP CAT: Anesthetic (intravenous).

47. Acetaminophen. [103-90-2] N-(4-Hydroxyphenyl)-acetamide; 4'-hydroxyacetanilide; p-hydroxyacetanilide; p-acetamidophenol; p-acetaminophenol; p-acetylaminophenol; N-acetyl-p-aminophenol; paracetamol; Acamol; Alpiny; Anaflon; Anhiba; Apamide; Ben-u-ron; Calpol; Captin; Dafalgan; Datril; Dirox; Disprol; Doliprane; Dolprone; Enelfa; Gelocatil; Hedex; Momentum; Ortensan; Panadol; Panaleve; Panodil; Paraspen; Pasolind N; Tempra; Tylenol; Valadol. $C_8H_9NO_2$; mol wt 151.16. C 63.57%, H 6.00%, N 9.27%, O 21.17%. Prepn from p-nitrophenol: Morse, *Ber.* **11,** 232 (1878); Tingle, Williams, *Am. Chem. J.* **37,** 63 (1907); from p-aminophenol: Lumière *et al., Bull. Soc. Chim. Fr.* [3] **33,** 785 (1905); Fierz-David, Kuster, *Helv. Chim. Acta* **22,** 94 (1939); Wilbert, De Angelis, **US 2998450** (1961 to Warner-Lambert); Bergmann, **DE 453577**; *Chem. Zentralbl.* **1928, I,** 2663; *Frdl.* **16,** 238; from p-hydroxyacetophenone hydrazone: Pearson *et al., J. Am. Chem. Soc.* **75,** 5907 (1953). Toxicity data: G. A. Starmer *et al., Toxicol. Appl. Pharmacol.* **19,** 20 (1971); D. C. Dahlin, S. D. Nelson, *J. Med. Chem.* **25,** 885 (1982). Evaluation of renal effects: D. P. Sandler *et al., N. Engl. J. Med.* **320,** 1238 (1989). Comprehensive description: J. E. Fairbrother, *Anal. Profiles Drug Subs.* **3,** 1-109 (1974). Review of pharmacology: B. Ameer, D. J. Greenblatt, *Ann. Intern. Med.* **87,** 202-209 (1977). Review of acetaminophen-induced hepatotoxicity: J. A. Hinson, *Rev. Biochem. Toxicol.* **2,** 103-129 (1980); *idem, Life Sci.* **29,** 107-116 (1981); and proposed protective agents: M. Davis, *Semin. Liver Dis.* **6,** 138-147 (1986). For proposed toxic metabolite *see* Acetimidoquinone.

Large monoclinic prisms from water, mp 169-170.5°. d_4^{21} 1.293. uv max (ethanol): 250 nm (ε 13800). Very slightly sol in cold water, considerably more sol in hot water. Sol in methanol, ethanol, dimethylformamide, ethylene dichloride, acetone, ethyl acetate. Slightly sol in ether. Practically insol in petr ether, pentane, benzene. LD$_{50}$ in mice (mg/kg): 338 orally (Starmer), 500 i.p. (Dahlin, Nelson).

USE: Manuf azo dyes, photographic chemicals.

THERAP CAT: Analgesic; antipyretic.

48. Acetaminosalol. [118-57-0] 2-Hydroxybenzoic acid 4-(acetylamino)phenyl ester; p-acetamidophenyl salicylate; acetylaminophenyl salicylate; acetyl-p-aminosalol; p-acetylaminophenol salicylic acid ester; phenetsal; Salophen; Phenosal. $C_{15}H_{13}NO_4$; mol wt 271.27. C 66.41%, H 4.83%, N 5.16%, O 23.59%. Prepn: Brewster, *J. Am. Chem. Soc.* **40,** 1136 (1918).

Crystals from hot ethanol, mp 187°. Practically insol in petr ether, cold water, more sol in warm water. Sol in alcohol, ether, benzene. Incompatible with alkalies and alkaline solns which dissolve it with decompn. The alkaline soln gradually becomes blue when boiled, the blue color being discharged upon continued boiling and again produced upon cooling and exposure to air.

THERAP CAT: Analgesic; antipyretic; anti-inflammatory.

THERAP CAT (VET): Analgesic; antipyretic.

49. Acetamiprid. [160430-64-8] (1E)-N-[(6-Chloro-3-pyridinyl)methyl]-N'-cyano-N-methylethanimidamide; N-cyano-N'-(2-chloro-5-pyridylmethyl)-N'-methylacetamidine; NI-25; Assail; Mospilan. $C_{10}H_{11}ClN_4$; mol wt 222.67. C 53.94%, H 4.98%, Cl 15.92%, N 25.16%. Neonicotinoid insecticide for use in food crops. Prepn: K. Ishimitsu et al., WO 9104965; eidem, US 5304566 (1991, 1994 both to Nippon Soda); of tritiated form: B. Latli et al., J. Labelled Compd. Radiopharm. 38, 971 (1996). Physical properties, biological activity and field trials: H. Takahashi et al., Proc. Br. Crop Prot. Conf. - Pests Dis. 1992, 89. HPLC determn in soil: M. Tokieda et al., J. Pestic. Sci. 23, 296 (1998). Stereochemistry and active conformation: A. Nakayama et al., Pestic. Sci. 51, 157 (1997). Efficacy against diamondback moth: H. Takahashi et al., J. Pestic. Sci. 24, 23 (1999); against green peach aphid: eidem, ibid. 270.

White crystals, mp 101.0-103.3°. Soly in water at 25°: 4200 mg/l. Sol in acetone, methanol, ethanol, dichloromethane, chloroform, acetonitrile, tetrahydrofuran. Vapor pressure at 25°: < 1 × 10^{-8} mmHg. LD$_{50}$ in male, female rats, male, female mice (mg/kg): 217, 146, 198, 184 orally (Takahashi).

USE: Insecticide.

50. Acetanilide. [103-84-4] N-Phenylacetamide; antifebrin; acetylaniline; acetylaminobenzene. C_8H_9NO; mol wt 135.16. C 71.09%, H 6.71%, N 10.36%, O 11.84%. p-Aminophenol deriv related to acetaminophen, q.v., with analgesic and antipyretic properties. Usually prepd from aniline and acetic acids: A. I. Vogel, Practical Organic Chemistry (London, 3rd ed., 1959) p 577. From aniline and acetyl chloride: Gattermann-Wieland, Praxis des Organischen Chemikers (Berlin, 40th ed., 1961) p 114. From aniline, acetone and ketene: Hurd, Org. Synth. coll. vol. I (New York, 2nd ed., 1941) p 332. Chemistry: G. C. Derick, J. H. Bornman, J. Am. Chem. Soc. 35, 1269 (1913). Toxicity data: P. K. Smith, W. E. Hambourger, J. Pharmacol. Exp. Ther. 54, (1935). Monograph: Gross, Acetanilid (Hillhouse Press, New Haven, 1946).

Orthorhombic plates, scales from water. mp 113-115°; bp 304-305°. Slightly burning taste. Appreciably volatile at 95°. d_4^{15} 1.219. pK (28°): 13.0. One gram dissolves in 185 ml water, 20 ml boiling water, 3.4 ml alcohol, 3 ml methanol, 0.6 ml boiling alcohol, 3.7 ml chloroform, 4 ml acetone, 5 ml glycerol, 8 ml dioxane, 18 ml ether, 47 ml benzene. Very sparingly sol in petr ether. Chloral hydrate increases the soly of acetanilide in water. LD$_{50}$ intragastric in rats: 800 mg/kg (Smith, Hambourger).

USE: Manuf of medicinals and dyes; stabilizer for H_2O_2 soln; as addition to cellulose ester varnishes.

51. p-Acetanisidine. [51-66-1] N-(4-Methoxyphenyl)-acetamide; p-acetanisidide; methacetin; p-methoxyacetanilide. $C_9H_{11}NO_2$; mol wt 165.19. C 65.44%, H 6.71%, N 8.48%, O 19.37%. $CH_3OC_6H_4NHCOCH_3$. Prepn by acetylation of p-anisidine: Reverdin, Bucky, Ber. 39, 2679 (1906); from p-acetylanisole and hydroxylamine-O-sulfonic acid: Sanford et al., J. Am. Chem. Soc. 67, 1941 (1945).

Cryst powder, feeble, bitter taste, mp 130-132°. Slightly sol in water; sol in alcohol, acetone, chloroform, dil acids, alkalies.

52. Acetarsone. [97-44-9] [3-(Acetylamino)-4-hydroxyphenyl]arsonic acid; N-acetyl-4-hydroxy-m-arsanilic acid; 3-acetamido-4-hydroxyphenylarsonic acid; 3-acetamido-4-hydroxybenzenearsonic acid; acetarsol; acetphenarsine; Ehrlich 594; Fourneau 190; F-190; Gynoplix; Orarsan; Spirocid; Stovarsol. $C_8H_{10}AsNO_5$; mol wt 275.09. C 34.93%, H 3.66%, As 27.24%, N 5.09%, O 29.08%. Pentavalent arsenical formerly used in the treatment of syphilis. Also used in combination with arecoline, q.v. Prepn: Raiziss, Fisher, J. Am. Chem. Soc. 48, 1323 (1926); Hewitt, King, J. Chem. Soc. 1926, 823. Toxicity data: H. H. Anderson, C. D. Leake, Proc. Soc. Exp. Biol. Med. 27, 267 (1930).

Stout prisms from water, dec 240-250°; slight acid taste. Slightly sol in water; freely sol in solns of alkalies and alkali carbonates. Stable at ordinary temps. MLD in rabbits, cats (mg/kg): 125-150, 150-175 orally (Anderson, Leake).

THERAP CAT: Antiprotozoal (Trichomonas).

THERAP CAT (VET): Antiprotozoal.

53. Acetazolamide. [59-66-5] N-[5-(Aminosulfonyl)-1,3,4-thiadiazol-2-yl]acetamide; 5-acetamido-1,3,4-thiadiazole-2-sulfonamide; 2-acetylamino-1,3,4-thiadiazole-5-sulfonamide; 6063; Acetamox; Atenezol; Défiltran; Diamox; Didoc; Diuriwas; Donmox; Edemox; Fonurit; Glaupax. $C_4H_6N_4O_3S_2$; mol wt 222.25. C 21.62%, H 2.72%, N 25.21%, O 21.60%, S 28.85%. Carbonic anhydrase inhibitor. Prepn: R. O. Roblin, J. W. Clapp, J. Am. Chem. Soc. 72, 4890 (1950); J. W. Clapp, R. O. Roblin, US 2554816 (1951 to Am. Cyanamid). HPLC determn in pharmaceuticals: Z. S. Gomaa, Biomed. Chromatogr. 7, 134 (1993). Effect on retinal circulation: S. M. B. Rassam et al., Eye 7, 697 (1993). Clinical trial in postoperative elevation of intraocular pressure: I. D. Ladas et al., Br. J. Ophthalmol. 77, 136 (1993). Comprehensive description: J. Parasrampuria, Anal. Profiles Drug Subs. Excip. 22, 1-32 (1993). Review of efficacy in acute mountain sickness: L. D. Ried et al., J. Wilderness Med. 5, 34-48 (1994).

Crystals from water, mp 258-259° (effervescence). Weak acid. pKa 7.2. Sparingly sol in cold water. Slightly sol in alcohol, acetone. Practically insol in carbon tetrachloride, chloroform, ether. Soly (mg/ml): polyethylene glycol-400 87.81; propylene glycol 7.44; ethanol 3.93; glycerin 3.65; water 0.72.

Sodium salt. [1424-27-7] Vetamox.

THERAP CAT: Antiglaucoma; diuretic; in treatment of acute mountain sickness.

THERAP CAT (VET): Diuretic.

54. Acetiamine. [299-89-8] Ethanethioic acid S-[1-[2-(acetyloxy)ethyl]-2-[[(4-amino-2-methyl-5-pyrimidinyl)methyl]-formylamino]-1-propenyl] ester; thioacetic acid S-ester with N-[(4-amino-2-methyl-5-pyrimidinyl)methyl]-N-(4-hydroxy-3-mercapto-1-methyl-1-butenyl)formamide acetate; N-[(4-amino-2-methyl-5-pyrimidinyl)methyl]-N-(4-hydroxy-2-mercapto-1-methyl-1-butenyl)formamide O,S-diacetate; 3-acetylthio-4-[(4-amino-2-methyl-5-pyrimidinyl)methyl-N-formylamino]-3-pentenyl acetate; 5-acetoxy-3-acetylthio-2-[(4-amino-2-methyl-5-pyrimidinyl)methyl-N-formylamino]-2-pentene; diacethiamine; O,S-diacetylthiamine; vitamin B$_1$ O,S-diacetate; D.A.T.; Thianeuron. $C_{16}H_{22}N_4O_4S$; mol wt 366.44. C 52.44%, H 6.05%, N 15.29%, O 17.46%, S 8.75%. A fat-soluble deriv. of vitamin B$_1$. Prepn: Matsukawa, Kawasaki, J. Pharm. Soc. Jpn. 23, 705, 709 (1953); C.A. 48, 7017e (1954); Takamizawa et al., Bull. Chem. Soc. Jpn. 36, 1214 (1963). Synthesis and pharmacology: Gauthier et al., Ann. Pharm. Fr. 21, 655 (1963). Clinical studies: Wagner, Wagner, Arzneim.-Forsch. 16, 1643 (1966); Blum, Thomas, Pharmacol. Clin. 2, 177 (1970).

cis-form

Colorless prisms from benzene-petr ether, mp 122-123° (dec); from water, mp 123-124°. Soluble in water, methanol, ethanol.

Hydrochloride. [28008-04-0] Nevriton. $C_{16}H_{22}N_4O_4S.HCl$; mol wt 402.90.

THERAP CAT: Vitamin (enzyme cofactor).

55. Acetic Acid Glacial. [64-19-7] Aci-Jel. $C_2H_4O_2$; mol wt 60.05. C 40.00%, H 6.71%, O 53.29%. CH_3COOH. Obtained in the destructive distillation of wood; from acetylene and water, via acetaldehyde by oxidation with air. Manuf processes: Bhattacharyya, Sourirajan, *J. Appl. Chem.* **6**, 442 (1956); *eidem, ibid.* **9**, 126 (1959); Elce *et al.,* **US 2800504** (1957 to Distillers Co.); Wirth, **US 2818428** (1957 to British Petroleum); McKusick and Hoover, **US 2940913** and **US 2940914** (both 1960 to Du Pont); *Faith, Keyes & Clark's Industrial Chemicals,* F. A. Lowenheim, M. K. Moran, Eds. (Wiley-Interscience, New York, 4th ed., 1975) pp 8-15. Toxicity data: H. F. Smyth *et al., Arch. Ind. Hyg. Occup. Med.* **4**, 119 (1951). *Review:* F. S. Wagner in *Kirk-Othmer Encyclopedia of Chemical Technology* vol. 1 (Wiley-Interscience, New York, 3rd ed., 1978) pp 124-147.

Liquid; pungent odor. *Produces burns of the skin!* $d^{16.67}$ (liq) 1.053; $d^{16.60}$ (solid) 1.266. d_{25}^{25} 1.049. bp 118°. mp 16.7°. n_D^{20} 1.3718. Flash pt, closed cup: 103°F (39°C). *Caution: Flammable!* Contracts slightly on freezing. It is an excellent solvent for many organic compounds; also dissolves phosphorus, sulfur and halogen acids. Miscible with water, alcohol, glycerol, ether, carbon tetrachloride. Practically insol in carbon disulfide. Weakly ionized in aq solns: pKa 4.74. pH of aq solns 1.0M = 2.4; 0.1M = 2.9; 0.01M = 3.4. LD_{50} in rats (g/kg): 3.53 orally (Smyth).

Incompat. Carbonates, hydroxides, many oxides, phosphates.

Caution: Ingestion may cause severe corrosion of mouth and G.I. tract, with vomiting, hematemesis, diarrhea, circulatory collapse, uremia, death. Chronic exposure may cause erosion of dental enamel, bronchitis, eye irritation, *cf. Patty's Industrial Hygiene and Toxicology* vol. 2C, G. D. Clayton, F. E. Clayton, Eds. (Wiley-Interscience, New York, 3rd ed., 1982) p 4909-4911.

USE: Manuf various acetates, acetyl compounds, cellulose acetate, acetate rayon, plastics and rubber in tanning; as laundry sour; printing calico and dyeing silk; as acidulant and preservative in foods; solvent for gums, resins, volatile oils and many other substances. Widely used in commercial organic syntheses. Pharmaceutic aid (acidifier).

THERAP CAT (VET): Vesicant, caustic, destruction of warts.

56. Acetic Anhydride. [108-24-7] Acetic oxide; acetyl oxide. $C_4H_6O_3$; mol wt 102.09. C 47.06%, H 5.92%, O 47.02%. $(CH_3CO)_2O$. Equivalent to 117.64% acetic acid. Made formerly from sod. acetate and acetyl or sulfuryl chloride; now usually obtained from acetaldehyde or acetic acid: *Faith, Keyes & Clark's Industrial Chemicals,* F. A. Lowenheim, M. K. Moran, Eds. (Wiley-Interscience, New York, 4th ed., 1975) pp 16-20. Of industrial importance is also the ketene process, starting with the thermal decomposition of acetone: Schmidlin, Bergmann, *Ber.* **43**, 2821 (1910). Toxicity study: H. F. Smyth *et al., Arch. Ind. Hyg. Occup. Med.* **4**, 119 (1951).

Very refractive liquid; strong acetic odor. *Readily combustible. Fire hazard.* Flash pt 130°F. d_4^{15} 1.080. mp −73°. bp 139°. n_D^{20} 1.3904. Slowly soluble in water, forming acetic acid; with alcohol forms ethyl acetate; sol in chloroform, ether. LD_{50} orally in rats: 1.78 g/kg (Smyth).

Caution: Potential symptoms of overexposure are conjunctivitis, lacrimation, corneal edema, opacity and photophobia; nasal, pharyngeal irritation; cough, dyspnea and bronchitis; skin burns, vesiculation and sensitization dermatitis. *See NIOSH Pocket Guide to Chemical Hazards* (DHHS/NIOSH 97-140, 1997) p 2.

USE: Manuf acetyl compounds, cellulose acetates. As acetulizer and solvent in examining wool fat, glycerol, fatty and volatile oils, resins; detection of rosin. Widely used in organic syntheses, e.g., as dehydrating agent in nitrations, sulfonations and other reactions where removal of water is necessary.

57. Acetimidoquinone. [50700-49-7] *N*-(4-oxo-2,5-cyclohexadien-1-ylidene)acetamide; *N*-acetyl-*p*-benzoquinonimine; *N*-acetylimidoquinone; NAPQI. $C_8H_7NO_2$; mol wt 149.15. C 64.42%, H 4.73%, N 9.39%, O 21.45%. Proposed "ultimate" toxic metabolite of acetaminophen, *q.v.* Initially prepared by oxidation of acetaminophen with lead tetraacetate and characterized as a Diels-Alder adduct: I. C. Calder *et al., J. Med. Chem.* **16**, 499 (1973). Electrochemical generation in buffer: D. J. Miner, P. T. Kissinger, *Biochem. Pharmacol.* **28**, 3285 (1979). Synthesis in stable benzene soln and reactivity: I. A. Blair *et al., Tetrahedron Lett.* **21**, 4947 (1980). Prepn in cryst form, decomposition kinetics, preliminary toxicological studies: D. C. Dahlin, S. D. Nelson, *J. Med. Chem.* **25**, 885 (1982). Microsomal reactivity study: G. B. Corcoran, *Adv. Exp. Med. Biol.* **136B**, 1085 (1982). Review of acetaminophen-induced hepatotoxicity: J. A. Hinson *et al., Life Sci.* **29**, 107-116 (1981).

Yellow cubic cryst, mp 74-75°. Sublimes at 45-50° (0.07 mm Hg). uv max (*n*-hexane): 263, 376 nm (ε 3.3×10^4, 1.6×10^2 M^{-1} cm^{-1}). LD_{50} i.p. in male BALB/c mice: 20 mg/kg (Dahlin, Nelson).

58. Acetoacetanilide. [102-01-2] 3-Oxo-*N*-phenylbutanamide; α-acetylacetanilide; acetoacetic anilide; β-ketobutyranilide. $C_{10}H_{11}NO_2$; mol wt 177.20. C 67.78%, H 6.26%, N 7.90%, O 18.06%. $C_6H_5NHCOCH_2COCH_3$. Prepd by the reaction of ketene dimer with aniline: Chick, Wilsmore, *J. Chem. Soc.* **1908**, 946; Boese, *Ind. Eng. Chem.* **32**, 16 (1940); Williams, Krynitsky, *Org. Synth.* **coll. vol. III**, 10 (1955). By the reaction of aniline with ethyl acetoacetate: Knorr, *Ann.* **26**, 69 (1886); Roos, *Ber.* **21**, 624 (1883); Knorr, Reuter, *Ber.* **27**, 1169 (1894). Enol form (unstable) prepd by pouring an alkaline soln of the keto form in cold, dilute H_2SO_4.

Ketone Form. Leaflets from dilute alcohol, mp 85°. Slightly soluble in water; sol in alcohol, chloroform, ether, hot benzene, hot petr ether, acids, or alkali hydroxide solns. Gives a violet color with ferric chloride.

USE: Manuf of yellow dyes, such as Hansa and benzidine yellows. In rubber compounding. In organic syntheses.

59. Acetoacetic Acid. [541-50-4] 3-Oxobutanoic acid; diacetic acid; acetylacetic acid; acetonecarboxylic acid; 3-ketobutyric acid; 2-ketobutyric acid. $C_4H_6O_3$; mol wt 102.09. C 47.06%, H 5.92%, O 47.02%. CH_3COCH_2COOH. Prepd by hydrolysis of ethyl acetoacetate: Krueger, *J. Am. Chem. Soc.* **74**, 5536 (1952).

Crystals from ether, mp 36-37°. A strong, but unstable acid. At 100° violently decomposes into acetone and CO_2. Miscible with water, alc.

Caution: Severely irritating to skin, mucous membranes.

USE: In organic syntheses.

60. Acetobromglucose. [572-09-8] α-D-Glucopyranosyl bromide 2,3,4,6-tetraacetate; α-acetobromoglucose; 2,3,4,6-tetra-acetyl-α-D-glucopyranosyl bromide. $C_{14}H_{19}BrO_9$; mol wt 411.20. C 40.89%, H 4.66%, Br 19.43%, O 35.02%. Prepd by the action of hydrogen bromide upon anhydrous glucose in acetic anhydride: Redemann, Niemann, *Org. Synth.* **coll. vol. III**, 11 (1955). See also Fischer, *Ber.* **49**, 584 (1916); Freudenberg, *Ber.* **60**, 241 (1927); Gattermann-Wieland, *Praxis des Organischen Chemikers* (de Gruyter, Berlin, 40th ed., 1961) p 340.

R = CCH$_3$

Crystals from isopropyl ether, mp 88-89°. $[\alpha]_D^{19}$ +199.3° (c = 3 in chloroform); $[\alpha]_D^{15}$ +230.3° (c = 9 in benzene). Best stored in a vacuum desiccator. Dec on contact with water. One gram dissolves in 20 ml absolute ethanol, more soluble in methanol. Freely sol in ether, chloroform, acetone, ethyl acetate, benzene. Slightly sol in petr ether.

61. Acetochlor. [34256-82-1] 2-Chloro-N-(ethoxymethyl)-N-(2-ethyl-6-methylphenyl)acetamide; 2-chloro-N-(ethoxymethyl)-6'-ethyl-o-acetotoluidide; 2'-ethyl-6'-methyl-N-(ethoxymethyl)-2-chloroacetanilide; MON-097; MG-02; Harness; Surpass; TopNotch; Trophy. $C_{14}H_{20}ClNO_2$; mol wt 269.77. C 62.33%, H 7.47%, Cl 13.14%, N 5.19%, O 11.86%. Pre-emergent herbicide. Prepn: J. F. Olin, US 3547620 (1970 to Monsanto). Description of physical and biological properties: R. P. Upchurch et al., Proc. North Cent. Weed Control Conf. **25**, 56 (1970). Synthesis: B. G. Zupancic, M. Sopcic, Synthesis **1982**, 942. Field trials on peanuts and soybeans: C. W. Derting et al., Proc. South. Weed Sci. Soc. **25**, 131 (1972); on peanuts: L. R. Hawf, K. R. Frost, Jr., ibid. **38**, 20 (1985). Soil adsorption and bioactivity: J. B. Weber, C. J. Peter, Weed Sci. **30**, 14 (1982). Soil transformation: P. C. C. Feng, Pestic. Biochem. Physiol. **40**, 136 (1991).

Pale straw-colored oil. $bp_{0.4\ torr}$ 134°. n_D^{20} 1.5272. Sol in water (25°): 400 ppm. LD_{50} orally in rats: 1160 mg/kg (Upchurch).

USE: Herbicide.

62. Acetohexamide. [968-81-0] 4-Acetyl-N-[(cyclohexylamino)carbonyl]benzenesulfonamide; 1-[(p-acetylphenyl)sulfonyl]-3-cyclohexylurea; 3-cyclohexyl-1-(p-acetylphenylsulfonyl)-urea; N-(p-acetylbenzenesulfonyl)-N'-cyclohexylurea; cyclamide; tsiklamid; Dimelor; Dymelor; Dimeline; Ordimel. $C_{15}H_{20}N_2O_4S$; mol wt 324.40. C 55.54%, H 6.21%, N 8.64%, O 19.73%, S 9.88%. Prepn: GB 912789 (1962 to Lilly); Marshall et al., J. Med. Chem. **6**, 60 (1963). Comprehensive description: C. E. Shafer, Anal. Profiles Drug Subs. **1**, 1-14 (1972); A. A. Al-Badr, H. A. El-Obeid, Anal. Profiles Drug Subs. Excip. **21**, 1-41 (1992).

Crystals from 90% aq ethanol, mp 188-190° (GB 912789); from dil ethanol, mp 175-177° (Marshall). uv max (methanol): 247, 283 nm. Sol in pyridine; slightly sol in alcohol, chloroform. Insol in water, ether.

THERAP CAT: Antidiabetic.

63. Acetohydroxamic Acid. [546-88-3] N-Hydroxyacetamide; N-acetylhydroxylamine; acetic acid oxime; AHA; Lithostat. $C_2H_5NO_2$; mol wt 75.07. C 32.00%, H 6.71%, N 18.66%, O 42.63%. $CH_3CONHOH$. Urease inhibitor. Prepn: A. Miolati, Ber. **25**, 699 (1892); W. M. Wise, W. W. Brandt, J. Am. Chem. Soc. **77**, 1058 (1955); H. A. Staab et al., Ber. **95**, 1275 (1962); G. Sosnovsky, J. A. Krogh, Synthesis **1980**, 654. Inhibition of urease activity: K. Kobashi et al., Biochim. Biophys. Acta **65**, 380 (1962); W. N. Fishbein et al., Nature **208**, 46 (1965); W. N. Fishbein, P. P. Carbone, J. Biol. Chem. **240**, 2407 (1965); D. P. Griffith et al., Invest. Urol. **11**, 234 (1973). Metabolism: E. Wolpert et al., Proc. Soc. Exp. Biol. Med. **136**, 592 (1971); W. N. Fishbein et al., J. Pharmacol. Exp. Ther. **186**, 173 (1973). Pharmacokinetics: S. Feldman et al., Invest. Urol. **15**, 498 (1978). Clinical studies in treatment of kidney stones: D. B. Griffith et al., J. Urol. **119**, 9 (1978); A. Martelli et al., Urology **17**, 320 (1981).

mp 89-92°. pKa 8.70. pH (aq soln): 9.39.

THERAP CAT: Antiurolithic. Antibacterial adjunct (urinary tract infection).

64. Acetoin. [513-86-0] 3-Hydroxy-2-butanone; 2,3-butanolone; acetyl methyl carbinol; dimethylketol; γ-hydroxy-β-oxobutane. $C_4H_8O_2$; mol wt 88.11. C 54.53%, H 9.15%, O 36.32%. $CH_3CH(OH)COCH_3$. A product of fermentation, also in cream ripened for churning. Obtained by the action of sorbose bacterium or Mycoderma aceti on 2,3-butanediol or by the action of fungi, such as Aspergillus, Penicillium, Mycoderma on sugar cane juice: Browne, J. Am. Chem. Soc. **28**, 467 (1906). By action of yeast on diacetyl: Nagelschmidt, Biochem. Z. **186**, 317 (1927). From diacetyl by partial reduction with Zn and acid: Diels, Stephan, Ber. **40**, 4338 (1907). Fermentation process: Vergnaud, US 2529061 (1950 to Usines de Melle).

Liquid. Pleasant odor. mp 15°. d_4^{17} 0.9972. bp_{760} 148°. $n_D^{17.3}$ 1.4190. Miscible with water, alcohol. Sparingly sol in ether, petr ether. Reduces Fehling's soln forming acetic acid. Forms a solid dimer $C_8H_{16}O_4$ on standing or on treatment with granulated zinc. The dimer is easily converted back to the monomer by melting, distilling or dissolving.

65. Acetol. [116-09-6] 1-Hydroxy-2-propanone; hydroxyacetone; acetone alcohol; acetylcarbinol; acetylmethanol; 2-oxopropanol. $C_3H_6O_2$; mol wt 74.08. C 48.64%, H 8.16%, O 43.19%. H_3CCOCH_2OH. Widely distributed in nature. Produced in animals as an intermediate in the intrahepatic metabolism of acetone. Also formed by the action of aldose reductase on methylglyoxal, q.v. and accumulates in uncontrolled diabetes. Prepn: W. H. Perkin, Jr., J. Chem. Soc. **59**, 786 (1891); T. Matsumoto et al., J. Org. Chem. **50**, 603 (1985). Isoln from coffee extract: M. Stoll et al., Helv. Chim. Acta **50**, 628 (1967). HPLC determn in serum: J. P. Casazza, J. L. Fu, Anal. Biochem. **148**, 344 (1985). Metabolism and potential role in diabetic complications: D. L. Vander Jagt et al., J. Biol. Chem. **267**, 4364 (1992). Use in peptide synthesis: B. Kundu, Tetrahedron Lett. **33**, 3193 (1992).

Colorless oil with peculiar odor. bp_{25} 50°; bp_{200} 105-106°; bp_{760} 147° (dec). n_D^{20} 1.4235. d_4^{20} 1.0872. Misc with water.

USE: Reagent in organic synthesis; protecting group for the synthesis of peptides.

66. Acetone. [67-64-1] 2-Propanone; dimethylformaldehyde; dimethyl ketone; β-ketopropane; pyroacetic ether. C_3H_6O; mol wt 58.08. C 62.04%, H 10.41%, O 27.55%. CH_3COCH_3. Obtained by fermentation (by-product of butyl alcohol manufacture) or by chemical synthesis from isopropanol (as chief product); from cumene (by-product in phenol manufacture); from propane (by-product of oxidation-cracking); Faith, Keyes & Clark's Industrial Chemicals, F. A. Lowenheim, M. K. Moran, Eds. (Wiley-Interscience, New York, 4th ed., 1975) pp 21-25. Toxicity: Smyth et al., Ind. Hyg. J. **23**, 95 (1962). Review: Weiss, Chem. Eng. News **36**, 79 (1958); W. L. Howard in Kirk-Othmer Encyclopedia of Chemical Technology vol. **1** (Wiley-Interscience, New York, 4th ed., 1991) pp 176-194. Review of toxicology and human exposure: Toxicological Profile for Acetone (PB95-100095, 1994) 276 pp.

Volatile, highly flammable liquid; characteristic odor; pungent, sweetish taste. d_4^{25} 0.788. bp 56.5°. mp −94°. n_D^{20} 1.3591. Flash pt, closed cup: 0°F (−18°C). Miscible with water, alcohol, dimethylformamide, chloroform, ether, most oils. Keep away from fire! Keep away from plastic eyeglass frames, jewelry, pens and pencils, rayon stockings and other rayon garments. LD_{50} in rats: 10.7 ml/kg orally (Smyth).

Caution: Potential symptoms of overexposure are irritation of eyes, nose and throat; headache, dizziness, CNS depression; dermatitis. See NIOSH Pocket Guide to Chemical Hazards (DHHS/NIOSH 97-140, 1997) p 2.

USE: Solvent for fats, oils, waxes, resins, rubber, plastics, lacquers, varnishes, rubber cements. Manuf methyl isobutyl ketone, mesityl oxide, acetic acid (ketene process), diacetone alcohol, chloroform, iodoform, bromoform, explosives, aeroplane dopes, rayon, photographic films, isoprene; storing acetylene gas (takes up about 24 times its vol of the gas); extraction of various principles from animal and plant substances; in paint and varnish removers; purifying paraffin; hardening and dehydrating tissues. Pharmaceutic aid (solvent).

67. Acetone Cyanohydrin. [75-86-5] 2-Hydroxy-2-methylpropanenitrile; 2-methyllactonitrile; α-hydroxyisobutyronitrile. C_4H_7NO; mol wt 85.10. C 56.45%, H 8.29%, N 16.46%, O 18.80%. $(CH_3)_2C(OH)CN$. Prepd by adding acetone to sodium or potassium cyanide in water and treating with H_2SO_4 at below 20°: Welch, Clemo, *J. Chem. Soc.* **1928**, 2629; Cox, Stormont, *Org. Synth.* **coll. vol. II**, 7 (1943). Continuous production from HCN and aq acetone: G. Barsky, **US 2731490** (1956). Toxicity study: H. F. Smyth *et al.*, *Am. Ind. Hyg. Assoc. J.* **23**, 95 (1962).

Liquid; d_4^{25} 0.9267; d_4^{19} 0.932. mp −19°. bp_{15} 81°; bp_{20} 88-90°; bp_{23} 82°; bp_{760} 95°. n_D^{19} 1.40002; n_D^{15} 1.3980. Freely sol in water and in the usual organic solvents. Practically insol in petr ether and carbon disulfide. Decomposes readily to form hydrogen cyanide, *q.v.*, which is highly toxic. LD_{50} orally in rats: 0.17 g/kg (Smyth).

Caution: Potential symptoms of overexposure are irritation of eyes, skin, respiratory system; dizziness, weakness, headache, confusion, convulsions; liver, kidney injury; pulmonary edema, asphyxia. *See NIOSH Pocket Guide to Chemical Hazards* (DHHS/NIOSH 97-140, 1997) p 4.

USE: In preparative organic chemistry for transcyanohydrination, such as preparing the 17-monocyanohydrin of a 3,17-diketo steroid by hydrogen cyanide exchange with the reagent, *e.g.* Ercoli, de Ruggieri, *J. Am. Chem. Soc.* **75**, 6113 (1953).

68. Acetonedicarboxylic Acid. [542-05-2] 3-Oxo-pentanedioic acid; 3-oxoglutaric acid; β-ketoglutaric acid. $C_5H_6O_5$; mol wt 146.10. C 41.10%, H 4.14%, O 54.75%. $CO_2HCH_2COCH_2CO_2H$. Prepd by the action of fuming sulfuric acid on citric acid: Willstätter, Pfannenstiel, *Ann.* **422**, 5 (1921); Ingold, Nickolls, *J. Chem. Soc.* **121**, 1642 (1922); R. Adams *et al.*, *Org. Synth.* **coll. vol. I**, 10 (2nd ed., 1941). By the action of *Aspergillus niger* on ammonium citrate mixed with some citric acid: Walker *et al.*, *J. Chem. Soc.* **1927**, 3050; also by *B. pyocyaneus*: Butterworth, Walker, *Biochem. J.* **23**, 931 (1929). Decomposition studies: Wiig, *J. Phys. Chem.* **32**, 961 (1928). Intermediate in synthesis of tropinone: R. Robinson, *J. Chem. Soc.* **111**, 762 (1917); C. Schöpf, G. Lehmann, *Ann.* **518**, 1 (1921).

Needles from ethyl acetate, mp 138° (dec). The pure compound may be stored over P_2O_5 for several months. Crude material dec after a few hours. Decomposed by hot water, acids or alkalies to CO_2 and acetone. pK (25°) 3.10. Very sol in water and alcohol; slightly sol in ethyl acetate, ether. Insol in chloroform, ligroin, benzene.

USE: In organic synthesis.

69. Acetone Sodium Bisulfite. [540-92-1] 2-Hydroxy-2-propanesulfonic acid sodium salt; acetone sulfite. $C_3H_7NaO_4S$; mol wt 162.14. C 22.22%, H 4.35%, Na 14.18%, O 39.47%, S 19.78%. $(CH_3)_2C(OH)SO_3Na$.

Crystals, fatty feel, slight SO_2 odor. Freely sol in water, sparingly in alcohol. Decomposed by acids.

USE: In photography; manuf of pure acetone; dyeing and printing texiles; in organic syntheses.

70. Acetonitrile. [75-05-8] Methyl cyanide; cyanomethane; ethanenitrile. C_2H_3N; mol wt 41.05. C 58.52%, H 7.37%, N 34.12%. CH_3CN. Small amounts occur in coal tar. Obtained commercially as a byproduct in manuf of acrylonitrile, *q.v.*: R. A. Smiley in *Kirk-Othmer Encyclopedia of Chemical Technology* vol. 15 (Wiley-Interscience, New York, 3rd ed., 1978) p 896. Prepn by dehydration of acetamide: Adkins, Nissen, *J. Am. Chem. Soc.* **46**, 143 (1924); A. I. Vogel, *Practical Organic Chemistry* (Longmans, London, 3rd ed., 1959) p 407; Gattermann-Wieland, *Praxis des Organischen Chemikers* (de Gruyter, Berlin, 40th ed., 1961) p 125; or from acetylene and ammonia: **DE 365432**; *Chem. Zentralbl.* **1924 I**, 2398; **1925 II**, 1563. Review of purification methods: *Techniques of Chemistry* vol. II, entitled "Organic Solvents", J. A. Riddick, W. B. Bunger, Eds. (Wiley-Interscience, New York, 3rd ed., 1970) pp 798-805. Toxicity: H. F. Smyth, C. P. Carpenter, *J. Ind. Hyg. Toxicol.* **30**, 63 (1968).

Liquid. Ether-like odor. *Poisonous!* Burns with a luminous flame. mp −45°. bp_{760} 81.6°. Flash pt 12.8°C (55°F). d_4^{15} 0.78745; d_4^{30} 0.77125. n_D^{15} 1.34604, n_D^{30} 1.33934. Dielectric constant at 20° = 38.8. Surface tension at 20° = 29.04 dynes/cm. Misc with water, methanol, methyl acetate, ethyl acetate, acetone, ether, acetamide, chloroform, carbon tetrachloride, ethylene chloride and many unsaturated hydrocarbons. Immiscible with many saturated hydrocarbons (petroleum fractions). Dissolves some in organic salts, *e.g.*, silver nitrate, lithium nitrate, magnesium bromide. Constant boiling mixture with water contains 16% H_2O and bp 76°. LD_{50} orally in rats: 3800 mg/kg (Smyth).

Caution: Potential symptoms of overexposure are irritation of nose, throat; asphyxia; nausea, vomiting; chest pain; weakness; stupor, convulsions. *See NIOSH Pocket Guide to Chemical Hazards* (DHHS/NIOSH 97-140, 1997) p 4.

USE: In organic synthesis as starting material for acetophenone, α-naphthaleneacetic acid, thiamine, acetamidine. To remove tars, phenols, and coloring matter from petroleum hydrocarbons which are not soluble in acetonitrile. To extract fatty acids from fish liver oils and other animal and vegetable oils. Can be used to recrystalize steroids. As an indifferent medium in physicochemical investigations. Wherever a polar solvent having a rather high dielectric constant is required. As medium for promoting reactions involving ionization. As a solvent in non-aqueous titrations. As a non-aqueous solvent for inorganic salts.

71. Acetonylacetone. [110-13-4] 2,5-Hexanedione; α,β-diacetylethane. $C_6H_{10}O_2$; mol wt 114.14. C 63.14%, H 8.83%, O 28.03%. $CH_3COCH_2CH_2COCH_3$. Prepn by decarboxylation of diacetosuccinic ester (from sodium acetoacetic ester and iodine): Paal, *Ber.* **18**, 58 (1885); Knorr, *Ber.* **22**, 2100 (1889); by hydrolysis of 2,5-dimethylfuran: Perkins, Toussaint, **US 2052652** (1936 to Union Carbide). Toxicity data: H. F. Smyth, C. P. Carpenter, *J. Ind. Hyg. Toxicol.* **26**, 269 (1944).

Liquid, gradually turns yellow. d_4^{20} 0.970. mp −9°. bp 188°, n_D^{20} 1.449. Misc with water, alcohol, ether. LD_{50} orally in rats: 2.7 g/kg (Smyth, Carpenter).

Caution: A mild local irritant. High concns cause narcosis.

72. Acetophenazine. [2751-68-0] 1-[10-[3-[4-(2-Hydroxyethyl)-1-piperazinyl]propyl]-10*H*-phenothiazin-2-yl]ethanone; 10-[3-[4-(2-hydroxyethyl)-1-piperazinyl]propyl]phenothiazin-2-yl methyl ketone; 2-acetyl-10-[3-[4-(β-hydroxyethyl)piperazinyl]propyl]phenothiazine; 1-(2-hydroxyethyl)-4-[3-(2-acetyl-10-phenothiazyl)propyl]piperazine. $C_{23}H_{29}N_3O_2S$; mol wt 411.56. C 67.12%, H 7.10%, N 10.21%, O 7.78%, S 7.79%. Prepd from 1-(2-hydroxyethyl)piperazine and 10-(3-chloropropyl)-2-acetyl-phenothiazine: Sherlock, Sperber, **US 2985654** (1961 to Schering). Toxicity study: E. W. Schafer, *Toxicol. Appl. Pharmacol.* **21**, 315 (1972).

Dimaleate. [5714-00-1] Tindal. $C_{23}H_{29}N_3O_2S.2C_4H_4O_4$; mol wt 643.70. Crystals from ethanol, mp 167-168.5°. LD_{50} orally in rats: 433 mg/kg (Schafer).

THERAP CAT: Antipsychotic.

73. Acetophenone. [98-86-2] 1-Phenylethanone; phenyl methyl ketone; acetylbenzene; hypnone. C_8H_8O; mol wt 120.15. C 79.97%, H 6.71%, O 13.32%. Made from benzene and acetyl-chloride in presence of aluminum chloride; catalytically from acetic and benzoic acids. Prepn from benzene and acetic anhydride: Adams, *J. Am. Chem. Soc.* **46**, 1889 (1924); A. I. Vogel, *Practical Organic Chemistry* (Longmans, London, 3rd ed., 1959) p 730; Gattermann-Wieland, *Die Praxis des Organischen Chemikers* (de Gruyter, Berlin, 40th ed., 1961) p 297. Toxicity study: H. F. Smyth, C. P. Carpenter, *J. Ind. Hyg. Toxicol.* **30**, 63 (1948).

Liquid. Forms laminar crystals at low temp. mp 20.5°. d_{15}^{15} 1.033. bp 202°. n_D^{20} 1.5339. Flash pt, closed cup: 221°F (105°C). Slightly sol in water; freely in alcohol, chloroform, ether, fatty oils, glycerol. Sol in concd H_2SO_4 with orange color. LD_{50} orally in rats: 0.90 g/kg (Smyth, Carpenter).

USE: In perfumery to impart an orange-blossom-like odor; catalyst for the polymerization of olefins; in organic syntheses, esp. as photosensitizer.

74. Acetotoluide. $C_9H_{11}NO$; mol wt 149.19. C 72.46%, H 7.43%, N 9.39%, O 10.72%. Prepn of *m-, o-,* and *p*-acetotoluidides, from *m-, o-,* or *p*-toluidine and acetic acid: Gasopoulos, *Ber.* **59B**, 2187 (1926).

m-**Acetotoluide.** [537-92-8] *N*-(3-Methylphenyl)acetamide; *m*-acetotoluidide; *m*-tolylacetamide; aceto-*m*-aminotoluene; *m*-methylacetanilide; *N*-acetyl-*m*-toluidine. Needles, mp 65.5°, bp 303°. Slightly sol in water; freely sol in alc, ether.

o-**Acetotoluide.** [120-66-1] Crystals, mp 110°, bp 296°. Slightly sol in water; sol in alc, chloroform, ether. Determn of soly at various temps: Hall *et al., J. Phys. Chem.* **37**, 1087 (1933).

p-**Acetotoluide.** [103-89-9] Crystals, mp 153°, bp 307°. Very slightly sol in water; sol in alc, ether, ethyl acetate, glacial acetic acid.

75. Acetoxime. [127-06-0] 2-Propanone oxime; acetone oxime; β-isonitrosopropane. C_3H_7NO; mol wt 73.09. C 49.30%, H 9.65%, N 19.16%, O 21.89%. $(CH_3)_2C=NOH$. Prepd by shaking an aqueous soln of hydroxylamine with acetone and extracting with ether: W. L. Semon, *Org. Synth.* **coll. vol. I,** 318 (2nd ed., 1941). Ionization constants: C. V. King, A. P. Marion, *J. Am. Chem. Soc.* **66**, 977 (1944).

Columnar prisms. Volatilizes quickly in air. Odor resembling that of chloral hydrate. d_4^{62} 0.9113. mp 60°. bp$_{728}$ 134.8°. Neutral reaction. pK (24.9°): 12.42. uv spectrum: Hartley, Dobbie, *J. Chem. Soc.* **77**, 326 (1900). Freely soluble in water, alcohol, ether, petr ether. Can be extracted with ether from neutral water solns, but not from alkaline or acidic solns.

76. Acetoxolone. [6277-14-1] (3β,20β)-3-(Acetyloxy)-11-oxoolean-12-en-29-oic acid; 3β-hydroxy-11-oxoolean-12-en-30-oic acid acetate; 3-O-acetyl-18β-glycyrrhetic acid; acetylglycyrrhetinic acid; glycyrrhetic acid acetate. $C_{32}H_{48}O_5$; mol wt 512.72. C 74.96%, H 9.44%, O 15.60%. Deriv of enoxolone, *q.v.;* homolog of carbenoxolone, *q.v.* Prepn: J. M. Beaton, F. S. Spring, *J. Chem. Soc.* **1955**, 3126. Prepn of the aluminum salt: A. Bonati, **ZA 7006901**; *idem,* **US 3764618** (1971, 1973 both to Dott. Inverni & Della Beffa). NMR study of the acetate: M. Mousseron-Canet *et al., Bull. Soc. Chim. Fr.* **12**, 4668 (1967). Pharmacology of the aluminum salt: C. Capra, *Fitoterapia* **40**, 8 (1969), *C.A.* **73**, 64754 (1970). Absorption in rats: B. D. Cameron *et al., Arzneim.-Forsch.* **26**, 1680 (1976). Analysis of gastric protective effect: P. Altmayer *et al., ibid.* **31**, 853 (1981).

Crystals, mp 322-325°. $[\alpha]_D^{20}$ +141°.

Aluminum salt. [29728-34-5] Almacet. $C_{96}H_{141}AlO_{15}$; mol wt 1562.12. White powder, mp 286-290°. $[\alpha]_D^{20}$ +126±2° (c = 1 in chloroform). Insol in water. Sol in most organic solvents. LD_{50} in male rats (mg/kg): >3300 orally, and i.p. (Bonati).

THERAP CAT: Antiulcerative.

77. 21-Acetoxypregnenolone. [566-78-9] (3β)-21-(Acetyloxy)-3-hydroxypregn-5-en-20-one; 3β,21-dihydroxypregn-5-en-20-one 21-acetate; 5-pregnene-3β,21-diol-20-one 21-acetate; 21-acetoxy-5-pregnen-3-ol-20-one; 3-hydroxy-21-acetoxy-5-pregnen-20-one; prebediolone acetate; A.O.P.; Acetoxanon; Artisone acetate. $C_{23}H_{34}O_4$; mol wt 374.51. C 73.76%, H 9.15%, O 17.09%. Intermediate product in the synthesis of desoxycorticosterone acetate: Steiger, Reichstein, *Helv. Chim. Acta* **20**, 1164 (1937). Prepd by reacting 5,6-pregnen-3-ol-20-one with bromine in chloroform and treating the obtained oily bromide with potassium acetate in alcohol: Herloff, Inhoffen, **US 2409043** (1946 to Schering).

Needles from acetone. Becomes opaque at about 80° or on prolonged standing. mp 184-185°. Very slightly sol in ether, in pentane; sol in chloroform, toluene. The esterified keto group is relatively stable to the action of chromic acid in cold and to such reducing agents as potassium iodide or zinc. On heating with aluminum isopropoxide in isopropyl alcohol it is reduced to 5-pregnene-3,20,21-triol.

THERAP CAT: Anti-inflammatory.

78. Acetozone. [644-31-5] Acetyl benzoyl peroxide; benzoyl acetyl peroxide; benzozone. $C_9H_8O_4$; mol wt 180.16. C 60.00%, H 4.48%, O 35.52%. Prepd from benzaldehyde and acetic anhydride in the presence of O-contg gas and dibenzoyl peroxide: Carruthers, **US 1985886** (1935 to Carbide & Carbon Chemicals); Appell, **US 3397245** (1968 to Koppers).

Crystals, mp 36-37°. bp$_{19}$ 130°. Decomposes on contact with moisture or in a warm place. Soluble in carbon tetrachloride, chloroform, ether, oils. Marketed as a mixture with an equal part of an absorbent powder. *Incompat.* Water, alkalies, heat.

Caution: Strong oxidizing agent. Can cause severe skin burns.

USE: Germicide; in bleaching of flour and food oils.

79. Acetrizoate Sodium. [129-63-5] 3-(Acetylamino)-2,4,6-triiodobenzoic acid sodium salt; 3-acetamido-2,4,6-triiodo-benzoic acid sodium salt; acetrizoic acid sodium salt; Cystokon; Diaginol; Pyelokon-R; Thixokon; Urokon Sodium. $C_9H_5I_3$-$NNaO_3$; mol wt 578.84. C 18.67%, H 0.87%, I 65.77%, N 2.42%, Na 3.97%, O 8.29%. Prepn: Wallingford *et al., J. Am. Chem. Soc.* **74**, 4365 (1952); Wallingford, *J. Am. Pharm. Assoc. Sci. Ed.* **42**, 721 (1953). Toxicity data: J. O. Hoppe *et al., J. Pharmacol. Exp. Ther.* **116**, 394 (1956).

Not isolated from soln. Marketed as a sterile 30% aq soln, pH between 4.8 and 5.2. The free acid is a white powder, decompn 278-283°. Sol in alcohol. Solubility in water at 25°: 94.2 g/100 ml. Very slightly sol in chloroform. Practically insol in benzene. LD_{50} in rabbits, cats, dogs (mg/kg): 5200, 5600, 6300 i.v. (Hoppe).

Mixture with meglumine acetrizoate. Opacoron.

THERAP CAT: Diagnostic aid (radiopaque medium).

80. Aceturic Acid. [543-24-8] N-Acetylglycine; acetamidoacetic acid; acetylaminoacetic acid; acetylglycocoll; ethanoylaminoethanoic acid. $C_4H_7NO_3$; mol wt 117.10. C 41.03%, H 6.03%, N 11.96%, O 40.99%. $CH_3CONHCH_2COOH$. Prepd by warming glycine with a slight excess of acetic anhydride in benzene: Radenhausen, *J. Prakt. Chem.* [2] **52**, 437 (1895); by warming glycine in glacial acetic acid with the stoichiometric amount of acetic anhydride: Dakin, *J. Biol. Chem.* **82**, 443 (1929).

Long needles from water, mp 206-208°. pK (25°) 3.64. Sol in water at 15° = 2.7%. Moderately soluble in alcohol. Slightly sol in acetone, chloroform, glacial acetic acid. Practically insol in ether, benzene. Forms stable salts with organic bases.

81. Acetylacetone. [123-54-6] 2,4-Pentanedione; diacetylmethane. $C_5H_8O_2$; mol wt 100.12. C 59.98%, H 8.05%, O 31.96%. $CH_3COCH_2COCH_3$. Made by the action of sodium on ethyl acetate and acetone or by the action of anhydrous aluminum chloride on acetyl chloride in the presence of an inert solvent: Combes, *Compt. Rend.* **103**, 814 (1886); *Ann. Chim. (Paris)* **12**, 199 (1887); Claisen, *Ber.* **38**, 695 (1905); Hunt, US 2737528 (1956 to Shawinigan Chem.); Georgieff, US 2834811 (1958); Gattermann-Wieland, *Praxis des Organischen Chemikers* (de Gruyter, Berlin, 40th ed., 1961) p 219. Toxicity data: Carpenter, *J. Ind. Hyg. Toxicol.* **31**, 343 (1949).

Colorless or slightly yellow, flammable liquid; pleasant odor. d 0.976. bp 140.5°. mp −23°. n_D^{20} 1.4512. One part dissolves in about 8 parts of water. Miscible with alcohol, benzene, chloroform, ether, acetone, glacial acetic acid. LC_{50} (4 hrs) in rats: 1000 ppm (Carpenter).

Caution: Mild irritant to skin, mucous membranes.

USE: Forms organometallic complexes which are used as gasoline additives, lubricant additives, driers for varnishes and printer's inks, fungicides, insecticides, colors.

82. Acetyl Bromide. [506-96-7] C_2H_3BrO; mol wt 122.95. C 19.54%, H 2.46%, Br 64.99%, O 13.01%. CH_3COBr. Prepd from phosphorus tribromide and glacial acetic acid or acetic anhydride: Burton, Degering, *J. Am. Chem. Soc.* **62**, 227 (1940).

Fuming liquid; *irritating to the eyes.* bp 76°. d^9 1.52. mp −96°. Violently decomposed by water, or by alcohol; miscible with ether, chloroform, benzene. *Protect from water.*

83. α-Acetylbutyrolactone. [517-23-7] 3-Acetyldihydro-2(3H)-furanone; α-(2-hydroxyethyl)acetoacetic acid γ-lactone; α-acetyl-γ-hydroxybutyric acid γ-lactone; α-acetobutyrolactone. $C_6H_8O_3$; mol wt 128.13. C 56.24%, H 6.29%, O 37.46%. Prepn from sodium acetoacetate and ethylene oxide in abs alcohol: Knunyantz *et al., Compt. Rend. Acad. Sci. (U.R.S.S.)* [N.S.] **1**, 312 (1934), *C.A.* **28**, 4383 (1934); Feofilaktov, Onishchenko, *J. Gen. Chem. USSR* **9**, 304 (1939), *C.A.* **34**, 378 (1940); Forman; Johnson, US 2397134 and US 2443827 (1946, 1948 both to U.S. Industrial Chemicals).

Liquid; ester-like odor. Soly in water: 20% v/v; soly of water in lactone: 12% v/v. d_4^{20} 1.1846; d_{20}^{20} 1.185-1.189; bp_{30} 142-143°; bp_{18} 130-132°; bp_5 107-108°. n_D^{20} 1.4562 (Knunyantz); n_D^{20} 1.4590 (Feofilaktov). Acquires a blue to bluish-purple color when in contact with iron.

Caution: Irritating to skin, mucous membranes.

USE: In synthesis of 3,4-disubstituted pyridines; of 5-(β-hydroxyethyl)-4-methylthiazole.

84. Acetylcarnitine. [3040-38-8]; [14992-62-2] (DL-form). (2R)-2-(Acetyloxy)-3-carboxy-N,N,N-trimethyl-1-propanaminium inner salt; L-(3-carboxy-2-hydroxypropyl)trimethylammonium hydroxide inner salt acetate; acetyl-L-carnitine; ALCAR. $C_9H_{17}NO_4$; mol wt 203.24. C 53.19%, H 8.43%, N 6.89%, O 31.49%. Natu-

rally occurring ester of carnitine, *q.v.*; important acetyl donor in metabolic processes. Prepn from carnitine extracted from meat: R. Engeland, *Ber.* **42**, 2457 (1909); R. Krimberg, W. Wittandt, *Biochem. Z.* **251**, 229 (1932); E. Strack *et al., Z. Physiol. Chem.* **238**, 183 (1936). Resolution of isomers: K. Brendel, R. Bressler, *Biochim. Biophys. Acta* **137**, 98 (1967). Extraction from calf brain tissue: E. A. Hosein, A. Orzeck, *Int. J. Neuropharmacol.* **3**, 71 (1964). Enzymatic determn in serum: K. Tomita *et al., J. Pharm. Biomed. Anal.* **24**, 1147 (2001). Clinical trial in cognitive impairment in the elderly: G. Salvioli, M. Neri, *Drugs Exp. Clin. Res.* **20**, 169 (1994). Review of pharmacology in the CNS: L. Janiri, E. Tempesta, *Int. J. Clin. Pharmacol. Res.* **3**, 295-306 (1983); of bioactivity and clinical studies in Alzheimer's disease and geriatric depression: J. W. Pettegrew *et al., Mol. Psychiatry* **5**, 616-632 (2000); of pharmacokinetics and metabolism: C. J. Rebouche, *Ann. N.Y. Acad. Sci.* **1033**, 30-41 (2004).

Hygroscopic crystals, mp 145° (dec). $[\alpha]_D^{20}$ −19.52° (c = 6). Very sol in water, alcohol. Practically insol in ether.

Hydrochloride. [5080-50-2] Acetyl-L-carnitine chloride; levacecarnine hydrochloride; ST-200; Branigen; Nicetile; Normobren; Zibren. $C_9H_{17}NO_4 \cdot HCl$; mol wt 239.70. Stable crystals, mp 187° (dec). Also reported as small rod-shaped crystals from butanol, mp 181° (Strack). $[\alpha]_D^{20}$ −26.9° (c = 9). $[\alpha]_D^{25}$ −28° (c = 2 in water). Very sol in water, sol in alcohol. Practically insol in ether.

THERAP CAT: Nootropic.

85. Acetyl Chloride. [75-36-5] C_2H_3ClO; mol wt 78.50. C 30.60%, H 3.85%, Cl 45.16%, O 20.38%. CH_3COCl. Prepd from acetic acid and chlorine in the presence of phosphorus; from acetic acid and salts of chlorosulfonic acid; from sodium acetate and sulfuryl chloride. Details of prepn: Gattermann-Wieland, *Praxis des Organischen Chemikers* (de Gruyter, Berlin, 40th ed., 1961) p 111; A. I. Vogel, *Practical Organic Chemistry* (Longmans, London, 3rd ed., 1959) p 367. Lab prepn from acetic anhydride and calcium chloride: Gmünder, *Helv. Chim. Acta* **36**, 2021 (1953).

Flammable liquid; pungent odor. *Extremely irritating to the eyes.* Imparts a green tinge to a colorless flame. d 1.104. mp −112°. bp 52°. n_D^{20} 1.3898. Decomposed violently by water or alc. Miscible with benzene, chloroform, ether, glacial acetic acid, petr ether. *Protect from water.*

Caution: Irritant, corrosive. Causes severe burns. Avoid contact with skin, eyes, mucous membranes.

USE: Acetylating agent; in testing for cholesterol, determination of H_2O in organic liquids.

86. Acetylcholine Bromide. [66-23-9] 2-(Acetyloxy)-N,N,N-trimethylethanaminium bromide; Pragmoline; Tonocholin B. $C_7H_{16}BrNO_2$; mol wt 226.11. C 37.18%, H 7.13%, Br 35.34%, N 6.19%, O 14.15%. $(CH_3)_3N(Br)CH_2CH_2OOCCH_3$. From trimethylamine and β-bromoethyl acetate: Fourneau, Page, *Bull. Soc. Chim. Fr.* [4] **15**, 544 (1914).

Deliquesc crystals. Very soluble in cold water; decomposed by hot water or alkalies; soluble in alcohol; practically insol in ether. *Keep tightly closed.*

THERAP CAT: Cholinergic.

87. Acetylcholine Chloride. [60-31-1] 2-(Acetyloxy)-N,N,N-trimethylethanaminium chloride; Acecoline; Arterocoline; Miochol; Ovisot. $C_7H_{16}ClNO_2$; mol wt 181.66. C 46.28%, H 8.88%, Cl 19.52%, N 7.71%, O 17.61%. $(CH_3)_3N(Cl)CH_2CH_2-OOCCH_3$. Prepd from trimethylamine and β-chloroethyl acetate: Fourneau, Page, *Bull. Soc. Chim. Fr.* [4] **15**, 544 (1914). Review of pharmacology: H. Molitor, *J. Pharmacol. Exp. Ther.* **58**, 337 (1936).

Crystalline powder, very deliquescent, mp 149-152°. Hygroscopic. Very sol in cold water, alcohol; decomposed by hot water or alkalies. Practically insol in ether. *Keep tightly closed.* LD_{50} in mice, rats (mg/kg): 20, 22 i.v., 170, 250 s.c., 3000, 2500 i.p. (Molitor).

THERAP CAT: Cholinergic.

88. Acetylcysteine. [616-91-1] *N*-Acetyl-L-cysteine; L-α-acetamido-β-mercaptopropionic acid; *N*-acetyl-3-mercaptoalanine; Acetadote; Brunac; Fabrol; Fluimucil; Fluprowit; Mucocedyl; Mucolator; Mucomyst; Muco Sanigen; Mucosil; Mucret; Neo-Fluimucil; Parvolex; Tixair. $C_5H_9NO_3S$; mol wt 163.19. C 36.80%, H 5.56%, N 8.58%, O 29.41%, S 19.65%. Thiol-containing antioxidant. Prepn: Smith, Gorin, *J. Org. Chem.* **26**, 820 (1961). Prepn and use in treatment of respiratory diseases: Martin, Waller, **US 3184505** (1965 to Mead Johnson). Effect in corneal healing: F. Menna *et al., Bull. Mem. Soc. Fr. Opthalmol.* **94**, 425 (1982); G. Petroutsos *et al., Ophthalmic Res.* **14**, 241 (1982). Toxicity: E. I. Goldenthal, *Toxicol. Appl. Pharmacol.* **18**, 185 (1971). Clinical trial in acetaminophen overdose: M. J. Smilkstein *et al., N. Engl. J. Med.* **319**, 1557 (1988); as renal protectant with radiocontrast agents: M. Tepel *et al., ibid.* **343**, 180 (2000). *Review:* G. R. McKinney, G. M. Sisson, in *Pharmacological and Biochemical Properties of Drug Substances* vol. 2, M. E. Goldberg, Ed. (Am. Pharm. Assoc., Washington, DC, 1979) pp 479-488. Review of use in clinical toxicology: R. J. Flanagan, T. J. Meredith, *Am. J. Med.* **91**, Suppl. 3C, 131S-139S (1991).

Crystals from water, mp 109-110°. LD_{50} orally in rats: 5050 mg/kg (Goldenthal).

THERAP CAT: Mucolytic; corneal vulnerary; antidote (acetaminophen poisoning).

THERAP CAT (VET): Expectorant.

89. Acetyldigitoxins. $C_{43}H_{66}O_{14}$; mol wt 806.98. C 64.00%, H 8.24%, O 27.76%. Obtained by enzymatic hydrolysis of lanatoside A, *q.v.* Composed of the aglycone digitoxigenin and 3 mols digitoxose, to one of which an acetyl group is attached. Acetyldigitoxin-α differs from acetyldigitoxin-β in the position of the acetyl group. The β-form is obtained either by splitting off the glucose residue from lanatoside A by means of enzymes, or by extraction from the leaves of *Digitalis ferruginea* L., *Scrophulariaceae.* The α-form can be obtained from acetyldigitoxin-β by heating in an anhydrous or aq organic solvent at pH 3.5 to 8: Stoll, Kreis, **US 2776963** (1957 to Sandoz).

α-Form. [1111-39-3] Acylanid. Platelets from methanol, mp 217-221°. $[\alpha]_D^{20}$ +5.0° (c = 0.7 in pyridine). Slightly sol in chloroform.

β-Form. Stout, solvated prisms from methanol losing their solvent of crystn in desiccator. When dry, dec 225°. $[\alpha]_D^{20}$ +16.7° (pyridine). One gram dissolves in 7 to 9 ml chloroform, in 150 ml methanol, in 220 ml amyl alc. Almost insol in ether, water (one gram dissolves in 200 liters H_2O at 20°).

THERAP CAT: Cardiotonic.

90. Acetylene. [74-86-2] Ethyne; ethine. C_2H_2; mol wt 26.04. C 92.25%, H 7.74%. HC≡CH. Manuf from calcium carbide and water: Eastman, **US 3017259** (1962 to Texaco); from methane: Anderson, **US 3051639** (1962 to Union Carbide). Toxicity data: Riggs, *Proc. Soc. Exp. Biol. Med.* **22**, 269 (1925). Review of manuf processes: *Faith, Keyes & Clark's Industrial Chemicals*, F. A. Lowenheim, M. K. Moran, Eds. (Wiley-Interscience, New York, 4th ed., 1975) pp 26-35. *Review:* Nieuwland, Vogt, *The Chemistry of Acetylene* (Reinhold, New York, 1945) pp 1-219. Comprehensive monograph in 2 vols: S. A. Miller, *Acetylene* (Academic Press, New York, 1965); several authors in *Kirk-Othmer Encyclopedia of Chemical Technology* vol. 1 (Wiley-Interscience, New York, 3rd ed., 1978) pp 192-243.

Gas; odor not unpleasant when pure, but disagreeable when impure (due to phosphine). mp −81° (subl). At 0° liquifies at 21.5 atm; below 37° (crit temp) liquifies at 68 atm. One liter at 0° and 760 mm weighs 1.165 g; d gas (air = 1) 0.90. Burns brilliantly in air with very sooty flame. Heat of combustion 313 cal. Not explosive at ordinary atmospheric pressure, but at 2 atms or more it is explo-

sive by spark or decomposition. Mixture with air containing more than 3% or less than 65% gas is explosive, max being 1 vol gas and 12.5 vol air. Forms insoluble explosive compounds with copper and silver; hence copper or brass containers must be avoided. One vol dissolves in 1 vol water, in 6 vols glacial acetic acid or alcohol; soluble in ether, benzene. Acetone dissolves 25 vols acetylene at 15° and 760 mm; but 300 vols at 12 atm. LC in rats: 900000 ppm (Riggs).

Caution: Potential symptoms of overexposure are headache, dizziness; asphyxia; direct contact with liquid may cause frostbite. *See NIOSH Pocket Guide to Chemical Hazards* (DHHS/NIOSH 97-140, 1997) p 4.

USE: Illuminant, oxyacetylene welding, cutting, and soldering metals, signalling; pptg metals, particularly Cu; manuf acetaldehyde, acetic acid; fuel for motor boats.

91. Acetylene Dibromide. [540-49-8] 1,2-Dibromoethene; 1,2-dibromoethylene; *sym*-dibromoethylene. $C_2H_2Br_2$; mol wt 185.85. C 12.93%, H 1.08%, Br 85.99%. BrCH=CHBr. Prepd by reaction of tetrabromoethylene with Zn and alc followed by sepn of *cis*- and *trans*-forms by fractional distillation: Noyes *et al., J. Am. Chem. Soc.* **72**, 33 (1950).

Liquid, gradually decomposed by air, moisture, or light. d_4^{17} 2.21. n_D^{20} 1.5428. Practically insol in water. Sol in many organic solvents.

cis-**Form.** n_D^{25} 1.5370.

trans-**Form.** n_D^{25} 1.5440.

Caution: Narcotic in high concns.

92. Acetylene Dichloride. [540-59-0] 1,2-Dichloroethene; 1,2-dichloroethylene; *sym*-dichloroethylene; dioform. $C_2H_2Cl_2$; mol wt 96.94. C 24.78%, H 2.08%, Cl 73.14%. ClCH=CHCl. Prepn: Bordner, **US 2504919** (1950 to du Pont). Prepn of *trans*-form: Adler, **US 2440997** (1948 to Stockholms Superfosfot Fabriks Aktiebolag). Sepn of *cis*- and *trans*-forms by fractional distillation: Wood, Dickinson, *J. Am. Chem. Soc.* **61**, 3259 (1939); Johnsen, Fitzpatrick, *Rec. Trav. Chim.* **70**, 823 (1951); Truce, Barney, *J. Org. Chem.* **27**, 128 (1962). Toxicity studies: D. Gradiski *et al., Eur. J. Toxicol.* **7**, 247 (1974); K. J. Freundt *et al., Toxicology* **7**, 141 (1977). *Review:* V. L. Stevens in *Kirk-Othmer Encyclopedia of Chemical Technology* **Vol. 5** (Wiley-Interscience, New York, 3rd ed., 1979) pp 742-745. Review of toxicology and human exposure: *Toxicological Profile for 1,2-Dichloroethene* (PB95-100152, 1996) 198 pp.

Liquid; ethereal, slightly acrid odor; gradually decomposed by air, light and moisture, forming HCl. d ~1.28. bp ~55°. *Highly flammable; extremely corrosive*. Insol in water. Sol in alc, ether and most other organic solvents. LD_{50} i.p. in mice: ~2150 mg/kg (Gradiski).

cis-**Form.** [156-59-2] mp −81.5°. bp_{745} 59.6°, bp_{760} 60°. n_D^{25} 1.4435.

trans-**Form.** [156-60-5] mp −49.4°. bp_{745} 47.2°. Noticeably subject to air oxidation. LD_{50} in rats (ml/kg): 1.0 orally; 60 i.p.; in mice (ml/kg): 3.2 i.p. (Freundt).

Caution: Potential symptoms of overexposure are irritation of eyes and respiratory system; CNS depression. *See NIOSH Pocket Guide to Chemical Hazards* (DHHS/NIOSH 97-140, 1997) p 98. *See also Patty's Industrial Hygiene and Toxicology* vol. 2B, G. D. Clayton, F. E. Clayton, Eds. (Wiley-Interscience, New York, 3rd ed., 1981) pp 3550-3553.

USE: Solvent for fats, phenol, camphor, etc. Intermediate in synthesis of chlorinated solvents and compounds.

93. Acetyleneurea. [496-46-8] Tetrahydroimidazo[4,5-*d*]imidazole-2,5-(1*H*,3*H*)-dione; glycoluril; acetylenediureine; glyoxaldiureine; acetylene carbamide. $C_4H_6N_4O_2$; mol wt 142.12. C 33.80%, H 4.26%, N 39.42%, O 22.52%. Prepd by the sodium amalgam reduction of allantoin: Biltz, Schiemann, *J. Prakt. Chem.* **113**, 77 (1926); from glyoxal and urea: Reibnitz, **US 2731472** (1956 to BASF).

Crystals, dec at about 300°. Slightly sol in cold, more sol in hot water; sol in warm mineral acids, warm ammonia.

94. Acetyl Iodide. [507-02-8] C_2H_3IO; mol wt 169.95. C 14.13%, H 1.78%, I 74.67%, O 9.41%. CH_3COI. Prepd from acetyl chloride and HI: Gustus, Stevens, *J. Am. Chem. Soc.* **55**, 374 (1933).

Liquid; suffocating odor; fumes and turns brown in air. bp 108°, bp$_{735}$ 104-106°; d_4^{20} 2.0674; n_D^{20} 1.5491. Dec by water or alcohol; sol in benzene, ether. *Keep tightly closed and protected from light.*

Caution: A strong irritant. Avoid contact with skin. Vapors can cause pulmonary edema.

95. Acetylleucine Monoethanolamine. [149-90-6] *N*-Acetyl-DL-leucine compd with 2-aminoethanol (1:1); monoethanolamine DL-acetylleucinate; DL-acetylleucine monoethanolamine salt; monoethanolamine salt of α-acetamidoisocaproic acid; RP-7452; Tanganil. $C_{10}H_{22}N_2O_4$; mol wt 234.29. C 51.26%, H 9.46%, N 11.96%, O 27.32%. Prepn: Gailliot *et al.*, **US 2941924** (1960 to Rhône-Poulenc).

Crystals, mp ~150°. Soly in water: >20%; slight soly in alcohol: ~1%. pH of 10% aq soln: ~6.

THERAP CAT: Antivertigo agent.

96. *N*-Acetylmethionine. [65-82-7] $C_7H_{13}NO_3S$; mol wt 191.25. C 43.96%, H 6.85%, N 7.32%, O 25.10%, S 16.77%. $CH_3SCH_2CH_2CH(NHCOCH_3)COOH$. Prepn of racemic mixture: Wheeler, Ingersoll, *J. Am. Chem. Soc.* **73**, 4604 (1951); Callanan, Patton, **US 2745873** (1956 to Distillers Products). Resolution: Wheeler, Ingersoll, *loc. cit.;* Gillingham, **US 3028395** (1962 to Parke, Davis); Tullar, **US 3056799** (1962 to Sterling Drug); **GB 1072876** (1967 to Tanabe Seiyaku), *C.A.* **67**, 114015x (1967).

DL-Form. Methionamine. Crystals from water, mp 114-115°.

D(+)-Form. Crystals from water or ethyl acetate, mp 104-105°. $[\alpha]_D^{25}$ +20.3° (c = 4 in water).

L(−)-Form. Crystals, mp 104°. $[\alpha]_D^{25}$ −20.3°.

THERAP CAT: DL-Form as lipotropic.

97. Acetyl Nitrate. [591-09-3] Acetic acid anhydride with nitric acid. $C_2H_3NO_4$; mol wt 105.05. C 22.87%, H 2.88%, N 13.33%, O 60.92%. CH_3COONO_2. Prepn from acetic anhydride and N_2O_5: Boh, *Ann. Chim.* [11] **20**, 437 (1945).

Fuming, mobile, hygroscopic liquid. Should be colorless. d_4^{15} 1.24. bp$_{70}$ 22°. Although it may be stored in the dark over P_2O_5 for the weekend, it should be used in *statu nascendi* to avoid explosions. Always explodes when heated suddenly over 60° or when in contact with HgO. Explosions have occurred upon contact with ground glass surfaces: König, *Angew. Chem.* **67**, 157 (1955).

Caution: Irritant, corrosive.

USE: In nitrations, especially to introduce a single nitro group in an ortho position on an aromatic ring.

98. *N*-Acetylpenicillamine. [15537-71-0] *N*-Acetyl-3-mercapto-D-valine. $C_7H_{13}NO_3S$; mol wt 191.25. C 43.96%, H 6.85%, N 7.32%, O 25.10%, S 16.77%. Prepn: Crooks in *The Chemistry of Penicillin* (Princeton Univ. Press, 1949) p 470; Sheehan *et al.*, **US 2477148** and **US 2496416** (1949, 1950, both to Merck & Co.).

*dl-*Form. Crystals from hot water, mp 183°.

*d-*Form. Crystals from water, mp 189-190°; $[\alpha]_D^{25}$ +18° (50% ethanol).

99. Acetylpheneturide. [13402-08-9] *N*-[(Acetylamino)-carbonyl]-α-ethylbenzeneacetamide; 1-acetyl-3-(2-phenylbutyryl)-urea; *N*-(α-ethylphenylacetyl)-*N'*-acetylurea; Crampol. $C_{13}H_{16}N_2O_3$; mol wt 248.28. C 62.89%, H 6.50%, N 11.28%, O 19.33%. Synthesis: Umemoto *et al.*, *Yakugaku Zasshi* **83**, 753 (1963), *C.A.* **59**, 13849d (1963); Takamatsu *et al.*, **US 3110728** (1963 to Dainippon). Pharmacology and toxicology: Nakamura *et al.*, *Arzneim.-Forsch.* **18**, 524 (1968).

Crystals from dil alcohol, mp 100-101°. LD$_{50}$ orally in mice: 4.73 mMole/kg (1.17 g/kg) (Nakamura).

THERAP CAT: Anticonvulsant.

100. Acetylsalicylsalicylic Acid. [530-75-6] 2-(Acetyloxy)benzoic acid 2-carboxyphenyl ester; 2-hydroxybenzoic acid acetate 2-carboxyphenyl ester; salicylacetylsalicylic acid; Diplosal Acetate. $C_{16}H_{12}O_6$; mol wt 300.26. C 64.00%, H 4.03%, O 31.97%. Prepd by treating salicylsalicylic acid *q.v.*, with acetic anhydride or by fractionating an acetylsalicylic acid melt: **DE 236196** (1908 to Boehringer).

Leaflets from dilute acetic acid, mp 159°; also reported as mp 152°, Rudoi, *Sov. Med.* **1941**, no. 12, 26-27. Practically insol in water, benzene. One part dissolves in 3 parts boiling alcohol, in 70 parts boiling ether, in 45 parts boiling benzene. Sol in alkaline solns, but is saponified by heating in alk soln. On acidification of the soln salicylic acid is precipitated.

THERAP CAT: Analgesic.

101. Acetyl Sulfamethoxypyrazine. [3590-05-4] *N*-[(4-Aminophenyl)sulfonyl]-*N*-(3-methoxypyrazinyl)acetamide; N^1-acetyl-N^1-(3-methoxypyrazinyl)sulfanilamide; 2-(N^1-acetylsulfanilamido)-3-methoxypyrazine; Acetylazide. $C_{13}H_{14}N_4O_4S$; mol wt 322.34. C 48.44%, H 4.38%, N 17.38%, O 19.85%, S 9.95%. Prepn: Camerino, Palamidessi, *Gazz. Chim. Ital.* **90**, 1815 (1960); *eidem*, **US 3098069** (1963 to Soc. Farmaceutici Italia).

Crystals, mp 199°.

THERAP CAT: Antibacterial.

102. *N*-Acetylsulfanilic Acid. [121-62-0] 4-(Acetylamino)benzenesulfonic acid; *N-p*-acetylanilinosulfonic acid; acetanilidsulfonic acid; 4-acetamidobenzenesulfonic acid. $C_8H_9NO_4S$; mol wt 215.23. C 44.64%, H 4.21%, N 6.51%, O 29.73%, S 14.90%. Prepd by the action of oleum or sulfuric acid on acetanilide in acetic anhydride: Junghahn, Neumann, *Ber.* **33**, 1366 (1900); Söll, Stutzer, *Ber.* **42**, 4539 (1909).

Dihydrate, crystals. Freely sol in water, sol in alcohol, sparingly sol in glacial acetic acid, insol in ether. Slowly hydrolyzes in aq soln.

Sodium salt. Cosaprin. $C_8H_8NNaO_4S$. Prisms, soluble in water, moderately sol in alcohol, insol in ether.

Ethyl ester. $C_{10}H_{13}NO_4S$. Needles from benzene, mp 115°.

103. *N*-Acetylsulfanilyl Chloride. [121-60-8] 4-(Acetylamino)benzenesulfonyl chloride; *p*-acetamidobenzenesulfonyl chloride; *p*-acetaminobenzenesulfonyl chloride; acetanilide-*p*-sulfonyl chloride; ASC. $C_8H_8ClNO_3S$; mol wt 233.67. C 41.12%, H 3.45%, Cl 15.17%, N 5.99%, O 20.54%, S 13.72%. Prepd by sulfonation of acetanilide: Stewart, *J. Chem. Soc.* **121**, 2558 (1922); Smiles, Stewart, *Org. Synth.* **coll. vol. I**, 8 (2nd ed., 1941).

Thick, light tan prisms from benzene, mp 149°. Has slight odor of acetic acid. Benzene and ether are poor solvents for purification by recrystn. Much better results are obtained using chloroform or ethylene dichloride. *Cf.* Northey, *Sulfonamides* (New York, 1948) p 12.

Caution: Irritant to skin, eyes, and mucous membranes of nose and throat.

USE: Intermediate in the prepn of sulfanilamide and its derivs.

104. Acetyltannic Acid. [1397-74-6] Diacetyltannic acid; tannyl acetate; Acetannin; Tannigen. Acetylation of tannin: Ciusa, Sollazzo, *Ann. Chim. Appl.* **33**, 72 (1942); *C.A.* **38**, 5794[4] (1944).

Yellowish- or grayish-white odorless powder; darkens on exposure to light. Softens under water at about 70°. Slightly soluble in water or alcohol; sol in ethyl acetate, solns of borax or sodium phosphate, or with gradual decompn in solns of alkali hydroxides and carbonates. *Incompat.* Alkalies, iron salts.

THERAP CAT: Astringent (intestinal).

THERAP CAT (VET): Astringent (intestinal) for foals, calves, dogs.

105. Achillea. Milfoil; yarrow; thousand-leaf. Flowering herb, *Achillea millefolium* L., *Compositae. Habit.* Europe, Asia, naturalized in U.S. Extensively used as herbal remedy by many cultures. Constituents of plant and of the volatile oil may vary depending on origin of plant. Identification of constituents: Pailer, Kump, *Monatsh. Chem.* **90**, 395 (1959); *eidem, Arch. Pharm.* **293**, 646 (1960); A. J. Falk *et al., J. Nat. Prod.* **37**, 598 (1974); R. F. Chandler *et al., J. Pharm. Sci.* **71**, 690 (1982). Isoln of anti-inflammatory constituents: A. S. Goldberg, *J. Pharm. Sci.* **58**, 938 (1969). Phytopharmacology: J. P. Tewari *et al., Indian J. Med. Sci.* **28**, 331 (1974). Review of medicinal uses and composition: R. F. Chandler *et al., Econ. Bot.* **36**, 203-223 (1982); J. Gruenwald *et al., PDR for Herbal Medicines* (Medical Economics, Montvale, 2nd Ed., 2000) pp 833-835.

Volatile oil. [8022-07-9] Oil of yarrow. Obtained by steam distillation of leaves and tops. *Constit.* Chamazulene (0-40%), camphor, β-pinene, cineol, caryophyllene. Blue liquid. d_{20}^{20} 0.905-0.925. Insol in water; very sol in alc, ether. *Keep well closed, cool and protected from light.*

USE: In hair preparations and skin lotions for cleansing and to promote healing.

THERAP CAT: Carminative; cholagogue; antiseptic.

106. Acibenzolar-*S*-methyl. [135158-54-2] 1,2,3-Benzothiadiazole-7-carbothioic acid *S*-methyl ester; 7-(methylthiocarbonyl)-benzo-1,2,3-thiadiazole; CGA-245704; Bion. $C_8H_6N_2$-OS_2; mol wt 210.28. C 45.69%, H 2.88%, N 13.32%, O 7.61%, S 30.50%. Crop protection agent which activates the natural plant response to infection, known as systemic aquired resistance (SAR). Prepn: R. Schurter *et al., EP 313512; eidem, US 5523311* (1989, 1996 both to Ciba-Geigy). Properties and biological activity: W. Ruess *et al., Brighton Crop Prot. Conf. - Pests Dis.* **1996**, 53. Mode of action: H. Kessman *et al. ibid.* 961. Use as a seed treatment: B. D. Jensen *et al., Pestic. Sci.* **52**, 63 (1998).

White to beige odorless powder, mp 132.9°. Vapor pressure at 25°: 4.6×10^{-4} Pa. Soly at 25°(g/l): *n*-hexane 1.3; toluene 36; *n*-octanol 5.4; acetone 28; dichloroethane 160. Soly in water (25°): 7.7 mg/l. Log P (*n*-octanol/water) at 25°: 3.1. LD_{50} in rats (mg/kg): >2000 orally; >2000 dermally (Ruess).

USE: Plant disease resistance activator.

107. Acid Fuchsin. [3244-88-0] 2-Amino-5-[(4-amino-3-sulfophenyl)(4-imino-3-sulfo-2,5-cyclohexadien-1-ylidene)methyl]-3-methylbenzenesulfonic acid disodium salt; C.I. Acid Violet 19; 2-amino-α^5-(4-amino-3-sulfophenyl)-α^5-(4-imino-3-sulfo-2,5-cyclohexadien-1-ylidene)-3,5-xylenesulfonic acid disodium salt; acid rubin; fuchsin(e) acid; acid roseine; C.I. 42685. $C_{20}H_{17}N_3$-$Na_2O_9S_3$; mol wt 585.54. C 41.02%, H 2.93%, N 7.18%, Na 7.85%, O 24.59%, S 16.43%. The trisulfonated derivative of rosanilin, or pararosanilin. *See: Colour Index* vol. **4** (3rd ed., 1971) p 4399. Use as stain: P. W. Benoit, *Stain Technol.* **48**, 177 (1973); E. Hals, *Scand. J. Dent. Res.* **85**, 542 (1977). Mechanism of action: L. F. Nielsen *et al., Biotech. Histochem.* **73**, 71(1998). Brief review: *H. J. Conn's Biological Stains*, R. D. Lillie, Ed. (Williams & Wilkins, Baltimore, 9th ed., 1977) pp 285-286.

Olive to dark olive-green coarse powder. Absorption max: 540-545 nm (10 mg/l of 0.01% HCl). Very sol in water, very slightly sol to insol in alcohol. Dil aq solns are purplish red. Very dil aq solns (1:10,000) are decolorized by drops of concd aq NaOH solns, but not returned by concd HCl. The decolorized soln neutralized with NaOH is called the **Andrade indicator**. Changes from red to colorless at pH 12-14.

USE: As pH indicator; biological stain.

108. Acid α-Glucosidase. Acid maltase; lysosomal α-glucosidase; GAA. Lysosomal enzyme that hydrolyzes α-1,4- and α-1,6-glucosidic linkages in oligosaccharides and α-glucans to liberate glucose at acid pH. Natural substrate is glycogen stored in lysosomes. Produced as a 110 kDa glycosylated precursor that is routed to lysosomes via the mannose-6-phosphate recognition marker and is proteolytically processed to the mature forms of 70 and 76 kDa. Genetic deficiency of the enzyme results in a glycogen storage disorder known as Pompe's disease. Identification and role in disease: H. G. Hers, *Biochem. J.* **86**, 11 (1963). Localization in liver lysosomes: N. Lejeune *et al., ibid.* 16. Purification: F. Auricchio, C. B. Bruni, *ibid.* **105**, 35 (1967); F. Auricchio *et al., ibid.* **108**, 161 (1968). *Review:* R. Hirschhorn in *The Metabolic and Molecular Bases of Inherited Disease*, C. R. Scriver *et al.,* Eds. (McGraw-Hill, New York, 7th Ed., 1995) pp 2443-2464.

Alglucosidase alfa. [420784-05-0] [199-arginine, 223-histidine]prepro-α-glucosidase (human); Myozyme. Recombinant human precursor form. Production in Chinese hamster ovary cells: J. L. K. Van Hove *et al., Proc. Natl. Acad. Sci. USA* **93**, 65 (1996). Clinical evaluation in Pompe patients: A. Amalfitano *et al., Genet. Med.* **3**, 132 (2001).

THERAP CAT: Enzyme replacement therapy for Pompe's disease.

109. Acifluorfen. [50594-66-6] 5-[2-Chloro-4-(trifluoromethyl)phenoxy]-2-nitrobenzoic acid. $C_{14}H_7ClF_3NO_5$; mol wt 361.66. C 46.49%, H 1.95%, Cl 9.80%, F 15.76%, N 3.87%, O 22.12%. Selective pre- and post-emergence herbicide. Prepn: H. O. Bayer *et al.,* **DE 2311638**; *eidem,* **US 3928416, US 4063929** (1973, 1975, 1977 all to Rohm & Haas). Synthesis, activity and toxicity: W. O. Johnson *et al., J. Agric. Food Chem.* **26**, 285 (1978). Carcinogenicity studies: J. A. Quest *et al., Regul. Toxicol. Pharmacol.* **10**, 149 (1989).

Off-white solid, mp 151.5-157°.

Sodium salt. Scifluorfen; RH-6201; Blazer. $C_{14}H_6ClF_3$-$NNaO_5$; mol wt 383.64. White powder, mp 124-125°. Soly in water >25%. LD_{50} orally in rats: 1300 mg/kg (Johnson).

Caution: Skin and eye irritant. Do not incorporate in soil. Do not mix with oils, surfactants, liquid fertilizers or other pesticides.

USE: Herbicide.

110. Acifran. [72420-38-3] 4,5-Dihydro-5-methyl-4-oxo-5-phenyl-2-furancarboxylic acid; 2-methyl-2-phenyl-3(2*H*)-furanone-5-carboxylic acid; AY-25712; Reductol. $C_{12}H_{10}O_4$; mol wt 218.21. C 66.05%, H 4.62%, O 29.33%. Prepd (not claimed): I. L. Jirkovsky *et al.,* **US 4169202**; prepn and resolution of enantiomers: *eidem,* **US 4244958** (1979, 1981 both to American Home); I. L. Jirkovsky, M. N. Cayen, *J. Med. Chem.* **25,** 1154 (1982). Metabolism and pharmacokinetics in dogs and rats: M. N. Cayen *et al., Xenobiotica* **16,** 251 (1986). LC determn in serum: R. Gonzalez, D. Thibeault, *Clin. Biochem.* **16,** 244 (1983). Clinical evaluation in hyperlipoproteinemia: D. B. Hunninghake *et al., Clin. Pharmacol. Ther.* **38,** 313 (1985); J. C. LaRosa *et al., Artery* **14,** 338 (1987).

Crystals, mp 176°. uv max (methanol): 281 nm (ε 7960). LD_{50} orally in rats: 3 g/kg (Jirkovsky, 1982).

(−)-Form. [77103-92-5] mp 87-89°. $[\alpha]_D^{25}$ −144.7° (c = 2 in methanol).

(+)-Form. [77103-91-4] mp 87-89°. $[\alpha]_D^{25}$ +146.4° (c = 2 in methanol).

THERAP CAT: Antilipemic.

111. Acipimox. [51037-30-0] 5-Methylpyrazinecarboxylic acid 4-oxide; 2-carboxy-5-methylpyrazine 4-oxide; K-9321; Olbemox; Olbetam. $C_6H_6N_2O_3$; mol wt 154.12. C 46.76%, H 3.92%, N 18.18%, O 31.14%. Prepn: V. Ambrogi *et al.,* **DE 2319834**; *eidem,* **US 4002750** (1973, 1977 both to Carlo Erba). Prepn and toxicology: *eidem, Eur. J. Med. Chem.* **15,** 157 (1980). Pharmacological profile: P. P. Lovisolo *et al., Pharmacol. Res. Commun.* **13,** 151, 163 (1981). Pharmacokinetics: L. M. Fuccella *et al., Clin. Pharmacol. Ther.* **28,** 790 (1980); L. Musatti *et al., J. Int. Med. Res.* **9,** 381 (1981). Mechanism of action: K. Aktories *et al., Arzneim.-Forsch.* **33,** 1525 (1983).

Crystals from water, mp 177-180°. LD_{50} orally in mice: 3500 mg/kg (Ambrogi).

THERAP CAT: Antilipemic.

112. Acitretin. [55079-83-9] (2*E*,4*E*,6*E*,8*E*)-9-(4-Methoxy-2,3,6-trimethylphenyl)-3,7-dimethyl-2,4,6,8-nonatetraenoic acid; etretin; Ro-10-1670; Neotigason; Soriatane. $C_{21}H_{26}O_3$; mol wt 326.43. C 77.27%, H 8.03%, O 14.70%. Synthetic retinoid; free acid form and major metabolite of etretinate, *q.v.* Prepn: W. Bollag *et al.,* **DE 2414619**; *eidem,* **US 4105681** (1974, 1978 both to Hoffmann-La Roche). Teratogenicity study: A. Kistler, H. Hummler, *Arch. Toxicol.* **58,** 50 (1985). HPLC determn in plasma: N. R. Al-Mallah *et al., Anal. Lett.* **21,** 1603 (1988). Pharmacokinetics in humans: F. G. Larsen *et al., Pharmacol. Toxicol.* **62,** 159 (1988). Clinical evaluation in cutaneous lupus erythematosus: T. Ruzicka *et al., Arch. Dermatol.* **124,** 897 (1988). Review of clinical pharmacology: A. Vahlquist, O. Rollman, *Dermatologica* **175,** Suppl. 1, 20-27 (1987). Review of clinical studies in psoriatic and nonpsori-

atic dermatoses: J.-M. Geiger, B. M. Czarnetzki, *ibid.* **176,** 182-190 (1988).

Crystals from hexane, mp 228-230°. LD_{50} i.p. in mice (mg/kg): >4000 (1 day), 700 (10 days), 700 (20 days) (Bollag, 1978).

THERAP CAT: Antipsoriatic.

113. Aclacinomycins. Antitumor antibiotic complex of the anthracycline group, produced by *Streptomyces galilaeus.* Thirteen yellow and seven red-colored components have been identified. Isoln of the major components, aclacinomycins A and B: H. Umezawa *et al.,* **DE 3532568**; *eidem,* **US 3988315** (1974, 1976 both to Microbiochem. Res. Found.). *See also:* T. Oki *et al., J. Antibiot.* **28,** 830 (1975). Structure, taxonomy, production, properties: *eidem, ibid.* **32,** 791, 801 (1979). The aglycone portion of aclacinomycin A is known as *aklavinone.* Isoln of aklavinone: J. J. Gordon *et al., Tetrahedron Lett.* **8,** 28 (1960). Synthesis of racemic aklavinone: B. A. Pearlman *et al., J. Am. Chem. Soc.* **103,** 4248 (1981); P. A. Confalone, G. Pizzolato, *ibid.* 4251; R. K. Boeckman, F. W. Sum, *ibid.* **104,** 4604 (1982). Synthesis of optically active aklavinone: A. S. Kende, J. P. Rizzi, *ibid.* **103,** 4247 (1981); J. M. McNamara, Y. Kishi, *ibid.* **104,** 7371 (1982). *In vitro* metabolism of aclacinomycins: T. Komiyama *et al., Gann* **70,** 395 (1979), *C.A.* **92,** 15143x (1980). HPLC determn of aclacinomycin A and its metabolites: T. Ogasawara *et al., J. Antibiot.* **34,** 47, 52 (1981). Pharmacokinetics: M. J. Egorin *et al., Cancer Chemother. Pharmacol.* **8,** 41 (1982). Series of articles on absorption, excretion, distribution and general pharmacology: *Jpn. J. Antibiot.* **33,** 169-213 (1980), *C.A.* **93,** 19316, 125326, 125649, 142986 (1980). Immunological study: M. Ishizuka *et al., J. Antibiot.* **34,** 331 (1981). Clinical studies: R. Maral, *Drugs Exp. Clin. Res.* **9,** 375 (1983); R. P. Warrell, Jr., S. J. Kempin, *Am. J. Clin. Oncol.* **6,** 81 (1983); A. Y. Bedikian *et al., ibid.* 187 (1983). Review of pharmacology of aclacinomycin A: T. Oki, *Anthracyclines [Proc. Workshop],* S. T. Crooke, S. D. Reich, Eds. (Academic Press, New York, 1980) pp 323-342, *C.A.* **93,** 160778h (1980).

Aclacinomycin A

Aclacinomycin A. [57576-44-0] [1*R*-(1α,2β,4β)]-2-Ethyl-1,2,-3,4,6,11-hexahydro-2,5,7-trihydroxy-6,11-dioxo-4-[[2,3,6-trideoxy-4-*O*-[2,6-dideoxy-4-*O*-[(2*R-trans*)-tetrahydro-6-methyl-5-oxo-2*H*-pyran-2-yl]-α-L-*lyxo*-hexopyranosyl]-3-(dimethylamino)-α-L-*lyxo*-hexopyranosyl]oxy]-1-naphthacenecarboxylic acid methyl ester; aclarubicin; antibiotic MA 144A1; NSC-208734; Jaclacin. $C_{42}H_{53}NO_{15}$; mol wt 811.87. Yellow microcryst powder from chloroform/hexane, mp 151-153° (dec). $[\alpha]_D^{24}$ −11.5° (c = 1 in methylene chloride). uv max (methanol): 229.5, 259, 289.5, 431 nm ($E_{1cm}^{1\%}$ 550, 326, 135, 161); (0.1*N* HCl) 229.5, 258.5, 290, 431 nm

($E_{1cm}^{1\%}$ 571, 338, 130, 161); (0.1N NaOH) 239, 287, 523 nm ($E_{1cm}^{1\%}$ 450, 113, 127). Sol in CHCl$_3$, ethyl acetate. Insol in ethyl ether, n-hexane, petr ether. Addn of alkali to aq solns gives an intense reddish-purple color; in conc HCl the soln is yellow. LD$_{50}$ in mice (mg/kg): 22.6 i.p., 33.7 i.v. (Oki).

Aclacinomycin A hydrochloride. Aclarubicin hydrochloride; Aclacin; Aclacinon; Aclaplastin. C$_{42}$H$_{53}$NO$_{15}$.HCl; mol wt 848.33.

Aclacinomycin B. [57596-79-9] [1R-(1α,2β,4β)]-4-[[[2′′′,3′′-Anhydro]-O-3,6-dideoxy-α-L-$erythro$-hexopyranos-4-ulos-1-yl-(1 → 4)-O-2,6-dideoxy-α-L-$lyxo$-hexopyranosyl-(1 → 4)-2,3,6-tri-deoxy-3-(dimethylamino)-α-L-$lyxo$-hexopyranosyl]oxy]-2-ethyl-1,-2,3,4,6,11-hexahydro-2,5,7-trihydroxy-6,11-dioxo-1-naphthacene-carboxylic acid methyl ester; antibiotic MA 144B1. C$_{42}$H$_{51}$NO$_{15}$; mol wt 809.85. Yellow microcryst powder from chloroform/hexane, mp 163-167° (dec). [α]$_D^{24}$ +3° (c = 1 in methylene chloride). Other physical properties similar to aclacinomycin A. LD$_{50}$ in mice (mg/kg): 13.7 i.p., 16.4 i.v. (Oki).

THERAP CAT: Antineoplastic.

114. Aclatonium Napadisilate. [55077-30-0] 2-[2-(Acetyloxy)-1-oxopropoxy]-N,N,N-trimethylethanaminium 1,5-naphthalenedisulfonate (2:1); 1,5-naphthalenedisulfonic acid bis [2-[2-(acetyloxy)-1-oxopropoxy]-N,N,N-trimethylethanaminium]ion (2$^-$); acetyllactoylcholine 1,5-naphthalenedisulfonate; choline 1,5-naphthalenedisulfonate (2:1), dilactate, diacetate; TM-723; Abovis. C$_{30}$H$_{46}$N$_2$O$_{14}$S$_2$; mol wt 722.82. C 49.85%, H 6.41%, N 3.88%, O 30.99%, S 8.87%. Spasmolytic agent related structurally to acetylcholine chloride, $q.v.$ Prepn: K. Miura $et al.$, **DE 2425983**; $eidem$, **US 3903137** (1973, 1975 both to Toyama). Synthesis and smooth muscle activity: $eidem$, $Yakugaku$ $Zasshi$ **99**, 1245 (1979), $C.A.$ **92**, 146197r (1980). Toxicity study: A. Takai $et al.$, Oyo $Yakuri$ **19**, 93 (1980), $C.A.$ **93**, 613367 (1980). Series of articles on metabolism, pharmacology, toxicity studies: Oyo $Yakuri$ **18**, 695-942 (1979), $C.A.$ **92**, 191015r, 191281z, 191282a, 208995k-7n (1980).

Crystals, mp 189-191°. LD$_{50}$ in mice: 15 g/kg orally, 826 mg/kg s.c. (Miura); in dogs: >10 g/kg orally (Takai).

THERAP CAT: Cholinergic.

115. Aconine. [509-20-6] (1α,3α,6α,14α,15α,16β)-20-Ethyl-1,6,16-trimethoxy-4-(methoxymethyl)aconitane-3,8,13,14,15-pentol. C$_{25}$H$_{41}$NO$_9$; mol wt 499.59. C 60.10%, H 8.27%, N 2.80%, O 28.82%. Obtained by hydrolysis of aconitine: Schulze, $Arch. Pharm.$ **244**, 165 (1906); Schneider, $Ber.$ **89**, 768 (1956). Structure: Schneider, Tausend, $Ann.$ **628**, 114 (1959); McCaldin, Marion, $Can. J. Chem.$ **37**, 1071 (1959).

Amorphous powder, mp 132°. Bitter taste. [α]$_D$ +23°. pK 9.52. Absorption spectrum: Nath, $J. Indian Chem. Soc.$ **32**, 75 (1955). Very sol in water, alcohol; moderately sol in chloroform; slightly sol in benzene. Practically insol in ether, petr ether.

Hydrochloride dihydrate. C$_{25}$H$_{42}$ClNO$_9$.2H$_2$O. Crystals, mp 175-176°. [α]$_D$ −8°.

Hydrobromide sesquihydrate. C$_{25}$H$_{42}$BrNO$_9$.1½H$_2$O. Crystals from water, mp 225°.

116. Aconite. Monkshood; wolf's-bane; friar's cowl; mouse-bane. Dried tuberous root of $Aconitum$ $napellus$ L., $Ranunculaceae.$ **Habit.** Mountainous regions of Europe, Asia, and North America. **Constit.** 0.4-0.8% aconitine; aconine; napelline (isoaconitine, pseudoaconitine); picraconitine; aconitic acid; itaconic acid; succinic acid; malonic acid; fat; levulose. $Quite$ $toxic.$ $Ref:$ Freudenberg, $Ber.$ **69**, 1962 (1936); Rogers, Freudenberg, $ibid.$ **70**, 349 (1937); Lascombes, $Ann. Pharm. Fr.$ **16**, 429 (1958). See $also$ "Aconite," A. Ph. A. Monograph No. 1 (Am. Pharm. Assoc., Washington, D.C., 1938).

THERAP CAT: Antipyretic.

THERAP CAT (VET): Formerly used as an antihypertensive.

117. Aconitic Acid. [499-12-7] 1-Propene-1,2,3-tricarboxylic acid; equisetic acid; citridic acid; achilleic acid. C$_6$H$_6$O$_6$; mol wt 174.11. C 41.39%, H 3.47%, O 55.14%. Found in leaves and tubers of $Aconitum$ $napellus$ L., $Ranunculaceae$, in various species of $Achillea$ ($Compositae$) and $Equisetum$ ($Equisetaceae$), in beet root, and in sugar cane. Can be prepd commercially from calcium magnesium aconitate recovered from sugar cane juice: McCalip, Seibert, $Ind. Eng. Chem.$ **33**, 637 (1941); from molasses: Regna, Bruins, $ibid.$ **48**, 1268 (1956). Most of the commercial aconitic acid is, however, manufactured by sulfuric acid dehydration of citric acid: Bruce, $Org. Synth.$ **coll. vol. II**, p 12 (1943); by using methanesulfonic acid instead of sulfuric: Cranston, **US 2727066** (1955 to Daniel F. Kelly). Aconitic acid prepd by any of the above methods has the $trans$-configuration which is the form described here.

$trans$-form

Leaflets, plates from water. Decompn 198-199° (capillary inserted in oil bath at 190°); decompn 204-205° (capillary in oil bath at 195°); decompn 209° (electrically heated bar). K$_1$ at 25° = 1.58 × 10^{-3}; K$_2$ = 3.5 × 10^{-5}. One gram dissolves in 5.5 ml water at 13°, in 2 ml water at 25°. Soluble in 2 parts of 88% alcohol at 12°. Slightly sol in ether.

Triethyl ester. bp$_5$ 155°.

Tributyl ester. bp$_3$ 190°.

USE: Manuf itaconic acid. As plasticizer for buna rubber and plastics. Used in form of triethyl or tributyl ester.

118. Aconitine. [302-27-2] (1α,3α,6α,14α,15α,16β)-20-Ethyl-1,6,16-trimethoxy-4-(methoxymethyl)aconitane-3,8,13,14,-15-pentol 8-acetate 14-benzoate. C$_{34}$H$_{47}$NO$_{11}$; mol wt 645.74. C 63.24%, H 7.34%, N 2.17%, O 27.25%. Several isomers from $Aconitum$ $napellus$ L., $Ranunculaceae$ and other aconites. Majima $et al.$, $Ber.$ **57**, 1456 (1924); $Proc. Imp. Acad. Tokyo$ **5**, 415 (1929); Freudenberg, $Ber.$ **69**, 1964 (1936); Swanson $et al.$, $Aconite$, A. Ph. A. Monograph no. 1 (1938); $Methods of Analysis, A.O.A.C.$, 8th ed., 598, 651 (1955). Structure: Wiesner $et al.$, $Collect. Czech. Chem. Commun.$ **28**, 2462 (1963); Wiesner $et al.$, $Can. J. Chem.$ **47**, 2734 (1969). Stereochemistry: Bachelor $et al.$, $Tetrahedron Lett.$ **1960**, no. 10, 1; Gilman, Marion, $ibid.$ **1961**, 923; Tsuda, Marion, $Can. J. Chem.$ **41**, 1634 (1963); Birnbaum $et al.$, $Tetrahedron Lett.$ **1971**, 867. Pharmacology: H. Sato $et al.$, $Tohoku J. Exp. Med.$ **128**, 175 (1979). Inotropic effects: P. Honerjäger, A. Meissner, $Arch. Pharmacol.$ **322**, 49 (1983). Toxicity: Dybing $et al.$, $Acta Pharmacol. Toxicol.$ **7**, 337 (1951).

Hexagonal plates, mp 204°. [α]$_D$ +17.3° (chloroform). Aq soln is alkaline to litmus. pK 5.88. One gram dissolves in 2 ml chloroform, 7 ml benzene, 28 ml abs alcohol, 50 ml ether, 3300 ml water. Slightly sol in petr ether. *Poisonous!* LD$_{50}$ in mice (mg/kg): 0.166 i.v.; 0.328 i.p.; approx 1 orally (Dybing) also reported as LD$_{50}$ in mice (mg/kg): 1.8 orally, 0.270 s.c.; 0.380 i.p.; 0.12 i.v. (Sato).

Hydrobromide hemipentahydrate. C$_{34}$H$_{47}$NO$_{11}$.HBr.2½H$_2$-O. Hexagonal tablets from water, mp 200-207° (sinters at 160°). Amorphous form mp 115-120°. Also crystallizes from ethanol + ether with ½H$_2$O, mp 206-207°; [α]$_D$ −30.8°. *Violent poison! Ref:* Paech, Tracey, *Modern Methods of Plant Analysis* **vol. IV** (Springer-Verlag, Berlin, 1955) p 375.

Hydrochloride hemipentahydrate. C$_{34}$H$_{47}$NO$_{11}$.HCl.2½H$_2$-O. Crystals, mp 149-153°. mp 194-195° (dry). [α]$_D$ −30.9°. *Violent poison! Ref:* Paech, Tracey.

Nitrate. C$_{34}$H$_{47}$NO$_{11}$.HNO$_3$. Crystals, mp about 200° (dec). [α]$_D^{20}$ −35° (c = 2 in water). *Violent poison!* One gram dissolves in 10 ml boiling water. Less sol in cold water. Sol in alcohol.

Caution: Potential symptoms of overexposure are nausea, vomiting, diarrhea due to CNS stimulation; restlessness, ataxia, vertigo, slow and dyspneic breathing, hypothermia, convulsions. Direct contact may cause warm tingling sensation with subsequent numbness on mouth and mucous membranes. *See Clinical Toxicology of Commercial Products*, R. E. Gosselin *et al.*, Eds. (Williams & Wilkins, Baltimore, 5th ed., 1984) Section II, p 249.

USE: Used in producing heart arrhythmia in experimental animals: Boyadzhiev, *C.A.* **73**, 86256e (1970).

THERAP CAT: Has been used topically in neuralgia.

119. Aconitine, Amorphous. Mild aconitine. Highly toxic mixture of amorphous alkaloids from *Aconitum napellus* L., *Ranunculaceae.* Contains aconitine, mesaconitine, hypaconitine, neopelline, *l*-ephedrine, sparteine, neoline and napelline. *Ref:* Rogers, Freudenberg, *Ber.* **70**, 349 (1937); *eidem, J. Am. Chem. Soc.* **59**, 2572 (1937). Toxicity data: Munch, *J. Am. Pharm. Assoc.* **18**, 17 (1929).

Yellowish-white, amorphous powder. *Violent poison!* Insol in water. Sol in alcohol, chloroform, ether, dil acids. MLD in rats (mg/kg): 0.175 s.c., 0.1 i.p. (Munch).

120. Aconitum Ferox. Indian aconite; bish; visha; bishma; bikhroot. Tuber of *Aconitum ferox* Wall., *Ranunculaceae. Habit.* Nepal, Himalaya Mountains, India. *Constit.* Pseudoaconitine. Most powerful of all the aconites. Used by natives as arrow poison in big game hunting; in neuralgia and rheumatism. *Ref: Aconite,* A. Ph. A. Monograph no. 1, p 78 and *passim* (Am. Pharm. Assoc., Washington, D.C., 1938); N. B. Dutt, *Indian J. Pharm.* **1**, 81-84 (1939); *C.A.* **34**, 6768 (1940).

Caution: Extremely toxic. A very small dose can cause fatal cardiac depression.

121. Acranil®. [1684-42-0] 1-[(6-Chloro-2-methoxy-9-acridinyl)amino]-3-(diethylamino)-2-propanol dihydrochloride; 5-[(γ-diethylamino-β-hydroxypropyl)amino]-3-methoxy-8-chloro-acridine dihydrochloride; SKF-16214-A2; SN-186. C$_{21}$H$_{28}$Cl$_3$N$_3$-O$_2$; mol wt 460.82. C 54.73%, H 6.12%, Cl 23.08%, N 9.12%, O 6.94%. Prepn: Mietzsch, Mauss, **DE 553072** *Frdl.* **19**, 1167; **GB 363392; US 2113357** (1930, 1930, 1938 all to I. G. Farben.); Maghidson, Grigorovski, *Ber.* **69**, 396 (1936); *J. Gen. Chem. USSR* **6**, 806 (1936). Antiviral activity: T. E. Gláz *et al.*, *Antimicrob. Agents Chemother.* **3**, 537 (1973). Interferon induction and radioprotective activity: T. E. Glaz, M. Talas, *Arch. Virol.* **48**, 375 (1975); M. Talas, E. Szolgay, *ibid.* **56**, 309 (1978).

Bitter, yellow crystals, mp 237-239° (dec). Sol in water. **Free base.** C$_{21}$H$_{26}$ClN$_3$O$_2$. Yellow crystals, mp 105-107°. Sparingly sol in ether.

THERAP CAT: Antiprotozoal (Giardia).

122. Acridine. [260-94-6] Dibenzo[*b,e*]pyridine; 10-aza-anthracene. C$_{13}$H$_9$N; mol wt 179.22. C 87.12%, H 5.06%, N 7.82%. Occurs in coal tar. Isoln: Graebe, Caro, *Ann.* **158**, 265 (1871); from high boiling tar oils: Wirth, **DE 440771** (1926). Prepn from *N*-phenylanthranilic acid: Perkin, Clemo, **GB 214756** (1923); from Ca-anthranilate: Koller, Krakauer, *Monatsh. Chem.* **50**, 51 (1928); by passing benzylaniline vapor over red-hot platinum wire: Meyer, Hofmann, *ibid.* **37**, 698 (1916); *cf.* Ullmann, *Ber.* **40**, 2521 (1907). Absorption spectrum: Pinnow, **GB 214756** (1923). Toxicity: S. D. Rubbo, *Br. J. Exp. Pathol.* **28**, 1 (1947). *Reviews:* A. Albert, *The Acridines* (St. Martin's Press, New York, 2nd ed., 1966); R. M. Acheson, *Acridines* (Interscience, New York, 2nd ed., 1973).

Pale yellow orthorhombic plates, needles from diluted alcohol. There are five crystalline forms of acridine all of which melt below 111°. Purified acridine mp 110-111°; commercial samples mp 107° or mp 109°. Begins to sublime at 100°. bp$_{760}$ 346°; also reported as bp$_{760}$ >360°. Volatile with steam. Slightly sol in boiling water, liquid ammonia, liquid sulphur dioxide; sparingly sol in light petroleum; freely sol in alcohol, ether, hydrocarbons, carbon disulfide. 1 gm sol in <1 ml boiling benzene or alcohol; 5 ml benzene (20°); 6 ml alcohol (20°); 16 ml of ether (20°); 1.8 ml boiling cyclohexane. d 1.27-1.28. Dilute solns of acridine and its salts have a violet and green fluorescence, respectively. Weak base, colors litmus paper blue, forms yellow crystalline salts with mineral acids. Forms colored quaternary ammonium compounds (acridinium compounds), by the action of alkyl and aryl halides and sulfates. LD$_{50}$ s.c. in mice: 0.40 g/kg (Rubbo).

Caution: Strongly irritating to skin, mucous membranes. *See: Clinical Toxicology of Commercial Products*, R. E. Gosselin *et al.*, Eds. (Williams & Wilkins, Baltimore, 5th ed., 1984) Section II, p 384.

USE: Manuf dyes and intermediates; some dyes derived from it are used as antiseptics, e.g. 9-aminoacridine, acriflavine and proflavine. The hydrochloride has been used as reagent for cobalt, iron and zinc.

123. Acriflavine. [8048-52-0] 3,6-Diamino-10-methyl-acridinium chloride mixt with 3,6-acridinediamine; neutral acriflavine; euflavine; trypaflavine; neutroflavine; gonacrine. Contains 30-40% unmethylated compd. Prepn: L. Benda, *Ber.* **45**, 1787 (1912); M. Gaillot, *Q. J. Pharm. Pharmacol.* **7**, 63 (1934); J. Marshall, *ibid.* 514. Activity studies: C. H. Browning, W. Gilmour, *J. Pathol. Bact.* **18**, 144 (1913); C. H. Browning *et al., Br. Med. J.* **1**, 73 (1917); H. Berry, *Q. J. Pharm. Pharmacol.* **14**, 149 (1941); H. McIlwain, *Biochem. J.* **35**, 1311 (1941). Toxicology: J. Ungar *et al., J. Pharmacol. Exp. Ther.* **80**, 217 (1944). *Reviews:* A. Adrien, *The Acridines* (St. Martin's Press, New York, 2nd ed., 1966); R. M. Acheson, *Acridines* (Interscience, New York, 2nd ed., 1973).

Deep orange, granular powder. One gram dissolves in about 3 ml water. Incompletely sol in alcohol; nearly insol in ether, chloroform, fixed oils. Aqueous solns are reddish orange and fluoresce on dilution. pH (1% soln) ~3.5.

Dihydrochloride. [8063-24-9] Acid acriflavine; acid trypaflavine; acriflavine hydrochloride; Panflavin. Deep reddish-brown, crystalline powder. pH (1% soln) ~1.5.

THERAP CAT: Anti-infective.

THERAP CAT (VET): Antiseptic; locally in wounds in trichomoniasis of bulls.

124. Acrilan®. A brand of acrylic fiber, a copolymer of acrylonitrile and of a minor constituent with mildly basic character. Prepn of such copolymers: Mowry, Craig, **US 2744086** and Craig, **US 2749325** (both 1956 to Chemstrand). *Review:* R. W. Moncrieff, *Man-Made Fibres* (John Wiley & Sons, New York, 4th ed., 1963) pp 471-482.

Solid, d^{25} 1.17. Fiber decomposes before it melts. Sticks at 245°. Prolonged exposure in air at elevated temps causes some yellowing. Fabrics are not readily ignited and their rate of burning is less than that of cotton, viscose rayon, or acetate rayon. Fiber is practically insoluble in, and unaffected by common solvents. Has fairly good resistance to weak alkalies, very good resistance to mineral acids, sunlight, weathering. Has good dyeing properties. Its wear resistance is better than that of wool, but generally greatly inferior to that of nylon or Terylene. It is unaffected by mildew, molds, moth and carpet beetle larvae.

USE: Fabrics, sweaters, blankets, carpets.

125. Acrinathrin. [101007-06-1] (1*R*,3*S*)-2,2-Dimethyl-3-[(1*Z*)-3-oxo-3-[2,2,2-trifluoro-1-(trifluoromethyl)ethoxy]-1-propenyl]cyclopropanecarboxylic acid (*S*)-cyano(3-phenoxyphenyl)-methyl ester; (*S*)-α-cyano-3-phenoxybenzyl (1*R-cis*)-2,2-dimethyl-3-[(*Z*)-3-oxo-3-[2-(1,1,1,3,3,3-hexafluoropropoxy)]-1-propenyl]-cyclopropanecarboxylate; RU-38702; Rufast. $C_{26}H_{21}F_6NO_5$; mol wt 541.44. C 57.68%, H 3.91%, F 21.05%, N 2.59%, O 14.77%. Synthetic pyrethroid acaricide. Prepn: J. Martel *et al.*, **FR 2486073**; *eidem*, **US 4542142** (1982, 1985 both to Roussel-UCLAF); J. R. Tessier *et al.*, in *Pesticide Chemistry: Human Welfare and the Environment* vol. 1, J. Miyamoto, P. C. Kearney, Eds. (Pergamon Press, Oxford, 1983) pp 95-100. Field trial vs spider mite: B. H. Labanowska, C. Tkaczuk, *Fruit Sci. Rep.* **18**, 185 (1991). *Review:* J. J. Heller *et al.*, *Meded. Fac. Landbouwwet. Univ. Gent* **57**, 931-939 (1992).

mp 82°. $[\alpha]_D^{20}$ +23.5° (c = 0.5% in benzene). LD_{50} in rats (mg/kg): >5000 orally; >2000 dermally (Heller).

USE: Insecticide.

126. Acrisorcin. [7527-91-5] 4-Hexyl-1,3-benzenediol compd with 9-acridinamine (1:1); 9-aminoacridine compd with 4-hexylresorcinol; 9-aminoacridinium 4-hexylresorcinolate; Sch-7056; Akrinol. $C_{25}H_{28}N_2O_2$; mol wt 388.50. C 77.29%, H 7.26%, N 7.21%, O 8.24%. Prepd from 9-aminoacridine and 4-hexylresorcinol: Seneca, *Antibiot. Chemother.* **11**, 587 (1961).

Yellow crystals.
THERAP CAT: Antifungal.

127. Acrivastine. [87848-99-5] (2*E*)-3-[6-[(1*E*)-1-(4-Methylphenyl)-3-(1-pyrrolidinyl)-1-propenyl]-2-pyridinyl]-2-propenoic acid; (*E*)-6-[(*E*)-3-(1-pyrrolidinyl)-1-*p*-tolylpropenyl]-2-pyridineacrylic acid; BW-270C; BW-825C; BW-A825C; Semprex. $C_{22}H_{24}N_2O_2$; mol wt 348.44. C 75.83%, H 6.94%, N 8.04%, O 9.18%. Nonsedating type histamine H_1-receptor antagonist; analog of triprolidine, *q.v.* Prepn: G. G. Coker, J. W. A. Findlay, **EP 85959** (1983 to Wellcome); J. W. A. Findlay, G. G. Coker, **US 4501893** (1985). Pharmacodynamics and pharmacokinetics in humans: A. F. Cohen *et al.*, *Eur. J. Clin. Pharmacol.* **28**, 197 (1985).

Evaluation of CNS effects: A. F. Cohen *et al.*, *Clin. Pharmacol. Ther.* **38**, 381 (1985). Clinical trials in idiopathic urticaria: J. G. Gibson *et al.*, *Dermatologica* **169**, 179 (1984); H. Neittaanmaki *et al., ibid.* **177**, 98 (1988); in allergic rhinitis: T. G. Gibbs *et al., J. Int. Med. Res.* **16**, 413 (1988). Review of pharmacology and therapeutic efficacy: R. N. Brogden, D. McTavish, *Drugs* **41**, 927-940 (1991).

Crystals from isopropanol, mp 222° (dec).
Combination with pseudoephedrine, *Duact*.
THERAP CAT: Antihistaminic.

128. Acrolein. [107-02-8] 2-Propenal; acrylic aldehyde; acrylaldehyde; acraldehyde; Aqualin; Magnacide. C_3H_4O; mol wt 56.06. C 64.27%, H 7.19%, O 28.54%. CH_2=CHCHO. Prepd industrially by passing glycerol vapors over magnesium sulfate heated to 330-340°. Lab prepn by heating a mixture of anhydr glycerol, acid potassium sulfate and potassium sulfate in the presence of a small amount of hydroquinone and distilling in the dark: H. Adkins, W. H. Hartung, *Org. Synth.* **coll. vol. I**, 15 (1941). Formation from glycerol by the action of *B. amaracrylus:* Voisenet, *Compt. Rend.* **188**, 941, 1271 (1929); by *B. welchii:* Humphreys, *J. Infect. Dis.* **35**, 282; *Chem. Zentralbl.* **1925, II**, 309. Toxicity study: H. F. Smyth *et al., Arch. Ind. Hyg. Occup. Med.* **4**, 119 (1951). *Review:* L. G. Hess *et al.*, in *Kirk-Othmer Encyclopedia of Chemical Technology* vol. 1 (Wiley-Interscience, New York, 3rd ed., 1978) pp 277-297. Review of toxicology and human exposure: *Toxicological Profile for Acrolein* (PB91-180307, 1990) 157 pp.

Flammable liquid with pungent odor. mp −88°. d^0 0.8621; d^{20} 0.8389; d^{50} 0.8075. bp_{760} 52.5°; bp_{200} 17.5°; bp_{100} 2.5°; bp_{60} −7.5°; $bp_{1.0}$ −64.5°. n_D^{19} 1.4022. Sol in 2 to 3 parts water; in alcohol, ether. Flash pt, open cup: <0°F (−18°C). Vapor pressure at 20°: 210 mm Hg. Unstable, polymerizes (especially under light or in the presence of alkali or strong acid) forming disacryl, a plastic solid. Absorption spectrum: Lüthy, *Z. Phys. Chem.* **107**, 291, 298 (1923). LD_{50} orally in rats: 0.046 g/kg (Smyth).

Caution: Potential symptoms of overexposure are irritation of eyes, skin and mucous membranes; decreased pulmonary function; delayed pulmonary edema; chronic respiratory disease. *See NIOSH Pocket Guide to Chemical Hazards* (DHHS/NIOSH 97-140, 1997) p 6. *See also Clinical Toxicology of Commercial Products*, R. E. Gosselin *et al.*, Eds. (Williams & Wilkins, Baltimore, 5th ed., 1984) Section II, p 186.

USE: Manuf colloidal forms of metals; making plastics, perfumes; warning agent in methyl chloride refrigerant. Has been used in military poison gas mixtures. Used in organic syntheses. Aquatic herbicide.

129. Acrylamide. [79-06-1] 2-Propenamide. C_3H_5NO; mol wt 71.08. C 50.69%, H 7.09%, N 19.71%, O 22.51%. CH_2=CHCONH₂. Prepd from acrylonitrile by treatment with H_2SO_4 or HCl: Bayer, *Angew. Chem.* **61**, 240 (1949); Weisgerber, **US 2535245** (1950 to Hercules). *Reviews:* Carpenter, Davis, *J. Appl. Chem.* **7**, 671 (1957); C. E. Habermann in *Kirk-Othmer Encyclopedia of Chemical Technology* vol. 1 (John Wiley & Sons, New York, 4th ed., 1991) pp 251-266. Toxicity: R. E. Peterson, N. K. Sheth, *Toxicol. Appl. Pharmacol.* **33**, 142 (1975). Review of carcinogenic risk: *IARC Monographs* **60**, 389-433 (1994). Identification in cooked carbohydrate-rich foods: E. Tareke *et al., J. Agric. Food Chem.* **50**, 4998 (2002). Proposed formation from asparagine, *q.v.*, during cooking: D. S. Mottram *et al., Nature* **419**, 448 (2002); R. H. Stadler *et al., ibid.* 449.

Monomer, flake-like crystals from benzene. d_4^{30} 1.122. mp 84.5°. bp_2 87°; bp_5 103°; bp_{25} 125°. Solubilities in g/100 ml solvent at 30°: water 215.5; methanol 155; ethanol 86.2; acetone 63.1; ethyl acetate 12.6; chloroform 2.66; benzene 0.346; heptane 0.0068. The solid may be stored in a cool, dark place. Readily polymerizes at the mp or under uv light. Commercial solns of the monomer may be stabilized with hydroquinone, *tert*-butylpyrocatechol, *N*-phenyl-2-naphthylamine or other antioxidants. LD$_{50}$ i.p. in mice: 170 mg/kg (Peterson, Sheth).

Polymer. Various forms, sol and insol in water, are obtained by heating with various polymerization catalysts: C. E. Schildknecht, *Vinyl and Related Polymers* (Wiley, New York, 1952) pp 314-322; D. Lipp, J. Kozakiewicz in *Kirk-Othmer Encyclopedia of Chemical Technology* vol. 1 (John Wiley & Sons, New York, 4th ed., 1991) pp 266-287.

Caution: Potential symptoms of overexposure to the monomer are ataxia, numbness of limbs, paresthesia; muscle weakness; absence of deep tendon reflex; sweating of hands; fatigue, lethargy; irritation of eyes and skin; reproductive effects. *See NIOSH Pocket Guide to Chemical Hazards* (DHHS/NIOSH 97-140, 1997) p 6. Readily absorbed through intact skin from aqueous solutions. *See Clinical Toxicology of Commercial Products,* R. E. Gosselin *et al.,* Eds. (Williams & Wilkins, Baltimore, 5th ed., 1984) Section II, p 409. This substance is reasonably anticipated to be a human carcinogen: *Report on Carcinogens, Eleventh Edition* (PB2005-104914, 2004) p III-4.

USE: Monomer as chemical intermediate in production of polyacrylamides; in synthesis of dyes; in copolymers for contact lenses; in construction of dam foundations, tunnels and sewers. Polymers as additives for water treatment, enhanced oil recovery, flocculants, papermaking aids, thickeners, soil conditioning agents, sewage and waste treatment, ore processing, permanent-press fabrics.

130. Acrylic Acid. [79-10-7] 2-Propenoic acid; vinylformic acid. $C_3H_4O_2$; mol wt 72.06. C 50.00%, H 5.60%, O 44.41%. $CH_2=CHCO_2H$. Prepd by hydrolysis of acrylonitrile: Kaszuba, *J. Am. Chem. Soc.* **67**, 1227 (1945); by oxidation of acrolein: **US 1911219** (1933 to Rohm & Haas); **US 2288566** (1942 to Acrolein Corp.); **US 2341339** (1944 to Distillers). Various other syntheses, *see Org. Synth.* **coll. vol. III**, 30-34 (1955). Toxicity study: H. F. Smyth *et al., Am. Ind. Hyg. Assoc. J.* **23**, 95 (1962). *Review:* J. W. Nemec, W. Bauer in *Kirk-Othmer Encyclopedia of Chemical Technology* vol. 1 (Wiley-Interscience, New York, 3rd ed., 1978) pp 330-354.

Corrosive liquid; acrid odor and fumes. d$_4^{16}$ 1.0621. mp 14°. bp 141.0°; bp$_{400}$ 122.0°; bp$_{200}$ 103.3°; bp$_{100}$ 86.1°; bp$_{40}$ 66.2°; bp$_{10}$ 39.0°; bp$_5$ 27.3°. n_D^{20} 1.4224. Flash pt, open cup: 155°F (68°C). pKa (25°): 4.25. Miscible with water, alc, ether. Polymerizes readily in the presence of oxygen. LD$_{50}$ orally in rats: 2.59 g/kg (Smyth).

Caution: Potential symptoms of overexposure are irritation of eyes, skin, respiratory system; eye, skin burns; skin sensitization. *See NIOSH Pocket Guide to Chemical Hazards* (DHHS/NIOSH 97-140, 1997) p 8.

USE: In the manuf of plastics.

131. Acrylonitrile. [107-13-1] 2-Propenenitrile; vinyl cyanide; cyanoethylene; Ventox. C_3H_3N; mol wt 53.06. C 67.91%, H 5.70%, N 26.40%. $CH_2=CHCN$. Prepn by dehydration of ethylene cyanohydrin or acrylamide: Moureu, *Ann. Chem. Phys.* [7] **2**, 186 (1893). Manuf by ammoxidation of propylene: *Faith, Keyes & Clark's Industrial Chemicals,* F. A. Lowenheim, M. K. Moran, Eds. (Wiley-Interscience, New York, 4th ed., 1975) pp 46-49. Toxicity: H. F. Smyth, C. P. Carpenter, *J. Ind. Hyg. Toxicol.* **30**, 63 (1948). Causes acute and chronic adrenocortical insufficiency: S. Szabo *et al., Lab. Invest.* **42**, 533 (1980); *eidem, J. Appl. Toxicol.* **4**, 131 (1984). Review of carcinogenic risk: *IARC Monographs* **19**, 73-133 (1979); of toxicology and human exposure: *Toxicological Profile for Acrylonitrile* (PB91-180489, 1990) 136 p. Comprehensive review: *The Chemistry of Acrylonitrile* (Am. Cyanamid, New York, 2nd ed., 1959) 272 pp; J. F. Brazdil in *Kirk-Othmer Encyclopedia of Chemical Technology* vol. 1 (John Wiley & Sons, New York, 4th ed., 1991) pp 352-369.

Volatile liquid. *Flammable and combustible.* Should be stored and used in closed systems whenever possible. Work areas should be adequately ventilated, and should be free from open lights, flames, and equipment that is not explosion-proof. *Handle in hood.* May polymerize spontaneously, particularly in the absence of oxygen or on exposure to visible light. Polymerizes violently in the presence of concentrated alkali. On standing may slowly develop a yellow color particularly after excessive exposure to light. bp$_{760}$ 77.3°; bp$_{500}$ 64.7°; bp$_{250}$ 45.5°; bp$_{100}$ 23.6°; bp$_{50}$ 8.7°. mp −83.55°. d$_4^{20}$ 0.8060; d$_4^{25}$ 0.8004. n_D^{25} 1.3888. Flash pt, open cup:

32°F (0°C). Explosive mixtures in air at 25°: 3.05% low limit; 17.0% upper limit. At 20° 7.35 parts dissolve in 100 parts water and 3.1 parts water dissolve in 100 parts acrylonitrile. Miscible with most organic solvents. LD$_{50}$ orally in rats: 0.093 g/kg (Smyth, Carpenter).

Caution: Potential symptoms of overexposure are asphyxia; irritation of eyes and skin; headache; sneezing; nausea, vomiting; weakness, lightheadedness; skin vesiculation; scaling dermatitis. *See NIOSH Pocket Guide to Chemical Hazards* (DHHS/NIOSH 97-140, 1997) p 8. *See also Clinical Toxicology of Commercial Products,* R. E. Gosselin *et al.,* Eds. (Williams & Wilkins, Baltimore, 5th ed., 1984) Section II, p 215. This substance is reasonably anticipated to be a human carcinogen: *Report on Carcinogens, Eleventh Edition* (PB2005-104914, 2004) p III-6.

USE: Manufacture of acrylic fibers. In the plastics, surface coatings, and adhesives industries. As a chemical intermediate in the synthesis of antioxidants, pharmaceuticals, dyes, surface-active agents, etc. In organic synthesis to introduce a cyanoethyl group. As a modifier for natural polymers. As a pesticide fumigant for stored grain. Experimentally to induce adrenal hemorrhagic necrosis in rats.

132. Actaplanins. A-4696; Kamoran. Complex of glycopeptide antibiotics produced by *Actinoplanes missouriensis*. Six actaplanins (A, B$_1$, B$_2$, B$_3$, C$_1$, G) have been isolated and characterized as having a central peptide core with the amino sugar *ristosamine* and up to four neutral sugars attached. Isoln: R. L. Hamill *et al.,* **DE 2209018** (1972 to Lilly), *C.A.* **77**, 138338n (1972); A. P. Raun, **US 3816618**; R. L. Hamill *et al.,* **US 4115552** (1974, 1978 to Lilly). Chemical characterization: M. Debono *et al., J. Antibiot.* **37**, 85 (1984). ^{1}H NMR studies and structures: A. H. Hunt *et al., J. Org. Chem.* **49**, 635 (1984); *eidem, ibid.* 641. Growth promotant activity: C. Tsaltos *et al., Bull. Hellenic Vet. Med. Soc.* **33**, 139 (1982). Use to increase milk production in ruminants: C. C. Scheifinger, **EP 63491**; *idem,* **US 4430328** (1982, 1984 to Eli Lilly). Determn in milk: K. H. Hahne *et al., Milchwissenschaft* **39**, 473 (1984).

	R	R'
Actaplanin A	mannosylglucose	mannose
Actaplanin B$_1$	rhamnosylglucose	mannose
Actaplanin B$_2$	glucose	mannose
Actaplanin B$_3$	mannosylglucose	H
Actaplanin C$_1$	rhamnosylglucose	H
Actaplanin G	glucose	H

Hydrochloride. White cryst solid, mp >220°. Approx mol wt 1158. [α]$_D^{25}$ −42.3° (c = 1 in water). uv max (acidic and neutral solns): 276 nm (E$_{1\ cm}^{1\%}$ 65). Sol in water. Insol in most organic solvents. Stable over pH 1.0 to 5.0 up to 27°.

THERAP CAT (VET): Growth stimulant.

133. Actarit. [18699-02-0] 4-(Acetylamino)benzeneacetic acid; (*p*-acetamidophenyl)acetic acid; MS-932; Mover; Orcl. $C_{10}H_{11}NO_3$; mol wt 193.20. C 62.17%, H 5.74%, N 7.25%, O 24.84%. Immunomodulator. Prepn: S. Gabriel, *Ber.* **15**, 834 (1882). *See also:* H. Munakata *et al.,* **DE 3317107**; *eidem,* **US 4720506** (1983, 1988 both to Mitsubishi Chem. Ind. and Nippon Shinyaku). Pharmacology: H. Fujisawa *et al., Arzneim.-Forsch.* **40**, 693 (1990). Pharmacokinetics: K. Sugihara *et al., ibid.* 800, 806. Antiarthritic effect in mice: H. Fujisawa *et al., ibid.* **44**, 64 (1994). Acute toxicity: K. Toshida *et al., Oyo Yakuri* **40**, 117 (1990), *C.A.* **114**, 17276q (1991).

Odorless, white crystals or crystalline powder. mp 173-175° (Munakata); also reported as mp 168-170° (Gabriel). Freely sol in methanol; sol in ethanol; sparingly sol in acetone; slightly sol in water; very slightly sol in ether. LD_{50} in male, female mice, male, female rats (mg/kg): 1.06, 1.30, 1.95, 2.03 i.p.; 5.68, 5.48, 5.48, 6.12 s.c.; 15.3, 14.7, 14.8, 15.4 orally (Toshida).

THERAP CAT: Antiarthritic.

134. ACTH. [9002-60-2] Corticotropin; adrenocorticotrop(h)in; corticotrophin; adrenocorticotrop(h)ic hormone of the pituitary gland; Acethropan; Acortan; Acthar; Acton; Cortiphyson; Cortrophin; Isactid. Pituitary hormone which stimulates the secretion of adrenal cortical steroids and induces growth of the adrenal cortex. Occurs also in female human urine and in serum of pregnant mares. Isoln procedure from swine pituitaries: Sayers *et al., J. Biol. Chem.* **149**, 425 (1943); *Proc. Soc. Exp. Biol. Med.* **52**, 199 (1943); from sheep pituitaries: Li *et al., J. Biol. Chem.* **149**, 413 (1943); Li, *J. Am. Chem. Soc.* **74**, 2124 (1952); from human pituitaries: Pickering *et al., Biochim. Biophys. Acta* **74**, 763 (1963). Purification: Johnson, US 3124509 (1964 to Upjohn). Corticotropin is a single chain polypeptide containing 39 amino acids. The first 24 residues are identical in all species. *In vivo* studies show that this portion of the peptide chain is responsible for the biological activity and that the remaining residues, while not necessary for the hormonal action, are essential in the species immunological specificity of ACTH. The term α-ACTH is used to distinguish it from the pepsin- or acid-degraded product, β-ACTH. Prepn of active cleavage products by hydrolysis and simultaneous dialysis: Wettstein, Benz, US 2734015 (1956 to Ciba). Amino acid sequence of bovine ACTH: Li *et al., J. Am. Chem. Soc.* **80**, 2587 (1958); proposed structure of human ACTH: Lee *et al., J. Biol. Chem.* **236**, 2970 (1961). Revised amino acid sequences of porcine and human ACTH: Riniker *et al., Nature New Biol.* **235**, 114 (1972). Revised sequences of ovine and bovine ACTH: Li, *Biochem. Biophys. Res. Commun.* **49**, 835 (1972). Synthesis of the revised human corticotropin: Sieber *et al., Helv. Chim. Acta* **55**, 1243 (1972); solid phase synthesis: Yamashiro, Li, *J. Am. Chem. Soc.* **95**, 1310 (1973).

White powder. Freely sol in water. Partly precipitated at the isoelectric point (pH 4.65-4.80). Appreciably soluble in 60 to 70% alcohol or acetone. Almost completely precipitated in 2.5% trichloroacetic acid soln. Also precipitated from dilute soln by 20% sulfosalicylic acid and by 5% lead acetate soln. Solns are stable to heat. An aq soln buffered to pH 7.5 may be put in a boiling water bath for at least 120 minutes. In 0.10 molar HCl an 0.2% soln retains its biological potency when kept at 100° for 60 min, but in 0.10 molar NaOH the activity is lost within 30 min. At 60° at 0.2% soln at pH 10.8 maintains its potency for 60 min. In general the substance is more stable in acid soln. Pure ACTH has 150 to 200 potency units per mg. The biological activity is not destroyed by digestion with pepsin, and hydrolysis products have the biological activity of ACTH. One U.S.P. unit or one international unit or one Armour unit or one potency unit denotes the same activity.

Corticotrophin zinc hydroxide suspension. Cortrophine-Z. ACTH absorbed on zinc hydroxide. Used as an aqueous suspension.

THERAP CAT: Adrenocorticotropic hormone.

THERAP CAT (VET): Stimulates glucocorticoid production.

135. Actimid. [19171-19-8] 4-Amino-2-(2,6-dioxo-3-piperidinyl)-1*H*-isoindole-1,3(2*H*)-dione; 3-amino-*N*-(2,6-dioxo-3-piperidyl)phthalamide; 1,3-dioxo-2-(2,6-dioxopiperidin-3-yl)-4-aminoisoindoline; CC-4047. $C_{13}H_{11}N_3O_4$; mol wt 273.24. C 57.14%, H 4.06%, N 15.38%, O 23.42%. Second generation immunomodulator and TNF-α inhibitor; analog of thalidomide, *q.v.* Prepn: G. W. Muller *et al.*, **WO 9803502**; *eidem*, **US 6335349** (1998, 2002 both to Celgene); *eidem, Bioorg. Med. Chem. Lett.* **9**, 1625 (1999). *In vivo* immunostimulant activity in cancer vaccine

model: K. Dredge *et al., J. Immunol.* **168**, 4914 (2002). Mechanism of action study: F. Payvandi *et al., Cell. Immunol.* **230**, 81 (2004). *In vitro* immunomodulation of hematopoietic stem cells: K.-R. Koh *et al., Blood* **105**, 3833 (2005). Clinical pharmacokinetics and clinical evaluation in multiple myeloma: S. A. Schey *et al., J. Clin. Oncol.* **22**, 3269 (2004).

Yellow solid from dioxane + ethyl acetate, mp 318.5 - 320.5°.
THERAP CAT: Immunomodulator.

136. Actin. One of the major proteins of muscle and an important component of all eukaryotic cells. Formerly believed to be a single, highly conserved protein in all cell types, but multiple forms have been shown to exist. Muscle actin, or *α-actin*, is found in differentiated muscle cells; *β-actin* and *γ-actin* are present in all non-muscle cell types. All three forms contain equimolar amounts of *N*-methylhistidine, although α-actin differs from β- and γ-actins by several peptides; the two "non-muscle" actins are nearly identical. Several "minor actins" are also known. The various forms, although similar in activity, mol wt and amino acid composition, show immunological differences and are considered to be synthesized under the control of different genes. In addition to its role in muscle relaxation and contraction (together with myosin, *q.v.*), actin is involved in a variety of cellular events: cell movement, cytokinesis, phagocytosis, exocytosis and chromosome movement. Identification in muscle: F. B. Straub, *Stud. Szeged* **2**, 3 (1942). Isoln: Feuer *et al., Hung. Acta Physiol.* **1**, 150 (1948). Separation of actin from muscle material: A. Szent-Gyorgyi, US 2742456 (1956 to Armour). In soln, actin and myosin combine to give *actomyosin*: Tonomura *et al., J. Biol. Chem.* **237**, 1074 (1962). Actin, in the absence of salts, exists in a globular form, designated as *G-actin*; in the presence of ATP and potassium, sodium, or magnesium chlorides it polymerizes to a fibrous form, *F-actin*. Removal of bound ATP results in complete loss of polymerizability: Straub, Feuer, *Biochim. Biophys. Acta* **4**, 455 (1950). Structure of G-actin: Nagy, Jencks, *Biochemistry* **1**, 987 (1962); of F-actin: Hanson, Lowy, *J. Mol. Biol.* **6**, 46 (1963). Complete amino acid sequence of rabbit skeletal muscle actin: Elzinga *et al., Proc. Natl. Acad. Sci. USA* **70**, 2687 (1973). Identification and characterization of multiple forms of actin: J. I. Garrels, W. Gibson, *Cell* **9**, 793 (1976). Partial amino acid sequence of calf brain actin: R. C. Lu, M. Elzinga, *Biochemistry* **16**, 5801 (1977). Comparison of actins from calf thymus, bovine brain, mouse cells and rabbit skeletal muscle: J. Vandeker, K. Weber, *Eur. J. Biochem.* **90**, 451 (1978). Isoln, characterization of porcine brain actin: J. P. Weir, D. W. Frederik, *Arch. Biochem.* **203**, 1 (1980). *In vivo* and *in vitro* synthesis of multiple forms of rat brain actin: E. Palmer, J. L. Saborio, *J. Biol. Chem.* **253**, 7482 (1978). Evidence for control of synthesis of human heart and platelet actins by different genes: M. Elzinga *et al., Science* **191**, 94 (1976). Immunological differences between cardiac muscle, skeletal muscle and brain actins: J. L. Morgan *et al., Proc. Natl. Acad. Sci. USA* **77**, 2069 (1980). History of discovery: Finck, *Science* **160**, 332 (1968). *Reviews:* Several authors, *Biochemistry of Muscle Contraction*, J. Gergely, Ed. (Little, Brown, Boston, 1964); Laki, "Actin" in *Contractile Proteins and Muscle*, K. Laki, Ed. (Marcel Dekker, New York, 1971) pp 97-133; E. D. Korn, *Proc. Natl. Acad. Sci. USA* **75**, 588-599 (1978); R. Kassab *et al., Biochimie* **63**, 273-289 (1981); S. Highsmith, *Biochim. Biophys. Acta* **639**, 31-39 (1981); E. D. Korn, *Physiol. Rev.* **62**, 672-737 (1982).

137. Actinium. [7440-34-8] Ac; at. no. 89; valence 3. Group IIIB (3). No stable nuclides; known isotopes (mass numbers): 209-233; naturally occurring isotopes: 227, 228. Longest-lived isotope: ^{227}Ac (T$_{1/2}$ 21.773 ±0.003 years, mode of decay α, β, γ-emission, rel. at. mass 227.0277). Daughter of ^{231}Pa; parent of ^{227}Th (radioactinium) and ^{223}Fr. Originally extracted from uranium ores where it occurs naturally as a member of the ^{235}U decay series; now prepd by neutron bombardment of ^{226}Ra in nuclear reactors.

[228]Ac or *mesothorium II* (MsTh$_2$) occurs naturally as a member of the [232]Th decay series. T$_{1/2}$ 6.13 ±0.03 hrs; decays by β and γ-emission. Daughter of [228]Ra (mesothorium I); parent of [228]Th (radiothorium). Discovery of [227]Ac: A. Debierne, *C.R. Hebd. Seances Acad. Sci.* **129**, 593 (1899); F. O. Geisel, *Ber.* **55**, 3608 (1902). Prepn of metal: J. G. Stites, Jr., *et al.*, *J. Am. Chem. Soc.* **77**, 237 (1955); J. D. Farr *et al.*, *J. Inorg. Nucl. Chem.* **18**, 42 (1961). Discovery of [228]Ac: O. Hahn, *Ber.* **40**, 1462 (1907). Review of actinium and the actinides: *Comprehensive Inorganic Chemistry* vol. 5, J. C. Bailar, Jr. *et al.*, Eds. (Pergamon Press, Oxford, 1973) *passim;* H. W. Kirby in *The Chemistry of the Actinide Elements* **vol. 1**, J. J. Katz *et al.*, Eds. (Chapman and Hall, New York, 1986) pp 14-40; G. T. Seaborg in *Kirk-Othmer Encyclopedia of Chemical Technology* vol. 1 (Wiley-Interscience, New York, 4th ed., 1991) pp 412-444.

Cubic crystal, d^{25} 10.07. mp 1050 ±50°. bp ~3300°. Homologous with lanthanum; more basic than lanthanum. Strong electropositive element. Forms insol salts, e.g. carbonate, oxalate, phosphate etc. just as the lanthanides. Rapidly oxidizes to AcO$_3$ in moist air.

Caution: Radiation hazard; handling requires special equipment and shielding facilities (Katz *et al.*, *loc. cit.* **vol. 2**, p 1128).

138. Actinobolin. [24397-89-5] (2*S*)-2-Amino-*N*-[(3*R*,4*R*,4a*R*,5*R*,6*R*)-3,4,4a,5,6,7-hexahydro-5,6,8-trihydroxy-3-methyl-1-oxo-1*H*-2-benzopyran-4-yl]propanamide; 4-(2-aminopropionamido)-3,4,4a,5,6,7-hexahydro-5,6,8-trihydroxy-3-methylisocoumarin. C$_{13}$H$_{20}$N$_2$O$_6$; mol wt 300.31. C 51.99%, H 6.71%, N 9.33%, O 31.97%. Antibiotic produced by *Streptomyces griseoviridus* var *atrofaciens;* (+)-form is naturally occurring. Isoln and characterization: T. H. Haskell, Q. R. Bartz, *Antibiot. Annu.* **1958-1959**, 505; T. H. Haskell *et al.*, *US 3043830* (1962 to Parke, Davis). Structural studies: Struck *et al.*, *Tetrahedron Lett.* **1967**, 1589; Munk *et al.*, *J. Am. Chem. Soc.* **89**, 4158 (1967). Structure: *eidem*, *ibid.* **90**, 1087 (1968). Absolute configuration and chemistry: Antosz *et al.*, *ibid.* **92**, 4933 (1970). Crystal structure: J. B. Wetherington, J. W. Moncrief, *Acta Crystallogr.* **B31**, 501 (1975). Total synthesis: M. Yoshioka *et al.*, *J. Am. Chem. Soc.* **106**, 1133 (1984); *eidem*, *Heterocycles* **21**, 151 (1984); R. S. Garigipati *et al.*, *J. Am. Chem. Soc.* **107**, 7790 (1985). Antibacterial activity and toxicity: R. F. Pittillo *et al.*, *Antibiot. Annu.* **1958-1959**, 497. Series of articles on antineoplastic activity: *ibid.* 515-532. Inhibition of protein synthesis: D. Smithers *et al.*, *Mol. Pharmacol.* **5**, 433 (1969). Experimental use as cariostat: D. E. Hunt *et al.*, *J. Dent. Res.* **50**, 371 (1971). Reduction of periodontal syndrome in mice, rats: J. H. Shaw, J. K. Ivimey, *Arch. Oral Biol.* **18**, 357 (1973).

Amorphous, fluffy, very hygroscopic powder. $[\alpha]_D^{28}$ +59° (c = 0.5 in pH 7 phosphate buffer). pKa: 7.5, 8.8. Freely sol in water; mod sol in methanol, ethanol. Unstable in aqueous solns pH >7. uv max: 262 nm (0.1*N* HCl); 288 nm (0.1*N* NaOH). LD$_{50}$ in mice, rats (mg/kg): 800 ±27, 1550 ±26 i.v. (Pittillo).

Acetate. C$_{13}$H$_{20}$N$_2$O$_6$.C$_2$H$_4$O$_2$. Needles from ethanol; softens at 130°, resolidifies at 145°, mp 263-266°. $[\alpha]_D^{26}$ +58°. pKa: 4.6, 7.5, 8.8. Very sol in water; sol in warm methanol, ethanol, acetone; sparingly sol in ethyl acetate. uv max: 264 nm (pH 7 phosphate buffer).

Hydrochloride. C$_{13}$H$_{20}$N$_2$O$_6$.HCl. Hygroscopic. $[\alpha]_D^{22}$ +59° (c = 0.41) (natural); $[\alpha]_D^{22}$ +55° (c = 0.47) (synthetic).

139. Actinodaphnine. [517-69-1] 6,7,7a,8-Tetrahydro-11-methoxy-5*H*-benzo[*g*]-1,3-benzodioxolo[6,5,4-*de*]quinolin-10-ol; 10-methoxy-1,2-(methylenedioxy)-6aα-noraporphin-9-ol; 1,2-methylenedioxy-9-hydroxy-10-methoxynoraporphine. C$_{18}$H$_{17}$-NO$_4$; mol wt 311.33. C 69.44%, H 5.50%, N 4.50%, O 20.56%.

In bark of *Actinodaphne hookeri* Meissn., *Lauraceae.* Isoln: Krishna, Ghose, *J. Indian Chem. Soc.* **9**, 429 (1932). Structure: Ghose *et al.*, *Helv. Chim. Acta* **17**, 919 (1934). Photolytic synthesis: M. S. Premila *et al.*, *Indian J. Chem.* **13**, 945 (1975).

Needles from alcohol, mp 211°. $[\alpha]_D^{20}$ +33° (ethanol). Sol in acetone, alcohol, benzene, chloroform. Moderately sol in ether. Practically insol in water.

Hydrochloride. C$_{18}$H$_{17}$NO$_4$.HCl. Needles from alcohol-ether, mp 281° (dec). $[\alpha]_D^{20}$ +9°.

Methyl ether. C$_{19}$H$_{19}$NO$_4$. Needles from ether + alc, mp 114-115°. Synthesis: Hey, Lobo, *J. Chem. Soc.* **1954**, 2246.

140. Actinomycetin. [1402-37-5] Bacteriolytic cell-free fluid of culture filtrates of actinomycetes. Produced by most species of *Streptomyces;* studied mostly in *Streptomyces albus.* Protein-like in nature. Stated to consist of a bactericidal fatty acid fraction and an enzyme: Welsch, *J. Bacteriol.* **42**, 801 (1941); **44**, 571 (1942); **53**, 101 (1947). Dissolves dead gram-negative, and, with more difficulty, dead gram-positive organisms. Also dissolves living organisms in aq suspensions, such as *Staph. aureus.* In answer to the question whether actinomycetin deserves the name "antibiotic", *see* the polemic between Hoogerheide and Welsch, *Bot. Rev.* **10**, 599 (1944) and *J. Bacteriol.* **53**, 101 (1947). Purification and prepn from *Streptomyces albus:* Ghuysen, **BE 517191** and **BE 521114** (both 1953 to Soc. Belge de l'Azote), *C.A.* **53**, 5600g, 12593e (1959). *Review:* Caltrider in *Antibiotics* **vol. 1**, D. Gottlieb, P. D. Shaw, Eds. (Springer Verlag, New York, 1967) pp 681-683.

Sol in water. Pptd by alcohol, acetone, ammonium sulfate and other protein precipitants. Destroyed by strong acid. More stable at pH 10 than at pH 4. Rapidly inactivated by heat, 60-70° destroys activity.

141. Actinomycin F$_1$. [1402-44-4] Actinomycin KS4; KS4. Antineoplastic antibiotic produced by cultures of actinomycin C-elaborating strains of Streptomyces, such as Streptomyces BOP 476 (NRRL 2580) and *Streptomyces chrysomallus* (NRRL 2250). Considered to be a derivative of actinomycin C$_2$; amino acid analysis indicates that the prolines present in actinomycin C$_2$ are substituted by sarcosine in actinomycin F$_1$. Production by controlled biosynthesis: Schmidt-Kastner, *Naturwissenschaften* **43**, 131 (1956); *idem, Ann. N.Y. Acad. Sci.* **89**, 299 (1960); Schmidt-Kastner, Hackmann, **US 3219544** (1965 to Bayer).

142. Actinorhodine. [1397-77-9] C$_{32}$H$_{26}$O$_{14}$; mol wt 634.54. C 60.57%, H 4.13%, O 35.30%. Antibiotic pigment produced by *Streptomyces coelicolor*, found in woods near Göttingen, Germany: Brockmann, Pini, *Naturwissenschaften* **34**, 190 (1947); Brockmann *et al.*, *Ber.* **83**, 161 (1950). Tentative structure: Brockmann, Hieronymus, *Ber.* **88**, 1379 (1955); Brockmann *et al.*, *Naturwissenschaften* **49**, 131 (1962). Structure: Brockmann, *Angew. Chem.* **76**, 863 (1964); Brockmann *et al.*, *Ann.* **698**, 209 (1966). Stereochemistry: Zeeck, Christiansen, *Ann.* **724**, 172 (1969). Biosynthesis and determn of point of dimerization: C. P. Gorst-Allman *et al.*, *J. Org. Chem.* **46**, 455 (1981).

Fine red needles from dioxane, dec 270°. Absorption max (dioxane): 560, 523 nm. Sol in pyridine, piperidine, tetrahydrofuran,

Actiphenol

dioxane, phenol; slightly sol in alcohol, acetic acid, acetone. Red soln with acetone, blue soln with pyridine. Practically insol in aq acid; sol in aq alkali with bright blue color.

143. Actiphenol. [526-02-3] 4-[2-(2-Hydroxy-3,5-dimethylphenyl)-2-oxoethyl]-2,6-piperidinedione; 3-(2-hydroxy-3,5-dimethylphenacyl)glutarimide; β-(3,5-dimethyl-2-hydroxybenzoylmethyl)glutarimide; C-73. $C_{15}H_{17}NO_4$; mol wt 275.30. C 65.44%, H 6.22%, N 5.09%, O 23.25%. Metabolic product found in culture filtrates of cycloheximide-producing actinomycetes (Streptomyces albulus): Highet, Prelog, Helv. Chim. Acta 42, 1523 (1959); Rao, J. Org. Chem. 25, 661 (1960). Synthesis: Johnson, ibid. 27, 3658 (1962). May be prepd from cycloheximide: Highet, Prelog, loc. cit. Structure-activity studies: Ennis, Biochem. Pharmacol. 17, 1197 (1968).

Fluffy needles from methylene chloride + methanol. mp 200-202°. Pure crystals are white or colorless. uv max: 262, 345 nm (ε 10870, 4550). Exhibits bright yellow fluorescence under u.v. Soluble in aqueous NaOH (forming bright yellow solns), in anhydr alcohol, tetrahydrofuran. Insol in aq solns of sodium bicarbonate.

Acetate. $C_{17}H_{19}NO_5$. Crystals from methylene chloride + ether, mp 155.5°.

144. Activin. Polypeptide hormone, identified in ovarian follicular fluid, which selectively stimulates secretion of FSH, q.v. Dimer composed of β subunits of inhibin, q.v. (either β_A or β_B), mol wt 24,000 daltons. Isolation and characterization of the heterodimer, activin AB: N. Ling et al., Nature 321, 779 (1986); of the homodimer, activin A: W. Vale et al., ibid. 776; N. Ling et al., Biochem. Biophys. Res. Commun. 138, 1129 (1986). Comparison of FSH stimulation with gonadotropin releasing hormone (LH-RH, q.v.): R. H. Schwall et al., ibid. 151, 1099 (1988). Approach to nonradiometric assays: R. H. Schwall et al., Prog. Clin. Biol. Res. 285, 205 (1988). Brief review of chemical properties and biological activity: S.-Y. Ying, Proc. Soc. Exp. Biol. Med. 186, 253-264 (1987). Review: S. A. Pangas, T. K. Woodruff, Trends Endocrinol. Metab. 11, 309-314 (2000).

145. ACV. [32467-88-2] N-[(5S)-5-Amino-5-carboxy-1-oxopentyl]-L-cysteinyl-D-valine; N-[N-(L-5-amino-5-carboxyvaleryl)-L-cysteinyl]-D-valine; δ-(L-α-aminoadipyl)-L-cysteinyl-D-valine. $C_{14}H_{25}N_3O_6S$; mol wt 363.43. C 46.27%, H 6.93%, N 11.56%, O 26.41%, S 8.82%. Biosynthetic precursor of penicillins and cephalosporins. Isoln from mycelial extracts of Penicillium chrysogenum: H. R. V. Arnstein et al., Biochem. J. 76, 353 (1960); structure determn of tripeptide: H. R. V. Arnstein, D. Morris, ibid. 357. Isoln from Cephalosporium sp., identification and optical configuration of constituent amino acids: P. B. Loder, E. P. Abraham, ibid. 123, 471 (1971). Configuration of peptide from P. chrysogenum, identity with peptide from Cephalosporium: P. Adriaens et al., Antimicrob. Agents Chemother. 8, 638 (1975). Synthesis of labelled tripeptide and role in penicillin biosynthesis: P. A. Fawcett et al., Biochem. J. 157, 651 (1976). Synthesis of ACV as the disulfide: S. Wolfe, M. G. Jokinen, Can. J. Chem. 57, 1388 (1979). Cellfree conversion of ACV directly into isopenicillin N: J. O'Sullivan et al., Biochem. J. 184, 421 (1979); T. Konomi et al., ibid. 427. Confirmation by ^{13}C NMR: J. E. Baldwin et al., Chem. Commun. 1980, 1271. Reviews: D. J. Aberhart, Tetrahedron 33, 1545-1559 (1977); E. P. Abraham, Jpn. J. Antibiot. 30, Suppl., S1-S26 (1977); S. Wolfe et al., Science 226, 1386-1392 (1984).

146. Acyclovir. [59277-89-3] 2-Amino-1,9-dihydro-9-[(2-hydroxyethoxy)methyl]-6H-purin-6-one; acycloguanosine; 9-[(2-hydroxyethoxy)methyl]guanine; BW-248U; Wellcome 248U; Acicloftal; Avirase; Cycloviran; Maynar; Virmen; Viruseen; Zoliparin; Zovir; Zovirax. $C_8H_{11}N_5O_3$; mol wt 225.20. C 42.67%, H 4.92%, N 31.10%, O 21.31%. Orally active acyclic nucleoside with inhibitory activity towards several herpes viruses. Prepn: H. J. Schaeffer, DE 2539963; idem, US 4199574 (1976, 1980 to Wellcome). Convenient synthesis from guanine: H. Matsumoto et al., Chem. Pharm. Bull. 36, 1153 (1988). Selectivity of action: G. B. Elion et al., Proc. Natl. Acad. Sci. USA 74, 5716 (1977). Chemistry, antiviral activity, metabolism: H. J. Schaeffer et al., Nature 272, 583 (1978). In vitro activity: P. Collins, D. J. Bauer, J. Antimicrob. Chemother. 5, 431 (1979). Effect on herpes simplex infections in mice: H. J. Field et al., Antimicrob. Agents Chemother. 15, 554 (1979); on herpes zoster in immunocompromised patients: H. H. Balfour et al., N. Engl. J. Med. 308, 1448 (1983). Treatment of primary episodes of genital herpes simplex infection: Y. J. Bryson et al., ibid. 916; of recurrent genital herpes: S. E. Straus et al., ibid. 310, 1545 (1984); J. M. Douglas et al., ibid. 1551. HPLC determn in serum and clinical pharmacokinetics: G. Bahrami et al., J. Chromatogr. B 816, 327 (2005). Symposia on pharmacology and clinical studies: Am. J. Med. 73, Suppl. 1A, 1-392 (1982); J. Antimicrob. Chemother. 12, Suppl. B, 1-202 (1983); Scand. J. Infect. Dis. Suppl. 47, 1-176 (1985). Review: R. J. Whitley, J. W. Gnann, Jr., N. Engl. J. Med. 327, 782-789 (1992).

Crystals from methanol, mp 256.5-257°. LD_{50} in mice (mg/kg): >10,000 orally; 1000 i.p. (Schaeffer).

THERAP CAT: Antiviral.

147. ADA. [26239-55-4] N-(2-Amino-2-oxoethyl)-N-(carboxymethyl)glycine; N-(2-acetamido)iminodiacetic acid. $C_6H_{10}N_2O_5$; mol wt 190.15. C 37.90%, H 5.30%, N 14.73%, O 42.07%. One of several zwitterionic N-substituted amino acids known as "Good" buffers. Active in the pH range 6-8. Prepn: G. Schwarzenbach et al., Helv. Chim. Acta 38, 1147 (1955); and description: N. E. Good et al., Biochemistry 5, 467 (1966). Thermodynamic behavior: C. D. McGlothlin, J. Jordan, Anal. Lett. 9, 245 (1976); F. Jumean, J. Indian Chem. Soc. 69, 237 (1992). Use as buffer: Z. Pietrzkowski, W. Korohoda, Folia Histochem. Cytobiol. 26, 143 (1988); as analytical reagent for chromium: C. Baluja-Santos et al., Rev. Roum. Chim. 39, 73 (1994); as chelator: M. C. Steele, J. Pichtel, J. Environ. Eng. 124, 639 (1998).

Crystals from chloroacetamide, dec 220°. Slightly sol in water. pKa_1: <2; pKa_2: 2-3; pKa_3 when 0.1M (0°): 6.85; (20°): 6.60; (37°): 6.45. ΔpKa/°C = −0.011.

USE: Buffer for biological systems and chelator for metals.

148. Adalimumab. [331731-18-1] Anti-(human tumor necrosis factor) immunoglobulin G1 (human monoclonal D2E7 heavy chain) disulfide with human monoclonal D2E7 light chain, dimer; D2E7; Humira. Fully human monoclonal antibody against tumor necrosis factor α (TNFα). Prepn: J. G. Salfeld et al., WO 9729131; eidem, US 6090382 (1997, 2000 both to BASF). Characterization: L. C. Santora et al., Anal. Biochem. 275, 98 (1999). Characterization of antigen binding: idem et al., ibid. 299, 119 (2001). Clinical trial in rheumatoid arthritis: A. A. den Broeder et al., Ann. Rheum. Dis. 61, 311 (2002); in combination with methotrexate: F. C. Breedveld et al., Arthritis Rheum. 54, 26 (2006); in psoriatic arthritis: P. J. Mease et al., ibid. 52, 3279 (2005). Review of pharmacology and clinical experience: K. P. Machold, J. S. Smolen, Expert Opin. Biol. Ther. 3, 351-360 (2003). Review of safety

and efficacy in psoriasis and rheumatoid arthritis: T. Patel, K. B. Gordon, *Dermatol. Ther.* **17**, 427-431 (2004); in psoriatic arthritis: P. J. Mease, *Expert Opin. Biol. Ther.* **5**, 1491-1504 (2005).
THERAP CAT: Anti-inflammatory.

149. Adamantane. [281-23-2] Tricyclo[3.3.1.1^{3,7}]decane; diamantane (obsolete). $C_{10}H_{16}$; mol wt 136.23. C 88.16%, H 11.84%. Isoln from petroleum from Moravia province in Czechoslovakia: Landa, Machacek, *Collect. Czech. Chem. Commun.* **3**, 1 (1933); from American petroleum: Mair *et al., Anal. Chem.* **31**, 2082 (1959). Synthesis: Prelog, Seiwerth, *Ber.* **74**, 1769 (1941); Stetter *et al., Ber.* **89**, 1922 (1956); by aluminum chloride-catalyzed isomerization of tetrahydrodicyclopentadiene: Yan, Shreh, *Bull. Inst. Chem. Acad. Sinica* **Dec. 1965**, no. 11, pp 79-81. Two step synthesis starting with dicyclopentadiene: Schleyer, *J. Am. Chem. Soc.* **79**, 3292 (1957); Schleyer, Donaldson, *ibid.* **82**, 4645 (1960); Ludwig US 2937211 (1960 to du Pont). *Reviews:* Stetter, *Angew. Chem.* **66**, 217 (1954); Fort, Schleyer, *Chem. Rev.* **64**, 277 (1964).

Crystallizes at −30°; can be purified by recrystallization from acetone or by sublimation. mp 269.6-270.8°.
Note: The name diamantane has been abandoned as a synonym for adamantane and proposed as the name for the second member of the adamantane series, congressane: Vogl, Anderson, *Tetrahedron Lett.* **1966**, 415.
USE: The diamine as curing agent for epoxy resins [US 3053907 (1962 to du Pont)].

150. Adapalene. [106685-40-9] 6-(4-Methoxy-3-tricyclo[3.3.1.1^{3,7}]dec-1-ylphenyl)-2-naphthalenecarboxylic acid; 6-[3-(1-adamantyl)-4-methoxyphenyl]-2-naphthoic acid; CD-271; Differin. $C_{28}H_{28}O_3$; mol wt 412.52. C 81.52%, H 6.84%, O 11.64%. Retinoid selective for retinoic acid receptor (RAR) subtypes β and γ. Prepn: B. Shroot *et al., EP 199636; eidem,* US 4717720 (1986, 1988 both to Cent. Int. Recher. Dermatol.); and structure-activity study: B. Charpentier *et al., J. Med. Chem.* **38**, 4993 (1995). Pilot-scale synthesis: Z. Liu, J. Xiang, *Org. Process Res. Dev.* **10**, 285 (2006). HPLC determn in plasma and tissue: R. Ruhl, H. Nau, *Chromatographia* **45**, 269 (1997). Clinical pharmacology: C. E. M. Griffiths *et al., J. Invest. Dermatol.* **101**, 325 (1993). Clinical trial in acne: A. Shalita *et al., J. Am. Acad. Dermatol.* **34**, 482 (1996). Reviews of pharmacology and clinical potential: B. A. Bernard, *Skin Pharmacol.* **6**, Suppl. 1, 61-69 (1993); R. N. Brogden, K. L. Goa, *Drugs* **53**, 511-519 (1997); of clinical use in acne vulgaris: J. Waugh *et al., Drugs* **64**, 1465-1478 (2004).

White crystals from THF and ethyl acetate, mp 319-322°. pK 4.2. Stable to light.
THERAP CAT: Antiacne.

151. Adefovir. [106941-25-7] [[2-(6-Amino-9*H*-purin-9-yl)ethoxy]methyl]phosphonic acid; 9-(2-phosphonylmethoxyethyl)adenine; PMEA; GS-393. $C_8H_{12}N_5O_4P$; mol wt 273.19. C 35.17%, H 4.43%, N 25.64%, O 23.43%, P 11.34%. Acyclic nucleoside phosphonate (ANP) analog. Prepn: A. Holy, I. Rosenberg, **EP 206459;** *eidem,* **US 4808716** (1986, 1989 both to Ceskoslov. Akad. Ved); *eidem, Collect. Czech. Chem. Commun.* **52**, 2801 (1987); of dipivoxil ester prodrug: J. E. Starrett, Jr. *et al., EP 481214* (1992 to Bristol-Myers Squibb); *eidem,* US 5663159 (1997 to Inst. Org. Chem. Biochem. Acad. Sci. Czech Rep.; Rega). Crystal structure: C. H. Schwalbe *et al., J. Chem. Soc.*

Perkin Trans. 1 **1991**, 1348. HPLC determn: P. Augustijns *et al., J. Liq. Chromatogr. Relat. Technol.* **19**, 2271 (1996). Clinical pharmacokinetics: K. C. Cundy *et al., Antimicrob. Agents Chemother.* **39**, 2401 (1995). Review of pharmacology and therapeutic potential: L. Naesens *et al., Antiviral Chem. Chemother.* **8**, 1-23 (1997). Clinical trial in HIV infected patients: J. Kahn *et al., J. Am. Med. Assoc.* **282**, 2305 (1999); in hepatitis B virus (HBV): R. J. C. Gilson *et al, J. Viral Hepat.* **6**, 387 (1999). Resistance surveillance in HBV infections: H. Yang *et al., Hepatology* **36**, 464 (2002).

Off-white crystalline solid, mp >250°. pKa$_1$ 2.0, pKa$_2$ 6.8. uv max (H_2O) 208, 260 nm (ε 19600, 14100); (0.1N HCl) 210, 260 nm (ε 19000, 13700); (0.1N NaOH) 216, 262 nm (ε 9600, 14500).
Di(pivaloyloxymethyl) ester. [142340-99-6] Adefovir dipivoxil; bis(POM)-PMEA; GS-840; Hepsera; Preveon. $C_{20}H_{32}N_5O_8P$; mol wt 501.47. Off-white crystalline powder. Soly in water (mg/ml): 19 (pH 2.0); 0.4 (pH 7.2). Log P (octanol/aq phosphate buffer): 1.91.
THERAP CAT: Antiviral.

152. Adenine. [73-24-5] 1*H*-Purin-6-amine; 6-aminopurine; 6-amino-1*H*-purine; 6-amino-3*H*-purine; 6-amino-9*H*-purine; 1,6-dihydro-6-iminopurine; 3,6-dihydro-6-iminopurine; Leuco-4. $C_5H_5N_5$; mol wt 135.13. C 44.44%, H 3.73%, N 51.83%. Also referred to as *vitamin B_4*: Lecoq, *Int. Z. Vitaminforsch.* **27**, 291 (1957). Widespread throughout animal and plant tissues combined with niacinamide, D-ribose, and phosphoric acids; a constituent of nucleic acids and coenzymes, such as codehydrase I and II, adenylic acid, coalaninedehydrase. Isoln from bovine pancreas: Kossel, *Ber.* **18**, 79, 1928 (1885). Syntheses: Fischer, *ibid.* **30**, 2226 (1897); Traube, *Ann.* **331**, 64 (1904); Hoffer, *Jubilee Vol. Emil Barell* **1946**, 428-434; Taylor *et al., Ciba Found. Symp. Chem. Biol. Purines* **1957**, 20, *C.A.* **53**, 6238b (1959); Bredereck *et al., Angew. Chem.* **71**, 524 (1959); Morita *et al., Chem. Ind. (London)* **1968**, 1117; Sekiya, Suzuki, *Chem. Pharm. Bull.* **20**, 209 (1972); N. J. Kos *et al., J. Org. Chem.* **44**, 3140 (1979). Toxicity study: Philips *et al., J. Pharmacol. Exp. Ther.* **104**, 20 (1952). *Review:* Ts'o, "Bases, Nucleosides and Nucleotides" in *Basic Principles in Nucleic Acid Chemistry* **vol. 1**, P. O. P. Ts'o, Ed. (Academic Press, New York, 1974) pp 453-584.

Trihydrate, orthorhombic needles. Anhydr at 110°, dec 360-365°; subl 220°. uv max (pH 7.0): 207, 260.5 nm (ε × 10^{-3} 23.2, 13.4). One gram of anhydr compd dissolves in 2000 ml water, 40 ml boiling water; slightly sol in alc. Practically insol in ether, $CHCl_3$. Aq solns are neutral. Combines with acids and bases. LD$_{50}$ orally in rats: 745 mg/kg (Philips).
Hydrochloride hemihydrate. Monoclinic prisms. One gram dissolves in 42 ml water.
Sulfate dihydrate. Crystals. One gram dissolves in 150 ml water; slightly sol in alc.
USE: In microbial determination of niacin; in research on heredity, virus diseases, and cancer.

153. Adenosine. [58-61-7] 9-β-D-Ribofuranosyl-9*H*-purin-6-amine; 6-amino-9-β-D-ribofuranosyl-9*H*-purine; 9-β-D-ribofuranosidoadenine; adenine riboside; Adenocard; Adenocor; Adenoscan. $C_{10}H_{13}N_5O_4$; mol wt 267.24. C 44.94%, H 4.90%, N 26.21%, O 23.95%. Nucleoside; widely distributed in nature. From yeast nucleic acid: Levene and Bass, *Nucleic Acids* (New York, 1931) p 163. Structure: Levene, Tipson, *J. Biol. Chem.* **94**,

809 (1932); Bredereck, *Ber.* **66,** 198 (1933); *Z. Physiol. Chem.* **223,** 61 (1934); Gulland, Holiday, *J. Chem. Soc.* **1936,** 765. *Cf.* Szent-Györgyi, *J. Physiol.* **68,** 213 (1930); Lythgoe *et al., J. Chem. Soc.* **1947,** 355; **1948,** 965. Synthesis: Davoll *et al., ibid.* **1948,** 967; H. Vorbrueggen, K. Krolikiewicz, *Angew. Chem. Int. Ed.* **14,** 421 (1975). Crystal structure: T. F. Lai, R. E. Marsh, *Acta Crystallogr.* **B28,** 1982 (1972). Conformational properties: D. B. Davies, A. Rabczenko, *J. Chem. Soc. Perkin Trans. 2* **1975,** 1703. Symposium on cardiac electrophysiology, pharmacology and clinical efficacy in supraventricular tachycardia: *Prog. Clin. Biol. Res.* **230,** 1-395 (1987). *Reviews: see* Adenine.

Crystals from water, mp 234-235°. $[\alpha]_D^{11}$ −61.7° (c = 0.706 in water); $[\alpha]_D^9$ −58.2° (c = 0.658 in water). uv max: 260 nm (ε 15100). Practically insol in alcohol.

THERAP CAT: Antiarrhythmic.

154. Adenosine Diphosphate. [58-64-0] Adenosine 5′-(trihydrogen diphosphate); ADP; adenosine 5′-pyrophosphoric acid; 5′-adenylphosphoric acid; adenosinediphosphoric acid. $C_{10}H_{15}N_5O_{10}P_2$; mol wt 427.20. C 28.11%, H 3.54%, N 16.39%, O 37.45%, P 14.50%. Formed from ATP in the muscle by the enzyme adenosinetriphosphatase upon stimulation of the muscle unless hydrolysis is prevented by injection of magnesium sulfate. Prepd by hydrolysis of ATP: LePage, *Biochem. Prep.* **I,** 1 (1949). Synthesis: Chambers *et al., J. Am. Chem. Soc.* **82,** 970 (1960). *See also* the ref and data *under* Adenosine Triphosphate.

Barium salt. $Ba_3(C_{10}H_{12}N_5O_{10}P_2)_2$. The purity of the prepns can be checked by analyses for nitrogen, ribose (orcinol reaction), total phosphorus, easily hydrolyzable phosphorus, and inorganic phosphorus. ADP should give a ratio of 2:1 for total organic phosphorus to easily hydrolyzable phosphorus. uv max (pH 7.0): 259 nm (a_M 15.4 × 10³).

155. Adenosine Triphosphate. [56-65-5] Adenosine 5′-(tetrahydrogen triphosphate); ATP; adenosine 5′-triphosphoric acid; Adetol; Atriphos; Striadyne; Triadenyl. $C_{10}H_{16}N_5O_{13}P_3$; mol wt 507.18. C 23.68%, H 3.18%, N 13.81%, O 41.01%, P 18.32%. Coenzyme valuable in the transfer of phosphate bond energy. Mammalian skeletal muscle at rest contains 350-400 mg ATP per 100 g. Upon stimulation of the muscle the ATP is hydrolyzed to ADP by the myosin-actin complex unless hydrolysis is prevented by injection of magnesium sulfate. Isoln from rabbit muscle: LePage, *Biochem. Prep.* **1,** 5 (1949); *cf.* Fiske, Subbarow, *Science* **70,** 381 (1929); Lohmann, *Biochem. Z.* **223,** 460 (1931); **254,** 381 (1932); Barrenscheen, Filz, *ibid.* **250,** 281 (1932); Kerr, *J. Biol. Chem.* **139,** 121 (1941); Needham, *Biochem. J.* **36,** 113 (1942). Synthetic routes: Tanaka, Honjo, **US 3079379** (1963 to Takeda). Reviews of biosynthesis: Racker, *Adv. Enzymol.* **23,** 323-399 (1961); Deamer, *J. Chem. Educ.* **46,** 198-206 (1971). Reviews of nucleotide coenzymes: Bock in *The Enzymes* **vol. 2A,** P. D. Boyer

et al., Eds. (Academic Press, New York, 2nd ed., 1960) pp 3-38; A. M. Michelson, *The Chemistry of Nucleosides and Nucleotides* (Academic Press, New York, 1963) pp 153-250; D. W. Hutchinson, *Nucleotides and Coenzymes* (John Wiley, New York, 1964) pp 36-82.

Free ATP, isolated as a glass (by treatment of the Ba salt with H_2SO_4 and treating the concd aq soln with acetone). $[\alpha]_D^{22}$ −26.7° (c = 3.095). uv max (pH 7.0): 259 nm (a_M 15.4 × 10³). Freely sol in water. A 1% aq soln has a pH of about 2 and is stable at 0° for several hrs. ATP is a tetrabasic acid and after hydrolytic cleavage it is hexabasic. It is usually pptd as the dibarium salt with 4 or 6 mols of water of crystn which can be removed by prolonged drying at 100° over P_2O_5 and in a vacuum. The anhydr salt is stable, but the hydrated salt slowly decomp forming 5′-adenylic acid and barium pyrophosphate. For use the barium salt is converted to the sodium or potassium salt by treatment with sodium or potassium sulfate in HCl soln. At pH 6.8-7.4 the Na salt is stable in aq soln provided the product is pure. Ba^{2+} catalyzes breakdown.

Disodium salt. [987-65-5] Adetphos; Atenen; Circulen; Trinosin. $C_{10}H_{14}N_5Na_2O_{13}P_3$; mol wt 551.14.

USE: In biochemical research. To inhibit enzymatic browning of raw edible plant materials, such as sliced apples, potatoes, etc.

THERAP CAT: Coenzyme.

156. S-Adenosylmethionine. [29908-03-0] 5′-[(3S)-(3-Amino-3-carboxypropyl)methylsulfonio]-5′-deoxyadenosine inner salt; S-(5′-desoxyadenosin-5′-yl)-L-methionine; active methionine; ademetionine; AdoMet; SAMe. $C_{15}H_{22}N_6O_5S$; mol wt 398.44. C 45.22%, H 5.57%, N 21.09%, O 20.08%, S 8.05%. Physiological methyl donor involved in enzymatic transmethylation reactions; present in all living organisms. Enzymatic prepn: G. L. Cantoni, *J. Am. Chem. Soc.* **74,** 2942 (1952). Synthesis of racemate: J. Baddiley, G. A. Jamieson, *J. Chem. Soc.* **1954,** 4280; of optically active chloride: C. H. Shunk, J. W. Richter, **US 2969353** (1961 to Merck & Co.). Review of enzymatic and microbial prepns: S. Shimizu, H. Yamada, *Trends Biotechnol.* **2,** 137-141 (1984). Pharmacology and toxicity: G. Stramentinoli *et al., Minerva Med.* **66,** 1541 (1975). Radioenzymatic determn in biological fluids: P. Giulidori, G. Stramentinoli, *Anal. Biochem.* **137,** 217 (1984). Cytoprotective effects against bile-acid induced apoptosis: C. R. L. Webster *et al., Vet. Ther.* **3,** 474 (2002). Clinical trial in arthritis: J. D. Bradley *et al., J. Rheumatol.* **21,** 905 (1994); in depression: M. Fava *et al., Psychiatry Res.* **56,** 295 (1995). Review of clinical efficacy in intrahepatic cholestasis: M. Coltorti *et al., Methods Find. Exp. Clin. Pharmacol.* **2,** 69-78 (1990); in neurological disorders: T. Bottiglieri *et al., Drugs* **48,** 137-152 (1994). Review of role in biological methylation: P. K. Chiang *et al., FASEB J.* **10,** 471-480 (1996). Symposium on use in treatment of alcoholic liver disease: *Alcohol* **27,** 149-198 (2002). Review of clinical use in canine hepatitis: A. Honeckman, *Clin. Tech. Small Anim. Pract.* **18,** 239-244 (2003); in management of heptobiliary disorders: S. A. Center, *Vet. Clin. Small Anim.* **34,** 67-172 (2004).

1,4-Butanedisulfonate. [200393-05-1] Donamet; Samyr. C_{15}-$H_{22}N_6O_5S.C_4H_{10}S_2O_6$.

Disulfate tosylate. [55722-12-8] 5'-[(3S)-(3-Amino-3-carboxypropyl)methylsulfonio]-5'-deoxyadenosine sulfate (salt) 4-methylbenzenesulfonate (salt) sulfate (salt) (1:1:2:1); Gumbaral; S-Amet; Zentonil. $C_{15}H_{23}N_6O_5S.2C_7H_8O_3S.H_2SO_4.HSO_4$; mol wt 939.00.

THERAP CAT: Antidepressant; antirheumatic; hepatoprotectant.

THERAP CAT (VET): Heptoprotectant.

157. 3'-Adenylic Acid. [84-21-9] Adenosine 3'-monophosphate; adenosine-3'-phosphoric acid; adenosine-3'-monophosphoric acid; adenylic acid b; yeast adenylic acid; synadenylic acid; h-adenylic acid. $C_{10}H_{14}N_5O_7P$; mol wt 347.22. C 34.59%, H 4.06%, N 20.17%, O 32.25%, P 8.92%. Early prepns from yeast nucleic acid: Levene, Bass, *Nucleic Acids* (Chemical Catalogue Co., New York, 1931). Early work probably done on mixtures of 2'- and 3'-adenylic acids; both compds isomerize readily to form an equilibrium mixture under acid conditions: Carter, Cohn, *Fed. Proc.* **8**, 190 (1949); Baddily, in *The Nucleic Acids* **vol. 1**, E. Chargaff, J. N. Davidson, Eds. (Academic Press, New York, 1955) pp 165-168; A. M. Michelson, *The Chemistry of Nucleosides and Nucleotides* (Academic Press, New York, 1963) pp 100-106. Synthesis: Brown, Todd, *J. Chem. Soc.* **1952**, 44. Structure of dihydrate: Brown *et al., Nature* **172**, 1184 (1953); Sundaralingam, *Acta Crystallogr.* **21**, 495 (1966). *Reviews: see* Adenosine.

Long, fine, colorless, needles. mp 197° (dec). Dihydrate, d (calc) 1.698. Absorption spectrum: Voet *et al., Biopolymers* **1**, 193 (1963). Difficultly sol in boiling water. Gives quantitative yield of furfural when distilled with 20% HCl for 3 hrs (different from 5'-adenylic acid which yields only traces). *cf.* Hoffman, *J. Biol. Chem.* **73**, 15 (1927); Embden, Schmidt, *Z. Physiol. Chem.* **181**, 130 (1929).

158. 5'-Adenylic Acid. [61-19-8] Muscle adenylic acid; ergadenylic acid; t-adenylic acid; adenosine 5'-monophosphate; adenosine phosphate; adenosine-5'-phosphoric acid; adenosine-5'-monophosphoric acid; A-5MP; AMP; NSC-20264; Adényl. C_{10}-$H_{14}N_5O_7P$; mol wt 347.22. C 34.59%, H 4.06%, N 20.17%, O 32.25%, P 8.92%. Nucleotide; widely distributed in nature. Prepn from tissues: Embden, Zimmerman, *Z. Physiol. Chem.* **167**, 137 (1927); Embden, Schmidt, *ibid.* **181**, 130 (1929); *cf.* Kalckar, *J. Biol. Chem.* **167**, 445 (1947). Prepn by hydrolysis of ATP with barium hydroxide: Kerr, *J. Biol. Chem.* **139**, 131 (1941). Synthesis: Baddiley, Todd, *J. Chem. Soc.* **1947**, 648. Commercial prepn by enzymatic phosphorylation of adenosine. Monograph on synthesis of nucleotides: G. R. Pettit, *Synthetic Nucleotides* vol. 1 (Van Nostrand-Reinhold, New York, 1972) 252 pp. Crystal structure: Kraut, Jensen, *Acta Crystallogr.* **16**, 79 (1963). *Reviews: see* Adenosine.

Crystals from water + acetone, mp 196-200°. $[\alpha]_D^{20}$ −47.5° (c = 2, 2% NaOH); $[\alpha]_D^{20}$ −26.0° (c = 2, 10% HCl). pK_1 = 3.8; pK_2 = 6.2. uv max (pH 7.0): 259 nm (a_M 15.4 × 10^3). Readily sol in boiling water. The compound is readily deaminated by nitrous acid to form inosinic acid; less rapidly hydrolyzed than 3'-adenylic acid by sulfuric acid. Furfural is formed only in traces on distillation with 20% HCl, *cf.* Levene, Bass, *Nucleic Acids* (New York, 1931) pp 230-232.

THERAP CAT: Nutrient.

159. Adhatoda. Malabar nut; arusa; adulsa; vasaca; adhatodai; bakash. Leaves of *Adhatoda vasica* Nees, *Acanthacae*. *Habit.* East India. *Constit.* Adhatodic acid, vasicine. *Ref:* Krishnaswami, David, *Indian J. Pharm.* **2**, 141 (1940).

THERAP CAT: Expectorant.

160. Adinazolam. [37115-32-5] 8-Chloro-N,N-dimethyl-6-phenyl-4H-[1,2,4]triazolo[4,3-a][1,4]benzodiazepine-1-methanamine; 8-chloro-1-[(dimethylamino)methyl]-6-phenyl-4H-s-triazolo[4,3-a][1,4]benzodiazepine; U-41123. $C_{19}H_{18}ClN_5$; mol wt 351.83. C 64.86%, H 5.16%, Cl 10.08%, N 19.91%. Triazolobenzodiazepine; dimethylamino derivative of alprazolam, *q.v.* Prepn: H. Allgeier, A. Gagneux, **DE 2201210**; **GB 1393256** (1972, 1975 both to Ciba-Geigy); J. B. Hester, Jr., **US 4250094** (1984 to Upjohn); *idem, J. Heterocycl. Chem.* **17**, 575 (1980). Chromatographic determn in human plasma: G. W. Peng, *J. Pharm. Sci.* **73**, 1173 (1984). Pharmacological profile: R. A. Lahti *et al., Neuropharmacology* **22**, 1277 (1983). Biological activity and metabolism: V. H. Sethy *et al., J. Pharm. Pharmacol.* **36**, 546 (1984). Preliminary clinical study in severe depression: R. E. Pyke *et al., Psychopharmacol. Bull.* **19**, 96 (1983).

Crystals from ethyl acetate, mp 171-172.5° (**US 4250094**). Also reported as mp 165-166° (**DE 2201210**).

Methanesulfonate. [57938-82-6] Adinazolam mesylate; Deracyn. $C_{19}H_{18}ClN_5.CH_3SO_3H$; mol wt 447.94. Crystals from methanol-ether, mp 230-244°.

THERAP CAT: Antidepressant.

161. Adiphenine. [64-95-9] α-Phenylbenzeneacetic acid 2-(diethylamino)ethyl ester; 2-diethylaminoethyl diphenylacetate; diphenylacetyldiethylaminoethanol; diphacil; spasmolytin. C_{20}-$H_{25}NO_2$; mol wt 311.42. C 77.14%, H 8.09%, N 4.50%, O 10.28%. Anticholinergic. Prepn: **DE 626539** (1936 to Ciba); and pharmacology: T. Wagner-Jauregg *et al., Ber.* **72**, 1551 (1939); R. R. Burtner, J. W. Cusic, *J. Am. Chem. Soc.* **65**, 262 (1943). Crystal and molecular structure: J. J. Guy, T. A. Hamor, *J. Chem. Soc. Perkin Trans.* 2 **1973**, 942. Effect on TSH release: D. Jordan *et al., Eur. J. Pharmacol.* **41**, 53 (1977). HPLC determn in tissues: J. Michelot *et al., J. Chromatogr.* **257**, 395 (1983). Pharmacokinetics: *idem et al., Xenobiotica* **11**, 123 (1981).

Hydrochloride. [50-42-0] Trasentine. $C_{20}H_{25}NO_2.HCl$; mol wt 347.88. Crystals, mp 113-114°. Readily sol in water; very sparingly sol in alcohol, ether. LD_{50} i.p. in mice: 0.24 g/kg (Burtner, Cusic).

THERAP CAT: Antispasmodic.

162. Adipic Acid. [124-04-9] Hexanedioic acid; 1,4-butanedicarboxylic acid. $C_6H_{10}O_4$; mol wt 146.14. C 49.31%, H 6.90%, O 43.79%. HOOC(CH$_2$)$_4$COOH. Found in beet juice. Prepn from cyclohexanol: Bouveault, Locquin, *Bull. Soc. Chim.* [4] **3**, 438 (1908); Ellis, *Org. Synth.* **coll. vol. I**, 18 (2nd ed., 1941); Feagen, Copenhaver, *J. Am. Chem. Soc.* **62**, 869 (1940); US 2191786 (1940); US 2196357 (1940); Zilberman *et al., J. Appl. Chem. (USSR)* **29**, 621 (1956). Convenient lab prepn from cyclohexanone: L. F. Fieser, *Organic Experiments* (Heath, Boston, 1964) pp 106-108. Prepn by one-step oxidation of cyclohexane: Onopchenko, Schulz, *J. Org. Chem.* **38**, 3729 (1973); Tanaka, 167th Am. Chem. Soc. Meet. (Los Angeles, March-April, 1974) *Abstracts of Papers,* p 29. Manuf: *Faith, Keyes & Clark's Industrial Chemicals,* F. A. Lowenheim, M. K. Moran, Eds. (Wiley-Interscience, New York, 4th ed., 1975) pp 50-54. *Review:* D. E. Danly, C. R. Campbell in *Kirk-Othmer Encyclopedia of Chemical Technology* vol. 1 (Wiley-Interscience, New York, 3rd ed., 1978) pp 510-531.

Monoclinic prisms from ethyl acetate, from water or from acetone + petr ether. d_4^{25} 1.360. mp 152°. bp$_{760}$ 337.5°; bp$_{100}$ 265°; bp$_{40}$ 240.5°; bp$_{20}$ 222°; bp$_{10}$ 205.5°; bp$_5$ 191°; bp$_{1.0}$ 159.5°. K_1 (25°) = 3.90×10^{-5}; $K_2 = 5.29 \times 10^{-6}$. Absorption spectrum: Ramart-Lucas, Salmon-Legagneur, *Compt. Rend.* **189**, 916 (1929). Freely soluble in methanol, ethanol; sol in acetone. 100 ml of a satd aq soln contains 1.44 g; 100 ml of boiling water dissolves 160 g; 100 parts of ether dissolve 0.633 parts (w/w) at 19°. Slightly sol in cyclohexane. Practically insol in benzene, petr ether. pH of satd aq soln at 25° = 2.7; pH of 0.1% soln = 3.2.

Dimethyl ester. $C_8H_{14}O_4$. Liquid, solidifies at 0°, bp$_{10}$ 112°.

Diethyl ester. Ethyl adipate. $C_{10}H_{18}O_4$. Liquid, bp 240-245°. d^{20} 1.009. Insol in water; sol in alcohol and many other organic solvents.

USE: Manuf artificial resins, plastics (nylon), urethan foams. Used as acidulant in baking powders instead of tartaric acid, cream of tartar, and phosphates because adipic acid is not hygroscopic. As an intermediate in lubricating oil additives.

163. Adiponectin. Acrp30; adipoQ; GBP28. Adipocyte hormone involved in glucose and lipid homeostasis. Consists of an N-terminal collagenous domain and a C-terminal globular domain with sequence homology to complement factor C1q. One of the most abundant proteins in human plasma, ranging from 0.5-30μg/ml; levels are reduced in diabetes and obesity. Discovery in murine adipocytes: P. E. Scherer *et al., J. Biol. Chem.* **270**, 26746 (1995); in human adipose tissue: K. Maeda *et al., Biochem. Biophys. Res. Commun.* **221**, 286 (1996). Isolation and characterization from human plasma: Y. Nakano *et al., J. Biochem. (Tokyo)* **120**, 803 (1996). Review of structure and physiology: T.-S. Tsao *et al., Eur. J. Pharmacol.* **440**, 213-221 (2002); of anti-inflammatory and atheroprotective effects in vascular tissue: B. J. Goldstein, R. Scalia, *J. Clin. Endocrinol. Metab.* **89**, 2563-2568 (2004); of role in insulin resistance: M. Haluzík *et al., Physiol. Res.* **53**, 123-129 (2004).

164. Adipsin. [104118-48-1] Serine protease homolog synthesized by mammalian adipocytes and secreted into the bloodstream; also produced by sciatic nerve. Developmentally regulated glycoprotein; mol wt ranges from 37-44 kilodaltons depending on the degree of glycosylation. Circulating levels of adipsin protein are reduced in certain genetic and experimental models of obesity. Originally identified as a 28 kDa protein encoded by a cDNA clone corresponding to messenger RNA specifically induced during adipocyte differentiation: B. M. Spiegelman *et al., J. Biol. Chem.* **258**, 10083 (1983). Nucleotide analysis and predicted amino acid sequence: K. S. Cook *et al., Proc. Natl. Acad. Sci. USA* **82**, 6480 (1985). Structure of adipsin gene: H. Y. Min, B. M. Spiegelman, *Nucleic Acids Res.* **14**, 8879 (1986). Isoln from adipose tissue, reportedly the primary site of synthesis, and from sciatic nerve: K. S. Cook *et al., Science* **237**, 402 (1987). Studies in murine disease models and potential biological role: J. S. Flier *et al., ibid.* 405.

165. Adlumidine. [550-49-2] (6S)-6-[(5S)-5,6,7,8-Tetrahydro-6-methyl-1,3-dioxolo[4,5-g]isoquinolin-5-yl]furo[3,4-e]-1,3-benzodioxol-8(6H)-one. $C_{20}H_{17}NO_6$; mol wt 367.35. C 65.39%, H 4.66%, N 3.81%, O 26.13%. An alkaloid present in the d-form in the entire plant of *Adlumia fungosa* (Ait.) Greene (*A. cirrhosa* Raf.), *Corydalis thalictrifolia* Franch. and *C. incisa* (Thumb.) Pers., *Fu-*

mariaceae. Schlotterbeck, Watkins, *J. Am. Chem. Soc.* **25**, 596 (1903); R. H. F. Manske, *Can. J. Res.* **21B**, 111 (1943). *l*-Adlumidine was isolated from *Corydalis sempervirens* (L.) Pers., *C. scouleri* Hook., and *C. crystallina* Engelm., *Fumariaceae:* R. H. F. Manske, *ibid.* **8**, 407 (1932); **14B**, 347 (1936); **17B**, 57 (1939). Structure: *idem, J. Am. Chem. Soc.* **72**, 3207 (1950). Stereochemistry: Blaha *et al., Collect. Czech. Chem. Commun.* **29**, 2328 (1964); Snatzke *et al., Tetrahedron* **25**, 5059 (1969). *Review:* Stanek, Manske in *The Alkaloids* vol. IV, R. H. F. Manske, H. L. Holmes, Eds. (Academic Press, New York, 1954) pp 167-198. Stereoisomer of bicuculline, *q.v.*

d-Adlumidine

Rhombic plates from chloroform + methanol, mp 236-237°. $[\alpha]_D^{25}$ +116.2° (c = 22 in chloroform). pKa 4.27. Practically insol in water. Very sparingly sol in alcohol, ether, hexane.

l-**Adlumidine.** [485-50-7] Capnoidine. Stout prisms from chloroform + methanol, mp 238°. $[\alpha]_D^{22}$ −113.2° (in chloroform). pKa 4.24. Practically insol in water. Sparingly sol in methanol; sol in chloroform.

166. Adlumine. [524-46-9] 6-(1,2,3,4-Tetrahydro-6,7-dimethoxy-2-methyl-1-isoquinolinyl)furo[3,4-e]-1,3-benzodioxol-8(6H)-one. $C_{21}H_{21}NO_6$; mol wt 383.39. C 65.79%, H 5.52%, N 3.65%, O 25.04%. An alkaloid present in the entire plant of some *Fumariaceae* species. *d*-Adlumine was isolated from *Adlumina fungosa* (Ait.) Greene (*A. cirrhosa* Raf.); *l*-adlumine was isolated from *Corydalis scouleri* Hook. and *C. sempervirens* (L.) Pers., *C. ophiocarpa* Hook. f. et Thoms *Fumariaceae:* Manske, *Can. J. Res.* **8**, 210 (1933); **14B**, 347 (1936); **16B**, 81 (1938); **17B**, 51 (1939). Preliminary stereochemical studies of *d*-form: Safe, Moir, *Can. J. Chem.* **42**, 160 (1964). Revised stereochemistry: Blaha *et al., Collect. Czech. Chem. Commun.* **29**, 2328 (1964); Snatzke *et al., Tetrahedron* **25**, 5059 (1969). *Review:* Stanek, Manske in *The Alkaloids* Vol. IV, R. H. F. Manske, H. L. Holmes, Eds. (Academic Press, New York, 1954) pp 167-198.

d-Adlumine

l-**Form.** Hexagonal plates from chloroform + methanol, mp 180°. $[\alpha]_D^{22}$ −42.5° (c = 0.8 in chloroform).

dl-**Form.** Stout short prisms, mp 190°.

167. Adonis vernalis. False hellebore; pheasant's eye; bird's eye. Herbaceous perennial, *Adonis vernalis* L., *Ranunculaceae,* used in traditional medicine as a cardiac stimulant. Medicinal formulations are derived from the aerial parts collected while flowering and dried. *Habit.* Central to eastern Europe and Siberia. *Constit.* Cardenolides, primarily adonitoxin, cymarin, k-strophanthoside, k-strophanthoside-β; flavonoids, including vitexin, luteolin. Isoln of constituents: F. W. Heyl *et al., J. Am. Chem. Soc.* **40**, 436

(1918); A. Pusz, S. Büchner, *Arzneim.-Forsch.* **13**, 409 (1963). Description and medicinal uses: J. Gruenwald *et al.*, *PDR for Herbal Medicines* (Medical Economics, Montvale, 2nd Ed., 2000) pp 5-6.

THERAP CAT: Cardiotonic.

168. Adonitol. [488-81-3] Ribitol; adonite. $C_5H_{12}O_5$; mol wt 152.15. C 39.47%, H 7.95%, O 52.58%. A pentitol from *Adonis vernalis* L., *Ranunculaceae; also* from *A. amurensis* L., *Ranunculaceae:* Santavy, Reichstein, *Pharm. Acta Helv.* **23**, 153 (1948).

Large, optically inactive crystals. mp 102°. Does not reduce Fehling's soln. Freely soluble in water, hot alcohol; insol in ether.

169. Adonitoxin. [17651-61-5] (3β,5β,16β)-3-[(6-Deoxy-α-L-mannopyranosyl)oxy]-14,16-dihydroxy-19-oxocard-20(22)-enolide. $C_{29}H_{42}O_{10}$; mol wt 550.64. C 63.26%, H 7.69%, O 29.06%. From *Adonis vernalis* L., *Ranunculaceae:* Katz, Reichstein, *Pharm. Acta Helv.* **22**, 437 (1947); *C.A.* **43**, 1790i (1949); Pitra, Cekan, *Collect. Czech. Chem. Commun.* **26**, 1551 (1961). Structure: Poláková, Cekan, *Chem. Ind. (London)* **1963**, 1766.

Crystals from chloroform + methanol + ether, decomp 251-258°.

3-O-Acetyladonitoxin. $C_{31}H_{44}O_{11}$. Needles from dil methanol, prisms from methanol+ ether, decomp 213-219°. $[\alpha]_D^{22}$ −19.9° (c = 0.33 in methanol).

170. Adrafinil. [63547-13-7] 2-[(Diphenylmethyl)-sulfinyl]-*N*-hydroxyacetamide; 2-(benzhydrylsulfinyl)acetohydroxamic acid; CRL-40028; Olmifon. $C_{15}H_{15}NO_3S$; mol wt 289.35. C 62.26%, H 5.23%, N 4.84%, O 16.59%, S 11.08%. α-Adrenergic agonist. Prepn, pharmacology: L. Lafon, **BE 846880**; **US 4066686** (1977, 1978 both to Lafon). Mode of action: J. Duteil *et al.*, *Eur. J. Pharmacol.* **59**, 121 (1979); C. Rozé *et al.*, *Arch. Int. Pharmacodyn. Ther.* **265**, 119 (1983). Psychopharmacology in mice: F. A. Rambert *et al., J. Pharmacol.* **17**, 37 (1986).

Crystals from ethyl acetate-isopropyl alcohol, mp 159-160°. Soly in water <1 g/l. LD_{50} in mice (mg/kg): <2048 i.p.; 1950 gastric admin (Lafon).

THERAP CAT: Treatment of depression.

171. Adrenalone. [99-45-6] 1-(3,4-Dihydroxyphenyl)-2-(methylamino)ethanone; 3′,4′-dihydroxy-2-(methylamino)-acetophenone; 3,4-dihydroxy-α-methylaminoacetophenone; adrenone; 4-methylaminocetopyrocatechol; Stryphnon. $C_9H_{11}NO_3$; mol wt 181.19. C 59.66%, H 6.12%, N 7.73%, O 26.49%. Intermediate in some epinephrine manuf processes. Prepd from 4-chloroacetylpyrocatechol and methylamine: **DE 152814** (Hoechst); Stolz, *Ber.* **37**, 4152 (1904); by heating α-(*p*-toluene sulfonyl-methylamino)-3,4-dimethoxyacetophenone with HCl under pressure: **DE 277540** (Bayer); *Frdl.* **12**, 764; *Chem. Zentralbl.* **1914**, **II**, 740.

Needles, dec 235-236°. Sparingly sol in water, alc, ether.

Hydrochloride. [62-13-5] Stryphnasal. $C_9H_{11}NO_3.HCl$; mol wt 217.65. Crystals, mp 243°. Freely sol in water; sol in alcohol. Insol in ether. Aq solns are neutral to litmus.

THERAP CAT: Hemostatic.

172. Adrenochrome. [54-06-8] 2,3-Dihydro-3-hydroxy-1-methyl-1*H*-indole-5,6-dione; 3-hydroxy-1-methyl-5,6-indolinedione. $C_9H_9NO_3$; mol wt 179.17. C 60.33%, H 5.06%, N 7.82%, O 26.79%. Pigment obtained by the oxidation of epinephrine. Prepn using Ag_2O as oxidizing agent: MacCarthy, *Chim. Ind. (Paris)* **55**, 435 (1946). Structure: D. E. Green, D. Richter, *Biochem. J.* **31**, 596 (1937); J. Harley-Mason, *Experientia* **4**, 307 (1948). Probably has the zwitterionic quinonimine structure shown here. Spectral data: A. Lund, *Acta Pharmacol. Toxicol.* **5**, 1218 (1949). *Review:* R. A. Heacock, *Chem. Rev.* **59**, 181-237 (1959). Review, as a psychotomimetic agent: R. A. Heacock, *Chim. Ther.* **6**, 300 (1971).

Brilliant red crystals may exist as hemihydrate from methanol-formic acid, dec 115-120°. Absorption max (1 mg % aq sol): 220, 300, 485 nm (log ε 4.33, 4.01, 3.64). Well-formed and well-dried crystals can be kept in a vacuum desiccator for several weeks. Easily oxidized to melanin. Freely sol in water; fairly sol in alcohol. Almost insol in benzene and ether. Solns are unstable. Optimum pH of water soln 4.0.

Oxime sesquihydrate. [6055-73-8] $C_9H_{10}N_2O_3.1\frac{1}{2}H_2O$. Orange needles from water, mp 278°. Much more stable than adrenochrome.

Monosemicarbazone. [69-81-8] Carbazochrome; Adrenoxyl; Cromosil. $C_{10}H_{12}N_4O_3$; mol wt 236.23. Prepn: Dechamps *et al.*, **US 2506294** (1950 to Société Belge de l'Azote). Orange-red crystals from dil alcohol, mp 203° (dec). *See also* Carbazochrome Salicylate.

Thiosemicarbazone. [113185-69-6] $C_{10}H_{12}N_4O_2S$. Description: Fleischhacker, Barsel, **US 2712024** (1955 to International Hormones). mp 215-220°.

THERAP CAT: Monosemicarbazone as hemostatic.

173. Adrenoglomerulotropin. [1210-56-6] 2,3,4,9-Tetrahydro-6-methoxy-1-methyl-1*H*-pyrido[3,4-*b*]indole; aldosterone-stimulating hormone; ASH; 1-methyl-6-methoxy-1,2,3,4-tetrahydro-2-carboline. $C_{13}H_{16}N_2O$; mol wt 216.28. C 72.19%, H 7.46%, N 12.95%, O 7.40%. Found in extracts of pineal gland tissue: Farrell, *Circulation* **21**, 1009 (1960); Farrell, McIsaac, *Arch. Biochem. Biophys.* **94**, 543 (1961). Synthesis from 5-methoxy-tryptamine and acetaldehyde: McIsaac, *Biochim. Biophys. Acta* **52**, 607 (1961); Meek *et al.*, *Chem. Ind. (London)* **1964**, 622.

Crystals, mp 150-151°. uv max (ethanol): 225, 280 nm (log ε 4.34, 3.86); (0.1N HCl): 220, 273 nm (log ε 4.40, 3.86).

174. Adrenolutin. [642-75-1] 1-Methyl-1H-indole-3,5,6-triol; N-methyl-5,6-dihydroxyindoxyl; 3,5,6-trihydroxy-N-methyl-indole. $C_9H_9NO_3$; mol wt 179.17. C 60.33%, H 5.06%, N 7.82%, O 26.79%. Alkaline rearrangement product of adrenochrome. Isoln and identification: Lund, Acta Pharmacol. Toxicol. **5**, 75 (1949). Structure and synthesis: Balsinger et al., Helv. Chim. Acta **36**, 708 (1953); Heacock, Mahon, Can. J. Chem. **36**, 1550 (1958). NMR studies and its existence in the ketonic form in solution: Powell, Heacock, Chim. Ther. **7**, 133 (1972).

Monohydrate, bright yellow prisms from water, mp 236° (dec); mp 195° (Balsinger). Anhydrous, bright yellow prisms, mp 245°.

175. Adrenomedullin. Hypotensive peptide originally isolated from human pheochromocytoma; subsequently found in all tissues with highest levels in heart, kidney, lung and adrenal gland. Highly conserved among species, human form is a 52-amino acid peptide; shares some sequence homology with calcitonin gene related peptide and amylin, q.v. Plasma levels are elevated in patients with hypertension and heart failure. Biological effects include vasodilation, diuresis and increased cardiac output; also exhibits antiproliferative and anti-apoptotic effects in the myocardium and stimulates angiogenesis. Isoln and hypotensive activity: K. Kitamura et al., Biochem. Biophys. Res. Commun. **192**, 553 (1993). RIA determn in plasma: L. K. Lewis et al., Clin. Chem. **44**, 571 (1998). Review of biosynthesis, pharmacology and bioactivities: J. P. Hinson et al., Endocr. Rev. **21**, 138-167 (2000). Series of articles on physiological roles: Regul. Pept. **112** 1-196 (2003). Review of clinical relevance and therapeutic potential: D. C. Bunton et al., Pharmacol.Ther. **103**, 179-201 (2004); S. A. Hamid, G. F. Baxter, ibid. **105**, 95-112 (2005).

176. Adrenosterone. [382-45-6] Androst-4-ene-3,11,17-trione; Reichstein's substance G. $C_{19}H_{24}O_3$; mol wt 300.39. C 75.97%, H 8.05%, O 15.98%. Prepn: Reichstein, Helv. Chim. Acta **19**, 29, 1107 (1936); Kendall et al., J. Biol. Chem. **116**, 267 (1936); Reichstein, Helv. Chim. Acta **20**, 817, 953 (1937). Total synthesis: Velluz et al., Compt. Rend. **250**, 1293 (1960). Crystal structure: Ohrt et al., Acta Crystallogr. **19**, 479 (1965). Metabolism: Bradlow et al., Steroids **10**, 233 (1967).

Needles from alcohol, mp 220-224°. Sublimes in high vacuum. Soly in water: 9.85 (23°), 15.2 (37°) mg/100 ml. Sol in alcohol, acetone, ether. $[\alpha]_D^{20}$ +262° (abs alcohol); $[\alpha]_{5461}^{25}$ +364 ± 5° (c = 0.18 in abs alc). uv max: 235 nm.

177. Aequorin. Photoprotein from the luminescent jellyfish Aequorea, mol wt 20,000 Da. Contains a single chromophore, **coelentrazine**, which emits a blue light via an intramolecular reaction when traces of Ca^{2+} are present. The protein is converted to **apoaequorin**, **coelenteramide**, and CO_2 with the emission of light.

Isolation and purification: O. Shimomura et al., J. Cell. Comp. Physiol. **59**, 223 (1962). Mechanism of luminescence: O. Shimomura et al., Biochemistry **13**, 3278 (1974). Verification of coelentrazine as chromophore: S. Inoue et al., Chem. Lett. **1975**, 141. Characterization and properties of isoforms: O. Shimomura, Biochem. J. **234**, 271 (1986); of semisynthetic aequorin: O. Shimomura et al., ibid. **251**, 405 (1988); and recombinant forms: eidem, ibid. **270**, 309 (1990). Crystal structure: J. F. Head et al., Nature **405**, 372 (2000). Use in measurement of cellular calcium: A. Azzi, B. Chance, Biochim. Biophys. Acta **189**, 141 (1969); J. M. Kendall et al., Anal. Biochem. **221**, 173 (1994); M. N. Badminton et al., Exp. Cell Res. **216**, 236 (1995). Review: O. Shimomura in Natural Products and Biological Activities, H. Imura et al., Eds (Elsevier Science Publishers, Amsterdam, 1986) p 33-44.

Sol in aq buffers >30 mg/ml. $E_{1cm}^{1\%}$ at 280 nm: 27.0; $E_{1cm}^{1\%}$ at 460 nm: 0.81. pI 4.2-4.9.

USE: For quantitation of free calcium in biological systems.

178. AET. [56-10-0] Carbamimidothioic acid 2-aminoethyl ester dihydrobromide; 2-(2-aminoethyl)-2-thiopseudourea dihydrobromide; S-(2-aminoethyl)isothiuronium bromide hydrobromide; β-aminoethylisothiuronium bromide hydrobromide; Antiradon. $C_3H_{11}Br_2N_3S$; mol wt 281.01. C 12.82%, H 3.95%, Br 56.87%, N 14.95%, S 11.41%. Prepd by refluxing thiourea with 2-bromoethylamine HBr in isopropanol: Clinton et al., J. Am. Chem. Soc. **70**, 950 (1948); Funahashi, Miyano, J. Agric. Chem. Soc. Jpn. **27**, 775 (1953), C.A. **49**, 15737b (1955); Doherty et al., J. Am. Chem. Soc. **79**, 5667 (1957). Toxicity study: J. Pospisil et al., Cas. Lek. Cesk. **105**, 1165 (1966), C.A. **67**, 72261s (1967).

Crystals from abs ethanol + ethyl acetate, mp 194-195°. Hygroscopic, cakes together, and is converted in significant amounts of 2-aminothiazoline, a transformation that can be detected by a drop in melting point by as much as 30°. The animal organism appears to convert it to 2-mercaptoethylguanidine hydrobromide. LD_{50} in mice (mg/kg): 100 i.v., 280 s.c., 480 i.p., 1600 orally (Pospisil).

THERAP CAT: Radioprotective agent.

179. Affinin. [25394-57-4] (2E,6Z,8E)-N-(2-Methylpropyl)-2,6,8-decatrienamide; (E,E,Z)-N-isobutyl-2,6,8-decatrienamide; N-isobutyldeca-trans-2-cis-6-trans-8-trienamide; spilanthol. $C_{14}H_{23}NO$; mol wt 221.34. C 75.97%, H 10.47%, N 6.33%, O 7.23%. Insecticidal lipid amide isolated from Heliopsis longipes (A. Gray) Blake, Compositae. Isoln and structure: Acree et al., J. Org. Chem. **10**, 236, 449 (1945). Identity with spilanthol: Jacobson, Chem. Ind. (London) **1957**, 50. Stereochemistry and synthesis: Crombie, Krasinski, ibid. **1962**, 983; Crombie et al., J. Chem. Soc. **1963**, 4970.

Pale yellow viscous oil, $bp_{0.2}$ 141°; $bp_{0.3-0.5}$ 160-165°. mp 23°. n_D^{25} 1.5134. Soluble in organic solvents. Practically insoluble in aq alkali and acid. uv max (95% ethanol): 228.5 nm (ε 33700).

USE: Insecticide synergist.

180. Aflatoxins B. Aflatoxins are a closely related group of secondary fungal metabolites shown to be mycotoxins. They are produced by Aspergillus flavus Link ex Fries, the causative principle of turkey "X" disease; and by Aspergillus parasiticus: Sargeant et al., Nature **192**, 1096 (1961); Hesseltine et al., Proc. 1st U.S. Japan Conf. Toxic Microorganisms, Honolulu, Hawaii 1968, p 202. Aflatoxins have been reported to naturally occur in peanuts, peanut meal, cottonseed meal, corn, dried chili peppers etc. However, the growth of the mold itself does not always indicate the presence of toxin since the yield of aflatoxin depends on growth conditions such as moisture, temperature, substrates, and aeration as well as genetic requirements. These heterocycles are now characterized as aflatoxins B_1, B_2, G_1, G_2, M_1 and M_2 (milk toxins) and B_{2a}, G_{2a}: Büchi, Rae in *Aflatoxin*, L. Goldblatt, Ed. (Academic Press, New York, 1969) pp 55-75. Toxic material is separated chromatographically into 4 distinct compounds based on fluorescent color (blue = B, green = G with subscripts relating to relative mobility): Nesbitt *et al.*, *Nature* **195**, 1062 (1962); Sargeant *et al.*, *Chem. Ind. (London)* **1963**, 53. B_1 is one of the most potent environmental mutagens and carcinogens known. B_2 and G_2 are the less toxic dihydro derivs of B_1 and G_1: Asao *et al.*, *J. Am. Chem. Soc.* **85**, 1706 (1963); **87**, 882 (1965), and B_{2a} and G_{2a} are the 2-hydroxy derivs of B_2 and G_2: Dutton, Heathcote, *Biochem. J.* **101**, 21P (1967); *Chem. Ind. (London)* **1968**, 418. Isoln of B_3 (*parasiticol*), a possible metabolite of G_1, from *A. flavus*: J. G. Heathcote, M. F. Dutton, *Tetrahedron* **25**, 1497 (1969). Aflatoxins R_0 (*aflatoxicol*), P_1, Q_1, RB_1, RB_2, and D_1 are also known: P. F. Schuda, *Top. Curr. Chem.* **91**, 77-106 (1980). Total syntheses of aflatoxins B_1 and G_1: Buchi *et al.*, *J. Am. Chem. Soc.* **88**, 4534 (1966); Knight *et al.*, *Chem. Commun.* **1966**, 706; Büchi, Weinreb, *J. Am. Chem. Soc.* **93**, 746 (1971). The extreme toxicity and carcinogenicity of aflatoxins may be due to their inhibition of nucleic acid synthesis by either direct interaction with enzymes involved or by a toxin-DNA template: Clifford, Rees, *Nature* **209**, 312 (1966); Sporn *et al.*, *Science* **151**, 1539 (1966). See also Wogan *et al.*, *Food Cosmet. Toxicol.* **12**, 681 (1974). Inhibition of salt-induced conversion of B-DNA to Z-DNA by aflatoxin B_1: A. Nordheim *et al.*, *Science* **219**, 1434 (1983). Prepn of the *exo*-8,9-epoxide of B_1, the metabolic deriv thought to be responsible for B_1's carcinogenicity: S. W. Baertschi *et al.*, *J. Am. Chem. Soc.* **110**, 7929 (1988). uv spectrum of B_2: Hartley *et al.*, *Nature* **198**, 1056 (1963). Physicochemical data for B_1: A. E. Pohland *et al.*, *Pure Appl. Chem.* **54**, 2219 (1982). Toxicity data: Carnaghan *et al.*, *ibid.* **200**, 1101 (1963); G. Büchi *et al.*, *Life Sci.* **13**, 1143 (1973). Symposium on toxicology and synthesis: *J. Toxicol. Toxin Rev.* **8**, 1-416 (1991). Review and evaluation of studies of carcinogenic action in laboratory animals and humans: *IARC Monographs* **10**, 51-72 (1976). Comprehensive reviews: Goldblatt, *Econ. Bot.* **22**, 51-62 (1968); Detroy *et al.*, "Aflatoxin and Related Compounds" in *Microbial Toxins* **Vol. VI**, A. Ciegler *et al.*, Eds. (Academic Press, New York, 1971) pp 3-178; W. F. Busby, Jr., G. N. Wogan in *ACS Monograph Series* **no. 182**, entitled "Chemical Carcinogens," vol. 2, C. E. Searle, Ed. (American Chemical Society, Washington DC, 2nd ed., 1984) pp 945-1136. Review of chemistry and syntheses: P. F. Schuda, *loc. cit.*; of biosynthesis: M. W. Sinz, W. T. Shier, *J. Toxicol. Toxin Rev.* **10**, 87-121 (1991).

Aflatoxin B_1

Aflatoxin B_1. [1162-65-8] (6a*R*-cis)-2,3,6a,9a-Tetrahydro-4-methoxycyclopenta[*c*]furo[3′,2′:4,5]furo[2,3-*h*][1]benzopyran-1,11-dione. $C_{17}H_{12}O_6$; mol wt 312.27. Crystals, mp 268-269°. Exhibits blue fluorescence. $[\alpha]_D$ −558° (c = 0.1 in CHCl$_3$). $[\alpha]_D$ −480° (c = 0.1 in DMF). uv max (ethanol): 223, 265, 362 nm (ε 25600, 13400, 21800). LD$_{50}$ orally in day old duckling: 18.2 μg/50 gm body wt (Carnaghan); i.p. in newborn mice: 9.50 mg/kg body wt (Büchi).

Aflatoxin B_2. [7220-81-7] (6a*R*-cis)-2,3,6a,8,9,9a-Hexahydro-4-methoxycyclopenta[*c*]furo[3′,2′:4,5]furo[2,3-*h*][1]benzopyran-1,11-dione. $C_{17}H_{14}O_6$; mol wt 314.29. The 8,9-dihydro deriv of aflatoxin B_1. Crystals, mp 286-289°. Exhibits blue fluorescence. $[\alpha]_D$ −492° (c = 0.1 in CHCl$_3$). uv max (ethanol): 265, 363 nm (ε 11700, 23400). LD$_{50}$ orally in day old duckling: 84.8 μg/50 gm body wt (Carnaghan).

Caution: The aflatoxins are listed as known human carcinogens: *Report on Carcinogens, Eleventh Edition* (PB2005-104914, 2004) p III-8.

181.   Aflatoxins G. Toxic metabolites of fungi *Aspergillus flavus* Link ex Fries and *Aspergillus parasiticus*. Total synthesis of

G_1: Büchi, Weinreb, *J. Am. Chem. Soc.* **93**, 746 (1971). Physical and chemical data: Hartley *et al.*, *Nature* **198**, 1056 (1963); Asao, *J. Am. Chem. Soc.* **87**, 882 (1965). Toxicity data: R. B. A. Carnaghan *et al.*, *Nature* **200**, 1101 (1963). For general refs *see* Aflatoxins B.

Aflatoxin G_1

Aflatoxin G_1. [1165-39-5] (7a*R*,10a*S*)-3,4,7a,10a-Tetrahydro-5-methoxy-1*H*,12*H*-furo[3′,2′:4,5]furo[2,3-*h*]pyrano[3,4-*c*][1]benzopyran-1,12-dione. $C_{17}H_{12}O_7$; mol wt 328.27. Crystals, mp 244-246°. Exhibits green fluorescence. $[\alpha]_D$ −556° (chloroform). uv max (ethanol): 243, 257, 264, 362 nm (ε 11500, 9900, 10000, 16100). LD$_{50}$ orally in day old duckling: 39.2 μg/50 gm body wt (Carnaghan).

Aflatoxin G_2. [7241-98-7] (7a*R*,10a*S*)-3,4,7a,9,10,10a-Hexahydro-5-methoxy-1*H*,12*H*-furo[3′,2′:4,5]furo[2,3-*h*]pyrano[3,4-*c*]-[1]benzopyran-1,12-dione. $C_{17}H_{14}O_7$; mol wt 330.29. The 9,10-dihydro deriv of aflatoxin G_1. Crystals, mp 237-240°. Exhibits green-blue fluorescence. $[\alpha]_D$ −473° (c = 0.084 in chloroform). uv max (ethanol): 265, 363 nm (ε 9700, 21000). LD$_{50}$ orally in day old duckling: 172.5 μg/50 gm body wt (Carnaghan).

Caution: The aflatoxins are listed as known human carcinogens: *Report on Carcinogens, Eleventh Edition* (PB2005-104914, 2004) p III-8.

182.   Aflatoxins M. Highly toxic 4-hydroxylated aflatoxin B derivs found in the milk of cows fed toxic meal. Initial reports: Allcroft, Carnaghan, *Vet. Rec.* **75**, 259 (1963). Isoln: De Iongh *et al.*, *Nature* **202**, 466 (1964); Allcroft *et al.*, *ibid.* **209**, 154 (1966). Isoln and structure of M_1 and M_2: C. W. Holzapfel, P. S. Steyn, *Tetrahedron Lett.* **1966**, 2799. Total synthesis of M_1: Büchi, Weinreb, *J. Am. Chem. Soc.* **91**, 5408 (1969); **93**, 746 (1971); G. Büchi *et al.*, *ibid.* **103**, 3497 (1981). Carcinogenicity studies: Wogan, Paglialunga, *Food Cosmet. Toxicol.* **12**, 381 (1974). For general refs *see* Aflatoxins B.

Aflatoxin M_1

Aflatoxin M_1. [6795-23-9] (6a*R*,9a*R*)-2,3,6a,9a-Tetrahydro-9a-hydroxy-4-methoxycyclopenta[*c*]furo[3′,2′:4,5]furo[2,3-*h*][1]benzopyran-1,11-dione; 4-hydroxyaflatoxin B_1. $C_{17}H_{12}O_7$; mol wt 328.27. Crystals from methanol, mp 299° (dec). Exhibits blue-violet fluorescence. $[\alpha]_D$ −280° (c = 0.1 in DMF). uv max (ethanol): 226, 265, 357 nm (ε 23100, 11600, 19000). LD$_{50}$ orally in day old Pekin ducklings: 16.6 μg/duckling (Holzapfel, Steyn).

Aflatoxin M_2. [6885-57-0] 2,3,6a,8,9,9a-Hexahydro-9a-hydroxy-4-methoxycyclopenta[*c*]furo[3′,2′:4,5]furo[2,3-*h*][1]benzopyran-1,11-dione; 4-hydroxyaflatoxin B_2. $C_{17}H_{14}O_7$; mol wt 330.29. The 8,9-dihydro deriv of aflatoxin M_1. Exhibits violet fluorescence. Crystals from methanol-chloroform, mp 293° (dec). uv max (ethanol): 221, 264, 357 nm (ε 20000, 10900, 21000). LD$_{50}$ orally in day old Pekin ducklings: 62 μg/duckling (Holzapfel, Steyn).

Caution: The aflatoxins are listed as known human carcinogens: *Report on Carcinogens, Eleventh Edition* (PB2005-104914, 2004) p III-8.

183.   Afloqualone. [56287-74-2] 6-Amino-2-(fluoromethyl)-3-(2-methylphenyl)-4(3*H*)-quinazolinone; 6-amino-2-fluoromethyl-3-(*o*-tolyl)-4(3*H*)-quinazolinone; HQ-495; Arofuto. C_{16}-

$H_{14}FN_3O$; mol wt 283.30. C 67.83%, H 4.98%, F 6.71%, N 14.83%, O 5.65%. A centrally acting muscle relaxant. Prepn: I. Inoue *et al.*, **DE 2449113**; *eidem*, **US 3966731** (1975, 1976 to Tanabe); J. Tani *et al.*, *J. Med. Chem.* **22**, 95 (1979). Pharmacology: T. Ochiai, R. Ishida, *Jpn. J. Pharmacol.* **31**, 491 (1981); **32**, 427 (1982). Metabolism: N. Otsuka *et al.*, *J. Pharmacobio-Dyn.* **5**, S-59 (1982); S. Furuuchi *et al.*, *Drug Metab. Dispos.* **11**, 371 (1983).

Pale yellow prisms from 2-propanol, mp 195-196°. LD_{50} in mice (mg/kg): 315.1 i.p. (Tani).

THERAP CAT: Muscle relaxant (skeletal).

184.   Agar. [9002-18-0] Agar-agar; gelose; Japan agar; Bengal isinglass; Ceylon isinglass; Chinese isinglass; Japan isinglass; Layor Carang. A polysaccharide complex extracted from the agarocytes of algae of the *Rhodophyceae*. Predominant agar-producing genera are *Gelidium, Gracilaria, Acanthopeltis, Ceramium, Pterocladia* found in the Pacific and Indian Oceans and Japan Sea. Can be separated into a neutral gelling fraction, *agarose*, and a sulfated non-gelling fraction, *agaropectin*: Araki, *J. Chem. Soc. Jpn.* **58**, 1338 (1937). Structure believed to be a complex range of polysaccharide chains having alternating α-(1 → 3) and β-(1 → 4) linkages and varying in total charge content; three extremes of structure noted, namely neutral agarose, pyruvated agarose having little sulfation, and a sulfated galactan: Duckworth *et al.*, *Carbohydr. Res.* **16**, 189, 435, 446 (1971). *Reviews:* V. J. Chapman, *Seaweeds and Their Uses* (Pitman Publ., New York, 1952) pp 89-123; Humm, *Econ. Bot.* **1**, 317 (1947); Mori, *Adv. Carbohydr. Chem.* **8**, 317 (1953); Selby, Wynne, in *Industrial Gums*, R. L. Whistler, Ed. (Academic Press, N.Y., 2nd ed., 1973) pp 29-48.

Transparent, odorless, tasteless strips or coarse or fine powder. Insol in cold water, alc; slowly sol in hot water to a viscid soln. A 1% soln forms a stiff jelly on cooling.

USE: Substitute for gelatin, isinglass, etc. in making emulsions including photographic, gels in cosmetics, and as thickening agent in foods esp. confectionaries and dairy products; in meat canning; in production of medicinal encapsulations and ointments; as dental impression mold base; as corrosion inhibitor; sizing for silks and paper; in the dyeing and printing of fabrics and textiles; in adhesives. In nutrient media for bacterial cultures.

THERAP CAT: Cathartic.

THERAP CAT (VET): Laxative in dogs, cats. Demulcent.

185.   Agaric. Larch agaric; touch wood; white agaric; purging agaric; amadou; German fungus. The dried fruit body of *Fomes laricis* (Jacq.) Murrill *(Polyporus officinalis* Fries), *Polyporaceae*, deprived of its outer rind. *Habit.* European and Asiatic Russia. Grows upon various species of *Pinus, Larix,* and *Picea. Constit.* 14-16% Agaricic acid; agaricoresin, agaricol, phytosterin, ricinoleic acid, cetyl alcohol, glucose, malic acid, carbohydrates. Isoln and separation of some constituents: Valentin, Knütter, *Pharm. Zentralhalle* **96**, 478 (1957). Impregnated with potassium nitrate and dried, it constitutes punk or tinder.

Light, fibrous, grayish-white to pale brown, spongy, friable pieces of irregular shape; feeble odor and bitter, acrid, yet somewhat sweetish taste.

USE: Anhidrotic.

186.   Agaricic Acid. [666-99-9] 2-Hydroxy-1,2,3-nonadecanetricarboxylic acid; agaric acid; agaricin; agaricinic acid; laricic acid; *n*-hexadecylcitric acid; α-cetylcitric acid. $C_{22}H_{40}O_7$; mol wt 416.55. C 63.43%, H 9.68%, O 26.89%. Active principle of *Fomes laricis* (Jacq.) Murrill *(Polyporus officinalis* Fries), *Polyporaceae:* Thoms, Vogelsang, *Ann.* **357**, 145 (1907). Attempted syntheses: Evans, *J. Chem. Soc.* **1959**, 1313; Graf, Liu, *Arch. Pharm.* **306**, 366 (1973). Activity studies: Bacchi *et al.*, *J. Bacteriol.* **98**, 23 (1969).

Sesquihydrate, odorless, almost tasteless, crystalline powder. Anhydrous, mp 142° (dec). $[\alpha]_D^{19}$ −9° (NaOH). Slightly sol in cold water, chloroform or ether; freely sol in boiling water, alkalies, hot glacial acetic acid. One gram dissolves in 180 ml cold, 10 ml boiling alcohol.

Note: The name agaric acid has also been used for a lanostane-like mixture [*C.A.* **68**, 29894j (1968)].

USE: Has been used as antiperspirant.

187.   Agaritine. [2757-90-6] L-Glutamic acid 5-[2-[4-(hydroxymethyl)phenyl]hydrazide]; β-*N*-[γ-L(+)-glutamyl]-4-hydroxymethylphenylhydrazine. $C_{12}H_{17}N_3O_4$; mol wt 267.28. C 53.92%, H 6.41%, N 15.72%, O 23.94%. Constituent of the commercial, edible mushroom *Agaricus bisporus* (Lange) Sing. *[Psalliota hortensis* Cooke var. *bispora], Agaricaceae (Agaricales).* Isoln and structure: Levenberg, *Fed. Proc.* **19**, 6 (1960); *J. Am. Chem. Soc.* **83**, 503 (1961); Daniels *et al.*, *ibid.* 3333; *see also* Levenberg in *Methods Enzymol.* **17** (Part A), 877 (1970). Synthesis: Kelly *et al.*, *J. Org. Chem.* **27**, 3229 (1962); Hinman, Kelly, **US 3274232**; **US 3288848** (both 1966 to Upjohn).

Glistening crystals from dil alcohol, dec 205-209°. $[\alpha]_D^{25}$ +7° (c = 0.8). uv max (water): 237.5, 280 nm (ε 12,000, 1,400). Very freely sol in water, practically insol in the usual anhydr organic solvents. pKa in water: 3.4 and 8.86.

188.   Agmatine. [306-60-5] 4-(Aminobutyl)guanidine; 1-amino-4-guanidobutane. $C_5H_{14}N_4$; mol wt 130.19. C 46.13%, H 10.84%, N 43.03%. Decarboxylated arginine. Found in pollen of *Ambrosia artemisifolia* L., *Compositae,* in ergot, in sponges, in herring sperm, in octopus muscle: F. W. Heyl, *J. Am. Chem. Soc.* **41**, 670 (1919); A. Kossel, *Z. Physiol. Chem.* **66**, 257 (1910); J. L. Irvin, D. W. Wilson, *J. Biol. Chem.* **127**, 565 (1939). Prepn of salts: **DE 463576** (1928 to Schering-Kahlbaum AG). Synthesis: A. Kossel, *Z. Physiol. Chem.* **68**, 170 (1910); K. Odo, *J. Chem. Soc. Jpn.* **67**, 132 (1946); K. Dose, *Ber.* **90**, 1251 (1957). Use as marker for tumor cells: F. S. Steven *et al., Anticancer Res.* **9**, 247 (1989); F. S. Steven *et al., J. Enzyme Inhib.* **4**, 63 (1990).

Sulfate. [2482-00-0] $C_5H_{14}N_4.H_2SO_4$. Needles from dil methanol, mp 231°. Fairly sol in water. Nearly insol in alcohol.

Gold chloride. $C_5H_{14}N_4.2HCl.2AuCl_3$. Yellow needles from water, dec 223°.

USE: Biochemical probe

189.   Agnus Castus. Chaste tree; monk's pepper. Deciduous shrub, *Vitex agnus-castus* L., *Verbenaceae.* Used medicinally since ancient times for treatment of female conditions and for suppression of sexual desire. Medicinal parts include the dried leaves and the dried ripe fruit, known as *chasteberry.* The dried fruits are similar in appearance and odor to black pepper. *Habit.* Indigenous to the Mediterranean region; widely distributed in central Asia, the tropics and southern Europe. *Constit.* Iridoid glycosides, agnoside and aucubin; flavonoids including casticin and vitexin; labdan diterpenoids, rotundifuran, vitexilactone, and $6\beta,7\beta$-diacetoxy-13-hydroxy-labda-8,14-diene; and volatile oil containing a complex mixture of monoterpenes and sesquiterpenes. Brief description: P. Houghton, *Pharm. J.* **253**, 720 (1994). Yield and composition of essential oil: J. M. Sorensen, S. T. Katsiotis, *Planta*

Med. **66**, 245 (2000). HPLC analysis of diterpenoids: E. Hoberg *et al., ibid.* 352. Inhibition of prolactin secretion: G. Sliutz *et al., Horm. Metab. Res.* **25**, 253 (1993). Dopaminergic activity: H. Jarry *et al., Exp. Clin. Endocrinol.* **102**, 448 (1994). Series of articles on phytochemistry, pharmacology and biological activity: *Z. Phytother.* **20**, 140-158 (1998). Historical overview: J. G. Mayer, F.-C. Czygan, *ibid.* 177. Clinical trial in treatment of hyperprolactinemia: A. Milewicz *et al., Arzneim.-Forsch.* **43**, 752 (1993); in treatment of premenstrual syndrome: R. Schellenberg *et al., Br. Med. J.* **322**, 134 (2001).

Dry extract. Agnolyt; Strotan; Valverde.

THERAP CAT: In treatment of premenstrual syndrome.

190. Agomelatine. [138112-76-2] *N*-[2-(7-Methoxy-1-naphthalenyl)ethyl]acetamide; S-20098; Valdoxan. $C_{15}H_{17}NO_2$; mol wt 243.30. C 74.05%, H 7.04%, N 5.76%, O 13.15%. Melatoninergic agonist and selective serotonin 5-HT$_{2B}$ and 5-HT$_{2C}$ receptor antagonist; metabolically stable analogue of melatonin, *q.v.* Prepn: J. Andrieux *et al.,* **EP 447285**; *eidem,* **US 5225442** (1991, 1993 both to Adir); and structure-activity studies: S. Yous *et al., J. Med. Chem.* **35**, 1484 (1992); P. Depreux *et al., ibid.* **37**, 3231 (1994). Mechanism of action: M. J. Millan *et al., J. Pharmacol. Exp. Ther.* **306**, 954 (2003). Clinical evaluation in major depressive disorder: H. Lôo *et al., Int. Clin. Psychopharmacol.* **17**, 239 (2002); S. H. Kennedy, R. Emsley, *Eur. Neuropsychopharmacol.* **16**, 93 (2006).

Crystals from toluene + hexane, 2:1, mp 109-110°.

THERAP CAT: Antidepressant.

191. Agroclavine. [548-42-5] 8,9-Didehydro-6,8-dimethylergoline. $C_{16}H_{18}N_2$; mol wt 238.33. C 80.63%, H 7.61%, N 11.75%. A non-peptide ergot alkaloid obtained from cultures of fungi parasitic on *Elymus mollis* Trin.: Abe *et al.,* **JP 49 178336** (1949 to Takeda), *C.A.* **45**, 6352c (1951); *Annu. Rep. Takeda Res. Lab.* **10**, 145, 167, 171 (1951); **JP 54 7498** (1954), *C.A.* **50**, 6000^b (1956); **US 2835675** (1958). Found in fungi parasitic on *Pennisetum typhoideum* Rich.: Stoll *et al., Helv. Chim. Acta* **37**, 1815 (1954). Structure and stereochemistry: Schreier, *ibid.* **41**, 1984 (1958). Biosynthesis: Floss *et al., J. Am. Chem. Soc.* **90**, 6500 (1968). Synthesis: Plieninger *et al., Ann.* **743**, 95 (1971). Metabolism: Ramstad, *Lloydia* **31**, 327 (1968).

Rods from ether, dec 198-203°; needles from acetone, dec 205-206°. $[\alpha]_D^{20}$ −155° (c = 0.9 in chloroform); $[\alpha]_D^{20}$ −182° (c = 0.5 in pyridine). uv max: 225, 284, 293 nm (ε 4.47, 3.88, 3.81). Freely sol in alc, chloroform, pyridine; sol in benzene, ether; very slightly sol in water.

192. Agrocybin. [544-44-5] 8-Hydroxy-2,4,6-octatriynamide. $C_8H_5NO_2$; mol wt 147.13. C 65.31%, H 3.43%, N 9.52%, O 21.75%. Phytotoxic acetylene responsible for killing of grass by fairy ring mushroom fungus. Isolation from basidiomycete *Agrocybe dura:* Kavanagh *et al., Proc. Natl. Acad. Sci. USA* **36**, 102 (1950); from *Marasmius oreades* and activity: W. A. Ayer, P. A. Craw, *Can. J. Chem.* **67**, 1371 (1989). Structure and synthesis:

Bu'Lock *et al., Chem. Ind. (London)* **1954**, 990; and spectrum: Ashworth *et al., J. Chem. Soc.* **1958**, 950. Origin of the carbon skeleton: E. R. H. Jones *et al., J. Chem. Res. Miniprint* **1977**, 744.

Crystals from 20% alc or ether, mp 140° (conflagrates). Stable in air for about one day after which the crystals turn black and become insol in ether. Sol in alc, acetone, ether, chloroform, methyl isobutyl ketone; slightly sol in water. Practically insol in hexane.

193. Ajaconine. [545-61-9] $C_{22}H_{33}NO_3$; mol wt 359.50. C 73.50%, H 9.25%, N 3.90%, O 13.35%. From seeds of larkspur, *Delphinium ajacis* L., *Ranunculaceae:* Keller, Volker, *Arch. Pharm.* **251**, 207 (1913); Goodson, *J. Chem. Soc.* **1945**, 245. Structure: Dvornik, Edwards, *Tetrahedron* **14**, 54 (1961); Nabors *et al., Tetrahedron Lett.* **1969**, 2445. Stereochemistry: Solo, Pelletier, *Chem. Ind. (London)* **1960**, 1108; Whalley, *Tetrahedron* **18**, 43 (1962). Synthetic studies: Nabors *et al., ibid.* **27**, 2385 (1971). Rearrangement: S. W. Pelletier, N. V. Mody, *J. Am. Chem. Soc.* **101**, 492 (1979).

Prisms from dil alcohol, mp 172°. $[\alpha]_D^{18}$ −119° (c = 2 in anhydr alcohol).

Sulfate heptahydrate. Hexagonal plates from dil acetone, mp 113°. $[\alpha]_D^{20}$ +5.5° (c = 2).

194. Ajmaline. [4360-12-7] Ajmalan-17,21-diol; rauwolfine; Aritmina; Gilurytmal; Ritmos; Tachmalin. $C_{20}H_{26}N_2O_2$; mol wt 326.43. C 73.59%, H 8.03%, N 8.58%, O 9.80%. From roots of *Rauwolfia serpentina* (L.) Benth. *(Ophioxylon serpentinum* L.), *Apocynaceae.* Isolation: S. Siddiqui, R. H. Siddiqui, *J. Indian Chem. Soc.* **8**, 667 (1931); **9**, 539 (1932); **12**, 37 (1935); L. van Itallie, A. J. Steenhauer, *Arch. Pharm.* **270**, 313 (1932). Structure: A. Chatterjee, S. Bose, *J. Indian Chem. Soc.* **31**, 17 (1954); F. A. L. Anet *et al., J. Chem. Soc.* **1954**, 1242. Stereochemistry: M. F. Bartlett *et al., J. Am. Chem. Soc.* **84**, 622 (1962). Synthesis: S. Masamune *et al., ibid.* **89**, 2506 (1967); E. E. Van Tamelen, L. K. Oliver, *ibid.* **92**, 2136 (1970); K. Mashimo, Y. Sato, *Chem. Pharm. Bull.* **18**, 353 (1970). Physico-chemical properties: A. Petter, *Arzneim.-Forsch.* **24**, 874 (1974). Antiarrhythmic activity: A. Petter, K. Engelmann, *ibid.* 876. *Reviews:* R. Robinson in *Festschrift Arthur Stoll* (Birkhäuser-Verlag, Basel, 1957) pp 457-467; A. Koskinen, M. Lounasmaa in *Progress in the Chemistry of Natural Products* **vol. 43**, W. Herz *et al.,* Eds. (Springer-Verlag, New York, 1983) pp 268-346.

Pale amber, solvated, tetragonal prisms from methanol, $C_{20}H_{26}$-N_2O_2·CH$_3$OH, mp 158-160°. $[\alpha]_D^{18}$ +131° (c = 0.4 in chloroform). Anhydr mp 205-207°. $[\alpha]_D^{20}$ +144° (c = 0.8 in chloroform). uv max (ethanol): 247, 295 nm (log ε 3.94, 3.49). Sol in methanol, ethanol, ether, chloroform; slightly sol in water.

Hydrochloride dihydrate. $C_{20}H_{26}N_2O_2$·2HCl·2H$_2$O. Hexagonal bipyramidal crystals from water, mp 140°. $[\alpha]_D^{18}$ +96.6°. One gram dissolves in 40 ml water.

THERAP CAT: Antihypertensive; antiarrhythmic.

195. Ajoene. [92285-01-3] 2-Propenyl 3-(2-propenylsulfinyl)-1-propenyl disulfide; 4,5,9-trithiadodeca-1,6,11-triene 9-oxide. $C_9H_{14}OS_3$; mol wt 234.40. C 46.12%, H 6.02%, O 6.83%, S 41.04%. Antithrombotic principle found in garlic (*Allium sativum* L., *Liliaceae*). Formed from allicin, *q.v.*, in the approximate ratio of 4:1 (*E:Z*). The (*Z*)-isomer appears to be more bioactive. Isoln and effect on human platelet aggregation *in vitro:* R. Apitz-Castro *et al., Thromb. Res.* **32**, 155 (1983). [*Note:* Structure initially assigned as *allyl 1,5-hexadienyltrisulfide.*] Structural study, isoln of isomers and synthesis of (*E,Z*)-form: E. Block *et al., J. Am. Chem. Soc.* **106**, 8295 (1984). Structure determn and structure-activity study: *eidem, ibid.* **108**, 7045 (1986). Synthesis, not claimed: E. Block, S. Ahmad, US 4643994 (1987 to Res. Found. SUNY). Mechanism of antiplatelet activity: R. Apitz-Castro *et al., Biochem. Biophys. Res. Commun.* **141**, 145 (1986). Synergism with other antiplatelet compounds: *eidem, Thromb. Res.* **42**, 303 (1986). *In vitro* antifungal activity: S. Yoshida *et al., Appl. Environ. Microbiol.* **53**, 615 (1987).

(Z)–Ajoene

(E)–Ajoene

(*E*)-Form. [92284-99-6] Colorless, odorless oil. uv max: 240 nm.

196. Ajowan Oil. Ptychotis oil. Obtained by distillation of seeds of *Carum copticum* (DC.) Benth. & Hook. (*Ptychotis ajowan* DC.), *Umbelliferae*. Contains thymol, α-pinene, *p*-cymene, dipentene, γ-terpinene; fixed oil content includes petroselenic acid, oleic acid, linoleic acid, resin acids, and palmitic acid. *Ref:* Farook *et al. J. Sci. Food Agric.* **4**, 132 (1953); E. Guenther, *The Essential Oils* **IV**, 551-2 (Van Nostrand, New York, 1950).

Almost colorless or brownish liquid; thyme odor; sharp burning taste. d 0.910-0.930. Rotation 0° to +5°. n_D^{20} 1.498-1.504. Sol in 1-2.5 vol and more of 80% alcohol. The oil is toxic to earthworms, while alcoholic extracts are toxic to staphylococci and *Escherichia coli*. Dil extracts are useful as expectorants: Umanskii, Krutik, *Farmatsiya* **8**, no. 6, 19 (1945), *C.A.* **41**, 2209 (1947).

197. Ajugarins. Diterpenes isolated from the leaves of *Ajuga remota (Labiatae)*. Five different ajugarins have been isolated and identified; of these ajugarins I-III possess antifeedant activity against the African army worm, ajugarin-IV has insecticidal activity, ajugarin V is inactive. Isoln and structure of ajugarins I-III: I. Kubo *et al., Chem. Commun.* **1976**, 949; of ajugarin IV: *eidem, ibid.* **1982**, 618; of ajugarin V: *eidem, Chem. Lett.* **1983**, 223. See also: JP Kokai 82 48979 (1982 to Otsuka). X-ray crystal structure of 12-bromoajugarin-I and absolute configuration: I. Kubo *et al., Chem. Commun.* **1980**, 897; ^{13}C-NMR shift data: J. M. Luteijn *et al., Org. Magn. Reson.* **19**, 95 (1982). Synthetic approaches: D. J. Goldsmith *et al., J. Org. Chem.* **43**, 3182 (1978); J. M. Luteijn, Ae. de Groot, *Tetrahedron Lett.* **1981**, 789. Total synthesis of ajugarin-I: S. V. Ley *et al., Chem. Commun.* **1983**, 503.

Ajugarin-I   R = CH2OCOCH3

Ajugarin-I. [62640-05-5] [1*R*-(1α,4aβ,5β,6α,8α,8aα)]-4-[2-[8-(Acetyloxy)-8a-[(acetyloxy)methyl]octahydro-5,6-dimethylspiro[naphthalene-1(2*H*),2'-oxiran]-5-yl]ethyl]-2(5*H*)furanone. $C_{24}H_{34}O_7$; mol wt 434.52. mp 155-157°. uv max (methanol): 212 nm (ε 10000).

Ajugarin-II. [62640-06-6] $C_{22}H_{32}O_6$; mol wt 392.49. 8-Hydroxy analog of ajugarin I. mp 188-189°.

Ajugarin-III. [62640-07-7] $C_{24}H_{36}O_8$; mol wt 452.54. 1,1-Dihydroxy analog of ajugarin I. mp 243-245°.

Ajugarin-IV. [82225-47-6] $C_{23}H_{34}O_6$; mol wt 406.51. mp 119-120.5°. $[\alpha]_D$ −57.5° (c = 0.06 in $CHCl_3$). uv max (ethanol): 215 nm (ε 17000).

Ajugarin-V. [82231-14-9] $C_{22}H_{32}O_5$; mol wt 376.49. mp 217-218°. $[\alpha]_D$ −13.5° (c = 0.18 in $CHCl_3$). uv max (ethanol): 210 nm (ε 11000).

198. Ajulemic Acid. [137945-48-3] (6a*R*,10a*R*)-3-(1,1-Dimethylheptyl)-6a,7,10,10a-tetrahydro-1-hydroxy-6,6-dimethyl-6*H*-dibenzo[*b,d*]pyran-9-carboxylic acid; 1′,1′-dimethylheptyl-Δ^8-tetrahydrocannabinol-11-oic acid; (3*R*,4*R*)-Δ^6-THC-DMH-7-oic acid; CT-3; IP-751. $C_{25}H_{36}O_4$; mol wt 400.55. C 74.96%, H 9.06%, O 15.98%. Cannabinoid receptor agonist; synthetic, non-psychoactive derivative of Δ^9-tetrahydrocannabinol, *q.v.* Prepn: S. H. Burstein *et al., J. Med. Chem.* **35**, 3135 (1992); S. H. Burstein, R. Mechoulam, WO 9401429; *eidem*, US 5338753 (both 1994). GC-MS determn in plasma: C. Batista *et al., J. Chromatogr. B* **820**, 77 (2005). Binding to CB-receptors: M.-H. Rhee *et al., J. Med. Chem.* **40**, 3228 (1997); to PPAR$_\gamma$ receptor: J. Liu *et al., Mol. Pharmacol.* **63**, 983 (2003). Clinical evaluation in chronic neuropathic pain: M. Karst *et al., J. Am. Med. Assoc.* **290**, 1757 (2003). Reviews of development and pharmacology: S. Burstein *et al., Life Sci.* **75**, 1513-1522 (2004); *idem, AAPS Journal* **7**, E143-E148 (2005); J. L. Wiley, *IDrugs* **8**, 1002-1011 (2005).

Crystals from acetonitrile, mp 112-114° (sintering). $[\alpha]_D$ −275° (c = 3.8 in chloroform). Sol in most organic solvents. Practically insol in hexane.

Acetate. $C_{25}H_{36}O_4 \cdot C_2H_2O$; mol wt 442.59. Crystals from pentane, mp 120-122°. $[\alpha]_D$ −265° (c = 9.0 in chloroform).

THERAP CAT: Anti-inflammatory.

199. Akuammicine. [639-43-0] 2,16,19-20-Tetradehydrocuran-17-oic acid methyl ester. $C_{20}H_{22}N_2O_2$; mol wt 322.40. C 74.51%, H 6.88%, N 8.69%, O 9.93%. From the seeds of *Picralima klaineana*, Pierre, *Apocynaceae* found in the Gold Coast: Henry, Sharp, *J. Chem. Soc.* **1927**, 1950; Henry, *ibid.* **1932**, 2759. Structure: Aghoramurthy, Robinson, *Tetrahedron* **1**, 172 (1957); Bernauer *et al., Helv. Chim. Acta* **43**, 717 (1960); Edwards, Smith, *J. Chem. Soc.* **1961** 152. Derivs: Robinson, Thomas, *ibid.* **1955**, 2049. Total synthesis: Kutney, Fuller, *Heterocycles* **3**, 197 (1975).

Plates from ethanol+ water, mp 182°. $[\alpha]_D^{16}$ −745° (c = 0.994 in ethanol). pKa 7.45. uv max (ethanol): 227, 300, 330 nm (log ε 4.09, 4.07, 4.24).

Hydrochloride dihydrate. $C_{20}H_{22}N_2O_2 \cdot HCl \cdot 2H_2O$. Leaflets from alcohol or water, mp 171°. $[\alpha]_D^{21}$ −610° (c = 1.430 in ethanol).

Consult the Name Index before using this section.

Perchlorate monohydrate. $C_{20}H_{22}N_2O_2.HClO_4.H_2O$. Needles from ethanol + water, mp 134-136°.

Hydriodide monohydrate. $C_{20}H_{22}N_2O_2.HI.H_2O$. Square plates from water, mp 128°.

Methiodide. Crystals from water, mp 252°.

Nitrate. Needles from hot water, mp 182.5°.

200. Alacepril. [74258-86-9] 1-[(2S)-3-(Acetylthio)-2-methyl-1-oxopropyl]-L-prolyl-L-phenylalanine; 1-(D-3-acetylthio-2-methylpropanoyl)-L-prolyl-L-phenylalanine; N-[1-[(S)-3-mercapto-2-methylpropionyl]-L-prolyl]-3-phenyl-L-alanine acetate (ester); DU-1219; Cetapril. $C_{20}H_{26}N_2O_5S$; mol wt 406.50. C 59.09%, H 6.45%, N 6.89%, O 19.68%, S 7.89%. Angiotensin-converting enzyme (ACE) inhibitor. Prepn: T. Sawayama *et al.*, **JP Kokai 80 9058**; *idem*, **US 4248883** (1980, 1981 both to Dainippon Pharm.). Pharmacology in animals: K. Takeyama *et al.*, *Arzneim.-Forsch.* **35**, 1502 (1985); *idem, ibid.* 1507. Series of articles on pharmacology, metabolism, enzyme inhibiting activity: *ibid.* **36**, 47-83 (1986). Metabolism to captopril, *q.v.:* K. Matsumoto *et al.*, *ibid.* 40. HPLC determn of metabolites in plasma and urine: K. Hayashi *et al., J. Chromatogr.* **338**, 161 (1985). Pharmacokinetics in humans: K. Onoyama *et al., Clin. Pharmacol.* **38**, 462 (1985). Preclinical evaluation in essential hypertension: K. Mizuno *et al., Res. Commun. Chem. Pathol. Pharmacol.* **49**, 175 (1985); H. Shionoiri *et al., Curr. Ther. Res.* **38**, 537 (1985). Series of articles on toxicology: M. Iida *et al., Yakuri to Chiryo* **13**, 7033-7121 (1985), *C.A.* **104**, 21888h-21890c; **105**, 396v (1986).

Crystals from ethanol/*n*-hexane, mp 155-156°. $[\alpha]_D^{25}$ −81.3° (c = 1.02 in ethanol). LD_{50} in rats, mice (mg/kg): >5000, >5000 orally; >3000, >3000 s.c.; ~2000, ~3000 i.p. (Iida, pp 7033-40).

THERAP CAT: Antihypertensive.

201. Alachlor. [15972-60-8] 2-Chloro-N-(2,6-diethylphenyl)-N-(methoxymethyl)acetamide; 2-chloro-2′,6′-diethyl-N-(methoxymethyl)acetanilide; metachlor; CP-50144; Lasso; Alanex. $C_{14}H_{20}ClNO_2$; mol wt 269.77. C 62.33%, H 7.47%, Cl 13.14%, N 5.19%, O 11.86%. Pre-emergence herbicide. Prepn: **NL 6602564** (1967 to Monsanto), *C.A.* **67**, 99832r (1967). Activity: D. M. Evans, *Chem. Ind. (London)* **1969**, 615. Soil degradn: R. S. Hargrove, M. G. Merkle, *Weed Sci.* **19**, 652 (1971). Mechanism of action: L. M. Deal, F. D. Hess, *ibid.* **28**, 168 (1980).

Cryst solid, mp 40-41°. $d_{15.6}^{25}$ 1.133. Soly in water at 23°: 140 mg/l. Sol in ether, acetone, benzene, ethanol, ethyl acetate. Hydrolyzed under strong acid or alkaline conditions. LD_{50} orally in rats: 1200 mg/kg (Evans).

USE: Herbicide.

202. Alafosfalin. [60668-24-8] [(1R)-1-[[(2S)-2-Amino-1-oxopropyl]amino]ethyl]phosphonic acid; 1R-1-(L-alanylamino)ethylphosphonic acid; alaphosphin; Ro-3-7008. $C_5H_{13}N_2O_4P$; mol wt 196.14. C 30.62%, H 6.68%, N 14.28%, O 32.63%, P 15.79%. Synthetic phosphonodipeptide with antibacterial activity. Prepn: F. R. Atherton *et al.*, **DE 2602193**; *idem*, **US 4016148** (1976, 1977 both to Hoffmann-La Roche); J. G. Allen *et al., Nature* **272**, 56 (1978); F. R. Atherton *et al., Antimicrob. Agents Chemother.* **15**, 677 (1979). Improved process: E. K. Baylis, **EP 10872**; *idem*, **US 4331591** (1980, 1982 both to Ciba-Geigy). Separation of diaster-

eoisomers: J. Szewczyk *et al., Experientia* **38**, 983 (1982). Antibacterial spectrum: F. R. Atherton *et al., Antimicrob. Agents Chemother.* **15**, 684 (1979); W. H. Traub, *Chemotherapy* **26**, 103 (1980). Synergism with β-lactams: H. B. Maruyama *et al., Antimicrob. Agents Chemother.* **16**, 444 (1979); F. R. Atherton *et al., ibid.* **20**, 470 (1981); M. Arisawa *et al., ibid.* **21**, 706 (1982). Pharmacokinetics: J. D. Allen, L. J. Lees, *ibid.* **17**, 973 (1980). Comprehensive review: C. H. Hassall in *Antibiotics* VI, F. E. Hahn, Ed. (Springer-Verlag, New York, 1983) pp 1-11.

Crystals from ethanol-water, mp 295-296° (dec). $[\alpha]_D^{20}$ −44.0° (c = 1 in H_2O).

203. Alagebrium Chloride. [341028-37-3] 4,5-Dimethyl-3-(2-oxo-2-phenylethyl)thiazolium chloride; ALT-711. $C_{13}H_{14}$-ClNOS; mol wt 267.77. C 58.31%, H 5.27%, Cl 13.24%, N 5.23%, O 5.98%, S 11.97%. Catalytically cleaves crosslinks between advanced glycation end products (AGE) and extracellular matrix proteins. Prepn: A. Cerami *et al.*, **EP 808163**; *idem*, **US 5853703** (1997, 1998 both to Alteon; Picower Inst. Med. Res.). *In vivo* AGE cross-link breaking activity: B. H. R. Wolffenbuttel *et al., Proc. Natl. Acad. Sci. USA* **95**, 4630 (1998). Clinical pharmacology and effect on vascular stiffening: D. A. Kass *et al., Circulation* **104**, 1464 (2001); in elderly patients with heart failure: W. C. Little *et al., J. Cardiac Failure* **11**, 191 (2005). Review of pharmacology and therapeutic potential: S. Vasan *et al., Arch. Biochem. Biophys.* **419**, 89-96 (2003); of clinical evaluations in cardiovascular disease: G. L. Bakris *et al., Am. J. Hypertens.* **17**, 23S-30S (2004).

THERAP CAT: In treatment of cardiovascular complications of diabetes and aging.

204. Alanine. [56-41-7] L-Alanine; Ala; A; L-α-alanine; L-α-aminopropionic acid; (S)-2-aminopropanoic acid. $C_3H_7NO_2$; mol wt 89.09. C 40.44%, H 7.92%, N 15.72%, O 35.92%. Nonessential amino acid for human development. First syllable of the name denotes its origin from aldehyde. First synthesized and named by: A. Strecker, *Ann.* **75**, 27 (1850); prior to identification in silk hydrolysate: P. Schützenberger, A. Bourgeous, *Compt. Rend.* **81**, 191 (1875); Th. Weyl, *Ber.* **21**, 1407 (1888). Early chemistry and biochemistry: *Amino Acids and Proteins*, D. M. Greenberg, Ed. (Charles C. Thomas, Springfield, IL, 1951) 950 pp., *passim*; J. P. Greenstein, M. Winitz, *Chemistry of the Amino Acids* vols 1-3 (John Wiley and Sons, Inc., New York, 1961) pp. 1819-1840, *passim*. Enantiomeric selective synthesis: R. Amoroso *et al., J. Org. Chem.* **57**, 1082 (1992). Review of metabolism in man: J. E. Liljenquist *et al., Clin. Nutr. Update*, H. L. Greene *et al.*, Eds. (American Medical Association, Chicago, IL, 1977) pp 22-34; T. N. Palmer *et al., Biosci. Rep.* **5**, 1015-1033 (1985). Review of industrial production by microorganisms: S. Takamatsu, T. Tosa, *Bioprocess Technol.* **16**, 25-35 (1993).

Orthorhombic crystals from water, dec 297°. d 1.401. $[\alpha]_D^{25}$ +2.42° (c = 10 in H_2O); +13.7° (c = 2.06 in 6N HCl). pK_1 2.34; pK_2 9.69. Soly (g/l) in water at 0°: 127.3; at 25°: 166.5; at 50°: 217.9; at 75°: 285.1; at 100°: 373.0. Soly in cold 80% ethanol: 0.2%. Insol in ether.

D-Form. [338-69-2] Occurs in bacterial cell walls and in some peptide antibiotics. *Review:* M. Bodanszky, D. Perlman, *Science* **163**, 352-358 (1969); C. T. Walsh, *J. Biol. Chem.* **264**, 2393-2396 (1989). Crystals, mp 289-291°. $[\alpha]_D$ −14.1° (c = 0.9 in 1*N* HCl).

DL-Form. [302-72-7] Orthorhombic bipyramidal needles or rods from water. d 1.424. Sublimes above 200°. Decomp 264-296° depending on rate of heating. pK$_1$ 2.35; pK$_2$ 9.87. Soly in water at 0°: 121 g/l, at 25°: 167 g/l, at 50°: 231 g/l, at 75°: 319 g/l, at 100°: 440 g/l; in ethanol 0.0087 g/100 g at 25°. Insol in ether.

205. β-Alanine. [107-95-9] β-Aminopropionic acid; 3-aminopropanoic acid; 3-aminopropionic acid; Abufène. $C_3H_7NO_2$; mol wt 89.09. C 40.44%, H 7.92%, N 15.72%, O 35.92%. NH_2-$CH_2CH_2CO_2H$. Prepd by the action of KOBr and KOH upon succinimide: Clarke, Behr, *Org. Synth.* **16**, 1 (1936). By the action of liq ammonia upon methyl acrylate: Morsch, *Monatsh. Chem.* **63**, 220 (1933), *cf. C.A.* **41**, 4104 (1947); by the addition of NH_4OH to acrylonitrile: Ford *et al., J. Am. Chem. Soc.* **69**, 844 (1947). By electrolytic oxidation of 3-amino-1-propanol in H_2SO_4 using Pb electrodes without diaphragm: *Jubilee Vol. Emil Barell* **1946**, 85-91. For industrial methods of prepn *see* several pats. by T. L. Gresham to B. F. Goodrich. Prepn from ethylene cyanohydrin (β-hydroxypropionitrile): Boatright, *US 2734081* (1956 to Am. Cyanamid); from β-aminopropionitrile: Ford, *Org. Synth.* **coll. vol. III**, 34 (1955). Improved process: Beutel, Klemchuk, *US 2956080* (1960 to Merck & Co.).

Orthorhombic bipyramidal crystals from water, decomp 207° (very rapid heating). Decomp 197-198° (Ford, *Org. Syn. loc. cit.*). Slightly sweet taste. pK$_1$ 3.60; pK$_2$ 10.19. pH of 5% aq soln: 6.0 to 7.3. Freely sol in water, slightly in alcohol. Practically insol in ether, acetone.

Hydrochloride. $C_3H_7NO_2$.HCl. Plates, leaflets, mp 122.5°. Freely sol in water, less sol in alcohol, insol in ether.

Platinichloride. $2C_3H_7NO_2$.2HCl.PtCl$_4$. Yellow leaflets from alcohol + HCl, decomp 210°. Freely sol in water, sparingly in abs alcohol.

USE: In the synthesis of pantothenic acid and derivatives; as buffer in electroplating.

206. L-Alanosine. [5854-93-3] 3-(Hydroxynitrosoamino)-L-alanine; L-2-amino-3-(hydroxynitrosoamino)propanoic acid; L-2-amino-3-[(*N*-nitroso)hydroxylamino]propionic acid. $C_3H_7N_3O_4$; mol wt 149.11. C 24.16%, H 4.73%, N 28.18%, O 42.92%. Antibiotic substance from the fermentation of *Streptomyces alanosinicus* n. sp. Prepn: *NL 6509543*; J. Thiemann, Y. S. K. Murthy, *US 3676490* (1966, 1972 both to Lepetit). The first natural product found to have a *N*-nitrosohydroxylamino group on an aliphatic chain. Isoln and structure: Coronelli *et al., Farmaco Ed. Sci.* **21**, 269 (1966). Characterization: Thiemann, Beretta, *J. Antibiot.* **19A**, 155 (1966). Structure and synthesis of L-, D- and DL-forms: Lancini *et al., Tetrahedron Lett.* **1966**, 1769; *eidem, Farmaco Ed. Sci.* **24**, 169 (1969). Synthesis of L-form: Isowa *et al., Bull. Chem. Soc. Jpn.* **46**, 1847 (1973). Improved synthesis of DL-form: Eaton *et al., J. Med. Chem.* **16**, 289 (1973). Pharmacology: Murthy *et al., Nature* **211**, 1198 (1966). Mode of action studies: Gale *et al., Biochem. Pharmacol.* **17**, 363, 1823 (1968). Effect on insect growth: E. E. Kenaga, *J. Econ. Entomol.* **62**, 1006 (1969); S. Matsumoto *et al., Agric. Biol. Chem.* **48**, 827 (1984).

Crystalline powder from slightly acidic water, dec 190°. $[\alpha]_D$ +8°, −46°, −37.8° (in 1*N* HCl, 0.1*N* NaOH, water). uv max (0.1*N* HCl): 228 nm (E$_{1cm}^{1\%}$ 505); in 0.1*N* NaOH: 250 nm (E$_{1cm}^{1\%}$ 630). pKa 4.8. Slightly sol in water; practically insol in the common organic solvents. Sol in alkaline and acidic solns, from which it ppts by adjusting the pH between 4 and 6. LD$_{50}$ in mice (mg/kg): 600 i.p.; 300 i.v. (Thiemann, Murthy).

D-Form. mp 183°. $[\alpha]_D$ +45° (c = 0.5*N* in 1*N* HCl).

USE: Experimental insect reproduction inhibitor.

207. Alantolactone. [546-43-0] [3a*R*-(3aα,5β,8aβ,9aα)]-3a,5,6,7,8,8a,9,9a-Octahydro-5,8a-dimethyl-3-methylenenaphtho[2,3-*b*]furan-2(3*H*)-one; 8β-hydroxy-4αH-eudesm-5-en-12-oic acid γ-lactone; helenin; alant camphor; elecampane camphor; inula camphor. $C_{15}H_{20}O_2$; mol wt 232.32. C 77.55%, H 8.68%, O 13.77%. A terpene from roots of *Inula helenium* L., *Compositae:* Kallen, *Ber.* **6**, 1506 (1873); **9**, 154 (1876); Ruzicka *et al., Helv. Chim. Acta* **14**, 397, 1090 (1931); **16**, 268 (1933). Structure: Marshall, Cohen, *J. Org. Chem.* **29**, 3727 (1964). Stereoselective synthesis: Marshall *et al., J. Am. Chem. Soc.* **88**, 3408 (1966).

Crystals from alcohol, mp 78-79°. bp 275°. $[\alpha]_D$ +175° (chloroform). uv max (ethanol): 212 nm (ε 9500). Volatile with steam. Freely sol in alcohol, chloroform, benzene, ether, oils. Practically insol in water.

208. Alazopeptin. [1397-84-8] L-Alanyl-(6-diazo-5-oxo)-L-norleucyl-(6-diazo-5-oxo)-L-norleucine. $C_{15}H_{20}N_6O_5$; mol wt 364.36. C 49.45%, H 5.53%, N 23.07%, O 21.96%. Tumor-inhibiting antibiotic produced by *Streptomyces griseoplanus* from soil near Williamsburg, Iowa: De Voe *et al., Antibiot. Annu.* **1956-7**, p 730. Peptide consisting of one mole α-alanine and two moles of a C$_6$ diazo keto amino acid oxidizable to glutamic acid: E. L. Patterson *et al., Antimicrob. Agents Chemother.* **1965**, 115-118. Antitumor activity: T. Hata *et al., J. Antibiot.* **26**, 181 (1973). Toxicity: J. B. Thiersch, *Proc. Soc. Exp. Biol. Med.* **97**, 888 (1958).

Monohydrate. Crystals from dilute acetone. Poor stability. Has no definite melting point. $[\alpha]_D^{25}$ +9.5° (c = 4.7 in H_2O). uv max (pH 7.0 phosphate buffer): 242, 274 nm (E$_{1cm}^{1\%}$ 321, 549). Freely sol in water. Somewhat sol in acetic acid, formamide, DMSO, aq solns of methanol, ethanol, acetone. Practically insol in anhyd alcohols, acetone, ethyl acetate, ether. LD$_{50}$ i.p. in rats: 150 mg/kg (Thiersch).

209. Albaspidin. [58409-52-2] 2,2′-Methylenebis[6-butyryl-3,5-dihydroxy-4,4-dimethyl-2,5-cyclohexadien-1-one]; polystichalbin; methylenebis(butyrylfilicinic acid); albaspidin-BB. C_{25}-$H_{32}O_8$; mol wt 460.52. C 65.20%, H 7.00%, O 27.79%. Found in the rhizomes of the male fern, *Aspidium filix mas* (L.) Schott., *Dryopteris filix mas* (L.) Schott., *A. spinulosum, Polypodiaceae* and other ferns. Isoln from *Aspidium* extract: Boehm, *Ann.* **318**, 305 (1901); McGookin *et al., J. Chem. Soc.* **1953**, 1828; *see also* Tryon *et al., Phytochemistry* **12**, 683 (1973). Isoln as one component of a homologous mixture: Penttila, Sundman, *Acta Chem. Scand.* **18**, 344 (1964). Synthesis: Riedl, Mitteldorf, *Ber.* **89**, 2595 (1956); Inagaki *et al., J. Pharm. Soc. Jpn.* **76**, 1258 (1956). Biosynthetic studies: Penttila, Fales, *J. Am. Chem. Soc.* **88**, 2327 (1966).

Crystals from ethanol or methanol, mp 149°. Freely sol in chloroform; moderately sol in ether, benzene; sparingly sol in alc, acetone, glacial acetic acid, sol in KOH solns; very sparingly sol in Na_2CO_3 solns. Practically insol in methanol.

Consult the Name Index before using this section.

210. Albendazole. [54965-21-8] [5-(Propylthio)-1H-benz-imidazol-2-yl]carbamic acid methyl ester; methyl 5-(propylthio)-2-benzimidazolecarbamate; 5-(propylthio)-2-carbomethoxyamino-benzimidazole; SKF-62979; Albenza; Eskazole; Valbazen; Zentel. $C_{12}H_{15}N_3O_2S$; mol wt 265.33. C 54.32%, H 5.70%, N 15.84%, O 12.06%, S 12.08%. Prepn: R. J. Gyurik, V. J. Theodorides, **US 3915986** (1975 to SmithKline). Anthelmintic spectrum: V. J. Theodorides, *Experientia* **32**, 702 (1976). Metabolism: R. J. Gyurik *et al., Drug Metab. Dispos.* **9**, 503 (1981). Efficacy in cattle vs gastrointestinal parasites: J. C. Williams *et al., Am. J. Vet. Res.* **38**, 2037 (1977); vs liver flukes: T. M. Craig *et al., ibid.* **53**, 1170 (1992). Clinical trial in mixed helminth infections: P. Pene *et al., Am. J. Trop. Med. Hyg.* **31**, 263 (1982); in echinococcosis: R. J. Horton, *Trans. R. Soc. Trop. Med. Hyg.* **83**, 97 (1989).

Colorless crystals, mp 208-210°. Sol in DMSO, strong acids, strong bases; slightly sol in methanol, chloroform, ethyl acetate, acetonitrile. Practically insol in water.

Sulfoxide. [54029-12-8] Albendazole oxide; ricobendazole; rycobendazole; RS-8852; Rycoben. $C_{12}H_{15}N_3O_3S$; mol wt 281.33. Active metabolite of albendazole. Bioavailability: L. Dominguez *et al., Farmaco* **50**, 697 (1995). mp 226-228° (dec).

THERAP CAT: Anthelmintic (Cestodes).
THERAP CAT (VET): Anthelmintic.

211. Albizziin. [1483-07-4] 3-[(Aminocarbonyl)amino]-L-alanine; 2-amino-3-ureidopropionic acid. $C_4H_9N_3O_3$; mol wt 147.13. C 32.65%, H 6.17%, N 28.56%, O 32.62%. NH_2-CONHCH$_2$CH(NH$_2$)COOH. Constituent of several plants belonging to the family *Mimosaceae*. First obtained from the seeds of *Albizzia julibrissin* Durazz., *Mimosaceae:* Gmelin *et al., Z. Naturforsch.* **13b**, 252 (1958); *Z. Physiol. Chem.* **314**, 28 (1959). Structure: Kjaer *et al., Experientia* **15**, 253 (1959). Synthesis: Kjaer, Larsen, *Acta Chem. Scand.* **13**, 1565 (1959); Rudinger *et al., Collect. Czech. Chem. Commun.* **25**, 2022 (1960).

Needles from dil alcohol, decomp 218-220°. $[\alpha]_D^{25}$ −66.2° (c = 4 in H$_2$O); $[\alpha]_D^{24}$ −22.2° (c = 4.24 in 1.0N HCl); $[\alpha]_D^{24}$ +3.2° (c = 4.7 in 1.0N NaOH). ORD data: Kjaer *et al., Acta Chem. Scand.* **18**, 2412 (1964).

212. Albofungin. [37895-35-5] [1S-(1α,4α,8aα)]-13-Amino-3,4,8a,13-tetrahydro-1,15,16-trihydroxy-4-methoxy-12-methyl-1H-xantheno[4',3',2':4,5][1,3]benzodioxino[7,6-g]isoquinoline-14,-17(2H,9H)-dione. $C_{27}H_{24}N_2O_9$; mol wt 520.49. C 62.30%, H 4.65%, N 5.38%, O 27.67%. Antifungal antibiotic produced by *Streptomyces albus* var *fungistaticus (fungatus)* Solovyeva et Rudaya. Isoln procedure: Khokhlov, Liberman, *Proc. Symp. Antibiotics Prague* (May 1959) p 81. Structure: A. I. Gurevich *et al., Tetrahedron Lett.* **1972**, 1751. Stereochemistry: A. I. Gurevich *et al., ibid.* **1974**, 2801. Thought to be identical with *Ba-180265* described by Liu *et al.,* in *Antimicrob. Agents Chemother.* **1962**, 767. Chemical and biological properties: A.I. Gurevich *et al., Antibiotiki* **17**, 771 (1972).

Crystals from nitromethane, mp 304-307°. Also reported as mp 190° (dec). $[\alpha]_D^{20}$ −670° (DMF). uv max (ethanol): 228, 254,

303, 376 nm (log ε 4.58, 4.58, 4.19, 4.42). Practically insol in water, petr ether. Sparingly sol in alcohol; quite sol in chloroform, dichloroethane, acetone, chlorobenzene, formamide, dimethylformamide, glacial acetic acid.

213. Albomycin. [1414-39-7] Iron-containing antibiotic produced by *Actinomyces subtropicus:* Gauze, Braznikova, *Nov. Med.* **23**, 3 (1951). Used as the sulfate. Consists of six components, α, β, γ, δ$_1$, δ$_2$, ε, of which δ$_1$ and δ$_2$ are the main components. δ$_2$ is the unstable, highly active albomycin A$_1$; the other components are its degradation products: Braznikova *et al., Biokhimiya* **22**, 111 (1959); Turkovà *et al., Antibiotiki* **7**, 878 (1962). Early studies proposed cyclic hexapeptide structures containing three serines and three ornithine derivatives for δ$_1$-, δ$_2$- and ε-albomycin (cf. Ferrichromes). Structural studies: *eidem., Collect. Czech. Chem. Commun.* **30**, 118 (1965); Poddubnaya, el'Naggar, *Zh. Obshch. Khim.* **38**, 450 (1968). Conflicting structural analysis shows a 3:1 ornithine : serine ratio: Maehr, Pitcher, *J. Antibiot.* **24**, 830 (1971). Similarity to or identity with grisein, q.v.: Stapley, Ormond, *Science* **125**, 587 (1957); Turková *et al., Collect. Czech. Chem. Commun.* **31**, 2444 (1966). Review and antibacterial spectrum of albomycin and other hydroxamic acids: Gauze, *Br. Med. J.* **2**, 1177 (1955); Bhuyan in *Antibiotics* **1**, D. Gottlieb, P. D. Shaw, Eds. (Springer-Verlag, New York, 1967) pp 153-155; Maehr, *Pure Appl. Chem.* **28**, 603-636 (1971); Emery, *Adv. Enzymol. Relat. Areas Mol. Biol.* **35**, 135-185 (1971).

Sulfate. Amorphous red powder. uv max: 283 nm (E$_{1cm}^{1\%}$ 880). Freely sol in water. Slightly sol in methanol. Practically insol in most other organic solvents. Aq solns have a bright orange color. Effective against penicillin-resistant pneumococci and staphylococci. The toxicity is comparable to that of penicillin.

Note: Not to be confused with albamycin.

214. Alborixin. [57760-36-8] Antibiotic S 14750A. C_{48}-$H_{84}O_{14}$; mol wt 885.17. C 65.13%, H 9.57%, O 25.30%. Polycyclic polyether antibiotic ionophore, isolated from a strain of *Streptomyces albus*. Initial description and x-ray structure: M. Allèaume *et al., Chem. Commun.* **1975**, 411. Production from *Streptomyces hygroscopicus* and use: M. Kuhn, H. D. King, **DE 2608337** (1976 to Sandoz), *C.A.* **86**, 28491k (1977). Isoln from *S. albus,* structure, properties: P. Gachon *et al., J. Antibiot.* **29**, 603 (1976); C. Delhomme *et al., ibid.* 692. NMR spectrum and solution conformation: N. A. Rodios, M. J. O. Anteunis, *Bull. Soc. Chim. Belg.* **88**, 279 (1979). Revised structure: H. Seto *et al., J. Antibiot.* **32**, 970 (1979). *In vitro* study: M. Chapel *et al., ibid.* 740. Effects on cardiovascular function and plasma cation concentration in the dog: N. Moins *et al., J. Cardiovasc. Pharmacol.* **1**, 659 (1979).

White amorphous powder, mp 100-105°. $[\alpha]^{20}$ −7° (c = 4 in acetone). pKa 10.02 (25° in methanol). LD$_{50}$ in mice: 15 mg/kg s.c. (Delhomme). LD$_{50}$ originally reported as 150 mg/kg, corrected in *J. Antibiot.* **30**, Suppl. (1977), facing p 77-12.

215. Albumen. Egg white; dried egg white. By convention the pure protein is spelled "albumin" and commercial egg white is called "albumen". The word "albumen" goes back to Roman times and is classical Latin for egg white: *Ref:* Plinius (Major), *Historia Naturalis* **28**, 6, 18 paragraph 66. Constitutes about six parts by weight of a hen's egg (wet basis). Average weight of raw egg white 32.9 g. Albumen contains 75% ovalbumin, (q.v.), ovoconalbumin, ovomucoid, ovomucin, ovoglobulin, lysozyme, (q.v.) and avidin, (q.v.). Monograph: A. L. Romanoff, A. J. Romanoff, *The Avian Egg* (Wiley, New York, 1949) 918 pp.

Raw egg albumen. Clear, colloidal, flowing, limpid mass. White rubbery solid when denatured. d$_{25}^{25}$ 1.035. n$_D^{25}$ 1.356. Coagulating temp 61°. mp −0.42°. pH 7.6.

Dried albumen. Yellow, transparent, amorphous lumps or scales, or yellow powder. Decomposes in moist air. In water it swells at first, then dissolves gradually. The soln coagulates at 61° (because of denaturation of the proteins). Albumen solns are also denatured on contact with the following chemicals: Salts of copper, iron, mercury and silver; H_2O_2, phenol, picric acid, alum, tannic acid, formaldehyde, ether, alcohol.

USE: For clarifying and refining wines and vinegars. As textile dye mordant, in lithography as vehicle for substances that sensitize plates, in gilding leather (Venetian decorations), stamping with gold and bronze powder (especially in book binding). In adhesives and veneers. Ingredient of compositions used in sizing and in making papers. In fine color preparations for artist's paints. As activating agent for certain enzymes. Formerly in sugar refining. Ingredient of bakery products, confectionery, food preparations. In pharmaceutical compounding, i.e. to make various albuminates. As analytical reagent in testing for ionic mercury, foreign oil in olive oil, candy or wine colorings.

THERAP CAT: Antidote to mercury poisoning.

216. Albuterol. [18559-94-9] α^1-[[(1,1-Dimethylethyl)-amino]methyl]-4-hydroxy-1,3-benzenedimethanol; α^1-[(tert-butyl-amino)methyl]-4-hydroxy-m-xylene-α,α'-diol; 2-(tert-butylamino)-1-(4-hydroxy-3-hydroxymethylphenyl)ethanol; 4-hydroxy-3-hy-droxymethyl-α-[(tert-butylamino)methyl]benzyl alcohol; salbuta-mol; AH-3365. $C_{13}H_{21}NO_3$; mol wt 239.31. C 65.25%, H 8.84%, N 5.85%, O 20.06%. β-Adrenergic agonist. Prepn: L. H. C. Lunts et al., ZA 6705591; eidem, US 3644353 (1968, 1972 both to Allen & Hanburys). Synthesis and structure-activity studies: D. T. Collin et al., J. Med. Chem. **13**, 674 (1970). Prepn of isomers: C. J. Hawkins, G. T. Klease, ibid. **16**, 856 (1973); R. P. Bakale, Spec. Chem. **15**, 249 (1995). Absolute configuration of isomers: D. Hartley, D. Middlemiss, J. Med. Chem. **14**, 895 (1971). Pharmacology: R. T. Brittain et al., Nature **219**, 862 (1968); V. A. Cullum et al., Br. J. Pharmacol. **35**, 141 (1969). Metabolism: L. E. Martin et al., Eur. J. Pharmacol. **14**, 183 (1971). Clinical comparison of levalbuterol with racemate: H. S. Nelson et al., J. Allergy Clin. Immunol. **102**, 943 (1998). Comprehensive description: H. Y. Aboul-Enein et al., Anal. Profiles Drug Subs. **10**, 665-689 (1981). Review of clinical experience in asthma and in preterm labor: A. H. Price, S. P. Clissold, Drugs **38**, 77-122 (1989); of toxicology: S. E. Libretto, Arch. Toxicol. **68**, 213-216 (1994). Review of clinical trials for add-on therapy to inhaled steroids: S. Shrewsbury et al., Br. Med. J. **320**, 1368-1373 (2000).

Crystalline powder from ethanol-ethyl acetate or ethyl acetate-cyclohexane, mp 151° (Lunts); 157-158° (Collin). Sol in most organic solvents.

Sulfate. [51022-70-9] Aerolin; Asmaven; Cobutolin; Ecovent; Loftan; Proventil; Salbulin; Salbumol; Salbutard; Salbuvent; Sultanol; Venetlin; Ventilastin; Ventodisks; Ventolin; Volmax. $(C_{13}H_{21}-NO_3)_2.H_2SO_4$; mol wt 576.70. White crystalline powder. Sol in water; slightly sol in ethanol.

(R)-Form. [34391-04-3] Levalbuterol; levosalbutamol.

(R)-Form hydrochloride. [50293-90-8] Xopenex. $C_{13}H_{21}-NO_3.HCl$; mol wt 275.77. Crystallized as the monohydrate; changes crystalline form at 175°; dec 188-195°. $[\alpha]_D^{20}$ $-32.2°$ (c = 0.1 in water).

THERAP CAT: Bronchodilator; tocolytic.

217. Albutoin. [830-89-7] 5-(2-Methylpropyl)-3-(2-pro-penyl)-2-thioxo-4-imidazolidinone; 3-allyl-5-isobutyl-2-thio-hydantoin; 3-allyl-5-sec-butyl-2-thiohydantoin; CO-ORD; Euprax. $C_{10}H_{16}N_2OS$; mol wt 212.31. C 56.57%, H 7.60%, N 13.19%, O 7.54%, S 15.10%. Prepn: Oba et al., C.A. **46**, 3885f (1952).

Crystals, mp 210-211°.

USE: Fog inhibitor in photography.

THERAP CAT: Anticonvulsant.

218. Alcian Blue. [12040-44-7] C.I. Ingrain Blue 1; C.I. 74240; alcian blue 8GX; michrome no. 24. When R = toluyl, the mol wt is about 1300. Discovered by Haddock and Wood in 1944: Haddock, Research **1**, 685 (1948); GB 586340 and GB 587636 (both to ICI). During dyeing the X groups split off. Prepn: Colour Index vol. **4** (3rd ed.) p 4620.

X = an onium group, e.g. $—CH_2S—$
(R = alkyl or aryl)

Greenish-black crystals with metallic sheen. When R = toluyl the solubility in water at 20° is about 9.5% w/w giving bright greenish-blue solutions. Soly in absolute ethanol about 6.0, Cellosolve 6.0, ethylene glycol 3.25. Practically insoluble in xylene.

USE: Gelling agent for lubricating fluids. As bacterial stain. To dye histiocytes and fibroblasts in vivo: McManus, Bailie, Fed. Proc. **22**, no. 2, part I, p 190 (March-April 1963).

219. Alclofenac. [22131-79-9] 3-Chloro-4-(2-propenyl-oxy)benzeneacetic acid; [4-(allyloxy)-3-chlorophenyl]acetic acid; W-7320; Allopydin; Epinal; Mervan; Reufenac. $C_{11}H_{11}ClO_3$; mol wt 226.66. C 58.29%, H 4.89%, Cl 15.64%, O 21.18%. Prepn: N. P. Buu-Hoi et al., BE 704368 (1968 to Madan). Pharmacology: eidem, Naturwissenschaften **56**, 330 (1969). Series of articles on pharmacology, toxicology and metabolism: Arzneim.-Forsch. **20**, 610-636 (1970). Toxicity data: G. Lambelin et al., ibid. 618. Clinical studies: F. Lambotte, ibid. 569; Van Hoek, Curr. Ther. Res. **12**, 551 (1970).

Prisms from cyclohexane, mp 92-93°. LD_{50} in mice, rats (mg/kg): 1100, 1050 orally; 600, 630 s.c.; 555, 530 i.p. (Lambelin).

Monoethanolamine complex. [22131-80-2] Mirvan. $C_{13}H_{18}-ClNO_4$; mol wt 287.74.

THERAP CAT: Analgesic; antipyretic; anti-inflammatory.

220. Alclometasone. [67452-97-5] (7α,11β,16α)-7-Chloro-11,17,21-trihydroxy-16-methylpregna-1,4-diene-3,20-dione; 7α-chloro-16α-methylprednisolone. $C_{22}H_{29}ClO_5$; mol wt 408.92. C 64.62%, H 7.15%, Cl 8.67%, O 19.56%. Non-fluorinated corticosteroid with low systemic effects. Prepn: M. J. Green et al., US 4076708; M. J. Green, H. J. Shue, US 4124707 (both 1978 to Schering); M. J. Green et al., J. Steroid Biochem. **11**, 61 (1979); H. J. Shue et al., J. Med. Chem. **23**, 430 (1980). Topical anti-inflammatory activity of the 17,21-dipropionate: B. Lutsky et al., Arzneim.-Forsch. **29**, 992 (1979); M. J. Green et al., ibid. **30**, 1618 (1980).

Crystals from acetone/hexane, mp 176-179°. $[\alpha]_D^{26}$ +47.5° (c = 0.3 in DMF). uv max (methanol): 242 nm (ε 15500).

17,21-Dipropionate. [66734-13-2] Sch-22219; Aclosone; Aclovate; Almeta; Delonal; Legederm; Modrasone; Perderm. $C_{28}H_{37}ClO_7$; mol wt 521.04. Crystals from acetone/methanol/isopropyl ether, mp 212-216°. $[\alpha]_D^{26}$ +42.6° (c = 0.3 in DMF). uv max (methanol): 242 nm (ε 15600).

THERAP CAT: Anti-inflammatory (topical).

221. Alcuronium. [23214-96-2] 4,4′-Didemethyl-4,4′-di-2-propenyltoxiferine I; N,N′-diallylnortoxiferinium; diallylbis(nortoxiferine); diallylnortoxiferine; diallyltoxiferine. $[C_{44}H_{50}N_4O_2]^{2+}$. Prepn of dichloride and diiodide: Boller et al., US 3080373 (1963 to Hoffmann-La Roche).

Dichloride. [15180-03-7] N,N′-Diallylnortoxiferinium dichloride; Ro-4-3816; Alloferin. $C_{44}H_{50}Cl_2N_4O_2$; mol wt 737.80. Crystals from methanol or ethanol. Compd contains 5 moles of water of crystn after equilibration in air; $[\alpha]_D^{22}$ −348° (methanol); uv max (methanol): 292 nm (ε 43000).

Diiodide. $C_{44}H_{50}I_2N_4O_2$. Solid. uv max (methanol): 291 nm (ε 39900).

THERAP CAT: Neuromuscular blocking agent.

THERAP CAT (VET): Neuromuscular blocking agent.

222. Aldicarb. [116-06-3] 2-Methyl-2-(methylthio)propanal O-[(methylamino)carbonyl]oxime; 2-methyl-2-(methylthio)propionaldehyde O-(methylcarbamoyl)oxime; UC-21149; Temik. $C_7H_{14}N_2O_2S$; mol wt 190.26. C 44.19%, H 7.42%, N 14.72%, O 16.82%, S 16.85%. Prepn: L. K. Payne, Jr., M. H. J. Weiden, FR 1377474; eidem, US 3217037 (1963, 1965 both to Union Carbide); L. K. Payne, Jr. et al., J. Agric. Food Chem. **14**, 356 (1966). Metabolism: W. J. Bartley et al., ibid. **18**, 446 (1970). Crystal and molecular structure: F. Takusagawa, R. A. Jacobson, ibid. **25**, 333 (1977). HPLC-APCI-MS determn in fruits and vegetables: G. S. Nunes et al., J. Chromatogr. A **888**, 113 (2000). Efficacy for control of nematodes on potato: S. L. Hafez et al., Nematol. Mediterranea **30**, 227 (2002); of thrips on cotton: K. H. Lohmeyer et al., J. Econ. Entomol. **96**, 748 (2003). Efficacy on citrus and economic analysis: L. Blakeley et al., HortTechnology **13**, 694 (2003). Review: R. R. Romine, Anal. Methods Pestic. Plant Growth Regul. **7**, 147-162 (1979). Review of persistence in soil and root crops: A. C. Maheshwari, V. S. Kavadia, Pesticides **19**, 30-31 (1985); of groundwater contamination: H. A. Moye, C. J. Miles, Rev. Environ. Contam. Toxicol. **105**, 99-146 (1988). Review of toxicology: R. L. Baron, T. L. Merriam, ibid. **105**, 1-70 (1988); idem, Environ. Health Perspect. **102**, Suppl. 11, 23-27 (1994).

Crystals from isopropyl ether, mp 99-100° with dec >100°. d_4^{25} 1.195. Vapor pressure (25°): 1×10^{-4} mmHg. Sparingly sol in

water and certain organic solvents, most sol in chloroform and acetone. Percent soly: acetone 28 (10°), 43 (30°), 50 (50°); benzene 9 (10°), 24 (30°), 49 (50°); carbon tetrachloride 2 (10°), 5 (30°), 25 (50°); chloroform 38 (10°), 44 (30°), 50 (50°); methyl isobutyl ketone 13 (10°), 24 (30°), 42 (50°); toluene 10 (10°), 12 (30°), 33 (50°); water 0.4 (10°), 0.9 (30°), 1.4 (50°). LD_{50} in male and female rats (mg/kg): 0.81-0.93, 0.67-1.20 orally. LC_{50} (96 hr) in rainbow trout, bluegill sunfish (ppb): 560-580, 50-100 (Baron, 1988).

USE: Insecticide, acaricide, nematocide.

223. Aldioxa. [5579-81-7] [(2,5-Dioxo-4-imidazolidinyl)ureato]dihydroxyaluminum; (allantoinato)dihydroxyaluminum; dihydroxy[(4,5-dihydro-2-hydroxy-5-oxo-1H-imidazol-4-yl)ureato]aluminum; aluminum dihydroxy allantoinate; RC-172; Alanetorin; Alusa; Arlanto; Ascomp; Chlokale; Isalon; Nische; Peptilate. $C_4H_7AlN_4O_5$; mol wt 218.10. C 22.03%, H 3.24%, Al 12.37%, N 25.69%, O 36.68%. Prepn: S. B. Mecca, US 2761867 (1956 to Schuylkill Chem.). Pharmacology: R. Cahen, J. F. Clement, Ann. Pharm. Fr. **20**, 693 (1962); R Cahen, A. Pessonnier, ibid. 704. Toxicology: R. Cahen, A. Pessonnier, ibid. 623. Metabolism studies: K. Fukawa et al., Oyo Yakuri **11**, 421 (1976), C.A. **88**, 130701g (1978). HPLC determn in plasma: K. Hirota et al., J. Chromatogr. **277**, 165 (1983). Clinical studies of combination therapy for peptic ulcer: M. Sakai et al., Jpn. Arch. Intern. Med. **31**, 275 (1984); idem et al., ibid. **33**, 61 (1986); idem et al., ibid. **36**, 357 (1989). Review of cosmetic use and safety assessment: S. N. J. Pang, J. Am. Coll. Toxicol. **12**, 237-242 (1993).

White powder. mp 230°. Insol in polar and nonpolar solvents.

USE: Astringent and skin conditioning agent in cosmetics.

THERAP CAT: Antiulcerative.

224. Aldol. [107-89-1] 3-Hydroxybutanal; 3-hydroxybutyraldehyde; acetaldol. $C_4H_8O_2$; mol wt 88.11. C 54.53%, H 9.15%, O 36.32%. $CH_3CH(OH)CH_2CHO$. Manuf by condensation of acetaldehyde in aq NaOH: Alhéritière, Gobron, US 2713598 (1955 to Usines de Melle). Toxicity study: H. F. Smyth et al., J. Ind. Hyg. Toxicol. **31**, 60 (1949).

Colorless, thick liquid. d^{16} 1.109. bp_{20} 83°; dec about 85°. Miscible with water, alcohol, ether. LD_{50} orally in rats: 2.18 g/kg (Smyth).

USE: Manuf rubber vulcanizers, accelerators and age resisters; in perfumes; ore flotation.

225. Aldosterone. [52-39-1] (11β)-11,21-Dihydroxy-3,20-dioxopregn-4-en-18-al; 3,20-diketo-11β,18-oxido-4-pregnene-18,21-diol; Aldocorten. $C_{21}H_{28}O_5$; mol wt 360.44. C 69.98%, H 7.83%, O 22.19%. Adrenocortical steroid which exerts regulatory influence on metabolism of electrolytes and water. Isoln: Simpson et al., Experientia **9**, 333 (1953); Helv. Chim. Acta **37**, 1163 (1954); Mattox et al., J. Am. Chem. Soc. **75**, 4869 (1953); Harman et al., ibid. **76**, 5035 (1954). Solutions contain an equilibrium mixture of the aldehyde and the hemiacetal, the equilibrium favoring the latter. Structure: Tait et al., Experientia **10**, 132 (1954); Helv. Chim. Acta **37**, 1200 (1954). Crystal structure and molecular conformation: Duax, Hauptmann, J. Am. Chem. Soc. **94**, 5467 (1972). ^{13}C-NMR spectrum: P. Gerard, Org. Magn. Reson. **11**, 478 (1978). Total synthesis: Schmidlin et al., Helv. Chim. Acta **40**, 1438 (1957); Johnson et al., J. Am. Chem. Soc. **80**, 2585 (1958); **85**, 1409 (1963). Three-step synthesis from corticosterone: Barton, Beaton, ibid. **82**, 2640 (1960); **83**, 4083 (1961). Alternate synthesis: D. H. R. Barton et al., J. Chem. Soc. Perkin Trans. 1 **1975**, 2243; M. Miyano, J. Org. Chem. **46**, 1846 (1981). Biosynthesized in the zona glomerulosa and transported chiefly by albumin. In man, 400 μg secreted normally in one day. Secretion influenced by ACTH, growth hormone, plasma sodium and potassium, and the renin-angiotensin system. Causes reabsorption of Na^+, Cl^-, and HCO_3^- and diuresis of K^+. Review: L. F. Fieser, M. Fieser, Steroids (Reinhold, New York, 1959) pp 701-720.

Hydrated crystals from dilute acetone, mp 108-112° (when anhydr mp 164°). $[\alpha]_D^{23}$ +152.2° (anhydr; c = 2 in acetone). $[\alpha]_D^{25}$ +161° (c = 0.1 in chloroform). uv max: 240 nm (log ε 4.20 for the monohydrate; ε_{mol} 15,000 for the anhydr).

21-Acetate. $C_{23}H_{30}O_6$. Synthesis: Wettstein *et al.*; Jeger, **US 3002972** and **US 3014029** (both 1958 to Ciba). Flat needles from acetone + ether, mp 198-199°. $[\alpha]_D^{24}$ +121.7° (c = 0.71 in chloroform).

THERAP CAT: Mineralocorticoid.

THERAP CAT (VET): Mineralocorticoid.

226.   Aldrin. [309-00-2] 1,2,3,4,10,10-Hexachloro-1,4,4a,-5,8,8a-hexahydro-1,4:5,8-dimethanonaphthalene; HHDN; compd 118; Octalene. $C_{12}H_8Cl_6$; mol wt 364.91. C 39.50%, H 2.21%, Cl 58.29%. Chlorinated hydrocarbon insecticide; readily metabolized to dieldrin, *q.v.* Activity: C. W. Kearns *et al.*, *J. Econ. Entomol.* **42**, 127 (1949). Prepn of aldrin and *endo,endo*-isomer: Lidov, **US 2635977** (1953 to Shell). Alternate syntheses: Schmerling, **US 2911447** (1959 to Universal Oil Prod.); Korte, Rechmeier, *Ann.* **656**, 131 (1962). Toxicity study: T. B. Gaines, *Toxicol. Appl. Pharmacol.* **14**, 515 (1969). Review of toxicology and human exposure: *Toxicological Profile for Aldrin/Dieldrin* (PB2003-100134, 2002) 354 pp.

Crystals, mp 104°. Vapor pressure at 20°: 7.5×10^{-5} mm Hg. Very sol in most organic solvents. Practically insol in water. Stable in presence of organic and inorganic alkalies; stable to the action of hydrated metal chlorides. LD_{50} in male, female rats (mg/kg): 39, 60 orally (Gaines).

*endo,endo-***Isomer.** Isodrin; compd 711. Crystals, mp 240-242°. LD_{50} in male, female rats (mg/kg): 15, 7.0 orally (Gaines).

Caution: Potential symptoms of overexposure by ingestion, inhalation, or skin absorption are headache, dizziness; nausea, vomitting, malaise; myoclinic limb jerks; clonic and tonic convulsions; coma; hematuria, azotemia. Potential occupational carcinogen. See *NIOSH Pocket Guide to Chemical Hazards* (DHHS/NIOSH 97-140, 2003) p 8; *Patty's Industrial Hygiene and Toxicology* vol. **2B**, G. D. Clayton, F. E. Clayton, Eds. (Wiley-Interscience, New York, 4th ed., 1994) pp 1517-1523.

USE: Formerly as insecticide.

227.   Alefacept. [222535-22-0] 1-92-LFA-3 (antigen) (human) fusion protein with immunoglobulin G1 (human hinge-C_H2-C_H3 γ1-chain), dimer; human LFA-3-IgG$_1$ fusion protein; LFA3 TIP; BG-9273; BG-9712; Amevive. Recombinant fusion protein consisting of the first extracellular domain of human leukocyte function-associated antigen-3 (LFA-3) fused to the hinge and C_H2 and C_H3 sequences of human IgG$_1$. Expressed in Chinese hamster ovary cells; secreted as a glycosylated dimer, mol wt ~110 kDa. Antagonist at the CD2 receptor on T-lymphocytes and NK cells; inhibits T-cell proliferation. Prepn: B. P. Wallner *et al.*, **EP 503648**; *eidem*, **US 5547853** (1992, 1996 both to Biogen); and binding study: G. T. Miller *et al.*, *J. Exp. Med.* **178**, 211 (1993). Pharmacology and ELISA determn in serum: P. L. Chisholm *et al.*, *Ther. Immunol.* **1**, 205 (1994). Effect of glycosylation on pharmacokinetics: W. Meier *et al.*, *ibid.* **2**, 159 (1995). Mechanism of action study: F. Chamian *et al.*, *Proc. Natl. Acad. Sci. USA* **102**,

2075 (2005). Clinical trial in psoriasis: C. N. Ellis *et al.*, *N. Engl. J. Med.* **345**, 248 (2001). Safety profile: B. Goffe *et al.*, *Clin. Ther.* **27**, 1912 (2005). Review of clinical development in psoriasis: R. G. Langley *et al.*, *Expert Opin. Pharmacother.* **6**, 2327-2333 (2005).

THERAP CAT: Antipsoriatic; immunosuppressant.

228.   Alemtuzumab. [216503-57-0] Anti-(human CD52 (antigen)) immunoglobulin G1 (human-rat monoclonal CAM-PATH-1H γ1-chain) disulfide with human-rat monoclonal CAM-PATH-1H light chain, dimer; Campath-1H; LDP-03; Campath; MabCampath. Humanized monoclonal antibody directed against the pan-lymphocyte antigen, CD52. Induces complement-mediated cytolysis resulting in lymphocyte depletion. Prepn: L. Riechmann *et al.*, *Nature* **322**, 323 (1988); H. Waldmann *et al.*, **WO 8907452** (1989 to Medical Research Council); *eidem*, **US 5846534** (1998 to British Technology Group). Structure-activity study: J. Greenwood *et al.*, *Eur. J. Immunol.* **23**, 1098 (1993). Crystal structure of the antibody combining site: G. M. T. Cheetham *et al.*, *J. Mol. Biol.* **284**, 85 (1998). Clinical evaluation in chronic lymphocytic leukemia: A. Osterborg *et al.*, *Br. J. Haematol.* **93**, 151 (1996); in renal transplant patients: R. Calne *et al.*, *Transplantation* **68**, 1613 (1999). *Review:* F. J. Dumont, *Curr. Opin. Invest. Drugs* **2**, 139-160 (2001).

THERAP CAT: Antineoplastic; immunosuppressant.

229.   Alendronic Acid. [66376-36-1] (4-Amino-1-hydroxybutylidene)bisphosphonic acid; α-hydroxy-δ-aminobutylidenediphosphonic acid; ABDP. $C_4H_{13}NO_7P_2$; mol wt 249.10. C 19.29%, H 5.26%, N 5.62%, O 44.96%, P 24.87%. Bisphosphonate antiresorptive agent. Prepn: M. I. Kabachnik *et al.*, *Bull. Acad. Sci. USSR*, **27**, 374 (1978). *See also:* **BE 903519**; G. Staibano, **US 4705651** (1986, 1987 both to Gentili). Improved prepn: G. R. Kieczykowski *et al.*, *J. Org. Chem.* **60**, 8310 (1995). Pharmacokinetics: J. H. Lin *et al.*, *Drug Metab. Dispos.* **19**, 926 (1991). Mechanism of action: M. Sato *et al.*, *J. Clin. Invest.* **88**, 2095 (1991). Determn by HPLC in urine: W. F. Kline *et al.*, *J. Chromatogr.* **534**, 139 (1990); by IC in pharmaceutical formulations: E. W. Tsai *et al.*, *ibid.* **596**, 217 (1992). Clinical evaluation in malignant hypercalcaemia: R. Rizzoli *et al.*, *Int. J. Cancer* **50**, 706 (1992). Clinical trial in postmenopausal osteoporosis: U. A. Liberman *et al.*, *N. Engl. J. Med.* **333**, 1437 (1995); in prevention of bone loss in women: D. Hosking *et al.*, *ibid.* **338**, 485 (1998). Clinical trial in men with osteoporosis: E. Orwoll *et al.*, *ibid.* **343**, 604 (2000).

Fine white powder, mp 233-235° (dec). pK$_1$ 2.72 ±0.05; pK$_2$ 8.73 ±0.05; pK$_3$ 10.5 ±0.1; pK$_4$ 11.6 ±0.1 at 25°, (0.1M KCl).

Monosodium salt trihydrate. [121268-17-5] Alendronate sodium; MK-217; G-704650; Adronat; Alendros; Bonalon; Dronal; Fosamac; Fosamax; Onclast. $C_4H_{12}NNaO_7P_2 \cdot 3H_2O$; mol wt 325.12. mp 257-262.5°. Sol in water; very slightly sol in alcohol. Practically insol in chloroform.

THERAP CAT: Bone resorption inhibitor.

230.   Aletris. Star grass; starwort; true unicorn root; blazing star; colic root. Rhizome of *Aletris farinosa* L., Liliaceae. Habit. Eastern U.S., Ontario. Constit. Starch, diosgenin. Isoln of sapogenin: Marker *et al.*, *J. Am. Chem. Soc.* **62**, 2620 (1940). Pharmacological studies: Butler, Costello, *J. Am. Pharm. Assoc. Sci. Ed.* **33**, 177 (1944).

THERAP CAT: Antiflatulent.

231.   Aleuritic Acid. [533-87-9] (9R,10S)-*rel*-9,10,16-Trihydroxyhexadecanoic acid; 9,10,16-trihydroxypalmitic acid; 8,9,15-trihydroxypentadecane-1-carboxylic acid. $C_{16}H_{32}O_5$; mol wt 304.42. C 63.13%, H 10.60%, O 26.28%. One of the constituent acids of shellac. Obtained in 43% yield from dewaxed shellac: Schaeffer, Gardner, *Ind. Eng. Chem.* **30**, 333 (1938); Gidvani, *J.*

Chem. Soc. **1944**, 306; Sengupta, Bose, *J. Sci. Ind. Res.* **11B**, 458 (1952). The acid obtained from shellac is optically inactive, although it contains two asymmetric carbon atoms. It has been shown to be the DL-*erythro* or *dl-cis* form, and is the only form described here. Synthesis of diastereoisomers: Mitter *et al., Sci. Cult.* **8**, 273 (1942); Hunsdiecker, *Ber.* **76**, 142 (1943); **77**, 185 (1944); Baudart, *Compt. Rend.* **221**, 205 (1945).

Crystals from dilute ethanol, mp 100-101°. Sol in methanol. Forms a crystalline sodium salt.

Methyl ester. $C_{17}H_{34}O_5$. Fine feathery needles, mp 72-73°; $bp_{0.1}$ 235°. Sol in methanol, ethanol, chloroform, acetone. Less sol in benzene. Insol in petr ether.

Ethyl ester. [6003-09-4] $C_{18}H_{36}O_5$. Needles from dil ethanol, mp 59°.

Hydrazide. [6003-10-7] $C_{16}H_{34}N_2O_4$. Crystals from abs ethanol, mp 139-140°.

232. Alexidine. [22573-93-9] *N,N″*-Bis(2-ethylhexyl)-3,12-diimino-2,4,11,13-tetraazatetradecanediimidamide; 1,1′-hexamethylenebis[5-(2-ethylhexyl)biguanide]; Win-21904; Sterwin 904; Bisguanide. $C_{26}H_{56}N_{10}$; mol wt 508.79. C 61.38%, H 11.09%, N 27.53%. Prepn from 1,1′-hexamethylenebis(3-cyanoguanide) and 2-ethylhexylamine hydrochloride: **FR 1463818** (1965 to Sterling Drug). Evaluation as antimicrobial agent: McNamara *et al., J. Soc. Cosmet. Chem.* **16**, 499 (1965).

Dihydrochloride. Crystals from methanol + ether, mp 220.6-223.4°.

THERAP CAT: Antibacterial.

233. Alfadolone Acetate. [23930-37-2] (3α,5α)-21-(Acetyloxy)-3-hydroxypregnane-11,20-dione; 3α,21-dihydroxy-5α-pregnane-11,20-dione 21-acetate; 21-acetoxy-3α-hydroxy-5α-pregnane-11,20-dione; alphadolone acetate; GR-2/1574. $C_{23}H_{34}O_5$; mol wt 390.51. C 70.74%, H 8.78%, O 20.49%. Prepn: Brown, Kirk, *J. Chem. Soc. C* **1969**, 1653; Davis *et al.,* **DE 2030402** and **ZA 7003861** (both 1971 to Glaxo), *C.A.* **75**, 20793n, 64114w (1971).

Crystals from acetone-hexane, mp 175-177°. $[\alpha]_D^{26}$ +97° (c = 1.02 in chloroform).

Mixture with alfaxalone *see* Alfaxalone.

THERAP CAT: Combination with alfaxalone as anesthetic (intravenous).

THERAP CAT (VET): Combination with alfaxalone as anesthetic (intravenous).

234. Alfaprostol. [74176-31-1] (5Z)-7-[(1R,2S,3R,5S)-2-[(3S)-5-Cyclohexyl-3-hydroxy-1-pentynyl]-3,5-dihydroxycyclopentyl]-5-heptenoic acid methyl ester; 18,19,20-trinor-17-cyclohexyl-13,14-didehydro-PGF$_{2\alpha}$ methyl ester; Ro-22-9000; K-11941; Alfavet; Alphacept. $C_{24}H_{38}O_5$; mol wt 406.56. C 70.90%, H 9.42%,

O 19.68%. Synthetic analog of prostaglandin $F_{2\alpha}$, *q.v.* Synthesis: C. Gandolfi *et al.,* **DE 2539116**; *eidem,* **US 4035415** (1976, 1977 both to Carlo Erba). Efficacy in bovine estrus synchronization: E. Schilling *et al., Theriogenology* **18**, 413 (1982). Treatment of infertility in cows caused by persistent corpus luteum: G. Maffeo *et al., Prostaglandins* **25**, 541 (1983).

THERAP CAT (VET): Estrus control.

235. Alfaxalone. [23930-19-0] (3α,5α)-3-Hydroxypregnane-11,20-dione; alphaxalone; GR-2/234. $C_{21}H_{32}O_3$; mol wt 332.48. C 75.86%, H 9.70%, O 14.44%. Prepn: Nagata *et al., Helv. Chim. Acta* **42**, 1399 (1959); Browne, Kirk, *J. Chem. Soc. C* **1969**, 1653; Davis *et al.,* **DE 2030402**; **ZA 7003861** (both 1971 to Glaxo), *C.A.* **75**, 20793n, 64114w (1971). Mass spectral data: Ende, Spiteller, *Monatsh. Chem.* **102**, 929 (1971). Review of pharmacology and clinical efficacy of mixture with alfadolone acetate, *q.v.: Postgrad. Med. J.* **48**, Suppl. 2, 1-139 (1972). *See also* Child *et al.;* Campbell *et al.; Br. J. Anaesth.* **43**, 2-24 (1971); *Lancet* **1**, 888 (1972). Pharmacology and toxicity data: M. I. Al-Khawashki *et al., J. Egypt. Med. Assoc.* **62**, 191 (1979).

Colorless prisms from ether, mp 172-174°. $[\alpha]_D^{26}$ +113.4° (c = 1.2 in chloroform). LD_{50} i.v. in mice: 43 mg/kg (Al-Khawashki).

Mixture with alfadolone acetate. [8067-82-1] Alphadione; alfadione; CT-1341; Alfatésin; Althesin; Saffan. LD_{50} in mice (mg/kg): 140 i.p., 47 i.v. (Al-Khawashki).

THERAP CAT: Combination with alfadolone acetate as anesthetic (intravenous).

THERAP CAT (VET): Combination with alfadolone acetate as anesthetic (intravenous).

236. Alfentanil. [71195-58-9] *N*-[1-[2-(4-Ethyl-4,5-dihydro-5-oxo-1H-tetrazol-1-yl)ethyl]-4-(methoxymethyl)-4-piperidinyl]-*N*-phenylpropanamide; *N*-[1-[2-(4-ethyl-5-oxo-2-tetrazolin-1-yl)ethyl]-4-(methoxymethyl)-4-piperidyl]propionanilide.$C_{21}H_{32}$-N_6O_3; mol wt 416.52. C 60.56%, H 7.74%, N 20.18%, O 11.52%. Tetrazole derivative of fentanyl, *q.v.* Prepn: F. Janssens, **DE 2819873**; *idem,* **US 4167574** (1978, 1979 both to Janssen); F. Janssens *et al., J. Med. Chem.* **29**, 2290 (1986). Determn in human plasma by GC: T. J. Gillespie *et al., J. Anal. Toxicol.* **5**, 133 (1981); by radioimmunoassay: M. Michaels *et al., J. Pharm. Pharmacol.* **35**, 86 (1983). Pharmacology in animals: C. J. E. Niemegeers, P. A. J. Janssen, *Drug Dev. Res.* **1**, 83 (1981); in humans: B. Kay, B. Pleuvry, *Anaesthesia* **35**, 952 (1980). Cardiovascular effects during surgery: P. S. Sebel *et al., Br. J. Anaesth.* **54**, 1185 (1982). Clinical evaluation as analgesic component of anesthesia: B. Kay *et al., Ann. R. Coll. Surg. Engl.* **65**, 316 (1983); as anesthetic induction agent: J. Nauta *et al., Anesth. Analg.* **61**, 267 (1982); M. E. Sinclair, G. M. Cooper, *Anaesthesia* **38**, 435 (1983). Review of clinical pharmacokinetics: L. E. Mather, *Clin. Pharmacokinet.* **8**, 422 (1983); of clinical trials of alfentanil and sufentanil: S. De Lange, *Mt. Sinai J. Med.* **50**, 312 (1983).

Hydrochloride monohydrate. [70879-28-6] Alfentanil hydrochloride; R-39209; Rapifen; Alfenta. $C_{21}H_{32}N_6O_3 \cdot HCl \cdot H_2O$; mol wt 470.99. Crystals from 2-propanone, mp 140.8° (Janssens, 1979); also reported as crystals from acetone, mp 138.4° (Janssens, 1986). Sol in water. LD_{50} in rats, dogs (mg/kg): 47.5, 20 i.v. (Niemegeers, Janssen).

Note: This is a controlled substance (opiate): **21 CFR,** 1308.12.

THERAP CAT: Analgesic (narcotic).

THERAP CAT (VET): Analgesic (narcotic).

237.   Alfimeprase. [259074-76-5] 3-203-Fibrolase [3-serine] (*Agkistrodon contortrix contortrix* recombinant). Truncated form of fibrolase, *q.v.,* containing 201 amino acid residues; mol wt ~22.6 kDa. Directly acting fibrinolytic metalloproteinase; preferentially degrades the Aα chain of fibrinogen, *q.v.* Inhibited by serum α2-macroglobulin. Prepn by recombinant technology in *Pichia pastoris:* T. C. Boone *et al.,* **WO 0125445;** *eidem,* **US 6261820** (both 2001 to Amgen). Disulfide structure: G. Jones *et al., Protein Sci.* **10,** 1264 (2001). Pharmacology: C. F. Toombs, *Haemostasis* **31,** 141 (2001). Review of biochemistry and pharmacology: *idem, Fundam. Clin. Cardiol.* **46,** 627-650 (2003). Clinical evaluation for peripheral arterial thrombolysis: K. Ouriel *et al., J. Vasc. Interv. Radiol.* **16,** 1075 (2005).

THERAP CAT: Thrombolytic.

238.   Alfuzosin. [81403-80-7] *N*-[3-[(4-Amino-6,7-dimethoxy-2-quinazolinyl)methylamino]propyl]tetrahydro-2-furancarboxamide; N^1-(4-amino-6,7-dimethoxyquinazol-2-yl)-N^1-methyl-N^2-(tetrahydrofuroyl-2)-propylenediamine; SL-77.499. $C_{19}H_{27}N_5O_4$; mol wt 389.45. C 58.60%, H 6.99%, N 17.98%, O 16.43%. α_1-Adrenoceptor antagonist structurally similar to prazosin, *q.v.* Prepn: P. M. J. Manoury, **DE 2904445;** *idem,* **US 4315007** (1979, 1982 both to Synthelabo); and antihypertensive activity in rats: P. M. Manoury *et al., J. Med. Chem.* **29,** 19 (1986). Pharmacology: A. G. Ramage, *Eur. J. Pharmacol.* **129,** 307 (1986). HPLC determn in biological fluids: P. Guinebault *et al., J. Chromatogr.* **353,** 361 (1986). Pharmacology in humans: A. H. Deering, *Br. J. Clin. Pharmacol.* **25,** 417 (1988). Clinical evaluation in essential hypertension: S. Leto Di Priolo *et al., Eur. J. Clin. Pharmacol.* **35,** 25 (1988); A. K. Ghosh, S. Ghosh, *Ger. Cardiovasc. Med.* **1,** 81 (1988). Clinical trial in benign prostatic hyperplasia (BPH): C. G. Roehrborn *et al., BJU Int.* **92,** 257 (2003). Review of clinical experience in BPH: D. M. Weiner, F. C. Lowe, *Expert Opin. Pharmacother.* **4,** 2057-2063 (2003).

Hydrochloride. [81403-68-1] SL-77.499-10; Mittoval; Urion; UroXatral; Xatral. $C_{19}H_{27}N_5O_4 \cdot HCl$; mol wt 425.91. Crystals from ethanol + ether, mp 225° (Manoury, 1986), also reported earlier as mp 235° (dec) (Manoury, 1982). pKa 8.13.

THERAP CAT: Antihypertensive. In treatment of benign prostatic hypertrophy.

239.   Algestone. [595-77-7] (16α)-16,17-Dihydroxypregn-4-ene-3,20-dione; 16α,17-dihydroxyprogesterone; 4-pregnene-16α,17α-diol-3,20-dione; alphasone. $C_{21}H_{30}O_4$; mol wt 346.46. C 72.80%, H 8.73%, O 18.47%. Prepn from 16-dehydroprogesterone: Inhoffen *et al., Ber.* **87,** 593 (1954); Cooley *et al., J. Chem. Soc.* **1955,** 4373; Allen, Bernstein, *J. Am. Chem. Soc.* **78,** 1909 (1956); Hydorn *et al., Steroids* **3,** 493 (1964). Manuf from 16-

dehydroprogesterone: Colton, **US 2727909** (1955 to Searle); Hydorn *et al.,* **US 3165541** (1965 to Olin Mathieson); from its 16α-acetate: Diassi, **US 3027384** (1962 to Olin Mathieson).

Needles from ethanol + dichloromethane, mp 225°. $[\alpha]_D^{22}$ +95° (c = 0.81 in $CHCl_3$). uv max: 240 nm (ε 16600).

Cyclic acetal with acetone. [4968-09-6] 16α,17-[(1-Methylethylidene)bis(oxy)]pregn-4-ene-3,20-dione; algestone acetonide; alphasone acetonide; 16α,17α-isopropylidenedioxyprogesterone. $C_{24}H_{34}O_4$. Prepn: Cooley *et al., loc. cit;* Fried *et al., Chem. Ind. (London)* **1961,** 465. Needles from aq ethanol, mp 210°. $[\alpha]_D^{20}$ +137° (c = 0.7 in $CHCl_3$).

16α-Methyl ether. 17-Hydroxy-16α-methoxypregn-4-ene-3,20-dione. $C_{22}H_{32}O_4$. Prepd from the free diol via 16α,17-dihydroxy-pregn-4-ene-3,20-dione cyclic borate: Fried, **US 3006930** (1961 to Olin Mathieson). Crystals from 95% ethanol, mp 142-143°. $[\alpha]_D^{23}$ +60° (c = 0.15 in $CHCl_3$). uv max: 234 nm (ε 15400).

THERAP CAT: Acetonide as anti-inflammatory (topical).

240.   Algestone Acetophenide. [24356-94-3] [16α(*R*)]-16,17-[(1-Phenylethylidene)bis(oxy)]pregn-4-ene-3,20-dione; 16α,17-dihydroxypregn-4-ene-3,20-dione cyclic acetal with acetophenone; 16α,17α-dihydroxyprogesterone acetophenide; alphasone acetophenide; P-DHP; SQ-15101; Deladroxone (obsolete); Droxone (obsolete); Neolutin Depositum. $C_{29}H_{36}O_4$; mol wt 448.59. C 77.65%, H 8.09%, O 14.27%. Progestogen. Prepn: J. Fried, **US 2941997** (1960 to Olin Mathieson); J. Fried *et al., Chem. Ind. (London)* **1961,** 465. Improved prepn: **IE 6800457;** S. J. Brancato *et al.,* **US 3488347** (1968, 1970 both to Smith Kline & French). In estrus synchronization: J. N. Wiltbank *et al., J. Anim. Sci.* **26,** 764 (1967). Clinical evaluations of combination with estradiol enanthate as injectable contraceptive: R. Plesner, *Acta Endocrinol.* **61,** 494 (1969); *idem, ibid.* **65,** 683 (1970); R. Recio *et al., Contraception* **33,** 579 (1986).

Crystals from 95% ethanol, mp 150-151°. $[\alpha]_D^{23}$ +51° ($CHCl_3$). Stable to boiling mineral acids; readily cleaved by warming with formic acid, with subsequent deformylation.

THERAP CAT: Antiacne.

241.   Algin. [9005-38-3] Alginic acid sodium salt; sodium alginate; sodium polymannuronate; Alto; Alman; Alloid; Allose. A gelling polysaccharide extracted from giant brown seaweed (giant kelp, *Macrocystis pyrifera* (L.) Ag., *Lessoniaceae)* or from horsetail kelp (*Laminaria digitata* (L.) Lamour, *Laminariaceae)* or from sugar kelp (*Laminaria saccharina* (L.) Lamour. Process of manuf: Tseng, *Chem. Metall. Eng.* **52,** 97 (1945); Mantell, *The Water-Soluble Gums* (New York, 1947); Green, **US 2036934** (1936 to Kelco); Gloahec, Herter, **US 2128551** (1938 to Algin Corp. of America). Wound healing properties and use in hemostatic dressings: J. H. M. Miller, **GB 1328088** (1973 to Wallace, Cameron & Co.), *C.A.* **80,** 6974u (1974). Series of articles on hemostatic effects: *Yakugaku Zasshi* **101,** 452-469 (1981), *C.A.* **95,** 35654e,

35655f, 35405z (1981). Immunoadjuvant effect: G. H. Scherr, A. S. Markowitz, **US 3075883** (1963 to Consolidated Labs.). Clinical comparison with alum immunoadjuvant: G. Bruno *et al., Ann. Allergy* **56,** 384 (1986). Review of structural studies: D. A. Rees, E. J. Welsh, *Angew. Chem. Int. Ed.* **16,** 214 (1977). Review of production, properties and use in the food industry: A. Askar, *Alimenta* **21,** 165-169 (1982). *Reviews:* McNeely, Pettitt, in *Industrial Gums,* R. L. Whistler, Ed. (Academic Press, New York, 2nd ed., 1973) pp 49-81; I. W. Cottrell, J. K. Baird, "Gums" in *Kirk-Othmer Encyclopedia of Chemical Technology* **vol. 12** (Wiley-Interscience, New York, 3rd ed., 1980) pp 48-51.

Cream-colored powder. Sol in water, forming a viscous, colloidal soln. Insol in alcohol and in hydro-alcoholic solns in which the alcohol content is >30% w/w. Insol in chloroform, ether, in aq acid solns when the pH is below 3.

USE: In the manufacture of ice cream where it serves as a stabilizing colloid, insuring creamy texture and preventing the growth of ice crystals; in drilling muds; in coatings; in the flocculation of solids in water treatment; as sizing agent; thickener; emulsion stabilizer; suspending agent in soft drinks; in dental impression preparations. Pharmaceutic aid (suspending agent).

THERAP CAT: Hemostatic.

242. Alginic Acid. [9005-32-7] Norgine; polymannuronic acid; Sazio. Mol wt over 240,000. A hydrophilic, colloidal polysaccharide obtained from seaweeds which, in the form of mixed salts of calcium, magnesium, and other bases, occurs as a structural component of the cell wall. Isoln from fronds of *Laminaria digitata* (L.) Edmonson, *Laminariaceae:* Stanford, *J. Chem. Soc.* **44,** 943 (1883); Bird, Haas, *Biochem. J.* **25,** 403 (1931); from *Macrocystis pyrifera* (L.) C. Ag., *Lessoniaceae:* Nelson, Cretcher, *J. Am. Chem. Soc.* **51,** 1914 (1929). Polysaccharides similar to alginic acid are also secreted by the bacteria *Pseudomonas aeruginosa* and *Azotobacter vinelandii:* G. H. Cohen, D. B. Johnstone, *J. Bacteriol.* **88,** 329 (1964); L. R. Evans, A. Linker, *ibid.* **116,** 915 (1973). Alginic acid is a linear polymer of β-(1 → 4)-D-mannosyluronic acid and α-(1 → 4)-L-gulosyluronic acid residues, the relative proportions of which vary with the botanical source and state of maturation of the plant. Clinical use of combination with antacid in gastric reflux esophagitis: D. Y. Graham *et al., Curr. Ther. Res.* **22,** 653 (1977). Clinical evaluation of calcium salt as hemostatic dressing: T. Gilchrist, A. M. Martin, *Biomaterials* **4,** 317 (1983); A. R. Groves, J. C. Lawrence, *Ann. R. Coll. Surg. Engl.* **68,** 27 (1986). Review of structure studies and of secondary and tertiary structure in solutions and gels: D. A. Rees, E. J. Welsh, *Angew. Chem. Int. Ed.* **16,** 214 (1977). Review of production, properties and use in the food industry: A. Askar, *Alimenta* **21,** 165-169 (1982).

Very slightly sol in water. Tasteless. Capable of absorbing 200-300 times its weight of water and salts to the extent of 60%. Resists hydrolysis. Sol in alkaline solns. pH of a 3 in 100 suspension in water is between 2.0 and 3.4.

Calcium salt. [9005-35-0] Sorbsan.

Sodium salt. *See* Algin.

USE: Sizing paper and textiles; as binder for briquettes; manuf artificial horn, ivory, celluloid; emulsionizing mineral oils; mucilage. Additional uses are described under Algin.

THERAP CAT: Calcium salt as hemostatic.

243. Alglucerase. [143003-46-7] Glucosylceramidase (human placental isoenzyme protein moiety reduced); mannose-terminated human placental glucocerebrosidase; macrophage-targeted β-glucocerebrosidase; Ceredase. Modified form of β-glucocerebrosidase, an enzyme involved in glycolipid metabolism, which is deficient in patients with Gaucher's disease. Designed to target the tissue macrophages in which the lipid accumulates. Monomeric glycoprotein of 497 amino acids. Prepd by sequential deglycosolation of the native placental-derived enzyme to expose terminal mannose residues that can be recognized by macrophage cell surface receptors. Prepn: F. S Furbish *et al., Biochim. Biophys. Acta* **673,** 425 (1981); G. J. Murray, *Methods Enzymol.* **149,** 25 (1987). Clinical evaluation in Gaucher's disease: N. W. Barton *et al., N. Engl. J. Med.* **324,** 1464 (1991); M. L. Figueroa *et al., ibid.* **327,** 1632 (1992). Review of pharmacology and therapeutic efficacy: R. Whittington, K. L. Goa, *Drugs* **44,** 72-93 (1992). Effect of long-term treatment: N. J. Weinreb *et al., Am. J. Med.* **113,** 112-119 (2002).

Imiglucerase. RGCR; Cerezyme. Mannose-terminated human glucocerebrosidase produced by recombinant DNA technology. Prepn: J. Rasmussen *et al.,* **WO 9007573**; *eidem,* **US 5236838** (1990, 1993 both to Genzyme).

THERAP CAT: Enzyme replacement therapy for Gaucher's disease.

244. Alibendol. [26750-81-2] 2-Hydroxy-*N*-(2-hydroxyethyl)-3-methoxy-5-(2-propenyl)benzamide; 5-allyl-2-hydroxy-*N*-(2-hydroxyethyl)-*m*-anisamide; 2-hydroxy-3-methoxy-5-allyl-*N*-(β-hydroxyethyl)benzamide; EB-1856; FC-54; H-3774; Cebera. $C_{13}H_{17}NO_4$; mol wt 251.28. C 62.14%, H 6.82%, N 5.57%, O 25.47%. Amide analog of eugenol, *q.v.* Prepn: **FR 1584715**; F. Clémence, O. Le Martret, **US 3668238** (1967, 1972 both to Roussel). Synthesis and pharmacologic activity: F. Clémence *et al., Chim. Ther.* **5,** 188 (1970).

Crystals from benzene, mp 95°. uv max (ethanol): 316, 218 nm. LD_{50} in Swiss male mice (mg/kg): >3000 orally; >2000 s.c.; 209 i.p.; 217 i.v. (Clémence).

THERAP CAT: Choleretic; antispasmodic.

245. Alicaforsen. [185229-68-9] d[(*R*)-*P*-Thio](G-C-C-C-A-A-G-C-T-G-G-C-A-T-C-C-G-T-C-A)deoxyribonucleic acid. Synthetic 20 base phosphorothioate antisense oligonucleotide designed to inhibit expression of intercellular adhesion molecule-1 (ICAM-1), a key mediator of inflammation. Prepn: C. F. Bennett, C. K. Mirabelli, **WO 9405333**; *eidem,* **US 5514788** (1994, 1996 both to Isis). Purifn and scale up: R. R. Deshmukh *et al., Nucleosides Nucleotides Nucleic Acids* **20,** 567 (2001). ICAM-1 inhibition in cell culture: C. F. Bennett *et al., J. Immunol.* **152,** 3530 (1994). Clinical pharmacokinetics: J. M. Glover *et al., J. Pharmacol. Exp. Ther.* **282,** 1173 (1997). ELISA determn in plasma: R. Z. Yu *et al., Anal. Biochem.* **304,** 19 (2002). Clinical evaluation in Crohn's disease: B. R. Yacyshyn *et al., Gut* **51,** 30 (2002); in ulcerative colitis: S. J. H. van Deventer *et al., ibid.* **53,** 1646 (2004). Review of toxicology: S. P. Henry *et al., Toxicol. Pathol.* **27,** 95-100 (1999); A. A. Levin, *Biochim. Biophys. Acta* **1489,** 69-84 (1999); of pharmacology and clinical development: W. R. Shanahan, Jr., *Expert Opin. Invest. Drugs* **8,** 1417-1429 (1999); C. F. Barish, *Expert Opin. Biol. Ther.* **5,** 1387-1391 (2005).

Sodium salt. [331257-52-4] ISIS-2302

THERAP CAT: Anti-inflammatory.

246. Alinidine. [33178-86-8] *N*-(2,6-Dichlorophenyl)-4,5-dihydro-*N*-2-propenyl-1*H*-imidazol-2-amine; 2-(*N*-allyl-2,6-dichloroanilino)-2-imidazoline; 2-[*N*-allyl-*N*-(2,6-dichlorophenyl)amino]-2-imidazoline; ST-567. $C_{12}H_{13}Cl_2N_3$; mol wt 270.16. C 53.35%, H 4.85%, Cl 26.25%, N 15.55%. Specific bradycardic agent; analog of clonidine, *q.v.* Prepn: H. Stähle *et al.,* **DE 1958201**; *eidem,* **US 3708485** (1971, 1973 both to Boehringer, Ing.); *eidem, J. Med. Chem.* **23,** 1217 (1980). Clinical pharmacology: D. W. G. Harron *et al., J. Cardiovasc. Pharmacol.* **4,** 213 (1982). Mode of action study: J. S. Millar, E. M. Vaughan Williams, *Lancet* **1,** 1291 (1981). HPLC determn in human plasma: U.-W. Wiegand *et al., J. Chromatogr.* **223,** 238 (1981). Clinical pharmacokinetics: *eidem, J. Cardiovasc. Pharmacol.* **4,** 59 (1982). Hemodynamic effects in angina or infarction: M. L. Simoons, P. G. Hugenholtz, *Eur. Heart J.* **5,** 227 (1984). Review of pharmacology and potential therapeutic uses: D. W. G. Harron, R. G. Shanks, *ibid.* **6,** 722-729 (1985).

Crystals, mp 130-131° (Stähle, 1973); also reported as mp 127-129° (Stähle, 1980). pKa 10.42.

Hydrobromide. $C_{12}H_{14}BrCl_2N_3$. Crystals from methanol + water, mp 193-194°.

247. Aliskiren. [173334-57-1] ($\alpha S,\gamma S,\delta S,\zeta S$)-δ-Amino-N-(3-amino-2,2-dimethyl-3-oxopropyl)-γ-hydroxy-4-methoxy-3-(3-methoxypropoxy)-α,ζ-bis(1-methylethyl)benzeneoctanamide; (2S,4S,5S,7S)-5-amino-N-(2-carbamoyl-2-methylpropyl)-4-hydroxy-2-isopropyl-7-[4-methoxy-3-(3-methoxypropoxy)benzyl]-8-methyl-nonanamide; 5S-amino-4S-hydroxy-2S,7S-diisopropyl-8-[4-methoxy-3-(3-methoxypropyloxy)phenyl]octanoic acid N-(2-carbamoyl-2,2-dimethylethyl)amide; CGP-60536. $C_{30}H_{53}N_3O_6$; mol wt 551.76. C 65.30%, H 9.68%, N 7.62%, O 17.40%. Orally active, synthetic nonpeptide renin inhibitor. Prepn: R. Göschke et al., EP **678503**; eidem, US **5559111** (1995, 1996 both to Ciba-Geigy); H, Rüeger et al., Tetrahedron Lett. **41**, 10085 (2000). Synthesis: A. Dondoni et al., ibid. **42**, 4819 (2001). Determn by HPLC in biological fluids: G. Lefevre, S. Gauron, J. Chromatogr. B **738**, 129 (2000); by RIA in plasma: G. Lefevre et al., J. Immunoassay **21**, 65 (2000). Structure activity study: J. M. Wood et al., Biochem. Biophys. Res. Commun. **308**, 698 (2003). Clinical pharmacology: J. Nussberger et al., Hypertension **39**, e1 (2002). Clinical study: A. H. Gradman et al., Circulation **111**, 1012 (2005). Review of development and therpaeutic potential: K. Allikmets, Curr. Opin. Invest. Drugs **3**, 1479-1482 (2002).

pKa 9.49. Log P (octanol/water): 2.45 (pH 7.4). Soly in water: >350 mg/ml (pH 7.4).
Hemifumarate. [173334-58-2] CGP-60536B; SPP-100; Rasilez. $2C_{30}H_{53}N_3O_6.C_4H_4O_4$; mol wt 1219.59.
THERAP CAT: Antihypertensive.

248. Alitame. [80863-62-3] L-α-Aspartyl-N-(2,2,4,4-tetramethyl-3-thietanyl)-D-alaninamide; L-aspartyl-N-(2,2,4,4-tetramethylthietan-3-yl)amide; 3-(L-aspartyl-D-alaninamido)-2,2,4,4-tetramethylthietane; CP-54802; Aclame. $C_{14}H_{25}N_3O_4S$; mol wt 331.43. C 50.73%, H 7.60%, N 12.68%, O 19.31%, S 9.67%. Dipeptide amide reported to be approx 2000 times sweeter than sucrose. Prepn: T. M. Brennan, M. E. Hendrick, EP **34876**; eidem, US **4411925** (1981, 1983 both to Pfizer). Conformational analysis: R. D. Feinstein et al., J. Am. Chem. Soc. **113**, 3467 (1991). Review of development and uses: R. C. Glowaky et al., ACS Symp. Ser. **450**, 57-67 (1991); of chemical and physical properties: M. E. Hendrick et al., in Advances in Sweeteners, T. H. Grenby, Ed. (Blackie, Glasgow, 1996) pp 226-239; M. H. Auerbach et al., in Alternative Sweeteners, L. O'Brien Nabors, Ed. (Marcel Dekker, Inc., New York, 2001) pp 31-40.

White, crystalline, non-hygroscopic powder, mp 136-147°. Faint, characteristic odor; intensely sweet taste. $[\alpha]_D^{25}$ +40 to +50° (c = 1 in water). pI 5.6. Soly at 25° (% w/v): water (pH 5.6) 13.1; methanol 41.9; ethanol 61.0; propylene glycol 53.7; chloroform 0.02; n-heptane 0.001.
USE: Non-nutritive sweetener.

249. Alitretinoin. [5300-03-8] 9-cis-Retinoic acid; 6-cis-retinoic acid; ALRT-1057; LGD-1057; Panretin. $C_{20}H_{28}O_2$; mol wt 300.44. C 79.95%, H 9.39%, O 10.65%. Naturally occurring derivative of vitamin A, q.v. Morphogenic agent that modulates cell growth and differentiation; activates both retinoic acid (RAR) and retinoid X (RXR) receptors. Prepn: C. D. Robeson et al., J. Am.

Chem. Soc. **77**, 4111 (1955); M. Matsui et al., J. Vitaminol. **4**, 178 (1958); M. F. Boehm et al., J. Med. Chem. **37**, 408 (1994). Identification as physiological ligand of RXR: R. A. Heyman et al., Cell **68**, 397 (1992); A. A. Levin et al., Nature **355**, 359 (1992). Role in morphogenesis: C. Thaller et al., Development **118**, 957 (1993). Biosynthesis from all-trans-retinoic acid: J. Urbach, R. R. Rando, Biochem. J. **299**, 459 (1994). HPLC determn in plasma: A. M. Dzerk et al., J. Pharm. Biomed. Anal. **16**, 1013 (1998). Clinical pharmacokinetics: C. Weber, E. Dumont, J. Clin. Pharmacol. **37**, 566 (1997). Clinical evaluation in acute promyelocytic leukemia: S. L. Soignet et al., Leukemia **12**, 1518 (1998); in advanced cancers: N. A. Rizvi et al., Clin. Cancer Res. **4**, 1437 (1998). Review of role as hormone: B. F. Tate et al., Trends Endocrinol. Metab. **5**, 189-194 (1994); of clinical development: J. Cell. Biochem. Suppl. **26**, 158-167 (1996).

Yellow fine needles from ethanol, mp 190-191°. uv max (methanol): 343 nm (ε 39000).
THERAP CAT: Antineoplastic.

250. Alizapride. [59338-93-1] 6-Methoxy-N-[[1-(2-propenyl)-2-pyrrolidinyl]methyl]-1H-benzotriazole-5-carboxamide; N-[(1-allyl-2-pyrrolidinyl)methyl]-6-methoxy-1H-benzotriazole-5-carboxamide. $C_{16}H_{21}N_5O_2$; mol wt 315.37. C 60.94%, H 6.71%, N 22.21%, O 10.15%. Prepn: BE **825605**; G. Bulteau et al., US **4039672** (1975, 1977 both to Soc. d'Etudes Sci. Ind. de l'Ile-de-France). Series of articles on pharmacology and clinical studies in chemotherapy induced emesis: Sem. Hop. **58**, 323-374 (1982).

Cryst from acetone, mp 139°. LD$_{50}$ i.v. in mice (5 days): 92.7 mg/kg (Bulteau).
Hydrochloride. [59338-87-3] Nausilen; Plitican; Vergentan. $C_{16}H_{21}N_5O_2.HCl$; mol wt 351.83. Cryst from methanol/methyl ethyl ketone, mp 206-208°.
THERAP CAT: Antiemetic.

251. Alizarin. [72-48-0] 1,2-Dihydroxy-9,10-anthracenedione; 1,2-dihydroxyanthraquinone; C.I. Mordant Red 11; C.I. Pigment Red 83; C.I. 58000. $C_{14}H_8O_4$; mol wt 240.21. C 70.00%, H 3.36%, O 26.64%. Occurs in the root of the madder plant (Rubia tinctorum L., Rubiaceae; Krappwurzel) in combination with 2 mols glucose, called ruberythric acid. Was known and used in ancient Egypt, Persia, and India. Synthesized from 2-anthraquinonesulfonic acid sodium salt : Caro et al., Ber. **3**, 359 (1870); Perkin, Ber. **9**, 281 (1876). Historical review: Fieser, J. Chem. Educ. **7**, 2609 (1930). Laboratory prepn: Gattermann-Wieland, Laboratory Methods of Organic Chemistry (New York, 1937). Modern methods of manufacture: Pohl, Ullmanns Encyklopädie der technischen Chemie vol. I, p 200; Fierz-David and Blangey, Grundlegende Operationen der Farbenchemie (Vienna, 5th ed., 1943). See also Colour Index vol. 4, (3rd ed., 1971) p 4513.

Orthorhombic, orange needles by sublimation or from abs alc. Solvated scales from dil alc or by evaporation from ether. Sublimes at 110° (2 mm Hg). mp 290°. bp 430°. Absorption spectrum: Moir, *J. Chem. Soc.* **1927**, 1810. Soly in water at 18°: 2.1×10^{-6} mols/l; at 25°: 2.5×10^{-6} mols/l. Sol in 300 parts boiling water; moderately sol in alcohol, freely in hot methanol and in ether at 25°. Also sol in benzene, toluene, xylene, pyridine, carbon disulfide, glacial acetic acid. Sol in water solns of alkalies with blue color, but without fluorescence. Fluorescent solns indicate unchanged 2-anthraquinone sodium sulfonate.

1-Methyl ether. $C_{15}H_{10}O_4$. Orange needles with $1H_2O$ from dil methanol. When dried at 100° mp 179°.

2-Methyl ether. $C_{15}H_{10}O_4$. Orange needles from alcohol, mp 231°.

Dimethyl ether. $C_{16}H_{12}O_4$. Golden-yellow needles from alcohol, mp 215°.

USE: In the manufacture of acid and chrome dyes for wool; acid-base indicator (in 0.5% alcoholic soln; pH: yellow 5.5, red 6.8); in spot tests as reagent for aluminum, indium, mercury, zinc, and zirconium; biological stain.

252. Alizarin Cyanine Green F. [4403-90-1] 2,2-[(9,10-Dihydro-9,10-dioxo-1,4-anthracenediyl)diimino]bis(5-methylbenzenesulfonic acid) disodium salt; 6,6'-(1,4-anthraquinonylenediimino)di-*m*-toluenesulfonic acid disodium salt; D & C Green No. 5; C.I. Acid Green 25; C.I. 61570. $C_{28}H_{20}N_2Na_2O_8S_2$; mol wt 622.58. C 54.02%, H 3.24%, N 4.50%, Na 7.39%, O 20.56%, S 10.30%. Discovered by R. E. Schmidt in 1894: *Colour Index* **vol. 4** (3rd ed., 1971) p 4541.

Green powder. Slightly sol in acetone, alc, pyridine. Insol in chloroform, toluene. Dull blue soln in conc H_2SO_4, turning turquoise on dilution. Absorption spectra: C. F. H. Allen *et al.*, *J. Org. Chem.* **7**, 63, 169 (1942).

USE: For nylon sutures: *Fed. Regist.* **42**, 52395 (1977). Permitted for use in drugs and cosmetics, excluding use in eye area: *ibid.* **47**, 49628 (1982).

253. Alizarine Blue. [568-02-5] 5,6-Dihydroxynaphtho-[2,3-*f*]quinoline-7,12-dione; 7,8-dihydroxy-5,6-phthalylquinoline; Alizarin Blue R; C.I. 67410. $C_{17}H_9NO_4$; mol wt 291.26. C 70.10%, H 3.11%, N 4.81%, O 21.97%. Prepn from 3-nitroalizarin, glycerol, and concd sulfuric acid: Auerbach, *J. Chem. Soc.* **35**, 799 (1879); *Colour Index* **vol. 4** (3rd ed., 1971) p 4567.

Lustrous brownish violet needles from benzene, mp 268-270°. Practically insol in water; sparingly sol in alc, ether; slightly sol in cold benzene; sol in amyl alcohol, glacial acetic acid, hot benzene.

USE: As indicator in saturated alcoholic soln. pH: pink 0.0 to yellow 1.6; yellow 6.0 to green 7.6.

254. Alizarine Orange. [568-93-4] 1,2-Dihydroxy-3-nitro-9,10-anthracenedione; 1,2-dihydroxy-3-nitroanthraquinone; 3-nitroalizarin; C.I. Mordant Orange 14; C.I. 58015. $C_{14}H_7NO_6$;

mol wt 285.21. C 58.96%, H 2.47%, N 4.91%, O 33.66%. From 3-bromoalizarin in acetic acid with nitric acid: Barnett, Cook, *J. Chem. Soc.* **121**, 1376 (1922). Additional prepns: *Colour Index* **vol. 4** (3rd ed., 1971) p 4514.

Orange needles or plates from acetic acid, dec 244°. Sublimes with partial decompn. Yellow in organic solvents, purple-red in dil aq alkali, orange in H_2SO_4.

USE: Dyes cloth mordanted with Al orange, with Fe red to violet. As indicator in satd alc soln. pH 2.0-4.0, color change from golden orange to flat yellow (in water). pH 5.0-6.5 from yellow to purplish red.

255. Alizarine Yellow R. [2243-76-7] 2-Hydroxy-5-[(4-nitrophenyl)azo]benzoic acid; 5-(*p*-nitrophenylazo)salicylic acid; *p*-nitrobenzeneazosalicylic acid; Alizarine Yellow RW; C.I. Mordant Orange 1; C.I. 14030. $C_{13}H_9N_3O_5$; mol wt 287.23. C 54.36%, H 3.16%, N 14.63%, O 27.85%. Prepd by coupling diazotized *p*-nitroaniline with salicylic acid: Armento, **US 2746955** (1956 to General Aniline and Film); *Colour Index* **vol. 4** (3rd ed., 1971) p 4058.

Orange-brown needles from dil glacial acetic acid, dec 253-254°. Sol in water, alc; slightly sol in acetone, Cellosolve; practically insol in other org solvents.

Sodium salt. Mordant Yellow 3R. $C_{13}H_8N_3NaO_5$. Brownish yellow powder. Sol in water.

USE: Sodium salt used as indicator in 0.1% aq soln pH: yellow to red, range 10.2 to 12.0.

256. Alkanet. Alkanna; orcanette; dyer's alkanet; anchusa; orkanet. The root of *Alkanna tinctoria* Tausch, *Boraginaceae*. *Habit.* Asia Minor, Hungary, Greece, Mediterranean region. *Constit.* Alkannin (the coloring principle) and tannin. Extraction of roots: Betrabet, Chakravarti, *J. Indian Inst. Sci.* **16A**, 51 (1933); *C.A.* **28**, 1038 (1934); Majamdar, Chakravarti, *J. Indian Chem. Soc.* **17**, 272 (1940); *C.A.* **34**, 6262 (1940).

Alkannin paper. Anchusin paper; Boettger's paper. White paper impregnated with a 1% alc tincture of alkanet root and dried. A blue paper can be made from the red paper by treating the latter with a 1% Na_2CO_3 soln. This paper acts nearly like litmus paper. Alkalies = green or blue; acids = red. pH: 8.0 red; 10.0 blue.

USE: For coloring wines, cosmetics, confectionery. Alkannin paper as indicator.

THERAP CAT: Astringent.

257. Alkannin. [517-88-4] 5,8-Dihydroxy-2-[(1*S*)-1-hydroxy-4-methyl-3-pentenyl]-1,4-naphthalenedione; (−)-5,8-dihydroxy-2-(1-hydroxy-4-methyl-3-pentenyl)-1,4-naphthoquinone; anchusa acid; anchusin; alkanna red; alkanet extract; 1-hydroxy-3-isohexenyl)naphthazarine; 2-(1-hydroxy-4-methyl-3-pentenyl)-5,8-dihydroxy-1,4-naphthoquinone; C.I. Natural Red 20; C.I. 75530. $C_{16}H_{16}O_5$; mol wt 288.30. C 66.66%, H 5.59%, O 27.75%. Isoln from the root of *Alkanna tinctoria* Tausch, *Boraginaceae*: Brockmann, *Ann.* **521**, 1 (1936); Toribara, Underwood, *Anal. Chem.* **21**, 1352 (1949). Absolute configuration: Arakawa, Nakagaki, *Chem. Ind. (London)* **1961**, 947. Toxicity study: L. Majlathova, *Nahrung* **15**, 505 (1971), *C.A.* **76**, 122513j (1972).

Brownish-red prisms with a metallic sheen from benzene, mp 149°. Can be sublimed in high vac at 140-150°. $[\alpha]_{Cd}^{20}$ −165° (benzene); −226° (chloroform). Also reported as −254 ± 7° (chloroform) (Toribara). Sol in organic solvents, sparingly sol in water. Buffered aq solns are red at pH 6.1; purple at pH 8.8; blue at pH 10.0. LD_{50} in male, female mice, rats (g/kg): 3.0 ± 1.0; 3.1 ± 0.1; >1.0 orally (Majlathova).

(+)-Form. Shikonin.

(±)-Form. Shikalkin.

USE: Red dye for cosmetics and food; spectrophotometric micro-determination of beryllium.

THERAP CAT: Astringent.

258. Allantoin. [97-59-6] (2,5-Dioxo-4-imidazolidinyl)-urea; 5-ureidohydantoin; glyoxyldiureide; cordianine. $C_4H_6N_4O_3$; mol wt 158.12. C 30.38%, H 3.82%, N 35.43%, O 30.36%. Product of purine metabolism. Prepd synthetically by the oxidation of uric acid with alkaline potassium permanganate: *Org. Synth.* **coll. vol. II,** 23 (1943). By heating urea with dichloroacetic acid: C. N. Zellner, J. R. Stevens, US 2158098 (1939 to Merck & Co.) Acetyl derivs: Biltz, Loewe, *J. Prakt. Chem.* **141,** 291 (1934). Optically active forms have been obtained by extraction procedures.

Racemic Form. Monoclinic plates or prisms from water, mp 238°. One gram dissolves in 190 ml water, 500 ml alcohol; more sol in hot water and hot alcohol. Almost insol in ether. pH of satd water soln: 5.5.

THERAP CAT: Vulnerary.

THERAP CAT (VET): Vulnerary; debriding agent.

259. Allenolic Acid. [553-39-9] 6-Hydroxy-2-naphtha-lenepropanoic acid; 2-hydroxy-6-naphthalenepropionic acid; amphihydroxynaphthyl-β-propionic acid. $C_{13}H_{12}O_3$; mol wt 216.23. C 72.21%, H 5.59%, O 22.20%. Prepn from the corresponding methoxy compd: Jacques, Horeau, *Bull. Soc. Chim. Fr.* **1948,** 714.

Crystals from aq methanol, mp 180-181°. Sol in alcohol, methanol, pyridine.

USE: In biochemical research, in the prepn of estrogenic compds.

260. Allethrins. Allyl cinerins. Synthetic analogs of the naturally occurring insecticides cinerins, jasmolins, and pyrethrins, *q.q.v. Review:* Barthel, *World Rev. Pest Control* **6,** 59 (1967); World Health Org., *Environ. Health Criter.* **87,** 1-75 (1989). Review of toxicology and human exposure: *Toxicological Profile for Pyrethrins and Pyrethroids* (PB2004-100004, 2003) 332 pp.

Allethrin I   R = CH₃
Allethrin II   R = COOCH₃

Allethrin I. [584-79-2] 2,2-Dimethyl-3-(2-methyl-1-propen-yl)cyclopropanecarboxylic acid 2-methyl-4-oxo-3-(2-propenyl)-2-cyclopenten-1-yl ester; allethrolone ester of chrysanthemummono-carboxylic acid; Pynamin. $C_{19}H_{26}O_3$; mol wt 302.41. Synthesis: M. S. Schechter *et al., J. Am. Chem. Soc.* **71,** 1517, 3165 (1949); H. A. Stansbury, H. R. Guest, US 2768965 (1956 to UCC). Commer-

cial process: H. J. Sanders, A. W. Taff, *Ind. Eng. Chem.* **46,** 414 (1954). The commercial product is a mixture of 8 optically active isomers. Clear, pale yellow oil. bp $_{0.1}$ 140°. Decomp by rapid pyrolysis at >400°. Vaporizes without dec when heated at 150°. Unstable in light, air, alkaline conditions. d_{20}^{20} 1.010; n_D^{20} 1.5040; n_D^{30} 1.5023. Practically insol in water. Sol in alcohol, petr ether, kerosene, carbon tetrachloride, ethylene dichloride, nitromethane. Incompatible with alkalies.

Allethrin II. [497-92-7] 3-(3-Methoxy-2-methyl-3-oxo-1-pro-penyl)-2,2-dimethylcyclopropanecarboxylic acid 2-methyl-4-oxo-3-(2-propenyl)-2-cyclopenten-1-yl ester; allethrolone ester of chrysanthemumdicarboxylic acid monomethyl ester; ENT-17510. C_{20}-$H_{26}O_5$; mol wt 346.42. Synthesis: M. Matsui, Y. Yamada, *Agric. Biol. Chem.* **27,** 373 (1963); M. Matsui, H. Meguro, *ibid.* **28,** 27 (1964); M. Elliott, N. F. Janes, *Chem. Ind. (London)* **1969,** 270; A. Kobayashi *et al., Agric. Biol. Chem.* **35,** 1961 (1971); T. Sugiyama *et al., ibid.* **36,** 565 (1972). Oily pale yellow liq. $n_D^{20.6}$ 1.5156. uv max (ethanol): 232 nm (ε 23000). Unstable in light, air, alkaline conditions. Sol in organic solvents. Practically insol in water.

Caution: Potential symptoms of toxicity are similar to those of the pyrethrins.

USE: Insecticide.

261. Allicin. [539-86-6] 2-Propene-1-sulfinothioic acid *S*-2-propenyl ester; thio-2-propene-1-sulfinic acid *S*-allyl ester; diallyl disulfide-oxide. $C_6H_{10}OS_2$; mol wt 162.27. C 44.41%, H 6.21%, O 9.86%, S 39.52%. A biologically active constit of freshly crushed garlic (*Allium sativum* L., *Liliaceae*). Naturally formed by the action of the enzyme allicinase on alliin, *q.v.,* when the tissue of the garlic bulb is disrupted. Isoln and antibacterial activity: C. J. Cavallito, J. H. Bailey, *J. Am. Chem. Soc.* **66,** 1950 (1944). Structure: Cavallito *et al., ibid.* 1952. Synthesis: Stoll, Seebeck, *Experientia* **6,** 330 (1950); Cavallito, Small, US 2508745 (1950 to Sterling Drug). Antifungal activity: Y. Yamada, K. Azuma, *Antimicrob. Agents Chemother.* **11,** 743 (1977). Pharmacological effects and prepn: P. R. Mayeux *et al., Agents Actions* **25,** 182 (1988). Stability in blood, solvents, and simulated physiological fluids: F. Freeman, Y. Kodera, *J. Agric. Food Chem.* **43,** 2332 (1995). Identification as the source of garlic's pungent burning and prickling sensations: L. J. Macpherson *et al., Curr. Biol.* **15,** 929 (2005).

Yellow liquid. True odor of garlic. Decomp on distilling. d_4^{20} 1.112. n_D^{20} 1.561. Soly in water at 10° about 2.5% w/w. pH about 6.5. Upon standing an oily precipitate forms from aq solns. Miscible with alcohol, ether, benzene; fairly insol in the Skellysolves; unstable to hot alkali; stable to acids. LD_{50} in mice (mg/kg): 60 i.v.; 120 s.c. (Cavallito, Bailey).

262. Alliin. [556-27-4] 3-[(*S*)-2-Propenylsulfinyl]-L-ala-nine; 3-((*S*)-allylsulfinyl)-L-alanine; *S*-allyl-L-cysteine sulfoxide. $C_6H_{11}NO_3S$; mol wt 177.22. C 40.66%, H 6.26%, N 7.90%, O 27.08%, S 18.09%. Constituent of garlic, *Allium sativum* L., *Liliaceae;* also found in other *Allium* spp. Degraded by alliinase to produce the garlic flavor component, allicin, *q.v.* Isoln: Stoll, Seebeck, *Helv. Chim. Acta* **31,** 189 (1948). Synthesis: *eidem, Experientia* **6,** 330 (1950); *Helv. Chim. Acta* **34,** 481 (1951). Extraction from *Allium* plants and LC determn: E. Mochizuki *et al., J. AOAC Int.* **80,** 1052 (1997). *In vitro* immunomodulatory effects on peripheral blood cells: H. Salman *et al., Int. J. Immunopharmacol.* **21,** 589 (1999). Biosynthesis in garlic tissue cultures: J. Hughes *et al., Phytochemistry* **66,** 187 (2005).

Hemihydrate, odorless, bunched needles from dil acetone, mp 164-166° (effervescence). $[\alpha]_D^{20}$ +63.5° (c = 2). Freely sol in water. Practically insol in abs ethanol, chloroform, acetone, ether, benzene.

263. Allobarbital. [52-43-7] 5,5-Di-2-propenyl-2,4,-6(1H,3H,5H)pyrimidinetrione; 5,5-diallylbarbituric acid; allobarbitone. $C_{10}H_{12}N_2O_3$; mol wt 208.21. C 57.69%, H 5.81%, N 13.45%, O 23.05%. Prepn: US 1042265 (1912). Acute toxicity: F. Sandberg, *Acta Physiol. Scand.* **24**, 7 (1951).

Crystals, leaflets. Slightly bitter taste, mp 171-173°. One part dissolves in about 300 parts water, 50 parts boiling water, 20 parts cold alcohol, 20 parts ether; very sol in hot alcohol and in acetone; sol in ethyl acetate. Insol in aliphatic hydrocarbons. A satd aq soln is acid to litmus. LD_{50} i.p. in rats: 127.3 mg/kg (Sandberg).

Note: This is a controlled substance (depressant): 21 CFR, 1308.13.

THERAP CAT: Sedative, hypnotic.

264. Allocholesterol. [517-10-2] (3β)-Cholest-4-en-3-ol; coprostenol; 4:5-coprosten-3-ol. $C_{27}H_{46}O$; mol wt 386.65. C 83.87%, H 11.99%, O 4.14%. Prepn: Windaus, *Ann.* **453**, 101 (1927); Schoenheimer, Evans, *J. Biol. Chem.* **114**, 567 (1936). Sepn from cholesterol: Stoll, *Z. Physiol. Chem.* **246**, 10 (1937).

Needles from ether-methanol, mp 132°. $[\alpha]_D^{23}$ +43.7° (c = 1 in benzene). Freely sol in benzene, acetone, ether, chloroform, dioxane, pyridine; less sol in methanol, alcohol. Pptd by digitonin. Deep-red color with 90% trichloroacetic acid.

Acetate. $C_{29}H_{48}O_2$. Long needles from dil methanol, mp 85°.

265. Allocryptopine. [485-91-6] 5,7,8,15-Tetrahydro-3,4-dimethoxy-6-methylbenzo[e][1,3]dioxolo[4,5-k][3]benzazecin-14(6H)-one. $C_{21}H_{23}NO_5$; mol wt 369.41. C 68.28%, H 6.28%, N 3.79%, O 21.66%. Isomeric with cryptopine, *q.v.* Obtained from *Chelidonium majus* L., *Bocconia cordata* Willd., *Sanguinaria canadensis* L. and allied *Papaveraceae:* Manske in Manske, Holmes, *The Alkaloids* **vol. IV** (Academic Press, New York, 1954) p 159. Structure: Gadamer, *Arch. Pharm.* **257**, 298 (1919). Exists in two isomeric modifications designated as α- and β-forms. Identity of α-form with α-fagarine: Redemann *et al., J. Am. Chem. Soc.* **71**, 1030 (1949). Synthesis: Haworth, Perkin, *J. Chem. Soc.* **1926**, 445; Bentley, Murray, *ibid.* **1963**, 2497.

α-Allocryptopine. α-Fagarine. Crystals from ethanol, mp 160-161°. Soluble in alcohol, chloroform, ether, ethyl acetate and dil acids.

β-Allocryptopine. Crystallizes with ½ mol of alcohol or ethyl acetate. Melts after expelling the solvent, at 169-171°.

266. Allopregnane. [641-85-0] (5α)-Pregnane. $C_{21}H_{36}$; mol wt 288.51. C 87.42%, H 12.58%. Prepn from corticosterone: Steiger, Reichstein, *Helv. Chim. Acta* **21**, 161 (1938); from allopregnan-3-one: Ruzicka *et al., ibid.* **22**, 1294 (1939); from 21-hydroxyallopregnane: Plattner *et al., ibid.* **27**, 1177 (1944); Casanova, Reichstein, *ibid.* **32**, 647 (1949); by degradation of conessine: Haworth *et al., J. Chem. Soc.* **1949**, 831; by Hofmann decomposition of 3β- and 3α-dimethylaminopregnanes: Haworth *et al., ibid.* **1953**, 1110.

Crystals from acetone + methanol, mp 84-85°. $[\alpha]_D^{19}$ +18.4° (c = 1.69 in chloroform).

267. Allopregnane-3α,20α-diol. [566-58-5] (3α,5α,20S)-Pregnane-3,20-diol; 5α-pregnane-3α,20α-diol; 3α,20α-dihydroxy-5α-pregnane. $C_{21}H_{36}O_2$; mol wt 320.51. C 78.69%, H 11.32%, O 9.98%. Progesterone metabolite. Isoln from human pregnancy urine: Beall, *Biochem. J.* **31**, 35 (1937); from bulls' urine: Marker *et al., J. Am. Chem. Soc.* **60**, 2931 (1938). Prepn by reduction of 5α-pregn-1-ene-3,20-dione with lithium aluminum hydride: Schütt, Tamm, *Helv. Chim. Acta* **41**, 1751 (1958).

Crystals from methanol, mp 243-245°. $[\alpha]_D^{20}$ +17° (c = 0.148 in ethanol).

Diacetate. $C_{25}H_{40}O_4$. Crystals, mp 139.5-140.5°. $[\alpha]_D^{20}$ +18° (c = 0.408 in benzene).

268. Allopregnane-3α,20β-diol. [566-57-4] (3α,5α,20R)-Pregnane-3,20-diol; 3α,20β-dihydroxy-5α-pregnane. $C_{21}H_{36}O_2$; mol wt 320.51. C 78.69%, H 11.32%, O 9.98%. Progesterone metabolite. Prepn by hydrogenation of progesterone: Marker, Lawson, *J. Am. Chem. Soc.* **61**, 694 (1939); by catalytic hydrogenation of epiallopregnane-3-ol-20-one: Marker, US 2231019 (1941 to Parke, Davis); by reduction of 5α-pregn-1-ene-3,20-dione with lithium aluminum hydride: Schütt, Tamm, *Helv. Chim. Acta* **41**, 1751 (1958).

Needles from acetone, mp 207-209°. $[\alpha]_D^{26}$ +12° (c = 1.132 in chloroform).

269. Allopregnane-3β,20α-diol. [566-56-3] (3β,5α,20S)-Pregnane-3,20-diol; 5α-pregnane-3β,20α-diol; 3β,20α-dihydroxy-5α-pregnane. $C_{21}H_{36}O_2$; mol wt 320.51. C 78.69%, H 11.32%, O 9.98%. Progesterone metabolite. Isoln from pregnant mares' urine: Brooks *et al., Biochem. J.* **51**, 694 (1952). Prepn by heating 3α,20α-dihydroxy-5α-pregnane with sodium, or by hydrogenation of 5α-pregnane-20-ol-3-one in acid: Marker, US 2196220 and US 2250962 (1940, 1941, both to Parke, Davis); by reduction of allopregnan-3β-ol-20-one acetate with sodium: Klyne, Barton, *J. Am. Chem. Soc.* **71**, 1500 (1949); by reduction of 5,16-pregnadien-3β-ol-20-one with Zn + acetic acid: Ercoli, De Ruggieri, *Farm. Sci. Tec.* **7**, 11 (1952), *C.A.* **46**, 10186b (1952).

Crystals from acetone, mp 218-219°. $[\alpha]_D^{22}$ +23° (c = 0.93 in chloroform).

Diacetate. $C_{25}H_{40}O_4$. Crystals from petr ether, mp 164-165°. $[\alpha]_D^{19}$ +0.8° (c = 1.2 in chloroform).

Dibenzoate. $C_{35}H_{44}O_4$. Crystals, mp 170.5-172°. $[\alpha]_D^{20}$ +27.7° (c = 0.84 in chloroform).

270. Allopregnane-3β,20β-diol. [516-53-0] (3β,5α,20R)-Pregnane-3,20-diol; 3β,20β-dihydroxy-5α-pregnane. $C_{21}H_{36}O_2$; mol wt 320.51. C 78.69%, H 11.32%, O 9.98%. Progesterone metabolite. Isoln from pregnant mares' urine: Brooks *et al., Biochem. J.* **51**, 694 (1952). Prepn by catalytic reduction of allopregnane-3,20-dione: Marker *et al.,* GB 512940 (1939 to Parke, Davis); by hydrogenation of pregn-5-ene-3β-ol-20-one: Klyne, Barton, *J.*

Am. Chem. Soc. **71,** 1500 (1949); by hydrogenation of pregn-5-ene-3β,20β-diol: Klyne, Miller, *J. Chem. Soc.* **1950,** 1972.

Leaflets from ethyl acetate + petr ether, mp 194.5-195.5°. $[\alpha]_D$ +4.4° (c = 1.04 in chloroform).

Diacetate. $C_{25}H_{40}O_4$. Needles from ethyl acetate + petr ether, mp 141-142.5°. $[\alpha]_D^{20}$ +21° (c = 1 in chloroform).

Dibenzoate. $C_{35}H_{44}O_4$. Crystals, mp 237.5-239°. $[\alpha]_D^{20}$ −10.1° (c = 2.08 in chloroform).

271. Allopregnane-3β,17α-diol-20-one. [570-54-7] (3β,5α)-3,17-Dihydroxypregnan-20-one; 3β,17-dihydroxy-5α-pregnan-20-one; 3β,17-dihydroxy-20-oxo-5α-pregnane; 17-(1-ketoethyl)androstane-3,17-diol; Reichstein's substance L; Wintersteiner's compound G. $C_{21}H_{34}O_3$; mol wt 334.49. C 75.41%, H 10.25%, O 14.35%. Isoln from adrenal cortex: Wintersteiner, Pfiffner, *J. Biol. Chem.* **116,** 291 (1936). Structure: Reichstein, Gätzi, *Helv. Chim. Acta* **21,** 1497 (1938). Prepn from allopregnan-3β-ol-20-one 3-acetate: Rosenkranz *et al., J. Am. Chem. Soc.* **72,** 4081 (1950); from pregn-5-ene-3β-ol-20-one: Ramirez, Stafie, *ibid.* **77,** 134 (1955).

Crystals from abs alcohol, mp 264-266°. $[\alpha]_D^{21}$ +30.6° (c = 0.54 in abs alcohol).

3-Acetate. $C_{23}H_{36}O_4$. Crystals from acetone, mp 187-189°. $[\alpha]_D^{20}$ +18° (acetone).

272. 3,20-Allopregnanedione. [566-65-4] (5α)-Pregnane-3,20-dione; 3,20-dioxo-5α-pregnane. $C_{21}H_{32}O_2$; mol wt 316.48. C 79.70%, H 10.19%, O 10.11%. From pregnancy urine: Hartmann, Locher, *Helv. Chim. Acta* **18,** 160 (1935); Lieberman *et al., J. Biol. Chem.* **172,** 263 (1948). Prepn from pregna-4,11-diene-3,20-dione: Shoppee, Reichstein, *Helv. Chim. Acta* **24,** 356 (1941); by oxidation of allopregnan-3β-ol-20-one with chromium trioxide: Billeter, Miescher, *ibid.* **30,** 1409 (1947); by hydrogenation of pregnenolone: Pappas, Nace, *J. Am. Chem. Soc.* **81,** 4556 (1959); from funtumine: Janot *et al., Bull. Soc. Chim. Fr.* **1960,** 1669.

Crystals from methylene chloride + hexane, mp 200°. $[\alpha]_D$ +125° (c = 1.2 in chloroform).

USE: In the synthesis of progesterone, **FR 845034** *C.A.* **34,** 8184² (1940).

273. Allopregnane-3α,11β,17α,21-tetrol-20-one. [302-91-0] (3α,5α,11β)-3,11,17,21-Tetrahydroxypregnan-20-one; 3α,11β,-17,21-tetrahydroxy-5α-pregnan-20-one; 3α,11β,17,21-tetrahydroxy-20-oxo-5α-pregnane; 17-(1-keto-2-hydroxyethyl)androstane-3,11,17-triol; 3α-allotetrahydrocortisol; Kendall's compound C; Reichstein's substance C; Wintersteiner's compound D. $C_{21}H_{34}-O_5$; mol wt 366.49. C 68.82%, H 9.35%, O 21.83%. Isoln from adrenal cortex: Mason *et al., J. Biol. Chem.* **124,** 459 (1938); Kuizenga, Cartland, *Endocrinology* **24,** 526 (1939); v. Euw, Reichstein, *Helv. Chim. Acta* **25,** 988 (1942); v. Euw *et al., ibid.* **41,** 1516 (1958). Prepn by hydrogenation of cortisol with rhodium: Caspi, *J. Org. Chem.* **24,** 669 (1959); from bismethylenedioxyhydrocortisone: Fukushima, Daum, *ibid.* **26,** 520 (1961).

Crystals from methanol, mp 244-245°. $[\alpha]_D^{21}$ +59.7° (c = 0.34 in methanol).

3,21-Diacetate. $C_{25}H_{38}O_7$. Crystals, dec 204-205°. $[\alpha]_D^{20}$ +73.8°; $[\alpha]_{542}^{20}$ +90.5° (dioxane).

274. Allopregnane-3β,11β,21-triol-20-one. [516-16-5] (3β,5α,11β)-3,11,21-Trihydroxypregnan-20-one; 3β,11β,21-trihydroxy-20-oxo-5α-pregnane; Reichstein's substance R. $C_{21}H_{34}O_4$; mol wt 350.49. C 71.96%, H 9.78%, O 18.26%. Isolation from adrenal glands: Reichstein, von Euw, *Helv. Chim. Acta* **21,** 1197 (1938); Reichstein, *ibid.* 1490. Partial synthesis by hydrogenation of corticosterone acetate: Pataki *et al., J. Biol. Chem.* **195,** 751 (1952). Prepn from 3β,11β-dihydroxyalloetiocholanic acid: Lardon, Reichstein, *Helv. Chim. Acta* **37,** 443 (1954); from hydrocortisone: Mancera *et al, J. Am. Chem. Soc.* **77,** 5669 (1955); from 3β,21-diacetoxy-17(20)-allopregnene + osmium tetroxide and triethylamine oxide peroxide: Schneider, Hanze, **US 2769823** (1956 to Upjohn).

Needles from alc, mp 202-204°. $[\alpha]_D$ +110° (ethanol).

3,21-Diacetate. $C_{25}H_{38}O_6$. Crystals from acetone + ether, mp 170-172°. $[\alpha]_D^{22}$ +82.5° (c = 1.38 in dioxane); $[\alpha]_D^{20}$ +101° (acetone).

275. Allopregnan-3α-ol-20-one. [516-54-1] 3α-Hydroxy-5α-pregnan-20-one; 5α-pregnan-3α-ol-20-one; epiallopregnanolone; allotetrahydroprogesterone. $C_{21}H_{34}O_2$; mol wt 318.49. C 79.19%, H 10.76%, O 10.05%. Naturally occurring metabolite of progesterone. Prototype of the neuroactive steroids known as *epalons* that allosterically modulate γ-aminobutyric acid type A (GABA$_A$) receptors in the CNS. Isoln from human pregnancy urine: R. E. Marker *et al., J. Am. Chem. Soc.* **59,** 616 (1937). Prepn from pregnenolone: G. Fleischer *et al., ibid.* **60,** 79 (1938). Chromatographic determn in urine: F. J. Bègue *et al., J. Chromatogr. Sci.* **12,** 763 (1974). Synthesis, metabolism and pharmacology: R. H. Purdy *et al., J. Med. Chem.* **33,** 1572 (1990). Review of pharmacology and therapeutic potential of epalons: K. W. Gee *et al., Crit. Rev. Neurobiol.* **9,** 207-227 (1995).

Crystals from abs alc, mp 176-178°. $[\alpha]_D$ +87.7° (abs alc).

Acetate. $C_{23}H_{36}O_3$. Crystals from aq ethanol, mp 141-142°. $[\alpha]_D^{22}$ +94.5° (abs ethanol).

276. Allopregnan-3β-ol-20-one. [516-55-2] (3β,5α)-3-Hydroxypregnan-20-one; 3β-hydroxy-20-oxo-5α-pregnane. $C_{21}-H_{34}O_2$; mol wt 318.49. C 79.19%, H 10.76%, O 10.05%. Isoln from adrenal cortex: von Euw, Reichstein, *Helv. Chim. Acta* **24,** 885 (1941); from corpus luteum: Butenandt, Mamoli, *Ber.* **68,** 1847 (1935); Prelog, Meister, *Helv. Chim. Acta* **32,** 2435 (1949); from human pregnancy urine: Lieberman *et al., J. Biol. Chem.* **172,** 263 (1948); from human placenta: Pearlman, Cerceo, *ibid.* **194,** 807 (1952). Prepn from 20-methyl-Δ²⁰-allopregnen-3β-ol: Koechlin, Reichstein, *Helv. Chim. Acta* **27,** 549 (1944); from pregnenolone: Mancera *et al., J. Org. Chem.* **16,** 192 (1951); Pappas, Nace, *J. Am. Chem. Soc.* **81,** 4556 (1959); by redn of allopregnane-3,20-dione with sodium borohydride: Mancera *et al., ibid.* **75,** 1286 (1953); from progesterone 20-cycloethylene ketal: Sondheimer, Klibansky, *Tetrahedron* **5,** 15 (1959).

Plates from dil methanol, mp 194-195°. $[\alpha]_D^{27}$ +91.2° (c = 0.4 in ethanol).

Acetate. $C_{23}H_{36}O_3$. Plates from methanol, mp 144-146°. $[\alpha]_D^{25}$ +69° (chloroform).

277. Allopregnan-20α-ol-3-one. [516-59-6] (5α,20S)-20-Hydroxypregnan-3-one; 20α-hydroxy-5α-pregnan-3-one; 20α-hydroxy-3-oxo-5α-pregnane. $C_{21}H_{34}O_2$; mol wt 318.49. C 79.19%, H 10.76%, O 10.05%. Prepn from funtumidine: Janot *et al., Bull. Soc. Chim. Fr.* **1960,** 1669.

Crystals, mp 179°. $[\alpha]_D$ +36.6° (c = 0.8 in chloroform).

Acetate. $C_{23}H_{36}O_3$. Crystals from ethanol, mp 155°. $[\alpha]_D$ +24° (c = 1.5 in chloroform).

278. Allopregnan-20β-ol-3-one. [516-58-5] (5α,20R)-20-Hydroxypregnan-3-one; 20β-hydroxy-5α-pregnan-3-one; 20β-hydroxy-3-oxo-5α-pregnane. $C_{21}H_{34}O_2$; mol wt 318.49. C 79.19%, H 10.76%, O 10.05%. Prepn from allopregnane-3β,20β-diol-3-acetate: Rubin *et al., J. Am. Chem. Soc.* **73,** 2338 (1951); from isofuntumidine: Janot *et al., Bull. Soc. Chim. Fr.* **1960,** 1669.

Crystals from heptane, mp 185°. $[\alpha]_D$ +20° (c = 1.2 in chloroform).

Acetate. $C_{23}H_{36}O_3$. Crystals from ethanol, mp 148°. $[\alpha]_D$ +57° (c = 1.9 in chloroform).

279. Allopurinol. [315-30-0] 1,5-Dihydro-4H-pyrazolo-[3,4-d]pyrimidin-4-one; 1H-pyrazolo[3,4-d]pyrimidin-4-ol; 4-hydroxypyrazolo[3,4-d]pyrimidine; HPP; BW-56158; Adenock; Allurit; Aloral; Alositol; Allo-Puren; Allozym; Allural; Anoprolin; Anzief; Apulonga; Apurol; Apurin; Bleminol; Caplenal; Cellidrin; Cosuric; Dabroson; Embarin; Epidropal; Foligan; Gichtex; Hamarin; Hexanurat; Ketanrift; Lopurin; Lysuron; Miniplanor; Monarch; Remid; Riball; Sigapurol; Suspendol; Takanarumin; Uricemil; Uripurinol; Urosin; Urtias; Zyloprim; Zyloric. $C_5H_4N_4O$; mol wt 136.11. C 44.12%, H 2.96%, N 41.16%, O 11.75%. Xanthine oxidase inhibitor; decreases uric acid production. Prepn: Robins, *J. Am. Chem. Soc.* **78**, 784 (1956); Schmidt, Druey, *Helv. Chim. Acta* **39**, 986 (1956); Druey, Schmidt, **US 2868803** (1959 to Ciba); **GB 798646** (1958 to Wellcome Found.); Hitchings, Falco, **US 3474098** (1969 to Burroughs Wellcome). Physiological and biochemical studies: Hitchings, in *Biochem. Aspects Antimetab. Drug Hydroxylation*, D. Shugar, Ed. (Academic Press, London, 1969) pp 11-22, *C.A.* **75**, 3531h (1971). Clinical trial in treatment of renal calculi: M. J. V. Smith, *J. Urol.* **117**, 690 (1977); B. Ettinger *et al., N. Engl. J. Med.* **315**, 1386 (1986). Use in hyperuricemia and gout: G. R. Boss, J. E. Seegmiller, *ibid.* **300**, 1459 (1977). Effect on renal function in treatment of gout: T. Gibson, *Ann. Rheum. Dis.* **41**, 59 (1982). Comprehensive description: S. A. Benezra, T. R. Bennett, *Anal. Profiles Drug Subs.* **7**, 1-17 (1978).

Crystals, mp above 350°. uv max (0.1*N* NaOH): 257 nm (ε 7200); (0.1*N* HCl): 250 nm (ε 7600); (methanol): 252 nm (ε 7600). Soly in mg/ml at 25°: water 0.48; *n*-octanol <0.01; chloroform 0.60; ethanol 0.30; DMSO 4.6. pKa 10.2.

Sodium salt. [17795-21-0] Aloprim. $C_5H_3N_4NaO$; mol wt 158.09. White amorphous mass. pKa 9.31.

THERAP CAT: Treatment of hyperuricemia and chronic gout. Antiurolithic.

280. D-Allose. [2595-97-3] β-D-Allopyranose. $C_6H_{12}O_6$; mol wt 180.16. C 40.00%, H 6.71%, O 53.28%. An aldohexose sugar. Obtained from leaves of *Protea rubropilosa*: Beylis, Perold, *Chem. Commun.* **1971**, 597. Prepd by reduction of D-allonic lactone with sodium amalgam: Levene, Jacobs, *Ber.* **43**, 3147 (1910). Synthesis: Hughes, Speakman, *J. Chem. Soc.* **1965**, 2236; Baker *et al., Carbohydr. Res.* **24**, 192 (1972).

Crystals from dilute methanol, mp 128-128.5°. Shows mutarotation: $[\alpha]_D^{20}$ +0.58° (4 min) → +3.26° (10 min) → +14.41° (final value, 20 hr; c = 5). Soluble in water. Practically insol in alcohol.

Phenylosazone. $C_{18}H_{22}N_4O_4$. mp 178°.

281. Allotetrahydrocortisone. [547-77-3] (3α,5α)-3,17,21-Trihydroxy-pregnane-11,20-dione; Reichstein's substance Dehydro-C; 11-dehydro C; allopregnane-3α,17α,21-triol-11,20-dione. $C_{21}H_{32}O_5$; mol wt 364.48. C 69.20%, H 8.85%, O 21.95%. Isoln from beef adrenals: v. Euw *et al., Helv. Chim. Acta* **41**, 1516 (1958). Synthesis of the 3α,21-diacetate: Nagata *et al., ibid.* **42**, 1399 (1959).

Rhombohedric leaflets from acetone + water, mp 212-214°.

3α,21-Diacetate. $C_{25}H_{36}O_7$. Rhombohedric platelets, mp 225-227°; $[\alpha]_D^{25}$ +94.2 ±1.5° (c = 1.45 in dioxane).

282. Alloxan. [50-71-5] 2,4,5,6(1*H*,3*H*)-pyrimidinetetrone; 2,4,5,6-tetraoxohexahydropyrimidine; mesoxalylurea; mesoxalylcarbamide. $C_4H_2N_2O_4$; mol wt 142.07. C 33.82%, H 1.42%, N 19.72%, O 45.05%. Found by Liebig in mucus excreted during dysentery. Prepn by direct oxidation of uric acid: G. Brugnatelli, *Ann. Chim. Phys.* [2] **8**, 201 (1818); J. Liebig, F. Wöhler, *Ann.* **26**, 241 (1838); H. Biltz, M. Hehn, *ibid.* **413**, 60 (1917). Prepd from alloxantin: J. Liebig, *ibid.* **147**, 366 (1868); W. W. Hartman, O. E. Sheppard, *Org. Synth.* **coll. vol. III**, 37 (1955). *See also* A. V. Holmgren, W. W. Wenner, *ibid.* **coll. vol. IV**, 23 (1963). Produces diabetes in animals by selective necrosis of pancreatic islet β-cells: J. S. Dunn, N. G. B. McLetchie, *Lancet* **2**, 384 (1943); W. B. Kennedy, F. D. W. Lukens, *Proc. Soc. Exp. Biol. Med.* **57**, 143 (1944). Mechanism of action study: L. Boquist, *Acta Pathol. Microbiol. Scand. Sect. A* **88**, 201 (1980). *In vitro* antineoplastic activity: P. Grobon, *C.R. Seances Acad. Sci. Ser. D* **280**, 2413 (1975). Antibacterial and antifungal activity: J. D. Douros, A. F. Kerst, **JP Kokai 72 4900**; *eidem*, **US 3728454** (1972, 1973 both to Gates Rubber Co.). Toxicological study in mice: B. A. Waisbren, *Proc. Soc. Exp. Biol. Med.* **67**, 154 (1948).

Anhydrous, orthorhombic crystals from anhydr acetone or glacial acetic acid or by sublimation in vacuo. Turns pink at 230° and dec at 256°. Acid to litmus. pK (25°) 6.63. Absorption spectrum: Hartley, *J. Chem. Soc.* **87**, 1802, 1808 (1905). Freely sol in water. Hot aqueous solns are yellow and become colorless on cooling. Aqueous solns, after being in contact with the human skin for some time, give it a red color and a disagreeable odor. Sol in acetone, alcohol, methanol, glacial acetic acid; slightly sol in chloroform, petr ether, toluene, ethyl acetate and acetic anhydride. Insol in ether.

Tetrahydrate. Large triclinic prisms or oblique monoclinic rhombs from water.

Monohydrate. By heating the tetrahydrate at 100° or by exposing it to the air. Forms triclinic pinacoidal crystals.

Compound with urea. $CH_4N_2O.C_4H_2N_2O_4.H_2O$. Minute, yellow needles; red at 170°, decomp at 185-186°.

USE: In production of diabetes in experimental animals; in nutrition experiments; in organic syntheses.

283. Alloxantin. [76-24-4] 5,5'-Dihydroxy-[5,5'-bipyrimidine]-2,2',4,4',6,6'(1*H*,1'*H*,3*H*,3'*H*,5*H*,5'*H*)-hexone; 5,5'-dihydroxy-5,5'-bibarbituric acid; uroxin. $C_8H_6N_4O_8$; mol wt 286.16. C 33.58%, H 2.11%, N 19.58%, O 44.73%. Prepd from uric acid: Nightingale, *Org. Synth.* **coll. vol. II**, 42 (1955); from alloxan monohydrate: Tipson, *ibid.* **coll. vol. IV**, 25 (1963). Structure: Singh, *Acta Crystallogr.* **19**, 767 (1965).

Dihydrate. Cryst powder. On exposure to air becomes red. Becomes yellow at 225°; dec at 253-255°. Sparingly sol in cold water, alcohol or ether. Its aq soln is acid; reduces Ag salts and gives a blue ppt with Ba(OH)$_2$ soln. *Keep tightly closed.* Emits toxic fumes upon decompn.

Caution: Ingestion causes disturbed carbohydrate metabolism leading to diabetes, *cf. Dangerous Properties of Industrial Materials*, N. I. Sax, Ed. (Van Nostrand Reinhold, New York, 4th ed., 1975) p 366.

284. Allura Red AC. [25956-17-6] 6-Hydroxy-5-[(2-methoxy-5-methyl-4-sulfophenyl)azo]-2-naphthalenesulfonic acid disodium salt; 6-hydroxy-5-[(6-methoxy-4-sulfo-*m*-tolyl)azo]-2-naphthalenesulfonic acid disodium salt; 1-[(6-methoxy-4-sulfo-*m*-tolyl)azo]-2-naphthol-6-sulfonic acid disodium salt; FD & C Red No. 40; C.I. 16035; C.I. Food Red 17. $C_{18}H_{14}N_2Na_2O_8S_2$; mol wt 496.42. C 43.55%, H 2.84%, N 5.64%, Na 9.26%, O 25.78%, S 12.92%. Prepn: **GB 1164249** *C.A.* **72,** 68195j (1970) corresp to Rast, Steiner, **US 3519617** (1969, 1970, both to Allied Chem.).

Dark red powder. Soly at 25°: water, 22.5%; 50% alcohol, 1.3%.

USE: Color additive in foods, drugs and cosmetics.

285. Allyl acetate. [591-87-7] Acetic acid 2-propenyl ester; 3-acetoxy-1-propene. $C_5H_8O_2$; mol wt 100.12. C 59.98%, H 8.05%, O 31.96%. $CH_2=CHCH_2OCOCH_3$. Prepn: N. Zinin, *Ann.* **1855,** 361; K. N. Gurudutt *et al., Tetrahedron* **38,** 1843 (1982); and physical properties: G. H. Jeffery, A. I. Vogel, *J. Chem. Soc.* **1948,** 658. Vibrational spectra and thermodynamic functions: B. Singh *et al., Proc. Indian Acad. Sci.* **89,** 201 (1980). Acute toxicity: H. F. Smyth, Jr. *et al., J. Ind. Hyg. Toxicol.* **31,** 60 (1949); P. M. Jenner *et al., Food Cosmet. Toxicol.* **2,** 327 (1964). Effect on respiratory function in mice: G. D. Nielsen *et al., Acta Pharmacol. Toxicol.* **54,** 292 (1984).

bp_{760} 104° (Gurudutt); also reported as bp_{773} 104° (Jeffery, Vogel), bp 105° (Zinin). n_D 1.40396. d_4^{20} 0.9277. LD_{50}: 0.13 g/kg orally in rats; 1.1 ml/kg dermally in rabbits (Smyth). LD_{50} in rats, mice (mg/kg): 142, 170 orally (Jenner).

286. Allyl Alcohol. [107-18-6] 2-Propen-1-ol; 1-propenol-3; vinyl carbinol. C_3H_6O; mol wt 58.08. C 62.04%, H 10.41%, O 27.55%. $CH_2=CHCH_2OH$. Prepd by heating glycerol with formic acid: O. Kamm, C. S. Marvel, *Org. Synth.* **coll. vol. I,** 42 (2nd ed., 1941); *cf.* Delaby, Dubois, *Compt. Rend.* **188,** 710 (1929). Toxicity study: Smyth, Carpenter, *J. Ind. Hyg. Toxicol.* **30,** 63 (1948).

Colorless liquid; pungent, mustard-like odor. d_4^{20} 0.8540. bp 96-97°. mp −50°. n_D^{20} 1.41345. Absorption spectrum: Lüthy, *Z. Phys. Chem.* **107,** 289 (1923). Flash pt 70°F (open cup); 75°F (closed cup); autoignition temp 713°F. 72.3% of the alcohol with 27.7% water forms a constant boiling mixture, bp at 87.5°. Miscible with water, alcohol, chloroform, ether, petr ether. *Keep tightly closed.* Upon storage for several years allyl alcohol polymerizes and a thick syrup is formed (insol in water, sol in chloroform) which on treatment with ether yields a brittle resinoid mass: Blicke, *J. Am. Chem. Soc.* **45,** 1563 (1923). LD_{50} orally in rats: 64 mg/kg (Smyth, Carpenter).

Caution: Potential symptoms of overexposure are eye irritation, tissue damage; irritation of upper respiratory system and skin; pulmonary edema. *See NIOSH Pocket Guide to Chemical Hazards* (DHHS/NIOSH 97-140, 1997) p 10.

USE: Manuf allyl compds, war gas, resins, plasticizers.

287. Allylamine. [107-11-9] 2-Propen-1-amine; 3-aminopropylene. C_3H_7N; mol wt 57.09. C 63.11%, H 12.36%, N 24.53%. $CH_2=CHCH_2NH_2$. Manuf from allyl chloride and ammonia: Ploetz, **US 2915385** (1959 to Feldmühle Papier und Zellstoffwerke). Toxicity study: C. H. Hine *et al., Arch. Environ. Health* **1,** 34 (1960).

Liquid; burning taste; strong ammonia odor causing sneezing and tears. d_{20}^{20} 0.760. bp 55-58°. n_D^{20} 1.4186. Flash pt, closed cup: 10°F (−12°C). Misc with water, alc, chloroform, ether. *Keep tightly closed.* LD_{50} i.p. in mice: 49 mg/kg (Hine).

Caution: A strong eye and respiratory tract irritant; intolerable at 14 ppm. *See Patty's Industrial Hygiene and Toxicology* **vol. 2B,** G. D. Clayton, F. E. Clayton, Eds. (Wiley-Interscience, New York, 3rd ed., 1981) pp 3157-3158.

USE: In the manuf of mercurial diuretics.

288. Allyl Bromide. [106-95-6] 3-Bromo-1-propene; 3-bromopropylene; bromallylene. C_3H_5Br; mol wt 120.98. C 29.78%, H 4.17%, Br 66.05%. $CH_2=CHCH_2Br$. Prepd from hydrobromic acid and allyl alcohol: O. Kamm, C. S. Marvel, *Org. Synth.* **coll. vol. I,** 27 (2nd ed., 1941); from triphenylphosphite, allyl alcohol and benzyl bromide: Landauer, Rydon, *J. Chem. Soc.* **1953,** 2224.

Colorless liquid; unpleasant, pungent odor. d_4^{20} 1.398. bp_{760} 71.3°. mp −119°. n_D^{20} 1.46545. Slightly sol in water; miscible with alcohol, chloroform, ether, carbon disulfide, carbon tetrachloride. *Keep tightly closed.*

Caution: Produces irritation of eyes, respiratory passages.

USE: Manuf synthetic perfumes, other allyl compounds.

289. Allyl Chloride. [107-05-1] 3-Chloro-1-propene; 3-chloropropylene; chlorallylene. C_3H_5Cl; mol wt 76.52. C 47.09%, H 6.59%, Cl 46.33%. $CH_2=CHCH_2Cl$. Manuf by chlorination of propylene: Samples, Hilbert, **US 3054831** (1962 to Union Carbide). Prepd from diphenylphosphite, allyl alcohol and benzyl chloride: Landauer, Rydon, *J. Chem. Soc.* **1953,** 2224. Toxicity data: H. F. Smyth, C. P. Carpenter, *J. Ind. Hyg. Toxicol.* **30,** 63 (1948).

Liquid; unpleasant, pungent odor. d_4^{20} 0.938. bp 44-45°. mp −134.5°. n_D^{20} 1.4154. Flash pt, closed cup: −25°F (−31°C). Slightly sol in water; misc with alcohol, chloroform, ether, petrol ether. *Keep tightly closed.* LD_{50} orally in rats: 0.7 g/kg (Smyth, Carpenter).

Caution: Potential symptoms of overexposure are irritation of eyes, nose, skin and mucous membranes; pulmonary edema. *See NIOSH Pocket Guide to Chemical Hazards* (DHHS/NIOSH 97-140, 1997) p 10.

USE: In the synthesis of allyl compds.

290. Allyl Cyanide. [109-75-1] 3-Butenenitrile; vinylacetonitrile; β-butenonitrile. C_4H_5N; mol wt 67.09. C 71.61%, H 7.51%, N 20.88%. $CH_2=CHCH_2CN$. Found in some mustard oils. Prepd by treating dry CuCN with allyl bromide: Bruylants, *Bull. Soc. Chim. Belg.* **31,** 175 (1922); Supniewski, Salzberg, *Org. Synth.* **coll. vol. I,** 46 (2nd ed., 1941). Toxicity study: H. F. Smyth *et al., Am. Ind. Hyg. Assoc. J.* **30,** 470 (1969).

Liquid. Agreeable onion-like odor. Stable to heat. d_4^{20} 0.8341. mp −87°. bp_{760} 119°; bp_{400} 98°; bp_{200} 78°; bp_{100} 60.2°; bp_{60} 48.8°; bp_{40} 40.0°; bp_{20} 26.6°; bp_{10} 14.1°; bp_5 2.9°; $bp_{1.0}$ −19.6°. n_D^{20} 1.4060. Absorption spectrum in hexane, water and dil alkali: Bruylants, Castille, *op. cit.* **34,** 265; *Chem. Zentralbl.* **1926, I,** 1962. LD_{50} orally in rats: 0.115 g/kg (Smyth).

291. Allylestrenol. [432-60-0] (17β)-17-(2-Propenyl)estr-4-en-17-ol; 17-allylestr-4-en-17β-ol; 17α-allyl-17-hydroxy-19-nor-4-androstene; 17-hydroxy-17α-allyl-4-estrene; Gestanin; Gestanon; Gestanyn; Orageston; Turinal. $C_{21}H_{32}O$; mol wt 300.48. C 83.94%, H 10.73%, O 5.32%. Prepn: **GB 841411** (1960 to Organon). Determn in pharmaceutical formulations: S. Görög *et al., Analyst* **104,** 196 (1979). Clinical experience in pregnancy: J. Cortés-Prieto *et al., Clin. Ther.* **3,** 200 (1980).

Crystals, mp 79.5-80°. Practically insol in water. Sol in alcohol, ether, acetone, chloroform. Sensitive to oxidizing agents.

THERAP CAT: Progestogen.

292. Allyl Ether. [557-40-4] 3,3'-Oxybis-1-propene; diallyl ether. $C_6H_{10}O$; mol wt 98.14. C 73.43%, H 10.27%, O

16.30%. $(CH_2=CHCH_2)_2O$. Prepn from allyl alcohol in the presence of $CuCl-H_2SO_4$: Stephenson, **GB 913919** (1962 to Monsanto); from allyl alcohol with K_2CO_3 and allyl bromide: Riemschneider, Kötzsch, *Monatsh. Chem.* **90**, 787 (1959). Toxicity: H. F. Smyth *et al., J. Ind. Hyg. Toxicol.* **31**, 60 (1949).

Liquid; radish-like odor. d_0^{18} 0.805. bp 94°. n_D^{20} 1.4240. Practically insol in water. Miscible with alc, ether. LD_{50} orally in rats: 0.32 g/kg (Smyth).

Caution: An irritant. Can be absorbed through skin.

293. Allyl Ethyl Ether. [557-31-3] 3-Ethoxy-1-propene; ethyl allyl ether. $C_5H_{10}O$; mol wt 86.13. C 69.72%, H 11.70%, O 18.58%. $CH_2=CHCH_2OCH_2CH_3$. Prepd from allyl bromide and sodium alcoholate: Brühl, *Ann.* **200**, 139 (1880).

Liquid. d 0.765. $bp_{742.9}$ 66-67°. n_D^{20} 1.3881. Practically insol in water. Miscible with alc, ether.

Caution: Irritating to eyes, skin, mucous membranes.

294. Allyl Iodide. [556-56-9] 3-Iodo-1-propene; 3-iodopropylene. C_3H_5I; mol wt 167.98. C 21.45%, H 3.00%, I 75.55%. $CH_2=CHCH_2I$. Prepd from allyl alcohol, methyl iodide, and triphenyl phosphite: Landauer, Rydon, *J. Chem. Soc.* **1953**, 2224; Rydon, Landauer, **GB 695468** (1953 to Nat. Res. Dev. Corp.).

Yellowish liquid; darkens on exposure to light and air, liberating iodine. Unpleasant, pungent odor. d^{12} 1.848. bp 103°. n_D^{21} 1.5540. Practically insol in water. Miscible with alc, chloroform, ether.

Caution: See Allyl Chloride. *Keep tightly closed and protected from light.*

295. Allyl Isothiocyanate. [57-06-7] 3-Isothiocyanato-1-propene; isothiocyanic acid allyl ester; allyl isosulfocyanate; "mustard oil"; allyl mustard oil. C_4H_5NS; mol wt 99.15. C 48.45%, H 5.08%, N 14.13%, S 32.34%. Principal constituent of *volatile oil of mustard*. Occurs in seeds as the glucoside, sinigrin, *q.v.* Isolated from *Brassica nigra* (L.) Koch, *Cruciferae* (black mustard seed), or prepd from allyl iodide and potassium thiocyanate: Dulière, *J. Pharm. Belg.* **2**, 981 (1920), *C.A.* **15**, 571⁴ (1921). Description: E. Guenther, D. Althausen, *The Essential Oils* vol. II (Van Nostrand, New York, 1949) pp. 734-7. Review of isolation: E. Guenther, *ibid.* vol VI, pp. 55-60 (1952); and synthesis: G. M. Dyson, *Perfum. Essent. Oil Rec.* **20**, 42 (1929). Evaluation in relieving muscle pain: J. G. Macarthur, S. Alstead, *Lancet* **2**, 1060 (1953). Toxicity study: P. M. Jenner *et al., Food Cosmet. Toxicol.* **2**, 327 (1964). HPLC determn in brown mustard: K. Kanemaru *et al., J. Jpn. Soc. Food Sci. Technol.* **37**, 565 (1990).

Colorless or pale yellow, very refractive liquid; very pungent, irritating odor; acrid taste. d_4^{15} 1.024. bp 152°. n_D^{25} 1.5248. Sparingly sol in water; misc with alcohol and most organic solvents. One ml dissolves in 8 ml 70% alcohol. LD_{50} orally in rats: 339 mg/kg (Jenner).

USE: Manuf flavors; war gas.

THERAP CAT: Counterirritant.

THERAP CAT (VET): Counterirritant.

296. Allylprodine. [25384-17-2] 1-Methyl-4-phenyl-3-(2-propenyl)-4-piperidinol propanoate; α-3-allyl-1-methyl-4-phenyl-4-propionoxypiperidine; α-3-allyl-1-methyl-4-phenyl-4-piperidinol propionate; NIH-7440; Ro-2-7113. $C_{18}H_{25}NO_2$; mol wt 287.40. C 75.22%, H 8.77%, N 4.87%, O 11.13%. Narcotic analgesic. Prepn: Ziering *et al., J. Org. Chem.* **22**, 1521 (1957); Lee, Ziering, **US 2798073** (1957 to Hoffmann-La Roche).

Hydrochloride. $C_{18}H_{25}NO_2.HCl$. Crystals from acetone + methanol, mp 186-187°.

Note: This is a controlled substance (opiate): **21 CFR,** 1308.11.

297. Allyl Sulfide. [592-88-1] 3,3'-Thiobis-1-propene; diallyl sulfide; thioallyl ether; "oil garlic". $C_6H_{10}S$; mol wt 114.21. C 63.10%, H 8.83%, S 28.08%. $(CH_2=CHCH_2)_2S$. Prepared from allyl bromide and sulfur in soln of Na in liquid NH_3: Brandsma, Wijers, *Rec. Trav. Chim.* **82**, 68 (1963).

Liquid, garlic odor. bp 139°. d_4^{27} 0.888. n_D^{27} 1.4877. Practically insoluble in water. Miscible with alc, chloroform, ether, carbon tetrachloride.

USE: Manuf flavors.

298. Allylurea. [557-11-9] N-2-Propenylurea; allylcarbamide. $C_4H_8N_2O$; mol wt 100.12. C 47.99%, H 8.05%, N 27.98%, O 15.98%. $CH_2=CHCH_2NHCONH_2$. Prepn: Neville, McGee, *Can. J. Chem.* **41**, 2123 (1963).

Crystals, mp 85°. Freely sol in water, alc. Practically insol in chloroform, ether, toluene, carbon disulfide.

USE: Manuf allylthiourea; corrosion inhibitors.

299. Almagate. [66827-12-1] [Carbonato(2)]heptahydroxy(aluminum)trimagnesium dihydrate; carbonic acid, aluminum-magnesium complex; Almax. $C_2H_{14}Al_2Mg_6O_{20}.4H_2O$; mol wt 629.97. C 3.81%, H 3.52%, Al 8.57%, Mg 23.15%, O 60.95%. $Al_2Mg_6(OH)_{14}(CO_3)_2.4H_2O$. A crystalline hydrated aluminum-magnesium hydroxycarbonate. Prepn: R. G. W. Spickett *et al.,* **BE 873843**; *eidem,* **US 4447417** (1979, 1984 both to Anphar). Crystal structure: J. Moragues *et al., Arzneim.-Forsch.* **34**, 1346 (1984). pH curves, acid consuming capacity: J. E. Beneyto *et al., ibid.* 1350. Effect of proteolytic enzymes, polypeptides: J. E. Beneyto, J. L. Fábregas, *ibid.* 1357. Serum levels of magnesium, aluminum not increased by high doses of almagate: J. Jauregui, J. Segura, *ibid.* 1364. Pharmacology: P. R. Beckett *et al., ibid.* 1367. Clinical trials: A. Suau *et al., ibid.* 1380.

Dehydrates at 510 K. USP acid neutralization capacity 28.3 mEq HCl/g.

THERAP CAT: Antacid.

300. Alminoprofen. [39718-89-3] α-Methyl-4-[(2-methyl-2-propenyl)amino]benzeneacetic acid; 2-(p-methylallylaminophenyl)propionic acid; EB-382; Minalfene. $C_{13}H_{17}NO_2$; mol wt 219.28. C 71.21%, H 7.81%, N 6.39%, O 14.59%. Prepn: **FR 2137211**; E. Bouchera, **US 3957850** (1971, 1976 both to Bouchera). Synthesis, pharmacology and toxicity data: B. Dumaitre *et al., Eur. J. Med. Chem.* **14**, 207 (1979). Pharmacokinetic study: A. Premel-Cabic *et al., Eur. J. Clin. Pharmacol.* **18**, 419 (1980).

Crystals from cyclohexane, mp 107°. LD_{50} orally in mice: 2400 mg/kg (Dumaitre).

THERAP CAT: Anti-inflammatory; analgesic.

301. Almitrine. [27469-53-0] 6-[4-[Bis(4-fluorophenyl)-methyl]-1-piperazinyl]-N,N'-di-2-propenyl-1,3,5-triazine-2,4-diamine; 2,4-bis[allylamino]-6-[4-[bis(p-fluorophenyl)methyl]-1-piperazinyl]-s-triazine; S-2620. $C_{26}H_{29}F_2N_7$; mol wt 477.55. C 65.39%, H 6.12%, F 7.96%, N 20.53%. Prepn: G. Regnier, R. Canevari, **DE 1947332**; *eidem,* **US 3647794** (1970, 1972 both to Sci. Union et Cie.-Soc. Franç. Recher. Méd.). Physical properties and toxicity: G. Regnier *et al., Experientia* **28**, 814 (1972). Pharmacology: M. Laubie, F. Diot, *J. Pharmacol.* **3**, 363 (1972); M. Laubie, H. Schmitt, *Eur. J. Pharmacol.* **61**, 125 (1980). Evaluation of combination with raubasine, *q.v.,* in cerebral ischemia in rats: M. G. Borzeix, J. Cahn, *Arzneim.-Forsch.* **37**, 491 (1987). Clinical effect on hypoxemia in chronic obstructive pulmonary disease: R. C. Bell *et al., Ann. Intern. Med.* **105**, 342 (1986); B. Gothe *et al., Am. J. Med.* **84**, 436 (1988).

Crystals, mp 181°.

Dimethanesulfonate. [29608-49-9] Almitrine dimesylate; Vectarion. $C_{26}H_{29}F_2N_7 \cdot 2CH_3SO_3H$; mol wt 669.76. mp 243° (dec). uv max (ethanol): 227, 246 nm (log ε 4.52, 4.53). LD_{50} in mice: 210 mg/kg i.v., 390 mg/kg i.p., >2 g/kg orally (Regnier).

THERAP CAT: Respiratory stimulant.

302. Almond, Bitter. Ripe seed of *Prunus amygdalus* Stokes var *amara* Focke (*P. communis* Arcang. var *amara* (Focke) Schneid.), *Rosaceae. Habit.* Italy, Spain, and Southern France. *Constit.* 35-50% fixed oil, about 3% amygdalin, proteins, emulsin (synaptase), sugar. *Ref:* E. W. Eckey, *Vegetable Fats and Oils* (Reinhold, New York, 1954) p 455.

Caution: Cyanide poisoning from ingestion of burnt bitter almonds has been reported: *C.A.* **50,** 6666a (1956).

USE: Preparing amygdalin, essential and expressed oils, almond and bitter-almond water; in perfumery and in manuf of liqueurs.

303. Almond, Sweet. Jordan almond. Ripe seed of *Prunus amygdalus* Stokes var *dulcis* (D.C.) Baill. (*P. communis* Arcang. var *dulcis* (Focke) Schneid.); *P. amygdalus* var *sativa* (Focke), *Rosaceae. Habit.* Italy, Spain and Southern France. *Constit.* About 50% fixed oil, proteins, emulsin, sugar. *Ref:* E. W. Eckey, *Vegetable Fats and Oils* (Reinhold, New York, 1954) p 455; Subrahmanyam, Achaya, *J. Sci. Food Agric.* **8,** 657 (1957).

USE: In perfumery and in confectionery; preparing expressed oil of almond, almond milk, almond meal, etc.

304. Almotriptan. [154323-57-6] 1-[[3-[2-(Dimethylamino)ethyl]-1*H*-indol-5-yl]methyl]sulfonyl]pyrrolidine; 1-[[3-(2-dimethylaminoethyl)-5-indolyl]methanesulphonyl]pyrrolidine; LAS-31416. $C_{17}H_{25}N_3O_2S$; mol wt 335.46. C 60.87%, H 7.51%, N 12.53%, O 9.54%, S 9.56%. Serotonin 5HT$_{1B/1D}$-receptor agonist. Prepn: D. F. Forner *et al.,* **WO 9402460;** *eidem,* **US 5565447** (1994, 1996 both to Almirall). Clinical pharmacokinetics: J. C. Fleishaker *et al., Clin. Pharmacol. Ther.* **67,** 498 (2000). Review of pharmacology: F. Kamali, *Curr. Opin. Cent. Peripher. Nerv. Syst. Invest. Drugs* **2,** 197-202 (2000); of clinical studies: D. W. Dodick, *Expert Opin. Pharmacother.* **4,** 1157-1163 (2003).

Maleate. [181183-52-8] PNU-180638E; Almogran; Axert. $C_{17}H_{25}N_3O_2S \cdot C_4H_6O_5$; mol wt 469.55. White to slightly yellow crystalline powder; sol in water.

THERAP CAT: Antimigraine.

305. Aloe. Genus of succulent plants (family *Liliaceae*) having triangular, spear-like leaves with thorny ridges. *Habit.* Africa, southern Arabia, Madagascar. Naturalized in the West Indies, southern U.S., Central America, Asia. Several species have been used medicinally, primarily *Aloe barbadensis* Miller (also known as *Aloe vera* Linné, Curaçao aloe, or Barbados aloe) and *Aloe ferox* Miller (also known as Cape aloe). "Drug aloe", used as a cathartic, is the dried latex or bitter, yellow exudate from the leaf bundle sheath cells. The latex contains varying amounts of aloin, aloe-emodin, chrysophanic acid, *q.q.v.,* volatile oil, and resins. Aloe vera gel is the fresh mucilaginous gel obtained from the parenchymatous

tissue in the leaf center, used for its emollient and wound healing activity. Physical and chemical properties of the gel: Y.-T. Wang, K. J. Strong, *Phytother. Res.* **7,** S1 (1993). Effects in wound healing: J. P. Heggers *et al., ibid.* S48. *Reviews:* D. Grindlay, T. Reynolds, *J. Ethnopharmacol.* **16,** 117-151 (1986); A. D. Klein *et al., J. Am. Acad. Dermatol.* **18,** 714-720 (1988); R. M. Shelton, *Int. J. Dermatol.* **30,** 679-683 (1991).

Aloeresin A

Aloeresin A. [74545-79-2] 7-Hydroxy-8-[2-O-[(2*E*)-3-(4-hydroxyphenyl)-1-oxo-2-propenyl]-β-D-glucopyranosyl]-5-methyl-2-(2-oxopropyl)-4*H*-1-benzopyran-4-one. $C_{28}H_{28}O_{11}$; mol wt 540.52. A major constituent of Cape aloe latex. Structure: P. Gramatica *et al., Tetrahedron Lett.* **23,** 2423 (1982). HPLC determn in plant and commerical preparations: N. Okamura *et al., J. Chromatogr. A* **746,** 225 (1996). mp 148-150°. uv max in methanol: 228, 252, 300 nm (ε 34250, 25000, 37960).

THERAP CAT: Latex as laxative; gel as emollient, vulnerary.

306. Aloe-Emodin. [481-72-1] 1,8-Dihydroxy-3-(hydroxymethyl)-9,10-anthracenedione; 1,8-dihydroxy-3-(hydroxymethyl)anthraquinone; 3-hydroxymethylchrysazin; rhabarberone. $C_{15}H_{10}O_5$; mol wt 270.24. C 66.67%, H 3.73%, O 29.60%. Occurs in the free state and as a glycoside in *Rheum* (rhubarb), in senna leaves and in various species of *Aloe (Liliaceae).* Isolation: Condo-Vissicchio, *Arch. Pharm.* **247,** 81 (1909); Mary *et al., J. Am. Pharm. Assoc.* **45,** 229 (1956). Prepn: Cahn, Simonsen, *J. Chem. Soc.* **1932,** 2573; Hay, Haynes, *ibid.* **1956,** 3141; Bapat *et al., Tetrahedron Letters* no. 5, 15 (1960). HPLC determn in plasma: M. Zaffaroni *et al., J. Chromatogr. B* **796,** 113 (2003).

Orange needles from toluene, mp 223-224°. Sublimes in CO_2 stream. Absorption spectrum: Stone, Furman, *J. Am. Chem. Soc.* **68,** 2742 (1946). Freely sol in hot alcohol, in ether, in benzene with yellow color, in ammonia water and in sulfuric acid with crimson color.

Trimethyl ether. $C_{18}H_{16}O_5$. Orange needles from acetic acid, mp 163°.

Triacetate. $C_{21}H_{16}O_8$. Yellow needles from benzene, mp 175-177°.

Note: See also Emodin.

THERAP CAT: Cathartic.

307. Aloin. [5133-19-7] 10-Glucopyranosyl-1,8-dihydroxy-3-(hydroxymethyl)-9(10*H*)-anthracenone; 1,8-dihydroxy-3-hydroxymethyl-10-(6-hydroxymethyl-3,4,5-trihydroxy-2-pyranyl)anthrone; 10-(1′,5′-anhydroglucosyl)-aloe-emodin-9-anthrone; barbaloin. $C_{21}H_{22}O_9$; mol wt 418.39. C 60.28%, H 5.30%, O 34.42%. Isoln from various species of aloe (Cape, Uganda and Socotrine): Léger, *Ann. Chim.* **6,** 318 (1916); **8,** 265 (1918); Cahn, Simonsen, *J. Chem. Soc.* **1932,** 2573; Rosenthaler, *Arch. Pharm.* **270,** 214 (1932); Mühlemann, *Pharm. Acta Helv.* **27,** 17 (1952); Böhme, Bertram, *Arch. Pharm.* **288,** 510 (1955). The molecule is built from aloe-emodin, *q.v.,* and from glucose. Structure: Hay, Haynes, *J. Chem. Soc.* **1956,** 3141.

Lemon-yellow crystals, mp 148-149°. Quickly forms a mono-hydrate, mp 70-80°. Slight odor of aloe; bitter taste. Solubility at 18°: 57% in pyridine, 7.3% in glacial acetic acid, 5.4% in meth-anol, 3.2% in acetone, 2.8% in methyl acetate, 1.9% in ethanol, 1.8% in water, 1.6% in propanol, 0.78% in ethyl acetate, 0.27% in isopropanol. Very slightly soluble in isobutanol, chloroform, car-bon disulfide, ether. Incompatible with alkali hydroxides, tannin, ferric chloride.

THERAP CAT: Cathartic.

THERAP CAT (VET): Purgative.

308. Alosetron. [122852-42-0] 2,3,4,5-Tetrahydro-5-methyl-2-[(5-methyl-1*H*-imidazol-4-yl)methyl]-1*H*-pyrido[4,3-*b*]indol-1-one; GR-68755. $C_{17}H_{18}N_4O$; mol wt 294.35. C 69.37%, H 6.16%, N 19.03%, O 5.44%. Serotonin 5HT$_3$-receptor antagonist. Prepn: I. H. Coates *et al.,* **EP 306323**; *eidem,* **US 5360800** (1989, 1994 both to Glaxo); of isotopically labelled compd: S. R. Prakash *et al., J. Labelled Compd. Radiopharm.* **36,** 993 (1995). HPLC determn in plasma: T. L. Lloyd *et al., J. Chromatogr. B* **678,** 261 (1996). Review of clinical pharmacology: M. D. Gunput, *Aliment. Pharmacol. Ther.* **13,** Suppl. 2, 70-76 (1999); of clinical studies: A. W. Mangel, A. R. Northcutt, *ibid.* 77-82. Clinical trial in irritable bowel syndrome: M. Camilleri *et al., Lancet* **355,** 1035 (2000).

Hydrochloride. [122852-69-1] GR-68755C; Lotronex. $C_{17}H_{18}N_4O \cdot HCl$; mol wt 330.81. mp 288-291°.

THERAP CAT: In treatment of irritable bowel syndrome.

309. Aloxiprin. [9014-67-9] 2-(Acetyloxy)benzoic acid polymer with aluminum oxide; polyoxyaluminum acetylsalicylate; Lyman; Palaprin; Rumatral. A polymeric condensation product of aluminum oxide and aspirin. Approx formula, $Al_3O_2[C_6H_4-(OOCCH_3)COO]_5$. Prepd from aluminum isopropoxide and as-pirin: Cummings *et al., J. Pharm. Pharmacol.* **15,** 56 (1963).

Powder with greater bulk density and relatively low free salicylic acid content as compared with other aluminum salicylates. Rates of soln of aspirin from aloxiprin in buffer solns of pH 2-8 are lower than those of aspirin, particularly in more acid buffers.

THERAP CAT: Analgesic.

310. Alphaprodine. [77-20-3] (*cis*)-1,3-Dimethyl-4-phen-yl-4-piperidinol propanoate; (±)-α-1,3-dimethyl-4-phenyl-4-piperi-dinyl propionate; *dl*-α-1,3-dimethyl-4-phenyl-4-propionoxypiperi-dine; (±)-α-prodine. $C_{16}H_{23}NO_2$; mol wt 261.36. C 73.53%, H 8.87%, N 5.36%, O 12.24%. Mixture of the two *cis* isomers of prodine; *betaprodine* is the mixture of *trans* isomers. Prepn: J. Lee, A. Ziering, **US 2498433** (1950 to Hoffmann-La Roche); A. H. Beckett *et al., J. Pharm. Pharmacol.* **9,** 939 (1957); A. Ziering *et al., J. Org. Chem.* **22,** 1521 (1957). Configurational studies: F. R. Ahmed *et al., Chem. Ind. (London)* **1959,** 485; *eidem, ibid.* **1962,**

97. Stereostructure-activity studies: M. M. Abdel-Monem *et al., J. Med. Chem.* **15,** 494 (1972). Pharmacology and toxicology: G. M. Gruber *et al., J. Pharmacol. Exp. Ther.* **99,** 312 (1950). Review of clinical experience: R. C. Lunt, H. E. Howard, *Pediatr. Dent.* **10,** 121-126 (1988).

(+)-form

Hydrochloride. [561-78-4] Nu-1196; Nisentil. $C_{16}H_{23}NO_2 \cdot$HCl; mol wt 297.82. Crystals from acetone, mp 220-221°. Slightly saline taste. Freely sol in water, alc, chloroform. Practically insol in ether. pH of 1% aq soln 4.5-5.2. LD$_{50}$ in mice: 54 mg/kg i.v., 73 mg/kg i.p.; in rats: 22 mg/kg i.p. (Gruber).

Betaprodine hydrochloride. [49638-23-5] (±)-β-Prodine hy-drochloride; Nu-1779. Crystals from methyl ethyl ketone, mp 195-196° (Beckett); from acetone + methanol, mp 199-200° (Ziering).

Note: These are controlled substances (opiates): **21 CFR,** 1308.11 (betaprodine) and 1308.12 (alphaprodine).

THERAP CAT: Analgesic (narcotic).

311. Alpiropride. [81982-32-3] 4-Amino-2-methoxy-5-[(methylamino)sulfonyl]-*N*-[[1-(2-propenyl)-2-pyrrolidinyl]meth-yl]benzamide; (±)-*N*-[(1-allyl-2-pyrrolidinyl)methyl]-4-amino-5-(methylsulfamoyl)-*o*-anisamide; *N*-(1-allyl-2-pyrrolidinylmethyl)-2-methoxy-4-amino-5-methylsulfamoylbenzamide; RIV-2093; Riv-istel. $C_{17}H_{26}N_4O_4S$; mol wt 382.48. C 53.38%, H 6.85%, N 14.65%, O 16.73%, S 8.38%. Dopamine D$_2$-receptor antagonist structurally similar to sulpiride, *q.v.* Prepn: J. Perrot, M. Thomi-net, **EP 47207**; *eidem,* **US 4550179** (1982, 1985 both to Soc. d'Etudes Sci. Ind. l'Ile-de-France). Dopamine receptor binding study: P. Sokoloff *et al., Arch. Pharmacol.* **327,** 221 (1984). HPLC determn in plasma and urine: F. Bressolle *et al., J. Chromatogr.* **343,** 443 (1985). Pharmacokinetics and metabolism in humans: F. Bressolle *et al., J. Pharm. Clin.* **4,** 261 (1985). Preliminary study in experimentally induced migraine: A. Bès *et al., Int. J. Clin. Phar-macol. Res.* **6,** 189 (1986).

Crystals from absolute ethanol, mp 168.5-169°. LD$_{50}$ in male mice (mg/kg): 44 i.v.; 184 i.p.; 204 s.c.; 3600 orally (Perrot, Thominet, 1985).

THERAP CAT: Antimigraine.

312. Alprazolam. [28981-97-7] 8-Chloro-1-methyl-6-phenyl-4*H*-[1,2,4]triazolo[4,3-*a*][1,4]benzodiazepine; 8-chloro-1-methyl-6-phenyl-4*H*-*s*-triazolo[4,3-*a*][1,4]benzodiazepine; D-65MT; U-31889; Alplax; Cassadan; Esparon; Tafil; Tranquinal; Trankimazin; Xanax. $C_{17}H_{13}ClN_4$; mol wt 308.76. C 66.13%, H 4.24%, Cl 11.48%, N 18.15%. Prepn: J. B. Hester, **DE 2012190**; *idem,* **US 3987052** (1970, 1976 both to Upjohn); J. B. Hester *et al., Tetrahedron Lett.* **1971,** 1609; A. Walser, G. Zenchoff, *J. Med. Chem.* **20,** 1694 (1977). Central depressant activity: R. Nakajima *et al., Jpn. J. Pharmacol.* **21,** 497 (1971). Pharmacology: V. H. Sethy, *Arch. Pharmacol.* **301,** 157 (1978). Clinical studies: L. F. Fabre, *Curr. Ther. Res.* **19,** 661 (1976); J. B. Cohn, *J. Clin. Psychia-try* **42,** 347 (1981). Pharmacokinetics: D. R. Abernethy *et al., ibid.* **44,** 45 (1983). Review of pharmacokinetics, clinical efficacy, and mechanism of action: J. A. Fawcett, H. M. Kravitz, *Pharmacother-*

apy **2**, 242-254 (1982); of pharmacology and efficacy in anxiety and depression: *Drugs* **27**, 132 (1984).

Crystals from ethyl acetate, mp 228-228.5°. Sol in alc. Insol in water. uv max (ethanol): 222 nm (ε 40250). LD_{50} in mice, rats (mg/kg): 1020, >2000 orally; 540, 610 i.p. (Nakajima).

Note: This is a controlled substance (depressant): **21 CFR**, 1308.14.

THERAP CAT: Anxiolytic.

313. Alprenolol. [13655-52-2] 1-[(1-Methylethyl)amino]-3-[2-(2-propenyl)phenoxy]-2-propanol; 1-(*o*-allylphenoxy)-3-(isopropylamino)-2-propanol; H-56/28. $C_{15}H_{23}NO_2$; mol wt 249.35. C 72.25%, H 9.30%, N 5.62%, O 12.83%. β-Adrenergic blocker. Prepn: Brandstrom *et al., Acta Pharm. Suec.* **3**, 303 (1966); **NL 6605692** (1966 to AB Hassle), *C.A.* **66**, 46214p (1967); **NL 6612958** (1967 to ICI), *C.A.* **67**, 99851w (1967). Pharmacology: Marmo, *Clin. Ter.* **56**, 121-176 (1971). Series of articles on clinical effect in myocardial infarction: *Acta Med. Scand.* **1984**, Suppl. 680, 1-64.

Hydrochloride. [13707-88-5] Apllobal; Aptine; Aptol Duriles; Gubernal; Regletin; Yobir. $C_{15}H_{23}NO_2$.HCl; mol wt 285.81. Crystals from ethyl acetate, mp 107-109°. LD_{50} in mice, rats, rabbits (mg/kg): 278.0, 597.0, 337.3 orally (Marmo).

THERAP CAT: Antihypertensive; antianginal; antiarrhythmic.

314. Alsactide. [34765-96-3] 1-β-Alanine-17-[*N*-(4-aminobutyl)-L-lysinamide]-α^{1-17}-corticotropin; 1-β-alanine-17-[L-2,6-diamino-*N*-(4-aminobutyl)hexanamide]-α^{1-17}-corticotropin; [β-ala^1,lys^{17}]corticotropin-(1-17)-heptadecapeptide-4-amino-*N*-butylamide; [β-ala^1,lys^{17}]ACTH$^{1-17}$-4-amino-*N*-butylamide; alisactide; HOE-433; Synchrodyn. $C_{99}H_{155}N_{29}O_{21}S$; mol wt 2119.54. C 56.10%, H 7.37%, N 19.16%, O 15.85%, S 1.51%. Short-chain ACTH analog. Synthesis: R. Geiger, H. G. Schroeder, **DE 1954794**; *eidem*, **US 3749704** (1971, 1973, both to Hoechst); R. Geiger, *Ann.* **750**, 165 (1971). Pharmacology: J. Sandow *et al., Arch. Pharmacol.* **297**, Suppl. 2, R41 (1977). Dose dependent effects on cortisol and aldosterone plasma levels in man: A. Angeli *et al., Horm. Metab. Res.* **13**, 24 (1981). Review of chronobiological activity: *idem et al., Chronobiologica* **14**, 99-143 (1987).

β-Ala–Tyr–Ser–Met–Glu–His–Phe–Arg–Trp–Gly–Lys–Pro–Val–Gly–Lys–Lys–LysNH(CH₂)₄NH₂

Acetate. [33194-27-3] $C_{99}H_{155}N_{29}O_{21}S$.x$C_2H_4O_2$. $[\alpha]_D^{20}$ −68.6° (c = 0.5 in 1% acetic acid).

THERAP CAT: Diagnostic aid (adrenal function).

315. Alstonidine. [25394-75-6] 3β-(Hydroxymethyl)-2α-methyl-4β-[(9-methyl-9*H*-pyrido[3,4-*b*]indol-1-yl)methyl]-2*H*-pyran-5-carboxylic acid methyl ester. $C_{22}H_{24}N_2O_4$; mol wt 380.44. C 69.46%, H 6.36%, N 7.36%, O 16.82%. From the bark or root of *Alstonia constricta* F. Muell., *Apocynaceae*: Hesse, *Ann.* **205**, 360 (1880); Svoboda, *J. Am. Pharm. Assoc.* **46**, 508 (1957). Structure: Boaz *et al., ibid.* 510. Stereochemistry: Crow *et al., Aust. J. Chem.* **23**, 2489 (1970).

Fine crystals from ether, mp 188-190°. Practically insol in water. Sol in alcohol, chloroform, ether, acetone, 5% HCl. uv max (methanol): 238, 291, 360 nm (log ε 4.66, 4.25, 3.74). The acid solutions are fluorescent.

Acetyl deriv trihydrate. $C_{24}H_{26}N_2O_5$.3H_2O. Fine needles from dil acetone, mp 92-96°.

316. Alstonine. [642-18-2] 3,4,5,6,16,17-Hexahydro-16-(methoxycarbonyl)-19α-methyl-20α-oxayohimbanium. C_{21}-$H_{20}N_2O_3$; mol wt 348.40. C 72.40%, H 5.79%, N 8.04%, O 13.78%. From *Alstonia constricta* F. Mull., *Rauwolfia vomitoria* Afzel., *Rauwolfia obscura* K. Schum., *Vinca rosea* L., and other *Apocynaceae*: Sharp, *J. Chem. Soc.* **1934**, 287; Schlittler *et al., Helv. Chim. Acta* **35**, 271 (1952); Pillay, Kumari, *J. Sci. Ind. Res.* **20B**, 458 (1961); *C.A.* **56**, 7425b (1962). Structure: Bader, *Helv. Chim. Acta* **36**, 215 (1953). Stereoisomer of serpentine (alkaloid), *q.v.* Stereochemistry: Wenkert, Roychaudhuri, *J. Am. Chem. Soc.* **79**, 1519 (1957); **80**, 1613 (1958); Shamma, Richey, *ibid.* **85**, 2507 (1963). Biosynthesis: Woodward, *Angew. Chem.* **68**, 13 (1956).

Fine, yellow needles from acetone, dec above 300° (brown at 200°, black at 260°). uv max (methanol): 252, 289, 309, 336, 369 nm (log ε 4.54, 4.08, 4.36, 3.39, 3.60). Quickly decomposes on standing in organic solvents, yielding red solns with blue fluorescence.

Hydrochloride. $C_{21}H_{20}N_2O_3$.HCl. Yellow plates from abs alcohol, dec 286°. $[\alpha]_D$ +132° (c = 1.06). Sol in water.

317. Althea. Marshmallow. Dried root of *Althaea officinalis* L., *Malvaceae* (marshmallow), deprived of brown, corky layer. *Habit.* Europe, Western and Northern Asia, naturalized in Eastern U.S. *Constit.* Asparagine, 25-35% mucilage, sugar, pectin.

USE: Demulcent.

318. Althiazide. [5588-16-9] 6-Chloro-3,4-dihydro-3-[(2-propenylthio)methyl]-2*H*-1,2,4-benzothiadiazine-7-sulfonamide 1,1-dioxide; 3-[(allylthio)methyl]-6-chloro-3,4-dihydro-2*H*-1,2,4-benzothiadiazine-7-sulfonamide 1,1-dioxide; 3-allylthiomethyl-6-chloro-7-sulfamoyl-3,4-dihydrobenzothiadiazine 1,1-dioxide; 6-chloro-3,4-dihydro-7-sulfamoyl-3-(2-thiapent-4-enyl)-2*H*-1,2,4-benzothiadiazine 1,1-dioxide; altizide; P-1779. $C_{11}H_{14}ClN_3O_4S_3$; mol wt 383.89. C 34.42%, H 3.68%, Cl 9.24%, N 10.95%, O 16.67%, S 25.06%. Prepn: **GB 902658**; W. M. McLamore, G. D. Laubach, **US 3111517** (1962, 1963 both to Pfizer). HPLC determn in tablets: F. DeCroo *et al., J. Chromatogr.* **329**, 422 (1985). Clinical evaluation in hypertension: G. Simon *et al., Curr. Ther. Res.* **46**, 44 (1989).

Solid, mp 206-207°.
Combination with spironolactone, *Aldactazine*.
THERAP CAT: Diuretic; antihypertensive.

319. Altrenogest. [850-52-2] (17β)-17-Hydroxy-17-(2-propenyl)estra-4,9,11-trien-3-one; 17α-allyl-17-hydroxyestra-4,9,11-trien-3-one; 13β-methyl-17α-allyl-Δ^{4,9,11}-gonatriene-17β-ol-3-one; allyltrenbolone; A-35957; RU-2267; Regu-Mate. $C_{21}H_{26}O_2$; mol wt 310.43. C 81.25%, H 8.44%, O 10.31%. Synthetic oral progestogen. Prepn: **NL 6401555**; G. Nomine *et al.*, **US 3257278** (1964, 1966 both to Roussel). Effect on estrous cycle and fertility of mares: E. L. Squires *et al.*, *J. Anim. Sci.* **49**, 729 (1979). Synchronization of estrus in swine: R. R. Kraeling *et al.*, *ibid.* **52**, 831 (1981); in gilts: V. G. Pursel *et al.*, *ibid.* 130.

Cryst, mp 120°. [α]$_D^{20}$ −72° (c = 0.5 in ethanol).
THERAP CAT (VET): Progestogen.

320. Altretamine. [645-05-6] *N,N,N',N',N",N"*-Hexamethyl-1,3,5-triazine-2,4,6-triamine; 2,4,6-tris(dimethylamino)-*s*-triazine; hemel; hexamethylmelamine; HMM; ENT-50852; NSC-13875; Hexalen; Hexastat. $C_9H_{18}N_6$; mol wt 210.28. C 51.41%, H 8.63%, N 39.97%. An antitumor agent which also acts as a chemosterilant for male houseflies and other insects. Synthesis: A. W. Hofmann, *Ber.* **18**, 2755 (1885); D. W. Kaiser *et al.*, *J. Am. Chem. Soc.* **73**, 2984 (1951); Y. Bessiere-Chretien, H. Serne, *Bull. Soc. Chim. Fr.* **6**, 2039 (1973). Production process: H. von Brachel, H. Kindler, **DE 1240870**; *eidem*, **US 3424752** (1967, 1969 both to Casella Farbwerke). Chemosterilant effect: S. C. Chang *et al.*, *Science* **144**, 57 (1964); A. De Milo *et al.*, *J. Econ. Entomol.* **65**, 1548 (1972). Chromatographic detn in plasma or serum: A. Hulshoff *et al.*, *J. Chromatogr.* **181**, 363 (1980). Disposition and metabolism in rabbits and humans: M. M. Ames *et al.*, *Cancer Res.* **39**, 5016 (1979). Evaluation in breast cancer: C. J. Fabian *et al.*, *Cancer Treat. Rep.* **63**, 1359 (1979); in ovarian cancer: J. T. Wharton *et al.*, *Am. J. Obstet. Gynecol.* **133**, 833 (1979). Mammalian toxicity study: R. L. Jasper *et al.*, *Fed. Proc.* **24**, 641 (1965). Toxicological studies in dogs and mice: D. C. Thake *et al.*, *Gov. Rep. Announce. Index (USA)* **79**, 92 (1979), *C.A.* **91**, 168372a (1979). *In vitro* cytotoxicity study: M. D'Incalci *et al.*, *Br. J. Cancer* **41**, 630 (1980).

Needles from abs ethanol, mp 172-174°. uv max (ethanol): 226 nm (ε 49400), H. J. Anderson *et al.*, *Can. J. Chem.* **49**, 2315 (1971). LD$_{50}$ in rats, guinea pigs (mg/kg): 350, 255 orally (Jasper).
USE: As exptl insect chemosterilant.
THERAP CAT: Antineoplastic.

321. D-Altrose. [1990-29-0] D-Altropyranose. $C_6H_{12}O_6$; mol wt 180.16. C 40.00%, H 6.71%, O 53.28%. Prepd by the reduction of D-altronic lactone with sodium amalgam: Levene, Jacobs, *Ber.* **43**, 3143 (1910).

Prisms from dilute alcohol, mp 103-105°. [α]$_D^{20}$ +32.6° (c = 7.6). Soluble in water. Practically insol in alcohol.
Phenylosazone. $C_{18}H_{22}N_4O_4$. mp 178°.

322. Aluminon. [569-58-4] 5-[(3-Carboxy-4-hydroxyphenyl)(3-carboxy-4-oxo-2,5-cyclohexadien-1-ylidene)methyl]-2-hydroxybenzoic acid triammonium salt; 3-[bis(3-carboxy-4-hydroxyphenyl)methylene]-6-oxo-1,4-cyclohexadiene-1-carboxylic acid triammonium salt; ammonium salt of aurintricarboxylic acid; Lysofon. $C_{22}H_{23}N_3O_9$; mol wt 473.43. C 55.81%, H 4.90%, N 8.88%, O 30.42%. Prepd by reacting sodium nitrite with salicylic acid and adding formaldehyde, then treating with ammonia: G. B. Heisig, W. M. Lauer, *Org. Synth.* **coll. vol. I**, 54 (2nd ed., 1941).

Yellowish-brown, glassy powder. Freely sol in water.
USE: Forms brilliantly colored lakes with aluminum, chromium, iron, beryllium. Generally used for the detection and colorimetric estimation of aluminum in water, foods, tissues. *Cf.* Scherrer, Mogerman, *J. Res. Natl. Bur. Stand.* **21**, 105 (1938).
THERAP CAT: Pharyngeal aerosol spray.

323. Aluminum. [7429-90-5] Aluminium. Al; at. wt 26.9815386; at. no. 13; valence 3. Group IIIA (13). Naturally occurring isotope (mass number): 27 (100%); known artificial radioactive isotopes: 22-25, 26 (T$_½$ 7.2×10^5 years, longest-lived known isotope, β$^+$ and γ emitter, found in meteors), 28-32. One of the most abundant metals in earth's crust: 8.3% by wt (83,000 ppm); occurs in nature primarily in combination with silica, also as oxide (*see* Aluminum Silicate; Aluminum Oxide). First obtained in impure form by Oersted in 1825; prepd as metal powder by Wöhler in 1827. Commercially important source is bauxite. Reviews of aluminum, its alloys and compds: Brandt, "Aluminum and Aluminum Alloys" in *Proc. Met. Soc. Conf.* **vol. 40**, E. D. Verink, Ed. (Gordon & Breach, New York, 1966); *Aluminum* 3 vols., K. R. Van Horn, Ed. (American Society for Metals, Metal Park, Ohio, 1967); Wade, Bannister, "Aluminum, Gallium, Indium and Thallium" in *Comprehensive Inorganic Chemistry* vol. 1, J. C. Bailar, Jr. *et al.*, Eds. (Pergamon Press, Oxford, 1973) pp 993-1064; *Chemistry of the Elements*, N. N. Greenwood, A. Earnshaw, Eds. (Pergamon Press, New York, 1984) pp 243-295; J. T. Stanley, W. Haupin in *Kirk-Othmer Encyclopedia of Chemical Technology* **vol. 2** (John Wiley & Sons, 4th ed., 1992) pp 184-251; W. C. Sleppy *et al.*, *ibid.* 252-345. Review of clinical toxicology: C. D. Hewitt *et al.*, *Clin. Lab. Med.* **10**, 403-422 (1990); of toxicology and human exposure: *Toxicological Profile for Aluminum* (PB99-166613, 1999) 393 pp. Book: *Chemistry of Aluminum, Gallium, Indium and Thallium*, A. J. Downs, Ed. (Blackie Academic & Professional, London, 1993) 515 pp.

Tin-white, malleable, ductile metal, with somewhat bluish tint; capable of taking brilliant polish which is retained in dry air. In moist air, oxide film forms which protects metal from corrosion. Available in bars, leaf, powder, sheets, or wire. d 2.70. mp 660°. bp 2327°. Does not vaporize even at high temps, but finely divided aluminum dust is easily ignited, and may cause explosions. Reacts with dil HCl, H_2SO_4, KOH and NaOH with evolution of hydrogen. Reduces the cations of many heavy metals to the metallic state E°(aq) Al^{3+}/Al −1.66 V. Solns of Al^{3+} in dil HCl or neutral or slightly acid solns of most aluminum salts, yield with Na$_2$S, a white ppt soluble in excess of Na$_2$S. Dil neutral soln of aluminum salts yields white gelatinous ppt on boiling with sodium acetate.

Caution: Potential symptoms of overexposure are irritation of eyes, skin and respiratory system. *See NIOSH Pocket Guide to Chemical Hazards* (DHHS/NIOSH 97-140, 1997) p 12. *See also Patty's Industrial Hygiene and Toxicology* vol. 2C, G. D. Clayton, F.

E. Clayton, Eds. (John Wiley & Sons, New York, 4th ed., 1994) pp 1881-1902.

USE: As pure metal or alloys (magnalium, aluminum bronze, etc.) for structural material in construction, automotive, electrical and aircraft industries. In cooking utensils, highway signs, fencing, containers and packaging, foil, machinery, corrosion resistant chemical equipment, dental alloys. The coarse powder in aluminothermics (thermite process); the fine powder as flashlight in photography; in explosives, fireworks, paints; for absorbing occluded gases in manuf of steel. In testing for Au, As, Hg; coagulating colloidal solns of As or Sb; pptg Cu; reducer for determining nitrates and nitrites; instead of Zn for generating hydrogen in testing for As. Forms complex hydrides with lithium and boron, such as $LiAlH_4$, which are used in preparative organic chemistry.

324. Aluminum Acetate Solution. [8006-13-1] Burow's Solution; Domeboro. Contains about 5% neutral aluminum acetate. $Al(C_2H_3O_2)_3 = 0.66\%$ Al, 4.4% acetic acid (1.25% Al_2O_3). Prepn from a dry mix consisting of an alkali metal acetate, acetic acid and a dibasic aluminum acetate stabilized with boric acid: Gibbons *et al.,* US 2824042 (1958).

Colorless liquid; slight odor of acetic acid. d ~1.002. pH of 1:20 aq soln 4.2.

THERAP CAT: Astringent, antiseptic.

THERAP CAT (VET): External astringent, antiseptic.

325. Aluminum Acetotartrate. Alsol; Essitol. Consists of approx 70% basic aluminum acetate and 30% tartaric acid. Prepn: *Gmelins, Aluminum* (8th ed.) **35B**, 304 (1934).

Crystals or powder; slight acetic odor; astringent, acidulous taste. On long keeping loses acetic acid and becomes incompletely sol. Slowly sol in cold water. Practically insol in alcohol.

THERAP CAT: Astringent, antiseptic.

326. Aluminum Alkyls. Highly reactive compounds of the form R_3Al, *trialkylaluminum*; $[R_nAlX_{3-n}]_2$, $n = 1, 2$, *alkylaluminum halide*; or $R_3Al_2X_3$, *alkylaluminum sesquihalide*. (The sesquihalides are actually equilibrium mixtures of $R_3Al_2X_3$, $[R_2AlX]_2$ and $[RAlX_2]_2$.) First prepn of aluminum alkyls: ethylaluminum sesquiiodide $[(C_2H_5)_3Al_2I_3]$ prepd by Hallwachs, Schaferik, *Ann.* **109**, 207 (1859); trimethylaluminum, $[(CH_3)_3Al]_2$, and triethylaluminum, $[(C_2H_5)_3Al]_2$, prepd by Buckton, Odling, *Ann. Suppl,* **4**, 109 (1865). The alkylaluminum halides are prepd from alkyl halides and aluminum, or by halogenation of trialkylaluminums. The trialkylaluminums are prepd from aluminum, hydrogen and olefins; this improved "direct synthesis" was developed by Ziegler and co-workers. Comprehensive reviews of prepn, properties and chemistry: Schultz in *Adv. Chem. Ser.* **23**, entitled "Metal-Organic Compounds," M. Sittig, Ed. (ACS, Washington DC, 1959) pp 163-171; Ziegler in *ACS Monograph Series* **no. 147**, entitled "Organometallic Chemistry," H. Zeiss, Ed. (Reinhold, New York, 1960) pp 194-269; Köster, Binger, *Adv. Inorg. Chem. Radiochem.* **7**, 263-348 (1965); T. Mole, E. A. Jeffery, *Organoaluminum Compounds* (Elsevier, New York, 1972) 465 pp; Wade, Banister in *Comprehensive Inorganic Chemistry* vol **1**, J. C. Bailar, Jr. *et al.,* Eds. (Pergamon Press, Oxford, 1973) pp 1058-1064.

Trialkylaluminum compounds. Colorless liquids at room temperature. Must be stored in an inert atm; sensitive to oxidation and hydrolysis in air; the lighter trialkylaluminums ignite spontaneously in air. The low mol wt, linear-chain alkyl compounds exist as dimers; the branched-chain alkyl compounds exist primarily as monomers. Among the industrially important trialkyl aluminums are **triethylaluminum**, dimeric liq, d^{25} 0.832, bp_{760} 194°, bp_{13} 100° and **triisobutylaluminum**, primarily monomeric liq, d^{25} 0.781; bp_{10} 86°, mp 6°.

Alkylaluminum halides. Low melting solids or colorless, volatile liquids. Strongly associated forming dimers; held together by bridging halogen bonds. Less sensitive than trialkylaluminums to oxidation upon exposure to air. Halogen aluminum bonds cleaved by water, alcohol. Industrially important halides include **chlorodiethylaluminum**, $[(C_2H_5)_2AlCl]_2$, liq, d^{25} 0.961, bp_{50} 127°, bp_{17} 100°, $bp_{1.9}$ 60° and **dichloroethylaluminum**, $[C_2H_5AlCl_2]_2$, solid, d^{50} 1.207, mp 32°, bp_{50} 113°, bp_{30} 100°, bp_5 60°.

USE: Catalyst; with compds of early transition metals as Ziegler-Natta polymerization catalysts; intermediates in organic syntheses.

327. Aluminum Ammonium Sulfate. [7784-25-0] Burnt ammonium alum; exsiccated ammonium alum. $AlH_4NO_8S_2$; mol

wt 237.15. Al 11.38%, H 1.70%, N 5.91%, O 53.97%, S 27.04%. $AlNH_4(SO_4)_2$. Prepn: *Gmelins, Aluminum* (8th ed) **35B**, pp 508-515 (1934). Crystal structure of dodecahydrate: Larson, Cromer, *Acta Crystallogr.* **22**, 793 (1967).

About 97-98% pure, the balance is chiefly excess Al_2O_3. White powder. One gram dissolves in about 20 ml cold, 1.5 ml boiling water, usually incompletely; practically insol in alcohol. *Keep well closed.*

Dodecahydrate. Ammonium alum. It is about 99.5% pure. Colorless crystals, white granules or powder; styptic taste. d 1.65. mp 94.5°. At about 250° becomes anhyd; decomposes above 280°. One gram dissolves in 7 ml water, 0.5 ml boil. water; freely soluble in glycerol; practically insol in alc. The aq soln is acid to litmus; pH of 0.05 molar soln 4.6.

USE: Purifying drinking water; in baking powders; dyeing and printing fabrics; manuf pigments, lakes, artificial gems, paper, vegetable glue, marble and porcelain cements; fireproofing; tanning; electrolytic copperplating. *See also* Aluminum Potassium Sulfate.

THERAP CAT: Astringent, styptic.

THERAP CAT (VET): Astringent, styptic.

328. Aluminum Antimonide. [25152-52-7] AlSb; mol wt 148.74. Al 18.14%, Sb 81.86%. Prepn of high purity crystals, resistance measurements, activation energies: Justi, Lautz, *Abh. Braunschw. Wiss. Ges.* **5**, 36 (1953); *C.A.* **48**, 1756i (1954). Electrical properties: Willardson *et al., J. Electrochem. Soc.* **101**, 354 (1954); and prepn: Kover, *Compt. Rend.* **243**, 648 (1956). Zone melting to remove impurities and to improve electr properties: Scheel, *Z. Metallkd.* **46**, 58 (1955), *C.A.* **49**, 4486f (1955). Oxidation by water: Rudorff, Kohlmeyer, *Z. Metallkd.* **45**, 608 (1954), *C.A.* **49**, 7432c (1955).

Lattice constant: 6.1361×10^{-8} cm. mp 1050°. Absorption const, n, width of forbidden zone (opt & electr) = 0.78; 3.4; 16; 1.65 e.v.: Oswald, Schade, *Z. Naturforsch.* **9a**, 611 (1954); *C.A.* **49**, 52a (1955). Width of forbidden band = 1.6 e.v. at 0 K: Blunt *et al., Phys. Rev.* **96**, 578 (1954); *C.A.* **49**, 2861b (1955).

USE: In semiconductor research.

329. Aluminum Benzoate. [555-32-8] $C_{21}H_{15}AlO_6$; mol wt 390.32. C 64.62%, H 3.87%, Al 6.91%, O 24.59%. $Al(C_6H_5-COO)_3$. Prepn: Kränzlein *et al.,* **DE 569946** (1933 to I. G. Farbenind.); *Frdl.* **19**, 597.

Cryst powder. Very slightly sol in water.

330. Aluminum Borate. [11121-16-7] Occurs in nature as the mineral **eremeyevite** or **jeremejevite**, $Al_2O_3 \cdot B_2O_3$. Prepd by heating Al_2O_3 with B_2O_3; when heated to 1000° $2Al_2O_3 \cdot B_2O_3$ is formed; when heated to 1100° $9Al_2O_3 \cdot 2B_2O_3$ is formed: Scholze, *Z. Anorg. Allg. Chem.* **284**, 272 (1956).

$2Al_2O_3 \cdot B_2O_3$. Needles, mp ~1050°. Practically insol in water.

$9Al_2O_3 \cdot 2B_2O_3$. Needles, mp ~1440°. Practically insol in water.

USE: Catalyst for polymerizations; in glass manuf.

331. Aluminum Borohydride. [16962-07-5] Aluminum tetrahydroborate. AlB_3H_{12}; mol wt 71.51. Al 37.73%, B 45.35%, H 16.91%. $Al(BH_4)_3$. Prepn from alkali metal hydride and aluminum halide: Schlesinger *et al., J. Am. Chem. Soc.* **75**, 209 (1953); Hinkamp, Hnizda, *Ind. Eng. Chem.* **47**, 1560 (1955); Kollonitsch, Fuchs, *Nature* **176**, 1081 (1955); Hinkamp, US **2854312** (1958 to Ethyl Corp.); Schechter, US **2913306** (1959 to Callery Chem.); from trimethylaluminum and diborane: Schlesinger *et al., J. Am. Chem. Soc.* **61**, 536 (1939).

Liquid. mp −64.5°; bp 44.5°; bp_{119} 0°. Reacts vigorously with water and hydrogen chloride to liberate hydrogen; ignites in air; decomposes slowly even at room temp evolving hydrogen. Forms addn products with dimethyl ether, trimethylamine and ammonia.

USE: Reducing agent; prepn of borohydrides of heavy metals; fuel for jet engines and rockets.

332. Aluminum Bromide. [7727-15-3] $AlBr_3$; mol wt 266.69. Al 10.12%, Br 89.88%. Prepd from aluminum and bromine: Nicholson *et al., Inorg. Synth.* **3**, 30 (1950).

White to yellowish-red very hygroscopic lumps, mp 97°; bp reported within the range 250-270°; d_4^{18} 3.205. Fumes strongly in air; combines with water *with violence. Keep tightly closed and protect from moisture.* Sol in many organic solvents such as benzene, nitrobenzene, toluene, xylene, simple hydrocarbons.

Hexahydrate. Colorless to slightly yellow deliquesc crystals. mp 93°; d 2.5. Sol in water, alcohol, ether, carbon disulfide. *Keep well closed.*

USE: *Anhydrous* form as acid catalyst in organic syntheses. It is similar to anhydr $AlCl_3$ but is more reactive and more sol in organic media.

333. Aluminum *tert*-Butoxide. [556-91-2] 2-Methyl-2-propanol aluminum salt. $C_{12}H_{27}AlO_3$; mol wt 246.32. C 58.51%, H 11.05%, Al 10.95%, O 19.49%. $Al[OC(CH_3)_3]_3$. Prepd from aluminum *tert*-butyl alcohol and mercuric chloride: Wayne, Adkins, *Org. Synth.* **coll. vol. III,** 48 (1955).

Powder; can be recryst from benzene. Sublimes at 180°. Pure compd does not melt or decomp upon heating up to 300° in a sealed tube, but traces of moisture or *tert*-butyl alc cause it to melt at 160-200°. Very sol in organic solvents; approx 9 g dissolves in 5 g ethyl propionate at 120°.

USE: Reagent for oxidation of alcohols to ketones; in dealcoholation of orthoesters.

334. Aluminum Calcium Hydride. [16941-10-9] Calcium tetrahydroaluminate; calcium aluminum hydride. Al_2CaH_8; mol wt 102.10. Al 52.85%, Ca 39.25%, H 7.90%. $Ca(AlH_4)_2$. Prepd by the interaction of aluminum chloride and calcium hydride in tetrahydrofuran: Schwab, Wintersberger, *Z. Naturforsch.* **8b,** 690 (1953); Conn, Taylor, **US 2999005** (1961 to Merck & Co.).

Slate-gray mass. The dry pulverized material can ignite spontaneously in moist air and is best handled under dry nitrogen. Reacts violently with water, the ensuing conflagration resembles a display of fireworks. Slightly less violent reaction with alcohols. Sol in dry tetrahydrofuran. Practically insol in dry ether, dioxane, benzene.

USE: Reducing agent for aldehydes, ketones, acid chlorides. Also in the reduction of esters to alcohols, nitriles to amines, aromatic nitro compounds to azo compounds.

335. Aluminum Carbide. [1299-86-1] C_3Al_4; mol wt 143.96. C 25.03%, Al 74.97%. Al_4C_3. Prepd by heating aluminum powder with carbon: Becher in *Handbook of Preparative Inorganic Chemistry* **vol. 1,** G. Brauer, Ed. (Academic Press, New York, 2nd ed., 1963) p 832.

Yellow hexagonal crystals or powder. mp 2100°; decomposes above 2200°. d 2.36. Decomposed by water with evolution of methane (fire hazard).

USE: In generating methane; reducing metal oxides; in manuf of aluminum nitride.

336. Aluminum Chlorate. [15477-33-5] Chloric acid, aluminum salt. $AlCl_3O_9$; mol wt 277.34. Al 9.73%, Cl 38.35%, O 51.92%. $Al(ClO_3)_3$. Occurs as hexahydrate and nonahydrate. Prepn: *Gmelins, Aluminum* (8th ed.) **35B,** 216-217 (1934).

Nonahydrate. [7784-15-8] Mallebrin. Deliquesc crystals. Freely sol in water; sol in alc. *Keep well closed.*

USE: Disinfectant; ClO_2 manuf; prevention of yellowing of acrylic fibers.

THERAP CAT: Antiseptic, astringent.

337. Aluminum Chloride. [7446-70-0] $AlCl_3$; mol wt 133.34. Al 20.24%, Cl 79.77%. Prepd from aluminum metal in a heated stream of HCl gas: Gattermann-Wieland, *Praxis des Organischen Chemikers* (de Gruyter, Berlin, 40th ed., 1961) p 295; H. J. Becher in *Handbook of Preparative Inorganic Chemistry* **vol. 1,** G. Brauer, Ed. (Academic Press, New York, 2nd ed., 1963) p 812. Manufacture: *Faith, Keyes & Clark's Industrial Chemicals,* F. A. Lowenheim, M. K. Moran, Eds. (Wiley-Interscience, New York, 4th ed., 1975) pp 72-75. Monograph: *ACS Monograph Series* **no. 87,** entitled "Anhydrous Aluminum Chloride in Organic Chemistry," C. A. Thomas, Ed. (Reinhold, New York, 1941).

White when pure; ordinarily gray or yellow to greenish. Fumes in air; strong odor of HCl; when heated in small quantities volatilizes without melting. Combines with water *with explosive violence* and liberation of much heat. Freely sol in many organic solvents, such as benzophenone, benzene nitrobenzene, carbon tetrachloride, chloroform. *Keep tightly closed and protected from moisture.* For physical properties *see* C. A. Thomas, *loc. cit.*

Hexahydrate. [7784-13-6] Anhydrol; Driclor; Drysol; Xerac. Colorless crystals, or white or slightly yellow deliquesc, cryst pow-

der; odorless or slight HCl odor. One gram dissolves in 0.9 ml water, 4 ml alc; sol in ether, glycerol, propylene glycol. *Keep well closed.*

Caution: Anhydrous form is a strong irritant.

USE: The *anhydrous* form suitable as an acid catalyst, esp in Friedel-Crafts type reactions; in cracking of petroleum; in manuf rubbers, lubricants. The *hexahydrate* form used in preserving wood; disinfecting stables, slaughterhouses, etc.; in deodorants and antiperspirant preparations; refining crude oil; dyeing fabrics; manuf parchment paper.

THERAP CAT: The *hexahydrate* as anhidrotic.

338. Aluminum Ethoxide. [555-75-9] Ethanol aluminum salt; aluminum ethylate. $C_6H_{15}AlO_3$; mol wt 162.16. C 44.44%, H 9.32%, Al 16.64%, O 29.60%. $Al(OC_2H_5)_3$. Prepd by reacting aluminum powder with absolute ethanol in xylene using small amounts of mercuric chloride and iodine as catalysts: Meerwein, Schmidt, *Ann.* **444,** 232 (1925); *Newer Methods of Preparative Organic Chemistry* (Interscience, New York, 1948) p 132; *see also* Farbwerke vorm. Meister, Lucius und Brüning, **DE 286596**; *J. Soc. Chem. Ind. London* **34,** 1168 (1915); Adkins, *J. Am. Chem. Soc.* **44,** 2178 (1922). Laboratory procedure: Gattermann-Wieland, *Praxis des Organischen Chemikers* (de Gruyter, Berlin, 40th ed., 1961) p 333.

Liquid. bp_{6-8} 200°; bp_3 175-180°. Slowly solidifies to a whole white solid, mp 140°. May crystallize with alcohol of crystallization. Decomposed by water. Slightly sol in hot xylene, chlorobenzene, other high boiling solvents.

USE: In the reduction of aldehydes and ketones; as catalyst for polymerizations.

339. Aluminum Fluoride. [7784-18-1] Aluminum trifluoride. AlF_3; mol wt 83.98. Al 32.13%, F 67.87%. Prepd by heating $(NH_4)_3AlF_6$ to red heat in a stream of nitrogen: Witt, Barrow, *Trans. Faraday Soc.* **55,** 730 (1959); Kwasnik in *Handbook of Preparative Inorganic Chemistry* **Vol. 1,** G. Brauer, Ed. (Academic Press, New York, 2nd ed., 1963) p 225. *Review:* Kemmitt, Sharp, *Adv. Fluorine Chem.* **4,** 154-155 (1965).

Hexagonal crystals. Sublimes (760 mm) 1272°. Soly in water (25°) 0.559 g/100 ml. Sparingly sol in acids and alkalies, even hot concd H_2SO_4 has little effect. Hydrolyzed by superheated steam at 300-400°.

Monohydrate. Fluellite. Orthorhombic crystals, d 2.17.

Trihydrate. Usually $AlF_3 \cdot 3.1H_2O$. Prepn: Ehret, Frere, *J. Am. Chem. Soc.* **67,** 64 (1945). Loses water at 100°, more at 200°. It does not seem possible to obtain the anhydrous compd free from oxides by dehydration of the hydrates.

Caution: Less toxic on ingestion than other fluorides because of slight solubility.

USE: In ceramics, as flux in metallurgy, in aluminum manufacture, as inhibitor of fermentation; as catalyst in organic reactions.

340. Aluminum Hexafluorosilicate. [17099-70-6] Aluminum fluosilicate; aluminum silicofluoride. $Al_2F_{18}Si_3$; mol wt 480.19. Al 11.24%, F 71.22%, Si 17.55%. $Al_2(SiF_6)_3$. Occurs in nature as *topaz*, $Al_2SiO_4(OH,F)_2$. Prepn: Sanfourche, Krapivine, *Compt. Rend.* **208,** 2080 (1939).

Nonahydrate. Hexagonal prisms. Easily sol in water; aq soln decomposes on heating or neutralization. Solid loses water on heating to temperatures below 500°, leaving a hexahydrate form; decomposes completely on heating to 1000°.

USE: Protection and preservation of construction materials; manuf of glass.

341. Aluminum Hydride. [7784-21-6] AlH_3; mol wt 30.01. Al 89.91%, H 10.08%. Mild, selective reducing agent. Prepd by treating lithium hydride with an ether solution of aluminum chloride: A. E. Finholt *et al., J. Am. Chem. Soc.* **69,** 1199 (1947). Brief review: K. Lopinti, *Synlett* **2005,** 2265-2266.

Colorless solid, nonvolatile, probably highly polymerized and containing residual ether which cannot be completely removed.

USE: As catalyst for polymerizations; reducing agent. Lithium aluminum hydride, *q.v.* is a more powerful reagent because of its greater soly.

342. Aluminum Hydroxide. [21645-51-2] Aluminum hydrate; aluminum trihydrate; hydrated alumina. AlH_3O_3; mol wt

78.00. Al 34.59%, H 3.88%, O 61.54%. Al(OH)$_3$. Prepn and properties: Dominé-Berges, *Ann. Chim.* [12] **5**, 106 (1950); Hennig, *Chem. Tech.* **1**, 66 (1949); *C.A.* **44**, 965f (1950); *Gmelins, Aluminum* (8th ed.) **35B**, pp 98-132 (1934); Becher in *Handbook of Preparative Inorganic Chemistry* vol. 1, G. Brauer, Ed. (Academic Press, New York, 2nd ed., 1963) pp 820-821; Wagner, *ibid.* vol. 2 (1965) pp 1652-1654. Comparative pharmacology and clinical use of antacids: F. W. Green, Jr. *et al.*, *Am. J. Hosp. Pharm.* **32**, 425 (1975). Clinical comparison with calcium carbonate as phosphate binder in chronic renal failure: R. H. K. Mak *et al.*, *Br. Med. J.* **291**, 623 (1985). Review of use as vaccine adjuvant: W. Nicklas, *Res. Immunol.* **143**, 489-494 (1992).

Usually obtained as a white, bulky, amorphous powder. Practically insol in water, but sol in alkaline aq solns or in HCl, H$_2$SO$_4$ and other strong acids in the presence of some water. Forms gels on prolonged contact with water. Absorbs acids, CO$_2$.

Aluminum hydroxide gel. Aldrox; ALternaGEL; Aludyal; Amphojel; Cremorin; Pepsamar; Uracid. White, viscous suspension. May also be used as the dried gel.

USE: Adsorbent; emulsifier; ion-exchanger; in chromatography; mordant in dyeing; filtering medium; manuf glass, fire clay, paper, pottery, printing inks, lubricating compositions, detergents; waterproofing fabrics; in antiperspirants, dentifrices. Vaccine adjuvant.

THERAP CAT: Antacid; antihyperphosphatemic.

THERAP CAT (VET): Antacid.

343. Aluminum Hydroxychloride. [1327-41-9] Basic aluminum chloride; aluminum chlorohydroxide; aluminum chlorohydrate; Chlorhydrol; Hyperdrol; Locron; Phosphonorm. The generally accepted empirical formula is Al$_2$(OH)$_5$Cl.2H$_2$O. Prepd by electrolyzing solns of suitable Al salts: **FR 837862** and **GB 509815** (both 1939 to I. G. Farben.); H. Huehn, W. Haufe, **US 2392531** (1946); Andersen, **US 2492085** (1949 to Elizabeth Arden). Structural studies and physicochemical properties: D. L. Teagarden *et al.*, *J. Pharm. Sci.* **70**, 758, 762 (1981). Phosphate binding activity and use in hyperphosphatemia: **DE 3147869** (1983 to Nefro-Pharma), *C.A.* **99**, 110747a (1983).

Glassy solid. Dissolves in water, forming slightly turbid colloidal solns (up to 55% w/w). pH of 15% aq soln ~4.3.

USE: In antiperspirants.

THERAP CAT: Astringent; antihyperphosphatemic.

344. Aluminum Hydroxydiacetate. [142-03-0] Bis(aceto-κO)hydroxyaluminum; hydroxybis(acetato)aluminum; basic aluminum acetate; aluminum diacetate; aluminum subacetate; aluminum hydroxyacetate; Lenicet. C$_4$H$_7$AlO$_5$; mol wt 162.08. C 29.64%, H 4.35%, Al 16.65%, O 49.36%. Al(OH)(CH$_3$CO$_2$)$_2$. Prepd from aluminum hydroxide and acetic acid or from sodium acetate and aluminum chloride hexahydrate: Hood, Ihde, *J. Am. Chem. Soc.* **72**, 2094 (1950). Other methods of prepn: *Gmelins, Aluminum* (8th ed.) **35B**, p 296 (1934). Also prepd in aq solution, see Aluminum Subacetate Solution.

White curdy precipitate or white amorphous powder. Material that has been oven-dried at 110° is practically insoluble in water. Freshly prepared material forms numerous hydrates and is quite sol in water. Greatest soly is obtained by formation in solution. The pharmacist's stock soln (see Aluminum Subacetate Solution) contains about 8% Al(OH)(CH$_3$CO$_2$)$_2$, while commercial solns used for waterproofing, contain 22 to 25% Al(OH)(CH$_3$CO$_2$)$_2$. When heated, the salt loses acetic acid, and aluminum to oxygen bonding occurs, resulting in a very insol compd of disputed nature, see Gmelin's, *loc. cit.* and Thomas, *Pap. Trade J.* **100**, 36 (1935). Aq solns are generally acid to litmus; gradually become turbid and gelatinous. Sometimes a more basic salt precipitates out and settles to the bottom of the container. Increasing the pH to a marked degree will clear up an old soln due to formation of sodium acetate and sodium aluminate. Urea and thiourea have been suggested as stabilizers for aq solns.

USE: Manuf color lakes; mordant in dyeing; in waterproofing and fireproofing fabrics (solns for these purposes are known as *red liquor* or *mordant rouge* because they were originally used for preparing red color lakes); in antiperspirant formulations; as disinfectant by embalmers. Dusting powder.

345. Aluminum Hypophosphite. [7784-22-7] AlH$_6$O$_6$P$_3$; mol wt 221.95. Al 12.16%, H 2.72%, O 43.25%, P 41.87%.

Al(PO$_2$H$_2$)$_3$. Prepd by heating Al(OH)$_3$ or a solution of an aluminum salt with hypophosphorous acid or sodium hypophosphite: Everest, *J. Chem. Soc.* **1952**, 2945.

Cryst powder; decomposes without melting at ~220° with evolution of phosphine. Practically insol in water. Sol in warm NaOH soln, dilute sulfuric and dilute or concd hydrochloric acid.

USE: In acrylonitrile polymer fiber finishes.

346. Aluminum Iodide. [7784-23-8] AlI$_3$; mol wt 407.69. Al 6.62%, I 93.38%. Prepn from aluminum and iodine: Watt, Hall, *Inorg. Synth.* **4**, 117 (1953); H. J. Becher in *Handbook of Preparative Inorganic Chemistry* vol. 1, G. Brauer, Ed. (Academic Press, New York, 2nd ed., 1963) p 814; Wilson, Worrall, *J. Chem. Soc. A* **1968**, 316.

White leaflets if pure; commercial grade yellowish- to blackish-brown lumps. mp 191°; bp 382°; d^{17} 3.948. Fumes in moist air; strong exothermic reaction with water. *Keep tightly closed and protected from light.* Sol in carbon disulfide, alcohol, ether, liquid ammonia.

Hexahydrate. Yellowish, deliquesc cryst powder. Sol in water, alcohol, ether. *Keep tightly closed.*

USE: Catalyst in organic reactions.

347. Aluminum Isopropoxide. [555-31-7] 2-Propanol aluminum salt; aluminum isopropylate. C$_9$H$_{21}$AlO$_3$; mol wt 204.24. C 52.93%, H 10.36%, Al 13.21%, O 23.50%. Al-[OCH(CH$_3$)$_2$]$_3$. Prepd from aluminum and isopropyl alcohol in the presence of mercuric chloride: Young *et al.*, *J. Am. Chem. Soc.* **58**, 100 (1936); by adding excess isopropyl alcohol to a benzene soln of AlCl$_3$ at 6°: Teichner, *Compt. Rend.* **237**, 810 (1953). Forms trimers and tetramers: Shiner *et al.*, *J. Am. Chem. Soc.* **85**, 2318 (1963); Oliver *et al.*, *J. Inorg. Nucl. Chem.* **31**, 1609 (1969); Worrall, *J. Chem. Educ.* **46**, 510 (1969). Toxicity: Smyth *et al.*, *Am. Ind. Hyg. Assoc. J.* **30**, 470 (1969). *Review:* Whitaker in *Adv. Chem. Ser.* **23**, entitled "Metal-Organic Compounds," M. Sittig, Ed. (ACS, Washington DC, 1959) pp 184-189.

Hygroscopic white solid, mp 119°. Solidifies rather slowly after distillation. bp$_{10}$ 135°; bp$_{7.5}$ 131°; bp$_{5.5}$ 125.5°; bp$_{2.5}$ 113°; bp$_{1.5}$ 106°; bp$_{0.5}$ 94°. Sol in ethanol, isopropanol, benzene, toluene, chloroform, carbon tetrachloride, petroleum hydrocarbons. Decomposed by water. LD$_{50}$ orally in rats: 11.3 g/kg (Smyth).

USE: Meerwein-Ponndorf reactions; alcoholysis and ester exchange; synthesis of higher alkoxides, chelates, and acylates; formation of aluminum soaps, formulation of paints; waterproofing finishes for textiles.

348. Aluminum Lactate. [18917-91-4] Tris[2-(hydroxy-κO)propanoato-κO]aluminum; Al(lact)$_3$. C$_9$H$_{15}$AlO$_9$; mol wt 294.19. C 36.74%, H 5.14%, Al 9.17%, O 48.95%. Prepn from lactic acid and aluminum isopropoxide or aluminum chloride: A. K. Rai *et al.*, *J. Prakt. Chem.* **20**, 105 (1963); from lactic acid and aluminum foil: R. W. Jones, J. E. Cluskey, *Cereal Chem.* **40**, 589 (1963). Partition coefficients: A. Tapparo, M. Perazzolo, *Int. J. Environ. Anal. Chem.* **36**, 13 (1989). Molecular structure: G. G. Bombi *et al.*, *Inorg. Chim. Acta* **171**, 79 (1990). Stability and NMR spectra: B. Corain *et al.*, *J. Chem. Soc. Dalton Trans.* **1992**, 169. Optical rotation isotherms: I. G. Bratu *et al.*, *COFrRoCA 2002, Actes Colloq. Fr.-Roum. Chim Appl.* **2**, 157 (2002). Reactant in sol-gel synthesis of aluminophosphate glass: L. Zhang *et al.*, *Chem. Mater.* **15**, 2702 (2003). Inhibition of the biological effects of silica quartz: R. Bégin *et al.*, *Exp. Lung Res.* **10**, 385 (1986); R. Duffin *et al.*, *Toxicol. Appl. Pharmacol.* **176**, 10 (2001). Clinical evaluation as antiseptic throat spray: W. Klingbeil, *Fortschr. Med.* **100**, 146 (1982); in dental hypersensitivity: Y. Higuchi *et al.*, *J. Clin. Dent.* **7**, 9 (1996).

White powder. $[\alpha]_{366}^{20}$ +48.31°; $[\alpha]_{436}^{20}$ +33.37°; $[\alpha]_{578}^{20}$ +10.20° (c = 0.1 M). $[\alpha]_{366}^{25}$ +48.40°; $[\alpha]_{436}^{25}$ +31.36°; $[\alpha]_{578}^{25}$ +10.22° (c = 0.1 M). Partition coefficient (n-octanol/water): 0.0037-0.0127. Soly in water (25°): 0.70 ±0.01 mol dm^{-3}. pH of saturated soln: 2.9.

USE: As a reagent in biological activity studies of aluminum; in sol-gel processing.

THERAP CAT: Antiseptic.

349. Aluminum Lithium Hydride. [16853-85-3] Lithium tetrahydroaluminate; lithium aluminum hydride; lithium aluminohydride; lithium alanate. AlH$_4$Li; mol wt 37.95. Al 71.10%, H 10.62%, Li 18.29%. LiAlH$_4$. Prepd by treating lithium hydride with an ether soln of AlCl$_3$: Finholt, et al., J. Am. Chem. Soc. **69**, 1199 (1947). Crystal structure: Sklar, Post, Inorg. Chem. **6**, 669 (1967). Review of chemistry: J. S. Pizey, Synthetic Reagents **Vol. 1** (John Wiley, New York, 1974) pp 101-294.

Microcrystalline white powder when pure; gray when aluminum impurity present. Monoclinic crystals. d 0.92. Stable in dry air at room temperature, decomp above 125°, slowly loses hydrogen at 120°, decomp in moist air, may ignite on grinding in air. Soly (parts/100 parts solvent): 30 (ether); 13 (tetrahydrofuran); 10 (dimethylcellosolve); 2 (dibutyl ether); 0.1 (dioxane). Reacts rapidly with water and alcohols; reduces aldehydes, ketones, acid chlorides and esters to alcohols; nitriles to amines; aromatic nitro compounds to azo compounds. Does not attack olefinic double bonds unless they are conjugated with a phenyl group and a carbonyl or nitrile group.

USE: Reducing agent; in preparation of other hydrides.

350. Aluminum Magnesium Silicate. [12511-31-8] Magnesium aluminum silicate. Al$_2$MgO$_8$Si$_2$; mol wt 262.43. Al 20.56%, Mg 9.26%, O 48.77%, Si 21.40%. MgAl$_2$(SiO$_4$)$_2$. Occurs in nature in the minerals: *colerainite, leuchtenbergite, pyrope, saponite, sapphirine, sheridanite, zebedassite*. Prepn: **GB 834517** (1960 to Fuji Chem.)

Hydrate. Ervasil.

USE: As suspending agent, thickening agent.

THERAP CAT: Antacid.

351. Aluminum Nicotinate. Nicalex. Pharmaceutical composition consisting of aluminum hydroxydinicotinate and nicotinic acid. Manufacturing process: J. P. Miale, **US 2970082** (1961 to Walker Labs.). Prepn, properties and clinical studies: idem, Curr. Ther. Res. **7**, 392 (1965). Clinical trial in hypercholesterolemia: E. S. McCabe, Del. Med. J. **38**, 49 (1966).

White, amorphous powder with very slight acidulous taste. Insol in water, alchol. Sol in diluted mineral acids.

THERAP CAT: Has been used as antilipemic.

352. Aluminum Nitrate. [13473-90-0] AlN$_3$O$_9$; mol wt 213.00. Al 12.67%, N 19.73%, O 67.60%. Al(NO$_3$)$_3$. Occurs in several states of hydration of which the nonahydrate is the most stable. Prepn: Gmelins, Aluminum (8th ed.) **35B**, pp 149-152 (1934). Toxicity data: Smyth et al., Am. Ind. Hyg. Assoc. J. **30**, 470 (1969).

Nonahydrate. Deliquesc crystals; mp 73°; dec at 135°. Very sol in water, alc; very slightly sol in acetone. Almost insol in ethyl acetate and pyridine. The aq soln is acid. Keep well closed. LD$_{50}$ orally in rats: 4.28 g/kg (Smyth).

USE: Tanning leather; antiperspirant; corrosion inhibitor; extraction of uranium; nitrating agent.

353. Aluminum Nitride. [24304-00-5] AlN; mol wt 40.99. Al 65.82%, N 34.17%. Semiconductor material. Prepn: F. Briegleb, A. Geuther, Ann. **123**, 228 (1862). Lattice structure: H. Ott, Z. Physik. **22**, 201 (1924). Crystal structure: G. A. Jeffrey, G. S. Parry, J. Chem. Phys. **23**, 406 (1953). Prepn of AlN films by laser-induced chemical vapor deposition: X. Li, T. L. Tansley, J. Appl. Phys. **68**, 5369 (1990). Review of growth of high purity crystals: G. A. Slack, T. F. McNelly, J. Cryst. Growth **34**, 263-279 (1976); of prepn and properties: D. D. Marchant, T. E. Nemecek, Adv. Ceram. **26**, 19-54 (1989); of properties and applications: B. H. Mussler, Am. Ceram. Soc. Bull. **79**, 45-47 (2000).

Colorless, translucent material; crystallizes with a hexagonal wurtzite structure. Bandgap at room temp: 6.2 eV. d 3.26. Hardness no. 8 on Mohs' scale. mp 2400° (dec). Thermal conductivity at 300 K: 3.19 W/cm K. Specific heat: 738 ±20 J/kgK.

USE: In semiconductor electronics; in steel manuf. AlN components and substrates are used in electrical engines, microelectronics, naval radio and defense systems, railway transport systems, telecommunications and research satellites, and emission control systems.

354. Aluminum Oleate. [688-37-9] (9Z)-9-Octadecenoic acid aluminum salt; oleic acid aluminum salt. C$_{54}$H$_{99}$AlO$_6$; mol wt 871.34. C 74.43%, H 11.45%, Al 3.10%, O 11.02%. Prepd from freshly pptd Al$_2$(OH)$_6$ and oleic acid: Stich, Pharm. Zentralhalle **63**, 261 (1922), C.A. **16**, 2755 (1922).

Yellowish, viscid mass. Practically insol in water. Sol in alcohol, benzene, ether, oil turpentine.

USE: In oil or turpentine soln as lacquer for metals, as size, waterproofing agent, drier, for paints, high-pressure and high-temp greases for thickening lubricating oils.

355. Aluminum Oxalate. [814-87-9] C$_6$Al$_2$O$_{12}$; mol wt 318.02. C 22.66%, Al 16.97%, O 60.37%. Al$_2$(C$_2$O$_4$)$_3$. Prepn: **GB 348789** and **GB 348790** (both 1930 to I.G. Farben).

Hydrate. Powder. Practically insol in water, alc. Sol in mineral acids.

USE: Mordant in printing textiles, dyeing cotton.

356. Aluminum Oxide. [1344-28-1] Alumina. Al$_2$O$_3$; mol wt 101.96. Al 52.93%, O 47.08%. Occurs in nature as the minerals: *bauxite, bayerite, boehmite, corundum, diaspore, gibbsite*. Prepn and properties: Mellor's **vol. V**, 263-273 (1929); Gmelins, Aluminum (8th ed.) **35B**, pp 7-98 (1934); Becher in Handbook of Preparative Inorganic Chemistry **vol. 1**, G. Brauer, Ed. (Academic Press, New York, 2nd ed., 1963) pp 822-823; Wagner, ibid. **vol. 2** (1965) pp 1660-1663. Use as column matrix in ion chromatography: W. Buchberger, K. Winsauer, J. Chromatogr. **482**, 401 (1989); in HPLC: M. T. Kelly, M. R. Smyth, J. Pharm. Biomed. Anal. **7**, 1757 (1989). Clinical evaluation in hip replacement: L. Sedel et al., J. Bone Joint Surg. Br. **72-B**, 658 (1990); of wear in hip replacement: L. P. Zichner, H.-G. Willert, Clin. Orthop. Relat. Res. **282**, 86 (1992). Review of properties, biocompatibility and clinical use: P. Boutin et al., J. Biomed. Mater. Res. **22**, 1203-1232 (1988); of biocompatibility: P. S. Christel, Clin. Orthop. Relat. Res. **282**, 10-18 (1992).

Approximate characteristics of native aluminum oxide: White cryst powder. Very hard, about 8.8 on Moh's scale. An electrical insulator; electrical resistivity at 300° about 1.2×10^{13} ohms-cm. When heated above 800° it becomes insol in acid and specific gravity increases from 2.8 to 4.0. Insol in water. Very hygroscopic.

Caution: Potential symptoms of overexposure by direct contact are irritation of eyes, skin and respiratory system. See NIOSH Pocket Guide to Chemical Hazards (DHHS/NIOSH 97-140, 1997) p 12.

USE: As adsorbent, desiccant, abrasive; as filler for paints and varnishes; in manuf of alloys, ceramic materials, electrical insulators and resistors, dental cements, glass, steel, artificial gems; in coatings for metals, etc.; as catalyst for organic reactions. As a chromotagraphic matrix; originally called *Brockmann aluminum oxide* when used for this purpose. The minerals *corundum* (hardness = 9) and *Alundum* (obtained by fusing bauxite in an electric furnace) are used as abrasives and polishes; in manuf of refractories.

357. Aluminum Palmitate. [555-35-1] Hexadecanoic acid aluminum salt; palmitic acid aluminum salt. C$_{48}$H$_{93}$AlO$_6$; mol wt 793.23. C 72.68%, H 11.82%, Al 3.40%, O 12.10%. [CH$_3$-(CH$_2$)$_{14}$COO]$_3$Al. Prepd from AlCl$_3$ and palmitic acid: Mehrotra, Rai, J. Indian Chem. Soc. **39**, 1 (1962).

White to yellow mass or powder. Practically insol in water or alcohol; when fresh, dissolves in petrol ether or oil turpentine.

USE: Thickening petroleum and lubricants; water-proofing fabrics; sizing and glazing paper and leather.

358. Aluminum Phosphate. [7784-30-7] Aluminum orthophosphate. AlO$_4$P; mol wt 121.95. Al 22.13%, O 52.48%, P

25.40%. AlPO$_4$. Occurs in nature as the minerals *angelite*; *co-eruleolactite*; *evansite*; *lucinite*; *metavariscite*; *sterretite*; *variscite*; *vashegyite*; *wavellite*; *zepharovicht*. Prepn from NaAlO$_2$ and H$_3$PO$_4$: Becher in *Handbook of Preparative Inorganic Chemistry* vol. 1, G. Brauer, Ed. (Academic Press, New York, 2nd ed., 1963) p 831.

White, infusible powder. mp >1460°; d^{23} 2.56. Practically insol in water or acetic acid. Very slightly sol in concentrated hydrochloric acid and nitric acid. Isomorphous with quartz.

Aluminum phosphate gel. Fosfalugel; Phosphaljel; Phosphalugel.

USE: As cement in admixture with calcium sulfate and sodium silicate; as flux for ceramics; dental cements; for special glasses.

THERAP CAT: Antacid.

359. Aluminum Phosphide. [20859-73-8] Celphos; Phostoxin; Quickphos. AlP; mol wt 57.96. Al 46.55%, P 53.44%. Prepd from red phosphorus and aluminum powder: White, Bushey, *J. Am. Chem. Soc.* **66**, 1666 (1944); *Inorg. Synth.* **4**, 23 (1953); Montignie, *Bull. Soc. Chim. Fr.* **1946**, 276; from Al and Zn$_2$P$_3$: Wang *et al.*, *J. Inorg. Nucl. Chem.* **25**, 326 (1963). Use as insecticidal fumigant: W. Freyberg, W. Haupt, US 2117158 (1938 to Freyberg).

Dark gray or dark yellow crystals. Cubic zinc blende structure. Must be protected from moist air since it reacts readily to produce phosphine which is highly toxic. d$_4^{15}$ 2.85 (Montignie); d 2.40 (Wang *et al.*). Does not melt or decompose thermally at temps up to 1000°. Treatment with water and acid produces phosphine in quantitative yields.

USE: Source of phosphine; in semiconductor research; as fumigant.

360. Aluminum Potassium Sulfate. [10043-67-1] AlK-O$_8$S$_2$; mol wt 258.21. Al 10.45%, K 15.14%, O 49.57%, S 24.84%. KAl(SO$_4$)$_2$. Prepn: *Gmelins, Aluminum* (8th ed.) **35B**, 453-477 (1934). Crystal structure: Manoli *et al.*, *Bull. Soc. Chim. Fr.* **1970**, 27; of dodecahydrate: Larson, Cromer, *Acta Crystallogr.* **22**, 793 (1967).

Anhydrous. Burnt alum; exsiccated alum. Usually about 97-98% pure. White powder; styptic taste; attracts moisture from the air. One gram dissolves in about 20 ml cold or 1 ml boiling water, usually incompletely; practically insol in alcohol. *Keep well closed.*

Dodecahydrate. Alum; potassium alum; kalinite. The technical product is also known as *alum flour*, *alum meal*, *cube alum*. It is about 99.5% pure. Colorless, odorless, hard, large, transparent crystals or cryst fragments or white, cryst powder; sweetish, astringent taste. Stable at ordinary temp; when kept for a long time at 60-65° (or over H$_2$SO$_4$) loses 9 H$_2$O which is reabsorbed on exposure to air. Becomes anhydr at about 200°; at higher temp loses SO$_3$ and becomes basic and incompletely sol in water. d 1.725. mp 92.5°. One gram dissolves in 7.2 ml water, in 0.3 ml boiling water; freely sol in glycerol. Insol in alcohol. The aq soln is acid; pH of 0.2 molar aq soln 3.3.

USE: In dyeing, printing fabrics; manuf dyes, lakes, paper, vegetable glue, marble cement, porcelain cement, explosives; in tanning, hardening gelatin, baking powders, purifying water, clarifying sugar, hardening plaster casts; electrolytic copperplating; as catalyst in synthesis of ammonia; as mordant in staining with carmine, eosine, hematoxylin; clarifier (as alumina cream); identifying coloring matters; hardening agent in microscopy.

THERAP CAT: Astringent.

THERAP CAT (VET): Astringent.

361. Aluminum Selenide. [1302-82-5] Al$_2$Se$_3$; mol wt 290.84. Al 18.55%, Se 81.45%. Prepn from aluminum and selenium: Waitkins, Shutt, *Inorg. Synth.* **2**, 184 (1946); Becher in *Handbook of Preparative Inorganic Chemistry* vol. 1, G. Brauer, Ed. (Academic Press, New York, 2nd ed., 1963) p 825.

Yellowish to light-brown powder. d$_4^{15}$ 3.437. Unstable in air. Decomp in water and acid.

USE: In prepn of hydrogen selenide; in semiconductor research.

362. Aluminum Silicate. [12141-46-7] Aluminum oxide silicate [Al$_2$O(SiO$_4$)]. Al$_2$O$_5$Si; mol wt 162.05. Al 33.30%, O 49.37%, Si 17.33%. Al$_2$SiO$_5$. Usually contains some water. Polymorphic; the three naturally occurring forms are *andalusite*,

cyanite, *sillimanite*. Other aluminum silicate minerals are *anauxite*, *dickite*, *kaolinite*, *kochite*, *mullite*, *newtonite*, *pyrophyllite*, *takizolite*, *termierite*, *ton*. For prepn and properties see *Gmelins, Aluminum* (8th ed.) **35B**, p 313-317 (1934).

USE: In dental cements, glass industry; manuf of semiprecious stones, enamels, ceramics, and colored lakes; paint filler; in washing compounds.

363. Aluminum Sodium Sulfate. [10102-71-3] AlNaO$_8$-S$_2$; mol wt 242.10. Al 11.14%, Na 9.50%, O 52.87%, S 26.49%. NaAl(SO$_4$)$_2$. Prepn: *Gmelins, Aluminum* (8th ed) **35B**, p 378-384 (1934).

Dodecahydrate. Sodium alum; soda alum. Colorless crystals or white granules or powder. d 1.61. mp about 60°. Sol in 1 part water. Practically insol in alc.

USE: Industrially, like aluminum potassium sulfate.

THERAP CAT: Astringent.

THERAP CAT (VET): Astringent.

364. Aluminum Stearate. [637-12-7] Octadecanoic acid aluminum salt; stearic acid aluminum salt; aluminum tristearate. C$_{54}$H$_{105}$AlO$_6$; mol wt 877.39. C 73.92%, H 12.06%, Al 3.08%, O 10.94%. [CH$_3$(CH$_2$)$_{16}$COO]$_3$Al. Prepn: Gilmour *et al.*, *J. Chem. Soc.* **1956**, 1972.

Hard material, passes into plastic form on heating. mp 117-120°. Practically insol in water. When freshly made, sol in alcohol, benzene, oil turpentine, mineral oils. Forms cryst pyridine complex.

USE: Waterproofing fabrics, ropes; in paint and varnish driers; thickening lubricating oils; in cements; in light-sensitive photographic compositions.

365. Aluminum Subacetate Solution. [8000-61-1] Essigsäure Tonerde. Contains about 8% aluminum diacetate, Al-(OH)(CH$_3$CO$_2$)$_2$. Prepd from aluminum sulfate, acetic acid, calcium carbonate and water. Details of prepn, *see* Aluminum Diacetate. *USP* **XVIII**, pp 29-30. Several other routes of prepn, *see* Aluminum Diacetate.

Clear, colorless liquid. Odor of acetic acid. d 1.045. Acid to litmus. Gradually becomes turbid and colloidal. Sometimes a more basic salt precipitates out and settles to the bottom of the container. Heat promotes the decomposition. *Keep in a cool place and discard when cloudy.*

Caution: Ingestion of large doses may cause severe nausea, vomiting, diarrhea, melena, hematemesis.

USE: As mordant in cotton dyeing, in printing fabrics, in water- and fireproofing fabrics, in waterproofing tissues, in formulations for antiperspirants and embalming fluids. *See also* Aluminum Diacetate.

THERAP CAT: Astringent, antiseptic.

THERAP CAT (VET): Astringent.

366. Aluminum Sulfate. [10043-01-3] Al$_2$O$_{12}$S$_3$; mol wt 342.15. Al 15.77%, O 56.11%, S 28.11%. Al$_2$(SO$_4$)$_3$. Occurs in nature as the mineral *alunogenite*. Prepn: *Gmelins, Aluminum* (8th ed.) **35B**, pp 267-269 (1934).

White, lustrous crystals, pieces, granules, or powder. d 1.61. Melts when gradually heated. At 250° loses its water; decomposes at red heat. Sol in 1 part water. Practically insol in alcohol. On long boiling of the aq soln, insol basic salt ppts. The aq soln is acid.

Octadecahydrate. The commercial product is also known as *cake alum* or *patent alum*. It is about 99.5% pure. The article of commerce usually contains 5 to 10% less water than theory.

USE: Tanning leather, sizing paper, mordant in dyeing; purifying water; manuf lakes, aluminum resinate; fireproofing and waterproofing cloth; clarifying oils and fats; treating sewage; waterproofing concrete; deodorizing and decolorizing petroleum; antiperspirants; agricultural pesticides; manuf aluminum salts.

THERAP CAT: Anti-infective.

367. Aluminum Sulfide. [1302-81-4] Al$_2$S$_3$; mol wt 150.16. Al 35.94%, S 64.06%. Prepd by heating aluminum with sulfur: Flahaut, *Compt. Rend.* **232**, 334 (1951); Becher in *Handbook of Preparative Inorganic Chemistry* vol. 1, G. Brauer, Ed. (Academic Press, New York, 2nd ed., 1963) p 823.

Yellowish-gray, compact lumps; H$_2$S odor; decomposes in moist air to a gray powder. d 2.02. mp 1100°. Hydrolyzed by water to Al(OH)$_3$ and H$_2$S. *Keep tightly closed.*

368. Aluminum Tartrate. [815-78-1] 2,3-Dihydroxybutanedioic acid aluminum salt. $C_{12}H_{12}Al_2O_{18}$; mol wt 498.18. C 28.93%, H 2.43%, Al 10.83%, O 57.81%. $Al_2(C_4H_4O_6)_3$. Usually contains some water. Prepn: Goldman, *Biochem. Z.* **133**, 459 (1922); **GB 348790** (1930 to I. G. Farben.).

Odorless granules. Slowly sol in cold, readily in hot water; sol in ammonia.

USE: In textile dyeing.

369. Aluminum Thiocyanate. [538-17-0] Aluminum sulfocyanate. $C_3AlN_3S_3$; mol wt 201.23. C 17.91%, Al 13.41%, N 20.88%, S 47.80%. $Al(CNS)_3$. Prepn: *Gmelins, Aluminum* (8th ed.) **35B**, p 306 (1934).

USE: Aq solution used as mordant in dye industry.

370. Aluminum Tris(8-hydroxyquinoline). [2085-33-8] Tris(8-quinolinolato-$\kappa N^1,\kappa O^8$)aluminum; tris(8-hydroxyquinoline)aluminium; Alq$_3$. $C_{27}H_{18}AlN_3O_3$; mol wt 459.43. C 70.59%, H 3.95%, Al 5.87%, N 9.15%, O 10.45%. Metal chelate; fluorescent solid-state material for organic light-emitting devices (OLED). Prepn: R. Berg, *Z. Anal. Chem.* **71**, 369 (1927); I. M. Kolthoff, E. B. Sandell, *J. Am. Chem. Soc.* **50**, 1900 (1928); of analogs: H. Jang *et al.*, *Synth. Metals* **121**, 1667 (2001); of solid state: A. K. Saxena, *Synth. React. Inorg. Met.-Org. Chem.* **29**, 1747 (1999). Exists as two geometric isomers *mer-* and *fac-* with several crytalline forms. Crystal structure and optical properties of α, β, and γ-forms: M. Brinkmann *et al.*, *J. Am. Chem. Soc.* **122**, 5147 (2000); of blue luminescent δ-form: M. Cölle *et al.*, *Adv. Funct. Mater.* **13**, 108 (2003). Photoemission at thin-film faces: W. Zhao *et al.*, *Chem. Mater.* **16**, 750 (2004). Reliability and degradation study: Z. D. Popovic, H. Aziz, *IEEE J. Sel. Top. Quantum Electron.* **8**, 362 (2002). Use in OLEDs: C. W. Tang, S. A. VanSlyke, *Appl. Phys. Lett.* **51**, 913 (1987); G. Baldacchini *et al.*, *Proc. 149th Int. School Phys. Enrico Fermi Rome 2002* 561-567; as functionalized polymer: A. Meyers, M. Werk, *Macromolecules* **36**, 1766 (2003). Review as emitting material for electroluminescence: C. H. Chen, J. Shi, *Coord. Chem. Rev.* **171**, 161-174 (1998).

Light yellow complex, 330° (dec) (Jang); also reported as mp 340° (dec) (Saxena). Sublimes >500 K. uv max (0.1 mg/ml): 316, 372 nm; uv max (THF): 391 nm. Fluorescence max (0.09 mg/ml): 509 nm. Photoluminescence (THF): 516 nm; electroluminescence: 528 nm. Luminance max: 3400 cd/m^2 at 13 V.

USE: In OLEDs as an electron transport and/or light emitting layer.

371. Alverine. [150-59-4] N-Ethyl-N-(3-phenylpropyl)benzenepropanamine; N-ethyl-3,3'-diphenyldipropylamine; bis(γ-phenylpropyl)ethylamine; di(phenylpropyl)ethylamine. $C_{20}H_{27}N$; mol wt 281.44. C 85.35%, H 9.67%, N 4.98%. Prepn: Külz *et al.*, *Ber.* **72**, 2165 (1939); Stühner, Elbrächter, *Arch. Pharm.* **287**, 139 (1954). Physical properties: E. F. Salim, W. R. Ebert, *J. Pharm. Sci.* **56**, 1162 (1967). Clinical trial in irritable bowel syndrome: G. J. Tudor, *Br. J. Clin. Pract.* **40**, 276 (1985).

Liquid, bp$_{0.3}$ 165-168°; bp$_{13}$ 210-215°.

Citrate. [5560-59-8] Spasmaverine; Spasmonal. $C_{20}H_{27}$-N.$C_6H_8O_7$; mol wt 473.56. White to off-white powder having a sweet odor and slightly bitter taste, mp 100-102°. Slightly sol in water, chloroform; sparingly sol in alcohol; very slightly sol in ether.

THERAP CAT: Antispasmodic.

372. Alvimopan. [156053-89-3] N-[(2S)-2-[[(3R,4R)-4-(3-Hydroxyphenyl)-3,4-dimethyl-1-piperidinyl]methyl]-1-oxo-3-phenylpropyl]glycine; [[2(S)-[[4(R)-(3-hydroxyphenyl)-3(R),4-dimethyl-1-piperidinyl]methyl]-1-oxo-3-phenylpropyl]amino]acetic acid; ADL-8-2698; LY-246736; Entereg. $C_{25}H_{32}N_2O_4$; mol wt 424.53. C 70.73%, H 7.60%, N 6.60%, O 15.07%. Peripheral mu-opioid receptor antagonist. Prepn: B. E. Cantrell *et al.*, **EP 506478**; *eidem*, **US 5250542** (1992, 1993 both to Lilly); D. M. Zimmerman *et al.*, *J. Med. Chem.* **37**, 2262 (1994). Improved synthesis: J. A. Werner *et al.*, *J. Org. Chem.* **61**, 587 (1996). Clinical pharmacology: S. S. Liu *et al.*, *Clin. Pharmacol. Ther.* **68**, 66 (2000). Clinical trial in postoperative ileus: A. Taguchi *et al.*, *N. Engl. J. Med.* **345**, 935 (2001); E. R. Viscusi *et al.*, *Surg. Endosc.* **20**, 64 (2006). Review of clinical experience: W. K. Schmidt, *Am. J. Surg.* **182**, Suppl., 27S-38S (2001); and pharmacology: P. Neary, C. P. Delaney, *Expert Opin. Invest. Drugs* **14**, 479-488 (2005).

Dihydrate. [170098-38-1] Crystals, mp 210-213°. $[\alpha]_D^{25}$ +51.8° (c = 1.0 in DMSO).

THERAP CAT: Gastroprokinetic.

373. Amanitin. [11030-71-0] Group 1 mushroom toxin from the poisonous mushroom *Amanita phalloides* (Fr.) Secr., *Agaricaceae*. Inhibits protein synthesis of mammalian cells. Comprised of α-, β-, γ-amanitin and **amanin**. α-Amanitin is the major poisonous constituent of *A. phalloides;* it is 10-20 times more toxic than phalloidin, *q.v.* Isoln of α- and β-amanitin: Wieland, *Ann.* **564**, 152 (1949). Prepn of α-amanitin from β-amanitin: Wieland, Boehringer, *ibid.* **635**, 178 (1960). Structure: Wieland, *Pure Appl. Chem.* **9**, 145 (1964); Wieland, Gebert, *Ann.* **700**, 157 (1967). Review of chemistry and toxicology of the toxins of *Amanita phalloides:* Wieland, Wieland, *Pharmacol. Rev.* **11**, 87-107 (1959); T. Wieland, *Fortschr. Chem. Org. Naturst.* **25**, 214-250 (1967); T. Wieland, H. Faulstich, *Crit. Rev. Biochem.* **5**, 185-260 (1978). Book: H. Faulstich *et al.*, *Amanita Toxins and Poisoning: International Amanita Symposium* (Lubrecht & Cramer, Heidelberg, 1980) 246 pp.

α-Amanitin R = NH$_2$
β-Amanitin R = OH

α-Amanitin. [23109-05-9] $C_{39}H_{54}N_{10}O_{14}S$; mol wt 918.97. Needles from methanol, mp 254-255°. $[\alpha]_D^{20}$ +191°. uv max: 302 nm. LD$_{50}$ i.p. in albino mice: 0.1 mg/kg (Wieland, Wieland).

β-Amanitin. [21150-22-1] $C_{39}H_{53}N_9O_{15}S$; mol wt 919.95. Needles from methanol, mp 300°. uv max: 302 nm. Sol in water, methanol, ethanol, aqueous butanol. LD$_{50}$ i.p. in albino mice: 0.4 mg/kg (Wieland, Wieland).

Caution: Highly toxic. Following a characteristic asymptomatic period of 6-15 hrs, potential symptoms of intoxication due to ingestion include violent gastroenteritis; fever, tachycardia, hyperglycemia, dehydration, electrolyte imbalance; liver dysfunction and necrosis; renal failure; may be fatal. *See Clinical Toxicology of Commercial Products*, R. E. Gosselin *et al.*, Eds. (Williams & Wilkins, Baltimore, 5th ed., 1984) Section II, p 246; M. J. Ellenhorn, D. G. Barceloux, *Medical Toxicology: Diagnosis and Treatment of Human Poisoning* (Elsevier, New York, 1988) pp 1331-1338.

USE: As a tool in molecular biology.

374. Amantadine. [768-94-5] Tricyclo[3.3.1.1³,⁷]decan-1-amine; 1-adamantanamine; 1-aminoadamantane; 1-aminodiamantane (obsolete); 1-aminotricyclo[3.3.1.1³,⁷]decane. $C_{10}H_{17}N$; mol wt 151.25. C 79.41%, H 11.33%, N 9.26%. NMDA-receptor antagonist; also active vs influenza A virus. Prepn: H. Stetter *et al.*, *Ber.* **93**, 226 (1960); W. Haaf, *ibid.* **97**, 3234 (1964); P. Kovacic, P. D. Roskos, *Tetrahedron Lett.* **1968**, 5833. Antiviral activity: W. L. Davies *et al.*, *Science* **144**, 862 (1964). GC determn in biological samples and pharmacodynamics: W. E. Bleidner *et al.*, *J. Pharmacol. Exp. Ther.* **150**, 484 (1965). Pharmacology and toxicology: V. G. Vernier *et al.*, *Toxicol. Appl. Pharmacol.* **15**, 642 (1969). Comprehensive description: J. Kirschbaum, *Anal. Profiles Drug Subs.* **12**, 1-36 (1983). Review of use vs influenza A: R. L. Tominack, F. G. Hayden, *Infect. Dis. Clin. North Am.* **1**, 459-478 (1987); of pharmacokinetics: F. Y. Aoki, D. S. Sitar, *Clin. Pharmacokinet.* **14**, 35-51 (1988). Review of NMDA receptor binding and neuroprotective properties: J. Kornhuber *et al.*, *J. Neural Transm.* **43**, Suppl., 91-104 (1994). Series of articles on clinical experience in Parkinson's disease: *ibid.* **46**, Suppl., 399-421 (1995).

Crystals by sublimation, mp 160-190° (closed tube) (Stetter). Also reported as mp 180-192° (Haaf). pKa: 10.1. Sparingly sol in water.

Hydrochloride. [665-66-7] EXP-105-1; NSC-83653; Adekin; Lysovir; Mantadan; Mantadine; Mantadix; Symmetrel; Virofral. $C_{10}H_{17}N \cdot HCl$; mol wt 187.71. Crystals from abs ethanol + anhyd ether, mp >360° (dec). Freely sol in water (at least 1:20); sol in alcohol, chloroform. Practically insol in ether. LD₅₀ orally in mice, rats: 700, 1275 mg/kg (Vernier).

Sulfate. [31377-23-8] PK-Merz. $C_{10}H_{17}N \cdot \frac{1}{2}H_2SO_4$; mol wt 200.29.

THERAP CAT: Antiviral; antiparkinsonian.

375. Amaranth (Dye). [915-67-3] 3-Hydroxy-4-[(4-sulfo-1-naphthalenyl)azo]-2,7-naphthalenedisulfonic acid trisodium salt; C.I. Acid Red 27; C.I. 16185; FD & C Red No. 2; Red no. 2; 1-(4-sulfo-1-naphthylazo)-2-naphthol-3,6-disulfonic acid trisodium salt. $C_{20}H_{11}N_2Na_3O_{10}S_3$; mol wt 604.47. C 39.74%, H 1.83%, N 4.63%, Na 11.41%, O 26.47%, S 15.91%. Azo dye. Prepn: Knecht, *J. Soc. Dyers Colour.* **2**, 24 (1886). *See also Colour Index* vol. 4 (3rd ed., 1971) p 4093. Metabolism: J. L. Radomski, T. J. Mellinger, *J. Pharmacol. Exp. Ther.* **136**, 259 (1962). Use as indicator: N. K. Murty, K. R. Rao, *J. Indian Chem. Soc.* **53**, 532 (1976). Stability studies: A. Motawi, S. El-Gamal, *Sci. Pharm.* **48**, 377 (1980). Effect of pH and concentration on reduction: J. Maslowska, J. Janiak, *Zesz. Nauk. Politech. Lodz.* **1994**, 150. Spectrophotometric analysis: C. C. Blanco *et al.*, *Talanta* **43**, 1019 (1996). Review of carcinogenic risk: *IARC Monographs* **8**, 41-60 (1975).

Dark, reddish-brown powder. Absorption max at 25°: 520 nm (water); 528 nm (acetone); 520 nm (DMF). One gram dissolves in about 15 ml water. Also reported as 7.20 g/100 ml H_2O at 26°.

Very slightly sol in ethanol, cellosolve. The aq soln is vivid red (1 cm layer). Discharge white by hydrosulfite on wool and silk. HCl does not change the color intensity of the soln, NaOH increases it. The aq soln is stable toward light.

USE: Dyeing wool and silk bright bluish-red from an acid bath. Food colorant. As indicator. In color photography.

376. Amaranth (Plant). Genus of the *Amaranthaceae* L. family which contains approx 60 species having worldwide distribution. Many species are considered weeds but *Amaranthus caudatus* L. (*love-lies-bleeding*), *A. hybridus* variety *hypochondriacus* L. (*prince's feather*), *A. tricolor* have been cultivated as ornamentals. *A. retroflexus* L. and some of the other weedy species are known as *pigweed*, *redroot* and *water hemp*. *A. spinosus* L. has been used in the treatment of gonorrhea: W. H. Brown, *Useful Plants of the Philippines* **1** (Philippines Dept. Agr. and Natl. Resources, Manila, 1951) pp 510-515; as a poultice in the treatment of inflammation, bruises and eczema: T. H. P. de Tavera, *The Medicinal Plants of the Philippines* (P. Blakiston's Son, Philadelphia, 1901) pp 200-202. Most species are hardy, herbaceous and fast-growing cereal-like plants. Leaves and grain are used for food in parts of South America, Africa and Asia. Plants are high in protein; the amino acid composition is complementary to that of wheat. The grain was a basic food in pre-Columbian South and Central America and was important in Aztec ritual. Grain amaranths (*A. hypochondriacus, A. cruentas, A. caudatus*) produce large seedheads containing many edible seeds. The seed can be made into low gluten flour, cooked into gruel or popped like corn. Compositional study of grain: R. Becker *et al.*, *J. Food Sci.* **46**, 1175 (1981); K. C. Pant, *Nutr. Rep. Int.* **28**, 1445 (1983). Properties of seed starches: P. V. S. Rao, J. K. Goering, *Cereal Chem.* **47**, 655 (1970); Y. Tomita *et al.*, *J. Nutr. Sci. Vitaminol.* **27**, 471 (1981); saccharides: K. Lorenz, M. Gross, *Nutr. Rep. Int.* **29**, 721 (1984); lipids: F. I. Opute, *J. Exp. Bot.* **30**, 601 (1979). Baking potential of flour: K. Lorenz, *Starch/Staerke* **33**, 149 (1981). Most amaranth species have edible leaves with mild spinach-like flavor. *A. cruentas, A. dubius, A. hybridus, A. lividus* and *A. tricolor* are some of the species grown as vegetables. Magnesium and copper content of leaf: N. M. Guttiker *et al.*, *J. Nutr. Diet.* **3**, 4 (1966); vitamin A content: C. N. Rao, *ibid.* **4**, 10 (1967); amino acids: I. G. Vasi, V. P. Kalintha, *J. Inst. Chem. (India)* **52**, 13 (1980). Nutritive value of leaf protein concentrate: P. R. Cheeke *et al.*, *Can. J. Anim. Sci.* **61**, 199 (1981). Toxicology: R. M. Hill, P. D. Rawate: *J. Agric. Food Chem.* **30**, 465 (1982). Book: J. N. Cole, *Amaranth, From the Past for the Future* (Rodale Press, Emmaus, Pennsylvania, 1979) 311 pp; Nat'l. Academy of Sciences Report: *Amaranth, Modern Prospects for an Ancient Crop* (Nat'l. Academy Press, Washington, D.C., 1984) 80 pp.

377. Amarogentin. [21018-84-8] [4aS-(4aα,5β,6α)]-3,3',5-Trihydroxy[1,1'-biphenyl]-2-carboxylic acid 2-ester with 5-ethenyl-6-(β-D-glucopyranosyloxy)-4,4a,5,6-tetrahydro-1H,3H-pyrano[3,4-c]pyran-1-one; sweroside-2'-(3'',5'',3'''-trihydroxy-diphenyl)-2''-carboxylic acid ester. $C_{29}H_{30}O_{13}$; mol wt 586.54. C 59.38%, H 5.16%, O 35.46%. Strongly bitter glucoside. Isoln from *Swertia chirata* Buch-Ham., *Gentianaceae*: Korte, *Ber.* **88**, 704 (1955); **89**, 2404 (1956); from *Swertia japonica* Makino: Inouye *et al.*, *Chem. Pharm. Bull.* **18**, 1856 (1970). Occurrence in gentianaceous plants: Inouye, Nakamura, *J. Pharm. Soc. Jpn.* **91**, 755 (1971), *C.A.* **75**, 95431b (1971). Structure: *eidem, Tetrahedron Lett.* **1968**, 4919; *eidem, Tetrahedron* **27**, 1951 (1971).

Colorless needles, mp 229-230° (monohydrate). $[\alpha]_D^{20}$ −116.6° (methanol). uv max: 230, 266, 306 nm (log ε 4.46, 4.07, 3.68). Slightly sol in benzene, water; freely sol in acetone, anhydr dioxane, tetrahydrofuran, methanol, ethanol. Practically insol in petr ether, ether, cyclohexane, CHCl₃.

378. Amarolide. [29913-86-8] (2α,11α)-2,11-Dihydroxy-picrasane-1,12,16-trione. $C_{20}H_{28}O_6$; mol wt 364.43. C 65.91%, H 7.74%, O 26.34%. Isoln from *Ailanthus altissima* (Mill.) Swingle (*A. glandulosa* Desf.), *Simaroubaceae,* and proposed structure: Casinovi *et al., Tetrahedron Lett.* **1965,** 2273. Isoln from *Castela nicholsoni* Hook, *Simaroubaceae,* and revised structure: Stöcklin *et al., ibid.* **1970,** 2399.

mp 253-255°. Practically insol in weak alkaline solns. Slightly sol in sodium carbonate, easily dissolved by sodium hydroxide.

Monoacetate. $C_{22}H_{30}O_7$. mp 264-265° for 11-acetate; mp 225° for 2-acetate.

Diacetate. $C_{24}H_{32}O_8$. mp 269-270° (from alcohol). Also reported as mp 260-262°.

379. Ambenonium Chloride. [115-79-7] *N,N'*-[(1,2-Di-oxo-1,2-ethanediyl)bis(imino-2,1-ethanediyl)]bis[2-chloro-*N,N*-diethylbenzenemethanaminium] dichloride; [oxalylbis(iminoethyl-ene)]bis[(*o*-chlorobenzyl)diethylammonium chloride]; *N,N'*-bis[2-diethylaminoethyl]oxamide bis[2-chlorobenzyl chloride]; Win-8077; Mytelase. $C_{28}H_{42}Cl_4N_4O_2$; mol wt 608.47. C 55.27%, H 6.96%, Cl 23.31%, N 9.21%, O 5.26%. Prepn: F. K. Kirchner, **DE 1024517** (1958 to Sterling Drug), *C.A.* **54,** 18366g (1960). Determn in serum: C. Tharasse-Bloch *et al., J. Chromatogr.* **421,** 407 (1987). Pharmacokinetics in dogs: *eidem, Arzneim.-Forsch.* **39,** 257 (1989).

2Cl⁻

Crystals, mp 196-199°. Freely soluble in water.

THERAP CAT: Cholinesterase inhibitor.

380. Amber. [9000-02-6] Baltic amber; bernstein; succinite. A fossil resin from the extinct pine tree *Pinites succinifera* (Goepp.) Conway, *Pinaceae.* Found along the Baltic coast, also mined in Samland (East Prussia). Baltic amber contains: C 79%, H 10.5%, O 10.5%; succinic acid 3-8%; α-amyrin 20-30%. *Refs:* Plonait, *Angew. Chem.* **48,** 184 (1935); Schmid and co-workers: *Ann.* **503,** 269 (1933); *Monatsh. Chem.* **63,** 210 (1933); **65,** 348 (1935); **72,** 290, 311 (1939). *Review:* Berthelot, *Chim. Ind. (Paris)* **50,** 78-9 (1943); Frondel, *Econ. Bot.* **22,** 371 (1968). Infrared spectroscopy of different varieties of powdered amber: C. W. Beck *et al., Nature* **201,** 256 (1964). Chemical constitution: J. B. Lambert, J. S. Frye, *Science* **217,** 55 (1982).

Pale-yellow to reddish-brown resin. Transparent or cloudy (due to enclosed air bubbles and free succinic acid). Brittle; conchoidal fracture. d 1.05 to 1.10. Harder than most other resins. n_D 1.539-1.545. Softens at 150°, mp 350-375° giving off a choking, aromatic odor. When rubbed it is a good generator of static electricity.

Oil of Amber, Rectified. Obtained by the destructive distillation of amber and purified by redistillation. Consists of a mixture of terpenes with resinous, oxygen-containing substances. Pale yellow to yellowish-brown, volatile oil; penetrating odor; burning acrid

taste. d 0.850-0.920. α_D^{20} +22 to +26°. Insol in water. Sol in about 10 vols alcohol; freely sol in chloroform, ether, carbon disulfide, oils.

USE: The best quality is machined into beads and other personal ornaments. For teething strings. Also used for making mouthpieces of tobacco pipes and cigarette holders. Small pieces are pressed into "ambroid" and then used for the same purpose. Impure material goes into the manufacture of "amber" varnishes.

381. Ambergris. [8038-65-1] Concretion from intestinal tract of the sperm whale, *Physeter catodon* L., *Physeteridae.* Found in tropical seas or seashores. Perfumers have used ambergris for centuries for its desirable odoriferous and fixative properties. Three major components isolated are the triterpene alcohol ambrein, epicoprostanol and coprostanone: Ruzicka, Lardon, *Helv. Chim. Acta* **29,** 912 (1946); Lederer *et al., ibid.,* 1354; Hardwick, Laws, *Analyst* **76,** 662 (1951). Ambergris falls under the Marine Mammal Protection Act of 1972 and is illegal to import in the U.S.A. Analytical method for the detection and identification of ambergris: T. F. Governo *et al., J. Assoc. Off. Anal. Chem.* **60,** 160 (1977). Hypothesis on the biological origin of ambergris: P. A. Dubois, *Parfums Cosmet. Aromes* **19,** 35 (1978).

Gray to black, waxy mass; characteristic odor. d 0.8-0.92. mp ~60°. Flammable; almost completely volatile by heat. Insoluble in water or in alkali hydroxides. Sol in hot alcohol, chloroform, ether, fats, volatile oils.

USE: Chiefly in perfumery as tincture and essence for fixing delicate odors.

382. Amberlite®. [9079-25-8] Synthetic, high capacity cation and anion exchange resins and ion exchange-impregnated papers. *Reviews:* Nachod, Schubert, *Ion Exchange Technology* (Academic Press, New York, 1956); Kunin, *Ion Exchange Resins* (John Wiley, New York, 1958); Kunin, *Elements of Ion Exchange* (Reinhold, New York, 1960); Rieman, Walton, *Ion Exchange in Analytical Chemistry* (Pergamon Press, 1970); Dorfner, *Ion Exchangers Properties and Applications* (Ann Arbor Science, 1972).

383. Amberlyst 15®. [9037-24-5] Macroreticular sulfonic acid cation exchange resin based on a styrene-divinylbenzene copolymer. Prepn and characterization: R. Kunin *et al., Ind. Eng. Chem. Prod. Res. Dev.* **1,** 140 (1962). Small-angle x-ray scattering structural study: B. Chu, D. M. T. Creti, *J. Phys. Chem.* **71,** 1943 (1967). Water sorption study: R. S. D. Toteja *et al., Langmuir* **13,** 2980 (1997). Review of catalytic applications in synthetic organic chemistry: M. Kalesse, *Acros Org. Acta* **1,** 67-68 (1995).

Opaque beads. Moisture holding capacity: 50% H_2O. Apparent density: 1.012. True skeletal density: 1.513. Surface area: 42.5 m²/g dry resin. Avg pore diameter: 288 Å.

USE: Ion exchange resin; reusable solid acid catalyst.

384. Ambrisentan. [177036-94-1] (αS)-α-[(4,6-Dimethyl-2-pyrimidinyl)oxy]-β-methoxy-β-phenylbenzenepropanoic acid; BSF-208075; LU-208075. $C_{22}H_{22}N_2O_4$; mol wt 378.42. C 69.83%, H 5.86%, N 7.40%, O 16.91%. Nonpeptide endothelin ETₐ receptor antagonist. Prepn: H. Riechers *et al.,* **WO 9611914**; *eidem,* **US 5932730** (1996, 1998 both to BASF); H. Riechers *et al., J. Med. Chem.* **39,** 2123 (1996). Pharmacology: H. Vatter *et al., Clin. Neuropharmacol.* **26,** 73 (2003). Clinical evaluation in pulmonary arterial hypertension: N. Galiè *et al., J. Am. Coll. Cardiol.* **46,** 529 (2005). Review of development and therapeutic potential: G. E. Billman, *Curr. Opin. Invest. Drugs* **3,** 1483-1486 (2002).

(±)-**Form.** [713516-99-5] Crystals from diethylether, mp 190-191°.

THERAP CAT: Antihypertensive.

385. Ambrosin. [509-93-3] 3,3a,4,5,6,6a,9a,9b-Octahydro-6,9a-dimethyl-3-methyleneazuleno[4,5-*b*]furan-2,9-dione; 6β-hydroxy-4-oxo-10α*H*-ambrosa-2,11(13)-dien-12-oic acid γ-lactone. $C_{15}H_{18}O_3$; mol wt 246.30. C 73.15%, H 7.37%, O 19.49%. From herb of *Ambrosia maritima* L., *Compositae:* Abu-Shady, Soine, *J. Am. Pharm. Assoc.* **42,** 387 (1953); **43,** 365 (1954). Structure: Bernardi, Büchi, *Experientia* **13,** 466 (1957); Sorm *et al., Collect. Czech. Chem. Commun.* **24,** 1548 (1959); Nerz *et al., J. Am. Chem. Soc.* **84,** 2601 (1962). Absolute configuration: Emerson *et al., Tetrahedron Lett.* **1966,** 6151. Stereospecific total synthesis of (±)-form: P. A. Grieco *et al., J. Am. Chem. Soc.* **99,** 7393 (1977).

Crystals from alc, mp 146°. $[\alpha]_D^{22}$ −154.50° (c = 2 in alcohol). uv max (95% ethanol): 217, 324 nm (ε 13465; 36). Very sol in chloroform; sol in alc, benzene, sparingly sol in ether, petr ether. Practically insol in water, cold dil NaOH, dil acids.

(±)-**Form.** mp 188-190°.

386. Ambroxol. [18683-91-5] 4-[[(2-Amino-3,5-dibromophenyl)methyl]amino]cyclohexanol; *N*-(*trans-p*-hydroxycyclohexyl)-(2-amino-3,5-dibromobenzyl)amine; NA-872. $C_{13}H_{18}Br_2N_2O$; mol wt 378.10. C 41.30%, H 4.80%, Br 42.27%, N 7.41%, O 4.23%. Metabolite of bromhexine, q.v. Structure: E. Schraven *et al., Eur. J. Pharmacol.* **7,** 445 (1967). Synthesis: J. Keck, *Ann.* **707,** 107 (1967); **FR 1522709**; J. Keck *et al.,* **US 3536713** (1968, 1970 both to Thomae). Toxicity: S. Püschmann, R. Engelhorn, *Arzneim.-Forsch.* **28,** 889 (1978). Series of articles on pharmacology, metabolism, and clinical studies: *ibid.* 889-935; on pharmacology and clinical efficacy of combination with amoxicillin, q.v., in bronchopulmonary disease: *ibid.* **37,** 965-971 (1987). Symposium on pharmacology and efficacy in multicenter studies: *Respiration* **51,** Suppl. 1, 1-68 (1987).

Hydrochloride. [23828-92-4] Abramen; Ambril; Bronchopront; Duramucal; Fluibron; Fluixol; Frenopect; Lindoxyl; Motosol; Mucofar; Mucosan; Mucosolvan; Mucoclear; Mucovent; Pect; Solvolan; Stas-Hustenlöser; Surbronc; Surfactal. $C_{13}H_{18}Br_2N_2O\cdot HCl$; mol wt 414.56. Crystals from ethanol, mp 233-234.5° (dec). LD_{50} in mice, rats (mg/kg): 268, 380 i.p.; 2720, 13400 orally (Püschmann, Engelhorn).

THERAP CAT: Expectorant.

387. Ambutonium Bromide. [115-51-5] γ-(Aminocarbonyl)-*N*-ethyl-*N*,*N*-dimethyl-γ-phenylbenzenepropanaminium bromide; 3-(carbamoyl-3,3-diphenylpropyl)ethyldimethylammonium bromide; 4-dimethylamino-2,2-diphenylbutyramide ethyl bromide; R-100. $C_{20}H_{27}BrN_2O$; mol wt 391.35. C 61.38%, H 6.95%, Br 20.42%, N 7.16%, O 4.09%. Anticholinergic. Prepn: Janssen *et al., Arch. Int. Pharmacodyn.* **103,** 82 (1955). Pharmacology: P. J. Southgate, *ibid.* **196,** 376 (1972).

Crystals, mp 228-229° (dec).
Combination with oxazepam. Praxiten SP.
THERAP CAT: Antispasmodic.

388. Amcinonide. [51022-69-6] (11β,16α)-21-(Acetyloxy)-16,17-[cyclopentylidenebis(oxy)]-9-fluoro-11-hydroxypregna-1,4-diene-3,20-dione; 9-fluoro-11β,16α,17,21-tetrahydroxypregna-1,4-diene-3,20-dione cyclic 16,17-acetal with cyclopentanone 21-acetate; CL-34699; Amciderm; Cyclocort; Penticort. $C_{28}H_{35}FO_7$; mol wt 502.57. C 66.92%, H 7.02%, F 3.78%, O 22.28%. Prepn: W. Shultz *et al.,* **DE 2437847** (1975 to Am. Cyanamid), *C.A.* **83,** 10608g (1975). Bioavailability study: R. Woodford, J. M. Haigh, *Curr. Ther. Res.* **26,** 301 (1979). Therapeutic use in eczematoid conditions: G. L. Rocha *et al., ibid.* **19,** 538 (1976); E. W. Rosenberg, *Cutis* **24,** 642 (1979).

THERAP CAT: Glucocorticoid.

389. Amdinocillin. [32887-01-7] (2S,5R,6R)-6-[[(Hexahydro-1*H*-azepin-1-yl)methylene]amino]-3,3-dimethyl-7-oxo-4-thia-1-azabicyclo[3.2.0]heptane-2-carboxylic acid; 6-[(hexahydro-1*H*-azepin-1-yl)methyleneamino]penicillanic acid; mecillinam; FL-1060; Ro-10-9070; Selexid (inj). $C_{15}H_{23}N_3O_3S$; mol wt 325.43. C 55.36%, H 7.12%, N 12.91%, O 14.75%, S 9.85%. Semi-synthetic antibiotic related to penicillin. Prepn: F. J. Lund, **DE 2055531**; *idem,* **US 3957764** (1971, 1976 both to Lövens Kemiske Fabrik). Synthesis and chemical properties: H. B. König *et al., Arzneim.-Forsch.* **33,** 88 (1983). X-ray structural study: J. W. Krajewski *et al., J. Antibiot.* **34,** 282 (1981). *In vitro* study: B. Chattopadhyay, I. Hall, *J. Antimicrob. Chemother.* **5,** 549 (1979). Activity against gram-negative bacteria: D. S. Reeves, *J. Antimicrob. Chemother.* **3,** Suppl. B, 5 (1977). Studies on mechanism of action: B. G. Spratt, *ibid.* **13.** Metabolism: A. P. Ball *et al., ibid.* **4,** 241 (1978). Use in urinary tract infections and septicemia: N. Frimodt-Miller, T. J. Ravn, *Infection* **7,** 35 (1979). Determn in plasma and urine by HPLC: T. L. Lee, M. A. Brooks, *J. Chromatogr.* **227,** 137 (1982). Pharmacokinetics in man: B. R. Meyers *et al., Antimicrob. Agents Chemother.* **23,** 827 (1983). Symposium on pharmacology, pharmacokinetics, clinical studies: *Am. J. Med.* **75,** no. 2A, 1-138 (1983). Review of pharmacology and clinical efficacy: H. C. Neu, *Pharmacotherapy* **5,** 1-10 (1985).

Crystals from methanol-acetone mp 156° (dec). $[\alpha]_D^{20}$ +285° (c = 1 in 0.1*N* HCl). Sol in water.
Pivaloyloxymethyl ester *see* Amdinocillin Pivoxil.
THERAP CAT: Antibacterial.

390. Amdinocillin Pivoxil. [32886-97-8] (2S,5R,6R)-6-[[(Hexahydro-1*H*-azepin-1-yl)methylene]amino]-3,3-dimethyl-7-oxo-4-thia-1-azabicyclo[3.2.0]heptane-2-carboxylic acid (2,2-dimethyl-1-oxopropoxy)methyl ester; pivaloyloxymethyl 6-[(hexahydro-1*H*-azepin-1-yl)methyleneamino]penicillanate; pivamdinocillin; pivmecillinam; FL-1039; Selexid (susp). $C_{21}H_{33}N_3O_5S$; mol wt 439.57. C 57.38%, H 7.57%, N 9.56%, O 18.20%, S 7.29%. Semi-synthetic antibiotic related to penicillin. Pivaloyloxymethyl ester of amdinocillin, q.v. Prepn: F. J. Lund, **DE 2055531**; *idem,* **US 3957764** (1971, 1976 both to Lövens Kemiske Fabrik). HPLC stability analysis: R. B. Hagel, E. H. Waysek, *J. Chromatogr.* **178,** 97 (1979). Bacteriological and pharmacokinetic study: T. Damsgaard *et al., J. Antimicrob. Chemother.* **5**, 267 (1979). Metabolism: J. D. Anderson, M. A. Adams, *Chemotherapy* **25**, 1 (1979). Clinical study: B. T. Andersen *et al., Infection* **8**, 27 (1980). Toxicity study: S. Sato *et al., Takeda Kenkyushoho* **35**, 179 (1976), *C.A.* **86**, 115154w (1977).

Crystals from cyclohexane, mp 118.5-119.5°. $[\alpha]_D^{20}$ +231° (c = 1 in 96% ethanol). LD$_{50}$ in mice, rats (mg/kg): 475-480, 465 i.v.; 1736-1930, 1935-2100 s.c.; 3020, 9500-10000 orally (Sato).

Hydrochloride. [32887-03-9] Selexid (tabl.); Melysin. $C_{21}H_{33}N_3O_5S.HCl$; mol wt 476.03. Crystals from methanol-diisopropyl ether, mp 172-173°. $[\alpha]_D^{20}$ +219° (c = 1 in 0.1*N* HCl).

THERAP CAT: Antibacterial.

391. Amediplase. [151912-11-7] [173-Serine,174-tyrosine,175-glutamine]-173-275-plasminogen activator (human tissue-type reduced) fusion protein with urokinase (human urine β-chain reduced); K₂tu-PA; CGP-42935; MEN-9063; Chimeric, recombinant single chain glycoprotein of 365 amino acid residues composed of the kringle-2 domain of human tissue plaminogen activator, *q.v.*, fused to the serine protease domain of single chain pro-urokinase, *q.v.* Prepn: B. Rajput *et al., EP 277313; eidem,* **US 5242819** (1988, 1993 both to Ciba-Geigy); and primary structure: A. A. Bergwerff *et al., Eur. J. Biochem.* **212**, 639 (1993). Characterization of glycoforms: D. Müller *et al., Biol. Mass Spectrom.* **23**, 330 (1994). CHO cell-based production system: F. A. M. Asselbergs *et al., J. Biotechnol.* **42**, 221 (1995). Thrombolytic activity *in vivo:* G. Agnelli *et al., Thromb. Haemostasis* **68**, 331 (1992). Review of development and therapeutic potential: S. A. Doggrell, *Curr. Opin. Invest. Drugs* **5**, 344-347 (2004).

THERAP CAT: Thrombolytic.

392. Americium. [7440-35-9] Am; at. no. 95; valences 3, 4, 5, 6. Man-made radioactive element. No stable nuclides; known isotopes (mass numbers): 234, 237-247. Longest-lived known isotope 243 (T$_{1/2}$ 7.38 × 10^3 years, rel. at. mass 243.0614, α-emitter. First isotope prepared: ^{241}Am (T$_{1/2}$ 432.7 years, α and γ-emitter, rel. at. mass 241.0568); prepd in 1944 by G. T. Seaborg *et al.* in *The Transuranium Elements*, G.T. Seaborg *et al.*, Eds., (McGraw-Hill, New York, 1949) p 1525-1553; *eidem, Phys. Rev.* **78**, 472 (1950). Isoln: Armstrong *et al., A. I. Ch. E. J.* **3**, 286 (1957); Coleman, *J. Inorg. Nucl. Chem.* **3**, 327 (1957). Prepn of metal: E. F. Westrum, Jr., L. Eyring, *J. Am. Chem. Soc.* **73**, 3396 (1951); Cunningham, Lohr, *ibid.* 2026. Superconducting properties: J. L. Smith, R. G. Haire, *Science* **200**, 535 (1978). Clinical application in bone mineral determn: E. G. De Puey *et al., J. Nucl. Med.* **16**, 891 (1975); in cancer radiotherapy: R. Nath *et al., Int. J. Radiat. Oncol. Biol. Phys.* **14**, 969 (1988). *Reviews:* C. Keller, *The Chemistry of the Transuranium Elements* (Verlag Chemie, Weinheim, English Ed., 1971) pp 485-527; *Comprehensive Inorganic Chemistry* vol. 5, J. C. Bailar, Jr. *et al.*, Eds. (Pergamon Press, Oxford, 1973) *passim; Handb. Exp. Pharmakol.* **36**, 689-940 (1973); W. W. Schulz, R. A. Penneman in *The Chemistry of the Actinide Elements* vol. 2, J. J. Katz *et al.*, Eds. (Chapman and Hall, New York, 1986) pp 887-961. *See also* metabolism study of internal contamination of ^{241}Am in man: N. Cohen *et al., Science* **206**, 64 (1979). Review of toxicology and human exposure: *Toxicological Profile for Americium* (PB2004-104396, 2004) 333 pp.

Silvery, ductile, very maleable, non-magnetic metal. Allotropic forms: double hexagonal close-packed α-form transforms to β-form at 658°; face-centered cubic β-form exists from 793-1004°; γ-form exists from ~1050° to mp. mp 1173°. bp (calc) 2067°. d 13.671. Dissolves readily in aq HCl; insol in liquid NH_3.

Trivalent americium. The most common in aq soln. Color light pink changing to yellow with increasing concn. Sharp absorption peak at 5027 Å. Americium dioxide, AmO_2, is obtained by ignition of most trivalent Am compounds.

Tetravalent americium. Known only in the solid state. When AmO_2 or AmF_3 is treated with fluoride, solid AmF_4 results.

Pentavalent and hexavalent americium compds. When obtained in soln are doubly oxygenated and have the general formula AmO_2^{+n}, where n = +1 for Am(V) and n = +2 for Am(VI). Hexavalent americium is yellow or light brown in dilute perchloric or nitric acid, green in fluoride solns and dark brown in sulfuric acid. A deep red ion complex is formed in bicarbonate-carbonate solns.

Caution: Radiation hazard; handling requires special equipment and shielding facilities (Katz *et al., loc. cit.* **vol. 2**, p 1128).

USE: ^{241}Am as radiation source for thickness gauging, density and radiographic measurements; parent for production of ^{242}Cf and ^{242}Pu; in ionization smoke detectors; for dissipation of static electrical charges. ^{241}Am-Be mixture as neutron source. ^{243}Am as target material for production of transcurium elements in high neutron-flux reactors.

THERAP CAT: ^{241}Am as diagnostic aid (bone mineral analyzer); as antineoplastic (radiation source).

393. Ametryn. [834-12-8] *N*-Ethyl-*N'*-(1-methylethyl)-6-(methylthio)-1,3,5-triazine-2,4-diamine; 2-(ethylamino)-4-(isopropylamino)-6-(methylthio)-*s*-triazine; 2-ethylamino-4-isopropylamino-6-methylmercapto-*s*-triazine; 2-methylthio-4-ethylamino-6-isopropylamino-*s*-triazine; ametryne; G-34162; Ametrex; Evik; Gesapax. $C_9H_{17}N_5S$; mol wt 227.33. C 47.55%, H 7.54%, N 30.81%, S 14.11%. Prepn: Gysin, Knuesli, **CH 337019** *C.A.* **57**, 14226c (1962); Rufener *et al.*, **US 3558622** (1959, 1971 both to Geigy). Acute toxicity: T. B. Gaines, R. E. Linder, *Fundam. Appl. Toxicol.* **7**, 299 (1986).

Crystals, mp 88-89°. Aqueous soly data: Ward, Weber, *J. Agric. Food Chem.* **16**, 959 (1968). LD$_{50}$ in adult male, female rats (mg/kg): 508, 590 orally (Gaines, Linder).

USE: Herbicide.

394. Amezinium Methyl Sulfate. [30578-37-1] 4-Amino-6-methoxy-1-phenylpyridazinium methyl sulfate; LU-1631; Regulton; Risumic; Supratonin. $C_{12}H_{15}N_3O_5S$; mol wt 313.33. C 46.00%, H 4.83%, N 13.41%, O 25.53%, S 10.23%. Sympathomimetic agent with vascular and cardiac activity. Prepn: F. Richenender, R. Kropp, **DE 1912941**; *eidem,* **US 3631038** (1970, 1971 both to BASF). Series of articles on synthesis, pharmacology, mechanism of action, metabolism, pharmacokinetics, bioavailability, clinical trials: *Arzneim.-Forsch.* **31**, 1527-1671 (1981). Acute toxicity data: H. J. Teschendorf, *ibid.* 1580. HPLC determn in human plasma: D. Hotz, E. Brode, *J. Chromatogr.* **277**, 217 (1983). Disposition and identification of major metabolites in rats: K. Nambu *et al., Arzneim.-Forsch.* **38**, 909 (1988).

Crystals from water, mp 176° (dec). LD$_{50}$ in mice, rats (mg/kg): 1630, 1410 orally; 40.4, 45.5 i.v. (Teschendorf).

THERAP CAT: Antihypotensive.

395. Amfenac. [51579-82-9] 2-Amino-3-benzoylbenzeneacetic acid; 2-amino-3-benzoylphenylacetic acid. $C_{15}H_{13}NO_3$; mol wt 255.27. C 70.58%, H 5.13%, N 5.49%, O 18.80%. Prepn: W. J. Welstead, H. W. Moran, **DE 2324768** *C.A.* **80**, 59708s (1974) and **US 4045576** (1973, 1977 both to A. H. Robbins). Synthesis and anti-inflammatory activity: W. J. Welstead *et al., J. Med. Chem.* **22**,

1074 (1979). Anti-inflammatory, analgesic, antipyretic activities: H. Fujimura *et al., Oyo Yakuri* **22,** 381 (1981), *C.A.* **97,** 49427m (1982). Platelet aggregation inhibition: *eidem, ibid.* 399, *C.A.* **97,** 49502g (1982). Effect on polymorphonuclear leukocytes: T. Matsumoto *et al., Pharmacol. Res. Commun.* **14,** 523 (1982). Toxicity data: L. F. Sancilio *et al.,* 170th Am. Chem. Soc. Meet. (Chicago, Aug. 1975), Abstracts of Papers, MEDI 17.

mp 121-123° (dec). LD_{50} in mice, rats (mg/kg): 615, 311 orally (Sancilio).

Sodium salt monohydrate. [61618-27-7] AHR-5850D; Fenazox. $C_{15}H_{12}NNaO_3 \cdot H_2O$; mol wt 295.27. Yellow solid from ethanol/isopropyl ether, mp 254-255.5°.

THERAP CAT: Anti-inflammatory.

396. Amicarbazone. [129909-90-6] 4-Amino-*N*-(1,1-dimethylethyl)-4,5-dihydro-3-(1-methylethyl)-5-oxo-1*H*-1,2,4-triazole-1-carboxamide; 4-amino-1-(*N-t*-butylcarbamoyl)-3-isopropyl-1,2,4-triazolin-5-one; 4-amino-*N-tert*-butyl-3-isopropyl-5-oxo-Δ^2-1,2,4-triazoline-1-carboxamide; BAY-314666; BAY MKH 3586; Dinamic. $C_{10}H_{19}N_5O_2$; mol wt 241.29. C 49.78%, H 7.94%, N 29.02%, O 13.26%. Triazolinone herbicide for use in food crops. Prepn: K.-H. Müller *et al.,* **DE 3839206**; M. Lindig *et al.,* **US 5194085** (1990, 1993 both to Bayer). Comprehensive description: B. D. Philbrook *et al., Brighton Crop Prot. Conf. - Weeds* 1999, 29-34.

Colorless crystals, mp 137.5°. d 1.12. Vapor pressure (Pa): 1.3 × 10^{-6} (20°); 3.0 × 10^{-6} (25°). Log P (octanol/water): 1.18 (pH 4); 1.23 (pH 7); 1.23 (pH 9). Soly in water (20°): 4.6 g/l (pH 4 - 9). LD_{50} in rats (mg/kg): 1015 orally; >2000 dermally. LC_{50} in rats (4 hr): 2.242 mg/l air. LC_{50} in bluegill sunfish, rainbow trout (96 hr): >129, >120 mg/l (Philbrook).

USE: Herbicide.

397. Amicetin. [17650-86-1] 4-[[(2*S*)-2-Amino-3-hydroxy-2-methyl-1-oxopropyl]amino]-*N*-[1-[(2*R*,5*S*,6*R*)-5-[[4,6-dideoxy-4-(dimethylamino)-α-D-glucopyranosyl]oxy]tetrahydro-6-methyl-2*H*-pyran-2-yl]-1,2-dihydro-2-oxo-4-pyrimidinyl]benzamide. $C_{29}H_{42}N_6O_9$; mol wt 618.68. C 56.30%, H 6.84%, N 13.58%, O 23.27%. Antibiotic substance produced by *Streptomyces vinaceus-drappus* isolated from soil near Kalamazoo, Mich.: C. DeBoer *et al., J. Am. Chem. Soc.* **75,** 499 (1953); J. W. Hinman *et al., ibid.* 5864; McKormich, Hoehn, *Antibiot. Chemother.* **3,** 718 (1953). Chemistry: E. H. Flynn *et al., J. Am. Chem. Soc.* **75,** 5867 (1953). Structural studies: C. L. Stevens *et al., J. Org. Chem.* **27,** 2991 (1962). Configuration: S. Hanessian, T. H. Haskell, *Tetrahedron Lett.* **5,** 2451 (1964). Inhibition of protein synthesis: A. Bloch, C. Coutsogeorgopoulos, *Biochemistry* **5,** 3345 (1966). Binding to 23S rRNA as mechanism of inhibition of peptide bond formation: I. G. Leviev *et al., EMBO J.* **13,** 1682 (1994).

Colorless granular crystals, mp 244-245°. pKa = 10.4, 7.0. $[\alpha]_D^{24}$ +116.5° (c = 0.5 in 0.1*N* HCl). uv max in water: 305 nm ($E_{1cm}^{1\%}$ 465); in 0.1*N* HCl: 316 nm ($E_{1cm}^{1\%}$ 433); in 0.1*N* NaOH: 322 nm ($E_{1cm}^{1\%}$ 470). Soly in water at 25° = 2 mg/ml. Slightly sol in common organic solvents. LD_{50} of citrate complex, pH 6 (mg/kg) in mice: ~90 i.v., 600-700 s.c.; in rats: ~200 i.v., ~600 s.c. (DeBoer).

398. Amicoumacin A. [78654-44-1] 3-Amino-2,3-dideoxy-N^6-[1-(3,4-dihydro-8-hydroxy-1-oxo-1*H*-2-benzopyran-3-yl)-3-methylbutyl]hexaramide. $C_{20}H_{29}N_3O_7$; mol wt 423.46. C 56.73%, H 6.90%, N 9.92%, O 26.45%. Major component of a complex of antibiotics produced by *Bacillus pumilus* BN-103. Also exhibits anti-inflammatory activity *in vivo*. Isoln and biol activity: **JP Kokai 83 18379** (1983 to Meiji Seika), *C.A.* **99,** 20906x (1983); J. Itoh *et al., J. Antibiot.* **34,** 611 (1981); *eidem, Agric. Biol. Chem.* **46,** 1255 (1982). Structure: *eidem, ibid.* 2659. Use as acaricide: **JP Kokai 83 216107** (1983 to Meiji Seika), *C.A.* **100,** 116494b (1984).

Hydrochloride. Colorless powder, mp 132-135° (dec). uv max (methanol): 208, 247, 315 nm (ε 27300, 6400, 4380). $[\alpha]_D^{23}$ −97.2° (c = 1.0 in methanol). LD_{50} orally in mice: 132 mg/kg (Itoh).

399. Amidephrine. [3354-67-4] *N*-[3-[1-Hydroxy-2-(methylamino)ethyl]phenyl]methanesulfonamide; 3′-[1-hydroxy-2-(methylamino)ethyl]methanesulfonanilide; MJ-1996. $C_{10}H_{16}N_2O_3S$; mol wt 244.31. C 49.16%, H 6.60%, N 11.47%, O 19.65%, S 13.12%. α_1 Adrenoceptor agonist. Prepn: Larsen, Uloth, **FR M3027** (1965 to Mead Johnson), *C.A.* **62,** 13091a (1965); Uloth *et al., J. Med. Chem.* **9,** 88 (1966). Pharmacology of the racemate: Dungan *et al., Int. J. Neuropharmacol.* **4,** 219 (1965); Stanton *et al., ibid.* 235; of the isomers: Larsen, Lish, *Nature* **203,** 1283 (1964); Buchthal, Jenkinson, *Eur. J. Pharmacol.* **10,** 293 (1970). Toxicology: J. H. Weikel, Jr., K. H. Harper, *Toxicol. Appl. Pharmacol.* **23,** 589 (1972).

Crystals, mp 159-161°. pKa 9.1.

Methanesulfonate. [1421-68-7] Amidephrine mesylate; MJ-5190; Fentrinol. $C_{10}H_{16}N_2O_3S \cdot CH_3SO_3H$; mol wt 340.42. Crystals from ethanol, mp 207-209°. LD_{50} in mice (mg/kg): 2284 orally, 780 i.p., 190 i.v., 1990 s.c.; in male, female Mead Johnson rats (mg/kg): 229, 36 orally; 144, 25 i.p.; in male, female Sprague-Dawley rats (mg/kg): 24, 13 orally; in rabbits (mg/kg): 12 orally, 7.5 intradermally (Weikel, Harper).

THERAP CAT: Vasoconstrictor; decongestant (nasal).

400. Amidinomycin. [3572-60-9] 3-Amino-*N*-(3-amino-3-iminopropyl)cyclopentanecarboxamide; *N*-(2′-amidinoethyl)-3-aminocyclopentanecarboxamide; myxoviromycin. $C_9H_{18}N_4O$; mol wt 198.27. C 54.52%, H 9.15%, N 28.26%, O 8.07%. Antibiotic substance produced by *Streptomyces flavochromogenes* isolated from Japanese soil (Shiuoka Prefecture). Isoln and structure: S. Nakamura *et al., J. Antibiot.* **14A,** 103 (1961); S. Nakamura, *Chem. Pharm. Bull.* **9,** 641 (1961). Identity with myxoviromycin: S. Nakamura *et al., J. Antibiot.* **14A,** 163 (1961). Prepn: Katsube, Saito, **JP 68 21418** (1968 to Sumitomo), *C.A.* **70,** 87135q (1969). Synthesis of amidinomycin and *trans* isomer: H. Paul *et al., Arch.*

Pharm. **301,** 512 (1968). Crystal and molecular structure: M. Kaneda *et al., J. Antibiot.* **33,** 778 (1980).

Sulfate. $C_9H_{18}N_4O.H_2SO_4$. Plates or needles from water + methanol, dec 285-288°. $[\alpha]_D^{21}$ −3.9° (c = 3). Absorption spectra: S. Nakamura, *loc. cit.* Soluble in water. Practically insol in ether, benzene, ethyl acetate, methanol, ethanol, butanol, acetone.

THERAP CAT: Antiviral.

401. Amido-G-Acid. [86-65-7] 7-Amino-1,3-naphthalenedisulfonic acid; 2-naphthylamine-6,8-disulfonic acid; amino-G-acid. $C_{10}H_9NO_6S_2$; mol wt 303.31. C 39.60%, H 2.99%, N 4.62%, O 31.65%, S 21.14%. Prepd by sulfonation of β-naphthylamine: Fierz-David, Braunschweig, *Helv. Chim. Acta* **6,** 1146 (1923).

Tetrahydrate. Fine monoclinic needles. Sol in water, less sol in alc. Soly in water at 20°: 9.24 g in 100 g of satd soln.

USE: Manufacture of dyes.

402. Amido-R-Acid. [92-28-4] 3-Amino-2,7-naphthalenedisulfonic acid; 2-naphthylamine-3,6-disulfonic acid. $C_{10}H_9NO_6S_2$; mol wt 303.31. C 39.60%, H 2.99%, N 4.62%, O 31.65%, S 21.14%. Prepd by treating 2-hydroxy-3,6-naphthalenedisulfonic acid with ammonium sulfite and ammonium hydroxide: Petitcolas, Josué, *Bull. Soc. Chim. Fr.* **1952,** 89.

Crystals or powder. Soluble in water. Solutions show a violet-blue fluorescence.

USE: Manufacture of dyes.

403. Amidosulfuron. [120923-37-7] N-(4,6-Dimethoxy-2-pyrimidinyl)-3-methyl-2,4-dithia-3,5-diazahexan-6-amide 2,2,4,-4-tetraoxide; 3-(4,6-dimethoxypyrimidin-2-yl-)-1-(N-methyl-N-methyl-sulfonyl)urea; HOE-75032; Gratil; Eagle. $C_9H_{15}N_5O_7S_2$; mol wt 369.37. C 29.27%, H 4.09%, N 18.96%, O 30.32%, S 17.36%. Post-emergence herbicide for broad-leaf weed control in cereals. Prepn: L. Willms *et al.,* **EP 131258**; *eidem,* **US 4601747** (1985, 1986 both to Hoechst). Degradation in soil: G. Fent *et al., Sci. Total Environ.* **132,** 201 (1993); K. L. Sagan *et al., J. Agric. Food Chem.* **46,** 1205 (1998). Field trial in cereal crops: D. S. M. D'Souza *et al., Brighton Crop Prot. Conf. - Weeds* **1993,** 567; for control of wild mustard in canola: K. J. Kirkland *Weed Technol.* **9,** 541 (1995).

mp 160-163°. Soly in water (mg/l): 3.3 at pH 3, 9.0 at pH 7, 13500 at pH 10. Vapor pressure at 20°: 1.3×10^{-5} Pa.

USE: Herbicide.

404. Amifostine. [20537-88-6] 2-[(3-Aminopropyl)-amino]ethanethiol dihydrogen phosphate (ester); phosphorothioic acid S-[2-[(3-aminopropyl)amino]ethyl] ester; aminopropylamino-

ethyl thiophosphate; ethiofos; gammaphos; SAPEP; NSC-296961; WR-2721; YM-08310; Ethyol. $C_5H_{15}N_2O_3PS$; mol wt 214.22. C 28.03%, H 7.06%, N 13.08%, O 22.41%, P 14.46%, S 14.97%. Thiophosphate derivative of cysteamine, *q.v.*; provides normal cells with selective protection against the toxic effects of cancer chemotherapy and radiation treatment. Prepn of monohydrate: J. R. Piper *et al., J. Med. Chem.* **12,** 236 (1969); J. R. Piper, T. P. Johnston, **US 3892824** (1975 to Southern Res. Inst.). Differential radioprotective activity: J. M. Yuhas, J. B. Storer, *J. Natl. Cancer Inst.* **42,** 331 (1969). Mechanism of action study: G. D. Smoluk *et al., Cancer Res.* **48,** 3641 (1988). Bioavailability: L. Fleckenstein *et al., Pharmacol. Ther.* **39,** 203 (1988). Clinical pharmacokinetics: L. M. Shaw *et al., ibid.* 195. HPLC determn in plasma: N. F. Swynnerton *et al., Int. J. Radiat. Oncol. Biol. Phys.* **12,** 1495 (1986). Review of development as radioprotector: D. Q. Brown *et al., Pharmacol. Ther.* **39,** 157-168 (1988); of role in chemotherapy: R. L. Capizzi *et al., Cancer* **72,** 3495-3501 (1993); M. Treskes, W. J. M. van der Vijgh, *Cancer Chemother. Pharmacol.* **33,** 93-106 (1993).

Monohydrate. [63717-27-1] White solid from methanol/ether, mp 160-161° (dec). LD_{50} in mice (mg/kg): 700 i.p. (Piper, Johnston).

Trihydrate. [112901-68-5] Soly in water: >9 g/100 ml. pKa_1 <2.0; pKa_2 4.2; pKa_3 9.0; pKa_4 11.7.

THERAP CAT: Radioprotective agent.

405. Amikacin. [37517-28-5] O-3-Amino-3-deoxy-α-D-glucopyranosyl-(1 → 6)-O-[6-amino-6-deoxy-α-D-glucopyranosyl-(1 → 4)]-N^1-[(2S)-4-amino-2-hydroxy-1-oxobutyl]-2-deoxy-D-streptamine; 1-N-[L-(−)-4-amino-2-hydroxybutyryl]kanamycin A. $C_{22}H_{43}N_5O_{13}$; mol wt 585.60. C 45.12%, H 7.40%, N 11.96%, O 35.52%. Semisynthetic aminoglycoside antibiotic derived from kanamycin A. Prepn: Kawaguchi *et al., J. Antibiot.* **25,** 695 (1972); H. Kawaguchi, T. Naito, **DE 2234315**; H. Kawaguchi *et al.,* **US 3781268** (both 1973 to Bristol-Myers). Biological formation from kanamycin A: L. M. Cappelletti, R. Spagnoli, *J. Antibiot.* **36,** 328 (1983). Microbiological evaluation: Price *et al., ibid.* **25,** 709 (1972). Pharmacokinetics: Cabana, Taggart, *Antimicrob. Agents Chemother.* **3,** 478 (1973). *In vitro* studies: Yu, Washington, *ibid.* **4,** 133 (1973); Bodey, Stewart, *ibid.* 186. Pharmacology in humans: Bodey *et al., ibid.* **5,** 508 (1974). Toxicity studies: Fujisawa *et al., J. Antibiot.* **27,** 677 (1974). *Review:* K. A. Kerridge in *Pharmacological and Biochemical Properties of Drug Substances* **vol. 1,** M. E. Goldberg, Ed. (Am. Pharm. Assoc., Washington, DC, 1977) pp 125-153. Comprehensive description: P. M. Monteleone *et al., Anal. Profiles Drug Subs.* **12,** 37-71 (1983).

White crystalline powder from methanol-isopropanol, mp 203-204° (sesquihydrate). $[\alpha]_D^{23}$ +99° (c = 1.0 in water). LD_{50} in mice of solns pH 6.6, pH 7.4 (mg/kg): 340, 560 i.v. (Kawaguchi).

Sulfate. [39831-55-5] Amiglyde-V; Amikin; Amiklin; BB-K8; Biklin; Lukadin; Mikavir; Novamin; Pierami. $C_{22}H_{43}N_5O_{13}.2H_2SO_4$; mol wt 781.76. Amorphous form, dec 220-230°. $[\alpha]_D^{22}$ +74.75° (water).

THERAP CAT: Antibacterial.

THERAP CAT (VET): Antibacterial.

406. Amiloride. [2609-46-3] 3,5-Diamino-N-(aminoiminomethyl)-6-chloropyrazinecarboxamide; N-amidino-3,5-diamino-6-chloropyrazinecarboxamide; N-amidino-3,5-diamino-6-chloropyrazinamide; 1-(3,5-diamino-6-chloropyrazinecarboxyl)guanidine; 1-(3,5-diamino-6-chloropyrazinoyl)guanidine; guanamprazine; amipramidin; amipramizide. $C_6H_8ClN_7O$; mol wt 229.63. C 31.38%, H 3.51%, Cl 15.44%, N 42.70%, O 6.97%. Sodium channel blocker. Prepn: E. J. Cragoe, Jr., **BE 639386**; *idem*, **US 3313813** (1964, 1967 both to Merck & Co.). NMR study on tautomerism and conformation: R. L. Smith *et al.*, *J. Am. Chem. Soc.* **101**, 191 (1979). Pharmacology: Baer *et al.*, *J. Pharmacol. Exp. Ther.* **157**, 472 (1967); Baba *et al.*, *Clin. Pharmacol. Ther.* **9**, 318 (1968); Lant *et al.*, *ibid.* **10**, 50 (1969). Metabolism: Weiss *et al.*, *ibid.* 401. Clinical evaluation in cystic fibrosis: M. R. Knowles *et al.*, *N. Engl. J. Med.* **322**, 1189 (1990); in combination with uridine 5'-triphosphate, *q.v.*: W. D. Bennett *et al.*, *Am. J. Respir. Crit. Care Med.* **153**, 1796 (1996). *Reviews*: H. L. Macfie *et al.*, *Drug Intell. Clin. Pharm.* **15**, 94-98 (1981); D. E. Hyams, *Int. Congr. Symp. Ser. - R. Soc. Med.* **44**, 65-73 (1981). Comprehensive description of hydrochloride: D. J. Mazzo, *Anal. Profiles Drug Subs.* **15**, 1-34 (1986). Review of mechanism of action: T. R. Kleyman, E. J. Cragoe, Jr., *Semin. Nephrol.* **8**, 242-248 (1988).

Solid, mp 240.5-241.5°.
Hydrochloride dihydrate. [17440-83-4] MK-870; Amikal; Midamor; Modamide. $C_6H_8ClN_7O.HCl.2H_2O$; mol wt 302.12. Crystalline solid, dec 285-288°. Anhydr, mp 293.5°. uv max (water): 212, 285, 362 nm ($E_{1cm}^{1\%}$ 642, 555, 617). pKa 8.7. Freely sol in DMSO, slightly sol in water, isopropanol, ethanol. Practically insol in acetone, chloroform, diethyl ether, ethyl acetate.
Hydrochloride dihydrate mixture with hydrochlorothiazide. Co-amilozide; Amil-Co; Aquaretic; Ecodurex; Grodurex; Hexarese; Moduretic; Moduretik; Normetic; Normorix.
THERAP CAT: Diuretic.

407. Aminacrine. [90-45-9] 9-Acridinamine; 5-aminoacridine; 9-aminoacridine. $C_{13}H_{10}N_2$; mol wt 194.23. C 80.39%, H 5.19%, N 14.42%. Prepn: A. Albert, B. Ritchie, *Org. Synth.* **coll. vol. III**, 53 (1955). Toxicity study: D. C. Brodie, E. Lowenhaupt, *J. Am. Pharm. Assoc.* **38**, 498 (1949). Spectrophotometric determn in pharmaceuticals: E. A. Bunch, *J. Assoc. Off. Anal. Chem.* **66**, 140 (1983). DNA intercalator used to induce exptl frameshift mutations: M. Conrad, M. D. Topal, *J. Biol. Chem.* **261**, 16226 (1986).

Sulfur-yellow needles from alcohol or acetone, mp 241°. Moderately strong base. pKa (25°): 4.53. Freely sol in alcohol; slightly sol in chloroform, toluene, pyridine; sol in acetone.
Hydrochloride. [134-50-9] Monacrin. $C_{13}H_{10}N_2.HCl$; mol wt 230.69. Pale yellow crystals. Neutral reaction. One of the most highly fluorescent substances. One gram dissolves in 300 ml water giving a faintly yellow soln showing bluish-violet fluorescence. LD_{50} orally in mice: 78 mg/kg (Brodie, Lowenhaupt).
THERAP CAT: Antiseptic.
THERAP CAT (VET): Antiseptic.

408. Amine 220. [95-38-5] 2-(8-Heptadecenyl)-4,5-dihydro-1*H*-imidazole-1-ethanol; 2-(8-heptadecenyl)-2-imidazoline-1-ethanol; 1-(2-hydroxyethyl)-2-(8-heptadecenyl)-2-imidazoline. $C_{22}H_{42}N_2O$; mol wt 350.58. C 75.37%, H 12.08%, N 7.99%, O 4.56%. Prepared from oleic acid and 2-[(2-aminoethyl)amino]-ethanol: Stromberg, Hughes, and Hughes, Stromberg, **US 2987515** and **US 3020276** (1961, 1962 both to Petrolite Corp.).

409. Amineptine. [57574-09-1] 7-[(10,11-Dihydro-5*H*-dibenzo[*a,d*]cyclohepten-5-yl)amino]heptanoic acid. $C_{22}H_{27}NO_2$; mol wt 337.46. C 78.30%, H 8.06%, N 4.15%, O 9.48%. Dopamine uptake blocker. Prepn: C. Malen *et al.*, **DE 2011806**; *eidem*, **US 3758528** (1970, 1973 both to Sci. Union et Cie Soc. Franc. Recher. Med.). Biochemical and pharmacological study: R. Samanin *et al.*, *J. Pharm. Pharmacol.* **29**, 555 (1977). Effect on dopamine uptake: N. B. Mercuri *et al.*, *Br. J. Pharmacol.* **104**, 700 (1991). Metabolism: L. Grislain *et al.*, *Eur. J. Drug Metab. Pharmacokinet.* **15**, 339 (1990). HPLC determn in plasma: P. P. Rop *et al.*, *J. Chromatogr.* **532**, 351 (1990). Clinical trial in depression: M. Paes de Sousa, J. Tropa, *Clin. Neuropharmacol.* **12**, Suppl. 2, S77 (1989).

Hydrochloride. [30272-08-3] S-1694; Maneon; Survector. $C_{22}H_{27}NO_2.HCl$; mol wt 373.92. Crystals from distilled water, mp 226-230°.
THERAP CAT: Antidepressant.

410. Aminitrozole. [140-40-9] *N*-(5-Nitro-2-thiazolyl)-acetamide; 2-acetamido-5-nitrothiazole; 2-acetylamino-5-nitrothiazole; acinitrazole; nithiamide; Tritheon; Trichorad; Enheptin-A. $C_5H_5N_3O_3S$; mol wt 187.18. C 32.08%, H 2.69%, N 22.45%, O 25.64%, S 17.13%. Prepd by nitration of 2-acetamidothiazole: Ganapathi, Venkataraman, *Proc. Indian Acad. Sci.* **22A**, 343 (1945); Bellavita, *Ann. Chim. Appl.* **38**, 449 (1948); Hurd, Wehrmeister, *J. Am. Chem. Soc.* **71**, 4007 (1949); Yamamoto, *J. Pharm. Soc. Jpn.* **72**, 1017 (1952). As an antihistomonad: Waletzky, Marson, **US 2531756** (1950 to Am. Cyanamid).

Needles from alc, elongated plates from acetic acid. mp 264-265°. The commercial product may be yellow. Sol in aq solns of NaOH and NH₃ with deep orange color.
THERAP CAT: Antiprotozoal (Trichomonas).
THERAP CAT (VET): Antihistomonad for turkeys.

411. p-Aminoacetanilide. [122-80-5] *N*-(4-Aminophenyl)acetamide; 4'-aminoacetanilide; acetyl-*p*-phenylenediamine. $C_8H_{10}N_2O$; mol wt 150.18. C 63.98%, H 6.71%, N 18.65%, O 10.65%. Prepd by catalytic hydrogenation of 4'-nitroacetanilide: Atkinson *et al.*, *J. Chem. Soc.* **1954**, 2023. Crystal and molecular structure: M. Haisa *et al.*, *Acta Crystallogr.* **33B**, 2449 (1977).

White or slightly reddish crystals, mp 163.5-166.0°; darkens in air. Slightly soluble in cold water; freely soluble in hot water, alc, ether.
USE: Intermediate in the manufacture of azo dyes, pharmaceuticals.

412. Aminoacetonitrile. [540-61-4] Glycinonitrile; cyanomethylamine; glycine nitrile. $C_2H_4N_2$; mol wt 56.07. C 42.84%, H 7.19%, N 49.96%. H_2NCH_2CN. Prepd by the action

Consult the Name Index before using this section.

of alcoholic HCl or H_2SO_4 on dimolecular or trimolecular methyleneaminoacetonitrile: Anslow, King, *J. Chem. Soc.* **1929**, 2465.

Oily liquid. bp_{15} 58° (partial decompn).

Hydrochloride. [6011-14-9] $C_2H_4N_2 \cdot HCl$. Hygroscopic crystals from alcohol, dec 165°.

Sulfate (1:1). [151-63-3] $C_2H_4N_2 \cdot H_2SO_4$. Prepn: H. Stephen, *J. Chem. Soc.* **1931**, 871. Hygroscopic leaflets from ethanol + ether, mp 121°.

Sulfate (2:1). [5466-22-8] $(C_2H_4N_2)_2 \cdot H_2SO_4$. Long flat prisms from water/ethanol, mp 166° (dec).

413. Aminoacetophenone. C_8H_9NO; mol wt 135.16. C 71.09%, H 6.71%, N 10.36%, O 11.84%. Prepn of *m*-, *o*-, and *p*-isomers: Grammaticakis, *Compt. Rend.* **235**, 546 (1952); Braude *et al., J. Chem. Soc.* **1954**, 3586. Prepn of *m*-isomer: Tinsley, **US 2797244** (1957 to Union Carbide); of *p*-isomer: Norman *et al., Can. J. Chem.* **40**, 1547 (1962). Toxicity studies: J. M. Vandenbelt *et al., J. Pharmacol. Exp. Ther.* **80**, 31 (1944); H. F. Smyth *et al., Arch. Ind. Hyg. Occup. Med.* **10**, 61 (1954).

m-**Aminoacetophenone.** 1-(3-Aminophenyl)ethanone; 3'-aminoacetophenone; *m*-aminoacetylbenzene. Yellow leaflets, mp 98-99°. Partly volatile in steam. LD_{50} orally in rats: 1.87 g/kg (Smyth).

o-**Aminoacetophenone.** Yellow oily liquid. bp_{760} 250-252° (some dec); bp_{17} 135°. Volatile with steam. Practically insol in water. Sol in alc.

p-**Aminoacetophenone.** Yellow needles, pleasant, characteristic odor. mp 106°. bp 293-295°. Sparingly sol in cold, freely in hot water; sol in alc, ether, HCl; sparingly sol in benzene. LD_{50} i.p. in rats: 260 mg/kg (Vandenbelt).

414. D-Amino Acid Oxidase. [9000-88-8] DAAO. Flavoprotein that catalyzes the oxidative deamination of D-amino acids to the corresponding α-keto acids. Found in the kidney and liver of nearly all mammals studied. Isoln from pig kidney: Krebs, *Enzymologia* **7**, 53 (1939); Straub, *Nature* **141**, 603 (1938); Negelein, Brömel, *Biochem. Z.* **300**, 225 (1939); Massey *et al., Biochim. Biophys. Acta* **48**, 1 (1961); from sheep kidney: Burton, *Methods Enzymol.* **2**, 199 (1955). Physical properties: Yagi *et al., J. Biochem.* **61**, 580 (1967). Partial structure: Kotaki *et al., ibid.* 598. Studies on specificity and inhibition: Dixon, Kleppe, *Biochim. Biophys. Acta* **96**, 368 (1965). Reaction intermediates: K. Yagi, *Front. Physicochem. Biol., Proc. Int. Symp.* **1977**, B. Pullman, Ed. (Academic Press, New York, 1978) pp 299-308. *Review:* Meister, Wellner in *The Enzymes* **7**, P. Boyer *et al.,* Eds. (Academic Press, New York, 1963) pp 634-648.

415. L-Amino Acid Oxidase. [9000-89-9] LAAO. Flavoprotein that catalyzes the oxidative deamination of L-amino acids to the corresponding α-keto acids. Found in microorganisms and in animal tissue, esp in kidney and liver. Occurs also in many snake venoms. Isoln from rat kidney: Blanchard *et al., J. Biol. Chem.* **161**, 583 (1945). Isoln of crystalline enzyme from the venom of the eastern diamondback rattlesnake (*Crotalus adamanteus*): Wellner, Meister, *J. Biol. Chem.* **235**, 2013 (1960). Structural studies: DeKok, Rawitch, *Biochemistry* **8**, 1405 (1969). Studies on inhibitors: DeKok, Veeger, *Biochim. Biophys. Acta* **167**, 35 (1968). Mechanism of reversible activation-deactivation: C. J. Coles *et al., Flavins Flavoproteins, Proc. Int. Symp. 6th* **1978**, K. Yagi, T. Yamano, Eds. (Japan Sci. Soc. Press, Tokyo, 1980) pp 101-105. Multiple conformational states: D. Wellner, L. A. Lichtenberg, *Dev. Biochem.* **21**, 78 (1982). *Review:* Meister, Wellner in *The Enzymes* **7**, P. Boyer *et al.,* Eds. (Academic Press, New York, 1963) pp 609-634.

416. α-Aminoadipic Acid. [542-32-5] 2-Aminohexanedioic acid. $C_6H_{11}NO_4$; mol wt 161.16. C 44.72%, H 6.88%, N 8.69%, O 39.71%. $HO_2CCH(NH_2)CH_2CH_2CH_2CO_2H$. An ami-

no acid isolated from *Cholera vibrio:* Blass, Macheboeuf, *Helv. Chim. Acta* **29**, 1315 (1946). Occurrence in proteins or protein containing material: Windsor, *J. Biol. Chem.* **192**, 595 (1951). Synthesis: Dieckmann, *Ber.* **38**, 1656 (1905); T. P. Waalkes *et al., J. Am. Chem. Soc.* **72**, 5760 (1952); A. I. Scott, T. J. Wilkinson, *Synth. Commun.* **10**, 127 (1980).

Forms a monohydrate if crystallized from water below 20°. Anhydrous platelets from water above 20°. mp 206° (effervescence). One gram dissolves in 450 ml water. Sparingly sol in alcohol, ether.

Diethyl ester. $C_{10}H_{19}NO_4$. bp_{13} 155-156°.

417. 1-Aminoanthraquinone. [82-45-1] 1-Amino-9,10-anthracenedione. $C_{14}H_9NO_2$; mol wt 223.23. C 75.33%, H 4.06%, N 6.27%, O 14.33%. Prepd by reduction of 1-nitroanthraquinone: Graham, Hort, **US 2874168** (1959 to General Aniline & Film).

Ruby-red crystals. mp ~250°; also reported as mp 243°. Practically insoluble in water. Freely soluble in alcohol, benzene, chloroform, ether, glacial acetic acid, HCl.

USE: In the mfg of dyes and pharmaceuticals.

418. 1-Aminoanthraquinone-2-carboxylic Acid. [82-24-6] 1-Amino-9,10-dihydro-9,10-dioxo-2-anthracenecarboxylic acid. $C_{15}H_9NO_4$; mol wt 267.24. C 67.42%, H 3.39%, N 5.24%, O 23.95%. Prepd by reduction of 1-nitroanthraquinone-2-carboxylic acid with sodium sulfide: Terres, *Ber.* **46**, 1639 (1913); by boiling 1-nitro-2-methylanthraquinone with alcoholic potassium hydroxide: Scholl, *Monatsh. Chem.* **34**, 1011 (1913); by heating 1-nitro-2-bromomethylanthraquinone with sodium acetate and *o*-dichlorobenzene: Locher, Fierz, *Helv. Chim. Acta* **10**, 667 (1927).

Red needles from nitrobenzene, mp 295-296°. Soluble in aniline, boiling nitrobenzene, in sodium hydroxide and aq pyridine with formation of a deep red soln, in concd sulfuric acid with formation of a yellowish-brown soln; slightly sol in ether, benzene, alcohol. Insol in water, ligroin.

Methyl ester. $C_{16}H_{11}NO_4$. Red needles from glacial acetic acid, mp 228°.

Ethyl ester. $C_{17}H_{13}NO_4$. mp 198°.

Phenyl ester. $C_{21}H_{13}NO_4$. Reddish-golden crystals from glacial acetic acid, mp 198°.

USE: For the detection of traces of aluminum, magnesium, or zinc.

419. *p*-Aminoazobenzene. [60-09-3] 4-(Phenylazo)-benzenamine; C.I. Solvent Yellow 1; *p*-(phenylazo)aniline; *p*-aminodiphenylimide; aniline yellow; C.I. 11000. $C_{12}H_{11}N_3$; mol wt 197.24. C 73.07%, H 5.62%, N 21.30%. Prepd from aniline, $NaNO_2$, and HCl: A. I. Vogel, *A Text-Book of Practical Organic Chemistry* (Longmans, Green & Co., New York, 3rd ed., 1956) p 627; W. R. Hydro, T. L. Willard, **US 2894942** (1959 to Goodrich); *Colour Index vol. 4* (3rd ed., 1971) p 4014.

Brownish-yellow needles with a bluish cast. mp 128°. bp above 360°. Slightly sol in water; freely sol in alc, benzene, chloroform, ether. Reduces alcoholic ammoniacal AgNO$_3$.

USE: In form of its salts in dyeing; intermediate in manuf of Acid Yellow, diazo dyes and indulines.

420. *o*-Aminoazotoluene. [97-56-3] 2-Methyl-4-[(2-methylphenyl)azo]benzenamine; C.I. Solvent Yellow 3; 4-(*o*-tolylazo)-*o*-toluidine; 4'-amino-2,3'-dimethylazobenzene; 5-(*o*-tolylazo)-2-aminotoluene; toluazotoluidine; C.I. 11160. C$_{14}$H$_{15}$N$_3$; mol wt 225.29. C 74.64%, H 6.71%, N 18.65%. Prepd from *o*-toluidine, NaNO$_2$, and HCl: Shulman, **US 2538431** (1951 to Pfister Chem. Works); *Colour Index* **vol. 4** (3rd ed., 1971) p 4017. Crystal and molecular structure: S. Kurosaki *et al.*, *Acta Crystallogr.* **32B**, 3160 (1976). Carcinogenic activity: Maini, Stich, *J. Natl. Cancer Inst.* **26**, 1413 (1961). *See also: H. J. Conn's Biological Stains*, R. D. Lillie, Ed. (Williams & Wilkins, Baltimore, 9th ed., 1977) p 87.

Golden crystals, mp 101-102°. Practically insoluble in water. Sol in alc, ether, chloroform, acetone, ethyl acetate, benzene, ligroin, linseed oil, oleic acid, stearic acid. Very sol in cellosolve. Absorption max (50% alcoholic 1*N* HCl): 326, 490 nm (ε 19000, 2500), Sawicki, *J. Org. Chem.* **21**, 605 (1956).

Caution: This substance is reasonably anticipated to be a human carcinogen: *Report on Carcinogens, Eleventh Edition* (PB2005-104914, 2004) p III-12.

USE: Coloring oils, fats and waxes; manuf of pigments. Chemical intermediate for the production of dyes.

421. *m*-Aminobenzoic Acid. [99-05-8] 3-Aminobenzoic acid. C$_7$H$_7$NO$_2$; mol wt 137.14. C 61.31%, H 5.14%, N 10.21%, O 23.33%. Prepn: Toland, Heaton, **US 2878281** (1959 to California Res. Corp.); Neilson *et al.*, *J. Chem. Soc.* **1962**, 371.

Cryst, mp 174°. d 1.51. Aq soln turns brown on standing in air. Forms soluble salts with mineral acids; slightly sol in cold, freely in boiling water or alcohol; sol in ether.

422. *o*-Aminobenzoic Acid. [118-92-3] 2-Aminobenzoic acid; anthranilic acid. C$_7$H$_7$NO$_2$; mol wt 137.14. C 61.31%, H 5.14%, N 10.21%, O 23.33%. Found to be the same as *vitamin L$_1$*: Nakahara *et al.*, *Sci. Papers Inst. Phys. Chem. Res. Jpn.* (Tokyo) **42**, 39 (1945), *C.A.* **41**, 6317d (1947). *See also* Vitamins L. Prepd by reduction of *o*-nitrobenzoic acid: Neilson *et al.*, *J. Chem. Soc.* **1962**, 371. Purification: Sugihara, Newman, *J. Org. Chem.* **21**, 1445 (1956).

White to pale yellow, cryst powder; sweetish taste. mp 144-146°. Sparingly sol in cold, freely in hot water, alcohol, ether. The solns in alcohol or ether and particularly in glycerol exhibit an amethyst fluorescence.

THERAP CAT (VET): The cadmium salt has been used as an ascaricide in swine.

423. *p*-Aminobenzoic Acid. [150-13-0] 4-Aminobenzoic acid; vitamin B$_x$; bacterial vitamin H^1; chromotrichia factor; antichromotrichia factor; trichochromogenic factor; anticanitic vitamin; PABA; Pabanol. C$_7$H$_7$NO$_2$; mol wt 137.14. C 61.31%, H 5.14%, N 10.21%, O 23.33%. Widely distributed in nature as a B complex

factor. Baker's yeast contains 5 to 6 ppm, brewer's yeast from 10 to 100 ppm. Occurs free and in ester form. Prepn: Toland, Heaton, **US 2878281** (1959 to Calif. Research Corp.); Spiegler, **US 2947781** (1960 to Du Pont); Nielson *et al.*, *J. Chem. Soc.* **1962**, 371. Purification: Lyding, **US 2735865** (1956 to Heyden Chem.). Antirickettsial activity: M. L. Robbins *et al.*, *J. Immunol.* **64**, 431 (1950). Toxicity studies: C. C. Scott, E. B. Robbins, *Proc. Soc. Exp. Biol. Med.* **49**, 184 (1942); R. K. Richards, *Fed. Proc.* **1**, 71 (1942); G. Cronheim, *ibid.* **10**, 289 (1952). Comprehensive description: H. A. El-Obeid, A. A. Al-Badr, *Anal. Profiles Drug Subs. Excip.* **22**, 33-106 (1993).

Monoclinic prisms from dil alcohol. May turn slightly yellow on prolonged exposure to light and air. mp 187.0-187.5°. pKa: 4.65, 4.80; pH (0.5% soln): 3.5. uv max (water): 266 nm (E$_{1cm}^{1\%}$ 1070); (isopropanol): 288 nm (E$_{1cm}^{1\%}$ 137). One gram dissolves in 170 ml water at 25°, in 90 ml boiling water; in 8 ml alcohol, in 50 ml ether. Sol in ethyl acetate, glacial acetic acid; slightly sol in benzene. Practically insol in petr ether. Incompatible with ferric salts and oxidizing agents. LD$_{50}$ in mice, rats (g/kg): 2.85, >6.0 orally (Scott, Robbins). LD$_{50}$ in rabbits (g/kg): 2.0 i.v. (Richards); 1.83 orally (Cronheim).

Diethylamine salt. [6018-84-4] C$_{11}$H$_{18}$N$_2$O$_2$. Crystals from acetone mp 170-173°. Very soluble in water.

Potassium salt *see* Potassium *p*-Aminobenzoate.

Note: p-Aminobenzoic acid is also known as ***anti-gray-hair factor*** (in rats only).

USE: Manuf various esters (local anesthetics), folic acid, and azo dyes; in sunburn preventives. Used in laboratories as sulfonamide antagonist.

THERAP CAT: Ultraviolet screen. Formerly as antirickettsial.

THERAP CAT (VET): Has been used in *eczema nasi* ("collie nose") in dogs.

424. 2-Aminobenzothiazole. [136-95-8] 2-Benzothiazolamine. C$_7$H$_6$N$_2$S; mol wt 150.20. C 55.98%, H 4.03%, N 18.65%, S 21.35%. Prepd from 2-chlorobenzothiazole by treatment with alcoholic ammonia at 150-160°: Hofmann, *Ber.* **12**, 1129 (1880); **13**, 11 (1881); from benzothiazole by boiling with hydroxylamine in water or in 2*N* NaOH: Skraup, *Ann.* **419**, 65 (1919). Toxicity study: E. F. Domino *et al.*, *J. Pharmacol. Exp. Ther.* **105**, 486 (1952).

Leaflets from water, mp 132°. Distills without decompn. Very sparingly sol in water; freely in alcohol, ether, chloroform; sol in concd acids. LD$_{50}$ i.v. in mice: 126 mg/kg (Domino).

USE: In the prepn of azo dyes.

425. 6-Aminobenzothiazole. [533-30-2] 6-Benzothiazolamine. C$_7$H$_6$N$_2$S; mol wt 150.20. C 55.98%, H 4.03%, N 18.65%, S 21.35%. Prepd from 2,5-diaminothiophenol by boiling with concd formic acid or from 6-nitrobenzothiazole by reduction with tin and HCl: Mylius, *Thesis* (Berlin, 1883).

Prisms from water, mp 87°. Sol in alcohol. Practically insol in water and ether.

USE: In the prepn of azo dyes.

426. *N*-(4-Aminobenzoyl)-L-glutamic acid. [4271-30-1] *N*-(*p*-aminobenzoyl)glutamic acid; PABG. C$_{12}$H$_{14}$N$_2$O$_5$; mol wt

266.25. C 54.13%, H 5.30%, N 10.52%, O 30.05%. Catabolite of folate. Prepn: J. Van der Scheer, K. Landsteiner, *J. Immunol.* **29**, 371 (1935). Improved synthesis: A. P. Reddy, C. P. R. Reddy, *Org. Prep. Proced. Int.* **22**, 117 (1990); P. Maunder *et al., J. Chem. Soc. Perkin Trans. I* 1311 (1999). HPLC determn: B. A. Allen, R. A. Newman, *J. Chromatogr.* **190**, 241 (1980); densitometric determn in folic acid tablets: J. Krzek, A. Kwiecien, *J. Pharm. Biomed. Anal.* **21**, 451 (1999). Use as marker of folate degradation: J. McPartlin, J. Scott, *Methods Enzymol.* **281**, 70 (1997); of turnover in pregnant women: J. F. Gregory, III *et al., J. Nutr.* **131**, 1928 (2001).

Off white solid, mp 173-174° (dec). $[\alpha]_D^{23}$ −15° (c = 2 in 0.1 M HCl).

USE: Marker in folate metabolism studies.

427. 2-Amino-1-butanol. [96-20-8] 2-Amino-*n*-butyl alcohol. $C_4H_{11}NO$; mol wt 89.14. C 53.90%, H 12.44%, N 15.71%, O 17.95%. $CH_3CH_2CH(NH_2)CH_2OH$. Prepd from 2-nitro-1-butanol by reduction or catalytic hydrogenation: Stiénon, *Chem. Zentralbl.* **1902**, I, 717; Vanderbilt, Haas, US 2174242 (1940); Johnson, Degering, *J. Org. Chem.* **8**, 7 (1943).

Liquid. d_{20}^{20} 0.944. mp −2°. bp_{760} 178°; bp_{10} 79-80°. n_D^{20} 1.453. Miscible with water. Sol in alcohols. pH of 0.1 molar aq soln 11.1.

Hydrochloride. $C_4H_{11}NO.HCl$. Deliquesc needles.

Platinichloride monohydrate. $(C_4H_{11}NO)_2.2HCl.PtCl_4.H_2O$. Yellow leaflets, dec 189-190°. Moderately sol in water, freely sol in alcohol.

Oxalate. $(C_4H_{11}NO)_2.C_2H_2O_4$. mp 176°.

USE: In the synthesis of surface-active agents, vulcanization accelerators, pharmaceuticals. As emulsifying agent for cosmetic creams and lotions, mineral oil and paraffin wax emulsions, leather dressings, textile specialties, polishes, cleaning compounds, so-called soluble oils.

428. α-Aminobutyric Acid. [80-60-4] 2-Aminobutanoic acid; α-amino-*n*-butyric acid. $C_4H_9NO_2$; mol wt 103.12. C 46.59%, H 8.80%, N 13.58%, O 31.03%. $CH_3CH_2CH(NH_2)$-COOH. Prepn of the DL-form from α-bromobutyric acid and ammonia: Fisher, Mounegrat, *Ber.* **33**, 2388 (1900); from potassium cyanide, ammonium chloride and propionaldehyde: Zelinsky, Stadnikow, *Ber.* **41**, 2062 (1908); by reduction of α-oxobutyric acid: Knoop, Oesterlin, *Z. Physiol. Chem.* **148**, 305 (1925); from α-ethylacetoacetic ester and hydrazoic acid: Schmidt, *Ber.* **57**, 706 (1924). The L(+)-form has been isolated from proteins: Oikawa, *Chem. Zentralbl.* **1926**, 1, 148. Configuration: Clough, *J. Chem. Soc.* **113**, 544, 591; Levene, *Chem. Rev.* **2**, 203 (1926); Vogler, *Helv. Chim. Acta* **30**, 1766 (1947).

DL-Form. Crystals, mp 304° (begins to sublime when heated above 300°). Sol in water. One liter of water will dissolve 210.5 g at 25°. Sparingly sol in alcohol. One liter of boiling ethanol dissolves about 1.8 g. Insol in ether.

DL-Form ethyl ester. Viscous liquid. bp_{11} 61°. Sol in water and in organic solvents.

L-Form. Leaflets from dil alc. Sweet taste. mp 270-280° (depending on speed of heating, *see* Vogler, *loc. cit.*). $[M]_D$ +21.2° (5N HCl); $[M]_D$ +43.3° (glacial acetic acid). $[\alpha]_D^{16}$ +8.40° (c = 4); $[\alpha]_D^{16}$ +18.65° (c = 4.8 in 6N HCl).

L-Form hydrochloride. Needles; $[\alpha]_D^{19}$ +12.90° (c = 3.64). Readily sol in water.

429. β-Aminobutyric Acid. [541-48-0] 3-Aminobutanoic acid; β-amino-*n*-butyric acid. $C_4H_9NO_2$; mol wt 103.12. C 46.59%, H 8.80%, N 13.58%, O 31.03%. $CH_3CH(NH_2)CH_2$-COOH. Prepd from pyrotartaric acid diamide: Weidel, Roithmer, *Monatsh. Chem.* **17**, 185 (1896); from β-chlorobutyric acid ethyl ester and alcoholic NH_3: Balbiano, *Ber.* **13**, 312 (1880); from crotonic acid and concd NH_3: Engel, *Bull. Soc. Chim.* [2] **50**, 102 (1888); Curtius, Gumlich, *J. Prakt. Chem.* [2] **70**, 204 (1904); Stadnikow, *Chem. Zentralbl.* **1909**, II, 1988; *see* Fischer, Roeder,

Ber. **34**, 3755 (1901) footnote; Stoermer, Robert, *Ber.* **55**, 1038 (1922). Prepn of HCl salt from β-aminobutyronitrile: Bruylants, *Bull. Soc. Chim. Belg.* **32**, 259 (1923); *Chem. Zentralbl.* **1924**, I, 1668. By reducing acetoacetic ester phenylhydrazone and saponifying the resulting ester: Fischer, Groh, *Ann.* **383**, 338 (1911). The D(−)-form has been obtained by hydrolysis of its ester: Fischer, Scheibler, *ibid.* 346.

DL-Form. Crystals from alcohol, mp 193-194°. Practically tasteless. Sol in water. One liter of water dissolves 1250 g. Insol in cold absolute alcohol and ether.

Methyl ester. $C_5H_{11}NO_2$. Odoriferous liquid; d^{20} 0.993; bp_{13} 54-55°. Sol in water, alcohol, ether, petr ether.

D-Form. Prisms from methanol. Dec near 220° without melting. $[\alpha]_D^{20}$ −35.20° (p = 10).

430. γ-Aminobutyric Acid. [56-12-2] 4-Aminobutanoic acid; γ-amino-*n*-butyric acid; piperidic acid; GABA; Gammalon. $C_4H_9NO_2$; mol wt 103.12. C 46.59%, H 8.80%, N 13.58%, O 31.03%. $H_2NCH_2CH_2CH_2COOH$. Nonprotein amino acid that functions as a neurotransmitter. Prepn from succinimide: Tafel, Stern, *Ber.* **33**, 2224 (1900); from piperylurethan and fuming nitric acid: Schotten, *Ber.* **16**, 643 (1883); Abderhalden, *Chem. Zentralbl.* **1926**, II, 779; from N-(β-bromoethyl)phthalimide and sodiomalonic ester: Aschan, *Ber.* **24**, 2450 (1891); from γ-chlorobutyronitrile and potassium phthalimide: Gabriel, *Ber.* **22**, 3335 (1889); **23**, 1771 (1890); DeWitt, *Org. Synth.* coll. vol. II, 25 (1943). Review of biochemical pharmacology: R. Tapia in *Handbook of Psychopharmacology*, L. L. Iversen *et al.*, Eds. (Plenum, New York, 1975) pp 1-58; L. L. Iversen in *Psychopharmacology: A Generation of Progress*, M. A. Lipton *et al.*, Eds. (Raven, New York, 1978) pp 25-38; C. C. Mao, E. Costa, *ibid.* pp 307-318.

Leaflets from methanol + ether, needles from water + alcohol, mp 202° (dec on rapid heating). Ka 3.7×10^{-11}; Kb 1.7×10^{-10} at 25°. Freely sol in water. Insol or poorly sol in other solvents. On melting it dec forming pyrrolidone and water.

Hydrochloride. $C_4H_9NO_2.HCl$. Crystals, mp 135-136°.

Ethyl ester. $C_6H_{13}NO_2$. Liquid, bp_{12} 76°.

THERAP CAT: Antihypertensive.

431. 9-Aminocamptothecin. [91421-43-1] (4S)-10-Amino-4-ethyl-4-hydroxy-1*H*-pyrano[3′,4′:6,7]indolizino[1,2-*b*]quinoline-3,14(4*H*,12*H*)-dione; 9-Amino-20(*S*)-camptothecin; 9-AC. $C_{20}H_{17}N_3O_4$; mol wt 363.37. C 66.11%, H 4.72%, N 11.56%, O 17.61%. Semisynthetic camptothecin which inhibits DNA topoisomerase I. Prepn: T. Miyasaka *et al.*, **JP Kokai 59 51289** (1984 to Yakult Honsha); M. C. Wani *et al., J. Med. Chem.* **29**, 2358 (1986); and activity: S. Sawada *et al., Chem. Pharm. Bull.* **39**, 3183 (1991). Synthesis: W. Cabri *et al., Tetrahedron Lett.* **36**, 9197 (1995). HPLC determn in plasma: W. J. Loos *et al., J. Chromatogr. B* **694**, 435 (1997). Structure/activity study: M.-L. Li *et al., Clin. Cancer Res.* **7**, 168 (2001). Clinical pharmacodynamics and pharmacokinetics: C. H. Takimoto *et al., J. Clin. Oncol.* **15**, 1492 (1997). Clinical evaluation in colorectal cancer: H. C. Pitot *et al., Cancer* **89**, 1699 (2000). Review of clinical developments: C. H. Takimoto, R. Thomas, *Ann. N.Y. Acad. Sci.* **922**, 224-236 (2000).

Orange-yellow solid from $CH_3OH/CHCl_3$ (13:87), mp 300° (dec). $[\alpha]_D^{23}$ +16° (c = 0.05 in $CH_3OH/CHCl_3$ 1:4). Insol in water.

THERAP CAT: Antineoplastic.

432. ε-Aminocaproic Acid. [60-32-2] 6-Aminohexanoic acid; epsilon-aminocaproic acid; epsilcapramin; EACA; CY-116; Amicar; Epsikapron; Hemocaprol. $C_6H_{13}NO_2$; mol wt 131.17. C 54.94%, H 9.99%, N 10.68%, O 24.39%. $H_2N(CH_2)_5COOH$. Antifibrinolytic; inhibits the activity of plasmin and plasminogen, *q.q.v.* Prepn: S. Gabriel, T. A. Maass, *Ber.* **32**, 1266 (1899); A. Galat, S. Mallin, *J. Am. Chem. Soc.* **68**, 2729 (1946); C. Y. Meyers, L. E. Miller, *Org. Synth.* **coll. vol. IV**, 39 (1963). Toxicity data: D. W. Hallesy *et al., Pharmacologist* **3**, 62 (1961). Crystal structure: G. Bodor *et al., Acta Crystallogr.* **23**, 482 (1967). Clinical trial and mode of action study: T. J. Vander Salm *et al., J. Thorac. Cardiovasc. Surg.* **112**, 1098 (1996).

Crystals from alcohol, mp 202-203°. pK_1 4.43; pK_2 10.75. Freely sol in water; sparingly in methanol. Practically insol in ethanol, chloroform. LD_{50} in rats (g/kg): 7.0 i.p.; ~3.3 i.v. (Hallesy).

Hydrochloride. [4321-58-8] $C_6H_{13}NO_2 \cdot HCl$. mp 128-129°.
THERAP CAT: Hemostatic.

433. Aminocarb. [2032-59-9] 4-(Dimethylamino)-3-methylphenol methylcarbamate (ester); methylcarbamic acid 4-(dimethylamino)-*m*-tolyl ester; 4-dimethylamino-*m*-tolyl methylcarbamate; A-363; Bay 44646; ENT-25784; Matacil. $C_{11}H_{16}N_2$-O_2; mol wt 208.26. C 63.44%, H 7.74%, N 13.45%, O 15.36%. Prepn: **GB 913439**, *C.A.* **58**, 10122e (1963); R. Heiss *et al.,* **DE 1145162**, *C.A.* **59**, 9885b (1963) (1962, 1963 both to Bayer). Metabolism: A. Strother, *Toxicol. Appl. Pharmacol.* **21**, 112 (1972). Photochemistry: J. B. Addison *et al., Bull. Environ. Contam. Toxicol.* **11**, 250 (1974); J. B. Addison, *ibid.* **27**, 250 (1981). Toxicity study: T. B. Gaines, *Toxicol. Appl. Pharmacol.* **14**, 515 (1969).

Crystals, mp 93-94°. uv max (ethanol): 248.5 nm (ε 6.67 $\times$ 10^4). Slightly sol in water; moderately sol in aromatic solvents; sol in most polar organic solvents. LD_{50} orally in male, female rats: 40, 38 mg/kg (Gaines).

USE: Insecticide.

434. 7-Aminocephalosporanic Acid. [957-68-6] (6*R*,7*R*)-3-[(Acetyloxy)methyl]-7-amino-8-oxo-5-thia-1-azabicyclo[4.2.0]-oct-2-ene-2-carboxylic acid; 7-amino-3-(hydroxymethyl)-8-oxo-5-thia-1-azabicyclo[4.2.0]oct-2-ene-2-carboxylic acid acetate ester; 3-acetoxymethyl-7-aminoceph-3-em-4-oic acid; 7-ACA. $C_{10}H_{12}N_2$-O_5S; mol wt 272.28. C 44.11%, H 4.44%, N 10.29%, O 29.38%, S 11.78%. Starting material for semi-synthetic cephalosporins. Obtained by mild acid hydrolysis of cephalosporin C, *q.v.*: Loder *et al., Biochem. J.* **79**, 408 (1961); Morin *et al., J. Am. Chem. Soc.* **84**, 3400 (1962); Morin *et al.,* **BE 615955** (1962 to Lilly), *C.A.* **58**, 11373c (1963); by enzymatic hydrolysis of cephalosporin C: Walton, **US 3239394** (1966 to Merck & Co.). Improved prepn: Fechtig *et al., Helv. Chim. Acta* **51**, 1108 (1968). Review of preparative methods: Huber *et al.,* in *Cephalosporins and Penicillins,* E. H. Flynn, Ed. (Academic Press, New York, 1972) pp 27-73.

Crystals. pI 3.5. R_f 0.14 in 1-butanol-ethanol-water (4:1:5 by vol).

435. 4-Amino-4′-chlorodiphenyl. [135-68-2] 4′-Chloro[1,1′-biphenyl]-4-amine; 4′-chloroxenylamine; 4′-chloro-4-aminodiphenyl; *p*′-chloro-*p*-phenylaniline; *p*-amino-*p*′-chloro-biphenyl. $C_{12}H_{10}ClN$; mol wt 203.67. C 70.77%, H 4.95%, Cl 17.41%, N 6.88%. Prepd from 4′-amino-4-biphenyldiazonium chloride by Sandmeyer's reaction: Gelmo, *Ber.* **39**, 4176 (1906); by chlorination of 4-nitrodiphenyl and reduction of 4-chloro-4′-nitrodiphenyl with iron and HCl in ethanol: Belcher *et al., J. Chem. Soc.* **1953**, 1334.

Crystals from light petroleum, mp 134° (Gelmo); mp 128° (Belcher). uv max (0.1*N* HCl): 254 nm (ε 22090). Sol in warm alcohol, ether, benzene, acetone, glacial acetic acid. Practically insol in water and alkalies.

USE: As a reagent in the determination of sulfur, in coal, rubber, etc.

436. Aminochromes. Family of highly colored 2,3-dihydroindole-5,6-quinones obtained by oxidative cyclization of catecholamines: Sobotka, Austin, *J. Am. Chem. Soc.* **73**, 3077 (1951). Best represented by a zwitterionic structure with the substituents determined by the catecholamine used, e.g. for epinephrine as starting material, R = CH_3, R′ = H, and R″ = OH. Numerous physiological activities, such as hallucinogenic, hemostatic, radioprotective, have been ascribed to aminochromes. *Reviews:* Sobotka *et al., Fortschr. Chem. Org. Naturst.* **14**, 217 (1957); Heacock, *Adv. Heterocycl. Chem.* **5**, 205 (1965); Heacock, Powell, *Prog. Med. Chem.* **9**, 275 (1972). Review of toxicity: A. Bindoli *et al., Toxicol. Lett.* **48**, 3-20 (1989).

See also adrenochrome, adrenolutin, carbazochrome salicylate.
THERAP CAT: Hemostatic.

437. 2-Amino-4,6-dichlorophenol. [527-62-8] 2,4-Dichloro-6-aminophenol; 4,6-dichloro-*o*-aminophenol. $C_6H_5Cl_2NO$; mol wt 178.02. C 40.48%, H 2.83%, Cl 39.83%, N 7.87%, O 8.99%. Prepd by reduction of the corresponding nitrophenol: F. Fischer, *Z. Chem.* [N.F.] **4**, 386 (1868); *Ann.* Suppl. **7**, 189 (1870); Katz, Cohen, *J. Org. Chem.* **19**, 758 (1954). Purification: J. Meyer, *Helv. Chim. Acta* **41**, 1890 (1958).

Long needles from carbon disulfide, warts from benzene, mp 95-96°. Sublimes (0.06 torr) 70-80° (bath temp). Freely sol in benzene, somewhat less in carbon disulfide, much less in petr ether. The stability of the free base (snow-white when pure) seems to be impaired by impurities.

Hydrochloride. $C_6H_5Cl_2NO \cdot HCl$. Crystals, dec 280-285°. Very stable when pure. The commercial product may be dark brown. Sol in water, alcohol. Precipitated from aq soln by the addition of concd HCl.

USE: Important azo-dye intermediate.

438. 1-[(2-Aminoethyl)amino]-2-propanol. [123-84-2] *N*-(2-Hydroxypropyl)ethylenediamine; Monolene. $C_5H_{14}N_2O$; mol wt 118.18. C 50.82%, H 11.94%, N 23.70%, O 13.54%. CH_3-$CH(OH)CH_2NHCH_2CH_2NH_2$. Prepn: Kitchen, Pollard, *J. Org. Chem.* **8**, 342 (1943).

Viscous liquid; mild ammoniacal odor. $bp_{3.0}$ 94°; $bp_{10.0}$ 112°. d_4^{25} 0.9837. n_D^{25} 1.4738.

Dihydrochloride. $C_5H_{16}Cl_2N_2O$. mp 184.7-185.0°.
USE: Rapid curing agent in the manuf of epoxy resins.

439. 2-Amino-2-ethyl-1,3-propanediol. [115-70-8] C_5-$H_{13}NO_2$; mol wt 119.16. C 50.40%, H 11.00%, N 11.75%, O 26.85%. An amino glycol prepd by reduction of catalytic hydrogenation of the corresp nitro compound: Vanderbilt, Hass, **US**

2174242 (1940); Johnson, Degering, *J. Org. Chem.* **8**, 7 (1943). Manuf: McMillan, **US 2485982** (1949 to Comm. Solvents).

Crystalline mass, mp 37.5-38.5°. (The commercial product may be a viscous liquid.) d_{20}^{20} 1.099. n_D^{20} 1.490. bp_{10} 152-153°. Miscible with water. Sol in alcohols. pH of 0.1 molar aq soln 10.8.

USE: In the synthesis of surface-active agents, vulcanization accelerators, pharmaceuticals. As emulsifying agent for cosmetic creams and lotions, mineral oil and paraffin wax emulsions, leather dressings, textile specialties, polishes, cleaning compounds, so-called soluble oils. For absorbing CO_2 and H_2S from industrial gases.

440. Aminoglutethimide. [125-84-8] 3-(4-Aminophenyl)-3-ethyl-2,6-piperidinedione; 2-(*p*-aminophenyl)-2-ethylglutarimide; 3-ethyl-3-(*p*-aminophenyl)-2,6-dioxopiperidine; Cytadren; Orimeten. $C_{13}H_{16}N_2O_2$; mol wt 232.28. C 67.22%, H 6.94%, N 12.06%, O 13.78%. Aromatase inhibitor; also blocks adrenal steroidogenesis. Formerly used as anticonvulsant. Prepn: K. Hoffmann, E. Urech, **US 2848455** (1958 to Ciba). Mass spectrum: G. Ruecker, G. Bohn, *Arch. Pharm.* **302**, 204 (1969). Resolution and abs config of antipodes: N. Finch *et al., Experientia* **31**, 1002 (1975). Comprehensive description: H. Y. Aboul-Enein, *Anal. Profiles Drug Subs.* **15**, 35-69 (1986). Review of pharmacology and clinical use in Cushing's disease and breast cancer: R. J. Santen, R. I. Misbin, *Pharmacotherapy* **1**, 95-120 (1981); in prostate cancer: K. A. Havlin, D. L. Trump, *Cancer Treat. Res.* **39**, 83-96 (1988).

Crystals from methanol or ethyl acetate, mp 149-150°. Freely sol in most organic solvents; poorly sol in ethyl acetate, 0.1*N* HCl and absolute ethanol; readily sol in acetone and 100% acetic acid. Practically insol in water.

THERAP CAT: Adrenocortical suppressant; antineoplastic.

441. Aminoguanidine. [79-17-4] Hydrazinecarboximidamide; guanylhydrazine; pimagedine. CH_6N_4; mol wt 74.09. C 16.21%, H 8.16%, N 75.62%. Nucleophilic hydrazine; inhibits the formation of advanced glycosylation end products (AGEs) that have been implicated in the etiology of diabetic complications. Prepn: J. Thiele, *Ann.* **270**, 1 (1892); G. B. L. Smith, E. Anzelmi, *J. Am. Chem. Soc.* **57**, 2730 (1935). Review of chemistry of aminoguanidine and related compounds: E. Lieber, G. B. L. Smith, *Chem. Rev.* **25**, 213-271 (1939); of preparative methods: F. Kurzer, L. E. A. Godfrey, *Chem. Ind. (London)* **1962**, 1584-1595. Prevention of glucose-derived aortic collagen cross-linking in diabetic rats: M. Brownlee *et al., Science* **232**, 1629 (1986). Mechanism of action study: D. Edelstein, M. Brownlee, *Diabetes* **41**, 26 (1992). Review of therapeutic potential: B. H. R. Wolffenbuttel, M. S. P. Huijberts, *Neth. J. Med.* **42**, 205-208 (1993).

Crystals. Sol in water, alc. Practically insol in ether. Aq soln is strongly alkaline and reddens on standing in air; ammonia is evolved on heating.

Hydrochloride. [1937-19-5] GER-11. CH_6N_4·HCl; mol wt 110.55. Large prisms from dil alc, mp 163°. Very sol in water; sol in alc. Practically insol in ether.

THERAP CAT: In prevention and treatment of chronic diabetic complications.

442. *p*-Aminohippuric Acid. [61-78-9] *N*-(4-Aminobenzoyl)glycine; *N*-(*p*-aminobenzoyl)aminoacetic acid; PAH. C_9H_{10}-N_2O_3; mol wt 194.19. C 55.67%, H 5.19%, N 14.43%, O 24.72%. Prepn: J. B. Muenzen *et al., J. Biol. Chem.* **67**, 469 (1926). Method to determine renal function: L. Schumann, P. W. Wüstenberg, *Clin. Nephrol.* **33**, 35 (1990); R. A. Gabel *et al., J. Pharmacol. Toxicol. Methods* **36**, 189 (1996).

Short, irregular prisms from hot water, mp 199°. Soluble in alc, chloroform, benzene, acetone. Practically insol in cold water, ether, carbon tetrachloride.

Sodium salt. [94-16-6] Nephrotest. $C_9H_9N_2NaO_3$; mol wt 216.17. Soluble in water.

THERAP CAT: Diagnostic aid (renal function).

443. 3-Amino-4-hydroxybutyric Acid. [589-44-6] 3-Amino-4-hydroxybutanoic acid; γ-hydroxy-β-aminobutyric acid; GOBAB. $C_4H_9NO_3$; mol wt 119.12. C 40.33%, H 7.62%, N 11.76%, O 40.29%. $HOCH_2CH(NH_2)CH_2COOH$. Prepn: Jollès, Fromageot, *Bull. Soc. Chim. Fr.* **1951**, 862; Chibnall *et al., Biochem. J.* **68**, 122 (1958); Piskov, *Zh. Obshch. Khim.* **32**, 3407 (1962); Nagai *et al., Arzneim.-Forsch.* **17**, 1575 (1967); Kondo, Tanaka, **JP 68 12127** (1968 to Kaken Kagaku), *C.A.* **70**, 77328r (1969).

Prismatic crystals, mp 216°. Also reported as mp 228° (Nagai); mp 232-233.5° (Chibnall).

Hydrochloride. $C_4H_9NO_3$·HCl. mp 156°.

THERAP CAT: Anti-inflammatory, antifungal.

444. 4-Amino-3-hydroxybutyric Acid. [352-21-6] 4-Amino-3-hydroxybutanoic acid; γ-amino-β-hydroxybutyric acid; buksamin; GABOB; Gabomade; Gamibetal. $C_4H_9NO_3$; mol wt 119.12. C 40.33%, H 7.62%, N 11.76%, O 40.29%. H_2NCH_2-$CH(OH)CH_2COOH$. Prepn of DL-form: Tomita, *Z. Physiol. Chem.* **124**, 255 (1923); Balenovic *et al., J. Org. Chem.* **19**, 1589 (1964); Hayashi *et al.,* **JP 58 772** *C.A.* **53**, 1172d (1959); Sakai *et al.,* **JP 62 12264** (to Kaken), *C.A.* **59**, 9805e (1963); **ES 278780** (1963 to Antonio Gallardo, S.A.), *C.A.* **60**, 2779a (1964); Hayashi, **FR 1348105** (1964 to Kaken), *C.A.* **60**, 11956b (1964); D'Alo, Masserini, *Farmaco Ed. Sci.* **19**, 30 (1964); M. Pinza, G. Pifferi, *J. Pharm. Sci.* **67**, 120 (1978). Prepn of L-form: Tomita, Sendju, *Z. Physiol. Chem.* **169**, 270 (1927); Kaneko, Yoshida, *Bull. Chem. Soc. Jpn.* **35**, 1153 (1962); M. E. Jung, T. J. Shaw, *J. Am. Chem. Soc.* **102**, 6304 (1980); of D-form: Tomita, Sendju, *loc. cit.* Improved synthesis of L-form: S. Takano *et al., Tetrahedron Lett.* **28**, 1783 (1987). Purification: Yamagiwa, Tanaka, **JP 63 24365** (to Kaken), *C.A.* **60**, 10515a (1964).

DL-Form. Crystals from dil alc, dec 218°. Fairly readily sol in water; very sparingly sol in methanol, alc, ether, chloroform, ethyl acetate.

D(+)-Form. Crystals from water, dec 214°. $[\alpha]_D^{20}$ +18.3° (c = 2 in H_2O).

L(−)-Form. Crystals from water or water + ethanol, dec 212°, also reported as dec 216-217°. $[\alpha]_D^{20}$ −21.06° (c = 2 in H_2O); −20.7° (c = 1.83 in H_2O).

THERAP CAT: Anticonvulsant.

445. α-Aminoisobutyric Acid. [62-57-7] 2-Methylalanine; 2-aminoisobutyric acid; 2-amino-2-methylpropanoic acid. $C_4H_9NO_2$; mol wt 103.12. C 46.59%, H 8.80%, N 13.58%, O 31.03%. $(CH_3)_2C(NH_2)COOH$. Prepd by the treatment of acetone with hydrocyanic acid and then with alcoholic ammonia (Strecker synthesis): Tiemann, Friedländer, *Ber.* **14**, 1970 (1881), *see also* p 1965; Marckwald *et al., Ber.* **24**, 3283 (1891); Bailey,

Randolph, *Ber.* **41**, 2507 (1908); Clarke, Bean, *Org. Synth.* **coll. vol. II**, 29 (1943); or directly with ammonium cyanide: Gulewitsch, *Ber.* **33**, 1900 (1900) or with a mixture of KCN and NH₄Cl: Zelinsky, Stadnikow, *Ber.* **39**, 1726 (1906); *cf.* Hellsing, *Ber.* **37**, 1921 (1904); and subsequent hydrolysis of the nitrile formed. By heating dimethylhydantoin (obtained from acetone, hydrocyanic and cyanic acids) with concd HCl: Urech, *Ann.* **164**, 268 (1872), *cf.* Heilpern, *Monatsh. Chem.* **17**, 241 (1896).

Monoclinic prisms, tables, mp 335° (sealed capillary). Begins to sublime at 280°. Sweetish taste. Absorption spectrum: Ley, Arends, *Ber.* **61**, 219 (1928); Abderhalden, Rossner, *Z. Physiol. Chem.* **176**, 253 (1928). Freely sol in water. Difficultly sol in alcohol; insol in ether.

Hydrochloride. $C_4H_9NO_2 \cdot HCl$. Platelets from water, dec 236-237°. Readily sol in water, methanol, alcohol.

446. **δ-Aminolevulinic Acid.** [106-60-5] 5-Amino-4-oxo-pentanoic acid; ALA. $C_5H_9NO_3$; mol wt 131.13. C 45.80%, H 6.92%, N 10.68%, O 36.60%. $H_2NCH_2COCH_2CH_2COOH$. Naturally occurring amino acid; precursor of tetrapyrroles in the biosynthesis of chlorophyll and heme. Prepn: R. W. Wynn, A. H. Corwin, *J. Org. Chem.* **15**, 203 (1950); A. A. Marei, R. H. Raphael, *J. Chem. Soc.* **1958**, 2624; C. Herdeis, A. Dimmerlung, *Arch. Pharm.* **317**, 304 (1984). Role in tetrapyrrole biosynthesis: D. Shemin, C. S. Russell, *J. Am. Chem. Soc.* **75**, 4873 (1953). Enhancement of chlorophyll formation: E. C. Sisler, W. H. Klein, *Physiol. Plant.* **16**, 315 (1963). HPLC determn in plasma: K. Miyajima *et al.*, *J. Chromatogr. B* **654**, 165 (1994). Review of role in chlorophyll biosynthesis and potential as photodynamic herbicide: C. A. Rebeiz *et al.*, *Enzyme Microb. Technol.* **6**, 390-401 (1984). Review of role in heme biosynthesis and clinical experience in photodynamic therapy: Q. Peng *et al.*, *Cancer* **79**, 2282-2308 (1997).

Hydrochloride. [5451-09-2] Levulan. $C_5H_{10}ClNO_3$; mol wt 167.59. Needles from methanol-ether, mp 144-147° (dec).

THERAP CAT: Antineoplastic (photosensitizer).

447. **β-Amino-α-methylphenethyl Alcohol.** [52500-61-5] β-Amino-α-methylbenzeneethanol; 1-amino-1-phenyl-2-propanol; 1-phenyl-1-amino-2-propanol. $C_9H_{13}NO$; mol wt 151.21. C 71.49%, H 8.67%, N 9.26%, O 10.58%. Prepn from α-isonitroso-α-phenylacetone: Sichner, Pankova, *Collect. Czech. Chem. Commun.* **20**, 1419 (1955); from an oxazole: Viscontini, *Helv. Chim. Acta* **44**, 636 (1961).

DL-*erythro*-Form. So called **dl-norisoephedrine**. Crystals, mp 85°.

DL-*erythro*-Hydrochloride. $C_9H_{13}NO \cdot HCl$. Crystals from ethanol + ether, mp 170-171°.

448. **2-Amino-2-methyl-1,3-propanediol.** [115-69-5] 1,1-Di(hydroxymethyl)ethylamine; 1,3-dihydroxy-2-methyl-2-propylamine; AMPD. $C_4H_{11}NO_2$; mol wt 105.14. C 45.69%, H 10.55%, N 13.32%, O 30.43%. An amino glycol prepd by reduction of the corresponding nitro compd: O. Piloty, O. Ruff, *Ber.* **30**, 2057 (1897); B. M. Vanderbilt, H. B. Hass, *Ind. Eng. Chem.* **32**, 34 (1940); Johnson, Degering, *J. Org. Chem.* **8**, 7 (1943). Review of uses: G. A. Bergy, *J. Am. Pharm. Assoc. Pract. Pharm. Ed.* **3**, 358-364 (1942). Toxicological evaluation and review: Cosmetic, Toiletry and Fragrance Assoc., *J. Am. Coll. Toxicol.* **9**, 203-228 (1990).

Crystalline mass, mp 109-111°. bp₁₀ 151-152°. 250 grams dissolve in 100 ml water at 20°. Sol in alcohols. pH of 0.1M aq soln 10.8.

USE: In the synthesis of surface-active agents, vulcanization accelerators, pharmaceuticals. As emulsifying agent for cosmetic

creams and lotions, mineral oil and paraffin wax emulsions, leather dressings, textile specialties, polishes, cleaning compounds, so-called sol oils. In hair sprays, wave sets and other noncoloring hair preparations. Absorbent for acidic gases. Biological buffer.

449. **2-Amino-2-methyl-1-propanol.** [124-68-5] 2,2-Diethylethanolamine; 2-hydroxymethyl-2-propylamine; AMP. $C_4H_{11}NO$; mol wt 89.14. C 53.90%, H 12.44%, N 15.71%, O 17.95%. An amino alcohol prepd by reduction of the corresp nitro compound: H. B. Hass, B. M. Vanderbilt, US 2139122 (1938 to Purdue Res. Found.); Johnson, Degering, *J. Org. Chem.* **8**, 7 (1943). Toxicological evaluation and review: Cosmetic, Toiletry and Fragrance Assoc. (CTFA), *J. Am. Coll. Toxicol.* **9**, 203-228 (1990).

Crystalline mass, mp 30-31°. (The commercial product may be a viscous liquid.) d²⁰₂₀ 0.934. n_D^{20} 1.449. bp₇₆₀ 165°; bp₁₀ 67.4°. Miscible with water. Sol in alcohols. pH of 0.1M aq soln 11.3. LD₅₀ in mice, rats (g/kg): 2.15 ± 0.2, 2.90 ± 0.14 orally (CTFA).

USE: In the synthesis of surface-active agents, vulcanization accelerators, pharmaceuticals. As emulsifying agent for cosmetic creams and lotions, mineral oil and paraffin wax emulsions, leather dressings, textile specialties, polishes, cleaning compounds, so-called soluble oils. In hair sprays, wave sets and hair dyes. Absorbent for acidic gases. For use as a drug *see* Pamabrom.

450. **2-Amino-4-methylthiazole.** [1603-91-4] 4-Methyl-2-thiazolamine; 4-methyl-2-thiazolylamine; aminomethiazole. $C_4H_6N_2S$; mol wt 114.17. C 42.08%, H 5.30%, N 24.54%, S 28.09%. Prepn: Sprague *et al.*, *J. Am. Chem. Soc.* **68**, 2155 (1946); Rossi, *Gazz. Chim. Ital.* **85**, 898 (1955). Use in gravimetric determn and extraction of mercury: S. N. Tandon *et al.*, *Anal. Chim. Acta* **59**, 311 (1972).

Crystals, mp 45-46°. bp₂₀ 124-126°; bp₀.₄ 70°. Very sol in water, alcohol, ether.

USE: Reagent.

451. **Aminometradine.** [642-44-4] 6-Amino-3-ethyl-1-(2-propenyl)-2,4(1H,3H)-pyrimidinedione; 1-allyl-6-amino-3-ethyluracil; 1-allyl-6-amino-3-ethyl-2,4(1H,3H)-pyrimidinedione; 1-allyl-3-ethyl-6-amino-1,2,3,4-tetrahydro-2,4-pyrimidinedione; aminometramide; Mictine; Mincard. $C_9H_{13}N_3O_2$; mol wt 195.22. C 55.37%, H 6.71%, N 21.52%, O 16.39%. Prepn: Papesch, Schroeder, US 2650922 (1953 to Searle).

Monohydrate, crystals from water, mp 75-115°. When anhydrous, mp 143-144°.

THERAP CAT: Diuretic.

452. **3-Amino-2-naphthoic Acid.** [5959-52-4] 3-Amino-2-naphthalenecarboxylic acid; 3-aminoisonaphthoic acid. $C_{11}H_9NO_2$; mol wt 187.19. C 70.58%, H 4.85%, N 7.48%, O 17.09%. Prepd from 3-hydroxy-2-naphthoic acid: C. F. H. Allen, A. Bell, *Org. Synth.* **coll. vol. III**, 78 (1955).

Yellow scales from dil alcohol, mp 214°. Sol in alcohol, ether. Solns are yellow with greenish fluorescence.

Sodium salt. $C_{11}H_8NNaO_2$. Leaflets, very sparingly sol in water, alcohol.

Ethyl ester. $C_{13}H_{13}NO_2$. Yellow needles from dil alcohol. Sol in the usual organic solvents, mp 115-115.5°.

USE: In the determination of copper, nickel, cobalt.

453. 4-Amino-1-naphthol. [2834-90-4] 4-Amino-1-naphthalenol; 4-hydroxy-α-naphthylamine. $C_{10}H_9NO$; mol wt 159.18. C 75.45%, H 5.70%, N 8.80%, O 10.05%. Prepd by treating α-naphthol with benzenediazonium chloride and reducing the benzeneazo-α-naphthol with sodium hydrosulfite: Conant *et al., Org. Synth.* **3**, 7 (1923); *cf.* Fieser, Fieser, *J. Am. Chem. Soc.* **57**, 493 (1935). From α-naphthylhydroxylamine by rearrangement in acetone: Neunhoffer, Liebich, *Ber.* **71B**, 2247 (1938).

Needles. Unless kept absolutely dry, it acquires a violet discoloration on storage and oxidizes to 1,4-naphthoquinone. Usually isolated as the hydrochloride, $C_{10}H_9NO.HCl$, needles, very sol in water.

N-Acetyl deriv. 4-Acetamido-1-naphthol; naphthacetol. $C_{12}H_{11}NO_2$. Needles from alcohol, mp 188°, sparingly sol in water, sol in alcohol.

USE: Polymerization inhibitor; prepn of 2-allyl-4-amino-1-naphthol hydrochloride (an antihemorrhagic cpd); prepn of 1,4-naphthoquinone.

454. 1-Amino-2-naphthol-4-sulfonic Acid. [116-63-2] 4-Amino-3-hydroxy-1-naphthalenesulfonic acid; 1,2,4-acid. $C_{10}H_9NO_4S$; mol wt 239.25. C 50.20%, H 3.79%, N 5.85%, O 26.75%, S 13.40%. Prepd by treatment of nitroso-β-naphthol with sodium bisulfite and sulfuric acid: L. F. Fieser, *Org. Synth.* **coll. vol. II**, 42 (1943); *cf. idem, J. Am. Chem. Soc.* **57**, 494 (1935).

White or gray needles, usually contg 0.5 H_2O. May turn pink on exposure to light, especially when moist. Insol in water, alcohol, ether, benzene; sol in hot sodium bisulfite soln; sol in alkaline soln but such solns oxidize quickly on exposure to air yielding a brown substance which is sol in hot water giving a green soln. Controlled oxidation with HNO_3 yields ammonium 1,2-naphthoquinone-4-sulfonate, *see* Fieser, *loc. cit.*

Sodium salt. $C_{10}H_8NNaO_4S$. Needles, sol in hot water with blue fluorescence.

USE: Manuf of azo dyes, 1,2-naphthoquinone-4-sulfonic acid.

455. 1-Amino-2-naphthol-6-sulfonic Acid. [5639-34-9] 5-Amino-6-hydroxy-2-naphthalenesulfonic acid. $C_{10}H_9NO_4S$; mol wt 239.25. C 50.20%, H 3.79%, N 5.85%, O 26.75%, S 13.40%. Prepd by reduction of sodium 1-nitroso-2-naphthol-6-sulfonate with zinc and acetic acid: Fierz-David *et al., Helv. Chim. Acta* **29**, 1765 (1946).

Needles or prisms. Slightly sol in boiling water, less sol in alc. Practically insol in ether.

Sodium salt hemipentahydrate. Eikonogen. $C_{10}H_8NNaO_4S.$-$2\frac{1}{2}H_2O$; mol wt 306.27. Powder. Sol in water. Practically insol in alc, ether. Strong reducing action on silver salts.

USE: Free acid formerly used in manuf of azo dyes. Sodium salt used as photographic developer and for detection of potassium.

456. 6-Aminonicotinic Acid. [3167-49-5] 6-Amino-3-pyridinecarboxylic acid; 6-amino-3-carboxypyridine. $C_6H_6N_2O_2$; mol wt 138.12. C 52.18%, H 4.38%, N 20.28%, O 23.17%. Prepd by heating 6-chloronicotinic acid with ammonia: Marckwald, *Ber.* **26**, 2188 (1893); **27**, 1319 (1894); Räth, Prauge, *Ann.* **467**, 4 (1928); Johnson *et al., J. Biol. Chem.* **153**, 37 (1944).

Dihydrate. Crystals from dil acetic acid. Dec above 300° yielding 2-aminopyridine and CO_2. Sparingly sol in most solvents.

Potassium salt. $C_6H_5KN_2O_2$. Crystals, freely sol in water, insol in alcohol.

Hydrochloride. $C_6H_6N_2O_2.HCl$. Needles, freely sol in water, slightly sol in alcohol.

457. 2-Amino-5-nitrothiazole. [121-66-4] 5-Nitro-2-thiazolamine; Enheptin. $C_3H_3N_3O_2S$; mol wt 145.14. C 24.83%, H 2.08%, N 28.95%, O 22.05%, S 22.09%. Prepd by deacetylation of 2-acetamido-5-nitrothiazole: Hubbard; Steahly, **US 2573641**; **US 2573656**; **US 2573657** (all 1951 to Monsanto).

Greenish-yellow to orange-yellow fluffy powder, dec 202°. Slightly bitter taste. uv max (0.0005% in water): 386 nm (ε 0.540); min: 295 nm. Very sparingly soluble in water. (To make a water soln, a 15% stock soln in propylene glycol should first be prepd.) One gram dissolves in 150 g of 95% alcohol; in 250 g ether. Almost insol in chloroform. Sol in dilute mineral acids.

THERAP CAT (VET): Antihistomonad in turkeys. For trichomoniasis in pigeons.

458. 6-Aminopenicillanic Acid. [551-16-6] (2S,5R,6R)-6-Amino-3,3-dimethyl-7-oxo-4-thia-1-azabicyclo[3.2.0]heptane-2-carboxylic acid; 6-APA; penicin; penin. $C_8H_{12}N_2O_3S$; mol wt 216.26. C 44.43%, H 5.59%, N 12.95%, O 22.19%, S 14.83%. Obtained from cultures of *Penicillium chrysogenum* in the absence of side chain precursors: F. R. Batchelor *et al., Nature* **183**, 257 (1959). Synthesis: J. C. Sheehan, K. R. Henery-Logan, *J. Am. Chem. Soc.* **81**, 5838 (1959); **84**, 2983 (1962). Intermediate in the manuf of synthetic penicillins: J. C. Sheehan, **US 3159617** (1964 to Arthur D. Little). HPLC determn: J. Haginaka, J. Wakai, *Anal. Biochem.* **158**, 146 (1986). Review of prepn: F. M. Huber *et al.* in *Cephalosporins Penicillins: Chem. Biol.*, E. H. Flynn, Ed. (Academic, New York, 1972) pp 27-73. Review of chemistry: E. J. Vandamme, J. P. Voets, *Adv. Appl. Microbiol.* **17**, 311-369 (1974). General review: G. N. Rolinson, *J. Antimicrob. Chemother.* **22**, 5-14 (1988).

Crystals from water + HCl, dec 208-209°, also reported as 207-208° (dried) (Sheehan). $[\alpha]_D^{31}$ +273° (c = 1.2 in 0.1*N* HCl).

USE: In manuf of synthetic penicillins.

459. Aminopentamide. [60-46-8] α-[2-(Dimethylamino)-propyl]-α-phenylbenzeneacetamide; 4-dimethylamino-2,2-diphenylvaleramide; α,α-diphenyl-γ-dimethylaminovaleramide; dimevamide; BL-139. $C_{19}H_{24}N_2O$; mol wt 296.41. C 76.99%, H 8.16%, N 9.45%, O 5.40%. Anticholinergic. Prepn similar ' that of methadone, starts by condensing diphenylmethyl cya'' with chlorodimethylaminopropane: Walton, *et al., J. Cher*

1949, 648; Cheney *et al.*, *J. Org. Chem.* **17**, 770 (1952); Specter, **US 2647926** (1953 to Bristol). Prepn of optical isomers: Wheatley *et al.*, *J. Org. Chem.* **19**, 794 (1954). *See also* Moffett, Aspergren, *J. Am. Chem. Soc.* **79**, 4451 (1957). Toxicity study: Cazort, *J. Pharmacol. Exp. Ther.* **100**, 325 (1950).

dl-Form. Long prisms from dilute alcohol, mp 183-184°. Practically insol in water.

d-Form. Crystals from petr ether, mp 136.5-137.5° (sintering). $[\alpha]_D^{23}$ +98.9° (methanol).

l-Form. Crystals from petr ether, mp 136.5-137.5° (sintering). $[\alpha]_D^{23}$ −101.9° (methanol).

dl-Form hydrochloride. $C_{19}H_{24}N_2O.HCl$. Slightly deliquescent leaflets from alcohol + ether, dec 190-191°. Bitter taste. Soluble in water, alcohol. A 1% aq soln has a pH of 6.8. LD_{50} in mice (mg/kg): 34.7 i.v.; 396 orally (Cazort).

dl-Form acid sulfate. Centrine. $C_{19}H_{24}N_2O.H_2SO_4$; mol wt 394.49. Deliquescent crystals from isopropanol + ethyl acetate, mp 185-187°. The commercial medicinal grade, mp 178-181°. Bitter taste. uv max (1% H_2SO_4): 258.5 nm ($A_{1cm}^{1\%}$ 10.3); min: 249 nm. Freely sol in water, alc. Very slightly sol in chloroform. Practically insol in ether. pH of 2.5% aq soln 1.3-2.2.

THERAP CAT: Antispasmodic.

THERAP CAT (VET): Antispasmodic; antiemetic.

460. *m*-Aminophenol. [591-27-5] 3-Amino-1-hydroxybenzene; 3-hydroxyaniline. C_6H_7NO; mol wt 109.13. C 66.04%, H 6.47%, N 12.83%, O 14.66%. Manuf by reduction of *m*-nitrophenol: Freifelder, Robinson, **US 3079435** (1963 to Abbott). Toxicity study: Koelzer, Giesen, *Z. Naturforsch.* **6b**, 183 (1951).

Crystals, mp 122-123°. Sol in 40 parts cold water, freely in hot water, alcohol, ether, amyl alcohol; slightly in benzene, very slightly in petr ether. LD_{50} i.p. in mice: 4.5 mg/20g (Koelzer, Giesen).

USE: Dye intermediate, manuf *p*-aminosalicylic acid.

461. *o*-Aminophenol. [95-55-6] 2-Aminophenol; 2-amino-1-hydroxybenzene; 2-hydroxyaniline. C_6H_7NO; mol wt 109.13. C 66.04%, H 6.47%, N 12.83%, O 14.66%. Manuf by reduction of *o*-nitrophenol: Freifelder, Robinson, **US 3079435** (1963 to Abbott).

Crystals, rapidly becoming brown, mp 170-174°; sublimes. One gram dissolves in 50 ml cold water, 23 ml alcohol; freely soluble in ether, very slightly in benzene. *Keep tightly closed and protected from light.*

Hydrochloride. $C_6H_7NO.HCl$; mol wt 145.59. Crystals readily becoming gray on exposure to light. Freely sol in water or alcohol.

USE: Manuf ... sulfur dyes; dyeing furs and hair. Hydro- ... ur, hair, leather, etc.

... ol. [123-30-8] *p*-Hydroxyaniline; 4- ...Azol; Rodinal; Unal; Ursol P. C_6H_7NO; ...%, H 6.47%, N 12.83%, O 14.66%. ...ction of *p*-nitrophenol: *BIOS Final Re-* ...on, **US 3079435** (1963 to Abbott).

Orthorhombic plates from water. *Deteriorates under the influence of air and light.* mp 189.6-190.2°. The commercial product is usually pink, mp 186°. Can be sublimed at 0.3 mm and 110° without decompn. bp_{760} 284° (dec); $bp_{8.0}$ 167°; $bp_{3.0}$ 150°; $bp_{0.3}$ 130.2°. Kb at 15° = 6.6 × 10^{-9}. Forms salts with acids and bases. Soly in water: 0.39% at 13°; 0.65% at 24°; 0.80% at 30°; 1.5% at 50°; 4.7% at 80°; 8.5% at 96°. Soly in ethyl methyl ketone: 9.3% at 58.5°; in abs ethanol: 4.5% at 0°. Practically insol in benzene, chloroform.

Hydrochloride. $C_6H_7NO.HCl$; mol wt 145.59. Cryst powder; gradually becomes darker. Dec about 306°. Very sol in water; sol in alc.

Caution: May cause skin sensitization, dermatitis. Inhalation can cause asthma, methemoglobin formation.

USE: Photographic developer; intermediate in the manufacture of sulfur and azo dyes; in dyeing furs and feathers.

463. *p*-Aminophenylacetic Acid. [1197-55-3] 4-Aminobenzeneacetic acid; *p*-amino-α-toluic acid. $C_8H_9NO_2$; mol wt 151.16. C 63.57%, H 6.00%, N 9.27%, O 21.17%. Prepd by the reduction of *p*-nitrophenylacetic acid with hydrogen sulfide in the presence of ammonia: G. R. Robertson, *Org. Synth.* **coll. vol. I**, 52 (2nd ed., 1941).

Plates, leaflets from water, mp 199-200° (dec). Moderately sol in hot water; sol in alcohol, in alkalies.

Hydrochloride. $C_8H_9NO_2.HCl$. Rods from HCl, freely sol in water, sol in alcohol (about 3% w/w).

Ethyl ester. $C_{10}H_{13}NO_2$. Platelets from water, mp 51°.

N-Benzoyl deriv. Needles from alcohol, mp 205-206°.

464. 4-Amino-3-phenylbutyric Acid. [1078-21-3] β-(Aminomethyl)benzenepropanoic acid; β-(aminomethyl)hydrocinnamic acid; 4-amino-3-phenylbutanoic acid; β-phenyl-γ-aminobutyric acid; fenibut; phenibut; phenigamma; phenygam; PhGABA. $C_{10}H_{13}NO_2$; mol wt 179.22. C 67.02%, H 7.31%, N 7.82%, O 17.85%. Prepn starting with α,γ-diamino-β-phenylpropane: Jackson, Kenner, *J. Chem. Soc.* **1928**, 1657. Alternate prepn: Cologne, Pouchol, *Bull. Soc. Chim. Fr.* **1962**, 598. Pharmacology: R. A. Khaunina, *Bull. Exp. Biol. Med.* **57**, 52 (1964). Structure-activity studies: *idem, Farmakol. Toksikol.* **31**, 202 (1968). Activity studies of the isomers: *eidem, Byull. Eksp. Biol. Med.* **72**, 49 (1971), *C.A.* **76**, 81208t (1972). Review of pharmacology and clinical experience: I. Lapin, *CNS Drug Rev.* **7**, 471-481 (2001).

mp 250-253° (dec).

Hydrobromide. [103095-38-1] $C_{10}H_{13}NO_2.HBr$; mol wt 260.13. Irregular platelets from benzene, mp 114°.

Hydrochloride. [3060-41-1] $C_{10}H_{13}NO_2.HCl$; mol wt 215.68. LD_{50} in mice, rats (mg/kg): 900, 700 i.p. (Khaunina, 1964).

THERAP CAT: Anxiolytic.

465. Aminophylline. [317-34-0] 3,7-Dihydro-1,3-dimethyl-1*H*-purine-2,6-dione compd with 1,2-ethanediamine (2:1); theophylline compd with ethylenediamine; theophylline ethylenediamine; theophyllamine; Afonilum; Aminodur; Cardophylin; Euphyllina; Pecram; Phyllocontin; Phyllotemp; Planphylline; Pulmovet; Tefamin. $C_{16}H_{24}N_{10}O_4$; mol wt 420.43. C 45.71%, H 5.75%, N 33.32%, O 15.22%. Prepn: Grüter, **US 919161** (1909 to Byk). Toxicity data: C. R. Thompson, M. R. Warren, *J. Lab. Clin. Med.* **31**, 1337 (1946). Comprehensive description: K. D. Thakker, L. T. Grady, *Anal. Profiles Drug Subs.* **11**, 1-44 (1982). Reviews of clinical experience: J. A. Stirt, S. F. Sullivan, *Anesth. Analg.* **60**, 587-602 (1981); A. G. Perry, *AACN Clin. Issues* **6**, 297-306 (1995).

Consult the Name Index before using this section.

Occurs as the dihydrate. White or slightly yellowish granules or powder. Slight ammoniacal odor. Bitter taste. Gradually absorbs carbon dioxide from the air and becomes incompletely sol due to liberation of theophylline. One gram dissolves in about 5 ml water, but the soln may become turbid on standing. Insol in alcohol, ether. *Keep tightly closed.* LD_{50} orally in mice: 540 mg/kg (Thompson, Warren).

Caution: Potential symptoms of overexposure include acute restlessness, anorexia, nausea, fever, vomiting, dehydration; followed by tremors, delirium, convulsions and coma; may result in cardiovascular and respiratory collapse, shock, cyanosis and death. See *Clinical Toxicology of Commercial Products*, R. E. Gosselin et al., Eds. (Williams & Wilkins, Baltimore, 5th ed., 1984) Section III, pp 17-21.

THERAP CAT: Bronchodilator.
THERAP CAT (VET): Bronchodilator.

466. 2-Amino-4-picoline. [695-34-1] 4-Methyl-2-pyridinamine; 2-amino-4-methylpyridine; α-amino-γ-picoline; 4-methyl-2-aminopyridine; W-45; Askensil. $C_6H_8N_2$; mol wt 108.14. C 66.64%, H 7.46%, N 25.90%. Prepd by heating 4-picoline with sodamide in xylene: Seide, *Ber.* **57**, 791 (1924); **58**, 1733 (1925); Räth, *ibid.* 347. Formulations: von Haxthausen et al., US **2937118** (1960 to Raschig). Pharmacology: von Haxthausen, *Arch. Exp. Pathol. Pharmakol.* **226**, 163; **227**, 234 (1955); Marchetti et al., *Arch. Int. Pharmacodyn. Ther.* **143**, 385 (1963).

Leaflets from petr ether, mp 100-100.5°. bp_{11} 115-117°. Sublimes on slow heating. Freely sol in water, lower alcohols, dimethylformamide, coal tar bases. Slightly sol in petr ether, aliphatic hydrocarbons.

THERAP CAT: Cardiotonic.

467. Aminopromazine. [58-37-7] N,N,N',N'-Tetramethyl-3-(10H-phenothiazin-10-yl)-1,2-propanediamine; 10-[2,3-bis(dimethylamino)propyl]phenothiazine; proquamezine; tetrameprozine; RP-3828. $C_{19}H_{25}N_3S$; mol wt 327.49. C 69.68%, H 7.69%, N 12.83%, S 9.79%. Prepn: Jacob et al., *Compt. Rend.* **243**, 1637 (1956); Horclois, GB **800635** (1958 to Rhône-Poulenc).

Fumarate. [3688-62-8] Lispamol; Sedofarmolo. $(C_{19}H_{25}N_3S)_2 \cdot C_4H_4O_4$; mol wt 771.05. Crystals, sensitive to light, dec 166-170°. Soly at 20° (g/100 ml): water 9.0; methanol 5.0; ethanol 0.5. Very slightly sol in isopropanol, acetone. Practically insol in benzene, ether. pH of a 2% aq soln 5.0 to 7.0.

THERAP CAT: Antispasmodic.
THERAP CAT (VET): Antispasmodic.

468. 2-Aminopropanol. [78-91-1] 2-Amino-1-propanol; 2-aminopropyl alcohol; β-propanolamine; 2-hydroxyisopropylamine. C_3H_9NO; mol wt 75.11. C 47.97%, H 12.08%, N 18.65%, O 21.30%. $CH_3CH(NH_2)CH_2OH$. Obtained together with isopropylamine on reduction of acetylcarbinoloxime with sodium amalgam in dilute acetic acid: Gabriel, *Ber.* **49**, 2121 (1916); from DL-alanylglycine by reduction with sodium and abs alcohol: Abderhalden, Schwab, *Z. Physiol. Chem.* **143**, 292 (1925); by boil-

ing the ethyl ester of DL-acetylalanine with sodium in abs alcohol: Karrer, *Helv. Chim. Acta* **4**, 98 (1921); as hydrolytic cleavage product of ergonovine and ergometrinine: Stoll, Hofmann, *ibid.* **26**, 956 (1943); by catalytic hydrogenation of the ethyl ester of alanine: Adkins, Pavlic, *J. Am. Chem. Soc.* **69**, 3039 (1947).

dl-**Form.** Liquid, fishy odor. bp 173-176°. Freely sol in water, alcohol, ether.

Hydrochloride. $C_3H_9NO \cdot HCl$. Leaflets from abs alcohol + acetone, dec 86-87.5°.

469. 3-Aminopropionitrile. [151-18-8] 3-Amino-propanenitrile; β-aminopropionitrile. $C_3H_6N_2$; mol wt 70.09. C 51.41%, H 8.63%, N 39.97%. $H_2NCH_2CH_2CN$. Prepd by the reaction of acrylonitrile with ammonia: Buc et al., *J. Am. Chem. Soc.* **67**, 93 (1945); *Org. Synth.* **coll. vol. III**, 93 (1955); Weijlard, Sullivan, US **2742491** (1956 to Merck & Co.).

Liquid. Amine odor. bp_{760} 185°; bp_{20} 87-89°; bp_5 66-69°; bp_3 50-55°. n_D^{20} 1.4396. The pure, anhydrous material may be stored in tightly stoppered bottles for several months. Storing under refrigeration is recommended to avoid development of pressure in the bottles. Polymerization takes place slowly during storage in an open container, or very rapidly in the presence of acid or acidic compds.

USE: Intermediate in the manufacture of β-alanine and pantothenic acid.

470. p-Aminopropiophenone. [70-69-9] 1-(4-Amino-phenyl)-1-propanone; ethyl p-aminophenyl ketone; PAPP. $C_9H_{11}NO$; mol wt 149.19. C 72.46%, H 7.43%, N 9.39%, O 10.72%. Pretreatment antidote to cyanide; activity probably through the formation of methemoglobin, which has a higher affinity for cyanide than mitochondrial cytochrome oxidase. Prepd by the action of propionyl chloride on aniline in carbon bisulfide in the presence of aluminum chloride: Kunckell, *Ber.* **33**, 2641 (1900); Derrick, Bornemann, *J. Am. Chem. Soc.* **35**, 1283 (1913); Hartung, Foster, *J. Am. Pharm. Assoc.* **35**, 15 (1946). Antidotal activity: C. L. Rose et al., *J. Pharmacol. Exp. Ther.* **89**, 109 (1947). Toxicity study: J. W. Scawin et al., *Toxicol. Lett.* **23**, 359 (1984). Review of pharmacology of cyanide detoxification: S. I. Baskin, R. F. Fricke, *Cardiovasc. Drug Rev.* **10**, 358-375 (1992).

Yellow needles from water, mp 140°. Sol in water, alc, DMSO. LD_{50} in male, female mice (mg/kg): 145, 200 i.v.; in female mice, guinea pigs, rats, male rats (mg/kg): >5000, 1020, 223.7, 475 orally (Scawin).

Hydrochloride. [6170-25-8] $C_9H_{11}NO \cdot HCl$. Needles, yellowish cast, mp 198-199°. Freely sol in water. LD_{50} i.v. in dogs: 7.15 ±0.89 mg/kg (Rose).

Sulfate. $(C_9H_{11}NO)_2 \cdot H_2SO_4$. Yellow plates from alcohol, dec 25°.

THERAP CAT: Antidote (cyanide).

471. α-(α-Aminopropyl)benzyl Alcohol. [5897-76-7] α-(1-Aminopropyl)benzenemethanol; 2-amino-1-phenyl-1-butanol; β-amino-α-phenylbutyl alcohol; 1-phenyl-1-hydroxy-2-amino-n-butane. $C_{10}H_{15}NO$; mol wt 165.23. C 72.69%, H 9.15%, N 8.48%, O 9.68%. Prepn of the *dl-threo*-form: Abrams, Kipping, *J. Chem. Soc.* **1936**, 1480; Rebstock et al., *J. Am. Chem. Soc.* **73**, 3666 (1951). Prepn of the *dl-erythro*-form: Hartung et al., *ibid.* **52**, 3317 (1930); Rebstock et al., loc. cit. See also Beilstein **13**, suppl. 3, 1791-1792 (1973).

dl-threo-**Form.** Thick, shiny plates from benzene + petr ether, mp 79-80° (Abrams, Kipping); 78-79° (Rebstock et al.). Freely sol in alcohol; moderately sol in chloroform, benzene; sparingly sol in petr ether.

dl-threo-**Form hydrochloride.** $C_{10}H_{15}NO \cdot HCl$. Lust prisms, mp 195-196° (Abrams, Kipping); 204-205° (Rebs al.). Freely sol in water; sol in alcohol; slightly sol in chlo

Consult the Name Index before using this section.

dl-erythro-Form. mp 80.5-81°.
dl-erythro-Form hydrochloride. mp 242°.

472. Aminopterin. [54-62-6] N-[4-[[(2,4-Diamino-6-pteridinyl)methyl]amino]benzoyl]-L-glutamic acid; 4-aminofolic acid; 4-aminopteroylglutamic acid; 4-amino-PGA. $C_{19}H_{20}N_8O_5$; mol wt 440.41. C 51.82%, H 4.58%, N 25.44%, O 18.16%. Prepd from 2,4,5,6-tetraminopyrimidine sulfate, 2,3-dibromopropionaldehyde and p-aminobenzoylglutamic acid: Seeger et al., J. Am. Chem. Soc. **69**, 2567 (1947); from 6-(bromomethyl)-2,4-diaminopteridine HBr: Piper, Montgomery, J. Heterocycl. Chem. **11**, 279 (1974). Purification: Loo, J. Med. Chem. **8**, 139 (1965). Inhibition of dihydrofolate reductase: J. S. Erickson et al., J. Biol. Chem. **247**, 5661 (1972). Use as rodenticide: **US 2575168** (1951 to Am. Cyanamid).

Dihydrate. Clusters of yellow needles. uv max of the 0.75 hydrate (0.1N NaOH): 261, 282, 373 (log ε 4.41, 4.39, 3.91).
USE: Rodenticide.

473. α-Aminopyridine. [504-29-0] 2-Pyridinamine; 2-aminopyridine. $C_5H_6N_2$; mol wt 94.11. C 63.81%, H 6.43%, N 29.77%. Prepd from pyridine and sodamide: Tschitschibabin, Chem. Zentralbl. **1915, I,** 1065; Wibaut, Rec. Trav. Chim. **42,** 240 (1923); A. I. Vogel, Practical Organic Chemistry (Longmans, London, 3rd ed., 1959) p 1007; Gattermann-Wieland, Praxis des Organischen Chemikers (de Gruyter, Berlin, 40th ed., 1961) p 316.

Leaflets, or large crystals. mp 58.1°. bp 210.6°. Soluble in water, alcohol, benzene, ether, hot petrol ether.
β-Aminopyridine. [462-08-8] 3-Pyridinamine. Prepn: Allen, Wolf, Org. Synth. coll. vol. IV, 45 (1963). Crystals, mp 64°. bp 250-252°. Sol in water, alcohol, benzene, ether. Insol in petr ether.
Caution: Potential symptoms of overexposure to α-aminopyridine are irritation of eyes, nose, throat; headache, dizziness; excitement; nausea; high blood pressure; respiratory distress; weakness; convulsions; stupor. See NIOSH Pocket Guide to Chemical Hazards (DHHS/NIOSH 97-140, 1997) p 14.
USE: Manuf pharmaceuticals and dyes.

474. Aminopyrine. [58-15-1] 4-(Dimethylamino)-1,2-dihydro-1,5-dimethyl-2-phenyl-3H-pyrazol-3-one; 4-(dimethylamino)antipyrine; dimethylaminophenyldimethylpyrazolone; 4-dimethylamino-2,3-dimethyl-1-phenyl-3-pyrazolin-5-one; aminophenazone; amidazophen; dipyrine; dimethylaminophenazone; amidopyrine; Mamallet-A; Pyramidon; Netsusarin. $C_{13}H_{17}N_3O$; mol wt 231.29. C 67.51%, H 7.41%, N 18.17%, O 6.92%. Prepn: Beilstein **25,** 452 (1936); T. Takahashi et al., J. Pharm. Soc. Jpn. **76,** 1180 (1956); T. Takahashi, K. Kenematsu, Chem. Pharm. Bull. **6,** 98 (1958). Metabolism: G. F. Lockwood, J. B. Houston, J. Pharm. Pharmacol. **31,** 787 (1979). Hepatotoxicity: E. Bien et al., Pharmazie **36,** 492 (1981). Toxicity studies: Hart, J. Pharmacol. Exp. Ther. **89,** 205 (1947); Tubaro et al., Arzneim.-Forsch. **20,** 1024 (1970). Use in breath test of hepatic function: G. W. Hepner, E. S. Vesell, N. Engl. J. Med. **291,** 1384 (1974).

Leaflets from ligroin, mp 107-109°. The aq soln is slightly alkaline to litmus. Soly in water is increased by the addition of sodium benzoate. One gram dissolves in 1.5 ml alcohol, 12 ml benzene, 1 ml chloroform, 13 ml ether, 18 ml water. Stable in air, but affected by light. Readily attacked by mild oxidizing agents in the presence of water. LD_{50} orally in rats: 1.7 g/kg (Hart).
Hydrochloride. [6170-29-2] $C_{13}H_{17}N_3O.HCl$. Deliquescent prisms, mp 143-144°. Freely sol in water with acid reaction.
Bicamphorate. [94442-12-3] $C_{13}H_{17}N_3O.2C_{10}H_{16}O_4$. Crystalline powder, mp 94°. Sol in water with gradual decompn; sol in alcohol.
Salicylate. [603-57-6] $C_{13}H_{17}N_3O.C_7H_6O_3$. Crystalline powder, mp 70°. One gram dissolves in 16 ml water, about 6 ml alcohol.
Caution: Agranulocytosis may occur: E. Urbach, H. L. Goldburgh, J. Am. Med. Assoc. **131,** 893 (1946); G. Discombe, Br. Med. J. **1,** 1270 (1952).
THERAP CAT: Antipyretic; analgesic. Diagnostic aid (hepatic function).

475. Aminoquinuride. [3811-56-1] N,N'-Bis(4-amino-2-methyl-6-quinolinyl)urea; bis(2-methyl-4-amino-6-quinolyl)urea; di(4-aminoquinald-6-yl)urea; aminoquincarbamide; aminochinuride; aminokinuride; Surfen. $C_{21}H_{20}N_6O$; mol wt 372.42. C 67.73%, H 5.41%, N 22.57%, O 4.30%. Prepn: Jensch, **DE 591480** (1934 to I. G. Farbenind). Oncogenic and heparin-neutralizing properties: D. T. Hunter, J. M. Hill, Nature **191,** 1378 (1961).

Crystals from butanol, dec 255° (effervescence).
THERAP CAT: Antiseptic.

476. Aminorex. [2207-50-3] 4,5-Dihydro-5-phenyl-2-oxazolamine; 2-amino-5-phenyl-2-oxazoline; aminoxafen; aminoxaphen; McN-742. $C_9H_{10}N_2O$; mol wt 162.19. C 66.65%, H 6.21%, N 17.27%, O 9.86%. Prepn: Poos et al., J. Med. Chem. **6,** 266 (1963); Poos, **US 3161650** (1964 to McNeil).

Crystals from benzene, mp 136-138°.
Fumarate. [13425-22-4] Menocil; Apiquel. $C_9H_{10}N_2O.C_4H_4O_4$; mol wt 278.26.
Note: This is a controlled substance (stimulant): **21 CFR,** 1308.11.
THERAP CAT: Anorexic.

477. p-Aminosalicylic Acid. [65-49-6] 4-Amino-2-hydroxybenzoic acid; 4-aminosalicylic acid; PAS; PASER; Rezipas. $C_7H_7NO_3$; mol wt 153.14. C 54.90%, H 4.61%, N 9.15%, O 31.34%. Prepn: **DE 50835** (1889); **US 427564** (1890); Sheehan, J. Am. Chem. Soc. **70,** 1665 (1948); Erlenmeyer et al., Helv. Chim. Acta **31,** 988 (1948); Wenis, Gardner, J. Am. Pharm. Assoc. **38,** 9 (1949); Centolella, **US 2844625** (1958 to Miles). Toxicity study: E. M. Bavin et al., J. Pharm. Pharmacol. **2,** 764 (1950). Comprehensive description: M. M. A. Hassan et al., Anal. Profiles Drug Subs. **10,** 1-27 (1981).

Minute crystals from alcohol, mp 150-151° with effervescence. uv max (0.1N HCl): 265, 300 nm. pKa 3.25. pH of 0.1% aq soln: 3.5. One gram dissolves in about 500 ml water, in 21 ml alcohol. Slightly sol in ether. Practically insol in benzene. Sol in dilute nitric acid, dil sodium hydroxide. At temps above 40°, aq solns of

PAS and its hydrochloride are readily decarboxylated to give brown solns consisting mainly of *m*-aminophenol. LD_{50} orally in mice: 4 g/kg (Bavin).

Hydrochloride. $C_7H_7NO_3$.HCl. Crystals, dec 224°.

Sodium salt dihydrate. [6018-19-5] Aminacyl; Nemasol Sodium; Pamisyl Sodium; Paramisan Sodium; Pasalon. $C_7H_6NNaO_3.2H_2O$; mol wt 211.15. pH of 1% soln ~7. One gram dissolves in 2 ml water. Very sparingly sol in acetone. Practically insol in ether, chloroform, benzene. Solns of the sodium salt are more resistant to heat than PAS, but sterilization by bacterial filtration is recommended.

Calcium salt. [133-15-3] Nippas Calcium. $C_{14}H_{12}CaN_2O_6$; mol wt 344.33. Bittersweet crystals. One gram dissolves in about 7 ml water, slightly sol in alc. Aq solns dec slowly and darken in color.

Potassium salt. [133-09-5] Paskalium. $C_7H_6NO_3K$; mol wt 191.23. Crystals, freely sol in water. pH of 1% soln about 7. Reported to cause less gastric irritation than the free acid or the sodium salt.

Ethyl ester. $C_9H_{11}NO_3$. Needles from alc, mp 115°. Prepd by reduction of the ethyl ester of 4-nitrosalicylic acid.

Phenyl ester *see* Phenyl Aminosalicylate.

THERAP CAT: Antibacterial (tuberculostatic).

478. p-Aminosalicylic Acid Hydrazide. [6946-29-8] 4-Amino-2-hydroxybenzoic acid hydrazide; Apacizin; Apacizina. $C_7H_9N_3O_2$; mol wt 167.17. C 50.29%, H 5.43%, N 25.14%, O 19.14%. Prepn: Drain *et al., J. Chem. Soc.* **1949**, 1498; Magrane, **ES 206645** (1952), *C.A.* **49**, 5529e (1955); **JP 54 7472** (1954), *C.A.* **50**, 9947c (1956).

Needles from alcohol, mp 190-200°. Slightly soluble in water, somewhat more in ethanol.

THERAP CAT: Antibacterial (tuberculostatic).

479. 2-Aminothiazole. [96-50-4] 2-Thiazolamine; Abadol; Basedol. $C_3H_4N_2S$; mol wt 100.14. C 35.98%, H 4.03%, N 27.97%, S 32.02%. Prepn from vinyl acetate: Christiansen, **US 2242237** (1941 to Squibb); Kyrides, **US 2330223** (1943 to Monsanto); *cf.* Skrimshire, **GB 540032** (1941 to B.D.H.). Prepd also by condensing tribromoparaldehyde with thiourea: Leitch, Brickman, **US 2230962** (1941); **US 2339083** (1944 to Mallinckrodt). Prepn from paraldehyde and thiourea: Erlenmeyer *et al., Helv. Chim. Acta* **38**, 1293 (1955). Toxicology: W. B. Deichmann *et al., J. Ind. Hyg. Toxicol.* **30**, 71 (1948).

Crystals from benzene + petr ether, mp 93°. Distills at 3 mm without decompn. Sol in hot water. Slightly sol in cold water, alc, ether. Freely sol in dil HCl and in 20% H_2SO_4. LD_{50} orally in rats: 0.48 g/kg (Deichmann).

Hydrochloride monohydrate. $C_3H_4N_2S$.HCl.H_2O. Needles, freely sol in water. Also used as the acid tartrate. Crystals, sol in water.

THERAP CAT: Thyroid inhibitor.

480. 2-Amino-1,1,3-tricyanopropene. [868-54-2] 2-Amino-1-propene-1,1,3-tricarbonitrile; 2-amino-1,3,3-tricyano-2-propene; malononitrile dimer. $C_6H_4N_4$; mol wt 132.12. C 54.54%, H 3.05%, N 42.41%. $(CN)_2C$═$C(NH_2)CH_2CN$. Prepn: Carboni *et al., J. Am. Chem. Soc.* **80**, 2838 (1958); Carboni, **US 2719861** (1955 to du Pont); Coenen, **DE 922531** (1955 to Bayer).

Rod-like crystals from water, mp 170-173°.

481. Amioca. [9037-22-3] Amylopectin. A non-linear polymer of glucose, obtained from waxy corn: Caldwell, *Converter* **17**, No. 11, 12, 14 (1943); *Manuf. Confect.* **33**, No. 12, 15, 17 (1943),

C.A. **38**, 1137[1] (1944); Schopmeyer, *Food Ind.* **17**, 1476 (1945), *C.A.* **40**, 2331[3] (1946). *Review:* Powell in *Industrial Gums*, R. L. Whistler, Ed. (Academic Press, New York, 2nd ed., 1973) pp 567-576.

482. Amiodarone. [1951-25-3] (2-Butyl-3-benzofuranyl)[4-[2-(diethylamino)ethoxy]-3,5-diiodophenyl]methanone; 2-butyl-3-benzofuranyl-4-[2-(diethylamino)ethoxy]-3,5-diiodophenyl ketone; 2-butyl-3-[3,5-diiodo-4-(β-diethylaminoethoxy)benzoyl]-benzofuran. $C_{25}H_{29}I_2NO_3$; mol wt 645.31. C 46.53%, H 4.53%, I 39.33%, N 2.17%, O 7.44%. Benzofuran derivative with multiple electrophysiological effects. Prepn: **FR 1339389**; R. Tondeur, F. Binon, **US 3248401** (1963, 1966 to Soc. Belge l'Azote Prod. Chim. Marly). Physicochemical properties: M. Bonati *et al., J. Pharm. Sci.* **73**, 829 (1984). HPLC determn in plasma: M. De Smet, D. L. Massart, *J. Pharm. Biomed. Anal.* **6**, 277 (1988). Comprehensive description: T. A. Plomp, *Anal. Profiles Drug Subs.* **20**, 1-120 (1991). Review of pharmacology, clinical efficacy and safety: M. Chow, *Ann. Pharmacother.* **30**, 637-643 (1996); B. N. Singh, *Clin. Cardiol.* **20**, 608-618 (1997). Clinical trial in cardiac resuscitation: P. J. Kudenchuk *et al., N. Engl. J. Med.* **341**, 871 (1999); to prevent atrial fibrillation: D. Roy *et al., ibid.* **342**, 913 (2000).

Hydrochloride. [19774-82-4] L-3428; Amiodar; Ancaron; Cordarex; Cordarone; Ortacrone; Pacerone; Tachydaron; Trangorex. $C_{25}H_{29}I_2NO_3$.HCl; mol wt 681.77. Crystalline powder, mp 156°. Also reported as crystals from acetone, mp 159 ±2° (Bonati). Soly at 25° (g/100ml): chloroform 44.51; methylene chloride 19.20; methanol 9.98; ethanol 1.28; benzene 0.65; tetrahydrofuran 0.60; acetonitrile 0.32; 1-octanol 0.30; ether 0.17; 1-propanol 0.13; water 0.07; hexane 0.03 petroleum ether 0.001. Sparingly sol in isopropanol; slightly sol in acetone, dioxane, and carbon tetrachloride. pH (5% soln) 3.4-3.9. pK_a (25°C) 6.56 ±0.06. uv max (methanol): 208, 242 nm ($E_{1cm}^{1\%}$ 662 ±8, 623 ±10).

THERAP CAT: Antiarrhythmic (class III).

483. Amiphenazole. [490-55-1] 5-Phenyl-2,4-thiazolediamine; 2,4-diamino-5-phenylthiazole; DAPT; phenamizole; Dizol; Daptazole; Daptazile; Fenamizol. $C_9H_9N_3S$; mol wt 191.25. C 56.52%, H 4.74%, N 21.97%, S 16.77%. Prepd by the interaction of thiourea and α-bromobenzyl cyanide *et al., J. Chem. Soc.* **1950**, 3491; from thiourea and α-cyanobenzyl sulfonate in acetone: Dodson, Turner, *J. Am. Chem. Soc.* **73**, 4517 (1951).

Flakes from water or dilute alcohol, dec 163-164°. Turns brown on exposure to light and air.

Hydrobromide. $C_9H_9N_3S$.HBr. Prisms from alc, dec >250°. Freely sol in hot water, moderately in cold water.

Benzenesulfonate. $C_{15}H_{15}N_3O_3S_2$. Crystals from alcohol + ether, dec 261-262°. Practically insol in water, most organic solvents. Slightly sol in alcohol.

THERAP CAT: Narcotic antagonist.

THERAP CAT (VET): Barbiturate and morphine antagonist.

484. Amiprilose. [56824-20-5] 3-O-[3-(Dimethylamino)-propyl]-1,2-O-(1-methylethylidene)-α-D-glucofuranose; 1,2-O-isopropylidene-3-O-[3'-(N,N-dimethylamino)propyl]-α-D-glucofuranose. $C_{14}H_{27}NO_6$; mol wt 305.37. C 55.06%, H 8.91%, N 4.59%, O 31.44%. Synthetic, substituted monosaccharide with immunomodulatory activity. Prepn: **BE 823313**; P. Gordon, **US 3939146** (1975, 1976 both to Strategic Med. Res.); E. R. Garrett *et al., J.*

Pharm. Sci. **71**, 387 (1982). Absolute configuration: R. J. Linhardt *et al., ibid.* **79**, 158 (1990). HPLC determn in plasma: S. T. Wu *et al., J. Chromatogr. B* **692**, 149 (1997). Clinical pharmacokinetics: E. R. Garrett *et al., J. Pharmacokinet. Biopharm.* **10**, 247 (1982). Clinical trial in rheumatoid arthritis: W. G. Riskin *et al., Ann. Intern. Med.* **111**, 455 (1989). Review of immunoregulatory effects: D. M. Chang, *Immunopharmacol. Immunotoxicol.* **17**, 437-450 (1995).

Colorless, viscous oil. n^{25} 1.4687.

Hydrochloride. [60414-06-4] SM-1213; Therafectin. C_{14}-$H_{27}NO_6 \cdot HCl$; mol wt 341.83. Crystals from methanol, mp 181-183°. Sol in water, methanol, hot ethanol.

THERAP CAT: Immunomodulator; anti-inflammatory.

485. Amisulpride. [71675-85-9] 4-Amino-*N*-[(1-ethyl-2-pyrrolidinyl)methyl]-5-(ethylsulfonyl)-2-methoxybenzamide; 4-amino-*N*-[(1-ethyl-2-pyrrolidinyl)methyl]-5-(ethylsulfonyl)-*o*-anisamide; aminosultopride; DAN-2163; Deniban; Socian; Solian; Sulamid. $C_{17}H_{27}N_3O_4S$; mol wt 369.48. C 55.26%, H 7.37%, N 11.37%, O 17.32%, S 8.68%. Dopamine receptor antagonist. Prepn: M. Thominet *et al., BE 872585; eidem, US 4401822* (1979, 1983 both to Soc. d'Etudes Sci. Ind. de l'Ile-de-France). Crystal structure: H. L. DeWinter *et al., Acta Crystallogr.* **C46**, 313 (1990). Psychopharmacology: G. Perrault *et al., J. Pharmacol. Exp. Ther.* **280**, 73 (1997). HPLC determn in plasma and urine: B. Malavasi *et al., J. Chromatogr. B* **676**, 107 (1996). Series of articles on pharmacology and clinical efficacy in schizophrenia: *Int. Clin. Psychopharmacol.* **12**, Suppl. 2, S11-S36 (1997).

Crystals from acetone, mp 126-127°. LD_{50} in male mice (mg/kg): 56-60 i.v.; 175-180 i.p.; 224-250 s.c.; 1024-1054 orally (Thominet).

THERAP CAT: Antipsychotic.

486. Amitraz. [33089-61-1] *N'*-(2,4-Dimethylphenyl)-*N*-[[(2,4-dimethylphenyl)imino]methyl]-*N*-methylmethanimidamide; *N*-methyl-*N'*-2,4-xylyl-*N*-(*N*-2,4-xylylformimidoyl)formamidine; *N,N*-di-(2,4-xylyliminomethyl)methylamine; 2-methyl-1,3-di-(2,4-xylylimino)-2-azapropane; 1,5-di-(2,4-dimethylphenyl)-3-methyl-1,3,5-triazapenta-1,4-diene; *N*-methylbis(2,4-xylyliminomethyl)-amine; BTS-27419; U-36059; ENT-27967; Aludex; Ectodex; Mitaban; Mitac; Taktic; Topline. $C_{19}H_{23}N_3$; mol wt 293.41. C 77.78%, H 7.90%, N 14.32%. Formamide insecticide for use on deciduous fruit and citrus mites, and tick eradication in cattle. Prepn: I. R. Harrison *et al., DE 2061132; eidem, US 3781355* (1971, 1973 both to Boots); and activity: *idem et al., Pestic. Sci.* **4**, 901 (1973). Prepn and characterization of polymorphs: M. M. de Villiers *et al., J. Agric. Food Chem.* **52**, 7362 (2004). Bacterial degradation: E. R. Allcock, D. R. Woods, *J. Appl. Bacteriol.* **44**, 383 (1978). Properties and use as insecticide: V. Labonne *et al. Def. Veg.* **33**, 66 (1979). Pharmacokinetics and metabolism in animals: M. A. Pass, T. D. Mogg, *J. Vet. Pharmacol. Ther.* **18**, 210 (1995). Use in treatment of demodicosis in dogs: L. Medleau, T. Willemse, *J. Small Anim. Pract.* **36**, 3 (1995).

White monoclinic needles, mp 86-87°. Unstable to acidic pH. Soly at 20° (g/100 cc): water $<10^{-4}$; methanol 2.5; xylene 33; acetone 50. LD_{50} in male rats, female mice, rabbits, guinea pigs, bobwhite quail (mg/kg): 800, >1600, >100, >400, 788 orally; LD_{50} in rabbits, male rats (mg/kg): >200, >1600 dermally; LC_{50} (48 hr) in rainbow trout, Japanese carp: 3.3, 1.2 ppm (Labonne).

USE: Acaricide; insecticide.

THERAP CAT (VET): Ectoparasiticide.

487. Amitriptyline. [50-48-6] 3-(10,11-Dihydro-5*H*-dibenzo[*a,d*]cyclohepten-5-ylidene)-*N,N*-dimethyl-1-propanamine; 10,11-dihydro-*N,N*-dimethyl-5*H*-dibenzo[*a,d*]cycloheptene-$\Delta^{5,\gamma}$-propylamine; 5-(γ-dimethylaminopropylidene)-5*H*-dibenzo[*a,d*]-10,11-dihydrocycloheptene; 10,11-dihydro-5-(γ-dimethylamino-propylidene)-5*H*-dibenzo[*a,d*]cycloheptene; 5-(3-dimethylamino-propylidene)dibenzo[*a,d*][1,4]cycloheptadiene. $C_{20}H_{23}N$; mol wt 277.40. C 86.59%, H 8.36%, N 5.05%. Prepn: Hoffsommer *et al., J. Org. Chem.* **27**, 4134 (1962); **28**, 1751 (1963); *J. Med. Chem.* **8**, 555 (1965); Engelhardt *et al., BE 584061* (1960 to Merck & Co.); **GB 858187; GB 858188** (both 1961 to Hoffmann-La Roche); Tristram, Tull, *US 3205264* (1965 to Merck & Co.). Toxicity data: A. Tobe *et al., Arzneim.-Forsch.* **31**, 1278 (1981). Comprehensive description: K. W. Blessel *et al., Anal. Profiles Drug Subs.* **3**, 127-148 (1974).

Hydrochloride. [549-18-8] Ro-4-1575; Adepril; Amineurin; Domical; Elavil; Endep; Euplit; Laroxyl; Lentizol; Redomex; Saroten; Sarotex; Triptizol; Tryptanol; Tryptizol. $C_{20}H_{23}$-N·HCl; mol wt 313.86. Minute crystals, mp 196-197°. Freely sol in water, chloroform, alc. uv max (methanol): 240 nm (ε 13800). pKa 9.4. LD_{50} in mice, rats (mg/kg): 350, 380 orally; 65, 75 i.p. (Tobe).

THERAP CAT: Antidepressant.

488. Amitriptylinoxide. [4317-14-0] 3-(10,11-Dihydro-5*H*-dibenzo[*a,d*]cyclohepten-5-ylidene)-*N,N*-dimethyl-1-propanamine *N*-oxide; 10,11-dihydro-*N,N*-dimethyl-5*H*-dibenzo[*a,-d*]cycloheptene-$\Delta^{5,\gamma}$-propylamine *N*-oxide; amitriptyline *N*-oxide; Ambivalon; Equilibrin. $C_{20}H_{23}NO$; mol wt 293.40. C 81.87%, H 7.90%, N 4.77%, O 5.45%. Centrally acting metabolite of amitriptyline, *q.v.* Prepn: J. B. Pedersen, *GB 991651; idem, US 3299103* (1965, 1967 both to Dumex). Series of articles on pharmacology, pharmacokinetics, metabolism, clinical studies, toxicity studies, teratological studies: *Arzneim.-Forsch.* **28**, 1873-1926 (1978). HPLC determn: K. M. Jensen, *J. Chromatogr.* **183**, 321 (1980). Neuropharmacology: J. Hyttel *et al., Acta Pharmacol. Toxicol.* **47**, 53 (1980). Toxicity study: H. Friehe, R. Fontaine, *Arzneim.-Forsch.* **28**, 1898 (1978).

Crystals, mp 228-230°. (Dihydrate, mp 102-103°.) LD_{50} in mice, guinea pigs, rabbits, dogs (mg/kg): between 330-460 orally; in mice, rats: 87, 25 i.v.; 320, 110 i.p. (Friehe, Fontaine).

THERAP CAT: Antidepressant.

489. Amitrole. [61-82-5] 1*H*-1,2,4-Triazol-3-amine; 3-amino-1*H*-1,2,4-triazole; aminotriazole; ATA; ENT-25445; Amizol; Cytrol; Weedazol. $C_2H_4N_4$; mol wt 84.08. C 28.57%, H 4.80%, N 66.64%. Non-selective post-emergence, translocated herbicide. Prepn: G. Sjostedt, L. Gringas, *Org. Synth.* **coll. vol. III**, 95 (1955). Use as herbicide: Allen, *US 2670282* (1954 to Am. Chemical Paint Co.). Antithyroid activity: T. H. Jukes, C. B.

Shaffer, *Science* **132**, 296 (1960). *Review:* E. Kröller, *Residue Rev.* **12**, 163-192 (1966). Review of carcinogenicity studies: *IARC Monographs* **7**, 31-43 (1974).

Crystals from abs ethanol, mp 159°. Soluble in water, methanol, ethanol, chloroform. Sparingly sol in ethyl acetate. Insol in ether, acetone. Aq solns are neutral. LD_{50} in mice, rats (g/kg): 14.7, 25.0 orally (Kröller).

Hydrochloride. $C_2H_4N_4$·HCl. Crystals from alcohol, mp 153°.

Caution: Potential symptoms of overexposure are irritation of eyes, skin; dyspnea, muscle spasms, ataxia, anorexia, salivation, increased body temperature; lassitude, skin dryness and depression associated with thyroid function suppression. *See NIOSH Pocket Guide to Chemical Hazards* (DHHS/NIOSH 97-140, 1997) p 14. Amitrole is reasonably anticipated to be a human carcinogen: *Report on Carcinogens, Eleventh Edition* (PB2005-104914, 2004) p III-16.

USE: Herbicide.

490. Amlexanox. [68302-57-8] 2-Amino-7-(1-methylethyl)-5-oxo-5*H*-[1]benzopyrano[2,3-*b*]pyridine-3-carboxylic acid; 2-amino-7-isopropyl-5-oxo-5*H*-[1]benzopyrano[2,3-b]pyridine-3-carboxylic acid; 2-amino-7-isopropyl-1-azaxanthone-3-carboxylic acid; amoxanox; AA-673; CHX-3673; Aphthasol; Elics; Solfa. $C_{16}H_{14}N_2O_4$; mol wt 298.29. C 64.42%, H 4.73%, N 9.39%, O 21.45%. Inhibits release of allergic mediators from mast cells. Prepn: A. Nohara *et al.*, **BE 864647**; **US 4143042** (1978, 1979 both to Takeda); *eidem, J. Med. Chem.* **28**, 559 (1985). Mode of action studies: T. Saijo *et al., Int. Arch. Allergy Appl. Immunol.* **79**, 231 (1986); H. Makino *et al., ibid.* **82**, 66 (1987). Pharmacodynamics: G. Rankov *et al., Ophthalmic Res.* **22**, 359 (1990). Clinical trial in aphthous ulcers: R. O. Greer, Jr. *et al., J. Oral Maxillofac. Surg.* **51**, 243 (1993).

Crystals from DMF, mp >300°.

THERAP CAT: Antiallergic; antiasthmatic.

491. Amlodipine. [88150-42-9] 2-[(2-Aminoethoxy)-methyl]-4-(2-chlorophenyl)-1,4-dihydro-6-methyl-3,5-pyridinedicarboxylic acid 3-ethyl 5-methyl ester; (±)-2-[(2-aminoethoxy)-methyl]-4-(2-chlorophenyl)-3-ethoxycarbonyl-5-methoxycarbonyl-6-methyl-1,4-dihydropyridine; UK-48340. $C_{20}H_{25}ClN_2O_5$; mol wt 408.88. C 58.75%, H 6.16%, Cl 8.67%, N 6.85%, O 19.56%. Dihydropyridine calcium channel blocker; activity resides mainly in the (−)-isomer. Prepn: S. F. Campbell *et al.*, **EP 89167**; *eidem,* **US 4572909** (1983, 1986 both to Pfizer). Synthesis and pharmacology of racemate and enantiomers: J. E. Arrowsmith *et al., J. Med. Chem.* **29**, 1696 (1986). Calcium antagonist activity: R. A. Burges *et al., J. Cardiovasc. Pharmacol.* **9**, 110 (1987). GC determn in plasma: A. P. Beresford *et al., J. Chromatogr.* **420**, 178 (1987). Metabolism: *idem et al., Xenobiotica* **18**, 245 (1988). Review of pharmacology and therapeutic efficacy: M. Haria, J. Wagstaff, *Drugs* **50**, 560-586 (1995). Clinical potential in severe heart failure: M. Packer *et al., N. Engl. J. Med.* **335**, 1107 (1996). Review of mechanism of plaque stabilization: R. P. Mason, *Atherosclerosis* **165**, 191-199 (2002); of clinical potential in combination with atorvastatin in atherosclerosis: J. W. Jukema, J. W. A. van der Hoorn, *Expert Opin. Pharmacother.* **5**, 459-468 (2004).

Maleate. [88150-47-4] UK-48340-11. $C_{20}H_{25}ClN_2O_5$·$C_4H_4O_4$; mol wt 524.95. White crystals from ethyl acetate, mp 178-179°.

Benzenesulfonate. [111470-99-6] Amlodipine besylate; UK-48340-26; Amlor; Antacal; Istin; Monopina; Norvasc. $C_{20}H_{25}ClN_2O_5$·$C_6H_5SO_3H$; mol wt 567.05. White crystalline powder. Slightly sol in water; sparingly sol in ethanol.

THERAP CAT: Antianginal; antihypertensive.

492. Ammonia. [7664-41-7] H_3N; mol wt 17.03. H 17.76%, N 82.25%. NH_3. Manufactured from water gas (obtained by blowing steam through incandescent coke) as source of hydrogen, and from producer gas (obtained from steam and air through incandescent coke), as source of nitrogen by the Haber-Bosch process. Manuf from natural gas: *Faith, Keyes & Clark's Industrial Chemicals*, F. A. Lowenheim, M. K. Moran, Eds. (Wiley-Interscience, New York, 4th ed., 1975) pp 83-92. Historical monograph: A. Mittasch, *Geschichte der Ammoniaksynthese* (Verlag Chemie, 1951). Reviews of prepn, properties and chemistry: Several authors in *Mellor's* Vol. **VIII**, supplement I, *Nitrogen* part 1 (1964) pp 240-369; Jones in *Comprehensive Inorganic Chemistry* Vol. **2**, J. C. Bailar, Jr. *et al.*, Eds. (Pergamon Press, Oxford, 1973) pp 199-227; J. R. LeBlanc *et al.*, in *Kirk-Othmer Encyclopedia of Chemical Technology* vol. **2** (Wiley-Interscience, New York, 3rd ed., 1978) pp 470-516. Review of toxicology and human exposure: *Toxicological Profile for Ammonia* (PB2004-107331, 2004) 269 pp.

Colorless gas; very pungent odor (characteristic of drying urine). Lower limit of human perception: 0.04 g/cubic meter or 53 ppm. One liter of the gas weighs 0.7714 g. d 0.5967 (air = 1). mp −77.7°. bp$_{760}$ −33.35°. Densities of liq NH_3 (temp; press.): 0.6818 (−33.35°; 1 atm); 0.6585 (−15°; 2.332 atm); 0.6386 (0°; 4.238 atm); 0.6175 (15°; 7.188 atm); 0.5875 (35°; 13.321 atm). Critical temp 132.4°; critical press. 111.5 atm. Heat capacity (25°) 8.38 cal/mole/deg. Mixtures of ammonia and air will explode when ignited under favorable conditions: *Angew. Chem.* **43**, 302 (1930), but ammonia is generally regarded as nonflammable. Corrosive, alkaline gas. pH of 1.0*N* aq soln 11.6; of 0.1*N* aq soln 11.1; of 0.01*N* aq soln 10.6. Water at 0° holds 47%, at 15° 38%, at 20° 34%, at 25° 31%, at 30° 28%, at 50° 18%. d_4^{20} (aq solns): 0.9939 (1%); 0.9811 (4%); 0.9651 (8%); 0.9362 (16%); 0.9229 (20%); 0.9101 (24%); 0.8980 (28%). fp (aq solns): −2.9° (4%); −8.1° (8%); −23.1° (16%); −34.9° (20%); −44.5° (24%); −69.2° (28%). Solution of NH_3 in water is exothermic. 95% alcohol at 20° holds 15%, at 30° 11%. Abs ethanol at 0° 20%, at 25° 10%. Methanol at 25° 16%. It is also sol in chloroform and ether. Liquid ammonia produces low temps by its own evaporation. Heat of vaporization: 5.581 kcal/mole. It is a good solvent for many elements and compds. Usually marketed in liquefied form in steel cylinders or as ammonia water (aqua ammonia, ammonium hydroxide) in drums and bottles.

Caution: Potential symptoms of overexposure are eye, nose and throat irritation; dyspnea, bronchospasm and chest pain; pulmonary edema; pink frothy sputum; skin burns, vesiculation; direct contact with liquid may cause frostbite. *See NIOSH Pocket Guide to Chemical Hazards* (DHHS/NIOSH 97-140, 1997) p 14. *See also Patty's Industrial Hygiene and Toxicology* vol. **2B**, G. D. Clayton, F. E. Clayton, Eds. (Wiley-Interscience, New York, 3rd ed., 1981) pp 3045-3052.

USE: Fertilizer, corrosion inhibitor, purification of water supplies, component of household cleaners, as refrigerant. Manuf nitric acid, explosives, synthetic fibers, fertilizers. In pulp and paper, metallurgy, rubber, food and beverage, textile and leather industries.

493. Ammoniacum. [9000-03-7] Gum ammoniac. A gum-resin exuded from the flowering and fruiting stem of *Dorema ammoniacum, D. Don*, and probably other *Umbelliferae. Habit.* Persia, Northern India, Southern Siberia, Africa. *Constit.* 1.3-6.7% volatile oil; 50-70% resin; 18-26% gum; ash content about 2%, may be as high as 10%; salicylic acid; aminoresinol. *Ref:* W. Sandermann, *Naturharze, Terpentinöl, Tallöl* (Springer, 1960) pp 82-83.

Irregular rounded tears, yellowish or brownish outside and whitish within; brittle when cold, but soft when warm; also masses, darker in color and less homogeneous; peculiar odor; slightly sweetish, bitter, somewhat acrid taste. mp 45-55°. Acid no. 60-80. Sapon no. 97-114. d 1.207. Partly soluble in water, alcohol, ether, vinegar or alkali soln; forms emulsions with water.

USE: Ingredient of porcelain cements.

THERAP CAT: Diaphoretic; emmenagogue.

494. Ammonia Water. Ammonium hydroxide; aqua ammonia; spirit of hartshorn. A soln of 28-29% NH_3 in water.

Colorless liquid; intense, pungent, suffocating odor; acrid taste; strong alkaline reaction. d_{25}^{25} ~0.90, 26°Bé. Dissolves copper, zinc. Fumes are formed when brought near volatile acids. *Keep cool in strong glass, plastic or rubber-stoppered bottles not completely filled.* Reaction with H_2SO_4 or other strong mineral acids is exothermic; mixture becomes boiling hot.

Ammonia Water—10%. Colorless liquid. Very pungent odor. d_{25}^{25} 0.957. *Irritating to skin and mucous membranes.*

USE: Detergent, removing stains, bleaching, calico printing, extracting plant colors (cochineal, archil, etc.) and alkaloids; manuf ammonium salts, aniline dyes, and a wide variety of other uses.

THERAP CAT: 10% Solution as reflex respiratory stimulant.

495. Ammonium Acetate. [631-61-8] Acetic acid ammonium salt. $C_2H_7NO_2$; mol wt 77.08. C 31.16%, H 9.15%, N 18.17%, O 41.51%. CH_3COONH_4. Commercial product contains 95-97% salt with acetic acid and some water. Prepd from acetic acid and NH_3: Zuffanti, *J. Am. Chem. Soc.* **63**, 3123 (1941). Toxicity data: Welch *et al., J. Lab. Clin. Med.* **29**, 809 (1944).

Deliquesc crystals or crystalline masses. Slight acetous odor. d 1.07. mp 114° (Zuffanti, *loc. cit.*). Tends to lose NH_3. Sol in less than 1 part water; freely sol in alc; slightly sol in acetone. Very concd aq soln is slightly acid; a 0.5 molar aq soln has pH 7.0. *Keep cool and tightly closed.* LD i.v. in mice: 1.8 mg (NH_4^+)/20g (Welch).

Ammonium acetate solution. [8013-61-4] Spirit of Mindererus. Colorless, clear liquid; acid reaction to litmus. Prepd from 1 g ammonium carbonate, 20 ml dil acetic acid (6%). Contains 6.5-7.5% CH_3COONH_4.

USE: Preserving meats, dyeing, stripping; as a reagent in anal. chemistry, *e.g.*, for determining Pb, Fe; separating $PbSO_4$ from other sulfates.

THERAP CAT: Diuretic.

THERAP CAT (VET): Formerly as diuretic, antipyretic.

496. Ammonium Benzoate. [1863-63-4] Benzoic acid, ammonium salt. $C_7H_9NO_2$; mol wt 139.15. C 60.42%, H 6.52%, N 10.07%, O 23.00%. $C_6H_5COONH_4$. It is about 99% pure. Manuf from benzoic acid and NH_3: Spina, **US 1704636** (1929 to Hooker Electrochem.).

Lamellar crystals or crystalline powder; odorless or faint benzoic acid odor; gradually loses NH_3 on exposure to air. d 1.26. mp 198°. One gram dissolves in 4.7 ml water, 1.2 ml boil. water, 36 ml alcohol, 8 ml boil. alcohol, 8 ml glycerol. The aq soln is slightly acid. *Keep well closed. Incompat.* Ferric salts, acids, alkali hydroxides or carbonates.

USE: To preserve glue and latex.

THERAP CAT: Urinary anti-infective.

497. Ammonium Bicarbonate. [1066-33-7] Acid ammonium carbonate; ammonium hydrogen carbonate. CH_5NO_3; mol wt 79.06. C 15.19%, H 6.37%, N 17.72%, O 60.71%. NH_4HCO_3. Occurs in the urine of alligators: Coulson, Hernandez, *Proc. Soc. Exp. Biol. Med.* **88**, 682 (1955). Usually prepd by passing an excess of carbon dioxide through concd ammonia water. Manuf: **GB 304872** (1927 to I.G. Farben.); Brooks, **GB 742386** (1955 to I.C.I.). *See also* Ammonium Carbonate.

Shiny, hard, colorless or white prisms or crystalline mass. Faint odor of ammonia. Comparatively stable at room temp. Volatile with decompn at about 60°. The white fumes given off consist of NH_3 21.5%, CO_2 55.7%, H_2O vapor 22.8%. Rate of decompn increases as temp rises. mp 107.5° (very rapid heating). Soly in water: 14% (10°); 17.4% (20°); 21.3% (30°). Decomposed by hot water. One gram dissolves in 10 ml glycerol (pharmaceutical grade). pH of 0.1N soln in water at 25° = 7.8. Insol in alcohol and acetone. Negative heat of solution.

Pharmaceutical Incompat: Acids, caustic alkalies.

USE: In baking powder formulations; in cooling baths (one kg dissolved in 5 liters H_2O at 17° lowers it to 7°); in fire extinguishers; manuf porous plastics, ceramics; manuf dyes, pigments; in compost heaps to accelerate decompn; as fertilizer; for defatting textiles; in cold wave solns; in chrome leather tanning; to remove gypsum from heat exchanges and other processing equipment.

THERAP CAT: Expectorant.

THERAP CAT (VET): Expectorant. Used in bloat, colic.

498. Ammonium Bifluoride. [1341-49-7] Acid ammonium fluoride; ammonium hydrogen fluoride. F_2H_5N; mol wt 57.04. F 66.61%, H 8.84%, N 24.56%. NH_4HF_2. Prepn from hydrofluoric acid and NH_3: Hassel, Luzanski, *Z. Kristallogr.* **A83**, 449 (1932); *Gmelins, Ammonium* (8th ed.) **23**, 148 (1936).

Orthorhombic crystals which readily etch glass. d 1.5. mp 124.6°. Freely sol in water. *Keep in plastic, rubber, wood or paraffined containers and well closed. See also* Ammonium Fluoride.

USE: In manuf of Mg and Mg alloys; in brightening of Al; for purifying and cleansing various parts of beer-dispensing apparatus, tubes, etc., sterilizing dairy and other food equipment; in glass and porcelain industries; as mordant for aluminum; as a "sour" in laundering cloth. In lab production of HF.

499. Ammonium Binoxalate. [5972-72-5] Ammonium acid oxalate; ammonium hydrogen oxalate. $C_2H_5NO_4$; mol wt 107.07. C 22.44%, H 4.71%, N 13.08%, O 59.77%. NH_4-OOCCOOH. Prepn of monohydrate: Dehn, Heuse, *J. Am. Chem. Soc.* **29**, 1137 (1907). *Review: Gmelins, Ammonium* (8th ed.) **23**, pp 405-406 (1936).

Monohydrate. Rhombic crystals. *Poisonous.* d 1.56. Sol in 25 parts water; slightly sol in alcohol.

USE: To remove ink stains.

500. Ammonium Bisulfate. [7803-63-6] Acid ammonium sulfate; ammonium hydrogen sulfate. H_5NO_4S; mol wt 115.11. H 4.38%, N 12.17%, O 55.60%, S 27.86%. NH_4HSO_4. Prepn: *Gmelins, Ammonium* (8th ed.) **23**, 293-298 (1936).

Deliquesc crystals. mp about 147°. d 1.787. Freely sol in water. Practically insol in alcohol, acetone, pyridine. *Keep well closed.*

USE: In hair-waving preparations; as catalyst for organic reactions.

501. Ammonium Bisulfide. [12124-99-1] Ammonium hydrogen sulfide; ammonium hydrosulfide; ammonium sulfhydrate. H_5NS; mol wt 51.11. H 9.86%, N 27.41%, S 62.74%. NH_4HS. Prepd by mixing stoichiometric amts of NH_3 and H_2S gases at 0°: Thomas, Riding, *J. Chem. Soc.* **123**, 1181 (1923).

White, tetragonal or orthorhombic crystals. d 1.17. Sublimes *in vacuo.* Decomposes into H_2S and NH_3 rather easily at room temp when in crystal form. The commercial product is furnished in porcelain-like lumps which are more stable and can be stored in a closed bottle at a cool place. Dissociation press. at room temp about 350 mm Hg. Freely sol in water or alcohol giving colorless solns which turn yellow rapidly. Decomposed by boiling water. Soly (0°): 128.1 g/100 g H_2O. Slightly sol in acetone; almost insol in ether, benzene.

Caution: Very irritating to skin; penetrates more rapidly than hydrogen sulfide and may be fatal.

USE: In lubricants.

502. Ammonium Bisulfite. [10192-30-0] H_5NO_3S; mol wt 99.11. H 5.08%, N 14.13%, O 48.43%, S 32.35%. NH_4HSO_3. Prepn: *Gmelins, Ammonium* (8th ed.) **23**, 259-260 (1936).

Crystals. Soly in water (g/100 ml H_2O): 267 (10°); 620 (60°). *Keep well closed.* Sold as solution only.

USE: Preservative.

503. Ammonium Bitartrate. [3095-65-6] (2*R*,3*R*)-2,3-Dihydroxybutanedioic acid monoammonium salt; L-tartaric acid monoammonium salt; ammonium acid tartrate; ammonium hydrogen tartrate. $C_4H_9NO_6$; mol wt 167.12. C 28.75%, H 5.43%, N 8.38%, O 57.44%. $NH_4OOCCH(OH)CH(OH)COOH$. Prepd from ammonium tartrate and tartaric acid: Dulk, *Ann.* **2**, 39 (1832).

Odorless crystals. d 1.68. Sol in 45.6 parts water at 15°; freely sol in hot water, alkalies, alkali carbonates. Practically insol in alc. $[\alpha]_D^{20}$ +26.0° (c = 1.5 in water): Long, *J. Am. Chem. Soc.* **23**, 813 (1901).

504. Ammonium Borate. [12007-58-8] Ammonium tetraborate; ammonium biborate; ammonium metaborate. $B_4H_8N_2O_7$; mol wt 191.32. B 22.60%, H 4.21%, N 14.64%, O 58.54%. $(NH_4)_2B_4O_7$. Prepn: *Gmelins, Ammonium* (8th ed.) **23**, 323 (1936).

Tetrahydrate. Tetragonal crystals. Sol in water. Practically insol in alcohol.

USE: Fireproofing wood and textiles; in electrolytic condensers.

505. Ammonium Bromide. [12124-97-9] BrH$_4$N; mol wt 97.94. Br 81.58%, H 4.12%, N 14.30%. NH$_4$Br. Contains 99-99.5% NH$_4$Br. Prepn and properties: *Gmelins, Ammonium* (8th ed.) **23**, 203-218 (1936); Richards, "Ammonium Bromide" in *Mellor's* Vol. VIII, supplement I, *Nitrogen* (part 1) 433-447 (1964).

White, odorless, slightly hygroscopic crystals or granules; pungent, saline taste; slowly becomes yellowish in air; sublimes at high temp without melting. d^{25} 2.429. Freely sol in water, methanol, ethanol, acetone; slightly sol in ether. Practically insol in ethyl acetate. *Keep well closed.*

Incompat. Acids, acid salts, spirit nitrous ether, alkaloids; salts of lead, mercury, silver.

USE: Manuf of photographic films, plates, and papers; in process engraving and lithography; fireproofing of wood; in corrosion inhibitors.

THERAP CAT: Sedative.

THERAP CAT (VET): Sedative.

506. Ammonium Caprylate. [5972-76-9] Octanoic acid ammonium salt; caprylic acid ammonium salt. C$_8$H$_{19}$NO$_2$; mol wt 161.24. C 59.59%, H 11.88%, N 8.69%, O 19.85%. C$_7$H$_{15}$-COONH$_4$. Prepn from the acid and ammonia: McMaster, Magill, *J. Am. Chem. Soc.* **38**, 1793 (1916); Stumpf, *Am. Paint J.* **38** (45), 60 (1954).

Monoclinic crystals from ether + alcohol. Somewhat hygroscopic. Decomposes on standing and develops odor of caprylic acid. mp 70-85°. Easily hydrolyzed by water. Freely sol in glacial acetic acid and ethanol; less sol in methanol; slightly sol in acetone and ethyl acetate. Practically insol in chloroform, benzene. *Keep well closed.*

USE: In photographic emulsions; as insecticide and nematocide; in manuf of zinc caprylate.

507. Ammonium Carbamate. [1111-78-0] "Anhydride" of ammonium carbonate; ammonium aminoformate. CH$_6$N$_2$O$_2$; mol wt 78.07. C 15.38%, H 7.75%, N 35.88%, O 40.99%. NH$_2$-COONH$_4$. Prepd from dry ice and liq ammonia: Brooks, Audrieth, *Inorg. Synth.* **2**, 85 (1946).

Cryst powder; ammonia odor; gradually loses ammonia in the air changing to ammonium carbonate. Volatilizes at about 60°. Freely sol in water; sol in alcohol.

USE: Ammoniating agent, less vigorous than NH$_3$.

508. Ammonium Carbonate. [10361-29-2] Hartshorn. A mixture of ammonium bicarbonate and ammonium carbamate, obtained by subliming a mixture of ammonium sulfate and calcium carbonate. Contains 30-34% NH$_3$, about 45% CO$_2$. *See USP* XVII, p 941. *Review:* Allen, "Ammonium Carbonate" in *Mellor's* Vol. VIII, supplement 1, *Nitrogen* (part 1) 459-468 (1964).

Colorless, hard, translucent, crystalline masses, white cubes or powder; strong odor of ammonia; sharp taste and alkaline reactions. Decomposes on exposure to air with loss of NH$_3$ and CO$_2$, becoming white and powdery and converting into ammonium bicarbonate. Volatilizes at about 60°. Slowly sol in 4 parts water; decomposed by hot water; the carbamate portion dissolves in alcohol. *Keep tightly closed in a cool place.*

Incompat. Acids and acid salts; salts of iron, zinc; alkaloids, alum, calomel, tartar emetic.

USE: In baking powders, for washing and defatting woolens, tanning; as mordant in dyeing; manuf rubber articles, casein glue, casein colors; in fire extinguishers, smelling salts; for separating cacao constituents; as a reagent in analytical chemistry. Pharmaceutic aid (source of ammonia).

THERAP CAT: Expectorant.

THERAP CAT (VET): Expectorant. Has been used as a carminative and stomachic.

509. Ammonium Chloride. [12125-02-9] Ammonium muriate; sal ammoniac; salmiac. ClH$_4$N; mol wt 53.49. Cl 66.28%, H 7.54%, N 26.19%. NH$_4$Cl. Contains 99.5-99.8% NH$_4$-Cl; principal impurity is NaCl; exists in two temperature dependent crystal modifications. Prepn and properties: *Gmelins, Ammonium* (8th ed.) **23**, pp 150-184 (1936); N. C. R. Kane, "Ammonium

Chloride" in *Mellor's* Vol. VIII, supplement 1, *Nitrogen* (part 1), 378-432 (1964). Manuf: A. W. Bamforth, S. R. S. Sastry, *Chem. Process Eng.* **53**, 72 (1972). NMR study: K. H. Michel, *Proc. Int. Sch. Phys.* **1976**, 392. Toxicity data: E. M. Boyd, K. G. W. Seymour, *Exp. Med. Surg.* **4**, 223 (1946). Brief review: C. W. Weston in *Kirk-Othmer Encyclopedia of Chemical Technology* **vol 2** (Wiley-Interscience, New York, 4th ed., 1992) pp 695-698. Review of properties and use in water treatment: P. Smeets, *Trib. Eau* **570**, 26-29 (1994).

Colorless, odorless crystals or cryst masses; or white, granular powder; cooling, saline taste; somewhat hygroscopic. Tendency to cake. Strongly endothermic. d$_4^{20}$ 1.5274. Sublimes without melting. Soly in water (w/w): 22.9% (0°); 26.0% (15°); 28.3% (25°); 39.6% (80°). HCl and NaCl decrease soly in water. Sol in methanol, ethanol. Almost insol in acetone, ether, ethyl acetate. pH of aq solns (25°): 1% 5.5; 3% 5.1; 10% 5.0. LD$_{50}$ in rats (mg/kg): 30 i.m. (Boyd, Seymour). LD$_{50}$ in rats (mg/kg): 1650 orally (Smeets).

Caution: Potential symptoms of overexposure to fumes are irritation of eyes, skin, respiratory system; cough, dyspnea, pulmonary sensitization. *See NIOSH Pocket Guide to Chemical Hazards* (DHHS/NIOSH 97-140, 1997) p 16.

USE: As a flux in zinc and tin plating; electroplating, electrolytic refining of zinc; etching solutions in manufacture of printed circuit boards; in dry and Leclanché batteries; as a nitrogen source for fertilization of rice and wheat, manufacturing of explosives; flame suppressant; hardener for formaldehyde-based adhesives; mordant for dyes and printing.

THERAP CAT: Acidifier.

THERAP CAT (VET): Expectorant; diaphoretic; acidifying diuretic.

510. Ammonium Chromate(VI). [7788-98-9] Neutral ammonium chromate. CrH$_8$N$_2$O$_4$; mol wt 152.07. Cr 34.19%, H 5.30%, N 18.42%, O 42.08%. (NH$_4$)$_2$CrO$_4$. Prepn: *Gmelins, Chromium* (8th ed.) **52**, part B, pp 707-712 (1962).

Yellow acicular crystals; loses some NH$_3$ in air; decomposes at 185°. d 1.8. Soly in water: 19.78% (0°); 41.20% (75°). Sparingly sol in liquid ammonia, acetone. Slightly sol in methanol. Practically insol in ethanol. The aq soln is alkaline. *Keep well closed.*

USE: Sensitizing gelatin in photography, in textile printing pastes, in fixing chromate dyes on wool, and as a reagent in analytical chemistry.

511. Ammonium Chromic Sulfate. [13548-43-1] Ammonium disulfatochromate(III); chromic ammonium sulfate. CrH$_4$-NO$_8$S$_2$; mol wt 262.16. Cr 19.83%, H 1.54%, N 5.34%, O 48.82%, S 24.46%. NH$_4$Cr(SO$_4$)$_2$. Prepd by crystallization from a soln contg equimolar amounts of Cr$_2$(SO$_4$)$_3$ and (NH$_4$)$_2$-SO$_4$: Howarth in *ACS Monograph Series* **no. 132**, entitled "Chromium," vol. 1, M. J. Udy, Ed. (Reinhold, New York, 1956) p 287; electrolytic prepn: Nishihara *et al.*, *JP 60 2164* (1960), *C.A.* **55**, 5200e (1961).

Dodecahydrate. Chrome alum ammonium. Small dark-violet or violet-blue, octahedral, cubic crystals; ruby-red by transmitted light. mp 94°; loses 9H$_2$O on melting and the remaining H$_2$O by 300°. d^{25} 1.72. Readily sol in water; slightly sol in alcohol. Aq soln is violet when cold, green when hot.

USE: Mordant in textile industry; in manuf of electrolytic Cr metal.

512. Ammonium Citrate, Dibasic. [3012-65-5] Diammonium citrate; citric acid diammonium salt. C$_6$H$_{14}$N$_2$O$_7$; mol wt 226.18. C 31.86%, H 6.24%, N 12.39%, O 49.52%. Prepn: Heldt, *Ann.* **47**, 157 (1843).

$$\begin{array}{c} COO^- \\ | \\ CH_2 \\ | \\ HO-C-COOH \qquad 2NH_4^+ \\ | \\ CH_2 \\ | \\ COO^- \end{array}$$

Granules or crystals; acid reaction. d 1.48. Sol in about 1 part water, slightly in alc. pH of 0.1M soln in H$_2$O = 4.3.

USE: For the determination of phosphate, esp in fertilizers.

513. Ammonium Cobaltous Phosphate. [14590-13-7] Cobaltous ammonium phosphate. CoH_4NO_4P; mol wt 171.94. Co 34.28%, H 2.34%, N 8.15%, O 37.22%, P 18.01%. NH_4CoPO_4. Prepd by reaction of a cobaltous salt with $(NH_4)_3PO_4$, $(NH_4)_2$-HPO_4, or H_3PO_4 and NH_3: Grat-Cabanac, *Bull. Microsc. Appl.* **8**, 97 (1958); Salutsky *et al.*; McCullogh, Salutsky, **US 3126254**; **US 3141732** (both 1964 to W. R. Grace).

Hydrate, red to violet powder, or monoclinic rectangular lamellae. Practically insol in water. Sol in acids.

USE: As pigment in ceramic glazes and vitreous enamels; as temp indicator in textile industry; in fertilizers for plant nutrition; in Co analysis.

514. Ammonium Cupric Chloride. [15610-76-1] Ammonium tetrachlorocuprate(II); ammonium chlorocuprate; cupric ammonium chloride. $Cl_4CuH_8N_2$; mol wt 241.43. Cl 58.74%, Cu 26.32%, H 3.34%, N 11.60%. $(NH_4)_2CuCl_4$. Prepd by evaporation of a 2:1 soln of NH_4Cl and $CuCl_2$: Chrobak, *Bull. Int. Acad. Polonaise* **1929A**, 361; *C.A.* **24**, 3688[7] (1930); Willet, *J. Chem. Phys.* **41**, 2243 (1964).

Yellow, hygroscopic, orthorhombic crystals. Sol in water. *Keep well closed.*

Dihydrate. Ammonium tetrachlorodiaquocuprate(II). Blue to bluish-green tetragonal, rhombododecahedral crystals. d 2.0. Becomes anhyd at 110-120°; decomposes on stronger heating. Sol in water, alcohol, liquid NH_3; the aq soln is acid to litmus.

USE: Analytical reagent; formerly for determining carbon in iron and steel.

515. Ammonium Dichromate(VI). [7789-09-5] Ammonium bichromate. $Cr_2H_8N_2O_7$; mol wt 252.06. Cr 41.26%, H 3.20%, N 11.11%, O 44.43%. $(NH_4)_2Cr_2O_7$. Prepd from ammonium sulfate and sodium dichromate or by the interaction of ammonia gas and chromic acid in soln: Hartford, *Ind. Eng. Chem.* **41**, 1993 (1949); *Chromium Chemicals* **Vol. 52** (Mutual Chem. Div., Allied Chem.) p. 34-39. *Review: ACS Monograph Series* **no. 132**, entitled "Chromium," vol. I, M. J. Udy, Ed. (Reinhold, New York, 1956) *passim.*

Bright orange-red crystals. *Flammable.* Odorless and non-hygroscopic. Crystal system: monoclinic. Crystal habit: prismatic. d_4^{25} 2.155. Bulk density: 82 lbs/cu ft. Dec at about 180°. Decomposition becomes self-sustaining at about 225° with spectacular swelling and evolution of heat and nitrogen, leaving Cr_2O_3. Heat of soln −23.0 cal/g. Very sol in water. Soly in water (w/w): 15.16% (0°); 26.67% (20°); 36.99% (40°); 46.14% (60°); 54.20% (80°); 60.89% (100°). Acid reaction. A 1% soln has a pH of 3.95 and a 10% soln has a pH of 3.45.

Caution: Causes skin irritation, ulceration, "chrome sores," perforation of nasal septum, pulmonary irritation.

USE: Source of pure nitrogen (esp in the laboratory); in pyrotechnics (Vesuvius fire); in lithography and photo engraving; in special mordant, catalysts, and porcelain finishes; intermediate in the manufacture of pigments; of magnetic recording materials.

516. Ammonium Dithiocarbamate. [513-74-6] Dithiocarbamic acid monoammonium salt; ammonium sulfocarbamate. $CH_6N_2S_2$; mol wt 110.20. C 10.90%, H 5.49%, N 25.42%, S 58.19%. NH_2CSSNH_4. Prepd from CS_2 and NH_3: Mathes, *Inorg. Synth.* **3**, 48 (1950); Redemann *et al., Org. Synth.* **coll. vol. III**, 763 (1955); Gatlow, Hahnkamm, *Z. Anorg. Allg. Chem.* **364**, 161 (1969). Crystal structure: Cappuchi *et al., Chem. Commun.* **1966**, 44l.

Yellow, lustrous almost odorless, orthorhombic crystals when fresh. Undergoes a reversible, exothermic transition at 63°; mp 99° (dec). d_4^{20} 1.451. Sol in water. Decomposes in air, and is then no longer clearly sol; acquires an odor of H_2S; the decomposition products contain ammonium thiocyanate, ammonium sulfide, etc. *Keep in tightly closed bottles.*

USE: Instead of H_2S or $(NH_4)_2S$ for pptg metals in chemical analysis; synthesis of heterocyclic compounds.

517. Ammonium Ferric Oxalate. [14221-47-7] Triammonium tris[ethanedioato(2−)-*O,O'*]ferrate(3−); ammonium trioxalatoferrate(III); ferric ammonium oxalate. $C_6H_{12}FeN_3O_{12}$; mol wt 374.02. C 19.27%, H 3.23%, Fe 14.93%, N 11.23%, O 51.33%. $(NH_4)_3Fe(C_2O_4)_3$. Prepn: *Gmelins, Iron* (8th ed.) **59**, part B, pp 1020-1021 (1932).

Hydrate, bright-green, monoclinic, prismatic crystals. $d^{17.5}$ 1.78. Affected by light. Loses 3 H_2O by 100°, decomp at 160-170°. Very sol in water; practically insol in alcohol. *Protect from light.*

USE: In photography, blueprints; in coloring of Al and Al alloys.

518. Ammonium Ferric Sulfate. [10138-04-2] Ferric ammonium sulfate. $FeH_4NO_8S_2$; mol wt 266.01. Fe 20.99%, H 1.52%, N 5.27%, O 48.12%, S 24.11%. $NH_4Fe(SO_4)_2$. Prepn: *Gmelins, Iron* (8th ed.) **59**, part B, pp 1010-1018 (1932).

Dodecahydrate. Ferric alum; iron alum. Colorless to pale-violet, transparent, efflorescent, octahedral crystals. Odorless; acid styptic taste. mp ~37°; d 1.71. Very sol in water; practically insol in alcohol; pH of 0.1*M* aq soln 2.5.

USE: As analytical reagent; mordant in dyeing and printing textiles.

THERAP CAT: Astringent, styptic.

519. Ammonium Ferricyanide. [14221-48-8] Triammonium hexakis(cyano-*C*)ferrate(3−); ammonium hexacyanoferrate(III). $C_6H_{12}FeN_9$; mol wt 266.06. C 27.09%, H 4.55%, Fe 20.99%, N 47.38%. $(NH_4)_3Fe(CN)_6$. Prepn: *Gmelins, Iron* (8th ed.) **59**, part B, p 1027 (1932).

Trihydrate, red crystals. Freely sol in water; practically insol in alcohol. *Protect from light.*

520. Ammonium Ferrocyanide. [14481-29-9] Triammonium hexakis(cyano-*C*)ferrate(4−); ammonium hexacyanoferrate (II). $C_6H_{16}FeN_{10}$; mol wt 284.10. C 25.37%, H 5.68%, Fe 19.66%, N 49.30%. $(NH_4)_4Fe(CN)_6$. Prepn: *Gmelins, Iron* (8th ed.) **59**, part B, p 1024 (1932); Lux in *Handbook of Preparative Inorganic Chemistry* **Vol. 2**, G. Brauer, Ed. (Academic Press, New York, 2nd ed., 1965) pp 1509-1510.

Trihydrate. Yellow cryst powder. Loses NH_3 on exposure to air and light. Decomposes on heating. Freely sol in water. Practically insol in alcohol. *Protect from light.*

521. Ammonium Ferrous Sulfate. [10045-89-3] Ferrous ammonium sulfate; Mohr's salt. $FeH_8N_2O_8S_2$; mol wt 284.05. Fe 19.66%, H 2.84%, N 9.86%, O 45.06%, S 22.58%. $(NH_4)_2$-$Fe(SO_4)_2$. Manuf from Fe, H_2SO_4 and NH_3: Demmerle *et al., Ind. Eng. Chem.* **42**, 9 (1950); from pickling waste: Brundin, **US 2694657** (1954 to Ekstrand and Tholand). Toxicity study: H. F. Smyth *et al., Am. Ind. Hyg. Assoc. J.* **30**, 470 (1969).

Hexahydrate. Pale blue-green crystals or crystalline powder. Slowly oxidizes and effloresces in air. d_4^{20} 1.86. Soluble in water. Practically insol in alcohol. *Keep well closed and protected from light.* LD_{50} orally in rats: 3.25 g/kg (Smyth).

USE: In photography; as analytical standard; as polymerization catalyst; in dosimeters.

522. Ammonium Fluoride. [12125-01-8] Neutral ammonium fluoride. FH_4N; mol wt 37.04. F 51.29%, H 10.88%, N 37.82%. NH_4F. Prepd by passing ammonia gas into ice-cooled 40% hydrofluoric acid or by heating 1 part NH_4Cl with 2.25 parts NaF and separatng the ammonium fluoride by sublimation: Kwasnik in *Handbook of Preparative Inorganic Chemistry* **vol. 1**, G. Brauer, Ed. (Academic Press, New York, 2nd ed., 1963) p 183. *Review:* Steele, "Ammonium Fluoride" in *Mellor's* **vol. VIII**, supplement I, *Nitrogen* (part 1), 370-377 (1964).

Deliquescent leaflets or needles. Hexagonal prisms by sublimation. Occurs commercially as a granular powder. d 1.015. On heating dec into NH_3 and HF. *Corrodes glass.* Soly in water (0°): 100 g/100 ml. Decomposed by hot water into NH_3 and ammonium bifluoride. $(NH_4F.HF)$. Cannot be obtained by evapn of its aq soln. Slightly sol in alcohol. The aq soln is acid. May be stored in iron vessels. *Incompat.* Quinine salts; soluble calcium salts.

Caution: Ingestion produces nausea, salivation, vomiting, abdominal pain, diarrhea, hemorrhagic gastroenteritis, muscular weakness, tremors, convulsions, vascular collapse. Increased respiration is followed by depression, death. *Chronic toxicity:* mottling of enamel, generalized osteosclerosis, calcification in tendons and ligaments; synostoses.

USE: Etching and frosting glass; as antiseptic in brewing beer; preserving wood; in printing and dyeing textiles; as mothproofing agent.

523. Ammonium Formate. [540-69-2] Formic acid ammonium salt. CH_5NO_2; mol wt 63.06. C 19.05%, H 7.99%, N

22.21%, O 50.74%. HCOONH$_4$. Prepd from formic acid and NH$_3$: Zuffanti, *J. Am. Chem. Soc.* **63**, 3123 (1941); from methylformate and NH$_3$: Kelly, Cuthbert, US 3122584 (1964 to Allied Chem.).

Deliquesc crystals or granules. d 1.27. mp 116°. Sol in less than its own wt of water; sol in alc. *Keep tightly closed.*

USE: In chemical analysis, especially to ppt base metals from salts of the "noble" metals.

524. Ammonium Hexafluoroaluminate. [7784-19-2] Triammonium hexafluoroaluminate(3−); ammonium cryolite; ammonium aluminum fluoride; ammonium fluoaluminate. AlF$_6$H$_{12}$N$_3$; mol wt 195.09. Al 13.83%, F 58.43%, H 6.20%, N 21.54%. (NH$_4$)$_3$AlF$_6$. Prepn from ammonium fluoride and aluminum hydroxide: v. Helmolt, *Z. Anorg. Allg. Chem.* **3**, 127 (1893); Petersen, *J. Prakt. Chem.* [2] **40**, 55 (1889); Kwasnik in *Handbook of Preparative Inorganic Chemistry* vol. 1, G. Brauer, Ed. (Academic Press, New York, 2nd ed. 1963) p 236.

Cubic crystals, d 1.78. Thermally stable to above 100°. Freely sol in water. Does not attack glass.

USE: Prepn of pure aluminum fluoride.

525. Ammonium Hexafluorogallate. [14639-94-2] Triammonium hexafluorogallate(3−); ammonium hexafluogallate. F$_6$GaH$_{12}$N$_3$; mol wt 237.83. F 47.93%, Ga 29.32%, H 5.09%, N 17.67%. (NH$_4$)$_3$GaF$_6$. Prepd from Ga(OH)$_3$, HF and NH$_4$F: Hannebohn, Klemm, *Z. Anorg. Allg. Chem.* **229**, 341 (1936); Kwasnik in *Handbook of Preparative Inorganic Chemistry* vol. 1, G. Brauer, Ed., (Academic Press, New York, 2nd ed., 1963) p 228.

Octahedra. On heating in air changes to Ga$_2$O$_3$; on heating *in vacuo* at 200° for several hours forms GaN.

USE: In the prepn of GaF$_3$.

526. Ammonium Hexafluorophosphate. [16941-11-0] Ammonium hexafluophosphate; ammonium phosphorus hexafluoride. F$_6$H$_4$NP; mol wt 163.00. F 69.93%, H 2.47%, N 8.59%, P 19.00%. NH$_4$PF$_6$. Prepn: Lange, Müller, *Ber.* **63**, 1063 (1930); v. Krueger, *Ber.* **65**, 1265 (1932); Woyski, *Inorg. Synth.* **3**, 111 (1950); Kwasnik in *Handbook of Preparative Inorganic Chemistry* **Vol. 1**, G. Brauer, Ed. (Academic Press, New York, 2nd ed., 1963) p 195.

Square leaflets or tables, seldom rectangular plates; cubic system. d$_4^{18}$ 2.180. Decomposes on heating to a relatively high temp without prior melting. Soly in water (20°): 74.8 g/100 ml. Sol in acetone, methanol, ethanol, methyl acetate. Does not etch glass at room temp. Slowly hydrolyzed by boiling with strong acids.

527. Ammonium Hexafluorosilicate. [16919-19-0] Diammonium hexafluorosilicate(2−); ammonium fluosilicate; ammonium silicofluoride. F$_6$H$_8$N$_2$Si; mol wt 178.15. F 63.99%, H 4.53%, N 15.72%, Si 15.77%. (NH$_4$)$_2$SiF$_6$. Occurs in nature as the mineral ***cryptohalite***. Prepn: *Gmelins, Ammonium* (8th ed.) **23**, pp 414-415 (1936). Crystal structure: Schlemper *et al.*, *J. Chem. Phys.* **44**, 2499 (1966); **45**, 408 (1966). Toxicity study: Simonin, Pierron, *C.R. Seances Soc. Biol. Ses Fil.* **124**, 133 (1937).

Odorless crystalline powder. Two modifications at room temp: stable, cubic phase; metastable, trigonal phase. Freely sol in water. Practically insol in alcohol, acetone. LD orally in guinea pigs: 150 mg/kg (Simonin, Pierron).

Caution: Toxic symptoms similar to sodium fluoride.

USE: In pesticides; in soldering flux; etching glass.

528. Ammonium Hypophosphite. [7803-65-8] H$_6$NO$_2$P; mol wt 83.03. H 7.28%, N 16.87%, O 38.54%, P 37.30%. NH$_4$-H$_2$PO$_2$. Prepn: *Gmelins, Ammonium* (8th ed.) **23**, 416 (1936).

Hygroscopic and deliquesc crystals or white granules. Decomposes when heated with evolution of phosphine which ignites spontaneously. One gram dissolves in about 1 ml water, 0.2 ml boiling water, 20 ml alcohol; freely sol in boiling alcohol, practically insol in acetone. The aq soln is practically neutral. *Keep well closed.*

USE: As catalyst in polyamide manuf.

529. Ammonium Iodide. [12027-06-4] H$_4$IN; mol wt 144.94. H 2.78%, I 87.56%, N 9.66%. NH$_4$I. Contains about 98% NH$_4$I; about 1% ammonium hypophosphite is usually added as a preservative. Prepd from ammonia, iodine and hydrogen peroxide; from ammonia and hydrogen iodide; or from ammonium carbonate and hydrogen iodide: Wulff, Cameron, *Z. Phys. Chem.* **B10**, 350 (1930); Schmeisser in *Handbook of Preparative Inorganic*

Chemistry **vol. 1**, G. Brauer, Ed. (Academic Press, New York, 2nd ed., 1963) p 289. *Review:* Richards "Ammonium Iodide" in *Mellor's* **vol. VIII**, Supplement I, *Nitrogen* (part 1) 448-458 (1964).

White, odorless, very hygroscopic, tetragonal crystals or granular powder, sharp saline taste. Becomes yellow to brown on exposure to air and light because of liberation of iodine. When heated it partly decomposes and partly sublimes. d^{25} 2.5142. One gram dissolves in 0.6 ml water, 0.5 ml boiling water, 3.7 ml alc, 1.5 ml glycerol, 2.5 ml methanol. Except in the presence of a stabilizer, such as ammonium hypophosphite, the aq soln will quickly become yellow. The aq soln is nearly neutral to litmus. pH of 0.1M soln about 4.6. *Keep tightly closed and protected from light.*

USE: In photographic chemicals.

530. Ammonium Lactate. [52003-58-4] DL-Lactic acid ammonium salt. C$_3$H$_9$NO$_3$; mol wt 107.11. C 33.64%, H 8.47%, N 13.08%, O 44.81%. CH$_3$CH(OH)COONH$_4$. Prepd by neutralizing DL-lactic acid with NH$_4$OH: Costello, Filachione, *J. Am. Chem. Soc.* **75**, 1242 (1953).

Crystals from propanol, mp 91-94°. Sol in water, glycerol, 95% alc; slightly sol in methanol; practically insol in ethyl, *n*-propyl, isopropyl, and *n*-butyl alcohols, ether, acetone, ethyl acetate. For a 78.8% by wt soln: n_D^{20} 1.4543, n_D^{25} 1.4536, n_D^{40} 1.4503; d$_4^{20}$ 1.2006, d$_4^{25}$ 1.1984, d$_4^{40}$ 1.1904.

THERAP CAT (VET): Has been used for bovine ketosis.

531. Ammonium Magnesium Chloride. [39733-35-2] Magnesium ammonium chloride. Cl$_3$H$_4$MgN; mol wt 148.70. Cl 71.53%, H 2.71%, Mg 16.34%, N 9.42%. MgNH$_4$Cl$_3$.

Hexahydrate, deliquesc crystals. Sol in 6 parts water. *Keep well closed.*

USE: Prepn of magnesia mixture and anhydrous magnesium chloride.

532. Ammonium Mandelate. [530-31-4] α-Hydroxybenzeneacetic acid monoammonium salt; mandelic acid ammonium salt. C$_8$H$_{11}$NO$_3$; mol wt 169.18. C 56.79%, H 6.55%, N 8.28%, O 28.37%. C$_6$H$_5$CH(OH)COONH$_4$. Prepd from mandelic acid and NH$_3$ or excess of strong NH$_3$-water: Tabern *et al.*, US 2220692 (1941 to Abbott); Baker, US 2209314 (1941 to Squibb).

Very deliquescent, cryst powder; odorless or with slight odor; discolors in light. Very sol in water, sparingly in alc. The aq soln is slightly acid to litmus. *Keep tightly closed and protected from light.*

THERAP CAT: Anti-infective (urinary).

THERAP CAT (VET): Has been used as a urinary antiseptic.

533. Ammonium Molybdate(VI). [12027-67-7] Hexaammonium molybdate (Mo$_7$O$_{24}^{6-}$); ammonium paramolybdate. H$_{24}$-Mo$_7$N$_6$O$_{24}$; mol wt 1163.80. H 2.08%, Mo 57.71%, N 7.22%, O 32.99%. (NH$_4$)$_6$Mo$_7$O$_{24}$. Prepn and structure: Guiter, *Compt. Rend.* **220**, 146 (1945); Lindqvist, *Acta Chem. Scand.* **2**, 88 (1948). Toxicity studies: L. T. Fairhall *et al.*, "The Toxicity of Molybdenum," *U.S. Public Health Service Bulletin No. 293*, Washington D.C. (1945) 39 pp.

Tetrahydrate. Colorless or slightly greenish or yellowish crystals. Sol in 2.3 parts water; practically insol in alcohol. pH of 5% aq soln 5.0 to 5.5.

USE: In photography and for decorating ceramics; for detecting and determining phosphates, arsenates, lead; also as reagent for alkaloids and many other substances.

534. Ammonium Nitrate. [6484-52-2] H$_4$N$_2$O$_3$; mol wt 80.04. H 5.04%, N 35.00%, O 59.97%. NH$_4$NO$_3$. Manuf: *Faith, Keyes & Clark's Industrial Chemicals*, F. A. Lowenheim, M. K. Moran, Eds. (Wiley-Interscience, New York, 4th ed., 1975) pp 97-102. Comprehensive description of manuf processes and physical data: B. T. Federoff *et al.*, *Encyclopedia of Explosives and Related Items* vol. I (Picatinny Arsenal, Dover, N.J., 1960) pp A311-A319. *Review:* Thatcher, "Ammonium Nitrate" in *Mellor's* **vol. VIII**, supplement I, *Nitrogen* (part 1) 506-562 (1964).

Odorless, transparent, hygroscopic, deliquesc crystals or white granules. Five solid phases exist at normal pressure. Orthorhombic at room temp. d 1.72. Dec at about 210°, mostly into H$_2$O and N$_2$O. One gram dissolves in 0.5 ml water, 0.1 ml boil. water, about 20 ml alc, about 8 ml methanol, pH of 0.1M soln in water: 5.43. *Keep well closed.*

Note: Disastrous explosions ascribed to ammonium nitrate occurred in 1947 at Texas City and at Brest.

USE: Making nitrous oxide (laughing gas); in freezing mixtures, safety explosives, matches; pyrotechnics; in fertilizers.

THERAP CAT (VET): Has been used as an expectorant, urinary acidifier.

535. Ammonium Oleate. [544-60-5] (Z)-9-Octadecenoic acid ammonium salt; oleic acid ammonium salt; ammonia soap. $C_{18}H_{37}NO_2$; mol wt 299.49. C 72.19%, H 12.45%, N 4.68%, O 10.68%. $CH_3(CH_2)_7CH=CH(CH_2)_7COONH_4$. Prepd from oleic acid and excess 28-30% NH_3 soln: Stumpf, *Am. Paint J.* **38**, no. 45, 60, 64, 68 (1954), *C.A.* **48**, 12428b (1954).

Yellowish-brown paste, softens at 50-55°F, mp 70-72°F. At 80°F: sol in water; slightly sol in acetone, ethanol, methanol, benzene, CCl_4, xylene, naphtha. Sol in water at 212°F, acetone at 134°F, ethanol at 172°F, methanol at 148°F, benzene at 176°F, CCl_4 at 170°F, xylene at 180°F, naphtha at 160°F.

USE: Detergent, solidifying alcohol, demonstrating liquid crystals according to Lehmann.

536. Ammonium Osmium Chloride. [12125-08-5] Ammonium hexachloroosmate(IV); ammonium chloroosmate; osmium ammonium chloride. $Cl_6H_8N_2Os$; mol wt 439.02. Cl 48.45%, H 1.84%, N 6.38%, Os 43.33%. $(NH_4)_2OsCl_6$. Prepn: Dwyer, Hogarth, *Inorg. Synth.* **5**, 206 (1957).

Red powder, or dark red, octahedral crystals. Soluble in water or alcohol.

537. Ammonium Oxalate. [1113-38-8] Ethanedioic acid diammonium salt. $C_2H_8N_2O_4$; mol wt 124.10. C 19.36%, H 6.50%, N 22.57%, O 51.57%. $NH_4OOCCOONH_4$. Commercial product is 98-99% pure. Prepn of monohydrate from aq oxalic acid and NH_3 or ammonium carbonate: Bérard, *Ann. Chim.* **73**, 277 (1810). *Review: Gmelins, Ammonium* (8th ed.) **23**, pp 400-407 (1936). Crystal structure of monohydrate: Robertson, *Acta Crystallogr.* **18**, 410, 417 (1965).

Monohydrate. Orthorhombic, odorless crystals or granules. *Poisonous!* d 1.50. One gram dissolves in 20 ml water, 2.6 ml boil water; slightly sol in alcohol. The aq soln is practically neutral. pH of 0.1 *M* soln 6.4.

USE: Manuf explosives; electrolytic detinning of iron; in dyeing, metal polishes; for detection and determination of Ca, Pb, and rare earth metals.

538. Ammonium Palmitate. [593-26-0] Hexadecanoic acid ammonium salt; palmitic acid ammonium salt. $C_{16}H_{35}NO_2$; mol wt 273.45. C 70.28%, H 12.90%, N 5.12%, O 11.70%. $CH_3-(CH_2)_{14}COONH_4$. Prepn from palmitic acid and excess 28-30% NH_3 soln: Stumpf, *Am. Paint J.* **38**, No. 45, 60, 64, 68 (1954), *C.A.* **48**, 12428b (1954); from palmitic acid and ammonium carbonate: Reiling, *US 3053867* (1962 to Boston Chem. Prods.).

Yellow-white powder, softens at 38-40°F, mp 70-73°F. At 80°F: sol in water; slightly sol in benzene, xylene; practically insol in acetone, ethanol, methanol, CCl_4, naphtha. Sol in water at 212°F, acetone at 134°F, ethanol at 172°F, methanol at 148°F, benzene at 176°F, CCl_4 at 170°F, xylene at 180°F, naphtha at 160°F.

USE: Waterproofing fabrics, thickening lubricants.

539. Ammonium Pentachlorozincate. [14639-98-6] Zinc ammonium chloride. $Cl_5H_{12}N_3Zn$; mol wt 296.79. Cl 59.73%, H 4.08%, N 14.16%, Zn 22.04%. $ZnCl_2.3NH_4Cl$. Prepn: Klug, Alexander, *J. Am. Chem. Soc.* **66**, 1056 (1944).

Hygroscopic, orthorhombic, bipyramidal crystals. d 1.81. Sublimes at 340° without melting if absolutely dry. Very sol in water.

USE: In manuf of dry cells; as flux for welding, soldering, galvanizing.

540. Ammonium Perchlorate. [7790-98-9] ClH_4NO_4; mol wt 117.49. Cl 30.18%, H 3.43%, N 11.92%, O 54.47%. NH_4-ClO_4. Prepn: *Gmelins, Ammonium* (8th ed.) **23**, pp 196-200 (1936). Review of decompn and combustion: Jacobs, Whitehead, *Chem. Rev.* **69**, 551-590 (1969).

Orthorhombic crystals. Dec on heating. d 1.95. Freely sol in water; sol in methanol; slightly sol in ethanol, acetone; almost insol in ethyl acetate, ether.

USE: In explosives, pyrotechnic compositions, jet and rocket propellants.

541. Ammonium Peroxydisulfate. [7727-54-0] Ammonium persulfate. $H_8N_2O_8S_2$; mol wt 228.20. H 3.53%, N 12.28%, O 56.09%, S 28.10%. $(NH_4)_2S_2O_8$. Available oxygen 7.01%. Contains, when recently made, 95 to 98% $(NH_4)_2S_2O_8$. Prepd by anodic oxidation of a satd $(NH_4)_2SO_4$ soln: Feher in *Handbook of Preparative Inorganic Chemistry* **Vol. 1**, G. Brauer, Ed. (Academic Press, New York, 2nd ed., 1963) p 390. Toxicity study: Smyth *et al., Am. Ind. Hyg. Assoc. J.* **30**, 470 (1969).

Odorless platelike or prismatic (monoclinic) crystals, or white granular powder. Stable for months when pure and dry; dec in presence of moisture, gradually evolving ozone-contg oxygen; dec on heating, evolving O_2 and forming $(NH_4)_2S_2O_7$. d 1.98. Strong oxidizing agent. Freely sol in water; aq soln is acid and dec slowly at room temp and rapidly at higher temp evolving O_2 and forming NH_4HSO_4. *Keep dry, in a cool place and protected from organic matter.* LD_{50} orally in rats: 820 mg/kg (Smyth).

USE: As oxidizer and bleacher; to remove hypo; reducer and retarder in photography; in dyeing, manuf aniline dyes; oxidizer for copper; etching zinc; decolorizing and deodorizing oils; electroplating; washing infected yeast; removing pyrogallol stains; making soluble starch; depolarizer in electric batteries; in anal. chemistry chiefly for detection and determination of manganese.

542. Ammonium Phosphate, Dibasic. [7783-28-0] Secondary ammonium phosphate; diammonium hydrogen phosphate; Fyrex. $H_9N_2O_4P$; mol wt 132.06. H 6.87%, N 21.21%, O 48.46%, P 23.45%. $(NH_4)_2HPO_4$. The grade used medicinally is 98-99% pure. Prepn: *Gmelins, Ammonium* (8th ed.) **23**, pp 422-426 (1936).

Odorless crystals or cryst powder; saline, cooling taste; gradually loses about 8% NH_3 on exposure to air. One gram dissolves in 1.7 ml water, 0.5 ml boil water; practically insol in alcohol, acetone. pH about 8. *Keep well closed.*

USE: Fireproofing textiles, paper, wood, and vegetable fibers; impregnating lamp wicks; preventing afterglow in matches; flux for soldering tin, copper, brass, and zinc; purifying sugar; in yeast cultures; in dentifrices; in corrosion inhibitors; in fertilizers.

543. Ammonium Phosphate, Monobasic. [7722-76-1] Ammonium biphosphate; ammonium dihydrogen phosphate; primary ammonium phosphate. H_6NO_4P; mol wt 115.03. H 5.26%, N 12.18%, O 55.64%, P 26.93%. $(NH_4)H_2PO_4$. Prepn: *Gmelins, Ammonium* (8th ed.) **23**, pp 426-429 (1936).

Odorless crystals or white, cryst powder; stable in air. d 1.80. One gram dissolves in about 2.5 ml water; slightly sol in alcohol; practically insol in acetone. pH of 0.2 molar aq soln 4.2.

USE: As baking powder with sodium bicarbonate; in fermentations (yeast cultures, etc.); fireproofing of paper, wood, fiberboard, etc.

544. Ammonium Phosphite. [51503-61-8] $H_9N_2O_3P$; mol wt 116.06. H 7.82%, N 24.14%, O 41.36%, P 26.69%. Prepn: *Gmelins, Ammonium* (8th ed.) **23**, pp 416-417 (1936).

$$NH_4^+ \quad {}^-O-\overset{\displaystyle OH}{\underset{\displaystyle O^-}{\overset{|}{\underset{|}{P}}}}\quad NH_4^+$$

Monohydrate, deliquesc crystals. Sol in water. *Keep tightly closed.*

USE: As reducing agent; corrosion inhibitor for lubricating grease.

545. Ammonium Phosphomolybdate. [12026-66-3] Ammonium molybdophosphate. $H_{12}Mo_{12}N_3O_{40}P$; mol wt 1876.35. H 0.64%, Mo 61.36%, N 2.24%, O 34.11%, P 1.65%. $(NH_4)_3-PO_4.12MoO_3$. Prepn and constitution: Illingworth, Keggin, *J. Chem. Soc.* **1935**, 575; Thistlewaite, *Analyst* **72**, 531 (1947); Healy, *Radiochim. Acta* **3**, 100 (1964).

Yellow, heavy, cryst powder. Solubility in water (20°): 0.2 ±0.1 g/l. Practically insol in nitric acid; sol in fixed alkali hydroxides.

USE: In phosphorus analysis; as cation-exchanger.

546. Ammonium Phosphotungstate. [1311-90-6] Ammonium tungstophosphate; ammonium phosphowolframate. $H_{12}-N_3O_{40}PW_{12}$; mol wt 2931.15. H 0.41%, N 1.43%, O 21.83%, P 1.06%, W 75.26%. $(NH_4)_3PO_4.12WO_3$. Prepn: Wu, *J. Biol. Chem.* **43**, 189 (1920); Healy. *Radiochim. Acta* **2**, 146 (1964).

Dihydrate, microcryst powder. Soly in water (20°): 0.15 g/l. Freely sol in fixed alkali hydroxide solns.

USE: As ion-exchanger.

547. Ammonium Picrate. [131-74-8] 2,4,6,-Trinitrophenol ammonium salt; picric acid ammonium salt; ammonium picronitrate; ammonium carbazoate. $C_6H_6N_4O_7$; mol wt 246.13. C 29.28%, H 2.46%, N 22.76%, O 45.50%. Prepn: Berl, Berl, **US 2350322** (1944). Crystal structure: Maartmann-Moe, *Acta Crystallogr.* **25B**, 1452 (1969).

Bright yellow, bitter scales or orthorhombic crystals. *Explodes easily from heat or shock.* d 1.72. Soly in water at 20°: about 1 g/100 ml. Slightly sol in alc. "Red modification" is not a distinct polymorph, but a slightly contaminated form of the yellow salt: Mitchell, Bryant, *J. Am. Chem. Soc.* **65**, 128 (1943). Physiologic effects and protective measures in cases of exposure to ammonium picrate: Foulger, *U.S. Armed Forces Med. J.* **4**, 1425 (1953).

USE: In explosives, fireworks, rocket propellants.

548. Ammonium Platinic Chloride. [16919-58-7] Ammonium hexachloroplatinate(IV); ammonium chloroplatinate; platinic ammonium chloride. $Cl_6H_8N_2Pt$; mol wt 443.88. Cl 47.92%, H 1.82%, N 6.31%, Pt 43.95%. $(NH_4)_2PtCl_6$.

Orange-red crystals or yellow powder. d 3.06. Slightly sol in water. Practically insol in alcohol.

USE: Platinum plating; manuf spongy platinum.

549. Ammonium Platinous Chloride. [13820-41-2] Ammonium tetrachloroplatinate(II); ammonium chloroplatinite; ammonium platinochloride; platinous ammonium chloride. $Cl_4H_8N_2Pt$; mol wt 372.97. Cl 38.02%, H 2.16%, N 7.51%, Pt 52.31%. $(NH_4)_2PtCl_4$.

Dark ruby-red crystals. Sol in water.

USE: In photography.

550. Ammonium Salicylate. [528-94-9] 2-Hydroxybenzoic acid monoammonium salt; salicylic acid monoammonium salt; Salicyl-Vasogen. $C_7H_9NO_3$; mol wt 155.15. C 54.19%, H 5.85%, N 9.03%, O 30.94%. Prepd from salicylic acid and aq NH_3: Cahours, *Ann.* **52**, 336 (1844).

Odorless, lustrous crystals or white, cryst powder. Discolors on exposure to light; loses some NH_3 on long exposure to air. Readily discolored by iron compounds. One gram dissolves in 1 ml water, 3 ml alcohol. The aq soln is slightly acid. *Keep in the dark and protected from contamination by iron.*

THERAP CAT: Analgesic; topically to loosen psoriatic scales.

551. Ammonium Selenate. [7783-21-3] $H_8N_2O_4Se$; mol wt 179.03. H 4.50%, N 15.65%, O 35.75%, Se 44.10%. Prepd by treating a soln of selenic acid with ammonia: Retgers, *Z. Phys. Chem.* **8**, 36 (1891); King, *J. Phys. Chem.* **41**, 797 (1937). Crystal structure: Gatlow, *Acta Crystallogr.* **15**, 419 (1962).

Monoclinic crystals. d_4^{20} 2.194. Decomposed by heat. 117 parts dissolve in 100 parts water at 7°, 197 parts in 100 parts at 160°; sol in glacial acetic acid. Insol in alcohol, acetone, ammonia.

552. Ammonium Selenite. [7783-19-9] $H_8N_2O_3Se$; mol wt 163.04. H 4.95%, N 17.18%, O 29.44%, Se 48.43%. Prepd by dissolving selenious acid in a slight excess of concd aqueous ammonia and evaporating: Berzelius, *Acad. Handl. Stockholm* **39**, 13 (1818); Nilson, *Bull. Soc. Chim.* [2] **21**, 253 (1874); *ibid.* [2] **23**, 262 (1875).

White or slightly reddish crystals. Sol in water. Dec by heat. Deliquescent.

USE: In manuf red glass; reagent for alkaloids.

553. Ammonium Stearate. [1002-89-7] Octadecanoic acid ammonium salt; stearic acid ammonium salt. $C_{18}H_{39}NO_2$; mol wt 301.51. C 71.70%, H 13.04%, N 4.65%, O 10.61%. $CH_3-(CH_2)_{16}COONH_4$. Prepn from stearic acid and excess 28-30% NH_3 soln: Stumpf, *Am. Paint J.* **38**, No. 45, 60, 64, 68 (1954), *C.A.* **48**, 12428b (1954); from stearic acid and ammonium carbonate: Reiling, **US 3053867** (1962 to Boston Chem. Prod.).

Yellow-white powder, softens at 35-40°F, mp 70-75°F. At 80°F: sol in methanol, ethanol; slightly sol in water, benzene, xylene, naphtha; practically insol in acetone, CCl_4. Sol in water at 212°F, acetone at 134°F, ethanol at 172°F, methanol at 148°F, benzene at 176°F, CCl_4 at 170°F, xylene at 180°F, naphtha at 160°F.

USE: In vanishing creams, in waterproofing cements.

554. Ammonium Sulfamate. [7773-06-0] Sulfamic acid monoammonium salt; AMS; Ammate. $H_6N_2O_3S$; mol wt 114.12. H 5.30%, N 24.55%, O 42.06%, S 28.10%. $NH_4SO_3NH_2$. Weedkilling prepn: Cupery, Tanberg, **US 2277744** (1941 to du Pont). Prepn from ammonia and sulfamic acid: Sisler, Audrieth, *Inorg. Synth.* **2**, 180 (1946). Toxicity study: Ambrose, *J. Ind. Hyg. Toxicol.* **25**, 26 (1943).

Hygroscopic crystals (large plates). mp 131°, dec 160°. Extremely soluble in water, liquid NH_3; slightly soluble in ethanol; moderately soluble in glycerol, glycol, formamide. pH of 0.27M soln in H_2O = 4.9. Aq solns are stable to boiling. LD_{50} orally in rats: 3.0 g/kg (Ambrose).

Caution: Potential symptoms of overexposure are irritation of eyes, nose and throat; coughing, dyspnea. *See NIOSH Pocket Guide to Chemical Hazards* (DHHS/NIOSH 97-140, 1997) p 16.

USE: In the manuf of fire-retardant compositions, for flameproofing textiles and paper products; in the manuf of weed killing compositions; in electroplating solns; for the generation of nitrous oxide gas.

555. Ammonium Sulfate. [7783-20-2] Sulfuric diammonium salt; mascagnite. $H_8N_2O_4S$; mol wt 132.14. H 6.10%, N 21.20%, O 48.43%, S 24.27%. $(NH_4)_2SO_4$. The "pure" grade of commerce contains at least 99% $(NH_4)_2SO_4$. Prepn: *Gmelins, Ammonium* (8th ed.) **23**, 261-280 (1936). Manuf: *Faith, Keyes & Clark's Industrial Chemicals*, F. A. Lowenheim, M. K. Moran, Eds. (Wiley-Interscience, New York, 4th ed., 1975) pp 103-108. *Review:* Call, "Ammonium Sulfate" in *Mellor's* **Vol. VIII**, Supplement I, *Nitrogen* (part 1) 473-505 (1964). Solubility studies: A. C. D. Rivett, *J. Chem. Soc.* **121**, 379 (1922); R. M. Caven, T. C. Mitchell, *ibid.* **125**, 1428 (1924).

Odorless, orthorhombic crystals or white granules. d 1.77. Dec above 280°. Soly in water (g $(NH_4)_2SO_4$ per 100 g of satd soln): 41.22 (0°); 43.47 (25°); 50.42 (100°) (Rivett). Soly in water (g/100 g H_2O): 70.6 (0°); 76.7 (25°); 103.8 (100°) (Caven, Mitchell). Insol in alcohol, acetone. pH of 0.1 molar aq soln 5.5.

USE: Manuf ammonia alum; in the manuf of H_2SO_4 to free it from nitrogen oxides; analytical uses; freezing mixtures, flameproofing fabrics and paper; manuf viscose silk; tanning, galvanizing iron; in fractionation of proteins. The commercial grade is used as fertilizer.

556. Ammonium Sulfide. [12135-76-1] True ammonium sulfide. H_8N_2S; mol wt 68.14. H 11.83%, N 41.11%, S 47.06%. $(NH_4)_2S$. Prepn: *Gmelins, Ammonium* (8th ed.) **23**, p 246 (1936). Prepn of high purity soln: Johnson *et al.*, *Chemist-Analyst* **53**, 46 (1964).

Forms crystals below $-18°$; at high temps it dec into NH_4HS, NH_3, polysulfides, etc.

USE: To apply patina to bronze, in photographic developers, in textile manufacture, in trace metal analysis.

557. Ammonium Sulfite. [10196-04-0] $H_8N_2O_3S$; mol wt 116.14. H 6.94%, N 24.12%, O 41.33%, S 27.61%. $(NH_4)_2SO_3$. Prepn: *Gmelins, Ammonium* (8th ed.) **23**, pp 256-258 (1936).

Monohydrate. Efflorescent crystals. Under the influence of air and heat loses all its water of crystallization and is gradually oxidized to $(NH_4)_2SO_4$. Sol in water; almost insol in alcohol, acetone. Its aq soln is alkaline to litmus. *Keep tightly closed and in a cool place.*

USE: In photography; as reducing agent; in bricks for blast-furnace linings; in lubricants for metal cold-working.

558. Ammonium Tetrachloroaluminate. [7784-14-7] Aluminum ammonium chloride; ammonium chloroaluminate. $AlCl_4H_4N$; mol wt 186.83. Al 14.44%, Cl 75.90%, H 2.16%, N 7.50%. NH_4AlCl_4. Prepn from $AlCl_3$ and NH_4Cl: Friedman, Taube, *J. Am. Chem. Soc.* **72**, 2236 (1950).

mp 304°. Sol in water and ether.

USE: In the processing of furs.

559. Ammonium Tetrachlorozincate. [14639-97-5] Cl_4-H_8N_2Zn; mol wt 243.30. Cl 58.29%, H 3.31%, N 11.51%, Zn 26.88%. $(NH_4)_2ZnCl_4$. Prepd by dissolving 70 g $ZnCl_2$ and 30 g NH_4Cl in 29 ml hot water and crystallizing: Meerburg, *Z. Anorg. Allg. Chem.* **37**, 199 (1903); Wagenknecht, Juza in *Handbook of Preparative Inorganic Chemistry* Vol. 1, G. Brauer, Ed. (Academic Press, New York, 2nd ed., 1963) p 1072.

White, thin, shiny platelets. Orthorhombic bipyramidal. Hygroscopic. d 1.879. mp $\sim150°$ (dec). Sublimes at 341° without melting, if absolutely dry. Very sol in water with absorption of heat.

560. Ammonium Tetrathiomolybdate. [15060-55-6]; [16330-92-0] (tetrathiomolybdate(2−)). (*T*-4)-Diammonium tetrathioxomolybdate(2−). $H_8MoN_2S_4$; mol wt 260.28. H 3.10%, Mo 36.86%, N 10.76%, S 49.28%. $(NH_4)_2MoS_4$. Forms a complex with copper *in vivo*, blocking intestinal absorption. Prepn: G. Krüss, *Ann.* **225**, 1 (1884); and characterization: J. W. McDonald *et al.*, *Inorg. Chim. Acta* **72**, 205 (1983). Thermal decomposition study: R. I. Walton *et al.*, *Chem. Mater.* **10**, 3737 (1998). Mechanism of action study: G. N. George *et al.*, *J. Am. Chem. Soc.* **125**, 1704 (2003). Use in treatment of copper poisoning in sheep: W. R. Humphries *et al.*, *Vet. Rec.* **123**, 51 (1988). Clinical evaluation in Wilson's disease: G. J. Brewer *et al.*, *Arch. Neurol.* **51**, 545 (1994); **53**, 1017 (1996); **60**, 379 (2003). Review of therapeutic potential: G. J. Brewer, *J. Cell. Mol. Med.* **7**, 11-20 (2003).

uv max (H_2O): 241, 316, 467 nm (ε 24700, 16750, 11850).

USE: In prepn of molybdenum disulfide, *q.v.*, and other transition metal sulfide clusters.

THERAP CAT: Chelating agent (copper); Wilson's Disease treatment.

THERAP CAT (VET): Antidote (copper poisoning).

561. Ammonium Thiocyanate. [1762-95-4] Thiocyanic acid ammonium salt; ammonium rhodanide; ammonium sulfocyanate; ammonium sulfocyanide. CH_4N_2S; mol wt 76.12. C 15.78%, H 5.30%, N 36.80%, S 42.12%. NH_4SCN. Commercial grade is 98-99% pure. Prepn: *Gmelins, Ammonium* (8th ed.) **23**, pp 372-383 (1936). Review of toxicology and human exposure: *Toxicological Profile for Cyanide* (PB98-101207, 1997) 291 pp.

Deliquesc crystals. mp $\sim149°$. Freely sol in water, ethanol; sol in methanol, acetone. Practially insol in $CHCl_3$, ethyl acetate. *Keep tightly closed.*

USE: In matches; double-dyeing fabrics; photography; improving and increasing strength of silks weighted with tin salts; producing grayish-black coating on Zn; manuf transparent artificial resins, thiourea; in pesticides. Detection and determn of small quantities of Fe; determn of Ag, Hg, etc.

562. Ammonium Thiosulfate. [7783-18-8] Ammonium hyposulfite. $H_8N_2O_3S_2$; mol wt 148.21. H 5.44%, N 18.90%, O 32.39%, S 43.27%. $(NH_4)_2S_2O_3$. Prepn: *Gmelins, Ammonium* (8th ed.) **23**, pp 304-306 (1936). Crystal structure: S. T. Teng *et al.*, *Acta Crystallogr.* **B35**, 1682 (1979).

Crystals, dec at 150°. Sol in water; insol in alc, ether.

USE: To clean "white" metal; in photography; in lubricants for metal cold-working.

563. Ammonium Titanium Oxalate. [10580-02-6] Ammonium oxodioxalatotitanate(IV); titanium ammonium oxalate; titanyl ammonium oxalate. $C_4H_8N_2O_9Ti$; mol wt 275.98. C 17.41%, H 2.92%, N 10.15%, O 52.18%, Ti 17.34%. $(NH_4)_2$-$TiO(C_2O_4)_2$.

Monohydrate, crystals or crystalline powder. Very sol in water.

USE: As mordant in dyeing cotton and leather.

564. Ammonium Tungstate(VI). [11120-25-5] Ammonium paratungstate. $H_{40}N_{10}O_{41}W_{12}$; mol wt 3042.44. H 1.33%, N 4.60%, O 21.56%, W 72.51%. $(NH_4)_{10}W_{12}O_{41}$. Prepn: Pilloton, *US 3077379* (1963 to Union Carbide).

Pentahydrate, plates. Freely sol in water; practically insol in alcohol.

USE: Manuf of tungsten alloys.

565. Ammonium Uranate(VI). [7783-22-4] Ammonium uranium oxide $((NH_4)2U_2O_7)$; ammonium diuranate. $H_8N_2O_7U_2$; mol wt 624.13. H 1.29%, N 4.49%, O 17.94%, U 76.28%. $(NH_4)_2U_2O_7$. Incorrectly called *"Uranium Yellow"*; the true uranium yellow is sodium uranate. Prepn: Miller, Armstrong, *US 2466118* (1949 to USAEC); Tridot, *Ann. Chim.* [12] **5**, 358 (1950).

Reddish-yellow, amorphous powder. Practically insol in water, alkalies. Sol in acids or in ammonium carbonate soln.

USE: Painting black on porcelain; as reagent for alkaloids; prepn of UO_2 and UF_4.

566. Ammonium Uranium Carbonate. [18077-77-5] (*HB*-8-22-111′1′1″1″)-Tetraammonium tris[carbonato(2−)-κO,-$\kappa O'$]dioxouranate(4−); ammonium dioxotricarbonatouranate(VI); uranium ammonium carbonate; uranyl ammonium carbonate. C_3-$H_{16}N_4O_{11}U$; mol wt 522.21. C 6.90%, H 3.09%, N 10.73%, O 33.70%, U 45.58%. May contain $2H_2O$.

Yellow crystals; decomposed on exposure to air. Sol in water.

USE: In uranium yellow glazes.

567. Ammonium Uranium Fluoride. [18433-40-4] Triammonium pentafluorodioxouranate; ammonium dioxopentafluorouranate(VI); uranium ammonium fluoride; uranyl ammonium fluoride. $F_5H_{12}N_3O_2U$; mol wt 419.14. F 22.66%, H 2.89%, N 10.03%, O 7.63%, U 56.79%. $UO_2(NH_4)_3F_5$. Usually contains some water of crystallization. Prepn and crystal structure: Nguyen-Quy-Dao, *Bull. Soc. Chim. Fr.* **1968**, 3543; *idem, Acta Crystallogr.* **25B**, 67 (1969).

Greenish-yellow, monoclinic, cryst powder. Freely sol in water; practically insol in alcohol.

USE: Has been used in x-ray work because of its fluorescence under these rays.

568. Ammonium Vanadate(V). [7803-55-6] Ammonium metavanadate. H_4NO_3V; mol wt 116.98. H 3.45%, N 11.97%, O 41.03%, V 43.55%. NH_4VO_3. Prepn: Baker *et al.*, *Inorg. Synth.* **3**, 117 (1950). Toxicity study: H. F. Smyth *et al.*, *Am. Ind. Hyg. Assoc. J.* **30**, 470 (1969).

White or slightly yellow, crystalline powder. Sol in 165 parts water; more sol in hot water, in dil ammonia. Loses water and ammonia on heating. LD_{50} orally in rats: 0.16 g/kg (Smyth).

USE: In dyeing and printing on woolens; staining wood black; manuf vanadium black and "indelible ink"; producing vanadium luster on pottery; as photographic developer; in hematoxylin staining in microscopy; as reagent in analytical chemistry.

569. Ammonium Zirconyl Carbonate. [12616-24-9] Ammonium tricarbonatozirconate. $C_3H_{13}N_3O_{10}Zr$; mol wt 342.37. C 10.52%, H 3.83%, N 12.27%, O 46.73%, Zr 26.64%. $(NH_4)_3ZrOH(CO_3)_3$. Prepd from $ZrO_2CO_2.8H_2O$, NH_4HCO_3 and $(NH_4)_2CO_3$: Blumenthal, *J. Chem. Educ.* **39**, 604 (1962).

Dihydrate. Large prisms from water. Unstable in air, gradually evolving carbon dioxide and ammonia. Sol in water. Marketed as aq soln: d_{24}^{24} 1.238. The aq soln is moderately stable at room temp, although when standing a month or so, it is likely to deposit hydrous zirconia. At temps above 60° aq solns dec rapidly.

USE: Water-repellent. Leaves a zirconium residue after the evaporation of ammonia and carbon dioxide, without leaving other cations or anions.

570. Amobarbital. [57-43-2] 5-Ethyl-5-(3-methylbutyl)-2,4,6-(1*H*,3*H*,5*H*)-pyrimidinetrione; 5-ethyl-5-isopentylbarbituric acid; 5-ethyl-5-isoamylbarbituric acid; barbamil; amylobarbitone; 5-isoamyl-5-ethylbarbituric acid; pentymal; Amal; Amasust; Amytal; Eunoctal; Isomytal; Mylodorm; Sednotic; Stadadorm. C$_{11}$H$_{18}$N$_2$O$_3$; mol wt 226.27. C 58.39%, H 8.02%, N 12.38%, O 21.21%. Prepn: **US 1514573** (1924). Metabolism: Frey, Magnussen, *Arzneim.-Forsch.* **16,** 612 (1966). Toxicity data: K. Irrgang, *ibid.* **15,** 688 (1965). Comprehensive description: N. A. A. Mian *et al.*, *Anal. Profiles Drug Subs.* **19,** 27-58 (1990).

Slightly bitter crystals, mp 156-158°. One gram dissolves in 1300 ml water, in 5 ml alc, in 17 ml chloroform, in 6 ml ether. Freely sol in benzene; sol in alkaline solns. Insol in petr ether, aliphatic hydrocarbons. A satd aq soln is acid to litmus paper. Dissolves in aq solns of alkali hydroxides and carbonates. pH of a saturated soln in water about 5.6. pKa (25°C) 8.0. LD$_{50}$ in mice (mg/kg): 212 s.c. (Irrgang).

Sodium salt. [64-43-7] Sodium Amytal. C$_{11}$H$_{17}$N$_2$NaO$_3$; mol wt 248.25. Hygroscopic, friable granules of powder. Slightly bitter taste. Very soluble in water; sol in alcohol (1:1). Practically insol in ether.

Note: This is a controlled substance (depressant): **21 CFR,** 1308.12 and 1308.13.

THERAP CAT: Sedative, hypnotic.

THERAP CAT (VET): Sedative, hypnotic.

571. Amocarzine. [36590-19-9] 4-Methyl-*N*-[4-[(4-nitrophenyl)amino]phenyl]-1-piperazinecarbothioamide; 4-nitro-4′-[(*N*-methylpiperazinyl)thiocarbonylamino]diphenylamine; CGP-6140. C$_{18}$H$_{21}$N$_5$O$_2$S; mol wt 371.46. C 58.20%, H 5.70%, N 18.85%, O 8.61%, S 8.63%. Orally active macrofilaricide; derivative of amoscanate, *q.v.* Prepn: **BE 772053** (1971 to Agripat); R. Spaun *et al.*, **US 3781290** (1973 to Ciba-Geigy). Mechanism of action study: K. P. Davies *et al.*, *Exp. Parasitol.* **68,** 382 (1989). HPLC determn in biological fluids: S. C. Bhatia *et al.*, *J. Chromatogr.* **434,** 288 (1988). Pharmacokinetics: J. B. Lecaillon *et al.*, *Br. J. Clin. Pharmacol.* **30,** 625, 629 (1990). Clinical trial in onchocerciasis: A. A. Poltera *et al.*, *Lancet* **337,** 583 (1991).

mp 191-196°. Sol in acetonitrile.

THERAP CAT: Anthelmintic (Nematodes).

572. Amodiaquin. [86-42-0] 4-[(7-Chloro-4-quinolinyl)-amino]-2-[(diethylamino)methyl]phenol; 4-[(7-chloro-4-quinolyl)-amino]-α-(diethylamino)-*o*-cresol; 7-chloro-4-(3-diethylamino-methyl-4-hydroxyanilino)quinoline; 7-chloro-4-(3-diethylamino-methyl-4-hydroxyphenylamino)quinoline; 4-(3′-diethylaminometh-yl-4′-hydroxyanilino)-7-chloroquinoline; SN-10751. C$_{20}$H$_{22}$ClN$_3$-O; mol wt 355.86. C 67.50%, H 6.23%, Cl 9.96%, N 11.81%, O 4.50%. Prepd from 4,7-dichloroquinoline and 4-acetamido-α-di-ethylamino-*o*-cresol: Burckhalter *et al.*, *J. Am. Chem. Soc.* **70,** 1363 (1948); **US 2474819; US 2474821** (1949 to Parke, Davis). Alternate synthesis from 2-aminomethyl-*p*-aminophenol and 4,7-dichloroquinoline: Natarajan, Lan, *Arzneim.-Forsch.* **22,** 1230 (1972). Spectral study: J. Kracmar *et al*, *Pharmazie* **29,** 773 (1974). HPLC determn in plasma, blood and urine: E. Pussard *et al.*, *J. Chromatogr.* **374,** 111 (1986). Comprehensive description: I. Ahmad *et al.*, *Anal. Profiles Drug Subs.* **21,** 43-73 (1992).

Crystals from abs. ethanol, mp 208° (dec).

Dihydrochloride dihydrate. [6398-98-7] CAM-AQ1; Camoquin; Flavoquine. C$_{20}$H$_{22}$ClN$_3$O.2HCl.2H$_2$O; mol wt 464.81. Yellow, bitter crystals, dec 150-160°. uv max (methanol): 342 nm (E$_{1cm}^{1\%}$ 349); (water): 341.5 nm (E$_{1cm}^{1\%}$ 389); (0.1*N* HCl): 342 nm (E$_{1cm}^{1\%}$ 396). Sol in water; sparingly sol in alc; very slightly sol in benzene, chloroform, ether. pH of 1% aq soln 4.0 to 4.8.

Dihydrochloride hemihydrate. Yellow crystals from methanol, mp 243°. Slightly sol in water, alc.

THERAP CAT: Antimalarial.

573. Amorolfine. [78613-35-1] *cis*-4-[3-[4-(1,1-Dimeth-ylpropyl)phenyl]-2-methylpropyl]-2,6-dimethylmorpholine; *cis*-4-[3-(4-*tert*-amylphenyl)-2-methylpropyl]-2,6-dimethylmorpholine; (±)-*cis*-2,6-dimethyl-4-[2-methyl-3-(*p-tert*-pentylphenyl)propyl]-morpholine; Ro-14-4767/000. C$_{21}$H$_{35}$NO; mol wt 317.51. C 79.44%, H 11.11%, N 4.41%, O 5.04%. Antimycotic morpholine derivative; inhibits fungal ergosterol biosynthesis. Prepn (unspec stereochem): A. Pfiffner, K. Bohnen, **DE 2752096**; A. Pfiffner, **US 4202894** (1978, 1980 both to Hoffmann-La Roche); of *cis*-form: **NL 8004537** (1980 to Hoffmann-La Roche). *In vitro* comparative antifungal spectrum: S. Shadomy *et al.*, *Sabouraudia* **22,** 7 (1984). Mechanism of action: A. Polak-Wyss *et al.*, *ibid.* **23,** 433 (1985); A. Polak, *Ann. N.Y. Acad. Sci.* **544,** 221 (1988). LC determn in pharmaceutical formulations: M. A. Czech *et al.*, *J. Pharm. Biomed. Anal.* **9,** 1019 (1991). Series of articles on mode of action and clinical trials: *Clin. Exp. Dermatol.* **17,** Suppl. 1, 1-70 (1992). Review of pharmacology and clinical efficacy: M. Haria, H. M. Bryson, *Drugs* **49,** 103-120 (1995).

bp$_{0.1}$ 120°.

Hydrochloride. [78613-38-4] Ro-14-4767/002; Loceryl. C$_{21}$-H$_{35}$NO.HCl; mol wt 353.97.

THERAP CAT: Antifungal (topical).

574. Amoscanate. [26328-53-0] 4-Isothiocyanato-*N*-(4-nitrophenyl)benzeneamine; isothiocyanic acid *p*-(*p*-nitroanilino)-phenyl ester; 4-isothiocyanato-4′-nitrodiphenylamine; nithiocya-mine; C-9333-Go; CGP-4540. C$_{13}$H$_9$N$_3$O$_2$S; mol wt 271.29. C 57.55%, H 3.34%, N 15.49%, O 11.80%, S 11.82%. Analog of nitroscanate, *q.v.* Prepn: K. Antos *et al.*, **DE 1932690** (1970 to Cesk. Akad. Ved), *C.A.* **72,** 100265 (1970); S. Rajappa *et al.*, *J. Chem. Soc. Perkin Trans. 1* **1979,** 2001; N. Viswanathan, R. C. Desai, *Indian J. Chem.* **20B,** 308 (1981). Anthelmintic activity: H. P. Striebel, *Experientia* **32,** 457 (1976); K. R. Middleton *et al.*, *ibid.* **35,** 243 (1979); H. G. Sen, B. N. Deb, *Am. J. Trop. Med. Hyg.* **30,** 992 (1981). HPLC determn in human plasma: W. M. Kofi-Tsekpo, C. W. Karekezi, *Drugs Exp. Clin. Res.* **14,** 31 (1988). Clinical pharmacology: A. B. Vaidya *et al.*, *Br. J. Clin. Pharmacol.* **4,** 463 (1977). Mutagenicity study: B. S. Reddy *et al.*, *Antimicrob. Agents Chemother.* **22,** 707 (1982). Brief review: J. I. Bruce, *Int. J. Parasitol.* **17,** 131-140 (1987).

Crystals from acetone, mp 196-198°.

THERAP CAT: Anthelmintic (Schistosoma).

575. Amosulalol. [85320-68-9] 5-[1-Hydroxy-2-[[2-(2-methoxyphenoxy)ethyl]amino]ethyl]-2-methylbenzenesulfonamide. $C_{18}H_{24}N_2O_5S$; mol wt 380.46. C 56.82%, H 6.36%, N 7.36%, O 21.03%, S 8.43%. Sulfonamide-substituted phenylethanolamine with α- and β-adrenergic blocking activity. Prepn: K. Imai et al., **DE 2843016**; eidem, **US 4217305** (1979, 1980 both to Yamanouchi). Pharmacology and receptor blocking activity: T. Takenaka et al., Eur. J. Pharmacol. **85**, 35 (1982); of isomers: K. Honda et al., J. Pharmacol. Exp. Ther. **236**, 776 (1986). GC determn in urine: H. Kamimura et al., J. Chromatogr. **275**, 81 (1983); HPLC determn in plasma: H. S. Gwak et al., J. Chromatogr. B **818**, 109 (2005). Clinical pharmacokinetics: M. Nakashima et al., Clin. Pharmacol. Ther. **36**, 436 (1984); metabolism: H. Kamimura et al., Xenobiotica **15**, 413 (1985). Clinical evaluation in hypertension: K. Ando et al., J. Cardiovasc. Pharmacol. **20**, 7 (1992).

Monohydrochloride. [93633-92-2] YM-09538; Lowgan. $C_{18}H_{24}N_2O_5S\cdot HCl$; mol wt 416.92. Colorless crystals, mp 158-160°. pK_1 7.4; pK_2 10.2.

R-(−)-**Form hydrochloride.** mp 158°. $[\alpha]_D^{20}$ −30.4° (c = 1 in methanol).

S-(+)-**Form hydrochloride.** mp 158°. $[\alpha]_D^{20}$ +30.7° (c = 1 in methanol).

THERAP CAT: Antihypertensive.

576. Amoxapine. [14028-44-5] 2-Chloro-11-(1-piperazinyl)dibenz[b,f][1,4]oxazepine; CL-67772; Asendin; Asendis; Defanyl; Demolox; Moxadil. $C_{17}H_{16}ClN_3O$; mol wt 313.78. C 65.07%, H 5.14%, Cl 11.30%, N 13.39%, O 5.10%. Prepn: J. Schmutz et al., Helv. Chim. Acta **50**, 245 (1967); eidem, Chim. Ther. **2**, 424 (1967); C. F. Howell et al., **FR 1508536**; eidem, **US 3663696** (1968, 1972 both to Am. Cyanamid). Analysis of amoxapine and its metabolites by GLC: T. B. Cooper, R. G. Kelly, J. Pharm. Sci. **68**, 216 (1979). X-ray crystallography: D. B. Cosulich, F. M. Lovell, Acta Crystallogr. **B33**, 1147 (1977). Pharmacology: E. N. Greenblatt et al., Arch. Int. Pharmacodyn. Ther. **233**, 107 (1978). Clinical study: R. Takahashi et al., J. Int. Med. Res. **7**, 7 (1979). Review: T. A. Ban, Psychopharmacol. Bull. **15**, 22-25 (1979); E. N. Greenblatt et al., in Pharmacological and Biochemical Properties of Drug Substances **vol. 2**, M. E. Goldberg, Ed. (Am. Pharm. Assoc., Washington, DC, 1979) pp 1-18. Review of pharmacology and therapeutic efficacy: S. G. Jue et al., Drugs **24**, 1-23 (1982).

Crystals from benzene/petr ether, mp 175-176°. LD_{50} in mice (mg/kg): 122 i.p.; 112 orally (Howell, 1972).

THERAP CAT: Antidepressant.

577. Amoxicillin. [26787-78-0] (2S,5R,6R)-6-[[(2R)-Amino(4-hydroxyphenyl)acetyl]amino]-3,3-dimethyl-7-oxo-4-thia-1-azabicyclo[3.2.0]heptane-2-carboxylic acid; (−)-6-[2-amino-2-(p-hydroxyphenyl)acetamido]-3,3-dimethyl-7-oxo-4-thia-1-azabicyclo[3.2.0]heptane-2-carboxylic acid; 6-[D(−)-α-amino-p-hydroxyphenylacetamido]penicillanic acid; α-amino-p-hydroxybenzylpenicillin; 6-(p-hydroxy-α-aminophenylacetamido)penicillanic acid; p-hydroxyampicillin; amoxycillin; AMPC; Helvamox; Pasetocin; Penimox; Supramox; Zamocilline. $C_{16}H_{19}N_3O_5S$; mol wt 365.40. C 52.59%, H 5.24%, N 11.50%, O 21.89%, S 8.78%.

Semi-synthetic antibiotic related to penicillin. Prepn: Nayler, Smith, **GB 978178** (1964 to Beecham); eidem, **US 3192198** (1965); Long, Nayler, **DE 1942693** and **GB 1241844** (1970 and 1971 to Beecham), C.A. **72**, 90447q (1970). Resolution of isomers: Long et al., J. Chem. Soc. C **1971**, 1920. Series of articles on activity, pharmacology, absorption and excretion: Antimicrob. Agents Chemother. **1970**, 407-430. Review of antibacterial activity, pharmacokinetics and therapeutic use: R. N. Brogden et al., Drugs **18**, 169-184 (1979). Comprehensive description: A. E. Bird, Anal. Profiles Drug Subs. Excip. **23**, 1-52 (1994).

Trihydrate. [61336-70-7] BRL-2333; Agram; Alfamox; Amocilline; Amodex; Amoram; Amoxidin; Amoxil; Amoxillat; Amoxypen; Ardine; Bactox; Betamox; Bristamox; Cuxacillin; Flemoxine; Gramidil; Hiconcil; Larotid; Ospamox; Polymox; Robamox; Sigamopen; Trimox; Velamox; Widecillin; Wymox; Zimox. Off-white crystalline powder. $[\alpha]_D^{20}$ +246° (c = 0.1). uv max (ethanol): 230, 274 nm (ε 10850, 1400); (0.1N HCl): 229, 272 nm (ε 9500, 1080); (0.1N KOH): 248, 291 (ε 2200, 3000). Solubility (mg/ml): water 4.0; methanol 7.5; abs ethanol 3.4. Insol in hexane, benzene, ethyl acetate, acetonitrile.

Sodium salt. [34642-77-8] Clamoxyl; Ibiamox. $C_{16}H_{18}N_3NaO_5S$; mol wt 387.39.

THERAP CAT: Antibacterial.

THERAP CAT (VET): Antibacterial.

578. AMPA. [77521-29-0] α-Amino-2,3-dihydro-5-methyl-3-oxo-4-isoxazolepropanoic acid; α-amino-3-hydroxy-5-methyl-4-isoxazolepropionic acid. $C_7H_{10}N_2O_4$; mol wt 186.17. C 45.16%, H 5.41%, N 15.05%, O 34.38%. Synthetic excitatory amino acid that characterizes a specific subset of ionotropic glutamate receptors in the CNS, consequently known as AMPA-receptors. The activity resides primarily in the L-isomer. Prepn: J. J. Hansen, P. Krogsgaard-Larsen, J. Chem. Soc. Perkin Trans. 1 **1980**, 1826; M. Begtrup, F. A. Slok, Synthesis **1993**, 861. Characterization of neuroexcitatory activity: P. Krogsgaard-Larsen et al., Nature **284**, 64 (1980). Resolution of enantiomers and stereospecific activity: J. J. Hansen et al., J. Med. Chem. **26**, 901 (1983). Review of AMPA receptors: K. Borges, R. Dingledine, Prog. Brain Res. **116**, 153-170 (1998); and potential for pharmacological intervention: G. J. Lees, Drugs **59**, 33-78 (2000).

L-AMPA

Crystals from water as the monohydrate, mp 252° (dec).

L-AMPA. [83643-88-3] S-AMPA. Crystals from water + ethanol as the hydrate, gradual decomp above ~200°. $[\alpha]_D^{28}$ −21 ±2° (c = 0.19 in water).

579. Ampelopsin. [27200-12-0] (2R-trans)-2,3-Dihydro-3,5,7-trihydroxy-2-(3,4,5-trihydroxyphenyl)-4H-1-benzopyran-4-one; 3,3',4',5,5',7-hexahydroxyflavanone; ampeloptin; dihydromyricetin. $C_{15}H_{12}O_8$; mol wt 320.25. C 56.26%, H 3.78%, O 39.97%. From leaves of Ampelopsis meliaefolia Kudo, Vitaceae: Kotake, Kubota, Ann. **544**, 253 (1940); from bark of Pinus contoria Dougl., Pinaceae: Hergert, J. Org. Chem. **21**, 534 (1956); **US 2870165** (1959 to Rayonier); from Erythrophleum africanum (Welw.) Harms, Caesalpiniaceae: Hansel, Klaffenbach, Arch. Pharm. **294**, 158 (1961). Synthesis from myricetin, q.v.: Kotake, Kubota, J. Inst. Polytech. Osaka City Univ. **1**, no. 2, 47 (1950), C.A. **46**, 2052e (1952).

Consult the Name Index before using this section.

Hemipentahydrate. Needles from water, mp 245-246°.
Hexaacetate. $C_{27}H_{24}O_{14}$. Needles from alc, mp 174-175°.
Hexabenzoate. $C_{57}H_{42}O_{14}$. Needles from alc, mp 174°.

580. Amperozide. [75558-90-6] 4-[4,4-Bis(4-fluorophenyl)butyl]-N-ethyl-1-piperazinecarboxamide; FG-5606; Hogpax. $C_{23}H_{29}F_2N_3O$; mol wt 401.49. C 68.81%, H 7.28%, F 9.46%, N 10.47%, O 3.99%. Piperazine deriv with effects on stress-induced disorders. Prepn: A. K. K. Björk et al., **DE 2941880**; **US 4308387** (1980, 1981 both to Ferrosan). Effects on psychosomatic disorders in man: E. Christensson et al., 3rd World Congr. Biol. Psychiatr., Abstr. F 78 (Stockholm, 1981). Clinical effects in pig prodn: A. Björk et al., Proc. Int. Pig Vet. Soc. Congr., pp 315, 316, 317 (Mexico, 1982).

Hydrochloride. $C_{23}H_{30}ClF_2N_3O$. mp 177-178°.
THERAP CAT (VET): Anti-aggressive.

581. Amphenone B. [2686-47-7] 3,3-Bis[4-aminophenyl]-2-butanone; amphenone; 2-oxo-3,3-bis[p-aminophenyl]butane. $C_{16}H_{18}N_2O$; mol wt 254.33. C 75.56%, H 7.13%, N 11.01%, O 6.29%. Prepn: Allen, Corwin, J. Am. Chem. Soc. **72**, 117 (1950); **US 2539388** (1951). Structure: Bencze, Allen, J. Org. Chem. **22**, 352 (1957). Shows antiestrogenic activity in the chick oviduct test: Hertz et al., Recent Prog. Horm. Res. **11**, 119-147 (1955). Decreases adrenal action. Review: Subsidia Med. **10**, 99-102 (1958).

Crystals, mp 137.5-138°.
Dihydrochloride. $C_{16}H_{20}Cl_2N_2O$. Crystals from ethanol, dec 272-275°. Soluble in water.
Note: Formerly a pinacolone structure was assigned to amphenone B: *1,2-Bis[p-aminophenyl]-2-methyl-1-propanone*.
USE: In biological research.

582. Amphetamine. [300-62-9] α-Methylbenzeneethanamine; (±)-α-methylphenethylamine; 1-phenyl-2-aminopropane; β-phenylisopropylamine; β-aminopropylbenzene; (±)-desoxynorephedrine. $C_9H_{13}N$; mol wt 135.21. C 79.95%, H 9.69%, N 10.36%. Prepn: L. Edeleano, Ber. **20**, 616 (1887); F. P. Nabenhauer, **US 1921424** (1933 to SK & F); W. H. Hartung, J. C. Munch, J. Am. Chem. Soc. **53**, 1875 (1931); N. Kornblum, D. C. Iffland, ibid. **71**, 2137 (1949). Demonstration of binding sites in hypothalamic membranes: S. M. Paul et al., Science **218**, 487 (1982). Toxicity data: M. R. Warren, H. W. Werner, J. Pharmacol. Exp. Ther. **85**, 119 (1945); W. A. Behrendt, R. Deininger, Arzneim.-Forsch. **13**, 711 (1963). Books: C. D. Leake, The Amphetamines: Their Actions

and Uses (Thomas, Springfield, 1958) 167 pp; O. J. Kalant, The Amphetamines: Toxicity and Addiction (Thomas, Springfield, 1966) 151 pp. Review of use and abuse: J. P. Morgan, Substance Abuse: Clinical Problems and Perspectives, J. H. Lowinson, P. Ruiz, Eds. (Williams & Wilkins, Baltimore, 1981) pp 167-184. Review of pharmacology, behavioral effects and therapeutic uses: L. S. Seiden et al., Annu. Rev. Pharmacol. Toxicol. **32**, 639-677 (1993). Review of HPLC determns in biological samples: P. Campins-Falco et al., J. Liq. Chromatogr. **17**, 731-747 (1994).

Mobile liquid. Amine odor. Acrid, burning taste. Volatilizes slowly at room temp. d_4^{25} 0.913. bp_{760} 200-203°; bp_{13} 82-85°. Slightly soluble in water; sol in alc, ether; readily sol in acids. Aq solns are alkaline to litmus. LD_{50} in rats (mg/kg): 180 s.c. (Warren, Werner).
Sulfate. [60-13-9] Benzedrine. $(C_9H_{13}N)_2.H_2SO_4$; mol wt 368.49. White, odorless crystalline powder with slightly bitter taste. mp above 300° (dec). Freely sol in water (1:9); slightly sol in alcohol (about 1:500). A soln of 1 g/10 ml water has a pH 5-6. LD_{50} in mice, rats (mg/kg): 24.2, 55 orally (Behrendt, Deininger).
Phosphate. [139-10-6] Actemin; Aktedron. $C_9H_{13}N.H_3PO_4$; mol wt 233.20. Prepn: Goggin, **US 2507468** (1950 to Clark & Clark). Crystals bitter taste. Sinters at about 150°. Dec around 300°. Freely sol in water. Slightly sol in alcohol. Practically insol in benzene, chloroform, ether. The pH of a 10% soln is about 4.6.
d-Form see Dextroamphetamine.
l-Form. [156-34-3] Levamphetamine; levamfetamine.
Note: This is a controlled substance (stimulant): **21 CFR, 1308.12.**
THERAP CAT: CNS stimulant; anorexic.

583. Amphetaminil. [17590-01-1] α-[(1-Methyl-2-phenylethyl)amino]benzeneacetonitrile; N-(α-methylphenethyl)-2-phenylglycinonitrile; α-phenyl-α-(β-phenylisopropylamino)acetonitrile; α-phenyl-α-(1-methyl-2-phenyl)ethylaminoacetonitrile; α-phenyl-α-N-(1-phenylisopropyl)aminoacetonitrile; AN 1; Aponeuron. $C_{17}H_{18}N_2$; mol wt 250.34. C 81.56%, H 7.25%, N 11.19%. Prepd by reaction of DL-β-phenylisopropylamine with sodium cyanide and benzaldehyde or with α-phenyl-α-bromoacetonitrile: Klosa, **DE 1112987** (1959), C.A. **56**, 3409d (1962); idem, J. Prakt. Chem. **20**, 275 (1963). Pharmacology: Dominok, Oelssner, Acta Biol. Med. Ger. **20**, 625 (1968); Beyer et al., Dtsch. Apoth. Ztg. **111**, 677, 680 (1971). Metabolic studies: Remberg et al., Arch. Toxicol. **29**, 153 (1972). Chemistry: Beyrich et al., Pharmazie **27**, 28 (1972); Gloeckl, Beyrich, ibid. 95.

Crystals from ethanol-water, mp 85-87°.
Hydrochloride. $C_{17}H_{19}ClN_2$. Sinters at 100-104°, mp 134-136°.
THERAP CAT: Psychotropic.

584. Amphomycin. [1402-82-0] Amfomycin; glumamycin. $C_{58}H_{91}N_{13}O_{20}$; mol wt 1290.42. C 53.98%, H 7.11%, N 14.11%, O 24.80%. Polypeptide antibiotic modified at the amino terminus with a fatty acid moiety; active against gram positive bacteria. Produced by Streptomyces canus from soil collected near Syracuse, N.Y.: B. Heinemann et al., Antibiot. Chemother. **3**, 1239 (1953). Production: eidem, **US 3126317** (1964 to Bristol-Myers). Structure and identity with glumamycin: M. Bodanszky et al., J. Am. Chem. Soc. **95**, 2352 (1973). Pharmacology and toxicity: D. E. Tisch et al., Antibiot. Annu. **1954-1955**, 1011. Mechanism of action: H. Tanaka et al., Biochem. Biophys. Res. Commun. **86**, 902 (1979). Use to improve feed efficiency in ruminant animals: M. Gordon, G. J. Christie, **DE 3027370**; *eidem*, **US 4414206** (1981, 1983 both to Bristol-Myers).

R–Asp–MeAsp–Asp–Gly–Asp–Gly–Dab^e–Val–Pro
|
Pip—Dab^t

Dab^e = D-*erythro*-α,β–diaminobutyric acid
Dab^t = L-*threo*-α,β–diaminobutyric acid
Pip = D-pipecolic acid
R   = (+)-3-anteisotridecenoic acid or (+)-3-isododecenoic acid

Acidic, surface-active polypeptide. $[\alpha]_D^{25}$ +7.5° (c = 1 at pH 6). Isoelectric point 3.5-3.6. Soluble in water and the lower alcohols. Insol in nonpolar solvents. Aq solns at neutral pH are stable at room temp for at least one month. Forms sodium and calcium salts. Induces hemolysis. Suggested as a topical agent for animal and plant infections.

Sodium salt. Amorphous solid, sol in water. LD$_{50}$ in mice (mg/kg): 177.8 i.v. (Tisch).

Calcium salt. Crystalline solid, sol in water, methyl alcohol. Used in combination with other antibiotics as antibacterial ingredient in topical anti-inflammatory preparations. LD$_{50}$ in mice (mg/kg): 120.2 i.v. (Tisch).

THERAP CAT: Antibacterial.

585. Amphotericin B. [1397-89-3] Fungizone; Fungilin; Ampho-Moronal. $C_{47}H_{73}NO_{17}$; mol wt 924.08. C 61.09%, H 7.96%, N 1.52%, O 29.43%. Polyene antibiotic produced by *Streptomycetes nodosus* M4575 obtained from soil of the Orinoco river region of Venezuela: Gold *et al., Antibiot. Annu.* **1955-1956**, 579; Vandeputte *et al., ibid.* 587; Dutcher *et al., ibid.* **1956-1957**, 866; Walters *et al., J. Am. Chem. Soc.* **79**, 5076 (1957); Dutcher *et al.*, **US 2908611** (1959 to Olin Mathieson). Structure studies: Borowski *et al., Tetrahedron Lett.* **1965**, 473. Carbon skeleton, ring size, and partial structure: Cope *et al., J. Am. Chem. Soc.* **88**, 4228 (1966). Complete structure: Mechlinski *et al., Tetrahedron Lett.* **1970**, 3873; Borowski *et al., ibid.* 3909; R. C. Pandey, K. L. Rinehart, *J. Antibiot.* **29**, 1035 (1976). Total synthesis: K. C. Nicolaou *et al., J. Am. Chem. Soc.* **109**, 2821 (1987). Toxicity: G. R. Keim *et al., Science* **179**, 584 (1973). Comprehensive description: I. M. Asher *et al., Anal. Profiles Drug Subs.* **6**, 1-42 (1977). Review of clinical experience: H. A. Gallis *et al., Rev. Infect. Dis.* **12**, 308-329 (1990); of lipid formulations: J. W. Hiemenz, T. J. Walsh, *Clin. Infect. Dis.* **22**, Suppl. 2, S133-S144 (1996). *Review:* K. M. Abu-Salah, *Br. J. Biomed. Sci.* **53**, 122-133 (1996).

Deep yellow prisms or needles from DMF. Dec gradually above 170°. uv max (methanol): 406, 382, 363, 345 nm. $[\alpha]_D^{24}$ +333° (acidic DMF); −33.6° (0.1N methanolic HCl). Insol in water at pH 6 to 7. Soly at pH 2 or pH 11 in water: about 0.1 mg/ml. Water soly increased by sodium desoxycholate. Soly in DMF 2 to 4 mg/ml; in DMF + HCl: 60 to 80 mg/ml; in DMSO: 30 to 40 mg/ml. Solids and solns appear stable for long periods between pH 4 and 10 when stored at moderate temps out of contact with light and air. LD$_{50}$ in mice (mg/kg): 88 i.p., 4 i.v. (Keim).

Compd with cholesteryl sulfate. [120895-52-5] Amphotericin B compd with (3β)-cholest-5-en-3-yl hydrogen sulfate (1:1); amphotericin B colloidal dispersion; ABCD; Amphocil. Reviews: L. S. S. Guo, P. K. Working, *J. Liposome Res.* **3**, 473-490 (1993); D. A. Stevens, *J. Infect.* **28**, Suppl.1, 45-49 (1994). Forms uniform disc-shaped particles in aq media.

Liposomal complex. AmBisome. Unilamellar liposomes containing phosphatidylcholine, cholesterol, distearoylphosphatidylglycerol and amphotericin B in a molar ratio of 2: 1:0.8:0.4. Review: R. J. Hay, *J. Infect.* **28**, Suppl. 1, 35-43.

Amphotericin B lipid complex. ABLC; Abelcet. Complex with 2 phospholipids, L-α-dimyristoyl phosphatidylcholine and L-α-dimyristoyl phosphatidylglycerol, which are present in a 7:3 molar ratio. Review: J. Lister, *Eur. J. Haematol. Suppl.* **57**, 18-23 (1996).

THERAP CAT: Antifungal.
THERAP CAT (VET): Antifungal.

586. Ampicillin. [69-53-4] (2S,5R,6R)-6-[[(2R)-Aminophenylacetyl]amino]-3,3-dimethyl-7-oxo-4-thia-1-azabicyclo[3.2.0]heptane-2-carboxylic acid; 6-[D-(−)-α-aminophenylacetamido]penicillanic acid; D(−)-α-aminobenzylpenicillin; AY-6108; BRL-1341; P-50; Albipen; Amfipen; Ampitab; Amplital; Omnipen; Pénicline. $C_{16}H_{19}N_3O_4S$; mol wt 349.40. C 55.00%, H 5.48%, N 12.03%, O 18.32%, S 9.18%. Orally active, semi-synthetic antibiotic; structurally related to penicillin. Prepn: Doyle *et al., US* **2985648** (1961); *eidem*, **GB 902703** (1962 to Beecham); Doyle *et al., J. Chem. Soc.* **1962**, 1440. Prepn of the trihydrate: D. A. Johnson, G. A. Hardcastle, **US 3157640** (1964 to Bristol-Myers); of the anhydrous crystalline form: N. H. Grant, H. E. Alburn, **US 3144445** (1964 to Am. Home Prods.). Alternate syntheses: Dane, Dockner, *Ber.* **98**, 789 (1965); F. Kajfez *et al., J. Heterocycl. Chem.* **13**, 561 (1976). LC determn: M. Margosis, *J. Assoc. Off. Anal. Chem.* **70**, 206 (1987). Series of articles on pharmacology and antibacterial activity: *Br. Med. J.* **2**, 193-206 (1961). Comprehensive description: E. Ivashkiv, *Anal. Profiles Drug Subs.* **2**, 1-61 (1973). Review of pharmacology and clinical efficacy in combination with sulbactam, *q.v.:* D. M. Campoli-Richards, R. N. Brogden, *Drugs* **33**, 577-609 (1987).

Crystals, dec 199-202°. $[\alpha]_D^{23}$ +287.9° (c = 1 in water). Sparingly sol in water.

Monohydrate. Crystals from water, dec 202°. $[\alpha]_D^{21}$ +281° (water). Sparingly sol in water at room temp.

Sesquihydrate. Dec 199-202°. $[\alpha]_D^{20}$ +283.1° (water).

Trihydrate. [7177-48-2] Amblosin; Amipenix; Ampilar; Cymbi; Doktacillin; Penbritin; Polycillin; Principen; Rosampline; Totapen; Vidopen.

Sodium salt. [69-52-3] Ampicin; Binotal; Cilleral; Penbristol; Pentrex; Pentrexyl; Polycillin-N; Synpenin; Totacillin N; Viccillin. $C_{16}H_{18}NaN_3O_4S$; mol wt 371.39.

L(+)-Form. Crystals, dec at about 205°. $[\alpha]_D^{20}$ +209° (c = 0.2 in water). Less active as an antibiotic than D(−)-form.

THERAP CAT: Antibacterial.
THERAP CAT (VET): Antibacterial.

587. Ampiroxicam. [99464-64-9] Carbonic acid ethyl 1-[[2-methyl-3-[(2-pyridinylamino)carbonyl]-2H-1,2-benzothiazin-4-yl]oxy]ethyl ester S,S-dioxide; (±)-4-(1-hydroxyethoxy)-2-methyl-N-2-pyridyl-2H-1,2-benzothiazine-3-carboxamide ethyl carbonate (ester) 1,1-dioxide; 4-[1-(ethoxycarbonyloxy)ethoxy]-2-methyl-N-(2-pyridyl)-2H-1,2-benzothiazine-3-carboxamide 1,1-dioxide; CP-65703; Flucam. $C_{20}H_{21}N_3O_5S$; mol wt 447.46. C 53.68%, H 4.73%, N 9.39%, O 25.03%, S 7.17%. Prodrug of piroxicam, *q.v.* Prepn: A. Marfat, **EP 147177**; *idem*, **US 4551452** (both 1985 to Pfizer). Clinical pharmacokinetics: F. C. Falkner *et al., Xenobiotica* **20**, 645 (1990). Toxicity study: M. Iijima *et al., Oyo Yakuri* **43**, 1 (1992); *C.A.* **116**, 187689k (1992). Pharmacology: T. J. Carty *et al., Agents Actions* **39**, 157 (1993). Clinical trial in oral postoperative pain: K. Kurita *et al., Oral. Ther. Pharmacol.* **10**, 138 (1991); in rheumatoid arthritis: S. Irimajiri *et al., Jpn. J. Inflammation* **12**, 81 (1992).

White crystals from toluene, mp 159-161°. LD_{50} orally in male, female rats: 1798, 747 mg/kg (Iijima).

THERAP CAT: Anti-inflammatory.

588. Ampligen. [38640-92-5] 5'-Inosinic acid homopolymer complex with 5'-cytidylic acid polymer with 5'-uridylic acid (1:1); poly I . poly $(C_{12}U)$; poly(rI) . poly[r$(C_{12}U)_n$]; rI$_n$. r$(C_{12}U)_n$. Synthetic, mismatched double-stranded RNA capable of inducing interferons, *q.v.* Consists of a strand of 5'-inosinic acid (I) units hydrogen bonded to a second strand of 5'-cytidylic- (C) 5'-uridylic- (U) acid units in a 12C:U ratio. Prepn and pharmacology: P. O. P. Ts'o *et al., Mol. Pharmacol.* **12,** 299 (1976). Antiviral activity: W. A. Carter *et al., ibid.* 440; against HIV: D. C. Montefiori, W. M. Mitchell, *Proc. Natl. Acad. Sci. USA* **84,** 2985 (1987); D. C. Montefiori *et al., Antiviral Res.* **9,** 47 (1988). Induction of interferon: D. A. Stringfellow, S. D. Weed, *Antimicrob. Agents Chemother.* **17,** 988 (1980). Mechanism of action study: W. G. Hearl, M. I. Johnston, *Biochem. Biophys. Res. Commun.* **138,** 40 (1986). Antitumor effects in comparison with interferon: H. R. Hubbell *et al., Cancer Res.* **44,** 3252 (1984); and immunomodulatory effects: H. R. Hubbell *et al., ibid.* **45,** 2481 (1985); W. A. Carter *et al., J. Biol. Response Modif.* **4,** 613 (1985). HPLC determn in plasma: M. G. Rosenblum, L. Cheung, *J. Liq. Chromatogr.* **9,** 2869 (1986). Clinical evaluation in metastatic cancers: I. Brodsky *et al., J. Biol. Response Modif.* **4,** 669 (1985). Clinical trial in chronic fatigue syndrome: D. R. Strayer *et al., Clin. Infect. Dis.* **18,** Suppl. 1, S88 (1994); in treatment of HIV: K. A. Thompson *et al., Eur. J. Clin. Microbiol. Infect. Dis.* **15,** 580 (1996).

THERAP CAT: Antiviral; immunomodulator.

589. Amprenavir. [161814-49-9] [(1S,2R)-3-[[(4-Amino-phenyl)sulfonyl](2-methylpropyl)amino]-2-hydroxy-1-(phenyl-methyl)propyl]carbamic acid (3S)-tetrahydro-3-furanyl ester; 4-amino-*N*-((2syn,3S)-2-hydroxy-4-phenyl-3-((S)-tetrahydrofuran-3-yloxycarbonylamino)-butyl)-*N*-isobutylbenzene sulfonamide; 141W94; KVX-478; VX-478; Agenerase; Prozei. $C_{25}H_{35}N_3O_6S$; mol wt 505.63. C 59.38%, H 6.98%, N 8.31%, O 18.99%, S 6.34%. Second generation HIV protease inhibitor. Prepn: R. D. Tung *et al.,* **WO 9405639**; *eidem,* **US 5585397** (1994, 1996 both to Vertex). Crystal structure of complex with HIV protease: E. E. Kim *et al., J. Am. Chem. Soc.* **117,** 1181 (1995). Review of design strategy: M. A. Navia *et al., Int. Antiviral News* **3,** 143-145 (1995); of pharmacology and clinical evaluation: J. C. Adkins, D. Faulds, *Drugs* **55,** 837-842 (1998).

White to cream-colored solid. Soly in water (25°): 0.04 mg/ml.

THERAP CAT: Antiviral.

590. Amprolium. [121-25-5] 1-[(4-Amino-2-propyl-5-pyrimidinyl)methyl]-2-methylpyridinium chloride; 1-[(4-amino-2-propyl-5-pyrimidinyl)methyl]-2-picolinium chloride; Corid. $C_{14}H_{19}ClN_4$; mol wt 278.78. C 60.32%, H 6.87%, Cl 12.72%, N 20.10%. Prepn: Rogers *et al., J. Am. Chem. Soc.* **82,** 2974 (1960); Rogers, Sarett, **US 3020277** (1962 to Merck & Co.), *see*

also **US 3020200**. Formulations as poultry feed: Rogers, Sarett, **US 3065132** (1962 to Merck & Co.).

Hydrochloride. Amprol. $C_{14}H_{19}ClN_4$.HCl; mol wt 315.24. Crystals from methanol + ethanol, dec 248-249°. Freely sol in water, methanol, 95% ethanol, dimethylformamide. Sparingly sol in abs ethanol. Practically insol in isopropanol, butanol, dioxane, acetone, ethyl acetate, acetonitrile, isooctane. pH of 10% aq soln 2.5-3.0.

THERAP CAT (VET): Coccidiostat.

591. Ampyrone. [83-07-8] 4-Amino-1,2-dihydro-1,5-di-methyl-2-phenyl-3*H*-pyrazol-3-one; 4-aminoantipyrine; 4-amino-2,3-dimethyl-1-phenyl-3-pyrazolin-5-one; 1,5-dimethyl-2-phenyl-4-aminopyrazolone. $C_{11}H_{13}N_3O$; mol wt 203.24. C 65.01%, H 6.45%, N 20.68%, O 7.87%. Prepn: Waser, *Helv. Chim. Acta* **8,** 117 (1925); Freedman, Sherndal, **US 1877166** (1933 to H. A. Metz Labs.); Turpechen, Kallro, *C.A.* **36,** 426 (1942); Takahashi, Ogyu, **JP 54 3663** (1954 to Nippon New Drug), *C.A.* **50,** 2687c (1956). Metabolite of aminopyrine, *q.v.*: E. S. Vessel *et al., Clin. Pharmacol. Ther.* **20,** 661 (1976); G. F. Lockwood, J. B. Houston, *J. Pharm. Pharmacol.* **31,** 787 (1979).

Pale yellow crystals from benzene, mp 109°. Sol in water, ethanol, benzene; sparingly sol in ether.

592. Amrinone. [60719-84-8] 5-Amino-(3,4'-bipyridin)-6(1*H*)-one; 3-amino-5-(4-pyridinyl)-2(1*H*)-pyridinone; Win-40680; Cartonic; Inocor; Vesistol; Wincoram. $C_{10}H_9N_3O$; mol wt 187.20. C 64.16%, H 4.85%, N 22.45%, O 8.55%. Selective cAMP phosphodiesterase (PDE-3) inhibitor with positive inotropic and vasodilatory activity. Prepn: G. Y. Lesher, C. J. Opalka, **US 4004012**; **US 4072746** (1977, 1978 both to Sterling). Clinical hemodynamic assessment: J. R. Benotti *et al., N. Engl. J. Med.* **21,** 1373 (1978). Review of pharmacology and clinical efficacy: A. Ward *et al., Drugs* **26,** 468 (1983); M. B. Bottorff *et al., Pharmacotherapy* **5,** 227-237 (1985). Series of articles on pharmacology, mechanism of action and clinical experience: *J. Cardiothorac. Anesth.* **6,** Suppl. 2, 1-57 (1989).

Crystals from DMF, mp 294-297° (dec).

THERAP CAT: Cardiotonic.

593. Amrubicin. [110267-81-7] (7S,9S)-9-Acetyl-9-ami-no-7-[(2-deoxy-β-D-*erythro*-pentopyranosyl)oxy]-7,8,9,10-tetrahy-dro-6,11-dihydroxy-5,12-naphthacenedione; (+)-9-amino-4-de-methoxy-9-deoxy-7-*O*-(2-deoxy-β-D-*erythro*-pentopyranosyl)-daunomycinone. $C_{25}H_{25}NO_9$; mol wt 483.47. C 62.11%, H 5.21%, N 2.90%, O 29.78%. Synthetic anthracycline antibiotic; inhibits DNA topoisomerase II. Prepn: K. Ishizumi *et al., EP*

107486; *eidem*, **US 4673668** (1984, 1987 both to Sumitomo); *eidem*, *J. Org. Chem.* **52**, 4477 (1987). NMR study of complex with DNA: J. Igarashi, M. Sunagawa, *Bioorg. Med. Chem. Lett.* **5**, 2923 (1995). Mechanism of action: M. Hanada *et al.*, *Jpn. J. Cancer Res.* **89**, 1229 (1998). Toxicology: S. Morisada *et al.*, *ibid.* **80**, 77 (1989). Clinical pharmacokinetics: K. Inoue *et al.*, *Invest. New Drugs* **7**, 213 (1989); Y. Matsunaga *et al.*, *Ther. Drug Monit.* **28**, 76 (2006). Clinical evaluation in lung cancer: T. Sugiura *et al.*, *Invest. New Drugs* **23**, 331 (2005); in combination with cisplatin: Y. Ohe *et al.*, *Ann. Oncol.* **16**, 430 (2005).

mp 172-174°. $[\alpha]_D^{20}$ +119° (c = 0.02 in CHCl$_3$).
Hydrochloride. [110311-30-3] SM-5887; Calsed. C$_{25}$H$_{25}$-NO$_9$.HCl; mol wt 519.93. mp 145-151°. LD$_{50}$ i.v. in mice: 32-50 mg/kg (Morisada).
THERAP CAT: Antineoplastic.

594. Amsacrine. [51264-14-3] N-[4-(9-Acridinylamino)-3-methoxyphenyl]methanesulfonamide; 4'-(9-acridinylamino)-methanesulfon-m-anisidide; m-AMSA; CI-880; NSC-249992; SN-11841; Amekrin; Amsidine; Amsidyl. C$_{21}$H$_{19}$N$_3$O$_3$S; mol wt 393.46. C 64.10%, H 4.87%, N 10.68%, O 12.20%, S 8.15%. Cytostatic agent with antiviral and immunosuppressive properties. Prepn: B. F. Cain *et al.*, *J. Med. Chem.* **18**, 1110 (1975). Synthesis and biological properties of spin-labeled amsacrine: B. K. Sinha *et al.*, *ibid.* **19**, 994 (1976). Mechanism of action: W. R. Wilson, *Chem. N. Z.* **37**, 148 (1973). Pharmacologic disposition: R. L. Cysyk *et al.*, *Drug Metab. Dispos.* **5**, 579 (1977). Antiviral activity: D. M. Byrd, *Ann. N.Y. Acad. Sci.* **284**, 463 (1977). Immunosuppressive properties: B. C. Baguley *et al.*, *Eur. J. Cancer* **10**, 169 (1974). Exptl antitumor properties: B. F. Cain, G. J. Atwell, *ibid.* 539. Efficacy in adult acute leukemia: S. S. Legha *et al.*, *Ann. Intern. Med.* **93**, 17 (1980). Toxicologic studies: K. L. Pavkov *et al.*, *U.S. NTIS Report* **PB-298106** (1979) 284 pp, *C.A.* **92**, 34335c (1980). Review of pharmacology and clinical efficacy: J. Hornedo, D. A. Van Echo, *Pharmacotherapy* **5**, 78-90 (1985).

LD$_{50}$ in male, female CDF$_1$ mice: 810 mg/m^2; 729 mg/m^2 orally (Pavkov).
Hydrochloride. NSC-141549. C$_{21}$H$_{19}$N$_3$O$_3$S.HCl; mol wt 429.92. Crystals, mp 197-199°. LD$_{50}$ i.p. in mice: ~60 mg/kg (Byrd).
Methanesulfonate. NSC-156303. C$_{21}$H$_{19}$N$_3$O$_3$S.CH$_3$SO$_3$H; mol wt 489.56. Crystals, mp 292-293°. LD$_{50}$ i.p. in mice: ~24 mg/kg (Byrd).
THERAP CAT: Antineoplastic.

595. Amsonic Acid. [81-11-8] 2,2'-(1,2-Ethenediyl)bis[5-aminobenzenesulfonic acid]; 4,4'-diamino-2,2'-stilbenedisulfonic acid. C$_{14}$H$_{14}$N$_2$O$_6$S$_2$; mol wt 370.40. C 45.40%, H 3.81%, N 7.56%, O 25.92%, S 17.31%. Prepn: Bender, Schultz, *Ber.* **19**, 3234 (1886); H. E. Fierz-David, L. Blangey, *Grundlegende Operationen der Farbenchemie* (Springer-Verlag, Vienna, 7th ed., 1947) p 161; Spiegler, **US 2784220** (1957 to du Pont).

Yellow needles; very slightly sol in water. Forms sparingly water-sol, crystalline salts with many bisquaternary ammonium bases.
USE: In manuf of dyes, bleaching agents.

596. Amtolmetin Guacil. [87344-06-7] N-[[1-Methyl-5-(4-methylbenzoyl)-1H-pyrrol-2-yl]acetyl]glycine 2-methoxyphenyl ester; N-[(1-methyl-5-p-toluoylpyrrol-2-yl)acetyl]glycine o-methoxyphenyl ester; 1-methyl-5-p-toluoylpyrrole-2-acetamidoacetic acid guaicil ester; ST-679; MED-15; Eufans. C$_{24}$H$_{24}$N$_2$O$_5$; mol wt 420.46. C 68.56%, H 5.75%, N 6.66%, O 19.03%. Ester prodrug of tolmetin, *q.v.* Prepn: A. Baglioni, **BE 896018**; *idem*, **US 4578481** (1983, 1986 both to Sigma-Tau). Pharmacology: E. Arrigoni-Martelli, *Drugs Exp. Clin. Res.* **16**, 63 (1990); A. Caruso *et al.*, *ibid.* **18**, 481 (1992). HPLC determn in plasma: A. Mancinelli *et al.*, *J. Chromatogr.* **553**, 81 (1991). Series of articles on pharmacokinetics and clinical trials: *Clin. Ter.* **142** (1 pt 2) 3-59 (1993).

Crystals from cyclohexane-benzene, mp 117-120°. Sol in common organic solvents. LD$_{50}$ in male mice, rats (mg/kg): 1370, 1100 i.p.; >1500, 1450 orally (Baglioni).
THERAP CAT: Analgesic; anti-inflammatory.

597. Amygdalin. [29883-15-6] [(6-O-β-D-Glucopyranosyl-β-D-glucopyranosyl)oxy]benzeneacetonitrile; amygdaloside; mandelonitrile-β-gentiobioside; D-mandelonitrile-β-D-glucosido-6-β-D-glucoside; NSC-15780. C$_{20}$H$_{27}$NO$_{11}$; mol wt 457.43. C 52.51%, H 5.95%, N 3.06%, O 38.47%. The name amygdalin is currently used interchangeably with **laetrile**. Cyanogenic glycoside which occurs in seeds of *Rosaceae;* principally in bitter almonds; also in peaches and apricots. Most common constituent of *Laetrile*® preparations. Structure and synthesis: W. N. Haworth, B. Wylam, *J. Chem. Soc.* **123**, 3120 (1923); Kuhn, *Ber.* **56**, 857 (1923); R. Campbell, W. N. Haworth, *J. Chem. Soc.* **125**, 1337 (1924); Hudson, *J. Am. Chem. Soc.* **46**, 483 (1924); Zemplén, Kunz, *Ber.* **57**, 1357 (1924); Kuhn, Sobotka, *ibid.* 1767; Baumann, Pigman, *The Carbohydrates*, W. Pigman, Ed. (Academic Press, New York, 1957) p 550. Enzymic hydrolysis studies: Haisman, Knight, *Biochem. J.* **103**, 528 (1967). The term Laetrile® has also been applied to **mandelonitrile β-glucuronide**. Purported prepn: E. T. Krebs, E. T. Krebs, Jr., **GB 788855** (1958) and **US 2985664** (1961). Synthesis, characterization and comparison of mandelonitrile β-glucuronide with amygdalin: C. Fenselau *et al.*, *Science* **198**, 625 (1977). Pharmacology and cyanide toxicity studies of amygdalin (laetrile): C. G. Moertel *et al.*, *J. Am. Med. Assoc.* **245**, 591 (1981); M. M. Ames *et al.*, *Cancer Chemother. Pharmacol.* **6**, 51 (1981). Pharmacokinetics: A. G. Rauws *et al.*, *Arch. Toxicol.* **49**, 311 (1982). Determn methods in tissues and fluids: J. Balkon, *J. Anal. Toxicol.* **6**, 244 (1982). Amygdalin (laetrile) is a toxic drug that is not effective as a cancer treatment: C. G. Moertel *et al.*, *N. Engl. J. Med.* **306**, 201 (1982). Review of the controversial use of amygdalin (laetrile): V. Herbert, *Am. J. Clin. Nutr.* **32**, 1121-1158 (1979).

Trihydrate. Orthorhombic columns from water, mp 200°; mp about 220° when anhydr. The once melted and solidif substance remelts at 125-130°. $[\alpha]_D^{20}$ −42° (anhydr basis). One gram dissolves in 12 ml water, in 900 ml alcohol, in 11 ml boiling alcohol.Very sol in boiling water; almost insol in ether. pH of satd aq soln ~7.

Note: The misleading term *vitamin B_{17}* has sometimes been applied to amygdalin.

598. *n*-Amylamine. [110-58-7] 1-Pentanamine; pentylamine; 1-aminopentane. $C_5H_{13}N$; mol wt 87.16. C 68.90%, H 15.03%, N 16.07%. $CH_3(CH_2)_3CH_2NH_2$. Prepd by reduction of valeronitrile with $LiAlH_4$ and with $LiAlH_4$-$AlCl_3$: Nystrom, *J. Am. Chem. Soc.* 77, 2544 (1955).

Liquid. d^{19} 0.766. bp 104°. mp −55°. Very sol in water; sol in alcohol; miscible with ether.

Caution: A strong irritant.

599. Amylase. [9000-92-4] Enzymes catalyzing the hydrolysis of α-1 → 4 glucosidic linkages of polysaccharides such as glycogen, starch, or their degradation products. *Endoamylases* attack the α-1 → 4 linkage at random. A single type of endoamylase is known, *i.e.*, α-amylases (*α-1,4-glucan 4-glucanohydrolases*), so named, because the reducing hemiacetal group liberated by the hydrolysis has α optical configuration and mutarotates downward. The more common α-amylases include those isolated from human saliva, human, hog and rat pancreas, *Bacillus subtilis, B. coagulans, Aspergillus oryzae, A. candidus, Pseudomonas saccharophila,* and barley malt. *Exoamylases* attack the α-1 → 4 linkages only from the non-reducing outer polysaccharide chain ends. Those breaking every glucosidic bond to produce solely α-glucose are known as *glucoamylases* (*γ-amylases*). Those breaking every alternate bond to produce maltose are known as β-amylases (*α-1,4-glucan malto-hydrolases*). Exoamylases are exclusively of vegetable or microbial origin. *Reviews:* Fischer, Stein, "α-Amylases" and French, "β-Amylases" in *The Enzymes* Vol. 4, P. D. Boyer *et al.,* Eds., (Academic Press, New York, 2nd ed., 1960) pp 313-343, 345-368; J. A. Thoma *et al., ibid.* Vol. V (3rd ed., 1971) pp 115-189; W. M. Fogarty, C. T. Kelly, *Microbial Enzymes and Bioconversions,* A. H. Rose, Ed. (Academic Press, New York, 1980) pp 115-170.

α-**Amylase (porcine).** [9000-90-2] Maxilase. Enzyme derived from swine pancrease. mol wt ~45,000. Prepn: Caldwell *et al., J. Am. Chem. Soc.* 74, 4033 (1952).

α-**Amylase (bacterial).** [9000-85-5] Usually derived from *Bacillus subtilis.* Purification: Stein, Fischer, *Helv. Chim. Acta* 40, 529 (1957).

β-**Amylase (sweet potato).** [9000-91-3] Mol wt ~152,000. Prepn: Balls *et al., J. Biol. Chem.* 173, 9 (1948).

USE: In starch processing, brewing, distilling, baking, animal feed, sewage treatment.

THERAP CAT: Enzyme (digestive aid).

600. Amylbenzene. [538-68-1] Pentylbenzene; *n*-amylbenzene; 1-phenylpentane. $C_{11}H_{16}$; mol wt 148.24. C 89.12%, H 10.88%. Prepd by the action of benzylmagnesium chloride on *n*-butyl *p*-toluenesulfonate: Rossander, Marvel, *J. Am. Chem. Soc.* 50, 1491 (1928); Gilman, Heck, *ibid.* 50, 2223 (1928); Gilman, Robinson, *Org. Synth.* coll. vol. II, 47, (1943).

Liquid. mp −78.25°. bp_{760} 202.2°; bp_{10} 81°. d_4^{20} 0.8594. n_D^{20} 1.48849: Vogel, *J. Chem. Soc.* 1948, 607. Insol in water. Sol in alcohol; miscible with ether, benzene.

601. *d*-Amyl Bromide. [534-00-9] 1-Bromo-2-methylbutane; *d*-pri-act-amyl bromide; L-1-bromo-2-methylbutane. C_5-$H_{11}Br$; mol wt 151.04. C 39.76%, H 7.34%, Br 52.90%. CH_3-$CH_2CH(CH_3)CH_2Br$. Prepn: W. Marckwald, *Ber.* 37, 1038 (1904); H. O. Jones, *J. Chem. Soc.* 87, 135 (1905); R. P. Frohardt *et al., J. Am. Chem. Soc.* 81, 5500 (1959).

Liquid. d_4^{20} 1.221. bp 120-121°. n_D^{25} 1.4425; $[\alpha]_D^{28}$ +4.69° (neat). Practically insol in water. Sol in alcohol, ether.

602. *n*-Amyl Bromide. [110-53-2] 1-Bromopentane. C_5-$H_{11}Br$; mol wt 151.04. C 39.76%, H 7.34%, Br 52.90%. CH_3-$(CH_2)_3CH_2Br$. Prepn: Fournier, *Bull. Soc. Chim. Fr.* 35, 623 (1906); Lindstone, Morris, *Chem. Ind. (London)* 1958, 560.

Liquid. d_4^{15} 1.2237. bp_{740} 129.7°. mp −95°. n_D^{20} 1.4444. Practically insol in water. Sol in alcohol; miscible with ether.

603. *tert*-Amyl Bromide. [507-36-8] 2-Bromo-2-methylbutane; 2-bromoisopentane. $C_5H_{11}Br$; mol wt 151.04. C 39.76%, H 7.34%, Br 52.90%. $(CH_3)_2CBrCH_2CH_3$. Prepd from trimethylethylene and dry HBr at −78°: Michael, Weiner, *J. Org. Chem.* 4, 531 (1939).

Liquid, bp 107.4°. d_0^0 1.2439. n_D^{20} 1.4430.

604. *n*-Amyl Butyrate. [540-18-1] Butanoic acid pentyl ester. $C_9H_{18}O_2$; mol wt 158.24. C 68.31%, H 11.47%, O 20.22%. $CH_3CH_2CH_2COOCH_2(CH_2)_3CH_3$. Prepn: Gartenmeister, *Ann.* 233, 269 (1886). Toxicity study: P. M. Jenner *et al., Food Cosmet. Toxicol.* 2, 327 (1964).

Liquid. Apricot-like odor. mp −73.2°. d_0^0 0.8832; d_4^{15} 0.8713. bp_{760} 185°. n_D^{20} 1.4110. Soly in water (50°): 0.54 g/l; very sol in alc, ether. LD_{50} orally in rats: 12210 mg/kg (Jenner).

USE: Has been used in such flavors as apricot, pineapple, pear, plum, and sparingly in some perfume compositions.

605. *n*-Amyl Caproate. [540-07-8] Hexanoic acid pentyl ester; pentyl hexanoate; *n*-caproic acid *n*-amyl ester. $C_{11}H_{22}O_2$; mol wt 186.29. C 70.92%, H 11.90%, O 17.18%. $CH_3(CH_2)_4$-$COOCH_2(CH_2)_3CH_3$. Prepn: Simonini, *Monatsh. Chem.* 13, 320 (1892).

Liquid, bp 222-227°.

606. Amyl Chloride. [543-59-9] 1-Chloropentane; *n*-amyl chloride; *n*-butylcarbonyl chloride. $C_5H_{11}Cl$; mol wt 106.59. C 56.34%, H 10.40%, Cl 33.26%. $CH_3(CH_2)_3CH_2Cl$. Prepd from 1-pentanol and concd HCl in sealed tube at 120°: Conant, Kirner, *J. Am. Chem. Soc.* 46, 245 (1924); with HCl and zinc chloride: Clark, Streight, *Trans. R. Soc. Can. Sect. 3* 23, III 77 (1929); Vogel, *J. Chem. Soc.* 1943, 638, 640; for prepn without admixed 2- and 3-chloropentanes *see* Whitmore's procedure from 1-pentanol with $SOCl_2$ and pyridine: Whitmore *et al., J. Am. Chem. Soc.* 60, 2540 (1938); Mixer, Young, *ibid.* 78, 3382 (1956).

Liquid. d_4^{20} 0.8828. mp −99°. bp_{760} 107.8°. n_D^{20} 1.41280. Flash pt, closed cup: 55°F (13°C). Miscible with alc, ether. Insol in water. Forms a constant boiling mixture with water, bp 82°, with ethanol bp 72.5°.

607. Amylene. [513-35-9] 2-Methyl-2-butene; β-isoamylene; trimethylethylene. C_5H_{10}; mol wt 70.13. C 85.63%, H 14.37%. $(CH_3)_2C=CHCH_3$. Prepd by dehydration of *tert*-amyl alcohol in the presence of *p*-toluenesulfonic acid: Applequist, Babad, *J. Org. Chem.* 27, 288 (1962); by disproportionation of isobutene with propylene or 2-butene: Banks, Regier, *Ind. Eng. Chem. Prod. Res. Dev.* 10, 46 (1971).

Liquid, bp 37.5-38.5°. Highly flammable, flash pt 0°F. d_4^{15} 0.66. Disagreeable odor. Polymerizes on long standing. Practically insol in water. Miscible with alc, ether.

Caution: A simple asphyxiant.

608. *n*-Amyl Ether. [693-65-2] 1,1'-Oxybispentane; pentyl ether; amyl oxide; diamyl ether. $C_{10}H_{22}O$; mol wt 158.28. C 75.88%, H 14.01%, O 10.11%. $[CH_3(CH_2)_3CH_2]_2O$. Prepn from amyl alcohol with concd H_2SO_4: Hinton, Nieuwland, *Proc. Indiana Acad. Sci.* 42, 109 (1933), *C.A.* 27, 5716 (1933).

Liquid, bp 186.75°. mp −69.43°. Flash pt, closed cup: 57°C. d_4^{20} 0.78326, d_4^{25} 0.77924. n_D^{20} 1.41195, n_D^{25} 1.40985: Dreisbach, Martin, *Ind. Eng. Chem.* 41, 2875 (1949). Practically insol in water. Miscible with alcohol, ether.

Caution: Vapors narcotic in high concns.

USE: Industrial solvent.

609. Amylin. [106602-62-4] Diabetes-associated peptide; insulinoma amyloid peptide; islet amyloid polypeptide; IAPP. Peptide hormone co-secreted with insulin by pancreatic beta cells in response to a meal or other nutrient stimuli. Affects carbohydrate absorption and disposition; modulates the effects of insulin. Major component of pancreatic amyloid deposits characteristic of non-insulin-dependent diabetes and thought to be involved in insulin resistance. Amylin deficiency occurs in insulin-dependent diabetes and may contribute to excessive insulin sensitivity and a heightened tendency to hypoglycemia. Structurally homologous with *calcito-*

nin gene related peptide, sharing certain bioactivities such as vasodilation, osteoclast inhibition, and appetite suppression. Isoln from human insulinoma amyloid: P. Westermark *et al., Biochem. Biophys. Res. Commun.* **140**, 827 (1986); from diabetic islet amyloid: *idem et al., Am. J. Pathol.* **127**, 414 (1987); G. J. S. Cooper *et al., Proc. Natl. Acad. Sci. USA* **84**, 8628 (1987). Review of bioactivities: B. J. Edwards, J. E. Morley, *Life Sci.* **51**, 1899-1912 (1992); T. J. Rink *et al., Trends Pharmacol. Sci.* **14**, 113-118 (1993). Review of role in insulin resistance: B. Leighton, G. J. S. Cooper, *Trends Biochem. Sci.* **15**, 295-299 (1990); in carbohydrate metabolism: A. Young *et al., Biochem. Soc. Trans.* **23**, 325 (1995). Effects on appetite regulation and memory: J. E. Morley *et al., Can. J. Physiol. Pharmacol.* **73**, 1042-1046 (1995). Review of role in age-related disease and therapeutic potential: G. J. S. Cooper, C. A. Tse, *Drugs Aging* **9**, 202-212 (1996).

Lys–Cys–Asn–Thr–Ala–Thr–Cys–Ala–Thr–Gln–Arg–Leu–Ala–Asn–Phe–Leu–Val–His
                                                                    Ser
                                                                    Ser
H₂N–Tyr–Thr–Asn–Ser–Gly–Val–Asn–Thr–Ser–Ser–Leu–Ile–Ala–Gly–Phe–Asn–Asn

Human Amylin

Human amylin. [122384-88-7] Amlintide; AC-001. C_{165}-$H_{261}N_{51}O_{55}S_2$; mol wt 3903.28. Composed of 37 amino acid residues; mol wt 3903.35.

THERAP CAT: In treatment of insulin-dependent diabetes.

610. *tert*-**Amyl Isovalerate.** [542-37-0] 3-Methylbutanoic acid 1,1-dimethylpropyl ester; isovaleric acid *tert*-pentyl ester; *tert*-pentyl isovalerate; isovaleric acid *tert*-amyl ester. $C_{10}H_{20}O_2$; mol wt 172.26. C 69.72%, H 11.70%, O 18.58%. $(CH_3)_2CHCH_2$-$COOC(CH_3)_2C_2H_5$. Prepd from trimethylethylene, isovaleric acid and zinc chloride: *Beilstein* **vol. 2**, 312.

Liquid, valerian odor and taste, bp 173-174°. d_4^0 0.8729, d_0^{14} 0.8608. Slightly sol in water; freely sol in alc; miscible with oils.

611. *n*-**Amyl Mercaptan.** [110-66-7] 1-Pentanethiol; amyl thioalcohol. $C_5H_{12}S$; mol wt 104.21. C 57.63%, H 11.61%, S 30.77%. $CH_3(CH_2)_3CH_2SH$. Prepn: Cossar *et al., J. Org. Chem.* **27**, 93 (1962).

Liquid, bp 123-124°, n_D^{25} 1.4439. Penetrating, unpleasant odor. d_4^{20} 0.857. Practically insol in water. Sol in alc.

Caution: Potential symptoms of overexposure are irritation of eyes, skin, nose, throat, respiratory system; headache, nausea, dizziness; vomiting, diarrhea; dermatitis, skin sensitization. *See NIOSH Pocket Guide to Chemical Hazards* (DHHS/NIOSH 97-140, 1997) p 244.

USE: In organic syntheses.

612. *tert*-**Amyl Methyl Ether.** [994-05-8] 2-Methoxy-2-methylbutane; methyl *tert*-pentyl ether; 1,1-dimethylpropyl methyl ether; methyl *tert*-amyl ether; TAME. $C_6H_{14}O$; mol wt 102.17. C 70.53%, H 13.81%, O 15.66%. Gasoline octane booster. Prepn: A. Reychler, *Bull. Soc. Chim. Belg.* **21**, 71 (1907); and properties: T. W. Evans, K. R. Edlund, *Ind. Eng. Chem.* **28**, 1186 (1936). Industrial synthesis and processing: H. Short, *Chem. Eng.* **93**, 34 (1986); S. Randriamahefa *et al., J. Mol. Catal.* **49**, 85 (1988); W. J. Reagan, *Prepr. Pap. - Am. Chem. Soc. Div. Fuel Chem.* **39**, 337 (1994). Reaction equilibria in synthesis: L. K. Rihko *et al., J. Chem. Eng. Data* **39**, 700 (1994). Chromatographic and spectroscopic analyses: J. S. Hardman *et al., Fuel* **72**, 1563 (1993). Comparison with MTBE, *q.v.*, of effects on emissions: W. J. Koehl *et al., Soc. Automot. Eng.* **SP-1000**, vol 2, 289 (1993). Reaction with nitrate radical (environmental implications): S. Langer, E. Ljungström, *J. Phys. Chem.* **98**, 5906 (1994).

Liquid, bp₇₆₀ mm 86.3°. d_4^{15} 0.7750; d_4^{20} 0.7703; d_4^{25} 0.7656; d_4^{30} 0.7607. n_D^{20} 1.3885. Vapor pressure (25°): 75 mm Hg. Soly in water (20°): 1.15g/100g soln.

USE: Fuel additive for gasoline.

613. **Amyl Nitrite.** Mixture of isomers containing not less than 97.0% and not more than 100.0% of $C_5H_{11}NO_2$. Consists chiefly of isoamyl nitrite $[(CH_3)_2CHCH_2CH_2ONO]$, but other isomers are also present.

The N.F. grade has d_{25}^{25} 0.870-0.876. *See* Isoamyl Nitrite.

614. **Amylocaine Hydrochloride.** [532-59-2] 1-(Dimethylamino)-2-methyl-2-butanol benzoate hydrochloride; 1-(dimethylaminomethyl)-1-methylpropyl benzoate hydrochloride; methylethyldimethylaminomethylcarbinol benzoyl ester hydrochloride; amyleine hydrochloride; Stovaine. $C_{14}H_{22}ClNO_2$; mol wt 271.78. C 61.87%, H 8.16%, Cl 13.04%, N 5.15%, O 11.77%. Prepd by benzoylation of 1-(dimethylamino)-2-methyl-2-butanol: Fourneau, Ribas, *Bull. Sci. Pharmacol.* **35**, 273 (1928), *C.A.* **22**, 2919¹ (1928).

Crystals, bitter taste, followed by temporary numbness of the tongue. Dec 177-179°. One gram dissolves in 2 ml water, in 3.3 ml abs ethanol. Practically insol in ether. A 5% aq soln is faintly acid to litmus and neutral to Congo red.

THERAP CAT: Anesthetic (local).

615. **Amyloid β Peptide.** Aβ; β/A4; β-amyloid protein. A 39-43 residue peptide deposited into the extracellular amyloid or senile plaques characterizing Alzheimer's disease and Down's syndrome. Mol wt approx 4,200. Multiple isoforms exist, the most predominant are 40 and 42 amino acids in length. Natural component of cerebrospinal fluid and blood plasma; sol under normal conditions. Forms insol, cytotoxic fibrillar plaques and aggregates in diseased brains. Derived from the proteolysis of *amyloid precursor protein* by proteases known as *secretases*. Purification and characterization: G. G. Glenner, C. W. Wong, *Biochem. Biophys. Res. Commun.* **120**, 885 (1984); C. L. Masters *et al., Proc. Natl. Acad. Sci. USA* **82**, 4245 (1985). Structure and neurotoxicity studies: L. K. Simmons *et al., Mol. Pharmacol.* **45**, 373 (1994); C. J. Pike *et al., J. Neurochem.* **64**, 253 (1995). Brain accumulation of Aβ during aging and in Alzheimer's disease: H. Funato *et al., Am. J. Pathol.* **152**, 1633 (1998). Role of soluble oligomers in Alzheimer's disease: R. Kayed *et al., Science* **300**, 486 (2003). Soly study of Aβ₄₀: P. Sengupta *et al., Biochemistry* **42**, 10506 (2003). Oligomerization study: G. Bitan *et al., J. Biol. Chem.* **278**, 34882 (2003). Clinical evaluation of immunization with aggregated Aβ₄₂ in Alzheimer's disease: C. Hock *et al., Neuron* **38**, 547 (2003). Series of articles: *J. Struct. Biol.* **130**, 87-371 (2000). Review of solid state NMR studies: R. Tycko, *Biochemistry* **42**, 3151-3159 (2003). Reviews of role in Alzheimer's disease: C. L. Joachim, D. J. Selkoe, *Alzheimer Dis. Assoc. Disord.* **6**, 7-34 (1992). D. H. Small, C. A. McLean, *J. Neurochem.* **73**, 443-449 (1999); D. A. Butterfield *et al., Trends Mol. Med.* **7**, 548-554 (2001); W. I. Rosenblum, *Neurobiol. Aging* **23**, 225-230 (2002); T. E. Golde *et al., Biochim. Biophys. Acta* **1502**, 172-187 (2002).

Aβ₄₀. [131438-79-4] Human β-amyloid peptide (1-40).

Aβ₄₂. [107761-42-2] Human β-amyloid peptide (1-42).

616. **Amylpenicillin.** [4493-18-9] (2S,5R,6R)-3,3-Dimethyl-7-oxo-6-[(1-oxohexyl)amino]-4-thia-1-azabicyclo[3.2.0]heptane-2-carboxylic acid; dihydropenicillin F; hexanoylpenicillin; penicillin DF. $C_{14}H_{22}N_2O_4S$; mol wt 314.40. C 53.48%, H 7.05%, N 8.91%, O 20.36%, S 10.20%. Antibiotic produced by the mold *Aspergillus flavus* from a Czapek-Dox medium supplemented with corn steep liquor or by *Penicillium chrysogenum* Q176 or by *P. notatum* strains: McKee, MacPhillamy, *Proc. Soc. Exp. Biol. Med.* **53**, 247 (1943); Bush, Goth, *J. Pharmacol. Exp. Ther.* **78**, 164 (1943); McKee *et al., J. Bacteriol.* **47**, 187 (1944); Bush *et al., J. Pharmacol. Exp. Ther.* **84**, 264 (1945); Fried *et al., J. Biol. Chem.* **163**, 341 (1946); *see also* Wintersteiner under "Flavacidin" in *Chemistry of Penicillin* (Princeton, 1949). Prepn by hydrogenation of 2-pentenylpenicillin: Catch *et al., GB 584852*; Cook, Heilbron in *Chemistry of Penicillin* (Princeton, 1949). Characterization and antibacterial activity: Leigh, *Nature* **163**, 95 (1949).

Sodium salt. [575-47-3] Sodium *n*-amylpenicillinate; flavacidin; flavicin. $C_{14}H_{21}N_2NaO_4S$. Flat, blunt-ended needles from moist acetone or moist ethyl acetate as the monohydrate. When anhydrous, mp 188° (dec). $[\alpha]_D^{23}$ +319°. Very soluble in water.

617. α-Amyrin. [638-95-9] (3β)-Urs-12-en-3-ol; α-amyrenol; viminalol. $C_{30}H_{50}O$; mol wt 426.72. C 84.44%, H 11.81%, O 3.75%. Occurs mostly as acetate in latex of rubber trees, in latex from *Ficus variegata* Blume, *Moraceae*, also in *Balanophora elongata* Blume, *Balanophoraceae*, and in *Erythroxylum coca* Lam. var. *novogranatense* Morris, and var. *spruceanum* Burck, *Erythroxylaceae*. Isoln from *Manila elemi*: Vesterberg, Westerlind, *Ann.* **428**, 247 (1922). Structural studies: Spring, Vickerstaff, *J. Chem. Soc.* **1937**, 249; Beynon *et al., ibid.* **1938**, 1233; Meisels *et al., Helv. Chim. Acta* **32**, 1075 (1949), **38**, 2355 (1955); Melera *et al., ibid.* **39**, 441 (1956). Identity with viminalol: Soldin, Marais, *J. Pharm. Soc.* **55**, 452 (1966). Formation from ursolic acid: Goodson, *J. Chem. Soc.* **1938**, 999; from boswellic acid: Ruzicka, Wirz, *Helv. Chim. Acta* **22**, 948 (1939). Partial synthesis from glycyrrhetic acid and stereochemistry: Corey, Cantrall, *J. Am. Chem. Soc.* **81**, 1745 (1959). *Review:* J. Simonsen, W. C. J. Ross, *The Terpenes* **vol. IV** (University Press, Cambridge, 1957) pp 116-148.

Needles from alcohol, mp 186°. $bp_{0.7}$ 243°. $[\alpha]_D^{17}$ +91.6° (c = 1.3 in benzene). Sol in 22 parts 98% alc. Sol in ether, benzene, chloroform, glacial acetic acid. Slightly sol in petr ether.

Acetate. $C_{32}H_{52}O_2$. Leaflets from petr ether, mp 227°. $[\alpha]_D^{20}$ +76.35° (c = 0.572 in $CHCl_3$).

Benzoate. $C_{37}H_{54}O_2$. Prisms from benzene + acetone, mp 195-196°. $[\alpha]_D^{10}$ +94.6° (c = 1.9 in $CHCl_3$).

618. β-Amyrin. [559-70-6] (3β)-Olean-12-en-3-ol; β-amyrenol. $C_{30}H_{50}O$; mol wt 426.72. C 84.44%, H 11.81%, O 3.75%. Occurs together with α-amyrin. Isoln and structural studies: *see* α-amyrin. *See also* Vesterberg, *Bull. Soc. Chim.* **37**, 742 (1925); Horrmann, Firzlaff, *Arch. Pharm.* **268**, 64 (1930); Ruzicka, Marxer, *Helv. Chim. Acta* **22**, 195 (1939); Jeger, Ruzicka, *ibid.* **28**, 209 (1945); Prelog *et al., ibid.* **29**, 360 (1946). Conversion of δ-amyrene to β-amyrin: Barton *et al., J. Chem. Soc. C* **1968**, 1031. Biogenetic-type total synthesis: van Tamelen *et al., J. Am. Chem. Soc.* **94**, 8229 (1972). Biosynthesis from squalene: Suga *et al., Chem. Lett.* **1972**, 129, 313.

Needles from petr ether or alc, mp 197-197.5°. $bp_{0.8}$ 260°. $[\alpha]_D^{19}$ +99.8° (c = 1.3 in benzene). Somewhat less soluble than the α-form. Soluble in 37 parts of 98% alc.

Acetate. $C_{32}H_{52}O_2$. Prisms from petr ether, mp 241°. $[\alpha]_D^{17}$ +79° (c = 0.9 in benzene).

Palmitate. Balanophorin. $C_{46}H_{80}O_2$. mp 77°. $[\alpha]_D^{15}$ +54.5° (c = 1.1 in benzene). Occurs in *Balanophora elongata* Blume, *Balanophoraceae*, in *Erythroxylum coca* Lam. var *novogranatense* Morris, and var *spruceanum* Burck, *Erythroxylaceae*, in latex from *Ficus variegata* Blume, *Moraceae*.

Di-β-amyrin ether. $C_{60}H_{98}O$. mp 135-136°: Rollett, *Monatsh. Chem.* **47**, 437 (1926).

619. Anabasine. [494-52-0] 3-(2-Piperidinyl)pyridine; 2-(3-pyridyl)piperidine; neonicotine. $C_{10}H_{14}N_2$; mol wt 162.23. C 74.04%, H 8.70%, N 17.27%. In *Anabasis aphylla* L., *Chenopodiaceae:* Orechoff, Menschikoff, *Ber.* **64**, 266 (1931); in *Nicotiana glauca* Graham, *Solanaceae:* Smith, *J. Am. Chem. Soc.* **57**, 959 (1935); Pyriki, Oehler, *Pharmazie* **9**, 685 (1954). Synthesis: Späth, *Ber.* **70B**, 70 (1937). Extracted on a large scale in Russia. Industrial extraction processes: Sadykov, Timbekov, *J. Appl. Chem. USSR* **29**, 148 (1956). Abs config: Lukes *et al., Collect. Czech. Chem. Commun.* **27**, 751 (1962).

Liquid, bp 270-272°; bp_{14} 145-147°; bp_2 105°. Freezes at 9°. d_4^{20} 1.0455. n_D^{20} 1.5430. $[\alpha]_D^{20}$ −83.1°. Sol in water and in most organic solvents.

Hydrochloride. $[\alpha]_D$ +16.5° (c = 10 in water).

Caution: Acute and *subacute toxicity:* increased salivation, vertigo, confusion, disturbed vision and hearing, photophobia, cold extremities, nausea, vomiting, diarrhea, syncope, clonic spasms.

USE: Insecticide.

620. Anabsinthin. [6903-12-4] (3S,3aS,6S,6aR,6bS,7R,-7aR,8S,10aS,11S,13aS,13bS,13cR,14bS,15S)-3,3a,4,5,6,6a,6b,7,7a,-8,9,10,10a,13a,13c,14b-Hexadecahydro-6-hydroxy-3,6,8,11,14,15-hexamethyl-2*H*-8,15-epoxy-7,13b-ethanopentaleno[1″,2″:6,7;5″,-4″:6′,7′]dicyclohepta[1,2-b:1′,2′-b′]difuran-2,12(11*H*)-dione; anabsynthin. $C_{30}H_{40}O_6$; mol wt 496.64. C 72.55%, H 8.12%, O 19.33%. A bitter principle isolated from *Artemisia absinthium* L., *Compositae* (wormwood). Isoln: F. Sorm *et al., Chem. Ind. (London)* **1955**, 569; V. Herout *et al., Collect. Czech. Chem. Commun.* **21**, 1485 (1956). Structure: L. Novotny *et al., Chem. Ind. (London)* **1958**, 465; V. Herout *et al., Collect. Czech. Chem. Commun.* **25**, 1492 (1960); J. Beauhaire *et al., Tetrahedron Lett.* **21**, 3191 (1980).

Anhydrous Form. Crystals from benzene or isopropanol + diisopropyl ether, or by drying over phosphorus pentoxide in vacuo, mp 267°. $[\alpha]_D^{20}$ +113° (c = 1.85 in chloroform).

Monohydrate. Crystals from methanol, mp 210°.

621. Anacardic Acid. Principal constituent of cashew nut-shell liquid, *Anacardium occidentalis* L., *Anacardiaceae*, member of the family of non-isoprenoid long-chain phenols. (*See also* Urushiol.) Anacardic acid is a mixture of **2-hydroxy-6-alkylbenzoic**

acids in which the alkyl chain (C_{11} or higher) is fully saturated (I) or is a monoene (II), a diene (III) or a triene (IV). The name anacardic acid is also used in the literature to designate one component of the mixture: *6-pentadecyl-2-hydroxybenzoic acid* (I) (*6-pentadecyl-salicylic acid*). Another component of the mixture *6-(8-pentade-cenyl)-2-hydroxybenzoic acid* (II), is also known as **ginkgoic acid**. Isoln and structure: Städeler, *Ann.* **63**, 137 (1847); Ruhemann, Skinner, *Ber.* **20**, 1861 (1887); Haagen, Smit, *K. Akad. Wetensch.* **34**, 165 (1931); Backer, Haack, *Rec. Trav. Chim.* **660**, 61 (1941); Kremers, **US 2431127** (1947). Structure of side chain: Sletzinger, Dawson, *J. Org. Chem.* **14**, 670, 849 (1949). Structure of unsaturated components: J. H. P. Tyman, N. Jacobs, *J. Chromatogr.* **54**, 83 (1971). GLC analysis of components: J. H. P. Tyman, *ibid.* **111**, 285 (1975). Synthesis and prostaglandin synthetase inhibiting activity of I and II: Y. Yamagiwa *et al., Tetrahedron* **43**, 3387 (1987); of I: I. Kubo *et al., Chem. Lett.* **1987**, 1101. Antitumor activity of I: H. Itokawa *et al., Chem. Pharm. Bull.* **35**, 3016 (1987). *Review:* J. H. P. Tyman, *Chem. Soc. Rev.* **8**, 499-537 (1979).

I   R = $(CH_2)_7CH_3$
II   R = $CH=CH(CH_2)_5CH_3$
III R = $CH=CHCH_2CH=CH(CH_2)_2CH_3$
IV R = $CH=CHCH_2CH=CHCH_2CH=CH_2$

Mixture, crystals from acetone, mp 34-37°. Sparingly sol in water; freely sol in alc, ether, petr ether. Forms a water-soluble sodium salt.
6-Pentadecyl component (I). Needles from hexane, mp 90.2-91.5°.
6-(8-Pentadecenyl) component (II). Needles, mp 45.3-48° (subl).

622. Anagrelide. [68475-42-3] 6,7-Dichloro-1,5-dihydro-imidazo[2,1-*b*]quinazolin-2(3*H*)-one; 6,7-dichloro-1,2,3,5-tetra-hydroimidazo[2,1-*b*]quinazolin-2-one. $C_{10}H_7Cl_2N_3O$; mol wt 256.09. C 46.90%, H 2.76%, Cl 27.69%, N 16.41%, O 6.25%. Phosphodiesterase inhibitor with antiplatelet activity. Prepn: W. N. Beverung, A. Partyka, **US 3932407**; **US RE 31617**; T. A. Jenks *et al.*, **US 4146718** (1976, 1984, 1979 all to Bristol-Myers); H. Yama-guchi, F. Ishikawa, *J. Heterocycl. Chem.* **18**, 67 (1981). Antithrom-botic and platelet aggregation inhibiting properties: J. S. Fleming, J. P. Buyniski, *Thromb. Res.* **15**, 373 (1979). Mode of action studies: S. S. Tang, M. M. Frojmovic, *J. Lab. Clin. Med.* **95**, 241 (1980); S. Seiler *et al., J. Pharmacol. Exp. Ther.* **243**, 767 (1987). GC-MS determn in human plasma: E. H. Kerns *et al., J. Chroma-togr.* **416**, 357 (1987). Clinical reduction of platelet counts: W. A. Andes *et al., Thromb. Haemostasis* **52**, 325 (1984). Clinical trials to control thrombocytosis in chronic myeloproliferative diseases: M. N. Silverstein *et al., N. Engl. J. Med.* **318**, 1292 (1988); Anagrelide Study Group, *Am. J. Med.* **92**, 69 (1992). Review of pharmacology and clinical experience: P. E. Petrides, *Expert Opin. Pharmacother.* **5**, 1781-1798 (2004).

Hydrochloride monohydrate. [58579-51-4] BL-4162A; BMY-26538-01; Agrylin; Thromboreductin; Xagrid. $C_{10}H_7Cl_2N_3$·O.HCl.H_2O; mol wt 310.56. Off-white powder. Very slightly sol in water; sparingly sol in DMSO, DMF. Also prepd as the hemi-hydrate; crystals from ethanolic HCl, mp >280°.
THERAP CAT: Antithrombocythemic.

623. Anagyrine. [486-89-5] [7*R*-(7α,7aβ,14α)]-7,7a,8,9,-10,11,13,14-Octahydro-7,14-methano-4*H*,6*H*-dipyrido[1,2-*a*:1′,2′-

e][1,5]diazocin-4-one; monolupine; rhombinin. $C_{15}H_{20}N_2O$; mol wt 244.33. C 73.74%, H 8.25%, N 11.47%, O 6.55%. Found in seeds of *Anagyris foetida* L., *Leguminosae* and in gorse *(Ulex euro-paeus* L., *Leguminosae*). Isoln: Ing, *J. Chem. Soc.* **1933**, 504; Orekhov *et al., Ber.* **67**, 1394 (1934); Couch, *J. Am. Chem. Soc.* **61**, 3327 (1939); Briggs, Russell, *J. Chem. Soc.* **1942**, 507; Galinsky, Stern, *Ber.* **77**, 132 (1944); Faugeras, *Ann. Pharm. Fr.* **29**, 241 (1971). Absolute configuration: Okuda *et al., Chem. Ind. (London)* **1961**, 1116; Okuda *et al., Chem. Pharm. Bull.* **13**, 491 (1965). Synthesis: van Tamelen, Baran, *J. Am. Chem. Soc.* **80**, 4659 (1958); Goldberg, Lipkin, *J. Org. Chem.* **37**, 1823 (1972).

Pale yellow glass. bp$_4$ 210-215°; bp$_{12}$ 260-270°. $[\alpha]_D^{25}$ −168° (c = 4.8 in ethanol). Sol in water, alcohol, chloroform; slightly sol in ether, benzene.
Hydrochloride trihydrate. $C_{15}H_{21}ClN_2O$·$3H_2O$. Crystals, mp 235-236° (mp 296° when dry). $[\alpha]_D^{25}$ −142.5° (c = 5). Freely sol in water.

624. Anandamide. [94421-68-8] *(5Z,8Z,11Z,14Z)-N-(2-Hydroxyethyl)-5,8,11,14-eicosatetraenamide; arachidonylethanol-amide; N-(2-hydroxyethyl)arachidonamide.* $C_{22}H_{37}NO_2$; mol wt 347.53. C 76.03%, H 10.73%, N 4.03%, O 9.21%. Endogenous ligand for the mammalian cannabinoid receptor; derivative of arach-idonic acid, *q.v.* Name coined from the Sanskrit word "ananda," meaning bliss. Identification in pig brain: W. A. Devane *et al., Science* **258**, 1946 (1992). Identification in chocolate and cocoa: E. di Tomaso *et al., Nature* **382**, 677 (1996). Pharmacology: P. B. Smith *et al., J. Pharmacol. Exp. Ther.* **270**, 219 (1994). Biosyn-thetic studies: W. A. Devane, J. Axelrod, *Proc. Natl. Acad. Sci. USA* **91**, 6698 (1994); V. Di Marzo *et al., Nature* **372**, 686 (1994). LC/MS/MS determn and distribution in human tissues: C. C. Felder *et al., FEBS Lett.* **393**, 231 (1996). *Review:* V. Di Marzo, A. Fontana, *Prostaglandins Leukotrienes Essent. Fatty Acids* **53**, 1-11 (1995).

625. Anastrozole. [120511-73-1] α,α,α′,α′-Tetramethyl-5-(1*H*-1,2,4-triazol-1-ylmethyl)-1,3-benzenediacetonitrile); 2,2′-[5-(1*H*-1,2,4-triazol-1-ylmethyl)-1,3-phenylene]di(2-methylpropio-nitrile); ZD-1033; ICI-D-1033; Arimidex. $C_{17}H_{19}N_5$; mol wt 293.37. C 69.60%, H 6.53%, N 23.87%. Aromatase inhibitor. Prepn: P. N. Edwards, M. S. Large, **EP 296749**; *eidem*, **US 4935437** (1989, 1990 both to ICI). Reviews of pharmacology, clinical pharmacokinetics: P. V. Plourde *et al., Breast Cancer Res. Treat.* **30**, 103-111 (1994); *idem et al., J. Steroid Biochem. Mol. Biol.* **53**, 175-179 (1995). Clinical trial in advanced breast cancer: A. U. Buzdar *et al., Cancer* **79**, 730 (1997).

Crystals from ethyl acetate/cyclohexane, mp 81-82°.
THERAP CAT: Antineoplastic.

626. Anatabine. [581-49-7] 1,2,3,6-Tetrahydro-2,3'-bipyr-idine; 2-(3-pyridyl)-1,2,3,6-tetrahydropyridine; 1,2,3,6-tetrahydro-2-(3-pyridyl)pyridine. $C_{10}H_{12}N_2$; mol wt 160.22. C 74.96%, H 7.55%, N 17.48%. The most abundant of the minor alkaloids of tobacco: Späth, Kesztler, *Ber.* **70**, 239, 704, 2450 (1937). Fresh *Nicotiana tabacum*, the species most commonly used for the production of cigarette tobacco, contains 3.9% anatabine. Configuration: Lukes *et al., Collect. Czech. Chem. Commun.* **27**, 751 (1962). Total synthesis of *dl*-form: Quan *et al., J. Org. Chem.* **30**, 2769 (1965). Biosynthesis: E. Leete, S. Slattery, *J. Am. Chem. Soc.* **98**, 6326 (1976). Biomimetic synthesis: E. Leete, M. E. Mueller, *ibid.* **104**, 6440 (1982).

l-Form. Liquid. d_4^{19} 1.091. bp$_{10}$ 145-146°. $[\alpha]_D^{17}$ −177.8°. n_D^{20} 1.5676. Misc with water. Sol in alc, ether, benzene.

dl-Form. Liquid. bp$_{6.5}$ 136°.

627. Anatoxins. ANTXS. First isolated, freshwater neuro-toxins present in algal blooms associated with a number of blue-green cyanobacteria including *Anabaena.* spp., *Aphanizomenon* spp. and *Oscillatoria* spp. Responsible for fatal poisoning of cattle and wildlife as well as human illness worldwide. *Review:* W. W. Carmichael *et al., ACS Symp. Ser.* **418**, 87-106 (1990). Review of occurence, chemistry and analysis: K. Sivonen, *Food Sci. Technol.* **103**, 567-581 (2000).

Anatoxin A   Anatoxin A(s)

Anatoxin a. [64285-06-9] 1-(1*R*,6*R*)-9-Azabicyclo[4.2.1]non-2-en-2-ylethanone; 2-acetyl-9-azabicyclo[4.2.1]non-2ene; (+)-ANTX-a; Very Fast Death Factor. $C_{10}H_{15}NO$; mol wt 165.23. C 72.69%, H 9.15%, N 8.48%, O 9.68%. Alkaloid post-synaptic depolarizing neuromuscular blocker acting as a nicotinic cholinergic receptor agonist. Isoln and purification: J. P. Devlin *et al., Can. J. Chem.* **55**, 1367 (1977). Improved purification: K. Harada *et al., Toxicon* **27**, 1289 (1989). Synthesis: H. F. Campbell *et al., Can. J. Chem.* **55**, 1372 (1977); stereoselective synthesis: M. Skrinjar *et al., Tetrahedron: Asymmetry* **3**, 1263 (1992). TLC determn in algal material: I. Ojanpera *et al., Analyst* **116**, 265 (1991); by LC/MS in cyanobacteria and drinking water: A. Furey *et al., Rapid Commun. Mass Spectrom.* **17**, 583 (2003). Review of syntheses: H. L. Mansell, *Tetrahedron* **52**, 6025-6061 (1996). $[\alpha]_D^{25}$ +39.8° (c = 0.676 in abs. ethanol). pKa: 9.4 Degrades readily in sunlight and high pH to non-toxic products. LD$_{50}$ i.p. in mice: 200 μg/kg (Carmichael).

Anatoxin a(s). [103170-78-1] (5*S*)-2-Amino-4,5-dihydro-1-[(hydroxymethoxyphosphinyl)oxy]-*N*,*N*-dimethyl-1*H*-imidazole-5-methanamine; ANTX-a(s). $C_7H_{17}N_4O_4P$; mol wt 252.21. C 33.34%, H 6.79%, N 22.21%, O 25.37%, P 12.28%. Irreversible acetylcholinesterase inhibitor; only known organophosphate toxin found in cyanobacteria. The (s) refers to the production of excess saliva upon ingestion. Identification and preliminary purification: N. A. Mahmood, W. W. Carmichael, *Toxicon* **24**, 425 (1986); anti-cholinesterase activity: *eidem, ibid.* **25**, 1221 (1987). Mechanism of action: E. G. Hyde, W. W. Carmichael, *J. Biochem. Toxicol.* **6**, 195 (1991). Pharmacology in rat: W. O. Cook *et al., J. Environ. Pathol. Toxicol. Oncol.* **9**, 393, (1989). Biosensor determn in water: F. Villatte *et al., Anal. Bioanal. Chem.* **372**, 322 (2002). Stable in neutral or acid conditions. LD$_{50}$ i.p. in mice: 20 μg/kg (Carmichael).

Caution: Overexposure in animals has caused muscle fascicula-tion, gasping and convulsions and death due to respiratory arrest. Anatoxin a(s) also causes salivation. (Carmichael).

628. Anazolene Sodium. [3861-73-2] 4-Hydroxy-5-[[4-(phenylamino)-5-sulfo-1-naphthalenyl]azo]-2,7-naphthalenedisul-fonic acid trisodium salt; 4'-anilino-8-hydroxy-1,1'-azonaphthalene-3,5',6-trisulfonic acid trisodium salt; trisodium 4'-anilino-8-hy-droxy-1,1'-azonaphthalene-3,6,5'-trisulfonate; 1-naphthol-3,6-di-sulfonic acid-8-azo-4'-[*N*-phenyl-1'-naphthylamine]-8'-sulfonic acid trisodium salt; C.I. Acid Blue 92; C.I. 13390; Sulfone Acid Blue R; Coomassie Blue RL. $C_{26}H_{16}N_3Na_3O_{10}S_3$; mol wt 695.58. C 44.89%, H 2.32%, N 6.04%, Na 9.92%, O 23.00%, S 13.83%. Prepn: Ulrich, **US 611664** (1897 to Bayer); **DE 108546** (1899 to Farbwerke Mülheim); *Frdl.* **5**, 497; *Beilstein* **16**, EII, 226; *Colour Index* **vol. 4** (3rd ed., 1971) p 4053. Properties and biological behavior: S. H. Taylor, J. M. Thorp, *Br. Heart J.* **21**, 492 (1959). Clinical applications: S. H. Taylor, J. P. Shillingford, *ibid.* 497; I. S. Menzies, *J. Clin. Pathol.* **19**, 179 (1966).

Reddish-black powder. Soluble in water, acetone, Cellosolve, giving a reddish-blue soln. Slightly sol in alc. Absorption max (water): 565-570 nm; in acetone 585 nm; in human plasma 580-590 nm (E$_{1cm}^{1\%}$ about 600). Aq solns are stable and are not affected by light. Solns up to 10% do not stain the skin appreciably. LD$_{50}$ i.v. in mice: 450 mg/kg (Taylor, Thorp).

THERAP CAT: Diagnostic aid (cardiac output, blood volume de-termination).

629. Ancitabine. [31698-14-3] [2*R*-(2α,3β,3aβ,9aβ)]-2,3,-3a,9a-Tetrahydro-3-hydroxy-6-imino-6*H*-furo[2',3':4,5]oxazolo[3,-2-*a*]pyrimidine-2-methanol; 2,2'-anhydro-(1β-D-arabinofuranosyl)-cytosine; 2,2'-*O*-cyclocytidine; $O^{2,2'}$-cyclocytidine; ancytidine; an-hydroara C. $C_9H_{11}N_3O_4$; mol wt 225.20. C 48.00%, H 4.92%, N 18.66%, O 28.42%. A cytostatic agent and intermediate in the synthesis of cytarabine, *q.v.* Prepn of the hydrochloride: E. R. Walwick *et al., Proc. Chem. Soc. London* **1959**, 84; T. Y. Shen, W. V. Ruyle, **US 3463850** (1969 to Merck & Co.); E. K. Hamamura *et al., J. Med. Chem.* **19**, 654 (1976). General pharmacological properties: H. Hirayama *et al., Oyo Yakuri* **6**, 1259 (1972), *C.A.* **79**, 49175f (1973). Metabolism: D. H. W. Ho, *Drug Metab. Dispos.* **1**, 752 (1973). Biochemical study: *idem, Biochem. Pharmacol.* **23**, 1235 (1974). Pharmacokinetic study: H. S. Chen, J. F. Gross, *Cancer Chemother. Pharmacol.* **2**, 85 (1979). Clinical studies: J. Z. Fin-klestein *et al., Cancer Treat. Rep.* **63**, 1331 (1979); T. Miale *et al., ibid.* 1913. Toxicity studies: K. Sugihara *et al., Oyo Yakuri* **8**, 1469 (1974); H. Hirayama *et al., ibid.* 1693, *C.A.* **83**, 71766, 37747 (1975). HPLC study: V. Reichelova *et al., J. Chromatogr.* **588**, 147 (1991).

Hydrochloride. [10212-25-6] NSC-145668; Cyclo-C. C_9H_{11}-N_3O_4·HCl; mol wt 261.66. Cryst, mp 248-250° (dec). $[\alpha]_D^{23}$ −21.8° (c = 2.0 in water). uv max (pH 1-7): 262, 231 nm (ε 10600, 9400).

THERAP CAT: Antineoplastic.

630. Ancrod. [9046-56-4] Agkistrodon serine proteinase; *Agkistrodon rhodostoma* venom proteinase; A-38414; Arvin; Arwin; Viprinex. Defibrinating enzyme isolated from the venom of the Malayan pit-viper, *Agkistrodon rhodostoma* Boie (*Calloselasma rhodostoma* Boie). Glycosylated serine protease composed of 234 amino acid residues; mol wt ~35,400. Cleaves fibrinogen to form soluble, non-cross-linked fibrin and enhances the local release of tissue plasminogen activator, *q.v.* Isoln: **NL 6502120**; H. A. Reid *et al.*, **US 3657416** (1965, 1972 to Nat. Res. Dev. Corp.); K. E. Chan *et al., Br. J. Haematol.* **11,** 646 (1965). Initial purification: M. P. Esnouf, G. W. Tunnah, *ibid.* **13,** 581 (1967). Improved purification, chemical composition: C. Nolan *et al., Methods Enzymol.* **45,** 205 (1976). Mechanism of action studies: W. R. Bell *et al., J. Lab. Clin. Med.* **91,** 592 (1978); C. R. M. Prentice *et al., Br. J. Haematol.* **83,** 276 (1993). Review of clinical pharmacology and efficacy: K. A. Illig, K. Ouriel, *Semin. Vasc. Surg.* **9,** 303-314 (1996). Review of use in anticoagulant therapy: R. L. Soutar, J. S. Ginsberg, *Crit. Rev. Oncol. Hematol.* **15,** 23-33 (1993); in acute ischemic stroke: R. P. Atkinson, *Drugs* **54,** Suppl. 3, 100-108 (1997).

Colorless substance when pure, having a light powdery texture when in the freeze-dried state. Soluble in physiological saline. Absorbable on weakly basic anion exchange materials.

THERAP CAT: Anticoagulant.

631. Ancymidol. [12771-68-5] α-Cyclopropyl-α-(4-methoxyphenyl)-5-pyrimidinemethanol; α-cyclopropyl-4-methoxy-α-(pyrimidin-5-yl)benzyl alcohol; EL-531; A-Rest; Reducymol. $C_{15}H_{16}N_2O_2$; mol wt 256.30. C 70.29%, H 6.29%, N 10.93%, O 12.48%. Prepn: J. D. Davenport *et al.*, **FR 1569940**; H. M. Taylor *et al.*, **US 3818009** (1969, 1974 to Lilly). Properties and efficacy: M. Snel, J. V. Gramlich, *Meded. Fac. Landbouwwet. Rijksuniv. Gent* **38,** 1033 (1973). GLC determn: R. Frank, E. W. Day, *Anal. Methods Pestic. Plant Growth Regul.* **8,** 475 (1976); S. D. West, E. W. Day, *J. Assoc. Off. Anal. Chem.* **60,** 904 (1977). Studies on the specificity and site of action: R. C. Coolbaugh *et al., Plant Physiol.* **62,** 571 (1978).

Cryst. solid, mp 110-111°. Vapor pressure at 50°: <1 × 10⁻⁶ mm Hg. Thermally stable. Soly in water at 25°: ~650 mg/l. Readily sol in acetone, methanol, ethyl acetate, chloroform, acetonitrile. Moderately sol in aromatic hydrocarbons; slightly sol in saturated hydrocarbons. LD50 in rats, mice (mg/kg): 4500, 5000 orally (Snel, Gramlich).

USE: Plant growth regulator.

632. Andrographis. Chuan-xin-lian; Kalmegh. Herbaceous plant, *Andrographis paniculata* Nees, *Acanthaceae*, which has been used in Asian traditional medicine as an antipyretic, anti-inflammatory, and hepatoprotectant. *Habit.* Tropical regions of Asia; common ground flora in dry deciduous forests of southeastern India. *Constit.* Andrographolide, *q.v.,* deoxyandrographolide, neoandrographolide, andrographidines, paniculides. Brief description: R. D. Girach *et al., Int. J. Pharmacognosy* **32,** 95 (1994). Review of constituents and pharmacology: W. Tang, G. Eisenbrand, *Chinese Drugs of Plant Origin* (Springer-Verlag, Berlin, 1992) pp 97-103. Chromatographic analysis of diterpenoids in leaves: S. Saxena *et al., Phytochem. Anal.* **11,** 34 (2000). Clinical evaluation in respiratory tract infections: J. Melchior *et al., Phytomedicine* **7,** 341 (2000); in familial Mediterranean fever: G. Amaryan *et al., ibid.* **10,** 271 (2003). *In vitro* anticancer and immunostimulatory activities: R. A. Kumar *et al., J. Ethnopharmacol.* **92,** 291 (2004).

THERAP CAT: In treatment of upper respiratory infections; hepatoprotectant.

633. Andrographolide. [5508-58-7] (3*E*,4*S*)-3-[2-[(1*R*,-4a*S*,5*R*,6*R*,8a*S*)-Decahydro-6-hydroxy-5-(hydroxymethyl)-5,8a-dimethyl-2-methylene-1-naphthalenyl]ethylidene]dihydro-4-hy-

droxy-2(3*H*)-furanone; 3α,14,15,18-tetrahydroxy-5β,9βH,10α-labda-8(20),12-dien-16-oic acid γ-lactone. $C_{20}H_{30}O_5$; mol wt 350.45. C 68.54%, H 8.63%, O 22.83%. Main bitter constituent and medicinally active principle isolated from the leaves of andrographis, *q.v.* Isoln: M. K. Gorter, *Rec. Trav. Chim.* **30,** 151 (1911). Rapid isoln method: M. Rajani *et al., Pharmaceut. Biol.* **38,** 204 (2000). Characterization: D. Chakravarti, R. N. Chakravarti, *J. Chem. Soc.* **1952,** 1697; R. Schwyzer *et al., Helv. Chim. Acta* **34,** 652 (1951). Structure: M. P. Cava, B. Weinstein, *Chem. Ind. (London)* **1959,** 851. Revised structure: M. P. Cava *et al., ibid.* **1963,** 167; M. P. Cava *et al., Tetrahedron* **21,** 2617 (1965). X-ray crystallographic analysis: T. Fujita *et al., Chem. Pharm. Bull.* **32,** 2117 (1984). HPLC determn in plant material: A. Sharma *et al., Phytochem. Anal.* **3,** 129 (1992). Determn in Chinese medicinal prepns: Z. Yanfang *et al., J. Pharm. Biomed. Anal.* **40,** 157 (2006). Mechanism of anti-inflammatory action: Y.-F. Xia *et al., J. Immunol.* **173,** 4207 (2004). Clinical pharmacokinetics and bioavailability from herbal preparations: A. Panossian *et al., Phytomedicine* **7,** 351 (2000).

Colorless plates from ethanol or methanol, mp 218° (dec) (Gorter). Also reported as mp 218-221° (Fujita). $[\alpha]_D^{25}$ −96.2° (c = 1.00 in C_5H_5N). d_4^{21} 1.2317. uv max (alcohol): 223 nm (log ε 4.09). Sparingly sol in water; sol in acetone, methanol, chloroform, ether.

Triacetyl derivative. $C_{26}H_{36}O_8$. Fine needles from alcohol + ether, mp 126-126.5°.

634. Androisoxazole. [360-66-7] (5α,17β)-17-Methylandrostano[3,2-*c*]isoxazol-17-ol; 2,3,3a,3b,4,5,5a,6,10,10a,10b,11,-12,12a-tetradecahydro-1,10a,12a-trimethyl-1*H*-cyclopenta[7,8]-phenanthro[2,3-*c*]isoxazol-1-ol; 17β-hydroxy-17α-methylandrostano[3,2-*c*]isoxazole; 17α-methylandrostan[3,2-*c*]isoxazol-17β-ol; Neo-Ponden. $C_{21}H_{31}NO_2$; mol wt 329.48. C 76.55%, H 9.48%, N 4.25%, O 9.71%. Prepn: Zderic *et al., Chem. Ind. (London)* **1960,** 1625.

Crystals, mp 169-170°. $[\alpha]_D$ +19°. uv max (ethanol): 226 nm (log ε 3.71).

THERAP CAT: Anabolic.

635. Androstane. [438-22-2] (5α)-Androstane; etioallocholane. $C_{19}H_{32}$; mol wt 260.46. C 87.62%, H 12.38%. From androstane-3,17-dione: Butenandt, Tscherning, *Z. Physiol. Chem.* **229,** 185 (1934). From androstane-3,17-diol: Steiger, Reichstein, *Helv. Chim. Acta* **20,** 817 (1937). From Δ¹⁶-androstene: Prelog *et al., ibid.* **27,** 66 (1944).

Leaflets from acetone-methanol, mp 50-50.5°. Sublimes at 60° and 0.003 mm Hg. $[\alpha]_D^{16}$ +2° (c = 1.2 in chloroform). Sol in acetone, alc, methanol, ether, petr ether, chloroform.

17-Amino-HCl. Dec 345°: Marker, *J. Am. Chem. Soc.* **58**, 480 (1936).

636. Androstane-3β,11β-diol-17-one. [514-17-0] (3β,-5α,11β)-3,11-Dihydroxyandrostan-17-one. $C_{19}H_{30}O_3$; mol wt 306.44. C 74.47%, H 9.87%, O 15.66%. First obtained by degradation of allopregnane-3β,11β,17α,20β,21-pentol (Reichstein's Substance A): Reichstein, *Helv. Chim. Acta* **19**, 402 (1936), but later isolated in small quantities directly from extracts of the adrenal cortex: Reichstein, von Euw, *ibid.* **21**, 1197 (1938); *ibid.* **24**, 879 (1941). It is uncertain whether this substance occurs in the fresh adrenal gland; it may possibly occur by oxidation or decompn during the isolation procedure: Reichstein, Shoppee, *Vitam. Horm.* **I**, 368 (1943). Structure-activity study: S. Sassa *et al., J. Biol. Chem.* **254**, 10011 (1979). Chromatographic studies: A. Kerebel *et al., J. Chromatogr.* **140**, 229 (1977); J. T. Lin, E. Heftmann, *ibid.* **237**, 215 (1982).

Needles from acetone + ether, mp 235-238°. $[\alpha]_D^{20}$ +84.5° (ethanol); $[\alpha]_D^{19}$ +81.3° (dioxane); $[\alpha]_{545}^{19}$ +105° (dioxane). Precipitated by digitonin.

3-Acetate. $C_{21}H_{32}O_4$. Needles from actone + ether, mp 230-231°. $[\alpha]_D^{19}$ +70.5° (dioxane); $[\alpha]_{546}^{19}$ +87.1° (dioxane).

Diacetate. $C_{23}H_{34}O_5$. Crystals, mp 154-156°.

637. Androstenediol. [521-17-5] (3β,17β)-Androst-5-ene-3,17-diol; Δ^5-androstene-3β,17β-diol. $C_{19}H_{30}O_2$; mol wt 290.44. C 78.57%, H 10.41%, O 11.02%. Obtained from dehydroandrosterone: Butenandt, Hanisch, *Ber.* **68**, 1859 (1935); *Z. Physiol. Chem.* **237**, 89 (1935); Ruzicka, Wettstein, *Helv. Chim. Acta* **18**, 1264 (1935); *FIAT Final Report* 996, 45 (1947); Levy, Kapp, **US 2521586** (1950 to Nopco Chem.).

Leaflets from acetone + petr ether, or from methanol or ethyl acetate. Sublimes in high vacuum. mp 184°. $[\alpha]_D^{18}$ −55.5° (c = 0.4 in isopropanol). Insol in water.

3-Acetate. [1639-43-6] $C_{21}H_{32}O_3$. Crystals from hexane, mp 147-148°.

17-Acetate. [5937-72-4] $C_{21}H_{32}O_3$. Crystals from hexane, mp 146.5-148.5°, $[\alpha]_D^{18}$ −62.4° (alc).

Diacetate. [2099-26-5] $C_{23}H_{34}O_4$. Leaflets from hexane, mp 165-166°, $[\alpha]_D^{18}$ −56.5° (alc).

17-Benzoate. $C_{26}H_{34}O_3$. Crystals from methanol, mp 220-222°.

3-Acetate-17-benzoate. [5953-63-9] $C_{28}H_{36}O_4$. Crystals, mp 180-182°.

Dipropionate. [2297-30-5] $C_{25}H_{38}O_4$; mol wt 402.57.

Note: This is a controlled substance (anabolic steroid): **21 CFR,** 1308.13, as defined in 1300.01.

USE: Dietary supplement for body building.

638. Androstenedione. [63-05-8] Androst-4-ene-3,17-dione; Δ^4-androstenedione; Δ^4-etiocholendione-3,17. $C_{19}H_{26}O_2$; mol wt 286.41. C 79.68%, H 9.15%, O 11.17%. Weak androgen

produced by the adrenal gland; converted in peripheral tissues to testosterone or estrone, *q.q.v.* Prepn: L. Ruzicka, A. Wettstein, *Helv. Chim. Acta* **18**, 986 (1935); E. S. Wallis, E. Fernholz, *J. Am. Chem. Soc.* **57**, 1511 (1935); and physiological activity: A. Butenandt, H. Kudszus, *Z. Physiol. Chem.* **237**, 75 (1935). Isoln from adrenal cortex: J. von Euw, T. Reichstein, *Helv. Chim. Acta* **24**, 879 (1941). Physiology: V. H. T. James, A. B. Goodall in *Proc. 9th Congr. Hung. Soc. Endocrinol. Metab.*, F. A. Laszlo, Ed. (Akad. Kiado, Budapest, 1979) pp 235-241. HPLC determn in plasma or serum: V. R. Walker *et al., Anal. Biochem.* **234**, 194 (1996). Discussion of use as dietary supplement: L. Schnirring, *Physician Sportsmed.* **26**, 15-18 (1998). Clinical effect of oral supplement on blood chemistry: D. S. King *et al., J. Am. Med. Assoc.* **281**, 2020 (1999).

Crystals from hexane, mp 173-174°. $[\alpha]_D^{30}$ +199° (in chloroform).

Note: This is a controlled substance (anabolic steroid): **21 CFR,** 1308.13, as defined in 1300.01.

639. (3α,5α)-Androst-16-en-3-ol. [1153-51-1] 3α-Hydroxy-5α-androst-16-ene; Δ^{16}-androsten-3-ol. $C_{19}H_{30}O$; mol wt 274.44. C 83.15%, H 11.02%, O 5.83%. A major constituent of boar pheromone, having a pronounced musk-like odor. Isoln from swine testes: V. Prelog, L. Ruzicka, *Helv. Chim. Acta* **27**, 61 (1944). Prepn: V. Prelog *et al., ibid.* 66; J. Fishman *et al., J. Org. Chem.* **28**, 1443 (1963). Physiological role as a sex attractant for pigs: D. B. Gower, *J. Steroid Biochem.* **3**, 45 (1972). Use in pig artificial insemination: D. R. Melrose *et al.,* **DE 1937264**; *eidem,* **US 3681490** (1970, 1972 both to Nat. Res. Dev. Corp.). *In vivo* metabolism in boar testes: Y. A. Saat *et al., Biochem. J.* **144**, 347 (1974). It has also been detected in human male axillary sweat, but has no androgenic activity: B. W. L. Brooksbank *et al., Experientia* **30**, 864 (1974). Radioimmunoassay: D. C. Bickell, D. B. Gower, *J. Steroid Biochem.* **7**, 451 (1976). Receptor studies: J. N. Gennings *et al., Biochim. Biophys. Acta* **496**, 547 (1977). Biosynthetic studies: E. L. Hurden *et al., J. Endocrinol.* **81**, 161P (1979); G. M. Cook, D. B. Gower, *ibid.* **88**, 409 (1981). Discovery of the presence of androst-16-en-3-ol in truffles (*Tuber melanosporum*) has been offered as an explanation for the ability of pigs to detect truffles growing as deep as 1 meter underground: R. Claus *et al., Experientia* **37**, 1178 (1981).

Crystals, mp 142.5-143°. Purified by sublimation in high vacuum and recryst from acetone. $[\alpha]_D^{20}$ +13.1° (c = 0.957 in chloroform). Gives a blue color in the Kägi-Miescher test, *cf. Helv. Chim. Acta* **22**, 683 (1939).

USE: As an aid to estrus determn in pig artificial insemination.

640. Androsterone. [53-41-8] (3α,5α)-3-Hydroxyandrostan-17-one; *cis*-androsterone; 3α-hydroxy-17-androstanone; andro-stan-3α-ol-17-one; 3α-hydroxyetioallocholan-17-one; 3-epihydroxy-etioallocholan-17-one. $C_{19}H_{30}O_2$; mol wt 290.44. C 78.57%, H 10.41%, O 11.02%. Isolation from male urine after removal of the phenolic estrogen fraction: Butenandt, Tscherning, *Z. Physiol. Chem.* **229**, 167 (1934); v. Euw, Reichstein, *Helv. Chim. Acta* **25**, 988 (1942). Prepn from cholesterol: Ruzicka, *ibid.* **17**, 1389 (1934); Marker, *J. Am. Chem. Soc.* **57**, 1755 (1935); Schoeller *et al.,* **US 2232735** (1941 to Schering).

Crystals from acetone-ether, mp 185-185.5°. Sublimes in high vacuum. $[\alpha]_D^{20}$ +94.6° (c = 0.7 in abs alc). $[\alpha]_D^{15}$ +87.8° (c = 1.5 in dioxane). Not precipitated by digitonin. Barely soluble in water. Sol in most organic solvents.

Acetate. $C_{21}H_{32}O_3$. Crystals from ether, sublimes in high vac, mp 165°, $[\alpha]_D^{14}$ +76.7° (c = 2.04 in dioxane); $[\alpha]_D^{25}$ +86° (c = 2 in ethanol).

Propionate. $C_{22}H_{34}O_3$. mp 151-152°.

Benzoate. $C_{26}H_{34}O_3$. mp 178°.

641.   Anecortave Acetate. [7753-60-8] 21-(Acetyloxy)-17-hydroxypregna-4,9(11)-diene-3,20-dione; $\Delta^{4,9(11)}$-pregnadien-17α,21-diol-3,20-dione-21-acetate; Al-3789; Retaane. $C_{23}H_{30}O_5$; mol wt 386.48. C 71.48%, H 7.82%, O 20.70%. Angiostatic steroid. Prepn: J. Fried, E. F. Sabo, *J. Am. Chem. Soc.* **75**, 2273 (1953); R. P. Graber *et al., ibid.* **4722**; J. Fried, E. F. Sabo, *ibid.* **79**, 1130 (1957). Angiostatic activity *in vitro:* L. G. McNatt *et al., J. Ocul. Pharmacol. Ther.* **15**, 413 (1999); *in vivo:* D. BenEzra *et al., Invest. Ophthalmol. Visual Sci.* **38**, 1954 (1997). Clinical study in age-related macular degeneration: J. S. Slakter *et al., Ophthalmology* **110**, 2372 (2003). Review of pharmacology: A. F. Clark, *Expert Opin. Invest. Drugs* **6**, 1867-1877 (1997); and clinical experience: S. A. Vinores, *IDrugs* **8**, 327-334 (2005).

Crystals from acetone, mp 236-237°. $[\alpha]$ +117° (c = 1.0 in CHCl$_3$). uv max (alcohol): 238 nm (ε 15500). Also reported as mp 231.5-234.5°. $[\alpha]_D^{22}$ +124° (c = 1.04 in CHCl$_3$).

THERAP CAT: In treatment of macular degeneration.

642.   Anemonin. [508-44-1] (5R,6R)-*rel*-1,7-Dioxadispiro[4.0.4.2]dodeca-3,9-diene-2,8-dione; β,β'-1,2-dihydroxy-1,2-cyclobutanediacrylic acid di-γ-lactone; Anemone camphor; Pulsatilla camphor. $C_{10}H_8O_4$; mol wt 192.17. C 62.50%, H 4.20%, O 33.30%. Found in *Anemone pulsatilla* L. and other *Ranunculaceae*. Its precursor in plants is protoanemonin. Isoln from *Ranunculus acer:* Zecher, Wohlmuth, *Sci. Pharm.* **22**, 95 (1954); *C.A.* **48**, 13169b (1954). Structure: Moriarty *et al., J. Am. Chem. Soc.* **87**, 3251 (1965); Romain, *Diss. Abstr. B* **27**, 3867 (1967). Synthesis: Sugiyama *et al., C.A.* **67**, 116604n (1967). Toxicity study: R. Brodersen, A. Kjaer, *Acta Pharmacol. Toxicol.* **2**, 109 (1946).

Crystals from petr ether, mp 157-158°. Volatile with steam. Slightly sol in cold, more in hot water; sol in hot alcohol, chloroform, alkalies with yellow color. Practically insol in ether. LD$_{50}$ i.p. in mice: 150 mg/kg (Brodersen, Kjaer).

Note: Not to be confused with anemonine which is 5-(carboxymethyl)-1,1-dimethylimidazolium hydroxide inner salt.

643.   Anethole. [4180-23-8]; [104-46-1] (unspecified). 1-Methoxy-4-(1E)-1-propenylbenzene; *trans-p*-propenylanisole; *trans*-1-*p*-anisylpropene; anise camphor; isoestragole; Monasirup. $C_{10}H_{12}O$; mol wt 148.20. C 81.04%, H 8.16%, O 10.80%. Chief constituent of anise, star anise and fennel oils; responsible for the characteristic odor and flavor of aniseed. Isoln: A. Cahours, *Ann.* **41**, 56 (1842). Description of prepns and properties: A. Wagner, *Manuf. Chem.* **23**, 56 (1952). Prepn from estragole, *q.v.*, and separation of isomers: Y.-R. Naves, *Compt. Rend.* **246**, 1734 (1958). Improved synthesis: R. J. DePasquale, *Synth. Commun.* **10**, 225 (1980). Characterization of isomers: Y.-R. Naves *et al., Bull. Soc. Chim. Fr.* **1958**, 566; and comparative pharmacology: J.-R. Boissier *et al., Therapie* **22**, 309 (1967). HPLC determn in alcoholic beverages: P. Curro *et al., J. Chromatogr.* **404**, 273 (1987). Isoln by supercritical fluid extraction: L. K. Liu, *Anal. Commun.* **33**, 175 (1996). Metabolism in humans: J. Caldwell, J. D. Sutton, *Food Chem. Toxicol.* **26**, 87 (1988). Review of use as aroma chemical: G. S. Clark, *Perfum. Flavor.* **18**, 11-18 (1993); of safety evaluation as flavoring substance: P. Newberne *et al., Food Chem. Toxicol.* **37**, 789-811 (1999).

Colorless, slightly oily liquid; sweet, characteristic odor and taste. mp 21.4°. d_4^{20} 0.9883. bp 231-237°; bp$_{2.3}$ 81-81.5°. n_D^{20} 1.56145. uv max (ethanol): 259 nm (ε 22300). Practically insol in water. Misc with ether, chloroform; sol in benzene, ethyl acetate, acetone, carbon disulfide, petr ether; 1 ml dissolves in 2 ml alc. LD$_{50}$ i.p. in rats: 900 mg/kg (Boissier).

cis-**Anethole.** [25679-28-1] Naturally occurs in trace amounts in oils of anise, star anise and fennel; by-product in prepn of synthetic anethole. Stereospecific prepn: Y.-R. Naves, *Helv. Chim. Acta* **43**, 230 (1960). Camphoraceous, unpleasant, fennel-like odor. mp −22.5°. d_4^{20} 0.9878. bp$_{2.3}$ 79-79.5°. n_D^{20} 1.55455. uv max (ethanol): 253.5 nm (ε 18500). LD$_{50}$ i.p. in rats: 93 mg/kg (Boissier).

USE: Flavoring agent in foods and beverages; in perfumery, particularly for soap and dentifrices; pharmaceutic aid (flavor).

THERAP CAT: Antitussive.

644.   Anethole Trithione. [532-11-6] 5-(4-Methoxyphenyl)-3H-1,2-dithiole-3-thione; 3-(*p*-anisyl)trithione; 3-(*p*-methoxyphenyl)-4,5-dithiacyclopent-2-ene-1-thione; trithio-*p*-methoxyphenylpropene; 5-(*p*-methoxyphenyl)-1,2-dithiacyclopent-4-ene-3-thione; 3-(*p*-methoxyphenyl)trithione; trithioanethole; anethole dithiolthione; ADT; Felviten; Mucinol; Sialor; Sulfarlem. $C_{10}H_8OS_3$; mol wt 240.36. C 49.97%, H 3.35%, O 6.66%, S 40.02%. Organosulfur compound that enhances glutathione synthesis and stimulates secretion of bile and saliva. Prepn: B. Böttcher, A. Lüttringhaus, *Ann.* **557**, 89 (1947); O. Gaudin, N. Lozac'h, *Compt. Rend.* **224**, 557 (1947); A. Thuillier, J. Vialle, *Bull. Soc. Chim. Fr.* **1959**, 1398. HPLC determn in urine: A. N. Masoud, E. Bueding, *J. Chromatogr.* **276**, 111 (1983). Clinical trial in xerostomia: J. B. Epstein *et al., Oral Surg. Oral Med. Oral Pathol.* **56**, 495 (1983). Clinical trial in chemoprevention of lung cancer: S. Lam *et al., J. Natl. Cancer Inst.* **94**, 1001 (2002). Review of mechanism of chemoprotective and antioxidant effects: M.-O. Christen, *Methods Enzymol.* **252**, 316-323 (1995).

Orange-colored prisms from butyl acetate. Very bitter taste. mp 111°. Practically insol in water. Sol in pyridine, chloroform, benzene, dioxane, carbon disulfide. Slightly sol in ether, acetone, ethyl acetate, acetic acid, alc, cyclohexane, petr ether.

THERAP CAT: Choleretic; sialogogue.

645.   Angelica. Tall, perennial, herbaceous plant, *Angelica archangelica* L., *Umbelliferae*. Habit. Europe, Asia. Medicinal parts are the seed, leaves and root. *Constit.* Root: Volatile oil (0.35-1.9%); more than 20 furanocoumarins including bergapten, angelicin, archangelicin, isoimperatorin, xanthotoxin; osthol, umbelliferone, flavonoids, sugars. Fruit: Volatile oil, furanocoumarins, fatty oil, phytosterols. Review of constituents and uses: V. E. Tyler, *The Honest Herbal* (Pharmaceutical Products Press, New York, 3rd Ed., 1993) pp 29-30; N. G. Bisset, M. Wichtl, *Herbal Drugs and Phytopharmaceuticals*, English Ed. (CRC Press, Boca Raton, 1994) pp 70-72; J. Gruenwald *et al.*, *PDR for Herbal Medicines* (Medical Economics, Montvale, 2nd Ed., 2000) pp 32-34.

Angelica root oil. [8015-64-3] Volatile oil obtained by steam distillation of the dried slender roots. *Constit.* Chiefly β-phellandrene (13-28%), α-phellandrene, α-pinene (14-31%). Pale yellow to deep amber liquid with warm, pungent odor and bittersweet taste. d_{25}^{25} 0.850-0.880. n_D^{20} 1.473-1.487. Acid value not more than 7.0. Rotation: 0° to +46°. Sol in most fixed oils, slightly sol in mineral oil. Relatively insol in glycerin, propylene glycol. *Keep well closed, cool, and protected from light.*

Angelica seed oil. Volatile oil obtained by steam distillation of the fresh seeds. Light yellow liquid having a sweet, delicate aroma. d_{25}^{25} 0.853-0.876. n_D^{20} 1.480-1.488. Rotation: +4° to +16°. Acid value not more than 3.0. *Keep well closed, cool, and protected from light.*

USE: Flavoring for liqueurs and gin.

THERAP CAT: Carminative, diaphoretic, diuretic.

646. Angelic Acid. [565-63-9] (Z)-2-Methyl-2-butenoic acid; *cis*-2-dimethylcrotonic acid; 2-methylisocrotonic acid; *cis*-2,3-dimethylacrylic acid. $C_5H_8O_2$; mol wt 100.12. C 59.98%, H 8.05%, O 31.96%. Stereoisomer of tiglic acid. Found in ester form in sumbul root, *Angelica archangelica* L., *Umbelliferae* and together with tiglic acid esters in the oil of the Roman camomile, *Anthemis nobilis* L., *Compositae*. Isoln from seeds of *Schoenocaulon officinale* (Lindl.) A. Gray, *Liliaceae* (cevadilla seeds) by alkaline hydrolysis of cevadine: Stoll, Seebeck, *Helv. Chim. Acta* **35**, 1275 (1952). Synthesis by *trans* addition of bromine to tiglic acid: Buckles, Mock, *J. Org. Chem.* **15**, 680 (1950). Review and bibliography: Buckles *et al.*, *Chem. Rev.* **55**, 659 (1955).

Monoclinic rods, needles, plates; mp 45°. Spicy odor. *Vesicant.* d_4^{47} 0.983. bp_{760} 185°; bp_{12} 86°. Sublimes. Volatile with steam. n_D^{47} 1.4434. pK (25°) 4.30. uv max (H_2O): 217 nm (ε 5.15 × 10^3). Molar heat of combustion 626.6 kcal. Sparingly soluble in cold water, freely sol in hot water. Sol in alcohol, ether. Prolonged boiling of aq soln causes isomerization to tiglic acid; the process is speeded up by traces of bromine and sunlight, also by strong mineral acids or alks. Dry crystals of angelic acid have been stored in bottles for years without evidence of isomerization.

Calcium salt dihydrate. $Ca(C_5H_7O_2)_2 \cdot 2H_2O$. Leaflets. Much more soluble in water than calcium tiglate: 100 parts of aq soln satd at 17.5° contains 23 parts of anhydr calcium angelate.

Amide. C_5H_9NO. Crystals, mp 127-128°.

Methyl ester. $C_6H_{10}O_2$. Liquid; d_4^{20} 0.9413; bp_{764} 128°; n_D^{20} 1.4321.

Ethyl ester. $C_7H_{12}O_2$. Liquid; $d_4^{19.5}$ 0.9178; bp_{760} 141.5°, bp_{11} 49°. n_D^{20} 1.4304. Heat of formn at constant vol 963.1 kcal, at constant press. 964.2 kcal.

647. Angelica Lactone. [1333-38-6] 5-Methyl-2-furanone. $C_5H_6O_2$; mol wt 98.10. C 61.22%, H 6.16%, O 32.62%. Exists in three forms. Prepn of α and β-forms: Wolff, *Ann.* **229**, 250 (1885); Thiele, *Ann.* **319**, 184 (1901); v. Auwers, *Ber.* **56**, 1672 (1923); J. H. Helberger *et al.*, *Ann.* **561**, 215 (1949). Prepn of α'-form: J. P. Wineburg *et al.*, *J. Heterocycl. Chem.* **12**, 749 (1975); V. Jäger, H. J. Günther, *Tetrahedron Lett.* **1977**, 2543; R.A. Amos, J. A. Katzenellenbogen, *J. Org. Chem.* **43**, 560 (1978). Toxicity data for α-form: E. J. Moran *et al.*, *Drug Chem. Toxicol.* **3**, 249 (1980).

| α-form | β-form | α'-form |

α-Form. 5-Methyl-2(3H)-furanone; Δ^2-angelica lactone; γ-methyl-β,γ-crotonolactone; 4-hydroxy-3-pentenoic acid γ-lactone. Volatile needles, mp 18°. d_4^{20} 1.084. bp_{12} 56°. n_{He}^{20} 1.4476. One gram dissolves in 20 ml water at 15°. Heating with triethylamine soln converts it to the β-form. LD$_{50}$ orally in mice: 2800 mg/kg (Moran).

β-Form. 5-Methyl-2(5H)-furanone; Δ^1-angelica lactone; γ-methyl-α,β-crotonolactone; 4-hydroxy-2-pentenoic acid γ-lactone. Liquid. Not solidified at $-17°$. d_4^{20} 1.076. bp_{751} 208-209°. bp_{10} 87°. n_{He}^{20} 1.4603. Sol in water. Forms a dimer. More stable than α-form.

α'-Form. Dihydro-5-methylene-2(3H)-furanone; γ-methylene-γ-butyrolactone. bp_{17} 80°.

648. Angeli's Salt. [13826-64-7] Hyponitric acid disodium salt; sodium *N*-nitrohydroxylaminate; sodium α-oxyhyponitrite; sodium trioxodinitrate. $N_2Na_2O_3$; mol wt 121.99. N 22.96%, Na 37.69%, O 39.35%. $Na_2(ONNO_2)$. Highly oxidizing compound; decomposes to produce nitroxyl (HNO). Prepn: A. Angeli, *Gazz. Chim. Ital.* **26**, 17 (1896); and uv spectrum: C. C. Addison *et al.*, *J. Chem. Soc.* **1952**, 338. Crystal structure of monohydrate: H. Hope, M. R. Sequeira, *Inorg. Chem.* **12**, 286 (1973). Reactivity studies: P. A. S. Smith, G. E. Hein, *J. Am. Chem. Soc.* **82**, 5731 (1960); L. Torun *et al.*, *Tetrahedron Lett.* **40**, 5279 (1999). Decomposition studies: F. T. Bonner, B. Ravid, *Inorg. Chem.* **14**, 558 (1975); C. M. Maragos *et al.*, *J. Med. Chem.* **34**, 3242 (1991). pH-dependent cytotoxicity: D. A. Stoyanovsky *et al.*, *ibid.* **47**, 210 (2004).

White, microcrystalline powder. Very sol in water. d 2.26 (monohydrate). uv max (0.1 *M* NaOH): 248 nm (ε 8300). uv max (pH 7.4 phosphate buffer): 237 nm (ε 6100).

USE: HNO/NO$^-$ donor in biochemical model studies.

649. Angiogenin. Single-chain, basic protein of 123 amino acids that induces the *in vivo* formation of blood vessels. Mol wt ~14,000 Da. First isolated from human adenocarcinoma cells; subsequently found in normal human plasma and shown to be produced by the liver. Angiogenin exhibits a characteristic ribonucleolytic activity toward 28S and 18S ribosomal RNA. Its amino acid sequence is 35% identical with that of human pancreatic ribonuclease. Isoln, characterization, and angiogenic activity: J. W. Fett *et al.*, *Biochemistry* **24**, 5480 (1985). Amino acid sequence: D. J. Strydom *et al.*, *ibid.* 5486. Cloning and DNA sequence of human angiogenin gene: K. Kurachi *et al.*, *ibid.* 5494. Structural study: K. A. Palmer *et al.*, *Proc. Natl. Acad. Sci. USA* **83**, 1965 (1986). Ribonucleolytic activity: R. Shapiro *et al.*, *Biochemistry* **25**, 3527 (1986). Isoln from normal human plasma: R. Shapiro *et al.*, *ibid.* **26**, 5141 (1987). Tissue distribution in neonatal and adult rats: H. L. Weiner *et al.*, *Science* **237**, 280 (1987); in human tumor and normal cells: S. M. Rybak *et al.*, *Biochem. Biophys. Res. Commun.* **146**, 1240 (1987). Inhibition of protein synthesis: D. K. St. Clair *et al.*, *Proc. Natl. Acad. Sci. USA* **84**, 8330 (1987). Inhibition of angiogenic and ribonucleolytic activities of angiogenin by placental ribonuclease inhibitor: R. Shapiro, B. L. Vallee, *ibid.* 2238; F. S. Lee, B. L. Vallee, *Biochemistry* **28**, 3556 (1989). Reviews: J. F. Riordan, B. L. Vallee, *Br. J. Cancer* **57**, 587-590 (1988); B. L. Vallee, J. F. Riordan, *Adv. Exp. Med. Biol.* **234**, 41-53 (1988).

650. Angiostatin. Naturally occurring inhibitor of angiogenesis that suppresses the growth of primary and metastatic tumors. 38 kDa protein generated by the cancer-mediated proteolysis of plasminogen, *q.v.*; amino acid sequence corresponds to the first four kringle domains. Isoln, amino acid sequence and bioactivity: M. S. O'Reilly *et al.*, *Cell* **79**, 315 (1994). Review of discovery: R. Vile, *Curr. Biol.* **5**, 10-13 (1995). Effect on human carcinomas in mice: M. S. O'Reilly *et al.*, *Nat. Med.* **2**, 689 (1996). Mechanism of angiostatin generation: S. Gately *et al.*, *Proc. Natl. Acad. Sci. USA* **94**, 10868 (1997).

651. Angiotensin. [1407-47-2] Formerly *hypertensin* and *angiotonin*. Pressor substance formed by the action of renin, *q.v.*, on a plasma substrate, *angiotensinogen* (*renin substrate*, *hypertensinogen*). The substance so formed is a decapeptide called *angiotensin I* which is converted to the active pressor agent, *angiotensin II*, by the splitting off of the *C*-terminal His-Leu residues by the *angiotensin converting enzyme* (ACE) or *angiotensinase*. The octapeptide angiotensin II differs among species only in the amino acid residue in position 5 being either Val or Ile. *See* reviews for refs to isoln and synthesis. Angiotensin II acts directly on the adrenal gland to stimulate the release of aldosterone, *q.v.* Rapid liquid phase synthesis of a protected angiotensin II: S. Nozaki, I. Muramatsu, *Bull. Chem. Soc. Jpn.* **55**, 2165 (1982). Extraction and characterization of angiotensins I and II from rat brain: D. Ganten *et al., Science* **221**, 869 (1983). *Reviews:* M. Bodanszky, M. A. Ondetti, *Peptide Synthesis* (John Wiley, New York, 1966) pp 215-223; E. Schröder, K. Lübe, *The Peptides* vol. II (English ed., New York, 1966) pp 4-62; Bumpus, Smeby, "Angiotensin" in *Renal Hypertension*, I. Page, J. McCubbin, Eds. (Year Book Medical Publishers, Chicago, 1968) pp 62-98; Lee, "Angiotensin" in *Renin and Hypertension* (Williams & Wilkins, Baltimore, 1969) pp 32-94; G. M. Molinatti, P. Limone, *Minerva Med.* **72**, 715-732 (1981); J. A. Oliver *et al., Ann. N.Y. Acad. Sci.* **394**, 275-277 (1982); M. Marin-Grez, *Biochem. Pharmacol.* **31**, 3941-3947 (1982). Symposium on hemodynamic effects of angiotensin II and its role in cardiovascular disease: *Am. J. Hypertens.* **15**, Suppl. 1, S1-S27 (2002). *See also* Tonin.

Asp–Arg–Val–Tyr–Ile–His–Pro–Phe

Angiotensin II (horse)

Angiotensins are very stable. Hydrolyzed by strong acids and bases and above pH 9.5. Sol in organic solvents, in aq solns pH 5-8. In high dilution, lost by absorption on walls of glass vessels.

Amide. [53-73-6] 5-Valine-angiotensin II amide; angiotensin II aspartic-β-amide 5-valine; 1-asparagine-5-valine-angiotensin II; val⁵-angiotensin II-asp¹-β-amide; Hypertensin. $C_{49}H_{70}N_{14}O_{11}$; mol wt 1031.17.

THERAP CAT: Amide as vasoconstrictor.

652. Angostura Bark. Cusparia bark; Carony bark; *Cortex Angosturae*; *Cortex Cuspariae*. The bark of the tree *Galipea officinalis* Hancock, habitat Venezuela, or the bark of the tree *Cusparia febrifuga* Humb., or *C. trifoliata* Engl., *Rutaceae*, habitat Brazil. *Ref:* Meyer, *Pharm. Ztg.* **80**, 120 (1935).

Unpleasant, musty odor. Bitter, slightly aromatic taste with pungent after-taste. The bitterness is due mainly to the bitter principle angosturin, $C_9H_{12}O_5$. The bark contains also the quinoline alkaloids cusparine, cuspareine; galipine, galipoidine, and galipoline.

THERAP CAT: Antipyretic.

653. Anhalamine. [643-60-7] 1,2,3,4-Tetrahydro-6,7-dimethoxy-8-isoquinolinol; 6,7-dimethoxy-8-hydroxy-1,2,3,4-tetrahydroisoquinoline. $C_{11}H_{15}NO_3$; mol wt 209.24. C 63.14%, H 7.23%, N 6.69%, O 22.94%. From *Lophophora williamsii* (Lemaire) Coutl. *(Anhalonium lewinii* Henn.), *Cactaceae:* Kauder, *Arch. Pharm.* **237**, 190 (1899); Späth, Becke, *Monatsh. Chem.* **66**, 327 (1935). Structure: *eidem, Ber.* **67**, 2100 (1934). Synthesis: Späth, Roder, *Monatsh. Chem.* **43**, 93 (1922); Brossi *et al., Helv. Chim. Acta* **47**, 2089 (1964); **49**, 403 (1966). Biosynthetic studies: Kapadia *et al., J. Am. Chem. Soc.* **92**, 6943 (1970). *Review:* Manske in R. H. F. Manske, H. L. Holmes, *The Alkaloids* vol. IV (Academic Press, New York, 1954) pp 8-14.

Crystals, mp 189-191°. uv max (ethanol): 274 nm (log ε 2.90). Almost insol in cold water, cold alcohol, ether. Sol in hot water, alcohol, acetone, dil acids.

Hydrochloride dihydrate. $C_{11}H_{15}NO_3 \cdot HCl \cdot 2H_2O$. Crystals from water, mp 258°.

654. Anhalonidine. [17627-77-9] 1,2,3,4-Tetrahydro-6,7-dimethoxy-1-methyl-8-isoquinolinol; 6,7-dimethoxy-8-hydroxy-1-methyl-1,2,3,4-tetrahydroisoquinoline. $C_{12}H_{17}NO_3$; mol wt 223.27. C 64.55%, H 7.67%, N 6.27%, O 21.50%. From mescal buttons, the buds of *Lophophora williamsii* (Lemaire) Coutl. *(Anhalonium lewinii* Henn.) *Cactaceae:* Heffter, *Ber.* **27**, 2975 (1894);

29, 221 (1896); Kauder, *Arch. Pharm.* **237**, 190 (1899). Structure and synthesis from 3-acetoxy-4,5-dimethoxy-*N*-acetylphenethyl-amine: Späth, Passl, *Ber.* **65**, 1778 (1932); from mescaline: Brossi *et al., Helv. Chim. Acta* **47**, 2089 (1964). Biosynthesis: Kapadia *et al., J. Am. Chem. Soc.* **92**, 6943 (1970).

Small octahedra from benzene, mp 160-161°. uv max (ethanol): 270 nm (log ε 2.81). Strong base. Freely sol in water, alcohol, chlorofom, hot benzene. Sparingly sol in ether. Insol in petr ether. Solns of anhalonidine acquire a reddish color on standing.

655. Anhalonine. [519-04-0] 6,7,8,9-Tetrahydro-4-methoxy-9-methyl-1,3-dioxolo[4,5-*h*]isoquinoline. $C_{12}H_{15}NO_3$; mol wt 221.25. C 65.14%, H 6.83%, N 6.33%, O 21.69%. From mescal buttons *[Lophophora williamsii* (Lemaire) Coult. *(Anhalonium lewinii* Henn.), *Cactaceae]* also in *Ariocarpus*, in *Gymnocalycium gibbosum*. Synthesis of *dl*-form and resolution: Späth, Kesztler, *Ber.* **68**, 1663 (1935); Brossi *et al., J. Am. Chem. Soc.* **93**, 6248 (1971). Configuration: Battersby, Edwards, *J. Chem. Soc.* **1960**, 1214.

Rhombic needles from petr ether, mp 86°, bp$_{0.02}$ 140°. $[\alpha]_D^{25}$ −63.8° (methanol); −56.3° (chloroform). Very sol in alcohol, ether, chloroform, benzene, petr ether.

Hydrochloride. $C_{12}H_{15}NO_3 \cdot HCl$. Orthorhombic prisms, dec 255°; freely sol in hot water. Aq soln is neutral.

656. Anidulafungin. [166663-25-8] 1-[(4*R*,5*R*)-4,5-Dihydroxy-*N*²-[[4″-(pentyloxy)[1,1′:4′,1″-terphenyl]-4-yl]carbonyl]-L-ornithine]echinocandin B; V-echinocandin; LY-303366; VER-002. $C_{58}H_{73}N_7O_{17}$; mol wt 1140.24. C 61.09%, H 6.45%, N 8.60%, O 23.85%. Semisynthetic echinocandin antifungal; inhibits 1,3-β-D-glucan synthase. Prepn: F. J. Burkhardt *et al.,* **EP 561639** (1993 to Lilly); M. Debono *et al., J. Med. Chem.* **38**, 3271 (1995). HPLC determn in plasma: L. L. Zornes, R. E. Stratford, *J. Chromatogr. B* **695**, 381 (1997). Comparative *in vitro* susceptibility: M. A. Pfaller *et al., Diagn. Microbiol. Infect. Dis.* **30**, 251 (1998); M. Cuenca-Estrella *et al., J. Antimicrob. Chemother.* **46**, 475 (2000). Pharmacokinetics and antifungal activity: A. H. Groll *et al., Antimicrob. Agents Chemother.* **45**, 2845 (2001). Clinical evaluation in invasive candidiasis: M. A. Pfaller *et al., ibid.* **49**, 4795 (2005). Review of clinical experience: M. A. Pfaller, *Expert Opin. Invest. Drugs* **13**, 1183-1197 (2004); of pharmacology: J. A. Vazquez, *Clin. Ther.* **27**, 657-673 (2005).

THERAP CAT: Antifungal.

657. Anilazine. [101-05-3] 4,6-Dichloro-N-(2-chloro-phenyl)-1,3,5-triazin-2-amine; 2,4-dichloro-6-(o-chloroanilino)-s-triazine; (o-chloroanilino)dichlorotriazine; Dyrene. $C_9H_5Cl_3N_4$; mol wt 275.52. C 39.23%, H 1.83%, Cl 38.60%, N 20.33%. Prepn: C. N. Wolf, **US 2720480** (1955 to Ethyl Corp.); E. G. Hill, E. Clinton, **US 2820032** (1958); K. H. Rattenburg *et al.,* **US 3074946** (1963 to Chemagro). Toxicity study: S. D. Cohen, S. D. Murphy, *J. Agric. Food Chem.* **21,** 140 (1973).

White to tan crystals, mp 159-160°. Insol in water. Soly at 30° (g/100 ml): toluene, 5; xylene, 4; acetone, 10. Subject to hydrolysis; not compatible with oils and alkaline materials. LD$_{50}$ orally in rats: >5000 mg/kg, Mobay Technical Information Sheet, Jan. 1979.
USE: Fungicide.

658. Anileridine. [144-14-9] 1-[2-(4-Aminophenyl)eth-yl]-4-phenyl-4-piperidinecarboxylic acid ethyl ester; 1-(p-amino-phenethyl)-4-phenylisonipecotic acid ethyl ester; ethyl 1-(4-amino-phenethyl)-4-phenylisonipecotate; N-[β-(p-aminophenyl)ethyl]-4-phenyl-4-carbethoxypiperidine; N-β-(p-aminophenyl)ethylnor-meperidine; Leritine. $C_{22}H_{28}N_2O_2$; mol wt 352.47. C 74.97%, H 8.01%, N 7.95%, O 9.08%. Synthesis: Weijlard *et al., J. Am. Chem. Soc.* **78,** 2342 (1956); **US 2966490** (1960 to Merck & Co.).

Mp 83°.
Dihydrochloride. [126-12-5] $C_{22}H_{28}N_2O_2 \cdot 2HCl$. Crystals from methanol + ether, mp 280-287° (dec). Freely soluble in water, methanol. Solubility in ethanol: 8 mg/g. pH of aq solns 2.0 to 2.5. Solns are stable at pH 3.5 and below. At pH 4 and higher the insol free base is precipitated. uv max (pH 7 in 90% methanol contg phosphate buffer): 235, 289 nm (A$_{1cm}^{1\%}$ 293, 34.5). Distribution coefficient (water, pH 3.6/n-butanol): 0.9.
Note: This is a controlled substance (opiate): **21 CFR,** 1308.12.
THERAP CAT: Analgesic (narcotic).

659. Aniline. [62-53-3] Benzenamine; aniline oil; phenyl-amine; aminobenzene; aminophen; kyanol. C_6H_7N; mol wt 93.13. C 77.38%, H 7.58%, N 15.04%. First obtained in 1826 by Unver-dorben from dry distillation of indigo. Runge found it in coal tar in 1834. Fritzsche, in 1841, prepared it from indigo and potash and gave it the name aniline. Manuf from nitrobenzene or chloroben-zene: *Faith, Keyes & Clark's Industrial Chemicals,* F. A. Low-enheim, M. K. Moran, Eds. (Wiley-Interscience, New York, 4th ed., 1975) pp 109-116. Procedures: A. I. Vogel, *Practical Organic Chemistry* (Longmans, London, 3rd ed., 1959) p 564; Gattermann-Wieland, *Praxis des Organischen Chemikers* (de Gruyter, Berlin, 40th ed., 1961) p 148. Brochure *"Aniline"* by Allied Chemical's National Aniline Division (New York, 1964) 109 pp, gives reactions and uses of aniline (877 references). Toxicity study: K. H. Jacob-son, *Toxicol. Appl. Pharmacol.* **22,** 153 (1972).

Oily liquid; colorless when freshly distilled, darkens on exposure to air and light. *Poisonous!* Characteristic odor and burning taste;

combustible; volatile with steam. d_{20}^{20} 1.022. bp 184-186°. Solidif −6°. Flash pt, closed cup: 169°F (76°C). n_D^{20} 1.5863. pKb 9.30. pH of 0.2 molar aq soln 8.1. One gram dissolves in 28.6 ml water, 15.7 ml boil. water; misc with alcohol, benzene, chloroform, and most other organic solvents. Combines with acids to form salts. It dissolves alkali or alkaline earth metals with evolution of hydrogen and formation of anilides, e.g., C_6H_5NHNa. *Keep well closed and protected from light. Incompat.* Oxidizers, albumin, solns of Fe, Zn, Al, acids, and alkalies. LD$_{50}$ orally in rats: 0.44 g/kg (Jacobson).

Hydrobromide. $C_6H_7N \cdot HBr$. White to slightly reddish, crys-talline powder, mp 286°. Darkens in air and light. Sol in water, alc. *Protect from light.*

Hydrochloride. $C_6H_7N \cdot HCl$. Crystals, mp 198°. d 1.222. Darkens in air and light. Sol in about 1 part water; freely sol in alc. *Protect from light.*

Hydrofluoride. $C_6H_7N \cdot HF$. Crystalline powder. Turns gray on standing. Freely sol in water; slightly sol in cold, freely in hot alc.

Nitrate. $C_6H_7N \cdot HNO_3$. Crystals, dec about 190°. d 1.36. Discolors in air and light. Sol in water, alc. *Protect from light.*

Hemisulfate. $C_5H_7N \cdot \frac{1}{2}H_2SO_4$. Crystalline powder. d 1.38. Darkens on exposure to air and light. One gram dissolves in about 15 ml water; slightly sol in alc. Practically insol in ether. *Protect from light.*

Acetate. $C_6H_5NH_2 \cdot HOOCCH_3$. Prepd from aniline and acetic acid: Vignon, Evieux, *Bull. Soc. Chim. Fr.* [4] **3,** 1012 (1908). Colorless liquid. d 1.070-1.072. Darkens with age; gradually converted to acetanilide on standing. Misc with water, alc.

Oxalate. $C_6H_5NH_2 \cdot HOOCCOOH.H_2NC_6H_5$. Prepd from ani-line and oxalic acid in alc soln: Hofmann, *Ann.* **47,** 37 (1843). Triclinic rods from water, mp 174-175°. Readily sol in water; sparingly sol in abs alc. Practically insol in ether.

Caution: Poisoning may occur from inhalation, skin penetration or ingestion. Potential symptoms of overexposure are navy blue to black lips, tongue, mucous membranes; slate gray skin; headache, nausea, vomiting, confusion, ataxia, vertigo, tinnitus, weakness, disorientation, cyanosis, coma; tachycardia, heart blocks, arryhthmia, shock; painful micturition, hematuria, hemoglobinuria, methemo-globinuria, oliguria, renal insufficiency; cirrhosis. Direct contact may cause eye irritation. Potential occupational carcinogen. *See* NIOSH *Pocket Guide to Chemical Hazards* (DHHS/NIOSH 97-140, 1997) p 18; *Clinical Toxicology of Commercial Products,* R. E. Gosselin *et al.,* Eds. (Williams & Wilkins, Baltimore, 5th ed., 1984) Section III, pp 31-36.

USE: Manuf dyes, medicinals, resins, varnishes, perfumes, shoe blacks; vulcanizing rubber; as solvent. Hydrochloride used in manuf of intermediates, aniline black and other dyes, in dyeing fabrics or wood black.

660. Aniline Mustard. [553-27-5] N,N-Bis(2-chloroeth-yl)benzenamine; N,N-bis(2-chloroethyl)aniline; phenylbis[2-chlo-roethylamine]; β,β'-dichlorodiethylaniline. $C_{10}H_{13}Cl_2N$; mol wt 218.12. C 55.06%, H 6.01%, Cl 32.51%, N 6.42%. Prepd by the action of phosphorus pentachloride on N,N-bis-[2-hydroxyethyl]-aniline (phenyldiethanolamine): Robinson, Watt, *J. Chem. Soc.* **1934,** 1538; Korshak, Strepikheev, *J. Gen. Chem. USSR* **14,** 312 (1944).

Stout prisms from methanol, mp 45°. bp$_{14}$ 164°; bp$_{0.5}$ 110°. Sol in hot methanol, ethanol. Very slightly sol in ether.

Hydrochloride. $C_{10}H_{14}Cl_3N$. Crystals. *Vesicant.* Freely sol in water. Sol in alcohol.

USE: In cancer research.

661. 1-Anilino-8-naphthalenesulfonate. [82-76-8] 8-(Phenylamino)-1-naphthalenesulfonic acid; 8-anilino-1-naphtha-lenesulfonic acid; ANS; phenylperi acid. $C_{16}H_{13}NO_3S$; mol wt

299.34. C 64.20%, H 4.38%, N 4.68%, O 16.03%, S 10.71%. Hydrophobic fluorescent probe for protein studies; originally used in prepn of aniline dyes. Prepd from 8-aminonaphthalenesulfonic acid, aniline and anilinium hydrochloride. Fluorescence spectrum: L. Stryer, *Science* **162,** 526 (1968). Binding to bovine serum albumin: G. Weber, L. B. Young, *J. Biol. Chem.* **239,** 1415 (1964); to lipoproteins: R. A. Muesing, T. Nishida, *Biochemistry* **10,** 2952 (1971); to chymotrypsin: J. D. Johnson *et al., ibid.* **18,** 1292 (1979); L. D. Weber *et al., ibid.* 1297. Interaction with rod outer segment membrane: U. P. Andley, B. Chakrabarti, *ibid.* **20,** 1687 (1981).

Magnesium salt. $C_{32}H_{24}MgN_2O_6S_2$. Green crystals from water. uv max: 350 nm (ε 4.95 × 10³).

Ammonium salt. $C_{16}H_{16}N_2O_3S$. mp 242-244°.

USE: Fluorescent probe. In protein conformation studies. Magnesium salt as visualization reagent for proteins.

662.　　Aniracetam. [72432-10-1] 1-(4-Methoxybenzoyl)-2-pyrrolidinone; 1-*p*-anisoyl-2-pyrrolidinone; Ro-13-5057; Draganon; Sarpul. $C_{12}H_{13}NO_3$; mol wt 219.24. C 65.74%, H 5.98%, N 6.39%, O 21.89%. Cognition enhancer related to piracetam, *q.v.* Prepn: **JP Kokai 79 117468;** E. Kyburz, W. Aschwanden, **US 4369139** (1979, 1983 both to Hoffmann-La Roche). Effects on learning and memory in rats: R. Cumin *et al., Psychopharmacology* **78,** 104 (1982); K. Yamada *et al., Pharmacol. Biochem. Behav.* **22,** 645 (1985); in monkeys and pigeons: M. J. Pontecorvo, H. L. Evans, *ibid.* 745. Clinical evaluation in geriatric patients: P. Foltyn *et al., Arzneim.-Forsch.* **33,** 865 (1983); in Alzheimer's disease: L. B. Sourander *et al., Psychopharmacology* **91,** 90 (1987). Review of toxicology: B. Schläppi *et al., Drug Invest.* **5,** Suppl. 1, 50-67 (1993).

Crystals from ethanol, mp 121-122°. LD₅₀ in rats, mice (mg/kg): ~4500, >5000 orally (Cumin).

THERAP CAT: Nootropic.

663.　　*p*-Anisaldehyde. [123-11-5] 4-Methoxybenzaldehyde; anisic aldehyde. $C_8H_8O_2$; mol wt 136.15. C 70.57%, H 5.92%, O 23.50%. Metabolic product of the odoriferous fungus *Lentinus lepidus* Fr.: Birkinshaw *et al., Biochem. J.* **38,** 131 (1944); of wood-rotting fungus *Polyporus benzoinus* (Wahl.) Fr.: Birkinshaw *et al., ibid.* **50,** 509 (1952); of *Daldalea juniperina* Murr.: Birkinshaw, Chaplen, *ibid.* **60,** 255 (1955). Prepn: Niedzielski, Nord, *J. Am. Chem. Soc.* **63,** 1462 (1941); Sisti *et al., J. Org. Chem.* **27,** 279 (1962). Toxicity study: P. M. Jenner *et al., Food Cosmet. Toxicol.* **2,** 327 (1964).

Oily liquid, bp 248°, bp₁.₅ 89-90°. mp 0°. d_4^{15} 1.119. n_D^{13} 1.5764. Volatile in steam. Very slightly sol in water; misc with alc, ether. LD₅₀ orally in rats: 1510 mg/kg (Jenner).

USE: Perfumery and toilet soaps; odor resembles that of coumarin, but the aldehyde must be mixed with other odorous substances to yield an agreeable odor. Also used in organic syntheses.

664.　　Anise. Aniseed. Dried ripe fruit of *Pimpinella anisum* L., *Umbelliferae. Habit.* Western Asia, Egypt; cultivated in Southern Europe, India and U.S. *Constit.* Coumarins including scopoletin, umbelliferone; flavonol and flavone glycosides; 2-6% volatile oil, 50% carbohydrate, 16% lipids, β-amyrin, stigmasterol. Description and uses: J. Barnes *et al., Herbal Medicines* (Pharmaceutical Press, London, 2nd Ed., 2002) pp 51-54.

Volatile oil. [8007-70-3] Aniseed oil; oil of anise. *Constit.* 80-95% *trans*-anethole, estragole (methylchavicol), anise ketone, β-caryophyllene, anisaldehyde. Colorless or pale yellow, refractive liquid. d_{25}^{25} 0.978-0.988. Solidif pt not below 15°. α_D +1 to −1°. n_D^{20} 1.553-1.560. Slightly sol in water; sol in about 3 vols alcohol, freely in chloroform, ether. *Keep cool in well-closed and well-filled containers, protected from light.*

USE: Pharmaceutic aid (flavor). As condiment and flavor in foods or beverages; in manuf of liqueurs.

THERAP CAT: Carminative; expectorant.

665.　　Anise Alcohol. [105-13-5] 4-Methoxybenzenemethanol; *p*-methoxybenzyl alcohol; anisyl alcohol. $C_8H_{10}O_2$; mol wt 138.16. C 69.55%, H 7.30%, O 23.16%. Prepd by reduction of anisaldehyde with triisobutyl aluminum and with amine boranes: Ziegler *et al., Ann.* **623,** 9 (1959); Chamberlain, Schechter, **US 2898379** (1959 to Callery Chemical). Toxicity study: Woodart *et al., J. Pharmacol. Exp. Ther.* **93,** 26 (1948).

Liquid, bp 259°. mp 24-25°, solidif 17°. d_{15}^{15} 1.113. Practically insoluble in water. Freely soluble in alc, ether. LD₅₀ orally in rats: 1.2 ml/kg (Woodart).

666.　　*p*-Anisic Acid. [100-09-4] 4-Methoxybenzoic acid. $C_8H_8O_3$; mol wt 152.15. C 63.15%, H 5.30%, O 31.55%. Prepd from methoxybenzene: Gross *et al., Ber.* **96,** 1382 (1963). Manuf by catalytic oxidation of *p*-methoxytoluene: **GB 798619** (1958 to General Electric); Cotterill *et al.,* **GB 842998** (1960 to I.C.I.).

Needles, mp 184° (subl). bp 275-280°. d 1.385. Soluble in 2500 parts water; more sol in boiling water; freely sol in alc, chloroform, ether, ethyl acetate.

667.　　Anisidine. C_7H_9NO; mol wt 123.15. C 68.27%, H 7.37%, N 11.37%, O 12.99%. Prepn of *p*-isomer: Cahours, *Ann.* **74,** 298 (1850); of *o*-isomer: Mühlhäuser, *Ann.* **207,** 235 (1881); of *m*-isomer: Kadaba, Massie, *J. Org. Chem.* **22,** 333 (1957).

m-**Anisidine.** 3-Methoxybenzenamine; 3-methoxyaniline; 3-aminoanisole. Pale yellow, oily liquid. Remains fluid even at −10°. bp 251°, bp₂ 81-86°. Sparingly sol in water; sol in alc, acids.

o-**Anisidine.** 2-Methoxybenzenamine. Yellowish liquid; becomes brownish on exposure to air. Volatile with steam. bp 225°. mp 5°. d_{15}^{15} 1.098. Practically insol in water. Miscible with alc, ether, acetone, benzene. *Keep well closed and protected from light.*

p-**Anisidine.** 4-Methoxybenzenamine. Crystals, mp 57°. bp 246°. Sparingly sol in water; freely sol in methanol, ethanol.

Caution: *o*-Anisidine hydrochloride is reasonably anticipated to be a human carcinogen: *Report on Carcinogens, Eleventh Edition* (PB2005-104914, 2004) p III-17.

USE: In the manuf of azo dyes.

668. Anisindione. [117-37-3] 2-(4-Methoxyphenyl)-1*H*-indene-1,3(2*H*)-dione; 2-*p*-anisyl-1,3-indandione; 2-(*p*-methoxyphenyl)-1,3-indandione; SPE-2792; Miradon; Unidone. $C_{16}H_{12}O_3$; mol wt 252.26. C 76.18%, H 4.79%, O 19.03%. Prepn: Koelsch, *J. Am. Chem. Soc.* **58,** 1331 (1936); Horeau, Jacques, *Bull. Soc. Chim. Fr.* **1948,** 53; Sperber, US 2899358 (1959 to Schering).

Pale yellow crystals from acetic acid or ethanol, mp 156-157°.

THERAP CAT: Anticoagulant.

669. Anisole. [100-66-3] Methoxybenzene. C_7H_8O; mol wt 108.14. C 77.75%, H 7.46%, O 14.80%. Prepn from phenol and dimethyl sulfate: Ullmann, *Ann.* **327,** 114 (1903); Graebe, *Ann.* **340,** 204 (1905); G. S. Hiers, F. D. Hager, *Org. Synth.* **coll. vol. I,** 58 (2nd ed., 1941); from bromobenzene: Agfa, DE 411052; *Chem. Zentralbl.* **1925, I,** 2411; *Frdl.* **15,** 193; by passing methyl chloride into a suspension of sodium phenolate in liquid ammonia: White *et al., J. Am. Chem. Soc.* **46,** 965 (1924); from phenol, methyl iodide and potassium carbonate in dimethylformamide: Brieger *et al., J. Chem. Eng. Data* **13,** 581 (1968). Forms oils or resins by condensation with formaldehyde: DE 403264; DE 406152; *Chem. Zentralbl.* **1925, I,** 307, 1816; *Frdl.* **14,** 626, 627. Absorption spectrum: Scheibe, *Ber.* **59,** 2625 (1926). Soly in glycerol, *see* McEwen, *J. Chem. Soc.* **123,** 2285 (1923). Toxicity studies: J. M. Taylor *et al., Toxicol. Appl. Pharmacol.* **6,** 378 (1964).

Liquid. Agreeable aromatic odor. d_4^{18} 0.9956; d_4^{45} 0.9701. mp −37.3°. bp_{760} 155.5°; bp_{100} 93.0°; bp_{40} 70.7°; bp_{20} 55.8°; bp_{10} 42.2°; bp_5 30.0°; $bp_{1.0}$ 5.4°. n_D^{20} 1.51791. Sol in alcohol and ether. Insol in water. LD_{50} orally in rats: 3700 mg/kg (Taylor).

USE: In perfumery, in organic syntheses.

670. Anisomycin. [22862-76-6] (2*R*,3*S*,4*S*)-2-[(4-Methoxyphenyl)methyl]-3,4-pyrrolidinediol 3-acetate; [2*R*-(2α,3α,4β)]-2-[(4-methoxyphenyl)methyl]-3,4-pyrrolidinediol 3-acetate; 2-*p*-methoxyphenylmethyl-3-acetoxy-4-hydroxypyrrolidine; 1,4,5-trideoxy-1,4-imino-5-(4-methoxyphenyl)-D-*xylo*-pentitol 3-acetate. $C_{14}H_{19}NO_4$; mol wt 265.30. C 63.38%, H 7.22%, N 5.28%, O 24.12%. Protein synthesis inhibiting antibiotic isolated from *Streptomyces*: B. A. Sobin, F. W. Tanner, Jr., *J. Am. Chem. Soc.* **76,** 4053 (1954); Tanner *et al.,* US 2691618 (1954 to Pfizer). Activity: J. E. Lynch *et al., Antibiot. Chemother.* **4,** 844, 899 (1954). Structure and stereochemistry: J. J. Beereboom *et al., J. Org. Chem.* **30,** 2334 (1965); J. P. Schaefer, P. J. Wheatley, *ibid.* **33,** 166 (1968); K. Butler, *ibid.* 2136. Biosynthesis: *idem, ibid.* **31,** 317 (1966). Total synthesis: Oida, Ohki, *Chem. Pharm. Bull.* **16,** 2086 (1968); *ibid.* **17,** 1405 (1969); I. Felner, K. Schenker, *Helv. Chim. Acta* **53,** 754 (1970). Chiral synthesis: J. P. H. Verheyden *et al., Pure Appl. Chem.* **50,** 1363 (1978). Stereospecific total synthesis: D. P. Schumacher, S. S. Hall, *J. Am. Chem. Soc.* **104,** 6076 (1982). Improved synthesis: A. N. Hulme, E. M. Rosser, *Org. Lett.* **4,** 265 (2002). Mechanism of action: A. Jiménez, D. Vázquez in *Antibiotics* **vol.**

5(pt. 2), F. E. Hahn, Ed. (Springer-Verlag, New York, 1979) pp 1-19. Soly and stability data: *Antibiot. Annu.* **1954-55,** pp 809-810. Memory impairment effects in mice: K. M. Lattal, T. Abel, *Proc. Natl. Acad. Sci. USA* **101,** 4667 (2004).

Long needles from ethyl acetate or water, mp 140-141°. $[\alpha]_D^{23}$ −30° (methanol). uv max: 224, 277, 283 nm (ε 10800, 1800, 1600). pKa 7.9. Base is moderately sol in water; sol in lower alcohols, esters, ketones, chloroform; slightly sol in benzene, toluene and hexane.

Hydrochloride. [1963-48-0] $C_{14}H_{19}NO_4$.HCl. Crystals from ethyl acetate + ethanol, mp 187-188°. Very sol in water.

Deacetylanisomycin. [27958-06-1] $C_{12}H_{17}NO_3$; mol wt 223.27. Prepn from anisomycin: Nickell *et al.,* US 2935444 (1960 to Pfizer). mp 176-179°. $[\alpha]_D^{25}$ −20.0° (methanol), pK 9.2.

USE: Agricultural fungicide.

671. Anisotropine Methylbromide. [80-50-2] *endo*-8,8-Dimethyl-3-[(1-oxo-2-propylpentyl)oxy]-8-azoniabicyclo[3.2.1]octane bromide; 3α-hydroxy-8-methyl-1α*H*,5α*H*-tropanium bromide 2-propylvalerate; 8-methyltropinium bromide 2-propylvalerate; 8-methyl-3-(2-propylpentanoyloxy)tropinium bromide; octatropine methylbromide; Valpin. $C_{17}H_{32}BrNO_2$; mol wt 362.35. C 56.35%, H 8.90%, Br 22.05%, N 3.87%, O 8.83%. Anticholinergic. Prepn: Weiner, Gordon, US 2962499 (1960 to Endo Labs.). Metabolism: Shindo *et al., Chem. Pharm. Bull.* **19,** 513 (1971). Clinical trial in ulcer: J. H. Bowers *et al., J. Clin. Pharmacol.* **18,** 365 (1978).

Crystals from acetone, mp 329°.

Methyl chloride. $C_{17}H_{32}ClNO_2$. Crystals from acetone, mp 289°.

THERAP CAT: Antispasmodic.

672. *o*-(*p*-Anisoyl)benzoic Acid. [1151-15-1] 2-(4-Methoxybenzoyl)benzoic acid; S-23/46. $C_{15}H_{12}O_4$; mol wt 256.25. C 70.31%, H 4.72%, O 24.97%. Prepn from phthalic anhydride and anisole: Meyer, Turnau, *Monatsh. Chem.* **30,** 486 (1909). Alternate route: Arcus, Marks, *J. Chem. Soc.* **1956,** 1627.

Leaflets from water. Stout crystals from alcohol or toluene, mp 146°. Very sparingly sol in water. Freely sol in alc, ether, toluene, chloroform, glacial acetic acid.

Sodium salt. $C_{15}H_{11}NaO_4$. Needles. Freely sol in water. Sol in alcohol. Rated approximately 150 times as sweet as cane sugar. Bitter taste if used in concns exceeding 0.2 g/liter. *Review:* Möhler, *Z. Lebensm.-Unters. Forsch.* **90,** 431 (1950), *C.A.* **44,** 8558d (1950).

USE: The sodium salt has been proposed as a sweetening agent.

673. *p*-Anisoyl Chloride. [100-07-2] 4-Methoxybenzoyl chloride. $C_8H_7ClO_2$; mol wt 170.59. C 56.33%, H 4.14%, Cl 20.78%, O 18.76%. Prepd from *p*-anisic acid and thionyl chloride: Vanderhaeghe *et al., J. Pharm. Pharmacol.* **6,** 119 (1954).

Crystals or liquid. mp 22°. bp ~262-263° with slight decompn. Dec by water or alcohol. Sol in acetone, benzene.

Caution: Vapors can cause serious eye burns. Sealed containers may explode, because slow decompn at room temp may build up pressure. *Ref:* Carroll, *Chem. Eng. News* **38,** 40 (Aug. 22, 1960).

674. Anistreplase. [81669-57-0] Anisoylated plasminogen streptokinase activator complex; APSAC; BRL-26921; Eminase; Multilase. Binary complex of streptokinase and human plasminogen in which the catalytic site is reversibly blocked by a *p*-methoxybenzoyl group without affecting the fibrin-binding site. Prepn and fibrinolytic activity: R. A. G. Smith, J. G. Winchester, **EP 28489;** *eidem, US 4808405* (1981, 1989 both to Beecham). Deacylation of the fibrin-bound complex initiates thrombolysis: R. A. G. Smith *et al., Nature* **290,** 505 (1981); D. Matsuo *et al., Thromb. Res.* **24,** 347 (1981). Effect on hemostasis in humans: D. H. Staniforth *et al., Eur. J. Clin. Pharmacol.* **24,** 751 (1983). Pharmacokinetics: M. Been *et al., Int. J. Cardiol.* **11,** 53 (1986). Evaluation of thrombolytic efficacy in myocardial infarction: W. Kasper *et al., Am. J. Cardiol.* **58,** 418 (1986); in major pulmonary embolism: J. H. Brett *et al., Aust. N.Z. J. Med.* **17,** 77 (1987). Controlled clinical trial in acute myocardial infarction: S. Ikram *et al., Br. Med. J.* **293,** 786 (1986). Review of mechanism of action, pharmacology and therapeutic use: J. P. Monk, R. C. Heel, *Drugs* **34,** 25-49 (1987).

THERAP CAT: Thrombolytic.

675. Annatto. [1393-63-1] C.I. Natural Orange 4; C.I. 75120; arnotta; annotta. Coloring matter from seeds of *Bixa orellana* L., *Bixaceae.* Extraction from seed: Barnett, Espoy, **US 2815287** (1957); Kocher, **US 2831775** (1958). Contains bixins, *q.v.,* and several other yellow to orange-red pigments which give carotene reactions: Diemair *et al., Naturwissenschaften* **39,** 211 (1933). Review of chemistry and applications: P. Collins, *Food Ingred. Proc. Int.* **13,** 23-27 (1992). *See also: Colour Index* vol. 3 (3rd ed., 1971) p. 3233.

Sol in alcohol, ether, oils.

USE: Food coloring in dairy products, esp butter and cheese, flour confectionary, fish, meat products, soft drinks, snack foods and dry mixes. In wood stains, polish, and varnishes. Spice or condiment. Insect repellent.

676. Annexins. Family of calcium and phopholipid binding proteins; virtually ubiquitous in both animal and plant cells. Characterized by a common structure composed of 4 or 8 homologous repeats of ~70 amino acids. Involved in membrane trafficking, transmembrane channel activity, inhibition of phospholipase A2, and inhibition of coagulation. Known variously by such names as *synexin, lipocortin, anchorin,* and *calpactin,* the term annexins was chosen for their ability to bind, or "annex", to cellular membranes. Description of nomenclature: M. J. Crumpton, J. R. Dedman, *Nature* **345,** 212 (1990). Isoln of synexin from bovine adrenal medullary tissue: C. E. Creutz *et al., J. Biol. Chem.* **253,** 2858 (1978). Review of discovery, molecular biology and bioactivites: P. Raynal, H. B. Pollard, *Biochim. Biophys. Acta* **1197,** 63-93 (1994); of annexins in plant cells: G. B. Clark, S. J. Roux, *Plant Physiol.* **109,** 1133-1139 (1995). Review of three-dimensional structure: S. Liemann, R. Huber, *Cell. Mol. Life Sci.* **53,** 516-521 (1997). Review of role in plasminogen binding: H.-M. Kang et al., *Trends Cardiovasc. Med.* **9,** 92-102 (1999); K. A. Hajjar, S. Krishman, *ibid.* 128-138; of role in membrane fusion: H. Kubista *et al., Subcell. Biochem.* **34,** 73-131 (2000); as nucleotide binding proteins: J. Bandorowicz-Pikula *et al., BioEssays* **23,** 170-178 (2001). Comprehensive description: V. Gerke, S. E. Moss, *Physiol. Rev.* **82,** 331-371 (2002).

677. Annotinine. [559-49-9] $C_{16}H_{21}NO_3$; mol wt 275.34. C 69.79%, H 7.69%, N 5.09%, O 17.43%. Isoln from *Lycopodium annotinum* L., *Lycopodiaceae:* Manske, Marion, *Can. J. Res.* **21B,** 92 (1943). Structure: Przybylska, Marion, *Can. J. Chem.* **35,** 1075 (1957); Wiesner *et al., Tetrahedron* **4,** 87 (1958); Przybylska, Ahmed, *Acta Crystallogr.* **11,** 718 (1958). Stereochemistry: Wiesner *et al., Tetrahedron Lett.* **1961,** 187; Ho, *ibid.* **1969,** 1307. Synthesis: Wiesner *et al., Can. J. Chem.* **47,** 433 (1969). Biogenesis: Leete, *Tetrahedron* **3,** 313 (1958).

Brilliant prisms from chloroform + methanol, mp 232°. Sol in chloroform, dil HCl. Sparingly sol in methanol.

678. *p*-Anol. [539-12-8] 4-(1-Propenyl)phenol; *p*-propenylphenol; 4-hydroxy-1-propenylbenzene. $C_9H_{10}O$; mol wt 134.18. C 80.56%, H 7.51%, O 11.92%. Prepn from anethole: Stoermer, Kahlert, *Ber.* **34,** 1812 (1901); from 4-propenylphenylmagnesium bromide: Quelet, *Bull. Chim. Soc.* [4] **45,** 268 (1929).

Leaflets from boiling water. Weak odor of cloves, resembling that of eugenol. Spicy, pungent taste. mp 93-94°. bp_{760} 250° (dec); bp_{14} 138-140°. Slightly sol in hot water. Freely sol in dimethylformamide, other organic solvents. Sol in aq solns of KOH and NaOH.

USE: Intermediate in the synthesis of estrogens.

679. Anserine. [584-85-0] *N*-β-Alanyl-3-methyl-L-histidine; α-(β-aminopropionylamino)-β-(1-methyl-5-imidazolyl)-propionic acid; 3-methyl-*N*,α-(β-alanyl)-L-histidine. $C_{10}H_{16}N_4O_3$; mol wt 240.26. C 49.99%, H 6.71%, N 23.32%, O 19.98%. First found in muscles of geese, later in many more animals, but not in man, cow, horse, or dog. Isoln: Ackermann, *Z. Physiol. Chem.* **183,** 1 (1929); Wolff, Wilson, *J. Biol. Chem.* **109,** 565 (1935). Synthesis: Behrens, du Vigneaud, *J. Biol. Chem.* **120,** 517 (1937); Rinderknecht *et al., J. Org. Chem.* **29,** 1968 (1964). Review: M. Guggenheim, *Die biogenen Amine* (Karger, Basel & New York, 4th ed., 1951) pp 439-446, 502.

L-Form. Needles from dil alc, dec 240-242°. $[\alpha]_D^{30}$ +12.3° (c = 5). pK_1 2.64; pK_2 7.04; pK_3 9.49. The dried material is very hygroscopic. Freely soluble in water. Slightly sol in methanol, even less in ethanol.

Nitrate. $C_{10}H_{16}N_4O_3 \cdot HNO_3$. Needles from dil methanol, mp 226-228°.

680. Antazoline. [91-75-8] 4,5-Dihydro-*N*-phenyl-*N*-(phenylmethyl)-1*H*-imidazole-2-methanamine; 2-(*N*-benzylanilino-methyl)-2-imidazoline; phenazoline; 2-(*N*-phenyl-*N*-benzyl-aminomethyl)imidazoline; imidamine; 5512-M. $C_{17}H_{19}N_3$; mol wt 265.35. C 76.95%, H 7.22%, N 15.84%. Prepn: Miescher, Klarer, *US 2449241* (1948 to Ciba). HPLC determn in ophthalmic solutions: S. C. Ruckmick *et al., J. Pharm. Sci.* **84,** 502 (1995). Clinical trial in combination with naphazoline in allergic conjunctivitis: M. B. Abelson *et al., Arch. Ophthalmol.* **108,** 520 (1990).

Crystals, mp 120-122°.

Hydrochloride. [2508-72-7] Antistine; Antasten. $C_{17}H_{19}N_3$·HCl; mol wt 301.81. Bitter crystals producing temporary numbness of the tongue. mp 237-241°. uv max: 242 nm ($E_{1cm}^{1\%}$ 495 to 515); min 222 nm. One gram dissolves in 40 ml water, in 25 ml alc. Practically insol in ether, benzene, chloroform. pH (1% aq soln): 6.3.

Phosphate. [154-68-7] $C_{17}H_{19}N_3$·H_3PO_4. Crystals. Bitter taste. mp 194-198°. Sol in water. Sparingly sol in methanol. Practically insol in benzene, ether. pH (2% aq soln): 4.5.

THERAP CAT: Antihistaminic.

THERAP CAT (VET): Antihistaminic.

681. Antheridiol. [22263-79-2] (3β,22S,23R)-3,22,23-Trihydroxy-7-oxostigmasta-5,24(28)-dien-29-oic acid γ-lactone; 3β,22,23-trihydroxy-24-(carboxymethylene)cholest-5-en-7-one 23,24-lactone. $C_{29}H_{42}O_5$; mol wt 470.64. C 74.01%, H 8.99%, O 17.00%. The first specific functioning sex hormone to be identified in the plant kingdom. A diffusible substance secreted by the female mycelium of the filamentous water molds *Achlya bisexualis* and *A. ambisexualis*, which induces the growth of antheridial hyphae in the male plant, thereby initiating sexual reproduction in the species. Isoln and preliminary chemical data: Raper, Haagen-Smit, *J. Biol. Chem.* **143**, 311 (1942). Isoln of crystalline material: McMorris, Barksdale, *Nature* **215**, 320 (1967). Structure: Arsenault *et al., J. Am. Chem. Soc.* **90**, 5635 (1968). Synthesis: J. A. Edwards *et al., ibid.* **91**, 1248 (1969); J. H. Fried, J. A. Edwards, **US 3547911** (1970 to Syntex). Stereochemical proposal: Green *et al., Tetrahedron* **27**, 1199 (1971). Absolute stereochemistry and alternate syntheses: Edwards *et al., Tetrahedron Lett.* **1972**, 791; T. C. McMorris *et al., ibid.* 2673; *eidem, J. Org. Chem.* **39**, 669 (1974). *Reviews:* Barksdale, *Ann. N.Y. Acad. Sci.* **144**, 313-319 (1967); *idem, Science* **166**, 831-837 (1969); T. C. McMorris, *Lipids* **13**, 716-722 (1978).

Colorless crystals from methanol, mp 250-255°. uv max (ethanol): 220 nm (ε 17,000). Sol in hot methanol. Slightly sol in chloroform; very slightly sol in water.

USE: Control and regulation of plant fertility.

682. Anthracene. [120-12-7] $C_{14}H_{10}$; mol wt 178.23. C 94.34%, H 5.66%. Obtained from coal tar, *q.v.*: Dumas, Laurent, *Ann.* **5**, 10 (1833); Laurent, *Ann.* **34**, 287 (1840); Anderson, *Ann.* **122**, 294 (1862); *J. Chem. Soc.* **15**, 44 (1862); Auerbach, *Das Anthracen und seine Derivate* (Braunschweig, 1880); Perkin, *J. Soc. Arts* **27**, 572 (1879); Lunge, *Coal Tar and Ammonia* (1916); Barnett, *Anthracene and Anthraquinone* (London, 1921); Nanson, *Text. Color.* **48**, 605, 678, 751 (1926); **49**, 19, 246, 557, 593 (1927); Houben, Fischer, *Das Anthracen und die Anthrachinone* (Leipzig, 1929); Borrmann, *Der Teer* (Leipzig, 1940); Schumann, *Kokereiteer* (Stuttgart, 1940). Extensive patent literature on purification. Prepn of very pure anthracene from synthetic anthraquinone: Clar, *Ber.* **72**, 1645 (1939). *Review:* E. Clar, *Polycyclic Hydrocarbons* Vol. 1 & 2 (Academic Press, New York, 1964). Review of toxicology and human exposure: *Toxicological Profile for Polycyclic Aromatic Hydrocarbons* (PB95-264370, 1995) 487 pp.

Monoclinic plates from alc. Sublimes. When pure, colorless with violet fluorescence; when impure (due to tetracene, naphthacene), yellow with green fluorescence. Strongly triboluminescent and triboelectric. d_4^{27} 1.25. mp 218°. bp$_{760}$ 342°. Absorption spectrum: Clar, *Ber.* **65**, 506 (1932). Less soluble than the isomeric phenanthrene. Insol in water; one gram dissolves in 67 ml abs alcohol, 70 ml methanol, 62 ml benzene, 85 ml chloroform, 200 ml ether, 31 ml carbon disulfide, 86 ml carbon tetrachloride, 125 ml toluene. Anthracene darkens in sunlight. According to Downs, **US 1303639** (1919), when solns of crude anthracene in coal tar naphtha are exposed to ultraviolet irradiation, the anthracene is precipitated as dianthracene (*para*-anthracene) which is reconverted to anthracene by sublimation. Forms molecular addn products with nitro compounds.

Picric acid complex. mp 139°.

sym-**Trinitrobenzene complex.** mp 164°.

Trinitrotoluene complex. mp 162°.

USE: Important source of dyestuffs (manuf anthraquinone, alizarin dyes).

683. Anthragallol. [602-64-2] 1,2,3-Trihydroxy-9,10-anthracenedione; 1,2,3-trihydroxyanthraquinone; anthragallic acid; anthracene brown. $C_{14}H_8O_5$; mol wt 256.21. C 65.63%, H 3.15%, O 31.22%. From gallic acid and benzoic acid with sulfuric acid at 125° or from phthalic anhydride and pyrogallol with sulfuric acid at 160°: Seuberlich, *Ber.* **10**, 39 (1877). Other methods: Kubota, Perkin, *J. Chem. Soc.* **127**, 1889 (1925); Perkin, Story, *ibid.* **1929**, 1399; Cross, Perkin, *ibid.* **1930**, 292. Absorption spectrum: Meyer, Fischer, *Ber.* **46**, 85 (1913).

Brown crystals, mp 312-313°. Sublimes 290°. Slightly sol in water, chloroform; sol in alcohol, ether, glacial acetic acid. Its soln in concd H_2SO_4 is reddish-brown. Greenish-brown soln in ammonia water changes to blue on heating. Forms salts with Na, K, Ba, Tl, Pb, La, Ce, Nd, Co.

Trimethyl ether. $C_{17}H_{14}O_5$. Yellow needles from benzene + petr ether, mp 168°. Insol in water solns of alkalies.

684. Anthralin. [1143-38-0] 1,8-Dihydroxy-9(10H)-anthracenone; 1,8-dihydroxyanthrone; dithranol; Anthraforte; Anthranol; Anthrascalp; Antraderm; Cignolin; Dithrocream; Drithocreme; Dritho-Scalp; Micanol; Psoradrate; Psoriderm. $C_{14}H_{10}O_3$; mol wt 226.23. C 74.33%, H 4.46%, O 21.22%. Prepn: Y. Hirosé, *Ber.* **45**, 2474 (1912); K. Zahn, H. Koch, *ibid.* **71B**, 172 (1938). Revised structure: H. M. Avdovich, G. A. Neville, *Can. J. Spectrosc.* **25**, 110 (1980); F. R. Ahmed, *Acta Crystallogr.* **B36**, 3184 (1980). Historical review: R. E. Ashton *et al., J. Am. Acad. Dermatol.* **9**, 173-192 (1983). Review of mechanism of action: L. Kemény *et al., Skin Pharmacol.* **3**, 1-20 (1990); of clinical pharmacology and efficacy in psoriasis: G. Mahrle, *Clin. Dermatol.* **15**, 723-737 (1997).

Lemon yellow leaflets or needles from ligroin, mp 176-181°. Practically insol in water. Sol in chloroform, acetone, benzene. Slightly sol in alcohol, ether, glacial acetic acid. Sol in dil NaOH with yellow color and green fluorescence, becoming orange-red on exposure to air.

THERAP CAT: Antipsoriatic.

685. Anthramycin. [4803-27-4] [11R-[2(E),11α,11aβ]]-3-(5,10,11,11a-Tetrahydro-9,11-dihydroxy-8-methyl-5-oxo-1H-pyrrolo[2,1-c][1,4]benzodiazepin-2-yl)-2-propenamide; 5,10,11,11a-tetrahydro-9,11-dihydroxy-8-methyl-5-oxo-1H-pyrrolo[2,1-c][1,4]-benzodiazepin-2-acrylamide. $C_{16}H_{17}N_3O_4$; mol wt 315.32. C 60.94%, H 5.43%, N 13.33%, O 20.30%. Antitumor antibiotic produced by *Streptomyces refuineus* var *thermotolerans*, NRRL 3143: Leimgruber *et al.*, *J. Am. Chem. Soc.* **87**, 5791 (1965); Berger *et al.*, US 3361742 (1968 to Hoffmann-La Roche). Also from *Streptomyces spadicogriseus*: N. Komatsu *et al.*, *J. Antibiot.* **33**, 54 (1980). Structure: Leimgruber *et al.*, *J. Am. Chem. Soc.* **87**, 5793 (1965). Synthesis: *eidem, ibid.* **90**, 5641 (1968); Batcho, Leimgruber, US 3524849 (1970 to Hoffmann-La Roche). Activity studies: Horwitz, Grollman, *Antimicrob. Agents Chemother.* **1968**, 21. Biosynthesis: L. H. Hurley *et al.*, *J. Am. Chem. Soc.* **97**, 4372 (1975). *Review:* Kohn in *Antibiotics* vol. 3, J. W. Corcoran, F. E. Hahn, Eds. (Springer-Verlag, New York, 1975) pp 3-11.

Yellow prisms from acetone + water, dec 188-194°. uv max (acetonitrile): 235, 333 nm (ϵ 18,200, 31,800). $[\alpha]_D^{25}$ +930° (DMF).

Methyl ether hydrate. $C_{17}H_{19}N_3O_4 \cdot H_2O$. Pale yellow needles from methanol + water, dec above 120°.

686. Anthranol. [529-86-2] 9-Anthracenol; 9-anthrol; 9-hydroxyanthracene. $C_{14}H_{10}O$; mol wt 194.23. C 86.57%, H 5.19%, O 8.24%. Prepd by dissolving anthrone in 5 to 10% boiling NaOH soln, cooling to −5° and pouring in cooled 5% H_2SO_4: Meyer, *Ann.* **379**, 56 (1911). Also prepared from anthraquinone.

Needles from glacial acetic acid, plates from dil alcohol. Orthorhombic, mp 120° (if bath is heated to 110°). Sinters at 120°, mp 152° (if bath is cold at start). Absorption spectrum (of acetate): Barnett *et al.*, *J. Chem. Soc.* **1928**, 885. Sol in most solvents with blue fluorescence. The solid is fairly stable when kept dry. In solution it changes quickly to anthrone. Recrystallizations of anthranol may lead to a less pure compound.

Acetate. $C_{16}H_{12}O_2$. Crystals from petr ether, mp 134°.
Benzoate. $C_{21}H_{14}O_2$. Crystals from pyridine + alcohol, mp 170-172°.
Methyl ether. $C_{15}H_{12}O$. Crystals from alcohol, mp 97-98°.
Ethyl ether. $C_{16}H_{14}O$. Crystals from methanol, mp 73°.
USE: In the manuf of dyes.

687. Anthraquinone. [84-65-1] 9,10-Anthracenedione; 9,10-anthraquinone; 9,10-dioxoanthracene; Flight Control. $C_{14}H_8O_2$; mol wt 208.21. C 80.76%, H 3.87%, O 15.37%. Prepn: A. Laurent, *Ann.* **34**, 287 (1840). Structural relationship with anthracene: C. Graebe, C. Liebermann, *Ber.* **2**, 332 (1869). Industrial prepn from phthalic anydride and benzene: Klipstein, *Ind. Eng. Chem.* **18**, 1327 (1926). From anthracene with vanadium pentoxide, sodium chlorate, glacial acetic and sulfuric acids: *Org. Synth.* coll. vol. II, 554 (1943). Convenient lab procedure: L. F. Fieser, *Organic Experiments* (Heath & Co., Boston, 1964) pp 195-200. Review of chemistry: M. Phillips, *Chem. Rev.* **6**, 157 (1929); of manufacture and uses: A. J. Cofrancesco in *Kirk-Othmer Encyclopedia of Chemical Technology* Vol. 2 (Wiley-Interscience, New York, 4th ed., 1992) pp 801-814. Development as bird repellent: R. M. Poché, *Proc. 18th Vertebr. Pest Conf.* **1998**, 338. Field trial to control Canadian geese: P. Devers *et al. ibid.* 345.

Light yellow, slender monoclinic prisms by sublimation *in vacuo*. Almost colorless, orthorhombic, bipyramidal crystals from H_2SO_4 + H_2O. d_4^{20} 1.42-1.44. mp 286°. bp_{760} 377°. Absorption spectrum: Flexser *et al.*, *J. Am. Chem. Soc.* **57**, 2103 (1935). Insol in water. Solubility (g/100 g) in alc at 18° 0.05; at 25° 0.44; in boiling alc 2.25; in ether at 25° 0.11; in chloroform at 20° 0.61; at 40° 1.00; at 60° 1.60; in benzene at 20° 0.26; at 40° 0.50; at 60° 1.00; at 80° 1.80; in toluene at 25° 0.30.

Caution: Low acute oral toxicity, but may cause skin irritation, sensitization. *See Clinical Toxicology of Commercial Products*, R. E. Gosselin *et al.*, Eds. (Williams & Wilkins, Baltimore, 5th ed., 1984) Section II, p 189.

USE: Starting material for the manufacture of dyes; bird repellent.

688. Anthrarobin. [577-33-3] 1,2,10-Anthracenetriol; 1,2,10-anthratriol; 3,4-dihydroxyanthranol; desoxyalizarin; leucoalizarin. $C_{14}H_{10}O_3$; mol wt 226.23. C 74.33%, H 4.46%, O 21.22%. Prepd from alizarin, ammonia, and zinc dust: *Hagers Handb. Pharm. Praxis* Vol. **1**, 466 (1930).

Yellow-brown to dark brown crystals; easily oxidized to alizarin. mp 208°; not sublimable. Slightly sol in water or benzene; freely sol in alcohol, ether, acetone, glacial acetic acid. Dissolves in alkalies with greenish-yellow color; in concd H_2SO_4 with golden-yellow color.

THERAP CAT: Parasiticide.

689. Anthrarufin. [117-12-4] 1,5-Dihydroxy-9,10-anthracenedione; 1,5-dihydroxyanthraquinone. $C_{14}H_8O_4$; mol wt 240.21. C 70.00%, H 3.36%, O 26.64%. Prepd from 1,5-anthraquinone potassium disulfonate: Fierz-David, Blangey, *Farbenchemie* (Vienna, 5th ed, 1943), pp 224-225.

Green to yellow crystals from acetic acid, mp 280°. Sublimes at 120°. Absorption spectrum in H_2SO_4: Meyer, Fischer, *Ber.* **46**, 85 (1913). Sol in concd H_2SO_4, in aq KOH soln (reddish color); insol in aq Na_2CO_3, NH_3, $Ba(OH)_2$. Moderately sol in alcohol, slightly in water.

USE: Important intermediate in the manuf of alizarin and indanthrene dyestuffs. Forms insol Ba and Ca lakes; has been proposed as analytical reagent for the detection of Ca.

690. Anthrimide. [82-22-4] 1,1′-Iminobis-9,10-anthracenedione; 1,1′-iminodianthraquinone; dianthraquinonylamine; dianthrimide. $C_{28}H_{15}NO_4$; mol wt 429.42. C 78.31%, H 3.52%, N 3.26%, O 14.90%. Prepd by heating 1-aminoanthraquinone with 1-chloroanthraquinone in nitrobenzene in the presence of copper: Bayer & Co., DE 162823; *Chem. Zentralbl.* **1905, II**, 1206; Eckert, Steiner, *Monatsh. Chem.* **35**, 1129 (1914); *FIAT Report* **no. 1313, vol. II** (1948), p 137.

Deep red needles from chlorobenzene, rhombs from nitrobenzene. Also described as coppery red needles with metallic sheen. Practically insol in low boiling organic solvents. Sparingly sol in aniline, nitrobenzene, chlorobenzene, quinoline. Sol in concd sulfuric acid first giving a scarlet-red color which turns olive-green on standing.

USE: Determination of boron. Used as a 0.02% soln in concd H_2SO_4. The olive-green soln turns blue in the presence of boron. The blue soln has an absorption max at 620 nm. Also used in the determination of silicon.

691. Anthrone. [90-44-8] 9(10*H*)-Anthracenone; 9,10-dihydro-9-oxoanthracene; Carbothrone. $C_{14}H_{10}O$; mol wt 194.23. C 86.57%, H 5.19%, O 8.24%. Prepn from anthraquinone by reduction with tin, glacial acetic and hydrochloric acid: *Org. Synth.* **coll. vol. I**, 60 (1941). By cyclization of *o*-benzylbenzoic acid with liquid HF: Fieser, Hershberg, *J. Am. Chem. Soc.* **61**, 1278 (1939).

Orthorhombic needles from benzene + petr ether, mp 155°. Absorption spectrum: Martin, *Ann. Combustibles Liq.* **12**, 967 (1937). Sol in most organic solvents without fluorescence. Any fluorescence present is due to anthranol. Tendency to change to anthraquinone. Equilibrium in abs alc: 89% anthrone; 11% anthranol.

Addition compound with 4 mols desoxycholic acid. $C_{110}H_{170}O_{17}$. mp 179°.

USE: In organic syntheses; in the colorimetric determination of sugar and animal starch in body fluids.

692. Antimony. [7440-36-0] Stibium; regulus of antimony. Sb; at. wt 121.60; at. no. 51; valence 3, 5. Group VA (15). Two naturally occurring isotopes: 121 (57.25%); 123 (42.75%); artificial radioactive isotopes: 112-120; 122; 124-135; isotopes 122 and 124 are useful radioactive tracers. First accurate description of antimony by Thölde (Basil Valentine) in 1604. Antimony ore is mined in China, Mexico, and Bolivia. The antimony of commerce is about 99% pure. Prepn in the laboratory by reduction of Sb_2O_5 with KCN: Schenk in *Handbook of Preparative Inorganic Chemistry* **vol. 1**, G. Brauer, Ed. (Academic Press, 2nd ed., 1963) p 606. Toxicity study: W. R. Bradley, W. G. Fredrick, *Ind. Med.* **10**, *Ind. Hyg. Sect.* **2**, 15 (1941). *Review:* Smith, "Arsenic, Antimony and Bismuth" in *Comprehensive Inorganic Chemistry* **vol. 2**, J. C. Bailar, Jr. *et al.*, Eds. (Pergamon Press, Oxford, 1973) pp 547-683; S. C. Carapella in *Kirk-Othmer Encyclopedia of Chemical Technology* **vol. 3** (Wiley-Interscience, New York, 3rd ed., 1978) pp 96-105. Review of toxicology and human exposure: *Toxicological Profile for Antimony and Compounds* (PB93-110641, 1992) 160 pp.

Silver-white, lustrous, hard, brittle metal; scale-like crystalline structure; or dark gray, lustrous powder. Is not tarnished in dry air and only slowly in moist air. d 6.68. mp 630°. bp 1635°; also reported to be 1440°: *Gmelins, Antimony* (8th ed.) **18B**, p 69 (1949). sp heat 0.049; electrical resistivity 39 μ-ohm-cm at 0°. Not affected by cold dil acids; attacked by hot concd H_2SO_4; readily by aqua regia. Nitric acid, depending on the concn, converts it to antimonous or antimonic oxide. When finely divided it reacts with hot concd HCl. Qualitative analysis for antimony: react with slight excess of HCl with aid of HNO_3; pour soln in large vol of water; white ppt forms which becomes orange-red on addn of H_2S and is sol in ammonium sulfide. LD_{50} in rats, guinea pigs (mg Sb/100 g): 10.0, 15.0 i.p. (Bradley, Fredrick).

Caution: Potential symptoms of overexposure are cough, dizziness, headache, nausea, vomiting, diarrhea, stomach cramps, insomnia, anorexia, inability to smell properly. Direct contact may cause irritation of eyes, skin, nose, throat and mouth. *See NIOSH Pocket Guide to Chemical Hazards* (DHHS/NIOSH 97-140, 2003) p 18.

USE: In manufacture of alloys, such as Britannia or Babbitt metal, hard lead, white metal, type, bullets and bearing metal; in fireworks; for thermoelectric piles, blackening iron, coating metals, etc.

693. Antimony Chloride Oxide. [7791-08-4] Antimony oxychloride; basic antimony chloride; powder of Algaroth; Mercurius vitae. ClOSb; mol wt 173.21. Cl 20.47%, O 9.24%, Sb 70.30%. SbOCl. Prepd from $SbCl_3$ and water: Schenk in *Handbook of Preparative Inorganic Chemistry* **vol 1**, G. Brauer, Ed. (Academic Press, N.Y., 2nd ed., 1963) p 611.

Monoclinic crystals or crystalline powder. Hydrolyzed by water to Sb_2O_3. Sol in HCl, tartaric acid, CS_2; practically insol in alcohol, ether. Heating to 250° results in formation of $Sb_2O_5Cl_2$; above 320° Sb_2O_3 is formed.

694. Antimony Dichlorotrifluoride. [7791-16-4] Antimony chloride fluoride; antimony dichlorofluoride; antimony trifluorodichloride. Cl_2F_3Sb; mol wt 249.66. Cl 28.40%, F 22.83%, Sb 48.77%. $SbCl_2F_3$. Prepd according to the exothermic reaction $SbF_3 + Cl_2 \rightarrow SbCl_2F_3$: Henne, *Org. React.* **2**, 61 (1944); Kwasnik in *Handbook of Preparative Inorganic Chemistry* **Vol. 1**, G. Brauer, Ed. (Academic Press, New York, 2nd ed., 1963) pp 200-201. Prepd from $SbCl_5$ and ClF_3: Dehnicke, Weidlein, *Z. Anorg. Allg. Chem.* **323**, 267 (1963).

Viscous liquid. Can be stored in iron vessels.

Caution: Highly toxic.

USE: As catalyst in the manufacture of organic fluorine compds: Slesser, Schram, *Preparation, Properties, and Technology of Fluorine and Organic Fluoro Compounds* (New York, 1951) *passim.*

695. Antimony Pentachloride. [7647-18-9] Cl_5Sb; mol wt 299.03. Cl 59.28%, Sb 40.72%. $SbCl_5$. Usually prepd by passing chlorine into molten antimony trichloride. Laboratory procedure: Schenk in *Handbook of Preparative Inorganic Chemistry* **Vol. 1**, G. Brauer, Ed. (Academic Press, New York, 2nd ed., 1963) p 610.

Colorless to yellow, oily liquid. Fumes in air. Cannot be distilled at atmospheric pressures without complete decompn. d_4^{16} 2.358; d_4^{36} 2.319; d_4^{52} 2.289; d_4^{78} 2.231. mp 3.5°. bp_{14} 68°; bp_{22} 79°; bp_{30} 92°; bp_{55} 85°; bp_{68} 102.5°. Dipole moment: 1.14 at 16.3° in CCl_4. Mono- and tetrahydrates are formed in the presence of small amounts of water. Large amounts of water cause hydrolysis to Sb_2O_5. Sol in hydrochloric acid, chloroform, carbon tetrachloride.

USE: As catalyst when replacing a fluorine substituent with chlorine in organic compounds.

696. Antimony Pentafluoride. [7783-70-2] F_5Sb; mol wt 216.75. F 43.83%, Sb 56.18%. SbF_5. Lewis acid. Prepd industrially (in aluminum apparatus) according to the equation $SbCl_5 + 5HF \rightarrow 5HCl + SbF_5$: Ruff, Plato, *Ber.* **37**, 673 (1904); Perkins, Irwin, *US* 2410358 (1946). Laboratory procedure using SbF_3 and F_2: Woolf, Greenwood, *J. Chem. Soc.* **1950**, 2200; Kwasnik in *Handbook of Preparative Inorganic Chemistry* **Vol. 1**, G. Brauer, Ed. (Academic Press, New York, 2nd ed., 1963) p 200. *Reviews:* Burg in *Fluorine Chemistry* **Vol. 1**, J. Simons, Ed. (Academic Press, New York, 1950) pp 104-106; Kemmitt, Sharp, *Adv. Fluorine Chem.* **4**, 210-211 (1965).

Hygroscopic, corrosive, moderately viscous liquid. *Poisonous, attacks skin.* mp 8.3°; bp 141°. $d^{25.8}$ 3.097; density data: Hoffman, Jolly, *J. Phys. Chem.* **61**, 1574 (1957). Reacts violently with water. Also forms a solid dihydrate, which reacts violently with more water to form a clear soln. Slowly hydrolyzed in NaOH solns forming $Sb(OH)_6^-$. Forms solids with sulfur chloride, carbon disulfide, benzene, toluene, petr ether (resin formation), ether, alc, acetone, ethyl acetate. Glacial acetic acid gives a clear soln. Slowly corrodes glass, copper, lead. May be stored in aluminum vessels.

USE: In the fluorination of organic compds, *see* the monograph *Preparation, Properties and Technology of Fluorine and Organic*

Fluoro Compounds, C. Slesser, S. R. Schram, Eds. (McGraw-Hill, New York, 1951) 868 pp.

697.   Antimony Pentasulfide. [1315-04-4] Golden antimony sulfide; antimonic sulfide; antimonial saffron; antimony red. S_5Sb_2; mol wt 403.85. S 39.70%, Sb 60.30%. Sb_2S_5. Prepn: *Gmelins, Antimony* (8th ed.) **18B**, pp 534-539 (1949). Existence of Sb^{5+} sulfide doubted: Birchall, Della Valle, *Chem. Commun.* **1970**, 675. Toxicity study: W. R. Bradley, W. G. Fredrick, *Ind. Med.* **10**, *Ind. Hyg. Sect.* **2**, 15 (1941).

Orange-yellow, odorless powder. Insol in water. Sol in concd HCl with evolution of H_2S; sol in solns of alkali hydroxides or sulfides, forming sulfantimoniates. *Incompat.* Acids, metal salts. LD_{50} i.p. in rats: 150.0 mg Sb/100 g (Bradley, Fredrick).

USE: As pigment; vulcanizing and coloring rubber; manuf matches and fireworks.

698.   Antimony Pentoxide. [1314-60-9] Antimonic oxide; "stibic" anhydride; antimonic "acid". O_5Sb_2; mol wt 323.52. O 24.73%, Sb 75.27%. Sb_2O_5. Prepn: Schenk in *Handbook of Preparative Inorganic Chemistry* **vol. 1**, G. Brauer, Ed. (Academic Press, New York, 2nd ed., 1963) p 616. Toxicity study: W. R. Bradley, W. G. Fredrick, *Ind. Med.* **10**, *Ind. Hyg. Sect.* **2**, 15 (1941).

Yellowish powder. Cubic. d 3.78. Loses oxygen at 300° or higher. Studies have shown that the compound does not correspond fully to Sb_2O_5, but that it is always somewhat hydrated. Slightly soluble in water. Practically insol in HNO_3. Slowly dissolves in warm HCl or in warm KOH soln. LD_{50} i.p. in rats: 400.0 mg Sb/100 g (Bradley, Fredrick).

USE: Fire retardant in clothing.

699.   Antimony Potassium Oxalate. [5965-33-3] Ethanedioic acid anhydride with antimonic acid (3:1) tripotassium salt; tripotassium tris(oxalato)antimonate(3−); potassium oxalatoantimonate(III); "antimony salt". $C_6K_3O_{12}Sb$; mol wt 503.11. C 14.32%, K 23.31%, O 38.16%, Sb 24.20%. $K_3[Sb(OOCCOO)_3]$. Prepn of trihydrate: Graddon, *J. Inorg. Nucl. Chem.* **3**, 308 (1956-1957).

Trihydrate, cryst powder. Sol in water. *Poisonous!*

USE: A mordant in dyeing and printing fabrics instead of tartar emetic.

700.   Antimony Potassium Tartrate. [28300-74-5] Dipotassium bis[$μ$-[2,3-dihydroxybutanedioato(4−)-01,02:03,04]]diantimonate(2−) trihydrate stereoisomer; tartar emetic; tartrated antimony; tartarized antimony; potassium antimonyltartrate. $C_8H_4K_2$-$O_{12}Sb_2$.$3H_2O$; mol wt 667.87. C 14.39%, H 1.51%, K 11.71%, O 35.93%, Sb 36.46%. Manuf from potassium bitartrate and metallic antimony in the presence of HNO_3 or solid antimony oxide: Davies, **US 2335585** (1943 to Am. Cream Tartar); **US 2391297** (1945 to Stauffer Chem.). Structural studies: P. Pfeiffer, E. Schmitz, *Pharmazie* **4**, 451 (1949); E. Chinoporos, N. Papathanasopoulos, *J. Phys. Chem.* **65**, 1643 (1961); D. Grdenic, B. Kamenar, *Acta Crystallogr.* **19**, 197 (1965); R. Iyer *et al., J. Inorg. Nucl. Chem.* **34**, 3351 (1972). Toxicity: N. Ercoli, *Proc. Soc. Exp. Biol. Med.* **129**, 284 (1968). Anthelmintic activity: Z. Farid *et al., Trans. R. Soc. Trop. Med. Hyg.* **66**, 119 (1972); R. R. C. New *et al., Nature* **272**, 56 (1978). Oxidimetric determn: Y. A. Gawargious *et al., Pharmazie* **41**, 59 (1980).

2K⁺ • 3H₂O

Transparent crystals (effloresce on exposure to air) or powder. Sweetish, metallic taste. *Poisonous!* d 2.6. $[\alpha]_D^{20}$ +140.69° (c = 2 in water), +139.25° (c = 2 in glycerol). One gram dissolves in 12 ml water, 3 ml boiling water, 15 ml glycerol. Insol in alcohol. The aq soln is slightly acid. LD_{50} in mice (mg/kg): 55 s.c.; 65 i.v. (Ercoli). *Incompat.* Mineral acids, tannic acid, gallic acids, alkali hydrox-

ides and carbonates, lead and silver salts, mercury bichloride, lime water, albumin, soap.

USE: As mordant in the textile and leather industry.

THERAP CAT: Anthelmintic (Schistosoma).

THERAP CAT (VET): Has been used as a parasiticide (gastrointestinal and blood parasites); as an expectorant, and as a ruminatoric.

701.   Antimony Sodium Gluconate. General term referring to either a trivalent or pentavalent antimony complex with sodium gluconate. Pentavalent compound may require reduction *in vivo* to the trivalent form to be bioactive. Determn in biological materials and pharmacodynamics: R. J. Ward *et al., Clin. Chim. Acta* **99**, 143 (1979). Mechanism of action study: J. C. Mottram, G. H. Coombs, *Exp. Parasitol.* **59**, 151 (1985).

Sodium antimonylgluconate. [12550-17-3] $C_6H_8NaO_7Sb$; mol wt 336.87. Trivalent antimony compound. Prepn: Das Gupta, *Indian J. Pharm.* **15**, 84 (1953); A. Axon *et al.,* **US 3306921** (1967 to Burroughs Wellcome). Antiparasitic activity: N. Ercoli *et al., Chemotherapy* **26**, 254 (1980). White, amorphous powder. Sol in water. Insol in organic solvents. pH of 2% aq soln 9-10; the soln at this pH is unstable.

Sodium stibogluconate. [16037-91-5] 2,4:2′,4′-O-(Oxydistibylidyne)bis[D-gluconic acid] Sb,Sb'-dioxide trisodium salt nonahydrate; Pentostam; Solustibosan. $C_{12}H_{17}Na_3O_{17}Sb_2$.$9H_2O$; mol wt 907.88. Pentavalent antimony compound. Prepn: Datta, Ghosh, *Sci. Cult.* **11**, 699 (1945-6); Bose, Ghosh, *Indian J. Pharm.* **11**, 155 (1949). Pharmacokinetics: J. D. Chulay *et al., Trans. R. Soc. Trop. Med. Hyg.* **82**, 69 (1988). Review of clinical safety and efficacy in leishmaniasis: B. L. Herwaldt, J. D. Berman, *Am. J. Trop. Med. Hyg.* **46**, 296 (1992). Crystals. Freely sol in water. pH of 10% aq soln 5.4-5.6.

THERAP CAT: Trivalent compd as an anthelmintic (Schistosoma); pentavalent compd as an antiprotozoal (Leishmania).

702.   Antimony Sodium Tartrate. [34521-09-0] Antimony sodium oxide L(+)-tartrate; sodium antimonyl tartrate; Stibnal. $C_4H_4NaO_7Sb$; mol wt 308.82. C 15.56%, H 1.31%, Na 7.44%, O 36.27%, Sb 39.43%. (SbO)$NaC_4H_4O_6$. Trivalent antimonial. Prepn: Fargher, Gray, *J. Pharmacol. Exp. Ther.* **18**, 341 (1921). Antiparasitic activity *in vitro:* N. Ercoli *et al., Chemotherapy (Basel)* **26**, 254 (1980).

Hygroscopic, transparent or whitish scales or powder. Sweetish taste. Sol in 1.5 parts water. Practically insol in 90% alc. Aq solns are slightly acid to litmus. LD i.v. in mice: 25 mg/kg (Fargher, Gray).

THERAP CAT: Anthelmintic (Schistosoma).

703.   Antimony Sodium Thioglycollate. [539-54-8] [(5-Oxo-1,3,2-oxathiostibolan-2-yl)thio]acetic acid sodium salt; mercaptoacetic acid antimony derivative sodium salt; antimony sodium thioacetate. $C_4H_4NaO_4S_2Sb$; mol wt 324.95. C 14.78%, H 1.24%, Na 7.07%, O 19.69%, S 19.74%, Sb 37.47%. Prepn of the free acid: Klason, Carlson, *Ber.* **39**, 732 (1906); of the salt: Myers, *J. Lab. Clin. Med.* **6**, 359 (1921).

Hygroscopic prismatic crystals turning pink under the influence of light. May develop slight odor of mercaptan on standing. Freely sol in water. Practically insol in alc. Decomposed by excess alkali; incompatible with alkalies.

THERAP CAT: Anthelmintic (Schistosoma).

704.   Antimony Sulfate. [7446-32-4] Antimonous sulfate; antimony trisulfate. $O_{12}S_3Sb_2$; mol wt 531.71. O 36.11%, S 18.09%, Sb 45.80%. $Sb_2(SO_4)_3$. Prepn: Schenk in *Handbook of Preparative Inorganic Chemistry* **vol. 1**, G. Brauer, Ed. (Academic Press, New York, 2nd ed., 1963) pp 618-619.

Crystalline powder or lumps; deliquesc in air. *Poisonous!* d 3.62. With a little water forms a solid mass which dissolves in more water, but excess of water changes it into an insol basic salt. Sol in dil acids. *Keep well closed.*

705.   Antimony Thioglycollamide. [6533-78-4] Thioantimonic acid tris(2-amino-2-oxoethyl) ester; mercaptoacetamide antimony derivative; antimony thioglycollic acid triamide. C_6H_{12}-$N_3O_3S_3Sb$; mol wt 392.13. C 18.38%, H 3.08%, N 10.72%, O 12.24%, S 24.53%, Sb 31.05%. $Sb(SCH_2CONH_2)_3$. Prepd by the action of ammonia on ethyl antimony thioglycollate in absolute alc. The ethyl antimony glycollate is prepd from ethyl thioglycollate and antimony trioxide: Rowntree, Abel, *J. Pharmacol.* **2**, 109 (1910). *cf.* Christiansen, *Organic Derivatives of Antimony*, A.C.S. Monograph Series No. **24**, (New York, 1925).

Crystals, mp 140°. One gram dissolves in about 200 ml water. Slightly sol in alc. Insol in ether. Incompatible with alkalies.

THERAP CAT: Anthelmintic (Schistosoma).

706. Antimony Tribromide. [7789-61-9] Br_3Sb; mol wt 361.47. Br 66.32%, Sb 33.68%. $SbBr_3$. Best prepd from the elements: Schenk in *Handbook of Preparative Inorganic Chemistry* **vol. 1**, G. Brauer, Ed. (Academic Press, New York, 2nd ed., 1963) p 613.

Orthorhombic bipyramidal needles. Less hygroscopic than $SbCl_3$. d_4^{23} 4.148. mp 96°. bp_{749} 288°. Cryoscopic constant: 26.7. Specific heat: 0.0709 at 33°. Critical temp: 904.5°; crit press. 56 atm. Dipole moment: 2.47. Dec by light, water, alc. Sol in dil HCl, HBr, carbon disulfide, acetone, benzene, chloroform.

707. Antimony Trichloride. [10025-91-9] Trichlorostibine; Butter of antimony. Cl_3Sb; mol wt 228.12. Cl 46.62%, Sb 53.38%. $SbCl_3$. Prepd from the elements: Hensgen, *Rec. Trav. Chim.* **9**, 301 (1890); Kendall *et al.*, *J. Am. Chem. Soc.* **45**, 967 (1923); Schenk in *Handbook of Preparative Inorganic Chemistry* **vol. 1**, G. Brauer, Ed. (Academic Press, New York, 2nd ed., 1963) p 608. Purification: Werner, *Z. Anorg. Allg. Chem.* **181**, 154 (1929); Schaafsma, *US 2324240* (1943 to Shell).

Orthorhombic, deliquesc needles from carbon disulfide or by sublimation at 100°. Fumes in air. *Poisonous!* d_4^{20} 3.14. mp 73°. bp 223.5°; bp_{70} 143.5°; bp_{11} 102°. Cryoscopic constant: 18.4. Heat of fusion at 73.2°: 13.29 cal/g. Specific heat at 33°: 0.110 cal/g/°C. Dipole moment: 3.12 at 25° in CS_2. One gram dissolves in 10.1 ml H_2O at 25°. Gradual hydrolysis to SbOCl. Considerably more sol in dil HCl. Sol in alcohol, benzene, carbon disulfide, dioxane, chloroform (about 22%), ether, acetone, carbon tetrachloride. A satd soln in carbon tetrachloride is about 1.1 molar. Insol in pyridine, quinoline, other organic bases.

Caution: Irritant, corrosive to skin.

USE: As of antimony trichloride soln; also as reagent for chloral, aromatic hydrocarbons, and vitamin A. For mol wt determinations. In chemical microscopy for the identification of drugs (forms adducts and addition compds). Commercially as a mordant, in making other antimony salts, in organic syntheses, as catalyst.

THERAP CAT (VET): Escharotic; dehorning agent (calves, goats).

708. Antimony Trichloride Solution. [10025-91-9] Antimony chloride solution; liquid butter of antimony. Contains 36-38% $SbCl_3$ and 10-12% free HCl.

Yellow to reddish-brown, clear, somewhat oily, strongly caustic liquid. d 1.5.

USE: Bronzing iron, especially gun barrels; mordant for patent leather and in dyeing; coloring zinc black; manuf lakes, particularly from dye woods; furniture polishes.

709. Antimony Trifluoride. [7783-56-4] Antimony fluoride; antimonous fluoride. F_3Sb; mol wt 178.76. F 31.88%, Sb 68.11%. SbF_3. Prepd by dissolving Sb_2O_3 in aq HF and evaporating the water: Berzelius, *Pogg. Ann.* **1**, 34 (1824); Söll, *FIAT-Review* **23**, 276 (1947); Andersen *et al.*, *Acta Chem. Scand.* **7**, 236 (1953); Kwasnik in *Handbook of Preparative Inorganic Chemistry* **Vol. 1**, G. Brauer, Ed. (Academic Press, New York, 2nd ed., 1963) p 199. Industrial prepn from $SbCl_3$ and HF: Midgeley *et al.*, *US 2024654* (1935). *Reviews:* Burg in *Fluorine Chemistry* **Vol. 1**, J. H. Simons, Ed. (Academic Press, New York, 1950) p 106; Kemmitt, Sharp, *Adv. Fluorine Chem.* **4**, 211 (1965).

Orthorhombic, deliquesc crystals. *Poisonous! Irritates the skin.* d_{20}^{20} 4.379. mp 292°. bp 376°. Also reported as bp 319° (Andersen). Soly in water (g/100 ml): 443 (20°); 562 (30°). Dissolves in water with limited hydrolysis, readily forms complexes such as $[SbF_4]^-$ and many sol salts. For the purpose of halogen exchange fluorination, the compd must be dry: Henne, *US 2082161* (1937). May be stored in glass vessels or steel drums. *Keep well closed.*

USE: To catalyze fluorinations by HF, manuf chlorofluorides, in dyeing, usually in form of double salts, e.g., antimony sodium fluoride or antimony fluoride and ammonium sulfate double salt, manuf pottery and porcelains.

710. Antimony Triiodide. [7790-44-5] I_3Sb; mol wt 502.47. I 75.77%, Sb 24.23%. SbI_3. Prepd by the interaction of antimony and iodine in boiling benzene or tetrachloroethane: Bailar, Cundy, *Inorg. Synth.* **1**, 104 (1939); Scattergood, *J. Chem. Educ.* **20**, 40 (1943).

Ruby-red, trigonal crystals (yellowish-green modifications have been observed). d_4^{17} 4.921. The tendency to sublime becomes noticeable at 100°. mp 168°. bp 420°. Critical temp 1101°; crit press. 55 atm. Dipole moment: 1.58. Dec by water and air to SbOI (antimony oxyiodide). Sol in alcohol, acetone, carbon disulfide, HCl, soln of KI. Insol in carbon tetrachloride.

711. Antimony Trioxide. [1309-64-4] Diantimony trioxide; flowers of antimony; exitelite; senarmontite; valentinite; weisspiessglanz. O_3Sb_2; mol wt 291.52. O 16.46%, Sb 83.53%. Sb_2O_3. Laboratory prepn from $SbCl_3$ and water: Schenk in *Handbook of Preparative Inorganic Chemistry* **vol. 1**, G. Brauer, Ed. (Academic Press, New York, 2nd ed., 1963) p 615. Obtained from antimony ore minerals by a volatilization (roasting) process: L. D. Freedman in *Kirk-Othmer Encyclopedia of Chemical Technology* **vol. 3** (Wiley-Interscience, New York, 3rd ed., 1978) pp 107-108. Toxicity study: H. F. Smyth *et al.*, *J. Ind. Hyg. Toxicol.* **30**, 63 (1948).

Crystals, polymorphic. mp 655°. bp 1425°; bp_{210} 870°. Sublimes in high vacuum at 400°. Exists in the vapor phase as Sb_4O_6. Heat capacity at 21° (294.4 K): 24.11 cal/g-atom/°C, Anderson, *J. Am. Chem. Soc.* **52**, 2712 (1930). Heat of vaporization: 17.82 kcal/mol. Slightly sol in water, dilute H_2SO_4, or dilute HNO_3. Soly in dil HCl (0.1 moles HCl/kg H_2O): ~1×10^{-4} g-atoms Sb/kg H_2O, Gayer, Garrett, *ibid.* **74**, 2353 (1952). Soly increases with increasing HCl concn: Lea, Wood, *J. Chem. Soc.* **125**, 137 (1924). Sol in solns of alkali hydroxides or sulfides, in warm soln of tartaric acid, or of bitartrates. LD_{50} orally in rats: >20 g/kg (Smyth).

USE: Manuf tartar emetic; as paint pigment; in enamels and glasses; as mordant; in flame-proofing canvas.

712. Antimony Triselenide. [1315-05-5] Antimony selenide. Sb_2Se_3; mol wt 480.40. Sb 50.69%, Se 49.31%. Prepd by the action of hydrogen selenide on a soln of potassium antimonyl tartrate: Moser, Atynsky, *Monatsh. Chem.* **45**, 235 (1924); Berzelius cited in *Mellor's* **Vol. 10**, 793 (1930); by direct union of the elements: Chretien, *Compt. Rend.* **142**, 1339, 1412 (1906); Parravano, *Gazz. Chim. Ital.* **43**, I, 210 (1913); Berzelius, *loc. cit. See also:* Chikashige, Fujita, *Mem. Coll. Sci. Kyoto Imp. Univ.* **2**, 233 (1917).

Gray powder. mp 605° (Berzelius); mp 611° (Chretien); mp 617° (Parravano); mp 572° (Chikashige, Fujite). Very slightly sol in water. Forms a brown soln with hot potash lye.

713. Antimony Trisulfide. [1345-04-6] Antimonous sulfide; antimony sulfide; needle antimony; antimony glance. S_3Sb_2; mol wt 339.72. S 28.32%, Sb 71.68%. Sb_2S_3. Occurs in nature as the mineral *stibnite*. Prepn: Donges, Fricke, *Z. Anorg. Chem.* **253**, 2 (1945); Gagliardi, Pilz, *Z. Anal. Chem.* **136**, 344 (1952); *Gmelins, Antimony* (8th ed.) **18B**, pp 503-524 (1949). Toxicity study: W. R. Bradley, W. G. Fredrick, *Ind. Med.* **10**, *Ind. Hyg. Sect.* **2**, 15 (1941).

Gray, lustrous, crystalline masses or grayish-black powder. Also exists in a red modification. mp 550°. Practically insol in water. Sol in concd HCl with evolution of H_2S; sol in solutions of the fixed alkali hydroxides. LD i.p. in rats: 100.0 mg Sb/100 g (Bradley, Fredrick).

USE: In pyrotechnics, Bengal fires; manuf ruby glass, matches, explosives; as a pigment in paints.

714. Antimycin A₁. [642-15-9] 3-Methylbutanoic acid 3-[[3-(formylamino)-2-hydroxybenzoyl]amino]-8-hexyl-2,6-dimethyl-4,9-dioxo-1,5-dioxonan-7-yl ester; isovaleric acid 8-ester with 3-formamido-*N*-(7-hexyl-8-hydroxy-4,9-dimethyl-2,6-dioxo-1,5-dioxonan-3-yl)salicylamide. $C_{28}H_{40}N_2O_9$; mol wt 548.63. C 61.30%, H 7.35%, N 5.11%, O 26.25%. Antibiotic substance produced by *Streptomyces* spp. Isoln: Dunshee *et al.*, *J. Am. Chem.*

Soc. **71**, 2436 (1949); Lockwood *et al., Phytopathology* **44**, 438 (1954); US 2657170 (1953 to Wisconsin Alumni Res. Found.). Structure: van Tamelen *et al., J. Am. Chem. Soc.* **83**, 1639 (1961); Birch *et al., J. Chem. Soc.* **1961**, 889. Absolute config.: Kinoshita *et al., J. Antibiot.* **25**, 373 (1972).

Crystals from ethyl acetate + Skellysolve B, mp 149-150°. $[\alpha]_D^{26}$ +76° (c = 1 in chloroform). uv max (alc): 226, 320 nm (log ε 4.54, 3.68). Freely sol in alc, ether, acetone, chloroform. Very slightly sol in petr ether, benzene, carbon tetrachloride. Practically insol in water and in 5% aq solns of hydrochloric acid, sodium carbonate and sodium bicarbonate. In aq sodium hydroxide a milky suspension is formed. This clears on warming, but all potency is lost.

USE: Experimentally as fungicide, insecticide, miticide.

715. Antimycin A₃. [522-70-3] [2R-(2R*,3S*,6S*,7R*,-8R*)]-3-Methylbutanoic acid 8-butyl-3-[[3-(formylamino)-2-hydroxybenzoyl]amino]-2,6-dimethyl-4,9-dioxo-1,5-dioxonan-7-yl ester; isovaleric acid 8-ester with N-(7-butyl-8-hydroxy-4,9-dimethyl-2,6-dioxo-1,5-dioxonan-3-yl)-3-formamidosalicylamide; blastmycin. $C_{26}H_{36}N_2O_9$; mol wt 520.57. C 59.99%, H 6.97%, N 5.38%, O 27.66%. Antifungal antibiotic substance produced by *Streptomyces blastmyceticus* from Japanese soil: Watanabe *et al., J. Antibiot.* **10A**, 39 (1957). Sepn from complex: Harada *et al., ibid.* **11**, 32 (1958). Identity of blastmycin with antimycin A₃: Liu, Strong, *J. Am. Chem. Soc.* **81**, 4387 (1959). Structural studies: Yonehara, Takeuchi, *J. Antibiot.* **11**, 254 (1958). Structure: van Tamelen *et al., J. Am. Chem. Soc.* **83**, 1639 (1961). Abs config: Kinoshita *et al., J. Antibiot.* **25**, 373 (1972). Total synthesis of diastereomeric mixture: *eidem, ibid.* **22**, 580 (1969); of natural form: *eidem, ibid.* **24**, 724 (1971); *eidem, Bull. Chem. Soc. Jpn.* **46**, 1279 (1973). Improved synthesis: S. Aburaki, M. Kinoshita, *ibid.* **52**, 198 (1979). Chemical studies: Endo, Yonehara, *J. Antibiot.* **23**, 91 (1970).

Needles from benzene + petr ether, mp 170.5-171.5° (Liu); 174-174.5° (Kinoshita). $[\alpha]_D^{26}$ +64.3° (chloroform) (Liu); $[\alpha]_D^{21}$ +80° (Kinoshita). uv max (methanol): 225, 320 nm (log ε 4.52, 3.86). Moderately sol in methanol, ethanol, ether; freely sol in acetone, ethyl acetate, benzene, chloroform, carbon tetrachloride. Slightly sol in hexane, cyclohexane; very sparingly sol in petr ether. Practically insol in water. LD₅₀ in mice (mg/kg): 1.8 i.p.; 1.6 s.c. (Watanabe).

716. Antipyrine. [60-80-0] 1,2-Dihydro-1,5-dimethyl-2-phenyl-3H-pyrazol-3-one; 2,3-dimethyl-1-phenyl-3-pyrazolin-5-one; phenazone; 1,5-dimethyl-2-phenyl-3-pyrazolone; phenyldimethylpyrazolon(e); dimethyloxychinizin; dimethyloxyquinazine; oxydimethylquinizine; Analgesine; Anodynine; Parodyne; Phenylone; Sedatine. $C_{11}H_{12}N_2O$; mol wt 188.23. C 70.19%, H 6.43%, N 14.88%, O 8.50%. Prepn: Müller *et al., Monatsh. Chem.* **89**, 23 (1958); *Hagers Handb. Pharm. Praxis* Vol. 6 (Springer Verlag, Berlin, 1977) p 571. Toxicity: Hart, *J. Pharmacol. Exp. Ther.* **89**, 205 (1947). Metabolism: H. Uchino *et al., Xenobiotica* **13**, 155 (1983). Clinical comparison with paracetamol: H. Quiding *et al., Int. J. Oral Surg.* **11**, 304 (1982). Use as indicator of hepatic drug metabolism: E. S. Vessel, *Clin. Pharm. Ther.* **26**, 275

(1979); G. C. Farrell, L. Zaluzny, *Br. J. Clin. Pharmacol.* **18**, 559 (1984). HPLC determn in urine: E. Brendel *et al., J. Pharm. Biomed. Anal.* **7**, 1783 (1989). Clinical pharmacokinetics: H. A. Ali *et al., Hum. Exp. Toxicol.* **13**, 658 (1994).

Tabular crystals or white powder; slightly bitter taste. mp 111-113°. One gram dissolves in less than 1 ml water, 1.3 ml alcohol, 1 ml chloroform, 43 ml ether. The aq soln is neutral to litmus. LD₅₀ orally in rats: 1.8 g/kg (Hart).

Acetylsalicylate. [569-84-6] Acetopyrine; Acopyrine; Acetasol. $C_{20}H_{20}N_2O_5$; mol wt 368.38. Crystals, mp 63-65°. One part dissolves in 400 parts of water, in 20 parts of 2% aq sod. bicarbonate soln. Freely sol in hot water, cold alc, chloroform; sparingly sol in ether. *Note:* Not to be confused with antipyrine salicylacetate.

Mandelate. [603-64-5] Antipyrine amygdalate. $C_{11}H_{12}N_2-O.C_8H_8O_3$. Cryst powder, mp 52-55°. One gram dissolves in 15 ml water, 4 ml alc, 26 ml ether.

Methylethylglycolate. [5794-16-1] Antipyrine 2-hydroxy-2-methylbutyrate; Astrolin. $C_{16}H_{22}N_2O_4$; mol wt 306.36. Crystalline powder, mp 64-65.5°. Soluble in water, alc.

Salicylacetate. [603-59-8] α-Carboxy-o-anisic acid compd with antipyrine; Pyrosal. $C_{20}H_{20}N_2O_6$; mol wt 384.38. Crystals, mp 149-150°. Bitter, acid taste. Sparingly soluble in water; soluble in alc. *Note:* Not to be confused with antipyrine acetylsalicylate.

THERAP CAT: Analgesic.

THERAP CAT (VET): Has been used as an antipyretic, analgesic and in laminitis of horses.

717. Antipyrine Salicylate. [520-07-0] 2-Hydroxybenzoic acid compd with 1,2-dihydro-1,5-dimethyl-2-phenyl-3H-pyrazol-3-one (1:1); Phenazone salicylate; Saliphenazon; Salazolon; Salipyrazolon; Salipyrine. $C_{18}H_{18}N_2O_4$; mol wt 326.35. C 66.25%, H 5.56%, N 8.58%, O 19.61%. Prepd by fusing antipyrine and salicylic acid: *Hagers Handb. Pharm. Praxis* Vol. 6, (Springer Verlag, Berlin, 1977) p 574.

Slightly sweet, cryst powder. mp 91-92°. One gram dissolves in 200 ml water, 40 ml boil. water; freely sol in alc, chloroform, sparingly in ether.

THERAP CAT: Analgesic.

THERAP CAT (VET): Has been used as an antipyretic, analgesic in dogs.

718. Antireticular Cytotoxic Serum. ACS; cytoxin-anticytotoxin serum; Bogomolets' serum; sarvinal. Biologic synthesis: Loiseleur, *Ann. Inst. Pasteur* **91**, 445 (1956). Purification: *C.A.* **52**, 6574e (1958). Stimulating effect on reticuloendothelial system: I. P. Miagkaia, *Zh. Mikrobiol. Epidemiol. Immunobiol.* **1978**, 82.

719. α₁-Antitrypsin. [9041-92-3] α₁-Trypsin inhibitor; α₁-proteinase inhibitor; α₁-protease inhibitor; alpha₁-antitrypsin; AAT; A1AT; A1PI; Aralast; Prolastin; Zemaira. Serum glycoprotein synthesized by the liver. Major serine protease inhibitor (serpin) in mammalian plasma; primarily inhibits neutrophil elastase. Consists of a single polypeptide chain of 394 amino acid residues and 3 carbohydrate side chains linked to asparagine residues. Mol wt ~52,000 daltons. Highly pleomorphic protein with a number of genetic variants. Characterization of trypsin inhibitor in alpha₁-

fraction of human serum: K. Jacobsson, *Scand. J. Clin. Invest.* **7**, Suppl. 14, 57-102 (1955). Isoln from human serum: F. C. Moll *et al., J. Biol. Chem.* **233**, 121 (1958); H. F. Bundy, J. W. Mehl, *ibid.* **234**, 1124 (1959). Purification: I. P. Crawford, *Arch. Biochem. Biophys.* **156**, 215 (1973); M. H. Coan, W. J. Brockway, **US 4379087** (1983 to Cutter). Structural study of active site: D. Johnson, J. Travis, *J. Biol. Chem.* **253**, 7142 (1978). Complete amino acid sequence and review of genetic variants: R. W. Carrell *et al., Nature* **298**, 329 (1982). Crystal structure: H. Loebermann *et al., J. Mol. Biol.* **177**, 531 (1984). Cloning and expression of human AAT gene: M. Courtney *et al., Proc. Natl. Acad. Sci. USA* **81**, 669 (1984). AAT deficiency has been associated with degenerative lung disease: C.-B. Laurell, S. Eriksson, *Scand. J. Clin. Lab. Invest.* **15**, 132 (1963); with hepatic cirrhosis: H. L. Sharp, *Gastroenterology* **70**, 611 (1976). Inhibition of leukocyte elastase: K. Ohlsson, *Scand. J. Clin. Lab. Invest.* **28**, 251 (1971); K. Beatty *et al., J. Biol. Chem.* **255**, 3931 (1980). Review of human phenotypes and relationship to disease: J. O. Morse, *N. Engl. J. Med.* **299**, 1045-1048; 1099-1105 (1978). Clinical evaluation in AAT deficiency: M. D. Werwers *et al., ibid.* **316**, 1055 (1987); N. Konietzko *et al., Dtsch. Med. Wochenschr.* **113**, 369 (1988); of the effect of cigarette smoking on the association rate constant with neutrophil elastase: F. Ogushi *et al., J. Clin. Invest.* **87**, 1060 (1991). Symposium on structure, function and clinical applications: *Am. J. Med.* **84**, Suppl. 6A, 1-90 (1988). Review of role in emphysema: P. J. Stone, *Clin. Chest Med.* **4**, 405-412 (1983); J. A. Pierce, *J. Am. Med. Assoc.* **259**, 2890-2895 (1988).

THERAP CAT: In treatment of emphysema associated with inherited α_1-antitrypsin deficiency.

720. Antivenin (Crotalidae) Polyvalent. North and South American antisnakebite serum. Immunoglobulin G (IgG) complex isolated from serum of horses that have been immunized with venoms of snakes from the *Crotalidae* family *(Crotalus atrox, C. adamanteus, C. durissus terrificus, Bothrops atrox)*. Ref: Gingrich, Hohenadel, in *Venoms*, E. E. Buckley, N. Porges, Eds. (Publ. 44 of Am. Assoc. Adv. of Sci., Washington, 1956) p 381; Keegan, *ibid.*, p 413. Purification: F. O. Cope, *Proc. Pa. Acad. Sci.* **53**, 43 (1979). Use in treatment of rattlesnake bites: T. M. Davidson, S. F. Schafer, *Postgrad. Med.* **96**, 107 (1994). ELISA determn in serum: C. L. Ownby *et al., South. Med. J.* **89**, 803 (1996).

THERAP CAT: Antidote to snake venom.

THERAP CAT (VET): Antidote to snake venom.

721. Antivenin (*Latrodectus mactans*). Antivenin. Black widow spider antivenin. Prepd from the serum of horses immunized against the venom of the New World spider *Latrodectus mactans* Fabr., *Araneae*. Review of clinical efficacy: R. F. Clark *et al., Ann. Emerg. Med.* **21**, 782-787 (1992).

THERAP CAT: In treatment of black widow spider bites.

722. ANTU. [86-88-4] 1-Naphthalenylthiourea; 1-(1-naphthyl)-2-thiourea; α-naphthylthiourea; *N*-1-naphthylthiourea; α-naphthylthiocarbamide; krysid; chemical 109; Anturat; Bantu; Rattrack. $C_{11}H_{10}N_2S$; mol wt 202.28. C 65.31%, H 4.98%, N 13.85%, S 15.85%. Prepd from α-naphthylamine and ammonium or potassium or sodium thiocyanate: de Clermont, Wehrlin, *Bull. Soc. Chim.* [2] **26**, 125 (1876); Alvarez, *C.A.* **42**, 4560 (1948); from α-naphthylisothiocyanate by treatment with alcoholic ammonia: Dyson, Hunter, *Chem. News* **134**, 4 (1927). Rodenticide activity: Richter, *J. Am. Med. Assoc.* **129**, 927 (1945). Review of carcinogenic risk: *IARC Monographs* **30**, 347-357 (1983).

Prisms from alc. Bitter taste. mp 198°. Solubility in water at 25°: 0.06 g/100 ml; in acetone: 2.43 g/100 ml; in triethylene glycol: 8.6 g/100 ml. Fairly sol in hot alc.

Caution: Potential symptoms of toxicity following ingestion of large doses are vomiting, dyspnea, cyanosis and coarse pulmonary rales; liver damage. *See NIOSH Pocket Guide to Chemical Hazards* (DHHS/NIOSH 97-140, 1997) p 20. May cause glomerular injury in nonlethal poisonings. *See Clinical Toxicology of Commercial Products*, R. E. Gosselin *et al.*, Eds. (Williams & Wilkins, Baltimore, 5th ed., 1984) Section III, p 40-42.

USE: Rodenticide. Specific control for the adult Norway rat; less toxic to other rat species.

723. Apafant. [105219-56-5] 4-[3-[4-(2-Chlorophenyl)-9-methyl-6*H*-thieno[3,2-*f*][1,2,4]triazolo[4,3-*a*][1,4]diazepin-2-yl]-1-oxopropyl]morpholine; 3-[4-(2-chlorophenyl)-9-methyl-6*H*-thieno[3,2-*f*][1,2,4]triazolo[4,3-*a*][1,4]diazepin-2-yl]-1-(4-morpholinyl)-1-propanone; WEB-2086. $C_{22}H_{22}ClN_5O_2S$; mol wt 455.96. C 57.95%, H 4.86%, Cl 7.78%, N 15.36%, O 7.02%, S 7.03%. Platelet activating factor (PAF) antagonist. Prepn: K. H. Weber *et al, DE 3502392; eidem, US 5082839* (1986, 1992 both to Boehringer, Ing.). Pharmacology: J. Casals-Stenzel *et al., J. Pharmacol. Exp. Ther.* **241**, 974 (1987). Clinical pharmacology, pharmacokinetics: H. M. Brecht *et al., Arzneim.-Forsch.* **41**, 51 (1991). Clinical effect vs PAF-induced bronchoconstriction: W. S. Adamus *et al., Clin. Pharmacol. Ther.* **47**, 456 (1990).

Viscous, almost colorless oil. LD_{50} in mice (mg/kg): 540 i.v.; 4600 orally (Casals-Stenzel).

USE: Tool to evaluate the role of PAF in exptl models of human disease.

724. Apalcillin. [63469-19-2] (2*S*,5*R*,6*R*)-6-[[(2*R*)-[[(4-Hydroxy-1,5-naphthyridin-3-yl)carbonyl]amino]phenylacetyl]amino]-3,3-dimethyl-7-oxo-4-thia-1-azabicyclo[3.2.0]heptane-2-carboxylic acid. $C_{25}H_{23}N_5O_6S$; mol wt 521.55. C 57.57%, H 4.44%, N 13.43%, O 18.41%, S 6.15%. Semi-synthetic antibiotic related to penicillin. Prepn of the potassium salt: H. Tobiki *et al., ZA 7205865; eidem, US 3864329* (1973, 1975 both to Sumitomo); of the sodium salt: Y. Hirotada *et al., US 4005075* (1977 to Sumitomo); H. Tobiki *et al., Yakugaku Zasshi* **100**, 49 (1980), *C.A.* **93**, 95179x (1980). Microbiological evaluation: H. Noguchi *et al., Antimicrob. Agents Chemother.* **9**, 262 (1976). Analytical studies: I. Umeda *et al., Yakugaku Zasshi* **99**, 717 (1979), *C.A.* **92**, 11287z (1980). Series of articles on pharmacology, exptl and clinical effects: *Chemotherapy (Tokyo)* **26**, Suppl. 2, 111-223 (1978). Pharmacokinetics in man: U. Busch *et al., Arzneim.-Forsch.* **32**, 1131 (1982).

Sodium salt. [58795-03-2] PC-904; Lumota. $C_{25}H_{22}N_5$-NaO_6S; mol wt 543.53. White cryst, sol in water.

THERAP CAT: Antibacterial.

725. Apamin. [24345-16-2] $C_{79}H_{131}N_{31}O_{24}S_4$; mol wt 2027.34. C 46.80%, H 6.51%, N 21.42%, O 18.94%, S 6.33%. Neurotoxic polypeptide consisting of 18 amino acid residues and 2 disulfide bridges. Comprises about 2% by wt of the dried venom of *Apis mellifica (mellifera)*, the honey bee. Isoln: E. Habermann, K. G. Reiz, *Naturwissenschaften* **51**, 61 (1964); *eidem, Biochem. Z.* **341**, 451 (1965). Structure: P. Haux *et al., Z. Physiol. Chem.* **348**,

737 (1967); R. Shipolini *et al.*, *Chem. Commun.* **1967**, 679. Conformation: R. C. Hider, U. Ragnarsson, *FEBS Lett.* **111**, 189 (1980); B. Busetta, *ibid.* **112**, 138 (1980). Solution structure: J. H. B. Pease, D. E. Wemmer, *Biochemistry* **27**, 8491 (1988). Solid-phase synthesis: J. van Rietschoten *et al.*, *Eur. J. Biochem.* **56**, 35 (1975); B. E. B. Sandberg, U. Ragnarsson, *Int. J. Pept. Protein Res.* **11**, 238 (1978). Pharmacology: Wellheoner, *Arch. Pharmakol. Exp. Pathol.* **262**, 29 (1969). Biochemistry: E. Habermann, K. G. Reiz, *Biochem. Z.* **343**, 192 (1965). Action on CNS: E. Habermann, D. Cheng-Raude, *Toxicon* **13**, 465 (1975). Binding and toxicity studies: C. Labbé-Jullié *et al.*, *Eur. J. Biochem.* **196**, 639 (1991). *Review:* E. Habermann, *Science* **177**, 314-322 (1972); C. Granier, J. van Rietschoten, in *Natural Toxins*, D. Eaker, T. Wadström, Eds. (Pergamon, New York, 1980) pp 481-486; E. Habermann, *Pharmacol. Ther.* **25**, 255-270 (1984).

Cys–Asn–Cys–Lys–Ala–Pro–Glu–Thr–Ala–Leu–Cys–Ala–Arg–Arg–Cys–Gln–Gln–HisNH$_2$

Highly basic compd. Pharmacologic activity destroyed by oxidn with performic acid. LD_{50} i.v. in mice: 4 mg/kg (Habermann, Reiz); LD_{50} intracerebroventricularly in mice: 12 ng/animal (Labbé-Jullié).

726. Apazone. [13539-59-8] 5-(Dimethylamino)-9-methyl-2-propyl-1*H*-pyrazolo[1,2-*a*][1,2,4]benzotriazine-1,3(2*H*)-dione; 3-dimethylamino-7-methyl-1,2-(*n*-propylmalonyl)-1,2-dihydro-1,2,4-benzotriazine; azapropazone; AHR-3018; MI-85; Cinnamin. $C_{16}H_{20}N_4O_2$; mol wt 300.36. C 63.98%, H 6.71%, N 18.65%, O 10.65%. Prepn: **FR 1440629**; I. Molnar *et al.*, **US 3349088** (1966, 1967, both to Siegfried); Mixich, *Helv. Chim. Acta* **51**, 532 (1968). Pharmacological and toxicological studies: Jahn, Adrian, *Arzneim.-Forsch.* **19**, 36 (1969). Metabolism: Mixich, *Helv. Chim. Acta* **55**, 1031 (1972). HPLC determn in plasma and urine: B. J. Kline *et al.*, *Arzneim.-Forsch.* **33**, 504 (1983).

mp 228°.

Dihydrate. [22304-30-9] MI-85Di; Prolixan; Rheumox; Tolyprin. Almost colorless crystals, mp 247-248°.

THERAP CAT: Anti-inflammatory; analgesic.

727. Aphidicolin. [38966-21-1] (3α,4α,5α,17α)-3,17-Dihydroxy-4-methyl-9,15-cyclo-*C*,18-dinor-14,15-secoandrostane-4,17-dimethanol; tetradecahydro-3,9-dihydroxy-4,11b-dimethyl-8,11a-methano-11a*H*-cyclohepta[*a*]naphthalene-4,9-dimethanol; ICI-69653; NSC-234714. $C_{20}H_{34}O_4$; mol wt 338.48. C 70.97%, H 10.12%, O 18.91%. Novel tetracyclic diterpene antibiotic with antiviral and antimitotic properties, isolated as (+)-form from *Cephalosporium aphidicola* Petch. Specific inhibitor of DNA α-polymerase. Description and x-ray crystallographic determn of structure: K. M. Brundret *et al.*, *Chem. Commun.* **1972**, 1027. Prepn and antiviral activity: A. Borrow *et al.*, **US 3761512** (1973 to ICI). Structure and abs config: W. Dalziel *et al.*, *J. Chem. Soc. Perkin Trans. I* **1973**, 2841. Total synthesis of (±)-aphidicolin: B. M. Trost *et al.*, *J. Am. Chem. Soc.* **101**, 1328 (1979); J. E. McMurry *et al.*, *ibid.* 1331; E. J. Corey *et al.*, *ibid.* **102**, 1743 (1980); J. E. McMurry *et al.*, *Tetrahedron* **37**, Suppl. 1, 319 (1981). Antiviral effects *in vitro* and *in vivo*: R. A. Bucknall *et al.*, *Antimicrob. Agents Chemother.* **4**, 294 (1973). Antimitotic activity: S. Ikegami *et al.*, *Nature* **275**, 458 (1978). Effects on DNA synthesis in mouse sarcoma: S. Seki *et al.*, *Biochim. Biophys. Acta* **610**, 413 (1980). Enzymatic determn method: G. Pedrali-Noy *et al.*, *J. Biochem. Biophys. Methods* **4**, 113 (1981). Induction of differentiation of human myeloid leukemia cells: J. Griffin *et al.*, *Exp. Hematol.* **10**,

774 (1982). Effects on cell proliferation: G. Iliakis *et al.*, *Int. J. Radiat. Biol.* **42**, 417 (1982); on γ-irradiated human fibroblasts: P. J. Smith, M. C. Paterson, *Biochim. Biophys. Acta* **739**, 17 (1983).

Needles from ethyl acetate, mp 227-232°. $[\alpha]_D^{27}$ +12° (c = 1 in methanol).

(±)-**Form.** White cryst, mp 218-220°.

USE: As a biological tool in studies of cell proliferation and differentiation.

728. Apholate. [52-46-0] 2,2,4,4,6,6-Hexakis(1-aziridinyl)-2,2,4,4,6,6-hexahydro-1,3,5,2,4,6-triazatriphosphorine; hexakis(1-aziridinyl)phosphonitrile; 1-aziridinylphosphonitrile trimer. $C_{12}H_{24}N_9P_3$; mol wt 387.30. C 37.21%, H 6.25%, N 32.55%, P 23.99%. Prepn: Rätz, Grundmann, **US 2858306** (1958 to Olin Mathieson). Toxicity study: T. B. Gaines, *Toxicol. Appl. Pharmacol.* **14**, 515 (1969).

Crystals from heptane, mp 147.5°. LD_{50} in male, female rats (mg/kg): 98, 113 orally (Gaines).

USE: Insect chemosterilant.

729. Aphylline. [577-37-7] [7*R*-(7α,7aβ,14α,14aα)]-Dodecahydro-7,14-methano-2*H*,6*H*-dipyrido[1,2-*a*:1′,2′-*e*][1,5]-diazocin-6-one. $C_{15}H_{24}N_2O$; mol wt 248.36. C 72.54%, H 9.74%, N 11.28%, O 6.44%. From *Anabasis aphylla* L., *Chenopodiaceae*. Extraction procedure and structure: Orechoff, Menschikoff, *Ber.* **64**, 266 (1931); **65**, 234 (1932). Structure: Galinovsky, Jarish, *Monatsh. Chem.* **84**, 199 (1953). Stereochemistry: Edwards *et al.*, *Can. J. Chem.* **32**, 235 (1954); Galinovsky *et al.*, *Monatsh. Chem.* **86**, 1014 (1955). Synthesis: Bohlmann *et al.*, *Ber.* **90**, 653 (1957).

Crystals, mp 52-57°. bp$_4$ 200°. $[\alpha]_D^{20}$ +10.3° (c = 20 in methanol). Soluble in the usual organic solvents.

Hydrochloride. $C_{15}H_{24}N_2O\cdot HCl$. Rhombohedra from alc, mp 209°. $[\alpha]_D^{20}$ +14° (c = 25). Freely soluble in water.

730. Apigenin. [520-36-5] 5,7-Dihydroxy-2-(4-hydroxyphenyl)-4*H*-1-benzopyran-4-one; 4′,5,7-trihydroxyflavone; 2-(*p*-hydroxyphenyl)-5,7-dihydroxychromone; pelargidenon 1449. $C_{15}H_{10}O_5$; mol wt 270.24. C 66.67%, H 3.73%, O 29.60%. The aglucon of apiin and of apigenin-7-glucoside. From apiin by boiling with acids, from apigenin-7-glucoside by enzymatic hydrolysis with emulsin or by boiling with 15% H_2SO_4. Isoln and structure: Czajkowski *et al.*, *Ber.* **33**, 1992 (1900); Schmid, Waschkau, *Monatsh. Chem.* **49**, 83 (1928); Baker *et al.*, *J. Chem. Soc.* **1963**, 1477.

Synthesis: Hutchins, Wheeler, *ibid.* **1939**, 91; Farooq *et al., Arch. Pharm.* **292**, 792 (1959).

Yellow needles from aqueous pyridine, mp 345-350°. uv max (ethanol): 269, 340 nm (ε 18,800; 20,900). Practically insoluble in water; moderately sol in hot alcohol. Sol in dil KOH with intense yellow color.

USE: Has been used to dye Cr mordanted wool yellow. The color is fast to soap.

731. Apigetrin. [578-74-5] 7-(β-D-Glucopyranosyloxy)-5-hydroxy-2-(4-hydroxyphenyl)-4*H*-1-benzopyran-4-one; apigenin-7-D-glucoside; 7-D-glycosylapigenin; cossmetin. $C_{21}H_{20}O_{10}$; mol wt 432.38. C 58.33%, H 4.66%, O 37.00%. Isoln from flowers of *Anthemis nobilis* L., *Compositae:* Power, Browning, *J. Chem. Soc.* **105**, 1833 (1914); from parsley: Nordström, Swain, *Chem. Ind. (London)* **1953**, 85; *J. Chem. Soc.* **1953**, 2764.

Pale yellow, cryst powder, dec 178-180°. Astringent taste. uv max (ethanol): 335, 268 nm. Sol in water, dil alcohol.

732. Apiin. [26544-34-3] 7-[(2-*O*-D-Apio-β-D-furanosyl-β-D-glucopyranosyl)oxy]-5-hydroxy-2-(4-hydroxyphenyl)-4*H*-1-benzopyran-4-one; 4′,5,7-trihydroxyflavone-7-apiosylglucoside; apigenin-7-apiosylglucoside; apioside. $C_{26}H_{28}O_{14}$; mol wt 564.49. C 55.32%, H 5.00%, O 39.68%. Isoln from parsley and from celery: Vongerichten, *Ber.* **33**, 2334, 2904 (1900); Gupta, Seshadri, *Proc. Indian Acad. Sci.* **35A**, 242 (1952), *C.A.* **47**, 3306c (1953); Rahman, *Z. Naturforsch.* **13b**, 201 (1958). Structure: Vongerichten, *Ann.* **318**, 121 (1901); Marchlewski, Skarzynski, *Biochem. Z.* **297**, 56 (1938); Hemming, Ollis, *Chem. Ind. (London)* **1953**, 85.

Crystals from ethanol, mp 230-232°. uv max (96% ethanol): 267.5, 342.5 nm (log ε 4.18, 4.30). Sol in hot water, hot alcohol; practically insol in ether. Sol in Na_2CO_3 or NH_3 solns with intense yellow color, in NaOH with pale yellow color.

733. Apiole (Dill). [484-31-1] 4,5-Dimethoxy-6-(2-propenyl)-1,3-benzodioxole; 1-allyl-2,3-dimethoxy-4,5-(methylenedioxy)benzene; dill apiole. $C_{12}H_{14}O_4$; mol wt 222.24. C 64.85%, H 6.35%, O 28.80%. Occurs in dill oil, *Anethum graveolus* L., *Umbelliferae.* Isoln: G. Ciamician, P. Silber, *Ber.* **29**, 1799 (1896); D. B. Spoelstra, *Rec. Trav. Chim.* **48**, 372 (1929). Structure: H. Thoms, *Arch. Pharm.* **242**, 344 (1904). Synthesis: W. Baker *et al., J. Chem. Soc.* **1934**, 1681; F. Dallacker, *Ber.* **102**, 2663 (1969); J. R. Cannon *et al., J. Sci. Soc. Thailand* **6**, 59 (1980). Synergistic activity with insecticides: E. P. Lichtenstein *et al., J. Agric. Food*

Chem. **22**, 658 (1974); S.S. Tomar *et al., Agric. Biol. Chem.* **43**, 1479 (1979).

Oil, mp 29.5°. bp 285°. n_D^{17} 1.5305; d_{15}^{15} 1.1598.

734. Apiole (Parsley). [523-80-8] 4,7-Dimethoxy-5-(2-propenyl)-1,3-benzodioxole; 1-allyl-2,5-dimethoxy-3,4-methylenedioxybenzene; parsley apiole; apiol; apioline; parsley camphor. $C_{12}H_{14}O_4$; mol wt 222.24. C 64.85%, H 6.35%, O 28.80%. Occurs in parsley oil, *Petroselinum sativum:* Blanchet, Sell, *Ann.* **6**, 259 (1833); Vongerichten, *Ber.* **9**, 1477 (1876); Kolesnikov *et al., Aptechnoe Delo* **7**(4), 27 (1958), *C.A.* **54**, 12491e (1960). Structure: Ciamician, Silber, *Ber.* **23**, 2283 (1890); Thoms, *ibid.* **36**, 1714 (1903). Synthesis: Baker, Savage, *J. Chem. Soc.* **1938**, 1602; F. Dallacker, *Ber.* **102**, 2663 (1969). Synergistic activity with insecticides: E. P. Lichtenstein *et al., J. Agric. Food Chem.* **22**, 658 (1974).

Crystals; faint parsley odor. mp 29.5°. bp 294°. n_D^{20} 1.536-1.538. Insol in water; sol in alcohol, benzene, chloroform, ether, acetone, oils. *Keep in a cool place.*

735. Apiose. [639-97-4] D-Apiose; tetrahydroxy-isovaleraldehyde; 3-*C*-(hydroxymethyl)-D-glyceroaldotetrose. $C_5H_{10}O_5$; mol wt 150.13. C 40.00%, H 6.71%, O 53.29%. First found in parsley in which it occurs as the flavinoid glycoside apiin, *q.v.* Isoln from apiin: Vongerichten, *Ann.* **318**, 126 (1901); **321**, 74 (1902); Hemming, Ollis, *Chem. Ind. (London)* **1953**, 85. From the rubber plant, *Hevea brasiliensis, Euphorbiaceae:* Patrick, *Nature* **178**, 216 (1956). Discussion of structure and isoln from the Australian marine plant *Posidonia australis* Kon., *Potamogetonaceae:* Bell, *Methods in Carbohydrate Chemistry* **vol. I** (Academic Press, New York, 1962) pp 260-263. Synthesis: Gorin, Perlin, *Can. J. Chem.* **36**, 480 (1958); Khalique, *J. Chem. Soc.* **1962**, 2515; Ezekiel *et al., Tetrahedron Lett.* **1969**, 1635. Synthesis of L-form: Weygand, Schmiechen, *Ber.* **92**, 535 (1959); of DL-form: Kinoshita, Miwa, *Carbohydr. Res.* **28**, 175 (1973); Y. Araki *et al., ibid.* **58**, C4 (1977); of D- and L-forms: P. Ho, *Can. J. Chem.* **57**, 381 (1979). Chemistry, configuration and synthesis studies: Williams, Jones, *ibid.* **42**, 69 (1964); Hulyalker *et al., ibid.* **43**, 2085 (1965). *Review:* Watson, Orenstein, *Adv. Carbohyd. Chem. Biochem.* **31**, 135-184 (1975).

Syrup. $[\alpha]_D^{15}$ +5.6°; $[\alpha]_D^{19}$ +9.1°. Soluble in water.

D-Apiose di-*O*-isopropylidene. $C_{11}H_{18}O_5$. Plates from water containing a trace of NH_3, mp 81-83°. $[\alpha]_D^{20}$ +55.5° (c = 1.1 in ethanol).

736. Aplasmomycin. [61230-25-9] ICI-122378. $C_{40}H_{60}$-$BNaO_{14}$; mol wt 798.70. C 60.15%, H 7.57%, B 1.35%, Na 2.88%, O 28.04%. Antibiotic produced by *Streptomyces griseus* strain SS-20, obtained from shallow sea mud: Y. Okami *et al., J. Antibiot.* **29**, 1019 (1976); *eidem,* **JP Kokai 77 108901** (1977 to Microbiochem. Res. Found.), *C.A.* **88**, 35843 (1978). It inhibits the growth of gram-positive bacteria *in vitro* and is active vs *Plasmodium berghei in vivo*. Aplasmomycin is a symmetrical dimer related to boromycin, *q.v.*, the only other known natural product that contains boron. Structure, x-ray crystallography: H. Nakamura *et al., J. Antibiot.* **30**, 714 (1977). Total synthesis of (+)-form: E. J. Corey *et al., J. Am. Chem. Soc.* **104**, 6816, 6818 (1982); T. Nakata *et al., Tetrahedron Lett.* **27**, 6341, 6345 (1986); J. D. White *et al., J. Am. Chem. Soc.* **108**, 8105 (1986). Use as growth promotant in ruminants: D. H. Davies *et al., EP 2893; eidem, US 4225593* (1979, 1980 both to ICI). Two minor components, aplasmomycins B and C, have also been isolated from the fermentation; both aplasmomycin and aplasmomycin B show ionophoric properties, mediating net K+ transport across a bulk phase: K. Sato *et al., J. Antibiot.* **31**, 632 (1978). NMR analysis of aplasmomycin and deboroaplasmomycin: T. S. S. Chen *et al., ibid.* **33**, 1316 (1980). Comparative anti-anaerobic activity of aplasmomycin: K. Watanabe *et al., Antimicrob. Agents Chemother.* **19**, 519 (1981). Structural studies: T. J. Stout *et al., Tetrahedron* **47**, 3511 (1991). Review of biosynthetic studies: H. G. Floss, C. Chang in *Antibiotics* IV, J. W. Corcoran, Ed. (Springer-Verlag, New York, 1981) pp 203-210.

(+)-Aplasmomycin

Colorless needles, mp 283-285° (dec). $[\alpha]_D^{22}$ +225° (c = 1.24 in chloroform). Very lipophilic. Practically insol in water. LD_{50} i.p. in mice: 125 mg/kg (Okami).

Silver salt. $C_{40}H_{60}AgBO_{14}$. Colorless needles, mp 218-220°. $[\alpha]_D^{23}$ +194° (c = 0.34 in chloroform).

USE: Growth promotant in ruminants.

737. Aplaviroc. [461443-59-4] 4-[4-[[(3R)-1-Butyl-3-[(R)-cyclohexylhydroxymethyl]-2,5-dioxo-1,4,9-triazaspiro[5.5]-undec-9-yl]methyl]phenoxy]benzoic acid; (3R)-1-butyl-2,5-dioxo-3-[(1R)-1-hydroxy-1-cyclohexylmethyl]-9-[4-(4-carboxyphenyloxy)phenylmethyl]-1,4,9-triazaspiro[5.5]undecane. $C_{33}H_{43}N_3O_6$; mol wt 577.71. C 68.61%, H 7.50%, N 7.27%, O 16.62%. CCR5 chemokine receptor antagonist; inhibits HIV entry by blocking interaction of viral coat protein gp120 with the receptor. Prepn: H. Habashita *et al.,* **WO 02074770** (2002 to Ono); *eidem,* **US 04082584** (2004). Study of CCR5 binding and mechanism of action: C. Watson *et al., Mol. Pharmacol.* **67**, 1268 (2005). Antiretroviral activity in immunodeficient mice: H. Nakata *et al., J. Virol.* **79**, 2087 (2005). Clinical pharmacokinetics: K. K. Adkison *et al., Antimicrob. Agents Chemother.* **49**, 2802 (2005).

Hydrochloride. [461023-63-2] AK-602; GW-873140; ONO-4128. $C_{33}H_{43}N_3O_6$·HCl; mol wt 614.17.

THERAP CAT: Antiviral.

738. Aplidine. [137219-37-5] *N*-[1-(1,2-Dioxopropyl)-L-prolyl]-didemnin A; dehydrodidemnin B; DDB; Aplidin. $C_{57}H_{87}$-

N_7O_{15}; mol wt 1110.34. C 61.66%, H 7.90%, N 8.83%, O 21.61%. Cyclic depsipeptide analog of the didemnins, *q.v.*, isolated from the marine tunicate, *Aplidum albicans*. Induces rapid apoptotic death with or without previous cell cycle arrest. Isoln and synthesis: K. Rinehart, A. M. Lithgow-Bertelloni, **WO 9104985** (1991 to PharmaMar); G. Jou *et al., J. Org. Chem.* **62**, 354 (1997). Antiproliferative effects on Ehrlich carcinoma: J. L. Urdiales *et al., Cancer Lett.* **102**, 31 (1996); cytotoxic effect on acute lymphoblastic leukemia cells: E. Erba *et al., Br. J. Cancer* **89**, 763 (2003). Mechanism of action study: *idem et al., ibid.* **86**, 1510 (2002). Degradation kinetics in solution: J. C. M. Waterval *et al., J. Chromatogr. B* **754**, 161 (2001). 2D-NMR conformational analysis in solution: F. Cárdenas *et al., J. Org. Chem.* **68**, 9554 (2003). LC/MS/MS determn in plasma: J. Yin *et al., Rapid Commun. Mass Spectrom.* **17**, 1909 (2003). *In vitro* toxicity on hematopoietic progenitors and stem cells: S. G. Gomez *et al., Exp. Hematol.* **31**, 1104 (2003). Clinical pharmacokinetics and evaluation in advanced malignancies: S. Faivre *et al., J. Clin. Oncol.* **23**, 7871 (2005).

White solid, mp 152-160°. $[\alpha]_D$ −95.9° (c = 1.8 in CHCl$_3$).
THERAP CAT: Antineoplastic.

739. Apoatropine. [500-55-0] *endo*-α-Methylenebenzeneacetic acid 8-methyl-8-azabicyclo[3.2.1]oct-3-yl ester; 1α*H*,5α*H*-tropan-3α-ol atropate; atropamine; atropyltropeine. $C_{17}H_{21}NO_2$; mol wt 271.35. C 75.25%, H 7.80%, N 5.16%, O 11.79%. Anticholinergic. Occurs in root of *Atropa belladonna* L., *Solanaceae*. Also obtained from atropine by splitting off water or by total synthesis: Ladenburg, *Ann.* **217**, 102 (1883); Merck, *Arch. Pharm.* **230**, 134 (1892); **231**, 110 (1893); Hesse, *Ann.* **261**, 87 (1891); **271**, 124 (1892); **277**, 290 (1893). Isoln by chromatography: Steinegger, Phokas, *Pharm. Acta Helv.* **31**, 284 (1956).

Prisms from chloroform, mp 62°. Absorption spectrum: Gompel, Henri, *Compt. Rend.* **156**, 1543 (1913). Freely sol in alcohol, ether, chloroform, benzene, carbon disulfide; slightly in petr ether, isoamyl alcohol. Almost insol in water.

Hydrochloride. $C_{17}H_{21}NO_2$·HCl. Scales, mp 239°. Sol in hot water; sparingly sol in alc, acetone. Nearly insol in ether.

Sulfate pentahydrate. $(C_{17}H_{21}NO_2)_2$·H_2SO_4·$5H_2O$. Crystals, sparingly sol in water.

740. Apocodeine. [641-36-1] (6a*R*)-5,6,6a,7-Tetrahydro-10-methoxy-6-methyl-4*H*-dibenzo[*de,g*]quinolin-11-ol; 10-methoxy-6aβ-aporphin-11-ol. $C_{18}H_{19}NO_2$; mol wt 281.35. C 76.84%, H 6.81%, N 4.98%, O 11.37%. A monomethyl ether of apomorphine, *q.v.* Prepd by heating codeine with oxalic acid: Folkers, *J. Am. Chem. Soc.* **58**, 1814 (1936); by heating codeine with phosphoric acid: Small *et al., J. Org. Chem.* **5**, 344 (1940). Configuration: Corrodi, Hardegger, *Helv. Chim. Acta* **38**, 2038 (1955). Total synthesis and pharmacology: Neumeyer *et al., J. Med. Chem.* **16**, 1223 (1973).

Small prisms from methanol (lose solvent at 80°/2 mm), mp 124° (dry). $[\alpha]_D^{24}$ −97° (c = 0.45). Slightly soluble in water; sol in alcohol, ether, dilute acids.

Hydrochloride. $C_{18}H_{20}ClNO_2$. Crystals from alcohol-ether, softening 140°, dec 260-263°. $[\alpha]_D^{22}$ −43° (c = 0.51). Very sol in water; sol in alcohol.

THERAP CAT: Emetic.

741. Apocynin. [498-02-2] 1-(4-Hydroxy-3-methoxyphenyl)ethanone; acetovanillon; 4-hydroxy-3-methoxyacetophenone. $C_9H_{10}O_3$; mol wt 166.17. C 65.05%, H 6.07%, O 28.88%. From rhizome of Canadian hemp, *Apocynum cannabinum* L., *Apocynaceae* and from *A. androsaemifolium:* Finnemore, *J. Chem. Soc.* **93**, 1513, 1520 (1908). Also from the essential oil (butter) of the rhizomes of *Iris* spp., *Iridaceae:* Naves, *Helv. Chim. Acta* **32**, 1351 (1949).

Fine needles from water, mp 115°. bp 295-300°. Faint vanilla odor. Slightly sol in cold, freely in hot water, alc, benzene, chloroform, ether. Practically insol in petr ether.

742. Apocynum androsaemifolium. Dogbane; bitter root; spreading dogbane; milk ipecac; wild ipecac; rheumatism weed. Root of *Apocynum androsaemifolium* L., *Apocynaceae. Habit.* North America. *Constit.* Apocynin, apocynein, apocynamarin, volatile oil.

THERAP CAT: Cardiotonic.

743. Apocynum cannabinum. Canadian hemp; American Indian hemp; black Indian hemp; Indian physic; Indian dogbane. Dried rhizome and roots of *Apocynum cannabinum* L., *Apocynaceae. Habit.* U.S. *Constit.* Cynotoxin, apocyncein, apocynin, cymarin, resin, tannin, bitter extractive, starch.

Note: Not to be confused with *Apocynum androsaemifolium* which has few of its properties.

THERAP CAT: Cardiotonic.

744. Apo-β-erythroidine. [478-85-3] 4,5,7,8,9,12-Hexahydro-11*H*-pyrano[3,4-*d*]pyrrolo[3,2,1-*jk*][1]benzazepin-11-one. $C_{15}H_{15}NO_2$; mol wt 241.29. C 74.67%, H 6.27%, N 5.80%, O 13.26%. A degradation product of β-erythroidine. Prepd by heating β-erythroidine to 120° with phosphoric or sulfuric acid: Sauvage *et al., Science* **109**, 627 (1947); by reacting β-erythroidine with concd hydrobromic acid at 100°: Koniuszy, Folkers, *J. Am. Chem. Soc.* **73**, 333 (1951). Synthesis and structure: Blake *et al., J. Am. Chem. Soc.* **87**, 1397 (1965).

Crystals, mp 128-129°, also reported as mp 132-132.5°. uv max (ethanol): 345, 240 nm (ε 3500, 24500).

745. Apolipoprotein E. ApoE. Protein component of several classes of lipoproteins; plays a central role in plasma lipoprotein metabolism and cholesterol transport. Also involved in lipid-transport in the development and repair of nervous tissue. Polymorphic glycoprotein containing 299 amino acid residues; mol wt 34.2 kDa. Three major isoforms have been identified in humans (apo-E2, E3, E4) which are the product of 3 independent alleles (ε2, ε3, ε4) at a single gene locus. The isoforms differ from each other only in cysteine-arginine interchanges at 2 substitution sites. Allele ε3 is the most common; inheritance of ε4 has been associated with increased risk of Alzheimer's disease. Primarily synthesized in the liver by parenchymal cells and in the brain by astrocytes. Also produced in significant amounts by mature macrophages. Discovery as component of VLDL: V. G. Shore, B. Shore, *Biochemistry* **12**, 502 (1973). Purification and characterization: V. I. Zannis, J. L. Breslow, *Mol. Cell. Biochem.* **42**, 3 (1982). Amino acid sequence: S. C. Rall, Jr. *et al., J. Biol. Chem.* **257**, 4171 (1982). Biosynthesis and activity: R. W. Mahley, *Science* **240**, 622 (1988). Association with Alzheimer's disease: A. M. Saunders *et al., Neurology* **43**, 1467 (1993); L. A. Farrer *et al., J. Am. Med. Assoc.* **278**, 1349 (1997). Review of role in lipoprotein metabolism: A. D. Dergunov, M. Rosseneu, *Biol. Chem. Hoppe-Seyler* **375**, 485-495 (1994); P. de Knijff *et al., Hum. Mutat.* **4**, 178-194 (1994). Review of role in the nervous system: J. Poirier, *Trends Neurosci.* **17**, 525-530 (1994); K. H. Weisgraber *et al., Curr. Opin. Lipidol.* **5**, 110-116 (1994); R. W. Mahley *et al., ibid.* **6**, 86-91 (1995).

746. Apomorphine. [58-00-4] (6a*R*)-5,6,6a,7-Tetrahydro-6-methyl-4*H*-dibenzo[*de,g*]quinoline-10,11-diol; 6aβ-aporphine-10,11-diol. $C_{17}H_{17}NO_2$; mol wt 267.32. C 76.38%, H 6.41%, N 5.24%, O 11.97%. Dopamine (D_1 and D_2) receptor agonist. Synthetic opiate obtained by treating morphine with concd HCl: A. Matthiessen, C. R. A. Wright, *Proc. R. Soc. London Ser. B* **17**, 455 (1869). Structure: R. Pschorr *et al., Ber.* **35**, 4377 (1902). Configuration: H. Corrodi, E. Hardegger, *Helv. Chim. Acta* **38**, 2038 (1955). Total synthesis of (±)-form: J. L. Neumeyer *et al., J. Pharm. Sci.* **59**, 1850 (1970); of (+)- and (−)-forms: V. J. Ram, J. L. Neumeyer, *J. Org. Chem.* **46**, 2830 (1981). Toxicity data: J. Z. Ginos *et al., J. Med. Chem.* **18**, 1194 (1975). Clinical evaluation in impotence: J. P. W. Heaton *et al., Urology* **45**, 200 (1995). Historical review: J. L. Neumeyer *et al.,* in *Apomorphine and Other Dopaminomimetics* vol. **1**, G. L. Gessa, G. U. Corsini, Eds. (Raven, New York, 1981) p 1-17. Comprehensive description: F. J. Muhtadi, M. S. Hifnawy, *Anal. Profiles Drug Subs.* **20**, 121-166 (1991). Review of pharmacology and clinical efficacy in Parkinson's disease: D. Muguet *et al., Biomed. Pharmacother.* **49**, 197-209 (1995); in erectile dysfunction: F. Giuliano, J. Allard, *Int. J. Impotence Res.* **14**, Suppl. 1, S53-S56 (2002).

Hexagonal plates from chloroform and petr ether, dec 195°; subl in high vacuum. Oxidizes rapidly in air and becomes green. Sol in alcohol, acetone, chloroform. Slightly sol in water, benzene, ether, petr ether. Solns darken rapidly. pKb 7.0; pKa 8.92. uv max (98% alc): 336, 399 nm.

Hydrochloride. [314-19-2]; [41372-20-7] (hemihydrate). Apokinon; Apokyn; Apomine; Britaject; Ixense; Uprima. $C_{17}H_{17}NO_2 \cdot HCl$; mol wt 303.78. Small crystals (usually hemihydrate). Dec and turn green on exposure to light and air. $[\alpha]_D^{25}$ −48° (c = 1.2). uv spectrum: Csokan, *Z. Anal. Chem.* **124**, 344 (1942). pH of aq soln (1 in 300) = 4.8. One gram dissolves in 50 ml water, 17 ml water at 80°, 50 ml alcohol. Very slightly sol in chloroform and ether. LD_{50} i.p. in mice: 145 μg/g (Ginos).

Diacetate (ester). [6191-56-6] Diacetylapomorphine. $C_{21}H_{21}NO_4$. mp 127-128°, $[\alpha]_D^{24}$ −88° (c = 1.12 in 0.1*N* HCl).

THERAP CAT: Antiparkinsonian; emetic. In treatment of male erectile dysfunction.

THERAP CAT (VET): Emetic.

747. Apoptolidin. [194874-06-1] O-2,6-Dideoxy-3-O-methyl-β-D-*arabino*-hexopyranosyl-(1 → 4)-2,6-dideoxy-3-C-methyl-α-L-*arabino*-hexopyranosyl-(1→8)-3,5,7-trideoxy-1-C-[(2S,4S,-5S,8E,10E,12R,13R,14E,16E,18E)-12-[(6-deoxy-4-O-methyl-α-L-glucopyranosyl)oxy]-5-hydroxy-4-methoxy-9,13,15,17,19-pentamethyl-20-oxooxacycloeicosa-8,10,14,16,18-pentaen-2-yl]-3,5-dimethyl-9-O-methyl-L-*glycero*-α-D-*galacto*-2-nonulopyranose; FU-40A. $C_{58}H_{96}O_{21}$; mol wt 1129.37. C 61.68%, H 8.57%, O 29.75%. Natural product isolated from *Nocardiopsis* sp.; specifically induces apoptosis in transformed tumor cells. Isoln, properties and bioactivity: J. W. Kim *et al.*, *J. Antibiot.* **50**, 628 (1997). Structure: Y. Hayakawa *et al.*, *J. Am. Chem. Soc.* **120**, 3524 (1998). Partial synthesis: J. Schuppan *et al.*, *Tetrahedron Lett.* **41**, 621 (2000); K. C. Nicolaou *et al.*, *Chem. Commun.* **2000**, 307. Review of synthetic methods: P. T. Daniel *et al.*, *Angew. Chem. Int. Ed.* **45**, 872-893 (2006).

Colorless powder, mp 128-130°. $[\alpha]_D^{21}$ −5.2° (c = 1.0 in methanol). uv max (methanol): 234, 320 nm (ε 28300, 22000).

748. Aporeine. [2030-53-7] (7aS)-6,7,7a,8-Tetrahydro-7-methyl-5H-benzo[g]-1,3-benzodioxolo[6,5,4-de]quinoline; aporheine; 1,2-methylenedioxyaporphine; (+)-roemerine. $C_{18}H_{17}NO_2$; mol wt 279.33. C 77.40%, H 6.13%, N 5.01%, O 11.46%. From *Papaver dubium* L., *Papaveraceae*: Pavesi, *Gazz. Chim. Ital.* **37 I**, 629 (1907); **44 I**, 398 (1914). Structure and identity with (+)-roemerine: Slavik, *Collect. Czech. Chem. Commun.* **28**, 1738 (1963). Synthesis of *dl*-roemerine: Marion, Grassie, *J. Am. Chem. Soc.* **66**, 1290 (1944).

Needles from ether + petroleum ether, mp 102°. $[\alpha]_D^{22}$ +80° (c = 0.50 in ethanol). uv max: 262, 315 nm (log ε 4.3, 3.7). pK 6.1. Sol in ether, methanol, ethanol, chloroform; slightly sol in petr ether. Practically insol in water, alkali.

Hydrochloride. $C_{18}H_{17}NO_2$.HCl. Leaflets from ethanol or water, mp 266-267°. Slightly sol in ethanol, water.

Methiodide. $C_{18}H_{17}NO_2$.CH$_3$I. Crystals from boiling methanol, mp 232-233°.

749. Appel's Salt. [75318-43-3] 4,5-Dichloro-1,2,3-dithiazol-1-ium chloride. $C_2Cl_3NS_2$; mol wt 208.52. C 11.52%, Cl 51.01%, N 6.72%, S 30.75%. Readily prepd from chloroacetonitrile and disulfur dichloride; 5-chloro position is reactive to nucleophilic substitution. Prepn: R. Appel *et al.*, **DE 2848221** (1980 to Bayer); *eidem et al.*, *Ber.* **118**, 1632 (1985). Synthetic applications: J. J. Folmer, S. M. Weinreb, *Tetrahedron Lett.* **34**, 2737 (1993); A. M. Cuadro, J. Alvarez-Builla, *Tetrahedron* **50**,

10037 (1994); G. L'abbé *et al.*, *J. Chem. Soc. Perkin Trans. 1* **1995**, 2379; and crystal structure: C. W. Rees *et al.*, *ibid.* **2002**, 1535. Review of chemistry of polysulfur-nitrogen heterocycles: C. W. Rees, *J. Heterocycl. Chem.* **29**, 639-651 (1992).

Pale yellow-green crystals, mp 172° (dec). Insol in organic solvents. *Sensitive to water and other nucleophiles.*

USE: Synthon in heterocyclic chemistry; in conversion of alcohols and carboxylic acids to esters.

750. Appetize®. Blended cholesterol-reduced animal fat and vegetable oil free of *trans* fatty acids, wherein the final weight ratio of linoleic acid and myristic acid is between about 2 and 9: D. Perlman, K. C. Hayes, **WO 9322933**; *eidem*, **US 5382442** (1993, 1995 both to Brandeis University). Historical perspective: K. Kevin, *Food Process.* **55**, 81-85 (1994).

Contains approx 8 mg cholesterol per 100 g and as many calories as natural fats.

USE: Low cholesterol fat alternative.

751. Apraclonidine. [66711-21-5] 2,6-Dichloro-N¹-(4,5-dihydro-1H-imidazol-2-yl)-1,4-benzenediamine; 2,6-dichloro-N'-2-imidazolidinylidene-1,4-benzenediamine; 2-[(4-amino-2,6-dichlorophenyl)imino]imidazolidine; *p*-aminoclonidine; aplonidine; NC-14. $C_9H_{10}Cl_2N_4$; mol wt 245.11. C 44.10%, H 4.11%, Cl 28.93%, N 22.86%. α₂-Adrenergic agonist; structural analog of clonidine, *q.v.* Synthesis: B. Rouot, G. LeClerc, *Bull. Soc. Chim. Fr.* **Pt. 2**, 520 (1979). Prepn (not claimed) and use in treatment of intraocular pressure: B. M. York, Jr., **US 4517199** (1985 to Alcon). Pharmacology: B. Rouot *et al.*, *C.R. Seances Acad. Sci. Ser. D* **286**, 909 (1978). Receptor binding studies: D. C. U'Prichard, *Prog. Clin. Biol. Res.* **71**, 53 (1981). D. C. Stump, D. E. MacFarlane, *J. Lab. Clin. Med.* **102**, 779 (1983). Clinical pharmacology: D. A. Abrams *et al.*, *Arch. Ophthalmol.* **105**, 1205 (1987). Clinical evaluation in treatment of intraocular pressure: A. L. Robin *et al.*, *ibid.* 1208; as additive to maximally tolerated medical therapy in glaucoma: A. L. Robin *et al.*, *Am. J. Ophthalmol.* **120**, 423 (1995).

Solid, mp >230°.

Hydrochloride. [73218-79-8] ALO-2145; Iopidine. $C_9H_{10}Cl_2N_4$.HCl; mol wt 281.57.

Dihydrochloride. [73217-88-6] $C_9H_{10}Cl_2N_4$.2HCl. uv max (ethanol): 254, 304 nm (ε 1800, 2500).

THERAP CAT: Treatment of post-surgical elevated intraocular pressure.

752. Apramycin. [37321-09-8] O-4-Amino-4-deoxy-α-D-glucopyranosyl-(1 → 8)-O-(8R)-2-amino-2,3,7-trideoxy-7-(methylamino)-D-glycero-α-D-*allo*-octodialdo-1,5:8,4-dipyranosyl-(1→4)-2-deoxy-D-streptamine; 4-O-[3α-amino-6α-[(4-amino-4-deoxy-α-D-glucopyranosyl)oxy]-2,3,4,4aβ,6,7,8aα-octahydro-8β-hydroxy-7β-(methylamino)pyranopyrano[3,2-b]pyran-2α-yl]-2-deoxy-D-streptamine; nebramycin factor 2; EL-857; EL-857/820; 47657; Apralan. $C_{21}H_{41}N_5O_{11}$; mol wt 539.58. C 46.74%, H 7.66%, N 12.98%, O 32.62%. Broad spectrum aminocyclitol antibiotic and component of the nebramycin complex, produced by a strain of *Streptomyces tenebrarius*: R. Q. Thompson, E. A. Presti, *Antimicrob. Agents Chemother.* **1967**, 332; W. M. Stark, **US 3691279** (1972 to Lilly). Structure, abs config and properties: S. O'Connor *et al.*, *J. Org. Chem.* **41**, 2087 (1976). ¹³C-NMR: E. Wenkert, E. W. Hagaman, *ibid.* 701. *In vitro* activity: R. Ryden *et al.*, *J. Antimicrob. Chemother.* **3**, 609 (1977). Synthetic studies: H. C. Jarrell, W. A. Szarek, *Carbohydr. Res.* **67**, 43 (1978); *eidem, Can. J. Chem.* **56**, 144 (1978); **57**, 924 (1979). *See also* tobramycin.

P. Zipes *et al.*, *Am. J. Cardiol.* **40**, 586 (1977); P. J. Troup, D. P. Zipes, *Am. Heart J.* **97**, 322 (1979). *Reviews:* P. Danilo, *ibid.* 119; I. Stoel, S. F. Hagemeijer, *Eur. Heart J.* **1**, 147 (1980).

Monohydrate. From aqueous ethanol, mp 245-247°. pKa (H$_2$O): 8.5, 7.8, 7.2, 6.2, 5.4. Very soluble in water; slightly sol in lower alcohols.

THERAP CAT (VET): Antibacterial.

753. Aprepitant. [170729-80-3] 5-[[(2R,3S)-2-[(1R)-1-[3,5-Bis(trifluoromethyl)phenyl]ethoxy]-3-(4-fluorophenyl)-4-morpholinyl]methyl]-1,2-dihydro-3H-1,2,4-triazol-3-one; (2R)-[(1R)-3,5-bis(trifluoromethyl)phenylethoxy]-(3S)-(4-fluoro)phenyl-4-(3-oxo-1,2,4-triazol-5-yl)methyl morpholine; MK-0869; Emend. C$_{23}$H$_{21}$F$_7$N$_4$O$_3$; mol wt 534.43. C 51.69%, H 3.96%, F 24.88%, N 10.48%, O 8.98%. Selective neurokinin-1 (NK-1) receptor antagonist. Prepn: C. P. Dorn *et al.*, **WO 9516679**; *eidem*, **US 5719147** (1995, 1998 both to Merck & Co.); and pharmacology: J. J. Hale *et al.*, *J. Med. Chem.* **41**, 4607 (1998). Improved synthesis: K. M. J. Brands *et al.*, *J. Am. Chem. Soc.* **125**, 2129 (2003). LC/MS/MS determn in plasma: C. M. Chavez-Eng *et al.*, *J. Pharm. Biomed. Anal.* **35**, 1213 (2004). Clinical trial in prevention of cisplatin-induced emesis: S. Van Belle *et al.*, *Cancer* **94**, 3032 (2002); with granisetron and/or dexamethasone: D. Campos *et al.*, *J. Clin. Oncol.* **19**, 1759 (2001). Clinical pharmacokinetics: A. K. Majumdar *et al.*, *J. Clin. Pharmacol.* **46**, 291 (2006). Review of clinical experience in prevention of chemotherapy-induced nausea and vomiting (CINV): T. M. Dando, C. M. Perry, *Drugs* **64**, 777-794 (2004); A. M. Massaro, K. L. Lenz, *Ann. Pharmacother.* **39**, 77-85 (2005).

mp 255°. [α]$_D^{25}$ +69° (c = 1.00 in methanol). Sparingly sol in ethanol, isopropyl acetate; slightly sol in acetonitrile. Practically insol in water.

Fosaprepitant dimeglumine. [265121-04-8]; [172673-20-0] (free acid). 1-Deoxy-1-(methylamino)-D-glucitol [3-[[(2R,3S)-2-[(1R)-1-[bis(trifluoromethyl)phenyl]ethoxy]-3-(4-fluorophenyl)-4-morpholinyl]methyl]-2,5-dihydro-5-oxo-1H-1,2,4-triazol-1-yl]phosphonate (2:1) (salt); MK-0517. C$_{23}$H$_{22}$F$_7$N$_4$O$_3$P.2C$_7$H$_{17}$NO$_5$; mol wt 1004.83. Water-soluble prodrug. Prepn: C. P. Dorn *et al.*, **WO 9523798**; *eidem*, **US 5691336** (1995, 1997 both to Merck & Co.); J. J. Hale *et al.*, *J. Med. Chem.* **43**, 1234 (2000).

THERAP CAT: Antiemetic.

754. Aprindine. [37640-71-4] N-(2,3-Dihydro-1H-inden-2-yl)-N'-,N'-diethyl-N-phenyl-1,3-propanediamine; N,N-diethyl-N'-2-indanyl-N''-phenyl-1,3-propanediamine; N-[3-(diethylamino)propyl]-N-phenyl-2-indanamine; compd 99170; AC-1802; Lilly 99170. C$_{22}$H$_{30}$N$_2$; mol wt 322.49. C 81.94% H 9.38%, N 8.69%. Membrane-stabilizing agent. Prepn: P. M. Vanhoof, P. M. Clarebout, **BE 760018**; *eidem*, **US 3923813** (1971, 1975 both to Christiaens). Toxicological study: A. Georges *et al.*, *Arzneim.-Forsch.* **23**, 519 (1973). Pharmacokinetics: T. Kobari *et al.*, *Eur. J. Clin. Pharmacol.* **26**, 129 (1984). HPLC determn in plasma: T. Kobari *et al.*, *J. Chromatogr.* **278**, 220 (1983). Clinical studies: D.

Hydrochloride. [33237-74-0] Compd 83846; Amidonal; Aspenon; Fiboran; Ritmusin. C$_{22}$H$_{30}$N$_2$.HCl; mol wt 358.95. Crystals from benzene, mp 120-121°.

THERAP CAT: Antiarrhythmic (class I).

755. Aprinocarsen. [151879-73-1] d(P-Thio)(G-T-T-C-T-C-G-C-T-G-G-T-G-A-G-T-T-T-C-A)deoxyribonucleic acid; CGP-64128A; ISI-641A; LY-900003; Synthetic 20 base phosphorothioate antisense oligonucleotide designed to inhibit protein kinase C-α (PKC-α) expression. Prepn: C. F. Bennett, N. Dean, **WO 9319203**; *eidem*, **US 5882927** (1993, 1999 both to Isis). Pharmacology: N. Dean *et al.*, *Cancer Res.* **56**, 3499 (1996). CGE determn in tissue: R. S. Geary *et al.*, *Anal. Biochem.* **274**, 241 (1999). Clinical pharmacology and evaluation in advanced cancer: J. Nemunaitis *et al.*, *J. Clin. Oncol.* **17**, 3586 (1999). Review of pharmacokinetics: P. L. Nicklin *et al.*, *Handb. Exp. Pharmacol.* **131**, 141-168 (1998). Review of development and clinical evaluations: J. T. Holmlund *et al.*, *Curr. Opin. Mol Ther.* **5**, 372-385 (1999); K. Li, J. Zhang, *Curr. Opin. Invest. Drugs* **2**, 1454-1461 (2001).

Sodium salt. [331257-53-5] ISIS-3521; Affinitac; Affinitak.

THERAP CAT: Antineoplastic.

756. Aprobarbital. [77-02-1] 5-(1-Methylethyl)-5-(2-propenyl)-2,4,6(1H,3H,5H)-pyrimidinetrione; 5-allyl-5-isopropylbarbituric acid; allypropymal; Alurate. C$_{10}$H$_{14}$N$_2$O$_3$; mol wt 210.23. C 57.13%, H 6.71%, N 13.33%, O 22.83%. Prepn: **US 1444802** (1923). Toxicity data: H. H. Frey, *Arzneim.-Forsch.* **12**, 389 (1962).

Slightly bitter crystals, mp 140-141.5°. Almost insoluble in water, petr ether, aliphatic hydrocarbons. Sol in alcohol, chloroform, ether, acetone, benzene, glacial acetic acid, also in solns of fixed alkali hydroxides. A satd aq soln is acid to litmus. LD$_{50}$ i.p. in mice: 200 mg/kg (Frey).

Sodium salt. [125-88-2] Aprobarbital sodium; sodium 5-allyl-5-isopropylbarbiturate. C$_{10}$H$_{13}$N$_2$NaO$_3$. Hygroscopic powder; slightly bitter taste. Very soluble in water; slightly sol in alc. Practically insol in ether. Aq solns are alkaline to litmus.

Note: This is a controlled substance (depressant): **21 CFR**, 1308.13.

THERAP CAT: Sedative, hypnotic.

757. Aprotinin. [9087-70-1] Pancreatic basic trypsin inhibitor; pancreatic trypsin inhibitor (Kunitz); Bayer A 128; Riker 52G; RP-9921; Antagosan; Antikrein; Fosten; Iniprol; Kir Richter; Repulson; Trasylol; Trazinin; Zymofren. C$_{284}$H$_{432}$N$_{84}$O$_{79}$S$_7$; mol wt 6511.44. C 52.39%, H 6.69%, N 18.07%, O 19.41%, S 3.45%. Serine protease inhibitor which inhibits kallikrein, plasmin, trypsin, chymotrypsin and various intracellular proteases. Single chain polypeptide containing 58 amino acids; found in tissues and blood, highest concentration in bovine parotid gland, pancreas and lung. Initial description: H. Kraut *et al.*, *Z. Physiol. Chem.* **192**, 1 (1930). Isoln from bovine pancreas: M. Kunitz, J. H. Northrup, *J. Gen. Physiol.* **19**, 991 (1936); from bovine parotid glands: H. Kraut, R.

Körbel, **US 2890986** (1959 to Bayer). Amino acid sequence: B. Kassell *et al., Biochem. Biophys. Res. Commun.* **18**, 255 (1965); F. A. Anderer, S. Hörnle, *Z. Naturforsch.* **20b**, 457, 462 (1965); B. Kassell, M. Laskowski, *Biochem. Biophys. Res. Commun.* **20**, 463 (1966). Two-dimensional ^{1}H-NMR studies: K. Nagayama, K. Wüthrich, *Eur. J. Biochem.* **114**, 365 (1981); G. Wagner *et al., ibid.* 375. Review of early literature: I. Trautschold *et al., Biochem. Pharmacol.* **16**, 59-72 (1957). Review of mechanism of therapeutic action: G. Haberland, R. McConn, *Fed. Proc.* **38**, 2760-2767 (1979). Review of use as a proteolytic inhibitor in radioimmunoassays of polypeptide hormones: E. S. Zyzner, *Life Sci.* **28**, 1861-1866 (1981). Review of biochemistry and applications: H. Fritz, G. Wunderer, *Arzneim.-Forsch.* **33**, 479-494 (1983); of pharmacology and therapeutic efficacy in reducing blood loss associated with cardiac surgery: R. Davis, R. Whittington, *Drugs* **49**, 954-983 (1995).

uv max (pH 5.9): 280 nm. Isoelec pt pH 10.5. Stable in neutral or acid media at high temp. Irreversible changes in molecular structure occur in strongly alkaline media (pH >12). Partially and reversibly denatured on treatment with 8*M* urea. May be kept at room temp in physiological saline soln for >1 yr without detrimental effects. LD_{50} i.v. in mice: 2500000 kallikrein inhibitor units/kg (Trautschold).

USE: Proteolytic inhibitor in radioimmunoassays of polypeptide hormones.

THERAP CAT: Protease inhibitor.

758. Aptiganel. [137159-92-3] *N*-(3-Ethylphenyl)-*N*-methyl-*N'*-1-naphthalenylguanidine; *N*-(1-naphthyl)-*N'*-(3-ethylphenyl)-*N'*-methylguanidine; aptaguanal. $C_{20}H_{21}N_3$; mol wt 303.40. C 79.17%, H 6.98%, N 13.85%. Noncompetitive NMDA-receptor antagonist. Prepn: E. Weber, J. F. W. Keana, **WO 9112797**; *eidem,* **US 5262568** (1991, 1993 both to State of Oregon); N. L. Reddy *et al., J. Med. Chem.* **37**, 260 (1994). Clinical pharmacology and kinetics: K. W. Muir *et al., Ann. N.Y. Acad. Sci.* **765**, 279 (1995). Review of theoretical basis for use in stroke: K. W. Muir, K. R. Lees, *Stroke* **26**, 503-513 (1995). Clinical trial in acute ischemic stroke: G. W. Albers *et al., J. Am. Med. Assoc.* **286**, 2673 (2001).

Hydrochloride. [137160-11-3] CNS-1102; Cerestat. $C_{20}H_{21}$-N_3.HCl; mol wt 339.86. Off-white needles from ethanol + diethyl ether, mp 223-225°.

THERAP CAT: Neuroprotective.

759. Apyrase. [9000-95-7] An enzyme found in plants, especially potatoes. Cofactor: Ca^{2+}. Hydrolyzes acid anhydride links. Substrate: Adenosine triphosphate, adenosine diphosphate (giving adenylate and phosphate). *Ref:* Krishnan, *Arch. Biochem.* **20**, 272 (1949). Partial purification and properties of potato apyrase: Liebecq *et al., Bull. Soc. Chim. Biol.* **45**, 573 (1963).

760. Aquaporins. Group of integral membrane proteins that function as molecular water channels to facilitate osmotic movement of water across the plasma membrane. Found in plant and animal cells characterized as having high osmotic water permeability. Part of the *MIP* family of channel proteins, typified by the major intrinsic protein of the eye, that are responsible for the per-

meability of ions and small molecules. Homologs exhibit ~40% sequence identity. Structure consists of six transmembrane domains with 5 connecting loops; the water pore is thought to be formed by the juxtaposition of 2 highly conserved Asn-Pro-Ala (NPA) sequences within the lipid bilayer. Isoln of aquaporin-1 from human erythrocytes and renal tubules: B. M. Denker *et al., J. Biol. Chem.* **263**, 15634 (1988). Cloning and sequence homology with MIP family: G. M. Preston, P. Agre, *Proc. Natl. Acad. Sci. USA* **88**, 11110 (1991). Identification of function as membrane water channel: G. M. Preston *et al., Science* **256**, 385 (1992). Nomenclature: P. Agre *et al., Am. J. Physiol.* **265**, F461 (1993). Molecular structure: J. S. Jung *et al., J. Biol. Chem.* **269**, 14648 (1994). Review of structure and tissue distribution: C. H. van Os *et al., Biochim. Biophys. Acta* **1197**, 291-309 (1994); M. J. Chrispeels, P. Agre, *Trends Biochem. Sci.* **19**, 421-425 (1994). Review of aquaporins in plants: M. J. Chrispeels, C. Maurel, *Plant Physiol.* **105**, 9-13 (1994). Review of role in renal water transport: A. F. van Lieburg *et al., Pediatr. Nephrol.* **9**, 228-234 (1995); of model for water permeation: T. Zeuthen, *Trends Biochem. Sci.* **26**, 77-79 (2001); of function and physiology in the kidney: S. Nielsen *et al., Physiol. Rev.* **82**, 205-244 (2002).

Aquaporin-1. AQP1; CHIP28; AQP-CHIP; aquaporin-CHIP; channel forming integral protein. 269 amino acid residues; mol wt 28 kDa. Constitutes 2.4% of the plasma membrane protein in red blood cells; also found in renal proximal tubules and in other water-permeable epithelia.

Aquaporin-2. AQP2; AQP-CD; WCH-CD; water channel of collecting duct. 271 amino acids; mol wt 29 kDa. Vasopressin-regulated water channel in the kidney; has a primary role in concentrating the urine.

γ-TIP. γ-Tonoplast intrinsic protein; AQP.At1. Found in plant vacuolar membrane (tonoplast); facilitates rapid exchange of water between the vacuole and the cytoplasm.

761. Arabinose. [147-81-9] L-Arabinose; pectin sugar. $C_5H_{10}O_5$; mol wt 150.13. C 40.00%, H 6.71%, O 53.29%. Widely distributed in plants, usually in the form of complex polysaccharides. Also in mycobacteria. Isoln from mesquite gum: Anderson, Sands, *J. Am. Chem. Soc.* **48**, 3172 (1926); *Org. Synth.* **coll. vol. I,** 16 (2nd ed., 1941); White, *J. Am. Chem. Soc.* **69**, 715 (1947); from western red cedar *(Thuja plicata* Don., *Cupressaceae):* Anderson, Erdtman, *ibid.* **71**, 2927 (1949); from sapote gum: White, *ibid.* **75**, 257 (1953); from heartwood of port orford cedar *(Chamaecyparis lawsoniana* (Murr.) Parl, *Cupressaceae):* Kritchevsky, Anderson, *ibid.* **77**, 3391 (1955). Structure: Wolfrom, Christman, *ibid.* **58**, 39 (1936). Synthesis: Hough, Jones, *J. Chem. Soc.* **1951**, 1122.

β-L-Arabinose

Orthorhombic bisphenoidal crystals, mp 157-160°. Shows mutarotation. $[\alpha]_D^{12}$ +173° (6 min) → $[\alpha]_D^{20}$ +105.1° (22½ hrs c = 3). One gram dissolves in about 1 ml water, about 250 ml 90% alc. Ka at 17°, -3.7×10^{-13}. Reduces Fehling's soln. Forms furfurol on heating to 200° in closed tube also contg water.

USE: As culture medium for certain bacteria.

762. Arabitol. [2152-56-9] Arabinitol; 1,2,3,4,5-pentanepentol; arabite. $C_5H_{12}O_5$; mol wt 152.15. C 39.47%, H 7.95%, O 52.58%. D-Form obtained by reduction of D-arabinose or D-lyxose with sodium amalgam: Ruff, *Ber.* **32**, 555 (1899); Ruff, Ollendorff, *Ber.* **33**, 1802 (1900); Bertrand, *Bull. Soc. Chim.* [3] **15**, 593 (1896). Production by fermentation from molasses using *Saccharomyces rouxii* and *Saccharomyces mellis:* Lavin, Holloway, **US 2934474** (1960 to Comm. Solvents). L-Form obtained by reduction of L-arabinose with sodium amalgam: Kiliani, *Ber.* **20**, 1234, 1571 (1887). DL-Form obtained from equal parts of D- and L-arabitol: Ruff, *loc. cit.* Synthesis: Lespian, *Compt. Rend.* **206**, 1773 (1938).

CH₂OH ... D-Arabitol | L-Arabitol

(Structures of D-Arabitol and L-Arabitol)

D-Form. Big prismatic crystals. Sweet taste. mp 103°. $[\alpha]_D^{20}$ +7.7° (c = 9.26 in satd borax soln). Freely sol in water. One part dissolves in 48 parts of 90% alc at 12°.

Pentanitrate. $C_5H_7N_5O_{15}$. Sirup, sol in alcohol, ether, acetone. Strongly reduces Fehling's soln.

L-Form. Wart-like crystals, sweet taste. mp 102°. Weakly levorotatory in satd borax soln. Freely sol in water and in boiling 90% alc. One part dissolves in 46 parts of 90% alc at 12°. Does not reduce Fehling's soln.

DL-Form. Prisms from 90% alc. mp 105-106°. One part dissolves in 66 parts of 90% alc at 12°.

763. D-Araboflavin. [5978-87-0] 1-Deoxy-1-(3,4-dihydro-7,8-dimethyl-2,4-dioxobenzo[g]pteridin-10(2H)-yl)-D-arabinitol; 7,8-dimethyl-10-(arabino-2,3,4,5-tetrahydroxypentyl)benzo[g]-pteridine-2,4(3H,10H)-dione; 6,7-dimethyl-9-D-araboflavin. $C_{17}H_{20}N_4O_6$; mol wt 376.36. C 54.25%, H 5.36%, N 14.89%, O 25.51%. An antagonist of riboflavine. Prepd from D-(2-amino-4,5-dimethylphenyl)arabinamine and alloxan: Kuhn, Weygand, *Ber.* **68**, 1286 (1935); Sahashi *et al., Bull. Inst. Phys. Chem. Res.* (Tokyo) **24**, 72 (1948), *C.A.* **42**, 5458 (1948).

(Structure)

Orange-yellow needles from dil acetic acid. Bitter taste, mp 302-303°. $[\alpha]_D^{20}$ +78.6° (c = 0.509 in 0.1N NaOH); $[\alpha]_D^{20}$ −441° (c = 0.253 in 0.2N NaOH satd with borax).

Tetraacetate. $C_{25}H_{28}N_4O_{10}$. Flat yellow prisms from ethyl acetate, mp 221-222°.

764. Arachidic Acid. [506-30-9] Eicosanoic acid; arachic acid. $C_{20}H_{40}O_2$; mol wt 312.53. C 76.86%, H 12.90%, O 10.24%. Fatty acid found in peanut oil, vegetable and fish oils, etc. Also obtained by hydrogenation of arachidonic acid: Ege *et al., J. Am. Chem. Soc.* **83**, 3080 (1961). Synthesis: Linstead *et al., J. Chem. Soc.* **1955**, 1097. Reviews: A. W. Ralston, *Fatty Acids and Their Derivatives* (Wiley & Sons, New York, 1948) pp 43-46; K. S. Markley, *Fatty Acids* Part I (Interscience, New York, 2nd ed., 1960) pp 164-167, 398-400.

(Structure) H₃C—(CH₂)₁₇—COOH

Crystals from alc, mp 75.5°. bp₇₆₀ ~328° with some decompn; $bp_{1.0}$ 205°. d_4^{100} 0.8240. n_D^{100} 1.4250. Practically insoluble in water; sparingly sol in cold water; freely sol in hot abs alcohol, benzene, chloroform, ether, petr ether.

Methyl ester. $C_{21}H_{42}O_2$. mp 47°; bp₁.₀ 180°.

Ethyl ester. $C_{22}H_{44}O_2$. mp 41°; bp₀.₃ 177°.

765. Arachidonic Acid. [506-32-1] (5Z,8Z,11Z,14Z)-5,8,-11,14-Eicosatetraenoic acid. $C_{20}H_{32}O_2$; mol wt 304.47. C 78.90%, H 10.59%, O 10.51%. An essential fatty acid and a precursor in the biosynthesis of prostaglandins, thromboxanes, and leukotrienes, q.q.v. Structure: Mowry *et al., J. Biol. Chem.* **142**, 679 (1942); Arcus, Smedley-Maclean, *Biochem. J.* **37**, 1 (1943). Occurs in liver, brain, glandular organs, and depot fats of animals, in small amounts in human depot fats, and is a constituent of animal phosphatides. Isolation from liver lipids: Brown, *J. Biol. Chem.* **80**, 455 (1928); from beef suprarenal phosphatides: Ault, Brown, *ibid.* **107**, 615 (1934); Shinowara, Brown, *ibid.* **134**, 331 (1940). *See also* Dolby *et al., Biochem. J.* **34**, 1422 (1940). Synthesis from 2-propargyloxytetrahydropyran and 1-heptyne: Goldberg, Rachlin, US 2934570 (1960 to Hoffmann-La Roche); Rachlin *et al., J. Org. Chem.* **26**, 2688 (1961). Alternate route: Osbond, Wickens, *Chem. Ind. (London)* **1959**, 1288; Ege *et al., J. Am. Chem. Soc.* **83**, 3080 (1961). *Reviews:* K. S. Markley, *Fatty Acids* Part I (Interscience, New York, 2nd ed., 1960) pp 164-167, 398-400; T. K. Schaaf, *Annu. Rep. Med. Chem.* **12**, 182-190 (1977); B. B. Weksler, *N. Engl. Soc. Allergy Proc.* **2**, 56-61 (1981); N. A. Nelson *et al., Chem. Eng. News* **60**, 30-44 (Aug. 16, 1982). Series of articles on metabolism, role in inflammation and therapeutic implications: *Drugs* **33**, Suppl. 1, 2-66 (1987).

(Structure)

Liquid. mp −49.5°. Neutralization value 184.20. Iodine value 333.50. n_D^{20} 1.4824.

Methyl ester. $C_{21}H_{34}O_2$. bp₂ 200-205°, bp₀.₀₀₁ 127-128°. n_D^{20} 1.4797 to 1.4810.

THERAP CAT: Nutrient (essential fatty acid).

THERAP CAT (VET): With linoleic and linolenic acids, in eczema and dermatitis in dogs and swine.

766. Aralia. Spikenard; American spikenard; spignet; petty-morrel; spice berry. Dried rhizome and roots of *Aralia racemosa* L., Araliaceae. Habit. Northeastern U.S. Constit. Starch, pectin, sugar, resin. The active constituent appears to be a volatile oil of unknown constitution.

Ingredient of Compound White Pine Syrup: N. F. XI.

767. Aranidipine. [86780-90-7] 1,4-Dihydro-2,6-dimethyl-4-(2-nitrophenyl)-3,5-pyridinedicarboxylic acid methyl 2-oxopropyl ester; (±)-methyl 2-oxopropyl 1,4-dihydro-2,6-dimethyl-4-(2-nitrophenyl)-3,5-pyridinedicarboxylate; (±)-acetonyl methyl 1,4-dihydro-2,6-dimethyl-4-(o-nitrophenyl)-3,5-pyridinedicarboxylate; MPC-1304; Sapresta. $C_{19}H_{20}N_2O_7$; mol wt 388.37. C 58.76%, H 5.19%, N 7.21%, O 28.84%. Calcium channel blocker. Prepn: S. Ohno *et al.*, FR 2514761; *eidem*, US 4446325 (1983, 1984 both to Maruko Seiyaku); *idem et al., Chem. Pharm. Bull.* **34**, 1589 (1986). Pharmacology and receptor binding studies: K. Miyoshi *et al., Eur. J. Pharmacol.* **238**, 139 (1993). Determn by GC-MS in plasma and urine: Y. Umeno *et al., J. Chromatogr.* **434**, 123 (1988); by HPLC in plasma: Y. Iida *et al., ibid.* **571**, 277 (1991). Cardiovascular profile: A. Kanda *et al., J. Cardiovasc. Pharmacol.* **22**, 167 (1993). Clinical pharmacology: S. Suzuki *et al., Arzneim.-Forsch.* **43**, 1152 (1993). Toxicity studies: S. Nakano *et al., Yakuri to Chiryo* **21**, S931 (1993), *C.A.* **119**, 131216 (1993).

(Structure)

Yellow prisms from ethyl acetate/hexane, mp 155°. LD₅₀ in male, female mice, rats (mg/kg): 143, 193, 1982, 1459 orally; LD₅₀ in male, female mice (mg/kg): 7.3, 9.1 i.p. (Nakano).

THERAP CAT: Antihypertensive.

768. Araroba. [1393-64-2] Goa powder; crude chrysarobin; Brazil powder; ringworm powder; "Arariba". Found in cavities in the trunk of *Andira araroba,* Aguiar *(Vouacapoua araroba* [Aguiar] Lyons), *Leguminosae* and freed as much as possible from fragments of wood. *Habit.* In damp forests of Brazil and Bahia. *Constit.* About 50% chrysarobin; chrysophanic acid, gum, about 2% resin, araRobinol—said to be the methyl ether of emodin.

Brown-yellow, slightly cryst, rough, odorless powder; becomes brownish on exposure to air.

THERAP CAT: Dermatologic.

769. Arbaprostil. [55028-70-1] (5Z,11α,13E,15R)-11,15-Dihydroxy-15-methyl-9-oxoprosta-5,13-dien-1-oic acid; (15R)-15-methylprostaglandin E₂; (15R)-15-methyl-PGE₂; (E,Z)-(1R,2R,3R)-7-[3-hydroxy-2-[(3R)-(3-hydroxy-3-methyl-1-octenyl)]-5-oxocyclopentyl]-5-heptenoic acid; U-42842. $C_{21}H_{34}O_5$; mol wt 366.49. C 68.82%, H 9.35%, O 21.83%. Antisecretory, cytoprotective derivative of prostaglandin E₂, *q.v.* Prepn: G. L. Bundy *et al.,* **DE 2121980**; G. L. Bundy, **US 3804889** (1971, 1974 both to Upjohn). Synthetic studies: G. Bundy *et al., Ann. N.Y. Acad. Sci.* **180,** 76 (1971); E. W. Yankee, G. Bundy, *J. Am. Chem. Soc.* **94,** 3651 (1972). Synthesis of *R*- and *S*-methyl esters: E. W. Yankee *et al., ibid.* **96,** 5865 (1974). HPLC separation of epimers: R. K. Lustgarten, *J. Pharm. Sci.* **65,** 1533 (1976); G. E. Peng, V. K. Sood, *J. Liq. Chromatogr.* **6,** 1499 (1983). Pharmacology: J. R. Weeks *et al., J. Pharmacol. Exp. Ther.* **186,** 67 (1973). Comparative activity of epimers: A. Robert, E. W. Yankee, *Proc. Soc. Exp. Biol. Med.* **148,** 1155 (1975). Kinetics of epimerization: M. V. Merritt, G. E. Bronson, *J. Am. Chem. Soc.* **100,** 1891 (1978). Clinical study in duodenal ulcers: G. Vantrappen *et al., Gastroenterology* **83,** 357 (1982); in prevention of aspirin-induced gastric mucosal injury: D. A. Gilbert *et al., ibid.* **86,** 339 (1984).

(15S)-Methyl ester. $C_{22}H_{36}O_5$. Colorless oil, $[\alpha]_D$ −79° (c = 1.3 in chloroform). uv max (basic ethanol): 278 nm (ε = 25250).

(15R)-Methyl ester. $C_{22}H_{36}O_5$. Colorless oil, $[\alpha]_D$ −74° (c = 1.0 in chloroform). uv max (basic ethanol): 278 nm (ε = 25200).

770. Arbekacin. [51025-85-5] *O*-3-Amino-3-deoxy-α-D-glucopyranosyl-(1 → 6)-*O*-[2,6-diamino-2,3,4,6-tetradeoxy-α-D-*erythro*-hexopyranosyl-(1 → 4)]-*N*¹-[(2S)-4-amino-2-hydroxy-1-oxobutyl]-2-deoxy-D-streptamine; 1-*N*-[(S)-4-amino-2-hydroxybutyryl]dibekacin; 1-*N*-[(S)-4-amino-2-hydroxybutyryl]-3′,4′-dideoxykanamycin B; HBK. $C_{22}H_{44}N_6O_{10}$; mol wt 552.62. C 47.82%, H 8.03%, N 15.21%, O 28.95%. Aminoglycoside antibiotic; derivative of kanamycin B, *q.v.* Prepn and antibacterial activity: S. Kondo *et al., J. Antibiot.* **26,** 412 (1973); H. Umezawa *et al., DE 2350169**; *eidem,* **US 4107424** (1974, 1978 both to Microbiochem. Res. Found.). Mechanism of action: N. Tanaka *et al., Antimicrob. Agents Chemother.* **24,** 797 (1983); K. Matsunaga *et al., J. Antibiot.* **37,** 596 (1984). Pharmacology: J. Stevens *et al., Arzneim.-Forsch.* **35,** 1440 (1985); M. Kurebe *et al., ibid.* **36,** 1511 (1986). Series of articles on antibacterial activity, pharmacology, pharmacokinetics, and clinical experience: *Chemotherapy* **34,** Suppl. 1, pp 1-670 (1986). *Review:* Y. Kobayashi *et al., Int. J. Antimicrob. Agents* **5,** 227-230 (1995).

Sulfate. [104931-87-5] 1665-RB; Habekacin. $C_{22}H_{44}N_6O_{10}\cdot H_2SO_4$; mol wt 650.70.

Dicarbonate. $C_{24}H_{48}N_6O_{16}$. Colorless, crystalline powder, mp 178° (dec). $[\alpha]_D^{24}$ +86.8° (c = 0.77 in water). LD₅₀ i.v. in mice: >150 mg/kg (Umezawa, 1978).

THERAP CAT: Antibacterial.

771. Arborescin. [6831-14-7] (3aR,4aS,6aS,7S,9aS,9bR)-5,6,6a,7,9a,9b-Hexahydro-1,4a,7-trimethyl-3H-oxireno[8,8a]azuleno[4,5-b]furan-8(4aH)-one; 1,10-epoxy-6β-hydroxy-1β,5β,7α-guiai-3-en-12-oic acid γ-lactone. $C_{15}H_{20}O_3$; mol wt 248.32. C 72.55%, H 8.12%, O 19.33%. Ancient Greek contraceptive. Isoln from *Artemisia arborescens* L. and *Matricaria globifera* (Thunb.) Druce, *Compositae:* Meisels, Weizmann, *J. Am. Chem. Soc.* **75,** 3865 (1953); Cekan *et al., Collect. Czech. Chem. Commun.* **25,** 2553 (1960). Structure: Bates *et al., Tetrahedron Lett.* **1963,** 1127; M. Suchy *et al., Collect. Czech. Chem. Commun.* **29,** 1829 (1964). Synthesis and revised structure: M. Ando *et al., Chem. Lett.* **1978,** 727. Stereochemistry: M. Ando *et al., J. Org. Chem.* **47,** 3909 (1982).

Crystals from ethanol, mp 140-142°. $[\alpha]_D^{20}$ +64° (c = 0.72 in chloroform).

772. Arbutamine. [128470-16-6] 4-[(1R)-1-Hydroxy-2-[[4-(4-hydroxyphenyl)butyl]amino]ethyl]-1,2-benzenediol; (R)-3,4-dihydroxy-α-[[[4-(p-hydroxyphenyl)butyl]amino]methyl]benzyl alcohol; 1-(3,4-dihydroxyphenyl)-2-(4-(4-hydroxyphenyl)butylamino)ethanol. $C_{18}H_{23}NO_4$; mol wt 317.38. C 68.12%, H 7.30%, N 4.41%, O 20.16%. Catecholamine cardiac stimulant. Prepn: R. R. Tuttle, C. E. Browne, III, **EP 329464**; *eidem,* **US 5395970** (1989, 1995 both to Gensia). Pharmacology and pharmacodynamics: M. Young *et al., Drug Dev. Res.* **32,** 19 (1994). Efficacy as exercise stimulating agent (ESA) in comparison with dobutamine, *q.v.:* H. K. Hammond, M. D. McKirnan, *J. Am. Coll. Cardiol.* **23,** 475 (1994).

Hydrochloride. [125251-66-3] GP-2-121-3; GenESA. Off-white, amorphous solid. mp 55-58°. $[\alpha]_D^{23}$ −18.5° (in ethanol). Freely sol in water, ethanol. Practically insol in diethyl ether, hexane.

THERAP CAT: Stress agent for diagnosis of coronary artery disease.

773. Arbutin. [497-76-7] 4-Hydroxyphenyl-β-D-glucopyranoside; hydroquinone-β-D-glucopyranoside; hydroquinone glucose; arbutoside; ursin. $C_{12}H_{16}O_7$; mol wt 272.25. C 52.94%, H 5.92%, O 41.14%. Naturally occurring glycoside of hydroquinone, *q.v.,* found in the bark and leaves of various plants, usually occurring together with methylarbutin. Principal antibacterial constituent of the traditional medicine, uva ursi, *q.v.* Isoln from bearberry leaves *(Arctostaphylos uva-ursi* Spreng., *Ericaceae):* A. Kawalier, *Ann.* **82,** 241 (1852); from leaves of blueberry, cranberry, and pear *(Pyrus communis* L., *Rosaceae):* G. Urban, M. Rogowski, *Arch. Exp. Pathol. Pharmakol.* **211,** 194 (1950). Synthesis: C. Mannich, *Arch. Pharm.* **250,** 547 (1912); A. Robertson, R. B. Waters, *J. Chem. Soc.* **1930,** 2729. Production by plant cell culture: S. Inomata *et al., Appl. Microbiol. Biotechnol.* **36,** 315 (1991). Physical properties: E. Lindpainter, *Arch. Pharm.* **277,** 398 (1940). Determn in drug prepns: L. Kraus, *Pharmazie* **19,** 41 (1964); E. Kenndler *et al., J. Chromatogr.* **514,** 383 (1990). Inhibition of human melanin synthesis *in vitro:* K. Maeda, M. Fukuda, *J. Pharmacol. Exp. Ther.* **276,** 765 (1996). Review of human exposure: P. J. Deisinger *et al., J. Toxicol. Environ. Health* **47,** 31-46 (1996).

Occurs as the monohydrate. Colorless elongated prisms from moist ethyl acetate, mp 199° after sintering at 163-164° (Robertson, Waters). Also reported as unstable form, mp 165°; stable form, mp 199.5-200° (Lindpaintner). $[\alpha]_D^{20}$ −60.3° (in water). Sol in water and in alc.

Methylarbutin. [6032-32-2] 4-Methoxyphenyl-β-D-glucopyranoside; methylarbutoside. $C_{13}H_{18}O_7$; mol wt 286.28. Crystallizes from water as the monohydrate, mp 158-160°; solidifies and melts again at 175° (Mannich). Also reported as unstable form, mp 160.5°; stable form, mp 176° (Lindpaintner). $[\alpha]_D^{20}$ −60.66° (in water). Sol in hot water or alcohol; slightly sol in ether.

USE: In cosmetics as skin lightening agent.

774. Arcitumomab. [154361-48-5] Anti-(human carcinoembryonic antigen) immunoglobulin G1 Fab' fragment (mouse monoclonal IMMU-4 γ_1-chain) disulfide with mouse monoclonal IMMU-4 light chain. Murine monoclonal antibody fragment Fab' directed against carcinoembryonic antigen (CEA), an antigen expressed by a majority of colorectal cancers and some adenocarcinomas. Radiolabeled form designed for imaging colorectal tumors. Series of articles on purifn and characterization of anti-CEA antibody: F. J. Primus *et al.*, *Cancer Res.* **43**, 679-701 (1983). Prepn of radiolabeled form: D. Shochat *et al.*, **EP 336678**; *eidem*, **US 5061641** (1989, 1991 both to Immunomedics); and preclinical evaluation: H. J. Hansen *et al.*, *Cancer Res.* Suppl. **50**, 794s (1990). Clinical study of diagnostic use in colorectal immunoscintigraphy: K. Hughes *et al.*, *Ann. Surg.* **226**, 621 (1997); in breast cancer: D. M. Goldenberg *et al.*, *Cancer* **89**, 104 (2000). Review of pharmacology: S. A. Eccles, *Curr. Opin. Mol. Ther.* **1**, 737-744 (1999); of technical prepn and clinical use: D. A. Erb, H. A. Nabi, *J. Nucl. Med. Technol.* **28**, 12-18 (2000).

⁹⁹ᵐTc-Labeled form. [154361-49-6] IMMU-4 ⁹⁹ᵐTc Fab'; CEA-Scan.

THERAP CAT: ⁹⁹ᵐTc-labeled form as diagnostic aid (radioactive tumor targeting agent).

775. Ardeparin. Low molecular weight heparin prepared by the depolymerization of porcine mucosal heparin in the presence of peroxides. Average mol wt 5500-6500 daltons. Manufacturing process: F. Fussi, **US 4281108** (1981 to Hepar Ind.). Description of properties and activity: *idem et al.*, *Dev. Biochem.* **12**, 535 (1981). Clinical pharmacokinetics: S. Troy *et al.*, *J. Clin. Pharmacol.* **35**, 1194 (1995). Clinical trials in prevention of postoperative venous thrombosis: M. N. Levine *et al.*, *Arch. Intern. Med.* **156**, 851 (1996); J. A. Heit *et al.*, *Thromb. Haemostasis* **77**, 32 (1997).

Sodium salt. WY-90493-RD; Normiflo. LD_{50} in mice, rats (mg/kg): >3000, >2000 i.p.; >1000, 354 ±30 i.v.; >6000, >6000 orally (Fussi *et al.*).

THERAP CAT: Antithrombotic.

776. Areca. Betel nuts; pinang. Nuts (seeds) of *Areca catechu* L., Palmaceae. *Habit.* East Indies. *Constit.* Arecoline, arecaidine, guvacine, guvacoline, arecolidine, choline, about 15% red tannin, about 14% fat. *Reviews:* L. Marion "The Alkaloids of Areca Nut" in Manske-Holmes, *The Alkaloids* **Vol. I** (Academic Press, New York, 1950) pp 171-175; Raghavan, Baruah, *Econ. Bot.* **12**, 315 (1958).

Hard and heavy; round-conical and depressed at base. Extern. brown, mottled with fawn color; intern. brownish-red with whitish veins; astringent taste; the fresh nuts have a faint, cheese-like odor.

THERAP CAT: Anthelmintic.

THERAP CAT (VET): Has been used for tapeworms, ascarids.

777. Arecaidine. [499-04-7] 1,2,5,6-Tetrahydro-1-methyl-3-pyridinecarboxylic acid; 1,2,5,6-tetrahydro-1-methylnicotinic acid; arecaine; methylguvacine. $C_7H_{11}NO_2$; mol wt 141.17. C 59.56%, H 7.85%, N 9.92%, O 22.67%. From seeds of *Areca catechu* L., Palmaceae (betel nuts). Synthesis: Wohl, Johnson,

Ber. **40**, 4712 (1907); Hess, Leibbrandt, *ibid.* **51**, 806 (1918); Freudenberg, *ibid.* 976; Maurit, Preobrazhenskii, *Zh. Obshch. Khim.* **28**, 968 (1958), *C.A.* **52**, 17263 (1958); Merck, **DE 485139** *C.A.* **24**, 919 (1930).

Plates from dil alc, dec 232° (after drying at 102°). pH of 0.1 molar soln 5.6. Freely soluble in water, and dilute alc; almost insol in abs alc, chloroform, ether, benzene.

Hydrochloride. $C_7H_{11}NO_2$.HCl. mp 251°; needles, dec 263° (rapid heating). Freely sol in water.

Hydrobromide. $C_7H_{11}NO_2$.HBr. Crystals from methanol, dec 249°.

778. Arecoline. [63-75-2] 1,2,5,6-Tetrahydro-1-methyl-3-pyridinecarboxylic acid methyl ester; methyl 1,2,5,6-tetrahydro-1-methylnicotinate; methyl 1-methyl-$\Delta^{3,4}$-tetrahydro-3-pyridinecarboxylate; methyl *N*-methyltetrahydronicotinate; arecaline; arecholine; methylarecaidin. $C_8H_{13}NO_2$; mol wt 155.19. C 61.91%, H 8.44%, N 9.03%, O 20.62%. Cholinergic alkaloid from seeds of the betel nut palm *Areca catechu* L., Palmaceae (catechu). Isoln: E. Johns, *Arch. Pharm.* **229**, 673 (1891). Synthesis: F. Chemnitius, *J. Prakt. Chem.* **117**, 147 (1926); Mannich, *Ber.* **75B**, 1480 (1942); Knox, **US 2506458** (1950 to Nopco). Improved synthesis from nicotinic acid: I. A. Kozello *et al.*, *Khim. Farm. Zh.* **10**, 90 (1976), *C.A.* **86**, 171205a (1977). Effect on human serial learning: N. Sitaram *et al.*, *Science* **201**, 274 (1978). Clinical evaluation in Alzheimer's disease: T. T. Soncrant *et al.*, *Psychopharmacology* **112**, 421 (1993). *Review:* R. B. Burrows, *Progress in Drug Research* **vol. 17**, E. Jucker, Ed. (Birkhaüser Verlag, Basel, 1973) pp 108-210.

Oily liquid, bp 209°, bp_7 92-93°, bp_{12} 105°. Volatile with steam. Strong base. pK 6.84. n_D^{20} 1.4302. d^{20} 1.0495. Miscible with water, alc, ether. Soluble in chloroform. LD_{50} in mice, dogs (mg/kg): 100, 5 s.c. (Burrows).

Hydrobromide. [300-08-3] $C_8H_{13}NO_2$.HBr. Bitter, optically inactive crystals, mp 169-171°. One gram dissolves in about 1 ml water, 10 ml alc, 2 ml boiling alc; slightly soluble in chloroform, ether. The aq soln is practically neutral.

Compd with acetarsone. [900-77-6] Arecoline-acetarsone; arecoline-acetarsol; drocarbil; Nemural. $C_8H_{13}NO_2.C_8H_{10}$-$AsNO_5$; mol wt 430.28. White to pale-yellow powder. Stable when kept dry. Freely sol in water.

Compd with *p*-stibonobenzoic acid. [17162-36-6] Arecoline *p*-stibonobenzoic acid; Anthelin. $C_8H_{13}NO_2.C_7H_7O_5Sb$; mol wt 448.08. Prepn: Kartsonis, Austin, **US 2557353** (1951 to Jensen-Salsbery Labs.).

THERAP CAT (VET): Anthelmintic (Cestodes); cathartic.

779. Argatroban. [74863-84-6] (2*R*,4*R*)-1-[(2*S*)-5-[(Aminoiminomethyl)amino]-1-oxo-2-[[(1,2,3,4-tetrahydro-3-methyl-8-quinolinyl)sulfonyl]amino]pentyl]-4-methyl-2-piperidinecarboxylic acid; (2*R*,4*R*)-4-methyl-1-[N^2-(3-methyl-1,2,3,4-tetrahydro-8-quinolinesulfonyl)-L-arginyl]-2-piperidinecarboxylic acid; (2*R*,4*R*)-4-methyl-1-[(*S*)-N^2-[[(*R*,*S*)-1,2,3,4-tetrahydro-3-methyl-8-quinolinyl]sulfonyl]arginyl]pipecolic acid; argipidine; MQPA. $C_{23}H_{36}N_6O_5S$; mol wt 508.63. C 54.31%, H 7.13%, N 16.52%, O 15.73%, S 6.30%. Synthetic thrombin inhibitor. Prepn of argatroban and stereoisomers: R. Kikumoto *et al.*, **EP 8746**; S. Okamoto *et al.*, **US 4258192** (1980, 1981 both to Mitsubishi Chem. Ind.); S. Okamoto *et al.*, *Biochem. Biophys. Res. Commun.* **101**, 440 (1981). Comparison with heparin, *q.v.*, of antithrombotic effect in animals: T. Kumada, Y. Abiko, *Thromb. Res.* **24**, 285 (1981). Stereoselective inhibition of thrombin: R. Kikumoto *et al., Biochemistry* **23**, 85 (1984). Clinical evaluation in hemodialysis: K. Ota *et al., Proc. Eur. Dial. Transplant. Assoc.* **20**, 144 (1983); in disseminated intravascular coagulation: K. Kumon *et al., Crit. Care Med.* **12**, 1039 (1984).

Crystals from ethanol, mp 188-191°.

Monohydrate. [141396-28-3] DK-7419; MCI-9038; MD-805; OM-805; Novastan; Slonnon. Crystals from aq ethanol, mp 176-180°. $[\alpha]_D^{27}$ +76.1° (c = 1 in 0.2N HCl).

THERAP CAT: Antithrombotic.

780.   Arginine. [74-79-3] L-Arginine; Arg; R; 2-amino-5-guanidinovaleric acid; (S)-2-amino-5-[(aminoiminomethyl)amino]-pentanoic acid. $C_6H_{14}N_4O_2$; mol wt 174.20. C 41.37%, H 8.10%, N 32.16%, O 18.37%. An essential amino acid for human development. Precursor for nitric oxide, *q.v.* Isoln from etiolated lupine seedlings: E. Schulze, E. Steiger, *Ber.* **19**, 1177 (1886). Early chemistry and biochemistry: *Amino Acids and Proteins,* D. M. Greenberg, Ed. (Charles C. Thomas, Springfield, IL, 1951) 950 pp., *passim;* J. P. Greenstein, M. Winitz, *Chemistry of the Amino Acids* vols 1-3 (John Wiley and Sons, Inc., New York, 1961) pp. 1841-1855, *passim.* Quick isoln from gelatin: R. M. Kothari, *J. Chromatogr.* **90**, 359 (1974). Fluorometric determn in serum: T. Miura *et al., Anal. Biochem.* **139**, 432 (1984). Review of biosynthesis: M. E. Jones, *Adv. Enzyme Regul.* **9**, 19-49 (1970). Review of biochemistry, physiology and therapeutic implication: A. Barbul, *J. Parenter. Enteral Nutr.* **10**, 227-238 (1986). Review of immune function: *idem, Nutrition* **6**, 53-62 (1990). Review of arginine:nitric oxide pathway: S. Moncada, A. Higgs, *N. Engl. J. Med.* **329**, 2002-2012 (1993); R. M. J. Palmer, *Curr. Opin. Nephrol. Hypertens.* **2**, 122-128 (1993). Review of structural role in proteins: C. L. Borders *et al., Protein Sci.* **3**, 541-548 (1994). Review of role in health and renal disease: A. A. Reyes *et al., Am. J. Physiol.* **267**, F331-F346 (1994).

Prisms containing 2 mol H_2O from water; anhydrous monoclinic plates from 66% alcohol. The dihydrate becomes anhydr at 105°, browns at 230°. Dec 244°. $[\alpha]_D^{20}$ +26.9° (c = 1.65 in 6.0N HCl); $[\alpha]_D^{20}$ +12.5° (c = 3.5 in water); $[\alpha]_D^{20}$ +11.8° (c = 0.87 in 0.5N NaOH). pK_1 2.17; pK_2 9.04; pK_3 12.48. Absorption spectrum: Castille, Ruppol, *Bull. Soc. Chim. Biol.* **10**, 643 (1928); *Chem. Zentralbl.* **1928, II**, 622. The satd aq soln contains 15% (w/w) at 21°. Sparingly sol in alc. Insol in ether. Strongly alkaline, its aq solns absorb CO_2 from the air.

Hydrochloride. [1119-34-2] R-Gene. $C_6H_{14}N_4O_2 \cdot HCl$. Plates, prisms from alc. Sinters at 218°, solidifies again at 225°. Dec 235°. $[\alpha]_D^{20}$ +12.0° (c = 4). $[\alpha]_D^{21}$ +21.9° (c = 12 in dil HCl). Sol in water, slightly sol in hot alc.

THERAP CAT: Ammonia detoxicant (hepatic failure); diagnostic aid (pituitary function).

781.   Arginine Glutamate. [4320-30-3] L-Glutamic acid compd with L-arginine; Modumate. $C_{11}H_{23}N_5O_6$; mol wt 321.33. C 41.12%, H 7.21%, N 21.79%, O 29.87%. Prepd from L-arginine and L-glutamic acid: Barker, Chang, US 2851482 (1958 to General Mills). Activity studies: Weisburger *et al., Toxicol. Appl. Phar-*

macol. **14**, 163 (1969); Yamamoto, Weisburger, *Life Sci.* **9(II)**, 285 (1970). Crystal and molecular structure: T. N. Bhat, M. Vijayan, *Acta Crystallogr.* **B33**, 1754 (1977). Reduction of blood ammonia: L. Zieve *et al., Metab. Brain Dis.* **4**, 113 (1989).

Crystals, dec 193-194.5°. Supplied as a 25% (w/v) soln in water for injection; each 100 ml represents 13.5 g of arginine and 11.5 g of glutamic acid.

THERAP CAT: Ammonia detoxicant (hepatic failure).

782.   Argol. [8007-14-5] Argilla vini; argil; arcilla; Weinstein; wine lees; crude cream of tartar; crude potassium bitartrate. Formed in the secondary fermentation of grapes for wine. Contains over 40% tartaric acid, potassium bitartrate, calcium. *Ref:* R. Pasternack in *Kirk-Othmer Encyclopedia of Chemical Technology* (Interscience, New York, 1954) **vol. 13**, p 649.

Gray or reddish-brown crystalline crusts.

USE: Mordant; manufacturing tartaric acid; vinegar from malt; in fertilizers.

783.   Argon. [7440-37-1] Ar; at. wt 39.948; at. no. 18. Group VIIIA (18), also known as Group 0. A noble gas characterized by an electronic structure in which the outer *p* subshell is entirely filled: $1s^2 2s^2 2p^6 3s^2 3p^6$. Stable naturally occurring isotopes (mass numbers): 36 (0.337%); 38 (0.063%); 40 (99.600%); known artificial radioactive isotopes: 32-35; 37; 39; 41-46. Longest-lived known isotope: 39 ($T_{1/2}$ 269 years, β-emitter). Abundance in igneous rock of the earth's crust: 4×10^{-2} ppm by wt; concentration in the atmosphere: 93.40 ppm by vol. Discovered in 1894 by Rayleigh and Ramsay. Obtained commercially from the atmosphere by distillation-liquefaction process. Monograph: *Argon, Helium and the Rare Gases* **Vols. 1, 2**, G. A. Cook, Ed. (Interscience, New York, 1961) 818 pp. *Reviews:* A. H. Cockett, K. C. Smith, "The Monatomic Gases" in *Comprehensive Inorganic Chemistry* **vol. 1**, J. C. Bailar, Jr. *et al.,* Eds. (Pergamon Press, Oxford, 1973) pp 139-211; S.-C. Hwang, W. R. Weltmer, Jr. in *Kirk-Othmer Encyclopedia of Chemical Technology* **vol. 13** (John Wiley & Sons, 4th ed., 1995) pp 1-38; *Chemistry of the Elements,* N. N. Greenwood, A. Earnshaw, Eds. (Pergamon Press, New York, 1984) pp 1042-1059. Review of use in inductively coupled plasma-mass spectrometry: S. F. Durrant, *Fresenius J. Anal. Chem.* **347**, 389-392 (1993).

Colorless, odorless, tasteless, monatomic, inert gas; will form compds with highly electronegative elements such as O, F, Cl. Atomic radius 1.92×10^{-8} cm. Triple pt temp 83.80 K, press 68.90 kPa. Critical temp 150.86 K, critical press 4898 kPa, critical d 535.7 kg/m^3. Gas: d^0 (101.3 kPa) 1.7838 kg/m^3, d (normal bp) 5.767 kg/m^3. Liquid: normal bp $-185.87°$, d (normal bp) 1393.9 kg/m^3, d (triple pt) 1415 kg/m^3, heat of vaporization (normal bp) 6469 J/mol. Solid: d (triple pt) 1623 kg/m^3, heat of vaporization (triple pt) 7.785 kJ/mol, heat of fusion (triple pt) 1.191 kJ/mol, exists as face-centered cubic crystals at normal pressure. Soly of gas in water (20°): 33.6 cc/kg water. Sol in organic liquids.

Caution: Can act as a simple asphyxiant by displacing air. *See: Matheson Gas Data Book* (Matheson Co., Inc., 4th ed., East Rutherford, NJ, 1966) pp 23-28.

USE: Gas as shield in gas metal-arc welding, in metal processing; carrier in gas-liquid and gas-solid chromatography; gas filler for incandescent light bulbs. Gas in fluorescent tubes analogous to neon lights, but produces a blue-purplish light; in rectifier tubes; in thermometers above mercury; in lasers; wherever an inert atmosphere is desired and the much cheaper nitrogen cannot be used; in ionization chambers and particle counters; in mixtures with He and Ne in Geiger counters; in argon-oxygen-decarburizing process for stainless steel; in manuf of semiconducting devices; in gas mixtures as the working fluid in plasma arc devices. Liquid as cryogen to produce low temps. The isotope ^{40}Ar is always found in minerals contg potassium, since it is a product of ^{40}K decay; measuring the amount of ^{40}Ar and ^{40}K can be used for determining the geologic age of minerals and meteors.

784. Aricine. [482-91-7] (19α,20α)-16,17-Didehydro-10-methoxy-19-methyloxayohimban-16-carboxylic acid methyl ester; quinovatine; cinchovatine; heterophylline. $C_{22}H_{26}N_2O_4$; mol wt 382.45. C 69.09%, H 6.85%, N 7.32%, O 16.73%. Originally found in Cusco bark, the bark of *Cinchona pelletierana* Wedd., *Rubiaceae*: Pelletier, Coriol, *J. Pharm. Chim.* [2] **15**, 565 (1829). Also from *Rauwolfia canescens* L., *R. heterophylla* Roem. & Schult., *R. sellowii* Muell. Argov. and *Aspidosperma marcgravianum* Woodson., *Apocynaceae*: Stoll *et al., Helv. Chim. Acta* **38**, 270 (1955); Hochstein *et al., J. Am. Chem. Soc.* **77**, 3551 (1955); Hochstein, *ibid.* **77**, 5744 (1955); Gilbert *et al., J. Org. Chem.* **27**, 4702 (1962). Structure: Stoll *et al., loc. cit.* Stereochemistry: Neuss, Boaz, *J. Org. Chem.* **22**, 1001 (1957); Shamma, Richey, *J. Am. Chem. Soc.* **85**, 2507 (1963).

Orthorhombic, elongated prisms from methanol, dec 188°. Sublimes at 0.01 mm and 180°. $[\alpha]_D^{20}$ −91° (c = 1.4 in chloroform); $[\alpha]_D^{20}$ −63° (c = 1.5 in pyridine); $[\alpha]_D^{20}$ −57° (ethanol). uv max (ethanol): 229, 281 nm (log ε 4.54, 3.97). pKa in 80% methyl cellosolve 5.80; in 1:1 DMF-water 6.8. Practically insol in water. Sol in 100 parts of 90% alcohol, 33 parts ether. Very sol in chloroform.

Hydrochloride. $C_{22}H_{26}N_2O_4$.HCl. Square plates from methanol + acetone, dec 241-254°. $[\alpha]_D^{20}$ −5° (c = 0.9 in 50% ethanol).

Hydrobromide. $C_{22}H_{26}N_2O_4$.HBr. Needles from methanol, dec 262-263°.

Note: Aricine does not seem to share the hypotensive and sedative properties of reserpine: Hochstein *et al., J. Am. Chem. Soc.* **77**, 3551 (1955).

785. Aripiprazole. [129722-12-9] 7-[4-[4-(2,3-Dichlorophenyl)-1-piperazinyl]butoxy]-3,4-dihydro-2(1*H*)-quinolinone; 7-[4-[4-(2,3-dichlorophenyl)-1-piperazinyl]butoxy]-3,4-dihydrocarbostyril; OPC-14597; OPC-31; Abilify; Abilitat. $C_{23}H_{27}Cl_2N_3O_2$; mol wt 448.39. C 61.61%, H 6.07%, Cl 15.81%, N 9.37%, O 7.14%. Dopamine-serotonin system stabilizer. Exhibits partial agonist activity at dopamine D_2-receptors and serotonin 5-HT$_{1A}$-receptors and antagonist activity at 5-HT$_{2A}$-receptors. Prepn: Y. Oshiro *et al.,* **EP 367141**; *eidem,* **US 5006528** (1990, 1991 both to Otsuka); and pharmacology: Y. Oshiro *et al., J. Med. Chem.* **41**, 658 (1998). Description of action on dopamine receptors: S. M. Stahl, *J. Clin. Psychiatry* **62**, 841, 923 (2001); on serotonin receptors: S. Jordan *et al., Eur. J. Pharmacol.* **441**, 137 (2002). Clinical trial in schizophrenia: J. M. Kane *et al., J. Clin. Psychiatry* **63**, 763 (2002). Review of pharmacology: J. K. McGavin, K. L. Goa, *CNS Drugs* **16**, 779-786 (2002); and clinical experience: P. E. Keck Jr., S. L. McElroy, *Expert Opin. Invest. Drugs* **12**, 655-662 (2003).

Colorless, flake crystals from ethanol, mp 139.0-139.5°.
THERAP CAT: Antipsychotic.

786. Aristolochic Acid. [313-67-7] 8-Methoxy-6-nitro-phenanthro[3,4-*d*]-1,3-dioxole-5-carboxylic acid; 3,4-methylenedioxy-8-methoxy-10-nitro-1-phenanthrenecarboxylic acid; aristolochic acid-I; aristolochine. $C_{17}H_{11}NO_7$; mol wt 341.27. C 59.83%, H 3.25%, N 4.10%, O 32.82%. One of a group of fourteen known, substituted 1-phenanthrenecarboxylic acids, aristolochic acids, that occur in *Aristolochiaceae* and in butterflies feeding on these plants. They are often accompanied by **aristololactams**, twelve of which have been characterized. Isoln: Gänshirt, *Pharmazie* **8**, 584 (1953); Pailer *et al., Monatsh. Chem.* **86**, 676 (1955); Coutts *et al., J. Pharm. Pharmacol.* **11**, 607 (1959); Kupchan, Doskotch, *J. Med. Pharm. Chem.* **5**, 657 (1962). Structure: Pailer *et al., Monatsh. Chem.* **87**, 249 (1956). Synthesis: Kupchan, Wormser, *J. Org. Chem.* **30**, 3792 (1965). Biosynthesis: Spenser, Tiwari, *Chem. Commun.* **1966**, 55. Acute toxicity: U. Mengs, *Arch. Toxicol.* **59**, 328 (1987). *Review:* D. B. Mix *et al., J. Nat. Prod.* **45**, 657-666 (1982).

Shiny brown leaflets from DMF + hot water, dec 281-286°. uv max (ethanol): 390, 318, 250 nm (ε 6500; 12000; 27000). Slightly sol in water; sol in alcohol, chloroform, ether, acetone, acetic acid, aniline, alkalies. Practically insol in benzene, carbon disulfide. LD$_{50}$ in male, female mice, male, female rats (mg/kg): 38.4, 70.1, 82.5, 74.0 i.v.; 55.9, 106.1, 203.4, 183.9 orally (Mengs).

Methyl ester. $C_{18}H_{13}NO_7$. Orange-yellow rods from hot methanol, mp 285-286°.

787. Armepavine. [524-20-9] 4-[[(1*R*)-1,2,3,4-Tetrahydro-6,7-dimethoxy-2-methyl-1-isoquinolinyl]methyl]phenol; (−)-6,7-dimethoxy-1-*p*-hydroxybenzyl-2-methyl-1,2,3,4-tetrahydroisoquinoline. $C_{19}H_{23}NO_3$; mol wt 313.39. C 72.82%, H 7.40%, N 4.47%, O 15.32%. Isoln from *Papaver armeniacum* (L.) DC., *Papaveraceae*: Konowalowa *et al., Ber.* **68**, 2161 (1935); from *Euonymus europaea* L., *Celastraceae*: Bishay *et al., J. Pharm. Pharmacol.* **23** (Suppl), 233S (1971); from *Rhamnus frangula* L., *Rhamnaceae*: Pailer, Haslinger, *Monatsh. Chem.* **103**, 1399 (1972). Structure: *eidem, J. Gen. Chem. USSR* **10**, 641 (1940). Synthesis: Marion *et al., J. Org. Chem.* **15**, 216 (1950); Gibson *et al., J. Heterocycl. Chem.* **3**, 99 (1966). Resolution: Knabe, Horn, *Arch. Pharm.* **300**, 547 (1967); Farber, Giacomazi, *Chem. Ind. (London)* **1968** (2), 57.

mp 149-150°. $[\alpha]_D^{20}$ −117.6° (CHCl$_3$) (Knabe); $[\alpha]_D^{27}$ −103.2° (Farber).

10-Camphorsulfonate hydrate. $C_{29}H_{39}NO_7S.H_2O$. mp 130°. $[\alpha]_D^{20}$ −65° (MeOH).

dl-Form hydrate. Needles from acetone + ether; loses its water around 100°, then melts at 140°. Freely sol in alc, acetone, chloroform; slightly sol in ether. Almost insol in water.

dl-Form hydrochloride. $C_{19}H_{23}NO_3$.HCl. Needles from alcohol + ether, mp 152°. Freely soluble in water and alc.

788. Armstrong's Acid. [81-04-9] 1,5-Naphthalenedisulfonic acid. $C_{10}H_8O_6S_2$; mol wt 288.30. C 41.66%, H 2.80%, O 33.30%, S 22.24%. Prepd by sulfonation of naphthalene: Lynch, Scanlan, *Ind. Eng. Chem.* **19**, 1010 (1927).

SO₃H structure (1,5-naphthalenedisulfonic acid)

Crystals. Soluble in water, alc; practically insol in ether.

789. Arnica. Arnica flowers; leopard's bane; wolf's bane; mountain tobacco. Dried flowerheads of *Arnica montana* L., *Compositae*. *Habit*. Northern Europe. *Constit*. 0.5-1% volatile oil; arnicin, arnisterol (arnidiol), anthoxanthine, tannin, resin. *Review:* Faber, *Pharmazie* **8**, 179, 286, 340 (1953).

THERAP CAT: Counterirritant (topical).
THERAP CAT (VET): Counterirritant.

790. Arogenic Acid. [53078-86-7] [1(*S*)-*cis*]-α-Amino-1-carboxy-4-hydroxy-2,5-cyclohexadiene-1-propanoic acid; L-(8*S*)-β-(1-carboxy-4-hydroxy-2,5-cyclohexadien-1-yl)alanine; arogenate; pretyrosine. $C_{10}H_{13}NO_5$; mol wt 227.21. C 52.86%, H 5.77%, N 6.16%, O 35.21%. Precursor in the biosynthesis of L-phenylalanine and L-tyrosine, distributed widely in nature. Pseudomonad bacteria and plants use both the prephenate and arogenate pathways for L-tyrosine biosynthesis. In cyanobacteria, coryniform bacteria and at least one yeast organism the arogenate pathway has been identified as the sole route of L-tyrosine biosynthesis. Identification of arogenate (pretyrosine) in blue-green algae biosynthesis of L-tyrosine: S. L. Stenmark *et al.*, *Nature* **247**, 290 (1974). Dual enzymic routes to L-tyrosine and L-phenylalanine via arogenate (pretyrosine) in *P. aeruginosa:* N. Patel *et al.*, *J. Biol. Chem.* **252**, 5839 (1977). Isoln and prepn: R. A. Jensen *et al.*, *J. Bacteriol.* **132**, 896 (1977). Confirmation that arogenate is an obligatory intermediate of L-tyrosine biosynthesis: A. M. Fazel *et al.*, *Proc. Natl. Acad. Sci. USA* **77**, 1270 (1980). Structure and config: L. O. Zamir *et al.*, *J. Am. Chem. Soc.* **102**, 4499 (1980). Synthesis via immobilized microbial proteins: *eidem, Bioorg. Chem.* **11**, 32 (1982). Arogenate pathway of tyrosine and phenylalanine biosynthesis in *P. aureofaciens:* B. Keller *et al.*, *J. Gen. Microbiol.* **128**, 1199 (1982).

Unstable. Quantitatively converted to phenylalanine at acidic pH. Forms a disodium salt that is stable in the lyophilized state at basic pH (7.5) and room temperature, but is thermally unstable.

791. Arotinolol. [68377-92-4] 5-[2-[[3-[(1,1-Dimethylethyl)amino]-2-hydroxypropyl]thio]-4-thiazolyl]-2-thiophenecarboxamide; 2-(3′-*tert*-butylamino-2′-hydroxypropylthio)-4-(5′-carbamoyl-2′-thienyl)thiazole. $C_{15}H_{21}N_3O_2S_3$; mol wt 371.54. C 48.49%, H 5.70%, N 11.31%, O 8.61%, S 25.89%. Propanolamine deriv with α- and β-adrenergic blocking activity. Prepn: T. Hibino *et al.*, **DE 2341753**; *eidem*, **US 3932400** (1974, 1976 both to Sumitomo); Y. Hara *et al., J. Pharm. Sci.* **67**, 1334 (1978). Characterization of adrenoceptor blocking effects *in vivo*: A. Miyagishi *et al., Arch. Int. Pharmacodyn. Ther.* **271**, 249 (1984). Possible antianginal effects: M. Sakanashi *et al., Oyo Yakuri* **28**, 709 (1984); *C.A.* **102**, 39669z (1985). Long-term antihypertensive effect in rats: K. Kishi *et al., J. Pharmacobio-Dyn.* **8**, 50 (1985). Comparison with timolol, *q.v.*, of effect on intraocular pressure and hemodynamics: M. Nakashima *et al., Eur. J. Clin. Pharmacol.* **28**, 391 (1985).

Crystals from chloroform/petroleum ether, mp 148-149°.

Hydrochloride. [68377-91-3] S-596; ARL; Almarl. $C_{15}H_{21}N_3O_2S_3$·HCl; mol wt 408.00. Crystals from methanol/water, mp 234-235.5° (dec). LD_{50} in mice (mg/kg): 86 i.v., >360 i.p., >5000 orally (Hara).

THERAP CAT: Antihypertensive; antianginal; antiarrhythmic.

792. Arsanilic Acid. [98-50-0] (4-Aminophenyl)arsonic acid; *p*-aminobenzenearsonic acid; atoxylic acid; AS-101. C_6H_8-$AsNO_3$; mol wt 217.05. C 33.20%, H 3.72%, As 34.52%, N 6.45%, O 22.11%. Prepd by heating aniline and arsenic acid: Lewis, Cheetham, *Org. Synth.* **coll. vol. I** (2nd ed., 1941) p 70; Hoffmann, Green, **US 3763201** (1973); from *p*-nitroaniline: Bart, *Ann.* **429**, 96 (1922); Gattermann-Wieland, *Praxis des Organischen Chemikers* (de Gruyter, Berlin, 40th ed., 1961) p 254. Toxicology in swine: Ledet *et al., Clin. Toxicol.* **6**, 439 (1973). Toxicity study: E. I. Goldenthal, *Toxicol. Appl. Pharmacol.* **18**, 185 (1971). Review of toxicology and human exposure: *Toxicological Profile for Arsenic* (PB2000-108021, 2000) 468 pp.

Needles from water or alcohol. Slightly sol in cold water, alcohol or acetic acid; sol in hot water, pentanol, in solns of alkali carbonates; moderately sol in concd mineral acids. Practically insol in acetone, benzene, chloroform, ether, and in moderately dil mineral acids. LD_{50} orally in male rats: >1000 mg/kg (Goldenthal).

USE: Manuf medicinal arsenicals.

THERAP CAT (VET): Growth promotant; to improve feed efficiency. To control swine dysentery.

793. Arsenamide. [531-72-6] 2,2′-[[[4-(Aminocarbonyl)-phenyl]arsinidene]bis(thio)]bisacetic acid; [[(*p*-carbamoylphenyl)-arsylene]dithio]diacetic acid; bis[carboxymethylmercapto](*p*-carbamylphenyl)-arsine; *p*-bis[(carboxymethylmercapto)arsino]benzamide; dithioglycolyl *p*-arsenobenzamide; 4-carbamylphenyl bis[carboxymethylthio]arsenite; thioarsenite; thiacetarsamide; Caparsolate; Caparside. $C_{11}H_{12}AsNO_5S_2$; mol wt 377.27. C 35.02%, H 3.21%, As 19.86%, N 3.71%, O 21.20%, S 17.00%. Prepd by the condensation of *p*-arsenosobenzamide and thioglycolic acid: Gough, King *J. Chem. Soc.* **1930**, 669; Maren, *J. Am. Chem. Soc.* **68**, 1864 (1946).

White crystalline powder. Sparingly sol in cold water; appreciably sol in water above 90°. Sparingly sol in cold methanol, ethanol; very sol in these solvents when they are warm. Insol in warm isopropyl ether. pKa = 4. The disodium salt is stoichiometrically formed in aq soln at pH 7-8.

THERAP CAT (VET): Anthelmintic for heartworm infection in dogs, especially the adult worm.

794. Arsenic. [7440-38-2] Grey arsenic; metallic arsenic; arsen (German). As; at. wt 74.92160; at. no. 33; valences 3, 5. Group VA (15) element, classified as a metalloid. Naturally occurring isotope (mass number): 75 (100%); known artificial, radioactive isotopes: 66-74; 76-87. Arsenic compds were described and used in antiquity, especially as poisons; their reduction to the element was known to medieval alchemists. Albertus Magnus credited with isolation of the element from the mineral orpiment in ~1250 A.D. First precise directions for the prepn of As found in Paracelsus' writings (*ca.* 1520). Arsenic probably occurs throughout the universe. Meteorites reported to contain from 0.0005 to 0.1% As. Occurrence in the earth's crust: 1.8 ppm. Found in nature to a small extent as the element; occurs mostly in minerals such as realgar (As_4S_4), orpiment (A_2S_3), arsenolite (As_2O_3). Commercial sources: as by-product in flue dusts from smelting copper, lead, cobalt and gold ores; by melting $FeAs_2$ or $FeAsS$ ores. Prepn of pure As by reduction with carbon (sugar charcoal) and sublimation in N_2: Krepelka, *Collect. Czech. Chem. Commun.* **2**, 255 (1930); E. H. Archibald, *The Preparation of Pure Inorganic Substances* (Wiley, New York, 1932) p 269. Other methods: Schenk in *Handbook of Preparative Inorganic Chemistry* vol. 1, G. Brauer, Ed. (Academic Press, New York, 2nd ed., 1963) pp 591-593. *Reviews: Gmelins, Arsenic* (8th ed.) **17**, 475 pp (1952); Smith, "Arsenic, Antimony and Bismuth" in *Comprehensive Inorganic Chemistry* vol. 2, J. C. Bailar, Jr. *et al.*, Eds. (Pergamon Press, Oxford, 1973) pp 547-683; *Chemistry of the Elements*, N. N. Greenwood, A. Earnshaw, Eds. (Pergamon Press, New York, 1984) pp 637-697; S. C. Carapella, Jr. in *Kirk-Othmer Encyclopedia of Chemical Technology* vol. 3 (John Wiley & Sons, 4th ed., 1992) pp 624-633; G. O. Doak *et al., ibid.* pp 633-659. Review of carcinogenicity studies: *IARC Monographs* **23**, 39-141 (1980); of toxicology and human exposure: *Toxicological Profile for Arsenic* (PB2000-108021, 2000) 468 pp. Book: "The Chemistry of Organic Arsenic, Antimony and Bismuth Compounds," S. Patai, Ed. (John Wiley & Sons, New York, 1994) 962 pp.

Allotropic forms: α-form, metallic, steel-gray, shiny, brittle, rhombohedral crystal structure; β-form, dark gray, amorphous sold, d 4.700, transforms to metallic form at 280°. Can be heated to burn in air with bluish flame, giving off an odor of garlic and dense white fumes of As_2O_3. Stable in dry air; loses its luster on exposure to humid air as surface oxidizes, forming a black modification + As_2O_3. Brinell hardness: 147; Mohs' scale: 3.5. d_4^{25} 5.778. Sublimes$_{760}$ 615° without melting. mp 818° at 36 atm. Heat of vaporization 11.2 kcal/g-atom. Heat of sublimation 30.5 kcal/g-atom. Heat of fusion: 22.4 kcal/g-atom (*Gmelins, loc. cit.* pp 135-136). Also reported as: heat of fusion: 6.620 kcal/g-atom; heat of sublimation 7.63 kcal/g-atom: D. R. Stull, G. C. Sinke, "Thermodynamic Properties of the Elements" in *Advances in Chemistry Series* **18** (A.C.S., Washington, 1956) pp 11, 44. Latent heat of fusion: 27,740 J/mol K. Latent heat of sublimation: 31,974 J/mol K (Carapella). Specific heat (25°) 24.6 J/mol K. Dielectric constant = 10.23 at 20° and 60 cycles. Electrical and magnetic properties of crystalline As: Taylor *et al., J. Phys. Chem. Solids* **26**, 69 (1965). Insol in water. Not attacked by cold H_2SO_4 or HCl; converted by HNO_3 or hot H_2SO_4 into arsenous or arsenic acid. A yellow modification which has no metallic properties has been reported from sudden cooling of As-vapor. This yellow arsenic is converted back to the gray modification upon very short exposure to ultraviolet light.

Note: In German and other languages *Arsenik* means arsenic trioxide.

Caution: Overexposure to arsenic and arsenic compounds has been associated with acute and chronic toxicity due to inhalation or ingestion. Organic forms are usually less harmful than inorganic forms. Direct contact can cause local irritation and dermatitis. Overexposure has been associated with an increased risk of skin, liver, bladder, kidney and lung cancer. *See Toxicological Profile, loc. cit.* Inorganic arsenic compounds are listed as known human carcinogens: *Report on Carcinogens, Eleventh Edition* (PB2005-104914, 2004) pp III-18.

USE: In metallurgy for hardening copper, lead, nonferrous alloys; automotive body solder. In semiconductor materials. In the manufacture of low-melting glass. As wood preservative, herbicide, pesticide.

795. Arsenic Acid. [7778-39-4] Orthoarsenic acid. AsH_3-O_4; mol wt 141.94. As 52.78%, H 2.13%, O 45.09%. H_3AsO_4. Exists only as the hemihydrate. Excessive drying produces As_2-$O_5.⅔H_2O$. Conveniently prepd from As_2O_3 and HNO_3: Simon, Thaler, *Z. Anorg. Allg. Chem.* **161**, 143 (1927); **246**, 19 (1941). Toxicity study: Joachimoglu, *Biochem. Z.* **70**, 144 (1915). Review of toxicology and human exposure: *Toxicological Profile for Arsenic* (PB2000-108021, 2000) 468 pp.

Hemihydrate. Hygroscopic crystals. *Poisonous!* Converted to As_2O_5 by heating above 300°. Freely sol in water, alcohol, glycerol. LD$_{50}$ i.v. in rabbits: 6 mg/kg (Joachimoglu).

USE: In the manuf of arsenates.

796. Arsenic Pentafluoride. [7784-36-3] AsF_5; mol wt 169.91. As 44.09%, F 55.91%. Prepd from As + F_2: Ruff *et al., Z. Anorg. Allg. Chem.* **206**, 59 (1932); Seel, Detmer, *ibid.* **301**, 113 (1959); Kwasnik in *Handbook of Preparative Inorganic Chemistry* vol. **1**, G. Brauer, Ed. (Academic Press, New York, 2nd ed., 1963) p 198. *Reviews:* Burg in *Fluorine Chemistry* vol. I, J.

Simons, Ed. (Academic Press, New York, 1950) p 102; Kemmitt, Sharp, *Adv. Fluorine Chem.* **4**, 208 (1965).

Colorless gas. Forms white clouds in moist air. $d_{liq}^{25.8}$ 2.33. mp −79.8°. bp −53.2°. Instantly hydrolyzed by water. Sol in alcohol, ether, benzene. Dry AsF_5 does not attack glass, but a minute trace of moisture or HF catalyzes the etching reaction to the point of total destruction.

797. Arsenic Pentasulfide. [1303-34-0] Diarsenic pentasulfide. As_2S_5; mol wt 310.17. As 48.31%, S 51.69%. Prepd from H_3AsO_4 and H_2S: Schenk in *Handbook of Preparative Inorganic Chemistry* vol 1, G. Brauer, Ed. (Academic Press, New York, 2nd ed., 1963) p 603.

Brownish-yellow, glassy, amorphous, highly refractive mass. Insol in water; sol in alkalies and alkali sulfides. Dec into As_2O_3, S, and As_2S_3 when boiled with water.

USE: In thin sheets as a light filter; in pigments.

798. Arsenic Pentoxide. [1303-28-2] Arsenic acid anhydride. As_2O_5; mol wt 229.84. As 65.19%, O 34.81%. Prepn: *Gmelins, Arsenic* (8th ed.) **17**, pp 273-277 (1952). Review of toxicology and human exposure: *Toxicological Profile for Arsenic* (PB2000-108021, 2000) 468 pp.

Amorphous lumps or powder. *Poisonous!* Gradually deliquesces on exposure to air. Freely sol in water or alc. Combines very slowly with H_2O to form H_3AsO_4. *Keep well closed.*

USE: Manuf of colored glass; in adhesives for metals; in wood preservatives; in weed control; as fungicide.

799. Arsenic Sulfide. [12279-90-2] 2,4,6,8-Tetrathia-1,3,-5,7-tetraarsatricyclo[3.3.0.0^{3,7}]octane; red arsenic sulfide; realgar; red orpiment; ruby arsenic; red arsenic glass; tetraarsenic tetrasulfide; C.I. Pigment Yellow 39; C.I. 77085. As_4S_4; mol wt 427.95. As 70.03%, S 29.97%. Prepn: *Gmelins, Arsenic* (8th ed.) **17**, pp 417-422 (1952); Schenk in *Handbook of Preparative Inorganic Chemistry* vol 1, G. Brauer, Ed. (Academic Press, New York, 2nd ed., 1963) p 603.

Deep red, lustrous monoclinic crystals. mp 320°; bp 565°; d 3.5. Ignites at high temp. Practically insol in water; sol in alkali hydroxides; decomposed by HNO_3; very slightly sol in hot CS_2 and benzene.

USE: As pigment in painting; in fireworks as blue fire and to give an intense white flame; manuf shot; calico printing and dyeing; tanning and depilating hides.

800. Arsenic Tribromide. [7784-33-0] $AsBr_3$; mol wt 314.63. As 23.81%, Br 76.19%. Prepn: Oddo, Giachery, *Gazz. Chim. Ital.* **53**, 56 (1923); Schenk in *Handbook of Preparative Inorganic Chemistry* vol. **1**, G. Brauer, Ed. (Academic Press, New York, 2nd ed., 1963) p 597.

Deliquescent, orthorhombic prisms. *Intensely poisonous!* d_4^{25} 3.397; d_4^{50} (liq) 3.3282; d_4^{75} 3.2623; d_4^{100} 3.1995. mp 31.1°. bp$_{760}$ 221°; bp$_{11}$ 89°. Dipole moment 1.66. Heat of fusion 8.93 cal/g. Fumes in moist air. Dec by water with the formation of As_2O_3 and HBr. Miscible with ether, benzene. Sol in hydrocarbons, chlorinated hydrocarbons, carbon disulfide, oils and fats.

801. Arsenic Trichloride. [7784-34-1] Butter of arsenic; fuming liquid arsenic. $AsCl_3$; mol wt 181.28. As 41.33%, Cl 58.67%. Prepn: Smith, *Ind. Eng. Chem.* **11**, 109 (1919); Reisener in *Ullmanns Encyklopädie der technischen Chemie* vol. 3, (Urban & Schwarzenberg, Munich, 1953) p 850; Schenk in *Handbook of Preparative Inorganic Chemistry* vol. **1**, G. Brauer, Ed. (Academic Press, New York, 2nd ed., 1963) p 596.

Oily liquid. *Intensely poisonous!* Fumes in air. d_4^{25} 2.1497. mp −16°. bp 130.21°; bp$_{11}$ 25°. Dipole moment: 2.17. Heat of vaporization 8.9 kcal/mol. Specific heat: 3.19 cal/mol/°C. n_D^{20} 1.6006. Dec by water to form $As(OH)_3$ and HCl. One mol $AsCl_3$ can be dissolved in 9 mols H_2O, this soln (d 1.53) may be diluted again with another 9 mols H_2O giving a soln with d 1.346. Further dilution results in the precipitation of As_2O_3. Also dec by ultraviolet light. Miscible with, or solvent for, chloroform, carbon tetrachloride, ether, iodine, phosphorus, sulfur, alkali iodides, oils and fats.

USE: In the ceramic industry; in syntheses of chlorine-contg arsenicals, e.g., chloro derivs of arsine.

802. Arsenic Trifluoride. [7784-35-2] AsF_3; mol wt 131.92. As 56.79%, F 43.20%. Prepn: Russell *et al.*, *J. Am. Chem. Soc.* **63**, 2825 (1941); Woolf, Greenwood, *J. Chem. Soc.* **1950**, 2200; Hoffman, *Inorg. Synth.* **4**, 151 (1953); Kwasnik in *Handbook of Preparative Inorganic Chemistry* **vol. 1**, G. Brauer, Ed. (Academic Press, New York, 2nd ed., 1963) pp 197-198. *Review:* Kemmitt, Sharp, *Adv. Fluorine Chem.* **4**, 208-209 (1965).

Mobile liquid. *Very poisonous!* Fumes in air. Etches glass. d_{15}^{15} 2.73. mp $-5.95°$. bp 57.8°. Also reported as mp $-8.5°$; bp 63° (Kwasnik). Hydrolyzed by water. Sol in alcohol, ether, benzene. May be stored in iron vessels.

Caution: Extremely toxic.

803. Arsenic Triiodide. [7784-45-4] AsI_3; mol wt 455.64. As 16.44%, I 83.56%. Prepd from the elements or from $AsCl_3$ and KI: Bailar, *Inorg. Synth.* **I**, 103 (1939).

Orange-red, trigonal rhombohedra from acetone. Reacts slowly with O_2 from air, liberating iodine. d_4^{25} 4.688. Some tendency to sublime below 100°. mp 140.9° forming a red liquid. bp_{760} ~400°. One gram dissolves in 12 ml water forming a yellow soln. Does not hydrolyze rapidly and may be recovered from the water soln unchanged within 5 hrs. Aqueous solns are strongly acid (pH of $0.1N$ soln about 1.1) and ultimately form HI and As_2O_3, although an equilibrium $AsI_3 + 3H_2O = H_3AsO_3 + 3HI$ has been observed. Freely sol in carbon disulfide, chloroform, benzene, toluene, xylene. Less sol in alc, ether.

THERAP CAT: Formerly in dermatitides.

804. Arsenic Trioxide. [1327-53-3] Arsenous acid; arsenous acid anhydride; arsenous oxide; arsenic sesquioxide; white arsenic; Trisenox. As_2O_3; mol wt 197.84. As 75.74%, O 24.26%. Commercially important form of arsenic, *q.v.* By-product in the smelting of copper. Has been used in traditional medicine; induces apoptosis in leukemic cells. Prepn: Schenk in *Handbook of Preparative Inorganic Chemistry* **vol. 1**, G. Brauer, Ed. (Academic Press, New York, 2nd ed., 1963) p 600. Studies of antileukemic mechanisms: Z. Chen *et al.*, *Pharmacol. Ther.* **76**, 141 (1997); J. Dai *et al.*, *Blood* **93**, 268 (1999). Clinical evaluation in acute promyelocytic leukemia: S. L. Soignet *et al.*, *N. Engl. J. Med.* **339**, 1341 (1998). Acute toxicity: J. Harrison *et al.*, *Arch. Ind. Health* **17**, 118 (1958). Review of production, properties and uses: S. C. Carapella, Jr. in *Kirk-Othmer Encyclopedia of Chemical Technology* **vol. 3** (John Wiley & Sons, 4th ed., 1992) pp 626-629; G. O. Doak, *ibid.* pp 633-638. Review of use in glass industry: J. T. Kohli, *Key Eng. Mater.* **94-95**, 363-378 (1994). Review of toxicology: A. K. Done, A. J. Peart, *Clin. Toxicol.* **4**, 343-355 (1971); *Cah. Notes Doc.* **136**, 543-548 (1989); and human exposure: *Toxicological Profile for Arsenic* (PB2000-108021, 2000) 468 pp.

Two crystalline modifications exist. **Claudetite**: thermodynamically stable, monoclinic form, mp 313°. **Arsenolite**: the commonly occurring, octahedral or cubic form; white solid, sublimes freely above 135°, mp 275°. bp 465°. *Extremely poisonous!* Sparingly and extremely slowly sol in cold water; sol in 15 parts boiling water, in dil HCl, in alkali hydroxide or carbonate solns. Practically insol in alc, chloroform, ether. LD_{50} in mice, rats (mg/kg): 39.4, 15.1 orally (Harrison).

USE: Starting material for various arsenic compounds. Decolorizer and fining agent in manuf of glass. In wood preservatives, weed killers, rodenticides.

THERAP CAT: Antineoplastic.

THERAP CAT (VET): Has been used as ectoparasiticide.

805. Arsenic Triselenide. [1303-36-2] Arsenious selenide; arsenous selenide. As_2Se_3; mol wt 386.72. As 38.75%, Se 61.25%. Prepd by melting arsenic and selenium in the correct proportions: Uelsmann, *Ueber Selenverbindungen*, Göttingen (1860); *Ann.* **116**, 122 (1860); by the action of an arsenic salt on a soln of hydrogen selenide: Moser, Atynsky, *Monatsh. Chem.* **45**, 235 (1925).

Dark brown solid. d 4.75. mp 260°. Sol in nitric acid, alkalilye, alkali sulfide solutions; insol in water.

806. Arsenic Trisulfide. [1303-33-9] Yellow arsenic sulfide; orpiment; auripigment; arsenic yellow; king's yellow; king's gold. As_2S_3; mol wt 246.04. As 60.90%, S 39.10%. The article of commerce contains much less sulfur than theory. Prepn: *Gmelins, Arsenic* (8th ed.) **17**, pp 422-433 (1952).

Yellow or orange powder. mp reported from 300 to 325°. d 3.46. Practically insol in water. Sol in alkalies, alkali sulfides or carbonates; slowly sol in hot HCl; dec by HNO_3.

USE: Manuf of glass, particularly infrared-transmitting glass; manuf of oil cloth, linoleum; in electrical semiconductors, photoconductors; as pigment; for depilating hides; in pyrotechnics.

807. Arsenious Acid Solution. Arsenic chloride solution. Prepared with 1 g As_2O_3, 5 ml dil HCl and water to 100 ml. *Poisonous!*

THERAP CAT (VET): Has been used in skin and blood disorders.

808. Arsenoacetic Acid. [544-27-4] 2,2'-(1,2-Diarsenediyl)bisacetic acid; arsenodiacetic acid; diarsenoacetic acid. C_4H_6-As_2O_4; mol wt 267.93. C 17.93%, H 2.26%, As 55.93%, O 23.89%. $HOOCCH_2As=AsCH_2COOH$. Prepd by dissolving sodium arsonoacetate and sodium hypophosphite in 15% H_2SO_4: Palmer, *J. Am. Chem. Soc.* **45**, 3023 (1923); *Org. Synth.* **coll. vol. I**, 73 (1941). *Compare* Arsonoacetic Acid.

Minute yellow needles, begin to dec at about 205°, but do not melt below 260°. Practically insol in water and common organic solvents. Readily sol in pyridine, dil sodium hydroxide and dil sodium carbonate solns.

Disodium salt. Disodium arsenoacetate. $C_4H_4As_2Na_2O_4$; mol wt 311.89. Yellow powder, freely sol in water.

THERAP CAT (VET): Disodium salt has been used as an injectable tonic for horses.

809. Arsine. [7784-42-1] Arsenic trihydride; hydrogen arsenide. AsH_3; mol wt 77.95. As 96.11%, H 3.88%. Prepn: Wendt, Landauer, *J. Am. Chem. Soc.* **42**, 930 (1920); Jolly, Drake, *Inorg. Synth.* **7**, 41 (1963); Schenk in *Handbook of Preparative Inorganic Chemistry* **vol 1**, G. Brauer, Ed. (Academic Press, New York, 2nd ed., 1963) pp 593-595. Toxicity: Doig, *Lancet* **2**, 88 (1958); Vallee *et al.*, *Arch. Ind. Health* **21**, 132 (1960).

Colorless, neutral gas. Disagreeable garlic odor. *Very poisonous!* mp $-117°$. bp $-62.5°$. Dissociation pressure at $0° = 0.806$ atm. Decomposes when heated at 300°, depositing arsenic which volatilizes at 400°. On exposure to light, moist arsine decomposes quickly depositing shiny black arsenic. Slightly sol in water. Aq solns are neutral. Traces are best removed by absorption in potassium permanganate soln or in bromine water.

Caution: Potential symptoms of overexposure are headache, malaise, weakness and dizziness; dyspnea; abdominal and back pain; nausea, vomiting; bronze skin; hematuria; jaundice; peripheral neuropathy; direct contact with liquid may cause frostbite. Potential occupational carcinogen. See *NIOSH Pocket Guide to Chemical Hazards* (DHHS/NIOSH 97-140, 1997) p 20.

810. Arsonoacetic Acid. [107-38-0] $C_2H_5AsO_5$; mol wt 183.98. C 13.06%, H 2.74%, As 40.72%, O 43.48%. H_2O_3-$AsCH_2COOH$. Prepn from sodium arsenite and sodium chloroacetate: Palmer, *J. Am. Chem. Soc.* **45**, 3023 (1923); *Org. Synth.* **coll. vol. I**, 73 (1941).

Shiny plates, mp 152°. Very sol in water, alc; sparingly sol in hot glacial acetic acid. Practically insol in petr ether, benzene, acetone, chloroform, ethyl acetate.

Barium salt. $C_4H_4As_2Ba_3O_{10}$. Feathery needles. Slightly sol in boiling water.

Sodium salt monohydrate. Disodium arsonoacetate; disodium acetarsinate; acetarsonic acid disodium salt; sodium acetoarsinate; Aricyl. $C_2H_3AsNa_2O_5 \cdot H_2O$; mol wt 245.96. Crystals. Freely sol in water.

THERAP CAT (VET): Disodium salt has been used to treat anaplasmosis, and as a stimulant in nervous diseases.

811. Arsphenamine. [139-93-5] salvarsan; Ehrlich 606; Originally introduced as an antisyphilitic. Initially characterized as *4,4'-(1,2-diarsenediyl)bis[2-aminophenol] dihydrochloride*; composition was later determined to be of a mixture of cyclic 3-amino-4-hydroxyphenylarsenic species. Prepn: P. Ehrlich, A. Bertheim, **US 986148** (1911 to Hoechst); *eidem, Ber.* **45**, 756 (1912); W. A. Christiansen, *J. Am. Chem. Soc.* **42**, 2402 (1920). Toxicity data: J. F. Schamberg *et al.*, *Am. J. Syph. Neurol.* **18**, 37 (1934). Review of structure: A. S. Levinson, *J. Chem. Educ.* **54**, 98-99 (1977). MS determn of chemical composition: N. C. Lloyd *et al.*, *Angew. Chem. Int. Ed.* **44**, 941 (2005).

Light yellow, somewhat hygroscopic powder. It is odorless, or has a slight odor of the precipitant used. Oxidizes on exposure to air, becoming darker and more toxic. *It is poisonous!* Sol in water, alc or glycerol, very slightly sol in chloroform or ether. Its aq soln is acid; pH about 3. LD$_{100}$ i.v. in rats: 140 mg/kg (Schamberg).

812. Arsthinol. [119-96-0] *N*-[2-Hydroxy-5-[4-(hydroxymethyl)-1,3,2-dithiarsolan-2-yl]phenyl]acetamide; 3-acetamido-4-hydroxydithiobenzenearsonous acid, cyclic (hydroxymethyl)ethylene ester; 2-(3'-acetamido-4'-hydroxyphenyl)-1,3-dithia-2-arsacyclopentane-4-methanol; 3-acetamido-4-hydroxydithiobenzenearsonous acid cyclic 3-hydroxypropylene ester; 2-acetylamino-4-(methylolcycloethylenedimercaptoarsine)phenol; Balarsen. C$_{11}$H$_{14}$AsNO$_3$S$_2$; mol wt 347.29. C 38.04%, H 4.06%, As 21.57%, N 4.03%, O 13.82%, S 18.47%. Trivalent arsenical; derivative of acetarsone, *q.v.* Prepn: Friedheim, **US 2593434** (1952); **US 2772303** (1956).

Minute crystals, mp 163-166°. Soly in 95% ethanol about 2.7% w/v. Very slightly sol in water, ether.

THERAP CAT: Antiamebic.

813. Arteether. [75887-54-6] (3*R*,5a*S*,6*R*,8a*S*,9*R*,10*S*,-12*R*,12a*R*)-10-Ethoxydecahydro-3,6,9-trimethyl-3,12-epoxy-12*H*-pyrano[4,3-*j*]-1,2-benzodioxepin; dihydroartemisinin ethyl ether; dihydroqinghaosu ethyl ether; artemotil; SM-227. C$_{17}$H$_{28}$O$_5$; mol wt 312.40. C 65.36%, H 9.03%, O 25.61%. Derivative of artemisinin, *q.v.* Prepn: Y. Li *et al., Acta Pharm. Sin.* **16**, 429 (1981). Synthesis and antimalarial activity: China Cooperative Research Group on Qinghaosu, *J. Tradit. Chin. Med.* **2**, 9 (1982); A. Brossi *et al., J. Med. Chem.* **31**, 645 (1988).

White crystalline solid, mp 80-82°. [*α*]$_D^{21}$ +154.5° (c = 1.0 in CHCl$_3$).

THERAP CAT: Antimalarial.

814. Arteflene. [123407-36-3] (Z-form) [1*S*-[1*α*,4*β*(*Z*),-5*α*,8*β*]]-4-[2-[2,4-Bis(trifluoromethyl)phenyl]ethenyl]-4,8-dimethyl-2,3-dioxabicyclo[3.3.1]nonan-7-one; (1*S*,4*R*,5*R*,8*S*)-4-[(*Z*)-2,4-bis(trifluoromethyl)styryl]-4,8-dimethyl-2,3-dioxabicyclo[3.3.1]-nonan-7-one; Ro-42-1611; Synthetic sesquiterpene peroxide; structurally derived from the natural peroxides artemisinin, *q.v.* and yingzhaosu. Prepn: W. Hofheinz *et al., EP 311955*; *eidem,* **US 4977184** (1989, 1990 both to Hoffmann-La Roche). Series of articles on prepn, biological activities, pharmacokinetics and clinical evaluations: *Trop. Med. Parasitol.* **45**, 261-291 (1994).

Crystalline stable material, mp 124°. Highly lipophilic, not sol in water. Stable in soln except in the presence of strong bases or strong reducing agents.

THERAP CAT: Antimalarial.

815. Artemether. [71963-77-4] (3*R*,5a*S*,6*R*,8a*S*,9*R*,10*S*,-12*R*,12a*R*)-Decahydro-10-methoxy-3,6,9-trimethyl-3,12-epoxy-12*H*-pyrano[4,3-*j*]-1,2-benzodioxepin; dihydroartemisinin methyl ether; dihydroqinghaosu methyl ether; *o*-methyldihydroartemisinin; SM-224; Paluther. C$_{16}$H$_{26}$O$_5$; mol wt 298.37. C 64.41%, H 8.78%, O 26.81%. Derivative of artemisinin, *q.v.* Prepn: Y. Li *et al., K'o Hsueh T'ung Pao* **24**, 667 (1979), *C.A.* **91**, 211376u (1979); *eidem, Acta Pharm. Sin.* **16**, 429 (1981). Absolute configuration: X.-D. Luo *et al., Helv. Chim. Acta* **67**, 1515 (1984). NMR spectral study: F. S. El-Feraly *et al., Spectrosc. Lett.* **18**, 843 (1985). Inhibition of protein synthesis: H. M. Gu *et al., Biochem. Pharmacol.* **32**, 2463 (1983). Antimalarial activity: S. Thaithong, G. H. Beale, *Bull. WHO* **63**, 617 (1985). Series of articles on chemistry, pharmacology and antimalarial efficacy: China Cooperative Research Group on Qinghaosu, *J. Tradit. Chin. Med.* **2**, 3-50 (1982). Toxicity data: *eidem, ibid.* 31. Clinical trial in cerebral malaria in children: M. B. van Hensbroek *et al., N. Engl. J. Med.* **335**, 69 (1996). *Review:* R. N. Price, *Expert Opin. Invest. Drugs* **9**, 1815-1827 (2000).

Crystals, mp 86-88°. [*α*]$_D^{19.5}$ +171° (c = 2.59 in CHCl$_3$). LD$_{50}$ i.m. in mice: 263 mg/kg (China Cooperative Research Group on Qinghaosu).

THERAP CAT: Antimalarial.

816. Artemisin. [481-05-0] (3*S*,3a*R*,4*S*,5a*S*,9b*S*)-3a,5,5a,-9b-Tetrahydro-4-hydroxy-3,5a,9-trimethylnaphtho[1,2-*b*]furan-2,-8(3*H*,4*H*)-dione; 6*α*,8*α*-dihydroxy-3-oxoeudesma-1,4-dien-12-oic acid 12,6-lactone; 8-hydroxysantonin. C$_{15}$H$_{18}$O$_4$; mol wt 262.30. C 68.68%, H 6.92%, O 24.40%. From the closed, unexpanded flower heads of several *Artemisia* spp. especially *Artemisia maritima* L., and *A. cina* Berg., *Compositae* ("wormseed"). Found in the mother liquors from the extraction of santonin. Isoln: E. Merck, *E. Merck's Jahresber.* **1894**, 3; *Chem. Zentralbl.* **1895**, I, 436. Structure: Sumi, *J. Am. Chem. Soc.* **80**, 4869 (1958); Cocker, McMurry, *Tetrahedron* **8**, 181 (1960). Stereochemistry: Bolt *et al., J. Chem. Soc.* **1963**, 5235. Synthesis of (+)-artemisin: Nakazaki, Naemura, *Tetrahedron Lett.* **1966**, 2615.

Crystals from abs ethanol or ethyl acetate. Bitter taste. Turns yellow on exposure to light. mp 203°. bp$_{0.1}$ 260°. Sublimes$_{760}$ 170-175°. [*α*]$_D^{23}$ −84.9° (c = 3 in 95% ethanol). One gram dissolves in 60 ml boiling water, in 3 ml boiling alc. Sol in ethyl acetate. Practically insol in petr ether. Somewhat sol in chloroform.

817. Artemisinin. [63968-64-9] (3*R*,5a*S*,6*R*,8a*S*,9*R*,12*S*,-12a*R*)-Octahydro-3,6,9-trimethyl-3,12-epoxy-12*H*-pyrano[4,3-*j*]-1,2-benzodioxepin-10(3*H*)-one; artemisine; arteannuin; huanghuahaosu; QHS; qinghaosu; qing hau sau. C$_{15}$H$_{22}$O$_5$; mol wt 282.33. C 63.81%, H 7.85%, O 28.33%. Active antimalarial constituent of the traditional Chinese medicinal herb *Artemisia annua* L., *Compositae*, which has been known for almost 2000 years as **Qinghao**. Isolated in 1972 and shown to be a sesquiterpene lactone with a peroxide moiety: *K'o Hsueh T'ung Pao* **22**, 142 (1977), *C.A.* **87**, 98788g (1977); L. Jing-Ming *et al., Acta Chim. Sin.* **37**, 129 (1979), *C.A.* **92**, 94594w (1980). Total synthesis and absolute configuration: G. Schmid, W. Hofheinz, *J. Am. Chem. Soc.* **105**, 624 (1983). NMR spectral study: F. S. El-Feraly *et al., Spectrosc. Lett.* **18**, 843 (1985). Antimalarial activity: Qinghaosu Antimalaria Coordinating Research Group, *Chin. Med. J.* **92**, 811 (1979); L. J. Bruce-Chwatt, *Br. Med. J.* **284**, 767 (1982). Clinical trials: J.-B. Jiang *et al., Lancet* **2**, 285 (1982); W. Tongyin, X. Ruchang, *J. Tradit. Chin. Med.* **5**, 240 (1985). Toxicity data: China Cooperative Research Group on Qinghaosu, *ibid.* **2**, 31 (1982). Series of articles on chemistry, pharmacology, and antimalarial efficacy: *ibid.* 3-50. Brief reviews: H. Koch, *Pharm. Int.* **2**, 184-185 (1981); D. L. Klayman, *Science* **228**, 1049-1055 (1985). *Review:* R. N. Price, *Expert Opin. Invest. Drugs* **9**, 1815-1827 (2000). Review of chemistry, pharmacology and clinical applications: X. D. Luo, C. C. Shen, *Med. Res. Rev.* **7**, 29-52 (1987). Review of mechanism of action: S. R. Meshnick, *Int. J. Parasitol.* **32**, 1655-1660 (2002).

Needles, mp 156-157°. $[\alpha]_D^{17}$ +66.3°. (c = 1.64 in $CHCl_3$). Sol in most aprotic solvents. Slightly sol in oil. LD_{50} in mice (mg/kg): 5105 orally; 2800 i.m.; 1558 i.p. (Koch). LD_{50} in mice, rats (mg/kg): 4228, 5576 orally; 3840, 2571 i.m. (China Cooperative Research Group on Qinghaosu).

Dihydroartemisinin. [71939-50-9] Dihydroqinghaosu. $C_{15}H_{24}O_5$. Main metabolite of artemisinin, arteether, artemether, artesunate, *q.q.v.* HPLC determn: X.-D. Luo *et al., Chromatographia* **23**, 112 (1987); in plasma: H. Naik *et al., J. Chromatogr. B* **816**, 233 (2005).

THERAP CAT: Antimalarial.

818. Artesunate. [88495-63-0] Butanedioic acid mono[(3R,5aS,6R,8aS,9R,10R,12R,12aR)-decahydro-3,6,9-trimethyl-3,12-epoxy-12H-pyrano[4,3-j]-1,2-benzodioxepin-10-yl] ester; artesunic acid; dihydroqinghaosu hemisuccinate. $C_{19}H_{28}O_8$; mol wt 384.42. C 59.36%, H 7.34%, O 33.30%. Derivative of artemisinin, *q.v.* Prepn: China Cooperative Research Group on Qinghaosu, *J. Tradit. Chin. Med.* **2**, 9 (1982). Absolute configuration: X.-D. Luo *et al., Helv. Chim. Acta* **67**, 1515 (1984). GC/MS determn.: A. D. Theoharides *et al., Anal. Chem.* **60**, 115 (1988); HPLC determn in plasma: H. Naik *et al., J. Chromatogr. B* **816**, 233 (2005). Pharmacology: Y. Zhao, *J. Trop. Med. Hyg.* **88**, 391 (1985). Antimalarial activity: W. Peters *et al., Ann. Trop. Med. Parasitol.* **80**, 483 (1986); A. J. Lin *et al., J. Med. Chem.* **30**, 2147 (1987). Inhibition of cytochrome oxidase: Y. Zhao *et al., J. Nat. Prod.* **49**, 139 (1986). Toxicology: China Cooperative Research Group on Qinghaosu, *J. Tradit. Chin. Med.* **2**, 31 (1982). Series of articles on chemistry, pharmacology, and antimalarial efficacy: *ibid.* 3-50. Clinical trial as add-on therapy in pediatric malaria: L. von Seidlein *et al., Lancet* **355**, 352 (2000). *Review:* R. N. Price, *Expert Opin. Invest. Drugs* **9**, 1815-1827 (2000).

Fine white crystalline powder.
Sodium salt. SM-804. $C_{19}H_{27}NaO_8$; mol wt 406.40. Poor stability in aqueous solutions. LD_{50} in mice (mg/kg): 520 i.v.;

475 i.m. (China Cooperative Research Group); also reported as 699 ± 58.5 i.v. (Zhao, 1985).

THERAP CAT: Antimalarial.

819. Arylsulfatase B. [55354-43-3] Acetylgalactosamine 4-sulfatase; sulfatase B; EC 3.1.6.12. Lysosomal enzyme that hydrolyzes the 4-sulfate ester of N-acetylgalactosamine at the nonreducing terminus of dermatan sulfate and chondroitin-4-sulfate. Genetic deficiency of the enzyme results in the lysosomal storage disorder, mucopolysaccharidosis-VI (MPS-VI), also known as Maroteaux-Lamy syndrome. Purification from ox liver: A. B. Roy, *Biochem. J.* **57**, 30 (1954); from human liver: K. S. Dodgson, C. H. Wynn, *ibid.* **68**, 387 (1958). Identification of role in disease: D. A. Stumpf, J. H. Austin, *Trans. Amer. Neurol. Assoc.* **97**, 29 (1972). Identification of natural substrate: A. A. Farooqui, *Experientia* **32**, 1242 (1976). Prepn of recombinant human form and uptake by human fibroblast cells: D. S. Anson *et al., Biochem. J.* **284**, 789 (1992). Molecular structure and characterization of active site: C. S. Bond *et al., Structure* **5**, 277 (1997).

Galsulfase. [552858-79-4] Acetylgalactosamine 4-sulfatase (human CSL4S-342 cell); aryplase; rhASB; BM-102; Naglazyme. Human arylsulfatase B produced by recombinant DNA technology in Chinese hamster ovary cells. Glycoprotein comprised of 495 amino acids; mol wt ~56 kDa. Prepn: C. M. Starr, **WO 0183722** (2001 to BioMarin). Clinical evaluation in children with MPS-VI: P. Harmatz *et al., J. Pediatr.* **144**, 574 (2004). *Review:* G. Yogalingam, *Curr. Opin. Invest. Drugs* **5**, 1111-1120 (2004).

THERAP CAT: Enzyme replacement therapy for mucopolysaccharidosis-VI.

820. Arzoxifene. [182133-25-1] 2-(4-Methoxyphenyl)-3-[4-[2-(1-piperidinyl)ethoxy]phenoxy]benzo[b]thiophene; [6-hydroxy-3-[4-[2-(1-piperidinyl)ethoxy]phenoxy]2-(4-methoxyphenyl)]benzo[b]thiophene; LY-353381. $C_{28}H_{29}NO_4S$; mol wt 475.60. C 70.71%, H 6.15%, N 2.95%, O 13.46%, S 6.74%. Selective estrogen receptor modulator (SERM). Prepn: A. D. Palkowitz, K. J. Thrasher, **EP 729956**; *idem*, **US 5981765** (1996, 1999 both to Eli Lilly). Pharmacology: M. Sato *et al., Endocrinology* **139**, 4642 (1998); N. Suh *et al., Cancer Res.* **61**, 8412 (2001). Clinical pharmacokinetics: P. N. Münster *et al., J. Clin. Oncol.* **19**, 2002 (2001). Review of clinical evaluations and therapeutic potential: S. Chan, *Semin. Oncol.* **29**, Suppl. 1, 129-133 (2002).

Solid from hexane, mp 174-176°.
Hydrochloride. [182133-27-3] $C_{28}H_{29}NO_4S.HCl$; mol wt 512.06. Crystals from ethanol/ethyl acetate, mp 156-160°.

THERAP CAT: Antineoplastic (hormonal).

821. Asafetida. [9000-04-8] Devil's dung; food of the gods; asafoetida; asant. Gum-resin obtained as an exudation of the decapitated rhizome and roots of *Ferula assafoetida* L., *F. foetida* Regel and some other species of *Ferula, Umbelliferae.* *Habit.* Iran, Turkestan, Afghanistan. *Constit.* 6-17% ethereal oil; 40-60% resin, consisting of ester of asaresinotannol and ferulic acid; pinene, vanillin, about 25% gum. Three sulfur-containing compounds isolated from asafetida resin are: *1-methylpropyl 1-propenyl disulfide, 1-(methylthio)propyl 1-propenyl disulfide* and *1-methylpropyl 3-(methylthio)-2-propenyl disulfide;* the latter two have pesticidal properties. Studies of various constituents: Bézanger-Beauquesne, Chosson, *Ann. Pharm. Fr.* **16**, 665 (1958); Caglioti *et al., Helv. Chim. Acta* **41**, 2278 (1958); **42**, 2557 (1959). Isoln and structure elucidation of three sulfur-containing components: H. Naimie *et al., Collect. Czech. Chem. Commun.* **37**, 1166 (1972). Synthesis and configuration of sulfur-containing constituents: J. Meijer, P. Vermeer, *Rec. Trav. Chim.* **93**, 242 (1974); A. Kjaer *et al., Acta Chem. Scand. B* **30**, 137 (1976). *Review:* Howes, *Econ.*

Bot. **4**, 313 (1950); Subrahmanyam *et al., J. Sci. Ind. Res.* **13A**, 382-386 (1954).

Soft mass or irregular lumps or "tears"; garlic-like odor; bitter acrid taste. When triturated with water, it makes a milky emulsion.

USE: In India, Iran, etc., as condiment and flavoring for foods; an ingredient in Worcestershire sauce. A 2% suspension as repellent against dogs, cats, rabbits, deer.

THERAP CAT: Carminative; expectorant.

THERAP CAT (VET): Has been used as a carminative, and externally to prevent bandage chewing by dogs.

822. Asaprol. [516-18-7] 2-Hydroxy-1-naphthalenesulfonic acid calcium salt; calcium 2-hydroxy-1-naphthalenesulfonate; calcium β-naphthol-α-monosulfonate; calcium 1-naphthol-1-sulfonate; 2-naphthol-1-sulfonic acid calcium salt; Abrastol; Calcinaphthol. $C_{20}H_{14}CaO_8S_2$; mol wt 486.53. C 49.37%, H 2.90%, Ca 8.24%, O 26.31%, S 13.18%. Prepn: *Hagers Handb. Pharm. Praxis* **Band 2**, 204 (Berlin, 1930).

Trihydrate. Reddish-white, odorless powder. Dec at about 50°. One gram dissolves in 1.5 ml water, 3 ml alc.

USE: Has been used instead of gypsum to plaster wines.

823. Asarinin. [133-04-0] [1R-(1α,3aα,4β,6aα)]-5,5'-(Tetrahydro-1H,3H-furo[3,4-c]furan-1,4-diyl)bis-1,3-benzodioxole; *l*-asarinin; (−)-episesamin; xanthoxylin S. $C_{20}H_{18}O_6$; mol wt 354.35. C 67.79%, H 5.12%, O 27.09%. Naturally occurring *l*-form isolated from *Xanthoxylum clava-herculis* L. (*X. carolinianum* Lam.), *Rutaceae; Asarum sieboldi* Miguel var. *seulensis* Nakai, *A. blumei* Duch., *Aristolochiaceae:* Colton, *Am. J. Pharm.* **52**, 191 (1880); Eberhardt, *ibid.* **62**, 231 (1890); Gordin, *J. Am. Chem. Soc.* **28**, 1649 (1906); H. Dieterle *et al., Arch. Pharm.* **269**, 384 (1931); Huang-Minlon, *Ber.* **70**, 951 (1937); T. Kaku *et al., Keijo J. Med.* **9**, 1 (1934); *C.A.* **32**, 9090¹ (1938). Structure: H. Dieterle, K. Schwenger, *Arch. Pharm.* **277**, 33 (1939). Synthesis of *dl*-form: M. Beroza, M. S. Schechter, *J. Am. Chem. Soc.* **78**, 1242 (1956); K. Freudenberg, E. Fischer, *Ber.* **89**, 1230 (1956); D. R. Stevens, D. A. Whiting, *Tetrahedron Lett.* **27**, 4629 (1986). Diastereoisomeric with sesamin, *q.v.* Stereochemistry of the *d*-form: K. Freudenberg, G. S. Sidhu, *ibid.* **94**, 851 (1961). Antitubercular activity: Ramaswamy, *Naturwissenschaften* **44**, 380 (1957).

Crystals from alc, mp 121°. $[\alpha]_D^{20}$ −118.6°; $[\alpha]_D^{23}$ −122° (chloroform). Practically insol in water. Freely sol in boiling methanol, alcohol, chloroform, acetone, benzene.

d-**Form.** Episesamin; (+)-episesamin. Crystals from ethanol, mp 121.5°. $[\alpha]_D^{25}$ +124° (chloroform).

dl-**Form.** Crystals, mp 134-135°.

824. Asarones. 1,2,4-Trimethoxy-5-(1-propenyl)benzene; 2,4,5-trimethoxy-1-propenylbenzene; asarin; asarum camphor; asarabacca camphor. $C_{12}H_{16}O_3$; mol wt 208.25. C 69.21%, H 7.74%, O 23.05%. From root of *Asarum europaeum* L., *Aristolochiaceae* by distillation with water. Also found in the ethereal oils of *A. europaeum* and *A. arifolium* L., *Aristolochiaceae* and in *Acorus calamus* L., *Araceae*. Occurs in nature as a mixture of two isomeric forms, **α-asarone** being the *(E)*- or trans-isomer, **β-asarone**, the *(Z)*-

or *cis*-isomer. The unqualified term asarone is often used synonymously with α-asarone. Isoln: Gattermann, Eggers, *Ber.* **32**, 289 (1899). Early syntheses: Seshadri, Thiruvengadam, *Proc. Indian Acad. Sci.* **32A**, 110 (1950); Sharma, Dandiya, *Indian J. Appl. Chem.* **32**, 236 (1969). Stereochemistry of isomers: Baxter *et al., Can. J. Chem.* **40**, 154 (1962). Insect chemosterilant activity of β-asarone: B. P. Saxena *et al., Nature* **270**, 512 (1977); *see also* G. Motolesy *et al., Z. Naturforsch.* **35B**, 1449 (1980). Stereospecific synthesis of β-asarone: M. T. S. Hsia *et al.*, 177th Am. Chem. Soc. Meet. (Honolulu, April 1979), *Abstracts of Papers*, PEST 98. Synthetic and HPLC study of α- and β-asarone: L. Gracza, *Arch. Pharm.* **314**, 972 (1981).

α-Asarone   β-Asarone

α-Asarone. Needles from light petroleum, mp 62-63°. bp 296°. n_D^{11} 1.5719. Practically insol in water; sol in alcohol, ether, glacial acetic acid, carbon tetrachloride, chloroform, petr ether.

825. Asarum. Wild ginger; Canada snakeroot. Rhizomatous perennial herb, *Asarum canadense* L., *Aristolochiaceae*. Medicinal parts include the rhizomes and roots; used in Native American medicine for gastrointestinal discomfort, respiratory ailments and fever. *Habit.* North America, esp. Eastern U.S. and Canada. *Constit.* Flavonoids incl. kaempferol and quercetin glycosides; chalcononaringenin glycosides; volatile oil; aristolochic acid. Identification of flavonal and chalcone glycosides: T. Iwashina, J. Kitajima, *Phytochemistry* **55**, 971 (2000). Determn of aristolochic acids and safety of extracts: B. T. Schaneberg *et al., Pharmazie* **57**, 10 (2002).

Volatile oil. [8016-69-1] *Constit.* Terpene (pinene), methyleugenol, borneol, linalool, geraniol. Yellowish-brown liq; aromatic odor and taste. d_{15}^{15} 0.93-0.96. α_D^{20} −1.4 to −3.5°. Practically insol in water. Sol in 2 vols 70% alc. *Keep well closed, cool and protected from light.*

USE: In perfumes; flavoring in foods.

826. Asbestos. Amianthus. A family of naturally occurring, flexible, fibrous mineral silicates. Divided into two groups: **serpentine** and **amphibole.** Most common form is **chrysotile** [$Mg_6(Si_4O_{10})(OH)_8$], the fibrous form of serpentine (*see also* magnesium silicates). Subdivisions of amphibole are **anthophyllite** [$(Mg,Fe)_7(Si_8O_{22})(OH)_2$] (low iron content); **amosite** [Fe_5Mg_2-$(Si_8O_{22})(OH)_2$]; **actinolite** [$Ca_2(Mg,Fe)_5(Si_8O_{22})(OH)_2$]; **tremolite** [$Ca_2Mg_5(Si_8O_{22})(OH)_2$]; **crocidolite** or **blue asbestos** [Na_2-$Fe_3^{2+}Fe_2^{3+}(Si_8O_{22})(OH)_2$]. Commercially important forms: chrysotile, anthophyllite, amosite, crocidolite. Review of occupational use and carcinogenic risk: *IARC Monographs* **14**, 1-106 (1977); of toxicology and human exposure: *Toxicological Profile for Asbestos* (PB2001-109101, 2001) 441 pp. Review of properties and industrial applications: C. R. Jolicoeur *et al.* in *Kirk-Othmer Encyclopedia of Chemical Technology* **vol. 3** (John Wiley & Sons, New York, 4th ed., 1992) pp 659-688; of electron microscopic analysis of airborne fibers: P. N. Breysse, *Crit. Rev. Anal. Chem.* **22**, 201-277 (1991). Symposium on asbestos-related disease: P. J. Landrigan, H. Kazemi, Eds., *Ann. N.Y. Acad. Sci.* **643**, 1-628 (1991).

Fire resistant fibers. Chrysotile attacked by acid; amphiboles, acid resistant.

Caution: The effects of respiratory exposure to asbestos are subacute or chronic and exhibit a latent period. Nonmalignant respiratory diseases attributable to asbestos exposure include chronic pulmonary fibrosis (asbestosis), fibrotic pleural plaques, pleuritis, and diffuse pleural thickening. Neoplastic diseases associated with occupational exposure to airborne asbestos include lung cancer and mesothelioma. *See Patty's Industrial Hygiene and Toxicology* vol. 2A, G. D. Clayton, F. E. Clayton, Eds. (Wiley-Interscience, New York, 4th ed., 1993) pp 849-864. Potential symptoms of overexposure are dyspnea, interstitial fibrosis, restricted pulmonary function and finger clubbing; eye irritation. *See NIOSH Pocket Guide to Chemical Hazards* (DHHS/NIOSH 97-140, 1997) p 22. Asbestos and all commercial forms of asbestos are listed as known human carcinogens: *Report on Carcinogens, Eleventh Edition* (PB2005-104914, 2004) p III-21.

USE: Heat-resistant insulators, cements, furnace and hot pipe coverings, inert filler medium (laboratory & commercial), fireproof gloves, clothing, brake linings. NaOH treated asbestos, *Ascarite*, has been used to absorb CO_2 in combustion analysis.

827. Ascaridole. [512-85-6] 1-Methyl-4-(1-methylethyl)-2,3-dioxabicyclo[2.2.2]oct-5-ene; 1,4-peroxido-*p*-menthene-2. $C_{10}H_{16}O_2$; mol wt 168.23. C 71.39%, H 9.59%, O 19.02%. An organic peroxide which constitutes 60-80% of oil of chenopodium. Synthesis from α-terpinene by treatment with oxygen, chlorophyll, and light: Schenck, Ziegler, *Naturwissenschaften* **1944**, 157. Purification: Beckett *et al., J. Pharm. Pharmacol.* **7**, 55 (1955). Isoln from *Chenopodium ambrosioides* L.: E. Okuyama *et al., Chem. Pharm. Bull.* **41**, 1309 (1993). Review of use as anthelmintic: M. M. Kliks, *Soc. Sci. Med.* **21**, 879-886 (1985).

Liquid; unstable; prone to explode when heated or when treated with organic acids. d_4^{20} 1.0103; d_{20}^{20} 1.0113. mp 3.3°. bp$_{0.2}$ 39-40°. Sol in hexane, pentane, ethanol, toluene, benzene, castor oil.

THERAP CAT: Has been used as anthelmintic (Nematodes).

THERAP CAT (VET): Anthelmintic.

828. Asclepias. Pleurisy root; butterfly weed. Dried root of *Asclepias tuberosa* L., *Asclepiadaceae. Habit.* Ontario to Minnesota. *Constit.* Asclepiadin, resins, volatile oil.

829. Asclepias syriaca. Milkweed; silkweed; wild cotton. Root of *Asclepias syriaca* L. (*A. cornuti* Decaisne), *Asclepiadaceae. Habit.* Canada to North Carolina and Kansas. *Constit.* Asclepiadin, asclepion—a bitter principle; tannin, volatile oil.

830. Ascorbic Acid. [50-81-7] L-Ascorbic acid; vitamin C; 3-oxo-L-gulofuranolactone; L-*threo*-hex-2-enonic acid γ-lactone; L-3-keto-*threo*-hexuronic acid lactone; L-*xylo*-ascorbic acid; antiscorbutic vitamin; cevitamic acid; Ascorbicap; Ascorbin; Ascorvit; Cantan; Cebion; Cecon; Celaskon; Celin; Cetebe; Cevalin; Ce-Vi-Sol; Cevitan; Cewin; C-Vimin; Hicee; Hybrin; Laroscorbine; Redoxon; Ribena; Vitacimin; Vitacin; Vitascorbol. $C_6H_8O_6$; mol wt 176.12. C 40.92%, H 4.58%, O 54.51%. Physiological antioxidant. Coenzyme for a number of hydroxylation reactions; required for collagen synthesis. Widely distributed in plants and animals. Most primates (including humans), guinea pigs, and some birds and fish cannot synthesize ascorbic acid. Inadequate intake results in deficiency syndromes such as scurvy. Dietary sources include citrus fruits, potatoes, peppers, broccoli, cabbage, and rose hips. First isolated from the adrenal cortex of ox and later from lemons and paprika (originally called hexuronic acid): A. Szent-Györgyi, *Biochem. J.* **22**, 1387 (1928); W. N. Haworth, A. Szent-Györgyi, *Nature* **131**, 24 (1933). Structure studies: R. W. Herbert *et al., J. Chem. Soc.* **1933**, 1270. Synthesis: R. G. Ault *et al., ibid.* 1419; T. Reichstein *et al., Helv. Chim. Acta* **16**, 561, 1019 (1933); **17**, 311, 510 (1934). Review of discovery, structure and synthesis: E. L. Hirst, *Fortschr. Chem. Org. Naturst.* **2**, 132-159 (1939). Crystal structure: J. Hvoself, *Acta Chem. Scand.* **18**, 841 (1964). Review of syntheses: T. C. Crawford, S. A. Crawford, *Adv. Carbohydr. Chem.* **37**, 79-155 (1980). HPLC determn in plasma: J. Lykkesfeldt *et al., Anal. Biochem.* **229**, 329 (1995). Discussion of use in the treatment of the common cold: L. Pauling, *Proc. Natl. Acad. Sci. USA* **68**, 2678 (1971); H. Hemilä, *Scand. J. Infect. Dis.* **26**, 1 (1994). Clinical applications in immunology, lipid metabolism and

cancer: *Int. J. Vitam. Nutr. Res.* **1982**, Suppl. 23, 294 pp. Comprehensive description: I. A. Al-Meshal, M. M. A. Hassan, *Anal. Profiles Drug Subs.* **11**, 45-78 (1982). Reviews: G. M. Jaffe in *Kirk-Othmer Encyclopedia of Chemical Technology* vol. 24 (John Wiley & Sons, New York, 3rd Ed., 1984) pp 8-40; "Vitamin C" in *Vitamins*, W. Friedrich, Ed. (Walter de Gruyter, Berlin, 1988) pp 929-1001. Review of pharmacology and clinical applications: M. Levine, *N. Engl. J. Med.* **314**, 892-902 (1986); H. E. Sauberlich, *Annu. Rev. Nutr.* **14**, 371-391 (1994).

Crystals (usually plates, sometimes needles, monoclinic system). Pleasant, sharp acidic taste. mp 190-192° (some dec). d 1.65. $[\alpha]_D^{25}$ +20.5 to +21.5° (c = 1 in water); $[\alpha]_D^{23}$ +48° (c = 1 in methanol). pH = 3 (5 mg/ml); pH = 2 (50 mg/ml); pK_1 = 4.17; pK_2 = 11.57. uv max at pH 2: 245 nm (E$_{1cm}^{1\%}$ 695); at pH 6.4: 265 nm (E$_{1cm}^{1\%}$ 940). Redox potential (first stage): E$_0^1$ +0.166 V (pH 4). One gram dissolves in about 3 ml water, 30 ml alc, 50 ml abs alc, 100 ml glycerol, 20 ml propylene glycol. Soly in water: 80.0% at 100°; 40.0% at 45°. Insol in ether, chloroform, benzene, petr ether, oils, fats, fat solvents. Strong reducing agent. Stable to air when dry; aq solns are rapidly oxidized by air.

Calcium hypophosphite. Asphocalcium; Calscorbat. C_6H_9-CaO$_8$P; mol wt 280.18.

Calcium salt. [5743-27-1] Calcium ascorbate. $C_{12}H_{14}CaO_{12}$. Prepn: Ruskin, Merrill, *Science* **105**, 504 (1947). Dihydrate, triclinic crystals, $[\alpha]_D^{20}$ +95.6° (c = 2.4). Freely sol in water. Practically insol in methanol, ethanol.

Sodium salt. [134-03-2] Sodium ascorbate; Cenolate; Xitix. $C_6H_7NaO_6$; mol wt 198.11. Prepn: Holland, **US 2442005** (1948). Minute crystals, dec 218°. $[\alpha]_D^{20}$ +104.4°. Soly in water: 62 g/100 ml at 25°; 78 g/100 ml at 75°.

USE: As antimicrobial and antioxidant in foodstuffs.

THERAP CAT: Vitamin (antiscorbutic).

THERAP CAT (VET): Vitamin (antiscorbutic).

831. Ascorbigen. [8075-98-7] 2-*C*-(1*H*-Indol-3-ylmethyl)-β-L-*lyxo*-3-hexulofuranosonic acid γ-lactone mixt with 2-*C*-(1*H*-indol-3-ylmethyl)-β-L-*xylo*-3-hexulofuranosonic acid γ-lactone. $C_{15}H_{15}NO_6$; mol wt 305.28. C 59.01%, H 4.95%, N 4.59%, O 31.45%. Isoln from savoy cabbage juice: Procházka, Sanda, *Collect. Czech. Chem. Commun.* **25**, 270 (1960). Prepn from L-ascorbic acid + glucobrassicin: Gmelin, Virtanan, *Suom. Kemistil.* **34B**, 15 (1961), *C.A.* **55**, 17774f (1961); from L-ascorbic acid + gramine methiodide: Procházka, *Collect. Czech. Chem. Commun.* **28**, 544 (1963). Prepn from L-ascorbic acid + 3-hydroxymethylindole; forms two diastereoisomers: **ascorbigen A** as the main product and **ascorbigen B** as a minor product: Kiss, Neukom, *Helv. Chim. Acta* **49**, 989 (1966); Kiss, *Angew. Chem.* **78**, 1066 (1966).

Ascorbigen A   Ascorbigen B

Ascorbigen A. Amorphous powder, sinters about 65°. $[\alpha]_D^{25}$ +11.0° (c = 2 in ethanol). uv max (ethanol): 220, 273-274, 280, 290 nm.

Ascorbigen B. Yellow amorphous powder, sinters about 70°. $[\alpha]_D^{20}$ +12.5° (methanol).

832. Asenapine. [65576-45-6] (3a*R*,12b*R*)-*rel*-5-Chloro-2,3,3a,12b-tetrahydro-2-methyl-1*H*-dibenz[2,3:6,7]oxepino[4,5-*c*]pyrrole. C$_{17}$H$_{16}$ClNO; mol wt 285.77. C 71.45%, H 5.64%, Cl 12.41%, N 4.90%, O 5.60%. Combined serotonin (5HT$_2$) and dopamine (D$_2$) receptor antagonist; structurally related to mianserin, *q.v.* Prepn: BE 854915 (1977 to Akzo); W. J. van der Burg, US 4145434 (1979 to Akzona). Synthesis of labelled compd: J. Vader *et al., J. Labelled Compd. Radiopharm.* **34**, 845 (1994). Series of articles on properties, metabolism and pharmacology: *Arzneim.-Forsch.* **40**, 536-554 (1990). Receptor binding study: E. Richelson, T. Souder, *Life Sci.* **68**, 29 (2000). Clinical pharmacology: B. Andrée *et al., Psychopharmacology* **131**, 339 (1997). Review of development and therapeutic potential: J. J. Miguel-Hidalgo, *Curr. Opin. Cent. Peripher. Nerv. Syst. Invest. Drugs* **2**, 85-92 (2000).

Log P at 37° (*n*-octanol/water): 6.33.

Maleate. [85650-56-2] Org-5222. C$_{17}$H$_{16}$ClNO.C$_4$H$_4$O$_4$; mol wt 401.84. Racemic mixture. Crystals, mp 141-145°. uv max (ethanol): 270 nm (ε 1900). Soly at 21° (g/l): water 3, ethanol 30, methanol 250, acetone 125, ethyl acetate 10, dichloromethane 250, hexane <1. pH at 20° (0.1% soln in water): 4.56 ±0.05. pH at 23° (saturated soln 5.8 g/l): 4.43. pK$_1$ <3, pK$_2$ 7.52, pK$_3$ 8.51.

THERAP CAT: Antipsychotic.

833. Asiaticoside. [16830-15-2] (2α,3β,4α)-2,3,23-Trihydroxyurs-12-en-28-oic acid *O*-6-deoxy-α-L-mannopyranosyl-(1 → 4)-*O*-β-D-glucopyranosyl-(1 → 6)-*O*-β-D-glucopyranosyl ester. C$_{48}$H$_{78}$O$_{19}$; mol wt 959.12. C 60.11%, H 8.20%, O 31.69%. Active principle of *Centella asiatica* (L.) Urban, *Umbelliferae.* Trisaccharide moiety linked to the aglycone: **asiatic acid.** Isoln: J.-E. Bontems, *Bull. Sci. Pharmacol.* **49**, 186 (1941), *C.A.* **38**, 4094 (1944); *idem, Gaz. Med. Madagascar* **5**, 29 (1942). Structure of asiatic acid: J. Polonsky, *Bull. Soc. Chim. Fr.* **1953**, 173. Structure of asiaticoside: P. Boiteau *et al., Nature* **163**, 258 (1949); J. Polonsky *et al., Bull. Soc. Chim. Fr.* **1959**, 880. Metabolism: L. F. Chasseaud *et al., Arzneim.-Forsch.* **21**, 1379 (1971). Wound healing properties: H. Rosen *et al., Proc. Soc. Exp. Biol. Med.* **125**, 279 (1967). Clinical study: J.-P. Bosse *et al., Ann. Plast. Surg.* **3**, 13 (1979). Review on asiatic acid: J. L. Simonsen, W. C. J. Ross, *The Terpenes* vol. **5** (University Press, Cambridge, 1957) pp 58-67.

Minute needles from 60% methanol, mp 230-233°. Insol in water. Sol in alcohol, pyridine. [α]$_D^{20}$ −14° (alc).

834. Asoprisnil. [199396-76-4] [*C*(*E*)]-4-[(11β,17β)-17-Methoxy-17-(methoxymethyl)-3-oxoestra-4,9-dien-11-yl]benzaldehyde-1-oxime; 11β-[4-(hydroxyiminomethyl)phenyl]-17β-methoxy-17α-(methoxymethyl)estra-4,9-dien-3-one; J-867. C$_{28}$H$_{35}$NO$_4$; mol wt 449.58. C 74.80%, H 7.85%, N 3.12%, O 14.23%. Selective progesterone receptor modulator. Prepn: G. Schubert *et al.,* EP 648778; *eidem,* US 5693628 (1995, 1997 both to Jenpharm). Clinical effects on menstrual and ovarian cyclicity in premenopausal women: K. Chwalisz *et al., Hum. Reprod.* **20**, 1090 (2005). Review of pharmacology and therapeutic potential: D. DeManno *et al., Steroids* **68**, 1019-1032 (2003); of early clinical experience: K. Chwalisz *et al., Semin. Reprod. Med.* **22**, 113-119 (2004).

Crystals from isopropanol + CH$_2$Cl$_2$, mp 118° (dec). [α]$_D$ +197° (CHCl$_3$). uv max (methanol): 264, 299 nm (ε 20366, 20228).

THERAP CAT: In treatment of uterine fibroids.

835. Asoxime Chloride. [34433-31-3]; [124051-64-5] (free base). 1-[[[4-(Aminocarbonyl)pyridinio]methoxy]methyl]-2-[(hydroxyimino)methyl]pyridinium dichloride; 4'-carbamoyl-2-formyl-1,1'-(oxydimethylene)dipyridinium chloride 2-oxime; 1-(2-hydroxyiminomethyl-1-pyridinio)-3-(4-carbamoyl-1-pyridinio)-2-oxapropane dichloride; HI-6. C$_{14}$H$_{16}$Cl$_2$N$_4$O$_3$; mol wt 359.21. C 46.81%, H 4.49%, Cl 19.74%, N 15.60%, O 13.36%. Cholinesterase reactivator. Prepn: I. Hagedorn, US 3773775 (1973 to E. Merck); L. Y. Y. Hsiao, H. A. Musallam, US 5130438 (1992 to U.S.A. Secy. of Army). Chemical stability study: P. Eyer *et al., Arch. Toxicol.* **59**, 266 (1986). Dissolution studies: H. Thiermann *et al., Int. J. Pharm.* **137**, 167 (1996). HPLC determn in plasma: M. P. McCluskey *et al., J. Anal. Toxicol.* **14**, 239 (1990). Metabolism study: D. J. Ecobichon *et al., Can. J. Physiol. Pharmacol.* **68**, 614 (1990). Clinical pharmacokinetics and safety: J. G. Clement *et al., Biopharm. Drug Dispos.* **16**, 415 (1995). Clinical evaluation in insecticide poisoning: R. Kusic *et al., Hum. Exp. Toxicol.* **10**, 113 (1991). Review of pharmacology: C. G. Rousseaux, A. K. Dua, *Can. J. Physiol. Pharmacol.* **67**, 1183-1189 (1989); of physical properties and acute toxicity: J. G. Clement *et al., Arch. Toxicol.* **62**, 220-223 (1988).

Monohydrate. [82504-20-9] Crystals from water/ethanol (20:75), mp 145-147°. uv max (H$_2$O): 350, 300, 270, 218 nm (log ε 3.093, 4.018, 3.966, 4.181).

Dimethanesulfonate. [144252-71-1] C$_{14}$H$_{16}$N$_4$O$_3$.2CH$_3$O$_3$S; mol wt 478.50. Comparative studies of *in vitro* reactivation: S. Krummer *et al., Arch. Toxicol.* **76**, 589 (2002); of *in vivo* pharmacokinetics and efficacy: P. M. Lundy *et al., Toxicology* **208**, 399 (2005).

THERAP CAT: Antidote (organophosphate poisoning).

836. L-Asparaginase. [9015-68-3] L-Asparagine amidohydrolase; colaspase; L-asnase; EC 3.5.1.1; MK-965; NSC-109229; Crasnitin; Elspar; Kidrolase; Leunase. Enzyme which catalyzes the hydrolysis of L-asparagine to L-aspartic acid and ammonia. Inhibits the growth of tumor cells requiring exogenous asparagine. Widely distributed; occurs in bacteria, fungi, yeasts, plants, animal tissues and guinea pig serum. Commonly obtained from *E. coli* and *Erwinia* sp. Asparaginase from *E. coli* has a mol wt of ~136,000 and is composed of four identical subunits. Identification of antitumor activity: J. D. Broome, *Nature* **191**, 1114 (1961); *idem, J. Exp. Med.* **118**, 99 (1963). Purif, chemical properties of asparaginase from *E. coli*: D. H. Ho *et al., J. Biol. Chem.* **245**, 3708 (1970). Structural studies: A. C. Greenquist, J. C. Wriston, *Arch. Biochem. Biophys.* **152**, 280 (1972). Amino acid sequence: T. Maita *et al., J. Biochem.* **76**, 1351 (1974). Pharmacology and clinical effects: R. H. Adamson, S. Fabro, *Cancer Chemother. Rep. Part 1* **52**, 617 (1968); R. L. Capizzi *et al., Annu. Rev. Med.* **21**, 433 (1970). *Reviews*: R. L. Capizzi, *Leuk. Lymphoma* **10**, Suppl., 147-150 (1993); M. J. Keating *et al., ibid.* 153-157.

White crystalline powder. Freely sol in water where it appears to be global in shape. $[\alpha]_D^{20}$ −30 to −32°. uv max (0.03*M* sodium phosphate, pH 7.3): 278 nm (A$_{1cm}^{1\%}$ 7.1 ±0.15). Active at pH 5-9. Practically insol in methanol, acetone, chloroform.

Compd with polyethylene glycol. [130167-69-0] Pegaspargase; PEG-asparaginase; (monomethoxypolyethylene glycol succinimidyl)$_{74}$-L-asparaginase; Oncaspar. L-Asparaginase from *E. coli* covalently coupled to polyethylene glycol moieties of mol wt ~5000 Da. Prepn: F. F. Davis *et al., DE 2433883* (1976 to Research Corp.); *eidem, US 4179337* (1979). Prepn, pharmacology and antitumor efficacy: A. Abuchowski *et al., Cancer Biochem. Biophys.* **7**, 175 (1984). Toxicology: A. T. Viau *et al., Am. J. Vet. Res.* **47**, 1398 (1986). Review of clinical experience: F. Fuertges, A. Abuchowski, *J. Controlled Release* **11**, 139 (1990).

THERAP CAT: Antineoplastic (acute leukemia).

837. Asparagine. [70-47-3] L-Asparagine; Asn; N; L-β-asparagine; α-aminosuccinamic acid; aspartic acid β-amide; altheine; asparamide; agedoite; (*S*)-2,4-diamino-4-oxobutanoic acid. $C_4H_8N_2O_3$; mol wt 132.12. C 36.36%, H 6.10%, N 21.20%, O 36.33%. Non-essential amino acid for human development. First amino acid noted in natural sources; it was named for the asparagus juice from which it was isolated: L. N. Vauquelin, P. J. Robiquet, *Ann. Chim.* **57**, 88 (1806). Due to ease of conversion to aspartic acid, *q.v.*, it was not isolated from protein until 1932: M. Damodoran, *Biochem. J.* **26**, 235 (1932). Early chemistry and biochemistry: *Amino Acids and Proteins*, D. M. Greenberg, Ed. (Charles C. Thomas, Springfield, IL, 1951) 950 pp, *passim*; J. P. Greenstein, M. Winitz, *Chemistry of the Amino Acids* **vols. 1-3** (John Wiley & Sons, Inc., New York, 1961) pp. 1856-1878, *passim*. As attachment point for saccharides: A. J. Mencke *et al., Methods Enzymol.* **138**, 409 (1987). Colorimetric assay: S. Sheng *et al., Anal. Biochem.* **211**, 242 (1993). Proposed formation of acrylamide, *q.v.*, in cooking: D. S. Mottram *et al., Nature* **419**, 448 (2002); R. H. Stadler *et al., ibid.* 449. Review of metabolism: D. A. Cooney, R. E. Handschumacher, *Annu. Rev. Pharmacol.* **10**, 421-440 (1970); in plants: K. A. Sieciechowicz *et al., Phytochemistry* **27**, 663-671 (1988). Review of deamidation in proteins: R. Bischoff, H. V. J. Kolbe, *J. Chromatogr. B* **662**, 261-278 (1994).

Orthorhombic bisphenoidal crystals, mp 234-235° (bath preheated to 226°). d$_4^{15}$ 1.543. Acid to litmus. pK$_1$ 2.02; pK$_2$ 8.80. $[\alpha]_D^{20}$ −5.30° (c = 1.41); $[\alpha]_D^{20}$ +34.26° (c = 2.24 in 3.4*N* HCl); $[\alpha]_D^{20}$ −6.35° (c = 11.23 in 2.5*N* NaOH). Practically insol in methanol, ethanol, ether, benzene. Sol in acids, alkalies.

D-Form. [2058-58-4] In peptidoglycans of bacterial cell walls: D. A. Reaveley, R. E. Burge, *Adv. Microb. Physiol.* **7**, 1-81 (1972).

D-Form monohydrate. Crystals, mp 215°. $[\alpha]_D^{20}$ +5.41° (c = 1.3).

838. Asparagus. Shoot of *Asparagus officinalis* L., *Liliaceae*. *Habit.* Europe, cultivated everywhere. *Constit.* Asparagine, tyrosine, succinic acid, arginine, α-aminodimethyl-γ-butyrothetin (a methylsulfonium deriv of methionine), fat, sugar. In some humans, ingestion of asparagus is followed by excretion of a substance that produces a characteristic strong odor in the urine: M.

Nencki, *Arch. Exp. Pathol. Pharmakol.* **28**, 206 (1891); C. Gautier, *C.R. Seances Soc. Biol. Ses Fil.* **89**, 239 (1923); A. C. Allison, K. G. McWhirter, *Nature* **178**, 748 (1956). The odor-causing substance was originally thought to be methyl mercaptan, but subsequent investigation using GC-mass spectrometry has suggested that *S*-methylthioacrylate and *S*-methyl 3-(methylthio)thiopropionate are the malodorous agents, *cf* R. H. White, *Science* **189**, 810 (1975).

839. Aspartame. [22839-47-0] *N*-L-α-Aspartyl-L-phenylalanine 1-methyl ester; 3-amino-*N*-(α-carboxyphenethyl)succinamic acid *N*-methyl ester; APM; SC-18862; Equal; NutraSweet; Sanecta. $C_{14}H_{18}N_2O_5$; mol wt 294.30. C 57.14%, H 6.16%, N 9.52%, O 27.18%. Dipeptide ester about 160 times sweeter than sucrose in aqueous solution. Prepn: Davey *et al., J. Chem. Soc. C* **1966**, 555; J. M. Schlatter, ZA **6702190**; *idem, US 3492131* (1968, 1970 both to Searle); H. Pietsch, *Tetrahedron Lett.* **1976**, 4053; K. J. Vinick, S. Jung, *ibid.* **23**, 1315 (1982); utilizing immobilized enzyme technology: C. Fuganti, P. Grasselli, *ibid.* **27**, 3191 (1986). Structure-taste relationship: Mazur *et al., J. Am. Chem. Soc.* **91**, 2684 (1969). Potential as a low-calorie sweetener: Cloninger, Baldwin, *Science* **170**, 81 (1970). Metabolism: Oppermann *et al., J. Nutr.* **103**, 1454, 1460 (1973).

Colorless needles from water, mp 246-247°. $[\alpha]_D^{22}$ −2.3° (1*N* HCl).

USE: Non-nutritive sweetener.

840. Aspartic Acid. [56-84-8] L-Aspartic acid; Asp; D; aminosuccinic acid; asparagic acid; asparaginic acid; (*S*)-aminobutanedioic acid; 1-amino-1,2-carboxyethane; asparaginsäure (German). $C_4H_7NO_4$; mol wt 133.10. C 36.10%, H 5.30%, N 10.52%, O 48.08%. Non-essential amino acid for human development. First identified as the acid hydrolysis product of asparagine, *q.v.*: A. Plisson, *J. Pharm.* **13**, 477 (1827); later isolated from protein: H. Ritthausen, *J. Prakt. Chem.* **103**, 233, 239 (1868). Early chemistry and biochemistry: *Amino Acids and Proteins*, D. M. Greenberg, Ed. (Charles C. Thomas, Springfield, IL, 1951) 950 pp., *passim*; J. P. Greenstein, M. Winitz, *Chemistry of the Amino Acids* **vol 1-3** (John Wiley and Sons, Inc., New York, 1961) pp. 1856-1878, *passim*. Synthesis of optically active forms: K. Harada, K. Matsumoto, *J. Org. Chem.* **31**, 2985 (1966); of labelled form: A. Ivanof *et al., Anal. Biochem.* **110**, 267 (1981). Crystal structure: B. Dawson, *Acta Crystallogr.* **33B**, 882 (1977). Excitatory neurotransmitter: H. McLennan, H. V. Wheal, *Can. J. Physiol. Pharmacol.* **54**, 70 (1976). Role in protein activity: D. W. Urry *et al., Biopolymers* **34**, 889 (1994); J. M. Denu *et al., Biochemistry* **34**, 3396 (1995). Racemization with age in dentin: N. Saleh *et al., Calcif. Tissue Int.* **53**, 103 (1993). Review of metabolism and pathology: L. D. Stegink, *J. Toxicol. Environ. Health* **2**, 215-242 (1976). Review of role as excitatory amino acid: P. J. Roberts, S. W. Davies, *Biochem. Soc. Trans.* **15**, 218-219 (1986); of use in forensics: E. R. Waite *et al., Forensic Sci. Int.* **103**, 113-124 (1999); of pathobiology of age-related racemization in proteins: S. Ritz-Timme, M. J. Collins, *Ageing Res. Rev.* **1**, 43-59 (2002).

Orthorhombic bisphenoidal leaflets or rods, mp 270-271° (sealed capillary, preheated bath). $[\alpha]_D^{20}$ +25.0° (c = 1.97 in 6*N* HCl). d$^{12.5}$ 1.661. pK$_1$ 1.88; pK$_2$ 3.65; pK$_3$ 9.60. Soly in water at 20°, 30°: 1 g/222.2 ml, 1 g/149.9 ml. Forms supersatd solns easily. More soluble in salt solns; sol in acids, alkalies. Insol in alcohol.

D-Form. [1783-96-6] D-Asp. Occurs naturally although to a lesser extent than the L-form. Formed by non-enzymatic racemization in ageing protein. Purification and characterization from bovine lens: N. Fujii *et al., Biochim. Biophys. Acta* **999**, 239

(1989); from tissue of the mollusc, *Aplysia kurodai:* M. Sato *et al., Biochem. J.* **263**, 617 (1989). Review of industrial production by microorganisms: S. Takamatsu, T. Tosa, *Bioprocess Technol.* **16**, 25-35 (1993). $[\alpha]_D^{25}$ −2.0° (c = 3.93 in 5*N* HCl).

Compound with L-arginine. [3054-35-1] Arginine L-aspartate; Sargenor. $C_{10}H_{21}N_5O_6$; mol wt 307.30.

Compound with L-ornithine *see* Ornithine.

N-**Acetyl-L-aspartic acid.** [997-55-7] NAA. $C_6H_9NO_5$; mol wt 175.14. Found in nervous system; second most abundant free amino acid in mammals. Review: D. L. Birken, W. H. Oldendorf, *Neurosci. Biobehav. Rev.* **13**, 23-31 (1989).

USE: Nutritional supplement; in forensic determn of age.

841. Aspergillic Acid. [490-02-8] 1-Hydroxy-6-(1-methylpropyl)-3-(2-methylpropyl)-2(1*H*)-pyrazinone; 6-*sec*-butyl-1-hydroxy-3-isobutyl-2(1*H*)-pyrazinone; 6-*sec*-butyl-3-isobutyl-pyrazinol 1-oxide; 2-hydroxy-3-isobutyl-6-(1-methylpropyl)-pyrazine 1-oxide; 3-isobutyl-6-*sec*-butyl-2-hydroxypyrazine 1-oxide. $C_{12}H_{20}N_2O_2$; mol wt 224.30. C 64.26%, H 8.99%, N 12.49%, O 14.27%. Antibiotic substance produced by *Aspergillus flavus:* White, Hill, *J. Bacteriol.* **45**, 433 (1943); Dunn *et al., J. Chem. Soc.* **1949**, Suppl. S126. Extraction and purification: Dutcher, *J. Biol. Chem.* **171**, 321 (1947). Structure: *idem, ibid.* **232**. 785 (1958). Biosynthesis: MacDonald, *ibid.* **236**, 512 (1961), **237**, 1977 (1962). Synthesis of racemate: Chigira *et al., Bull. Chem. Soc. Jpn.* **39**, 632 (1966); Masaki *et al., J. Org. Chem.* **31**, 4143 (1966); Ohta, Fujii, *Chem. Pharm. Bull.* **17**, 851 (1969). Industrial prepn: Omata, Ueno, **JP 65 13794** (1965 to Dainippon), *C.A.* **63**, 11589b (1965). Proposed as a hypotensive: Jones, Martin, **US 3720768** (1973 to Abbott). *Reviews:* MacDonald, "Aspergillic Acid and Related Compounds" in *Antibiotics* vol. II, D. Gottlieb, P. Shaw, Eds. (Springer-Verlag, New York, 1967) pp 43-51; Wilson, "Miscellaneous Aspergillus Toxins" in *Microbial Toxins* vol. VI, A. Ciegler *et al.*, Eds. (Academic Press, New York, 1971) pp 207-235.

Pale yellow needles having odor similar to black walnuts, mp 97-99° (methanol). pK'a 5.5. $[\alpha]_D^{18}$ +13.3° (c = 3.9 in ethanol). uv max (water pH 8): 328, 235 nm (ε 8500, 10500). Slightly sol in cold water; sol in dil acids and alkalies, alcohol, ether, acetone, benzene, chloroform, pyridine.

842. Aspergillin. The inappropriate designation of a number of different antibacterial agents produced by *Aspergilli* as "aspergillin" has resulted in confusion. The legitimate contender for this name by prior use is an allomelanin produced by mature spores of *A. niger:* Hugouneng, Florence, *Bull. Soc. Chim. Biol.* **2**, 133 (1920). This pigment is a mixture of chemically similar macromolecules of which the fundamental monomer is probably the perylene unit substituted with several oxygenated functions. *Review:* R. A. Nicolaus, *Melanins* (Hermann, Paris, 1968) pp 130-142.

Dried pigment, as shiny black blocks, does not melt but decomposes above 200°. Slightly sol in polar solvents. uv max (2% aqueous soln): 295, 450 nm.

843. Asperlicin. [93413-04-8] (7*S*)-6,7-Dihydro-7-[[(2*S*,-9*S*,9a*S*)-2,3,9,9a-tetrahydro-9-hydroxy-2-(2-methylpropyl)-3-oxo-1*H*-imidazo[1,2-*a*]indol-9-yl]methyl]quinazolino[3,2-*a*][1,4]-benzodiazepine-5,13-dione. $C_{31}H_{29}N_5O_4$; mol wt 535.59. C 69.52%, H 5.46%, N 13.08%, O 11.95%. Naturally occurring, nonpeptide cholecystokinin (CCK) antagonist. Produced by several strains of *Aspergillus alliaceus* along with minor related compounds known as asperlicin B, C, D and E. Isoln from fermentation cultures of *A. alliaceus* Thom and Church, ATCC 20655 and ATCC 20656: R. L. Monaghan *et al.*, **EP 116150**; *idem,* **US 4530790** (1984, 1985 both to Merck & Co.). Fermentation, isoln and bioactivity: M. A. Goetz *et al., J. Antibiot.* **38**, 1633 (1985); of asperlicins B, C, D and E: *idem, ibid.* **41**, 875 (1988). Structure elucidation: J. M. Liesch *et al., ibid.* **38**, 1638 (1985); of asperlicins B, C, D and E: *idem, ibid.* **41**, 878 (1988). Biosynthetic study: D. R. Houck *et al., ibid.* 882. Total synthesis of asperlicins C and E:

M. G. Bock *et al., J. Org. Chem.* **52**, 1644 (1987). Pharmacology of asperlicin: R. S. L. Chang *et al., Science* **230**, 177 (1985). Effect on pancreatic enzyme secretion *in vitro:* K. A. Zucker *et al., Surgery* **102**, 163 (1987). Effect in exptl pancreatitis in rats: J. R. Wisner, Jr., I. G. Renner, *Pancreas* **3**, 174 (1988).

White crystals, mp 211-213°. $[\alpha]_D^{26.5}$ −185.3° (c = 1.10 in methanol). uv max (methanol): 310.5 nm (ε 4075). Sol in methylene chloride, acetone and lower alcohols. Insol in water.

Asperlicin B. [93413-08-2] $C_{31}H_{29}N_5O_5$; mol wt 551.59. Colorless powder. uv max (methanol): 310 nm (ε 4000).

Asperlicin C. [93413-06-0] $C_{25}H_{18}N_4O_2$; mol wt 406.44. Off-white powder. uv max (methanol): 222, 268, 278, 310 nm (ε 56300, 15100, 14000, 4650).

Asperlicin D. [93413-07-1] $C_{25}H_{18}N_4O_2$; mol wt 406.44. Colorless powder. uv max (methanol): 222, 290, 310 nm (ε 61060, 14600, 5920).

Asperlicin E. [93413-05-9] $C_{25}H_{18}N_4O_3$; mol wt 422.44. Off-white powder. uv max (methanol): 227, 268, 324 nm (ε 38450, 8680, 3200).

844. Asperuloside. [14259-45-1] [2a*S*-(2aα,4aα,5α,7bα)]-4-[(Acetyloxy)methyl]-5-(β-D-glucopyranosyloxy)-2a,4a,5,7b-tetrahydro-1*H*-2,6-dioxacyclopent[*cd*]inden-1-one; rubichloric acid. $C_{18}H_{22}O_{11}$; mol wt 414.36. C 52.18%, H 5.35%, O 42.47%. From herb of *Asperula odorata* L., *Galium aparine* L., *Rubiaceae*. Occurs also in *Coprosma* spp. Isoln: Hérissey, *Compt. Rend.* **180**, 1695 (1925); Briggs, Nicholls, *J. Chem. Soc.* **1954**, 3940. Structure: Grimshaw, *Chem. Ind. (London)* **1961**, 403; Briggs *et al., J. Chem. Soc.* **1965**, 2595.

Needles from alcohol or acetone, mp 131-132°. $[\alpha]_D^{25}$ −198.6° (c = 1.44 in water). Absorption spectra: Briggs, Cain, *J. Chem. Soc.* **1954**, 4182. Sol in water, methanol, ethanol, acetone, ethylacetate, dioxane, pyridine, acetic acid. Practically insol in ether, benzene, chloroform, ligroin.

845. Asphalt. Asphaltum; mineral pitch; Judean pitch; bitumen. Bituminous substance resulting from petroleum by evaporation of lighter hydrocarbons and partial oxidation of the residue. Occurs in West Indies (chiefly Trinidad), Venezuela, Dead Sea, Switzerland, etc.

The "Syriac" asphalt (from the Dead Sea) forms deep black, shining, brittle masses of conchoidal fracture; faint, pitch-like odor and luster. Burns with a bright flame. d 1.00-1.18. Insol in water, alc, acids, alkalies. Sol in oil turpentine, petroleum, CS_2, chloroform, ether, acetone.

Caution: Potential symptoms of overexposure to fumes are irritation of eyes and respiratory system. Potential occupational carcinogen. *See NIOSH Pocket Guide to Chemical Hazards* (DHHS/-NIOSH 97-140, 1997) p 22.

USE: Making roads, roofs; making tanks watertight.

846. Aspidin. [584-28-1] 2-[[2,6-Dihydroxy-4-methoxy-3-methyl-5-(1-oxobutyl)phenyl]methyl]-3,5-dihydroxy-4,4-dimethyl-6-(1-oxobutyl)-2,5-cyclohexadien-1-one; 3′-[(5-butyryl-2,4-dihydroxy-3,3-dimethyl-6-oxo-1,4-cyclohexadien-1-yl)methyl]-2′,4′-dihydroxy-6′-methoxy-5′-methylbutyrophenone;polystichin.$C_{25}H_{32}O_8$; mol wt 460.52. C 65.20%, H 7.00%, O 27.79%. Active principle of fern root: Boehm, *Ann.* **302**, 171 (1898); **329**, 321 (1903); from *Dryopteris austriaca* (Jacq.) Woynar, *Polypodiaceae:* Aebi *et al., Helv. Chim. Acta* **40**, 266 (1957). Structure: *eidem, ibid.* 569. Synthesis: Riedl, Mitteldorf, *Ber.* **89**, 2595 (1956).

Crystals from ethanol, mp 124-125°. uv max (cyclohexane): 230, 290 nm (ε 25500, 21300). Soluble in ether, benzene, chloroform; less sol in petr ether; sparingly sol in methanol, ethanol, acetone.

THERAP CAT: Anthelmintic (Cestodes).

847. Aspidinol. [519-40-4] 1-(2,6-Dihydroxy-4-methoxy-3-methylphenyl)-1-butanone; 2′,6′-dihydroxy-4′-methoxy-3′-methyl-1-butyrophenone; 4-butyryl-2-methylphloroglucinol 1-methyl ether; 4-butyryl-3,5-dihydroxy-1-methoxy-2-methylbenzene. $C_{12}H_{16}O_4$; mol wt 224.25. C 64.27%, H 7.19%, O 28.54%. Occurs in extracts of male fern: Boehm, *Ann.* **318**, 247 (1901); Hausmann, *Arch. Pharm.* **237**, 559 (1899). Isoln from *Dryopteris austriaca* (Jacq.) Woynar, *Polypodiaceae:* Aebi *et al., Helv. Chim. Acta* **40**, 266 (1957). Synthesis from 2-methylphloroglucinol 1-methyl ether: Karrer, Widmer, *Helv. Chim. Acta* **3**, 392 (1920); Riedl, Mittledorf, *Ber.* **89**, 2589 (1956).

Needles or prisms from benzene. mp 156-161°. Freely sol in alc, ether, chloroform, acetone; sparingly sol in water, benzene. Less soluble in ligroin than pseudoaspidinol, mp 116.5°. Sol in NaOH solns. Practically insol in Na_2CO_3 solns.

THERAP CAT: Anthelmintic (Cestodes).

848. Aspidium. Male fern; male shield-fern; filix mas (B.P.). Rhizome and stipes of *Dryopteris filix-mas* (L.) Schott., *Polypodiaceae. Habit.* North America, Northern Asia, Europe, Northern Africa. *Constit.* Filicic and flavaspidic acids, volatile oil, asbaspidin, filicin, filmaron, filix red, resin. It yields not less than 6.5% oleoresin (U.S.P.).

Oleoresin of Aspidium. Oleoresin of male fern. An ether extract of male fern containing not less than 24% crude filicin. Dark green, thick liq, usually depositing a granular, cryst substance. Bitter, unpleasant taste. d not less than 1.0. Insoluble in water. Partly sol in alcohol or chloroform. Almost completely sol in ether; not less than 85% sol in petr ether. *Shake well before dispensing.*

THERAP CAT: Anthelmintic (Cestodes).

THERAP CAT (VET): Anthelmintic (Cestodes).

849. Aspidosperma. Quebracho. Dried bark of *Aspidosperma quebracho-blanco* Schlecht., *Apocynaceae. Habit.* Argentina. *Constit.* 0.3-1.4% alkaloids —aspidospermine, aspidospermatine, aspidosamine, quebrachine, quebrachamine, hypoquebrachine, quebrachol, quebrachit; tannin.

USE: Chlorinated quebracho can be used to control nematodes and other parasitic worms in soils: Santmyer, **US 2799612** (1957 to Monsanto).

THERAP CAT: Respiratory stimulant.

850. Aspidospermine. [466-49-9] 1-Acetyl-17-methoxyaspidospermidine. $C_{22}H_{30}N_2O_2$; mol wt 354.49. C 74.54%, H

8.53%, N 7.90%, O 9.03%. In *Aspidosperma quebracho-blanco* Schlect., *Vallesia dichotoma* Ruiz & Pav., and *Vallesia glabra* (Cav.) Link, *Apocynaceae:* G. Fraude, *Ber.* **11**, 2189 (1878); Hesse, *Ann.* **211**, 249 (1882); Ewins, *J. Chem. Soc.* **105**, 2738 (1914); Deulofeu *et al., ibid.* **1940**, 1051; Holker *et al., J. Org. Chem.* **24**, 314 (1959). Structure: Conroy *et al., Tetrahedron Lett.* no. 11, 4 (1959). Crystal structure: Mills, Nyburg, *J. Chem. Soc.* **1960**, 1458. Stereochemistry: Smith, Wrobel, *ibid.* 1463; Craven, Zacharias, *Experientia* **24**, 770 (1968). Biogenesis: Robinson, *Tetrahedron Lett.* no. 18, 1F4 (1959). Synthesis of *dl*-form: Stork, Dolfini, *J. Am. Chem. Soc.* **85**, 2872 (1963); Ban *et al., Tetrahedron Lett.* **1965**, 2261; Stevens *et al., Chem. Commun.* **1971**, 857; S. F. Martin *et al., J. Am. Chem. Soc.* **102**, 3294 (1980). Aspidospermine has been reported as having a wide variety of pharmacological properties, including diuretic and respiratory stimulant activity. Biological and phytochemical evaluation: R. L. Lyon *et al., J. Pharm. Sci.* **62**, 218 (1973). Microbial transformation: S. K. Lin *et al., ibid.* **64**, 2021 (1975). NMR study: W. E. Campbell *et al., Spectrosc. Lett.* **26**, 707 (1993). Isoln: H. F. Deutsch *et al., J. Pharm. Biomed. Anal.* **12**, 1283 (1994). Acute toxicity data: V. Plzak, J. Doull, *Further Survey of Compounds for Radiation Protection* (AD691490, USAF Radiation Lab., 1969) 82 pp.

Needles or prisms from alc, needles from petr ether. mp 208°. Sublimes 180°. bp_2 220°. $[\alpha]_D^{15}$ −100.2° (alc); $[\alpha]_D$ −93° (chloroform). uv max (methanol): 218, 255, 280-290 nm (log ε 4.52, 4.04, 3.53-3.40). One gram dissolves in 60 ml water, 50 ml alc, 100 ml ether. Also sol in benzene, chloroform, petr ether. LD_{50} i.p. in mice: 40 mg/kg (Plzak, Doull).

N-Formyl-N-deacetylaspidospermine. Vallesine. $C_{21}H_{28}N_2O_2$. Structure: Taylor *et al., Helv. Chim. Acta* **42**, 2750 (1959). Long, fine needles from acetone, mp 154-156°. $[\alpha]_D^{24}$ −91 ± 2° (c = 1.814 in abs alc). uv max: 211, 250 nm (log ε 4.47, 3.94).

851. Aspirin. [50-78-2] 2-(Acetyloxy)benzoic acid; salicylic acid acetate; 2-acetoxybenzoic acid; acetylsalicylic acid; Acylpyrin; Angettes; Asatard; Aspro; Cardioaspirin; Cardiprin; Cemirit; Claragine; Ecotrin; Empirin; Encaprin; Rhonal; Solprin. $C_9H_8O_4$; mol wt 180.16. C 60.00%, H 4.48%, O 35.52%. Prepn: C. Gerhardt, *Ann.* **87**, 149 (1853). Manuf from salicylic acid and acetic anhydride: *Faith, Keyes & Clark's Industrial Chemicals,* F. A. Lowenheim, M. K. Moran, Eds. (Wiley-Interscience, New York, 4th ed., 1975) pp 117-120. Crystallization from acetone: Hamer, Phillips, **US 2890240** (1959 to Monsanto). Novel process involving distillation: Edmunds, **US 3235583** (1966 to Norwich Pharm.). Crystal structure: P. J. Wheatley, *J. Chem. Soc. (Suppl.)* **1964**, 6036. Characterization of a second polymorphic form: P. Vishweshwar *et al., J. Am. Chem. Soc.* **127**, 16802 (2005). Toxicity data: E. R. Hart, *J. Pharmacol. Exp. Ther.* **89**, 205 (1947). Evaluation as a risk factor in Reye's syndrome: P. J. Waldman *et al., J. Am. Med. Assoc.* **247**, 3089 (1982). Review of clinical trials in prevention of myocardial infarction and stroke: P. C. Elwood, *Drugs* **28**, 1-5 (1984). Symposium on aspirin therapy: *Am. J. Med.* **74**, no. 6A, 1-109 (1983). Clinical trials in prevention of colorectal cancer: R. S. Sandler *et al., N. Engl. J. Med.* **348**, 883 (2003); J. A. Baron *et al., ibid.* 891. Comprehensive description: K. Florey, *Anal. Profiles Drug Subs.* **8**, 1-46 (1979). Monograph: M. J. H. Smith, P. K. Smith, *The Salicylates* (Interscience, New York, 1966) 313 pp. Book: *Acetylsalicylic Acid,* H. J. M. Barnett *et al.,* Eds. (Raven, New York, 1982) 278 pp.

Monoclinic tablets or needle-like crystals. d 1.40. mp 135° (rapid heating); the melt solidifies at 118°. uv max (0.1N H_2SO_4): 229 nm ($E_{1cm}^{1\%}$ 484); ($CHCl_3$): 277 nm ($E_{1cm}^{1\%}$ 68). Is odorless, but in moist air it is gradually hydrolyzed into salicylic and acetic acids and acquires the odor of acetic acid. Stable in dry air. pK (25°) 3.49. One gram dissolves in 300 ml water at 25°, in 100 ml water at 37°, in 5 ml alcohol, 17 ml chloroform, 10-15 ml ether. Less soluble in anhydr ether. Decomp by boiling water or when dissolved in solns of alkali hydroxides and carbonates. Inorganic salts of acetylsalicylic acid are soluble in water (esp the Ca salt, $q.v.$), but are decomposed quickly. LD_{50} orally in mice, rats: 1.1, 1.5 g/kg (Hart).

Guaiacol ester. [55482-89-8] Guacetisal; Guaiaspir. $C_{16}H_{14}O_5$; mol wt 286.28.

Methyl ester *see* Methyl Acetylsalicylate.

Phenyl ester *see* Phenyl Acetylsalicylate.

Caution: Potential symptoms of overexposure are increased blood clotting time; nausea, vomiting; liver, kidney injury. Direct contact may cause eye, skin and upper respiratory irritation. *See NIOSH Pocket Guide to Chemical Hazards* (DHHS/NIOSH 97-140, 1997) p 6.

THERAP CAT: Analgesic; antipyretic; anti-inflammatory; antithrombotic.

THERAP CAT (VET): Analgesic; antipyretic; anti-inflammatory; antithrombotic.

852. Aspoxicillin. [63358-49-6] (2R)-N-Methyl-D-asparaginyl-N-[(2S,5R,6R)-2-carboxy-3,3-dimethyl-7-oxo-4-thia-1-azabicyclo[3.2.0]hept-6-yl]-D-2-(4-hydroxyphenyl)glycinamide; 6-[D-2-(D-2-amino-3-N-methylcarbamoylpropionamido)-2-p-hydroxyphenylacetamido]penicillanic acid; (2S,5R,6R)-6-[(2R)-2-[(2R)-2-amino-3-(methylcarbamoyl)propionamido]-2-(p-hydroxyphenyl)acetamido]-3,3-dimethyl-7-oxo-4-thia-1-azabicyclo[3.2.0]heptane-2-carboxylic acid; N^4-methyl-D-asparaginylamoxicillin; ASPC; TA-058; Doyle. $C_{21}H_{27}N_5O_7S$; mol wt 493.53. C 51.11%, H 5.51%, N 14.19%, O 22.69%, S 6.50%. Semisynthetic penicillin. Prepn: M. Kawazu *et al.*, **DE 2638067**; *eidem*, **US 4053609** (both 1977 to Tanabe); prepn and antibacterial activity: M. Wagatsuma *et al.*, *J. Antibiot.* **36**, 147 (1985). Mechanism of action study: T. Nishino *et al.*, *Chemotherapy (Tokyo)* **33**, 132 (1985), *C.A.* **103**, 34792v (1985). Toxicological study: M. Takeshita *et al.*, *Oyo Yakuri* **30**, 687 (1985), *C.A.* **104**, 101990u (1986). HPLC determn in serum: J. Knöller *et al.*, *Zentralbl. Bakteriol. Mikrobiol. Hyg.* **265**, 176 (1987). Clinical evaluation in ocular infections: M. Ooishi *et al.*, *Acta Med. Biol.* **34**, 1 (1986). Series of articles on antibacterial activity, pharmacology and clinical efficacy: *Chemotherapy (Tokyo)* **32**, Suppl. 2, 1-791 (1984).

Colorless crystalline powder, mp 195-198° (dec). THERAP CAT: Antibacterial.

853. Astacin. [514-76-1] β,β-Carotene-3,3',4,4'-tetrone; 3,4,3',4'-tetraketo-β-carotene; 3,3'-dihydroxy-2,3,2',3'-tetradehydro-β,β-carotene-4,4'-dione; astacene. $C_{40}H_{48}O_4$; mol wt 592.81. C 81.04%, H 8.16%, O 10.80%. Red carotenoid pigment isolated from biological material originating from crustacea, algae, sponges, protozoa, fish and reptiles. Small amounts were isolated from the fat of mammals (whales, *Balaenoptera musculus*). Occurs together with astaxanthin from which it is formed by autoxidation. Appears to be an artifact rather than a natural product. Isoln from lobster shells: Kuhn, Lederer, *Ber.* **66**, 488 (1933). Structure: Karrer *et al.*, *Helv. Chim. Acta* **17**, 412, 745 (1934); **18**, 96 (1935); **19**, 479 (1936). Total synthesis: J. B. Davis, B. C. L. Weedon, *Proc. Chem. Soc. London* **1960**, 182; E. Widmer *et al.*, *Helv. Chim. Acta* **65**, 671 (1982). Prepn by autoxidation of canthaxanthin: R. D. G. Cooper *et al.*, *J. Chem. Soc. Perkin Trans. 1* **1975**, 2195.

Purple needles or leaflets with metallic luster, sometimes bent into sickle shape, esp when crystallized from pyridine + water, mp 240-243° (slow heating in evac tube, Karrer), mp 228° (Kuhn). Absorption max (pyridine): 500 nm. Practically insol in water; freely sol in chloroform, pyridine, dioxane, carbon disulfide and dil aq alkali; slightly sol in benzene, ethyl acetate, glacial acetic acid; nearly insol in ether, petr ether, methanol.

Diacetate. $C_{44}H_{52}O_6$. Black to violet needles from pyridine + water, dec 235°.

Dipalmitate (astacein). $C_{72}H_{108}O_6$. Almost square red leaflets from petr ether, mp 121°.

854. Astatine. [7440-68-8] At; at. no. 85. Radioactive halogen; Group VIIA (17). One of the rarest elements in nature. Known oxidation states: −1, 0, +5; existence of +1, +3, +7 oxidation states uncertain. No stable nuclides; radioisotopes range in mass numbers from 194 to 223. Naturally occurring isotopes produced in the natural decay series of uranium: 215, 218, 219 (longest-lived natural isotope, $T_{1/2}$ 56 sec). Most stable artificial isotopes: 209 ($T_{1/2}$ 5.41 hr); 210 ($T_{1/2}$ 8.1 hr, longest-lived isotope, rel. at. mass 209.9871); 211 ($T_{1/2}$ 7.21 hr, rel. at. mass 210.9875). Prepn and characterization of ^{211}At by cyclotron reaction ^{209}Bi (α,2n): D. R. Corson *et al.*, *Phys. Rev.* **58**, 672 (1940); of other artificial isotopes by α-particle bombardment of bismuth: E. L. Kelley, E. Segre, *Phys. Rev.* **75**, 999 (1949); Johnson *et al.*, *J. Chem. Phys.* **17**, 1, (1949); Neumann, *J. Inorg. Nucl. Chem.* **4**, 349 (1957). Prepn, purifn and nuclear decay data for ^{211}At: R. M. Lambrecht, S. Mirzadeh, *Int. J. Appl. Radiat. Isot.* **36**, 443 (1985). Inorganic chemistry: G. W. M. Visser, E. L. Diemer, *Radiochim. Acta* **33**, 145 (1983); *idem, ibid.* **47**, 97 (1989). Toxicity studies of ^{211}At: L. M. Cobb *et al.*, *Hum. Toxicol.* **7**, 529 (1988). Review: A. J. Downs, C. J. Adams, "Chlorine, Bromine, Iodine and Astatine" in *Comprehensive Inorganic Chemistry* vol. 2, J. C. Bailar, Jr. *et al.*, Eds. (Pergamon Press, Oxford, 1973) pp 1573-1594. Review of organic chemistry and potential biomedical applications: I. Brown, *Adv. Inorg. Chem.* **31**, 43-88 (1987); K. Berei, L. Vasáros in *The Chemistry of Halides, Pseudo-halides and Azides*, S. Patai, Z. Rappaport, Eds. (John Wiley & Sons, Chichester, 1995) pp 787-819.

More metallic than iodine. Soluble in organic solvents. E^0(aq) At/At⁻ 0.3 V.

855. Astaxanthin. [472-61-7] 3,3'-Dihydroxy-β,β-carotene-4,4'-dione; 3,3'-dihydroxy-4,4'-diketo-β-carotene; ovoester. $C_{40}H_{52}O_4$; mol wt 596.84. C 80.50%, H 8.78%, O 10.72%. Carotenoid pigment found mostly in animal organisms, but also occurring in plants; thought to be the precursor of astacin, *q.v.* Structure and isoln from lobster eggs: Kuhn, Sörensen, *Angew. Chem.* **51**, 465 (1938); *Ber.* **71**, 1879 (1938). Isoln from other animal organisms: Kuhn *et al.*, *Ber.* **72**, 1688 (1939). Occurrence in plants: Tischer, *Z. Physiol. Chem.* **267**, 281 (1941); in the flower petals of *Adonis annua* L., *Ranunculaceae:* Seybold, Goodwin, *Nature* **184**, 1714 (1959). Occurs also in the red feathers of birds of the *Laniarius* spp: *Z. Physiol. Chem.* **288**, 20 (1951). Stereochemistry and spectra: Grangaud, *Compt. Rend.* **242**, 1767 (1956). Abs config: Andrewes *et al.*, *Acta Chem. Scand. B* **28**, 730 (1974). *See also* T. W. Goodwin, *Carotenoids* (Chemical Publ. Co., New York, 1954) pp 167-172. Synthesis: R. D. G. Cooper *et al.*, *J. Chem. Soc. Perkin Trans. 1* **1975**, 2195; F. Kienzle, H. Mayer, *Helv. Chim. Acta* **61**, 2609 (1978); E. Widmer *et al., ibid.* **64**, 2405 (1981); H. Mayer *et al., ibid.* 2419.

Needles from acetone/light petroleum, mp 182-183°. uv max: (CS_2) 503 nm; (methanol) 472 nm; (hexane) 466-467 nm; (chloroform) 485 nm (Cooper *et al.*). Also reported as shiny purple platelets with gold luster from pyridine, mp 216° (some decompn). Readily sol in pyridine, from which it can be cryst by the addn of water (Kuhn, Sörensen).

Diacetate. $C_{44}H_{56}O_6$. Stout, blue-black needles, mp 203-205° (vac).

856. Astemizole. [68844-77-9] 1-[(4-Fluorophenyl)methyl]-*N*-[1-[2-(4-methoxyphenyl)ethyl]-4-piperidinyl]-1*H*-benzimidazol-2-amine; 1-(*p*-fluorobenzyl)-2-[[1-(*p*-methoxyphenethyl)-4-piperidyl]amino]benzimidazole; R-43512; Astemisan; Hismanal; Histamen; Histaminos; Kelp; Laridal; Metodik; Novo-Nastizol A; Paralergin; Retolen; Waruzol. $C_{28}H_{31}FN_4O$; mol wt 458.57. C 73.34%, H 6.81%, F 4.14%, N 12.22%, O 3.49%. Nonsedating-type histamine H_1-receptor antagonist. Prepn: F. Janssens *et al.*, **EP 5318**; *eidem*, **US 4219559** (1979, 1980 both to Janssen). Pharmacology: J. Van Wauwe *et al.*, *Arch. Int. Pharmacodyn. Ther.* **251**, 39 (1981); A. Wauquier, C. J. E. Niemegeers, *Eur. J. Pharmacol.* **72**, 245 (1981). *In vitro* and *in vivo* binding characteristics: P. M. Laduron *et al.*, *Mol. Pharmacol.* **21**, 294 (1982). Effect on human psychomotor performance: T. Seppala, K. Savolainen, *Curr. Ther. Res.* **31**, 638 (1982). Clinical study in treatment of hay fever: J. Callier *et al.*, *ibid.* **29**, 24 (1981). Mutagenicity study: P. Vanparys *et al.*, *Arch. Toxicol.* **50**, 167 (1982). Review of pharmacology and clinical trials: D. M. Richards *et al.*, *Drugs* **28**, 38-61 (1984). Comprehensive description: A. M. Al-Obaid, M. S. Mian, *Anal. Profiles Drug Subs.* **20**, 173-208 (1991).

Crystals from 2,2'-oxybispropane, mp 172.9°. Freely sol in organic solvents. Practically insol in water. uv max (ethanol): 219, 249, 286 nm (ε 27250.229, 6480.293, 8634.280); (0.1*N* HCl): 209, 277 nm (ε 57889.908, 18073.394).

THERAP CAT: Antihistaminic.

857. Asulam. [3337-71-1] [(4-Aminophenyl)sulfonyl]carbamic acid methyl ester; N^1-methoxycarbonylsulfanilamide; sulfanilylcarbamic acid methyl ester; methyl *p*-aminobenzenesulfonylcarbamate; M & B 9057; Asulox. $C_8H_{10}N_2O_4S$; mol wt 230.24. C 41.73%, H 4.38%, N 12.17%, O 27.80%, S 13.93%. Carbamate herbicide; folic acid biosynthesis inhibitor. Prepn: **BE 622214** (1963 to May & Baker). Description of herbicidal properties: H. J. Cottrell, B. J. Heywood, *Nature* **207**, 655 (1965). Persistence in soil: A. E. Smith, A. Walker, *Pestic. Sci.* **8**, 449 (1977). Mode of action: P. Veerasekaran *et al.*, *Pestic. Sci.* **12**, 325, 330 (1981). Field study on sugarcane and torpedograss: M. A. Hossain *et al.*, *J. Weed Sci. Tech.* **43**, 10 (1998); in bracken control: R. J. Pakeman *et al.*, *J. Environ. Management* **53**, 255 (1998). Review of properties and analytical methods: C. H. Brockelsby, D. F. Muggleton, *Anal. Methods Pestic. Plant Growth Regul.* **7**, 497 (1973); A. Guardigli *et al.*, *ibid.* **13**, 197 (1984).

White crystals, mp 143-144° (dec). Soly: water 0.5%, hydrocarbons <2%, chlorinated hydrocarbons <2%, acetone 34%, methanol 28%. pKa 4.82. LD_{50} in rats, mice, dogs, rabbits (mg/kg): >5000, >5000, >5000, >2000 orally; in rats (mg/kg): >1200 dermally (Brockelsby).

USE: Herbicide.

858. Atazanavir. [198904-31-3] (3*S*,8*S*,9*S*,12*S*)-3,12-Bis(1,1-dimethylethyl)-8-hydroxy-4,11-dioxo-9-(phenylmethyl)-6-[[4-(2-pyridinyl)phenyl]methyl]-2,5,6,10,13-pentaazatetradecanedioic acid dimethyl ester; 1-[4-(pyridin-2-yl)phenyl]-5*S*-2,5-bis[[*N*-

(methoxycarbonyl)-L-*tert*-leucinyl]amino]-4*S*-hydroxy-6-phenyl-2-azahexane; BMS-232632; CGP-73547. $C_{38}H_{52}N_6O_7$; mol wt 704.86. C 64.75%, H 7.44%, N 11.92%, O 15.89%. Azapeptide HIV protease inhibitor. Prepn: A. Fässler *et al.*, **WO 9740029**; *eidem*, **US 5849911** (1997, 1998 both to Novartis); G. Bold *et al.*, *J. Med. Chem.* **41**, 3387 (1998); of bisulfate salt: J. Singh *et al.*, **WO 9936404**; *eidem*, **US 6087383** (1999, 2000 both to Bristol-Myers Squibb); Z. Xu *et al.*, *Org. Process Res. Dev.* **6**, 323 (2002). Comparative anti-HIV activity: B. S. Robinson *et al.*, *Antimicrob. Agents Chemother.* **44**, 2093 (2000). HPLC determn in plasma: E. Cateau *et al.*, *J. Pharm. Biomed. Anal.* **39**, 791 (2005). Clinical evaluation in HIV: I. Sanne *et al.*, *J. Acquired Immune Defic. Synd.* **32**, 18 (2003). Review of pharmacology and clinical efficacy in HIV: C. Le Tiec *et al.*, *Clin. Pharmacokinet.* **44**, 1035-1050 (2005); T. S. Harrison, L. J. Scott, *Drugs* **65**, 2309-2336 (2005).

Crystals from ethanol/water, mp 207-209°. $[\alpha]_D$ −47° (c = 1 in ethanol). Insol in water (<1 μg/ml at 24°).

Sulfate. [229975-97-7] Reyataz. $C_{38}H_{52}N_6O_7 \cdot H_2SO_4$; mol wt 802.93. Crystals from ethanol + heptane, mp 195.0°, or acetone, mp 198-199° (dec). $[\alpha]_D^{22}$ −46.1° (c = 1 in 1:1 CH_3OH/H_2O, pH = 2.6). Soly in water: 4-5 mg/ml.

THERAP CAT: Antiviral.

859. Atenolol. [29122-68-7] 4-[2-Hydroxy-3-[(1-methylethyl)amino]propoxy]benzeneacetamide; 2-[*p*-[2-hydroxy-3-(isopropylamino)propoxy]phenyl]acetamide; 1-*p*-carbamoylmethylphenoxy-3-isopropylamino-2-propanol; ICI-66082; Atehexal; Ateno basan; Atenol; Cuxanorm; Myocord; Prenormine; Seles Beta; Tenoblock; Tenormin; Uniloc. $C_{14}H_{22}N_2O_3$; mol wt 266.34. C 63.13%, H 8.33%, N 10.52%, O 18.02%. Cardioselective β-adrenergic blocker. Prepn: Barrett *et al.*, **DE 2007751**; *eidem*, **US 3663607** and **US 3836671** (1970, 1972, 1974 all to I.C.I.). Pharmacology and clinical studies: Giudicelli *et al.*, *C.R. Seances Soc. Biol. Ses Fil.* **167**, 232 (1973); Hansson *et al.*, *Acta Med. Scand.* **194**, 549 (1973); Amery *et al.*, *N. Engl. J. Med.* **290**, 284 (1974). Clinical trial in treatment of alcohol withdrawal syndrome: M. L. Kraus *et al.*, *ibid.* **313**, 905 (1985). HPLC determn of enantiomers in plasma and urine: S. K. Chin *et al.*, *J. Chromatogr.* **489**, 438 (1989). Comprehensive description: V. Caplar *et al.*, *Anal. Profiles Drug Subs.* **13**, 1-25 (1984). *Review:* J. D. Fitzgerald in *Pharmacological and Biochemical Properties of Drug Substances* **vol. 2**, M. E. Goldberg, Ed. (Am. Pharm. Assoc., Washington, DC, 1979) pp 98-147; E. Marmo, *Drugs Exp. Clin. Res.* **6**, 639-663 (1980). Symposium on clinical studies: *Drugs* **25**, Suppl. 2, 1-346 (1983).

Crystals from ethyl acetate, mp 146-148°. Also reported as mp 150-152° (Caplar). Freely sol in methanol; sol in acetic acid, DMSO; sparingly sol in 96% ethanol; slightly sol in water, isopropanol; very slightly sol in acetone, dioxane. Practically insol in acetonitrile, ethylacetate, chloroform. pKa 9.6. Partition coefficient (*n*-octanol/phosphate buffer): 0.008 (pH 7.0); 0.052 (pH 8.0). Dipole moment: 5.71 ±0.20 D at 20° in propionic acid. uv max (methanol): 225, 275, 283 nm. LD$_{50}$ in mice, rats (mg/kg): 2000, 3000 orally; 98.7, 59.24 i.v. (Fitzgerald).

THERAP CAT: Antihypertensive, antianginal, antiarrhythmic (class II).

860. Athamantin. [1892-56-4] (8S-cis)-3-Methylbutanoic acid 8,9-dihydro-8-[1-methyl-1-(3-methyl-1-oxobutoxy)ethyl]-2-oxo-2H-furo[2,3-h]-1-benzopyran-9-yl ester; isovaleric acid diester with 8,9-dihydro-9-hydroxy-8-(1-hydroxy-1-methylethyl)-2H-furo[2,3-h]-1-benzopyran-2-one; 2,3-dihydro-3,4-dihydroxy-2-(1-hydroxy-1-methylethyl)-5-benzofuranacrylic acid δ-lactone diisovalerate. C$_{24}$H$_{30}$O$_7$; mol wt 430.49. C 66.96%, H 7.02%, O 26.02%. From *Peucedanum oreoselinum* (L.) Moench (*Athamanta oreoselinum* L.), *Ammi visnaga* Lam., *Umbelliferae*. Isoln: Schnedermann, Winckler, *Ann.* **51**, 315 (1844). Structure: Halpern *et al.*, *Helv. Chim. Acta* **40**, 758 (1957). Absolute configuration: Nakazaki *et al.*, *Tetrahedron Lett.* **1966**, 4735.

Fine needles from petr ether, mp 58-60°; sublimes in high vacuum at 180-200°. [α]$_D^{20}$ +88° (c = 1.145 in glacial acetic acid); [α]$_{546}^{22}$ +129° (c = 0.5575 in methanol); [α]$_{546}^{21}$ +73.9° (c = 1.024 in chloroform). [M]$_D$ +440° (methanol); +258° (chloroform). uv max (96% ethanol): 217, 322 nm (log ε 4.18, 4.17). Practically insol in water; sol in alc, ether, chloroform.

861. Atipamezole. [104054-27-5] 4-(2-Ethyl-2,3-dihydro-1H-inden-2-yl)-1H-imidazole; 4(5)-(2-ethyl-2-indanyl)imidazole. C$_{14}$H$_{16}$N$_2$; mol wt 212.29. C 79.21%, H 7.60%, N 13.20%. Specific α$_2$-adrenoceptor antagonist. Prepn: A. J. Karjalainen *et al.*, **EP 183492**; *eidem*, **US 4689339** (1986, 1987 both to Farmos). Behavioral and neurochemical effects: H. Scheinin *et al.*, *Eur. J. Pharmacol.* **151**, 35 (1988). Pharmacodynamics and pharmacokinetics: X. Fargetton, T. Vähä-Vahe, *Tijdschr. Diergeneeskd* **114**, Suppl. 1, 91S (1989). Binding study in comparison with yohimbine, *q.v.*: R. Virtanen *et al.*, *Arch. Int. Pharmacodyn.* **297**, 190 (1989). Attenuation of ethanol effects in mice: M. J. Durcan *et al.*, *Alcohol* **6**, 189 (1989). Preliminary report as detomidine, *q.v.*, antagonist in horses: L. Nilsfors, C. Kvart, *Acta Vet. Scand.* **82**, 121 (1986). Use as medetomidine, *q.v.*, antagonist in zoo animals: H. Jalanka, *ibid.* **85**, 193 (1989).

Hydrochloride. [104075-48-1] MPV-1248; Antisedan. C$_{14}$-H$_{16}$N$_2$.HCl; mol wt 248.75. Crystals from dry HCl in ethyl acetate, mp 211-215°. LD$_{50}$ in male, female rats (mg/kg): >50, 44 s.c. (Scheinin).

THERAP CAT (VET): Antidote to α$_2$-adrenoceptor induced sedation.

862. Atisine. [466-43-3] Anthorine. C$_{22}$H$_{33}$NO$_2$; mol wt 343.50. C 76.92%, H 9.68%, N 4.08%, O 9.32%. From roots of the "atis" plant, *Aconitum heterophyllum* Wall., and from *A. anthora* L., *Ranunculaceae*: Broughton, *Blue Book of East India Cinchona Cultivation* **1877**, 133; Goris, Metin, *Compt. Rend.* **180**, 968 (1925); Lawson, Topps, *J. Chem. Soc.* **1937**, 1640. Structure: Wiesner *et al.*, *Chem. Ind. (London)* **1954**, 132; Pelletier, Jacobs, *J. Am. Chem. Soc.* **76**, 4496 (1954). Structure and stereochemistry: Dvornik, Edwards, *Can. J. Chem.* **42**, 137 (1964). Partial synthesis: Pelletier, Jacobs, *J. Am. Chem. Soc.* **78**, 4144 (1956); Pelletier, Parthasarathy, *Tetrahedron Lett.* **1963**, 205. Racemic synthesis and resolution: Nagata *et al.*, *J. Am. Chem. Soc.* **85**, 2342 (1963); **89**, 1499 (1967); Masamune, *ibid.* **86**, 291 (1964); Guthrie *et al.*,

Tetrahedron Lett. **1966**, 4645. ^{13}C-NMR study of C-20 epimers: N. V. Mody, S. W. Pelletier, *Tetrahedron* **34**, 2421 (1978).

Solid, mp 57-60°. Distills in high vacuum at a bath temp of 140°. Strong base: pK 12.2.

Hydrochloride. C$_{22}$H$_{33}$NO$_2$.HCl. Flat needles from dil alc, dec 311-312°. [α]$_D^{25}$ +28°.

863. Atomoxetine. [83015-26-3] (γR)-N-Methyl-γ-(2-methylphenoxy)benzenepropanamine; (−)-N-methyl-3-(o-tolyloxy)-3-phenylpropylamine; tomoxetine. C$_{17}$H$_{21}$NO; mol wt 255.35. C 79.96%, H 8.29%, N 5.49%, O 6.27%. Norepinephrine reuptake inhibitor. Prepn (stereochem unspec): B. B. Molloy, K. K. Schmiegel, **DE 2500110**; *eidem*, **US 4314081** (1975, 1982 both to Lilly). Prepn of (R)-form: B. J. Foster, E. R. Lavagnino, **EP 52492** (1982 to Lilly); Y. Gao, K. B. Sharpless, *J. Org. Chem.* **53**, 4081 (1988). Clinical pharmacokinetics: N. A. Farid *et al.*, *J. Clin. Pharmacol.* **25**, 296 (1985). Binding study: D. R. Gehlert *et al.*, *J. Neurochem.* **64**, 2792 (1995). Biotransformation by human liver microsomes: B. J. Ring *et al.*, *Drug Metab. Dispos.* **30**, 319 (2002). Evaluation of abuse potential: S. H. Heil *et al.*, *Drug Alcohol Depend.* **67**, 149 (2002). Clinical trial in pediatric ADHD: C. J. Kratochvil *et al.*, *J. Am. Acad. Child Adolesc. Psychiatry* **41**, 776 (2002); and comorbid tic disorders: A. J. Allen *et al.*, *Neurology* **65**, 1941 (2005). Review of clinical pharmacokinetics: J.-M. Sauer *et al.*, *Clin. Pharmacokinet.* **44**, 571-590 (2005).

Hydrochloride. [82248-59-7] LY 139603; Strattera. C$_{17}$H$_{21}$-NO.HCl; mol wt 291.82. Crystals, mp 166-168° (Foster, Lavagnino). [α]$_D^{25}$ −38.01°; [α]$_{365}^{25}$ −177.26° (c = 1 in methanol). Also reported as white solid from acetonitrile, mp 162-164° (Gao, Sharpless). [α]$_D^{23}$ −41.37° (c = 1.02 in methanol); [α]$_D^{25}$ −40.3° (c = 0.94 in ethanol). Soly in water: 27.8 mg/ml. pKa 10.13.

THERAP CAT: In treatment of attention deficit hyperactivity disorder (ADHD).

864. Atorvastatin. [134523-00-5] (βR,δR)-2-(4-Fluorophenyl)-β,δ-dihydroxy-5-(1-methylethyl)-3-phenyl-4-[(phenylamino)carbonyl]-1H-pyrrole-1-heptanoic acid. C$_{33}$H$_{35}$FN$_2$O$_5$; mol wt 558.64. C 70.95%, H 6.31%, F 3.40%, N 5.01%, O 14.32%. HMG-CoA reductase inhibitor. Prepn: B. D. Roth, **EP 409281**; *idem*, **US 5273995** (1991, 1993 both to Warner-Lambert); K. L. Baumann *et al.*, *Tetrahedron Lett.* **33**, 2283 (1992). Solubility and kinetic studies: A. S. Kearney *et al.*, *Pharm. Res.* **10**, 1461 (1993). LC/MS/MS determn in serum: M. Jemal *et al.*, *Rapid Commun. Mass Spectrom.* **13**, 1003 (1999). Clinical pharmacokinetics: D. D. Cilla, Jr. *et al.*, *Clin. Pharmacol. Ther.* **60**, 687 (1996). Review of pharmacology and clinical experience: H. S. Yee, N. T. Fong, *Ann. Pharmacother.* **32**, 1030-1043 (1998); of efficacy in diabetic patients: K. F. Croom, G. L. Plosker, *Drugs* **65**, 137-152 (2005).

Calcium salt trihydrate. [344423-98-9]; [134523-03-8] (anhydrous). CI-981; Lipitor; Sortis; Torvast; Totalip. $C_{66}H_{68}CaF_2N_4$-$O_{10}.3H_2O$; mol wt 1209.39. White to off-white crystalline powder. $[\alpha]_D$ $-7.4°$ (c = 1 in DMSO). Freely sol in methanol; slightly sol in ethanol; very slightly sol in acetonitrile, distilled water, phosphate buffer (pH 7.4). Insol in aq solns of pH 4 and below.

Sodium salt. [134523-01-6] $C_{33}H_{34}FN_2NaO_5$. pKa 4.46. Soly in water (30°): 20.4 μg/ml (pH 2.1); 1.23 mg/ml (pH 6.0).

Lactone. [125995-03-1] 5-(4-Fluorophenyl)-2-(1-methylethyl)-N,4-diphenyl-1-[2-[(2R,4R)-tetrahydro-4-hydroxy-6-oxo-2H-pyran-2-yl]ethyl]-1H-pyrrole-3-carboxamide. $C_{33}H_{33}FN_2O_4$; mol wt 540.62. mp 159.2-160.7°. $[\alpha]_D$ +26.05° (c = 1 in chloroform).

THERAP CAT: Antilipemic.

865. Atosiban. [90779-69-4] 1-(3-Mercaptopropanoic acid)-2-(O-ethyl-D-tyrosine)-4-L-threonine-8-L-ornithineoxytocin; 1-(3-mercaptopropionic acid)-2-[3-(p-ethoxyphenyl)-D-alanine]-4-L-threonine-8-L-ornithineoxytocin; 1-deamino-2-D-tyr-(OEt)-4-thr-8-orn-oxytocin; antocin; dTVT; ORF-22164; F-314; RWJ-22164; CAP-440; Tractocile. $C_{43}H_{67}N_{11}O_{12}S_2$; mol wt 994.19. C 51.95%, H 6.79%, N 15.50%, O 19.31%, S 6.45%. Oxytocin antagonist. Prepn: P. O. R. Melin, J. A. Trojnar, **EP 112809**; *eidem*, **US 4504469** (1984, 1985 both to Ferring). Mechanism of action: A. Lopez Bernal *et al.*, *Br. J. Obstet. Gynaecol.* **96**, 1108 (1989). Effect on *in vitro* contractility of myometrium: V. A. Kinsler *et al.*, *ibid.* **103**, 373 (1996). Clinical pharmacokinetics: T. M. Goodwin *et al.*, *Am. J. Obstet. Gynecol.* **173**, 913 (1995). Clinical trial: T. M. Goodwin *et al.*, *ibid.* **170**, 474 (1994).

THERAP CAT: Tocolytic.

866. Atovaquone. [95233-18-4] 2-[trans-4-(4-Chlorophenyl)cyclohexyl]-3-hydroxy-1,4-naphthalenedione; trans-2-[4-(4-chlorophenyl)cyclohexyl]-3-hydroxy-1,4-naphthoquinone; 566C80; BW-566C; BW-566C-80; Mepron; Wellvone. $C_{22}H_{19}$-ClO_3; mol wt 366.84. C 72.03%, H 5.22%, Cl 9.66%, O 13.08%. Hydroxynaphthoquinone derivative that inhibits mitochondrial electron transport. Prepn: A. T. Hudson, A. W. Randall, **EP 123238**; *eidem*, **US 5053432** (1984, 1991 both to Burroughs Wellcome). Antiprotozoal activity, metabolism, and pharmacokinetics: A. T. Hudson *et al.*, *Drugs Exp. Clin. Res.* **17**, 427 (1991). Mechanism of action study: M. Fry, M. Pudney, *Biochem. Pharmacol.* **43**, 1545 (1992). Clinical trial for prevention of pneumocystis pneumonia in AIDS patients: W. M. El-Sadr *et al.*, *N. Engl. J. Med.* **339**, 1889 (1998).

Crystals from acetonitrile, mp 216-219°. Practically insol in water.

THERAP CAT: Antipneumocystic.

867. Atractyloside. [17754-44-8] (2β,4α,15α)-15-Hydroxy-2-[[2-O-(3-methyl-1-oxobutyl)-3,4-di-O-sulfo-β-D-glucopyranosyl]oxy]-19-norkaur-16-en-18-oic acid dipotassium salt; potassium atractylate; atractylin (C_{30} glucoside). $C_{30}H_{44}K_2O_{16}S_2$; mol wt 802.99. C 44.87%, H 5.52%, K 9.74%, O 31.88%, S 7.99%.

Toxic principle isolated from the thistle *Atractylis gummifera* L., *Compositae:* M. Lefranc, *Compt. Rend.* **67**, 954 (1868). Structure and stereochemistry of the aglycone, *atractyligenin:* F. Piozzi *et al.*, *Tetrahedron* Suppl. 8 **II**, 515 (1966); total synthesis of (±)-form: A. K. Singh *et al.*, *J. Am. Chem. Soc.* **109**, 6187 (1987). Structure and stereochemistry of atractyloside: *eidem*, *Gazz. Chim. Ital.* **97**, 935 (1967). Toxicity studies: G. Cascio *et al.*, *Boll. Soc. Ital. Biol. Sper.* **44**, 253 (1968). *Review: Atractyloside: Chemistry, Biochemistry, and Toxicology*, R. Santi, S. Luciani, Eds. (Piccin Medical Books, Padova, Italy, 1978) 136 pp.

Crystals, dec 174°. $[\alpha]_D^{20}$ $-53°$ (water). *Highly toxic!* Has strychnine-like action; produces convulsion of a hypoglycemic nature: R. Santi, G. Cascio, *C.A.* **50**, 7320i (1956); R. Santi, *C.A.* **52**, 15733c (1958). LD_{50} i.m. in rats: 431 mg/kg (Cascio).

868. Atracurium Besylate. [64228-81-5] 2,2′-[1,5-Pentanediylbis[oxy(3-oxo-3,1-propanediyl)]]bis[1-[(3,4-dimethoxyphenyl)methyl]-1,2,3,4-tetrahydro-6,7-dimethoxy-2-methylisoquinolinium] dibenzenesulfonate; 2-(2-carboxyethyl)-1,2,3,4-tetrahydro-6,7-dimethoxy-2-methyl-1-veratrylisoquinolinium benzenesulfonate pentamethylene ester; N,N′-dimethyl-N,N′-(4,10-dioxa-3,11-dioxotridecylene)-1,13-bis-tetrahydropapaverinium dibesylate; BW-33A; Wellcome 33-A-74; Tracrium. $C_{65}H_{82}N_2O_{18}S_2$; mol wt 1243.48. C 62.78%, H 6.65%, N 2.25%, O 23.16%, S 5.16%. Benzylisoquinolinium, competitive neuromuscular blocker. Prepn: J. B. Stenlake *et al.*, **DE 2655883**; *eidem*, **US 4179507** (1977, 1979 both to Burroughs Wellcome). Pharmacology: R. Hughes, D. J. Chapple, *Br. J. Anaesth.* **53**, 31 (1981). Clinical pharmacology: S. J. Basta *et al.*, *Anesth. Analg.* **61**, 723 (1982). Neuromuscular effects in man: R. L. Katz *et al.*, *ibid.* 730. Metabolic studies: E. A. Neill, D. J. Chapple, *Xenobiotica* **12**, 203 (1982). Pharmacokinetics: S. Ward *et al.*, *Br. J. Anaesth.* **55**, 113 (1983). Use during halothane anesthesia in humans: J. A. Stirt *et al.*, *Anesth. Analg.* **62**, 207 (1983). Symposium on pharmacology, metabolism, and clinical studies: *Br. J. Anaesth.* **55**, Suppl. 1, 1S-139S (1983); on pharmacokinetics and clinical experience: *ibid.* **58**, Suppl. 1, 1S-113S (1986).

Off-white powder, mp 85-90°. Softens at 60°.

Cisatracurium besylate. [96946-42-8] (1R,1′R,2R,2′R)-2,2′-[1,5-Pentanediylbis[oxy(3-oxo-3,1-propanediyl)]]bis[1-[(3,4-dimethoxyphenyl)methyl]-1,2,3,4-tetrahydro-6,7-dimethoxy-2-methylisoquinolinium] dibenzenesulfonate; 51W89; Nimbex. Prepn: D. A. Hill, G. L. Turner, **WO 9200965** (1992 to Wellcome Found.). Clinical pharmacology: C. A. Lien *et al.*, *Anesthesiology* **82**, 1131 (1995); M. R. Belmont *et al.*, *ibid.* 1139. White solid.

THERAP CAT: Neuromuscular blocking agent.

THERAP CAT (VET): Neuromuscular blocking agent.

869. Atranorin. [479-20-9] 3-Formyl-2,4-dihydroxy-6-methylbenzoic acid 3-hydroxy-4-(methoxycarbonyl)-2,5-dimethylphenyl ester; atranoric acid. $C_{19}H_{18}O_8$; mol wt 374.34. C 60.96%, H 4.85%, O 34.19%. From a number of lichens. Belongs to the group of lichen acids. Isoln: Paterno, Ogliarori, *Gazz. Chim. Ital.*

1877, 189; Hesse, *Ber.* **30,** 357, 1983 (1897); St. Pfau, *Helv. Chim. Acta* **9,** 650 (1926). Synthesis: Neelakantan *et al., Tetrahedron Lett.* **1962,** 287. TLC analysis: R. Klee, L. Steubing, *J. Chromatogr.* **129,** 478 (1976); J. L. Ramaut *et al., ibid.* **155,** 450 (1978).

Bitter crystals or cryst powder from chloroform, mp 195°. Practically insol in water; slightly sol in alc; sol in boiling benzene or in chloroform; also sol in alkalies giving a yellow soln.

870. Atrasentan. [173937-91-2] (2*R*,3*R*,4*S*)-4-(1,3-Benzodioxol-5-yl)-1-[2-(dibutylamino)-2-oxoethyl]-2-(4-methoxyphenyl)-3-pyrrolidinecarboxylic acid; *trans,trans*-2-(4-methoxyphenyl)-4-(1,3-benzodioxol-5-yl)-1-[[(dibutylamino)carbonyl]-methyl]pyrrolidine-3-carboxylic acid; (+)-A-127722. $C_{29}H_{38}N_2O_6$; mol wt 510.62. C 68.21%, H 7.50%, N 5.49%, O 18.80%. Endothelin (ET) antagonist with selectivity for the ET_A subtype. Prepn: M. Winn *et al.,* **WO 9606905;** *eidem,* **US 5767144** (1996, 1998 both to Abbott); *eidem, J. Med. Chem.* **39,** 1039 (1996). Synthesis: S. J. Wittenberger, M. A. McLaughlin, *Tetrahedron Lett.* **40,** 7175 (1999). HPLC determn in pharmaceutical formulations: J. A. Morley *et al., J. Pharm. Biomed. Anal.* **19,** 777 (1999); in plasma: P. D. Bryan *et al., Biomed. Chromatogr.* **15,** 525 (2001). *In vitro* inhibition of ovarian carcinoma: D. Salani *et al., Clin. Sci.* **103,** Suppl. 48, 318S (2002). Clinical pharmacokinetics and dynamics: M. C. Verhaar *et al., Br. J. Clin. Pharmacol.* **49,** 562 (2000); and safety: M. A. Carducci *et al., J. Clin. Oncol.* **20,** 2171 (2002). Clinical evaluation in prostate cancer: M. Fisher, *Clin. Prostate Cancer* **1,** 79 (2002). Review of clinical development in prostate cancer: A. Jimeno, M. Carducci, *Expert Opin. Invest. Drugs* **13,** 1631-1640 (2004).

mp 122-124°.

Hydrochloride. [195733-43-8] ABT-627; A-147627.1; Xinlay. $C_{29}H_{38}N_2O_6 \cdot HCl$; mol wt 547.08. Crystalline, non-hygroscopic solid. Readily sol in water.

THERAP CAT: Antineoplastic.

871. Atrazine. [1912-24-9] 6-Chloro-*N*-ethyl-*N'*-(1-methylethyl)-1,3,5-triazine-2,4-diamine; 2-chloro-4-ethylamino-6-isopropylamine-*s*-triazine; G-30027; AAtrex; Atranex; Gesaprim. $C_8H_{14}ClN_5$; mol wt 215.68. C 44.55%, H 6.54%, Cl 16.44%, N 32.47%. Prepn: Gysin, Knüsli, **CH 342784, CH 342785** (both 1960 to Geigy), *C.A.* **55,** 5552d (1961); Mel'nikov *et al., Khim. Prom.* **1961,** 703, *C.A.* **58,** 526c (1963); Andriska *et al.,* **HU 149189** (1962 to Nehézvegyipari Kutato Intézet), *C.A.* **58,** 13972c (1963); Mildner, **FR 1317812** (1963 to Radonja Kemijska Ind.), *C.A.* **59,** 8765h (1963). Toxicity study: S. Dalgaard-Mikkelsen, E. Poulsen, *Pharmacol. Rev.* **14,** 225 (1962). Review of toxicology and human exposure: *Toxicological Profile for Atrazine* (PB2004-100001, 2003) 262 pp.

Crystals, mp 171-174°. Soly at 25° in water 70 ppm; ether 12,000 ppm; chloroform 52,000 ppm; methanol 18,000 ppm. Stable in slightly acidic or basic media; hydrolyzed to inactive hydroxy deriv by alkali or mineral acids. LD_{50} orally in mice: 1750 mg/kg (Dalgaard-Mikkelsen, Poulsen).

Caution: Potential symptoms of overexposure are irritation of eyes and skin; dermatitis, skin sensitization; dyspnea, weakness, incoordination, salivation; hypothermia; liver injury. *See NIOSH Pocket Guide to Chemical Hazards* (DHHS/NIOSH 97-140, 1997) p 22.

USE: Selective herbicide.

872. Atrial Natriuretic Peptide. [85637-73-6] Atriopeptin; ANF; ANP; atrial natriuretic factor; cardionatrin. Peptide hormone involved in the regulation of salt and fluid balance and blood pressure homeostasis. Endogenous antagonist of the renin angiotensin aldosterone system; physiological effects include vasodilation, natriuresis and diuresis. Produced primarily by the cardiac atrium; also identified in the lung, brain and kidney. Synthesized as a species dependent, 149-153 residue precursor (preproANP) which is cleaved to produce a 126 residue prohormone that is stored in myocyte granules. The major circulating form, known as α-ANP, is a 28 amino acid peptide derived from the carboxy terminus of the prohormone. The amino acid sequence is highly conserved across species. Several bioactive forms of varying length have been identified. Removal of ANP from circulation is effected by clearance receptors and by *neutral endopeptidase*, also known as *atriopeptidase* or *enkephalinase*, that cleaves the disulfide bond required for activity. Demonstration of physiological effect: A. J. de Bold *et al., Life Sci.* **28,** 89 (1981). Purification and amino acid sequence of rat ANP peptides: T. G. Flynn *et al., Biochem. Biophys. Res. Commun.* **117,** 859 (1983); of human: K. Kangawa, H. Matsuo, *ibid.* **118,** 131 (1984). Synthesis of bioactive forms of ANP: N. G. Seidah *et al., Proc. Natl. Acad. Sci. USA* **81,** 2640 (1984); S. A. Atlas *et al., Nature* **309,** 717 (1984). Series of articles on cloning and sequence analysis: *ibid.* 719-726. Identification of storage form: K. Kangawa *et al., ibid.* **312,** 152 (1984); of major circulating form: A. Miyata *et al., Biochem. Biophys. Res. Commun.* **129,** 248 (1985); D. Schwartz *et al., Science* **229,** 397 (1985). Clinical pharmacology of synthetic peptide: A. M. Richards *et al., Lancet* **1,** 545 (1985). Identification of clearance receptors: T. Maack *et al., Science* **238,** 675 (1987). Role of endopeptidase to inactivate ANP: A. J. Kenny, S. L. Stephenson, *FEBS Lett.* **232,** 1 (1988). Determn in plasma by RIA: L. M. Burrell *et al., J. Immunoassay* **11,** 159 (1990). Review of early literature: A. J. de Bold, *Science* **230,** 767-770 (1985); of physiological effects: P. Needleman, J. E. Greenwald, *N. Engl. J. Med.* **314,** 828-834 (1986); J. D. Baxter *et al., Biotechnology* **6,** 529-546 (1988). Review of biosynthesis, release and metabolism: H. Ruskoaho, *Pharmacol. Rev.* **44,** 479-602 (1992). Review of clinical pharmacology and therapeutic potential: A. Deutsch *et al., J. Clin. Pharmacol.* **34,** 1133-1147 (1994). Role in lung physiology and pathology: T. Perreault, J. Gutkowska, *Am. J. Respir. Crit. Care Med.* **151,** 226-242 (1995).

```
1
Ser–Leu–Arg–Arg–Ser–Ser–Cys–Phe–Gly–Gly–Arg–Met–Asp–Arg
                                 \                      |
                                  \                    Ile
                                   \                    |
    28                              \                   |
Tyr–Arg–Phe–Ser–Asn–Cys–Gly–Leu–Gly–Ser–Gln–Ala–Gly
```

α-hANP

Carperitide. [89213-87-6] Human atriopeptin (1-28); human α-ANP; α-hANP; SUN-4936; Hanp. $C_{127}H_{203}N_{45}O_{39}S_3$; mol wt 3080.44. Peptide corresponding to the major circulating form of human ANP. Pharmacology: M. Yoshioka *et al., Res. Commun. Chem. Pathol. Pharmacol.* **77,** 55 (1992).

Anaritide. [95896-08-5] Human atriopeptin (4-28); human atriopeptin (102-126); human α-ANP (4-28); Wy-47663; Auriculin. $C_{112}H_{175}N_{39}O_{35}S_3$; mol wt 2724.02. Peptide corresponding to residues 4-28 of human α-ANP. Clinical effects in congestive heart failure: M. A. Fifer *et al., Am. J. Cardiol.* **65,** 211 (1990).

THERAP CAT: In treatment of acute heart failure; antihypertensive.

873. Atrolactic Acid. [515-30-0] α-Hydroxy-α-methylbenzeneacetic acid; α-methylmandelic acid; 2-phenyllactic acid; α-hydroxy-α-phenylpropionic acid; 2-hydroxy-2-phenylpropionic acid; 2-phenyl-2-hydroxypropionic acid. $C_9H_{10}O_3$; mol wt 166.17. C 65.05%, H 6.07%, O 28.88%. Prepd from acetophenone cyanohydrin: McKenzie, Clough, *J. Chem. Soc.* **101,** 393 (1912); Freudenberg *et al., Ann.* **501,** 213 (1932); Eliel, Freeman, *Org. Synth. coll. vol. IV,* 58 (1963).

DL-Form, hemihydrate. Orthorhombic crystals from water, mp 88-90° (softening at 75°). Anhydr, mp 94.5° (obtained by drying the hemihydrate at 55° and 0.5 mm Hg). pKa (25°): 3.467. Soly of the anhydr acid in one liter of water at 18° = 17.04 g, at 25° = 21.17 g, at 30° = 25.65 g. Much more sol in boiling water. Slightly sol in petr ether.

874. Atropic Acid. [492-38-6] α-Methylenebenzeneacetic acid; α-phenylacrylic acid. $C_9H_8O_2$; mol wt 148.16. C 72.96%, H 5.44%, O 21.60%. Prepn: Normant, Maitte, *Bull. Soc. Chim. Fr.* **1956,** 1439.

Tabular or acicular crystals; volatilizes in steam. mp 106-107°. bp ~267° with partial decompn. Sol in 790 parts water; sol in alc, benzene, chloroform, ether, CS_2.

Caution: Irritating to skin, mucous membranes.

875. Atropine. [51-55-8] α-(Hydroxymethyl)benzeneacetic acid (3-*endo*)-8-methyl-8-azabicyclo[3.2.1]oct-3-yl ester; 1αH,-5αH-tropan-3α-ol (±)-tropate (ester); *dl*-hyoscyamine; tropic acid ester with tropine; *dl*-tropyl tropate; tropine tropate. $C_{17}H_{23}NO_3$; mol wt 289.37. C 70.56%, H 8.01%, N 4.84%, O 16.59%. Parasympatholytic alkaloid isolated from *Atropa belladonna* L., *Datura stramonium* L., and other *Solanaceae.* Extraction procedure: Chemnitius, *J. Prakt. Chem.* **116,** 276 (1927). During extraction, partial racemization of the *l*-hyoscyamine takes place which is completed by treatment with dil alkali on heating in chloroform soln: Schneider, *Arch. Pharm.* **284,** 306 (1951). Structure and synthesis: Ladenburg, *Ann.* **217,** 75 (1883); Willstätter, *Ber.* **31,** 1537 (1898); *idem., Ann.* **326,** 23 (1903); Schwenker *et al., Ber.* **99,** 2407 (1966). Prepn of the sulfate: **DE 247455** (1912 to Hoffmann-La Roche), *Frdl.* **11,** 1022. Use as antidote to cholinesterase inhibitors: R. V. Brown, *Br. J. Pharmacol.* **15,** 170 (1960). Effect on cardiac arrhythmias: P. Schweitzer, H. Mark, *Am. Heart J.* **100,** 119, 255 (1980). Pharmacokinetics and pharmacodynamics: P. H. Hinderling *et al., J. Pharm. Sci.* **74,** 703, 711 (1985). Toxicity: R. L. Cahen, K. Tvede, *J. Pharmacol. Exp. Ther.* **105,** 166 (1952); Goldenthal, *Toxicol. Appl. Pharmacol.* **18,** 185 (1971). Review of clinical use in anesthesia: L. E. Shutt, J. B. Bowes, *Anaesthesia* **34,** 476-490 (1979). Comprehensive description: A. A. Al-Badr, F. J. Muhtadi, *Anal. Profiles Drug Subs.* **14,** 325-389 (1985). Review of clinical toxicology: J. D. Truwit, *Crit. Care Clin.* **7,** 639-657 (1991).

Long, orthorhombic prisms from acetone, mp 114-116°. Sublimes in high vacuum at 93-110°. pK 4.35; pH of 0.0015 molar soln 10.0. Absorption spectra: Dobbie, Fox, *J. Chem. Soc.* **103,** 1194 (1913); Fischer, *Arch. Exp. Pathol. Pharmakol.* **170,** 623 (1933). One gram dissolves in 455 ml water, 90 ml water at 80°, 2 ml alc, 1.2 ml alc at 60°, 27 ml glycerol, 25 ml ether, 1 ml chloroform; also sol in benzene, dil acids. LD_{50} orally in rats: 750 mg/kg (Cahen, Tvede).

Methylbromide. [2870-71-5] Methylatropine bromide; Tropin. $C_{17}H_{23}NO_3 \cdot CH_3Br$; mol wt 384.31. Crystals, mp 222-223°. Sol in 1 part water; slightly sol in alc. Almost insol in chloroform, ether.

Methylnitrate. [52-88-0] Methylatropine nitrate; Eumydrin. $C_{17}H_{23}NO_3 \cdot CH_3NO_3$; mol wt 366.41. Crystals, mp 163°. Freely sol in water or alc, very slightly in chloroform, ether.

Sulfate monohydrate. [5908-99-6]; [55-48-1] (anhydrous). Atropisol; Atropt. $(C_{17}H_{23}NO_3)_2 \cdot H_2SO_4 \cdot H_2O$; mol wt 694.83. Granules or powder, mp 190-194°. Almost inactive optically. Very bitter. pH ~5.4. One gram dissolves in 0.4 ml water; 5 ml cold, 2.5 ml boil. alc; in 2.5 ml glycerol, 420 ml chloroform, 3000 ml ether. Bitterness threshold 1:10,000. Incompatible with alkalies, tannin, salts of mercury or gold, vegetable decoctions or infusions, borax, bromides, iodides, benzoates. LD_{50} orally in rats: 622 mg/kg (Goldenthal).

N-Oxide. [4438-22-6] Atropine aminoxide; aminoxytropine tropate; genatropine. $C_{17}H_{23}NO_4$; mol wt 305.37. C 66.86%, H 7.59%, N 4.59%, O 20.96%. Prepn: Polonovski, Polonovski, *Bull. Soc. Chim. Fr.* **39,** 1147 (1926). Crystalline powder, mp 127-128°, dec 135°. Very hygroscopic. Soluble in alc, chloroform. Practically insol in ether.

Caution: Causes blurred vision, suppressed salivation, vasodilation, hyperpyrexia, excitement, agitation, and delirium. See: *Clinical Toxicology of Commercial Products,* R. E. Gosselin *et al.,* Eds. (Williams & Wilkins, Baltimore, 5th Ed., 1984) Section III, pp 47-50.

THERAP CAT: Mydriatic; antispasmodic. In preanesthetic medication.

THERAP CAT (VET): Mydriatic; antispasmodic. Antidote to organophosphorus insecticides.

876. Attacins. Immune protein P5. A major class of nonspecific antibacterial proteins induced in the hemolymph of the pupae of silk moths, particularly *Hyalophora cecropia,* as part of the immune response. (See also Cecropins.) Originally designated as immune ***protein P5,*** attacins are a heterogeneous family consisting of four basic (A,B,C,D) and two acidic (E,F) forms with similar amino acid sequences and mol wts of 20,000-23,000 daltons. Initial identification and isolation of immune response proteins: I. Faye *et al., Infect. Immun.* **12,** 1426 (1975). Purification and preliminary characterization: A. E. Pye, H. G. Boman, *ibid.* **17,** 408 (1977). Amino acid sequences and antibacterial activity: D. Hultmark *et al., EMBO J.* **2,** 571 (1983). Structural study on attacin F: Å. Engström *et al., ibid.* **3,** 2065 (1984). Mode of action: P. Engström *et al., ibid.* 3347.

877. Aucubin. [479-98-1] [1S-(1α,4aα,5α,7aα)]-1,4a,5,7a-Tetrahydro-5-hydroxy-7-(hydroxymethyl)cyclopenta[c]pyran-1-yl-β-D-glucopyranoside; rhinanthin; aucuboside. $C_{15}H_{22}O_9$; mol wt 346.33. C 52.02%, H 6.40%, O 41.58%. From leaves, roots, stalks and seeds of *Aucuba japonica* Thunb., *Cornaceae;* also occurs in 75 different plants: Paris, Chaslot, *Ann. Pharm. Fr.* **13,** 648 (1955). Isoln: Trim, Hill, *Biochem. J.* **50,** 310 (1952); Rombouts, Links, *Experientia* **12,** 78 (1956). Structure: Haegele *et al., Tetrahedron*

Lett. **1961**, 110; Birch et al., J. Chem. Soc. **1961**, 5194. Abs config: A. Bianco et al., Gazz. Chim. Ital. **106**, 725 (1976). Brief review of structural studies: J. M. Bobbitt, K.-P. Segebarth, "The Iridoid Glycosides and Similar Substances" in *Cyclopentanoid Terpene Derivatives*, W. I. Taylor, A. R. Battersby, Eds. (Marcel Dekker, New York, 1969) pp 25-31.

Crystals from ethanol + ether, mp 181°. $[\alpha]_D^{21}$ −163.1° (c = 1.6). Soluble in water, alc, methanol; practically insol in chloroform, ether, petr ether. Absorption spectrum: Trim, Hill, *loc. cit.*

878. Auranofin. [34031-32-8] (1-Thio-β-D-glucopyranose-2,3,4,6-tetraacetato-S)(triethylphosphine)gold; (2,3,4,6-tetra-O-acetyl-1-thio-β-D-glucopyranosato-S)(triethylphosphine)gold; (1-thio-β-D-glucopyranosato)(triethylphosphine)gold 2,3,4,6-tetraacetate; SKF-39162; Crisinor; Crisofin; Ridaura; Ridauran. $C_{20}H_{34}AuO_9PS$; mol wt 678.48. C 35.40%, H 5.05%, Au 29.03%, O 21.22%, P 4.57%, S 4.73%. Disease modifying antirheumatic drug (DMARD); orally active gold coordination complex. Prepn: E. R. McGusty, B. M. Sutton, DE 2051495; *eidem*, US 3635945 (1971, 1972 both to SKF). Toxicity study: B. H. Payne, D. T. Walz, *Vet. Pathol.* **15**, Suppl. 5, 1 (1978). HPLC determn in urine: R. Kizu *et al.*, *Chem. Pharm. Bull.* **41**, 1261 (1993). Symposium on pharmacology and clinical experience: *J. Rheumatol.* **9**, Suppl. 8, 1-209 (1982). Clinical trial in rheumatoid arthritis: M. Itokazu *et al.*, *Clin. Ther.* **17**, 60 (1995); in steroid-dependent asthma: I. L. Bernstein *et al.*, *J. Allergy Clin. Immunol.* **98**, 317 (1996). *Review:* W. F. Kean *et al.*, *Br. J. Rheumatol.* **36**, 560-572 (1997).

R = COCH₃

White, odorless, crystalline powder, mp 112-115°. Insol in water. Unstable to light and heat. LD_{50} in rats, mice (mg/kg): 265, 310 orally (Payne, Walz).

THERAP CAT: Antirheumatic.

879. Aureothin. [2825-00-5] (Z,E)-2-Methoxy-3,5-dimethyl-6-[tetrahydro-4-[2-methyl-3-(4-nitrophenyl)-2-propenylidene]-2-furanyl]-4H-pyran-4-one; mycolutein. $C_{22}H_{23}NO_6$; mol wt 397.42. C 66.49%, H 5.83%, N 3.52%, O 24.15%. Antibiotic by-product of aureothricin, *q.v.*, isolated from the culture of *Streptomyces thioluteus*. Isoln: K. Maeda, J. Antibiot. **6A**, 137 (1953); (as mycolutein): H. Schmitz, R. Woodside, *Antibiot. Chemother.* **5**, 652 (1955). Structure: Y. Hirata *et al.*, *Tetrahedron* **14**, 252 (1961). Identity with mycolutein: J. L. Schwartz *et al.*, *J. Antibiot.* **29**, 236 (1976). Biosynthesis: R. Cardillo *et al.*, *Tetrahedron* **30**, 459 (1974); M. Yamazaki *et al.*, *Chem. Pharm. Bull.* **23**, 569 (1975). Synthesis: Y. Shizuri *et al.*, *Chem. Lett.* **1987**, 1381.

Yellow prisms, mp 158°. $[\alpha]_D^{18}$ +51° (chloroform). Sol in methanol, ethanol, acetone, chloroform, tetrahydrofuran. Practically insol in water, nonpolar solvents. uv max (ethanol): 257, 346 nm (log ε 4.39, 4.27).

880. Aureothricin. [574-95-8] N-(4,5-Dihydro-4-methyl-5-oxo-1,2-dithiolo[4,3-b]pyrrol-6-yl)propanamide; 4-methyl-6-propionamido-1,2-dithiolo[4,3-b]pyrrol-5(4H)-one; 5-methyl-3-propionamidopyrrolin-4-one[4,3-d]-1,2-dithiole; propionopyrrothine. $C_9H_{10}N_2O_2S_2$; mol wt 242.32. C 44.61%, H 4.16%, N 11.56%, O 13.21%, S 26.47%. Antibiotic substance produced by *Streptomyces sp* 26A (Mitaka, Tokyo, June 1947) which resembles *Nocardia farcinicus* or *Streptomyces lipmanii*: Umezawa *et al., Jpn. Med. J.* **1**, 512 (1948); Umezawa *et al., J. Antibiot.* **2**, Suppl. A, 105 (1949); Maeda, *ibid.* **2**, 793 (1949); Maeda, *Jpn. Med. J.* **2**, 85 (1949); Celmer *et al., J. Am. Chem. Soc.* **74**, 6304 (1952). Structure: Celmer, Solomons, *ibid.* **77**, 2861 (1955). Prepn: Celmer, US 2752359 (1956 to Pfizer). Total synthesis: Schmidt, Geiger, *Angew. Chem.* **74**, 328 (1962).

Crystals, usually solvated. Stable in air. When anhydr dec 260-270° (sublimes near 200°). uv max: 248, 312, 388 nm (ε 6100, 3900, 11000). Practically insol in water; slightly sol in ethyl acetate, butyl acetate, acetone, benzene, ether, alc.

881. Aurin. [603-45-2] 4-[Bis(4-hydroxyphenyl)methylene]-2,5-cyclohexadien-1-one; 4-(p,p'-dihydroxybenzhydrylidene)-2,5-cyclohexadien-1-one; p-rosolic acid; corallin; C.I. 43800. $C_{19}H_{14}O_3$; mol wt 290.31. C 78.61%, H 4.86%, O 16.53%. Prepd by heating a mixture of phenol, oxalic and sulfuric acids: Zulkowsky, *Ann.* **194**, 109, 122 (1878); **202**, 179 (1880); *Monatsh. Chem.* **16**, 358 (1895); *Colour Index* vol. 4 (3rd ed., 1971) pp 4407. By heating phenol with formic acid and stannous chloride: Nencki, Schmid, *J. Prakt. Chem.* [2] **23**, 549 (1881). By heating phenol and carbon tetrachloride to 140-160° in presence of $AlCl_3$ or $ZnCl_2$ and treating the reaction product with water: Heumann, DE 68976 (*Frdl.* **3**, 103).

Deep red (garnet-like) crystals with metallic luster. Orthorhombic bipyramidal. Technical product may occur as yellowish-brown pieces with dark green metallic fracture. Dec 308-310°. Not volatile in vacuo at 180°. Absorption max (KOH): 534.6, 479.5 nm. Practically insol in water (0.12%) and in benzene. Freely sol in alc, giving a golden yellow solution, in aq or alc NaOH and KOH giving a carmine-red solution, in concd or 70% H_2SO_4, in HCl, in $HClO_4$ giving a yellow to orange soln. Moderately soluble in glacial acetic acid; slightly sol in ether, chloroform.

Sodium salt (yellow corallin). Yellowish pieces with greenish, metallic luster; sol in water, giving a carmine-red soln.

USE: Dye intermediate.

882. Aurodox. [12704-90-4] 1-Methylmocimycin; antibiotic X-5108; goldinodox; goldinomycin; X-5108. $C_{44}H_{62}N_2O_{12}$; mol wt 810.97. C 65.17%, H 7.71%, N 3.45%, O 23.67%. Antibiotic produced by *Streptomyces goldiniensis* var. *goldiniensis*: J. Berger, DE 2140322; *idem*, US 3708577 (1972, 1973 both to Hoffmann-La Roche). Isoln, production, properties and toxicity data: J. Berger *et al.*, *J. Antibiot.* **26**, 15 (1973). Improved production: J.

Unowsky, D. C. Hoppe, *ibid.* **31,** 662 (1978). Structure: H. Maehr *et al., J. Am. Chem. Soc.* **95,** 8449 (1973). Absolute stereochemistry: *eidem, ibid.* **96,** 4034 (1974). Biosynthesis: C.-M. Liu *et al., J. Antibiot.* **30,** 416 (1977); **32,** 414 (1979). Stereospecific total synthesis: R. E. Dolle, K. C. Nicolaou, *J. Am. Chem. Soc.* **107,** 1691, 1695 (1985). Growth promoting activity: W. L. Marusich *et al., Poult. Sci.* **53,** 636 (1974). Review of chemistry: H. Maehr *et al., Can. J. Chem.* **58,** 501 (1980).

Yellow amorphous solid. Weakly acidic. Sol in methanol, ethyl acetate, CHCl$_3$, acetone, methylene chloride. Insol in water. pKa = 6.1. Unstable in acidic or basic soln, but can be kept in aq soln at pH 7-9 for 4 hrs at 25° without significant loss of activity. Solns kept at 25° or heated to 56° are 2-10 times more stable in methanol than in water or pH 9 borate buffer. LD$_{50}$ in mice (mg/kg): >1000 s.c., >4000 orally (Berger *et al.*).

Sodium salt. C$_{44}$H$_{61}$N$_2$NaO$_{12}$. Yellow solid. $[\alpha]_D^{25}$ −82.8° (c = 0.52 in ethanol). uv max (0.1N HCl): 334, 233, 206 nm (E$_{1cm}^{1\%}$ 403, 610, 500); (0.1N KOH): 327, 231 nm (E$_{1cm}^{1\%}$ 416, 647). Sol in water, methanol, ethanol, isopropanol, butanol, DMF. Slightly sol in amyl alcohol, THF, dioxane. Insol in benzene, chloroform, ethyl ether, petr ether.

THERAP CAT (VET): Poultry growth promotant.

883. Aurothioglucose. [12192-57-3] (1-Thio-D-glucopyranosato-*O2,S1*)gold; (1-D-glucosylthio)gold; gold thioglucose; Aureotan; Solganal. C$_6$H$_{11}$AuO$_5$S; mol wt 392.18. C 18.38%, H 2.83%, Au 50.22%, O 20.40%, S 8.18%. Disease modifying antirheumatic drug (DMARD). Prepn: Lebeau-Janot, *Traité Pharm. Chim.* **II,** 661 (1956). Induction of obesity in exptl animals: A. F. Debons *et al., Fed. Proc.* **36,** 143 (1977). Clinical comparison with auranofin, *q.v.,* in rheumatoid arthritis: P. L. C. M. Van Riel *et al., Clin. Rheumatol.* **5,** 359 (1986); P. E. Prete *et al., Clin. Rheumatol.* **13,** 60 (1994).

Yellow crystals. Slight mercaptan-like odor. Sol in water with decompn; slightly sol in propylene glycol. Practically insol in acetone, alcohol, chloroform, ether.

USE: To produce obesity in exptl animals.

THERAP CAT: Antirheumatic.

884. Avasimibe. [166518-60-1] [[2,4,6-Tris(1-methylethyl)phenyl]acetyl]sulfamic acid 2,6-bis(1-methylethyl)phenyl ester; 2,6-diisopropylphenyl[(2,4,6-triisopropylphenyl)acetyl]sulfamate; CI-1011; PD-148515. C$_{29}$H$_{43}$NO$_4$S; mol wt 501.72. C 69.42%, H 8.64%, N 2.79%, O 12.76%, S 6.39%. Acyl-coenzyme A:cholesterol *O*-acyltransferase (ACAT) inhibitor. Prepn: H. T. Lee *et al.,* **WO 9426702**; *eidem,* **US 5491172** (1994, 1996 both to Warner Lambert). Scale up synthesis: G. J. Dozeman *et al, Org. Process Res. Dev.* **1,** 137 (1997). ACAT inhibition studies: H. T. Lee *et al., J. Med. Chem.* **39,** 5031 (1996). HPLC/MS/MS determn in plasma: W. W. Bullen *et al., J. Pharm. Biomed. Anal.* **17,** 1399 (1998). Clinical evaluation in hyperlipidemia: W. Insull Jr. *et al., Atherosclerosis* **157,** 137 (2001). Toxicology: D. G. Robertson *et al., Toxicol. Sci.* **59,** 324 (2001). Reviews of development and therapeutic potential: R. Jones, *Curr. Opin. Cardiovasc. Pulmon. Renal Invest. Drugs* **1,** 263-269 (1999); *idem, ibid.* **2,** 274-278 (2000).

White solid, mp 178-180° (Lee). Also reported as white powder, mp 169.5-170.4° (Dozeman).

Sodium salt. [166518-61-2] White solid, mp 250-252°.

THERAP CAT: Antilipemic.

885. Avermectins. AVM. A group of broad-spectrum antiparasitic antibiotics which are derivs of pentacyclic 16-membered lactones related to the milbemycins, *q.v.* Isoln from a novel actinomycete, *Streptomyces avermitilis,* and separation of major components A$_{1a}$, A$_{2a}$, B$_{1a}$, B$_{2a}$ and minor components A$_{1b}$, A$_{2b}$, B$_{1b}$, B$_{2b}$: G. Albers-Schönberg *et al.,* **DE 2717040**; *eidem,* **US 4310519** (1977, 1982 both to Merck & Co.); R. W. Burg *et al., Antimicrob. Agents Chemother.* **15,** 361 (1979); T. W. Miller *et al., ibid.* 368. Antiparasitic activity: S. R. Egerton *et al., ibid.* 372. Mechanism of action: L. C. Fritz *et al., Proc. Natl. Acad. Sci. USA* **76,** 2062 (1979). Pesticidal activity: I. Putter *et al., Experientia* **37,** 963 (1981). Structure determn: G. Albers-Schönberg *et al., J. Am. Chem. Soc.* **103,** 4216 (1981). Absolute configuration of avermectin B$_{1a}$ and aglycon B$_{2a}$: J. P. Springer *et al., ibid.* 4221. Prepn of aglycons: H. Mrozik *et al., J. Org. Chem.* **47,** 489 (1982). Total synthesis of A$_{1a}$ (C$_{49}$H$_{74}$O$_{14}$): S. J. Danishefsky *et al., J. Am. Chem. Soc.* **109,** 8119 (1987). Biosynthetic studies: D. E. Cane *et al., ibid.* **105,** 4110 (1983); M. D. Schulman *et al., J. Antibiot.* **39,** 541 (1986); T. S. Chen *et al., Arch. Biochem. Biophys.* **269,** 544 (1989). *Reviews:* W. C. Campbell *et al., ACS Symp. Ser.* **255,** 1-20 (1984); M. H. Fisher, H. Mrozik, "The Avermectin Family of Macrolide Antibiotics" in *Macrolide Antibiotics,* S. Omura, Ed. (Academic Press, New York, 1984) pp 553-606; *Southwest. Entomol.* **1985,** Suppl. 7, 1-51; J. R. Babu, *ACS Symp. Ser.* **380,** 91-108 (1988). Review of syntheses: T. Blizzard *et al.,* in *Recent Prog. Synth. Antibiotics,* G. Lukacs, M. Ohno, Eds (Springer-Verlag, Berlin, 1990) pp 66-102. Review of structure-activity relationships: W. L. Shoop *et al., Vet. Parasitol.* **59,** 139-156 (1995). For related structures *see* abamectin, ivermectin.

Avermectin A$_{1a}$

Avermectin A$_{1a/b}$. $[\alpha]_D^{27}$ +68.5 ± 2° (c = 0.77 in chloroform). uv max (methanol): 237, 243, 252 nm (ε 28700, 31275, 20290).
Avermectin A$_{2a/b}$. $[\alpha]_D^{27}$ +48.8 ± 2° (c = 1.64 in chloroform). uv max (methanol): 237, 243, 245 nm (ε 28800, 31740, 20425).
Avermectin B$_{1a/b}$ *see* Abamectin.
Avermectin B$_{2a/b}$. $[\alpha]_D^{27}$ +38.3 ± 2° (c = 0.87 in chloroform). uv max (methanol): 237, 243, 252 nm (ε 27580, 30590, 20060).

886. Avidin. Basic glycoprotein isolated from raw egg white. Exhibits high binding affinity for biotin and is capable of producing biotin deficiency in rats and chicks. Occurs in the white portion of eggs and the oviducts of birds and amphibia. Destroyed by cooking or irradiation. Isoln: Eakin *et al., J. Biol. Chem.* **136,**

801 (1940); Pennington *et al., J. Am. Chem. Soc.* **64**, 469 (1942); Fraenkel-Conrat *et al., Arch. Biochem. Biophys.* **39**, 80, 97 (1952). Improved purification and crystallization: Green *et al., Biochem. J.* **118**, 67, 71 (1970). Structure is a glycoprotein containing four essentially identical subunits: Green, *ibid.* **92**, 16c (1964). The combined mol wt of the subunits is about 66,000. Each subunit is a single polypeptide chain containing 128 amino acid residues with alanine at the *N*-terminal, glutamic acid at the *C*-terminal, and a carbohydrate moiety attached at the asparaginyl residue, position 17. Complete amino acid sequence of the protein subunit: De-Lange, Huang, *J. Biol. Chem.* **246**, 698 (1971). Studies on biotin inactivation by avidin: Becker, Wilchek, *Biochim. Biophys. Acta* **264**, 165 (1972). Review of chemistry and binding properties: N. M. Green, *Adv. Protein Chem.* **29**, 85-133 (1975). Review of use of avidin-biotin complex in molecular biology: E. A. Bayer, M. Wilchek, *Methods Biochem. Anal.* **26**, 1-45 (1980); in immunoassays: M. Wilchek, E. A. Bayer, *Immunol. Today* **5**, 39-43 (1984).

USE: Biochemical tool for affinity chromatography, affinity cytochemistry and immunoassay.

887. Avilamycin. [11051-71-1] LY-048740; Maxus; Surmax. Polyether antibiotic complex produced by *Streptomyces viridochromogenes,* ETH 23575 (NRRL 2860); belongs to the orthosomycin family of antibiotics, members of which contain one or more ortho ester linkages associated with carbohydrate residues. Isoln: E. Gaeumann *et al.,* **DE 1116864**; *eidem,* **US 3131126** (1961, 1964 both to Ciba-Geigy); and characterization: F. Buzzetti *et al., Experientia* **24**, 320 (1968). Mechanism of action studies: H. Wolf, *FEBS Lett.* **36**, 181 (1973). Avilamycin A is the main component; avilamycins B through N are also known and are derivatives of A differing at the C-45 linkage and/or the C-56 ketone adduct. Isoln of avilamycin C: W. Heilman *et al., Helv. Chim. Acta* **62**, 1 (1979). Structural study of A and C: *eidem, ibid.*; W. Keller-Schierlein *et al., ibid.* 7; E. Kupfer *et al., ibid.* **65**, 3 (1982). Isoln and structure of avilamycins F through N: J. L. Mertz *et al., J. Antibiot.* **39**, 877 (1986). GC determn of avilamycin residues in swine tissue and fluids: G. Formica, C. Giannone, *J. Assoc. Off. Anal. Chem.* **69**, 763 (1986). Synthesis of the A-B fragment of avilamycins A and C: P. Jütten *et al., Tetrahedron* **43**, 4133 (1987); of the disaccharide C-D fragment: J.-M. Beau *et al., Tetrahedron Lett.* **28**, 1105 (1987). Use as a feed additive: F. Knusel *et al.,* **US 4185091** (1980 to Ciba-Geigy); in prevention of swine dysentery: E. E. Ose, **US 4436734** (1984 to Lilly). Effect on feed conversion efficiency in swine: D. J. Jones *et al., J. Anim. Sci.* **65**, 881 (1987). Metabolism in swine: J. D. Magnussen *et al., J. Agric. Food Chem.* **39**, 306 (1991).

Avilamycin A

Colorless, needle-shaped crystals from acetone/ether, mp 188-189.5°. $[\alpha]_D^{20}$ +0.8° (c = 1.165 in abs ethanol) and −7.7° (c = 1.083 in chloroform).

Avilamycin A. $C_{61}H_{88}Cl_2O_{32}$; mol wt 1404.24. Colorless needles from chloroform/petr ether, mp 181-182° (1-2.H_2O). uv max (methanol): 227, 286 nm (log ε 4.15, 3.33).

Avilamycin C. $C_{61}H_{90}Cl_2O_{32}$; mol wt 1406.25. Dihydrate, colorless fine plates from acetone/ether, mp 188-189°. $[\alpha]_D^{20}$ −4.8° (c = 1.44 in chloroform). uv max (methanol): 228, 284 nm (log ε 4.12, 3.33).

THERAP CAT (VET): Growth promotant.

888. Avobenzone. [70356-09-1] 1-[4-(1,1-Dimethylethyl)phenyl]-3-(4-methoxyphenyl)-1,3-propanedione; butyl methoxydibenzoylmethane; 4-*tert*-butyl-4′-methoxydibenzoylmethane; Eusolex 9020; Neo Heliopan 357; Parsol 1789. $C_{20}H_{22}O_3$; mol wt 310.39. C 77.39%, H 7.14%, O 15.46%. UV-A blocker. Prepn: K.-F. De Polo, **DE 2945125**; *idem,* **US 4387089** (1980, 1983 both to Givaudan). Clinical efficacy as sunscreen: R. W. Gange *et al., J. Am. Acad. Dermatol.* **15**, 494 (1986); K. Kaidbey, R. W. Gange, *ibid.* **16**, 346 (1987); N. J. Lowe *et al., ibid.* **17**, 224 (1987). Assessment of photostability: A. Deflandre, G. Lang, *Int. J. Cosmet. Sci.* **10**, 53 (1988). Photodecomposition: N. M. Roscher *et al., J. Photochem. Photobiol. A* **80**, 417 (1994). Photochemistry in solution: W. Schwack, T. Rudolph, *ibid. B* **28**, 229 (1995). HPLC determn in cosmetic products: L. Gagliardi *et al., J. Chromatogr.* **408**, 409 (1987); P. Wallner, *Dtsch. Lebensm. Rundsch.* **89**, 375 (1993). Effect of reflectance of light on protection of skin: G. J. Smith *et al., Photochem. Photobiol.* **75**, 122 (2002).

Crystals from methanol, mp 83.5°.

THERAP CAT: Ultraviolet screen.

889. Avoparcin. [37332-99-3] AV-290; C-254; CL-81588; LL-AV290; Avotan. Animal feed glycopeptide antibiotic complex produced by *Streptomyces candidus.* Prodn: M. P. Kunstmann, J. N. Porter, **US 3338786** (1967 to Am. Cyanamid). Fermentation, isoln, characterization: M. P. Kunstmann *et al., Antimicrob. Agents Chemother.* **8**, 242 (1968). Isoln, purif of major components: W. J. McGahren *et al., J. Antibiot.* **36**, 1671 (1983). HPLC separation of α-, β-avoparcin: F. Sztaricskai *et al., ibid.* 1691. Structural studies: J. J. Hlavka *et al., Tetrahedron Lett.* **1974**, 175; W. J. McGahren *et al., J. Am. Chem. Soc.* **101**, 2237 (1979). Structure: *eidem, ibid.* **102**, 1671 (1980). Stereochemistry and epimerization: G. A. Ellestad *et al., J. Antibiot.* **36**, 1683 (1983). Relationship between structure, antibacterial activity: S.W. Fesik *et al., Mol. Pharmacol.* **25**, 275 (1984). Effect on resistance patterns in chickens: J. R. Walton, *Zentralbl. Veterinaermed. (B)* **25**, 290 (1978), *C.A.* **89**, 173507 (1978). Prevention of exptly induced necrotic enteritis in chickens: J. F. Prescott, *Avian Dis.* **23**, 1072 (1979). Effect on feedlot performance: R. J. Johnson *et al., J. Anim. Sci.* **48**, 1338 (1979).

α-Avoparcin R = H
β-Avoparcin R = Cl

White, hygroscopic, amorphous solid; no definitive mp. uv max: 280 nm in neutral or acidic solns; 300 nm in basic solns. Sol in water, DMF, DMSO. Max stability of aq solns is at pH 4-8. Moderately sol in methanol. LD_{50} in mice, rats, and chickens: >10000 mg/kg orally (Am. Cyanamid, company literature).

α-Avoparcin. [73957-86-5] $C_{89}H_{102}ClN_9O_{36}$. $[\alpha]_D^{25}$ −96 ±2° (c = 0.62 in 0.1*N* HCl). uv max (0.1*N* HCl): 280 nm ($E_{1cm}^{1\%}$ 42.0).

β-Avoparcin. [73957-87-6] $C_{89}H_{101}Cl_2N_9O_{36}$. $[\alpha]_D^{25}$ −102 ±2° (c = 0.65 in 0.1*N* HCl). uv max (0.1*N* HCl): 280 nm ($E_{1cm}^{1\%}$ 44.0).

THERAP CAT (VET): Antibacterial; growth promotant.

890. Azacitidine. [320-67-2] 4-Amino-1-β-D-ribofurano-syl-1,3,5-triazin-2(1*H*)-one; 5-azacytidine; 5-AzaC; ladakamycin; U-18496; NSC-102816; Mylosar (formerly); Vidaza. $C_8H_{12}N_4O_5$; mol wt 244.20. C 39.35%, H 4.95%, N 22.94%, O 32.76%. DNA methylation inhibitor; analog of the pyrimidine nucleoside, cytidine, *q.v.* Chemical synthesis: A. Piskala, F. Sorm, *Collect. Czech. Chem. Commun.* **29,** 2060 (1964); M. W. Winkley, R. K. Robins, *J. Org. Chem.* **35,** 491 (1970). Production by fermentation of *Streptoverticillium ladakanus* and activity: L. J. Hanka *et al., Antimicrob. Agents Chemother.* **1966,** 619; M. E. Bergy, R. R. Herr, *ibid.* 625. HPLC determn in pharmaceutical prepns: L. D. Kissinger, N. L. Stemm, *J. Chromatogr.* **353,** 309 (1986). Toxicology study: P. E. Palm, C. J. Kensler, *U.S. Clearinghouse Fed. Sci. Tech. Inform.* (PB-194791, 1970) 191 pp., *C.A.* **75,** 33704j (1971). Review of clinical experience in acute nonlymphocytic leukemia: A. B. Glover *et al., Cancer Treat. Rep.* **71,** 737-746 (1987); of mechanism of action: A. B. Glover, B. Leyland-Jones, *ibid.* 959-964. Review of carcinogenic risk: *IARC Monographs* **50,** 47-63 (1990). Clinical efficacy in β-thalassemia: C. H. Lowrey, A. W. Nienhuis, *N. Engl. J. Med.* **329,** 845 (1993); in myelodysplastic syndrome: L. R. Silverman *et al., J. Clin. Oncol.* **20,** 2429 (2002); A. B. Kornblith *et al., ibid.* 2441.

Crystals from aq ethanol, mp 235-237° (dec). $[\alpha]_D^{26}$ +22.4° (c = 1 in water). uv max (water): 241 nm (ε 8767); (0.01*N* HCl): 249 nm (ε 3077); (0.01*N* KOH): 223 nm (ε 24200). Soly (mg/ml): 40 warm water, 14 cold water, 28 0.1*N* HCl, 43 0.1*N* NaOH, 52.7 DMSO, 1 acetone, 1 chloroform, 1 hexane. LD_{50} in mice (mg/kg): 115.9 i.p.; 572.3 orally (Palm, Kensler).

Caution: This substance is reasonably anticipated to be a human carcinogen: *Report on Carcinogens, Eleventh Edition* (PB2005-104914, 2004) p III-24.

THERAP CAT: Antineoplastic.

891. Azaconazole. [60207-31-0] 1-[[2-(2,4-Dichlorophen-yl)-1,3-dioxolan-2-yl]methyl]-1*H*-1,2,4-triazole; R-28644; Rode-wod; Safetray. $C_{12}H_{11}Cl_2N_3O_2$; mol wt 300.14. C 48.02%, H 3.69%, Cl 23.62%, N 14.00%, O 10.66%. Steroid demethylation inhibitor. Prepn: G. Van Reet *et al., DE 2551660; eidem,* **US 4079062** (1975, 1978 both to Janssen). Wood fungicide for mushroom cultivation: L. Van Leemput *et al., Med. Fac. Landbouww. Rijksuniv. Gent* **52,** 703 (1987); A. Eicker, E. Strydom, *Bot. Bull. Acad. Sinica* **31,** 51 (1990). Use as a preservative for composite wood products: E. L. Schmidt, R. O. Gertjejansen, *Forest Prod. J.* **38,** 19 (1988); A. Jeihooni *et al., Wood Fiber Sci.* **26,** 178 (1994).

Crystals from diisopropylether. mp 109.9°.

USE: Fungicide for cultivation on wood; preservative for composite wood products.

892. Azacosterol. [313-05-3] (3β,17β)-17-[[3-(Dimethyl-amino)propyl]methylamino]androst-5-en-3-ol; *N*-methyl-*N*-[3-(di-methylamino)propyl]-17β-aminoandrost-5-en-3β-ol; 20,25-diaza-cholesterol; diazasterol. $C_{25}H_{44}N_2O$; mol wt 388.63. C 77.26%, H 11.41%, N 7.21%, O 4.12%. Prepn: Counsell *et al., J. Med. Pharm. Chem.* **5,** 1224 (1962); Counsell, Klimstra, **US 3084156** (1963 to Searle).

Crystals from acetone + methanol, mp 146-148°. $[\alpha]_D$ −54.5°.

Dihydrochloride. [1249-84-9] SC-12937; Ornitrol. $C_{25}H_{44}$-$N_2O.2HCl$; mol wt 461.55. $[\alpha]_D$ −32°.

THERAP CAT (VET): Avian chemosterilant.

893. Azadirachtin. [11141-17-6] $C_{35}H_{44}O_{16}$; mol wt 720.71. C 58.33%, H 6.15%, O 35.52%. A tetranortriterpinoid isolated from the seeds of the neem tree, *Azadirachta indica* A. Juss. *(Melia azadirachta* L.), *Meliaceae,* and the chinaberry tree, *M. azedarach* L. Highly active insect feeding deterrent and growth regulator. Isoln from *A. indica* and identification as feeding inhibitor in locusts: J. H. Butterworth, E. D. Morgan, *Chem. Commun.* **1968,** 23; from *M. azedarach:* E. D. Morgan, M. D. Thornton, *Phytochemistry* **12,** 391 (1973). Partial synthesis: D. Pflieger *et al., Tetrahedron Lett.* **28,** 1519 (1987). Structural studies: J. H. Butterworth *et al., J. Chem. Soc. Perkin Trans.* 2 **1972,** 2445. ^{1}H- and ^{13}C-NMR data and structure: P. R. Zanno *et al., J. Am. Chem. Soc.* **97,** 1975 (1975); K. Nakanishi in *Recent Advances in Phyto-chemistry* vol. 9, V. C. Runeckles, Ed. (Plenum Press, New York, 1975) pp 283-298. Revised structure: W. Kraus *et al., Tetrahedron Lett.* **26,** 6435 (1985); H. B. Broughton *et al., Chem. Commun.* **1986,** 46. Isoln by HPLC: E. C. Uebel *et al., J. Liq. Chromatogr.* **2,** 875 (1979); J. D. Warthen, Jr. *et al., ibid.* **7,** 591 (1984). Antifeedant activity in locusts: J. S. Gill, C. T. Lewis, *Nature* **232,** 402 (1971); in fall army worms, cotton bollworms: J. A. Klocke, I. Kubo, *Entomol. Exp. Appl.* **32,** 299 (1982). Insect ecdysis and growth inhibition: H. Rembold, K. P. Sieber, *Z. Naturforsch.* **36C,** 466 (1981); I. Kubo, J. A. Klocke, *Agric. Biol. Chem.* **46,** 1951 (1982); K. P. Sieber, H. Rembold, *J. Insect Physiol.* **29,** 523 (1983). Series of articles on chemistry and activity: *Natural Pesticides from the Neem Tree,* Proc. 1st Int. Neem Conf., 1980, H. Schmutterer *et al.,* Eds. (German Agency for Technical Cooperation, Eschborn, 1981) 291 pp.

Microcrystalline powder from carbon tetrachloride, mp 154-158°. $[\alpha]_D$ −53° (c = 0.5 in CHCl₃). uv max (methanol): 217 nm (ε 9100).

USE: Experimentally as insect control agent.

894. Azafenidin. [68049-83-2] 2-[2,4-Dichloro-5-(2-pro-pynyloxy)phenyl]-5,6,7,8-tetrahydro-1,2,4-triazolo[4,3-*a*]pyridin-3(2*H*)-one; DPX-R6447; Milestone; Evolus. $C_{15}H_{13}Cl_2N_3O_2$; mol wt 338.19. C 53.27%, H 3.87%, Cl 20.97%, N 12.42%, O 9.46%. Porphyrin biosynthesis inhibitor. Prepn: A. D. Wolf, **BE 862884**; *idem*, **US 4213773** (1978, 1980 both to Du Pont). Review of physical properties, mode of action, and activity: K. Amuti *et al.*, *Brighton Crop Prot. Conf. - Weeds* **1997**, 59-66.

White powdered solid, mp 168-168.5°. Vapor pressure at 20°: 1.0×10^{-11} torr. Partition coefficient (octanol/water): 229. LD_{50} in rats, mice, bobwhite quail, mallard duck (mg/kg): >5000, >5000, >2500, >2500 orally; in rabbits (mg/kg): >2000 dermally. LC_{50} in rats, rainbow trout, blue gill sunfish (mg/l): >5.3, 33, 48 (Amuti).

USE: Herbicide.

895. Azafrin. [507-61-9] (5R,6R)-5,6-Dihydro-5,6-dihydroxy-10′-*apo*-β,ψ-carotenoic acid; escobedin. $C_{27}H_{38}O_4$; mol wt 426.59. C 76.02%, H 8.98%, O 15.00%. Carotenoid-carboxylic acid from roots of the South American plant "Azafranillo," *Escobedia scabrifolia* Ruiz & Pav., and *Escobedia laevis* Cham. & Schlecht., *Scrophulariaceae*. Isoln: R. Kuhn *et al.*, *Ber.* **64**, 333 (1931); *ibid.* **65**, 1873 (1932). Structure: R. Kuhn, A. Deutsch, *ibid.* **66**, 883 (1933); R. Kuhn, H. Brockmann, *ibid.* **67**, 885 (1934); *Ann.* **516**, 104 (1935). Absolute configuration (5R:6R): W. Eschenmoser, C. H. Eugster, *Helv. Chim. Acta* **58**, 1722 (1975).

Orange-colored prisms from toluene, mp 213°. $[\alpha]_{6438}^{20}$ −75° (c = 0.28 in alcohol). Absorption max (chloroform): 458, 428 nm. Practically insol in water. Sol in dil NaOH or Na_2CO_3 solns, in chloroform, alc, acetic acid and benzene; sparingly sol in ether. **Methyl ester.** $C_{28}H_{40}O_4$. Reddish-yellow leaflets from ether, mp 191°. $[\alpha]_{6438}^{22}$ −32° (chloroform).

896. 8-Azaguanine. [134-58-7] 5-Amino-1,4-dihydro-7H-1,2,3-triazolo[4,5-d]pyrimidin-7-one; 5-amino-1,6-dihydro-7H-ν-triazolo[4,5-d]pyrimidine-7-one; 5-amino-1H-ν-triazolo[d]pyrimidin-7-ol; 5-amino-7-hydroxy-1H-ν-triazolo[d]pyrimidine; pathocidin; guanazolo. $C_4H_4N_6O$; mol wt 152.11. C 31.58%, H 2.65%, N 55.25%, O 10.52%. Triazolo analog of guanine. Prepd from 2,4,5-triamino-6-hydroxypyrimidine: Roblin, Jr. *et al.*, *J. Am. Chem. Soc.* **67**, 290 (1945); from 2-amino-5-nitro-4-oxopyrimidine: H. U. Blank *et al.*, *J. Org. Chem.* **35**, 1131 (1970). Formation from guanine by *Streptomyces albus* and identity with pathocidin: K. Hirasawa, K. Isono, *J. Antibiot.* **31A**, 628 (1978). The first purine analog to show carcinostatic effects in murine malignancies; is readily incorporated into ribonucleic acids. *Review:* R. E. Parks, Jr., K. C. Agarwal, *Handb. Exp. Pharmacol.* **38**, pt. 2, 458 (1975); D. Grunberger, G. Grunberger in *Antibiotics* vol. **5**(pt. 2), F. E. Hahn, Ed. (Springer-Verlag, New York, 1979) pp 110-123.

Crystals from dil aq NaOH. Dec above 300° without melting. Absorption spectrum: L. F. Cavalieri *et al.*, *J. Am. Chem. Soc.* **70**, 3875 (1948). Soluble in dil caustic, in dil acids. Practically insol in water, alcohol, ether.

USE: Purine antimetabolite.

897. Azanidazole. [62973-76-6] (E)-4-[2-(1-Methyl-5-nitro-1H-imidazol-2-yl)ethenyl]-2-pyrimidinamine; (E)-2-amino-4-[2-(1-methyl-5-nitroimidazol-2-yl)vinyl]pyrimidine; nitromidine; F-4; Triclose. $C_{10}H_{10}N_6O_2$; mol wt 246.23. C 48.78%, H 4.09%, N 34.13%, O 13.00%. Prepn and use: A. Garzia, **DE 2358483**; *eidem*, **US 3882105**; **US 3969520** (1974, 1975, 1976 all to Chemoterapico). Toxicological and teratological studies: R. Tammiso *et al.*, *Arzneim.-Forsch.* **28**, 2251 (1978).

Bright yellow odorless powder, mp 232-235°. Sol in DMF, DMSO, mineral oils and acids. Slightly sol in dioxane and acetone. LD_{50} in mice, rats (mg/kg): 5100, 7600 orally; 590, 860 i.p. (Tammiso).

THERAP CAT: Antiprotozoal (Trichomonas).

898. Azaperone. [1649-18-9] 1-(4-Fluorophenyl)-4-[4-(2-pyridinyl)-1-piperazinyl]-1-butanone; 4′-fluoro-4-[4-(2-pyridyl)-1-piperazinyl]butyrophenone; 1-[3-(4-fluorobenzoyl)propyl]-4-(2-pyridyl)piperazine; R-1929; Stresnil; Suicalm. $C_{19}H_{22}FN_3O$; mol wt 327.40. C 69.70%, H 6.77%, F 5.80%, N 12.83%, O 4.89%. Prepn: Janssen, **US 2979508** (1961). Synthesis of labeled compound: Soudijn, van Wijngaarden, *J. Lab. Comp.* **4**, 159 (1968). Distribution and metabolism studies in rat and pig: Heykants *et al.*, *Arzneim.-Forsch.* **21**, 982, 1263, 1357 (1971). Veterinary clinical studies: Symoens, van den Brande, *Vet. Rec.* **85**, 64 (1969). Crystal structure: M. H. J. Koch *et al.*, *Acta Crystallogr.* **33B**, 1975 (1977).

Crystals, mp 73-75°.
THERAP CAT (VET): Sedative; tranquilizer.

899. Azaserine. [115-02-6] L-Serine diazoacetate (ester); O-diazoacetyl-L-serine; CL-337; CN-15757; P-165. $C_5H_7N_3O_4$; mol wt 173.13. C 34.69%, H 4.08%, N 24.27%, O 36.97%. Antitumor antibiotic produced by *Streptomyces* sp. Isoln, characterization, and antitumor activity: C. C. Stock *et al.*, *Nature* **173**, 71 (1954); J. Ehrlich *et al.*, *ibid.* 72; Q. R. Bartz *et al.*, *ibid.* 72; S. A. Fusari *et al.*, *J. Am. Chem. Soc.* **76**, 2878 (1954). Structural studies: *idem et al.*, *ibid.* 2881. Synthetic studies: J. A. Moore *et al.*, *ibid.*, 2884; E. D. Nicolaides *et al.*, *ibid.*, 2887; T. J. Curphey, D. S. Daniel, *J. Org. Chem.* **43**, 4666 (1978). Pathology and pharmacology studies: S. S. Sternberg, F. S. Philips, *Cancer* **10**, 889 (1957). Crystal and molecular structure: A. Fitzgerald, L. H. Jensen, *Acta Crystallogr.* **B34**, 828 (1978). Review of carcinogenicity studies: *IARC Monographs* **10**, 73-77 (1976). *Review:* Pettillo, Hunt, *Antibiotics* vol. **1**, D. Gottlieb, P. Shaw, Eds. (Springer-Verlag, New York, 1967) pp 481-493. Use in study of the progression of pancreatic adenocarcinoma in rat models: K. Nagy *et al.*, *Histochem. Cell Biol.* **119**, 405 (2003).

Light yellow-green needles from aq ethanol, mp 146-162° (dec). $[\alpha]_D^{27.5}$ −0.5° (c = 8.46% in H_2O at pH 5.18). uv max (pH 7): 250.5 nm ($E_{1cm}^{1\%}$ 1140); in 0.1N NaOH: 252 nm ($E_{1cm}^{1\%}$ 1230). Very sol in water; slightly sol in abs methanol, abs ethanol, acetone, but sol in warm aq solns of these solvents. pKa 8.55. LD$_{50}$ in mice, rats (mg/kg/day): 150, 170 orally (Sternberg, Philips).

USE: Reagent used to induce pancreatic cancer in experimental animal models.

900. Azasetron. [123040-69-7] *N*-1-Azabicyclo[2.2.2]oct-3-yl-6-chloro-3,4-dihydro-4-methyl-3-oxo-2*H*-1,4-benzoxazine-8-carboxamide; (±)-6-chloro-3,4-dihydro-4-methyl-3-oxo-*N*-(3-quinuclidinyl)-2*H*-1,4-benzoxazine-8-carboxamide; nazasetron. C$_{17}$H$_{20}$ClN$_3$O$_3$; mol wt 349.81. C 58.37%, H 5.76%, Cl 10.13%, N 12.01%, O 13.72%. Serotonin 5-HT$_3$ receptor antagonist. Prepn: T. Tahara *et al., EP 313393; eidem,* **US 4892872** (1989, 1990 both to Yoshitomi); T. Kawakita *et al., Chem. Pharm. Bull.* **40,** 624 (1992). Receptor binding study: N. Sato *et al., Jpn. J. Pharmacol.* **59,** 443 (1992). Pharmacology: K. Haga *et al., ibid.* **63,** 377 (1993). Toxicity study: S. Takagi *et al., Oyo Yakuri* **42,** 255 (1991), *C.A.* **117,** 40208q (1991).

Hydrochloride. [123040-16-4] Y-25130; Serotone. C$_{17}$H$_{20}$-ClN$_3$O$_3$.HCl; mol wt 386.27. Crystals from ethanolic HCl, mp 281° (dec). Also reported as crystals from ethanol, mp 305° (dec) (Kawakita). LD$_{50}$ in male, female rats (mg/kg): 135, 132 i.v. (Takagi).

THERAP CAT: Antiemetic.

901. Azatadine. [3964-81-6] 6,11-Dihydro-11-(1-methyl-4-piperidinylidene)-5*H*-benzo[5,6]cyclohepta[1,2-*b*]pyridine; 11-aza-5-(*N*-methyl-4-piperidinylidene)-10,11-dihydro-5*H*-dibenzo[*a,d*]cycloheptene. C$_{20}$H$_{22}$N$_2$; mol wt 290.40. C 82.72%, H 7.64%, N 9.65%. Prepn: F. J. Villani, **BE 647043** (1964 to Scherico); *idem,* **US 3326924** (1967 to Schering); *idem et al., J. Med. Chem.* **15,** 750 (1972). Pharmacology: S. Tozzi *et al., Agents Actions* **4,** 264 (1974). Toxicity studies: H. Tanaka *et al., Jitchuken Zenrinsho Kenkyuho* **1,** 173 (1975), *C.A.* **84,** 25951h (1976). Clinical evaluation in allergic rhinitis: J. D. Wilson *et al., N. Z. Med. J.* **94,** 79 (1981).

Crystals from isopropyl ether, mp 124-126°.

Dimaleate. [3978-86-7] Sch-10649; Bonamid; Idulian; Optimine; Zadine. C$_{20}$H$_{22}$N$_2$.2C$_4$H$_4$O$_4$; mol wt 522.55. Crystals from ethyl acetate-methanol, mp 152-154°.

THERAP CAT: Antihistaminic.

902. Azathioprine. [446-86-6] 6-[(1-Methyl-4-nitro-1*H*-imidazol-5-yl)thio]-1*H*-purine; 6-(1-methyl-4-nitro-5-imidazolyl)-mercaptopurine; azothioprine; BW-57-322; NSC-39084; Azanin; Imuran; Imurek; Imurel; Zytrim. C$_9$H$_7$N$_7$O$_2$S; mol wt 277.26. C 38.99%, H 2.54%, N 35.36%, O 11.54%, S 11.56%. Immunosuppressive antimetabolite; also active as disease modifying antirheumatic drug (DMARD). Metabolized *in vivo* to 6-mercaptopurine, *q.v.* Prepn: G. H. Hitchings, G. B. Elion, **US 3056785**

(1962 to Burroughs Wellcome). Metabolism and pharmacokinetics: T. L. Ding, L. Z. Benet, *Drug Metab. Dispos.* **7,** 373 (1979). Carcinogenicity studies: P. S. Mitrou *et al., Arzneim.-Forsch.* **29,** 483, 662 (1979). HPLC determn in plasma: E. C. Van Os *et al., J. Chromatogr. B* **679,** 147 (1996). Clinical trial in rheumatoid arthritis: R. F. Wilkens, D. Stablein, *J. Rheumatol.* **23,** Suppl. 44, 64 (1996). Comprehensive description: W. P. Wilson, S. A. Benezra, *Anal. Profiles Drug Subs.* **10,** 29-53 (1981). Review of clinical efficacy in renal transplantation: G. L. C. Chan *et al., Pharmacotherapy* **7,** 165-177 (1987); in multiple sclerosis: C. Confavreux, T. Moreau, *Mult. Scler.* **1,** 379-384 (1996); in inflammatory bowel disease: W. J. Sandborn, *Scand. J. Gastroenterol.* **33,** Suppl. 225, 92-99 (1998).

Pale yellow crystals from 50% aq acetone, dec 243-244°. uv max (methanol): 276 nm (ε 1.82 × 10^4); (0.1*N* HCl): 280 nm (ε 1.73 × 10^4); (0.1*N* NaOH): 285 nm (ε 1.55 × 10^4). pKa$_2$ 8.2. Slightly sol in chloroform, ethanol. Practically insol in water.

Sodium salt. [55774-33-9] C$_9$H$_6$N$_7$NaO$_2$S. Soly in water: 10 mg/ml.

Caution: Azathioprine is listed as a known human carcinogen: *Report on Carcinogens, Eleventh Edition* (PB2005-104914, 2004) p III-25.

THERAP CAT: Immunosuppressant; antirheumatic.

903. 6-Azathymine. [932-53-6] 6-Methyl-1,2,4-triazine-3,5(2*H*,4*H*)-dione; 5-methyl-6-azauracil; 3,5-dihydroxy-6-methyl-1,2,4-triazine. C$_4$H$_5$N$_3$O$_2$; mol wt 127.10. C 37.80%, H 3.97%, N 33.06%, O 25.18%. Prepn: Thiele, Bailey, *Ann.* **303,** 82 (1898); Bailey, *Am. Chem. J.* **28,** 386 (1902); Bougault, Daniel, *Compt. Rend.* **186,** 1216 (1928); Chang, *J. Org. Chem.* **23,** 1951 (1958).

Crystals from water. mp 210-212°. pKa 7.6. uv max (0.1*N* HCl): 261 nm (ε 5200); in 0.1*N* NaOH: 246 nm (ε 4770).

904. 6-Azauridine. [54-25-1] 2-β-D-Ribofuranosyl-1,2,4-triazine-3,5(2*H*,4*H*)-dione; 6-azauracil riboside; 3,5-dioxo-2,3,4,5-tetrahydro-1,2,4-triazine riboside; AzUR. C$_8$H$_{11}$N$_3$O$_6$; mol wt 245.19. C 39.19%, H 4.52%, N 17.14%, O 39.15%. Cytostatic nucleoside analog; inhibits orotidyl decarboxylase and blocks *de novo* pyrimidine biosynthesis. Production by *E. coli* in the presence of 6-azauracil: J. Skoda *et al., Experientia* **13,** 150 (1957). Chemical synthesis: M. Prystas *et al., Chem. Ind. (London)* **1961,** 947. Crystal structure and conformation: C. H. Schwalbe *et al., Biochem. Biophys. Res. Commun.* **44,** 57 (1971). Degradation kinetics: C. M. Riley *et al., Pharm. Res.* **12,** 1361 (1995). Clinical evaluation in recalcitrant psoriasis: J. C. Alper *et al., J. Am. Acad. Dermatol.* **13,** 567 (1985). Toxicity study: J. Plevova *et al., Toxicol. Appl. Pharmacol.* **17,** 511 (1970). Review of effect on vitamin B$_6$ and homocystinemia: W. Drell, A. D. Welch, *Pharmacol. Ther.* **41,** 195-206 (1989).

Crystals from ethanol, ether, mp 160-161°. $[\alpha]_D^{24}$ −132° (pyridine). uv max (water): 262 nm (ε 6100). pK 6.70.

2′,3′,5′-Triacetate. [2169-64-8] Azaribine; 2-(2,3,5-tri-O-acetyl-β-D-ribofuranosyl)-as-triazine-3,5(2H,4H)-dione; CB-304; Triazure. $C_{14}H_{17}N_3O_9$; mol wt 371.30. pKa (25°): 6.42. LD_{50} in mice, rats (g/kg): 7.8, 12.0 orally (Plevova).

THERAP CAT: Antipsoriatic.

905. Azelaic Acid. [123-99-9] Nonanedioic acid; 1,7-heptanedicarboxylic acid; lepargylic acid; anchoic acid; Azelex; Finacea; Skinoren. $C_9H_{16}O_4$; mol wt 188.22. C 57.43%, H 8.57%, O 34.00%. HOOC$(CH_2)_7$COOH. Prepd by disruptive oxidation of ricinoleic acid: Hill, McEwen, *Org. Synth.* **coll. vol. II**, 53 (1943). Occurs in rancid oleic acid. Clinical comparison with tetracycline in acne: P. T. Bladon *et al., Br. J. Dermatol.* **114**, 493 (1986). Review of clinical studies in hyperpigmentary disorders: A. S. Breathnach, M. Nazzaro-Porro, *ibid.* **111**, 115-120 (1984); of pharmacology and clinical uses: M. Nazzaro-Porro, *J. Am. Acad. Dermatol.* **17**, 1033-1041 (1987). Clinical comparison with metronidazole, *q.v.*, in rosacea: S. Maddin, *J. Am. Acad. Dermatol.* **40**, 961 (1999).

Monoclinic prismatic needles, mp 106.5°. Distills above 360° with partial anhydride formation. bp_{100} 286.5°; bp_{50} 265°; bp_{15} 237°; bp_{10} 225°. $d_4^{110.6}$ 1.0291. One liter of water dissolves 1.0 g at 1.0°; 2.4 g at 20°; 8.2 g at 50°; 22 g at 65°. Freely sol in boiling water, in alcohol. 1000 g of ether dissolves 18.8 g at 11° and 26.8 g at 15°. pK_1 (25°) 4.53; pK_2 5.33.

Dimethyl ester. $C_{11}H_{20}O_4$. Liquid, d_4^{20} 1.0026. mp −3.9°. bp_8 140°.

THERAP CAT: Antiacne.

906. Azelastine. [58581-89-8] 4-[(4-Chlorophenyl)methyl]-2-(hexahydro-1-methyl-1H-azepin-4-yl)-1(2H)-phthalazinone; 4-(p-chlorobenzyl)-2-(hexahydro-1-methyl-1H-azepin-4-yl)-1(2H)-phthalazinone; 4-(p-chlorobenzyl)-2-(N-methylperhydroazepin-4-yl)-1(2H)-phthalazinone. $C_{22}H_{24}ClN_3O$; mol wt 381.90. C 69.19%, H 6.33%, Cl 9.28%, N 11.00%, O 4.19%. Orally active H_1-histamine receptor antagonist. Prepn: **BE 778269**; D. Vogelsang *et al.*, **US 3813384** (1972, 1974 both to Asta-Werke AG). Synthesis and x-ray structure determn: G. Scheffler *et al., Arch. Pharm.* **321**, 205 (1988). Pharmacology: K. Tasaka, M. Akagi, *Arzneim.-Forsch.* **29**, 488 (1979). Pharmacology and toxicology: H. J. Zechel *et al., ibid.* **31**, 1184 (1981). Series of articles on pharmacokinetics, pharmacology and toxicology: *ibid.* 1184-1238. Mechanism of action studies: N. Chand *et al., Int. J. Immunopharmacol.* **7**, 833 (1985); *eidem, Br. J. Pharmacol.* **87**, 443 (1986). HPLC determn in plasma: J. Pivonka *et al., J. Chromatogr.* **420**, 89 (1987). Clinical evaluations in asthma: H. Magnussen, *Chest* **91**, 855 (1987); M. K. Albazzaz, K. R. Patel, *Thorax* **43**, 306 (1988); in allergic conjunctivitis: G. W. Canonica *et al., Curr. Med. Res. Opin.* **19**, 321-329 (2003).

Oil. Sol in methylene chloride.

Monohydrate. $C_{22}H_{24}ClN_3O \cdot H_2O$. Crystals from alcohol/water. Two distinct crystal forms have been identified (Scheffler).

Hydrochloride. [79307-93-0] A-5610; E-0659; W-2979M; Afluon; Allergodil; Astelin; Azeptin; Optilast; Rhinolast. $C_{22}H_{24}ClN_3O \cdot HCl$; mol wt 418.36. Crystals from alcohol, mp 225-229°. LD_{50} in male, female mice, male, female rats (mg/kg): 36.5, 35.5, 26.9, 30.3 i.v.; 56.4, 42.8, 43.2, 46.6 i.p.; 63.0, 54.2, 66.5, 59.6 s.c.; 124, 139, 310, 417 orally (Zechel).

THERAP CAT: Antihistaminic.

907. Azelnidipine. [123524-52-7] 2-Amino-1,4-dihydro-6-methyl-4-(3-nitrophenyl)-3,5-pyridinedicarboxylic acid 3-[1-(diphenylmethyl)-3-azetidinyl] 5-(1-methylethyl) ester; (±)-3-(1-diphenylmethylazetidin-3-yl) 5-isopropyl 2-amino-1,4-dihydro-6-methyl-4-(3-nitrophenyl)-3,5-pyridinedicarboxylate; CS-905; RS-9054; Calblock. $C_{33}H_{34}N_4O_6$; mol wt 582.65. C 68.03%, H 5.88%, N 9.62%, O 16.48%. Dihydropyridine L-type calcium channel blocker. Prepn: H. Koike *et al.*, **EP 266922**; *eidem,* **US 4772596** (both 1988 to Sankyo); T. Kobayashi *et al., Chem. Pharm. Bull.* **43**, 797 (1995). Clinical evaluation in hypertension: M. Arita *et al., J. Cardiovasc. Pharmacol.* **33**, 186 (1999). Review of pharmacology: Y. Yagil, A. Lustig, *Cardiovasc. Drug Rev.* **13**, 137-148 (1995); of development, pharmacokinetics, safety, and clinical experience: H. Koike *et al., Annu. Rep. Sankyo Res. Lab.* **54**, 1-64 (2002); of pharmacology and clinical experience: K. Wellington, L. J. Scott, *Drugs* **63**, 2613-2621 (2003).

Pale yellow to yellow crystalline powder, mp 122-123°. Insol in water. pKa 7.89. LD_{50} in female, male mice, female, male rats (mg/kg): 785, 979, 1267, 1971 orally (Koike).

THERAP CAT: Antihypertensive.

908. 2-Azetidinecarboxylic Acid. [2517-04-6] $C_4H_7NO_2$; mol wt 101.10. C 47.52%, H 6.98%, N 13.85%, O 31.65%. From *Convallaria majalis* L. (lily-of-the-valley) and *Polygonatum officinale* Moensh., *Liliaceae*: Fowden, *Biochem. J.* **64**, 323 (1956); Fowden, Bryant, *ibid.* **70**, 626 (1958). Structure: Virtanen, *Angew. Chem.* **67**, 619 (1955); Fowden, *loc. cit.* Biosynthesis: Linko, *Acta Chem. Scand.* **12**, 101 (1958); Fowden, Bryant, *Biochem. J.* **71**, 210 (1959); Fowden, *ibid.* **71**, 643 (1959); Leete, *J. Am. Chem. Soc.* **86**, 3162 (1964). Shows growth-inhibitory activity on cultures of *Escherichia coli* and on germinating seeds of different species in which it does not normally occur; Fowden, Richmond, *Biochim. Biophys. Acta* **71**, 459 (1963). Acts as a proline analog where a stoichiometric replacement of proline occurred with production of abnormal proteins having impaired biological activity: Peterson, Fowden, *Nature* **200**, 148 (1963).

Crystals from 95% hot methanol, discolors at 200° and darkens until 310° when heating stopped. $[\alpha]_D^{20}$ −108° (c = 3.6). Unstable to mineral acids. Soluble in cold and hot water. Practically insol in abs ethanol.

909. Azidamfenicol. [13838-08-9] 2-Azido-N-[2-hydroxy-1-(hydroxymethyl)-2-(4-nitrophenyl)ethyl]acetamide; D-(−)-threo-1-p-nitrophenyl-2-azidoacetylaminopropane-1,3-diol; D-(−)-threo-2-azidoacetamido-1-p-nitrophenyl-1,3-propanediol; azidoamphenicol; Berlicetin; Leukomycin-N; Posifenicol; Thilocanfol. $C_{11}H_{13}N_5O_5$; mol wt 295.25. C 44.75%, H 4.44%, N 23.72%, O 27.09%. Semi-synthetic antibiotic related to chloramphenicol, *q.v.* Prepn: Meiser, Domagk, **US 2882275** (1959 to Bayer).

Crystals from ethylene chloride, mp 107°. $[\alpha]_D^{20}$ −20° (c = 1.6 in ethyl acetate). pH 7.1. Sol in water up to 2%.

THERAP CAT: Antibacterial.

910.   Azidocillin. [17243-38-8] (2S,5R,6R)-6-[[(2R)-Azidophenylacetyl]amino]-3,3-dimethyl-7-oxo-4-thia-1-azabicyclo[3.2.0]heptane-2-carboxylic acid; α-azidobenzylpenicillin; 6-[D-α-azidophenylacetamido]penicillanic acid; SPC-97D; BRL-2351. $C_{16}H_{17}N_5O_4S$; mol wt 375.40. C 51.19%, H 4.56%, N 18.66%, O 17.05%, S 8.54%. Semi-synthetic antibiotic related to penicillin. Prepn: B. O. H. Sjöberg, B. A. Ekström, **GB 940488**; *eidem*, **US 3293242** (1963, 1966 to Beecham); Ekström *et al.*, *Acta Chem. Scand.* **19**, 281 (1965). Pharmacology: Hanssen *et al.*, *Antimicrob. Agents Chemother.* **1967**, 568; Tunevall, Frisk, *ibid.* 573. Chemistry: Sjöberg *et al.*, *ibid.* 560. Metabolic studies: Ramsey *et al.*, *Arzneim.-Forsch.* **22**, 1962 (1972).

Sodium salt. [35334-12-4] Globacillin; Longatren; Syncillin. $C_{16}H_{16}N_5NaO_4S$; mol wt 397.38.

THERAP CAT: Antibacterial.

THERAP CAT (VET): Antimicrobial. (In mastitis, as feed supplement).

911.   Azimilide. [149908-53-2] 1-[[[5-(4-Chlorophenyl)-2-furanyl]methylene]amino]-3-[4-(4-methyl-1-piperazinyl)butyl]-2,4-imidazolidinedione. $C_{23}H_{28}ClN_5O_3$; mol wt 457.95. C 60.32%, H 6.16%, Cl 7.74%, N 15.29%, O 10.48%. Potassium channel blocker. Prepn: S. S. Pelosi *et al.*, **WO 9304061** (1993 to Procter & Gamble); C.-N. Yu *et al.*, **US 5462940** (1995 to Norwich Eaton). Clinical pharmacokinetics: A. Corey *et al.*, *J. Clin. Pharmacol.* **37**, 946 (1997). Clinical trial to improve post-infarct survival: A. J. Camm *et al.*, *Am. J. Cardiol.* **81**, Suppl. 6A, 35D (1998). Review of electrophysiologic properties and pharmacology: R. Karam *et al.*, *ibid.* 40D-46D.

Dihydrochloride. [149888-94-8] NE-10064; Stedicor. $C_{23}H_{28}ClN_5O_3 \cdot 2HCl$; mol wt 530.88. Crystals from ethanol/water.

THERAP CAT: Antiarrhythmic (class III).

912.   Azimsulfuron. [120162-55-2] N-[[(4,6-Dimethoxy-2-pyrimidinyl)amino]carbonyl]-1-methyl-4-(2-methyl-2H-tetrazol-5-yl)-1H-pyrazole-5-sulfonamide; 1-(4,6-dimethoxypyrimidin-2-yl)-3-[1-methyl-4-(2-methyl-2H-tetrazol-5-yl)-pyrazol-5-ylsulfonyl]urea; DPX-A8947; IN-A8947. $C_{13}H_{16}N_{10}O_5S$; mol wt 424.40. C 36.79%, H 3.80%, N 33.00%, O 18.85%, S 7.56%. Broad spectrum, post-emergent sulfonylurea herbicide which inhibits acetolactate synthase. Prepn: G. Levitt, **US 4746353** (1988 to Du Pont). Description of chemical properties and biological activities: T. Marquez *et al.*, *Brighton Crop Prot. Conf. - Weeds* **1995**, 65. Environmental fate: A. C. Barefoot *et al.*, *ibid.* 713. Absorption, translocation and metabolism: S. Shirakura *et al.*, *Weed Res. Jpn.* **40**, 299 (1995). Efficacy in combination with bensulfuron methyl: *eidem*, *ibid.* 29.

Solid, mp 170°. Soly at 25° (ppm): methylene chloride 65900; acetone 26400; methanol 2100; acetonitrile 13900; ethyl acetate 13000. Aqueous soly at 20° (ppm): pH 5 72.3; pH 7 1050; pH 9 6540. pKa 3.6. Vapor pressure at 25°: 3.0×10^{-11} mm Hg. Partition coefficient (*n*-octanol/ water): 4.43 (pH 5); 0.043 (pH 7); 0.0083 (pH 9). LD$_{50}$ in rats, bobwhite quail, mallard duck (mg/kg): >5000, >2250, >2250 orally; in rats (mg/kg): >2000 dermally (Marquez). LC$_{50}$ (96 hr) in carp, bluegill sunfish, rainbow trout (ppm): >300, >1000, 154 (Marquez).

USE: Herbicide.

913.   Azinphos-methyl. [86-50-0] Phosphorodithioic acid O,O-dimethyl S-[(4-oxo-1,2,3-benzotriazin-3(4H)-yl)methyl]ester; phosphorodithioic acid O,O-dimethyl ester, S-ester with 3-mercaptomethyl-1,2,3-benzotriazin-4(3H)-one; Bayer 17147; ENT-23233; R-1582; Cotnion-methyl; Gusathion M; Guthion. PS_2; mol wt 317.32. C 37.85%, H 3.81%, N 13.24%, O 15.13%, P 9.76%, S 20.21%. Cholinesterase inhibitor. Prepn: Lorenz, **US 2758115** (1956 to Bayer). Activity: E. E. Ivy *et al.*, *J. Econ. Entomol.* **48**, 293 (1955). Toxicity study: T. B. Gaines, *Toxicol. Appl. Pharmacol.* **14**, 515 (1969).

Crystals from methanol, mp 73-74°. d_4^{20} 1.44; n_D^{76} 1.6115. Soly in water at 25°: 33 mg/l. Sol in methanol, ethanol, propylene glycol, xylene, other organic solvents. Solns in ethanol and propylene glycol are stable for at least 3 weeks. Unstable at temperatures >200°. Hydrolyzes in acid or cold alkali. LD$_{50}$ in female rats (mg/kg): 11 orally; 220 dermally (Gaines).

O,O-Diethyl analog. Azinphos-ethyl; Bayer 16259; ENT-22014; R-1513. $C_{12}H_{16}N_3O_3PS_2$; mol wt 345.38. Colorless needles, mp 53°, bp$_{0.001}$ 111°. d_4^{20} 1.284; n_D^{53} 1.5928. Vapor pressure at 20°: 2.2×10^{-7} mm Hg.

Caution: Potential symptoms of overexposure to azinphos-methyl are miosis; aching eyes; blurred vision, lacrimation and rhinorrhea; headache; chest tightness, wheezing, laryngeal spasms; salivation; cyanosis; anorexia; nausea, vomiting and diarrhea; sweating; twitching, paralysis and convulsions; low blood pressure, cardiac irregularities. *See NIOSH Pocket Guide to Chemical Hazards* (DHHS/NIOSH 97-140, 1997) p 22.

USE: Insecticide; acaricide.

914.   Azintamide. [1830-32-6] 2-[(6-Chloro-3-pyridazinyl)thio]-N,N-diethylacetamide; N,N-diethyl-2-[6-(3-chloropyridazinyl)thio]acetamide; N,N-diethyl-2-[6-(3-chloropyridazinyl)mercapto]acetamide; (3-chloro-6-pyridazinylthio)acetic acid diethylamide; ST-9067; Ora-Gallin purum. $C_{10}H_{14}ClN_3OS$; mol wt 259.76. C 46.24%, H 5.43%, Cl 13.65%, N 16.18%, O 6.16%, S 12.34%. Prepn: E. Kloimstein *et al.*, *Arzneim.-Forsch.* **14**, 261 (1964); *eidem*, **DE 1188604** (1965 to Lentia). Pharmacology and acute toxicity: H. Stormann, *Arzneim.-Forsch.* **14**, 266 (1964). Toxicology: I. Lindner *et al.*, *ibid.* 271. Clinical pharmacology: G. Hitzenberger, *ibid.* 279. Comprehensive description: E. M. Abdel-Moety, H. A. Al-Khamees, *Anal. Profiles Drug Subs.* **18**, 1-32 (1989).

Colorless, bitter tasting microcrystals, mp 97-98°. Freely sol in benzene, chloroform, ethyl acetate, acetone. Sol in water 0.5%. uv max (ethanol): 316, 306, 258 nm (ε 1.404 × 10³, 1.492 × 10³, 1.421 × 10⁴). LD$_{50}$ in mice, rats (g/kg): 2.34, 1.55 orally (Stormann).

THERAP CAT: Choleretic.

915.   Azithromycin. [83905-01-5] (2R,3S,4R,5R,8R,10R,-11R,12S,13S,14R)-13-[(2,6-Dideoxy-3-C-methyl-3-O-methyl-α-L-

ribo-hexopyranosyl)oxy]-2-ethyl-3,4,10-trihydroxy-3,5,6,8,10,12,-14-heptamethyl-11-[[3,4,6-trideoxy-3-(dimethylamino)-β-D-*xylo*-hexopyranosyl]oxy]-1-oxa-6-azacyclopentadecan-15-one; *N*-methyl-11-aza-10-deoxo-10-dihydroerythromycin A; 9-deoxo-9a-methyl-9a-aza-9a-homoerythromycin A. $C_{38}H_{72}N_2O_{12}$; mol wt 748.98. C 60.94%, H 9.69%, N 3.74%, O 25.63%. Semi-synthetic macrolide antibiotic; related to erythromycin A, *q.v.* Prepn: **BE 892357**; G. Kobrehel, S. Djokic, **US 4517359** (1982, 1985 both to Sour Pliva); of the crystalline dihydrate: D. J. M. Allen, K. M. Nepveux, **EP 298650**; *eidem*, **US 6268489** (1989, 2001 both to Pfizer). Antibacterial spectrum: S. C. Aronoff *et al.*, *J. Antimicrob. Chemother.* **19**, 275 (1987); and mode of action: J. Retsema *et al.*, *Antimicrob. Agents Chemother.* **31**, 1939 (1987). Series of articles on pharmacology, pharmacokinetics, and clinical experience: *J. Antimicrob. Chemother.* **31**, Suppl. E, 1-198 (1993). Clinical trial in prevention of *Pneumocystis carinii* pneumonia in AIDS patients: M. W. Dunne *et al.*, *Lancet* **354**, 891 (1999). Review of pharmacology and clinical efficacy in pediatric infections: H. D. Langtry, J. A. Balfour, *Drugs* **56**, 273-297 (1998).

Amorphous solid, mp 113-115°. $[\alpha]_D^{20}$ −37° (c = 1 in $CHCl_3$).
Dihydrate. [117772-70-0] CP-62993; XZ-450; Azitrocin; Ribotrex; Sumamed; Trozocina; Zithromax; Zitromax. White crystalline powder. mp 126°. $[\alpha]_D^{26}$ −41.4° (c = 1 in $CHCl_3$).
THERAP CAT: Antibacterial.

916. Azlocillin. [37091-66-0] (2*S*,5*R*,6*R*)-3,3-Dimethyl-7-oxo-6-[[(2*R*)-[[(2-oxo-1-imidazolidinyl)carbonyl]amino]phenylacetyl]amino]-4-thia-1-azabicyclo[3.2.0]heptane-2-carboxylic acid; D-α-[(imidazolidin-2-on-1-yl)carbonylamino]benzylpenicillin; Bay e 6905. $C_{20}H_{23}N_5O_6S$; mol wt 461.49. C 52.05%, H 5.02%, N 15.18%, O 20.80%, S 6.95%. Semi-synthetic, broad-spectrum acylureido penicillin. Prepn: H. Disselnkotter, K. G. Metzger, **FR 2100682**; *eidem*, **US 3933795** (1971, 1976 both to Bayer); H. B. Konig *et al.*, *Eur. J. Med. Chem. - Chim. Ther.* **17**, 59 (1982). *In vitro* studies: D. Stewart *et al.*, *Antimicrob. Agents Chemother.* **11**, 865 (1977). *In vitro* and *in vivo* activity: G. K. Daikos *et al.*, *Curr. Chemother., Proc. 10th Int. Congr. Chemother.*, 1977 (Amer. Soc. Microbiol., Washington, D.C., 1978) **1**, pp 626-8. Pharmacokinetics: P. Fiegel, K. Becker, *Antimicrob. Agents Chemother.* **14**, 288 (1978). Comparison with other penicillins: J. M. Andrews, K. A. Bedford, *ibid.* 559. Clinical studies: H. Lode *et al.*, *Infection* **5**, 163 (1977); E. B. Helm *et al.*, *Dtsch. Med. Wochenschr.* **102**, 1211 (1977). Series of articles on antibacterial activity, pharmacology, and clinical trials: *Arzneim.-Forsch.* **29**, 1915-2032 (1979); *Infection* **10**, Suppl. 3, S121-S266 (1982); *J. Antimicrob. Chemother.* **11**, Suppl. B, 1-239 (1983).

Sodium salt. [37091-65-9] Azlin; Securopen. $C_{20}H_{22}N_5$-NaO_6S; mol wt 483.47. Pale yellow crystals, sol in water, methanol, DMF. Slightly sol in ethanol, isopropanol.
THERAP CAT: Antibacterial.

917. Azobenzene. [103-33-3] Diphenyldiazene; diphenyl diimide; azobenzide; azobenzol; benzeneazobenzene. $C_{12}H_{10}N_2$; mol wt 182.22. C 79.10%, H 5.53%, N 15.37%. Parent compound of azobenzene disperse dyes. Prepn: A. I. Vogel, *Practical Organic Chemistry* (Longmans, London, 3rd ed., 1959) p 631. Toxicity data: E. W. Schafer, Jr., W. A. Bowles, Jr., *Arch. Environ. Contam. Toxicol.* **14**, 111 (1985). Review of carcinogenicity studies: *IARC Monographs* **8**, 75 (1975). Review of photochemistry: G. S. Kumar, D. C. Neckers, *Chem. Rev.* **89**, 1915-1925 (1989). Review of use in artificial membranes: J.-I. Anzai, T. Osa, *Tetrahedron* **50**, 4039-4070 (1994); as modeling ligand: A. A. Pasynskii *et al.*, *Bull. Pol. Acad. Sci. Chem.* **42**, 23-33 (1994); in polymers: A. Natansohn, P. Rochon, *ACS Symp. Ser.* **672**, 236-250 (1997).

Orange-red leaflets. d 1.20. mp 68°. bp 293°. Insol in water. Sol in alcohol, ether, glacial acetic acid.
USE: Precursor for dyes, for polymers.

918. 2,2′-Azobisisobutyronitrile. [78-67-1] 2,2′-Azobis[2-methylpropanenitrile]; AIBN; α,α′-azodiisobutyronitrile; 2,2′-dicyano-2,2′-azopropane; Porofor-57. $C_8H_{12}N_4$; mol wt 164.21. C 58.51%, H 7.37%, N 34.12%. Prepn by oxidation of α,α′-hydrazobutyric acid dinitrile: Overberger *et al.*, *J. Am. Chem. Soc.* **71**, 2661 (1949); Horner, Schwenk, *Ann.* **566**, 69 (1950); from 2-aminoisobutyronitrile + NaOCl: **GB 672106** (1952 to Rohm & Haas); Anderson, **US 2711405** (1955 to du Pont); from 2,2′-dichloro-2,2′-azopropane: Benzing, *Ann.* **631**, 1 (1960); **GB 929182** (1963 to Monsanto).

Crystals from ethanol + water, dec 107°. uv max (ethanol): 345 nm. Soly in methanol at 0°, 20°, 40°: 1.8, 4.96, 16.06 g/100 ml. Soly in ethanol at 0°, 20°, 40°: 0.58, 2.04, 7.15 g/100 ml. Can explode when dissolved in acetone: Carlisle, *Chem. Eng. News* **27**, 150 (1949).
Caution: In the organism, forms HCN which is found in blood, liver and brain: Rusin, *C.A.* **56**, 2682f (1962).
USE: Blowing agent for elastomers and plastics. Initiator for free radical reactions: Griesbaum *et al.*, *J. Org. Chem.* **30**, 261 (1965).

919. Azodicarbonamide. [123-77-3] Diazenedicarboxamide; 1,1′-azobisformamide; azodicarboxamide; azobiscarbonamide; azobiscarboxamide; 1,1′-azobiscarbamide. $C_2H_4N_4O_2$; mol wt 116.08. C 20.69%, H 3.47%, N 48.27%, O 27.57%. NH_2-$CON{=}NCONH_2$. Prepn: J. Thiele, *Ann.* **270**, 1 (1892); **271**, 127 (1892); T. Curtis, K. Heindenreich, *J. Prakt. Chem.* [2] **52**, 454 (1895); J. P. Picard, J. L. Boivin, *Can. J. Chem.* **29**, 223 (1951). Crystal structure: D. T. Cromer, A. C. Larson, *J. Chem. Phys.* **60**, 176 (1974). Safety assessment as a flour-maturing agent: B. L. Oser *et al.*, *Toxicol. Appl. Pharmacol.* **7**, 445 (1965).
Orange-red crystals, mp 225° (dec). *Flammable!* Sol in hot water; insol in cold water, alc.
USE: As blowing and foaming agent for plastics; as maturing and bleaching agent in cereal flour.

920. Azolitmin. [1395-18-2] Purified coloring matter from litmus: I. M. Kolthoff, C. Rosenblum, *Acid-Base Indicators* (MacMillan Co., New York, 1937) pp 160-162, 174, 208, 355, 361, 365-366, 368-369, 373, 377, 387.
Dark violet scales or dark red powder. Sparingly soluble in water; insol in alc; freely sol in dil alkali hydroxides or carbonates. The indicator solution is prepared by dissolving 0.5 g in 80 ml of warm H_2O, then adding 20 ml alcohol.
USE: Indicator instead of litmus. pH: 4.5 red, 8.3 blue. Usable with most mineral, some organic acids (not hydroxy acids) and some alkaloids; also used for preparing litmus media for bacteriologic purposes.

921. Azomycin. [527-73-1] 2-Nitro-1*H*-imidazole. C_3-$H_3N_3O_2$; mol wt 113.07. C 31.87%, H 2.67%, N 37.16%, O 28.30%. Antibiotic substance produced by an unidentified *Streptomyces* sp. (resembling *Nocardia mesenterica* in some aspects) from soil collected at Shiba Shirokane Daimachi (Japan): Maeda *et al., J. Antibiot.* **6A**, 182 (1953); Okami *et al., ibid.* **7A**, 53 (1954); Nakamura, Umezawa, *ibid.* **8A**, 66 (1955). Structure: Nakamura, *Pharm. Bull.* **3**, 379 (1955). Synthesis: Beaman *et al., J. Am. Chem. Soc.* **87**, 389 (1965); Lancini, Lazzari, *Experientia* **21**, 83 (1965).

Crystals from methanol, dec 283°. uv max (ethanol): 313 nm ($E_{1cm}^{1\%}$ 915); in 0.1*N* NaOH: 374 nm (ε 12750). Soluble in methanol, ethanol, acetone, ethyl acetate, butyl acetate, alkaline water. Practically insol in ether, petr ether, chloroform, acidic water. LD_{50} i.v. in mice: 80 mg/kg (Maeda).
Caution: Irritating to skin.

922. Azosemide. [27589-33-9] 2-Chloro-5-(1*H*-tetrazol-5-yl)-4-[(2-thienylmethyl)amino]benzenesulfonamide; 2-chloro-5-(2*H*-tetrazol-5-yl)-*N*⁴-2-thenylsulfanilamide; 5-(4′-chloro-2′-thenylamino-5′-sulfamoylphenyl)tetrazole; Ple-1053; Diart; Luret. C_{12}-$H_{11}ClN_6O_2S_2$; mol wt 370.84. C 38.87%, H 2.99%, Cl 9.56%, N 22.66%, O 8.63%, S 17.29%. Prepn: A. Popelak *et al., DE 1815922; eidem, US 3665002* (1968, 1972 both to Boehringer, Mann.). Separation and analysis in blood and urine by HPLC: R. Seiwell, C. Brater, *J. Chromatogr.* **182**, 257 (1980). Sites of action: C. Brater, *Clin. Pharmacol. Ther.* **25**, 428 (1979). Clinical and pharmacological studies: F. Krueck *et al., Eur. J. Clin. Pharmacol.* **14**, 153 (1978). Diuretic effect in animals: J. Greven, O. Heidenreich, *Arzneim.-Forsch.* **31**, 346, 350 (1981).

Crystals, mp 218-221°.
THERAP CAT: Diuretic.

923. Azoxybenzene. [495-48-7] Diphenyldiazene 1-oxide; azoxybenzide. $C_{12}H_{10}N_2O$; mol wt 198.22. C 72.71%, H 5.08%, N 14.13%, O 8.07%. Prepd by reduction of nitrobenzene with sodium arsenite: Bigelow, Palmer, *Org. Synth.* **coll. vol. II**, 57 (1943); also by treatment of nitrobenzene with glucose in alkaline medium: Opolonick, *Ind. Eng. Chem.* **27**, 1045 (1935). Industrial prepn by heating nitrobenzene with molasses and NaOH in high flash naphtha: **DE 228722**. Also prepd by catalytic reduction of nitrobenzene: Busch, Schulz, *Ber.* **62**, 1458 (1929). By peracetic acid oxidation of azobenzene: D'Ans, Kneip, *Ber.* **48**, 1145 (1915); *cf.* Greenspan, *Ind. Eng. Chem.* **39**, 847 (1947). Prepn of *cis*- and *trans*-forms by perbenzoic acid oxidation of azobenzene: G. M. Badger *et al., J. Chem. Soc.* **1953**, 2143.

trans-Azoxybenzene

trans-Form. [20972-43-4] Pale yellow orthorhombic needles. d_4^{26} 1.1590. d_4^{50} 1.1373. mp 36°. Slightly volatile with steam; easily volatile in superheated steam at 140-150°. Absorption spec-

trum: Müller, *Ann.* **493**, 166 (1932). Insol in water. Sol in alcohol, ether. 100 parts of abs alc satd at 16° contain 17.5 parts (w/w) azoxybenzene. At 15° 100 g ligroin dissolves 43.5 g azoxybenzene.
cis-Form. [21650-65-7] mp 87°.
USE: In organic syntheses.

924. Azoxystrobin. [131860-33-8] (α*E*)-2-[[6-(2-Cyanophenoxy)-4-pyrimidinyl]oxy]-α-(methoxymethylene)benzeneacetic acid methyl ester; methyl (*E*)-2-[2-[6-(2-cyanophenoxy)pyrimidin-4-yloxy]phenyl]-3-methoxyacrylate; ICI-A-5504; Amistar; Heritage; Quadris. $C_{22}H_{17}N_3O_5$; mol wt 403.39. C 65.50%, H 4.25%, N 10.42%, O 19.83%. Strobilurin fungicide; inhibits mitochondrial respiration by blocking electron transfer between cytochromes b and c_1. Prepn: J. M. Clough *et al., EP 382375* (1990 to I.C.I.); *eidem, US 5395837* (1995 to Zeneca). Comprehensive description: J. R. Godwin *et al., Brighton Crop Prot. Conf. - Pests Dis.* **1992**, 435-442. Field trials in turfgrass: J. A. Frank, P. L. Sanders, *ibid.* **1994**, 871. Environmental fate: E. D. Pilling *et al., ibid.* **1996**, 315.

White crystalline solid, mp 118-119°. d 1.33. Partition coefficient (*n*-octanol/water): 440. Vapor pressure (20°): $<10^{-5}$ Pa. Soly in water (25°): 10 mg/l. LD_{50} in rats (mg/kg): >5000 orally; >2000 dermally (Godwin).
USE: Agricultural fungicide.

925. Aztreonam. [78110-38-0] [2*S*-[2α,3β(*Z*)]]-2-[[[1-(2-Amino-4-thiazolyl)-2-[(2-methyl-4-oxo-1-sulfo-3-azetidinyl)-amino]-2-oxoethylidene]amino]oxy]-2-methylpropanoic acid; azthreonam; SQ-26776; Azactam; Primbactam. $C_{13}H_{17}N_5O_8S_2$; mol wt 435.43. C 35.86%, H 3.94%, N 16.08%, O 29.40%, S 14.73%. The first totally synthetic monocyclic β-lactam (monobactam) antibiotic. It has a high degree of resistance to β-lactamases and shows specific activity vs aerobic gram-negative rods. Prepn: R. B. Sykes *et al., NL 8100571* (1981 to Squibb), *C.A.* **96**, 181062x (1982). Fast-atom-bombardment mass spectra: A. I. Cohen *et al., J. Pharm. Sci.* **71**, 1065 (1982). Activity vs gram-negative bacteria: R. B. Sykes *et al., Antimicrob. Agents Chemother.* **21**, 85 (1982). Series of articles on structure-activity, *in vitro* and *in vivo* properties, pharmacokinetics: *J. Antimicrob. Chemother.* **8**, Suppl. E, 1-148 (1981). Toxicology: G. R. Keim *et al., ibid.* 141. Mechanism of action study: A. D. Russell, J. R. Furr, *ibid.* **9**, 329 (1982). Comparative stability to renal dipeptidase: H. Mikami *et al., Antimicrob. Agents Chemother.* **22**, 693 (1982). Human pharmacokinetics: E. A. Swabb *et al., ibid.* **21**, 944 (1982). Clinical evaluation in urinary tract infection: C. Donadio *et al., Drugs Exp. Clin. Res.* **13**, 167 (1987). Clinical efficacy in neonatal sepsis: S. Sklavunu-Tsurutsoglu *et al., Rev. Infect. Dis.* **13**, Suppl. 7, S591 (1991). Comprehensive description: K. Florey, *Anal. Profiles Drug Subs.* **17**, 1-39 (1988).

White crystalline, odorless powder, dec 227°. Very slightly sol in ethanol, slightly sol in methanol, sol in DMF, DMSO. Practically insol in toluene, chloroform, ethyl acetate.
Disodium salt. $C_{13}H_{15}N_5Na_2O_8S_2$. LD_{50} (mg/kg): 3300 i.v. in mice; 6600 i.p. in rats (Keim).
THERAP CAT: Antibacterial.

926. Azulene. [275-51-4] Cyclopentacycloheptene; bicyclo-[5.3.0]-deca-2,4,6,8,10-pentaene; bicyclo-[0.3.5]-deca-1,3,5,7,-9-pentaene. $C_{10}H_8$; mol wt 128.17. C 93.71%, H 6.29%. Prepn from octahydronaphthalene: Plattner, Pfau, *Helv. Chim. Acta* **20,** 224 (1937); from indan: Plattner, Magyar, *ibid.* **25,** 581 (1942).

Intensely blue leaflets or monoclinic plates from alc. Odor of naphthalene. mp 98.5-99°. Absorption spectrum: Susz *et al., Helv. Chim. Acta* **20,** 469 (1937); Plattner, *ibid.* **24,** 283 (1941). Insol in water; sol in the usual organic solvents, in concd mineral acids with decompn.

Sodium sulfonate. [51873-93-9] Azunol; Azusalen.

THERAP CAT: Sodium sulfonate as antacid.

927. Azure A. [531-53-3] 3-Amino-7-(dimethylamino)-phenothiazin-5-ium chloride; 7-(dimethylamino)-3-imino-3*H*-phenothiazine hydrochloride; 3-amino-7-dimethylaminophenazathionium chloride; *asym*-dimethyl-3,7-diaminophenazathionium chloride; *asym*-dimethylthionine chloride; methylene azure A; C.I. 52005. $C_{14}H_{14}ClN_3S$; mol wt 291.80. C 57.63%, H 4.84%, Cl 12.15%, N 14.40%, S 10.99%. One of the main constituents of methylene azure. Prepn: Bernthsen, *Ann.* **230,** 169 (1885); Kehrmann, *Ber.* **39,** 1804 (1906); MacNeal, Killian, *J. Am. Chem. Soc.* **48,** 740 (1926). *Review: H. J. Conn's Biological Stains,* R. D. Lillie, Ed. (Williams & Wilkins, Baltimore, 9th ed., 1977) pp 420-421, 603. *See also: Colour Index* vol. 4 (3rd ed., 1971) p 4469.

Green glistening crystals or dark green powder. Soluble in water (blue soln); sparingly sol in alc. Absorption max: 620-634 nm (3 ml of a soln of 50 mg in 250 ml H_2O diluted to 200 ml; read in a Beckman spectrophotometer 1 cm cell).

USE: Biological stain.

928. Azure B. [531-55-5] 3-(Dimethylamino)-7-(methylamino)phenothiazin-5-ium chloride; 7-(dimethylamino)-3-(methylimino)-3*H*-phenothiazine hydrochloride; 3-methylamino-7-dimethylaminophenazathonium chloride; trimethyldiaminophenazathonium chloride; trimethylthionine chloride; methylene azure B; C.I. 52010. $C_{15}H_{16}ClN_3S$; mol wt 305.83. C 58.91%, H 5.27%, Cl 11.59%, N 13.74%, S 10.48%. One of the main constituents of methylene azure. Prepn: Bernthsen, *Ann.* **230,** 169 (1885); Kehrmann, *Ber.* **39,** 1804 (1906); Kehrmann, Duttenhöfer, *ibid.* 925, 1403; Kehrmann *et al., ibid.* **46,** 2137 (1913); MacNeal, Killian, *J. Am. Chem. Soc.* **48,** 740 (1926). *Review: H. J. Conn's Biological Stains,* R. D. Lillie, Ed. (Williams & Wilkins, Baltimore, 9th ed., 1977) pp 421-423, 603-604. *See also: Colour Index* vol. 4 (3rd ed., 1971) p 4470.

Green glistening crystals or dark green powder. Sol in water (blue soln); sparingly sol in alc. Absorption max: 648-655 nm (3 ml of a soln of 50 mg in 250 ml H_2O dil to 200 ml; read in a Beckman spectrophotometer 1 cm cell).

USE: Biological stain.

929. Azure C. [531-57-7] 3-Amino-7-(methylamino)-phenothiazin-5-ium chloride; 3-imino-7-(methylamino)-3*H*-phenothiazine hydrochloride; 3-amino-7-methylaminophenazathonium chloride; monomethyldiaminodiphenazothionium chloride; monomethylthionine chloride; C.I. 52002. $C_{13}H_{12}ClN_3S$; mol wt 277.77. C 56.21%, H 4.35%, Cl 12.76%, N 15.13%, S 11.54%. Prepn: Holmes, French, *Stain Technol.* **1,** 17 (1926). *Review: H. J. Conn's Biological Stains,* R. D. Lillie, Ed. (Williams & Wilkins, Baltimore, 9th ed., 1977) pp 419-420, 604. *See also: Colour Index* vol. 4 (3rd ed., 1971) p 4469.

Green glistening crystals or dark green powder. Sol in water (blue soln); sparingly sol in alc. Absorption max: 608-622 nm (3 ml of a soln of 50 mg in 250 ml H_2O dil to 200 ml; read in a Beckman spectrophotometer 1 cm cell).

USE: Biological stain.

B

930. Babbitt Metal. Originally an alloy of 69% Zn, 19% Sn, 4% Cu, 3% Sb, and 5% Pb. This name now covers a variety of formulations, such as lead base babbitt, silver base babbitt, tin base babbitt, cadmium base babbitt, arsenic base babbitt. Generally and better described as "white metal bearing alloys".

USE: For machinery bearings.

931. Bacampicillin. [50972-17-3] (2S,5R,6R)-6-[[(2R)-Aminophenylacetyl]amino]-3,3-dimethyl-7-oxo-4-thia-1-azabicyclo[3.2.0]heptane-2-carboxylic acid 1-[(ethoxycarbonyl)oxy]ethyl ester; (2S,5R,6R)-6-[(R)-(2-amino-2-phenylacetamido)]-3,3-dimethyl-7-oxo-4-thia-1-azabicyclo[3.2.0]heptane-2-carboxylic acid ester with ethyl 1-hydroxyethyl carbonate; 6-[(R)-2-amino-2-phenylacetamido]penicillanic acid [1-(ethoxycarbonyloxy)ethyl] ester; 1'-ethoxycarbonyloxyethyl 6-(D-α-aminophenylacetamido)-penicillanate. $C_{21}H_{27}N_3O_7S$; mol wt 465.52. C 54.18%, H 5.85%, N 9.03%, O 24.06%, S 6.89%. Semi-synthetic antibiotic related to penicillin. Prepn: B. A. Ekstrom, B. O. H. Sjoberg, **DE 2144457**; *eidem*, **US 3873521** and **US 3939270** (1972, 1975 and 1976 all to Astra). *In vitro* and *in vivo* study: N. O. Bodin *et al.*, *Antimicrob. Agents Chemother.* **8**, 518 (1975). Pharmacokinetics: M. Rozencweig *et al.*, *Clin. Pharmacol. Ther.* **19**, 592 (1976); T. Bergan, *Antimicrob. Agents Chemother.* **13**, 971 (1978). Animal studies: C. Carbon *et al.*, *Scand. J. Infect. Dis. Suppl.* **14**, 127 (1978); T. Bergan, I. Versland, *ibid.* 135; U. Forsgren *et al.*, *ibid.* 207. Clinical studies: P. V. Maesen *et al.*, *J. Antimicrob. Chemother.* **2**, 279 (1976); J. Sjövall, *J. Int. Med. Res.* **5**, 313 (1977); C. Ekedahl *et al.*, *Scand. J. Infect. Dis. Suppl.* **14**, 279 (1978). Toxicology: M. Edanaga *et al.*, *Chemotherapy (Tokyo)* **27**, Suppl. 4, 17 (1979).

Hydrochloride. [37661-08-8] Ambacamp; Ambaxin; Bacacil; Bacampicine; Penglobe. $C_{21}H_{27}N_3O_7S\cdot HCl$; mol wt 501.98. White crystals from acetone-petr ether, mp 171-176° (dec). $[\alpha]_D^{20}$ +161.5°, also reported as +173° (Bodin). Sol in water. LD_{50} in mice (mg/kg): 8529 orally; 176 i.p.; 9475 s.c.; 184 i.v. (Edanaga).

THERAP CAT: Antibacterial.

932. Bacillus thuringiensis. Bt; Sporeine. A gram-positive spore-forming bacterium which during sporulation forms a parasporal protein crystal with insecticidal properties. Various subspecies are used as bioinsecticides against Lepidoptera, Diptera, and Coleoptera pests. First isolated by Ishiwata in 1902 from dying silkworm larvae. Later isolated as *B. thuringiensis*, Berliner, from the larvae of the flour moth, *Ephestia kuehniella* Zell: Berliner, *Z. Angew. Entomol.* **2**, 29 (1915). Characterization of the protein crystal: K. W. Nickerson, *Biotechnol. Bioeng.* **22**, 1305 (1950); C. L. Hannay, *Nature* **172**, 1004 (1953). The protein crystals consist of one or more types of protoxin subunits known as δ-endotoxins. Bt also produces an exotoxin which is released in the culture medium during bacterial growth. Isoln and structure of the exotoxin: Sebesta *et al.*, *Collect. Czech. Chem. Commun.* **34**, 891 (1969); Farkas *et al.*, *ibid.* 1118. Review of ultrastructure, physiology and biochemistry: L. A. Bulla *et al.*, *Crit. Rev. Microbiol.* **8**, 147-204 (1980); of industrial production: X.-M. Yang, S. S. Wang, *Biotechnol. Appl. Biochem.* **28**, 95-98 (1998). Review of persistence in soil and effects on non-target organisms: J. A. Addison, *Can. J. For. Res.* **23**, 2329-2342 (1993); of mammalian safety and toxicity studies: J. T. McClintock *et al.*, *Pestic. Sci.* **45**, 95-105 (1995). Review of expression of toxin genes in plant cells: M. Mazier *et al.* in *Biotechnology Annual Review* **vol. 3**, M. R. El-Gewely, Ed. (Elsevier Science, Amsterdam, 1997) pp 313-347; of

use in transgenic plants for insect resistance: L. Jouanin *et al.*, *Plant Sci.* **131**, 1-11 (1998).

Bacillus thuringiensis subsp. israelensis. Skeetal; Teknar.

Bacillus thuringiensis subsp. kurstaki. Deliver; DiPel; Javelin; Thuricide.

USE: Bioinsecticide.

933. Bacilysin. [29393-20-2] [1R-(1α,2β,6α)]-N-L-Alanyl-3-(5-oxo-7-oxabicyclo[4.1.0]hept-2-yl)-L-alanine; α-[(2-amino-1-oxopropyl)amino]-5-oxo-7-oxabicyclo[4.1.0]heptane-2-propanoic acid; α-(2-aminopropionamido)-5-oxo-7-oxabicyclo[4.1.0]heptane-2-propionic acid, stereoisomer; bacillin; tetaine. $C_{12}H_{18}N_2O_5$; mol wt 270.28. C 53.33%, H 6.71%, N 10.36%, O 29.60%. Antibiotic produced by the soil bacillus NCTC 7197: Gilliver *et al.*, in *Antibiotics* **vol. I**, Florey *et al.*, Eds. (Oxford, 1949) p 458. Production by *Bacillus subtilis* and purification: Rogers *et al.*, *Biochem. J.* **97**, 573 (1965). Identity with tetaine: K. Kaminski, T. Sololowska, *J. Antibiot.* **26**, 184 (1973). Identity with bacillin: K. Atsumi *et al.*, *ibid.* **28**, 77 (1975). Improved isoln: Walker, Abraham, *Biochem. J.* **118**, 557 (1970). Structural study: Rogers *et al.*, *ibid.* **97**, 579 (1965). Final structure: Walker, Abraham, *ibid.* **118**, 563 (1970).

White amorphous powder. Freely sol in water; sol in 80% alc; sparingly sol in abs alc. Stable in aq soln at 100° for 5 min at pH 7; becomes inactive at pH 2 or pH 9.

934. Bacitracin. [1405-87-4] Ak-Tracin; Baciim; Fortracin; Ocu-Tracin. Antibiotic polypeptide complex produced by *Bacillus subtilis* and *B. licheniformis*; mixture of at least nine bacitracins of which **bacitracin A** is the major component. Isoln: Johnson *et al.*, *Science* **102**, 376 (1945); Anker *et al.*, *J. Bacteriol.* **55**, 249 (1948). Purification of bacitracin by carrier displacement method: Porath, *Acta Chem. Scand.* **6**, 1237 (1952). Purification with ion exchange resin: Chaiet, Cochrane, **US 2915432** (1959 to Merck & Co.). Production: Johnson, Meleney, **US 2498165** (1950 to the U.S. Secy. of War); Freaney, Allen, **US 2828246** (1958 to Commercial Solvents). Solubilities: Weiss *et al.*, *Antibiot. Chemother.* **7**, 374 (1957). Preliminary structure studies: Hausmann *et al.*, *J. Am. Chem. Soc.* **77**, 723 (1955); Lockhart *et al.*, *Biochem. J.* **61**, 534 (1955); Stoffel, Craig, *J. Am. Chem. Soc.* **83**, 145 (1961). Structure of bacitracin A: Ressler, Kashelikar, *ibid.* **88**, 2025 (1966); Galardy *et al.*, *Biochemistry* **10**, 2429 (1971). Synthetic studies: Munekata *et al.*, *Bull. Chem. Soc. Jpn.* **46**, 3187, 3835 (1973). Mechanism of action: Storm, *Ann. N.Y. Acad. Sci.* **235**, 387 (1974). Comprehensive description: G. A. Brewen, *Anal. Profiles Drug Subs.* **9**, 1-69 (1980). *Reviews:* Craig *et al.*, "Bacitracin" in G. E. W. Wolstenholme, C. M. O'Connor, *Ciba Foundation Symposium on Amino Acids and Peptides with Antimetabolic Activity* (Little, Brown, Boston, 1958) pp 226-246; E. D. Weinberg in *Antibiotics*, D. Gottlieb, P. D. Shaw, Eds. (Springer-Verlag, New York, 1967) **I**, pp 90-99; **II**, pp 240-245; D. R. Storm, W. A. Toscano, Jr. in *Antibiotics* **vol. 5**, pt. 1, F. E. Hahn, Ed. (Springer-Verlag, New York, 1979) pp 1-17.

Bacitracin A

Grayish-white powder. Very bitter taste. Sol in water, alcohol. Practically insol in ether, chloroform, acetone. Stable in acid soln; unstable in alkaline solns. Potency loss probably due to transformation of bacitracin A to bacitracin F, latter having little antimicrobial activity.

THERAP CAT: Antibacterial.

THERAP CAT (VET): Antibacterial.

935. Bacitracin Methylenedisalicylate. [1405-88-5] Bacitracin methylenebis[2-hydroxybenzoate] (salt); bacitracin methylenedisalicylic acid; BMD; Solu-Tracin. Prepn: Baron, US 2774712 (1956 to S. B. Penick & Co.). LC determn in animal feed: G. K. Webster, *J. AOAC Int.* **80,** 732 (1997). Efficacy as growth promotant: A. L. Izat *et al., Poult. Sci.* **69,** 1787 (1990); in combination with anticoccidial agents: H. D. Chapman *et al., Avian Pathol.* **27,** 498 (1998).

White to grayish-brown powder. Slightly disagreeable odor. Somewhat less bitter than bacitracin. uv max (dil acetic acid): 318 nm, min: 280 nm. Solubility in water about 50 mg/ml. pH of satd aq soln 3.5 to 5.0. Sol in pyridine, ethanol, less sol to insol in acetone, ether, chloroform, pentane, benzene. Sol in dil aq alkali at pH 6 and higher, increasingly insol at pH 6 to 3.

Sodium salt. Creamy-white powder. Sol in water. pH 2% aq soln 9.5.

THERAP CAT (VET): Animal growth promotant; antibacterial.

936. Bacitracin Zinc. [1405-89-6] Zinc bacitracin; Albac; Baciferm. Prepn: H. S. Anker *et al., J. Bacteriol.* **55,** 249 (1948). Review of properties and formulatory characteristics: H. M. Gross, *Drug Cosmet. Ind.* **75,** 612 (1954); *idem et al., J. Am. Pharm. Assoc. Sci. Ed.* **45,** 447 (1956). Solubility data: P. J. Weiss *et al., Antibiot. Chemother.* **7,** 374 (1957). ELISA determn in animal feed: C. Williams *et al., Analyst* **119,** 427 (1994). Field trials as performance enhancer in pigs: S. C. Kyriakis *et al., Vet. Rec.* **138,** 489 (1996); in chickens: G. Huyghebaert, G. De Groote, *Poult. Sci.* **76,** 849 (1997). Clinical trial in giardiasis: B. J. Andrews *et al., Am. J. Trop. Med. Hyg.* **52,** 318 (1995); in prevention of wound infection: D. J. Dire *et al., Acad. Emerg. Med.* **2,** 4 (1995).

Creamy powder contg 1-4% H_2O. Less bitter and more stable than bacitracin. Soly at about 28° (mg/ml): water 5.1; methanol 6.55; ethanol 2.0; isopropanol 0.16; ethyl acetate 1.3; chloroform 0.01; petr ether 0.025.

THERAP CAT: Antibacterial.

THERAP CAT (VET): Antibacterial; growth promotant.

937. Baclofen. [1134-47-0] β-(Aminomethyl)-4-chlorobenzenepropanoic acid; β-(aminomethyl)-*p*-chlorohydrocinnamic acid; γ-amino-β-(*p*-chlorophenyl)butyric acid; β-(4-chlorophenyl)-GABA; Ba-34647; Baclon; Clofen; Lioresal. $C_{10}H_{12}ClNO_2$; mol wt 213.66. C 56.21%, H 5.66%, Cl 16.59%, N 6.56%, O 14.98%. Specific GABA-B receptor agonist. Prepn: **NL 6407755;** H. Keberle *et al.,* **US 3471548** (1965, 1969 both to Ciba). Toxicity study: T. Tadokoro *et al., Osaka Daigaku Igaku Zasshi* **28,** 265 (1976), *C.A.* **88,** 183016u (1978). Comprehensive description: S. Ahuja, *Anal. Profiles Drug Subs.* **14,** 527-548 (1985). Review of pharmacology and therapeutic efficacy in spasticity: R. N. Brogden *et al., Drugs* **8,** 1-14 (1974); of intrathecal use in spinal cord injury: K. S. Lewis, W. M. Mueller, *Ann. Pharmacother.* **27,** 767-774 (1993). Clinical evaluation in reflex sympathetic dystrophy: B. J. van Hilten *et al., N. Engl. J. Med.* **343,** 625 (2000).

Crystals from water, mp 206-208° (Keberle); 189-191°, (Uchimaru). LD_{50} in male mice, rats (mg/kg): 45, 78 i.v.; 103, 115 s.c.; 200, 145 orally (Tadokoro).

Hydrochloride. $C_{10}H_{13}Cl_2NO_2$. mp 179-181°.

THERAP CAT: Muscle relaxant (skeletal).

938. Bactericidal Permeability-Increasing Protein. BPI. Antibacterial protein found in azurophilic granules of mammalian neutrophils; plays a predominant role during phagocytosis. Selectively cytotoxic for gram negative bacteria; binds to both soluble and membrane lipopolysaccharide (LPS) and neutralizes endotoxin activity. Cationic protein containing 456 amino acid residues having a characteristic "boomerang" shape; mol wt ~55 kDa. Antibacterial activity resides in the amino terminal half while the C-terminal domain facilitates phagocytosis. Isoln from human polymorphonuclear leukocytes: J. Weiss *et al., J. Biol. Chem.* **253,** 2664 (1978). Cloning and primary structure: P. W. Gray *et al., ibid.* **264,** 9505 (1989). Crystal structure: L. J. Beamer *et al., Science* **276,** 1861 (1997); *eidem, Biochem. Pharmacol.* **57,** 225 (1999). ELISA determn in body fluids: M. L. White *et al., J. Immunol. Methods* **167,** 227 (1994). Review of role in host defense: P. Elsbach, *J. Leukocyte Biol.* **64,** 14-18 (1998); P. Elsbach, J. Weiss, *Curr. Opin. Immunol.* **10,** 45-49 (1998).

Opebacan. [158113-60-1] 1-193-Bactericidal/permeability-increasing protein [132-alanine] (human reduced); rBPI₂₁; Neuprex. Amino-terminal fragment of human BPI produced by recombinant DNA technology in Chinese hamster ovary cells. Biologically active mutein in which the cysteine at position 132 has been replaced with alanine; mol wt 25 kDa. Prepn: G. Theofan *et al.,* **WO 9418323;** *eidem,* **US 5420019** (1994, 1995 both to Xoma); A. H. Horwitz *et al., Protein Expression Purif.* **8,** 28 (1996). Clinical trial in meningococcal sepsis: M. Levin *et al., Lancet* **356,** 961 (2000). Review of development and clinical potential in meningococcemia and hemorrhagic trauma: P. J. Scannon *et al., J. Endotoxin Res.* **5,** 209-212 (1999); O. Levy, *Expert Opin. Invest. Drugs* **11,** 159-167 (2002).

THERAP CAT: Antisepsis; in treatment of meningococcemia.

939. Bacteriorhodopsin. BR. The only protein of the purple membrane of *Halobacterium halobium* and other halophilic bacteria. It is a rhodopsin-like pigment containing retinal linked to lysine through a Schiff's base and has a mol wt of approx 26,000. Bacteriorhodopsin functions as an energy transducer or "proton pump"; unlike animal rhodopsins, it uses light energy to generate an electrochemical gradient and this stored energy is used by the cell for ATP synthesis and other important energy-requiring functions. Discovery in the purple membrane of *Halobacterium halobium:* D. Oesterhelt, W. Stoekenius, *Nature New Biol.* **233,** 149 (1971); A. E. Blaurock, W. Stoekenius, *ibid.* 152. Isoln and identification in *H. cutirubrum:* S. C. Kushwaha, M. Kates, *Biochim. Biophys. Acta* **316,** 235 (1973). Description of functions: D. Oesterhelt, W. Stoekenius, *Proc. Natl. Acad. Sci. USA* **70,** 2853 (1973). Proposed mechanism of the "proton pump": K. Schulten, P. Tavan, *Nature* **272,** 85 (1978). Structural elucidation: Y. A. Ovchinnikov *et al., FEBS Lett.* **100,** 219 (1979); H. G. Khorana *et al., Proc. Natl. Acad. Sci. USA* **76,** 5046 (1979). Three-dimensional crystallographic study: H. Michel, D. Oesterhelt, *ibid.* **77,** 1283 (1980). Series of articles on structure, biosynthesis, and energy transduction: *Photochem. Photobiol.* **33,** 417-608 (1981). Review of energy transduction: H. V. Westerhoff, Z. Dancshazy, *Trends Biochem. Sci.* **9,** 112 (1984). Comprehensive reviews: W. Stoekenius *et al., Biochim. Biophys. Acta* **505,** 215-278 (1979); W. Stoekenius, R. A. Bogomolni, *Annu. Rev. Biochem.* **51,** 587-616 (1982). Review of crystallization, structure and function: J. Deisenhoffer, H. Michel, *Science* **245,** 1463-1473 (1989). Review of photophysical properties and optimization for use in bioelectronic devices: K. J. Wise *et al., Trends Biotechnol.* **20,** 387-394 (2002).

Bacteriorhodopsin is not bleached by light in the same fashion as animal rhodopsins; only small spectral changes are caused by transfer from light to dark. When exposed to light, BR has a broad light absorption maximum at 568 nm that slowly shifts back to 558 nm in the dark. The 558 and 568 nm states are known as the dark-adapted and light-adapted states, respectively. Light-adapted BR, upon absorption of a light quantum, undergoes a series of reversible changes, having intermediate forms with absorption maxima of 590, 550, and 412 nm. uv max (2M HCl): 565 nm. Slow bleaching occurs when membrane suspensions are illuminated in the presence of hydroxylamine or sodium borohydride. When hydroxylamine is used, the uv max is shifted to 360 nm. The bleached membrane is called the "apomembrane"; the protein after loss of the chromophore is termed ***bacterio-opsin.***

USE: As a tool in biological energy transduction research.

940. Badische Acid. [86-60-2] 7-Amino-1-naphthalenesulfonic acid; 2-naphthylamine-8-sulfonic acid. $C_{10}H_9NO_3S$;

mol wt 223.25. C 53.80%, H 4.06%, N 6.27%, O 21.50%, S 14.36%. Prepd by sulfonation of 2-naphthylamine: Green, Vakil, *J. Chem. Soc.* **113**, 35 (1918); Hennion, Schmidle, *J. Am. Chem. Soc.* **65**, 2468 (1943).

Needles or prisms. Sol in 1680 parts water, in alkalies; slightly sol in alc.

941. Bagasse. Fibrous residue from cane sugar mfg operations, which contains 50% cellulose, 25% pentosans, and 25% lignin: Wiggins, *Sugar J.* **16**, No. 8, pp 18, 22, 24 (1954), *C.A.* **48**, 9729h (1954). Review of properties and uses: Vo Tong Xuan, Samaniego, *Sugar News* **46**, 276, 284 (1970); M. A. Clarke in *Kirk-Othmer Encyclopedia of Chemical Technology* **vol. 3** (Wiley-Interscience, New York, 3rd ed., 1978) pp 434-438.

Caution: Inhalation of bagasse dust may cause pneumonitis, asthma.

USE: Raw material for pulp, paper and board.

942. Baicalein. [491-67-8] 5,6,7-Trihydroxy-2-phenyl-4*H*-1-benzopyran-4-one; 5,6,7-trihydroxyflavone; noroxylin. C_{15}-$H_{10}O_5$; mol wt 270.24. C 66.67%, H 3.73%, O 29.60%. From roots of *Scutellaria baicalensis*. Isoln and structure: Bargellini, *Gazz. Chim. Ital.* **49**, II, 47 (1919); Shibata *et al., Acta Phytochim.* **1**, 109 (1923). Synthesis: Sastri, Seshadri, *Proc. Indian Acad. Sci.* **23A**, 262 (1946), *C.A.* **41**, 449 (1947); Schönberg *et al., J. Am. Chem. Soc.* **77**, 5390 (1955); Jouanne, Mentzer, *Compt. Rend.* **254**, 727 (1962); Agasimundin, Siddappa, *J. Chem. Soc. Perkin Trans. 1* **1973**, 503. Pharmacology: Koda *et al., C.A.* **75**, 47200d (1971).

Yellow prisms from alc, dec 264-265°. uv max (ethanol): 324, 276 nm (log ε 4.18, 4.42). Sol in alcohol, methanol, ether, acetone, ethyl acetate, hot glacial acetic acid. Sparingly sol in chloroform, nitrobenzene. Practically insol in water. Sol in dil NaOH with greenish-brown color. Concd H_2SO_4 gives yellow color, green fluorescence.

THERAP CAT: Astringent.

943. Bakankosin. [1398-17-0] [3*S*-(3α,4β,4aα)]-4-Ethenyl-3-(β-D-glucopyranosyloxy)-3,4,4a,5,6,7-hexahydro-8*H*-pyrano[3,4-*c*]pyridin-8-one; bacancosin; Bakankoside. $C_{16}H_{23}$-NO_8; mol wt 357.36. C 53.78%, H 6.49%, N 3.92%, O 35.82%. Nitrogenous glucoside from seed of *Strychnos vacacoua* Baill., *Loganiaceae*. Ref: E. Bourquelot, H. Hérissey, *Compt. Rend.* **144**, 575 (1907); **147**, 750 (1908); *Arch. Pharm.* **247**, 56 (1909); K. Balenovic *et al., Helv. Chim. Acta* **35**, 2519 (1952). Proposed structure: G. Büchi, R. E. Manning, *Tetrahedron Letters* no. 26, 5 (1960); H. C. Beyerman *et al., Bull. Soc. Chim. Fr.* **1961**, 1812; H. Inouye *et al., Chem. Pharm. Bull.* **24**, 1406 (1976). Synthesis and structure: L. F. Tietze, *Tetrahedron Lett.* **29**, 2535 (1976).

Hydrate. Bitter crystals, mp 157°; when anhydr mp 200°, also reported as mp 211-212°. $[\alpha]_D$ −197°. uv max (alcohol): 235 nm (log ε 4.2). Freely sol in water, alc; slightly sol in ethyl acetate.

944. Balofloxacin. [127294-70-6] 1-Cyclopropyl-6-fluoro-1,4-dihydro-8-methoxy-7-[3-(methylamino)-1-piperidinyl]-4-oxo-3-quinolinecarboxylic acid; Q-35; Baloxin. $C_{20}H_{24}FN_3O_4$; mol wt 389.42. C 61.69%, H 6.21%, F 4.88%, N 10.79%, O 16.43%. Fluorinated quinolone antibacterial. Prepn: H. Nagano *et al.,* **EP 342675**; *eidem,* **US 5051509** (1989, 1991 both to Chugai). Photostability: K. Marutani *et al., Antimicrob. Agents Chemother.* **37**, 2217 (1993). Comparative antibacterial activity: H. Iwasaki *et al., Chemotherapy (Basel)* **41**, 100 (1995). Pharmacokinetics: T. Nakagawa *et al., Arzneim.-Forsch.* **45**, 719 (1995). HPLC determn in biological fluids: T. Nakagawa *et al., ibid.* 716. Clinical evaluation in respiratory tract infection: O. Kunii, F. Matsumoto, *Proc. 18th Int. Congr. Chemother., Stockholm 1993*, 22-23; in urinary tract infection: J. Kumazawa, F. Matsumoto, *ibid.,* 69-70.

Colorless needles from acetonitrile-water, mp 134-135°.
THERAP CAT: Antibacterial.

945. Balsalazide. [80573-04-2] 5-[(1*E*)-[4-[[(2-Carboxyethyl)amino]carbonyl]phenyl]azo]-2-hydroxybenzoic acid; *(E)*-5-[[*p*-[(2-carboxyethyl)carbamoyl]phenyl]azo]-2-salicylic acid. C_{17}-$H_{15}N_3O_6$; mol wt 357.32. C 57.14%, H 4.23%, N 11.76%, O 26.87%. Analog of sulfasalazine, *q.v.* Prodrug of 5-aminosalicylic acid where carrier molecule is 4-aminobenzoyl-β-alanine. Prepn: R. P. K. Chan, **GB 2080796**; *idem,* **US 4412992** (1982, 1983 both to Biorex). Toxicology study and clinical metabolism: *idem et al., Dig. Dis. Sci.* **28**, 609 (1983). Review of pharmacology and clinical efficacy in ulcerative colitis: A. Prakash, C. M. Spencer, *Drugs* **56**, 83 (1998).

Crystals from hot ethanol, mp 254-255°.
Disodium salt dihydrate. [150399-21-6]; [82101-18-6] (anhydrous). BX-661A; Colazal; Colazide. $C_{17}H_{13}N_3Na_2O_6.2H_2O$; mol wt 437.31. Orange to yellow microcrystalline powder, mp >350°. Nonhygroscopic. Freely sol in water, isotonic saline; sparingly sol in methanol, ethanol. Practically insol in organic solvents.
THERAP CAT: Anti-inflammatory (gastrointestinal).

946. Balsam Canada. Canada turpentine; balsam of fir. Improperly **"Balm of Gilead"**. Liquid oleoresin from *Abies balsamea* (L.), Mill., *Pinaceae. Habit.* Canada and Northern U.S. to Va., west to Minnesota. *Constit.* 27.5% Volatiles (pinene, nopinene, β-phellandrene), 44.5% resin acid (13% abietic, 8% neoabietic), 27% neutral resinous compounds. *Ref:* Lombard *et al., Peint. Pigm. Vernis* **34**, 106 (1958), *C.A.* **52**, 12420 (1958).

Yellowish to greenish, viscid, transparent, slightly fluorescent liquid; agreeable, aromatic pine-like odor; bitter taste; on exposure to air gradually solidifies to a solid, noncryst mass. d 0.987-0.994. n_4^{20} 1.52-1.54. $[\alpha]_D^{20}$ +1 to +4°. Acid no. 84-87. Sapon no. 89.4-95.7 (2 g in xylene for 1 hr). Insoluble in water; miscible with benzene, chloroform, xylene, ethyl acetate, oil of cedar; completely sol or almost sol in ether, oil turpentine; about 90% dissolves in alcohol or petr ether.

USE: Cement for lenses; manuf fine lacquers; for mounting in microscopy.

947. Balsam Gurjun. Wood oil; "East Indian Copaiba". Oleoresin from various species of *Dipterocarpus, Dipterocarpaceae*. *Habit.* Eastern India, Burma. *Constit.* About 75% volatile oil, boiling at about 255°; gurjunic acid, resin, bitter substance sol in water. Isoln of an optically inactive sesquiterpene δ-elemene, from gurjun balsam: Gough, Powell, *Tetrahedron Lett.* **1961,** 763.

Clear liquid, light brown by transmitted light with greenish fluorescence; somewhat bitter, but not very acrid taste. Acid no. 5-15. Sapon no. 10-20 (2 g in 20 g xylene for 1 hr); d 0.95-0.97; $[\alpha]_D$ −23 to −70°; n_D^{28} 1.510-1.516. Insol in water. Completely sol in benzene, chloroform; incompletely in alcohol, ether, carbon disulfide, petr ether.

USE: As of copaiba; adapted for varnishes and lacquers, particularly for articles to be exposed to a temp of 80° or so.

948. Balsam Mecca. Balm of Gilead; balsam of Gilead; balsán-Katél; Duhnul-balsan. Balsam obtained from twigs of *Commiphora opobalsamum* (Kunth.) Engl. (*Balsamodendrum gilaedense* Kunth.), *Burseraceae.*

Light-colored, mobile to viscid, turbid, brownish-red liquid; aromatic odor. Insoluble in water; sol in alcohol, benzene, chloroform, acetone, glacial acetic acid, carbon disulfide, oil turpentine, ether.

USE: In perfumery.

949. Balsam Peru. Peruvian balsam; Indian balsam; China oil; Black balsam; Honduras balsam; Surinam balsam. From *Toluifera pereirae* (Klotzsch) Baill. (*Myroxylon pereirae* Klotzsch), *Leguminosae. Habit.* Central America (San Salvador) in forests near Pacific coast. *Constit.* 50-60% cinnamein—esters of cinnamic and benzoic acid; about 28% resin, styracine, vanillin. *Ref:* Bergemann, *Pharmazie* **5,** 494 (1950); Cortesi, *Bull. Soc. Pharm. Bordeaux* **89,** 141 (1951), *C.A.* **46,** 1718b (1952).

Dark brown, viscid liquid; pleasant aromatic odor; warm, bitter taste and persistent aftertaste. d 1.150-1.170. Insol in water, olive oil; sol in alcohol, chloroform and glacial acetic acid, usually with a slight opalescence. Partly sol in ether, petr ether.

USE: In perfumery and some chocolate flavorings; also in masking of odors.

THERAP CAT: Vulnerary; ectoparasiticide (scabies).

THERAP CAT (VET): Vulnerary; miticide.

950. Balsam Tolu. Thomas balsam; opobalsam; resin Tolu. From *Toluifera balsamum* L. (*Myroxylon toluiferum* H. B. K.), *Leguminosae. Habit.* South America (Venezuela, Colombia, Peru) on elevated plains and mountains. *Constit.* 12-15% free cinnamic and benzoic acids; about 40% benzyl, etc., esters of these acids (5.2-13.4% cinnamein); 1.5-3% volatile oil. *Ref:* Rosenthaler, *Pharm. Ztg.-Nachr.* **88,** 716 (1952), *C.A.* **47,** 5076 (1953).

Yellowish-brown or brown, semifluid or nearly solid, resinous mass; aromatic odor and taste; brittle when cold. Insol in water; almost insol in petr ether. Sol in alcohol, benzene, chloroform, ether, glacial acetic acid, partially in carbon disulfide or NaOH.

USE: In perfumery, confectionery and chewing gums. In pharmacy, as ingredient and vehicle for expectorants.

THERAP CAT: Expectorant.

THERAP CAT (VET): Has been used as an expectorant.

951. Balsam Traumatic. Friar's balsam; Turlington's balsam. Composed of 100 parts benzoin, 35 storax, 35 balsam Tolu, 16 balsam Peru, 8 aloe, 8 myrrh, 4 angelica, and alcohol to make 1000.

THERAP CAT: Topical protectant; expectorant.

THERAP CAT (VET): Has been used for chronic bronchitis. Wound antiseptic and styptic.

952. Bambermycins. [11015-37-5] Moenomycin; flavophospholipol; Flavomycin. Antibiotic complex comprised of at least 4 active components, moenomycins A, B$_1$, B$_2$ and C, with **moenomycin A** being the major component. Obtained from cultures of *Streptomyces bambergiensis, S. ghanaensis, S. ederensis, S. geysiriensis* and related strains: Wallhäuser *et al., Antimicrob. Agents Chemother.* **1965,** 734 *sqq.; NL 6602132* *C.A.* **66,** 74946x (1967) and Lindner, Wallhäuser, *US 3674866* (1966, 1972 both to Hoechst). Structural studies: Tschesche *et al., Ann.* **720,** 58

(1968); *Tetrahedron Lett.* **1968,** 2905; **1969,** 141; Huber, *J. Antibiot.* **25,** 1226 (1972); P. Welzel *et al., Tetrahedron Lett.* **1973,** 227; F. J. Witteler *et al., ibid.* **1979,** 3493; P. Welzel *et al., Tetrahedron* **39,** 1583 (1983). Structure of moenomycin A: P. Welzel *et al., Angew. Chem. Int. Ed.* **20,** 121 (1981). Synthesis of **moenocinol,** the lipid moiety: Tschesche, Reden, *Ann.* **1974,** 853; P. J. Kocienski, *J. Org. Chem.* **45,** 2037 (1980); R. M. Coates, M. W. Johnson, *ibid.* 2685. *Review:* G. Huber in *Antibiotics* **vol. 5,** pt. 1, F. E. Hahn, Ed. (Springer-Verlag, New York, 1979) pp 135-153.

Moenomycin A

Complex is a colorless, amorphous solid, no definite mp, decompn starting at 200°C. uv max (water pH 7): 258 nm ($E_{1cm}^{1\%}$ 60). Sol in water, methanol, DMF; less sol in ethanol, propanol; slightly sol in ether, ethyl acetate. Insol in benzene, chloroform. Stable in neutral aq and methanolic solns; slowly decomp in acid and alkaline solns. LD$_{50}$ in mice (mg/kg): >2000 orally, s.c. and i.p.; 1400 i.v. (Lindner, Wallhäuser).

THERAP CAT: Antibacterial.

THERAP CAT (VET): Antibacterial; feed additive (poultry, swine and calves).

953. Bambuterol. [81732-65-2] Dimethylcarbamic acid 5-[2-[(1,1-dimethylethyl)amino]-1-hydroxyethyl]-1,3-phenylene ester; 1-[bis(3',5'-N,N-dimethylcarbamoyloxy)phenyl]-2-N-tert-butyl-aminoethanol; (±)-5-[2-(*tert*-butylamino)-1-hydroxyethyl]-*m*-phenylene bis(dimethylcarbamate); terbutaline bisdimethylcarbamate. C$_{18}$H$_{29}$N$_3$O$_5$; mol wt 367.44. C 58.84%, H 7.96%, N 11.44%, O 21.77%. Ester prodrug of the β$_2$-adrenergic agonist terbutaline, *q.v.* Prepn: O. A. T. Olsson *et al., EP 43807; eidem, US 4419364* (1982, 1983 both to AB Draco). Pharmacology: O. A. T. Olsson, L.-A. Svensson, *Pharm. Res.* **1984,** 19. Review of pharmacology and metabolism: L.-A. Svensson, *Acta Pharm. Suec.* **24,** 333 (1987). LC determn: O. Wannerberg, B. Persson, *J. Chromatogr.* **435,** 199 (1988). Clinical evaluation in asthma: T. Sandström *et al., Respiration* **53,** 31 (1988). Clinical comparison with terbutaline: G. Persson *et al., Eur. Respir. J.* **1,** 223 (1988).

Hydrochloride. [81732-46-9] KWD-2183; Bambec. C$_{18}$H$_{29}$-N$_3$O$_5$.HCl; mol wt 403.90.

THERAP CAT: Bronchodilator.

954. Bamethan. [3703-79-5] α-[(Butylamino)methyl]-4-hydroxybenzenemethanol; α-[(butylamino)methyl]-*p*-hydroxybenzyl alcohol; 1-(*p*-hydroxyphenyl)-2-butylaminoethanol; 1-(4-hydroxyphenyl)-1-hydroxy-2-butylaminoethane; 2-butylamino-1-*p*-hydroxyphenylethanol. $C_{12}H_{19}NO_2$; mol wt 209.28. C 68.87%, H 9.15%, N 6.69%, O 15.29%. Prepn: Corrigan *et al., J. Am. Chem. Soc.* **67**, 1894 (1945); Kovács, *Pharm. Zentralhalle* **92**, 193 (1953), *C.A.* **49**, 936 (1955). Metabolism of sulfate: Hajos, Szporny, *Arzneim.-Forsch.* **18**, 1212 (1968).

Crystals, mp 123.5-125°.
Hydrochloride. $C_{12}H_{19}NO_2$.HCl. mp 109-110°.
Sulfate. [5716-20-1] Vasculat; Vasculit; Bupatol; Garmian. $(C_{12}H_{19}NO_2)_2.H_2SO_4$; mol wt 516.65.
THERAP CAT: Vasodilator (peripheral).

955. Bamifylline. [2016-63-9] 7-[2-[Ethyl(2-hydroxyethyl)amino]ethyl]-3,7-dihydro-1,3-dimethyl-8-(phenylmethyl)-1*H*-purine-2,6-dione; 8-benzyl-7-[2-[ethyl(2-hydroxyethyl)amino]-ethyl]theophylline; 8-benzyl-7-[*N*-ethyl-*N*-(β-hydroxyethyl)amino-ethyl]theophylline; benzetamophylline; bamiphylline; 8102 CB. $C_{20}H_{27}N_5O_3$; mol wt 385.46. C 62.32%, H 7.06%, N 18.17%, O 12.45%. Prepn: BE 602888 (1961 to Christiaens), *C.A.* **56**, 5981c (1962). Pharmacology: Georges *et al., Therapie* **17**, 211 (1962). Metabolism: Dodion *et al., Arzneim.-Forsch.* **19**, 785 (1969). Toxicological studies: Georges *et al., ibid.* **18**, 460 (1968).

Crystals, mp 80-80.5°.
Hydrochloride. [20684-06-4] AC-3810; BAX-2739Z; Briofil; Trentadil. $C_{20}H_{27}N_5O_3$.HCl; mol wt 421.92. Crystals, mp 185-186°. LD$_{50}$ in mice, rats (mg/kg): 246, 1139 orally; 89, 131 i.p.; 67, 65 i.v. (Georges).
THERAP CAT: Bronchodilator.

956. Bamipine. [4945-47-5] 1-Methyl-*N*-phenyl-*N*-(phenylmethyl)-4-piperidinamine; 4-*N*-benzylanilino-1-methylpiperidine; *N*-phenyl-*N*-benzyl-4-amino-1-methylpiperidine. $C_{19}H_{24}N_2$; mol wt 280.41. C 81.38%, H 8.63%, N 9.99%. Prepn: Kallischnigg, US 2683714 (1954 to Knoll). Toxicity studies: Hanna, *Toxicol. Appl. Pharmacol.* **3**, 393 (1961). Determn in pharmaceutical preparations: M. H. Barary, *Pharmazie* **39**, 706 (1984).

Crystals from butanone or methanol, mp 115°.
Hydrochloride. [1229-69-2] Soventol. $C_{19}H_{24}N_2$.HCl; mol wt 316.87.
THERAP CAT: Antihistaminic.

957. BAPTA. [85233-19-8] *N,N*´-[1,2-Ethanediylbis(oxy-2,1-phenylene)]bis[*N*-(carboxymethyl)glycine]; 1,2-bis(2-aminophenoxy)ethane-*N,N,N*´,*N*´-tetraacetic acid. $C_{22}H_{24}N_2O_{10}$; mol wt 476.43. C 55.46%, H 5.08%, N 5.88%, O 33.58%. Calcium (Ca^{2+}) chelator derived from EGTA. Ca^{2+} binding causes a shift in the uv absorbance and fluorescence of the molecule. Parent com-

pound of second generation fluorescent imaging agents such as Indo-1, Fura-2, *q.q.v.* Prepn: R. Y. Tsien, *Biochemistry* **19**, 2396 (1980). Dissociation constants: R. Pethig *et al., Cell Calcium* **10**, 491 (1989). Use as chelator: P. W. Marks, F. R. Maxfield, *Anal. Biochem.* **193**, 61 (1991). Binding constants and fluorescence with heavy metals: A. Yuchi *et al., Bull. Chem. Soc. Jpn.* **66**, 3377 (1993). Prepn of ^{19}F-forms and use for intracellular Ca^{2+} measurement: G. A. Smith *et al., Proc. Natl. Acad. Sci. USA* **80**, 7178 (1983); L. A. Levy *et al., Am. J. Physiol.* **252**, C441 (1987). NMR determn of Ca^{2+} in brain by **5F-BAPTA**: H. S. Bachelard *et al., J. Neurochem.* **51**, 1311 (1988).

uv max (free dye): 209, 254 nm (ε 3.8 × 10^4, 1.6 × 10^4). uv max (complexed form): 203, 274 nm (ε 4.1 × 10^4, 4.2 ×10^3).
USE: As calcium chelator; ^{19}F labelled forms for measurement of intracellular calcium.

958. Baptigenin. [5908-63-4] 7-Hydroxy-3-(3,4,5-trihydroxyphenyl)-4*H*-1-benzopyran-4-one; 7,3´,4´,5´-tetrahydroxy-isoflavone. $C_{15}H_{10}O_6$; mol wt 286.24. C 62.94%, H 3.52%, O 33.54%. The aglucon of baptisin. From baptisin by acid hydrolysis or vacuum sublimation. From *radix Baptisiae:* Fischer, Ehrlich, *C.A.* **31**, 4449^3 (1937). Structure: Böhm, *Arzneim.-Forsch.* **10**, 472 (1960). Synthesis: Farkas *et al., Ber.* **96**, 1865 (1963). *See also* Pseudobaptigenin.

Needles from dil ethanol, mp 284-285°. Begins to sublime at 240°. Sublimes in oil pump vacuum at 180-200°. uv max (ethanol): 270.2, 247 nm. Practically insol in water, ammonia water; slightly sol in dil alc, hot glacial acetic acid; sol in acetone, in NaOH solns.
Tetraacetylbaptigenin. $C_{23}H_{18}O_{10}$. Needles from methanol, mp 214°.
Tetrabenzoylbaptigenin. $C_{43}H_{26}O_{10}$. Prisms from methanol, mp 191-192°.
Tetramethylbaptigenin. $C_{19}H_{18}O_6$. Crystals from methanol, mp 144-145°.

959. Baptisia. Wild indigo; indigo weed; false indigo; yellow indigo. Perennial herb. *Habit.* North America. Medicinal baptisia, from root of *Baptisia tinctoria* R. Br., *Leguminosae. Constit.* Baptin—a purgative glucoside, baptisin—a bitter glucoside, baptitoxine (identical with cytisine), an alkaloid. Also contains a blue dye which has been used as a substitute for indigo.
THERAP CAT: Anti-infective.

960. Barbasco. Name applied in the Spanish-speaking countries of the New World to many unrelated plants used to poison or stun fish. In Mexico it usually means roots of *Dioscorea composita* Hemsl., or of *Dioscorea tepinapensis* Uline, *Dioscoreaceae* which yield up to 5% of their dry weight in diosgenin: *Chem. Week* **79**, no. 2, p 20 (July 14, 1956). Isoln procedure: Julian, US 3019220 (1962 to Julian Labs.). Book: D. G. Coursey, *Yams* (Longmans, London, 1967) 230 pp, an account of the nature, origins, cultivation and utilization of the useful members of the *Dioscoreaceae. Compare* Yam, Mexican.

961. Barberry Bark. Berberis bark; jaundice berry; wood-sour; sowberry; pepperidge bush; sour-spine. Root bark of *Berberis vulgaris* L., *Berberidaceae*. *Habit*. Europe and Western Asia; also U.S. (New England States, Pennsylvania and Virginia). *Constit*. Berberine, berbamine, oxyacanthine, tannin, wax, fat, resin. *Ref:* Neugebauer, Brunner, *Pharm. Zentralhalle* **80**, 113 (1939).

962. Barbital. [57-44-3] 5,5-Diethyl-2,4,6($1H,3H,5H$)-pyrimidinetrione; 5,5-diethylbarbituric acid; barbitone; diethyl-malonylurea; Veronal. $C_8H_{12}N_2O_3$; mol wt 184.19. C 52.17%, H 6.57%, N 15.21%, O 26.06%. Prototype of the barbiturate hypnotics. Prepn: M. Conrad, M. Guthzeit, *Ber.* **15**, 2841 (1882); E. Fischer, A. Dilthey, *Ann.* **335**, 334 (1904). Use as physiological buffer: L. Michaelis, *J. Biol. Chem.* **87**, 33 (1930); in enzyme determn: J. Bergerman, *Clin. Chem.* **12**, 797 (1966).

Faintly bitter needles (trigonal in the stable phase) from water, mp 188-192°. Can be sublimed *in vacuo*. pK (25°) 7.43. One gram dissolves in about 130 ml water, 13 ml boiling water, 14 ml alcohol, 75 ml chloroform, 35 ml ether. Sol in acetone, ethyl acetate, alkalies, petr ether, acetic acid, amyl alcohol, pyridine, aniline, nitrobenzene.

Sodium salt. [144-02-5] Barbital sodium; sodium 5,5-diethyl-barbiturate; barbitone sodium; soluble barbital; sodium diethyl-malonylurea; Veronal sodium; Medinal. $C_8H_{11}N_2NaO_3$; mol wt 206.17. Bitter crystals or powder. One gram dissolves in 5 ml water, 2.5 ml boiling water, 400 ml alc. Aq soln is alkaline to litmus and phenolphthalein. pH of 0.1 molar aq soln, 9.4.

Note: This is a controlled substance (depressant): **21 CFR**, 1308.14.

USE: Biological buffer.

THERAP CAT: Sedative, hypnotic.

THERAP CAT (VET): Sedative, hypnotic.

963. Barbituric Acid. [67-52-7] 2,4,6($1H,3H,5H$)-pyrimidinetrione; malonylurea; 2,4,6-trioxohexahydropyrimidine. $C_4H_4N_2O_3$; mol wt 128.09. C 37.51% H 3.15%, N 21.87%, O 37.47%. Prepn from hydurilic acid + nitric acid: Baeyer, *Ann.* **127**, 199 (1863); *ibid.* **130**, 129 (1864). Structure: Mulder, *Ber.* **6**, 1233 (1873). Prepd from ethyl malonate and urea using sodium ethoxide as a condensing agent: Dickey, Gray, *Org. Synth.* **coll. vol. II**, 60 (1943). Crystal structure: Bolton, *Nature* **201**, 987 (1964). Toxicity study: E. I. Goldenthal, *Toxicol. Appl. Pharmacol.* **18**, 185 (1971). Unsubstituted barbituric acid has no hypnotic properties. *Review:* Carter, *J. Chem. Educ.* **28**, 524 (1951).

Dihydrate. Rhombs from water. mp ~248° when anhydrous, with some decompn. Strong acid. K at 25° = 9.9 × 10^{-5}. uv spectrum: Hartley, *J. Chem. Soc.* **87**, 1808 (1905). Difficultly sol in cold water; freely sol in hot water, in dil acids. Forms salts with metals. LD$_{50}$ orally in male rats: >5000 mg/kg (Goldenthal).

USE: Manuf plastics, pharmaceuticals.

964. Barium. [7440-39-3] Ba; at. wt. 137.327; at. no. 56; valence 2. Group IIA (2). Alkaline earth metal. Abundance in earth's crust 0.05% by wt. Naturally occurring isotopes: 138 (71.70%); 137 (11.23%); 136 (7.85%); 135 (6.593%); 134 (2.42%); 132 (0.101%); 130 (0.106%). Known radioactive isotopes: 117, 119-129, 131, 133, 139-149. Does not occur free in nature as metal. Compds occur in minerals barite and witherite. Commercial production by thermal reduction of barium oxide with aluminum. First prepared as a mercury amalgam by Davy in 1808.

Toxicity studies of barium compds: Syed, Hosain, *Toxicol. Appl. Pharmacol.* **22**, 150 (1972). *Reviews: Gmelins, Barium* (8th ed.) **30**, (1960); Goodenough, Stenger, "Magnesium, Calcium, Strontium, Barium and Radium" in *Comprehensive Inorganic Chemistry* **Vol. 1**, J. C. Bailar, Jr. *et al.*, Eds. (Pergamon Press, Oxford, 1973) pp 591-664; *Chemistry of the Elements*, N. N. Greenwood, A. Earnshaw, Eds. (Pergamon Press, New York, 1984) pp 117-154; C. Boffito in *Kirk-Othmer Encyclopedia of Chemical Technology* **vol. 3** (Wiley-Interscience, New York, 4th ed., 1992) pp 902-908. Review of toxicology and human exposure: *Toxicological Profile for Barium and Compounds* (PB93-110658, 1992) 163 pp.

Silvery-white, slightly lustrous metal when pure; yellowish-white when contaminated with nitrogen. Body-centered cubic structure at atm pressure. Soft, ductile. Fairly volatile; extremely reactive, very easily oxidizable; must be kept under petroleum or other oxygen-free liquid to exclude air. Reacts vigorously with water, liberating hydrogen and creating an explosion hazard. Keep dry and tightly sealed. Pyrophoric when finely divided; store powder under dry argon or helium. d 3.6. mp ~710°. bp ~1600°. E^0 (aq) Ba^{2+}/Ba −2.91 V. Emits characteristic yellow-green color in flame. Dissolves in liq NH$_3$ to give deep blue-black solns. Solns of sol barium salts give a white ppt with H$_2$SO$_4$ or sol sulfates.

Caution: Potential symptoms of overexposure to soluble barium compounds are excessive salivation, vomiting, colic, diarrhea, convulsive tremors, slow, hard pulse, elevated blood pressure, confusion; hemorrhages in stomach, intestines, kidneys; respiratory failure, cardiac arrest. *See: Clinical Toxicology of Commercial Products*, R. E. Gosselin *et al.*, Eds. (Williams & Wilkins, Baltimore, 5th ed., 1984) Section III, pp 61-63; *Patty's Industrial Hygiene and Toxicology* **vol. 2C**, G. D. Clayton, F. E. Clayton, Eds. (Wiley-Interscience, New York, 4th ed., 1994) pp 1925-1930.

USE: Alloys with Al or Mg as "getters" to remove residual gases from vacuum systems and electronic tubes. Deoxidizer for steel and other metals. Carrier for radium. The β- and γ-radiation emitted by ^{140}Ba + ^{140}La makes a large contribution to the activity of the fission products of uranium rods during the first few weeks after their withdrawal from the reactor. The emissions from ^{133}Ba and ^{137m}Ba as standards in γ-spectrometry: Haissinsky, Adloff, *Radiochemical Survey of the Elements* (Elsevier, 1965) pp 12-14.

965. Barium Acetate. [543-80-6] $C_4H_6BaO_4$; mol wt 255.42. C 18.81%, H 2.37%, Ba 53.77%, O 25.06%. Ba($C_2H_3O_2$)$_2$. Prepn: *Gmelins, Barium* (8th ed.) **30**, 315 (1932) and supplement, 478 (1960). Toxicity study: Syed, Hosain, *Toxicol. Appl. Pharmacol.* **22**, 150 (1972).

Monohydrate. *Poisonous!* d 2.19. Loses its H$_2$O of hydration at 110°. One gram dissolves in 1.5 ml cold or boiling water, in 700 ml alc. The aq soln is neutral or slightly acid to litmus. LD$_{50}$ i.v. in ICR mice: 23.31 mg Ba^{2+}/kg (Syed, Hosain).

USE: Mordant for printing fabrics; in lubricating oil and grease; as catalyst for organic reactions.

966. Barium Benzenesulfonate. [515-72-0] Benzenesulfonic acid barium salt. $C_{12}H_{10}BaO_6S_2$; mol wt 451.66. C 31.91%, H 2.23%, Ba 30.40%, O 21.25%, S 14.20%. Prepn: Freund, *Ann.* **120**, 76 (1861).

Monohydrate. White, nacreous leaflets. *Poisonous!* Freely sol in water; slightly sol in alc.

USE: Lubricating oil additives.

967. Barium Bromate. [13967-90-3] BaBr$_2$O$_6$; mol wt 393.13. Ba 34.93%, Br 40.65%, O 24.42%. Ba(BrO$_3$)$_2$. Prepd from potassium bromate and barium chloride: Pearce, Russell, *Inorg. Synth.* **2**, 20 (1946).

Monohydrate. Monoclinic crystals from hot water. *Poisonous!* May develop slight odor of bromine on long standing. d 3.99. Dec. at 260°. Sol in water (g/100 ml): 0.44 (10°); 0.96 (30°); 5.39 (100°). Sol in acetone. Practically insol in alc, most other organic solvents.

USE: In the prepn of rare earth bromates; as corrosion inhibitor for low-C steel.

968. Barium Bromide. [10553-31-8] BaBr$_2$; mol wt 297.14. Ba 46.22%, Br 53.78%. Prepn: *Gmelins, Barium* (8th ed.) **30**, 223 (1932) and supplement 380-381 (1960).

Dihydrate, crystals or granules; loses 1H$_2$O at 75° and all the H$_2$O at 120°. *Poisonous!* mp ~850° when anhydr. Very sol in water;

sol in methanol. Almost insol in ethanol, ethyl acetate, acetone, dioxane.

USE: In the manuf of other bromides; in the prepn of phosphors.

969. Barium Carbonate. [513-77-9] $CBaO_3$; mol wt 197.34. C 6.09%, Ba 69.59%, O 24.32%. $BaCO_3$. Occurs in nature as the mineral *witherite*. Prepn: *Gmelins, Barium* (8th ed) **30**, 301-303 (1932) and supplement, 186-188, 461-466 (1960). Manuf: *Faith, Keyes & Clark's Industrial Chemicals*, F. A. Lowenheim, M. K. Moran, Eds. (Wiley-Interscience, New York, 4th ed., 1975) pp 121-125.

White, heavy powder. *Poisonous!* d (witherite) 4.2865. At about 1300° dec into BaO and CO_2. Almost insol in water, 0.024 g in a liter. Slightly sol (1:1000) in CO_2-water; sol in dil HCl, HNO_3 or acetic acid; also sol in soln NH_4Cl or NH_4NO_3.

Caution: Potential symptoms of overexposure are excessive salivation, vomiting, severe abdominal pain, violent diarrhea; increased blood pressure; tinnitis, giddiness, vertigo; muscle twitching, convulsions, paralysis; dilated pupils; confusion, somnolence; cardiac arrest; death due to respiratory failure. *See Clinical Toxicology of Commercial Products*, R. E. Gosselin *et al.*, (Williams & Wilkins, Baltimore, 5th ed., 1984) Section III, pp 61-63.

USE: Rat poison; in ceramics, paints, enamels, marble substitutes, rubber; manuf of paper, barium salts, electrodes, optical glasses; as an analytical reagent.

970. Barium Chlorate. [13477-00-4] $BaCl_2O_6$; mol wt 304.23. Ba 45.14%, Cl 23.31%, O 31.55%. $Ba(ClO_3)_2$. Prepn: Vanino, *Handb. Präp. Chem., Anorgan. Teil* (2.Aufl., Stuttgart, 1925) p 297; Schmeisser in *Handbook of Preparative Inorganic Chemistry* Vol. 1, G. Brauer, Ed. (Academic Press, New York, 2nd ed., 1963) p 314. Large-scale process: Munroe, *Chem. Metall. Eng.* **23**, 188 (1920). Also prepd by electrolysis of barium chloride.

Monohydrate. Monoclinic prismatic crystals. *Poisonous!* d 3.179. Loses its water of hydration at 120°, begins to give off oxygen at 250°, mp 414°. Freely sol in water; sol in hydrochloric acid; moderately sol in ethylamine; very sparingly sol in alc, somewhat more in acetone. Practically insol in ethyl acetate, pyridine. Fire hazard when in contact with combustible material.

USE: In pyrotechnics (green fire); manuf of explosives and matches; mordant in dyeing.

971. Barium Chloride. [10361-37-2] $BaCl_2$; mol wt 208.23. Ba 65.95%, Cl 34.05%. Prepn: *Gmelins, Barium* (8th ed) **30**, 171-175 (1932) and supplement, 179-181, 324-325 (1960). Toxicity studies: I. B. Syed, F. Hosain, *Toxicol. Appl. Pharmacol.* **22**, 150 (1972). Induction of arrhythmia in exptl animals: F. W. Eichbaum, *Basic Res. Cardiol.* **68**, 73 (1973).

Dihydrate. Crystals or granules or powder; bitter salty taste. d 3.86; mp 963°. *Poisonous!* Very sol in water; sol in methanol. Practically insol in ethanol, acetone, ethyl acetate. LD_{50} i.v. in ICR mice: 19.2 mg Ba^{2+}/kg (Syed, Hosain).

Caution: Potential symptoms of overexposure are irritation of eyes, skin and upper respiratory system; gastroenteritis; muscle spasm; slow pulse, extrasystoles; hypokalemia; skin burns. *See NIOSH Pocket Guide to Chemical Hazards* (DHHS/NIOSH 97-140, 1997) p 24.

USE: Manuf pigments, color lakes, glass, mordant for acid dyes; weighting and dyeing textile fabrics; in Al refining; as pesticide; boiler compds for softening water; tanning and finishing leather.

THERAP CAT (VET): Formerly used as purgative in horses, ruminatoric in cattle.

972. Barium Chromate(VI). [10294-40-3] C.I. 77103; C.I. Pigment Yellow 31; Baryta yellow; lemon yellow; permanent yellow; Steinbühl yellow; ultramarine yellow. $BaCrO_4$; mol wt 253.32. Ba 54.21%, Cr 20.53%, O 25.26%. Prepn: Beyer, Rieman, *J. Am. Chem. Soc.* **65**, 971 (1943); *Colour Index* vol. 4 (3rd ed., 1971) p 4656.

Yellow, heavy, monoclinic, orthorhombic crystals. *Poisonous!* d 4.50. Practically insol in water, dil acetic or chromic acids. Dissolved or dec by mineral acids.

USE: As a pigment almost entirely in anticorrosion jointing pastes to prevent electro-chemical corrosion at junctions of dissimilar metals; some use in artists' colors and in coloring glass, ceramics, porcelain. Also used in metal primers, pyrotechnic compositions.

973. Barium Cyanide. [542-62-1] C_2BaN_2; mol wt 189.36. C 12.69%, Ba 72.52%, N 14.79%. $Ba(CN)_2$. Prepn: **GB 602393** (1948 to I.C.I.); *Gmelins, Barium* (8th ed.) **30**, 327 (1932) and supplement 483 (1960).

Crystals; slowly dec in air. *Very poisonous!* Very sol in water; sol in alcohol.

USE: In electroplating processes; in metallurgy.

974. Barium Fluoride. [7787-32-8] BaF_2; mol wt 175.32. Ba 78.33%, F 21.67%. Prepd by dissolving $BaCO_3$ in excess HF, evaporating to dryness, and heating to red heat: W. Olbrich, *Thesis* (Technische Hochschule, Breslau, 1929), p 2; Kwasnik in *Handbook of Preparative Inorganic Chemistry* vol. 1, G. Brauer, Ed., (Academic Press, New York, 2nd ed., 1963) p 234.

Transparent cubic crystals (fluorite lattice). *Poisonous!* d 4.83. mp 1353°. bp 2260°. Soly in water (g/l): 1.586 (10°); 1.607 (20°); 1.620 (30°). Also sol in hydrochloric, nitric, hydrofluoric acids and in aq solns of ammonium chloride. May be stored in glass bottles.

USE: As a flux and opacifier in vitreous enamels; in the manuf of carbon brushes for DC motors and generators; in heat-treating metals; in embalming; in glass manuf.

975. Barium Formate. [541-43-5] $C_2H_2BaO_4$; mol wt 227.36. C 10.57%, H 0.89%, Ba 60.40%, O 28.15%. $Ba(HCOO)_2$. Prepn: *Gmelins, Barium* (8th ed) **30**, 311 (1932), and supplement, 477 (1960).

Crystals. *Poisonous!* d 3.21. Soluble in 4 parts cold, 3 parts boiling water. Practically insol in alcohol.

976. Barium Hexafluorosilicate. [17125-80-3] Barium fluosilicate; barium silicofluoride. BaF_6Si; mol wt 279.40. Ba 49.15%, F 40.80%, Si 10.05%. $BaSiF_6$. Prepd from $BaCl_2$ and H_2SiF_6: Truchot, *Compt. Rend.* **98**, 821 (1884); Hoffmann, Gutowsky, *Inorg. Synth.* **4**, 145 (1953).

Orthorhombic needles. d_4^{21} 4.29. Dec at 300°. Heat of formation (solid) -677.42 kcal/mol. Soly in water (g/100 ml H_2O): 0.015 (0°); 0.0235 (25°); 0.091 (100°). Prolonged contact with water produces hydrolysis which is much accelerated by the presence of alkali. Slightly sol in dil acids; sol in ammonium chloride soln; practically insol in alc.

Caution: Highly toxic, especially when brought into soln by alkali.

USE: Prepn of silicon tetrafluoride; as pesticide.

977. Barium Hydroxide. [17194-00-2] Barium dihydroxide; activated barium hydroxide; caustic baryta. BaH_2O_2; mol wt 171.34. Ba 80.15%, H 1.18%, O 18.68%. $Ba(OH)_2$. Reacts as base/nucleophile in organic syntheses. Prepn: *Gmelins, Barium* (8th ed) **30**, 106-111 and suppl. 175-177, 289 (1960). Thermal dehydration and decomposition study: G. M. Habashy, G. A. Kolta, *J. Inorg. Nucl. Chem.* **34**, 57 (1972). Use as a catalyst in organic synthesis: J. Barrios *et al.*, *J. Catal.* **112**, 528 (1988); I. Paterson *et al.*, *Synlett* **1993**, 774; Y.-D. Gong *et al.*, *J. Org. Chem.* **63**, 4854 (1998); R. S. Varma *et al.*, *Tetrahedron Lett.* **39**, 8437 (1998). Review of synthetic applications: S. Jeanmart, *Synlett* **2002**, 1739-1740. Review of toxicology and human exposure: *Toxicological Profile for Barium and Compounds* (PB93-110658, 1992) 163 pp.

Monohydrate. [22326-55-2] Dried barium hydroxide. $BaH_2O_2.H_2O$; mol wt 189.36. Ba 72.52%, H 2.13%, O 25.35%. Obtained by heating commercial $Ba(OH)_2.8H_2O$ at 200°. White powder. *Poisonous!* d 3.743. Slightly sol in water; sol in dil acids.

Octahydrate. [12230-71-6] $BaH_2O_2.8H_2O$; mol wt 315.46. Ba 43.53%, H 5.75%, O 50.72%. Most common form of the hydroxide, readily available commerically. Transparent crystals or white masses. Very alkaline; rapidly absorbs CO_2 from air, becoming incompletely sol in water. *Poisonous!* mp 78°. Freely sol in water, methanol; slightly sol in ethanol. Practically insol in acetone. *Keep tightly closed.*

USE: In manuf of alkali, glass; in synthetic rubber vulcanization, in corrosion inhibitors, pesticides, sugar industry; boiler scale remedy; refining animal and vegetable oils; softening water. Catalyst in organic synthesis.

978. Barium Hypophosphite. [14871-79-5] $BaH_4O_4P_2$; mol wt 267.30. Ba 51.38%, H 1.51%, O 23.94%, P 23.18%. $Ba(H_2PO_2)_2$. Prepd by treating white phosphorus with barium hydroxide: $8P + 3Ba(OH)_2.8H_2O + H_2O \rightarrow 3Ba(H_2PO_2)_2.H_2O + 2PH_3$: Rose, *Pogg. Ann.* **9**, 370 (1827); Klement in *Handbook of Preparative Inorganic Chemistry* **Vol. 1**, G. Brauer, Ed. (Academic Press, New York, 2nd ed., 1963) p 557.

Monohydrate. Monoclinic platelets with nacreous sheen from hot water. *Poisonous!* d_4^{17} 2.90. Soly (g/100 ml H_2O): 28.6 (17°); 33.3 (100°). Practically insol in alcohol.

USE: In nickel plating.

979. Barium Iodate. [10567-69-8] BaI_2O_6; mol wt 487.13. Ba 28.19%, I 52.10%, O 19.71%. $Ba(IO_3)_2$. Prepn: Lambert, Yasada, *Inorg. Synth.* **7**, 13 (1963).

Monohydrate, crystals; becomes anhyd at 130°. d 5.00. *Poisonous!* Sol in 3350 parts water at 25°, 625 parts boiling water; sol in HCl or HNO_3; practically insol in alcohol.

980. Barium Iodide. [13718-50-8] BaI_2; mol wt 391.14. Ba 35.11%, I 64.89%. Prepn: *Gmelins, Barium* (8th ed) **30**, 238-239 (1932) and supplement, 394 (1960).

Dihydrate, colorless, odorless, transparent crystals or white granules; rapidly becomes reddish in the air due to liberation of iodine. *Poisonous!* d 5.15. Freely sol in water; the aq soln is neutral or slightly alkaline. Sol in alcohol, acetone. *Keep well closed and protected from light.*

USE: In the manuf of other iodides.

981. Barium Manganate(VI). [7787-35-1] Manganese green; Cassel's green; Rosenstiehl's green. $BaMnO_4$; mol wt 256.26. Ba 53.59%, Mn 21.44%, O 24.97%. Prepn: Schlesinger, Stems, *J. Am. Chem. Soc.* **46**, 1965 (1924); Jellinek, *J. Inorg. Nucl. Chem.* **13**, 329 (1960); R. S. Nyholm, P. R. Woolliams, *Inorg. Synth.* **11**, 56 (1968); Bayan, Aymonino, *Ber.* **101**, 3337 (1968); H. Firouzabadi, Z. Mostafavipoor, *Bull. Chem. Soc. Jpn.* **56**, 914 (1983).

Dark blue-green crystals. d 4.85. Disproportionates in water or dil acid to form $Ba(MnO_4)_2$ and MnO_2.

USE: As pigment in fresco painting instead of Scheele's green because not so poisonous as latter. As mild oxidizing agent in organic synthesis.

982. Barium Mercuric Iodide. [10048-99-4] Barium tetraiodomercurate(II); mercuric barium iodide. $BaHgI_4$; mol wt 845.53. Ba 16.24%, Hg 23.72%, I 60.04%.

Yellow or reddish, deliquesc crystals; said to become red even when kept in sealed tubes. d 3.5 (conc aq soln). *Poison!* Very sol in water or alc. *Keep well closed!*

USE: As an aq soln known as *Rohrbach's Soln,* for separating minerals of different densities; also for microchemical detection of alkaloids.

983. Barium Nitrate. [10022-31-8] BaN_2O_6; mol wt 261.34. Ba 52.55%, N 10.72%, O 36.73%. $Ba(NO_3)_2$. Prepn: *Gmelins, Barium* (8th ed) **30**, 149-151 (1932) and supplement, 178-179, 305 (1960). Toxicity study: Syed, Hosain, *Toxicol. Appl. Pharmacol.* **22**, 150 (1972).

Crystals or crystalline powder. *Poisonous!* d 3.24. mp ~590°; dec at higher temp. Freely sol in water; very slightly sol in alcohol, acetone. LD_{50} i.v. in ICR mice: 20.10 mg Ba^{2+}/kg (Syed, Hosain).

Caution: Potential symptoms of overexposure are upper respiratory irritation; gastroenteritis; muscle spasm; slow pulse, extrasystoles; hypokalemia; irritation of eyes and skin; skin burns. *See NIOSH Pocket Guide to Chemical Hazards* (DHHS/NIOSH 97-140, 1997) p 24.

USE: Manuf BaO_2; pyrotechnics for green fire; green signal lights; in the vacuum-tube industry.

984. Barium Nitrite. [13465-94-6] BaN_2O_4; mol wt 229.34. Ba 59.88%, N 12.21%, O 27.91%. $Ba(NO_2)_2$. Prepn: *Gmelins, Barium* (8th ed) **30**, 144-147 (1932) and suppl, 303 (1960).

Monohydrate, crystals. *Poisonous!* d 3.187. Sol in water; practically insol in alc.

USE: In diazotization reactions; prevention of corrosion of steel bars; in explosives.

985. Barium Oxalate. [516-02-9] Ethanedioic acid barium salt. C_2BaO_4; mol wt 225.35. C 10.66%, Ba 60.94%, O 28.40%. BaC_2O_4. Prepn: *Gmelins, Barium* (8th ed) **30**, 320-323 (1932) and supplement, 480-482 (1960).

Monohydrate. Cryst powder. *Poisonous!* d 2.66. Sol in 10,000 parts cold, 5000 parts boiling water; sol in dil HNO_3 or HCl.

986. Barium Oxide. [1304-28-5] Barium monoxide; barium protoxide; calcined baryta. BaO; mol wt 153.33. Ba 89.56%, O 10.43%. Prepn: Ehrlich in *Handbook of Preparative Inorganic Chemistry* **vol. 1**, G. Brauer, Ed. (Academic Press, New York, 2nd ed., 1963) p 933.

White to yellowish-white powder or lumps. Very alkaline; absorbs moisture and CO_2 on exposure to air. *Poisonous!* On contact with water it forms $Ba(OH)_2$ with evolution of much heat. At 450° combines with oxygen to form BaO_2, which is reduced to BaO above 600°. d 5.7. mp ~1920°. Sol in water, dil acids. Slowly, but considerably sol in methanol, ethanol forming barium alcoholate. *Keep tightly closed.*

USE: Porous grades are marketed especially for drying gases and solvents (particularly alcohols, aldehydes and petroleum solvents). Swells, but does not become sticky upon absorption of moisture. Used in manuf of lubricating oil detergents. Also used for making barium methoxide.

987. Barium Perchlorate. [13465-95-7] $BaCl_2O_8$; mol wt 336.23. Ba 40.84%, Cl 21.09%, O 38.07%. $Ba(ClO_4)_2$. Prepn: *Gmelins, Barium* (8th ed) **30**, 218 (1932) and supplement, 373 (1960).

Trihydrate, crystals. *Poisonous!* Sol in water, methanol; slightly sol in ethanol, ethyl acetate, acetone; practically insol in ether.

USE: In the determination of ribonuclease; as absorbent for water in C and H analysis.

988. Barium Permanganate. [7787-36-2] Barium manganate(VII). $BaMn_2O_8$; mol wt 375.20. Ba 36.60%, Mn 29.28%, O 34.11%. $Ba(MnO_4)_2$. Prepn: Lux in *Handbook of Preparative Inorganic Chemistry* **vol. 1**, G. Brauer, Ed. (Academic Press, New York, 2nd ed., 1963) p 1462.

Brownish-violet to black crystals. *Poisonous!* d 3.77. Sparingly sol in water; dec by alcohol.

USE: As dry cell depolarizer.

989. Barium Peroxide. [1304-29-6] Barium dioxide; barium superoxide. BaO_2; mol wt 169.33. Ba 81.10%, O 18.90%. Prepn: *Gmelins, Barium* (8th ed) **30**, 92-98 (1932) and supplement, 177, 296 (1960).

White or grayish-white, heavy powder. *Poisonous!* Dec slowly in air. Insol in water, but slowly dec by contact with it; dec by dil acid or CO_2 in presence of H_2O forming H_2O_2. Combines with water to form octahydrate. *Keep well closed.* The article of commerce contains about 85% BaO_2; the remainder is chiefly BaO.

USE: Bleaching animal substances, vegetable fibers and straw; glass decolorizer; manuf H_2O_2 and oxygen; dyeing and printing textiles; with powdered aluminum in welding; in cathodes; in igniter compositions. Oxidizing agent in organic synthesis.

990. Barium Phosphate, Dibasic. [10048-98-3] Secondary barium phosphate. $BaHO_4P$; mol wt 233.31. Ba 58.86%, H 0.43%, O 27.43%, P 13.28%. $BaHPO_4$. Prepn: *Gmelins, Barium* (8th ed) **30**, 340 (1932) and supplement, 492 (1960).

Crystals. *Poisonous!* d 4.16. Practically insol in water; sol in dil HCl or HNO_3.

USE: In fireproofing compositions; in prepn of phosphors.

991. Barium Platinous Cyanide. [562-81-2] Barium tetracyanoplatinate(II); barium cyanoplatinate(II); barium platinocyanide; platinous barium cyanide. C_4BaN_4Pt; mol wt 436.48. C 11.01%, Ba 31.46%, N 12.84%, Pt 44.69%. $BaPt(CN)_4$.

Tetrahydrate. Large dichroic crystals; yellowish-green by transmitted, bluish-violet by reflected light. *Poison!* d 3.05. Sol in about 35 parts water; more sol in hot water.

USE: An aq soln mixed with some adhesive and painted on paper or wood exhibits luminescence when exposed to the invisible ultraviolet rays of the spectrum or to Roentgen, radium, or cathode rays; hence used in radiography for making x-ray screens.

992. Barium Selenide. [1304-39-8] BaSe; mol wt 216.29. Ba 63.49%, Se 36.51%. Prepn: Henglein, *Z. Anorg. Chem.* **120**, 77 (1921); *Z. Elektrochem.* **30**, 11 (1924); *Gmelins, Barium* (8th ed) **30**, 290 (1932) and supplement, 453 (1960).

Cubic microcrystalline powder. d 5.02. Turns red on exposure to air. Dec in water.

USE: In photocells, semiconductors.

993. Barium Silicide. [1304-40-1] $BaSi_2$; mol wt 193.50. Ba 70.97%, Si 29.03%. Prepn: *Gmelins, Barium* (8th ed) **30**, 330 (1932) and supplement, 486 (1960).

Metal-like, gray lumps; quite permanent in dry air, but dec by moisture with evolution of H_2. Melts at white heat.

USE: Deoxidizing and desulfurizing steel and for other metallurgical purposes.

994. Barium Sulfate. [7727-43-7] Blanc fixe; Baritop; Barosperse; Esophotrast; E-Z-Paque; Intestibar; Micropaque; Microtrast; Mixobar; Neobar; Oratrast; Prontobario; Radiopaque; Telebar; Tixobar. BaO_4S; mol wt 233.39. Ba 58.84%, O 27.42%, S 13.74%. $BaSO_4$. Occurs in nature as the mineral *barite*; also as *barytes*, *heavy spar*. Prepn: *Gmelins, Barium* (8th ed.) **30**, 262-267 (1932) and supplement, 182-186, 412-414 (1960). Review of clinical use: R. F. Theoni, A. R. Margulis, *Radiology* **167**, 7 (1988).

Fine, white, odorless powder or polymorphous crystals, d 4.25-4.5. Dec above 1600°. Practically insol in water (one gram dissolves in 400,000 parts), dil acids, alc. Sol in hot concd H_2SO_4.

Caution: Potential symptoms of overexposure by direct contact are irritation of eyes, nose and upper respiratory system; inhalation may cause benign pneumoconiosis. *See NIOSH Pocket Guide to Chemical Hazards* (DHHS/NIOSH 97-140, 1997) p 24.

USE: Manuf photographic papers, artificial ivory, cello-phane; filler for rubber, linoleum, oil cloth, polymeric fibers and resins, paper, lithographic inks; as a water-color pigment for colored paper, in wallpaper; as a size for modifying the colors of other pigments; in heavy concrete for radiation shield.

THERAP CAT: Diagnostic aid (radiopaque medium).

THERAP CAT (VET): X-ray contrast medium.

995. Barium Sulfide. [21109-95-5] BaS; mol wt 169.39. Ba 81.07%, S 18.93%. The commercial article contains 80-90% BaS. Prepn: Ehrlich in *Handbook of Preparative Inorganic Chemistry* **vol. 1**, G. Brauer, Ed. (Academic Press, New York, 2nd ed., 1963) p 938.

Heavy, grayish-white or pale yellow powder. d 4.36. mp >2000°. *Poisonous!* Oxidizes in dry air; slowly dec in damp air into carbonate, etc., with evolution of H_2S. Slightly sol in cold, more in hot water; sol in NH_4Cl soln; decomposed by acids, even CO_2, forming H_2S. *Keep in well-closed containers.*

USE: As depilatory; in luminous paints; manuf lithopone; vulcanizing rubber, generating H_2S.

996. Barium Sulfide, Black. [8011-62-9] Black ash. This is the crude barium sulfide obtained by strong heating of a mixture of barium sulfate mineral (barite) and charcoal. Contains 60-70% BaS; the remainder is chiefly barium sulfate and carbon.

USE: Prepn of barium salts.

997. Barium Sulfite. [7787-39-5] BaO_3S; mol wt 217.39. Ba 63.17%, O 22.08%, S 14.75%. $BaSO_3$. Prepn: *Gmelins, Barium* (8th ed.) **30**, 261 (1932) and supplement, 411 (1960).

Odorless crystals or powder; gradually oxidizes in air to $BaSO_4$. *Poisonous!* Slightly sol in water. Practically insol in alcohol; dec by acids with liberation of SO_2.

USE: In paper manufacture.

998. Barium Thiocyanate. [2092-17-3] Barium sulfocyanate; barium sulfocyanide; barium rhodanide. $C_2BaN_2S_2$; mol wt 253.49. C 9.48%, Ba 54.17%, N 11.05%, S 25.30%. $Ba(SCN)_2$. Prepn: Herstein, *Inorg. Synth.* **3**, 24 (1950).

Deliquesc crystals. *Poisonous!* Very sol in water, sol in acetone, methanol, ethanol. *Keep well closed.*

Trihydrate. Needle-shaped crystals (from water).

USE: In dyeing; in photography; as dispersing agent for cellulose; in prepn of thiocyanates of other metals.

999. Barium Thiosulfate. [35112-53-9] Barium hyposulfite. BaO_3S_2; mol wt 249.46. Ba 55.05%, O 19.24%, S 25.71%. BaS_2O_3. Prepn: *Gmelins, Barium* (8th ed.) **30**, 283 (1932) and supplement, 449 (1960).

Monohydrate. Cryst powder. *Poisonous!* Very slightly sol in water. Practically insol in alc, ether, acetone, CCl_4, CS_2.

USE: Manuf explosives, matches; as an iodometry standard; in photographic diffusion-transfer process.

1000. Barium Titanate(IV). [12047-27-7] Barium titanium oxide ($BaTiO_3$); barium metatitanate. BaO_3Ti; mol wt 233.19. Ba 58.89%, O 20.58%, Ti 20.53%. $BaTiO_3$. Usually prepd by calcining (at about 1300°) an intimate mixture of titanium dioxide and barium carbonate. Prepn from Ti oxalate and a barium compd: Lynd, Merker, **US 2758911** (1956 to National Lead). Wet process by the addn of a titanium ester, such as tetrapropyl titanate, to an aq soln of barium hydroxide: Flaschen, *J. Am. Chem. Soc.* **77**, 6194 (1955). Prepn of high purity material by ignition of barium titanyloxalate: Clabaugh *et al., J. Res. Natl. Bur. Stand.* **56**, 289 (1956). Prepn by ignition of Ba and Ti alcoholates in an organic solvent: DiVita, Fischer, **US 2985504** (1961 to U.S. Dept. of the Army).

Exists in five cryst modifications. The tetragonal form (obtained by the wet process) appears to have the most desirable electric properties and is described here: d 6.08. mp 1625°. Curie point 120°. Has ferroelectric and piezoelectric properties. Becomes permanently polarized when exposed to high voltage direct current, provided the temperature is never allowed to rise above Curie pt. Has high dielectric properties which can be influenced by temp, voltage, and frequency.

USE: In electronic devices, e.g., as voltage-sensitive dielectric in so-called dielectric amplifiers, in computer elements, magnetic amplifiers, memory devices.

1001. Barium Uranium Oxide. [10380-31-1] Barium uranate(VI); barium diuranate; uranium barium oxide. BaO_7U_2; mol wt 725.38. Ba 18.93%, O 15.44%, U 65.63%. BaU_2O_7. Prepn: Allpress, *J. Inorg. Nucl. Chem.* **26**, 1847 (1964); Klima *et al., ibid.* **28**, 1861 (1966).

Orange or yellow powder. Practically insol in water. Sol in acids.

USE: In painting on porcelain.

1002. Barnidipine. [104713-75-9] (4S)-1,4-Dihydro-2,6-dimethyl-4-(3-nitrophenyl)-3,5-pyridinedicarboxylic acid methyl (3S)-1-(phenylmethyl)-3-pyrrolidinyl ester; (+)-(3'S,4S)-1-benzyl-3-pyrrolidinyl methyl 1,4-dihydro-2,6-dimethyl-4-(*m*-nitrophenyl)-3,5-pyridinedicarboxylate; (3S)-1-benzyl-3-pyrrolidinyl methyl (4S)-2,6-dimethyl-4-(*m*-nitrophenyl)-1,4-dihydropyridine-3,5-dicarboxylate; mepirodipine. $C_{27}H_{29}N_3O_6$; mol wt 491.54. C 65.97%, H 5.95%, N 8.55%, O 19.53%. Dihydropyridine calcium channel blocker. Prepn (stereochemistry unspecified): T. Kojima, T. Takenaka, **DE 2904552**; *eidem*, **US 4220649** (1979, 1980 both to Yamanouchi). Prepn and bioactivity of enantiomers: K. Tamazawa *et al., J. Med. Chem.* **29**, 2504 (1986). GC-MS determn in plasma: T. Teramura *et al., J. Chromatogr.* **528**, 191 (1990). Review of pharmacology and therapeutic efficacy: H. Satoh, *Cardiovasc. Drug Rev.* **9**, 340-356 (1991).

mp 137-139°. $[\alpha]_D^{20}$ +64.8° (c = 1 in methanol).

Hydrochloride. [104757-53-1] YM-09730-5; Hypoca. $C_{27}H_{29}N_3O_6 \cdot HCl$; mol wt 528.00. mp 226-228°. $[\alpha]_D^{20}$ +116.4° (c = 1 in methanol). Insol in water. LD_{50} orally in male, female rats: 105, 113 mg/kg (Satoh).

THERAP CAT: Antihypertensive; antianginal.

1003. Barthrin. [70-43-9] 2,2-Dimethyl-3-(2-methyl-1-propenyl)cyclopropanecarboxylic acid (6-chloro-1,3-benzodioxol-5-yl) methyl ester; 2,2-dimethyl-3-(2-methylpropenyl)cyclopropanecarboxylic acid 6-chloropiperonyl ester; 6-chloropiperonyl

2,2-dimethyl-3-(2-methylpropenyl)cyclopropanecarboxylate; 6-chloropiperonyl chrysanthemumate; chrysanthemummonocarboxylic acid 6-chloropiperonyl ester. $C_{18}H_{21}ClO_4$; mol wt 336.81. C 64.19%, H 6.28%, Cl 10.53%, O 19.00%. Prepn: Barthel, Alexander, *J. Org. Chem.* **23**, 1012 (1958); Barthel *et al.*, **US 2886485** (1959).

trans-form

Oily liquid, $bp_{0.2}$ 155-171°, $bp_{0.7}$ 184-206°. n_D^{25} 1.5383. Sol in kerosine.

USE: Insecticide.

1004. Basic Aluminum Carbonate Gel. [1339-92-0] Basaljel. An aluminum hydroxide/aluminum carbonate gel.

THERAP CAT: Phosphorus binding agent in prevention of recurrent renal phosphatic calculi; antacid.

1005. Basic Lead Carbonate. [1319-46-6] C.I. Pigment White 1; C.I. 77597; lead subcarbonate; white lead; flake lead; ceruse; cerussa; bleiweiss (German). $C_2H_2O_8Pb_3$; mol wt 775.63. C 3.10%, H 0.26%, O 16.50%, Pb 80.14%. $(PbCO_3)_2$·$Pb(OH)_2$. Occurs in nature as the mineral *hydrocerussite*. See: *Mellor's* **vol. VII**, 837 (1927); *Colour Index* **vol. 4** (3rd ed., 1971) p 4676. Review of chemistry and use as pigment: E. J. Dunn, Jr., *Pigment Handbook* **1**, 65-84 (1973). Microdetermn by nuclear microprobe for use in analysis of masterpieces: B. Nens *et al.*, *Nucl. Instruments Methods Phys. Res.* **B14**, 148 (1986); by laser breakdown: D. Anglos, *Appl. Spectrosc.* **55**, 186A (2001).

White, heavy powder. *Poisonous!* Dec at 400°, leaving a residue of PbO. Insol in water or alcohol. Sol in acetic acid or dil HNO_3 with effervescence.

USE: Pigment in oil paints and water colors; in cements; for making putty and lead carbonate paper; in the processing of parchment.

1006. Basiliximab. [179045-86-4] Anti-(human interleukin 2 receptor) immunoglobulin G1 (human-mouse monoclonal CHI621 γ_1-chain) disulfide with human-mouse monoclonal CHI621 light chain, dimer; chRFT5; SDZ-CHI-621; Simulect. Human-murine chimeric monoclonal antibody directed against the interleukin-2 receptor α-chain (IL-2Rα), also known as CD25 antigen, on the surface of activated T cells. Prepn: P. L. Amlot *et al.*, **EP 449769** (1991 to Sandoz; Roy. Free Hosp. Sch. Med.). Clinical pharmacology: *idem et al.*, *Transplantation* **60**, 748 (1995). Clinical pharmacokinetics: J. Kovarik *et al.*, *ibid.* **64**, 1701 (1997). Clinical trial in kidney transplantation: B. Nashan *et al.*, *Lancet* **350**, 1193 (1997).

THERAP CAT: Immunosuppressant.

1007. Basswood. Linden tree. Also called *Tilia americana* L., *Tiliaceae*. Grows in mountainous woods from Canada to Georgia and west to Texas. Various decoctions of flowers, trees, bark and wood are used in American folk medicine for disorders of the bile and liver. Preparation of active extracts from the obscure *"Tilia alburnum"*: Lafon, **US 3030271** (1962 to S. A. Orsymonde).

1008. Batimastat. [130370-60-4] $(2R,3S)$-N^4-Hydroxy-N^1-[(1S)-2-(methylamino)-2-oxo-1-(phenylmethyl)ethyl]-2-(2-methylpropyl)-3-[(2-thienylthio)methyl]butanediamide; (2S,3R)-5-methyl-3-[[(αS)-α-(methylcarbamoyl)phenethyl]carbamoyl]-2-[(2-thienylthio)methyl]hexanohydroxamic acid; [4-(N-hydroxyamino)-2R-isobutyl-3S-(2-thienylthiomethyl)succinyl]-L-phenylalanine-N-methylamide; BB-94. $C_{23}H_{31}N_3O_4S_2$; mol wt 477.64. C 57.84%, H 6.54%, N 8.80%, O 13.40%, S 13.43%. Synthetic matrix metalloproteinase inhibitor. Prepn: C. Campion *et al.*, **WO 9005719**; *eidem*, **US 5240958** (1990, 1993 both to British Biotech.). Effect on transplanted human ovarian carcinoma: B. Davies *et al.*, *Cancer Res.* **53**, 2087 (1993). Inhibition of metastasis of transplanted human colorectal carcinoma: X. Wang *et al.*, *ibid.* **54**, 4726 (1994).

Fine white powder. mp 236-238°.

THERAP CAT: Antineoplastic adjunct (antimetastatic agent).

1009. Batrachotoxin. [23509-16-2] Batrachotoxinin A 20-(2,4-dimethyl-1*H*-pyrrole-3-carboxylate); 3α,9α-epoxy-14β,18β-(epoxyethano-*N*-methylimino)-5β-pregna-7,16-diene-3β,11α,20α-triol 20α-ester with 2,4-dimethylpyrrole-3-carboxylic acid. C_{31}-$H_{42}N_2O_6$; mol wt 538.67. C 69.12%, H 7.86%, N 5.20%, O 17.82%. One of a group of toxic steroidal alkaloids consisting of batrachotoxin, *pseudobatrachotoxin*, homobatrachotoxin, and batrachotoxinin A. Extracted orginally from the skin of South American poison-dart frogs, genus *Phyllobates*. Its name is derived from the Greek word "batrachos" meaning frog. Isoln: F. Märki, B. Witkop, *Experientia* **19**, 329 (1963); and preliminary characterization: J. W. Daly *et al.*, *J. Am. Chem. Soc.* **87**, 124 (1965). Structure: T. Tokuyama *et al.*, *ibid.* **91**, 3931 (1969). Synthetic studies: J. F. W. Keana, R. R. Schumaker, *J. Org. Chem.* **41**, 3840 (1976); P. Magnus *et al.*, *Chem. Commun.* **1985**, 1185; P. Hudson, *Tetrahedron Lett.* **34**, 7295 (1993). Mode of action: E. X. Albuquerque, *Fed. Proc.* **31**, 1133 (1972). Kinetics and gating action on Na^+ channels: J. A. Wasserstrom *et al.*, *Biophys. J.* **65**, 386 (1993). Review: J. Daly, B. Witkop, *Clin. Toxicol.* **4**, 331-342 (1971); of chemistry and pharmacology: E. X. Albuquerque *et al.*, *Science* **72**, 995-1002 (1971); J. W. Daly, *Fortschr. Chem. Org. Naturst.* **41**, 206-227 (1982). Review of sodium channel activation: G. B. Brown, *Int. Rev. Neurobiol.* **29**, 77-116 (1988).

$[\alpha]_{584}^{24}$ -5 To $-10°$; $[\alpha]_{300}^{24}$ $-260°$ (c = 0.23 in methanol). uv max (0.1N HCl-MeOH): 234, 262 nm (log ε 3.99, 3.70). pKa 7.45. LD_{50} s.c. in mice: 2 μg/kg (Tokuyama).

Batrachotoxinin A. [19457-37-5] $C_{24}H_{35}NO_5$; mol wt 417.54. Abs config: R. D. Gilardi, *Acta Crystallogr.* **B 26**, 440 (1970). LD_{50} s.c. in mice: 1000 μg/kg (Tokuyama).

Homobatrachotoxin. [23509-17-3] Isobatrachotoxin. C_{32}-$H_{44}N_2O_6$; mol wt 552.70. Also isolated from the feathers and skin of hooded pitohui bird of New Guinea. First demonstration of chemical defense in birds: J. P. Dumbacher *et al.*, *Science* **258**, 799 (1992). uv max (0.1N HCl-MeOH): 233, 264 nm (log ε 3.95, 3.70). LD_{50} s.c. in mice: 3 μg/kg (Tokuyama).

USE: Biochemical tool for study of Na^+ channels.

1010. Batroxobin. [9039-61-6] *Bothrops atrox* serine proteinase; Bothrops venom proteinase; Botropase; Defibrase. Thrombin-like enzyme from the venom of *Bothrops atrox* (Linn.), a pit viper found in several varieties in Southern and Central America. Prepn of conc extract from *B. jararaca* venom and coagulative properties: D. von Klobusitzky, *Arch. Exp. Pathol. Pharmakol.* **179**, 204 (1935). The enzyme from *B. atrox* venom is hemostatic at low doses and acts as a blood anti-coagulant at higher doses.

Composition and manuf: E. E. Percs *et al., DE 2201993; eidem,* US 3849252 (1972, 1974 both to Pentapharm). Studies on the subunit structure of fibrin produced by batroxobin: P. Mattock, M. P. Esnouf, *Nature New Biol.* 233, 277 (1971). *In vitro* blood-clotting activity: K. O. Wik *et al., Br. J. Haematol.* 23, 37 (1972). Electron microscopic study: S. Ishimaru *et al., Thromb. Haemostasis* 45, 276 (1981). Clinical pharmacology: K. Fukutake *et al., Nippon Ketsueki Gakkai Zasshi* 44, 1178 (1981), *C.A.* 96, 62775x (1982). Review of characterization, properties: K. G. Stocker, G. H. Barlow, *Aktuel. Probl. Angiol.* 26, 45-62 (1975).

Rectangular crystals. Sol in physiological saline. Practically insol in distilled water. Forms complexes with phenol and phenol derivs that are practically insol in water.

Mixture with factor-X activator. Hemocoagulase; Reptilase.

THERAP CAT: Hemostatic.

1011. Batyl Alcohol. [544-62-7] 3-(Octadecyloxy)-1,2-propanediol; monooctadecyl ether of glycerol. $C_{21}H_{44}O_3$; mol wt 344.57. C 73.20%, H 12.87%, O 13.93%. $CH_2OHCHOHCH_2-O(CH_2)_{17}CH_3$. Isoln from shark liver oils: Heilbron, Owens, *J. Chem. Soc.* **1928**, 942; Davies *et al., ibid.* **1933**, 165; Nakamiya, *C.A.* 33, 8175 (1939); from yellow bone marrow: Holmes *et al., J. Am. Chem. Soc.* 63, 2607 (1941); from coral-reef-building animals: Kind, Bergmann, *J. Org. Chem.* 7, 424 (1942). Synthesis from allyl octadecyl ether: Davies *et al., J. Chem. Soc.* **1930**, 2542: Kornblum, Holmes, *J. Am. Chem. Soc.* 64, 3045 (1942). Synthesis of optically active batyl alc: Baer, Fischer, *J. Biol. Chem.* 140, 397 (1941).

Glistening plates from dilute acetone, mp 70.5-71°. $[\alpha]_D^{20} +1.14°$ (c = 6.6 in $CHCl_3$). Sol in the usual fat solvents.

Bis(*p*-nitrobenzoate). $C_{35}H_{50}N_2O_9$. Pale yellow needles from methanol, soft at 63°, mp 65-66°.

THERAP CAT (VET): Has been recommended for bracken fern poisoning in cattle.

1012. Bayberry Bark. Candleberry bark; myrica; myrtle wax; berry wax; tallow shrub. Dried root bark of *Myrica cerifera* L., *Myricaceae. Habit.* Maryland to Florida, west to Texas and Arkansas. *Constit.* Acrid and astringent resin, myricic acid, tannin, red coloring matter, gum, starch. Bayberry wax consists of palmitic, myristic and lauric acid esters.

THERAP CAT: Astringent; emetic.

1013. Bazedoxifene. [198481-32-2] 1-[[4-[2-(Hexahydro-1*H*-azepin-1-yl)ethoxy]phenyl]methyl]-2-(4-hydroxyphenyl)-3-methyl-1*H*-indol-5-ol; 1-[4-(2-azepan-1-ylethoxy)benzyl]-2-(4-hydroxyphenyl)-3-methyl-1*H*-indol-5-ol. $C_{30}H_{34}N_2O_3$; mol wt 470.60. C 76.57%, H 7.28%, N 5.95%, O 10.20%. Nonsteroidal selective estrogen receptor modulator (SERM). Prepn: C. P. Miller *et al.,* EP 802183; *eidem,* US 5998402 (1997, 1999 both to American Home); C. P. Miller *et al., J. Med. Chem.* 44, 1654 (2001). Pharmacology and receptor binding study: B. S. Komm *et al., Endocrinology* 146, 3999 (2005). Clinical pharmacology: S. Ronkin *et al., Obstet. Gynecol.* 105, 1397 (2005). Review of development: B. S. Komm, C. R. Lyttle, *Ann. N.Y. Acad. Sci.* 949, 317-326 (2001); and therapeutic potential: C. Gruber, D. Gruber, *Curr. Opin. Invest. Drugs* 5, 1086-1093 (2004).

mp 98-102°.

Acetate. [198481-33-3] TSE-424; WAY-140424; WAY-TSE-424. $C_{30}H_{34}N_2O_3.C_2H_4O_2$; mol wt 530.65. Crystals from acetone + acetic acid, mp 174-178°.

THERAP CAT: Antiosteoporotic.

1014. BBOT. [7128-64-5] 2,2'-(2,5-Thiophenediyl)bis[5-(1,1-dimethylethyl)benzoxazole]; 2,5-bis(5-*tert*-butyl-2-benzoxazolyl)thiophene; C.I. Fluorescent Brightener 184; Uvitex OB.

$C_{26}H_{26}N_2O_2S$; mol wt 430.56. C 72.53%, H 6.09%, N 6.51%, O 7.43%, S 7.45%. High mol wt fluorescent whitening agent. Prepn: P. Liechti *et al.,* CH 427822 (1967 to Ciba); Z. Seha, C. D. Weis, *Helv. Chim. Acta* 63, 413 (1980). Fluorescence depolarization studies: G. R. Fleming *et al., Chem. Phys. Lett.* 51, 399 (1977). Photostability study: G. Tury *et al., J. Photochem. Photobiol. A* 114, 51 (1998).

Yellow to green powder, mp 196-202°. Flash pt: >350°C. d^{20} 1.26. Vapor pressure (20°): 2.6×10^{-8} Pa. Soly at 20° (%w/w): water <0.01; acetone 0.5; chloroform 14; ethyl acetate 1; *n*-hexane 0.2; methanol <0.1. Absorption max (cyclohexane): 374 nm. Emission max (cyclohexane): 435 nm.

USE: Optical brightener additive in polymers, fibers, films, inks, laquers, and paints. In liquid scintillators.

1015. BCG. An abbreviation for *Bacillus Calmette-Guérin,* a strain of *Mycobacterium tuberculosis.* Prepn of BCG labeled with C^{14}: Pasquier, Kurylowicz, *Rev. Immunol.* 20, 245 (1956). Has the potential to act as a non-specific immunopotentiating agent that stimulates the whole range of immune responses. Role as an immunotherapeutic agent: Bartlett and Zbar *et al., J. Natl. Cancer Inst.* 48, 245, 1441, 1709 (1972); 49, 119 (1972). Comparison of potentiation of specific tumor immunity in mice: M. T. Scott, R. Bomford, *ibid.* 57, 555 (1976). Review of use in Hodgkin's disease: H. Zywicka-Lopaciuk *et al., Arch. Immunol. Ther. Exp.* 29, 739-755 (1981); in operable lung cancer: B. H. Stack *et al., Thorax* 37, 588-593 (1982). Review of use as anti-tumor agent and of the interaction of BCG with cells of the mammalian immune system: M. Davies, *Biochim. Biophys. Acta* 651, 143-174 (1982). Review of pathogenesis of tuberculosis and the effectiveness of BCG vaccination: H. G. ten Dam, A. Pio, *Tubercle* 63, 225-233 (1982).

THERAP CAT: BCG vaccine as active immunizing agent.

THERAP CAT (VET): Vaccination vs. tuberculosis (cattle). Use prohibited where bovine tuberculosis eradication programs are in progress.

1016. Bebeerine. [477-60-1] (13a*S*,25a*S*)-2,3,13a,14,15,-16,25,25a-Octahydro-18,29-dimethoxy-1,14-dimethyl-13*H*-4,6:21,24-dietheno-8,12-metheno-1*H*-pyrido[3',2':14,15][1,11]-dioxacycloeicosino[2,3,4-*ij*]isoquinoline-9,19-diol; 1'α-6,6'-dimethoxy-2,2'-dimethyltubocuraran-7',12'-diol; *d*-bebeerine; chondodendrine; pelosine. $C_{36}H_{38}N_2O_6$; mol wt 594.70. C 72.71%, H 6.44%, N 4.71%, O 16.14%. From bark of *Nectandra rodioei* Hook., *Lauraceae:* Maclagan, *Ann.* 48, 106 (1843). From root of *Chondodendron microphyllum* (Eichl.) Moldenke and stem of *Ch. candicans* (Rick ex. D.C.) Sandwith, *Menispermaceae* and *radix pareirae bravae:* King, *J. Chem. Soc.* **1940**, 737. Structure: Faltis *et al., Ber.* 69, 1269 (1936); King, *J. Chem. Soc.* **1939**, 1157. Stereochemistry: King, *ibid.* **1948**, 265.

Needles from methanol, mp 215°. $[\alpha]_D^{20} +345.7°$ (c = 0.4 in 1*N* HCl). Sol in benzene, chloroform, pyridine.

Hydrochloride. $C_{36}H_{38}N_2O_6.HCl.$ mp 260°. $[\alpha]_D^{20} +294°$ (c = 0.7). Sol in water and chloroform.

THERAP CAT: Antimalarial.

1017. Bebeeru Bark. Greenheart; bibiru bark; sipiri bark. From *Nectandra rodioei* Hook., *Lauraceae. Habit.* British Guiana. *Constit.* Bebeerine, sipirine, bebeeric acid, tannin, resin.

1018. Beclamide. [501-68-8] 3-Chloro-*N*-(phenylmethyl)-propanamide; *N*-benzyl-3-chloropropionamide; *N*-benzyl-β-chloropropanamide; benzchlorpropamide; chloroethylphenamide; Neuracen; Nidrane; Posedrine; Seclar. $C_{10}H_{12}ClNO$; mol wt 197.66. C 60.76%, H 6.12%, Cl 17.94%, N 7.09%, O 8.09%. $ClCH_2CH_2$-$CONHCH_2C_6H_5$. Prepd by the action of β-chloropropionyl chloride on benzylamine in cooled water at pH 8: Cassell, Kushner, **US 2569288** (1951 to Am. Cyanamid); Kushner *et al., J. Org. Chem.* **16**, 1283 (1951).

Large crystals from methanol, mp 94°. Slightly sol in water (0.005 to 0.01%). Moderately sol in the lower alcs. Dec in hot aq acid soln and in hot aq alkaline soln.

THERAP CAT: Anticonvulsant.

1019. Beclomethasone. [4419-39-0] (11β,16β)-9-Chloro-11,17,21-trihydroxy-16-methylpregna-1,4-diene-3,20-dione; 9α-chloro-16β-methyl-1,4-pregnadiene-11β,17α,21-triol-3,20-dione; 9α-chloro-16β-methylprednisolone. $C_{22}H_{29}ClO_5$; mol wt 408.92. C 64.62%, H 7.15%, Cl 8.67%, O 19.56%. Glucocorticoid. Prepn of free alcohol and 21-acetate: **GB 912378** (1962 to Merck & Co.); of 21-acetate: **GB 901093** (1962 to Schevico); of mono and diesters: J. Elks *et al.,* **BE 649170**; *eidem,* **US 3312590** (1964, 1967 both to Glaxo). Symposium on clinical studies: *Br. J. Clin. Pharmacol.* **4**, Suppl. 3, 249S-312S (1977). Use in chronic asthma in children: M. Rao *et al., J. Asthma* **19**, 21 (1982); in treatment of asthma in steroid-independent adults: V. A. Malfitan, *Clin. Ther.* **4**, 472 (1982). Review of use in rhinitis: P. Small *et al., Ann. Allergy* **49**, 127 (1982); of pharmacology, side effects and use in asthma and allergic rhinitis: R. N. Brogden *et al., Drugs* **28**, 99-126 (1984).

Dipropionate. [5534-09-8] Sch-18020W; Aerobec; Aldecin; Anceron; Andion; Beclacin; Becloforte; Beclomet; Beclorhinol; Beclovent; Becodisks; Beconase; Beconasol; Becotide; Clenil-A; Entyderma; Inalone; Korbutone; Propaderm; Qvar; Rino-Clenil; Sanasthmax; Vancenase; Vanceril; Viarex; Viarox. $C_{28}H_{37}ClO_7$; mol wt 521.04. Crystals from acetone + ether, mp 117-120° (dec). $[\alpha]_D$ +98.0° (c = 1.0 in dioxane). uv max (ethanol): 238 nm (ε 15990).

THERAP CAT: Antiallergic, antiasthmatic (inhalant). Anti-inflammatory (topical).

1020. Beeswax. [8012-89-3] Yellow beeswax. A substance obtained from bee honeycombs. Consists of esters of straight-chain monohydric alcohols with even-numbered carbon chains from C_{24} to C_{36} esterified with straight-chain acids also having even numbers of C atoms up to C_{36} (some C_{18} hydroxy acids). Examples of such esters are triacontanol hexadecanoate and hexacosanol hexacosanoate. These esters are mixed with about 20% (w/w) of hydrocarbons having odd-numbered straight carbon chains from C_{21} to C_{33}. Propolis, pigments and unidentified substances amount to about 6%. Composition: D. T. Downing *et al., Aust. J. Chem.* **14**, 253 (1961); Callow, *Bee World* **44**, 95 (1963). Brief review: C. S. Letcher in *Kirk-Othmer Encyclopedia of Chemical Technology* Vol. **24** (Wiley-Interscience, New York, 3rd ed., 1984) pp 466-467.

Yellowish to brownish-yellow, soft to brittle; honey-like odor; slight balsamic taste. d 0.95-0.960. mp 62-65°. Saponification number 84. Acid number 20. Practically insol in water. Slightly sol in cold alc; sol in hot alc, chloroform, benzene, ether, carbon disulfide.

White beeswax. White wax; bleached yellow wax; bleached beeswax. Prepd by oxidizing yellow beeswax cakes with peroxide or in sunlight. Yellowish-white. Properties similar to those of yellow beeswax, except for a slightly different taste. Preferred to yellow beeswax in cosmetics.

USE: Manuf of wax paper, candles, cosmetics; modeling artificial fruits and flowers; in process engraving; shoe polish. Pharmaceutic aid (in ointments, plasters).

1021. Befloxatone. [134564-82-2] (5R)-5-(Methoxymethyl)-3-[4-[(3R)-4,4,4-trifluoro-3-hydroxybutoxy]phenyl]-2-oxazolidinone; MD-370503. $C_{15}H_{18}F_3NO_5$; mol wt 349.30. C 51.58%, H 5.19%, F 16.32%, N 4.01%, O 22.90%. Reversible monoamine oxidase type A (MAO-A) inhibitor. Prepn: F. X. Jarreau *et al.,* **EP 424244**; *eidem,* **US 5036091** (1990, 1991 both to Delalande). Pharmacology: D. Caille *et al., J. Pharmacol. Exp. Ther.* **277**, 265 (1996). Biochemical profile: O. Curet *et al., ibid.* 253. Structure-activity study: J. Wouters *et al., Bioorg. Med. Chem.* **7**, 1683 (1999). Review of clinical pharmacology: P. Rosenzweig *et al., J. Affective Disord.* **51**, 305-312 (1998).

Crystals from ethanol + isopropyl ether, mp 101°. $[\alpha]_D^{20}$ −11.5° (c = 1 in methylene chloride).

THERAP CAT: Antidepressant.

1022. Befunolol. [39552-01-7] 1-[7-[2-Hydroxy-3-[(1-methylethyl)amino]propoxy]-2-benzofuranyl]ethanone; 7-[2-hydroxy-3-(isopropylamino)propoxy]-2-benzofuranyl methyl ketone; 2-acetyl-7-(2-hydroxy-3-isopropylaminopropoxy)benzofuran. $C_{16}H_{21}NO_4$; mol wt 291.34. C 65.96%, H 7.27%, N 4.81%, O 21.97%. β-Adrenergic blocker. Prepn: K. Ito *et al.,* **DE 2223184**; *eidem,* **US 3853923** (1972, 1974 both to Kakenyaku Kako). Prepn and activity of optical isomers: J. Nakano *et al., Chem. Pharm. Bull.* **36**, 1399 (1988). Determn of befunolol and metabolites in human plasma: K. Kawahara, T. Ofuji, *J. Chromatogr.* **168**, 266 (1979). Absorption, distribution, excretion in rats: H. Kitagawa *et al., Oyo Yakuri* **17**, 383, 393 (1979), *C.A.* **91**, 13374w-5x (1979). General pharmacology: S. Masumoto *et al., Iyakuhin Kenkyu* **10**, 741 (1979), *C.A.* **92**, 88015s (1980). Pharmacodynamics: S. Harada *et al., Arch. Int. Pharmacodyn. Ther.* **252**, 262 (1981).

Crystals from cyclohexane/acetone, mp 115°. LD_{50} in mice: 100-105 mg/kg i.v. (Ito).

Hydrochloride. [39543-79-8] BFE-60; Benfuran; Bentos; Glauconex. $C_{16}H_{21}NO_4$.HCl; mol wt 327.80. Crystals from ethyl acetate, mp 163°.

(S)-(−)-Form hydrochloride. [66717-59-7] Pale yellow prisms from isopropyl alcohol, mp 151-152°. $[\alpha]_D$ −15.5° (c = 1 in methanol).

(R)-(+)-Form hydrochloride. [66685-79-8] Pale yellow prisms from isopropyl alcohol, mp 151°. $[\alpha]_D$ +15.3° (c = 1 in methanol).

THERAP CAT: Antiglaucoma.

1023. Behenic Acid. [112-85-6] Docosanoic acid. $C_{22}H_{44}O_2$; mol wt 340.58. C 77.58%, H 13.02%, O 9.40%. $CH_3(CH_2)_{20}$-CO_2H. Minor constituent of most seed fats, animal milk fats and marine animal oils. Large amts (~50%) are found in (hydrogenated?) jamba oil, mustard seed oil and rape oil: Sudborough *et al., J. Indian Inst. Sci.* **9A**, 25 (1926). Prepn from erucic acid by catalytic reduction: Morgan, Holmes, *J. Soc. Chem. Ind. London Trans. Commun.* **44**, 491 (1925). Brief review: E. S. Lower, *Manuf. Chem.* **56**(7), 44-46 (1985).

Waxy solid, mp 79.95°. Neutralization value 164.73. bp_{60} 306°. d_4^{100} 0.8221; n_D^{100} 1.4270. One hundred grams of 90% ethanol dissolve 0.102 g of behenic acid at 17°; at 25° 0.218 g of the acid dissolves in 100 ml of 91.5% ethanol, 0.116 g in 100 ml of 86.2%

ethanol, 0.011 g in 100 ml of 63.07% ethanol. One hundred grams of ether dissolves 0.1922 g of behenic acid at 16°.

Methyl ester. $C_{23}H_{46}O_2$. mp 54°.

Ethyl ester. $C_{24}H_{48}O_2$. mp 50°. bp$_{0.2}$ 185°.

Amide. $C_{22}H_{45}NO$. mp 111-112°.

USE: In lubricating oils, as solvent evaporation retarder in paint removers. Amide as anti-foam in the manuf of detergents, in floor polishes, in dripless candles.

1024. Belatacept. [706808-37-9] [29-Tyrosine,104-glutamic acid] CTLA-4 (antigen) (human extracellular domain-containing fragment) fusion protein with immunoglobulin G1 (human monoclonal Fc domain-containing fragment), bimol. (120 → 120')-disulfide; LEA29Y; BMS-224818; Selective costimulation blocker similar to abatacept, *q.v.* Soluble fusion protein combining a modified form of the extracellular portion of cytotoxic T-lymphocyte-associated antigen 4 (CTLA-4) with the constant region of human IgG1. Prepn: R. J. Peach *et al.*, *WO 0192337*; *eidem US 05214313* (2001, 2005 both to Bristol-Myers Squibb). Pharmacology and development: C. P. Larsen *et al.*, *Am. J. Transpl.* **5**, 443 (2005). Clinical trial in rheumatoid arthritis: L. W. Moreland *et al.*, *Arthritis Rheum.* **46**, 1470 (2002); in renal transplantation: F. Vincenti *et al.*, *N. Engl. J. Med.* **353**, 770 (2005).

THERAP CAT: Immunosuppressant.

1025. Belladonna. Deadly nightshade; banewort; death's herb; dwale; poison black cherry. Dried leaves and root of *Atropa belladonna* L., *Solanaceae*. Habit. Southern and Central Europe, Asia Minor, Algeria; cultivated in North America. On extraction it yields atropine, hyoscyamine, scopolamine, asparagine, choline, chrysatropic acid, atroscine, leucatropic acid, phytosterol. Leaves usually contain 0.3-0.5% total alkaloids; dried root contains 0.4-0.7% total alkaloids. *See:* Romeike, *Pharmazie* **8**, 729 (1953); Phokas, Steinegger, *ibid.* **11**, 652 (1956); *Pharm. Acta Helv.* **31**, 284 (1956).

Caution: Toxicity based on content of atropine, *q.v.*, and related alkaloids.

THERAP CAT: Anticholinergic.

THERAP CAT (VET): Anticholinergic; antispasmodic.

1026. Belleau's Reagent. [88816-02-8] 2,4-Bis(4-phenoxyphenyl)-1,3,2,4-dithiadiphosphetane 2,4-disulfide. $C_{24}H_{18}O_2P_2S_4$; mol wt 528.61. C 54.53%, H 3.43%, O 6.05%, P 11.72%, S 24.26%. *p*-Phenoxy derivative of Lawesson's reagent, *q.v.* Prepn: G. Lajoie *et al.*, *Tetrahedron Lett.* **24**, 3815 (1983). Synthetic applications: B. Yde *et al.*, *Tetrahedron* **40**, 2047 (1984); M. Caron, *J. Org. Chem.* **51**, 4075 (1986); M. M. Campbell *et al.*, *Tetrahedron Lett.* **30**, 1997 (1989); A. G. M. Barrett, A. C. Lee, *J. Org. Chem.* **57**, 2818 (1992); R. Shabana *et al.*, *Tetrahedron* **49**, 1271 (1993); *eidem, ibid.* **50**, 6975 (1994); S. V. Ley *et al.*, *Org. Lett.* **4**, 711 (2002).

Yellow crystals from toluene, mp 187-190°. Sol in CHCl$_3$, THF, toluene, acetonitrile.

USE: Mild thionation reagent in organic synthesis.

1027. Bemegride. [64-65-3] 4-Ethyl-4-methyl-2,6-piperidinedione; 3-ethyl-3-methylglutarimide; 4-ethyl-4-methyl-2,6-dioxopiperidine; 2,6-dioxo-4-methyl-4-ethylpiperidine; methetharimide; β,β-methylethylglutarimide; NP-13; Eukraton; Megimide. $C_8H_{13}NO_2$; mol wt 155.19. C 61.91%, H 8.44%, N 9.03%, O 20.62%. Prepn: Thole, Thorpe, *J. Chem. Soc.* **99**, 439 (1911); Sircar, *ibid.* **1937**, 602, 604; Benica, Wilson, *J. Am. Pharm. Assoc. Sci. Ed.* **39**, 451 (1950); Lukes, Ferles, *Chem. Listy* **49**, 510 (1955), *C.A.* **49**, 10290 (1955). Pharmacology: Delay *et al.*, *Presse Med.* **64**, 1525 (1956); Oberdorf, Meyer, *Arch. Exp. Pathol. Pharmakol.* **238**, 128 (1960); Kretzschmar *et al.*, *Arch. Int. Pharmacodyn. Ther.* **174**, 318 (1968). Metabolism: Nicholls, *Nature* **185**, 927 (1960). Toxicity study: F. Hahn, A. Oberdorf, *Arch. Int. Pharmacodyn. Ther.* **135**, 9 (1962). Reduction of barbiturate anesthesia in mice: V. K. Patel *et al.*, *Psychopharmacology* **71**, 21 (1980). Postsynaptic effects: P. W. Gage, P. Sah, *Br. J. Pharmacol.* **75**, 493 (1982).

Platelets from water or from acetone + ether, mp 127°. Sublimes at 100° and 2 mm press. Sol in water, acetone. LD$_{50}$ in male mice (mg/kg): 20.1 ±1.41 i.v., 43.0 ±1.8 s.c.; LD$_{50}$ in male rats (mg/kg): 16.3 ±1.24 i.v., 23.5 ±1.67 i.p (Hahn, Oberdorf).

THERAP CAT: CNS stimulant. Antidote (barbiturate poisoning).

THERAP CAT (VET): CNS stimulant. Antidote (barbiturate poisoning).

1028. Bemotrizinol. [187393-00-6] 2,2'-[6-(4-Methoxyphenyl)-1,3,5-triazine-2,4-diyl]bis[5-[(2-ethylhexyl)oxy]phenol]; 2,4-bis-[4-(2-ethylhexyloxy)-2-hydroxy]phenyl-6-(4-methoxyphenyl)-1,3,5-triazine; bis-ethylhexyloxyphenol methoxyphenyl triazine; BEMT; Tinosorb S. $C_{38}H_{49}N_3O_5$; mol wt 627.81. C 72.70%, H 7.87%, N 6.69%, O 12.74%. Broad spectrum, photostable UV-A and UV-B filter in cosmetics and sunscreens. Prepn: D. Hüglin *et al.*, *EP 775698*; *eidem, US 5955060* (1997, 1999 both to Ciba Specialty Chem.). Lack of estrogenic or androgenic activity: J. Ashby *et al.*, *Regul. Toxicol. Pharmacol.* **34**, 287 (2001). Photostabilizing effects on avobenzone and ethylhexyl methoxycinnamate, *q.q.v.*: E. Chatelain, B. Gabard, *Photochem. Photobiol.* **74**, 401 (2001). Comprehensive review: S. Mongiat *et al.*, *Cosmet. Toiletries* **118**, 47-54 (2003).

Slightly yellow crystals, mp 83-85° (Hüglin); also reported as mp 80° (Mongiat). Sol in oil. Absorption max (ethanol): 343 nm (ε 47000). Absorption max (isopropanol): 341 nm (E$_{1cm}^{1\%}$ ≥ 790).

THERAP CAT: Ultraviolet screen.

1029. Benactyzine. [302-40-9] α-Hydroxy-α-phenylbenzeneacetic acid 2-(diethylamino)ethyl ester; benzilic acid β-diethylaminoethyl ester; β-diethylaminoethyl benzilate; 2-diethylaminoethyl diphenylglycolate. $C_{20}H_{25}NO_3$; mol wt 327.42. C 73.37%, H 7.70%, N 4.28%, O 14.66%. An antagonist of acetylcholine in the central and peripheral nervous systems. Prepn: Horenstein, Pahlicke, *Ber.* **71**, 1654 (1938); Blicke, Maxwell, *J. Am. Chem. Soc.* **64**, 428 (1942); Hill, Holmes, *US 2394770* (1946 to Am. Cyanamid). Toxicity and pharmacodynamics: Fournier, Petit, *Therapie* **17**, 1245 (1962). Metabolism: Eldeson *et al.*, *Arch. Int. Pharmacodyn. Ther.* **187**, 139 (1970). Crystal and molecular structure determn by x-ray diffraction: T. J. Petcher, *J. Chem. Soc. Perkin Trans. 2* **1974**, 1151.

Crystals, mp 51°.

Hydrochloride. [57-37-4] AY-5406-1; Cedad; Nutinal; Parasan; Suavitil. $C_{20}H_{25}NO_3 \cdot HCl$; mol wt 363.88. Crystals from acetone, mp 177-178°. Soly in water (25°): 14.9/100 ml. Practically insol in ether.

Methobromide. [3166-62-9] Spatomac. $C_{20}H_{25}NO_3.CH_3Br$; mol wt 422.36. Crystals from alcohol + ether, mp 169-170°.

THERAP CAT: Antispasmodic.

1030. Benalaxyl. [71626-11-4] N-(2,6-Dimethylphenyl)-N-(phenylacetyl)-DL-alanine methyl ester; methyl N-phenylacetyl-N-2,6-xylyl-DL-alaninate; N-(2,6-dimethylphenyl)-N-(1-carbomethoxyethyl)phenylacetamide; M-9834; Galben. $C_{20}H_{23}NO_3$; mol wt 325.40. C 73.82%, H 7.12%, N 4.30%, O 14.75%. Acylalanine fungicide systemically active against phytopathogens of the order *Peronosporales*. Prepn: E. Boson *et al.*, *DE 2903612*; *eidem*, *US 4425357* (1978, 1984 both to Montedison). Activity and toxicology: P. Bergamaschi *et al.*, *Proc. Br. Crop Prot. Conf. - Pests Dis.* **1981**, 19. Residue accumulation in edible crops: P. Cabras *et al.*, *J. Agric. Food Chem.* **33**, 86 (1985). GC-MS study: B. D. Ripley, *ibid.* 560.

Crystals from ligroin, mp 78-80°. LD_{50} in rats (mg/kg): 4200 orally; 1100 i.p. LC_{50} (96 hr) in rainbow trout: 3.75 mg/l (Bergamaschi).

USE: Agricultural fungicide.

1031. Benazepril. [86541-75-5] (3S)-3-[[(1S)-1-(Ethoxycarbonyl)-3-phenylpropyl]amino]-2,3,4,5-tetrahydro-2-oxo-1H-1-benzazepine-1-acetic acid; (3S)-1-(carboxymethyl)-[[(1S)-1-(ethoxycarbonyl)-3-phenylpropyl]amino]-2,3,4,5-tetrahydro-1H-[1]-benzazepin-2-one; (3S)-3-[[(1S)-1-carboxy-3-phenylpropyl]amino]-2,3,4,5-tetrahydro-2-oxo-1H-1-benzazepine-1-acetic acid 3-ethyl ester. $C_{24}H_{28}N_2O_5$; mol wt 424.49. C 67.91%, H 6.65%, N 6.60%, O 18.85%. Angiotensin converting enzyme (ACE) inhibitor. Hydrolyzed *in vivo* to the active diacid metabolite. Prepn: J. W. H. Watthey, *EP 72352*; *idem*, *US 4410520* (both 1983 to Ciba-Geigy); J. W. H. Watthey *et al.*, *J. Med. Chem.* **28**, 1511 (1985). Clinical pharmacology: M. D. Schaller *et al.*, *Eur. J. Clin. Pharmacol.* **28**, 267 (1985). GC-MS determn in plasma and urine: A. Sioufi *et al.*, *J. Chromatogr.* **434**, 239 (1988). Pharmacokinetics of benazepril and benazeprilat: G. Kaiser *et al.*, *Biopharm. Drug Dispos.* **10**, 365 (1989). Multicenter clinical trial in hypertension: M. Moser *et al.*, *ibid.* **49**, 322 (1991); in congestive heart failure: H. T. Colfer *et al.*, *Am. J. Cardiol.* **70**, 354 (1992).

mp 148-149°. $[\alpha]_D$ −159° (c = 1.2 in ethanol).

Hydrochloride. [86541-74-4] CGS-14824A; Briem; Cibacen; Fortekor; Lotensin. $C_{24}H_{28}N_2O_5.HCl$; mol wt 460.95. Crystals from 3-pentanone + methanol (10:1), mp 188-190°. $[\alpha]_D$ −141.0° (c = 0.9 in ethanol). Sol in water, ethanol, methanol.

Diacid. [86541-78-8] Benazeprilat; CGS-14831. $C_{22}H_{24}N_2$-O_5; mol wt 396.44. mp 270-272°. $[\alpha]_D$ −200.5° (c = 1 in 3% aqueous NH_4OH).

THERAP CAT: Antihypertensive.

THERAP CAT (VET): In treatment of congestive heart failure in dogs.

1032. Bence-Jones Proteins. Low molecular weight, heat-sensitive proteins isolated from urine of multiple myeloma patients: Caputo, *Aminoacidosi* **7**, 163-77 (1957), *C.A.* **54**, 6841 (1960). Used as a model in structural studies of immunoglobulins, they are structurally homogeneous within each patient and antigenically related. Crystallographic structural study: E. E. Aeola *et al.*, *Biochemistry* **19**, 432 (1980). They constitute the light-chain compo-

nent of myeloma globulin and have been implicated in the pathogenesis of amyloidosis, *cf.* G. G. Glenner, *N. Engl. J. Med.* **302**, 1283 (1980); G. G. Glenner *et al.*, *Amyloid and Amyloidosis* (Excerpta Medica, Amsterdam, 1980) p 351.

Coagulates on heating at 45-55°. Redissolves partially or wholly on boiling. Amino acid composition in g-%: Arginine 5.6, histidine 3.3, lysine 9.5, tyrosine 6.4, tryptophan 3.4, phenylalanine 4.2, cystine 2.6, methionine 1.9, serine 8.4, threonine 8.1, leucine 7.3, isolecine 2.2, valine 9.8, glycine 8.6, alanine 3.1, proline 6.9, glutamic acid 7.5, aspartic acid 9.2. The molecule also shows a carbohydrate content of 9.4% (mostly glucose, mannose, and glucosamine).

1033. Bencyclane. [2179-37-5] N,N-Dimethyl-3-[[1-(phenylmethyl)cycloheptyl]oxy]-1-propanamine; 3-[(1-benzylcycloheptyl)oxy]-N,N-dimethylpropylamine; 1-benzyl-1-(3-dimethylaminopropoxy)cycloheptane; N-[3-(1-benzylcycloheptyloxy)propyl]-N,N-dimethylamine; benzcyclan. $C_{19}H_{31}NO$; mol wt 289.46. C 78.84%, H 10.79%, N 4.84%, O 5.53%. Prepn: Pallos *et al.*, *HU 151865* (1965 to EGYT), *C.A.* **62**, 16125b (1965). Series of articles on pharmacology: *Arzneim.-Forsch.* **20**, 1337-1460 (1970). Toxicity: E. Komlos, L. E. Petöcz, *ibid.* 1338.

bp_3 146-156°.

Fumarate. [14286-84-1] EGYT-201; Angiociclan; Dantrium; Dilangio; Fludilat; Fluxema; Halidor; Vasorelax. $C_{19}H_{31}NO.C_4$-H_4O_4; mol wt 405.53. Crystals from 25% ethanol, mp 131-133°. Soly in water at 25°: 1 g/100 ml; in hot water: 2 g/100 ml. Poorly sol in acetone, easily in alc. uv spectrum: Simonyi *et al.*, *Acta Pharm. Hung.* **36**, 257 (1966). At pH 3.4-6.6, uv max (ethanol): 207 nm. LD_{50} in mice, rats (mg/kg): 445.6, 414 orally; 49.9, 41.3 i.v.; 132, 86.3 i.p.; 203, 257 s.c. (Komlos, Petöcz).

THERAP CAT: Vasodilator (peripheral, cerebral).

1034. Bendamustine. [16506-27-7] 5-[Bis(2-chloroethyl)-amino]-1-methyl-1H-benzimidazole-2-butanoic acid; γ-[1-methyl-5-[bis(β-chloroethyl)amino]-2-benzimidazolyl]butyric acid. C_{16}-$H_{21}Cl_2N_3O_2$; mol wt 358.26. C 53.64%, H 5.91%, Cl 19.79%, N 11.73%, O 8.93%. Bifunctional alkylating agent. Prepn: W. Ozegowski, D. Krebs, *J. Prakt. Chem.* **20**, 178 (1963); *eidem*, *Zentralbl. Pharm. Pharmakother. Laboratoriumsdiagn.* **110**, 1013 (1971). Antitumor activity: W. Jungstand *et al.*, *ibid.* 1021. Capillary GC determn in plasma: H. Weber *et al.*, *J. Chromatogr.* **525**, 459 (1990). Toxicity study: U. Horn *et al.*, *Arch. Toxicol.* **Suppl. 8**, 504 (1985). Clinical evaluation in non-Hodgkin's lymphomas: K. Bremer, *J. Cancer Res. Clin. Oncol.* **128**, 603 (2002); in chronic lymphocytic leukemia: T. Lissitchkov *et al.*, *ibid.* **132**, 99 (2006); with prednisone in multiple myeloma: W. Pönisch *et al.*, *ibid* 205. Review of pharmacology and clinical development: K. Bremer, W. Roth, *Tumordiagn. Ther.* **17**, 1-6 (1996); J. A. Barman Balfour, K. L. Goa, *Drugs* **61**, 631-638 (2001).

Hydrochloride. [3543-75-7] IMET-3393; SDX-105; Cytostasan; Ribomustin; Treanda. $C_{16}H_{21}Cl_2N_3O_2.HCl$; mol wt 394.72. Monohydrate mp 152-156°. Sol in water. LD_{50} (monohydrate) in mice, rats (mg/kg): 400-500, 200-300 orally; 80, 40 i.v. (Horn).

THERAP CAT: Antineoplastic.

1035. Bendazac. [20187-55-7] [[1-(Phenylmethyl)-1H-indazol-3-yl]oxy]acetic acid; [(1-benzyl-1H-indazol-3-yl)oxy]acetic acid; bendazolic acid; bindazac; AF-983; Zildasac. $C_{16}H_{14}N_2O_3$;

mol wt 282.29. C 68.08%, H 5.00%, N 9.92%, O 17.00%. Principle action is inhibition of protein denaturation. Prepn: **BE 699226**; G. Palazzo, **US 3470194** (1967, 1969 both to Francesco Angelini). Pharmacology: B. Silvestrini *et al., Inflammation Biochem. Drug Interaction, Proc. Int. Symp.* **1968**, A. Bertelli, Ed. (Excerpta Med., Amsterdam, 1970) p 283. Mechanism of action: *eidem, Arzneim.-Forsch.* **20**, 250 (1970). Photoprotective capacity: Fuga *et al., Ann. Ital. Dermatol. Clin. Sper.* **24**, 205 (1970). NMR study of albumin, *q.v.*, binding: M. Delfini *et al., Bioorg. Chem.* **31**, 378 (2003). Toxicity: *Rx Bulletin* **3**, 147 (1972).

Odorless, crystalline powder, mp 158-159°. Insol in water. Sol in chloroform, ethanol, acetone. uv max: 306 nm ($E_{1cm}^{1\%}$ 191). LD_{50} in mice, rats (mg/kg): 380, 304 i.v.; 355, 388 i.p.; 440, 910 s.c.; 1105, ~1200 orally (*Rx Bulletin*).

Lysine salt. [81919-14-4] bendaline; bendazac lysine; Bendalina; Dogalina. $C_{16}H_{13}N_2O_3 \cdot C_6H_{14}N_2O_2$; mol wt 427.47. HPLC determn: S. Scalia, M. Massaccesi, *Int. J. Pharm.* **82**, 179 (1992). Clinical evaluation in senile cataract: P. Baraldi *et al., Graefe's Arch. Clin. Exp. Opthalmol.* **228**, 105 (1990); in *in vivo* contact lens cleaning: T. C. Evans *et al., Optom. Vis. Sci.* **70**, 210 (1993). Review of pharmacology and therapeutic potential: J. A. Balfour, S. P. Clissold, *Drugs* **39**, 575-596 (1990).

Sodium salt. [23255-99-4] Versus. $C_{16}H_{13}N_2NaO_3$; mol wt 304.28.

USE: Contact lens cleaning and wetting solution.

THERAP CAT: Anti-inflammatory; in treatment of cataracts.

THERAP CAT (VET): In treatment of cataracts.

1036. Bendiocarb. [22781-23-3] 2,2-Dimethyl-1,3-benzodioxol-4-ol methylcarbamate; methylcarbamic acid 2,3-(isopropylidenedioxy)phenyl ester; NC-6897; Ficam. $C_{11}H_{13}NO_4$; mol wt 223.23. C 59.18%, H 5.87%, N 6.27%, O 28.67%. Acetylcholinesterase inhibitor. Prepn: Gates, Gillon, **ZA 6800736** *C.A.* **71**, 38941m (1969), corresp to **US 3736338** (1968, 1973 both to Fisons). Insecticidal activity: Story, *Int. Pest Control* **14**, 6 (1972).

White solid, mp 129-130°. Soly in water: 40 ppm; in hexane: 350 ppm.

USE: Contact insecticide.

1037. Bendroflumethiazide. [73-48-3] 3,4-Dihydro-3-(phenylmethyl)-6-(trifluoromethyl)-2H-1,2,4-benzothiadiazine-7-sulfonamide 1,1-dioxide; 3-benzyl-6-trifluoromethyl-3,4-dihydro-7-sulfamoyl-2H-1,2,4-benzothiadiazine 1,1-dioxide; 3-benzyl-3,4-dihydro-7-sulfamyl-6-trifluoromethyl-1,2,4-benzothiadiazine 1,1-dioxide; bendrofluazide; benzydroflumethiazide; benzylhydroflumethiazide; Aprinox; Berkozide; Centyl; Naturetin; Neo-Naclex; Salures; Sinesalin. $C_{15}H_{14}F_3N_3O_4S_2$; mol wt 421.41. C 42.75%, H 3.35%, F 13.52%, N 9.97%, O 15.19%, S 15.22%. Prepn: C. T. Holdrege *et al., J. Am. Chem. Soc.* **81**, 4807 (1959); F. Lund, W. O. Godtfredsen, **GB 863474**; *eidem,* **US 3392168** (1961, 1968 both to Lövens Kemiske Fabrik). Comprehensive description: K. Florey, F. M. Russo-Alesi, *Anal. Profiles Drug Subs.* **5**, 1-19 (1976).

Crystals from dioxane, mp 224.5-225.5° (U.S. patent). Also reported as mp 221-223° (Holdrege). uv max (methanol): 208, 273, 326 nm ($E_{1cm}^{1\%}$ 745, 565, 96). Insol in water, chloroform, benzene, ether. Sol in acetone, alcohol.

THERAP CAT: Diuretic, antihypertensive.

1038. Benexate Hydrochloride. [78718-25-9] 2-[[[*trans*-4-[[(Aminoiminomethyl)amino]methyl]cyclohexyl]carbonyl]-oxy]benzoic acid phenylmethyl ester monohydrochloride; benzyl salicylate *trans*-4-(guanidinomethyl)cyclohexanecarboxylate hydrochloride; (2'-benzyloxycarbonyl)phenyl *trans*-4-(guanidinomethyl)cyclohexanecarboxylate hydrochloride. $C_{23}H_{28}ClN_3O_4$; mol wt 445.94. C 61.95%, H 6.33%, Cl 7.95%, N 9.42%, O 14.35%. Synthetic protease inhibitor with antiulcer activity. Prepn: **BE 885263**; M. Muramatsu *et al.,* **US 4348410** (1981, 1982 to Nippon Chemiphar; Teikoku Chem. Ind.). Prepn and protease inhibition: T. Satoh *et al., Chem. Pharm. Bull.* **33**, 647 (1985). Prepn of the clathrate compound with β-cyclodextrin: **JP Kokai 83 38250**; M. Shinoda *et al.,* **US 4478995** (1983, 1984 both to Teikoku Chem. Ind.). Effect on gastric secretion and exptl ulcers in rats: S. Okabe *et al., Oyo Yakuri* **27**, 829 (1984), *C.A.* **101**, 143881c (1984); I. Tanaka, H. Tagami, *Nippon Yakurigaku Zasshi* **85**, 167 (1985), *C.A.* **103**, 64660t (1985); F. Hirose *et al., Yakuri to Chiryo* **15**, 4749 (1987), *C.A.* **108**, 137769a (1988).

Crystals from methanol + ether, mp 83°.

Compd with β-cyclodextrin (1:1). [91574-91-3] Benexate-CD; TA-903; Lonmiel; Ulgut. $C_{65}H_{98}ClN_3O_{39}$; mol wt 1580.92.

THERAP CAT: Antiulcerative.

1039. Benfluorex. [23602-78-0] 2-[[1-Methyl-2-[3-(trifluoromethyl)phenyl]ethyl]amino]ethanol benzoate (ester); 2-[[α-methyl-*m*-(trifluoromethyl)phenethyl]amino]ethanol benzoate (ester); 1-(*m*-trifluoromethylphenyl)-2-(β-benzoyloxyethyl)aminopropane; N-(2-benzoyloxyethyl)norfenfluramine; benfluramate; S-780; SE-780. $C_{19}H_{20}F_3NO_2$; mol wt 351.36. C 64.95%, H 5.74%, F 16.22%, N 3.99%, O 9.11%. Prepn from 1-(*m*-trifluoromethylphenyl)-2-(β-hydroxyethyl)aminopropane and benzoyl chloride: L. Beregi *et al.,* **FR 1517587**; *eidem,* **US 3607909** (1968, 1971 both to Sci. Union et Cie, Soc. Franc. Rech. Med.). Metabolism studies: A. H. Beckett *et al., J. Pharm. Pharmacol.* **23**, 950 (1971); **24**, 281 (1972). Pharmacology: D. N. Brindley *et al., ibid.* **28**, 670 (1976); P. Pritchard *et al., ibid.* **29**, 343 (1977); *eidem, Biochem. J.* **166**, 639 (1977).

Colorless oil.

Hydrochloride. [23642-66-2] S-992; JP-992; Minolip; Mediator; Mediaxal. $C_{19}H_{20}F_3NO_2 \cdot HCl$; mol wt 387.82. Crystals from ethyl acetate, mp 161-162°.

THERAP CAT: Antilipemic.

1040. Benfluralin. [1861-40-1] N-Butyl-N-ethyl-2,6-dinitro-4-(trifluoromethyl)benzenamine; N-butyl-N-ethyl-α,α,α-trifluoro-2,6-dinitro-p-toluidine; N-butyl-N-ethyl-2,6-dinitro-4-trifluoromethylaniline; benefin; bethrodine; EL-110; Balan; Balfin; Benefex; Quilan. $C_{13}H_{16}F_3N_3O_4$; mol wt 335.28. C 46.57%, H 4.81%, F 17.00%, N 12.53%, O 19.09%. Selective pre-emergence herbicide. Prepn: Q. F. Soper, **US 3257190** (1966 to Lilly). Activity: E. F. Alder *et al., Proc. Northeast. Weed Control Conf.* **15**, 298 (1961). Environmental fate: T. Golab *et al., J. Agric. Food Chem.* **18**, 838 (1970). Soil degradn: J. H. Miller *et al., Weed Sci.* **23**, 211 (1975); R. L. Zimdahl, S. M. Gwynn, *ibid.* **25**, 247 (1977). Toxicity study: E. I. Goldenthal, *Toxicol. Appl. Pharmacol.* **18**, 185 (1971).

Yellow-orange crystalline solid, mp 65-66.5°. Vapor pressure at 30°: 3.89×10^{-4} mm Hg. Soly in water at 25°: <1 mg/l. Sol in most organic solvents; less sol in ethanol. Decomp in uv light. LD_{50} orally in female rats: >10,000 mg/kg (Goldenthal).

USE: Herbicide.

1041. Benfotiamine. [22457-89-2] Benzenecarbothioic acid S-[2-[[(4-amino-2-methyl-5-pyrimidinyl)methyl]formylamino]-1-[2-(phosphonooxy)ethyl]-1-propenyl] ester; thiobenzoic acid S-ester with N-[(4-amino-2-methyl-5-pyrimidinyl)methyl]-N-(4-hydroxy-2-mercapto-1-methyl-1-butenyl)formamide O-phosphate; S-benzoylthiamine monophosphate; BTMP; Biotamin; Vitanevril. $C_{19}H_{23}N_4O_6PS$; mol wt 466.45. C 48.92%, H 4.97%, N 12.01%, O 20.58%, P 6.64%, S 6.87%. Vitamin B_1 source. Prepn: A. Ito et al., **DE 1130811** (1962), C.A. **57**, 13764h (1962). Exists as 3 temperature dependent crystalline forms, α, γ, δ: A. Ito et al., Takamine Kenkyusho Nempo **14**, 64 (1962); C.A. **59**, 3920a (1963). Pharmacokinetics: H. Nogami et al., Chem. Pharm. Bull. **18**, 1937 (1970). Clinical bioequivalence to thiamine: R. Bitsch et al., Ann. Nutr. Metab. **35**, 292 (1991).

(Z)-form

Crystals, dec 165° (δ-form).

THERAP CAT: Vitamin (enzyme cofactor).

1042. Benfuracarb. [82560-54-1] N-[[[(2,3-Dihydro-2,2-dimethyl-7-benzofuranyl)oxy]carbonyl]methylamino]thio]-N-(1-methylethyl)-β-alanine ethyl ester; 2-methyl-4-(1-methylethyl)-7-oxo-8-oxa-3-thia-2,4-diazadecanoic acid 2,3-dihydro-2,2-dimethyl-7-benzofuranyl ester; 2,3-dihydro-2,2-dimethylbenzofuran-7-yl N-(N-isopropyl-N-ethoxycarbonylethylaminosulfenyl)-N-methylcarbamate; 2,3-dihydro-2,2-dimethyl-7-benzofuranyl N-[N-[2-(ethoxycarbonyl)ethyl]-N-isopropylsulfenamoyl]-N-methylcarbamate; ethyl N-[2,3-dihydro-2,2-dimethylbenzofuran-7-yloxycarbonyl(methyl)aminothio]-N-isopropyl-β-alaninate; OK-174; Oncol. $C_{20}H_{30}N_2O_5S$; mol wt 410.53. C 58.51%, H 7.37%, N 6.82%, O 19.49%, S 7.81%. Broad spectrum soil and foliar insecticide; cholinesterase inhibitor. Prepn and insecticidal properties: A. Tanaka et al., **BE 890162**; T. Goto et al., **US 4413005** (1982, 1983 both to Otsuka). Biological activity and field trials: T. Goto et al., Proc. 10th Conf. Int. Congr. Plant Prot. **1**, 360 (1983). Absorption and metabolism in plants: A. Tanaka et al., J. Agric. Food Chem. **33**, 1049 (1985). Brief review, field trials: P. Cagnieul, Def. Veg. **38**, 3-10 (1984).

Viscous brown-red liquid. d^{20} 1.17. Almost insol in water (8 mg/l at 20°). Sol in organic solvents. LD_{50} in male rats, mice, dogs (mg/kg): 138, 175, 300 orally (Goto).

USE: Insecticide.

1043. Benidipine. [105979-17-7] (4R)-rel-1,4-Dihydro-2,6-dimethyl-4-(3-nitrophenyl)-3,5-pyridinedicarboxylic acid methyl (3R)-1-(phenylmethyl)-3-piperidinyl ester; (±)-(R*)-3-[(R*)-1-benzyl-3-piperidyl] methyl 1,4-dihydro-2,6-dimethyl-4-(m-nitrophenyl)-3,5-pyridinedicarboxylate; (±)-2,6-dimethyl-4-(3-nitrophenyl)-1,4-dihydropyridine-3,5-dicarboxylic acid-3-(1-benzyl-3-piperidyl) ester-5-methyl ester. $C_{28}H_{31}N_3O_6$; mol wt 505.56. C 66.52%, H 6.18%, N 8.31%, O 18.99%. Dihydropyridine calcium channel blocker. Prepn (stereochemistry unspecified): K. Muto et al., **EP 63365**; eidem, **US 4448964** (1982, 1984 both to Kyowa). Prepn: eidem, **EP 106275** (1984 to Kyowa); and toxicity data: eidem, Arzneim.-Forsch. **38**, 1662 (1988). Structural studies: N. Hirayama, E. Shimizu, Acta Crystallogr. **C47**, 458 (1991). Series of articles on properties, pharmacology, determn and clinical evaluation: Arzneim.-Forsch. **38**, 1666-1763 (1988). Review: H. Suzuki, T. Saruta, Cardiovasc. Drug Rev. **7**, 25-38 (1989).

Hydrochloride. [91599-74-5] KW-3049; Coniel. $C_{28}H_{31}N_3$-$O_6 \cdot HCl$; mol wt 542.02. Yellow crystalline powder, mp 199.4-200.4°. uv max (ethanol): 238, 359 nm (ε 2.80 × 10^4, 6.68 × 10^3). Soly at 25° (%): methanol 6.9; ethanol 2.2; water 0.19; chloroform 0.16; acetone 0.13; ethyl acetate 0.0056; toluene 0.0019; n-heptane 0.00009. pKa 7.34. Partition coefficient (n-octanol/water): 1230 (pH 6.4, 22°). LD_{50} orally in male mice: 218 mg/kg (Muto, 1988).

THERAP CAT: Antihypertensive.

1044. Benomyl. [17804-35-2] [1-[(Butylamino)carbonyl]-1H-benzimidazol-2-yl]carbamic acid methyl ester; 1-(butylcarbamoyl)-2-benzimidazolecarbamic acid methyl ester; methyl 1-(butylcarbamoyl)-2-benzimidazolecarbamate; F-1991; Benlate. C_{14}-$H_{18}N_4O_3$; mol wt 290.32. C 57.92%, H 6.25%, N 19.30%, O 16.53%. Prepn: H. L. Klopping, **FR 1523597**; eidem, **US 3631176** (1968, 1971 both to du Pont). The degradation product, methyl 2-benzimidazolecarbamate, is thought to be the active component; see carbendazim. Antifungal activity and mode of action studies: Kilgore, White, Bull. Environ. Contam. Toxicol. **5**, 67 (1970); Maxwell, Brody, Appl. Microbiol. **21**, 944 (1971); Bartels-Schooley, MacNeill, Phytopathology **61**, 816 (1971). Activity as catalyst in biological oxidation of sewage and fertilizers: Kouba, **US 3649530** (1972 to du Pont). Toxicity: E. W. Schafer, Toxicol. Appl. Pharmacol. **21**, 315 (1972). Metabolism: J. A. Gardiner et al., J. Agric. Food Chem. **22**, 419 (1974). Mutagenicity study: J. P. Seiler, Mutat. Res. **32**, 151 (1975); H. Sherman et al., Toxicol. Appl. Pharmacol. **32**, 305 (1975). Review: W. E. Bleidner et al., Anal. Methods Pestic. Plant Growth Regul. **10**, 157-171 (1978).

White crystalline solid. Sol in chloroform. Insol in water or oil. LD_{50} orally in rats: >9590 mg/kg (Schafer).

Caution: Potential symptoms of overexposure are irritation of eyes, skin and upper respiratory system; skin sensitization; possible reproductive and teratogenic effects. See NIOSH Pocket Guide to Chemical Hazards (DHHS/NIOSH 97-140, 1997) p 24.

USE: Fungicide; ascaricide.

THERAP CAT (VET): Anthelmintic.

1045. Benorylate. [5003-48-5] 2-(Acetyloxy)benzoic acid 4-(acetylamino)phenyl ester; salicylic acid acetate, ester with 4-

hydroxyacetanilide; 2-acetoxy-4'-(acetamino)phenylbenzoate; *p*-acetamidophenyl acetylsalicylate; 4'-(acetamido)phenyl-2-acetoxybenzoate; fenasprate; Win-11450; Benoral; Benortan; Salipran. $C_{17}H_{15}NO_5$; mol wt 313.30. C 65.17%, H 4.83%, N 4.47%, O 25.53%. Prepn: **NL 6504517** (1965 to Sterwin), *C.A.* **64**, 8097c (1966), corresp to **GB 1101747** (1968); Robertson, **US 3431293** and Miller, **GB 1168289** (both 1969 to Sterling Drug). Pharmacological investigations: Rosner *et al., Therapie* **23**, 525 (1968); Raab, *Arzneim.-Forsch.* **21**, 1662 (1971). Pharmacokinetic studies in animals: Liss, Palme, *ibid.* **19**, 1177 (1969). Clinical evaluation: Bain, Burt, *Clin. Trials J.* **7**, 307 (1970); Cardoe, *ibid.* 313.

Crystals from methanol or ethanol, mp 175-176°. LD_{50} in mice, rats (mg/ml): 2000, ~10000 orally; 1255, 1830 i.p. (Robertson).

THERAP CAT: Analgesic; anti-inflammatory; antipyretic.

1046. Benoxacor. [98730-04-2] 4-(Dichloroacetyl)-3,4-dihydro-3-methyl-2*H*-1,4-benzoxazine; CGA-154281. $C_{11}H_{11}Cl_2$-NO_2; mol wt 260.12. C 50.79%, H 4.26%, Cl 27.26%, N 5.38%, O 12.30%. Protects maize from toxic effects of chloroacetanilide herbicides. Increases the expression of glutathione *S*-transferase (GST) isozymes in plants, accelerating herbicide metabolism. Prepn: H. Moser, **EP 149974**; *idem,* **US 4618361** (1985, 1986 both to Ciba-Geigy). Effects on metolachlor, *q.v.,* metabolism in corn: C. K. Cottingham, K. K. Hatzios, *Z. Naturforsch.* **46c**, 846 (1991). Efficacy and mode of action studies: L. Rowe *et al., Weed Sci.* **39**, 78 (1991); E. P. Fuerst *et al., Pestic. Sci.* **43**, 242 (1995). Metabolism studies: K. D. Miller *et al., J. Agric. Food Chem.* **44**, 3326, 3335 (1996). Environmental tolerances: *Fed. Regist.* **63**, 7299 (1998).

Crystals from diisopropyl ether, mp 105-107°. LD_{50} (mg/kg): >5000 orally in rats; >2010 dermally in rabbits. LC_{50} in rats (mg/l): >2000 by inhalation (*Fed. Regist.*).

USE: Herbicide safener.

1047. Benoxinate. [99-43-4] 4-Amino-3-butoxybenzoic acid 2-(diethylamino)ethyl ester; 3-butoxy-4-aminobenzoic acid 2-(diethylamino)ethyl ester; 2-(diethylamino)ethyl 4-amino-3-*n*-butoxybenzoate; oxibuprokain; oxybuprocaine. $C_{17}H_{28}N_2O_3$; mol wt 308.42. C 66.20%, H 9.15%, N 9.08%, O 15.56%. Prepn: **GB 654484** (1951 to Wander).

bp$_2$ 215-218°.

Hydrochloride. [5987-82-6] Conjuncain; Cebesine; Novesine; Benoxil; Lacrimin. $C_{17}H_{28}N_2O_3$·HCl; mol wt 344.88. Crystals, mp ~155° (*U.S.P.* **XVI**, 1960), also reported as mp 157-160° (*N.N.R.* 1955). Very sol in water, chloroform; sol in alc. Practically insol in ether. pH of aq solns, 4.5-5.2.

THERAP CAT: Anesthetic (local).

1048. Benperidol. [2062-84-2] 1-[1-[4-(4-Fluorophenyl)-4-oxobutyl]-4-piperidinyl]-1,3-dihydro-2*H*-benzimidazol-2-one; 1-

[1-[3-(*p*-fluorobenzoyl)propyl]-4-piperidyl]-2-benzimidazolinone; 1-[1-[4-(*p*-fluorophenyl)-4-oxobutyl]piperidin-4-yl]-2-benzimidazolinone; benzperidol; McN-JR-4584; R-4584; Anquil; Frénactil; Glianimon. $C_{22}H_{24}FN_3O_2$; mol wt 381.44. C 69.27%, H 6.34%, F 4.98%, N 11.02%, O 8.39%. Prepn: **BE 626307** (1963 to Janssen), *C.A.* **60**, 10690c (1964), corresp. to **GB 989755**.

Solid, mp 170-171.8°.

Hydrochloride hydrate. Solid, mp 134-142°.

THERAP CAT: Antipsychotic.

1049. Benproperine. [2156-27-6] 1-[1-Methyl-2-[2-(phenylmethyl)phenoxy]ethyl]piperidine; 1-[1-methyl-2-[(α-phenyl-*o*-tolyl)oxy]ethyl]piperidine; 1-[2-(2-benzylphenoxy)-1-methylethyl]-piperidine. $C_{21}H_{27}NO$; mol wt 309.45. C 81.51%, H 8.79%, N 4.53%, O 5.17%. Prepn: **GB 914008**; Rubinstein, **US 3117059** (1962, 1964 to Aktieselskabet Pharmacia). Pharmacology: Yamatsu *et al., Jpn. J. Pharmacol.* **17**, 538 (1967); N. Tellini, V. De Fina, *Boll. Chim. Farm.* **109**, 476 (1970).

Liquid. bp$_{0.2}$ 159-161°. LD_{50} orally in mice: 1087 mg/kg (Tellini, De Fina).

Trihydrogen phosphate. [19428-14-9] Tussafug. $C_{21}H_{27}$-$NO.H_3PO_4$. Crystals from abs ethanol, mp 150-152°. LD_{50} orally in mice: 1431 mg/kg (Tellini, De Fina).

Pamoate. [64238-92-2] Benzproperine embonate; Blascorid; Pirexyl. $(C_{21}H_{27}NO)_2.C_{23}H_{16}O_6$; mol wt 1007.26.

THERAP CAT: Antitussive.

1050. Benserazide. [322-35-0] DL-Serine 2-[(2,3,4-trihydroxyphenyl)methyl] hydrazide; *N*-(DL-seryl)-*N*'-(2,3,4-trihydroxybenzyl) hydrazine. $C_{10}H_{15}N_3O_5$; mol wt 257.24. C 46.69%, H 5.88%, N 16.33%, O 31.10%. Prepn: **BE 619015**; Hegedüs, Zeller, **US 3178476** (1962, 1965 both to Hoffmann-La Roche). Inhibition of dopa decarboxylase *in vitro* and *in vivo:* W. P. Burkard *et al., Experientia* **18**, 411 (1962); *eidem, Arch. Biochem. Biophys.* **107**, 187 (1964). Synergy with dopa *in vivo:* G. Bartholini *et al., Nature* **215**, 852 (1967); G. Bartholini, A. Pletscher, *J. Pharmacol. Exp. Ther.* **161**, 14 (1968). Clinical comparison with carbidopa, *q.v.:* I. Kuruma *et al., J. Pharm. Pharmacol.* **24**, 289 (1972). Clinical and pharmacokinetic profile: M.-H. Marion *et al., Adv. Neurol.* **45**, 493 (1987). Review of pharmacology and clinical efficacy of decarboxylase inhibitors: R. M. Pinder *et al., Drugs* **11**, 329-377 (1976).

Hydrochloride. [14919-77-8] Ro-4-4602. $C_{10}H_{15}N_3O_5$·HCl; mol wt 293.70. White crystalline powder, mp 146-148°. Sol in water.

Combination with levodopa. [37270-69-2] Co-beneldopa; Madopar; Madopark; Prolopa.

THERAP CAT: In combination with levodopa as antiparkinsonian.

1051. Bensuldazic Acid. [1219-77-8] 5-Benzyldihydro-6-thioxo-2H-1,3,5-thiadiazine-3(4H)-acetic acid; ujothion; D-4720. $C_{12}H_{14}N_2O_2S_2$; mol wt 282.38. C 51.04%, H 5.00%, N 9.92%, O 11.33%, S 22.71%. Prepn: A. Rieche et al., Arch. Pharm. **296**, 770 (1963); W. Schade et al., **DD 31793** (1964), C.A. **63**, 16370g (1965). Antimicrobial activity: M. Schorr et al., Arzneim.-Forsch. **19**, 1807 (1969). Efficacy vs ringworm in cattle: B. Vujic, Berl. Muench. Tieraerztl. Wochenschr. **84**, 144 (1971).

Crystals, mp 152°.
Sodium salt. [1950-15-8] Defungit. $C_{12}H_{13}N_2NaO_2S_2$; mol wt 304.36.
THERAP CAT (VET): Antifungal.

1052. Bensulfuron-methyl. [83055-99-6] 2-[[[[[(4,6-Dimethoxy-2-pyrimidinyl)amino]carbonyl]amino]sulfonyl]methyl]-benzoic acid methyl ester; methyl 2-[(4,6-dimethoxypyrimidin-2-yl)ureidosulfonylmethyl]benzoate; DPX-F5384; Londax; Mariner. $C_{16}H_{18}N_4O_7S$; mol wt 410.40. C 46.83%, H 4.42%, N 13.65%, O 27.29%, S 7.81%. Sulphonylurea herbicide primarily used on rice and aquatic weeds. Prepn: R. F. Sauers, **EP 51466**; idem, **US 4420325** (1982, 1983 both to DuPont). Conformation study: Y. K. Kang, D. W. Kim, Bull. Korean Chem. Soc. **11**, 144 (1990). Environmental persistence: A. Ferrero et al., Mobility Degrad. Xenobiot., Proc. 9th Simp. Pestic. Chem. **1993**, 257. HPLC determn in soil: C. Salardi et al., Meded. Fac. Landbouwwet. Univ. Gent **61**, 617 (1996). LC determn in rice and crayfish; M. Zhou et al., J. AOAC Int. **79**, 791 (1996). Control of aquatic weeds: G. McCorkelle et al., Proc. 9th Aust. Weeds Conf. **1990**, 549. Field trials on rice: J. L. Pacheco, C. L. Pope, Proc. West. Soc. Weed Sci. **39**, 147 (1986); M. P. Braverman, Weed Technol. **9**, 494 (1995).

Mp 179-183°.
USE: Herbicide.

1053. Bentazon. [25057-89-0] 3-(1-Methylethyl)-1H-2,1,3-benzothiadiazin-4(3H)-one 2,2-dioxide; 3-isopropyl-1H-2,1,3-benzothiadiazin-4(3H)-one 2,2-dioxide; bentazone; bendioxide; Basagran. $C_{10}H_{12}N_2O_3S$; mol wt 240.28. C 49.99%, H 5.03%, N 11.66%, O 19.98%, S 13.34%. Selective post-emergence herbicide. Prepn: A. Zeidler et al., **ZA 6705164**; idem, **US 3708277** (1968, 1973 both to BASF). Weed control: C. E. G. Mulder, G. B. Wortmann, Proc. 3rd Natl. Weeds Conf. S. Afr. **1980**, 159. HPLC determn in sugar maize and surface water: E. A. Hogendoorn, C. E. Goewie, J. Chromatogr. **475**, 432 (1989); in soil: F. S. Rasero et al., Sci. Total Environ. **123/124**, 57 (1992). Stability in ground, surface, soil waters: C. Mouvet et al., Chemosphere **35**, 1083 (1997). Toxicity data: G. Ugazio et al., Res. Commun. Chem. Pathol. Pharmacol. **74**, 349 (1991). Review of synthesis: G. Hamprecht et al., Kem. - Kemi **1**, 590-592 (1974); of environmental behavior: R. Huber, S. Otto, Rev. Environ. Contam. Toxicol. **137**, 111-134 (1994).

White crystalline powder, mp 137-139°. Soly (w/w) at 20°: water 0.05%; acetone 150.7%; benzene 3.3%; chloroform 18%; ethanol 86.1%. pKa (24°): 3.3. Vapor pressure at 20°: 1.7 × 10^{-6} hPa. Log P (octanol/water) at 22°: −0.456 (pH 7). LD_{50} in male, female rats (mg/kg): 383.2, 433.6 orally (Ugazio).
USE: Herbicide.

1054. Bentiromide. [37106-97-1] 4-[[(2S)-2-(Benzoylamino)-3-(4-hydroxyphenyl)-1-oxopropyl]amino]benzoic acid; (S)-p-(α-benzamido-p-hydroxyhydrocinnamamido)benzoic acid; N-benzoyl-L-tyrosyl-p-aminobenzoic acid; BTPABA; E-2663; Chymex; PFT Roche. $C_{23}H_{20}N_2O_5$; mol wt 404.42. C 68.31%, H 4.98%, N 6.93%, O 19.78%. Synthetic chymotrypsin-labile peptide, used in diagnosis of exocrine pancreatic disease. Prepn: P. L. De Benneville, N. J. Greenberger, **DE 2156835**; eidem, **US 3801562** (1972, 1974 both to Rohm & Haas). Synthesis, in vitro and in vivo data: P. L. De Benneville et al., J. Med. Chem. **15**, 1098 (1972). Early clinical studies: K. Gyr et al., Schweiz. Med. Wochenschr. **105**, 1717 (1975); W. Bornschein et al., Clin. Chim. Acta **67**, 21 (1976). Pediatric study: G. Dockter et al., Eur. J. Pediatr. **135**, 277 (1981). Human toxicity study, effects of renal insufficiency on pancreatic function test: C. Lang et al., J. Clin. Chem. Clin. Biochem. **18**, 551 (1980).

Cryst from methanol/water, mp 240-242°. $[\alpha]_D^{25}$ +72.3° (c = 1 in DMF) (**US 3801562**); also reported as $[\alpha]_D^{25}$ +87° (c = 1 in DMF) (De Benneville).
THERAP CAT: Diagnostic aid (pancreatic function).

1055. Bentonite. [1302-78-9] Wilkinite. A colloidal native hydrated aluminum silicate (clay) found in the midwest of the U.S.A. and in Canada. Consists principally of montmorillonite, $Al_2O_3.4SiO_2.H_2O$. Usually contains some magnesium, iron, and calcium carbonate. Review: J. Alexander, Ind. Eng. Chem. **16**, 1140 (1924).

The color in the massive condition varies from yellowish-white to almost black. The powder is cream colored to pale brown. It has the property of forming highly viscous suspensions or gels with not less than ten times its weight of water. The property of forming gels is very much increased by the addition of small amounts of alkaline substances such as magnesium oxide.
USE: As of Fuller's earth; as emulsifier for oils; as a base for plasters. Pharmaceutic aid (suspending agent).

1056. Bentoquatam. [1340-69-8] Quaternium 18-bentonite; bis(hydrogenated tallow alkyl)dimethylammonium complex with sodium bentonite; Bentone 34; Ivy Block; Tixogel VP. Ion exchange addition product of the montmorillonite clay, bentonite, q.v., and quaternium-18, a dimethyl, ditallow quaternary ammonium salt containing predominantly C_{18} alkyl chains. Acts as a barrier to block urushiol, q.v., from the skin. Prepn of aliphatic ammonium bentonites: E. A. Hauser, **US 2531427** (1950); and organophilic properties: J. W. Jordan, J. Phys. Colloid Chem. **53**, 294 (1949); idem et al., ibid. **54**, 1196 (1950). Use as stationary phase in GSC and HPLC: D. W. Grant et al., J. Chromatogr. **99**, 721 (1974). Description of properties, toxicology and use in cosmetics: J. Am. Coll. Toxicol. **1**, 71-83 (1982). Clinical trial in poison ivy/oak dermatitis: J. G. Marks, Jr. et al., J. Am. Acad. Dermatol. **33**, 212 (1995).

Hydrophobic, thixotropic organoclay with gel-like consistency. Expansible in water, methanol, ethanol, isopropanol, sorbitol, glycerine, acetone. Heat stable up to 500°. Resists base or acid attacks over pH range of 3-11.
USE: Emulsion stabilizer in cosmetics. Stationary phase in chromatography.
THERAP CAT: Barrier for the prevention of allergic contact dermatitis.

1057. Benzal Chloride. [98-87-3] (Dichloromethyl)benzene; benzylidene chloride; benzyl dichloride; α,α-dichlorotoluene; benzylene chloride. $C_7H_6Cl_2$; mol wt 161.03. C 52.21%, H

3.76%, Cl 44.03%. $C_6H_5CHCl_2$. Obtained by chlorination of toluene. Lab procedure: A. I. Vogel, *Practical Organic Chemistry* (Longmans, London, 3rd ed., 1959) p 539; Gattermann-Wieland, *Praxis des Organischen Chemikers* (de Gruyter, Berlin, 40th ed., 1961) p 184.

Very refractive liquid; fumes in air; vapors irritate the eyes; pungent odor. d 1.26. bp 205°. mp −17°. Insol in water; freely sol in alcohol, ether.

USE: Manuf benzaldehyde, cinnamic acid.

1058. Benzaldehyde. [100-52-7] Benzoic aldehyde; artificial essential oil of almond. C_7H_6O; mol wt 106.12. C 79.23%, H 5.70%, O 15.08%. Occurs in kernels of bitter almonds; made synthetically from benzal chloride and lime or by oxidation of toluene. Laboratory prepn from benzal chloride: A. I. Vogel, *Practical Organic Chemistry* (Longmans, London, 3rd ed., 1959) p 693; Gattermann-Wieland, *Praxis des Organischen Chemikers* (de Gruyter, Berlin, 40th ed., 1961) p 184. Toxicity data: P. M. Jenner *et al., Food Cosmet. Toxicol.* **2**, 327 (1964). *Review:* A. E. Williams in *Kirk-Othmer Encyclopedia of Chemical Technology* **vol. 3** (Wiley-Interscience, New York, 3rd ed., 1978) pp 736-743.

Strongly refractive liquid, becoming yellowish on keeping; characteristic odor of volatile oil of almond; burning aromatic taste. Oxidizes in air to benzoic acid; volatile with steam. d_4^{15} 1.050; 1.043 at 25°. bp 179°. mp −56.5°. Flash pt 62°C. n_D^{20} 1.5456. Sol in 350 parts water; miscible with alcohol, ether, oils. It reduces ammoniacal $AgNO_3$, but not Fehling's soln. *Keep tightly closed and protected from light.* LD_{50} in rats, guinea pigs (mg/kg): 1300, 1000 orally (Jenner).

Note: Benzaldehyde FFC designates a grade of benzaldehyde free from chlorine.

Caution: Narcotic in high concns. May cause contact dermatitis.

USE: Manufacture of dyes, perfumery, cinnamic and mandelic acids, as solvent; in flavors.

1059. Benzalkonium Chloride. [8001-54-5] Alkylbenzyldimethyl quaternary ammonium compounds chlorides; alkyldimethyl(phenylmethyl)ammonium chloride; Baktonium; Benirol; Bradosol; Callusolve; Capitol; Laudamonium; Osvan; Pharmatex; Roccal; Sagrotan; Zephiran; Zephirol. A mixture of alkyldimethylbenzylammonium chlorides; three major homologues consist of C_{12}, C_{14} and C_{16} straight chain alkyls. Prepn and biological activity: R. A. Cutler *et al., Proc. Annu. Meet. Chem. Spec. Manuf. Assoc.* **1966**, 102. Acute toxicity data: L. M. Cummins, E. T. Kimura, *Toxicol. Appl. Pharmacol.* **20**, 89 (1971). Capillary electrophoretic determn in formulations: M. Jimidar *et al., Biomed. Chromatogr.* **12**, 128 (1998); MS determn on skin: S. Kawakami *et al., Analyst* **123**, 489 (1998). Efficacy as disinfecting wound irrigant: B. B. Tarbox *et al., Clin. Orthop. Relat. Res.* **1998**, 255. Use as disinfectant against viruses: A. Wood, D. Payne, *J. Hosp. Infect.* **38**, 283 (1998). Brief review: A. C. S. Parr *et al., Spec. Chem.* **16**, 157-160 (1996).

$R = C_8H_{17}$ to $C_{18}H_{37}$

White or yellowish-white, amorphous powder or gelatinous pieces. Very sol in water, alcohol, acetone; slightly sol in benzene. Almost insol in ether. The aq soln is slightly alkaline to litmus and foams strongly when shaken. LD_{50} orally in rats: 400 mg/kg (Cummins, Kimura).

USE: Cationic surface active agent and germicide. Pharmaceutic aid (preservative). Algicide.

THERAP CAT: Antiseptic, disinfectant.

THERAP CAT (VET): Antiseptic for skin preoperatively or for wounds, burns, etc. Udder wash.

1060. Benzamide. [55-21-0] Benzoylamide. C_7H_7NO; mol wt 121.14. C 69.40%, H 5.82%, N 11.56%, O 13.21%. $C_6H_5CONH_2$. Prepd from benzoyl chloride and ammonium carbonate. Lab prepn: Gattermann-Wieland, *Praxis des Organischen Chemikers* (de Gruyter, Berlin, 40th ed., 1961) p 119. Alternate procedure using concd ammonia soln: A. I. Vogel, *Practical Organic Chemistry* (Longmans, London, 3rd ed., 1959) p 797.

Crystals. d^4 1.341. mp 130°. bp 288°. One gram dissolves in 74 ml water, more sol in boiling water, in 6 ml alc, 3.3 ml pyridine. Sol in hot benzene, slightly in ether; sol in ammonia with formation of a small quantity of benzonitrile.

N-Chloro deriv. mp 116°. Sol in water; insol in alcohol or benzene.

1061. Benzanilide. [93-98-1] *N*-Phenylbenzamide; *N*-benzoylaniline. $C_{13}H_{11}NO$; mol wt 197.23. C 79.17%, H 5.62%, N 7.10%, O 8.11%. $C_6H_5CONHC_6H_5$. Prepd by the treatment of aniline with benzoic acid: Hübner, *Ann.* **208**, 291 (1881); Nägeli, *Bull. Soc. Chim.* [3] **11**, 892 (1894); Webb, *Org. Synth.* **7**, 6 (1927); **coll. vol. I** (2nd ed., 1941) p 82.

Leaflets from alc. d 1.315. mp 163°. Sublimes. Distills without decompn. bp_{10} 117-119°. Absorption spectrum: Crymble, *J. Chem. Soc.* **99**, 459 (1911). Insoluble in water. One gram dissolves in 60 ml alc, 7 ml boiling alc. Slightly sol in ether.

USE: Manuf dyes and perfumes.

1062. 1,2-Benzanthracene. [56-55-3] Benz[*a*]anthracene; 2,3-benzphenanthrene; tetraphene; benzanthrene; naphthanthracene. $C_{18}H_{12}$; mol wt 228.29. C 94.70%, H 5.30%. Occurs in coal tar, *q.v.*: Cook *et al., J. Chem. Soc.* **1933**, 395. Synthesis from naphthalene and phthalic anhydride: Elbs, *Ber.* **19**, 2209 (1886). From *o*-toluylnaphthalene: Fieser, Dietz, *Ber.* **62**, 1827 (1929). From phenanthrene and succinic anhydride: Haworth, Mavin, *J. Chem. Soc.* **1933**, 1012. Absorption spectrum: Capper, Marsh, *J. Chem. Soc.* **1926**, 726; Clar, *Ber.* **65**, 507 (1932); Mayneord, Roe, *Proc. Roy. Soc. London* **A152**, 299 (1935). *Review:* E. Clar, *Polycyclic Hydrocarbons* **Vol. 1 & 2** (Academic Press, New York, 1964). Review of toxicology and human exposure: *Toxicological Profile for Polycyclic Aromatic Hydrocarbons* (PB95-264370, 1995) 487 pp.

Plates from glacial acetic acid or alc. Greenish-yellow fluorescence. Sublimes. mp 155-157° (Fieser, Dietz); mp 160° [Fieser, Hershberg, *J. Am. Chem. Soc.* **59**, 2502 (1937)]; mp 167° (I. G. Farbenind., DE 481819; DE 486766). Difficultly sol in boiling alc; sol in most other organic solvents. Insol in water.

Caution: This substance is reasonably anticipated to be a human carcinogen: *Report on Carcinogens, Eleventh Edition* (PB2005-104914, 2004) p III-220.

1063. Benzanthrone. [82-05-3] 7*H*-Benz[*de*]anthracen-7-one. $C_{17}H_{10}O$; mol wt 230.26. C 88.67%, H 4.38%, O 6.95%. Prepd by heating a reduction product of anthraquinone with sulfuric acid and glycerol: Macleod, Allen, *Org. Synth.* **14**, 4 (1934); *cf.* US 1626392 (1927). Review of toxicology: G. B. Singh *et al., J. Sci. Ind. Res.* **49**, 288-296 (1990).

Pale yellow needles from alcohol or xylene. mp 170°. Absorption spectrum: Clar, *Ber.* **65**, 846 (1932). Solubility at 20° = 0.52 g in 100 g glacial acetic acid; 1.61 g in 100 g benzene; 2.05 g in 100 g chlorobenzene. Solution in H_2SO_4 is orange with green fluorescence. LD_{50} in albino rabbits: >3 g/kg dermally; LD_{50} in rats, mice (g/kg): 1.5, 0.29 i.p. (Singh).

USE: Manufacture of dyes.

1064. Benzathine. [140-28-3] N,N'-Bis(phenylmethyl)-1,2-ethanediamine; N,N'-dibenzylethylenediamine; 1,2-bis(benzylamino)ethane; DBED. $C_{16}H_{20}N_2$; mol wt 240.34. C 79.96%, H 8.39%, N 11.66%. Prepd from N,N'-dibenzenesulfonyl-N,N'-dibenzylethylenediamine by heating with concd HCl in bomb tube at 170-180°: Bleier, *Ber.* **32,** 1829 (1899); from ethylene chloride and benzylamine: Frost *et al., J. Am. Chem. Soc.* **71,** 3842 (1949); by reduction of N,N'-dibenzylideneethylenediamine: **DE 98031** (1898 to Schering); *Chem. Zentralbl.* **1898, II,** 743; Van Alphen, *Rec. Trav. Chim.* **54,** 93 (1935); Lob, *ibid.* **55,** 859 (1936); Szabo *et al., Antibiot. Chemother.* **1,** 499 (1951); Rebenstorf, **US 2773098** (1956 to Upjohn).

Oily liquid, mp 26°. d_4^{20} 1.024. bp_{12} 212-213°; bp_4 195°. n_D^{20} 1.5624. Insol in water. Freely sol in the usual organic solvents except CS_2, with which it gives a solid addition product.

Diacetate. $C_{20}H_{28}N_2O_4$. Needles, mp 111°. Soly in water: 253 mg/ml.

Dihydrobromide. $C_{16}H_{22}Br_2N_2$. Shiny leaflets, dec 300°. Soly in water: 30 mg/ml.

Dihydrochloride. $C_{16}H_{22}Cl_2N_2$. Shiny leaflets, dec 298°. Soly in water: 23.9 mg/ml.

Sulfate. $C_{16}H_{22}N_2O_4S$. Crystals, dec 247-250°. Soly in water: 15.8 mg/ml.

Disalicylate. $C_{30}H_{34}N_2O_6$. Crystals, mp 85°. Soly in water: 2.43 mg/ml.

USE: Manuf of a repository form of penicillins G and V, *q.q.v.*

1065. Benzbromarone. [3562-84-3] (3,5-Dibromo-4-hydroxyphenyl)(2-ethyl-3-benzofuranyl)methanone; 3,5-dibromo-4-hydroxyphenyl 2-ethyl-3-benzofuranyl ketone; 3-(3,5-dibromo-4-hydroxybenzoyl)-2-ethylbenzofuran; 2-ethyl-3-benzofuranyl 4-hydroxy-3,5-dibromophenyl ketone; 2-ethyl-3-(3,5-dibromo-4-hydroxybenzoyl)benzofuran; 2-ethyl-3-(3,5-dibromo-4-hydroxybenzoyl)oxaindene; 2-ethyl-3-benzofuryl 3,5-dibromo-4-hydroxyphenyl ketone; L-2214; MJ-10061; Azubromaron; Desuric; Max-Uric; Minuric; Narcaricin; Normurat; Uricovac; Urinorm. $C_{17}H_{12}Br_2O_3$; mol wt 424.08. C 48.15%, H 2.85%, Br 37.68%, O 11.32%. Prepn: **BE 553621** (1957 to Labaz); Buu-Hoi *et al., J. Chem. Soc.* **1957,** 625; Buu-Hoi, Beaudet, **US 3012042** (1961 to Soc. Belge l'Azote Prod. Chim. Marly). Structure-activity study: Delbarre *et al., Chim. Ther.* **3,** 470 (1968). Pharmacology of hypouricemic effect: D. S. Sinclair, I. H. Fox, *J. Rheumatol.* **2,** 437 (1975). Pharmacokinetic and clinical studies: T. F. Yu, *ibid.* **3,** 305 (1976). Pharmacokinetics and biotransformation in man: H. Ferber *et al., Eur. J. Clin. Pharmacol.* **19,** 431 (1981). HPLC determn in serum: H. Vergin *et al., J. Chromatogr.* **183,** 383 (1980).

Yellowish prisms, mp 151°.
THERAP CAT: Uricosuric.

1066. Benzene. [71-43-2] Benzol; cyclohexatriene. C_6H_6; mol wt 78.11. C 92.26%, H 7.74%. Natural component of petroleum, usually <1.0% by weight. Discovered by Faraday in compressed oil gas in 1825. Obtained in the coking of coal and in the

production of illuminating gas from coal. Manuf by catalytic reforming and separation of aromatic compounds, thermal or catalytic dealkylation of toluene, toluene disproportionation; from pyrolysis gasoline. Purification by washing with water: **GB 863711** (1961 to Schloven-Chemie and H. Koppers GmbH), *C.A.* **55,** 16971f (1961). Lab prepn from aniline: Gattermann-Wieland, *Praxis des Organischen Chemikers* (de Gruyter, Berlin, 40th ed., 1961) p 247. Production of pure benzene: French, *Ind. Chem.* **39,** 9-12 (1963). Manuf: *Faith, Keyes & Clark's Industrial Chemicals,* F. A. Lowenheim, M. K. Moran, Eds. (Wiley-Interscience, New York, 4th ed., 1975) pp 126-137. Physical properties: Thorne *et al., Ind. Eng. Chem. Anal. Ed.* **17,** 481 (1945). Solubility studies: F. P. Schwarz, *Anal. Chem.* **52,** 10 (1980). Toxicity data: Kimura *et al., Toxicol. Appl. Pharmacol.* **19,** 699 (1971). *Review:* W. Fruscella in *Kirk-Othmer Encyclopedia of Chemical Technology* **vol. 4** (Wiley-Interscience, New York, 4th ed., 1992) pp 73-103. Reviews of toxicology: R. Snyder *et al., Rev. Biochem. Toxicol.* **3,** 123-154 (1981); D. J. Paustenbach *et al., Environ. Health Perspect.* **101,** Suppl. 6, 177-200 (1993); and human exposure: *Toxicological Profile for Benzene* (PB98-101157, 1997) 463 pp. Symposia on metabolism, toxicity and carcinogenesis: *Environ. Health Perspect.* **82,** 3-310 (1989); *ibid.* **104,** Suppl. 6, 1121-1441 (1996).

Clear, colorless, volatile, highly flammable liquid; characteristic odor. d_4^{15} 0.8787. bp 80.1°. mp 5.5°. n_D^{20} 1.50108. Flash pt, closed cup: 12°F (−11°C). Soly in water at 23.5°C (w/w): 0.188%. Miscible with alcohol, chloroform, ether, carbon disulfide, carbon tetrachloride, glacial acetic acid, acetone, oils. *Keep in well-closed containers in a cool place and away from fire.* LD_{50} orally in young adult rats: 3.8 ml/kg (Kimura).

Sodium deriv. Phenyl sodium. C_6H_5Na. Prepn: Schlosser, *Angew. Chem.* **76,** 267 (1964). Solid mass, dec by water, acids, alkalies. Sol in liquid ammonia, tetrahydrofuran.

Caution: Potential symptoms of overexposure by inhalation or ingestion are dizziness, headache, vomiting, visual disturbances, staggering gait, hilarity, fatigue, anorexia, lassitude, CNS depression, loss of consciousness, respiratory arrest. Chronic exposure has been associated with bone marrow depression and leukemia. Direct contact may cause irritation of eyes, nose, respiratory system and skin; dermatitis may develop due to defatting action. Aspiration into the lung may lead to chemical pneumonitis. *See Patty's Industrial Hygiene and Toxicology* vol. 2B, G. D. Clayton, F. E. Clayton, Eds. (Wiley-Interscience, New York, 4th ed., 1994) pp 1306-1326; *NIOSH Pocket Guide to Chemical Hazards* (DHHS/NIOSH 97-140, 1997) p 26. Benzene is listed as a known human carcinogen: *Report on Carcinogens, Eleventh Edition* (PB2005-104914, 2004) p III-26.

USE: Manuf of industrial chemicals such as polymers, detergents, pesticides pharmaceuticals, dyes, plastics, resins. Solvent for waxes, resins, oils, natural rubber, etc. Gasoline additive.

THERAP CAT (VET): Has been used as a disinfectant.

1067. Benzenearsonic Acid. [98-05-5] Phenylarsonic acid. $C_6H_7AsO_3$; mol wt 202.04. C 35.67%, H 3.49%, As 37.08%, O 23.76%. $C_6H_5AsO(OH)_2$.

Cryst powder. mp 158-162° with dec. Sol in 40 parts water, 50 parts alcohol; insol in chloroform.

USE: Reagent for tin.

1068. Benzeneboronic Acid. [98-80-6] Phenylboronic acid; phenylboric acid; phenylboron dihydroxide. $C_6H_7BO_2$; mol wt 121.93. C 59.10%, H 5.79%, B 8.87%, O 26.24%. Prepd by the reaction of phenylmagnesium bromide with methyl borate: Washburn *et al.* in *Adv. Chem. Ser.* **23,** entitled "Metal-Organic Compounds," M. Sittig, Ed. (ACS, Washington DC, 1959) pp 102-128. Crystal and molecular structure: S. J. Rettig, J. Trotter, *Can. J. Chem.* **55,** 3071 (1977).

Crystals from water. Spontaneous conversion to C_6H_5BO, **benzene boronic anhydride** or **phenylboroxide** on standing in dry air, although the best method is by azeotropic dehydration with toluene. mp 215-216° (anhydride). pKa 13.7. Dipole moment 1.72 (dioxane). Soly in water at 25°: 2.5%, benzene: 1.75%, xylene: 1.2%, ether: 30.2%, methanol: 178%.

1069. Benzenestibonic Acid. [535-46-6] Dihydroxyphenylstibine oxide; phenylstibonic acid; phenylstibinic acid. $C_6H_7O_3Sb$; mol wt 248.88. C 28.96%, H 2.83%, O 19.29%, Sb 48.92%. $C_6H_5SbO(OH)_2$. Arylstibonic acids exist in the solid state as polymers of high mol wt, associated by H-bonds. The ions exist probably in the form $[ArSb(OH)_5]^-$. Benzenestibonic acid is prepd from benzenediazonium chloride and antimony trioxide in the presence of alkali: Schmidt, *Ann.* **421**, 176, 188 (1920); **DE 254421**; *Chem. Zentralbl.* **1913**, I, 345; *Frdl.* **11**, 1084. From the double compd of benzenediazonium chloride and antimony trichloride by the action of alkali: May, *J. Chem. Soc.* **101**, 1033 (1912); **US 1260707**.

Minute crystals from acetic acid, larger diamond-shaped, glistening crystals from alcohol-chloroform mixture on the addition of water. Not melted at 250°, dec at higher temps. Insol in water; slightly sol in alc; more sol in acetone, in alcohol + benzene, alcohol + ether, alcohol + chloroform; sol in warm chloroform or amyl acetate; freely sol in aq soln of sodium hydroxide, sodium carbonate, and ammonia.

1070. Benzenesulfonic Acid. [98-11-3] $C_6H_6O_3S$; mol wt 158.18. C 45.56%, H 3.82%, O 30.34%, S 20.27%. $C_6H_5SO_3H$. Made by treating benzene with fuming H_2SO_4: Gattermann-Wieland, *Praxis des Organischen Chemikers* (de Gruyter, Berlin, 40th ed., 1961) p 168.

Sesquihydrate. Deliquescent plates, tablets, mp 43-44°. When anhydrous mp 50-51°, also reported as mp 65-66°. pKa (25°): 0.699. Freely sol in water, alc; slightly sol in benzene; insol in ether, carbon disulfide. *Keep well closed.*

Ethyl ester. Ethyl benzenesulfonate. $C_8H_{10}O_3S$. Colorless to slightly yellow, almost odorless liq. bp$_{15}$ 156°. d$_4^{17}$ 1.219. Slightly sol in water; misc with alc, benzene, chloroform, ether.

Sodium salt. Sodium benzenesulfonate; sodium benzosulfonate. $C_6H_5NaO_3S$. Crystals. Sol in water.

Caution: Highly irritant to skin, eyes, mucous membranes.

USE: Manuf phenol by fusion with NaOH.

1071. Benzenesulfonic Anhydride. [512-35-6] $C_{12}H_{10}O_5S_2$; mol wt 298.33. C 48.31%, H 3.38%, O 26.81%, S 21.50%. $(C_6H_5SO_2)_2O$. Prepd by heating benzenesulfonic acid with excess phosphorus pentoxide mixed with inert support: Field, *J. Am. Chem. Soc.* **74**, 394 (1952).

Light tan solid, mp 60-85° (softens about 55°); may be recrystallized from ether, mp 88-91° (softens about 75°). Liquefies upon exposure to air for 2.5 hrs. Explosion occurs when mixed with 90-95% H_2O_2.

USE: In Friedel-Crafts sulfone synthesis; in other sulfonylation reactions.

1072. Benzenesulfonyl Chloride. [98-09-9] Benzene sulfonechloride; benzenesulfonic (acid) chloride. $C_6H_5ClO_2S$; mol wt 176.62. C 40.80%, H 2.85%, Cl 20.07%, O 18.12%, S 18.15%. Prepd from benzene and chlorosulfonic acid or from the sodium salt of benzenesulfonic acid and PCl$_5$ or POCl$_3$: R. Adams, C. S. Marvel, *Org. Synth.* **coll. vol. I**, (2nd ed., 1964) p 84; H. T. Clarke *et al., ibid.* p 85.

Colorless, oily liquid. d$_{15}^{15}$ 1.3842. Solidifies 0°, mp 14.5°. bp$_{760}$ 251-252° (decompn); bp$_{100}$ 177°; bp$_{10}$ 120°. Insol in and stable toward cold water; sol in ether, alc.

1073. 1,2,4-Benzenetriol. [533-73-3] Hydroxyhydroquinone; hydroxyquinol. $C_6H_6O_3$; mol wt 126.11. C 57.14%, H 4.80%, O 38.06%. Prepd by hydrolysis of the triacetate with H_2SO_4 in methanol, the triacetate being formed by the action of acetic

anhydride on quinone: Vliet, *Org. Synth.* **coll. vol. I** (2nd ed, 1941) p 317.

Monoclinic prismatic leaflets from ether, mp 141°. Freely sol in water, alcohol, ether, ethyl acetate; almost insol in chloroform, carbon disulfide, ligroin, benzene.

Trimethyl ether. $C_9H_{12}O_3$. bp 247°.

Triacetate. $C_{12}H_{12}O_6$. Needles from abs alc, mp 96.5-97.0°. Readily hydrolyzed by acids or alkalies.

USE: In gas analysis; 1,2,4-benzenetriol in alkaline soln is just as good an absorbent for oxygen as is pyrogallol.

1074. Benzethonium Chloride. [121-54-0] *N,N*-Dimethyl-*N*-[2-[2-[4-(1,1,3,3-tetramethylbutyl)phenoxy]ethoxy]ethyl]benzenemethanaminium chloride; benzyldimethyl[2-[2-(*p*-1,1,3,3-tetramethylbutylphenoxy)ethoxy]ethyl]ammonium chloride; diisobutylphenoxyethoxyethyl dimethyl benzyl ammonium chloride; Hyamine 1622; Phemeride; Phemerol Chloride. $C_{27}H_{42}ClNO_2$; mol wt 448.08. C 72.37%, H 9.45%, Cl 7.91%, N 3.13%, O 7.14%. Quaternary ammonium salt with antimicrobial activity. Prepn: H. A. Bruson, **US 2115250** (1938 to Rohm & Haas). Germicidal activity and toxicity data: P. Weiss *et al., J. Am. Pharm. Assoc. Sci. Ed.* **40**, 267 (1951). HPLC determn in fish: T. B. A. Reuvers *et al., J. Chromatogr.* **467**, 321 (1989). Use for determn of total protein in cerebrospinal fluid (CSF): R. W. Luxton *et al., Clin. Chem.* **35**, 1731 (1989). Review of properties, commercial uses and toxicology studies: *J. Am. Coll. Toxicol.* **4**, 65-106 (1985).

Odorless, colorless crystals with very bitter taste. mp 160-165°. Sol in water giving a foamy, soapy soln. Sol in alcohol, chloroform; slightly sol in ether. Incompatible with soap, anionic detergents. LD$_{50}$ i.v. in mice: 29.5 mg/kg (Weiss).

USE: In cosmetics as preservative; cationic surfactant. As disinfectant in dairies and food industries. Clinical reagent for determn of protein in CSF; pharmaceutic aid (preservative).

THERAP CAT: Antiseptic, disinfectant.

THERAP CAT (VET): Antiseptic, disinfectant.

1075. Benzetimide. [14051-33-3] 3-Phenyl-1'-(phenylmethyl)-[3,4'-bipiperidine]-2,6-dione; 2-(1-benzyl-4-piperidyl)-2-phenylglutarimide; 1-benzyl-4-(2,6-dioxo-3-phenyl-3-piperidyl)-piperidine. $C_{23}H_{26}N_2O_2$; mol wt 362.46. C 76.21%, H 7.23%, N 7.73%, O 8.83%. Anticholinergic. Prepn: Janssen, **US 3125578** (1964 to Janssen); Hermans *et al., J. Med. Chem.* **11**, 797 (1968). Synthesis of labelled compound: van Wijngaarden, Soudijn, *J. Labelled Compd.* **1**, 207 (1965). Resolution of isomers and pharmacology: van Wijngaarden, *Life Sci.* **8**, 517 (1969); *ibid.* **9**, part 1, 489 (1970); Janssen *et al., Arzneim.-Forsch.* **21**, 1365 (1971). Metabolism: van Wijngaarden, Soudijn, *Life Sci.* **7**, 225 (1968).

Crystals, mp 156-159°.

Hydrochloride. [5633-14-7] R-4929; Dioxatrine; Spasmentral. $C_{23}H_{26}N_2O_2 \cdot HCl$; mol wt 398.93. Crystals, mp 299-301.5°. LD$_{50}$ in rats, mice (mg/kg): 37.6, 46.0 i.v. (Janssen).

l-Form. mp 180.5-182° (from toluene). $[\alpha]_D^{20}$ −124° (chloroform). LD$_{50}$ i.v. in mice: 38.5 mg/kg (Janssen).

d-Form see Dexetimide.

THERAP CAT: Antiparkinsonian.

THERAP CAT (VET): Antidiarrheal.

1076. Benzhydrylamine. [91-00-9] α-Phenylbenzenemethanamine; 1,1-diphenylmethylamine; α-aminodiphenylmethane. C$_{13}$H$_{13}$N; mol wt 183.25. C 85.21%, H 7.15%, N 7.64%. Prepd by boiling benzophenone oxime with zinc dust and ammonia: Scholl, *Ber.* **60**, 1247 (1927).

Hexagonal plates from water, mp 34°. d$_4^{22}$ 1.0635 (supercooled liq). bp$_{763}$ 304.1°; bp$_{12}$ 166°. n$_D^{99}$ 1.59631 (supercooled liq). Strong base. Absorbs CO$_2$ from the air forming a substance that melts at 91°. Slightly sol in water.

Hydrochloride. C$_{13}$H$_{13}$N.HCl. Needles, mp 293°. Sparingly sol in cold water.

1077. Benzidine. [92-87-5] [1,1'-Biphenyl]-4,4'-diamine; *p*-diaminodiphenyl. C$_{12}$H$_{12}$N$_2$; mol wt 184.24. C 78.23%, H 6.56%, N 15.20%. Discovered by Zinin in 1845. Produced by reduction of nitrobenzene with Zn and NaOH; the resultant hydrazobenzene is heated with acid. Lab proc: A. I. Vogel, *Practical Organic Chemistry* (Longmans, London, 3rd ed., 1959) p 633; Gattermann-Wieland, *Praxis des Organischen Chemikers* (de Gruyter, Berlin, 40th ed., 1961) p 165. Review of carcinogenic risk: *IARC Monographs* **1**, 80-86 (1972); *ibid.* **29**, 149-183 (1982); M. Boeniger, *Carcinogenicity and Metabolism of Azo Dyes, Especially Those Derived from Benzidine* (DHHS/NIOSH 80-119, 1980) 141 pp. Review of toxicology and human exposure: *Toxicological Profile for Benzidine* (PB2001-109102, 2001) 242 pp.

White or slightly-reddish, cryst powder; darkens on exposure to air and light. *Poisonous!* mp 115-120° when slowly heated; 128° when anhydr and rapidly heated. bp ~400°. Soly: one gram dissolves in 2500 ml cold, 107 ml boiling water, 5 ml boiling alcohol, 50 ml ether. *Keep well closed and protected from light.*

Dihydrochloride. C$_{12}$H$_{12}$N$_2$.2HCl. Crystals. Sol in water, alcohol.

Caution: Potential symptoms of overexposure are hematuria; secondary anemia from hemolysis; acute cystitis; acute liver disorders; dermatitis; painful and irregular urination. *See NIOSH Pocket Guide to Chemical Hazards* (DHHS/NIOSH 97-140, 1997) p 26. Benzidine and dyes metabolized to benzidine are listed as known human carcinogens: *Report on Carcinogens, Eleventh Edition* (PB2005-104914, 2004) p III-28, III-29.

USE: Manuf direct azo dyes; as a reagent for H$_2$O$_2$ in milk; for detection of blood. Dihydrochloride used for quantitative determn of sulfates, and as reagent for metals.

1078. Benzil. [134-81-6] Diphenylethanedione; bibenzoyl; dibenzoyl; diphenylglyoxal; diphenyl-α,β-diketone. C$_{14}$H$_{10}$O$_2$; mol wt 210.23. C 79.98%, H 4.79%, O 15.22%. Prepd by the oxidation of benzoin, C$_6$H$_5$CH(OH)COC$_6$H$_5$, with HNO$_3$ or with a copper sulfate-pyridine mixture: Adams, Marvel, *Org. Synth.* **vol. I**, p 25 (1921); Clarke, Dreger, *ibid.* **coll. vol. I**, 80 (87, 2nd ed); Hatt et al., *J. Chem. Soc.* **1936**, 93; L. F. Fieser, *Experiments in Organic Chemistry* (Boston, 3rd ed, 1955) p 173; *Organic Experiments* (Boston, 1964) p 214.

Yellow prisms (trigonal trapezohedral) from alcohol. d$_4^{15}$ 1.23. mp 95°. bp$_{760}$ 346-348°; bp$_{12}$ 188°. Absorption spectrum: Hantzsch, Schwiete, *Ber.* **49**, 216 (1916). uv max (ethanol): 260 nm (ε 22000). Infrared in chloroform: 5.93; 6.22; 6.85 μ. Insol in water; sol in alcohol, ether, chloroform, ethyl acetate, benzene, toluene, nitrobenzene.

α-Benzilmonoxime. C$_{14}$H$_{11}$NO$_2$. Leaflets from 30% alc, mp 137-138°.

β-Benzilmonoxime. C$_{14}$H$_{11}$NO$_2$. Solvated needles from benzene, when dry mp 113-114°.

Disemicarbazone. C$_{16}$H$_{16}$N$_6$O$_2$. Leaflets from alc, dec 243-244°.

USE: In organic syntheses.

1079. Benzil Dioxime. [23873-81-6] Diphenylethanedione dioxime; diphenylglyoxime. C$_{14}$H$_{12}$N$_2$O$_2$; mol wt 240.26. C 69.99%, H 5.03%, N 11.66%, O 13.32%. Three isomers occur: α or *anti*, β or *syn*, γ or *amphi*. Prepn of α-form from benzil and hydroxylamine hydrochloride: Brady, Perry, *J. Chem. Soc.* **127**, 2874 (1925); F. J. Welcher, *Organic Analytical Reagents* **vol. III** (Van Nostrand, New York, 1947) pp 224-227; Boyer et al., *J. Am. Chem. Soc.* **77**, 5688 (1955). Prepn of β-form: Brady, Perry, *loc. cit.*; Boyer et al., *loc. cit.* Prepn of γ-form: Welcher, *loc. cit.*, pp 227-228; *see also* Boyer et al., *loc. cit.*

α-Form. Crystals from methanol, mp 238-240°, Boyer et al., *loc. cit.*, also reported as mp 243-244°, Meisenheimer, Lamparter, *Ber.* **57**, 276 (1924). Practically insol in water, ether, glacial acetic acid; slightly sol in alc; readily sol in NaOH solns.

β-Form. Crystals, mp 212-214°, Meisenheimer, Lamparter, *loc. cit.*

1080. Benzilic Acid. [76-93-7] α-Hydroxy-α-phenylbenzeneacetic acid; diphenylglycolic acid. C$_{14}$H$_{12}$O$_3$; mol wt 228.24. C 73.67%, H 5.30%, O 21.03%. Prepd from benzil by the action of concd aq or alc KOH: Adams, Marvel, *Org. Synth.* **vol. 1**, p 29 (1921); Ballard, Dehn, *ibid.* **coll. vol. I**, 82; Kao, Ma, *J. Chem. Soc.* **1931**, 443.

Monoclinic needles from water. Bitter taste. mp 150°. Melt is deep red at higher temp. pKa (25°): 3.036. Slightly sol in cold water; freely sol in hot water, alc, ether.

Potassium salt. C$_{14}$H$_{11}$O$_3$K. Crystals, very sol in water, alc.

Lead salt. (C$_{14}$H$_{11}$O$_3$)$_2$Pb. Amorphous precipitate. Upon heating it becomes a red liquid.

Methyl ester. C$_{15}$H$_{14}$O$_3$. mp 74-75°. bp$_{13}$ 187°.

1081. Benzimidazole. [51-17-2] Benziminazole; 1,3-benzodiazole; azindole; benzoglyoxaline; *N,N'*-methenyl-*o*-phenylenediamine. C$_7$H$_6$N$_2$; mol wt 118.14. C 71.17%, H 5.12%, N 23.71%. Prepd by reaction of *o*-phenylenediamine with formic acid: Wundt, *Ber.* **11**, 826 (1878); Wagner, Millett, *Org. Synth.* **coll. vol. II**, 65 (1943). *Reviews*: J. B. Wright, *Chem. Rev.* **48**, 397-541 (1951); K. Hofmann, *Imidazole and Its Derivatives* (Interscience, New York, 1953) p 247 sqq.

Tabular crystals. Orthorhombic and monoclinic modifications. mp 170.5°. bp$_{760}$ >360°. Weak base. pKa = 5.48 at 25°. Absorption spectrum: Steck *et al.*, *J. Am. Chem. Soc.* **70**, 3406 (1948). Dipole moment: 3.93 (dioxane). Sparingly sol in cold water, more sol in hot water. Freely sol in alcohol, sparingly sol in ether. Practically insol in benzene, petr ether. One gram dissolves in 2 g of boiling xylene. Sol in aq solns of acids and strong alkalies. High degree of chemical stability.

1082.   2-Benzimidazolethiol. [583-39-1] 1,3-Dihydro-2*H*-benzimidazole-2-thione; 2-mercaptobenzimidazole. $C_7H_6N_2S$; mol wt 150.20. C 55.98%, H 4.03%, N 18.65%, S 21.35%. Prepn from *o*-phenylenediamine and potassium ethyl xanthate: Van Allan, Deacon, *Org. Synth.* **coll. vol. IV**, 569 (1963).

Glistening platelets from 95% ethanol, mp 303-304°. Slightly sol in water; sol in methanol, ethanol.

1083.   Benziodarone. [68-90-6] (2-Ethyl-3-benzofuranyl)(4-hydroxy-3,5-diiodophenyl) methanone; 2-ethyl-3-(3′,5′-diiodo-4′-hydroxybenzoyl)benzofuran; 2-ethyl-3-(3′,5′-diiodo-4′-hydroxybenzoyl)oxaindene; 2-ethyl-3-benzofuryl 3′,5′-diiodo-4′-hydroxyphenyl ketone; 2-ethyl-3-(3,5-diiodo-4-hydroxybenzoyl)coumarone; 2-ethyl-3-(4-hydroxy-3,5-diiodobenzoyl)benzofuran; 2329 Labaz; L-2329; Amplivix; Dilafurane. $C_{17}H_{12}I_2O_3$; mol wt 518.08. C 39.41%, H 2.33%, I 48.99%, O 9.26%. Description: Charlier, *Acta Cardiol. Suppl.* **7**, 1-60 (1959). Synthesis: Beaudet, Henaux, **BE 553621**; **GB 836272** (1957, 1960, both to Labaz); Buu-Hoi, Beaudet, **US 3012042** (1961 to Soc. Belge Azote Prod. Chim. Marly). Clinical trial in hyperuricemia in renal transplant patients: F. Perez-Ruiz *et al.*, *Nephrol. Dial. Transplant.* **18**, 603 (2003).

Yellowish powder, mp 167°. Soly in water at 25° about 0.2%, at 45° about 1.0%. Sol in chloroform, acetone.

THERAP CAT: Uricosuric.

1084.   Benznidazole. [22994-85-0] 2-Nitro-*N*-(phenylmethyl)-1*H*-imidazole-1-acetamide; *N*-benzyl-2-nitroimidazole-1-acetamide; Ro-7-1051; Radanil. $C_{12}H_{12}N_4O_3$; mol wt 260.25. C 55.38%, H 4.65%, N 21.53%, O 18.44%. Prepn: **GB 1138529**; A. G. Beaman *et al.*, **US 3679698** (1966, 1972 both to Hoffmann-La Roche). *In vitro* effect on *T. cruzi*: S. Yoneda *et al.*, *Experientia* **33**, 1201 (1977). Pharmacokinetics: J. Raaflaub, W. H. Ziegler, *Arzneim.-Forsch.* **29**, 1611 (1979). Antibacterial activity and electron affinity: A. V. Reynolds, *J. Pharm. Pharmacol.* **31**, Suppl., 29P (1979). Mutagenicity study: C. E. Voogd *et al.*, *Mutat. Res.* **66**, 207 (1979). *In vitro* toxicity study: G. E. Adams *et al.*, *J. Natl. Cancer Inst.* **64**, 555 (1980).

Crystals from ethanol, mp 188.5-190°. uv max (ethanol): 313 nm (ε 7,600). Soly in water at 37°: 40 mg/100 ml, J. Raaflaub, W. H. Ziegler, *loc. cit.*

THERAP CAT: Antiprotozoal (Trypanosoma).

1085.   Benzo Azurine G. [2429-71-2] 3,3′-[(3,3′-Dimethoxy[1,1′-biphenyl]-4,4′-diyl)bis(azo)]bis[4-hydroxy-1-naphthalenesulfonic acid] disodium salt; disodium *o*-dianisidinediazobis(1-naphthol-4-sulfonate); C.I. Direct Blue 8; C.I. 24140. $C_{34}H_{24}N_4$-$Na_2O_{10}S_2$; mol wt 758.68. C 53.83%, H 3.19%, N 7.38%, Na 6.06%, O 21.09%, S 8.45%. Prepared from diazotized *o*-dianisi-

dine and sodium 4-hydroxy-1-naphthalenesulfonate: F. J. Welcher, *Organic Analytical Reagents* **vol. 4** (D. Van Nostrand Co., New York, 1948) pp 337-338. *See also Colour Index* **vol. 4** (3rd ed., 1971) p 4202.

Bluish-black powder. Sol in water, aq sodium hydroxide (red soln), sulfuric acid (blue soln), Cellosolve; very slightly sol in ethanol. Practically insol in other organic solvents.

USE: As a dye: *Colour Index* **vol. 2** (3rd ed., 1971) p 2223. As analytical reagent in detection of Mg.

1086.   Benzocaine. [94-09-7] 4-Aminobenzoic acid ethyl ester; ethyl aminobenzoate; Americaine; Anaesthesin; Flavamed; Subcutin. $C_9H_{11}NO_2$; mol wt 165.19. C 65.44%, H 6.71%, N 8.48%, O 19.37%. Prepd by the esterification of *p*-aminobenzoic acid: Salkowski, *Ber.* **28**, 1921 (1895); Vorländer, Meyer, *Ann.* **320**, 135 (1902); by the reduction of ethyl *p*-nitrobenzoate: Limpricht, *ibid.* **303**, 278 (1898); R. Adams, F. L. Cohen, *Org. Synth.* **coll. vol. I**, 240 (2nd ed., 1941). In industrial practice the reducing agent is usually iron and water in the presence of a little acid. Comprehensive description: S. L. Ali, *Anal. Profiles Drug Subs.* **12**, 73-104 (1983).

Rhombohedra from ether, mp 88-90°. Stable in air. One gram dissolves in about 2500 ml water, 5 ml alcohol, 2 ml chloroform, in about 4 ml ether, and in 30 to 50 ml of expressed almond oil or olive oil. Also sol in dil acids. pKa 2.5.

THERAP CAT: Anesthetic (local).

THERAP CAT (VET): Local (usually surface) anesthetic.

1087.   Benzoctamine. [17243-39-9] *N*-Methyl-9,10-ethanoanthracene-9(10*H*)-methanamine; 1-(methylaminomethyl)dibenzo[*b,e*]bicyclo[2.2.2]octadiene; 9-(methylaminomethyl)-9,10-dihydro-9,10-ethanoanthracene. $C_{18}H_{19}N$; mol wt 249.35. C 86.70%, H 7.68%, N 5.62%. Prepn: **BE 610863**; P. Schmidt *et al.*, **US 3399201** (1962, 1968 to Ciba); Wilhelm, Schmidt, *Helv. Chim. Acta* **52**, 1385 (1969). Pharmacology: Keberle *et al.*, *Present Status Psychotropic Drugs* (Excerpta Medica, New York, 1969) p 123; Baltzer, Bein, *Arch. Int. Pharmacodyn. Ther.* **201**, 25 (1973). Toxicity: E. I. Goldenthal, *Toxicol. Appl. Pharmacol.* **18**, 185 (1971).

Hydrochloride. [10085-81-1] Ba-30803; Tacitin. $C_{18}H_{19}$-N.HCl; mol wt 285.81. Crystals, mp 320-322°. pKa: 7.6. LD_{50} orally in rats: 700 ±170 mg/kg (Goldenthal).

THERAP CAT: Anxiolytic.

1088.   Benzofuran. [271-89-6] Coumarone; cumarone. C_8H_6O; mol wt 118.13. C 81.34%, H 5.12%, O 13.54%. Constituent of coal tar, *q.v.* Isoln from coal tar oils: Kraemer, Spilker, *Ber.* **23**, 78 (1890); **33**, 2261 (1900); Breston, Gauger, *Am. Gas Assoc. Proc.* **28**, 492 (1946). Synthesis by heating phenoxyacetaldehyde with zinc chloride and acetic acid: Stoermer, *Ber.* **30**, 1703 (1897); *Ann.* **312**, 261 (1900). Review of toxicology and human exposure: *Toxicological Profile for 2,3-Benzofuran* (PB93-110666, 1992) 95 pp.

Oil. Aromatic odor. Not solid at $-18°$. bp_{760} 173-175°; bp_{15} 62-63°. Volatile with steam. $d_4^{22.7}$ 1.0913. $n_D^{16.3}$ 1.56897; $n_D^{22.7}$ 1.565. Insol in water, aq alkaline solns; miscible with benzene, petr ether, abs alcohol, ether. Slowly polymerizes on standing. For additional physical data *see* Breston, Gauger, *loc. cit.*

USE: Manuf of coumarone-indene resins.

1089. Benzoguanamine. [91-76-9] 6-Phenyl-1,3,5-triazine-2,4-diamine; 2,4-diamino-6-phenyl-*s*-triazine; 4,6-diamino-2-phenyl-*s*-triazine. $C_9H_9N_5$; mol wt 187.20. C 57.74%, H 4.85%, N 37.41%. Prepd from benzonitrile and dicyandiamide in the presence of Na and liquid ammonia: Jones, **US 2735850** (1956 to British Oxygen Co.); from benzonitrile and dicyandiamide in the presence of KOH and methyl Cellosolve: Simons, Saxton, *Org. Synth.* **33**, 13 (1953).

Crystals. d_4^{25} 1.40. mp 227-228°. uv max (ethanol): 249 nm (ε 25,000). Sol in alcohol, ether, dil HCl; partially sol in dimethylformamide. Practically insol in acetone, chloroform, ethyl acetate. Soly in water at 22° 0.06%; at 100° 0.6%.

USE: In the manuf of thermosetting resins, pesticides, pharmaceuticals and dyestuffs.

1090. Benzohydrol. [91-01-0] α-Phenylbenzenemethanol; benzhydrol; diphenylcarbinol. $C_{13}H_{12}O$; mol wt 184.23. C 84.75%, H 6.57%, O 8.68%. $(C_6H_5)_2CHOH$. Prepd by reducing benzophenone with zinc dust in strongly alkaline soln: Wiselogle, Sonneborn, *Org. Synth.* **coll. vol. I** (2nd ed, 1941) p 90. By reducing benzophenone with magnesium in methanol: Zechmeister, Rom, *Ann.* **468**, 123 (1929).

Needles from ligroin, mp 69°. bp_{748} 298°; bp_{20} 180°; bp_{13} 176°. Absorption spectrum: Orndorff *et al., J. Am. Chem. Soc.* **49**, 1542 (1927). One gram dissolves in 2 liters of water at 20°. Freely sol in alcohol, ether, chloroform and carbon bisulfide; almost insol in cold ligroin.

Diphenylmethyl ether. $(C_6H_5)_2CHOCH(C_6H_5)_2$. Monoclinic crystals from benzene, mp 110°; bp_{15} 267°.

USE: In organic syntheses.

1091. Benzoic Acid. [65-85-0] Benzenecarboxylic acid; phenylformic acid; dracylic acid. $C_7H_6O_2$; mol wt 122.12. C 68.85%, H 4.95%, O 26.20%. Occurs in nature in free and combined forms. Gum benzoin may contain as much as 20%. Most berries contain appreciable amounts (around 0.05%). Excreted mainly as hippuric acid by almost all vertebrates, except fowl. Mfg processes include the air oxidation of toluene, the hydrolysis of benzotrichloride, and the decarboxylation of phthalic anhydride: *Faith, Keyes & Clark's Industrial Chemicals*, F. A. Lowenheim, M. K. Moran, Eds. (Wiley-Interscience, New York, 4th ed., 1975) pp 138-144. Lab prepn from benzyl chloride: A. I. Vogel, *Practical Organic Chemistry* (Longmans, London, 3rd ed, 1959) p 755; from benzaldehyde: Gattermann-Wieland, *Praxis des Organischen Chemikers* (de Gruyter, Berlin, 40th ed, 1961) p 193. Prepn of ultra-pure benzoic acid for use as titrimetric and calorimetric standard: Schwab, Wicher, *J. Res. Natl. Bur. Stand.* **25**, 747 (1940). *Review:* A. E. Williams in *Kirk-Othmer Encyclopedia of Chemical Technology* vol. 3 (Wiley-Interscience, New York, 3rd ed., 1978) pp 778-792.

Monoclinic tablets, plates, leaflets. d 1.321 (also reported as 1.266). mp 122.4°. Begins to sublime at $\sim$100°. bp_{760} 249.2°; bp_{400} 227°; bp_{200} 205.8°; bp_{100} 186.2°; bp_{60} 172.8°; bp_{40} 162.6°; bp_{20} 146.7°; bp_{10} 132.1°. Volatile with steam. Flash pt 121°C. pK (25°) 4.19. pH of satd soln at 25°: 2.8. Soly in water (g/l) at 0° = 1.7; at 10° = 2.1; at 20° = 2.9; at 25° = 3.4; at 30° = 4.2; at 40° = 6.0; at 50° = 9.5; at 60° = 12.0; at 70° = 17.7; at 80° = 27.5; at 90° = 45.5; at 95° = 68.0. Mixtures of excess benzoic acid and water form two liquid phases beginning at 89.7°. The two liquid phases unite at the critical soln temp of 117.2°. Composition of critical mixture: 32.34% benzoic acid, 67.66% water: *see* Ward, Cooper, *J. Phys. Chem.* **34**, 1484 (1930). One gram dissolves in 2.3 ml cold alc, 1.5 ml boiling alc, 4.5 ml chloroform, 3 ml ether, 3 ml acetone, 30 ml carbon tetrachloride, 10 ml benzene, 30 ml carbon disulfide, 23 ml oil of turpentine; also sol in volatile and fixed oils, slightly in petr ether. The soly in water is increased by alkaline substances, such as borax or trisodium phosphate, *see also* Sodium Benzoate.

Barium salt dihydrate. Barium benzoate. $C_{14}H_{10}BaO_4.2H_2O$. Nacreous leaflets. *Poisonous!* Soluble in about 20 parts water; slightly sol in alc.

Calcium salt trihydrate. Calcium benzoate. $C_{14}H_{10}CaO_4.3H_2O$. Orthorhombic crystals or powder. d 1.44. Soluble in 25 parts water; very sol in boiling water.

Cerium salt trihydrate. Cerous benzoate. $C_{21}H_{15}CeO_6.3H_2O$. White to reddish-white powder. Sol in hot water or hot alc.

Copper salt dihydrate. Cupric benzoate. $C_{14}H_{10}CuO_4.2H_2O$. Light blue, cryst powder. Slightly soluble in cold water, more in hot water; sol in alc or in dil acids with separation of benzoic acid.

Lead salt dihydrate. Lead benzoate. $C_{14}H_{10}O_4Pb.2H_2O$. Cryst powder. *Poisonous!* Slightly sol in water.

Manganese salt tetrahydrate. Manganese benzoate. $C_{14}H_{10}MnO_4.4H_2O$. Pale-red powder. Sol in water, alc. Also occurs with $3H_2O$.

Nickel salt trihydrate. Nickel benzoate. $C_{14}H_{10}NiO_4.3H_2O$. Light-green odorless powder. Slightly sol in water; sol in ammonia; dec by acids.

Potassium salt trihydrate. Potassium benzoate. $C_7H_5KO_2.3H_2O$. Crystalline powder. Sol in water, alc.

Silver salt. Silver benzoate. $C_7H_5AgO_2$. Light-sensitive powder. Sol in 385 parts cold water, more sol in hot water; very slightly sol in alc.

Uranium salt. Uranium benzoate; uranyl benzoate. $C_{14}H_{10}O_6U$. Yellow powder. Slightly sol in water, alc.

Caution: Mild irritant to skin, eyes, mucous membranes.

USE: Preserving foods, fats, fruit juices, alkaloidal solns, etc; manuf benzoates and benzoyl compds, dyes; as a mordant in calico printing; for curing tobacco. As standard in volumetric and calorimetric analysis. Pharmaceutic aid (antifungal).

THERAP CAT (VET): Has been used with salicylic acid as a topical antifungal.

1092. Benzoic Anhydride. [93-97-0] Benzoic acid anhydride. $C_{14}H_{10}O_3$; mol wt 226.23. C 74.33%, H 4.46%, O 21.22%. $(C_6H_5CO)_2O$. Prepd by heating benzoic acid with acetic anhydride in the presence of a trace of phosphoric acid: Clarke, Rahrs, *Org. Synth.* **3**, 2 (1923); **coll. vol. I** (Wiley, New York, 2nd ed., 1941) p 91.

Orthorhombic bipyramidal prisms from benzene + petr ether. d_4^{15} 1.1989. mp 42°. bp_{760} 360°; bp_{200} 299.1°; bp_{60} 252.7°; bp_{40} 239.8°; bp_{20} 218°; bp_{10} 198°; bp_5 180°; $bp_{1.0}$ 143.8°. n_D^{15} 1.57665. Almost insol in water (0.01 g/l). Sol in alcohol, chloroform, acetone, ethyl acetate, benzene, toluene, xylene, ether, glacial acetic acid, acetic anhydride; moderately sol in petr ether; stable in water and in cold alkaline solns.

USE: In organic syntheses, as benzoylating agent in the manufacture of pharmaceuticals, dyes, and intermediates.

1093. Benzoin. [119-53-9] 2-Hydroxy-1,2-diphenylethanone; benzoylphenylcarbinol; α-hydroxy-α-phenylacetophenone; bitter-almond-oil camphor. $C_{14}H_{12}O_2$; mol wt 212.24. C 79.23%, H 5.70%, O 15.08%. Prepd by treating an alcoholic soln of benzaldehyde with an alkali cyanide: Adams, Marvel, *Org. Synth.* **vol. 1**, p 33 (1921); **coll. vol. I**, 88; Arnold, Fuson, *J. Am. Chem. Soc.* **58**, 1295 (1936); L. F. Fieser, *Organic Experiments* (D. C. Heath & Co., Boston, 1964) pp 211-214.

Colorless to faintly yellow oil. Soluble in most organic solvents except aliphatic hydrocarbons.

THERAP CAT: Antitussive.

1097. Benzonitrile. [100-47-0] Phenyl cyanide; cyano-benzene. C_7H_5N; mol wt 103.12. C 81.53%, H 4.89%, N 13.58%. C_6H_5CN. Prepd by heating Na benzenesulfonate with NaCN or by adding benzenediazonium chloride soln to a hot aq NaCN soln contg $CuSO_4$ and distilling. Lab prepn: A. I. Vogel, *Practical Organic Chemistry* (Longmans, London, 3rd ed, 1959) p 608.

Liquid, odor of volatile oil of almond. bp_{760} 190.7°, bp_{100} 123.5°, bp_{10} 69.2°, bp_1 28.2°. mp $-12.75°$. d_{15}^{15} 1.010. n_D^{20} 1.5289. Fire pt 167°F. Slightly sol in cold water; sol to the extent of 1% in water at 100°; miscible with common organic solvents.

USE: Solvent.

1098. Benzophenone. [119-61-9] Diphenylmethanone; diphenyl ketone; benzoylbenzene. $C_{13}H_{10}O$; mol wt 182.22. C 85.69%, H 5.53%, O 8.78%. $C_6H_5COC_6H_5$. Prepd by the Friedel-Crafts ketone synthesis from benzene and benzoyl chloride in the presence of $AlCl_3$: Marvel, Sperry, *Org. Synth.* **coll. vol. I** (Wiley, New York, 2nd ed., 1941) p 95. By decarboxylation of *o*-benzoylbenzoic acid in the presence of copper catalyst: L. F. Fieser, *Organic Experiments* (D. C. Heath & Co., Boston, 1964) pp 201-203.

Stable form (there are two other labile forms), orthorhombic bisphenoidal prisms from alcohol or ether. Geranium-like odor. d_4^{18} 1.1108. d_4^{50} 1.0869. $n_D^{45.2}$ 1.5975. Absorption spectrum: Purvis, McCleland, *J. Chem. Soc.* **101**, 1516 (1912). mp 48.5°. bp_{760} 305.4°; bp_{400} 276.8°; bp_{200} 249.8°; bp_{100} 224.4°; bp_{60} 208.2°; bp_{40} 195.7°; bp_{20} 175.8°; bp_{10} 157.6°; bp_5 141.7°; $bp_{1.0}$ 108.2°. Insoluble in water. One gram dissolves in 7.5 ml alcohol, 6 ml ether; sol in chloroform.

Oxime. $C_{13}H_{11}NO$. For prepn *see Org. Synth.* **10**, 10. Crystals from ligroin, mp 143-144°. Freely sol in ether, acetone.

USE: Fixative for heavy perfumes, such as geranium, new-mown hay, especially when used in soaps. In the manuf of antihistamines, hypnotics, insecticides.

1099. Benzophenone-6. [131-54-4] Bis(2-hydroxy-4-methoxyphenyl)methanone; 2,2'-dihydroxy-4,4'-dimethoxybenzophenone; Uvinul D49. $C_{15}H_{14}O_5$; mol wt 274.27. C 65.69%, H 5.14%, O 29.17%. Prepn: Grover *et al., J. Chem. Soc.* **1955**, 3982; Hardy, Forster, **US 2773903** (1956 to Am. Cyanamid); Dayan, Roberts; Hahn, Stanley, **US 2853522** and **US 2853523** (both 1958 to Gen. Aniline); Hosler, Storfer, **US 2928878** (1960 to Am. Cyanamid).

Crystals, mp 139-140°. uv max: 284, 340 nm (log ε 4.12, 4.12).

USE: As ultraviolet light absorber, esp in paints, plastics.

1100. Benzopinacol. [464-72-2] 1,1,2,2-Tetraphenyl-1,2-ethanediol; benzpinacone; tetraphenylethylene glycol. $C_{26}H_{22}O_2$; mol wt 366.45. C 85.22%, H 6.05%, O 8.73%. $(C_6H_5)_2$-C(OH)C(OH)$(C_6H_5)_2$. Prepd by photochemical reduction of benzophenone: Bachmann, *Org. Synth.* **coll. vol. II**, 71 (1943); L. F. Fieser, *Organic Experiments* (D. C. Heath & Co., Boston, 1964) p 203. By the action of phenylmagnesium bromide on benzil: Acree, *Ber.* **37**, 2761 (1904).

Monoclinic prisms, may contain 1 mol C_6H_6 when crystallized from benzene. mp 197° (open capillary, rapid heating); mp 222° (copper block). On heating to mp it dec to benzophenone and benzohydrol. Soluble in 11.5 parts boiling glacial acetic acid; in 26 parts boiling benzene; in 39 parts boiling 95% alcohol. Freely sol in ether, carbon bisulfide, chloroform.

1101. Benzopurpurine 4B. [992-59-6] 3,3'-[(3,3'-Dimethyl[1,1'-biphenyl]-4,4'-diyl)bis(azo)]bis[4-amino-1-naphthalenesulfonic acid] disodium salt; disodium *o*-tolidinediazobis(1-naphthylamine-4-sulfonate); C.I. Direct Red 2; C.I. 23500; azamin 4B; eclipse red; fast scarlet; Paper Red 4B; Sultan Red 4B; Cotton

---

dl-**Form.** Six-sided monoclinic prisms from alcohol, mp 137°. bp_{768} 344°. bp_{12} 194°. Reduces Fehling's soln. uv max (ethanol): 247 nm (ε 14500); infrared in chloroform: 2.88; 5.93; 6.21; 6.28, 6.85 μ. Soluble in 3335 parts water, more in hot water, in 5 parts pyridine; sol in acetone, in boiling alc; slightly in ether.

Methyl ether. $C_{15}H_{14}O_2$. Needles, mp 49°.
Ethyl ether. $C_{16}H_{16}O_2$. Needles, mp 62°.
l-**Form.** Needles, mp 132°. $[\alpha]_D^{12}$ $-118°$ (c = 1.2 in acetone).
d-**Form.** Needles, mp 132°. $[\alpha]_D^{12}$ $+120.5°$ (c = 1.2 in acetone).
Note: Not to be confused with Gum Benzoin.

USE: In organic syntheses.

1094. Benzoin Oxime. [441-38-3] 2-Hydroxy-1,2-diphenylethanone oxime; 2-hydroxy-2-phenylacetophenone oxime. C_{14}-$H_{13}NO_2$; mol wt 227.26. C 73.99%, H 5.77%, N 6.16%, O 14.08%. Two isomers occur: α or *anti* and β or *syn*. Both have been prepd from benzoin and hydroxylamine hydrochloride. Prepn of α-form: Werner, Detscheff, *Ber.* **38**, 69 (1905); F. J. Welcher, *Organic Analytical Reagents* **vol. III** (Van Nostrand, New York, 1947) pp 239-251. Prepn of β-form: Werner, Detscheff, *loc. cit.* Configuration of α- and β-forms: Meisenheimer, Meis, *Ber.* **57**, 289 (1924).

α-form   β-form

α-**Form.** Cupron. Prisms from benzene, mp 151-152°. Darkens on exposure to light. Slightly sol in water; sol in alc, aq ammonium hydroxide soln. *Protect from light.*

β-**Form.** Prismatic crystals from ether. Ether of crystn is lost on standing in air. Ether-free compd, mp 99°.

USE: The α-form is used in the detection and determination of Cu, Mo, and W: Welcher, *loc. cit.*

1095. 6,7-Benzomorphan. [575-19-9] 1,2,3,4,5,6-Hexahydro-2,6-methano-3-benzazocine; 6,7-benzmorphan. $C_{12}H_{15}N$; mol wt 173.25. C 83.19%, H 8.73%, N 8.08%. Parent compound of a series of potent analgetics. Synthesis: Kanematsu *et al., J. Am. Chem. Soc.* **90**, 1064 (1968); Kanematsu *et al., J. Med. Chem.* **12**, 405 (1969). Review of derivative syntheses and pharmacology: May, Sargent, "Morphine and its Modifications", in *Analgetics*, G. de Stevens, Ed. (Academic Press, New York, 1965) pp 145-171.

Hydrochloride. $C_{12}H_{15}N.HCl$. Needles from methanol-acetone, mp 261-262°.

1096. Benzonatate. [104-31-4] 4-(Butylamino)benzoic acid 3,6,9,12,15,18,21,24,27-nonaoxaoctacos-1-yl ester; nonaethyleneglycol monomethyl ether *p-n*-butylaminobenzoate; *p*-butylaminobenzoic acid ω-O-methylnonaethyleneglycol ester; benzononatine; Exangit; Tessalon. $C_{30}H_{53}NO_{11}$; mol wt 603.74. C 59.68%, H 8.85%, N 2.32%, O 29.15%. Prepn: Matter, **US 2714608** (1955 to Ciba).

Red 4B. $C_{34}H_{26}N_6Na_2O_6S_2$; mol wt 724.72. C 56.35%, H 3.62%, N 11.60%, Na 6.34%, O 13.25%, S 8.85%. Prepn from diazotized *o*-tolidine and sodium 4-amino-1-naphthalenesulfonate: **DE 35615** (1885 to A. G. für Anilinfabrikation Berlin), *Frdl.* **1**, 473; F. J. Welcher, *Organic Analytical Reagents* vol. **4** (Van Nostrand Co., New York, 1948) pp 338-339; *Colour Index* vol. **4** (3rd ed., 1971) p 4189. *See also:* H. J. Conn's *Biological Stains*, R. D. Lillie, Ed. (Williams & Wilkins, Baltimore, 9th ed., 1977) p 154.

Brown powder. Soluble in water, sodium hydroxide, sulfuric acid, ethanol, acetone, Cellosolve. Practically insol in other organic solvents.

USE: For dyeing primarily cotton and viscose rayon: *Colour Index* vol. **2** (3rd ed., 1971) p 2101. As an analytical reagent in detection of Al, Mg, Hg, Ag, U; as a biological stain; as pH indicator, violet 1.2 to red 4.0.

1102. 1,2-Benzopyran. [254-04-6] 2*H*-1-Benzopyran; α-5:6-benzopyran; 1,2-chromene; 3-chromene. C_9H_8O; mol wt 132.16. C 81.79%, H 6.10%, O 12.11%. Prepn from *cis-o*-hydroxycinnamyl alcohol: Chatterjea, *J. Indian Chem. Soc.* **36**, 76 (1959), *C.A.* **54**, 519b (1960); from phenyl propargyl ether in diethylphenylamine: Iwai, Ide, *Chem. Pharm. Bull.* **11**, 1042 (1963); Iwai, Iwade, **JP 63 22587** (1963 to Sankyo), *C.A.* **60**, 2901e (1964). Earlier prepns: Maitte, *Ann. Chim. (Paris)* **9**, 431 (1954); Normant, Maitte, *Compt. Rend.* **234**, 1787 (1952).

Liquid; bp_{102} 132°, bp_{15} 92-92.5°, bp_{13} 91°, bp_9 77°. d^{16} 1.0993. n_D^{24} 1.5869; n_D^{16} 1.5923 (Maitte); also reported as n_D 1.5837 (**JP 63 22587**).

1103. Benzo[a]pyrene. [50-32-8] 3,4-Benzpyrene. C_{20}-H_{12}; mol wt 252.31. C 95.21%, H 4.79%. Formerly called *1,2-benzpyrene*. Occurs in coal tar, *q.v.* Isoln by fractionation: Cook *et al., J. Chem. Soc.* **1933**, 395; by adsorption and fluorimetric determn: Hieger, *Am. J. Cancer* **29**, 705 (1937); Winterstein *et al., Z. Physiol. Chem.* **230**, 158, 169 (1934); *Naturwissenschaften* **22**, 237 (1934). Synthesis from pyrene and succinic anhydride: Cook, Hewett, *J. Chem. Soc.* **1933**, 398; Fieser, Fieser, *J. Am. Chem. Soc.* **57**, 782 (1935); Winterstein *et al., Ber.* **68**, 1079 (1935); Fieser *et al., J. Am. Chem. Soc.* **57**, 1509 (1935). Absorption spectrum: Mayneord, Roe, *Proc. Roy. Soc. London* **A152**, 299 (1935). *Review:* Clar, *Polycyclic Hydrocarbons* Vol. **1 & 2** (Academic Press, New York, 1964). Review of carcinogenicity studies: *IARC Monographs* **3**, 91-136 (1973). Inhibition of the mutagenicity of the ultimate carcinogenic metabolite of benzo[a]pyrene by ellagic acid: A. W. Wood *et al., Proc. Natl. Acad. Sci. USA* **79**, 5513 (1982). Study of the reaction between this metabolite (*benzo[a]-pyrene-7,8-diol 9,10-epoxide*) and ellagic acid: J. M. Sayer *et al., J. Am. Chem. Soc.* **104**, 5562 (1982). *Review:* D. H. Phillips, *Nature* **303**, 468-472 (1983). Review of toxicology and human exposure: *Toxicological Profile for Polycyclic Aromatic Hydrocarbons* (PB95-264370, 1995) 487 pp.

Yellowish plates, needles from benzene + methanol, mp 179-179.3°. Crystals may be monoclinic or orthorhombic. bp_{10} 310-312°. Violet fluorescence of dil benzene solns: Hieger, *loc. cit.* Soluble in benzene, toluene, xylene; sparingly sol in alc, methanol. Practically insol in water.

Caution: This substance is reasonably anticipated to be a human carcinogen: *Report on Carcinogens, Eleventh Edition* (PB2005-104914, 2004) p III-220.

1104. Benzo[e]pyrene. [192-97-2] 1,2-Benzpyrene; 4,5-benzpyrene. $C_{20}H_{12}$; mol wt 252.31. C 95.21%, H 4.79%. Constituent of coal tar, *q.v.* Isoln: Cook *et al., J. Chem. Soc.* **1933**, 396. Synthesis: Cook, Hewett, *ibid.* 398; Clar, *Ber.* **76**, 609 (1943); Buchta, Kröger, *Ann.* **705**, 190 (1967). NMR spectra: Cobb, Memory, *J. Chem. Phys.* **47**, 2020 (1967). *Review:* Clar, *Polycyclic Hydrocarbons* Vol. **2**, (Academic Press, New York, 1964) p 127. Review of toxicology and human exposure: *Toxicological Profile for Polycyclic Aromatic Hydrocarbons* (PB95-264370, 1995) 487 pp.

Prisms or plates from benzene, mp 178-179°.

1105. Benzo[f]quinoline. [85-02-9] β-Naphthoquinoline; 5,6-benzoquinoline; naphthopyridine. $C_{13}H_9N$; mol wt 179.22. C 87.12%, H 5.06%, N 7.82%. Prepn from from β-naphthylamine by the Skraup reaction: Knueppel, *Ber.* **29**, 703 (1896); Clem, Hamilton, *J. Am. Chem. Soc.* **62**, 2349 (1940); Uhle, Jacobs, *J. Org. Chem.* **10**, 76 (1945).

Crystals from alcohol + water, mp 93°. bp_{721} 349-350°. uv max (ethanol): 347, 331, 316, 266, nm (log ε 3.54, 3.41, 3.18, 4.06). Practically insol in water. Sol in dil acids; very sol in alcohol, ether, benzene.

USE: As a reagent for the determination of cadmium which is pptd as $(C_{13}H_9N)_2H_2(CdI_4)$ from dil nitric or sulfuric acid soln in the presence of potassium iodide.

1106. Benzoresorcinol. [131-56-6] (2,4-Dihydroxyphenyl)phenylmethanone; 2,4-dihydroxybenzophenone; 4-benzoylresorcinol; resbenzophenone; benzophenone-1; Uvinul 400. C_{13}-$H_{10}O_3$; mol wt 214.22. C 72.89%, H 4.71%, O 22.41%. Prepd from benzoyl chloride and resorcinol: Dobner, *Ann.* **210**, 246 (1881); by Fries rearrangement: Amin, Shah, *J. Indian Chem. Soc.* **29**, 351 (1952).

Needles from hot water, mp 144-145°. Practically insol in cold water. Easily sol in alcohol, ether, glacial acetic acid; scarcely sol in cold benzene.

USE: Ultraviolet light absorber, esp in paints and plastics.

1107. Benzothiazole. [95-16-9] C_7H_5NS; mol wt 135.19. C 62.19%, H 3.73%, N 10.36%, S 23.72%. Prepd from *N,N*-dimethylaniline and sulfur: Knowles, Watt, *J. Org. Chem.* **7**, 56 (1942). Chemistry of benzothiazoles, their use as carbonyl equivalents and in carbon-carbon bond formation: E. J. Corey, D. L. Boger, *Tetrahedron Lett.* **1978**, 5, 9, 13. Toxicity study: E. F. Domino *et al., J. Pharmacol. Exp. Ther.* **105**, 486 (1952).

Liquid. Odor similar to that of quinoline. Volatile with steam. d_4^{20} 1.246. bp_{765} 227-228°; bp_{34} 131°. n_D^{20} 1.6379. Slightly sol in water. Freely sol in alcohol, carbon disulfide. LD_{50} i.v. in mice: 95±3 mg/kg (Domino).

USE: In organic synthesis.

1108. 1*H*-Benzotriazole. [95-14-7] 1,2,3-Benzotriazole; benztriazole; azimidobenzene; benzisotriazole. $C_6H_5N_3$; mol wt 119.12. C 60.50%, H 4.23%, N 35.28%. Prepd by the action of nitrous acid on *o*-phenylenediamine: Ladenburg, *Ber.* **9**, 219 (1876); Damschroder, Peterson, *Org. Synth.* **coll. vol. III**, 106 (1955).

Needles from benzene, mp 98.5°. bp_{15} 204°; $bp_{2.0}$ 159°. *Caution:* May explode during vacuum distillation, *see Chem. Eng. News* **34**, 2450 (1956). Sparingly sol in water. Sol in alc, benzene, toluene, chloroform, DMF.

1109. Benzotrichloride. [98-07-7] (Trichloromethyl)-benzene; α,α,α-trichlorotoluene; phenylchloroform; ω,ω,ω-trichlorotoluene; benzenyl trichloride; toluene trichloride. $C_7H_5Cl_3$; mol wt 195.47. C 43.01%, H 2.58%, Cl 54.41%. Produced by chlorination of boiling toluene in the presence of light and of 2% phosphorus trichloride: Swarts, *Bull. Soc. Chim. Belg.* **31**, 375 (1922); Conklin, **US 1828858**; **US 1828859** (both 1931 to Solvay Process Co.). Commercial grades may contain hydrochloric acid, benzylidene chloride, and benzyl chloride. Purification procedures: Holleman, deMooy, *Rec. Trav. Chim.* **33**, 25, 33 (1914); Britton, **US 1804458** (1931 to Dow); *Chem. Zentralbl.* **1931**, II, 497. Toxicity data: H. F. Smyth *et al.*, *Arch. Ind. Hyg. Occup. Med.* **4**, 119 (1951). *Review:* H. C. Lin in *Kirk-Othmer Encyclopedia of Chemical Technology* **vol. 6** (John Wiley & Sons, New York, 4th ed., 1993) pp 113-126.

Colorless, oily liquid with pungent odor. Fumes in air. mp −5.0°. d_4^{20} 1.3756. bp_{760} 220.8°. bp_{60} 129°; bp_{25} 105°; bp_{10} 89°. n_D^{20} 1.55789. Autoignition temp: 211°. Unstable. Hydrolyzes in the presence of moisture, forming benzoic and hydrochloric acids. Insol in water. Sol in alcohol, benzene, ether, many other organic solvents. LD_{50} orally in rats: 6.0 g/kg (Smyth).

Caution: Vapors may be stongly irritating and lacrimatory (Lin). This substance is reasonably anticipated to be a human carcinogen: *Report on Carcinogens, Eleventh Edition* (PB2005-104914, 2004) p III-31.

USE: In dye chemistry. In organic syntheses (source of benzenyl group).

1110. Benzotrifluoride. [98-08-8] (Trifluoromethyl)benzene; α,α,α-trifluorotoluene; phenylfluoroform. $C_7H_5F_3$; mol wt 146.11. C 57.54%, H 3.45%, F 39.01%. Prepd by the action of hydrogen fluoride on benzotrichloride: Simons, Lewis, *J. Am. Chem. Soc.* **60**, 492 (1938); Simons, *Ind. Eng. Chem.* **32**, 178 (1940); by the action of antimony trifluoride on benzotrichloride: Swarts, *Bull. Sci. Acad. R. Belg.*, [4] **35**, 375 (1898); [5] **6**, 389 (1920); [5] **13**, 175 (1927); Holt *et al.*, **US 2058453** (1937 to Kinetic Chemicals).

Liquid. mp −29.05°. d^{20} 1.1886. bp 103.46°. $n_D^{13.3}$ 1.41486. Soluble in many organic solvents.

USE: In dye chemistry; in the manuf of substituted benzotrifluorides contg an ethylenic group, used in high polymer chemistry; in dielectric fluids, such as transformer oils.

1111. Benzoxonium Chloride. [19379-90-9] *N*-Dodecyl-*N*,*N*-bis(2-hydroxyethyl)benzenemethanaminium chloride; benzyl-

dodecylbis(2-hydroxyethyl)ammonium chloride; dodecyldi(β-hydroxyethyl)benzylammonium chloride; D-301; ZY-15021; Absonal; Bactofen; Bialcol. $C_{23}H_{42}ClNO_2$; mol wt 400.04. C 69.05%, H 10.58%, Cl 8.86%, N 3.50%, O 8.00%. Quaternary ammonium salt with antimicrobial activity. Prepn: **CH 306648** (1955 to Ciba), *C.A.* **51**, 2023g (1957). Antimicrobial activity and toxicology: H. Goeth *et al.*, *Arzneim.-Forsch.* **9**, 622 (1959). Potentiometric determn: S. Pinzauti, E. La Porta, *Analyst* **102**, 938 (1977). Clinical evaluation in dental plaque control: U. P. Saxer *et al.*, *J. Clin. Periodontol.* **9**, 162 (1982). *In vitro* antibacterial spectrum: M. Cortat, P. Fels, *Arzneim.-Forsch.* **37**, 463 (1987). Clinical evaluation in pharyngeal infections: M. A. Weibel *et al.*, *ibid.* 467.

Colorless powder from ethyl ether, mp 107-109°. Sol in water, alcohol, benzene, toluene, chlorobenzene. LD_{50} orally in rats: 750 mg/kg (Goeth).

THERAP CAT: Antiseptic.

THERAP CAT (VET): Antiseptic.

1112. Benzoyl Chloride. [98-88-4] Benzenecarbonyl chloride. C_7H_5ClO; mol wt 140.57. C 59.81%, H 3.59%, Cl 25.22%, O 11.38%. Prepd by partial hydrolysis of benzotrichloride: Davies, Dick, *J. Chem. Soc.* **1932**, 2808; by chlorination of benzaldehyde: Wöhler, *Ann.* **3**, 262 (1832); from benzoic acid and PCl_5 or from benzoic acid and phosgene: Uwarow, Stepanow, **SU 56693** (1936). Lab prepn from benzoic acid and thionyl chloride: A. I. Vogel, *Practical Organic Chemistry* (Longmans, London, 3rd ed., 1959) p 792; Gattermann-Wieland, *Praxis des Organischen Chemikers* (de Gruyter, Berlin, 40th ed., 1961) p 112.

Liquid. Penetrating odor. d_4^{25} 1.2070. mp −1.0°. bp_{760} 197.2°; bp_{35} 100°; bp_{15} 82.3°; bp_9 71°; bp_3 49°. n_D^{20} 1.55369. Dipole moment 3.28. Flash pt 88°C (190.4°F). Parachor 289.8. Dec by water and alc. Miscible with ether, benzene, carbon disulfide, oils.

Caution: Lacrimator. Irritating to skin, eyes, mucous membranes.

USE: For acylation, i.e., introduction of the benzoyl group into alcohols, phenols, and amines (Schotten-Baumann reaction); in the manuf of benzoyl peroxide and of dye intermediates. In organic analysis for making benzoyl derivatives for identification purposes.

1113. Benzoylecgonine. [519-09-5] 3-(Benzoyloxy)-8-methyl-8-azabicyclo[3.2.1]octane-2-carboxylic acid; 3β-hydroxy-1αH,5αH-tropane-2β-carboxylic acid benzoate; ecgonine benzoate. $C_{16}H_{19}NO_4$; mol wt 289.33. C 66.42%, H 6.62%, N 4.84%, O 22.12%. Cocaine metabolite. Isoln from coca leaves: De Jong, *Rec. Trav. Chim.* **42**, 980 (1923). Prepn from *l*-ecgonine and benzoic anhydride: *idem, ibid.* **66**, 544 (1947).

Tetrahydrate. Orthorhombic prisms or needles from water, mp 86-92° (dec 195°, dry). $[\alpha]_D^{15}$ −45° (c = 3 in abs alc). Soluble in alc, hot H_2O.

1114. Benzoyl Isothiocyanate. [532-55-8] Benzoylthiocarbimide. C_8H_5NOS; mol wt 163.20. C 58.88%, H 3.09%, N 8.58%, O 9.80%, S 19.65%. C_6H_5CONCS. Prepd by refluxing a mixture of KSCN and benzoyl chloride in benzene at 110-120°: Ambelang, Johnson, *J. Am. Chem. Soc.* **61**, 632 (1939). From NH_3SCN, acetone and benzoyl chloride: Frank, Smith, *Org. Synth.* **28**, 89 (1948).

Liquid; bp_{18} 133-137°; bp_{10} 119°. $d_4^{18.3}$ 1.2142; d_4^{16} 1.197. $n_D^{18.3}$ 1.6382. Reacts with a primary or secondary amine to form a benzoylthiourea, which is readily hydrolyzed by alkalies to the free thiourea.

1115. Benzoylpas. [13898-58-3] 4-(Benzoylamino)-2-hydroxybenzoic acid; N-benzoyl-p-aminosalicylic acid; 4-benzamidosalicylic acid. $C_{14}H_{11}NO_4$; mol wt 257.24. C 65.37%, H 4.31%, N 5.44%, O 24.88%. Prepn: Drain *et al., J. Chem. Soc.* **1949**, 1498; **GB 676363** (1952 to Wander). Prepn of sodium and calcium salts: Suddaby, Sumpter, **GB 711163** (1954 to Herst).

Crystals, mp 260-261°.

Calcium salt pentahydrate. [5631-00-5] Benzoylpas calcium; Therapas. $C_{28}H_{20}CaN_2O_8 \cdot 5H_2O$; mol wt 642.62. White powder or crystals.

Mixture of calcium salt with isoniazid. Iso-Benzacyl.

THERAP CAT: Antibacterial (tuberculostatic).

1116. Benzoyl Peroxide. [94-36-0] Dibenzoyl peroxide; benzoyl superoxide; Acetoxyl; Acnegel; Akneroxid L; Benoxyl; Benzac; Benzagel; Benzaknen; Brevoxyl; Debroxide; Desanden; Lucidol; Nericur; Oxy-5; PanOxyl; Peroxyderm; Persa-gel; Sanoxit; Theraderm; Xerac BP. $C_{14}H_{10}O_4$; mol wt 242.23. C 69.42%, H 4.16%, O 26.42%. $(C_6H_5CO)_2O_2$. Prepd by interaction of benzoyl chloride and a cooled soln of sodium peroxide. Laboratory procedure: A. I. Vogel, *Practical Organic Chemistry* (Longmans, London, 3rd ed., 1954) p 807; Gattermann-Wieland, *Praxis des Organischen Chemikers* (de Gruyter, Berlin, 40th ed., 1961) p 115. Comparative clinical study with clindamycin, *q.v.*, in acne vulgaris: L. J. Swinyer *et al., Br. J. Dermatol.* **119**, 615 (1988). Review of carcinogenic and allergenic potential: D. J. Hogan, *Int. J. Dermatol.* **30**, 467-470 (1991).

Crystals. mp 103-106°. *May explode when heated.* Sparingly sol in water or alcohol; sol in benzene, chloroform, ether. One gram dissolves in 40 ml carbon disulfide, in about 50 ml olive oil.

Caution: Potential symptoms of overexposure are irritation of skin, eyes and mucous membranes; sensitization dermatitis. *See NIOSH Pocket Guide to Chemical Hazards* (DHHS/NIOSH 97-140, 1997) p 26.

USE: Source of free radicals for industrial processes. Oxidizing agent in bleaching oils, flour, etc.; catalyst in the plastics industry; initiator in polymerization.

THERAP CAT: Keratolytic.

THERAP CAT (VET): Keratolytic.

1117. 3,4-Benzphenanthrene. [195-19-7] Benzo[c]phenanthrene. $C_{18}H_{12}$; mol wt 228.29. C 94.70%, H 5.30%. Synthesis by a Pschorr reaction from diazotized α-(2-naphthyl)-2-aminocinnamic acid: Cook, *J. Chem. Soc.* **1931**, 2524. From diphenylmethylsuccinic anhydride: Hewett, *J. Chem. Soc.* **1936**, 599. By double ring closure of β-benzohydrylglutaric acid: Newman, Joshel, *J. Am. Chem. Soc.* **60**, 487 (1938). From 4-keto-1,2,3,4-tetrahydrophenanthrene: Bachmann, Edgerton, *ibid.* **62**, 2970 (1940).

Needles from alcohol, mp 68° (needles or leaflets from petr ether, fine needles from alcohol + acetone). Absorption maxima: Mayneord, Roe, *Proc. Roy. Soc. London* **A158**, 63 (1937).

1118. Benzphetamine. [156-08-1] (αS)-N,α-Dimethyl-N-(phenylmethyl)benzeneethanamine; N-benzyl-N,α-dimethylphenethylamine; d-N-methyl-N-benzyl-β-phenylisopropylamine. $C_{17}H_{21}N$; mol wt 239.36. C 85.30%, H 8.84%, N 5.85%. Prepd from d-desoxyephedrine: Heinzelman, Aspergren, **US 2789138** (1957 to Upjohn).

Liquid. $bp_{0.02}$ 127°. n_D^{19} 1.5515. Practically insol in water. Sol in methanol, ethanol, ether, chloroform, acetone, benzene.

Hydrochloride. [5411-22-3] Didrex; Inapetyl. $C_{17}H_{21}N \cdot HCl$; mol wt 275.82. Crystals from ethyl acetate, mp 129-130°. Dextrorotatory. Sol in water, 95% ethanol.

Note: This is a controlled substance (stimulant): **21 CFR**, 1308.13.

THERAP CAT: Anorexic.

1119. Benzquinamide. [63-12-7] 2-(Acetyloxy)-N,N-diethyl-1,3,4,6,7,11b-hexahydro-9,10-dimethoxy-2H-benzo[a]quinolizine-3-carboxamide; N,N-diethyl-1,3,4,6,7,11b-hexahydro-2-hydroxy-9,10-dimethoxy-2H-benzo[a]quinolizine-3-carboxamide acetate; 2-acetoxy-3-(N,N-diethylcarboxamido)-9,10-dimethoxy-1,2,3,4,6,7-hexahydro-11bH-benzopyridocoline; 2-hydroxy-3-diethylcarbamyl-9,10-dimethoxy-1,2,3,4,6,7-hexahydro-11bH-benzoquinolizine acetate; BZQ; NSC-64375; P-2647; Emete-Con; Promecon; Quantril. $C_{22}H_{32}N_2O_5$; mol wt 404.50. C 65.32%, H 7.97%, N 6.93%, O 19.78%. Prepn: Trettner, **US 3053845** (1962 to Pfizer). Pharmacology: Scriabine *et al., J. Am. Med. Assoc.* **184**, 276 (1963); Kadzielawa, Gumulka, *Arch. Int. Pharmacodyn. Ther.* **163**, 139 (1966). Metabolic studies: Koe, Pinson, *J. Med. Chem.* **7**, 635 (1964); Wiseman *et al., Biochem. Pharmacol.* **13**, 1421 (1964). Toxicity: E. I. Goldenthal, *Toxicol. Appl. Pharmacol.* **18**, 185 (1971).

Crystals from diisopropyl ether, mp 130-131.5°. LD_{50} orally in rats: 990 mg/kg; i.p. in mice: 376 mg/kg (Goldenthal).

THERAP CAT: Antipsychotic, antiemetic.

1120. Benzthiazide. [91-33-8] 6-Chloro-3-[[(phenylmethyl)thio]methyl]-2H-1,2,4-benzothiadiazine-7-sulfonamide 1,1-dioxide; 3-[(benzylthio)methyl]-6-chloro-2H-1,2,4-benzothiadiazine-7-sulfonamide 1,1-dioxide; 3-[(benzylthio)methyl]-6-chloro-7-sulfamoyl-2H-benzo-1,2,4-thiadiazine 1,1-dioxide; 6-chloro-7-sulfamoyl-3-benzylthiomethyl-2H-1,2,4-benzothiadiazine 1,1-dioxide; benzothiazide; Exna; Fovane. $C_{15}H_{14}ClN_3O_4S_3$; mol wt 431.94. C 41.71%, H 3.27%, Cl 8.21%, N 9.73%, O 14.82%, S 22.27%. Prepn: J. M. McManus *et al., 136th Am. Chem. Soc. Meet.* (Atlantic City, Sept. 1959) *Abstr. of Papers*, pp 13-O; W. M. McLamore, G. D. Laubach, **DE 1137740**; *eidem,* **US 3440244** (1962, 1969 both to Pfizer). Pharmacology, toxicity: S. Y. P'an *et al., J. Pharmacol. Exp. Ther.* **128**, 122 (1960).

Crystals from acetone, mp 231-232° (U.S. patent); also reported as mp 238-239° (P'an). Bitter taste. Practically insol in water. Sol in alkaline solns. LD_{50} in mice, rats (mg/kg): >5000, >10000 orally; 410, 422 i.v. (P'an).

THERAP CAT: Diuretic, antihypertensive.

1121. Benztropine Mesylate. [132-17-2] 3-(Diphenylmeth-oxy)-8-methyl-8-azabicyclo[3.2.1]octane methanesulfonate; 3α-(di-phenylmethoxy)-1αH,5αH-tropane methanesulfonate; benztropine methanesulfonate; tropine benzohydryl ether methanesulfonate; Co-gentin; Cogentinol. $C_{22}H_{29}NO_4S$; mol wt 403.53. C 65.48%, H 7.24%, N 3.47%, O 15.86%, S 7.95%. Anticholinergic. Prepd by the action of diphenyldiazomethane on tropine: Phillips, US 2595405 (1952 to Merck & Co.). Crystal structure: P. G. Jones et al., Acta Crystallogr. **B34**, 3125 (1978).

Crystals from acetone + ether, mp 143°. uv max: 259 nm (E_M = 437). Soluble in water. pH about 6.

THERAP CAT: Antiparkinsonian.

1122. Benzydamine. [642-72-8] N,N-Dimethyl-3-[[1-(phenylmethyl)-1H-indazol-3-yl]oxy]-1-propanamine; 1-benzyl-3-[3-(dimethylamino)propoxy]-1H-indazole; 1-benzyl-1H-indazol-3-yl 3-(dimethylamino)propyl ether; benzindamine. $C_{19}H_{23}N_3O$; mol wt 309.41. C 73.75%, H 7.49%, N 13.58%, O 5.17%. Prepn: FR 1382855; Palazzo, US 3318905 (1964, 1967 both to Angelini Francesco); Palazzo et al., J. Med. Chem. **9**, 38 (1966). Pharma-cology: Lisciani et al., Eur. J. Pharmacol. **3**, 157 (1968). Metab-olism: Catanese et al., Arzneim.-Forsch. **16**, 1354 (1966); Kataoka et al., Chem. Pharm. Bull. **19**, 1511 (1971). Toxicology: B. Sil-vestrini et al., Toxicol. Appl. Pharmacol. **10**, 148 (1967). Series of articles on pharmacology: Arzneim.-Forsch. **37**, 587-646 (1987).

$bp_{0.05}$ 160°.
Hydrochloride. [132-69-4] Afloben; Andolex; Benzyrin; Dif-flam; Enzamin; Imotryl; Opalgyne; Riripen; Salyzoron; Saniflor; Tamas; Tantum; Verax. $C_{19}H_{23}N_3O.HCl$; mol wt 345.87. Crys-tals, mp 160°. uv max: 306 nm ($E_{1cm}^{1\%}$ 160). Very sol in water; rather sol in ethanol, chloroform, n-butanol. LD_{50} in mice, rats (mg/kg): 110, 100 i.p.; 515, 1050 orally (Silvestrini).

THERAP CAT: Analgesic; anti-inflammatory; antipyretic.

THERAP CAT (VET): Anti-inflammatory.

1123. Benzyl Acetate. [140-11-4] Acetic acid phenylmeth-yl ester; acetic acid benzyl ester. $C_9H_{10}O_2$; mol wt 150.17. C 71.98%, H 6.71%, O 21.31%. $C_6H_5CH_2OOCCH_3$. Occurs in a number of plants, particularly jasmine: S. Arctander, Perfume and Flavor Materials of Natural Origin (Elizabeth, N.J., 1960) pp 313-314. Prepd from benzyl chloride, acetic acid or sodium acetate and triethylamine: Merker, Scott, J. Org. Chem. **26**, 5180 (1961); Hen-nis et al., Ind. Eng. Chem. Prod. Res. Dev. **6**, 193 (1967). Toxicity study: P. M. Jenner et al., Food Cosmet. Toxicol. **2**, 327 (1964).

Liquid; pear-like odor. bp 213°, bp_{102} 134°. mp −51°. d_4^{25} 1.050. n_D^{20} 1.5232, n_D^{25} 1.4998. Flash pt, closed cup: 216°F (102°C). Practically insol in water. Misc with alcohol, ether. LD_{50} orally in rats: 2490 mg/kg (Jenner).

Caution: Ingestion can cause G.I. irritation with vomiting and diarrhea. Also irritating to skin, eyes, respiratory tract.

USE: In perfumery, solvent for cellulose acetate and nitrate.

1124. Benzyl Alcohol. [100-51-6] Benzenemethanol; phen-ylcarbinol; phenylmethanol; α-hydroxytoluene. C_7H_8O; mol wt 108.14. C 77.75%, H 7.46%, O 14.80%. $C_6H_5CH_2OH$. Constit-uent of jasmine, hyacinth, ylang-ylang oils, Peru and Tolu balsams, storax, where it occurs in ester form also. Originally prepd by the Cannizzaro reaction from benzaldehyde + KOH: Cannizzaro, Ann. **88**, 129 (1853); cf. Hickinbottom, Reactions of Organic Compds. (Longmans, London, 3rd ed., 1957) p 251; A. I. Vogel, Practical Organic Chemistry (Longmans, London, 3rd ed., 1959) p 711; Gattermann-Wieland, Praxis des Organischen Chemikers (de Gruyter, Berlin, 40th ed., 1961) p 193. Produced on a large scale by the action of sodium or potassium carbonate on benzyl chloride: DE 484662; Chem. Zentralbl. **1930**, I, 1052; Frdl. **16**, 426; cf. Kirk-Othmer Encyclopedia of Chemical Technology vol. 3 (Interscience, New York, 1964) pp 442-449. Toxicity: Smyth et al., Arch. Ind. Hyg. Occup. Med. **4**, 119 (1951).

Liquid. Faint aromatic odor. Sharp burning taste. d_4^{20} 1.04535; d_4^{25} 1.04156. mp −15.19°. bp_{760} 204.7°; bp_{400} 183.0°; bp_{200} 160.0°; bp_{100} 141.7°; bp_{60} 129.3°; bp_{40} 119.8°; bp_{20} 105.8°; bp_{10} 92.6°; bp_5 80.8°; $bp_{1.0}$ 58.0°. n_D^{20} 1.54035; n_D^{25} 1.53837: Dreisbach, Martin, Ind. Eng. Chem. **41**, 2875 (1941). Absorption spectrum: Brode, J. Phys. Chem. **30**, 61 (1926). Vapor density 3.72 (air = 1.00). Flash pt, closed cup 213°F, open cup 220°F. Autoignition temp 817°F. One gram dissolves in about 25 ml water. One volume dissolves in 1.5 vols of 50% ethyl alcohol. Misc with abs and 94% alcohol, ether, chloroform. LD_{50} orally in rats: 3.1 g/kg (Smyth).

USE: Manuf other benzyl compds. Pharmaceutic aid (antimicro-bial). Solvent for gelatin, casein (when hot), solvent for cellulose acetate, shellac. Used in perfumery and in flavoring (mostly in form of its aliphatic esters). In microscopy as embedding material.

THERAP CAT (VET): Has been used for relief from pruritis.

1125. Benzylamine. [100-46-9] Benzenemethanamine; aminotoluene; phenylmethylamine; moringine. C_7H_9N; mol wt 107.15. C 78.46%, H 8.47%, N 13.07%. Prepn from benzyl-chloride and ammonia: Mason, J. Chem. Soc. **63**, 1311 (1893); by redn of benzonitrile: Carothers, Jones, J. Am. Chem. Soc. **47**, 3051 (1925); from benzyl bromide + acetamide: Erikson, Ber. **59**, 2665 (1926); from N-benzylphthalimide + hydrazine hydrate: Ing, Manske, J. Chem. Soc. **129**, 2348 (1926). Identity with moringine: Chakravarti, Bull. Calcutta Sch. Trop. Med. **3**, 162 (1955); C.A. **50**, 16891e (1956).

Liquid; strongly alkaline reaction. bp 185°; bp_{12} 90°. d_4^{19} 0.983. n_D^{20} 1.5401. Miscible with water, alcohol, ether.
Hydrochloride. $C_7H_9N.HCl$. Crystals, mp 253°.
Hydroiodide. $C_7H_9N.HI$. Leaflets, mp 162°.
Caution: Highly irritating to skin, mucous membranes.
USE: In organic synthesis.

1126. Benzylaniline. [103-32-2] N-Phenylbenzenemethan-amine; N-phenylbenzylamine; benzylphenylamine. $C_{13}H_{13}N$; mol wt 183.25. C 85.21%, H 7.15%, N 7.64%. $C_6H_5CH_2NHC_6H_5$. Prepn from benzyl alc and aniline in the presence of KOH: Sprin-zak, J. Am. Chem. Soc. **78**, 3207 (1956); from benzaldehyde and aniline in the presence of $NaBH_4$: Schellenberg, J. Org. Chem. **28**, 3259 (1963).

Prisms, mp 37-38°. bp 306-307°. Practically insol in water; sol in alcohol, chloroform, ether.

1127. Benzyl Benzoate. [120-51-4] Benzoic acid phenyl-methyl ester; benzoic acid benzyl ester; benzylbenzenecarboxylate; Acarosan; Antiscabiosum; Ascabiol. $C_{14}H_{12}O_2$; mol wt 212.24. C 79.23%, H 5.70%, O 15.08%. $C_6H_5COOCH_2C_6H_5$. Contained in

Peru and Tolu balsams. Prepd by the action of sodium benzylate on benzaldehyde: Kamm, Kamm, *Org. Synth.* **coll. vol. I,** 104 (2nd ed., 1941); by the dry esterification of sodium benzoate and benzyl chloride in the presence of triethylamine: Thorp, Nottorf, *Ind. Eng. Chem.* **39,** 1300 (1947). Toxicity studies: Graham, Kuizenga, *J. Pharmacol. Exp. Ther.* **84,** 358 (1945); Draize *et al., J. Pharmacol. Exp. Ther.* **93,** 26 (1948). Comprehensive description: M. M. A. Hassan, J. S. Mossa, *Anal. Profiles Drug Subs.* **10,** 55-74 (1981).

Leaflets or oily liq; faint, pleasant, aromatic odor; sharp burning taste. mp 21°. d_4^{25} 1.118. bp 323-324°. bp_{16} 189-191°. $bp_{4.5}$ 156°. Sparingly volatile with steam. n_D^{21} 1.5681. Insol in water or glycerol. Miscible with alc, chloroform, ether, oils. LD_{50} in rats, mice, rabbits, guinea pigs (g/kg): 1.7, 1.4, 1.8, 1.0 orally (Draize).

Caution: Direct contact may cause skin irritation. Potential symptoms of overexposure by ingestion in exptl animals are progressive incoordination, CNS excitation, convulsions. *See Clinical Toxicology of Commercial Products,* R. E. Gosselin *et al.,* Eds. (Williams & Wilkins, Baltimore, 5th ed., 1984) Section II, p 203.

USE: As solvent of cellulose acetate, nitrocellulose and artificial musk; substitute for camphor in celluloid and plastic pyroxylin compds; perfume fixative; in confectionery and chewing gum flavors.

THERAP CAT: Scabicide, pediculicide.

THERAP CAT (VET): Acaricide, pediculicide. *Contraindicated* in cats.

1128. Benzyl Bromide. [100-39-0] (Bromomethyl)benzene; α-bromotoluene; ω-bromotoluene. C_7H_7Br; mol wt 171.03. C 49.16%, H 4.13%, Br 46.72%. $C_6H_5CH_2Br$. Prepd by the action of bromine on toluene in ultraviolet light: v. Konek, Loczka, *Ber.* **57,** 679 (1924); Zelinsky, *DE 478084; Chem. Zentralbl.* **1929 II,** 1216; *Frdl.* **16,** 335; by the action of bromine on dibenzyl ether: Lachman, *J. Am. Chem. Soc.* **45,** 2359 (1923).

Lacrimatory liquid. mp −3.9°. bp 198-199°. bp_{80} 127°. d_0^2 1.4380; d^{17} 1.443; d_4^{64} 1.3886. Slowly decomp by water.

Caution: Intensely irritating to skin, eyes, mucous membranes. Large doses cause CNS depression.

1129. Benzyl Chloride. [100-44-7] (Chloromethyl)benzene; α-chlorotoluene. C_7H_7Cl; mol wt 126.58. C 66.42%, H 5.57%, Cl 28.01%. $C_6H_5CH_2Cl$. Made by cautious chlorination of toluene: A. I. Vogel, *Practical Organic Chemistry* (Longmans, London, 3rd ed., 1959) p 538; Gattermann-Wieland, *Praxis des Organischen Chemikers* (de Gruyter, Berlin, 40th ed., 1961) p 92. Manuf: *Faith, Keyes & Clark's Industrial Chemicals,* F. A. Lowenheim, M. K. Moran, Eds. (Wiley-Interscience, New York, 4th ed., 1975) pp 145-148.

Very refractive liquid; rather unpleasant, irritating odor. d_{20}^{20} 1.100. bp 179°. mp −48 to −43°. n_D^{15} 1.5415. Insol in water. Miscible with alcohol, chloroform, ether. Rapidly dec when heated in the presence of iron.

Caution: Potential symptoms of overexposure are irritation of eyes, skin and nose; weakness; irritability; headache; skin eruption; pulmonary edema. *See NIOSH Pocket Guide to Chemical Hazards* (DHHS/NIOSH 97-140, 1997) p 28.

USE: Manuf benzyl compds, perfumes, pharmaceutical products, dyes, synthetic tannins, artificial resins.

1130. Benzyl Cinnamate. [103-41-3] 3-Phenyl-2-propenoic acid phenylmethyl ester; *trans*-cinnamic acid benzyl ester; cinnamein. $C_{16}H_{14}O_2$; mol wt 238.28. C 80.65%, H 5.92%, O 13.43%. $C_6H_5CH=CHCOOCH_2C_6H_5$. Constituent of storax, Peru and Tolu balsams: Tschirch, Trog, *Arch. Pharm.* **232,** 70 (1894); Tschirch, Oberländer, *ibid.* 559. Prepn: Volwiler, Vliet, *J. Am. Chem. Soc.* **43,** 1672 (1921); Eliel, Anderson, *ibid.* **74,** 547 (1952); Bender, Zerner, *ibid.* **84,** 2550 (1962). Toxicity study: P. M. Jenner *et al., Food Cosmet. Toxicol.* **2,** 327 (1964).

Crystals from 95% ethanol; sweet odor of balsam. mp 39°; also reported as mp 33-34° (Volwiler, Vliet). Dec on distillation at ordinary pressure; $bp_{0.5}$ 154-157°, bp_5 195-200°, bp_{22} 228-230°. Practically insol in water, propylene glycol and glycerin. Sol in alc, ether, oils. LD_{50} orally in rats: 5530 mg/kg (Jenner).

USE: In artificial flavors, in perfumes, mainly as a fixative.

1131. Benzyl Cyanide. [140-29-4] Benzeneacetonitrile; phenylacetonitrile; α-tolunitrile; ω-cyanotoluene. C_8H_7N; mol wt

117.15. C 82.02%, H 6.02%, N 11.96%. $C_6H_5CH_2CN$. Occurs in garden cress and other plants; made from benzyl chloride, and NaCN: Adams, Thal, *Org. Synth.* **vol. 2,** 9 (1922); **coll. vol. I,** 101 (107 in 2nd ed.).

Oily liquid, aromatic odor. d_{15}^{15} 1.0214. mp −23.8°. bp_{760} 233.5°; bp_{100} 161.8°; bp_{20} 119.4°; $bp_{1.0}$ 60°. n_D^{25} 1.52105. Insoluble in water, miscible with alc, ether.

1132. Benzyl Ether. [103-50-4] 1,1'-[Oxybis(methylene)]-bis[benzene]; dibenzyl ether. $C_{14}H_{14}O$; mol wt 198.26. C 84.81%, H 7.12%, O 8.07%. $(C_6H_5CH_2)_2O$. Prepd: Lachman, *J. Am. Chem. Soc.* **45,** 2356 (1923); Staab, Wendel, *Ber.* **93,** 2902 (1960); Lichtenberger, Tritsch, *Bull. Soc. Chim. Fr.* **1961,** 363. Manuf by reduction of benzaldehyde in the presence of $[Co(CO)_4]_2$: Wender, Orchin, *US 2614107* (1952 to U.S.A. as represented by the Secy. of Agr.). Physical properties: Svirbely *et al., J. Am. Chem. Soc.* **71,** 507 (1949); Dreisbach, Martin, *Ind. Eng. Chem.* **41,** 2875 (1949). Miscibility: Jackson, Drury, *ibid.* **51,** 1491 (1959).

Unstable liquid, bp 295-298° (with dec), bp_{21} 173-174°; bp_2 125.5-126.5°. Appears to dec slowly at ordinary temps. d^{35} 1.0341; d_4^{25} 0.99735; d_4^{20} 1.00142; d^{15} 1.0482. n_D^{25} 1.5601 (Svirbely *et al.*), 1.53851 (Dreisbach, Martin); n_D^{20} 1.54057 (Dreisbach, Martin), 1.566 (Lichtenberger, Tritsch). Practically insol in water; miscible with ethanol, ether, chloroform, acetone.

USE: Plasticizer for nitrocellulose; solvent in perfumery.

1133. Benzyl Ethyl Ether. [539-30-0] (Ethoxymethyl)benzene. $C_9H_{12}O$; mol wt 136.19. C 79.37%, H 8.88%, O 11.75%. $C_6H_5CH_2OC_2H_5$. Preparation from sodium ethoxide and benzyl bromide: Letsinger, Pollart, *J. Am. Chem. Soc.* **78,** 6079 (1956); by reduction of benzaldehyde diethyl acetal with $LiAlH_4$-$AlCl_3$: Eliel, Rerick, *J. Org. Chem.* **23,** 1088 (1958).

Oily liquid, aromatic odor. bp 186°; bp_{10} 65°. d 0.949, n_D^{20} 1.4955. Volatile with steam. Practically insol in water; miscible with alcohol, ether.

1134. Benzyl Formate. [104-57-4] Formic acid phenylmethyl ester; formic acid benzyl ester. $C_8H_8O_2$; mol wt 136.15. C 70.57%, H 5.92%, O 23.50%. $HCOOCH_2C_6H_5$. Prepn from formic acid and benzyl alcohol: Mailhe, *Chem. Ztg.* **35,** 508 (1911).

Liquid; pleasant fruity odor. d 1.081. bp 203°. Practically insol in water. Sol in alcohol.

USE: Solvent for cellulose esters; in perfumery.

1135. Benzyl Fumarate. [538-64-7] (*E*)-2-Butenedioic acid bis(phenylmethyl) ester; fumaric acid dibenzyl ester; dibenzyl fumarate. $C_{18}H_{16}O_4$; mol wt 296.32. C 72.96%, H 5.44%, O 21.60%. $C_6H_5CH_2OOCCH=CHCOOCH_2C_6H_5$. Prepd from fumaric acid and benzyl alcohol: Volwiler, Vliet, *J. Am. Chem. Soc.* **43,** 1672 (1921).

Cryst powder, mp 58.5-59.5°. bp_5 210-211°. Practically insol in water. Sol in alcohol, chloroform, ether, oils.

USE: In room spray deodorant: Kulka, *US 3077457* (1963 to Fritzsche Bros.).

1136. Benzylhydrochlorothiazide. [1824-50-6] 6-Chloro-3,4-dihydro-3-(phenylmethyl)-2*H*-1,2,4-benzothiadiazine-7-sulfonamide 1,1-dioxide; 3-benzyl-6-chloro-3,4-dihydro-2*H*-1,2,4-benzothiadiazine-7-sulfonamide 1,1-dioxide; 6-chloro-7-sulfamoyl-3-benzyl-3,4-dihydro-1,2,4-benzothiadiazine 1,1-dioxide; 3-benzyl-6-chloro-3,4-dihydro-7-sulfamoyl-1,2,4-benzothiadiazine 1,1-dioxide; Behyd. $C_{14}H_{14}ClN_3O_4S_2$; mol wt 387.86. C 43.35%, H 3.64%, Cl 9.14%, N 10.83%, O 16.50%, S 16.53%. Prepn: Werner *et al., J. Am. Chem. Soc.* **82,** 1161 (1960); Novello *et al., J. Org. Chem.* **25,** 970 (1960); Ugi, *US 3108097* (1963).

Crystals from acetic acid + water, mp 260-262°. Also reported as crystals from water, mp 269°.

THERAP CAT: Antihypertensive; diuretic.

1137. Benzylideneacetone. [122-57-6] 4-Phenyl-3-buten-2-one; benzalacetone; methyl styryl ketone; cinnamyl methyl ketone; acetocinnamone. $C_{10}H_{10}O$; mol wt 146.19. C 82.16%, H 6.89%, O 10.94%. $C_6H_5CH=CHCOCH_3$. Prepd by condensing acetone and benzaldehyde by means of aq alkali: Drake, Allen, *Org. Synth.* **3**, 17 (1923).

Lustrous plates on vacuum distillation. Coumarin type odor. Purification by steam distillation: Fromm, Haas, *Ann.* **394**, 291 (1912). mp 41.5°. d_{15}^{15} 1.0377; $d_4^{45.2}$ 1.0097. bp_{760} 261°; bp_{200} 211°; bp_{100} 187.8°; bp_{40} 161.3°; bp_{20} 143.8°; bp_{10} 127.4°; bp_5 112.2°; $bp_{1.0}$ 81.7°. $n_D^{45.9}$ 1.5836. Absorption spectrum: Baker, *J. Chem. Soc.* **91**, 1492 (1907); Baly, Schafer, *ibid.* **93**, 1813 (1908). Freely sol in alcohol, benzene, chloroform, ether; sparingly sol in water, petr ether.

USE: In perfumery, organic syntheses.

1138. Benzylideneaniline. [538-51-2] N-(Phenylmethylene)benzenamine; benzalaniline. $C_{13}H_{11}N$; mol wt 181.23. C 86.16%, H 6.12%, N 7.73%. $C_6H_5N=CHC_6H_5$. Prepd by the action of aniline on benzaldehyde: Bigelow, Eatough, *Org. Synth.* **coll. vol. I** (2nd ed., 1941) p 80. Molecular structure: M. Traetteberg *et al.*, *J. Mol. Struct.* **48**, 395 (1978).

Plates from 85% alc. Has been obtained as the yellow modification (needles from CS_2). The colorless form melts at 48°, after solidifying melts again at 56°. d_4^{50} 1.045. bp_{760} 300°. Absorption spectrum: Baly *et al.*, *J. Chem. Soc.* **97**, 590 (1910). Sol in alcohol, chloroform, acetic anhydride, carbon disulfide.

1139. Benzylimidobis(p-methoxyphenyl)methane. [524-96-9] N-[Bis(4-methoxyphenyl)methylene]benzenemethanamine. $C_{22}H_{21}NO_2$; mol wt 331.41. C 79.73%, H 6.39%, N 4.23%, O 9.66%. Prepd by heating p,p′-dimethoxybenzophenone, thionyl chloride and benzylamine: Schönberg, Urban, *Ber.* **67**, 1999 (1934).

Pale-yellow crystals, mp 89-91°. Soluble in ether, chloroform. Slightly sol in petr ether.

USE: Detection of elementary sulfur.

1140. Benzyl Methyl Ether. [538-86-3] (Methoxymethyl)benzene; methyl benzyl ether. $C_8H_{10}O$; mol wt 122.16. C 78.66%, H 8.25%, O 13.10%. $C_6H_5CH_2OCH_3$. Prepd from benzyl chloride, methanol, and NaOH: Olson *et al.*, *J. Am. Chem. Soc.* **69**, 2451 (1947).

Liquid. d 0.987. bp 174°. Practically insol in water. Sol in alcohol, ether.

1141. Benzylmorphine. [14297-87-1] 7,8-Didehydro-4,5-epoxy-17-methyl-3-(phenylmethoxy)morphinan-6-ol. $C_{24}H_{25}NO_3$; mol wt 375.46. C 76.77%, H 6.71%, N 3.73%, O 12.78%. Prepn from morphine and benzyl chloride in the presence of sodium ethylate: **DE 91813** (1897 to E. Merck), *Frdl.* **4**, 1245; from morphine and benzyldimethylphenylammonium hydroxide: Rodionow, *Bull. Soc. Chim. Fr.* [4] **45**, 109 (1929). Properties of hydrochloride: Dott, *Pharm. J.* **115**, 757 (1925).

Needles from water, prisms or platelets from ether, chloroform. mp 132°. Soluble in 2500 parts cold water, more sol in boiling water; 1.6 parts dissolves in 100 parts ether; readily sol in 50% alcohol, benzene.

Hydrochloride. Peronine. $C_{24}H_{25}NO_3 \cdot HCl$. Monohydrate, needles from water. Sol at 15° in 133 parts water, 218 parts 95% alcohol, 390 parts chloroform, 100 parts methanol; slightly sol in abs alcohol; very slightly sol in ether, acetone, isoamyl alcohol.

Note: This is a controlled substance (opium derivative): **21 CFR,** 1308.11.

THERAP CAT: Analgesic (narcotic).

1142. o-Benzylphenol. [28994-41-4] 2-(Phenylmethyl)phenol; α-phenyl-o-cresol; (2-hydroxydiphenyl)methane. $C_{13}H_{12}O$; mol wt 184.23. C 84.75%, H 6.57%, O 8.68%. Prepn from benzyl bromide and sodium phenoxide: Kornblum, Lurie, *J. Am. Chem. Soc.* **81**, 2711 (1959).

Crystals or liquid. mp 20.2-20.9°. bp_{10} 154-156°; $bp_{1.0}$ 121-123°. n_D^{20} 1.59945. Practically insol in water. Sol in organic solvents, in fixed alkali hydroxide solns.

1143. p-Benzylphenol. [101-53-1] 4-(Phenylmethyl)phenol; α-phenyl-p-cresol; (4-hydroxydiphenyl)methane. $C_{13}H_{12}O$; mol wt 184.23. C 84.75%, H 6.57%, O 8.68%. Prepd from phenol and benzyl chloride in the presence of zinc chloride: Ziegenbein *et al.*, *Ber.* **88**, 1906 (1955).

Crystals, mp 84°. bp 322°; bp_4 154-157°. Slightly sol in cold water; moderately sol in hot water; sol in organic solvents, glacial acetic acid, alkali hydroxide solns.

USE: Germicide, antiseptic, preservative; also in organic syntheses.

1144. Benzyl Salicylate. [118-58-1] 2-Hydroxybenzoic acid phenylmethyl ester; salicylic acid benzyl ester. $C_{14}H_{12}O_3$; mol wt 228.24. C 73.67%, H 5.30%, O 21.03%. Prepd from sodium salicylate and benzyl chloride: Volwiler, Vliet, *J. Am. Chem. Soc.* **43**, 1672 (1921).

Thick liquid, slight, pleasant odor. d^{20} 1.175. bp_{25} 208°. Slightly sol in water; miscible with alcohol or ether.

USE: As fixer in perfumery; in sunscreen preparations.

1145. Benzyl Sulfide. [538-74-9] 1,1′-[Thiobis(methylene)]bisbenzene; dibenzylsulfide. $C_{14}H_{14}S$; mol wt 214.33. C 78.45%, H 6.58%, S 14.96%. $(C_6H_5CH_2)_2S$. Prepn: Runge *et al.*, *J. Prakt. Chem.* **11**, 284 (1960). Manuf from benzyl chloride and Na_2S: Stucker, Brennan, **US 2755305** (1956 to Pure Oil Co.).

Plates, mp 49°. Practically insol in water. Sol in alc, ether.

1146. S-Benzylthiuronium Chloride. [538-28-3] Carbamimidothioic acid phenylmethyl ester monohydrochloride. $C_8H_{11}ClN_2S$; mol wt 202.70. C 47.40%, H 5.47%, Cl 17.49%, N 13.82%, S 15.82%. Prepd by refluxing a mixture of 126 g benzyl chloride, 76 g thiourea, and 200 ml alcohol for 0.5 hr: Donleavy, *J. Am. Chem. Soc.* **58**, 1004 (1936).

Crystals from alc or dil HCl, mp 172-174°. Metastable form, mp 146-148°. Can be converted to the higher melting form by dissolving in alcohol and seeding with crystals, mp 172-174°.

USE: Reagent for cobalt and nickel; identification and separation of carboxylic, sulfinic, and sulfonic acid.

1147. Benzylurea. [538-32-9] (Phenylmethyl)urea; benzyl-carbamide. $C_8H_{10}N_2O$; mol wt 150.18. C 63.98%, H 6.71%, N 18.65%, O 10.65%. $C_6H_5CH_2NHCONH_2$. Prepn: Neville, McGee, *Can. J. Chem.* **41**, 2123 (1963).

Crystals, mp 147-148°; dec at 200°. One gram dissolves in 60 ml warm water, 33 ml acetone; slightly sol in benzene, ether.

1148. Bephenium Hydroxynaphthoate. [3818-50-6] *N,N*-Dimethyl-*N*-(2-phenoxyethyl)benzenemethanaminium salt with 3-hydroxy-2-naphthalene carboxylic acid (1:1); bephenium embonate; Lecibis. $C_{28}H_{29}NO_4$; mol wt 443.53. C 75.82%, H 6.59%, N 3.16%, O 14.43%. Prepn: F. C. Copp, US 2918401 (1959 to Burroughs Wellcome). Mode of action: G. C. Coles *et al.*, *Experientia* **30**, 1265 (1974). Spectrophotometric determn: C. S. P. Sastry, M. Aruna, *Pharmazie* **43**, 361 (1988). Efficacy against strongylosis in elephants: K. Chandrasekharan *et al.*, *Kerala J. Vet. Sci.* **13**, 15 (1982). Clinical trial in hookworm infections: J. Nahmias *et al.*, *Ann. Trop. Med. Parasitol.* **83**, 625 (1989).

Crystals, mp 170-171°. Absorption max (water): 600 nm.
THERAP CAT: Anthelmintic (Nematodes).
THERAP CAT (VET): Anthelmintic (Nematodes).

1149. Bepotastine. [190786-43-7] 4-[(*S*)-(4-Chlorophen-yl)-2-pyridinylmethoxy]-1-piperidinebutanoic acid; betotastine. $C_{21}H_{25}ClN_2O_3$; mol wt 388.89. C 64.86%, H 6.48%, Cl 9.12%, N 7.20%, O 12.34%. Histamine H_1-receptor antagonist. Prepn (stereochem. unspec.): A. Koda *et al.*, EP 335586; *eidem*, US 4929618 (1989, 1990 both to Ube). Prepn of optically active salts: J. Kita *et al.*, EP 949260 (1999 to Ube; Tanabe Seiyaku). Pharmacology: M. Kato *et al.*, *Arzneim.-Forsch.* **47**, 1116 (1997). Suppression of IL-5 production: O. Kaminuma *et al.*, *Biol. Pharm. Bull.* **21**, 411 (1998). Antiallergic activity in animal models: M. Ueno *et al.*, *Pharmacology* **57**, 206 (1998).

Benzenesulfonate salt. [190786-44-8] Bepotastine besilate; TAU-284; Talion. $C_{21}H_{25}ClN_2O_3 \cdot C_6H_6O_3S$; mol wt 547.06. Pale grey prisms from acetonitrile, mp 161-163°. $[\alpha]_D^{20}$ +6.0° (c = 5 in methanol).
THERAP CAT: Antihistaminic.

1150. Bepridil. [64706-54-3] β-[(2-Methylpropoxy)meth-yl]-*N*-phenyl-*N*-(phenylmethyl)-1-pyrrolidineethanamine; 1-[2-(*N*-benzylanilino)-1-(isobutoxymethyl)ethyl]pyrrolidine; 1-isobutoxy-2-pyrrolidino-3-*N*-benzylanilinopropane; 3-isobutoxy-2-pyrrolidino-*N*-phenyl-*N*-benzylpropylamine. $C_{24}H_{34}N_2O$; mol wt 366.54. C 78.64%, H 9.35%, N 7.64%, O 4.36%. Calcium channel blocker with antianginal and antiarrhythmic properties. Prepn: R. Y. Mauvernay *et al.*, DE 2310918; *eidem*, US 3962238; reissued with structure correction: N. Busch *et al.*, US RE 30577 (1973, 1976, 1981 all to CERM). *See also:* R. Y. Mauvernay *et al.*, DE 2802864 (1978 to CERM), *C.A.* **89**, 179852s (1978). Cardiovascular pharmacology in dogs: M.-T. Michelin *et al.*, *Therapie* **32**, 485 (1977). Mechanism of action studies: S. Vogel *et al.*, *J. Pharmacol. Exp. Ther.* **210**, 378 (1979); C. Labrid *et al.*, *ibid.* **211**, 546 (1979). Clinical comparison of hemodynamic and coronary changes: J. P. Merillon *et al.*, *Therapie* **36**, 123 (1981). Clinical evaluation in angina: M. K. Sharma *et al.*, *Am. J. Cardiol.* **61**, 1210 (1988).

Viscous liquid, $bp_{0.1}$ 184°, $bp_{0.5}$ 192°. n_D^{20} 1.5538.
Hydrochloride monohydrate. [74764-40-2] CERM-1978; Cordium; Vascor; Unicordium. $C_{24}H_{34}N_2O \cdot HCl \cdot H_2O$; mol wt 421.02. Crystals, mp 91 ±2°. LD_{50} in mice (mg/kg): 1955 orally, 23.5 i.v. (Mauvernay, 1978).
THERAP CAT: Antianginal.

1151. Beractant. [108778-82-1] Surfactant TA; A-60386X; Surfacten; Survanta. Organic solvent extract of bovine lung, consisting mostly of phospholipids, modified by the addition of colfosceril palmitate, palmitic acid and tripalmitin. Prepn: JP 83 45299; Y. Tanaka *et al.*, US 4397839 (both 1983 to Tokyo Tanabe). Effect of protein component on surface activity: S. B. Hall *et al.*, *Am. Rev. Respir. Dis.* **145**, 24 (1992). Pharmacology: J. J. Cummings *et al.*, *ibid.* 999. Metabolism in rabbits: J. F. Lewis *et al.*, *ibid.* 19. Evaluation of establishment of normal surfactant function in comparison with Exosurf: E. M. Scarpelli *et al.*, *Am. J. Perinatol.* **9**, 414 (1992). Clinical trial in neonatal respiratory distress syndrome: M. D. Reller *et al.*, *Am. J. Dis. Child.* **145**, 1017 (1991); E. M. Zola *et al.*, *Pediatrics* **91**, 546 (1993).
THERAP CAT: Pulmonary surfactant.

1152. Beraprost. [88430-50-6] 2,3,3a,8b-Tetrahydro-2-hydroxy-1-(3-hydroxy-4-methyl-1-octen-6-ynyl)-1*H*-cyclopenta(*b*)-benzofuran-5-butanoic acid; *dl*-16-methyl-18,19-tetradehydro-5,6,7-trinor-4,8-inter-*m*-phenyleneprostaglandin I_2; *dl*-4-[(1*R*,2*R*,-3a*S*,8b*S*)-1,2,3a,8b-tetrahydro-2-hydroxy-[(3*S*,4*RS*)-3-hydroxy-4-methyl-oct-6-yne-(*E*)-1-enyl]-5-cyclopenta(*b*)benzofuranyl]butanoic acid; befaprost; ML-1229. $C_{24}H_{30}O_5$; mol wt 398.49. C 72.34%, H 7.59%, O 20.08%. Platelet aggregation inhibitor; stable analog of prostacyclin, *q.v.* Prepn: K. Ohno *et al.*, EP 84856; *eidem*, US 4474802 (1983, 1984 both to Toray); *eidem*, Adv. Prostaglandin Thromboxane Leukotriene Res. **15**, 279 (1985). PGI_2 receptor binding: N. Kajikawa *et al.*, *Arzneim.-Forsch.* **39**, 495 (1989). Series of articles on pharmacology: *ibid.* 856-876. Clinical pharmacokinetics: J.-L. Demolis *et al.*, *J. Cardiovasc. Pharmacol.* **22**, 711 (1993). Clinical trial in intermittent claudication: M. Lievre *et al.*, *ibid.* **27**, 788 (1996); in diabetic angiopathy: Y. Okuda *et al.*, *Prostaglandins* **52**, 375 (1996).

Sodium salt. [88475-69-8] ML-1129; TRK-100; Dorner; Procylin. $C_{24}H_{29}NaO_5$; mol wt 420.47.
THERAP CAT: Antithrombotic; vasodilator (peripheral).

1153. Berbamine. [478-61-5] (4a*S*,16a*R*)-3,4,4a,5,16a,17,-18,19-Octahydro-21,22,26-trimethoxy-4,17-dimethyl-16*H*-1,24:6,9-dietheno-11,15-metheno-2*H*-pyrido[2',3':17,18][1,-11]dioxacycloeicosino[2,3,4-*ij*]isoquinolin-12-ol; 6,6',7-trimethoxy-2,2'-dimethylberbaman-12-ol; berbenine. $C_{37}H_{40}N_2O_6$; mol wt 608.72. C 73.00%, H 6.62%, N 4.60%, O 15.77%. Alkaloid found in various members of Berberis family. Used as a traditional medicine in China as antipyretic, antidiarrhoea and as a tonic. Identification in *Berberis vulgaris*: C. Rüdel, *Arch. Pharm.* **229**, 631 (1895); isoln from *Atherosperma moschatum* Labill., *Monimiaceae*: I. R. C. Bick *et al.*, *Aust. J. Chem.* **9**, 111 (1956). Structure: F. von Bruchhausen, *Ann.* **507**, 144 (1933); configuration: Y.

Inubishi, *J. Pharm. Soc. Jpn.* **72**, 220 (1952), *C.A.* **47**, 6429e (1953). Immunopharmacology and toxicology: C. W. Wong *et al., Int. J. Immunopharmacol.* **13**, 579 (1991). Brief review: C.-X. Liu *et al., Phytother. Res.* **5**, 228-230 (1991).

Colorless plates from aq ethanol as the monohydrate, sinters 147°. pKa (20°): 7.33 in aq methanol. $[\alpha]_D^{20}$ +114.6° (c = 1.0 in chloroform). uv max (ethanol): 282 nm (log ε 3.89; E $^{1\%}_{1cm}$ 126).

1154. Berberine. [2086-83-1] 5,6-Dihydro-9,10-dimethoxybenzo[*g*]-1,3-benzodioxolo[5,6-*a*]quinolizinium; 7,8,13,13a-tetradehydro-9,10-dimethoxy-2,3-(methylenedioxy)berbinium; umbellatine. $[C_{20}H_{18}NO_4]^+$. Tautomeric alkaloid widely distributed in nine or more botanical families but occurs most frequently in *Berberidaceae*. A component of many traditional medicines, first isolated in 1826. Structure: Perkin, Robinson, *J. Chem. Soc.* **97**, 305 (1910). Biosynthesis: J. R. Gear, I. D. Spenser, *Can. J. Chem.* **41**, 783 (1963). Pharmacology: Fukuda *et al., Chem. Pharm. Bull.* **18**, 1299 (1970). Total synthesis: Kametani *et al., J. Chem. Soc. C* **1969**, 2036. NMR: G. Blasko *et al., Heterocycles* **27**, 911 (1988). HPLC determn in biological fluids: C.-M. Chen, H.-C. Chang, *J. Chromatogr.* B **665**, 117 (1995). Clinical evaluation in malaria: W. D. Sheng *et al., East Afr. Med. J.* **74**, 283 (1997). Review of biological activities: F. E. Hahn, J. Ciak, in *Antibiotics* **vol. 3**, D. Gottlieb *et al.*, Eds. (Springer-Verlag, New York, 1975) pp 577-584; of chemistry, distribution and use: R. S. Thakur, S. K. Srivastava, *Curr. Res. Med. Aromat. Plants* **4**, 249-272 (1982). Review of antidiarrheal action: A. W. Baird *et al., Adv. Drug Delivery Rev.* **23**, 111-120 (1997).

Yellow needles from ether, mp 145°: Gadamer, *Arch. Pharm.* **243**, 33 (1905). uv max: 265, 343 nm. pK 2.47.

Acid sulfate. Berberine bisulfate. $C_{20}H_{19}NO_8S$. Yellow needles. Sol in about 100 parts water; slightly sol in alc.

Chloride dihydrate. $C_{20}H_{18}NO_4.Cl.2H_2O$. Yellow crystals. Slightly sol in cold, freely in boiling water. Practically insol in cold alcohol, chloroform, ether.

Sulfate trihydrate. Yellow needles. Sol in about 30 parts water; sol in alcohol. Activity studies: Amin *et al., Can. J. Microbiol.* **15**, 1067 (1969). Pharmacology: Sabir, Bhide, *Indian J. Physiol. Pharmacol.* **15**, 111 (1971).

THERAP CAT: Antiprotozoal (Leishmania); antimalarial; antibacterial; antidiarrheal.

1155. Berberis. Holly-leaved barberry; Oregon grape root; mountain grape. Dried rhizome and roots of species of section of *Mahonia* DC. of the genus *Berberis* L., *Berberidaceae. Habit.* U.S. and British Columbia. *Constit.* Berberine, berbamine, oxyacanthine, phytosterol, sugar.

THERAP CAT: Bitter. Antipyretic.

1156. Berberis Aristata. Indian barberry; ruswut; rusat. Dried stem of *Berberis aristata* DC., *Berberidaceae. Habit.* India, Ceylon. *Constit.* Berberine and other alkaloidal substances, tannin, resin, starch.

THERAP CAT: Bitter. Antipyretic.

1157. Bergapten. [484-20-8] 4-Methoxy-7*H*-furo[3,2-*g*][1]benzopyran-7-one; 5-methoxypsoralen; bergaptan; bergaptene; heraclin; majudin; 5-MOP; Psoraderm-5. $C_{12}H_8O_4$; mol wt 216.19. C 66.67%, H 3.73%, O 29.60%. Naturally occurring analog of psoralen and isomer of methoxsalen, *q.q.v.*, found in a wide variety of plants. It was first isolated from oil of bergamot from *Citrus bergamia* Risso, *Aurantiodiae:* Pomeranz, *Monatsh. Chem.* **12**, 379 (1891), **14**, 28 (1893). Isoln from *Fagara xanthoxyloides* Lam., *Rutaceae:* H. Thoms, E. Baetcke, *Ber.* **44**, 3326 (1911); **45**, 3705 (1912). Synthesis: E. Späth *et al., Ber.* **70**, 478 (1937); W. N. Howell, R. Robertson, *J. Chem. Soc.* **1937**, 293; G. Caporale, *Farmaco Ed. Sci.* **13**, 784 (1958); V. K. Ahluwalia *et al., Indian J. Chem.* **7**, 831 (1969). Use in photochemotherapy of psoriasis: H. Hönigsmann *et al., Br. J. Dermatol.* **101**, 369 (1979). Mutagenicity studies: B. R. Scott *et al., Mutat. Res.* **39**, 29 (1976); M. J. Ashwood-Smith *et al., Nature* **285**, 407 (1980). Phototoxicity study: A. Kornhauser *et al., Science* **217**, 733 (1982).

Needles from alcohol, mp 188° (sublimes). Practically insol in boiling water. Slightly sol in glacial acetic acid, chloroform, benzene, warm phenol. Sol in abs alcohol: 1 part in 60. Its soln in sulfuric acid is yellow-gold.

USE: Has been used to promote tanning in suntan preparations.

THERAP CAT: Antipsoriatic.

1158. Berkelium. [7440-40-6] Bk; at. no. 97; valence 3, 4. Man-made radioactive element; second element in the curide series. No stable nuclides, known isotopes (mass numbers): 240, 242-251. Longest-lived known isotope: 247 ($T_{1/2}$ 1.38 × 10^3 years, α-decay, rel. at. mass 247.0703). Prepn of first isotope, ^{243}Bk ($T_{1/2}$ 4.5 hrs, electron capture and α-decay) by helium ion bombardment of ^{241}Am: S. G. Thompson *et al., Phys. Rev.* **77**, 838 (1950); *eidem, ibid.* **80**, 781. Prepn of macroscopic quantities as ^{249}Bk ($T_{1/2}$ 320 days, β-decay, rel. at. mass 249.0750): B. B. Cunningham, *J. Chem. Educ.* **36**, 32-37 (1959). Prepn of metal and determn of crystal structure: J. A. Fahey, *U.S. Atomic Energy Commission* **TID-25741** (1971) 119 pp, *C.A.* **76**, 9882r (1972); J. R. Peterson *et al., J. Inorg. Nucl. Chem.* **33**, 3345 (1971). Reviews: M. Haissinsky, J.-P. Adloff, *Radiochemical Survey of the Elements* (Elsevier, New York, 1965) pp 14-15; C. Keller, *The Chemistry of the Transuranium Elements* (Verlag Chemie, Weinheim, English Ed., 1971) pp 553-566; Silva, "Trans-Curium Elements" in *MTP Int. Rev. Sci.: Inorg. Chem., Ser. One* **vol. 8**, A. G. Maddock, Ed. (University Park Press, Baltimore, 1972) pp 71-105; *Comprehensive Inorganic Chemistry* **vol. 5**, J. C. Bailar, Jr. *et al.*, Eds. (Pergamon Press, Oxford, 1973) *passim; Handb. Exp. Pharmakol.* **36**, 689-928 (1973); D. E. Hobart, J. R. Peterson in *The Chemistry of the Actinide Elements* **vol. 1**, J. J. Katz *et al.*, Eds. (Chapman and Hall, New York, 1986) pp 989-1024.

Metal. Two allotropic forms: double hexagonal close-packed α-form, d (calc) 14.78, transforms to β-form at 930°; face-centered cubic β-form, d (calc) 13.25, exists from 930-986°. mp 986 ± 25° (Fahey). Also reported as mp 1050° (Katz *et al., loc. cit.* **vol. 2**, p 1150). Changes from the trivalent to the tetravalent state under the influence of oxidizing agents. In the trivalent state, its chemical properties are very close to those of curium. Can be separated from other transuranium elements by ion-exchange or by extraction of Bk(IV) with dioctylphosphonic acid in heptane (Haissinsky, Adloff). Metal dissolves rapidly in aqueous mineral acids.

Caution: Radiation hazard; handling requires special equipment and shielding facilities (Katz *et al., loc. cit.* **vol. 2**, p 1128).

1159. Bermoprofen. [78499-27-1] 10,11-Dihydro-α,8-dimethyl-11-oxodibenz[*b,f*]oxepin-2-acetic acid; 2-(8-methyl-10,11-dihydro-11-oxodibenz[*b,f*]oxepin-2-yl)propionic acid; AD-1590; AJ-1590; Dibenon. $C_{18}H_{16}O_4$; mol wt 296.32. C 72.96%, H

5.44%, O 21.60%. Prostaglandin synthetase inhibitor. Prepn: H. Uno *et al.*, **EP 3893**; *eidem*, **US 4238620** (1979, 1980 both to Dainippon); Y. Nagai *et al.*, *J. Med. Chem.* **25**, 1065 (1982). Pharmacology: H. Nakamura *et al.*, *Arzneim.-Forsch.* **33**, 1555 (1983). Mechanism of action: K. Ishii *et al.*, *Yakugaku Zasshi* **108**, 1001 (1988), *C.A.* **110**, 33462v (1989).

Crystals from toluene, mp 128-129°. LD$_{50}$ in mice, rats (mg/kg): 500, 147 orally (Nakamura).

THERAP CAT: Anti-inflammatory; analgesic; antipyretic.

1160. Berninamycin. [58798-97-3] Berninamycin A. C$_{51}$-H$_{51}$N$_{15}$O$_{15}$S; mol wt 1146.11. C 53.45%, H 4.49%, N 18.33%, O 20.94%, S 2.80%. Major component of cyclic peptide antibiotic complex also containing minor component **Berninamycin B** (C$_{51}$-H$_{51}$N$_{15}$O$_{14}$S). Isoln from *Streptomyces bernesis* Dietz: M. E. Bergy *et al.*, **US 3689639** (1972). Inhibition of protein synthesis: F. Reusser, *Biochemistry* **8**, 3303 (1969); J. Thompson *et al.*, *J. Gen. Microbiol.* **128**, 875 (1982). Structural studies and characterization of degradation product berninamycinic acid, a novel sulfur containing moiety: J. M. Liesch *et al.*, *J. Am. Chem. Soc.* **98**, 299 (1976); J. M. Liesch *et al.*, *ibid.* 8237; J. M. Liesch, K. L. Rinehart, Jr., *ibid.* **99**, 1645 (1977). Revised structure: H. Abe *et al.*, *Tetrahedron Lett.* **29**, 1401 (1988). Confirmation of structures: R. C. M. Lau, K. L. Rinehart, *J. Antibiot.* **47**, 1466 (1994). Biosynthetic study: C. J. Pearce, K. L. Rinehart, Jr., *J. Am. Chem. Soc.* **101**, 5069 (1979). Use as growth permittant: R. M. Pellegrino, **EP 112233** (1984 to Merck & Co.). Synthesis of berninamycinic acid: T. R. Kelly *et al.*, *Tetrahedron Lett.* **25**, 2127 (1984).

Berninamycin A

White crystals, mp >290°. Sol in DMF, methanol, ethanol, propanol, butanol. Relatively insol in water, ether, cyclohexane, benzene, acetone, ethyl acetate. uv max (methanol): 208, 236 nm (A = 62.4, 64.4).

Berninamycinic acid. C$_{12}$H$_6$N$_2$O$_5$S. Golden needles, mp 210° (dec). pKa 5.8. Insol in water. uv max (0.01*N* HCl): 228, 272 nm (ε 13500, 13500); uv max (0.01*N* NaOH): 232, 294 nm (ε 9500, 13000).

Note: The characteristics of berninamycin are similar to those previously reported in the literature for **theiomycetin**: M. Shibata, *Takeda Kenkyusho Nempo* **18**, 44 (1959), *C.A.* **54**, 19840c (1960).

1161. Beryllium. [7440-41-7] Glucinium. Be; at. wt 9.012182; at. no. 4; valence 2. Group IIA (2). Alkaline earth metal. Estimated abundance in earth's crust 2 to 6 ppm. Natural isotopes (mass number): 9 (100%); known artificial radioactive isotopes: 6-8; 10-12. Oxide discovered by Vauquelin in 1797;

free metal isolated by Wöhler and Bussy in 1828. Produced industrially from *beryl* (3BeO.Al$_2$O$_3$.6SiO$_2$) and *bertrandite* (4BeO-.2SiO$_2$.H$_2$O); also found in *phenacite* (Be$_2$SiO$_4$), *chrysoberyl* (BeO.Al$_2$O$_3$). Precious forms of beryl: *emerald, aquamarine*. Reviews of beryllium and its compounds: Kjellgren, "Beryllium" in *Rare Metals Handbook*, C. A. Hampel, Ed. (Reinhold, New York, 1954) pp 31-55; D. A. Everest, *Chemistry of Beryllium* (Elsevier, New York, 1964) 151 pp. Review of properties and use: N. P. Pinto, J. Greenspan, "Beryllium" in *Modern Materials* vol. 6, B. W. Gonser, Ed. (Academic Press, New York, 1968) pp 319-372; D. A. Everest, "Beryllium" in *Comprehensive Inorganic Chemistry*, J. C. Bailar, Jr. *et al.*, Eds. (Pergamon Press, Oxford, 1973) pp 531-590; A. J. Stonehouse *et al.*, in *Kirk-Othmer Encyclopedia of Chemical Technology* vol. 4 (Wiley-Interscience, New York, 4th ed., 1992) pp 126-146; A. J. Stonehouse, M. N. Emly, *ibid.* 147-153. Review of carcinogenic risk of beryllium and its compds: *IARC Monographs* **1**, 17-28 (1972); *ibid.* **23**, 143-204 (1980); of toxicology and human exposure: *Toxicological Profile for Beryllium* (PB2003-100135, 2002) 290 pp.; of immunotoxicology: A. L. Reeves, O. P. Preuss in *Immunotoxicology and Immunopharmacology*, J. H. Dean *et al.*, Eds. (Raven Press, New York, 1985) pp 441-455; of human and environmental toxicology: WHO, *Environ. Health Criter.* **106**, 1-210 (1990).

Gray, brittle metal; close-packed hexagonal structure; anisotropic; high permeability to X-rays; can serve as a neutron source through either (α,n) or (n,2n) reactions. Lightest of all solid and chemically-stable substances. Displays excellent electrical and thermal conductivities. mp 1287°. bp 2500° (extrapolated). d 1.8477. Heat capacity at constant pressure (30°) 0.437 cal/g/°C: Walker *et al.*, *J. Chem. Eng. Data* **7**, 595 (1962). Latent heat of fusion: 3.5 kcal/ mole. Brinell hardness: 60-125. Chemical properties similar to aluminum; metal resistant to attack by acid due to the formation of a thin oxide film. E° (aq) Be/Be^{2+} 1.85 V (calc.). Finely divided or amalgamated metal reacts with HCl, dil H$_2$SO$_4$ and dil HNO$_3$; attacked by strong bases with evolution of H$_2$.

Caution: Overexposure to beryllium and beryllium compounds has been associated with acute and chronic toxicity. Toxicity due to chronic exposure is called "berylliosis" and appears after a latent period as an immunologically mediated, progressive, systemic disease leading to the formation of a characteristic granulomatous lesion. Potential symptoms of overexposure are anorexia, weight loss, weakness, chest pains, cough, clubbing of fingers, cyanosis, pulmonary insufficiency; direct contact may cause eye irritation. Dermal exposure may cause acute contact dermatitis; chronic dermal exposure may cause granulomatous skin ulceration. See *Patty's Industrial Hygiene and Toxicology* vol. 2C, G. D. Clayton, F. E. Clayton, Eds. (John Wiley & Sons, Inc., New York, 4th ed., 1994) pp 1930-1948; *NIOSH Pocket Guide to Chemical Hazards* (DHHS/ NIOSH 97-140, 1997) p 28. Beryllium and beryllium compounds are listed as known human carcinogens: *Report on Carcinogens, Eleventh Edition* (PB2005-104914, 2004) p III-32.

USE: Source of neutrons when bombarded with alpha particles according to the equation $^9_4Be + ^4_2He \rightarrow ^{12}_6C + ^1_0n$. This yields about 30 neutrons per million alpha particles. Also as neutron reflector and neutron moderator in nuclear reactors. In beryllium copper and beryllium aluminum alloys (by direct reduction of beryllium oxide with carbon in the presence of Cu or Al). In aerospace, aircraft and satellite structures; x-ray transmission windows; missile parts; nuclear weapons; fuel containers; precision instruments; rocket propellants; navigational systems; heat shields; and mirrors. For fiber optics and cellular network communications systems.

1162. Beryllium Acetate. [543-81-7] Acetic acid beryllium salt. C$_4$H$_6$BeO$_4$; mol wt 127.10. C 37.80%, H 4.76%, Be 7.09%, O 50.35%. (CH$_3$COO$^-$)$_2$Be^{2+}. Prepn: Besson, Hardt, *Compt. Rend.* **237**, 1525 (1953).

Crystals, dec at 60-100° when heated slowly, 150-180° when heated rapidly. Dissolves slowly with hydrolysis in boiling water. Practically insol in abs alc and other common organic solvents.

1163. Beryllium Acetylacetonate. [10210-64-7] (*T*-4)-Bis(2,4-pentanedionato-O,O′)beryllium. C$_{10}$H$_{14}$BeO$_4$; mol wt 207.23. C 57.96%, H 6.81%, Be 4.35%, O 30.88%. Prepd by the action of 2,4-pentanedione on an soln of beryllium hydroxide in dil acetic acid or on a soln of beryllium chloride in presence of ammonia: Biltz, *Ann.* **331**, 336 (1904); Parsons, *J. Am. Chem. Soc.* **26**, 732 (1904); Arch, Young, *Inorg. Synth.* **2**, 17 (1946); from 2,4-pentanedione and beryllium sulfate in NaOH soln: Jones, *J. Am. Chem. Soc.* **81**, 3188 (1959).

Monoclinic crystals. mp 108°. bp 270°. d_4^{20} 1.168. Practically insol in water; hydrolyzed by boiling water. Freely sol in alc, acetone, ether, benzene, CS_2, other organic solvents.

1164. Beryllium Bromide. [7787-46-4] $BeBr_2$; mol wt 168.82. Be 5.34%, Br 94.66%. Prepn: Ehrlich in *Handbook of Preparative Inorganic Chemistry* **vol. 1**, G. Brauer, Ed. (Academic Press, New York, 2nd ed., 1963) p 891. Review of beryllium halides: Bell, *Adv. Inorg. Chem. Radiochem.* **14**, 255-332 (1972).

Orthorhombic crystals, d 3.465. mp 506-509°; also reported as 488°: Bell, *loc. cit.* Sublimes at 473°. bp 520°. Very hygroscopic. Freely sol in water. By saturating the concd viscous soln with HBr, the tetrahydrate is formed. Sol in ethanol, in pyridine (185.6 g/l), in ethyl bromide (1.0 g/l). Forms addition compounds with amines, alcohols. *Keep tightly closed.*

1165. Beryllium Carbide. [506-66-1] CBe_2; mol wt 30.04. C 39.98%, Be 60.00%. Be_2C. Prepn: Coobs, Koshuba, *J. Electrochem. Soc.* **99**, 115 (1952); Mallett *et al.*, *ibid.* **101**, 298 (1954); Ehrlich in *Handbook of Preparative Inorganic Chemistry* **vol. 1**, G. Brauer, Ed. (Academic Press, New York, 2nd ed., 1963) p 899.

Brick-red or yellow-red octahedra, d 1.90, dec above 2100°. Very slowly dec by water, somewhat faster by mineral acids and quickly by alkalies with the evolution of methane.

USE: Nuclear reactor core material: Schwartz, *US 3170812* (1965 to USAEC).

1166. Beryllium Chloride. [7787-47-5] $BeCl_2$; mol wt 79.92. Be 11.28%, Cl 88.72%. Prepn from the elements: Tannenbaum, *Inorg. Synth.* **5**, 22 (1957); from BeO, Cl_2 and C: Ehrlich in *Handbook of Preparative Inorganic Chemistry* **vol. 1**, G. Brauer, Ed. (Academic Press, New York, 2nd ed., 1963) p 889. Toxicity data: K. W. Cochran *et al.*, *Fed. Proc.* **9**, 264 (1950). Review of beryllium halides: Bell, *Adv. Inorg. Chem. Radiochem.* **14**, 255-332 (1972).

White to faintly yellow, very deliquesc, orthorhombic crystals or cryst mass. Reported mp ranges from 399.2° to 440°, 399.2° is considered to be the most reliable (Bell). bp 482.3°. Sublimes *in vacuo* at 300°. d 1.90. Very sol in water with evolution of heat; the aq soln is strongly acid. Sol in alcohol, ether, pyridine, CS_2. Insol in benzene, toluene. *Keep tightly closed.*

Tetrahydrate. Monoclinic deliquesc platelets. Has been reported to have $4\frac{1}{2}H_2O$: Semenenko, Turova, *Russ. J. Inorg. Chem.* **10**, 42 (1965). LD_{50} in guinea pigs, rats (mg Be/kg): 63, 0.6 i.p. (Cochran).

Caution: Beryllium and beryllium compounds are listed as known human carcinogens: *Report on Carcinogens, Eleventh Edition* (PB2005-104914, 2004) p III-32.

USE: Manuf of beryllium. *Anhydrous* form used as acid catalyst in organic reactions, similar to $AlCl_3$.

1167. Beryllium Fluoride. [7787-49-7] BeF_2; mol wt 47.01. Be 19.17%, F 80.83%. Prepd by heating ammonium fluoroberyllate $(NH_4)_2BeF_4$: Lebeau, *Compt. Rend.* **126**, 1418 (1898); Kwasnik in *Handbook of Preparative Inorganic Chemistry* **vol. 1**, G. Brauer, Ed. (Academic Press, New York, 2nd ed., 1963) p 231. Review of prepn and properties of beryllium halides: Bell, *Adv. Inorg. Chem. Radiochem.* **14**, 255-332 (1972).

Glassy hygroscopic mass (tetragonal system). True mp 555°; becomes free-flowing about 800°. Sublimes at 1036° under 1 mm press. in the presence of beryllium: d_4^{25} 1.986. Very freely sol in water; sparingly sol in alc; more sol in a mixture of alc and ether; insol in anhydr HF.

Caution: Beryllium and beryllium compounds are listed as known human carcinogens: *Report on Carcinogens, Eleventh Edition* (PB2005-104914, 2004) p III-32.

USE: Manuf of Be and Be alloys; manuf of glass; in nuclear reactors.

1168. Beryllium Hydride. [7787-52-2] BeH_2; mol wt 11.03. Be 81.71%, H 18.28%. Lower purity material prepd by treating dimethylberyllium with $LiAlH_4$ in ether: Barbaras *et al.*, *J. Am. Chem. Soc.* **73**, 4585 (1951); higher purity by pyrolysis of di-*tert*-butylberyllium: Coates, Glocking, *J. Chem. Soc.* **1954**, 2526; Head *et al.*, *J. Am. Chem. Soc.* **79**, 3687 (1957); from triphenyl phosphine and beryllium borohydride: Banford, Coates, *J. Chem. Soc.* **1964**, 5591.

White solid. Higher purity material is inert to laboratory air. Loss of hydrogen at 190-200° negligible, rapid at 220°. Reacts slowly with water, rapidly with dil acids. Insol in ether, toluene, isopentane. Reacts with diborane to form beryllium borohydride.

1169. Beryllium Hydroxide. [13327-32-7] BeH_2O_2; mol wt 43.03. Be 20.94%, H 4.68%, O 74.36%. $Be(OH)_2$. Prepn: Ehrlich in *Handbook of Preparative Inorganic Chemistry* **vol. 1**, G. Brauer, Ed. (Academic Press, New York, 2nd ed., 1963) p 894.

Amorphous powder or crystals. d 1.92. Amphoteric. Very slightly sol in water and dil alkali. Sol in hot concd NaOH soln and acids.

Caution: Beryllium and beryllium compounds are listed as known human carcinogens: *Report on Carcinogens, Eleventh Edition* (PB2005-104914, 2004) p III-32.

USE: Manuf of beryllium and beryllium oxide.

1170. Beryllium Nitrate. [13597-99-4] BeN_2O_6; mol wt 133.02. Be 6.78%, N 21.06%, O 72.17%. $Be(NO_3)_2$. Prepn: *Gmelins, Beryllium* (8th ed.) **26**, 102-104 (1930). Review of toxicology: B. Venugopal, T. D. Luckey, *Environ. Qual. Saf.* **1**, Suppl. 1, 4-73 (1975); of toxicity: *Dangerous Prop. Ind. Mater. Rep.* **9**, 29-37 (1989).

Trihydrate. [7787-55-5] White to slightly yellow, deliquesc cryst mass. mp ~60°. Very sol in water, ethanol. *Keep well closed in a cool place.* LD_{50} i.p. in mice: 0.5 mg/kg (Venugopal, Luckey).

USE: Stiffening mantles in gas and acetylene lamps.

1171. Beryllium Nitride. [1304-54-7] Be_3N_2; mol wt 55.05. Be 49.11%, N 50.89%. Prepn: Ehrlich in *Handbook of Preparative Inorganic Chemistry* **vol. 1**, G. Brauer, Ed. (Academic Press, New York, 2nd ed., 1963) p 898; Langsdorf, Jr., *US 2567518* (1951 to USAEC).

White crystals to grayish white powder; mp 2200 ±40°. Volatile at bp, on further heating it dissociates into Be and N_2. Oxidized in air at 600°. Dec slowly by water, quickly by acids and alkalies with the evolution of ammonia.

1172. Beryllium Oxide. [1304-56-9] Beryllia. BeO; mol wt 25.01. Be 36.03%, O 63.97%. Prepn: *Gmelins, Beryllium* (8th ed.) **26**, 82-91 (1930); Ehrlich in *Handbook of Preparative Inorganic Chemistry* **vol. 1**, G. Brauer, Ed. (Academic Press, New York, 2nd ed., 1963) p 893. *Review:* Lillie, *USAEC* **UCRL 6457**, 23 pp (1961).

Light, amorphous powder. mp 2530°. Very sparingly sol in water; slowly sol in concd acids or solns of fixed alkali hydroxides. After ignition it is almost insol in these solvents. Pure (100%) BeO insulates electrically like a ceramic, but conducts heat like a metal. Electrical resistivity in ohm-cm: $>10^{16}$. Dielectric const at 8.5 gigacycles: 6.57.

Caution: Beryllium and beryllium compounds are listed as known human carcinogens: *Report on Carcinogens, Eleventh Edition* (PB2005-104914, 2004) p III-32.

USE: Manuf of beryllium oxide ceramics, glass; in nuclear reactor fuels and moderators; catalyst for organic reactions.

1173. Beryllium Potassium Sulfate. [53684-48-3] $BeK_2O_8S_2$; mol wt 279.33. Be 3.23%, K 27.99%, O 45.82%, S 22.96%. $BeSO_4 \cdot K_2SO_4$. Prepn: *Gmelins, Beryllium* (8th ed) **26**, 174 (1930).

Dihydrate. Brilliant crystals. Sol in water, concd K_2SO_4 solns; practically insol in alc.

USE: In chromium- and silver-plating.

1174. Beryllium Sodium Fluoride. [13871-27-7] Sodium tetrafluoroberyllate. BeF_4Na_2; mol wt 130.99. Be 6.88%, F 58.01%, Na 35.10%. Na_2BeF_4. Prepn: *Gmelins, Beryllium* (8th ed.) **26,** 169 (1930). Review of prepn and properties of beryllium halides: Bell, *Adv. Inorg. Chem. Radiochem.* **14,** 255-332 (1972). Orthorhombic or monoclinic crystals. mp ~350°. Sol in water.

1175. Beryllium Sulfate. [13510-49-1] BeO$_4$S; mol wt 105.07. Be 8.58%, O 60.91%, S 30.52%. BeSO$_4$. Prepn: *Gmelins, Beryllium* (8th ed.) **26,** 130-141 (1930). Toxicity study: White *et al., J. Pharmacol. Exp. Ther.* **102,** 88 (1951).

Tetrahydrate. Crystals. d 1.71. At about 100° loses 2H$_2$O. Very sol in water. Practically insol in alc. LD$_{50}$ i.v. in mice: 0.5 mg Be/kg (White).

Caution: Beryllium and beryllium compounds are listed as known human carcinogens: *Report on Carcinogens, Eleventh Edition* (PB2005-104914, 2004) p III-32.

1176. Besipirdine. [119257-34-0] *N*-Propyl-*N*-4-pyridinyl-1*H*-indol-1-amine; 1-(propyl-4-pyridylamino)indole. C$_{16}$H$_{17}$N$_3$; mol wt 251.33. C 76.46%, H 6.82%, N 16.72%. Cholinomimetic agent with noradrenergic activity. Prepn: R. C. Effland, J. T. Klein, **EP 287982** (1988 to Hoechst); *idem et al.,* **US 4970218** (1990 to Hoechst-Roussel); of hydrochloride: S. Kongsamut *et al.,* **US 5356910** (1994 to Hoechst-Roussel). HPLC determn in plasma: R. S. Hsu *et al., J. Chromatogr.* **572,** 352 (1991). Mechanism of action study: C. P. Smith *et al., Drug Dev. Res.* **32,** 13 (1994). Pharmacokinetics: J. W. Hubbard *et al., J. Clin. Pharmacol.* **35,** 688 (1995).

Hydrochloride. [130953-69-4] HP-749. C$_{16}$H$_{17}$N$_3$.HCl; mol wt 287.79. Crystals from methanol, mp 212-214°.

Maleate. [119257-40-8] C$_{16}$H$_{17}$N$_3$.C$_4$H$_4$O$_4$. Crystals from methanol/ether, mp 115-116°.

THERAP CAT: Nootropic.

1177. Bestmann-Ohira Reagent. [90965-06-3] (1-Diazo-2-oxopropyl)phosphonic acid dimethyl ester; dimethyl (1-diazo-2-oxopropyl)phosphonate. C$_5$H$_9$N$_2$O$_4$P; mol wt 192.11. C 31.26%, H 4.72%, N 14.58%, O 33.31%, P 16.12%. Diazoalkylphosphonate reagent; converted *in situ* to the Seyferth-Gilbert reagent, *q.v.* Prepn: P. Callant *et al., Synth. Commun.* **14,** 155 (1984). Synthetic applications: S. Ohira, *ibid.* **19,** 561 (1989); S. Müller *et al., Synlett* **1996,** 521; G. J. Roth *et al., Synthesis* **2004,** 59; E. Quesada, R. J. K. Taylor, *Tetrahedron Lett.* **46,** 6473 (2005).

USE: Reagent for transformation of aldehydes to terminal alkynes and ketones to methyl enol ethers.

1178. Betahistine. [5638-76-6] *N*-Methyl-2-pyridineethanamine; 2-[2-(methylamino)ethyl]pyridine; [2-(2-pyridyl)ethyl]methylamine. C$_8$H$_{12}$N$_2$; mol wt 136.19. C 70.55%, H 8.88%, N 20.57%. Prepn: Löffler, *Ber.* **37,** 161 (1904); Walter *et al., J. Am. Chem. Soc.* **63,** 2771 (1941).

Liquid. bp$_{30}$ 113-114°. Soluble in water, alcohol, ether, chloroform.

Dihydrochloride. [5579-84-0] Betaserc; Serc; Vasomotal. C$_8$H$_{12}$N$_2$.2HCl; mol wt 209.12. Crystals from alc, mp 148-149°.

Maleate. Suzutolon. C$_8$H$_{12}$N$_2$.C$_4$H$_4$O$_4$; mol wt 252.27.

Mesylate. Medan; Menitazine; Merislon; Remark; Tenyl. C$_8$H$_{12}$N$_2$.CH$_3$SO$_3$H; mol wt 232.30.

Dimesylate. Aequamen; Melopat; Ribrain. C$_8$H$_{12}$N$_2$.(CH$_3$SO$_3$H)$_2$; mol wt 328.41.

THERAP CAT: Vasodilator.

1179. Betaine. [107-43-7] 1-Carboxy-*N,N,N*-trimethylmethanaminium inner salt; (carboxymethyl)trimethylammonium hydroxide inner salt; glycine betaine; glycocoll betaine; lycine; oxyneurine; trimethylglycine hydroxide inner salt; trimethylglycocoll anhydride; Cystadane. C$_5$H$_{11}$NO$_2$; mol wt 117.15. C 51.26%, H 9.46%, N 11.96%, O 27.31%. Widely distributed in plants and animals: M. Guggenheim, *Die biogenen Amine* (S. Karger, Basel, 4th ed., 1951) pp 240-242. Prepn via or from hydrochloride: Stoltzenberg, *Z. Physiol. Chem.* **92,** 445 (1914); Edsall, *J. Am. Chem. Soc.* **65,** 1767 (1943). Prepn of the hydrochloride: Kuhn, Ruelius, *Ber.* **83,** 420 (1950); of the hydrate: Vassel, **US 2800502** (1957 to IMC). Structure of hydrate: Leifer, Lippincott, *J. Am. Chem. Soc.* **79,** 5098 (1957). HPLC determn in urine: M. D. Laryea *et al., Clin. Chim. Acta* **230,** 169 (1994). Clinical evaluations in homocystinuria: D. E. Wilcken *et al., N. Engl. J. Med.* **309,** 448 (1983); N. P. B. Dudman *et al., J. Nutr.* **126,** Suppl. 4, 1295S (1996).

Deliquescent scales or prisms dec around 310°. (Isomerizes at the mp to methyl ester of dimethylaminoacetic acid.) Sweet taste. Solubility (g/100 g solvent): water, 160; methanol, 55; ethanol, 8.7. Sparingly sol in ether. Betaine yields trimethylamine with concd KOH.

Monohydrate. [590-47-6] (Carboxymethyl)trimethylammonium hydroxide; trimethylglycine hydroxide. Formed by crystn of betaine from aq solvents. pH of satd soln about 8.0. Loses water at 100° forming inner salt again.

Hydrochloride. [590-46-5] 1-Carboxy-*N,N,N*-trimethylmethanaminium chloride; (carboxymethyl)trimethylammonium chloride; pluchine; Acidol. C$_5$H$_{11}$NO$_2$.HCl; mol wt 153.61. Monoclinic crystals from alc, dec 227-228° (Stoltzenberg); also reported as dec 232° (Kuhn, Ruelius). Soly in water at 25° = 64.7 g/100 ml, in ethanol 5.0 g/100 ml. pH of 5% aq soln 1.0. Practically insol in chloroform, ether.

Sodium aspartate. [93227-64-6] Somatyl. C$_9$H$_{17}$N$_2$NaO$_6$; mol wt 272.23. Prepn: R. Cote, **FR 1356945** (1964), *C.A.* **61,** 7098 (1964). Prepd as trihydrate, dec 160-170°. Hygroscopic. Sol in water.

USE: In soldering, resin curing fluxes, organic synthesis.

THERAP CAT: In treatment of homocystinuria; hepatoprotectant. Hydrochloride as gastric acidifier.

1180. Betamethasone. [378-44-9] (11β,16β)-9-Fluoro-11,17,21-trihydroxy-16-methylpregna-1,4-diene-3,20-dione; 9α-fluoro-16β-methylprednisolone; 16β-methyl-9α-fluoro-Δ^1-hydrocortisone; 16β-methyl-9α-fluoroprednisolone; betadexamethasone; flubenisolone; β-methasone; Sch-4831; NSC-39470; beta-Corlan; Becort; Betasolon; Betnelan; Celestene; Celestone; Dermabet; Visubeta. C$_{22}$H$_{29}$FO$_5$; mol wt 392.46. C 67.33%, H 7.45%, F 4.84%, O 20.38%. Prepn: Taub *et al., J. Am. Chem. Soc.* **80,** 4435 (1958); Oliveto *et al., ibid.* 6688; Taub *et al., ibid.* **82,** 4012 (1960); **US 3053865** (1962 to Merck & Co.); Amiard *et al.,* **US 3104246** (1963 to Roussel-UCLAF). Also prepared from hecogenin. Comprehensive description of the dipropionate ester: M. G. Ferrante, B. C. Rudy, *Anal. Profiles Drug Subs.* **6,** 43-60 (1977).

Crystals from ethyl acetate, mp 231-234° (dec). [α]$_D$ +108° (acetone). uv max (methanol): 238 nm (ε 15200).

21-Acetate. [987-24-6] Betafluorene; Celestovet. $C_{24}H_{31}FO_6$; mol wt 434.50. Hexagonal prisms from acetone + ether, mp 205-208° (Taub); also reported as mp 196-201° (Oliveto). $[\alpha]_D$ +140° (chloroform). uv max (methanol): 238 nm (ε 14800).

17-Benzoate. [22298-29-9] W-5975; Bebate; Beben; Benisone; Euvaderm; Flurobate; Uticort. $C_{29}H_{33}FO_6$; mol wt 496.57. Crystals from acetone-ether, mp 225-228°. $[\alpha]_D^{24}$ +63.5° (dioxane). Synthesis and activity: Ercoli et al., J. Med. Chem. **15**, 783 (1972). See also Cullen, Curr. Ther. Res. **15**, 243 (1973).

17,21-Dipropionate. [5593-20-4] Sch-11460; Diproderm; Diprolene; Diprophos; Diprosis; Diprosone; Maxivate; Rinderon-DP. $C_{28}H_{37}FO_7$; mol wt 504.59. Powder, mp 170-179° (dec). $[\alpha]_D$ +65.7° (dioxane). uv max (methanol): 238 nm (ε 15700). Insol in water.

17-Valerate. [2152-44-5] Bedermin; Betnesol-V; Betneval; Betnovate; Bextasol; Celestan-V; Celestoderm-V; Dermosol; Dermovaleas; Ecoval 70; Hormezon; Tokuderm; Valisone. $C_{27}H_{37}$-FO_6; mol wt 476.58. Needles from acetone + petr ether, mp 183-184°. $[\alpha]_D$ +77° (dioxane). uv max: 239 nm (ε 15920). **NL 6406615** (1964 to Glaxo).

21-Phosphate disodium salt. [151-73-5] Betamethasone 21-(dihydrogen phosphate) disodium salt; Bentelan; Betnesol; Celestan; Durabetason; Vista-Methasone. $C_{22}H_{28}FNa_2O_8P$; mol wt 516.40.

THERAP CAT: Glucocorticoid.

THERAP CAT (VET): Glucocorticoid.

1181. Betamipron. [3440-28-6] N-Benzoyl-β-alanine; 3-(benzoylamino)propionic acid; β-benzamidopropionic acid; CS-443. $C_{10}H_{11}NO_3$; mol wt 193.20. C 62.17%, H 5.74%, N 7.25%, O 24.84%. Acyl amino acid that inhibits active transport of carbapenem antibiotics in the renal cortex. See also panipenem. Prepn: F. H. Holm, Arch. Pharm. **242**, 590 (1904); C. C. Barker, J. Chem. Soc. **1954**, 317; J. Barluenga et al., Tetrahedron **45**, 2183 (1989). Use as renal protectant: T. Shiokari et al., **EP 226304**; eidem, **US 4757066** (1987, 1988 both to Sankyo). Crystal structure: N. Feeder, W. Jones, Acta Crystallogr. **C50**, 813 (1994). Nephroprotective effect: Y. Hirouchi et al., Jpn. J. Pharmacol. **63**, 487 (1993). Mode of action: eidem, ibid. **66**, 1 (1994). Pharmacokinetics: A. Kurihara et al., Antimicrob. Agents Chemother. **36**, 1810 (1992).

Colorless prisms from hot water, mp 120° (Holm); also reported as crystals from water, mp 133° (Barker). Readily sol in warm water, chloroform. Very easily sol in alcohol, ether, acetone. LD_{50} in rats (mg/kg): >3000 i.v. (Hirouchi, 1994).

THERAP CAT: Antibacterial adjunct (renal protectant).

1182. Betaxolol. [63659-18-7] 1-[4-[2-(Cyclopropylmethoxy)ethyl]-phenoxy]-3-[(1-methylethyl)amino]-2-propanol; ($\pm$)-1-(isopropylamino)-3-[p-(cyclopropylmethoxyethyl)phenoxy]-2-propanol. $C_{18}H_{29}NO_3$; mol wt 307.43. C 70.32%, H 9.51%, N 4.56%, O 15.61%. Cardioselective β_1-adrenergic blocker. Prepn: P. M. J. Manoury et al., **DE 2649605**; eidem, **US 4252984** (1977, 1981 both to Synthelabo). Blood concn and pharmacodynamic effects: S. J. Warrington et al., Br. J. Clin. Pharmacol. **10**, 449 (1980). Pharmacokinetics: G. Bianchetti et al., Arzneim.-Forsch. **30**, 1912 (1980). Cardiovascular effects in normal volunteers: P. J. Cadigan et al., Br. J. Clin. Pharmacol. **9**, 569 (1980). Efficacy and pharmacokinetics: K. Balnave et al., ibid. **11**, 171 (1981). Use in treatment of glaucoma: A. R. Berrospi, H. M. Leibowitz, Arch. Ophthalmol. **100**, 943 (1982). Antihypertensive effect: M. Pathe et al., Therapie **37**, 75 (1982). Book: Betaxolol and Other β_1-Adrenoceptor Antagonists, P. L. Morselli et al., Eds. (Raven Press, New York, 1983) 385 pp.

Crystals from petr ether, mp 70-72°.

Hydrochloride. [63659-19-8] SLD-212; SL-75.212; Betoptic; Betoptima; Kerlone. $C_{18}H_{29}NO_3$.HCl; mol wt 343.89. Crystals from acetone, mp 116°. LD_{50} in mice (mg/kg): 944 orally; 37 i.v. (Manoury).

THERAP CAT: Antihypertensive; antiglaucoma.

1183. Betazole. [105-20-4] 1H-Pyrazole-3-ethanamine; 3-(2-aminoethyl)pyrazole; 3-(β-aminoethyl)pyrazole; ametazole; gastramine. $C_5H_9N_3$; mol wt 111.15. C 54.03%, H 8.16%, N 37.80%. Prepd by the catalytic reduction of 3-pyrazoleacetaldehyde hydrazone: Jones, Mann, J. Am. Chem. Soc. **75**, 4048 (1953); Jones, **US 2785177** (1957 to Lilly).

Viscous liquid. $bp_{0.5}$ 118-123°.

Dihydrochloride. [138-92-1] Histimin; Histalog. $C_5H_9N_3$.2 HCl; mol wt 184.07. Crystals from ethanol, mp 224-226°. Sol in water. Practically insol in chloroform. Aq solns are acid to litmus.

THERAP CAT: Diagnostic aid (gastric secretion stimulant).

1184. Betel. Dried leaves of Piper betle L., Piperaceae. Habit. India, Ceylon, Malay Archipelago. Constit. 0.2-1% volatile oil, chavibetol, chavicol, cadinene, allylpyrocatechol. Ref: Ueda, Sasaki, J. Pharm. Soc. Jpn. **71**, 559 (1951), C.A. **45**, 9137g (1951).

THERAP CAT: Counterirritant.

1185. Bethanechol Chloride. [590-63-6] 2-[(Aminocarbonyl)oxy]-N,N,N-trimethyl-1-propanaminium chloride; (2-hydroxypropyl)trimethylammonium chloride carbamate; 2-carbamoyloxypropyltrimethylammonium chloride; carbamylmethylcholine chloride; β-methylcholine chloride urethan; Duvoid; Myocholine; Myotonine; Urecholine. $C_7H_{17}ClN_2O_2$; mol wt 196.68. C 42.75%, H 8.71%, Cl 18.03%, N 14.24%, O 16.27%. Prepn: Dalmer, Diehl, **US 1894162** (1933); Major, Bonnett, **US 2322375** (1943 to Merck & Co.). ^{1}H-NMR determn in tablets: G. M. Hanna, C. A. Lau-Cam, J. Assoc. Off. Anal. Chem. **70**, 557 (1987). Clinical trial in postoperative urinary retention: L. Gottesman et al., Dis. Colon Rectum **32**, 867 (1989).

Hygroscopic crystals, slight amine odor, dec 218-219°. One gram dissolves in 0.6 ml of water, in 12.5 ml of 95% alc. pH of an 0.5% aq soln 5.5-6.0. Aq solns may be sterilized by autoclaving at 120° for 20 minutes.

THERAP CAT: Cholinergic; in treatment of urinary retention.

THERAP CAT (VET): Cholinergic.

1186. Bethanidine. [55-73-2] N,N'-Dimethyl-N''-(phenylmethyl)guanidine; 1-benzyl-2,3-dimethylguanidine; N-benzyl-N',N''-dimethylguanidine. $C_{10}H_{15}N_3$; mol wt 177.25. C 67.76%, H 8.53%, N 23.71%. Adrenergic neuron blocking agent. Prepn: Walton, Ruffell, **US 3168562** (1965 to Wellcome Found.); **GB 1084461** and **GB 1111564** (1967 and 1968 to Wellcome Found.). Pharmacology: A. L. A. Boura, A. F. Green, Br. J. Pharmacol. **20**, 36 (1963); J. A. Oates et al., Ann. N.Y. Acad. Sci. **179**, 302 (1971). Pharmacokinetics: C. N. Corder, J. Clin. Pharmacol. **19**, 428 (1979). HPLC determn in plasma: J. R. Shipe et al., Clin. Chem. **29**, 1793 (1983). Anti-arrhythmic activity: M. B. Bacaner, D. G. Benditt, Am. J. Cardiol. **50**, 728 (1982); J. C. Somberg et al., ibid. **54**, 343 (1984). Review: A. F. Green, Br. J. Clin. Pharmacol. **13**, 25-34 (1982).

Crystals from methanol + ether, mp 195-197°.

Hydriodide. $C_{10}H_{15}N_3$.HI. Crystals from ethanol + ether, mp 141-146°.

Sulfate. [114-85-2] Benzaidin; BW-467C60; Bendogen; Benzoxine; Betaling; Betanidol; Esbatal; Eusmanid; Hypersin; Tenathan. $(C_{10}H_{15}N_3)_2.H_2SO_4$; mol wt 452.57. LD_{50} in mice (mg/kg): 12 i.v.; 150 i.p.; 260 s.c.; 520 by stomach intubation (Boura, Green).

THERAP CAT: Antihypertensive.

1187. Betoxycaine. [3818-62-0] 3-Amino-4-butoxybenzoic acid 2-[2-(diethylamino)ethoxy]ethyl ester; 2-diethylaminoethoxyethyl 3-amino-4-butoxybenzoate. $C_{19}H_{32}N_2O_4$; mol wt 352.47. C 64.74%, H 9.15%, N 7.95%, O 18.16%. Prepn and properties: E. Cuingnet, **US 3209022** (1965 to Corbiere). Ionization potential: A. Cier et al., Therapie **26**, 941 (1971). Investigations of possible antifibrillatory properties: P. Amaud et al., C.R. Seances Soc. Biol. Ses Fil. **159**, 2427 (1965); G. Faucon et al., Therapie **21**, 1253 (1966).

Monohydrochloride. [5003-47-4] Millicaine. $C_{19}H_{32}N_2O_4$.-HCl; mol wt 388.93. White crystals from acetone, mp 117°. Soluble in methanol.

THERAP CAT: Anesthetic (local).

1188. Betula. European white birch. Bark and leaves of *Betula alba* L., *Betulaceae*. *Habit*. Europe and Northern Asia, also America, north of Pennsylvania. *Constit*. 10-15% Betulin (betula camphor), betuloresinic acid, essential oil, saponins, betulol (sesquiterpene alcohol), apigenin dimethyl ether, betuloside, gaultherin, methyl salicylate, ascorbic acid. *Ref*: Kreitmair, *Pharmazie* **8**, 534 (1953).

USE: Pharmaceutic aid (flavor).

1189. Betulin. [473-98-3] (3β)-Lup-20(29)-ene-3,28-diol; lup-20(30)-ene-3β,28-diol; trochol; betulinol; betulol. $C_{30}H_{50}O_2$; mol wt 442.72. C 81.39%, H 11.38%, O 7.23%. In the outer portion of the bark of white birch (up to 24%), in other barks, and in lignite. Isoln: Lowitz, *Crell's Chem. Ann.* **1**, 312 (1788); L. Ruzicka, O. Isler, *Helv. Chim. Acta* **19**, 506 (1936); and botanical distribution: Steiner, *Molisch Festschrift* (1936). Isoln from *Lemaireocereus griseus* Britton et Rose, *Cactaceae*: C. Djerassi et al., *J. Am. Chem. Soc.* **78**, 2312 (1956). Structure: Ames et al., *J. Chem. Soc.* **1951**, 450; Davy et al., ibid. **1951**, 2696, 2702. Stereochemistry: Guider et al., ibid. **1953**, 3024; Das, *Chem. Ind. (London)* **1971**, 1331. Reviews: J. Simonsen, W. C. J. Ross, *The Terpenes* **vol. IV** (Cambridge Univ. Press, 1957) pp 187-328; E. W. H. Hayek et al., *Phytochemistry* **28**, 2229-2242 (1989).

Crystals from methanol-chloroform, mp 248-251°; sublimes at 240° at 0.01 mm. Solvated needles from alc contg one mol EtOH. After drying sublimes at 170-180° (bath temp) at 0.08 mm. uv max (H_2SO_4): 316 nm. $[\alpha]_D^{15}$ +20° (c = 2 in pyridine). Sparingly sol in cold water, petr ether, carbon disulfide. One part is sol in 149 parts alc, 251 ether, 113 chloroform, 417 benzene. Sol in acetic acid.

Diacetate. [1721-69-3] $C_{34}H_{54}O_4$. mp 223-224°. $[\alpha]_D^{20}$ +22° (c = 1.2 in $CHCl_3$). $d_4^{228.5}$ 0.9635; $n_D^{228.5}$ 1.4661.

USE: Light stabilizer for cellulose and wood pulp. In mfr of resins, laquers, emulsifiers and polyurethanes. Cosmetics additive.

1190. Betulinic Acid. [472-15-1] (3β)-3-Hydroxylup-20(29)-en-28-oic acid; betulic acid; ALS-357. $C_{30}H_{48}O_3$; mol wt 456.70. C 78.90%, H 10.59%, O 10.51%. Naturally occurring triterpene found in many plant sources, notably the bark of white birch trees, *Betula alba* L. *Betulaceae*. Melanoma-specific cytotoxic agent. Isoln: L. Ruzicka et al., *Helv. Chim. Acta* **21**, 1706 (1938); and characterization: A. Robertson et al., *J. Chem. Soc.* **1939**, 1267. Synthesis from betulin, q.v.: D. S. H. Kim et al., *Synth. Commun.* **27**, 1607 (1997). Isoln and crystal structure of benzyl ester: G. Bringmann et al., *Planta Med.* **63**, 255 (1997). Inhibition of HIV replication: T. Fujioka et al., *J. Nat. Prod.* **57**, 243 (1994). Induction of apoptosis in human melanoma cells: E. Pisha et al., *Nat. Med.* **1**, 1046 (1995). Mechanism of action study: S. Fulda et al., *Cancer Res.* **57**, 4956 (1997). Pharmacokinetics in mice: G. O. Udeani et al., *Biopharm. Drug Dispos.* **20**, 379 (1999). Tumor cell-specific cytotoxicity: V. Zuco et al., *Cancer Lett.* **175**, 17 (2002). LC/MS determn in plasma: X. Cheng et al., *Rapid Commun. Mass Spectrom.* **17**, 2089 (2003). Review of natural distribution: G. Pavanasasivam, M. U. S. Sultanbawa, *Phytochemistry* **13**, 2002-2006 (1974); of anticancer activity: D. A. Eiznhamer, Z.-Q. Xu, *IDrugs* **7**, 359-373 (2004); of chemistry, biology and therapeutic potential: R. H. Cichewicz, S. A. Kouzi, *Med. Res. Rev.* **24**, 90-114 (2004); of biological properties: P. Yogeeswari, D. Sriram, *Curr. Med. Chem.* **12**, 657-666 (2005).

Colorless needles from methanol, mp 290-293°. $[\alpha]_D^{25}$ +7.5° (c = 0.37 in pyridine). Highly sol in pyridine, acetic acid. Limited soly in methanol, ethanol, $CHCl_3$, ether. Low soly in H_2O, petroleum ether, DMF, DMSO, benzene.

1191. Bevacizumab. [216974-75-3] Anti-(human vascular endothelial growth factor) immunoglobulin G1 (human-mouse monoclonal rhuMAb-VEGF γ$_1$-chain) disulfide with human-mouse monoclonal rhuMAb-VEGF light chain, dimer; rhuMAb-VEGF; Avastin. Recombinant humanized monoclonal antibody directed against vascular endothelial growth factor (VEGF). Prepn: L. G. Presta et al., *Cancer Res.* **57**, 4593 (1997); M. Baca et al., **WO 9845331** (1998 to Genentech). Biodistribution study: Y. S. Lin et al., *J. Pharmacol. Exp. Ther.* **288**, 371 (1999). Clinical pharmacokinetics: M. S. Gordon et al., *J. Clin. Oncol.* **19**, 843 (2001). Clinical trial in renal cancer: J. C. Yang et al., *N. Engl. J. Med.* **349**, 427 (2003); in combination therapy in colorectal cancer: F. Kabbinavar et al., *J. Clin. Oncol.* **21**, 60 (2003). Symposium on antiangiogenic and antitumor activity: *Semin. Oncol.* **29**, Suppl. 16, 1-18 (2002). Review of development and clinical experience: N. Ferrara et al., *Nat. Rev. Drug Disc.* **3**, 391-400 (2004).

THERAP CAT: Antineoplastic.

1192. Bevantolol. [59170-23-9] 1-[[2-(3,4-Dimethoxyphenyl)ethyl]amino]-3-(3-methylphenoxy)-2-propanol; 1-[(3,4-dimethoxyphenethyl)amino]-3-(m-tolyloxy)-2-propanol. $C_{20}H_{27}$-NO_4; mol wt 345.43. C 69.54%, H 7.88%, N 4.05%, O 18.53%. Cardioselective β$_1$-adrenergic blocker. Prepn: **BE 790165**; A. Holmes, R. F. Meyer, **US 3857891** (1973, 1974 both to Parke, Davis & Co.); M. L. Hoefle et al., *J. Med. Chem.* **18**, 148 (1975). Pharmacology in animals: S. G. Hastings et al., *Arch. Int. Pharmacodyn. Ther.* **226**, 81 (1977). Cardiovascular effects in animals: I. D. Dukes, E. M. Vaughan Williams, *Br. J. Pharmacol.* **84**, 365 (1985). Cardioselectivity in asthmatic patients: C.-G. Löfdahl et al., *Pharmacotherapy* **4**, 205 (1984). GC determn in plasma: E. J. Randinitis et al., *J. Chromatogr.* **308**, 345 (1984). Pharmacokinetics in humans: P. Vermeij, P. van Brummelen, *Eur. J. Clin. Pharmacol.* **30**, 375 (1986). Comparative clinical trial with hydrochlorothiazide in hypertension: C. P. Lucas et al., *Clin. Ther.* **8**, 49 (1985).

Symposium on pharmacology and clinical efficacy: *Am. J. Cardiol.* **58**, 1E-44E (1986).

Hydrochloride. [42864-78-8] CI-775; Ranestol; Sentiloc; Vantol. $C_{20}H_{27}NO_4 \cdot HCl$; mol wt 381.89. Crystals from acetonitrile, mp 137-138°.

THERAP CAT: Antianginal; antihypertensive; antiarrhythmic.

1193. Bevonium Methyl Sulfate. [5205-82-3] 2-[[(Hydroxydiphenylacetyl)oxy]methyl]-1,1-dimethylpiperidinium methyl sulfate (salt); 2-(hydroxymethyl)-1,1-dimethylpiperidinium methyl sulfate benzilate; piribenzil methyl sulfate; benzilic acid ester with 2-(hydroxymethyl)-1,1-dimethylpiperidinium methyl sulfate; CG-201; Acabel. $C_{23}H_{31}NO_7S$; mol wt 465.56. C 59.34%, H 6.71%, N 3.01%, O 24.06%, S 6.89%. Anticholinergic. Prepn: BE 616951 (1962 to Grünenthal), *C.A.* **58**, 7914d (1963); Beckmann, *Arzneim.-Forsch.* **16**, 910 (1966). Series of publications on pharmacology, toxicology, clinical trials, *see ibid.* 901-988.

Crystals from petr ether, mp 134-135°.
THERAP CAT: Antispasmodic.

1194. Bexarotene. [153559-49-0] 4-[1-(5,6,7,8-Tetrahydro-3,5,5,8,8-pentamethyl-2-naphthalenyl)ethenyl]benzoic acid; SR-11247; LGD-1069; Targretin. $C_{24}H_{28}O_2$; mol wt 348.48. C 82.72%, H 8.10%, O 9.18%. Selective retinoid X receptor (RXR) agonist. Prepn: M. F. Boehm *et al.*, WO 9321746 (1993 to Ligand Pharm.); M. L. Dawson *et al.*, US 5466861 (1995 to SRI Int.; La Jolla Cancer Res. Found.); and structure-activity study: M. F. Boehm *et al.*, *J. Med. Chem.* **37**, 2930 (1994); M. I. Dawson *et al.*, *ibid.* **38**, 3368 (1995). Chemopreventive effect in rat mammary carcinoma: M. M. Gottardis *et al.*, *Cancer Res.* **56**, 5566 (1996). Effect on glucose homeostasis in exptl diabetes: R. Mukherjee *et al.*, *Nature* **386**, 407 (1997). Clinical pharmacokinetics and evaluation in advanced cancers: V. A. Miller *et al.*, *J. Clin. Oncol.* **15**, 790 (1997). Clinical evaluation in cutaneous T-cell lymphoma: D. Breneman *et al.*, *Arch. Dermatol.* **138**, 325 (2002).

White solid from methylene chloride, mp 230-231° (Dawson, 1995); also reported as white crystals, mp 234° (Boehm, 1994). uv max (methanol): 264 nm (ε 16400).
THERAP CAT: Antineoplastic.

1195. Bezafibrate. [41859-67-0] 2-[4-[2-[(4-Chlorobenzoyl)amino]ethyl]phenoxy]-2-methylpropanoic acid; 2-[p-[2-(p-chlorobenzamido)ethyl]phenoxy]-2-methylpropionic acid; α-[4-(4-chlorobenzoylaminoethyl)phenoxy]isobutyric acid; BM-15075; Befizal; Bezalip; Bezatol; Cedur; Difaterol. $C_{19}H_{20}ClNO_4$; mol wt 361.82. C 63.07%, H 5.57%, Cl 9.80%, N 3.87%, O 17.69%. Prepn: E. Witte *et al.*, DE 2149070; *eidem*, US 3781328 (both 1973 to Boehringer, Mann.). Pharmacology: R. Zimmerman *et al.*, *Atherosclerosis* **29**, 477 (1978). Clinical studies: A. G. Olsson, P.

D. Lang, *ibid.* **31**, 421, 429 (1978); P. Wahl *et al.*, *Dtsch. Med. Wochenschr.* **103**, 1233 (1978). Review of pharmacodynamics and therapeutic use: J. P. Monk, P. A. Todd, *Drugs* **33**, 539-576 (1987).

Crystals from acetone, mp 186°.
THERAP CAT: Antilipemic.

1196. Bezitramide. [15301-48-1] 1-[1-(3-Cyano-3,3-diphenylpropyl)-4-piperidinyl]-1,3-dihydro-3-(1-oxopropyl)-2H-benzimidazol-2-one; 1-[1-(3-cyano-3,3-diphenylpropyl)-4-piperidyl]-3-propionyl-2-benzimidazolinone; 1-(3-cyano-3,3-diphenylpropyl)-4-(2-oxo-3-propionyl-1-benzimidazolinyl)piperidine; benzitramide; R-4845; Burgodin. $C_{31}H_{32}N_4O_2$; mol wt 492.61. C 75.58%, H 6.55%, N 11.37%, O 6.50%. Prepn: BE 633495; P. A. J. Janssen, US 3196157 (1963, 1965 both to Janssen). Pharmacology and clinical data: P. A. J. Janssen *et al.*, *Arzneim.-Forsch.* **21**, 862 (1971); W. K. P. Amery *et al.*, *ibid.* 868; H. Knape, *Anaesthesist* **21**, 251 (1972).

White crystalline powder, mp 145-149°. Also reported as pale yellow amorphous powder, mp 124.5-126°. Solubility of >1 g/100 ml in ethyl acetate, acetone, benzene, chloroform. Almost insol in water, dilute acids. LD_{50} orally in mice, rats: 2101, 141 mg/kg (Janssen).

Note: This is a controlled substance (opiate): **21 CFR,** 1308.12.
THERAP CAT: Analgesic (narcotic).

1197. Biapenem. [120410-24-4] 6-[[(4R,5S,6S)-2-Carboxy-6-((1R)-1-hydroxyethyl)-4-methyl-7-oxo-1-azabicyclo[3.2.0]-hept-2-en-3-yl]thio]-6,7-dihydro-5H-pyrazolo[1,2-a][1,2,4]triazol-4-ium inner salt; (1R,5S,6S)-2-[(6,7-dihydro-5H-pyrazolo[1,2-a][1,2,4]-triazolium-6-yl)thio]-6-[(R)-1-hydroxyethyl]-1-methyl-carbapen-2-em-3-carboxylate; LJC-10627; L-627; CL-186815. $C_{15}H_{18}N_4O_4S$; mol wt 350.39. C 51.42%, H 5.18%, N 15.99%, O 18.26%, S 9.15%. 1-β-methyl-carbapenem antibiotic. Prepn: T. Kumagai *et al.*, EP 289801; *eidem*, US 4990613 (1988, 1991 both to Lederle). Total synthesis: Y. Nagao *et al.*, *J. Org. Chem.* **57**, 4243 (1992). Renal dehydropeptidase stability: M. Hikida *et al.*, *Antimicrob. Agents Chemother.* **36**, 481 (1992). *In-vitro* antimicrobial spectrum: H. M. Wexler *et al.*, *J. Antimicrob. Chemother.* **33**, 629 (1994); H. Y. Chen, D. M. Livermore, *ibid.* 949. Clinical pharmacokinetics: M. Nakashima *et al.*, *Int. J. Clin. Pharmacol. Ther. Toxicol.* **31**, 70 (1993). Clinical evaluation: H. Meguro *et al.*, *Jpn. J. Antibiot.* **47**, 903 (1994).

Amorphous, pale yellow powder from acetone/water, occurs as hemihydrate. $[\alpha]_D^{20}$ −32.9° (c = 0.5).
THERAP CAT: Antibacterial.

1198. Bibenzyl. [103-29-7] 1,1'-(1,2-Ethanediyl)bisbenzene; dibenzyl; *sym*-diphenylethane; 1,2-diphenylethane. $C_{14}H_{14}$; mol wt 182.26. C 92.26%, H 7.74%. Prepn by the reduction of benzil or benzoin: Clemmensen, *Ber.* **47,** 688 (1914); Gattermann-Wieland, *Praxis des Organischen Chemikers* (de Gruyter, Berlin, 40th ed., 1961) p 333; from stilbene, Kleiderer, Kornfeld, *J. Org. Chem.* **13,** 455 (1948).

Monoclinic prisms from methanol, mp 52.0-52.5°. bp_{760} 284°. d_4^0 1.104; d_4^{25} 0.9782; d_4^{58} 0.958. Heat of combustion (25°): 9909.9 cal (15°)/g. Moderately sol in alcohol; freely sol in carbon disulfide, ether, chloroform, amyl acetate; sol in liquid sulfur dioxide. Practically insol in water, liquid ammonia.

1199. Bibrocathol. [6915-57-7] 4,5,6,7-Tetrabromo-2-hydroxy-1,3,2-benzodioxabismole; tetrabromopyrocatechol bismuth derivative; bismuth tetrabromopyrocatechol; bibrocathin; Noviform; Posiformin. $C_6HBiBr_4O_3$; mol wt 649.67. C 11.09%, H 0.16%, Bi 32.17%, Br 49.20%, O 7.39%. Prepn: Hundrup, *Arch. Pharm. Chemi* **54,** 537 (1947), *C.A.* **42,** 2727a (1948). Antibacterial activity: Frank, Stark, *Pharm. Acta Helv.* **29,** 283 (1954). Identity tests: Hakkesteegt, *Pharm. Weekbl.* **99,** 922 (1964).

Yellow, odorless, tasteless powder. Practically insol in water. Slightly sol in alcohol, ether. Dec in acid, alkalies.

THERAP CAT: Antiseptic.

1200. Bicalutamide. [90357-06-5] *N*-[4-Cyano-3-(trifluoromethyl)phenyl]-3-[(4-fluorophenyl)sulfonyl]-2-hydroxy-2-methylpropanamide; 4-cyano-3-trifluoromethyl-*N*-(3-*p*-fluorophenylsulfonyl-2-hydroxy-2-methylpropionyl)aniline; (±)-4'-cyano-α,α,-α-trifluoro-3-[(*p*-fluorophenyl)sulfonyl]-2-methyl-*m*-lactotoluidide; ICI-176334; Casodex. $C_{18}H_{14}F_4N_2O_4S$; mol wt 430.37. C 50.23%, H 3.28%, F 17.66%, N 6.51%, O 14.87%, S 7.45%. Non-steroidal peripherally active antiandrogen. Prepn: H. Tucker, **EP 100172**; *idem,* **US 4636505** (1984, 1987 both to ICI); and structure-activity: H. Tucker *et al., J. Med. Chem.* **31,** 954 (1988). Resolution and activity of enantiomers: H. Tucker, G. J. Chesterson, *ibid.* 885. Pharmacokinetics: I. D. Cockshott *et al., Eur. Urol.* **18,** Suppl. 3, 10 (1990). Clinical trials in prostate cancer: G. Lunglmayr, *Horm. Res.* **32,** Suppl. 1, 77 (1989); D. W. W. Newling, *Eur. Urol.* **18** Suppl. 3, 18 (1990). Review of pharmacology: B. J. A. Furr in *Hormonal Therapy of Prostatic Diseases: Basic and Clinical Aspects,* M. Motta, M. Serio, Eds. (Mediocom Europe, Milan, 1987) 148-161.

Crystals from a 1:1 (v/v) mix of ethyl acetate and petroleum ether, mp 191-193°.

THERAP CAT: Antiandrogen; antineoplastic (hormonal).

1201. Bicine. [150-25-4] *N,N*-Bis(2-hydroxyethyl)glycine; di(hydroxyethyl)glycine; *N,N*-bis(hydroxyethyl)aminoacetic acid; *N,N*-di(hydroxyethyl)aminoacetic acid; diethylolglycine; 2-HxG. $C_6H_{13}NO_4$; mol wt 163.17. C 44.17%, H 8.03%, N 8.58%, O 39.22%. $(HOCH_2CH_2)_2NCH_2COOH$. One of the zwitterionic amino acids known as "Good" buffers, active in the pH range 6-8.5. Prepn by hydrolysis of its lactone (obtained from glycine and ethylene oxide): Pascal, *Compt. Rend.* **245,** 1318 (1957); from diethanolamine and bromoacetic acid: N. E. Good *et al., Biochemistry* **5,** 467 (1966). Crystal structure: V. Cody *et al., Acta Crystallogr.* **33B,** 905 (1977). Use as sequestering agent: A. Grawitz, *Rev. Tech. Ind. Cuir* **65,** 187, 190 (1973), *C.A.* **80,** 49281h (1974). Temperature effects on pKa: M. L. Soni, R. C. Kapoor, *Int. J. Quantum Chem.* **20,** 385 (1981). Use as a buffer: A. L. Remisov, *Biokhimiya* **25,** 323 (1960); S. Ito *et al., Histochem. J.* **16,** 489 (1984).

Crystals from dil ethanol, mp 193-195° (slight decompn). pKa (20°): 8.35. pKa$_2$ (0.1*M*): 0°, 8.7; 20°, 8.35; 37°, 8.2. ΔpKa/°C −0.018. Saturated aq soln is 1.1*M* at 0°. Slightly sol in water. Forms a water-soluble sodium salt.

USE: Biological buffer and chelating agent.

1202. Bicozamycin. [38129-37-2] Bicyclomycin; aizumycin; 8,10-diaza-6-hydroxy-5-methylene-1-(2-methyl-1,2,3-trihydroxypropyl)-2-oxabicyclo[4.2.2]decan-7,9-dione; antibiotic 5879; WS-4545 antibiotic; Bacfeed. $C_{12}H_{18}N_2O_7$; mol wt 302.28. C 47.68%, H 6.00%, N 9.27%, O 37.05%. Cyclic peptide antibiotic substance. Prepn by fermentation of *Streptomyces sapporensis*: T. Miyoshi *et al.,* **DE 2150593**; H. Imanaka *et al.,* **US 3923790** (1972, 1975 both to Fujisawa). Isoln and characterization: T. Miyoshi *et al., J. Antibiot.* **25,** 569 (1972). Isoln from *S. aizunensis* and identity with antibiotic 5879: S. Miyamura *et al., ibid.* **26,** 479 (1973). Bicyclomycin has a unique chemical structure which bears no relation to any group of known antibiotics. Structural elucidation: T. Kamiya *et al., ibid.* **25,** 576 (1972). Crystal and molecular structure: Y. Tokuma *et al., Bull. Chem. Soc. Jpn.* **47,** 18 (1974). *In vitro* and *in vivo* activity studies: M. Nishida *et al., J. Antibiot.* **25,** 582 (1972). Metabolism: *eidem, ibid.* 594. Mechanism of action: N. Tanaka *et al., ibid.* **29,** 155 (1976); N. Tanaka in *Antibiotics* vol. 5(pt. 1), E. Hahn, Ed. (Springer, New York, 1979) p 18. Synthetic approaches: L. V. Dunkerton, R. M. Ahmed, *Tetrahedron Lett.* **21,** 1803 (1980); R. M. Williams, *ibid.* **22,** 2341 (1981); S. Nakatsuka *et al., ibid.* 4973; J. H. Hoare, P. Yates, *Chem. Commun.* **1981,** 1126. Total synthesis of (±)-bicyclomycin: S. Nakatsuka *et al., Tetrahedron Lett.* **24,** 5627 (1983); of (+)-bicyclomycin: R. M. Williams *et al., J. Am. Chem. Soc.* **106,** 5749 (1984); *eidem, ibid.* **107,** 3253 (1985). Review of synthetic, mechanistic and biological studies: R. M. Williams, C. A. Durham, *Chem. Rev.* **88,** 511-540 (1988).

Monoclinic crystals from ethanol, mp 188-191° (dec); rhombic crystals from methanol + acetone, mp 187-189° (dec) (Imanaka), also reported as mp 166-170° (Nakatsuka *et al.*). $[\alpha]_D^{23}$ +63.5° (methanol). Weakly basic substance. Soly in water: 192 mg/ml. Sol in methanol; sparingly sol in ethanol. Slightly sol in acetone. Practically insol in chloroform, ethyl acetate, benzene, *n*-hexane. Unstable in alkaline soln. LD_{50} in mice: >4 g/kg (Williams, Durham).

THERAP CAT (VET): Antibacterial; feed additive (livestock).

1203. Bicuculline. [485-49-4] (6*R*)-6-[(5*S*)-5,6,7,8-Tetrahydro-6-methyl-1,3-dioxolo[4,5-g]isoquinolin-5-yl]furo[3,4-*e*]-1,3-benzodioxol-8(6*H*)-one. $C_{20}H_{17}NO_6$; mol wt 367.35. C 65.39%, H 4.66%, N 3.81%, O 26.13%. Alkaloid naturally occurring in the *d*-form; found in *Dicentra cucullaria* (L.) Bernh., *Adlumia fungosa* (Ait.) Greene, *Fumariaceae,* and several *Corydalis* species: Manske, *Can. J. Res.* **7,** 265 (1932); **8,** 210, 407 (1933); **9,** 436 (1933); Edwards, Handa, *Can. J. Chem.* **39,** 1801 (1961). Synthesis of *dl*-form: Groenewoud, Robinson, *J. Chem. Soc.* **1936,** 199. Resolution of isomers: Haworth *et al., Nature* **165,** 529 (1950). Stereoisomer of adlumidine, *q.v.,* and of capnoidine: Manske, *J. Am. Chem. Soc.* **72,** 3207 (1950). Preliminary stereochemical studies: Safe, Moir, *Can. J. Chem.* **42,** 160 (1964). Revised stereochemistry: Blaha *et al., Collect. Czech. Chem. Commun.* **29,** 2328 (1964); Snatzke *et al., Tetrahedron* **25,** 5059 (1969). Crystal and molecular structure: Gorinsky, Moss, *J. Cryst. Mol. Struct.* **3,** 299

(1973). Shows GABA *(q.v.)* antagonist activity: Curtis *et al., Nature* **226,** 1222 (1970).

Elongated plates from chloroform-methanol, mp 215°; also reported as mp 177°, solidifies and remelts 193-195°: Manske, *Can. J. Res.* **21B,** 13 (1943). uv max (acidified ethanol): 225, 296, 324 nm (ε 36700, 6390, 5870). $[\alpha]_D^{25}$ +130.5° (CHCl₃). pKa 4.84. Sol in benzene, chloroform, ethyl acetate. Sparingly sol in alc and ether.

1204. Bidisomide. [116078-65-0] α-[2-[Acetyl(1-methylethyl)amino]ethyl]-α-(2-chlorophenyl)-1-piperidinebutanamide; (±)-α-(*o*-chlorophenyl)-α-[2-(*N*-isopropylacetamido)ethyl]-1-piperidinebutyramide; SC-40230. C₂₂H₃₄ClN₃O₂; mol wt 407.98. C 64.77%, H 8.40%, Cl 8.69%, N 10.30%, O 7.84%. Sodium channel blocker. Prepn: B. N. Desai *et al., EP 170901; eidem, US 4639524* (1986, 1987 both to Searle); *eidem, J. Med. Chem.* **31,** 2158 (1988). Cardiovascular pharmacology: L. G. Frederick *et al., Cardiovasc. Res.* **23,** 897 (1989). Electrophysiologic study: S. M. Garthwaite *et al., Drug Dev. Res.* **27,** 329 (1992). Bioavailability and tolerability in humans: R. L. Page *et al., Clin. Pharmacol. Ther.* **51,** 371 (1992). Clinical pharmacokinetics: C. S. Cook *et al., Pharm. Res.* **10,** 1675 (1993).

Crystals from ethyl acetate, mp 140-141°.
THERAP CAT: Antiarrhythmic (class I).

1205. Bietamiverine. [479-81-2] α-Phenyl-1-piperidineacetic acid 2-(diethylamino)ethyl ester; β-diethylaminoethyl phenylpiperidinoacetate; β-diethylaminoethyl α-(1-piperidyl)phenylacetate. C₁₉H₃₀N₂O₂; mol wt 318.45. C 71.66%, H 9.50%, N 8.80%, O 10.05%. Prepd by reacting piperidine with phenylchloroacetic acid ethyl ester in chloroform: Reetz, **DE 859892** (1952 to Nordmark-Werke); from β-diethylaminoethyl phenylbromoacetate and piperidine in chloroform: Blicke *et al., J. Am. Chem. Soc.* **76,** 3161 (1954); from ethyl α-(1-piperidyl)phenylacetate and β-diethylaminoethyl chloride: Moffett, Hart, *J. Am. Pharm. Assoc. Sci. Ed.* **42,** 717 (1953). Clinical tests: Ciravegna *et al., Clin. Ter.* **57,** 227 (1971).

Liquid, d₄²⁵ 1.0184. bp₁ 65°. n_D²⁵ 1.5070.
Hydrochloride. [1477-10-7] Novosparol. C₁₉H₃₀N₂O₂.HCl; mol wt 354.91. Crystals from methyl isobutyl ketone, mp 187-189°.
Dihydrochloride. [2691-46-5] C₁₉H₃₀N₂O₂.2HCl. Crystals from ethanol + ether, mp 194-195°.
THERAP CAT: Antispasmodic.

1206. Bifemelane. [90293-01-9] *N*-Methyl-4-[2-(phenylmethyl)phenoxy]-1-butanamine; 4-(*o*-benzylphenoxy)-*N*-methylbutylamine; 2-(4-methylaminobutoxy)diphenylmethane; 2-benzyl-1-[4-(methylamino)butoxy]benzene. C₁₈H₂₃NO; mol wt 269.38. C 80.26%, H 8.61%, N 5.20%, O 5.94%. Monoamine oxidase inhibitor. Prepn: R. Kikumoto *et al., DE 2627227; eidem, US 4091114* (1976, 1978 both to Mitsubishi); and antidepressant activity: R. Kikumoto *et al., J. Med. Chem.* **24,** 145 (1981). Pharmacology: A. Tobe *et al., Arzneim.-Forsch.* **31,** 1278 (1981). Effects on experimental amnesia in rats: A. Tobe *et al., Jpn. J. Pharmacol.* **39,** 153 (1985). Effects on neuronal activity in cats: M. Egawa *et al., Neuropharmacology* **26,** 379 (1987). Inhibition of MAO: M. Naoi *et al., J. Neurochem.* **50,** 243 (1988).

Hydrochloride. [62232-46-6] E-0687; MCI-2016; Alnert; Celeport. C₁₈H₂₃NO.HCl; mol wt 305.84. Crystals from acetone, mp 117-121°. LD₅₀ in mice, rats (mg/kg): 1000, 1080 orally; 173, 130 i.p. (Tobe, 1981).
THERAP CAT: Nootropic.

1207. Bifenazate. [149877-41-8] 2-(4-Methoxy[1,1'-biphenyl]-3-yl)hydrazinecarboxylic acid 1-methylethyl ester; isopropyl 3-(4-methoxy-3-biphenylyl)carbazate; D-2341; Floramite. C₁₇H₂₀N₂O₃; mol wt 300.35. C 67.98%, H 6.71%, N 9.33%, O 15.98%. Hydrazinecarboxylate miticide for use on fruits and ornamentals. Prepn: M. A. Dekeyser, P. T. McDonald, **WO 9310083**; *eidem, US 5367093* (1993, 1994 both to Uniroyal). Review of physical properties, biological activity, and field trials: M. A. Dekeyser *et al., Brighton Crop Prot. Conf. - Pests Dis.* **1996,** 487-492.

White crystals, mp 120-121°. Soly in water at 20°: 3.76 mg/l. Log P (*n*-octanol/water) at 25°: 3.4 (pH 7). LD₅₀ in rats (mg/kg): 5000 orally, >2000 dermally (Dekeyser).
USE: Acaricide.

1208. Bifenox. [42576-02-3] 5-(2,4-Dichlorophenoxy)-2-nitrobenzoic acid methyl ester; methyl 5-(2,4-dichlorophenoxy)-2-nitrobenzoate; 2,4-dichlorophenyl 3-(methoxycarbonyl)-4-nitrophenyl ether; MC-4379; Modown. C₁₄H₉Cl₂NO₅; mol wt 342.13. C 49.15%, H 2.65%, Cl 20.72%, N 4.09%, O 23.38%. Pre-emergence herbicide. Prepn and herbicidal activity: **BE 749444**; R. J. Thiessen, **US 3652645** (1970, 1972 both to Mobil). Comparison with other herbicides in corn: W. M. Dest *et al., Proc. Annu. Meet. Northeast. Weed Sci. Soc.* **27,** 31 (1973). Metabolism in soil, plants: G. R. Leather, C. L. Foy, *Pestic. Biochem. Physiol.* **7,** 437 (1977). Brief description: R. H. Dreger, *Weeds Today* **8**(2), 18 (1977). *Review:* P. J. Kruger *et al., Proc. 12th Br. Weed Control Conf.* **2,** 839-845 (1974).

Yellow tan crystals, mp 84-86°. Practically insol in water (0.35 ppm at 25°). Soly in xylene at 25°: 30%. Vapor pressure at 30°: 2.4 × 10⁻⁶ mm Hg. LD₅₀ orally in rats, mice: >6400, 4556 mg/kg; LC₅₀ in pheasants, wild ducks: >5000 ppm (Kruger).
USE: Herbicide.

1209. Bifenthrin. [82657-04-3] [1α,3α(Z)-(±)-3-(2-Chloro-3,3,3-trifluoro-1-propenyl)-2,2-dimethylcyclopropanecarboxylic acid (2-methyl[1,1'-biphenyl]-3-yl)methyl ester; 2-methylbiphenyl-3-ylmethyl-(Z)-(1RS)-cis-3-(2-chloro-3,3,3-trifluoroprop-1-enyl)-2,2-dimethylcyclopropanecarboxylate; biphenate; biphenthrin; biphentrin; FMC-54800; Brigade; Talstar; Capture; Wisdom. C_{23}-$H_{22}ClF_3O_2$; mol wt 422.87. C 65.33%, H 5.24%, Cl 8.38%, F 13.48%, O 7.57%. Third generation synthetic pyrethroid. Prepn: J. F. Engel, **EP 3336**; idem, **US 4238505** (1979, 1980 both to FMC); E. L. Plummer et al., Pestic. Sci. **14**, 560 (1983). Physical properties, toxicology and review of field studies: H. J. H. Doel et al., Meded. Fac. Landbouwwet. Rijksuniv. Gent **49**, 929 (1984). Insecticidal activity: M. S. Mulla, H. A. Darwazeh, Bull. Soc. Vector Ecol. **10**, 1 (1985); M. S. Hamed, C. O. Knowles, J. Econ. Entomol. **81**, 1295 (1988). Field studies: Y. Antignus et al., Ann. Appl. Biol. **110**, 557 (1987); J. T. Trumble et al., J. Econ. Entomol. **81**, 608 (1988). Review of toxicology and human exposure: Toxicological Profile for Pyrethrins and Pyrethroids (PB2004-100004, 2003) 332 pp.

Light brown viscous oil, mp 51-66°. d^{25} 1.212 g/ml. Vapor pressure at 25°: 1.81×10^{-7} Torr. Sol in methylene chloride, chloroform, acetone, ether, toluene. Slightly sol in heptane, methanol. Soly in water: <0.1 ppb. LD_{50} orally in rats: 54.5 mg/kg; LD_{50} dermally in rabbits: >2000 mg/kg (Doel).
USE: Insecticide, acaricide.

1210. Bifeprunox. [350992-10-8] 7-[4-([1,1'-Biphenyl]-3-ylmethyl)-1-piperazinyl]-2(3H)-benzoxazolone. $C_{24}H_{23}N_3O_2$; mol wt 385.46. C 74.78%, H 6.01%, N 10.90%, O 8.30%. Exhibits partial agonist activity at dopamine D_2 and serotonin 5-HT$_{1A}$ receptors. Prepn: R. W. Feenstra et al., **WO 9736893**; idem, **US 6225312** (1997, 2001 both to Duphar); and receptor binding studies: idem et al., Bioorg. Med. Chem. Lett. **11**, 2345 (2001). Analysis of binding affinity vs in vitro efficacy: A. Newman-Tancredi et al., Int. J. Neuropsychopharmacol. **8**, 341 (2005). Review of development: W. Wolf, Curr. Opin. Invest. Drugs **4**, 72-76 (2003).

Methanesulfonate. [350992-13-1] Bifeprunox mesylate; DU-127090. $C_{24}H_{23}N_3O_2.CH_4O_3S$; mol wt 481.56.
THERAP CAT: Antipsychotic.

1211. Bifidus Factor. [9007-03-8] Lactobacillus bifidus factor; Lactobacillus bifidus growth factor. A factor found in human milk and causing a predominant occurrence of L. bifidus in the intestinal tract of breast-fed infants: Petuely, Kristen, Oesterr. Z. Kinderheilkd. Kinderfuersorge **6**, 173 (1951); Petuely, Naturwissenschaften **40**, 349 (1953). Essential growth factor for L. bifidus var Penn: György in Ciba Found. Symp., Chemistry and Biology of Mucopolysaccharides (Little, Brown, Boston, 1958) pp 140-156. Isoln from human milk: György et al., Arch. Biochem. Biophys. **48**, 193, 202, 209, 214 (1954); György, **US 2786051** (1957 to Am. Home Prod.); from L. bifidus cultured together with Escherichia coli: Kludas, **US 2962424** (1960 to J. Carl Pflüger). Isoln from carrots and identification of the major and minor bifidus factor: Samejima et al., Chem. Pharm. Bull. **19**, 166, 178, 186 (1971); Z. Tamura et al., Proc. Jpn. Acad. **48**, 138, 144 (1972). Prepn from porcine gastric mucosa and use as dietetic adjuvant in infant food: **FR 2101032** C.A. **78**, 28221g (1970); P. C. Wirth, **DE 2040268** C.A. **78**, 41859r (1970) (both 1972 to Sogeras).
USE: As adjuvant in powdered milk formulas for infants.

1212. Bifluranol. [34633-34-6] rel-4,4'-[(1R,2S)-1-Ethyl-2-methyl-1,2-ethanediyl]bis[2-fluorophenol]; erythro-3,3'-difluoro-4,4'-dihydroxy-α-ethyl-α'-methyldibenzyl; BX-341; Prostarex. $C_{17}H_{18}F_2O_2$; mol wt 292.32. C 69.85%, H 6.21%, F 13.00%, O 10.95%. Orally active antiprostatic agent. Prepn: J. C. Turner, R. P. Chan, **DE 2110428**; eidem, **US 4051263** (1971, 1977 both to Biorex). Antiprostatic activity: J. B. Dekanski, Br. J. Pharmacol. **71**, 11 (1980). Chemistry, disposition in animals: D. J. Pope et al., J. Pharm. Pharmacol. **33**, 297 (1981). Metabolism: eidem, ibid. 302.

Cryst from toluene, mp 158-159°.
THERAP CAT: Antiandrogen.

1213. Bifonazole. [60628-96-8] 1-([1,1'-Biphenyl]-4-yl-phenylmethyl)-1H-imidazole; (±)-1-(p,α-diphenylbenzyl)imidazole; Bay h 4502; Amycor; Azolmen; Bedriol; Mycospor; Mycosporan. $C_{22}H_{18}N_2$; mol wt 310.39. C 85.13%, H 5.85%, N 9.03%. Antimycotic deriv of imidazole. Prepn: E. Regel et al., **DE 2461406**; eidem, **US 4118487** (1976, 1978 both to Bayer). Series of articles on in vitro and in vivo antimycotic efficacy, microscopic studies, pharmacokinetics, efficacy in dermatomycoses and comparison with clotrimazole and miconazole, q.q.v.: Arzneim.-Forsch. **33**, 517-551, 745-754 (1983). Toxicology: G. Schlüter, ibid. 739.

Crystals from acetonitrile, mp 142°. Very lipophilic. Sol in alcohols, DMF, DMSO. Soly in water at pH 6: <0.1 mg/100 ml. Stable in aq soln at pH 1-12. LD_{50} in male mice, rats (mg/kg): 2629, 2854 orally (Schlüter).
THERAP CAT: Antifungal.

1214. BIGCHAP. [86303-22-2] (3α,5β,7α,12α)-N,N-Bis[3-(D-gluconoylamino)propyl]-3,7,12-trihydroxycholan-24-amide. $C_{42}H_{75}N_3O_{16}$; mol wt 878.06. C 57.45%, H 8.61%, N 4.79%, O 29.15%. Homogeneous nonionic detergent; derivative of cholic acid, q.v. Prepn: L. M. Hjelmeland et al., Anal. Biochem. **130**, 485 (1983). QSAR study as surfactant: P. Campbell et al., Biotechnol. Bioeng. **64**, 527 (1999). Use in protein purification via hydrophobic interaction displacement chromatography: K. M. Sunasara et al., ibid. **82**, 330 (2003). Clinical evaluation as a transduction enhancing agent in gene therapy: J. Kuball et al., J. Clin. Oncol. **20**, 957 (2002).

BigChap   R = OH
deoxyBigChap R =H

Crystals at 0° from 2-propanol. Critical micelle conc: 2.9 mM; also reported as 3.4 mM. Log P (octanol/water): 2.450. Dipole moment: 7.44 D.

Deoxy-BIGCHAP. [86303-23-3] N,N'-[[[(3α,5β,12α)-3,12-Di-hydroxy-24-oxocholan-24-yl]imino]di-3,1-propandiyl]bis-D-gluconamide. $C_{42}H_{75}N_3O_{15}$; mol wt 862.06. Use as mobile phase additive in microcolumn LC: W. Hu *et al.*, *J. High Resolut. Chromatogr.* **15**, 275 (1992). Critical micelle conc: 1.4 mM.
   USE: Surfactant and solubilizer for biological systems.

1215. Biguanide. [56-03-1] Imidodicarbonimidic diamide; guanylguanidine; amidinoguanidine; diguanide. $C_2H_7N_5$; mol wt 101.11. C 23.76%, H 6.98%, N 69.26%. Preparation from dicyanodiamide: Rackmann, *Ann.* **376**, 169 (1910); Karipides, Fernelius, *Inorg. Synth.* **7**, 56, 58 (1963). Crystal structure: S. R. Ernst, F. W. Cagle, *Acta Crystallogr.* **33B**, 235 (1977); S. R. Ernst, *ibid.* 237.

   Crystals from alc, mp 130°; dec rapidly at about 142°. Sol in water, alcohol. Insol in ether, benzene, chloroform. The aq soln dec on standing or heating. Aq solns are alkaline. Biguanide is a stronger base (pK$_1$ = 11.52; pK$_2$ = 2.93) than ammonia (pK = 9.61).
   Hydrochloride. $C_2H_7N_5$.HCl. Needles, mp 235°, very sol in water, slightly sol in alc.
   Neutral sulfate. $(C_2H_7N_5)_2$.H$_2$SO$_4$.2H$_2$O. Large crystals, sol in water.
   Acid sulfate. $C_2H_7N_5$.H$_2$SO$_4$.H$_2$O. Rhombic prisms, sol in water, the soln giving an acid reaction.
   USE: Sulfates in the determination of copper and nickel.

1216. Bikhaconitine. [6078-26-8] (1α,6α,14α,16β)-20-Ethyl-1,6,16-trimethoxy-4-(methoxymethyl)aconitane-8,13,14-triol 8-acetate 14-(3,4-dimethoxybenzoate); acetylveratroylbikhaconine. $C_{36}H_{51}NO_{11}$; mol wt 673.79. C 64.17%, H 7.63%, N 2.08%, O 26.12%. From roots of *Aconitum spicatum* Stapf., *Ranunculaceae*: Dunstan, Andrews, *J. Chem. Soc.* **87**, 1636 (1905). Structure: Tsuda, Marion, *Can. J. Chem.* **41**, 3055 (1963).

   Prisms from *n*-hexane, mp 163.5-164°.
   Monohydrate. Needles from ether or dil methanol, mp 105-110°. [α]$_D$ +16° (c = 1.6 in ethanol). Sol in alcohol, chloroform, ether, dil acids. Practically insol in water, petr ether.

1217. Bilberry. Heidelberry; huckleberry; European blueberry; whortleberry. Deciduous, dwarf shrub, *Vaccinium myrtillus* L., *Ericaceae*, bearing edible blue-black berries. Medicinal parts include the leaves and fruit. *Habit.* Northern and central Europe. *Constit.* Berries: anthocyanins, particularly glycosides of delphinidin, cyanidin, petunidin, peonidin, malvidin; quercetin, catechin, epicatechin, tannins, pectins, vitamin C. Leaves: Catechol tannins (0.8-6.7%); leucoanthocyans; flavonoids esp. quercetin glycosides; phenolic acids incl. caffeic, *p*-coumaric, *p*-hydroxybenzoic, protocatechuic, melilotic; iridoids; manganese; chromium. Berries have been used in traditional medicine to treat diarrhea and mouth and throat inflammations; leaves used in antidiabetic teas. Comprehensive description and medicinal uses: J. Barnes *et al.*, *Herbal Medicines* (Pharmaceutical Press, London, 2nd Ed., 2002) pp 73-77. Anthocyanin content and radical scavenging activity: J. Nakajima *et al.*, *J. Biomed. Biotechnol.* **5**, 241-247 (2004). Phenolic profile and antioxidant activity: S. Ehala *et al.*, *J. Agric. Food Chem.* **53**, 6484 (2005). Review of clinical trials in impaired night vision: P. H. Carter, E. Ernst, *Surv. Ophthalmol.* **49**, 38-50 (2004).
   Bilberry extract. [84082-34-8] Alcodin; Difrarel; Tegens. Anthocyanin enriched extract from the fruit.

   USE: In jams and jellies; food flavoring. Extracts as astringent and capillary protectant in eyecare and skin products.
   THERAP CAT: In treatment of night blindness.

1218. Bilirubin. [635-65-4] 2,17-Diethenyl-1,10,19,22,23,-24-hexahydro-3,7,13,18-tetramethyl-1,19-dioxo-21*H*-biline-8,12-dipropanoic acid; 1,10,19,22,23,24-hexahydro-2,7,13,17-tetramethyl-1,19-dioxo-3,18-divinylbiline-8,12-dipropionic acid; 1,3,6,7-tetramethyl-4,5-dicarboxyethyl-2,8-divinyl-(*b*-13)-dihydrobilenone; bilirubin IXα. $C_{33}H_{36}N_4O_6$; mol wt 584.66. C 67.79%, H 6.21%, N 9.58%, O 16.42%. Principal pigment of bile and constituent of many biliary calculi. Major end-product of the biological breakdown of heme, *q.v.* Bilirubin is the chromophore responsible for coloration in various forms of jaundice. Also found in blood serum, where it exists in four major forms: unconjugated bilirubin, the monoglucuronide, the diglucuronide, and albuminbound bilirubin. Most easily obtained from ox gallstones which are largely calcium bilirubinate: Städeler, *Ann.* **132**, 323 (1864); Küster, *Z. Physiol. Chem.* **94**, 136 (1915); **99**, 86 (1917); **121**, 80 (1922); Küster, Haas, *ibid.* **141**, 279 (1924); Fischer, *ibid.* **3**, 204 (1911); Fischer, Hess, *ibid.* **194**, 193 (1931). Isoln from pig bile: Gibson, Lowe, *J. Biol. Chem.* **XLI** (1938); Gray *et al.*, *J. Chem. Soc.* **1961**, 2264, 2268; from ox bile: Libowitzky, *Z. Physiol. Chem.* **263**, 267 (1940). Industrial isoln from ox bile using chlorobenzene as extractant: US 2166073; US 2331574; US 2363471; US 2386716. Structure and synthesis: Fischer, Plieninger, *Naturwissenschaften* **30**, 382 (1942); *Z. Physiol. Chem.* **274**, 231 (1942); *cf.* Fischer-Orth, *Die Chemie des Pyrrols* **II**, 1, 621 (Leipzig, 1937); Gray *et al.*, *Nature* **181**, 183 (1958); *eidem, J. Chem. Soc.* **1961**, 2276. Structure: Fog, Jellum, *Nature* **198**, 88 (1963). Configuration: Kuenzle *et al.*, *Biochem. J.* **133**, 364 (1973). X-ray analysis and structure: Bonnett *et al., J. Chem. Soc. Perkin Trans. 2* **1972**, 902, 1335; *Nature* **262**, 326 (1976). NMR conformation studies: D. Kaplan, G. Navon, *J. Chem. Soc. Perkin Trans. 2* **1981**, 1374. Separation of bilirubin species in serum and bile by reversed-phase HPLC: J. J. Lauff *et al.*, *J. Chromatogr.* **226**, 391 (1981); *eidem, Clin. Chem.* **29**, 800 (1983). Clinical importance of albumin-bound bilirubin: J. S. Weiss *et al.*, *N. Engl. J. Med.* **309**, 148 (1983). Comprehensive reviews: Lemberg, Legge, *Hematin Compounds and Bile Pigments* (New York, 1949); With, *Bile Pigments* (Academic Press, New York, 1968). Reviews of toxicity: D. Bratlid, *N. Y. State J. Med.* **91**, 489-493 (1991); R. P. Wennberg, *ibid.* 493-496.

   Light orange to deep reddish-brown monoclinic rhomboid, prisms, plates from chloroform. Gradually blackens on heating and does not melt. The greenish solns show a red fluorescence in ultraviolet light. A 0.001% soln in chloroform shows selective abs from 490 to 400 nm with a max at 453 nm; ε mM 60.7 ± 0.8. Practically insol in water. Sol in benzene, chloroform, chlorobenzene, carbon disulfide, acids, alkalies; slightly sol in alcohol, ether. Spreads on water. Penetrates into cholesterol, octadecylamine, and protein monolayers: Stenhagen, Rideal, *Biochem. J.* **33**, 1591 (1939).

1219. Biliverdine. [114-25-0] 3,18-Diethenyl-1,19,22,24-tetrahydro-2,7,13,17-tetramethyl-1,19-dioxo-21*H*-biline-8,12-dipropanoic acid; 1,19,22,24-tetrahydro-2,7,13,17-tetramethyl-1,19-dioxo-3,18-divinylbiline-8,12-dipropionic acid; 1,3,6,7-tetramethyl-4,5-dicarboxyethyl-2,8-divinylbilatriene; dehydrobilirubin; uteroverdine; oöcyan. $C_{33}H_{34}N_4O_6$; mol wt 582.65. C 68.03%, H 5.88%, N 9.62%, O 16.48%. Precursor of bilirubin. Formed in the body from hemoglobin. The bile of amphibia and of birds contains biliverdine only. Does not occur in normal human bile or normal human serum, but regularly accompanies bilirubin in the serum of patients with carcinomatous obstruction of the bile duct, and frequently in that of patients with liver cirrhosis, catarrhal jaundice, and bile duct occlusion by gallstones. Can be obtained by autooxidation of bilirubin in alkaline soln but the yield is poor: Lemberg, *Biochem. J.* **28**, 978 (1934); better yields by oxidation of bilirubin with ferric chloride in glacial acetic acid: Lemberg, *Ann.* **499**, 25 (1932); by coupled oxidation of hemoglobin and ascorbic acid: Lemberg *et al.*, *Biochem. J.* **35**, 363 (1941); by oxidation of bilirubin with ferric chloride in methanol: Gray *et al.*, *J. Chem. Soc.* **1961**, 2264. Crystal and molecular structure: W. S. Sheldrick, *J. Chem. Soc. Perkin Trans. 2* **1976**, 1457. Comprehensive reviews: Lemberg, Legge, *Hematin Compounds and Bile Pigments* (New York, 1949); With, *Bile Pigments* (Academic Press, New York, 1968).

Dark green plates or prisms with violet surface color from methanol. Does not melt, blackens and dec above 300°. Absorption spectrum: Gray *et al.*, *loc. cit.* Soluble in methanol, ether, chloroform, carbon disulfide, benzene, soln of alkali hydroxides. Gives the later color changes of the Gmelin test starting with green.

Dimethyl ester. $C_{35}H_{38}N_4O_6$. Green crystals from chloroform + petr ether. When produced from bilirubin, mp 215-223°; synthetic 206-209°; from hemin 208°; from hemoglobin 216°.

Dimethyl ester ferrichloride. $C_{35}H_{39}Cl_4FeN_4O_6$. (Green hemin ester), pleochroitic elongated platelets, no definite mp. Ferric chloride and HCl can be removed by washing the chloroform soln with water.

1220. Bilobalide. [33570-04-6] (3aS,5aR,8R,8aS,9R,10aS)-9-(1,1-Dimethylethyl)-10,10a-dihydro-8,9-dihydroxy-4H,5aH,9H-furo[2,3-b]furo[3′,2′:2,3]cyclopenta[1,2-c]furan-2,4,7(3H,8H)trione. $C_{15}H_{18}O_8$; mol wt 326.30. C 55.21%, H 5.56%, O 39.23%. Sesquiterpene isolated from the leaves of *Ginko biloba* L., *Ginkgoaceae*; closely related to the ginkgolides, *q.v.* Component of the *Ginkgo biloba* extract, EGb 761, *q.v.* Isoln: K. Weinges, W. Bähr, *Ann.* **724**, 214 (1969). NMR and MS analysis: *eidem*, *ibid.* **759**, 158 (1972). Structure determn: K. Nakanishi *et al.*, *J. Am. Chem. Soc.* **93**, 3544 (1971). Total synthesis of (±)-form: E. J. Corey, W. Su, *ibid.* **109**, 7534 (1987). Enantioselective synthesis of (−)-form: *eidem*, *Tetrahedron Lett.* **29**, 3423 (1988). Separation from *Ginkgo biloba* extracts: S. Jaracz *et al.*, *Phytochemistry* **65**, 2897 (2004). Neuroprotective effects in animal models of brain ischemia: K. Chandrasekaran *et al.*, *Brain Res.* **922**, 282 (2001). GABA$_A$ antagonist activity: S. H. Huang *et al.*, *Eur. J. Pharmacol.* **464**, 1 (2003). Review of neuroprotective properties: F. V. Defeudis, *Pharmacol. Res.* **46**, 565-568 (2002); of physical properties: T. A. van Beek, *Bioorg. Med. Chem.* **13**, 5001-5012 (2005).

Colorless crystals from water, mp >300°. $[\alpha]_{578}^{20}$ −64.3° (c = 2 in acetone).

1221. Bimatoprost. [155206-00-1] (5Z)-7-[(1R,2R,3R,5S)-3,5-Dihydroxy-2-[(1E,3S)-3-hydroxy-5-phenyl-1-pentenyl]cyclopentyl]-N-ethyl-5-heptenamide; (5Z,9α,11α,13E,15S)-9,11,15-trihydroxy-17-phenyl-18,19,20-trinorprosta-5,13-dienoicacidethylamide; 17-phenyl-18,19,20-trinorprostaglandin $F_{2\alpha}$ ethylamide; AGN-192024; Lumigan. $C_{25}H_{37}NO_4$; mol wt 415.57. C 72.25%, H 8.97%, N 3.37%, O 15.40%. Synthetic prostamide; structurally related to prostaglandin $F_{2\alpha}$, *q.v.* Prepn: D. F. Woodward *et al.*, **WO 9406433**; *eidem*, **US 6403649** (1994, 2002 both to Allergan). Series of articles on pharmacology and clinical experience: *Surv. Ophthalmol.* **45**, Suppl. 4, S335-S368 (2001). Pharmacology: D. F. Woodward *et al.*, *J. Pharmacol. Exp. Ther.* **305**, 772 (2003). Clinical comparison with timolol in glaucoma and ocular hypertension: J. D. Brandt *et al.*, *Ophthalmology* **108**, 1023 (2001). Clinical trial in glaucoma and ocular hypertension: R. Quinones *et al.*, *J. Ocul. Pharmacol. Ther.* **20**, 115 (2004). Review of pharmacology and clinical efficacy: L. B. Cantor, *Expert Opin. Invest. Drugs* **10**, 721-731 (2001); of mechanism of action: A. H.-P. Krauss, D. F. Woodward, *Surv. Ophthalmol.* **49**, Suppl. 1, S5-S11 (2004): of pharmacoeconomics of use: G. L. Plosker, S. J. Keam, *Pharmacoeconomics* **24**, 297-314 (2006).

Powder. Very sol in ethanol, methanol; slightly sol in water.
THERAP CAT: Antiglaucoma.

1222. Bimosiamose. [187269-40-5] 3′,3′″-(1,6-Hexanediyl)bis[6′-(α-D-mannopyranosyloxy)[1,1′-biphenyl]]-3-acetic acid; 1,6-bis[3-(3-carboxymethylphenyl)-4-(2-α-D-mannopyranosyloxy)phenyl]hexane; TBC-1269. $C_{46}H_{54}O_{16}$; mol wt 862.91. C 64.03%, H 6.31%, O 29.67%. Pan-selectin receptor antagonist. Prepn: T. P. Kogan *et al.*, **WO 9701335**; *eidem*, **US 5919768** (1997, 1999 both to Texas Biotechnol.); *eidem*, *J. Med. Chem.* **41**, 1099 (1998). Stereospecific synthesis: I. L. Scott *et al.*, *Carbohydr. Res.* **317**, 210 (1999). Review of pharmacology and clinical development: L. Pradella, *Curr. Opin. Anti-Inflam. Immunomod. Invest. Drugs* **1**, 56-60 (1999); E. Aydt, G. Wolff, *Pathobiology* **70**, 297-301 (2003). Clinical pharmacokinetics: M. Meyer *et al.*, *Int. J. Clin. Pharmacol. Ther.* **43**, 463 (2005). Clinical evaluation in allergic asthma: K. M. Beeh *et al.*, *Pulm. Pharmacol. Ther.* **19**, 233 (2006).

White solid, mp 115-117°.
Disodium salt. [187269-60-9] TBC-1269z. $C_{46}H_{52}Na_2O_{16}$; mol wt 906.88. Slightly hygroscopic white powder, mp 243-245°.
THERAP CAT: Anti-inflammatory

1223. BINAP. [98327-87-8] [1,1′-Binaphthalene]-2,2′-diylbis[diphenylphosphine]; 2,2′-bis(diphenylphosphino)-1,1′-binaphthyl. $C_{44}H_{32}P_2$; mol wt 622.67. C 84.87%, H 5.18%, P 9.95%. Axially dissymmetric bis(triaryl)phosphine ligand. Synthesis: A. Miyashita *et al.*, *J. Am. Chem. Soc.* **102**, 7932 (1980); preparative scale synthesis of enantiomers: *eidem*, *Tetrahedron* **40**, 1245 (1984). Review of asymmetric synthesis by metal-BINAP catalysts: S. Akutagawa, *Appl. Catal. A* **128**, 171-207 (1995). Review of industrial applications: H. Kumobayashi, *Rec. Trav. Chim.* **115**, 201-210 (1996); *idem et al.*, *Synlett* **2001**, S1 1055-1064.

(R)-form

(R)-(+)-Form. [76189-55-4] Crystals from benzene/ethanol, mp 240-241°. $[\alpha]_D^{25}$ +229° (c = 0.32 in benzene).

(S)-(−)-Form. [76189-56-5] Crystals from benzene/ethanol, mp 241-242°. $[\alpha]_D^{25}$ −229° (c = 0.31 in benzene).

USE: Chiral ligand for metal mediated asymmetric catalysis.

1224. Binifibrate. [69047-39-8] 3-Pyridinecarboxylic acid 2-[2-(4-chlorophenoxy)-2-methyl-1-oxopropoxy]-1,3-propanediyl ester; trihydroxypropane 2-p-chlorophenoxyisobutyrate-1,3-dinicotinate; 2-(p-chlorophenoxy)-2-methylpropionic acid ester with 1,3-dinicotinoyloxy-2-propanol; glyceryl 2-p-chlorophenoxyisobutyrate-1,3-dinicotinate; WAC-104; Biniwas. $C_{25}H_{23}ClN_2O_7$; mol wt 498.91. C 60.18%, H 4.65%, Cl 7.11%, N 5.61%, O 22.45%. Antilipemic agent structurally related to clofibrate, *q.v.* Prepn: R. Andreoli, X. Cicera, **ES 463218** (1978 to Soc. Espan. Espec. Farm.-Ter.), *C.A.* **90**, 72067h (1979); and pharmacology: *eidem*, **BE 884722** (1980 to Soc. Espan. Espec. Farm.-Ter.). Microhemorheological properties in animals: L. Bruseghini *et al., Arzneim.-Forsch.* **33**, 854 (1983); in patients: M. Dalmau *et al., ibid.* 858. Clinical evaluation: M. Labios *et al., Clin. Hemorheol. Microcirc.* **21**, 79 (1999).

Yellowish-white crystals from alcohol-isopropyl ether, mp 100°. Saponification number 166. LD_{50} orally in mice and rats: >4000 mg/kg (Andreoli).

THERAP CAT: Antilipemic.

1225. Binodenoson. [144348-08-3] 2-[(Cyclohexylmethylene)hydrazino]adenosine; MRE-0470; WRC-0470. $C_{17}H_{25}N_7O_4$; mol wt 391.42. C 52.16%, H 6.44%, N 25.05%, O 16.35%. A_{2A}-adenosine receptor agonist, more selective than adenosine, *q.v.* Prepn: R. A. Olsson, R. D. Thompson, **EP 567094**; *eidem*, **US 5278150** (1993, 1994 both to Whitby Research); K. Niiya *et al., J. Med. Chem.* **35**, 4557 (1992). Dose ranging and clinical evaluation as coronary vasodilator in myocardial imaging: J. E. Udelson *et al., Circulation* **109**, 457 (2004). Clinical pharmacokinetics: R. J. Barrett *et al., J. Nucl. Cardiol.* **12**, 166 (2005). Review: A. Zaza, *Curr. Opin. Cardiovasc. Pulm. Renal Invest. Drugs* **1**, 301-306 (1999).

Crystals from methanol/water, mp 154-157°.

THERAP CAT: Diagnostic aid (cardiac stress testing).

1226. BINOL. [602-09-5] [1,1′-Binaphthalene]-2,2′-diol; β-binaphthol; 2,2′-dihydroxy-1,1′-binaphthyl. $C_{20}H_{14}O_2$; mol wt 286.32. C 83.90%, H 4.93%, O 11.18%. C_2-symmetric ligand for metal-mediated stereoselective catalysis. Prepn: H. Walder, *Ber.* **15**, 2166 (1882). Resolution of enantiomers: E. P. Kyba *et al., J. Org. Chem.* **42**, 4173 (1977). Elucidation of catalyst structure: H. Sasai *et al., J. Am. Chem. Soc.* **115**, 10372 (1993). Effect of substituents on enantioselectivity: C. Qian *et al., J. Chem. Soc. Perkin Trans. 1* **1998**, 2097. Photochromism: M. Cavazza *et al., J. Am. Chem. Soc.* **118**, 9990 (1996). Review of role in catalysis: R. Zimmer, J. Suhrbier, *J. Prakt. Chem.* **339**, 758-762 (1997); with titanium: K. Mikami, *Pure Appl. Chem.* **68**, 639-644 (1996); with rare-earth metals: H. Sasai *et al., Chemtracts: Org. Chem.* **11**, 264-267 (1998); of synthesis and use as a chiral reagent and ligand: J. M. Brunel, *Chem. Rev.* **105**, 857-897 (2005).

Long flat lustrous white needles from alcohol, mp 216-218°.

(R)-(+)-Form. [18531-94-7] Crystals from benzene, mp 207.5-208.5°. $[\alpha]_{546}^{25}$ +50.9°; $[\alpha]_{589}^{25}$ +34.3° (c = 1.0 in THF).

(S)-(−)-Form. [18531-99-2] Crystals from benzene, mp 207-208°. $[\alpha]_{546}^{25}$ −51.3°; $[\alpha]_{589}^{25}$ −33.3° (c = 1.1 in THF).

USE: Chiral ligand.

1227. Biocytin. [576-19-2] N^6-[5-(Hexahydro-2-oxo-1H-thieno[3,4-d]imidazol-4-yl)-1-oxopentyl]-L-lysine; ε-N-biotinyl-L-lysine; biotin complex of yeast. $C_{16}H_{28}N_4O_4S$; mol wt 372.48. C 51.59%, H 7.58%, N 15.04%, O 17.18%, S 8.61%. A naturally occurring complex of biotin. Isoln: Wright *et al., J. Am. Chem. Soc.* **72**, 1048 (1950); **74**, 1996 (1952). Structure: Peck *et al., ibid.* **72**, 1048 (1950); **74**, 1999 (1952). Synthesis: Wolf *et al., ibid.* **74**, 2002 (1952); Weijlard *et al., ibid.* **76**, 2505 (1954); Wolf, Folkers, **US 2710298** (1955 to Merck & Co.). Purification: McCormick, Föry, *Methods Enzymol.* **18** (pt A), 413 (1970). *Review:* A. F. Wagner, K. Folkers, *Vitamins and Coenzymes* (Wiley, New York, 1964) pp 138-159.

Crystals, mp 241-243°. Upon rapid crystn from dil methanol or dil acetone, mp 228-230° (dec); upon slow crystn sinters at 227°. mp 245-252° (dec, microblock). Crystals from water, mp 228.5°. $[\alpha]_D^{25}$ +53° (c = 1.05 in 0.1N NaOH). Infrared absorption spectrum: *J. Am. Chem. Soc.* **74**, 2001 (1952). Freely sol in water, glacial acetic acid. Less sol in alc. Practically insol in acetone and most other organic solvents. When subjected to strong acid hydrolysis (at least 3N at 120° for one hour) biocytin yields biotin and L-lysine. Forms a crystalline hydrochloride. Biocytin is characterized microbiologically by its availability as a source of biotin to *Lactobacillus casei, L. delbrückii* LD 5, *L. acidophilus, Streptococcus fecalis* R, *Neurospora crassa,* and *Saccharomyces carlsbergensis* and by its unavailability as a source of biotin to *Lactobacillus arabinosus, L. pentosus,* and *Leuconostoc mesenteroides* P-60.

1228. Bioflavonoids. Vitamin P complex; citrus flavonoid compounds; Arliflav; Pecitrol Veinogène; C.V.P.. A group of compounds which contribute to the maintenance of normal blood vessel conditions by decreasing capillary permeability and fragility. Widely distributed among plants: J. B. Harborne, *Comparative Biochemistry of the Flavonoids* (Academic Press, New York, 1967). Biosynthesis: Grisebach, Barz, *Naturwissenschaften* **56**, 538 (1969). High concentrates can be obtained from all citrus fruits, rose hips, and black currants. Commercial methods extract the rinds of oranges, tangerines, lemons, limes, kumquats, and grapefruits. Solvents used in the extraction processes are aqueous alkalies, hot water, or water-miscible organic solvents, such as iso-propanol: Freedman *et al.,* **US 2888381** (1959 to U.S. Vitamin). Early interest in the compounds developed because of their syner-gistic effect with ascorbic acid. Other pharmacologic effects such as inhibition of adrenaline autooxidation and of enzyme action are also under study: several authors in *The Pharmacology of Plant Phenolics,* J. W. Fairbairn, Ed. (Academic Press, New York, 1959); several authors in *Angiologica* **9,** 133-446 (1972). Metabolism: DeEds, "Flavonoid Metabolism" in *Comprehensive Biology* **Vol. 20,** M. Florkin, E. H. Stotz, Eds. (Elsevier, New York, 1968). *Reviews:* Scarborough, Bacharach, *Vitam. Horm.* **7,** 1-55 (1949); Baier *et al., Ann. N.Y. Acad. Sci.* **61,** (Art. 3), 637-736 (1955); T. Robinson, *The Organic Constituents of Higher Plants* (Burgess, Minneapolis, 1967) pp 178-209; H. Geiger, C. Quinn in *Flavonoids,* J. B. Harborne *et al.,* Eds. (Academic Press, New York, 1975) pp 692-742.

THERAP CAT: Capillary protectant.

1229. Biopterin. [22150-76-1] 2-Amino-6-[(1*R*,2*S*)-1,2-di-hydroxypropyl]-4(1*H*)-pteridinone; 1-(2-amino-4-hydroxy-6-pteri-dinyl)-1,2-propanediol; 2-amino-4-hydroxy-6-(1,2-dihydroxypro-pyl)pteridine; pterin HB$_2$. C$_9$H$_{11}$N$_5$O$_3$; mol wt 237.22. C 45.57%, H 4.67%, N 29.52%, O 20.23%. A pteridine widely dis-tributed in nature; naturally occurring as the L-*erythro*-form. Con-sidered as a growth factor for some insects; *see also* Neopterin. Isoln from human urine: Patterson *et al., J. Am. Chem. Soc.* **77,** 3167 (1955); **78,** 5871 (1956); **GB 814462** (1959 to Am. Cyana-mid); from drosophila: H. S. Forrest, H. K. Mitchell, *J. Am. Chem. Soc.* **77,** 4865 (1955); from queen bee jelly: Butenandt, Rembold, *Z. Physiol. Chem.* **311,** 79 (1958). Absolute configuration: E. L. Patterson *et al., J. Am. Chem. Soc.* **78,** 5871 (1956). Synthesis: E. L. Patterson *et al., ibid.* 5868; Tschesche *et al., Ann.* **658,** 193 (1962); Rembold, Metzger, *Ber.* **96,** 1395 (1963); Viscontini *et al., Helv. Chim. Acta* **55,** 570, 574 (1972); B. Schircks *et al., ibid.* **60,** 211 (1977); T. Sugimoto *et al., Bull. Chem. Soc. Jpn.* **53,** 2344 (1980). Synthesis from neopterin: A. Kaiser, H. P. Wessel, *Helv. Chim. Acta* **70,** 766 (1987). Biosynthesis: G. Kapatos *et al., Science* **213,** 1129 (1981).

Minute, yellow, spherical crystals from water. Chars without melting at 250-280°. $[\alpha]_D^{24}$ −50° (c = 0.4 in 0.1*N* HCl); $[\alpha]_D^{24}$ −26° (c = 0.92 in 0.1*N* NaOH). uv max (0.08*N* HCl): 247 nm (ε 11000). Soly in water: 0.7 mg/ml (20°); 4 mg/ml (90°). Soly in alc, ether, acetone, benzene: <0.1 mg/ml; in 1*N* NaOH, 1*N* HCl: >25 mg/ml. Fluoresces with a blue color in alkaline soln.

1230. Bioresmethrin. [28434-01-7] (1*R*,3*R*)-2,2-Dimethyl-3-(2-methyl-1-propenyl)cyclopropanecarboxylic acid [5-(phenyl-methyl)-3-furanyl]methyl ester; *trans*-(+)-2,2-dimethyl-3-(2-meth-ylpropenyl)cyclopropanecarboxylic acid (5-benzyl-3-furyl)methyl ester; 5-benzyl-3-furylmethyl-(+)-*trans*-chrysanthemate; *d-trans*-[(5-benzyl-3-furyl)methyl]chrysanthemumate; (+)-*trans*-resmeth-rin; NRDC-107; NIA-18739; SBP-1390; Resbuthrin; Biobenzyfuro-line. C$_{22}$H$_{26}$O$_3$; mol wt 338.44. C 78.07%, H 7.74%, O 14.18%. Synthetic pyrethroid insecticide. Prepn: M. Elliott, N. F. Janes, **FR 1503260;** *eidem,* **US 3465007** and **US 3542928** (1967, 1969, 1970, all to Nat. Res. Dev. Corp.). Insecticidal activity: M. Elliott *et al., Nature* **213,** 493 (1967); *idem, et al., Pestic. Sci.* **2,** 243 (1971). Mammalian metabolism: C. O. Abernathy, J. E. Casida, *Science* **179,** 1235 (1973). Control of cockroaches: P. R. Chadwick *et al., J. Med. Entomol.* **13,** 625 (1977). Acute toxicity: T. B. Gaines, R. E. Linder, *Fundam. Appl. Toxicol.* **7,** 299 (1986). Brief review: D. S. Gunew, *Anal. Methods Pestic. Plant Growth Regul.* **10,** 19-29 (1978). Review of toxicology and human exposure: *Toxicological Profile for Pyrethrins and Pyrethroids* (PB2004-100004, 2003) 332 pp.

bp$_{0.0008}$ 174°. n_D^{20} 1.5346. $[\alpha]_D^{20}$ −7.8° (c = 5 in acetone). Sol in most organic solvents. Insol in water. LD$_{50}$ in adult male, female rats (mg/kg): 1244, 1721 orally (Gaines, Linder).

USE: Insecticide.

1231. Biotin. [58-85-5] Hexahydro-2-oxo-1*H*-thieno[3,4-*d*]imidazole-4-pentanoic acid; *cis*-tetrahydro-2-oxothieno[3,4-*d*]imidazoline-4-valeric acid; *cis*-hexahydro-2-oxo-1*H*-thieno[3,-4]imidazole-4-valeric acid; vitamin H; coenzyme R; bios II; Bio-dermatin. C$_{10}$H$_{16}$N$_2$O$_3$S; mol wt 244.31. C 49.16%, H 6.60%, N 11.47%, O 19.65%, S 13.12%. Growth factor present in minute amounts in every living cell. Plays an indispensable role in numer-ous naturally occurring carboxylation reactions. Occurs mainly bound to proteins or polypeptides. The richest sources are liver, kidney, pancreas, yeast, and milk. The biotin content of cancerous tumors is higher than that of normal tissue. Biotin combines with the proteinaceous substance, avidin, in raw egg-white and becomes inactive. When on diets contg large amounts of raw egg-white the rat or chick develops characteristic skin lesions and growth is re-tarded; these symptoms can be prevented by feeding additional biotin. Isoln from egg yolk: Kögl, Tönnis, *Z. Physiol. Chem.* **242,** 43 (1936); from liver: György *et al., J. Biol. Chem.* **131,** 745 (1939); du Vigneaud *et al., ibid.* **140,** 643 (1941). Identity of biotin with vitamin H: du Vigneaud *et al., Science* **92,** 62 (1940). Structure: du Vigneaud *et al., J. Biol. Chem.* **146,** 475 (1942). First synthesis: Harris *et al., J. Am. Chem. Soc.* **67,** 2096 (1945). Con-figuration: Traub, *Nature* **178,** 649 (1956). Stereospecific total synthesis of the naturally occurring *d*-form: P. N. Confalone *et al., J. Am. Chem. Soc.* **97,** 5936 (1975); *eidem, J. Org. Chem.* **42,** 1630 (1977); T. Ogawa *et al., Carbohydr. Res.* **57,** C31 (1977); F. G. M. Vogel *et al., Ann.* **1980,** 1972; R. R. Schmidt, M. Maier, *Synthesis* **1982,** 747. Synthesis of the *dl*-form: P. N. Confalone *et al., Helv. Chim. Acta* **59,** 1005 (1976); M. Marx *et al., J. Am. Chem. Soc.* **99,** 6794 (1977); A. Fliri, K. Hohenlohe-Oehringen, *Ber.* **113,** 607 (1980); Ph. Rossy *et al., Tetrahedron Lett.* **22,** 3493 (1981). Bio-synthetic studies: R. J. Parry, M. G. Kunitani, *J. Am. Chem. Soc.* **98,** 4024 (1976); R. J. Parry, M. V. Naidu, *Tetrahedron Lett.* **1980,** 4783. Coordination properties: H. Siegel, *Experientia* **37,** 789 (1981). Mechanism of action: M. J. Cravey, H. Kohn, *J. Am. Chem. Soc.* **102,** 3928 (1980); D. L. Vesely, *Science* **216,** 1329 (1982). *Re-views:* A. F. Wagner, K. Folkers, *Vitamins and Coenzymes* (Wiley, New York, 1964) pp 138-159; Harris in *The Vitamins* **vol. II,** W. H. Sebrell, R. S. Harris, Eds. (Academic Press, New York, 2nd ed., 1968) pp 261-359; D. B. McCormick, *Nutr. Rev.* **33,** 97-102 (1975). Review of assay methods: P. György, *The Vitamins* **vol. VII,** P. Gyorgy, W. N. Pearson, Eds. (1967) pp 303-313.

Characteristics of biotin isolated from liver or milk (Kögl's *β*-biotin): fine long needles, mp 232-233°. $[\alpha]_D^{21}$ +91° (c = 1 in 0.1*N* NaOH). Isoelec pt pH 3.5. pH of 0.01% aq soln 4.5. Soly at 25° (mg/100 ml): water ~22; 95% alc ~80. More sol in hot water and in dil alkali. Insol in other common organic solvents. The pure compd is stable to air and temp. Moderately acid and neutral solns are stable several months; alkaline solns are less stable, but appear reasonably stable up to a pH of about 9. Aq solns are very suscep-tible to mold growth. Acidic solns can be heat sterilized.

THERAP CAT: Vitamin (enzyme cofactor).

THERAP CAT (VET): Vitamin (enzyme cofactor).

1232. Biotin *l*-Sulfoxide. [3376-83-8] [3a*S*-(3aα,4β,5β,-6aα)]-Hexahydro-2-oxo-1*H*-thieno[3,4-*d*]imidazole-4-pentanoic acid 5-oxide; AN factor. C$_{10}$H$_{16}$N$_2$O$_4$S; mol wt 260.31. C

46.14%, H 6.20%, N 10.76%, O 24.59%, S 12.32%. Isolated from *Aspergillus niger* culture filtrate where growth had taken place in the presence of pimelic acid; also from milk residue concentrates or by synthesis: Melville, *J. Biol. Chem.* **208**, 495 (1954); Wright *et al., J. Am. Chem. Soc.* **76**, 4163 (1954).

Polymorphic plates from water, mp 238° (some dec). $[\alpha]_D^{20}$ $-39.5°$ (c = 1.01 in 0.1N NaOH). Ineffective in curing the biotin deficiency syndrome when administered to rats at a level 100 times the effective dose of biotin.

1233. Biperiden. [514-65-8] α-Bicyclo[2.2.1]hept-5-en-2-yl-α-phenyl-1-piperidinepropanol; α-5-norbornen-2-yl-α-phenyl-1-piperidinepropanol; 3-piperidino-1-phenyl-1-bicycloheptenyl-1-propanol; 1-bicycloheptenyl-1-phenyl-3-piperidinopropanol; 3-piperidino-1-phenyl-(Δ^5-bicyclo[2.2.1]hepten-2-yl)-1-propanol; KL-373. $C_{21}H_{29}NO$; mol wt 311.46. C 80.98%, H 9.38%, N 4.50%, O 5.14%. Prepn: W. Klavehn, US 2789110 (1957 to Knoll). Toxicology study: C. Hanna, *Toxicol. Appl. Pharmacol.* **2**, 379 (1960).

Crystals, mp 101°. Difficultly sol in water; slightly sol in ethanol; readily sol in methanol. LD$_{50}$ in mice (mg/kg): 195 s.c., 56 i.v. (Klavehn).

Hydrochloride. [1235-82-1] Akineton; Akinophyl. $C_{21}H_{29}$-NO.HCl; mol wt 347.92. Fluffy white powder, mp 238°. Soly in water (mg/100 ml) at 30°: 220 (pH 3.8), 280 (pH 5.5), 290 (pH 6.7), 264 (pH 7.9), 244 (9.2-10.1). LD$_{50}$ in rats, dogs (mg/kg): 750, 340 orally (Hanna).

THERAP CAT: Antiparkinsonian.

1234. Biphenamine. [3572-52-9] β-Diethylaminoethyl 2-hydroxy-3-phenylbenzoate; 2-diethylaminoethyl 3-phenylsalicylate; 2-diethylaminoethyl 2-hydroxy-3-biphenylcarboxylate; 3-phenylsalicylic acid 2-diethylaminoethyl ester; xenysalate. C_{19}-$H_{23}NO_3$; mol wt 313.39. C 72.82%, H 7.40%, N 4.47%, O 15.32%. Prepn: Sahyun, US 2594350 (1952).

Oily liquid. Sol in water.
Hydrochloride. [5560-62-3] Sebaclen; Sebaklen. $C_{19}H_{23}$-NO$_3$.HCl; mol wt 349.85.

THERAP CAT: Anesthetic (local); antibacterial; antifungal.

1235. *p*-Biphenylamine. [92-67-1] [1,1'-Biphenyl]-4-amine; 4-aminobiphenyl; *p*-aminodiphenyl; anilinobenzene; xenylamine. $C_{12}H_{11}N$; mol wt 169.22. C 85.17%, H 6.55%, N 8.28%. Prepn from diazoaminobenzene: Heusler, *Ann.* **260**, 232 (1890). Review of carcinogenicity studies: *IARC Monographs* **1**, 74-79 (1972).

Leaflets from alc or water. mp 53°. Volatile with steam. Slightly sol in cold water, readily sol in hot water, alcohol, chloroform.

Caution: Potential symptoms of overexposure are headache, dizziness; lethargy, dyspnea; ataxia, weakness; methemoglobinemia; urinary burning; acute hemorrhagic cystitis. *See NIOSH Pocket Guide to Chemical Hazards* (DHHS/NIOSH 97-140, 1997) p 14. This substance is listed as a known human carcinogen: *Report on Carcinogens, Eleventh Edition* (PB2005-104914, 2004) p III-13.

USE: In the detection of sulfates. Formerly as rubber antioxidant. As carcinogen in cancer research.

1236. 2,4'-Biphenyldiamine. [492-17-1] Diphenyline; 2,4'-diphenyldiamine; *o,p'*-dianiline; 2,4'-diaminodiphenyl. $C_{12}H_{12}N_2$; mol wt 184.24. C 78.23%, H 6.56%, N 15.20%. Preparation by reducing azobenzene with tin and hydrochloric acid: Fischer, *Monatsh. Chem.* **6**, 547 (1885).

Needles from dil alc, mp 45°. bp 363°. Very slightly sol in alc or ether.

USE: Detection of tungsten; manuf azo dyes.

1237. Bipiperidyl Mustard. [6802-93-3] 1,1'-Bis(2-chloro-ethyl)-4,4'-bipiperidine; BPM. $C_{14}H_{26}Cl_2N_2$; mol wt 293.28. C 57.33%, H 8.94%, Cl 24.18%, N 9.55%. Obesifying agent causing rapid lipid deposition in mice: Rutman *et al., Science* **153**, 1000 (1966). Activity shown only by the active form, prepd by neutralizing the conjugate acid form and generating a bicyclic ammonium deriv at pH 10. Metabolic studies: *eidem, Trans. N.Y. Acad. Sci.* **30**, 244 (1967). Research use for obesity-producing brain lesions: H.-R. Berthoud, T. L. Powley, *Am. J. Physiol.* **248**, R46 (1985); A. C. Scallet, J. W. Olney, *Brain Res.* **374**, 380 (1986). Toxicity study: E. W. Schafer, Jr. *et al., Ecotoxicol. Environ. Saf.* **6**, 149 (1982).

LD$_{50}$ orally in male quail: 75.0 mg/kg (Schafer).

1238. Birch Tar Oil, Empyreumatic. Oil white birch; oleum rusci. Obtained by destructive distillation of the bark and wood of *Betula alba* L., *Betulaceae* (white birch). *Constit.* Oil turpentine, other isomeric hydrocarbons, various empyreumatic resins, guaiacol, cresol, pyrocatechol, betulin.

Black, viscid liquid; characteristic odor. d 0.926-0.955. Partly sol in alcohol; sol in chloroform, fats, oils.

USE: For preserving leather and wood.

1239. Birch Tar Oil, Rectified. "Essential oil of birch wood". Obtained from the empyreumatic oil by steam distillation. *Constit.* Phenol, cresol, xylenol, guaiacol, creosol, pyrocatechol.

Dark brown liquid. d 0.886-0.950. One ml dissolves in about 3 ml abs alcohol; sol in benzene, chloroform, ether, glacial acetic acid, carbon disulfide, oil turpentine.

THERAP CAT: Dermatologic.

THERAP CAT (VET): Has been used extern. in skin diseases.

1240. Biricodar. [159997-94-1] (2S)-1-[Oxo(3,4,5-trimethoxyphenyl)acetyl]-2-piperidinecarboxylic acid 4-(3-pyridinyl)-1-[3-(3-pyridinyl)propyl]butyl ester. $C_{34}H_{41}N_3O_7$; mol wt 603.71. C 67.64%, H 6.85%, N 6.96%, O 18.55%. Chemosensitizer that restores sensitivity to cytotoxic agents in multidrug resistant (MDR) cells. Prepn: D. M. Armistead *et al.,* WO 9407858; *eidem,* US 5620971 (1994, 1997 both to Vertex). Effect on MDR mediated by P-glycoprotein: U. A. Germann *et al., Anti-Cancer Drugs* **8**, 125 (1997); by multidrug resistance-associated protein (MRP): *eidem, ibid.* 141. Clinical pharmacology, pharmacokinetics: E. K. Rowinsky *et al., J. Clin. Oncol.* **16**, 2964 (1998).

Dicitrate. [174254-13-8] VX-710; Incel. $C_{34}H_{41}N_3O_7.2C_6$-H_8O_7; mol wt 987.95. Sol in water.

THERAP CAT: Antineoplastic adjunct (chemosensitizer).

1241. α-Bisabolol. [515-69-5] ($\alpha R,1R$)-*rel*-α,4-Dimethyl-α-(4-methyl-3-pentenyl)-3-cyclohexene-1-methanol; 6-methyl-2-(4-methyl-3-cyclohexen-1-yl)-5-hepten-2-ol; 1-methyl-4-(1,5-dimethyl-1-hydroxyhex-4(5)-enyl)cyclohexen-1; Camilol; Dragosantol; Hydagen B. $C_{15}H_{26}O$; mol wt 222.37. C 81.02%, H 11.79%, O 7.19%. Fragrant sesquiterpene isolated from the essential oils of a variety of plants, shrubs and trees. Both isomers occur in nature; the (−)-form is the most widespread and is an active anti-inflammatory component of chamomile. The (+) and (−)-epi isomers are also naturally occurring. Isoln of (−)-form from *Matricaria chamomilla*: F. Sorm *et al., Collect. Czech. Chem. Commun.* **16**, 626 (1951); of (+)-form from Populus balsamifera: *idem et al., Chem. Listy* **46**, 364 (1952). Synthesis of racemic mixture: L. Ruzicka, M. Liguori, *Helv. Chim. Acta* **15**, 3 (1932); C. D. Gutsche *et al., Tetrahedron* **24**, 859 (1968). Enantioselective synthesis of (−)-form: H. Nemoto *et al., Tetrahedron Lett.* **34**, 4939 (1993). Separation of four stereoisomers: K. Günther *et al., Fresenius J. Anal. Chem.* **345**, 787 (1993). Pharmacology and toxicology of (−)-form: V. Jakovlev, A. von Schlichtegroll, *Arzneim.-Forsch.* **19**, 615 (1969); S. Habersang *et al., Planta Med.* **37**, 115 (1979). Comparative pharmacology of racemate and enantiomers: V. Jakovlev *et al., ibid.* **35**, 125 (1979). Determn by HPLC in chamomile extracts: R. Herrmann, *Dtsch. Apoth. Ztg.* **36**, 1797 (1982); by GC in cosmetic products: D. Andre *et al., Int. J. Cosmet. Sci.* **13**, 137 (1991). Evaluation of use as dermal penetration enhancer: R. Kadir, B. W. Barry, *Int. J. Pharm.* **70**, 87 (1991). Review of anti-inflammatory activity and use in cosmetics: N. Jellinek, *Parfums Cosmet. Aromes* **57**, 55-57 (1984); of absolute configuration studies: G. W. O'Donnell, M. D. Sutherland, *Aust. J. Chem.* **42**, 2021-2034 (1989).

(−)-form

bp$_{12}$ 155-157°. d$_4^{23}$ 0.9223. n$_D^{23}$ 1.4917. Also reported as colorless oil, bp$_{1.5}$ 128-130° (Gutsche). Miscible with alcohols, oils and lipophilic substances.

(−)-Form. [23089-26-1] ($\alpha S,1S$)-α-Bisabolol; levomenol. bp$_{12}$ 153°. d^{20} 0.9211. n$_D^{20}$ 1.4936. [α]$_D$ −55.7°. Also reported as [α]$_D^{20}$ −51.02° (Günther). LD$_{50}$ in mice, rats (mg/kg): 11350, 14850 orally (Jakovlev, von Schlichtegroll). LD$_{50}$ in male, female mice, rats (ml/kg): 15.2, 15.0, 14.9, 15.6 orally (Habersang).

(+)-Form. [23178-88-3] ($\alpha R,1R$)-α-Bisabolol. bp$_{1.0}$ 120-122°. d^{20} 0.9213. n$_D^{20}$ 1.4919. [α]$_D^{20}$ +51.7°. Also reported as [α]$_D^{20}$ +57.04° (Günther).

(−)-Epi-α-bisabolol. [78148-59-1] ($\alpha R,1S$)-α-Bisabolol; anymol. Isoln from *Myoporum crassifolium*: K. G. O'Brien *et al., Aust. J. Chem.* **6**, 166 (1953). [α]$_D^{20}$ −67.6°. Also reported as [α]$_D^{20}$ −67.48° (Günther).

(+)-Epi-α-bisabolol. [76738-75-5] ($\alpha S,1R$)-α-Bisabolol. Isoln from *Salvia stenophylla*: E. J. Brunke, F. J. Hammerschmidt, *Proc.*

15th Int. Symp. Essent. Oils Aromat. Plants **1985**, 145. [α]$_D^{20}$ +67.4°. Also reported as [α]$_D^{20}$ +70.11° (Günther).

USE: In cosmetics.

THERAP CAT: Anti-inflammatory.

1242. Bisacodyl. [603-50-9] 4,4'-(2-Pyridylmethylene)bis-phenol diacetate; bis(*p*-acetoxyphenyl)-2-pyridylmethane; (4,4'-diacetoxydiphenyl)(2-pyridyl)methane; 2-(4,4'-diacetoxydiphenyl-methyl)pyridine; Contalax; Correctol; Dulcolax; Durolax; Ex-Lax Ultra; Gentlax; Laxadin; Perilax; Pyrilax; Stadalax. $C_{22}H_{19}NO_4$; mol wt 361.39. C 73.12%, H 5.30%, N 3.88%, O 17.71%. Prepn: **GB 730243**; A. Kottler, E. Seeger, **US 2764590** (1955, 1956 both to Thomae). Pharmacology and toxicology: Schmidt, *Arzneim.-Forsch.* **3**, 19 (1953). Comparison of efficacy and safety with other stimulant laxatives: A. Wald, *J. Clin. Gastroenterol.* **36**, 386 (2003).

Tasteless crystals, mp 138°. Practically insol in water and alkaline solns. Sol in acids, alc, acetone, propylene glycol, and other organic solvents. LD$_{50}$ orally in rats: >3 g/kg (Schmidt).

Complex with tannin. [1336-29-4] Bisacodyl tannex; Clysodrast.

THERAP CAT: Cathartic.

1243. Bis(4-amino-1-anthraquinonyl)amine. [128-87-0] 1,1'-Iminobis[4-amino-9,10-anthracenedione]; 4,4'-diamino-1,1'-dianthraquinonylamine; 4,4'-diamino-1,1'-anthrimide; 4,4'-diamino-1,1'-iminobisanthraquinone. $C_{28}H_{17}N_3O_4$; mol wt 459.45. C 73.20%, H 3.73%, N 9.15%, O 13.93%. Prepn: **DE 255822** (1913); *Frdl.* **11**, 615; Tinker, Stallmann, **US 2420022** (1947), *C.A.* **41**, 5730 (1947).

On heating with fuming sulfuric acid (30% SO$_3$) at 100° yields a dark powder, sol in water or alc with bluish-black coloration, used as dyestuff for wool. On heating with molten potassium hydroxide at 190° and oxidizing the reaction product with sodium hypochlorite, an olive-green vat dye is obtained.

USE: In the textile industry; in the determination of boron: Beckett, Webster, *Analyst* **68**, 306 (1943), *C.A.* **38**, 38 (1944).

1244. Bisantrene. [78186-34-2] 9,10-Anthracenedicarboxaldehyde bis[[(4,5-dihydro-1*H*-imidazol-2-yl)hydrazone]; 9,10-anthracenedicarboxaldehyde bis(2-imidazolin-2-ylhydrazone). $C_{22}H_{22}N_8$; mol wt 398.46. C 66.31%, H 5.57%, N 28.12%. Prepn: K. C. Murdock *et al.*, **DE 2850822**; K. C. Murdock, F. E. Durr, **US 4258181** (1979, 1981 both to Am. Cyanamid); and antitumor activity: K. C. Murdock *et al., J. Med. Chem.* **25**, 505 (1982). Crystallographic characterization of hydrochloride: R. B. Bates *et al., Acta Crystallogr.* **C42**, 186 (1986); C. G. Pierpont, S. A. Lang, Jr., *ibid.* 1085. HPLC determn in plasma: Y.-M. Peng *et al., J. Chromatogr.* **233**, 235 (1982). Antitumor activity *in vitro*: J. D. Cowan *et al., Invest. New Drugs* **1**, 139 (1983); *in vivo*: R. V. Citarella *et al., Cancer Res.* **42**, 440 (1982). Clinical pharmacokinetics: K. Lu *et al., Cancer Chemother. Pharmacol.* **16**, 156 (1986). Clinical trials in breast cancer: H.-Y. Yap *et al., Cancer Res.* **43**, 1402 (1983); C. K. Osborne *et al., Cancer Treat. Rep.* **68**, 357 (1984).

Dihydrochloride. [71439-68-4] ADAH; ADCA; NSC-337766; CL-216942; Orange Crush; Zantrène. $C_{22}H_{22}N_8 \cdot 2HCl$; mol wt 471.39. Crystalline orange solid from ethanol. Hemihydrate, mp 288-289° (dec). uv max (H_2O) 260, 415 nm (ε 72700, 16300).

THERAP CAT: Antineoplastic.

1245. 2,5-Bis(1-aziridinyl)-3,6-bis(2-methoxyethoxy)-1,4-benzoquinone. [800-24-8] 2,5-Bis(1-aziridinyl)-3,6-bis(2-methoxyethoxy)-2,5-cyclohexadiene-1,4-dione; Bayer E 39 soluble. $C_{16}H_{22}N_2O_6$; mol wt 338.36. C 56.79%, H 6.55%, N 8.28%, O 28.37%. Prepn: Gauss, Petersen, *Angew. Chem.* **69**, 252 (1957); **GB 793796** (1958 to Bayer). Antineoplastic activity *in vitro:* M. Akhtar *et al., Can. J. Chem.* **53**, 2891 (1975); J. S. Driscoll *et al., J. Pharm. Sci.* **68**, 185 (1979).

Gray needles from petr ether, mp 79-80.5°: Gauss, Petersen, *Med. Chem.* (Bayer) **7**, 649 (1963), *C.A.* **60**, 2875i (1964).

1246. Bisbentiamine. [2667-89-2] *N,N'*-[Dithiobis[2-[2-(benzoyloxy)ethyl]-1-methyl-2,1-ethenediyl]]bis[*N*-[(4-amino-2-methyl-5-pyrimidinyl)methyl]formamide]; *N,N'*-[dithiobis[2-(2-hydroxyethyl)-1-methylvinylene]]bis[*N*-[(4-amino-2-methyl-5-pyrimidinyl)methyl]formamide] dibenzoate; *O*-benzoylthiamine disulfide; Béprocin; Beston. $C_{38}H_{42}N_8O_6S_2$; mol wt 770.92. C 59.20%, H 5.49%, N 14.54%, O 12.45%, S 8.32%. Prepn: **GB 922444** (1963 to Tanabe Seiyaku) corresp to **US 3109000** (1963); Yurugi *et al., Annu. Rep. Takeda Res. Lab.* **27**, 25 (1968), *C.A.* **70**, 96741m (1968); Imai, Miyaji, **DE 1954519** (1971 to Hitachi), *C.A.* **75**, 63821n (1971).

cis-form

Prisms from alc, mp 146-147°.
THERAP CAT: Vitamin B_1 source.

1247. Bis(*p*-chlorophenoxy)methane. [555-89-5] 1,1'-[Methylenebis(oxy)]bis[4-chloro]benzene; di-(*p*-chlorophenoxy)methane; DCPM; K-1875; Neotran. $C_{13}H_{10}Cl_2O_2$; mol wt 269.12. C 58.02%, H 3.75%, Cl 26.35%, O 11.89%. Prepd from *p*-chlorophenol and dichloromethane: Moyl, **US 2503207** (1950 to Dow); from sodium phenolate and dichloromethane: Miron, Lowry, *J. Am. Chem. Soc.* **73**, 1872 (1951). Toxicology: H. C. Spencer *et al., Arch. Ind. Hyg. Occup. Med.* **1**, 341 (1950).

Crystals from petr ether. mp 69.7-70.2°. bp$_6$ 189-194°. Solubilities at 25° in g/100 ml: acetone 189; benzene 40; carbon tetrachloride 28; methanol 0.5; ether 87. Very sol in ethyl ether. Practically insol in water, petr oils, naphtha. LD$_{50}$ orally in rats: 5.8 g/kg (Spencer).

USE: Miticide.

1248. Bisdequalinium Chloride. [52951-36-7] 6,7,8,9,10,-11,12,13,14,15,16,17,24,25,26,27,28,29,30,31,32,33-Docosahydro-35,37-dimethyl-5,34:18,23-diethenodibenzo[*b,r*][1,5,16,20]tetraazacyclotriacontine-23,34-diium dichloride; $N^1,N^{1'}$-decamethylene-$N^4,N^{4'}$-decamethylenebis[4-aminoquinaldinium chloride]; 1,1'-decamethylene-4,4'-(1,10-decamethylenediimino)bis[quinaldinium chloride]; Salvizol. $C_{40}H_{58}Cl_2N_4$; mol wt 665.82. C 72.16%, H 8.78%, Cl 10.65%, N 8.41%. Prepn: Stark, **GB 895090** (1960).

THERAP CAT: Antiseptic, disinfectant.

1249. Bis(*p*-dimethylaminobenzylidene)benzidine. [6001-51-0] *N,N'*-Bis[[4-(dimethylamino)phenyl]methylene][1,1'-biphenyl]-4,4'-diamine; 4,4'-di(4-dimethylaminobenzylideneamino)-biphenyl;bis(4-dimethylaminobenzylidene)-*p,p'*-diaminodiphenyl; *N,N'*-bis(*p*-dimethylaminobenzal)benzidine. $C_{30}H_{30}N_4$; mol wt 446.59. C 80.68%, H 6.77%, N 12.55%. Prepn from hydrazobenzene and *p*-dimethylaminobenzaldehyde: Sachs, Whittaker, *Ber.* **35**, 1435 (1902).

Yellow crystals from nitrobenzene; mp 318°. Reacts with solutions of the alkali tungstates to give a cinnabar-red precipitate.

USE: Determination of tungsten: Hovorka, *Collect. Czech. Chem. Commun.* **10**, 518 (1938), *C.A.* **33**, 1624 (1939).

1250. Bis(1,2-dimethylpropyl)borane. [1069-54-1] Disiamylborane; di-*sec*-isoamylborine; bis(3-methyl-2-butyl)borane. $C_{10}H_{23}B$; mol wt 154.10. C 77.94%, H 15.04%, B 7.02%. Prepn: Brown, Zweifel, *J. Am. Chem. Soc.* **83**, 1241 (1961). Use in selective reductions: G. W. Kabalka, C. F. Lane, *Chem. Tech.* **6**, 324 (1976).

Crystals, mp 35-40°. Unstable to air.
USE: Selective reagent for steric control of hydroboration of olefins.

1251. Bis(2-ethylhexyl) Sebacate. [122-62-3] Decanedioic acid bis(2-ethylhexyl) ester; di(2-ethylhexyl) sebacate; Octoil S; Plexol 201. $C_{26}H_{50}O_4$; mol wt 426.67. C 73.19%, H 11.81%, O 15.00%. Prepn: Bruno, **US 2628249** (1953 to Pittsburgh Coke & Chemical); **GB 747260** (1956 to Chemische Werke Hüls).

Liquid, d_{25}^{25} 0.9119, n_D^{25} 1.4496.
USE: In vacuum pumps.

1252. Bismark Brown R. [8005-78-5] 4,4′-[(4-Methyl-1,3-phenylene)bis(azo)]bis[6-methyl-1,3-benzenediamine] dihydrochloride; C.I. Basic Brown 4; 5,5′-[(4-methyl-*m*-phenylene)-bis(azo)]bis[toluene-2,4-diamine] dihydrochloride; C.I. 21010; Bismark Brown 53; Vesuvine. $C_{21}H_{26}Cl_2N_8$; mol wt 461.39. C 54.67%, H 5.68%, Cl 15.37%, N 24.29%. Prepd by reaction of toluene-2,4-diamine HCl with nitrous acid: *Colour Index* **vol. 4** (3rd ed., 1971) p 4154.

2HCl

Dark brown solid. Very sol in water (yellowish-brown soln); sol in ethanol, Cellosolve; slightly sol in acetone; practically insol in benzene. In concd H_2SO_4 gives brown soln which on dilution turns reddish-brown; in concd HNO_3 gives violet soln which turns brown.

Free base. C.I. Solvent Brown 12; C.I. 21010:1. $C_{21}H_{24}N_8$. mp 130-135°. Very slightly sol in water; sol in ethanol, acetone.

USE: As textile dye, leather dye, biological stain.

1253. Bismark Brown Y. [10114-58-6] 4,4′-[1,3-Phenylenebis(azo)]bis[1,3-benzenediamine] dihydrochloride; C.I. Basic Brown 1; 4,4′-[*m*-phenylenebis(azo)]bis[*m*-phenylenediamine] dihydrochloride; C.I. 21000; phenylene brown. $C_{18}H_{20}Cl_2N_8$; mol wt 419.31. C 51.56%, H 4.81%, Cl 16.91%, N 26.72%. Prepd by reaction of *m*-phenylenediamine HCl and nitrous acid: F. J. Welcher, *Organic Analytical Reagents* (D. Van Nostrand Co., New York, 1948) p 339; *Colour Index* **vol. 4** (3rd ed., 1971) p 4154.

2 HCl

Blackish-brown powder. Very sol in water; slightly sol in ethanol, Cellosolve. Practically insol in acetone, benzene carbon tetrachloride. In concd H_2SO_4 gives brown soln; in concd nitric acid gives orange soln which turns yellow.

USE: As a textile dye, biological stain.

1254. Bis(2-mercaptoethyl)sulfone. [145626-87-5] 2,2′-Sulfonylbis(ethanethiol); BMS. $C_4H_{10}O_2S_3$; mol wt 186.32. C 25.79%, H 5.41%, O 17.17%, S 51.63%. Reducing agent for proteins. Prepn: G. V. Lamoureux, G. M. Whitesides, *J. Org. Chem.* **58**, 633 (1993). Enhanced reduction rate in comparison with dithiothreitol, *q.v.*: R. Singh, G. M. Whitesides, *Bioorg. Chem.* **22**, 109 (1994). Use in reduction of disulfide bonds: D. Winitz *et al., J. Biol. Chem.* **271**, 27645 (1996); A. Brunella, O. Ghisalba, *J. Mol. Catal. B* **10**, 215 (2000); S. Lee, J. P. N. Rosazza, *Org. Lett.* **6**, 365 (2004).

White fluffy crystals from hexane, mp 57-58°. pKa (aqueous soln at 25°): 7.9, 9.0. Keq (for the reduction of DTT): 0.35

USE: Reagent for reduction of disulfide bonds in aqueous solutions.

1255. Bis(1-methylamyl) Sodium Sulfosuccinate. [6001-97-4] Sulfobutanedioic acid 1,4-bis(1-methylpentyl) ester sodium salt; dihexyl sodium sulfosuccinate; Aerosol MA; Alphasol MA. $C_{16}H_{29}NaO_7S$; mol wt 388.45. C 49.47%, H 7.52%, Na 5.92%, O 28.83%, S 8.25%. The bis(1-methylamyl) ester of sulfosuccinic acid monosodium salt, perhaps in admixture with the dihexyl ester. Prepd by the action of the appropriate alcohols on maleic anhydride followed by addition of sodium bisulfite: A. O. Jaeger, US 2028091; US 2176423 (1936, 1939 both to Am. Cyanamid); **FR** 776495 (1935 to Selden Co.).

Available as white, slightly hygroscopic, wax-like pellets. Must be soaked to dissolve in cold water. Dissolves rapidly in hot water. Solubility in water at 25° = 343 g/l; at 70° = 447 g/l. Maximum concn of electrolyte soln in which 1% of the wetting agent is sol: 2% NaCl; 2% NH_4Cl; 14% $(NH_4)_2HPO_4$; 3% $NaNO_3$ (slightly turbid); 3% Na_2SO_4. Also sol in pine oil, oleic acid, acetone, kerosene, carbon tetrachloride, 2B ethanol, benzene, hot olive oil, glycerol. Insol in liquid petrolatum. Stable in acid and neutral solns, hydrolyzes in alkaline solns.

USE: Wetting agent.

1256. Bis[methylthio]methane. [1618-26-4] Bis[methyl-mercapto]methane; methylenebis[methyl sulfide]. $C_3H_8S_2$; mol wt 108.23. C 33.29%, H 7.45%, S 59.25%. $(CH_3S)_2CH_2$. Odorous principle of the white truffle *Tuber magnatum* (Pico) Vitt., *Tuberaceae*. Isoln: Fiecchi *et al., Tetrahedron Lett.* **1967**, 1681. Synthesis from methyl mercaptan: Böhme, Marx, *Ber.* **74**, 1672 (1941).

Oily liquid. Odor in high dilutions reminiscent of white truffles. The odor of the neat liquid resembles that of freshly prepd mustard without its acrid and irritating qualities. bp 148-149°. Mass spectra: Fiecchi, *loc. cit.*

1257. Bismuth. [7440-69-9] Bi; at. wt 208.98040; at. no. 83; valence 3, 5. Group VA (15). One naturally occurring isotope: 209; artificial radioactive isotopes: 199-208; 210-215. Confused with tin until 1450. First isolated by Hillot in 1737. It was, however, Geoffrey the Younger who clearly proved its individuality in 1753. Pott and Bergmann are named as the scientific discoverers. Occurrence in the earth's crust: approx 0.2 ppm. Obtained as a byproduct from the processing of lead, copper, and tin ores. *Reviews: Nouveau Traité de Chimie Minérale*, tome **11**, P. Pascal, Ed. (Masson, Paris, 1958); *Gmelins, Bismuth* (8th ed.) **19**, pp 1-104 (1927); supplement, pp 1-621 (1964); Smith, "Arsenic, Antimony and Bismuth" in *Comprehensive Inorganic Chemistry* **vol. 2**, J. C. Bailar, Jr. *et al.*, Eds. (Pergamon Press, Oxford, 1973) pp 547-683; S. C. Carapella, H. E. Howe in *Kirk-Othmer Encyclopedia of Chemical Technology* **vol. 3** (Wiley-Interscience, New York, 3rd ed., 1978) pp 912-921.

Grayish-white with reddish tinge and bright metallic luster; soft and brittle; superficially oxidized by air, frequently becoming iridescent. mp 271°; contracts when melted. bp 1420°; bp 1490°: *Gmelins*, p. 43. d_4^{20} 9.78; d_4^{271} 10.07. Poor conductor of electricity. Has the greatest Hall effect of any metal, *i.e.,* its resistance increases when placed in a magnetic field. Attacked by dil HNO_3, hot H_2-SO_4, concd HCl. Cold solns of Bi give a white ppt with NaOH, turning yellow on boiling; with HCl a white ppt sol in excess of acid. The solns in HCl or HNO_3 yield with much water a white ppt blackened by H_2S (different from Sb).

Precipitated bismuth. Prepd by treating a soln of bismuth chloride in HCl with hypophosphorous acid, washing and drying. Contains not less than 98.5% metallic bismuth. Dull gray powder. The particles are of no greater diameter than 15 microns (0.015 mm). Easily dispersed in water.

D'Arcet metal-fusible. An alloy of 49.2% Bi, 32.2% Pb and 18.4% Sn. Whitish-gray metal, mp 96-97°.

USE: Manuf Bi salts, fusible alloys, stereotype metal, fusible boiler plugs, electric fuses, low-melting solders; tempering baths for steel; "silvering" mirrors; in dental technique.

THERAP CAT (VET): Has been used externally in dusting powders for indolent, moist or suppurating lesions; internally as a protectant of the gastrointestinal lining, and as an x-ray contrast medium. Has also been recommended to treat buccal warts in dogs.

1258. Bismuth Aluminate. [12284-76-3] Aluminum bismuth oxide; almuth; Bisminat. $Al_6Bi_2O_{12}$; mol wt 771.84. Al 20.97%, Bi 54.15%, O 24.87%. $Bi_2(Al_2O_4)_3$. Prepn: Roques, **US** 2901316 (1959 to Etablissements Roques).

Decahydrate. Extremely light powder. Practically insol in water.

THERAP CAT: Antacid.

1259. Bismuth Bromide. [7787-58-8] Bismuth tribromide. BiBr$_3$; mol wt 448.69. Bi 46.58%, Br 53.42%. Prepn from the elements: Schenk in *Handbook of Preparative Inorganic Chemistry* vol. 1, G. Brauer, Ed. (Academic Press, New York, 2nd ed., 1963) p 623.

Yellowish crystals; odor of HBr. d 5.7. mp 218°. bp 441°. Dec by water, forming BiOBr; sol in solns of KI, KBr, KCl, and in dil HCl. Practically insol in alc. *Keep tightly closed.*

1260. Bismuth Bromide Oxide. [7787-57-7] Basic bismuth bromide; bismuth oxybromide; bismuthyl bromide; bismuth "subbromide". BiBrO; mol wt 304.88. Bi 68.55%, Br 26.21%, O 5.25%. BiOBr. Prepn: Schenk in *Handbook of Preparative Inorganic Chemistry* vol. 1, G. Brauer, Ed. (Academic Press, New York, 2nd ed., 1963) p 624.

Crystals or amorphous powder. Very stable, melts at red heat. Practically insol in water, alc; sol in HCl, HBr, HNO$_3$.

USE: Manuf of dry cell cathodes.

1261. Bismuth Butylthiolaurate. [53897-25-9] 2-(Butylthio)dodecanoic acid bismuth basic salt; Bispecia; Neocardyl. C$_{16}$H$_{33}$BiO$_4$S; mol wt 530.48. C 36.23%, H 6.27%, Bi 39.39%, O 12.06%, S 6.04%. CH$_3$(CH$_2$)$_9$CH(SC$_4$H$_9$)COOBi(OH)$_2$. Prepn: P. Lebeau, M. M. Janot, *Traité Pharm. Chim.* **Vol. II** (Masson, Paris, 4th ed., 1955-1956) p 435.

Yellowish powder. Practically insol in water; sol in oils. Dec in acids, liberating hydrogen sulfide.

THERAP CAT: Formerly as antisyphilitic.

1262. Bismuth Chloride. [7787-60-2] Bismuth trichloride. BiCl$_3$; mol wt 315.34. Bi 66.27%, Cl 33.73%. Prepn from the elements: Schenk in *Handbook of Preparative Inorganic Chemistry* vol. 1, G. Brauer, Ed. (Academic Press, New York, 2nd ed., 1963) p 621.

White to yellowish, deliquesc crystals; HCl odor. d 4.75. mp ~230°. Sublimes at about 430°. bp 447°. Dec by water or aq alc into BiOCl; sol in HCl, HNO$_3$, abs alcohol, acetone, ethyl acetate. *Keep tightly closed.*

USE: In the manuf of other bismuth salts; as catalyst for organic reactions.

1263. Bismuth Chloride Oxide. [7787-59-9] Basic bismuth chloride; bismuth oxychloride; bismuthyl chloride; bismuth "subchloride"; pearl white; blanc d'Espagne; blanc de perle; Chlorbismol. BiClO; mol wt 260.43. Bi 80.24%, Cl 13.61%, O 6.14%. BiOCl. Prepn: Schenk in *Handbook of Preparative Inorganic Chemistry* vol. 1, G. Brauer, Ed. (Academic Press, New York, 2nd ed., 1963) p 622.

Fine powder or tetragonal crystals. Melts at low red heat; d 7.72. Practically insol in water, alc; sol in HCl, HNO$_3$.

USE: In face powders; as pigment; manuf artificial pearls, dry-cell cathodes.

THERAP CAT: Formerly as antisyphilitic.

1264. Bismuth Ethyl Camphorate. [52951-37-8] *d*-Camphoric acid ethyl ester bismuth salt; bismuth(III) salt of *d*-camphoric acid monoethyl ester. C$_{36}$H$_{57}$BiO$_{12}$; mol wt 890.81. C 48.54%, H 6.45%, Bi 23.46%, O 21.55%. Prepd from sodium ethyl camphorate and bismuth nitrate: W. M. Lauter, H. A. Braun, *J. Am. Pharm. Assoc.* **25**, 394 (1936).

Amorphous solid, faint aromatic odor. Softens at 55°. mp 61-67° (clear melt). Practically insol in water. Sol in chloroform,

ether, ethylene dichloride, oils. The soly in vegetable oils is increased by the addition of camphor. MLD i.m. in rats: 250 mg Bi/kg (Lauter, Braun).

THERAP CAT: Formerly as antisyphilitic.

1265. Bismuth Fluoride. [7787-61-3] Bismuth trifluoride. BiF$_3$; mol wt 265.98. Bi 78.57%, F 21.43%. Prepd by dissolving bismuth oxide or hydroxide in aqueous HF. May also be prepd by reduction of BiF$_5$ with CO$_2$ in very dil H$_2$ at 80-150° in a Pt tube: Muir *et al., J. Chem. Soc.* **39**, 33 (1881); v. Wartenberg, *Z. Anorg. Allg. Chem.* **244**, 344 (1940); Aurivillius, *Acta Chem. Scand.* **9**, 1206 (1955). *Review:* Kemmitt, Sharp, *Adv. Fluorine Chem.* **4**, 213 (1965).

White to gray dimorphic crystals. d 8.3. mp 725-730°. Volatilizes at higher temps slowly and without decompn. Practically insol in water. Sol in concd HF with the formation of complexes.

USE: In the prepn of bismuth pentafluoride, *q.v.*

1266. Bismuth Germanate. [12233-56-6] Bismuth germanium oxide (Bi$_4$Ge$_3$O$_{12}$); BGO. Bi$_4$Ge$_3$O$_{12}$; mol wt 1245.83. Bi 67.10%, Ge 17.49%, O 15.41%. Bi$_4$(GeO$_4$)$_3$. High density scintillation material; γ-ray absorber. Single crystal growth and characterization: R. Nitsche, *J. Appl. Phys.* **36**, 2358 (1965); R. V. A. Murthy *et al., J. Cryst. Growth* **197**, 865 (1999); J. B. Shim *et al., ibid.* **243**, 157 (2002). Luminescence properties: M. J. Weber, R. R. Monchamp, *J. Appl. Phys.* **44**, 5495 (1973). Temperature-dependent scintillation properties: H. V. Piltingsrud, *J. Nucl. Med.* **20**, 1279 (1979). Laser-excited optical properties: F. Rogemond *et al., J. Luminescence* **33**, 455 (1985). Optical and photoelastic properties: P. A. Williams *et al., Appl. Optics* **35**, 3562 (1996). Thermophysical properties: V. D. Golyshev *et al., J. Cryst. Growth* **262**, 202, 212 (2004). Performance in PET applications: G. Gervino, E. Monticone, *Sensors Actuators A* **41-42**, 487 (1994); in radiation detectors: Z. S. Macedo *et al., Nucl. Instrum. Methods Phys. Res. B* **218**, 153 (2004).

Colorless, non-hygroscopc, cubic crystals, mp ~1050°. n_{550} 2.1204. n_{600} 2.1058. n_{750} 2.0786. d 7.13. Emission max: 480 nm.

USE: Scintillator crystal in nuclear physics, high-energy physics, geology, and nuclear medical imaging applications including PET, X-ray CT and positron CT; in electromagnetic calorimeters.

1267. Bismuth Hydroxide. [10361-43-0] Bismuth hydrate. BiH$_3$O$_3$; mol wt 260.00. Bi 80.38%, H 1.16%, O 18.46%. Bi(OH)$_3$. Prepn: *Gmelins, Bismuth* (8th ed.) **19**, pp 119-122 (1927).

White to yellowish-white, amorphous powder. d^{15} 4.962. Practically insol in water. When freshly pptd it is soluble in glycerol in presence of NaOH; sol in acids. Readily loses one mol H$_2$O forming the metahydroxide which is yellow.

USE: As absorbent for rutin and quercetin; in hydrolysis of ribonucleic acid; in separation of plutonium from irradiated uranium.

1268. Bismuthine. [18288-22-7] Bismuth trihydride; Bismutan. BiH$_3$; mol wt 212.00. Bi 98.58%, H 1.43%. Prepn: Wiberg, Mödritzer, *Z. Naturforsch.* **12b**, 123 (1957); Amberger, *Ber.* **94**, 1447 (1961).

Thermally unstable liquid, bp 16.8° (est).

USE: In manuf of Ge or Si semiconductors, Scott *et al., US* **2910394** (1959 to Int'l Standard Electric).

1269. Bismuth Iodide. [7787-64-6] Bismuth triiodide. BiI$_3$; mol wt 589.69. Bi 35.44%, I 64.56%. Best prepd from the elements: Watt *et al., Inorg. Synth.* **4**, 114 (1953).

Black, minute, hexagonal crystals with metallic sheen. d$_4^{17}$ 5.778, also reported as d 5.64. Sublimes at 439° (760 mm), dec at 500°. Practically insol in cold water, dec slowly in hot water. Sol in liquid ammonia, abs ethanol (about 3.5% at 20°), in aq solns of KI, HI, and HCl. The solid is slowly converted to Bi(IO$_3$)$_3$ upon prolonged exposure to air.

1270. Bismuth Iodide Oxide. [7787-63-5] Basic bismuth iodide; bismuth oxyiodide; bismuthyl iodide; bismuth "subiodide". BiIO; mol wt 351.88. Bi 59.39%, I 36.06%, O 4.55%. BiOI. Prepn: *Gmelins, Bismuth* (8th ed) **19**, p 159 (1927); Schenk in

Handbook of Preparative Inorganic Chemistry **vol. 1**, G. Brauer, Ed. (Academic Press, New York, 2nd ed., 1963) p 625.

Brick-red, heavy, odorless powder or copper-colored crystals. d 7.92. Fuses at red heat with partial decompn. Practically insol in water, alcohol, $CHCl_3$; sol in HCl; dec by HNO_3 or alkali.

USE: Manuf of dry cell cathodes.

THERAP CAT: Anti-infective.

1271. Bismuth Nitrate. [10361-44-1] Bismuth trinitrate. BiN_3O_9; mol wt 395.00. Bi 52.91%, N 10.64%, O 36.45%. $Bi(NO_3)_3$. Prepn: *Gmelins, Bismuth* (8th ed.) **19**, pp 126-129 (1927).

Pentahydrate, lustrous, hygroscopic crystals; acid reaction; odor of nitric acid. d 2.83. Sol in water containing nitric acid; dec by water alone into subnitrate; sol in glycerol, dil acids including acetic acid, acetone. Practically insol in alcohol, ethyl acetate.

USE: Prepn of other bismuth salts, luminous paints; pptn of alkaloids.

1272. Bismuth Oxalate. [6591-55-5] Oxalic acid bismuth salt. $C_6Bi_2O_{12}$; mol wt 682.02. C 10.57%, Bi 61.28%, O 28.15%. $Bi_2(C_2O_4)_3$. Prepn: Vanino, Zumbusch, *Ber.* **41**, 3994 (1908); Soerbye, Kruse, *Acta Chem. Scand.* **16**, 1662 (1962).

Powder. *Poisonous!* Practically insol in water or alcohol. Sol in moderately dil HCl or HNO_3.

1273. Bismuth Oxide. [1304-76-3] Bismuth trioxide; bismuthous oxide; bismuth yellow. Bi_2O_3; mol wt 465.96. Bi 89.70%, O 10.30%. Occurs in nature as the mineral *bismite*. Prepn: *Gmelins, Bismuth* (8th ed.) **19**, p 109-113 (1927).

Yellow, heavy, odorless powder or monoclinic crystals; stable in air. Practically insol in water; sol in HCl or HNO_3.

USE: In disinfectants, magnets, glass, rubber vulcanization; in fireproofing of papers and polymers; in catalysts.

THERAP CAT: Astringent.

1274. Bismuth Pentafluoride. [7787-62-4] BiF_5; mol wt 303.97. Bi 68.75%, F 31.25%. Prepd according to the equation $BiF_3 + F_2 \rightarrow BiF_5$: v. Wartenberg, *Z. Anorg. Allg. Chem.* **244**, 344 (1940); Kwasnik in *Handbook of Preparative Inorganic Chemistry* **vol. 1**, G. Brauer Ed. (Academic Press, New York, 2nd ed., 1963) pp 202-203. Prepn from Bi and F_2: Fischer, Rodzitis, *J. Am. Chem. Soc.* **81**, 6375 (1959); Kemmitt, Sharp, *Adv. Fluorine Chem.* **4**, 212 (1965); Hebecker, *Z. Anorg. Allg. Chem.* **384**, 111 (1971).

Body-centered tetragonal crystals, sublimes at 120°. d 5.55. Very sensitive to moisture, discolors quickly in moist air. Violent reaction with water forming BiF_3 and ozone. Reacts with liquid petrolatum above 50°.

Caution: Highly toxic and irritating to mucous membranes, skin, eyes, respiratory tract.

USE: Fluorinating agent.

1275. Bismuth Phosphate. [10049-01-1] Bismugel. BiO_4-P; mol wt 303.95. Bi 68.75%, O 21.06%, P 10.19%. $BiPO_4$. Prepn: Schenk in *Handbook of Preparative Inorganic Chemistry* **vol. 1**, G. Brauer, Ed. (Academic Press, New York, 2nd ed., 1963) p 626.

Odorless powder or monoclinic crystals. Does not melt on heating. d^{15} 6.323. Slightly sol in water and dil acids; not hydrolyzed by boiling water. Practically insol in alcohol, acetic acid; sol in concd HNO_3 and HCl.

USE: In the separation of plutonium from fission products; manuf of optical flint glass.

THERAP CAT: Antacid; protectant.

1276. Bismuth Potassium Iodide. [41944-01-8] Potassium heptaiodobismuthate(4−). BiI_7K_4; mol wt 1253.70. Bi 16.67%, I 70.86%, K 12.47%. K_4BiI_7. Prepn: *Gmelins, Potassium* (8th ed.) **22**, p 1068 (1936).

Red crystals. Partly dec by water; completely sol in alkali iodide solns.

USE: Pptn of vitamins, particularly thiamine HCl, and antibiotics from soln.

1277. Bismuth Potassium Tartrate. [5798-41-4] Potassium bismuthotartrate; potassium bismuth tartrate; potassium bismuthyl tartrate; tartaric acid bismuth complex potassium salt. The bismuth content of the complex salts of bismuth and alkali

tartrate may be made to range within wide limits (35-75% Bi). The medicinal grade contains 60-64% bismuth. Prepn: Kober, **US 1663201** (1928 to Searle); *Hagers Handb. Pharm. Praxis* **1st Suppl.**, 316 (Berlin, 1949).

Odorless powder; sweetish taste; darkens on exposure to light. Sol in 2 parts water. Practically insol in alc or other organic solvents. The aq soln is slightly alkaline. Dec by mineral acids.

THERAP CAT: Formerly as antisyphilitic.

1278. Bismuth Selenide. [12068-69-8] Bismuth triselenide. Bi_2Se_3; mol wt 654.84. Bi 63.83%, Se 36.17%. Prepn by heating a stoichiometric mixture at 475° in evacuated tube: Dönges, *Z. Anorg. Allg. Chem.* **265**, 56 (1951); Konorov, *Zh. Tekh. Fiz.* **26**, 1394 (1956); from BiO, Se and sodium oxalate at high press.: Cambi, Elli, *Chim. Ind. (Milan)* **50**, 94 (1968).

Black crystals. Rhombohedral and hexagonal crystal structure. d_4^{20} 7.70 (also reported as 6.82). mp 710°. Heat of formation: −13.9 kcal/mol. Heat of combustion: 296.4 kcal/mol. Dec when heated in air. Dec by concd nitric acid and aqua regia. Insol in water.

USE: In semiconductor research.

1279. Bismuth Sodium Tartrate. [31586-77-3] Sodium bismuth tartrate; sodium bismuthyl tartrate; tartaric acid bismuth complex sodium salt; Natrol; Tartrol. The bismuth content of the complex salts of bismuth and alkali tartrate may be made to range within wide limits (35-75% Bi). The article generally used contains 70-74% bismuth. Prepn: Kober, **US 1663201** (1928 to Searle); *Hagers Handb. Pharm. Praxis* **1st Suppl.**, 316 (Berlin, 1949).

Odorless, tasteless powder; discolors in light. Sol in about 3 parts water. Insol in alc or other organic solvents. The aq soln is slightly alkaline.

THERAP CAT: Formerly as antisyphilitic.

THERAP CAT (VET): See Bismuth.

1280. Bismuth Sodium Triglycollamate. [5798-43-6] Nitrilotriacetic acid bismuth complex sodium salt; Bistrimate. C_{24}-$H_{28}BiN_4Na_7O_{25}$; mol wt 1142.40. C 25.23%, H 2.47%, Bi 18.29%, N 4.90%, Na 14.09%, O 35.01%. A double salt of sodium bismuthyl triglycollamate and disodium triglycollamate. Prepn: Lehman, Sproull, **US 2348984** (1944).

Crystals. Slightly salty taste. Very sol in water. Insol in acetone, ether, benzene. pH of 2% aq soln is between 7 and 8.

THERAP CAT: Lupus erythematosus suppressant.

1281. Bismuth Subacetate. [5142-76-7] (Acetyloxy)-oxobismuthine; acetic acid basic bismuth salt; bismuth acetate basic; bismuth acetate oxide; bismuth oxide acetate; bismuthyl acetate. $C_2H_3BiO_3$; mol wt 284.02. C 8.46%, H 1.06%, Bi 73.58%, O 16.90%. $CH_3COOBiO$. Prepn: Hofmann, *Ann.* **223**, 110 (1884); Aurivillius, *Acta Chem. Scand.* **9**, 1213 (1955). Crystal structure: Aurivillius, *loc. cit.*

Thin crystal plates. Slight acetic odor. Practically insol in water. Sol in glacial acetic acid, dil HCl or HNO_3.

1282. Bismuth Subcarbonate. [5892-10-4] Bismuth carbonate oxide ($Bi_2(CO_3)O_2$); bismuth oxycarbonate; bismutite. CBi_2O_5; mol wt 509.97. C 2.36%, Bi 81.96%, O 15.69%. $(BiO)_2CO_3$. Prepn: *Gmelins, Bismuth* (8th ed.) **19**, p 178 (1927). Crystal structure, stability and spectral studies: P. Taylor *et al., Can. J. Chem.* **62**, 2863 (1984). Thermal decompn study: H. Henmi *et al., Thermochim. Acta* **114**, 393 (1987). Powder neutron diffraction structural study: C. Greaves, S. K. Blower, *Mater. Res. Bull.* **23**, 1001 (1988). Vibrational spectrum of hemihydrate: G. E. Tobon-Zapata *et al., J. Mater. Sci. Lett.* **16**, 656 (1997). *In vitro* efficacy vs *Campylobacter pylori*: K. Vogt *et al., Zentralbl. Bakteriol.* **273**, 33 (1990). Review of pharmaceutical prepns: M. Wesolowski, *Arzneim.-Forsch.* **28**, 372-378 (1978).

Insol in water.

Hemihydrate. [5798-45-8] Odorless, tasteless powder. Practically insol in water or alc. Sol in mineral acids, in concd acetic acid.

USE: In admixture with other substances in glazes on ceramics; for pearly surfaces for plastics.

THERAP CAT: Antacid; antidiarrheal.

THERAP CAT (VET): Antidiarrheal.

1283.   Bismuth Subgallate. [22650-86-8] Gallic acid bismuth basic salt; bismuth gallate, basic; B.S.G.; Dermatol. C_7H_5-BiO_6; mol wt 394.09. C 21.33%, H 1.28%, Bi 53.03%, O 24.36%. Prepd from bismuth nitrate and gallic acid in an acetic acid medium. The acetic acid may be replaced with a glycol or mannitol: Pfeiffer, Schmitz, *Pharmazie* **5**, 517 (1950).

Hydrate. Bright yellow, odorless, tasteless powder. Practically insol in water, alc, chloroform, ether; sol in dil alkali hydroxide solns, in hot mineral acids with decompn. Forms a water-sol sodium salt which has an alkaline reaction.

Note: Major active ingredient of *Bongast.*

THERAP CAT: Astringent; antacid; protective.

THERAP CAT (VET): See Bismuth.

1284.   Bismuth Subnitrate. [1304-85-4] Bismuth hydroxide nitrate oxide ($Bi_5(OH)_9(NO_3)_4O$); bismuth nitrate basic; bismuth oxynitrate; bismuth subnitricum; bismuthyl nitrate; bismuth white; magistery of bismuth; novismuth; paint white; Spanish white. $Bi_5H_9N_4O_{22}$; mol wt 1461.99. Bi 71.47%, H 0.62%, N 3.83%, O 24.08%. A basic salt, the compn of which varies with the conditions of preparation. Contains 70 to 74% Bi or 79 to 82% Bi_2O_3. Prepd by partial hydrolysis of $Bi(NO_3)_3$: *Gmelins, Bismuth* (8th ed.) **19**, pp 132-135 (1927); *Traité Pharm. Chim.* **vol. 1,** P. Lebeau, M. M. Janot, Eds. (Masson, Paris, 1956) p 371; *Handbuch der Pharmazie* **vol. 4**(1), H. Thoms, Ed. (Urban & Schwarzenberg, Berlin, 1927) p 325. Mechanism of action study: S. Pugh, M. R. Lewin, *J. Gastroenterol. Hepatol.* **5**, 382 (1990). Clinical studies in ulcer caused by *Helicobacter pylori* infection: A. F. Carvalho *et al., Aliment. Pharmacol. Ther.* **12**, 557 (1998); M. W. Whitehead *et al., Helicobacter* **5**, 169 (2000); R. H. Phillips *et al., ibid.* 176.

Odorless, tasteless, heavy, slightly hygroscopic, microcrystalline powder. Dec to Bi_2O_3 and nitrogen oxides when heated to red heat. Practically insol in water, alc. Sol in dil HCl and HNO_3. *Keep well closed and protect from light. Incompat.* Alkaline bicarbonates, soluble iodides, gallic acid, calomel, salicylic acid, tannin, sulfur.

USE: Manuf bismuth fluxes for enamels; in cosmetics.

THERAP CAT: Antacid; antiulcerative.

THERAP CAT (VET): See Bismuth.

1285.   Bismuth Subsalicylate. [14882-18-9] 2-Hydroxy-$4H$-1,3,2-benzodioxabismin-4-one; (2-hydroxybenzoato-O^1,O^2)-oxobismuth; oxo(salicylato)bismuth; basic bismuth salicylate; bismuth oxysalicylate; Bismed; Jatrox; Pepto-Bismol. $C_7H_5BiO_4$; mol wt 362.09. C 23.22%, H 1.39%, Bi 57.72%, O 17.67%. Prepn: Fischer, Grützner, *Arch. Pharm.* **231**, 680 (1893). Clinical trial in infant diarrhea: D. Figueroa-Quintanilla *et al., N. Engl. J. Med.* **328**, 1653 (1993). Symposium on pharmacology and therapeutic use in gastrointestinal infections: *Rev. Infect. Dis.* **12**, Suppl. 1, S1-S119 (1990). Mechanism of gastroprotection: D. Bagchi *et al., Dig. Dis. Sci.* **44**, 2419 (1999).

White or nearly white amorphous or microcrystalline, odorless powder. Practically insol in water.

THERAP CAT: Antidiarrheal; antiemetic.

THERAP CAT (VET): Antidiarrheal.

1286.   Bismuth Sulfate. [7787-68-0] $Bi_2O_{12}S_3$; mol wt 706.15. Bi 59.19%, O 27.19%, S 13.62%. $Bi_2(SO_4)_3$. Prepn: *Gmelins, Bismuth* (8th ed.) **19**, p 170 (1927).

White crystals. Dec by water or alc into a basic salt; sol in acids.

USE: In analysis of other metallic sulfates.

1287.   Bismuth Sulfide. [1345-07-9] Bi_2S_3; mol wt 514.16. Bi 81.29%, S 18.71%. Occurs in nature as the mineral *bismuthinite.* Prepn: *Gmelins, Bismuth* (8th ed.) **19**, pp 162-167 (1927).

Blackish-brown, orthorhombic, bipyramidal crystals. Practically insol in water, ethyl acetate. Sol in HNO_3, HCl.

1288.   Bismuth Tannate. Tanbismuth; tannic acid bismuth derivative. Contains about 36% bismuth equivalent to 40% Bi_2O_3. Prepd from freshly pptd bismuth hydroxide and tannin: *Hagers Handb. Pharm. Praxis* **Band 1,** 685 (Berlin, 1930).

Yellow or brownish-yellow powder. Practically insol in water, alcohol, ether.

THERAP CAT: Astringent; protective.

1289.   Bismuth Telluride. [1304-82-1] Tellurobismuthite. Bi_2Te_3; mol wt 800.76. Bi 52.20%, Te 47.80%. Prepd by heating stoichiometric amounts of the elements to 475° for several days in an evacuated glass or quartz tube: Dönges, *Z. Anorg. Allg. Chem.* **265**, 56 (1951). Prepn of single crystals: Ainsworth, *Proc. Phys. Soc. London* **B69**, 606 (1956); in zone-melting apparatus: Harmon *et al., J. Phys. Chem. Solids* **2**, 181 (1957). Review of different methods: Minden, *Sylvania Technol.* **11** (no. 1), 13-25 (1958).

Gray hexagonal platelets. d 7.642. mp 585°. Single crystals have been grown by the Czochralski technique in which a hydrogen atmosphere was used to minimize the evaporation of tellurium. Since the crystals cleave readily along the (0001) basal hexagonal plane, it is mechanically easier to orient the seed so that the growth direction is in this plane rather than normal to it. The resulting crystals grow more readily along the basal plane, so that they have an oval cross section, often with a characteristic notch. All crystals so pulled are the *P* type. Heat of formation: -8 kcal/mol. Resistivity: 0.00033 ohm-cm. Thermal conductivities at room temp: $\lambda_0 = 0.015$ watt/cm-deg; $\lambda_e = 1.4 \times 10^{-3}$ watt/cm-deg. Energy gap: 0.15 ev. Electron mobility: 800 cm²/volt-sec. Hole mobility: 400 cm²/volt-sec.

Caution: Potential symptoms of overexposure are irritation of eyes, skin, upper respiratory system; garlic breath. *See NIOSH Pocket Guide to Chemical Hazards* (DHHS/NIOSH 97-140, 1997) p 28.

USE: In electronics as semiconductor.

1290.   Bismuth Tetroxide. [12048-50-9] "Bismuth peroxide". Bi_2O_4; mol wt 481.96. Bi 86.72%, O 13.28%. It may contain 1 or 2 mols of H_2O. Prepn: *Gmelins, Bismuth* (8th ed.) **19**, 115 (1927); Schenk in *Handbook of Preparative Inorganic Chemistry* **vol. 1**, G. Brauer, Ed. (Academic Press, New York, 2nd ed., 1963) p 629.

Orange-red to yellowish-brown heavy powder. Slowly dec by water without dissolving. Dec and dissolved by hot mineral acids.

USE: In lubricants for metal extrusion.

1291.   Bismuth Tribromophenate. [5175-83-7] Tris(2,4,6-tribromophenoxy)bismuthine; bismuth tribromophenol; tribromophenolbismuth; Sigmaform; Xeroform. $C_{18}H_6BiBr_9O_3$; mol wt 1198.35. C 18.04%, H 0.50%, Bi 17.44%, Br 60.01%, O 4.01%. $(Br_3C_6H_2O)_3Bi$. Prepd from sodium tribromophenolate and bismuth nitrate: Kollo, *Pharm. Post.* **45**, 1013-1014, *C.A.* **7**, 2831[1] (1913); *Hagers Handb. Pharm. Praxis* **Band 1,** 686 (Berlin, 1930); *N.N.R.* **1951**, pp 66, 505. [In early publications bismuth tribromophenate was described as a basic bismuth salt ($Br_3C_6H_2O)_2$-$BiOH.Bi_2O_3$: *Hagers Handb., loc. cit.*]

Amorphous yellow powder. Stable below 120°. Neutral to moistened litmus paper. Slightly sol in water, alcohol, chloroform, vegetable oils. Dec by alkalies and strong acid. *Ref: N.N.R.* **1951**, p 505.

THERAP CAT: Anti-infective.

THERAP CAT (VET): See Bismuth.

1292.   Bismuth Triflate. [88189-03-1] Trifluoromethanesulfonic acid bismuth (3+) salt; Bismuth(III) tris(trifluoromethanesulfonate); Bi(OTf)₃. $C_3BiF_9O_9S_3$; mol wt 656.19. C 5.49%, Bi 31.85%, F 26.06%, O 21.94%, S 14.66%. Lewis acid catalyst. Prepn: S. Singh *et al., Indian J. Chem.* **22A**, 814 (1983); M. Labrouillère *et al., Tetrahedron Lett.* **40**, 285 (1999). Catalysis of large scale acetylations of alcohols and diols: M. D. Carrigan *et al., Synthesis* **2001**, 2091; of Biginelli Reaction: R. Varala *et al., Synlett* **2003**, 67; of epoxide opening with aromatic amines: T. Ollevier, G. Lavie-Compin, *Tetrahedron Lett.* **45**, 49 (2004). Review as catalyst for acylations and sulfonylations: C. Le Roux, J. Dubac, *Synlett*

2002, 181-200; brief review of catalytic use in a variety of organic reactions: S. Antoniotti, *ibid.* **2003**, 1566-1567.

White hygroscopic solid, stable in air to 100 °C. Decomposes in two steps: between 100-400 °C to $Bi_2O_2SO_4$; between 400-600 °C to Bi_2O_3. Sol in DMSO and DMF.

USE: Catalyst for organic syntheses.

1293. Bis(1-naphthylmethyl)amine. [5798-49-2] *N*-(1-Naphthalenylmethyl)-1-naphthalenemethanamine; di(α-naphthylmethyl)amine; α-dinaphthomethylamine. $C_{22}H_{19}N$; mol wt 297.39. C 88.85%, H 6.44%, N 4.71%. Prepd by catalytic hydrogenation of α-naphthonitrile: Rupe, Becherer, *Helv. Chim. Acta* **6**, 880 (1923).

Pale yellow crystals from petr ether, mp 62°.

USE: In determination of nitrates in fertilizers: Konek, *Z. Anal. Chem.* **97**, 416 (1934), *C.A.* **28**, 5779 (1934). The acetate has been proposed as a sensitive reagent for nitric acid.

1294. Bisoctrizole. [103597-45-1] 2,2′-Methylenebis[6-(2*H*-benzotriazol-2-yl)-4-(1,1,3,3-tetramethylbutyl)phenol]; MBBT; Tinosorb M; Tinuvin 360. $C_{41}H_{50}N_6O_2$; mol wt 658.87. C 74.74%, H 7.65%, N 12.76%, O 4.86%. UV-A filter with dual mechanism of action. Photostable organic molecule with broad UV absorption; microfine structure causes light scattering and reflection. Prepn and use in light stabilizer formulations: N. Kubota, A. Nishimura, *EP 180992; eidem*, **US 4681905** (1986, 1987 both to Adeka Argus). Light stabilization of polymers: G. Rytz *et al., Angew. Makromol. Chem.* **247**, 213 (1997). Skin photoprotection study: C. Gélis *et al., Photodermatol. Photoimmunol. Photomed.* **19**, 242 (2003). HPLC determn in suncare formulations: C. G. Smyrniotakis, H. A. Archontaki, *J. Chromatogr. A* **1031**, 319 (2004). UV attenuating properties of microparticles: B. Herzog *et al., J. Colloid Interface Sci.* **276**, 354 (2004).

Slightly yellow powder, mp 195°. Flash pt: >200°C. d^{20} 1.2. Vapor pressure (25°): 6×10^{-13} Pa. Soly at 20° (%w/w): water < 0.001; acetone 0.05; chloroform 100; *n*-hexane 0.03; methylene chloride 75; toluene 34. Absorption max (chloroform): 308, 349 nm (ε 31895). Absorption max (*n*-heptane): 348 nm (ε 31600).

USE: Light stabilizer in polymers and resins.

THERAP CAT: Ultraviolet screen.

1295. Bisoprolol. [66722-44-9] 1-[4-[[2-(1-Methylethoxy)-ethoxy]methyl]phenoxy]-3-[(1-methylethyl)amino]-2-propanol; ($\pm$)-1-[[α-(2-isopropoxyethoxy)-*p*-tolyl]oxy]-3-(isopropylamino)-2-propanol; ($\pm$)-1-[*p*-(2-isopropoxyethoxymethyl)phenoxy]-3-(isopropylamino)-2-propanol; EMD-33512. $C_{18}H_{31}NO_4$; mol wt 325.44. C 66.43%, H 9.60%, N 4.30%, O 19.66%. Cardioselective β_1-adrenergic blocker. Prepn: **BE 859425**; R. Jonas *et al.*, **US 4258062** (1978, 1981 both to E. Merck). Clinical pharmacology:

A. E. Tattersfield *et al., Br. J. Clin. Pharmacol.* **18**, 343 (1984); P. Dorow, U. Tönnesmann, *Eur. J. Clin. Pharmacol.* **27**, 135 (1984). Binding study of (−)-form: A. J. Kaumann, H. Lemoine, *Arch. Pharmacol.* **331**, 27 (1985). HPLC determn of enantiomers in plasma and urine: T. Suzuki *et al., J. Chromatogr.* **619**, 267 (1993). Clinical evaluation in angina: R. S. Kohli *et al., Eur. Heart J.* **6**, 845 (1985); in hypertension: F. R. Bühler *et al., J. Cardiovasc. Pharmacol.* **8**, Suppl. 11, S122 (1986). Review of pharmacokinetics: J. Grevel *et al., Clin. Pharmacokinet.* **17**, 53-63 (1989); of clinical efficacy in combination with hydrochlorothiazide: P. K. Zachariah *et al., Clin. Ther.* **15**, 779-787 (1993). Clinical trial in chronic heart failure: CIBIS-II Investigators, *Lancet* **353**, 9 (1999).

Hemifumarate. [104344-23-2] Concor; Detensiel; Emconcor; Emcor; Euradal; Isoten; Monocor; Soprol; Zebeta. $C_{18}H_{31}$-$NO_4 \cdot \frac{1}{2}C_4H_4O_4$; mol wt 383.48. Crystals, mp 100°. Sol in ethanol.

Mixture with hydrochlorothiazide. Ziac.

THERAP CAT: Antihypertensive.

1296. Bisoxatin Acetate. [14008-48-1] 2,2-Bis[4-(acetyloxy)phenyl]-2*H*-1,4-benzoxazin-3(4*H*)-one; 2,2-bis(4-acetoxyphenyl)-3-oxo-2,3-dihydrobenz-1,4-oxazine; Wy-8138; Laxonalin; Maratan; Talsis; Tasis. $C_{24}H_{19}NO_6$; mol wt 417.41. C 69.06%, H 4.59%, N 3.36%, O 23.00%. Prepd from 2,2-dichloro-3-oxo-2,3-dihydrobenz-1,4-oxazine and phenylacetate or by acetylation of the diphenol: Seeger, **US 3006917** (1961 to Thomae). Toxicity: E. I. Goldenthal, *Toxicol. Appl. Pharmacol.* **18**, 185 (1971).

Crystals from ethanol, mp 190°. LD_{50} orally in rats, mice: 8000, >10,000 mg/kg (Goldenthal).

THERAP CAT: Cathartic.

1297. Bisphenol A. [80-05-7] 4,4′-(1-Methylethylidene)-bisphenol; 4,4′-isopropylidenediphenol; 2,2-bis(4-hydroxyphenyl)-propane. $C_{15}H_{16}O_2$; mol wt 228.29. C 78.92%, H 7.06%, O 14.02%. Monomer used for polycarbonate and epoxy resins; exhibits estrogenic activity. Manuf from phenol and acetone: Jansen, **US 2468982** (1949); *Faith, Keyes & Clark's Industrial Chemicals*, F. A. Lowenheim, M. K. Moran, Eds. (Wiley-Interscience, New York, 4th ed., 1975) pp 149-152. Identification as xenoestrogen released from polycarbonate: A. V. Krishnan *et al., Endocrinology* **132**, 2279 (1993). HPLC determn in serum: K. Inoue *et al., J. Chromatogr. B* **749**, 17 (2000); in food: H. Petersen *et al., Eur. Food Res. Technol.* **216**, 355 (2003). Review of bioactivity and uses: N. Ben-Jonathan, R. Steinmetz, *Trends Endocrinol. Metab.* **9**, 124-128 (1998); of properties and environmental fate: C. A. Staples *et al., Chemosphere* **36**, 2149-2173 (1998).

Crystals or flakes. Mild phenolic odor. mp 150-155° (solidification range). bp_4 220°. Dec above 8 mm pressure when heated above 220°. Log P (*n*-octanol/water): 3.40. Soly in water: 120-

300 mg/l. Sol in aq alkaline solns, alcohol, acetone. Slightly sol in carbon tetrachloride. LC$_{50}$ (96 hr) in fathead minnow, rainbow trout: 4600, 3000-3500 μg/l (Staples).

Diglycidyl ether. [1675-54-3] BADGE. C$_{21}$H$_{24}$O$_4$; mol wt 340.41. Monohydrate as white solid, mp 40°. uv max (acetonitrile/water): 226.5, 277.1 nm.

USE: In the manuf of epoxy resins and polycarbonates for food packaging.

1298. Bisphenol B. [77-40-7] 4,4′-(1-Methylpropylidene)-bisphenol; *p,p′-sec*-butylidenediphenol; 2,2-bis(4-hydroxyphenyl)-butane. C$_{16}$H$_{18}$O$_2$; mol wt 242.31. C 79.31%, H 7.49%, O 13.21%. May be prepd from phenol and ethyl methyl ketone: Jansen, US 2468982 (1949 to Goodrich).

Crystals or tan granules, mp 118.9-121.7°. Approximate soly per 100 g: acetone 266 g; benzene 2.3 g; carbon tetrachloride <0.1 g; ether 133 g; methanol 166 g; V.M.P. naphtha <0.1 g; water <0.1 g.

USE: In the manufacture of phenolic resins.

1299. 9,10-Bis(phenylethynyl)anthracene. [10075-85-1] BPEA. C$_{30}$H$_{18}$; mol wt 378.46. C 95.21%, H 4.79%. Fluorescent dye. Prepn: W. Ried *et al., Ber.* **94**, 1051 (1961). Scintillation and fluorescence properties: A. Heller, G. Rio, *Bull. Soc. Chim. Fr.* **1963**, 1707. Absorption and emission properties: D. R. Maulding, B. G. Roberts, *J. Org. Chem.* **34**, 1734 (1969). ^{1}H NMR and ^{13}C NMR of dianion: M. Hirayama *et al., Bull. Chem. Soc. Jpn.* **61**, 1501 (1988). Photophysics and electronic spectroscopy: M. Levitus, M. A. Garcia-Garibay, *J. Phys. Chem. A* **104**, 8632 (2000).

Orange needles from benzene + petroleum ether, mp 249-250°. Absorption max (benzene): 439, 455 nm (log ε 4.50, 4.52).

USE: Bright yellow-green fluorescer in chemiluminescent formulations including *Cyalume* light sticks.

1300. Bis(pinacolato)diborane. [73183-34-3] 4,4,4′,4′,5,-5,5′,5′-Octamethyl-2,2′-bi-1,3,2-dioxaborolane; Miyaura's reagent; pinacol diborane; 4,4,5,5-tetramethyl-1,3,2-dioxaborolan-1-yl-4′,-4′,5′,5′-tetramethyl-1′,3′,2′-dioxaborolan; B$_2$pin$_2$. C$_{12}$H$_{24}$B$_2$O$_4$; mol wt 253.94. C 56.76%, H 9.53%, B 8.51%, O 25.20%. Boron source for organic syntheses. Prepn and crystal structure: H. Nöth, *Z. Naturforsch.* **39b**, 1463 (1984). Synthesis: T. Ishiyama *et al., Org. Synth.* **77**, 176 (2000). NMR spectroscopic data: W. Biffar *et al., Ber.* **113**, 333 (1980). First use as boron source in Pt-catalyzed diboration of alkynes: T. Ishiyama *et al., J. Am. Chem. Soc.* **115**, 11018 (1993). Stereospecific synthesis via cross coupling with aromatic amine: C. Malan, C. Morin, *J. Org. Chem.* **63**, 8019 (1998). Rh-catalyzed activation of the C-H bond: Y. Kondo *et al., J. Am. Chem. Soc.* **124**, 1164 (2002). Brief review: X. Liu, *Synlett* **2003**, 2442-2443.

Colorless plates, mp 138°. Crystalline form can be handled in air and stored in capped bottle.

USE: As a boron source in Pt-mediated diborations, coupling reactions; in Rh-or Ir-mediated borylations of alkanes and arenes, and in carbenoid chemistry.

1301. Bispyribac. [125401-75-4] 2,6-Bis[(4,6-dimethoxy-2-pyrimidinyl)oxy]benzoic acid. C$_{19}$H$_{18}$N$_4$O$_8$; mol wt 430.37. C 53.02%, H 4.22%, N 13.02%, O 29.74%. Post-emergence herbicide; turfgrass growth regulator. Prepn: N. Wada *et al.*, **EP 321846**; *eidem*, US 4906285 (1989, 1990 both to Kumiai Chem. Ind. and Ihara Chem. Ind.). Metabolism in rats: Y. Fukai *et al., J. Pestic. Sci.* **20**, 479 (1995). Field studies in rice: M. P. Braverman, D. L. Jordan, *Weed Technol.* **10**, 876 (1996); in turfgrass: M. J. Fagerness, D. Penner, *Weed Technol.* **12**, 436 (1998). Review of physical properties, mode of action and efficacy: M. Yokoyama *et al., Brighton Crop Prot. Conf. - Weeds* **1993**, 61-66.

White powder, mp 148-150°.

Sodium salt. [125401-92-5] KIH-2023; KUH-911; V-10029; Nominee. C$_{19}$H$_{17}$N$_4$NaO$_8$; mol wt 452.35. White powder, mp 228.0° (dec). Soly in water at 25°: 733 g/l. Vapor pressure at 25°: 5.05 × 10^{-9} Pa. LD$_{50}$ in male, female rats (mg/kg): 4111, 2635 orally; in rats (mg/kg): >2000 dermally. LC$_{50}$ in bluegill sunfish, rainbow trout (ppm): >100, >100 (Yokoyama).

USE: Herbicide.

1302. Bis(pyridine)iodonium Tetrafluoroborate. [15656-28-7] Bis(pyridine)iodine(1+) tetrafluoroborate(1−); Barluenga's reagent; IPy$_2$BF$_4$. C$_{10}$H$_{10}$IN$_2$.BF$_4$; mol wt 371.91. C 32.29%, H 2.71%, I 34.12%, N 7.53%, B 2.91%, F 20.43%. Mild source of iodonium ions in organic synthesis. Prepn: J. Barluenga *et al., Angew. Chem. Int. Ed.* **24**, 319 (1985). Oxidation of alcohols: *idem et al., Chem. Eur. J.* **10**, 4206 (2004). Brief review: K. Muñiz, *Synlett* **1999**, 1679. Review of iodination chemistry: J. Barluenga, *Pure Appl. Chem.* **71**, 431-436 (1999).

Crystals from dichloromethane, mp 149-151° (dec). *Store under inert atmosphere at 4° in the dark.*

USE: Iodination and oxidation reagent.

1303. 1,4-Bis(trichloromethyl)benzene. [68-36-0] α,α,α,-α′,α′,α′-Hexachloro-*p*-xylene; *p*-bis(perchloromethyl)benzene; Bitriben; Hetol. C$_8$H$_4$Cl$_6$; mol wt 312.84. C 30.71%, H 1.29%, Cl 68.00%. Usually obtained by photochlorination of *p*-xylene: McBee *et al., Ind. Eng. Chem.* **39**, 298 (1947); *eidem* in Slesser, Schram, *Preparation, Properties, and Technology of Fluorine and Organic Fluoro Compounds* (McGraw-Hill, New York, 1951) pp 207-221; Ross *et al., J. Am. Chem. Soc.* **75**, 4697 (1953); Rabjohn, *ibid.* **76**, 5479 (1954); Harvey *et al., J. Appl. Chem.* **4**, 319 (1954); Ligett, US 2654789 (1953 to Ethyl Corp.).

Crystals from hexane or ether, mp 108-110°.

Note: The name Hetol was previously used to designate sodium cinnamate.

USE: Insecticide.

THERAP CAT (VET): Anthelmintic (Trematodes).

1304. Bis(triphenylphosphine)dicarbonylnickel. [13007-90-4] Dicarbonylbis(triphenylphosphine)nickel; dicarbonyl-di(triphenylphosphino)nickel. C$_{38}$H$_{30}$NiO$_2$P$_2$; mol wt 639.28. C 71.39%, H 4.73%, Ni 9.18%, O 5.01%, P 9.69%. [((C$_6$H$_5$)$_3$P]$_2$-Ni(CO)$_2$. Obtained by reacting one mole of nickel carbonyl with two moles of triphenylphosphine: Reppe, Schweckendiek, *Ann.* **560**, 104 (1948); Rose, Statham, *J. Chem. Soc.* **1950**, 69. Also by reacting CO with a methanol soln of triphenylphosphine and reduced Ni at 170° and 60 atm: Yamamoto, Oku, *Bull. Chem. Soc. Jpn.* **27**, 382 (1954), *C.A.* **49**, 6856 (1955).

Crystals from benzene, mp 210-215° (Rose); mp 206-209° (Reppe). Catalytic activity decreases with storage.

USE: Catalyst in polymerization of acetylene to benzene and styrene, trimerization of ethynyl compds, cyclization of butadiene.

1305. Bitertanol. [55179-31-2] β-[(1,1'-Biphenyl)-4-yl-oxy]-α-(1,1-dimethylethyl)-1*H*-1,2,4-triazol-1-ethanol; 1-(biphenyl-4-yloxy)-3,3-dimethyl-1-(1*H*-1,2,4-triazol-1-yl)butan-2-ol; biloxazol; BAY KWG 0599; Baycor; Sibutol. $C_{20}H_{23}N_3O_2$; mol wt 337.42. C 71.19%, H 6.87%, N 12.45%, O 9.48%. Prepn: **BE 814831**; W. Kramer *et al.*, **US 3952002** (1974, 1976 both to Bayer AG). Physical properties and fungicidal activity: W. Brandes *et al.*, *Pflanzenschutz-Nachr.* **32**, 1 (1979). Mechanism of action: P. Kraus, *ibid.* 17; S. V. Overton *et al.*, *J. Hortic. Sci.* **63**, 183 (1988). GC determn in plants, soil and water: R. Brennecke, *Pflanzenschutz-Nachr.* **38**, 33 (1985). Resolution of diastereomers: R. S. Burden *et al.*, *J. Chromatogr.* **391**, 273 (1987). *In vitro* activity: T. B. Sutton *et al.*, *Plant Dis.* **69**, 700 (1985). Field use in control of apple diseases: K. S. Yoder, *ibid.* **66**, 580 (1982); W. F. S. Schwabe, *Pflanzenschutz-Nachr.* **35**, 125 (1982); in wheat seed pretreatment: J. A. Hoffmann, D. V. Sisson, *Plant Dis.* **71**, 839 (1987).

The marketed product is a mixture of diastereomers. Colorless crystals, mp 125-129°. Vapor pressure at 20°: 10^{-5}mbar. Soly at 20° (g/100 g solvent): water 0.0005, ligroin (80-110°) 0-1, propan-2-ol 1-5, toluene 1-5, cyclohexane 5-10, methylene chloride 10-20. Stable in aqueous acid and alkaline solns. LD_{50} in rats, male and female mice (mg/kg): >5000, 4488, 4202 orally (Brandes).

USE: Agricultural fungicide.

1306. Bithionol. [97-18-7] 2,2'-Thiobis[4,6-dichlorophenol]; TBP; bis(2-hydroxy-3,5-dichlorophenyl)sulfide; XL-7; Bithin; Lorothidol. $C_{12}H_6Cl_4O_2S$; mol wt 356.05. C 40.48%, H 1.70%, Cl 39.83%, O 8.99%, S 9.01%. Prepn from 2,4-halo substituted phenol with S halides: Muth, **DE 583055** (1933 to I. G. Farbenind.), *C.A.* **28**, 179 (1934); Copper, Godfrey, **US 2849494** (1958 to Monsanto). Comprehensive review and bibliography: Shumard *et al.*, *Soap Sanit. Chem.* **29**, no. 1, 34-37, 90 (1953). Anthelmintic activity of the sulfoxide: J. Guilhon, M. Graber, *Bull. Acad. Vet. Fr.* **52**, 225 (1979). Metabolism of the sulfoxide in humans: M. Sakamoto *et al.*, *J. Toxicol. Sci.* **6**, 307 (1981).

Crystals, mp 188°. d_4^{25} 1.73. pK_1 4.82; pK_2 10.50. Vapor press. at 37°: 1.1×10^{-9} mm Hg. Practically insol in water (0.0004% at 25°). Sol in dil caustic solns. A 4% NaOH soln will dissolve 16.2% bithionol. Soly (g/100 ml): acetone 15.0; polysorbate 80 19.0; dimethylacetamide 72.5; lanolin at 42° 5.0; pine oil 4.0; corn oil 1.0; propylene glycol 0.5; 70% ethanol 0.3.

Sodium salt. [6385-58-6] Bithionolate sodium; Vancide BN. $C_{12}H_4Cl_4Na_2O_2S$; mol wt 400.02. Harvey *et al.*, **US 3024163** (1962 to Vanderbilt Co.).

Sulfoxide. BTS; Bitin-S; Disto-5. $C_{12}H_6Cl_4O_3S$; mol wt 372.05.

USE: Surfactant-formulated antimicrobial against bacteria, molds and yeast. In cosmetics. Proposed as agricultural fungicide.

THERAP CAT: Anti-infective (topical).

THERAP CAT (VET): Anthelmintic; antiseptic.

1307. Bitolterol. [30392-40-6] 4-Methylbenzoic acid 4-[2-[(1,1-dimethylethyl)amino]-1-hydroxyethyl]-1,2-phenylene ester;

p-toluic acid 4-[2-(*t*-butylamino)-1-hydroxyethyl]-*o*-phenylene ester; α-[(*tert*-butylamino)methyl]-3,4-dihydroxybenzyl alcohol 3,4-di-*p*-toluate. $C_{28}H_{31}NO_5$; mol wt 461.55. C 72.86%, H 6.77%, N 3.03%, O 17.33%. β_2-Adrenergic agonist; a diester of *N-tert*-butylnorepinephrine. Prepn: H. Minatoya *et al.*, **DE 2015573**; *eidem*, **US 4138581** (1970, 1979 both to Sterling); B. F. Tullar *et al.*, *J. Med. Chem.* **19**, 834 (1976). Pharmacology: H. Minatoya, *J. Pharmacol. Exp. Ther.* **206**, 515 (1978). Metabolism and excretion: T. Aimoto *et al.*, *Xenobiotica* **9**, 173 (1979). Comparative clinical studies with isoproterenol, *q.v.*, in asthma: J. L. Pinnas *et al.*, *J. Allergy Clin. Immunol.* **79**, 768 (1987); R. A. Nathan *et al.*, *ibid.* 822. *Review:* S. B. Walker *et al.*, *Pharmacotherapy* **5**, 127-137 (1985).

Methanesulfonate. [30392-41-7] Bitolterol mesylate; Win-32784; Biterol; Effectin; Tornalate. $C_{28}H_{31}NO_5 \cdot CH_3SO_3H$; mol wt 557.66. White crystalline powder, mp 170-172°. Sol in DMSO.

THERAP CAT: Bronchodilator.

1308. Bitoscanate. [4044-65-9] 1,4-Diisothiocyanatobenzene; phenylene-1,4-diisothiocyanate; isothiocyanic acid *p*-phenylene ester; Jonit. $C_8H_4N_2S_2$; mol wt 192.26. C 49.98%, H 2.10%, N 14.57%, S 33.36%. Prepn: Lieber, Slutkin, *J. Org. Chem.* **27**, 2214 (1962). Prepn and use as anthelmintic: **FR M1652** and **GB 1001314** (1963, 1965 to Hoechst). Purification: Soeder, Laemmer, **DE 1172664** (1964 to Hoechst). Series of articles on clinical studies: *Progress in Drug Research* **vol. 19**, E. Jucker, Ed. (Birkhäuser Verlag, Basel and Stuttgart, 1975) pp 2-107.

Tasteless, odorless, colorless needles, from acetic acid or acetone, mp 132°.

THERAP CAT: Anthelmintic (Nematodes).

1309. Biuret. [108-19-0] Imidodicarbonic diamide; carbamylurea. $C_2H_5N_3O_2$; mol wt 103.08. C 23.30%, H 4.89%, N 40.76%, O 31.04%. $NH_2CONHCONH_2$. Prepd on a large scale by the action of heat on urea. Other syntheses are based on the treatment of urea with inorganic halides, such as thionyl chloride, on the interaction of urea and cyanic acid, and on the ammonolysis of allophanic esters and related compds. Has weak bacteriostatic and diuretic properties in rats, also causes a fall in blood pressure, but produces strong irritation of the urinary tract. Increases the activity of pepsin. Comprehensive review and bibliography: Kurzer, *Chem. Rev.* **56**, 95-197 (1956).

Hygroscopic, elongated plates from ethanol. d_4^{-5} 1.467. When crystallized from water, $5C_2H_5N_3O_2.4H_2O$ is formed, which becomes anhydr at 110°, then dec at about 193°. Pyrolysis at higher temps yields melamine. Soly (g/100 g soln) in water at 25° = 2.01; at 50° = 7; at 75° = 20; at 105.5° = 53.5. Freely sol in alc, very slightly sol in ether. Aq solns treated with cupric sulfate and NaOH give a reddish-violet color (biuret reaction, details: Kurzer, *loc. cit.*, p 181).

1310. Bivalirudin. [128270-60-0] Hirulog-1; hirulog-8; BG-8967; Angiomax; Angiox; Hirulog. $C_{98}H_{138}N_{24}O_{33}$; mol wt 2180.29. C 53.99%, H 6.38%, N 15.42%, O 24.22%. Synthetic peptide of 20 amino acids; member of a novel class of bivalent direct thrombin inhibitors. Characterized by an anion binding exosite (ABE) derived from hirudin, *q.v.*, linked to a thrombin catalytic site inhibitor moiety by tetraglycine. Prepn and structure activity study: J. M. Maraganore *et al.*, **WO 9102750**; *eidem*, **US 5196404** (1991, 1993 both to Biogen); *eidem*, *Biochemistry* **29**, 7095 (1990). Determn in plasma and whole blood: T. J. Reid, B. M. Alving, *Thromb. Haemostasis* **70**, 608 (1993). Clinical pharmacology: I. Fox *et al.*, *ibid.* **69**, 157 (1993). Clinical study in myocardial infarction: P. Théroux *et al., Circulation* **91**, 2132 (1995); during coronary angioplasty: J. A. Bittl *et al., N. Engl. J. Med.* **333**, 764 (1995). Clinical trial with provisional glycoprotein IIb/IIIa inhibition during percutaneous coronary intervention: A. M. Lincoff *et al., J. Am. Med. Assoc.* **289**, 853 (2003). Review of pharmacology and clinical development: T. D. Gladwell, *Clin. Ther.* **24**, 38-58 (2002); of clinical experience in acute coronary syndromes: J. S. Kalus, M. F. Caron, *Expert Opin. Invest. Drugs* **13**, 465-477 (2004).

D-Phe–Pro–Arg–Pro–Gly–Gly–Gly–Gly–Asn–Gly–Asp
|
Phe
|
Leu–Tyr–Glu–Glu–Pro–Ile–Glu–Glu

THERAP CAT: Antithrombotic.

1311. Bixins. Carotenoid carboxylic acids isolated from seeds of *Bixa orellana* L., *Bixaceae*; principal pigments of the crude coloring extract, annatto, *q.v.* The natural product is the *cis*-form. Isomerization to the more stable all-*trans*-form occurs upon heating or commercial extraction. Isoln: J. B. Boussingault, *Ann. Chim. Phys.* **28**, 440 (1825). Isomerization studies: J. Herzig, F. Faltis, *Ann.* **431**, 40 (1923); P. Karrer *et al., Helv. Chim. Acta* **12**, 741 (1929). Structural studies: R. Kuhn *et al., ibid.* **11**, 427 (1928); **12**, 64, 904 (1929); *Ber.* **64**, 1732 (1931); **65**, 646, 1873 (1932). NMR determn of stereochemistry: M. S. Barber *et al., J. Chem. Soc.* **1961**, 1625. Properties of bixin and norbixin: J. F. Reith, J. W. Gielen, *J. Food Sci.* **36**, 861 (1971). ^{1}H and ^{13}C NMR, MS, and x-ray crystal structure determn: D. R. Kelly *et al., J. Chem. Res. Miniprint* **10**, 2640 (1996). HPLC analysis of food coloring formulations: M. J. Scotter *et al., J. Agric. Food Chem.* **46**, 1031 (1998). Biosynthesis and prodn in genetically engineered *E. coli* (stereo unspecified): F. Bouvier *et al., Science* **300**, 2089 (2003). Review of *cis-trans* isomerization and stereochemistry: L. Zechmeister, *Chem. Rev.* **34**, 267-344 (1944); of chemistry and extraction from annatto: H. D. Preston, M. D. Rickard, *Food Chem.* **5**, 47-56 (1980).

all-*trans* Bixin

cis Bixin

***cis*-Form.** [6983-79-5] (2*E*,4*Z*,6*E*,8*E*,10*E*,12*E*,14*E*,16*E*,18*E*)-4,8,13,17-Tetramethyl-2,4,6,8,10,12,14,16,18-eicosanonaenedioic acid monomethyl ester; 9-*cis*-6,6′-diapo-ψ,ψ-carotenedioic acid monomethyl ester; 6′-methyl hydrogen (9′*Z*)-6,6′-diapocarotene-6,6′-dioate; α-bixin; labile bixin. $C_{25}H_{30}O_4$; mol wt 394.50. C 76.11%, H 7.66%, O 16.22%. Dark purple, lustrous crystals from ethanol + chloroform or dichloromethane + acetone, mp 190 ± 1°; dec 200.3 ± 0.6°. Absorption max (chloroform): 502, 471 nm (log ε = 5.02, 5.07).

***trans*-Form.** [39937-23-0] (2*E*,4*E*,6*E*,8*E*,10*E*,12*E*,14*E*,16*E*,18*E*)-4,8,13,17-Tetramethyl-2,4,6,8,10,12,14,16,18-eicosanonaenedioic acid monomethyl ester; all-*trans* bixin; β-bixin; isobixin; stable bixin. $C_{25}H_{30}O_4$; mol wt 394.50. Orange to purple plates from acetone, mp 204-206° (dec). Absorption max (chloroform): 507, 476 nm ($E_{1cm}^{1\%}$ 2970 ±40, 3240 ±50). Sol in oil.

α-Norbixin. [626-76-6] (2*E*,4*E*,6*E*,8*E*,10*E*,12*E*,14*E*,16*Z*,18*E*)-4,8,13,17-Tetramethyl-2,4,6,8,10,12,14,16,18-eicosanonaenedioic acid; 9-*cis*-6,6′-diapo-ψ,ψ-carotenedioic acid. $C_{24}H_{28}O_4$; mol wt 380.48. No melting observed ≤280°; yellow coloring observed at 240°; black coloring (carbonization) at ≥280°. Absorption max (chloroform): 499, 468 nm ($E_{1cm}^{1\%}$ 2200 ±30, 2470 ±30).

β-Norbixin. [542-40-5] (All-*E*)-4,8,13,17-tetramethyl-2,4,6,8,10,12,14,16,18-eicosanonaenedioic acid; 6,6′-diapo-ψ,ψ-carotenedioic acid; all-trans norbixin. $C_{24}H_{28}O_4$; mol wt 380.48. No

melting observed ≤300°; red color darkens ≥250°. Absorption max (chloroform): 506, 475 nm; (0.1 N NaOH): 486, 457 nm. Sol in H_2O.

USE: Food coloring; imparts a golden yellow color to butter and cheese.

1312. Black Cohosh. Black snake root; bugbane; bugwort; cimicifuga; rattle weed. Flowering perennial plant, *Actaea racemosa* L., also known as *Cimicifuga racemosa* (L.) Nutt., *Ranunculaceae*. Traditionally used in Native American medicine for gynecological disorders, rheumatism and snake bite. Medicinal formulations are prepared from the dried rhizome and roots. *Habit.* Eastern North America; cultivated in Europe. *Constit.* Triterpene glycosides such as actein, 27-deoxyactein, cimicifugosides; isoferulic and salicylic acids; 15-20% cimicifugin; tannin, volatile oils, resin. Description of botany, constituents and medical uses: D. J. McKenna *et al., Altern. Ther. Health Med.* **7**, 93 (2001). LC/MS determn of active triterpene glycosides in commercial formulations: K. He *et al., Planta Med.* **66**, 635 (2000). *Review*: J. Barnes *et al., Herbal Medicines* (Pharmaceutical Press, London, 2nd Ed., 2002) pp 141-146.

Alcoholic aqueous extract. Remifemin. Review of clinical experience: E. Liske, *Adv. Ther.*, **15**, 45-53 (1998).

Note: Should not be confused with blue cohosh, *q.v.*

THERAP CAT: In treatment of menopausal symptons.

1313. Black Pepper. Dried, unripe fruit of *Piper nigrum* L., *Piperaceae*. White pepper consists of the seed only, with the ripe fruit removed. Widely used as a cooking spice and in traditional medicine for dyspepsia. *Habit.* Southern India; cultivated in tropical Asia and the Caribbean. *Constit.* Pungent principles, predominantly piperine, *q.v.*, piperylin, piperolein A and B, cumaperine; 3,4-dihydroxyphenylethanol glycosides; volatile oil. HPLC determn of piperine content: M. Rathnawathie, K. A. Buckle, *J. Chromatogr.* **264**, 316 (1983). GC-MS analysis of constituents and antifungal and antioxidant properties: G. Singh *et al., J. Sci. Food Agric.* **84**, 1878 (2004). Insecticidal activity: H. C. F. Su, *J. Econ. Entomol.* **70**, 18 (1977); W. P. Scott, G. H. McKibben, *ibid.* **71**, 343 (1978). Review of medicinal uses: J. Gruenwald *et al., PDR for Herbal Medicines* (Medical Economics, Montvale, 3rd Ed., 2004) pp 105-106.

Volatile oil. [8006-82-4] Black pepper oil; oil of pepper. Obtained from dried, unripened fruit. *Constit.* Complex mixture containing predominantly β-caryophyllene, limonene, sabinene, β-bisabolene, α-copaene, β-pinene. Colorless or slightly green liquid. d_{25}^{25} 0.864-0.884. Angular rotation: −1 to −23°. n_D^{20} 1.479-1.488. Sol in most fixed oils, mineral oil, propylene glycol; sparingly sol in glycerin. Sol in 3 vols 95% alcohol.

USE: Pungently aromatic condiment in foods.

1314. Blackstrap Molasses. The final, unpurified mother liquor in the cane sugar industry from which no more sugar can be crystallized by factory methods. Rich in inorganic constituents, may analyze as much as 10% ash upon ignition. Sucrose content about 30%.

1315. Blankophor® R. [2606-93-1] 2,2′-(1,2-Ethenediyl)-bis[5-[[(phenylamino)carbonyl]amino]benzenesulfonic acid] disodium salt; 4,4′-bis(3-phenylureido)-2,2′-stilbenedisulfonic acid disodium salt; [stilbene-(4,4′)]bis[ω-phenylurea]-2,2′-disulfonic acid disodium salt; C.I. Fluorescent Brightener 30; C.I. 40600; Blancol C; Leucophor R; Lumisol RV; Phorwite RN; Photine R; Pontamine White BR; Tintophen X. $C_{28}H_{22}N_4Na_2O_8S_2$; mol wt 652.61. C 51.53%, H 3.40%, N 8.59%, Na 7.05%, O 19.61%, S 9.83%. Prepd by treating 4,4′-diamino-2,2′-stilbenedisulfonic acid with phenyl isocyanate in aq soln at 40°: **DE 746569** and **FR 878155** (to I. G. Farbenind.); **GB 683895** (1952 to Bayer); *FIAT Final Rept.* No. 1302 (Sept. 15, 1947); *Colour Index* Vol. 4 (3rd ed., 1971) p 4371.

trans-form

USE: Fluorescent dye for cellulose, protein fibers, nylon, wool or paper.

1316. Blasticidin S. [2079-00-7] 4-[[3-Amino-5-[(amino-iminomethyl)methylamino]-1-oxopentyl]amino]-1-(4-amino-2-oxo-1(2H)-pyrimidinyl)-1,2,3,4-tetradeoxy-β-D-erythro-hex-2-eno-pyranuronic acid; 4-[3-amino-5-(1-methylguanidino)valeramido]-1-(4-amino-2-oxo-1(2H)-pyrimidinyl)-1,2,3,4-tetradeoxy-β-D-erythro-hex-2-enopyranuronic acid; 1-(1'-cytosinyl)-4-[L-3'-amino-5'-(1''-N-methylguanidino)-valerylamino]-1,2,3,4-tetradeoxy-β-D-erythro-hex-2-enuronic acid. $C_{17}H_{26}N_8O_5$; mol wt 422.44. C 48.33%, H 6.20%, N 26.53%, O 18.94%. Nucleoside antibiotic produced by Streptomyces griseochromogenes: Isoln and antimicrobial activity: Takeuchi et al., J. Antibiot. **11A,** 1 (1958); Sumiki, Umezawa, **JP 60 16449** (1960 to Japan Antibiot. Res. Assoc.), C.A. **55,** 21474e (1961). Structure: Otake et al., Agric. Biol. Chem. **30,** 132 (1966); Fox, Watanabe, Tetrahedron Lett. **1966,** 897. Abs config: Yonehara et al., ibid. **1966,** 3785. Synthesis of the unsaturated carbohydrate: Goody et al., ibid. **1970,** 293; of the cytosinine moiety: Fox, Watanabe, Pure Appl. Chem. **28,** 475 (1971); Kondo et al., Tetrahedron Lett. **1972,** 1881; eidem, Tetrahedron **29,** 1801 (1973). Crystal and molecular structure: V. Swaminathan et al., Biochim. Biophys. Acta **655,** 335 (1981).

Blastidic Acid   Cytosinine

Needles from water, dec 235-236°. $[\alpha]_D^{11}$ +108.4° (water). uv max (0.1N HCl): 275 nm ($E_{1cm}^{1\%}$ 349); (0.1N NaOH): 266-270 nm ($E_{1cm}^{1\%}$ 266). Sol in water, acetic acid. Practically insol in methanol, ethanol, acetone, benzene, ether, ethyl acetate, chloroform, carbon tetrachloride, cyclohexane, xylene, pyridine, dioxane. LD_{50} i.v. in mice: 2.82 mg/kg (Takeuchi).

Hydrochloride. Crystals, dec 224-225°.

USE: Antifungal against rice blast disease in Japan.

1317. Blebbistatin. [674289-55-5] 1,2,3,3a-Tetrahydro-3a-hydroxy-6-methyl-1-phenyl-4H-pyrrolo[2,3-b]quinolin-4-one; 1-phenyl-1,2,3,4-tetrahydro-4-hydroxypyrrolo[2,3-b]-7-methyl-quinolin-4-one. $C_{18}H_{16}N_2O_2$; mol wt 292.33. C 73.95%, H 5.52%, N 9.58%, O 10.95%. Small molecule inhibitor of the ATPase activity of myosin II; affects cell blebbing during cell division. Prepn and inhibition of non-muscle myosin II: A. F. Straight et al., Science **299,** 1743 (2003). Prepn and crystal structure of (−)-form: C. Lucas-Lopez et al., Eur. J. Org. Chem. **2005,** 1736. Crystal structure in complex with myosin II: J. S. Allingham et al., Nat. Struct. Mol. Biol. **12,** 378 (2005). Kinetics of non-muscle myosin IIB inhibition: B. Ramamurthy et al., Biochemistry **43,** 14832 (2004). Mechanism of myosin II inhibition: M. Kovács et al., J. Biol. Chem. **279,** 35557 (2004). Photochemistry studies: J. Kolega, Biochem. Biophys. Res. Commun. **320,** 1020 (2004); T. Sakamoto et al., Biochemistry **44,** 584 (2005).

(S)-Form

Bright yellow solid, mp 192-193°. Absorption max (phosphate-buffered saline): 265, 430 nm.

(S)-Form. (−)-Blebbistatin. Crystals from acetonitrile, $[\alpha]_D^{26}$ −464° (c = 0.2 in dichloromethane).

USE: In studies of cytoskeletal dynamics and the biological roles of class-II myosins.

1318. Bleomycins. NSC-125066; A group of related glyco-peptide antibiotics. Variations in the terminal amine account for differing activities. Isolated from Streptomyces verticillus: Umezawa, Antimicrob. Agents Chemother. **1965,** 1079. Purification and separation into bleomycins A and B and their components: Umezawa et al., J. Antibiot. **19,** 200, 210 (1966); T. Takita et al., ibid. **21,** 79 (1968); **22,** 237 (1969). Bleomycin A_2 is the main component of the bleomycin employed clinically. Total structure elucidation: T. Takita et al., ibid. **25,** 755 (1972). Revised structure: eidem, ibid. **31,** 801 (1978). Terminal amines: Fujii et al., ibid. **26,** 398 (1973). Synthesis of new bleomycins: T. Takita et al., ibid. 254. Total synthesis of bleomycin A_2: eidem, Tetrahedron Lett. **23,** 521 (1982). Improved total synthesis: S. Saito et al., J. Antibiot. **36,** 92 (1983). Biosynthesis: Fujii et al., ibid. **27,** 73 (1974). Bleomycins are believed to react with DNA and cause strand scission; they have also been shown to have a type of oxygen transferase activity. Mechanism of action studies: R. M. Burger et al., Life Sci. **28,** 715 (1981); N. Marugesan et al., J. Biol. Chem. **257,** 8600 (1982). Coordination chemistry: J. C. Dabrowiak, J. Inorg. Biochem. **13,** 317 (1980). Clinical pharmacology: S. T. Crooke, Cancer Chemother. **3,** 343 (1981). Characterization of analogs: N. J. Oppenheimer et al., J. Biol. Chem. **257,** 1606 (1982). Reviews: H. Umezawa, Pure Appl. Chem. **28,** 665-680 (1971); C. W. Haidle, R. S. Lloyd, Antibiotics vol. 5(pt. 2), F. E. Hahn, Ed. (Springer-Verlag, New York, 1979) pp 124-154; H. Umezawa, Anticancer Agents Based on Natural Product Models, J. M. Cassady, J. D. Douros, Eds. (Academic Press, New York, 1980) pp 147-166.

R = terminal amine

Colorless or yellowish powder which becomes bluish depending on Cu content. Very sol in water, methanol; slightly sol in ethanol. Practically insol in acetone, ethyl acetate, butyl acetate, ether. uv max: 244-248, 289-294 nm ($E_{1cm}^{1\%}$ 121-148, 102-121.5).

Sulfate. [9041-93-4] Blenoxane; Bleo.

Bleomycin A_2. [11116-31-7] N^1-[3-(Dimethylsulfonio)propyl]bleomycinamide. $C_{55}H_{84}N_{17}O_{21}S_3$; mol wt 1415.55.

THERAP CAT: Antineoplastic.

1319. Blonanserin. [132810-10-7] 2-(4-Ethyl-1-piperazin-yl)-4-(4-fluorophenyl)-5,6,7,8,9,10-hexahydrocycloocta[b]pyridine; AD-5423; Lonasen. $C_{23}H_{30}FN_3$; mol wt 367.50. C 75.17%, H 8.23%, F 5.17%, N 11.43%. Dopamine D_2 and serotonin 5-HT_2 receptor antagonist. Prepn: K. Hino et al., **EP 385237**; eidem, **US 5021421** (1990, 1991 both to Dainippon). HPLC determn in plasma: M. Matsuda et al., J. Pharm. Biomed. Anal. **15,** 1449 (1997). X-ray crystal structure: K. Suzuki et al., Anal. Sci. **18,** 1289 (2002). In vitro receptor binding study and in vivo pharmacology in animals: M. Oka et al., J. Pharmacol. Exp. Ther. **264,** 158 (1993). Evaluation in mouse models of schizophrenia: T. Nagai et al., NeuroReport **14,** 269 (2003). Review of development and clinical experience: C. E. Heading, Curr. Opin. Cent. Peripher. Nerv. Syst. Invest. Drugs **2,** 79-84 (2002).

Crystals from acetonitrile, mp 123-124°.
THERAP CAT: Antipsychotic.

1320. Blue Cohosh. Caulophyllum; papoose root; squaw root. Perennial herb, *Caulophyllum thalictroides* Michx., *Berberidaceae*. Mature plant is a peculiar bluish green color and bears dark blue fruit. Traditionally used in Native American medicine as a uterine stimulant, emmenagogue, antispasmodic. Medicinal formulations are prepared from the dried rhizome and roots. *Habit.* Damp woods of eastern North America. *Constit.* Alkaloids, primarily baptifoline, methylcytisine, anagyrine, magnoflorine, *q.q.v.*; 2 glycosides, caulosaponin, cauloside D; citrullol, gum, resins, phosphoric acid, phytosterol. GC determn of alkaloids: J. M. Betz *et al.*, *Phytochem. Anal.* **9**, 232 (1998). Tetratogenicity study of constituents: E. J. Kennelly *et al.*, *J. Nat. Prod.* **62**, 1385 (1999). Brief review of clinical use in labor stimulation: B. L. McFarlin *et al.*, *J. Nurse-Midwifery* **44**, 205-216 (1999). Reviews of medicinal uses: V. E. Tyler, *Herbs of Choice* (Pharmaceutical Products Press, New York, 1994) pp 47-48; J. Barnes *et al.*, *Herbal Medicines* (Pharmaceutical Press, London, 2nd Ed., 2002) pp 147-148.
Note: Do not confuse with black cohosh, *q.v.*
THERAP CAT: Emmenagogue; oxytocic.

1321. Bohrium. [54037-14-8] Element 107; nielsbohrium; unnilseptium. Bh, Ns, Uns; at. no. 107. Group VIIB(7). No stable nuclides. Known isotopes: 261, 262, 262m, 266, 267. Prepn of α-emitting isotope ^{261}107 by ^{209}Bi (^{54}Cr,2n); decay by spontaneous fission, $T_{1/2}$ 1-2 msec: Y. T. Organessian *et al.*, *Nucl. Phys. A* **273**, 505 (1976); G. N. Flerov, *C.A.* **87**, 173830v (1977); A. S. Iljinov *et al.*, *Report* **JINR-E-7-9686** (1976), *C.A.* **90**, 62354k (1979). Prepn of isotopes including ^{262}107 ($T_{1/2}$ 102 ±26 msec, α-emitter) by ^{209}Bi (^{54}Cr,1n): G. Münzenberg, *et al.*, *Z. Phys.* **A300**, 107 (1981); and revised $T_{1/2}$ 11.8 msec for ^{261}107: *eidem, ibid.* **A333**, 163 (1989). Chemical characterization of 6 isotopes as bohrium oxychloride: R. Eichler *et al.*, *Nature* **407**, 63 (2000). Review of history, prepn and properties: R. J. Silva in *The Chemistry of the Actinide Elements* vol. **2**, J. J. Katz *et al.*, Eds. (Chapman and Hall, New York, 1986) pp 1110-1112; N. Flerov, G. M. Ter-Akopian *Prog. Particle Nucl. Phys.* **19**, 197-239 (1987); G. T. Seaborg, W. D. Loveland, *The Elements Beyond Uranium* (John Wiley & Sons, Inc., New York, 1990) p 56-57. Brief review of properties and prepn of ^{267}Bh ($T_{1/2}$ 17 sec): R. F. Service, *Science* **289**, 1270 (2000).

1322. Bolandiol. [19793-20-5] (3β,17β)-Estr-4-ene-3,17-diol; 3β,17β-dihydroxyestr-4-ene. $C_{18}H_{28}O_2$; mol wt 276.41. C 78.21%, H 10.21%, O 11.58%. Prepn: Colton, **US 2843608** (1958 to Searle).

Crystals from dil acetone and from ethyl acetate + petr ether, mp 169-172°.
Dipropionate. [1986-53-4] Norpropandrolate; 3β,17β-dipropionyloxy-4-estrene; SC-7525; Anabiol; Storinal. $C_{24}H_{36}O_4$; mol wt 388.54.
THERAP CAT: Anabolic.

1323. Bolasterone. [1605-89-6] (7α,17β)-17-Hydroxy-7,17-dimethylandrost-4-en-3-one; 7α,17α-dimethyltestosterone. $C_{21}H_{32}O_2$; mol wt 316.48. C 79.70%, H 10.19%, O 10.11%. Synthetic anabolic; epimeric with calusterone, *q.v.* Prepn: **BE 610385**; Babcock, Campbell, **US 3341557** (1962, 1967 both to Upjohn); Campbell, Babcock, *Hormonal Steroids*, Proc. 1st Int. Congr., **2**, L. Martini, A. Pecile, Eds. (Academic Press, New York, 1965) pp 59-67. Activity studies: Stucki *et al., ibid.* 119-132. HPLC determn in urine: R. Gonzalo-Lumbreras, R. Izquierdo-Hornillos, *J. Chromatogr. B* **742**, 47 (2000).

Crystals, mp 163-165°.
Note: This is a controlled substance (anabolic steroid): **21 CFR**, 1308.13, as defined in 1300.01.

1324. Boldenone. [846-48-0] (17β)-17-Hydroxyandrosta-1,4-dien-3-one; 1,4-androstadien-17β-ol-3-one; 3-oxo-17β-hydroxy-1,4-androstadiene; dehydrotestosterone. $C_{19}H_{26}O_2$; mol wt 286.41. C 79.68%, H 9.15%, O 11.17%. Anabolic steroid. Prepn: Meystre *et al., Helv. Chim. Acta* **39**, 734 (1956); Florey, **US 2875196** (1949 to Olin Mathieson); Nobile, **US 2837464** (1958 to Schering). Metabolism in humans and GC/MS determn in urine: W. Schänzer, M. Donike, *Biol. Mass Spectrom.* **21**, 3 (1992). LC/MS determn in horse urine: F. Pu *et al., J. Chromatogr. B* **813**, 241 (2004). Review of metabolism in animal species: H. F. De Brabander *et al., Food Addit. Contam.* **21**, 515-525 (2004).

Crystals, mp 164-166°. $[\alpha]_D^{25}$ +25° (in chloroform).
Acetate. $C_{21}H_{28}O_3$. Crystals, mp 151-153°.
10-Undecenoate. [13103-34-9] Boldenone undecylenate; Ba-29038; Equipoise; Parenabol. $C_{30}H_{44}O_3$; mol wt 452.67.
Note: This is a controlled substance (anabolic steroid): **21 CFR**, 1308.13, as defined in 1300.01.
THERAP CAT (VET): Anabolic.

1325. Boldine. [476-70-0] 5,6,6a,7-Tetrahydro-1,10-dimethoxy-6-methyl-4*H*-dibenzo[*de,g*]quinoline-2,9-diol; 1,10-dimethoxy-6aα-aporphine-2,9-diol; 1,10-dimethoxy-2,9-dihydroxyaporphine; 2,6-dihydroxy-3,5-dimethoxyaporphine. $C_{19}H_{21}NO_4$; mol wt 327.37. C 69.71%, H 6.47%, N 4.28%, O 19.55%. Isoln from boldo (*Peumus boldus* Molina, *Monimiaceae*): Bourgoin, Verne, *J. Pharm. Chim.* **16**, 191 (1872); from *Laurelia novaezelandiae* A. Cunn.: Bernauer, *Helv. Chim. Acta* **50**, 1583 (1967). Structure: Warnat, *Ber.* **58**, 2768; **59**, 85 (1926); Späth, Tharrer, *ibid.* **66**, 904 (1933); Schlittler, *ibid.* 988. Synthesis of *dl*-form: S. M. Kupchan *et al., Chem. Commun.* **1976**, 91. Biosynthetic study: D. S. Bhakuni *et al., J. Chem. Soc. Perkin Trans. 1* **1977**, 706. Detailed description of the boldo brush, its ingredients and pharmacological properties: H. Schindler, *Arzneim.-Forsch.* **7**, 747 (1957).

***d*-Form.** Crystals from ether. mp 162-164°. $[\alpha]_D^{25}$ +127° (c = 0.1 in alcohol). Very slightly sol in water or ether; sol in alcohol, chloroform, dil acids.

***d*-Form hydrochloride.** Crystals from methanol-ether and methanol, mp 212-220°.

***dl*-Form.** mp 159-162°.

Dimethyl ether *see* Glaucine.

Note: Boldine is used as an ingredient in choleretics and laxatives. The total alkaloids from boldo are also marketed as a grayish-white to grayish-yellow, bitter powder; almost insol in water. Sol in alc, chloroform, slightly in ether.

1326. Boldo. Boldu; boldea; boldus; boldoa. Leaves of *Peumus boldus* Molina *(Boldu boldus* [Molina] Lyons, *Boldea fragrans* Gay), *Monimiaceae*. *Habit.* Peru, Chile. *Constit.* About 2% volatile oil, about 0.1% boldine. *Ref:* Schindler, *Arzneim.-Forsch.* **7**, 747 (1957).

THERAP CAT: In hepatic dysfunction, cholelithiasis.

1327. Bole, Armenian. Bolus armena; bolus rubra; red bole. A red variety of clay (aluminum silicate) contg naturally occurring ferric oxide (hematite). Originally found in Armenia.

Reddish, soft, unctuous pieces; adheres to the tongue; easily reduced to powder. Insol in usual solvents. d 1.9-2.0.

USE: For coloring powders, cements, and as a pigment.

THERAP CAT: Adsorbant; protectant.

1328. Boleko Oil. Isano oil. Oil extracted from the nuts of the tree *Ongokea gore* (Hua) Pierre, *Olacaceae*, growing in equatorial Africa. Contains fatty acids (as glycerides): isanic acid 46%, isanolic acid 44%. *Refs:* Scher, *Arch. Pharm.* **287**, 548 (1954); Dupont *et al., Bull. Soc. Chim. Fr.* **1957**, 1495; De Vries, *Oleagineux* **12**, 427 (1957); Kneeland *et al., J. Am. Oil Chem. Soc.* **35**, 361 (1958). Extraction procedure: Lambert, **US 2800492** (1957 to UCB). Structure of acids: Gunstone, Sealy, *J. Chem. Soc.* **1963**, 5772; Morris, *ibid.* 5779.

Typical characteristics: Acid no. 1-10; ester no. 183.5; sapon no. 185-200; iodine no. 254-259; d_4^{20} 0.973-0.983; n_D^{20} 1.505-1.509; viscosity (25°): 7-10 P. Soluble in acetone, benzene, ethyl ether, carbon tetrachloride, chloroform. Slightly insol in petr ether, ethanol, hexane. The viscosity increases upon heating and the oil is transformed into a rubber-like mass. Does not polymerize when heated to a moderate temp; when heated rapidly to temp above 200° polymerization becomes so rapid as to become explosive. Polymerization is explained by the acetylenic structure of isanic acid.

USE: In fire retardant paints.

1329. Bombesin. [31362-50-2] 2-L-Glutamine-6-L-asparaginealytesin. $C_{71}H_{110}N_{24}O_{18}S$; mol wt 1619.85. C 52.64%, H 6.84%, N 20.75%, O 17.78%, S 1.98%. Pharmacologically active tetradecapeptide found in skins of European amphibians of the family Discoglossidae, principally *Bombina bombina* and *Bombina variegata variegata*. Isoln and structure: A. Anastasi *et al., Experientia* **27**, 166 (1971). Pharmacological activity: V. Erspamer *et al., J. Pharm. Pharmacol.* **22**, 875 (1970). Synthesis: L. Bernardi *et al., Experientia* **27**, 873 (1971). It is a potent stimulant of gastric and pancreatic secretions in mammals; a bombesin-like immunoreactive peptide is found in both brain and gut, *cf.* J. M. Polak *et al., Lancet* **1**, 1109 (1976). Other actions include hypertensive reactions, antidiuresis, and hyperglycemic activity. Bombesin has been shown to have a strong effect on core temperature lowering in rats: M. Brown *et al., Science* **196**, 996 (1977). High levels of intracellular bombesin have also been found in human small-cell lung carcinoma: T. W. Moody *et al., ibid.* **214**, 1246 (1981). Brief review of chemistry, isoln, purification: V. Mutt, *Biochem. Soc. Trans.* **8**, 11 (1980). Effect on suppression of food intake: J. Gibbs *et al., Nature* **282**, 208 (1979). Pharmacological reviews: G. Bertaccini, *Pharmacol. Rev.* **28**, 127 (1976); S. R. Bloom, J. M. Polak, *Adv. Clin. Chem.* **21**, 177 (1980).

5-oxoPro–Gln–Arg–Leu–Gly–Asn–Gln–Trp–Ala–Val–Gly–His–Leu–MetNH₂

Hydrochloride. $C_{71}H_{112}Cl_2N_{24}O_{18}S$. Cryst from 99% ethanol, mp 185° (dec). $[\alpha]_D^{24}$ −20.6° (c = 0.65 in DMF-HMPT 8:2).

1330. Bomyl®. [122-10-1] 3-[(Dimethoxyphosphinyl)oxy]-2-pentenedioic acid dimethyl ester; 3-hydroxy-2-pentenedioic acid dimethyl ester dimethyl phosphate; 3-hydroxyglutaconic acid di-

methyl ester dimethyl phosphate; dimethyl 1,3-bis(carbomethoxy)-1-propen-2-yl phosphate; dimethyl 3-hydroxyglutaconate dimethyl phosphate; ENT-24833; GC-3707; Swat. $C_9H_{15}O_8P$; mol wt 282.18. C 38.31%, H 5.36%, O 45.36%, P 10.98%. Prepn: Gilbert, **US 2891887** (1959 to Allied). Activity: P. E. Newallis *et al., J. Agric. Food Chem.* **15**, 940 (1967). Toxicity: E. W. Schafer, *Toxicol. Appl. Pharmacol.* **21**, 315 (1972).

Liquid; bp_{17} 155-164°; bp_2 155-165° (tech grade). Miscible with methanol, ethanol, acetone, xylene. Practically insol in water, petr ether, kerosene. LD_{50} orally in rats: 32 mg/kg (Schafer).

USE: Insecticide.

1331. Bone Morphogenetic Proteins. Bone morphogenic factors; bone morphogenic proteins; BMPs. Multifunctional cytokines that induce formation of cartilage and bone; originally isolated from demineralized bone matrix. Structurally related to the transforming growth factor-β (TGF-β) superfamily; at least 15 closely related forms exist. All are dimers linked by 7 disulfide bonds. Prepn from rabbit bone: M. R. Urist *et al., Proc. Natl. Acad. Sci. USA* **76**, 1828 (1979); from human bone: *idem et al., Proc. Soc. Exp. Biol. Med.* **173**, 194 (1983). Clinical evaluations in bone repair: E. E. Johnson *et al., Clin. Orthop. Relat. Res.* **230**, 249, 257 (1988). Review of purification and structures of BMP-1 through BMP-7: J. M. Wozney, *Prog. Growth Factor Res.* **1**, 267-280 (1989); and osteogenic activity: *idem, Mol. Reprod. Dev.* **32**, 160-167 (1992). Review of potential clinical applications and delivery strategies: C. A. Kirker-Head, *Adv. Drug Delivery Rev.* **43**, 65-92 (2000); of clinical studies in human bone regeneration: E. H. J. Groeneveld, E. H. Burger, *Eur. J. Endocrinol.* **142**, 9-21 (2000); of clinical efficacy and safety: P. J. Harwood, P. V. Giannoudis, *Expert Opin. Drug Safety* **4**, 75-89 (2005).

BMP-2. BMP-2A. Mature human form is a homodimer, mol wt 32 kDa. Each monomer consists of 114 amino acid residues. Review of bioactivity: E. H Riley *et al., Clin. Orthop. Relat. Res.* **324**, 39-46 (1996).

BMP-7. Osteogenic protein-1; OP-1. Mature human form is a homodimer, mol wt 32-36 kDa. Each monomer consists of 139 amino acid residues. Prepn of recombinant human BMP-7 (*rhBMP-7*): T. K. Sampath *et al., J. Biol. Chem.* **267**, 20352 (1992). Review of bioactivity and potential clinical applications: S. D. Cook, D. C. Rueger, *Clin. Orthop. Relat. Res.* **324**, 29-38 (1996).

Dibotermin alfa. [246539-15-1] Bone morphogenetic protein 2 (human recombinant rhBMP-2). Glycosylated, disulfide-linked dimer, mol wt ~28-33 kDa. Prepn: E. A. Wang *et al.,* **WO 8800205**; *eidem,* **US 5013649** (1988, 1991 both to Genetics Institute); E. A. Wang *et al., Proc. Natl. Acad. Sci. USA* **87**, 2220 (1990). Clinical trial of collagen sponge implant in tibial fractures: S. Govender *et al., J. Bone Joint Surg.* **84-A**, 2123 (2002). Review of clinical trials in spinal fusion: S. N. Khan, J. M. Lane, *Expert Opin. Biol. Ther.* **4**, 741-748 (2004).

THERAP CAT: Osteoinductive agent.

1332. Bongkrekic Acid. [11076-19-0] (2*E*,4*Z*,6*R*,8*Z*,10*E*,-14*E*,17*S*,18*E*,20*Z*)-20-(Carboxymethyl)-6-methoxy-2,5,17-trimethyl-2,4,8,10,14,18,20-docosaheptaenedioic acid; 3-carboxymethyl-17-methoxy-6,18,21-trimethyldocosa-2,4,8,12,14,18,20-heptaenedioic acid; BA. $C_{28}H_{38}O_7$; mol wt 486.60. C 69.11%, H 7.87%, O 23.02%. One of the two toxic antibiotic principles produced by *Pseudomonas cocovenenans* on partially defatted coconut; the other being toxoflavin, *q.v.* Name derived from "bongkrek", a molded coconut product from Indonesia which becomes highly poisonous when *P. cocovenenans* outgrows the mold. Isoln: van Veen, Mertens, *Rec. Trav. Chim.* **53**, 257 (1934); **54**, 373 (1935); Nugteren, Berends, *ibid.* **76**, 13 (1957). Purification and properties: Lijmbach *et al., Tetrahedron* **26**, 5993 (1970). Structural studies: *idem, ibid.* **27**, 1839 (1971). Revised structure: De Bruijn *et al., ibid.* **29**, 1541 (1973). Absolute configuration: Zylber *et al., Experientia* **29**, 387, 648 (1973). Influence on carbohydrate metabolism: van Veen, Mertens, *Arch. Neerl. Physiol.* **21**, 73 (1936), *C.A.* **30**, 3880[9] (1936); inhibition of adenine nucleotide translocation: Henderson, Lardy, *J. Biol. Chem.* **245**, 1319 (1970); Klingenberg *et al., Biochem. Biophys. Res. Commun.* **39**, 363 (1970).

White, amorphous solid, mp 50-60°. uv max (methanol): 237, 267 nm (ε 32000, 36700). $[\alpha]_D^{25}$ +162.5°. LD_{50} i.v. in mice: 1.41 mg/kg (Lijmbach).

1333. Bopindolol. [62658-63-3] 1-[(1,1-Dimethylethyl)-amino]-3-[(2-methyl-1*H*-indol-4-yl)oxy]-2-propanol benzoate ester; ($\pm$)-1-(*tert*-butylamino)-3-[(2-methylindol-4-yl)oxy]-2-propanol benzoate (ester). $C_{23}H_{28}N_2O_3$; mol wt 380.48. C 72.60%, H 7.42%, N 7.36%, O 12.62%. Nonselective β-adrenergic blocker. Prepn: F. Troxler, F. Seemann, **DE 2635209**; *eidem*, **US 4340541** (1977, 1982 both to Sandoz). Clinical pharmacology: P. van Brummelen *et al., Eur. J. Clin. Pharmacol.* **22**, 491 (1982). HPLC determn in plasma: C. J. Oddie *et al., J. Chromatogr.* **273**, 469 (1983). Effect on plasma lipid fractions: P. van Brummelen *et al., Br. J. Clin. Pharmacol.* **17**, 86 (1984). Pharmacokinetics: R. Platzer *et al., Clin. Pharmacol. Ther.* **36**, 5 (1984). Clinical trials in hypertension: U. L. Hulthen *et al., J. Cardiovasc. Pharmacol.* **5**, 426 (1983); W. J. Schiess *et al., Eur. J. Clin. Pharmacol.* **27**, 529 (1984).

Sol in ether, methylene chloride. LD_{50} i.v. in mice: 17 mg/kg (Troxler, Seemann, 1977).

Maleate. [62658-64-4] Sandonorm. $C_{23}H_{28}N_2O_3 \cdot C_4H_4O_4$; mol wt 496.55.

Malonate. [82857-38-3] LT-31-200; Wandonorm. $C_{23}H_{28}N_2-O_3 \cdot C_3H_4O_4$; mol wt 484.54.

THERAP CAT: Antihypertensive.

1334. Borazine. [6569-51-3] Inorganic benzene; hexahydro-*s*-triazaborine; borazane; borazole; triborine triamine; triboron nitride; *s*-triazaborane. $B_3H_6N_3$; mol wt 80.50. B 40.29%, H 7.51%, N 52.20%. Isoelectronic with benzene. Prepn: Stock, Pohland, *Ber.* **59**, 2215 (1926); Wiberg, Bolz, *Ber.* **73**, 209 (1940). Structural study: H. Watanabe, W. Kubo, *J. Am. Chem. Soc.* **82**, 2428 (1960); W. Harshbarger *et al., Inorg. Chem.* **8**, 1683 (1969). Electronic structure: A. Lötz *et al., Chem. Phys.* **103**, 317 (1986). Raman spectroscopy: J. V. Kainnady, A. Weber, *J. Raman Spectrosc.* **5**, 35 (1976). Electric and magnetic properties: G. R. Dennis, G. L. D. Ritchie, *J. Phys. Chem.* **97**, 8403 (1993). Use in synthesis of ceramic composites: K. Su *et al., Chem. Mater.* **5**, 547 (1993). *Review:* E. M. Smolin, L. Rapoport, *s-Triazines and Derivatives* (Interscience, New York, 1959) pp 597-626.

Mobile liquid; mp −58°; bp 53°. Stable up to 500° when pure and totally anhydrous. d_4^0 0.824; d_4^{57} 0.898. n_D^{20} 1.3821. Critical temp 252°. Heat of vaporization 7.0 kcal. Mol vol at bp = 99.7 ml. Surface tension at mp = 31.09 dynes/cm. Parachor 207.9. Trou-

ton's constant 21.4. Eötvös' constant 2.0. Dipole moment in benzene (25°) = 0.50. Dissolves in water, giving a soln with strong reducing properties. Hydrolyzes slowly in aq soln yielding hydrogen, boric acid, and ammonia.

1335. Bordeaux Mixture. [8011-63-0] Mixture of calcium hydroxide (hydrated lime) and copper(II) sulfate, *q.q.v.* Prepn and use vs downy mildew on grapes: Millardet, *Ann. Agric. Prat. (Paris)* **49**, 513 (1885); *see also:* D. E. H. Frear, *Pesticide Index* (College Science, 4th ed., 1969) p 72. Field trial vs pink disease in mandarin oranges: P. M. Pradhanang, *Crop Prot.* **13**, 550 (1994); vs Persian walnut blight: A. Belisario, A. Zoina, *Eur. J. Forest Pathol.* **25**, 224 (1995). Effects on Sauvignon grape composition and wine aroma: E. Hatzidimitriou *et al., J. Int. Sci. Vigne Vin* **30**, 133 (1996).

Fine, blue pptd powder. Insol in water.

Burgundy Mixture. [11125-96-5] Carbonic acid disodium salt, mixt. with copper(2+) sulfate (1:1). Analog to Bordeaux mixture produced from copper(II) sulfate and sodium carbonate, *q.q.v.* Prepn and use vs downy mildew on grapes: E. Masson, *J. Agric. Prat. (Paris)* **51**, 814 (1887); *see also:* Frear, *Chemistry of the Pesticides* (Van Nostrand, 3rd ed., 1955) p 322. Review of chemistry: R. L. Mond, C. Heberlein, *J. Chem. Soc.* **115**, 908-922 (1919). Blue to green colloidal ppt. Practically insol in water.

USE: Fungicide.

1336. Boric Acid. [10043-35-3] Boracic acid; orthoboric acid; Borofax. BH_3O_3; mol wt 61.83. B 17.49%, H 4.89%, O 77.63%. H_3BO_3. Occurs in nature as the mineral *sassolite*. Manuf: *Faith, Keyes & Clark's Industrial Chemicals*, F. A. Lowenheim, M. K. Moran, Eds. (Wiley-Interscience, New York, 4th ed., 1975) pp 153-158. Toxicity study: Smyth *et al., Am. Ind. Hyg. Assoc. J.* **30**, 470 (1969). Review of toxicology and human exposure: *Toxicological Profile for Boron* (PB93-110674, 1992) 110 pp.

Colorless, odorless, transparent crystals, or white granules or powder; slightly unctuous to the touch. mp ~171°. Phase diagram for the $B_2O_3 \cdot H_2O$ system: Kracek *et al., Am. J. Sci.* **35A**, 143 (1938). Volatile with steam. pH: 5.1 (0.1 molar). One gram dissolves in 18 ml cold, 4 ml boiling water, in 18 ml cold, 6 ml boiling alcohol, in 4 ml glycerol; soly in water is increased by HCl, citric or tartaric acids. Soly of boric acid in glycerol solns of various concns: Sciarra, Elliott, *J. Am. Pharm. Assoc. Sci. Ed.* **49**, 116 (1960). LD_{50} orally in rats: 5.14 g/kg (Smyth).

Caution: Potential symptoms of overexposure by ingestion or absorption are vomiting, diarrhea, abdominal cramps, erythematous lesions on skin and mucous membranes, circulatory collapse, tachycardia, cyanosis, delirium, convulsions, coma. Chronic use may cause borism (dry skin, eruptions, gastric disturbances). *See* E. Browning, *Toxicity of Industrial Metals* (Appleton-Century-Crofts, New York, 2nd ed., 1969) pp 90-97.

USE: For weatherproofing wood and fireproofing fabrics; as a preservative; manuf cements, crockery, porcelain, enamels, glass, borates, leather, carpets, hats, soaps, artificial gems; in nickeling baths; cosmetics; printing and dyeing; painting; photography; for impregnating wicks; electric condensers; hardening steel. Also used as insecticide for cockroaches and black carpet beetles.

THERAP CAT: Astringent, antiseptic.

THERAP CAT (VET): Antibacterial and antifungal. Used chiefly in aqueous solution or powders for external use.

1337. Boric Anhydride. [1303-86-2] Boron oxide; boron trioxide; boric oxide; boron sesquioxide. B_2O_3; mol wt 69.62. B 31.06%, O 68.94%. Prepn of crystalline form: McCulloch, *J. Am. Chem. Soc.* **59**, 2650 (1937). Review of toxicology and human exposure: *Toxicological Profile for Boron* (PB93-110674, 1992) 110 pp.

Colorless, brittle, vitreous, semitransparent, hygroscopic lumps or hard, white crystals. d (amorph) 1.8; d (cryst) 2.46. mp (cryst) 450°. Slowly sol in 30 parts cold, or 5 parts boiling water; sol in alcohol, glycerol. *Keep dry*.

Note: Has been improperly called **anhydrous boric acid** or **fused boric acid**.

Caution: Potential symptoms of overexposure are irritation of eyes, skin, respiratory system; cough; conjunctivitis; skin erythema. *See NIOSH Pocket Guide to Chemical Hazards* (DHHS/NIOSH 97-140, 1997) p 30.

USE: In metallurgy; in analysis of silicates to determine SiO_2 and alkalies; in blowpipe analysis.

1338. Borneol. [507-70-0] *endo*-1,7,7-Trimethylbicy-clo[2.2.1]heptan-2-ol; *endo*-2-bornanol; *endo*-2-camphanol; *endo*-2-hydroxycamphane; bornyl alcohol; Baros camphor; Sumatra camphor; Borneo camphor; Dryobalanops camphor; Bhimsaim camphor; Malayan camphor; camphol. $C_{10}H_{18}O$; mol wt 154.25. C 77.87%, H 11.76%, O 10.37%. The dextrorotatory form which predominates occurs in the oil from *Dryobalanops aromatica* Gaertn., *Dipterocarpaceae,* and in many other plants; the levorotatory form comes from *Blumea balsamifera* (L.) DC., *Compositae:* E. Gildemeister, F. Hoffman, *Die ätherischen Ole* (Schimmel, Leipzig, 3rd ed., 1928) pp 475-481. Racemic borneol is prepd synthetically by reduction of camphor: Truett, Moulton, *J. Am. Chem. Soc.* **73,** 5913 (1951); Ziegler *et al., Ann.* **623,** 9 (1959); Ziegler, **GB 803178** (1958); from pinene: Schwyzer, *Pharm. Ztg.* **75,** 1275 (1930). Configuration (isoborneol = *exo*-form; borneol = *endo*-form): Toivonen *et al., Acta Chem. Scand.* **3,** 991 (1949). Toxicity data: R. C. Beier, *Rev. Environ. Contam. Toxicol.* **113,** 47-127 (1990). *Review:* J. L. Simonsen, *The Terpenes* vol. II (University Press, Cambridge, 2nd ed., 1949) pp 349-365.

d-Borneol

d-**Form.** Hexagonal plates from petr ether, mp 208°. Peculiar peppery odor and burning taste somewhat resembling that of mint. Sublimes, but is less volatile than samphor. d_4^{20} 1.011. bp 212°. $[\alpha]_D^{20}$ +37.7° (c = 5 in alc); $[\alpha]_{546}^{22}$ +44.4° (c = 0.5 in toluene). Almost insol in water. Sol in alc (176 parts dissolve in 100 parts w/w of abs alc), ether, petr ether (about 1:6), benzene (about 1:5), toluene, acetone, decalin, tetralin. LD orally in rabbits: 2000 mg/kg (Beier).

l-**Form.** Hexagonal plates, mp 204°. bp$_{779}$ 210°. $[\alpha]_D^{20}$ −37.7° (c = 5 in alc); $[\alpha]_{546}^{22}$ −44.4° (c = 0.5 in toluene).

dl-**Form.** mp 206-207°.

Caution: May cause nausea, vomiting, mental confusion, dizziness, convulsions.

USE: Primarily in the manuf of its esters. Some free borneol and isoborneol is used in perfumery and in incense making.

1339. Bornyl Acetate. [76-49-3] 1,7,7-Trimethylbicy-clo[2.2.1]heptan-2-ol acetate; borneol acetate. $C_{12}H_{20}O_2$; mol wt 196.29. C 73.43%, H 10.27%, O 16.30%. $CH_3COOC_{10}H_{17}$. Prepn of the *d*-form by acylation of *d*-borneol: Shishido *et al., J. Am. Chem. Soc.* **82,** 125 (1960).

d-**Form.** Crystals, mp 29°, also reported as mp 26.5°, Considine, *J. Org. Chem.* **25,** 671 (1960). bp 225-226°, bp$_8$ 92-93°. d 0.99. n_D^{22} 1.4623. $[\alpha]_D$ +44.38°, Haller, *Compt. Rend.* **109,** 29 (1889); $[\alpha]_D$ +41.2°, Considine, *loc. cit.;* α_D^{14} +44.72° (neat), Shishido, *loc. cit.* Very slightly sol in water; sol in alcohol, ether.

l-**Form.** Crystals, mp 27°. bp$_{14}$ 103°. $[\alpha]_D$ −44.45°, Haller, *loc. cit.;* $[\alpha]_D$ −42.0°, Considine, *loc. cit.*

dl-**Form.** Crystals, mp 7.0°, Considine, *loc. cit.*

1340. Bornyl Chloride. [464-41-5] *endo*-2-Chloro-1,7,7-trimethylbicyclo[2.2.1]heptane; pinene hydrochloride; 2-chlorobornane; 2-chlorocamphane; "terpene" hydrochloride; "turpentine camphor". $C_{10}H_{17}Cl$; mol wt 172.69. C 69.55%, H 9.92%, Cl 20.53%. Prepd from α-pinene: Zeiss, Zwanzig, *J. Am. Chem. Soc.* **79,** 1733 (1957); Hückel, Gelchsheimer, *Ann.* **625,** 12 (1959); by chlorination of camphane: Gandini, *Gazz. Chim. Ital.* **66,** 357 (1936). Configuration: Kwart, *J. Am. Chem. Soc.* **75,** 5942 (1953); Kwart, Null, *ibid.* **78,** 5943 (1956). *Review:* J. L. Simonsen, *The Terpenes* vol. II (University Press, Cambridge, 2nd ed., 1949) pp 340-349.

Crystals from alc, mp 132°. Odor resembling camphor. bp 207-208°. When prepd from optically active sources it has the same sign

as the hydrocarbon from which it is prepd: Thurber, Thielke, *J. Am. Chem. Soc.* **53,** 1032 (1931). Practically insol in water; sol in alc, ether.

THERAP CAT: Antiseptic.

1341. Bornyl Salicylate. [560-88-3] 2-Hydroxybenzoic acid 1,7,7-trimethylbicyclo[2.2.1]hept-2-yl ester; salicylic acid bornyl ester; borneol salicylate; Salit. $C_{17}H_{22}O_3$; mol wt 274.35. C 74.42%, H 8.08%, O 17.50%. $HOC_6H_4COOC_{10}H_{17}$. Prepd from borneol and salicylic acid: *Hagers Handb. Pharm. Praxis* **Band 1,** 210 (Berlin, 1930).

Brown, oily liquid. Slight odor and taste. Practically insol in water; miscible with alcohol, ether, chloroform, oils; slightly sol in glycerol; dec by alkalies and the intestinal fluids into its constituents.

THERAP CAT: Counterirritant.

1342. Boromycin. [34524-20-4] $C_{45}H_{74}BNO_{15}$; mol wt 879.88. C 61.43%, H 8.48%, B 1.23%, N 1.59%, O 27.28%. Antibiotic produced by *Streptomyces antibioticus* ETH 28829: Hütter *et al., Helv. Chim. Acta* **50,** 1533 (1967). The first known natural product in which boron has been found. It is a complex of boric acid with a tetradentate organic complexing agent and yields D-valine, boric acid and a polyhydroxy macrolide-type compound upon hydrolysis. Structure: Dunitz *et al., ibid.* **54,** 1709 (1971). Mechanism of action studies: Pache, Zähner, *Arch. Mikrobiol.* **67,** 156 (1969). Activity as a coccidiostat: Miller, Burg, **US 3864479** (1975 to Merck & Co.). Biosynthesis: T. S. S. Chen *et al., J. Org. Chem.* **46,** 2661 (1981). Partial synthesis: M. A. Avery *et al., Tetrahedron Lett.* **22,** 3123 (1981). Synthesis of C-3′ to C-17: S. Hanessian *et al., J. Am. Chem. Soc.* **103,** 6243 (1981); of C-3 to C-17: *eidem, Can. J. Chem.* **61,** 634 (1983); of C-1 to C-17: J. D. White *et al., J. Am. Chem. Soc.* **105,** 6517 (1983). Total synthesis: *eidem, ibid.* **111,** 790 (1989). *Review:* Pache in *Antibiotics* vol. 3, J. W. Corcoran, F. E. Hahn, Eds. (Springer-Verlag, New York, 1975) pp 585-587.

Colorless crystals from methanol, mp 223-228° (dec). $[\alpha]_D$ +63.5° (c = 0.55 in CHCl$_3$). No uv absorption between 210 and 400 nm. LD$_{50}$ orally in mice: 180 mg/kg (Hütter).

1343. Boron. [7440-42-8] B; at. no. 5; at. wt 10.811; valence 3. Group IIIA (13). Two naturally-occurring isotopes: 10; 11; three short-lived, artificial isotopes: 8, 12, 13. Occurrence in the earth's crust about 0.001% in the form of its compounds, never as the element. First obtained by Moissan in 1895 by reduction of boric anhydride (B_2O_3) with magnesium in a thermite-type reaction: Moissan, *Ann. Chim. Phys.* [7] **6,** 296 (1895), still a good method for large quantities of relatively impure boron. Prepn of high purity crystalline boron by vapor phase reduction of boron trichloride with hydrogen on electrically heated filaments in a flow system: Stern, Lynds, *J. Electrochem. Soc.* **105,** 676 (1958). Reviews of prepn and properties of boron and its compds: *Boron, Metallo-Boron Compounds and Boranes,* R. M. Adams, Ed. (Interscience, New York, 1964) 765 pp; *The Chemistry of Boron and Its Compounds,* E. L. Muetterties, Ed. (John Wiley, New York, 1967) 699 pp; Greenwood, "Boron" in *Comprehensive Inorganic Chemistry* vol. 1, J. C. Bailar, Jr. *et al.,* Eds. (Pergamon Press, Oxford, 1973) pp 655-991; J. G. Bower in *Kirk-Othmer Encyclopedia of*

Chemical Technology **vol. 4** (Wiley-Interscience, New York, 3rd ed., 1978) pp 62-66. Review of synthesis and applications of vinylic organoboranes: H. C. Brown, J. B. Campbell, *Aldrichim. Acta* **14**, 3-11 (1981). Review of toxicology and human exposure: *Toxicological Profile for Boron* (PB93-110674, 1992) 110 pp.

Polymorphic; α-rhombohedral form, clear red crystals, 12 atoms/unit cell, d 2.46; β-rhombohedral form, black, 105 atoms/unit cell, d 2.35; α-tetragonal form, black, opaque crystals with metallic luster, 50 atoms/unit cell, d 2.31; other crystal forms known but not entirely characterized. Amorphous form, black or dark brown powder, d 2.350. Crystals are almost as hard as diamond. mp ~2200°. Vapor pressure at 2413 K (2140°): 1.56×10^{-5} atm, Searcy, Myers, *J. Phys. Chem.* **61**, 957 (1957). Heat capacity at 25° of amorphous form: 2.858 cal/g-atom/°C; of β-rhombohedral form: 2.650 cal/g-atom/°C. Feeble conductor of electricity at room temp, good conductor at high temps. Admixture of traces of carbon improves conductivity. Self-limiting reaction with oxygen due to formation of B_2O_3 film; oxide coating evaporates above 1000°. Reacts with fluorine at room temp. Insol in water. Unaffected by aq hydrochloric and hydrofluoric acids. When finely divided, it is sol in boiling nitric and sulfuric acids and in most molten metals, such as copper, iron, magnesium, aluminum, calcium. Reacts vigorously with fused sodium peroxide, or with a fusion mixture of sodium carbonate and potassium nitrate.

USE: In nuclear chemistry as neutron absorber, in Ignitron rectifiers, in alloys, usually to harden other metals.

1344. Boron Carbide. [12069-32-8] Norbide. CB_4; mol wt 55.25. C 21.74%, B 78.27%. B_4C. Usually prepd in an electric furnace at 2500° according to the equation $2B_2O_3 + 7C \rightarrow B_4C + 6CO$: Ridgway, *Trans. Electrochem. Soc.* **66**, 117-133 (1934); also formed by reducing boric anhydride with magnesium in the presence of carbon: Dawihl, **DE 752324** (1942 to Krupp); *BIOS* rept. no. 925, p 22 (1947). Lab prepn by the reduction of boron trichloride with hydrogen in the presence of carbon or hydrocarbons: *Bell Labs. Record* **28**, 477 (1950). Comprehensive monograph: P. W. Gilles in *Adv. Chem. Ser.* **32**, entitled "Borax to Boranes," D. L. Martin, Ed. (ACS, Washington, DC, 1961).

Black shiny rhombohedra or octahedra. d_4^{25} 2.508-2.512. mp 2350° (no decompn); bp >3500°. Its hardness is less than that of industrial diamonds, but higher than the hardness of silicon carbide: ca 5,000 kg/mm², on Mohs' hardness scale = 9.3. Less brittle than most ceramics. Remarkably resistant to chemical action. Not attacked by hot HF, HNO_3 or $HCrO_4$. Decomposed by molten alkalis at red heat. Does not burn in oxygen flame.

USE: Abrasive. In the manuf of hard and chemicals-resistant ceramics or wear-resistant tools. Finely pulverized B_4C can be molded under (considerable) pressure and heat.

1345. Boron Monoxide. [12505-77-0] Boron oxide (BO). BO; mol wt 26.81. B 40.32%, O 59.68%. Exists in multiple polymeric forms, $(BO)_x$. Prepn: E. Zintl *et al.*, *Z. Anorg. Allg. Chem.* **245**, 8 (1940); T. Wartik, E. F. Apple, *J. Am. Chem. Soc.* **77**, 6400 (1955); and proposed structure: A. L. McCloskey *et al.*, *ibid.* **83**, 4750 (1961). VUV absorption spectrum: H. Bredohl *et al.*, *Mol. Phys.* **101**, 2145 (2003).

Fluffy white solid. Hygroscopic, converts back to tetrahydroxyboron on reaction with water. Sol in methanol, warm absolute ethanol, warm isopropyl alcohol. Sparingly sol in water. Insol in dimethylamine and methyl borate.

1346. Boron Nitride. [10043-11-5] BN; mol wt 24.82. B 43.56%, N 56.43%. Prepd by igniting compds of boron with compds of nitrogen: Taylor, **US 2855316** (1958 to Carborundum Co.). *Reviews:* Giardini, *Bur. Mines Inf. Circ.* No. **7664**, 13 pp (1953); K. Niedenzu, J. W. Dawson, *Boron-Nitrogen Compounds* (Academic Press, New York, 1965) pp 147-153.

Crystals with hexagonal, graphite lattice is most common form. *Borazon*, cubic crystalline modification, is probably the hardest substance known. There exists also an amorphous modification. mp 3000°. Begins to sublime at a temp slightly below 3000°. Begins to dissociate *in vacuo* at about 2700°. The chemical behavior of BN is dependent on the method of prepn. Not attacked by mineral acids, water; in general resistant to chemical attack. Hot concd alkali cleaves boron-nitrogen bond. Oxidation in air begins above 1200°. *See* Niedenzu, Dawson, *loc. cit.*

USE: Manuf of alloys; in semiconductors, nuclear reactors, lubricants.

1347. Boron Tribromide. [10294-33-4] BBr_3; mol wt 250.52. B 4.32%, Br 95.69%. Prepn: Gamble, *Inorg. Synth.* **3**, 27 (1950); Becher in *Handbook of Preparative Inorganic Chemistry* **Vol. 1**, G. Brauer, Ed. (Academic Press, New York, 2nd ed., 1963) p 781. Review of boron halides: Massey, *Adv. Inorg. Chem. Radiochem.* **10**, 1-152 (1967). Review of toxicology and human exposure: *Toxicological Profile for Boron* (PB93-110674, 1992) 110 pp. Brief review of synthetic applications: E. G. Doyagüez, *Synlett* **2005**, 1636-1637.

Colorless, fuming liquid; dec by water or alcohol. mp −46.0°; bp 90°. d^0 2.698. Vapor pressure data: Barber *et al.*, *J. Chem. Eng. Data* **9**, 137 (1964). *Store under dry inert atmosphere. Reacts violently with water, alcohols.*

Caution: Potential symptoms of overexposure are irritation of eyes, skin, respiratory system; skin and eye burns; dyspnea, pulmonary edema. *See NIOSH Pocket Guide to Chemical Hazards* (DHHS/NIOSH 97-140, 1997) p 32.

USE: Manuf of diborane; ultra high purity boron. Reagent for cleavage of ethers, amines, thiols; addition of allenes and alkynes.

1348. Boron Trichloride. [10294-34-5] BCl_3; mol wt 117.17. B 9.23%, Cl 90.77%. Prepn: Gamble, *Inorg. Synth.* **3**, 27 (1950). *Reviews:* Gerrard, Lappert, *Chem. Rev.* **58**, 1081-1111 (1958); Massey, *Adv. Inorg. Chem. Radiochem.* **10**, 1-152 (1967).

Colorless, fuming liquid at low temp; dec by water or alcohol. bp 12.5°. mp −107°. d_4^{12} 1.35. d^0 1.3728: Ward, *J. Chem. Eng. Data* **14**, 167 (1969).

USE: Manuf and purification of boron; as catalyst for organic reactions; in semiconductors; in bonding of iron, steels; in purification of metal alloys to remove oxides, nitrides and carbides.

1349. Boron Trifluoride. [7637-07-2] BF_3; mol wt 67.81. B 15.94%, F 84.05%. A strong Lewis acid. Prepn: Swinehart, **US 2148514**, **US 2196907** (1939, 1940 both to Harshaw Chemical); Booth, Wilson, *Inorg. Synth.* **1**, 21 (1939); Kwasnik in *Handbook of Preparative Inorganic Chemistry* **Vol. 1**, G. Brauer, Ed. (Academic Press, New York, 2nd ed., 1963) pp 219-222; Wiesboeck, **US 3690821** (1972 to U.S. Steel). Dihydrate: McGrath *et al.*, *J. Am. Chem. Soc.* **66**, 1263 (1944). *Reviews:* Booth, Martin, *Boron Trifluoride and Its Derivatives* (John Wiley & Sons, 1949), 296 pp; Booth in *Fluorine Chemistry* **Vol. 1**, J. Simons, Ed. (Academic Press, New York, 1950) pp 201-224; Topchiev *et al.*, *Boron Fluoride and Its Compounds as Catalysts in Organic Chemistry* (Pergamon Press, 1959) 326 pp; Martin in *Kirk-Othmer Encyclopedia of Chemical Technology* **Vol. 9** (Interscience, New York, 2nd ed., 1966) pp 554-562; Massey, *Adv. Inorg. Chem. Radiochem.* **10**, 1-152 (1967). Review of toxicology and human exposure: *Toxicological Profile for Boron* (PB93-110674, 1992) 110 pp.

Colorless gas. Pungent, suffocating odor. Forms dense white fumes in moist air. bp −127.1°. bp −100.4°. d_4 (−100.4°; liq) 1.57. d (gas at STP) 3.07666 g/l. Soly in water (0°): 332 g/100 g; some hydrolysis occurs to form fluoboric and boric acids. Soly in anhydrous H_2SO_4: 1.94 g/100 g acid. Forms solid complex with nitric acid ($HNO_3 . 2BF_3$). Sol in most saturated and halogenated hydrocarbons and in aromatic compds. Polymerizes unsaturated molecules. Easily forms coordination complexes with molecules having at least one unshared pair of electrons. Reacts with incandescence when heated with alkali metals or alkaline earth metals except magnesium.

Caution: Potential symptoms of overexposure are irritation of eyes, skin, nose, respiratory system; epistaxis; burns to eyes and skin. *See NIOSH Pocket Guide to Chemical Hazards* (DHHS/-NIOSH 97-140, 1997) p 32. *See also Patty's Industrial Hygiene and Toxicology* vol. **2B**, G. D. Clayton, F. E. Clayton, Eds. (Wiley-Interscience, New York, 3rd ed., 1981) pp 2996-2999.

USE: To protect molten magnesium and its alloys from oxidation; as a flux for soldering magnesium; as a fumigant; in ionization chambers for the detection of weak neutrons. By far the largest application of boron trifluoride is in catalysis with and without promoting agents.

1350. Boron Trifluoride Etherate. [109-63-7] Boron fluoride ethyl ether; boron fluoride etherate; ethyl ether-boron trifluoride complex. $C_4H_{10}BF_3O$; mol wt 141.93. C 33.85%, H 7.10%, B 7.62%, F 40.16%, O 11.27%. $(CH_3CH_2)_2O.BF_3$. Prepd by vapor-phase reaction of anhydr ether with BF_3: Laubengayer, Finlay, *J. Am. Chem. Soc.* **65**, 884 (1943).

Fuming liquid, immediately hydrolyzed by moisture in air. d_4^{25} 1.125. bp 125.7°. mp −60.4°. n_D^{20} 1.348. Heat of formation: 12.5 kcal. Heat of soln at 0° in ether: 2.7 kcal.

Caution: On decomposition forms highly toxic fumes of fluorides.

USE: Catalyst in acetylation, alkylation, polymerization, dehydration, and condensation reactions.

1351. Bortezomib. [179324-69-7] [(1*R*)-3-Methyl-1-[[(2*S*)-1-oxo-3-phenyl-2-[(pyrazinylcarbonyl)amino]propyl]amino]butyl]-boronic acid; *N*-(2-pyrazine)carbonyl-L-phenylalanine-L-leucine boronic acid; MG-341; PS-341; Velcade. $C_{19}H_{25}BN_4O_4$; mol wt 384.24. C 59.39%, H 6.56%, B 2.81%, N 14.58%, O 16.66%. Dipeptide boronic acid proteasome inhibitor. Prepn: J. Adams *et al., WO 9613266; eidem, US 5780454* (1996, 1998 both to ProScript); *idem et al., Bioorg. Med. Chem. Lett.* **8**, 333 (1998). Pharmacology and cytotoxic activity: *idem et al., Cancer Res.* **59**, 2615 (1999). Crystal structure in complex with the yeast 20S proteasome: M. Groll *et al., Structure* **14**, 451 (2006). Mechanism of action study: J. Codony-Servat *et al., Mol. Cancer Ther.* **5**, 665 (2006). Clinical trial in refractory myeloma: P. G. Richardson *et al., N. Engl. J. Med.* **348**, 2609 (2003). Review of clinical development: *idem et al., Annu. Rev. Med.* **57**, 33-47 (2006).

Soly in water: 3.3-3.8 mg/ml (pH 2-6.5).
THERAP CAT: Antineoplastic.

1352. Boscalid. [188425-85-6] 2-Chloro-*N*-(4′-chloro[1,1′-biphenyl]-2-yl)-3-pyridinecarboxamide; 2-chloro-*N*-(4′-chloro-biphenyl-2-yl)nicotinamide; nicobifen; BAS-510F; Cantus; Endura. $C_{18}H_{12}Cl_2N_2O$; mol wt 343.21. C 62.99%, H 3.52%, Cl 20.66%, N 8.16%, O 4.66%. Broad spectrum carboxamide fungicide used to control diseases in turf, field, row, orchard, and vineyard crops. Prepn: K. Eicken *et al., EP 545099; eidem, US 5589493* (1993, 1996 both to BASF). Terrestrial field dissipation study: S. H. Jackson, *Pest Manage. Sci.* **60**, 8 (2003). Comparative field trial vs sclerotinia drop in lettuce: M. E. Matheron, M. Porchas, *Plant Dis.* **88**, 665 (2004). Review of chemistry and toxicology: *Boscalid Pesticide Fact Sheet* (U.S. EPA, July 2003) 18 pp.

White crystalline solid, mp 142.8-143.8°. d 1.381. Partition coefficient (octanol/water): 915 at 21°. Soly at 20° (g/100 ml): acetone 16-20; acetonitrile 4-5; methanol 4-5; ethyl acetate 6.7-8; dichloromethane 20-25; toluene 2-2.5; 1-octanol <1. Soly in water at 20°: 6 mg/l. Vapor pressure (hPa): 7×10^{-9} at 20°; 2×10^{-8} at 25°. pH 5.5 at 23° (1% soln). LD_{50} in rats (mg/kg): >5000 orally; >2000 dermally (U.S. EPA).
USE: Fungicide.

1353. Bosentan. [147536-97-8] 4-(1,1-Dimethylethyl)-*N*-[6-(2-hydroxyethoxy)-5-(2-methoxyphenoxy)[2,2′-bipyrimidin]-4-yl]benzenesulfonamide; *p-tert*-butyl-*N*-[6-(2-hydroxyethoxy)-5-(*o*-methoxyphenoxy)-2-(2-pyrimidinyl)-4-pyrimidinyl]benzenesulfon-amide; Ro-47-0203. $C_{27}H_{29}N_5O_6S$; mol wt 551.61. C 58.79%, H 5.30%, N 12.70%, O 17.40%, S 5.81%. Mixed endothelin receptor antagonist. Prepn: K. Burri *et al., CA 2071193; eidem, US*

5292740 (1992, 1994 both to Hoffmann-La Roche). Receptor binding study: M. Clozel *et al., J. Pharmacol. Exp. Ther.* **270**, 228 (1994). LC-MS determn in plasma: B. Lausecker, G. Hopfgartner, *J. Chromatogr. A* **712**, 75 (1995). Clinical pharmacology: G. Sütsch *et al., Cardiovasc. Drugs Ther.* **10**, 717 (1996). Clinical pharmacokinetics: C. Weber *et al., Clin. Pharmacol. Ther.* **60**, 124 (1996). Clinical trial in hypertension: H. Krum *et al., N. Engl. J. Med.* **338**, 784 (1998); in pulmonary arterial hypertension: L. J. Rubin *et al., ibid.* **346**, 896 (2002).

Monohydrate. [157212-55-0] Tracleer. $C_{27}H_{29}N_5O_6S.H_2O$; mol wt 569.63. White to yellowish powder. Soly (mg/100 ml): water 1.0; aq soln 0.1 (pH 1.1); 0.1 (pH 4.0); 0.2 (pH 5.0); 43 (pH 7.5).

Sodium salt. [150726-52-6] $C_{27}H_{28}N_5NaO_6S$. mp 195-198°.
THERAP CAT: Antihypertensive.

1354. Bostrycoidin. [4589-33-7] 6,9-Dihydroxy-7-meth-oxy-3-methylbenz[*g*]isoquinoline-5,10-dione; 5,8-dihydroxy-6-methoxy-3-methyl-2-aza-9,10-anthraquinone. $C_{15}H_{11}NO_5$; mol wt 285.25. C 63.16%, H 3.89%, N 4.91%, O 28.04%. Antibiotic substance produced by *Fusarium bostrycoides:* Hamilton *et al., Antibiot. Chemother.* **3**, 853 (1953); Cajori *et al., J. Biol. Chem.* **208**, 107 (1954). Structure: Arsenault, *Tetrahedron Lett.* **1965**, 4033. Synthesis: D. W. Cameron *et al., ibid.* **21**, 5089 (1980).

Dark red crystals; mp 243-244°, changes to purple in alkaline medium, yellow in acid medium. Stable at room temp and withstands autoclaving. Insol in water; sol in abs ethanol and in 60% ethanol; moderately sol in dioxane, benzene, acetone, chloroform, carbon tetrachloride. Soluble in aq sodium carbonate solns. Partly sol in corn oil. Active *in vitro* against *Mycobacterium tuberculosis.* Serum seems to interfere.

1355. β-Boswellic Acid. [631-69-6] (3α,4β)-3-Hydroxyurs-12-en-23-oic acid. $C_{30}H_{48}O_3$; mol wt 456.70. C 78.90%, H 10.59%, O 10.51%. Occurs as the acetate in frankincense *(olibanum)* from *Boswellia carterii, Burseraceae.* The β-form is predominant and is accompanied by small amounts of α- and γ-boswellic acid. Isoln from olibanum tears: Winterstein, Stein, *Z. Physiol. Chem.* **208**, 9 (1932). Early structural studies: Simpson, Williams, *ibid.* **1938**, 686, 1712; Ruzicka, Wirz, *Helv. Chim. Acta* **22**, 948 (1939); **23**, 132 (1940); Ruzicka *et al., ibid.* **27**, 1859 (1944). Revised structure and stereochemistry: Beton *et al., J. Chem. Soc.* **1956**, 2904; Allan, *Chimia* **17**, 382 (1963); *idem, Phytochemistry* **7**, 963 (1968). *Review:* J. Simonsen, W. C. J. Ross, *The Terpenes* vol. 5 (University Press, Cambridge, 1957) pp 68-74.

Long prisms from methanol, mp 228-232° with preliminary sintering. $[\alpha]_D$ +107° (c = 0.75 in $CHCl_3$). 100 ml of boiling methanol will dissolve 8 grams of β-boswellic acid. Sol in chloroform, ether, acetone, alc.

Acetate. $C_{32}H_{50}O_4$. Prisms, mp 275-278°, $[\alpha]_D$ +63° (c = 1.88 in $CHCl_3$).

Methyl ester. $C_{31}H_{50}O_3$. mp 195-196°, $[\alpha]_D$ +111° (c = 1.6 in $CHCl_3$).

1356.   Bottromycin. [1393-68-6] B-mycin. A complex of five antibiotics of which the main active component is bottromycin A_2. Produced by *Streptomyces bottropensis* and *S. canadensis*: Waisvisz *et al., J. Am. Chem. Soc.* **79**, 4520, 4522, 4524 (1957); Miller *et al., Antimicrob. Agents Chemother.* **1967**, 407. Production: GB 762736 (1956 to Koninklijke Nederlandsche Gist en Spiritus-Fabriek); Umesawa *et al.,* JP 68 10998 (1968 to Microbiochem. Res. Found.), *C.A.* **69**, 85439x (1968); Hata *et al.,* US 3650904 (1972). Partial structure: Waisvisz, Hoeven, *J. Am. Chem. Soc.* **80**, 38 (1958). Sepn and structures of bottromycins A_1, A_2, and B: Nakamura *et al., J. Antibiot.* **18A**, 47, 60 (1965); **19A**, 10 (1966). Isoln and characterization of bottromycins A_2, B_2, C_2: Nakamura *et al., ibid.* **20A**, 1 (1967). Revised structure of bottromycin A_2: Takahashi *et al., ibid.* **29A**, 1120 (1976); D. Schipper, *ibid.* **36A**, 1076 (1983). Mode of action of bottromycin A_2: T. Otaka, A. Kaji, *J. Biol. Chem.* **251**, 2299 (1976); *eidem, FEBS Lett.* **123**, 173 (1981).

Bottromycin A_2

Bottromycin A_2. Bottromycic A_2 acid methyl ester. $C_{42}H_{62}N_8O_7S$; mol wt 823.06.

1357.   Botulin Toxins. Botulinum toxins; botulinus toxins. Potent neurotoxins produced by *Clostridium botulinum*. Seven serologically distinct types are known, designated A-G; mol wt ~150 kDa. Zinc-proteases synthesized as non-toxic single-chain precursors which become toxic upon proteolytic cleavage. Active form consists of one heavy and one light chain linked by a disulfide bond. Prevents release of acetylcholine from presynaptic nerve terminals at the neuromuscular junction. Identification of the causative agent of botulism: E. P. Van Ermengem, *Z. Hyg. Infektionskrankh.* **26**, 1 (1897). Isoln: P. T. Snipe, H. Sommer, *J. Infect. Dis.* **43**, 152 (1928). Review of isoln and purification: L. L. Simpson *et al., Methods Enzymol.* **165**, 76-85 (1988); of structure and function: K. Oguma *et al., Microbiol. Immunol.* **39**, 161-168 (1995). Review of pharmacology: J. L. Middlebrook, *J. Toxicol. Toxin Rev.* **5**, 177-190 (1986); of mode of action and detection: M. Wictome, C. C. Shone, *J. Appl. Microbiol. Symp. Suppl.* **84**, 87S-97S (1998). Review of clinical uses in focal dystonias: K. R. Kessler, R. Benecke, *Neurotoxicology* **18**, 761-770 (1997); in cosmetic dermatology: A. Carruthers, J. Carruthers, *Basic Clin. Dermatol.* **15**, 207-236 (1998). MLD in mouse: 0.0003 μg/kg (Middlebrook).

Botulin A. [93384-43-1] Botulinum toxin type A; oculinum; AGN-191622; BoTox; Dysport. Clinical trial in blepharospasm: B. Arthurs *et al., Can. J. Ophthalmol.* **22**, 24 (1987); in achalasia: P. J. Pasricha *et al., N. Engl. J. Med.* **332**, 774 (1995); in hyperhidrosis: M. Heckmann *et al., ibid.* **344**, 488 (2001); in spasticity following stroke: A. Brashear *et al., ibid.* **347**, 395 (2002).

Botulin B. [93384-44-2] Botulinum toxin type B; NeuroBloc. Clinical trial in cervical dystonia: P. A. Cullis *et al., Adv. Neurol.* **78**, 227 (1998).

THERAP CAT: Muscle relaxant (skeletal).

1358.   Bradycor. [140661-97-8] CP-0127. $C_{128}H_{194}N_{40}O_{28}S_2$; mol wt 2805.29. C 54.80%, H 6.97%, N 19.97%, O 15.97%, S 2.29%. Bradykinin antagonist. Dimer of D-Arg[0]-[Hyp[3], Cys[6], D-Phe[7], Leu[8]]-bradykinin joined by a bissuccinimidohexane linker via the sulfhydryl moieties of the cysteine residues. Prepn: J. C. Cheronis *et al.,* WO 9217201 (1992 to Cortech); *eidem, J. Med. Chem.* **35**, 1563 (1992). Effect on survival in endotoxin shock in animals: E. T. Whalley *et al., Agents Actions Suppl.* **38 (3)**, 413 (1992).

D-Arg–Arg–Pro–Hyp–Gly–Phe–Cys–D-Phe–Leu–Arg

D-Arg–Arg–Pro–Hyp–Gly–Phe–Cys–D-Phe–Leu–Arg

THERAP CAT: In treatment of systemic inflammatory response syndrome.

1359.   Bradykinin. [58-82-2] Kallidin I; kallidin-9; callidin I; BRS-640. $C_{50}H_{73}N_{15}O_{11}$; mol wt 1060.21. C 56.64%, H 6.94%, N 19.82%, O 16.60%. A tissue hormone belonging to a group of hypotensive peptides known as plasma kinins. First obtained by incubation with the venom of *Bothrops jararaca* or with crystalline trypsin: Rocha e Silva *et al., Cien Cult. (Sao Paulo)* **1**, 32 (1949); *eidem, Am. J. Physiol.* **156**, 261 (1949); Prado *et al., Arch. Biochem.* **27**, 410 (1950); Werle *et al., Biochem. Z.* **320**, 372 (1950). Large scale prepn from whole bovine plasma: Hamberg, Deutsch, *Arch. Biochem. Biophys.* **76**, 262 (1958). Formed by proteolysis of a precursor in the globulin fraction of plasma referred to as kininogen by the action of enzymes such as trypsin, plasmin, and plasma kallikrein, *q.q.v.* Acts on smooth muscle, dilates peripheral vessels, increases capillary permeability. Also is a potent pain-producing agent. Structure: Elliott *et al., Biochem. Biophys. Res. Commun.* **3**, 87 (1960); Werle *et al., Z. Physiol. Chem.* **326**, 174 (1961). Synthesis: Boissonnas *et al., Helv. Chim. Acta* **43**, 1349 (1960); **45**, 170 (1962); Merrifield, *Biochemistry* **3**, 1385 (1964); Young *et al., J. Chem. Soc. C* **1971**, 46; Bajusz *et al.,* HU 3840 (1972 to Gyogyszerkutato Intézet), *C.A.* **77**, 20027g (1972); F. Sipos, DE 2212787; *idem,* US 3714140 (1972, 1973 both to Squibb); Corley *et al., Biochem. Biophys. Res. Commun.* **47**, 1353 (1972); N. S. S. Kumari *et al., Indian J. Chem.* **17B**, 152 (1979). Review: Schröder, Hempel, *Experientia* **20**, 529 (1964).

Arg–Pro–Pro–Gly–Phe–Ser–Pro–Phe–Arg

Amorphous precipitate. $[\alpha]_D^{25}$ −76.5° (c = 1.37 in 1N acetic acid). Sol in glacial acetic acid, in a 10% soln of trichloroacetic acid, 70% ethanol, in hot methanol; less sol in 90% ethanol or cold methanol. Almost insol in acetone, chloroform, ethyl ether, ethyl methyl ketone, petr ether, butanol, amyl alcohol, ethyl acetate.

THERAP CAT: Vasodilator.

1360.   Brain Natriuretic Peptide. [114471-18-0] Brain natriuretic factor; B-type natriuretic peptide; BNP. Peptide hormone structurally and physiologically similar to atrial natriuretic peptide, *q.v.* Originally discovered in mammalian brain, subsequently found to be produced primarily by the cardiac ventricle in response to hemodynamic stress. Amino acid sequence shows a marked interspecies diversity; the normal circulating form in humans contains 32 amino acid residues. Isoln from porcine brain: T. Sudoh *et al., Nature* **332**, 78 (1988). Cloning of human BNP precursor: *idem et al., Biochem. Biophys. Res. Commun.* **159**, 1427 (1989). Direct isoln from human heart: Y. Kambayashi *et al., FEBS Lett.* **259**, 341 (1990). Use in prognosis of risk in acute coronary syndromes: J. A. de Lemos *et al., N. Engl. J. Med.* **345**, 1014 (2001); in diagnosis of congestive heart failure: A. S. Maisel *et al., ibid.* **347**, 161 (2002). *Review:* N. C. Davidson, A. D. Struthers, *J. Hypertens.* **12**, 329-336 (1994); T. Takeda, M. Kohno, *Hypertens. Res.* **18**, 259-266 (1995); of pathophysiological significance: M. Yoshibayashi *et* *al., Eur. J. Endocrinol.* **135**, 265-268 (1996); of clinical experience: N. Valli *et al., J. Lab. Clin. Med.* **134**, 437-444 (1999).

```
 1
Ser–Pro–Lys–Met–Val–Gln–Gly–Ser–Gly–Cys–Phe–Gly–Arg–Lys–Met–Asp–Arg
                                              |                    |
                                              |                   Ile
                                              |                    |
      32                                      |                    |
     His–Arg–Arg–Leu–Val–Lys–Cys–Gly–Leu–Gly–Ser–Ser–Ser–Ser
```

human BNP

Nesiritide. [124584-08-3] Human brain natriuretic peptide-32; natriuretic factor-32 (human brain clone λhBNP57); Natrecor. Clinical hemodynamic effects: L. S. Marcus *et al., Circulation* **94**, 3184 (1996). Clinical trial in congestive heart failure: W. S. Colucci *et al., N. Engl. J. Med.* **343**, 246 (2000).

THERAP CAT: In treatment of congestive heart failure.

1361. Brallobarbital. [561-86-4] 5-(2-Bromo-2-propenyl)-5-(2-propenyl)-2,4,6($1H,3H,5H$)-pyrimidinetrione; 5-allyl-5-(2-bromoallyl)barbituric acid; Vesperone. $C_{10}H_{11}BrN_2O_3$; mol wt 287.11. C 41.83%, H 3.86%, Br 27.83%, N 9.76%, O 16.72%. Prepn: Morren, BE 497501 (1950), *C.A.* **49**, 1100e (1955). Metabolism: Keding, Schmidt, *Arzneim.-Forsch.* **19**, 342 (1969).

Solid, mp 168-169°.
Note: This is a controlled substance (depressant): **21 CFR,** 1308.13.

THERAP CAT: Sedative, hypnotic.

1362. Brandy. A potable alcoholic liquid distilled from wine or from the fermented juices of peaches, cherries, apples, or other fruit.

To meet the specifications of the National Formulary, brandy must have been obtained by distillation of fermented juice from sound ripe grapes and contain between 48 and 54% ethanol (v/v), d_4^{15} 0.921-0.933. It must have been stored in wooden containers for a period of not less than 2 years. Unlike whisky, brandy is never made from cereal mash or from potatoes (as some brands of vodka).

THERAP CAT: Sedative, vasodilator (peripheral).

1363. Brassard's Diene. [90857-62-8] (*E*-form); [74272-66-5] (stereo unspecified). [[(1*E*)-1,3-Dimethoxy-1,3-butadienyl]-oxy]trimethylsilane; 1,3-dimethoxy-1-trimethylsiloxy-1,3-buta-diene. $C_9H_{18}O_3Si$; mol wt 202.32. C 53.43%, H 8.97%, O 23.72%, Si 13.88%. Highly reactive nucleophilic silyloxydiene; *cf.* Danishefsky's diene. Prepn: J. Savard, P. Brassard, *Tetrahedron Lett.* **20**, 4911 (1979); *eidem, Tetrahedron* **40**, 3455 (1984). Synthetic applications: M. M. Midland, R. W. Koops, *J. Org. Chem.* **55**, 5058 (1990); T. Ito *et al., Tetrahedron Lett.* **34**, 6583 (1993); Q. Fan *et al., Eur. J. Org. Chem.* **2005**, 3542; of polymer-supported derivatives: C. Pierres *et al., Tetrahedron Lett.* **44**, 3645 (2003).

Oil. $bp_{0.5}$ 54°. $bp_{0.8}$ 57-62°.
USE: Electron-rich diene in hetero Diels-Alder reactions.

1364. Brassidic Acid. [506-33-2] (13*E*)-13-Docosenoic acid. $C_{22}H_{42}O_2$; mol wt 338.57. C 78.04%, H 12.50%, O 9.45%. $CH_3(CH_2)_7CH=CH(CH_2)_{11}COOH$. Prepn by isomerization of its *cis*-isomer (erucic acid): Reimer, Will, *Ber.* **19**, 3320 (1886); Skellon, *Manuf. Chem.* **33**, 405 (1962). Synthesis and separation from erucic acid by crystn: Bowman, *Nature* **163**, 95 (1949).

Thin, cryst plates from alc, mp 61-62°. bp_{30} 282°. n_D^{57} 1.448. Practically insol in water; sparingly sol in cold alcohol; sol in ether.

Solubility at 10°, 0°, −10°, −20°, and −30° in methanol, ethyl acetate, ether, acetone, toluene, *n*-heptane: Kobl, *Diss. Abstr.* **20**, 82 (1959).

1365. Brassinolide. [72962-43-7] (2α,3α,5α,22*R*,23*R*,24*S*)-2,3,22,23-Tetrahydroxy-*B*-homo-7-oxaergostan-6-one; 2α,3α,22,-23-tetrahydroxy-24-methyl-B-homo-7-oxa-5α-cholestan-6-one. $C_{28}H_{48}O_6$; mol wt 480.68. C 69.96%, H 10.07%, O 19.97%. Plant hormone; natural steroid containing a seven-membered B-ring lactone, that promotes both cell elongation and cell division. Over ten brassinosteroids have been isolated and characterized from sources such as pollen, seedling, leaf. Isoln, structure and activity of brassinolide from rape pollen, *Brassica napus* L.: M. D. Grove *et al., Nature* **281**, 216 (1979). Stereoselective synthesis: S. Fung, J. B. Siddall, *J. Am. Chem. Soc.* **102**, 6580 (1980). Synthesis of two stereoisomers: M. J. Thompson *et al., J. Org. Chem.* **44**, 5002 (1979). Improved synthesis: T. Kametani *et al., J. Org. Chem.* **53**, 1982 (1988). Structure-activity relationship of brassinosteroids: S. Takatsuto *et al., Phytochemistry* **22**, 2437 (1983); interaction with cytokinin: C. Schlagnhaufer *et al., Physiol. Plant.* **60**, 347 (1984); bioassay: K. Wada *et al., Agric. Biol. Chem.* **48**, 719 (1984).

Crystals from methanol, mp 274-275°. $[\alpha]_D^{27}$ +16°.
USE: Plant growth regulator.

1366. Brayera. Kousso; kosso; cusso; koso; cousso; kouso; kusso. Dried panicles of pistillate flowers of *Hagenia abyssinica* J. F. Gmel. (*Brayera anthelmintica* Kunth), Rosaceae. Habit. Abyssinia. *Constit.* Kosin, kossein, kosidin, protokosin, kosotoxin, volatile oil, tannin. *Ref:* Leisenring, *Arch. Pharm.* **232**, 50 (1894); Kondakow, *ibid.* **237**, 481 (1899); Hess, Todd, *J. Chem. Soc.* **1937**, 562; Birch, Todd, *ibid.* **1952**, 3102.

THERAP CAT: Anthelmintic (Cestodes).
THERAP CAT (VET): Has been used as a teniacide.

1367. Brazilin. [474-07-7] (6a*S-cis*)-7,11b-Dihydrobenz-[*b*]indeno[1,2-*d*]pyran-3,6a,9,10(6*H*)-tetrol; brasilin; C.I. Natural Red 24; C.I. 75280. $C_{16}H_{14}O_5$; mol wt 286.28. C 67.13%, H 4.93%, O 27.94%. (May crystallize as the mono- or hemihydrate). From *Caesalpinia echinata* Lam. (Brazil-wood), or *C. sappan* L. (sappan-wood), Leguminosae. Isoln and structure: Perkin *et al., J. Chem. Soc.* **1928**, 1504; Pfeiffer *et al., Ber.* **63**, 1301 (1930). Synthesis of (±)-form: Dann, Hofmann, *Ann.* **667**, 116 (1963); Kirkiacharian, Billet, *Bull. Soc. Chim. Fr.* **1972**, 3292. Synthesis, resolution: Morsingh, Robinson, *Tetrahedron* **26**, 281 (1970). Stereochemistry: Craig *et al., J. Org. Chem.* **30**, 1573 (1965); *Colour Index* vol. 4 (3rd ed., 1971) p 4628. *Review:* Robinson, *Bull. Soc. Chim. Fr.* **1958**, 125-134.

Amber-yellow crystals; turn orange in air and light. Dec above 130°. Sol in water, freely in alcohol, ether, also in alkali hydroxide solns with carmine-red color. *Protect from air and light.*

USE: Chiefly as a dye. Has also been recommended as indicator in acid-base titrations; acids = yellow, alkalies = carmine-red.

1368. Bredereck's Reagent. [5815-08-7] 1-(1,1-Dimethyl-ethoxy)-*N,N,N',N'*-tetramethylmethanediamine; bis(dimethylami-no)-*tert*-butyloxymethane; *tert*-butoxybis(dimethylamino)methane; *tert*-butoxy-*N,N,N',N'*-tetramethylmethanediamine. $C_9H_{22}N_2O$; mol wt 174.28. C 62.02%, H 12.72%, N 16.07%, O 9.18%. Aminal ester used in condensation reactions. Prepn: H. Bredereck *et al., Angew. Chem. Int. Ed.* **6**, 356 (1967); *idem et al., Ber.* **101**, 41 (1968). Synthetic applications: B. M. Trost, M. Preckel, *J. Am. Chem. Soc.* **95**, 7862 (1973); W. Haefliger, H. Knecht, *Tetrahedron Lett.* **25**, 285 (1983); J.-P. Vors, *J. Heterocycl. Chem.* **28**, 1043 (1991); A. C. Spivey *et al., J. Org. Chem.* **65**, 5253 (2000); E. Morera *et al., Org. Lett.* **4**, 1139 (2002); S. Csihony *et al., Adv. Synth. Catal.* **346**, 1081 (2004). *Review*: W. Kantlehner, *J. Prakt. Chem. Chem.-Ztg.* **337**, 418-421 (1995).

bp$_{10-12}$ 48-52°. bp$_{15}$ 50-55°. n_D^{20} 1.4260.

USE: Mild enamination reagent; catalyst in ring-opening poly-merization reactions.

1369. Brefeldin A. [20350-15-6] 1,6,7,8,9,11a,12,13,14,-14a-Decahydro-1,13-dihydroxy-6-methyl-4*H*-cyclopent[*f*]oxacy-clotridecin-4-one; γ,4-dihydroxy-2-(6-hydroxy-1-heptenyl)-4-cy-clopentanecrotonic acid λ-lactone; ascotoxin; cyanein; decumbin. $C_{16}H_{24}O_4$; mol wt 280.36. C 68.54%, H 8.63%, O 22.83%. A fungal metabolite which is a macrocyclic lactone exhibiting a wide range of antibiotic activity. Produced by *Penicillium brefeldianum* Dodge: E. Haerri *et al., Helv. Chim. Acta* **46**, 1235 (1963). Also produced by *P. decumbens*: V. L. Singleton *et al., Nature* **181**, 1072 (1958); *P. cyaneum*: V. Betina *et al., Folia Microbiol.* **7**, 353 (1962). Structure: H. P. Sigg, *Helv. Chim. Acta* **47**, 1401 (1964). Abs configuration: H. P. Weber *et al., ibid.* **54**, 2763 (1971). Synthesis of (±)-form: E. J. Corey, R. H. Wollenberg, *Tetrahedron Lett.* **1976**, 4705; E. J. Corey *et al., ibid.* **1977**, 2243; R. Baudouy *et al., ibid.* 2973; P. A. Bartlett, F. R. Green, *J. Am. Chem. Soc.* **100**, 4548 (1978); A. E. Greene *et al., ibid.* **102**, 7583 (1980); M. Honda *et al., Tetrahedron Lett.* **1981**, 2679. Total synthesis of (+)-form: T. Kitahara *et al., ibid.* **1979**, 3021. Biosynthesis: B. E. Cross, P. Hendley, *Chem. Commun.* **1975**, 124; C. R. Hutchinson *et al., J. Am. Chem. Soc.* **103**, 2474, 2477 (1981); M. Sunagawa *et al., J. Antibiot.* **36**, 25 (1983). Antifungal activity: V. Betina *et al., ibid.* **17A**, 93 (1964); anti-HeLa cell effect: *eidem, Naturwissenschaften* **49**, 241 (1962). *See also* W. Keller-Schierlein, "Chemistry of Macrolide Antibiotics" in *Fortschr. Chem. Org. Naturst.* **30**, 313-445 (1973).

Colorless prisms from methanol/ether, mp 204-205°. uv max (ethanol): 215 nm (log ε 4.05). [α]$_D^{22}$ +96 ±2° (c = 1.08 in methanol). LD$_{50}$ i.p. in mice: >200 mg/kg (Haerri).

1370. Brequinar. [96187-53-0] 6-Fluoro-2-(2'-fluoro[1,1'-biphenyl]-4-yl)-3-methyl-4-quinolinecarboxylic acid. $C_{23}H_{15}F_2$NO$_2$; mol wt 375.37. C 73.59%, H 4.03%, F 10.12%, N 3.73%, O 8.52%. Inhibitor of dihydroorotate dehydrogenase, the fourth enzyme in the *de novo* pyrimidine biosynthetic pathway; depresses lymphocyte proliferation. Prepn: D. P. Hesson, **EP 133244**; *idem*, **US 4680299** (1985, 1987 both to DuPont). Mechanisms of action: T. L. Forrest *et al., Transplantation* **58**, 920 (1994). Clinical phar-macokinetics: M. de Forni *et al., Eur. J. Cancer* **29A**, 983 (1993). Symposium on pharmacology, toxicology: *Transplant. Proc.* **25**, Suppl. 2, 1-83 (1993). Review of development and clinical expe-rience: L. Makowka *et al., Immunol. Rev.* **136**, 51-70 (1993).

White crystals from DMF + water, mp 315-317°.
Sodium salt. [96201-88-6] DUP-785; NSC-368390. $C_{23}H_{14}$-F$_2$NNaO$_2$; mol wt 397.35. White solid, mp >360°. Sol in water.
THERAP CAT: Immunosuppressant.

1371. Bretylium Tosylate. [61-75-6] 2-Bromo-*N*-ethyl-*N,N*-dimethylbenzenemethanaminium salt with 4-methylbenzene-sulfonic acid (1:1); (*o*-bromobenzyl)ethyldimethylammonium *p*-tol-uenesulfonate; *N*-ethyl-*N*-*o*-bromobenzyl-*N,N*-dimethylammonium tosylate; Bretylate; Bretylol. $C_{18}H_{24}BrNO_3S$; mol wt 414.36. C 52.18%, H 5.84%, Br 19.28%, N 3.38%, O 11.58%, S 7.74%. Prepn: Copp, Stephenson, **US 3038004** (1962 to Burroughs Well-come). Metabolism: R. Kuntzman *et al., Clin. Pharmacol. Ther.* **11**, 829 (1970). Toxicity study: E. I. Goldenthal, *Toxicol. Appl. Pharmacol.* **18**, 185 (1971). Review of pharmacology: R. H. Heissenbuttel, J. T. Bigger, *Ann. Intern. Med.* **91**, 229-238 (1979); R. J. Lee *et al.*, in *Pharmacological and Biochemical Properties of Drug Substances* vol. 2, M. E. Goldberg, Ed. (Am. Pharm. Assoc., Washington, DC, 1979) pp 148-164. Comprehensive description: J. E. Carter *et al., Anal. Profiles Drug Subs.* **9**, 71-86 (1980).

Crystalline powder, mp 97-99°. Extremely bitter taste. uv max: 278, 271, 264 nm. Freely sol in water, methanol, ethanol. Practi-cally insol in ether, ethyl acetate, hexane. LD$_{50}$ in mice (mg/kg): 400 orally; 250 i.m. (Goldenthal).

THERAP CAT: Antiadrenergic; antiarrhythmic (class III).

1372. Brevetoxins. BTX. Structurally unique marine neuro-toxins produced by the "red-tide" dinoflagellate *Ptychodiscus bre-vis* Davis (*Karenia brevis*, formerly *Gymnodinium breve* Davis). Dense growths of these algae have been responsible for massive fish kills, mollusk poisoning and human food poisoning in the Gulf of Mexico and along the Florida coast, *cf. Marine Natural Products*, P. J. Scheuer, Ed. (Academic Press, New York, 1978). Unlike previously isolated dinoflagellate toxins, such as saxitoxin, *q.v.*, which are water-soluble sodium channel blockers, the brevetoxins are lipid-soluble sodium channel activators. Isoln of brevetoxins A, B, and C and structure of B, the major component: Y. Y. Lin *et al., J. Am. Chem. Soc.* **103**, 6773 (1981). Structure of C: J. Golik *et al., Tetrahedron Lett.* **23**, 2535 (1982). Structure of A, the most potent toxin: Y. Shimizu *et al., J. Am. Chem. Soc.* **108**, 514 (1986). Synthetic approaches to brevetoxin B: K. C. Nicolau *et al., Chem. Commun.* **1985**, 1359. Absolute configuration: Y. Shimizu *et al., Chem. Commun.* **22**, 1656 (1987). Biosynthetic study: H. N. Chou, Y. Shimizu, *J. Am. Chem. Soc.* **109**, 2184 (1987). ELISA determn in seawater, shellfish and biological fluids: J. Naar *et al., Environ. Health Perspect.* **110**, 179 (2002). Series of articles on pharmacology of brevetoxins: *Toxicon* **23**, 469-524 (1985); on exposures and health effects of aerosolized toxins: *Environ. Health Perspect.* **113**, 618-657 (2005). Review of chemistry: K. Naka-nishi, *ibid.* 473; of pharmacology, toxicokinetics and determn: M. A. Poli, *Recent Adv. Marine Biotechnol.* **7**, 1-3 (2002). For addi-tional information on red tide algae, *see Toxic Dinoflagellate Blooms*, D. L. Taylor, H. H. Seliger, Eds. (Elsevier, New York, 1979) pp 327-354.

Exp. Dermatol. **224**, 90 (1966); *idem, Arch. Dermatol. Forsch.* **243**, 1 (1972). *Review: H. J. Conn's Biological Stains,* R. D. Lillie, Ed. (Williams & Wilkins, Baltimore, 9th ed., 1977) pp 251-252, 580.

Brevetoxin A. GB-1. $C_{49}H_{70}O_{13}$; mol wt 867.07. Fine prisms from acetonitrile, mp 197-199°; 218-220° (double melting point). LC_{100} in guppies: 4 ng/ml (Shimizu).

Brevetoxin B. BTX-B; GB-2; T-34; T-47. $C_{50}H_{70}O_{14}$; mol wt 895.08. Needles from acetonitrile, mp 270° (dec). uv max (methanol): 208 nm (ε 16000, enal). LC_{50} (1 hr) in fresh water "zebra" fish, *Brachydanio rerio*: 16 ng/ml (Lin).

Brevetoxin C. BTX-C. $C_{49}H_{69}ClO_{14}$; mol wt 917.52. uv max (methanol): 208 nm (ε 11300, ene-lactone). LC_{50} (1 hr) in fresh water "zebra" fish: 30 ng/ml (Lin).

USE: As tools in neurochemical research.

1373. Brilliant Blue FCF. [3844-45-9] *N*-Ethyl-*N*-[4-[[4-[ethyl[(3-sulfophenyl)methyl]amino]phenyl](2-sulfophenyl)-methylene]-2,5-cyclohexadien-1-ylidene]-3-sulfobenzenemethan-aminium inner salt, disodium salt; FD & C Blue No. 1; C.I. Acid Blue 9; C.I. Food Blue 2; C.I. 42090. $C_{37}H_{34}N_2Na_2O_9S_3$; mol wt 792.85. C 56.05%, H 4.32%, N 3.53%, Na 5.80%, O 18.16%, S 12.13%. Discovered by Sandmeyer in 1896: *Colour Index* **vol. 4** (3rd ed., 1971) p 4385. Also prepared as the diammonium salt. Metabolism: S. M. Hess, O. G. Fitzhugh, *J. Pharmacol. Exp. Ther.* **114**, 38 (1955); J. P. Brown *et al., Food Cosmet. Toxicol.* **18**, 1 (1980). Toxicology: E. Gross, *Z. Krebsforsch.* **64**, 287 (1961); W. A. Mannell, H. C. Grice, *J. Pharm. Pharmacol.* **16**, 56 (1964); W. H. Hansen *et al., Toxicol. Appl. Pharmacol.* **8**, 29 (1966). Chronic toxicity and carcinogenicity: J. F. Borzelleca *et al., Food Chem. Toxicol.* **28**, 221 (1990). Review of carcinogenicity studies: *IARC Monographs* **16**, 171-186 (1978).

Reddish-violet powder or granules with a metallic lustre. Absorption max: 630 nm. Sol in water, ethanol. Practically insol in vegetable oils. Pale amber soln in conc H_2SO_4, changing to yellow then greenish blue on dilution. LD_{50} s.c. in mice: 4.6 g/kg (Gross).

USE: Colorant in food, drugs and cosmetics. Biological stain; textile dye; wood stain; indicator.

1374. Brilliant Green. [633-03-4] *N*-[4-[[4-(Diethylamino)phenyl]phenylmethylene]-2,5-cyclohexadien-1-ylidene]-*N*-ethylethanaminium sulfate (1:1); C.I. Basic Green 1; C.I. 42040; Malachite Green G; Emerald Green; Diamond Green G; Fast Green J; Solid Green. $C_{27}H_{34}N_2O_4S$; mol wt 482.63. C 67.19%, H 7.10%, N 5.80%, O 13.26%, S 6.64%. Prepn: Doebner, *Ber.* **13**, 2222 (1880); Fischer, *ibid.* **14**, 2521 (1881); *Colour Index* **vol. 4** (3rd ed., 1971) p 4382. Toxicity: Anderson, *Proc. Soc. Exp. Biol. Med.* **31**, 825 (1934). Antibacterial activity: O. H. Paetzold, *Arch. Klin.*

Minute, glistening, golden crystals. Soluble in water or alcohol with green color. Absorption max: 623 nm. Soln changes color from yellow to green at pH 0.0 to 2.6. LD_{100} i.v. in mice: 3 mg/kg (Anderson).

USE: Dyeing silk, wool, leather, jute and cotton yellowish-green; manuf green ink; biological stain; indicator.

THERAP CAT: Antiseptic.

THERAP CAT (VET): Antiseptic for external and internal (oral) use. In wounds and scours.

1375. Brimonidine. [59803-98-4] 5-Bromo-*N*-(4,5-dihydro-1*H*-imidazol-2-yl)-6-quinoxalinamine; 5-bromo-6-(2-imidazolin-2-ylamino)quinoxaline; UK-14304; AGN-190342. $C_{11}H_{10}$-BrN_5; mol wt 292.13. C 45.23%, H 3.45%, Br 27.35%, N 23.97%. α_2-Adrenoceptor agonist. Prepn: J. C. Danielewicz *et al.,* **DE 2309160**; *eidem,* **US 3890319** (1973, 1975 both to Pfizer). HPLC determn in serum and aqueous humour of the eye: N. K. Karamanos *et al., Biomed. Chromatogr.* **13**, 86 (1999). Clinical study in control of intraocular pressure: R. David *et al., Arch. Ophthalmol.* **111**, 1387 (1993); L. J. Katz *et al., Am. J. Ophthalmol.* **127**, 20 (1999). Review of pharmacology and mechanisms of action: J. C. Adkins, J. A. Balfour, *Drugs Aging* **12**, 225-241 (1998); of pharmacotherapeutic profile: L. B. Cantor, *Expert Opin. Pharmacother.* **1**, 815-834 (2000).

Yellow crystals from ethanol, mp 252°.

D-Tartrate. [70359-46-5] UK-14304-18; AGN-190342-LF; Alphagan. $C_{11}H_{10}BrN_5 \cdot C_4H_6O_6$; mol wt 442.22. White crystals from acetone, mp 207.5°.

THERAP CAT: Antiglaucoma.

1376. Brinzolamide. [138890-62-7] (4*R*)-4-(Ethylamino)-3,4-dihydro-2-(3-methoxypropyl)-2*H*-thieno[3,2-*e*]-1,2-thiazine-6-sulfonamide 1,1-dioxide; AL-4682; Azopt. $C_{12}H_{21}N_3O_5S_3$; mol wt 383.51. C 37.58%, H 5.52%, N 10.96%, O 20.86%, S 25.08%. Carbonic anhydrase inhibitor. Prepn: T. R. Dean *et al.,* **WO 9115486**; *eidem,* **US 5378703** (1991, 1995 both to Alcon). Clinical trial: L. H. Silver, *Am. J. Ophthalmol.* **126**, 400 (1998).

Sol in ethanol.

Hydrochloride. [150937-43-2] $C_{12}H_{21}N_3O_5S_3 \cdot HCl$. Crystals from methanol + methylene chloride, mp 175-177°. $[\alpha]_D$ +10.35° (c = 1 in water).

THERAP CAT: Antiglaucoma agent.

1377.   Brivaracetam. [357336-20-0] ($\alpha S,4R$)-α-Ethyl-2-oxo-4-propyl-1-pyrrolidineacetamide; (2S)-2-[(4R)-2-oxo-4-propylpyrrolidinyl]butanamide; UCB-34714. $C_{11}H_{20}N_2O_2$; mol wt 212.29. C 62.23%, H 9.50%, N 13.20%, O 15.07%. Orally active synaptic vesicle protein 2 (SV2A) ligand; analog of levetiracetam, $q.v.$ Prepn: E. Differding $et\ al.,$ **WO 0162726**; $eidem,$ **US 6911461** (2001, 2005 both to UCB); B. M. Kenda $et\ al., J.\ Med.\ Chem.$ **47**, 530 (2004). Review of pharmacology and clinical experience: B. Malawska, K. Kulig, $Curr.\ Opin.\ Invest.\ Drugs$ **6**, 740-746 (2005).

Colorless, monoclinic crystals from isopropyl ether, mp 76.38°. $[\alpha]_D^{25}$ −60.57° (c = 1 in methanol). Crystal density: 1.093. Log P (octanol/water, pH 7.4 PBS): 1.00. Soly in water: 681 mg/ml.

THERAP CAT: Anticonvulsant; in treatment of progressive myoclonic epilepsies.

1378.   Brivudine. [69304-47-8] 5-[(1E)-2-Bromoethenyl]-2′-deoxyuridine; (E)-5-(2-bromovinyl)-2′-deoxyuridine; brivudin; BVDU; Brivex; Brivirac; Nervinex; Zecovir; Zostex. $C_{11}H_{13}BrN_2O_5$; mol wt 333.14. C 39.66%, H 3.93%, Br 23.99%, N 8.41%, O 24.01%. Analog of thymidine, $q.v.$, with selective activity against herpes simplex virus type 1 and varicella-zoster virus. Prepn: A. S. Jones $et\ al.,$ **DE 2915254**; $eidem,$ **US 4424211** (1979, 1984 both to University of Birmingham and Rega Institut); and antiviral activity: E. De Clercq $et\ al,\ Proc.\ Natl.\ Acad.\ Sci.\ USA$ **76**, 2947 (1979). Mechanism of action studies: H. S. Allaudeen $et\ al., ibid.$ **78**, 2698 (1981); J. Balzarini, E. De Clercq, $Methods\ Find.\ Exp.\ Clin.\ Pharmacol.$ **11**, 379 (1989). Cytotoxic properties vs viral tumor cells: C. Grignet-Debrus $et\ al.,\ Cancer\ Gene\ Ther.$ **7**, 215 (2000). CE determn in plasma and urine: J. Olgemöller $et\ al., J.\ Chromatogr. B$ **726**, 261 (1999). Clinical evaluation in herpetic keratitis: P. C. Maudgal, E. De Clercq, $Curr.\ Eye\ Res.$ **10**, Suppl., 193 (1991). Clinical comparison with acyclovir, $q.v.$, in herpes zoster: S. W. Wassilew $et\ al., Antiviral\ Res.$ **59**, 49, 57 (2003). Review of pharmacology and clinical efficacy in herpes zoster: S. J. Keam $et\ al.,$ $Drugs$ **64**, 2091-2097 (2004); of antiviral activity, mechanism of action, and clinical efficacy: E. De Clercq, $Med.\ Res.\ Rev.$ **25**, 1-20 (2005).

White needles from methanol-water, mp 123-125° (dec). uv max: 253, 295 nm (ε 13100, 10300).

THERAP CAT: Antiviral.

1379.   Brodifacoum. [56073-10-0] 3-[3-(4′-Bromo[1,1′-biphenyl]-4-yl)-1,2,3,4-tetrahydro-1-naphthalenyl]-4-hydroxy-2H-1-benzopyran-2-one; 3-[3-(4′-bromobiphenyl-4-yl)-1,2,3,4-tetrahydro-1-naphthyl]-4-hydroxycoumarin; PP-581; WBA-8119; Talon. $C_{31}H_{23}BrO_3$; mol wt 523.42. C 71.13%, H 4.43%, Br 15.27%, O 9.17%. Coumarin analog. Prepn: M. R. Hadler, R. S. Shadbolt, **DE 2424806**; $eidem,$ **US 3957824** (1975, 1976 to Ward, Blenkinsop & Co.); $eidem; J.\ Chem.\ Soc.\ Perkin\ Trans.\ 1$ **1976**, 1190. Anticoagulant activity: M. R. Hadler, R. S. Shadbolt, $Nature$ **253**, 275 (1975). Field trials: B. D. Rennison, A. C. Dubock, $J.\ Hyg.$ **80**, 77 (1978); F. P. Rowe $et\ al., ibid.$ **81**, 197 (1978). Efficacy and toxicity: L. Yuet-Ming, $Malays.\ Agric.\ J.$ **52**, 1 (1980).

Off-white powder, mp 228-230°. Insol in water. Slightly sol in alc, benzene; sol in acetone, chloroform. LD_{50} orally in male, female field rats: 0.16, 0.18 mg/kg (Yuet-Ming).

USE: Rodenticide.

1380.   Brodimoprim. [56518-41-3] 5-[(4-Bromo-3,5-dimethoxyphenyl)methyl]-2,4-pyrimidinediamine; 2,4-diamino-5-(4-bromo-3,5-dimethoxybenzyl)pyrimidine; Ro-10-5970. $C_{13}H_{15}BrN_4O_2$; mol wt 339.19. C 46.03%, H 4.46%, Br 23.56%, N 16.52%, O 9.43%. Dihydrofolate reductase inhibitor; structural analog of trimethoprim, $q.v.$ Prepn: M. Hoffer, I. Kompis, **DE 2452889** (1975 to Hoffmann-La Roche), $C.A.$ **83**, 97361 (1975); I. Kompis, **US 4024145** (1977 to Hoffmann-La Roche); I. Kompis, A. Wick, $Helv.\ Chim.\ Acta$ **60**, 3025 (1977). Antibacterial activity: G. Giammanco $et\ al., Drugs\ Exp.\ Clin.\ Res.$ **9**, 721 (1983). Comparison with trimethoprim as inhibitor of dihydrofolate reductase: R. L. Then $et\ al., Rev.\ Infect.\ Dis.$ **4**, 372 (1982); R. L. Then, F. Hermann, $Chemotherapy\ (Basel)$ **30**, 18 (1984). Antimycobacterial activity $in\ vitro$: J. K. Seydel $et\ al., ibid.$ **29**, 249 (1983). Pharmacokinetics in human serum, skin blister fluid: T. Kalager $et\ al.,$ $Chemotherapy\ (Basel)$ **31**, 405 (1985). Clinical evaluation in respiratory infections: H. A. Salmi $et\ al., Drugs\ Exp.\ Clin.\ Res.$ **12**, 349 (1986); in urinary tract infections: F. Scaglione $et\ al., Int. J.\ Clin.\ Pharmacol.\ Res.$ **15**, 121 (1995); in bacterial cystitis: E. V. Cosmi $et\ al., Eur.\ J.\ Obstet.\ Gynecol.\ Reprod.\ Biol.$ **64**, 207 (1996).

Crystals from methanol, mp 225-228°. pKa 7.15.

THERAP CAT: Antibacterial.

1381.   Bromacil. [314-40-9] 5-Bromo-6-methyl-3-(1-methylpropyl)-2,4(1H,3H)-pyrimidinedione; 5-bromo-3-sec-butyl-6-methyluracil; 5-bromo-6-methyl-3-(1-methylpropyl)uracil; Du Pont Herbicide 976; Hyvar; Uragon; Urox B. $C_9H_{13}BrN_2O_2$; mol wt 261.12. C 41.40%, H 5.02%, Br 30.60%, N 10.73%, O 12.25%. Prepn: H. M. Loux, **US 3235357** (1966 to du Pont). Mode of action: C. E. Hoffman, $Pestic.\ Chem.,\ Proc.\ 2nd\ Int.\ Congr.\ Pestic.$ **5**, A. S. Tahori, Ed, (Gordon and Breach Science Publishers, New York, 1972) pp 65-85. Toxicology: H. Sherman, A. M. Kaplan, $Toxicol.\ Appl.\ Pharmacol.$ **34**, 189 (1975). $Review$: Pease, Deye, $Anal.\ Methods\ Pestic.\ Plant\ Growth\ Regul.\ Food\ Addit.$ **5**, 335 (1967).

White crystalline solid, mp 157.5-160°. Vapor pressure at 100°: 8×10^{-4} mm Hg. Soly in water at 20°: 815 mg/l. Moderately sol in strong aq bases, acetone, acetonitrile, ethanol. LD_{50} orally in rats: 5200 mg/kg (Sherman, Kaplan).

Caution: Potential symptoms of overexposure are irritation of eyes, skin and upper respiratory system. *See NIOSH Pocket Guide to Chemical Hazards* (DHHS/NIOSH 97-140, 1997) p 32.

USE: Herbicide.

1382. Bromadiolone. [28772-56-7] 3-[3-(4′-Bromo[1,1′-biphenyl]-4-yl)-3-hydroxy-1-phenylpropyl]-4-hydroxy-2*H*-1-benzopyran-2-one; 3-[α-[*p*-(*p*-bromophenyl)-β-hydroxyphenethyl]-benzyl]-4-hydroxycoumarin; LM-637; Maki; Bromone; Super-Caid; Super-Rozol. $C_{30}H_{23}BrO_4$; mol wt 527.41. C 68.32%, H 4.40%, Br 15.15%, O 12.13%. Anticoagulant rodenticide. Prepn: E. Boschetti *et al.,* **DE 1959317**; *eidem,* **US 3764693** (1970, 1973 both to Lipha). Activity studies: *eidem, Chim. Ther.* **7,** 20 (1972); M. Grand, *Phytiatr.-Phytopharm.* **25,** 69 (1976); R. E. Marsh, *Bull. OEPP* **7,** 495 (1977); R. Redfern, J. E. Gill, *J. Hyg.* **84,** 263 (1980). Pharmacokinetics: K. Nahas, *Pharmacol. Res. Commun.* **19,** 767 (1987). HPLC determn of diastereoisomers in animal tissues: K. Hunter *et al., J. Chromatogr.* **435,** 83 (1988).

White to offwhite powder, mp 200-210°. uv max (ethanol): 260 nm ($E_{1cm}^{1\%}$ 538-582). pKa (21°) 4.04. Soly at 20-25° (g/l): dimethylformamide 730.0; ethyl acetate 25.0; acetone 22.3; chloroform 10.1; ethanol 8.2; methanol 5.6; ethyl ether 3.7; hexane 0.2; water 0.019. LD_{50} in rats, mice (mg/kg): 1.125, 1.75 orally (Grand).

USE: Rodenticide.

1383. Bromal. [115-17-3] Tribromoacetaldehyde. C_2-HBr_3O; mol wt 280.74. C 8.56%, H 0.36%, Br 85.39%, O 5.70%. Br_3CCHO. Preparation from ethanol and bromine: Löwig, *Ann.* **3,** 288 (1832); from chloral and a bromide: Müller, **US 2053964** (1936 to Winthrop); from paraldehyde and bromine: Long, Howard, *Org. Synth.* **17,** 18 (1937).

Yellowish, oily liquid; forms with water bromal hydrate which is solid at temps below 50°. d 2.66. bp ~174° with decompn. Sol in water, alcohol or ether.

1384. Bromal Hydrate. [507-42-6] 2,2,2-Tribromo-1,1-ethanediol; tribromoacetaldehyde hydrate. $C_2H_3Br_3O_2$; mol wt 298.76. C 8.04%, H 1.01%, Br 80.24%, O 10.71%. Br_3-$CCH(OH)_2$. Prepd from bromal and water: Löwig, *Ann.* **3,** 288 (1832). Structure: Jain, Soundararajan, *Tetrahedron* **20,** 1589 (1964).

Deliquescent crystals, mp 53.5°. Odor of chloral and pungent taste. Dipole moment in benzene, 2.56D. Sol in water, alcohol, chloroform, ether, glycerol. *Keep tightly closed in a cool place.*

1385. Bromazepam. [1812-30-2] 7-Bromo-1,3-dihydro-5-(2-pyridinyl)-2*H*-1,4-benzodiazepin-2-one; 7-bromo-5-(2-pyridyl)-3*H*-1,4-benzodiazepin-2(1*H*)-one; Ro-5-3350; Compendium; Creosedin; Durazanil; Lectopam; Lexomil; Lexotan; Lexotanil; Normoc. $C_{14}H_{10}BrN_3O$; mol wt 316.15. C 53.19%, H 3.19%, Br 25.27%, N 13.29%, O 5.06%. Prepn: Berger *et al.,* **BE 619101**; *eidem,* Fryer *et al.,* **US 3100770** (1962, 1963 to Hoffmann-La Roche); *eidem, J. Pharm. Sci.* **53,** 264 (1964); **US 3182065; US 3182067** (both 1965 to Hoffmann-La Roche). Pharmacology: Korol, Brown, *Pharmacology* **1,** 115 (1968). Metabolism: M. A. Schwartz *et al., J. Pharm. Sci.* **62,** 1776 (1973); *Drug Metab. Dispos.* **2,** 31 (1974). Evaluation as pre-anesthesia medication: P. Chalmers, J. N. Horton, *Anesthesia* **39,** 370 (1984). Multicenter clinical comparison with lorazepam, *q.v.:* G. J. Cordingley *et al., Curr. Med. Res. Opin.* **9,** 505 (1985). Evaluation of adverse effects and withdrawal reactions: R. Fontaine *et al., Psychopharmacol. Bull.* **21,** 91 (1985). Toxicity: E. I. Goldenthal, *Toxicol. Appl. Pharmacol.* **18,** 185 (1971). Comprehensive description: M. M. Hassan, M. A. Abounassif, *Anal. Profiles Drug Subs.* **16,** 1-51 (1987).

Colorless prisms from acetone, mp 237-238.5° (dec). LD_{50} orally in rats: 3050 ±405 mg/kg (Goldenthal).

Note: This is a controlled substance (depressant): **21 CFR,** 1308.14.

THERAP CAT: Anxiolytic.

1386. Bromcresol Green. [76-60-8] 4,4′-(3*H*-2,1-Benzoxathiol-3-ylidene)bis[2,6-dibromo-3-methylphenol] *S,S*-dioxide; α,α-bis(3,5-dibromo-4-hydroxy-*o*-tolyl)-α-hydroxytoluenesulfonic acid, γ-sultone; 3,3′,5,5′-tetrabromo-*m*-cresolsulfonphthalein. $C_{21}H_{14}$-Br_4O_5S; mol wt 698.01. C 36.13%, H 2.02%, Br 45.79%, O 11.46%, S 4.59%. Prepd by adding bromine to a suspension of *m*-cresolsulfonphthalein in glacial acetic acid: Clark, Lubs, *J. Wash. Acad. Sci.* **5,** 610 (1915); **6,** 481 (1916); *J. Bacteriol.* **2,** 110 (1917); Cohen, *Biochem. J.* **16,** 31 (1922); **17,** 535 (1923); Cohen, *Public Health Rep.* **38,** 814 (1923); **41,** 3051 (1926); *Proc. Soc. Exp. Biol. Med.* **20,** 124 (1922); Orndorff, Purdy, *J. Am. Chem. Soc.* **48,** 2216 (1926).

Minute, slightly yellow crystals from acetic acid, mp 218-219°. Sparingly sol in water. Readily sol in alcohol, ether, ethyl acetate. Fairly sol in benzene. Very sensitive to alkalies, tap water being sufficiently alkaline to give the characteristic blue-green color. pK = 4.7. To prepare a soln for use as pH indicator, dissolve 0.10 g in 7.15 ml *N*/50 NaOH and dil with water to 250 ml. To prepare a soln for use as indicator in volumetric work, dissolve 0.1 g in 250 ml alc.

USE: As indicator, pH 3.8 yellow; pH 5.4 blue-green.

1387. Bromcresol Purple. [115-40-2] 4,4′-(3*H*-2,1-Benzoxathiol-3-ylidene)bis[2-bromo-6-methylphenol] *S,S*-dioxide; α-(5-bromo-4-hydroxy-*m*-tolyl)-α-(3-bromo-5-methyl-4-oxo-2,5-cyclohexadien-1-ylidene)-*o*-toluenesulfonic acid; 5,5′-dibromo-*o*-cresolsulfonphthalein. $C_{21}H_{16}Br_2O_5S$; mol wt 540.22. C 46.69%, H 2.99%, Br 29.58%, O 14.81%, S 5.94%. Prepd by treating *o*-cresol red with bromine in glacial acetic acid: *See refs* under Bromcresol Green.

Minute, slightly yellow crystals, mp 241-242°. Practically insol in water. Sol in alcohol, dil alkalies. pK 6.3. To prepare a soln for use as pH indicator, dissolve 0.10 g in 9.25 ml *N*/50 NaOH and dil with water to 250 ml. To prepare a soln for use as indicator in volumetric work, dissolve 0.05 g in 250 ml alc.

USE: As indicator, pH 5.2 yellow; pH 6.8 purple.

1388. Bromelain. [9001-00-7] Bromelin; Ananase; Extranase; Inflamen; Traumanase. Protein-digesting and milk-clotting enzymes found in pineapple fruit juice and stem tissue. Enzymes from the two sources are distinguished as fruit bromelain and stem bromelain. First isolns of fruit bromelain: Marcano, *Bull. Pharm.* **5,** 77 (1891); Chittenden, *Trans. Conn. Acad. Sci.* **8,** 281 (1892). From pineapple juice by precipitation with acetone and also with ammonium sulfide: Heinicke, US 3002891 (1961 to Pineapple Res. Inst.). Discovery in stem tissue: *idem, Science* **118,** 753 (1953). Stem bromelain has mol wt of about 33,000 and is probably the first proteolytic enzyme of plant origin to be established as a glycoprotein: Murachi *et al., Biochemistry* **3,** 48 (1964); Ota *et al., ibid.* 180. Purification of crude prepns: Gibian, Bratfisch, US 2950227 (1960 to Schering AG). *Reviews:* Balls *et al., Ind. Eng. Chem.* **33,** 950 (1941); of stem bromelain: Murachi, "Structure and Function of Stem Bromelain," in *Proteins, Structure and Function* **vol. 2,** M. Funatsu *et al.,* Eds. (Kodansha, Tokyo, Wiley, New York, 1972) pp 47-101.

Unlike papain, fruit bromelain does not disappear as the fruit ripens. Fruit and stem bromelains are acidic and basic proteins, resp. uv max (stem): 280 nm ($A_{1cm}^{1\%}$ 20.1).

USE: Tenderizing meat, chill-proofing beer, production of protein hydrolyzates.

THERAP CAT: Anti-inflammatory.

1389. Bromethalin. [63333-35-7] *N*-Methyl-2,4-dinitro-*N*-(2,4,6-tribromophenyl)-6-(trifluoromethyl)benzenamine; EL-614; Vengeance. $C_{14}H_7Br_3F_3N_3O_4$; mol wt 577.93. C 29.10%, H 1.22%, Br 41.48%, F 9.86%, N 7.27%, O 11.07%. Rodenticide which acts by uncoupling oxidative phosphorylation. Single-feed toxicant, effective against warfarin-resistant strains of mice, rats. Prepn and identification as rodenticide: B. A. Dreikorn, US 4187318 (1980 to Eli Lilly). Toxicology and activity: B. A. Dreikorn *et al., Proc. Br. Crop Prot. Conf. - Pests Dis.* **1979,** 491. *Review:* B. A. Dreikorn, G. O. P. O'Doherty, *ACS Symp. Ser.* **255,** 45-63 (1984).

Pale yellow odorless crystals from ethanol, mp 150-151°. Sol in chloroform, acetone; moderately sol in aromatic hydrocarbons. Insol in water. LD50 in mice, rats, cats, dogs (mg/kg): 2, 5, 2, 5 orally (Dreikorn).

USE: Rodenticide.

1390. Bromfenac. [91714-94-2] 2-Amino-3-(4-bromobenzoyl)benzeneacetic acid; AHR-10282. $C_{15}H_{12}BrNO_3$; mol wt 334.16. C 53.91%, H 3.62%, Br 23.91%, N 4.19%, O 14.36%. Prostaglandin synthetase inhibitor; analog of amfenac, *q.v.* Prepn: D. A. Walsh *et al., J. Med. Chem.* **27,** 1379 (1984). *See also:* R. G. Poser, US 4683242 (1987 to A. H. Robins). HPLC determn in plasma: M. A. Osman *et al., J. Chromatogr.* **489,** 452 (1989). Pharmacology: L. F. Sancilio *et al., Arzneim.-Forsch.* **37,** 513 (1987). Clinical pharmacokinetics: P. Högger, P. Rohdewald, *ibid.* **43,** 1114 (1993). *Review:* J. S. Wajdula *et al.* in *Nonsteroidal Anti-inflammatory Drugs,* A. J. Lewis, D. E. Furst, Eds. (Marcel Dekker, Inc., New York, 1994) 267-284. Evaluation of hepatotoxicity: R. J. Fontana *et al., Liver Transpl. Surg.* **5,** 480 (1999). Clinical trial in allergic conjunctivitis: M. Miyake-Kashima *et al., Jpn. J. Ophthalmol.* **48,** 587 (2004).

Monosodium salt sesquihydrate. [120638-55-3]; [91714-93-1] (monosodium salt). AHR-10282B; Duract; Xibrom. $C_{15}H_{11}BrN-NaO_3 \cdot 1\frac{1}{2}H_2O$; mol wt 365.15. Bright orange-yellow crystalline powder, mp 284-286° (dec). pKa 4.29. Sol in water, methanol, dilute base. Insol in chloroform, dilute acid.

THERAP CAT: Anti-inflammatory (ophthalmic).

1391. Bromhexine. [3572-43-8] 2-Amino-3,5-dibromo-*N*-cyclohexyl-*N*-methylbenzenemethanamine; 3,5-dibromo-*N*$^\alpha$-cyclohexyl-*N*$^\alpha$-methyltoluene-α,2-diamine; *N*-cyclohexyl-*N*-methyl-2-(2-amino-3,5-dibromo)benzylammonium; *N*-(2-amino-3,5-dibromobenzyl)-*N*-methylcyclohexylammonium. $C_{14}H_{20}Br_2N_2$; mol wt 376.13. C 44.71%, H 5.36%, Br 42.49%, N 7.45%. Prepn: Keck, *Ann.* **662,** 171 (1963); K. Thomae, **BE 625022** (1963), *C.A.* **61,** 5564 (1964). Pharmacology: R. Engelhorn, S. Püschmann, *Arzneim.-Forsch.* **13,** 474 (1963). Metabolism: R. Jauch *et al., ibid.* **25,** 1954 (1975). Toxicity: Boyd, Sheppard, *Arch. Int. Pharmacodyn. Ther.* **163,** 284 (1966).

Crystals from abs ethanol, dec 237.5-238°. One gram dissolves in 250 ml of water or 10% ethanol. Approx LD50 orally in rabbits: >10 g/kg (Boyd, Sheppard).

Hydrochloride. [611-75-6] NA-274; Auxit; Bisolvon; Ophtosol; Quentan. $C_{14}H_{20}Br_2N_2 \cdot HCl$; mol wt 412.59.

THERAP CAT: Expectorant; mucolytic.

THERAP CAT (VET): Expectorant.

1392. Bromic Acid. [7789-31-3] $BrHO_3$; mol wt 128.91. Br 61.98%, H 0.78%, O 37.23%. $HBrO_3$. Prepd from $Ba(BrO_3)_2$ and H_2SO_4: Burchard, *Z. Phys. Chem.* **2,** 814 (1888); Schmeisser in *Handbook of Preparative Inorganic Chemistry* **vol. 1,** G. Brauer, Ed. (Academic Press, 2nd ed, 1963) p 315.

Known in aq soln only. *Keep refrigerated!* Colorless soln, turns yellow on standing at room temp, even in the dark. Careful evapn *in vacuo* at −12° yields about a 50% soln. Dec on heating to 100°. Can be dil with cold water.

Caution: Highly irritating to skin, eyes, mucous membranes.

USE: Oxidizing agent.

1393. Bromindione. [1146-98-1] 2-(4-Bromophenyl)-1*H*-indene-1,3(2*H*)-dione; 2-(4-bromophenyl)-1,3-dioxohydrindene; HL-255; MG-2555; Fluidane; Halinone. $C_{15}H_9BrO_2$; mol wt 301.13. C 59.83%, H 3.01%, Br 26.53%, O 10.63%. Prepn: Cavallini *et al., Farmaco Ed. Sci.* **10,** 710 (1955); Freedman *et al.,* US 2847474 (1958 to U.S. Vitamin).

Crystals from ligroin, mp 137-139°.

THERAP CAT: Anticoagulant.

1394. Bromine. [7726-95-6] Br; at. wt 79.904; at. no. 35; valences 1, 3, 5, 7. A halogen; Group VIIA (17). Does not occur as elemental state, Br_2, in nature. Abundance in igneous rock: 1.6 × 10^{-4}% by wt; in seawater: 0.0065% by wt. Extracted commercially from natural brines (salt lakes) and seawater. Naturally occurring stable isotopes (mass numbers): 79 (50.69%), 81 (49.31%); known artificial radioactive isotopes: 69-76, 77 (longest-lived known isotope, $T_{1/2}$ 57.036 hr; EC decay), 78, 79m, 80, 80m, 82-94. Discovery: A. J. Balard, *Ann. Chim. Phys.* **32,** 337 (1826). Books: *Bromine and its Compounds,* Z. E. Jolles, Ed. (E. Benn, London, 1966) 940 pp; *Bromine Compounds: Chemistry and Applications,* D. Price *et al.,* Eds. (Elsevier, Amsterdam, 1988) 422 pp. *Reviews: MTP Int. Rev. Sci.: Inorg. Chem., Ser. One* vol. **3**, V. Gutmann, Ed. (Butterworths, London, 1972); A. J. Downs, C. J. Adams, "Chlorine, Bromine, Iodine and Astatine" in *Comprehensive Inorganic Chemistry* vol. **2**, J. C. Bailar, Jr. *et al.*, Eds. (Pergamon Press, Oxford, 1973) pp 1107-1573; *Chemistry of the Elements*, N. N. Greenwood, A. Earnshaw, Eds. (Pergamon Press, New York, 1984) pp 920-1041; P. F. Jackish in *Kirk-Othmer Encyclopedia of Chemical Technology* vol. **4** (Wiley-Interscience, New York, 4th ed., 1992) pp 536-560.

Dark reddish-brown, volatile, mobile, diatomic liquid; suffocating odor; vaporizes rapidly at room temp. Only nonmetallic element liquid at standard conditions. Nonflammable, but may ignite combustibles on contact. Corrosive material. mp $-7.25°$ (265.90 K); bp $59.47°$ *(JANAF Thermochemical Tables)*; $58.78°$ (Mellor's Suppl. II, Part I, "The Halogens"); d_4^{25} 3.1023; crit temp: $315°$; crit pressure: 102 atm. Heat capacity at constant pressure (liq, $25°$) 18.089 cal/mole deg: Hildenbrand *et al.*, *J. Am. Chem. Soc.* **80**, 4129 (1958). Vapor pressure data: A. N. Nesmeyanov, *Vapor Pressure of the Chemical Elements*, R. Gary, Ed. (Elsevier, New York, 1963) pp 354-58. Total soly in water ($25°$): 0.2141 moles/l with formation of 0.00115 moles/l of HOBr; freely sol in alc, ether, $CHCl_3$, CCl_4, CS_2, concd HCl, aq solns of bromides. Oxidizing agent; less reactive than chlorine; E^0 (aq) $½Br_2/Br^-$ 1.065 V; dissociation energy ($25°$): 46.072 kcal. *Keep sealed or glass-stoppered.*

Caution: Potential symptoms of overexposure are dizziness, headache; lacrimation, epistaxis; coughing, feeling of oppression, pulmonary edema and pneumonia; abdominal pain, diarrhea; measle-like eruptions; direct contact may cause severe burns of eyes and skin. *See NIOSH Pocket Guide to Chemical Hazards* (DHHS/-NIOSH 97-140, 1997) p 32. *See also Patty's Industrial Hygiene and Toxicology* vol. **2B**, G. D. Clayton, F. E. Clayton, Eds. (Wiley-Interscience, New York, 4th ed., 1994) pp 4505-4513.

USE: Manuf of organic and inorganic chemicals, such as fuel additives, fire retardants, pesticides, oil well drilling fluids, pharmaceuticals, dyestuffs. In water disinfection; as bleaching agent, surface disinfectant.

1395.   Bromine Pentafluoride. [7789-30-2] BrF_5; mol wt 174.90. Br 45.69%, F 54.31%. Prepd by fluorination of bromine at $200°$ in iron or Monel metal apparatus: Ruff, Menzel, *Z. Anorg. Allg. Chem.* **202**, 49 (1931); Kwasnik in *Handbook of Preparative Inorganic Chemistry* Vol. **1**, G. Brauer, Ed. (Academic Press, New York, 2nd ed., 1963) pp 158-159; from F_2 and KBr: Hyde, Boudakian, *Inorg. Chem.* **7**, 2648 (1968). *Reviews:* Kemmitt, Sharp, *Adv. Fluorine Chem.* **4**, 243-244 (1965); Stein, "Physical and Chemical Properties of Halogen Fluorides" in *Halogen Chemistry* Vol. **1**, V. Gutmann, Ed. (Academic Press, New York, 1967) pp 133-224; Meinert, *Z. Chem.* **7**, 41-57 (1967).

Liquid. Fumes in air. mp $-60.5°$. bp $40.76°$. d^{25} 2.4604. Trouton constant 23.7. Thermostable up to $460°$. Does not attack quartz when dry. *Produces an explosion on contact with water.* Very reactive, usually with conflagration.

Caution: Potential symptoms of overexposure are irritation of eyes, skin, respiratory system; corneal necrosis; skin burns; cough, dyspnea, pulmonary edema; liver, kidney injury. *See NIOSH Pocket Guide to Chemical Hazards* (DHHS/NIOSH 97-140, 1997) p 34.

1396.   Bromine Trifluoride. [7787-71-5] BrF_3; mol wt 136.90. Br 58.37%, F 41.63%. Prepd by fluorination of bromine at $+80°$: Lebeau, *Compt. Rend.* **141**, 1018 (1905); Prideaux, *J. Chem. Soc.* **89**, 316 (1906); Ruff, Braida, *Z. Anorg. Allg. Chem.* **206**, 59 (1932); **214**, 91 (1933); Simons, *Inorg. Synth.* **3**, 184 (1950); Kwasnik in *Handbook of Preparative Inorganic Chemistry* Vol. **1**, G. Brauer, Ed. (Academic Press, 2nd ed., 1963) pp 156-157. *Reviews:* Kemmitt, Sharp, *Adv. Fluorine Chem.* **4**, 244-245 (1965); Stein, "Physical and Chemical Properties of Halogen Fluorides" in *Halogen Chemistry* Vol. **1**, V. Gutmann, Ed. (Academic Press, New York, 1967) pp 133-224; Meinert, *Z. Chem.* **7**, 41-57 (1967).

Colorless liquid; also reported to be pale yellow. Long prisms when solid. mp $8.77°$. bp $125.75°$. d^{25} 2.8030. *Smokes in air. Attacks skin. Very reactive.*

Caution: Corrosive and irritating to skin, eyes, mucous membranes, respiratory tract.

USE: Solvent for fluorides.

1397.   Bromisovalum. [496-67-3] *N*-(Aminocarbonyl)-2-bromo-3-methylbutanamide; ($α$-bromoisovaleryl)urea; 2-mono-bromoisovalerylurea; $α$-bromo-$β$-dimethylpropanoylurea; bromvaletone; B.V.U.; Bromural; Bromisoval; Uvaleral; Bromuvan; Somnurol; Brovalurea; Dormigene; Isobromyl; Alluval; Pivadorm. $C_6H_{11}BrN_2O_2$; mol wt 223.07. C 32.31%, H 4.97%, Br 35.82%, N 12.56%, O 14.34%. $(CH_3)_2CHCHBrCONHCONH_2$. Prepn from urea and $α$-bromoisovaleryl bromide: US 914518 (1909). Toxicity: R. I. Mrongovius *et al.*, *Clin. Exp. Pharmacol. Physiol.* **3**, 443 (1976).

Practically tasteless needles, mp 147-149°. Sublimes. Slightly sol in cold water, but freely sol in hot water. Readily sol in alcohol, ether and in alkaline solns. LD_{50} in male mice (mmoles/kg): 3.25 i.p. (Mrongovius).

THERAP CAT: Sedative, hypnotic.

1398.   *N*-Bromoacetamide. [79-15-2] Acetobromamide. C_2H_4BrNO; mol wt 137.96. C 17.41%, H 2.92%, Br 57.92%, N 10.15%, O 11.60%. $CH_3CONHBr$. Prepd by treating a cooled (0-5°) soln of acetamide dissolved in bromine with ice cold aq 50% KOH, allowing to stand for 2-3 hr at 0-5°, treating with NaCl, and extracting with chloroform: Oliveto, Gerold, *Org. Synth.* **31**, 17 (1951).

Needles from chloroform + hexane, mp 102-105°. Sol in warm water, freely sol in cold ether. Unstable to light and heat.

Monohydrate. Rectangular plates from hydr ether, mp 70-80°. Freely sol in cold water, alcohol, ether, less freely in chloroform.

USE: Brominating agent; in oxidation of primary and secondary alcohols.

1399.   *p*-Bromoacetanilide. [103-88-8] *N*-(4-Bromophenyl)acetamide; 4'-bromoacetanilide; monobromoacetanilide; bromoanilide; Antisepsin; Asepsin; Bromoantifebrin. C_8H_8BrNO; mol wt 214.06. C 44.89%, H 3.77%, Br 37.33%, N 6.54%, O 7.47%. Prepd by bromination of acetanilide: Remmers, *Ber.* **7**, 346 (1874); Merker, Vona, *J. Chem. Educ.* **26**, 613 (1949); Knowles, Alt, US 3012035 (1959 to Monsanto).

Crystals, from 95% alc, mp 168° (with previous softening). d 1.72. Practically insol in cold water. Sparingly sol in hot water; sol in benzene, chloroform, ethyl acetate; moderately sol in alcohol.

THERAP CAT: Analgesic, antipyretic.

1400.   Bromoacetic Acid. [79-08-3] $C_2H_3BrO_2$; mol wt 138.95. C 17.29%, H 2.18%, Br 57.51%, O 23.03%. $BrCH_2$-COOH. Prepn by bromination of acetic acid: Perkin, Duppa, *Ann.* **108**, 106 (1858); from chloroacetic acid and HBr: Lake, Asadorian; Asadorian, Burk, US 2553518; US 3130222 (1951, 1964, both to Dow); from glycolic acid and HBr: Johnston, US 2876255 (1959 to Ethyl Corp.).

Hygroscopic crystals, mp 50°. bp 208°. d 1.93. Very sol in water, alcohol. *Protect from air and moisture.*

Caution: Irritant and corrosive to skin, mucous membranes.

1401.   Bromoacetone. [598-31-2] 1-Bromo-2-propanone. C_3H_5BrO; mol wt 136.98. C 26.30%, H 3.68%, Br 58.33%, O 11.68%. CH_3COCH_2Br. Prepn by bromination of acetone: Emmerling, Wagner, *Ann.* **204**, 29 (1880); Catch *et al.*, *J. Chem. Soc.* **1948**, 272; Ross US 2452154 (1948 to Colgate-Palmolive-Peet); by bromination acetone enol acetate: Magerlein, US 2752341 (1956 to Upjohn).

Liquid, mp $-36.5°$. bp 137°, bp_{50} 63.5-64°. d^{23} 1.634. n_D^{15} 1.4697. Turns violet rapidly even in absence of air. Sparingly sol in water; sol in alcohol, acetone. *Keep tightly closed and protected from light.*

Caution: Violent lacrimator.

USE: Chemical war gas.

1402.   *ω*-Bromoacetophenone. [70-11-1] 2-Bromo-1-phenylethanone; phenacyl bromide. C_8H_7BrO; mol wt 199.04. C 48.27%, H 3.54%, Br 40.14%, O 8.04%. $C_6H_5COCH_2Br$. Prepn from acetophenone and bromine: Rother, Reid, *J. Am. Chem. Soc.* **41**, 77 (1919); Cowper, Davidson, *Org. Synth.* **19**, 24 (1939); Shevchuk, Dombrovskii, *Zh. Obshch. Khim.* **33**(4), 1135 (1963).

Crystals, mp 50°. d 1.65. bp$_{20}$ 133-135°. Irritating vapors. *Lacrimator!* Practically insol in water. Freely sol in alcohol, benzene, chloroform, ether.

Caution: Highly irritating to skin, eyes, mucous membranes.

1403. *p*-Bromoacetophenone. [99-90-1] 1-(4-Bromophenyl)ethanone; methyl *p*-bromophenyl ketone. C_8H_7BrO; mol wt 199.04. C 48.27%, H 3.54%, Br 40.14%, O 8.04%. BrC_6H_4-$COCH_3$. Prepd from bromobenzene and acetic anhydride in CS_2 in the presence of anhyd $AlCl_3$: Adams, Noller, *Org. Synth.* **5**, 17 (1925).

Leaflets from alc. mp 54°. bp$_{736}$ 255.5°; bp$_{15}$ 130°; bp$_7$ 117°. Easily volatile with steam. Sol in alcohol, ether, glacial acetic acid, benzene, petr ether, carbon disulfide.

Oxime. C_8H_8BrNO. Needles from dil alc, mp 128.5°.

1404. *p*-Bromoaniline. [106-40-1] 4-Bromobenzeneamine; 4-bromoaniline. C_6H_6BrN; mol wt 172.02. C 41.89%, H 3.52%, Br 46.45%, N 8.14%. Prepd by steam distilling sodium hydroxide and *p*-bromoacetanilide: Scott, *J. Chem. Soc.* **123**, 3199 (1923); by direct bromination of aniline: Kosolapoff, *J. Am. Chem. Soc.* **75**, 3596 (1953).

Rhombic crystals from dil alc; mp 66-66.5°. d$_4^{99.6}$ 1.4970 (liq). Very sol in alcohol and ether. Insol in cold water. pKb (25°): 10.28 also reported as 9.98.

USE: In prepn of azo dyes; condensed with formaldehyde in prepn of dihydroquinazolines.

1405. 5-Bromoanthranilic Acid. [5794-88-7] 2-Amino-5-bromobenzoic acid; 5-bromo-2-aminobenzoic acid. $C_7H_6BrNO_2$; mol wt 216.03. C 38.92%, H 2.80%, Br 36.99%, N 6.48%, O 14.81%. Prepd by bromination of anthranilic acid: Wheeler, *J. Am. Chem. Soc.* **31**, 565 (1909); Wheeler, Oates, *ibid.* **32**, 771 (1910).

Crystals, mp 218-219°. Very slightly sol in water, moderately sol in alcohol, ether, chloroform, benzene, acetic acid, freely sol in acetone.

USE: Determination of cobalt, copper, nickel, and zinc.

1406. Bromobenzene. [108-86-1] Monobromobenzene; phenyl bromide. C_6H_5Br; mol wt 157.01. C 45.90%, H 3.21%, Br 50.89%. Prepd industrially by the action of bromide on benzene in the presence of iron powder: Gattermann-Wieland, *Praxis des Organischen Chemikers* (de Gruyter, Berlin, 40th ed., 1961) p 95; alternate procedure using pyridine as halogen carrier: A. I. Vogel, *Practical Organic Chemistry* (Longmans, London, 3rd ed., 1959) p 535.

Mobile liquid. Aromatic odor. d$_4^0$ 1.5220; d$_4^{10}$ 1.5083; d$_4^{15}$ 1.5017; d$_4^{20}$ 1.4952; d$_4^{30}$ 1.4815; d$_4^{71}$ 1.426. mp −30.6°. bp$_{760}$ 156.2°; bp$_{400}$ 132.3°; bp$_{200}$ 110.1°; bp$_{40}$ 68.6°; bp$_{20}$ 53.8°; bp$_{10}$ 40.0°; bp$_5$ 27.8°; bp$_{1.0}$ 2.9°. n$_D^{15}$ 1.5625; n$_D^{20}$ 1.5602. Flash pt 51°C. Fire pt 155°. Critical temp 397°; crit press. 33,912 mm (44.6 atm). Viscosity at 20° = 1.124 cP. Vapor density (air = 1): 5.41. Specific heat at 26.84° = 0.2368. Heat of melting 16.186 cal/g at 15°. Practically insol in water (0.045 g/100 g at 30°). Miscible with chloroform, benzene, petr hydrocarbons. Sol in alc (10.4 g/100 g at 25°), in ether (71.3 g/100 g at 25°).

Caution: Irritating to skin.

USE: In organic synthesis, especially to make phenyl magnesium bromide; as solvent, especially for crystns on a large scale and where a heavy liquid is desirable; as additive to motor oils.

1407. *p*-Bromobenzenesulfonyl Chloride. [98-58-8] C_6-H_4BrClO_2S; mol wt 255.52. C 28.20%, H 1.58%, Br 31.27%, Cl 13.87%, O 12.52%, S 12.55%. Prepd from sodium *p*-bromobenzenesulfonate and phosphorus pentachloride: Marvel, Smith, *J. Am. Chem. Soc.* **45**, 2696 (1923).

Needles from ligroin, mp 74.5°.

USE: Identification of amines.

1408. *p*-Bromobenzoic Acid. [586-76-5] $C_7H_5BrO_2$; mol wt 201.02. C 41.82%, H 2.51%, Br 39.75%, O 15.92%. Prepd by oxidation of *p*-bromotoluene with potassium permanganate: Hale, Thorp, *J. Am. Chem. Soc.* **35**, 269 (1913).

Needles from ether, leaflets from water or 90% alcohol. mp 251-253°. Slightly sol in hot water. Sol in alc, ether.

Methyl ester. $C_6H_4BrCO_2CH_3$. Needles from ether or leaflets from dil alcohol, mp 81°. d 1.689. Sol in alc, ether.

Ethyl ester. $C_6H_4BrCO_2C_2H_5$. Liquid; bp$_{737.4}$ 262°.

Phenyl ester. $C_{13}H_9BrO_2$. Scales, mp 117°. Sol in alc, ether, chloroform, CS_2, benzene; less sol in petr ether.

USE: For the detection of strontium; in org syntheses.

1409. *p*-Bromobenzyl Bromide. [589-15-1] 1-Bromo-4-(bromomethyl)benzene; *p*,α-dibromotoluene. $C_7H_6Br_2$; mol wt 249.93. C 33.64%, H 2.42%, Br 63.94%. Prepd by photo-bromination of *p*-bromotoluene: Weizmann, Patai, *J. Am. Chem. Soc.* **68**, 150 (1946). Alternate procedure: Goerner, Nametz, *ibid.* **73**, 2940 (1951).

Crystals from alc. Agreeable aromatic odor. mp 61°. bp$_{12}$ 115-124°. Sol in water, cold alc, more sol in hot alc, ether, carbon disulfide, benzene, glacial acetic acid.

Caution: Irritating to eyes, mucous membranes of nose and throat. Action similar to, but less intense than, benzylbromide, *q.v.*

USE: Identification of aromatic carboxylic acids.

1410. *p*-Bromobenzyl Chloride. [589-17-3] 1-Bromo-4-(chloromethyl)benzene; *p*-bromo-α-chlorotoluene; α-chloro-4-bromotoluene. C_7H_6BrCl; mol wt 205.48. C 40.92%, H 2.94%, Br 38.89%, Cl 17.25%. Prepd from *p*-bromobenzene, paraformaldehyde and $SnCl_4$: Quelet, *Bull. Soc. Chim.* **41**, 329 (1927); by benzoyl peroxide catalyzed chlorination of *p*-bromotoluene with sulfhydryl chloride: Goerner, Nametz, *J. Am. Chem. Soc.* **73**, 2940 (1951).

Needles from alc, mp 40-41°. bp$_{12}$ 105-115°; bp$_{27}$ 136-139°. Freely sol in hot alc.

1411. *p*-Bromobenzyl Chloroformate. [5798-78-7] Carbonochloridic acid (4-bromophenyl)methyl ester; chloroformic acid *p*-bromobenzyl ester. $C_8H_6BrClO_2$; mol wt 249.49. C 38.51%, H 2.42%, Br 32.03%, Cl 14.21%, O 12.83%. A stable, low-melting cryst product obtained from *p*-bromobenzyl alcohol. In the carbobenzyloxy method of prepn of amino acids and peptides, gives higher melting and better cryst products than the corresp carbobenzyloxy compds: Channing *et al.*, *Nature* **167**, 487 (1951).

USE: In the prepn of amino acids and peptides.

1412. α-Bromobenzyl Cyanide. [5798-79-8] α-Bromobenzeneacetonitrile; α-bromophenylacetonitrile; α-bromo-α-toluinitrile; B.B.C.; C.A.; Camite. C_8H_6BrN; mol wt 196.04. C 49.01%, H 3.08%, Br 40.76%, N 7.14%. $C_6H_5CHBrCN$. The practical industrial prepn consists of three steps: (1) Chlorination of toluene to form benzyl chloride, (2) conversion of benzyl chloride to benzyl cyanide by the action of sodium cyanide in alcoholic soln, (3) bromination of the benzyl cyanide with bromine vapor in the presence of sunlight: Steinkopf *et al., Ber.* **53,** 1146 (1920); Nekrassov, *J. Prakt. Chem.* **119,** 108 (1928).

Crystalline mass, mp 29°. Odor of soured fruit. bp_{760} 242° (dec); bp_{12} 132-134°. d_4^{29} 1.539. Vapor density 6.8 (air = 1). Vapor pressure at 20° = 0.012 mm; at 30° = 0.028 mm. Slightly sol in water. Freely sol in alcohol, ether, chloroform, acetone, and other common organic solvents; also sol in phosgene, chloropicrin, benzyl cyanide. LC (30 min.): 0.90 mg/l (A. M. Prentiss, *Chemicals in War* (McGraw-Hill, New York, 1937) p 141).

Caution: Highly potent lacrimator. *See Patty's Industrial Hygiene and Toxicology* **vol. 2D,** G. D. Clayton, F. E. Clayton, Eds. (Wiley-Interscience, New York, 4th ed., 1994) p 3163.

USE: War gas.

1413. α-Bromobutyric Acid. [80-58-0] 2-Bromobutanoic acid; *dl*-2-bromobutyric acid. $C_4H_7BrO_2$; mol wt 167.00. C 28.77%, H 4.22%, Br 47.85%, O 19.16%. $CH_3CH_2CHBrCOOH$. Prepd by bromination of butyric acid: Naumann, *Ann.* **119,** 115 (1861); Stevens, Holland, *J. Org. Chem.* **18,** 1112 (1953); Smissman, *J. Am. Chem. Soc.* **76,** 5805 (1954). Toxicity study: J. L. Morrison, *J. Pharmacol. Exp. Ther.* **86,** 336 (1946).

Oily liquid, mp −4°. bp_{250} 181-182°, bp_{25} 127-128°. d_4^4 1.5855, d_{15}^{15} 1.5735, d_{20}^{20} 1.5669, d_{25}^{22} 1.5620: Perkin, *J. Chem. Soc.* **65,** 402 (1894). Boils with decompn at ordinary pressure. Sol in 15 parts water; sol in alcohol, ether. *Corrosive!* LD_{50} orally in mice: 310 mg/kg (Morrison).

Ethyl ester. Ethyl α-bromobutyrate. $C_6H_{11}BrO_2$. Liquid, bp 177-178° with slight dec. d_{20}^{20} 1.329. Insol in water. Misc with alc, ether. *Protect from light. Lacrimator!*

1414. 3-Bromo-*d*-camphor. [76-29-9] 3-Bromo-1,7,7-trimethylbicyclo[2.2.1]heptan-2-one; 3-bromo-*d*-2-bornanone. $C_{10}H_{15}BrO$; mol wt 231.13. C 51.97%, H 6.54%, Br 34.57%, O 6.92%. Of the two configurations found, the *endo*-form is more stable than the *exo*-form: Lowry *et al., J. Chem. Soc.* **121,** 633 (1922); Cookson, *ibid.* **1954,** 282. Prepn of the *endo*-form by bromination of *d*-camphor: Kipping, Pope, *ibid.* **63,** 548 (1893); *cf.* Woods, Roberts, *J. Org. Chem.* **22,** 1124 (1957). Prepn of *exo*-form by isomerization of *endo*-form: Lowry *et al., loc. cit.* Configuration: Wiebenga, Krom, *Rec. Trav. Chim.* **65,** 663 (1946); Cookson, *loc. cit.* Review: J. L. Simonsen, Ed., *The Terpenes* **vol. II** (University Press, Cambridge, 2nd ed., 1949), pp 401-404.

endo-form   exo-form

endo-Form. α-Bromo-*d*-camphor; 3α-bromo-*d*-camphor; bromated camphor; camphor monobromated. Crystals from benzene, mp 76°. Camphor-like odor and taste. Discolors on prolonged exposure to light. d 1.449. $[\alpha]_D^{20}$ +122.7° (14.5 g/100 g benzene soln), Cutter *et al., J. Chem. Soc.* **127,** 1260 (1925). uv max (cyclohexane): 307.5 nm (log ε 1.98), Cookson, *loc. cit.* Sublimes, bp 274°. Almost insol in water: 1 g dissolves in 6.5 ml alcohol, 0.5 ml chloroform, 1.6 ml ether; sol in olive oil, slightly in glycerol.

When phenol, chloral hydrate, salol, menthol, or thymol is triturated with bromocamphor the mixture melts; these compds, however, are not incompatible.

exo-Form. α′-Bromo-*d*-camphor; 3β-bromo-*d*-camphor. Needles from methanol or ethanol, mp 78.5°. d 1.484. $[\alpha]_D^{20}$ −42.1° (14.5 g/100 g ethanol soln), Cutter *et al., loc. cit.* uv max (cyclohexane): 312 nm (log ε 1.95), Cookson, *loc. cit.*

THERAP CAT: Topical counterirritant.

1415. α-Bromo-*n*-caproic Acid. [616-05-7] 2-Bromohexanoic acid. $C_6H_{11}BrO_2$; mol wt 195.05. C 36.95%, H 5.68%, Br 40.97%, O 16.41%. $CH_3(CH_2)_3CHBrCOOH$. Prepd by heating bromine with *n*-caproic acid in the presence of phosphorus trichloride as catalyst: Clarke, Taylor, *Org. Synth.* **4,** 9 (1924). Resoln into optically active forms by means of the strychnine salt: Levene *et al., J. Biol. Chem.* **75,** 352 (1927); Levene, Mardashew, *ibid.* **117,** 707 (1937).

Liquid. bp_{760} 240°; bp_{30} 148-153°; bp_{17} 128-136°; bp_8 116-125°. Soluble in alcohol, ether.

Ethyl ester. $C_8H_{15}BrO_2$. Liquid, odor of anise oil. bp_{760} 205-210°; bp_{32} 99-102°; bp_{11} 103°; bp_9 95-96°.

1416. Bromocriptine. [25614-03-3] (5′α)-2-Bromo-12′-hydroxy-2′-(1-methylethyl)-5′-(2-methylpropyl)ergotaman-3′,6′,18-trione; 2-bromoergocryptine; 2-bromo-α-ergokryptin; CB-154. $C_{32}H_{40}BrN_5O_5$; mol wt 654.59. C 58.71%, H 6.16%, Br 12.21%, N 10.70%, O 12.22%. Dopamine receptor agonist; derivative of the ergotoxin group of ergot alkaloids. Prepn: E. Flückiger *et al., DE 1926045; eidem, US 3752814* (1969, 1973 both to Sandoz). Pharmacology: E. Flückiger, H. R. Wagner, *Experientia* **24,** 1130 (1968); E. Del Pozo *et al., Schweiz. Med. Wochenschr.* **103,** 847 (1973). Relationship of stereochemistry and biological activity: H. P. Weber, *Adv. Biochem. Psychopharmacol.* **23,** 25 (1980); N. Camerman, A. Camerman, *Mol. Pharmacol.* **19,** 517 (1981). Long term clinical trial in Parkinson's disease: T. Nakanishi *et al., Eur. Neurol.* **32,** Suppl. 1, 9 (1992). Clinical effect on body weight and glucose tolerance in obesity: A. H. Cincotta, A. H. Meier, *Diabetes Care* **19,** 667 (1996). Comprehensive description: D. A. Giron-Forest, W. D. Schönleber, *Anal. Profiles Drug Subs.* **8,** 47-81 (1979). Review of pharmacology, toxicology and therapeutic uses: D. Parkes, *Adv. Drug Res.* **12,** 247-344 (1977); of therapeutic applications in endocrine and neurological diseases: K. Y. Ho, M. O. Thorner, *Drugs* **36,** 67-82 (1988).

Crystals from methyl ethyl ketone-isopropyl ether, mp 215-218° (dec). $[\alpha]_D^{20}$ −195° (c = 1 in methylene chloride).

Methanesulfonate. [22260-51-1] CB-154 mesylate; Parlodel; Pravidel. $C_{32}H_{40}BrN_5O_5.CH_3SO_3H$; mol wt 750.70. Crystals from methyl ethyl ketone, mp 192-196° (dec). $[\alpha]_D^{20}$ +95° (c = 1 in methanol-methylene chloride). Soly at 25° (mg/ml): methanol 910; ethanol 23.0; water 0.8; chloroform 0.45; benzene <0.1; hexane <0.1. pKa 4.90. LD_{50} in mice, rats, rabbits (mg/kg): 190, 72, 12.5 i.v. (Parkes).

THERAP CAT: Prolactin inhibitor; antiparkinsonian.

1417. Bromodichloromethane. [75-27-4] Dichlorobromomethane; BDCM; NCI-C55243. $CHBrCl_2$; mol wt 163.83. C 7.33%, H 0.62%, Br 48.77%, Cl 43.28%. Trihalomethane contaminant found in chlorinated water. Prepn: O. Jacobsen, R. Neumeister, *Ber.* **15,** 599 (1882); M. Fedorynski *et al., Synth. Commun.* **7,** 287 (1977). Disposition and metabolism: J. M. Mathews *et al.,*

Consult the Name Index before using this section.

J. Toxicol. Environ. Health **30**, 15 (1990). Toxicity studies: F. J. Bowman *et al., Toxicol. Appl. Pharmacol.* **44**, 213 (1978); Y. Aida *et al., J. Toxicol. Sci.* **17**, 51 (1992). Review of quantitative analyses, toxicity and carcinogenicity: *IARC Monographs* **52**, 179-212 (1991); of toxicology and human exposure: *Toxicological Profile for Bromodichloromethane* (PB90-167461, 1989) 89 pp.

Colorless liquid. bp 88.4-88.6° (Fedorynski); also reported as bp 91-92° (Jacobsen). d^{15} 1.9254. n_D^{20} 1.4967. LD$_{50}$ in male, female mice (mg/kg): 450, 900 orally (Bowman).

Caution: Potential symptoms of acute oral overexposure in animals are liver and kidney damage; CNS depression, incoordination, sleepiness, lethargy, sedation. Chronic exposure has been associated with cancer of liver, kidney and intestines. *See: Toxicological Profile for Bromodichloromethane* (PB90-167461, 1989) 77 pp. This substance is reasonably anticipated to be a human carcinogen: *Report on Carcinogens, Eleventh Edition* (PB2005-104914, 2004) p III-35.

USE: Chemical reagent, intermediate in organic synthesis.

1418. Bromodiphenhydramine. [118-23-0] 2-[(4-Bromophenyl)phenylmethoxy]-*N,N*-dimethylethanamine; 2-(*p*-bromo-α-phenylbenzyloxy)-*N,N*-dimethylethylamine; β-(*p*-bromobenzhydryloxy)ethyldimethylamine; β-dimethylaminoethyl *p*-bromobenzhydryl ether; bromdiphenhydramine; bromazine; bromanautine; Bromo-Benadryl; Deserol; Histabromamine. $C_{17}H_{20}BrNO$; mol wt 334.25. C 61.09%, H 6.03%, Br 23.91%, N 4.19%, O 4.79%. Prepn: Rieveschl, **US 2527963** (1950 to Parke, Davis).

Hydrochloride. [1808-12-4] Ambodryl. $C_{17}H_{20}BrNO.HCl$; mol wt 370.71. Crystals from isopropanol, mp 144-145°.

THERAP CAT: Antihistaminic.

1419. Bromofenofos. [21466-07-9] 3,3',5,5'-Tetrabromo-(1,1'-biphenyl)-2,2'-diolmono(dihydrogenphosphate);3,3',5,5'-tetrabromo-2,2'-biphenyldiol mono(dihydrogen phosphate); 4,4',6,6'-tetrabromobiphenyl-2,2'-diol mono(dihydrogen phosphate); bromophenophos; bromphenphos; PH-1882; Acedist. $C_{12}H_7Br_4O_5P$; mol wt 581.77. C 24.77%, H 1.21%, Br 54.94%, O 13.75%, P 5.32%. Prepn: **NL 6505635**; S. Van der Meer *et al.,* **US 3662035** (1966, 1972 both to Chemiefarma); S. Van der Meer, H. Pouwels, *J. Med. Chem.* **12**, 534 (1969). Activity: J. Guilhon *et al., Bull. Acad. Vet. Fr.* **43**, 67 (1970). Toxicology: J. M. Poul, M. Dagorn, *Recl. Med. Vet.* **158**, 363 (1982).

Cryst, no mp, dec >350°.

THERAP CAT (VET): Anthelmintic (Trematodes).

1420. Bromoform. [75-25-2] Tribromomethane. $CHBr_3$; mol wt 252.73. C 4.75%, H 0.40%, Br 94.85%. Prepd from acetone and sodium hypobromite: Günther, *Jahresber. Fortschr. Chem.* **1887**, 741 (*Beilstein* **vol. 1**, 68); Kergomard, *Bull. Soc. Chim. Fr.* **1961**, 2360. Toxicity data: Kutob, Plaa, *Toxicol. Appl. Pharmacol.* **4**, 354 (1962). Review of toxicology and human exposure: *Toxicological Profile for Bromoform and Dibromochloromethane* (PB2006-100001, 2005) 273 pp.

Heavy liquid; chloroform odor; sweetish taste. bp 149-150°. mp 7.5°. d_4^{15} 2.9035. n_D^{15} 1.6005. Sol in about 800 parts water; mis-

cible with alc, benzene, chloroform, ether, petr ether, acetone, oils. Gradually dec, acquiring a yellow color; air and light accelerate the decompn. May be preserved by the addition of 3-4% alc. d 2.6-2.7. *Keep in well-closed containers, protected from light. Incompat.* Caustic alkalies. LD$_{50}$ s.c. in mice: 7.2 mmol/kg (Kutob, Plaa).

Caution: Potential symptoms of overexposure are irritation of skin, eyes and respiratory system; CNS depression; liver, kidney damage. *See NIOSH Pocket Guide to Chemical Hazards* (DHHS/NIOSH 97-140, 1997) p 34.

USE: In separating mixtures of minerals.

THERAP CAT: Has been used as sedative, hypnotic; antitussive.

1421. α-Bromoisobutyric Acid. [2052-01-9] 2-Bromo-2-methylpropanoic acid. $C_4H_7BrO_2$; mol wt 167.00. C 28.77%, H 4.22%, Br 47.85%, O 19.16%. $(CH_3)_2CBrCOOH$. Prepd by bromination of isobutyric acid: Markownikow, *Ann.* **153**, 228 (1870); Smissman, *J. Am. Chem. Soc.* **76**, 5805 (1954).

Crystals, mp 48-49°. bp 198-200°, bp$_{20}$ 110-116°. d 1.52. Sparingly sol in cold water; sol in alcohol, ether. Dec by hot water into the hydroxy acid.

1422. α-Bromoisovaleric Acid. [565-74-2] 2-Bromo-3-methylbutanoic acid. $C_5H_9BrO_2$; mol wt 181.03. C 33.17%, H 5.01%, Br 44.14%, O 17.68%. $(CH_3)_2CHCHBrCOOH$. Prepn of *dl*-form: Ley, Popow, *Ann.* **174**, 61 (1874); Smissman, *J. Am. Chem. Soc.* **76**, 5805 (1954); Marvel, *Org. Synth.* **coll. vol. III**, 848 (1955). Prepn of *d*- and *l*-forms: Berlingozzi, Furia, *Gazz. Chim. Ital.* **56**, 82 (1926); Berlingozzi, Lenoci, *ibid.* **68**, 721 (1938). Configuration of *d*-form: Brewster *et al., Nature* **166**, 179 (1950).

dl-**Form.** Prisms from ether or chloroform, mp 44°. bp ~230° with some decomp. Sparingly sol in water; sol in alcohol, ether.

d-**Form.** Crystals from petroleum ether, mp 43-44°. $[\alpha]_D^{20}$ +22.6° (c = 4 in benzene).

l-**Form.** Crystals from petroleum ether, mp 43-44°. $[\alpha]_D^{20}$ −22.4° (c = 4 in benzene).

1423. Bromolysergide. [478-84-2] (8β)-2-Bromo-9,10-didehydro-*N,N*-diethyl-6-methylergoline-8-carboxamide; D-2-bromolysergic acid diethylamide; 2-bromo-*N,N*-diethyl-D-lysergamide; bromo-LSD; BOL-148. $C_{20}H_{24}BrN_3O$; mol wt 402.33. C 59.71%, H 6.01%, Br 19.86%, N 10.44%, O 3.98%. Prepd by bromination of lysergide, *q.v.*: Troxler, Hofmann, *Helv. Chim. Acta* **40**, 2160 (1957). Serotonin antagonist without the hallucinogenic activity of LSD: J. P. Bennett, S. H. Snyder, *Brain Res.* **94**, 523 (1975).

Needles from ether, mp 120-127°. $[\alpha]_D^{20}$ +15° (c = 0.5 in pyridine); $[\alpha]_D^{20}$ +53° (c = 0.5 in chloroform). uv max: 240, 301 nm (log ε 4.28, 3.95).

1424. *p*-Bromomandelic Acid. [6940-50-7] 4-Bromo-α-hydroxybenzeneacetic acid; *p*-bromophenylglycolic acid. $C_8H_7BrO_3$; mol wt 231.04. C 41.59%, H 3.05%, Br 34.58%, O 20.77%. Prepd by condensing bromobenzene with ethyl oxomalonate in presence of boron trifluoride: Riebsomer *et al., J. Am. Chem. Soc.* **60**, 2974 (1938).

Crystals, mp 117-118°. Slightly sol in water.
Zirconium salt. Soly in water at 25°: 0.0446 g/l.
USE: Analytical reagent for zirconium.

1425.   1-Bromonaphthalene. [90-11-9] α-Bromonaphthalene. $C_{10}H_7Br$; mol wt 207.07. C 58.00%, H 3.41%, Br 38.59%. Prepd by dropping bromine into a mixture of naphthalene and carbon tetrachloride, distilling the CCl_4, heating the residue with NaOH, and fractionating the liquid under reduced pressure: Clarke, Schram, *Org. Synth.* **1**, 35 (1921); Clarke, Brethen, *ibid.* **coll. vol. I**, 121 (2nd ed., 1941). Also prepd by heating naphthalene (liquid or gaseous) with bromine; 2-bromonaphthalene also being produced, esp with increasing temps: Wibaut, *Chem. Weekbl.* **39**, 326, 328 (1942); Suyver, Wibaut, *Rec. Trav. Chim.* **64**, 65 (1945).

Oily liquid at room temp. More pungent odor than naphthalene. d_4^{20} 1.4834; d_4^{25} 1.4785; d_4^{30} 1.4732. When solid it exists in two forms: mp 0.2-0.7° and mp 6.2°. Darkens on standing when distilled at 760 mm, but remains colorless when distilled at 16 mm. Volatile with steam. bp_{760} 281.1°; bp_{400} 252.0°; bp_{200} 224.2°; bp_{100} 198.8°; bp_{60} 183.5°; bp_{40} 170.2°; bp_{20} 150.2°; bp_{10} 133.6°; bp_5 117.5°; $bp_{1.0}$ 84.2°. $n_D^{16.5}$ 1.66011. Slightly sol in water; miscible with alcohol, ether, benzene, chloroform. Absorption spectrum: DeLaszlo, *Proc. R. Soc. London Ser. A* **111**, 356 (1926).
Compd with 1,3,5-trinitrobenzene. $C_{10}H_7Br.C_6H_3N_3O_6$. Lemon-yellow needles, mp 137°.
USE: Immersion fluid in the determination of the refractive index of crystals. For the determination of water in alc by the cloud point method. For refractometric fat determinations. Mixed with polymerized castor oil as a general immersion oil in microscopy.

1426. 2-Bromonaphthalene. [580-13-2] β-Bromonaphthalene. $C_{10}H_7Br$; mol wt 207.07. C 58.00%, H 3.41%, Br 38.59%. Prepn: Liebermann, Palm, *Ann.* **183**, 267 (1876); Vingiello *et al.*, *J. Chem. Educ.* **40**, 544 (1963).

Crystals from alcohol, mp 59°; also reported as mp 54-56° (Vingiello *et al.*, *loc. cit.*). bp 281-282°, $bp_{4.5}$ 122-127°. d 1.60. Slightly sol in water; sol in 8 parts alcohol; very sol in ether, chloroform, benzene.

1427. p-Bromophenacyl Bromide. [99-73-0] 2-Bromo-1-(4-bromophenyl)ethanone; 2,4'-dibromoacetophenone; *p,α*-dibromoacetophenone. $C_8H_6Br_2O$; mol wt 277.94. C 34.57%, H 2.18%, Br 57.50%, O 5.76%. Prepd by adding bromine to *p*-bromoacetophenone in glacial acetic acid at below 20°: Langley, *Org. Synth.* **coll. vol. I**, 127 (2nd ed., 1941).

Crystals from ethanol, mp 109-110°. Very sol in warm alcohol.
USE: Identification of carboxylic acids.

1428. Bromophenol. C_6H_5BrO; mol wt 173.01. C 41.65%, H 2.91%, Br 46.18%, O 9.25%. Prepn of *m*-isomer: Wurster, Nölting, *Ber.* **7**, 904 (1874); Carpenter *et al.*, *J. Org. Chem.* **16**, 586 (1951); of *o*- and *p*-isomers: Medola, Streatfield, *J. Chem. Soc.* **73**, 681 (1898); Kaeding, Lindstrom, US 2805263 (1957 to Dow).

m-Bromophenol. [591-20-8] Crystals, mp 33°, also reported as mp 31°. bp 235-236°, bp_3 88-89°. Sol in alcohol, ether, alkalies.
o-Bromophenol. [95-56-7] Yellow to red oily liquid; unpleasant odor. d ~1.5. bp 194°. mp 6°. Sol in water; miscible in chloroform, ether. Fusion with NaOH gives resorcinol.
p-Bromophenol. [106-41-2] Tetragonal bipyramidal crystals from chloroform or ether. mp 64°. bp 238°. d^{15} 1.840; d^{80} 1.5875. Small amounts of water depress the mp considerably and may prevent crystallization. Absorption spectrum: Ley, *Z. Phys. Chem.* **94**, 412 (1920). Soluble in about 7 parts water; freely sol in alc, chloroform, ether, glacial acetic acid.
***p*-Form methyl ether.** *p*-Bromoanisole. C_7H_7BrO. Crystals, mp 9-10°. bp 223°.
***p*-Form ethyl ether.** *p*-Bromophenetole. C_8H_9BrO. Crystals, mp 4°. bp 233°.
USE: *p*-Bromophenol as disinfectant.

1429.   p-Bromophenylhydrazine. [589-21-9] $C_6H_7BrN_2$; mol wt 187.04. C 38.53%, H 3.77%, Br 42.72%, N 14.98%. Prepn from 4-bromophenyldiazonium chloride by modified Fischer phenylhydrazine synthesis: Chattaway, Humphrey, *J. Chem. Soc.* **1927**, 1323.

Needles from water, mp 108-109°. Sol in alcohol, ether, chloroform, benzene; moderately sol in ligroin; slightly sol in water.
USE: In prepn of indoleacetic acid derivatives; in the study of transosazonation of sugar phenylosazones.

1430.   p-Bromophenyl Isocyanate. [2493-02-9] 1-Bromo-4-isocyanatobenzene; 4-bromophenylcarbimide; *p*-bromophenylcarbonimide; *p*-bromocarbanil. C_7H_4BrNO; mol wt 198.02. C 42.46%, H 2.04%, Br 40.35%, N 7.07%, O 8.08%. Prepd by heating phenyl isocyanate dibromide: Curtius, *J. Prakt. Chem.* **87**, 517 (1913); by distilling *p*-bromophenylurethan and P_2O_5: Dennstedt, *Ber.* **13**, 228 (1880).

Needles, pungent odor, mp 42°. bp_{14} 158°. Very sol in ether.
USE: Prepn of bromophenylurea and urethan derivatives.

1431.   Bromophos. [2104-96-3] Phosphorothioic acid O-(4-bromo-2,5-dichlorophenyl) O,O-dimethyl ester; O-(4-bromo-2,5-dichlorophenyl)-O,O-dimethylphosphorothioate; bromophos-methyl; ENT-27162; OMS-658; S-1942; Nexion. $C_8H_8BrCl_2O_3PS$; mol wt 366.00. C 26.25%, H 2.20%, Br 21.83%, Cl 19.37%, O 13.11%, P 8.46%, S 8.76%. Prepn: BE 625198 *C.A.* **60**, 13187a (1964); R. Sehring, K. Zeile, US 3227610, US 3275718 (1963, 1966, 1966 all to Boehringer, Ing.). Metabolism in rats: M. Stiasni *et al.*, *J. Agric. Food Chem.* **15**, 474 (1967). Toxicity study: T. B. Gaines, *Toxicol. Appl. Pharmacol.* **14**, 515 (1969). *Review:* D. Eichler, *Residue Rev.* **41**, 65-112 (1972).

Yellow crystals, mp 53-54°. $bp_{0.01}$ 140-142°. Vapor pressure at 20°C: 1.3×10^{-4} mm Hg. Soly in water at 25°: 40 mg/l. Sol in CCl_4, ether, toluene. Stable in soln up to pH 9. Non-corrosive. LD_{50} in male, female rats (mg/kg): 1600, 1730 orally (Gaines).
O,O-Diethyl analog. Bromophos-ethyl; ENT-27258; OMS-659; S-2225; Nexagan. $C_{10}H_{12}BrCl_2O_3PS$; mol wt 394.05. Colorless to pale yellow oil, $bp_{0.001}$ 122-133°. Vapor pressure at 30°: 4.6×10^{-5} mm Hg. Soly in water at 25°: 2 mg/l.
USE: Insecticide, acaricide.

1432. Bromopride. [4093-35-0] 4-Amino-5-bromo-*N*-[2-(diethylamino)ethyl]-2-methoxybenzamide; 4-amino-5-bromo-*N*-[2-(diethylamino)ethyl]-*o*-anisamide; Emepride; Emoril; Viadil. $C_{14}H_{22}BrN_3O_2$; mol wt 344.25. C 48.85%, H 6.44%, Br 23.21%, N 12.21%, O 9.30%. Prepn: M. L. Thominet, **BE 620543**; *idem*, **US 3177252** (1962, 1965 both to Soc. d'Etudes Sci. Ind. de l'Ile-de-France); H. Mori, K. Shibata, **DE 2119724** (1971 to Teikoku Hormone Manuf. Co.), *C.A.* **76**, 99375e (1972). Action on guinea-pig ileum: J. Fontaine, J. J. Reuse, *Arch. Int. Pharmacodyn. Ther.* **213**, 322 (1975). Effects on intestinal peristalsis in dogs: P. Sava *et al.*, *Arzneim.-Forsch.* **29**, 799 (1979). Clinical study: M. Fischer *et al.*, *Fortschr. Med.* **97**, 883 (1979). Pharmacokinetics: P. W. Lücker *et al.*, *Arzneim.-Forsch.* **33**, 453 (1983).

Hydrochloride. [52423-56-0] Cascapride; Plesium; Praiden; Valopride; Viaben. $C_{14}H_{22}BrN_3O_2$.HCl; mol wt 380.71.

Dihydrochloride monohydrate. Opridan. $C_{14}H_{22}BrN_3O_2$.2-HCl.H_2O; mol wt 435.18.

THERAP CAT: Antiemetic.

1433. β-Bromopropionic Acid. [590-92-1] 3-Bromopropanoic acid. $C_3H_5BrO_2$; mol wt 152.97. C 23.56%, H 3.29%, Br 52.24%, O 20.92%. BrCH₂CH₂COOH. Prepd by the action of hydrobromic acid on acrylic acid, on hydracrylic acid, and on ethylene cyanohydrin: Kendall, McKenzie, *Org. Synth.* **3**, 25 (1923). Prepn of the ethyl ester: *eidem, ibid.* 51; of the methyl ester: Mozingo, Patterson, *ibid.* **20**, 64 (1940).

Plates from CCl_4. mp 62.5°. pK (25°): 4.00. Sol in water, alcohol, ether, chloroform, benzene. Aq alkalies hydrolyze β-bromopropionic acid to hydracrylic acid.

Ethyl ester. $C_5H_9BrO_2$. Liquid. Pungent odor. Becomes yellow on exposure to light. d_4^{18} 1.4123. bp_{44} 112°; bp_{12} 70°. n_D^{18} 1.4569. Insol in water; miscible with alchol, ether. *Protect from light.*

Methyl ester. $C_4H_7BrO_2$. Liquid. d^{15} 1.4897. bp_{27} 80°. bp_{18} 65°.

1434. Bromopropylate. [18181-80-1] 4-Bromo-α-(4-bromophenyl)-α-hydroxybenzeneacetic acid 1-methyl ethyl ester; 4,4'-dibromobenzilic acid isopropyl ester; isopropyl 4,4'-dibromobenzilate; phenisobromolate; ENT-27552; GS-19851; Acarol; Folbex VA; Neoron. $C_{17}H_{16}Br_2O_3$; mol wt 428.12. C 47.69%, H 3.77%, Br 37.33%, O 11.21%. Contact acaricide with residual activity. Prepn: **FR 1504969**; K. Gubler, **US 3639446** (1967, 1972 to Geigy). Toxicity data: E. E. Kenaga, W. E. Allison, *Bull. Entomol. Soc. Am.* **15**, 85 (1969). Persistence in soil: W. B. Wheeler *et al.*, *J. Environ. Qual.* **2**, 115 (1973). Control of bee mites: A. Rojahn, *Dtsch. Tieraerztl. Wochenschr.* **92**, 103 (1985). GC determn in honey: L. Torreti, A. Simonella, *J. High Resolut. Chromatogr.* **13**, 142 (1990).

Cryst solid, mp 77°. Vapor pressure at 20°: 5.1 × 10^{-8} mm Hg. Soly in water at 20°: <5 mg/l. Readily sol in most organic solvents. LD_{50} orally in rats: 5000 mg/kg (Kenaga, Allison).

USE: Acaricide.

1435. Bromosalicylchloranilide. [3679-64-9] 5-Bromo-*N*-(4-chlorophenyl)-2-hydroxybenzamide; 5-bromo-4'-chlorosalicylanilide; *N*-5-bromosalicyloyl-*p*-chloroaniline; Multifungin. $C_{13}H_9BrClNO_2$; mol wt 326.57. C 47.81%, H 2.78%, Br

24.47%, Cl 10.86%, N 4.29%, O 9.80%. Prepn: Schuler, **US 2802029** (1957 to Knoll); Lemaire *et al., J. Pharm. Soc.* **50**, 831 (1961).

Crystals, mp 238-243°.

THERAP CAT: Antifungal.

1436. 5-Bromosalicylhydroxamic Acid. [5798-94-7] 5-Bromo-*N*,2-dihydroxybenzamide; Brosalamid; Bromocyl. $C_7H_6BrNO_3$; mol wt 232.03. C 36.23%, H 2.61%, Br 34.44%, N 6.04%, O 20.69%. Prepd by direct bromination of salicylhydroxamic acid in acetic acid: Urbanski *et al., Nature* **170**, 753 (1952); *Bull. Acad. Pol. Sci. Cl. 3* **1**, 319 (1953); Hornung, Krakowska, *Gruzlica* **20**, 469 (1952).

Crystals from alcohol, dec 232°. Very sparingly sol in water. Forms a water-soluble sodium salt.

THERAP CAT: Antibacterial (tuberculostatic).

1437. Bromosuccinic Acid. [923-06-8] Bromobutanedioic acid; monobromosuccinic acid. $C_4H_5BrO_4$; mol wt 196.98. C 24.39%, H 2.56%, Br 40.56%, O 32.49%. HOOCCH₂CHBr-COOH. Prepn of *dl*-form by bromination of succinic acid: Kekulé, *Ann.* **117**, 120 (1861); from fumaric acid and HBr: Fittig, *Ann.* **188**, 42 (1877); by bromination of succinyl bromide or succinic anhydride: Hughes, Watson, *J. Chem. Soc.* **1930**, 1733. Prepn of *l*-form from *l*-aspartic acid: Walden, *Ber.* **29**, 133 (1896); Karrer *et al., Helv. Chim. Acta* **30**, 271 (1947).

dl-Form. Crystals, mp 161°. d 2.07. Soluble in 5.5 parts water; sol in alc.

d-Form. Crystals, mp 172°. $[\alpha]_D^{15}$ +41.9° (c = 5); $[\alpha]_D^{20}$ +67.9° (ether). *Ref:* Levene, Mikeska, *J. Biol. Chem.* **55**, 795 (1923); Clough, *J. Chem. Soc.* **129**, 1674 (1926).

l-Form. Crystals, dec 177-178°. $[\alpha]_D$ −43.8° (c = 6), −65.0° (c = 6 in abs alc), −73.5° (c = 6 in acetone).

1438. *N*-Bromosuccinimide. [128-08-5] 1-Bromo-2,5-pyrrolidinedione; succinbromimide; NBS. $C_4H_4BrNO_2$; mol wt 177.98. C 26.99%, H 2.27%, Br 44.89%, N 7.87%, O 17.98%. Prepn: K. Ziegler *et al., Ann.* **551**, 109 (1942). In bromination of olefins: *eidem, ibid.* 80. The method has been extended to other classes of compds by the use of catalysts: H. Schmid, P. Karrer, *Helv. Chim. Acta* **29**, 573 (1946); H. Schmid, *ibid.* 1144. In oxidation of aldehydes: Y. F. Cheung, *Tetrahedron Lett.* **1979**, 3809. Review of uses: C. Djerassi, *Chem. Rev.* **43**, 271-317 (1948); R. Filler, *ibid.* **63**, 21-43 (1963); J. S. Pizey, *Synthetic Reagents* **vol. 2** (John Wiley, New York, 1974) pp 1-63.

Orthorhombic bisphenoidal crystals, mp 173-175° (slight decompn). Faint odor of bromine. d 2.098. Soly (g/100 g of solvent at 25°): water 1.47; *tert*-butanol 0.73; acetone 14.40; carbon tetrachloride 0.02; hexane 0.006; glacial acetic acid 3.10.

Caution: Highly irritating to eyes, skin, mucous membranes.

USE: In bromination of olefins; in oxidation of alcohols to aldehydes and ketones and of aldehydes to acid bromides.

1439. Bromotoluene. C_7H_7Br; mol wt 171.03. C 49.16%, H 4.13%, Br 46.72%. Prepn of *o*-isomer: Bourgeois, *Ber.* **28**, 2312 (1895). Prepn of *m*-isomer: Acree, *Ber.* **37**, 994 (1904). Kohn, Bum, *Monatsh. Chem.* **33**, 924 (1912); Feitler, *Z. Phys. Chem.* **4**, 77

(1889). Prepn of *m*-, *o*- and *p*-isomers: Bigelow *et al., Org. Synth.* **coll. vol. I** (2nd ed., 1941) pp 133, 135, 136 resp. Isomerization of *p*-isomer yields mixture of monobromotoluenes containing 48.2% of *o*-isomer: Crump, **US 3077503** (1963 to Dow). Separation of *o*- and *p*-isomers by clathration: Coscia, **US 3114784** (1963 to Am. Cyanamid).

m-**Bromotoluene.** 1-Bromo-3-methylbenzene; 3-bromotoluene; *m*-tolylbromide. Liquid. d_4^{20} 1.4099; d_4^{58} 1.309; d_4^{184} 1.201. mp $-39.8°$. bp_{760} 183.7°; bp_{400} 160°; bp_{200} 138°; bp_{100} 117.8°; bp_{60} 104.1°; bp_{40} 93.9°; bp_{20} 78.1°; bp_{10} 64.0°; bp_5 50.8°; $bp_{1.0}$ 14.8°. n_D^{20} 1.551. Absorption spectrum: Purvis, *J. Chem. Soc.* **99**, 1706, 1710 (1911). Sol in alc, ether, benzene.

o-**Bromotoluene.** Colorless liq. d_{15}^{15} 1.431. bp 181°. mp $-26°$. n_D^{20} 1.555. Practically insol in water; misc with alc, benzene.

p-**Bromotoluene.** Crystals from abs alc. d_{35}^{35} 1.3959; d_{50}^{50} 1.3856; d_{100}^{100} 1.3637; d^{184} 1.1931. mp 28.5°. bp_{760} 184.5°; bp_{100} 116.4°; bp_{60} 102.3°; bp_{40} 91.8°; bp_{20} 75.2°; bp_{10} 61.1°; bp_5 47.5°; $bp_{1.0}$ 10.3°. n_D^{20} 1.5490. Sol in alc, ether, benzene.

Caution: Irritants!

1440. 5-Bromouracil. [51-20-7] 5-Bromo-2,4(1*H*,3*H*)-pyrimidinedione. $C_4H_3BrN_2O_2$; mol wt 190.98. C 25.16%, H 1.58%, Br 41.84%, N 14.67%, O 16.76%. Major chemical mutagen; incorporates into DNA by replacing thymine. Prepn: H. L. Wheeler, H. F. Merriam, *Am. Chem. J.* **29**, 478 (1903); P. A. Levene, F. B. LaForge, *Ber.* **45**, 608 (1912). UV effects on DNA containing 5-bromouracil: A. G. Skavronskaya *et al., Mutat. Res.* **6**, 319 (1968); F. Hutchinson, *Q. Rev. Biophys.* **6**, 201 (1973). Mechanisms of mutagenesis: I. Pietrzykowska, *Mutat. Res.* **19**, 1 (1973); E. M. Witkin, E. C. Parisi, *ibid.* **25**, 407 (1974); B. Rydberg, *Mol. Gen. Genet.* **152**, 19 (1977). Crystal structure and base stacking properties: H. Sternglanz, C. E. Bugg, *Biochim. Biophys. Acta* **378**, 1 (1975).

Prisms from water, mp 293°.
USE: Exptly as mutagen.

1441. Bromoxynil. [1689-84-5] 3,5-Dibromo-4-hydroxybenzonitrile; 3,5-dibromo-4-hydroxyphenyl cyanide; 2,6-dibromo-4-cyanophenol; broxynil; ENT-20852; MB-10064. $C_7H_3Br_2NO$; mol wt 276.91. C 30.36%, H 1.09%, Br 57.71%, N 5.06%, O 5.78%. Selective contact herbicide. Prepn: K. Auwers, J. Reis, *Ber.* **29**, 2359 (1896); E. Müller *et al., Ber.* **92**, 2278 (1959); K. Carpenter *et al., Weed Res.* **4**, 175 (1964); **FR 1375311** (1964 to May & Baker), *C.A.* **62**, 3982h (1965). Herbicidal activity: K. Carpenter, B. J. Heywood, *Nature* **200**, 28 (1963). HPLC analysis: J. C. Van Damme, M. Galoux, *J. Chromatogr.* **190**, 401 (1980). Persistence in soil: A. E. Smith, *Pestic. Sci.* **11**, 341 (1980).

Colorless solid, mp 194-195°. pKa 4.06. Subl at 135° (0.15 mm Hg). Slightly volatile in steam. Soly in (g/l) at 25°: water 0.13; methanol 90; acetone 170; tetrahydrofuran 410. LD50 orally in mice: 111 mg/kg (Carpenter, 1964).

Octanoate. [1689-99-2] MB-10731; NPH-1320; RP-16272; Brominal; Buctril. $C_{15}H_{17}Br_2NO_2$; mol wt 403.11. Waxy solid, mp 45-46°. Low volatility; subl at 90° (0.1 mm Hg). Insol in water.
USE: Herbicide.

1442. Bromperidol. [10457-90-6] 4-[4-(4-Bromophenyl)-4-hydroxy-1-piperidinyl]-1-(4-fluorophenyl)-1-butanone; 4-[4-(*p*-bromophenyl)-4-hydroxypiperidino]-4′-fluorobutyrophenone; R-11333; Azurene; Impromen; Tesoprel. $C_{21}H_{23}BrFNO_2$; mol wt 420.32. C 60.01%, H 5.52%, Br 19.01%, F 4.52%, N 3.33%, O 7.61%. Bromine analog of haloperidol, *q.v.* Prepn (no data): P. A. J. Janssen, **GB 895309**; *idem*, **US 3438991** (1962, 1969 both to Janssen); C. J. E. Niemegeers, P. A. J. Janssen, *Arzneim.-Forsch.* **24**, 45 (1974). Prepn of ^{82}Br bromperidol and preliminary tissue distribution studies: S. H. Vincent *et al., J. Med. Chem.* **23**, 75 (1980). Pharmacological study: C. J. E. Niemegeers, P. A. J. Janssen, *Life Sci.* **24**, 2201 (1979). Preliminary clinical study: B. Woggon *et al., Int. Pharmacopsychiatry* **14**, 213 (1979). Radioimmunoassay: E. Van Den Eeckhout *et al., Eur. J. Drug Metab. Pharmacokinet.* **5**, 45 (1980).

Off-white amorphous or microcrystalline powder, mp 155-158°. uv max: 245 nm. pKa 8.6-8.7. Soly in water: 0.09 mg/ml; in 0.1*M* tartaric, lactic, citric and acetic acids: greater than or equal to 10 mg/ml.
THERAP CAT: Antipsychotic.

1443. Brompheniramine. [86-22-6] γ-(4-Bromophenyl)-*N*,*N*-dimethyl-2-pyridinepropanamine; 2-[*p*-bromo-α-(2-dimethylaminoethyl)benzyl]pyridine; 1-(*p*-bromophenyl)-1-(2-pyridyl)-3-dimethylaminopropane; 3-(*p*-bromophenyl)-3-(2-pyridyl)-*N*,*N*-dimethylpropylamine; parabromdylamine. $C_{16}H_{19}BrN_2$; mol wt 319.24. C 60.20%, H 6.00%, Br 25.03%, N 8.78%. Prepn from α-(*p*-bromophenyl)-α-(β-dimethylaminoethyl)-2-pyridylacetonitrile: Sperber *et al.*, **US 2567245** (1951); **US 2676964** (1954 to Schering). Prepn of *d*-form: L. A. Walter, **US 3061517** (1962 to Schering).

Oily liquid. Slightly yellow color. Characteristic amine-like odor. $bp_{0.5}$ 147-152°. Soluble in dilute acids.

Maleate. [980-71-2] Dimegan; Dimetane; Dimotane; Ilvin; Nagemid; Symptom 3; Veltane. $C_{16}H_{19}BrN_2 \cdot C_4H_4O_4$; mol wt 435.31. Crystals, mp 132-134°. Sol in water, somewhat less sol in alcohol. pH of a 2% aq soln about 5.

d-**Form.** [132-21-8] Dexbrompheniramine; (+)-parabromdylamine. Oily liquid. $[\alpha]_D^{25}$ +42.7° (c = 1 in DMF).

d-**Form maleate.** [2391-03-9] Disomer; Ebalin. $C_{16}H_{19}BrN_2 \cdot C_4H_4O_4$; mol wt 435.31. Crystals, mp 103-113°.
THERAP CAT: Antihistaminic.

1444. Bromphenol Blue. [115-39-9] 4,4′-(3*H*-2,1-Benzoxathiol-3-ylidene)bis[2,6-dibromophenol] *S,S*-dioxide; α,α-bis(3,5-dibromo-4-hydroxyphenyl)-α-hydroxy-*o*-toluenesulfonic acid γ-sultone; 3,3′,5,5′-tetrabromophenolsulfonphthalein; Albutest. $C_{19}H_{10}Br_4O_5S$; mol wt 669.96. C 34.06%, H 1.50%, Br 47.71%, O 11.94%, S 4.79%. Prepd by slow addition of excess bromine to a hot soln of phenolsulfonphthalein in glacial acetic acid: White, Acree, *J. Am. Chem. Soc.* **41**, 1205 (1919); Orndorff, Sherwood, *ibid.* **45**, 495 (1923). *See also* ref given *under* Bromcresol Green.

Elongated hexagonal prisms from acetic acid + acetone. Dec 279°. (An orange discoloration with formation of a green sublimate sets in at 210°). Soluble in water (about 0.4 g/100 ml); more sol in methyl and ethyl alcohol, and in benzene. Freely sol in NaOH solns with the formation of a water-sol sodium salt. pK = 4.0. To prepare a soln for use as pH indicator, dissolve 0.10 g in 7.45 ml *N*/50 NaOH and dil with water to 250 ml.

USE: As indicator, pH 3.0 yellow; pH 4.6 purple.

1445. Bromthymol Blue. [76-59-5] 4,4′-(3*H*-2,1-Benzoxathiol-3-ylidene)bis[2-bromo-3-methyl-6-(1-methylethyl)phenol] *S,S*-dioxide; α,α-bis(6-bromo-5-hydroxycarvacryl)-α-hydroxy-*o*-toluenesulfonic acid γ-sultone; 3,3′-dibromothymolsulfonphthalein. $C_{27}H_{28}Br_2O_5S$; mol wt 624.38. C 51.94%, H 4.52%, Br 25.59%, O 12.81%, S 5.14%. Prepd by the action of bromine on thymol blue in glacial acetic acid: Clark, Lubs, *J. Wash. Acad. Sci.* **5**, 609 (1915); **6**, 482 (1916); *Chem. Zentralbl.* **1916, I,** 175; **II,** 1068. *See also* ref *under* Bromcresol Green.

Cream-colored crystals. Sparingly sol in water; sol in alcohol and in aq solns of alkalies. Also sol in ether. Less sol in benzene, toluene, xylene. Practically insol in petr ether. pK = 7.0. To prepare a soln for use as pH indicator, dissolve 0.10 g in 8.0 ml *N*/50 NaOH and dil with water to 250 ml. To prepare a soln for use as indicator in volumetric work, dissolve 0.1 g in 100 ml of 50% alc.

USE: As indicator, pH 6.0 yellow; pH 7.6 blue.

1446. Bromuconazole. [116255-48-2] 1-[[4-Bromo-2-(2,4-dichlorophenyl)tetrahydro-2-furanyl]methyl]-1*H*-1,2,4-triazole; 1-[(2*RS*,4*RS*;2*RS*,4*SR*)-4-bromo-2-(2,4-dichlorophenyl)tetrahydrofurfuryl]-1*H*-1,2,4-triazole; LS-860263; Granit. $C_{13}H_{12}BrCl_2N_3O$; mol wt 377.06. C 41.41%, H 3.21%, Br 21.19%, Cl 18.80%, N 11.14%, O 4.24%. Ergosterol biosynthesis inhibiting triazole. Prepn: A. Greiner, R. Pepin, **EP 258161** (1988 to Rhone Poulenc), *C.A.* **109**, 110440v (1988). Properties and antifungal activity: R. Pepin *et al., Brighton Crop Prot. Conf. - Pests Dis.* **1990**, 439. Effect on fungus ultrastructure: M. Mangin-Peyrard, R. Pepin, *Z. Pflanzenkrankh. Pflanzenschutz* **103**, 142 (1996). Determn by TLC in water: S. Butz, H.-J. Stan, *Anal. Chem.* **67**, 620 (1995); by GC with atomic emission detection in foodstuffs: H.-J. Stan, M. Linkerhägner, *J. Chromatogr. A* **750**, 369 (1996). Field trials in combination with iprodione, *q.v.*: P. Duvert *et al., Agro-Food-Ind. Hi-Tech* **7**, 34 (1996); in combination with prochloraz, *q.v.*: *eidem, Phytoma* **490**, 32 (1997).

White to off-white odorless powder, mp 84°. Moderate to high soly in organic solvents; soly in water 50 mg/l. Vapor pressure (25°): 0.3×10^{-7} mm Hg. LD$_{50}$ orally in rats, mice: 365, 1151 mg/kg; LD$_{50}$ dermally in rats: >2000 mg/kg; LD$_{50}$ by inhalation in rabbits: >5 mg/l; LC$_{50}$(96 hr) in rainbow trout, bluegill sunfish (mg/l): 1.7, 3.1 (Pepin).

USE: Agricultural fungicide.

1447. Bronopol. [52-51-7] 2-Bromo-2-nitro-1,3-propanediol; β-bromo-β-nitrotrimethyleneglycol; Bronosol. $C_3H_6BrNO_4$; mol wt 199.99. C 18.02%, H 3.02%, Br 39.95%, N 7.00%, O 32.00%. HOCH$_2$CBr(NO$_2$)CH$_2$OH. Prepn: E. Schmidt, R. Wilkendorf, *Ber.* **52**, 389 (1919); R. Wessendorf, **DE 1804068**; *idem*, **DE 1954173**; *idem*, **US 3658921**; *idem*, **US 3711561** (1970, 1971, 1972, 1973 all to Henkel & Cie). Antibacterial, antifungal and toxic properties: Z. Eckstein *et al., Bull. Acad. Pol. Sci. Ser. Sci. Chim.* **11**, 687 (1963); B. Croshaw *et al., J. Pharm. Pharmacol.* **16** (Suppl), 127T (1964); N. G. Clark *et al.*, **GB 1057131**; *eidem*, **US 3558788** (1967, 1971 both to Boots); R. J. Stretton, T. W. Mason, *J. Appl. Bacteriol.* **36**, 61 (1973). Biotransformation and distribution in rats: H. S. Buttar, R. H. Downie, *Toxicol. Lett.* **6**, 101 (1980). As a nitrosating agent for diethanolamine: I. Schmeltz, A. Wenger, *Food Cosmet. Toxicol.* **17**, 105 (1979); R. L. Elder, *J. Environ. Pathol. Toxicol.* **4**, 47 (1980). Review of bronopol and other preservatives: B. Croshaw, *J. Soc. Cosmet. Chem.* **28**, 3-16 (1977).

Odorless crystals from ethyl acetate-chloroform, mp 120-122°. Sol in water, alcohol, ethyl acetate. Slightly sol in chloroform, acetone, ether, benzene. Insol in ligroin. LD$_{50}$ in mice, rats (mg/kg): 350, 400 orally (Croshaw).

USE: Preservative in cosmetics and toiletries. Antiseptic.

1448. Broparoestrol. [479-68-5] 1-(2-Bromo-1,2-diphenylethenyl)-4-ethylbenzene; 1-bromo-2-(*p*-ethylphenyl)-1,2-diphenylethylene; 1-bromo-2-(4-ethylphenyl)-1,2-diphenylethene; α-bromo-α,β-diphenyl-β-(*p*-ethylphenyl)ethylene; 1-(*p*-ethylphenyl)-1,2-diphenyl-2-bromoethylene; B.D.P.E.; LN-107; Acnestrol; Longestrol. $C_{22}H_{19}Br$; mol wt 363.29. C 72.73%, H 5.27%, Br 21.99%. Prepn: Dvolaitsky, Jacques, *Bull. Soc. Chim. Biol.* **40**, 939 (1958).

cis - form

***cis-trans* Mixture.** Crystals, mp 89°. (Isomer A, needles from ethanol, mp 112-113.5°; isomer B, mp 111.5-112°). The commercial medicinal product is the *cis-trans* mixture. Soluble in ether, benzene, chloroform; less sol in ethanol.

THERAP CAT: Estrogen. Used in dermatology.

1449. Brostallicin. [203258-60-0] *N*-[5-[[[5-[[[2-[(Amino-iminomethyl)amino]ethyl]amino]carbonyl]-1-methyl-1*H*-pyrrol-3-yl]amino]carbonyl]-1-methyl-1*H*-pyrrol-3-yl]-4-[[[4-[(2-bromo-1-oxo-2-propenyl)amino]-1-methyl-1*H*-pyrrol-2-yl]carbonyl]amino]-1-methyl-1*H*-pyrrole-2-carboxamide. $C_{30}H_{35}BrN_{12}O_5$; mol wt 723.58. C 49.80%, H 4.88%, Br 11.04%, N 23.23%, O 11.06%. DNA minor groove binder; bromoacryloyl derivative of distamycin A, *q.v.* Prepn: P. Cozzi *et al.*, **WO 9804524**; *eidem*, **US 6482920** (1998, 2002 both to Pharmacia & Upjohn). LC/MS/MS determn in plasma: S. Calderoli *et al., J. Pharm. Biomed. Anal.* **32**, 601 (2003). Mechanism of action studies: C. Geroni *et al., Cancer Res.* **62**, 2332 (2002); A. Fedier *et al., Br. J. Cancer* **89**, 1559 (2003). Clinical pharmacokinetics and evaluation in advanced solid tumors: A. J. ten Tije *et al., Clin. Cancer Res.* **9**, 2957 (2003); A. C. Lockhart *et al., ibid.* **10**, 468 (2004). Review of clinical development: M. Broggini *et al., Anti-Cancer Drugs* **15**, 1-6 (2004).

Hydrochloride. [203258-38-2] PNU-166196. $C_{30}H_{35}BrN_{12}$-O_5.HCl; mol wt 760.04. Yellow solid. uv max (95% ethanol): 312.0 nm (ε 48792).

THERAP CAT: Antineoplastic.

1450. Brotizolam. [57801-81-7] 2-Bromo-4-(2-chlorophenyl)-9-methyl-6H-thieno[3,2-f][1,2,4]triazolo[4,3-a][1,4]diazepine; 2-bromo-4-(o-chlorophenyl)-9-methyl-6H-thieno[3,2-f]-s-triazolo[4,3-a][1,4]diazepine; 8-bromo-6-(o-chlorophenyl)-1-methyl-4H-s-triazolo[3,4-c]thieno[2,3-e]-1,4-diazepine; WE-941-BS; Lendorm; Lendormin; Mederantil; Nimbisan; Sintonal. C_{15}-$H_{10}BrClN_4S$; mol wt 393.69. C 45.76%, H 2.56%, Br 20.30%, Cl 9.01%, N 14.23%, S 8.14%. One of a class of triazolo-1,4-thienodiazepines having psychotropic activity. Prepn: K. H. Weber *et al.*, **DE 2410030**; *eidem*, **US 4094984** (1975, 1978 to Boehringer, Ing.); *eidem*, *Ann.* **8**, 1257 (1978). Pharmacodynamics: J. Gruenberger *et al.*, *Curr. Ther. Res.* **24**, 427 (1978). Bioavailability: B. Saletu *et al.*, *Arzneim.-Forsch.* **29**, 700 (1979). Pharmaco-EEG study: M. Fink, P. Irwin, *Clin. Pharmacol. Ther.* **30**, 319 (1981). Toxicity studies: C. Hewett *et al.*, *Arzneim.-Forsch.* **36**, 592 (1986). Series of articles on pharmacology, pharmacokinetics, toxicology: *ibid.* 517-620. Veterinary trial as appetite stimulant: A. van Miert *et al.*, *J. Vet. Pharmacol. Ther.* **12**, 147 (1989). Review of pharmacology and clinical efficacy: M. S. Langley, S. P. Clissold, *Drugs* **35**, 104-122 (1988).

Colorless crystals from ethanol, mp 212-214°. LD_{50} in mice, rats (mg/kg): >10000, >10000 orally; 920, 1000 i.p. (Hewett).

THERAP CAT: Sedative, hypnotic.

THERAP CAT (VET): Appetite stimulant.

1451. Brovincamine. [57475-17-9] (3α,14β,16α)-11-Bromo-14,15-dihydro-14-hydroxyeburnamenine-14-carboxylic acid methyl ester; *cis*-11-bromovincamine. $C_{21}H_{25}BrN_2O_3$; mol wt 433.34. C 58.20%, H 5.81%, Br 18.44%, N 6.46%, O 11.08%. Cerebrovascular agent, vincamine deriv. Prepn: P. Pfaeffli, **DE 2458164**; *idem*, **US 4146643** (1975, 1979 both to Sandoz). HPLC determn in plasma: R. R. Brodie, L. F. Chasseaud, *J. Chromatogr.* **228**, 413 (1982). Effect on autonomic nervous system in laboratory animals: K. Kushiku *et al.*, *J. Pharmacobio-Dyn.* **7**, 177 (1984). Cardiovascular effects, mechanistic studies: *eidem*, *Clin. Exp. Pharmacol. Physiol.* **12**, 121 (1985). Mode of action studies: T. Katsuragi *et al.*, *Gen. Pharmacol.* **15**, 43 (1984). Clinical trials in patients with multi-infarct dementia: S. Hagstadius *et al.*, *Psychopharmacology* **83**, 321 (1984).

Crystals from isopropanol, mp 214° (dec). $[\alpha]_D^{20}$ +8.7° (1% in CHCl$_3$).

Hydrogen fumarate. [84964-12-5] BV-26-723; Sabromin; Zabromin. $C_{21}H_{25}BrN_2O_3$.$C_4H_4O_4$; mol wt 549.41. mp 144°. $[\alpha]_D^{20}$ +4.7° (0.388% in H$_2$O).

THERAP CAT: Vasodilator (peripheral).

1452. Broxuridine. [59-14-3] 5-Bromo-2'-deoxyuridine; 5-bromouracil deoxyriboside; BrdUrd; BUdR; NSC-38297; Broxine; Neomark; Radibud. $C_9H_{11}BrN_2O_5$; mol wt 307.10. C 35.20%, H 3.61%, Br 26.02%, N 9.12%, O 26.05%. Thymidine, *q.v.*, analog. Preferentially incorporated into cellular DNA in place of thymidine during replication causing increased radiosensitivity of the cell. Prepn and inhibition of DNA biosynthesis: R. E. Beltz, D. W. Visser, *J. Am. Chem. Soc.* **77**, 736 (1955); T. J. Bardos *et al.*, *ibid.* 4279. X-ray crystallography: J. Iball *et al.*, *Nature* **209**, 1230 (1966). HPLC determn in plasma: D. A. Ganes, J. G. Wagner, *J. Chromatogr.* **432**, 233 (1988). Clinical studies in brain tumors: H. S. Greenberg *et al.*, *Neurology* **44**, 1715 (1994); T. L. Phillips *et al.*, *Int. J. Radiat. Oncol. Biol. Phys.* **21**, 709 (1991). Review of radiobiology and therapeutic potential: T. J. Kinsella *et al.*, *ibid.* **10**, 1399-1406 (1984); of genetic toxicology: S. M. Morris, *Mutat. Res.* **258**, 161-188 (1991); of role in management of CNS tumors: A. Freese *et al.*, *J. Neuro-Oncol.* **20**, 81-95 (1994). Series of reviews on diagnostic and research use: F. Dolbeare, *Histochem. J.* **27**, 339-369, 923-964 (1995); **28**, 531-575 (1996).

Crystals from abs ethanol, mp 187-189° (Beltz, Visser); also reported as mp 181-183° (Bardos). uv max (in HCl): 280 nm (ε 9.9×10^{-3}); uv max (in NaOH): 277 nm (ε 7.2×10^{-3}).

USE: Research tool for measuring DNA synthesis.

THERAP CAT: Antineoplastic adjunct (radiosensitizer); diagnostic aid (tumor cell label for cytokinetic analysis).

1453. Broxyquinoline. [521-74-4] 5,7-Dibromo-8-quinolinol; 5,7-dibromo-8-hydroxyquinoline; Brodiar; Broxykinolin; Colepur; Fenilor; Intensopan. $C_9H_5Br_2NO$; mol wt 302.95. C 35.68%, H 1.66%, Br 52.75%, N 4.62%, O 5.28%. Prepn by bromination of 5-formyl-8-quinolinol: Matsumura, Ito, *J. Am. Chem. Soc.* **77**, 6671 (1955); by bromination of 8-hydroxyquinaldine: Irving, Pinnington, *J. Chem. Soc.* **1957**, 285; by bromination of 8-quinolinol: Luis, Palomo, *Afinidad* **28**, 163 (1951), *C.A.* **47**, 10533d (1953); Zinnei, Fiedler, *Arch. Pharm.* **291**, 493 (1958); Aristov, Kostina, *Zh. Obshch. Khim.* **34**, 3421 (1964). Crystal structure: Kashino, Haisa, *Bull. Chem. Soc. Jpn.* **46**, 1094 (1973). Metabolism: Rodriguez, Close, *Biochem. Pharmacol.* **17**, 1647 (1968).

Monoclinic needles from alc. d 2.189. mp 196°. Freely sol in chloroform, alcohol, benzene, acetic acid; slightly sol in ether. Practically insol in water.

USE: In testing for Cu, Fe, Ti.

THERAP CAT: Antiseptic; disinfectant.

1454. Bruceantin. [41451-75-6] [11β,12α,15β(E)]-15-[(3,4-Dimethyl-1-oxo-2-pentenyl)oxy]-13,20-epoxy-3,11,12-trihydroxy-2,16-dioxopicras-3-en-21-oic acid methyl ester; NSC-

165563. $C_{28}H_{36}O_{11}$; mol wt 548.58. C 61.30%, H 6.61%, O 32.08%. Antileukemic quassinoid from the simaroubaceous tree *Brucea antidysenterica* J. F. Mill. Isoln and structure: S. M. Kupchan, **DE 2347576**; S. M. Kupchan, R. W. Britton, **US 3969369** (1975, 1976 both to Research Corp.); S. M. Kupchan *et al., J. Org. Chem.* **40,** 648 (1975). Mode of action: L. L. Liao *et al., Mol. Pharmacol.* **12,** 167 (1976). *In vivo* study: R. K. Johnson *et al., Cancer Treat. Rep.* **62,** 1535 (1978). Pharmacology: S. M. Sieber *et al., ibid.* **60,** 1127 (1976); M. Fresno *et al., Biochim. Biophys. Acta* **518,** 104 (1978). Clinical study: A. Y. Bedikian *et al., Proc. Am. Assoc. Cancer Res.* **20,** 193 (1979). Toxicologic evaluation: T. R. Castles *et al., U.S. NTIS Report* **PB-257175** (1976) 348 pp. Synthetic studies: O. D. Dailey, P. L. Fuchs, *J. Org. Chem.* **45,** 216 (1980); R. J. Pariza, P. L. Fuchs, *ibid.* **48,** 2306 (1983). Total synthesis: M. Sasaki *et al., ibid.* **55,** 528 (1990).

Crystals from ether, mp 225-226°. $[\alpha]_D^{25}$ −43° (c = 0.31 in pyridine). uv max (ethanol): 280, 221 nm (ε 8680, 18000); (ethanol, NaOH): 328, 221 nm (ε 7290, 28600). LD_{50} in male, female mice (mg/kg): 1.95, 2.58 i.v. (Castles).

1455. Brucine. [357-57-3] 2,3-Dimethoxystrychnidin-10-one; 10,11-dimethoxystrychnine. $C_{23}H_{26}N_2O_4$; mol wt 394.46. C 70.03%, H 6.64%, N 7.10%, O 16.22%. Toxic alkaloid resembling strychnine. Isoln from Strychnos seeds *(Strychnos nux-vomica* L. and *S. ignatii* Berg., *Loganiaceae):* C. Hartwick, P. Geiger, *Arch. Pharm.* **239,** 491 (1901). Prepn from strychnine, *q.v.:* E. Tedeschi *et al., Tetrahedron* **24,** 4573 (1968). ^{13}C-NMR study: E. Wenkert *et al., J. Org. Chem.* **43,** 1099 (1978). Electrophoretic determn in seeds: Y.-Y. Zong, C. Che, *Planta Med.* **61,** 456 (1995). Toxicity data: M. H. Malone *et al., J. Ethnopharmacol.* **35,** 295 (1992). Use as reagent for sulfur compounds: M. K. Tummuru *et al., Analyst* **109,** 1105 (1984); for nitrates: J. Masini *et al., Anal. Chem.* **69,** 1077 (1997). Review of structural elucidation: H. L. Holmes, Elucidation of the Structure of Strychnine and Brucine in *The Alkaloids* vol. I, R. H. F. Manske, Ed. (Academic Press, New York, 1950) pp 377-420.

Needles from acetone + water, mp 178°. $[\alpha]_D$ −127° (chloroform), −85° (in abs alcohol). uv max (ethanol): 263, 301 nm (log ε 4.09, 3.93).

Tetrahydrate. Monoclinic prisms. Also forms a dihydrate. Very bitter taste. Bitterness threshold 1:220,000. *Very poisonous! Handle dry powder in hood only.* Becomes anhyd at 100°. One gram dissolves in 0.8 ml methanol, 1.3 ml alcohol, 5 ml chloroform, 25 ml ethyl acetate, 36 ml glycerol, about 100 ml benzene, 187 ml ether, 1320 ml water, 750 ml boiling water. pH of satd water soln 9.5. pK_1 6.04, pK_2 11.7. LD_{50} in mice (mg/kg): 12.0 i.v.; 62.0 i.p.; 150.0 orally (Malone).

USE: Denaturing alcohol and oils; in analytical chemistry; for separating racemic mixtures. Addition agent to lubricants.

THERAP CAT: CNS stimulant.

1456. Bryonia. Bryony. Dried root of *Bryonia alba* L., or of *B. dioica* Jacq., *Cucurbitaceae. Habit.* Europe. *Constit.* Bryonin, bryonidin, bryonicine, bryoamarid glycoside, Δ^7-stigmastenol,

volatile oil, resin. Isoln of constituents: Tunmann, Wienecke, *Arch. Pharm.* **293,** 195 (1960); Biglino, *Farmaco Ed. Sci.* **14,** 673 (1959). Bryogenine structure studies: Biglino *et al., Tetrahedron Lett.* **1963,** 1651. *Poisonous!*

THERAP CAT: Cathartic.

THERAP CAT (VET): Formerly as a purgative.

1457. Bryostatins. Family of seventeen biologically active macrolides, bryostatins 1 through 15, A and B. Isolated from the marine bryozoans, *Bugula neritina,* L. and related organisms. Protein kinase C activators. Isoln and structure of bryostatin 1, one of the most abundant of the series: G. R. Pettit *et al., J. Am. Chem. Soc.* **104,** 6846 (1982). Large-scale isoln of 1: D. E. Schaufelberger *et al., J. Nat. Prod.* **54,** 1265 (1991). Abs config of 1, 2 and 3: G. R. Pettit *et al., J. Org. Chem.* **56,** 1337 (1991). ^{1}H- and ^{13}C-NMR analyses of 1: D. E. Schaufelberger *et al., Magn. Reson. Chem.* **29,** 366 (1991). Approaches to synthesis: R. Roy *et al., Chem. Commun.* **1989,** 1308; K. Ohmori *et al., Tetrahedron Lett.* **34,** 4981 (1993). Total synthesis of 7: M. Kageyama *et al., J. Am. Chem. Soc.* **112,** 7407 (1990). Conversion of 2 to 1: G. R. Pettit *et al., Can. J. Chem.* **69,** 856 (1991). Pharmacodynamics: R. L. Berkow *et al., Cancer Res.* **53,** 2810 (1993); C. Stanwell *et al., Int. J. Cancer* **56,** 585 (1994). Clinical evaluation of 1 in advanced cancer: J. Prendiville *et al., Br. J. Cancer* **68,** 418 (1993). Review of pharmacology: P. M. Blumberg, G. R. Pettit, "The Bryostatins, a Family of Protein Kinase C Activators with Therapeutic Potential", in *New Leads and Targets in Drug Research,* P. Krogsgaard-Larsen *et al.,* Eds. (Munksgaard, Copenhagen, 1992) pp 273-285. Review of isolation, structure elucidation and biological activity: G. R. Pettit, *Fortschr. Chem. Org. Naturst.* **57,** 153-195 (1991).

Bryostatin 1

Bryostatin 1. [83314-01-6] $C_{47}H_{68}O_{17}$. Colorless crystals from methylene chloride/methanol, mp 230-235°. $[\alpha]_D^{25}$ +34.1° (c = 0.044 in methanol). uv max (methanol): 233, 263 nm (ε 25700, 28700). Relatively insol in water. Soly in ethanol >4000 μg/ml. LD_{50} in mice, rats (mg/kg): 0.038, 0.068 i.v. (Prendiville).

1458. Bucetin. [1083-57-4] *N*-(4-Ethoxyphenyl)-3-hydroxybutanamide; 3-hydroxy-*p*-butyrophenetidide; β-hydroxybutyric acid *p*-phenetidide; *p*-ethoxy-*N*-(β-hydroxybutyryl)aniline; Betadid. $C_{12}H_{17}NO_3$; mol wt 223.27. C 64.55%, H 7.67%, N 6.27%, O 21.50%. Phenetidine derivative with analgesic and antipyretic activity. Prepn: G. Ehrhart *et al., US 2830087* (1958 to Hoechst); and pharmacology: *eidem, Arzneim.-Forsch.* **15,** 727 (1965). Toxicity data: H. Fujimura, *Folia Pharmacol. Jpn.* **62,** 123 (1966). Metabolism in rabbits: J. Shibasaki *et al., Chem. Pharm. Bull.* **16,** 1726, 2269 (1968). Synergistic effect with ethenzamide, *q.v.:* H. Kojima *et al., Oyo Yakuri* **16,** 549 (1978), *C.A.* **90,** 81035y (1979). TLC determn in saliva: P. Rohdewald, G. Drehsen, *J. Chromatogr.* **225,** 427 (1981).

Crystals from isopropanol, mp 160°. Sparingly sol in water. LD$_{50}$ in mice (mg/kg): 790 i.p., 2800 orally (Fujimura).

Note: Component in combination analgesics containing ethenzamide, caffeine and vitamin B$_1$, e.g. **Butylon, Bucetalon**.

THERAP CAT: Analgesic.

1459. Buchu. Bucco; bucku; buku. Dried leaves of *Barosma betulina* Bartl. & Wendl. (short buchu) or of *B. crenulata* (Linné) Hooker (oval buchu), or of *B. seratifolia* Willd. (long buchu), *Rutaceae. Habit.* Southern Africa (Cape of Good Hope). *Constit.* Diosphenol (barosma camphor), diosmin, bitter extractive, resin, *l*-menthone, mucilage, hesperidin, 1-2% volatile oil. *Review:* Feldman, Youngken, *J. Am. Pharm. Assoc.* **33**, 277 (1944).

THERAP CAT: Antiseptic (urinary).

THERAP CAT (VET): Has been used as a urinary antiseptic, diuretic.

1460. Bucillamine. [65002-17-7] *N*-(2-Mercapto-2-methyl-1-oxopropyl)-L-cysteine; *N*-(2-mercapto-2-methylpropanoyl)-L-cysteine; *N*-(2-mercaptoisobutyryl)-L-cysteine; tiobutarit; thiobutarit; DE-019; SA-96; Rimatil. C$_7$H$_{13}$NO$_3$S$_2$; mol wt 223.31. C 37.65%, H 5.87%, N 6.27%, O 21.49%, S 28.72%. Disease modifying antirheumatic drug (DMARD) which modulates the immune response; structurally related to tiopronin, *q.v.* Prepn: T. Fujita *et al.*, **DE 2709820**; *eidem*, **US 4305958** (1977, 1981 both to Santen); M. Oya *et al.*, *Chem. Pharm. Bull.* **29**, 940 (1981). GC-MS determn in blood: K. Matsuura *et al.*, *J. Mass Spectrom. Soc. Jpn.* **46**, 25 (1998). Clinical immunopharmacology: H. Matsuno *et al.*, *Drugs Exp. Clin. Res.* **19**, 205 (1993). Clinical trials in rheumatoid arthritis: M. Yasuda *et al.*, *Clin. Rheumatol.* **13**, 446 (1994); H. A. Kim, Y. W. Song, *Rheumatol. Int.* **17**, 5 (1997).

Crystals from ethyl acetate, mp 139-140°. [α]$_D^{25}$ +32.3° (c = 1.0 in ethanol). LD$_{50}$ in mice (mg/kg): 2285 i.p.; 989.6 i.v. (Fujita, 1981).

THERAP CAT: Antirheumatic.

1461. Bucindolol. [71119-11-4] 2-[2-Hydroxy-3-[[2-(1*H*-indol-3-yl)-1,1-dimethylethyl]amino]propoxy]benzonitrile. C$_{22}$H$_{25}$N$_3$O$_2$; mol wt 363.45. C 72.70%, H 6.93%, N 11.56%, O 8.80%. Non-selective β-adrenergic blocker with vasodilating activity. Prepn: **BE 868943** (1979 to Bristol-Myers); W. E. Kreighbaum, W. T. Comer, **US 4234595** (1980 to Mead Johnson); W. E. Kreighbaum *et al., J. Med. Chem.* **23**, 285 (1980). Crystal structure: J.-M. Léger *et al., Acta Crystallogr.* **C40**, 706 (1984). Conformation: E. Coutinho, *Indian J. Chem.* **34B**, 553 (1995). Review of chemistry and pharmacology: D. Deitchman *et al.*, in *New Drugs Annual: Cardiovascular Drugs* vol. 1, A. Scriabine, Ed. (Raven Press, New York, 1983) pp 1-18. Clinical pharmacokinetics: P. A. Meredith *et al, Xenobiotica* **15**, 979 (1985). Clinical pharmacology: N. Bett *et al., Am. J. Cardiol.* **57**, 678 (1986). GC-MS determn in plasma: M. J. Bartek *et al., J. Chromatogr.* **377**, 183 (1986). Evaluation in congestive heart failure: M. R. Bristow *et al., Circulation* **89**, 1632 (1994).

White crystals from abs ethanol, mp 125-127°.

Hydrochloride. [70369-47-0] MJ-13105-1. C$_{22}$H$_{25}$N$_3$O$_2$·HCl; mol wt 399.91. White crystals from abs ethanol, mp 185-187°. Sol in water. Nonhygroscopic. pKa 8.86. Partition coefficient (chloroform/0.01*M* phosphate buffer): 83.4 (pH 7.19); 361 (pH 7.78). LD$_{50}$ in mice, rats (mg/kg): ~100, ~100 orally (Deitchmann).

THERAP CAT: Antihypertensive; in treatment of congestive heart failure.

1462. Buckminsterfullerene. [99685-96-8] [5,6]Fullerene-C$_{60}$-Ih; buckyball; soccerballene. C$_{60}$; mol wt 720.64. C 100.00%. Named after R. Buckminster Fuller, the American engineer, whose geodesic domes possess the same symmetry as the C$_{60}$ truncated icosahedron typified by a soccerball. The most abundant of a class of carbon molecules characterized by a hollow cage structure and known as the *fullerenes*. One of the allotropic forms of carbon, *q.v.*, and the only molecular form, these molecules, described by C$_{20+2m}$, form stable closed nets composed of 12 pentagons and 'm' hexagons. Prepn: H. W. Kroto *et al., Nature* **318**, 162 (1985); in macroscopic quantities: W. Krätschmer *et al., ibid.* **347**, 354 (1990). Rational synthesis: L. T. Scott *et al., Science* **295**, 1500 (2002). Identification in shungite, a carbonaceous rock: P. R. Buseck *et al., Science* **257**, 215 (1992). Review of early work: R. F. Curl, R. E. Smalley, *Sci. Am.* **265**, 54-63 (1991). Review of synthesis, properties, chemistry including metal-doping: *Acc. Chem. Res.* **25**, 98-175 (1992); *Fullerenes*, G. S. Hammond, V. J. Kuck, Eds. *ACS Symp. Ser.* **481**, 1-195 (1992). Review of solids chemistry: A. Penicaud, *Fullerene Sci. Tech.* **6**, 731-741 (1998). Book: *The Chemical Physics of Fullerenes 10 (and 5) Years Later*, W. Andreoni, Ed. (Kluwer Academic Publishers, Dordrecht, 1996) 498 pp.

1463. Bucladesine. [362-74-3] *N*-(1-Oxobutyl)adenosine cyclic 3′,5′-(hydrogen phosphate) 2′-butanoate; *N*-(9-β-D-ribofuranosyl-9*H*-purin-6-yl)butyramide cyclic 3′,5′-(hydrogen phosphate) 2′-butyrate; *N*^{6},2′-*O*-dibutyryladenosine 3′,5′-cyclic monophosphate; *N*^{6},2′-*O*-dibutyryl cAMP; DBcAMP. C$_{18}$H$_{24}$N$_5$O$_8$P; mol wt 469.39. C 46.06%, H 5.15%, N 14.92%, O 27.27%, P 6.60%. Vasodilating cyclic nucleotide derivative which can permeate the cell membrane. Mimics the action of endogenous cyclic AMP, *q.v.* Prepn: Th. Posternak *et al., Biochim. Biophys. Acta* **65**, 558 (1962); O. Nagase *et al.*, **JP Kokai 76 113896**, *C.A.* **86**, 140409r (1977); T. Hirayama *et al.*, **JP Kokai 77 39698**; **JP 77 39699**, *C.A.* **87**, 136330m-136331n (1977) (1976, 1977, 1977 all to Daiichi Seiyaku). Pharmacology: H. S. White *et al., Eur. J. Pharmacol.* **57**, 107 (1979); J. D. Johnson *et al., ibid.* **91**, 343 (1983); N. Bondar *et al., J. Physiol.* **355**, 33 (1984). Clinical trial in congestive heart failure: S. Matsui *et al., Am. J. Cardiol.* **51**, 1364 (1983); after cardiopulmonary bypass surgery: T. Yoshitake *et al., Prog. Clin. Biol. Res.* **111**, 211 (1983).

Sodium salt. [16980-89-5] DC-2797; Actosin. C$_{18}$H$_{23}$N$_5$NaO$_8$P; mol wt 491.37.

Barium salt. [18837-96-2] C$_{36}$H$_{46}$BaN$_{10}$O$_{16}$P$_2$. uv max (ethanol-0.5*M* ammonium acetate, 5:2) 270 nm.

THERAP CAT: Cardiotonic.

Consult the Name Index before using this section.

1464. Buclizine. [82-95-1] 1-[(4-Chlorophenyl)phenyl-methyl]-4-[[4-(1,1-dimethylethyl)phenyl]methyl]piperazine; 1-(*p*-*tert*-butylbenzyl)-4-(*p*-chloro-α-phenylbenzyl)piperazine; 1-(*p*-chlorobenzhydryl)-4-(*p*-*tert*-butylbenzyl)diethylenediamine; 1-(*p*-*tert*-butylbenzyl)-4-(*p*-chlorodiphenylmethyl)piperazine; histabuty-zine; histabutizine. $C_{28}H_{33}ClN_2$; mol wt 433.03. C 77.66%, H 7.68%, Cl 8.19%, N 6.47%. Prepn: Morren, **US 2709169** (1955 to U.C.B.), see also **DE 964040**, Lui et al., C.A. **62**, 2776a (1965). Clinical evaluation as antiemetic in migraine: P. B. Jorgensen et al., Curr. Ther. Res. **16**, 1276 (1974); E. I. Adam, J. Int. Med. Res. **15**, 71 (1987).

bp$_{0.001}$ 217-220°.
Dihydrochloride. [129-74-8] UCB-4445; Aphilan; Buclina; Longifene; Postafen. $C_{28}H_{33}ClN_2 \cdot 2HCl$; mol wt 505.95. mp 230-240°.
THERAP CAT: Antiemetic.

1465. Buclosamide. [575-74-6] *N*-Butyl-4-chloro-2-hy-droxybenzamide; *N*-butyl-4-chlorosalicylamide; 4-chloro-2-hy-droxybenzoic acid *n*-butylamide. $C_{11}H_{14}ClNO_2$; mol wt 227.69. C 58.03%, H 6.20%, Cl 15.57%, N 6.15%, O 14.05%. Prepn: Ruschig et al., **US 2923737** (1960 to Hoechst).

Crystals from chloroform, mp 90-92°.
Combination with salicylic acid. [75199-98-3] Jadit.
THERAP CAT: Antifungal.

1466. Bucolome. [841-73-6] 5-Butyl-1-cyclohexyl-2,4,-6(1*H*,3*H*,5*H*)pyrimidinetrione; 5-butyl-1-cyclohexylbarbituric acid; 5-*n*-butyl-1-cyclohexyl-2,4,6-trioxoperhydropyrimidine; BCP; Paramidin. $C_{14}H_{22}N_2O_3$; mol wt 266.34. C 63.13%, H 8.33%, N 10.52%, O 18.02%. Prepn: Senda et al., **US 3243344** and **US 3274195** (both 1966 to Takeda). Metabolic studies in man: Yashiki et al., Chem. Pharm. Bull. **19**, 468, 869 (1971).

Needles from methanol, mp 84°. bp$_{0.8}$ 185-187°.
THERAP CAT: Anti-inflammatory.

1467. Bucumolol. [58409-59-9] 8-[3-[[(1,1-Dimethylethyl)-amino]-2-hydroxypropoxy]-5-methyl-2*H*-1-benzopyran-2-one; (±)-8-[3-(*t*-butylamino)-2-hydroxypropoxy]-5-methylcoumarin; *dl*-8-(2-hydroxy-3-*tert*-butylaminopropoxy)coumarin. $C_{17}H_{23}$-NO$_4$; mol wt 305.37. C 66.86%, H 7.59%, N 4.59%, O 20.96%. β-Adrenergic blocker. Prepn: Y. Sato et al., **DE 2021958**; eidem, **US 3663570** (1970, 1972 both to Sankyo); eidem, Chem. Pharm. Bull. **20**, 905 (1972). Pharmacology: T. Oshima et al., Jpn. J. Pharmacol. **23**, 497 (1973). Metabolic studies: R. Hayashi et al., Chem. Pharm. Bull. **23**, 1173 (1975). Antiarrhythmic activity in dogs: K. Nakayama et al., Jpn. J. Pharmacol. **29**, 935 (1979). Early clinical study: H. Kishida et al., Rinsho Yakuri **11**, 99 (1980), C.A. **93**, 107380w (1980).

Hydrochloride. [36556-75-9] CS-359; Bucumarol. $C_{17}H_{23}$-NO$_4 \cdot HCl$; mol wt 341.83. Colorless crystals from isopropanol, mp 226-228° (dec). LD$_{50}$ in male, female mice (mg/kg): 676, 692 orally; 33.1, 31.6 i.v. (Oshima).
THERAP CAT: Antianginal, antiarrhythmic.

1468. Budesonide. [51333-22-3] (11β,16α)-16,17-[Butyli-denebis(oxy)]-11,21-dihydroxypregna-1,4-diene-3,20-dione; (R,S)-11β,16α,17,21-tetrahydroxypregna-1,4-diene-3,20-dione cyclic 16,17-acetal with butyraldehyde; S-1320; Bidien; Budeson; Corti-vent; Entocort; Novopulmon; Preferid; Pulmicort; Rhinocort; Spi-rocort. $C_{25}H_{34}O_6$; mol wt 430.53. C 69.74%, H 7.96%, O 22.30%. Non-halogenated glucocorticoid related to triamcinolone hexaceto-nide, q.v. with a high ratio of topical to systemic activity. Prepn: R. L. Brattsand et al., **DE 2323215**; eidem, **US 3929768** (1973, 1975 both to Bofors). Synthesis and anti-inflammatory properties: A. Thalén, R. L. Brattsand, Arzneim.-Forsch. **29**, 1787 (1979). Phar-macokinetic study: A. Ryrfeldt et al., J. Steroid Biochem. **10**, 317 (1979). HPLC determn of epimers, impurities, content: G. Roth et al., J. Pharm. Sci. **69**, 766 (1980). Review of pharmacodynamics and efficacy in asthma and rhinitis: S. P. Clissold, R. C. Heel, Drugs **28**, 485-518 (1984).

Crystals, mp 221-232° (dec). Mixture of two isomers; the con-tent of the *S*-isomer in the mixture varies between 40-51%. [α]$_D^{25}$ +98.9° (c = 0.28 in methylene chloride).
THERAP CAT: Anti-inflammatory.

1469. Budipine. [57982-78-2] 1-(1,1-Dimethylethyl)-4,4-diphenylpiperidine; 1-*tert*-butyl-4,4-diphenylpiperidine. $C_{21}H_{27}N$; mol wt 293.45. C 85.95%, H 9.27%, N 4.77%. Centrally acting deriv of diphenylpiperidine. Prepn: H. G. Menge, J. Klosa, **DE 1936452**; eidem, **US 4016280** (1969, 1977 both to Byk Gulden). Pharmacological studies: U. Brand, H. G. Menge, Arzneim.-Forsch. **30**, 1242 (1980); M. Eltze, ibid. 1129; H. G. Menge, U. Brand, ibid. **32**, 85 (1982). Comparison to other drugs in treatment of dyskinesias: J. Siegfried, Can. J. Neurol. Sci. **6**, 89 (1979). Clinical evaluation with levodopa in Parkinson's disease: K. Jel-linger, H. Bliesath, J. Neurol. **234**, 280 (1987).

Hydrochloride. [63661-61-0] Parkinsan. $C_{21}H_{27}N \cdot HCl$; mol wt 329.91. LD$_{50}$ in male mice, rats (mg/kg): 120, 165 orally; 33, 28 i.v. (Menge, Brand).
THERAP CAT: Antiparkinsonian.

1470. Budralazine. [36798-79-5] 1(2*H*)-Phthalazinone (1,3-dimethyl-2-butenylidene)hydrazone; 4-methyl-3-penten-2-one (1-phthalazinyl)hydrazone; mesityl oxide (1-phthalazinyl)hydrazone; DJ-1461; Buterazine. $C_{14}H_{16}N_4$; mol wt 240.30. C 69.97%, H 6.71%, N 23.32%. Deriv of hydralazine, *q.v.* Prepn: K. Ueno *et al.*, **DE 2145359**; *eidem*, **US 3840539** (1972, 1974 both to Daiichi Seiyaku); *eidem, Chem. Pharm. Bull.* **24**, 1068 (1976). Pharmacology: A. Akashi *et al., Eur. J. Pharmacol.* **29**, 161 (1974); *eidem, Arch. Int. Pharmacodyn. Ther.* **235**, 134 (1978). Metabolism: R. Moroi *et al., Chem. Pharm. Bull.* **24**, 2850 (1976); K. Ono *et al., Xenobiotica* **9**, 227 (1979). Toxicity study: T. Onodera *et al., Toxicol. Appl. Pharmacol.* **44**, 431 (1978). Reproduction studies: *Oyo Yakuri* **21**, 313-350 (1981), *C.A.* **95**, 73764y-7b (1981). Series of articles on cardiovascular action, α-adrenergic effects, antihypertensive and general pharmacological properties: *Arzneim.-Forsch.* **31**, 1072-1087 (1981). Characterization of vasodilator action: T. Chiba *et al., ibid.* **33**, 112 (1983).

Crystals from isopropyl ether, mp 132-133°. uv max (methanol): 208, 240, 289, 357 nm (ε 27000, 89000, 20000, 15000). LD_{50} in mice, rats (mg/kg): 1820, 620 orally; 4020, 3570 i.p. (Onodera).

THERAP CAT: Antihypertensive.

1471. Bufalin. [465-21-4] (3β,5β)-3,14-Dihydroxybufa-20,22-dienolide. $C_{24}H_{34}O_4$; mol wt 386.52. C 74.58%, H 8.87%, O 16.56%. Cardiotonic steroid constituent of Ch'an Su (also called Senso), a galenical preparation of the dried venom of the Chinese toad, *Bufo bufo gargarizans.* Isoln and characterization: M. Kotake, K. Kuwada, *Sci. Papers Inst. Phys. Chem. Res. Jpn.* **36**, 106 (1939), *C.A.* **33**, 7304⁹ (1939); K. Meyer, *Helv. Chim. Acta* **32**, 1238 (1949). Structure: K. Kuwada, *J. Chem. Soc. Jpn.* **60**, 335 (1939), *C.A.* **35**, 51123⁹ (1941). Prepn from resibufogenin, *q.v.*: H. Kondo, S. Ohno, **US 3134772** (1964); from digitoxigenin, *q.v.*: G. R. Pettit *et al.*, **US 3687944** (1972). Total synthesis: F. Sondheimer *et al., J. Am. Chem. Soc.* **91**, 1228 (1969). Additional syntheses: G. R. Pettit *et al., J. Org. Chem.* **35**, 2895 (1970); Y. Kamano, G. R. Pettit, *ibid.* **38**, 222 (1973); E. Yoshii *et al., Chem. Pharm. Bull.* **25**, 2249 (1977); K. Wiesner *et al., Helv. Chim. Acta* **66**, 2632 (1983). Pharmacology: S. Yoshida, T. Sakai, *Jpn. J. Pharmacol.* **23**, 859 (1973); **24**, 97 (1974).

Needles from methanol/chloroform, mp 242-243°. $[\alpha]_D$ −20°. uv max (ethanol): 298 nm (log ε 3.77).

Sodium sulfate. Sodium bufalin-3-sulfate. $C_{24}H_{33}NaO_7S$. Isoln from Japanese toad *Bufo vulgaris formosus*: K. Shimada *et al., Tetrahedron Lett.* **1974**, 2767. Colorless amorphous solid, mp 165.5-166.5°. $[\alpha]_D^{23}$ −33.1° (c = 0.05 in methanol).

1472. Bufeniode. [22103-14-6] 4-Hydroxy-3,5-diiodo-α-[1-[(1-methyl-3-phenylpropyl)amino]ethyl]benzenemethanol; 1-(4-hydroxy-3,5-diiodophenyl)-2-(1-methyl-3-phenylpropylamino)-propanol; diiodobuphenine; Diastal; Proclival. $C_{19}H_{23}I_2NO_2$; mol wt 551.20. C 41.40%, H 4.21%, I 46.05%, N 2.54%, O 5.81%. Prepn: J. P. Fourneau, J. M. Delourme, **ZA 6800046**; *eidem*, **US 3542870** (1968, 1970 both to Lab. Houdé). Metabolism: Veyre *et al., C.R. Seances Soc. Biol. Ses Fil.* **163**, 136 (1969).

Crystals, mp (slow heating) 185° (dec), mp (fast heating) 212°. LD_{50} in mice: >600 mg/kg i.p., >2 g/kg orally (Fourneau, Delourme).

THERAP CAT: Antihypertensive; vasodilator (peripheral).

1473. Bufetolol. [53684-49-4] 1-[(1,1-Dimethylethyl)-amino]-3-[2-[(tetrahydro-2-furanyl)methoxy]phenoxy]-2-propanol; 1-(*tert*-butylamino)-3-[*o*-[(tetrahydrofurfuryl)oxy]phenoxy]-2-propanol. $C_{18}H_{29}NO_4$; mol wt 323.43. C 66.84%, H 9.04%, N 4.33%, O 19.79%. β-Adrenergic blocker. Prepn: M. Nakanishi *et al.*, **DE 2024001**; *eidem*, **US 3723476** (1970, 1973, both to Yoshitomi); *eidem, J. Med. Chem.* **15**, 45 (1972). Pharmacology: M. Nakanishi *et al., Yakugaku Zasshi* **91**, 1037 (1971); *ibid.* **92**, 375 (1972); Imamura *et al., ibid.* 1039. Metabolism: M. Nakanishi *et al., ibid.* 299; *Oyo Yakuri* **6**, 479 (1972), *C.A.* **78**, 66785b (1973). Toxicology: *eidem, ibid.* 485, 1267, *C.A.* **78**, 66945d; **79**, 337w (1973).

$bp_{0.07}$ 180-186°.

Hydrochloride. [35108-88-4] Y-6124; Adobiol. $C_{18}H_{29}$-NO_4.HCl; mol wt 359.89. White crystals from methanol-isopropanol, mp 153.5-157°; also reported as mp 151-154°. (Diastereoisomer, mp 118°). Freely sol in water, methanol, glacial acetic acid. Very slightly sol in benzene. Practically insol in ether. Unstable on exposure to light.

THERAP CAT: Antiarrhythmic; antianginal.

1474. Bufexamac. [2438-72-4] 4-Butoxy-*N*-hydroxyben-zeneacetamide; 2-(*p*-butoxyphenyl)acetohydroxamic acid; 2-[*p*-(butyloxy)phenyl]acetohydroxamic acid; CP-1044-J3; Droxarol; Droxaryl; Feximac; Malipuran; Mofenar; Norfemac; Parfenal. $C_{12}H_{17}NO_3$; mol wt 223.27. C 64.55%, H 7.67%, N 6.27%, O 21.50%. Synthesis: N. P. Buu-Hoï *et al., Compt. Rend.* **261**, 2259 (1965); *eidem*, **BE 661226**; *eidem*, **US 3479396** (1965, 1969 to Madan). Pharmacology and toxicology: Lambelin *et al., Med. Pharmacol. Exp.* **15**, 545 (1966).

Needles from acetone, mp 153-155°. Practically insol in water. LD_{50} orally in mice, rats: >8, >4 g/kg (Lambelin).

THERAP CAT: Anti-inflammatory, analgesic, antipyretic.

1475. Buflomedil. [55837-25-7] 4-(1-Pyrrolidinyl)-1-(2,4,6-trimethoxyphenyl)-1-butanone; 2′,4′,6′-trimethoxy-4-(1-pyrrolidinyl)butyrophenone; (2,4,6-trimethoxyphenyl)-(3-pyrrolidino-propyl) ketone. $C_{17}H_{25}NO_4$; mol wt 307.38. C 66.43%, H 8.20%, N 4.56%, O 20.82%. Prepn: L. Lafon, **DE 2122144**; *idem*, **US 3895030** (both 1971 to Orsymonde). Pharmacology: J. Duteil *et al., Therapie* **30**, 207 (1975); C. Debray *et al., ibid.* 259. HPLC determn: J. A. Badmin *et al., J. Chromatogr.* **172**, 319 (1979). Clinical pharmacokinetics: U. Gundert-Remy *et al., Eur. J. Clin. Pharmacol.* **20**, 459 (1981). Comparative safety and efficacy study: G. Rosas *et al., Angiology* **32**, 291 (1981). Review of pharmacology and therapeutic effects: S. P. Clissold *et al., Drugs* **33**, 430-460 (1987).

Hydrochloride. [35543-24-9] LL-1656; Bufedil; Buflan; Buflocit; Buflonat; Fonzylane; Irrodan; Lofton; Loftyl; Provas. C_{17}-$H_{25}NO_4$.HCl; mol wt 343.85. White crystals from isopropanol, mp 192-193°. LD_{50} in mice (mg/kg): 80 ±4.6 i.v. (Lafon).

THERAP CAT: Vasodilator (peripheral).

1476. Buformin. [692-13-7] N-Butylimidodicarbonimidic diamide; 1-butylbiguanide; n-butylbiguanide; butyldiguanide; butformin; W-37. $C_6H_{15}N_5$; mol wt 157.22. C 45.84%, H 9.62%, N 44.54%. Prepn: Shapiro et al., J. Am. Chem. Soc. **81**, 3728 (1959); Shapiro, Freedman, US 2961377 (1960 to USV). Toxicity study: Rikimaru et al., J. Antibiot. **18A**, 196 (1965).

Strong base. Very sol in water.
Hydrochloride. [1190-53-0] Andere; Biforon; Bigunal; Bufonamin; Bulbonin; Diabrin; Dibetos; Gliporal; Insulamin; Krebon; Panformin; Silubin; Sindiatil; Tidemol; Ziavetine. $C_6H_{15}N_5$.HCl; mol wt 193.68. Crystals, mp 174-177°. Freely sol in water, alcohol. LD_{50} i.p. in mice: 380 mg/kg (Rikimaru).
Nitrate. $C_6H_{15}N_5$.HNO$_3$. Crystals from ethanol, dec 125-126°.

THERAP CAT: Antidiabetic.

1477. Bufotalin. [471-95-4] $(3\beta,5\beta,16\beta)$-16-(Acetyloxy)-3,14-dihydroxybufa-20,22-dienolide; $3\beta,14,16\beta$-trihydroxy-5β-bufa-20,22-dienolide 16-acetate. $C_{26}H_{36}O_6$; mol wt 444.56. C 70.24%, H 8.16%, O 21.59%. One of the genins found in the venom of the common European toad (Bufo vulgaris). Isoln and structure: Faust, Arch. Exp. Pathol. Pharmakol. **47**, 279 (1902); **49**, 1 (1902); Wieland, Weil, Ber. **46**, 3315 (1913); Wieland, Weyland, Sitzungsber. Bayer. Akad. Wiss. (math.-physikal. Klasse) **1920**, 329; Wieland et al., Ann. **524**, 203 (1936); Meyer, Helv. Chim. Acta **32**, 1993 (1949); Pettit et al., Chem. Commun. **1970**, 1566. Synthesis: G. R. Pettit et al., J. Org. Chem. **52**, 3573 (1987).

Solvated crystals from alc. Sinters at 154°, dec 223°. Sublimes in high vacuum at 225-230°. uv max: 300 nm. $[\alpha]_D^{20}$ +5.4° (c = 0.5 in chloroform). Sol in alcohol, chloroform.
3-Acetate. mp 269-272°.

1478. Bufotenine. [487-93-4] 3-[2-(Dimethylamino)ethyl]-1H-indol-5-ol; 3-(2-dimethylaminoethyl)-5-indolol; 5-hydroxy-N,N-dimethyltryptamine; N,N-dimethylserotonin; 3-(β-dimethylaminoethyl)-5-hydroxyindole; mappine. $C_{12}H_{16}N_2O$; mol wt 204.27. C 70.56%, H 7.89%, N 13.71%, O 7.83%. Isoln from toads: Wieland et al., Ann. **513**, 1 (1934); Wieland, Wieland, ibid. **528**, 239 (1937); from toadstools: Wieland, Motzel, ibid. **581**, 10 (1953). Isoln from Piptadenia peregrina Benth., Leguminosae: Stromberg, J. Am. Chem. Soc. **76**, 1707 (1954). Synthesis: Hoshino, Shimodaira, Ann. **520**, 19 (1935); Harley-Mason, Jackson, Chem. Ind. (London) **1952**, 954; see also Serotonin; and Speetor, US 2708197 (1955 to Upjohn); Stoll et al., Helv. Chim. Acta **38**,

1452 (1955). Activity: Bhattacharya, Sanyal, Indian J. Physiol. Pharmacol. **15**, 133 (1971). Crystal and molecular structure: G. Falkenberg, Acta Crystallogr. **28B**, 3219 (1972).

Stout prisms from ethyl acetate, mp 146-147°. bp$_{0.1}$ 320°. uv max: 220, 265 nm (log ε 4.0, 3.7). Almost insol in water. Freely sol in alcohol, less sol in ether. Sol in dil acids and alkalies.
Methyliodide. $C_{13}H_{19}IN_2O$. Stout prisms from methanol, dec 214-215°.
Note: This is a controlled substance (hallucinogen): **21 CFR**, 1308.11.

1479. Bufotoxin. [464-81-3] $[3\beta(S),5\beta,16\beta]$-16-(Acetyloxy)-3-[[8-[[4-[(aminoiminomethyl)amino]-1-carboxybutyl]amino]-1,8-dioxooctyl]oxy]-14-hydroxybufa-20,22-dienolide; bufotalin 3-suberoylarginine ester. $C_{40}H_{60}N_4O_{10}$; mol wt 756.93. C 63.47%, H 7.99%, N 7.40%, O 21.14%. Principal toxin of the venom of the common European toad, Bufo vulgaris. Isoln and structure: Wieland, Alles, Ber. **55**, 1789 (1922); Wieland et al., Ann. **524**, 203 (1936); Meyer, Helv. Chim. Acta **32**, 1993 (1949); Urscheler et al., ibid. **38**, 883 (1955). Alternate structure: Kamano et al., Tetrahedron Lett. **1968**, 5673; Linde-Tempel, Helv. Chim. Acta **53**, 2188 (1970). Partial synthesis: Pettit, Kamano, Chem. Commun. **1972**, 45.

Monohydrate, bitter needles from alc, dec 205°. uv max: 295 nm (log ε 3.74). Freely sol in methanol, pyridine, sparingly sol in abs alc. Practically insol in water, ether, acetone, chloroform, petr ether.

1480. Bufuralol. [54340-62-4] α-[[(1,1-Dimethylethyl)-amino]methyl]-7-ethyl-2-benzofuranmethanol; α-[(tert-butylamino)methyl]-7-ethyl-2-benzofuranmethanol; 2-(2-tert-butylamino-1-hydroxyethyl)-7-ethylbenzofuran; 1-(7-ethylbenzofuran-2-yl)-2-tert-butylamino-1-hydroxyethane. $C_{16}H_{23}NO_2$; mol wt 261.36. C 73.53%, H 8.87%, N 5.36%, O 12.24%. β-Adrenergic blocker with peripheral vasodilating activity. Prepn: NL 6606441; G. A. Fothergill et al., US 3929836 (1966, 1975 both to Hoffmann-La Roche). Prepn and resolution of isomers: eidem, Experientia **31**, 1322 (1975); eidem, Arzneim.-Forsch. **27**, 981 (1977). Pharmacology: T. C. Hamilton, M. W. Parkes, ibid. 1410. HPLC determn in plasma: P. Haefelfinger, J. Chromatogr. **221**, 327 (1980). Metabolism of isomers and racemate: R. J. Francis et al., Eur. J. Clin. Pharmacol. **23**, 529 (1982). Pharmacokinetics in hypertensive patients: M. Eckert et al., ibid. **24**, 479 (1983). Hemodynamic effects in patients with angina: M. Pfisterer et al., J. Cardiovasc. Pharmacol. **6**, 417 (1984).

Hydrochloride. [59652-29-8] Ro-3-4787; Angium. $C_{16}H_{23}$-NO_2.HCl; mol wt 297.82. Fine, white powder from acetone, mp

146°. LD$_{50}$ in mice (mg/kg): 29.7 i.v.; 88.0 i.p.; 177 orally; in rats (mg/kg): 1400 s.c.; 750 orally (Hamilton, Parkes).

(+)-Hydrochloride. [57704-11-7] Crystals from ethyl acetate-ether, mp 122-123°. [α]$_{365}^{20}$ +135.0° (c = 1.0 in ethanol).

(−)-Hydrochloride. [57704-10-6] Crystals from ethyl acetate-ether, mp 122-123°. [α]$_{365}^{20}$ −136.0° (c = 1.0 in ethanol).

THERAP CAT: Antianginal; antihypertensive.

1481. Bulbocapnine. [298-45-3] (7aS)-6,7,7a,8-Tetrahydro-11-methoxy-7-methyl-5H-benzo[g]-1,3-benzodioxolo[6,5,4-de]quinolin-12-ol; 10-methoxy-1,2-(methylenedioxy)-6aα-aporphin-11-ol. C$_{19}$H$_{19}$NO$_4$; mol wt 325.36. C 70.14%, H 5.89%, N 4.30%, O 19.67%. From root of *Corydalis cava* (L.) Schweigg. & Körte (*C. tuberosa* DC), *Fumariaceae* and *Dicentra canadensis* Walp., *Papaveraceae*. Isoln: Freund, Josephi, *Ber.* **25**, 2411 (1892); Manske, *Can. J. Res.* **7**, 258 (1932). Pharmacology and toxicity study: H. Molitar, *J. Pharmacol. Exp. Ther.* **56**, 85 (1936). Structure: Gadamer, *Chem. Ztg.* **34**, 1004 (1910). Configuration: Ayer, Taylor, *J. Chem. Soc.* **1956**, 472; Corrodi, Hardegger, *Helv. Chim. Acta* **39**, 889 (1956). Synthesis: Kikkawa, *C.A.* **54**, 4649b (1960). Peripheral-dopamine-receptor blocking activity: R. G. Pendleton *et al.*, *Arch. Pharmacol.* **289**, 171 (1975).

dl-**Form.** Columns, mp 213-214°. Absorption max: Brustier, *C.A.* **49**, 12127b (1955).

l-**Form.** Columns, mp 202-203°. [α]$_D^{22}$ −239°.

d-**Form.** Columns, mp 201-203°. [α]$_D^{22}$ +231°. Practically insol in water, sol in alcohol, chloroform. LD$_{50}$ s.c. in mice: 195 mg/kg (Molitar).

Methyl ether. C$_{20}$H$_{21}$NO$_4$. Crystals from petr ether, mp 129°. [α]$_D^{20}$+260°. Absorption max: Girardet, *J. Chem. Soc.* **1931**, 2630.

1482. Bullvalene. [1005-51-2] Tricyclo[3.3.2.0^{2,8}]deca-3,6,9-triene; tricyclo[3.3.2.0^{4,6}]deca-2,7,9-triene. C$_{10}$H$_{10}$; mol wt 130.19. C 92.26%, H 7.74%. Molecular structure is highly fluxional; spontaneously undergoes a 3-fold structurally degenerate Cope rearrangement at room temp, resulting in 10!/3 structurally equivalent geometric isomers. ^{1}H NMR spectrum is a sharp singlet peak at high temp. Predicted as a hypothetical molecule: W. von E. Doering, W. R. Roth, *Tetrahedron* **19**, 715 (1963). Prepn: G. Schröder, *Angew. Chem.* **75**, 722 (1963). ^{1}H NMR spectrum: R. Merényi *et al.*, *Ber.* **97**, 3150 (1964). Vapor phase structure determn: B. Andersen, A. Marstrander, *Acta Chem. Scand.* **25**, 1271 (1971). Microwave and vibrational spectral study: W. M. Stigliani, V. W. Laurie, *J. Mol. Spectrosc.* **60**, 188 (1976). Calorimetry study: M. Mansson, S. Sunner, *J. Chem. Thermodyn.* **13**, 671 (1981). Review of chemistry: G. Schröder, J. F. M. Oth, *Angew. Chem. Int. Ed.* **6**, 414-423 (1967); of discovery and characterization: A. Ault, *J. Chem. Educ.* **78**, 924-927 (2001).

mp 96°.

1483. Bumadizon. [3583-64-0] Butylpropanedioic acid mono(1,2-diphenylhydrazide); butylmalonic acid mono(1,2-diphenylhydrazide); N-(2-carboxycaproyl)hydrazobenzene; α-carboxycaproyl-N,N'-diphenylhydrazine. C$_{19}$H$_{22}$N$_2$O$_3$; mol wt 326.39. C 69.92%, H 6.79%, N 8.58%, O 14.71%. Prepn: **NL 6406412**; Pfister *et al.*, **US 3455999** (1964, 1969 to Geigy); **NL 6600685** (1966 to Byk-Gulden). Main product of the hydrolysis of phenylbutazone, *q.v.*: Schmid, *Helv. Chim. Acta* **53**, 2239 (1970). Chemical characterization: Pawelczyk, Wachowiak, *Acta Pol. Pharm.* **26**,

433 (1969), *C.A.* **72**, 136355p (1970). Series of articles on pharmacology: *Arzneim.-Forsch.* **23**, 1226-1251, 1813-1822 (1973). Toxicity: R. Riedel, W. Schoetensack, *ibid.* 1215.

Crystals from ether-petr ether, mp 116-117°. Also reported as mp 77-79° (dependent on speed of crystallization). uv max (0.1N NaOH): 234, 264 nm (ε 16200, 3700).

Calcium salt hemihydrate. [69365-73-7] Bumaflex; Eumotol; Rheumatol. C$_{38}$H$_{42}$CaN$_4$O$_6$·½H$_2$O; mol wt 699.85. Dec 154°. Sol in chloroform, alcohol, ether. Slightly sol in water. LD$_{50}$ in mice, rats (mg/kg): 2500, 1250 orally; 258, 263 i.v. (Riedel, Schoetensack).

THERAP CAT: Analgesic; antipyretic; anti-inflammatory.

1484. Bumetanide. [28395-03-1] 3-(Aminosulfonyl)-5-(butylamino)-4-phenoxybenzoic acid; 3-(butylamino)-4-phenoxy-5-sulfamoylbenzoic acid; PF-1593; Ro-10-6338; Bumex; Burinex; Butinat; Fontego; Fordiuran; Lunetoron. C$_{17}$H$_{20}$N$_2$O$_5$S; mol wt 364.42. C 56.03%, H 5.53%, N 7.69%, O 21.95%, S 8.80%. Prepn: P. W. Feit, **DE 1964503** and **DE 1964504**; *idem*, **US 3806534** (1970, 1970, 1974 all to Lövens Kemiske Fabrik); *idem*, *J. Med. Chem.* **14**, 432 (1971). Pharmacology: E. H. Oestergaard *et al.*, *Arzneim.-Forsch.* **22**, 66 (1972). HPLC and GC/MS determn in urine: C. Y. Gradeen *et al.*, *J. Anal. Toxicol.* **14**, 123 (1990). Review of pharmacology and therapeutic use: A. Ward, R. C. Heel, *Drugs* **28**, 426-464 (1984). Series of articles on pharmacokinetics and comparative clinical studies in combination therapy: *Curr. Ther. Res.* **50**, Suppl. A, 1-82 (1991). Comprehensive description: P. N. V. Tata *et al.*, *Anal. Profiles Drug Subs. Excip.* **22**, 107-144 (1993).

Crystals from aq ethanol, mp 230-231°. pK$_1$ 3.6, pK$_2$ 7.7. Soly (mg/ml): water 0.1; ethanol 30.6; propylene glycol 18.7; dimethylacetamide >500; methanol 76.5; benzene 0.4; benzyl alcohol 21.6; acetone 50.2. Sol in alkaline solns. uv max (water): 260, 220 nm (E$^{1\%}$ 18.9, 17.1); (0.1 N NaOH): 326 nm; (methanol): 270, 345 nm. LD$_{50}$ i.v. in mice: 330 mg/kg (Oestergaard).

THERAP CAT: Diuretic.

1485. Bunaftine. [32421-46-8] N-Butyl-N-[2-(diethylamino)ethyl]-1-naphthalenecarboxamide; N-butyl-N-[2-(diethylamino)ethyl]-1-naphthamide; bunaphtide; bunaphtine. C$_{21}$H$_{30}$N$_2$O; mol wt 326.48. C 77.26%, H 9.26%, N 8.58%, O 4.90%. Prepn: M. Giannini, **DE 2099894** (1971 to Malesci), *C.A.* **75**, 20222a (1971); M. Giannini *et al.*, *Farmaco Ed. Sci.* **28**, 429 (1973). Pharmacology: A. Ferroni, G. Monticelli, *Pharmacol. Res. Commun.* **5**, 151 (1973). Clinical pharmacokinetics: B. Flouvat *et al.*, *Therapie* **37**, 143 (1982).

$bp_{0.1}$ 178°. LD_{50} i.p. in mice: 122 mg/kg (Giannini *et al.*).

Citrate. [94157-87-6] Meregon. $C_{21}H_{30}N_2O.C_6H_8O_7$; mol wt 518.60.

THERAP CAT: Antiarrhythmic (class III).

1486. Bunamiodyl Sodium. [1923-76-8] 2-[[2,4,6-Triiodo-3-[(1-oxobutyl)amino]phenyl]methylene]butanoic acid monosodium salt; 3-butyramido-α-ethyl-2,4,6-triiodocinnamic acid sodium salt; 3-(3-butyrylamino-2,4,6-triiodophenyl)-2-ethylacrylic acid sodium salt; α-ethyl-β-(2,4,6-triiodo-3-butyramidophenyl)acrylic acid sodium salt; α-(2,4,6-triiodo-3-butyrylaminobenzylidene)butyric acid sodium salt; sodium 3-butyramido-α-ethyl-2,4,6-triiodocinnamate; buniodyl; Bunaiod; Orabilex; Orabilix. $C_{15}H_{15}I_3$-$NNaO_3$; mol wt 660.99. C 27.26%, H 2.29%, I 57.60%, N 2.12%, Na 3.48%, O 7.26%. Prepn: Cassebaum, Dierbach, *Pharmazie* **16**, 389 (1961). Acute toxicity: J. O. Hoppe *et al.*, *J. Med. Chem.* **13**, 997 (1970).

Crystals from water (free acid, mp 105-120°). Slightly sol in water. LD_{50} in mice: 418 mg/kg i.v.; 2.78 g/kg orally (Hoppe).

THERAP CAT: Diagnostic aid (radiopaque medium).

1487. Bunazosin. [80755-51-7] 1-(4-Amino-6,7-dimethoxy-2-quinazolinyl)hexahydro-4-(1-oxobutyl)-1*H*-1,4-diazepine; 1-(4-amino-6,7-dimethoxy-2-quinazolinyl)-4-butyrylhexahydro-1*H*-1,4-diazepine; 4-amino-6,7-dimethoxy-2-[4-(*n*-butyryl)homopiperazin-1-yl]quinazoline; DDQ. $C_{19}H_{27}N_5O_3$; mol wt 373.45. C 61.11%, H 7.29%, N 18.75%, O 12.85%. Aminoquinazoline derivative with potent hypotensive properties. Prepn: T. Takahashi, H. Sugimoto, **BE 806626**; *eidem*, **US 3920636** (1974, 1975 to Eisai); alternative prepn: *eidem*, **JP Kokai 75 140474** (1975 to Eisai), *C.A.* **85**, 46769r (1976). *In vitro* and *in vivo* studies of adrenergic blocking action and antihypertensive properties: T. Shoji *et al.*, *Jpn. J. Pharmacol.* **30**, 763 (1980); K. Hoshi, S. Fujino, *ibid.* 427. Antihypertensive effect in volunteers: T. Kawasaki *et al.*, *Eur. J. Clin. Pharmacol.* **20**, 399 (1981). Pharmacokinetics: C. Yamato *et al.*, *Xenobiotica* **12**, 549 (1982).

Hydrochloride. [52712-76-2] E-643; Detantol. $C_{19}H_{27}N_5$-O_3.HCl; mol wt 409.91. Crystals from methanol/ethanol, mp 280-282°.

THERAP CAT: Antihypertensive.

1488. Bungarotoxins. Constituent proteins of the venom of the *Elapidae* snake, *Bungarus multicinctus* (Southeast Asian banded krait). Separation of the crude venom yields several fractions, the most important being **α-bungarotoxin (α-Bgt)** and **β-bungarotoxin (β-BuTX)**: C. C. Chang, C. Y. Lee, *Arch. Int. Pharmacodyn. Ther.* **144**, 241 (1963). α-Bgt is a single polypeptide chain of mol wt about 8,000 containing 74 amino acid residues with 5 disulfide bridges: D. Mebs *et al.*, *Biochem. Biophys. Res. Commun.* **44**, 711 (1971); *eidem*, *Z. Physiol. Chem.* **353**, 243 (1972). Purification, characterization, immunochemical studies: D. G. Clark *et al.*, *Biochemistry* **11**, 1663 (1972). It is a post-synaptic neurotoxin with curare-like action that binds irreversibly to acetylcholine receptor sites, producing neuromuscular blockade and skeletal muscle paralysis. Activity and use as a probe for acetylcholine receptors: C. C. Chang, *Nature* **215**, 1177 (1967); J. P. Changeux *et al.*, *Proc. Natl. Acad. Sci. USA* **67**, 1241 (1970); R. E. Oswald, J. A. Freeman,

Neuroscience **6**, 1 (1981). β-Bungarotoxin has been shown to contain several components, the major protein being designated as $β_1$- or β-bungarotoxin. It is composed of 2 subunits of mol wts of about 13,000 and 7,000, linked by disulfide bonds. The larger chain contains 120 amino acid residues including 13 half-cystine; the smaller chain contains 60 residues including 7 half cystine. Purification: T. Abe *et al.*, *Eur. J. Biochem.* **80**, 1 (1977); *eidem*, *Proc. R. Soc. London Ser. B* **207**, 487 (1980). Chemical properties, and amino acid sequence of the two polypeptide chains: K. Kondo *et al.*, *J. Biochem.* **83**, 91, 101 (1978). Complete purification and characterization of its action on synaptosomal accumulation and release of acetylcholine: J. W. Spokes, J. O. Dolly, *Biochim. Biophys. Acta* **596**, 81 (1980). β-BuTX is a pre-synaptic neurotoxin that prevents acetylcholine release at skeletal neuromuscular junctions without affecting the sensitivity of the post-synaptic membrane. Its proposed phospholipase A_2 activity is believed to be responsible for some of its effects at motor nerve terminals. Activity studies: P. N. Strong *et al.*, *Proc. Natl. Acad. Sci. USA* **75**, 1029 (1976); T. Abe, R. Miledi, *Proc. R. Soc. London Ser. B* **200**, 225 (1978); M. T. Alderdice, R. L. Volle, *Arch. Pharmacol.* **316**, 126 (1981). *Review*: A. T. Tu, *Venoms: Chemistry and Molecular Biology* (Wiley, New York, 1977) pp 185-187, 240-251.

The crude venom of *Bungarus multicinctus* is quite toxic, having an LD_{50} in mice (μg/g): 0.16 s.c. (Chang, Lee); also reported as 0.33 s.c. (Mebs, 1972). LD_{50} of α-Bgt in mice (μg/g): 0.21 s.c.; 0.15 i.p. (Mebs, 1972). LD_{50} of β-BuTX in mice (μg/g): 0.019 i.p. (Kondo).

USE: As exptl tools in investigating neuromuscular processes.

1489. Bunitrolol. [34915-68-9] 2-[3-[(1,1-Dimethylethyl)amino]-2-hydroxypropoxy]benzonitrile; *o*-[3-(*tert*-butylamino)-2-hydroxypropoxy]benzonitrile; 1-(2-cyanophenoxy)-2-hydroxy-3-*tert*-butylaminopropane; Ko-1366. $C_{14}H_{20}N_2O_2$; mol wt 248.32. C 67.71%, H 8.12%, N 11.28%, O 12.89%. β-Adrenergic blocker. Prepn: H. Koeppe *et al.*, **ZA 6803783**; *eidem*, **US 3541130** (1968, 1970 both to Boehringer, Ing.). Pharmacology: T. Kimura, *Experientia* **28**, 813 (1972). Studies on absorption, distribution, metabolism, excretion in rats and mice: T. Suzuki, T. Rikihisa, *Arzneim.-Forsch.* **29**, 1707 (1979). Clinical studies: A. Reale *et al.*, *J. Int. Med. Res.* **4**, 338 (1976); J. J. C. Jonker *et al.*, *Arzneim.-Forsch.* **31**, 1140 (1981). Toxicology study: M. Kanda *et al.*, *Oyo Yakuri* **9**, 457, 465, 499 (1975), *C.A.* **83**, 172616 (1975).

Hydrochloride. [23093-74-5] Betriol; Stresson. $C_{14}H_{20}N_2$-O_2.HCl; mol wt 284.78. Crystals from ethanol, mp 163-165°. LD_{50} in mice, rats (mg/kg): 1344-1440, 639-649 orally; 264-265, 222-225 i.p. (Kanda).

THERAP CAT: Antihypertensive, antiarrhythmic, antianginal.

1490. Bunte Salts. Water-sol salts of certain alkyl or aralkyl thiosulfuric acids of the general formula: $RSSO_2ONa$. Prepn: Lecher, Hardy, **US 2712547** (1955 to Am. Cyanamid); El-Heweki, Taeger, *J. Prakt. Chem.* **7**, 191 (1958); Tabushi *et al.*, *Kogyo Kagaku Zasshi* **67**, 478 (1964).

THERAP CAT (VET): Have been used as coccidiostats.

1491. Buparvaquone. [88426-33-9] 2-[[4-(1,1-Dimethylethyl)cyclohexyl]methyl]-3-hydroxy-1,4-naphthalenedione; 2-[(4-*tert*-butylcyclohexyl)methyl]-3-hydroxy-1,4-naphthoquinone; 3-(4-*t*-butylcyclohexyl)methyl-2-hydroxy-1,4-naphthoquinone; BW-720C; Butalex. $C_{21}H_{26}O_3$; mol wt 326.43. C 77.27%, H 8.03%, O 14.70%. Analog of antimalarial hydroxynaphthoquinones; *t*-butyl deriv of parvaquone, *q.v.* Prepn: A. T. Hudson, A. W. Randall, **EP 77550**; *eidem*, **US 4485117** (1983, 1984 both to Wellcome). *In vivo* and *in vitro* antiprotozoal activity: A. T. Hudson *et al.*, *Parasitology* **90**, 45 (1985); N. McHardy *et al.*, *Res. Vet. Sci.* **39**, 29 (1985). Treatment of bovine theileriosis: S. Dhar *et al.*, *Vet. Rec.* **119**, 635 (1986). Efficacy as a chemoimmunoprophylactic of theileriosis: *eidem*, *ibid.* **120**, 375 (1987).

Crystals, mp 124-125°. LD$_{50}$ orally in rats: >2 g/kg (Hudson).
THERAP CAT (VET): Antiprotozoal (Theileria).

1492. Buphanamine. [6793-24-4] (1α)-2,3-Didehydro-7-methoxycrinan-1-ol. C$_{17}$H$_{19}$NO$_4$; mol wt 301.34. C 67.76%, H 6.36%, N 4.65%, O 21.24%. Isoln from bulb of *Buphane (Boö-phane) disticha* Herb., Appleg. *(Haemanthus toxicarius* Herb.*) Amaryllidaceae:* Humber, Taylor, *Can. J. Chem.* **33**, 1268 (1955); Hauth, Stauffacher, *Helv. Chim. Acta* **44**, 491 (1961). From *B. fischeri* Baker: Renz *et al., ibid.* **38**, 1209 (1955). Identity with "oily" haemanthine: Goosen, Warren, *J. Chem. Soc.* **1960**, 1094. Structure and stereochemistry: Fales, Wildman, *J. Org. Chem.* **26**, 881 (1961). Revised structure: Wildman in *The Alkaloids* vol. **XI**, R. H. F. Manske, Ed. (Academic Press, New York, 1968) p 361. NMR of revised structure: Crain *et al., J. Am. Chem. Soc.* **93**, 990 (1971). High-resolution mass spectrum: P. Longevialle *et al., Org. Mass Spectrom.* **7**, 401 (1973).

Prisms from ethyl acetate, mp 183-185° (Fales); from acetone, mp 192-194° (Goosen). [α]$_{589}^{24}$ −195°; [α]$_{436}^{24}$ −408° (c = 0.97); [α]$_D^{20}$ −205° (c = 0.69, 95% ethanol); [α]$_D^{21}$ −194° (c = 0.247, chloroform). uv max: 287 nm (ε 1495).
Hydrochloride. C$_{17}$H$_{19}$NO$_4$.HCl. Prisms from ethanol + ether, mp 180°.

1493. Buphanitine. [4673-18-1] (1α,3α)-7-Methoxycrinan-1,3-diol; hemanthine; nerbowdine. C$_{17}$H$_{21}$NO$_5$; mol wt 319.35. C 63.94%, H 6.63%, N 4.39%, O 25.05%. Major alkaloid from *Buphane (Boöphane) disticha* Herb., Appleg. *(Haemanthus toxicarius* Herb.), *Amaryllidaceae.* Isoln: Lewin, *Arch. Exp. Pathol. Pharmakol.* **68**, 333 (1912); Tutin, *ibid.* **69**, 314 (1912). Identity with hemanthine: Goosen, Warren, *Chem. Ind.* **1957**, 267; with nerbowdine: Lyle *et al., J. Am. Chem. Soc.* **82**, 2620 (1960). Structure studies: Goosen, Warren, *J. Chem. Soc.* **1960**, 1097; Goosen *et al., ibid.* **1961**, 4038. High-resolution mass spectrum: P. Longevialle *et al., Org. Mass Spectrom.* **7**, 401 (1973).

Needles from chloroform + ether (changes crystalline form at 210°), mp 232°. Prisms from acetone. [α]$_D^{20}$ −102° (c = 1 in chloroform).
Hydrochloride. C$_{17}$H$_{22}$ClNO$_5$. mp 265°.
Nitrate. C$_{17}$H$_{22}$N$_2$O$_8$. mp 222-224°.

1494. Bupirimate. [41483-43-6] Dimethylsulfamic acid 5-butyl-2-(ethylamino)-6-methyl-4-pyrimidinyl ester; 5-butyl-2-(ethylamino)-6-methyl-4-pyrimidinyl dimethylsulfamate; PP-588; Nimrod. C$_{13}$H$_{24}$N$_4$O$_3$S; mol wt 316.42. C 49.35%, H 7.65%, N 17.71%, O 15.17%, S 10.13%. Prepn: A. M. Cole *et al., DE* **2246645**; *eidem,* **US 3880852** (1973, 1975 both to ICI). Activity:

J. R. Finney *et al., Proc. 8th Br. Insectic. Fungic. Conf.* **2**, 667 (1975).

Pale tan waxy solid, mp 50-51°. Vapor pressure at 20°: 5 × 10^{-7} mm Hg. Soly in water at 25°: 22 mg/l. Sol in most organic solvents except paraffins. Easily hydrolyzed by dil acids. LD$_{50}$ orally in rats: 4000 mg/kg (Finney).
USE: Fungicide.

1495. Bupivacaine. [2180-92-9] 1-Butyl-*N*-(2,6-dimethylphenyl)-2-piperidinecarboxamide; *dl*-1-butyl-2′,6′-pipecoloxylidide; 1-*n*-butyl-2′,6′-dimethyl-2-piperidinecarboxanilide; *dl*-N-*n*-butylpipecolic acid 2,6-xylidide; 1-butyl-2-(2,6-xylylcarbamoyl)-piperidine; *dl*-1-*n*-butylpiperidine-2-carboxylic acid 2,6-dimethylanilide. C$_{18}$H$_{28}$N$_2$O; mol wt 288.43. C 74.95%, H 9.78%, N 9.71%, O 5.55%. Prepn: B. Ekenstam *et al., Acta Chem. Scand.* **11**, 1183 (1957); B. T. Ekenstam, B. G. Pettersson, **US 2955111** (1960 to AB Bofors). Resolution of isomers: B. F. Tullar, *J. Med. Chem.* **14**, 891 (1971). Stereospecific synthesis: B. Adger *et al., Tetrahedron Lett.* **37**, 6399 (1996). Pharmacology of racemate: F. Henn, R. Brattsand, *Acta Anaesthesiol. Scand. Suppl.* **21**, 9 (1966), *C.A.* **66**, 17863u (1967); of isomers: F. P. Luduena *et al., Arch. Int. Pharmacodyn.* **200**, 359 (1972). Clinical pharmacokinetics: D. W. Blake *et al., Anaesth. Intensive Care* **22**, 522 (1994). Comprehensive description: T. D. Wilson, *Anal. Profiles Drug Subs.* **19**, 59-94 (1990). Review of use in spinal anesthesia: *Acta Anaesthesiol. Scand.* **35**, 1-10 (1991). Review of pharmacology and clinical efficacy of levobupivacaine: K. J. McClellan, C. M. Spencer, *Drugs* **56**, 355-362 (1998).

mp 107.5-108°. pKa 8.09; also reported as 8.17. Partition coefficient: (oleyl alcohol/water) 1565; (*n*-heptane/pH 7.4 buffer) 27.5.
Hydrochloride monohydrate. [14252-80-3] AH-2250; LAC-43; Carbostesin; Marcaine; Sensorcaine. C$_{18}$H$_{28}$N$_2$O.HCl.H$_2$O; mol wt 342.90. White, odorless crystalline powder. mp 258.5°. Slightly sol in acetone, chloroform, ether. Soly (mg/ml): water 40; alcohol 125. LD$_{50}$ in mice (mg/kg): 7.8 i.v., 82 s.c. (Henn, Brattsand).
(−)-Form. [27262-47-1] Levobupivacaine; (*S*)-bupivacaine. Crystals from isopropanol, mp 135-137°. [α]$_D^{25}$ −80.9° (c = 5 in methanol).
(−)-Form hydrochloride. [27262-48-2] Chirocaine. C$_{18}$H$_{28}$-N$_2$O.HCl; mol wt 324.89. mp 255-257°. [α]$_D^{25}$ −12.3° (c = 2 in water).
THERAP CAT: Anesthetic (local).

1496. Bupranolol. [14556-46-8] 1-(2-Chloro-5-methylphenoxy)-3-[(1,1-dimethylethyl)amino]-2-propanol; 1-(*tert*-butylamino)-3-[(6-chloro-*m*-tolyl)oxy]-2-propanol; 1-(6-chloro-3-methylphenoxy)-3-*tert*-butylaminopropan-2-ol; 1-*tert*-butylamino-3-(2-chloro-5-methylphenoxy)-2-propanol; bupranol; Ophtorenin. C$_{14}$-H$_{22}$ClNO$_2$; mol wt 271.78. C 61.87%, H 8.16%, Cl 13.04%, N 5.15%, O 11.77%. β-Adrenergic blocker. Prepn: Kunz *et al., DE* **1236523** (1967 to Sanol-Arzneimittel Dr. Schwarz), *C.A.* **67**, 64046k (1967) and **US 3309406** (1967). Pharmacology: Waterloh *et al., Arzneim.-Forsch.* **19**, 153, 330, 1710 (1969); Pendleton *et al., Arch. Int. Pharmacodyn. Ther.* **187**, 75 (1970); P. Montastruc *et al., Arch. Farmacol. Toxicol.* **3**, 93 (1977).

Hydrochloride. [15148-80-8] KL-255; Betadran; Betadrenol; Looser; Panimit. $C_{14}H_{22}ClNO_2 \cdot HCl$; mol wt 308.24. Crystals, mp 220-222°.

THERAP CAT: Antihypertensive; antianginal; antiarrhythmic; antiglaucoma.

1497. Buprenorphine. [52485-79-7] [5α,7α(S)]-17-(Cyclopropylmethyl)-α-(1,1-dimethylethyl)-4,5-epoxy-18,19-dihydro-3-hydroxy-6-methoxy-α-methyl-6,14-ethenomorphinan-7-methanol; 21-cyclopropyl-7α-[(S)-1-hydroxy-1,2,2-trimethylpropyl]-6,14-endo-ethano-6,7,8,14-tetrahydrooripavine; 21-cyclopropyl-7α-(2-hydroxy-3,3-dimethyl-2-butyl)-6,14-endo-ethano-6,7,8,14-tetrahydrooripavine; RX-6029-M. $C_{29}H_{41}NO_4$; mol wt 467.64. C 74.48%, H 8.84%, N 3.00%, O 13.69%. Analgesic that demonstrates narcotic agonist-antagonist properties. Prepn: K. W. Bentley, **GB 1136214**; idem, idem, 1968, 1969 to Reckitt & Sons). See also: K. W. Bentley, "The Morphine Alkaloids" in The Alkaloids vol. 13, R. F. Manske, Ed. (Academic Press, New York, 1971) pp 75-120. NMR and stereochemistry: B. C. Uff et al., Magn. Reson. Chem. **23**, 454 (1985). Pharmacokinetics and HPLC determn in whole blood: S.-Y. Liu et al., J. Chromatogr. B **818**, 233 (2005). Pharmacology: A. Cowan in Advan. Biochem. Psychopharmacol. **vol. 8**, M. C. Braude et al., Eds. (Raven Press, New York, 1974) pp 427-438; idem, J. Pharm. Pharmacol. **28**, 177 (1976); W. R. Martin et al., J. Pharmacol. Exp. Ther. **197**, 517 (1976). Metabolism: M. J. Rance, J. S. Shillingford, Biochem. Pharmacol. **25**, 735 (1976). Clinical study in chronic pain: M. Kjaer et al., Br. J. Clin. Pharmacol. **13**, 487 (1982). Clinical trial in treatment of opioid addiction: J. Kakko et al., Lancet **361**, 662 (2003). Review: J. W. Lewis, "Ring C-Bridged Derivatives of Thebaine and Oripavine" in Advan. Biochem. Psychopharmacol. **vol. 8**, M. C. Braude et al., Eds. (Raven Press, New York, 1974) pp 123-137. Review of pharmacology and therapeutic efficacy: R. C. Heel et al., Drugs **17**, 81-110 (1979).

Crystals, mp 209°.

Hydrochloride. [53152-21-9] CL-112302; NIH-8805; UM-952; Buprenex; Lepetan; Subutex; Temgesic. $C_{29}H_{41}NO_4 \cdot HCl$; mol wt 504.10. White powder. Slightly acidic. Limited solubility in water.

Note: This is a controlled substance (narcotic): **21 CFR**, 1308.13.

THERAP CAT: Analgesic (narcotic); in treatment of opioid dependence.

1498. Buprofezin. [69327-76-0] 2-[(1,1-Dimethylethyl)-imino]tetrahydro-3-(1-methylethyl)-5-phenyl-4H-1,3,5-thiadiazin-4-one; 2-tert-butylimino-3-isopropyl-5-phenylperhydro-1,3,5-thiadiazin-4-one; NNI-750; NNK-758; NN-29285; PP-618; Applaud. $C_{16}H_{23}N_3OS$; mol wt 305.44. C 62.92%, H 7.59%, N 13.76%, O 5.24%, S 10.50%. Insect growth regulator which inhibits chitin synthesis. Prepn: Z. Grünecker et al., **DE 2824126**; K. Ikeda et al., **US 4159328** (1978, 1979 both to Nihon Nohyaku); H. Kanno, Pure Appl. Chem. **59**, 1027 (1987). Mode of action study: T. Asai et al., Appl. Entomol. Zool. **20**, 111 (1985). Control of whiteflies and scale insects: I. Ishaaya et al., Meded. Fac. Landbouwwet. Univ. Gent **54**, 1003 (1989). GC-MS determn in clementine citrus: P.

Cabras et al., J. Agric. Food Chem. **46**, 4255 (1998). Persistence in olives and olive oil: idem et al., Food Addit. Contam. **17**, 855 (2000). Review of physical properties, activity and field trials: H. Kanno et al., Proc. Br. Crop Prot. Conf. - Pests Dis. **1981**, 59-66.

Crystals from isopropyl alcohol, mp 106.1°. Soly at 25° (g/l): acetone 240, chloroform 520, ethanol 80, toluene 320; water 0.9 mg/l. Vapor pressure at 25°: 9.4×10^{-6} mmHg. LD_{50} in mice, rats (mg/kg): 10000, 8740 orally. LC_{50} (48 hr) in carp: 2-10 mg/l (Kanno, 1981).

USE: Insecticide.

1499. Bupropion. [34911-55-2] 1-(3-Chlorophenyl)-2-[(1,1-dimethylethyl)amino]-1-propanone; (±)-2-(tert-butylamino)-3'-chloropropiophenone; m-chloro-α-(tert-butylamino)propiophenone; amfebutamone. $C_{13}H_{18}ClNO$; mol wt 239.74. C 65.13%, H 7.57%, Cl 14.79%, N 5.84%, O 6.67%. Unicyclic aminoketone with noradrenergic and dopaminergic activity. Prepn: N. B. Mehta, D. A. Yeowell, **DE 2059618** (1971 to Wellcome Found.); N. B. Mehta, **US 3819706** (1974 to Burroughs Wellcome). Pharmacology: F. Soroko et al., J. Pharm. Pharmacol. **29**, 767 (1977). Preclinical toxicology: W. E. Tucker, J. Clin. Psychiatry **44**, 60-62 (1983). Pharmacokinetics in smokers: P.-H. Hsyu et al., J. Clin. Pharmacol. **37**, 737 (1997). Clinical trial in attention deficit disorder with hyperactivity: C. K. Conners et al., J. Am. Acad. Child Adolesc. Psychiatry **34**, 1314 (1996); in smoking cessation: D. E. Jorenby et al., N. Engl. J. Med. **340**, 685 (1999). Review of pharmacology and clinical efficacy in depression: S. G. Bryant et al., Clin. Pharm. **2**, 525-537 (1983); of mechanism of action studies: J. A. Ascher et al., J. Clin. Psychiatry **56**, 395-401 (1995); of clinical use in smoking cessation: R. West, Expert Opin. Pharmacother. **4**, 533-540 (2003).

Pale yellow oil, $bp_{.005}$ 52°. Sol in methanol, ethanol, acetone, ether, benzene. Very hygroscopic and susceptible to decompn.

Hydrochloride. [31677-93-7] Budepion; Wellbutrin; Zyban. $C_{13}H_{18}ClNO \cdot HCl$; mol wt 276.20. Crystals from isopropanol and abs ethanol, mp 233-234°. Bitter, anesthetizing taste. Soly (mg/ml): water 312; alcohol 193; $0.1N$ HCl 333. pKa: 7.9. LD_{50} in mice, rats (mg/kg): 230, 210 i.p.; 575, 600 orally (Soroko).

THERAP CAT: Antidepressant; aid in smoking cessation.

1500. Buquinolate. [5486-03-3] 4-Hydroxy-6,7-bis(2-methylpropoxy)-3-quinolinecarboxylic acid ethyl ester; 4-hydroxy-6,7-diisobutoxy-3-quinolinecarboxylic acid ethyl ester; ethyl 6,7-diisobutoxy-4-hydroxyquinoline-3-carboxylate; Bonaid. $C_{20}H_{27}NO_5$; mol wt 361.43. C 66.46%, H 7.53%, N 3.88%, O 22.13%. Prepn: Watson, **BE 659237** (1965 to Norwich), C.A. **64**, 2071c (1966); corresp to **US 3267106** (1964).

Crystals, mp 288-291°.

THERAP CAT (VET): Coccidiostat.

1501. Buramate. [4663-83-6] (Phenylmethyl)carbamic acid 2-hydroxyethyl ester; benzylcarbamic acid 2-hydroxyethyl ester; 2-hydroxyethyl benzylcarbamate; glycol benzylcarbamate; AC-

601; Hyamate. $C_{10}H_{13}NO_3$; mol wt 195.22. C 61.52%, H 6.71%, N 7.17%, O 24.59%. Prepn from glycol cyclic carbonate and benzylamine: Viard, **GB 689705** (1953 to Chauny & Cirey).

Crystals, mp 40°.

THERAP CAT: Anticonvulsant; antipsychotic.

1502. Burgess Reagent. [29684-56-8] N,N-Diethyl-N-[[(methoxycarbonyl)amino]sulfonyl]ethanaminium inner salt; (methoxycarbonylsulfamoyl)triethylammonium hydroxide inner salt; methyl(carboxysulfamoyl)triethylammonium hydroxide inner salt; methyl-N-(triethylammoniumsulfonyl)carbamate. $C_8H_{18}N_2$-O_4S; mol wt 238.30. C 40.32%, H 7.61%, N 11.76%, O 26.86%, S 13.46%. Dehydrating agent. Synthesis method: G. M. Atkins, Jr., E. M. Burgess, *J. Am. Chem. Soc.* **90**, 4744 (1968). Prepn and applications in dehydration reactions: E. M. Burgess *et al.*, *ibid.* **92**, 5224 (1970); *eidem*, *J. Org. Chem.* **38**, 26 (1973). Prepn and reaction with primary alcohols to form urethanes: E. M. Burgess *et al.*, *Org. Synth.* **56**, 40 (1977). Reaction with epoxides: U. Rinner *et al.*, *Synlett* **2003**, 1247. Review of chemistry: C. Lamberth, *J. Prakt. Chem. Chem.-Ztg.* **342**, 518-522 (2000); K. C. Nicolaou *et al.*, *Chem. Eur. J.* **10**, 5581-5606 (2004).

Colorless needles from toluene, mp 71-72°.

USE: Reagent for dehydration of secondary and tertiary alcohols; source of heteroatoms (N, O, S) in organic synthesis.

1503. Buserelin. [57982-77-1] 6-[O-(1,1-dimethylethyl)-D-serine]-9-(N-ethyl-L-prolinamide)-10-deglycinamideluteinizing hormone-releasing factor (pig). $C_{60}H_{86}N_{16}O_{13}$; mol wt 1239.42. C 58.14%, H 6.99%, N 18.08%, O 16.78%. Synthetic nonapeptide agonist analog of LH-RH, *q.v.* Synthesis: W. Konig *et al.*, **DE 2438350**; *eidem*, **US 4024248** (1976, 1977 both to Hoechst); A. S. Dutta *et al.*, *J. Med. Chem.* **21**, 1018 (1978). Clinical pharmacology: A. Lemay *et al.*, *Fertil. Steril.* **37**, 193 (1982). Radioimmunoassay in plasma and urine: S. Saito *et al.*, *J. Immunol. Methods* **79**, 173 (1985). Veterinary use to increase conception rate: K. Moller, E. D. Fielden, *N. Z. Vet. J.* **29**, 214 (1981). Clinical evaluation in prostatic carcinoma: J. H. Waxman, *Br. J. Urol.* **55**, 737 (1983); as ovulatory stimulant for *in vitro* fertilization: V. MacLachlan *et al.*, *N. Engl. J. Med.* **320**, 1233 (1989). Review of pharmacokinetics and clinical profile: R. N. Brogden *et al.*, *Drugs* **39**, 399-437 (1990); of efficacy in prostatic carcinoma: H. J. de Voogt *et al.*, *Scand. J. Urol. Nephrol.* **Suppl 138**, 131-136 (1991).

5-oxoPro–His–Trp–Ser–Tyr–D-Ser(t-Bu)–Leu–Arg–ProNHCH₂CH₃

$[\alpha]_D^{20}$ −40.4° (c = 1 in dimethylacetamide).

Monoacetate. [68630-75-1] HOE-766; Receptal; Suprecur; Suprefact. $C_{60}H_{86}N_{16}O_{13}$·$C_2H_4O_2$; mol wt 1299.48.

THERAP CAT: Antineoplastic (hormonal). Gonad-stimulating principle.

THERAP CAT (VET): Gonad-stimulating principle.

1504. Buspirone. [36505-84-7] 8-[4-[4-(2-Pyrimidinyl)-1-piperazinyl]butyl]-8-azaspiro[4.5]decane-7,9-dione. $C_{21}H_{31}N_5O_2$; mol wt 385.50. C 65.43%, H 8.11%, N 18.17%, O 8.30%. Non-benzodiazepine anxiolytic; 5-hydroxytryptamine (5-HT₁) receptor agonist. Prepn: Y. H. Wu *et al.*, *J. Med. Chem.* **15**, 477 (1972); Y. H. Wu, J. W. Rayburn, **DE 2057845** (1971 to Bristol-Myers); *eidem*, **US 3717634** (1973 to Mead-Johnson). Pharmacology: L. E. Allen *et al.*, *Arzneim.-Forsch.* **24**, 917 (1974). Comparison with diazepam in treatment of anxiety: H. L. Goldberg, R. J. Finnerty, *Am. J. Psychiatry* **136**, 1184 (1979); A. F. Jacobson *et al.*, *Pharmacotherapy* **5**, 290 (1985). Nonsynergistic effect with alcohol: T. Seppala

et al., *Clin. Pharmacol. Ther.* **32**, 201 (1982). Disposition and metabolism: S. Caccia *et al.*, *Xenobiotica* **13**, 147 (1983). Series of articles on chemistry, pharmacology, addictive potential, and clinical trials: *J. Clin. Psychiatry* **43**, pp 1-116 (1982); on pharmacology, safety and clinical comparison with clorazepate: *Am. J. Med.* **80**, Suppl. 3B, 1-51 (1986). Review of pharmacology and therapeutic efficacy: K. L. Goa, A. Ward, *Drugs* **32**, 114-129 (1986). *Review:* M. W. Jann, *Pharmacotherapy* **8**, 100-116 (1988); D. P. Taylor, *FASEB J.* **2**, 2445-2452 (1988).

Hydrochloride. [33386-08-2] Ansial; Ansiced; Axoren; Bespar; Buspar; Buspimen; Buspinol; Buspisal; Narol. $C_{21}H_{31}N_5$-O_2·HCl; mol wt 421.96. Crystals from abs ethanol, mp 201.5-202.5°. LD₅₀ i.p. in rats: 136 mg/kg (Allen).

THERAP CAT: Anxiolytic.

1505. Busulfan. [55-98-1] 1,4-Butanediol dimethanesulfonate esters; 1,4-bis(methanesulfonoxy)butane; 1,4-di(methanesulfonyloxy)butane; 1,4-di(methylsulfonoxy)butane; methanesulfonic acid tetramethylene ester; tetramethylene bis(methanesulfonate); busulphan; CB-2041; GT-41; Busulfex; Misulban; Myleran. $C_6H_{14}O_6S_2$; mol wt 246.30. C 29.26%, H 5.73%, O 38.98%, S 26.04%. $CH_3SO_2O(CH_2)_4OSO_2CH_3$. Alkylating agent with antileukemic activity. Discovery: A. Haddow, G. M. Timmis, *Lancet* **1**, 207 (1953). Prepn: G. M. Timmis, **US 2917432** (1959 to Burroughs Wellcome). Chemosterilant effect in boll weevils: J. W. Haynes *et al.*, *J. Econ. Entomol.* **66**, 619 (1973); J. W. Haynes, J. E. Wright, *Southwest. Entomol.* **7**, 56 (1982). Pharmacokinetics: H. Ehrsson *et al.*, *Clin. Pharmacol. Ther.* **34**, 86 (1983). HPLC determn in human plasma: W. D. Henner *et al.*, *J. Chromatogr.* **416**, 426 (1987). Clinical pretreatment with cyclophosphamide, *q.v.*, for bone marrow transplants: G. W. Santos *et al.*, *N. Engl. J. Med.* **309**, 1347 (1983). Comparative clinical trial with mitobronitol, *q.v.*, in chronic myeloid leukemia: R. T. Silver *et al.*, *Cancer* **60**, 1442 (1987). Toxicity data: H. R. Scherf *et al.*, *Arzneim.-Forsch.* **20**, 1467 (1970). Review of pharmacology: C. D. R. Dunn, *Exp. Hematol.* **2**, 101-117 (1974); of toxicology: J. B. Bishop, J. S. Wassom, *Mutat. Res.* **168**, 15-45 (1986). Comprehensive description: M. Tariq, A. A. Al Badr, *Anal. Profiles Drug Subs.* **16**, 53-83 (1987).

Crystals, mp 114-118°. Soly in acetone at 25°: 2.4 g/100 ml; in alcohol: 0.1 g/100 ml. Practically insol in water, but will dissolve slowly as hydrolysis takes place. LD₅₀ i.v. in rats: 1.8 mg/kg (Scherf).

Caution: This substance is listed as a known human carcinogen: *Report on Carcinogens, Eleventh Edition* (PB2005-104914, 2004) p III-39.

USE: Insect sterilant.

THERAP CAT: Antineoplastic.

1506. Butabarbital Sodium. [143-81-7] 5-Ethyl-5-(1-methylpropyl)-2,4,6(1H,3H,5H)-pyrimidinetrione sodium salt; 5-*sec*-butyl-5-ethylbarbituric acid sodium salt; 5-ethyl-5-(1-methylpropyl)barbituric acid sodium salt; sodium 5-*sec*-butyl-5-ethylbarbiturate; sodium 5-ethyl-5-(1-methylpropyl)barbiturate; secbutobarbitone sodium; Asturidon; Bubarbital Sodium; Butabarbitone Sodium; Busodium; Busotran; Butabon; Butabar; Butak; Buta-Kay; Butrate; Butte; Buticaps; Butalan; Butanotic; Butex; Butatran; Butazem; Carrbutabarb; Butased; Butisol Sodium; Loubarb; Neravan; Prelital; Sarisol. $C_{10}H_{15}N_2NaO_3$; mol wt 234.23. C 51.28%, H 6.45%, N 11.96%, Na 9.82%, O 20.49%. Prepn: Shonle, **US 1856792** (1932 to Lilly).

Bitter powder. (The free acid mp 165-168°.) One gram dissolves in 2 ml water, in about 7 ml alcohol. Practically insol in ether, benzene. The pH of 10% aq soln 10.0-11.2 (USP XXI, 1985).

Note: This is a controlled substance (depressant): **21 CFR,** 1308.13.

THERAP CAT: Sedative, hypnotic.

1507. Butacaine. [149-16-6] 3-(Dibutylamino)-1-propanol 4-aminobenzoate; 3-(*p*-aminobenzoxy)-1-di-*n*-butylaminopropane; dibutylaminopropyl-*p*-aminobenzoate; *p*-aminobenzoyldibutyl-aminopropanol; Butelline. $C_{18}H_{30}N_2O_2$; mol wt 306.44. C 70.55%, H 9.87%, N 9.14%, O 10.44%. Prepd from *p*-nitrobenzoyl chloride and γ-di-*n*-butylaminopropanol followed by reduction of the NO_2 group to NH_2: O. Kamm *et al.*, **US 1358751**; Adams, Volwiler, **US 1676470**; A. Weston, **US 2437984** (1920, 1928, 1948 all to Abbott); Burnett *et al.*, *J. Am. Chem. Soc.* **59**, 2248 (1937); Kaye, Roberts, *ibid.* **73**, 4762 (1951). Toxicity study: Schmidt *et al.*, *Toxicol. Appl. Pharmacol.* **1**, 454 (1956).

Liquid, $bp_{0.11}$ 178-182°.

Sulfate. [149-15-5] Butyn Sulfate. $(C_{18}H_{30}N_2O_2)_2 \cdot H_2SO_4$; mol wt 710.96. Crystals from *n*-propanol, mp 138.5-139.5°. Also reported as mp 100-103°. Produces numbness of tongue on tasting. Affected by light. One gram dissolves slowly in somewhat less than 1 ml water, more rapidly on heating. Quite sol in warm alc, in acetone; slightly sol in chloroform. Practically insol in ether. Aq soln is practically neutral to litmus and may be boiled for sterilization without dec. LD_{50} i.v. in mice: 12.4 mg/kg (Schmidt). *Pharmaceutical Incompat.* Alkalies and alkaline-reacting substances liberate the free base as an oily liquid from solns. Bicarbonates produce a precipitate of butacaine carbonate. Iodine gives a brown precipitate. Chlorides form the almost insol butacaine chloride which may precipitate.

Hydrochloride. $C_{18}H_{30}N_2O_2 \cdot HCl$. Crystals from ethanol, mp 157-158.5°.

THERAP CAT: Anesthetic (local).

THERAP CAT (VET): Anesthetic (local).

1508. Butachlor. [23184-66-9] *N*-(Butoxymethyl)-2-chloro-*N*-(2,6-diethylphenyl)acetamide; *N*-(butoxymethyl)-2-chloro-2′,6′-diethylacetanilide; 2-chloro-2,6-diethyl-*N*-(butoxymethyl)acetanilide; CP-53619; Machete; Butanex. $C_{17}H_{26}ClNO_2$; mol wt 311.85. C 65.47%, H 8.40%, Cl 11.37%, N 4.49%, O 10.26%. Selective pre-emergent and pre-plant herbicide. Prepn: J. F. Olin, **US 3442945** (1969 to Monsanto). Toxicity data: A. Strateva, *Exp. Med. Morphol.* **13**, 123 (1974). Degradation: Y.-L. Chen, T.-C. Wu, *J. Pestic. Sci.* **3**, 411 (1978). Environmental persistence: T. Ohyama *et al.*, *Bull. Environ. Contam. Toxicol.* **39**, 555 (1987); and soil absorption: H.-C. Chiang *et al.*, *ibid.* **58**, 758 (1997). HPLC determn in soil: X. Weibing, *J. Environ. Sci. (China)* **8**, 504 (1996). Control of barnyardgrass: T. C. Miller *et al.*, *MAFES Res. Highlights* **46**, 4 (1983); in rice: B. S. Azad *et al.*, *Seed Farms* **15**, 29 (1989).

Light yellow oil, $bp_{0.5}$ 196°. d_4^{30} 1.0695. Soly in water at 20°: 20 mg/l. Sol in most organic solvents. LD_{50} orally in rats: 1740 mg/kg (Strateva).

USE: Herbicide.

1509. 1,3-Butadiene. [106-99-0] α,γ-Butadiene; bivinyl; divinyl; erythrene; vinylethylene; biethylene; pyrrolylene. C_4H_6; mol wt 54.09. C 88.82%, H 11.18%. $CH_2{=}CHCH{=}CH_2$. Manuf as a coproduct of hydrocarbon steam cracking to produce

ethylene. Also produced from ethanol; from petroleum gases, i.e., by catalytic dehydrogenation of butene or butene-butane mixtures; by cracking naphtha and light oil. Manuf: *Faith, Keyes & Clark's Industrial Chemicals*, F. A. Lowenheim, M. K. Moran, Eds. (Wiley-Interscience, New York, 4th ed., 1975) pp 164-172. Toxicity study: Carpenter *et al.*, *J. Ind. Hyg. Toxicol.* **26**, 69 (1944). *Reviews:* Norton, *Chem. Rev.* **31**, 319 (1942); Alder, "The Diene Synthesis" in *Newer Methods of Preparative Organic Chemistry* (Interscience, New York, 1948); Konrad, *Angew. Chem.* **62**, 491 (1950); Hillyer, Stallings, *Pet. Refin.* **35**(12), 157 (1956); A. S. Onishchenko, *Diene Synthesis* (New York, 1964); Bailey, "Butadiene" in *Vinyl and Diene Monomers* (part 2), E. C. Leonard, Ed. (Interscience, New York, 1971) pp 757-995; H. N. Sun, J. P. Wristers in *Kirk-Othmer Encyclopedia of Chemical Technology* vol. 4 (John Wiley & Sons, New York, 4th ed., 1992) pp 663-690. Review of toxicology: L. S. Birnbaum, *Environ. Health Perspect.* **101**, Suppl. 6, 161-167 (1993); and human exposure: *Toxicological Profile for 1,3-Butadiene* (PB93-110690, 1992) 148 pp; of carcinogenic risk: *IARC Sci. Publ.* **127**, 1-412 (1993).

Colorless gas. Mild aromatic odor. *Flammable and combustible.* mp −108.966°: Glasgow *et al.*, *Anal. Chem.* **22**, 1521 (1950). bp_{760} −4.5°. d_4^{-6} 0.650. Freezing pt −108.902°. Densities from −17.8° to 60°: *Ind. Eng. Chem. Anal. Ed.* **16**, 7 (1944). n_D^{-6} 1.4223. bp (at pressures greater than 1 atm): 2 atm: 15.3°; 5 atm: 47.0°; 10 atm: 76.0°; 20 atm: 114.0°; 30 atm: 139.8°; 40 atm: 160.0°. Critical temperature 161.8°; critical pressure 42.6 atm. Infrared absorption spectrum: *ibid.* 422. Stability: *Ind. Eng. Chem.* **36**, 3 (1944). Stabilization with *o*-dihydroxybenzene: **GB 569412**; with aliphatic mercaptans: **US 2373754.** Explosion limits in air, vol%: lower 2.0, upper 11.5. Polymerizes and copolymerizes easily, e.g. under the influence of sodium, thereby forming synthetic rubbers. Sparingly soluble in water; slightly soluble in methanol, ethanol; soluble in organic solvents such as diethyl ether, benzene, carbon tetrachloride. Alcohol dissolves about 40 vols at room temp. LC_{50} in rats (4 hr inhalation): 129,000 ppm; in mice (2 hr inhalation): 122,000 ppm (Birnbaum).

Caution: Potential symptoms of overexposure are irritation of eyes, nose and throat; drowsiness, lightheadedness; teratogenic and reproductive effects; direct contact with liquid may cause frostbite. See *NIOSH Pocket Guide to Chemical Hazards* (DHHS/NIOSH 97-140, 1997) p 34; *Patty's Industrial Hygiene and Toxicology* vol. 2B, G. D. Clayton, F. E. Clayton, Eds. (John Wiley & Sons, Inc., New York, 4th ed., 1994) p 1242, 1250-1252. This substance is listed as a known human carcinogen: *Report on Carcinogens, Eleventh Edition* (PB2005-104914, 2004) p III-37.

USE: As component in the manuf of polymers such as synthetic rubbers, plastics, resins. As a chemical intermediate for the production of many industral materials; in the manuf of adiponitrile.

1510. Butalamine. [22131-35-7] *N,N*-Dibutyl-*N′*-(3-phenyl-1,2,4-oxadiazol-5-yl)-1,2-ethanediamine; 5-[[2-(dibutylamino)ethyl]amino]-3-phenyl-1,2,4-oxadiazole; 3-phenyl-5-(dibutylaminoethylamino)-1,2,4-oxadiazole. $C_{18}H_{28}N_4O$; mol wt 316.44. C 68.32%, H 8.92%, N 17.71%, O 5.06%. Prepn: **FR M3334**; Aron-Samuel, Sterne, **US 3338899** (1965, 1967 to Aron-Samuel). Pharmacology and toxicity studies: J. Sterne *et al.*, *Therapie* **24**, 735 (1969); J. Sterne, *ibid.* 745; J. L. Fontaine, R. Fontaine, *ibid.* **25**, 961 (1970).

Hydrochloride. [56974-46-0] LA-1221; Adrevil; Hemotrope; Surem; Surheme. $C_{18}H_{28}N_4O \cdot HCl$; mol wt 352.90. mp 145°. LD_{50} in mice (mg/kg): 43 i.v., 2500 s.c., 625 orally; LD_{50} in rats (mg/kg): >4000 s.c., 1600 orally (Sterne).

THERAP CAT: Vasodilator (peripheral).

1511. Butalbital. [77-26-9] 5-(2-Methylpropyl)-5-(2-propenyl)-2,4,6(1*H,3H,5H*)-pyrimidinetrione; 5-allyl-5-isobutyl-barbituric acid; 5-allyl-5-(2-methylpropyl)barbituric acid; 5-isobutyl-5-allylbarbituric acid; alisobumal; allylbarbital; itobarbital; tet-rallobarbital; Sandoptal. $C_{11}H_{16}N_2O_3$; mol wt 224.26. C 58.91%, H 7.19%, N 12.49%, O 21.40%. Prepn: Volwiler, *J. Am. Chem. Soc.* **47**, 2236 (1925).

Prisms, mp 138-139°. Slightly bitter taste. Practically insol in water and petr ether. Sol in alcohol, chloroform, ether, acetone, glacial acetic acid, also in solns of fixed alkali hydroxides. A satd aq soln is acid to litmus.

Note: This is a controlled substance (depressant): **21 CFR,** 1308.13.

THERAP CAT: Sedative, hypnotic.

1512. Butamben. [94-25-7] 4-Aminobenzoic acid butyl ester; butyl aminobenzoate; *n*-butyl *p*-aminobenzoate; Butesin; Butoform; Planoform; Scuroforme. $C_{11}H_{15}NO_2$; mol wt 193.24. C 68.37%, H 7.82%, N 7.25%, O 16.56%. Prepn: Brill, *J. Am. Chem. Soc.* **43**, 1322 (1921); Adams, Volwiler, **US 1440652** (1923 to Abbott); **GB 252870**; *C.A.* **17**, 1243 (1923); *C.A.* **21**, 2478 (1927).

Crystals from alc, mp 57-59°. bp$_8$ 174°. One gram dissolves in about 7 liters of water. Sol in dil acids, alcohol, chloroform, ether, and fatty oils. It is hydrolyzed slowly when boiled with water.

THERAP CAT: Anesthetic (local).

THERAP CAT (VET): Anesthetic (local).

1513. Butamirate. [18109-80-3] α-Ethylbenzeneacetic acid 2-[2-(diethylamino)ethoxy]ethyl ester; 2-phenylbutyric acid 2-[2-(diethylamino)ethoxy]ethyl ester; 2-[2-(diethylamino)ethoxy]ethyl 2-phenylbutyrate; butamyrate. $C_{18}H_{29}NO_3$; mol wt 307.43. C 70.32%, H 9.51%, N 4.56%, O 15.61%. Prepd by the esterification of phenylethylacetyl chloride with diethylaminoethoxyethanol: **DE 1151515**; Heusser, **US 3349114** (1963, 1967, both to Hommel A.G.).

Practically colorless liquid with peculiar odor. bp$_1$ 140-155°. Practically insol in water. Very sol in alcohol, acetone, ether.

Citrate. [18109-81-4] Abbott 36581; HH-197; Acodeen; Panatus; Sincodix; Sinecod. $C_{18}H_{29}NO_3 \cdot C_6H_8O_7$; mol wt 499.55. White, hygroscopic crystals from acetone, mp 75°.

THERAP CAT: Antitussive.

1514. Butamisole. [54400-59-8] 2-Methyl-*N*-[3-(2,3,5,6-tetrahydroimidazo[2,1-*b*]thiazol-6-yl)phenyl]propanamide; (−)-2-methyl-3'-(2,3,5,6-tetrahydroimidazo[2,1-*b*]thiazol-6-yl)propion-anilide. $C_{15}H_{19}N_3OS$; mol wt 289.40. C 62.25%, H 6.62%, N 14.52%, O 5.53%, S 11.08%. Prepn: L. D. Spicer, J. J. Hand, **ZA 7105803** (1972 to Am. Cyanamid), *C.A.* **78**, 72151h (1973). Prepn and resolution of isomers: *eidem,* **FR 2199979**; *eidem,* **US 3899583** (1974, 1975 both to Am. Cyanamid). Efficacy and safety in dogs: B. T. Alford *et al., Vet. Med. Small Anim. Clin.* **74**, 487 (1979). Evaluation in horses and ponies: R. B. Grieve *et al., Am. J. Vet. Res.* **40**, 139 (1979).

Hydrochloride. [54400-62-3] CL-206214; Styquin. $C_{15}H_{19}$-$N_3OS \cdot HCl$; mol wt 325.86.

THERAP CAT (VET): Anthelmintic.

1515. Butane. [106-97-8] *n*-Butane. C_4H_{10}; mol wt 58.12. C 82.66%, H 17.34%. $CH_3CH_2CH_2CH_3$. Occurrence: in petroleum, Mabery, *J. Am. Chem. Soc.* **30**, 143 (1908); in natural gas and in refinery cracking products. Prepd from C_2H_5I and sodium amalgam: Löwig, *Jahresber. Fortschr. Chem.* **1860**, 397, *Beilstein* **vol. 1,** 118. Recovery of butanes from natural and refinery gases: Kirkbride, Bertelli, *Ind. Eng. Chem.* **35**, 1242 (1943); Walters, *ibid.* **47**, 2544 (1955); Gilmore, Bauer, *Oil Gas J.* **50**, 84, 90, 94, 119 (1951), *C.A.* **46**, 1743d (1952). Separation of butane and isobutane: Stone, *Pet. Refin.* **25**(4), 164 (1946), *C.A.* **43**, 2414 (1949). Handbook: *Butane-Propane Gases,* L. C. Denny *et al.,* Eds. (Chilton Co., Los Angeles, 4th ed., 1962) 383 pp.

Flammable gas. bp −0.50°. d(gas) 2.046 (air = 1). One vol of water dissolves 0.15 vol and 1 vol of alcohol 18 vols of the gas at 17° and 770 mm; 1 vol of ether or chloroform at 17° dissolves 25 or 30 vols of the gas, resp.

Caution: Potential symptoms of overexposure are drowsiness, narcosis, asphyxia; direct contact with liquid may cause frostbite. *See NIOSH Pocket Guide to Chemical Hazards* (DHHS/NIOSH 97-140, 1997) p 34.

USE: As producer gas; raw material for motor fuels, in the manuf of synthetic rubbers.

1516. Butaperazine. [653-03-2] 1-[10-[3-(4-Methyl-1-piperazinyl)propyl]-10*H*-phenothiazin-2-yl]-1-butanone; 2-butyryl-10-[3-(4-methyl-1-piperazinyl)propyl]phenothiazine; *N*-[γ-(4'-methyl-1'-piperazinyl)propyl]-3-butyrylphenothiazine; butyrylperazine; Bayer 1362; Repoise; Tyrylen. $C_{24}H_{31}N_3OS$; mol wt 409.59. C 70.38%, H 7.63%, N 10.26%, O 3.91%, S 7.83%. Prepn: Hoerlein *et al.,* **DE 1120451** (1961 to Bayer), *C.A.* **57**, 4677c (1962).

bp$_{0.05}$ 270-280°.

Dimaleate. [1063-55-4] Randolectil. $C_{24}H_{31}N_3OS \cdot 2C_4H_4O_4$; mol wt 641.73.

Maleate. $C_{24}H_{31}N_3OS \cdot C_4H_4O_4$. Crystals from carbon tetrachloride, mp 180-182°.

THERAP CAT: Antipsychotic.

1517. Butedronic Acid. [51395-42-7] (Diphosphonomethyl)butanedioic acid; (diphosphonomethyl)succinic acid; 2,3-dicarboxypropane-1,1-diphosphonic acid; DPD. $C_5H_{10}O_{10}P_2$; mol wt 292.07. C 20.56%, H 3.45%, O 54.78%, P 21.21%. Prepn: A. Heins *et al.,* **DE 2217692** (1973 to Henkel); *eidem,* **US 3923876** (1975 to Bayer A.G.); K. H. Worms, H. Blum, *Z. Anorg. Allg. Chem.* **457**, 219 (1979); and physical-chemical properties: N. Vanlic-Razumenic *et al., J. Serb. Chem. Soc.* **51**, 63 (1986). Clinical pharmacokinetics of ^{99m}Tc complex: C. Schümichen, H. Schmidt, *Nuklearmedizin Suppl.* **19**, 930 (1982). Clinical evaluation of ^{99m}Tc complex as skeletal imaging agent: G. Godart *et al., Clin. Nucl. Med.* **11**, 92 (1986).

Monohydrate. White crystalline powder from glacial acetic acid and water (15:1), mp 150°. uv max (water): 208 nm (ε 274).

Tetrasodium salt. [97772-98-0] Tc-924 (DPD); Teceos. $C_5H_6Na_4O_{10}P_2$; mol wt 380.00.

THERAP CAT: ^{99m}Tc complex as diagnostic aid (radioactive imaging agent).

1518. Butenafine. [101828-21-1] *N*-[[4-(1,1-Dimethylethyl)phenyl]methyl]-*N*-methyl-1-naphthalenemethanamine; *N*-(*p*-tert-butylbenzyl)-*N*-methyl-1-naphthalenemethylamine. $C_{23}H_{27}N$; mol wt 317.47. C 87.01%, H 8.57%, N 4.41%. Benzylamine antifungal; squalene epoxidase inhibitor. Prepn: T. Maeda *et al.*, **EP 164697**; *eidem*, **US 5021458** (1985, 1991 both to Kaken). Antifungal activity *in vivo*: T. Arika *et al.*, *Antimicrob. Agents Chemother.* **34**, 2250 (1990). Review of antifungal activity, mechanism of action, and clinical trials: R. Fukushiro *et al.*, in *Recent Progress in Antifungal Chemotherapy*, H. Yamaguchi *et al.*, Eds. (Dekker, New York, 1992) pp. 147-157. Clinical trial in treatment of athlete's foot: T. A. Syed *et al.*, *Clin. Drug Invest.* **9**, 393 (2000).

Hydrochloride. [101827-46-7] KP-363; Mentax. $C_{23}H_{27}$N.HCl; mol wt 353.93. Crystals from acetone + ethanol, mp 211-213°. Easily sol in methanol, ethanol, dichloromethane, chloroform. Slightly sol in water.

THERAP CAT: Antifungal.

1519. 1-Butene. [106-98-9] α-Butylene; ethylethylene. C_4H_8; mol wt 56.11. C 85.62%, H 14.37%. $CH_3CH_2CH=CH_2$. Occurs in oil and coal gas. Obtained by cracking of petr oils and by thermal decompn of butane or pentane or isopentane: Egloff *et al.*, *Ind. Eng. Chem.* **28**, 1283 (1936); Calingaert, *J. Am. Chem. Soc.* **45**, 130 (1923); from butyl alcohol by treatment with conc H_2SO_4: *Compt. Rend.* **176**, 813 (1923).

Gas. Not solid at −190°. bp$_{760}$ −6.47°. d$_4^{-6.47}$ 0.6255. Explodes in mixtures with oxygen. Description of properties: *Oil Gas J.* **44**, 119 (1945), *C.A.* **39**, 3783; *J. Am. Chem. Soc.* **50**, 1427 (1928).

Caution: May be narcotic in high concns. A simple asphyxiant.

1520. 2-Butene. [107-01-7] Pseudo-butylene; *sym*-dimethylethylene; β-butylene. C_4H_8; mol wt 56.11. C 85.62%, H 14.37%. $CH_3CH=CHCH_3$. Occurs in coal gas. Obtained by cracking of petroleum oils. From isobutanol by the action of hot $ZnCl_2$: LeBel, Greene, *Am. Chem. J.* **2**, 24 (1880). Configuration of the stereoisomeric forms: Kistiakowsky, *J. Am. Chem. Soc.* **57**, 879 (1935).

Flammable gas.

cis-**Form.** mp −139.3°; bp$_{760}$ 3.73°.

trans-**Form.** mp −105.8°; bp$_{744}$ 0.3-0.4°.

1521. Butethal. [77-28-1] 5-Butyl-5-ethyl-2,4,6(1*H*,3*H*,5*H*)-pyrimidinetrione; 5-butyl-5-ethylbarbituric acid; butobarbitone; Soneryl; Neonal; Butobarbital; Etoval. $C_{10}H_{16}N_2O_3$; mol wt 212.25. C 56.59%, H 7.60%, N 13.20%, O 22.61%. Prepn: **US 1609520** (1926). Pharmacology and toxicity: G. A. Alles *et al.*, *J. Pharmacol. Exp. Ther.* **89**, 356 (1947).

Crystals. Slightly bitter taste. mp 124-127°. One gram dissolves in about 5 ml alcohol, 10 ml ether. Practically insol in water;

insol in petr ether, aliphatic hydrocarbons. LD$_{50}$ i.p. in mice: 1.506 mM/kg (Alles).

Note: This is a controlled substance (depressant): **21 CFR**, 1308.13.

THERAP CAT: Sedative, hypnotic.

1522. Butethamate. [14007-64-8] Benzeneacetic acid α-ethyl-2-(diethylamino)ethyl ester; 2-phenylbutyric acid 2-(diethylamino)ethyl ester; β-diethylaminoethyl ethylphenylacetate; 2-diethylaminoethyl 2-phenylbutyrate. $C_{16}H_{25}NO_2$; mol wt 263.38. C 72.96%, H 9.57%, N 5.32%, O 12.15%. Prepn: Di Paco, Tauro, *Farmaco Ed. Sci.* **11**, 540 (1956); **CH 291375** (1953 to AG Hommel's Haematogen) and **CH 292596** (1953 to Chem. Fabrik "PARA"), *C.A.* **49**, 2505a,c (1955). Pharmacology: Jordan, *Arzneim.-Forsch.* **8**, 716 (1958); Fleisch *et al.*, *ibid.* **11**, 1119 (1961).

bp$_{11}$ 167-169°. n_D^{20} 1.4909.

Citrate. [3639-12-1] Abuphenine; Convenil; Hicoseen; Phenesin; Phenetin; Phenetin. $C_{16}H_{25}NO_2.C_6H_8O_7$; mol wt 455.50. Crystals from abs alcohol, mp 109-110°. Freely sol in water, alcohol.

THERAP CAT: Antitussive.

1523. Butethamine. [2090-89-3] 2-[(2-Methylpropyl)amino]ethanol 4-aminobenzoate (ester); 2-(isobutylamino)ethanol *p*-aminobenzoate (ester); 2-(isobutylamino)ethyl *p*-aminobenzoate. $C_{13}H_{20}N_2O_2$; mol wt 236.31. C 66.07%, H 8.53%, N 11.85%, O 13.54%. Prepn of the hydrochloride: Goldberg, **US 2139818** (1938 to Novocol Chem.); J. Büchi *et al.*, *Arzneim.-Forsch.* **14**, 161 (1964); **16**, 1657 (1966).

Formate. $C_{13}H_{20}N_2O_2.CH_2O_2$. mp 136-139°. Freely sol in water and alcohol. Slightly sol in chloroform, ether; very slightly sol in benzene. pH (1% aq soln): about 6.1.

Hydrochloride. [553-68-4] Ibylcaine; Monocaine. $C_{13}H_{20}N_2O_2.HCl$; mol wt 272.77. mp 192-196°. Sol in water, slightly sol in alcohol, chloroform, benzene. Practically insol in ether. pH (1% aq soln): about 4.7.

meta-**Isomer hydrochloride.** [553-58-2] Metabutethamine hydrochloride. $C_{13}H_{20}N_2O_2.HCl$. Bitter crystals, mp 181-184°. Sol in water. pH of 1:50 aq soln about 6.2. Slightly sol in alcohol, acetone, chloroform.

THERAP CAT: Anesthetic (local).

THERAP CAT (VET): Local anesthetic for nerve block.

1524. Buthalital Sodium. [510-90-7] Dihydro-5-(2-methylpropyl)-5-(2-propenyl)-2-thioxo-4,6(1*H*,5*H*)-pyrimidinedione monosodium salt; 5-allyl-5-isobutyl-2-thiobarbituric acid sodium salt; sodium 5-allyl-5-isobutyl-2-thiobarbiturate; 5-allyl-5-(2-methylpropyl)-2-thiobarbituric acid sodium salt; thialbutone sodium; Baytinal; Buthalitone Sodium; Thialisobumalnatrium; Transithal; Ulbreval. $C_{11}H_{15}N_2NaO_2S$; mol wt 262.30. C 50.37%, H 5.76%, N 10.68%, Na 8.76%, O 12.20%, S 12.22%. Prepn: Miller *et al.*, *J. Am. Chem. Soc.* **58**, 1090 (1936). Pharmacology: Schildt, Schildt, *Acta Pharmacol. Toxicol.* **19**, 377 (1962).

Pale yellow, hygroscopic powder. Freely sol in water, yielding alkaline solns. Partly sol in ethanol. Insol in ether, benzene.

Free acid. [468-65-5] $C_{11}H_{16}N_2O_2S$. Crystals, mp 147°.

Note: This is a controlled substance (depressant): **21 CFR,** 1308.13.

THERAP CAT: Anesthetic (intravenous).

1525. Buthiazide. [2043-38-1] 6-Chloro-3,4-dihydro-3-(2-methylpropyl)-2*H*-1,2,4-benzothiadiazine-7-sulfonamide 1,1-dioxide; 6-chloro-3,4-dihydro-3-isobutyl-7-sulfamoyl-1,2,4-benzothiadiazine 1,1-dioxide; thiabutazide; butizide; isobutylhydrochlorothiazide; Su-6187; S-3500; Eunephran; Saltucin. $C_{11}H_{16}ClN_3O_4S_2$; mol wt 353.85. C 37.34%, H 4.56%, Cl 10.02%, N 11.88%, O 18.09%, S 18.12%. Prepd from 5-chloro-2,4-disulfamoylaniline and isovaleraldehyde: Werner *et al., J. Am. Chem. Soc.* **82,** 1161 (1960); **GB 861367; GB 885078;** G. de Stevens, L. H. Werner, **US 3163645** (1961, 1961, 1964 all to Ciba); Topliss *et al., J. Org. Chem.* **26,** 3842 (1961).

Crystals, mp 241-245° (Werner, 1960); from methanol + chloroform, mp 228° (Topliss). An ingredient of *Modenol*.

THERAP CAT: Diuretic, antihypertensive.

1526. Buthionine Sulfoximine. [5072-26-4] 2-Amino-4-(*S*-butylsulfonimidoyl)butanoic acid; *S*-(3-amino-3-carboxypropyl)-*S*-butylsulfoximine; *S*-(*n*-butyl)homocysteine sulfoximine; BSO. $C_8H_{18}N_2O_3S$; mol wt 222.31. C 43.22%, H 8.16%, N 12.60%, O 21.59%, S 14.42%. Selective inhibitor of γ-glutamyl cysteine synthetase, an enzyme in the glutathione, *q.v.,* biosynthetic pathway. BSO-mediated depletion of intracellular glutathione has been associated with increased sensitivity of tumor cells to antineoplastic agents. Prepn: K. Hayashi, *Chem. Pharm. Bull.* **8,** 177 (1960). Synthesis and *in vitro* and *in vivo* enzyme inhibition: O. W. Griffith, A. Meister, *J. Biol. Chem.* **254,** 7758 (1979). Mechanism of action and metabolism in animals O. W. Griffith, *ibid.* **257,** 13704 (1982). Chemosensitization by BSO of melphalan-resistant murine leukemia cells *in vivo:* S. Somfai-Relle *et al., Biochem. Pharmacol.* **33,** 485 (1984); R. A. Kramer *et al., Cancer Res.* **47,** 1593 (1987). Enhanced melphalan, *q.v.,* cytotoxicity in human cancer cells *in vitro:* J. A. Green *et al., ibid.* **44,** 5427 (1984); and in mice bearing human tumor xenografts: H. S. Friedman *et al., J. Natl. Cancer Inst.* **81,** 524 (1989).

Crystals from aq ethanol, mp 214-215.5° (dec). Sol in water. Partition coefficient (octanol/water): 4.34 ±0.0004.

USE: Biological tool for depletion of glutathione.

1527. Butibufen. [55837-18-8] α-Ethyl-4-(2-methylpropyl)benzeneacetic acid; 2-(4-isobutylphenyl)butyric acid; Butilopan. $C_{14}H_{20}O_2$; mol wt 220.31. C 76.32%, H 9.15%, O 14.52%. Prepn: L. Aparicio *et al., DE 2505813; eidem, US 4031243* (1976, 1977 both to Juste); J. M. Carretero *et al., Eur. J. Med. Chem.* **13,** 77 (1978). Pharmacology: L. Aparicio, *Arch. Int. Pharmacodyn. Ther.* **227,** 130 (1977). Pharmacokinetics: R. Revilla De Granda *et al., An. R. Acad. Farm.* **43,** 419 (1977), *C.A.* **88,** 83349 (1978). HPLC determination: L. González Tavares *et al., Arzneim.-Forsch.* **42,** 818 (1992).

Solid, mp 51-53°. LD_{50} orally in mice: 810 mg/kg (Carretero).

THERAP CAT: Anti-inflammatory.

1528. Butirosin. [12772-35-9] Ambutyrosin. $C_{21}H_{41}N_5-O_{12}$; mol wt 555.58. C 45.40%, H 7.44%, N 12.61%, O 34.56%. Aminoglycosidic antibiotic complex obtained from fermentation filtrates of mucoid strains of *Bacillus circulans* (NRRL B-3312 and B-3313). Consists of two components, butirosin A (80-85%) and butirosin B (15-20%), isomers which differ only in the configuration at one carbon atom in the pentose moiety. Prepn: P. W. K. Woo *et al., DE 1914527; eidem, US 3541078* (1969, 1970 both to Parke, Davis). Isoln and characterization: Dion *et al., Antimicrob. Agents Chemother.* **2,** 84 (1972). Structures: Woo *et al., Tetrahedron Lett.* **1971,** 2617, 2621, 2625. Activity: Howells *et al., Antimicrob. Agents Chemother.* **2,** 79 (1972); Heifetz *et al., ibid.* 89. Synthesis of butirosin B: Ikeda *et al., J. Antibiot.* **25,** 741 (1972); Akita *et al., ibid.* **26,** 365 (1973). Proposed biosynthetic pathway to the butirosins: K. Takeda *et al., ibid.* **31,** 250 (1978).

| | Butirosin A : | R = OH | R' = H |
| | Butirosin B : | R = H | R' = OH |

Butirosin sulfate dihydrate. [51022-98-1] $C_{21}H_{41}N_5O_{12}.2-H_2SO_4.2H_2O$. No sharp mp, dec ~225°. $[\alpha]_D^{25}$ +29° (c = 2 in water). pKa' (water): 5.5, 7.2, 8.5, 9.4. Very sol in water; moderately sol in methanol; slightly sol in ethanol. LD_{50} i.v. in mice: 450-500 mg/kg (Howells).

Butirosin A. [34291-02-6] (*S*)-*O*-2,6-Diamino-2,6-dideoxy-α-D-glucopyranosyl-(1 → 4)-*O*-[β-D-xylofuranosyl-(1 → 5)]-*N*¹-(4-amino-2-hydroxy-1-oxobutyl)-2-deoxystreptamine. White, amorphous solid, melts with dec over wide range, beginning at ~149°. $[\alpha]_D^{25}$ +26° (c = 1.46 in water). pKa' (water): 5.6, 7.3, 8.7, 9.8.

Butirosin B. [34291-03-7] 1-*N*-[(*S*)-4-Amino-2-(hydroxybutyryl)]ribostamycin. Occurs as a dihydrate, melts over wide range beginning at 146°. $[\alpha]_D^{25}$ +33° (c = 1.5 in water). pKa' (water): 5.3, 7.1, 8.6, 9.8.

THERAP CAT: Antibacterial.

1529. Butoconazole. [64872-76-0] 1-[4-(4-Chlorophenyl)-2-[(2,6-dichlorophenyl)thio]butyl]-1*H*-imidazole. $C_{19}H_{17}Cl_3N_2S$; mol wt 411.78. C 55.42%, H 4.16%, Cl 25.83%, N 6.80%, S 7.79%. Imidazole derivative with antifungal properties. Prepn: K. A. M. Walker, **US 4078071** (1978 to Syntex). Prepn, toxicity, activity vs *Candida albicans* in mice: K. A. M. Walker *et al., J. Med. Chem.* **21,** 840 (1978). *In vitro* comparison with other antifungal agents: F. C. Odds *et al., J. Antimicrob. Chemother.* **14,** 105 (1984). Clinical trials in treatment of vulvovaginal candidiasis: W. Droegemueller *et al., Obstet. Gynecol.* **64,** 530 (1984); J. B. Jacobson *et al., Acta Obstet. Gynecol. Scand.* **64,** 241 (1985). Comparison with miconazole, *q.v.:* C. S. Bradbeer *et al., Genitourin. Med.* **61,** 270 (1985).

Crystals from cyclohexane, mp 68-70.5°.

Nitrate. [64872-77-1] RS-35887; Femstat; Gynomyk. $C_{19}-H_{17}Cl_3N_2S.HNO_3$; mol wt 474.79. Colorless blades from acetone/ethyl acetate, mp 162-163°. LD_{50} in mice, male, female rats (mg/kg): >3200, >3200, 1720 orally; >1600, 940, 940 i.p. (Walker).

THERAP CAT: Antifungal (topical).

1530. Butorphanol. [42408-82-2] 17-(Cyclobutylmethyl)-morphinan-3,14-diol; (−)-*N*-cyclobutylmethyl-3,14-dihydroxymorphinan; *levo*-BC-2627. $C_{21}H_{29}NO_2$; mol wt 327.46. C 77.02%, H 8.93%, N 4.28%, O 9.77%. Mixed opioid agonist-antagonist. Prepn: I. Pachter *et al., DE 2243961; eidem,* **US 3819635** (1973, 1974 to Bristol-Myers); I. Monkovic, T. Thomas, **US 3775414** (1973 to Bristol-Myers). Total synthesis and pharmacology: I. Monkovic *et al., J. Am. Chem. Soc.* **95,** 7910 (1973); *eidem, Can. J. Chem.* **53,** 3094 (1975). Clinical study: F. Vargas-Arreola *et al., Curr. Ther. Res.* **22,** 186 (1977). Antitussive effect: R. L. Cavanaugh *et al., Arch. Int. Pharmacodyn. Ther.* **220,** 258 (1976). *Review:* R. C. Heel *et al., Drugs* **16,** 473-505 (1978); F. S. Caruso *et al.,* in *Pharmacological and Biochemical Properties of Drug Substances* vol. **2,** M. E. Goldberg, Ed. (Am. Pharm. Assoc., Washington, DC, 1979) pp 19-57.

Solid, mp 215-217°. $[\alpha]_D$ −70.0° (c = 0.1 in methanol).
Tartrate. [58786-99-5] Stadol; Torbugesic; Torbutrol. $C_{21}H_{29}NO_2 \cdot C_4H_6O_6$; mol wt 477.55. Solid. mp 217-219°. $[\alpha]_D^{22}$ −64.0° (c = 0.4 in methanol). LD_{50} in mice, rats (mg/kg): 40-57, 17-20 i.v.; 395-527, 570-756 orally (Heel).
Note: This is a controlled substance: **21 CFR,** 1308.14.
THERAP CAT: Analgesic (narcotic).
THERAP CAT (VET): Analgesic (narcotic); antitussive.

1531. Butoxycaine. [3772-43-8] 4-Butoxybenzoic acid 2-(diethylamino)ethyl ester; 2-diethylaminoethyl *p*-butoxybenzoate. $C_{17}H_{27}NO_3$; mol wt 293.40. C 69.59%, H 9.28%, N 4.77%, O 16.36%. Prepd from *p*-butoxybenzoyl chloride and β-diethylaminoethanol: Christiansen, Harris, **US 2412966** (1946 to Squibb). Alternate prepn and activity: Reynaud *et al., Chim. Ther.* **2,** 25 (1967). *See also* Büchi *et al., Arzneim.-Forsch.* **18,** 610 (1968).

Hydrochloride. [2350-32-5] Stadacain. $C_{17}H_{27}NO_3 \cdot HCl$; mol wt 329.86. Heavy crystals, mp 146°.
THERAP CAT: Anesthetic (local).

1532. Butralin. [33629-47-9] 4-(1,1-Dimethylethyl)-*N*-(1-methylpropyl)-2,6-dinitrobenzenamine; *N-sec*-butyl-4-*tert*-butyl-2,6-dinitroaniline; dibutalin; Amchem 70-25; A-820; Amexine; Tamex. $C_{14}H_{21}N_3O_4$; mol wt 295.33. C 56.94%, H 7.17%, N 14.23%, O 21.67%. Pre-emergence herbicide. Prepn: J. J. Damiano, **DE 2058201;** *idem,* **US 3672866** (1971, 1972 both to Amchem). Activity: S. R. McLane *et al., Proc. South. Weed Sci. Soc.* **24,** 58 (1971). Soil persistence and metabolism: P. C. Kearney *et al., J. Agric. Food Chem.* **22,** 856 (1974). Photochemistry: J. R. Plimmer, U. I. Klingebiel, *ibid.* 689.

Yellow-orange crystals, mp 60-61°, bp$_{0.5}$ 134-136°. Vapor pressure at 25°: 1.3 × 10^{-5} mm Hg. Flash pt, open cup: 97°F (36°C). Soly in water at 25°: 1 mg/l. Soly at 25° (kg/kg): methanol 0.125; acetone 4.48; benzene 2.7; xylene 3.88; butanone 9.55; carbon tetrachloride 1.46. LD_{50} orally in rats: 2500 mg/kg (McLane).
USE: Herbicide.

1533. Butriptyline. [35941-65-2] 10,11-Dihydro-*N,N,β*-trimethyl-5*H*-dibenzo[*a,d*]cycloheptene-5-propanamine; 5-(3-dimethylamino-2-methylpropyl)-10,11-dihydro-5*H*-dibenzo[*a,d*]cycloheptene; 5-(2-methyl-3-dimethylaminopropyl)dibenzo[*a,d*][1,4]cycloheptadiene; butriptylene. $C_{21}H_{27}N$; mol wt 293.45. C 85.95%, H 9.27%, N 4.77%. Prepn: Winthrop, Davis, **BE 613750** (1962 to Ayerst, McKenna & Harrison), *C.A.* **57,** 15036c (1962); *eidem, J. Org. Chem.* **27,** 230 (1962); Villani, **US 3409640** (1968 to Schering). Review of pharmacology and clinical data: *see J. Med.* **2,** 249-343 (1971). Metabolic studies: Cameron *et al., Arzneim.-Forsch.* **24,** 93 (1974). Toxicity: Voith, Herr, *Arch. Int. Pharmacodyn. Ther.* **182,** 318 (1969).

Oil, bp$_1$ 180-185°.
Hydrochloride. [5585-73-9] AY-62014; Evadene; Evadyne. $C_{21}H_{27}N \cdot HCl$; mol wt 329.91. Crystals from isopropyl alcohol-ether, mp 188-190° (dec). uv max (methanol): 273, 270, 266 nm (ε 460, 441, 552). Freely sol in water; moderately sol in aliphatic alc, chloroform. Insol in ether, paraffinic hydrocarbons. LD_{50} in mice (mg/kg): 120 i.p.; 345 orally (Voith, Herr).
THERAP CAT: Antidepressant.

1534. Butropium Bromide. [29025-14-7] [3(*S*)-*endo*]-8-[(4-Butoxyphenyl)methyl]-3-(3-hydroxy-1-oxo-2-phenylpropoxy)-8-methyl-8-azoniabicyclo[3.2.1]octane bromide; 8-(*p*-butoxybenzyl)-3α-hydroxy-1α*H*,5α*H*-tropanium bromide (−)-tropate; *l*-[1-(*p*-*n*-butoxybenzyl)hyoscyaminium] bromide; BHB; Coliopan. $C_{28}H_{38}BrNO_4$; mol wt 532.51. C 63.15%, H 7.19%, Br 15.01%, N 2.63%, O 12.02%. Anticholinergic. Prepn: S. Tanaka, K. Hashimoto, **DE 1950378;** *eidem,* **US 3696110** (1970, 1972 both to Eisai); Tanaka *et al., J. Pharm. Soc. Jpn.* **92,** 510 (1972). Prepn of the labelled compound: Fujita *et al., J. Labelled Compd.* **9,** 149, 555 (1972). Activity: Akutsu, Ichikawa, *Showa Igakkai Zasshi* **32,** 494 (1972), *C.A.* **78,** 119243g (1973).

Crystals from ethanol-acetone, mp 166-168°; also reported as white needles from isopropanol, mp 158-160° (Tanaka, Hashimoto). $[\alpha]_D^{20}$ −21.7° (c = 0.5 in water). Freely sol in glacial acetic acid; sol in chloroform, DMF. Sparingly sol in ethanol; slightly sol in water, 0.1*N* HCl, 0.1*N* NaOH. Practically insol in acetone, ether, benzene. LD_{50} in male mice (mg/kg): 1500 orally; 660 s.c.; 12.0 i.v. (Tanaka, Hashimoto, 1972).
THERAP CAT: Antispasmodic.

1535. *n*-Butyl Acetate. [123-86-4] Acetic acid butyl ester. $C_6H_{12}O_2$; mol wt 116.16. C 62.04%, H 10.41%, O 27.55%. $CH_3COO(CH_2)_3CH_3$. Prepd from acetic acid and butyl alcohol: Leyes, Othmer, *Ind. Eng. Chem.* **37,** 968 (1945); Vogel, *J. Chem. Soc.* **1948,** 624; Zettlemoyer *et al.,* **US 2644839** (1953 to FMC); *Faith, Keyes & Clark's Industrial Chemicals,* F. A. Lowenheim, M. K. Moran, Eds. (Wiley-Interscience, New York, 4th ed., 1975) pp 171-177. Toxicity data: H. F. Smyth *et al., Arch. Ind. Hyg. Occup. Med.* **10,** 61 (1954).

Liquid. d_{20}^{20} 0.8826. bp 125-126°. mp −77°. n_D^{20} 1.3951. Flash pt, closed cup: 72°F (22°C). Sol in about 120 parts water at 25°; misc with alcohol, ether; sol in most hydrocarbons. LD_{50} orally in rats: 14.13 g/kg (Smyth).
Caution: Potential symptoms of overexposure are headache, drowsiness, narcosis; irritation of eyes, upper respiratory system

and skin. *See NIOSH Pocket Guide to Chemical Hazards* (DHHS/-NIOSH 97-140, 1997) p 36.

USE: Manuf lacquer, artificial leather, photographic films, plastics, safety glass.

1536. *sec*-Butyl Acetate. [105-46-4] Acetic acid 1-methylpropyl ester; acetic acid *sec*-butyl ester. $C_6H_{12}O_2$; mol wt 116.16. C 62.04%, H 10.41%, O 27.55%. $CH_3COOCH(CH_3)CH_2CH_3$. Prepd from *sec*-butanol and acetic anhydride: Altschul, *J. Am. Chem. Soc.* **68**, 2605 (1946). Prepn of *d*-form: Kenyon *et al., J. Chem. Soc.* **1935**, 1072; Bird, *Tetrahedron* **18**, 1 (1962). Prepn of *l*-form: Kenyon *et al., loc. cit.* Manuf: *Faith, Keyes & Clark's Industrial Chemicals,* F. A. Lowenheim, M. K. Moran, Eds. (Wiley-Interscience, New York, 4th ed., 1975) pp 171-177.

***dl*-Form.** Liquid. d_4^{25} 0.865. bp 112-113°. n_D^{25} 1.3866. Flash pt, open cup: 88°F (31°C). Slightly sol in water; sol in alcohol, ether.

***d*-Form.** Liquid, bp 116-117°. d_4^{19} 0.873. n_D^{18} 1.3899.

Caution: Potential symptoms of overexposure are irritation of eyes; headache; drowsiness; narcosis; dryness of upper respiratory system and skin. *See NIOSH Pocket Guide to Chemical Hazards* (DHHS/NIOSH 97-140, 1997) p 38.

1537. *tert*-Butyl Acetate. [540-88-5] Acetic acid 1,1-dimethylethyl ester; acetic acid *tert*-butyl ester. $C_6H_{12}O_2$; mol wt 116.16. C 62.04%, H 10.41%, O 27.55%. $CH_3COOC(CH_3)_3$. Prepn: Baker, Bordwell; Hauser *et al., Org. Synth.* coll. vol. III, 141, 142 (1955). Manuf from acetic acid and isobutylene: Young, Pare, US **3031495** (1962 to Sinclair); Wheeler *et al.,* US **3102905** (1963 to Celanese); Heisler *et al.,* US **3096365** (1963 to Texaco); *Faith, Keyes & Clark's Industrial Chemicals,* F. A. Lowenheim, M. K. Moran, Eds. (Wiley-Interscience, New York, 4th ed., 1975) pp 171-177.

Liquid, bp 97.8°. d_4^{20} 0.8665, d_4^{25} 0.8593. n_D^{20} 1.3870. Practically insol in water. Miscible with alcohol, ether.

Caution: Potential symptoms of overexposure are itching and inflammation of eyes; irritation of upper respiratory tract; headache; narcosis; dermatitis. *See NIOSH Pocket Guide to Chemical Hazards* (DHHS/NIOSH 97-140, 1997) p 38.

USE: As gasoline additive (Wheeler *et al.*).

1538. *tert*-Butylacetic Acid. [1070-83-3] 3,3-Dimethylbutanoic acid; 3,3-dimethylbutyric acid. $C_6H_{12}O_2$; mol wt 116.16. C 62.04%, H 10.41%, O 27.55%. $(CH_3)_3CCH_2COOH$. Prepn: Homeyer *et al., J. Am. Chem. Soc.* **55**, 4209 (1933); Botterson, Shulman, *J. Org. Chem.* **27**, 1059 (1962); A. Nilsson, R. Carlson, *Acta Chem. Scand.* **B34**, 621 (1980).

Liquid, bp$_{26}$ 96°, bp$_{739}$ 183.0-183.3°, bp 190°. mp 6-7°. n_D^{20} 1.4115 (Botterson, Shulman), also reported as 1.4096 (Homeyer *et al.*). d_4^{20} 0.9124.

1539. *n*-Butyl Acrylate. [141-32-2] 2-Propenoic acid butyl ester; acrylic acid *n*-butyl ester. $C_7H_{12}O_2$; mol wt 128.17. C 65.60%, H 9.44%, O 24.97%. $CH_2=CHCOOC_4H_9$. Prepn from *n*-butanol and methyl acrylate: Rehberg, *Org. Synth.* coll. vol. III, 146 (1955). Toxicity study: H. F. Smyth *et al., Arch. Ind. Hyg. Occup. Med.* **4**, 119 (1951).

Liquid. d_4^{20} 0.8986; d_4^{15} 0.9110; d_4^{12} 0.9117; d_4^{0} 0.9202. bp$_{760}$ 145°; also reported bp$_{760}$ 138°; bp$_{101}$ 84-86°; bp$_{25}$ 59°; bp$_{10}$ 39°; bp$_8$ 35°. n_D^{20} 1.4190; n_D^{12} 1.4254. Sp heat (−60°): 0.467 cal/g/°C; heat of vaporization 8.11 kcal/mol; heat of combustion 974.46 kcal/mol. Soly in water at 20°: 0.14 g/100 ml; at 40°: 0.12 g/100 ml. Soly of water in *n*-butyl acrylate at 20°: 0.8 ml/100 g. LD_{50} orally in rats: 3.73 g/kg (Smyth).

Polymer. Elastic, tacky substance. Brittle temp −45°.

Caution: Potential symptoms of overexposure to the monomer are irritation of eyes, skin, upper respiratory system; sensitization dermatitis; dyspnea. *See NIOSH Pocket Guide to Chemical Hazards* (DHHS/NIOSH 97-140, 1997) p 38.

USE: The monomer in the manuf of polymers and resins for textile and leather finishes, paint formulations, etc.

1540. *n*-Butyl Alcohol. [71-36-3] 1-Butanol; butyl alcohol; propyl carbinol. $C_4H_{10}O$; mol wt 74.12. C 64.82%, H 13.60%, O 21.59%. $CH_3CH_2CH_2CH_2OH$. Prepn by reduction of butyraldehyde with sodium borohydride: Chaikin, Brown, *J. Am. Chem. Soc.* **71**, 122 (1949). Manuf from ethylene oxide and triethylaluminum: Rudner, US **3091627** (1963 to Koppers); by oxidation of tributyl-

borane: Mirviss, US **3067235** (1962 to Esso). Manuf by carbohydrate fermentation, by hydrogenation of butyraldehyde, from crotonaldehyde: *Faith, Keyes & Clark's Industrial Chemicals,* F. A. Lowenheim, M. K. Moran, Eds. (Wiley-Interscience, New York, 4th ed., 1975) pp 178-185. Purification and vapor pressure: Biddiscombe *et al., J. Chem. Soc.* **1963**, 1954. Toxicity study: H. F. Smyth *et al. Arch. Ind. Hyg. Occup. Med.* **4**, 119 (1951).

Highly refractive liquid; burns with a strongly luminous flame; leaves a transitory greasy spot on paper. Odor similar to that of fusel oil, but weaker. d_4^{20} 0.810. bp 117-118°. mp −90°. Flash pt 36-38°C. n_D^{20} 1.3993. A mixture of 63% of the alcohol and 37% water forms a constant boiling mixture, boiling at 92°. Soly at 25°, 9.1 ml/100 ml H_2O: Booth, Everson, *Ind. Eng. Chem.* **40**, 1491 (1948). Sol in alc, ether and many other organic solvents. LD_{50} orally in rats: 4.36 g/kg (Smyth).

Caution: Potential symptoms of overexposure are irritation of eyes, nose and throat; headache, vertigo and drowsiness; corneal inflammation, blurred vision, lacrimation and photophobia; dermatitis; possible auditory nerve damage, hearing loss; CNS depression. *See NIOSH Pocket Guide to Chemical Hazards* (DHHS/NIOSH 97-140, 1997) p 38.

USE: As solvent for fats, waxes, resins, shellac, varnish, gums etc.; manuf lacquers, rayon, detergents, other butyl compds; in microscopy for preparing paraffin imbedding materials.

1541. *sec*-Butyl Alcohol. [78-92-2] 2-Butanol; butylene hydrate; 2-hydroxybutane; methyl ethyl carbinol. $C_4H_{10}O$; mol wt 74.12. C 64.82%, H 13.60%, O 21.59%. $CH_3CH_2CH(OH)CH_3$. Prepn by reduction of 2-butanone: Chaikin, Brown, *J. Am. Chem. Soc.* **71**, 122 (1949); Nystrom *et al., ibid.* 3245. Manuf by hydration of 2-butene or hydrocarbons contg butene: Dale *et al., Ind. Eng. Chem.* **48**, 913 (1956); Archibald, Mottern, US **2543820** (1951 to Standard Oil); Limerick, Wylie, US **2776324** (1957 to Shell). Purification and vapor pressure: Biddiscombe *et al., J. Chem. Soc.* **1963**, 1954. Prepn of *l*-form or *d*-form by hydroboration of *cis*-2-butene: Brown, US **3078313** (1963); Brown *et al., J. Am. Chem. Soc.* **86**, 397 (1964). Resolution of *dl*-form: Kantor, Hauser, *ibid.* **75**, 1744 (1953). Absolute configuration of *l*-form: Brown *et al., ibid.* **86**, 1071 (1964). Toxicity: H. F. Smyth *et al., Arch. Ind. Hyg. Occup. Med.* **10**, 61 (1954).

***dl*-Form.** Liquid, bp 99.5°. mp −114.7°. d_4^{20} 0.808. n_D^{20} 1.3949. Flash pt, open cup: 88°F (31°C). Sol in 12 parts water; misc with alcohol, ether. LD_{50} orally in rats: 6.48 g/kg (Smyth).

***d*-Form.** *Ref:* Leroux, Lucas, *J. Am. Chem. Soc.* **73**, 41 (1951). Liquid, d_4^{27} 0.8025. n_D^{27} 1.3954. $[\alpha]_D^{27}$ +13.52°.

***l*-Form.** *Ref:* Leroux, Lucas, *loc. cit.* Liquid, bp$_{744}$ 98°. d_4^{25} 0.8042. n_D^{25} 1.3970, n_D^{25} 1.3949. $[\alpha]_D^{25}$ −13.51°.

Caution: Potential symptoms of overexposure are eye, skin, nose, throat irritation; narcosis. *See NIOSH Pocket Guide to Chemical Hazards* (DHHS/NIOSH 97-140, 1997) p 40.

USE: In the synthesis of flotation agents, flavors, perfumes, dyestuffs, wetting agents. In industrial cleaners, paint removers. Solvent for many natural resins, linseed and castor oils.

1542. *tert*-Butyl Alcohol. [75-65-0] 2-Methyl-2-propanol; trimethyl carbinol. $C_4H_{10}O$; mol wt 74.12. C 64.82%, H 13.60%, O 21.59%. $(CH_3)_3COH$. Prepd from acetyl chloride and dimethylzinc: Butlerow, *Ann.* **144**, 1 (1867). Manuf by catalytic hydration of isobutylene: Kreps, Nachod, US **2477380** (1949 to Atlantic Refining); Serniuk, Vanderbilt, US **2534304** (1950 to Standard Oil); by reduction of *tert*-butyl hydroperoxide: Lorand, US **2484841** (1949 to Hercules Powder); De Jong, US **2853532** (1958 to Shell). Purification: Biddiscombe *et al., J. Chem. Soc.* **1963**, 1954. Physical properties: *eidem, ibid.;* Dreisbach, Martin, *Ind. Eng. Chem.* **41**, 2875 (1949). Toxicity: Schaffarzick, Brown, *Science* **116**, 663 (1952).

Crystals, camphor-like odor, mp 25.6°. At 99.69 mol-% purity, bp 82.41°. mp 25.7°. d_4^{20} 0.78581, d_4^{25} 0.78086, d_4^{25} (calcd) 0.78080; n_D^{20} 1.38468, n_D^{25} 1.38231. Flash pt, closed cup: 52°F (11.1°C). Sol in water. Miscible with alcohol, ether. LD_{50} orally in rats: 3.5 g/kg (Schaffarzick, Brown).

Caution: Potential symptoms of overexposure are drowsiness, narcosis; irritation of skin, eyes, nose, throat. *See NIOSH Pocket Guide to Chemical Hazards* (DHHS/NIOSH 97-140, 1997) p 40.

USE: Denaturant for ethanol, mfg flotation agents, flavors, perfumes; as solvent; in paint removers. Octane booster in gasoline.

1543. *n*-Butylamine. [109-73-9] 1-Butanamine; 1-amino-butane. $C_4H_{11}N$; mol wt 73.14. C 65.69%, H 15.16%, N 19.15%. $CH_3CH_2CH_2CH_2NH_2$. Prepn by reduction of butyral-doxime: Lycan *et al., Org. Synth.* **coll. vol. II,** 319 (1943). Usually manuf by catalytic alkylation of ammonia with butyl alcohol: Davies *et al.,* **US 2609394** (1952 to I.C.I.); Hindley, Fisher, **US 2782237** (1957 to British Celanese); Lemon, Myerly, **US 3022349** (1962 to Union Carbide); Shirley, Speranza, **US 3128311** (1964 to Jefferson Chem.). Manuf from butyraldehyde and ammonia in the presence of Raney nickel: Brimer *et al.,* **US 2518659** (1950 to Eastman Kodak). Toxicity study: C. H. Hine *et al., Arch. Environ. Health* **1,** 343 (1960).

Liquid, ammoniacal odor, bp 78°. mp $-50°$. d_4^2 0.7327. n_D^{20} 1.4010. Flash pt, open cup: 30°F ($-1°$C). Misc with water, alcohol, ether. LD_{50} orally in rats: 500 mg/kg (Hine).

Caution: Potential symptoms of overexposure are irritation of eyes, skin, nose and throat; headache; skin flushing and burns. See *NIOSH Pocket Guide to Chemical Hazards* (DHHS/NIOSH 97-140, 1997) p 40.

USE: Intermediate for pharmaceuticals, dyestuffs, rubber chemicals, emulsifying agents, insecticides, synthetic tanning agents.

1544. *sec*-Butylamine. [13952-84-6] 2-Butanamine; 2-aminobutane; Frucote; Deccotane; Tutane. $C_4H_{11}N$; mol wt 73.14. C 65.69%, H 15.16%, N 19.15%. $CH_3CH_2CH(NH_2)CH_3$. Prepn by reduction of ethyl methyl ketoxime: Lycan *et al., Org. Synth.* **coll. vol. II,** 319 (1943). Manuf: Taylor *et al.,* **US 2636902** (1953 to I.C.I.); Thurston, **US 2689868** (1954 to Am. Cyanamid). Resolution of *dl*-form: Leithe, *Ber.* **63,** 800 (1930); Bruck *et al., J. Chem. Soc.* **1956,** 921. Toxicity: Goldenthal, *Toxicol. Appl. Pharmacol.* **18,** 204 (1971).

***dl*-Form.** Liquid, bp 63°. mp $-104°$. d_4^{20} 0.724. n_D^{20} 1.394. Miscible with water, alc. LD_{50} orally in rats: 380 mg/kg (Goldenthal).

***d(S)*-Form.** Liquid, bp 63°. d_4^{15} 0.7308. n_4^{15} 1.3963. $[\alpha]_D^{15}$ +7.80° (neat).

***l*-Form.** Liquid, bp 63°. d_4^{19} 0.728. $[\alpha]_D^{19}$ $-7.64°$.

Caution: Irritating to skin and mucous membranes.

USE: Agricultural fungistat.

1545. *tert*-Butylamine. [75-64-9] 2-Methyl-2-propanamine; 2-aminoisobutane; 2-amino-2-methylpropane. $C_4H_{11}N$; mol wt 73.14. C 65.69%, H 15.16%, N 19.15%. $(CH_3)_3CNH_2$. Prepn: Campbell *et al., Org. Synth.* **coll. vol. III,** 148 (1955). Manuf: Gresham *et al.,* **US 2501509** (1950 to du Pont); Albert, Kibler, **US 2773097** (1956 to Firestone Tire & Rubber).

Liquid, bp 44-46°. mp $-72.65°$. d_4^{20} 0.6951, d_4^{25} 0.6867. n_D^{20} 1.37. Miscible with alcohol.

Hydrochloride. mp 310°. Sol in cold methanol, in boiling isopropyl alcohol.

1546. Butylate. [2008-41-5] Bis(2-methylpropyl)carbamo-thioic acid *S*-ethyl ester; diisobutylthiocarbamic acid *S*-ethyl ester; *S*-ethyl *N,N*-diisobutylthiocarbamate; butilate; diisocarb; R-1910; Sutan Plus; Anelda. $C_{11}H_{23}NOS$; mol wt 217.37. C 60.78%, H 10.67%, N 6.44%, O 7.36%, S 14.75%. Selective pre-planting herbicide. Prepn: H. Tilles, *J. Am. Chem. Soc.* **81,** 714 (1959); H. Tilles, J. Antognini, **US 2913327** (1959 to Stauffer). Metabolism: J. P. Hubbell, J. E. Casida, *J. Agric. Food Chem.* **25,** 404 (1977). Soil degradation: F. W. Roeth *et al., Weed Technol.* **3,** 24 (1989). HPLC determn in water: C. H. Marvin *et al., Anal. Chem.* **62,** 1495 (1990). Weed control in alfalfa: N. Sarpe *et al., Meded. Fac. Landbouwwet. Univ. Gent* **57,** 1117 (1992); in combination with atrazine, *q.v.,* in corn: G. D. Hoyt, *Crop Prot.* **14,** 75 (1995).

Clear liquid, bp_{21} 138°. n_D^{30} 1.4701; d 0.9417. Vapor press at 25°: 1.3×10^{-3} mm Hg. Soly in water at 25°: 45 mg/l.

USE: Herbicide.

1547. Butylated Hydroxyanisole. [25013-16-5] (1,1-Di-methylethyl)-4-methoxyphenol; 2(3)-*tert*-butyl-4-hydroxyanisole; BHA; Antrancine 12; Embanox; Nipantiox 1-F; Sustane 1-F; Tenox BHA. $C_{11}H_{16}O_2$; mol wt 180.24. C 73.30%, H 8.95%, O 17.75%. A mixture of **2-*tert*-butyl-4-methoxyphenol** (also called 3-*tert*-butyl-4-hydroxyanisole) and **3-*tert*-butyl-4-methoxyphenol** (also called 2-*tert*-butyl-4-hydroxyanisole). Prepn from *p*-methoxy-phenol and isobutene: R. H. Rosenwald, **US 2459540**; **US 2470902** (both 1949 to Universal Oil Products). Toxicity study: A. J. Lehman *et al., Adv. Food Res.* **3,** 197 (1951). Review of carcinogenic risk: *IARC Monographs* **40,** 123-159 (1986); antimicrobial activity: M. Riccach, *J. Food Saf.* **6,** 141-170 (1984); of physicochemical properties, antioxidant activity and toxicology: H. Verhagen *et al., Chem. Biol. Interact.* **80,** 109-134 (1991); of safety assessment as food additive: G. M. Williams *et al., Food Chem. Toxicol.* **37,** 1027-1038 (1999).

Waxy solid, mp 48-55°. bp_{733} 264-270°. Practically insol in water. Sol in petr ether (Skellysolve H), in 50% alcohol (or higher), in propylene glycol; alcohols. Sol in fats and oils. Exhibits antioxidant properties and synergism with acids, BHT, propyl gallate, hydroquinone, methionine, lecithin, thiodipropionic acid, etc. LD_{50} in mice, rats (mg/kg): 2000, 2200 orally (Lehman).

Caution: This substance is reasonably anticipated to be a human carcinogen: *Report on Carcinogens, Eleventh Edition* (PB2005-104914, 2004) p III-40.

USE: Antioxidant and preservative, esp in foods, cosmetics, pharmaceuticals; also rubber and petroleum products.

1548. Butylated Hydroxytoluene. [128-37-0] 2,6-Bis(1,1-dimethylethyl)-4-methylphenol; 2,6-di-*tert*-butyl-*p*-cresol; 2,6-di-*tert*-butyl-4-methylphenol; BHT; Antrancine 8; Tenox BHT; Ionol CP; Sustane; Dalpac; Impruvol; Vianol. $C_{15}H_{24}O$; mol wt 220.35. C 81.76%, H 10.98%, O 7.26%. Prepn from *p*-cresol and isobutylene: Stillson, **US 2428745** (1947 to Gulf); McConnell, Davis, **US 3082258** (1963 to Eastman Kodak). Toxicity study: W. A. McOmie *et al., J. Am. Pharm. Assoc.* **38,** 366 (1949). Review of physicochemical properties, antioxidant activity and toxicology: H. Babich, *Environ. Res.* **29,** 1-29 (1982); of antimicrobial activity: M. Raccach, *J. Food Saf.* **6,** 141-170 (1984); of safety assessment as food additive: G. M. Williams *et al., Food Chem. Toxicol.* **37,** 1027-1038 (1999).

Crystals, mp 70°. d_4^{20} 1.048. bp 265°. Flash pt (open cup): 260°F (127°C). Insol in water. Freely sol in toluene, sol in methanol, ethanol, isopropanol, methyl ethyl ketone, acetone, Cellosolve, petr ether, benzene, most other hydrocarbon solvents. Soly in liquid petrolatum (white oil): 0.5% w/w. More sol in food oils and fats than butylated hydroxyanisole. Good soly in linseed oil. LD_{50} orally in mice: 1040 mg/kg (McOmie).

Caution: Potential symptoms of overexposure are irritation of eyes and skin. See *NIOSH Pocket Guide to Chemical Hazards* (DHHS/NIOSH 97-140, 1997) p 124.

USE: Antioxidant for food, animal feed, petroleum products, synthetic rubbers, plastics, animal and vegetable oils, soaps. Anti-skinning agent in paints and inks.

1549. *n*-Butylbenzene. [104-51-8] 1-Phenylbutane. $C_{10}H_{14}$; mol wt 134.22. C 89.49%, H 10.51%. $C_6H_5(CH_2)_3CH_3$. Prepn: Radziszewski, *Ber.* **9,** 261 (1876); Balbiano, *Ber.* **10,** 296 (1877); Read, Foster, *J. Am. Chem. Soc.* **48,** 1606 (1926).

Liquid, mp −88.5°. d_4^{20} 0.8604. bp_{760} 183.1°; bp_{400} 159.2°; bp_{200} 136.9°; bp_{100} 116.2°; bp_{60} 102.6°; bp_{40} 92.4°; bp_{20} 76.3°; bp_{10} 62.0°; bp_5 48.8°; $bp_{1.0}$ 22.7°. n_D^{20} 1.49040. Flash pt, open cup: 160°F (71°C). Insol in water. Miscible with alcohol, ether, benzene.

1550. sec-Butylbenzene. [135-98-8] (1-Methylpropyl)benzene; 2-phenylbutane. $C_{10}H_{14}$; mol wt 134.22. C 89.49%, H 10.51%. $C_6H_5CH(CH_3)CH_2CH_3$. Prepd from benzene and n-butyl chloride in presence of $AlCl_3$: Schramm, *Monatsh. Chem.* **9**, 621 (1888); by the action of sodium on γ-chloro-sec-butylbenzene: Braun et al., *Ber.* **46**, 1277 (1913); with other products by heating n- or sec-butyl alcohol with 80% H_2SO_4: Meyer, Bernhauer, *Monatsh. Chem.* **53**, 727 (1929).

Liquid, mp −82.7°. d_4^{20} 0.8608. bp_{760} 173.5°; bp_{400} 150.3°; bp_{200} 128.8°; bp_{100} 109.5°; bp_{60} 96.0°; bp_{40} 86.2°; bp_{20} 70.6°; bp_{10} 57.0°; bp_5 44.2°; $bp_{1.0}$ 18.6°. n_D^{20} 1.48980. Flash pt, closed cup: 126°F (52°C). Insol in water. Misc with alcohol, ether, benzene.

d-Form. $[\alpha]_D^{25}$ +26.6°: Bonner, Greenlee, *J. Am. Chem. Soc.* **81**, 3336 (1959).

l-Form. $[\alpha]_D^{25}$ −27.3°.

USE: Solvent; in organic syntheses.

1551. tert-Butylbenzene. [98-06-6] (1,1-Dimethylethyl)-benzene; 2-methyl-2-phenylpropane; trimethylphenylmethane; pseudobutylbenzene. $C_{10}H_{14}$; mol wt 134.22. C 89.49%, H 10.51%. Prepn: Konowalow, *Bull. Soc. Chim.* [3] **16**, 865 (1896); Shoesmith, Mackie, *J. Chem. Soc.* **1928**, 2336; Meyer, Bernhauer, *Monatsh. Chem.* **53**, 727 (1929); Wilt, Abegg, *J. Org. Chem.* **33**, 923 (1968). *See also* Groose, Ipatieff, *J. Am. Chem. Soc.* **57**, 2415 (1935); Ipatieff, Pines, *ibid.* **58**, 1056 (1936).

Liquid, mp −58.1°. d_4^{20} 0.8669. bp_{760} 168.5°; bp_{400} 145.8°; bp_{200} 123.7°; bp_{100} 103.8°; bp_{60} 90.6°; bp_{40} 80.8°; bp_{20} 65.6°; bp_{10} 51.7°; bp_5 39.0°; $bp_{1.0}$ 13.0°. n_D^{20} 1.49235. Flash pt, open cup: 140°F (60°C). Insol in water. Misc with alcohol, ether, benzene.

1552. n-Butyl Benzoate. [136-60-7] Benzoic acid butyl ester. $C_{11}H_{14}O_2$; mol wt 178.23. C 74.13%, H 7.92%, O 17.95%. $C_6H_5COO(CH_2)_3CH_3$. Prepn: Newman, Fones, *J. Am. Chem. Soc.* **69**, 1046 (1947); Justoni, *GB 719891* (1954 to Vismara). Toxicity study: H. F. Smyth et al., *Arch. Ind. Hyg. Occup. Med.* **10**, 61 (1954).

Thick, oily liquid. d 1.00. mp −22°. bp 250°. Practically insoluble in water. Sol in alcohol or ether. LD_{50} orally in rats: 5.14 g/kg (Smyth).

1553. n-Butyl Bromide. [109-65-9] 1-Bromobutane. C_4H_9Br; mol wt 137.02. C 35.06%, H 6.62%, Br 58.32%. $CH_3-(CH_2)_3Br$. Prepd from n-butyl alc and a hydrobromic-sulfuric acid mixture: Kamm, Marvel, *Org. Synth.* **vol. 1**, 5 (1921); Skau, McCullough, *J. Am. Chem. Soc.* **57**, 2440 (1935).

Colorless liquid. d_4^{25} 1.2686. bp_{760} 101.3°. mp −112°. n_D^{20} 1.4398. Insol in water. Sol in alcohol, ether.

1554. sec-Butyl Bromide. [78-76-2] 2-Bromobutane; methylethylbromomethane. C_4H_9Br; mol wt 137.02. C 35.06%, H 6.62%, Br 58.32%. $CH_3CH_2CHBrCH_3$. Prepn: Levene, Marker, *J. Biol. Chem.* **91**, 405 (1931); Kenyon et al., *J. Chem. Soc.* **1935**, 1080; Skau, McCullough, *J. Am. Chem. Soc.* **57**, 2440 (1935); Colson et al., *J. Chem. Soc.* **1965**, 2364. Prepn of optically pure isomers: Goodwin, Hudson, *J. Chem. Soc. B* **1968**, 1333.

dl-Form. Colorless liquid, pleasant odor. d_4^{25} 1.2530. bp 91.2°. mp −112°. n_D^{25} 1.4344. Insol in water. Freely sol in alcohol, ether.

d-Form. n_D^{20} 1.4359-1.4362. α_D^{20} +42.64°.

l-Form. n_D^{20} 1.4368. α_D^{20} −43.7°.

Caution: Narcotic in high concns.

1555. tert-Butyl Bromide. [507-19-7] 2-Bromo-2-methylpropane; 2-bromoisobutane; trimethylbromomethane. C_4H_9Br; mol wt 137.02. C 35.06%, H 6.62%, Br 58.32%. $(CH_3)_3CBr$. Prepn: Brunel, *J. Am. Chem. Soc.* **39**, 1978 (1917); Bryce-Smith, Howlett, *J. Chem. Soc.* **1951**, 1141; Coe et al., *ibid.* **1954**, 2281.

Colorless liquid. d_4^{25} 1.2125. bp 73.3°. mp −16.3°. At 210° changes to isobutyl bromide. n_D^{25} 1.4249. Insol in water. Miscible with organic solvents.

1556. n-Butyl n-Butyrate. [109-21-7] Butanoic acid butyl ester; butyric acid butyl ester. $C_8H_{16}O_2$; mol wt 144.21. C 66.63%, H 11.18%, O 22.19%. $CH_3(CH_2)_2COO(CH_2)_3CH_3$. Prepn from butyl alcohol: Robertson, *Org. Synth.* **coll. vol. I**, 138 (1941); Horton, *US 2522676* (1950 to Socony-Vacuum Oil).

Liquid, bp 165°. d_4^{20} 0.8692. n_D^{20} 1.4064. Practically insol in water. Miscible with alcohol, ether.

1557. Butyl Carbitol®. [112-34-5] 2-(2-Butoxyethoxy)ethanol; diethylene glycol monobutyl ether; butyl digol; Butyl Diicinol. $C_8H_{18}O_3$; mol wt 162.23. C 59.23%, H 11.18%, O 29.59%. $HOCH_2CH_2OCH_2CH_2OC_4H_9$. Prepn: Riemschneider, Gross, *Monatsh. Chem.* **90**, 783 (1959). Purification: Miller, Yonan, *J. Am. Chem. Soc.* **79**, 5931 (1957); Ridley, Ridley, *GB 795866* (1958 to Esso). Toxicity data: Smyth et al., *J. Ind. Hyg. Toxicol.* **23**, 259 (1941).

Practically odorless liquid, bp 230.4°. mp −68.1°. d_{20}^{20} 0.9536. n_D^{27} 1.4258. Miscible in water, oils. Miscibility in other organic solvents: Jackson, Drury, *Ind. Eng. Chem.* **51**, 1491 (1959). LD_{50} orally in rats, guinea pigs: 6.56, 2.00 g/kg (Smyth).

USE: Solvent.

1558. n-Butyl Carbonate. [542-52-9] Carbonic acid dibutyl ester; dibutyl carbonate. $C_9H_{18}O_3$; mol wt 174.24. C 62.04%, H 10.41%, O 27.55%. $(C_4H_9O)_2CO$. Prepn from ethyl carbonate, butyl alcohol and ethylmagnesium bromide: Frank et al., *J. Am. Chem. Soc.* **66**, 1509 (1944); from butyl alcohol and CO in the presence of Pd and $CuCl_2$: Mador, Blackham, *US 3114762* (1963 to National Distillers).

Liquid, bp 206.6°. d_4^{20} 0.9251, d_4^{25} 0.9388. n_D^{20} 1.4117. Practically insol in water. Miscible with ethanol, benzene, chloroform, acetone, ether and other organic solvents, *see:* Jackson, Drury, *Ind. Eng. Chem.* **51**, 1491 (1959).

1559. Butyl Cellosolve®. [111-76-2] 2-Butoxyethanol; ethylene glycol monobutyl ether. $C_6H_{14}O_2$; mol wt 118.17. C 60.98%, H 11.94%, O 27.08%. $HOCH_2CH_2OC_4H_9$. Prepn: L. H. Cretcher, W. H. Pittenger, *J. Am. Chem. Soc.* **46**, 1503 (1924); W. W. Carlson, *US 2448767* (1948 to Mellon Inst. Ind. Res.); R. Riemschneider, P. Gross, *Monatsh. Chem.* **90**, 783 (1959). Toxicity: H. F. Smyth et al., *J. Ind. Hyg. Toxicol.* **23**, 259 (1941); C. P. Carpenter et al., *Arch. Ind. Health* **14**, 114 (1956). Series of articles on toxicology: *Environ. Health Perspect.* **57**, 1-275 (1984). Review of toxicology and human exposure: *Toxicological Profile for 2-Butoxyethanol and 2-Butoxyethanol Acetate* (PB99-102527, 1998) 404 pp.

Liquid, bp 171-172°. d_4^{20} 0.9012, d_{20}^{20} 0.9019. n_D^{20} 1.4196. Flash pt, closed cup: 141°F (60°C). Sol in water, mineral oil, most organic solvents. LD_{50} orally in rats: 1.48 g/kg (Smyth).

Caution: Potential symptoms of overexposure are hemolysis, hemoglobinuria; CNS depression, headache; vomiting. Direct contact may cause irritation of skin, eyes, nose and throat. *See NIOSH Pocket Guide to Chemical Hazards* (DHHS/NIOSH 97-140, 1997) p 36. *See also Patty's Industrial Hygiene and Toxicology* **vol. 2D**, G. D. Clayton, F. E. Clayton, Eds. (Wiley-Interscience, New York, 4th ed., 1994) pp 2765, 2795-2804.

USE: Solvent for nitrocellulose, resins, grease, oil, albumin; dry cleaning.

1560. n-Butyl Chloride. [109-69-3] 1-Chlorobutane; n-propylcarbinyl chloride; butyl chloride. C_4H_9Cl; mol wt 92.57. C 51.90%, H 9.80%, Cl 38.30%. $CH_3CH_2CH_2CH_2Cl$. Prepd from n-butyl alcohol by heating with HCl and anhydr $ZnCl_2$: Whaley, Copenhaver, *J. Am. Chem. Soc.* **60**, 2497 (1938); *Org. Synth.* **coll. vol. I**, 142 (2nd ed., 1941). Toxicity study: H. F. Smyth et al., *Arch. Ind. Hyg. Occup. Med.* **10**, 61 (1954).

Liquid. *Highly flammable.* d_4^{15} 0.89197; d_4^{20} 0.88648; d_4^{25} 0.88098. One gallon weighs 7.35 pounds. bp_{760} 78.5°. n_D^{20} 1.40223. Flash pt −6.7°C (20°F). Dipole moment: 1.95. Practically insol in water (0.066% at 12°). Misc with alcohol, ether. LD_{50} orally in rats: 2.67 g/kg (Smyth).

USE: As butylating agent in organic synthesis, e.g., in the manuf of butyl cellulose.

THERAP CAT (VET): Anthelmintic.

1561. *sec*-**Butyl Chloride.** [78-86-4] 2-Chlorobutane; 2-chloro-3-methylpropane. C_4H_9Cl; mol wt 92.57. C 51.90%, H 9.80%, Cl 38.30%. $CH_3CH_2CHClCH_3$. Prepn from *sec*-butyl alcohol, hydrochloric acid and $ZnCl_2$: Norris, Taylor, *J. Am. Chem. Soc.* **46**, 756 (1924); Copenhaver, Whaley, *Org. Synth.* **coll. vol. I**, 143 (1941); from *sec*-butyl alcohol and PCl_3: Coulson *et al.*, *J. Chem. Soc.* **1965**, 2364. Prepn of optically pure isomers: Goodwin, Hudson, *J. Chem. Soc. B* **1968**, 1333. Toxicity data: H. F. Smyth *et al.*, *Am. Ind. Hyg. Assoc. J.* **30**, 470 (1969).

dl-**Form.** Liquid; pleasant, ethereal odor. d_4^{20} 0.871. bp 68°. n_D^{20} 1.3960; n_D^{25} 1.3953. One gram dissolves in 1000 ml water at 25°; misc with alcohol, ether. LD_{50} orally in rats: 20.0 ml/kg (Smyth).

d-**Form.** n_D^{20} 1.3963. α_D^{20} +30.8°.
l-**Form.** n_D^{20} 1.3968. α_D^{20} −31.0°.

1562. *tert*-**Butyl Chloride.** [507-20-0] 2-Chloro-2-methylpropane; 2-chloroisobutane; trimethylchloromethane. C_4H_9Cl; mol wt 92.57. C 51.90%, H 9.80%, Cl 38.30%. $(CH_3)_3CCl$. Prepd by shaking *tert*-butyl alcohol with concd HCl and distilling: Norris, Olmsted, *Org. Synth.* **8**, 50 (1928). Prepn from *tert*-butyl alcohol and PCl_3: Gerrard *et al.*, *J. Chem. Soc.* **1953**, 1920.

Liquid. d_4^{15} 0.847. n_D^{18} 1.38686. mp −26.5°. bp_{760} 51.0°; bp_{400} 32.6°; bp_{200} 14.6°; bp_{100} −1.0°; bp_{60} −11.4°; bp_{40} −19.0°. Sparingly sol in water, miscible with alcohol and ether. Boiling with water yields *tert*-butyl alcohol.

1563. *tert*-**Butyl Chloroacetate.** [107-59-5] Chloroacetic acid 1,1-dimethyl ester; *t*-butyl chloroacetate; chloroacetic acid *tert*-butyl ester. $C_6H_{11}ClO_2$; mol wt 150.60. C 47.85%, H 7.36%, Cl 23.54%, O 21.25%. $ClCH_2COOC(CH_3)_3$. Prepd by reacting monochloroacetic acid and isobutylene in dioxane in the presence of sulfuric acid: Johnson *et al.*, *J. Am. Chem. Soc.* **75**, 4995 (1953); from *tert*-butyl alcohol, chloroacetyl chloride and dimethylaniline: Baker, *Org. Synth.* **24**, 21 (1944).

Liquid, bp 155° (dec); bp_{11} 48-49°; bp_{16-17} 56-57°. n_D^{25} 1.4204-1.4210; n_D^{20} 1.4259-1.4260. Hydrolyzes to *tert*-butyl alcohol and chloroacetic acid.

USE: In the glycidic ester condensation.

1564. **Butyl Citrate.** [77-94-1] 2-Hydroxy-1,2,3-propanetricarboxylic acid tributyl ester; citric acid tributyl ester; *n*-butyl citrate; tributyl citrate. $C_{18}H_{32}O_7$; mol wt 360.44. C 59.98%, H 8.95%, O 31.07%. Prepn: Fodor, *Arch. Biochem.* **28**, 274 (1950). Synthesis from *n*-butyl alcohol and citric acid: Benedict, *Chemistry* **47**, 27 (1974).

Colorless or pale yellow, odorless liquid. d_{20}^{20} 1.045. bp_{22} about 233°. mp −20°. n_D^{20} 1.4460 (Benedict). Insol in water. Miscible with most organic liquids.

USE: Plasticizer and solvent for nitrocellulose lacquers; in polishes, inks and similar prepns; also as anti-foam agent.

1565. *n*-**Butyl Cyanoacrylate.** [6606-65-1] 2-Cyano-2-propenoic acid butyl ester; enbucrilate; NBCA; *n*-butyl 2-cyanoacrylate; Histoacryl; Indermil; Liquiband; Tisuacryl; Vetbond. $C_8H_{11}NO_2$; mol wt 153.18. C 62.73%, H 7.24%, N 9.14%, O 20.89%. Monomer rapidly polymerizes upon contact with fluid or tissue to form a strong, biodegradable adhesive. Preparative methods: A. E. Ardis, *US 2467927* (1949 to B. F. Goodrich); C. H. McKeever, *US 2912454* (1959 to Rohm & Haas). Prepn, polymerization and degradation: F. Leonard *et al.*, *J. Appl. Polym. Sci.* **10**, 259 (1966). Mechanism of polymerization and nanoparticle formation: N. Behan *et al.*, *Biomaterials* **22**, 1335 (2001). Characterization of polymer nanoparticles by particle size analysis: A. Bootz *et al.*, *Eur. J. Pharm. Biopharm.* **57**, 369 (2004); by MS: *idem et al.*, *ibid.* **60**, 391 (2005). Clinical experience in ophthalmic applications: A. B. Leahey *et al.*, *Ophthalmology* **100**, 173 (1993); in closure of surgical incisions: G. E. Amiel *et al.*, *J. Am. Coll. Surg.* **189**, 21 (1999). Clinical evaluation in augmentation rhinoplasty: M. E. Sachs, *Arch. Otolaryngol.* **111**, 389 (1985); in management of

bleeding gastric varices: B. D. Greenwald *et al.*, *Am. J. Gastroenterol.* **98**, 1982 (2003). Review of biomedical applications: C. Vauthier *et al.*, *Adv. Drug Delivery Rev.* **55**, 519-548 (2003).

Colorless liquid. $bp_{1.8}$ 68°. d^{20} 0.989. n_D^{20} 1.4424. n_D^{25} 1.4410. Insol in water. Flash pt, closed cup: >176°F (>80°C). Vapor pressure (25°): <0.5 mmHg. Surface tension: 31.11 dynes/cm. *Highly reactive with water and weak bases.*

Polymer. [25154-80-7] Poly(butyl 2-cyanoacrylate).

USE: Adhesive. Polymer nanoparticles as pharmaceutic aid for controlled release drug delivery.

THERAP CAT: Tissue adhesive.

THERAP CAT (VET): Tissue adhesive.

1566. *α*-**Butylene Dibromide.** [533-98-2] 1,2-Dibromobutane. $C_4H_8Br_2$; mol wt 215.91. C 22.25%, H 3.73%, Br 74.02%. $CH_3CH_2CHBrCH_2Br$. Prepn by bromination of butene: Wurtz, *Ann.* **152**, 21 (1869); of bromobutane: Kharasch *et al.*, *J. Org. Chem.* **20**, 1430 (1955).

Yellowish liquid, bp 166°. mp −65°. d_4^{20} 1.7946. n_D^{20} 1.5144. Practically insol in water; miscible with alcohol.

1567. **1,3-Butylene Glycol.** [107-88-0] 1,3-Butanediol; 1,3-dihydroxybutane; *β*-butyleneglycol; methyltrimethylene glycol; butane-1,3-diol. $C_4H_{10}O_2$; mol wt 90.12. C 53.31%, H 11.18%, O 35.51%. $CH_3CHOHCH_2CH_2OH$. Usually prepd by catalytic hydrogenation of aldol using Raney nickel: Hancock, Henson, *Ind. Eng. Chem.* **45**, 629 (1953); **GB 853266** (1960 to Celanese); F. S. Wagner in *Kirk-Othmer Encyclopedia of Chemical Technology* **vol. 11** (Wiley-Interscience, New York, 3rd ed., 1980) pp 956-962. Toxicity: Smyth *et al.*, *Arch. Ind. Hyg. Occup. Med.* **4**, 119 (1951).

Viscous liquid. The pure compd is colorless. d_{20}^{20} 1.004-1.006. One gallon weighs 8.398 lbs at room temp. Viscosity (cSt): 24.6 (50°); 96 (25°); 590 (0°); 3253 (−17.7°); 6059 (−23°). mp < 50°. Because of the high viscosity at low temps heating is necessary for pumping. Very hygroscopic: Will absorb 38.5 wt % of water within 144 hrs. at 81% relative humidity. bp 207.5°. n_D^{20} 1.4401. Flash pt (tag open cup): 250°F (121°C). Dielectric constant 28.8 at 25°. Surface tension: 37.8 dynes/cm at 25°. Sol in water, acetone, methyl ethyl ketone, ethanol, dibutyl phthalate, castor oil. Practically insol in aliphatic hydrocarbons, benzene, toluene, carbon tetrachloride, ethanolamines, mineral oil, linseed oil. LD_{50} orally in rats: 22.8 g/kg (Smyth).

USE: Intermediate in the manufacture of polyester plasticizers, humectant for cellophane, tobacco. Has some mold inhibiting action.

1568. **2,3-Butylene Glycol.** [513-85-9] 2,3-Butanediol; 2,3-dihydroxybutane; dimethylethylene glycol. $C_4H_{10}O_2$; mol wt 90.12. C 53.31%, H 11.18%, O 35.51%. $CH_3CH(OH)CH(OH)CH_3$. Occurs in 3 isomeric forms: *meso*- or *erythro*-, D(−)-*threo*-, and L(+)-*threo*-forms. The commercial product is usually either the *meso*- or the D(−)-form. Prepn of *meso*-form from *trans*-2,3-epoxybutane and of DL-form from *cis*-2,3-epoxybutane: Wilson, Lucas, *J. Am. Chem. Soc.* **58**, 2396 (1936). Prepn of D(−)- and L(+)-forms from corresponding D- and L-mannitols: Rubin *et al.*, *ibid.* **74**, 425 (1952). Manuf of D(−)-form by fermentation of carbohydrate solns with organisms of the *Bacillus subtilis* group: Vergnaud, *US 2529061* (1950 to Usines de Melle). Manuf from 2-butene: Cosby *et al.*, *US 2808429* (1957 to Allied Chem.); Keith *et al.*, *US 2974161* (1961 to Sinclair); from 2-butyne: Saegebarth, *US 3157704* (1964 to du Pont). Configuration: Morell, Auernheimer, *J. Am. Chem. Soc.* **66**, 792 (1944); Leroux, Lucas, *ibid.* **73**, 41 (1951); Rubin *et al.*, *loc. cit.*

meso-**Form** (*erythro*-**Form**). Hygroscopic crystals from dry diisopropyl ether, mp 34.4°. bp_{742} 181.7°, bp_{16} 89°. d_4^{25} 0.9939. n_D^{35} 1.4324. Moderately sol in diisopropyl ether.

DL-*threo*-**Form.** Hygroscopic crystals from diisopropyl ether, mp 7.6°. bp_{742} 172.7°, bp_{16} 86°. n_D^{25} 1.4310. Very sol in diisopropyl ether.

D(−)-*threo*-Form. mp 19.7°. bp$_{745}$ 179-180°, bp$_{10}$ 77.5-78°. d$_4^{25}$ 0.9869. n$_D^{25}$ 1.4315. [α]$_D^{25}$ −13.0° (neat).

L(+)-*threo*-Form. bp 179-182°. d^{25} 0.9872. n$_D^{25}$ 1.4306.

1569. n-Butyl Ether. [142-96-1] 1,1'-Oxybisbutane; butyl ether; *n*-dibutyl ether. C$_8$H$_{18}$O; mol wt 130.23. C 73.78%, H 13.93%, O 12.29%. (CH$_3$CH$_2$CH$_2$CH$_2$)$_2$O. Prepn: Smyth, *J. Chem. Educ.* **39**, 212 (1962); d'Engenieres *et al.*, *Bull. Soc. Chim. Fr.* **1964**(10), 2471. Toxicity study: H. F. Smyth *et al.*, *Arch. Ind. Hyg. Occup. Med.* **10**, 61 (1954).

Liquid. d$_{20}^{20}$ 0.769. mp −98°. bp 142-143°. Flash pt, closed cup: 100°F (37°C). Almost insol in water. Misc with alcohol or ether. Tends to form explosive peroxides, especially when anhydr. LD$_{50}$ orally in rats: 7.4 g/kg (Smyth).

1570. tert-Butyl Hydroperoxide. [75-91-2] 1,1-Dimethylethylhydroperoxide. C$_4$H$_{10}$O$_2$; mol wt 90.12. C 53.31%, H 11.18%, O 35.51%. Prepn from *tert*-butyl alcohol and 30% H$_2$O$_2$: N. A. Milas, S. A. Harris, *J. Am. Chem. Soc.* **60**, 2434 (1938); N. A. Milas, Surgenor, *ibid.* **68**, 205 (1946); US 2573947 (1951 to Shell). By oxidation of *tert*-butylmagnesium chloride: Walling, Buckler, *J. Am. Chem. Soc.* **75**, 4372 (1953); **77**, 6032 (1955).

Liquid. Stable to 75°. d$_4^{20}$ 0.896. mp −8°. bp$_{20}$ 35°. n$_D^{20}$ 1.4007. Sol in organic solvents. *Flammable*. Slow first-order decompn can be accelerated by the presence of 1 mol-% of Cu, Co and Mn salts.

USE: Catalyst in polymerization reactions. To introduce peroxy group into org molecules, in radical substitution reactions: Kharasch, Fono, *J. Org. Chem.* **23**, 325 (1948); *see also* Kharasch, Sosnovsky, *Tetrahedron* **3**, 97, 105 (1958).

1571. tert-Butyl Hypochlorite. [507-40-4] Hypochlorous acid 1,1-dimethylethyl ester; *t*-butyl hypochlorite. C$_4$H$_9$ClO; mol wt 108.57. C 44.25%, H 8.36%, Cl 32.65%, O 14.74%. (CH$_3$)$_3$-COCl. Prepd by adding *tert*-butyl alcohol to a cooled aq soln of NaOH and passing chlorine into the mixture: Teeter, Bell, *Org. Synth.* **32**, 20 (1952). By adding CO$_2$ to neutral aq *tert*-butyl alcohol and NaOCl satd with NaCl: Katz, US 2694722 (1954 to Bjorksten Res. Labs.).

Pale yellow liquid, irritating odor. d$_{20}^{20}$ 0.910; d$_4^{18}$ 0.9583. bp 77-78°. n$_D^{20}$ 1.403. Hydrolyzes in presence of aq alkali but not aq acid. Dec upon exposure to bright light to methyl chloride and acetone with considerable evolution of heat. Should be stored in an inert atmosphere in a dark, refrigerated place. Violent reaction occurs if exposed to rubber, strong light or overheating. Has far greater stability than the corresponding *n*-butyl and *sec*-butyl hypochlorites.

USE: Dehydration of alcohols; *N*- and *C*-chlorinations.

1572. Butylidene Chloride. [541-33-3] 1,1-Dichlorobutane. C$_4$H$_8$Cl$_2$; mol wt 127.01. C 37.83%, H 6.35%, Cl 55.83%. CH$_3$CH$_2$CH$_2$CHCl$_2$. Prepn from butyraldehyde and PCl$_5$: Henne *et al.*, *J. Am. Chem. Soc.* **61**, 938 (1939).

Oily liquid. bp$_{752}$ 114.8-115.1°. d^{25} 1.0797; n$_D^{25}$ 1.4305: Brown, Ash, *J. Am. Chem. Soc.* **77**, 4019 (1955). Practically insol in water. Sol in alcohol, chloroform, ether.

1573. n-Butyl Iodide. [542-69-8] 1-Iodobutane. C$_4$H$_9$I; mol wt 184.02. C 26.11%, H 4.93%, I 68.96%. CH$_3$CH$_2$CH$_2$-CH$_2$I. Prepn: Franzen, *Ber.* **87**, 1148 (1954); Landauer, Rydon, *J. Chem. Soc.* **1954**, 2281; Stone, Shechter, *Org. Synth.* **coll. vol. IV**, 321 (1963). Manuf: Huber, Schenck, US 2899471 and US 3053910 (1959 and 1962, both to GAF).

Liquid, bp 130.4°. mp −103.0°. d$_4^{20}$ 1.616. n$_D^{20}$ 1.4998: Vogel, *J. Chem. Soc.* **1943**, 636. Practically insol in water. Sol in alcohol, ether. *Protect from light.*

1574. sec-Butyl Iodide. [513-48-4] 2-Iodobutane. C$_4$H$_9$I; mol wt 184.02. C 26.11%, H 4.93%, I 68.96%. CH$_3$CH$_2$CHICH$_3$. Prepn of *dl*-form from 2-butanol: Kornblum *et al.*, *J. Am. Chem. Soc.* **77**, 5528 (1955); from dibutyl ether: Long, Freeguard, *Chem. Ind. (London)* **1965**, 223. Prepn of *d*-form from *l*-butanol: Kenyon *et al.*, *J. Chem. Soc.* **1935**, 1072. Prepn of *l*-form from *d*-2-butanol:

Levene, Rothen, *J. Biol. Chem.* **115**, 415 (1936); Kornblum *et al.*, *J. Am. Chem. Soc.* **70**, 746 (1948).

dl-Form. Liquid, rapidly turns brown on exposure to light. bp 120°. mp −104°. d$_4^{20}$ 1.592, n$_D^{20}$ 1.4991: Vogel, *J. Chem. Soc.* **1943**, 636. Practically insol in water. Sol in alc, ether. *Protect from light.*

l-Form. Liquid, bp 118°. d$_4^{20}$ 1.596, n$_D^{20}$ 1.495, [α]$_D^{24}$ −15.9° (neat); also reported as [α]$_D^{17}$ −31.98° (Kornblum *et al.*).

1575. Butyl Isocyanate. [111-36-4] 1-Isocyanatobutane; isocyanic acid butyl ester; *n*-butyl isocyanate; BIC. C$_5$H$_9$NO; mol wt 99.13. C 60.58%, H 9.15%, N 14.13%, O 16.14%. CH$_3$-(CH$_2$)$_3$N═C═O. Prepn: R. J. Slocombe *et al.*, *J. Am. Chem. Soc.* **72**, 1888 (1950); T. I. Bieber, *ibid.* **74**, 4700 (1952); E. T. Shawl *et al.*, EP 408277 (1991 to Arco). Toxicity study: J. Pauluhn, A. Eben, *Arch. Toxicol.* **66**, 118 (1992). Analytical methods development: R. J. Rando *et al.*, *J. Liq. Chromatogr.* **16**, 3977 (1993).

Flammable liquid. bp 113-116°. n$_D^{20}$ 1.4060. d$_4^{20}$ 0.880. LC$_{50}$ (4hr) in male, female rats (mg/m^3): 60, 55 by inhalation (Pauluhn, Eben).

USE: Reagent in organic synthesis.

1576. n-Butylmalonic Acid. [534-59-8] Butylpropanedioic acid; pentane-1,1-dicarboxylic acid. C$_7$H$_{12}$O$_4$; mol wt 160.17. C 52.49%, H 7.55%, O 39.96%. CH$_3$(CH$_2$)$_3$CH(COOH)$_2$. Prepd by the interaction of sodium *n*-amyl chloride and carbon dioxide under pressure with ligroin as solvent: Morton *et al.*, *J. Am. Chem. Soc.* **58**, 754 (1936).

Prisms from water, mp 102°. pK (5°): 2.96. Sol in water: 100 g of a satd aq soln contain 11.6 g at 0°; 79.3 g at 50°. Sol in alc, ether. Heating to 150° yields caproic acid.

Diethyl ester. C$_{11}$H$_{20}$O$_4$. Prepared by the interaction of *n*-butyl bromide, diethyl malonate, and sodium alcoholate: Adams, Kamm, *Org. Synth.* **4**, 11 (1925). Liquid, bp$_{760}$ 235-240°; bp$_{40}$ 140-145°; bp$_{20}$ 130-135°. n$_D^{20}$ 1.425. Very sol in alcohol, ether.

1577. n-Butyl Mercaptan. [109-79-5] 1-Butanethiol; normal butyl thioalcohol; thiobutyl alcohol. C$_4$H$_{10}$S; mol wt 90.19. C 53.27%, H 11.18%, S 35.55%. CH$_3$(CH$_2$)$_2$CH$_2$SH. Formed by the action of yeast on a product obtained when hydrogen sulfide is made to react with butyraldehyde in alcoholic ammonia: Nord, *Ber.* **52**, 1209 (1919); by passing vapors of butanol and hydrogen sulfide over thorium oxide catalyst: Kramer, Reid, *J. Am. Chem. Soc.* **43**, 880 (1921); together with dibutyl sulfide in distilling an aq soln of sodium butyl sulfate and sodium sulfide: Gray, Gutekunst, *J. Am. Chem. Soc.* **42**, 858 (1920); by slightly warming dithiocarbamic butyl ester with aq KOH: v. Braun, Engelbertz, *Ber.* **56**, 1574 (1923); the sodium salt is formed when dibutyl disulfide is treated with sodium in ether or alcohol: Moses, Reid, *J. Am. Chem. Soc.* **48**, 777 (1926). Physical properties: Mathias, *ibid.* **72**, 1897 (1950); W. E. Haines *et al.*, *J. Phys. Chem.* **60**, 549 (1956). Once cited to occur in "skunk" fluid, see Beckmann, *Pharm. Zentralhalle* **37**, 557 (1896); T. B. Aldrich, *J. Exp. Med.* **1**, 323 (1896); however, recent literature rebuts this: K. K. Anderson, D. T. Bernstein, *J. Chem. Ecol.* **1**, 493 (1975); *eidem*, *J. Chem. Educ.* **55**, 559 (1978).

Mobile liquid. Heavy skunk odor. mp −115.9°. bp$_{766}$ 98.2°; bp$_{760}$ 98.4°. Flammable. d$_4^{25}$ 0.83679. n$_D^{25}$ 1.44014. Slightly sol in water. Very sol in alcohol, ether, liquid hydrogen sulfide. Forms azeotropic mixtures with butyl alcohol (bp 97.8°; 85.16% butanethiol) and with butyl alcohol and water.

Caution: Potential symptoms of overexposure are irritation of eyes, skin; muscle weakness, malaise, sweating, nausea, vomiting, headache, confusion. See *NIOSH Pocket Guide to Chemical Hazards* (DHHS/NIOSH 97-140, 1997) p 42.

1578. sec-Butyl Mercaptan. [513-53-1] 2-Butanethiol; *sec*-butyl thioalcohol. C$_4$H$_{10}$S; mol wt 90.19. C 53.27%, H 11.18%, S 35.55%. CH$_3$CH$_2$CH(SH)CH$_3$. Prepd from 2-iodobutane by means of alcoholic KSH soln: Reymann, *Ber.* **7**, 1287 (1874); from 2-bromobutane in the same manner: Ellis, Reid, *J. Am. Chem. Soc.* **54**, 1674 (1932).

Mobile liq. Heavy skunk odor. mp −165°. bp 84-85°. Flammable. d^{17} 0.8299; d$_4^{25}$ 0.8246. n$_D^{25}$ 1.4338. Slightly sol in water. Very sol in alc, ether, liquid H$_2$S.

1579. tert-Butyl Mercaptan. [75-66-1] 2-Methyl-2-propanethiol. C$_4$H$_{10}$S; mol wt 90.19. C 53.27%, H 11.18%, S 35.55%. (CH$_3$)$_3$CSH. Prepd from *tert*-butyl iodide, ZnS and alcohol: Dobbin, *J. Chem. Soc.* **57,** 641 (1890). *See also* US 2020421 *C.A.* **30,** 489 (1936) and **US 2051806** *C.A.* **30,** 6760 (1936).

Mobile liquid. Heavy skunk odor. mp $-0.5°$. bp$_{760}$ 63.7-64.2°. d$_4^{25}$ 0.79426; n$_D^{25}$ 1.41984: Mathias, *J. Am. Chem. Soc.* **72,** 1897 (1950). Flammable. Remarkably stable to oxidizing agents. Slightly sol in water. Very sol in alcohol, ether, liquid H$_2$S.

1580. *n*-Butylmercuric Chloride. [543-63-5] Butyl-chloromercury. C$_4$H$_9$ClHg; mol wt 293.16. C 16.39%, H 3.09%, Cl 12.09%, Hg 68.42%. CH$_3$CH$_2$CH$_2$CH$_2$HgCl. **Prepn:** Slotta, Jacobi, *J. Prakt. Chem.* [2] **120,** 249 (1929); R. C. Larock, H. C. Brown, *J. Am. Chem. Soc.* **92,** 2467 (1970). Distribution in mice: M. Yonaha *et al., Chem. Pharm. Bull.* **23,** 1718 (1975). For the prepn of the bromide *see* Slotta, Jacobi, *loc. cit.;* Marvel *et al., J. Am. Chem. Soc.* **47,** 3009 (1925). Review and bibliography: Krause, von Grosse, *Die Chemie der Metallorganischen Verbindungen* (Berlin, 1937).

White needles from ethanol, sometimes leaflets, mp 130°. Soly (g/100 ml) in water at 18°: 1.4×10^{-4}; at 100°: 3.3×10^{-4}; soly (g/100 g) in ethanol at 18°: 1.5; at 78°: 9.0; in chloroform at 18°: 5.6.

1581. Butylmethylimidazolium. [80432-08-2] 1-Butyl-3-methyl-1*H*-imidazolium; BMIM; C$_4$mim. C$_8$H$_{15}$N$_2$+. Cation used in prepn of room temperature ionic liquids, *q.v.* Prepn of hexafluorophosphate and tetrafluoroborate: Y. Chauvin *et al., Angew. Chem. Int. Ed.* **34,** 2698 (1995); and physical properties: P. A. Z. Suarez *et al., J. Chim. Phys.* **95,** 1626 (1998). Prepn and properties of ionic liquids containing the imidazolium cation: J. G. Huddleston *et al., Green Chem.* **3,** 156 (2001).

Chloride. [79917-90-1] C$_8$H$_{15}$ClN$_2$; mol wt 174.67. **Prepn:** J. S. Wilkes *et al., Inorg. Chem.* **21,** 1263 (1982). Slightly yellow, may be crystalline at room temp depending on water content. mp 41° (dried) (Huddleston). Also reported as mp 65-69° (Wilkes). d^{25} 1.08 (dried). Miscible with water.

Hexafluorophosphate. [174501-64-5] C$_8$H$_{15}$F$_6$N$_2$P; mol wt 284.18. Use as extraction medium: J. G. Huddleston *et al., Chem. Commun.* **16,** 1765 (1998); as a solvent for alkylation reactions: M. J. Earle *et al., ibid.* **20,** 2245 (1998). Use in environmentally benign manufacturing processes: L. A. Blanchard *et al., Nature* **339,** 28 (1999). Microscopic solvent properties: S. N. Baker *et al., Green Chem.* **4,** 165 (2002). Viscous liquid, mp 4° (water equilibrated); 10° (dried). Glass transition temperature: $-83°$ (water equilibrated), $-80°$ (dried). Viscosity (25°): 397 cP (water equilibrated), 450 cP (dried). d^{25} 1.35 (water equilibrated), 1.36 (dried). n^{25} 1.409 (dried). Miscible with water. Imiscible with toluene, hexane, other non-polar solvents.

Tetrafluoroborate. [174501-65-6] C$_8$H$_{15}$BF$_4$N$_2$; mol wt 226.02. Use as solvent for nucleophilic substitution reactions: D. W. Kim *et al., J. Org. Chem.* **68,** 4281 (2003). Viscous liquid. Glass transition temperature: $-97°$ (dried). Viscosity (25°): 219 cP (dried). d^{25} 1.12(dried). Miscible with water. Sol in methanol, ethanol. Insol in hydrocarbons.

USE: Solvent for organic reactions.

1582. *n*-Butyl Nitrite. [544-16-1] Nitrous acid butyl ester. C$_4$H$_9$NO$_2$; mol wt 103.12. C 46.59%, H 8.80%, N 13.58%, O 31.03%. CH$_3$CH$_2$CH$_2$CH$_2$ONO. Prepd by the action of nitrous acid on butyl alcohol: Noyes, *Org. Synth.* **coll. vol. II,** 108 (1943); Miller, Audrieth, *Inorg. Synth.* **2,** 139 (1946).

Oily liquid. Characteristic odor. Breathing of vapor causes headache and vasodilation. d$_4^0$ 0.9114. bp$_{760}$ 78.2° (some decompn). Miscible with alcohol, ether. Dec on storage. Polymerization products of butyraldehyde have been found in five-month-old samples.

Caution: Lowers blood pressure through vasodilation, causing headache, throbbing, weakness. Effects resemble those produced by amyl nitrate.

USE: In the manuf of rare earth azides.

1583. *tert*-Butyl Nitrite. [540-80-7] Nitrous acid 1,1-dimethyl ethyl ester; α,α-dimethylethyl nitrite; nitrous acid *tert*-butyl ester. C$_4$H$_9$NO$_2$; mol wt 103.12. C 46.59%, H 8.80%, N 13.58%,

O 31.03%. (CH$_3$)$_3$CONO. Prepd by adding *t*-butyl chloride to a cooled slurry of silver nitrite and anhydr ether: Kornblum *et al., J. Am. Chem. Soc.* **77,** 5528 (1955); by passing NO$_2$ or NO$_2$ + NO into *t*-butyl alcohol at 25-30°: Treacy, **US 2739166** (1956); from *t*-butanol, sodium nitrite and sulfuric acid: Coe, Doumani, *J. Am. Chem. Soc.* **70,** 1516 (1948).

Yellow liquid, agreeable odor. d$_4^0$ 0.8941; d$_4^{20}$ 0.8671. bp$_{760}$ 63°; bp$_{250}$ 34°; n$_D^{20}$ 1.3687. Very sol in alcohol, ether, chloroform, carbon disulfide; slightly sol in water; practically insol in glycerol.

USE: Jet propellant.

1584. Butylparaben. [94-26-8] 4-Hydroxybenzoic acid butyl ester; *n*-butyl *p*-hydroxybenzoate; Butyl Chemosept; Butyl Parasept; Tegosept B. C$_{11}$H$_{14}$O$_3$; mol wt 194.23. C 68.02%, H 7.27%, O 24.71%. Prepn of calcium and magnesium salts: Engels, Weijlard, **US 2046324** and **US 2056176** (both 1936 to Merck & Co.). Prepn of analogous derivatives: *See* ethyl-, methyl- and propyl-paraben.

Crystalline powder, mp 68-69°. Very slightly soluble in water (1:6500), glycerin; freely sol in acetone, alc, ether, chloroform, propylene glycol. Preserve in well-closed containers.

Calcium salt. C$_{22}$H$_{26}$CaO$_6$. Cryst powder. Soly in water: approx 1:125.

Magnesium salt. C$_{22}$H$_{26}$MgO$_6$. Cryst powder. Soly in water: approx 1:110.

USE: Pharmaceutic aid (antifungal). Preservative in foods.

1585. *p-tert*-Butylphenol. [98-54-4] 4-(1,1-Dimethylethyl)phenol; butylphen. C$_{10}$H$_{14}$O; mol wt 150.22. C 79.95%, H 9.39%, O 10.65%. Prepd by heating phenol with isobutanol in the presence of zinc chloride: **DE 17311;** *Frdl.* **1,** 22; also from phenol, *tert*-butyl chloride and excess alkali in alcohol: Lewis, *J. Chem. Soc.* **83,** 329 (1903). *See also* Smith, *J. Am. Chem. Soc.* **55,** 3718 (1933); Natelson, *ibid.* **56,** 1583 (1934); Huston, Hsieh, *ibid.* **58,** 439 (1936); **US 2039344** (1936 to Dow); Isagulyants, Bagryantseva, *C.A.* **33,** 8183 (1939). Toxicity study: H. F. Smyth *et al., Am. Ind. Hyg. Assoc. J.* **30,** 470 (1969).

Needles from water, mp 98°. d$_4^{114}$ 0.9081. bp 237°. Volatile with steam. Practically insol in cold water. Sol in alcohol, ether. LD$_{50}$ orally in rats: 3.25 ml/kg (Smyth).

Sodium salt. C$_{10}$H$_{13}$NaO. Deliquescent leaflets. Sol in water.

USE: Intermediate in the manuf of varnish and lacquer resins; as a soap antioxidant; ingredient in de-emulsifiers for oil field use; in motor oil additives.

1586. 4-*tert*-Butylphenyl Salicylate. [87-18-3] 2-Hydroxybenzoic acid 4-(1,1-dimethylethyl)phenyl ester; salicylic acid *p-tert*-butylphenyl ester; TBS. C$_{17}$H$_{18}$O$_3$; mol wt 270.32. C 75.53%, H 6.71%, O 17.76%. Prepd from salicylic acid and *p-tert*-butylphenol in the presence of POCl$_3$: Stoesser, Sommerfield, **US 2606920** (1952 to Dow).

Crystals, slight odor resembling that of salol, mp 62-64°. Maximum light absorption at 290-330 nm. Soly (w/w): in water <0.1%; abs ethanol 79%; ethyl acetate 153%; methyl ethyl ketone 197%; toluene 158%; Stoddard solvent 39%.

USE: Light absorber in plastic food wrappings.

1587. n-Butyl Propionate. [590-01-2] Propanoic acid butyl ester; propionic acid butyl ester. $C_7H_{14}O_2$; mol wt 130.18. C 64.58%, H 10.84%, O 24.58%. $CH_3CH_2COOC_4H_9$. Prepn from 1-butanol and propionic acid: Vogel, *J. Chem. Soc.* **1948**, 616; Spindt, Stevens, US 2470876 (1949 to Gulf).

Liquid, bp 146.8°. mp −89°. d_4^{20} 0.8754. n_D^{20} 1.401. Very slightly sol in water; very sol in alcohol, ether.

1588. N-Butylscopolammonium Bromide. [149-64-4] [7(S)-(1α,2β,4β,5α,7β)]-9-Butyl-7-(3-hydroxy-1-oxo-2-phenyl-propoxy)-9-methyl-3-oxa-9-azoniatricyclo[3.3.1.0²·⁴]nonane bromide; α-(hydroxymethyl)benzeneacetic acid 9-butyl-9-methyl-3-oxa-9-azoniatricyclo[3.3.1.0²·⁴]non-7-yl ester bromide; 8-butyl-6β,7β-epoxy-3α-hydroxy-1αH,5αH-tropanium bromide (−)-tropate; butylscopolamine bromide; hyoscine-N-butyl bromide; scopolamine-N-butyl bromide; scopolamine bromobutylate; Amisepan; Buscapina; Buscol; Buscolysin; Buscopan; Butylmin; Donopon; Monospan; Scobro; Scobron; Scobutil; Sparicon; Sporamin; Stibron; Tirantil. $C_{21}H_{30}BrNO_4$; mol wt 440.37. C 57.28%, H 6.87%, Br 18.14%, N 3.18%, O 14.53%. Anticholinergic. Prepn: F. Adickes *et al.*, DE 856890; *eidem*, US 2872452 (1952, 1959 both to Boehringer Ing.). Biological activity studies: Bauer *et al.*, *Arzneim.-Forsch.* **18**, 1132 (1968). Toxicological studies: K. Stockhaus, H. Wick, *Arch. Int. Pharmacodyn. Ther.* **180**, 155 (1969). Use in endoscopic examinations: J. R. Lee, *Clin. Radiol.* **33**, 273 (1982); D. N. Hupscher, O. Dommerholt, *Diagn. Imag. Clin. Med.* **53**, 77 (1984); A. C. Steger *et al.*, *Am. J. Gastroenterol.* **81**, 615 (1986).

Crystals from methanol, mp 142-144°. $[\alpha]_D^{20}$ −20.8° (c = 3 in water). LD_{50} in mice (mg/kg): 15.6 i.v.; 74 i.p.; 570 s.c.; 3000 orally (Stockhaus, Wick).

THERAP CAT: Antispasmodic.

1589. Butyl Stearate. [123-95-5] Octadecanoic acid butyl ester. $C_{22}H_{44}O_2$; mol wt 340.58. C 77.58%, H 13.02%, O 9.40%. $CH_3(CH_2)_{16}COOC_4H_9$. Prepn from silver stearate and n-butyl iodide: Whitby, *J. Chem. Soc.* **1926**, 1458; from stearic acid and n-butanol: Smith, *ibid.* **1931**, 802. Physical properties: *Beilstein* vol. **2**, Suppl. 3, 1016; Smith, *loc. cit.*; *Ind. Eng. Chem.* **32**, 880 (1940).

Crystals from alcohol, propanol, or ether, mp 27°. Also reported as mp 16°. bp 343°. Closed-cup flash pt 160°C (320°F). d_{25}^{25} 0.855-0.875. Slightly sol in water; sol in alcohol, ether.

USE: Solvent, spreading and softening agent in plastics, textiles, cosmetics, rubber industries.

1590. n-Butyl Sulfide. [544-40-1] 1,1'-Thiobisbutane; butylthiobutane; dibutyl sulfide. $C_8H_{18}S$; mol wt 146.29. C 65.68%, H 12.40%, S 21.92%. $(CH_3CH_2CH_2CH_2)_2S$. Prepd by refluxing a soln contg sodium sulfide and sodium n-butyl sulfate for several hrs: Gray, Gutekunst, *J. Am. Chem. Soc.* **42**, 856 (1920).

Liquid. mp −79.7°. d_0^{16} 0.839. d_4^0 0.852. bp 182°. Insol in water. Very sol in alcohol, ether.

1591. Butyraldehyde. [123-72-8] Butanal. C_4H_8O; mol wt 72.11. C 66.62%, H 11.18%, O 22.19%. $CH_3CH_2CH_2CHO$. Prepn from butyryl chloride: Brown, Tsukamoto, *J. Am. Chem. Soc.* **83**, 2016 (1961); by reduction of corresponding nitrile: Gaiffe, Pallaud, *Compt. Rend.* **254**, 496 (1962); by alkali aluminum hydride reduction of methyl butyrate: Zakharkin *et al.*, *Tetrahedron Lett.* **1963**, 208; by oxidation of butanol: Harrison, *Proc. Chem. Soc. London* **1964**, 110. Usually manuf by catalytic dehydrogenation of butanol, catalytic hydrogenation of crotonaldehyde, or by the oxo process from propene, *e.g., see:* Dunbar, Arnold, *J. Chem. Soc.* **10**, 501 (1945); Horn, *Ind. Eng. Chem.* **51**, 655 (1959); W. L. Faith *et al.*,

Industrial Chemicals (John Wiley, New York, 3rd ed., 1965) pp 183, 304-305. Toxicity study: Smyth *et al.*, *Arch. Ind. Hyg. Occup. Med.* **4**, 119 (1951). *Review:* P. D. Sherman in *Kirk-Othmer Encyclopedia of Chemical Technology* vol. **4** (Wiley-Interscience, New York, 3rd ed., 1978) pp 376-386.

Flammable liquid. bp 74.8°. mp −99°. Closed-cup flash pt −6.67°C (20°F). d_4^{20} 0.8016. n_D^{20} 1.379. Soly in water at 25°, 7.1 (wt-%): Smith, Bonner, *Ind. Eng. Chem.* **43**, 1169 (1951). Miscible with ethanol, ether, ethyl acetate, acetone, toluene, many other organic solvents and oils. Single-dose LD_{50} orally in rats: 5.89 g/kg (Smyth).

Caution: May act as irritant, narcotic.

USE: Chiefly in the manuf of rubber accelerators, synthetic resins, solvents, plasticizers.

1592. n-Butyramide. [541-35-5] Butanamide. C_4H_9NO; mol wt 87.12. C 55.15%, H 10.41%, N 16.08%, O 18.36%. $CH_3CH_2CH_2CONH_2$. Prepn by a modified Willgerodt reaction: Jelinek, US 2572809; US 2572810 (both 1951 to GAF); from butyryl chloride: Philbrook, *J. Org. Chem.* **19**, 623 (1954); from butyraldoxime: Huber, US 2721199 (1955 to du Pont); from butyric acid: Rahman, *Rec. Trav. Chim.* **79**, 188 (1960); from butyronitrile: Gilbert, Rumanowski, US 3062883 (1962 to Allied Chem.).

Crystals, mp 115-116°. bp 216°. Sol in water, alcohol; slightly sol in ether.

1593. Butyric Acid. [107-92-6] Butanoic acid; n-butyric acid; ethylacetic acid. $C_4H_8O_2$; mol wt 88.11. C 54.53%, H 9.15%, O 36.32%. $CH_3CH_2CH_2COOH$. Discovered by Lieben and Rossi in 1869. Present in butter as an ester to the extent of 4-5%. Obtained by suitable fermentation of carbohydrates; prepn from n-propanol + CO at 200 atm in the presence of $Ni(CO)_4$ and NiI_2: Reppe *et al.*, *Ann.* **582**, 83 (1953); lab prepn from ethyl-malonic acid: Gattermann-Wieland, *Praxis des Organischen Chemikers* (de Gruyter, Berlin, 40th ed., 1961) p 221. Toxicity study: Smyth *et al.*, *Arch. Ind. Hyg. Occup. Med.* **10**, 61 (1954).

Oily liq; unpleasant, rancid odor. d_4^{20} 0.959. bp 163.5°. mp −7.9°. n_D^{20} 1.3991. Flash pt, closed cup: 170°F (77°C). Neutralization value 636.79. Miscible with water, alcohol, ether. The calcium salt of this acid is less soluble in hot than in cold water (difference from isobutyric acid). LD_{50} orally in rats: 8.79 g/kg (Smyth).

Magnesium salt. Magnesium butyrate. $C_8H_{14}MgO_4$. Deliquesc leaflets. Sol in water. *Keep well closed.*

USE: Manuf of esters, some of which serve as bases of artificial flavoring ingredients of certain liqueurs, soda-water syrups, candies; also for varnishes; as decalcifier of hides.

1594. Butyric Anhydride. [106-31-0] Butanoic acid anhydride; butyryl oxide. $C_8H_{14}O_3$; mol wt 158.19. C 60.74%, H 8.92%, O 30.34%. $CH_3CH_2CH_2COOCOCH_2CH_2CH_3$. Prepn from butyric acid: Williams, Krynitsky, *Org. Synth.* **coll. vol. III**, 165 (1955); Kuwajima, Mukaiyama, *J. Org. Chem.* **29**, 1385 (1964). Manuf by catalytic hydrogenation of crotonic acid: Smith, Hunter, US 2492403 (1949 to Celanese); by catalytic carbonylation of the corresponding acid ester: Reppe, Friederich, US 2730546 (1956 to BASF).

Liq, bp 199.4-201.4°. mp −75°. d_4^{20} 0.9668. n_D^{20} 1.4070. Flash pt, open cup: 190°F (88°C). Sol in water and in alc with decompn; sol in ether.

1595. Butyroin. [496-77-5] 5-Hydroxy-4-octanone; 5-octanol-4-one. $C_8H_{16}O_2$; mol wt 144.21. C 66.63%, H 11.18%, O 22.19%. $CH_3(CH_2)_2CH(OH)CO(CH_2)_2CH_3$. Prepd by the reaction between an ether soln of ethyl butyrate and sodium or potassium: Bouveault, Locquin, *Bull. Soc. Chim.* [3] **35**, 629 (1906); Corson *et al.*, *J. Am. Chem. Soc.* **52**, 3988 (1930); Scheibler, Emden, *Ann.* **434**, 265 (1923); Snell, McElvain, *Org. Synth.* **coll. vol. II**, 114 (1943).

Liquid. d_4^0 0.9367; $d_4^{16.7}$ 0.91075. bp_{760} 180-190°; bp_{155} 150-154°; bp_{20} 95°; bp_{10} 85°. $n_D^{16.7}$ 1.43455. Reduces Fehling's soln.

Oxime. $C_8H_{17}NO_2$. Viscous liquid, bp_{10} 143°.

1596. Butyrolactone. [96-48-0] Dihydro-2(3H)-furanone; γ-butyrolactone; 1,2-butanolide; 1,4-butanolide; γ-hydroxybutyric acid lactone; 3-hydroxybutyric acid lactone; 4-hydroxybutanoic acid lactone. $C_4H_6O_2$; mol wt 86.09. C 55.81%, H 7.02%, O

37.17%. Prepd from acetylene and formaldehyde: Reppe, *Chem. Ing. Tech.* **1950**, 365; *Chem. Eng.* **58**, no. 6, 176 (1951); also prepd from ethylene chlorohydrin, glutaric acid, ν-hydroxybutyric acid solns, tetrahydrofuran, or vinylacetic acid: F. C. Whitmore, *Organic Chemistry* (Van Nostrand, New York, 2nd ed., 1951). Alternate synthesis: Y. Ogata *et al., J. Org. Chem.* **45**, 1320 (1980). Physical properties: McKinley, Copes *J. Am. Chem. Soc.* **72**, 5331 (1950). Toxicity: H. F. Smyth *et al., Am. Ind. Hyg. Assoc. J.* **30**, 470 (1969).

Oily liquid. d_0^0 1.1441; d_0^{15} 1.1286. mp −43.53°. bp_{760} 204°. bp_{12} 89°. n_D^{25} 1.4348. Flash pt, open cup: 209°F (98°C). Volatile with steam. Misc with water. Sol in methanol, ethanol, acetone, ether, benzene. Hydrolyzed by hot alkaline solns. LD_{50} orally in rats: 17.2 ml/kg (Smyth).

USE: Intermediate in the synthesis of polyvinylpyrrolidone, DL-methionine, piperidine, phenylbutyric acid, thiobutyric acids. Solvent for polyacrylonitrile, cellulose acetate, methyl methacrylate polymers, polystyrene. Constituent of paint removers, textile aids, drilling oils.

1597. Butyronitrile. [109-74-0] Butanenitrile; propyl cyanide; butyric acid nitrile. C_4H_7N; mol wt 69.11. C 69.52%, H 10.21%, N 20.27%. $CH_3CH_2CH_2CN$. Prepd from 1-butanol by controlled cyanation with NH_3 at 300° in the presence of Ni—Al_2O_3 catalysts: Popov, Shuikin, *Izv. Akad. Nauk SSSR Otd. Khim. Nauk* **1958**, 713-718, *C.A.* **52**, 19924 (1958). Toxicity: H. F. Smyth *et al., Am. Ind. Hyg. Assoc. J.* **23**, 95 (1962).

Liquid. d_4^0 0.8091; d_4^{15} 0.7954; d_4^{30} 0.7817. mp −112°. bp_{760} 117.5°; bp_{400} 96.8°; bp_{200} 76.7°; bp_{100} 59.0°; bp_{60} 47.3°; bp_{40} 38.4°; bp_{20} 25.7°; bp_{10} 13.4°; bp_5 2.1°; $bp_{1.0}$ −20.0°. n_D^{20} 1.38385. Flash pt, open cup: 85°F (29°C). Viscosity ($\eta \times 10^5$) at 15° = 624; at 30° = 515. Dipole moment 3.5. Sparingly sol in water. Misc with alcohol, ether, dimethylformamide. LD_{50} orally in rats: 0.14 g/kg (Smyth).

Caution: Potential symptoms of overexposure are irritation of eyes, skin, respiratory system; headache, dizziness, weakness, giddiness, confusion, convulsions; dyspnea; abdominal pain, nausea, vomiting. *See NIOSH Pocket Guide to Chemical Hazards* (DHHS/NIOSH 97-140, 1997) p 44.

1598. n-Butyryl Chloride. [141-75-3] Butanoyl chloride; butyryl chloride. C_4H_7ClO; mol wt 106.55. C 45.09%, H 6.62%, Cl 33.27%, O 15.02%. $CH_3CH_2CH_2COCl$. Prepn from butyric acid: Helferich, Schaefer, *Org. Synth.* **coll. vol. I**, 147 (1941).

Liquid, bp 101-102°. mp −89°. $d_4^{20.6}$ 1.0263. n_D^{20} 1.412. Dissolves slowly with decompn in water, alcohol. Miscible with ether.

1599. Buzepide. [3691-21-2] Hexahydro-α,α-diphenyl-1*H*-azepine-1-butanamide; 2,2-diphenyl-4-hexamethyleneiminobutyramide; R-658. $C_{22}H_{28}N_2O$; mol wt 336.47. C 78.53%, H 8.39%, N 8.33%, O 4.76%. Anticholinergic. Prepn: Janssen *et al., J. Med. Pharm. Chem.* **1**, 187 (1959); of methiodide as well as free base: Janssen, de Jongh, US 2881165 (1959 to N.V. Nederlandsche Combinatie Chem. Ind.). Clinical trial in irritable bowel syndrome: J. Ph. Barbier *et al., Ann. Gastroenterol. Hepatol.* **25**, 123 (1989).

Crystals from isopropanol, mp 141.5-143.5°.

Methiodide. [15351-05-0] Metazepium iodide; 1-(3-carbamoyl-3,3-diphenylpropyl)hexahydro-1-methylazepinium iodide; *N*-(3,3-diphenyl-3-carbamoylpropyl)-*N*-methylperhydroazepinium iodide; diphexamide methiodide. $C_{22}H_{28}N_2O.CH_3I$. Crystals, dec 212-213°.

Mixture with haloperidol. Vésadol.

THERAP CAT: Antispasmodic.

C

1600. Cabenegrins. Orally active antidotes against snake venoms; isolated from the root of a South American plant called "Cabeca de Negra" and structurally related to pterocarpin, *q.v.* Isoln: L. L. Darko *et al., EP 89229; eidem, US 4429141* (1983, 1984 both to Richter, Budapest). Structure determn: M. Nakagawa *et al., Tetrahedron Lett.* **1982**, 3855. Synthesis of (±)-cabenegrins A-I and A-II: M. Ishiguro *et al., ibid.* 3859.

Cabenegrin A-I   Cabenegrin A-II

Cabenegrin A-I. [84297-59-6] [6aR-[4(E),6aα,12aα]]-6a,12a-Dihydro-4-(4-hydroxy-3-methyl-2-butenyl)-6H-[1,3]dioxolo[5,-6]benzofuro[3,2-c][1]benzopyran-3-ol. $C_{21}H_{20}O_6$; mol wt 368.38. White crystalline solid, mp 167-168°. uv max (ethanol): 309 nm (ε 13000); uv max (methanol): 209, 233, 309 nm (ε 75000, 24000, 13000).

Cabenegrin A-II. [84297-60-9] 6a,12a-Dihydro-3-hydroxy-β-methyl-6H-[1,3]dioxolo[5,6]benzofuro[3,2-c][1]benzopyran-2-butanol. $C_{21}H_{22}O_6$; mol wt 370.40. uv max (methanol): 204, 230, 292, 308 nm (ε 116000, 8000, 9400, 11800).

1601. Cabergoline. [81409-90-7] (8β)-N-[3-(Dimethylamino)propyl]-N-[(ethylamino)carbonyl]-6-(2-propenyl)ergoline-8-carboxamide; 1-ethyl-3-(3'-dimethylaminopropyl)-3-(6'-allylergoline-8'β-carbonyl)urea; 1-[(6-allylergoline-8β-yl)carbonyl]-1-[3-(dimethylamino)propyl]-3-ethylurea; FCE-21336; Dostinex. $C_{26}H_{37}$-N_5O_2; mol wt 451.60. C 69.15%, H 8.26%, N 15.51%, O 7.09%. Dopamine D_2-receptor agonist. Prepn: P. Salvati *et al., BE 888243; eidem, US 4526892* (1981, 1985 both to Farmitalia Carlo Erba). Prepn and bioactivity: E. Brambilla *et al., Eur. J. Med. Chem.* **24**, 421 (1989). Clinical pharmacology: C. Ferrari *et al., J. Clin. Endocrinol. Metab.* **63**, 941 (1986). Veterinary trial as abortifacient in dogs: K. Post *et al., Theriogenology* **29**, 1233 (1988). Clinical evaluation to prevent puerperal lactation: G. B. Melis *et al., Obstet. Gynecol.* **71**, 311 (1988); in hyperprolactinemic disorders: C. Ferrari *et al., J. Clin. Endocrinol. Metab.* **68**, 1201 (1989). Clinical trial in Parkinson's disease: J. T. Hutton *et al., Neurology* **46**, 1062 (1996).

White crystals from diethyl ether, mp 102-104°. Sol in ethyl alcohol, chloroform, DMF; slightly sol in 0.1 *N* HCl; very slightly sol in *n*-hexane. Insol in water. LD_{50} orally in male mice: >400 mg/kg (Brambilla).

Diphosphate. [85329-89-1] $C_{26}H_{37}N_5O_2 \cdot 2H_3PO_4$. mp 153-155°.

THERAP CAT: Prolactin inhibitor; antiparkinsonian.

THERAP CAT (VET): Prolactin inhibitor.

1602. Cacao Shell. Cocoa shells. Shells of the seed of *Theobroma cacao* L., *Sterculiaceae. Habit.* Brazil, Central America, Mexico, West Indies, and most tropical countries. *Constit.* Theobromine, caffeine, cacao red, protein, pentosans, pectic acid, starch. *Ref:* Dittmar, *Engenharia e quim* **5**, no. 1, 1 (1953), *C.A.* **48**, 2949e (1954). *Monographs:* E. M. Chatt, *Cocoa* (Interscience, New York, 1953); D. H. Urquhart, *Cocoa* (Longmans, London, 1961); Powell, Harris, *Chocolate and Cocoa* in *Kirk-Othmer Encyclopedia of Chemical Technology* **vol. 5** (Interscience, New York, 2nd ed., 1964) pp 363-402.

Thin, papery, reddish-brown, concavo-convex shells; weak chocolate-like odor and taste.

Caution: Occasionally causes allergic dermatitis from handling.

USE: In the manuf of caffeine, theobromine.

1603. Cacodyl. [471-35-2] Tetramethyldiarsine; dicacodyl. $C_4H_{12}As_2$; mol wt 209.98. C 22.88%, H 5.76%, As 71.36%. $(CH_3)_2AsAs(CH_3)_2$. Prepn from cacodyl chloride by heating with zinc in an atm of carbon dioxide: Bunsen, *Ann.* **42**, 14 (1842); from dimethylarsine by the action of oxides of nitrogen, aqueous chromic acid, lead peroxide, cacodyl chloride or potassium ferricyanide: Dehn, Wilcox, *Am. Chem. J.* **35**, 1 (1906); by the action of free methyl on arsenic: Paneth, Loleit, *J. Chem. Soc.* **1935**, 366; by reduction of cacodyl oxide: Witten, **US 2531487** (1950 to U.S.A.); Fuson, Shive, **US 2756245** (1956 to U.S.A.).

Oily liquid. Solidifies to large quadratic plates, mp −6°. Almost intolerable garlicky odor. Inflames spontaneously in dry air. bp₇₆₀ 165°. Slightly sol in water. Controlled oxidation with moist air yields cacodyl oxide and cacodylic acid. Reduction with tin and HCl yields **Erytrarsin** $(CH_3As)_4As_2O_3$.

1604. Cacodylic Acid. [75-60-5] Dimethylarsinic acid; hydroxydimethylarsine oxide; Phytar. $C_2H_7AsO_2$; mol wt 138.00. C 17.41%, H 5.11%, As 54.29%, O 23.19%. $(CH_3)_2As(O)OH$. Prepn: Guinot, *J. Pharm. Chim.* **27**, 55 (1923), *C.A.* **17**, 2103[8] (1923); Inverni, *Boll. Chim. Farm.* **62**, 129 (1923), *C.A.* **17**, 2413[7] (1923); Challenger, Ellis, *J. Chem. Soc.* **1935**, 396; Fioretti, Portelli, *Ann. Chim. (Rome)* **53**, 1869 (1963), *C.A.* **60**, 10712c (1964). Use as herbicide: Sprague, **US 3056668** (1962 to Ansul). Toxicity study: G. W. Bailey, J. L. White, *Residue Rev.* **10**, 97 (1965). Review of toxicology and human exposure: *Toxicological Profile for Arsenic* (PB2000-108021, 2000) 468 pp.

Crystals from alcohol + ether. mp 195-196°. Hygroscopic. *Poisonous!* Sol in 0.5 part water; very sol in alcohol; sol in acetic acid. Practically insol in ether. *Keep well closed.* LD_{50} orally in rats: 1350 mg/kg (Bailey, White).

Mercury salt. Mercuric cacodylate. $C_4H_{12}As_2HgO_4$. Hygroscopic, somewhat unstable cryst powder. Soluble in water, alcohol. Practically insol in ether. *Keep well closed.*

USE: Herbicide.

THERAP CAT: Dermatologic.

THERAP CAT (VET): Has been used in chronic eczema, anemia and as a tonic.

1605. Cacotheline. [561-20-6] 2,3-Dihydro-4-nitro-2,3-dioxo-9,10-secostrychnidin-10-oic acid. $C_{21}H_{21}N_3O_7$; mol wt 427.41. C 59.01%, H 4.95%, N 9.83%, O 26.20%. A nitro derivative of brucine made by treating brucine with 10% nitric acid at 60-70°: Leuchs *et al., Ber.* **43**, 1042 (1910). Structure: Teuber, *ibid.* **86**, 232 (1953). Used as reversible redox indicator for Sn^{+2} titrations: P. Szarvas, J. Lantos, *Talanta* **10**, 477 (1963).

Yellow crystals; sparingly sol in water.

USE: Indicator.

1606. Cactinomycin. [8052-16-2] Actinomycin C; HBF-386; Sanamycin. Antibiotic complex produced by *Streptomyces* *chrysomallus:* Brockmann, Grubhofer, *Naturwissenschaften* **36**, 376 (1949); **37**, 494 (1950); *Ber.* **84**, 260 (1951); *US 2953495* (1960 to Shenley Inds.); Lindenbein, *Arch. Mikrobiol.* **17**, 361 (1952). Mixture of actinomycins C_1 (dactinomycin, *q.v.*), C_2 and C_3, 10%, 45% and 45%, resp: Brockmann, Pfennig, *Naturwissenschaften* **39**, 429 (1952); Brockmann, Gröne, *ibid.* **40**, 222 (1953). Description of other actinomycins: Waksman *et al., Proc. Natl. Acad. Sci. USA* **44**, 602 (1958). Structures: Brockmann *et al., Angew. Chem.* **68**, 70 (1956); Brockmann, Boldt, *Naturwissenschaften* **50**, 19 (1963). Synthesis of actinomycin C_3: Brockmann, Lackner, *ibid.* **47**, 230 (1960); **48**, 555 (1961); **51**, 407 (1964); Brockmann *et al., DE 1172680* (1964 to Bayer); Brockmann, Lackner, *Ber.* **100**, 353 (1967); **101**, 1312 (1968). Synthesis of actinomycin C_2: Brockmann, Lackner, *Tetrahedron Lett.* **1964**, 3517. Comprehensive review: H. Brockmann, in *Fortschr. Chem. Org. Naturst.* **18**, 1-54 (1960).

Actinomycin C_2 R = D-Valine R' = D-Alloisoleucine
Actinomycin C_3 R = D-Alloisoleucine R' = D-Alloisoleucine

Alizarin-red hexagonal bipyramids from ethyl acetate, mp 252°. $[\alpha]_D^{25}$ −325 to −349° (c = 0.25 in ethanol). Sparingly sol in water; moderately sol in ethanol; sol in chloroform, ethyl acetate, benzene, acetone. *Protect from light.*

Actinomycin C_2. $C_{63}H_{88}N_{12}O_{16}$; mol wt 1269.44. Red bipyramids, prisms or needles from ethyl acetate, mp 237-239°. $[\alpha]_D^{21}$ −325 ±10° (c = 0.23 in methanol). Abs max (methanol): 443 nm (ε 25400).

Actinomycin C_3. $C_{64}H_{90}N_{12}O_{16}$; mol wt 1283.47. Red hexagonal bipyramids from ethyl acetate or methanol, dec 235°. $[\alpha]_D^{17}$ −328° (c = 0.5 in ethanol). Absorption max (methanol): 443 nm (ε 24100). Weak base.

THERAP CAT: Antineoplastic.

1607. Cactus Grandiflorus. Night-blooming cereus; large-flowered cereus. Fresh, succulent stems of *Selenicereus grandiflorus* (L.) Britt. and Rose, *Cactaceae.* Habit. Tropical America. *Constit.* Cactine(?), acrid resinous glucoside, fat, wax. Extract containing combined principles from freshly tinctured stems and petals is known as *cactoid.*

THERAP CAT: Cardiotonic.

THERAP CAT (VET): Has been used as circulatory stimulant.

1608. Cadalene. [483-78-3] 1,6-Dimethyl-4-(1-methylethyl)naphthalene; 4-isopropyl-1,6-dimethylnaphthalene; cadalin. $C_{15}H_{18}$; mol wt 198.30. C 90.85%, H 9.15%. Obtained from cadinene and other sesquiterpenes or sesquiterpene alcohols by dehydrogenation: Ruzicka, Meyer, *Helv. Chim. Acta* **4**, 505 (1921); Ruzicka, Stoll, *ibid.* **7**, 84 (1924). Synthesis: Ruzicka, Seidel, *ibid.* **5**, 369 (1922); Barnett, Cook, *J. Chem. Soc.* **1933**, 22; Johnson, Jones, *J. Am. Chem. Soc.* **69**, 792 (1947); Kohli *et al., Experientia* **28**, 131 (1972).

Liquid. d_4^{25} 0.9667. bp_{720} 291-292°; bp_{10} 149°. n_D^{25} 1.5785. uv max: 228, 232, 280, 284, 295, 310, 317, 325 nm. Insol in water. Sol in fat solvents, oils.

1609. Cadaverine. [462-94-2] 1,5-Pentanediamine; pentamethylenediamine; animal coniine. $C_5H_{14}N_2$; mol wt 102.18. C 58.77%, H 13.81%, N 27.42%. $NH_2(CH_2)_5NH_2$. Biogenic polyamine and homolog of putrescine, *q.v.*, produced by decarboxylation of lysine. Found in cholera discharge. Isoln: Bocklisch, *Ber.* **18**, 1922 (1885); Ackermann, *Z. Physiol. Chem.* **54**, 16 (1907). Prepn: Ladenburg, *Ber.* **18**, 2956 (1885). GC determn in foods: W. F. Staruszkiewicz, J. F. Bond, *J. Assoc. Off. Anal. Chem.* **64**, 584 (1981). Metabolism study of ^{14}C-cadaverine in rat brain: S. K. Salzman, M. Stepita-Klauco, *J. Neurochem.* **37**, 1308 (1981). Biosynthetic study in *S. ruminantium:* Y. Kamio *et al., J. Biol. Chem.* **257**, 3326 (1982).

Colorless, syrupy liquid; characteristic odor. Strong base, fumes and attracts CO_2 on exposure to air. pKa_1 10.25; pKa_2 9.13. *Poisonous!* d_4^{25} 0.873. mp 9°. bp 178-180°. n_D^{20} 1.463. Sol in water, alcohol; slightly sol in ether. *Keep well closed.*

Dihydrochloride. $C_5H_{14}N_2 \cdot 2HCl$. Needles from water, mp 225-230°. Sol in water. Practically insol in abs alc.

Caution: Skin irritant and possible sensitizer.

1610. Cadexomer Iodine. Iodosorb. A hydrophilic modified starch polymer containing 0.9% (w/w) iodine within a helical matrix. Produced by the reaction of dextrin with epichlorohydrin coupled with ion exchange groups and iodine. Clinical use in venous ulcers: E. Skog *et al., Br. J. Dermatol.* **109**, 77 (1983); M. C. Ormiston *et al., Br. Med. J.* **291**, 308 (1985); L. Hillström, *Acta Chir. Scand. Suppl.* **544**, 53 (1988).

THERAP CAT: Vulnerary.

1611. Cadherins. Family of calcium-dependent cell adhesion molecules thought to be key regulators of morphogenesis in vertebrates. Transmembrane glycoproteins; mol wt ~120-140 kDa. Mediate tissue development by connecting cells bearing identical cadherin types via homophilic interactions. Loss of cadherin function has been associated with tumor metastasis. Two subfamilies have been identified: classic cadherins and the desmosomal cadherins, known as *desmocollins* and *desmogleins*, which differ from the classic cadherins primarily in the structure of the cytoplasmic domains. A number of classic cadherins have been identified; nomenclature is based on the cell from which they were first identified, *e.g.* E-, N- and P-cadherins from epithelial, neural, and placental cells, resp. Among subclasses, ~50% of amino acids are conserved within a particular species. Classic cadherins are complexed with cytoplasmic proteins known as *catenins* which anchor them to the actin-based cytoskeleton and are required for adhesive function. Review of discovery and characterization of cadherins: M. Takeichi, *Development* **102**, 639-655 (1988); *idem, Annu. Rev. Biochem.* **59**, 237-252 (1990); of properties and role in morphogenesis: *idem, Science* **251**, 1451-1455 (1991); J. Behrens, *Acta Anat.* **149**, 165-169 (1994). Review of interaction with catenins: R. Kemler, *Trends Genet.* **9**, 317-321 (1993); L. Hinck *et al., Trends Biochem. Sci.* **19**, 538-542 (1994). Review of role in tumor metastasis: M. Takeichi, *Curr. Opin. Cell Biol.* **5**, 806-811 (1993); W. Birchmeier, J. Behrens, *Biochim. Biophys. Acta* **1198**, 11-26 (1994); O. W. Blaschuk *et al., Endocrine* **3**, 83-89 (1995). Review of desmosomal cadherins: P. J. Koch, W. W. Franke, *Curr. Opin. Cell Biol.* **6**, 682-687 (1994).

1612. Cadinenes. $C_{15}H_{24}$; mol wt 204.35. C 88.16%, H 11.84%. Sesquiterpenes occurring in essential oils from Juniper species and cedars (oil of cade). Nine possible isomers differing in stereochemistry and position of the double bonds, the principal isomer being β-cadinene: Sykora *et al., Chem. Listy* **52**, 1314 (1958). Prepn and structure: Campbell, Soffer, *J. Am. Chem. Soc.* **64**, 417 (1942); Campbell *et al., ibid.* 425; Rao *et al., Tetrahedron Lett.* **1960**, 27; Herout *et al., Collect. Czech. Chem. Commun.* **31**, 3012 (1966). Synthesis: Soffer, Günay, *Tetrahedron Lett.* **1965**, 1355. Of the nine possible isomers, all able to yield (−)-cadinene dihydrochloride, six are known: Herout, Sykora, *Tetrahedron* **4**, 246 (1958); Kartha *et al., ibid.* **19**, 241 (1963). Structure and configuration of isomers: Sykora *et al., Collect. Czech. Chem. Commun.* **23**, 2181 (1958). Isoln of *α-cadinene* from Japanese hop: Y. Naya, M. Kotake, *Bull. Chem. Soc. Jpn.* **42**, 1468 (1969). Synthesis: O. P. Vig, *Indian J. Chem.* **21B**, 145 (1982). Brief review in *Rodd's Chemistry of Carbon Compounds* vol. 2, part C, S. Coffey, Ed. (Elsevier, New York, 1969) pp 268-270.

β-form

β-Cadinene. Oil. Slight pleasant odor. bp$_9$ 124°. d$_4^{20}$ 0.9239. n$_D^{20}$ 1.5059. [α]$_D^{20}$ −251°.

1613. Cadmium. [7440-43-9] Cd; at. wt 112.411; at. no. 48; valence 2. Group IIB (12) element. Abundance in earth's crust: 0.1 to 0.2 ppm. Naturally occurring isotopes (mass numbers): 114 (28.73%); 112 (24.13%); 111 (12.80%); 110 (12.49%); 113 (12.22%), T$_{1/2}$ 9.3 × 10^{15} yrs, β-emitter; 116 (7.49%); 106 (1.25%); 108 (0.89%); known artificial radioactive isotopes: 97-105, 107, 109, 115, 117-122, 124, 126. Found in zinc ores; also as CdS, greenockite; CdCO$_3$, otavite. Obtained in vapor form when roasting zinc ores, as sludge from zinc sulfate purification. Lab prepns from CdSO$_4$: Treadwell, *Helv. Chim. Acta* **4**, 551 (1921). Implicated as causative agent in Itai-Itai ("ouch-ouch") disease in Japan: Flick *et al.*, *Environ. Res.* **4**, 71-85 (1971); Fassett, *Annu. Rev. Pharmacol.* **15**, 425-435 (1975). *Review:* Aylett "Group IIB" in *Comprehensive Inorganic Chemistry* **vol. 3**, J. C. Bailar Jr. *et al.*, Eds. (Pergamon Press, Oxford, 1973) pp 187-328; D. S. Carr in *Kirk-Othmer Encyclopedia of Chemical Technology* **vol. 4** (John Wiley & Sons, New York, 4th ed., 1992) pp 748-760; N. Herron, *ibid.* 760-776. Review of carcinogenic risk: *IARC Monographs* **11**, 39-74 (1976); and toxicity: *Cadmium in the Human Environment: Toxicity and Carcinogenicity, IARC Scientific Publ.* **118**, G. F. Nordberg *et al.*, Eds. (1992) 469 pp; of toxicology and human exposure: *Toxicological Profile for Cadmium* (PB99-166621, 1999) 439 pp.

Silver-white, blue-tinged, lustrous metal; distorted hexagonal close-packed structure; easily cut with a knife; available in the form of bars, sheets or wire or a gray, granular powder. mp 321°. bp 765°. d^{25} 8.65. Specific heat at constant pressure (25°) 6.22 cal/mole deg. Slowly oxidized by moist air to form CdO. E° (aq) Cd/Cd^{2+} 0.4025 V. Insol in water. Reacts readily with dil HNO$_3$; reacts slowly with hot HCl; does not react with alkalies. Other reactions similar to those of zinc. Solns of cadmium salts and H$_2$S or Na$_2$S yield a yellow ppt insol in excess Na$_2$S.

Caution: Overexposure to cadmium and cadmium compounds has been associated with acute and chronic toxicity. Potential symptoms of acute poisoning from the inhalation of cadmium dusts or fumes include headache, chest pains, cough, metal fume fever, weakness. Potential symptoms of acute poisoning from ingestion of cadmium salts are GI disturbances, headache, muscular cramps, vertigo, convulsions. Chronic inhalation may cause pulmonary emphysema and chronic bronchitis. *See Clinical Toxicology of Commercial Products*, R. E. Gosselin *et al.*, Eds. (Williams & Wilkins, Baltimore, 5th ed., 1984) Section II, p 99; Section III, p 77-84. Potential toxic effects due to chronic overexposure by inhalation or ingestion are anemia; kidney damage; osteomalacia and osteoporosis. Itai-itai disease is a skeletal disease associated with a cadmium-induced renal disorder and is attributed to high oral intake of cadmium in food and water; characterized by progressive bone demineralization with painful joints and bones. *See Patty's Industrial Hygiene and Toxicology* **vol. 2C**, G. D. Clayton, F. E. Clayton, Eds. (John Wiley & Sons, New York, 4th ed., 1994) p 1954-1967. *See also NIOSH Pocket Guide to Chemical Hazards* (DHHS/NIOSH 97-140, 1997) p 44. Cadmium and cadmium compounds are listed as known human carcinogens: *Report on Carcinogens, Eleventh Edition* (PB2005-104914, 2004) p III-42.

USE: Batteries, including Ni-Cd storage batteries; coating and electroplating steel and cast iron; pigments; plastic stabilizers; constituent of low melting or easily fusible alloys, e.g., Lichtenberg's, Abel's, Lipowitz', Newton's, and Wood's metal; electronics and optics; soft solder and solder for aluminum; reactor control rods; hardener for copper; catalytsts.

THERAP CAT (VET): Many cadmium salts, especially the oxide and anthranilate, are used or have been suggested as anthelmintics in swine and poultry.

1614. Cadmium Acetate. [543-90-8] C$_4$H$_6$CdO$_4$; mol wt 230.50. C 20.84%, H 2.62%, Cd 48.77%, O 27.76%. Cd(CH$_3$-COO)$_2$. Prepd by treating cadmium nitrate with acetic anhydride: Späth, *Monatsh. Chem.* **33**, 241 (1912); Wagenknecht, Juza, in *Handbook of Preparative Inorganic Chemistry* **vol. 2**, G. Brauer, Ed. (Academic Press, New York, 2nd ed., 1965) p 1105.

Dihydrate. Crystals. Slight acetic acid odor; becomes anhyd at about 130°. d 2.01. d (anhydr) 2.341. mp (anhydr) 255°. Freely sol in water; sol in alcohol. pH of 0.2 molar aq soln 7.1.

USE: Producing iridescent effects on porcelains and pottery; as a reagent for determination of S, Se, and Te; in cadmium electroplating.

1615. Cadmium Bromide. [7789-42-6] Br$_2$Cd; mol wt 272.22. Br 58.71%, Cd 41.29%. CdBr$_2$. Usually prepd from the elements: Honigschmid, Schlee, *Z. Anorg. Allg. Chem.* **227**, 184 (1936); Wagenknecht, Juza, in *Handbook of Inorganic Chemistry* **vol. 2**, G. Brauer, Ed. (Academic Press, New York, 2nd ed., 1965) p 1096.

Hexagonal, pearly flakes; highly hygroscopic. mp 566°; bp 963°; d 5.192. Freely sol in water, alc; moderately sol in acetone; slightly sol in ether. Crystallizes as the monohydrate below 36°, as the tetrahydrate above 36°.

USE: In photography, process engraving, and lithography.

1616. Cadmium Carbonate. [513-78-0] CCdO$_3$; mol wt 172.42. C 6.97%, Cd 65.20%, O 27.84%. CdCO$_3$. Occurs in nature as the mineral, *otavite*. Prepn: de Schulten, *Bull. Soc. Chim. Fr.* [3] **19**, 34 (1898); Biltz, *Z. Anorg. Allg. Chem.* **220**, 312 (1934).

Powder or rhombohedral leaflets. d 4.26. Practically insol in water. Sol in concd solns of ammonium salts, dil acids.

1617. Cadmium Chloride. [10108-64-2] Caddy; Vi-Cad. CdCl$_2$; mol wt 183.32. Cd 61.32%, Cl 38.68%. Prepn: *Gmelins, Cadmium* (8th ed.) **33**, pp 82-83 (1925); supplement, pp 464-465 (1959); Pray, *Inorg. Synth.* **5**, 153 (1957). Book: *Cadmium in the Environment, Part I: Ecological Cycling*, J. O. Nriagu, Ed. (Wiley-Interscience, New York, 1980) 696 pp. Evaluation of carcinogenic risk: *IARC Monographs* **58**, 119-237 (1993).

Hygroscopic, rhombohedral crystals. mp 568°; bp 960°; d 4.05. Freely sol in water; sol in acetone; slightly sol in methanol, ethanol. Practically insol in ether. LD$_{50}$ orally in rats: 88 mg/kg (Nriagu).

Hemipentahydrate. Efflorescent granules or rhombohedral leaflets. d^{25} 3.33. Freely sol in water.

Caution: Cadmium and cadmium compounds are listed as known human carcinogens: *Report on Carcinogens, Eleventh Edition* (PB2005-104914, 2004) p III-42.

USE: Photography; dyeing and calico printing; in the vacuum tube industry; manuf of cadmium yellow; galvanoplasty; manuf of special mirrors; as ice-nucleating agent; as lubricant; in analysis of sulfides to absorb the H$_2$S; in testing for pyridine bases; as fungicide; in pyrotechnics; in electroplating.

1618. Cadmium Cyanide. [542-83-6] C$_2$CdN$_2$; mol wt 164.45. C 14.61%, Cd 68.36%, N 17.03%. Cd(CN)$_2$. Prepn from Cd(OH)$_2$ and HCN: Biltz, *Z. Anorg. Allg. Chem.* **170**, 161 (1928); Wagenknecht, Juza in *Handbook of Preparative Inorganic Chemistry* **vol. 2**, G. Brauer, Ed. (Academic Press, New York, 2nd ed., 1965) p 1105.

Crystals or white powder. Turns brown on heating in air. *Very poisonous!* d 2.226. Soly in water (15°) 1.71 g/100 ml. Slightly sol in alc; sol in solns of alkali cyanides or hydroxides; not appreciably attacked by organic acids, but readily dec by dil mineral acids with evolution of hydrogen cyanide. Readily forms complex cyanides.

USE: In copper bright electroplating.

1619. Cadmium Fluoride. [7790-79-6] CdF$_2$; mol wt 150.41. Cd 74.74%, F 25.26%. Prepn from CdCl$_2$ and NH$_4$F: Kurtenacker *et al.*, *Z. Anorg. Chem.* **211**, 89 (1933); from CdCO$_3$ and HF: Kwasnik in *Handbook of Preparative Inorganic Chemistry* **vol. 1**, G. Brauer, Ed. (Academic Press, New York, 2nd ed., 1963) p 243.

Cubic crystals. mp 1049°; bp 1748°; d 6.33. *Poisonous!* Soly in water (25°) 4.3 g/100 ml. Sol in HF and other mineral acids; practically insol in alcohol and liquid ammonia.

USE: Manufacture of phosphors, glass; in nuclear reactor controls.

1620. Cadmium Hydroxide. [21041-95-2] Cadmium hydrate. CdH_2O_2; mol wt 146.43. Cd 76.77%, H 1.38%, O 21.85%. $Cd(OH)_2$. Usually prepd from a Cd salt by treatment with KOH: de Schulten, *Compt. Rend.* **101**, 72 (1885); Fricke, Blaschke, *Z. Elektrochem.* **46**, 46 (1940); Scholder, Staufenbiel, *Z. Anorg. Allg. Chem.* **247**, 271 (1941).

Powder or trigonal and hexagonal crystals. d 4.79. Dehydration starts at 130° and is complete at 200°. Absorbs CO_2 from the air. Practically insol in water; slightly sol in NaOH soln; sol in dil acids, in NH_4OH or NH_4Cl solns.

USE: In storage battery electrodes.

1621. Cadmium Iodide. [7790-80-9] CdI_2; mol wt 366.22. Cd 30.69%, I 69.31%. Prepd from the elements or from the sulfate and KI: Wagenknecht, Juza in *Handbook of Preparative Inorganic Chemistry* **vol. 2**, G. Brauer, Ed. (Academic Press, New York, 2nd ed., 1965) p 1096.

Hexagonal, lustrous, flake-like crystals; becomes yellow on long exposure to air and light. mp 388°; bp 787°; d 5.67. Sol in water, alc, ether, acetone.

USE: In electrodeposition of Cd; as nematocide; in manuf of phosphors; as lubricant; in photoconductors; in photography, process engraving; lithography; in analytical chemistry.

1622. Cadmium Nitrate. [10325-94-7] CdN_2O_6; mol wt 236.42. Cd 47.55%, N 11.85%, O 40.60%. $Cd(NO_3)_2$. Prepn: *Gmelins, Cadmium* (8th ed.) **33**, pp 76-78 (1925); suppl. p 446 (1959).

Tetrahydrate. Hygroscopic, orthorhombic crystals. mp 59.5°. Sol in 0.6 part water; sol in alc, acetone, ethyl acetate; practically insol in concd HNO_3. *Keep well closed in a cool place.*

Caution: Cadmium and cadmium compounds are listed as known human carcinogens: *Report on Carcinogens, Eleventh Edition* (PB2005-104914, 2004) p III-42.

USE: In making other Cd salts; in photographic emulsions.

1623. Cadmium Oxide. [1306-19-0] Aska-Rid. CdO; mol wt 128.41. Cd 87.54%, O 12.46%. Prepn: *Gmelins, Cadmium* (8th ed.) **33**, pp 69-70 (1925); supplement, pp 419-420 (1959). Toxicity data: Barrett *et al.*, *J. Ind. Hyg. Toxicol.* **29**, 279 (1947).

Dark-brown, infusible powder or cubic crystals. d 8.15. Practically insol in water. Sol in dil acids; slowly sol in ammonium salts. LC_{50} in rats, monkeys (mg/m³): 500, ~15000 (Barrett).

Caution: Potential symptoms of overexposure to fumes are pulmonary edema, dyspnea, cough, chest tightness, substernal pain; headache; chills, muscle aches; nausea, vomiting, diarrhea; emphysema, proteinuria, anosmia; mild anemia. *See NIOSH Pocket Guide to Chemical Hazards* (DHHS/NIOSH 97-140, 1997) p 44. Cadmium and cadmium compounds are listed as known human carcinogens: *Report on Carcinogens, Eleventh Edition* (PB2005-104914, 2004) p III-42.

USE: In phosphors, semiconductors; manuf of silver alloys, glass; in storage battery electrodes; as nematocide; as catalyst for organic reactions, in cadmium electroplating; in ceramic glazes.

THERAP CAT (VET): Has been used as an ascaricide in swine.

1624. Cadmium Potassium Cyanide. [14402-75-6] Potassium tetracyanocadmate. $C_4CdK_2N_4$; mol wt 294.68. C 16.30%, Cd 38.15%, K 26.54%, N 19.01%. $K_2Cd(CN)_4$. Prepn: Dickinson, *J. Am. Chem. Soc.* **44**, 774 (1922); Biltz, *Z. Anorg. Allg. Chem.* **170**, 161 (1928).

Highly refractive, cubic crystals. d 1.846. mp ~450°. When heated, melts to a colorless liquid solidifying to a gray, cryst mass on cooling. Sol in 3 parts cold, 1 part boiling water; slightly sol in alc.

1625. Cadmium Salicylate. [19010-79-8] $C_{14}H_{10}CdO_6$; mol wt 386.64. C 43.49%, H 2.61%, Cd 29.07%, O 24.83%. $Cd(C_7H_5O_3)_2$. Prepn: Prasad *et al.*, *J. Indian Chem. Soc.* **35**, 267 (1958).

Monohydrate. Small needles or plates. mp 242° (dec). Slightly sol in cold water, freely sol in boiling water; very slightly sol in methanol, ethanol.

THERAP CAT: Antiseptic.

1626. Cadmium Selenide. [1306-24-7] CdSe; mol wt 191.37. Cd 58.74%, Se 41.26%. Prepd by heating cadmium in a current of hydrogen selenide and subliming the product in hydrogen at a dull red heat: Margottet, *Recherches sur les Sulfures, les Séléniures, et les Tellures Métalliques,* Paris (1879); by passing hydrogen selenide over heated cadmium chloride and washing with warm water: Grzenkowsky, *Ueber Selenide und Erdalkaliferrocyanide* (Danzig, 1925); from cadmium sulfate and hydrogen selenide: Wagenknecht, Juza in *Handbook of Preparative Inorganic Chemistry* **vol. 2**, G. Brauer, Ed. (Academic Press, New York, 2nd ed., 1965) p 1099. Prepn of high purity CdSe: Taylor, Conn, *US 3540859* (1970 to Merck & Co.).

White to brown cubic or hexagonal crystals; turns red in sunlight. d 5.8; mp 1350°. Dec in air or acids. Practically insol in water.

USE: In photoconductors, semiconductors, photoelectric cells, and rectifiers; in phosphors.

1627. Cadmium Sulfate. [10124-36-4] CdO_4S; mol wt 208.47. Cd 53.92%, O 30.70%, S 15.38%. $CdSO_4$. Prepn: *Gmelins, Cadmium* (8th ed.) **33**, p 121 (1925); suppl. pp 609-610. Book: *Cadmium in the Environment, Part I: Ecological Cycling*, J. O. Nriagu, Ed. (Wiley-Interscience, New York, 1980) 696 pp. Evaluation of carcinogenic risk: *IARC Monographs* **58**, 119-237 (1993).

Hydrate. [7790-84-3] 8/3 Moles water per mole cadmium sulfate, odorless, monoclinic crystals. On heating loses water above 40°, forming monohydrate by 80°. Does not become anhydrous on further heating. d 3.08. Freely sol in water. Almost insol in ethanol, acetone, ammonia, ethyl acetate.

Caution: Cadmium and cadmium compounds are listed as known human carcinogens: *Report on Carcinogens, Eleventh Edition* (PB2005-104914, 2004) p III-42.

USE: In electrodeposition of Cd, Cu, and Ni; in phosphors; manuf of standard cadmium elements; catalyst in the Marsh test for As, determining H_2S and detecting fumaric acid; as nematocide, fungicide, bactericide; lubricant; electrolyte in Weston cell.

1628. Cadmium Sulfide. [1306-23-6] C.I. 77199; Capsebon. CdS; mol wt 144.48. Cd 77.80%, S 22.19%. Occurs in nature as the mineral *greenockite*. Prepd from $CdSO_4 + H_2S$: Milligan, *J. Phys. Chem.* **38**, 797 (1934); Frerichs, *Naturwissenschaften* **33**, 281 (1946); prepn of single crystals: Grillot, *Compt. Rend.* **230**, 1280 (1950); Czyzak *et al.*, *J. Appl. Phys.* **23**, 932 (1952); Wagenknecht, Juza in *Handbook of Preparative Inorganic Chemistry* **vol. II**, G. Brauer, Ed. (Academic Press, New York, 2nd ed., 1965) pp 1098-1099. *See also Colour Index* **vol. 4** (3rd ed., 1971) p 4659.

Light-yellow or orange-colored cubic or hexagonal crystals. Cubic structure: d 4.50; hexagonal structure: d 4.82. The light-yellow variety is also known as *Cadmium Yellow* or *Jaune Brilliant*. d 4.82. Sublimes at 980°. Soly in water (18°): 0.13 mg/100 g. Sol in concd or warm dil mineral acids with evolution of H_2S; readily dec and dissolved by moderately dil HNO_3.

Caution: Cadmium and cadmium compounds are listed as known human carcinogens: *Report on Carcinogens, Eleventh Edition* (PB2005-104914, 2004) p III-42.

USE: As a pigment being fast to light and not affected by H_2S; color for soaps; coloring glass yellow; coloring textiles, paper, rubber; in printing inks, ceramic glazes, fireworks; in phosphors and fluorescent screens; in scintillation counters, semiconductors, photoconductors.

THERAP CAT: Dermatologic.

1629. Cadmium Telluride. [1306-25-8] CdTe; mol wt 240.01. Cd 46.84%, Te 53.16%. Prepd by fusion of the elements or by the action of H_2Te on $CdCl_2$ solns: Dennis, Anderson, *J. Am. Chem. Soc.* **36**, 887 (1914); Kroger, de Nobel, *J. Electron.* **1**, 190 (1955); Kretschmar, Schilberg, *J. Appl. Phys.* **28**, 865 (1957); from aluminum telluride and a cadmium salt: Nitsche, *US 2767049* (1956 to du Pont). Prepn of high purity CdTe: Taylor, Conn, *US 3540859* (1970 to Merck & Co.); prepn of single crystals: Kyle, *US 3519399* (1970 to Hughes Aircraft).

Brownish-black, cubic crystals by sublimation in hydrogen. d_4^{15} 6.2. mp 1041°. Oxidizes upon prolonged exposure to moist air. Practically insol in water and acids, except nitric, in which it is sol with decomp.

USE: In semiconductor research, in phosphors.

1630. Cadmium Tungstate(VI). [7790-85-4] CdO_4W; mol wt 360.25. Cd 31.20%, O 17.76%, W 51.03%. $CdWO_4$. Prepn: Karl, *Compt. Rend.* **196**, 1403 (1933); prepn of single crystals: Uitert, Soden, *J. Appl. Phys.* **31**, 328 (1960).

White or yellowish monoclinic crystals or powder. Practically insol in water or dil acids. Sol in solns of alkali cyanides.

USE: In x-ray screens; in scintillation counters; in phosphors; as catalyst for organic reactions.

1631. Cadralazine. [64241-34-5] 2-[6-[Ethyl(2-hydroxy-propyl)amino]-3-pyridazinyl]hydrazinecarboxylic acid ethyl ester; ethyl 6-[ethyl(2-hydroxypropyl)amino]-3-pyridazinecarbazate; 3-(2-carbethoxyhydrazino)-6-[N-(2-hydroxypropyl)ethylamino]-pyridazine; DC-826; ISF-2469; Cadral; Cadraten; Cadrilan; Presmode. $C_{12}H_{21}N_5O_3$; mol wt 283.33. C 50.87%, H 7.47%, N 24.72%, O 16.94%. Peripheral vasodilator similar to hydralazine, *q.v.* Prepn: C. Carpi *et al.,* **BE 811847**; *eidem,* **US 3925381**; **US 4002753** (1974, 1975, 1977 all to ISF); F. Parravicini *et al., Farmaco Ed. Sci.* **34**, 299 (1979). Analytical profile: L. Citerio *et al., Boll. Chim. Farm.* **120**, 222 (1981). Pharmacology: C. Semeraro *et al., J. Cardiovasc. Pharmacol.* **3**, 455 (1981). HPLC determn in plasma and urine: T. Crolla *et al., J. Chromatogr.* **310**, 139 (1984). Hemodynamic effects in dogs: L. Dorigotti *et al., Arzneim.-Forsch.* **34**, 984 (1984); in humans: B. Persson *et al., Eur. J. Clin. Pharmacol.* **31**, 513 (1987). Pharmacokinetics and metabolism in humans: H. Schütz *et al., Eur. J. Drug Metab. Pharmacokinet.* **10**, 147 (1985); S. A. Hauffe *et al., ibid.* 217. Preliminary clinical evaluations: R. Buoninconti, M. Motolese, *Int. J. Clin. Pharmacol. Ther. Toxicol.* **23**, 613 (1985); A. Salvadeo *et al., Arzneim.-Forsch.* **35**, 623 (1985).

Crystals from acetone, mp 160-162°. pKa 6.0. uv max: 248, 340 nm (ε 22100, 2250). Soly (mg/ml): water 1.3; HCl 235.0; DMSO 323.0; methanol 21.0; dioxane 18.6; chloroform 8.5; diethyl ether, benzene, cyclohexane <0.1. LD₅₀ in rats, dogs (mg/kg): 269, approx 400 i.v.; 2060, >2000 orally (Semeraro); in mice (mg/kg): 700 i.p. (Parravicini).

THERAP CAT: Antihypertensive.

1632. Cadusafos. [95465-99-9] Phosphorodithioic acid O-ethyl S,S-bis(1-methylpropyl) ester; S,S-di-*sec*-butyl O-ethyl phosphorodithioate; ebufos; FMC-67825; Apache; Rugby; Taredan. $C_{10}H_{23}O_2PS_2$; mol wt 270.39. C 44.42%, H 8.57%, O 11.83%, P 11.46%, S 23.72%. Organophosphate insecticide structurally similar to ethoprop, *q.v.* Manufacturing process: J. M. Brochard *et al.,* **EP 235056** (1987 to Rhone-Poulenc Agrochimie). Field trial as nematocide for bananas: P. Quénéhervé *et al., Rev. Nematol.* **14**, 251 (1991). Behavior in soils: S. Q. Zheng *et al., Sci. Total Environ.* **156**, 1 (1994).

Colorless to yellow liquid. Vapor press (25°): 120 mPa. Soly in water: 248 mg/l.

USE: Insecticide; nematocide.

1633. Cafaminol. [30924-31-3] 3,7-Dihydro-8-[(2-hydroxyethyl)methylamino]-1,3,7-trimethyl-1H-purine-2,6-dione; 8-[(2-hydroxyethyl)methylamino]caffeine; 8-(β-oxyethyl)methylaminocaffeine; methylcoffanolamine; Rhinoptil. $C_{11}H_{17}N_5O_3$; mol wt 267.28. C 49.43%, H 6.41%, N 26.20%, O 17.96%. Alkanolamine deriv of caffeine, *q.v.* Prepn: J. Klosa, **DE 1085530**; *eidem,* **US 3094531** (1958, 1963 both to Delmar Chemicals Ltd.). Efficacy studies: E. Szirmai, *Praxis* **13**, 412 (1969); R.

Leypoldt, *Therapiewoche* **26**, 3381 (1976). Bioavailability and absorption kinetics in humans: H. Walther, K. Kochler, *Pharmazie* **34**, 375 (1979).

Colorless crystals from ethanol, mp 162-164°. Soly in water is about 6%; pH of aq solns is 6.9. LD₅₀ s.c. in male mice: 700 mg/kg (Klosa).

THERAP CAT: Decongestant (nasal).

1634. Cafestol. [469-83-0] [3bS-(3bα,5aβ,7β,8β,10aα,-10bβ)]-3b,4,5,6,7,8,9,10,10a,10b,11,12-Dodecahydro-7-hydroxy-10b-methyl-5a,8-methano-5aH-cyclohepta[5,6]naphtho[2,1-*b*]furan-7-methanol; cafesterol. $C_{20}H_{28}O_3$; mol wt 316.43. C 75.91%, H 8.92%, O 15.17%. Diterpenoid constituent of coffee. Isoln from green coffee oil: Slotta, Neisser, *Ber.* **71**, 1991, 2342 (1938); C. Djerassi *et al., J. Org. Chem.* **18**, 1449 (1953). Prepn and purification: R. Bertholet, **US 4692534** (1987 to Nestec). Structure: C. Djerassi *et al., J. Am. Chem. Soc.* **81**, 2386 (1959); R. A. Finnegan, C. Djerassi, *ibid.* **82**, 4342 (1960). Stereochemical studies: R. A. Finnegan, *J. Org. Chem.* **26**, 3057 (1961); A. I. Scott *et al., J. Am. Chem. Soc.* **84**, 3197 (1962); A. I. Scott *et al., Tetrahedron* **20**, 1339 (1964). Stereospecific total synthesis of (±)-form: E. J. Corey *et al., J. Am. Chem. Soc.* **109**, 4717 (1987).

Crystals from hexane, mp 158°-160°. [α]$_D$ −101°. uv max: 222 nm (log ε 3.78).

Acetate. $C_{22}H_{30}O_4$. Needles from petr ether, mp 167-168°. [α]$_D$ −89°. uv max: 222 nm (log ε 3.80).

Tetrahydrocafestol. $C_{20}H_{32}O_3$. Crystals from dil methanol, mp 154.5-157°.

1635. Caffeic Acid. [331-39-5] 3-(3,4-Dihydroxyphenyl)-2-propenoic acid; 3,4-dihydroxycinnamic acid. $C_9H_8O_4$; mol wt 180.16. C 60.00%, H 4.48%, O 35.52%. Constituent of plants, probably occurs in plants only in conjugated forms, e.g., chlorogenic acid. Isoln from green coffee: Wolfrom *et al., J. Agric. Food Chem.* **8**, 58 (1960); from roasted coffee: Krasemann, *Arch. Pharm.* **293**, 721 (1960). Formation by acid hydrolysis of chlorogenic acid: Fiedler, *Arzneim.-Forsch.* **4**, 41 (1954); Whiting, Carr, *Nature* **180**, 1479 (1957); Guern, *C.A.* **61**, 9965h (1964). Synthesis: Hayduck, *Ber.* **36**, 2935 (1903); Posner, *J. Prakt. Chem.* **82**, 432 (1910); Mauthner, *ibid.* **142**, 33 (1935); Pandya *et al., Proc. Indian Acad. Sci.* **9A**, 511 (1939); Neish, *Can. J. Biochem. Physiol.* **37**, 1431 (1959). *Review:* Herrmann, *Pharmazie* **11**, 433 (1956).

Yellow crystals from concd aq solns. Monohydrate from dil solns. Dec 223-225° (softens at 194°). R$_f$ values: Fiedler, *loc. cit.* Sparingly sol in cold water. Freely sol in hot water, cold alc. Alkaline solns turn from yellow to orange.

Methyl ester. $C_{10}H_{10}O_4$. Colorless needles from water, mp 152-153°.

1636. Caffeine. [58-08-2] 3,7-Dihydro-1,3,7-trimethyl-1H-purine-2,6-dione; 1,3,7-trimethylxanthine; 1,3,7-trimethyl-2,6-dioxopurine; coffeine; thein; guaranine; methyltheobromine; No-

Doz. $C_8H_{10}N_4O_2$; mol wt 194.19. C 49.48%, H 5.19%, N 28.85%, O 16.48%. Naturally occurring alkaloid commonly found in tea leaves, coffee beans, cocoa beans, maté leaves, guarana paste and kola nuts. Originally isolated from coffee in 1821. Synthesis: E. Fischer, *Ber.* **15**, 453 (1882); E. Fischer, L. Ach, *ibid.* **28**, 3135 (1895); W. Traube, *ibid.* **33**, 1371, 3035 (1900); H. Bredereck *et al.*, *ibid.* **83**, 201 (1950). Crystal structure: D. J. Sutor, *Acta Crystallogr.* **11**, 453 (1958). Arrhythmogenic effects in humans: D. J. Dobmeyer *et al.*, *N. Engl. J. Med.* **308**, 814 (1983). Teratogenicity study: P. E. Palm *et al.*, *Toxicol. Appl. Pharmacol.* **44**, 1 (1978). HPLC determn in serum: D. T. Holland *et al.*, *J. Chromatogr. B* **707**, 105 (1998). Comprehensive description: M. U. Zubair *et al.*, *Anal. Profiles Drug Subs.* **15**, 71-150 (1986). Review of dietary sources: D. M. Graham, *Nutr. Rev.* **36**, 97-102 (1978); of clinical pharmacology: N. L. Benowitz, *Annu. Rev. Med.* **41**, 277-288 (1990); of CNS effects: A. Nehlig *et al.*, *Brain Res. Rev.* **17**, 139-170 (1992); of therapeutic uses: J. Sawynok, *Drugs* **49**, 37-50 (1996).

Hexagonal prisms by sublimation, mp 238°. Odorless with bitter taste. Sublimes 178°. Fast sublimation is obtained at 160-165° under 1 mm press. at 5 mm distance. d_4^{18} 1.23. pH of 1% soln 6.9. Absorption spectrum: Hartley, *J. Chem. Soc.* **87**, 1802 (1905). One gram dissolves in 46 ml water, 5.5 ml water at 80°, 1.5 ml boiling water, 66 ml alcohol, 22 ml alcohol at 60°, 50 ml acetone, 5.5 ml chloroform, 530 ml ether, 100 ml benzene, 22 ml boiling benzene. Freely sol in pyrrole; in tetrahydrofuran contg about 4% water; also sol in ethyl acetate; slightly in petr ether. Soly in water is increased by alkali benzoates, cinnamates, citrates or salicylates. LD_{50} orally in mice, hamsters, rats, rabbits (mg/kg): 127, 230, 355, 246 (males); 137, 249, 247, 224 (females) (Palm).

Monohydrate. Felted needles, contg 8.5% H_2O. Efflorescent in air; complete dehydration takes place at 80°.

Mixture with citric acid. [69-22-7] Caffeine citrate; citrated caffeine; Cafcit. Clinical trial in treatment of apnea in premature neonates: P. B. Larsen *et al.*, *Acta Paediatr.* **84**, 360 (1995). White, crystalline powder; acid reaction. Sol in about 4 parts warm water.

THERAP CAT: CNS stimulant; respiratory stimulant.

THERAP CAT (VET): Cardiac and respiratory stimulant; diuretic.

1637. Calamus. Sweet flag; calmus; sweet cane; sweet grass. Perennial, iris-like plant, *Acorus calamus* L., *Araceae*. *Habit*. Europe, North America, Western Asia; cultivated in Burma and Ceylon. Several varieties exist and are characterized based on β-asarone content. Medicinal portion is the rhizome. *Constit*. Volatile oil (1.5-3.5%), resins (2.5%), tannins (1.5%); bitter principles such as acorin; mucilage, starch, sugars. Review of toxicology: M. J. Cupp, *Toxicology and Clinical Pharmacology of Herbal Products* (Humana Press, Totowa, 2000) pp 171-175; of medicinal uses and constituents: J. Barnes *et al.*, *Herbal Medicines* (Pharmaceutical Press, London, 2nd Ed., 2002) pp 100-102.

Volatile oil. [8015-79-0] Oil of sweet flag. Obtained by steam distillation of the fresh or unpeeled dried rhizome. *Constit*. β-Asarone, highly variable, 90-96% in Indian variety; calamenol (5%), calamene (4%), calamone, methyl eugenol, eugenol, sesquiterpenes. Toxicity study: J. M. Taylor *et al.*, *Toxicol. Appl. Pharmacol.* **10**, 405 (1967). Fragrance monograph: *Food Cosmet. Toxicol.* **15**, 623-626 (1977). Review of composition and uses: C. Singh *et al.*, *J. Med. Aromat. Plant Sci.* **23**, 687-708 (2001). Yellow to yellowish-brown viscid liquid; bitter taste. Soft, mellow fragrance reminiscent of patchouli. d_{20}^{20} 0.960-0.970. α_D^{20} +9 to +31°. n_D^{20} 1.507-1.515. Sapon no. 16-20. Very slightly sol in water; miscible with alcohol. LD_{50} orally in rats (Jammu variety): 777 mg/kg (Taylor). *Keep well closed, cool and protected from light.*

USE: In perfumery; as moisturizer in skin and hair preparations. Has been used as a flavoring ingredient and cooking spice.

THERAP CAT: Carminative, spasmolytic, diaphoretic.

1638. Calcifediol. [19356-17-3] (3β,5Z,7E)-9,10-Secocholesta-5,7,10(19)-triene-3,25-diol; 25-hydroxyvitamin D_3; 25-hydroxycholecalciferol; 25-HCC; U-32070E; Dedrogyl; Didrogyl; Hidroferol. $C_{27}H_{44}O_2$; mol wt 400.64. C 80.94%, H 11.07%, O 7.99%. The principal circulating form of vitamin D_3, formed in the liver by hydroxylation at C-25: Ponchon, DeLuca, *J. Clin. Invest.* **48**, 1273 (1969). It is the intermediate in the formation of 1α,25-dihydroxycholecalciferol, *q.v.*, the biologically active form of vitamin D_3 in the intestine. Identification in rat as an active metabolite of vitamin D_3: Lund, DeLuca, *J. Lipid Res.* **7**, 739 (1966); Morii *et al.*, *Arch. Biochem. Biophys.* **120**, 513 (1967). Evaluation of biological activity in comparison with vitamin D_3: Blunt *et al.*, *Proc. Natl. Acad. Sci. USA* **61**, 717 (1968); *ibid.* 1503. Isoln from porcine plasma and establishment of structure: Blunt *et al.*, *Biochemistry* **7**, 3317 (1968). Synthesis: Blunt, DeLuca, *ibid.* **8**, 671 (1969). Review of isoln, identification and synthesis: DeLuca, *Am. J. Clin. Nutr.* **22**, 412 (1969). Review of bioassays: J. G. Haddad Jr., *Basic Clin. Nutr.* **2**, 579-597 (1980).

uv max (ethanol): 265 nm (ε 18000) (Blunt, DeLuca).

THERAP CAT: Calcium regulator.

1639. Calcimycin. [52665-69-7] 5-(Methylamino)-2-[[(2R,3R,6S,8S,9R,11R)-3,9,11-trimethyl-8-[(1S)-1-methyl-2-oxo-2-(1H-pyrrol-2-yl)ethyl]-1,7-dioxaspiro[5.5]undec-2-yl]methyl]-4-benzoxazolecarboxylic acid; antibiotic A-23187; A-23187. $C_{29}H_{37}N_3O_6$; mol wt 523.62. C 66.52%, H 7.12%, N 8.02%, O 18.33%. Polyether antibiotic produced by a strain of *Streptomyces chartreusensis* Calhoun and Johnson NRRL 3882. Activity as a divalent cation ionophore in isolated mitochondria: P. W. Reed, H. A. Lardy, *J. Biol. Chem.* **247**, 6970 (1972). Prepn and antimicrobial activity: R. M. Gale *et al.*, *US 3923823* (1975 to Lilly). Elucidation of structure: M. O. Chaney *et al.*, *J. Am. Chem. Soc.* **96**, 1932 (1974). Spectral studies of ionophore and metal ion complexes: D. R. Pfeiffer *et al.*, *Biochemistry* **13**, 4007 (1974). Total synthesis and absolute configuration: D. A. Evans *et al.*, *J. Am. Chem. Soc.* **101**, 6789 (1979); P. A. Grieco *et al.*, *J. Org. Chem.* **45**, 3537 (1980). Stereospecific synthesis: G. R. Martinez *et al.*, *J. Am. Chem. Soc.* **104**, 1436 (1982); D. P. Negri, Y. Kishi, *Tetrahedron Lett.* **28**, 1063 (1987). Review of cation binding and transport properties: D. R. Pfeiffer *et al.*, *Ann. N.Y. Acad. Sci.* **307**, 402-423 (1978). Use in model systems of calcium transport: M. Takamori *et al.*, *J. Neurol. Sci.* **50**, 89 (1981); M. Takamori *et al.*, *ibid.* **51**, 207 (1981); M. H. Freedman *et al.*, *Cell. Immunol.* **58**, 134 (1981); G. Thomas, *Eur. J. Pharmacol.* **81**, 35 (1982); V. L. Lew, J. Garcia-Sancho, *Cell Calcium* **6**, 15 (1985).

Crystalline solid, mp 181-182°. $[\alpha]_D^{25}$ −56° (c = 1 in chloroform). uv max (ethanol): 204, 225, 278, 378 nm (E 28200, 26200, 18200, 8200). pKa_1 6.9 in 90% DMSO. Slightly sol in water, readily sol in ethyl acetate, chloroform, methanol, DMSO. Also reported as mp 184.5-186° (Evans, 1979). LD_{50} i.p. in mice: 10 mg/kg (Gale).

Mixed calcium-magnesium salt. Colorless crystalline solid, mp 230-250° (dec). uv max (ethanol, neutral): 202, 228, 303, 370 nm ($E_{1cm}^{1\%}$ 425, 490, 278, 109). Insol in water, pentane, hexane, heptane. Very slightly sol in methanol, DMSO. Very sol in methylene chloride, chloroform, acetone, methyl ethyl ketone, diethyl ketone, ethyl acetate.

USE: Biochemical tool used to study the role of divalent cations in various biological systems.

1640. Calcineurin. [9025-75-6] Phosphoprotein phosphatase. Ca^{2+}/calmodulin dependent ser-thr phosphatase that participates in many signalling pathways involved in gene regulation or biological responses to external stimuli in various organisms and cell types. Highly conserved heterodimer from yeast to humans comprised of a 58-69 kDa catalytic and calmodulin binding subunit A, *calcineurin A*, and a 16-19 kDa regulatory subunit B, *calcineurin B*. Isoln: J. H. Wang, R. Desai, *Biochem. Biophys. Res. Commun.* **72**, 926 (1976). Purification: C. B. Klee, M. H. Krinks, *Biochemistry* **17**, 120 (1978); and phosphatase activity: C. B. Klee *et al., Proc. Natl. Acad. Sci. USA* **76**, 6270 (1979). Review of early work: C. B. Klee, J. Haiech, *Ann. N.Y. Acad. Sci.* **1980**, 43-54; of role in neuronal cells and brain injury: M. Morioka *et al., Prog. Neurobiol.* **58**, 1-30 (1999). Review of structure and function: C. B. Klee *et al., J. Biol. Chem.* **273**, 13367-13370 (1998); J. Aramburu *et al., Curr. Top. Cell. Regul.* **36**, 237-295 (2000).

1641. Calcipotriene. [112965-21-6] (1α,3β,5Z,7E,22E,-24S)-24-Cyclopropyl-9,10-secochola-5,7,10(19),22-tetraene-1,3,24-triol; (1S,1'E,3R,5Z,7E,20R)-9,10-seco-20-(3'-cyclopropyl-3'-hydroxyprop-1'-enyl)-1,3-dihydroxypregna-5,7,10(19)-triene; calcipotriol; MC-903; Daivonex; Dovonex; Psorcutan. $C_{27}H_{40}O_3$; mol wt 412.60. C 78.60%, H 9.77%, O 11.63%. Vitamin D_3 analog with low calcemic activity. Prepn: M. J. Calverley, E. T. Binderup, **WO 8700834**; *eidem,* **US 4866048** (1987, 1989 both to Leo Pharm.); M. J. Calverley, *Tetrahedron* **43**, 4609 (1987). Pharmacology: L. Binderup, E. Bramm, *Biochem. Pharmacol.* **37**, 889 (1988); P. J. Marie *et al., Bone* **11**, 171 (1990). Receptor binding: T. Valaja *et al., Biochem. Pharmacol.* **40**, 1827 (1990). Review of clinical trials in psoriasis: D. M. Ashcroft *et al., Br. Med. J.* **320**, 963-967 (2000).

Crystals from methyl formate, mp 166-168°. uv max (96% ethanol): 264 nm (ε 17200).

THERAP CAT: Antipsoriatic.

1642. Calciseptine. [134710-25-1] Peptide toxin, 60 amino acids long with 4 disulfide bridges, isolated from the venom of the black mamba snake (*Dendroaspis polylepis polylepis*); specific blocker of L-type Ca^{2+} channels. Isoln and characterization: J. R. De Weille *et al., Proc. Natl. Acad. Sci. USA* **88**, 2437 (1991). Solution synthesis: H. Kuroda *et al., Peptide Res.* **5**, 265 (1992). NMR 3d structure determn: H. Haruyama *et al., Bull. Magn. Reson.* **18**, 125 (1996). Analysis of residues involved in binding: R. M. Kini *et al., Biochemistry* **37**, 9058 (1998). Differential sensitivities to L-channel subtypes: C. M. Rogers, E. R. Brown, *Exp. Physiol.* **86**, 689 (2001). Comparison with 1,4-dihydropyridines of effects on smooth muscle: T. X. Watanbe *et al., Jpn. J. Pharmacol.* **68**, 305 (1995); on skeletal muscle: M. C. Garcia *et al., J. Membr. Biol.* **184**, 121 (2001).

USE: Biochemical probe for L-type Ca^{2+} channels.

1643. Calcitonin. [9007-12-9] Thyrocalcitonin; TCA; TCT. Calcium regulating hormone secreted from the mammalian thyroid gland and in non-mammalian species from the ultimobranchial gland. Postulation of a plasma-calcium lowering substance: Copp *et al., Endocrinology* **70**, 638 (1962). Recognition as a hormone: Hirsch *et al., ibid.* **73**, 244 (1963); of thyroid origin: Foster *et al., Nature* **202**, 1303 (1964). Over-all action is to oppose the bone and renal effects of parathyroid hormone, *q.v.;* inhibits bone resorption of Ca^{2+}, with accompanying hypocalcemia and hypophosphatemia and decreased urinary Ca^{2+} concentrations. Also abolishes the osteolytic effect of toxic doses of vitamins A and D. Calcitonin is highly active biologically, *e.g.* 50 mγ/min infused into a 100 g rat leads to a significant (1 mg/100 ml) decrease in the concn of the plasma calcium within 60 min (together with a corresponding fall in plasma phosphate). Activity is destroyed by trypsin, chymotrypsin, pepsin, polyphenol oxidase; also by hydrogen peroxide oxidation, photooxidation, and treatment with *N*-bromosuccinimide. Calcitonin structures are single polypeptide chains containing 32 amino acid residues. Structure of porcine: Neher *et al., Helv. Chim. Acta* **51**, 917 (1968); Potts *et al., Proc. Natl. Acad. Sci. USA* **59**, 1321 (1968); Bell *et al., J. Am. Chem. Soc.* **90**, 2704 (1968); *eidem, Biochemistry* **9**, 1665 (1970). Synthesis of porcine: Rittel *et al., Helv. Chim. Acta* **51**, 924 (1968); Guttmann *et al., ibid.* 1155. Isoln of human calcitonin from non-pathological thyroid glands: Haymovits, Rosen, *Endocrinology* **81**, 993 (1967); from medullary carcinoma of the thyroid: Neher *et al., Nature* **220**, 984 (1968); *Helv. Chim. Acta* **51**, 1738 (1968); Neher, Riniker, **DE 1929957** (1970 to Ciba), *C.A.* **73**, 28902b (1970). Structure of human: Neher *et al., Helv. Chim. Acta* **51**, 1900 (1968). Synthesis of human: Sieber *et al., ibid.* 2057; J. Hirt *et al., Rec. Trav. Chim.* **98**, 143 (1979). Biosynthetic studies: J. W. Jacobs *et al., J. Biol. Chem.* **254**, 10600 (1979); S. G. Amara *et al., ibid.* **255**, 2645 (1980). Amino acid sequence differs among mammalian species, salmon calcitonin showing a marked difference from that of the higher vertebrae as well as a more potent biological activity. Mechanism of action: E. M. Brown, G. D. Aurbach, *Vitam. Horm.* **38**, 236 (1980). Anorectic activity in rats: W. J. Freed *et al., Science* **206**, 850 (1979). Growth inhibition of human breast cancer cells *in vitro:* Y. Iwasaki *et al., Biochem. Biophys. Res. Commun.* **110**, 235 (1983). Review of early literature: Munson, Hirsch, *Clin. Orthop.* **49**, 209 (1966). Review of isoln, structure, synthesis: Behrens, Grinnan, *Annu. Rev. Biochem.* **38**, 83 (1969); Potts *et al., Vitam. Horm.* **29**, 41 (1971). Comprehensive review: *Calcitonin, Proc. Symp. on Thyrocalcitonin and the C Cells,* S. Taylor, Ed. (Springer-Verlag, New York, 1968); Foster *et al.,* "Calcitonin" in *Clinics in Endocrinology and Metabolism,* I. MacIntyre, Ed. (W. B. Saunders, Philadelphia, 1972) pp 93-124. Review of pharmacology and therapeutic use: J. C. Stevenson, I. M. A. Evans, *Drugs* **21**, 257-272 (1981).

  Calcitonin, porcine. [12321-44-7] Calcitar(e); Staporos.
  Calcitonin, human synthetic. [21215-62-3] Cibacalcin.
  Calcitonin, salmon synthetic. [47931-85-1] Salcatonin; Calciben; Calcimar; Calsyn; Calsynar; Catonin; Karil; Miacalcic; Miacalcin; Miadenil; Osteocalcin; Prontocalcin; Rulicalcin; Salmotonin; Stalcin; Tonocalcin. Clinical trial in postmenopausal osteoporosis: C. H. Chesnut *et al., Am. J. Med.* **109**, 267 (2000). LC determn in biological fluids: M. Aguiar *et al., J. Chromatogr. B* **818**, 301 (2005). *See also* Elcatonin.

  THERAP CAT: Calcium regulator.

1644. Calcitriol. [32222-06-3] (1α,3β,5Z,7E)-9,10-Seco-cholesta-5,7,10(19)-triene-1,3,25-triol; 1α,25-dihydroxycholecalciferol; 1α,25-dihydroxyvitamin D_3; 1,25-DHCC; Ro-21-5535; Calcijex; Rocaltrol; Silkis. $C_{27}H_{44}O_3$; mol wt 416.64. C 77.83%, H 10.64%, O 11.52%. The biologically active form of vitamin D_3, *q.v.,* in intestinal calcium transport and bone calcium resorption. First obtained from chick intestine and designated as metabolite 4B: J. F. Myrtle *et al., J. Biol. Chem.* **245**, 1190 (1970); M. R. Haussler *et al., Proc. Natl. Acad. Sci. USA* **68**, 177 (1971). Isoln and identification: M. F. Holick *et al., ibid.* 803; D. E. M. Lawson *et al., Nature* **230**, 228 (1971); A. W. Norman *et al., Science* **173**, 51 (1971). Synthesis: D. H. R. Barton *et al., J. Chem. Soc. Chem. Commun.* **1974**, 203; T. Sato *et al., Chem. Pharm. Bull.* **26**, 2933 (1978). Effect of calcium on *in vivo* synthesis: I. T. Boyle *et al., Proc. Natl. Acad. Sci. USA* **68**, 2131 (1971). Stimulation of bone resorption in tissue culture: L. G. Raisz *et al., Science* **175**, 768

(1972). Classification as a steroid hormone: J. S. Emtage *et al., Nature* **246**, 100 (1973). Pharmacokinetics: J. R. Muindi *et al., Clin. Pharmacol. Ther.* **72**, 648 (2002). Clinical evaluation in prostate cancer: C. Gross *et al., J. Urol.* **159**, 2035 (1998); in secondary hyperparathyroidism: S. Koshikawa *et al., Nephron* **90**, 413 (2002). Comprehensive description: T. Suda, *Vitamins* **45**, 175-188 (1972); E. Debesis, *Anal. Profiles Drug Subs.* **8**, 83-100 (1979). Review of clinical efficacy in osteoporosis: K. L. Dechant, K. L. Goa, *Drugs Aging* **5**, 300-317 (1994); of mechanism of action in renal failure: C. H. Hsu *et al., Kidney Int.* **46**, 605-612 (1994); of clinical experience in treatment of psoriasis: L. Kowalzick, *Br. J. Dermatol.* **144**, Suppl. 58, 21-25 (2001).

White crystalline powder, mp 111-115°. uv max (abs ethanol): 264 nm (ε 19000). [α]$_D^{25}$ +48° (methanol). Slightly sol in methanol, ethanol, ethyl acetate, THF. Air and light sensitive.

THERAP CAT: Calcium regulator; vitamin (antirachitic); antihyperparathyroid; antineoplastic; antipsoriatic.

1645. Calcium. [7440-70-2] Ca; at. wt 40.078; at. no. 20; valence 2. Group IIA (2). Alkaline earth metal. Occurrence in the earth's crust 3.64% (fifth element in order of abundance). Sea water contains about 400 g/ton. Naturally occurring isotopes: 40 (96.941%), 44 (2.086%), 42 (0.647%), 48 (0.187%), 43 (0.135%), 46 (0.004%). Known radioactive isotopes: 35-39, 41, 45, 47-51. Found naturally only in the form of its compds, never uncombined, in minerals such as limestone, dolomite, marble, chalk, iceland spar, gypsum, anhydrite, fluorite, apatite. Principal commercial source is limestone, *q.v.* Major commercial production by high temperature vacuum reduction of calcium oxide in aluminothermal process; less commonly by electrolysis followed by redistillation. Essential constituent of bones, shells, teeth, coral, pearls. Essential nutrient for animal life. First isolated by Davy in 1808. Produced by electrolysis of calcium chloride: Rathenau, Suter, **DE 155433** (1903); *Z. Elektrochem.* **10**, 502 (1904); Goodwin, *J. Am. Chem. Soc.* **27**, 1403 (1905); also by thermal reduction of lime with silicon, or with aluminum. Prepn of the pure metal for laboratory use: Whaley, *Inorg. Synth.* **6**, 18 (1960). Purifn of commercial material: Marshall, Whaley, *ibid.* 24. *Reviews:* Schaufler in *Ullmanns Encyklopädie der technischen Chemie* vol. 4 (Munich, 3rd ed., 1953) pp 830-836; Mantell in C. A. Hampel, *Rare Metals Handbook* (Reinhold, New York, 1954) p 17-29. Review of calcium and its compounds: Goodenough, Stenger, "Magnesium, Calcium, Strontium, Barium and Radium" in *Comprehensive Inorganic Chemistry* **Vol. 1**, J. C. Bailar Jr. *et al.*, Eds. (Pergamon Press, Oxford, 1973) pp 591-664; *Chemistry of the Elements*, N. N. Greenwood, A. Earnshaw, Eds. (Pergamon Press, New York, 1984) pp 117-154; R. L. Petersen, M. B. Freilich in *Kirk-Othmer Encyclopedia of Chemical Technology* vol. 4 (Wiley-Interscience, New York, 4th ed., 1992) pp 777-796. Book: R. P. Rubin, *Calcium and Cellular Secretion* (Plenum, New York, 1982) 276 pp.

Lustrous, silver-white surface (when freshly cut); face-centered cubic structure, transforms to body-centered cubic form at 428 ±2°. Soft, ductile. Brinell hardness: 17. Much harder than sodium, but softer than aluminum or magnesium. Oxidizes and acquires bluish-gray tarnish on exposure to moist air. d$_4^{20}$ 1.54. mp 839°. bp 1484°. Electrical resistivity at 20°: 3.5 μohm cm. Heat of combustion 151.9 cal/g. Specific heat (0-100°) 0.149 cal/g. Considerably less reactive than sodium. E° (aq) Ca^{2+}/Ca −2.87 V. Reacts with water, alcohols, and dil acids with evolution of hydrogen, creating explosion hazard. Reacts with halogens. Dissolves in liquid ammonia to form a blue black soln. Ignites in air when finely divided. Emits characteristic orange-red color in flame. Insol in and inert towards benzene, kerosene.

USE: Reducing agent for production of less common metals; alloying agent to increase strength and corrosion resistance in lead, to improve mechanical and electrical properties in aluminum; refining agent to remove bismuth from lead. In metallurgy as scavenger to deoxidize, desulfurize and degas steel and cast iron; to control non-metallic inclusions in steel; to promote uniform microstructure in gray iron. As anode material in thermal batteries; as "getter" for oxygen and nitrogen.

1646. Calcium Acetate. [62-54-0] Acetic acid calcium salt; Phos-ex; PhosLo. C$_4$H$_6$CaO$_4$; mol wt 158.17. C 30.37%, H 3.82%, Ca 25.34%, O 40.46%. Ca(CH$_3$COO)$_2$. The technical product was originally known as *brown acetate of lime* or *gray acetate of lime*. Prepn and analysis of acetate of lime: Stillwell, Gladding, *J. Am. Chem. Soc.* **4**, 94 (1882); T. S. Gladding, *Ind. Eng. Chem.* **1**, 250 (1909). Distillation to produce acetone: E. G. R. Ardagh *et al., ibid.* **16**, 1133 (1924). Electrolytic prepn: H. Schmidt, *Z. Anorg. Allg. Chem.* **270**, 188 (1952). Analysis of hydrated forms: J. Panzer, *J. Chem. Eng. Data* **7**, 140 (1962). Toxicity study: Smyth *et al., Am. Ind. Hyg. Assoc. J.* **30**, 470 (1969). Clinical evaluation in hyperphosphatemia: W. Y. Qunibi *et al., Kidney Int.* **65**, 1914 (2004).

Very hygroscopic, rod-shaped crystals. On heating above 160° dec to acetone and CaCO$_3$. d 1.50. Sol in water; slightly sol in methanol. Practically insol in ethanol, acetone, benzene. *Keep well closed.*

Monohydrate. [5743-26-0] Needles, granules or powder. Does not lose all its water below 150°. Sol in water; slightly sol in alcohol. pH of 0.2 molar aq soln 7.6. LD$_{50}$ orally in rats: 4.28 g/kg (Smyth).

USE: Manuf of acetic acid, acetone; in dyeing, tanning, and curing skins; in lubricants; as food stabilizer; as corrosion inhibitor.

THERAP CAT: Antihyperphosphatemic.

1647. Calcium Acetylsalicylate. [69-46-5] 2-(Acetyloxy)benzoic acid calcium salt; salicylic acid acetate calcium salt; acetylsalicylic acid calcium salt; calcium aspirin; soluble aspirin; Cal-Aspirin; Dispril; Disprin; Kalmopyrin; Kalsetal; Solaspin; Tylcalsin. C$_{18}$H$_{14}$CaO$_8$; mol wt 398.38. C 54.27%, H 3.54%, Ca 10.06%, O 32.13%. Ca(OOCC$_6$H$_4$OCOCH$_3$)$_2$. Prepd from calcium carbonate and acetylsalicylic acid: Lawrence, US 2003374 (1935 to Lee Labs.).

Dihydrate. Amorphous, nonhygroscopic powder. One gram dissolves in 6 ml water, 80 ml alcohol.

Complex with urea. [5749-67-7] Carbasalate calcium; acetylsalicylic acid calcium salt complex with urea; calcium acetylsalicylate carbamide; urea calcium acetylsalicylate; carbaspirin calcium; Alcacyl; Ascal; Calurin; Cardiosolupsan; Solupsan. C$_{19}$H$_{18}$CaN$_2$O$_9$; mol wt 458.43. Description and hydrolytic stability: Parrott, *J. Pharm. Sci.* **51**, 897 (1962). Clinical trial in migraine: C. Le Jeune *et al., Eur. Neurol.* **41**, 37 (1999). Amorphous powder, dec 243-245°. Soly in water at 37°: 231 mg/ml, pH 4.8.

THERAP CAT: Analgesic; antipyretic; anti-inflammatory.

1648. Calcium Aluminosilicate. [1327-39-5] Aluminum calcium silicate. Many different forms of calcium aluminosilicate are known, the most common of which are CaAl$_2$Si$_2$O$_8$ and Ca$_2$-Al$_2$SiO$_7$. It occurs in nature as the minerals: *anorthite, bavenite, clinozoisite, didymolite, epistilbite, gehlenite, gismondite, grossularite, heulandite, hibschite, laubanite, laumontite, lawsonite, levynite, margarite, meionite, plazolite, pumpellyite, scolecite, stellerite, vesuvianite, zoisite.* Prepn and properties: Gmelins, *Aluminum* (8th ed.) **35B**, 576-586 (1934). Summary and references for minerals: Hey, *An Index of Mineral Species and Varieties* (British Museum, London, 2nd ed., 1962) pp 159-162.

USE: Constituent of cement; in refractories.

1649. Calcium Arsenate. [7778-44-1] Tricalcium arsenate. As$_2$Ca$_3$O$_8$; mol wt 398.07. As 37.64%, Ca 30.20%, O 32.15%. Ca$_3$(AsO$_4$)$_2$. Prepn: Les Veaux, US 2715562 (1955 to FMC). Toxicity study: T. B. Gaines, *Toxicol. Appl. Pharmacol.* **14**, 515 (1969). *Review:* Guerin, *Chim. Ind. (Paris)* **77**, 1288 (1957). Review of toxicology and human exposure: *Toxicological Profile for Arsenic* (PB2000-108021, 2000) 468 pp.

Powder. *Poisonous!* Slightly sol in water; sol in dil acids. LD_{50} orally in female rats: 298 mg/kg (Gaines).

Caution: Potential symptoms of overexposure are weakness; GI disturbance; peripheral neuropathy; skin hyperpigmentation, palmar planter hyperkeratoses; dermatitis. Potential occupational carcinogen. *See NIOSH Pocket Guide to Chemical Hazards* (DHHS/-NIOSH 97-140, 1997) p 46.

USE: Insecticide; molluscicide.

1650. Calcium Arsenite. [52740-16-6] Variable composition. Prepd by passing steam over a dry mixture of CaO and As_2O_3: Altwegg, Dutel, **US 1700756** (1929).

White, granular powder. *Poisonous!* Slightly sol in water; sol in acids.

USE: As insecticide, germicide, molluscicide.

1651. Calcium Bisulfite, Solution. [13780-03-5] Ca-$(HSO_3)_2$ is known only in soln. Prepn from sulfite liquor: Arend, *Chem. Prod.* **10**, 53 (1947); Lougheed, *Pulp Paper Mag. Can.* **49**(3), 215 (1948); Schoeffel, **US 2696424** (1954 to Sterling Drug). The product here described is substantially a soln of calcium sulfite in an aq sulfur dioxide soln.

Colorless or slightly yellow liquid; strong SO_2 odor. On standing in the air, crystals of $CaSO_3.2H_2O$ form. d about 1.06. This soln corrodes metals.

USE: As germicide, preservative, and disinfectant; for washing (1:1000) casks in brewing to prevent souring and cloudiness of beer and to prevent secondary fermentation; as antichlor in bleaching fabrics; largely in manuf sulfite cellulose from wood for paper-making.

1652. Calcium Borate. [12007-56-6] Calcium pyroborate; calcium tetraborate. B_4CaO_7; mol wt 195.32. B 22.14%, Ca 20.52%, O 57.34%. CaB_4O_7. Prepn by direct fusion of B_2O_3 with $CaCO_3$: Griveau, *Compt. Rend.* **166**, 993 (1918). Various calcium borate minerals occur in nature. These include: *colemanite, ginorite, inyoite, meyerhofferite, pandermite, priceite.*

Hexahydrate. Powder. Almost insol in cold, moderately sol in hot water; sol in dil acids.

USE: As flux in heavy-metal metallurgy; mfr of forsterite porcelain insulators; in glycol antifreeze; in fire-retardant paint.

1653. Calcium Borogluconate. [5743-34-0] D-Gluconic acid cyclic 4,5-ester with boric acid calcium salt (2:1); calcium diborogluconate. $C_{12}H_{20}B_2CaO_{16}$; mol wt 481.98. C 29.90%, H 4.18%, B 4.49%, Ca 8.32%, O 53.11%. Prepn and use in milk fever: H. Dryerre, J. R. Greig, *Vet. Rec.* **15**, 456 (1935); H. T. Macpherson, J. Stewart, *Biochem. J.* **32**, 76 (1938). Physical properties: L. Seekles, E. Havinga, *Nor. Veterinaertidsskr.* **58**, No. 11, 433-445 (1946), *C.A.* **43**, 1907 (1949). Effect on plasma calcium concentration in sheep: D. A. H. Farningham, *Res. Vet. Sci.* **39**, 70 (1985). Spectrophotometric determn in plasma: D. J. Lyons, K. P. Spann, *J. Assoc. Off. Anal. Chem.* **68**, 160 (1985). Evaluation in bovine milk fever: P. A. Mullen, *Vet. Rec.* **97**, 87 (1975).

Crystals, freely sol in water. Soly in water 1:1 at 15°: 2.8:1 at 100°. A 20% aq soln has a pH of 3.5. If desired, the pH may be adjusted to 7.0 by the addition of CaO which is very sol in Ca borogluconate solns.

THERAP CAT (VET): In hypocalcemic states including bovine milk fever.

1654. Calcium Bromide. [7789-41-5] Br_2Ca; mol wt 199.89. Br 79.95%, Ca 20.05%. $CaBr_2$. Prepn: *Gmelins, Calcium* (8th ed.) **28B**, 100-102, 584-599 (1958). The N.F. article is a

hydrated salt, contg not less than 84% and not more than 94% $CaBr_2$.

Odorless, deliquesc granules or rhombic crystals; sharp, saline taste. Becomes yellow on long exposure to air. When anhydr mp 730°; d_4^{25} 3.353. When strongly heated in air, becomes alkaline due to loss of bromine and formation of lime. Very sol in water, methanol, ethanol; sol in acetone; practically insol in dioxane, chloroform, ether. The aq soln is neutral or only slightly alkaline to litmus. *Keep well closed.*

USE: In photography for making dry plates and light-sensitive papers; manuf mineral waters, NH_4Br, fire-extinguishing compositions.

THERAP CAT: Sedative, anticonvulsant.

THERAP CAT (VET): Has been used in hypocalcemic states such as canine eclampsia.

1655. Calcium N-Carbamoylaspartate. [16649-79-9] N-(Aminocarbonyl)-L-aspartic acid calcium salt (1:1); N-carbamoyl-aspartic acid calcium salt; calcium ureidosuccinate. $C_5H_6CaN_2O_5$; mol wt 214.19. C 28.04%, H 2.82%, Ca 18.71%, N 13.08%, O 37.35%. Prepn of optically active forms: Miyazaki *et al., Chem. Pharm. Bull.* **15**, 1604 (1967); Yoshimura *et al.,* **JP 68 14205** (1968 to Dainippon Pharm.), *C.A.* **71**, 112456a (1969); of DL-form: Clemence, **FR M6376** (1968 to Roussel-UCLAF), *C.A.* **74**, 76655r (1971).

$[\alpha]_D^{20}$ +32.2° (c = 2.53).
DL-Form. [30905-63-6] Pacilan. mp >350°.
D-Form. [16649-82-4] $[\alpha]_D^{20}$ −31.5° (c = 1.54).

1656. Calcium Carbide. [75-20-7] Acetylenogen. C_2Ca; mol wt 64.10. C 37.47%, Ca 62.52%. CaC_2. Prepn: Ehrlich in *Handbook of Preparative Inorganic Chemistry* **Vol. 1**, G. Brauer, Ed. (Academic Press, New York, 2nd ed., 1963) p 943. *Review:* Brennan, *J. Electrochem. Soc.* **99**, 61c (1952).

Grayish-black, irregular lumps or orthorhombic crystals; dec by water with evolution of acetylene leaving a residue of lime. d 2.22; mp 2300°.

USE: Generating acetylene gas for lighting purposes (1 kg of carbide yields ~300 liters acetylene); as reducing agent, e.g., for direct reduction of copper sulfide to metallic copper; signal fires for marine service; manuf of calcium, iron, alloys, lampblack, cyanamide; welding and cutting metals.

1657. Calcium Carbonate. [471-34-1] Carbonic acid calcium salt (1:1); Cacit; Calcichew; Calcidia; Caltrate; Citrical; Fixical; Maalox Quick Dissolve; Maalox Regular Strength; Os-Cal; Tums Smooth Dissolve. $CCaO_3$; mol wt 100.09. C 12.00%, Ca 40.04%, O 47.96%. $CaCO_3$. Exists in nature as the minerals *aragonite, calcite* and *vaterite.* Solubility and scale formation study: J.-Y. Gal *et al., Talanta* **43**, 1497 (1996). Clinical evaluation in protease inhibitor-induced diarrhea in HIV: M. J. Turner *et al., HIV Clin. Trials* **5**, 19 (2004). Review of commercial applications in paints, coatings and adhesives: R. D. Athey, *Eur. Coatings J.* **5**, 256-263 (1994).

Odorless, tasteless powder or crystals. Two crystal forms are of commercial importance: Aragonite, orthorhombic, mp 825° (dec), d 2.83, formed at temps above 30°; Calcite, hexagonal-rhombohedral, mp 1339° (102.5 atm), $d^{25.2}$ 2.711, formed at temps below 30°. At about 825° is dec into CaO and CO_2. Practically insol in water. Sol in dil acids.

Precipitated calcium carbonate. Precipitated chalk; Aeromatt; Albacar; Purecal. Commercial $CaCO_3$ produced by chemical means. It is 98-99% pure. The byproduct process, the carbonation process, and the calcium chloride process of manuf from limestone are outlined in *Kirk-Othmer Encyclopedia of Chemical Technology* **vol. 4** (Interscience, New York, 2nd ed., 1964) pp 7-11. *Review:* Woerner in *Pigment Handbook* **vol. 1**, T. C. Patton, Ed. (John Wiley, New York, 1973) pp 119-128.

Prepared calcium carbonate. Drop chalk; prepared chalk; whiting; English white; Paris white. Native $CaCO_3$ purified by elutriation.

Caution: Potential symptoms of overexposure are irritation of eyes, skin, respiratory system; cough. *See NIOSH Pocket Guide to Chemical Hazards* (DHHS/NIOSH 97-140, 1997) p 46.

USE: Manuf of paint, rubber, plastics, paper, dentifrices, ceramics, putty, polishes, insecticides, inks, shoe dressings; as a filler in production of adhesives, matches, pencils; crayons, linoleum, insulating compds, welding rods. In foods, cosmetics, pharmaceuticals, antibiotics; removing acidity of wines. In anal. chem for detecting and determining halogens in organic combinations; with NH_4Cl for decomposing silicates; preparing $CaCl_2$ soln for standardizing soap solns; for water analyses.

THERAP CAT: Antacid. Calcium supplement.

THERAP CAT (VET): Antacid, calcium supplement, antidiarrheal agent.

1658. Calcium Chlorate. [10137-74-3] $CaCl_2O_6$; mol wt 206.98. Ca 19.36%, Cl 34.26%, O 46.38%. $Ca(ClO_3)_2$. Prepn: Wilderman, **GB 183671** (1921); Duveau, *Bull. Soc. Chim.* **10**, 374 (1943).

Dihydrate. [10035-05-9] Monoclinic, hygroscopic crystals. d 2.711. mp 100° when rapidly heated. Sol in 0.6 part water; sol in alcohol. *Keep well closed.*

USE: Herbicide, insecticide, seed disinfectant.

1659. Calcium Chloride. [10043-52-4] Intergravin-orales. $CaCl_2$; mol wt 110.98. Ca 36.11%, Cl 63.89%. Forms mono-, di-, tetra- and hexahydrates. Obtained as a byproduct of the ammonia-soda (Solvay) process and as a joint product from natural salt brines: *Faith, Keyes & Clark's Industrial Chemicals,* F. A. Lowenheim, M. K. Moran, Eds. (Wiley-Interscience, New York, 4th ed., 1975) pp 186-190. Acute toxicity: I. B. Syed, F. Hosain, *Toxicol. Appl. Pharmacol.* **22**, 150 (1972).

Cubic crystals, granules or fused masses. Very hygroscopic. mp 772°. bp >1600°; d_4^{15} 2.152. Freely sol in water (with liberation of much heat), alcohol. The commercial product is about 94-97% $CaCl_2$, the chief impurity being $Ca(OH)_2$. *Keep well closed.* LD_{50} i.v. in mice: 42.2 mg/kg (Syed, Hosain).

Dihydrate. Hygroscopic granules, flakes or powder. Apparent (bulk) density: 0.835. Freely sol in water, alcohol. Commercial grades contain 73-80% $CaCl_2$. *Keep well closed.*

Hexahydrate. Deliquesc trigonal crystals. mp 30°. d^{17} 1.68. Loses all H_2O at 200°. Extremely sol in water, alcohol. *Keep well closed.*

USE: The *anhydrous* form used as a drying and dehydrating agent for organic liquids and gases, and in desiccators. The *dihydrate* and *hexahydrate* forms are used for antifreeze and refrigerating solns, in fire extinguishers, etc. (a 40% soln freezes at −41°); to preserve wood, stone; manuf ice, glues, cements; fireproofing fabrics; automobile antifreeze mixtures; to melt ice and snow; as coagulant in rubber manuf, as size in admixture with starch paste; in concrete mixes to give quicker initial set and greater strength; freezeproofing of coal and ores; dust control on unpaved roads; sizing and finishing cotton fabrics; as brine for filling inflatable tires on tractors to increase traction.

THERAP CAT: Electrolyte replacement. Has been used as diuretic, urinary acidifier, antiallergic.

THERAP CAT (VET): May be used intravenously in hypocalcemic states such as milk fever.

1660. Calcium Chromate(VI). [13765-19-0] Calcium chrome yellow; gelbin; yellow ultramarine; C.I. 77223; C.I. Pigment Yellow 33. $CaCrO_4$; mol wt 156.07. Ca 25.68%, Cr 33.32%, O 41.01%. Prepn: Mylius, Wrochem, *Ber.* **33**, 3689 (1900); Udy, **US 2493789**; **US 2494215** (both 1950); Dunn, O'Brien, **US 2745764/5** (both 1956 to Vanadium Corp. of America).

Yellow monoclinic or rhombic crystals. Sparingly sol in water; sol in dil acids; practically insol in alcohol. Also occurs as hemihydrate, monohydrate, and dihydrate.

Caution: Chromium hexavalent compounds are listed as known human carcinogens: *Report on Carcinogens, Eleventh Edition* (PB2005-104914, 2004) p III-63.

USE: As a pigment, corrosion inhibitor; manuf of chromium; in oxidizing reactions; in battery depolarization.

1661. Calcium Citrate. [813-94-5] 2-Hydroxy-1,2,3-propanetricarboxylic acid calcium salt (2:3). $C_{12}H_{10}Ca_3O_{14}$; mol wt 498.43. C 28.92%, H 2.02%, Ca 24.12%, O 44.94%. $Ca_3(C_6H_5-O_7)_2$. Prepn from citrus fruit: Cole, **US 2389766** (1945 to California Fruit Growers Exchange). Use in foods: R. Labin-Goldscher, S. Edelstein, *Food Technol.* **50**, 96 (1996). Bioavailability compared with calcium carbonate: K. Sakhaee *et al., Am. J. Ther.* **6**, 313 (1999). Clinical effect on bone density: L. A. Ruml *et al., ibid.* 303; on serum lipid concentrations: I. R. Reid *et al., Am. J. Med.* **112**, 343 (2002).

Tetrahydrate. [5785-44-4] Calcimax; Citracal. Odorless powder. Loses most of its water at 100° and all at 120°. Sol in 1050 parts cold water; somewhat more sol in hot water. Insol in alcohol.

USE: In foods as calcium fortifier; as anticaking agent in dry mixes.

THERAP CAT: Calcium supplement.

1662. Calcium Cyanamide. [156-62-7] Calcium carbimide; "cyanamide"; nitrolime. $CCaN_2$; mol wt 80.10. C 14.99%, Ca 50.03%, N 34.97%. N≡CN=Ca. Prepn: Kastens, McBurney, *Ind. Eng. Chem.* **43**, 1020 (1951); Franck, Heimann, *Angew. Chem.* **44**, 372 (1931); Owen, *Trans. Faraday Soc.* **57**, 670 (1961); Dedman, Owen, *ibid.* 678.

Commercial grades may occur as grayish-black lumps of powder. While pure calcium cyanamide is nonvolatile and noncombustible, commercial grades may contain small amounts of calcium carbide which will produce acetylene in containers and processing vessels. Other contaminants are carbon, $Ca(OH)_2$, CaO, and $CaCO_3$. Pure calcium cyanamide occurs as glistening, hexagonal crystals belonging to the rhombohedral system. mp ~1340°; d_4^{20} 2.29. Sublimes at 1150-1200°. Heat of formn from $CaC_2 + N_2$: −69.0 kcal/mole (25°). Heat of fusion 1.29 cal/g. Essentially insol in water, but undergoes partial hydrolysis to the sol calcium hydrogen cyanamide, a source of cyanamide ions. No known solvent will bring about soln without decompn.

Caution: Potential symptoms of overexposure are irritation of eyes, skin, respiratory system; headache, vertigo, rapid breathing, low blood pressure, nausea, vomiting; skin burns and sensitization; cough; Antabuse-like effects. *See NIOSH Pocket Guide to Chemical Hazards* (DHHS/NIOSH 97-140, 1997) p 46.

USE: As fertilizer, defoliant, herbicide, pesticide; manuf and refining of iron; manuf of calcium cyanide, melamine, dicyandiamide.

THERAP CAT (VET): Has been used as an anthelmintic.

1663. Calcium Cyanamide Citrated. [8013-88-5] Citrated calcium carbimide; CCC; carbimide; Colme; Dipsan; Abstem; Temposil. Contains citric acid in two parts by weight to one part of calcium cyanamide suitably purified for drug use. Used in treatment of alcoholism. Formulations: de Grunigen, Ferguson, **US 2998350** (1961 to Cyanamid and Alcoholism Res. Found., Toronto). Acts by inhibiting aldehyde dehydrogenase: J. A. Smith *et al., J. Am. Med. Assoc.* **165**, 2181 (1957). Effect on cardiovascular system: J. E. Peachey *et al., Clin. Pharmacol. Ther.* **29**, 40 (1981); on liver cells: J. J. Vázquez, S. Cervera, *Lancet* **1**, 361 (1980). Comparison with disulfiram, *q.v.:* M. S. Levy *et al., Am. J. Psychiatry* **123**, 1018 (1967). Review of drug therapy for alcoholism: E. M. Sellers *et al., N. Engl. J. Med.* **305**, 1255 (1981).

THERAP CAT: Alcohol deterrent.

1664. Calcium Cyanide. [592-01-8] Cyanogas. C_2CaN_2; mol wt 92.11. C 26.08%, Ca 43.51%, N 30.41%. $Ca(CN)_2$. Prepn: *Gmelins, Calcium* (8th ed.) **28B**, 173-178, 958-960 (1958). Commercial prepns contain 40-50% $Ca(CN)_2$. Toxicity study: H. F. Smyth *et al., Am. Ind. Hyg. Assoc. J.* **30**, 470 (1969). Review of toxicology and human exposure: *Toxicological Profile for Cyanide* (PB98-101207, 1997) 291 pp.

Rhombohedric crystals or powder; dec in moist air liberating hydrogen cyanide. *Very poisonous!* Sol in water with gradual liberation of HCN; even very weak acid (CO_2) liberates HCN; sol in alc. *Keep dry.* LD_{50} orally in rats: 39 mg/kg (Smyth).

USE: Fumigant; rodenticide; in stainless-steel manuf; in leaching ores of precious metals; stabilizer for cement.

1665. Calcium Cyclamate. [139-06-0] Cyclohexylsulfamic acid calcium salt; cyclohexanesulfamic acid calcium salt; calcium cyclohexanesulfamate; calcium cyclohexylsulfamate; cyclamate calcium; Cyclan; Sucaryl Calcium. $C_{12}H_{24}CaN_2O_6S_2$; mol wt 396.54. C 36.35%, H 6.10%, Ca 10.11%, N 7.06%, O 24.21%, S 16.17%. $[C_6H_{11}NHSO_3^-]_2Ca^{2+}$. Prepn: Cummins, Johnson; McQuaid, **US 2799700; US 2804477** (both 1957 to du Pont); Freifelder, **US 3082247** (1963 to Abbott); Birsten, Rosin, **US 3361798; US 3366670** (both 1968 to Baldwin-Montrose). Metabolism: Wallace *et al., J. Pharmacol. Exp. Ther.* **175,** 325 (1970); Prosky, O'Dell, *J. Pharm. Sci.* **60,** 1341 (1971); Renwick, Williams, *Biochem. J.* **129,** 869 (1972). *See also* Cyclamic Acid.

Dihydrate. Crystals with pleasant, very sweet taste. Freely sol in water. Practically insol in alc, benzene, chloroform, ether. pH of 10% aq soln 5.5-7.5. Said to be more resistant to cooking temps than saccharin.

Note: Consult latest Government regulations on use in foods.
USE: Non-nutritive sweetener.

1666. Calcium Dichromate(VI). [14307-33-6] Calcium bichromate. $CaCr_2O_7$; mol wt 256.07. Ca 15.65%, Cr 40.61%, O 43.74%. Prepn: Hartford *et al., J. Am. Chem. Soc.* **72,** 3353 (1950).

Trihydrate. Bipyramidal orange-red crystals. Nonhygroscopic if pure. Dec on heating above 100° to $CaCrO_4$ and CrO_3. d_4^{30} 2.370. Very sol in water; insol in ether, CCl_4, hydrocarbons; dissolves in alc with immediate reduction of the dichromate and pptn of brown hydrous chromic chromate; dissolves in acetone with subsequent pptn of $CaCrO_4$.

USE: As catalyst; in manuf of $CrCl_3$ and CrO_3; corrosion inhibitor.

1667. Calcium Fluoride. [7789-75-5] CaF_2; mol wt 78.07. Ca 51.34%, F 48.67%. Occurs in nature as the mineral *fluorite* or *fluorspar*. Prepd from $CaCO_3$ + HF: O. Ruff, *Die Chemie des Fluors* (Berlin, 1920) p 89; Emeleus in *Fluorine Chemistry* vol. I, J. H. Simons, Ed. (Academic Press, 1950) p 36; Kwasnik in *Handbook of Preparative Inorganic Chemistry* Vol. 1, G. Brauer, Ed. (Academic Press, New York, 2nd ed., 1963) p 233. Toxicity study: K.-R. Stratmann, *Dtsch. Zahnaerztl. Z.* **34,** 484 (1979).

White powder or cubic crystals. When F ions are pptd with Ca $^{2+}$ in the absence of CO_3 ions, a gel is obtained. For the crystals: d 3.18; mp 1403°; bp 2500°; Mohs' hardness: 4. Becomes luminous when heated. Practically insol in water (soly at 18°: 0.0015 g/100 ml). Slightly sol in dil mineral acids; dissolved by concd mineral acids with liberation of HF. LD_{50} i.p. in mice: 2638.27 mg/kg (Stratmann).

USE: Fluorspar is the main primary source of fluorine and its compds. In ferrous metallurgy it is used as a flux to increase the fluidity of the slag. The steel industry is the largest consumer; the chemical industry, second and glass and ceramics, third. Synthetic fluorspar is used in the optical industry (transmits u.v. rays), and pure calcium fluoride is used as catalyst in dehydration and dehydrogenations. Used to fluoridate drinking water.

1668. Calcium Formate. [544-17-2] $C_2H_2CaO_4$; mol wt 130.11. C 18.46%, H 1.55%, Ca 30.80%, O 49.19%. $Ca(HCOO)_2$. Prepn from $Ca(OH)_2$ and CO at high temp and pressure: Enderli, **US 1920851; US 1995607** (1933, 1935 to Rudulf Koepp); Erasmus, Hamby, **US 2913318** (1959 to Union Carbide); from $CaCl_2$ and formic acid: Funk, Romer, *Z. Anorg. Allg. Chem.* **239,** 288 (1938).

Orthorhombic crystals or cryst powder. Slight acetic acid-like odor. d 2.02. Sol in water, practically insol in alc.

USE: Preservative for food, silage; as binder for fine-ore briquets; in drilling fluids and lubricants.

1669. Calcium Gluconate. [299-28-5] D-Gluconic acid calcium salt (2:1); Calciofon; Calglucon; Ebucin; Glucal; Glucobiogen. $C_{12}H_{22}CaO_{14}$; mol wt 430.37. C 33.49%, H 5.15%, Ca 9.31%, O 52.05%. $Ca[HOCH_2(CHOH)_4COO]_2$. Description of injectable solns with sodium ascorbate: **GB 495675; DE 702185.** General directions and stability data: Siegrist, *Pharm. Acta Helv.* **24,** 430 (1949).

Odorless, tasteless crystals, granules, or powder. $[\alpha]_D^{20}$ about +6°. Does not lose its water on drying without some decomposition. Slowly sol in 30 parts cold, about 5 parts boiling water; insol in alc or other organic solvents. pH aq soln: 6-7. More concd (20 to 30%) aq solns are easily obtained by the addition of boric acid or

similar complex-forming acids. Supersatd injectable solns prepd with calcium D-saccharate.

USE: In sewage purification; in coffee powders to prevent caking.
THERAP CAT: Calcium replenisher.
THERAP CAT (VET): In hypocalcemic states, including bovine milk fever.

1670. Calcium Glycerophosphate. [27214-00-2] 1,2,3-Propanetriol, mono(dihydrogen phosphate) calcium salt (1:1); calcium glycerinophosphate; calcium phosphoglycerate; Neurosin. $C_3H_7CaO_6P$; mol wt 210.14. C 17.15%, H 3.36%, Ca 19.07%, O 45.68%, P 14.74%. Three isomers exist: The *β-glycerophosphoric acid calcium salt*, D(+)- and L(−)-*α-glycerophosphoric acid calcium salt*. Commercial product is a mixture of calcium *β*- and DL-*α*-glycerophosphates: Toal, Phillips, *J. Pharm. Pharmacol.* **1,** 869 (1949). Prepn of the calcium salt of the *α*- and *β*-acids: King, Pyman, *J. Chem. Soc.* **105,** 1238 (1914); Toal, Phillips, *loc. cit.* Sepn of the *α*-acid from *β*- and polyglycerophosphoric acids via the *α*-acid calcium salt: Carrara, **IT 460219** (1950), *C.A.* **46,** 5077a (1952). Protective action against demineralization of dental enamel: T. H. Grenby, J. M. Bull, *Caries Res.* **14,** 210 (1980).

Commercial product, fine, odorless, almost tasteless, slightly hygroscopic powder; dec >170°. Sol in about 50 parts water; almost insol in alc, boiling water. Soly in water is increased by citric or lactic acid. The aq soln is alkaline.

Mixture with calcium lactate. Calphosan.
USE: In dentifrices, baking powder, as food stabilizer.
THERAP CAT: Calcium and phosphorus source. Tonic.
THERAP CAT (VET): Has been used as dietary supplement.

1671. Calcium Hexafluorosilicate. [16925-39-6] Calcium fluosilicate; calcium silicofluoride. CaF_6Si; mol wt 182.15. Ca 22.00%, F 62.58%, Si 15.42%. $CaSiF_6$. Prepn from Ca salt and H_2SiF_6: Moller, Kreth, **GB 263780** (1925). Review of toxicology of fluoride compounds: G. L. Waldbott, *Acta Med. Scand. Suppl.* **400,** 1-44 (1963).

Dihydrate, powder. d 2.25. Almost insol in cold water. Partially dec by hot water. Practically insol in acetone. LD in guinea pigs (mg/kg): 250 orally, 450 s.c. (Waldbott).

USE: In wood, rubber, textile industries; flotation agent; insecticide.

1672. Calcium Hydride. [7789-78-8] CaH_2; mol wt 42.09. Ca 95.22%, H 4.79%. Prepd by direct combination of calcium and hydrogen at 300-400°: **GB 597055** (1948); by reduction of lime with magnesium in the presence of hydrogen: Gibb, *Trans. Electrochem. Soc.* **93,** 198-211 (1948); from $CaCl_2$ and hydrogen in the presence of sodium: Wade, Alexander, **US 2702740** (1955 to Metal Hydrides). *Reviews:* Halls, *Ind. Chem.* **22,** 680 (1946); Kilb, *USAEC* APEX-485, 57 pp (1959).

Orthorhombic crystals or powder; the commercial product is gray. d 1.7. mp 1.86°. Decomposes with water, lower alcohols and carboxylic acids to form hydrogen; moderately powerful condensing agent with ketones and acid esters; more powerful reducing agent toward metal oxides than lithium or sodium hydrides.

USE: To prepare rare metals by reduction of their oxides; as a drying agent for liquids and gases; to generate hydrogen: 1 g of calcium hydride in water liberates 1 liter of hydrogen at STP; in organic syntheses.

1673. Calcium Hydroxide. [1305-62-0] Calcium hydrate; slaked lime. CaH_2O_2; mol wt 74.09. Ca 54.09%, H 2.72%, O 43.19%. $Ca(OH)_2$. Contains at least 95% $Ca(OH)_2$. Commercial prepn by hydration of lime: W. L. Faith *et al., Industrial Chemicals* (John Wiley, New York, 3rd ed., 1965) pp 483-484. Laboratory prepn by treating an aq soln of a calcium salt with alkali: Ehrlich in *Handbook of Preparative Inorganic Chemistry* vol. 1, G. Brauer (Academic Press, New York, 2nd ed., 1963) p 934. Toxicity study: Smyth *et al., Am. Ind. Hyg. Assoc. J.* **30,** 470 (1969).

Crystals or soft, odorless, granules or powder. Slightly bitter, alkaline taste. Readily absorbs CO_2 from air forming $CaCO_3$. Loses water when ignited; forms CaO. d 2.08-2.34. Slightly sol in water; sol in glycerol, sugar or NH_4Cl solns; sol in acids with evolution of much heat. pH of aq soln satd at 25°: 12.4. *Keep well closed.* LD_{50} orally in rats: 7.34 g/kg (Smyth).

Caution: Potential symptoms of overexposure are irritation of eyes, skin, upper respiratory system; eye and skin burns; skin vesiculation; cough, bronchitis, pneumonia. *See NIOSH Pocket Guide to Chemical Hazards* (DHHS/NIOSH 97-140, 1997) p 46.

USE: In mortar, plaster, cement and other building and paving materials; in lubricants, drilling fluids, pesticides, fireproofing coatings, water paints; as egg preservative; manuf of paper pulp; in SBR rubber vulcanization; in water treatment; dehairing hides.

THERAP CAT: Astringent.

1674. Calcium Hypochlorite. [7778-54-3] Losantin. $CaCl_2O_2$; mol wt 142.98. Ca 28.03%, Cl 49.59%, O 22.38%. $Ca(OCl)_2$. Pure product has not been prepd. Commercial product usually contain 50% or more $Ca(OCl)_2$. Preparation of solid product contg 90-94% $Ca(OCl)_2$: Cady, *Inorg. Synth.* **5**, 161 (1957). Impurities include: $Ca(ClO_4)_2$, $CaCl_2$, $CaCO_3$, $Ca(OH)_2$ and water.

USE: Algicide, bactericide, deodorant, disinfectant, fungicide; in sugar refining; oxidizing agent; bleaching agent. Ingredient of *Camporit* which also contains NaCl. Also ingredient of *HTH* and *Perchloron*.

1675. Calcium Hypophosphite. [7789-79-9] $CaH_4O_4P_2$; mol wt 170.05. Ca 23.57%, H 2.37%, O 37.63%, P 36.43%. $Ca(H_2PO_2)_2$. Prepn: *Gmelins, Calcium* (8th ed.) **28B**, 1119-1121 (1958).

Monoclinic, prismatic crystals or granular powder. When heated above 300° it evolves spontaneously-inflammable phosphine. Sol in water; slightly sol in glycerol. Practically insol in alcohol. The aq soln is slightly acid.

USE: As corrosion inhibitor; in nickel plating. Pharmaceutic aid (retards oxidation of ferrous salts).

THERAP CAT: Calcium source.

THERAP CAT (VET): Has been used as a dietary supplement and also as a "nerve tonic".

1676. Calcium Iodate. [7789-80-2] Lautarite. CaI_2O_6; mol wt 389.88. Ca 10.28%, I 65.10%, O 24.62%. $Ca(IO_3)_2$. Prepd by passing chlorine into a hot soln of lime in which iodine has been dissolved: Bahl, Singh, *J. Indian Chem. Soc.* **17**, 397 (1940).

Nonhygroscopic, monoclinic-prismatic crystals. d_4^{15} 4.519. Stable up to 540°. Sensitive to reducing agents. Soly in water (g/100 ml): 0.10 (0°); 0.95 (100°). More sol in aq solns of iodides and in amino acid solns. Sol in nitric acid. Insol in alcohol.

Monohydrate. Cubic crystals. Slightly sol in water.

Hexahydrate. Orthorhombic crystals. Slightly sol in water.

USE: Nutritional source of iodine in foods and feedstuffs. More stable in table salts than iodides: *Food Field Reporter*, Aug. 8, 1956; Daum, *C.A.* **51**, 5324 (1957); to improve properties of yeast-leavened bakery products.

THERAP CAT: Antiseptic.

1677. Calcium Iodide. [10102-68-8] CaI_2; mol wt 293.89. Ca 13.64%, I 86.36%. Prepn: Farr, **US 2415346** (1947 to Mallinckrodt); Chaigneau, *Bull. Soc. Chim. Fr.* **1957**, 886; *Gmelins, Calcium* (8th ed.) **28B**, 102, 610-622 (1958). The commercial product usually contains 16-20% water.

Very hygroscopic hexagonal lamella. Becomes yellow and completely insol on exposure to air due to liberation of I_2 and absorption of CO_2. mp 740°; bp 1100°. Very sol in water, methanol, ethanol, acetone; practically insol in ether, dioxane. The aq soln is neutral or slightly alkaline. *Keep tightly closed and protected from light.*

Hexahydrate. Hexagonal, thick needles, or plates, or lumps or powder. Very hygroscopic; becomes yellow in air, mp ~42°. Freely sol in water, alcohol. *Keep tightly closed and protected from light.*

THERAP CAT: Expectorant.

1678. Calcium Lactate. [814-80-2] 2-Hydroxypropanoic acid calcium salt. $C_6H_{10}CaO_6$; mol wt 218.22. C 33.02%, H

4.62%, Ca 18.37%, O 43.99%. $Ca[CH_3CH(OH)COO]_2$. Commercial prepn usually contains about 25% water, and on the anhydr basis it is at least 98% pure. Prepd commercially by neutralization of lactic acid, from fermentation of dextrose, molasses, starch, sugar or whey, with $CaCO_3$: Inskeep *et al., Ind. Eng. Chem.* **44**, 1955 (1952). Clinical use as a supplement: G. M. Day *et al., Pediatr. Res.* **9**, 568 (1975). Evaluation as anticaries agent: B. M. Shrestha *et al., Caries Res.* **16**, 12 (1982); M. J. M. Schaeken, J. S. van der Hoeven, *ibid.* **24**, 376 (1990). Clinical pharmacology: M. Goddard *et al., Am. J. Clin. Nutr.* **44**, 653 (1986).

Pentahydrate, odorless, white, slightly efflorescent granules or powder. Becomes anhydr at 120°. pH: 6-8. Sol water. Practically insol in alcohol.

USE: As a preservative in foods and beverages; in dentifrices.

THERAP CAT: Calcium replenisher.

THERAP CAT (VET): Calcium replenisher.

1679. Calcium Levulinate. [591-64-0] 4-Oxopentanoic acid calcium salt; levulinic acid calcium salt. $C_{10}H_{14}CaO_6$; mol wt 270.29. C 44.44%, H 5.22%, Ca 14.83%, O 35.52%. $(CH_3-COCH_2CH_2COO)_2Ca$. Prepn: Cox, Dodds, **US 2033909** (1936 to Niacet Chemicals).

Dihydrate, crystals or granular powder. mp 125°. Loses 1 H_2O on drying *in vacuo* at room temp and all H_2O at 50°. Very sol in water; the aq soln is practically neutral.

THERAP CAT: Calcium replenisher.

THERAP CAT (VET): May be used in hypocalcemic states.

1680. Calcium Magnesium Acetate. [76123-46-1] Acetic acid, calcium magnesium salt; CMA; Ice-B-Gon. $C_2H_4O_2$.-xCa.xMg. Prepn and use as deicer: S. A. Dunn, R. U. Schenk, *Transport. Res. Rec.* **776**, 12 (1980); *eidem, U.S. Federal Highway Administration Report* **FHWA-RD-79-109** (1980) pp 17. Prepn by fermentation: C. W. Marynowski *et al., Ind. Eng. Chem. Prod. Res. Dev.* **24**, 457 (1985); via extraction and sorption: H. Reisinger, C. J. King, *Ind. Eng. Chem. Res.* **34**, 845 (1995). Acute toxicity: G. A. Rausina *et al., Acute Toxic. Data* **1**, 87 (1990). Environmental and toxicological evaluation: B. L. McFarland, K. T. O'Reilly, *Chemical Deicers and the Environment*, F. M. D'Itri, Ed. (Lewis Publishers, Chelsea, MI, 1992) pp 193-227. Anti-icing effect: E. E. Adams *et al., ibid.*, pp. 481-493. Degradation in soil: D. W. Ostendorf *et al., J. Environ. Qual.* **22**, 299 (1993). Effects on cement mortar: O. Peterson, *Cem. Concr. Res.* **25**, 617 (1995). Book: *Calcium Magnesium Acetate*, D. L. Wise *et al.,* Eds. (Elsevier Science Publishers, Amsterdam, 1991) pp 511.

Non-flammable. Shows no significant corrosion of steel, aluminum or zinc. LD_{50} orally in male, female rats: 3240, 3071 mg/kg (Rausina).

USE: Deicing agent for roadways; in fossil fuel combustion for removal of sulfur.

1681. Calcium Molybdate(VI). [7789-82-4] (T-4)-Calcium (1:1) molybdate (MoO_4^{2-}); calcium molybdenum oxide. $CaMoO_4$; mol wt 200.02. Ca 20.04%, Mo 47.97%, O 32.00%. Prepn from sodium molybdate and $CaSO_4$: Carosella, **US 2460974** (1949 to U.S. Vanadium); by heating a stoichiometric mixture of CaO or $CaCO_3$ and molybdic acid: Kroger, *Nature* **159**, 674 (1947). Toxicity studies: L. T. Fairhall *et al.*, "The Toxicity of Molybdenum," *U.S. Public Health Service Bulletin No. 293*, Washington D.C. (1945) 36 pp.

Tetragonal crystals. d. 4.35. Practically insol in water, alcohol. Sol in concd mineral acids.

USE: In phosphors and luminescent materials.

1682. Calcium Nitrate. [10124-37-5] CaN_2O_6; mol wt 164.09. Ca 24.42%, N 17.07%, O 58.50%. $Ca(NO_3)_2$. Prepn: *Gmelins, Calcium* (8th ed.) **28B**, 59-69, 341-382 (1956).

Deliquesc granules, mp ~560°. Very sol in water, heat being evolved; freely sol in methanol, ethanol, acetone. Almost insol in concd HNO_3. pH of 5% aq soln 6.0. *Keep well closed. Note:* $Ca(NO_3)_2$ crystallizes also with $4H_2O$ (30.5%), mp 45°. Technical flake usually contains 28.6% H_2O.

USE: In explosives, fertilizers, matches, pyrotechnics; manuf of incandescent mantles, radio tubes, HNO_3; corrosion inhibitor in diesel fuels.

1683. Calcium Nitrite. [13780-06-8] CaN_2O_4; mol wt 132.09. Ca 30.34%, N 21.21%, O 48.45%. $Ca(NO_2)_2$. Prepd by reaction of nitric oxide with a mixture of calcium ferrate(III) and calcium nitrate: Ray, Ogg, Jr., *J. Am. Chem. Soc.* **79**, 265 (1957). White or yellowish, deliquesc, hexagonal crystals. d 2.23. Freely sol in water; slightly sol in alc. *Keep well closed.*

USE: Corrosion inhibitor in lubricants, concrete.

1684. Calcium Oleate. [142-17-6] 9-Octadecenoic acid calcium salt; oleic acid calcium salt. $C_{36}H_{66}CaO_4$; mol wt 602.98. C 71.71%, H 11.03%, Ca 6.65%, O 10.61%. Ca($C_{18}H_{33}$-O_2)$_2$. Prepn: Harrison, *Biochem. J.* **18**, 1222 (1924); Pink, *J. Chem. Soc.* **1939**, 619.

Pale-yellow transparent solid. Dec above 140°. Slowly absorbs moisture from the air to form the monohydrate. Practically insol in water, alcohol, ether, acetone, petr ether; sol in chloroform, benzene.

USE: Thickening lubricating grease; waterproofing concrete; emulsifier for benzene, kerosene, etc.; in modeling waxes to vary hardness.

1685. Calcium Oxalate. [563-72-4] Ethanedioic acid calcium salt. C_2CaO_4; mol wt 128.10. C 18.75%, Ca 31.29%, O 49.96%. CaC$_2$O$_4$. Prepn from calcium formate: Bredt, **US 1622991** (1927); from calcium cyanamide: Barsky, Buchanan, *J. Am. Chem. Soc.* **53**, 1270 (1931).

Monohydrate. Cubic crystals. Loses all of its water at 200°. When ignited is converted into CaCO$_3$ or CaO without appreciable charring. d 2.2. Practically insol in water and acetic acid; sol in dil HCl or HNO$_3$.

USE: In ceramic glazes; as carrier for separation of rare earth metals; analysis for calcium: Ingols, Murray, *Anal. Chem.* **21**, 525 (1949).

1686. Calcium Oxide. [1305-78-8] Lime; burnt lime; calx; quicklime. CaO; mol wt 56.08. Ca 71.47%, O 28.53%. Properly stored lime of commerce contains 90-95% free CaO. Commercial production from limestone: W. L. Faith *et al.*, *Industrial Chemicals* (John Wiley, New York, 3rd ed., 1965) pp 482-487. Lab prepn by ignition of CaCO$_3$: Ehrlich in *Handbook of Preparative Inorganic Chemistry* vol. **1**, G. Brauer, Ed. (Academic Press, New York, 2nd ed., 1963) p 931. *Review:* R. S. Boynton in *Kirk-Othmer Encyclopedia of Chemical Technology* vol. **14** (Wiley-Interscience, New York, 3rd ed., 1981) pp 343-382.

Crystals, white or grayish-white lumps, or granular powder; commercial material sometimes has a yellowish or brownish tint, due to iron. mp 2572°; bp 2850°; d 3.32-3.35. Readily absorbs CO$_2$ and H$_2$O from air, becoming air-slaked. Sol in water forming Ca(OH)$_2$ and generating a large quantity of heat; sol in acids, glycerol, sugar soln; practically insol in alc. *Keep tightly closed and dry.*

Caution: Potential symptoms of overexposure are irritation of eyes, skin, upper respiratory tract; ulceration or perforation of nasal septum; pneumonia; dermatitis. *See NIOSH Pocket Guide to Chemical Hazards* (DHHS/NIOSH 97-140, 1997) p 48.

USE: In bricks, plaster, mortar, stucco and other building and construction materials; manuf of steel, aluminum, magnesium, and flotation of non-ferrous ores; manuf of glass, paper, Na$_2$CO$_3$ (Solvay process), Ca salts and many other industrial chemicals; dehairing hides; clarification of cane and beet sugar juices; in fungicides, insecticides, drilling fluids, lubricants; water and sewage treatment; in laboratory to absorb CO$_2$ (the combination with NaOH is known as soda-lime, *q.v.*).

1687. Calcium Palmitate. [542-42-7] Hexadecanoic acid calcium salt; palmitic acid calcium salt. $C_{32}H_{62}CaO_4$; mol wt 550.91. C 69.77%, H 11.34%, Ca 7.27%, O 11.62%. Ca($C_{16}H_{31}$-O_2)$_2$. Prepn: Harrison, *Biochem. J.* **18**, 1222 (1924).

Powder or rhombic crystals. Dec above 155°. Practically insol in water, alcohol, ether, acetone, petr ether; slightly sol in chloroform, benzene, acetic acid.

USE: Thickening lubricating oils; waterproofing fabrics and lubricating greases; as corrosion inhibitor in halohydrocarbons.

1688. Calcium Permanganate. [10118-76-0] CaMn$_2$O$_8$; mol wt 277.95. Ca 14.42%, Mn 39.53%, O 46.05%. Ca(MnO$_4$)$_2$. Prepn from KMnO$_4$ and CaCl$_2$: **GB 624885** (1949 to Boots Pure Drug Co. and T. Hagyard); from Al(MnO$_4$)$_3$ and Ca(OH)$_2$: Jaskowiak, **US 2504130** (1950 to Carus Chemical).

Violet or dark-purple, deliquesc crystals. Freely sol in water; dec in alcohol. *Keep tightly closed.*

USE: Antiseptic, disinfectant, deodorizer; with CaF$_2$ as binder for welding electrode coatings and fluxes.

1689. Calcium Peroxide. [1305-79-5] Calcium dioxide. CaO$_2$; mol wt 72.08. Ca 55.60%, O 44.39%. The commercial product usually contains about 60% CaO$_2$, water, and some Ca(OH)$_2$ and CaCO$_3$. Prepn: Young, **US 2533660** (1950 to du Pont); Ehrlich in *Handbook of Preparative Inorganic Chemistry* vol. **1**, G. Brauer, Ed. (Academic Press, New York, 2nd ed., 1963) p 936.

White or yellowish, odorless, almost tasteless powder. Dec in moist air. Slightly sol in water; sol in acids with formation of H$_2$O$_2$. *Keep well closed.*

USE: Stabilizer for rubber.

THERAP CAT: Antiseptic.

1690. Calcium Phenolsulfonate. [127-83-3] *p*-Hydroxybenzenesulfonic acid calcium salt; calcium sulfocarbolate; calcium sulfophenolate. $C_{12}H_{10}CaO_8S_2$; mol wt 386.41. C 37.30%, H 2.61%, Ca 10.37%, O 33.12%, S 16.60%. Ca[C_6H_4(OH)SO$_3$]$_2$. Prepn: *Hagers Handb. Pharm. Praxis* vol. **2**, 420 (Berlin, 1930).

Hydrate, odorless cryst powder. Sol in water or alcohol. The aq soln is neutral, and has a bitter, astringent taste.

THERAP CAT (VET): Has been used as an intestinal antiseptic, in dusting powders for ulcers and in ophthalmic solns.

1691. Calcium Phenoxide. [5793-84-0] Calcium carbolate; calcium phenate; calcium phenolate; calcium phenylate. $C_{12}H_{10}$-CaO$_2$; mol wt 226.28. C 63.69%, H 4.45%, Ca 17.71%, O 14.14%. Ca(OC$_6$H$_5$)$_2$. Prepn: Kluge, Drake, **US 2870134** (1959 to Texas Co.).

Reddish powder. Dec in air. Slightly sol in water or alcohol. *Keep well closed.*

USE: Detergent; additive for motor oils.

1692. Calcium Phosphate, Dibasic. [7757-93-9] Calcium monohydrogen phosphate; dicalcium orthophosphate; secondary calcium phosphate. CaHO$_4$P; mol wt 136.06. Ca 29.46%, H 0.74%, O 47.04%, P 22.76%. CaHPO$_4$. Occurs in nature as the mineral *monetite*. Prepn from CaCl$_2$ and Na$_2$HPO$_4$: Jensen, Rathley, *Inorg. Synth.* **4**, 19, 20 (1953); from Ca$_3$(PO$_4$)$_2$ and H$_3$PO$_4$: Perloff, Posner, *ibid.* **6**, 16 (1960), where it is an intermediate in the preparation of hydroxyapatite.

Triclinic crystals. At red heat dehydrated to calcium pyrophosphate. Practically insol in water, alcohol.

Dihydrate. Brushite. Monoclinic crystals. Loses water of crystn slowly below 100°. Dehydr at red heat to calcium pyrophosphate. d 2.31. Practically insol in water, alcohol; sol in dil HCl or HNO$_3$; slightly sol in dil acetic acid.

USE: Chiefly in animal feeds; mineral supplement in cereals and other foods; manuf of glass; in dental products, fertilizers (*see also* Calcium Phosphate, Monobasic).

THERAP CAT: Calcium replenisher.

THERAP CAT (VET): Has been used as a dietary supplement, and as an antacid.

1693. Calcium Phosphate, Monobasic. [7758-23-8] Acid calcium phosphate; calcium biphosphate; monocalcium orthophosphate; monocalcium phosphate; primary calcium phosphate; "calcium superphosphate". CaH$_4$O$_8$P$_2$; mol wt 234.05. Ca 17.12%, H 1.72%, O 54.69%, P 26.47%. Ca(H$_2$PO$_4$)$_2$. Commercial prepn for fertilizers by treating pulverized phosphate rock with H$_2$SO$_4$ or H$_3$-PO$_4$: *Faith, Keyes & Clark's Industrial Chemicals*, F. A. Lowenheim, M. K. Moran, Eds. (Wiley-Interscience, New York, 4th ed., 1975) pp 191-200. Laboratory prepn from CaCO$_3$ and H$_3$PO$_4$: Jensen, Kathley, *Inorg. Synth.* **4**, 18 (1953).

Monohydrate, large, shining, triclinic plates, cryst powder or granules. Non-hygroscopic when pure, but traces of impurities such as H$_3$PO$_4$ cause material to be deliquesc. Strong acid taste. Loses H$_2$O at 100°, dec at 200°. d$_4^{18}$ 2.220. Moderately sol in water; sol in dil HCl or HNO$_3$ or acetic acid.

Note: The products obtained from commercial processes are not pure monobasic calcium phosphate. The superphosphate obtained from the H$_2$SO$_4$ treatment is about 30% CaH$_4$(PO$_4$)$_2$.H$_2$O, 10% CaHPO$_4$, 45% CaSO$_4$, 10% iron oxide, silica, alumina, etc. and 5% water; it contains 18-21% available P$_2$O$_5$. The triple superphosphate obtained from the H$_3$PO$_4$ treatment contains from 43 to 50% available P$_2$O$_5$.

USE: Chiefly in fertilizers; as acidulant in baking powders and in wheat flours; mineral supplement for foods and feeds; in enameling.

1694. Calcium Phosphate, Tribasic. [7758-87-4] Tricalcium orthophosphate; tricalcium phosphate; tertiary calcium phosphate; Calcigenol Simple. $Ca_3O_8P_2$; mol wt 310.18. Ca 38.76%, O 41.26%, P 19.97%. $Ca_3(PO_4)_2$. It is about 96% pure, usually contg an excess of CaO. Occurs in nature as the minerals: *oxydapatit, voelicherite, whitlockite*. The technical product is also known as *"bone ash"*. Commercial prepn from phosphate rock: Hignett, Hubbard, *Ind. Eng. Chem.* **38**, 1208 (1946); Elmore, **US 2474831** (1949 to T.V.A.); Hollingsworth, **US 2556541** and **US 2562718** (both 1951 to Coronet Phosphate); Brosheer, Hignett, *Chem. Eng. Rept.* no. 7, 143 pp (1953).

Amorphous, odorless, tasteless powder. mp 1670°. d 3.14. Practically insol in water, alcohol or acetic acid; sol in dil HCl or HNO_3.

USE: Manuf of fertilizers, H_3PO_4 and P compds; manuf milk-glass, polishing and dental powders, porcelains, pottery; enameling; clarifying sugar syrups; in animal feeds; as noncaking agent; in the textile industry.

THERAP CAT: Calcium replenisher.

THERAP CAT (VET): Has been used as a dietary supplement, and as an antacid.

1695. Calcium Phosphide. [1305-99-3] Photophor. Ca_3P_2; mol wt 182.18. Ca 66.00%, P 34.00%. Prepn: Ehrlich in *Handbook of Preparative Inorganic Chemistry* vol. 1, G. Brauer, Ed. (Academic Press, New York, 2nd ed., 1963) p 943.

Red-brown cryst powder or gray lumps. Dec by moist air or water, evolving spontaneously-flammable phosphine. d 2.51; mp ~1600°. *Keep dry and tightly closed.*

USE: For signal fires; in purification of Cu and Cu alloys; as rodenticide.

1696. Calcium Phosphite. [21056-98-4] $CaHO_3P$; mol wt 120.06. Ca 33.38%, H 0.84%, O 39.98%, P 25.80%. $CaHPO_3$. Prepn: *Gmelins, Calcium* (8th ed.) **28B**, 1121 (1958).

Monohydrate. Crystals. Loses water at 200°; dec above 300°. Slightly sol in water; practically insol in alcohol.

USE: Fertilizers; polymerization catalyst.

1697. Calcium Polycarbophil. [9003-97-8] WL-140; Carbofil; Mitrolan; Quival; Sorboquel. Calcium salt of a synthetic loosely crosslinked hydrophilic resin of the polycarboxylic type. Review of pharmacology, toxicology, clinical efficacy, and adverse effects: I. E. Danhof, *Pharmacotherapy* **2**, 18-28 (1982).

THERAP CAT: Cathartic.

1698. Calcium Propionate. [4075-81-4] Propionic acid calcium salt. $C_6H_{10}CaO_4$; mol wt 186.22. C 38.70%, H 5.41%, Ca 21.52%, O 34.37%. $Ca(CH_3CH_2COO)_2$. Occurs as mono- or trihydrate. Prepn: *Beilstein* vol. 2, 238, 2nd suppl., 218, 3rd suppl., 516.

Powder or monoclinic crystals. Sol in water; slightly sol in methanol, ethanol; practically insol in acetone, benzene.

USE: As an inhibitor of molds and other microorganisms in foods, tobacco, pharmaceuticals; in butyl rubber to improve processability and scorching resistance.

THERAP CAT: Antifungal.

1699. Calcium Pyrophosphate. [35405-51-7] Calcium diphosphate. $Ca_2O_7P_2$; mol wt 254.10. Ca 31.55%, O 44.08%, P 24.38%. $Ca_2P_2O_7$. Prepn by ignition of $CaHPO_4$: St. Pierre, *J. Am. Chem. Soc.* **77**, 2197 (1955).

Polymorphous crystals or powder. d 3.09. mp 1353°. Practically insol in water. Sol in dil HCl or HNO_3.

USE: Abrasive; fertilizer; feed supplement; in dentifrices, ceramic ware, china, glass, phosphors.

1700. Calcium D-Saccharate. [5793-88-4] D-Glucaric acid calcium salt. $C_6H_8CaO_8$; mol wt 248.20. C 29.03%, H 3.25%, Ca 16.15%, O 51.57%. $CaC_6H_8O_8$. The normal calcium salt of D-saccharic acid, a dicarboxylic sugar acid derived from the oxidation of D-gluconic acid. Calcium D-saccharate is a true chemical compd and should not be confused with saccharated lime, formerly called "calcium saccharate" and produced by the action of lime upon sugar. Prepn: *Beilstein* vol. **3**, 2nd suppl., 378; *Hagers Handb. Pharm. Praxis* vol. **1**, 755 (Berlin, 1930).

Tetrahydrate. Odorless, tasteless crystals or fine white powder. Stable to air. Becomes anhydr upon heating at 100° *in vacuo*. Practically insol in water, alcohol, ether. Sol in dil mineral acids and in calcium gluconate solns.

USE: Pharmaceutic aid (stabilizer for calcium gluconate solns). As plasticizer in cement, concrete, mortar.

1701. Calcium Selenide. [1305-84-6] CaSe; mol wt 119.04. Ca 33.67%, Se 66.33%. Prepd by reducing $CaSeO_4$ in a stream of H_2 at 400-500°: Ehrlich in *Handbook of Preparative Inorganic Chemistry* vol. 1, G. Brauer, Ed. (Academic Press, New York, 2nd ed, 1963) p 939.

White powder. In air may turn red within a few minutes and light brown in a few hours. d 3.82. Decomposed by water. Treatment with HCl produces H_2Se gas, and red Se separates.

USE: In electron emitters.

1702. Calcium Silicate. [1344-95-2] Many different forms of calcium silicate are known. Among the most common forms are $CaSiO_3$, Ca_2SiO_4 and Ca_3SiO_5. Usually occur in hydrated form contg various percentages of water of crystallization. Names of calcium silicate minerals are: *afwillite; akermanite; calcium pectolith; centrallasite; crestmoreite; eaklite; foshagite; foshallasite; gjellebaekite; grammite; gyrolite; hillebrandite; larnite; okenite; parawollastonite; pseudo-wollastonite; riversideite; table spate; tobermorite; wollastonite; xonaltite; xonotlite*. Commercial calcium silicate sold for industrial use, such as *Micro-Cell* and *Silene*, is prepared synthetically to control its absorbing power. The usual method of prepn is from lime and diatomaceous earth under carefully controlled conditions: Boss, *Chem. Eng. News* **27**, 677 (1949); Steinour, *Chem. Rev.* **40**, 391 (1947). The commercial product is described here.

White or slightly cream-colored, free-flowing powder. Approximate analysis: CaO 19%, SiO_2 67%, H_2O 6 to 8%. d^{25} 2.10. Bulk density: 15-16 lb/cu ft. Absorbs 1 to 2.5 times its weight of liquids and still remains a free-flowing powder. Total absorption power for water about 600%, for mineral oil about 500%. Available surface area: 95 to 175 m^2/g. Ultimate particle size: 0.02 to 0.07 μ. pH of aq slurry 8.0 to 10.0. Practically insol in water. Forms a siliceous gel with mineral acids.

Caution: Potential symptoms of overexposure are irritation of eyes, skin, upper respiratory system. *See NIOSH Pocket Guide to Chemical Hazards* (DHHS/NIOSH 97-140, 1997) p 48.

USE: Constituent (produced *in situ*) of lime glass, portland cement; reinforcing filler in elastomers and plastics; absorbent for liquids, gases, vapors; as anti-caking agent, suspension agent, pigment and pigment extender; binder for refractory material; in chromatography; in road construction.

1703. Calcium Stearate. [1592-23-0] Octadecanoic acid calcium salt; stearic acid calcium salt. $C_{36}H_{70}CaO_4$; mol wt 607.02. C 71.23%, H 11.62%, Ca 6.60%, O 10.54%. The commercial prepn also contains palmitate. Prepn: Harrison, *Biochem. J.* **18**, 1222 (1924); Kebrich, Petrot, **US 2650932** (1953 to National Lead).

Granular, fatty powder. Bulk density ~20 lb/cu ft, mp 147-149° (determined by gradient bar). Practically insol in water, ether, chloroform, acetone, cold alcohol; slightly sol in hot alcohol, in hot vegetable and mineral oils; quite sol in hot pyridine.

USE: For waterproofing fabrics, cement, stucco, explosives; as a releasing agent for plastic molding powders; as a stabilizer for polyvinyl chloride resins; lubricant; in pencils and wax crayons. Food grade calcium stearate, derived from edible tallow, is used as a conditioning agent in certain food and pharmaceutical products.

1704. Calcium Stearyl-2 Lactylate. [5793-94-2] Octadecanoic acid 2-(1-carboxyethoxy)-1-methyl-2-oxoethyl ester, calcium salt; stearic acid ester with lactate of lactic acid calcium salt; calcium stelate; Verv-Ca. $C_{48}H_{86}CaO_{12}$; mol wt 895.27. C 64.40%, H 9.68%, Ca 4.48%, O 21.45%. Use in improving the mixing characteristics of flour: Thompson, Buddemeyer, *Cereal Chem.* **31**, 296 (1954); in improving whipping and baking properties of dried egg whites: Gorman, Keith, **US 2919992** (1960 to Seymour Foods). Metabolism: J. C. Phillips *et al., Food Cosmet. Toxicol.* **19**, 7 (1981).

Free flowing, nonhygroscopic powder. Sparingly sol in water. pH of a 2% aq suspension 4.7.

USE: Dough conditioner in yeast-leavened bakery products; emulsifier in cosmetic and pharmaceutical industry.

1705. Calcium Succinate. [140-99-8] Butanedioic acid calcium salt; succinic acid calcium salt; Artume. $C_4H_4CaO_4$; mol wt 156.15. C 30.77%, H 2.58%, Ca 25.67%, O 40.98%. $CaC_4H_4O_4$. Prepn: *Beilstein* vol. 2, 607, 2nd suppl., 548, 3rd suppl., 1657.

Trihydrate. Needles or granules. Slightly sol in water; practically insol in alcohol; sol in dil acids.

THERAP CAT: Combined with salicylates for rheumatic fever and rheumatoid arthritis.

1706. Calcium Sulfate. [7778-18-9] CaO_4S; mol wt 136.14. Ca 29.44%, O 47.01%, S 23.55%. $CaSO_4$. *Review:* R. J. Wenk, P. L. Henkels in *Kirk-Othmer Encyclopedia of Chemical Technology* vol. 4 (Wiley-Interscience, New York, 3rd ed., 1978) pp 437-448.

The natural form of anhydrous calcium sulfate is known as the mineral *anhydrite*; also as *karstenite, muriacite, anhydrous sulfate of lime, anhydrous gypsum.* Crystals are orthorhombic, color varies, e.g., white with blue, gray or reddish tinge, or brick red. d 2.96. Hardness 3-3.5 (Mohs'). Sol in water (18.75°) 0.2 pts/100 pts. *Insoluble anhydrite* or *dead-burned gypsum* which has the same crystal structure as the mineral is obtained upon complete dehydration of gypsum at above 650°. *Soluble anhydrite* is obtained in granular or powder form by complete dehydration of gypsum at below 300° in an electric oven. Estimated pore space is 38% by volume. Possesses high affinity for water and will absorb 6.6% of its weight of water forming the stable hemihydrate.

Hemihydrate. [26499-65-0] Dried calcium sulfate; dried gypsum; plaster of Paris; Annalin. Fine, odorless, tasteless powder. When mixed with water, sets to a hard mass. *Keep well closed.*

Dihydrate. [13397-24-5] Native calcium sulfate; precipitated calcium sulfate; gypsum; alabaster; selenite; terra alba; satinite; mineral white; satin spar; light spar. Lumps or powder. d 2.32. It loses only part of its water at 100-150°. Sol in water; very slowly sol in glycerol. Practically insol in most organic solvents.

Caution: Potential symptoms of overexposure to anhydrous compd, dihydrate or hemihydrate are irritation of eyes, skin, mucous membranes, respiratory system; cough. Potential symptoms of overexposure to anhydrous compd also include conjunctivitis; rhinitis, epistaxis. Potential symptoms of overexposure to dihydrate also include sneezing, rhinorrhea. *See NIOSH Pocket Guide to Chemical Hazards* (DHHS/NIOSH 97-140, 1997) pp 48, 154, 260.

USE: *Anhydrous:* Insol anhydrite is used in cement formulations and as a paper filler. Soluble anhydride, because of its strong tendency to absorb moisture, is useful as a drying agent for solids, organic liquids and gases; the desiccant used in laboratory and industry is known under the name **Drierite**. This material can be regenerated repeatedly and reused without noticeable decrease in its desiccating efficiency. The *hemihydrate* is used for wall plasters; wallboard; tiles and blocks for the building industry; moldings; statuary; in the paper industry. The *dihydrate* is used in the manuf of portland cement; in soil treatment to neutralize alkali carbonates and to prevent loss of volatile and dissolved nitrogenous compounds by volatilization and leaching; for the manuf of plaster of Paris, artificial marble; as a white pigment, filler or glaze in paints, enamels, pharmaceuticals, paper, insecticide dusts, yeast manuf, water treatment, polishing powders; in the manuf of sulfuric acid, CaC_2, $(NH_4)_2SO_4$, porous polymers. Pharmaceutic aid (in plaster casts).

1707. Calcium Sulfide. [20548-54-3] CaS; mol wt 72.14. Ca 55.56%, S 44.45%. Pure CaS prepd in the laboratory by heating pure $CaCO_3$ in a stream of $H_2S + H_2$ at 1000°: Ehrlich in *Handbook of Preparative Inorganic Chemistry* vol. 1, G. Brauer, Ed. (Academic Press, New York, 2nd ed., 1963) p 938. Crude calcium sulfide, erroneously called *sulfurated lime, calcic liver of sulfur, liver of lime, hepar calcis*, made by igniting calcium sulfate with carbonaceous matter. Contains not less than 55% CaS; the balance is calcium sulfate, sulfite and carbonate, and the "ash" from the carbonaceous material. *See Mellor's* vol III, p 740 (1928). *Luminous calcium sulfide* or *Canton's phosphorus* made by igniting a mixture of $CaCO_3$ and S with very small quantities of Bi or Mn salts, etc.: Verneuil, *Compt. Rend.* **103**, 600 (1886); *Mellor's, loc. cit.*

White powder if pure; crude and luminous calcium sulfide may be yellowish to pale-gray. Odor of H_2S in moist air; unpleasant alkaline taste. Oxidizes in dry air and dec in moist air. mp >2000°. d 2.59. Slightly sol in cold, more sol in hot water with partial decompn; freely sol in solns of ammonium salts; practically insol in alcohol; dec even by weak acids, evolving H_2S. *Keep well closed.*

USE: In phosphors; as lubricant additive. Pure CaS used in electron emitters. Luminous CaS used for making luminous paints or varnishes.

THERAP CAT (VET): Has been used in chronic suppurative lesions.

1708. Calcium Sulfite. [10257-55-3] CaO_3S; mol wt 120.14. Ca 33.36%, O 39.95%, S 26.69%. $CaSO_3$. Prepn: *Gmelins, Calcium* (8th ed.) **28B**, 107-108, 660-674 (1958).

Dihydrate. Crystals or powder. Slowly oxidizes in air to $CaSO_4$. Slightly sol in water, alcohol; sol in SO_2 solns, acids with liberation of SO_2.

USE: Preserving cider and other fruit juices; as disinfectant of brewing vats; antichlor in bleaching textiles; in sugar manuf; in paper pulp cooking; in cement.

1709. Calcium Tartrate. [3164-34-9] 2,3-Dihydroxybutanedioic acid calcium salt. $C_4H_4CaO_6$; mol wt 188.15. C 25.53%, H 2.14%, Ca 21.30%, O 51.02%. $CaC_4H_4O_6$. A byproduct of the wine industry. Prepn from wine dregs: Dabul, **US 3114770** (1963 to Orandi & Massera). *See also* the processes mentioned under L-tartaric acid.

Tetrahydrate. Powder. Slightly sol in water (from about 0.04% at 10° to about 0.2% at 85°) or in alcohol; sol in dil HCl or HNO_3.

USE: As preservative for fruits, vegetables, seafoods; in deodorization of fish; as antacid.

1710. Calcium Thiocyanate. [2092-16-2] Calcium rhodanate; calcium sulfocyanate. $C_2CaN_2S_2$; mol wt 156.24. C 15.37%, Ca 25.65%, N 17.93%, S 41.05%. $Ca(SCN)_2$. Prepn: *Gmelins, Calcium* (8th ed.) **28B**, 972-976 (1958).

Tetrahydrate. Hygroscopic crystals or cryst powder. Dec on heating above 160°. Very sol in water; sol in methanol, ethanol, acetone. *Keep well closed.*

USE: In manuf of acrylonitrile polymers; for parchmentizing; for stiffening of textiles; soln as a solvent for textiles.

1711. Calcium Thioglycollate. [814-71-1] Mercaptoacetic acid calcium salt (2:1); Depil. $C_4H_6CaO_4S_2$; mol wt 222.30. C 21.61%, H 2.72%, Ca 18.03%, O 28.79%, S 28.85%. Prepn: Hoshall, *J. Assoc. Off. Agric. Chem.* **23**, 727 (1940).

Trihydrate. [5793-98-6] Prismatic rod crystals. Odorless or faint mercaptan odor; somewhat astringent and fetid taste. Slowly loses H_2O above 95°, darkens at 220° and partially fuses with decompn at 280-290°. Sol in water; very slightly sol in alcohol, chloroform; practically insol in ether, petr ether, benzene. Solns readily absorb CO_2 from air, pptg $CaCO_3$. *Keep well closed.*

USE: Depilatory; tanning leather; in hair-waving prepns.

1712. Calcium Tungstate(VI). [7790-75-2] CaO_4W; mol wt 287.92. Ca 13.92%, O 22.23%, W 63.85%. $CaWO_4$. Occurs in nature as the mineral *scheelite*. The article of commerce is usually made by pptn: Boericke, Boericke, **US 2390687** (1945); prepn by heating a stoichiometric mixture of CaO or $CaCO_3$ and tungstic acid: Kroger, *Nature* **159,** 674 (1947); prepn of single crystals: Uitert, Soden, *J. Appl. Phys.* **31,** 328 (1960).

Tetragonal crystals. d 6.06. Practically insol in water. Dec by hot HCl or HNO$_3$.

USE: Very small crystals have been used for injection into malignant tumors, etc., thus affording by transillumination a means of x-ray treatment; for preparing screens for x-ray observations and photographs; in luminous paints; in scintillation counters.

1713.   Calendula. Marigold; Mary-bud; gold-bloom; holligold. Dried, ligulate florets of *Calendula officinalis* L., *Compositae. Habit.* Southern Europe and Levant; cultivated everywhere in gardens. *Constit.* Volatile oil; calendulin, carotenoid pigments, a saponin which on hydrolysis yields oleanolic acid, bitter principle (caledin). *Refs:* Zimmerman, *Helv. Chim. Acta* **29,** 445 (1946); Gedeon, *Pharmazie* **6,** 547 (1951); **9,** 922 (1954), Kasprzyk, *C.A.* **47,** 6918c (1953); Suchy, Herout, *Collect. Czech. Chem. Commun.* **26,** 890 (1961).

THERAP CAT: Anti-inflammatory (topical).

1714.   Calfactant. [183325-78-2] CLSE; CLL; Infasurf. Chloroform/methanol extract of calf lung lavage fluid. Consists of 35 mg/ml phospholipid, 55-70% of which is dipalmitoylphosphatidylcholine, and of low mol wt surfactant proteins. Also contains 0.9 mg/ml fatty acids and 1.8 mg/ml neutral lipids. *See also:* Beractant, Poractant Alfa. Prepn: R. H. Notter *et al., Pediatr. Res.* **16,** 515 (1982). Physiologic effects in preterm lambs: J. J. Cummings *et al., Am. Rev. Respir. Dis.* **145,** 999 (1992). Surface tension: E. M. Scarpelli *et al., Am. J. Perinatol.* **9,** 414 (1992). Separation of hydrophobic constituents: S. B. Hall *et al., J. Lipid Res.* **35,** 1386 (1994). Clinical trial in neonates: M. S. Kwong *et al., Pediatrics* **76,** 585 (1985). Efficacy of prophylactic administration to neonates: J. Kattwinkel *et al., ibid.* **92,** 90 (1993). Clinical trial in pediatric acute lung injury: D. F. Wilson *et al., J. Am. Med. Assoc.* **293,** 470 (2005).

THERAP CAT: Pulmonary surfactant. In treatment of respiratory distress syndrome.

1715.   Calicheamicins. LL-E33288; CLM. Family of 15-20 enediyne antitumor antibiotics produced by *Micromonospora echinospora* ssp. *calichensis,* a bacterium isolated from chalky soil or a caliche. Naming based on TLC mobility using Greek letters with subscripts and on the halogen substitution which is indicted by the superscript. Binds to the minor groove of DNA and initiates double stranded DNA cleavage via a radical abstraction process. This type of damage is usually lethal as it is not repairable by the cell. Isoln: W. M. Maiese *et al., J. Antibiot.* **42,** 558 (1989). Structure elucidation: M. D. Lee *et al., J. Am. Chem. Soc.* **109,** 3464, 3466 (1987); and NMR studies: *eidem, ibid.* **114,** 985 (1992). DNA cleavage behavior: N. Zein *et al., Science* **240,** 1198 (1988); S. Walker *et al., Proc. Natl. Acad. Sci. USA* **89,** 4608 (1992); M. Chatterjee *et al., J. Am. Chem. Soc.* **118,** 1938 (1996). Series of articles on total synthesis of γ_1^I: *ibid.* **115,** 7593-7635 (1993). Book on calicheamicins and related compounds: *Enediyne Antibiotics As Antitumor Agents,* D. B. Borders, T. W. Doyle, Eds. (Marcel Dekker, Inc., New York, 1995) 478 pp.

Calicheamicin γ$_1$

Calicheamicin γ$_1^I$. [108212-75-5] CLM γ$_1^I$. C$_{55}$H$_{74}$IN$_3$O$_{21}$S$_4$; mol wt 1368.35. White amorphous powder, [α]$_D^{26}$ −124° (c = 0.98%, EtOH).

1716.   Californium. [7440-71-3] Cf; at. no. 98; valence 4, 3, 2. Man-made, radioactive element. No stable nuclides; known isotopes (mass numbers): 239-256. Longest-lived known isotope: 251 (T$_{1/2}$ 898 years, α-emitter, rel. at. mass 251.0796). Prepn of isotope ^{245}Cf (T$_{1/2}$ 43.6 min) by bombarding ^{242}Cm with helium ions: S. G. Thompson *et al., Phys. Rev.* **78,** 298 (1950); *eidem, ibid.* **80,** 790. Prepn of ^{249}Cf metal (T$_{1/2}$ 351 years, α-emitter, rel. at. mass 249.0748) by reduction of Cf$_2$O$_3$ with lanthanum metal: Haire, Baybarz, *J. Inorg. Nucl. Chem.* **36,** 1295 (1974). Medical uses of ^{252}Cf (α-decay, T$_{1/2}$ half-life 2.645 years, rel. at. mass 252.0816; spontaneous fission T$_{1/2}$ half-life 85.5 years): Seaborg, *Handb. Exp. Pharmakol.* **36,** 929 (1973). *Reviews:* Cunningham, *J. Chem. Educ.* **36,** 32-37 (1959); M. Haissinsky, J. P. Adloff, *Radiochemical Survey of the Elements* (Elsevier, New York, 1965) pp 28-29; C. Keller, *The Chemistry of the Transuranium Elements* (Verlag Chemie, Weinheim, English Ed., 1971) pp 567-581; Silva, "Trans-Curium Elements" in *MTP Int. Rev. Sci.: Inorg. Chem., Ser. One* **vol. 8,** A. G. Maddock, Ed. (University Park Press, Baltimore, 1972) pp 71-105; *Comprehensive Inorganic Chemistry* **vol.5,** J. C. Bailar, Jr. *et al.,* Eds. (Pergamon Press, Oxford, 1973) *passim; Handb. Exp. Pharmakol.* **36,** 689-928 (1973); R. G. Haire in *The Chemistry of the Actinide Elements* vol. 2, J. J. Katz *et al.,* Eds. (Chapman and Hall, New York, 1986) pp 1025-1070. Review of radiobiology and therapeutic applications: Y. Maruyama *et al., Oncology* **35,** 172 (1978); of use in brachytherapy for cervical cancer: *idem et al., Cancer* **68,** 1189-1197 (1991). Review of production, distribution and uses of ^{252}Cf: R. C. Martin *et al., Appl. Radiat. Isot.* **53,** 785-792 (2000).

Metal; two crystalline forms: double hexagonal close-packed α-form, d 15.10, exists below 900°; face-centered cubic β-form, d 8.74 (Katz *et al., loc. cit.* vol. 2, p. 1150). mp 900±30° (Haire, Baybarz). Slowly oxidized in air at room temp; rate increases with increased moisture in air. Oxidized when warmed in air; reacts when heated with nitrogen, hydrogen or a chalogen. Reacts rapidly with dry hydrogen halides and with aq mineral acids.

Caution: Radiation hazard; handling requires special equipment and shielding facilities (Katz *et al., loc. cit.* vol. 2, p. 1128).

USE: ^{252}Cf as neutron source; startup source for nuclear reactors; in nuclear reactor fuel rod scanners; for neutron radiography of weapons components.

THERAP CAT: ^{252}Cf as antineoplastic (radiation source).

1717.   Calixarenes. Molecular baskets into which smaller molecules can fit. Name is derived from the Greek "calix" for "chalice" or "cup" and arene for the aryl residues; the name originally referred to the phenolic tetramer linked by methylene groups. The nomenclature uses calix[*n*]arene where *n* is the number of the aryl groups. Modifications to the phenol are indicated by prefixes; whereas total changes of the aryl group are indicated in front of the "arene". Prepn: A. Zinke, E. Ziegler, *Ber.* **77,** 264 (1944); A. Zinke *et al., Monatsh. Chem.* **79,** 438 (1948). Modification of basic structures: J. L. Atwood *et al., Angew. Chem. Int. Ed.* **32,** 1093 (1993). Book: *Calixarenes,* C. D. Gutsche, Ed. (Royal Society of Chemistry, Cambridge, U.K., 1989) 222 pp.

1718.   Calmagite. [3147-14-6] 3-Hydroxy-4-[(2-hydroxy-5-methylphenyl)azo]-1-naphthalenesulfonic acid; 1-(1-hydroxy-4-methyl-2-phenylazo)-2-naphthol-4-sulfonic acid. C$_{17}$H$_{14}$N$_2$O$_5$S; mol wt 358.37. C 56.98%, H 3.94%, N 7.82%, O 22.32%, S 8.95%. Prepn from 1-amino-2-naphthol-4-sulfonic acid and *p*-cresol: Lindstrom, Diehl, *Anal. Chem.* **32,** 1123 (1960).

Red crystals from acetone. Sol in water. Absorption max (pH 10.10): 610 nm (ε 20300). Functions as acid-base indicator: Aq solns are bright red at low pH, red at pH 7.1 to 9.1, blue at pH 9.1 to

11.4. The blue color at pH 10 is changed to red by the addition of calcium or magnesium.

USE: As indicator in titration of Ca or Mg with EDTA.

1719. Calmodulin. [77107-46-1] CaM; calcium-dependent regulator protein; CDR. A calcium-binding multifunctional regulatory protein, ubiquitously distributed in eukaryotic cells. It functions as an intracellular intermediary for calcium ions and activates a number of enzymes involved in fundamental cell processes, such as protein phosphorylation, contractile processes, and metabolism of cyclic nucleotides, of glycogen and of calcium, as well as in other metabolic reactions. Originally discovered as a protein activator of cyclic 3',5'-nucleotide phosphodiesterase: W. Y. Cheung, *Biochem. Biophys. Res. Commun.* **29,** 478 (1967); *idem, Biochim. Biophys. Acta* **191,** 303 (1969); *idem, Biochem. Biophys. Res. Commun.* **38,** 533 (1970); S. Kakiuchi *et al., ibid.* **41,** 1104 (1970). Calcium-binding activity: T. S. Teo, J. H. Wang, *J. Biol. Chem.* **248,** 5950 (1973). Calmodulin is a relatively small, acidic, stable monomer of mol wt 15,000-19,000, lacking cysteine, hydroxyproline, and tryptophan. It has a high content of acidic amino acids and low tyrosine content; almost all calmodulins isolated also contain a single, fully trimethylated lysyl residue. Purification from bovine brain: Y. M. Lin *et al., ibid.* **249,** 4943 (1974); *eidem, Methods Enzymol.* **39,** Pt. C, 262 (1974). Amino acid sequence of CaM from bovine brain: T. C. Vanaman in *Calcium Binding Proteins and Calcium Function,* R. H. Wasserman *et al.,* Eds. (Elsevier, New York, 1977) pp 107-116; D. M. Watterson *et al., J. Biol. Chem.* **255,** 962 (1980); from rat testis: J. R. Dedman *et al., ibid.* **253,** 343 (1978); from sea invertebrate, *Renilla reniformis:* T. C. Vanaman, F. Sharief, *Fed. Proc.* **38,** 788 (1979). Radioimmunoassay: R. W. Wallace, W. Y. Cheung, *J. Biol. Chem.* **254,** 6564 (1979); J. C. Chafouleas *et al., ibid.* 10262. CaM has four Ca^{2+}-binding sites; binding to any one of the sites results in a conformational change, which is required for calmodulin to regulate enzyme systems. Conformational transition study: C. B. Klee, *Biochemistry* **16,** 1017 (1977). An important feature of calmodulin's structure is the presence of four homologous internal amino acid sequences, called domains. Each of these domains (one for each bound calcium) are reportedly "E-F Hands", a structural concept described by R. H. Kretsinger in *Calcium Transport in Contraction and Secretions,* E. Carafoli *et al.,* Eds. (Elsevier, Amsterdam, 1975) pp 469-478. Calmodulins obtained from a wide range of phylogenetically different sources are similar in amino acid sequence and in physicochemical and biological properties; hence, the protein lacks both species and tissue specificity and appears to be structurally and functionally conserved throughout evolution. *Reviews:* W. Y. Cheung, *Science* **207,** 19-27 (1980); A. R. Means, J. R. Dedman, *Nature* **285,** 73-77 (1980); C. B. Klee *et al., Annu. Rev. Biochem.* **49,** 489-515 (1980); A. R. Means, *Recent Prog. Horm. Res.* **37,** 333-367 (1981); Y. M. Lin, *Mol. Cell. Biochem.* **45,** 101-112 (1982). Books: *Ann. N.Y. Acad. Sci.* **356,** entitled "Calmodulin and Cell Functions", D. M. Watterson, F. F. Vincenzi, Eds. (1980) 455 pp; *Calcium and Cell Function* vol. 1, W. Y. Cheung, Ed. (Academic Press, New York, 1980) 395 pp.

Isoelectric pt 3.9-4.3. $\varepsilon^{1\%}_{276nm}$ 1.8; $\varepsilon^{1\%}_{280nm}$ 2.1. Stable when subjected to heat at neutral or acidic pH.

1720. Calotropin. [1986-70-5] [2α(2S,3S,4S,6R),3β,5α]-14-Hydroxy-19-oxo-3,2-[(tetrahydro-3,4-dihydroxy-6-methyl-2H-pyran-2,3-diyl)bis(oxy)]card-20(22)-enolide. $C_{29}H_{40}O_9$; mol wt 532.62. C 65.40%, H 7.57%, O 27.04%. African arrow poison isolated from milk sap of *Calotropis procera* Dryand., *Asclepiadaceae.* Isolation: Lewin, *Arch. Exp. Pathol. Pharmakol.* **71,** 142 (1913); Hesse *et al., Ann.* **526,** 252 (1936); **566,** 130 (1950); Rajagopalan *et al., Helv. Chim. Acta* **38,** 1809 (1955). Isoln from *Asclepias curassavica* L., *Asclepiadaceae:* S. M. Kupchan *et al., Science* **146,** 1685 (1964). Structure: G. Hesse, G. Lettenbauer, *Ann.* **623,** 142 (1959); Hesse *et al., ibid.* **625,** 157, 161 (1959); D. G. H. Crout *et al., Tetrahedron Lett.* **1963,** 63; *J. Chem. Soc.* **1964,** 2187. Extraction from *C. procera* R.Br. and toxicity: F. Brüschweiler *et al., Helv. Chim. Acta* **52,** 2086 (1969). Revised structure: *eidem, ibid.* 2276. Sequestration by larvae of Monarch butterfly *Danaus plexippus* L.: J. N. Sieber *et al., J. Chem. Ecol.* **6,** 321 (1980). Quantitative analysis of cardenolides in latex and leaves of *C. procera: eidem, Phytochemistry* **21,** 2343 (1982). Biosynthesis of labelled compd: M. S. Lee, J. N. Sieber, *ibid.* **22,** 923 (1983).

Rectangular platelets from alcohol or ethyl acetate, mp 223° (dec). $[\alpha]_D^{18}$ +66.8° (in methanol). Sol in water, alc. Practically insol in ether. uv max: 217, 310 nm (log ε 4.21, 1.49). MLD i.v. in cats: 0.12 mg/kg (Brüschweiler).

1721. Calumba. Colombo. Root of *Jatrorrhiza palmata* (DC.) Miers (*J. columba* Miers), *Menispermaceae.* Habit. Eastern Africa. *Constit.* Columbin, chasmanthin, palmarin (isomer of chasmanthin), jatrorrhizine, columbic acid, columbamine; contains no tannin: Barton, Elad, *J. Chem. Soc.* **1956,** 2085, 2090. *Review:* Feist, *Arzneim.-Forsch.* **1,** 418 (1951).

THERAP CAT (VET): Has been used as a stomachic.

1722. Calusterone. [17021-26-0] (7β,17β)-17-Hydroxy-7,17-dimethylandrost-4-en-3-one; 7β,17α-dimethyltestosterone; methosarb; U-22550. $C_{21}H_{32}O_2$; mol wt 316.48. C 79.70%, H 10.19%, O 10.11%. Synthetic androgen epimeric with bolasterone, *q.v.* Has been used in treatment of breast cancer. Prepn: Campbell, Babcock, US 3029263; US 3341557 (1962, 1967 both to Upjohn). Clinical studies: Gordan *et al., J. Am. Med. Assoc.* **219,** 483 (1972).

Crystals from acetone, mp 127-129°. $[\alpha]_D$ +57° (CHCl$_3$). uv max (alcohol): 243 nm.

Note: This is a controlled substance (anabolic steroid): **21 CFR,** 1308.13, as defined in 1300.01.

1723. Calycanthine. [595-05-1] $C_{22}H_{26}N_4$; mol wt 346.47. C 76.27%, H 7.56%, N 16.17%. In *Calycanthus floridus* L., *C. glaucus* Willd.; *Chimonanthus praecox* (L.) Link, *Calycanthaceae.* First isoln: Eccles, *Proc. Am. Pharm. Assoc.* **84,** 382 (1888). Extraction procedure: Manske-Marion, *Can. J. Res.* **17B,** 293 (1939). Structure: Woodward *et al., Proc. Chem. Soc. London* **1960,** 76; Hamor *et al., ibid.* 78; Hamor, Robertson, *J. Chem. Soc.* **1962,** 194. Configuration: Clayton *et al., Tetrahedron* **18,** 1495 (1962). Synthesis of DL-form: Hendrickson *et al., ibid.* **20,** 565 (1964); Hall *et al., ibid.* **23,** 4131 (1967).

Crystals, mp 245° (evac tube). $[\alpha]_D^{18}$ +684° (c = 1.2 in abs alc). uv max (95% ethanol): 250, 309 nm (log ε 4.28, 3.80). Alkaline reaction to litmus. Freely sol in alc, chloroform; sol in ether, acetone, pyridine; slightly sol in water.

Monohydrate. Orthorhombic bipyramidal crystals from water, mp 220°.

Caution: Highly toxic. Can cause violent convulsions, paralysis, cardiac depression.

1724. Calyculin A. [101932-71-2] *N*-[(3*S*)-3-[4-[[(1*E*)-3-[(2*R*,3*R*,5*R*,7*S*,8*S*,9*R*)-2-[(1*S*,3*S*,4*S*,5*R*,6*R*,7*E*,9*E*,11*E*,13*Z*)-14-cyano-3,5-dihydroxy-1-methoxy-4,6,8,9,13-pentamethyl-7,9,11,13-tetradecatetraenyl]-9-hydroxy-4,4,8-trimethyl-3-(phosphonooxy)-1,6-dioxaspiro[4.5]dec-7-yl]-1-propenyl]-2-oxazolyl]butyl]-4-deoxy-4-(dimethylamino)-5-*O*-methyl-L-ribonamide;(−)-calyculin A. $C_{50}H_{81}N_4O_{15}P$; mol wt 1009.17. C 59.51%, H 8.09%, N 5.55%, O 23.78%, P 3.07%. One of a family of antitumor marine toxins which inhibits protein phosphatases 1 and 2a. Isoln from the marine sponge, *Discodermia calyx,* and structure determn: Y. Kato *et al., J. Am. Chem. Soc.* **108**, 2780 (1986); of calyculins B-D: *eidem, J. Org. Chem.* **53**, 3930 (1988); of E-H: S. Matsunaga *et al., Tetrahedron* **47**, 2999 (1991). Revised stereochemistry: S. Matsunaga, N. Fusetani, *Tetrahedron Lett.* **32**, 5605 (1991). Synthesis: N. Tanimoto *et al., Angew. Chem. Int. Ed.* **33**, 673 (1994). Inhibition of protein phosphatases: H. Ishihara *et al., Biochem. Biophys. Res. Commun.* **159**, 871 (1989); selectivity *in vivo:* B. Favre *et al., J. Biol. Chem.* **272**, 13856 (1997). Binding model: M. K. Lindvall *et al., ibid.* 23312. Use as inhibitor in biological studies: M. C. Arufe *et al., Endocrine* **11**, 235 (1999); I. Bize *et al., Am. J. Physiol.* **277**, C926 (1999).

Colorless needles from a mixture of hexane, ether and acetone, mp 247-249°. $[\alpha]_D$ −60° (c = 0.1 in ethanol). uv max (ethanol): 230, 342 nm (ε 12000, 19000).

USE: Inhibitor of phosphatases 1 and 2a.

1725. Camazepam. [36104-80-0] Dimethylcarbamic acid 7-chloro-2,3-dihydro-1-methyl-2-oxo-5-phenyl-1*H*-1,4-benzodiazepin-3-yl ester; 7-chloro-1,3-dihydro-3-hydroxy-1-methyl-5-phenyl-2*H*-1,4-benzodiazepine-carbamate (ester); 7-chloro-1,3-dihydro-3-(*N,N*-dimethylcarbamoyl)-1-methyl-5-phenyl-2*H*-1,4-benzodiazepin-2-one; SB-5833; Albego. $C_{19}H_{18}ClN_3O_3$; mol wt 371.82. C 61.37%, H 4.88%, Cl 9.53%, N 11.30%, O 12.91%. Prepn: G. Ferrari, C. Casagrande, **DE 2142181**; *eidem,* **US 3799920** (1972, 1974 both to Siphar). Metabolism: F. Marcucci *et al., J. Pharm. Sci.* **67**, 1470 (1978). Pharmacology: L. Merlo *et al., Arzneim.-Forsch.* **24**, 1759 (1974); R. Ferrini *et al., ibid.* 2029. Clinical studies: A. Tammaro *et al., ibid.* **27**, 2177 (1978); S. Carrara *et al., Eur. J. Clin. Pharmacol.* **13**, 335 (1978).

White crystalline powder from ethyl acetate, mp 173-174°. Sol in alcohol, moderately sol in water. LD_{50} in mice, rats (mg/kg): 970, >4000 orally (Ferrini).

Note: This is a controlled substance (depressant): **21 CFR,** 1308.14.

THERAP CAT: Anxiolytic.

1726. Cambendazole. [26097-80-3] [2-(4-Thiazolyl)-1*H*-benzimidazol-5-yl]carbamic acid 1-methylethyl ester; 2-(4-thiazolyl)-5-benzimidazolecarbamate isopropyl ester; 5-isopropoxycarbonylamino-2-(4-thiazolyl)benzimidazole; 5-isopropoxycarbonylaminothiabendazole; isopropyl 2-(4-thiazolyl)-5-benzimidazolecarbamate; MK-905; Camvet; Noviben. $C_{14}H_{14}N_4O_2S$; mol wt 302.35. C 55.61%, H 4.67%, N 18.53%, O 10.58%, S 10.61%. Prepn and activity studies: Hoff, Fisher, **ZA 6800351** (1969 to Merck & Co.), *C.A.* **72**, 90461q (1970); Hoff *et al., Experientia* **26**, 550 (1970). Clinical studies with sheep, cattle and swine: Egerton *et al., Res. Vet. Sci.* **11**, 193, 495, 590 (1970).

Odorless, white crystalline solid, mp 238-240° (dec). Sol in alcohol, dimethylformamide; sparingly sol in acetone; slightly sol in benzene; very slightly sol in 0.1*M* HCl. Practically insol in isooctane and water (0.02 mg/ml). Stable in acid and base in range of pH 1 to 12. uv max (0.1*N* HCl): 319, 232 nm ($A_{1cm}^{1\%}$ 740, 670).

THERAP CAT (VET): Anthelmintic.

1727. Cameleons. [205599-45-7] Yellow cameleons; YCs. Engineered proteins designed to measure intracellular calcium concentrations via FRET. Characterized by four domains: a modified green fluorescent protein, *q.v.*; a calmodulin; a cyan fluorescent protein; the calmodulin binding peptide, M13. Prepn: A. Miyawaki *et al., Nature* **388**, 882 (1997); modification: *eidem, Proc. Natl. Acad. Sci. USA* **96**, 2135 (1999). Use in monitoring calcium changes at vesicle surface: E. Emmanouilidou *et al., Curr. Biol.* **9**, 915 (1999); in the endoplasmic reticulum: R. Yu, P. M. Hinkle, *J. Biol. Chem.* **275**, 23648 (2000). Use as a tool for nervous system function in model organisms: R. Kerr *et al., Neuron* **26**, 583 (2000).

USE: Indicator for intracellular calcium.

1728. Camostat. [59721-28-7] 4-[[4-[(Aminoiminomethyl)amino]benzoyl]oxy]benzeneacetic acid 2-(dimethylamino)-2-oxoethyl ester; *N,N*-dimethylcarbamoylmethyl-*p*-(*p*-guanidinobenzoyloxy)phenylacetate. $C_{20}H_{22}N_4O_5$; mol wt 398.41. C 60.29%, H 5.57%, N 14.06%, O 20.08%. Orally active, non-peptide proteolytic enzyme inhibitor with anti-trypsin and anti-plasmin activities, related structurally to gabexate, *q.v.* Prepn: S. Fujii *et al.,* **DE 2548886**; *eidem,* **US 4021472** (1976, 1977 both to Ono). Enzyme inhibition study: Y. Tamura *et al., Biochim. Biophys. Acta* **484**, 417 (1977). Inhibition of exptl tumors in mice: M. Ohkoshi, *Gann* **72**, 959 (1981), *C.A.* **96**, 97304v (1982); M. Ohkoshi, S. Fujii, *ibid.* **73**, 108 (1982), *C.A.* **96**, 155182s (1982). Prevention of acute exptl pancreatitis: S. Takasugi *et al., Digestion* **24**, 36 (1982). Absorption and excretion: S. Hiraku *et al., Iyakuhin Kenkyu* **13**, 756 (1982), *C.A.* **97**, 120038t (1982).

Methanesulfonate. [59721-29-8] Camostat mesylate; FOY-305; Foipan. $C_{20}H_{22}N_4O_5 \cdot CH_3SO_3H$; mol wt 494.52. Solid from methanol/ether, mp 150-155°. Sol in water.

THERAP CAT: Protease inhibitor.

1729. Campesterol. [474-62-4] (3*β*,24*R*)-Ergost-5-en-3-ol. $C_{28}H_{48}O$; mol wt 400.68. C 83.93%, H 12.07%, O 3.99%. Small amounts are found in rape-seed oil derived from *Brassica campestris* L., *Cruciferae,* in soybean oil, and in wheat germ oil. Isoln: Fernholz, MacPhillamy, *J. Am. Chem. Soc.* **63**, 1155 (1941). Structure: Fernholz, Ruigh, *ibid.* 1157. Synthesis: Tarzia *et al., Gazz. Chim. Ital.* **97**, 102 (1967), *C.A.* **67**, 32883q (1967).

Crystals from acetone, mp 157-158°. $[\alpha]_D^{23}$ −33° (22.5 mg in 5 ml chloroform).

Acetate. $C_{30}H_{50}O_2$. Crystals from alc, mp 137-138°. $[\alpha]_D^{23}$ −35° (28.8 mg in 1 ml chloroform).

1730. Camphene. [79-92-5] 2,2-Dimethyl-3-methylenebicyclo[2.2.1]heptane; 2,2-dimethyl-3-methylenenorbornane; 3,3-dimethyl-2-methylenenorcamphane. $C_{10}H_{16}$; mol wt 136.23. C 88.16%, H 11.84%. Occurs in many essential oils, such as turpentine (*levo* and *dextro* forms), in cypress oil (*dextro* form), in camphor oil from species of *Lauraceae* (*dextro*), in bergamot oil, in oil of citronella, neroli, ginger, valerian. Reviews on isolation, preparation and properties: J. L. Simonsen, *The Terpenes* vol. **II** (Cambridge Univ. Press, 1949) pp 280-322; E. Guenther, *The Essential Oils* vol. **II** (Van Nostrand, 1949) pp 66-70. Synthesis: G. W. Hana, H. Koch, *Ber.* **111**, 2527 (1968).

dl-Form. Cubic crystals from alcohol. Large dodecahedra by slow sublimation. Volatilizes on exposure to air. Insipid odor. mp 51-52°. bp$_{760}$ 158.5-159.5°; bp$_{100}$ 92.4°; bp$_{16}$ 55-56°. d_4^{54} 0.8422. n_D^{54} 1.45514. Practically insol in water. Moderately sol in alcohol; sol in ether, cyclohexane, cyclohexene, dioxane, chloroform.

d-Form. mp 52°. $[\alpha]_D^{17}$ +103.5° (c = 9.67 in ether). d_4^{50} 0.8486. n_D^{50} 1.4605.

l-Form. mp 52°. $[\alpha]_D^{21}$ −119.11° (c = 2.33 in benzene). d_4^{54} 0.8422. n_D^{40} 1.4620.

1731. d-Camphocarboxylic Acid. [18530-30-8] 4,7,7-Trimethyl-3-oxobicyclo[2.2.1]heptane-2-carboxylic acid; d-2-oxo-3-bornanecarboxylic acid; d-3-camphorcarboxylic acid; d-2-oxo-3-camphanecarboxylic acid; d-3-carboxy-2-bornanone; d-3-carboxy-2-camphanone. $C_{11}H_{16}O_3$; mol wt 196.24. C 67.32%, H 8.22%, O 24.46%. Prepd by carboxylation of d-camphor: Brühl, *Ber.* **24**, 3373 (1891).

Crystals from benzene, water, ether, or 50% alcohol. mp 127-128°. Sparingly sol in cold water, more sol in warm water; sol in alcohol, ether, chloroform, in about 2 parts boiling benzene. Sparingly sol in cold benzene. Practically insol in cold petr ether; very slightly sol in boiling petr ether. For soln contg 0.38 g in 25 ml solvent: $[\alpha]_D$ +18° (benzene), +60° (alcohol), +73.3° (water).

Ammonium salt. [6799-26-4] Camphydryl; camphor solubilized; Canfoxil. $C_{11}H_{19}NO_3$; mol wt 213.27.

Basic bismuth salt. [4154-53-4] Angimuth. $C_{33}H_{46}Bi_2O_{11}$; mol wt 1036.67. Prepn: Raiziss, Clemence, US **1921638** (1933 to Abbott). Powder. Odor of camphor. Practically insoluble in water. Soluble in methanol, ether, benzene, oils.

THERAP CAT: Basic bismuth salt formerly as antisyphilitic.

1732. Camphor. [76-22-2] 1,7,7-Trimethylbicyclo[2.2.1]-heptan-2-one; 2-bornanone; 2-camphanone; 2-keto-1,7,7-trimethyl-

norcamphane; gum camphor; Japan camphor; Formosa camphor; laurel camphor. $C_{10}H_{16}O$; mol wt 152.23. C 78.90%, H 10.59%, O 10.51%. Naturally occuring in both the d- and l-forms; orginally obtained commercially as the d-form from the camphor tree, *Cinnamomum camphora* T. Nees & Ebermeier, *Lauraceae*. Primarily manufactured from pinene as the racemate. History of isolation and production of natural and synthetic forms: I. Gubelmann, H. W. Elley, *Ind. Eng. Chem.* **26**, 589 (1934); J. M. Derfer, M. M. Derfer in *Kirk-Othmer Encyclopedia of Chemical Technology* vol. 23 (John Wiley & Sons, New York, 4th ed., 1997) pp 865-866. Enantiomeric composition in oils of coriander, sage, and basil: F. Tateo *et al.*, *Anal. Commun.* **36**, 149 (1999). GC determn in human plasma: J. S. Valdez *et al.*, *J. Chromatogr. B* **729**, 163 (1999); in pharmaceutical formulation: E. González-Penas *et al.*, *Chromatographia* **52**, 245 (2000). *Review: Camphor and Camphor Containing Products* (PB293503, 1979) 65 pp; J. S. Mossa, M. M. A. Hassan, *Anal. Profiles Drug Subs.* **13**, 28-93 (1984). Review of use as starting material for syntheses: T. Money, *Org. Synth.* **3**, 1-83 (1996).

l-form   *d-form*

White or colorless crystals or crystalline masses; also colorless to white translucent masses. Characteristic fragrant and penetrating odor. Pungent, aromatic taste. d_4^{25} 0.992. mp 179°. bp$_{101.3\ kPa}$ 209°. Volatilizes slowly. uv max (CHCl$_3$): 292 nm. At 25° one gram dissolves in about 800 ml water, in 1 ml alcohol, 1 ml ether, 0.5 ml chloroform. Freely sol in carbon disulfide, petr. benzin, fixed and volatile oils. Also sol in concd mineral acids, in phenol, in liquid NH$_3$ and in liquid SO$_2$. LD$_{50}$ orally in mice: 1.3 g/kg (PB293505).

D-Form. [464-49-3] (1R)-(+)-Camphor. Colorless, transparent crystals, mp 179.8°, sublimes 204°. $[\alpha]_D^{25}$ +41 to +43° (c = 10 in U.S.P. alcohol) according to U.S.P. specif.

L-Form. [464-48-2] (1S)-(−)-Camphor.

Spirit of Camphor. A soln of camphor in alcohol contg 10 g camphor per 100 ml soln. Colorless liquid; camphor odor.

Caution: Potential symptoms of overexposure to synthetic camphor are irritation of eyes, skin, mucous membranes; nausea, vomiting, diarrhea; headache, dizziness, confusion, vertigo, excitement, restlessness, delerium, hallucinations; epileptic convulsions; CNS depression, coma. *See NIOSH Pocket Guide to Chemical Hazards* (DHHS/NIOSH 97-140, 1997) p 48; *Clinical Toxicology of Commercial Products*, R. E. Gosselin *et al.*, Eds. (Williams & Wilkins, Baltimore, 5th ed., 1984) Section III, pp 84-86.

USE: Starting reagent for organic syntheses. Used as an odorant and flavorant and as a moth repellant. Plasticizer in cosmetics and as a preservative.

THERAP CAT: Topical analgesic; topical antipruritic.

THERAP CAT (VET): Has been used internally as a stimulant and carminative; externally as an antipruritic, counterirritant and antiseptic.

1733. Camphoric Acid. [5394-83-2] 1,2,2-Trimethyl-1,3-cyclopentanedicarboxylic acid; dextrocamphoric acid. $C_{10}H_{16}O_4$; mol wt 200.23. C 59.98%, H 8.05%, O 31.96%. By oxidation of camphor: Bredt, *Ber.* **26**, 3047 (1893). Synthesis: Perkin, Thorpe, *J. Chem. Soc.* **89**, 799 (1906); Toivonan, *Acta Chem. Scand.* **2**, 597 (1948).

Leaflets from water, monoclinic prisms from alc, mp 186-188°. d 1.186. $[\alpha]_D^{20}$ +47 to +48° (alc). One gram dissolves in 125 ml water, 10 ml boiling water, 1 ml alc, 20 ml glycerol; sol in chloroform, ether, fats, oils.

1734. *d*-Camphorsulfonic Acid. [3144-16-9] 7,7-Dimethyl-2-oxobicyclo[2.2.1]heptane-1-methanesulfonic acid; 2-oxo-10-bornanesulfonic acid; 10-camphorsulfonic acid; camsylate; camphostyl; β-camphorsulfonic acid; Reychler's acid. $C_{10}H_{16}O_4S$; mol wt 232.30. C 51.70%, H 6.94%, O 27.55%, S 13.80%. Prepn from powdered camphor, concd H_2SO_4 and acetic anhydride: Reychler, *Bull. Soc. Chim. Fr.* [3] **19**, 120 (1898); Armstrong, Lowry, *J. Chem. Soc.* **81**, 1447 (1902); Lipp, Knapp, *Ber.* **73B**, 915 (1940). Structure: Loudon, *J. Chem. Soc.* **1933**, 823; Komppa, *J. Prakt. Chem.* **162**, 19 (1943).

Prisms from glacial acetic acid or ethyl acetate, dec 193-195°. $[\alpha]_D^{20}$ +43.5° (c = 4.3 in alcohol); $[\alpha]_D^{20}$ +21.5° (c = 4.3 in water). Deliquesc in moist air. Practically insol in ether; slightly sol in glacial acetic acid, ethyl acetate.

Ammonium salt. $C_{10}H_{19}NO_4S$. Needles from water. $[\alpha]_D^{16}$ +20.5° (c = 5 in water). Very sol in water.

Potassium salt. $C_{10}H_{15}KO_4S$. Needles from alcohol. $[\alpha]_D^{16}$ +18.4° (c = 4.4 in water).

USE: Resolution of optically active isomers.

1735. Camptothecin. [7689-03-4] (*S*)-4-Ethyl-4-hydroxy-1*H*-pyrano[3′,4′:6,7]indolizino[1,2-*b*]quinoline-3,14(4*H*,12*H*)-dione. $C_{20}H_{16}N_2O_4$; mol wt 348.35. C 68.96%, H 4.63%, N 8.04%, O 18.37%. Antitumor alkaloid; prototype DNA topoisomerase I inhibitor. Isoln from the stem wood of the Chinese tree, *Camptotheca acuminata* Decsne., *Nyssaceae,* and structure: M. E. Wall *et al., J. Am. Chem. Soc.* **88**, 3888 (1966). Approach to synthesis: Kepler *et al., J. Org. Chem.* **34**, 3853 (1969). Total synthesis: E. J. Corey *et al., ibid.* **40**, 2140 (1975). Total synthesis of racemate: Stork, Schultz, *J. Am. Chem. Soc.* **93**, 4074 (1971); Volkmann *et al., ibid.* 5576; Tang *et al., ibid.* **97**, 159 (1975); J. C. Bradley, G. Buchi, *J. Org. Chem.* **41**, 699 (1976); T. Kametani *et al., J. Chem. Soc. Perkin Trans. 1* **1981**, 1563. Pharmacologic and clinical evaluation: Gottlieb *et al., Cancer Chemother. Rep. Part 1* **54**, 461 (1970); Gallo *et al., J. Natl. Cancer Inst.* **46**, 789 (1971); S. M. Sieber *et al., Cancer Treat. Rep.* **60**, 1127 (1976). Mechanism of action: Y. H. Hsiang *et al., J. Biol. Chem.* **260**, 14873 (1985). HPLC determn in plasma: J. H. Beijnen *et al., J. Chromatogr.* **617**, 111 (1993). *Reviews:* M. Potmesil, *Cancer Res.* **54**, 1431-1439 (1994); M. E. Wall, M. C. Wani, *ibid.* **55**, 753-760 (1995).

Pale yellow needles from methanol + acetonitrile, dec 264-267°. Also reported as mp 275-277° (Volkmann); 287-288° (Stork, Schultz). $[\alpha]_D^{25}$ +31.3° (in chloroform-methanol, 8:2). Exhibits intense blue fluorescence under uv light. uv max: 220, 254, 290, 370 nm (ε 37320, 29230, 4980, 19900). Does not form stable salts with acids. Poorly sol in water.

Acetate. $C_{22}H_{18}N_2O_5$. Crystals, dec 271-274°. uv max: 220, 254, 290, 360-370 nm (ε 39010, 28740, 6160, 22000).

Chloroacetate. $C_{22}H_{17}ClN_2O_5$. Crystals, dec 245-248°.

1736. Canadine. [522-97-4] 5,8,13,13a-Tetrahydro-9,10-dimethoxy-6*H*-benzo[*g*]-1,3-benzodioxolo[5,6-*a*]quinolizine; 9,10-dimethoxy-2,3-(methylenedioxy)berbine; 5,6,13,13a-tetrahydro-9,10-dimethoxy-2,3-(methylenedioxy)-8*H*-dibenzo[*a,g*]quinolizine; tetrahydroberberine; xanthopuccine. $C_{20}H_{21}NO_4$; mol wt 339.39. C 70.78%, H 6.24%, N 4.13%, O 18.86%. A protoberberine alkaloid from *Corydalis cava* (L.), Schweigg & Korte (*C. tuberosa* DC.), *Fumariaceae:* Späth, Julian, *Ber.* **64**, 1131 (1931). Prepn by reduction of berberine: Bersch, Seufert, *ibid.* **70**, 1121 (1937); Awe, Hertel, *Arch. Pharm.* **288**, 516 (1955); Russell, *J. Am. Chem. Soc.* **78**, 3115 (1956). Configuration: Corrodi, Hardegger, *Helv. Chim. Acta* **39**, 889 (1956). Other syntheses: Kametani *et al., J. Chem. Soc. C* **1969**, 2036; **1971**, 2709; M. Cushman, F. W. Dekon, *J. Org. Chem.* **44**, 407 (1979); K. Iwasa *et al., ibid.* **46**, 4744 (1981); N. S. Narasimhan *et al., Tetrahedron Lett.* **22**, 2797 (1981). Pharmacology: F. Sadritdinov, M. B. Sultanov, *C.A.* **66**, 74714v (1967). *Review:* R. H. F. Manske, H. L. Holmes, *The Alkaloids* vol. 4 (Academic Press, New York, 1954) pp 91-92.

LD_{50} in mice (in mg/kg): 940 orally; 790 s.c.; 100 i.v. (Sadritdinov, Sultanov).

d-Form. [2086-96-0] mp 132°. $[\alpha]_D^{15}$ +299° (chloroform). Sol in aq methanol.

l-Form. [5096-57-1] Crystals from methanol, mp 135°. $[\alpha]_D^{22}$ −308°; −317° (c = 0.28; 0.4, both in methanol). Sol in aq methanol.

dl-Form. [29074-38-2] mp 172° (Späth, Julian), also reported as 163-165° (Cushman, Dekon). uv max (95% ethanol): 209, 284 nm (ε 28,300; 5200). Sol in aq methanol.

1737. Canavanine. [543-38-4] *O*-[(Aminoiminomethyl)amino]homoserine; 2-amino-4-(guanidinooxy)butyric acid. $C_5H_{12}N_4O_3$; mol wt 176.17. C 34.09%, H 6.87%, N 31.80%, O 27.25%. $H_2NC(NH)NHOCH_2CH_2CH(NH_2)COOH$. Basic amino acid isolated as L-canavanine from jack beans, *Canavalia ensiformis* (L.) DC., *Leguminosae:* Kitagawa, Tomiyama, *J. Biochem. (Tokyo)* **11**, 265 (1929). Constitutes about 1.5% of the dry weight of alfalfa seeds and sprouts: E. A. Bell *Biochem. J.* **75**, 618 (1960). Distribution in the plant kingdom: Turner, Harborne, *Phytochemistry* **6**, 863 (1967). Structure: Gulland, Morris, *J. Chem. Soc.* **1935**, 763; Kitagawa, Takani, *J. Biochem. (Tokyo)* **23**, 181 (1936). Configuration: Cadden, *Proc. Soc. Exp. Biol. Med.* **45**, 224 (1940). Synthesis of racemate: Nyberg, Christensen, *J. Am. Chem. Soc.* **79**, 1222 (1957); Frankel *et al., J. Chem. Soc.* **1963**, 3127. Alternate synthesis: Yamada *et al., Agric. Biol. Chem.* **37**, 2201 (1973). Bears resemblance to arginine, *q.v.* and is often used as substrate to some enzymes normally acting on arginine. Accordingly it is a potent growth inhibitor of many organisms: Pilcher *et al., Proc. Soc. Exp. Biol. Med.* **88**, 79 (1955). Toxic to mammals: B. Tschiersch, *Pharmazie* **17**, 621 (1962). L-Canavanine induces certain hematologic and serologic abnormalities characteristic of systemic lupus erythematosus in monkeys: M. R. Malinow *et al., Science* **216**, 415 (1982).

Crystals from abs alcohol, mp 184°. $[\alpha]_D^{20}$ +7.9° (c = 3.2).

Sulfate. $C_5H_{14}N_4O_7S$. Crystals from dil alcohol, dec 172°. $[\alpha]_D^{17}$ +19.4° (c = 2). Freely sol in water.

DL-Form. Crystals from ethanol, mp 180-182°. Soluble in water. Practically insol in alcohol. Forms a monohydrochloride, mp 190°.

1738. Candelilla Wax. [8006-44-8] Obtained from the candelilla plants; *Euphorbia antisyphilitica* Zucc., *Euphorbiaceae* and *E. cerifera* Alcocer (which is only doubtfully distinct from *E. antisyphilitica*) are now the principal sources of candelilla wax. *Pedilanthus pavonis* Boiss. and *P. aphyllus* Boiss. are secondary sources, yielding a wax of lower melting range and lower saponification number. Most of the wax is produced in Mexico by immersing the plants in boiling water containing sulfuric acid and skimming off the wax which rises to the surface as described by Dickinson, *Am. J. Pharm.* **91**, 808 (1919); Hodge, Sineath, *Econ. Bot.* **10**, 134 (1956). The main constituent is the hydrocarbon hentriacontane. Brief review: C. S. Letcher in *Kirk-Othmer Encyclopedia of Chemical Technology* vol. 24 (Wiley-Interscience, New York, 3rd ed., 1984) pp 468-469.

Consult the Name Index before using this section.

Brownish to yellowish-brown, hard, brittle, easily pulverizable lumps. d 0.950-0.990. mp 68-70°. Saponification number 50-65. Acid number 10-20. Iodine number 30-35. Practically insoluble in water. Sparingly sol in alcohol; sol in acetone, benzene, carbon disulfide, decalin, hot petr ether, gasoline, oils, turpentine, hot chloroform, carbon tetrachloride.

USE: Manuf cosmetics, rubber substitutes, furniture and leather polishes, candles, sealing wax, phonograph records; for waterproofing boxes and fabrics; electric insulations; lithographic, printing, stamping and writing inks; molding compositions; sizing paper; hardening other waxes; protective coating for citrus fruits; formerly in chewing gum.

1739. Candesartan. [139481-59-7] 2-Ethoxy-1-[[2'-(1*H*-tetrazol-5-yl)[1,1'-biphenyl]-4-yl]methyl]-1*H*-benzimidazole-7-carboxylic acid; 2-ethoxy-1-[4-[2-(1*H*-tetrazol-5-yl)phenyl]benzyl]-7-benzimidazolecarboxylic acid; CV-11974. $C_{24}H_{20}N_6O_3$; mol wt 440.45. C 65.45%, H 4.58%, N 19.08%, O 10.90%. Angiotensin II type-1 receptor antagonist. Prepn: T. Naka *et al., EP 459136; eidem,* **US 5196444** (1991, 1993 both to Takeda); K. Kubo *et al., J. Med. Chem.* **36,** 2182, 2343 (1993). Pharmacology: Y. Shibouta *et al., J. Pharmacol. Exp. Ther.* **266,** 114 (1993). Clinical pharmacology, pharmacokinetics: T. Ogihara *et al., Clin. Ther.* **16,** 74 (1994). Pilot study of cilexetil ester in essential hypertension: *idem et al., ibid.* **15,** 684 (1993). Series of clinical trials in chronic heart failure: *Lancet* **362,** 759-781 (2003).

Colorless crystals from ethyl acetate + methanol, mp 183-185°.
1-[[(Cyclohexyloxy)carbonyl]oxy]ethyl ester. [145040-37-5] Candesartan cilexetil; TCV-116; Atacand; Amias; Kenzen. $C_{33}H_{34}N_6O_6$; mol wt 610.66. Ester prodrug; hydrolyzed *in vivo* to the active carboxylic acid. Colorless crystals from ethanol + water, mp 163° (dec). Also reported as white to off-white powder, sparingly sol in methanol. Practically insol in water.

THERAP CAT: Antihypertensive. In treatment of congestive heart failure.

1740. Candicidin. [1403-17-4] Levorin; Vanobid. Heptaene macrolide antifungal antibiotic complex composed of candicidins A, B, C and D (major component). Produced by a strain of *Streptomyces griseus* (Rutgers no. 3570): Lechevalier *et al., Mycologia* **45,** 155 (1953). Methods of isoln: Siminoff, **US 2872373** (1959 to Penick); Waksman, Lechevalier, **US 2992162** (1961 to Rutgers Res. & Ed. Found.). Activity: Kligman, Lewis, *Proc. Soc. Exp. Biol. Med.* **82,** 399 (1953); *Lancet* **1,** 507 (1954); Lechevalier, *Presse Med.* **61,** 1327 (1953). Structure of candicidin D: J. Zielinski *et al., Tetrahedron Lett.* **1979,** 1791. Biosynthesis studies: Liu *et al., J. Antibiot.* **25,** 116 (1972). Anticholesteremic property and mode of action studies: I. H. Kwon, H. Fisher, *Nutr. Rep. Int.* **9,** 245 (1974); A. K. Singhal *et al., Lipids* **16,** 423 (1981). HPLC comparison of candicidin, hamycin, trichomycin, *q.q.v.*: P. Helboe *et al., J. Chromatogr.* **189,** 249 (1980). Toxicity study: L. C. Vining *et al., Antibiot. Annu.* **1954-55,** 980.

Candicidin D

Small yellow needles or rosettes from aq tetrahydrofuran or pyridine/acetic acid/water soln (when pure). Absorption max: 403, 380 ($E_{1cm}^{1\%}$ 1150), 360 nm. Practically insol in water, alcohols, ketones, esters, ethers, hydrocarbons, and other lipophilic solvents. Sol in DMSO, DMF, and lower aliphatic acids. Very sol in 80% aq tetrahydrofuran soln. The addn of 5%-25% water to alcohols greatly increases soly. Forms sol salts in alkaline solns. Soly: Marsh, Weiss, *J. Assoc. Off. Anal. Chem.* **50,** 457 (1967). LD_{50} i.p. in mice: 14 mg/kg (Vining).
Candicidin D. Levorin A_2. $C_{59}H_{84}N_2O_{18}$; mol wt 1109.30. Identity with levorin A_2: Bosshardt, Bickel, *Experientia* **24,** 422 (1968); J. Zielinski *et al., loc. cit.*

THERAP CAT: Antifungal (topical).

1741. Candidin. [1405-90-9] $C_{47}H_{71}NO_{17}$; mol wt 922.06. C 61.22%, H 7.76%, N 1.52%, O 29.50%. Main component of an antifungal antibiotic complex produced by the soil actinomycete *Streptomyces viridoflavus:* W. A. Taber *et al., Antibiot. Chemother.* **4,** 455 (1954); L. C. Vining *et al., Antibiot. Annu.* **2,** 980 (1954-1955); L. C. Vining, W. A. Taber, *Can. J. Chem.* **34,** 1163 (1956). The two other active principles are designated as **candidinin** and **candidoin.** Prepn of pure crystalline candidin: Preud'hamme, Vuillemin, **FR 1298345** (1962 to Rhone-Poulenc), *C.A.* **58,** 420c (1963). Synthesis: M. Subramanian *et al., J. Nat. Prod.* **55,** 1213 (1992). Structure: Borowski *et al., Tetrahedron Lett.* **1971,** 1987; and NMR characterization: J. Pawlak *et al., J. Antibiot.* **46,** 1598 (1993). Antifungal activity studies: Solotorovsky *et al., Antibiot. Chemother.* **8,** 364 (1958).

Golden-yellow needles from methanol + chloroform + water. Does not melt, but darkens slowly above 180°. $[\alpha]_D^{27}$ +363° (c = 0.3 in DMF); $[\alpha]_D^{27}$ +205° (c = 0.3 in glacial acetic acid). uv max (methanol): 406, 383, 362, 347 nm. Practically insol in water and most organic solvents. Moderately sol in glacial acetic acid, pyridine, DMF. LD_{50} in mice (mg/kg): 1.5 i.v., >100 orally, 30 s.c. (Vining *et al.*).

1742. Candoxatril. [123122-55-4] [4(*S*)-*cis*]-4-[[[1-[3-[(2,3-Dihydro-1*H*-inden-5-yl)oxy]-2-[(2-methoxyethoxy)methyl]-3-oxopropyl]cyclopentyl]carbonyl]amino]cyclohexanecarboxylic acid; (α*S*)-1-[[(*cis*-4-carboxycyclohexyl)carbamoyl]-α-[(2-methoxyethoxy)methyl]cyclopentanepropionic acid α-5-indanyl ester; (*S*)-*cis*-4-[1-[2-(5-indanyloxycarbonyl)-3-(2-methoxyethoxy)propyl]-1-cyclopentanecarboxamido]-1-cyclohexanecarboxylic acid; UK-79300. $C_{29}H_{41}NO_7$; mol wt 515.64. C 67.55%, H 8.01%, N 2.72%, O 21.72%. Neutral endopeptidase inhibitor. Prepn: I. T. Barnish *et al., EP 274234; eidem,* **US 5030654** (1988, 1991 both to Pfizer). Enzyme inhibition and pharmacology: J. C. Danilewicz *et al., Biochem. Biophys. Res. Commun.* **164,** 58 (1989). Clinical pharmacokinetics and effect on plasma ANP: J. G. Motwani *et al., Clin. Pharmacol. Ther.* **54,** 661 (1993). Clinical evaluation in congestive heart failure: C. D. Kimmelstiel *et al., Cardiology* **87,** 46 (1996).

White crystals, mp 107-109°. $[\alpha]_D$ −5,8° (c = 1 in methanol).
Diacid. [123122-54-3] Candoxatrilat; UK-73967. $C_{20}H_{33}NO_7$; mol wt 399.48. White crystals from ethyl acetate, mp 108.5-109.1°. $[\alpha]_D$ +1.4° (c = 1 in methanol).

THERAP CAT: In treatment of congestive heart failure.

1743. Canella. White cinnamon; wild cinnamon; false Winter's bark; Bahama white wood; wild canilla. Bark of *Canella alba* Murr. (*C. winterana* Gaertn.), *Canellaceae*. *Habit.* W. Indies and Florida. *Constit.* Eugenol, cineol, terpenes, caryophyllene, mannitol, resin, cancellin.

USE: As spice and as an addition to smoking tobacco.

1744. Canertinib. [267243-28-7] *N*-[4-[(3-Chloro-4-fluorophenyl)amino]-7-[3-(4-morpholinyl)propoxy]-6-quinazolinyl]-2-propenamide; *N*-[4-(3-chloro-4-fluorophenylamino)-7-(3-morpholin-4-ylpropoxy)quinazolin-6-yl]acrylamide. $C_{24}H_{25}ClFN_5O_3$; mol wt 485.94. C 59.32%, H 5.19%, Cl 7.30%, F 3.91%, N 14.41%, O 9.88%. Irreversible pan-erbB tyrosine kinase inhibitor. Prepn: A. J. Bridges *et al.,* **WO 0031048**; *eidem,* **US 6344455** (2000, 2002 both to Warner-Lambert); J. B. Smaill *et al., J. Med. Chem.* **43**, 1380 (2000). Clinical pharmacokinetics in patients with solid malignancies: E. Calvo *et al., Clin. Cancer Res.* **10**, 7112 (2004); and tolerability in refractory cancer: J. Nemunaitis *et al., ibid.* **11**, 3846 (2005). Review of pharmacology and mechanism of action: L. F. Allen *et al., Semin. Oncol.* **30**, Suppl. 16, 65-78 (2003); of development and clinical experience: C. M. Galmarini, *IDrugs* **7**, 58-63 (2004).

Crystals from methanol, mp 188-190°.

Dihydrochloride. [289499-45-2] CI-1033. $C_{24}H_{25}ClFN_5$-O_3.2HCl; mol wt 558.86. Sol in water.

THERAP CAT: Antineoplastic.

1745. Canfosfamide. [158382-37-7] (2*R*)-L-γ-Glutamyl-3-[[2-[[bis[bis(2-chloroethyl)amino]phosphinyl]oxy]ethyl]sulfonyl]-L-alanyl-2-phenylglycine; γ-glutamyl-α-amino-β-((2-ethyl-*N,N,N*′,-*N*′-tetrakis(2-chloro)ethylphosphoramidate)sulfonyl)propionyl-(*R*)-(−)phenylglycine; TER-286. $C_{26}H_{40}Cl_4N_5O_{10}PS$; mol wt 787.47. C 39.66%, H 5.12%, Cl 18.01%, N 8.89%, O 20.32%, P 3.93%, S 4.07%. Nitrogen mustard prodrug preferentially activated by glutathione *S*-transferase P1-1. Prepn: M. H. Lyttle *et al., J. Med. Chem.* **37**, 1501 (1994); L. M. Kauvar *et al.,* **WO 9509866**; *eidem,* **US 5556942** (1995, 1996 both to Terrapin). Mechanism of activation: A. Satyam *et al., J. Med. Chem.* **39**, 1736 (1996). *In vitro* and *in vivo* antitumor and myelosuppressive effects: A. S. Morgan *et al., Cancer Res.* **58**, 2568 (1998). Clinical pharmacokinetics and toxicology in advanced solid malignancies: L. S. Rosen *et al., Clin. Cancer Res.* **9**, 1628 (2003); *idem et al., ibid.* **10**, 3689 (2004).

White solid, mp 82-90°.

Hydrochloride. [439943-59-6] TLK-286; Telcyta. $C_{26}H_{40}$-$Cl_4N_5O_{10}PS$.HCl; mol wt 823.94.

THERAP CAT: Antineoplastic.

1746. Cangrelor. [163706-06-7] *N*-[2-(Methylthio)ethyl]-2-[(3,3,3-trifluoropropyl)thio]-5′-adenylic acid monoanhydride with (dichloromethylene)bis[phosphonic acid]; *N*⁶-(2-methylthio-

ethyl)-2-(3,3,3-trifluoropropylthio)-β,γ-dichloromethylene ATP; AR-C69931XX. $C_{17}H_{25}Cl_2F_3N_5O_{12}P_3S_2$; mol wt 776.36. C 26.30%, H 3.25%, Cl 9.13%, F 7.34%, N 9.02%, O 24.73%, P 11.97%, S 8.26%. Specific $P2Y_{12}$ purinoceptor antagonist; inhibits ADP-induced platelet aggregation. Prepn: A. H. Ingall *et al.,* **WO 9418216** (1994 to Fisons); *eidem,* **US 5721219** (1998 to Astra); and *in vivo* antithrombotic activity: *idem et al., J. Med. Chem.* **42**, 213 (1999). *In vivo* antithrombotic effects in canine arterial thrombosis: J. Huang *et al., J. Pharmacol. Exp. Ther.* **295**, 492 (2000). Mechanism of action study: A. Ishii-Watabe *et al., Biochem. Pharmacol.* **59**, 1345 (2000). Clinical safety assessment and evaluation in acute coronary syndromes: R. F. Storey *et al., Thromb. Haemostasis* **85**, 401 (2001); in angina pectoris and non-Q-wave myocardial infarction: F. Jacobsson *et al., Clin. Ther.* **24**, 752 (2002). Clinical pharmacodynamics compared with clopidogrel: R. F. Storey *et al., Platelets* **13**, 407 (2002). Review of clinical development: S. C. Chattaraj, *Curr. Opin. Invest. Drugs* **2**, 250-255 (2001).

Tetrasodium salt. [163706-36-3] AR-C69931MX. $C_{17}H_{21}$-$Cl_2F_3N_5Na_4O_{12}P_3S_2$; mol wt 864.29. Freely sol in water.

THERAP CAT: Antithrombotic.

1747. Cannabidiol. [13956-29-1] 2-[(1*R*,6*R*)-3-Methyl-6-(1-methylethenyl)-2-cyclohexen-1-yl]-5-pentyl-1,3-benzenediol; *trans*-(−)-2-*p*-mentha-1,8-dien-3-yl-5-pentylresorcinol. $C_{21}H_{30}$-O_2; mol wt 314.46. C 80.21%, H 9.62%, O 10.18%. Major non-psychoactive constituent of cannabis, *q.v.* (*Cannabis sativa* L., *Cannabinaceae*). Exhibits multiple bioactivities including anticonvulsant, anxiolytic and anti-inflammatory effects. Isoln from wild hemp: R. Adams *et al., J. Am. Chem. Soc.* **62**, 196, 2194 (1940); from hashish: A. Jacob, A. R. Todd, *J. Chem. Soc.* **1940**, 649. Structure: R. Mechoulam, Y. Shvo, *Tetrahedron* **19**, 2073 (1963). Crystal and molecular structure: T. Ottersen *et al., Acta Chem. Scand. B* **31**, 807 (1977). Abs config: Y. Gaoni, R. Mechoulam, *J. Am. Chem. Soc.* **93**, 217 (1971). Synthesis of (±)-form: *eidem, ibid.* **87**, 3273 (1965); of (−)-form: T. Petrzilka *et al., Helv. Chim. Acta* **52**, 1102 (1969); H. J. Kurth *et al., Z. Naturforsch.* **36B**, 275 (1981). LC-IT-MS determn in cannabis products: A. A. M. Stolker *et al., J. Chromatogr. A* **1058**, 143 (2004). Review of isoln, chemistry and metabolism: R. Mechoulam, L. Hanus, *Chem. Phys. Lipids* **121**, 35-43 (2002); of pharmacology and bioactivity: R. Mechoulam *et al., J. Clin. Pharmacol.* **42**, 11S-19S (2002).

Pale yellow resin or crystals, mp 66-67°. bp_2 187-190° (bath temp 220°). $bp_{0.001}$ 130°. d_4^{40} 1.040. n_D^{20} 1.5404. $[\alpha]_D^{27}$ −125° (0.066 g in 5 ml 95% ethanol). $[\alpha]_D^{18}$ −129° (c = 0.45 in ethanol). uv max (ethanol): 282, 274 nm (log ε 3.10, 3.12). Practically insol in water or 10% NaOH. Sol in ethanol, methanol, ether, benzene, chloroform, petr ether.

1748. Cannabinol. [521-35-7] 6,6,9-Trimethyl-3-pentyl-6*H*-dibenzo[*b,d*]pyran-1-ol; 3-amyl-1-hydroxy-6,6,9-trimethyl-6*H*-dibenzo[*b,d*]pyran; CBN. $C_{21}H_{26}O_2$; mol wt 310.43. C 81.25%,

H 8.44%, O 10.31%. Nonpsychoactive constituent of cannabis, *q.v.* (*Cannabis sativa* L. *Cannabinaceae*); weak cannabinoid receptor ligand. Isoln from cannabis resin: T. B. Wood *et al., J. Chem. Soc.* **69**, 539 (1896); R. S. Cahn, *J. Chem. Soc.* **1931**, 630; T. S. Work *et al., Biochem. J.* **33**, 123 (1939). Structural studies: R. S. Cahn, *J. Chem. Soc.* **1932**, 1342; **1933**, 1400; F. Bergel, K. Vögele, *Ann.* **493**, 250 (1932). Structure and synthesis: R. Adams *et al., J. Am. Chem. Soc.* **62**, 2204 (1940). Crystal structure: T. Ottersen *et al., Acta Chem. Scand. B* **31**, 781 (1977). Improved syntheses: P. C. Meltzer *et al., Synthesis* **1981**, 985; J. Novák, C. A. Salemink, *Tetrahedron Lett.* **23**, 253 (1982). Pharmacology: I. Yamamoto *et al., Chem. Pharm. Bull.* **35**, 2144 (1987); F. Petitet *et al., Life Sci.* **63**, 1 (1998). Review of chromatographic determn methods in biological samples: C. Staub, *J. Chromatogr. B* **733**, 119-126 (1999). Comparison of pharmacology with other cannabinoids: I. Yamamoto *et al., J. Toxicol. Toxin Rev.* **22**, 577-589 (2003).

Leaflets from petr ether, mp 76-77°. Sublimes at 4 mm with a bath temp of 180-190°. bp$_{0.05}$ 185°. Insol in water. Sol in methanol, ethanol, aq alkaline solns.

1749. Cannabis. Hemp; Indian hemp. Annual, dioecious plant, *Cannabis sativa* L. *Cannabinaceae*. Used since antiquity for its edible seed, fiber to produce rope and cloth, and medicinally as an analgesic, anti-emetic, hypnotic and intoxicant. *Habit.* Temporate to tropical regions, originally in central Asia, China and India. *Constit.* More than 60 known cannabinoids, primarily isomeric tetrahydrocannabinols, cannabidiol, cannabinol, *q.q.v.*; other constituents include alkaloids, proteins, sugars, steroids, flavonoids and vitamins. Seeds and seed oil contain fatty acids, including linoleic, oleic, stearic, and palmetic acids, vitamin E, phytosterols, carotenes. Pistillate plants secrete a cannabinoid containing resin from which **hashish** or **charas** is prepared. Preparations of dried flowering tops from these plants are known as **bhang**, **ganja**, or **marijuana**. Comprehensive description of constituents: C. E. Turner *et al., J. Nat. Prod.* **43**, 169-234 (1980). Review of analytical methods: T. J. Raharjo, R. Verpoorte, *Phytochem. Anal.* **15**, 79-94 (2004); of pharmacology and toxicology: I. B. Adams, B. R. Martin, *Addiction* **91**, 1585-1614 (1996). Series of articles on psychiatric effects, pharmacology and therapeutic uses: *Br. J. Psychiatry* **178**, 101-128 (2001). Book: *Cannabis and Cannabinoids: Pharmacology, Toxicology, and Therapeutic Potential*, F. Grotenhermen, E. Russo, Eds. (Haworth Press, New York, 2002) 439 pp.

Extract. GW-1000; Sativex. Medicinal preparation containing approximately equal amounts of Δ^9-tetrahydrocannabinol and cannabidiol. Prepn of extracts from dried leaf and flowerhead: B. Whittle, G. Guy, **WO 02064109** (2002 to GW Pharma); *eidem,* **US 04192760** (2004). Clinical evaluation for relief of neuropathic pain: J. S. Berman *et al., Pain* **112**, 299 (2004); in multiple sclerosis: C. M. Brady *et al., Mult. Scler.* **10**, 425 (2004). Review of development and clinical experience: P. F. Smith, *Curr. Opin. Invest. Drugs* **5**, 748-754 (2004).

Caution: This is a controlled substance (hallucinogen): **21 CFR**, 1308.11. Acute intoxication is frequently due to recreational use by ingestion or by inhalation of smoke. Psychological responses include euphoria, feelings of detachment and relaxation, visual and auditory hallucinations, anxiety, panic, paranoia, depression, drowsiness, psychotic symptoms. Other effects include impairment of cognitive and psychomotor performance, tachycardia, vasodilation, reddening of the conjuctivae, dry mouth, increased appetite. Chronic inhalation of smoke causes respiratory tract irritation and bronchoconstriction, and may be a significant risk factor for lung cancer. See Grotenhermen, Russo, *loc. cit.*

THERAP CAT: Analgesic.

1750. Canrenone. [976-71-6] (17α)-17-Hydroxy-3-oxopregna-4,6-diene-21-carboxylic acid γ-lactone; 17α-(2-carboxyeth-

yl)-17β-hydroxyandrosta-4,6-dien-3-one lactone; 17α-(2-carboxyethyl)-17β-hydroxy-3-oxoandrosta-4,6-diene lactone; 6-dehydrotestosterone-17α-propionic acid γ-lactone; 3-(3-oxo-17β-hydroxy-4,6-androstadien-17α-yl)propionic acid γ-lactone; Phanurane. C$_{22}$-H$_{28}$O$_3$; mol wt 340.46. C 77.61%, H 8.29%, O 14.10%. Aldosterone antagonist. Prepd by dehydrogenation of 17-hydroxy-3-oxo-17α-pregn-4-ene-21-carboxylic acid γ-lactone: Cella, Tweit, *J. Org. Chem.* **24**, 1109 (1959); Cella, **US 2900383** (1959 to Searle).

Crystals from ethyl acetate, mp 149-151°, solidifies and remelts at 165°. [α]$_D$ +24.5° (chloroform). uv max: 283 nm (ε 26700).

Free acid potassium salt. [2181-04-6] Potassium canrenoate; Kanrenol; Soldactone; Venactone. C$_{22}$H$_{29}$KO$_4$; mol wt 396.56.

THERAP CAT: Diuretic.

1751. Cantharides. Spanish fly; blistering fly; blistering beetle. Preparation of dried blister beetles, *Lytta vesicatoria*, also known as *Cantharis vesicatoria*, *Meloidae*; traditionally used as a vesicant, rubifacient, and aphrodisiac. *Habit.* Southern and Central Europe, mainly on plants of the family *Oleaceae* and *Caprifoliaceae*. *Constit.* 0.6-1% cantharidin, *q.v.*, 10-15% fat, resinous substances, acetic and uric acids. *Review:* Ude, Heeger, *Pharm. Zentralhalle* **82**, 193 (1941); A. Kar, *Pharmacognosy and Pharmacobiotechnology* (New Age Intl., New Delhi, 2003) pp 199-200.

Caution: Extreme irritant and vesicant. Direct contact with skin may cause intense blister formation. Potential symptoms of overexposure are burning sensation of oral cavity and throat; diarrhea, hemorrhagic necrosis in upper GI tract, abdominal pain; urinary urgency, strangury, hematuria, priapism, oliguria, tubular necrosis, renal failure. *See Clinical Toxicology of Commercial Products*, R. E. Gosselin *et al.*, Eds. (Williams & Wilkins, Baltimore, 5th ed., 1984) Section II, p 270.

1752. Cantharidin. [56-25-7] Hexahydro-3a,7a-dimethyl-4,7-epoxyisobenzofuran-1,3-dione; 2,3-dimethyl-7-oxabicyclo-[2.2.1]heptane-2,3-dicarboxylic anhydride; *exo*-1,2-*cis*-dimethyl-3,6-epoxyhexahydrophthalic anhydride; cantharides camphor. C$_{10}$-H$_{12}$O$_4$; mol wt 196.20. C 61.22%, H 6.16%, O 32.62%. Defensive toxin produced by blister beetles of the family *Meloidae*. Active principle of cantharides, *q.v.* and notorious **"Spanish Fly"** aphrodisiac. Synthesis and stereochemistry: Woodward, Loftfield, *J. Am. Chem. Soc.* **63**, 3167 (1941); Ziegler *et al., Ann.* **551**, 1 (1942). Stereospecific synthesis: Stork, Van Tamelen *et al., J. Am. Chem. Soc.* **75**, 384 (1953). Simple efficient synthesis: W. G. Dauben *et al., ibid.* **102**, 6893 (1980). Crystal structure: M. Zehnder, U. Thewalt, *Helv. Chim. Acta* **60**, 740 (1977). Review of biological source and medicinal uses: L. Moed *et al., Arch. Dermatol.* **137**, 1357-1360 (2001).

Orthorhombic plates, scales, mp 218°. Sublimes at about 110° (12 mm Hg, 3-5 mm distance). Insol in cold water, somewhat sol in hot water. One gram dissolves in 40 ml acetone, 65 ml chloroform, 560 ml ether, 150 ml ethyl acetate. Sol in oils.

Caution: Extreme irritant and vesicant. Direct contact may cause intense blister formation. Potential symptoms of overexposure are burning sensation of throat and oral cavity; diarrhea, hemorrhagic necrosis of upper GI tract, abdominal pain; urinary urgency, strangury, hematuria, priapism, oliguria, tubular necrosis, renal failure. *See Clinical Toxicology of Commercial Products*, R. E. Gosselin *et al.*, Eds. (Williams & Wilkins, Baltimore, 5th ed., 1984) Section II, 270.

THERAP CAT: Vesicant; in treatment of warts and molluscum.

THERAP CAT (VET): Rubefacient, vesicant, counterirritant.

1753. Canthaxanthin. [514-78-3] β,β-Carotene-4,4'-dione; 4,4'-dioxo-β-carotene; Food Orange 8; C.I. 40850; Carophyll Red; Orobronze; Roxanthin Red 10; Carotaben plus. $C_{40}H_{52}O_2$; mol wt 564.84. C 85.06%, H 9.28%, O 5.67%. All *trans*-carotenoid pigment widely distributed in nature. Isoln from the edible mushroom *Cantharellus cinnabarinus* Adans. ex Fr., *Agaricaceae*: Haxo, *Bot. Gaz.* **112**, 228 (1950); also isolated from flamingo feathers. Structure and synthesis: Isler *et al.*, *Verh. Naturforsch. Ges. Basel* **67**, 379 (1956); Zeller *et al.*, *Helv. Chim. Acta* **42**, 841 (1959). Alternate syntheses: M. Akhtar, B. C. L. Weedon, *J. Chem. Soc.* **1959**, 4058; R. Rüegg, G. Saucy, **US 2983752** and J. D. Surmatis, **US 3311656** (1961, 1967 both to Hoffmann-La Roche); J. D. Surmatis *et al.*, *Helv. Chim. Acta* **53**, 974 (1970); M. Rosenberger *et al.*, *Pure Appl. Chem.* **51**, 871 (1979); *eidem, J. Org. Chem.* **47**, 2130 (1982).

Violet crystals from methylene chloride, dec 217°. Absorption max (cyclohexane): 470 nm ($E_{1cm}^{1\%}$ 2250). Sol in chloroform, oils. Oil solns are more red than those of β-carotene.

USE: Permissible color additive for food and drugs (exempt from certification): *Fed. Regist.* **34**, no. 5 (Jan. 8, 1969). Oral suntanning agent.

1754. Capecitabine. [154361-50-9] 5'-Deoxy-5-fluoro-*N*-[(pentyloxy)carbonyl]cytidine; [1-(5-deoxy-β-D-ribofuranosyl)-5-fluoro-1,2-dihydro-2-oxo-4-pyrimidinyl]carbamic acid pentyl ester; pentyl 1-(5-deoxy-β-D-ribofuranosyl)-5-fluoro-1,2-dihyro-2-oxo-4-pyrimidinecarbamate; Ro-9-1978; Xeloda. $C_{15}H_{22}FN_3O_6$; mol wt 359.35. C 50.14%, H 6.17%, F 5.29%, N 11.69%, O 26.71%. Orally active fluoropyrimidine. Prodrug of doxifluridine, *q.v.*, designed to be metabolized to 5-fluorouracil, *q.v.*, at the tumor site. Prepn: M. Arasaki *et al.*, **EP 602454**; *eidem,* **US 5472949** (1994, 1995 both to Hoffmann-La Roche). Metabolism by tumor enzymes: T. Ishikawa *et al.*, *Cancer Res.* **58**, 685 (1998). Clinical comparison with i.v. fluorouracil in colorectal cancer: P. M. Hoff *et al.,J. Clin. Oncol.* **19**, 2282 (2001); E. Van Cutsem *et al., ibid.* 4097. Review of pharmacology and clinical experience: J. K. McGavin, K. L. Goa, *Drugs* **61**, 2309-2326 (2001).

Crystals from ethyl acetate, mp 110-121°. Soly in water (20°): 26 mg/ml.

THERAP CAT: Antineoplastic.

1755. Capravirine. [178979-85-6] 5-[(3,5-Dichlorophenyl)thio]-4-(1-methylethyl)-1-(4-pyridinylmethyl)-1*H*-imidazole-2-methanol carbamate ester; 2-carbamoyloxymethyl-5-(3,5-dichlorophenylthio)-4-isopropyl-1-(pyridin-4-yl)methyl-1*H*-imidazole; AG-1549; S-1153. $C_{20}H_{20}Cl_2N_4O_2S$; mol wt 451.37. C 53.22%, H 4.47%, Cl 15.71%, N 12.41%, O 7.09%, S 7.10%. Imidazole type non-nucleoside HIV-1 reverse transcriptase inhibitor (NNRTI).

Prepn: H. Sugimoto, T. Fujiwara, **WO 9610019**; *eidem,* **US 5910506** (1996, 1999 both to Shionogi). Antiviral activity: T. Fujiwara *et al., Antimicrob. Agents Chemother.* **42**, 1340 (1998). Crystal structure in complex with target enzyme: J. Ren *et al.,J. Biol. Chem.* **275**, 14316 (2000). Review of pharmacology and clinical evaluation: W. M. Brown, *Curr. Opin. Anti-Infect. Invest. Drugs* **2**, 286-294 (2000).

Crystals from diethylether as hemihydrate, mp 88° (dec).

THERAP CAT: Antiviral

1756. Caprenin. [138184-95-9] Reduced calorie fat with functional properties similar to cocoa butter. Synthetic triglyceride composed primarily of caprylic and capric acids (derived from coconut and palm-kernel oils) and behenic acid (derived from rapeseed oil). Prepn: A. M. Erhman *et al.*, **US 4888196** and **US 5066510** (1989, 1991, both to Procter & Gamble). Digestion and absorption in rats: D. R. Webb, R. A. Sanders, *J. Am. Coll. Toxicol.* **10**, 325 (1991). Toxicology and metabolism in animals: D. R. Webb *et al., ibid.* 341. Absorption and caloric value in humans: J. C. Peters *et al., ibid.* 357. Brief description: C. O'Donnell, D. Best, *Prepared Foods* **162**, 41-42 (February, 1993).

Caloric value in humans: 3-5 kcal/g.

USE: Reduced calorie fat substitute in soft candies and confectionary coatings.

1757. Capreomycin. [11003-38-6] Capastat. Cyclic peptide antibiotic similar to viomycin; produced by *Streptomyces capreolus* NRRL 2773; Herr *et al.*, 140th Am. Chem. Soc. Meet. (Chicago, Sept. 1961), *Abstracts of Papers*, p 49C; *Chem. Eng. News* **39**, 57 (Sept. 18, 1961); **GB 920563**; **US 3143468** (1963, 1964 both to Lilly). Mixture of capreomycins IA, IB, IIA, and IIB in the approx percentages, 25%, 67%, 3%, 6%, resp.: Herr, Redstone, *Ann. N.Y. Acad. Sci.* **135**, 940 (1966). Activity studies: Sutton *et al., ibid.* 947; Lucchesi, *Antibiot. Chemother.* **16**, 27 (1970). Proposed structure: Bycroft *et al., Nature* **231**, 301 (1971). Revised structure and total synthesis: T. Shiba *et al., Tetrahedron Lett.* **1976**, 3907; S. Nomoto *et al., Tetrahedron* **34**, 921 (1978). Structure of IA and IB: *eidem, J. Antibiot.* **30**, 955 (1977). Toxicity study: Welles *et al., Ann. N.Y. Acad. Sci.* **135**, 960 (1966).

Capreomycin IA   R = OH
Capreomycin IB   R = H

The mixture is a white solid. Sol in water. Practically insol in most organic solvents. pKa in 66% aq DMF: 6.2, 8.2, 10.1, 13.3. Stable in aq soln at pH 4-8; unstable in strongly acidic or strongly basic solns.

Disulfate. [1405-36-3] Caprocin; Ogostal. Solubility data: March, Weiss, *J. Assoc. Off. Anal. Chem.* **50**, 457 (1967). LD$_{50}$ in mice, rats (mg/kg): 250, 325 i.v.; 514, 1191 s.c. (Welles).

Capreomycin IA. [37280-35-6] $C_{25}H_{44}N_{14}O_8$; mol wt 668.71. mp 246-248° (dec). $[\alpha]_D^{22}$ −21.9° (c 0.5 in water). uv max (0.1*N* HCl): 269 nm (ε 24000); (H$_2$O): 268 nm (ε 23900); (0.1*N* NaOH): 287 nm (ε 15900) (all for hydrochloride ethanolate).

Capreomycin IB. [33490-33-4] $C_{25}H_{44}N_{14}O_7$; mol wt 652.71. mp 253-255° (dec). $[\alpha]_D^{21}$ −44.6° (c 0.5 in water). uv max (0.1*N* HCl): 268 nm (ε 22700); (H$_2$O): 268 nm (ε 22300); (0.1*N* NaOH): 290 nm (ε 14400) (all for hydrochloride ethanolate).

*Note: **Capreomycin IIA**, **capreomycin IIB**.* Structures corresp to capreomycins IA and IB but lack β-lysine residues.

THERAP CAT: Antibacterial (tuberculostatic).

1758. *n*-**Capric Acid.** [334-48-5] Decanoic acid. $C_{10}H_{20}$-O_2; mol wt 172.26. C 69.72%, H 11.70%, O 18.58%. $CH_3(CH_2)_8$-COOH. Prepn from octyl bromide: Shishido *et al., J. Am. Chem. Soc.* **81**, 5817 (1959); Closson, De Pree, US **2918494** (1959 to Ethyl Corp.). Recovery from *Cuphea llavea* Llave et Lex, *Lythaceae* seed oil: Miwa *et al.,* US **2964546** (1960 to U.S.D.A.). Toxicity study: L. Orö, A. Wretlind, *Acta Pharmacol. Toxicol.* **18**, 141 (1961). *Review: Fatty Acids* Part I, K. S. Markley, Ed. (Interscience, New York, 2nd ed., 1960) pp 34, 39.

Crystalline solid, mp 31.4°. Rancid odor. bp 270°. d_4^{50} 0.8782. n_D^{40} 1.4288. Practically insol in water (0.015 g/100 g at 20°). Sol in ethanol, ether, chloroform, benzene, carbon disulfide. Also sol in dil HNO$_3$ from which it precipitates unchanged by addition of water. LD$_{50}$ i.v. in mice: 129 ±5.4 mg/kg (Orö, Wretlind).

USE: Manuf of esters for artificial fruit flavors and perfumes; as an intermediate in other chemical syntheses.

1759. *n*-**Caproic Acid.** [142-62-1] Hexanoic acid. C_6H_{12}-O_2; mol wt 116.16. C 62.04%, H 10.41%, O 27.55%. $CH_3(CH_2)_4$-COOH. Occurs in milk fats (about 2%), in coconut oil (<1%), various palm and other oils. Prepn: Vliet *et al., Org. Synth.* **coll. vol. II**, 417 (1943); Reid, Ruhoff, *ibid.*, 475. Manuf by catalytic reduction of corresponding β-lactone: Caldwell, US **2484486** (1949 to Kodak); from oleic acid: Follett, Murray, US **2580417** (1952 to Arthur D. Little); from castor oil or a ricinoleate: Steadman, Peterson, US **2847432** (1958 to National Res. Corp.); by ozonolysis of tall oil unsaturated fatty acids: Maggiolo, US **2865937** (1958 to Welsbach); from 1,3-butadiene and potassium acetate in presence of NaNH$_2$: Schmerling, Toekelt, US **3075010** (1963 to Universal Oil Prod.); from cyclohexanol: Bartlett, Lippincott, US **3121728** (1964 to Esso); by catalytic oxidation of *n*-hexanol: Hay, US **3173933** (1965 to General Electric). Toxicity study: H. F. Smyth, C. P. Carpenter, *J. Ind. Hyg. Toxicol.* **26**, 269 (1944). *Review: Fatty Acids* Part 1, K. S. Markley, Ed. (Interscience, New York, 2nd ed., 1960) pp 34, 37.

Oily liquid, bp 205°. Characteristic goat-like odor. mp −3.4°. d_4^{20} 0.9265. n_D^{20} 1.4163. Slightly soluble in water (1.082 g/100 g); readily soluble in ethanol, ether. LD$_{50}$ orally in rats: 3.0 g/kg (Smyth, Carpenter).

USE: Manuf of esters for artificial flavors, and of hexyl derivatives, especially hexylphenols, hexylresorcinol, etc.

1760. **Caproic Aldehyde.** [66-25-1] Hexanal; caproaldehyde; hexaldehyde. $C_6H_{12}O$; mol wt 100.16. C 71.95%, H 12.08%, O 15.97%. $CH_3(CH_2)_4CHO$. Prepn: Bagard, *Bull. Soc. Chim.* **1**, 307 (1907). Toxicity study: Smyth *et al., Arch. Ind. Hyg. Occup. Med.* **10**, 61 (1954).

Liquid. d_4^{20} 0.8335. bp$_{760}$ 131°; bp$_{12}$ 28°. Autooxidizes and polymerizes, especially in the presence of traces of acid. LD$_{50}$ orally in rats: 4.89 g/kg (Smyth).

1761. **Caprolactam.** [105-60-2] Hexahydro-2*H*-azepin-2-one; ε-caprolactam; 2-oxohexamethylenimine; 2-ketohexamethylenimine; aminocaproic lactam. $C_6H_{11}NO$; mol wt 113.16. C 63.68%, H 9.80%, N 12.38%, O 14.14%. Prepn: Wallach, *Ann.* **312**, 187 (1900); **343**, 43 (1905); Ruzicka *et al., Helv. Chim. Acta* **4**, 477 (1921); Eck, Marvel, *J. Biol. Chem.* **106**, 387 (1934); Marvel, Eck, *Org. Synth.* **coll. vol. II**, 371 (1943); Lazier, Rigby, US **2234566** (1941 to du Pont); Schlack, US **2249177** (1941 to I. G. Farben); **DE 739953** (1943); **DE 745224** (1943); P. Smith, *J. Am. Chem. Soc.* **70**, 320 (1948); E. Schmitz *et al., J. Prakt. Chem.* **319**,

274 (1977). Environmentally benign synthesis from cyclohexanone: J. M. Thomas, R. Raja, *Proc. Natl. Acad. Sci. USA* **102**, 13732 (2005). Purification: Kampschmidt, US **2786052** (1957 to Stamicarbon N. V.). Stabilization with alkalies: Indest *et al.,* US **2884414** (1959 to Vereinigte Glanzstoff-Fabriken). Toxicity study: H. F. Smyth *et al., Am. Ind. Hyg. Assoc. J.* **30**, 470 (1969). *Reviews: CIOS Repts.* no. **22** and **31**, File XXXIII/Synthetic Fiber Developments in Germany, parts I & II; K. Kahr *et al.* in *Ullmanns Encyklopädie der technischen Chemie* vol. **9**, E. Bartholome *et al.,* Eds. (Verlag Chemie, Weinheim, 4th ed., 1975) pp 96-114.

Hygroscopic leaflets from petr ether, mp 70°. d_4^{75} (liq) 1.02. bp$_{50}$ 180°; bp$_3$ 100°. Viscosity (78°): 9 cP. Flash pt, open cup: 257°F (125°C). Freely sol in water, methanol, ethanol, ether, tetrahydrofurfuryl alcohol, dimethylformamide. Also sol in chlorinated hydrocarbons, cyclohexene, petroleum fractions. A 70% aq soln has d_4^{25} 1.05; n_D^{31} 1.4965; n_D^{40} 1.4935. LD$_{50}$ orally in rats: 2.14 g/kg (Smyth).

Caution: Potential symptoms of overexposure are irritation of eyes, skin, respiratory system; epistaxis; dermatitis, skin sensitization; asthma; irritability, confusion, dizziness, headache; abdominal cramps, diarrhea, nausea, vomiting; liver and kidney injury. *See NIOSH Pocket Guide to Chemical Hazards* (DHHS/NIOSH 97-140, 1997) p 50.

USE: Manuf of synthetic fibers of the polyamide type (Perlon); solvent for high mol wt polymers; precursor of nylon-6, *q.v.*

1762. **Capromab.** [151763-64-3] Anti-(human prostatic carinoma cell) immunoglobulin G1 (mouse monoclonal 7E11-C5.3 γ_1-chain) disulfide with mouse monoclonal 7E11-C5.3 light chain, dimer. Murine monoclonal antibody directed against prostate specific membrane antigen (PSMA), a transmembrane glycoprotein expressed by prostate epithelium. Designed for the detection of primary and metastatic prostate carcinoma. Prepn: J. S. Horoszewicz *et al., Anticancer Res.* **7**, 927 (1987); *idem,* US **5162504** (1992 to Cytogen). Characterization and specificity of immunoconjugate: A. D. Lopes *et al., Cancer Res.* **50**, 6423 (1990). Diagnostic use of labeled form in metastatic prostate cancer: M. J. Manyak *et al., Urology* **54**, 1058 (1999). Review of clinical studies: R. T. Maguire *et al., Cancer* **72**, 3453-3462 (1993); and pharmacology: H. M. Lamb, D. Faulds, *Drugs Aging* **12**, 293-304 (1998). Review of diagnostic use: M. K. Haseman *et al., Cancer Biother. Radiopharm.* **15**, 131-140 (2000).

Capromab pendetide. [145464-28-4] 7E11-C5.3-GYK-DTPA; 7E11-C5.3-glycyl-tyrosyl-(*N*-ε-diethylenetriaminepentaacetic acid)-lysine; CYT-356; ProstaScint. Monoclonal antibody conjugated to a linker-chelator to enable radiolabeling. Prepd as hydrochloride and labeled with Indium ^{111}In immediately before administration.

THERAP CAT: ^{111}In-labeled form as diagnostic aid (radioactive tumor-targeting agent).

1763. **Caproyl Chloride.** [142-61-0] Hexanoyl chloride. $C_6H_{11}ClO$; mol wt 134.60. C 53.54%, H 8.24%, Cl 26.34%, O 11.89%. $CH_3(CH_2)_4COCl$. Prepn: Brown, *J. Am. Chem. Soc.* **60**, 1325 (1938). Manuf: Wygant, US **2806061** (1957 to Monsanto).

Liquid, bp 151-153°. mp −87.3°. d_4^{15} 0.9805. n_D^{15} 1.4286. Dec by water or alcohol. Sol in ether, chloroform.

1764. **Caprylene.** [111-66-0] 1-Octene; octylene. C_8H_{16}; mol wt 112.21. C 85.63%, H 14.37%. $CH_3(CH_2)_5CH=CH_2$. Prepn from appropriate alkylmagnesium bromide and allyl bromide or chloride: Geisler, Pilz, *Ber.* **95**, 96 (1962); from formaldehyde or paraformaldehyde and triphenyl(phenylmethylene)phosphorane: Hauser *et al., J. Org. Chem.* **28**, 372 (1963); by catalytic dehydration of 2-octanol: Lundeen, Hoozer, *J. Am. Chem. Soc.* **85**, 2180 (1963).

Liquid, bp 121°, bp$_{100}$ 61.5-61.7°. mp −102°. d_4^{20} 0.7149, d_4^{25} 0.7109. n_D^{20} 1.4087, n_D^{25} 1.4062. Flash pt, open cup: 70°F (21°C). Practically insol in water; misc with alcohol, ether.

1765. Caprylic Acid. [124-07-2] Octanoic acid. $C_8H_{16}O_2$; mol wt 144.21. C 66.63%, H 11.18%, O 22.19%. $CH_3(CH_2)_6$-COOH. Prepn from 1-heptene: Dupont *et al.*, *Compt. Rend.* **240**, 628 (1955); by oxidation of octanol: Langenbeck, Richter, *Ber.* **89**, 202 (1956). Manuf: Alexander, US 2821534 (1958 to GAF); McAlister *et al.*, US 3053869 (1962 to Standard Oil Co., Indiana). Antifungal properties: O. Wyss *et al.*, *Arch. Biochem.* **7**, 418 (1945). Toxicity: P. M. Jenner *et al.*, *Food Cosmet. Toxicol.* **2**, 327 (1964). *Review: Fatty Acids* Part 1, K. S. Markley, Ed. (Interscience, New York, 2nd ed., 1960) pp 34, 38.

Oily liquid, bp 239.7°. Slightly unpleasant rancid taste. mp 16.7°. d_4^{20} 0.910. n_D^{20} 1.4280. Very slightly sol in water (0.068 g/100 g at 20°); freely sol in alcohol, chloroform, ether, carbon disulfide, petr ether, glacial acetic acid. LD_{50} orally in rats: 10,080 mg/kg (Jenner).

USE: An intermediate in manuf of esters used in perfumery; in manuf of dyes, etc.

1766. Caprylic Aldehyde. [124-13-0] Octanal; caprylaldehyde; octaldehyde. $C_8H_{16}O$; mol wt 128.21. C 74.94%, H 12.58%, O 12.48%. $CH_3(CH_2)_6CHO$. Prepn: Stephen, *J. Chem. Soc.* **127**, 1874 (1925).

Liquid. d_4^{20} 0.821. bp_{760} 163.4°; bp_{20} 72°; bp_9 60°. n_D^{26} 1.41667. Slightly sol in water; misc with alc, ether.

1767. CAPS. [1135-40-6] 3-(Cyclohexylamino)-1-propanesulfonic acid. $C_9H_{19}NO_3S$; mol wt 221.32. C 48.84%, H 8.65%, N 6.33%, O 21.69%, S 14.49%. One of the zwitterionic amino acids known as "Good" buffers; active in the pH range of 9.7-11.1. Prepn: H. Dorn, K. Walter, *Z. Chem.* **7**, 151 (1967). Thermodynamic parameters: C. D. McGlothlin, J. Jordan, *Anal. Lett.* **9**, 245 (1976). Effects on protein measurement: V. Kaushal, L. D. Barnes, *Anal. Biochem.* **157**, 291 (1986); H. M. Himmel, W. Heller, *J. Clin. Chem. Clin. Biochem.* **25**, 909 (1987). Use as buffer: I. I. Koukli *et al.*, *Analyst* **113**, 603 (1988); R. M. Smith *et al.*, *J. Chromatogr.* **514**, 97 (1990).

Colorless needles from methanol, mp 302-303°. pK (25°): 10.35.

USE: Biological buffer.

1768. Capsaicin. [404-86-4] (6*E*)-*N*-[(4-Hydroxy-3-methoxyphenyl)methyl]-8-methyl-6-nonenamide; *trans*-8-methyl-*N*-vanillyl-6-nonenamide; *N*-(4-hydroxy-3-methoxybenzyl)-8-methyl-non-*trans*-6-enamide; Axsain; Mioton; Zacin; Zostrix. $C_{18}H_{27}$-NO_3; mol wt 305.41. C 70.79%, H 8.91%, N 4.59%, O 15.72%. Pungent principle in fruit of various species of *Capsicum*, *Solanaceae*. Isoln from paprika and cayenne: Thresh, *Pharm. J. Trans.* **7**, 21 (1876); Micko, *Z. Nahr. Genussm.* **1**, 818 (1898). *See Beilstein* **13**, suppl. I, 322. Early structure study: Nelson, *J. Am. Chem. Soc.* **42**, 597 (1920). Synthesis: Späth, Darling, *Ber.* **63**, 737 (1930); L. Crombie *et al.*, *J. Chem. Soc.* **1955**, 1025; O. P. Vig *et al.*, *Indian J. Chem.* **17B**, 558 (1979). Constitution and biosynthesis: D. J. Bennet, E. W. Kirby, *J. Chem. Soc. C* **1968**, 442. Pharmacology: J. Molnar *et al.*, *Acta Physiol. Acad. Sci. Hung.* **35**, 369 (1969). Capsaicin is a powerful irritant; initial administration causes intense pain. Prolonged treatment causes insensitivity to painful stimuli and induces selective degeneration of certain primary sensory neurons: G. Jancso *et al.*, *Nature* **270**, 741 (1977); R. Gamse, *Arch. Pharmacol.* **320**, 205 (1982); P. Holzer *et al.*, *Neurosci. Lett.* **31**, 253 (1982). Neuronal depletion of substance P, *q.v.*: T. M. Jessell *et al.*, *Brain Res.* **152**, 183 (1978); T. L. Yaksh *et al.*, *Science* **206**, 481 (1979). Capsaicin pretreatment also induces long-lasting desensitization of airway mucosa to various mechanical and chemical irritants: J. M. Lundberg, A. Saria, *Nature* **302**, 251 (1983). Preliminary clinical evaluation in chronic postherpetic neuralgia: J. E. Bernstein *et al.*, *J. Am. Acad. Dermatol.* **17**, 93 (1987). *Reviews:* Molnar, *Arzneim.-Forsch.* **15**, 718 (1965); Walker, Gavern, *Manuf. Chem. Aerosol News* **39** (6), 35 (1968); R. M. Virus, G. F. Gebhart, *Life Sci.* **25**, 1273 (1979); Y. Monsereenusorn *et al.*, *Crit. Rev. Toxicol.* **10**, 321-339 (1982).

Monoclinic, rectangular plates, scales from petr ether, mp 65°. $bp_{0.01}$ 210-220° (air-bath temp). uv max: 227, 281 nm (ε 7000, 2500). Burning taste, one part in 100,000 can be detected by tasting. Practically insol in cold water. Freely sol in alc, ether, benzene, chloroform; slightly sol in CS_2.

USE: As a tool in neurobiological research.

THERAP CAT: Topical analgesic.

THERAP CAT (VET): Topical analgesic.

1769. Capsanthin. [465-42-9] (3*R*,3′*S*,5′*R*)-3,3′-Dihydroxy-β,κ-caroten-6′-one. $C_{40}H_{56}O_3$; mol wt 584.87. C 82.14%, H 9.65%, O 8.21%. Carotenoid pigment isolated from paprika *(Capsicum annuum* L., *Solanaceae)*: L. Zechmeister, L. Cholnoky, *Ann.* **454**, 54 (1927); L. Cholnoky *et al.*, *Ann.* **606**, 194 (1957); Warren, Weedon, *J. Chem. Soc.* **1958**, 3972. Structure: Entschel, Karrer, *Helv. Chim. Acta* **43**, 89 (1960); Faigle, Karrer, *ibid.* **44**, 1257, 1904 (1961). Absolute configuration: Bartlett *et al.*, *J. Chem. Soc. C* **1969**, 2527. Crystal structure: I. Ueda, W. Nowacki, *Verh. Schweiz. Naturforsch. Ges.* **1971**, 152, *C.A.* **77**, 106449h (1972).

Deep carmine-red needles from petr ether, mp 181-182°. Absorption max 483 nm (ε × 10^{-3} 121). $[α]_{Cd}$ +36° (chloroform). Freely sol in acetone, chloroform. Sol in methanol, ethanol, ether, benzene. Slightly sol in petr ether, CS_2.

Diacetate. $C_{44}H_{60}O_5$. Red plates from methanol, mp 150°.

Dipalmitate. $C_{72}H_{116}O_5$. Bordeaux-red plates from benzene + methanol, mp 95°.

1770. Capsicum. Cayenne Pepper. The dried ripe fruit of *Capsicum frutescens* L., *Solanaceae*, known commercially as *African Chillies*, or of *Capsicum annuum* L., var. *conoides* Irish, known as **Tabasco Pepper** or of *Capsicum annuum* var. *longum* Sendt, known as **Louisiana Long Pepper**, or of a hybrid between the Honka variety of Japanese Capsicum and the Old Louisiana Sport Capsicum known as **Louisiana Sport Pepper** (Fam. *Solanaceae*). Constit. Fixed oils; 0.1-1% capsaicin, capsanthin, *q.q.v.* Store in a cool place. Protect from light.

THERAP CAT (VET): Has been used externally as a counterirritant; internally as a carminative and stomachic.

1771. Captafol. [2425-06-1] 3a,4,7,7a-Tetrahydro-2-[(1,1,-2,2-tetrachloroethyl)thio]-1*H*-isoindole-1,3(2*H*)-dione; *N*-(1,1,2,2-tetrachloroethylthio)-4-cyclohexene-1,2-dicarboximide; *N*-(1,1,2,2-tetrachloroethylmercapto)-4-cyclohexene-1,2-dicarboximide; *N*-(1,1,2,2-tetrachloroethylthio)-Δ⁴-tetrahydrophthalimide; *N*-(1,1,2,2-tetrachloroethylsulfenyl)-*cis*-4-cyclohexene-1,2-dicarboximide; Difolatan. $C_{10}H_9Cl_4NO_2S$; mol wt 349.06. C 34.41%, H 2.60%, Cl 40.63%, N 4.01%, O 9.17%, S 9.19%. *N*-tetrachloroethyl analog of captan, *q.v.* Prepn: Kohn, BE 633205 (1963 to California Res. Corp.), *C.A.* **60**, 15789cd (1964). Toxicology: R. Ben-Dyke *et al.*, *World Rev. Pest Control* **9**, 119 (1970); G. L. Kennedy, Jr. *et al.*, *Food Cosmet. Toxicol.* **13**, 55 (1975). Carcinogenicity study: S. Tamano *et al.*, *Jpn. J. Cancer Res.* **81**, 1222 (1990).

Crystals, mp 160-161°. LD_{50} in rats, rabbits (mg/kg): 2500-6200 orally; 15400 dermally (Ben-Dyke).

Caution: Potential symptoms of overexposure are irritation of eyes, skin, respiratory system; dermatitis, skin sensitization; conjunctivitis; bronchitis, wheezing; diarrhea, vomiting; liver and kidney injury; high blood pressure. *See NIOSH Pocket Guide to Chemical Hazards* (DHHS/NIOSH 97-140, 1997) p 50.

USE: Agricultural fungicide, especially for potatoes.

1772. Captan. [133-06-2] 3a,4,7,7a-Tetrahydro-2-[(trichloromethyl)thio]-1*H*-isoindole-1,3(2*H*)-dione; *N*-(trichloromethylthio)-4-cyclohexene-1,2-dicarboximide; *N*-trichloromethylthio-3a,4,7,7a-tetrahydrophthalimide; *N*-trichloromethylmercapto-4-cyclohexene-1,2-dicarboximide; *N*-(trichloromethylmercapto)-Δ⁴-tetrahydrophthalimide; ENT-26538; SR-406; Merpan; Orthocide-406; Vancide 89. $C_9H_8Cl_3NO_2S$; mol wt 300.59. C 35.96%, H 2.68%, Cl 35.38%, N 4.66%, O 10.65%, S 10.67%. Prepn: A. R. Kittleson, US 2553771; US 2653155; US 2713058 (1951, 1953, 1955 all to Standard Oil); *idem, Science* **115,** 84 (1952); *idem, J. Agric. Food Chem.* **1,** 677 (1953). Colorimetric determination: A. R. Kittleson, *Anal. Chem.* **24,** 1173 (1952). Review of mutagenicity studies: B. A. Bridges, *Mutat. Res.* **32,** 3 (1975); of carcinogenic risk: *IARC Monographs* **30,** 295-318 (1983).

Odorless crystals from CCl_4, mp 178°. d 1.74. Practically insol in water. Soly at 26° in g/100 ml: chloroform 7.78; tetrachloroethane 8.15; cyclohexanone 4.96; dioxane 4.70; benzene 2.13; toluene 0.69; heptane 0.04; ethanol 0.29; ether 0.25. LD_{50} orally in rats: 9000 mg/kg (Bridges).
Caution: Potential symptoms of overexposure are irritation of eyes, skin, upper respiratory system; blurred vision; dermatitis, skin sensitization; dyspnea; diarrhea, vomiting. Potential occupational carcinogen. *See NIOSH Pocket Guide to Chemical Hazards* (DHHS/NIOSH 97-140, 1997) p 50.

USE: Fungicide; bacteriostat in soap.

1773. Captodiamine. [486-17-9] 2-[[[4-(Butylthio)phenyl]phenylmethyl]thio]-*N,N*-dimethylethanamine; 2-[*p*-(butylthio)-α-phenylbenzylthio]-*N,N*-dimethylethylamine; *p*-butylmercaptobenzhydryl β-dimethylaminoethyl sulfide; β-butylthiodiphenylmethyl 2-dimethylaminoethyl sulfide; captodiam; captodramin. $C_{21}H_{29}NS_2$; mol wt 359.59. C 70.14%, H 8.13%, N 3.90%, S 17.83%. Prepn: Hübner, Petersen, US 2830088 (1958). Pharmacological studies: R. Kopf, I. Moller-Nielsen, *Arzneim.-Forsch.* **8,** 154 (1958).

Hydrochloride. [904-04-1] Covatine; Covatix; Suvren. $C_{21}H_{29}NS_2.HCl$; mol wt 396.05. Crystals, mp 131-132°. LD_{50} (96 hr) in mice, rats (mg/kg): 180, 343 i.p.; 1630, 3800 orally (Kopf, Moller-Nielsen).

THERAP CAT: Anxiolytic.

1774. Captopril. [62571-86-2] 1-[(2*S*)-3-Mercapto-2-methyl-1-oxopropyl]-L-proline; (2*S*)-1-(3-mercapto-2-methylpropionyl)-L-proline; D-2-methyl-3-mercaptopropanoyl-L-proline; SQ-14225; Acediur; Acepril; Alopresin; Acepress; Capoten; Captolane; Captoril; Cesplon; Dilabar; Garranil; Hipertil; Lopirin; Lopril; Tensobon; Tensoprel. $C_9H_{15}NO_3S$; mol wt 217.29. C 49.75%, H 6.96%, N 6.45%, O 22.09%, S 14.76%. First orally active angiotensin-converting enzyme (ACE) inhibitor. Prepn: M. A. Ondetti, D. W. Cushman, DE 2703828; *eidem,* US 4046889 and US 4105776 (1977, 1977, 1978 all to Squibb). Design and synthesis: M. A. Ondetti *et al., Science* **196,** 441 (1977); D. W. Cush-

man *et al., Biochemistry* **16,** 5484 (1977). Improved synthesis: D. H. Nam *et al., J. Pharm. Sci.* **73,** 1843 (1984). Pharmacology: B. Rubin *et al., Eur. J. Pharmacol.* **51,** 377 (1978); *eidem, Prog. Cardiovasc. Dis.* **21,** 183 (1978). Clinical studies: D. B. Case *et al., ibid.* 195; H. R. Brunner *et al., Ann. Intern. Med.* **90,** 19 (1979). Toxicology and metabolism: G. R. Keim in *Captopril and Hypertension,* D. B. Case, Ed. (Plenum, New York, 1980) p 137. GC/MS determn in biological fluids: T. Ito, Y. Matsuki, *J. Chromatogr.* **417,** 79 (1987). Historical review and comprehensive bibliography: Z. P. Horovitz in *Pharmacological and Biochemical Properties of Drug Substances* vol. 3, M. E. Goldberg, Ed. (Am. Pharm. Assoc., Washington, DC, 1981) pp 148-175. Comprehensive description: H. Kadin, *Anal. Profiles Drug Subs.* **11,** 79-137 (1982). *Reviews: Am. Heart J.* **104,** pt. 2, 1125-1228 (1982); *Br. J. Clin. Pharmacol.* **14,** Suppl. 2, 69S-252S (1982). Series of articles on pharmacology and therapeutic efficacy: *Postgrad. Med. J.* **62,** Suppl. 1, 1-191 (1986).

Crystals from ethyl acetate/hexane, mp 103-104° (Ondetti, Cushman). Generally regarded as polymorphic: stable form, mp 106°; unstable form, mp 86° (Florey); also reported as mp 87-88°, resolidifies, second mp 104-105° (Cushman). $[\alpha]_D^{22}$ −131.0° (c 1.7 in ethanol). pK_1 3.7, pK_2 9.8. Freely sol in water, alc, chloroform, methylene chloride. LD_{50} in mice (mg/kg): 1040 i.v.; 6000 orally (Keim).
Combination with hydrochlorothiazide. [110075-07-5] Aceplus; Acezide; Capozide; Captea; Ecazide.

THERAP CAT: Antihypertensive.

1775. Caramel. Burnt sugar coloring; burnt sugar. Made by heating sugar or glucose, adding small quantities of alkali, alkaline carbonate or a trace of mineral acid during the heating.

Dark-brown, thick liq; pleasant, bitter taste; odor of burnt sugar. d about 1.35. Sol in water, dil alc. Insol in benzene, chloroform, ether, acetone, petr ether, oil turpentine.

USE: Coloring foods, confectionery, galenicals.

1776. Caramiphen. [77-22-5] 1-Phenylcyclopentanecarboxylic acid 2-(diethylamino)ethyl ester; diethylaminoethyl 1-phenylcyclopentane-1-carboxylate. $C_{18}H_{27}NO_2$; mol wt 289.41. C 74.70%, H 9.40%, N 4.84%, O 11.06%. Anticholinergic. Prepn: CH 234452; H. Martin, F. Häfliger, US 2404588 (1945, 1946 both to Geigy). Prepn of the ethanedisulfonate: CH 272708 (1951 to Geigy), *C.A.* **46,** 4563i (1952); *Chem. Zentralbl.* **1952,** 1571. Pharmacology and toxicology of the hydrochloride: C. P. Kraatz *et al., J. Pharmacol. Exp. Ther.* **96,** 42 (1949); of the ethanedisulfonate: J. J. Toner, E. Macko, *ibid.* **106,** 246 (1952). GLC determn in blood: P. Levandoski, T. Flanagan, *J. Pharm. Sci.* **69,** 1353 (1980). Mechanism of antitussive action: E. F. Domino *et al., J. Pharmacol. Exp. Ther.* **233,** 249 (1985).

$bp_{0.07}$ 112-115°.
Ethanedisulfonate. [125-86-0] $(C_{18}H_{27}NO_2)_2.C_2H_6O_6S_2$; mol wt 769.02. Crystals from acetone, mp 115-116°. More sol in water than the hydrochloride. Sol in alc, pharmaceutical syrups. Mixture with phenylpropanolamine hydrochloride, *Tuss-Ornade.*
Hydrochloride. [125-85-9] $C_{18}H_{27}NO_2.HCl$; mol wt 325.87. Crystals, mp 145-146°. Sol in alc; slightly sol in water. LD_{50} i.p. in rats: 209 mg/kg (Kraatz).

THERAP CAT: Antitussive.

1777. Caraway. Dried ripe fruit of *Carum carvi* L., *Umbelliferae. Habit.* Europe, Central and Western Asia; cultivated in England, Russia, U.S. *Constit.* 3-7% volatile oil; terpenes, chiefly *d*-limonene; 10-18% fixed oil; protein; carbohydrate; flavonoids. Composition studies: Von Schantz, Ek, *Sci. Pharm.* **39,** 82

(1971). *Review:* Arctander, *Perfume and Flavor Materials of Natural Origin* (S. Arctander, Elizabeth, N.J., 1960) pp 124-125; of medicinal uses: N. G. Bisset, M. Wichtl, *Herbal Drugs and Phytopharmaceuticals*, English Ed. (CRC Press, Boca Raton, 1994) pp 128-129.

Volatile oil. [8000-42-8] Oil of caraway. *Constit.* 53-63% carvone (by vol), *d*-limonene. Colorless or pale yellow liq; darkens and thickens with age. d_{25}^{25} 0.900-0.910. α_D^{25} +70 to +80°. n_D^{20} 1.484-1.488. Almost insol in water. Sol in 8 vols 80% or in 1 vol 90% alcohol. *Keep well closed, cool, and protected from light.*

USE: Pharmaceutic aid (flavor). In manuf liqueurs and perfuming soaps; as a spice in baking.

THERAP CAT: Carminative.

1778. Carazolol. [57775-29-8] 1-(9*H*-Carbazol-4-yloxy)-3-[(1-methylethyl)amino]-2-propanol; BM-51052; Conducton; Suacron. $C_{18}H_{22}N_2O_2$; mol wt 298.38. C 72.46%, H 7.43%, N 9.39%, O 10.72%. β-Adrenergic blocker. Prepn: H. Leinert *et al., DE 2240599* (1974 to Boehringer, Mann.), *C.A.* **80**, 133455a (1974). Comparative study of cardiac action: W. Bartsch *et al., Arzneim.-Forsch.* **27**, 1022 (1977). Initial clinico-pharmacological study: E. Chorianopoulos *et al., Herz/Kreislauf* **9**, 965 (1977), *C.A.* **88**, 164460t (1978). Receptor binding studies: G. Kaiser *et al., Arch. Pharmacol.* **305**, 41 (1978); R. B. Innis *et al., Life Sci.* **24**, 2255 (1979). Use in treatment of stress syndrome in pigs: G. Ballarini, F. Guizzardi, *Tieraerztl. Umsch.* **36**, 171 (1981).

Hydrochloride. $C_{18}H_{23}ClN_2O_2$. Crystals, mp 234-235°.

THERAP CAT: Antihypertensive, antianginal, antiarrhythmic.

THERAP CAT (VET): Treatment of stress in pigs.

1779. Carbachol. [51-83-2] 2-[(Aminocarbonyl)oxy]-*N,N,N*-trimethylethanaminium chloride; (2-hydroxyethyl)trimethyl ammonium chloride carbamate; choline chloride carbamate; carbamylcholine chloride; carbocholine; Doryl; Isopto Carbachol; Jestryl; Miostat. $C_6H_{15}ClN_2O_2$; mol wt 182.65. C 39.45%, H 8.28%, Cl 19.41%, N 15.34%, O 17.52%. Parasympathomimetic. Prepn: O. Dalmer, C. Diehl, **DE 539329** (1930 to E. Merck); *eidem,* **US 1894162** (1933); Kreitmair, *Arch. Exp. Pathol. Pharmakol.* **164**, 346 (1932); R. D. Haworth *et al., J. Chem. Soc.* **1947**, 176. Toxicity: Molitor, *J. Pharmacol. Exp. Ther.* **58**, 337 (1936). Evaluation in bronchoprovocation test for asthma: G. Rosati *et al., Eur. J. Respir. Dis.* **64**, Suppl. 128, 417 (1983). Clinical effect on postsurgical intraocular pressure: R. S. Ruiz *et al., Am. J. Ophthalmol.* **107**, 7 (1989).

Prismatic crystals from alcohol-ether, mp 207° (Haworth); also reported as mp 204-205° (Kreitmair). Hygroscopic. Odorless or slight amine-like odor. One gram dissolves in 1 ml water, 50 ml alcohol. Practically insol in chloroform, ether. LD_{50} in mice (mg/kg): 15 orally, 0.3 i.v. (Molitor).

THERAP CAT: Cholinergic; miotic.

THERAP CAT (VET): Cholinergic; miotic.

1780. Carbadox. [6804-07-5] (2-Quinoxalinylmethylene)-hydrazinecarboxylic acid methyl ester *N,N'*-dioxide; 3-(2-quinoxalinylmethylene)carbazic acid methyl ester *N,N'*-dioxide; methyl 3-(2-quinoxalinylmethylene)carbazate *N¹,N⁴*-dioxide; 2-formyl-quinoxaline-1,4-dioxide carbomethoxyhydrazone; GS-6244; Fortigro; Mecadox. $C_{11}H_{10}N_4O_4$; mol wt 262.22. C 50.38%, H 3.84%, N 21.37%, O 24.41%. Prepn: Johnston, **BE 669353**; *idem,* **US 3371090**; **US 3433871** (1964, 1968, 1969, all to Pfizer). Animal

studies: Thrasher *et al., J. Anim. Sci.* **26**, 911 (1967); Kornegay *et al., ibid.* **27**, 1134 (1968).

Minute yellow crystals, mp 239.5-240°. uv max (water): 236, 251, 303, 366, 373 nm (ε 11000, 10900, 36400, 16100, 16200). Practically insol in water.

THERAP CAT (VET): Antimicrobial.

1781. Carbamazepine. [298-46-4] 5*H*-Dibenz[*b,f*]-azepine-5-carboxamide; 5-carbamoyl-5*H*-dibenz[*b,f*]azepine; G-32883; Biston; Calepsin; Carbatrol; Epitol; Finlepsin; Sirtal; Stazepine; Tegretol; Telesmin; Timonil. $C_{15}H_{12}N_2O$; mol wt 236.27. C 76.25%, H 5.12%, N 11.86%, O 6.77%. Prepn: W. Schindler, **US 2948718** (1960 to Geigy). Toxicity: E. G. Stenger, F. C. Roulet, *Med. Exp.* **11**, 191 (1964). Review of GLC methods, pharmacokinetics and metabolism: S. Pynnönen, *Ther. Drug Monit.* **1**, 409-431 (1979). Comprehensive description: H. Y. Aboul-Enein, A. A. Al-Badr, *Anal. Profiles Drug Subs.* **9**, 87-106 (1980). Review of clinical use in pediatric seizures: J. T. Gilman, *DICP Ann. Pharmacother.* **25**, 1109-1112 (1991); in trigeminal neuralgia: A. Sidebottom, S. Maxwell, *J. Clin. Pharm. Ther.* **20**, 31-35 (1995).

Crystals from abs ethanol + benzene, mp 190-193°. Sol in alcohol, acetone, propylene glycol. Practically insol in water. LD_{50} orally in mice, rats: 3750, 4025 mg/kg (Stenger, Roulet).

THERAP CAT: Anticonvulsant. In treatment of pain associated with trigeminal neuralgia.

1782. Carbamide Peroxide. [124-43-6] Urea compd with hydrogen peroxide (1:1); urea hydrogen peroxide; Debrox; Exterol; Gly-Oxide; Hyperol; Ortizon (obsolete). $CH_6N_2O_3$; mol wt 94.07. C 12.77%, H 6.43%, N 29.78%, O 51.02%. $CO(NH_2)_2 \cdot H_2O_2$. Prepn: **GB 1555** (1911 to Bayer); M. Strauss, *Chem. Zentralbl.* **11**, 820 (1913). Use for prepn of H_2O_2: J. Milbauer, *Chem. Ztg.* **35**, 871 (1911), *C.A.* **5**, 3391 (1911). Clinical trial in aphthous stomatitis: M. F. Miller, N. W. Chilton, *Pharmacol. Ther. Dent.* **5**, 55 (1980); as cerumenolytic: S. Fahmy, M. Whitefield, *Br. J. Clin. Pract.* **36**, 197 (1982); as dental bleach: V. B. Haywood *et al., J. Am. Dent. Assoc.* **125**, 1219 (1994).

White crystals or cryst powder. Dec in air into urea, oxygen, and water. Sol in 2.5 parts water; partly dec by alcohol and ether into H_2O_2 and urea.

USE: For extemporaneous prepn of H_2O_2.

THERAP CAT: Antiseptic; cerumenolytic; dental bleach.

1783. Carbamyl Chloride. [463-72-9] Carbamic chloride; chloroformamide. CH_2ClNO; mol wt 79.49. C 15.11%, H 2.54%, Cl 44.60%, N 17.62%, O 20.13%. H_2NCOCl. Prepd by passing HCl gas over heated cyanuric acid: Gattermann, Rossolymo, *Ber.* **23**, 1190 (1890); Gattermann, *Ber.* **32**, 1117 (1899). From ammonia and phosgene at 400°: Rupe, Labhard, *Ber.* **33**, 236 (1900), *cf.* Gattermann, *Ann.* **244**, 30 (1888).

Liquid. Acrid, offensive odor. Has been obtained cryst, mp about 50°, bp 61-62° (decompn). Reacts violently on contact with water, forming ammonium chloride and carbon dioxide. During storage it gives off HCl and slowly changes to cyanuric acid.

1784. Carbanilic Acid. [501-82-6] Phenylcarbamic acid; *N*-carboxyaniline. $C_7H_7NO_2$; mol wt 137.14. C 61.31%, H 5.14%, N 10.21%, O 23.33%. $C_6H_5NHCOOH$. Known only by its derivatives (esters, etc.).

1785. Carbanilide. [102-07-8] N,N'-Diphenylurea; diphenylcarbamide; 1,3-diphenylurea; sym-diphenylurea. $C_{13}H_{12}N_2O$; mol wt 212.25. C 73.56%, H 5.70%, N 13.20%, O 7.54%. C_6H_5-NHCONHC$_6$H$_5$. Obtained during the preparation of phenylurea from aniline hydrochloride and urea: Davis, Blanchard, *Org. Synth.* **coll. vol. I,** 453 (2nd ed., 1941). Crystal structure: W. Dannecker *et al., Cryst. Struct. Commun.* **8,** 429 (1979).

Orthorhombic prisms from alc. d 1.239. mp 238°. bp 260° (decompn). Sublimes in current of hydrogen at 220°. Sol in ether, glacial acetic acid. Sparingly sol in water (0.15 g/l), acetone, alcohol, chloroform. Moderately sol in pyridine (69.0 g/l).

1786. Carbarsone. [121-59-5] [4-[(Aminocarbonyl)amino]phenyl]arsonic acid; N-carbamoylarsanilic acid; p-ureidobenzenearsonic acid; N-carbamylarsanilic acid; p-carbamidobenzenearsonic acid; 4-ureido-1-phenylarsonic acid; 4-carbamylaminophenylarsonic acid; p-arsonophenylurea; Amabevan; Ameban; Amibiarson; Arsambide; Carb-O-Sep; Histocarb; Fenarsone; Leucarsone; Aminarsone; Amebarsone. $C_7H_9AsN_2O_4$; mol wt 260.08. C 32.33%, H 3.49%, As 28.81%, N 10.77%, O 24.61%. Prepd from the sodium salt of arsanilic acid by treatment with potassium cyanate or cyanogen bromide: **DE 213155**; Stickings, *J. Chem. Soc.* **1928,** 3131; from arsanilic acid by treatment with phosgene: Nakatsu, Kawase, *Annu. Rep. Takamine Lab.* **8,** 44-47 (1956); **JP 58 4418** (1958 to Sankyo). Toxicity study: N. A. David *et al., Proc. Soc. Exp. Biol. Med.* **29,** 125 (1931).

White powder. mp 174°. Slightly sol in water, alcohol; sol in solns of alkali hydroxides and carbonates. The satd aq soln is acid to litmus. Nearly insol in ether or chloroform.

THERAP CAT: Antiamebic.

THERAP CAT (VET): Antihistomonad in turkeys.

1787. Carbaryl. [63-25-2] 1-Naphthalenol methylcarbamate; methyl carbamic acid 1-naphthyl ester; 1-naphthyl N-methylcarbamate; ENT-23969; OMS-29; UC-7744; Carylderm; Derbac; Ravyon; Sevin. $C_{12}H_{11}NO_2$; mol wt 201.22. C 71.63%, H 5.51%, N 6.96%, O 15.90%. Cholinesterase inhibitor. Prepn and description: Haynes *et al., Contrib. Boyce Thompson Inst.* **18,** 507 (1957); Lambrech, **US 2903478** (1959 to Union Carbide). Metabolism: W. E. Whitehurst *et al., J. Agric. Food Chem.* **11,** 167 (1963); J. B. Houston *et al., Xenobiotica* **5,** 637 (1975). Degradation: D. G. Crosby *et al., J. Agric. Food Chem.* **13,** 204 (1965); D. L. Heywood, *Environ. Qual. Saf.* **4,** 128 (1975). Toxicology: I. Nisbet, D. Miner, *Environment* **13,** 10 (1971). Toxicity: M. Vandekar *et al., Bull. WHO* **44,** 241 (1971). Clinical trial in pediculosis: J. W. Maunder, *Clin. Exp. Dermatol.* **6,** 605 (1981). *Review: Carbamate Insecticides: Chemistry, Biochemistry and Toxicology,* R. J. Kuhr, H. W. Dorough, Eds. (CRC Press, Cleveland, 1976) 301 pp.

Crystals, mp 142°. d_{20}^{20} 1.232. Moderately sol in DMF, acetone, isophorone, cyclohexanone. Soly in water at 30°: 120 mg/l. Vapor pressure at 25°: $<4 \times 10^{-5}$ mm Hg. Stable to heat, light, acids; hydrolyzed in alkalies; noncorrosive. LD_{50} orally in rats: 250 mg/kg (Vandekar).

Caution: Potential symptoms of overexposure are skin irritation; miosis, blurred vision, tearing; rhinorrhea, excessive salivation, sweating; abdominal cramps, nausea, vomiting, diarrhea; tremor, muscle twitching; slurred speech; cyanosis, convulsions; coma, respiratory failure; possible reproductive effects. *See NIOSH Pocket Guide to Chemical Hazards* (DHHS/NIOSH 97-140, 1997) p 50; *Clinical Toxicology of Commercial Products,* R. E. Gosselin *et al.,* Eds. (Williams & Wilkins, Baltimore, 5th ed., 1984) Section II p 305, Section III, pp 86-90.

USE: Contact insecticide.

THERAP CAT: Ectoparasiticide.

THERAP CAT (VET): Ectoparasiticide.

1788. Carbazochrome Salicylate. [13051-01-9] 2-Hydroxybenzoic acid monosodium salt compd with 2-(1,2,3,6-tetrahydro-3-hydroxy-1-methyl-6-oxo-5H-indol-5-ylidene)hydrazinecarboxamide (1:1); 3-hydroxy-1-methyl-1,5,6-indolinedione semicarbazone compd with sodium salicylate; adrenochrome semicarbazone compd with sodium salicylate; adrenochrome monosemicarbazone sodium salicylate complex; Adenogen; Adrestat-F. $C_{17}H_{17}$-N$_4$NaO$_6$; mol wt 396.33. C 51.52%, H 4.32%, N 14.14%, Na 5.80%, O 24.22%. $C_{10}H_{12}N_4O_3 \cdot C_7H_5NaO_3$. Prepd by refluxing adrenochrome semicarbazone and Na salicylate in 30% methanol: Iwao *et al., JP 57 546* (1957 to Tanabe), *C.A.* **52,** 4693 (1958).

Orange-red powder, mp 196-197.5° (dec). Soly in water (25°): 0.61 mg/ml. Practically insol in ether, chloroform. pH of 10% aq soln 6.7 to 7.3. *See also* Adrenochrome.

THERAP CAT: Hemostatic.

THERAP CAT (VET): Systemic hemostatic for capillary bleeding from increased capillary permeability.

1789. Carbazochrome Sodium Sulfonate. [51460-26-5] 5-[(Aminocarbonyl)hydrazono]-2,3,5,6-tetrahydro-1-methyl-6-oxo-1H-indole-2-sulfonic acid monosodium salt; 5,6-dihydro-1-methyl-5,6-dioxo-2-indolinesulfonic acid 5-semicarbazone sodium salt; epinochrome-2-sulfonic acid 5-monosemicarbazone sodium salt; 1-methyl-5-semicarbazono-2,3,5,6-tetrahydroindole-2-sulfonic acid sodium salt; sodium 5,6-dihydro-1-methyl-5,6-dioxo-2-indolinesulfonate 5-semicarbazone; AC-17; Adenaron; Adona; Carbazon; Donaseven; Emex; Odanon; Tazin. $C_{10}H_{11}N_4NaO_5S$; mol wt 322.27. C 37.27%, H 3.44%, N 17.39%, Na 7.13%, O 24.82%, S 9.95%. Prepn: Iwao, *Pharm. Bull.* **4,** 251 (1956), *C.A.* **51,** 6860f (1957); **GB 795184** (1958 to Gohei Tanabe). Revision of structure from a 3- to a 2-sulfonic acid: Kawazu *et al., J. Heterocycl. Chem.* **10,** 1059 (1973).

Yellow-orange needles from aq methanol, dec 227-228° (free acid dec 195°). Soluble in water.

THERAP CAT: Hemostatic.

1790. Carbazole. [86-74-8] 9H-Carbazole; 9-azafluorene; dibenzopyrrole; diphenylenimine. $C_{12}H_9N$; mol wt 167.21. C 86.20%, H 5.43%, N 8.38%. Prepn: Bunyan, Cadogan, *J. Chem. Soc.* **1963,** 42. Manuf from 2-biphenylamine: Conover, **US 2481292** (1949 to Monsanto); Voltz *et al.,* **US 2891965** (1959 to Houdry Process Corp.); Nevitt, Seelig, **US 3085095** (1963 to Standard Oil, Indiana); from 2-nitrobiphenyl: Larrison, **US 2508791** (1950 to Allied Chem.); by hydrogenolysis of coal-hydrogenation products: Murray *et al.,* **US 2913397** (1959 to Union Carbide); from diphenylamine: Grotta, **US 2921942** (1960 to American-Marietta); Bearse *et al.,* **US 3041349** (1962 to Martin-Marietta); Nevitt, Seelig, *loc. cit.* Purification: Rottschaefer, **US 2459135** (1949 to GAF); Insinger, **US 2464811** (1949 to Koppers Co.). Toxicity study: Eagle, Carlson, *J. Pharmacol. Exp. Ther.* **99,** 450 (1950). Review of prepn and properties: W. C. Sumpter, F. M. Miller, *Heterocyclic Compounds* (Interscience, New York, 1954) pp 70-109.

Crystals from alcohol, benzene, toluene, glacial acetic acid, mp 245°. Sublimes. bp 355°; bp$_{147}$ 200°. d$_4^{18}$ 1.10. Exhibits strong fluorescence and long phosphorescence on exposure to ultraviolet light. Extremely weak base. Insol in water. One gram dissolves in 3 ml quinoline, 6 ml pyridine, 9 ml acetone, 2 ml acetone at 50°, 35 ml ether, 120 ml benzene, 135 ml abs alcohol. Slightly sol in petr ether, chlorinated hydrocarbons, acetic acid. Dissolves in concd H$_2$SO$_4$ without dec. KOH fusion yields N-potassium salt. LD$_{50}$ orally in rats: >5 g/kg (Eagle, Carlson).

USE: Important dye intermediate. Used in making photographic plates sensitive to ultraviolet light. Reagent for lignin, carbohydrates, and formaldehyde.

1791. Carbendazim. [10605-21-7] 1H-Benzimidazol-2-yl-carbamic acid methyl ester; 2-benzimidazolecarbamic acid methyl ester; 2-(methoxycarbonylamino)benzimidazole; methyl 2-benzimidazolecarbamate; carbendazim; BMC; MBC; BCM; BAS-3460; BAS-67054; CTR-6669; HOE-17411; Bavistin; Derosal; Delsene. C$_9$H$_9$N$_3$O$_2$; mol wt 191.19. C 56.54%, H 4.74%, N 21.98%, O 16.74%. Degradn product of benomyl, *q.v.* Prepn: H. M. Loux, US 3010968 (1961 to du Pont); H. A. Selling *et al., Chem. Ind. (London)* **1970**, 1625. Activity: G. P. Clemons, H. D. Sisler, *Pestic. Biochem. Physiol.* **1**, 32 (1971). Degradn in soil: A. Helweg, *Pestic. Sci.* **8**, 71 (1977). Efficacy in controlling powdery mildew: G. R. Singh, T. B. Anilkumar, *Indian J. Mycol. Plant Pathol.* **16**, 30 (1986). Review of environmental and toxicological effects: *Carbendazim: Environ. Health Criteria* **149**, (World Health Organization, Geneva, 1993) 132 pp.

White powder, mp 302-307° (dec). pKa 4.48. Soly 20° (mg/ml): water, pH 7 8; pH 4 29. Soly 20° (mg/l): hexane 0.5; benzene 36; dichloromethane 68; ethanol 300; dimethylformamide 5000, chloroform 100, acetone 300. Slowly decomp in alkaline soln.

USE: Fungicide.

1792. Carbenicillin. [4697-36-3] (2S,5R,6R)-6-[(Carboxyphenylacetyl)amino]-3,3-dimethyl-7-oxo-4-thia-1-azabicyclo[3.2.0]heptane-2-carboxylic acid; N-(2-carboxy-3,3-dimethyl-7-oxo-4-thia-1-azabicyclo[3.2.0]hept-6-yl)-2-phenylmalonamic acid; α-carboxybenzylpenicillin; 6-(α-carboxyphenylacetamido)penicillanic acid; α-phenyl(carboxymethylpenicillin). C$_{17}$H$_{18}$N$_2$O$_6$S; mol wt 378.40. C 53.96%, H 4.79%, N 7.40%, O 25.37%, S 8.47%. Semi-synthetic antibiotic related to penicillin. Prepn of monopotassium salt: Hobbs, US 3142673 (1964 to Pfizer); of disodium salt: BE 646991; Brain, Nayler, US 3282926 (1964, 1966 both to Beecham). Activity studies and pharmacology: Naumann, Kempf, *Arzneim.-Forsch.* **19**, 1222 (1969). Chemistry and mode of action: Butler *et al., J. Infect. Dis.* **122**, *Suppl.*, 81 (1970). Clinical data: Hoffler *et al., ibid.* 1233; Gritz, Naumann, *ibid.* 1237. Toxicity data: E. I. Goldenthal, *Toxicol. Appl. Pharmacol.* **18**, 185 (1971).

Disodium salt. [4800-94-6] Carbenicillin disodium; BRL-2064; CP-15639-2; Carbapen; Carbecin; Geopen; Hyoper; Microcillin; Pyocianil; Pyopen. C$_{17}$H$_{16}$N$_2$Na$_2$O$_6$S; mol wt 422.36. White powder. LD$_{50}$ i.p. in rats: >2000 mg/kg (Goldenthal).

Phenyl sodium. [21649-57-0] Carfecillin sodium; BRL-3475; Gripenin-O; Urocarf. C$_{23}$H$_{21}$N$_2$NaO$_6$S; mol wt 476.48. Prepn and activity studies: Clayton *et al., J. Med. Chem.* **18**, 172 (1975). Crystals from ethanol, [α]$_D^{20}$ +216.2° (H$_2$O).

THERAP CAT: Antibacterial.

1793. Carbenoxolone. [5697-56-3] (3β,20β)-3-(3-Carboxy-1-oxopropoxy)-11-oxoolean-12-en-29-oic acid; 3β-hydroxy-

11-oxoolean-12-en-30-oic acid hydrogen succinate; 3-O-(β-carboxypropionyl)-11-oxo-18β-olean-12-en-30-oic acid; 18β-glycyrrhetic acid hydrogen succinate; carbenoxalone. C$_{34}$H$_{50}$O$_7$; mol wt 570.76. C 71.55%, H 8.83%, O 19.62%. Anti-inflammatory glucocorticoid related to enoxolone, *q.v.* Prepn: Gottfried, Baxendale, GB 843133; US 3070623 (1960, 1961 to Biorex). Monograph: *Carbenoxolone Sodium,* J. M. Robson, F. M. Sullivan, Eds. (Butterworths, London, 1969) 263 pp. Symposium on clinical efficacy: *Scand. J. Gastroenterol.* **15**, Suppl. 65, 1-121 (1980). Effect on gastric prostaglandin levels in humans: J. Rask-Madsen *et al., Eur. J. Clin. Invest.* **13**, 351 (1983); P. Minuz *et al., Pharmacol. Res. Commun.* **16**, 875 (1984). Comprehensive description: S. Pindado *et al., Anal. Profiles Drug Subs. Excip.* **24**, 1-43 (1996).

Cream-colored crystals, mp 291-294°. [α]$_D^{20}$ +128° (chloroform).

Disodium salt. [7421-40-1] Bioplex; Bioral; Neogel; Sanodin; Ulcus-Tablinen. C$_{34}$H$_{48}$Na$_2$O$_7$; mol wt 614.72. Creamy-white solid. Freely sol in water. Insol in chloroform, ether. pKa$_1$ 4.18; pKa$_2$ 5.52. uv max (water): 260 nm (E$_{cm}^{1\%}$ 172). LD$_{50}$ in male mice (mg/kg): 198 i.v.; 120 i.p.; in male rats (mg/kg): 3200 orally (Robson, Sullivan).

THERAP CAT: Antiulcerative.

1794. Carbetapentane. [77-23-6] 1-Phenylcyclopentanecarboxylic acid 2-(2-diethylaminoethoxy)ethyl ester; 2-(diethylaminoethoxy)ethyl 1-phenyl-1-cyclopentanecarboxylate; 2-(diethylaminoethoxy)ethyl 1-phenylcyclopentyl-1-carboxylate; 1-phenylcyclopentane-1-carboxylic acid diethylaminoethoxyethyl ester; pentoxyverine; pentoxiverin. C$_{20}$H$_{31}$NO$_3$; mol wt 333.47. C 72.03%, H 9.37%, N 4.20%, O 14.39%. Prepn: H. G. Morren, GB 753779; *idem,* US 2842585 (1956, 1958 both to Union Chimique Belge). Antispasmodic activity: D. Wellens, *Arzneim.-Forsch.* **17**, 495 (1967). Clinical effect on lung function: E. Krieger, *ibid.* **22**, 389 (1972).

bp$_{0.01}$ 165-170°.

Citrate. [23142-01-0] UCB-2543; Antees; Calnathal; Carbetane; Cossym; Fustpentane; Germapect; Pencal; Sedotussin; Toclase; Tosnone; Tuclase. C$_{20}$H$_{31}$NO$_3$.C$_6$H$_8$O$_7$; mol wt 525.59. Crystals, mp 93°. Freely sol in water, chloroform; sol in alcohol, acetone, ethyl acetate. Practically insol in ether, petr ether, benzene.

THERAP CAT: Antitussive.

1795. Carbetocin. [37025-55-1] 1-Butanoic acid-2-(O-methyl-L-tyrosine)-1-carbaoxytocin; 1-butyric acid-2-[3-(p-methoxyphenyl)-L-alanine]oxytocin; deamino-2-O-methyltyrosine-1-carbaoxytocin; 1-thia-4,7,10,13,16-pentaazacycloeicosane cyclic peptide deriv; 1-desamino-1-monocarba-[2-tyr(OMe)]-OT; (2-O-methyltyrosine)deamino-1-carbaoxytocin; d(COMOT); Decomoton; Depotocin. C$_{45}$H$_{69}$N$_{11}$O$_{12}$S; mol wt 988.16. C 54.70%, H 7.04%, N 15.59%, O 19.43%, S 3.24%. Synthetic carba-analog of oxytocin, *q.v.* Prepn: I. Fric *et al., Collect. Czech. Chem. Commun.* **39**, 1290 (1974); J. H. Cort *et al.,* DE 2732175 (1976 to Czech. Akad. Ved.). Chromatographic properties: M. Lebl, *Collect. Czech. Chem. Commun.* **45**, 2927 (1980). Uterotonic and galactogogic activity: T. Barth *et al., ibid.* 3045; T. Barth *et al., ibid.* **46**,

2441 (1981). Pharmacokinetics in lactating sows: N. Cort *et al.*, *Am. J. Vet. Res.* **42**, 1804 (1981). Use in regulation of bovine labor: Z. Veznik *et al.*, *ibid.* **40**, 425 (1979). Effect on milk let-down in sows: N. Cort *et al.*, *ibid.* **43**, 1283 (1982).

Solid from methanol with ether $[\alpha]_D$ −69.0° (c 0.25 in 1*M* acetic acid).

THERAP CAT (VET): Oxytocic, stimulates milk let-down.

1796. Carbic Anhydride. [129-64-6] 3aα,4,7,7aα-Tetrahydro-4α,7α-methanoisobenzofuran-1,3-dione; *cis-endo*-5-norbornene-2,3-dicarboxylic anhydride; *endo-cis*-bicyclo[2.2.1]hept-5-ene-2,3-dicarboxylic anhydride; 3,6-*endo*-methylene-1,2,3,6-tetrahydro-*cis*-phthalic anhydride; 3,6-*endo*-methylene-Δ^4-tetrahydrophthalic anhydride; nadic anhydride. $C_9H_8O_3$; mol wt 164.16. C 65.85%, H 4.91%, O 29.24%. Prepd by the reaction of maleic anhydride with cyclopentadiene in benzene: Diels, Alder, *Ann.* **460**, 98 (1928). Crystal structure: Destro *et al.*, *Acta Crystallogr.* **25B**, 2465 (1969).

Shiny, orthorhombic crystals from petr ether, mp 164-165°. d 1.417. Converted to equilibrium mixtures with *exo-cis* isomers when heated above mp. Sol in benzene, toluene, acetone, carbon tetrachloride, chloroform, ethanol, ethyl acetate. Slightly sol in petr ether. Reacts with water to form the corresponding acid. Forms the γ-lactone of 5-hydroxy-2,3-norcamphanedicarboxylic acid in 50% H_2SO_4.

1797. Carbidopa. [28860-95-9] (αS)-α-Hydrazino-3,4-dihydroxy-α-methylbenzenepropanoic acid monohydrate; (−)-L-α-hydrazino-3,4-dihydroxy-α-methylhydrocinnamic acid monohydrate; α-hydrazino-α-methyl-β-(3,4-dihydroxyphenyl)propionic acid monohydrate; L-α-(3,4-dihydroxybenzyl)-α-hydrazinopropionic acid monohydrate; α-methyldopahydrazine; HMD; MK-486; Lodosyn. $C_{10}H_{14}N_2O_4 \cdot H_2O$; mol wt 244.24. C 49.18%, H 6.60%, N 11.47%, O 32.75%. Peripheral decarboxylase inhibitor. Prepn of DL-form: Pfister, **FR M1553** (1962 to Merck & Co.), *C.A.* **59**, 12921e (1963); Sletzinger *et al.*, *J. Med. Chem.* **6**, 101 (1963); **GB 940596**; Chemerda *et al.*, **US 3462536** (1963, 1969 both to Merck & Co.). Synthesis of the L-form: Karady *et al.*, **DE 2062285**; **DE 2062332** (both 1971 to Merck & Co.), *C.A.* **75**, 118122t, 118120r (1971); *eidem, J. Org. Chem.* **36**, 1946, 1949 (1971). Inhibition of dopa decarboxylase: Porter *et al.*, *Biochem. Pharmacol.* **11**, 1067 (1962); Moran, Sourkes, *J. Pharmacol. Exp. Ther.* **148**, 252 (1962); Watanabe *et al.*, *Clin. Pharmacol. Ther.* **11**, 740 (1970). Only the L-form is pharmacologically active: Lotti, Porter, *J. Pharmacol. Exp. Ther.* **172**, 406 (1970).

Crystals from hot water, mp 203-205° (dec). $[\alpha]_D$ −17.3° (methanol). Also reported as mp 208°.

Combination with levodopa. [57308-51-7] Co-careldopa; Isicom; Nacom; Sinemet.

DL-Form. Tan fluffy crystals, mp 206-208° (dec). uv max (methanol): 282.5 nm (ϵ 2940).

THERAP CAT: In combination with levodopa as antiparkinsonian.

1798. Carbimazole. [22232-54-8] 2,3-Dihydro-3-methyl-2-thioxo-1*H*-imidazole-1-carboxylic acid ethyl ester; 1-ethoxycarbonyl-3-methyl-2-thio-4-imidazoline; ethyl 3-methyl-2-thioimidazoline-1-carboxylate; 1-methyl-3-carbethoxy-2-thioglyoxalone; athyromazole; Neo-mercazole; Neo-Thyreostat. $C_7H_{10}N_2O_2S$; mol wt 186.23. C 45.15%, H 5.41%, O 17.18%, S 17.22%. Thyroid inhibitor. Prepn: Rimington *et al.*, **US 2671088**, reissued as **US RE 24505**; **US 2815349** (1954, 1958, 1957, all to Natl. Res. Dev. Corp.); Baker, *J. Chem. Soc.* **1958**, 2387. Clinical efficacy in Graves' disease: J. Duprey *et al.*, *Presse Med.* **17**, 1124 (1988).

Crystalline powder with characteristic odor; tasteless at first, followed by bitter taste; mp 122-125°. Sol (at 20°) in 500 parts of water; in 50 parts of ethanol; in 330 parts of ether; in 3 parts of chloroform; in 17 parts of acetone. uv max in 0.1*N* HCl : water (1:8): 291 nm; in 0.1*N* H_2SO_4: 227 nm and 291 nm ($E_{1cm}^{1\%}$ 557).

THERAP CAT: Antihyperthyroid.

1799. Carbinoxamine. [486-16-8] 2-[(4-Chlorophenyl)-2-pyridinylmethoxy]-*N*,*N*-dimethylethanamine; 2-[*p*-chloro-α-(2-dimethylaminoethoxy)benzyl]pyridine; paracarbinoxamine. $C_{16}H_{19}$-ClN_2O; mol wt 290.79. C 66.09%, H 6.59%, Cl 12.19%, N 9.63%, O 5.50%. Prepn: Tilford, Shelton, **US 2606195** (1952 to Wm. S. Merrell); Swain, **US 2800485** (1957 to McNeil Labs.). Prepn of *l*-form: **GB 905993** (1962 to McNeil Labs.), *C.A.* **58**, 5644a (1962). Abs config of *l*-form: V. Barouh *et al.*, *J. Med. Chem.* **14**, 834 (1971). Pharmacology and toxicology: R. Cahen, *Ann. Pharm. Fr.* **20**, 463 (1962). GLC determn in serum: D. J. Hoffman *et al.*, *J. Pharm. Sci.* **72**, 1342 (1983).

Liquid, bp$_{0.1}$ 158-162°.

Hydrochloride. $C_{16}H_{19}ClN_2O \cdot HCl$. Crystals from isopropanol + ethyl acetate, dec 162-164°. Sol in water.

Maleate. [3505-38-2] Allergefon; Clistin; Ciberon; Lergefin; Polistin T-Caps. $C_{16}H_{19}ClN_2O \cdot C_4H_4O_4$; mol wt 406.86. Bitter crystals from ethyl acetate, mp 117-119°. Freely sol in water, alcohol, chloroform. Very slightly sol in ether. pH of 1% aq soln 4.6-5.1. LD_{50} in mice (mg/kg): 166 i.p. (Cahen).

l-**Form.** Levocarbinoxamine; rotoxamine; McN-R-73-Z. bp$_{0.5}$ 143-144°. n_D^{20} 1.5522. $[\alpha]_D^{25}$ −6.8° (c 2 in methanol).

l-**Form d-tartrate.** [49746-00-1] Twiston. $C_{16}H_{19}ClN_2O \cdot C_4H_6O_6$; mol wt 440.87. Crystals from isopropanol, mp 143-144.5°. $[\alpha]_D^{25}$ +37.2° (c 20 in methanol).

THERAP CAT: Antihistaminic.

1800. Carbitol®. [111-90-0] 2-(2-Ethoxyethoxy)ethanol; diethylene glycol monoethyl ether; ethyl digol. $C_6H_{14}O_3$; mol wt 134.17. C 53.71%, H 10.52%, O 35.77%. $CH_3CH_2OCH_2CH_2$-OCH_2CH_2OH. Prepn from ethylene oxide and 2-ethoxyethanol in the presence of SO_2: Britton, Sexton, **US 2807651** (1957 to Dow). Toxicity data: Smyth, Carpenter, *J. Ind. Hyg. Toxicol.* **30**, 63 (1948).

Very hygroscopic liquid, bp 196°. d_4^{25} 0.9855, d_{20}^{20} 1.0273. n_D^{20} 1.4273. Flash pt 96°C (Tag open cup). Miscible with acetone, benzene, chloroform, ethanol, ether, pyridine, etc.: Jackson, Drury, *Ind. Eng. Chem.* **51**, 1491 (1959). Also miscible with water. LD_{50} orally in rats: 8.69 g/kg (Smyth, Carpenter).

Acetate. $C_8H_{16}O_4$. Liquid, bp 218.5°. mp −25°. d_{20}^{20} 1.0114. n_D^{20} 1.4213. Flash pt 110°C (Tag open cup). Miscible with water, alc, ether, most oils. LD_{50} orally in rats: 11 g/kg (Smyth, Carpenter).

USE: As solvent for cellulose esters, in lacquer and thinner formulations, in quick-drying varnishes and enamels, for dyestuffs and wood stains. Acetate is used as a solvent and plasticizer for cellulose esters, gums, resins, etc.

1801. Carbobenzoxy Chloride. [501-53-1] Carbonochloridic acid phenylmethyl ester; benzyl chloroformate; chloroformic acid benzyl ester; benzylcarbonyl chloride. $C_8H_7ClO_2$; mol wt 170.59. C 56.33%, H 4.14%, Cl 20.78%, O 18.76%. Prepn by action of phosgene absorbed in toluene on benzyl alcohol: Carter *et al., Org. Synth.* **23,** 13 (1943); by reacting carbonyl chloride and benzyl alcohol at −20 to −30°: Farthing, *J. Chem. Soc.* **1950,** 3213.

Oily liquid; acrid odor; lacrimator. bp_{20} 103°; bp_7 85-87°. Dec to CO_2 and benzyl chloride upon heating at 100-155°.
USE: In peptide synthesis to block the amino group.

1802. Carbocysteine. [638-23-3] *S*-(Carboxymethyl)-L-cysteine; 3-[(carboxymethyl)thio]alanine; *S*-carboxymethyl-cysteine; AHR-3053; LJ-206; Carbocit; Fluifort; Lisomucil; Loviscol; Muciclar; Mucocis; Mucodyne; Mucolase; Mucolex; Mucopront; Pectox; Pulmoclase; Reomucil; Rhinathiol; Siroxyl; Transbronchin. $C_5H_9NO_4S$; mol wt 179.19. C 33.51%, H 5.06%, N 7.82%, O 35.71%, S 17.89%. HOOCCH$_2$SCH$_2$CH(NH$_2$)COOH. Prepn: Armstrong, Lewis, *J. Org. Chem.* **16,** 749 (1951); Schöberl, Wagner, *Z. Physiol. Chem.* **304,** 97 (1956); Foye, Verderame, *J. Am. Pharm. Assoc.* **46,** 273 (1957); Goodman *et al., J. Org. Chem.* **23,** 1251 (1958). Pharmacology: Huyen-Vu-Ngoc *et al., C.R. Seances Soc. Biol. Ses Fil.* **160,** 1849 (1966); Quevauviller *et al., Therapie* **22,** 485 (1967). Clinical trial in chronic bronchitis: M. Grillage, K. Bernard-Jones, *Br. J. Clin. Pract.* **39,** 395 (1985). Review of pharmacology and clinical uses: D. T. Brown, *Drug Intell. Clin. Pharm.* **22,** 603-608 (1988).
L-**Form.** mp 204-207°. $[\alpha]_D^{24}$ +0.5° (*1N* HCl).
DL-**Form.** Spherical aggregates of needles.
THERAP CAT: Mucolytic; expectorant.

1803. Carbofuran. [1563-66-2] 2,3-Dihydro-2,2-dimethyl-7-benzofuranol methylcarbamate; methyl carbamic acid 2,3-dihydro-2,2-dimethyl-7-benzofuranyl ester; 2,2-dimethyl-2,3-dihydro-7-benzofuranyl-*N*-methylcarbamate; 2,2-dimethyl-7-coumaranyl *N*-methylcarbamate; Bay 70143; NIA-10242; Furadan. $C_{12}H_{15}$-NO_3; mol wt 221.25. C 65.14%, H 6.83%, N 6.33%, O 21.69%. Cholinesterase inhibitor. Prepn and use as insecticide: **NL 6407316** (1964 to Bayer), *C.A.* **63,** 583a (1965); **NL 6500340;** W. G. Scharpf, **US 3474170; US 3474171** (1965, 1969, 1969 all to FMC); E. F. Orwoll, **US 3356690** (1967 to FMC). Metabolism: H. W. Dorough, *J. Agric. Food Chem.* **16,** 319 (1968); J. B. Knaak, *ibid.* **18,** 832 (1970). Toxicity studies: J. S. Tobin, *J. Occup. Med.* **12,** 16 (1970); M. A. Fahmy *et al., J. Agric. Food Chem.* **18,** 793 (1970). Teratogenicity study: K. D. Courtney *et al., J. Environ. Sci. Health* **B20,** 373 (1985).

White crystalline solid, mp 150-153°. Soly in water at 25°: 700 ppm. Unstable in alk. LD_{50} orally in mice: 2 mg/kg (Fahmy, 1970).
Caution: Potential symptoms of overexposure are miosis, blurred vision; sweating, salivation, abdominal cramps, diarrhea, headache, nausea, vomiting, weakness; muscle twitching, incoordination, convulsions. *See NIOSH Pocket Guide to Chemical Hazards* (DHHS/-NIOSH 97-140, 1997) p 52; *Clinical Toxicology of Commercial Products,* R. E. Gosselin *et al.,* Eds. (Williams & Wilkins, Baltimore, 5th ed., 1984) Section II, p 305.
USE: Systemic insecticide, acaricide, nematocide.

1804. Carbohydrazide. [497-18-7] Carbonic dihydrazide; 1,3-diaminourea. CH_6N_4O; mol wt 90.08. C 13.33%, H 6.71%, N 62.20%, O 17.76%. NH$_2$NHCONHNH$_2$. Prepd by refluxing diethyl carbonate with hydrazine hydrate: Mohr *et al., Inorg. Synth.* **4,** 32 (1953).

Crystals from water + ethanol, dec 153-154°. Freely sol in water. pH of 1% aq soln ~7.4. Practically insol in alcohol, ether, chloroform, benzene. Forms salts with acids. With nitrous acid it forms the highly explosive carbonyl azide $CO(N_3)_2$.

1805. γ-Carboline. [244-69-9] 5*H*-Pyrido[4,3-*b*]indole; 2*H*-pyrid[4,3-*b*]indole; 5-carboline. $C_{11}H_8N_2$; mol wt 168.19. C 78.55%, H 4.79%, N 16.66%. Prepn: Robinson, Thornley, *J. Chem. Soc.* **125,** 2169 (1924). Prepn of derivs: Hörlein, *Ber.* **87,** 463 (1954); C. Ducrocq *et al., J. Heterocycl. Chem.* **12,** 963 (1975). NMR studies: F. Balkau, M. L. Heffernan, *Aust. J. Chem.* **26,** 1501, 1523 (1973).

Monoclinic needles from water, mp 225°. d 1.352. Can be distilled at atmospheric pressure without dec. Strong base. Freely sol in methanol; somewhat less sol in ethanol. Slightly sol in benzene, water.

1806. Carbomycin. Sixteen-membered-ring macrolide antibiotic complex similar to leucomycin, *q.v.* and erythromycin, *q.v.,* produced by *Streptomyces halstedii.* Isoln and antibacterial activity: F. W. Tanner *et al., Antibiot. Chemother.* **2,** 441 (1952). Two components have been isolated: Carbomycin A (major) and carbomycin B. Isoln of A: Friedman *et al.,* **US 2960438** (1960 to Pfizer); of B: F. A. Hochstein, K. Murai, *J. Am. Chem. Soc.* **76,** 5080 (1954). Structure of A and B: R. B. Woodward, *Angew. Chem.* **69,** 50 (1957); revised structure: M. Kuehne, B. W. Benson, *J. Am. Chem. Soc.* **87,** 4660 (1965); R. B. Woodward *et al., ibid.* 4662. Abs config of A and B: W. D. Celmer, *ibid.* **88,** 5028 (1966). Identity of A with deltamycin A$_4$: Y. Shimauchi *et al., J. Antibiot.* **31,** 270 (1978). Synthesis of B: K. Tatsuta *et al., J. Am. Chem. Soc.* **99,** 5826 (1977). Stereospecific total synthesis of B: *eidem, Tetrahedron Lett.* **1980,** 2837. Retrosynthetic studies: K. C. Nicolaou *et al., J. Am. Chem. Soc.* **103,** 1222 (1981). *Reviews:* D. Vazquez, in *Antibiotics* **Vol. 1,** D. Gottlieb, P. D. Shaw, Eds. (Springer-Verlag, New York, 1967) pp 366-377; W. Keller-Schierlein in *Fortschr. Chem. Org. Naturst.* **30,** 314-460 (1973).

Carbomycin A

Carbomycin A. [4564-87-8] (12*S*,13*S*)-9-Deoxy-12,13-epoxy-12,13-dihydro-9-oxoleucomycin V 3-acetate 4^B-(3-methylbutanoate); deltamycin A$_4$; M-4209. $C_{42}H_{67}NO_{16}$; mol wt 841.98. Blunt needles from ethanol, mp 214°. $[\alpha]_D^{25}$ −58.6° (chloroform). uv max (abs ethanol): 238, 327 nm ($E_{1cm}^{1\%}$ 185, 0.9). Carbomycin standard is the free base having a potency of 1080 units/mg. For stability of soln data *see* H. L. Martin, *Antibiot. Chemother.* **3,** 865 (1953). Weak base, pKb 7.2. Solubilities determined by Weiss *et al., ibid.* **7,** 374 (1957) in mg/ml at about 28°: water 0.295; methanol >20; ethanol >20. LD_{50} i.v. in mice: 550 mg/kg (Tanner).

Carbomycin B. [21238-30-2] 9-Deoxy-9-oxoleucomycin V 3-acetate 4^B-(3-methylbutanoate). $C_{42}H_{67}NO_{15}$; mol wt 825.98. Colorless anisotropic plates from acetone/water, mp 141-144° (dec), softens at 138°. $[\alpha]_D^{25}$ −35° (c 1 in chloroform). uv max (abs ethanol): 278 nm ($E_{1cm}^{1\%}$ 276). pKb 7.56. Solubilities in mg/ml at 25°: ethanol 450; water 0.1-0.2.

1807. Carbon. [7440-44-0] C; at. wt 12.0107; at. no. 6; valence 4. Group IVA(14). Stable isotopes: 12 (98.892%); 13 (1.108%); radioactive isotopes: 9-11; 14-16. Abundance in earth's crust: approx 0.027%. Cosmic abundance: 6 atoms/atom Si. Occurs in 4 allotropic forms: (1) diamond, *q.v.*; (2) graphite, *q.v.* or black lead; (3) amorphous carbon such as coal, lampblack; (4) fullerenes, *see* Buckminsterfullerene, the only molecular form. Comprehensive reviews: P. L. Walker, *Am. Sci.* **50**, 259-293 (June 1962); Holliday *et al.* in *Comprehensive Inorganic Chemistry* **vol. 1,** J. C. Bailar, Jr. *et al.*, Eds. (Pergamon Press, Oxford, 1973) pp 1173-1294; several authors in *Kirk-Othmer Encyclopedia of Chemical Technology* **vol. 4** (Wiley-Interscience, New York, 3rd ed., 1978) pp 556-709.

^{14}**C isotope.** Continuously formed in the earth's atm by the bombardment of nitrogen with cosmic neutrons according to the reaction $^{14}_7N + ^1_0n \rightarrow ^{14}_6C + ^1_1H$. The ^{14}C is rapidly oxidized to CO_2, in this form it penetrates into animals and plants by photosynthesis and metabolism. The ^{14}C content of living matter is estimated at 15.3 disintegrations per minute and per gram of carbon, corresponding to the equilibrium reached between formation of ^{14}C and its exchange with ^{12}C. This equilibrium stops when the plant or animal dies, and the ^{14}C content begins to decrease, because the ^{14}C decays with a half-life of 5760 years. This fact can be used to date organic matter (not more than 40,000 years old) by comparison with the standard 15.3 disintegrations per min per gram: M. Haissinsky, J. P. Adloff, *Radiochemical Survey of the Elements* (Elsevier, New York, 1965) pp 30-32.

1808. Carbon, Amorphous. Carbon black; activated carbon; decolorizing carbon. A quasi-graphitic form of carbon of small particle size. By the term "carbon black" several forms of artificially prepared carbon or charcoal are designated, *e.g.*: (1) *Animal charcoal*, obtained by charring bones, meat, blood, etc.; (2) *Gas black*; *furnace black*; *channel black*; *C.I. 77266*, obtained by incomplete combustion of natural gas; (3) *Lamp black*, obtained by burning various fats, oils, resins, etc., under suitable conditions; (4) *Activated charcoal*, *e.g.* *Carbomix*, *Carboraffin*, *Medicoal*, *Norit*, *Opocarbyl*, *Ultracarbon*, prepd from wood and vegetables. Monograph: H. W. Davidson *et al.*, *Manufactured Carbon* (Pergamon Press, New York, 1968). *Reviews:* Cohan in *Science of Petroleum* **vol. V**, Pt 2, B. T. Brooks, A. E. Dunstan, Eds. (Oxford Univ. Press, 1953), pp 79-89; Smisek, Cerny, *Active Carbon* (Elsevier Publishing Co., Amsterdam, 1970).

Caution: Potential symptoms of overexposure are cough; eye irritation. Potential occupational carcinogen in the presence of polycyclic aromatic hydrocarbons. *See NIOSH Pocket Guide to Chemical Hazards* (DHHS/NIOSH 97-140, 1997) p 52.

USE: Pigment for rubber tires; for printing, stenciling and drawing inks; for leather; stove polish, phonograph records, electrical insulating apparatus. Activated charcoal for clarifying, deodorizing, decolorizing and filtering. As a color additive in foods and cosmetics.

THERAP CAT: Activated charcoal as antidote; adsorptive.

THERAP CAT (VET): Internally as an adsorptive in diarrhea; externally in foul wounds.

1809. Carbon Dioxide. [124-38-9] Carbonic acid gas; carbonic anhydride. CO_2; mol wt 44.01. C 27.29%, O 72.71%. Occurs in the atms of many planets. In our solar system, e.g., on Venus, the optical layer thickness due to CO_2 is 100,000 cm/atm, but only 220 cm/atm on Earth. Analyses of air in the temperate zones of the Earth show 0.027 to 0.036% (v/v) of CO_2: G. P. Kuiper, *The Atmospheres of the Earth and the Planets* (Univ. of Chicago Press, 1949); Landolt-Bornstein, *Zahlenwerte* **vol. III** (Springer-Verlag, 6th ed., 1952) pp 59 and 585. Constituent of carbonate type of minerals and products of animal metabolism. Necessary for the respiration cycle of plants and animals. Obtained industrially as a by-product in the manuf of lime during the "burning" of limestone ($CaCO_3$). Also produced by burning coke or other carbonaceous material. In the U.S.A. large amounts are produced by fermentation

(Backus process and Reich process). When glucose is fermented by yeast, the chief products are ethyl alcohol and CO_2. Prepd in the laboratory by dropping acid on a carbonate: E. H. Archibald, *The Preparation of Pure Inorganic Substances* (Wiley, New York, 1932) p 196; Loomis, Walters, *J. Am. Chem. Soc.* **48**, 3103 (1926). Purification: Glemser in *Handbook of Preparative Inorganic Chemistry* G. Brauer, Ed. (Academic Press, New York, 2nd ed., 1963) p 647. Discovery of a second polymorph of dry ice: L.-G. Liu, *Nature* **303**, 508 (1983). *Reviews:* E. L. Quinn, *J. Chem. Educ.* **7**, 151-162 and 403-419 (1930); J. Kuprianoff, *Die feste Kohlensäure (Trockeneis)* (Enke, Stuttgart, 1939); E. L. Quinn, C. L. Jones, *Carbon Dioxide* (Reinhold, New York, 1947); W. R. Ballou, in *Kirk-Othmer Encyclopedia of Chemical Technology* **vol. 4** (Interscience, New York, 3rd ed., 1978) pp 725-742. Reviews of supercritical CO_2 (*scCO$_2$*) solvent uses and environmental benefits in polymer chemistry: S. L. Wells, J. DeSimone, *Angew. Chem. Int. Ed.* **40**, 518-527 (2001); in catalysis: W. Leitner, *Acc. Chem. Res.* **35**, 746-756 (2002).

Colorless, odorless, noncombustible gas. Faint acid taste. Usually a nonsupporter of combustion, although burning magnesium continues to burn when transferred into a CO_2 atm. Usually marketed in steel cylinders (under sufficient pressure to keep it liquid) or in solid form as *Dry Ice* (compressed carbon dioxide snow, d 1.35). When shipped in steel cylinders, CO_2 is in the form of gas over liquid and at 20° exerts a pressure of 830 psi. Use gloves when handling dry ice, as its temp is at least −78.5°; momentary skin contact with dry ice has caused serious frostbites and blisters. At atmospheric pressures the solid form changes into the gaseous phase without liquefaction. d (gas) 1.527 (air 1); d (gas) 1.557 ($N_2 = 1$); abs d 0.1146 lb/cu ft at 25°; vol at 25°: 8.76 cu ft/lb. d (gas, 0°) 1.976 g/l at 760 mm; d (liq, 0°) 0.914 at 34.3 atm; d (solid, −56.6°) 1.512. Sublimes at −78.48° (760 mm). mp$_{5.2\ atm}$ −56.6°. The gas is not affected by heat until temp reaches about 2000°. Crit temp 31.3°; crit press 72.9 atm; crit density 0.464. Triple point −56.6° at 5.11 atm. Vapor press at −120°: 10.5 mm; at −100°: 104.2 mm; at −82°: 569.1 mm. Heat of formation 94.05 kcal/mol. Latent heat of vaporization 83.12 g cal/g. Specific heat 0.19 to 0.21 Btu/lb. Soly in water (ml CO_2/100 ml H_2O at 760 mm): 0° 171; 20° 88; 60° 36. More sol at higher pressures. Less sol in alcohol, other neutral organic solvents. Absorbed by alkaline solns with the formation of carbonates.

Caution: Potential symptoms of overexposure are headache, dizziness, restlessness and paresthesia; dyspnea; sweating, malaise; increased heart rate and cardiac output; elevated blood pressure; coma; asphyxia; convulsions; direct contact with liquid or dry ice may cause frostbite. *See NIOSH Pocket Guide to Chemical Hazards* (DHHS/NIOSH 97-140, 1997) p 52.

USE: In the carbonation of beverages; manuf of carbonates; in fire prevention and extinction; for inerting flammable materials during manuf, handling and transfer; as propellant in aerosols; as dry ice for refrigeration; to produce harmless smoke or fumes on stage; as rice fumigant; as antiseptic in bacteriology and in the frozen food industry. Supercritical or liquid CO_2 used in extraction of caffeine and hops aroma; dry cleaning; metal degreasing; cleaning semiconductor chips; paint spraying; polymer modification. Environmentally benign alternative to potentially hazardous solvents in organic and polymer chemistry.

THERAP CAT: Respiratory stimulant.

THERAP CAT (VET): Respiratory stimulant (inhalant).

1810. Carbon Diselenide. [506-80-9] Carbon selenide. CSe_2; mol wt 169.93. C 7.07%, Se 92.93%. Prepd by the action of methylene chloride vapor on heated selenium: Ives *et al., J. Chem. Soc.* **1947**, 1080; or from a mixture of CCl_4 and H_2Se in a stream of N_2 at 500°: Grimm, Metzger, *Ber.* **69**, 1356 (1936); from the elements by electrical discharge on Se vapor in the presence of sugar charcoal: Steudel, *Z. Anorg. Allg. Chem.* **361**, 195 (1968).

Light-sensitive, golden yellow, strongly refractive, liquid. Odor of rotten radishes. Turns brown to black on storage. d_4^{20} 2.6824; d_4^{25} 2.6626. mp −45.5°. bp 125-126°; bp$_{8.0}$ 10.0°. n_D^{20} 1.845. Heat of formation: 34 kcal/mol. Miscible with carbon tetrachloride, carbon disulfide, toluene, other organic solvents. Practically insol in water. Dec by alc, pyridine.

1811. Carbon Disulfide. [75-15-0] Carbon bisulfide; dithiocarbonic anhydride. CS_2; mol wt 76.14. C 15.77%, S

84.23%. Minute amounts occur in coal tar and in crude petroleum. Prepd on an industrial scale by heating charcoal with vaporized sulfur; from sulfur and natural gas: *Faith, Keyes & Clark's Industrial Chemicals,* F. A. Lowenheim, M. K. Moran, Eds. (Wiley-Interscience, New York, 4th ed., 1975) pp 224-229. Laboratory purification: Glemser in *Handbook of Preparative Inorganic Chemistry* vol. 1, G. Brauer, Ed. (Academic Press, New York, 2nd ed., 1963) p 652. Review of production and uses: Bushell, *Chem. Ind. (London)* **1961**, 1465; R. W. Timmerman in *Kirk-Othmer Encyclopedia of Chemical Technology* vol. 4 (Wiley-Interscience, New York, 3rd ed., 1978) pp 742-757; of toxicology and human exposure: *Toxicological Profile for Carbon Disulfide* (PB97-121073, 1996) 252 pp.

Highly refractive, mobile, very flammable liq. *Poisonous!* The purest distillates ever obtained are reported to have a sweet, pleasing, and ethereal odor, while the usual commercial and reagent grades are foul smelling. Dec on standing for a long time. Burns with a blue flame to CO_2 and SO_2. *Acute fire and explosion hazard,* can be ignited by hot steam pipes. Flash pt, closed cup: $-30°C$. Ignition pt: $100°$. Explosive range: 1 to 50% (v/v) in air. d_4^0 1.29272; d_4^{15} 1.27055; d_4^{20} 1.2632; d_4^{30} 1.24817. Vapors sink to the ground. Vapor density 2.67 (air 1). mp $-111.6°$. $bp_{1.0}$ $-73.8°$; bp_{10} $-44.7°$; bp_{100} $-5.1°$; bp_{400} 28.0°; bp_{760} 46.5°; $bp_{(2 atm)}$ 69.1°; $bp_{(5 atm)}$ 104.8°. Crit temp 280.0°; crit press. 72.9 atm. n_D^{15} 1.63189; $n_D^{20.1}$ 1.62803; $n^{23.5}$ 1.62543. Surface tension at 20°: 32.25. Coefficient of viscosity at 20°: 0.363. Heat of vaporization at bp: 84.1 cal/g. Heat of fusion: 1.049 kcal/mole. Heat capacity at 24.3°: 18.17 cal/mole/deg: Brown, Manov, *J. Am. Chem. Soc.* **59**, 500 (1937). Ebullioscopic constant: 2.35°. Dielectric constant at low frequencies: 2.641. Dipole moment: 0.0. Soly in water at 20°: 0.294%. Soly of water in CS_2: <0.005%. Azeotrope with water bp 42.6°, contains 97.2% CS_2. Misc with anhydr methanol, ethanol, ether, benzene, chloroform, carbon tetrachloride, oils. Can be stored in iron, aluminum, glass, porcelain, Teflon.

Caution: Poisoning usually occurs from inhalation but also may be caused by ingestion and skin absorption. Direct contact with liquid or concentrated vapors may cause irritation of skin, eyes, mucous membranes; eye and skin burns; dermatitis. Potential symptoms of acute overexposure are headache, garlicky breath, nausea, vomiting, diarrhea, fatigue, weakness, vertigo, dizziness, poor sleep; CNS depression with respiratory paralysis. Potential symptoms of chronic overexposure are nervousness, anorexia, weight loss; psychosis; polyneuropathy; Parkinson-like syndrome; ocular changes; coronary heart disease; gastritis; kidney and liver injury; reproductive effects; marked psychic disturbances ranging from extreme irritability to mania with hallucinations, tremors, auditory and visual disturbances. *See NIOSH Pocket Guide to Chemical Hazards* (DHHS/NIOSH 97-140, 1997) p 52; *Clinical Toxicology of Commercial Products,* R. E. Gosselin *et al.,* Eds. (Williams & Wilkins, Baltimore, 5th ed., 1984) Section III, pp 90-93.

USE: In the manuf of rayon, carbon tetrachloride, xanthogenates, soil disinfectants, electronic vacuum tubes. Solvent for phosphorus, sulfur, selenium, bromine, iodine, fats, resins, rubbers.

1812. Carbonic Anhydrase. [9001-03-0] Carbonate dihydratase; carbonate hydro-lyase. Mol wt ~30,000. A small zinc-contg enzyme which catalyzes the hydration of CO_2. Found in higher concns in erythrocytes, renal cortex, and gastric mucosa of mammals; also found in other animal tissues, in plants and in some bacteria. Isoln from bovine erythrocytes: Lindskog, *Biochim. Biophys. Acta* **39**, 218 (1960); from human erythrocytes: Nyman, *ibid.* **52**, 1 (1961); from renal cortex: Höber, *Proc. Soc. Exp. Biol. Med.* **49**, 87 (1942); from gastric mucosa: Davenport, *Physiol. Rev.* **26**, 560 (1946). Human carbonic anhydrase consists of two isoenzymes with distinctly different amino acid sequences and specific activities. The high activity form is called carbonic anhydrase C; the low activity form is called B; modified forms of these two isoenzymes exist: Funakoshi, Deutsch, *J. Biol. Chem.* **243**, 6474 (1968); **244**, 3438 (1969). Amino acid sequence of carbonic anhydrase B: Anderson *et al., Biochem. Biophys. Res. Commun.* **48**, 670 (1972); Lin, Deutsch, *J. Biol. Chem.* **248**, 1885 (1973); sequence of carbonic anhydrase C: Henderson, Henriksson, *Biochem. Biophys. Res. Commun.* **52**, 1388 (1973); Lin, Deutsch, *J. Biol. Chem.* **249**, 2329 (1974). Crystal structure of carbonic anhydrase C: Liljas *et al.,*

Nature New Biol. **235**, 131 (1972). Catalyzes the reversible reaction of CO_2 and H_2O to HCO_3^- and H^+. Permits CO interchange between blood and tissues. In gastric mucosa, reaction rate is sufficient to neutralize the excess alkalinity produced by the ionization of water and secretion of hydrogen ions: Roughton, Clark in *The Enzymes* vol. 1, part 2, J. B. Sumner, K. Myrbäck, Eds. (Academic Press, New York, 1951) pp 1250-1265. In the kidney, participates in Na^+ transport. Review of physiology: Maren in *Oxygen Affinity of Hemoglobin and Red Cell Acid Base Status, Alfred Benzon Symposium IV,* P. Astrup, M. Roerth, Eds. (Academic Press, New York, 1972) pp 418-433. Review of metal ion function: Prince, Woolley, *Angew. Chem. Int. Ed.* **11**, 408-417 (1972). *Review:* Lindskog *et al.,* "Carbonic Anhydrase" in *The Enzymes* vol. 5, P. D. Boyer, Ed. (Academic Press, New York, 1971) pp 587-665.

1813. Carbon Monoxide. [630-08-0] CO; mol wt 28.01. C 42.88%, O 57.12%. Produced on an industrial scale by partial oxidation of hydrocarbon gases from natural gas or by the gasification of coal and coke. Conveniently prepd in the laboratory by heating calcium carbonate with Zn dust: Weinhouse, *J. Am. Chem. Soc.* **70**, 442 (1948); by dehydration of formic acid with H_2SO_4: Gilliland, Blanchard, *Inorg. Synth.* **2**, 81 (1946). Purification of carbon monoxide bought in steel cylinders: A. Klemenc, *Die Behandlung und Reindarstellung von Gasen* (Vienna, 1948) p 160; Glemser in *Handbook of Preparative Inorganic Chemistry* vol. 1, G. Brauer, Ed. (Academic Press, New York, 2nd ed., 1963) p 646. *Review:* R. Pierantozzi in *Kirk-Othmer Encyclopedia of Chemical Technology* vol. 5 (Wiley-Interscience, New York, 4th ed., 1993) pp 97-122. Review of clinical toxicology: Stewart, *Annu. Rev. Biochem.* **15**, 409-423 (1975); D. Gorman *et al., Toxicology* **187**, 25-38 (2003); of industrial toxicology: *Patty's Industrial Hygiene and Toxicology* vol. 2F, G. D. Clayton, F. E. Clayton, Eds. (Wiley-Interscience, New York, 4th ed., 1994) pp 4523-4552.

Highly poisonous, odorless, colorless, tasteless gas. Very flammable, burns in air with a bright blue flame. Ignition pt in air: 700°. mp $-205.0°$. bp $-191.5°$. d_4^{-195} (liq) 0.814. d (gas) 0.968 (air 1.000). d_4^0 at 760 mm: 1.250 g/liter. The top pressure is 1500 psi. Flammable limits in air: 12 to 75 vol %. Crit press 35 atm, crit temp $-139°$. Heat capacity at 20°: 6.95 cal/mole/°C. Heat value per m^3: 3033 kcal. Heat of formation: -26.39 kcal/mol. Dec into carbon and carbon dioxide between 400 and 700°, at lower temp when in contact with catalytic surfaces. Above 800° the equilibrium reaction favors CO formation. Hopcalite, a mixture of the oxides of manganese and copper, catalyzes the decompn at room temp, as does Pd on silica gel. Sparingly sol in water: 3.3 ml/100 ml H_2O at 0°; 2.3 ml/100 ml H_2O at 20°; freely absorbed by a concd soln of cuprous chloride in HCl or in NH_4OH. Appreciably sol in some organic solvents, such as ethyl acetate, $CHCl_3$, acetic acid. The soly in methanol and ethanol is about 7 times as great as the soly in water.

Caution: Combines with the hemoglobin in the blood to form carboxyhemoglobin which disrupts oxygen transport and delivery throughout the body. Potential symptoms of overexposure by inhalation are headache, tachypnea, nausea, vomiting, lassitude, fatigue, dizziness, confusion, hallucinations; dimness of vision; irritability, impaired judgement; cyanosis; depression of S-T segment of electrocardiogram, angina, syncope; coma. *See NIOSH Pocket Guide to Chemical Hazards* (DHHS/NIOSH 97-140, 2003) p 54; *Clinical Toxicology of Commercial Products,* R. E. Gosselin *et al.,* Eds. (Williams & Wilkins, Baltimore, 5th ed., 1984) Section III, pp 94-101.

USE: As reducing agent in metallurgical operations especially in the Mond process for the recovery of nickel; in organic synthesis especially in the Fischer-Tropsch processes for petroleum-type products and in the oxo reaction; in the manuf of metal carbonyls.

1814. Carbon Nitride. [143334-20-7] C_3N_4; mol wt 92.06. C 39.14%, N 60.86%. Covalent crystalline solid which exists in two forms α and β. β-form may be harder than diamond. Model of structure and hardness: A. Y. Liu, M. L. Cohen, *Science* **245**, 841 (1989). Synthesis: E. E. Haller *et al.,* **WO 9116196**; *eidem,* **US 5110679** (1991, 1992 both to Regents U. California, Berkeley); C. Niu *et al., Science* **261**, 334 (1993). Hardness evaluation: O. Fukunaga, *Kagaku to Kyoiku* **41**, 325 (1993), *C.A.* **119**, 54572g (1993).

1815. Carbon Suboxide. [504-64-3] 1,2-Propadiene-1,3-dione; tricarbon dioxide. C_3O_2; mol wt 68.03. C 52.97%, O 47.04%. O=C=C=C=O. Prepn by thermal decompn of malonic acid: Glemser in *Handbook of Preparative Inorganic Chemistry* vol. 1, G. Brauer, Ed. (Academic Press, New York, 2nd ed., 1963) p 648. Reactions in organic synthesis: Dashkevich, Beilin, *Russ. Chem. Rev.* **36**, 391 (1967). Comprehensive reviews: Reyerson, Kobe, *Chem. Rev.* **7**, 479 (1930); Vol'kenshtein, *Usp. Khim.* **4**, 610 (1935); Grauer, *Chimia* **14**, 11 (1960); T. Kappe, E. Ziegler, *Angew. Chem. Int. Ed.* **13**, 491-504 (1974), reprinted in *New Synthetic Methods* vol. 1 (Verlag Chemie, Weinheim, 1975) pp 29-69.

Colorless, highly refractive liquid or colorless gas which burns with a blue, sooty flame. Odor like acrolein and mustard oil. mp −111.3°. bp$_{760}$ 6.8°. d$_4^0$ 1.114. n_D^0 1.45384; n_D^{-12} 1.46757. Vapor pressure at 0°: 587-589 mm. Explosive limits, 6 to 30 vol % in air. Dipole moment: 0.7D. Thermodynamic constants: Thompson, *Trans. Faraday Soc.* **37**, 249 (1941). The gas can be stored at pressures of up to 100 mm, but even at these pressures polymerization may occur, giving a red, water-sol product. This invariably occurs at higher pressure or in the liquid state. Polymerization facilitated by presence of P_2O_5. Dec when passed through heated glass tubes, forming a mirror surface. Difficultly sol in carbon disulfide, xylene. With water forms malonic acid quantitatively. Forms malonamide with ammonia.

Caution: In small amounts acts as a lacrimator; in high concns attacks eyes, nose, respiratory organs, producing a feeling of suffocation.

USE: Prepn of malonates; improving dye affinity of fibers.

1816. Carbon Tetrachloride. [56-23-5] Tetrachloromethane; perchloromethane; Necatorina; Benzinoform. CCl_4; mol wt 153.82. C 7.81%, Cl 92.19%. Obtained from carbon disulfide and chlorine in presence of a catalyst, e.g., $SbCl_5$, Fe filings, or by the chlorination of hydrocarbons: *Faith, Keyes & Clark's Industrial Chemicals*, F. A. Lowenheim, M. K. Moran, Eds. (Wiley-Interscience, New York, 4th ed., 1975) pp 230-234; H. D. DeShon in *Kirk-Othmer Encyclopedia of Chemical Technology* vol. 5 (Wiley-Interscience, New York, 3rd ed., 1979) pp 704-714. Toxicity data: Svirbely, *J. Ind. Hyg. Toxicol.* **29**, 382 (1947); E. Browning, *Toxicity and Metabolism of Industrial Solvents* (Elsevier, New York, 1965) pp 173-188. Use in induction of experimental liver damage: P. Trivedi, A. P. Mowat, *Br. J. Exp. Pathol.* **64**, 25 (1983). Review of carcinogenic risk: *IARC Monographs* **20**, 371-399 (1979); of toxicity studies: R. O. Recknagel *et al., Pharmacol. Ther.* **43**, 139-154 (1989); of toxicology and environmental exposure: *Environ. Health Criter.* **208**, 1-177 (1999); of toxicology and human exposure: *Toxicological Profile for Carbon Tetrachloride* (PB2006-100002, 2005) 361 pp.

Colorless, clear, nonflammable, heavy liquid; characteristic odor. May form phosgene when used to put out electrical fires. *Use only when adequate ventilation is possible.* d$_{25}^{25}$ 1.589. bp 76.7°. mp −23°. n_D^{20} 1.4607. One ml dissolves in 2000 ml water; misc with alcohol, benzene, chloroform, ether, carbon disulfide, petr ether, oils. LC$_{50}$ for mice: 9528 ppm (Svirbely). LD$_{50}$ in rats, mice, dogs (g/kg): 2.92, 12.1-14.4, 2.3 orally; LD$_{50}$ in mice (g/kg): 4.1 i.p., 30.4 s.c. (IARC, 1979).

Caution: Potential symptoms of overexposure are CNS depression; drowsiness, dizziness, incoordination; nausea, vomiting; liver and kidney injury. Direct contact may cause skin and eye irritation; dermatitis through defatting action. *See NIOSH Pocket Guide to Chemical Hazards* (PB2003-100121, 2003) p 54; *Patty's Industrial Hygiene and Toxicology* vol. 2E, G. D. Clayton, F. E. Clayton, Eds. (Wiley-Interscience, New York, 4th ed., 1994) p 4071-4080. This substance is reasonably anticipated to be a human carcinogen: *Report on Carcinogens, Eleventh Edition* (PB2005-104914, 2004) p III-44.

USE: As solvent for oils, fats, lacquers, varnishes, rubber waxes, resins; starting material in manuf of organic compds. Pharmaceutic aid (solvent). Formerly used as dry cleaning agent, fire extinguisher and grain fumigant.

THERAP CAT: Formerly as anthelmintic (Nematodes).

THERAP CAT (VET): Anthelmintic.

1817. Carbon Tetrafluoride. [75-73-0] Tetrafluoromethane; Freon 14. CF_4; mol wt 88.00. C 13.65%, F 86.36%. Prepd from carbon or carbon monoxide and fluorine: Yost, *Inorg. Synth.*

1, 34 (1939); Simons, Block, *J. Am. Chem. Soc.* **61**, 2962 (1939); Kwasnik in *Handbook of Preparative Inorganic Chemistry* vol 1, G. Brauer, Ed. (Academic Press, New York, 2nd ed., 1963) p 203. May also be prepd from SiC + F_2: Priest, *Inorg. Synth.* **3**, 178 (1950).

Colorless, odorless gas. Thermally stable. Chemically very inert. d (solid, −195°) 1.98. d (liq, −183°) 1.89. mp −183.6°. bp −127.8°. May be stored in steel cylinders.

Caution: Narcotic in high concns.

USE: Low temp refrigerant; gaseous insulator.

1818. Carbon Tetraiodide. [507-25-5] Tetraiodomethane. CI_4; mol wt 519.63. C 2.31%, I 97.69%. Prepd by the interaction of carbon tetrachloride and aluminum or calcium iodide: Gustavson, *Ann.* **172**, 173 (1874); boron iodide: Moissan, *C.R. Hebd. Seances Acad. Sci.* **113**, 19 (1891); lithium or calcium iodide: Lantenois, *ibid.* **156**, 1385 (1913); ethyl iodide in the presence of aluminum chloride: Walker, *J. Chem. Soc.* **85**, 1090 (1904); McArthur, Simons, *Inorg. Synth.* **3**, 37 (1950).

Red cubic crystals. Odor of iodine. Dec to iodine and tetraiodoethylene under the influence of light or heat. d$_4^{20}$ 4.32. mp 171°. Sol in benzene, chloroform. Dec by hot alcohol. Practically insol in water, but hydrolyzes slowly in contact with water, forming iodoform and iodine.

1819. N,N′-Carbonyldiimidazole. [530-62-1] 1,1′-Carbonylbis-1*H*-imidazole. $C_7H_6N_4O$; mol wt 162.15. C 51.85%, H 3.73%, N 34.55%, O 9.87%. Prepd from phosgene and imidazole in dry tetrahydrofuran or dry benzene: Staab, *Ann.* **609**, 75 (1957); Anderson, Paul, *J. Am. Chem. Soc.* **80**, 4423 (1958).

Crystals from tetrahydrofuran or benzene, mp 115.5-116°. Should be handled under exclusion of atmospheric moisture. Hydrolyzed by water in a few sec with evolution of CO_2.

USE: In the synthesis of peptides. Reacts readily with carboxylic acids to form acyl imidazoles; subsequent reaction with amines to form amides goes smoothly.

1820. Carbonyl Fluoride. [353-50-4] Carbonic difluoride; fluophosgene. CF_2O; mol wt 66.01. C 18.20%, F 57.56%, O 24.24%. COF$_2$. Prepd from CO and F_2 or BrF$_3$ and CO: Ruff, Miltschitzky, *Z. Anorg. Allg. Chem.* **221**, 154 (1935); Kwasnik in *Handbook of Preparative Inorganic Chemistry* vol. 1, G. Brauer, Ed. (Academic Press, New York, 2nd ed., 1963) p 206. Alternate route from CO + AgF$_2$: Farlow *et al., Inorg. Synth.* **6**, 155 (1960).

Pungent, very hygroscopic gas. d (solid, −190°): 1.388. d (liq, −114°): 1.139. mp −114.0°. bp −83.1°. Heat of formation: 166.6 kcal. Instantly hydrolyzed by water.

Caution: Potential symptoms of overexposure are irritation of eyes, skin, mucous membranes, respiratory system; eye, skin burns; lacrimation; cough, pulmonary edema, dyspnea; direct contact with liquid may cause frostbite. Chronic exposure may cause GI pain, muscular fibrosis, skeletal fluorosis. *See NIOSH Pocket Guide to Chemical Hazards* (DHHS/NIOSH 97-140, 1997) p 54.

1821. Carbonyl Sulfide. [463-58-1] Carbon oxide sulfide (COS); carbon oxysulfide. COS; mol wt 60.08. C 19.99%, O 26.63%, S 53.37%. O=C=S. Fluid found in petroleum and coal refinery gases and in coal gasification streams; impurity in commercial sources of propane. Prepn: C. Than, *Ann.* **5**, 236 (1867). Thermodynamic properties: J. D. Kemp, W. F. Giauque, *J. Am. Chem. Soc.* **59**, 79 (1937). Photolysis and extinction coefficient measurements: G. S. Forbes, J. E. Cline, *ibid.* **61**, 151 (1939). Potentiometric determn in petroleum gases: D. B. Bruss *et al., Anal. Chem.* **29**, 807 (1957). Hydrolysis in water-propane systems: W. C. Andersen, T. J. Bruno, *Ind. Eng. Chem. Res.* **42**, 963 (2003). Use as a grain fumigant: H. J. Banks *et al.,* WO 9313659; *eidem,* US 6203824 (1993, 2001 both to CSIRO). Uptake in grain products: P. C. Annis *et al., J. Agric. Food Chem.* **48**, 3646 (2000). Review of chemistry: R. J. Ferm, *Chem. Rev.* **57**, 621-640 (1957); P. D. N. Svoronos, T. J. Bruno, *Ind. Eng. Chem. Res.* **41**, 5321-5336 (2002); of development as a fumigant: E. J. Wright, *Proc. Austral.*

Postharvest Tech. Conf., Canberra 2003 224-229 (2003); of toxicology: A. R. Bartholomaeus, V. S. Haritos, *Food Chem. Toxicol.* **43**, 1687-1701 (2005).

Colorless gas, bp −50.2°. mp −138.8°. Odorless when very pure. n 1.3785. Liquid density (174 K): 1.274 g/cm^3. Vapor density (25°, 1 atm): 2.4849 ±0.0005 g/l. Critical temp 105°. Critical press 61 atm. Soly at 1 atm (ml/ml): water 0.80 (13.5°); toluene 15.0 (22.0°). Log P (octanol/water): ~0.8. uv max: 208, 225 nm. *Flammable in air at conc. of 12-28.5% (v/v).* LD$_{50}$ i.p. in rats: 22.5 mg/kg. LC$_{50}$ by inhalation (mg/m^3): 2940 in mice (35 min); 2650 in rats (4 h) (Bartholomaeus, Haritos).

Caution: Potential symptoms of overexposure are related to carbonyl sulfide hydrolysis to form hydrogen sulfide, *q.v.*

USE: Grain fumigant.

1822. Carboplatin. [41575-94-4] (*SP*-4-2)-Diammine[1,1-cyclobutanedi(carboxylato-κO)(2−)]platinum; 1,1-cyclobutanedicarboxylic acid platinum complex; *cis*-diammine(1,1-cyclobutanedicarboxylato)platinum(II); CBDCA; JM-8; NSC-241240; Paraplatin. C$_6$H$_{12}$N$_2$O$_4$Pt; mol wt 371.25. C 19.41%, H 3.26%, N 7.55%, O 17.24%, Pt 52.55%. Analog of cisplatin, *q.v.*, with reduced nephrotoxicity. Prepn and antitumor activity: NL 7307863; M. J. Cleare *et al.*, US 4140707 (1973, 1979 both to Research Corp.). Improved prepn: R. C. Harrison *et al., Inorg. Chim. Acta* **46**, L15 (1980). Crystal structure: S. Neidle *et al., J. Inorg. Biochem.* **13**, 205 (1980). Comparison with other antitumor platinum complexes: M. J. Cleare *et al., Biochimie* **60**, 835 (1978). Early clinical studies: A. H. Calvert *et al., Cancer Chemother. Pharmacol.* **9**, 140 (1982). Clinical pharmacokinetics: S. J. Harland *et al., Cancer Res.* **44**, 1693 (1984); M. J. Egorin *et al., ibid.* 5432. Toxicity, activity in mice, rats, dogs: P. Lelieveld *et al., Eur. J. Cancer Clin. Oncol.* **20**, 1087 (1984). Comparison with cisplatin chemotherapy in advanced seminoma: M. J. Peckham *et al., Br. J. Cancer* **52**, 7 (1985). In treatment of small cell lung cancer: I. E. Smith *et al., Cancer Treat. Rep.* **69**, 43 (1985).

White crystals, sol in water. LD$_{50}$ in mice (mg/kg): 150 i.p., 140 i.v.; in rats (mg/kg): 85 i.v. (Lelieveld).

THERAP CAT: Antineoplastic.

1823. Carboprost. [35700-23-3] (5*Z*,9α,11α,13*E*,15*S*)-9,11,15-Trihydroxy-15-methylprosta-5,13-dien-1-oic acid; 7-[3,5-dihydroxy-2-(3-hydroxy-3-methyl-1-octenyl)cyclopentyl]-5-heptenoic acid; (15*S*)-15-methyl PGF$_{2\alpha}$; U-32921. C$_{21}$H$_{36}$O$_5$; mol wt 368.51. C 68.44%, H 9.85%, O 21.71%. Analog of prostaglandin F$_{2\alpha}$, *q.v.* Prepn: G. L. Bundy *et al.*, DE 2121980; G. L. Bundy, US 3728382 (1971, 1973 both to Upjohn); *eidem, Ann. N.Y. Acad. Sci.* **180**, 76 (1971); E. W. Yankee *et al., J. Am. Chem. Soc.* **96**, 5865 (1974). Biological activity: J. R. Weeks *et al., J. Pharmacol. Exp. Ther.* **186**, 67 (1973). Mechanism of action: A. I. Csapo, M. O. Pulkkinen, *Prostaglandins* **18**, 479 (1979). Clinical studies: P. C. Schwallie, K. R. Lamborn, *J. Reprod. Med.* **23**, 289 (1979); M. P. Mapa *et al., Int. J. Gynaecol. Obstet.* **20**, 125 (1982). Teratological study: G. M. Szczech *et al., Adv. Prostaglandin Thromboxane Res.* **4**, 157 (1978).

Tromethamine salt. [58551-69-2] Carboprost trometamol; U-32921E; Hemabate; Prostin/15M. C$_{25}$H$_{47}$NO$_8$; mol wt 489.64.

Methyl ester. [35700-21-1] Carboprost methyl; U-36384. C$_{22}$H$_{38}$O$_5$; mol wt 382.53. Crystals from ether/hexane, mp 55-56°. [α]$_D$ +24° (c 0.81 in ethanol).

THERAP CAT: Oxytocic.

1824. Carboquone. [24279-91-2] 2-[2-[(Aminocarbonyl)-oxy]-1-methoxyethyl]-3,6-bis(1-aziridinyl)-5-methyl-2,5-cyclo-hexadiene-1,4-dione; 2,5-bis(1-aziridinyl)-3-(2-hydroxy-1-meth-oxyethyl)-6-methyl-*p*-benzoquinone carbamate (ester); 2,5-bis(1-aziridinyl)-3-(2-carbamoyloxy-1-methoxyethyl)-6-methyl-1,4-ben-zoquinone; carbazilquinone; Esquinon. C$_{15}$H$_{19}$N$_3$O$_5$; mol wt 321.33. C 56.07%, H 5.96%, N 13.08%, O 24.90%. Prepn and antitumor activity: Nakao *et al., Chem. Pharm. Bull.* **20**, 1968 (1972); T. Nakamura *et al.*, DE 1905224; H. Nakao *et al.*, US 3631026 (1969, 1971 both to Sankyo). Effect on tumors in mice: Arakawa *et al., Gann* **61**, 535 (1970). Acute toxicity: H. Masuda, Y. Suzuki, *Oyo Yakuri* **8**, 501 (1974), *C.A.* **81**, 163349g (1974).

Red to reddish-brown crystals, mp 202° (dec). Slightly sol in chloroform, acetone, abs alcohol. Practically insol in water. LD$_{50}$ in male mice, male rats (mg/kg): 6.09, 3.88 i.v.; 3.84, 3.16 i.p.; 30.8, 28.0 orally (Masuda, Suzuki).

THERAP CAT: Antineoplastic.

1825. Carbostyril. [59-31-4] 2(1*H*)-Quinolinone; 2-hy-droxyquinoline; 2-quinolinol; 2(1*H*)-quinolone; *o*-aminocinnamic acid lactam. C$_9$H$_7$NO; mol wt 145.16. C 74.47%, H 4.86%, N 9.65%, O 11.02%. Prepn from quinoline by heating with potassium hydroxide to 225° under anhyd conditions: Tschitschibabin, *Ber.* **56**, 1883 (1923); DE 406208; *Chem. Zentralbl.* **1925, I**, 1536; *Frdl.* **14**, 515.

Prisms from methanol, mp 199-200°. Sublimes at atmospheric pressure without dec. A monohydrate has been obtained from a satd aq soln. pKb (18°) 8.71. Very sparingly sol in water: One gram dissolves in 950 ml H$_2$O at 22°. Sol in alcohol, ether, dil HCl. Forms easily hydrolyzed Na and K salts.

Compd with 1,3,5-trinitrobenzene. (C$_9$H$_7$NO)$_2$·C$_6$H$_3$N$_3$O$_6$. Yellow needles, mp 178°.

1826. Carbosulfan. [55285-14-8] [(Dibutylamino)thio]-methylcarbamic acid 2,3-dihydro-2,2-dimethyl-7-benzofuranyl es-ter; FMC-35001; Marshal; Posse. C$_{20}$H$_{32}$N$_2$O$_3$S; mol wt 380.54. C 63.12%, H 8.48%, N 7.36%, O 12.61%, S 8.43%. Carbamate cholinesterase inhibitor which is hydrolyzed to carbofuran in soil. Prepn: A. L. Black, T. R. Fukuto, BE 817517; *eidem*, US 4006231 (1975, 1977 both to Regents Univ. Calif.). Metabolism in orange tree leaves and fruit: V. E. Clay, T. R. Fukuto, *Arch. Environ. Contam. Toxicol.* **13**, 53 (1984). Degradation and persistence in soil: A. Sahoo *et al., Bull. Environ. Contam. Toxicol.* **50**, 29 (1993). HPLC determn in oranges: M.W. Brooks, A. Barros, *Analyst* **120**, 2479 (1995). Spectrophotometric determn in formulations and water samples: K. R. Mohan *et al., Asian J. Chem.* **10**, 457 (1998). Review of physical properties and field trials: E. G. Mait-len, N. A. Sladen, *Proc. Br. Crop Prot. Conf. - Pests Dis.* **1979**, 557-564.

Viscous, brown liquid. Soly in water at 25°: 0.3 ppm. Soly in organic solvents: > 50%. Vapor pressure: 0.31 × 10^{-6} mmHg.

LD$_{50}$ in male, female rats (mg/kg): 250, 185 orally; in male, female rabbits (mg/kg): >2000, >2000 dermally; in pheasant, mallard, quail (ppm): 26.2, 8.1, 81.6 orally. LC$_{50}$ (96 hr) in bluegill, trout (ppb): 14.9, 42.4 (Maitlen).

USE: Insecticide.

1827. Carboxin. [5234-68-4] 5,6-Dihydro-2-methyl-*N*-phenyl-1,4-oxathiin-3-carboxamide; 2,3-dihydro-5-carboxanilido-6-methyl-1,4-oxathiin; carbathiin; DCMO; Vitavax. C$_{12}$H$_{13}$NO$_2$-S; mol wt 235.30. C 61.25%, H 5.57%, N 5.95%, O 13.60%, S 13.63%. Systemic fungicide, effective against loose smut in cereals. Prepn: B. von Schmeling *et al.*, US 3249499 (1966 to U.S. Rubber); M. Kulka *et al.*, US 3393202 (1968 to Uniroyal). Fungicidal activity: B. von Schmeling, M. Kulka, *Science* 152, 659 (1966). Inhibitor of succinate oxidation: D. E. Mathre, *Phytopathology* 60, 671 (1970); G. A. White, *Biochem. Biophys. Res. Commun.* 44, 1212 (1971); P. C. Mowery *et al.*, *ibid.* 71, 354 (1976). Residue determn in crops: J. R. Lane, *J. Agric. Food Chem.* 18, 409 (1970); H. R. Sisken, J. E. Newell, *ibid.* 19, 738 (1971). Toxicity studies: T. V. Dyadicheva, *Gig. Tr. Prof. Zabol.* 1979(2), 55, *C.A.* 90, 146673b (1979).

Crystals, from ethanol or methanol, mp 93-95°. LD$_{50}$ in rats, mice (mg/kg): 430, 3200 orally (Dyadicheva).

USE: Systemic plant fungicide.

1828. γ-Carboxyglutamic Acid. [53861-57-7] 3-Amino-1,1,3-propanetricarboxylic acid; γ-carboxy-L-glutamic acid; L-γ-carboxyglutamic acid; Gla. C$_6$H$_9$NO$_6$; mol wt 191.14. C 37.70%, H 4.75%, N 7.33%, O 50.22%. Amino acid found in blood coagulation proteins (prothrombin, Factor VII, Factor IX, Factor X, *q.q.v.*), plasma proteins and proteins from calcified tissue. Presence of Gla confers metal binding properties to the protein. Discovery in prothrombin: J. Stenflo, *Proc. Natl. Acad. Sci. USA* 71, 2730 (1974); G. L. Nelsestuen *et al.*, *J. Biol. Chem.* 249, 6347 (1974). Synthesis: S. Danishefsky *et al.*, *J. Am. Chem. Soc.* 101, 4385 (1979); of DL-form: H. R. Morris *et al.*, *Biochem. Biophys. Res. Commun.* 62, 856 (1975); W. Märki, R. Schwyzer, *Helv. Chim. Acta* 58, 1471 (1975); B. Weinstein *et al.*, *J. Org. Chem.* 41, 3634 (1976). Resolution of D- and L-forms: W. Märki *et al.*, *Helv. Chim. Acta* 60, 798 (1977). Biosynthesis by vitamin K-dependent carboxylation of glutamic acid: C. T. Esmon *et al.*, *J. Biol. Chem.* 250, 4744 (1975). Metal binding properties: G. L. Nelsestuen *et al.*, *Biochem. Biophys. Res. Commun.* 65, 233 (1975); G. L. Nelsestuen, *J. Biol. Chem.* 251, 5648 (1976); R. Robertson *et al.*, *ibid.* 253, 5880 (1978); S. P. Bajaj *et al.*, *ibid.* 257, 3726 (1982). HPLC determn in proteins, bone, urine: M. Kuwada, K. Katayama, *Anal. Biochem.* 117, 259 (1981). *Reviews:* J. Stenflo, J. W. Suttie, *Annu. Rev. Biochem.* 46, 157-172 (1977); R. E. Olson, J. W. Suttie, *Vitam. Horm.* 35, 59-108 (1977); J. W. Suttie, *Crit. Rev. Biochem.* 8, 191-223 (1980); J. P. Burnier *et al.*, *Mol. Cell. Biochem.* 39, 191-207 (1981).

Crystals, mp 167-167.5° (dec). [α]$_D^{20}$ +35.3° (c = 1 in 6*N* HCl). **DL-Form.** White powder, mp 90-92°.

1829. Carboxymethylcellulose Sodium. [9004-32-4] Carboxymethyl ether cellulose sodium salt; sodium carboxymethylcellulose; sodium cellulose glycolate; Cethylose; CMC; Cel-O-Brandt; Glykocellon; Carbose D; Xylo-Mucine; Tylose MGA; Cellolax; Polycell. R$_n$OCH$_2$COONa. Prepd by treating alkali cellulose with sodium chloroacetate: *Faith, Keyes & Clark's Industrial Chemicals*, F. A. Lowenheim, M. K. Moran, Eds. (Wiley-Inter-

science, New York, 4th ed., 1975) pp 235-238. Review and bibliography: Ott, *Cellulose and Cellulose Derivatives,* New York, 1946 (2nd ed., 1955).

White granules. Soly in water depends on degree of substitution. Water-soluble CMC is available in various viscosities (5-2000 cP in 1% soln), and the soly is equally good in hot and cold water (difference from methyl cellulose). Also the presence of metal salts has little effect on the viscosity. Solns are stable between pH 2 and 10. Below pH 2 precipitation of a solid occurs, above pH 10 the viscosity decreases rapidly. pKa 4.30. The free acid is obtained from aq soln at pH 2.5 and may be precipitated with alcohol.

USE: In drilling muds, in detergents as a soil-suspending agent, in resin emulsion paints, adhesives, printing inks, textile sizes, as protective colloid in general. As stabilizer in foods. Pharmaceutic aid (suspending agent; tablet excipient; viscosity-increasing agent).

1830. Carboxypolymethylene. [9007-20-9] Carbomer; carbopol; carboxyvinyl polymer. A vinyl polymer with active carboxyl groups. Description: *Chem. Eng. News* 36, 64 (Sept. 29, 1958).

White powder. Highly ionic and slightly acidic. Reacts with fatty amines to form thick and stable emulsions of oils in water.

USE: Thickening, suspending, dispersing, emulsifying agent. In the cosmetic and textile printing fields, in printing inks, in emulsion-based lubricants, in pharmaceuticals, polishes, waxes, paints, waterproof and oil-proof coatings, in industrial specialties.

1831. Carbromal. [77-65-6] *N*-(Aminocarbonyl)-2-bromo-2-ethylbutanamide; (α-bromo-α-ethylbutyryl)urea; (α-bromo-α-ethylbutyryl)carbamide; bromodiethylacetylurea; bromodiethylacetylcarbamide; Tildin; Adalin; Planadalin; Diacid; Addisomnol; Bromadal; Uradal; Nyctal. C$_7$H$_{13}$BrN$_2$O$_2$; mol wt 237.09. C 35.46%, H 5.53%, Br 33.70%, N 11.82%, O 13.50%. (C$_2$H$_5$)$_2$CBr-CONHCONH$_2$. Prepd by heating urea (to ~50°) with α-bromo-α-ethylbutyryl bromide (C$_2$H$_5$)$_2$CBrCOBr, *see* DE 225710 (1910); *Frdl.* 10, 1160; *Chem. Zentralbl.* 1910, II, 1008. Patent literature: Slotta, *Grundriss der modernen Arzneistoff-Synthese* (Stuttgart, 1931); H. P. Kaufmann, *Arzneimittel-Synthese* (Berlin, 1953).

Crystals, mp 116-119°. One gram dissolves in about 3000 ml water, 18 ml alcohol, 3 ml chloroform, 14 ml ether. Very sol in boiling alcohol; dissolves in concd sulfuric, nitric and hydrochloric acids, from which it is precipitated on dilution with water. Dissolved by solns of alkali hydroxides.

THERAP CAT: Sedative, hypnotic.

1832. Carbutamide. [339-43-5] 4-Amino-*N*-[(butylamino)carbonyl]benzenesulfonamide; 1-butyl-3-sulfanilylurea; *N*^{1}-(butylcarbamoyl)sulfanilamide; *N*^{1}-sulfanilyl-*N*^{2}-butylurea; *N*^{1}-sulfanilyl-*N*^{2}-butylcarbamide; *N*-(4-aminobenzenesulfonyl)-*N*'-butylurea; aminophenurobutane; BZ-55; U-6987; Bucarban; Glucidoral; Glucofren; Invenol; Nadisan. C$_{11}$H$_{17}$N$_3$O$_3$S; mol wt 271.34. C 48.69%, H 6.31%, N 15.49%, O 17.69%, S 11.82%. *Ref:* Achelis, Hardebeck, *Dtsch. Med. Wochenschr.* 80, 1452 (1955); Achelis *et al.*, *Arch. Exp. Pathol. Pharmakol.* 228, 163 (1956). Prepn from butylurea and sulfanilamide: Samaniego, ES 229696 (1956), *C.A.* 51, 7413 (1957); E. Haack, A. Hagedorn, US 2907692 (1959 to Boehringer, Mann.).

Crystals, mp 144-145°. Sol in water at pH 5 to 8. LD$_{50}$ s.c. in mice: 3 g/kg (Haack, Hagedorn).

THERAP CAT: Antidiabetic.

1833. Carbuterol. [34866-47-2] [5-[2-[(1,1-Dimethylethyl)amino]-1-hydroxyethyl]-2-hydroxyphenyl]urea; α-(*t*-butylaminomethyl)-4-hydroxy-3-ureidobenzyl alcohol. C$_{13}$H$_{21}$N$_3$O$_3$; mol wt 267.32. C 58.41%, H 7.92%, N 15.72%, O 17.96%. A β-adrenergic agonist related to isoproterenol, *q.v.*, with selectivity for airway smooth muscle receptors. Prepn: C. Kaiser, S. T. Ross, DE 2106620; *eidem*, US 3763232 (1971, 1973 both to SKF); C. Kaiser *et al.*, *J. Med. Chem.* 17, 49 (1974). Pharmacology, mechanism of action, toxicity study: J. R. Wardell *et al.*, *J. Pharmacol. Exp. Ther.*

189, 167 (1974). Analysis in aq soln: L. J. Ravin *et al.*, *J. Pharm. Sci.* **67**, 1523 (1978). Clinical study: T. D. James, H. A. Lyons, *J. Am. Med. Assoc.* **241**, 704 (1979).

Crystals, mp 174-176°. LD$_{50}$ in mice (mg/kg): 32.8 i.v.; 3134.6 orally; in rats: 77.2 i.v. (Wardell).

Hydrochloride. [34866-46-1] SKF-40383; Bronsecur; Pirem. C$_{13}$H$_{21}$N$_3$O$_3$·HCl; mol wt 303.79. Crystals from ethanol/ether, mp 205-207° (dec).

THERAP CAT: Bronchodilator.

1834. Cardamom. Perennial, ginger-like plant, *Elettaria cardamomum* L. Maton, *Zingiberaceae*; seeds and volatile oil have been used since ancient times in cooking and traditional medicine. Numerous cultivars are grown, paticularly the Malabar and Mysore varieties. Plants of *Amomum sp.* and *Afromomum sp.* yield seeds of similar flavor, but are considered inferior to true cardamom. *Habit:* India; cultivated in Sri Lanka, Guatemala, Tanzania. *Constit:* Mature seeds contain volatile oil (6.5-10.5%); crude fiber (6.7-12.8%); protein (8.8-10.5%); starch (38-47%); ash (3.8-6.7%); fixed oil containing glycerides of oleic, stearic, linoleic, palmitic, caprylic and caproic acids. Comprehensive review: V. S. Govindarajan *et al.*, *Crit. Rev. Food Sci. Nutr.* **16**, 229-326 (1982). Review of medicinal uses: A. Y. Leung, S. Foster, *Encyclopedia of Common Natural Ingredients*, (Wiley-Interscience, Hoboken, 2nd Ed., 2003) pp 121-122; J. Gruenwald *et al.*, *PDR for Herbal Medicines* (Medical Economics, Montvale, 3rd Ed., 2004) pp 157-158.

Volatile oil. [8000-66-6] Oil of cardamom. Usually obtained by steam distillation from the ripe seeds. *Constit.* Complex mixture, mainly α-terpinyl acetate (28-42%); 1,8-cineole (21-41%), linalyl acetate, limonene, linalool. Description: E. Guenther, *The Essential Oils* vol. V (New York, 1952) pp 85-106. Composition studies: Y. S. Lewis *et al.*, *Perfum. Essent. Oil Rec.* **57**, 623 (1966). Supercritical fluid extraction and analysis: B. Marongiu *et al.*, *J. Agric. Food Chem.* **52**, 6278 (2004). Colorless or pale yellow liquid. Warm and spicy flavor with camphoraceous and lemony undertones. d$_4^{25}$ 0.917-0.947. Angular rotation: +22 to +44°. n$_D^{20}$ 1.462-1.466. Sapon. value: 91.6 to 144.7. Acid value: 1.7 to 7.1. Sol in benzyl alcohol, diethyl phthalate, fixed oil, mineral oil, in 5 vols 70% alcohol. Insol in glycerin, propylene glycol. *Keep well closed, cool and protected from light.*

USE: Flavoring in baked goods, confectionery, coffee, tea; component of curry powder and garam masala. Pharmaceutic aid (flavor). Fragrance component of perfumes, soaps, lotions.

THERAP CAT: Carminative.

1835. Cardiotoxin. [11061-96-4] One of the toxic principles from cobra venom. Isoln: Sarkar, *J. Indian Chem. Soc.* **21**, 227 (1947). A single peptide chain composed of 60 amino acid residues cross-linked by four disulfide bridges with leucine and asparagine at the N and C terminals respectively: Narita, Lee, *Biochem. Biophys. Res. Commun.* **41**, 339 (1970). Causes irreversible depolarization of cell membrane and contraction of skeletal and smooth muscle. Shows direct lytic and marked cardiotoxic activities, potentiated by phospholipase A and prevented by polyanions (heparin, RNA, gangliosides). Pharmacology: Lee *et al.*, *Arch. Exp. Pathol. Pharmakol.* **259**, 360 (1968).

1836. 3-Carene. [13466-78-9] 3,7,7-Trimethylbicyclo[4.1.0]hept-3-ene; Δ^3-carene; 4,7,7-trimethyl-3-norcarene; isodiprene. C$_{10}$H$_{16}$; mol wt 136.23. C 88.16%, H 11.84%. Constituent of turpentine. The turpentine from *Pinus sylvestris* L. may contain as much as 42%, turpentine from *Pinus longifolia* Roxb., *Pinaceae* about 30%. Isoln and structure: Simonsen, *The Terpenes* vol. II (Cambridge, 1949) pp 64-72; Guenther, *The Essential Oils* vol. II (Van Nostrand, 1949) pp 49-51. Conformation: Acharya, *Tetrahedron Lett.* **1966**, 4117. Absorption spectrum: Cole, *J. Chem. Soc.* **1954**, 3807.

d-Form. Mobile liquid. Readily oxidized on exposure to air. Sweet and pungent odor, more agreeable than the odor of turpentine. d$_{15}^{15}$ 0.8668; d$_{30}^{30}$ 0.8586. bp$_{705}$ 168-169°. bp$_{200}$ 123-124°. [α]$_D^{20}$ +7.69°. n$_D^{30}$ 1.468. Practically insol in water. Miscible with fat solvents and oils.

d-Form nitrosate. C$_{10}$H$_{16}$N$_2$O$_4$. Prepd from *d*-Δ^3-carene with amyl nitrite, acetic and nitric acid, prisms, dec 147.5°.

1837. Carfentrazone-ethyl. [128639-02-1] α-2-Dichloro-5-[4-(difluoromethyl)-4,5-dihydro-3-methyl-5-oxo-1H-1,2,4-triazol-1-yl]-4-fluorobenzenepropanoic acid ethyl ester; ethyl 2-chloro-3-[2-chloro-4-fluoro-5-(4-difluoromethyl-4,5-dihydro-3-methyl-5-oxo-1H-1,2,4-triazol-1-yl)phenyl]propionate; F8426; Aurora. C$_{15}$H$_{14}$Cl$_2$F$_3$N$_3$O$_3$; mol wt 412.19. C 43.71%, H 3.42%, Cl 17.20%, F 13.83%, N 10.19%, O 11.64%. Cereal herbicide that disrupts membranes by inhibiton of protoporphyrinogen oxidase. Prepn: K. M. Poss, **WO 9002120** (1990 to FMC). Properties: W. A. Van Saun *et al.*, *Brighton Crop Prot. Conf. - Weeds* **1993**, 19. Synthesis and structure-activity: G. Theodoridis *et al.*, *ACS Symp. Ser.* **584**, 90 (1995). Mode of action: F. E. Dayan *et al.*, *Pestic. Sci.* **51**, 65 (1997). Control of broadleaf weeds in maize: S. F. Tutt *et al.*, *Brighton Crop Prot. Conf. - Weeds* **1995** 731; in wheat and barley: S. W. Shires *et al.*, *ibid.* **1997**, 117.

Viscous yellow liquid, mp −22.1°. bp$_{760}$ 350-355°. d^{20} 1.457 g/cm^3. Flash point: >110°C. log P (octanol/water): 3.36. Soly in water (μg/ml): 12 (20°); 22 (25°); 23 (30°). Vapor pressure at 25°: 1.2 × 10^{-7} mm Hg; at 20°: 5.4 × 10^{-8} mm Hg. LD$_{50}$ in rats (mg/kg): 5143 orally (female); >4000 dermally (Van Saun).

USE: Post-emergent herbicide.

1838. Carglumic acid. [1188-38-1] N-(Aminocarbonyl)-L-glutamic acid; carbamylglutamic acid; N-carbamoyl-L-glutamic acid; *l*-uramidoglutaric acid; ureidoglutaric acid; Carbaglu. C$_6$H$_{10}$N$_2$O$_5$; mol wt 190.15. C 37.90%, H 5.30%, N 14.73%, O 42.07%. Metabolically stable analog of N-acetylglutamate, a physiological activator of the first enzyme of the urea cycle, carbamylphosphate synthetase (CAPS). Prepn: H. McIlwain, *Biochem. J.* **33**, 1942 (1939). Effect on blood urea and ammonia levels and potential clinical application: J.-E. O'Connor *et al.*, *Eur. J. Pediatr.* **143**, 196 (1985). Evaluation in treatment of CAPS deficiency: G. Kuchler *et al.*, *J. Inher. Metab. Dis.* **19**, 220 (1996); of N-acetylglutamate synthetase (NAGS) deficiency: B. Plecko *et al.*, *Eur. J. Pediatr.* **157**, 996 (1998).

mp 174°.

THERAP CAT: In treatment of inherited urea cycle disorders.

1839. Cargutocin. [33605-67-3] 1-Butanoic acid-7-glycine-1,6-dicarbaoxytocin; 1-butyric acid-6-(L-2-aminobutyric acid)-7-glycineoxytocin; 7-glycine-1,6-aminosuberic acid-oxytocin; [Gly^7,Asu^{1,6}]oxytocin; Y-5350; Statocin. C$_{42}$H$_{65}$N$_{11}$O$_{12}$;

mol wt 916.03. C 55.07%, H 7.15%, N 16.82%, O 20.96%. Analog of oxytocin, *q.v.* Prepn: S. Sakakibara *et al.,* **DE 2056298**; *eidem,* **US 3749705** (1971, 1973 both to Yoshitomi). Synthesis and uterotonic activity: T. Yamanaka, S. Sakakibara, *Bull. Chem. Soc. Jpn.* **47**, 1228 (1974). Pharmacological and biochemical properties: T. Oka *et al., Jpn. J. Pharmacol.* **25**, 15 (1975). Comparison with prostaglandin $F_{2\alpha}$ as oxytocic: T. Hashimoto, *Iryo* **30**, 1121 (1976), *C.A.* **87**, 554e (1977). Distribution, metabolism, excretion: Y. Kato *et al., Iyakuhin Kenkyu* **12**, 433 (1981), *C.A.* **95**, 126386k (1981). Teratogenicity studies: Y. Hamada *et al., ibid.* **10**, 26, 41 (1979), *C.A.* **91**, 639u, 83856m (1979).

$[\alpha]_D^{25}$ −44.0° (c = 0.55 in water).

THERAP CAT: Oxytocic.

1840. Carindacillin. [35531-88-5] (2*S*,5*R*,6*R*)-6-[[3-[(2,3-Dihydro-1*H*-inden-5-yl)oxy]-1,3-dioxo-2-phenylpropyl]amino]-3,3-dimethyl-7-oxo-4-thia-1-azabicyclo[3.2.0]heptane-2-carboxylic acid; *N*-(2-carboxy-3,3-dimethyl-7-oxo-4-thia-1-azabicyclo[3.2.0]-hept-6-yl)-2-phenylmalonamic acid 1-(5-indanyl) ester; 6-[2-(5-indanyloxycarbonyl)phenylacetamido]-3,3-dimethyl-7-oxo-4-thia-1-azabicyclo[3.2.0]heptane-2-carboxylic acid; 1-(5-indanyl) *N*-(2-carboxy-3,3-dimethyl-7-oxo-4-thia-1-azabicyclo[3.2.0]hept-6-yl)-2-phenylmalonamate; 6-[2-phenyl-2-(5-indanyloxycarbonyl)acetamido]penicillanic acid; 6-(2-carboxy-2-phenylacetamido)-3,3-dimethyl-7-oxo-4-thia-1-azabicyclo[3.2.0]heptane-2-carboxylic acid 6-(5-indanyl ester); α-(5-indanyloxycarbonyl)benzylpenicillin; carbenicillin indanyl ester; CP-15464. $C_{26}H_{26}N_2O_6S$; mol wt 494.56. C 63.14%, H 5.30%, N 5.66%, O 19.41%, S 6.48%. Semi-synthetic antibiotic related to penicillin. Prepn: K. Butler, **ZA 6900060**; *idem,* **US 3679801** (1969, 1972 both to Pfizer). New process: S. Nakanishi, **US 3759898** (1973 to Pfizer). Activity studies: Butler, *Del. Med. J.* **43**, 366 (1971); English *et al., Antimicrob. Agents Chemother.* **1**, 185 (1972). Clinical evaluation: Wallace *et al., Antimicrob. Agents Chemother.* **1970**, 223; Bran *et al., Clin. Pharmacol. Ther.* **12**, 525 (1971); *Indanyl Carbenicillin,* H. Swarz, F. E. Storari, Eds. (Am. Elsevier, New York, 1974) 100 pp.

Sodium salt. [26605-69-6] CP-15464-2; Carindapen; Geocillin; G.U.-Pen. $C_{26}H_{25}N_2NaO_6S$; mol wt 516.54. mp 207-213°.

THERAP CAT: Antibacterial.

1841. Cariporide. [159138-80-4] *N*-(Aminoiminomethyl)-4-(1-methylethyl)-3-(methylsulfonyl)benzamide; 4-isopropyl-3-(methanesulfonylbenzoyl)guanidine. $C_{12}H_{17}N_3O_3S$; mol wt 283.35. C 50.87%, H 6.05%, N 14.83%, O 16.94%, S 11.32%. Selective inhibitor of the sodium-hydrogen exchanger subtype 1 (NHE-1); protects against myocardial injury following ischemia and reperfusion. Prepn: H. J. Lang *et al.,* **EP 589336**; *eidem,* **US 5591754** (1994, 1997 both to Hoechst); A. Weichert *et al., Arzneim.-Forsch.* **47**, 1204 (1997). Pharmacology: W. Scholz *et al., Cardiovasc. Res.* **29**, 260 (1995). Symposium on pharmacology and clinical experience: *Am. J. Cardiol.* **83**, Suppl. 10A, 1G-25G (1999). *Review:* W. Scholz *et al., J. Thromb. Thrombolysis* **8**, 61-70 (1999).

Colorless solid, mp 90-94° (dec).

Methanesulfonate. [159138-81-5] Cariporide mesylate; HOE-642. $C_{12}H_{17}N_3O_3S.CH_3SO_3H$; mol wt 379.45. Colorless needles from isopropanol + water, mp 227-230°.

THERAP CAT: Cardioprotective.

1842. Carisoprodol. [78-44-4] (1-Methylethyl)carbamic acid 2-[[(aminocarbonyl)oxy]methyl]-2-methylpentyl ester; *N*-isopropyl-2-methyl-2-propyl-1,3-propanediol dicarbamate; isopropyl meprobamate; isobamate; carisoprodate; Carisoma; Flexartal; Rela; Sanoma; Soma; Somadril; Somalgit. $C_{12}H_{24}N_2O_4$; mol wt 260.33. C 55.36%, H 9.29%, N 10.76%, O 24.58%. Prepn: Berger, Ludwig, **US 2937119** (1960 to Carter Prod.). Pharmacology: Berger *et al., J. Pharmacol. Exp. Ther.* **127**, 66 (1959).

Crystals, mp 92-93°. Slightly bitter taste. Very sparingly sol in water: 30 mg/100 ml at 25°; 140 mg/100 ml at 50°. Sol in many common organic solvents. Practically insol in vegetable oils. Stable in dil acids and alkalies. LD_{50} in mice, rats (mg/kg): 2340, 1320 orally; 980, 450 i.p. (Berger).

THERAP CAT: Muscle relaxant (skeletal).

1843. Carminic Acid. [1260-17-9] 7-α-D-Glucopyranosyl-9,10-dihydro-3,5,6,8-tetrahydroxy-1-methyl-9,10-dioxo-2-anthracenecarboxylic acid; C.I. Natural Red 4; C.I. 75470. $C_{22}H_{20}O_{13}$; mol wt 492.39. C 53.66%, H 4.09%, O 42.24%. Glucosidal coloring matter from the scale insect *Coccus cacti* L., *Homoptera* (cochineal). The essential constituent of carmine. Isoln: Schunk, Marchlewski, *Ber.* **27**, 2979 (1894); Dimroth, Scheuer, *Ann.* **399**, 43 (1913). Structure: Dimroth, Kammerer, *Ber.* **53**, 471 (1920); Ali, Haynes, *J. Chem. Soc.* **1959**, 1033; revised structure: Bhatia, Venkataraman, *Indian J. Chem.* **3** (2), 92 (1965). *See also Colour Index* vol. 4 (3rd ed., 1971) p 4632.

Red prisms from alc, no distinct melting point, darkens at 120°. Has a deep red color in water and is yellow to violet in acid solns. uv max (water): 500 nm (ε 6800); (0.02*N* HCl): 490-500 nm (ε 5800); (0.0001*N* NaOH): 540 nm (ε 3450). $[\alpha]_{654}^{15}$ +51.6° (water). Sol in water, alc, concd H_2SO_4; slightly sol in ether. Practically insol in petr ether, benzene, chloroform.

Methyl tetra-*O*-methylcarminate. $C_{27}H_{30}O_{13}$. Yellow needles from benzene + petr ether, mp 185-188°.

Aluminum calcium lake. Carmine. Bright-red, light pieces; easily reduced to powder. Practically insol in cold water or dil acids. Partly sol in hot water; sol in solns of alkali hydroxides or their carbonates giving deep red solns; also sol in borax.

USE: Free acid in color photography; pigment for artists' paints; as bacterial. stain; rarely now as acid-base indicator or as oxidimetric indicator; as a reagent for aluminum; as a complexing agent for cations. Aluminum calcium lake as dye; in inks; coloring foods, drugs and galenicals; in microscopy for making various stains.

1844. Carmofur. [61422-45-5] 5-Fluoro-*N*-hexyl-3,4-dihydro-2,4-dioxo-1(2*H*)-pyrimidinecarboxamide; 1-(*n*-hexylcarbamoyl)-5-fluorouracil; HCFU; Mifurol; Yamaful. $C_{11}H_{16}FN_3O_3$; mol wt 257.26. C 51.36%, H 6.27%, F 7.38%, N 16.33%, O 18.66%. Orally active cytostatic deriv of fluorouracil, *q.v.* Prepn: S. Ozaki *et al.,* **JP Kokai 77 78886**, *C.A.* **87**, 152265 (1977); *eidem,* **US 4071519** (1977, 1978 both to Mitsui); *eidem, Bull. Chem. Soc. Jpn.* **50**, 2406 (1977). Anti-tumor activity: A. Hoshi *et al., Chem.*

Pharm. Bull. **26,** 161 (1978). Determn in body fluids: S. Watanabe *et al., Chemotherapy (Tokyo)* **27,** 778 (1979); O. Nakajima *et al., J. Chromatogr.* **225,** 91 (1981). General pharmacology: Z. Henmi *et al., Oyo Yakuri* **19,** 369 (1980), *C.A.* **93,** 125639s (1980). Pharmacokinetics: M. Iigo *et al., Cancer Chemother. Pharmacol.* **4,** 189 (1980). Metabolism: *eidem, Xenobiotica* **10,** 847 (1980); T. Kobari *et al., ibid.* **11,** 57 (1981). Phase I clinical study: Y. Koyama, Y. Koyama, *Cancer Treat. Rep.* **64,** 861 (1980). Mutagenicity study: Y. Seino *et al., Cancer Res.* **38,** 2148 (1978). *Review:* T. Taguchi, *Recent Results Cancer Res.* **70,** 125-132 (1980).

White cryst from ethanol, mp 110-111°. uv max (chloroform): 258 nm (ε 1.16 × 10⁴) (S. Ozaki *et al., Bull. Chem. Soc. Japan*). Also reported as mp 283° (dec) (**US 4071519**).

THERAP CAT: Antineoplastic.

1845. Carmustine. [154-93-8] *N,N'*-Bis(2-chloroethyl)-*N*-nitrosourea; BCNU; NSC-409962; Becenun; Bicnu; Carmubris. $C_5H_9Cl_2N_3O_2$; mol wt 214.05. C 28.06%, H 4.24%, Cl 33.13%, N 19.63%, O 14.95%. Chloroethylnitrosourea derivative with antitumor activity. Similar to chlorozotocin, lomustine, nimustine, ranimustine, *q.q.v.* Synthesis: Johnston *et al., J. Med. Chem.* **6,** 669 (1963). Properties: Loo *et al., J. Pharm. Sci.* **55,** 492 (1966). Decompn studies as related to antileukemic activity: Montgomery *et al., J. Med. Chem.* **10,** 668 (1967). Antifungal action: Hunt, Pittilo, *Antimicrob. Agents Chemother.* **1965,** 710. Toxicology studies: Thompson, Larson, *Toxicol. Appl. Pharmacol.* **21,** 405 (1972). Review of pulmonary toxicity: A. C. Smith, *Pharmacol. Ther.* **41,** 443-460 (1989).

Light yellow powder that melts to an oily liquid; mp 30-32°. Both powder and liquid are stable. Dec rapidly in acid and in soln above pH 7. Most stable in petroleum ether or aqueous soln at pH 4. Non-ionized at pH 7 with consequent high lipid solubility. Sol in water up to 4 mg/ml and in 50% ethanol up to 150 mg/ml: DeVita *et al., Cancer Res.* **25,** 1876 (1965). LD₅₀ in mice (mg/kg): 19-25 orally, 26 i.p., 24 s.c.; in rats (mg/kg): 30-34 orally (Thompson, Larson).

Caution: This substance is reasonably anticipated to be a human carcinogen: *Report on Carcinogens, Eleventh Edition* (PB2005-104914, 2004) p III-53.

THERAP CAT: Antineoplastic.

1846. Carnauba Wax. [8015-86-9] Brazil wax. An exudate from the pores of the leaves of the Brazilian wax palm tree *Copernicia prunifera* (Muell.) H. E. Moore [*Copernicia cerifera* (Arruda da Camara) Mart.], *Palmae.* The botany of the tree and the native wax-collecting procedures are described adequately by A. H. Warth, *The Chemistry and Technology of Waxes* (Reinhold, New York, 1947). The hardness and high-polish capability of this important wax can be ascribed to the presence of esters of hydroxylated unsaturated fatty acids having about 12 carbon atoms in the acid chain. The usual names for the constituents, *i.e.* cerotic acid, melissyl cerotate, carnaubic acid etc., are meaningless. Brief review: C. S. Letcher in *Kirk-Othmer Encyclopedia of Chemical Technology* **vol. 24** (Wiley-Interscience, New York, 3rd ed., 1984) pp 469-470.

Hard greenish solid, cryst fracture. Sharp, characteristic, not unpleasant odor upon melting. mp 82-85.5°. d 0.990 to 0.999. Saponification number 78 to 89. Iodine number about 13. n_D^{90} 1.4500. Sparingly soluble in fat solvents at 25°, quite sol at 45°.

USE: Wherever a hard, high-polish wax is desired, *e.g.* in automobile waxes, floor wax emulsions, high quality shoe polishes, in the paper industry (especially for making carbon papers). As a plasticizer in dental impression compounds. To raise the melting point of other waxes; often used together with candelilla wax. The presence of the lower-melting ouricury wax is considered as an adulteration. Purified and bleached carnauba wax is used for cosmetic materials, such as depilatories and deodorant sticks. In pharmacy as the last stage in tablet coating. Skin sensitization or irritation by carnauba wax seems infrequent.

1847. Carnegine. [490-53-9] 1,2,3,4-Tetrahydro-6,7-dimethoxy-1,2-dimethylisoquinoline; 6,7-dimethoxy-1,2-dimethyl-1,2,3,4-tetrahydroisoquinoline; pectenine. $C_{13}H_{19}NO_2$; mol wt 221.30. C 70.56%, H 8.65%, N 6.33%, O 14.46%. In *Carnegiea gigantea* (Engelm.) Britt. & Rose *(Cereus giganteus* Engelm.), *Cactaceae,* a cactus of Arizona and Mexico. Extraction procedure: Heyl, *Arch. Pharm.* **266,** 668 (1928). Synthesis: Späth, *Ber.* **62,** 1021 (1929); Nakada, Nisgihara, *J. Pharm. Soc. Jpn.* **64,** 74 (1944). Pharmacology: E. Santi-Soncin, M. Furlanut, *Fitoterapia* **43,** 21 (1972), *C.A.* **80,** 66667f (1974). Review of synthetic methods: A. B. J. Bracca, T. S. Kaufman, *Tetrahedron* **60,** 10575-10610 (2004).

Viscous liquid, dec on standing. Distills at 1 mm pressure and 170° air bath temp. Sol in ether, alc, chloroform. LD₅₀ i.p. in mice: 15.23 mg/kg (Santi-Soncin, Furlanut).

Hydrochloride monohydrate. [5864-18-6] $C_{13}H_{19}NO_2$.-HCl.H₂O. Clusters from dil alc, mp 207° (mp 211° when anhydr). Sol in water, slightly sol in alc.

Hydrobromide monohydrate. [5853-25-8] $C_{13}H_{19}NO_2$.-HBr.H₂O. Needles from alc, mp 228°.

Methyliodide. [5911-58-0] $C_{13}H_{19}NO_2$.CH₃I. Needles from methanol, mp 211° (evac tube) after drying at 100° and 10 mm.

1848. Carnidazole. [42116-76-7] [2-(2-Methyl-5-nitro-1*H*-imidazol-1-yl)ethyl]carbamothioic acid *O*-methyl ester; *O*-methyl [2-(2-methyl-5-nitroimidazol-1-yl)ethyl]thiocarbamate; R-25831; Spartrix; $C_8H_{12}N_4O_3S$; mol wt 244.27. C 39.34%, H 4.95%, N 22.94%, O 19.65%, S 13.13%. Prepn and antiprotozoal activity: J. Heeres *et al.,* **DE 2429755**; *eidem,* **US 3928374** (both 1975 to Janssen); *eidem, Eur. J. Med. Chem. - Chim. Ther.* **11,** 237 (1976). Crystal structure of monohydrate: N. M. Blaton *et al., Acta Crystallogr.* **B35,** 753 (1979). Clinical efficacy in vaginal trichomoniasis: A. Notowicz *et al., Br. J. Vener. Dis.* **53,** 129 (1977); P. Chaudhuri, A. C. Drogendijk, *Eur. J. Obstet. Gynecol. Reprod. Biol.* **10,** 325 (1980).

Crystals from ethanol, mp 142.4° (dec).

THERAP CAT (VET): Antiprotozoal (Trichomonas).

1849. Carnitine. [541-15-1] (2*R*)-3-Carboxy-2-hydroxy-*N,N,N*-trimethyl-1-propanaminium inner salt; L-(3-carboxy-2-hydroxypropyl)trimethylammonium hydroxide inner salt; (−)-β-hydroxy-γ-trimethylaminobutyric acid; L-carnitine; levocarnitine; vitamin B_T; Cardiogen; Carnicor; Carnitor; L-Carn; Lefcar; Levocarnil; Miocor; Miotonal; Nefrocarnit. $C_7H_{15}NO_3$; mol wt 161.20. C 52.16%, H 9.38%, N 8.69%, O 29.78%. Essential cofactor of fatty acid metabolism; required for the transport of fatty acids through the inner mitochondrial membrane. Synthesized primarily in the liver and kidney; highest concentrations found in heart and skeletal muscle. Named derived from the Latin word, *carnis,* meaning meat or flesh. Dietary sources include red meat, dairy products, beans, avocado. Isoln from meat extract: W. Gulewitsch, R. Krimberg, *Z. Physiol. Chem.* **45,** 326 (1905); H. E. Carter, P. K. Bhattacharyya, *Methods Enzymol.* **III,** 660 (1957). Identification as vitamin B_T: H. E. Carter *et al., Arch. Biochem. Biophys.* **38,** 405 (1952). Synthesis: M. Tomita, Y. Sendju, Z. *Physiol. Chem.* **169**, 263 (1927); R. Voeffray *et al., Helv. Chim. Acta* **70**, 2058 (1987). Enantioselective synthesis from glycerol: M. Marzi *et al., J. Org. Chem.* **65**, 6766 (2000). Biosynthesis: G. Wolf, C. R. A. Berger, *Arch. Biochem. Biophys.* **92**, 360 (1961). Absolute configuration: T. Kaneko, R. Yoshida, *Bull. Chem. Soc. Jpn.* **35**, 1153 (1962). Metabolism in humans: M. E. Mitchell, *Am. J. Clin. Nutr.* **31**, 293 (1984). Historical review: G. Fraenkel, S. Friedman, *Vitam. Horm.* **XV**, 73-118 (1957). Review of physiological significance and deficiency syndromes: C. J. Rebouche, D. J. Paulson, *Annu. Rev. Nutr.* **6**, 41-66 (1986); of clinical pharmacology: J. J. Bahl, R. Bressler, *Annu. Rev. Pharmacol. Toxicol.* **27**, 257-277 (1987); of biosynthesis in mammals: F. M. Vaz, R. J. A. Wanders, *Biochem. J.* **361**, 417-429 (2002). Review of effect on myocardial metabolism and clinical experience in ischemic heart disease: R. Lango *et al., Cardiovasc. Res.* **51**, 21-29 (2001); of use as dietary supplement in athletes: H. Karlic, A. Lohninger, *Nutrition* **20**, 709-715 (2004). Symposium on physiology, pharmacology and therapeutic potential: *Ann. N.Y. Acad. Sci.* **1033**, 1-197 (2004).

Crystals from anhydrous ethanol + acetone, dec 196-198° (Carter, Bhattacharyya); also reported as crystals from isopropanol, mp 200° (dec) (Marzi). Very hygroscopic solid. $[\alpha]_D^{25}$ −31.3° (c = 10 in water); $[\alpha]_{546}^{25}$ −37.0° (c = 10 in water). Sol in water, hot alcohol. Practically insol in acetone, ether, benzene.

Hydrochloride. [6645-46-1] Levocarnitine chloride; Flatistine. $C_7H_{15}NO_3 \cdot HCl$; mol wt 197.66. Crystals, dec 142°.

DL-Form. [406-76-8] γ-Amino-β-hydroxybutyric acid trimethylbetaine; γ-trimethyl-β-hydroxybutyrobetaine. Synthesis: E. Strack *et al., Ber.* **86**, 525 (1953); H. E. Carter, P. K. Bhattacharyya, *J. Am. Chem. Soc.* **75**, 2503 (1953). Hygroscopic crystalline solid, dec 195-197°. Sol in water, ethanol.

DL-Form hydrochloride. [461-05-2] Needles from ethanol, mp 196° (dec). Very sol in water; sol in hot ethanol; slightly sol in cold ethanol. Practically insol in acetone, ether.

D-Form. [541-14-0] Prepn: S. Friedman *et al., Arch. Biochem. Biophys.* **66**, 10 (1957). Crystals, dec 210-212°. $[\alpha]_D$ +30.9°. Very sol in water and alcohol. Practically insol in acetone and ether.

D-Form hydrochloride. [10017-44-4] Crystals, dec 142°.

THERAP CAT: Vitamin (enzyme cofactor).

1850. Carnosine. [305-84-0] β-Alanyl-L-histidine; ignotine. $C_9H_{14}N_4O_3$; mol wt 226.23. C 47.78%, H 6.24%, N 24.77%, O 21.22%. Naturally occurring dipeptide found in large amounts in skeletal muscle. Also present in other tissues such as brain, cardiac muscle, kidney. Water soluble antioxidant; functions as a free-radical scavenger. Isoln: Gulewitsch, Amiradzibi, *Ber.* **33**, 1902 (1900); Wolff, Wilson, *J. Biol. Chem.* **95**, 495 (1932); **109**, 565 (1935). Synthesis from histidine and β-iodo- or β-nitropropionyl chloride: Baumann, Ingvaldsen, *ibid.* **35**, 271 (1918); Barger, Tutin, *Biochem. J.* **12**, 406 (1918). Later syntheses: Sifford, du Vigneaud, *J. Biol. Chem.* **108**, 753 (1935); R. A. Turner, *J. Am. Chem. Soc.* **75**, 2388 (1953); F. J. Vinick, S. Jung, *J. Org. Chem.* **48**, 392 (1983). Crystal structure: H. Itoh *et al., Acta Crystallogr.* **33B**, 2959 (1977). Possible role in wound healing: D. E. Fischer *et al., Proc. Soc. Exp. Biol. Med.* **158**, 402 (1978). Review of physiological properties and therapeutic potential: S. E. Gariballa, A. J. Sinclair, *Age Ageing* **29**, 207-210 (2000).

Crystals from aqueous ethanol, mp 262° (dec) (Vinick, Jung); also reported as mp 260° (capillary tube) and as mp 308-309° (Dennis bar) (Sifford, du Vigneaud). $[\alpha]_D^{25}$ +21.0° (c = 1.5 in water). pK$_1$ 2.64; pK$_2$ 6.83; pK$_3$ 9.51. Alkaline reaction. One gram dissolves in 3.1 ml water at 25°.

Nitrate. [5852-98-2] $C_9H_{15}N_5O_6$. Crystals, dec 222°. $[\alpha]_D^{20}$ +24.1° (c = 1.5 in water). Very sol in water.

Hydrochloride. [5852-99-3] $C_9H_{15}ClN_4O_3$. Crystals, dec 245°. Very sol in water.

D-Form. [5853-00-9] Crystals, mp 260°. $[\alpha]_D^{28}$ −20.4° (c = 1.5).

1851. Caro's Acid. [7722-86-3] Peroxymonosulfuric acid; sulfomonoperacid; persulfuric acid. H_2O_5S; mol wt 114.08. H 1.77%, O 70.12%, S 28.11%. Dry reagent is prepd by stirring 10 g potassium persulfate into 11 g concd H_2SO_4 for 10 min and adding 30 g finely powdered potassium sulfate; liquid reagent is obtained by triturating potassium persulfate with three times as much (by weight) of H_2SO_4; dil reagent is prepd by stirring 10 g potassium persulfate into 11 g concd H_2SO_4 and adding 50 cc ice: Baeyer, Villiger, *Ber.* **32**, 3625 (1899); another prepn by reacting 90% H_2O_2 with chlorosulfonic acid at −40 to −50°: Ball, Edwards, *J. Am. Chem. Soc.* **78**, 1125 (1956).

The product is a sirupy liquid consisting of about equal amounts of Caro's acid and H_2SO_4. pK$_2$ of Caro's acid 9.4 ± 0.1. Oxygen is evolved at room temp; should be stored at dry ice temp.

Caution: Can be dangerously unstable, like most peroxides. Description of explosion at Brown University: J. O. Edwards, *Chem. Eng. News* **33**, 3336 (1955). Explosion at Sun Oil, *ibid.* **38**, 59 (Nov. 21, 1960). May be highly irritating to skin, eyes, mucous membranes.

USE: In prepn of dyes; oxidation of olefins to α-glycols; oxidation of ketones to lactones or esters; treating woolens to prevent felting and shrinking; in bleaching compositions.

1852. α-Carotene. [7488-99-5] $C_{40}H_{56}$; mol wt 536.87. C 89.49%, H 10.51%. About as widely distributed as its β-isomer, but in smaller amounts. Best sources for both the α- and β-isomers are carrots, palm oil, and green leaves of various species. As a provitamin A it is half as active as β-carotene. Found in the mother liquors after crystallizing β-carotene. Isoln by chromatography: Karrer, Walker, *Helv. Chim. Acta* **16**, 641 (1933); Kuhn, Lederer, *Ber.* **64**, 1349 (1931); Karrer *et al., Helv. Chim. Acta* **14**, 614 (1931); **16**, 975 (1933). Natural (+)-α-carotene has 6'R configuration: Eugster *et al., ibid.* **52**, 1729 (1969). Synthesis of dl-α-carotene: Eugster, Karrer, *ibid.* **38**, 610 (1955); Tscharner *et al., ibid.* **40**, 1676 (1957); Ruegg *et al., ibid.* **44**, 985 (1961).

Deep purple prisms, polyhedra from petr ether or from benzene + methanol, mp 187.50° (evacuated tube). $[\alpha]_{643}^{18}$ +385° (c = 0.08 in benzene). Absorption max (CHCl$_3$): 485, 454 nm. More sol than β-carotene. Freely sol in carbon disulfide, chloroform; sol in ether, benzene. Slightly sol in petr ether, alcohol. 100 ml hexane dissolves 294 mg at 0°. Practically insol in water, acids, alkalies. Absorbs oxygen from the air, giving rise to inactive colorless oxidation products. The oxidation in light is autocatalytic. *Store in darkness in sealed ampoules and at low temp (−20°C).*

THERAP CAT: Vitamin A precursor.

THERAP CAT (VET): Vitamin A precursor for all species except cats.

1853. β-Carotene. [7235-40-7] β,β-Carotene; Carotaben; Provatene; Solatene. $C_{40}H_{56}$; mol wt 536.87. C 89.49%, H 10.51%. Most important of the provitamins A. Widely distributed in the plant and animal kingdom. In plants it occurs almost always together with chlorophyll. Isoln from carrots: Willstätter, Escher, Z. *Physiol. Chem.* **64**, 47 (1910); Kuhn, Lederer, *Ber.* **64**, 1349 (1931); Barnett *et al.*, US **2848508** (1958). Chromatography: Karrer, Walker, *Helv. Chim. Acta* **16**, 641 (1933). Structure: Willstätter, Mieg, *Ann.* **355**, 1 (1907); Zechmeister *et al., Ber.* **61**, 566 (1928); **66**, 123 (1933); Karrer *et al., Helv. Chim. Acta* **12**, 1142 (1929); **13**, 1084 (1930); **14**, 1033 (1931); Kuhn, Brockmann, *Ber.* **65**, 894 (1932); **66**, 1319 (1933); **67**, 1408 (1934); *Ann.* **516**, 95 (1935). Crystal structure: Sterling, *Acta Crystallogr.* **17**, 1224 (1964). Synthesis: Milas *et al., J. Am. Chem. Soc.* **72**, 4844

(1950); Karrer, Eugster, *Compt. Rend.* **250**, 1920 (1950); Inhoffen *et al., Chem. Ztg.* **74**, 285, 309 (1950); Surmatis, Ofner, *J. Org. Chem.* **26**, 1171 (1961); Rüegg *et al., Helv. Chim. Acta* **44**, 985 (1961); Bestmann *et al., Ann.* **1973**, 760; Fischli, Mayer, *Helv. Chim. Acta* **58**, 1584 (1975). Industrial mfg procedure: Isler *et al., Helv. Chim. Acta* **39**, 249 (1956); Isler *et al.*, US 2917539 (1959 to Hoffmann-La Roche). Microbial production by *Choanephora trispora:* Zajic, US 2959521; US 2959522 and US 3128236 (1960, 1960 and 1964, all to Grain Processing); Miescher, US 3001912 (1961 to C.S.C.). *Review:* Fleming, *Selected Organic Syntheses* (John Wiley, London, 1973) pp 70-74.

Deep-purple, hexagonal prisms from benzene + methanol. Red, rhombic, almost square leaflets from petr ether. mp 183° (evacuated tube). Absorption max (chloroform): 497, 466 nm. Less sol than α-carotene. Sol in CS_2, benzene, chloroform. Moderately sol in ether, petr ether, oils. 100 ml hexane dissolve 109 mg at 0°. Very sparingly sol in methanol and ethanol. Practically insol in water, acids, alkalies. Dil solns are yellow. Absorbs oxygen from the air giving rise to inactive, colorless oxidation products. *Keep tightly closed and protected from light. Store at low temp (−20°C).* Commercial crystalline β-carotene has a vitamin A activity of 1.67 million U.S.P. units per gram. The I.U. of 0.6 μg β-carotene is almost exactly equivalent to 0.3 μg vitamin A.

USE: Yellow coloring agent for foods.

THERAP CAT: Vitamin A precursor. Ultraviolet screen.

THERAP CAT (VET): Vitamin A precursor for all species except cats.

1854. γ-Carotene. [472-93-5] $C_{40}H_{56}$; mol wt 536.87. C 89.49%, H 10.51%. A rare carotenoid. Has provitamin A activity. Best source is *Penicillium sclerotiorum:* Mase *et al., Arch. Biochem. Biophys.* **68**, 150 (1957). Also present in small proportions in many plant materials, esp fruits containing β-carotene. Chromatographic isoln from crude carotenes: Kuhn, Brockmann, *Ber.* **66**, 407 (1933); Winterstein, *Z. Physiol. Chem.* **219**, 249 (1933). Structure: Kuhn, Brockmann, *loc. cit.; Naturwissenschaften* **21**, 44 (1933). Synthesis: Garbers *et al., Helv. Chim. Acta* **36**, 1783 (1953); Ruegg *et al., ibid.* **44**, 985 (1961).

Probably crystallizes in polymorphous forms. Synthetic form: red plates, mp 152-153.5°. Absorption max (petr ether): 437, 462, 494 nm ($E_{1cm}^{1\%}$ 2055, 3100, 2720). Natural form: minute, deep-red prisms with bluish luster from benzene + methanol. mp 177.5°. Absorption max (chloroform): 508.5, 475, 446 nm. Somewhat less sol than β-carotene. *Store in darkness in sealed ampoules at low temps (0°C).*

THERAP CAT: Vitamin A precursor.

THERAP CAT (VET): Vitamin A precursor for all species except cats.

1855. δ-Carotene. [472-92-4] ε,ψ-Carotene. $C_{40}H_{56}$; mol wt 536.87. C 89.49%, H 10.51%. Extracted from the fruit of *Gonocaryum pyriforme* Mig., *Icacinaceae:* Winterstein, *Z. Physiol. Chem.* **219**, 249 (1933). Occurs also in carrots and certain varieties of tomatoes. Isoln from tomato mutants: Porter, Murphey, *Arch. Biochem. Biophys.* **32**, 21 (1951). Structure: Kargl, Quackenbush, *ibid.* **88**, 59 (1960). Synthesis: Manchand *et al., J. Chem. Soc.* **1965**, 2019. Absolute configuration: Buchecker, Eugster, *Helv. Chim. Acta* **54**, 327 (1971).

Long orange-red needles from CS_2 + hexane + ethanol, mp 140.5°. $[\alpha]_{Cd}$ +317°; $[\alpha]_D^{25}$ +352° ±16% (hexane). Absorption spectrum: Kargl, Quackenbush, *loc. cit.*

1856. Carotol. [465-28-1] [3R-(3α,3aα,8aα)]-2,3,4,5,8,8a-Hexahydro-6,8-dimethyl-3-(1-methylethyl)-3a(1H)-azulenol; 2,3,-4,5,8,8a-hexahydro-3-isopropyl-6,8-dimethyl-3a(1H)-azulenol. $C_{15}H_{26}O$; mol wt 222.37. C 81.02%, H 11.79%, O 7.19%. From oil of carrot seeds, *Daucus carota* L., *Umbelliferae:* Asahina, Tsukamoto, *J. Pharm. Soc. Jpn.* **525**, 961 (1925), *C.A.* **20**, 2845 (1926); Sorm *et al., Collect. Czech. Chem. Commun.* **16**, 47 (1951); Pigulevskii, Kovaleva, *Zh. Prikl. Khim.* **32**, 2703 (1959). Structure: Sykora *et al., Collect. Czech. Chem. Commun.* **26**, 788 (1961); Zalkow *et al., J. Org. Chem.* **26**, 981 (1961). Stereochemistry: Levisalles, Rudler, *Bull. Soc. Chim. Fr.* **1964**, 2020; **1967**, 2059. Synthesis of (+)-form: DeBroissia *et al., ibid.* **1972**, 4314; *eidem, Chem. Commun.* **1972**, 855.

(+) - Carotol

Liquid. $bp_{2.5}$ 126°. $[\alpha]_D^{20}$ +30.4°. n_D^{20} 1.4964. d^{20} 0.9624.

1857. Caroverine. [23465-76-1] 1-[2-(Diethylamino)ethyl]-3-[(4-methoxyphenyl)methyl]-2(1H)-quinoxalinone; 1-(diethylaminoethyl)-3-(p-methoxybenzyl)dihydro-2-quinoxalone; Spasmium. $C_{22}H_{27}N_3O_2$; mol wt 365.47. C 72.30%, H 7.45%, N 11.50%, O 8.76%. Prepn: Zellner *et al.*, US 3028384 (1962 to Donau-Pharm.). Polarographic study: P. Pflegel, *Pharmazie* **24**, 667 (1969). Pharmacological study: F. Hahn *et al., Arch. Int. Pharmacodyn. Ther.* **199**, 108 (1972).

Crystals from isopropyl alcohol, mp 69°. $bp_{0.01}$ 202°.
Hydrochloride. Dec 188°.

THERAP CAT: Antispasmodic.

1858. Carpaine. [3463-92-1] $C_{28}H_{50}N_2O_4$; mol wt 478.71. C 70.25%, H 10.53%, N 5.85%, O 13.37%. Found in *Carica papaya* L. and in *Vasconcellosia hastata* Caruel, *Caricaceae.* Isoln from papaya leaves: Greshoff, *Mededeel. uit's Lands. Plant., Buitenzorg.* **No. 7**, 5 (1890); Rapoport, Baldridge, *J. Am. Chem. Soc.* **73**, 343 (1951). Reportedly causes bradycardia, CNS depression: Kakowski, *Arch. Int. Pharm.* **15**, 84 (1905). Structure and stereochemistry: Govindachari *et al., Tetrahedron Lett.* **1965**, 1907. Absolute configuration: Coke, Rice, *J. Org. Chem.* **30**, 3420 (1965). Review of structural studies: Govindachari, *J. Indian Chem. Soc.* **45**, 945 (1968).

Monoclinic prisms from acetone, mp 119-120°. Sublimes at 120° under 0.05 mm pressure. $[\alpha]_D^{12}$ +24.7° (c = 1.07 in ethanol). Slightly sol in water. Sol in most organic solvents except petr ether.

Consult the Name Index before using this section.

1859. Carpetimycins. Carbapenem antibiotics related to thienamycin and olivanic acids, q.q.v. Carpetimycins A, B, C and D are known. Prodn of A and B by *Streptomyces* strain No. C-19393, now named *Streptomyces griseus* subsp. *cryophilus*, and antibacterial properties: **NL 8000628**; A. Imada *et al.*, **US 4518529** (1980, 1985 to Takeda); A. Imada *et al.*, *J. Antibiot.* **33**, 1417 (1980); by *Streptomyces* strain KC-6643: M. Nakayama *et al.*, *ibid.* 1388. Structure and abs config: S. Harada *et al.*, *J. Antibiot.* **33**, 1425 (1980); M. Nakayama *et al.*, *ibid.* **34**, 818 (1981). Mode of action study: Y. Nozaki *et al.*, *ibid.* 206. Total synthesis of (±)-carpetimycin A: H. Natsugari *et al.*, *J. Chem. Soc. Perkin Trans. 1* **1983**, 403; M. Ihara *et al.*, *Heterocycles* **20**, 2182 (1983); J. D. Buynak, M. N. Rao, *J. Org. Chem.* **51**, 1571 (1986). Synthesis of (−)-carpetimycin A: T. Iimori *et al.*, *J. Am. Chem. Soc.* **105**, 1659 (1983); M. Aratani *et al.*, *Tetrahedron Lett.* **26**, 223 (1985); M. Shibasaki *et al.*, *ibid.* 2217.

Carpetimycin A: R = H
Carpetimycin B: R = SO₃H

Carpetimycin A. [76025-73-5] (5R,6R)-3-[(R)-[(1E)-2-(Acetylamino)ethenyl]sulfinyl]-6-(1-hydroxy-1-methylethyl)-7-oxo-1-azabicyclo[3.2.0]hept-2-ene-2-carboxylic acid; antibiotic Ab 651; antibiotic C-19393-H₂; antibiotic KA-6643-A; C-19393-H₂. $C_{14}H_{18}N_2O_6S$; mol wt 342.37. Colorless solid, mp >145° (dec). $[\alpha]_D^{24}$ −27° (c = 1.7 in water). uv max (water): 240, 288 nm ($E_{1cm}^{1\%}$ 369, 300) (Nakayama, 1980).

Carpetimycin B. [76094-36-5] Antibiotic C-19393-S₂; antibiotic KA-6643-B; C-19393-S₂. $C_{14}H_{18}N_2O_9S_2$; mol wt 422.43. Colorless solid melting above 130° (dec). $[\alpha]_D^{24}$ −145° (c = 1 in water). uv max (water): 240, 285 nm ($E_{1cm}^{1\%}$ 357, 305) (Nakayama, 1980).

1860. Carphenazine. [2622-30-2] 1-[10-[3-[4-(2-Hydroxyethyl)-1-piperazinyl]propyl]-10H-phenothiazin-2-yl]-1-propanone; 10-[3-[4-(2-hydroxyethyl)-1-piperazinyl]propyl]-3-propionylphenothiazine; 2-propionyl-10-[γ-(N′-β-hydroxyethylpiperazino)propyl]phenothiazine; Proketazine. $C_{24}H_{31}N_3O_2S$; mol wt 425.59. C 67.73%, H 7.34%, N 9.87%, O 7.52%, S 7.53%. Prepn: M. H. Sherlock, N. Sperber, **US 2985654** (1961 to Schering); R. F. Tislow *et al.*, **US 3023146** (1962 to Am. Home Products).

Dimaleate. [2975-34-0] $C_{24}H_{31}N_3O_2S.2C_4H_4O_4$. Yellow crystals from isopropanol, mp 175–177° (Tislow). Also reported as crystals from methanol, mp 165–167° (Sherlock, Sperber).

THERAP CAT: Antipsychotic.

1861. Carpipramine. [5942-95-0] 1′-[3-(10,11-Dihydro-5H-dibenz[b,f]azepin-5-yl)propyl]-[1,4′-bipiperidine]-4′-carboxamide; 5-[3-(4-piperidino-4-carbamoylpiperidino)propyl]-10,11-dihydro-5H-dibenz[b,f]azepine; carbadipimidine; Bay b 4343 b. $C_{28}H_{38}N_4O$; mol wt 446.63. C 75.30%, H 8.58%, N 12.54%, O 3.58%. Prepn: M. Nakanishi, T. Munakata, **JP 66 6752**; **GB 1017986**; Nakanishi *et al.*, **US 3329683** (1966, 1966, 1967 all to Yoshitomi);

Nakanishi *et al.*, *J. Med. Chem.* **13**, 644 (1970). Pharmacology: Nakanishi *et al.*, *Arzneim.-Forsch.* **18**, 1435 (1968). Metabolism: Nakanishi *et al.*, *J. Pharm. Soc. Jpn.* **90**, 204 (1970).

Dihydrochloride monohydrate. [7075-03-8] Defekton; Prazinil. $C_{28}H_{38}N_4O.2HCl.H_2O$; mol wt 537.56. Crystals from 90% methanol, mp 260°. Sparingly sol in water. LD_{50} in mice, rats (mg/kg): 28.2, 37.0 i.v.; 136.0, 76.0 i.p.; 2180, 1025 orally (Nakanishi, 1968).

THERAP CAT: Antipsychotic.

1862. Carprofen. [53716-49-7] 6-Chloro-α-methyl-9H-carbazole-2-acetic acid; C-5720; Ro-20-5720/000; Imadyl; Rimadyl. $C_{15}H_{12}ClNO_2$; mol wt 273.71. C 65.82%, H 4.42%, Cl 12.95%, N 5.12%, O 11.69%. Prepn: L. Berger, A. J. Corraz, **DE 2337340**; *eidem*, **US 3896145** (1974, 1975 both to Hoffmann-La Roche). Pharmacology: L. O. Randall, H. Baruth, *Arch. Int. Pharmacodyn.* **220**, 94 (1976). Stereospecific assay and disposition: J. M. Kemmerer *et al.*, *J. Pharm. Sci.* **68**, 1274 (1979). Metabolism: F. Rubio *et al.*, *ibid.* **69**, 1245 (1980). Pharmacokinetic and clinical studies in gout: T. F. Yu, J. Perel, *J. Clin. Pharmacol.* **20**, 347 (1980). Use in treatment of rheumatoid arthritis: S. Jalava, *Scand. J. Rheumatol.* **1983**, Suppl. 48, 5-12. Review of pharmacology and clinical efficacy: W. M. O'Brien, G. F. Bagby, *Pharmacotherapy* **7**, 16 (1987).

Cryst from chloroform, mp 197-198°. LD_{50} orally in mice: 400 mg/kg (Berger, Corraz).

THERAP CAT: Anti-inflammatory.

THERAP CAT (VET): Anti-inflammatory.

1863. Carpropamid. [104030-54-8] 2,2-Dichloro-N-[1-(4-chlorophenyl)ethyl]-1-ethyl-3-methylcyclopropanecarboxamide; KTU 3616; Win. $C_{15}H_{18}Cl_3NO$; mol wt 334.67. C 53.83%, H 5.42%, Cl 31.78%, N 4.19%, O 4.78%. Melanin inhibiting fungicide for control of rice blast. Prepn: Y. Kurahashi *et al.*, **EP 170842**; *eidem*, **US 4710518** (1985, 1987 both to Nihon Tokushu Noyaku Seizo). Synthesis of stereoisomers: U. Kraatz, M. Littmann, *Pflanzenschutz-Nachr.* **51**, 201 (1998). Inhibition of melanin biosynthesis: G. Tsuji *et. al.*, *Pestic. Biochem. Physiol.* **57**, 211 (1997). Suppression of secondary infection in rice: Y. Kurahashi *et. al.*, *Pestic. Sci.* **55**, 31 (1999). Review of physical properties, mode of action, and field trials: T. Hattori *et. al.*, *Brighton Crop Prot. Conf. - Pests Dis.* **1994**, 517-524.

Technical grade is a mixture of (1RS, 3SR, 1′RR) isomers, mp 152°. Sol in dichloromethane, slightly sol in toluene, very low sol in water. Vapor pressure at 20°: 2.70×10^{-7} Pa.

USE: Fungicide.

1864. Carrageenan. [9000-07-1] Carrageen; carrageenin. Mixture of sulfated polysaccharides extracted from red seaweed *(Rhodophyceae)*. Chief sources are *Chondrus crispus* (L.) Stackhouse, and *Gigartina stellata (G. mammillosa)* (Goodenough and Woodward) J. Aghardh, *Gigartinaceae*, found most abundantly in North Atlantic coastal regions from Norway to North Africa. The name carrageenan is derived from the Irish coastal town of Carragheen. The κ and λ structural families are identified based on position of sulfate and the presence/absence of anhydrogalactose. Kappa (κ) family consists of κ,ι,μ,ν carrageenans of which κ and ι are the most prevalent. Characterized by a repeating unit of 4-sulfate-β-D-galactopyranosyl(1 → 4)-α-D-galactose linked (1 → 3). The galactose unit varies: 3,6-anhydro-α-D-galactose for κ-form; 3,6-anhydro-α-D-galactose-2-sulfate for ι-form. Due to helical tertiary structure which allows for gelling, κ-family is of major commercial importance. Lambda (λ) family consists of λ and ξ; characterized by a repeating (1 → 3) linked disaccharide of 2-sulfate-β-D-galactopyranosyl(1 → 4)-α-D-galactose. The galactose residue is 2,6-sulfated for λ form and 2-sulfated for ξ form. These carrageenans are non-gelling. Conformational study: N. S. Anderson *et al.*, *J. Mol. Biol.* **45**, 85 (1969); and structural analysis: D. A. Rees, E. J. Welsh, *Angew. Chem. Int. Ed.* **16**, 214 (1977); C. Bodeau-Bellion, *Physiol. Veg.* **21**, 785 (1983). Use as phlogistic agent: C. A. Winter *et al.*, *Proc. Soc. Exp. Biol. Med.* **111**, 544 (1962); L. Levy, *Life Sci.* **8**, 601 (1969). IR determn of κ, ι, and λ forms: E. Tojo, J. Prado, *Carbohydr. Res.* **338**, 1309 (2003). Review of effect on inflammation and immunity: H. J. Schwartz in *Inadvert. Modif. Immune Resp.* **FDA-80-1074**, 109-114 (1980); S. Nicklin, K. Miller, *Food Addit. Contam.* **6**, 425-436 (1989). Review of toxicology: M. L. Weiner, *Agents Actions* **32**, 46-51 (1991). Review of industrial and non-food uses: R. J. Tye, *Carbohydr. Polym.* **10**, 259-280 (1989). *General Reviews:* G. H. Therkelsen in *Industrial Gums*, R. L. Whistler, J. N. BeMiller, Eds. (Academic Press, New York, 3rd ed., 1993) pp 145-180; J. K. Baird, "Gums" in *Kirk-Othmer Encyclopedia of Chemical Technology* vol. 12 (Wiley-Interscience, New York, 4th ed., 1994) pp 842-862.

κ-Form. Ability to form thermoreversible gels. Gelation depends on temperature, concentration of counterions and other polysaccharides. Sol in very polar solvents. Sol in hot milk, hot conc. sugar soln; above 60° in water, as Na⁺ salt in cold water. K⁺ and Ca²⁺ salts are insol in cold water. Insol in in conc. salt soln; 35% alcohol soln; insol with swelling in cold milk. Optimum stablility occurs in pH 9. Degree of sulphation varys from 25-30%.

ι-Form. Ability to form thermoreversible gels. Gelation depends on temperature, concentration of counterions and other polysaccharides. Sol in very polar solvents. Sol in hot milk, hot conc. salt soln; above 60° in water, as Na⁺ salt in cold water; slightly sol hot conc. sugar soln. K⁺ and Ca²⁺ salts are insol in cold water. Insol in 35% alcohol soln; insol in cold milk. Optimum stablility occurs in pH 9. Degree of sulfation varies from 28-35%. LD₅₀ orally in rat: >5000 mg/kg; dermally in rabbit: >2000 mg/kg (Weiner). LC50 (4 hr) in rat: >930.8 ±74.4 mg/m³ (Weiner).

λ-Form. Sol in very polar solvents. Sol in water, milk, hot conc. sugar soln, conc. salt soln., as Na⁺salt in 35% alcohol soln. Optimum stablility occurs in pH 9. The most highly sulfated from 32-39%.

USE: Gelling, emulsifying, and stabilizing agent and viscosity builder in foods and non-foods, but esp in milk or water systems. Demulcent. To induce experimental edema in laboratory animals.

1865. Cartap. [15263-53-3] Carbamothioic acid, *S,S'*-[2-(dimethylamino)-1,3-propanediyl] ester; 1,3-bis(carbamoylthio)-2-*N*,*N*-(dimethylamino)propane. $C_7H_{15}N_3O_2S_2$; mol wt 237.34. C 35.42%, H 6.37%, N 17.70%, O 13.48%, S 27.02%. Insecticide modeled on a toxin isolated from the marine annelid *Lumbrineris heteropoda*. Prepn and insecticidal activity: K. Konishi *et al.*, **FR 1452338**; *eidem*, **US 3332943** (1966, 1968 both to Takeda); K. Konishi, *Agric. Biol. Chem.* **34**, 935 (1970). Crystal structure of hydrochloride: C. J. Cheer, F. J. Pickles, *J. Chem. Soc. Perkin Trans. 2* **1980**, 1805. Comparative study of insecticidal activity: B. Gumey, N. W. Hussey, *Plant Pathol.* **23**, 127 (1974). Effect on soil enzyme activity: T. Endo *et al.*, *J. Pestic. Sci.* **7**, 101 (1982). Aquatic toxicity study: S. Lakota *et al.*, *Acta Hydrobiol.* **23**, 183

(1981). Chronic toxicity study in mice: Y. Tsubura *et al.*, *Nara Igaku Zasshi* **26**, 368 (1975), *C.A.* **84**, 174837c (1976). *Review:* Y. Kono, *Jpn. Pestic. Inf.* **34**, 22 (1978).

Colorless prisms from ethyl acetate, mp 130.5-131° (dec).
Monohydrochloride. NTD-2; Padan. $C_7H_{16}ClN_3O_2S_2$; mol wt 273.80. Colorless rods from methanol, mp 176° (dec). Sol in water. LD₅₀ in mice, rats (mg/kg): 165, 250 orally (Konishi, 1970).
USE: Insecticide.

1866. Carteolol. [51781-06-7] 5-[3-[(1,1-Dimethylethyl)-amino]-2-hydroxypropoxy]-3,4-dihydro-2(1*H*)-quinolinone; 5-[3-(*tert*-butylamino)-2-hydroxypropoxy]-3,4-dihydrocarbostyril. $C_{16}H_{24}N_2O_3$; mol wt 292.37. C 65.73%, H 8.27%, N 9.58%, O 16.42%. β-Adrenergic blocker. Prepn: K. Nakagawa *et al.*, **DE 2302027**; Y. Tamura *et al.*, **US 3910924** (1973, 1975 both to Otsuka); K. Nakagawa, *J. Med. Chem.* **17**, 529 (1974). Pharmacological evaluation in rats: S. Morita *et al.*, *Biochem. Pharmacol.* **25**, 1836 (1976). HPLC determn in plasma and urine: S. Y. Chu, *J. Pharm. Sci.* **67**, 1623 (1978). *In vitro* study: S. Chiba, *Arzneim.-Forsch.* **29**, 895 (1979). Carcinogenicity study: M. Kurosomi *et al.*, *Farmaco Ed. Prat.* **34**, 202 (1979). Series of articles on pharmacology, toxicology and clinical studies: *Arzneim.-Forsch.* **33**, 277-345 (1983). Acute toxicity data: W. Lang, *ibid.* 290. Review of clinical experience in glaucoma and ocular hypertension: P. Chrisp, E. M. Sorkin, *Drugs Aging* **2**, 58-77 (1992).

Hydrochloride. [51781-21-6] Abbott 43326; OPC-1085; Arteoptic; Carteol; Endak; Mikelan; Ocupress; Teoptic. $C_{16}H_{24}N_2O_3 \cdot HCl$; mol wt 328.83. Crystals from ethanol, mp 278°. LD₅₀ in male mice, rats (mg/kg): 810, 1380 orally; 54.5, 158 i.v.; 380, 400 i.p. (Lang).
THERAP CAT: Antihypertensive; antianginal; antiarrhythmic; antiglaucoma.

1867. Carthamin. [36338-96-2] (2*Z*,6*S*)-6-β-D-Glucopyranosyl-2-[[(3*S*)-3-β-D-glucopyranosyl-2,3,4-trihydroxy-5-[(2*E*)-3-(4-hydroxyphenyl)-1-oxo-2-propenyl]-6-oxo-1,4-cyclohexadien-1-yl]methylene]-5,6-dihydroxy-4-[(2*E*)-3-(4-hydroxyphenyl)-1-oxo-2-propenyl]-4-cyclohexene-1,3-dione; carthamic acid; safflor carmine; safflor red; C.I. Natural Red 26; C.I. 75140. $C_{43}H_{42}O_{22}$; mol wt 910.78. C 56.71%, H 4.65%, O 38.65%. Coloring principle from safflower, *Carthamus tinctorius* L., *Compositae*. Purification and review of early efforts: T. Kametaka, A. G. Perkin, *J. Chem. Soc.* **97**, 1415 (1910). Structure: C. Kuroda, *J. Chem. Soc.* **1930**, 752, 765. Revised structure: H. Obara, J. Onodera, *Chem. Lett.* **1979**, 201. Absolute configuration: S. Sato *et al.*, *ibid.* **1996**, 833. Total synthesis as acetate: S. Sato *et al.*, *ibid.* **2001**, 1318. Biogenesis: M. Shimokoriyama, S. Hattori, *Arch. Biochem. Biophys.* **54**, 93 (1955). Determn of levels in *Carthamus Red*: T. Morimoto *et al.*, *Nippon Shokuhin Kagaku Gakkaishi* **5**, 236 (1998). Color stability in aqueous soln: J.-B. Kim, Y.-S. Paik, *Arch. Pharmacal Res.* **20**, 643 (1997); with polysaccharides: K. Saito, *Acta Bot. Croat.* **57**, 123 (1998). Review of prepn protocols: K. Saito, Y. Fukaya, *Acta Alimentaria* **26**, 141-152 (1997). *See also: Colour Index* vol. 4 (3rd ed., 1971) p 4625.

Bright scarlet prismatic needles, mp 228-230° (dec). Hygroscopic. uv max (ethanol): 244, 373, 515 nm (log ε 4.33, 4.48, 4.99). Absorption max (DMF): 530 nm; $E_{1cm}^{1\%}$ 992 (ε 90370). Sparingly sol in water, ethanol and methanol; sol in dil alkali hydroxides, sodium carbonate and ammonia with an orange color. Insol in acetone.

USE: Food color and dye in cosmetics.

1868. Carthamus. Safflower; African saffron; thistle saffron; American saffron; false saffron; bastard saffron; Dyer's saffron. Florets of *Carthamus tinctorius* L. *Compositae. Habit.* Levant; Orient; cultivated extensively in Europe and America. *Constit.* Carthamin, safflor yellow.

USE: In dyeing; surrogate for Spanish saffron; coloring butter, liqueurs, confectionery, cosmetics.

THERAP CAT: Dietary supplement.

1869. Carticaine. [23964-58-1] 4-Methyl-3-[[1-oxo-2-(propylamino)propyl]amino]-2-thiophenecarboxylic acid methyl ester; 3-propylamino-α-propionylamino-2-carbomethoxy-4-methyl-thiophene; methyl 4-methyl-3-(2-propylaminopropionamido)thiophene-2-carboxylate; articaine. $C_{13}H_{20}N_2O_3S$; mol wt 284.37. C 54.91%, H 7.09%, N 9.85%, O 16.88%, S 11.28%. Prepn: H. Ruschig *et al., ZA 6804265; eidem, US 3855243* (1969, 1974 both to Farbwerke Hoechst). Pharmacological studies: R. Muschaweck, R. Rippel, *Prakt. Anaesth.* **9**, 135 (1974); H. Hofer *et al., ibid.* 157; A. Den Hertog, *Eur. J. Pharmacol.* **26**, 175 (1974). Toxicity studies: C. Baeder *et al., Prakt. Anaesth.* **9**, 147 (1974). Mechanism of action: U. Borchard, H. Drouin, *Eur. J. Pharmacol.* **62**, 73 (1980). *Review:* H. Schneider, *Schweiz. Monatsschr. Zahnheilkd.* **86**, 1188-1194 (1976).

bp$_{0.3}$ 162-167°.
Hydrochloride. [23964-57-0] HOE-045; HOE-40045; Ultracain. $C_{13}H_{20}N_2O_3S$·HCl; mol wt 320.84. White, fine crystals, mp 177-178°. LD$_{50}$ i.v. in mice: 37 mg/kg (Muschaweck, Rippel).
THERAP CAT: Anesthetic (local).

1870. Carubicin. [50935-04-1] (8S-cis)-Acetyl-10-[(3-amino-2,3,6-trideoxy-α-L-*lyxo*-hexopyranosyl)oxy]-7,8,9,10-tetrahydro-1,6,8,11-tetrahydroxy-5,12-naphthacenedione; (1S,3S)-3-acetyl-1,2,3,4,6,11-hexahydro-3,5,10,12-tetrahydroxy-6,11-dioxo-1-naphthacenyl 3-amino-2,3,6-trideoxy-α-L-*lyxo*-hexopyranoside; 4-O-demethyldaunorubicin; carminomycin; carminomycin I; karminomycin. $C_{26}H_{27}NO_{10}$; mol wt 513.49. C 60.81%, H 5.30%, N 2.73%, O 31.16%. Anthracycline antitumor antibiotic, related to daunorubicin and doxorubicin, *q.q.v.* Isoln from *Actinomadura carminata:* G. F. Gauze *et al., Antibiotiki* **18**, 675 (1973); M. G. Brazhnikova *et al., ibid.* 678. Antitumor activity: V. A. Shorin *et al., ibid.* 681. Physico-chemical characteristics, structure: M. G. Brazhnikova *et al., J. Antibiot.* **27**, 254 (1974). Pharmacokinetics, pharmacodynamics, toxicity study: L. E. Goldberg *et al., Antibiotiki* **19**, 57 (1974). Production: M. G. Brazhnikova *et al., SU 508076* (1976 to Inst. Antibiot. Res., USSR), *C.A.* **86**, 15215 (1977). Stereochemistry: *eidem, J. Antibiot.* **29**, 469 (1976). Synthesis from daunomycinone: G. Cassinelli *et al., ibid.* **31**, 178

(1978). Molecular pharmacology: V. H. DuVernay *et al., Cancer Res.* **40**, 387 (1980). Analysis in human serum: S. E. Fandrich, K. A. Pittman, *J. Chromatogr.* **223**, 155 (1981). Early clinical studies: L.H. Baker *et al., Cancer Treat. Rep.* **63**, 899 (1979). Embryotoxicity and teratogenicity study: I. Damjanov, A. Celluzzi, *Res. Commun. Chem. Pathol. Pharmacol.* **28**, 497 (1980).

Hydrochloride. [52794-97-5] NSC-180024. $C_{26}H_{27}NO_{10}$·HCl; mol wt 549.95. Crystals from ethanol/benzene. $[\alpha]_D^{20}$ +289°. uv max (ethanol): 236, 255, 462, 478, 492 (E$_{1cm}^{1\%}$ 300), 510, 525 nm. pKa$_1$ 8.00; pKa$_2$ 10.16. Sol in water, methanol. Practically insol in other organic solvents. LD$_{50}$ in mice (mg/kg): 7.3 orally; 1.3 i.v.; 3.7 s.c. (Goldberg).
THERAP CAT: Antineoplastic.

1871. Carumonam. [87638-04-8] [[(Z)-2-[[(2S,3S)-2-[[(Aminocarbonyl)oxy]methyl]-4-oxo-1-sulfo-3-azetidinyl]amino]-1-(2-amino-4-thiazolyl)-2-oxoethylidene]amino]oxy]acetic acid; (Z)-[[[(2-amino-4-thiazolyl)[[(2S,3S)-2-(hydroxymethyl)-4-oxo-1-sulfo-3-azetidinyl]carbamoyl]methylene]amino]oxy]acetic acid carbamate(ester);(3S,4S)-cis-3-[2-(2-amino-4-thiazolyl)-2-(Z)-carboxymethoxyiminoacetamido]-4-carbamoyloxymethyl-2-azetidinone-1-sulfonic acid. $C_{12}H_{14}N_6O_{10}S_2$; mol wt 466.40. C 30.90%, H 3.03%, N 18.02%, O 34.30%, S 13.75%. Synthetic monocyclic β-lactam (monobactam) antibiotic. Prepn: S. Kishimoto *et al., EP 93376;* T. Matsuo *et al., US 4572801* (1983, 1986 both to Takeda); M. Sendai *et al., J. Antibiot.* **38**, 346 (1985). Alternate synthesis: P. S. Manchard *et al., J. Org. Chem.* **53**, 5507 (1988). Comparative *in vitro* antimicrobial activity: R. J. Fass, V. L. Helsel, *Antimicrob. Agents Chemother.* **28**, 834 (1985); B. R. Smith *et al., ibid.* **29**, 346 (1986); I. M. Hoepelman *et al., Chemotherapy (Basel)* **33**, 103 (1987). β-Lactamase stability: R. L. Then, *ibid.* **30**, 398 (1984). Pharmacokinetics in humans: E. Weidekamm *et al., Antimicrob. Agents Chemother.* **26**, 898 (1984); C. A. M. McNulty *et al., ibid.* **28**, 425 (1985).

Colorless powder. $[\alpha]_D^{26}$ −45° (c = 1 in DMSO).
Disodium salt. [86832-68-0] AMA-1080; Ro-17-2301; Amasulin; Mobactam. $C_{12}H_{12}N_6Na_2O_{10}S_2$; mol wt 510.37.
THERAP CAT: Antibacterial.

1872. Carvacrol. [499-75-2] 2-Methyl-5-(1-methylethyl)-phenol; 2-p-cymenol; 2-hydroxy-p-cymene; isopropyl-o-cresol; isothymol. $C_{10}H_{14}O$; mol wt 150.22. C 79.95%, H 9.39%, O 10.65%. Found in oil of origanum, thyme, marjoram, summer savory: E. Guenther, *The Essential Oils* **vol. 2** (Van Nostrand, New York, 1949) p 503; Carpenter, Easter, *J. Org. Chem.* **20**, 401 (1955). Prepn by chlorination of α-pinene with *tert*-butyl hypochlorite: Ritter, Ginsburg, *J. Am. Chem. Soc.* **72**, 2381 (1950); from 2-bromo-p-cymol: Strubell, Baumgartel, *Arch. Pharm.* **291**, 66

(1958). Toxicity data: Kochmann, *Arch. Exp. Pathol. Pharmakol.* **161,** 196 (1931).

Liquid; thymol odor. d_4^{20} 0.976; d_{25}^{25} 0.9751. bp_{760} 237-238°; bp_{18} 118-122°; bp_3 93°. mp ~0°. n_D^{20} 1.52295. uv max (95% ethanol): 277.5 nm (log ε 3.262). Volatile with steam. Practically insol in water. Freely soluble in alc or ether. LD orally in rabbits: 100 mg/kg (Kochmann).

USE: As disinfectant; in organic syntheses.

THERAP CAT: Has been used as anti-infective; anthelmintic (Nematodes).

1873. Carvedilol. [72956-09-3] 1-(9*H*-Carbazol-4-yloxy)-3-[[2-(2-methoxyphenoxy)ethyl]amino]-2-propanol; BM-14190; DQ-2466; Coreg; Dilatrend; Dimitone; Eucardic; Kredex; Querto. $C_{24}H_{26}N_2O_4$; mol wt 406.47. C 70.92%, H 6.45%, N 6.89%, O 15.74%. Nonselective β-adrenergic blocker with $α_1$-blocking activity. Prepn: F. Wiedemann *et al.*, **DE 2815926**; *eidem*, **US 4503067** (1979, 1985 both to Boehringer Mannheim). General pharmacological profile: M. Hirohashi *et al.*, *Arzneim.-Forsch.* **40,** 735 (1990). HPLC determn in biological fluids: K. Reiff, *J. Chromatogr.* **413,** 355 (1987). Series of articles on clinical pharmacology and efficacy in hypertension: *J. Cardiovasc. Pharmacol.* **19,** Suppl. 1, S1-S146 (1992). Clinical trial in chronic heart failure: M. Packer *et al.*, *N. Engl. J. Med.* **334,** 1349 (1996). *Review:* W. H. Frishman, *ibid.* **339,** 1759-1765 (1998).

Colorless crystals from ethyl acetate, mp 114-115°. Freely sol in DMSO; sol in methylene chloride, methanol; sparingly sol in ethanol, isopropanol; slightly sol in ethyl ether. Practically insol in water.

THERAP CAT: Antihypertensive; in treatment of congestive heart failure.

1874. Carvone. [99-49-0] 2-Methyl-5-(1-methylethenyl)-2-cyclohexene-1-one; *p*-mentha-6,8-dien-2-one; 1-methyl-4-isopropenyl-$Δ^6$-cyclohexen-2-one; carvol. $C_{10}H_{14}O$; mol wt 150.22. C 79.95%, H 9.39%, O 10.65%. *d*-Carvone is found in caraway seed and dill seed oils: Schweizer, *J. Prakt. Chem.* **24,** 257 (1841); Gladstone, *J. Chem. Soc.* **25,** 1 (1872). Isoln of *d*-carvone from mandarin peel oil *(Citrus reticulata* Blanco, *Rutaceae): Kugler, Kováts, Helv. Chim. Acta* **46,** 1480 (1963). *l*-Carvone is found in spearmint and kuromoji oils: Kwaenick, *Ber.* **24,** 82 (1891). *dl*-Carvone is found in gingergrass oil: Walbaum, Hüthig, *J. Prakt. Chem.* **71,** 459 (1905). Prepn from α-pinene: Booth, Klein, **US 2796428** (1957 to Glidden). Structure: Wagner, *Ber.* **27,** 2270 (1894); Tiemann, Semmler, *ibid.* **28,** 2147 (1895). Synthesis of *l*-carvone: Royals, Horne, *J. Am. Chem. Soc.* **73,** 5856 (1951); Shono *et al.*, *Chem. Lett.* **1975,** 4330. Synthesis of *dl*-carvone: Suga, *Bull. Chem. Soc. Jpn.* **31,** 569 (1958); I. Fleming, I. Patterson, *Synthesis* **1979,** 736. Toxicity study: P. M. Jenner *et al.*, *Food Cosmet. Toxicol.* **2,** 327 (1964). *Review:* J. L. Simonsen, *The Terpenes* vol. I (University Press, Cambridge, 2nd ed., 1947) pp 394-408; B. Singaram, J. Verghese, *Perfum. Flavor.* **2,** 47 (1977).

d-Form. Liquid, bp_{755} 230°; $bp_{5.6}$ 91°. d_4^{20} 0.965. n_D^{20} 1.4989. $[α]_D^{20}$ +61.2°.
l-Form. Liquid, bp_{763} 230-231°. d_{15}^{15} 0.9652. n_D^{20} 1.4988. $[α]_D^{20}$ −62.46°.
dl-Form. Liquid, bp 230-231°. d_{15}^{15} 0.9645. n_D^{20} 1.5003. Practically insol in water. Misc with alc. LD_{50} orally in rats: 1640 mg/kg (Jenner).

USE: As oil of caraway; also for flavoring liqueurs; in perfumery and soaps.

THERAP CAT: Carminative.

1875. Caryophyllene. [87-44-5] (1*R*,4*E*,9*S*)-4,11,11-Trimethyl-8-methylenebicyclo[7.2.0]undec-4-ene; β-caryophyllene; *trans*-caryophyllene. $C_{15}H_{24}$; mol wt 204.35. C 88.16%, H 11.84%. Sesquiterpenoid occurring in many essential oils and especially in clove oil, the oils from stems and flowers of *Syzygium aromaticum* (L.) Merrill & Perry *(Jambrosa caryophyllus* Niedenzu; *Eugenia caryophyllata* Thunb.), *Myrtaceae.* Occurs in nature as a mixture with isocaryophyllene and α-caryophyllene (humulene, *q.v.*). Isolation of mixture: Schreiner, Kremers, *Pharm. Arch.* **2,** 273, 293 (1899). Existence of isomers: Deussen, *Ann.* **356,** 1 (1907). Structural studies: A. Aebi *et al.*, *J. Chem. Soc.* **1953,** 3124; G. R. Ramage, R. Whitehead, *ibid.* **1954,** 4336. Abs config: D. H. R. Barton, A. Nickon, *ibid.* 4665. Total synthesis of racemic *trans/cis*-forms: E. J. Corey *et al.*, *J. Am. Chem. Soc.* **86,** 485 (1964). Rearrangement to isocaryophyllene: Rachlin, **DE 2044018** (1971 to I.F.F.), *C.A.* **75,** 49364j (1971). *Reviews:* Simonsen, *The Terpenes* vol. III (University Press, Cambridge, 1952) pp 39-71; Barton, de Mayo, *Q. Rev. Chem. Soc.* **11,** 197 (1957); Halsall, *ibid.* **16,** 101 (1962).

Caryophyllene   Isocaryophyllene

Liquid. Has a terpene odor about midway between odor of cloves and turpentine. bp_{14} 129-130°; $bp_{9.7}$ 118-119°. $[α]_D$ −8 to −9° (chloroform). n_D^{17} 1.5009; n_D^{15} 1.5030. d_4^{17} 0.9052.
Isocaryophyllene. [118-65-0] γ-Caryophyllene; *cis*-caryophyllene. Liquid. bp_{19} 130°; $bp_{14.5}$ 125-125.5°. $[α]_D$ −24° (chloroform). n_D^{19} 1.4966. d^{19} 0.8995.

USE: In perfumery.

1876. Carzenide. [138-41-0] 4-(Aminosulfonyl)benzoic acid; *p*-sulfamoylbenzoic acid; 4-carboxybenzenesulfonamide; *p*-sulfonamidobenzoic acid; benzoic acid 4-sulfamide. $C_7H_7NO_4S$; mol wt 201.20. C 41.79%, H 3.51%, N 6.96%, O 31.81%, S 15.94%. Byproduct in the production of saccharin. Prepn from toluene *p*-sulfonamide: W. A. Noyes, *Am. Chem. J.* **7,** 145 (1885); A. A. Goldberg, A. H. Wragg, *J. Chem. Soc.* **1960,** 1408. Metabolism: L. M. Ball *et al.*, *Xenobiotica* **8,** 183 (1978). HPLC determn in saccharin samples: A. E. Mooser, *J. Chromatogr.* **287,** 113 (1984). Toxicity data: D. Appenroth, H. Bräunlich, *Pharmazie* **38,** 102 (1983).

Flat, shiny prisms from water, dec 280°. pKa 3.50. Practically insol in cold water, ether, benzene. Freely sol in alcohol. LD_{50} i.p. in rats: 350 ± 22 mg/kg (Appenroth, Bräunlich).

Sodium salt. $C_7H_6NNaO_4S$. Crystals. Neutral. Soly in water: ~20 g/100 ml.

1877. Carzinophilin A. [106486-76-4] 3-Methoxy-5-methyl-1-naphthalenecarboxylic acid (1S)-2-[[(1E)-1-[(3R, 4R,5S)-3-(acetyloxy)-4-hydroxy-1-azabicyclo[3.1.0]hex-2-ylidene]-2-[[(1Z)-1-(hydroxymethylene)-2-oxopropyl]amino]-2-oxoethyl]amino]-1-[(2S)-2-methyloxiranyl]-2-oxoethyl ester; cardinophyllin; CZ; azinomycin B. $C_{31}H_{33}N_3O_{11}$; mol wt 623.61. C 59.71%, H 5.33%, N 6.74%, O 28.22%. Antitumor antibiotic; alkylates DNA by interstrand crosslinking of the major groove. Isoln from *Streptomyces sahachiroi*: T. Hata *et al., J. Antibiot.* **7A**, 107 (1954). Purification: H. Kamada *et al., ibid.* **8A**, 187 (1955). Mechanism of action: J. W. Lown, K. C. Majumdar, *Can. J. Biochem.* **55**, 630 (1977); T. Fujiwara, I. Saito, *Tetrahedron Lett.* **40**, 315 (1999). Proposed structure: J. W. Lown, C. C. Hanstock, *J. Am. Chem. Soc.* **104**, 3213 (1982). Identity with azinomycin B: E. J. Moran, R. W. Armstrong, *Tetrahedron Lett.* **32**, 3807 (1991). Purification: K. Nagaoka *et al., J. Antibiot.* **39**, 1527 (1986). Total structure as azinomycin B: K. Yokoi *et al., Chem. Pharm. Bull.* **34**, 4554 (1986).

Amorphous white solid, mp 190° (dec). $[\alpha]_D^{20}$ +48° (c = 0.48 in $CHCl_3$). uv max (methanol): 217, 250, 340 nm (ε 65500, 30400, 8500). Sol in acetone, chloroform, ethyl acetate, methanol. Insol in diethyl ether, *n*-hexane, water.

1878. Casanthranol. Cantralax; Peristim. Complex mixture of the purified anthranol glycosides derived from *Cascara sagrada, q.v.*, practically devoid of free anthraquinones. Two active fractions have been identified as **casanthranol A** and **casanthranol B**. Upon oxidative hydrolysis, casanthranol A yields emodin, while casanthranol B under similar treatment yields the aglycone, aloe-emodin, and traces of chrysophanic acid. Prepn: Lee, Berger, **US 2552896** (1951 to Hoffmann-La Roche).

Component of **Peri-Colace**, **Casakol**.

THERAP CAT: Cathartic.

1879. Cascara Amara. Honduras bark. Bark of *Picramnia antidesma* Sw., *Simaroubaceae* and related species. *Habit.* West Indies, Mexico.

1880. Cascara Sagrada. Sacred bark; Chittem bark; Chittim bark; Purshiana bark; Persian bark; bearberry bark; bearwood. Dried bark of *Rhamnus purshiana* DC., *Rhamnaceae*, from which a naturally occurring cathartic is extracted. *Habit.* Northern Idaho, west to Northern California. The cathartic properties are primarily due to the presence of *cascarosides*, anthraglycosides which are related to glycosides found in aloe, *q.v.* and buckthorn. *See* A. Y. Leung, *Drug Cosmet. Ind.* **121**, 42 (December, 1977). Other constituents are aloins (*C*-glycosides), *O*-glycosides, and free anthraquinones: *Analyst* **93**, 749 (1968); *ibid.* **98**, 830 (1973) (Joint Committee Reports). Isoln of anthraquinone aglycones and glycosides: S. C. Yung Su, N. M. Ferguson, *J. Pharm. Sci.* **63**, 899 (1973). Structure of cascarosides A and B: J. W. Fairbairn *et al., J. Pharm. Pharmacol.* **15** (Suppl.) 292T, (1963); F. J. Evans *et al., ibid.* **27** (Suppl.), 91P (1975). Biological evaluation of cascara bark prepns: J. W. Fairbairn, G. E. D. H. Mahran, *ibid.* **5**, 827 (1953).

Commercial prepn, **Cas-Evac**.

THERAP CAT: Cathartic.

THERAP CAT (VET): Laxative.

1881. Cascarilla. Eleuthera bark; sweet-wood bark. Dried bark of *Croton eluteria* (L.) Sw., *Euphorbiaceae. Habit.* Bahama Islands, Cuba, Haiti. *Constit.* About 25% resins, 1.5-3% volatile oil, diterpene bitter principles including cascarillin A (15%). Description and medicinal use: J. Gruenwald *et al., PDR for Herbal Medicines* (Medical Economics, Montvale, 2nd Ed., 2000) p 156.

Volatile oil. [8007-06-5] Oil of cascarilla; oil of sweetwood bark. *Constit. l*-Limonene, *p*-cymene, dipentene, eugenol, cascarillic acid. Chromatographic separation of constituents: A. Claude-Lafontaine *et al., Bull. Soc. Chim. Fr.* **1973** (part 2), 2866. Fragrance monograph: D. L. J. Opdyke, *Food Cosmet. Toxicol.* **14**, Suppl. 1, 707 (1976). Light yellow to brown amber liquid with a pleasant, spicy odor. d_{25}^{25} 0.892-0.914. n_D^{20} 1.488-1.494. Rotation +2° to +5° in a 100-mm tube at 20°. Very sol in alcohol, ether. Sol in most fixed oils, mineral oil. Practically insol in glycerin, propylene glycol. *Keep well closed, cool, and protected from light.*

USE: Flavoring agent; as an addition to smoking tobacco for flavoring.

THERAP CAT: Aromatic bitter.

1882. Cascarillin. [10118-56-6] 3-(Acetyloxy)-1-[2-(3-furanyl)-2-hydroxyethyl]decahydro-5,6-dihydroxy-2,4a,5-trimethyl-1-naphthalenecarboxaldehyde. $C_{22}H_{32}O_7$; mol wt 408.49. C 64.69%, H 7.90%, O 27.42%. From bark of *Croton eluteria* (L.) Sw., *Euphorbiaceae.* Isoln: Duval, *J. Pharm.* **8**, 91 (1845); Mylius, *Ber.* **6**, 1051 (1873); Naylor, Littlefield, *Pharm. J.* **57**, 95 (1896). Structure and stereochemistry: McEachan *et al., J. Chem. Soc. B* **1966**, 633.

Needles from alc, mp 205°. Very bitter taste. Freely sol in ether, hot alc; slightly sol in water, cold alc, chloroform.

THERAP CAT: Aromatic bitter.

1883. Casein. [9000-71-9] A mixture of related phosphoproteins occurring in milk and cheese. Present to the extent of 3% in bovine milk. One of the most nutritive milk proteins in that it contains all of the common amino acids and is rich in the essential ones. Produced in mammary tissue from amino acids supplied by the blood. Obtained from milk by removing the cream and acidifying the skimmed milk which causes casein to precipitate. In cheese manufacture, casein is precipitated by the lactic acid formed from the same milk by fermentation. Precipitation by rennet is favored for casein intended for plastics manuf. Curdling by electricity has been described. The prepn of pure casein is described by Hammarsten, *Textbook of Physiological Chemistry* (New York, 7th ed., 1911) p 619; *Abderhalden's Handbuch* **vol. II** (Berlin, 1910) p 384. Alternate prepn: van Slyke, Baker, *J. Biol. Chem.* **35**, 127 (1918); *cf.* Cohn, Hendry, *Org. Synth.* **coll. vol. II**, 120 (1943). Prepn of casein free from vitamin B_{12} for nutrition experiments: Kissel, **US 2853479** (1958 to Natl. Dairy Prods.). The major casein components may be distinguished by electrophoresis and are designated as α-, β-, γ- and K-caseins, in order of decreasing mobility at pH 7. The complete amino acid sequence of bovine β-casein is known and contains 209 residues with an approx. mol wt of 23,600: Ribadeaudumas *et al., Eur. J. Biochem.* **25**, 505 (1972). *Review:* McKenzie, *Adv. Protein Chem.* **22**, pp 75-135 (1967).

White, amorphous powder or granules without odor or taste. Very sparingly sol in water and in nonpolar organic solvents; sol in aqueous solns of alkalies, levorotatory. The isoelectric zone is around pH 4.7; sol in concd HCl with light violet color. Amphoteric; forms salts with both acids and bases. Present in bovine milk as neutral calcium caseinate and in human milk as potassium caseinate. Precipitated from solns satd with metallic salts. Forms a hard, insol plastic with formaldehyde.

Casamino acids. Commercial acid-hydrolyzed casein. Hydrolysis is carried out until all the nitrogen in the casein is converted to amino acids or other compounds of relative chemical simplicity. Prepn: Mueller, Miller, *J. Immunol.* **40,** 21 (1941); Mueller, Johnson, *ibid.* 33. Typical analysis: N 10%, NaCl 14%, ash 20%, phosphorus as PO_4 2%, Fe 15 mg/3 g.

Note: Legumin, also known as *avenin* or *vegetable casein,* occurring in beans and nuts, is a globulin resembling casein. Isoln from *Avena sativa* L., *Graminea:* Sanson, *Compt. Rend.* **96,** 75 (1883). Structure: C. J. Bailey, D. Boulter, *Eur. J. Biochem.* **17,** 460 (1970).

USE: In the manuf of molded plastics, adhesives, paints, textile finishes, paper coatings, man-made fibers. Vitamin-free casein is used in diets of animals employed for the biological assay of vitamins. Medicinal grades are used in dietetic prepns and for determining the effectiveness of digestive enzyme prepns contg. pepsin, trypsin, papain. Casamino acids are used in microbial assays and in the prepn of microbiological media.

THERAP CAT: Nutrient.

1884. Caspase-1. [122191-40-6] Interleukin 1β precursor proteinase; interleukin-1β converting enzyme; IL-1β converting enzyme; ICE. Primary protease responsible for cleavage of the proinflammatory cytokines *interleukin-1β (IL-1β)* and *interleukin-18 (IL-18)* from their biologically inactive precursors. IL-1β is the predominant form of interleukin-1, *q.v.,* produced by human monocytes. Caspase-1 is synthesized as an inactive 45 kDa precursor protein, *procaspase-1,* that is cleaved to form an active heterodimer composed of 10 and 20 kDa subunits. Identification in monocytes and IL-1β activation: M. J. Kostura *et al., Proc. Natl. Acad. Sci. USA* **86,** 5227 (1989); R. A. Black *et al., FEBS Lett.* **247,** 386 (1989). Purification, primary structure and catalytic mechanism: N. A. Thornberry *et al., Nature* **356,** 768 (1992). Molecular cloning of human cDNA: D. P. Cerretti *et al., Science* **256,** 97 (1992). Induction of apoptosis in fibroblasts: M. Miura *et al., Cell* **75,** 653 (1993). Crystal structure of recombinant human form: N. P. C. Walker *et al., ibid.* **78,** 343 (1994); and mechanism of action: K. P. Wilson *et al., Nature* **370,** 270 (1994). Activation of IL-18 (*interferon-γ-inducing factor*): T. Ghayur *et al., ibid.* **386,** 619 (1997). Overexpression in chronic pancreatitis: M. Ramadani *et al., Pancreas* **22,** 383 (2001); in multiple sclerosis plaques: X. Ming *et al., J. Neurol. Sci.* **197,** 9 (2002). Review of assay methods, purification and inhibition: N. A. Thornberry, *Methods Enzymol.* **244,** 615-631 (1994); of structure and function: M. J. Tocci, *Vitam. Horm.* **53,** 27-63 (1997), of role in intestinal inflammation: B. Siegmund, *Biochem. Pharmacol.* **64,** 1-8 (2002).

1885. Caspase-3. [169592-56-7] Apopain; cysteine protease P32; CPP32. Primary effector caspase required for certain distinctive biochemical and morphological events in cells undergoing apoptosis. Necessary for the dATP/cytochrome *c, q.v.,* inducible cleavage of many cellular targets, including activation of an endonuclease, *caspase-activated DNase (CAD),* that is responsible for DNA fragmentation. CAD activation is achieved by caspase-3 cleavage and inactivation of the *inhibitor of CAD (ICAD).* Synthesized as a 32 kDa inactive zymogen, *procaspase-3,* that is activated by a proteolytic event generating a heterodimer consisting of a 20 kDa (*N*-terminal) and a 12 kDa (*C*-terminal) subunit. Identification: T. Fernandes-Alnemri *et al., J. Biol. Chem.* **269,** 30761 (1994). Identification of poly(ADP-ribose) polymerase (PARP)-cleaving activity: M. Tewari *et al., Cell* **81,** 801 (1995); and characterization of caspase-3: D. W. Nicholson *et al., Nature* **376,** 37 (1995). Role in Fas-mediated apoptosis: J. Schlegel *et al., J. Biol. Chem.* **271,** 1841 (1996). Crystal structure in complex with a tetrapeptide inhibitor: P. R. E. Mittl *et al., ibid.* **272,** 6539 (1997). Cleavage of ICAD: H. Sakahira *et al., Nature* **391,** 96 (1998); and activation of DNA fragmentation: B. B. Wolf *et al., J. Biol. Chem.* **274,** 30651 (1999). Role in the execution phase of apoptosis: R. U. Jänicke *et al., ibid.* **273,** 9357 (1998); E. A. Slee *et al., ibid.* **276,** 7320 (2001). Effect of pH, ionic charge, and osmolality on activity: M. S. Segal, E. Beem, *Am. J. Physiol. Cell Physiol.* **281,** C1196 (2001). Fluorescence studies characterizing the active site: M. Kyoung *et al., Biochim. Biophys. Acta* **1598,** 74 (2002). Review of role in apoptosis: A. G. Porter, R. U. Jänicke, *Cell Death Differ.* **6,** 99-104 (1999).

1886. Caspase-8. [179241-78-2] FADD-like ICE; FLICE; MACH; MORT1-associated CED-3 homolog; Mch5. Initiator caspase required for Fas/CD95/APO-1-mediated apoptosis. Synthesized as a 55 kDa inactive zymogen, *procaspase-8.* Activated by association with the *death-inducing signaling complex (DISC),* leading to the release of active ~12 and ~20 kDa subunits into the cytosol. Isoln, characterization, and apoptotic function: M. P. Boldin *et al., Cell* **85,** 803 (1996); M. Muzio *et al., ibid.* 817. DISC binding and activation: J. P. Medema *et al., EMBO J.* **16,** 2794 (1997). Expression and characterization of isoforms: C. Scaffidi *et al., J. Biol. Chem.* **272,** 26953 (1997). Activation of caspase-3, *q.v.:* H. R. Stennicke *et al., ibid.* **273,** 27084 (1998). Cleavage of the proapoptotic Bcl2 protein, *BID:* H. Li *et al., Cell* **94,** 491 (1998). Role in Fas-mediated apoptosis: P. Juo *et al., Curr. Biol.* **8,** 1001 (1998). X-ray crystal structure of complexes with peptide inhibitors: H. Blanchard *et al., Structure Fold. Des.* **7,** 1125 (1999); W. Watt *et al., ibid.* 1135. Role in lymphocyte activation: H. J. Chun *et al., Nature* **419,** 395 (2002). *Review:* M. Kruidering, G. I. Evan, *IUBMB Life* **50,** 85-90 (2000).

1887. Caspase-9. [180189-96-2] ICE-LAP6; Mch6. Central initiator caspase. Synthesized as an inactive 46 kDa precursor protein, *procaspase-9,* which consists of three domains: an *N*-terminal pro-domain, a 20 kDa large subunit, and a 10 kDa small subunit. Activated in the cytoplasm by cleavage of the prodomain, in response to mitochondrial damage. Activation occurs by binding to an Apaf-1/cytochrome *c* complex known as the apoptosome, in the presence of dATP. Isoln and characterization: H. Duan *et al., J. Biol. Chem.* **271,** 16720 (1996); S. M. Srinivasula *et al., ibid.* 27099. Purification, binding to Apaf-1, and activation of caspase-3, *q.v.:* P. Li *et al., Cell* **91,** 479 (1997). Role in initiation of the caspase cascade: E. A. Slee *et al., J. Cell Biol.* **144,** 281 (1999). Crystal structure of the prodomain in complex with the prodomain of Apaf-1: H. Qin *et al., Nature* **399,** 549 (1999). Human gene structure and chromosomal location: S. Hadano *et al., Mammal. Genome* **10,** 757 (1999). Activation mechanism: J. Rodriguez, Y. Lazebnik, *Genes Dev.* **13,** 3179 (1999); E. N. Shiozaki *et al., Proc. Natl. Acad. Sci. USA* **99,** 4197 (2002). Review of structure and function: K. Kuida, *Int. J. Biochem. Cell Biol.* **32,** 121-124 (2000); of activation mechanism: Y. Shi, *Structure* **10,** 285-288 (2002).

1888. Caspases. Class of cysteine proteases present as inactive zymogens (procaspases) in cytosol of healthy cells. Activated during apoptosis to cleave specific protein targets, usually after aspartic acid residues, leading to organized cellular destruction. At least 14 distinct mammalian caspases have been identified. Apoptotic caspases are divided into two categories, initiator caspases: caspase-2, -8, -9, and -10, and effector caspases: caspase-3, -6, and -7. Caspase-1, and likely caspases-4, -5, -11 and -12, are cytokine activators, responsible for generation of inflammatory response. Identification of interleukin-1β-converting enzyme (caspase-1) as a cysteine protease: N. A. Thornberry *et al., Nature* **356,** 768 (1992). Isolation and apoptotic role of *CED-3,* a caspase homolog from *Caenorhabditis elegans:* J. Yuan *et al., Cell* **75,** 641 (1993). Nomenclature: E. S. Alnemri *et al., Cell* **87,** 171 (1996). Substrate specificites: N. A. Thornberry *et al., J. Biol. Chem.* **272,** 17907 (1997). Induced proximity activation mechanism: G. S. Salvesen, V. M. Dixit, *Proc. Natl. Acad. Sci. USA* **96,** 10964 (1999). Analysis of active sites: D. Chéreau *et al., Biochemistry* **42,** 4151 (2003). Review of role in apoptosis: N. A. Thornberry, Y. Lazebnik, *Science* **281,** 1312-1316 (1998); V. Cryns, J. Yuan, *Genes Dev.* **12,** 1551-1570 (1998); of mammalian caspases: W. C. Earnshaw *et al., Annu. Rev. Biochem.* **68,** 383-424 (1999); of activation pathways: I. Budihardjo *et al., Annu. Rev. Cell Dev. Biol.* **15,** 269-290 (1999); of structure, function and inhibition: J.-B. Denault, G. S. Salvesen, *Chem. Rev.* **102,** 4489-4499 (2002); of mechanisms of activation and inhibition: Y. Shi, *Mol. Cell* **9,** 459-470 (2002); of apoptotic role in neurodegenerative diseases: R. M. Friedlander, *N. Engl. J. Med.* **348,** 1365-1375 (2003).

1889. Caspofungin. [162808-62-0] 1-[(4*R*,5*S*)-5-[(2-Aminoethyl)amino]-*N*^{2}-(10,12-dimethyl-1-oxotetradecyl)-4-hydroxy-L-ornithine]-5-[(3*R*)-3-hydroxy-L-ornithine]-pneumocandin B$_0$. C$_{52}$H$_{88}$N$_{10}$O$_{15}$; mol wt 1093.31. C 57.13%, H 8.11%, N 12.81%, O 21.95%. Semisynthetic echinocandin antifungal that inhibits 1,3-β-D-glucan synthase which is required for cell wall synthesis. Prepn:

J. M. Balkovec *et al.*, **WO 9421677**; *eidem*, **US 5378804** (1994, 1995 both to Merck & Co.). HPLC/MS determn in plasma: C. M. Chavez-Eng *et al.*, *J. Chromatogr. B* **721**, 229 (1999). Clinical study vs amphotericin B, *q.v.* in *Candida* esophagitis: A. Villanueva *et al.*, *Clin. Infect. Dis.* **33**, 1529 (2001). Review of *in vitro* antifungal activity, pharmacology and clinical development: A. H. Groll, T. J. Walsh, *Expert Opin. Invest. Drugs* **10**, 1545-1558 (2001); A. Hoang, *Am. J. Health-Syst. Pharm.* **58**, 1206-1214 (2001).

Acetate. [179463-17-3] MK-0991; Cancidas. $C_{52}H_{88}N_{10}$-$O_{15}.2C_2H_4O_2$; mol wt 1213.42. Hygroscopic white to off-white powder. Freely sol in water, methanol; slightly sol in ethanol.
THERAP CAT: Antifungal.

1890. Cassaidine. [26296-41-3] [1R-(1α,2E,4aα,7β,-8aα,10β,10aβ)]-(Dodecahydro-7,10-dihydroxy-1,4b,8,8-tetramethyl-2(1H)-phenanthrenylidene)acetic acid 2-(dimethylamino)ethyl ester; (E)-3β,7β-dihydroxy-14α-methyl-8β-podocarpane-Δ^{13,α}-acetic acid 2-(dimethylamino)ethyl ester. $C_{24}H_{41}NO_4$; mol wt 407.59. C 70.72%, H 10.14%, N 3.44%, O 15.70%. Cardiotonic principle from the bark of *Erythrophleum guineense* G. Don., *Leguminosae*. Isoln and structure: Ruzicka, Dalma, *Helv. Chim. Acta* **23**, 753 (1940); Engel, *ibid.* **42**, 1127 (1959). Synthesis: Turner *et al.*, *J. Am. Chem. Soc.* **88**, 1766 (1966). Stereochemistry: Clarke *et al.*, *ibid.* **88**, 5865 (1966).

Prisms from acetone + ether, mp 139.5°. $[\alpha]_D^{20}$ −98° (ethanol); $[\alpha]_D^{20}$ −104° (0.1N HCl). Slightly sol in methanol, ethanol, acetone, acetic, chloroform. Practically insol in ether, benzene.
Oxalate. $C_{24}H_{41}NO_4.(COOH)_2$. Crystals from methanol + acetone, mp 198-201°. $[\alpha]_D^{17}$ −84° (c = 1.39 in water).

1891. Cassaine. [468-76-8] [1R-(1α,2E,4aα,4bβ,7β,8aα,-10aβ)]-(Dodecahydro-7-hydroxy-1,4b,8,8-tetramethyl-10-oxo-2(1H)-phenanthrenylidene)acetic acid 2-(dimethylamino)ethyl ester; (E)-3β-hydroxy-14α-methyl-7-oxopodocarpane-Δ^{13,α}-acetic acid 2-(dimethylamino)ethyl ester. $C_{24}H_{39}NO_4$; mol wt 405.57. C 71.07%, H 9.69%, N 3.45%, O 15.78%. Cardiotonic principle

from the bark of *Erythrophleum guineense* G. Don., *Leguminosae*: Dalma, *Helv. Chim. Acta* **22**, 1497 (1939). Structure: Turner *et al.*, *Tetrahedron Lett.* **1959**, 7; Gensler *et al.*, *J. Am. Chem. Soc.* **81**, 5217 (1959). Absolute configuration: Hauth *et al.*, *Helv. Chim. Acta* **48**, 1087 (1965); Clarke *et al.*, *J. Am. Chem. Soc.* **88**, 5865 (1966). Synthesis: Turner *et al.*, *ibid.* 1766.

Glossy flakes from ether, mp 142.5°. $[\alpha]_D^{23}$ −110.5° (alc); $[\alpha]_D^{23}$ −101° (0.1N HCl). Absorption spectrum: Ruzicka, Dalma, *Helv. Chim. Acta* **22**, 1516 (1939). Sol in methanol, ethanol, acetone, acetic acid, chloroform, ether, benzene.
Hydrochloride hydrate. $C_{24}H_{40}ClNO_4.H_2O$. Minute crystals from alcohol + methyl ethyl ketone + ether (1:1:4), mp 220°.

1892. Cassella's Acid. 7-Hydroxy-2-naphthalenesulfonic acid; 2-naphthol-7-sulfonic acid; β-naphthol-δ-monosulfonic acid; β-naphtholsulfonic acid F; F Acid. $C_{10}H_8O_4S$; mol wt 224.23. C 53.56%, H 3.60%, O 28.54%, S 14.30%. Prepn: Bayer, Duisberger, *Ber.* **20**, 1426 (1887); Green, *J. Chem. Soc.* **55**, 33 (1889).

Needles from HCl, mp 89°. Readily sol in water, alcohol; practically insol in ether, benzene.
USE: Dyestuff intermediate.

1893. Cassella's Acid F. [494-44-0] 7-Amino-2-naphthalenesulfonic acid; 2-naphthylamine-7-sulfonic acid; β-naphthylamine-δ-sulfonic acid. $C_{10}H_9NO_3S$; mol wt 223.25. C 53.80%, H 4.06%, N 6.27%, O 21.50%, S 14.36%. Prepn by sulfonation of β-naphthylamine and separation from the 6-amino isomer: Green, *J. Chem. Soc.* **55**, 33 (1889); from 7-hydroxy-2-naphthalenesulfonic acid and ammonia: Green, *loc. cit.*; Wait, **US 1492497** (1924).

Monohydrate. Crystals. Sol in 5040 parts cold water, 350 parts boiling water; sol in glacial acetic acid.
Copper salt. Orange-yellow crystals. Sparingly sol in water.
Ref: Green, Vakil, *J. Chem. Soc.* **113**, 35 (1918).
Note: ***Bronner's acid*** was first described as *6-amino-2-naphthalenesulfonic acid* or *2-naphthylamine-6-sulfonic acid*. However, this product obtained by sulfonation of β-naphthylamine, was subsequently shown to be a mixture of about equal parts of 6- and 7-amino-2-naphthalenesulfonic acids: Green, *loc. cit.*
USE: Both the title compd and its 6-amino isomer are used in the manuf of azo dyes, *e.g.*, **GB 810246** (1959 to Bayer).

1894. Cassia Fistula. Cassia pods; drumstick; Indian laburnum; pudding-stick; pudding pipe; purging cassia. Dried fruit of *Cassia fistula* L. (*Cathartocarpus fistula* [L.] Pers.), *Leguminosae*. *Habit.* Upper Egypt, E. India; cultivated in tropical America and Africa. The pulp of the ripe fruit, ***cassia pulp***, is an almost black, viscid mass with a sweetish taste. *Constit.* Hydroxymethylanthraquinones, gum, tannin, albuminoids, about 60% sugars.
THERAP CAT: Cathartic.

1895. Castanea. Chestnut. Leaves of *Castanea dentata* (Marsh.) Borkh., *Fagaceae*, collected in September and October. *Habit.* Southern Europe. There are hardly any chestnut trees left in the U.S. *Constit.* Tannin, gum, albumin, resin.

1896. Castanospermine. [79831-76-8] (1S,6S,7R,8R,8aR)-Octahydro-1,6,7,8-indolizinetetrol; 1,6,7,8-tetrahydroxyoctahydroindolizine; (1S,6S,7R,8R,8aR)-1,6,7,8-tetrahydroxyindolizidine. $C_8H_{15}NO_4$; mol wt 189.21. C 50.78%, H 7.99%, N 7.40%, O 33.82%. Polyhydroxy alkaloid isolated from the seeds of the Australian leguminous tree, *Castanospermum australe*. Inhibits enzymatic glycoside hydrolysis. Isoln of the naturally occurring (+)-form: L. D. Hohenschutz *et al.*, *Phytochemistry* **20**, 811 (1981). Total synthesis and absolute configuration: R. C. Bernotas, B. Ganem, *Tetrahedron Lett.* **25**, 165 (1984). Alternate synthesis: H. Hamana *et al.*, *J. Org. Chem.* **52**, 5492 (1987). Inhibition of α- and β-glucosidases: R. Saul *et al.*, *Arch. Biochem. Biophys.* **221**, 593 (1983); *eidem, ibid.* **230**, 668 (1984). Insect antifeedant activity: D. L. Dreyer *et al.*, *J. Chem. Ecol.* **11**, 1045 (1985). Inhibition of HIV infectivity *in vitro*: B. D. Walker *et al.*, *Proc. Natl. Acad. Sci. USA* **84**, 8120 (1987); R. A. Gruters *et al.*, *Nature* **330**, 74 (1987).

Crystals from aq ethanol, mp 212-215° (dec). $[\alpha]_D^{25}$ +79.7° (c = 0.93 in water). pK 6.09.

1897. Castle's Intrinsic Factor. Intrinsic factor; IF. A thermolabile mucoprotein with mol wt about 60,000. Promotes vitamin B_{12} absorption by transporting it through the intestinal wall. Occurs in normal gastric juice, but is deficient in patients with pernicious anemia. Prepd from hog mucosa: Castle *et al.*, *Am. J. Med. Sci.* **178**, 748, 764 (1929); **180**, 305 (1930); Glass *et al.*, *Science* **115**, 101 (1952); Heinle *et al.*, *Trans. Assoc. Am. Physicians* **65**, 214 (1952); Latner *et al.*, *Biochem. J.* **55**, XXIII (1953); Callender *et al.*, *Br. Med. J.* **I**, 10 (1954); Latner *et al.*, *Lancet* **I**, 497 (1954); Baum, Federman, **US 2912360** (1959 to Lilly). Purification: Robbins, **US 3008877** (1961 to Armour); Highley, Ellenbogen, **US 3434927** and **US 3591678** (1969, 1971, both to Am. Cyanamid). In approx 30% of pernicious anemia patients, antibodies are produced in the serum which combine with IF, thus inhibiting its biological activity. In clinical tests diminished excretion of vitamin B_{12} in the feces is taken as evidence of intrinsic factor activity. Function in the metabolism of vitamin B_{12}: Glass, *Physiol. Rev.* **43**, 529 (1963). *Review:* Gräsbeck, *Prog. Hematol.* **6**, 233 (1969).

Combination with vitamin B_{12}: Gastrhéma.

THERAP CAT: Adjuvant in vitamin B_{12} utilization.

1898. Castor Oil. Ricinus oil; oil of Palma Christi; tangantangan oil; Neoloid. Fixed oil obtained by cold-pressing the seeds of *Ricinus communis* L., *Euphorbiaceae*. Triglyceride of fatty acids. Fatty acid composition is approx ricinoleic 87%, oleic 7%, linoleic 3%, palmitic 2%, stearic 1% and dihydroxystearic trace amounts: Binder *et al.*, *J. Am. Oil Chem. Soc.* **39**, 513 (1962). Review and bibliography: Anderson, *J. Philipp. Pharm. Assoc.* **42**, 5-16 (1955); Dominguez *et al.*, *J. Chem. Educ.* **20**, 446 (1952); F. C. Naughton *et al.*, in *Kirk-Othmer Encyclopedia of Chemical Technology* vol. 5 (Wiley-Interscience, New York, 3rd ed., 1979) pp 1-15.

Pale yellow, viscous oil. Slight somewhat characteristic odor. The crude oil tastes slightly acrid with a decidedly nauseating aftertaste. Has excellent keeping qualities, does not turn rancid unless subjected to excessive heat. Dextrorotatory (undil. in sodium light). $d_{15.5}^{15.5}$ 0.961-0.963. Wt of tech grades: 8.1 to 8.9 lbs/gallon. n_D^{25} 1.473-1.477. n_D^{40} 1.466-1.473. Solidif −10° to −18°. Viscosity (25°): 6-8 P, also expressed as U ± ½ (Gardner-Holdt Scale). Flash pt 445°F (230°C); ignition temp 840°F (449°C). Surface tension (dynes/cm): at 20°, 39.0; at 80°, 35.2. Acid value <4. Sapon no. 176-187. Iodine no. (Wijs') 81-91. Reichert-Meissl value <0.5. Polenske value <0.5. Acetyl value 144-150. Hydroxyl value 161-169. Miscible with abs ethanol, methanol, ether, chloroform, glacial acetic acid. Dissolves in its own vol of petr ether or 95% alcohol. Does not dissolve to any extent in mineral oil, unless mixed with another vegetable oil. When heated to 300° for several hours it polymerizes and becomes miscible with mineral oil.

USE: As an industrial raw material for the prepn of chemical derivs used in coatings, urethane derivs, surfactants and dispersants, cosmetics, lubricants; chief raw material for the production of sebacic acid, a basic ingredient in the production of synthetic resins and fibers; as lubricant in metal drawing, machine lubrication and 2-cycle engine fuels, in hydraulic fluids, rubber preservative and mold lubricants; constituent of embalming fluids; in soap manuf; to impart emollient and lubricant properties to cosmetic prepns; as Turkey-red oil (sulfated castor oil) for dyeing and finishing textiles; as dehydrated castor oil in alkyds, resinous copolymers, varnishes, oil-based paints, enamels, calks and putties; as blown oil (oxidized oil) for plasticizing oilcloth, artificial leather, coated fabrics, and lacquers; to plasticize rosin in the manuf of sticky fly-paper, for nitrocellulose and similar coating systems, hot melts, duplicating and stencil inks, adhesives and laminants; as release and anti-sticking agent in hard candy manuf.

THERAP CAT: Cathartic.

THERAP CAT (VET): Mild purgative, but considered unreliable in adult horses. Emollient.

1899. Castor Oil, Hydrogenated. Opalwax; Castorwax. Mol wt about 932. A hard, white wax, mp 86-88°. Iodine number (Wijs') <5.0. Extremely insol in water and in the more common organic solvents.

USE: In water-repellent coatings, candles, shoe polish, carbon paper, ointments and cosmetics; for impregnating paper, wood, cloth; for electrical condenser impregnation; as solid lubricant; as a pressure mold release agent in the manuf of formed plastics and rubber goods.

1900. Catalase. [9001-05-2] Caperase; Equilase; Optidase. Enzymes which promote reactions involving the decompn of hydrogen peroxide to water and oxygen. Although widely distributed among animals, plants, bacteria, and fungi, catalase in mammalian liver and blood has been most intensively studied. Catalase for commercial use obtained from animal liver, bacterial (*Micrococcus lysodeikticus*), and fungal (*Aspergillus niger*) sources. Isoln from mammalian livers and kidneys: Lolli, Cavanaugh, **US 2703779** (1955 to Armour); Schroeder *et al.*, *Biochim. Biophys. Acta* **58**, 611 (1962); Dan, **US 2992167** (1961 to Chr. Hansen's Lab.); from *Aspergillus niger*: Faucett *et al.*, **US 3102081** (1963 to Miles Labs.). All catalases so far isolated contain four tetrahedrally arranged subunits of equal size giving an approximate mol wt of 240,000. Each subunit consists of a single polypeptide chain associated with a single prosthetic group, ferric protoporphyrin IX. Amino acid sequence of bovine liver catalase subunit: Schroeder *et al.*, *Arch. Biochem. Biophys.* **131**, 653 (1969). Bovine *hepatocatalase*, a term for catalase obtained from liver, was reported to lower serum cholesterol; the active form was found to contain a catalytic amount of zinc (0.32%): Azarnoff, Curran, *J. Lab. Clin. Med.* **60**, 856 (1962); cf. Laporte *et al.*, *Biochem. Pharmacol.* **11**, 670 (1962). *Reviews:* Nicholls, Schonbaum, in *The Enzymes* vol. 8, P. D. Boyer *et al.*, Eds. (Academic Press, New York, 1963) pp 147-225; Deisseroth, Daunce, *Physiol. Rev.* **50**, 319 (1970); Schonbaum, Chance, in *The Enzymes* vol. 13 (part C), P. D. Boyer, Ed. (Academic Press, New York, 3rd ed., 1976) pp 363-408.

USE: In combination with glucose oxidase, for treatment of food wrappers to prevent oxidative deterioration of food: Sarett, Scott, **US 2765233** (1956 to Ben L. Sarett). In the removal of traces of peroxide in the process of cold sterilization (preservation of milk and cheese by treatment with hydrogen peroxide). With glucose oxidase, *q.v.*, in food preservation.

1901. Catalposide. [6736-85-2] [1aS-(1aα,1bβ,2β,5aβ,6β,-6aα)]-1a,1b,2,5a,6,6a-Hexahydro-6-[(4-hydroxybenzoyl)oxy]-1a-(hydroxymethyl)oxireno[4,5]cyclopenta[1,2-c]pyran-2-yl-β-D-glucopyranoside; Catalpin. $C_{22}H_{26}O_{12}$; mol wt 482.43. C 54.77%, H 5.43%, O 39.80%. From unripe fruit of *Catalpa bignonioides* Walt. or *C. ovata* G. Don, *Bignoniaceae*: Claassen, *Am. Chem. J.* **10**, 228 (1888). Historical summary: Bobbitt *et al.*, *J. Org. Chem.* **26**, 3090 (1961). Structure: Lunn *et al.*, *Can. J. Chem.* **40**, 104 (1962). Stereochemistry: Bobbitt *et al.*, *J. Org. Chem.* **31**, 500 (1966); **32**, 1459 (1967).

Crystals from methanol + ethyl acetate, mp 215-216.5°. $[\alpha]_D^{23.2}$ $-184°$ (c = 0.87 in methanol). uv max (ethanol): 260 nm (log ε 4.27); in sodium hydroxide: 303 nm (log ε 4.35). Soluble in water, alcohol; slightly sol in benzene, chloroform, ether.

Hexaacetate. $C_{34}H_{38}O_{18}$. Crystals from ethanol, mp 141.5°. $[\alpha]_D^{21.7}$ $-106°$ (c = 0.75 in chloroform).

1902. Catechin. [154-23-4] (2R-trans)-2-(3,4-Dihydroxy-phenyl)-3,4-dihydro-2H-1-benzopyran-3,5,7-triol; catechol; 3,3',4',-5,7-flavanpentol; catechinic acid; catechuic acid; (+)-cyanidanol-3; dexcyanidanol; cyanidol; Catergen. $C_{15}H_{14}O_6$; mol wt 290.27. C 62.07%, H 4.86%, O 33.07%. Flavonoid found primarily in higher woody plants as (+)-catechin along with (−)-epicatechin (cis form). From catechu (gambir and acacia), mahogany wood, etc.: Perkin, Yoshitake, J. Chem. Soc. 81, 1160 (1902); Freudenberg et al., Ber. 55, 1734 (1922). Structure: Freudenberg et al., Ann. 444, 135 (1925). Stereochemistry: Clark-Lewis, Chem. Ind. (London) 1955, 1218; Hardegger et al., Helv. Chim. Acta 40, 1819 (1957); Clark-Lewis, J. Chem. Soc. 1960, 2433. Pharmacology: Van Cauwenberge et al., C.R. Seances Soc. Biol. Ses Fil. 165, 1195 (1971). Metabolism: Das, Sothy, Biochem. J. 125, 417 (1971); and absorption in human: N. P. Das, Biochem. Pharmacol. 20, 3435 (1971). Biosynthesis of epicatechins: Zaprometov, Grisebach, Z. Naturforsch. 28c, 113 (1973). Other catechins such as **afzelechin** and **gallocatechin** and catechin oligomers (**procyanidins**) also exist in nature: Thompson et al., J. Chem. Soc. Perkin Trans. 1 1972, 1287. See also Bioflavonoids.

Needles from water + acetic acid, occurs as hydrate. mp 93-96°; 175-177° when anhydr. $[\alpha]_D^{18}$ +16 to +18.4°.

dl-Form. [7295-85-4] Needles from water + acetic acid, mp 212-216°. Slightly sol in cold water, ether; sol in hot water, alcohol, glacial acetic acid, acetone. Practically insol in benzene, chloroform, petr ether.

l-Form. [18829-70-4] Needles from water + acetic acid, mp 93-96°; 175-177° when anhydr. $[\alpha]_D$ $-16.8°$.

Note: Catechin is also called catechol (flavan) to distinguish it from catechol (pyrocatechol, q.v.).

USE: In dyeing and tanning.

THERAP CAT: Antidiarrheal.

1903. Catechu Black. Cutch; cachou; pegu catechu; cashoo. Extract prepd from heartwood of Acacia catechu Willd., Leguminosae. Habit. India, Hindustan, Ceylon; naturalized in Jamaica. Constit. 25-35% catechutannic acid, 2-10% catechin; catechu red, quercetin, gum.

Incompat. Iron compds, gelatin, lime water, zinc sulfate.

USE: Tanning, dyeing fabrics brown and black; staining wood; in toilet preparations.

THERAP CAT: Astringent (diarrheal).

THERAP CAT (VET): Has been used as intestinal astringent.

1904. Catharanthine. [2468-21-5] 3,4-Didehydroibogamine-18-carboxylic acid methyl ester; 7-ethyl-9,10,12,13-tetrahydro-6,9-methano-5H-pyrido[1',2':1,2]azepino[4,5-b]indole-6(6aH)-carboxylic acid methyl ester. $C_{21}H_{24}N_2O_2$; mol wt 336.43. C 74.97%, H 7.19%, N 8.33%, O 9.51%. Precursor of vinblastine-type alkaloids. Isoln from Vinca rosea Linn. (Catharanthus roseus G. Don.) Apocynaceae: M. Gorman et al., J. Am. Pharm. Assoc. Sci. Ed. 48, 256 (1959); G. H. Svoboda et al., ibid. 659. Structure: N. Neuss, M. Gorman, Tetrahedron Lett. 1961, 206. Abs config: K. Bláha et al., ibid. 1972, 2763. Synthesis of (±)-form: A. A. Qureshi, A. I. Scott, Chem. Commun. 1968, 947, 948; A. R. Battersby et al., ibid. 951; G. Büchi et al., J. Am. Chem. Soc. 92, 999 (1970); J. P. Kutney, F. Bylsma, Helv. Chim. Acta 58, 1672 (1975); B. M. Trost et al., J. Org. Chem. 44, 2052 (1979); T. Imanishi et al., Tetrahedron Lett. 21, 3285 (1980).

Crystals from methanol, mp 126-128°. uv max (ethanol): 226, 284, 292 nm (log ε 4.56, 3.92, 3.88). $[\alpha]_D^{27}$ +29.8° (CHCl₃). pKa' 6.8.

1905. Cathepsins. Intracellular proteinases obtained from animal tissue extracts, the richest sources being liver, kidney and spleen. Located primarily in the lysosomal fraction within the cell. Part of the general enzymic apparatus of animal cells; in most cases they do not specialize in functions characteristic of individual tissues. Review of cathepsins A-C: J. S. Fruton in The Enzymes vol. 4, P. D. Boyer et al., Eds. (Academic Press, New York, 1960) pp 233-241; of cathepsins A-E: M. J. Mycek, Methods Enzymol. 19, 285-315 (1970); of cathepsins B, D and G: several authors, Res. Monogr. Cell Tissue Physiol. 2, 57-89, 181-248 (1977); of cathepsins B, D, G, H, L, N and S: several authors, Ciba Found. Symp. 75, 1-68 (1980).

Cathepsin C. Dipeptidyl transferase; dipeptidyl amino peptidase I. Isoln from beef spleen: Tallan et al., J. Biol. Chem. 194, 793 (1952); de la Haba et al., ibid. 234, 316 (1959). Hydrolyzes dipeptidyl amides or esters bearing a free α-amino (or α-imino) group in the N-terminal position, esp. those containing an aromatic amino acid adjacent to the free α-amino group: Planta, Gruber, Biochim. Biophys. Acta 53, 443 (1961); Wurz et al., Biochemistry 1, 19 (1962). Enhances the proteolysis of prothrombin to thrombin and thus plays an important role in blood clotting: Purcell, Barnhart, Biochim. Biophys. Acta 78, 800 (1963).

Cathepsin D. Isoln from bovine spleen: Press et al., Biochem. J. 74, 501 (1960); Webb, ibid. 76, 538 (1960); 84, 455 (1962). Involved in the catabolism of cartilage and connective tissue: Weston et al., Nature 222, 285 (1969).

Cathepsin G. Isoln from human spleen: G. Starkey et al., Biochem. J. 155, 255 (1976). Chymotrypsin-like enzyme. Catalytic and immunological properties: P. M. Starkey, A. J. Barrett, ibid. 273.

1906. Cathinone. [71031-15-7] (2S)-2-Amino-1-phenyl-1-propanone; (−)-α-aminopropiophenone; norephedrone. C_9H_{11}-NO; mol wt 149.19. C 72.46%, H 7.43%, N 9.39%, O 10.72%. Psychoactive alkaloid found in the leaves of the khat plant, Catha edulis Forsk., Celastraceae. Prepn of racemic compd: L. Behr-Bergowski, Ber. 30, 1515 (1897); S. Gabriel, ibid. 41, 1127 (1908). Isoln from C. edulis: X. Schorno, E. Streinegger, Experientia 35, 572 (1979); and identification as active constituent of khat: D. W. Peterson et al., Life Sci. 27, 2143 (1980). Stereospecific synthesis from norephedrine: B. D. Berrang et al., J. Org. Chem. 47, 2643 (1982). Metabolism in humans: R. Brenneisen et al., J. Pharm. Pharmacol. 38, 298 (1986). HPLC determn in urine: K. Mathys, R. Brenneisen, J. Chromatogr. 593, 79 (1992). Quantitative determn in khat: A. M. Al-Obaid et al., J. Pharm. Biomed. Anal. 17, 321 (1998). Review of pharmacology: P. Kalix, Pharmacol. Toxicol. 70, 77-86 (1992).

Sol in methanol (with racemization), methylene chloride. $[\alpha]_D$ $-46.8°$ (c = 0.24 in methanol).

Hydrochloride. [76333-53-4] $C_9H_{11}NO.HCl$. Crystals from isopropanol-THF, mp 189-190°.

Note: This is a controlled substance (stimulant): **21 CFR,** 1308.11.

1907. Catnep. Cataria; catnip; catmint. Herb of *Nepeta cataria* L., *Labiatae*. *Habit.* Europe, Asia; naturalized in U.S. *Constit.* Volatile oil, nepetalactone, *q.v.,* nepetalic acid and related compds, tannin: McElvain, Eisenbraun, *J. Am. Chem. Soc.* **77,** 1599 (1955). Its odor is very attractive to all members of the cat family.

THERAP CAT: Aromatic.

1908. 2C-B. [66142-81-2] 4-Bromo-2,5-dimethoxybenz-eneethanamine; 4-bromo-2,5-dimethoxyphenethylamine; α-des-methyl DOB; BDMPEA; MFT; nexus. $C_{10}H_{14}BrNO_2$; mol wt 260.13. C 46.17%, H 5.42%, Br 30.72%, N 5.38%, O 12.30%. Psychoactive analog of mescaline, *q.v.* Synthesis and activity: A. T. Shulgin, M. F. Carter, *Psychopharmacol. Commun.* **1,** 93 (1975). Qualitative analysis: F. A. Ragan, Jr. *et al., J. Anal. Toxicol.* **9,** 91 (1985). Pharmacology: R. A. Glennon *et al., Pharmacol. Biochem. Behav.* **30,** 597 (1988); M. Lobos *et al., Gen. Pharmacol.* **23,** 1139 (1992).

Hydrochloride. [56281-37-9] $C_{10}H_{14}BrNO_2.HCl$. Pale pink crystals from ethanol, mp 237-239° (dec). uv max (dil H_2SO_4): 294 nm.

Note: This is a controlled substance (hallucinogen): **21 CFR,** 1308.11.

1909. Ceanothic Acid. [21302-79-4] (2α,3β)-3-Hydroxy-A(1),28-dinorlup-20(29)-ene-2,17-dicarboxylic acid; emmolic acid. $C_{30}H_{46}O_5$; mol wt 486.68. C 74.04%, H 9.53%, O 16.44%. From *Ceanothus americanus* L., *Rhamnaceae* (New Jersey tea). Isoln: Julian *et al., J. Am. Chem. Soc.* **60,** 77 (1938). Identity of ceanothic acid and emmolic acid: Mechoulam, *Chem. Ind. (London)* **1961,** 1835. Structure: de Mayo, Starratt, *Tetrahedron Lett.* **1961,** 259; Mechoulam, *J. Org. Chem.* **27,** 4070 (1962). Stereochemistry: de Mayo, Starratt, *Can. J. Chem.* **40,** 788 (1962). Revised stereochemistry: Eade *et al., Aust. J. Chem.* **24,** 621 (1971).

Crystals from methanol + ether, mp 356-357°. $[\alpha]_D$ +38° (c = 1.20 in ethanol).

Dimethyl ester. $C_{32}H_{50}O_5$. Crystals from ether + petr ether, mp 221-223°. $[\alpha]_D$ +41° (chloroform).

1910. Cecropins. A major class of non-specific antibacterial proteins induced in hemolymph of some insects as part of the immune response. First characterized in *Lepidoptera,* particularly *Hyalophora cecropia.* (*See also* attacins.) Small, basic polypeptides which possess similar amino acid sequences with relatively long hydrophobic regions, mol wt approx 4000 Da. Originally designated *protein P9,* three major peptides have been characterized, cecropins A, B, D; three minor peptides C, E, F are also known. Identification of cell free immune response in *Lepidoptera:* H. Boman *et al., Infect. Immun.* **10,** 136 (1974). Initial identification and isolation of immune response proteins in *H. cecropia:* I. Faye *et al., ibid.* **12,** 1426 (1975). Purification and preliminary characterization of cecropins A and B: D. Hultmark *et al., Eur. J. Biochem.* **106,** 7 (1980); antibacterial spectrum and amino acid sequence: H. Steiner *et al., Nature* **292,** 246 (1981). Partial synthesis of A: R. B. Merrifield *et al., Biochemistry* **21,** 5020 (1982). Total synthesis of A: D. Andreu *et al., Proc. Natl. Acad. Sci. USA* **80,** 6475 (1983); of B: P. van Hofsten *et al., ibid.* **82,** 2240 (1985). Isolation, characterization of cecropins C, D, E, F, and comparison with A and B: D. Hultmark *et al., Eur. J. Biochem.* **127,** 207 (1982); X. Qu *et al., ibid.* 219. Isoln of cecropin-like proteins from flesh fly larvae: M. Okada, S. Natori, *Biochem. J.* **211,** 727 (1983); from tsetse fly: G. P. Kaaya *et al., Insect Biochem.* **17,** 309 (1987). Cecropin-like proteins designated as *lepidopterans* have been isolated from *Bombyx mori* silkworms: T. Teshima *et al., Tetrahedron Lett.* **28,** 4705 (1987). Mechanism of action: H. Steiner *et al., Biochim. Biophys. Acta* **939,** 260 (1988); B. Christensen *et al., Proc. Natl. Acad. Sci. USA* **85,** 5072 (1988). Review of cecropins A and B: H. G. Boman, H. Steiner in *Current Topics in Microbiology and Immunology* **94/95,** W. Henle *et al.,* Eds. (Springer-Verlag, N.Y., 1981) pp 75-91.

1911. Cedrol. [77-53-2] [3*R*-(3α,3aβ,6α,7β,8aα)]-Octahydro-3,6,8,8-tetramethyl-1*H*-3a,7-methanoazulen-6-ol; 8β*H*-cedran-8-ol; cedar camphor; cypress camphor. $C_{15}H_{26}O$; mol wt 222.37. C 81.02%, H 11.79%, O 7.19%. Occurs in cedar wood oil from *Juniperus virginiana* L. (*J. sabina* Kook), *Cupressaceae,* in cypress oil from *Cupressus sempervirens: Schimmel's Report* **1904,** II, 20; in the oil from *Juniperus chinensis:* Kondo, *J. Pharm. Soc. Jpn.* **1907,** 236; and from *Origanum smyrnaeum* L., *Labiatae: Schimmel's Report* **1906,** Oct., 72. Structure: Stork, Breslow, *J. Am. Chem. Soc.* **75,** 3291, 3292 (1953). Stereochemistry and total synthesis: Stork, Clarke, *ibid.* **83,** 3114 (1961). Synthesis of *dl*-form: Corey *et al., ibid.* **91,** 1557 (1969); *eidem, Tetrahedron Lett.* **1973,** 3153; E. G. Breitholle, A. G. Fallis, *J. Org. Chem.* **43,** 1964 (1978).

Needles from dil methanol, mp 86-87°. $[\alpha]_D^{28}$ +9.9° (c = 5 in chloroform).

USE: In fragrances.

1912. Cefaclor. [70356-03-5] (6*R*,7*R*)-7-[[(2*R*)-Amino-phenylacetyl]amino]-3-chloro-8-oxo-5-thia-1-azabicyclo[4.2.0]oct-2-ene-2-carboxylic acid monohydrate; 7-(D-2-amino-2-phenylacet-amido)-3-chloro-3-cephem-4-carboxylic acid monohydrate; 3-chloro-7-D-(2-phenylglycinamido)-3-cephem-4-carboxylic acid monohydrate; compd 99638; Alfacet; Alfatil; Ceclor; Distaclor; Panacef; Panoral. $C_{15}H_{14}ClN_3O_4S.H_2O$; mol wt 385.82. C 46.70%, H 4.18%, Cl 9.19%, N 10.89%, O 20.73%, S 8.31%. Semi-synthetic cephalosporin antibiotic, related to cephalexin, *q.v.* Prepn: R. R. Chauvette, DE 2408698 (1974 to Lilly), *C.A.* **82,** 4278n (1975); US 3925372 (1975 to Lilly); R. R. Chauvette, P. A. Pennington, *J. Med. Chem.* **18,** 403 (1975). *In vitro* studies: M. S. Silver *et al., Antimicrob. Agents Chemother.* **12,** 591 (1977); R. N. Jones, *J. Antibiot.* **30,** 753 (1977); B. R. Meyers, S. Z. Hirschman, *J. Clin. Pharmacol.* **18,** 85 (1978). Metabolism: N. G. Waterman, L. F. Sharfenberger, *Antimicrob. Agents Chemother.* **14,** 614 (1978). Human pharmacology: G. R. Hodges *et al., ibid.* 454; A. Glynne *et al., J. Antimicrob. Chemother.* **4,** 343 (1978). Clinical studies: J. D. Nelson *et al., Am. J. Dis. Child.* **132,** 992 (1978); B. M. Gray *et al., Antimicrob. Agents Chemother.* **13,** 988 (1978). Comprehensive description: L. J. Lorenz, *Anal. Profiles Drug Subs.* **9,** 107-123 (1980).

Crystalline solid. uv max (pH 7 buffer): 265 nm (ε 6800). Sol in water. Practically insol in methanol, chloroform, benzene. Solns are stable at pH 2.5-4.5.

THERAP CAT: Antibacterial.

1913. Cefadroxil. [66592-87-8] (6R,7R)-7-[[(2R)-Amino-(4-hydroxyphenyl)acetyl]amino]-3-methyl-8-oxo-5-thia-1-azabicy-clo[4.2.0]oct-2-ene-2-carboxylic acid monohydrate; 7-[D-(-)-α-amino-α-(4-hydroxyphenyl)acetamido]-3-methyl-3-cephem-4-car-boxylic acid monohydrate; p-hydroxycephalexine monohydrate; BL-S578; MJF-11567-3; Baxan; Bidocef; Cefa-Drops; Cefamox; Ceforal; Cephos; Duracef; Duricef; Kefroxil; Oracéfal; Sedral; Ul-tracef. $C_{16}H_{17}N_3O_5S.H_2O$; mol wt 381.40. C 50.39%, H 5.02%, N 11.02%, O 25.17%, S 8.41%. Semi-synthetic cephalosporin antibiotic. Prepn: NL 6812382; L. B. Crast, Jr., US 3489752 (1969, 1970 both to Bristol-Myers); T. Takahashi et al., DE 2216113; eidem, US 3816253 (1972, 1974, both to Takeda). Prepn of crystalline monohydrate: D. Bouzard et al., US 4504657 (1985 to Bristol-Myers). Antimicrobial activity: R. E. Buck, K. E. Price, Antimicrob. Agents Chemother. 11, 324 (1977). Pharmacology: M. Pfeffer et al., ibid. 331; A. I. Hartstein et al., ibid. 12, 93 (1977). Review: J. Antimicrob. Chemother. 10, Suppl. B, 1-162 (1982). Series of articles on clinical trials in respiratory tract infections: Drugs 32, Suppl. 3, 1-56 (1986).

White crystals, mp 197° (dec).

THERAP CAT: Antibacterial.

THERAP CAT (VET): Antibacterial.

1914. Cefamandole. [34444-01-4] (6R,7R)-7-[[(2R)-Hy-droxyphenylacetyl]amino]-3-[[(1-methyl-1H-tetrazol-5-yl)thio]-methyl]-8-oxo-5-thia-1-azabicyclo[4.2.0]oct-2-ene-2-carboxylic acid; 7-mandelamido-3-[[(1-methyl-1H-tetrazol-5-yl)thio]methyl]-8-oxo-5-thia-1-azabicyclo[4.2.0]oct-2-ene-2-carboxylic acid; 7-D-mandelamido-3-[[(1-methyl-1H-tetrazol-5-yl)thio]methyl]-3-ceph-em-4-carboxylic acid; 7-D-mandelamido-3-(1-methyl-1,2,3,4-tetra-zole-5-thiomethyl)-Δ³-cephem-4-carboxylic acid; CMT; compd 83405. $C_{18}H_{18}N_6O_5S_2$; mol wt 462.50. C 46.74%, H 3.92%, N 18.17%, O 17.30%, S 13.87%. Broad-spectrum semi-synthetic cephalosporin antibiotic. Prepn: C. W. Ryan, DE 2018600; idem, US 3641021 (1970, 1972 to Lilly); J. M. Greene, DE 2312997; idem, US 3840531 (1973, 1974 to Lilly). Biological properties: W. E. Wick, D. A. Preston, Antimicrob. Agents Chemo-ther. 1, 221 (1972). Antibacterial activity: S. Eykyn et al., ibid. 3, 657 (1973); H. C. Neu, ibid. 6, 177 (1974); A. D. Russell, J. Antimicrob. Chemother. 1, 97 (1975). Pharmacologic studies: B. R. Meyers et al., Antimicrob. Agents Chemother. 9, 140 (1976); R. S. Griffith et al., ibid. 10, 814 (1976). Comprehensive description: R. H. Bishara, E. C. Rickard, Anal. Profiles Drug Subs. 9, 125-154 (1980).

Nafate. [42540-40-9] Bergacef; Cedol; Cefam; Cefiran; Ce-mado; Cemandil; Fado; Kefadol; Kefandol; Lampomandol; Man-dokef; Mandol; Mandolsan; Neocefal; Pavecef. $C_{19}H_{17}N_6NaO_6$-S_2; mol wt 512.49. White, odorless needles, mp 190° (dec). uv max (H₂O): 269 nm (ε 10800). pKa 2.6-3.0. Sol in water, meth-anol. Practically insol in ether, chloroform, benzene, cyclohexane.

THERAP CAT: Antibacterial.

1915. Cefatrizine. [51627-14-6] (6R,7R)-7-[[(2R)-Amino-(4-hydroxyphenyl)acetyl]amino]-8-oxo-3-[(1H-1,2,3-triazol-4-yl-thio)methyl]-5-thia-1-azabicyclo[4.2.0]oct-2-ene-2-carboxylic acid; 7-[D-α-amino-α-(4-hydroxyphenyl)acetamido]-3-(1,2,3-tria-zol-4(5)-ylthiomethyl)-3-cephem-4-carboxylic acid; BL-S640; SKF-60771; S-640P; Cefaperos. $C_{18}H_{18}N_6O_5S_2$; mol wt 462.50. C 46.74%, H 3.92%, N 18.17%, O 17.30%, S 13.87%. Orally active semi-synthetic cephalosporin antibiotic. Prepn: G. L. Dunn, J. R. E. Hoover, DE 2316866; eidem, US 3867380 (1974, 1975 both to SK&F); D. Willner, L. B. Crast, DE 2364192 (1974 to Bristol-Myers), C.A. 81, 105538 (1974); G. L. Dunn et al., J. Antibiot. 29, 65 (1976). Prepn of the propylene glycolate: M. A. Kaplan, A. P. Granatek, DE 2500385; eidem, US 3970601 (1975, 1976 both to Bristol-Myers). In vitro and in vivo antibacterial activity and phar-macokinetic behavior: P. Actor et al., ibid. 28, 594 (1975); F. Leitner et al., Antimicrob. Agents Chemother. 7, 298 (1975). Gen-eral pharmacological properties: M. Matsuzaki et al., Jpn. J. Anti-biot. 29, 107 (1976), C.A. 85, 311g (1976). Determn in serum and urine by HPLC: E. Crombez et al., J. Chromatogr. 173, 165 (1979). Disposition of ¹⁴C-cefatrizine in man: R. C. Gaver, G. Deeb, Drug Metab. Dispos. 8, 157 (1980). Activity and clinical use: A. J. Weinstein, Drugs 20, 137 (1980). Acute toxicity: M. Matsuzaki et al., Jpn. J. Antibiot. 29, 612 (1976), C.A. 85, 171724y (1976). Toxicological studies: ibid. 639-686, C.A. 85, 171722w-171723x (1976). Series of articles on pharmacokinetics and clinical efficacy: Drugs Exp. Clin. Res. 11, 441-462 (1985).

Zwitterionic. LD₅₀ in male, female mice, male, female rats (mg/kg): 6880, 6410, 4325, 4325 i.p. (Matsuzaki).

Compd with propylene glycol. [64217-62-5] Bricef; Cepticol; Cefotrizin; Faretrizin; Kefoxina; Tamyl; Zitrix. $C_{18}H_{18}N_6O_5S_2$.-$C_3H_8O_2$; mol wt 538.60. Rod-like crystals. $[\alpha]_D^{23}$ +55.9° (c = 1% in 1N HCl). uv max: 227, 272 nm.

THERAP CAT: Antibacterial.

1916. Cefazedone. [56187-47-4] (6R,7R)-7-[[(3,5-Di-chloro-4-oxo-1(4H)-pyridinyl)acetyl]amino]-3-[[(5-methyl-1,3,4-thiadiazol-2-yl)thio]methyl]-8-oxo-5-thia-1-azabicyclo[4.2.0]oct-2-ene-2-carboxylic acid; 3-(5-methyl-1,3,4-thiadiazolyl-2-mercapto-methyl)-7-(3,5-dichloro-4-pyridon-1-ylacetamido)-3-cephem-4-carboxylic acid; EMD-30087. $C_{18}H_{15}Cl_2N_5O_5S_3$; mol wt 548.44. C 39.42%, H 2.76%, Cl 12.93%, N 12.77%, O 14.59%, S 17.54%. Semi-synthetic cephalosporin antibiotic. Prepn: R. Gerike et al., DE 2345402; eidem, US 4153693 (1975, 1979 both to E. Merck, W. Ger.). See also eidem, DE 2621011, DE 2626026, DE 2627204 (all 1977 to E. Merck, W. Ger.), C.A. 88, 5093, 105383, 121213 (1978). Series of articles on prepn, in vitro and in vivo activity, kinetics, pharmacology, toxicology, and clinical trials: Arzneim.-Forsch. 29, 361-462 (1979). Toxicity data: M. von Eberstein et al., ibid. 424.

Crystals from acetonitrile.

Sodium salt. [63521-15-3] Refosporin. $C_{18}H_{14}Cl_2N_5NaO_5$-S_3; mol wt 570.43. LD_{50} in mice, rats, rabbits, dogs (mg/kg): 6800, 4225, 3200, 3000 i.v. (von Eberstein).

THERAP CAT: Antibacterial.

1917. Cefazolin. [25953-19-9] (6*R*,7*R*)-3-[[(5-Methyl-1,3,4-thiadiazol-2-yl)thio]methyl]-8-oxo-7-[(1*H*-tetrazol-1-ylacetyl)amino]-5-thia-1-azabicyclo[4.2.0]oct-2-ene-2-carboxylic acid; 7-(1-(1*H*)-tetrazolylacetamido)-3-[2-(5-methyl-1,3,4-thiadiazolyl)-thiomethyl]-Δ³-cephem-4-carboxylic acid; CEZ. $C_{14}H_{14}N_8O_4S_3$; mol wt 454.51. C 37.00%, H 3.10%, N 24.65%, O 14.08%, S 21.16%. Semi-synthetic antibiotic derived from 7-aminocephalosporanic acid, *q.v.* Prepn: T. Takano *et al.*, **ZA 6804513**; *eidem*, **US 3516997** (1969, 1970 to Fujisawa). Synthesis and properties: Kariyone *et al.*, *J. Antibiot.* **23**, 131 (1970). Activity and clinical studies: Nishida *et al., ibid.* **137**, 184; Shibata, Fujii, *Antimicrob. Agents Chemother.* **1970**, 467. Metabolic studies: Kozatani *et al., Chem. Pharm. Bull.* **20**, 1105 (1972). Toxicology: H. A. Birkhead *et al., J. Infect. Dis.* **128**, Suppl., 379 (1973). Comprehensive description: A. E. Zappala *et al., Anal. Profiles Drug Subs.* **4**, 1-20 (1975). *Review:* H. Nakano in *Pharmacological and Biochemical Properties of Drug Substances* **vol. 1**, M. E. Goldberg, Ed. (Am. Pharm. Assoc., Washington, DC, 1977) pp 155-182.

Needles from aq acetone, mp 198-200° (dec). uv max (buffer pH 6.4): 272 nm (ε 13150). Easily sol in DMF, pyridine; sol in aq acetone, aq dioxane, aq ethanol; slightly sol in methanol. Practically insol in chloroform, benzene, ether.

Sodium salt. [27164-46-1] Sodium CEZ; SKF-41558; Acef; Ancef; Atirin; Biazolina; Bor-Cefazol; Cefacidal; Cefamedin; Cefamezin; Cefazil; Cefazina; Elzogram; Firmacef; Gramaxin; Kefzol; Lampocef; Liviclina; Totacef; Zolicef. $C_{14}H_{13}N_8NaO_4S_3$; mol wt 476.49. White to yellowish-white, odorless crystalline powder with a bitter, salty taste. Crystallizes in α, β, and γ-forms (Kariyone). Easily sol in water, slightly sol in methanol, ethanol. Practically insol in benzene, acetone, chloroform. LD_{50} in mice, rats (mg/kg): 3.9, 3.18 i.v.: 6.2, 7.4 i.p. (Birkhead).

THERAP CAT: Antibacterial.

1918. Cefbuperazone. [76610-84-9] (6*R*,7*S*)-7-[[(2*R*,3*S*)-2-[[(4-Ethyl-2,3-dioxo-1-piperazinyl)carbonyl]amino]-3-hydroxy-1-oxobutyl]amino]-7-methoxy-3-[[(1-methyl-1*H*-tetrazol-5-yl)-thio]methyl]-8-oxo-5-thia-1-azabicyclo[4.2.0]oct-2-ene-2-carboxylic acid; (6*R*,7*S*)-7-[(2*R*,3*S*)-2-(4-ethyl-2,3-dioxo-1-piperazinecarboxamido)-3-hydroxybutyramido]-7-methoxy-3-[[(1-methyl-1*H*-tetrazol-5-yl)thio]methyl]-8-oxo-5-thia-1-azabicyclo[4.2.0]oct-2-ene-2-carboxylic acid; 7β-[D-α-(4-ethyl-2,3-dioxo-1-piperazinecarboxamido)-β-(*S*)-hydroxybutanamido]-7α-methoxy-3-[5-(1-methyl-1,2,3,4-tetrazolyl)thiomethyl]-Δ³-cephem-4-carboxylic acid. $C_{22}H_{29}N_9O_9S_2$; mol wt 627.65. C 42.10%, H 4.66%, N 20.08%, O 22.94%, S 10.22%. Broad spectrum injectable cephamycin. Prepn: I. Saikawa *et al., BE 879217; eidem,* US 4263292 (1980, 1981 both to Toyama). Distribution of ¹⁴C-cefbuperazone in mice: *eidem, Jpn. J. Antibiot.* **35**, 2159 (1982), *C.A.* **98**, 11062w (1982). *In vitro* and *in vivo* antibacterial activity: M. Tai *et al., Antimicrob. Agents Chemother.* **22**, 728 (1982). General pharmacology: A. Takai *et al., Jpn. J. Antibiot.* **35**, 2139 (1982), *C.A.* **98**, 65142r (1982). Absorption, distribution, excretion: I. Saikawa *et al., ibid.* 2163, *C.A.* **98**, 100691t (1982). Series of articles on cefbuperazone: *Chemotherapy (Tokyo)* **30**, Suppl. 3 (1982) 986 pp. Stability and degradation studies: S. Takano *et al., Yakugaku Zasshi* **103**, 62 (1983).

Solid, mp 118-120° (dec).

Sodium salt. [76648-01-6] T-1982; Keiperazon; Tomiporan. $C_{22}H_{28}N_9NaO_9S_2$; mol wt 649.63.

THERAP CAT: Antibacterial.

1919. Cefcapene Pivoxil. [105889-45-0] (6*R*,7*R*)-3-[[(Aminocarbonyl)oxy]methyl]-7-[[(2*Z*)-2-(2-amino-4-thiazolyl)-1-oxo-2-pentenyl]amino]-8-oxo-5-thia-1-azabicyclo[4.2.0]oct-2-ene-2-carboxylic acid (2,2-dimethyl-1-oxopropoxy)methyl ester; (6*R*,7*R*)-7-[(*Z*)-2-(2-aminothiazol-4-yl)-2-pentenoylamino]-3-(carbamoyloxymethyl)-3-cephem-4-carboxylic acid pivaloyloxymethyl ester; S-1108; Flumax. $C_{23}H_{29}N_5O_8S_2$; mol wt 567.64. C 48.67%, H 5.15%, N 12.34%, O 22.55%, S 11.30%. Orally absorbed cephalosporin; ester prodrug of the active free acid metabolite, cefcapene. Prepn: Y. Hamashima *et al., BE 904517; idem et al.,* US 4731361 (1986, 1988 both to Shionogi); K. Ishikura *et al., J. Antibiot.* **47**, 466 (1994). *In vitro* activity and stability of the free acid: H. C. Neu *et al., Antimicrob. Agents Chemother.* **36**, 1336 (1992). Metabolism: K. Totsuka *et al., ibid.* 757. Safety and pharmacokinetics: M. Nakashima *et al., ibid.* 762.

Free acid. [135889-00-8] S-1006. $C_{17}H_{19}N_5O_6S_2$; mol wt 453.49.

THERAP CAT: Antibacterial.

1920. Cefdinir. [91832-40-5] (6*R*,7*R*)-7-[[(2*Z*)-(2-Amino-4-thiazolyl)(hydroxyimino)acetyl]amino]-3-ethenyl-8-oxo-5-thia-1-azabicyclo[4.2.0]oct-2-ene-2-carboxylic acid; *syn*-7-[2-(2-amino-4-thiazolyl)-2-hydroxyiminoacetamido]-3-vinyl-3-cephem-4-carboxylic acid; FK-482; BMY-28488; Omnicef. $C_{14}H_{13}N_5O_5S_2$; mol wt 395.41. C 42.53%, H 3.31%, N 17.71%, O 20.23%, S 16.22%. Cephalosporin antibiotic structurally similar to cefixime, *q.v.* Prepn: T. Takaya *et al., BE 897864; eidem,* US 4559334 (1984, 1985 both to Fujisawa); Y. Inamoto *et al., J. Antibiot.* **41**, 828 (1988); H. Kamachi *et al., ibid.* 1602. Improved prepn: M. González *et al., Farmaco* **58**, 409 (2003). Clinical trial in children with acute otitis media: S. L. Block *et al., Pediatr. Infect. Dis. J.* **23**, 834 (2004). Review of pharmacokinetics and *in vitro* antimicrobial activity: D. R. P. Guay, *ibid.* **19**, S141-S146 (2000); of antibacterial activity, pharmacology and clinical efficacy: C. M. Perry, L. J. Scott, *Drugs* **64**, 1433-1464 (2004).

White to slightly brownish-yellow solid, mp 170° (dec). uv max (pH 7 phosphate buffer): 223, 286 nm (ε 17400, 19700). pKa 9.70. Slightly sol in dilute HCl; sparingly sol in 0.1 M pH 7.0 phosphate buffer.

THERAP CAT: Antibacterial.

1921. Cefditoren. [104145-95-1] (6R,7R)-7-[[(2Z)-(2-Amino-4-thiazolyl)(methoxyimino)acetyl]amino]-3-[(1Z)-2-(4-methyl-5-thiazolyl)ethenyl]-8-oxo-5-thia-1-azabicyclo[4.2.0]oct-2-ene-2-carboxylic acid; (+)-(6R,7R)-7-[2-(2-amino-4-thiazolyl)glyoxylamido]-3-[(Z)-2-(4-methyl-5-thiazolyl)vinyl]-8-oxo-5-thia-1-azabicyclo[4.2.0]oct-2-ene-2-carboxylic acid 7^2-(Z)-(O-methyloxime); ME-1206. $C_{19}H_{18}N_6O_5S_3$; mol wt 506.58. C 45.05%, H 3.58%, N 16.59%, O 15.79%, S 18.99%. Broad spectrum, third generation cephalosporin; active metabolite of orally absorbed pivaloyloxymethyl ester prodrug. Prepn: K. Atsumi et al., **EP 175610**; eidem, **US 4839350** (1986, 1989 both to Meiji); K. Sakagami et al., J. Antibiot. **43**, 1047 (1990); idem et al., Chem. Pharm. Bull. **39**, 2433 (1991). In vitro and in vivo activities: A. Tamura et al., Antimicrob. Agents Chemother. **32**, 1421 (1988). Extensive in vitro activity study: D. Felmingham et al., Drugs Exp. Clin. Res. **20**, 127 (1994). Clinical pharmacokinetics and efficacy in pediatrics: N. Iwai et al., Jpn. J. Antibiot. **47**, 181 (1994), C.A. **120**, 260636e (1994).

Sodium salt, sesquihydrate. $C_{19}H_{17}N_6NaO_5S_3 \cdot 1\frac{1}{2}H_2O$. Pale yellow crystals from water, mp 195-200° (dec). $[\alpha]_D^{20}$ +121.6° (c = 0.5 in methanol).

Pivaloyloxymethyl ester. [117467-28-4] Cefditoren pivoxil; ME-1207; Meiact. $C_{25}H_{28}N_6O_7S_3$; mol wt 620.72. Pale yellow powder, mp 127-129°. $[\alpha]_D^{20}$ −48.5° (c = 0.5 in methanol).

THERAP CAT: Antibacterial.

1922. Cefepime. [88040-23-7] 1-[[(6R,7R)-7-[[(2Z)-(2-Amino-4-thiazolyl)(methoxyimino)acetyl]amino]-2-carboxy-8-oxo-5-thia-1-azabicyclo[4.2.0]oct-2-en-3-yl]methyl]-1-methylpyrrolidinium inner salt; 1-[[(6R,7R)-7-[2-(2-amino-4-thiazolyl)glyoxylamido]-2-carboxy-8-oxo-5-thia-1-azabicyclo[4.2.0]oct-2-en-3-yl]methyl]-1-methylpyrrolidinium hydroxide inner salt 7^2-(Z)-2-(O-methyloxime); 7-[(Z)-2-(2-methoxyimino-2-(2-aminothiazol-4-yl)-2-methoxyimino-acetamido]-3-(1-methylpyrrolidinio)methyl-3-cephem-4-carboxylate; BMY-28142. $C_{19}H_{24}N_6O_5S_2$; mol wt 480.56. C 47.49%, H 5.03%, N 17.49%, O 16.65%, S 13.34%. Semisynthetic, fourth generation cephalosporin antibiotic. Prepn: S. Aburaki et al., **DE 3307550**; eidem, **US 4406899** (both 1983 to Bristol-Myers); and antibacterial activity: T. Naito et al., J. Antibiot. **39**, 1092 (1986). In vitro comparative antimicrobial spectrum: N. J. Khan et al., Antimicrob. Agents Chemother. **26**, 585 (1984); and β-lactamase stability: H. C. Neu et al., J. Antimicrob. Chemother. **17**, 441 (1986). HPLC determn in plasma and urine: R. H. Barbhaiya et al., Antimicrob. Agents Chemother. **31**, 55 (1987). Clinical evaluations in infection: N. Clynes et al., Diagn. Microbiol. Infect. Dis. **12**, 257 (1989); S. Oster et al., Antimicrob. Agents Chemother. **34**, 954 (1990). Review of clinical pharmacokinetics: M. P. Okamoto et al., Clin. Pharmacokinet. **25**, 88-102 (1993).

Colorless powder, mp 150° (dec). uv max (pH 7 phosphate buffer): 235, 257 nm (ε 16700, 16100).

Sulfate. $C_{19}H_{24}N_6O_5S_2 \cdot H_2SO_4$. mp 210° (dec). uv max (pH 7 phosphate buffer): 236, 258 nm (ε 17200, 16900).

Hydrochloride monohydrate. [123171-59-5] 1-[[(6R,7R)-7-[[(2Z)-(2-Amino-4-thiazolyl)(methoxyimino)acetyl]amino]-2-carboxy-8-oxo-5-thia-1-azabicyclo[4.2.0]oct-2-en-3-yl]methyl]-1-

methylpyrrolidinium chloride monohydrochloride monohydrate; cefepime hydrochloride; Axepim; Cepimex; Maxipime. $C_{19}H_{25}ClN_6O_5S_2 \cdot HCl \cdot H_2O$; mol wt 571.50.

THERAP CAT: Antibacterial.

1923. Cefetamet. [65052-63-3] (6R,7R)-7-[[(2Z)-(2-Amino-4-thiazolyl)(methoxyimino)acetyl]amino]-3-methyl-8-oxo-5-thia-1-azabicyclo[4.2.0]oct-2-ene-2-carboxylic acid; (6R,7R)-7-[2-(2-aminothiazol-4-yl)-(Z)-2-(methoxyimino)acetamido]-3-methyl-3-cephem-4-carboxylic acid; (6R,7R)-7-[2-(2-amino-4-thiazolyl)-glyoxylamido]-3-methyl-8-oxo-5-thia-1-azabicyclo[4.2.0]oct-2-ene-2-carboxylic acid 7^2-(Z)-(O-methyloxime); deacetoxycefotaxime; LY-097964; Ro-15-8074. $C_{14}H_{15}N_5O_5S_2$; mol wt 397.43. C 42.31%, H 3.80%, N 17.62%, O 20.13%, S 16.14%. Third generation cephalosporin antibiotic. Prepn: R. Heymes, A. Lutz, **DE 2713272**; eidem, **US 4396618** (1977, 1983 both to Roussel-UCLAF); R. Bucourt et al., Tetrahedron **34**, 2233 (1978). Prepn of the pivaloyloxymethyl ester: M. Ochiai et al., **DE 2715385**; eidem, **US 4680390** (1977, 1987 both to Takeda). Antibacterial spectrum: M. G. Thomas, S. D. R. Lang, Antimicrob. Agents Chemother. **29**, 945 (1986). HPLC determn in biological fluids: R. Wyss, F. Bucheli, J. Chromatogr. **430**, 81 (1988). Pharmacokinetics: K. Stoeckel et al., Curr. Med. Res. Opin. **11**, 432 (1989). Multicenter clinical trial: L. Bernstein-Hahn et al., ibid. 442.

Pivaloyloxymethyl ester. [65243-33-6] Cefetamet pivoxil; Ro-15-8075; Cefyl; Globocef. $C_{20}H_{25}N_5O_7S_2$; mol wt 511.57.

THERAP CAT: Antibacterial.

THERAP CAT (VET): Antibacterial.

1924. Cefixime. [79350-37-1] (6R,7R)-7-[[(2Z)-(2-Amino-4-thiazolyl)[(carboxymethoxy)imino]acetyl]amino]-3-ethenyl-8-oxo-5-thia-1-azabicyclo[4.2.0]oct-2-ene-2-carboxylic acid; 7-[2-(2-amino-4-thiazolyl)-2-(carboxymethoxyimino)acetamido]-3-vinyl-3-cephem-4-carboxylic acid; FK-027; FR-17027; CL-284635; Cefixoral; Cefspan; Cephoral; Oroken; Suprax; Unixime. $C_{16}H_{15}N_5O_7S_2$; mol wt 453.45. C 42.38%, H 3.33%, N 15.44%, O 24.70%, S 14.14%. Orally active, third generation cephalosporin antibiotic. Prepn: T. Takaya et al., **EP 30630**; eidem, **US 4409214** (1981, 1983 both to Fujisawa); H. Yamanaka et al., J. Antibiot. **38**, 1738 (1985). Synthesis and activity of (E)-isomer: K. Kawabata et al., Chem. Pharm. Bull. **34**, 3458 (1986). Mechanism of action: Y. Shigi et al., J. Antibiot. **37**, 790 (1984). Comparative antibacterial spectrum in vitro and in vivo: T. Kamimura et al., Antimicrob. Agents Chemother. **25**, 98 (1984). In vitro activity and β-lactamase stability: H. C. Neu et al., ibid. **26**, 174 (1984). HPLC determn in human plasma and urine: Y. Tokuma et al., J. Chromatogr. **311**, 339 (1984). Pharmacokinetics in humans: D. R. P. Guay et al., Antimicrob. Agents Chemother. **30**, 485 (1986). Clinical trial in urinary tract infections: J. Levenstein et al., S. Afr. Med. J. **70**, 455 (1986); A. Irvani et al., Am. J. Med. **85**, Suppl. 3A, 17 (1988); in respiratory infections: R. Kiani et al., ibid. 6.

(Z)-Form disodium salt. $C_{16}H_{13}N_5Na_2O_7S_2$. mp >250°.

(E)-Form trihydrate. Pale yellow solid, mp 218-225° (dec).

THERAP CAT: Antibacterial.

1925. Cefmenoxime. [65085-01-0] (6R,7R)-7-[[(2Z)-(2-Amino-4-thiazolyl)(methoxyimino)acetyl]amino]-3-[[(1-methyl-1H-tetrazol-5-yl)thio]methyl]-8-oxo-5-thia-1-azabicyclo[4.2.0]oct-2-ene-2-carboxylic acid; (6R,7R)-7-[2-(2-amino-4-thiazolyl)glyoxylamido]-3-[[(1-methyl-1H-tetrazol-5-yl)thio]methyl]-8-oxo-5-thia-1-azabicyclo[4.2.0]oct-2-ene-2-carboxylic acid 7^2-(Z)-(O-methyloxime); SCE-1365. $C_{16}H_{17}N_9O_5S_3$; mol wt 511.56. C 37.57%, H 3.35%, N 24.64%, O 15.64%, S 18.80%. Third generation cephalosporin antibiotic; related structurally to cefotaxime and ceftizoxime, q.q.v. The name cefmenoxime applies to the isomer having a syn-methoxyimino group. Prepn (unspecified stereochemistry): M. Ochiai et al., **DE 2556736**; eidem, **US 4098888** (1976, 1978 both to Takeda); syn-isomer: R. Heymes, A. Lutz, **DE 2713272**; eidem, **US 4476122** (1983, 1984 both to Roussel-Uclaf). Series of articles on antibacterial activity, absorption, excretion, metabolism, mechanism of action, clinical studies: *Chemotherapy (Tokyo)* **29**, Suppl. 1, 1-998 (1979). *In vitro* and *in vivo* study: K. Tsuchiya et al., *Antimicrob. Agents Chemother.* **19**, 56 (1981). β-Lactamase stability: K. Okonogi et al., ibid. **20**, 171 (1981). Clinical pharmacokinetics study: D. Höffler, P. Koeppe, *Arzneim.-Forsch.* **33**, 269 (1983). Symposium: *Am. J. Med.* **77**(6A), 1-59 (1984).

Hydrochloride (syn-isomer). [75738-58-8] Abbott 50192; Bestcall; Cefmax; Cemix; Tacef. $(C_{16}H_{17}N_9O_5S_3)_2 \cdot HCl$; mol wt 1059.58.

Sodium salt (syn-isomer). [65085-02-1] $C_{16}H_{16}N_9NaO_5S_3$. $[\alpha]_D^{20} -13.5 \pm 1°$ (c = 1 in water).

THERAP CAT: Antibacterial.

1926. Cefmetazole. [56796-20-4] (6R,7S)-7-[[[(Cyanomethyl)thio]acetyl]amino]-7-methoxy-3-[[(1-methyl-1H-tetrazol-5-yl)thio]methyl]-8-oxo-5-thia-1-azabicyclo[4.2.0]oct-2-ene-2-carboxylic acid; CS-1170; SKF-83088. $C_{15}H_{17}N_7O_5S_3$; mol wt 471.53. C 38.21%, H 3.63%, N 20.79%, O 16.97%, S 20.40%. Semi-synthetic antibiotic derived from cephamycin C, q.v. Prepn: H. Nakao et al., **DE 2455884** (1975 to Sankyo), C.A. **83**, 97330g (1975); eidem, J. Antibiot. **29**, 554 (1976). See also: J. E. Dolfini, **US 3920639** (1975 to Squibb). In vitro study: J. V. Uri et al., ibid. **31**, 82 (1978). Immunological study: M. Iwata, T. Matuhasi, *Jpn. J. Exp. Med.* **48**, 401 (1978). Absorption, distribution, excretion, metabolism in various species: H. Shindo et al., *Chemotherapy (Tokyo)* **27**, Suppl. 1, 64 (1979). Pharmacology: S. Kobayashi et al., ibid. **26**, Suppl. 5, 115 (1978). Toxicological studies: H. Masuda et al., Sankyo Kenkyusho Nempo **30**, 112 (1978), C.A. **90**, 180268h (1979). Comparative clinical study: M. Nishida et al., J. Antibiot. **32**, 1319 (1979).

Sodium salt. [56796-39-5] Cefmetazon; Metafar; Zefazone. $C_{15}H_{16}N_7NaO_5S_3$; mol wt 493.52. White solid. Very sol in water, methanol, sol in acetone. Practically insol in chloroform. LD_{50} i.v. in rats: >5000 mg/kg (Masuda).

THERAP CAT: Antibacterial.

1927. Cefminox. [84305-41-9] (6R,7S)-7-[[[[(2S)-2-Amino-2-carboxyethyl]thio]acetyl]amino]-7-methoxy-3-[[(1-methyl-1H-tetrazol-5-yl)thio]methyl]-8-oxo-5-thia-1-azabicyclo[4.2.0]oct-2-ene-2-carboxylic acid; 7β-(2-D-amino-2-carboxyethylthioacetamido)-7α-methoxy-3-[[(1-methyl-1H-tetrazol-5-yl)thio]methyl]-3-cephem-4-carboxylic acid. $C_{16}H_{21}N_7O_7S_3$; mol wt 519.58. C 36.99%, H 4.07%, N 18.87%, O 21.56%, S 18.51%. Semisynthetic

broad spectrum cephamycin antibiotic. Prepn: **BE 880656**, K. Iwamatsu et al., **US 4357331** (1980, 1982 both to Meiji Seika). Synthesis, biological activity: eidem, J. Antibiot. **36**, 229 (1983). Structure-activity studies: S. Inouye et al., ibid. **37**, 1403 (1984). Proposed mechanism of action: T. Tsuruoka et al., Eur. J. Biochem. **151**, 209 (1985). In vitro, in vivo antibacterial activity compared with that of other cephalosporins: S. Inouye et al., Antimicrob. Agents Chemother. **26**, 722 (1984). Activity against gram-negative infections in mice: T. Watanabe et al., Drugs Exp. Clin. Res. **10**, 293 (1984). Toxicity studies: M. Kurebe et al., Jpn. J. Antibiot. **37**, 847 (1984). Series of articles on pharmacokinetics, early clinical trials, treatment of urinary tract and respiratory infections: *Chemotherapy (Tokyo)* **32**, Suppl. 5 (1984) 561 pp.

Sodium salt heptahydrate. MT-141; Meicelin. $C_{16}H_{20}N_7 \cdot NaO_7S_3 \cdot 7H_2O$; mol wt 667.66. Crystals from ethanol-water, mp 90-91°. LD_{50} in male, female mice (mg/kg): 6100, 5200 i.v.; in male, female rats (mg/kg): 6600, 5700 i.v.; 8600, 8550 i.p.; >15000, >15000 s.c. or orally (Kurebe).

THERAP CAT: Antibacterial.

1928. Cefodizime. [69739-16-8] (6R,7R)-7-[[(2Z)-(2-Amino-4-thiazolyl)(methoxyimino)acetyl]amino]-3-[[[5-(carboxymethyl)-4-methyl-2-thiazolyl]thio]methyl]-8-oxo-5-thia-1-azabicyclo[4.2.0]oct-2-ene-2-carboxylic acid; (6R,7R)-7-[2-(2-amino-4-thiazolyl)glyoxylamido]-3-[[[5-(carboxymethyl)-4-methyl-2-thiazolyl]thio]methyl]-8-oxo-5-thia-1-azabicyclo[4.2.0]oct-2-ene-2-carboxylic acid 7^2(Z)-(O-methyloxime). $C_{20}H_{20}N_6O_7S_4$; mol wt 584.67. C 41.09%, H 3.45%, N 14.37%, O 19.16%, S 21.94%. Third generation cephalosporin antibiotic with immunomodulating activity; derivative of cefotaxime, q.v. Prepn: **BE 865632**; W. Dürckheimer et al., **US 4278793** (1978, 1981 both to Hoechst AG); and antibacterial activity: J. Blumbach et al., J. Antibiot. **40**, 29 (1987). In vitro comparative antibacterial spectrum: R. N. Jones et al., Antimicrob. Agents Chemother. **20**, 760 (1981); and β-lactamase stability: M. Limbert et al., J. Antibiot. **37**, 892 (1984). In vivo antibacterial activity: N. Klesel et al., ibid. 1712. Enhancement of immune response in vivo: M. Limbert et al., ibid. 1719; and ex vivo: A. Fietta et al., Chemotherapy (Basel) **34**, 430 (1988). HPLC determn in biological fluids: T. Marunaka et al., J. Chromatogr. **420**, 329 (1987). Pharmacokinetics: N. Klesel et al., J. Antibiot. **37**, 901 (1984); in humans: E. E. Dagrosa et al., Clin. Ther. **10**, 18 (1987). Clinical study in urogenital gonorrhea: H. van der Willigen et al., Antimicrob. Agents Chemother. **32**, 426 (1988). Physical properties, toxicology and structure-activity relationships: A. Bryskier et al., J. Antimicrob. Chemother. **26**, Suppl. C, 1 (1990). Series of articles on pharmacology, pharmacokinetics and clinical studies: *Chemotherapy (Tokyo)* **36**, Suppl. 5, 1-980 (1988); and immunomodulating activity: J. Antimicrob. Chemother. **26**, Suppl. C, 1-134 (1990).

$[\alpha]_D^{25} -55.9°$. pK_1 2.85; pK_2 3.37; pK_3 4.18. uv max (water): 228, 260, 288 nm (log ε 4.25, 4.25, 4.20).

Disodium salt. [86329-79-5] HR-221; THR-221; Kenicef; Neucef; Timecef. $C_{20}H_{18}N_6Na_2O_7S_4$; mol wt 628.63. White to yellow crystalline powder. Soly (g/l): water ~270. LD_{50} in mice, rabbits (mg/kg): 4000-8000 i.v. both species; in rats (mg/kg): 4000-8000 i.v., 15000-17500 s.c., 8000-11000 i.p. (Bryskier).

THERAP CAT: Antibacterial.

1929. Cefonicid. [61270-58-4] (6R,7R)-7-[[(2R)-Hydroxyphenylacetyl]amino]-8-oxo-3-[[[1-(sulfomethyl)-1H-tetrazol-5-yl]thio]methyl]-5-thia-1-azabicyclo[4.2.0]oct-2-ene-2-carboxylic acid; (6R,7R)-7-[(R)-mandelamido]-8-oxo-3-[[[1-(sulfomethyl)-1H-tetrazol-5-yl]thio]methyl]-5-thia-1-azabicyclo[4.2.0]oct-2-ene-2-carboxylic acid. $C_{18}H_{18}N_6O_8S_3$; mol wt 542.57. C 39.85%, H 3.34%, N 15.49%, O 23.59%, S 17.73%. Injectable semi-synthetic cephalosporin antibiotic related to cefamandole, q.v. Prepn: D. A. Berges, **DE 2611270**; idem, **US 4048311** (1976, 1977 both to Smith Kline); **US 4093723, US 4159373** (1978, 1979 both to Smith Kline). Antibacterial activity, pharmacokinetics: P. Actor et al., Antimicrob. Agents Chemother. **13**, 784 (1978). Series of articles on stability, comparative in vitro activity, serum levels: Curr. Chemother. Infect. Dis., Proc. 11th Int. Congr. Chemother. vol. 1 (Am. Soc. Microbiol., Washington, D.C., 1979) pp 246-254. Stability towards β-lactamases: R. Mehta et al., J. Antibiot. **34**, 202 (1981). Kinetics and renal handling: D. Pitkin et al., Clin. Pharmacol. Ther. **30**, 587 (1981). In vitro evaluation vs Group B streptococci: A. S. Bayer et al., Antimicrob. Agents Chemother. **21**, 344 (1982). Review of antibacterial activity, pharmacology, therapeutic use: E. Saltiel, R. N. Brogden, Drugs **32**, 222-259 (1986).

Disodium salt. [61270-78-8] SKF-75073; Cefodie; Monocid; Monocidur; Praticef. $C_{18}H_{16}N_6Na_2O_8S_3$; mol wt 586.53.
THERAP CAT: Antibacterial.

1930. Cefoperazone. [62893-19-0] (6R,7R)-7-[[(2R)-[[(4-Ethyl-2,3-dioxo-1-piperazinyl)carbonyl]amino](4-hydroxyphenyl)acetyl]amino]-3-[[(1-methyl-1H-tetrazol-5-yl)thio]methyl]-8-oxo-5-thia-1-azabicyclo[4.2.0]oct-2-ene-2-carboxylic acid; 7-[D-(−)-α-(4-ethyl-2,3-dioxo-1-piperazinecarboxamido)-α-(4-hydroxyphenyl)acetamido]-3-[[(1-methyl-1H-tetrazol-5-yl)thio]methyl]-3-cephem-4-carboxylic acid. $C_{25}H_{27}N_9O_8S_2$; mol wt 645.67. C 46.50%, H 4.21%, N 19.52%, O 19.82%, S 9.93%. Broad spectrum third generation cephalosporin antibiotic. Prepn: I. Saikawa et al., **BE 837682**; idem, **US 4410522** (1976, 1983 both to Toyama); idem, Yakugaku Zasshi **99**, 929 (1979). Stability in aq soln: idem, ibid. 1207. In vitro activity: M. V. Borobio et al., Antimicrob. Agents Chemother. **17**, 129 (1980). Kinetics in rats: J. Fabre et al., Schweiz. Med. Wochenschr. **110**, 264 (1980); in humans: A. F. Allaz, ibid. **109**, 1999 (1979). Review of pharmacology and therapeutic efficacy: R. N. Brogden et al., Drugs **22**, 423-460 (1981). Symposium on clinical studies: ibid. Suppl. 1, 1-124.

Crystals from acetonitrile/water, mp 169-171° (hydrated). Stable at pH 4.0-7.0; slightly unstable in acid; highly unstable in alkaline soln.
Sodium salt. [62893-20-3] CP-52640-2; T-1551; Bioperazone; Cefazone; Cefobid; Cefobine; Cefobis; Cefogram; Cefoneg; Cefosint; Dardum; Farecef; Kefazon; Novobiocyl; Pathozone; Peracef; Perocef; Tomabef. $C_{25}H_{26}N_9NaO_8S_2$; mol wt 667.65.
THERAP CAT: Antibacterial.
THERAP CAT (VET): Antibacterial.

1931. Ceforanide. [60925-61-3] (6R,7R)-7-[[[2-(Aminomethyl)phenyl]acetyl]amino]-3-[[[1-(carboxymethyl)-1H-tetrazol-5-yl]thio]methyl]-8-oxo-5-thia-1-azabicyclo[4.2.0]oct-2-ene-2-carboxylic acid; (6R,7R)-7-[2-(α-amino-o-tolyl)acetamido]-3-[[[1-

(carboxymethyl)-1H-tetrazol-5-yl]thio]methyl]-8-oxo-5-thia-1-azabicyclo[4.2.0]oct-2-ene-2-carboxylic acid; 7-[o-(aminomethyl)phenylacetamido]-3-[[[1-(carboxymethyl)-1H-tetrazol-5-yl]thio]methyl]-3-cephem-4-carboxylic acid; BL-S786. $C_{20}H_{21}N_7O_6S_2$; mol wt 519.55. C 46.24%, H 4.07%, N 18.87%, O 18.48%, S 12.34%. Injectable, semi-synthetic cephalosporin antibiotic. Prepn: M. A. Kaplan et al., **DE 2538804**; W. J. Gottstein et al., **US 4100346, US 4172196** and **US 4182863** (1976, 1978, 1979, 1980 all to Bristol-Myers); W. J. Gottstein et al., J. Antibiot. **29**, 1226 (1976). Laboratory evaluation: F. Leitner et al., Antimicrob. Agents Chemother. **10**, 426 (1976). In vitro susceptibility comparisons: R. N. Jones et al., J. Antibiot. **30**, 576, 583 (1977). Comparative tissue distribution: F. H. Lee et al., Antimicrob. Agents Chemother. **19**, 625 (1981). Pharmacokinetics: E. H. Estey et al., Clin. Pharmacol. Ther. **30**, 396 (1981); S. S. Hawkins et al., ibid. 468. Clinical study: R. J. Wallace et al., Antimicrob. Agents Chemother. **20**, 648 (1981).

White solid, mp >150° (dec).
L-Lysine salt. [63767-79-3] Precef. $C_{20}H_{21}N_7O_6S_2 \cdot C_6H_{14}N_2O_2$; mol wt 665.74.
THERAP CAT: Antibacterial.

1932. Cefoselis. [122841-10-5] (6R,7R)-7-[[(2Z)-(2-Amino-4-thiazolyl)(methoxyimino)acetyl]amino]-3-[[2,3-dihydro-2-(2-hydroxyethyl)-3-imino-1H-pyrazol-1-yl]methyl]-8-oxo-5-thia-1-azabicyclo[4.2.0]oct-2-ene-2-carboxylic acid; (syn)-7β-[2-(2-aminothiazol-4-yl)-2-methoxyiminoacetamido]-3-[3-amino-2-(2-hydroxyethyl)-1-pyrazolio]methyl-3-cephem-4-carboxylate; (−)-5-amino-2-[[(6R,7R)-7-[2-(2-amino-4-thiazolyl)glyoxylamido]-2-carboxy-8-oxo-5-thia-1-azabicyclo[4.2.0]oct-2-en-3-yl]methyl]-1-(2-hydroxyethyl)pyrazolium hydroxide inner salt 7^2-(Z)-(O-methyloxime). $C_{19}H_{22}N_8O_6S_2$; mol wt 522.56. C 43.67%, H 4.24%, N 21.44%, O 18.37%, S 12.27%. Fourth generation cephalosporin antibiotic. Prepn: K. Sakane et al., **EP 307804**; eidem, **US 4952578** (1989, 1990 both to Fujisawa); H. Ohki et al., J. Antibiot. **46**, 359 (1993). In vitro activity and β-lactamase stability: H. C. Neu et al., Antimicrob. Agents Chemother. **37**, 566 (1993). Clinical pharmacokinetics: R. Wise et al., ibid. **38**, 2369 (1994). Series of articles on activity, clinical pharmacology and therapeutic efficacy: Chemotherapy (Tokyo) **42**, Suppl. 3, 1-464 (1994).

Sulfate. [122841-12-7] FK-037; Wincef. $C_{19}H_{22}N_8O_6S_2 \cdot H_2SO_4$; mol wt 620.64.
THERAP CAT: Antibacterial.

1933. Cefotaxime. [63527-52-6] (6R,7R)-3-[(Acetyloxy)methyl]-7-[[(2Z)-(2-amino-4-thiazolyl)(methoxyimino)acetyl]amino]-8-oxo-5-thia-1-azabicyclo[4.2.0]oct-2-ene-2-carboxylic acid; (6R,7R)-7-[2-(2-amino-4-thiazolyl)glyoxylamido]-3-(hydroxymethyl)-8-oxo-5-thia-1-azabicyclo[4.2.0]oct-2-ene-2-carboxylate 7^2-(Z)-(O-methyloxime) acetate; 7-[2-(2-amino-4-thiazolyl)-2-methoxyiminoacetamido]cephalosporanic acid. $C_{16}H_{17}N_5O_7S_2$; mol wt 455.47. C 42.19%, H 3.76%, N 15.38%, O 24.59%, S 14.08%. Broad spectrum third generation cephalosporin antibiotic. The name cefotaxime applies to the isomer having a syn-methoxyimino group. Prepn (unspecified stereochemistry): M. Ochiai et al., **DE 2556736**; eidem, **US 4098888** (1976, 1978 both to Takeda); syn-isomer: R. Heymes, A. Lutz, **DE 2702501**; eidem, **US 4152432**

(1977, 1979 both to Roussel-UCLAF). Antibacterial activity: R. Wise, *Antimicrob. Agents Chemother.* **14**, 807 (1978); H. W. Van handuyt, M. Pyckavet, *ibid.* **16**, 109 (1979). Human pharmacology: R. Lüthy *et al.*, *ibid.* 127. Symposia: *Drug Ther.* **Suppl.**, 1-108 (Jan. 1981); *Rev. Infect. Dis.* **4**, Suppl., S281-S488 (1982); *Diagn. Microbiol. Infect. Dis.* **2**(3), Suppl., 1S-92S (1984); *Infection* **13**, Suppl. 1, S1-S162 (1985). Comprehensive description: F. J. Muhtadi, M. M. A. Hassan, *Anal. Profiles Drug Subs.* **11**, 139-168 (1982). Series of articles on clinical efficacy: *J. Antimicrob. Chemother.* **26**, Suppl. A, 1-83 (1990).

Sodium salt (*syn*-isomer). [64485-93-4] HR-756; RU-24756; Cefotax; Chemcef; Claforan; Pretor; Tolycar. $C_{16}H_{16}N_5NaO_7S_2$; mol wt 477.45. $[\alpha]_D^{20}$ +55±2° (c = 0.8 in water).

THERAP CAT: Antibacterial.

1934. Cefotetan. [69712-56-7] (6R,7S)-7-[[[4-(2-Amino-1-carboxy-2-oxoethylidene)-1,3-dithietan-2-yl]carbonyl]amino]-7-methoxy-3-[[(1-methyl-1*H*-tetrazol-5-yl)thio]methyl]-8-oxo-5-thia-1-azabicyclo[4.2.0]oct-2-ene-2-carboxylic acid; (6R,7S)-7-[4-(carbamoylcarboxymethylene)-1,3-dithietane-2-carboxamido]-7-methoxy-3-[[(1-methyl-1*H*-tetrazol-5-yl)thio]methyl]-8-oxo-5-thia-1-azabicyclo[4.2.0]oct-2-ene-2-carboxylic acid. $C_{17}H_{17}N_7$-O_8S_4; mol wt 575.62. C 35.47%, H 2.98%, N 17.03%, O 22.24%, S 22.28%. Broad-spectrum injectable semi-synthetic antibiotic derived from cephamycin C, *q.v.* Prepn: M. Iwanami *et al.*, **DE 2824559**; *eidem*, **US 4263432** (1979, 1981 both to Yamanouchi); *eidem*, *Chem. Pharm. Bull.* **28**, 2629 (1980). Commercial-scale synthesis: M. Fujimoto *et al.*, *Org. Process Res. Dev.* **8**, 915 (2004). *In vitro* comparison of antibacterial activity: B. Chattopadhyay, J. C. Teli, *J. Antimicrob. Chemother.* **10**, 151 (1982). Toxicity study: K. Imamura *et al.*, *Chemotherapy (Tokyo)* **30**, Suppl. 1, 212 (1982). Series of articles on pharmacology, clinical studies, toxicology: *ibid.* 1-947; *J. Antimicrob. Chemother.* **11**, Suppl. A, 1-236 (1983). Review of antibacterial activity, pharmacokinetics, therapeutic use: A. Ward, D. M. Richards, *Drugs* **30**, 382-426 (1985).

Disodium salt. [74356-00-6] ICI-156834; YM-09330; Apatef; Cefotan; Ceftenon; Cepan; Darvilen. $C_{17}H_{15}N_7Na_2O_8S_4$; mol wt 619.58. LD_{50} in male mice, rats (g/kg): 6.35, 8.48 i.v.; 8.12, 8.37 i.p.; >10 orally and s.c. both species (Imamura).

THERAP CAT: Antibacterial.

1935. Cefotiam. [61622-34-2] (6R,7R)-7-[[(2-Amino-4-thiazolyl)acetyl]amino]-3-[[[1-[2-(dimethylamino)ethyl]-1*H*-tetrazol-5-yl]-thio]methyl]-8-oxo-5-thia-1-azabicyclo[4.2.0]oct-2-ene-2-carboxylic acid; 7β-[2-(aminothiazol-4-yl)acetamido]-3-[[[1-[2-(dimethylaminoethyl)-1*H*-tetrazol-5-yl]thio]methyl]ceph-3-em-4-carboxylic acid; SCE-963. $C_{18}H_{23}N_9O_4S_3$; mol wt 525.63. C 41.13%, H 4.41%, N 23.98%, O 12.18%, S 18.30%. Semi-synthetic cephalosporin antibiotic. Prepn: S. Terao *et al.*, **DE 2458695**; M. Numata *et al.*, **US 4080498** (1975, 1978 both to Takeda); *eidem*, *J. Antibiot.* **31**, 1262 (1978). Prepn of the crystalline dihydrochloride: K. Naito *et al.*, **DE 2738711**; *eidem*, **US 4146710** (1978, 1979 both to Takeda). Pharmacodynamics: K. Tsuchiya *et al.*, *ibid.*, 1272. Antibacterial spectrum: *eidem*, *Antimicrob. Agents Chemother.* **14**, 557 (1978). Clinical trial in respiratory infections: H. M. Beumer *et al.*, *Int. J. Clin. Pharmacol. Ther. Toxicol.* **23**, 105 (1985).

Dihydrochloride. [66309-69-1] Abbott 48999; CGP-14221/E; Halospor; Pansporin; Pansporine; Spizef; Sporidyn. $C_{18}H_{23}N_9O_4$-S_3.2HCl; mol wt 598.55. White to light yellow crystals. Sol in methanol. Slightly sol in ethanol.

1-(Cyclohexyloxycarbonyloxy)ethyl ester dihydrochloride. [95789-30-3] Cefotiam hexetil hydrochloride; SCE-2174; Pansporin T; Taketiam; Texodil. $C_{27}H_{37}N_9O_7S_3$.2HCl; mol wt 768.76. Prepn: T. Nishimura *et al.*, **EP 128029**; *eidem*, **US 5120841** (1984, 1992 both to Takeda); *eidem et al.*, *J. Antibiot.* **40**, 81 (1987). Acute toxicity: S. Chiba *et al.*, *Oyo Yakuri* **35**, 179 (1988), *C.A.* **109**, 31615c (1988). Clinical trial: H. Maier *et al.* *Arzneim.-Forsch.* **42**, 980 (1992). Colorless powder. Soly in water at pH 4.5: >1 mg/ml. LD_{50} in male, female mice, male, female rats (mg/kg): 1290, 1150, 1470, 1620 i.p.; >2000 s.c.; >5000 orally (Chiba).

THERAP CAT: Antibacterial.

1936. Cefoxitin. [35607-66-0] (6R,7S)-3-[[(Aminocarbonyl)oxy]methyl]-7-methoxy-8-oxo-7-[(2-thienylacetyl)amino]-5-thia-1-azabicyclo[4.2.0]oct-2-ene-2-carboxylic acid; 3-(hydroxymethyl)-7-methoxy-8-oxo-7-[2-(2-thienyl)acetamido]-5-thia-1-azabicyclo[4.2.0]oct-2-ene-2-carboxylic acid carbamate (ester); 3-carbamoyloxymethyl-7α-methoxy-7-[2-(2-thienyl)acetamido]-3-cephem-4-carboxylic acid. $C_{16}H_{17}N_3O_7S_2$; mol wt 427.45. C 44.96%, H 4.01%, N 9.83%, O 26.20%, S 15.00%. Semi-synthetic antibiotic derived from cephamycin C, *q.v.*, possessing high resistance to β-lactamase inactivation. Synthesis: B. G. Christensen *et al.*, **DE 2129675**; **DE 2203653**; eidem, **US 4297488** (1971, 1972, 1981 all to Merck & Co.); Karady *et al.*, *J. Am. Chem. Soc.* **94**, 1410 (1972); Ratcliffe, Christensen, *Tetrahedron Lett.* **1973**, 4653. Biological evaluation: Wallick, Hendlin, *Antimicrob. Agents Chemother.* **5**, 25 (1974); Miller *et al.*, *ibid.* 33; Onishi *et al.*, *ibid.* 38; Hamilton, Miller *et al.*, *J. Antibiot.* **27**, 42 (1974). Mode of action: Onishi *et al.*, *Ann. N.Y. Acad. Sci.* **235**, 406 (1974). Toxicity: S. Takayama *et al.*, *Chemotherapy (Tokyo)* **26**, Suppl. 1, 150 (1978). Comprehensive reviews: *J. Antimicrob. Chemother.* **4**, Suppl. B, 1-256 (1978); R. N. Brogden *et al.*, *Drugs* **17**, 1-37 (1979); E. O. Stapley, K. R. Brown, in *Pharmacological and Biochemical Properties of Drug Substances* **vol. 3**, M. E. Goldberg, Ed. (Am. Pharm. Assoc., Washington, DC, 1981) pp 262-290. Comprehensive description: G. S. Brenner, *Anal. Profiles Drug Subs.* **11**, 169-195 (1982). Symposium on therapeutic use in anaerobic and aerobic infectons: *Hosp. Pract.* **25**, Suppl. 4, 1-56 (1990).

Crystals, mp 149-150° (dec). pKa 2.2. Very sol in acetone; sol in aq $NaHCO_3$; very slightly sol in water. Practically insol in ether and chloroform.

Sodium salt. [33564-30-6] MK-306; Betacef; Farmoxin; Mefoxin; Mefoxitin; Cenomycin. $C_{16}H_{16}N_3NaO_7S_2$; mol wt 449.43. White crystals with characteristic odor. $[\alpha]_{589nm}^{25}$ +210° (c = 1 in methanol). Very sol in water; sol in methanol; sparingly sol in ethanol and acetone. Insol in aromatic and aliphatic hydrocarbons. LD_{50} in mice, rats, dogs (g/kg): 5.10, 8.98, >10.0 i.v. (Takayama).

THERAP CAT: Antibacterial.

1937. Cefozopran. [113359-04-9] 1-[[(6R,7R)-7-[[(2Z)-(5-Amino-1,2,4-thiadiazol-3-yl)(methoxyimino)acetyl]amino]-2-carboxy-8-oxo-5-thia-1-azabicyclo[4.2.0]oct-2-en-3-yl]methyl]imidazo[1,2-*b*]pyridazinium inner salt; 7β-[2-(5-amino-1,2,4-thiadiazol-3-yl)-2(Z)-methoxyiminoacetamido]-3-[(imidazo[1,2-*b*]pyridazinium-1-yl)methyl]-3-cephem-4-carboxylate. $C_{19}H_{17}N_9O_5S_2$; mol wt 515.53. C 44.27%, H 3.32%, N 24.45%, O 15.52%, S 12.44%. Prepn: A. Miyake *et al.*, **WO 8605183**; *eidem*, **US 4864022** (1986, 1989 both to Takeda); A. Miyake *et al.*, *J. Antibiot.* **45**, 709 (1992). Antibacterial spectrum: T. Iwahi *et al.*, *Antimicrob. Agents Chemother.* **36**, 1358 (1992). *In vivo* activity: Y. Iizawa *et al.*, *ibid.* **37**, 100 (1993). Pharmacokinetics: W. Paulfeuerborn *et al.*, *ibid.* 1835. HPLC determn in serum and urine: K. Borner, E. Borner, *J. Chromatogr.* **615**, 174 (1993).

Hydrochloride. SCE-2787; Firstcin. $C_{19}H_{17}N_9O_5S_2$.HCl; mol wt 551.99.

THERAP CAT: Antibacterial.

1938. Cefpimizole. [84880-03-5] 1-[[(6R,7R)-2-Carboxy-7-[[(2R)-[[(5-carboxy-1H-imidazol-4-yl)carbonyl]amino]phenyl-acetyl]amino]-8-oxo-5-thia-1-azabicyclo[4.2.0]oct-2-en-3-yl]meth-yl]-4-(2-sulfoethyl)pyridinium inner salt; 1-[(6R,7R)-2-carboxy-7-[(R)-2-(5-carboxy-4-imidazolylcarboxamido)-2-phenylacetamido]-8-oxo-5-thia-1-azabicyclo[4.2.0]oct-2-en-3-ylmethyl]pyridino-4-ethylsulfonate; 7-β-[D-(−)-α-(4-carboxyimidazole-5-carbox-amido)phenylacetamido]-3-(4-β-sulfoethylpyridinium)methyl-3-cephem-4-carboxylic acid; U-63196; AC-1370. $C_{28}H_{26}N_6O_{10}S_2$; mol wt 670.67. C 50.14%, H 3.91%, N 12.53%, O 23.86%, S 9.56%. Third generation injectable cephalosporin antibiotic. Prepn: N. Yasuda *et al.*, **DE 2826546**; *eidem*, **US 4217450** (1979, 1980 both to Ajinomoto); N. Yasuda *et al.*, *J. Antibiot.* **36**, 242 (1983). *In vitro* antibacterial activity and β-lactamase stability: H. C. Neu, P. Labthavikul, *Antimicrob. Agents Chemother.* **24**, 375 (1983). Potentiating effect on phagocyte functions: H. Ohnishi *et al.*, *ibid.* **23**, 874 (1983). Toxicity study: S. Hashimoto *et al.*, *Toxicol. Lett.* **23**, 135 (1984). Therapeutic efficacy in mice: Y. Obana *et al.*, *J. Antimicrob. Chemother.* **16**, 727 (1985). HPLC determn in human plasma and urine: D. B. Lakings, J. M. Wozniak, *J. Chromatogr.* **308**, 261 (1984). Pharmacokinetics in humans: D. B. Lakings *et al.*, *Antimicrob. Agents Chemother.* **29**, 271 (1986). Efficacy and tolerance in gonorrhea in men: E. T. Sandberg *et al.*, *ibid.* 849.

Monosodium salt. [85287-61-2] U-63196E; Ajicef; Renilan. $C_{28}H_{25}N_6NaO_{10}S_2$; mol wt 692.65. $[\alpha]_D^{20}$ −28.2° (c = 0.5 in water). uv max (water): 257 nm (ε 22400). Sol in water. LD_{50} in male mice, male, female rats (g/kg): 2.7, 2.9, 4.2, 3.5 i.v.; 8.2, 6.8, 12.2, 11.5 s.c.; all >15.0 orally (Hashimoto).

THERAP CAT: Antibacterial.

1939. Cefpiramide. [70797-11-4] (6R,7R)-7-[[(2R)-[[(4-Hydroxy-6-methyl-3-pyridinyl)carbonyl]amino](4-hydroxyphen-yl)acetyl]amino]-3-[[(1-methyl-1H-tetrazol-5-yl)thio]methyl]-8-oxo-5-thia-1-azabicyclo[4.2.0]oct-2-ene-2-carboxylic acid; 7-[(R)-2-(4-hydroxy-6-methylnicotinamido)-2-(p-hydroxyphenyl)-acetamido]-3-[[(1-methyl-1H-tetrazol-5-yl)thio]methyl]-8-oxo-5-thia-1-azabicyclo[4.2.0]oct-2-ene-2-carboxylic acid; D-7-[(4-hy-droxy-6-methylnicotinamido)-4-hydroxyphenylacetamido]-3-(1-methyltetrazol-5-yl)thiomethylcephem-4-carboxylic acid. $C_{25}H_{24}$-$N_8O_7S_2$; mol wt 612.64. C 49.01%, H 3.95%, N 18.29%, O 18.28%, S 10.47%. Broad spectrum semi-synthetic cephalosporin antibiotic. Prepn: H. Yamada *et al.*, **BE 833063**; *eidem*, US

4156724; **US 4160087** (1975, 1979, 1979 all to Sumitomo); *eidem*, **JP Kokai 79 119497** (1979 to Sumitomo), *C.A.* **92**, 11042j (1980); I. Isaka *et al.*, **JP Kokai 79 30197** (1979 to Yamanouchi), *C.A.* **91**, 57037a (1979); **JP Kokai 84 65094** (1984 to Sumitomo), *C.A.* **101**, 110641w (1984). Prepn, NMR data, antibacterial activity: H. Yamada *et al.*, *J. Antibiot.* **36**, 522, 543 (1983). Pharmacokinetics: H. Matsui *et al.*, *Antimicrob. Agents Chemother.* **22**, 213 (1982); K. Sata *et al.*, *ibid.* **26**, 578 (1984). Metabolism: H. Imasaki *et al.*, *ibid.* **24**, 42 (1983). In vitro activity: H. Wexler *et al.*, *ibid.* **25**, 162 (1984); M. A. Pfaller *et al.*, *ibid.* 368. Comparison with other cephalosporins: N. J. Khan *et al.*, *ibid.* **26**, 585 (1984). Series of articles on *in vitro, in vivo* activity, determn in body fluids, pharmacokinetics, clinical studies: *Chemotherapy (Tokyo)* **31**, Suppl. 1, 1-842 (1983).

Yellow crystals, mp 213-215° (dec).

Sodium salt. [74849-93-7] SM-1652; Wy-44635; Cefpiran; Suncefal; Sepatren. $C_{25}H_{23}N_8NaO_7S_2$; mol wt 634.62.

THERAP CAT: Antibacterial.

1940. Cefpirome. [84957-29-9] 1-[[(6R,7R)-7-[[(2Z)-(2-Amino-4-thiazolyl)(methoxyimino)acetyl]amino]-2-carboxy-8-oxo-5-thia-1-azabicyclo[4.2.0]oct-2-en-3-yl]methyl]-6,7-dihydro-5H-cyclopenta[b]pyridinium inner salt; 3-[(2,3-cyclopenteno-1-pyridinium)methyl]-7-[2-syn-methoxyimino-2-(2-aminothiazol-4-yl)acetamido]ceph-3-em-4-carboxylate; 1-[[(6R,7R)-7-[2-(2-ami-no-4-thiazolyl)glyoxylamido]-2-carboxy-8-oxo-5-thia-1-azabicy-clo[4.2.0]oct-2-en-3-yl]methyl]-6,7-dihydro-5H-1-pyrinidinium hy-droxide, inner salt, 7^2-(Z)-(O-methyloxime); HR-810. $C_{22}H_{22}N_6$-O_5S_2; mol wt 514.58. C 51.35%, H 4.31%, N 16.33%, O 15.55%, S 12.46%. Fourth generation cephalosporin antibiotic. Prepn: R. Lattrell *et al.*, **GB 2098216** (1982 to Hoechst). Prepn of crystalline salts: W. Dürckheimer, R. Lattrell, **US 4609653** (1986 to Hoechst); and *in vitro* antibacterial activity: G. Seibert *et al.*, *Arzneim.-Forsch.* **33**, 1084 (1983). Physical properties: R. Lattrell *et al.*, *Proc. 13th Int. Congr. Chemother.* **4**, part 99, 1 (1983). Comparative *in vitro* antibacterial spectrum and β-lactamase stability: H. C. Neu *et al.*, *Infection* **13**, 146 (1985). HPLC determn in serum and urine: H. Uihlein *et al.*, *ibid.* **16**, 135 (1988). Clinical pharmacokinetics: J. Kavi *et al.*, *J. Antimicrob. Chemother.* **22**, 911 (1988). Series of articles on laboratory and clinical evaluations: *ibid.* **29**, Suppl A 1-104 (1992). Toxicity studies: G. Horstmann, K. Engelbart, *Arz-neim.-Forsch.* **40**, 1250 (1990); H. H. Donaubauer, D. Mayer, *J. Antimicrob. Chemother.* **29**, Suppl. A, 71 (1992).

LD_{50} in mice, rats (g/kg): 1.9-2.4, 1.9-2.15 i.v.; 3.8-4.2, 5.8-6.55 i.p. (Donaubauer, Mayer).

Sulfate. [98753-19-6] Broact; Cefrom; Keitin. $C_{22}H_{22}N_6O_5$-$S_2.H_2SO_4$; mol wt 612.66. Occurs as the monohydrate, crystals, dec 198-202°. $[\alpha]_D^{25}$ −4.7° (c = 5 in H_2O). uv max: 265 nm (ε 21100). Soly (aq buffer, pH 6.5) >50%.

THERAP CAT: Antibacterial.

1941. Cefpodoxime Proxetil. [87239-81-4] (6R,7R)-7-[[(2Z)-(2-Amino-4-thiazolyl)(methoxyimino)acetyl]amino]-3-(methoxymethyl)-8-oxo-5-thia-1-azabicyclo[4.2.0]oct-2-ene-2-carboxylic acid 1-[[(1-methylethoxy)carbonyl]oxy]ethyl ester; 1-(iso-propoxycarbonyloxy)ethyl ester (6*R*,7*R*)-7-[2-(2-amino-4-thiazolyl)-(*Z*)-2-(methoxyimino)acetamido]-3-methoxymethyl-3-cephem-4-car-boxylate; CS-807; U-76252; Cefodox; Orelox; Otreon; Vantin. $C_{21}H_{27}N_5O_9S_2$; mol wt 557.60. C 45.23%, H 4.88%, N 12.56%, O 25.82%, S 11.50%. Broad spectrum, orally absorbed third generation cephalosporin, ester prodrug of the active free acid metabolite, cefpodoxime. Prepn: H. Nakao *et al., EP 49118; eidem,* **US 4486425** (1982, 1984 both to Sankyo). Prepn, pharmacokinetics and NMR analysis: K. Fujimoto *et al., J. Antibiot.* **40**, 370 (1987). *In vitro* and *in vivo* antibacterial activity: Y. Utsui *et al., Antimicrob. Agents Chemother.* **31**, 1085 (1987). *In vitro* antibacterial spectrum and susceptibility testing of free acid: R. N. Jones, A. L. Barry, *ibid.* **32**, 443 (1988). Series of articles on antibacterial spectrum, pharmacokinetics, toxicology and clinical studies: *Chemotherapy (Tokyo)* **36**, Suppl. 1, 1-1126 (1988). Symposium on pharmacokinetics and clinical efficacy: *J. Antimicrob. Chemother.* **26**, Suppl. E, 1-101 (1990). Review of chemistry, antibacterial activity, toxicity and clinical studies: H. Nakao *et al., Sankyo Kenkyusho Nempo* **39**, 1-44 (1987), *C.A.* **109**, 27503x (1988).

LD$_{50}$ in male, female mice, male, female rats (mg/kg): >10000, >10000, >2000, >2000 s.c., 3502, 2535, >4000, >4000 i.p.; >8000, >8000, >4000, >4000 orally (Nakao, 1988).

Free acid. Cefpodoxime; R-3763; U-76253. $C_{15}H_{17}N_5O_6S_2$; mol wt 427.46.

Free acid sodium salt. U-76253A; R-3746. $C_{15}H_{16}N_5NaO_6$-S_2; mol wt 449.44.

THERAP CAT: Antibacterial.

1942. **Cefprozil.** [92665-29-7] (anhydrous); [121123-17-9] (monohydrate). (6*R*,7*R*)-7-[[(2*R*)-Amino(4-hydroxyphenyl)acetyl]amino]-8-oxo-3-(1-propenyl)-5-thia-1-azabicyclo[4.2.0]oct-2-ene-2-carboxylic acid monohydrate; (6*R*,7*R*)-7-[(*R*)-2-amino-2-(*p*-hydroxyphenyl)acetamido]-8-oxo-3-propenyl-5-thia-1-azabicyclo[4.2.0]oct-2-ene-2-carboxylic acid monohydrate; BMY-28100-03-800; Cefzil; Procef. $C_{18}H_{19}N_3O_5S.H_2O$; mol wt 407.44. C 53.06%, H 5.20%, N 10.31%, O 23.56%, S 7.87%. Semisynthetic oral cephalosporin consisting of ~90:10 *Z/E* isomeric mixture. Prepn and antibacterial activity: H. Hoshi *et al.,* **DE 3402642;** *eidem,* **US 4520022** (1984, 1985 both to Bristol-Myers); T. Naito *et al., J. Antibiot.* **40**, 991 (1987). Separation of isomers: M. A. Kaplan *et al.,* **US 4727070** (1988 to Bristol-Myers). Comparative *in vitro* antibacterial spectrum and β-lactamase stability: R. N. Jones *et al., Diagn. Microbiol. Infect. Dis.* **9**, 11 (1988). Clinical pharmacokinetics and tissue penetration: R. H. Barbhaiya *et al., Antimicrob. Agents Chemother.* **34**, 1204 (1990). Comparative clinical trials: A. Iravani, *ibid.* **35**, 1940 (1991); A. G. Arguedas *et al., Pediatr. Infect. Dis. J.* **10**, 375 (1991). HPLC determn in plasma and urine: W. C. Shyu *et al., Pharm. Res.* **8**, 992 (1991). Symposium on clinical use: *Clin. Infect. Dis.* **14**, Suppl. 2, S183-S272 (1992).

Z- isomer

Z-Form. [121412-77-9] BMY-28100. Isolated as the hemihydrate, crystals from acetone, mp 218-220° (dec). uv max (pH 7 phosphate buffer): 228, 279 nm (ε 12300, 9800).

E-**Form.** [92676-86-3] BMY-28167; BBS-1067. Colorless prisms from methanol, mp 230° (dec). uv max (pH 7 phosphate buffer): 228, 292 nm (ε 13000, 16900).

THERAP CAT: Antibacterial.

1943. **Cefquinome.** [84957-30-2] 1-[[(6*R*,7*R*)-7-[[(2*Z*)-(2-Amino-4-thiazolyl)(methoxyimino)acetyl]amino]-2-carboxy-8-oxo-5-thia-1-azabicyclo[4.2.0]oct-2-en-3-yl]methyl]-5,6,7,8-tetra-hydroquinolinium inner salt; HOE-111. $C_{23}H_{24}N_6O_5S_2$; mol wt 528.60. C 52.26%, H 4.58%, N 15.90%, O 15.13%, S 12.13%. Broad-spectrum fourth generation injectable aminothiazolyl cephalosporin. Prepn: **BE 893163;** R. Lattrell *et al.,* **US 5071979** (1982, 1991 both to Hoechst); R. F. Brown *et al., J. Med. Chem.* **33**, 2114 (1990). Antibacterial spectrum and pharmacokinetics in animals: M. Limbert *et al., Antimicrob. Agents Chemother.* **35**, 14 (1991). *In vitro* activity against bovine bacterial isolates: A. Böttner *et al., J. Vet. Med. B* **42**, 377 (1995). Efficacy in the treatment of mastitis in dairy cows: N. Y. Shpigel *et al., J. Dairy Sci.* **80**, 318 (1997).

Sulfate. [118443-89-3] HR-111V; Cobactan. $C_{23}H_{24}N_6O_5$-$S_2.H_2SO_4$; mol wt 626.68.

THERAP CAT (VET): Antibacterial.

1944. **Cefroxadine.** [51762-05-1] (6*R*,7*R*)-7-[[(2*R*)-Amino-1,4-cyclohexadien-1-ylacetyl]amino]-3-methoxy-8-oxo-5-thia-1-azabicyclo[4.2.0]oct-2-ene-2-carboxylic acid; 7-[D-2-amino-2-(1,4-cyclohexadienyl)acetamide]-3-methoxy-3-cephem-4-carboxylic acid; CGP-9000; Oraspor. $C_{16}H_{19}N_3O_5S$; mol wt 365.40. C 52.59%, H 5.24%, N 11.50%, O 21.89%, S 8.78%. Orally active cephalosporin deriv. Prepn: R. Scartazzini, H. Bickel, **DE 2331133;** *eidem,* **US 4073902** (1974, 1978 both to Ciba-Geigy). Antibiotic activity: O. Zak *et al., J. Antibiot.* **29**, 653 (1976). *In vivo* and *in vitro* microbiological evaluation: K. Yasuda *et al., Antimicrob. Agents Chemother.* **18**, 105 (1980). Pharmacokinetics: T. Bergan, *Chemotherapy* **26**, 225 (1980). Series of articles on activity, toxicity, reproduction studies: *Chemotherapy (Tokyo)* **28**, Suppl 3, 1-335 (1980).

Internal salt, mp 170° (dec). $[\alpha]_D^{20}$ +87° (c = 1.093 in 0.1*N* HCl). uv max (0.1*N* HCl): 267 nm (ε 6100). LD$_{50}$ in mice (mg/kg): >6000 orally; 7090 i.p. (Scartazzini, Bickel, 1978).

THERAP CAT: Antibacterial.

1945. **Cefsulodin.** [62587-73-9] 4-(Aminocarbonyl)-1-[[(6*R*,7*R*)-2-carboxy-8-oxo-7-[[(2*R*)-phenylsulfoacetyl]amino]-5-thia-1-azabicyclo[4.2.0]oct-2-en-3-yl]methyl]pyridinium inner salt; 7-(α-sulphophenylacetamido)-3-(4'-carbamoylpyridinium)methyl-3-cephem-4-carboxylic acid. $C_{22}H_{20}N_4O_8S_2$; mol wt 532.55. C 49.62%, H 3.79%, N 10.52%, O 24.03%, S 12.04%. Third generation cephalosporin antibiotic. Prepn: S. Morimoto *et al.,* **DE 2234280;** *eidem,* **US 4065619** (1973, 1977 both to Takeda). Prepn and separation of isomers: H. Nomura *et al., J. Med. Chem.* **17**, 1312 (1974). *In vitro* and *in vivo* antibacterial activity: K. Tsuchiya *et al., Antimicrob. Agents Chemother.* **13**, 137 (1978). Absorption, distribution, excretion in mice, rats, dogs: *eidem, J. Antibiot.* **31**, 593 (1978). Activity and susceptibility to β-lactamases: A. King *et al., Antimicrob. Agents Chemother.* **17**, 165 (1980). *In vitro* comparison with other antibacterials: H. Grimm, *Arzneim.-Forsch.* **30**, 1478 (1980). Clinical pharmacology: J. Fuellhaas *et* *al., Curr. Chemother., Proc. 10th Int. Congr. Chemother.* (Washington, D.C., 1978) **2**, 848-851. Review of activity: H. C. Neu, B. E. Scully, *Rev. Infect. Dis.* **6**, Suppl. 3, S667-S677 (1984). *Review:* A. Bryskier, *Lyon Pharm.* **34**, 343-355 (1983); D. B. Wright, *Drug Intell. Clin. Pharm.* **20**, 845-849 (1986).

Sodium salt. [52152-93-9] Sulcephalosporin; Abbott 46811; CGP-7174/E; SCE-129; Cefomonil; Monaspor; Pseudocef; Pyocefal; Takesulin; Tilmapor; Ulfaret. $C_{22}H_{19}N_4NaO_8S_2$; mol wt 554.53. Colorless needles from ethanol/water, mp 175° (dec). LD_{50} in mice (mg/kg): >4000 i.p.; >15000 orally (Bryskier).
d-Form sodium salt. $[\alpha]_D^{23}$ +16.5° (c = 1.08 in water). uv max (water): 263 nm (ε 14600).
l-Form sodium salt. $[\alpha]_D^{23}$ −16.8° (c = 1.01 in water).
THERAP CAT: Antibacterial.

1946. Ceftazidime. [72558-82-8] 1-[[(6*R*,7*R*)-7-[[(2*Z*)-(2-Amino-4-thiazolyl)[(1-carboxy-1-methylethoxy)imino]acetyl]amino]-2-carboxy-8-oxo-5-thia-1-azabicyclo[4.2.0]oct-2-en-3-yl]methyl]pyridinium inner salt; 1-[[(6*R*,7*R*)-7-[2-(2-amino-4-thiazolyl)-glyoxylamido]-2-carboxy-8-oxo-5-thia-1-azabicyclo[4.2.0]oct-2-en-3-yl]methyl]pyridinium hydroxide inner salt 7^2-(*Z*)-[*O*-(1-carboxy-1-methylethyl)oxime]; GR-20263. $C_{22}H_{22}N_6O_7S_2$; mol wt 546.58. C 48.34%, H 4.06%, N 15.38%, O 20.49%, S 11.73%. Third generation cephalosporin antibiotic. Prepn: C. H. O'Callaghan *et al.*, **DE 2921316**; *eidem*, **US 4258041** (1979, 1981 both to Glaxo). Prepn of crystalline pentahydrate: A. Brodie, L. A. Wetherill, **DE 3037102**; *eidem*, **US 4329453** (1981, 1982 both to Glaxo). Chemical and antibacterial properties: *eidem, Antimicrob. Agents Chemother.* **17**, 876 (1980). Activity vs *Pseudomonas* and *Enterobacteriaceae:* L. Verbist, J. Verhaegen, *ibid.* 807. *In vitro* comparison with other β-lactams: R. Wise *et al., ibid.* 884; L. Verbist, *ibid.* **19**, 407 (1981). Symposium on clinical studies: *J. Antimicrob. Chemother.* **12**, Suppl. A, 1-414 (1983). Review of antibacterial activity, pharmacokinetics and therapeutic use: D. M. Richards, R. N. Brogden, *Drugs* **29**, 105-161 (1985). Comprehensive description: M. A. Abounassif *et al., Anal. Profiles Drug Subs.* **19**, 95-121 (1990).

Pentahydrate. [78439-06-2] Fortam; Fortaz; Fortum; Fortumset; Glazidim; Kefadim; Kefamin; Kefazim; Modacin; Panzid; Spectrum; Starcef; Tazicef; Tazidime. $C_{22}H_{22}N_6O_7S_2 \cdot 5H_2O$; mol wt 636.65. Crystalline solid. uv max (pH 6): 257 nm ($E_{1cm}^{1\%}$ 348).
THERAP CAT: Antibacterial.

1947. Cefteram. [82547-58-8] (6*R*,7*R*)-7-[[(2*Z*)-(2-Amino-4-thiazolyl)(methoxyimino)acetyl]amino]-3-[(5-methyl-2*H*-tetrazol-2-yl)methyl]-8-oxo-5-thia-1-azabicyclo[4.2.0]oct-2-ene-2-carboxylic acid; (+)-(6*R*,7*R*)-7-[(*Z*)-2-(2-amino-4-thiazolyl)-2-(methoxyimino)acetamido]-3-[(5-methyl-2*H*-tetrazol-2-yl)methyl]-8-oxo-5-thia-1-azabicyclo[4.2.0]oct-2-ene-2-carboxylic acid; 7-[2-(2-aminothiazol-4-yl)-2-*syn*-methoxyiminoacetamido]-3-[2-(5-methyl-1,2,3,4-tetrazolyl)methyl]-Δ³-cephem-4-carboxylic acid; (+)-(6*R*,7*R*)-7-[2-(2-amino-4-thiazolyl)glyoxylamido]-3-[(5-methyl-2*H*-tetrazol-2-yl)methyl]-8-oxo-5-thia-1-azabicyclo[4.2.0]oct-2-ene-2-carboxylic acid 7^2-(*Z*)-(*O*-methyloxime); ceftetrame; Ro-19-

5247; T-2525. $C_{16}H_{17}N_9O_5S_2$; mol wt 479.49. C 40.08%, H 3.57%, N 26.29%, O 16.68%, S 13.37%. Third generation, orally active cephalosporin antibiotic. Prepn: **BE 890499**; H. Sadaki *et al.*, **US 4489072** (1982, 1984 both to Toyama). *In vitro* antibacterial activity: R. Wise *et al., Antimicrob. Agents Chemother.* **29**, 1067 (1986); *in vitro* activity vs *Neisseria gonorrhoeae:* W. R. Bowie *et al., ibid.* **31**, 470 (1987). General pharmacology in animals: S. Hirai *et al., Jpn. J. Antibiot.* **39**, 958 (1986), *C.A.* **105**, 183450a (1986). Pharmacokinetics and tissue distribution in animals: I. Saikawa *et al., ibid.* 979, *C.A.* **105**, 183338v (1986). Series of articles on activity, toxicology, pharmacology and clinical efficacy: *Chemotherapy (Tokyo)* **34**, Suppl. 2, 1-984 (1986). Acute toxicity: S. Sato *et al., ibid.* 166.

Crystals from acetone, mp >200°.
Pivaloyloxymethyl ester. [82547-81-7] Cefteram pivoxil; T-2588; Tomiron. $C_{22}H_{27}N_9O_7S_2$; mol wt 593.64. Oral prodrug of cefteram. Crystals, mp 127-128° (dec). LD_{50} in male, female mice, rats (g/kg): >6.00, 5.86, 5.63, 5.09 i.p.; in both species >6.00 s.c.; in male mice, rats, dogs (g/kg): >6.00, >6.00, >2.00 orally (Sato).
THERAP CAT: Antibacterial.

1948. Ceftezole. [26973-24-0] (6*R*,7*R*)-8-Oxo-7-[(1*H*-tetrazol-1-ylacetyl)amino]-3-[(1,3,4-thiadiazol-2-ylthio)methyl]-5-thia-1-azabicyclo[4.2.0]oct-2-ene-2-carboxylic acid; 7-(1*H*-tetrazol-1-yl)acetamido-3-(1,3,4-thiadiazol-2-ylthio)methylceph-3-em-4-carboxylic acid; CTZ; CG-B3Q. $C_{13}H_{12}N_8O_4S_3$; mol wt 440.48. C 35.45%, H 2.75%, N 25.44%, O 14.53%, S 21.84%. Broad spectrum antibiotic similar to cefazolin, *q.v.* Prepn: T. Takano *et al.*, **ZA 6804513**; *eidem*, **US 3516997** (1969, 1970 both to Fujisawa). *In vitro* and *in vivo* activity: T. Noto *et al., J. Antibiot.* **29**, 1058 (1976). Pharmacology: Y. Harada *et al., ibid.* 1071; M. Kakimoto *et al., Chemotherapy (Tokyo)* **24**, 722 (1976). Metabolism: K. Koyama *et al., ibid.* 619; Y. Tohira *et al., ibid.* 655. Clinical study: S. Ishiyama *et al., ibid.* 1006. Toxicity and teratogenicity studies: R. Niki *et al., ibid.* 671.

Solid, mp 155° (dec). uv max (phosphate buffer pH 6.4): 273 nm ($E_{1cm}^{1\%}$ 274).
Sodium salt. [41136-22-5] FR-10123; Celoslin; Falomesin. $C_{13}H_{11}N_8NaO_4S_3$; mol wt 462.46. White solid, freely sol in water.
THERAP CAT: Antibacterial.

1949. Ceftibuten. [97519-39-6] (6*R*,7*R*)-7-[[(2*Z*)-2-(2-Amino-4-thiazolyl)-4-carboxy-1-oxo-2-butenyl]amino]-8-oxo-5-thia-1-azabicyclo[4.2.0]oct-2-ene-2-carboxylic acid; 7β-[(*Z*)-2-(2-aminothiazol-4-yl)-4-carboxy-2-butenoylamino]-3-cephem-4-carboxylic acid; 7432-S; Sch-39720. $C_{15}H_{14}N_4O_6S_2$; mol wt 410.42. C 43.90%, H 3.44%, N 13.65%, O 23.39%, S 15.63%. Orally active third generation cephalosporin antibiotic. Prepn: Y. Hamashima, **EP 136721**; *idem*, **US 4634697** (1985, 1987 both to Shionogi); and *in vitro* antibacterial activity: Y. Hamashima *et al., J. Antibiot.* **40**, 1468 (1987). Industrial synthesis utilizing penicillin G: M. Yoshioka, *Pure Appl. Chem.* **59**, 1041 (1987). Comparative antibacterial spectrum: R. N. Jones, A. L. Barry, *Antimicrob. Agents Chemother.* **32**, 1576 (1988). Pharmacokinetics in humans: M. Nakashima *et al., J. Clin. Pharmacol.* **28**, 246 (1988).

Dihydrate. [118081-34-8] Cedax; Isocef; Seftem. $C_{15}H_{14}N_4$-$O_6S_2.2H_2O$; mol wt 446.46.

THERAP CAT: Antibacterial.

1950.   Ceftiofur. [80370-57-6] (6*R*,7*R*)-7-[[(2*Z*)-(2-Amino-4-thiazolyl)(methoxyimino)acetyl]amino]-3-[[[(2-furanylcarbonyl)-thio]methyl]-8-oxo-5-thia-1-azabicyclo[4.2.0]oct-2-ene-2-carboxylic acid; (6*R*,7*R*)-7-[2-(2-amino-4-thiazolyl)glyoxylamido]-3-(mercaptomethyl)-8-oxo-5-thia-1-azabicyclo[4.2.0]oct-2-ene-2-carboxylic acid 7²-(*Z*)-(*O*-methyloxime) 2-furoate (ester); Excede. $C_{19}H_{17}N_5O_7S_3$; mol wt 523.56. C 43.59%, H 3.27%, N 13.38%, O 21.39%, S 18.37%. Broad spectrum, third generation cephalosporin antibiotic. Prepn: B. Labeeuw, A. Salhi, **EP 36812**; *eidem*, **US 4464367** (1981, 1984 both to Sanofi). *In vivo* and *in vitro* antibacterial activity and β-lactamase stability: R. J. Yancey *et al., Am. J. Vet. Res.* **48**, 1050 (1987).

Monosodium salt. [104010-37-9] CM-31916; U-64279E; Naxcel. $C_{19}H_{16}N_5NaO_7S_3$; mol wt 545.54.
Monohydrochloride. [103980-44-5] U-67279A; Excenel. $C_{19}H_{17}N_5O_7S_3.HCl$; mol wt 560.02.

THERAP CAT (VET): Antibacterial.

1951.   Ceftizoxime. [68401-81-0] (6*R*,7*R*)-7-[[(2*Z*)-(2-Amino-4-thiazolyl)(methoxyimino)acetyl]amino]-8-oxo-5-thia-1-azabicyclo[4.2.0]oct-2-ene-2-carboxylic acid; (6*R*,7*R*)-7-[2-(2-imino-4-thiazolyl)glyoxylamido]-8-oxo-5-thia-1-azabicyclo[4.2.0]oct-2-ene-2-carboxylic acid 7²-(*Z*)-(*O*-methyloxime). $C_{13}H_{13}N_5O_5S_2$; mol wt 383.40. C 40.72%, H 3.42%, N 18.27%, O 20.87%, S 16.73%. Injectable third generation cephalosporin antibiotic related to cefotaxime, *q.v.* Exhibits broad spectrum activity and resistance to β-lactamase hydrolysis. Prepn: T. Takaya *et al.*, **DE 2810922**; *eidem*, **US 4427674** (1978, 1984 both to Fujisawa). *In vitro* and *in vivo* antibacterial activity: T. Kamimura *et al., Antimicrob. Agents Chemother.* **16**, 540 (1979). Comparison with other cephalosporins: M. Nishida *et al., J. Antibiot.* **32**, 1319 (1979). Pharmacokinetics: T. Murakawa *et al., Antimicrob. Agents Chemother.* **17**, 157 (1980). Series of articles on metabolism, pharmacology, laboratory evaluation: *Arzneim.-Forsch.* **30**, 1662-1687 (1980). Toxicity and reproduction studies: K. Fukuhara *et al., ibid.* 1669. Phase I clinical study: N. Nakashima *et al., J. Clin. Pharmacol.* **21**, 388 (1981). *Reviews: J. Antimicrob. Chemother.* **10**, Suppl. C, 1-355 (1982); D. M. Richards, R. C. Heel, *Drugs* **29**, 281-329 (1985).

Crystals, mp 227° (dec).
Sodium salt. [68401-82-1] FK-749; FR-13479; SKF-88373; Cefizox; Ceftix; Ceftizon; Epocelin; Eposerin. $C_{13}H_{12}N_5NaO_5S_2$; mol wt 405.38. LD_{50} in mice, rats (mg/kg): ~6000 i.v. (Fukuhara).

THERAP CAT: Antibacterial.

1952.   Ceftobiprole Medocaril. [376653-43-9] (6*R*,7*R*)-7-[[(2*Z*)-(5-Amino-1,2,4-thiadiazol-3-yl)(hydroxyimino)acetyl]amino]-3-[(*E*)-[(3′*R*)-1′-[[(5-methyl-2-oxo-1,3-dioxol-4-yl)methoxy]Carbonyl]-2-oxo[1,3′-bipyrrolidin]-3-ylidene]methyl]-8-oxo-5-thia-1-azabicyclo[4.2.0]oct-2-ene-2-carboxylic acid. $C_{26}H_{26}N_8O_{11}S_2$; mol wt 690.66. C 45.21%, H 3.79%, N 16.22%, O 25.48%, S 9.29%. Fourth generation cephalosporin antibiotic prodrug; rapidly cleaved in plasma to the active metabolite, ceftobiprole. Prepn: P. Hebeisen *et al.,* **WO 9965920**; *eidem,* **US 6232306** (1999, 2001 both to Hoffmann-La Roche). *In vitro* and *in vivo* activity against methicillin-resistant *Staphylococcus aureus* (MRSA): *idem et al., Antimicrob. Agents Chemother.* **45**, 825 (2001). Comparative antibacterial spectrum *in vitro:* R. N. Jones *et al., J. Antimicrob. Chemother.* **50**, 915 (2002). *In vivo* activity ine experimental pneumococcal pneumonia: E. Azoulay-Dupuis *et al., Antimicrob. Agents Chemother.* **48**, 1105 (2004). Clinical pharmacokinetics and safety: A. Schmitt-Hoffmann *et al., ibid.* **48**, 2576 (2004).

Sodium salt. [252188-71-9] BAL-5788; Ro-65-5788. $C_{26}H_{25}$-$N_8NaO_{11}S_2$; mol wt 712.64. Sol in water.
Ceftobiprole. [209467-52-7] (6*R*,7*R*)-7-[[(2*Z*)-(5-Amino-1,2,4-thiadiazol-3-yl)(hydroxyimino)acetyl]amino]-8-oxo-3[(*E*)-[(3′*R*)-2-oxo[1,3′-bipyrrolidin]-3-ylidene]methyl]-5-thia-1-azabicyclo[4.2.0]oct-2-ene-2-carboxylic acid. $C_{20}H_{22}N_8O_6S_2$; mol wt 534.57. Prepn: P. Angehrn *et al.*, **EP 849269**; *eidem,* **US 5981519** (1997, 1999 both to Hoffmann-La Roche).

THERAP CAT: Antibacterial.

1953.   Ceftriaxone. [73384-59-5] (6*R*,7*R*)-7-[[(2*Z*)-(2-Amino-4-thiazolyl)(methoxyimino)acetyl]amino]-8-oxo-3-[[(1,2,5,6-tetrahydro-2-methyl-5,6-dioxo-1,2,4-triazin-3-yl)thio]methyl]-5-thia-1-azabicyclo[4.2.0]oct-2-ene-2-carboxylic acid; (6*R*,7*R*)-7-[2-(2-amino-4-thiazolyl)glyoxylamido]-3-[[(2,5-dihydro-6-hydroxy-2-methyl-5-oxo-*as*-triazin-3-yl)thio]methyl]-8-oxo-5-thia-1-azabicyclo[4.2.0]oct-2-ene-2-carboxylic acid 7²-(*Z*)-(*O*-methyloxime); cefatriaxone. $C_{18}H_{18}N_8O_7S_3$; mol wt 554.58. C 38.98%, H 3.27%, N 20.21%, O 20.19%, S 17.35%. Parenteral third generation cephalosporin antibiotic. Prepn: M. Montavon, R. Reiner, **GB 2022090**; *eidem,* **US 4327210** (1979, 1982 both to Hoffmann-La Roche); R. Reiner *et al., J. Antibiot.* **33**, 783 (1980). *In vitro* and *in vivo* studies: P. Angehrn *et al., Antimicrob. Agents Chemother.* **18**, 913 (1980). Pharmacokinetics: M. Seddon *et al., ibid.* 240. Determn in plasma, urine, bile: K. H. Trautman, P. Haefelfinger, *J. High Resolut. Chromatogr. Chromatogr. Commun.* **4**, 54 (1981), *C.A.* **94**, 202437 (1981). Mechanism of action study: R. B. Wright *et al., J. Antibiot.* **34**, 590 (1981). Kinetics in humans: K. Stoekel *et al., Clin. Pharmacol. Ther.* **29**, 650 (1981). Toxicity data: K. Teelman *et al.,* "Experimentelle Toxikologie von Ceftriaxon", in *Ceftriaxon ein neues parenterales Cephalosporin, Proc. Hahnenklee Symp., 1981*, R. Grieshalber, Ed. (Editiones Roche, Basel, 1982) pp 91-111. Review of antibacterial activity, toxicology, pharmacology and clinical studies: D. M. Richards *et al., Drugs* **27**, 469 (1984); T. R. Beam, *Pharmacotherapy* **5**, 237-253 (1985).

Disodium salt hemiheptahydrate. [104376-79-6] Ro-13-9904/001; Rocefin; Rocephin(e). $C_{18}H_{16}N_8Na_2O_7S_3.3½H_2O$;

mol wt 661.60. White cryst powder, mp >155° (dec). $[\alpha]_D^{25}$ −165° (c = 1 in water) (calc for water-free substance). uv max (water): 242, 272 nm (ε 32300, 29530). pKa: ~3 (COOH), 3.2 (NH_3^+), 4.1 (enolic OH). Soly in water at 25°: ~40 g/100 ml. LD_{50} in male, female, mice, rats (mg/kg): 3000, 2800, 2175, 2175 i.v.; >10000 all species orally; >5000 all species s.c. (Teelman).

THERAP CAT: Antibacterial.

1954. Cefuroxime. [55268-75-2] (6R,7R)-3-[[(Aminocarbonyl)oxy]methyl]-7-[[(2Z)-2-furanyl(methoxyimino)acetyl]amino]-8-oxo-5-thia-1-azabicyclo[4.2.0]oct-2-ene-2-carboxylic acid; (6R,7R)-3-carbamoyloxymethyl-7-[2-(2-furyl)-2-(methoxyimino)-acetamido]-8-oxo-5-thia-1-azabicyclo[4.2.0]oct-2-ene-2-carboxylic acid; (6R,7R)-3-carbamoyloxymethyl-7-[2-(2-furyl)-2-(methoxyimino)acetamido]ceph-3-em-4-carboxylic acid. $C_{16}H_{16}N_4O_8S$; mol wt 424.39. C 45.28%, H 3.80%, N 13.20%, O 30.16%, S 7.56%. Prepn: M. C. Cook et al., **DE 2439880**; eidem, **US 3974153** (1973, 1976 both to Glaxo). Prepn of the 1-acetoxyethyl ester: M. Gregson, B. Sykes, **DE 2706413**; eidem, **US 4267320** (1977, 1981 both to Glaxo). In vitro studies: C. H. O'Callaghan et al., Antimicrob. Agents Chemother. **9**, 511 (1976); R. N. Jones et al., ibid. **12**, 47 (1977). In vitro antibacterial activity, human pharmacokinetics: C. H. O'Callaghan et al., J. Antibiot. **29**, 29 (1976). Pharmacology: H. Freiesleben et al., Proc. 10th Int. Congr. Chemother., Zürich, 1977 (Am. Soc. for Microbiol., Washington, 1978) **II**, pp 873-874. Pharmacokinetics: P. E. Gower, ibid. 877-878; J. Kosmidis et al., ibid. 875-876. Clinical studies: P. F. Wood et al., ibid. 1042-1044; R. Norrby et al., J. Antimicrob. Chemother. **3**, 355 (1977). Review of antibacterial activity, pharmacology and therapeutic efficacy: R. N. Brogden et al., Drugs **17**, 233-266 (1979). Comprehensive description: T. J. Wozniak, J. R. Hicks, Anal. Profiles Drug Subs. **20**, 209-236 (1991).

White crystalline solid. $[\alpha]_D^{20}$ +63.7° (c = 1.0 in 0.2M pH 7 phosphate buffer). uv max (pH 6 phosphate buffer): 274 nm (ε 17600).

Sodium salt. [56238-63-2] Anaptivan; Biociclin; Biofurex; Bioxima; Cefamar; Cefoprim; Cefumax; Cefurex; Cefurin; Curocef; Curoxim; Duxima; Gibicef; Ipacef; Kefurox; Kesint; Lampsporin; Medoxim; Novocef; Spectrazole; Ultroxim; Zinacef. $C_{16}H_{15}N_4$-NaO_8S; mol wt 446.37. White solid. $[\alpha]_D^{20}$ +60° (c = 0.91 in water). uv max (water): 274 nm (ε 17400). Freely sol in water and buffered solutions; sol in methanol; very slightly sol in ethyl acetate, diethyl ether, octanol, benzene and chloroform. Soly in water: 500 mg/2.5 ml. pKa (water): 2.5; (DMF): 5.1. Solns are stable at room temp for 13 hrs; <10% decompn in 48 hrs at 25° (O'Callaghan, J. Antibiot.).

1-Acetoxyethyl ester. Cefuroxime axetil; CCI-15641; Ceftin; Cefurax; Cepazine; Elobact; Oraxim; Zinat; Zinnat. $C_{20}H_{22}N_4$-$O_{10}S$; mol wt 510.47.

THERAP CAT: Antibacterial.

THERAP CAT (VET): Antibacterial.

1955. Cefuzonam. [82219-78-1] (6R,7R)-7-[[(2Z)-(2-Amino-4-thiazolyl)(methoxyimino)acetyl]amino]-8-oxo-3-[[(1,2,3-thiadiazol-5-ylthio)methyl]-5-thia-1-azabicyclo[4.2.0]oct-2-ene-2-carboxylic acid; (−)-(6R,7R)-7-[2-(2-amino-4-thiazolyl)glyoxylamido]-8-oxo-3-[(1,2,3-thiadiazol-5-ylthio)methyl]-5-thia-1-azabicyclo[4.2.0]oct-2-ene-2-carboxylic acid 7^2-(Z)-(O-methyloxime); 7β-[2-(2-aminothiazol-4-yl)-(Z)-2-methoxyiminoacetamido]-3-[(1,2,3-thiadiazol-5-yl)thiomethyl]ceph-3-em-4-carboxylic acid; CL-118523. $C_{16}H_{15}N_7O_5S_4$; mol wt 513.59. C 37.42%, H 2.94%, N 19.09%, O 15.58%, S 24.97%. Semi-synthetic third generation cephalosporin. Prepn and bactericidal activity: W. V. Curran, A. S. Ross, **FR 2488258**; eidem, **US 4399132** (1982, 1983 both to Am.

Cyanamid); eidem, J. Antibiot. **36**, 179 (1983). Improved prepn of sodium salt: K. Naito et al., **EP 145395** (1985 to Takeda). In vitro antibacterial spectrum: M. Hikada et al., J. Antimicrob. Chemother. **18**, 585 (1986). Toxicity study: S. Takita, Chemotherapy (Tokyo) **34**, Suppl. 3, 96 (1986). Conference proceedings: Recent Adv. Chemother., Antimicrobial Sect. 2., Proc. 14th Int. Congr. Chemother., Kyoto 1985, J. Ishigami, Ed. (Univ. Tokyo Press, Tokyo, 1985) pp 887-908. Series of articles: Chemotherapy (Tokyo) **34**, Suppl. 3, 1-732 (1986).

White amorphous solid. LD_{50} in female, male mice, female, male rats (mg/kg): 4117, >4800, 4281, 4222 i.v.; 6424, 6783, >8000, >8000 i.p.; all >10000 orally (Takita).

Sodium salt dihydrate. L-105 (Lederle); CL-251931; LJC-10305; Cosmosin. $C_{16}H_{14}N_7NaO_5S_4.2H_2O$; mol wt 571.61. Yellowish crystalline powder. Sol in water.

THERAP CAT: Antibacterial.

1956. Celecoxib. [169590-42-5] 4-[5-(4-Methylphenyl)-3-(trifluoromethyl)-1H-pyrazol-1-yl]benzenesulfonamide; SC-58635; YM-177; Celebrex; Onsenal. $C_{17}H_{14}F_3N_3O_2S$; mol wt 381.37. C 53.54%, H 3.70%, F 14.94%, N 11.02%, O 8.39%, S 8.41%. Selective cyclooxygenase-2 (COX-2) inhibitor. Prepn: J. J. Talley et al., **WO 9515316**; eidem, **US 5466823** (both 1995 to Searle); T. D. Penning et al., J. Med. Chem. **40**, 1347 (1997). Clinical pharmacology: P. E. Lipsky, P. C. Isakson, J. Rheumatol. **24**, Suppl. 49, 9 (1997). Clinical trials in arthritis: L. S. Simon et al., Arthritis Rheum. **41**, 1591 (1998). Evaluation of risk of gastrointestinal toxicity in patients with arthritis: F. E. Silverstein et al., J. Am. Med. Assoc. **284**, 1247 (2000). Clinical trial in familial adenomatous polyposis: G. Steinbach et al., N. Engl. J. Med. **342**, 1946 (2000).

Pale yellow solid, mp 157-159°.

THERAP CAT: Anti-inflammatory. In treatment of familial adenomatous polyposis.

1957. Celery Seed. Dried, ripe fruit of Apium graveolens L., Umbelliferae. Habit. Southern Europe; cultivated everywhere. Constit. Volatile and fixed oils; bitter extractive; resin.

1958. Celesticetin. [2520-21-0] 2-[(2-Hydroxybenzoyl)-oxy]ethyl 6,8-dideoxy-7-O-methyl-6-[[[(2S)-1-methyl-2-pyrrolidinyl]carbonyl]amino]-1-thio-D-erythro-α-D-galacto-octopyranoside; α-2-hydroxyethyl 6,8-dideoxy-7-O-methyl-6-(1-methyl-L-2-pyrrolidinecarboxamido)-1-thio-D-erythro-D-galacto-octopyranoside monosalicylate; S-demethyl-3'-depropyl-S-[2-[(2-hydroxybenzoyl)oxy]ethyl]-7-O-methyllincomycin. $C_{24}H_{36}N_2O_9S$; mol wt 528.62. C 54.53%, H 6.86%, N 5.30%, O 27.24%, S 6.07%. Antibiotic substance produced by Streptomyces caelestis from a soil obtained from Emigration Canyon near Salt Lake City: DeBoer et al., Antibiot. Annu. **1954-1955**, 831; Hoeksema et al., ibid. 837. Structure: Hoeksema, J. Am. Chem. Soc. **86**, 4224 (1964); **90**, 755 (1968).

Amphoteric, amorphous base. $[\alpha]_D^{24}$ +126.6° (c = 0.5 in chloroform). uv max (0.01N alcoholic H_2SO_4): 240, 310 nm ($E_{1cm}^{1\%}$ 183.7, 80.6). Soluble in acidic or strongly basic aq solns, practically insol in the pH range of 7 to 10. Soluble in the more polar organic solvents, but not in ether or light hydrocarbons. Active against gram-positive organisms and plant pathogens such as *B. stewartii, P. fascians, X. pruni* at 0.5 γ/ml. The antibacterial activity is rapidly destroyed in aq solns above pH 9 at 24°, but remains at pH 5 to 7 for at least 60 days. Celesticetin is more stable in acid than in basic solns, but is destroyed rapidly in 1N HCl at 100°. Cross resistance with erythromycin.

Salicylate. Monoclinic tablets, mp 139°. $[\alpha]_D^{24}$ +90.2° (c = 0.5 in H_2O). Sol in water.

Oxalate. Crystals, mp 149-154°. $[\alpha]_D^{24}$ +106.6° (c = 5 in H_2O). Sol in water.

1959. Celestin Blue. [1562-90-9] 1-(Aminocarbonyl)-7-(diethylamino)-3,4-dihydroxyphenoxazin-5-ium chloride; 1-carbamoyl-7-(diethylamino)-3,4-dihydroxyphenazoxonium chloride; C.I. Mordant Blue 14; C.I. 51050; michrome no. 66; Corein 2R. $C_{17}H_{18}ClN_3O_4$; mol wt 363.80. C 56.12%, H 4.99%, Cl 9.75%, N 11.55%, O 17.59%. Prepd by the action of gallamide on *N,N*-diethyl-*p*-nitrosoaniline HCl: Gnehm, Bauer, *J. Prakt. Chem.* **72**, 249 (1905); Grandmougin, Bodmer, *ibid.* **77**, 502 (1908). *See also:* US 534809 (1895); US 1227407 (1917); *Colour Index* vol. **4** (3rd ed., 1971). *Review:* H. J. *Conn's Biological Stains*, R. D. Lillie, Ed. (Williams & Wilkins, Baltimore, 9th ed., 1977) pp 407-408.

Greenish-black powder. With water it yields a reddish-purple soln, which appears blue on extreme diln. The alcoholic soln is blue in all concns. Approximate soly in water 2.0%, abs ethanol 1.5%, Cellosolve 2.25%, ethylene glycol 6.5%, xylene 0.005%.

USE: To dye fabrics a navy-blue color with faint reddish tinge. As nuclear and connective tissue stain. One of the ingredients of Picro-Mallory stain: Lendrum, McFarlane, *J. Pathol. Bacteriol.* **50**, 381 (1940).

1960. Celiprolol. [56980-93-9] *N'*-[3-Acetyl-4-[3-[(1,1-dimethylethyl)amino]-2-hydroxypropoxy]phenyl]-*N,N*-diethylurea; N-[3-acetyl-4-(3'-*tert*-butylamino-2'-hydroxy)propoxy]phenyl-*N'*-diethylurea; ST-1396. $C_{20}H_{33}N_3O_4$; mol wt 379.49. C 63.30%, H 8.76%, N 11.07%, O 16.86%. Cardioselective β_1-adrenergic blocker. Prepn: BE 823411; G. Zölss *et al.,* US 4034009 (1975, 1977 both to Chemie Linz). Hemodynamic effects: J. Bonelli *et al., Wien. Klin. Wochenschr.* **90**, 350 (1978); H. Pittner, *Arch. Pharmacol.* **311**, Suppl., 180 (1980). Series of articles on determn in biological material, pharmacology, toxicology, clinical studies: *Arzneim.-Forsch.* **33**, 1-79 (1983). Toxicity: W. Wendtlandt, H. Pittner, *ibid.* 41. Symposium on pharmacology, clinical efficacy and comparison with other β-blockers: *J. Cardiovasc. Pharmacol.* **8**, Suppl. 4, S1-S152 (1986). Comprehensive description: D. J. Mazzo *et al., Anal. Profiles Drug Subs.* **20**, 237-301 (1991).

Crystals, mp 110-112°.

Hydrochloride. [57470-78-7] Celectol; Corliprol; Selectol. $C_{20}H_{33}N_3O_4$·HCl; mol wt 415.95. White, odorless crystals, mp 197-200° (dec). Soly at ~25°C (g/100 ml): water 15.1, methanol 18.2, ethanol 1.61, chloroform 0.42. uv max (water): 231, 324 nm ($E_{1\%}$ 652, 57); (0.01N HCl): 231, 324 nm ($E_{1\%}$ 660, 60); (0.01N NaOH): 231, 324 nm ($E_{1\%}$ 640, 60); (methanol): 232, 329 nm ($E_{1\%}$ 775, 58). LD_{50} in male mice, rats (mg/kg): 56.2, 68.3 i.v.; 1834, 3826 orally (Wendtlandt, Pittner).

THERAP CAT: Antihypertensive, antianginal.

1961. Cellobiose. [528-50-7] 4-O-β-D-Glucopyranosyl-D-glucose; β-cellobiose; cellose; 4-(β-D-glucosido)-D-glucose. $C_{12}H_{22}O_{11}$; mol wt 342.30. C 42.11%, H 6.48%, O 51.41%. Unit of cellulose and lichenin. Does not occur free in nature, or as glucoside. Prepn from cotton: Braun, *Org. Synth.* coll. vol. II, 122, 124 (1943). Prepn from cell-free enzymatic hydrolyzate of cellulose: Whistler, Smart, *J. Am. Chem. Soc.* **75**, 1916 (1953). Structure: Haworth, Hirst, *J. Chem. Soc.* **119**, 193 (1923); Charlton *et al., ibid.* **1926**, 89; Zemplén, *Ber.* **59**, 1254 (1926); Haworth *et al., J. Chem. Soc.* **1927**, 2809; Peterson, Spencer, *J. Am. Chem. Soc.* **49**, 2822 (1927); Helferich *et al., Ber.* **63**, 992 (1930); Hess, Dziengel, *ibid.* **68**, 1594 (1935); Hassid, Ballou in *The Carbohydrates,* W. Pigman, Ed. (Academic Press, New York, 1957) p 490. Synthesis: Haskins *et al., J. Am. Chem. Soc.* **64**, 1289 (1942). *Review:* Pazur in *The Carbohydrates* vol. 2A, W. Pigman *et al.,* Eds. (Academic Press, New York, 2nd ed., 1970) pp 109-110; R. G. Edwards, *Dev. Food Carbohydr.* **2**, 229-273 (1980).

Minute crystals from dil alcohol which retain 0.25 to 0.50 mol water after drying in vacuo. Indifferent taste. Dec 225°. Shows mutarotation. $[\alpha]_D^{20}$ +14.2° → +34.6° (15 hrs, c = 8). One gram dissolves in 8 ml water, in 1.5 ml boiling water. Almost insol in abs alc and ether. Reduces Fehling's soln. Hydrolysis with acid or emulsin yields 2 mols β-D-glucose. Not fermented by brewers' yeast, maltase, or invertase.

Octaacetyl-aldehydo-cellobiose. $C_{28}H_{38}O_{19}$; mol wt 678.59. mp 105-110°. $[\alpha]_D^{20}$ +17.7° (c = 3 in chloroform).

Octaacetyl-α-cellobiose. $C_{28}H_{38}O_{19}$; mol wt 678.59. mp 229°. $[\alpha]_D^{20}$ +41° (c = 6 in chloroform).

Octaacetyl-β-cellobiose. mp 202°. $[\alpha]_D^{20}$ −14.7° (c = 5 in chloroform).

1962. Cellocidin. [543-21-5] 2-Butynediamide; acetylenedicarboxamide; acetylenedicarboxylic acid diamide; aquamycin; lenamycin. $C_4H_4N_2O_2$; mol wt 112.09. C 42.86%, H 3.60%, N 24.99%, O 28.55%. $H_2NCOC≡CCONH_2$. Antibiotic substance with antibacterial activity. Produced by *Streptomyces chibaensis* from soil collected at Chiba City, Japan: Suzuki *et al., J. Antibiot.* **11**, 81 (1958). Synthesis from dimethyl acetylenedicarboxylate and concd ammonium hydroxide at −10°: Saggiomo, *J. Org. Chem.* **22**, 1171 (1957); Suzuki, Okuma, *J. Antibiot.* **11**, 84 (1958). Identity with lenamycin: Y. Sekizawa, *Meiji Seika Kenkyu Nempo* **1960**, 42, *C.A.* **56**, 14609a (1962). Biosynthesis: E. R. H. Jones, *J. Chem. Soc. Perkin Trans. 1* **1973**, 148.

Crystals from dil methanol, dec. 216-218°. uv max (0.1N NaOH): 299 nm ($E_{1cm}^{1\%}$ 290). Sparingly sol in water, methanol, ethanol, acetone, chloroform, glacial acetic acid. Relatively stable in neutral or acid solns, showing no loss of activity at pH 2 to 7 when heated for 10 min at 100°. Unstable in alkaline soln evolving ammonia. LD_{50} i.v. in mice: 11 mg/kg (Suzuki).

1963. **Cellophane.** Francephane. Transparent, flexible cellulose sheeting made from viscose. The word "cellophane" is not a trademark in the U.S.

1964. **Celluloid.** [8050-88-2] Pyralin; Zylonite. Prepd from nitrocellulose and camphor.

Colorless, amorphous mass. *Flammable.* Prone to spontaneous decompn which is retarded or prevented by the addition of urea, ZnO, MgCO₃, diphenylamine, etc. It is rendered less flammable by addition of ammonium phosphate. Softens in boiling water; sol in acetone.

USE: Plastic material for manuf of toilet articles, toys, photographic films; substitute for amber, ivory, ebonite, tortoise shell; also in surgery for bandages and in dentistry as substitute for rubber.

1965. **Cellulose.** [9004-34-6] $(C_6H_{10}O_5)_n$. Polysaccharide with the glucose units linked as in cellobiose. Chief constituent of the fiber of plants; cotton is the purest natural form, contg about 90%. Rayon is regenerated cellulose. Books: C. Dorée, *The Methods of Cellulose Chemistry* (Chapman & Hall, London, 1947); T. Lieser, *Kurzes Lehrbuch der Cellulosechemie* (Gebrüder Borntraeger, Berlin, 1953); S. D. Antonovskii, *Chemistry of Wood and Cellulose* (Vsesoyuz. Zaochnyi Lesotekh Instit., Leningrad, 1954); E. Ott *et al.*, *Cellulose and Cellulose Derivatives* vols. **1-3** (Interscience, New York, 1954, 1955). *Reviews:* Several authors in *Encyclopedia of Polymer Science and Technology* vol. **3**, N. M. Bikales, Ed. (Interscience, New York, 1965) pp 131-539; Shafizadeh, *Pure Appl. Chem.* **35**, 195-208 (1973); A. F. Turbak *et al.* in *Kirk-Othmer Encyclopedia of Chemical Technology* vol. **5** (Wiley-Interscience, New York, 3rd ed., 1979) pp 70-89. Comprehensive review on constitution, conformation, size of molecule, structure and superstructure: H. Krässig, *Papier (Darmstadt)* **33**, 9-20 (1979). Review of toxicity studies: R. L. Anderson *et al.*, *Cancer Lett.* **63**, 83-92 (1992).

White substance. Practically insol in water or other usual solvents. Dissolved by concd soln of zinc chloride, by ammoniacal copper hydroxide soln; also by caustic alkali with carbon disulfide.

Microcrystalline Form. Avicel. Prepn and manuf of crystallite cellulosic aggregates: Battista, *Ind. Eng. Chem.* **42**, 502 (1950); Battista, Smith, *US 2978446* (1961 to Am. Viscose); *US 3141875* (1964 to FMC). Non-fibrous powder. Particle shape: rigid rods. Refractive index: 1.55. Bulk density: 18-19 lb/cubic foot. Practically insol, but dispersible in water; practically insol in and resistant to dil acid; practically insol and inert in organic acids. Partially sol with swelling in dil alkali.

Caution: Potential symptoms of overexposure are irritation of eyes, skin, mucous membranes. *See NIOSH Pocket Guide to Chemical Hazards* (DHHS/NIOSH 97-140, 1997) p 56.

USE: Fibrous form is the basic material for the textile and paper industries. Nitrated it yields nitrocellulose used for manuf of explosives, collodion, lacquers. Basic material also for cellulose acetate, cellulose xanthate. Also used in chromatography and as ion exchange material especially in the form of derivatives such as *DEAE-cellulose* (diethylaminoethyl cellulose) and ECTEOLA-cellulose, *q.v.* Microcrystalline forms of cellulose are used as combination binder-disintegrants in tableting, as separatory medium in thin-layer and column chromatography. Colloidal cellulose particles aid in stabilization and emulsification of liquid and foam systems. May be used as pure cellulose raw-material. Incorporation of cellulose crystallite aggregates in foods to reduce caloric content: Battista, *US 3023104* (1962 to American Viscose); also used in food industry as stabilizer, thickener, texturizer.

1966. **Cellulose Acetates.** Partially acetylated cellulose, *q.v.* Several acetates of cellulose are known, which differ from one another only in the degree of acetylation. In triacetates, no less than 92% of the hydroxyl groups are acetylated. In characterizing the degree of acetylation, percent acetyl value and percent combined acetic acid are used. All cellulose acetates are obtained by treating cellulose with acetic anhydride at various temps for different lengths of time to produce amorphous white solid material in granular, flake, or powder form from which fibers may be formed by extrusion. In the plastics industry, it is usual to acetylate fully and then to lower the acetyl value to 52-56% by partial hydrolysis. Such material when compounded with suitable plasticizers gives a tough thermoplastic product. Manuf: *Faith, Keyes & Clark's Industrial Chem-*

icals, F. A. Lowenheim, M. K. Moran, Eds. (Wiley-Interscience, New York, 4th ed., 1975) pp 239-243. Toxicity studies: W. C. Thomas *et al.*, *Food Chem. Toxicol.* **29**, 453 (1991). *Review:* G. A. Serad, J. R. Sanders, "Cellulose Acetate and Triacete Fibers" in *Kirk-Othmer Encyclopedia of Chemical Technology* Vol. **5** (Wiley-Interscience, New York, 3rd ed., 1979) pp 89-117.

R = —OOCCH₃

Cellulose Triacetate

Commercial products do not have sharp melting points. Solubility is affected by the acetyl value; the triacetate is insol in water, alcohol, ether, but sol in glacial acetic acid; the tetraacetate is insol in water, alcohol, ether, glacial acetic acid, methanol; the pentaacetate is insol in water, but sol in alcohol.

USE: Manuf rubber and celluloid substitutes, nonflammable photographic and cinema films, airplane dopes, varnishes and lacquers, filaments, phonograph records; waterproofing fabrics and rendering balloons gas-tight; sizing and finishing fabrics; coating skins; insulating electric wires; tow for cigarette smoke filters.

1967. **Cellulose Ethyl Hydroxyethyl Ether.** [9004-58-4] Ethyl 2-hydroxyethyl ether cellulose; ethyl hydroxyethyl cellulose; Etulos. Prepn: Jullander, *C.A.* **48**, 6114g (1954); idem, **DE 1000367** (1957 to Mo och Domsjö Ab.), *C.A.* **54**, 5088f (1960). Use as laxative: Alm, *C.A.* **50**, 2122i (1956); idem, *Am. J. Dig. Dis.* [NS] **2**, 493 (1957).

R is H, –CH₂CH₃, or –CH₂CH₂OH

THERAP CAT: Cathartic.

1968. **Centaurein.** [35595-03-0] 7-(β-D-Glucopyranosyloxy)-5-hydroxy-2-(3-hydroxy-4-methoxyphenyl)-3,6-dimethoxy-4H-1-benzopyran-4-one; 3′,5,7-trihydroxy-3,4′,6-trimethoxyflavone 7-β-D-glucoside. $C_{24}H_{26}O_{13}$; mol wt 522.46. C 55.17%, H 5.02%, O 39.81%. Isoln from root of *Centaurea jacea* L., *Compositae:* Bridel, Charaux, *Compt. Rend.* **175**, 833, 1168 (1922). Structure: Farkas *et al.*, *Ber.* **97**, 1666 (1964).

Monohydrate. Yellow crystals, mp 208-209°. $[\alpha]_D^{20}$ −76.6° (c = 1.4 in methanol). uv max (methanol): 349, 258 nm (log ε 4.31, 4.30). Sol in hot water, hot alcohol, and hot acetone; practically insol in cold water, chloroform, ether.

1969. **Centaury.** Minor centaury; lesser centaury; bitter herb. Dried flowering plant of *Centaurium erythracea* Rafn. (syn. *C. umbellatum* Gilib., *Erythraea centaurium* Pers.), Gentianaceae.

Habit. Europe, North America, Middle East, North Africa. *Constit.* Gentiopicrin, amarogentin, gentisin: Korte, *Ber.* **87,** 1357 (1954); **88,** 704 (1955). *Review:* A. Y. Leung, *Encyclopedia of Common Natural Ingredients* (John Wiley & Sons, New York, 1980) pp 109-110.

Chilean centaury. Chanchalagua; canchalagua. Dried flowering plant of *C. cachanlahuen* (Mol) Robins (syn *Gentiana peruviana* Lam.). *Habit.* Chile, Peru.

THERAP CAT: Bitter tonic.

1970. Centaury, American. Rose-pink; bitter-bloom; square-stem rose-gentian. Dried flowering plant of *Sabatia angularis* (L.) Pursh, *Gentianaceae.* *Habit.* Florida to Louisiana and Oklahoma, northern to southeastern New York; southern Ontario, Michigan, Wisconsin, Missouri. *Constit.* Gentiopicrin, amarogentin, gentisin: Korte, *Ber.* **87,** 1357 (1954); **88,** 704 (1955). Prepn of sedative extracts: Huneker, *Am. J. Pharm.* **43,** 207 (1871).

THERAP CAT: Bitter tonic.

1971. Centchroman. [31477-60-8] *rel*-1-[2-[4-[(3*R*,4*R*)-3,4-Dihydro-7-methoxy-2,2-dimethyl-3-phenyl-2*H*-1-benzopyran-4-yl]phenoxy]ethyl]pyrrolidine; *(trans)*-1-[2-[*p*-(7-methoxy-2,2-dimethyl-3-phenyl-4-chromanyl)phenoxy]ethyl]pyrrolidine; 3,4-*trans*-2,2-dimethyl-3-phenyl-4-[*p*-(β-pyrrolidinoethoxy)phenyl]-7-methoxychroman; *trans*-centchroman; ormeloxifene; Centron; Saheli. $C_{30}H_{35}NO_3$; mol wt 457.60. C 78.74%, H 7.71%, N 3.06%, O 10.49%. Estrogen antagonist; synthetic nonsteroidal postcoital antifertility agent. Pharmacology: V. P. Kamboj *et al., Indian J. Exp. Biol.* **9,** 103 (1971); *idem et al., ibid.* **15,** 1144 (1977). Prepd (not claimed): J. W. Bolger, *DE* **2329201** (1974 to Riker); *idem, US* **3822287** (1974 to Rexall); S. Ray *et al., J. Med. Chem.* **19,** 276 (1976). Mechanism of action: M. S. Sankaran, M. R. N. Prasad, *Contraception* **9,** 279 (1974). Clinical pharmacology: R. Vaidya *et al., ibid.* **1173.** Physicochemical properties: R. K. Seth *et al., Indian J. Pharm. Sci.* **45,** 14 (1983). Resolution and stereoselective binding of enantiomers: M. Salman *et al., J. Med. Chem.* **29,** 1801 (1986). Absolute configuration: N. Srivastava *et al., Bioorg. Med. Chem. Lett.* **6,** 1747 (1996). HPLC determn in serum and milk: J. Lal *et al., J. Chromatogr. B* **658,** 193 (1994). Clinical pharmacokinetics: *idem et al., Contraception* **52,** 297 (1995). Toxicity: I. M. Chak *et al., Indian J. Exp. Biol.* **15,** 1159 (1977). Review of clinical experience: M. M. Singh, *Med. Res. Rev.* **21,** 302-347 (2001).

Crystals from ether/petr ether, mp 99-101°, sinters ~50°.

Hydrochloride. [51023-56-4] 6720 CDRI. $C_{30}H_{35}NO_3 \cdot HCl$; mol wt 494.06. White crystals, mp 165-166°. uv max (methanol): 232, 278 nm (ε 3701 at 278 nm). pKa 2.1. Sol in 10 parts chloroform, 20 parts acetone, 60 parts 95% ethanol, 20 parts methanol. Practically insol in water, isobutanol, 0.1*N* HCl, 0.1*N* NaOH. LD_{50} i.p. in mice: 400 mg/kg (Chak).

(−)-Form. [78994-23-7] Levormeloxifene. Prepd as hydrochloride, mp 197°. [α]$_D^{20}$ −192.9° (c = 1.0 in CHCl$_3$).

THERAP CAT: Oral contraceptive.

1972. Cephacetrile Sodium. [23239-41-0] (6*R*,7*R*)-3-[(Acetyloxy)methyl]-7-[(cyanoacetyl)amino]-8-oxo-5-thia-1-azabicyclo[4.2.0]oct-2-ene-2-carboxylic acid monosodium salt; sodium 7-(2-cyanoacetamido)-3-(hydroxymethyl)-8-oxo-5-thia-1-azabicyclo[4.2.0]oct-2-ene-2-carboxylate (ester); sodium 7-(2-cyanoacetamido)cephalosporanic acid; Ciba 36278-Ba; Celospor; Ubrocef; Vetimast. $C_{13}H_{12}N_3NaO_6S$; mol wt 361.31. C 43.21%, H 3.35%, N 11.63%, Na 6.36%, O 26.57%, S 8.87%.

Semi-synthetic cephalosporin antibiotic. Prepn: **NL 6600586**; Bickel *et al., US* **3483197** (1966, 1969 both to Ciba). Activity studies: Knüsel *et al., Antimicrob. Agents Chemother.* **1970,** 140; Neu *et al., J. Antibiot.* **25,** 400 (1972). Pharmacokinetics and clinical results: Kradolfer *et al., Schweiz. Med. Wochenschr.* **103,** 711 (1973); Riess *et al., ibid.* 718. Toxicology: Kradolfer *et al., Antimicrob. Agents Chemother.* **1970,** 150. *Review: Arzneim.-Forsch.* **24,** 1446-1533 (1974).

White crystalline powder. LD_{50} in mice (mg/kg): 4500 ± 540 i.v.; 9100 ± 1500 s.c. (Kradolfer).

Free acid. Needles from acetone + ether, mp 168-170° (dec). uv max (0.1*N* NaHCO$_3$): 260 nm (ε 9300).

THERAP CAT: Antibacterial.

THERAP CAT (VET): Antibacterial.

1973. Cephaeline. [483-17-0] 7′,10,11-Trimethoxyemetan-6′-ol; desmethylemetine; dihydropsychotrine. $C_{28}H_{38}N_2O_4$; mol wt 466.61. C 72.07%, H 8.21%, N 6.00%, O 13.72%. Next to emetine the most important alkaloid of ipecac, the ground roots of *Uragoga ipecacuanha* (Brot.) Baill. [*Cephaelis ipecacuanha* (Brot.) A. Rich.], *Rubiaceae:* Carr, Pyman, *J. Chem. Soc.* **105,** 1591 (1914); Hesse, *Ann.* **405,** 1 (1914). Structure: Pailer, Porschinski, *Monatsh. Chem.* **80,** 101 (1914). Stereochemistry: Van Tamelen *et al., J. Am. Chem. Soc.* **79,** 4817 (1957). Partial synthesis: A. K. Garg, J. R. Gear, *Tetrahedron Lett.* **50,** 4377 (1969). Biosynthetic studies: *eidem, ibid.* **1968,** 141. HPLC determn in biological fluids: D. J. Crouch *et al., J. Anal. Toxicol.* **8,** 63 (1984). *Review:* M. Janot in Manske, Holmes, *The Alkaloids* vol. 3 (Academic Press, New York, 1953) pp 363-394.

Needles from ether. Faintly bitter taste. mp 115-116°. [α]$_D^{20}$ −43.4° (c = 2 in chloroform). Practically insol in water. Freely sol in dil hydrochloric acid, dil sulfuric acid, acetic acid, methanol, ethanol, acetone, chloroform. Less sol in ether, petr ether.

Dihydrochloride heptahydrate. $C_{28}H_{40}Cl_2N_2O_4 \cdot 7H_2O$. Prisms, sinters at 245°, slowly melts up to 270°. [α]$_D^{20}$ +25.0° (c = 2). Sol in water. Solns turn yellow. Less sol in alc, acetone, chloroform. Practically insol in benzene, ligroin.

Dihydrobromide heptahydrate. $C_{28}H_{40}Br_2N_2O_4 \cdot 7H_2O$. Prisms from dil hydrobromic acid, sinters at 266°, slowly melts up to 293°. Sol in water; moderately sol in alcohol, acetone. Practically insol in benzene.

Methyl ether *see* Emetine.

THERAP CAT: Emetic; antiamebic.

THERAP CAT (VET): Has been used as an emetic and expectorant.

1974. Cephalexin. [15686-71-2] (6*R*,7*R*)-7-[[(2*R*)-Aminophenylacetyl]amino]-3-methyl-8-oxo-5-thia-1-azabicyclo[4.2.0]-oct-2-ene-2-carboxylic acid; 7-(D-α-aminophenylacetamido)desacetoxycephalosporanic acid; 7-(D-2-amino-2-phenylacetamido)-3-methyl-Δ³-cephem-4-carboxylic acid; Cefadros; Cefaloto; Cefanex; Cefaseptin; Cex; Derantel; Efalexin; Farexin; Fergon 500; Garasin; Ibilex; Iwalexin; Larixin; Lexibiotico; Llonexina; Madlexin; Mamalexin; Mecilex; Ohlexin; Oracocin; Rinesal; Sencephalin; Sintolexyn; Syncl; Taicelexin; Tokiolexin; Xahl. $C_{16}H_{17}N_3O_4S$; mol wt 347.39. C 55.32%, H 4.93%, N 12.10%, O 18.42%, S 9.23%. Semi-synthetic cephalosporin antibiotic. Prepn: R. B. Morin, B. G. Jackson, **US 3275626**; **US 3507861** (1966, 1970 both to Lilly); Ryan *et al., J. Med. Chem.* **12**, 310 (1969). Pharmacology and toxicology: Muggleton *et al., Antimicrob. Agents Chemother.* **1968**, 353; Kind *et al.*, Welles *et al., ibid.* 361, 489. Comprehensive description: L. P. Marrelli, *Anal. Profiles Drug Subs.* **4**, 21-46 (1975). Clinical pharmacology, efficacy, adverse reactions: *Postgrad. Med. J.* **59**, Suppl. 5, 1-56 (1983).

Crystals. uv max: 260 nm (ε 7750). pKa 5.2, 7.3.

Monohydrate. [23325-78-2] Cefa-Iskia; Cefibacter; Ceporex; Ceporexin; Keforal; Keflet; Keflex; Oracef; Ortisporina; Sartosona; Servispor. LD_{50} in mice, rats (g/kg): 1.6-4.5, >5.0 orally; 0.4-1.3, >3.7 i.p. (Welles).

Monohydrochloride monohydrate. [105879-42-3] LY-061188; Keftab. $C_{16}H_{17}N_3O_4S.HCl.H_2O$; mol wt 401.87.

Sodium salt. [38932-40-0] Alfaspoven. $C_{16}H_{16}N_3NaO_4S$; mol wt 369.37.

Pivalate ester *see* Pivcefalexin.

THERAP CAT: Antibacterial.

THERAP CAT (VET): Antibacterial.

1975. Cephalins. Kephalins; phosphatidylethanolamine. Group of phospholipids found in all living organisms. Significant constituent of nervous tissue and brain substance. Cephalins consist of glycerophosphoric acid in which the two free hydroxyls are esterified with long-chain fatty acid residues, and ethanolamine forms an ester linkage with the phosphate group. α-Isomers are derivatives of α-glycerophosphoric acid, *q.v.*; β-isomers are derivatives of β-glycerophosphoric acid, *q.v.* Natural products occur in the α-form, while the β-form is now recognized to be an artifact. Prepn from commercial "soybean lecithin": Scholfield, Dutton, *Biochem. Prep.* **5**, 5 (1957); **US 2801255** (1957 to USDA). Diagnostic use: C. R. Ratliff *et al., Am. J. Gastroenterol.* **55**, 589 (1971). Reviews on natural and synthetic cephalins: E. Baer in *Progress in the Chemistry of Fats and Other Lipids* vol. **6**, (MacMillan, New York, 1963) pp 39-44; Van Deenen, de Haas in *Advances in Lipid Research* vol. **2** (Academic Press, New York, 1964) pp 183-189; Verkade, *Bull. Soc. Chim. Fr.* **1963**, 1993.

α - Cephalin

Yellowish amorphous substances; characteristic odor and taste. Practically insol in water, acetone. Freely sol in chloroform, ether; slightly sol in ethanol.

USE: Clinical reagent (liver function test).

THERAP CAT: Hemostatic (local).

1976. Cephaloglycin. [3577-01-3] (6R,7R)-3-[(Acetyloxy)-methyl]-7-[[(2R)-aminophenylacetyl]amino]-8-oxo-5-thia-1-azabi-cyclo[4.2.0]oct-2-ene-2-carboxylic acid; 7-(2-amino-2-phenylacet-amido)-3-(hydroxymethyl)-8-oxo-5-thia-1-azabicyclo[4.2.0]oct-2-ene-2-carboxylic acid acetate (ester); 7-(D-2-amino-2-phenylacet-amido)-3-acetoxymethyl-Δ^3-cephem-4-carboxylic acid; 7-(D-α-aminophenylacetamido) cephalosporanic acid; Kefglycin. $C_{18}H_{19}$-N_3O_6S; mol wt 405.42. C 53.33%, H 4.72%, N 10.36%, O 23.68%, S 7.91%. Semi-synthetic cephalosporin antibiotic. Prepn: **BE 635137**; F. W. Wall *et al.*, **US 3422103** (1964, 1969 both to Glaxo); **GB 1017624** (1966 to Merck & Co.); Spencer *et al., J. Med. Chem.*

9, 746 (1966); of D- and DL-forms: **GB 985747** (1965 to Lilly); Kurita *et al., J. Antibiot.* **19A**, 243 (1966). Metabolism and pharmacokinetics in man: J. Haginaka *et al., J. Antibiot.* **33**, 236 (1980).

Dihydrate. [22202-75-1] Kafocin. Crystalline powder, mp 223-250° (dec). uv max (2% DMF): 258 nm ($E_{1cm}^{1\%}$ 166). Isoelectric point and pH of maximum stability: 4.5.

THERAP CAT: Antibacterial.

1977. Cephalonic Acid. [18456-04-7] 8-Hydroxy-5-oxo-ophiobola-3,6,19-trien-25-oic acid; ophiobolin D. $C_{25}H_{36}O_4$; mol wt 400.55. C 74.96%, H 9.06%, O 15.98%. Minor antibiotic metabolite produced by *Cephalosporium caerulens*. Exhibits weak activity against *Staphylococcus aureus*. Isolation, structure elucidation and physical data: Itai *et al., Tetrahedron Lett.* **1967**, 4111; Nozoe *et al., ibid.* 4113. Crystal structure: Itai *et al., Acta Crystallogr.* **25B**, 872 (1969). Synthetic studies on related compounds: P. C. Dutta, T. K. Das, *Synth. Commun.* **6**, 253 (1976); W. G. Dauben, D. S. Hart, *J. Org. Chem.* **42**, 922 (1977); R. K. Boeckman *et al., ibid.* 3630.

Solid, mp 139°. $[\alpha]_D$ +76.2° (c = 0.54 in chloroform). uv max: 259 nm (ε 11700).

1978. Cephalonium. [5575-21-3] 4-(Aminocarbonyl)-1-[[(6R,7R)-2-carboxy-8-oxo-7-[(2-thienylacetyl)amino]-5-thia-1-azabicyclo[4.2.0]oct-2-en-3-yl]methyl]pyridinium inner salt; cefalonium; 2-thienylmethyl isonicotinamide cephalosporin C_A; Cepravin Dry Cow. $C_{20}H_{18}N_4O_5S_2$; mol wt 458.51. C 52.39%, H 3.96%, N 12.22%, O 17.45%, S 13.99%. Cephalosporin antibiotic. Prepn: E. H. Flynn, **GB 1067644** (1967 to Lilly); and antibacterial activity: J. L. Spencer *et al., Antimicrob. Agents Chemother.* **1966**, 573. Determn in milk samples: J. E. Hillerton *et al., J. Dairy Sci.* **82**, 704 (1999). Prophylactic use in dry udder infections: R. Curtis *et al., Vet. Rec.* **100**, 557 (1977); in mastitis: J. H. Williamson *et al., N. Z. Vet. J.* **43**, 228 (1995); in combination with a teat sealer: M. W. Woolford *et al., ibid.* **46**, 12 (1998).

Crystals from hot water, mp 147-150° (dec). uv max: 233, 262 nm (ε 16650, 13550). pKa: 3.3.

THERAP CAT (VET): Prophylactic use in mastitis and dry udder therapy.

1979. Cephaloridine. [50-59-9] 1-[[(6R,7R)-2-Carboxy-8-oxo-7-[(2-thienylacetyl)amino]-5-thia-1-azabicyclo[4.2.0]oct-2-en-3-yl]methyl]pyridinium inner salt; 1-[(7'-β-[2-(2-thienyl)acet-amido]-8'-oxo-1'-aza-5'-thiabicyclo[4.2.0]oct-2'-en-3'-yl)methyl]-pyridinium-2'-carboxylate; *N*-[7-[(2-thienyl)acetamido]ceph-3-em-3-ylmethyl]pyridinium-4-carboxylate; *N*-[7-(2'-thienylacetamido-ceph-3-ylmethyl)]pyridinium-2-carboxylate; cefaloridin; Ceflorin; Cepaloridin; Cer; Faredina; Ceporan; Ceporin; Cilifor; Intrasporin;

Keflodin; Keflordin (obsolete); Lloncefal; Sefacin; Cepalorin; Deflorin; Kefspor; Loridine; Ampligram; Floridin. $C_{19}H_{17}N_3O_4S_2$;
mol wt 415.49. C 54.92%, H 4.12%, N 10.11%, O 15.40%, S
15.43%. Semi-synthetic cephalosporin antibiotic. Prepn: **FR
1384197** (1965 to Glaxo), *C.A.* **63**, 11591c (1965); E. H. Flynn,
US 3449338 (1969 to Lilly). Toxicity studies: Atkinson *et al.*,
Toxicol. Appl. Pharmacol. **8**, 398 (1966).

Crystals. Soluble in water. Aq solns are slightly acid (pH 4.5-5);
$[\alpha]_D$ +47.7° (c = 1.25 in water). uv max: 239, 252 nm (ε 15160,
13950). pKa 3.2. Aq solns (20% w/v) are stable for four weeks at
4° in the dark. Exposure to sunlight causes discoloration. LD_{50}
mice, rats (g/kg): >15, 2.5-4 orally; in monkeys (g/kg): >0.2 i.m.
(Atkinson).

THERAP CAT: Antibacterial.

THERAP CAT (VET): Antibacterial.

1980. Cephalosporin C. [61-24-5] (6*R*,7*R*)-3-[(Acetyloxy)methyl]-7-[[(5*R*)-5-amino-5-carboxy-1-oxopentyl]amino]-8-
oxo-5-thia-1-azabicyclo[4.2.0]oct-2-ene-2-carboxylic acid; 7-(D-5-
amino-5-carboxyvaleramido)-3-(hydroxymethyl)-8-oxo-5-thia-1-
azabicyclo[4.2.0]oct-2-ene-2-carboxylic acid acetate. $C_{16}H_{21}N_3$-
O_8S; mol wt 415.42. C 46.26%, H 5.10%, N 10.12%, O 30.81%,
S 7.72%. Antibiotic substance produced along with penicillin N by
a *Cephalosporium* sp. cultivated from sea water near a sewage outlet
on the coast of Sardinia: G. Brotzu, *Lav. Ist. Igiene Cagliari* (1948);
Newton, Abraham, *Nature* **175**, 548 (1955); *eidem, Biochem. J.* **62**,
651 (1956); *eidem*, **DE 1014711** (1957 to Natl. Res. Dev. Corp.); **GB
810196** (1959); Kelly *et al.*, **US 3082155** (1963 to Natl. Res. Dev.
Corp.); Demain, **US 3116216**; **US 3116217** (both 1963 to Merck &
Co.). Biosynthesis: Demain, Newkirk, *Appl. Microbiol.* **10**, 321
(1962). Has the same side chain as penicillin N, but the nucleus is
different and is named 7-aminocephalosporanic acid: Jago, Heatley, *Br. J. Pharmacol.* **16**, 170 (1961). Structure: Abraham, Newton, *Biochem. J.* **79**, 377 (1961); Hodgkin, Maslen, *ibid.* 393. In
cephalosporin C_A the acetoxy group is replaced by a pyridinium
group: Hale *et al.*, *ibid.* 403. Transformation to *cephalosporin C_C*
for which greater activity is claimed: Abraham *et al.*, **US 3049541**
(1962 to Natl. Res. Dev. Corp.). Total synthesis: Woodward *et al.*,
J. Am. Chem. Soc. **88**, 852 (1966). Review of cephalosporin C and
related compounds: Abraham, *Q. Rev. Chem. Soc.* **21**, 231 (1967);
Abraham, Loder, in *Cephalosporins and Penicillins*, E. H. Flynn,
Ed. (Academic Press, New York, 1972) pp 1-26.

Sodium salt, dihydrate. $C_{16}H_{20}N_3NaO_8S.2H_2O$. Monoclinic
crystals from dil alc. $[\alpha]_D^{20}$ +103° (H_2O). uv max: 260 nm ($E_{1cm}^{1\%}$
200). pKa values: <2.6, 3.1, 9.8. Sol in water. Practically insol in
ethanol, ether. Aq solns are stable at pH 2.5 to 8. Low toxicity.
Shows *in vitro* activity against penicillin-resistant staphylococci.

THERAP CAT: Antibacterial.

1981. Cephalosporin P_1. [28393-42-2] (3α,4α,6α,7β,8α,-
9β,13α,14β,16β,17Z)-6,16-Bis(acetyloxy)-3,7-dihydroxy-29-nor-
dammara-17(20),24-dien-21-oic acid. $C_{33}H_{50}O_8$; mol wt 574.75.
C 68.96%, H 8.77%, O 22.27%. Antibiotic substance produced by
a *Cephalosporium* sp. cultivated from the sea near Sardinia. Crude
cephalosporin P contains at least 5 components: P_1, P_2, P_3, P_4, P_5,
the major active substance being cephalosporin P_1. Isoln: Burton,
Abraham, *Biochem. J.* **50**, 168 (1951). Structure: Baird *et al.*,
Proc. Chem. Soc. London **1961**, 257; Halsall *et al.*, *ibid.* **1963**, 16;

Melera, *Experientia* **19**, 565 (1963); Halsall *et al., Chem. Commun.*
1966, 685.

Orthorhombic crystals from 50% aq ethanol, $C_{33}H_{50}O_8.H_2$-
$O.\frac{1}{2}C_2H_5OH$. mp 147°. $[\alpha]_D^{20}$ +28° (c = 2.7 in chloroform).
uv max: 211 nm (ε 9140). Readily sol in chloroform and ethanol;
sparingly sol in hexane and water.

1982. Cephalothin. [153-61-7] (6*R*,7*R*)-3-[(Acetyloxy)-
methyl]-8-oxo-7-[(2-thienylacetyl)amino]-5-thia-1-azabicy-
clo[4.2.0]oct-2-ene-2-carboxylic acid; 3-(hydroxymethyl)-8-oxo-7-
[2-(2-thienyl)acetamido]-5-thia-1-azabicyclo[4.2.0]oct-2-ene-2-
carboxylic acid acetate; 7-(2-thienylacetamido)cephalosporanic
acid; 7-(thiophene-2-acetamido)cephalosporanic acid. $C_{16}H_{16}N_2$-
O_6S_2; mol wt 396.44. C 48.47%, H 4.07%, N 7.07%, O 24.21%, S
16.18%. Semi-synthetic cephalosporin antibiotic. Prepn: Chauvette *et al., J. Am. Chem. Soc.* **84**, 3401 (1962); E. H. Flynn, **US
3218318** (1965 to Lilly); **FR 1384197** (1965 to Glaxo), *C.A.* **63**,
11591c (1965). Bacteriology and pharmacology: Lee, Anderson,
Antimicrob. Agents Chemother. **1962**, 695; Walters *et al., ibid.* 706;
Naumann, *Arzneim.-Forsch.* **16**, 1099 (1966). Acute toxicity: M.
Kuramoto *et al., Jpn. J. Antibiot.* **27**, 746 (1974), *C.A.* **83**, 71972t
(1975). Comprehensive description: R. J. Simmons, *Anal. Profiles
Drug Subs.* **1**, 319-341 (1972).

mp 160-160.5°. $[\alpha]_D^{20}$ +50° (c = 1.03 in acetonitrile), *see* R. B.
Woodward *et al., J. Am. Chem. Soc.* **88**, 852 (1966).

Sodium salt. [58-71-9] Averon-1; Cefalotin; Cemastin; Cephation; Ceporacin; Cepovenin; Chephalotin; Coaxin; Keflin; Lospo-
ven; Synclotin; Toricelocin. $C_{16}H_{15}N_2NaO_6S_2$; mol wt 418.42.
mp 204-205°. $[\alpha]_D$ +135° (c = 1.0 in water). uv max: 236, 260
nm (ε 12950, 9350). LD_{50} in mice, rats (mg/kg): >20000, >10000
orally; 5670, 7716 i.p. (Kuramoto).

THERAP CAT: Antibacterial.

THERAP CAT (VET): Antibacterial.

1983. Cephamycins. A family of β-lactam antibiotics produced by various *Streptomyces* species. Detection and production:
Stapley *et al., Antimicrob. Agents Chemother.* **2**, 122 (1972). Chemical characterization: Miller *et al., ibid.* 132. Cephamycins A, B,
and C have been isolated, the latter being identical to a *Streptomyces
clavuligerus* metabolite: Nagarajan *et al., J. Am. Chem. Soc.* **93**,
2308 (1971). Structures: Albers-Schoenberg *et al., Tetrahedron
Lett.* **1972**, 2911. Antibacterial activity studies: Miller *et al.,
Antimicrob. Agents Chemother.* **2**, 281, 287 (1972); Daoust *et al.,
ibid.* **3**, 254 (1973). Review of syntheses: T. Hiraoka *et al., Heterocycles* **8**, 719 (1977).

Cephamycin C

Consult the Name Index before using this section.

1984. Cephapirin Sodium. [24356-60-3] (6R,7R)-3-[(Acetyloxy)methyl]-8-oxo-7-[[[(4-pyridinylthio)acetyl]amino]-5-thia-1-azabicyclo[4.2.0]oct-2-ene-2-carboxylic acid monosodium salt; 3-(hydroxymethyl)-8-oxo-7-[2-(4-pyridylthio)acetamido]-5-thia-1-azabicyclo[4.2.0]oct-2-ene-2-carboxylic acid acetate monosodium salt; 7-[α-(4-pyridylthio)acetamido]cephalosporanic acid sodium salt; sodium 7-(pyrid-4-ylthioacetamido)cephalosporanate; BL-P-1322; Ambrocef; Brisfirina; Bristocef; Cefadyl; Cefa-Lak; Piricef; ToDay. $C_{17}H_{16}N_3NaO_6S_2$; mol wt 445.45. C 45.84%, H 3.62%, N 9.43%, Na 5.16%, O 21.55%, S 14.40%. A cephalosporin C antibiotic effective against gram-pos. and gram-neg. bacteria including *Staphylococcus aureus, Escherichia coli, Klebsiella pneumoniae* and *Proteus mirabilis.* Prepn: L. B. Crast, **ZA 6707783**; *eidem,* **US 3422100** (1968, 1970 both to Bristol-Myers). Alternate processes: H. H. Silvestri, D. A. Johnson, **US 3503967**; R. E. Havranek, L. B. Crast, **US 3578661** (1970, 1971 both to Bristol-Myers); L. B. Crast *et al., J. Med. Chem.* **16,** 1413 (1973). Activity studies: Chisholm *et al., Antimicrob. Agents Chemother.* **1969,** 244; Axelrod *et al., Appl. Microbiol.* **22,** 904 (1971); Bran *et al., Antimicrob. Agents Chemother.* **1,** 35 (1972); Wiesner *et al., ibid.* 303.

White crystalline powder, sol in water.
THERAP CAT: Antibacterial.
THERAP CAT (VET): Antibacterial.

1985. Cepharanthine. [481-49-2] 6',12'-Dimethoxy-2,2'-dimethyl-6,7-[methylenebis(oxy)]oxyacanthan. $C_{37}H_{38}N_2O_6$; mol wt 606.71. C 73.25%, H 6.31%, N 4.62%, O 15.82%. From tubers of *Stephania cephalantha* Hayata, and *Stephania sasahii* Hayata, *Menispermaceae:* Kondo *et al.,* **US 2206407** (1940); Kondo, Hasegawa, **US 2248241** (1941). Structure: Kondo, Keimatsu, *Ber.* **71,** 2553 (1938); Tomita, Sasaki, *Pharm. Bull.* **2,** 89, 375 (1954). Total synthesis (*dl*-form): Tomita *et al., Tetrahedron Lett.* **1967,** 1201.

Yellow powder, mp 145-155°. Obtained by drying solvated needles from acetone + benzene. $[\alpha]_D^{20}$ +277° (c = 2 in chloroform). Soluble in the usual organic solvents except petr ether.

1986. Cephradine. [38821-53-3] (6R,7R)-7-[[(2R)-Amino-1,4-cyclohexadien-1-ylacetyl]amino]-3-methyl-8-oxo-5-thia-1-azabicyclo[4.2.0]oct-2-ene-2-carboxylic acid; 7-[D-2-amino-2-(1,4-cyclohexadienyl)acetamido]desacetoxycephalosporanic acid; cefradine; SQ-11436; Cefro; Dexef; Eskacef; Velocef; Zeefra. $C_{16}H_{19}N_3O_4S$; mol wt 349.40. C 55.00%, H 5.48%, N 12.03%, O 18.32%, S 9.18%. A semisynthetic cephalosporin antibiotic. Prepn and activity data: Weisenborn *et al.,* **US 3485819** (1969 to Squibb); Dolfini *et al., J. Med. Chem.* **14,** 117 (1971). Clinical trials: Limson *et al., Curr. Ther. Res.* **14,** 101 (1972); Landa, *ibid.* 496. Comprehensive description: K. Florey, *Anal. Profiles Drug Subs.* **5,** 21-59 (1976). *Review:* W. E. Brown, J. R. Knill, in *Pharmacological and Biochemical Properties of Drug Substances* **vol. 2,** M. E. Goldberg, Ed. (Am. Pharm. Assoc., Washington, DC, 1979) pp 279-304.

Monohydrate. [75975-70-1] Small, colorless crystals. mp 140-142° (dec). pK_1 2.63; pK_2 7.27. Sol in propylene glycol; slightly sol in acetone, ethanol. Insol in ether, chloroform, benzene, hexane.

Dihydrate. [31828-50-9] SQ-22022. mp 183-185°.
THERAP CAT: Antibacterial.

1987. Ceresin. [8001-75-0] Purified ozokerite; earth wax; mineral wax; cerosin; cerin. A mixture of hydrocarbons of complex composition purified by treatment with concd H_2SO_4 and filtration through bone-black. Found in Ukraine, Lake Baikal, also in Utah, Texas.

White or yellow, tasteless, waxy cakes. The white is odorless, the yellow has a slight odor. Fracture is very much like that of white wax. d 0.91-0.92. mp 61-78°. It is very stable toward oxidizing agents. Insol in water; sol in 30 parts abs alcohol; sol in benzene, chloroform, petr ether, hot oils.

USE: Substitute for beeswax; for making candles, wax figures; for waxed paper and cloth; in polishes, electrical insulators; waterproofing fabrics; for bottles for hydrofluoric acid; in dentistry for impression and inlay waxes and modeling compounds.

1988. Ceric Fluoride. [10060-10-3] CeF_4; mol wt 216.11. Ce 64.84%, F 35.16%. Prepd from CeF_3 and F_2: Klemm, Henkel, *Z. Anorg. Allg. Chem.* **220,** 181 (1934); von Wartenberg, *ibid.* **244,** 343 (1940); Kwasnik in *Handbook of Preparative Inorganic Chemistry* **vol. 1,** G. Brauer, Ed. (Academic Press, New York, 2nd ed., 1963) pp 247-248; from CeO_2 and F_2: Asker, Wylie, *Aust. J. Chem.* **18,** 959 (1965).

Minute crystals, d 4.77. mp >650°. Practically insol in water; very slowly hydrolyzed by cold water. Thermally stable below 550°. May be reduced to CeF_3 by H_2 at 300°.
Monohydrate. White powder. Sol in acids.
USE: Fluorinating agent.

1989. Ceric Oxide. [1306-38-3] Ceria. CeO_2; mol wt 172.11. Ce 81.41%, O 18.59%. Prepn from Ce salts: Duval, *Anal. Chim. Acta* **1,** 341 (1947); other prepns: Warf, **US 2564241** (1951 to USAEC); Wilke, *Z. Anorg. Allg. Chem.* **330,** 164 (1964). Purification: Wetzel in *Handbook of Preparative Inorganic Chemistry* **vol. 2,** G. Brauer, Ed. (Academic Press, New York, 2nd ed., 1965) pp 1132-1135. *Review:* Davis, Wayman, *Can. Chem. Process Ind.* **29,** 230 (1945). Toxicity data: C. E. Lambert *et al., J. Am. Coll. Toxicol.* **12,** 617 (1993).

Heavy powder or cubic crystals; white if pure, but usually pale yellow; traces of lanthanum, praseodymium, etc., give a pink to reddish-brown color. Practically insol in water, acids. LD_{50} orally in rats: >5.0 g/kg (Lambert).

USE: Polishing and decolorizing glass; as opacifier for vitreous enamels; in heat-resistant alloy coatings; in coatings for infrared filters to prevent reflection; in analysis for Ce and oxidimetry; as catalyst for organic reactions.

1990. Ceric Sulfate. [13590-82-4] CeO_8S_2; mol wt 332.24. Ce 42.17%, O 38.52%, S 19.30%. $Ce(SO_4)_2$. Prepd by heating CeO_2 with concd H_2SO_4: Vanino, *Handbuch der Präparativen Chemie* **vol. 1** (Stuttgart, 3rd ed., 1925) p 755. *Review:* Smith, *Ceric Sulfate* (G. Frederick Smith Chem. Co., Columbus, Ohio, 2nd ed., 1935) 51 pp. The commercial salt usually contains small amounts of associated rare earths.

Tetrahydrate. Yellow to orange powder or orthorhombic crystals. On heating loses water, becoming anhyd at 180-200°; dec above 350°, forming $CeOSO_4$. Sol in a small quantity of water, but dec with much water with separation of a basic salt. Slowly sol in cold, more readily sol in hot mineral acids; sol in dil H_2SO_4.

USE: Oxidizing agent; analytical reagent; in radiation dosimeters.

1991. Cerium. [7440-45-1] Ce; at. wt 140.116; at. no. 58; valences 3, 4. A rare earth metal, most abundant member of the lanthanide series. Naturally occurring isotopes (mass numbers): 140 (88.48%); 142 (11.08%), radioactive, $T_{1/2} >5 \times 10^{16}$ years; 138 (0.25%); 136 (0.19%). Known artificial radioactive isotopes: 124-135; 137; 139; 141; 143-152. Estimated abundance in the earth's crust: 46-66 ppm. Commercially important sources are the rare earth minerals monazite and bastnaesite; also found in cerite. Discovered by Klaproth, Hisinger and Berzelius in 1803. Can be separated from other rare earths by selective precipitation of ceric (4+) salts from buffered solns (pH 3-4); also by ion exchange techniques. Prepn of metal: Spedding *et al., Ind. Eng. Chem.* **44**, 553 (1952). Review of prepn, properties and compds: *The Rare Earths,* F. H. Spedding, A. H. Daane, Eds. (Krieger, Huntington, N.Y., 1971, reprint of 1961 ed.) 641 pp; Hulet, Bode, "Separation Chemistry of the Lanthanides and Transplutonium Actinides" in *MTP Int. Rev. Sci.: Inorg. Chem., Ser. One* vol. 7, K. W. Bagnall, Ed. (University Park Press, Baltimore, 1972) pp 1-45; Moeller, "The Lanthanides" in *Comprehensive Inorganic Chemistry* vol. 4, J. C. Bailar, Jr. *et al.,* Eds. (Pergamon Press, Oxford, 1973) pp 1-101; B. T. Kilbourn in *Kirk-Othmer Encyclopedia of Chemical Technology* vol. 5 (John Wiley & Sons, New York, 4th ed., 1993) pp 728-749; *Chemistry of the Elements,* N. N. Greenwood, A. Earnshaw, Eds. (Pergamon Press, New York, 1984) pp 1423-1449. Brief review of properties: G. T. Seaborg, *Radiochim. Acta* **61**, 115-122 (1993).

Iron-gray, ductile, malleable metal. Only material known to have a solid-solid critical point. Crystalline forms: face-centered cubic α-form, d 6.770, transforms to β-form at −150°; hexagonal β-form transforms to γ-form at −10°; face-centered cubic γ-form transforms to δ-form at 730°; body-centered cubic δ-form exists at >730°. mp 798°. bp 3433°. Heat of fusion: 5.179 kJ/mol. Heat of sublimation (25°): 422.6 kJ/mol. $E^0(aq)$ Ce^{3+}/Ce −2.48 V (calc). Stable in dry air, but superficially oxidized in moist air; when finely divided may ignite spontaneously. Slowly dec by cold, rapidly by hot water; sol in dil mineral acids. Ceric salts usually are yellow to orange-red in color and liberate iodine from KI. Cerous salts are usually white and give a white ppt with alkali hydroxides or sulfides, insol in excess of reagent; they also are pptd by ammonium oxalate from cold dil acid sols.

USE: In metallurgy as stabilizers in alloys and as an alternative to thorium oxide in welding electrodes. In glass as polishing agent, decolorizer to stabilize impurities, to render glass opaque to near uv radiation, to resist discoloration from strong light or high energy electron bombardment (as in television screens). In ceramics as an opacifying and strengthening agent. Catalysts to impart high cracking activity for crude oil processing, in automotive exhaust control devices, as combustion additive, polymerization initiator, paint drier, polymer stabilizer. As phosphor in fluorescent lamps, cathode ray tubes and thorium dioxide gas mantles.

1992. Cerium(IV) Ammonium Nitrate. [16774-21-3]; [10139-51-2] nitric acid ammonium cerium salt. (*OC*-6-11)-Hexakis(nitrato-κO)-diammonium cerate(2−); ammonium ceric nitrate; ammonium hexanitratocerate; ammonium nitratocerate. $CeH_8N_8O_{18}$; mol wt 548.22. Ce 25.56%, H 1.47%, N 20.44%, O 52.53%. $(NH_4)_2Ce(NO_3)_6$. Versatile one-electron oxidizing agent. Prepn: G. F. Smith *et al., Ind. Eng. Chem. Anal. Ed.* **8**, 449 (1936). Use as a primary standard in oxidimerty: G. F. Smith, W. H. Fly, *Anal. Chem.* **21**, 1233 (1949). Improved prepn: G. F. Smith, *Talanta* **10**, 709 (1963). Review of synthetic applications: J. R. Hwu, K.-Y. King, *Curr. Sci.* **81**, 1043-1053 (2001); V. Nair *et al., Acc. Chem. Res.* **37**, 21-30 (2004).

Orange, non-hygroscopic solid. Soly in water (g/ml): 1.41 at 25°; 2.27 at 80°. Sol in sulfuric, nitric, perchloric, and hydrochloric acids. Extremely limited soly in organic solvents.

USE: As a standard in oxidimetry. Oxidant in redox reactions. In reactions involving carbon-carbon bond formation, oxidative carbon-carbon bond cleavage, nitration, and removal of protecting groups. Soln in dilute perchloric acid as etchant for prepn of printed circuits, metal samples, and surface cleaning prior to fabrication by soldering.

1993. Cerivastatin. [145599-86-6] (3*R*,5*S*,6*E*)-7-[4-(4-Fluorophenyl)-5-(methoxymethyl)-2,6-bis(1-methylethyl)-3-pyridinyl]-3,5-dihydroxy-6-heptenoic acid; (3*R*,5*S*,6*E*)-7-[4-(*p*-fluorophenyl)-2,6-diisopropyl-5-(methoxymethyl)-3-pyridyl]-3,5-dihydroxy-6-heptenoic acid. $C_{26}H_{34}FNO_5$; mol wt 459.55. C 67.95%, H 7.46%, F 4.13%, N 3.05%, O 17.41%. HMG-CoA reductase inhibitor. Prepd and claimed as methyl ester: R. Angerbauer *et al.,*

EP 325130; *eidem,* **US 5006530**; as (+)-form sodium salt: *eidem,* **US 5177080** (1989, 1991, 1993 all to Bayer). Determn in plasma by fluorescence linked LC: G. J. Krol *et al., J. Pharm. Biomed. Anal.* **11**, 1269 (1993); by HPLC: *eidem, Methodol. Surv. Bioanal. Drugs* **23**, 147 (1994). Effects on LDL receptor levels: G. C. Ness *et al., Arch. Biochem. Biophys.* **325**, 242 (1996). Pharmacokinetics in dogs and rats: W. Steinke *et al., Jpn. Pharmacol. Ther.* **24** Suppl. 9, S1217 (1996). Clinical trial in hyperlipidemia: N. Nakaya *et al., ibid.* S1381.

Sodium salt. [143201-11-0] Rivastatin; Bay w 6628; Baycol; Lipobay. $C_{26}H_{33}FNNaO_5$; mol wt 481.53. Solid, $[\alpha]_D^{20}$ +24.1° (c = 1 in ethanol).

THERAP CAT: Antilipemic.

1994. Ceronapril. [111223-26-8] 1-[(2*S*)-6-Amino-2-[[hydroxy(4-phenylbutyl)phosphinyl]oxy]-1-oxohexyl]-L-proline; 1-[(2*S*)-6-amino-2-hydroxyhexanoyl]-L-proline, hydrogen (4-phenylbutyl)phosphonate (ester); ceranapril; SQ-29852. $C_{21}H_{33}N_2O_6P$; mol wt 440.47. C 57.26%, H 7.55%, N 6.36%, O 21.79%, P 7.03%. Hydroxylphosphonate angiotensin converting enzyme (ACE) inhibitor. Prepn: D. S. Karanewsky, E. W. Petrillo, Jr., **EP 97534**; *eidem,* **US 4452790** (both 1984 to Squibb); *eidem et al., J. Med. Chem.* **31**, 204 (1988). HPLC determn in body fluids: H. Kadin *et al., J. Chromatogr.* **487**, 135 (1989). Pharmacology: J. M. DeForrest *et al., J. Cardiovasc. Pharmacol.* **16**, 121 (1990). Radioimmunoassay and pharmacokinetics: J. Tu *et al., Ther. Drug Monit.* **14**, 209 (1992). Clinical evaluation in hypertension: J. Sasaki *et al., Int. J. Clin. Pharmacol. Ther. Toxicol.* **31**, 83 (1993).

Prepd as the monohydrate. Crystals from water, mp 190-195° (dec). $[\alpha]_D$ −47.5° (c = 1 in methanol).

THERAP CAT: Antihypertensive.

1995. Cerous Bromide. [14457-87-5] Br_3Ce; mol wt 379.83. Br 63.11%, Ce 36.89%. $CeBr_3$. Prepn: Jantsch, Wein, *Monatsh. Chem.* **69**, 161 (1936).

Heptahydrate. Colorless, deliquesc needles. mp 732°. Sol in water, alcohol. *Keep well closed.*

1996. Cerous Carbonate. [537-01-9] $C_3Ce_2O_9$; mol wt 460.26. C 7.83%, Ce 60.89%, O 31.29%. $Ce_2(CO_3)_3$. Prepn: Head, Holley, Jr., *USAEC* LADC-5579, 8 pp (1962).

Pentahydrate. Powder, or microcryst prisms. Almost insol in water; sol in dil mineral acids and in soln of ammonium salts.

1997. Cerous Chloride. [7790-86-5] $CeCl_3$; mol wt 246.48. Ce 56.85%, Cl 43.15%. Prepn: Kleinheksel, Kremers, *J. Am. Chem. Soc.* **50**, 959 (1928); Didtschenko, **US 2932553** (1960 to Union Carbide); Harmon, Wickers, **US 2982603** (1961 to USAEC); Taylor, Carter, *J. Inorg. Nucl. Chem.* **24**, 387 (1962). Toxicity study: Graca *et al., Arch. Environ. Health* **5**, 437 (1962).

Very fine powder, mp 822°. d^{25} 3.97. Sol in water, alcohol (exothermic). LD_{50} in mice, guinea pigs (mg/kg): 352, 110 i.p. (Graca).

Heptahydrate. Colorless to yellow deliquesc orthorhombic crystals. Begins to lose water above 90°, becomes anhydr by 230°. Very sol in H_2O, alcohol. *Keep well closed.*

USE: In manuf of Ce and Ce salts; with Al or Mg salts as catalyst in the polymerization of olefins.

1998. Cerous Fluoride. [7758-88-5] CeF_3; mol wt 197.11. Ce 71.09%, F 28.92%. Prepd by the action of HF on CeO_2: von Wartenberg, *Z. Anorg. Allg. Chem.* **244**, 343 (1940); by the action of F_2 or concd HF on $CeSi_2$: Sterba, *Ann. Chim. Phys.* [8] **2**, 193 (1904); from CCl_2F_2 and CeO_2: Pausewang, Rüdorff, *Z. Anorg. Allg. Chem.* **369**, 89 (1969).

Hexagonal crystals or powder. d 6.157. mp 1460°. Practically insol in, but slowly hydrolyzed by water.

1999. Cerous Iodide. [7790-87-6] CeI_3; mol wt 520.83. Ce 26.90%, I 73.10%. Prepn from Ce and HgI_2: Asprey *et al., Inorg. Chem.* **3**, 1137 (1964); from the oxide and HI in the presence of NH_4I: Taylor, Curtis, *J. Inorg. Nucl. Chem.* **24**, 387 (1962).

Bright yellow, orthorhombic crystals. mp 752°. Dec in moist air. Sol in water.

Nonahydrate. White to reddish-white crystals. Very sol in water, the soln readily decomposing with separation of iodine; sol in alc. *Keep well closed and protected from light.*

2000. Cerous Nitrate. [10108-73-3] CeN_3O_9; mol wt 326.13. Ce 42.96%, N 12.88%, O 44.15%. $Ce(NO_3)_3$. Prepn from Ce sulfate and $Ca(NO_3)_2$: Blumenfeld, *US 2166702* (1939 to Soc. de Produits Chimiques des Terres Rares); in separation of cerium from other rare earths: Pierce, Butler, *Inorg. Synth.* **2**, 51 (1946); Scargill *et al., J. Inorg. Nucl. Chem.* **4**, 304 (1957). For physical and chemical properties *see USAEC* **IDO-14504**, 126 pp (1961). Toxicity study: Bruce *et al., Toxicol. Appl. Pharmacol.* **5**, 750 (1963).

Hexahydrate. LD_{50} in rats: 290 mg/kg i.p.; 4.2 g/kg orally (Bruce).

USE: Separation of Ce from other rare earths; catalyst in hydrolysis of phosphoric acid esters; mixture with $Th(NO_3)_4$ (1:99) formerly used in manuf incandescent mantles.

2001. Cerous Oxalate. [139-42-0] Sedemesis. $C_6Ce_2O_{12}$; mol wt 544.29. C 13.24%, Ce 51.49%, O 35.27%. $Ce_2(C_2O_4)_3$. Prepn from $Ce(NO_3)_3.6H_2O$ and oxalic acid: Wylie, *J. Chem. Soc.* **1947**, 1687. The article of commerce contains variable amounts of the oxalates of cerium, lanthanum, and other associated elements.

Nonahydrate. White or slightly pink, tasteless powder. Practically insol in water; sol in hot, moderately dil H_2SO_4 or HCl.

THERAP CAT: Antiemetic.

2002. Cerous Sulfate. [13454-94-9] $Ce_2O_{12}S_3$; mol wt 568.42. Ce 49.30%, O 33.78%, S 16.92%. $Ce_2(SO_4)_3$. Prepn: Blandin, Rerat, *Compt. Rend.* **239**, 1055 (1954); Wendlandt, *J. Inorg. Nucl. Chem.* **7**, 51 (1958).

Octahydrate. Orthorhombic octahedral crystals. d 2.87. Loses water on heating, becoming anhyd by 250°; loses SO_3 to form a basic salt above 650°. Soluble in water.

USE: Developing aniline black; said to be superior to vanadium for this purpose.

2003. Certolizumab Pegol. [428863-50-7]; [339184-10-0] Fab fragment. Pegylated anti-(human tumor necrosis factor α) Fab' fragment (human-mouse monoclonal CDP870 heavy chain) immunoglobulin disulfide with human-mouse monoclonal CDP870 light chain; CDP-870; Cimzia. Recombinant humanized monoclonal antibody Fab fragment linked to polyethylene glycol, *q.v.;* directed against tumor necrosis factor α (TNF-α). Prepn: D. S. Athwal *et al., WO 0194585; eidem, US 02151682* (2001, 2002 both to Celltech). Clinical evaluation in rheumatoid arthritis: E. H. S. Choy *et al., Rheumatology* **41**, 1133 (2002); in Crohn's disease: S. Schreiber *et al., Gastroenterology* **129**, 807 (2005). Review of development and therapeutic potential: S. Rose-John, H. Schooltink, *Curr. Opin. Invest. Drugs* **4**, 588-592 (2003); of clinical evaluation in rheumatoid arthritis: V. V. Kaushik, R. J. Moots, *Expert Opin. Biol. Ther.* **5**, 601-606 (2005).

THERAP CAT: Anti-inflammatory.

2004. Cerulenin. [17397-89-6] (2*R*,3*S*)-3-[(4*E*,7*E*)-1-Oxo-4,7-nonadienyl]oxiranecarboxamide; 2,3-epoxy-4-oxo-7,10-dodecadienamide; 2,3-epoxy-4-oxo-7,10-dodecadienoylamide; helicocerin. $C_{12}H_{17}NO_3$; mol wt 223.27. C 64.55%, H 7.67%, N 6.27%, O 21.50%. Antifungal antibiotic isolated from *Cephalo-*

sporium caerulens; Acryocylindrium oryzae; Helicoceras oryzae: T. Hata *et al., Jpn. J. Bacteriol.* **15**, 1075 (1960); Matsumae *et al., J. Antibiot.* **16A**, 236, 239 (1963); Sano *et al., ibid.* **20A**, 344 (1967); Furuya, Shirasaka, **JP 70 21638** (1970 to Sankyo), *C.A.* **73**, 108271k (1970). Biological characteristics: Matsumae *et al., J. Antibiot.* **17A**, 1 (1964). Structure: Omura *et al., ibid.* **20A**, 349 (1967). Abs config: *eidem, Chem. Pharm. Bull.* **17**, 2361 (1969); Arison, Omura, *J. Antibiot.* **27**, 28 (1974). Stereoselective synthesis of (+)- and (−)-*tetrahydrocerulenin* and corrected abs config of (+)-cerulenin: H. Ohrui, S. Emoto, *Tetrahedron Lett.* **1978**, 2095; J.-R. Pougny, P. Sinay, *ibid.* 3301. Stereoselective synthesis of the (+)-form from D-glucose: N. Sueda *et al., ibid.* **1979**, 2039; M. Pietraszkiewicz, P. Sinay, *ibid.* 4741. Interrupts yeast-type fungi growth by inhibiting the biosynthesis of sterols and fatty acids. Mechanism of action studies: Nomura *et al., J. Biochem.* **71**, 783 (1972); *eidem, J. Antibiot.* **25**, 365 (1972); *see also* D. Vance, *Biochem. Biophys. Res. Commun.* **48**, 649 (1972). Total synthesis of (±)-cerulenin: R. K. Boeckman, Jr., E.W. Thomas, *J. Am. Chem. Soc.* **99**, 2805 (1977); A. A. Jakubowski *et al., Tetrahedron Lett.* **1977**, 2399; E. J. Corey, D. R. Williams, *ibid.* 3847; K. Mikami *et al., Chem. Lett.* **1981**, 1721; A. A. Jakubowski *et al., J. Org. Chem.* **47**, 1221 (1982).

White needles from benzene, mp 93-94°. bp 120° (10^{-8} mm). $[\alpha]_D^{16}$ +63° (c = 2 in methanol). Stable in neutral and acidic solns. Sol in ethanol, acetone, benzene and most common solvents. Slightly sol in water. Practically insol in petr ether. LD_{50} in mice (mg/kg): 154 i.v.; 211 i.p.; 547 orally (Matsumae 1964).

DL-Form. mp 40-43°.

USE: Biochemical tool.

2005. Ceruletide. [17650-98-5] Caerulein; cerulein; FI-6934. $C_{58}H_{73}N_{13}O_{21}S_2$; mol wt 1352.40. C 51.51%, H 5.44%, N 13.46%, O 24.84%, S 4.74%. Cholecystokinin analog; decapeptide discovered in the skins of Australian amphibians: V. Erspamer *et al., Nature* **212**, 204 (1966). Isoln from *Hyla caerulea* and structure: A. Anastasi *et al., Experientia* **23**, 699 (1967); *eidem, Arch. Biochem. Biophys.* **125**, 57 (1968). Synthesis: L. Bernardi *et al., Experientia* **23**, 700 (1967); *eidem, ZA 6704716; eidem, US 3472832* (1968, 1969 to Soc. Farm. Italia). Shows hypotensive activity, stimulates smooth muscle and increases gastric, pancreatic, and biliary secretions: V. Erspamer *et al., Experientia* **23**, 702 (1967). Series of articles on metabolism: *Eur. J. Biochem.* **91**, 21-48 (1978). Pharmacodynamics: N. Iwatsuki, O. H. Petersen, *J. Cell Biol.* **79**, 533 (1978); T. Fujita *et al., Adv. Exp. Med. Biol.* **106**, 147 (1978). Diagnostic use: R. Fujita *et al., Acta Gastroenterol. Belg.* **40**, 167 (1977); C. Monti *et al., Radiology* **129**, 611 (1978). Toxicology: T. Chieli *et al., Toxicol. Appl. Pharmacol.* **23**, 480 (1972). Reviews of pharmacology and clinical applications: G. Bertaccini, *Pharmacol. Rev.* **28**, 127 (1976); and toxicology: M. E. Vincent *et al., Pharmacotherapy* **2**, 223 (1982).

5-oxoPro–Gln–Asp–Tyr–Thr–Gly–Trp–Met–Asp–PheNH$_2$
|
SO$_3$H

mp 224-226° (dec). $[\alpha]_D^{20}$ −26° (c = 1 in DMF).

Diethylamine salt. [71247-25-1] Ceosunin; Takus; Tymtran. Off-white hygroscopic powder. Sol in DMF and DMSO. Insol in acetone, diethyl ether. LD_{50} i.v. in mice: 1012 mg/kg (Chieli).

THERAP CAT: Stimulant (gastric secretory). Diagnostic aid (pancreatic function; cholecystokinetic agent in cholecystography).

2006. Ceruloplasmin. [9031-37-2] Caeruloplasmin; ferroxidase. Intensely blue colored copper-containing glycoprotein of the α_2-globulin fraction of mammalian blood; it is the principal copper transport protein and is believed to play an important role in iron mobilization via its ferroxidase activity. First reported by C. G. Holmberg, *Acta Physiol. Scand.* **8**, 227 (1944). Isoln, purification and description of properties of porcine and human ceruloplasmin: C. G. Holmberg, C. B. Laurell, *Acta Chem. Scand.* **2**, 550 (1948). Ceruloplasmin accounts for 90-95% of the circulating copper in normal mammals. Its concentration increases by a factor of 2 to 3 during pregnancy and varies significantly in several diseases and hormonal conditions. Prepd by Cohn cold ethanol fractionation: Cohn *et al., J. Am. Chem. Soc.* **68**, 459 (1946); Steinbuch, Quentin, *Nature* **183**, 323 (1959); and further purified from fraction IV: Sanders *et al., Arch. Biochem. Biophys.* **84**, 60 (1959); US **3003918** (1961 to Merck & Co.). Different mol wts have been reported for human ceruloplasmin, ranging from 126,000 to 160,000; the most generally accepted is 134,000 ±3000, *cf.* L. Ryder, I. Björk, *Biochemistry* **15**, 3411 (1976). Chemical and structural studies of porcine ceruloplasmin: Osaki *et al., J. Biochem. (Tokyo)* **48**, 190 (1960); **50**, 24, 29 (1961); Mukasa *et al., Biochim. Biophys. Acta* **168**, 132 (1968); Matsunaga, Nosoh, *ibid.* **215**, 280 (1970); of human: Kasper, Deutsch, *J. Biol. Chem.* **238**, 2325 (1963); Jamieson, *ibid.* **240**, 2019 (1965); Poillon, Bearn, *Biochim. Biophys. Acta* **127**, 407 (1966); Simons, Bearn, *ibid.* **175**, 260 (1969); Ryden, *Eur. J. Biochem.* **26**, 380 (1972); T. G. Samsonidze *et al., Int. J. Pept. Protein Res.* **14**, 161 (1979); V. N. Zaitsev *et al., Kristallografiya* **25**, 174 (1980), *C.A.* **92**, 210415q (1980). Human metabolism: Kekki *et al., Nature* **209**, 1252 (1966). Reviews of biological role: E. Frieden, H. S. Hsieh, *Adv. Exp. Med. Biol.* **74**, 505-529 (1976); J. M. C. Gutteridge, *Ann. Clin. Biochem.* **15**, 293-296 (1978). Comprehensive review: S. H. Laurie, E. S. Mohammed, *Coord. Chem. Rev.* **33**, 279-312 (1980).

Absorption max: 280, 610 nm ($E_{1cm}^{1\%}$ 14.9, 0.68). Electrophoretic mobility (cm/volt/sec): -5.05×10^{-5} at pH 7.0 ($0.1M$ phosphate buffer); -5.32×10^{-5} at pH 8.6 ($0.1M$ barbital sodium buffer).

2007. Cervicarcin. [18700-78-2] 1,2,3,4-Tetrahydro-1,3,4,-5,10-pentahydroxy-2-methyl-3-[(3-methyloxiranyl)carbonyl]-4a,9a-epoxyanthracen-9(10*H*)-one; 4a,9a-epoxy-3-(2,3-epoxybutyryl)-1,2,3,4,4a,9a-hexahydro-1,3,4,5,10-pentahydroxy-2-methylanthrone. $C_{19}H_{20}O_9$; mol wt 392.36. C 58.16%, H 5.14%, O 36.70%. Antineoplastic antibiotic produced by *Streptomyces ogaensis*: Okuma *et al., J. Antibiot.* **15A**, 152, 247 (1962). Prepn: Sumiki *et al.*, **JP 64 7400** (1964 to Inst. Phys. & Chem. Res.). Structure: Marumo *et al., J. Am. Chem. Soc.* **86**, 4507 (1964); *eidem, Agric. Biol. Chem.* **32**, 209 (1968). Stereochemistry: *eidem, ibid.* **35**, 1931 (1971). Activity studies: C. Itakura *et al., J. Antibiot.* **16A**, 231 (1963).

Needles, mp 203-205° (dec). $[\alpha]_D^{20}$ −144° (in ethanol). uv max: 227, 264, 323 nm (ε 14200, 7800, 2600). pKa 9.0. Sol in acetone, lower alcohols, acetic acid, pyridine. Moderately sol in ethyl acetate, ethyl ether, chloroform, carbon tetrachloride. Slightly sol in water, benzene. Insol in petr ether, ligroin. Stable in neutral or acidic soln; unstable in alkaline soln. LD₅₀ i.p. in mice: 48.5 mg/kg (Itakura).

2008. Cesium. [7440-46-2] Caesium. Cs; at. wt 132.9054519; at. no. 55; valence 1. Group IA (1). Alkali metal. Occurrence in earth's crust: 2.6 ppm. Naturally occurring isotope: ^{133}Cs (100%); artificial isotopes (mass nos.): 112-132, 134-148. Occurs in nature in the aluminosilicates, *pollucite* and *lepidolite* and in the borate, *rhodizite*. Acid digestion of pollucite ore is primary commercial source. Discovered by Bunsen and Kirchhoff in 1860. Prepn from pollucite: *Inorg. Synth.* **4**, 5 (1953). ^{137}Cs (T½ 30.07 years; β^- 0.514, 1.176 MeV) is a product of atomic fission of uranium and an important constituent of radioactive fallout; decays to and reaches radioactive equilibrium with ^{137m}Ba (T½ 2.552 min; γ 0.662 MeV). Review of cesium and its compounds: Whaley, "Sodium, Potassium, Rubidium, Cesium, and Francium" in *Comprehensive Inorganic Chemistry* vol. 1, J. C. Bailar, Jr. *et al.*, Eds. (Pergamon Press, Oxford, 1973) pp 369-529; *Chemistry of the Elements*, N. N. Greenwood, A. Earnshaw, Eds. (Pergamon Press, New York, 1984) pp 75-116; R. O. Burt in *Kirk-Othmer Encyclopedia of Chemical Technology* vol. 5 (Wiley-Interscience, New York, 4th ed., 1993) pp 749-764. Review of toxicology and human

exposure: *Toxicological Profile for Cesium* (PB2004-104397, 2004) 310 pp.

Silver-white, ductile metal; body-centered cubic structure. mp 28.5°. bp 705°. d²⁰ 1.90. Specific heat (25°) 0.057 cal/g/°C. E°/v (aq) Cs/Cs⁺ −2.92. Electrical resistivity 36.6 micro-ohm cm at 30°. Mohs' hardness 0.2. Oxidizes rapidly in air; in moist air may ignite spontaneously to produce nonluminous reddish-violet flame. Emits characteristic blue color (455.5 nm) in flame. Reacts with water to form hydroxide with evolution of hydrogen which ignites spontaneously. Sol in liquid ammonia. *Keep immersed in mineral oil.*

USE: In photoelectric cells, as a "getter" in vacuum tubes; in photoemitter devices, scintillation counters. Adsorbent in CO_2 purifn; scavenger of gases and impurities in metallurgy. For doping catalysts. For construction and operation of one type of atomic clock based on the vibrational frequency (9,192.76 megacycles/sec) of ^{133}Cs. ^{137}Cs in process control instruments, sewage and sludge sterilization.

2009. Cesium Bromide. [7787-69-1] BrCs; mol wt 212.81. Br 37.55%, Cs 62.45%. CsBr. Prepn from pollucite: Thomas, Steton, *Compt. Rend.* **241**, 56 (1955). Toxicity study: Cochran *et al., Arch. Ind. Hyg.* **1**, 637 (1950).

Crystals. d 4.44. mp 636°. bp ~1300°. Very sol in water; sol in alc. Practically insol in acetone. LD₅₀ i.p. in rats: 1.4 g/kg (Cochran).

USE: In x-ray fluorescent screens, spectrometer prisms, absorption-cell windows.

2010. Cesium Carbonate. [534-17-8] CCs_2O_3; mol wt 325.82. C 3.69%, Cs 81.58%, O 14.73%. Cs_2CO_3. Prepn: Suhrmann, Clusius, *Z. Anorg. Allg. Chem.* **152**, 52 (1926); Thomas, *Ann. Chim.* **6**, 367 (1957); Bernard, *Compt. Rend.* **243**, 1528 (1956).

Very deliquesc crystals; melts at red heat. Extremely sol in water, alcohol; sol in ether.

USE: Catalyst in ethylene oxide polymerization; in coating for spatter-free welding of steel in CO_2; in oxide cathode.

2011. Cesium Chloride. [7647-17-8] ClCs; mol wt 168.36. Cl 21.06%, Cs 78.94%. CsCl. Prepn from carnallite and from pollucite: Donges in *Handbook of Preparative Inorganic Chemistry* vol. 1, G. Brauer, Ed. (Academic Press, New York, 2nd ed., 1963) pp 951, 955. Toxicity study: Cochran *et al., Arch. Ind. Hyg.* **1**, 637 (1950).

Deliquesc cubic crystals. d 3.99. mp 646°. bp 1303°. Very sol in water; sol in alc. *Keep well closed.* LD₅₀ i.p. in rats: 1.5 g/kg (Cochran).

^{131}CsCl. Cescan-131.

USE: In the final evacuation of radio and television vacuum tubes; in x-ray fluorescent screens; as radiographic contrast medium; in manuf of cesium.

2012. Cesium Fluoride. [13400-13-0] CsF; mol wt 151.90. Cs 87.50%, F 12.51%. Basic catalyst in fluoride chemistry and oxidation reactions. Prepn from pulverized pollucite: R. V. Winsor, G. H. Cady, *J. Am. Chem. Soc.* **70**, 1500 (1948). Properties as a scintillator: M. Moszynski *et al., Nucl. Instrum. Methods* **179**, 271 (1981); and use as a detector in positron cameras: R. Allemand *et al., J. Nucl. Med.* **21**, 153 (1980). Vapor pressure determn: H. Kawano *et al., Bull. Chem. Soc. Jpn.* **57**, 581 (1984). Infrared spectroscopy: A. G. Maki, W. B. Olson, *J. Mol. Spectrosc.* **140**, 185 (1990). Use in malonic ester synthesis: T. Sato, J. Otera, *J. Org. Chem.* **60**, 2627 (1995); in trifluoromethylation of esters, aldehydes and ketones: R. P. Singh *et al., ibid.* **64**, 2873 (1999); in synthesis of esters and ethers: S. T. A. Shah *et al., Tetrahedron* **61**, 6652 (2005); in Stille coupling reactions: S. P. H. Mee *et al., Chem. Eur. J.* **11**, 3294 (2005).

Hygroscopic crystalline solid, mp 682°. d 4.61.

USE: Catalyst in oxidation reactions; as a solid base when adsorbed onto Celite, *q.v.* Fluoride source in organic synthesis. Inorganic scintillator.

2013. Cesium Hydroxide. [21351-79-1] Cesium hydrate. CsHO; mol wt 149.91. Cs 88.66%, H 0.67%, O 10.67%. CsOH. Prepd by electrolysis of Cs salts: Winslow *et al., J. Phys. Colloid Chem.* **51**, 967 (1947); Jolibois, Berger, *Compt. Rend.* **224**, 78 (1947). Alternate prepn: H. Jacobs, B. Harbrecht, *Z. Naturforsch.*

B36, 270 (1981). Toxicity study: Cochran *et al., Arch. Ind. Hyg.* **1,** 637 (1950).

White or yellowish, fused, very deliquescent, crystalline mass; strongly alkaline reaction. mp 272°. d 3.68. *Corrosive!* Sol in about 0.25 part water, much heat being evolved; sol in alcohol. *Keep tightly closed.* LD$_{50}$ i.p. in rats: 100 mg/kg (Cochran).

Caution: Potential symptoms of overexposure are irritation of eyes, skin, upper respiratory tract; eye and skin burns. *See NIOSH Pocket Guide to Chemical Hazards* (DHHS/NIOSH 97-140, 1997) p 56.

USE: In storage-battery electrolytes; as catalyst in the polymerization of cyclic siloxanes.

2014. Cesium Iodide. [7789-17-5] CsI; mol wt 259.81. Cs 51.15%, I 48.85%. Prepn: *Gmelins, Cesium* (8th ed.) **25,** pp 188-204 (1938). Toxicity study: Cochran *et al., Arch. Ind. Hyg.* **1,** 637 (1950).

Deliquesc crystals or crystalline powder. d 4.5. mp 621°. bp about 1280°. Very sol in water; sol in ethanol; slightly sol in methanol. Practically insol in acetone. *Keep well closed.* LD$_{50}$ i.p. in rats: 1.4 g/kg (Cochran).

USE: Prisms for infrared spectroscopy; in x-ray fluorescent screens, scintillation counters.

2015. Cesium Nitrate. [7789-18-6] CsNO$_3$; mol wt 194.91. Cs 68.19%, N 7.19%, O 24.63%. Prepn from pollucite: Watt, *Inorg. Synth.* **4,** 6 (1953). Toxicity study: Cochran *et al., Arch. Ind. Hyg.* **1,** 637 (1950).

White, lustrous hexagonal or cubic prisms; saltpeter taste. d$_4^{20}$ 3.64-3.68. mp 414°; dec at higher temp. Sol in 5 parts cold, 0.5 part boiling water; sol in acetone; very slightly sol in alc. LD$_{50}$ i.p. in rats: 1.2 g/kg (Cochran).

USE: Prepn of other Cs salts.

2016. Cesium Sulfate. [10294-54-9] Cs$_2$O$_4$S; mol wt 361.87. Cs 73.45%, O 17.69%, S 8.86%. Cs$_2$SO$_4$. Prepn: *Gmelins, Cesium* (8th ed.) **25,** pp 218-225 (1938).

Orthorhombic or hexagonal prisms. d 4.24. mp 1019°. Very sol in water. Practically insol in alc, acetone, pyridine.

USE: With V or V$_2$O$_5$ as catalyst for SO$_2$ oxidation.

2017. Cetalkonium Chloride. [122-18-9] *N*-Hexadecyl-*N,N*-dimethylbenzenemethanaminium chloride; benzylhexadecyldimethylammonium chloride; cetyldimethylbenzylammonium chloride; hexadecyldimethylbenzylammonium chloride; Banicol; Acetoquat CDAC; Acquat CDAC; Ammonyx G; Zettyn; Ammonyx T; Cetol. C$_{25}$H$_{46}$ClN; mol wt 396.09. C 75.81%, H 11.71%, Cl 8.95%, N 3.54%. Prepn: **FR 771746** (1934 to I. G. Farben); Piggott, **US 2075958** (1937 to I.C.I.); Westphal, Jerchel, *Ber.* **73,** 1011 (1940). *Review* of this type of quaternary ammonium compounds: J. P. Sisley, P. J. Wood, *Encyclopedia of Surface-Active Agents* (Chem. Publishing Co., New York, 1952) p 96 sqq.

Leaflets from ethyl acetate + petr ether, mp 59°. Sol in water, alc, acetone, ethyl acetate, propylene glycol, sorbitol solns, glycerol, ether, CCl$_4$. pH of aq solns 7.2.

USE: Cationic quaternary ammonium surfactant germicide and fungicide. Used in leather processing, textile dyeing. A mildew preventive in silicone-based water repellents. Compatible with many nonionic detergents. Active in moderately alkaline solns.

THERAP CAT: Anti-infective (topical).

2018. Cetamolol. [34919-98-7] 2-[2-[3-[(1,1-Dimethylethyl)amino]-2-hydroxypropoxy]phenoxy]-*N*-methylacetamide; 2-[*o*-[3-(*t*-butylamino)-2-hydroxypropoxy]phenoxy]-*N*-methylacetamide; (±)-1-*t*-butylamino-3-(*o*-*N*-methylcarbamoylmethoxyphenoxy)propan-2-ol. C$_{16}$H$_{26}$N$_2$O$_4$; mol wt 310.39. C 61.91%, H 8.44%, N 9.03%, O 20.62%. Cardioselective β_1-adrenergic blocker. Prepn: **BE 767781;** D. J. Lecount, C. J. Squire, **US 4059622** (1971, 1977 both to ICI). Cardiovascular effects in dogs: G. Beaulieu *et al., Can. J. Physiol. Pharmacol.* **63,** 610 (1984). Determn in human serum: M. D. Stern, *Clin. Biochem.* **17,** 162 (1984). Pharmacology and pharmacodynamics in humans: M. A. Klausner *et al., Curr. Ther. Res.* **36,** 379 (1984); J. Coelho *et*

al., Br. J. Clin. Pharmacol. **19,** 411 (1985). Evaluation in hypertensive patients: W. B. White *et al., Clin. Pharmacol. Ther.* **39,** 664 (1986).

Crystals from benzene-petr ether, mp 96-97°.

Hydrochloride. [77590-95-5] AI-27303; ICI-72222; Betacor. C$_{16}$H$_{26}$N$_2$O$_4$.HCl; mol wt 346.85.

THERAP CAT: Antihypertensive.

2019. Cethexonium Bromide. [1794-74-7] *N*-Hexadecyl-2-hydroxy-*N,N*-dimethylcyclohexanaminium bromide; hexadecyl(2-hydroxycyclohexyl)dimethylammonium bromide; cetyldimethyl(2-hydroxycyclohexyl)ammonium bromide; dimethylcetyl-2-cyclohexanolammonium bromide; *N*-cetyl-*N,N*-dimethyl-2-cyclohexanolammonium bromide; Biocidan. C$_{24}$H$_{50}$BrNO; mol wt 448.56. C 64.26%, H 11.24%, Br 17.81%, N 3.12%, O 3.57%. Prepd by the action of cetyl bromide upon 2-dimethylaminocyclohexanol: Mousseron *et al., Bull. Soc. Chim. Biol.* **33,** 369 (1951).

White powder, mp 75°. Sol in water, alcohol, chloroform. Practically insol in petr ether.

THERAP CAT: Antiseptic.

2020. Cethromycin. [205110-48-1] (3a*S*,4*R*,7*R*,9*R*,10*R*,-11*R*,13*R*,15*R*,15a*R*)-4-Ethyloctahydro-3a,7,9,11,13,15-hexamethyl-11-[[3-(3-quinolinyl)-2-propenyl]oxy]-10-[[3,4,6-trideoxy-3-(dimethylamino)-β-D-xylohexopyranosyl]oxy]-2*H*-oxacyclotetradecino[4,3-*d*]oxazole-2,6,8,14(1*H*,7*H*,9*H*)-tetrone; A-195773; ABT-773. C$_{42}$H$_{59}$N$_3$O$_{10}$; mol wt 765.93. C 65.86%, H 7.76%, N 5.49%, O 20.89%. Semisynthetic macrolide antibiotic of the ketolide class; structurally similar to telithromycin, *q.v.* Prepn: Y. S. Or *et al.,* **WO 9809978;** *eidem,* **US 5866549** (1998, 1999 both to Abbott); *eidem, J. Med. Chem.* **43,** 1045 (2000). Improved prepn: D. J. Plata *et al., Tetrahedron* **60,** 10171 (2004). Comparative *in vitro* antibacterial spectrum: A. M. Nilius *et al., Antimicrob. Agents Chemother.* **45,** 2163 (2001). Mechanism of action study: W. S. Champney, J. Pelt, *Curr. Microbiol.* **45,** 155 (2002). HPLC-MS determn in biological samples: Q. Ren *et al., J. Chromatogr. Sci.* **41,** 494 (2003). Clinical pharmacokinetics: M. W. Pletz *et al., Antimicrob. Agents Chemother.* **47,** 1129 (2003). Reviews of development and therapeutic potential: L. E. Lawrence, *Curr. Opin. Invest. Drugs* **2,** 766-772 (2001); T. J. Dougherty, J. F. Barrett, *Expert Opin. Invest. Drugs* **10,** 343-351 (2001).

White crystalline solid, mp 211-213°.

THERAP CAT: Antibacterial.

2021. Cetiedil. [14176-10-4] α-Cyclohexyl-3-thiophene-acetic acid 2-(hexahydro-1*H*-azepin-1-yl)ethyl ester; α-cyclohexyl-α-(3-thienyl)acetic acid 2-hexamethyleneiminoethyl ester. $C_{20}H_{31}$-NO_2S; mol wt 349.53. C 68.72%, H 8.94%, N 4.01%, O 9.15%, S 9.17%. Prepn: Pons, Robba, **FR 1460571** and Pons *et al.*, **FR M5504** (1966, 1967, both to Innothera), *C.A.* **68**, 59429d (1968); **71**, 91286c (1969). Prepn and activity: Robba, LeGuen, *Chim. Ther.* **2**, 120 (1967). Antisickling effect: T. Asakura *et al.*, *Proc. Natl. Acad. Sci. USA* **77**, 2955 (1980); L. R. Berkowitz, E. P. Orringer, *J. Clin. Invest.* **68**, 1215 (1981).

Citrate. [16286-69-4] Stratene; Vasocet. $C_{20}H_{31}NO_2S.C_6H_8$-O_7; mol wt 541.65. Crystals from ethanol-ether, mp 115°.

Hydrochloride. $C_{20}H_{31}NO_2S.HCl$. Crystals from acetonitrile, mp 152° (Robba, LeGuen); also mp 143° (Pons, Robba).

THERAP CAT: Vasodilator (peripheral).

2022. Cetirizine. [83881-51-0] [2-[4-[(4-Chlorophenyl)-phenylmethyl]-1-piperazinyl]ethoxy]acetic acid; [2-[4-(*p*-chloro-α-phenylbenzyl)-1-piperazinyl]ethoxy]acetic acid. $C_{21}H_{25}ClN_2$-O_3; mol wt 388.89. C 64.86%, H 6.48%, Cl 9.12%, N 7.20%, O 12.34%. Nonsedating type histamine H_1-receptor antagonist; major metabolite of hydroxyzine, *q.v.* Pharmacological activity resides primarily in the (*R*)-isomer. Prepn: E. Baltes *et al.*, **EP 58146**; *eidem*, **US 4525358** (1982, 1985 both to UCB); of enantiomers: E. Cossement *et al.*, **GB 2225321** (1989 to UCB). *See also*: *eidem*, **US 5478941** (1995 to UCB). Enantioselective HPLC determn in urine: S. O. Choi *et al.*, *Arch. Pharmacal Res.* **23**, 178 (2000). Stereoselective binding study: M. Gillard *et al.*, *Mol. Pharmacol.* **61**, 391 (2002). Clinical pharmacokinetics: E. Baltes *et al.*, *Fundam. Clin. Pharmacol.* **15**, 269 (2001). Clinical comparison with enantiomers on cutaneous response: J. L. Devalia *et al.*, *Allergy* **56**, 50 (2001); on nasal response: D. Y. Wang *et al.*, *ibid.* 339. Review of pharmacology and clinical experience in allergic disorders: J. M. Portnoy, C. Dinakar, *Expert Opin. Pharmacother.* **5**, 125-135 (2004).

Crystals from ethanol, mp 110-115°.

Dihydrochloride. [83881-52-1] P-071; Alerlisin; Formistin; Reactine; Virlix; Zirtek; Zyrtec; Zyrlex. $C_{21}H_{25}ClN_2O_3.2HCl$; mol wt 461.81. Crystals from isopropanol, mp 225°. Sol in water.

(*R*)-**Form.** [130018-77-8] Levocetirizine; (−)-cetirizine.

(*R*)-**Form dihydrochloride.** [130018-87-0] Levocetirizine hydrochloride; UCB-28556; Xusal; Xyzal. mp 229.3°. $[\alpha]_D^{25}$ −12.79° (c = 1 in water).

THERAP CAT: Antihistaminic.

2023. Cetotiamine. [137-76-8] Thiocarbonic acid *O*-ethyl ester, *S*-ester with *N*-[(4-amino-2-methyl-5-pyrimidinyl)methyl]-*N*-(4-hydroxy-2-mercapto-1-methyl-1-butenyl)formamide ethyl carbonate (ester); *O*,*S*-bis(ethoxycarbonyl)thiamine; *O*,*S*-dicarbethoxy-thiamine; DCET. $C_{18}H_{26}N_4O_6S$; mol wt 426.49. C 50.69%, H 6.14%, N 13.14%, O 22.51%, S 7.52%. Prepn: Takamizawa, Hirai, *Chem. Pharm. Bull.* **10**, 1102 (1962); Takamizawa *et al.*, *ibid.* 1107; Yamamoto *et al.*, *Bitamin* **25**, 472 (1962), *C.A.* **60**, 9773e (1964); **GB 944641** (1963 to Shionogi).

cis-form

Prisms from ethyl acetate + petr ether, mp 113.5-114.5°.

Hydrochloride monohydrate. Dicethiamin; Dicetamin. C_{18}-$H_{26}N_4O_6S.HCl.H_2O$; mol wt 480.96. Crystals from ethyl acetate, dec 122-124°. Sol in water, methanol. Practically insol in ether, benzene.

THERAP CAT: Vitamin B_1 source.

2024. Cetraxate. [34675-84-8] 4-[[[*trans*-4-(Aminomethyl)cyclohexyl]carbonyl]oxy]benzenepropanoic acid; *p*-hydroxyhydrocinnamic acid *trans*-(4-aminomethyl)cyclohexanecarboxylate; tranexamic acid *p*-(2-carboxyethyl)phenyl ester. $C_{17}H_{23}NO_4$; mol wt 305.37. C 66.86%, H 7.59%, N 4.59%, O 20.96%. Deriv of tranexamic acid, *q.v.* Prepn: Y. Yamamura *et al.*, **DE 1951061**; *eidem*, **US 3699149** (1970, 1972 both to Daiichi); O. Atsuji *et al.*, *J. Med. Chem.* **15**, 247 (1972); S. Kitahara, **JP Kokai 73 75547** (1973 to Daiichi), *C.A.* **80**, 59727x (1974). Mechanism of action: Y. Suzuki *et al.*, *Jpn. J. Pharmacol.* **29**, 829 (1979), *C.A.* **92**, 88029 (1980). Anti-ulcer effects in rats: T. Hashizume *et al.*, *Arch. Int. Pharmacodyn. Ther.* **240**, 314 (1979). Clinical study: A. Ishimori *et al.*, *Arzneim.-Forsch.* **29**, 1625 (1979); S. Yamagata, K. Miura, *ibid.* **33**, 1191 (1983).

Crystals from methanol, melts over a range of 200-280°.

Hydrochloride. [27724-96-5] DV-1006; Neuer. $C_{17}H_{23}NO_4$.-HCl; mol wt 341.83. Crystals from methanol/ether, mp 238-240°.

THERAP CAT: Antiulcerative.

2025. Cetrimonium Bromide. [57-09-0] *N*,*N*,*N*-Trimethyl-1-hexadecanaminium bromide; hexadecyltrimethylammonium bromide; cetyltrimethylammonium bromide; Bromat; Cetab; Cetavlon; Cetylamine; C.T.A.B.; Lissolamine V; Micol; Quamonium. C_{19}-$H_{42}BrN$; mol wt 364.45. C 62.62%, H 11.62%, Br 21.92%, N 3.84%. $[CH_3(CH_2)_{15}N(CH_3)_3]Br$. Prepd from cetyl bromide and trimethylamine: Shelton *et al.*, *J. Am. Chem. Soc.* **68**, 753 (1946). Toxicity and pharmacology: B. Isomaa, K. Bjondahl, *Acta Pharmacol. Toxicol.* **47**, 17 (1980). RP-HPLC determn in commercial formulations: A. Malenovic *et al.*, *Farmaco* **60**, 157 (2005).

Crystals, mp 237-243°. Soluble in about 10 parts water. Freely sol in alc; sparingly sol in acetone. Practically insol in ether, benzene. Stable in acid soln. LD_{50} in mice, rats (mg/kg): 32.0, 44.0 i.v. (Isomaa, Bjondahl).

p-**Toluenesulfonate analog.** [138-32-9] Cetrimonium tosylate; Cetats. $C_{26}H_{49}NO_3S$; mol wt 455.74.

Note: **Cetrimide** is a mixture consisting chiefly of tetradecyltrimethylammonium bromide together with smaller amounts of dodecyltrimethylammonium bromide and cetrimonium bromide.

USE: As cationic detergent and antiseptic; as laboratory reagent.

THERAP CAT: Antiseptic, disinfectant.

THERAP CAT (VET): Antiseptic, cleansing agent.

2026. Cetrorelix. [120287-85-6] *N*-Acetyl-3-(2-naphthalenyl)-D-alanyl-4-chloro-D-phenylalanyl-3-(3-pyridinyl)-D-alanyl-L-seryl-L-tyrosyl-N^5-(aminocarbonyl)-D-ornithyl-L-leucyl-L-arginyl-L-prolyl-D-alaninamide; Ac-D-Nal(2)[1]-D-Phe(4Cl)[2]-D-Pal(3)[3]-D-Cit[6]-D-Ala[10]-LH-RH; SB-75. $C_{70}H_{92}ClN_{17}O_{14}$; mol wt 1431.04. C 58.75%, H 6.48%, Cl 2.48%, N 16.64%, O 15.65%. Decapeptide LH-RH antagonist. Prepn: A. V. Schally, S. Bajusz, **EP 299402** (1989 to Asta); *eidem*, **US 4800191** (1989); S. Bajusz *et al.*, *Int. J. Pept. Protein Res.* **32**, 425 (1988). Structural study: A. Müller *et al.*, *ibid.* **43**, 264 (1994). HPLC determn in plasma: H. H. Raffel *et al.*, *J. Chromatogr. B* **653**, 102 (1994). Pharmacology: T. Reissmann *et al.*, *Eur. J. Cancer* **32A**, 1574 (1996). Clinical evaluation in prostatic cancer: D. Gonzalez-Barcena *et al.*, *Urology* **45**, 275 (1995); in assisted fertilization: C. Albano *et al.*, *Fertil. Steril.* **67**, 917 (1997).

Acetate. [145672-81-7] D-20761; Cetrotide. Sol in water.

THERAP CAT: Antineoplastic (hormonal). In treatment of infertility.

2027. Cetuximab. [205923-56-4] Anti-(human epidermal growth factor receptor) immunoglobulin G1 (human-mouse monoclonal C225 γ₁-chain), disulfide with human-mouse monoclonal C225 κ-chain, dimer; C225; IMC-C225; Erbitux. Chimeric monoclonal antibody directed against human epithelial growth factor receptor (EGFR). Prepn: N. I. Goldstein *et al.*, **WO 9640210** (1995 to Imclone and MRC); *eidem, Clin. Cancer Res.* **1**, 1311 (1995). Antitumor activity: J. Mendelson, *ibid.* **6**, 747 (2000). Clinical pharmacokinetics: F. Robert *et al.*, *J. Clin. Oncol.* **19**, 3234 (2001); in combination with irinotecan: C. Delbaldo *et al.*, *Eur. J. Cancer* **41**, 1739 (2005). Clinical trial in head and neck cancer: B. Burtness *et al.*, *J. Clin. Oncol.* **23**, 8646 (2005); in combination with radiotherapy: J. A. Bonner *et al.*, *N. Engl. J. Med.* **354**, 567 (2006). Review of mechanism of action: R. S. Herbst *et al.*, *Expert Opin. Biol. Ther.* **1**, 719-732 (2001); J. Baselga, *Eur. J. Cancer* **37**, S16-S22 (2001); of pharmacology and clinical studies: R. S. Herbst, C. J. Langer, *Semin. Oncol.* **29**, Suppl. 4, 27-36 (2002); of use in colorectal cancer: S.-F. Wong, *Clin. Ther.* **27**, 684-694 (2005).

THERAP CAT: Antineoplastic.

2028. Cetyl Alcohol. [36653-82-4] 1-Hexadecanol; ethal; ethol; palmityl alcohol. $C_{16}H_{34}O$; mol wt 242.44. C 79.27%, H 14.14%, O 6.60%. $CH_3(CH_2)_{14}CH_2OH$. Discovered by Chevreul in 1813. Obtained from spermaceti by saponification: Spada, Gavioli, *Farm. Sci. Tec.* (Pavia) **7**, 435 (1952), *C.A.* **47**, 891c (1953). Prepn from palmitoyl chloride + NaBH₄: Caikin, Brown, *J. Am. Chem. Soc.* **71**, 122 (1949); from methylthiopalmitate + Raney Ni: Ruzicka, Prelog, **US 2509171** (1950 to Ciba); from hexadecyl bromide: Levine, Clippinger, **US 3018308** (1962 to California Res. Corp.).

White crystals. d 0.811. mp 49°. bp 344°; bp₁₅ 190°. n_D^{79} 1.4283. Practically insol in water. Sol in alcohol, chloroform, ether.

Hexadecyl alcohol. Primary, branched chain, C₁₆ alcohol, made up of an array of isomeric compds maintained in constant proportion by a complex manufacturing process (not from spermaceti): Edman, Lowden, *Drug Cosmet. Ind.* **93**, 631 (Nov. 1963). Liquid, d_{20}^{20} 0.842. bp₅₀ 195-205°. Freezes at <−60°. Miscible with most alcohols, glycols, esters, ketones, cosmetic oils and aromatics. Immiscible with water.

USE: In cosmetics as emollient, emulsion modifier, coupling agent. Pharmaceutic aid (emulsifying and stiffening agent).

2029. Cetyldimethylethylammonium Bromide. [124-03-8] *N*-Ethyl-*N*,*N*-dimethyl-1-hexadecanaminium bromide; ethylhexadecyldimethylammonium bromide; ethyl cetab; CDA; Ammonyx DME. $C_{20}H_{44}BrN$; mol wt 378.47. C 63.47%, H 11.72%, Br 21.11%, N 3.70%. Cationic germicidal detergent. Prepn and antibacterial activity: R. S. Shelton *et al.*, *J. Am. Chem. Soc.* **68**, 753 (1946).

White powder, mp 178-186°. Soluble in water, alcohol; slightly sol in chloroform, benzene, ether.

USE: Disinfectant; laboratory reagent.

2030. Cetyl Lactate. [35274-05-6] 2-Hydroxypropanoic acid hexadecyl ester; 1-hexadecanol lactate; lactic acid cetyl ester; lactic acid hexadecyl ester; Ceraphyl 28. $C_{19}H_{38}O_3$; mol wt 314.50. C 72.56%, H 12.18%, O 15.26%. $CH_3CHOHCOOC_{16}$-H_{33}. Preparation: Rehberg, Marion, *J. Am. Chem. Soc.* **72**, 1918 (1950).

Waxy solid. mp 41°. bp₀.₁ 132°; bp₁ 170°; bp₁₀ 219°. n_D^{40} 1.4410; n_D^{50} 1.4370.

USE: Nonionic emollient. To improve feel and texture of cosmetic and pharmaceutical prepns.

2031. Cetyl Palmitate. [540-10-3] Hexadecanoic acid hexadecyl ester; palmitic acid hexadecyl ester; hexadecyl palmitate. $C_{32}H_{64}O_2$; mol wt 480.85. C 79.93%, H 13.42%, O 6.65%. CH_3-$(CH_2)_{14}COOCH_2(CH_2)_{14}CH_3$. Prepn from palmitoyl chloride and cetyl alcohol in the presence of Mg: Paquot, Bouquet, *Bull. Soc. Chim. Fr.* **1947**, 321; by $CrO_3H_2SO_4$ oxidation of cetyl alcohol: Cymerman-Craig, Horning, *J. Org. Chem.* **25**, 2098 (1960). Biosynthesis using inoculum of *Nocardia salmonicolor:* Davis, **US 3169099** (1965 to Socony Mobil Oil).

Monoclinic leaflets, mp 54°. d²⁰ 0.989. n_D^{70} 1.4398. Practically insol in water. Sol in abs alc, ether.

2032. Cetylpyridinium Chloride. [123-03-5] 1-Hexadecylpyridinium chloride; Ceepryn; Medilave; Merocet; Pristacin; Pyrisept. $C_{21}H_{38}ClN$; mol wt 339.99. C 74.19%, H 11.27%, Cl 10.43%, N 4.12%. Pharmacology and toxicology: *J. Pharmacol. Exp. Ther.* **74**, 401 (1942). Review of early literature: C. L. Huyck, *Am. J. Pharm.* **116**, 50 (1944). Toxicity data: J. W. Nelson, S. C. Lyster, *J. Am. Pharm. Assoc.* **35**, 89 (1946).

Monohydrate. [6004-24-6] Dobendan; Halset. White powder, mp 77-83°. Freely sol in water, alcohol, chloroform; very slightly sol in benzene, ether. pH (1% aq soln): 6.0 to 7.0. Surface tension (25°): 43 dyn/cm (0.1% aq soln); 41 dyn/cm (1.0%); 38 dyn/cm (10%). LD₅₀ in rats (mg/kg): 250 s.c.; 6 i.p.; 30 i.v.; 200 orally (Nelson, Lyster).

USE: Pharmaceutic aid (preservative).

THERAP CAT: Antiseptic; disinfectant.

THERAP CAT (VET): Topical antiseptic; disinfectant.

2033. Cevadine. [62-59-9] [3β(Z),4α,16β]-4,9-Epoxy-cevane-3,4,12,14,16,17,20-heptol 3-(2-methyl-2-butenoate); veratrine. $C_{32}H_{49}NO_9$; mol wt 591.73. C 64.95%, H 8.35%, N 2.37%, O 24.33%. From seeds of *Schoenocaulon officinale* (Schlecht & Cham.) A. Gray (*Sabadilla officinarum* Brandt), *Liliaceae:* Poetsch *et al.*, *J. Am. Pharm. Assoc.* **38**, 525 (1949); Ringel, *ibid.* **45**, 433 (1956). Evaluation as insecticide: Ikawa, Link *et al.*, *J. Biol. Chem.* **159**, 517 (1945). Structure: Kupchan, Alfonso, *ibid.* **49**, 242 (1960). Toxicity study: Swiss, Bauer, *Proc. Soc. Exp. Biol. Med.* **76**, 847 (1951). *Review:* Wintersteiner in Graff, *Essays in Biochemistry* (Wiley, New York, 1956) pp 308-321.

Flat needles from ether, decomp 213-214.5°. $[α]_D^{20}$ +12.8° (c = 3.2 in alc). One gram dissolves in about 15 ml alc or ether; slightly sol in water. LD₅₀ i.p. in mice: 3.5 mg/kg (Swiss, Bauer).

Aurichloride. Fine yellow needles from alc, dec 190°.

Mercurichloride. $C_{32}H_{49}NO_9 \cdot HCl \cdot HgCl_2$. Silvery scales, dec 172°.

Caution: Extremely irritating locally, particularly to mucous membranes. Serious poisoning has resulted from local application. Caution must be used in handling. *See also* Veratrine (Mixture).

2034. Cevimeline. [107233-08-9] (2′R,3R)-*rel*-2′-Methylspiro[1-azabicyclo[2.2.2]octane-3,5′-[1,3]oxathiolane]; (±)-*cis*-2-methylspiro[1,3-oxathiolane-5,3′-quinuclidine]. $C_{10}H_{17}NOS$; mol wt 199.31. C 60.26%, H 8.60%, N 7.03%, O 8.03%, S 16.09%. Muscarinic M_1 and M_3 receptor agonist. Prepn: A. Fisher *et al.*, **JP Kokai 61 280497**; *eidem*, **US 4855290**; (1986, 1989 both to State of Israel). Improved process: K. Hayashi *et al.*, **US 5571918** (1996 to Ishihara Sangyo Kaisha). Sialogogic effect in animals: H. Masunaga *et al.*, *Eur. J. Pharmacol.* **339**, 1 (1997). General pharmacology: H. Arisawa *et al.*, *Arzneim.-Forsch.* **52**, 14, 81 (2002). Clinical experience in Sjögren's syndrome dry eye: M. Ono *et al.*, *Am. J. Ophthalmol.* **138**, 6 (2004); in dry mouth: K. Suzuki *et al.*, *Pharmacology* **74**, 100 (2005). Review of clinical pharmacokinetics and efficacy in Sjögren's syndrome: H. Yasuda, H. Niki, *Clin. Drug Invest.* **22**, 67-73 (2002).

(R,R)-Form

Hydrochloride hemihydrate. [153504-70-2]; [107220-28-0] anhydrous. AF-102B; SNI-2011; Evoxac. $C_{10}H_{17}NOS \cdot HCl \cdot \frac{1}{2}H_2O$; mol wt 244.78. White to off white crystalline powder, mp 201-203°. Freely sol in alcohol, chloroform; very sol in water. Virtually insol in ether.

THERAP CAT: Sialagogue.

2035. Cevine. [124-98-1] (3α,4α,16β)-4,9-Epoxycevane-3,-4,12,14,16,17,20-heptol. $C_{27}H_{43}NO_8$; mol wt 509.63. C 63.63%, H 8.50%, N 2.75%, O 25.12%. By hydrolysis of cevadine. Structure and stereochemistry: Barton *et al.*, *Experientia* **10**, 81 (1954); Kupchan *et al.*, *J. Am. Chem. Soc.* **80**, 1769 (1958); Kupchan *et al.*, *Tetrahedron* **7**, 47 (1959); Eeles, *Tetrahedron Letters* no. 7, 24 (1960). Comparative toxicity: O. Krayer *et al.*, *J. Pharmacol. Exp. Ther.* **82**, 167 (1944); K. Tanaka, *ibid.* **113**, 89 (1955).

Occurs as the hemiheptahydrate, triclinic prisms from dil alc. After drying at 110° it sinters at 165° and becomes a transparent resin at 165-170°: M. Ikawa *et al.*, *J. Biol. Chem.* **159**, 517 (1945). $[\alpha]_D^{17}$ −17.5° (aq alc). Sol in water, alc; slightly sol in ether. LD_{50} i.p. in rats: 87.0 mg/kg (Krayer). LD_{50} s.c. in male mice: 160 mg/kg (Tanaka).

Hydrochloride. mp 247°.

2036. Chalcomycin. [20283-48-1] $C_{35}H_{56}O_{14}$; mol wt 700.81. C 59.98%, H 8.05%, O 31.96%. Antibiotic substance produced from *Streptomyces bikiniensis* NRRL 2737: Frohardt *et al.*, **DE 1109835** (1960 to Parke, Davis). Structure: Woo *et al.*, *J. Am. Chem. Soc.* **86**, 2726 (1964). *Review:* Jordan, "Chalcomy-

cin" in *Antibiotics* **I**, D. Gottlieb, P. Shaw, Eds. (Springer-Verlag, New York, 1967) pp 446-450.

Crystals from butanol, mp 121-123°. $[\alpha]_D^{27}$ −43.5° (ethanol). uv max: 218 nm (ε 22770). Sol in ethyl acetate, methanol, ethanol, benzene, toluene, chloroform; sparingly sol in carbon tetrachloride, ether, water. Practically insol in petr ether.

2037. Chalcone. [94-41-7] 1,3-Diphenyl-2-propen-1-one; chalkone; benzylideneacetophenone; benzalacetophenone; phenyl styryl ketone. $C_{15}H_{12}O$; mol wt 208.26. C 86.51%, H 5.81%, O 7.68%. $C_6H_5CH{=}CHCOC_6H_5$. Prepd by the action of NaOH on an alcoholic soln of benzaldehyde and acetophenone: E. P. Kohler, H. M. Chadwell, *Org. Synth.* **coll. vol. I**, 78 (1941).

Pale-yellow orthorhombic prisms from petr ether. mp 57-58°. d_4^{62} 1.0712. bp_{760} 345-348° (slight decompn). bp_{25} 208°. n_D^{62} 1.6458. Freely sol in ether, chloroform, carbon bisulfide, benzene; slightly sol in alcohol; very sparingly in cold petr ether.

Caution: Skin irritant.

Note: Exists in other forms (polymorphic) with different mps. Irradiation produces four forms of dimers.

2038. Chalcopyrite. [1308-56-1] Cupric ferrous sulfide; copper pyrites; yellow copper; Chalkopyrite; Kupferkies. $CuFeS_2$; mol wt 183.52. Cu 34.63%, Fe 30.43%, S 34.94%. Occurs as a mineral. It is an important copper ore found in Canada, Montana, Utah, Arizona, Tennessee, Chile, Peru, Bolivia, Europe, Japan. Prepd synthetically by treating $KFeS_2$ with an ammoniacal soln of Cu^+ ions: Schneider, *J. Prakt. Chem.* [2] **38**, 569 (1888); **56**, 415 (1897); Boon, *Rec. Trav. Chim.* **63**, 69 (1954).

Yellow brass-colored or bronze-colored crystals. Metallic, greenish sheen. Tetragonal crystal system. d 4.1-4.3. mp 950°. Specific heat 0.1291. Hardness 3.5-4.0. Soluble in nitric acid, but dissolves faster in aqua regia. Practically insol in hydrochloric acid.

Note: Copper iron sulfide of the formula $FeS \cdot 2Cu_2S \cdot CuS$ occurs as the mineral *bornite*.

USE: The ore as source of copper. The synthetic material in semiconductor research.

2039. D-Chalcose. [3150-28-5] 4,6-Dideoxy-3-*O*-methyl-D-*xylo*-hexose; 4,6-dideoxy-3-*O*-methyl-D-glucose; lankavose. $C_7H_{14}O_4$; mol wt 162.18. C 51.84%, H 8.70%, O 39.46%. Component of chalcomycin and lankamycin, *q.q.v.* Prepn from chalcomycin and structure: Woo *et al.*, *J. Am. Chem. Soc.* **83**, 3352 (1961). Stereochemistry: Woo *et al.*, *ibid.* **84**, 1066 (1962); Foster *et al.*, *J. Chem. Soc.* **1965**, 2318. Synthesis: Kochetkov, Usov, *Tetrahedron Lett.* **1963**, 519; McNally, Overend, *Chem. Ind. (London)* **1964**, 2021; Lawton *et al.*, *Can. J. Chem.* **47**, 2899 (1969). Synthesis of DL-form: R. M. Srivastava, R. K. Brown, *Can. J. Chem.* **48**, 830 (1970); K. Torssell, M. P. Tyagi, *Acta Chem. Scand. B* **31**, 1 (1977); S. Danishefsky, J. F. Kerwin, *J. Org. Chem.* **47**, 1597 (1982).

Crystals, mp 96-99°. $[\alpha]_D^{24}$ +120° (2 min) → +97° (10 min) → +76° (3 hr and 26 hr) (c = 1.5 in water).

Methyl chalcoside. $C_8H_{16}O_4$. Crystals, mp 101.5-102°. $[\alpha]_D^{27}$ −21° (c = 2.04 in chloroform).

2040. Chamazulene. [529-05-5] 7-Ethyl-1,4-dimethyl-azulene; 1,4-dimethyl-7-ethylazulene; dimethulene. $C_{14}H_{16}$; mol wt 184.28. C 91.25%, H 8.75%. Anti-inflammatory principle obtained from chamazulenogenic compds found in chamomile (*Matricaria chamomilla* L.), wormwood (*Artemisia absinthium* L.), and yarrow (*Achillea millefolium* L., *Compositae*). Isoln: Ruzicka, Rudolph, *Helv. Chim. Acta* **9**, 118 (1926); Ruzicka, Haagen-Smit, *ibid.* **14**, 1104 (1931). Structure: Sorm *et al.*, *Collect. Czech. Chem. Commun.* **18**, 527 (1953); Meisels, Weizmann, *J. Am. Chem. Soc.* **75**, 3865 (1953); Suchy *et al.*, *Collect. Czech. Chem. Commun.* **21**, 477 (1956). Synthesis: Mangoni, Bandiera, *Gazz. Chim. Ital.* **90**, 947 (1960); White, Winter, *Tetrahedron Lett.* **1963**, 137; D. Mukherjee *et al.*, *J. Am. Chem. Soc.* **101**, 251 (1979). Pharmacology: I. G. Boldina, *Farmakol. Toksikol.* **29**, 672 (1966); I. G. Boldina, M. V. Nazarenko, *C.A.* **67**, 42441h (1967).

Blue oil. bp_{12} 161°; bp_{11} 145°. d_4^{20} 0.9883. uv max: 370 nm (log ε 3.7). LD_{50} i.m. in white mice: 3 g/kg (Boldina, Nazarenko). **Trinitrobenzene derivative.** $C_{20}H_{19}N_3O_6$. Dark violet needles from abs ethanol, mp 131.5-132.5°.

2041. Chamomile. Camomile. The term chamomile refers to the dried flowerheads of either of two distinct plants of the family *Asteraceae (Compositae):* German chamomile, *Chamomilla recutita* (L.) Rauschert, also known as *Matricaria recutita* L. or *M. chamomilla*, and Roman chamomile, *Chamaemelum nobile* (L.) All. (formerly *Anthemis nobilis* L.). Both chamomiles have been used in traditional medicines as antispasmodic and anti-inflammatory agents. Evaluation of hydroalcoholic extracts for antispasmodic activity: H. B. Forster *et al.*, *Planta Med.* **40**, 309 (1980); for anti-inflammatory activity: A. Tubaro *et al.*, *ibid.* **50**, 359 (1984). Stability of extracts: R. Carle *et al.*, *ibid.* **55**, 540 (1989). HPLC determn of flavones and coumarins in extracts: P. Pietta *et al.*, *J. Chromatogr.* **404**, 279 (1987). Reviews: A. Y. Leung, *Encyclopedia of Common Natural Ingredients* (Wiley-Interscience, New York, 1980) pp 110-112; C. Mann, E. J. Staba in *Herbs, Spices, and Medicinal Plants: Recent Advances in Botany, Horticulture, and Pharmacology* vol. 1 (Oryx Press, 1986) pp 235-280.

German chamomile. Hungarian chamomile; wild chamomile; Matricaria. *Habit.* Europe, northern and western Asia; naturalized in North America. Cultivated in Hungary, Romania, Germany. *Constit.* 0.24-1.9% volatile oil; flavonoids including apigenin, luteolin, quercetin; coumarins such as herniarin, umbelliferone; proazulenes (matricin, matricarin, etc.); phenolic carboxylic acids (anisic, vanillic, syringic, caffeic); polysaccharide mucilage.

German chamomile oil. [8002-66-2] Matricaria oil. Extracted from flower heads by steam distillation. *Constit.* (−)-α-bisabolol (up to 50%), bisabolol oxides, chamazulene, farnesene. Review of constituents: B. M. Lawrence, *Perfum. Flavor.* **12**, 35-52 (1987). Deep ink-blue oil. d 0.91-0.95. Ester value: <40. Acid value: 5 to 50. Sol in propylene glycol. Insol in glycerin, mineral oil.

Roman chamomile. English chamomile; garden chamomile. *Habit.* Southern and western Europe; naturalized in North America. Cultivated in Great Britain, Belgium, France, U.S. *Constit.* up to 1.75% volatile oil; up to 0.6% sesquiterpene lactones of the germacranolide type (mainly nobilin, 3-epinobilin); flavonoids (apigenin, luteolin, apiin, etc.); phenolic carboxylic acids (caffeic, ferulic); coumarins; and thiophene derivatives.

Roman chamomile oil. [8015-92-7] Oil of anthemis. Extracted from flowerheads by steam distillation. *Constit.* esters of angelic and tiglic acids (~85%), chamazulene, α-pinene, farnesol. Blue oil. n^{20} 1.44-1.45. $[α]^{20}$ −1 to +4°. Ester value: 250 to 310. Acid value <15. Sol in mineral oil and most fixed oils; sol with haziness in propylene glycol. Practically insol in glycerin.

USE: Flowers in herbal teas. Extracts and oils in perfumery; as flavor in foods and alcoholic beverages; hair dye.

THERAP CAT: Carminative; vulnerary. Extracts and oils as topical anti-inflammatory.

2042. Chanoclavine. [2390-99-0] [4R-[4α,5β(E)]]-2-Methyl-3-[1,3,4,5-tetrahydro-4-(methylamino)benz[cd]indol-5-yl]-2-propen-1-ol; (E)-8,9-didehydro-6-methyl-6,7-secoergoline-8-methanol; chanoclavin-I; secaclavine. $C_{16}H_{20}N_2O$; mol wt 256.34. C 74.97%, H 7.86%, N 10.93%, O 6.24%. Precursor of the tetracyclic ergolines, agroclavine, elymoclavine, and lysergic acid amide, *q.q.v.*: Gröger *et al.*, *Z. Naturforsch.* **21b**, 827 (1966); Floss *et al.*, *Chem. Commun.* **1967**, 105. Occurs in sclerotia of *Claviceps purpurea* (Fries) Tul., *Hypocreaceae*, in *Ipomea tricolor* Cav., *Convolvulaceae* and is one of the active principles of the ancient Aztec drug "Ololiuqui," *Rivea corymbosa* (L.) Hall. f., *Convolvulaceae:* Hofmann, Tscherter, *Experientia* **16**, 414 (1960). Isoln and structure: Hofmann *et al.*, *Helv. Chim. Acta* **40**, 1358 (1957). Isoln of stereoisomers: Stauffacher, Tscherter, *ibid.* **47**, 2186 (1964). Stereochemistry: Acklin *et al.*, *Chem. Commun.* **1966**, 799. Biosynthetic studies: Floss *et al.*, *J. Am. Chem. Soc.* **90**, 6500 (1968). Total synthesis of (±)-chanoclavine: H. Plieninger *et al.*, *Tetrahedron Lett.* **1975**, 1827; H. Plieninger, D. Schmalz, *Ber.* **109**, 2140 (1976); M. Natsume, H. Muratake, *Heterocycles* **16**, 375 (1981).

Thick prisms and polyhedra from acetone or methanol, mp 220-222°. $[α]_D^{20}$ −240° (pyridine), $[α]_D^{20}$ −205° (c = 0.75 in alcohol). uv max: 225, 284, 293 nm (ε 4.44, 3.82, 3.72). One gram dissolves in 25 ml boiling methanol, 140 ml boiling acetone, 170 ml boiling ethyl acetate or 350 ml boiling chloroform. Practically insol in water.

Epimer at position 10. Chanoclavine II.

2043. Chaperonins. Cpns. Subset of molecular chaperone proteins, including the nucleoplasmins and heat shock proteins, that guide the in-vivo transport, folding and assembly of other protein structures but are not themselves components of these structures as part of their biological function. The term "chaperonin" was coined by S. M. Hemmingsen *et al.*, *Nature* **333**, 330 (1988) to describe the function of these proteins. Characterized by large oligomeric cage-like structures with multiple rings of subunits possessing 7,8 or 9-fold symmetry. Ubiquitous conserved proteins which have been identified in most microorganisms and cellular compartments, requires the interaction of two chaperonins to ensure correct folding: J. Martin *et al.*, *Nature* **366**, 228, 279 (1993). Molecular study of mechanism: S. G. Burston *et al.*, *J. Mol. Biol.* **249**, 138 (1995). Review: R. J. Ellis, S. M. van der Vies, *Annu. Rev. Biochem.* **60**, 321-347 (1991). Review of structures and conformations: H. Saibil, S. Wood, *Curr. Opin. Struct. Biol.* **3**, 207-213 (1993). Review of *E. coli* chaperonins, cpn60-cpn10: F. Baneyx, *Ann. N.Y. Acad. Sci.* **745**, 383-394 (1994).

2044. CHAPS. [75621-03-3] *N,N*-Dimethyl-*N*-(3-sulfopropyl)-3-[[(3α,5β,7α,12α)-3,7,12-trihydroxy-24-oxocholan-24-yl]-amino]-1-propanaminium inner salt; 3-[(3-cholamidopropyl)dimethylammonio]-1-propanesulfonate. $C_{32}H_{58}N_2O_7S$; mol wt 614.88. C 62.51%, H 9.51%, N 4.56%, O 18.21%, S 5.21%. Sulfobetaine zwitterionic derivative of cholic acid, *q.v.* Prepn: L. M. Hjelmeland, *Proc. Natl. Acad. Sci. USA* **77**, 6368 (1980); idem, US 4372888 (1983 to U.S. Secy. Health and Human Services); and physical properties: L. M. Hjelmeland *et al.*, *Anal. Biochem.* **130**, 72 (1983). Physical characterization: R. E. Stark *et al.*, *J. Phys. Chem.* **88**, 6063 (1984). Micellar properties: M. A. Partearroyo *et al.*, *Biochem. Int.* **16**, 259 (1988). Solubilization of membrane proteins: A. J. Bitonti *et al.*, *Biochemistry* **21**, 3650 (1982); W. Wouters *et al.*, *Eur. J. Pharmacol.* **115**, 1 (1985); L. Bancells *et al.*,

Biochem. Pharmacol. **36**, 2539 (1987); of opioid receptors: J. Simon et al., J. Neurochem. **46**, 695 (1986).

Crystals from absolute methanol at 0°.

Hydroxy analog. [82473-24-3] CHAPSO. $C_{32}H_{58}N_2O_8S$. White granular detergent.

USE: Nondenaturing biological detergent.

2045. Chartreusin. [6377-18-0] 10-[[6-Deoxy-2-O-(6-de-oxy-3-O-methyl-α-D-galactopyranosyl)-β-D-galactopyranosyl]-oxy]-6-hydroxy-1-methylbenzo[h][1]benzopyrano[5,4,3-cde][1]-benzopyran-5,12-dione; antibiotic X-465A; lambdamycin; NSC-5159. $C_{32}H_{32}O_{14}$; mol wt 640.59. C 60.00%, H 5.04%, O 34.97%. Antibiotic substance produced by Streptomyces chartreusis from African soil, also by another Streptomyces sp. from North American soil: B. E. Leach et al., J. Am. Chem. Soc. **75**, 4011 (1953). Identity with Antibiotic X-465A: J. Berger et al., ibid. **80**, 1636 (1958). Structure: L. H. Sternbach et al., ibid. 1639; E. Simonitsch et al., Helv. Chim. Acta **47**, 1459 (1964); W. Eisenhuth et al., ibid. 1475. Anticancer activity: J. P. McGovern et al., Cancer Res. **37**, 1666 (1977). Synthesis of **chartarin**, the chartreusin aglycone: T. R. Kelly et al., J. Am. Chem. Soc. **102**, 798 (1980); F. M. Hauser, D.W. Combs, J. Org. Chem. **45**, 4071 (1980).

Yellow plates from acetone or methylene chloride + ethanol, mp 184-186°. Weak acid. $[\alpha]_D^{25}$ +132.5° (c = 0.2 in pyridine); $[\alpha]_D^{25}$ −33° (c = 0.3 in glacial acetic acid). uv max: 237, 262, 332, 382, 405, 422 nm. Practically insol in water. Sol in acetone.

Sodium salt. Gold-colored needles or plates from water. Soly in water: at least 20 mg/ml (pH 9.5). LD_{50} i.v. in mice: 250 mg/kg (Leach).

2046. Charybdotoxin. [95751-30-7] ChTX; CTX. C_{176}-$H_{277}N_{57}O_{55}S_7$; mol wt 4295.89. C 49.21%, H 6.50%, N 18.58%, O 20.48%, S 5.22%. Peptide inhibitor of K^+ channels isolated from the venom of the scorpion Leiurus quinquestriatus var. hebraeus. Single chain of 4.3 kDa comprised of 37 amino acids with 3 disulfide linkages. Identification: C. Miller et al., Nature **313**, 316 (1985). Purification and amino acid sequence: G. Gimenez-Gallego et al., Proc. Natl. Acad. Sci. USA **85**, 3329 (1988). Synthesis: E. E. Sugg et al., J. Biol. Chem. **265**, 18745 (1990); P. Lambert et al., Biochem. Biophys. Res. Commun. **170**, 684 (1990). NMR structural study: F. Bontems et al., Eur. J. Biochem. **196**, 19 (1991). Mechanism of channel block: R. MacKinnon, C. Miller, J. Gen. Physiol. **91**, 335 (1988). Characterization of binding sites: J. Vázquez et al., J. Biol. Chem. **264**, 20902 (1989); J. Vázquez et al., ibid. **265**, 15564 (1990). Use as probe for K^+ channels: M. Garcia, G. Gimenez-Gallego, US 4960867 (1990 to Merck & Co.).

pyroE-F-T-N-V-S-C-T-T-S-K-E-C-W-S-V-C-Q-R-L-H-N-T-S-R-G-K-C-M-N-K-K-C-R-C-Y-S

Extinction coefficient: 1.52 $(mg/ml)^{-1}cm^{-1}$ at 280 nm; 15.05 $(mg/ml)^{-1}cm^{-1}$ at 215 nm.

USE: Biochemical probe.

2047. Chaulmoogra Oil. Hydnocarpus oil; gynocardia oil. Fixed oil expressed from chaulmoogra, the seeds of Taraktogenos kurzii King, Bixaceae; Hydnocarpus wightiana Blume or H. anthelmintica Pierre, Flacourtiaceae. The seeds contain about 50% chaulmoogra oil. Constit. Glycerides of chaulmoogric and hydnocarpic acids with small amounts of glycerides of palmitic acid, etc.

Yellow or brownish-yellow oil. Below 25° it is a soft solid; characteristic odor. About d_{25}^{25} 0.95; d_{15}^{45} 0.940. $[\alpha]_D^{20}$ +48 to +60°. Sol in benzene, chloroform, ether, petr ether, slightly in cold alcohol; almost entirely sol in hot alcohol, carbon disulfide.

THERAP CAT: Antibacterial (leprostatic).

2048. Chaulmoogric Acid. [29106-32-9] (1S)-2-Cyclopentene-1-tridecanoic acid; D-13-(2-cyclopenten-1-yl)tridecanoic acid; hydnocarpylacetic acid. $C_{18}H_{32}O_2$; mol wt 280.45. C 77.09%, H 11.50%, O 11.41%. Isoln from chaulmoogra oil and characterization: Power, Gornall, J. Chem. Soc. **85**, 838, 851 (1904); Barrowcliff, Power, ibid. **91**, 557 (1907); Hashimoto, J. Am. Chem. Soc. **47**, 2325 (1925); Cole, Cardoso, ibid. **61**, 2349, 2351, 3442 (1939). Structure: Shriner, Adams, ibid. **47**, 2727 (1925). Synthesis: Noller, Adams, ibid. **48**, 1080 (1926); Perkins, Cruz, ibid. **49**, 1070 (1927). Synthesis and stereochemistry: Mislow, Steinberg, ibid. **77**, 3807 (1955). Activity against Mycobacterium leprae: L. Levy, Am. Rev. Respir. Dis. **111**, 703 (1975). Biosynthesis: T. Kaneda, Biochem. Biophys. Res. Commun. **99**, 1226 (1981).

Shiny leaflets from petr ether or alcohol. mp 68.5°. bp_{20} 247-248°. $[\alpha]_D^{20}$ +60.3° (c = 4 in chloroform). Iodine value 90.5. Freely sol in ether, chloroform, ethyl acetate; sol in other organic fat solvents.

Methyl ester. [24828-59-9] $C_{19}H_{34}O_2$. Prepd by passing HCl gas into a methanol soln of the acid. Needles, mp 22°. bp_{20} 227°. d_{25}^{25} 0.9119. $[\alpha]_D^{15}$ +50° (c = 5 in chloroform).

Ethyl ester. [623-32-5] Chaulmestrol; Moogrol; $C_{20}H_{36}O_2$; mol wt 308.50. Essentially a mixt of the ethyl esters of the unsaturated fatty acids (chaulmoogric and hydnocarpic) of chaulmoogra oil. Pale yellow, clear liquid; slight fruity odor; not unpleasant taste. Iodine no. 90-100. d_{25}^{25} ~0.904. $[\alpha]_D^{25}$ +4.5° (chloroform). Insol in water; misc with alc, chloroform.

THERAP CAT: Ethyl ester in treatment of leprosy, sarcoidosis.

2049. Chavicine. [495-91-0] (Z,Z)-1-[5-(1,3-Benzodioxol-5-yl)-1-oxo-2,4-pentadienyl]piperidine; (Z,Z)-1-piperoylpiperidine. $C_{17}H_{19}NO_3$; mol wt 285.34. C 71.56%, H 6.71%, N 4.91%, O 16.82%. One of the most active constituents of black pepper: Buchheim, Arch. Exp. Pathol. Pharmakol. **5**, 455 (1876); Ott, Eichler, Ber. **55**, 2653 (1922); Ott, Lüdemann, Ber. **57**, 214 (1924). Stereoisomer of piperine: Lohaus, Gall, Ann. **517**, 282 (1935). Loss of pungency of ground pepper during storage attributed to gradual isomerization of chavicine into piperine, q.v.: Newman, Chem. Prod. **16**, 379 (1953). Synthesis of chavicine and pungency of its existence as constituent of black pepper: R. Grewe et al., Ber. **103**, 3752 (1970). Spectroscopic structural elucidation and prepn: R. DeCleyn, M. Verzele, Bull. Soc. Chim. Belg. **84**, 435 (1975).

Yellowish, oily mass; sharp, peppery taste. Sol in alc, ether, petr ether. uv max (methanol): 318 nm (ε 16200).

2050. Chavicol. [501-92-8] 4-(2-Propenyl)phenol; p-allylphenol; γ-(p-hydroxyphenyl)-α-propylene. $C_9H_{10}O$; mol wt 134.18. C 80.56%, H 7.51%, O 11.92%. Found together with terpenes in volatile betel oils (from leaves of Piper betle L., Piperaceae): Eijkman, Ber. **22**, 2739 (1889). Prepd from a mixture of estragole, ethyl bromide and magnesium in benzene: Grignard,

Compt. Rend. **151,** 323 (1910); from 4-allylphenylmagnesium bromide in ether by the action of oxygen: Quelet, *Bull. Soc. Chim. Fr.* [4] **45,** 265 (1929).

HO — CH₂

Liquid. mp 15.8°. d_4^{15} 1.0203; d_4^{20} 1.0175. bp₇₆₀ 238°; bp₁₆ 123°. n_D^{18} 1.5441. Miscible with alcohol, ether, chloroform, petr ether.

Methyl ether see Estragole.

2051. Chelerythrine. [34316-15-9] 1,2-Dimethoxy-12-methyl[1,3]benzodioxolo[5,6-c]phenanthridinium; toddaline. $[C_{21}H_{18}NO_4]^+$. From root of *Chelidonium majus* L., *Papaveraceae:* Kratzmann, *Pharm. Monatsh.* **5,** 161 (1924), *C.A.* **18,** 3406² (1924); Platonova *et al., J. Gen. Chem. USSR* **26,** 181 (1956). Structure: Späth, Kuffner, *Ber.* **64,** 1123 (1931); N. Decaudain *et al., Ann. Pharm. Fr.* **35,** 521 (1977). Identity with toddaline: Govindachari, Thyagarajan, *J. Chem. Soc.* **1956,** 769. Synthesis of chelerythrine chloride: Bailey, Worthing, *ibid.* 4535; S. V. Kessar *et al., J. Org. Chem.* **53,** 1708 (1988). Pharmacology: Chelombit'o, Murav'eva, *Aktual. Probl. Farmakol. Farm. Vses. Nauchn. Konf.* **1971,** 183, *C.A.* **76,** 112g (1972).

Crystals from chloroform + methanol, mp 207° [Manske, *Can. J. Res.* **21B,** 140 (1943)]. The free base is colorless, but its quaternary salts are yellow. Aq solns of base and salts show violet fluorescence. uv spectrum of chelerythrine chloride: Hruban *et al., Collect. Czech. Chem. Commun.* **35,** 3420 (1970).

2052. Chelidonic Acid. [99-32-1] 4-Oxo-4*H*-pyran-2,6-dicarboxylic acid; 4-oxo-1,4-pyran-2,6-dicarboxylic acid; Jerva acid; jervasic acid. $C_7H_4O_6$; mol wt 184.10. C 45.67%, H 2.19%, O 52.14%. Presence in various plants: Stransky, *Arch. Pharm.* **258,** 56 (1920); Ramstad, *Pharm. Acta Helv.* **28,** 45 (1953). Structure: Verkade, *Recl. Trav. Chim. Pays-Bas* **43,** 879 (1924). Synthesis: Riegel, Reinhard, *J. Am. Chem. Soc.* **48,** 1334 (1926); Riegel, Zwilgmeyer, *Org. Synth.* coll. vol. II, 126 (1943); Toomey, Riegel, *J. Org. Chem.* **17,** 1492 (1952).

HOOC — O — COOH

Crystals, dec 257°. uv max (water): 270 nm (ε 11500). One gram dissolves in 65 ml water, 26 ml boiling water. Sparingly sol in alc.

Monohydrate. Monoclinic crystals from hot alcohol + water. The water of crystn is given up when heated at 102° and then at 160° to constant weight.

Sodium salt. Sparingly sol in water.

2053. Chelidonine. Stylophorin. $C_{20}H_{19}NO_5$; mol wt 353.37. C 67.98%, H 5.42%, N 3.96%, O 22.64%. Hexahydro-benzophenanthridine alkaloid. Occurs in nature in (+)-form, (−)-form and racemic form. Isoln of (+)-form from root of *Chelidonium majus* L., *Stylophorum diphyllum* (Michx.) Nutt., and *Dicranostigma franchetianum* (Prain) Fedde, *Papaveraceae:* J. M. Probst, *Ann.* **29,** 113 (1839); E. Schmidt, F. Selle, *Arch. Pharm.* **228,** 441 (1890); F. Selle, *ibid.* 96; Manske, *Can. J. Res.* **20B,** 53 (1942); J. Slavik, *Collect. Czech. Chem. Commun.* **20,** 198 (1955); from *Symphoricarpos albus* L., Blake, *Caprifoliaceae:* M. Szaufer *et al., Phytochemistry* **17,** 1446 (1978). Isoln of (−)-form from *Glaucium*

corniculatum Curt., *Papaveraceae:* J. Slavik, L. Slavikova, *Collect. Czech. Chem. Commun.* **22,** 279 (1957). Structure: F. von Bruchhausen, H. W. Bersch, *Ber.* **63,** 2520 (1930); E. Späth, F. Kuffner, *ibid.* **64,** 370 (1931); H. W. Bersch, *Arch. Pharm.* **291,** 491 (1958). Identity of (±)-form with diphylline: J. Slavik, *Collect. Czech. Chem. Commun.* **26,** 2933 (1961). Absolute configuration of (+)-*p*-bromobenzoate: N. Takao *et al., Tetrahedron Lett.* **1979,** 495. Conformation: M. Cushman, T.-C. Choong, *Heterocycles* **14,** 1935 (1980); M. Sugiura *et al., J. Chem. Soc. Perkin Trans. 2* **1986,** 175. Chiroptic properties and absolute configuration of (+)-chelidonine: N. Takao *et al., Arch. Pharm.* **317,** 223 (1984). Biosynthesis: E. Leete, *J. Am. Chem. Soc.* **85,** 473 (1963). Total synthesis of (±)-form: W. Oppolzer, K. Keller, *ibid.* **93,** 3836 (1971); M. Cushman *et al., J. Org. Chem.* **45,** 5067 (1980); W. Oppolzer, C. Rabbiani, *Helv. Chim. Acta* **66,** 1119 (1983); M. Hanaoka *et al., Chem. Lett.* **1986,** 736. Effect on smooth muscle: P. J. Hanzlik: *J. Pharmacol. Exp. Ther.* **7,** 99 (1915). Inhibition of reverse transcriptase activity: M. L. Sethi, *Can. J. Pharm. Sci.* **16,** 29 (1981). Cytotoxic effects: M. Cushman *et al., loc. cit.* Review of pharmacological effects: V. Preininger, "The Biology of Papaveraceae Alkaloids" in *The Alkaloids* **vol. 15,** R. H. F. Manske, Ed. (Academic Press, Orlando, 1975) pp 241-242. General review: V. Simanek, "Benzophenanthridine Alkaloids" *ibid.* **vol. 26,** A. Brossi, Ed. (1985) pp 185-240. Toxicity data: R. C. Anderson, K. K. Chen, *Fed. Proc.* **5,** 163 (1946).

(+)-form

(+)-Form. [476-32-4] [5b*R*-(5bα,6β,12bα)]-5b,6,7,12b,13,14-Hexahydro-13-methyl[1,3]benzodioxolo[5,6-c]-1,3-dioxolo[4,5-i]-phenanthridin-6-ol. Monoclinic prisms from methanol, ethanol or ethanol + chloroform, mp 135-136°. bp₀.₀₀₂ 220° (air-bath temp). $[\alpha]_D^{22}$ +115 ±3° (ethanol); $[\alpha]_D^{20}$ +117° (c = 3 in CHCl₃). uv max (methanol): 289, 239, 208 nm (log ε 3.89, 3.88, 4.69). Sol in alc, chloroform, ether, amyl alc. Practically insol in water. LD₅₀ in mice (mg/kg): 34.6 ±2.44 i.v. (Anderson, Chen).

(+)-O-Acetylchelidonine. $C_{22}H_{21}NO_6$. Crystals from chloroform, mp 184-186°. $[\alpha]_D$ +110°.

(+)-Benzoylchelidonine. $C_{27}H_{23}NO_6$. Crystals from chloroform, mp 210-211°.

(−)-Form. [88200-01-5] Crystals from aqueous ethanol, mp 136°. $[\alpha]_D^{22}$ −112 ±3° (c = 0.47 in ethanol).

(±)-Form. [20267-87-2] Diphylline. Crystals from ethanol, mp 215-216°.

2054. Chenodiol. [474-25-9] (3α,5β,7α)-3,7-Dihydroxy-cholan-24-oic acid; 3α,7α-dihydroxy-5β-cholanic acid; anthropodesoxycholic acid; gallodesoxycholic acid; 17β-(1-methyl-3-carboxypropyl)etiocholane-3α,7α-diol; chenic acid; chenodeoxycholic acid; CDC; Chendol; Chenocol; Chenofalk; Chenossil; Cholanorm; Fluibil. $C_{24}H_{40}O_4$; mol wt 392.57. C 73.43%, H 10.27%, O 16.30%. A major bile acid in many vertebrates, occurring as the *N*-glycine and/or *N*-taurine conjugate. With other bile acids, forms mixed micelles with lecithin in bile which solubilize cholesterol and thus facilitates its excretion. Facilitates fat absorption in the small intestine by micellar solubilization of fatty acids and monoglicerides. Has cathartic properties since it induces fluid secretion from large intestine. Main constituent of the bile of hens, geese and other fowl; occurs in appreciable amounts in the bile of hamster, hog, guinea pig, bear and man. Epimeric with ursodiol, *q.v.* Isoln: Windhaus *et al., Z. Physiol. Chem.* **140,** 177 (1924); Wieland, Reveney, *ibid.* 186. Configuration: Lettré, *Ber.* **68,** 766 (1935). Prepn from cholic acid: Fieser, Rajagopalan, *J. Am. Chem. Soc.* **72,** 5530 (1950); Hauser *et al., Helv. Chim. Acta* **43,** 1595 (1960); Hofmann, *Acta Chem. Scand.* **17,** 173 (1963). Alternate prepns: Sato, Ikekawa, *J. Org. Chem.* **24,** 1367 (1959); T. Iida, F. C. Chang, *ibid.* **46,** 2786 (1981). Stereoselective total synthesis: T. Kametani *et al., J.*

Am. Chem. Soc. **103,** 2890 (1981). Asymmetric total synthesis of (+)-form: *eidem, J. Org. Chem.* **47,** 2331 (1982). Dissolution of cholesterol gallstones: Danzinger *et al., N. Engl. J. Med.* **286,** 1 (1972); Bell *et al., Lancet* **II,** 1213 (1972). Use in long-term treatment of cerebrotendinous xanthomatosis: V. M. Berginer *et al., N. Engl. J. Med.* **311,** 1649 (1984). Monograph on bile acids: *The Bile Acids,* 2 vols., P. P. Nair, D. Kritchevsky, Eds. (Plenum Press, New York, 1971, 1973). Review of pharmacology and therapeutic use of chenodeoxycholic acid: J. H. Iser, A. Sali, *Drugs* **21,** 90-119 (1981). Effect on cholesterol and bile acid metabolism: G. S. Tint *et al., Gastroenterology* **91,** 1007 (1986).

Needles from ethyl acetate + heptane, mp 119°. $[\alpha]_D^{20}$ +11.5° (dioxane). Freely sol in methanol, alc, acetone, acetic acid; more sol in ether and ethyl acetate than deoxycholic acid. Practically insol in water, petr ether, benzene. High solvent power for alkali soaps, but does not form "choleic" acid addition compds as does deoxycholic acid. Forms beautiful cryst salts of Na, K and Ba. While the acid is tasteless, the Na salt tastes slightly sweet at first, then bitter.

Diformate. $C_{25}H_{40}O_6$. Clusters of needles from alc; mp with slight effervescence at 137°, upon further heating solidifies again, and finally melts around 172°.

Methyl ester. $C_{25}H_{42}O_4$. Fine needles from benzene + heptane, mp 90-91°. $[\alpha]_D^{25}$ +20°.

THERAP CAT: Anticholelithogenic.

2055. CHES. [103-47-9] 2-(Cyclohexylamino)ethanesulfonic acid; *N*-cyclohexyltaurine. $C_8H_{17}NO_3S$; mol wt 207.29. C 46.35%, H 8.27%, N 6.76%, O 23.16%, S 15.47%. Zwitterionic *N*-substituted aminosulfonic acid in the style of the "Good" buffers; active in the pH range 8.6-10.0. Synthesis: A. Champseix *et al., Bull. Soc. Chim. Fr.* **1985,** 463. Effects of freezing on buffering: D. L. Williams-Smith *et al., Biochem. J.* **167,** 593 (1977). Effects on Lowry protein assay: C. Cookson, *Anal. Biochem.* **88,** 340 (1978). Dissociation constants and buffering capacity: M. J. Taylor, Y. Pignat, *Cryobiology* **19,** 99 (1982). Use as buffer: M. G. N. Hartmanis, T. C. Stadtman, *Proc. Natl. Acad. Sci. USA* **84,** 76 (1987); C. Engstrand *et al., Biochim. Biophys. Acta* **1122,** 321 (1992).

Crystals, mp 320°. pKa in water (25°) 9.27 ±0.01; in 20% (w/w) DMSO (25°) 9.10, (0°) 9.76, (−5.5°) 10.01; in 30% (w/w) DMSO (25°) 9.11, (0°) 9.89, (−12°) 10.27.

USE: Biological buffer.

2056. Chicle. The partially evaporated, milky juice from *Manilkara zapotilla* (Jacq.) Gilly *(Achras sapota* L.*), Sapotaceae. Habit.* West Indies, Mexico and Central America.

USE: In the chewing gum industry.

2057. Chimaphila. Pipsissewa; Prince's pine; bitter wintergreen; rheumatism weed; ground holly; pyrola; pine tulip. Dried leaves of *Chimaphila umbellata* (L.) Nutt., *Ericaceae. Habit.* Europe, Asia, North America. *Constit.* Chimaphilin, arbutin, ericolin, urson, tannin, resin.

THERAP CAT: Urinary antiseptic.

2058. Chimaphilin. [482-70-2] 2,7-Dimethyl-1,4-naphthalenedione; 2,7-dimethyl-1,4-naphthoquinone. $C_{12}H_{10}O_2$; mol wt

186.21. C 77.40%, H 5.41%, O 17.18%. From *Chimaphila carymbosa* Pursh. and *Pyrola incarnata* (Fisch.) Fernald, *Ericaceae:* DiModica *et al., Gazz. Chim. Ital.* **83,** 393 (1953); Inouye, *J. Pharm. Soc. Jpn.* **76,** 976 (1956). Structure: DiModica, Tira, *Gazz. Chim. Ital.* **86,** 234 (1956).

Yellow needles, mp 113.5-114.5°. uv max (alc): 233, 256, 339 nm. Polymerizes in sunlight to needles, mp 232-233°.

Diacetate. Crystals from ethanol + water, mp 90.5-91.5°.

2059. Chimonanthine. [5545-89-1] 1-Demethylcalycanthidine. $C_{22}H_{26}N_4$; mol wt 346.47. C 76.27%, H 7.56%, N 16.17%. From leaves of *Chimonanthus fragrans* Lindle, *Calicanthaceae:* Hodson *et al., Proc. Chem. Soc. London* **1961,** 465. Structure: Clayton *et al., Tetrahedron* **18,** 1495 (1962). Synthesis: Hendrickson *et al., Proc. Chem. Soc. London* **1962,** 383; Scott *et al., J. Am. Chem. Soc.* **86,** 302 (1964); Hall *et al., Tetrahedron* **23,** 4131 (1967).

Crystals, mp 188-189°. Weak diacidic base of equivalent weight 173. uv max: 246, 304 nm.

Dimethiodide. Crystals, dec 235-236°.

2060. Chimyl Alcohol. [506-03-6] (+)-3-(Hexadecyloxy)-1,2-propanediol; α-hexadecylglyceryl ether; testriol. $C_{19}H_{40}O_3$; mol wt 316.52. C 72.10%, H 12.74%, O 15.16%. $CH_3(CH_2)_{15}$-$OCH_2CHOHCH_2OH$. Isoln from bull and boar testes: Hirano, *J. Pharm. Soc. Jpn.* **56,** 122 (1936); Prelog *et al., Helv. Chim. Acta* **27,** 674 (1944). Synthesis: Baer, Fischer, *J. Biol. Chem.* **140,** 397 (1941).

Leaflets from hexane, mp 64°. $bp_{0.005}$ 120°. $[\alpha]_D^{20}$ +3.0° (c = 1.16 in chloroform). Sol in acetone, hexane, chloroform.

Bis(phenylurethan). $C_{33}H_{50}N_2O_5$. Leaflets from petr ether, mp 97.5-98.5°.

2061. Chinese Wax. The excretion of an insect, *Coccus ceriferus* Fabr., or *C. pela* Westwood, deposited on the twigs and branches of a species of ash tree in Western China. Chief constituent is ceryl cerotate.

White to yellowish-white, practically odorless, tasteless solid. d ~0.93. mp ~92°. Solidif 80-81°. Sapon no. 80-92. Iodine no. 1.4. Acid no. 63. Insol in water; freely sol in benzene, slightly in alcohol or ether.

USE: Manuf candles, leather and furniture polish; treating silk and cotton fabrics; sizing and glazing papers.

2062. Chirald. [38345-66-3] (αS)-α-[(1R)-2-(Dimethylamino)-1-methylethyl]-α-phenylbenzeneethanol; (+)-oxyphene; (2S,3R)-(+)-4-dimethylamino-3-methyl-1,2-diphenyl-2-butanol; Darvon alcohol. $C_{19}H_{25}NO$; mol wt 283.41. C 80.52%, H 8.89%, N 4.94%, O 5.65%. Asymmetric reducing agent. Prepn of racemate: W. G. Stoll *et al., Helv. Chim. Acta* **33,** 1194 (1950). Resolution of enantionmers: A. Pohland, H. R. Sullivan, *J. Am. Chem. Soc.* **77,** 3400 (1955). Asymmetric synthesis: T. J. Erickson, *J. Org. Chem.* **51,** 934 (1986). HPLC determn as an impurity in dextropropoxyphene, *q.v.*: S. Kryger, P. Helboe, *J. Chromatogr.* **539,** 186 (1991). Use as an enantioselective reducing agent: M. N.

Nefedova *et al., J. Organomet. Chem.* **425,** 125 (1992); D. R. Williams *et al., Tetrahedron Lett.* **41,** 9397 (2000).

mp 55-57°. bp$_{0.1\ mm}$ 138-139°. Flash point: >230°F. $[\alpha]^{21}$ +8.2° (c = 10 in ethanol).

Note: Also referred to in the literature as Mosher's reagent, *q.v.*

USE: Reducing reagent in organic synthesis.

2063. (S,S)-Chiraphos. [64896-28-2] [(1S,2S)-1,2-Dimethyl-1,2-ethanediyl]bis[diphenylphosphine]; (2S,3S)-(−)-bis(diphenylphosphino)butane. $C_{28}H_{28}P_2$; mol wt 426.47. C 78.86%, H 6.62%, P 14.53%. Chiral, bidentate phosphine ligand in asymmetric catalysis. Prepn: M. D. Fryzuk, B. Bosnich, *J. Am. Chem. Soc.* **99,** 6262 (1977); J. F. G. Jansen, B. L. Feringa, *Tetrahedron: Asymmetry* **1,** 719 (1990); S. H. Bergens *et al., Inorg. Synth.* **31,** 131 (1997). ^{1}H and ^{31}P NMR of platinum complexes: N. C. Payne, D. W. Stephan, *J. Organomet. Chem.* **221,** 203 (1981). Synthetic applications: C. Moinet, J.-C. Fiaud, *Tetrahedron Lett.* **36,** 2051 (1995); H. Frauenrath *et al., Tetrahedron: Asymmetry* **9,** 1103 (1998); K. Akiyama *et al., Adv. Synth. Catal.* **347,** 1569 (2005).

Large, colorless plates from absolute ethanol, mp 108-109°. $[\alpha]_D^{27}$ −211° (c = 1.5 in CHCl$_3$). Sol in acetone, THF, dichloromethane, chloroform, diethyl ether, toluene, hot ethanol. Insol in hexanes, methanol, cold ethanol.

USE: Ligand for palladium-catalyzed carbon-carbon bond formation.

2064. Chirata. Chiretta; chirayita; bitter stick; East Indian balmony. Dried plant, *Swertia (Ophelia) chirata* (Roxb.) Buch.-Ham., *Gentianaceae. Habit.* India (Himalaya). *Constit.* Chiratin, ophelic acid.

THERAP CAT: Bitter tonic, antimalarial.

2065. Chitin. [1398-61-4] $(C_8H_{13}NO_5)_n$. C 47.29%, H 6.45%, N 6.89%, O 39.37%. Cellulose-like biopolymer consisting predominantly of unbranched chains of β-(1 → 4)-2-acetamido-2-deoxy-D-glucose (also named *N*-acetyl-D-glucosamine) residues. Found in fungi, yeasts, marine invertebrates and arthropods, where it is a principal component in the exoskeletons. May be regarded as a derivative of cellulose, in which the C-2 hydroxyl groups have been replaced by acetamido residues. Occurrence in lower animals: A. G. Richards, *The Integument of Arthropods* (University of Minnesota Press, Minneapolis, 1951). Occurrence in the plant kingdom: F. von Wettstein, *Handbuch der systematischen Botanik* (F. Deuticke, Leipzig and Vienna, 4th ed., 1933). Typical isoln: Hackman, *Aust. J. Biol. Sci.* **7,** 168 (1954); Horowitz *et al., J. Am. Chem. Soc.* **79,** 5046 (1957). Occurrence in the anthozoan *Stylobates aeneus* Dall, the first sea anemone proved capable of synthesizing chitin: D. F. Dunn, M. H. Liberman, *Science* **221,** 157 (1983). Structure: Dweltz, *Biochim. Biophys. Acta* **44,** 416 (1960); **51,** 283 (1961); Carlstrom, *ibid.* **59,** 361 (1962); Ramachadran, Ramakrishman, *ibid.* **63,** 307 (1962). *Review:* Foster, Webber, *Adv. Carbohydr. Chem.* **15,** 371-393 (1960); C. Jeuniaux, "Chitinous Structures" in *Comprehensive Biochemistry* **vol. 26c,** M. Florkin, E. H. Stotz, Eds. (Elsevier, New York, 1971) pp 595-632. Book: R. A.

A. Muzzarelli, *Chitin* (Pergamon Press, New York, 1977). Review of properties and possible novel applications: P. R. Austin *et al., Science* **212,** 749-753 (1981).

Amorphous solid. Practically insol in water, dil acids, dil and concd alkalies, alcohol and other organic solvents; sol in concd HCl, H_2SO_4, 78-97% H_3PO_4, anhyd HCOOH. There are substantial variations in solubility, molecular weight, acetyl values, specific rotation among chitins of different origins and prepared by different methods.

Acetate. Prepn: Shorigin, Hait, *Ber.* **68,** 971 (1935). Sol in HCOOH, 50% resorcinol, concd HCl, H_2SO_4, HNO$_3$; practically insol in organic solvents.

Sulfate. Process for sulfating chitin: Cushing, Kratovil, **US 2755275** (1956 to Abbott). Sulfated chitin has been found to possess anticoagulant properties in laboratory animals: Roth *et al., Am. J. Physiol.* **171,** 761 (1952); *Proc. Soc. Exp. Biol. Med.* **86,** 315 (1954).

USE: Deacylated chitin, *chitosan,* used in water treatment; in photographic emulsions; in improving the dyeability of synthetic fibers and fabrics.

THERAP CAT: Vulnerary.

2066. Chlophedianol. [791-35-5] 2-Chloro-α-[2-(dimethylamino)ethyl]-α-phenylbenzenemethanol; 2-chloro-α-(2-dimethylaminoethyl)benzhydrol; 1-*o*-chlorophenyl-1-phenyl-3-dimethylamino-1-propanol; 1-phenyl-1-(*o*-chlorophenyl)-3-dimethylaminopropanol; α-(dimethylaminoethyl)-*o*-chlorobenzhydrol; clofedanol; Tussistop. $C_{17}H_{20}ClNO$; mol wt 289.80. C 70.46%, H 6.96%, Cl 12.23%, N 4.83%, O 5.52%. Prepn: Henecka, Lorenz, **DE 1083277** (1960); Lorenz *et al.,* **US 3031377** (1962, both to Bayer).

mp 120°. LD$_{50}$ i.v. in mice: 70 mg/kg (Lorenz).

Hydrochloride. [511-13-7] Coldrin; Pectolitan; Refugal; Ulone; ULO. $C_{17}H_{20}ClNO\cdot HCl$; mol wt 326.26. Crystals, mp 190-191°. Freely sol in water, methanol, ethanol. Sparingly sol in ether, benzene, ethyl acetate. LD$_{50}$ orally in rats: 350 mg/kg; s.c. in mice: 95 mg/kg (Lorenz).

THERAP CAT: Antitussive.

2067. Chloracetyl Chloride. [79-04-9] $C_2H_2Cl_2O$; mol wt 112.94. C 21.27%, H 1.78%, Cl 62.78%, O 14.17%. ClCH$_2$COCl. Prepn from chloroacetic acid and benzoyl chloride: Brown, *J. Am. Chem. Soc.* **60,** 1325 (1938); by chlorination of ketene: Erickson, Prill, *J. Org. Chem.* **23,** 141 (1958); Prill, **US 2889365** (1959 to Monsanto); from chloroacetic acid and pyrocatechylphosphorus trichloride: Gross, Gloede, *Ber.* **96,** 1387 (1963). Manuf from chloroacetic acid and POCl$_2$: MacKenzie, Morris, **US 2848491** (1958 to Dow); from ketene: Prill, **US 2889365** (1959 to Monsanto). Physical data: McDonald *et al., J. Chem. Eng. Data* **4,** 311 (1959).

Liquid, very pungent odor. bp 106°. mp −21.77°. d$_4^{20}$ 1.4202. n_D^{20} 1.4541. Dec by water. *Protect from moisture.*

Caution: Potential symptoms of overexposure are irritation of eyes, skin, respiratory system; eye and skin burns; cough, wheezing, dyspnea, lacrimation. *See NIOSH Pocket Guide to Chemical Hazards* (DHHS/NIOSH 97-140, 1997) p 60.

USE: In the synthesis of organic compounds.

2068. Chloracizine. [800-22-6] 2-Chloro-10-[3-(diethylamino)-1-oxopropyl]-10*H*-phenothiazine; 2-chloro-10-(*N*,*N*-diethyl-β-alanyl)phenothiazine; 10-(β-diethylaminopropionyl)-2-chlorophenothiazine; 2-chloro-10-(β-diethylaminopropionyl)phenothiazine; chloracysin; chlorocyzine; chlorocizin; khloratsizin; G-020. $C_{19}H_{21}ClN_2OS$; mol wt 360.90. C 63.23%, H 5.86%, Cl 9.82%, N 7.76%, O 4.43%, S 8.88%. Prepn: Horclois, Metivier, **FR 1060715** (1954 to Rhône Poulenc); **GB 740932** (1955); Zhuravlev, Gritsenko, *Zh. Obshch. Khim.* **26**, 3385 (1956), *C.A.* **51**, 9623h (1957). For other prepns in Russian journals *see C.A.* **55**, 6484b, 9425a (1961).

Hydrochloride. $C_{19}H_{21}ClN_2OS.HCl$. Crystals from isopropanol, mp 168-169°. Sol in water.

THERAP CAT: Vasodilator (coronary).

2069. Chloral Alcoholate. [515-83-3] 2,2,2-Trichloro-1-ethoxyethanol; chloral ethylalcoholate; trichloroacetaldehyde monoethylacetal. $C_4H_7Cl_3O_2$; mol wt 193.46. C 24.83%, H 3.65%, Cl 54.98%, O 16.54%. Prepd by refluxing trichloroacetaldehyde or chloral hydrate with alcohol: Personne, *Compt. Rend.* **69**, 1363 (1869); Magnani, McElvain, *J. Am. Chem. Soc.* **60**, 2212 (1938); Post, *J. Org. Chem.* **6**, 830 (1941).

Crystals, d 1.143. mp 47.5°. bp₇₆₀ 116°. Less sol in water than chloral hydrate. Sol in organic solvents. With concd H_2SO_4 it forms trichloroacetaldehyde and ethyl sulfate.

2070. Chloral Formamide. [515-82-2] *N*-(2,2,2-Trichloro-1-hydroxyethyl)formamide; chloralamide; chloramide. $C_3H_4Cl_3$-NO_2; mol wt 192.43. C 18.72%, H 2.10%, Cl 55.27%, N 7.28%, O 16.63%. $HCONHCH(OH)CCl_3$. Prepn or manuf from chloral and formamide: Bennett, Campbell, *Q. J. Pharm. Pharmacol.* **8**, 398 (1955); and herbicidal activity: Reuter, Sehring, **DE 1168161** (1964 to Boehringer, Ing.), *C.A.* **62**, 1024g (1965).

Crystals from water of 30% alc, mp 124-126°, also reported as 115-116° (Bennett, Campbell). Soluble in water; readily sol in alcohol, ether, glycerol, acetone, ethyl acetate. Dec by hot solvents.

THERAP CAT: Sedative, hypnotic.

2071. Chloral Hydrate. [302-17-0] 2,2,2-Trichloro-1,1-ethanediol; trichloroacetaldehyde monohydrate; Escre; Noctec; Nycton; Somnos; Chloraldurat. $C_2H_3Cl_3O_2$; mol wt 165.40. C 14.52%, H 1.83%, Cl 64.30%, O 19.35%. Made by adding the required amount of water to trichloroacetaldehyde, *q.v.* First synthesized by Liebig in 1832. Introduced as hypnotic by Liebreich in 1869. Comprehensive description: J. E. Fairbrother, *Anal. Profiles Drug Subs.* **2**, 85-143 (1973). Toxicity data: E. Goldenthal, *Toxicol. Appl. Pharmacol.* **18**, 185 (1971). Evaluation of mutagenicity: J. Leuschner, F. Leuschner, *Arzneim.-Forsch.* **41**, 1101 (1991).

Monohydrate. Large, monoclinic plates. Perfect 001 cleavage. Skin irritant. Aromatic, penetrating and sightly acrid odor, slightly bitter, caustic taste. Slowly volatilizes on exposure to air. d 1.91. mp 57° when heated in an open vessel. bp 98° with dissociation into chloral and water. Freely sol in water. One ml of water dissolves the following amounts of chloral hydrate: 2.4 g at 0°; 8.3 g at 25°, 14.3 g at 40°. One gram of chlorate hydrate dissolves in 1.3 ml

alcohol, in 2 ml chloroform, in 1.5 ml ether, in 1.4 ml olive oil, in 0.5 glycerol, in 68 g carbon disulfide. Freely sol in acetone, methyl ethyl ketone. Moderately or sparingly sol in turpentine, petr ether, carbon tetrachloride, benzene, toluene. Dissociation in water: Piguet *et al.*, *Helv. Chim. Acta* **46**, 406 (1963). An alcoholic soln of chloral hydrate (1 in 20) does not at once redden moistened blue litmus paper. Dec by NaOH into chloroform. Reduces ammoniacal $AgNO_3$. Liquefies when triturated with an equal quantity of menthol, camphor or thymol. LD₅₀ orally in rats: 479 mg/kg (Goldenthal).

Note: This is a controlled substance (depressant): **21 CFR, 1308.14**.

USE: Manuf DDT.

THERAP CAT: Sedative, hypnotic.

THERAP CAT (VET): Anesthetic, sedative, hypnotic.

2072. α-Chloralose. [15879-93-3] 1,2-*O*-[(1*R*)-2,2,2-Trichloroethylidene]-α-D-glucofuranose; α-D-glucochloralose; glucochloral; anhydroglucochloral; chloralosane; Alphakil; Somio. $C_8H_{11}Cl_3O_6$; mol wt 309.53. C 31.04%, H 3.58%, Cl 34.36%, O 31.01%. Prepd from anhydr glucose and trichloroacetaldehyde (anhydr chloral); β-chloralose is also formed. Prepn: M. Hanroit, C. Richet, *C.R. Hebd. Seances Acad. Sci.* **116**, 63 (1893); and structure: Pictet, Reichel, *Helv. Chim. Acta* **6**, 621 (1923); Freudenberg, Vajda, *J. Am. Chem. Soc.* **59**, 1955 (1937); *cf.* Coles *et al.*, *ibid.* **51**, 519 (1929); White, Hixon, *ibid.* **55**, 2438 (1933). Crystal structure: T. Taga *et al.*, *Acta Crystallogr.* **B38**, 1874 (1982). Immobilizing agent in control of depredating birds: Redpath *et al.*, *Ann. Appl. Biol.* **49**, 77 (1961). Anesthetic for dogs in experimental work: B. G. Bass, N. M. Buckley, *Am. J. Physiol.* **210**, 854 (1966); R. H. Cox, *ibid.* **223**, 660 (1972). CNS depressant activity: J. L. Barker, *Nature* **252**, 52 (1974). GLC determn in rodenticides: J. Theobald, *J. Chromatogr.* **129**, 444 (1976); in tissue: E. Odam *et al.*, *Analyst* **109**, 1335 (1984). Acute toxicity: E. W. Schafer, *Toxicol. Appl. Pharmacol.* **21**, 315 (1971). Review of pharmacology: G. U. Balis, R. R. Monroe, *Psychopharmacologia* **6**, 1-30 (1964); and toxicology: P. Lees, *Vet. Rec.* **91**, 330-333 (1972). Review as canine anesthetic: H. Holzgrefe *et al.*, *Lab. Anim. Sci.* **37**, 587-595 (1987).

Needles from alcohol or ether, mp 187°. $[\alpha]_D^{22}$ +19° (c = 5 in 98% alc). One gram dissolves in 225 ml water at 15°, in 120 ml at 37°, in 15 ml alc at 25°. Sol in ether, glacial acetic acid; slightly in chloroform. Almost insol in petr ether. LD₅₀ orally in mice: 400 mg/kg (Schafer).

β-Chloralose. mp 227-230°, is much less sol in water, alcohol, and ether.

USE: Rodenticide. Control of avian pests.

THERAP CAT: Sedative, hypnotic.

THERAP CAT (VET): Surgical anesthetic for laboratory animals.

2073. Chlorambucil. [305-03-3] 4-[Bis(2-chloroethyl)amino]benzenebutanoic acid; 4-[*p*-[bis(2-chloroethyl)amino]phenyl]butyric acid; γ-[*p*-di(2-chloroethyl)aminophenyl]butyric acid; *N*,*N*-di-2-chloroethyl-γ-*p*-aminophenylbutyric acid; chloraminophene; chloroambucil; CB-1348; Leukeran. $C_{14}H_{19}Cl_2NO_2$; mol wt 304.21. C 55.27%, H 6.30%, Cl 23.31%, N 4.60%, O 10.52%. Nitrogen mustard deriv. Prepn: W. C. J. Ross *et al.*, **GB 727336**; *eidem*, **US 2944079** (1955, 1960 both to Nat. Res. Dev. Corp.); Everett *et al.*, *J. Chem. Soc.* **1953**, 2390. Improved process: Phillips, Mentha, **US 3046301** (1962 to Burroughs Wellcome). Chemotherapeutic activity: Van Putten *et al.*, *Eur. J. Cancer* **7**, 11 (1971). Toxicity: W. C. J. Ross, *Biochem. Pharmacol.* **13**, 969 (1964). Review of carcinogenicity studies: *IARC Monographs* **9**, 125-134 (1975). Comprehensive description: M. Tariq, A. A. Al-Badr, *Anal. Profiles Drug Subs.* **16**, 85-118 (1987).

Flattened needles from petr ether, mp 64-66°. Sol in ether. Sol (20°) in 1.5 parts alcohol, in 2.5 parts chloroform, in 2 parts acetone. Practically insol in water. LD$_{50}$ i.p. in rats: 58.2 μmole/kg (Ross).

Caution: This substance is listed as a known human carcinogen: *Report on Carcinogens, Eleventh Edition* (PB2005-104914, 2004) p III-47.

THERAP CAT: Antineoplastic.

THERAP CAT (VET): Antineoplastic agent, esp for leukemia.

2074. Chloramine-B. [127-52-6] *N*-Chlorobenzenesulfonamide sodium salt; (*N*-chlorobenzenesulfonamido)sodium; sodium benzenesulfochloramine; Neomagnol. C$_6$H$_5$ClNNaO$_2$S; mol wt 213.62. C 33.73%, H 2.36%, Cl 16.60%, N 6.56%, Na 10.76%, O 14.98%, S 15.01%. C$_6$H$_5$SO$_2$NNaCl. Prepd via benzenesulfonate: Chattaway, *J. Chem. Soc.* **87,** 145 (1905); Cuiban *et al., Pharmazie* **13,** 407 (1958).

Trihydrate. Prisms. Soluble in 20 parts of water, more sol in hot water. Sol in 25 parts of ethanol, yielding a turbid soln. Very sparingly sol in ether, chloroform. An aq soln first turns red litmus paper blue, then gradually bleaches it. Gives a red color wth phenolphthalein.

THERAP CAT: Antibacterial.

THERAP CAT (VET): Antiseptic (topical).

2075. Chloramine-T. [127-65-1] *N*-Chloro-4-methylbenzenesulfonamide sodium salt; (*N*-chloro-*p*-toluenesulfonamido)-sodium; sodium *p*-toluenesulfonchloramide; chloramine; tosylchloramide sodium; Chlorazene; Euclorina; Halamid. C$_7$H$_7$-ClNNaO$_2$S; mol wt 227.64. C 36.93%, H 3.10%, Cl 15.57%, N 6.15%, Na 10.10%, O 14.06%, S 14.09%. Prepd via *p*-toluenesulfonate: Chattaway, *J. Chem. Soc.* **87,** 145 (1905); Inglis, *J. Soc. Chem. Ind. London* **37,** 288 (1918); F. J. Welcher, *Organic Analytical Reagents* **vol. 4** (Van Nostrand, New York, 1948) pp 316-320. Brief review of synthetic applications: G. Agnihotri, *Synlett* **2005,** 2857-2858.

Trihydrate. [7080-50-4] Prisms. Loses water on drying. Dec slowly on exposure to air. *Keep well closed.* Fairly sol in water. Practically insol in benzene, chloroform, ether. Dec by alc.

USE: Detection of bromate and halogens. Source of halonium ions and nitrogen anions in organic synthesis.

THERAP CAT: Antibacterial.

THERAP CAT (VET): Antiseptic (topical).

2076. Chloraminophenamide. [121-30-2] 4-Amino-6-chloro-1,3-benzenedisulfonamide; 4-amino-6-chloro-*m*-benzenedisulfonamide; 5-chloro-2,4-bis(sulfonamido)aniline; 6-amino-4-chlorobenzene-1,3-disulfonamide; 5-chloro-2,4-disulfamylaniline; Idorese. C$_6$H$_8$ClN$_3$O$_4$S$_2$; mol wt 285.73. C 25.22%, H 2.82%, Cl 12.41%, N 14.71%, O 22.40%, S 22.44%. Prepn: Novello, Sprague, *J. Am. Chem. Soc.* **79,** 2028 (1957); Novello, **US 2809194; US 2965655; US 2965656** (1957, 1960, 1960 all to Merck & Co.); Novello *et al., J. Org. Chem.* **25,** 965 (1960).

Crystals from aq ethanol, mp 251-252°. uv max (ethanol): 223.5-224.5, 265-266, 312-314 nm (ε 41776, 18633, 3874). Slightly sol in water; more freely sol in alkalies.

THERAP CAT: Diuretic.

2077. Chloramphenicol. [56-75-7] 2,2-Dichloro-*N*-[(1*R*,2*R*)-2-hydroxy-1-(hydroxymethyl)-2-(4-nitrophenyl)ethyl]-acetamide; D-*threo*-*N*-dichloroacetyl-1-*p*-nitrophenyl-2-amino-1,3-propanediol; D(−)-*threo*-2-dichloroacetamido-1-*p*-nitrophenyl-1,3-propanediol; D-*threo*-*N*-(1,1′-dihydroxy-1-*p*-nitrophenylisopropyl)dichloroacetamide; Aquamycetin; Chlorocid; Chloromycetin; Chloroptic; Fenicol; Pantovernil; Paraxin; Quemicetina; Sintomicetina; Tifomycine; Viceton. C$_{11}$H$_{12}$Cl$_2$N$_2$O$_5$; mol wt 323.13. C 40.89%, H 3.74%, Cl 21.94%, N 8.67%, O 24.76%. Broad spectrum antibiotic obtained from cultures of the soil bacterium *Streptomyces venezuelae:* Bartz, *J. Biol. Chem.* **172,** 445 (1948); Gottlieb *et al., J. Bacteriol.* **55,** 409 (1948); Ehrlich *et al., ibid.* **56,** 467 (1948). Isoln from the moon snail, *Lunatia heros:* C. A. Price *et al., J. Antibiot.* **34,** 118 (1981). Structure: Rebstock *et al., J. Am. Chem. Soc.* **71,** 2458 (1949). Synthesis: Controulis *et al., ibid.* 2463; Long, Troutman, *ibid.* 2469, 2473. *See also* **US 2483871; US 2483884; US 2483892.** Alternate synthesis: Ehrhart *et al., Ber.* **90,** 2088 (1957); **GB 795131; GB 796901** *C.A.* **53,** 2161 (1959) (both to Chinoin); **US 2839577** (1958 to Chinoin). Review and evaluation of toxicity studies: *IARC Monographs* **10,** 85-98 (1976). Review of pharmacology and clinical efficacy: I. Shalit, M. I. Marks, *Drugs* **28,** 281-291 (1984). Comprehensive description: D. Szulczewski, F. Eng, *Anal. Profiles Drug Subs.* **4,** 47-90 (1975); A. A. Al-Badr, H. A. El-Obeid, *ibid.* **15,** 701-760 (1986). *Reviews:* Hahn in *Antibiotics* **vol. 1,** D. Gottlieb, P. D. Shaw, Eds. (Springer-Verlag, New York, 1967) pp 308-330; Pestka, *ibid.* **vol. 3,** J. W. Corcoran, F. E. Hahn, Eds. (1975) pp 370-395; O. Pongs, *ibid.* **vol. 5,** pt. 1, F. E. Hahn, Ed. (1979) pp 26-42.

Needles or elongated plates from water or ethylene dichloride. mp 150.5-151.5°. Sublimes in high vacuum. [α]$_D^{27}$ +18.6° (c = 4.86 in ethanol). [α]$_D^{25}$ −25.5° (ethyl acetate). uv max: 278 nm (E$_{1cm}^{1\%}$ 298). Soly (25°) in water: 2.5 mg/ml; in propylene glycol: 150.8 mg/ml. Very sol in methanol, ethanol, butanol, ethyl acetate, acetone. Fairly sol in ether. Insol in benzene, petr ether, vegetable oils. Soly in 50% acetamide soln about 5%. Additional soly data: Weiss *et al., Antibiot. Chemother.* **7,** 374 (1957). Aq solns are neutral. Neutral and acid solns are stable on heating.

Monosuccinate sodium salt. [982-57-0] Globenicol; Kemicetine. C$_{15}$H$_{15}$Cl$_2$N$_2$NaO$_8$; mol wt 445.18. Freely sol in water (about 50% w/w).

Palmitate. [530-43-8] Chloropal. Prepn: Edgerton, **US 2662906** (1953 to Parke, Davis). Structure: Edgerton *et al., J. Am. Chem. Soc.* **77,** 27 (1955). Description: Glazko *et al., Antibiot. Chemother.* **2,** 234 (1952). Soly data: Weiss *et al., ibid.* **7,** 374 (1957). Crystals from benzene, mp 90°. Practically tasteless. [α]$_D^{26}$ +24.6° (c = 5 in ethanol). uv max (ethanol): 271 nm (E$_{1cm}^{1\%}$ 179). Very slightly sol in water (1.05 mg/ml at 28°); petr ether (0.225 mg/ml). Freely sol in methanol, ethanol, chloroform, ether, benzene.

Monosuccinate arginine salt. [34327-18-9] Chloramphenicol arginine succinate. C$_{21}$H$_{30}$Cl$_2$N$_6$O$_{10}$; mol wt 597.40. mp 135-145° (dec). *See Jpn. Med. Gaz.* **7**(10), 15 (1970).

Pantothenate calcium complex (4:1). [31342-36-6] Chloramphenicol pantothenate. C$_{62}$H$_{80}$CaCl$_4$N$_{10}$O$_{30}$; mol wt 1769.05. Prepn: I. Villax, **GB 866787; GB 866788; GB 866789** (all 1961); I. Villax, **US 3078300** (1963).

Caution: Chloramphenicol is reasonably anticipated to be a human carcinogen: *Report on Carcinogens, Eleventh Edition* (PB2005-104914, 2004) p III-48.

THERAP CAT: Antibacterial; antirickettsial.

THERAP CAT (VET): Antibacterial.

2078. Chloranil. [118-75-2] 2,3,5,6-Tetrachloro-2,5-cyclohexadiene-1,4-dione; 2,3,5,6-tetrachloro-*p*-benzoquinone; tetrachloroquinone; Spergon; Vulklor. C$_6$Cl$_4$O$_2$; mol wt 245.88. C 29.31%, Cl 57.68%, O 13.01%. Prepd from *p*-phenylenediamine or phenol by treating with KClO$_3$ and HCl. Because of its great resistance to further oxidation, chloranil is formed as the final product of the chlorate-HCl oxidation of many aromatic compds. For comprehensive list *see* Huntress, *Organic Chlorine Compounds* (New York, 1948). Laboratory procedure starting with phenol or *p*-chlorophenol: Fierz-David, Blangey, *Grundlegende Operationen der Farbenchemie* (Vienna, 5th ed., 1943) p 140. Use as reagent for pamaquine, *q.v.*, in urine: Schulemann *et al., Chem. Zentralbl.* **1928,** I, 2193. Aqueous decomposition study: D. H. Sarr *et al., Environ. Sci. Technol.* **29,** 2735 (1995). *Review: Health and Environmental Effects Profile for Chloranil* (EPA PB88-219696, 1986) 59 pp.

Golden-yellow platelets from acetic acid or acetone. Monoclinic prisms from benzene or toluene or by sublimation *in vacuo,* mp 290°. Absorption spectrum in chloroform: Lifschitz *et al., Rec. Trav. Chim.* **43,** 276, 658 (1924). Insol in water; almost insol in cold petr ether, cold alcohol. Sol in ether; sparingly sol in chloroform, carbon tetrachloride, carbon disulfide. Solubility data: Dimroth, Bamberger, *Ann.* **438,** 103, 106 (1924).

Caution: Potential symptoms of overexposure are watery diarrhea, CNS depression, coma. Not absorbed percutaneously; direct contact may cause skin irritation. *See Clinical Toxicology of Commercial Products,* R. E. Gosselin *et al.,* Eds. (Williams & Wilkins, Baltimore, 5th ed., 1984) p II-317.

USE: Agricultural fungicide, dye intermediate, reagent. Manuf of electrodes for pH measurement.

2079. Chloranilic Acid. [87-88-7] 2,5-Dichloro-3,6-dihydroxy-2,5-cyclohexadiene-1,4-dione; 2,5-dichloro-3,6-dihydroxy-*p*-benzoquinone. $C_6H_2Cl_2O_4$; mol wt 208.98. C 34.48%, H 0.96%, Cl 33.93%, O 30.62%. Prepd from chloranil by alkaline hydrolysis: Conant, Fieser, *J. Am. Chem. Soc.* **46,** 1866 (1924).

Red crystals, mp 283-284°. Tendency to sublime. Relatively strong dibasic acid. Absorption max (pH 4 in water): 290-340 nm, 520-555 nm.

USE: Reacts with metal cations to form stable salts. Used in spectrophotometry: Hart, *Org. Chem. Bull.* **33,** no. 3 (1961).

2080. Chlorbenzoxamine. [522-18-9] 1-[2-[(2-Chlorophenyl)phenylmethoxy]ethyl]-4-[(2-methylphenyl)methyl]piperazine; 1-[2-(*o*-chloro-α-phenylbenzyloxy)ethyl]-4-*o*-methylbenzyl-piperazine; 1-[2′-(*o*-chlorobenzhydryloxy)ethyl]-4-(*o*-methylbenzyl)diethylenediamine; 1-(*o*-chlorobenzhydryloxyethyl)-4-(*o*-methylbenzyl)piperazine; chlorbenzoxyethamine; chlorobenzoxamine. $C_{27}H_{31}ClN_2O$; mol wt 435.00. C 74.55%, H 7.18%, Cl 8.15%, N 6.44%, O 3.68%. Anticholinergic. Prepn: Morren *et al., Ind. Chim. Belge* **22,** 409 (1957); Morren, *GB 837986* (1960). Toxicity study: Levis *et al., Arch. Int. Pharmacodyn. Ther.* **118,** 167 (1959).

bp$_{0.01}$ 234-236°; bp$_{0.005}$ 235°.

Dihydrochloride. [5576-62-5] UCB-1474; Libratar; Gastomax. $C_{27}H_{31}ClN_2O.2HCl$; mol wt 507.92. Bitter crystals, mp 197-200°. Freely sol in methanol; sol in ethanol, chloroform, acetic acid; slightly sol in water, acetone. Practically insol in acetonitrile, ether, benzene. LD$_{50}$ in rats (mg/kg): 4000 s.c., 66 i.v.; in mice (mg/kg): 1400 orally (Levis).

THERAP CAT: Antispasmodic.

2081. Chlorcyclizine. [82-93-9] 1-[(4-Chlorophenyl)phenylmethyl]-4-methylpiperazine; 1-(*p*-chloro-α-phenylbenzyl)-4-methylpiperazine; 1-(4-chlorobenzhydryl)-4-methylpiperazine; *N*-methyl-*N*′-(4-chlorobenzhydryl)piperazine; chlorocyclizine; compd 47-282; Alergicide; Perazyl; Trihistan. $C_{18}H_{21}ClN_2$; mol wt 300.83. C 71.87%, H 7.04%, Cl 11.79%, N 9.31%. Prepn: Baltzly *et al., J. Org. Chem.* **14,** 775 (1949); Murfitt, Dewing, **GB 656043** (1951 to Wellcome Found.); US 2630435 (1953 to Burroughs Wellcome). Toxicity study: Castillo *et al., J. Pharmacol. Exp. Ther.* **96,** 388 (1949).

Oil, bp$_{0.1-0.15}$ 137-145°.

Hydrochloride. [1620-21-9] AH-289; Di-Paralene; Perazil; Histantin. $C_{18}H_{21}ClN_2.HCl$; mol wt 337.29. Crystalline powder, mp 226-227°. One gram dissolves in about 2 ml water, in 11 ml alc, in about 4 ml chloroform. Practically insol in ether, benzene.

Dihydrochloride. $C_{18}H_{21}ClN_2.2HCl$. Prisms from alc + ether, mp 216-216.5°. Freely sol in water; sol in alc. Aq soln is acid to litmus. LD$_{50}$ i.p. in mice: 137 mg/kg (Castillo).

Di[(*tert*-butyl)naphthalene sodium sulfonate]. Bexedan. C_{18}-$H_{21}ClN_2.2C_{14}H_{15}NaOS$; mol wt 809.47.

THERAP CAT: Antihistaminic.

THERAP CAT (VET): The hydrochloride as antihistaminic.

2082. Chlordan(e). [57-74-9] 1,2,4,5,6,7,8,8-Octachloro-2,3,3a,4,7,7a-hexahydro-4,7-methano-1*H*-indene; 1,2,4,5,6,7,8,8-octachloro-3a,4,7,7a-tetrahydro-4,7-methanoindan; 1,2,4,5,6,7,8,8-octachloro-4,7-methane-3a,4,7,7a-tetrahydroindane; CD-68; Velsicol 1068; Toxichlor; Niran; Octachlor; Ortho-Klor; Synklor; Corodane; Belt. $C_{10}H_6Cl_8$; mol wt 409.78. C 29.31%, H 1.48%, Cl 69.21%. The commercial product is a mixture containing 60 to 75% of the pure compound and 25 to 40% of related compds. Chlorine content: 64-67%. Prepn: Hyman, **GB 618432** (1949); Kleiman, **US 2598561** (1952 to Velsicol). Insecticidal activity: Bussart, Schor, *Soap Sanit. Chem.* **24,** 126 (1948). Toxicity study: R. B. Harbison, *Toxicol. Appl. Pharmacol.* **32,** 443 (1975). Review of toxicology and human exposure: *Toxicological Profile for Chlordane* (PB95-100111, 1994) 262 pp.

Viscous, amber-colored liquid. Viscosity (25°): 69 P (about that of 95% glycerol). Viscosity reduced considerably by heating to 120-140°F when it may be sprayed directly. d^{25} 1.59-1.63. n$_D^{25}$ 1.56-1.57. Insol in water. Miscible with aliphatic and aromatic hydrocarbon solvents, including deodorized kerosene. Loses its chlorine in presence of alkaline reagents, and should not be formulated with any solvent, carrier, diluent or emulsifier, which has an alkaline reaction. LD$_{50}$ i.p. in male rats: 343 mg/kg (Harbison).

Caution: Potential symptoms of overexposure are blurred vision; confusion; ataxia, delirium; coughing; abdominal pain, nausea, vomiting and diarrhea; irritability, tremor, convulsions; anuria. *See NIOSH Pocket Guide to Chemical Hazards* (DHHS/NIOSH 97-140, 1997) p 56. Direct contact may cause skin, eye and mucous membrane irritation. *See Patty's Industrial Hygiene and Toxicology* vol. 2B, G. D. Clayton, F. E. Clayton, Eds. (Wiley-Interscience, New York, 3rd ed., 1981) pp 3718-3725. *See also Clinical Toxicology of Commercial Products,* R. E. Gosselin *et al.,* Eds. (Williams & Wilkins, Baltimore, 5th ed., 1984) Section III, p 108-109.

USE: Insecticide, fumigant.

THERAP CAT (VET): Insecticide, acaricide.

2083. Chlordecone. [143-50-0] 1,1a,3,3a,4,5,5,5a,5b,6-Decachlorooctahydro-1,3,4-metheno-2*H*-cyclobuta[*cd*]pentalen-2-one; GC-1189; Kepone. $C_{10}Cl_{10}O$; mol wt 490.64. C 24.48%, Cl 72.26%, O 3.26%. Prepn: Gilbert, Giolito, **US 2616825** and **US 2616928** (1952 to Allied Chem.); reissued as **US RE 24435** (1958). Structure: McBee *et al., J. Am. Chem. Soc.* **78,** 1511 (1956). *Review:* Ungnade, McBee, *Chem. Rev.* **58,** 249-320 (1958). Toxicity data: T. B. Gaines, *Toxicol. Appl. Pharmacol.* **14,** 515 (1969). Occupational exposure: *Chem. Eng. News* **54,** 19 (Feb. 2, 1976). Comparative toxicity in man and animals: P. S. Guzelian, *Annu. Rev. Pharmacol. Toxicol.* **22,** 89-113 (1982). Review of toxicology and human exposure: *Toxicological Profile for Mirex and Chlordecone* (PB95-264354, 1995) 362 pp.

Crystals, dec 350°. Slightly sol in water and hydrocarbon solvents. Sol in alcohols, ketones, acetic acid. LD_{50} orally in rats: 125 mg/kg (Gaines).

Caution: Potential symptoms of overexposure are headache, nervousness, tremor; liver and kidney damage; visual disturbances; ataxia, chest pain, skin erythema; testicular atrophy, low sperm count. *See NIOSH Pocket Guide to Chemical Hazards* (DHHS/NIOSH 97-140, 1997) p 184. *See also Patty's Industrial Hygiene and Toxicology* vol. **2B,** G. D. Clayton, F. E. Clayton, Eds. (John Wiley & Sons, New York, 4th ed., 1994) 1504-1506, 1545-1550. This substance is reasonably anticipated to be a human carcinogen: *Report on Carcinogens, Eleventh Edition* (PB2005-104914, 2004) p III-158.

USE: Formerly as insecticide, fungicide.

2084. Chlordiazepoxide. [58-25-3] 7-Chloro-*N*-methyl-5-phenyl-3*H*-1,4-benzodiazepin-2-amine 4-oxide; 7-chloro-2-methyl-amino-5-phenyl-3*H*-1,4-benzodiazepine 4-oxide; methaminodiazepoxide; clopoxide; Helogaphen; Libritabs; Multum; Risolid; Silibrin; Tropium. $C_{16}H_{14}ClN_3O$; mol wt 299.75. C 64.11%, H 4.71%, Cl 11.83%, N 14.02%, O 5.34%. Prototype of the benzodiazepine anxiolytics. Prepn: Sternbach, **US 2893992** (1959 to Hoffmann-La Roche); Sternbach, Reeder, *J. Org. Chem.* **26,** 1111 (1961). Comprehensive description: A. MacDonald *et al., Anal. Profiles Drug Subs.* **1,** 15-51 (1972). Review of pharmacokinetics: D. J. Greenblatt *et al., Clin. Pharmacokinet.* **3,** 381-394 (1978); of pharmacology and effect on cognitive function: J. B. Murray, *Genet. Psychol. Monogr.* **109** (2), 167-197 (1984). Clinical trial in alcohol withdrawal: A. K. Burroughs *et al., Alcohol Alcohol.* **20,** 263 (1985).

Light yellow plates from ethanol, mp 236-236.5°. pK 4.8.

Hydrochloride. [438-41-5] Ansiacal; A-Poxide; Balance; Benzodiapin; Cebrum; Corax; Disarim; Elenium; Equibral; Labican; Lentotran; Librium; O.C.M.; Psichial; Psicoterina; Reliberan; Seren Vita; SK-Lygen; Viansin. $C_{16}H_{14}ClN_3O \cdot HCl$; mol wt 336.22. Crystals from methanol, mp 213°. Sol in water.

Note: This is a controlled substance (depressant): **21 CFR,** 1308.14.

THERAP CAT: Anxiolytic.

THERAP CAT (VET): Tranquilizer.

2085. Chlordimeform. [6164-98-3] *N'*-(4-Chloro-2-methylphenyl)-*N,N*-dimethylmethanimidamide; *N'*-(4-chloro-*o*-tolyl)-*N,N*-dimethylformamidine; chlorophenamidine; chlorphenamidine; spanon; CDM; Ciba 8514; Schering 36268; Fundal; Galecron. $C_{10}H_{13}ClN_2$; mol wt 196.68. C 61.07%, H 6.66%, Cl 18.03%, N 14.24%. Member of a class of insecticides possessing the formamidine moiety, effective vs many organophosphate and carbamate resistant pests. Prepn: H. Arndt, W. Steinhausen, **DE 1172081;** *eidem,* **US 3502720** (1964, 1970, both to Schering AG). Acts by interfering with amine regulatory mechanisms: Beeman, Matsumura, *Nature* **242,** 273 (1973); Aziz, Knowles, *ibid.* 417. Review of metabolism: Knowles, *J. Agric. Food Chem.* **18,** 1038 (1970); Degradation products: Witkonton, Ercegovich, *ibid.* **20,** 569 (1972). Toxicity data: C. P. Robinson, P. W. Smith, *J. Toxicol. Environ. Health* **3,** 565 (1977). Toxicological studies: D. S. Folland *et al., J. Am. Med. Assoc.* **13,** 1052 (1978); K. T. Maddy *et al., Toxicol. Lett.* **33,** 37 (1986). Review of carcinogenicity studies: *IARC Monographs* **30,** 61-72 (1983).

Colorless crystals, mp 35°. $bp_{0.4}$ 156-157°. n_D^{25} 1.5885. d_4^{25} 1.105. Vapor pressure at 20°: 3.5×10^{-4} mm. Slightly sol in water; easily sol in organic solvents. LD_{50} i.p. in rats: 238 mg/kg (Robinson, Smith).

USE: Acaricide, insecticide.

2086. Chlorendic Anhydride. [115-27-5] 4,5,6,7,8,8-Hexachloro-3a,4,7,7a-tetrahydro-4,7-methanoisobenzofuran-1,3-dione; 1,4,5,6,7,7-hexachloro-*endo*-5-norbornene-2,3-dicarboxylic anhydride; hexachloroendomethylenetetrahydrophthalic anhydride; 1,4,5,6,7,7-hexachloro-*endo*-bicyclo[2.2.1]hept-5-ene-2,3-dicarboxylic anhydride. $C_9H_2Cl_6O_3$; mol wt 370.83. C 29.15%, H 0.54%, Cl 57.36%, O 12.94%. Prepd from hexachlorocyclopentadiene and maleic anhydride: Herzfeld *et al.,* **US 2606910** (1952 to Velsicol); Baranauckas *et al.,* **US 2903463** (1959 to Hooker Chem.). Purification: Zimmer *et al.,* **DE 1113451** (1961 to Hooker Chem.), *C.A.* **57,** 697a (1962).

Crystals, mp 231-235°.

USE: In prepn of polyester resins.

2087. Chlorethoxyfos. [54593-83-8] Phosphorothioic acid *O,O*-diethyl *O*-(1,2,2,2-tetrachloroethyl) ester; *O,O*-diethyl *O*-(1,2,-2,2-tetrachloroethyl)thionophosphate; DPX-43898; SD-208304; Fortress. $C_6H_{11}Cl_4O_3PS$; mol wt 336.00. C 21.45%, H 3.30%, Cl 42.21%, O 14.29%, P 9.22%, S 9.54%. Soil insecticide for use in corn. Prepn: M. Schnell *et al.,* **DD 107581** (1974); *eidem, J. Prakt. Chem.* **319,** 723 (1977). Physical properties and field trials: I. A. Watkinson, D. W. Sherrod, *Brit. Crop Prot. Conf. - Pests Dis.* **1986,** 107. Persistence in soil: R. A. Chapman *et al., J. Environ Sci. Health* **B28,** 151 (1993). Assessment of volatility losses from soil:

B. W. Fuller *et al., J. Agric. Entomol.* **14,** 399 (1997). Field trials for control of corn rootworm: *eidem, J. Econ. Entomol.* **90,** 1332 (1997).

Colorless liquid, $bp_{0.05 torr}$ 80°. n_D^{25} 1.4980. d_4^{20} 1.464. Also reported as white, crystalline, powder (Watkinson). Soly in water <1 mg/l. Sol in hexane, ethanol, xylene, acetonitrile, chloroform. Vapor pressure at 20°: 8×10^{-4} mm Hg. LD_{50} in rats, mice (mg/kg): 1-10, 20-50 orally; in rabbits (mg/kg): 20-200 dermally (Watkinson).

USE: Insecticide.

2088. Chlorfenapyr. [122453-73-0] 4-Bromo-2-(4-chlorophenyl)-1-(ethoxymethyl)-5-(trifluoromethyl)-1*H*-pyrrole-3-carbonitrile; AC-303630; CL-303630; Pirate; Stalker. $C_{15}H_{11}BrClF_3$-N_2O; mol wt 407.61. C 44.20%, H 2.72%, Br 19.60%, Cl 8.70%, F 13.98%, N 6.87%, O 3.93%. Halogenated pyrrole mitochondrial uncoupler. Prepn: D. G. Brown *et al.,* **BR 8803788;** *eidem,* **US 5010098** (1988, 1991 both to Am. Cyanamid). Chemical and biological properties: J. B. Lovell *et al., Brighton Crop Prot. Conf. - Pests Dis.* **1990,** 37. Summary of field trials: T. P. Miller *et al., ibid.,* 43. Field trials on apples: Y.-J. Ahn *et al., Appl. Entomol. Zool.* **31,** 67 (1996). Mechanism of action: B. C. Black *et al., Pestic. Biochem. Physiol.* **50,** 115 (1994).

White solid, mp 91-92°. Sol in acetone, diethyl ether, DMSO, THF, acetonitrile, alcohols. Insol in water. Log P ~5. LD_{50} (single dose) in male, female rats (mg/kg): 223, 459 orally; in rabbits: >2000 dermally (Lovell). LC_{50} in Japanese carp: 0.5 ppm (Lovell).

USE: Insecticide. Acaricide.

2089. Chlorfenvinphos. [470-90-6] Phosphoric acid 2-chloro-1-(2,4-dichlorophenyl)ethenyl diethyl ester; *O,O*-diethyl *O*-[2-chloro-1-(2,4-dichlorophenyl)vinyl] phosphate; 2,4-dichloro-α-(chloromethylene)benzyl alcohol diethyl phosphate; CVP; SD-7859; Compd 4072; Birlane; Steladone; Supona. $C_{12}H_{14}Cl_3O_4P$; mol wt 359.57. C 40.08%, H 3.92%, Cl 29.58%, O 17.80%, P 8.61%. Organophosphorous insecticide; acetylcholinesterase inhibitor. Commercial prepn contains at least 90% of the active Z-isomer. Prepn: E. E. Gilbert *et al.,* **US 3003916** (1961 to Allied Chemical); Phillips *et al.,* **US 3102842** (1963 to Shell); Whetstone, Phillips *et al., J. Agric. Food Chem.* **14,** 352 (1966). Metabolism: W. F. Chamberlain, D. E. Hopkins, *J. Econ. Entomol.* **55,** 86 (1962); D. H. Hotson *et al., Biochem. J.* **102,** 133 (1967). Toxicity studies: A. M. Ambrose *et al., Toxicol. Appl. Pharmacol.* **17,** 323 (1970); Bunyan *et al., Pestic. Sci.* **2,** 148 (1971). Review of toxicology and human exposure: *Toxicological Profile for Chlorfenvinphos* (PB98-101116, 1997) 220 pp.

Z- isomer

Amber liquid, mild odor, $bp_{0.001}$ 120°, $bp_{0.5}$ 167-170°. Vapor press at 25°C: 7.5×10^{-6} mm Hg. n_D^{25} 1.5272. Soly in water at 23°: 145 ppm. Miscible with acetone, ethanol, propylene glycol.

Slowly hydrolyzed by water. Corrosive to metal. LD_{50} in rats (mg/kg): 6.6 i.v.; 9.66 orally (Ambrose).

Caution: Potential symptoms of overexposure are headache, dizziness, weakness, feeling of anxiety, confusion, runny nose, constriction of pupils, blurred vision, nausea, vomiting, abdominal cramps, slow pulse, diarrhea, difficulty breathing, fainting (PB98-101116).

USE: Insecticide; acaricide.

2090. Chlorguanide. [500-92-5] *N*-(4-Chlorophenyl)-*N'*-(1-methylethyl)imidodicarbonimidic diamide; 1-(*p*-chlorophenyl)-5-isopropylbiguanide; N^1-*p*-chlorophenyl-N^5-isopropyldiguanide; chloroguanide; proguanil. $C_{11}H_{16}ClN_5$; mol wt 253.73. C 52.07%, H 6.36%, Cl 13.97%, N 27.60%. Prepn: Curd, Rose, *J. Chem. Soc.* **1946,** 729; Curd *et al., ibid.* **1948,** 1630; Ainley *et al., ibid.* **1949,** 98. Manuf of acetate: Gailliot, **FR 1001548** (1952 to Rhône-Poulenc), *C.A.* **51,** 7411e (1957). Toxicity study: Schmidt *et al., J. Pharmacol. Exp. Ther.* **90,** 233 (1947).

Rectangular plates from toluene, mp 129°.

Acetate. $C_{11}H_{16}ClN_5 \cdot C_2H_4O_2$. Crystals from acetone, mp 189-190°.

Hydrochloride. [637-32-1] M-4888; RP-3359; SN-12837; Paludrine. $C_{11}H_{16}ClN_5 \cdot HCl$; mol wt 290.19. Crystals from water or aq ethanol, mp 243-244°. uv max (alc): 259 nm. Sol in alc; slightly sol in water. Practically insol in chloroform and ether. pH of satd aq soln 5.8-6.3. LD_{50} orally in rats: 200 mg/kg (Schmidt).

THERAP CAT: Antimalarial.

2091. Chlorhexidine. [55-56-1] *N,N''*-Bis(4-chlorophenyl)-3,12-diimino-2,4,11,13-tetraazatetradecanediimidamide; 1,1'-hexamethylenebis[5-(*p*-chlorophenyl)biguanide]; 1,6-bis[*N'*-(*p*-chlorophenyl)-N^5-biguanido]hexane; 1,6-bis(N^5-*p*-chlorophenyl-*N'*-diguanido)hexane; 1,6-di(4'-chlorophenyldiguanido)hexane; 10040. $C_{22}H_{30}Cl_2N_{10}$; mol wt 505.45. C 52.28%, H 5.98%, Cl 14.03%, N 27.71%. Bisbiguanide with bacteriostatic activity. Prepn: Rose, Swain, *J. Chem. Soc.* **1956,** 4422; *eidem,* **US 2684924** (1954 to I.C.I.). Antibacterial activity and acute toxicity: G. E. Davies *et al., Br. J. Pharmacol.* **9,** 192 (1954). Review of toxicology and clinical uses: D. M. Foulkes, *J. Periodontal Res.* **8,** Suppl. 12, 55-60 (1973). Series of articles on clinical efficacy in gingivitis and plaque control: *ibid.* **21,** Suppl. 16, 1-89 (1986).

Crystals from methanol, mp 134°. Strong alkaline reaction. Soly in water at 20°: 0.08% (w/v).

Dihydrochloride. [3697-42-5] Lisium. $C_{22}H_{30}Cl_2N_{10} \cdot 2HCl$; mol wt 578.37. Crystals, dec 260-262°. Soly in water at 20°: 0.06 g/100 ml.

Diacetate. [56-95-1] Chlorasept 2000; Nolvasan. $C_{22}H_{30}Cl_2$-$N_{10} \cdot 2C_2H_4O_2$; mol wt 625.55. Crystals, mp 154-155°. Neutral reaction. Soly in water at 20°: 1.9 g/100 ml. Aq solns dec when heated above 70°. Soluble in alcohol, glycerol, propylene glycol, polyethylene glycols. LD_{50} orally in mice: 2 g/kg (Davies).

D-Digluconate. [18472-51-0] Chlorhexamed; Bacticlens; Corsodyl; Gingisan; Hibiclens; Hibident; Hibidil; Hibiscrub; Hibital; Hibitane; Peridex; pHiso-Med; Plac Out; Rotersept; Secalan; Sterilon; Unisept. Soly in water at 20°: >50% (w/v). LD_{50} in mice (mg/kg): 22 i.v.; 1800 orally (Foulkes).

THERAP CAT: Antiseptic; disinfectant.

THERAP CAT (VET): Antiseptic; disinfectant.

2092. Chloric Acid. [7790-93-4] $ClHO_3$; mol wt 84.46. Cl 41.98%, H 1.19%, O 56.83%. $HClO_3$. Prepd from barium chlorate and sulfuric acid: Lamb *et al., J. Am. Chem. Soc.* **42,** 1643 (1920); from sodium chlorate using ion-exchange resins: Klement, *Z. Anorg. Allg. Chem.* **260,** 271 (1949).

Known in aq soln only. Aq solns are stable if pure and protected from light. 1% aq soln d_4^{18} 1.0044; 6% soln d_4^{18} 1.0344; 10% soln d_4^{18} 1.0594; 16% soln d_4^{18} 1.0991; 20% soln d_4^{18} 1.1273; 24% soln d_4^{18} 1.1568. A 40% soln corresponds to $HClO_3 \cdot 7H_2O$, d_4^{20} 1.282. If higher concns are attempted by evaporation the soln begins to dec with evolution of chlorine and oxygen and formation of perchloric acid.

Caution: Strongly irritating to skin, mucous membranes.

USE: Oxidizing agent; with H_2SO_3 as catalyst in acrylonitrile polymerization.

2093. Chlorimuron-ethyl. [90982-32-4] 2-[[[[(4-Chloro-6-methoxy-2-pyrimidinyl)amino]carbonyl]amino]sulfonyl]benzoic acid ethyl ester; ethyl 2-[[[[(4-chloro-6-methoxypyrimidin-2-yl)-amino]carbonyl]amino]sulfonyl]benzoate; DPX-F6025; Classic. $C_{15}H_{15}ClN_4O_6S$; mol wt 414.82. C 43.43%, H 3.64%, Cl 8.55%, N 13.51%, O 23.14%, S 7.73%. Selective sulfonylurea herbicide. Prepn: A. D. Wolf, **AT 8316181**; *idem,* **US 4547215** (1984, 1985 both to Du Pont). Effect on plant growth and pigment synthesis: R. M. Devlin, Z. K. Koszanski, *Proc. Annu. Meet. Northeast. Weed Sci. Soc.* **40,** 115 (1986). Metabolism by plants: H. M. Brown, S. M. Neighbors, *Pestic. Biochem. Physiol.* **29,** 112 (1987). Field trial in soybeans: G. N. Rhodes *et al., Tenn. Farm Home Sci.* **142,** 21 (1987). HPLC determn in crops: J. L. Prince, R. A. Guinivan, *J. Agric. Food Chem.* **36,** 63 (1988). Brief review: J. S. Claus, *Weed Technol.* **1,** 114-115 (1987).

Crystals from butyl chloride, mp 198-201°. Soly (ppm): acetone 71000, acetonitrile 31000, benzene 8000, methylene chloride 153000, water (pH 7) 1200, (pH 6.5) 450, (pH 5) 11. LD_{50} in male, female rats (mg/kg): 4102, 4236 orally (Claus).

USE: Herbicide.

2094. Chlorinated Lime. [7778-54-3] Bleaching powder. Improperly called *"chloride of lime"* or *"calcium oxychloride".* A relatively unstable chlorine carrier in solid form; a complex chemical compd of indefinite composition, presumably consisting of varying proportions of $Ca(OCl)_2$, $CaCl_2$, $Ca(OH)_2$ and H_2O in its molecular structure. Maximum available chlorine content approaches 39%. Commercial products usually range between 24% and 37% of available chlorine.

White or grayish-white powder; strong odor of chlorine. On exposure to air it becomes moist and rapidly decomposes. Most of it dissolves in water or alcohol. *Keep dry and tightly closed.*

Caution: Strong solns irritate skin. Inhalation of fumes may cause laryngeal and pulmonary irritation, pulmonary edema, death. Ingestion may produce severe oral, esophageal, gastric irritation.

USE: Bleaching of wood pulp, linen, cotton, straw, oils, soaps, and in laundering; oxidizer in calico printing to obtain white designs on a colored ground; destroying caterpillars; disinfecting drinking water, sewage, etc.; as a decontaminant for mustard gas and similar substances.

THERAP CAT: Disinfectant.

THERAP CAT (VET): Disinfectant for premises. Has been used as a topical antiseptic for superficial wounds.

2095. Chlorine. [7782-50-5] Cl; at. wt 35.4527; at. no. 17; valences 1, 3, 5, 7. A halogen; Group VIIA (17). Does not occur as elemental state, Cl_2, in nature. Abundance in igneous rock (95% of earth's crust): 0.031% by wt; in seawater: 1.9% by wt (primarily as NaCl). Naturally occurring stable isotopes (mass numbers): 35 (75.77%), 37 (24.23%); known artificial radioactive isotopes: 31-34, 36 (longest-lived known isotope, $T_{1/2}$ 3.0×10^5 yrs; β^-, EC decay), 38-46, 48. Discovered in 1774 by C. W. Scheele; recognized as an element in 1810 by H. Davy. Commercial sources:

seawater, ocean derived mineral deposits, brines from lakes, wells and springs. Industrial prepn from brine in electrolytic cells. Lab prepn from MnO_2 and HCl: Schmeisser in *Handbook of Preparative Inorganic Chemistry* **vol. 1,** G. Brauer, Ed. (Academic Press, New York, 2nd ed., 1963) p 272. Cosmogenic production and determn of ^{36}Cl for geological dating: H. E. Gove, *Philos. Trans. R. Soc. London Ser. A* **323,** 103 (1987); M. G. Zreda *et al., Earth Planet. Sci. Lett.* **105,** 94 (1991). *Reviews: Ciba Review* **vol. 12,** no. 139 (Aug. 1960); *ACS Monograph Series* **no. 154,** entitled "Chlorine," J. S. Sconce, Ed. (Reinhold, New York, 1962) 901 pp; *MTP Int. Rev. Sci.: Inorg. Chem., Ser. One* **vol. 3,** V. Gutmann, Ed. (Butterworths, London, 1972); A. J. Downs, C. J. Adams, "Chlorine, Bromine, Iodine and Astatine" in *Comprehensive Inorganic Chemistry* **vol. 2,** J. C. Bailar, Jr. *et al.,* Eds. (Pergamon Press, Oxford, 1973) pp 1107-1594; *Chemistry of the Elements,* N. N. Greenwood, A. Earnshaw, Eds. (Pergamon Press, New York, 1984) pp 920-1041; L. C. Curlin, T. V. Bommaraju in *Kirk-Othmer Encyclopedia of Chemical Technology* **vol. 1** (Wiley-Interscience, New York, 4th ed., 1994) pp 938-1025. Review of potential human health and environmental adverse effects of chlorine and its compounds: E. Delzell *et al., Regul. Toxicol. Pharmacol.* **2,** S1-S1056 (1994).

Greenish-yellow, diatomic gas; suffocating odor. mp $-101.00°$. bp $-34.05°$. d^{20} at 6.864 atm 1.4085 (liq); d^{-35} at 0.9949 atm 1.5649 (liq). d (relative to air) 2.48. Heat capacity at constant pressure (gas, 25°) 8.11 cal/mole/°C. Vapor pressure data: Giauque, Powell, *J. Am. Chem. Soc.* **61,** 1970 (1939). Critical temp 144°; critical pressure 76.1 atm; critical density 0.573. Sol in water (25°) with formation of aqueous Cl_2 (0.062 moles/l), HOCl (0.030 moles/l) and Cl^- (0.030 moles/l); total soly: 0.092 moles/l. More sol in alkalies. Oxidizing agent. Very reactive; E^0 (aq) $\frac{1}{2}Cl_2/Cl^-$ 1.356 V; dissociation energy (25°): 57.978 kcal. Forms halides with all elements except the rare gases helium, neon and argon. Noncombustible in air; most combustible materials will burn in chlorine. Forms explosive mixtures with flammable gases and vapors. Reacts explosively or forms explosive compounds with many common chemicals, especially acetylene, turpentine, ether, ammonia gas, fuel gas, hydrocarbons, hydrogen and finely divided metals. LC_{50} (1 hr) in rats, mice (ppm): 293, 137 (K. C. Back *et al., Reclassification of Materials Listed as Transportation Health Hazards* (TSA-20-72-3; PB 214-270, 1972) pp A-182-183).

Caution: Potential symptoms of overexposure are burning of eyes, nose and mouth; lacrimation, rhinorrhea; coughing, choking and substernal pain; nausea, vomiting; headache, dizziness; syncope; pulmonary edema; pneumonia; hypoxemia; dermatitis; direct contact with liquid may cause frostbite. *See NIOSH Pocket Guide to Chemical Hazards* (DHHS/NIOSH 97-140, 1997) p 58. *See also Patty's Industrial Hygiene and Toxicology* **vol. 2F,** G. D. Clayton, F. E. Clayton, Eds. (Wiley-Interscience, New York, 4th ed., 1994) pp 4483-4505.

USE: Manuf of organic and inorganic chemicals. As oxidizing and bleaching agent in pulp and paper industry, and for textiles. As disinfectant for water purification, industrial waste, sewage, swimming pools. In the extraction and refining of metals. ^{36}Cl for determining geological age of natural samples such as meteorites, surface rocks, polar ice and ground water. Has been used as a military poison gas under the name **bertholite.**

2096. Chlorine Dioxide. [10049-04-4] Chlorine peroxide. ClO_2; mol wt 67.45. Cl 52.56%, O 47.44%. Prepn from chlorine and sodium chlorite: Derby, Hutchinson, *Inorg. Synth.* **4,** 152 (1953); from potassium chlorate and sulfuric acid: Bodenstein *et al., Z. Anorg. Allg. Chem.* **147,** 233 (1925); by passing NO_2 through a column of sodium chlorate: Hutchinson, Derby, *Cereal Chem.* **24,** 372 (1947); alternate methods of prepn: Schmeisser in *Handbook of Preparative Inorganic Chemistry* **vol. 1,** G. Brauer, Ed. (Academic Press, New York, 2nd ed., 1963) p 301. *Review:* Bedumeau, *Rev. Prod. Chim.* **57,** 173-177, 257-261 (1954). Book: W. J. Masschelein, *Chlorine Dioxide,* R. G. Rice, Ed (Ann Arbor Science Publishers Inc., Ann Arbor, MI, 1979) 189 pp. Review of toxicology and human exposure: *Toxicological Profile for Chlorine Dioxide and Chlorite* (PB2003-101465, 2002) 182 pp.

Strongly oxidizing, yellow to reddish-yellow gas at room temp. Unpleasant odor similar to that of chlorine and reminiscent of that of nitric acid. Unstable in light; stable in dark if pure, but chlorides catalyze its decompn even in the dark. *Reacts violently with organic materials.* In concns in excess of 10% at atm pressure easily detonated by sunlight, heat, contact with mercury or carbon monoxide. mp −59°; bp 11°; d^0(liq) 1.642: Cheesman, *J. Chem. Soc.* **1930**, 35. Sol in water (3.01 g/l at 25° and 34.5 mm Hg), with slight hydrolysis to chlorous and chloric acid; sol in alkaline and sulfuric acid solns. Solid is yellowish-red crystalline mass; liquid is reddish-brown.

Caution: Potential symptoms of overexposure are irritation of eyes, nose and throat; coughing, wheezing, bronchitis, pulmonary edema; chronic bronchitis. *See NIOSH Pocket Guide to Chemical Hazards* (DHHS/NIOSH 97-140, 1997) p 58.

USE: Bleaching cellulose, paper-pulp, flour, leather, fats and oils, textiles, beeswax; purification of water; taste and odor control of water; cleaning and detanning leather; manuf of chlorite salts; oxidizing agent; bactericide, antiseptic and deodorizer.

2097. Chlorine Heptoxide. [10294-48-1] Dichlorine heptoxide; perchloric anhydride. Cl_2O_7; mol wt 182.90. Cl 38.77%, O 61.23%. Prepd by dehydration of perchloric acid with P_2O_5: Michael, Conn, *Am. Chem. J.* **23**, 445 (1900); **25**, 92 (1901); Meyer, Kessler, *Ber.* **54**, 566 (1921); Goodeve, Powney, *J. Chem. Soc.* **1932**, 2078.

Colorless, very volatile oily liquid. d_4^0 1.86. mp −91.5°; bp 82°; $bp_{23.7}$ 0°. Trouton constant 23.4. The most stable oxide of chlorine. *Explodes violently upon concussion or on contact with a flame or iodine.* Dipole moment in CCl_4 at 20° is 0.72. Does not attack wood or paper. Slowly hydrolyzed by water, forming perchloric acid.

Caution: May be irritating to skin, mucous membranes.

USE: Catalyst in cellulose esterification.

2098. Chlorine Monofluoride. [7790-89-8] Chlorine fluoride. ClF; mol wt 54.45. Cl 65.11%, F 34.89%. Prepd from Cl_2 and F_2 at 400°: Ruff *et al.*, *Z. Anorg. Allg. Chem.* **176**, 256 (1928); Kwasnik in *Handbook of Preparative Inorganic Chemistry* vol. 1, G. Brauer, Ed. (Academic Press, New York, 2nd ed., 1963) p 153.

Colorless gas. Slightly yellow when liquid. mp −155.6°. bp −100.1°. Crit temp −14°. d (liq; −108°) 1.67. *Extremely reactive.* Destroys glass instantly, attacks quartz readily in presence of moisture; organic matter bursts into flame on contact; violent reaction with water.

Caution: Extremely corrosive and irritating to skin, eyes, mucous membranes, respiratory tract.

2099. Chlorine Monoxide. [7791-21-1] Dichlorine monoxide; dichloromonoxide; dichloroxide; hypochlorous anhydride. Cl_2O; mol wt 86.91. Cl 81.59%, O 18.41%. First preparation by J. L. Gay-Lussac in 1842 from yellow mercuric oxide and chlorine. See also: Cady, *Inorg. Synth.* **5**, 156 (1957); Schmeisser in *Handbook of Preparative Inorganic Chemistry* vol. 1, G. Brauer, Ed. (Academic Press, New York, 2nd ed., 1963) p 299. Use as a powerful and selective chlorinating agent: F. D. Marsh *et al.*, *J. Am. Chem. Soc.* **104**, 4680 (1982).

Yellowish-brown gas. Disagreeable, penetrating odor. *Explodes on contact with organic matter.* Can also be caused to explode by a spark or by heating. Dec at moderate rate at room temp. mp −120.6°. bp 2.2°. Trouton constant: 22.5. Suffers photochemical and thermal decompn: at 100-140° there is an induction period, followed by a second order reaction, *see* N. V. Sidgwick, *The Chemical Elements and Their Compounds* vol. II (Oxford, 1950) p 1201. One vol of water at 0° dissolves more than 100 vols Cl_2O with formation of HClO; sol in CCl_4. Stored as a liquid or solid at temps below −80°.

Caution: Intensely irritating to eyes, skin, mucous membranes, respiratory tract.

USE: Chlorinating agent.

2100. Chlorine Trifluoride. [7790-91-2] ClF_3; mol wt 92.45. Cl 38.35%, F 61.65%. Prepd from F_2 and Cl_2 or ClF. May be purified by distillation in suitable steel apparatus: Ruff, Krug, *Z. Anorg. Allg. Chem.* **190**, 270 (1930); Grisard *et al.*, *J. Am. Chem. Soc.* **73**, 5724 (1951); Kwasnik in *Handbook of Preparative Inorganic Chemistry* vol. 1, G. Brauer, Ed. (Academic Press, New York, 2nd ed., 1963) p 156. *Reviews:* Kemmitt, Sharp, *Adv. Fluorine Chem.* **4**, 240-241 (1965); Stein, "Physical and Chemical Prop-

erties of Halogen Fluorides" in *Halogen Chemistry* **vol. 1**, V. Gutmann, Ed. (Academic Press, New York, 1967) pp 133-224; Meinert, *Z. Chem.* **7**, 41-57 (1967).

Corrosive, colorless gas. Somewhat sweet, suffocating odor. mp −76.34°. bp 11.75°. *Extremely reactive.* Glass wool and organic matter burst into flames on contact even with dil vapors. Violently hydrolyzed by water. Attacks quartz if traces of moisture are present. Liquid is yellow-green in color and solid is white.

Caution: Potential symptoms of overexposure to liquid or high vapor concentrations are eye and skin burns; respiratory irritation. *See NIOSH Pocket Guide to Chemical Hazards* (DHHS/NIOSH 97-140, 1997) p 60.

USE: Fluorinating agent; in nuclear reactor fuel processing; incendiary; igniter and propellant for rockets; pyrolysis inhibitor for fluorocarbon polymers.

2101. Chlorisondamine Chloride. [69-27-2] 4,5,6,7-Tetrachloro-2,3-dihydro-2-methyl-2-[2-(trimethylammonio)ethyl]-2*H*-isoindolium dichloride; 4,5,6,7-tetrachloro-2-(2-dimethylaminoethyl)-2-methylisoindolinium chloride methochloride; 4,5,6,7-tetrachloro-2-(2-dimethylaminoethyl)isoindoline dimethylchloride; *N*-[(2-dimethylammonium)ethyl]-4,5,6,7-tetrachloroisoindolinium dimethochloride; chlorisondamine dimethochloride; Ecolid. $C_{14}H_{20}$-Cl_6N_2; mol wt 429.04. C 39.19%, H 4.70%, Cl 49.58%, N 6.53%. Nicotinic receptor antagonist of the ganglion blocking class. Prepn: Allen, Ocampo, *J. Electrochem. Soc.* **103**, 452, 682 (1956); Huebner, **US 3025294** (1962 to Ciba). Pharmacology: P. B. S. Clarke *et al.*, *Br. J. Pharmacol.* **111**, 397 (1994). Use in studies of neuronal nicotinic acetylcholine receptors: A. S. Woods *et al.*, *J. Proteome Res.* **2**, 207 (2003).

Non-hygroscopic crystals contg ethanol of crystallization, mp 258-265° (dec). Sol in water, methanol, ethanol. pH of aq solns 4.7 to 6.2. Forms yellow, chloroform-soluble complex with bromcresol green, absorption max 420 nm.

USE: Biochemical probe in nicotinic receptor studies.

2102. Chlormadinone Acetate. [302-22-7] 17-(Acetyloxy)-6-chloropregna-4,6-diene-3,20-dione; 6-chloro-17-hydroxypregna-4,6-diene-3,20-dione acetate; 6-chloro-6-dehydro-17α-hydroxyprogesterone; 17α-acetoxy-6-chloro-6,7-dehydroprogesterone; Chronosyn; Cyclonorm; Fertiletten; Gestafortin; Lormin; Luteran; Matrol; Normenon; Menstridyl; Prostal; Traslan. $C_{23}H_{29}ClO_4$; mol wt 404.93. C 68.22%, H 7.22%, Cl 8.76%, O 15.80%. Orally active progestogen with antiandrogenic activity; has been used in combinations as an oral contraceptive. Prepn: Brückner, **DE 1075114** (1960 to E. Merck, AG); Brückner *et al.*, *Ber.* **94**, 1225 (1961); Sciaky, *Gazz. Chim. Ital.* **91**, 545 (1961); **GB 932153**; H. J. Ringold, A. Bowers, **US 3485852** (1963, 1969 both to Syntex). Endocrinological activities: D. M. Brennan, R. J. Kraay, *Acta Endocrinol.* **44**, 367 (1963). Metabolism: S. Honma *et al.*, *Chem. Pharm. Bull.* **25**, 2019 (1977). Clinical evaluation in prostatic carcinoma: R. Nishimura, K. Shida, *Prostate*, Suppl. 1, 27 (1981); in benign prostatic hypertrophy: T. Usui *et al.*, *Acta Urol. Jpn.* **27**, 327 (1981), *B.A.* **73**, 27225 (1982). Review of carcinogenicity studies: *IARC Monographs* **21**, 365-375 (1979).

Crystals from methanol or ether, mp 212-214°. $[\alpha]_D$ +6° (c = 1 in CHCl$_3$). uv max: 283.5, 286 nm (ε 23400, 22100).

Mixture with ethinyl estradiol. [37301-55-6] Amenyl; Lutestral; Menova.

Mixture with mestranol. [8065-91-6] C-Quens; Gestamestrol; Sequens.

THERAP CAT: Progestogen; antineoplastic (hormonal).

THERAP CAT (VET): Progestogen; estrus regulator.

2103. Chlormephos. [24934-91-6] S-(Chloromethyl)-phosphorodithioic acid O,O-diethyl ester; chlormethylfos; O,O-diethyl S-(chloromethyl)dithiophosphate; MC-2188; Dotan; Sherman. $C_5H_{12}ClO_2PS_2$; mol wt 234.70. C 25.59%, H 5.15%, Cl 15.11%, O 13.63%, P 13.20%, S 27.32%. Prepn: O. Scherer et al., **DE 1015794**; eidem, **GB 817360** (1957, 1959 both to Hoechst); W. W. Brand et al., Phosphorus Sulfur **10**, 183 (1981). Photodegradation: S. J. Buckland, R. S. Davidson, Pestic. Sci. **19**, 61 (1987). TLC/MS determn in biological samples: H. Brzezinka, N. Bertram, J. Chromatogr. Sci. **40**, 609 (2002). Review of physical properties and field trials: F. Colliot et al., Proc. Br. Insect. Fungic. Conf. 7th **2**, 557-565 (1973); physical properties and residue analysis: V. P. Lynch, Anal. Methods Pestic. Plant Growth Regul. **10**, 49-55 (1978).

Water-white oil. bp$_{1mm}$ 93-95°; bp$_{0.1\,Torr}$ 81-85°. Vapor pressure (30°): 5.7 x 10^{-2}. Miscible with most organic solvents. Soly in water (20°): 60 ppm. d^{20} 1.260. n_{D2}^{20} 1.5244. uv max (ethanol): 208 nm. LD$_{50}$ in rats (mg/kg): 7 orally; 27 dermally. LC$_{50}$ in fish: 1.5 mg/l (Lynch).

USE: Insecticide primarily for soil applications.

2104. Chlormequat Chloride. [999-81-5] 2-Chloro-N,N,N-trimethylethanaminium chloride; (2-chloroethyl)trimethylammonium chloride; chlorocholine chloride; choline dichloride; CCC; AC-38555; Cycocel; Cycogan. $C_5H_{13}Cl_2N$; mol wt 158.07. C 37.99%, H 8.29%, Cl 44.86%, N 8.86%. [ClCH$_2$CH$_2$N$^+$(CH$_3$)$_3$]-Cl$^-$. Prepn: Kauffmann, Vorlander, Ber. **43**, 2740 (1910); Freiss, Carville, J. Am. Chem. Soc. **76**, 2260 (1954); H. Linser et al., **AT 222145** (1962 to OSSW), C.A. **57**, 7660f (1962). Activity: N. E. Tolbert, J. Biol. Chem. **235**, 475 (1960); J. Namokar, Pesticides **11**, 53 (1977). Metabolism: R. C. Blinn, J. Agric. Food Chem. **15**, 984 (1967). Toxicity study: G. Hennighausen, B. Wiegershausen, Acta Biol. Med. Ger. **27**, 663 (1971).

White crystalline solid, mp 245° (dec). Fish-like odor; very hygroscopic. Sol in water, lower alcs. Insol in ether, hydrocarbons. Aq solns corrosive to metal. LD$_{50}$ in mice (mg/kg): 7 i.v., 54 orally (Hennighausen, Wiegershausen).

USE: Plant growth regulator.

2105. Chlormerodrin. [62-37-3] [3-[(Aminocarbonyl)amino]-2-methoxypropyl]chloromercury; 1-[3-(chloromercuri)-2-methoxypropyl]urea; chlormeroprin; Katonil; Mercoral; Diurone; Mercloran; Percapyl; Merilid; Oricur. $C_5H_{11}ClHgN_2O_2$; mol wt 367.20. C 16.35%, H 3.02%, Cl 9.65%, Hg 54.63%, N 7.63%, O 8.71%. Prepn: R. L. Rowland, **US 2635982** (1953 to Lakeside); R. L. Rowland et al., J. Am. Chem. Soc. **72**, 3595 (1950); E. L. Foreman, **US 2635983** (1953 to Lakeside). Toxicity data: E. I. Goldenthal, Toxicol. Appl. Pharmacol. **18**, 185 (1971).

Crystals from ethanol, mp 152-153°. Bitter, metallic taste. Stable to light and air. Soly in water, methanol: both 1.1 g/100 ml; in ethanol: 0.56 g/100 ml. Sparingly sol in chloroform.

Freely sol in alkaline solns. pH of a 0.5% aq soln 4.3-5.0. LD$_{50}$ orally in rats: ~82 mg/kg (Goldenthal).

THERAP CAT: Diuretic.

THERAP CAT (VET): Diuretic.

2106. Chlormezanone. [80-77-3] 2-(4-Chlorophenyl)-tetrahydro-3-methyl-4H-1,3-thiazin-4-one 1,1-dioxide; 2-(p-chlorophenyl)perhydro-3-methyl-1,3-thiazin-4-one 1,1-dioxide; 2-(4-chlorophenyl)-3-methyl-4-metathiazanone 1,1-dioxide; dichloromethazanone; chlormethazanone; Alinam; Banabin-Sintyal; Fenarol; Lobak; Mio-Sed; Rexan; Rilansyl; Rilaquil; Rilassol; Supotran; Suprotan; Tanafol; Trancopal; Trancote; Transanate. $C_{11}H_{12}$-ClNO$_3$S; mol wt 273.74. C 48.26%, H 4.42%, Cl 12.95%, N 5.12%, O 17.53%, S 11.71%. Prepn starting with 4-chlorobenzylidenemethylamine: Surrey et al., J. Am. Chem. Soc. **80**, 3469 (1958); **GB 815203** (1959 to Sterling Drug).

Crystals, mp 116.2-118.2°. Soly in water at 25° less than 0.25% (w/v); in 95% ethanol at 25° less than 1.0% (w/v).

THERAP CAT: Anxiolytic; muscle relaxant (skeletal).

2107. Chlormidazole. [3689-76-7] 1-[(4-Chlorophenyl)-methyl]-2-methyl-1H-benzimidazole; 1-(p-chlorobenzyl)-2-methylbenzimidazole; 2-methyl-1-(p-chlorobenzyl)benzimidazole; clomidazole. $C_{15}H_{13}ClN_2$; mol wt 256.73. C 70.18%, H 5.10%, Cl 13.81%, N 10.91%. Prepn: Herrling et al., **US 2876233** (1959 to Grünenthal).

bp$_{12}$ 240-242°.

Monohydrate. mp 67-68°.

Hydrochloride. [74298-63-8] H-115; Diamyceline; Futrican. $C_{15}H_{13}ClN_2$·HCl; mol wt 293.19. mp 227-228°.

THERAP CAT: Antifungal.

2108. Chlornaphazine. [494-03-1] N,N-Bis(2-chloroethyl)-2-naphthylamine; dichloroethyl-β-naphthylamine; β-naphthyl-di(2-chloroethyl)amine; β-naphthylbis(β-chloroethyl)amine; di(2-chloroethyl)-β-naphthylamine; CB-1048; R-48; Cloronaftina; Erysan. $C_{14}H_{15}Cl_2N$; mol wt 268.18. C 62.70%, H 5.64%, Cl 26.44%, N 5.22%. Prepd from 2-C$_{10}$H$_7$N(C$_2$H$_4$OH)$_2$ by treatment with POCl$_3$: Ross, J. Chem. Soc. **1949**, 183; Ghielmetti, Farmaco Ed. Sci. **5**, 275 (1950); **11**, 603 (1956). Mechanism of action studies: Jeney et al., Kiserl. Orvostud. **20**, 369 (1968), C.A. **70**, 18766j (1969). Review of carcinogenicity studies: IARC Monographs **4**, 119-124 (1974).

Platelets from petr ether, mp 54-56°. bp$_5$ 210°. Very sparingly sol in water, glycerol. More sol (in ascending degree) in petr ether, ethanol, olive oil, ether, acetone, benzene.

Caution: This substance has been listed as a known carcinogen: Fourth Annual Report on Carcinogens (NTP 85-002, 1985) p 44;

delisted because no U.S. residents exposed: *Fifth Annual Report on Carcinogens* (NTP 89-239, 1989) p 340.

THERAP CAT: Antineoplastic.

2109. Chloroacetaldehyde. [107-20-0] 2-Chloro-1-ethanal; monochloroacetaldehyde. C_2H_3ClO; mol wt 78.50. C 30.60%, H 3.85%, Cl 45.16%, O 20.38%. $ClCH_2CHO$. Prepd industrially by carefully controlled chlorination of acetaldehyde: Söll, **DE 844595** (1943 to Knapsack-Griesheim); Shawinigan Chem. Ltd., **GB 644914** (1947); Guinot, Tabuteau, *Compt. Rend.* **231,** 234 (1950); **FR 1012991** (1950 to Comp. des Prod. Chim. et Electrometallurg.).

Liquid. Acrid, penetrating odor. bp$_{760}$ 85-86°. The anhydr substance polymerizes on standing but reverts to the monomer on distillation.

Hemihydrate. Probably $ClCH_2CH(OH)OCH(OH)CH_2Cl$, platelets from water, mp 43-50°, bp 85.5° with decompn into water and chloraldehyde. Sol in water, alcohol, ether.

Caution: Potential symptoms of overexposure are irritation of eyes, skin and mucous membranes; skin burns; eye damage; pulmonary edema; skin, respiratory system sensitization. *See NIOSH Pocket Guide to Chemical Hazards* (DHHS/NIOSH 97-140, 1997) p 60.

USE: In the manufacture of 2-aminothiazole; to facilitate bark removal from tree trunks.

2110. Chloroacetamide. [79-07-2] 2-Chloroacetamide. C_2H_4ClNO; mol wt 93.51. C 25.69%, H 4.31%, Cl 37.91%, N 14.98%, O 17.11%. $ClCH_2CONH_2$. Prepn from ethyl chloroacetate and ammonia: Jacobs, Heidelberger, *Org. Synth.* **coll. vol. I,** 153 (2nd ed., 1941); from chloroacetyl chloride and ammonium acetate: Finan, Fothergill, *J. Chem. Soc.* **1962,** 2824.

Crystals from water, mp 119-120°. bp ~225° (dec). Sol in 10 parts water, 10 parts abs alc; very slightly sol in ether. Two isomorphous crystalline modifications: α-form, "stable form", obtained by sublimation and by crystallization from nonpolar solvents; β-form, "unstable form", obtained by quenching the melt or by crystallization from polar solvents, *see* Katayama, *Acta Crystallogr.* **9,** 986 (1956); **10,** 468 (1957); B. Kalyanaraman *et al., J. Cryst. Mol. Struct.* **8,** 175 (1978).

2111. Chloroacetanilide. C_8H_8ClNO; mol wt 169.61. C 56.65%, H 4.75%, Cl 20.90%, N 8.26%, O 9.43%. Prepn of *m-, o-* and *p-*isomers: Roberts *et al., J. Org. Chem.* **24,** 654 (1959). Sepn of *o-* and *p-*isomers: Orton, Bradford, *J. Chem. Soc.* **1927,** 986.

*m-***Chloroacetanilide.** *N-*(3-Chlorophenyl)acetamide; 3'-chloroacetanilide. Needles from 50% glacial acetic acid, mp 77-78°. Readily sol in alcohol, benzene, carbon disulfide; very slightly sol in ligroin. uv max (95% ethanol): 245 nm (log ε 4.19).

*o-***Chloroacetanilide.** Needles from dil glacial acetic acid, mp 87-88°. Sublimes at about 50-60°. Practically insol in water, alkalies; sol in alc; more sol in benzene than corresponding *p-*isomer. uv max (95% ethanol): 240 nm (log ε 4.02).

*p-***Chloroacetanilide.** Orthorhombic crystals from aq glacial acetic acid, alc, or acetone. mp 178-179°. d$_4^{22}$ 1.385. Practically insol in water; readily sol in alc, ether, carbon disulfide; slightly sol in CCl$_4$, benzene. uv max (95% ethanol): 249 nm (log ε 4.25).

2112. Chloroacetic Acid. [79-11-8] Chloroethanoic acid; monochloroacetic acid; MCA. $C_2H_3ClO_2$; mol wt 94.50. C 25.42%, H 3.20%, Cl 37.52%, O 33.86%. $ClCH_2COOH$. Made by chlorination of glacial acetic acid in presence of small amount of sulfur or iodine; also by hydrolysis of trichlorethylene with 90% H_2SO_4. Lab prepn: Gattermann-Wieland, *Praxis des Organischen Chemikers* (de Gruyter, Berlin, 40th ed., 1961) pp 109, 110. Manuf: *Faith, Keyes & Clark's Industrial Chemicals,* F. A. Lowenheim, M. K. Moran, Eds. (Wiley-Interscience, New York, 4th ed., 1975) pp 254-257. Toxicity: Woodward *et al., J. Ind. Hyg. Toxicol.* **23,** 78 (1941).

Colorless or white, deliquesc crystals. d 1.580. Exists in α, β and γ forms having mp 63°, 55-56° and 50° respectively. mp for acid of commerce is 61-63°. bp for all forms is 189°. Very sol in water; sol in alcohol, benzene, chloroform, ether. *Keep well closed and in a cool place.*

Sodium salt. Somon. $C_2H_2ClNaO_2$; mol wt 116.48. White crystalline solid. Soly in water at 20°: 85 g/100 ml. LD$_{50}$ in rats, mice, guinea pigs (mg/kg): 76, 255, 80 orally (Woodward).

Caution: Irritating to skin, mucous membranes.

USE: Herbicide. Manuf various dyes and other organic chemicals.

2113. Chloroacetic Anhydride. [541-88-8] Chloroacetic acid anhydride; monochloroacetic acid anhydride; *sym-*dichloroacetic anhydride. $C_4H_4Cl_2O_3$; mol wt 170.98. C 28.10%, H 2.36%, Cl 41.47%, O 28.07%. $(ClCH_2CO)_2O$. Prepd by treating monochloroacetic acid in tetrahydrofuran with methoxyacetylene at 15° and distilling the mixture: Eglinton *et al., J. Chem. Soc.* **1954,** 1860; by mixing monochloroacetic acid and HCN with 1,4-dioxane satd with HCl and fractionating the mixture: Krieble, Smellie, **US 2390106** (1945); by heating chloroacetyl chloride with monochloroacetic acid in the presence of AlCl$_3$: Strosacker, Schwegler, **US 1713104** (1929 to Dow).

Prisms from benzene; d$_4^4$ 1.5494; mp 46°. bp$_{760}$ 203°; bp$_{116}$ 163°; bp$_{62}$ 149°; bp$_{24}$ 126°; bp$_{10}$ 109-110°; bp$_{0.05}$ 118-120°. Freely sol in ether, chloroform; slightly sol in benzene, practically insol in cold ligroin.

USE: In *N-*acetylation of amino acids in alkaline soln; prepn of cellulose chloroacetates.

2114. Chloroacetone. [78-95-5] 1-Chloro-2-propanone; chloracetone; monochloroacetone; monochloracetone; acetonyl chloride; chloropropanone; 1-chloro-2-ketopropane; 1-chloro-2-oxopropane. C_3H_5ClO; mol wt 92.52. C 38.95%, H 5.45%, Cl 38.32%, O 17.29%. $ClCH_2COCH_3$. Prepn by the action of chlorine upon diketene: A. B. Boese, Jr., **US 2209683** (1940 to Carbide and Carbon Chem.); by chlorination of acetone: E. J. Rahrs, **US 2235562** (1941 to Eastman Kodak); G. H. Morey, **US 2243484** (1941 to Commercial Solvents Corp.). Stabilization: *idem,* **US 2229651** (1941 to Commercial Solvents Corp.); E. J. Rahrs, **US 2263010** (1941 to Eastman Kodak). Forms binary azeotropes with many organic liquids: L. H. Horsley, *Azeotropic Data,* Advances in Chemistry Series No. 6 (Washington, 1952) p 73. Reacts with aryl Grignard reagents to form stilbenes: Huang, *J. Chem. Soc.* **1954,** 2539. Toxicology: E. V. Sargent *et al., Am. Ind. Hyg. Assoc. J.* **47,** 375 (1986).

Liquid. Pungent odor. Lacrimator. Turns dark and resinifies on prolonged exposure to light. May be stabilized by addition of 0.1% H$_2$O or 1.0% CaCO$_3$. d$_4^{25}$ 1.123; d$_4^{15}$ 1.135. mp −44.5°. bp 119.7°, bp$_{50}$ 61°, bp$_{12}$ 20°. Volatile with steam. Surface tension at 20° = 35.27 dyn/cm. Dipole moment in hexane, 2.36D. Sol in 10 parts water (w/w). Miscible with alcohol, ether, chloroform. LD$_{50}$ (14 day) in mice, rats (mg/kg): 127, 100 orally; LC$_{50}$ (1 hr) in rats (ppm): 262 by inhalation (Sargent).

2,4-Dinitrophenylhydrazone. Yellow needles from alc, mp 124°.

Caution: Intensely irritating to eyes, skin, mucous membranes.

USE: Has been proposed as tear gas component for police and military use; in the manuf of couplers for color photography; as enzyme inactivator; intermediate in the manuf of perfumes, antioxidants, drugs; in insecticide formulations; in photopolymerization of vinyl compds. Proposed as catalyst in tetraethyllead production, as selective solvent for separating diolefins.

2115. ω-Chloroacetophenone. [532-27-4] 2-Chloro-1-phenylethanone; 2-chloroacetophenone; α-chloroacetophenone; phenacyl chloride; Chemical Mace; CN. C_8H_7ClO; mol wt 154.59. C 62.16%, H 4.56%, Cl 22.93%, O 10.35%. C_6H_5-COCH$_2$Cl. Chemical warfare agent with lacrimatory properties. Prepn: R. Scholl, H. Korten, *Ber.* **34,** 1902 (1901); H. Rheinboldt, M. Perrier, *J. Am. Chem. Soc.* **69,** 3148 (1947); Schaefer, Sonnenberg, *J. Org. Chem.* **28,** 1128 (1963). Purification: Lofton, **US 2414418** (1947 to Pennsylvania Coal Prod.). Melting point determination and review of prepn: Macy, *J. Chem. Educ.* **24,** 222 (1947). Comparative toxicity with *o-*chlorobenzylidenemalononitrile, *q. v.:* B. Ballantyne, D. W. Swanston, *Arch. Toxicol.* **40,** 75 (1978).

Crystals from dil alcohol, carbon tetrachloride, or light petr. mp 58-59°; also reported as 54° (Macy) and 56.5° (Rheinboldt, Perrier). bp 244-245°. d^{15} 1.324. Vapor pressure at 20°: 5.4 × 10^{-3} mm Hg. Practically insol in water. Freely sol in alcohol, ether, benzene. LD$_{50}$ in rats (mg/kg): 41 i.v., 36 i.p., 127 orally; LC$_{50}$ in rats: 8750 mg/min/m^3 (Ballantyne, Swanston).

Caution: Potential symptoms of overexposure are irritation of eyes, skin and respiratory system; pulmonary edema. *See NIOSH Pocket Guide to Chemical Hazards* (DHHS/NIOSH 97-140, 1997) p 60.

USE: Riot control agent.

2116. *p*-Chloroacetophenone. [99-91-2] 1-(4-Chlorophenyl)ethanone; 4'-chloroacetophenone. C$_8$H$_7$ClO; mol wt 154.59. C 62.16%, H 4.56%, Cl 22.93%, O 10.35%. Prepd from chlorobenzene and acetic anhydride in the presence of AlCl$_3$: Adams, Noller, *Org. Synth.* **coll. vol. I,** 109 (1941). Physical properties: *eidem, ibid.;* Dreisbach, Martin, *Ind. Eng. Chem.* **41,** 2875 (1949).

Liquid, bp$_{24}$ 124-126°, bp 237°. mp 20-21° (Adams, Noller); also reported as 18.4° (Dreisbach, Martin). d$_4^4$ 1.192, d$_4^{25}$ 1.188. n$_D^{20}$ 1.555, n$_D^{25}$ 1.553. Practically insol in water. Miscible with alcohol, ether.

Caution: Highly irritating to eyes, mucous membranes.

2117. Chloroacetyl Isocyanate. [4461-30-7] Chloroacetic acid anhydride with isocyanic acid. C$_3$H$_2$ClNO$_2$; mol wt 119.51. C 30.15%, H 1.69%, Cl 29.67%, N 11.72%, O 26.77%. ClCH$_2$-CONCO. Obtained by the reaction of chloroacetamide with oxalyl chloride: Speziale, Smith, *J. Org. Chem.* **28,** 1808 (1963).

Liquid. bp$_{20}$ 50-55°. n$_D^{21.5}$ 1.4580.

2118. Chloroaniline. C$_6$H$_6$ClN; mol wt 127.57. C 56.49%, H 4.74%, Cl 27.79%, N 10.98%. Prepn of *m*-, *o*- and *p*-isomers: Sidgwick, Rubie, *J. Chem. Soc.* **119,** 1013 (1921). Manufacture of *m*- and *p*-isomers by catalytic hydrogenation of chloronitrobenzene: Pray, Trager, **US 2791613** (1957 to Columbia-Southern Chem.); by reduction of chloronitrobenzene with NaHS: Latourette *et al.,* **US 2894035** (1959 to Food Machinery & Chem.). Properties of *o*-isomer: Dreisbach, Martin, *Ind. Eng. Chem.* **41,** 2875 (1949). Toxicity data: H. F. Smyth *et al., Am. Ind. Hyg. Assoc. J.* **23,** 95 (1962).

***m*-Chloroaniline.** [108-42-9] 3-Chlorobenzenamine. Liquid, bp 230.5°. mp −10.4°. d$_4^{22}$ 1.2150. n$_D^{20}$ 1.5931. Practically insol in water. Sol in most common organic solvents.

***o*-Chloroaniline.** [95-51-2] Liquid. At 99.61 mol-% purity, bp 208.84°; mp −1.94°. d$_4^{22}$ 1.2114. n$_D^{20}$ 1.5895. Practically insol in water. Sol in acid and in most organic solvents.

***p*-Chloroaniline.** [106-47-8] Orthorhombic crystals from alcohol or petr ether, mp 72.5°. bp 232°. d$_4^{77}$ 1.169. Sol in hot water; freely sol in alcohol, ether, acetone, carbon disulfide. LD$_{50}$ orally in rats: 0.31 g/kg (Smyth).

2119. Chloroarsenol. [151-07-5] (2-Chloro-1-heptenyl)-arsonic acid; 2-chloro-1-heptene-1-arsonic acid. C$_7$H$_{14}$AsClO$_3$; mol wt 256.56. C 32.77%, H 5.50%, As 29.20%, Cl 13.82%, O 18.71%. Prepn: **DE 296915** (1917 to Bayer).

Needles from water, mp 115°.

Ammonium salt. Ammonium chloroheptenearsonate. C$_7$H$_{17}$-AsClNO$_3$. Freely sol in water.

2120. Chloroazodin. [502-98-7] *N,N''*-Dichlorodiazenedicarboximidamide; α,α'-azobis[chloroformamidine]; chlorazodin; dichloroazodicarbonamidine; azochloramide. C$_2$H$_4$Cl$_2$N$_6$; mol wt 183.00. C 13.13%, H 2.20%, Cl 38.75%, N 45.92%. Prepd by treating an AcOH-NaOAc soln of guanidine nitrate with sodium hypochlorite in the cold: Braz *et al., Appl. Chem. USSR* **17,** 565 (1944), *C.A.* **40,** 2267 (1946). Structure and uv spectra: Kumler, *J. Am. Chem. Soc.* **75,** 3092 (1953).

Bright yellow needles, plates, flakes. Faint chlorine odor, burning taste. Dec explosively at ~155°. Decompn is accelerated by contact with metals. Very slightly sol in water; sparingly sol in alcohol; slightly sol in glycerol, glyceryl triacetate (1:100), vegetable oils, ether, chloroform. Practically insol in carbon tetrachloride and liquid petrolatum. Oil solns are generally made by diluting a triacetin (glyceryl triacetate) soln of chloroazodin with oil. Solns of chloroazodin in glycerol and in alcohol dec rapidly on warming; all solns dec on exposure to light.

THERAP CAT: Antiseptic, disinfectant.

THERAP CAT (VET): Antiseptic, disinfectant.

2121. Chlorobenzene. [108-90-7] Monochlorobenzene; benzene chloride. C$_6$H$_5$Cl; mol wt 112.56. C 64.02%, H 4.48%, Cl 31.50%. Produced by the chlorination of benzene in the presence of a catalyst. Review of manuf, properties, and use: *Faith, Keyes & Clark's Industrial Chemicals,* F. A. Lowenheim, M. K. Moran, Eds. (Wiley-Interscience, New York, 4th ed., 1975) pp 258-265. Review of toxicology and human exposure: *Toxicological Profile for Chlorobenzene* (PB91-180505, 1990) 100 pp.

Colorless, very refractive liquid; faint, not unpleasant odor. d$_D^{20}$ 1.107. bp 131-132°. Solidif −55°. mp −45°. Flash pt 28°C. n$_D^{20}$ 1.5248. Insol in water. Freely sol in alcohol, benzene, chloroform, ether.

Caution: Potential symptoms of overexposure are irritation of skin, eyes and nose; drowsiness, incoordination; CNS depression. *See NIOSH Pocket Guide to Chemical Hazards* (DHHS/NIOSH 97-140, 1997) p 62.

USE: Manuf phenol, aniline, DDT; solvent for paints; heat transfer medium.

2122. *p*-Chlorobenzenesulfonic Acid. [98-66-8] 4-Chlorobenzenesulfonic acid; closylate. C$_6$H$_5$ClO$_3$S; mol wt 192.62. C 37.41%, H 2.62%, Cl 18.41%, O 24.92%, S 16.65%. Prepd by heating chlorobenzene with concd sulfuric acid or oleum under dehydrating conditions: Meyer, *Ann.* **433,** 327, 333 (1923).

Monohydrate. Crystals from water, mp 67°. The anhydr material is usually obtained as a syrup, bp$_{25}$ 148°. Sol in water, alc. Practically insol in ether, benzene.

Sodium salt monohydrate. C$_6$H$_4$ClNaO$_3$S.H$_2$O. Cubic crystals from water. Sol in water.

2123. *m*-Chlorobenzoic Acid. [535-80-8] 3-Chlorobenzoic acid. C$_7$H$_5$ClO$_2$; mol wt 156.57. C 53.70%, H 3.22%, Cl 22.64%, O 20.44%. Prepn by catalytic oxidation of 1-chloro-3-ethylbenzene: Emerson *et al., J. Am. Chem. Soc.* **71,** 1742 (1949); by chlorination of benzoic acid: Gorvin, *Chem. Ind. (London)* **1951,** 910; by the von Richter reaction from 1-chloro-4-nitrobenzene and alcoholic KCN: Samuel, *J. Chem. Soc.* **1960,** 1318.

Crystals, mp 158°. d$_4^{25}$ 1.496. Sol in 2850 parts cold water; more sol in hot water; freely sol in alcohol, ether.

Methyl ester. Methyl *m*-chlorobenzoate. $C_8H_7ClO_2$. mp 21°, bp 231°.

2124. *o*-Chlorobenzoic Acid. [118-91-2] 2-Chlorobenzoic acid. $C_7H_5ClO_2$; mol wt 156.57. C 53.70%, H 3.22%, Cl 22.64%, O 20.44%. Prepd by $KMnO_4$ oxidation of *o*-chlorotoluene: Clarke, Taylor, *Org. Synth.* **coll. vol. II**, 135 (1943). Crystal structure: Ferguson, Sim, *Acta Crystallogr.* **12**, 941 (1959), *C.A.* **55**, 24188i (1961).

Monoclinic crystals, mp 142°. d_4^{20} 1.544. Sol in 900 parts cold water; more sol in hot water, freely in alc, ether.

USE: Preservative for glues, paints. Intermediate in the manufacture of fungicides and dyes.

2125. *p*-Chlorobenzoic Acid. [74-11-3] 4-Chlorobenzoic acid; chlorodracylic acid. $C_7H_5ClO_2$; mol wt 156.57. C 53.70%, H 3.22%, Cl 22.64%, O 20.44%. Prepn by catalytic oxidation of 1-chloro-4-ethylbenzene: Emerson *et al., J. Am. Chem. Soc.* **71**, 1742 (1949). Manuf by oxidation of *p*-chlorobenzaldehyde: Shipman, US 3124611 (1964 to ICI). Crystal structure: Toussaint, *Acta Crystallogr.* **4**, 71 (1951), *C.A.* **45**, 6604e (1951); Pollock, Woodward, *ibid.* **7**, 605 (1954), *C.A.* **48**, 13331e (1954).

Triclinic crystals, mp 243°. Sol in 5290 parts water; freely sol in alcohol, ether.

Methyl ester. Methyl *p*-chlorobenzoate. $C_8H_7ClO_2$. mp 44°.

Sodium salt. Sodium *p*-chlorobenzoate. $C_7H_4ClNaO_2$. White, odorless, crystalline powder, freely sol in water.

USE: Sodium salt as a preservative.

2126. *p*-Chlorobenzotrifluoride. [98-56-6] 1-Chloro-4-(trifluoromethyl)benzene; (4-chlorophenyl)trifluoromethane; 4-chloro-α,α,α-trifluorotoluene; PCBTF; Oxsol 100. $C_7H_4ClF_3$; mol wt 180.55. C 46.57%, H 2.23%, Cl 19.64%, F 31.57%. Environmentally friendly solvent. Prepn: H. S. Booth *et al., J. Am. Chem. Soc.* **57**, 2066 (1935). Mass spectrum: F. Belsito *et al., Ann. Chim.* **69**, 259 (1979). Photochemical reactivity: M. Khan *et al., Atmos. Environ.* **33**, 1085 (1999). Use as chemical intermediate: E. R. Lavagnino *et al., Org. Prep. Proced. Int.* **11**, 23 (1979); M. Beller, A. Zapf, *Synlett* **1998**, 792. GLC/MS determn in fish: M. P. Yurawecz, *J. Assoc. Off. Anal. Chem.* **62**, 36 (1979). Toxicology: P. E. Newton *et al., Inhalation Toxicol.* **10**, 33 (1998). *Review:* C. H. Hare, *Mod. Paint Coat.* **88**, 30-36 (1998).

Liquid, strong though not unpleasant aromatic odor. bp 139°. Freezing pt: −36°. mp −34°. Flash point (closed cup): 109°F (43°C). d^{20} 1.34. d_4^{25} 1.334. n_D^{21} 1.4469. Vapor pressure (20°): 5.3 mm Hg. Soly in water (25°): 29 ppm.

USE: Chemical intermediate for dinitroaniline herbicides, dyes. As dielectric fluid and as solvent.

2127. *o*-Chlorobenzylidenemalononitrile. [2698-41-1] [(2-Chlorophenyl)methylene]propanedinitrile; *o*-chlorobenzalmalononitrile; β,β-dicyano-*o*-chlorostyrene; CS. $C_{10}H_5ClN_2$; mol wt 188.61. C 63.68%, H 2.67%, Cl 18.80%, N 14.85%. Lacrimatory chemical warfare agent. Prepn: B.B. Corson, R. W. Stoughton, *J. Am. Chem. Soc.* **50**, 2825 (1928). Pharmacology: R. W. Brimblecombe *et al., Br. J. Pharmacol.* **44**, 561 (1972). Toxicology: C. L. Punte *et al., Toxicol. Appl. Pharmacol.* **4**, 656 (1962); J. R. Gaskins *et al., Arch. Environ. Health* **24**, 449 (1972); B. Ballantyne, S. Callaway, *Med. Sci. Law* **12**, 43 (1972). Comparative

toxicity of CS and ω-chloroacetophenone, *q.v.:* B. Ballantyne, D. W. Swanston, *Arch. Toxicol.* **40**, 75 (1978).

White crystalline solid, mp 95-96°, bp 310-315°. Vapor pressure at 20°: 3.4×10^{-5} mm Hg. Sparingly sol in water; sol in acetone, dioxane, methylene chloride, ethyl acetate, benzene. LD_{50} in rats (mg/kg): 28 i.v., 48 i.p.; LC_{50} in rats: 88,480 mg/min/m^3 (Ballantyne, Swanston).

Caution: Potential symptoms of overexposure are pain, burning of eyes, lacrimation and conjunctivitis; erythemic eyelids, blepharospasm; irritation of throat, coughing and chest constriction; headache; erythema and vesiculation of skin. *See NIOSH Pocket Guide to Chemical Hazards* (DHHS/NIOSH 97-140, 1997) p 62.

USE: Riot control agent.

2128. *p*-Chlorobenzylpseudothiuronium Chloride. [544-47-8] Carbamimidothioic acid (4-chlorophenyl)methyl ester monohydrochloride. $C_8H_{10}Cl_2N_2S$; mol wt 237.15. C 40.52%, H 4.25%, Cl 29.90%, N 11.81%, S 13.52%. Prepd by refluxing a mixture of *p*-chlorobenzyl chloride and thiourea in ethanol: Dewey, Sperry, *J. Am. Chem. Soc.* **61**, 3251 (1939).

Crystals from concd HCl + water, mp 197°.

USE: Identification of organic acids.

2129. Chlorobutanol. [57-15-8] 1,1,1-Trichloro-2-methyl-2-propanol; β,β,β-trichloro-*tert*-butyl alcohol; acetone chloroform; chlorbutol; Chloretone; Coliquifilm; Methaform; Sedaform. $C_4H_7Cl_3O$; mol wt 177.46. C 27.07%, H 3.98%, Cl 59.93%, O 9.02%. Chlorobutanol may be anhydrous or it may contain up to about one-half molecule of water. Prepn: Fishburn, Watson, *J. Am. Pharm. Assoc.* **28**, 491 (1939); E. Bergman, US 2446453 (1948 to Polymerisable Products Ltd.); P. Riegger, H. Richtzenbain, DE 1271697 (1968 to Dynamit Nobel A.-G.), *C.A.* **69**, 95967g (1968); M. Saljoughian, *Monatsh. Chem.* **114**, 813 (1983). Toxicity studies: E. Impens, *Arch. Int. Pharmacodyn. Ther.* **8**, 77 (1901).

Crystals. Camphor odor and taste. A crystal of chlorobutanol placed on a water surface "dances" like a camphor crystal. Sublimes easily. The anhydrous form mp 97° (the hemihydrate mp 78°). bp_{760} 167°; bp_{246} 135°. Easily sol in hot water; one gram dissolves in 1 ml alcohol, 10 ml glycerol; sol in chloroform, ether, acetone, petr ether, glacial acetic acid, oils. MLD orally in dogs, rabbits (mg/kg): 238, 213 (Impens).

Compd with chloral hydrate. Ref: DE 151188 (1904). mp 65°.

USE: Plasticizer for cellulose esters and ethers. Preservative for biological fluids, hypodermic solns, and solns of alkaloids. Pharmaceutic aid (antimicrobial).

THERAP CAT: Analgesic (dental).

THERAP CAT (VET): Has been used as a mild sedative, antipruritic, and antiseptic.

2130. 1-Chloro-2-butene. [591-97-9] α-Chloro-β-butylene; crotyl chloride; γ-methallyl chloride; γ-methylallyl chloride. C_4H_7Cl; mol wt 90.55. C 53.06%, H 7.79%, Cl 39.15%. $CH_3CH=CHCH_2Cl$. Prepn of *cis*- and *trans*-isomers: Hatch, Nesbitt, *J. Am. Chem. Soc.* **72**, 727 (1950). Manuf: Carlson, US 2494034 (1950 to Shell); Montagna, Hess, US 3055954 (1962 to Union Carbide). Equilibrium constant for isomerization of 3-chloro-1-

butene to 1-chloro-2-butene: Dittmer, Marcantonio, *J. Org. Chem.* **29**, 3473 (1964).

trans-Isomer. Liquid, bp$_{752}$ 84.8°. n_D^{20} 1.4350, n_D^{25} 1.4327. d$_4^{20}$ 0.9295.

cis-Isomer. Liquid, bp$_{758}$ 84.1°. n_D^{20} 1.4390. d$_4^{20}$ 0.9426.

Caution: Irritates eyes, respiratory passages.

2131. 3-Chloro-1-butene. [563-52-0] γ-Chloro-α-butylene; α-methallyl chloride; α-methylallyl chloride. C$_4$H$_7$Cl; mol wt 90.55. C 53.06%, H 7.79%, Cl 39.15%. CH$_2$=CHCHClCH$_3$. Prepn of DL-form: Böhme, *Ber.* **71**, 2372 (1938), Curtin, Gerber, *J. Am. Chem. Soc.* **74**, 4052 (1952); of D(−)-form: Böhme, *loc. cit.;* of L(+)-form: Young, Caserio, *J. Org. Chem.* **26**, 245 (1961). Absolute configuration: Young, Caserio, *loc. cit.* Equilibrium constant for isomerization to 1-chloro-2-butene: Dittmer, Marcantonio, *J. Org. Chem.* **29**, 3473 (1964).

DL-Form. Liquid, bp 63.9-64.2°, bp$_{26}$ −5°. d$_4^{20}$ 0.9001. n_D^{20} 1.4150.

D(−)-Form. Liquid, bp$_{26}$ −5°. α_D^{20} −2.52° (neat).

L(+)-Form. Liquid, α_D^{25} +5.87° (neat).

2132. 3-Chloro-d-camphor. [508-29-2] 3-Chloro-1,7,7-tri-methylbicyclo[2.2.1]heptan-2-one; 3-chloro-d-2-bornanone. C$_{10}$-H$_{15}$ClO; mol wt 186.68. C 64.34%, H 8.10%, Cl 18.99%, O 8.57%. Of the two isomers, the *endo*-form is more stable than the *exo*-form: Cookson, *J. Chem. Soc.* **1954**, 282. Prepn of *endo*-form: Kipping, Pope, *ibid.* **63**, 548 (1893). Prepn of *exo*-form by isomerization of *endo*-form: Lowry, Steele, *ibid.* **107**, 1382 (1915). uv spectra: Lowry, Owen, *J. Chem. Soc.* **129**, 606 (1926). Crystal structure of *endo*-form: Wiebenga, Krom, *Rec. Trav. Chim.* **65**, 663 (1946). Configuration: Cookson, *loc. cit.;* Kumler *et al., J. Am. Chem. Soc.* **83**, 2711 (1961). *Review: The Terpenes* **vol. II**, J. L. Simonsen, Ed. (University Press, Cambridge, 2nd ed., 1949) p 397.

endo-form   exo-form

endo-Form. α-Chloro-d-camphor; 3α-chloro-d-camphor; camphor monochlorated. Monoclinic prisms from alc, mp 94°. Volatile with steam. [α]$_D$ +96.2° (c = 5 in alc). Practically insol in water. Sol in alcohol, chloroform, ether. uv max (cyclohexane): 305 nm (log ε 1.72).

exo-Form. α'-Chloro-d-camphor; 3β-chloro-d-camphor. Crystals from alc, mp 117°. [α]$_D$ +35° (c = 5 in alc). Readily sol in all ordinary solvents, except water and formamide. Much more sol in 96% alc than *endo*-form. On standing, loses HCl. uv max (cyclohexane): 306 nm (log ε 1.75).

2133. Chlorocresol. [59-50-7] 4-Chloro-3-methylphenol; 3-methyl-4-chlorophenol; 4-chloro-m-cresol; 6-chloro-m-cresol; 6-chloro-3-hydroxytoluene; 2-chloro-5-hydroxytoluene; parachloro-metacresol. C$_7$H$_7$ClO; mol wt 142.58. C 58.97%, H 4.95%, Cl 24.87%, O 11.22%. Prepd by chlorination of *m*-cresol: **DE 90847** (1897 to Kalle), *Frdl.* **4**, 94; Laschinger, **US 1847566** (1932), *C.A.* **26**, 2471 (1932); Sah, Anderson, *J. Am. Chem. Soc.* **63**, 3165 (1941). HPLC determn in pharmaceutical formulations: R. Gatti *et al., J. Pharm. Biomed. Anal.* **16**, 405 (1997).

Dimorphous crystals, mp 55.5° and mp 66° (ligroin). Said to be odorless when very pure, but usually a phenolic odor persists. bp 235°. Volatile with steam. One gram dissolves in 260 ml water at 20°, more sol in hot water. Freely sol in alcohol, benzene, chloroform, ether, acetone, petr ether, fixed oils, terpenes, aq alkaline solns. Aq solns turn yellow on exposure to light and air.

USE: Disinfectant; pharmaceutic aid (preservative).

THERAP CAT: Antiseptic, disinfectant.

2134. Chlorocyanohydrin. [513-96-2] 3,3,3-Trichloro-2-hydroxypropanenitrile; 3,3,3-trichlorolactonitrile; 3,3,3-trichloro-2-hydroxypropionitrile; chloral hydrocyanide. C$_3$H$_2$Cl$_3$NO; mol wt 174.41. C 20.66%, H 1.16%, Cl 60.98%, N 8.03%, O 9.17%. Cl$_3$CCH(OH)CN. Prepd from chloral hydrate and HCN: Chwala, Wassmuth, *Monatsh. Chem.* **81**, 843 (1950).

Crystals, mp 61°. Odor of HCN and chloral. Sublimes easily. bp 220°. Freely sol in water, alcohol, ether, and most other common organic solvents; moderately sol in carbon tetrachloride. Practically insol in petr ether.

2135. Chlorodibromomethane. [124-48-1] Dibromo-chloromethane; chlorobromoform; monochlorodibromomethane; DBCM; NCI-C55254. CHBr$_2$Cl; mol wt 208.28. C 5.77%, H 0.48%, Br 76.73%, Cl 17.02%. Trihalomethane contaminant found in chlorinated water. Prepn: O. Jacobsen, R. Neumeister, *Ber.* **15**, 599 (1882); M. Fedorynski *et al., Synth. Commun.* **7**, 287 (1977). Toxicity studies: F. J. Bowman *et al., Toxicol. Appl. Pharmacol.* **44**, 213 (1978); Y. Aida *et al., J. Toxicol. Sci.* **17**, 119 (1992). Review of toxicology and human exposure: *Toxicological Profile for Bromoform and Dibromochloromethane* (PB2006-100001, 2005) 273 pp. Review of carcinogenic risk: *IARC Monographs* **52**, 243-268 (1991).

Liquid. bp 121.3-121.8° (Fedorynski); also reported as bp 123-125° (Jacobsen). d^{15} 2.4450. n_D^{20} 1.5471. Sol in ethanol, ether, acetone. LD$_{50}$ in male, female rats (mg/kg): 370, 760 orally (Aida); in male, female mice (mg/kg): 800, 1200 by gavage (Bowman).

USE: Chemical reagent/intermediate in organic synthesis.

2136. 1-Chloro-2,4-dinitrobenzene. [97-00-7] 2,4-Dinitro-1-chlorobenzene; 4-chloro-1,3-dinitrobenzene; 6-chloro-1,3-dini-trobenzene. C$_6$H$_3$ClN$_2$O$_4$; mol wt 202.55. C 35.58%, H 1.49%, Cl 17.50%, N 13.83%, O 31.60%. Obtained by nitrating *o*-nitro-chlorobenzene: Borsche, Rantscheff, *Ann.* **379**, 152 (1911); Hodgson, Dodgson, *J. Chem. Soc.* **1948**, 1006. The mixture of 2,4- and 2,6-dinitrochlorobenzenes (of which the 2,4-compd is present in largest amount) can be separated with an alkaline ethanol-water soln: Molard, Vaganay, *Mem. Poudres* **39**, 111 (1957). Toxicity study: H. F. Smyth *et al., Am. Ind. Hyg. Assoc. J.* **23**, 95 (1962).

Yellow crystals. *Skin irritant.* d ~1.7. mp 52-54°. bp 315°. Practically insol in water. Sparingly sol in cold, freely sol in hot alc; sol in ether, benzene, CS$_2$. LD$_{50}$ orally in rats: 1.07 g/kg (Smyth).

Caution: May cause dermatitis of both primary and allergic types.

USE: As a reagent for the detection and determination of nicotinic acid, nicotinamide, and other pyridine compds.

2137. 2-Chloro-1,3-dinitrobenzene. [606-21-3] 1-Chloro-2,6-dinitrobenzene; 2,6-dinitro-1-chlorobenzene. C$_6$H$_3$ClN$_2$O$_4$; mol wt 202.55. C 35.58%, H 1.49%, Cl 17.50%, N 13.83%, O 31.60%. Prepd from 2,6-dinitroaniline by the Sandmeyer reaction: Gunstone, Tucker, *Org. Synth.* **coll. vol. IV**, 160 (1963).

Yellow crystals from benzene + petr ether or from acetic acid. *Skin irritant.* mp 86-87°. d$_4^{16.5}$ 1.6867. bp 315°. Moderately sol in ether, benzene. Sol in alc. Practically insol in water.

Caution: See 1-Chloro-2,4-dinitrobenzene.

2138. N-(2-Chloroethyl)dibenzylamine Hydrochloride. [55-43-6] N-(2-Chloroethyl)-N-(phenylmethyl)benzenemethan-amine hydrochloride; N,N-dibenzyl-β-chloroethylamine hydrochloride; *N,N*-dibenzylaminoethyl chloride hydrochloride; Dibenamine hydrochloride. $C_{16}H_{19}Cl_2N$; mol wt 296.23. C 64.87%, H 6.46%, Cl 23.94%, N 4.73%. $(C_6H_5CH_2)_2NCH_2CH_2Cl \cdot HCl$. α-Adrenergic blocker. Prepn: Rabald, Dimroth, **DE 824208** (1951 to Boehringer, Mann.), *C.A.* **47**, 2206 (1953). Pharmacology and toxicity: M. Nickerson, G. M. Nomaguchi, *J. Pharmacol. Exp. Ther.* **101**, 379 (1951). Use in adrenergic receptor differentiation: R. F. Furchgott, *ibid.* **111**, 265 (1954); in specific receptor labelling: R. D. Green *et al., ibid.* **187**, 524 (1973). *In vivo* studies of protection against hepatotoxic agents: H. M. Maling *et al., Toxicol. Appl. Pharmacol.* **27**, 380 (1974); E. K. Weisburger *et al., ibid.* **28**, 477 (1974); H. M. Maling *et al., Biochem. Pharmacol.* **23**, 1479 (1974).

Crystals, mp 192°, also given as 180-181° (the free base is an oily liquid). Practically insol in water near neutrality. Sol in dil acids (2% at pH 2.1, 1% at pH 2.4 and 0.5% at pH 2.7), in 95% alcohol and in propylene glycol. Stable in acid soln, but rapidly loses activity in neutral or alkaline solns. LD_{50} s.c. in mice: 800 mg/kg (Nickerson, Nomaguchi).

2139. 2-Chloroethyl Vinyl Ether. [110-75-8] (2-Chloroethoxy)ethene. C_4H_7ClO; mol wt 106.55. C 45.09%, H 6.62%, Cl 33.27%, O 15.02%. $ClCH_2CH_2OCH=CH_2$. Prepd by the action of solid NaOH + triethanolamine upon β,β'-dichlorodiethyl ether: Chitwood, Perkins, **US 2104717** (1938 to Carbide and Carbon Chem.); *cf.* Cretcher *et al., J. Am. Chem. Soc.* **47**, 1175 (1926). Toxicity study: Smyth *et al., J. Ind. Hyg. Toxicol.* **31**, 60 (1949).

Liquid. d_{15}^{15} 1.0525. bp_{740} 109°. Quite stable to NaOH solns. Even dil acids produce hydrolysis to acetaldehyde and ethylene chlorohydrin [2-chloroethanol]. LD_{50} orally in rats: 250 mg/kg (Smyth).

USE: Mfg anesthetics, sedatives, cellulose ethers.

2140. Chlorofluorocarbons. CFCs; FCCs. Chemically stable series of chlorinated and fluorinated compounds usually with methane or ethane skeleton, marketed under general names such as *Arcton, Freon, Frigen, Genetron.* Known collectively as CFCs, individually identified by a CFC code based on the "rule of 90". (To derive the chemical formula for CFC-12, e.g., add "90" to 12; the resulting number "102" indicates 1 carbon, 0 hydrogen, 2 fluorine yielding the formula CCl_2F_2.) Initial report on suitability as refrigerants: T. Midgley, Jr., A. L. Henne, *Ind. Eng. Chem.* **22**, 542 (1930). Review including physical and chemical properties of various CFCs: E. Heiskel, *Aerosol Rep.* **22**, 403-415 (1983). CFCs do not decompose in the lower atmosphere. Photodecomposition occurs in the stratosphere via absorption of uv radiation and subsequent release of atomic chlorine which can catalyze ozone breakdown. CFC-ozone depletion hypothesis: M. J. Molina, F. S. Rowland, *Nature* **249**, 810 (1974). Reviews focusing on atmospheric chemistry of CFCs, uses, potential hydrogen-substituted replacements, environmental and regulatory issues: J. P. Cohn, *BioScience* **37**, 647-650 (1987); R. Pool, *Science* **242**, 666-668 (1988); F. S. Rowland, *Environ. Conserv.* **15**, 101-115 (1988); L. B. Weisfeld, *Plast. Compd.* **1988**, 15-22, 40-43; F. S. Rowland, *Am. Sci.* **77**, 36-45 (1989). For prepn information *see* dichlorodifluoromethane (CFC-12), trichlorofluoromethane (CFC-11), cryofluorane (CFC-114).

Colorless, essentially odorless, nonflammable, noncorrosive. Miscible with aliphatic, alicyclic and aromatic hydrocarbons, halogenated hydrocarbons, monovalent low molecular alcohols.

Note: Consult latest Government regulations on use as aerosol propellant.

USE: In aerosol propellants (CFC-11, 12, 113); air conditioning; refrigeration (CFC-12); blowing agents for making foam (CFC-11, 12); cleaning fluids (CFC-113); solvents for the electronics industry, bedding and packaging.

2141. Chloroform. [67-66-3] Trichloromethane. $CHCl_3$; mol wt 119.38. C 10.06%, H 0.84%, Cl 89.09%. Improperly called "formyl trichloride". From the addition of sulfuric acid to acetone and bleaching powder: $2CH_3COCH_3 + 6CaOCl_2 \cdot H_2O \rightarrow 2CHCl_3 + (CH_3COO)_2Ca + 2Ca(OH)_2 + 3CaCl_2 + 6H_2O$. May also be prepd by carefully controlled chlorination of methane: *Faith, Keyes & Clark's Industrial Chemicals,* F. A. Lowenheim, M. K. Moran, Eds. (Wiley-Interscience, New York, 4th ed., 1975) pp 266-269. Has been used as an anesthetic and in pharmaceutical preparations. Toxicity data: H. F. Smyth *et al., Am. Ind. Hyg. Assoc. J.* **23**, 95 (1962); E. T. Kimura *et al., Toxicol. Appl. Pharmacol.* **19**, 699 (1971). Review of toxicology: L. R. Pohl, *Rev. Biochem. Toxicol.*

1, 79-108 (1979); of carcinogenic risk: *IARC Monographs* **20**, 401-427 (1979); of toxicology and human exposure: *Toxicological Profile for Chloroform* (PB98-101140, 1997) 343 pp. Review: M. T. Holbrook in *Kirk-Othmer Encyclopedia of Chemical Technology* **vol. 5** (John Wiley & Sons, New York, 4th ed., 1993) pp 1051-1062.

Highly refractive, nonflammable, heavy, very volatile, sweet-tasting liquid; characteristic odor. d_{20}^{20} 1.484. bp 61-62°. mp −63.5°. n_D^{20} 1.4476. Forms a constant boiling mixture with 7% alc, boiling at 59°. d 1.474-1.478 for U.S.P. chloroform contg 0.5-1% ethanol as stabilizer. One ml dissolves in about 200 ml water at 25°. Misc with alcohol, benzene, ether, petr ether, carbon tetrachloride, carbon disulfide, oils. Pure chloroform is light sensitive and reagent grade chloroform usually contains 0.75% ethanol as stabilizer. *Protect from light and keep cool.* LD_{50} (14 day) orally in rats: 2.18 ml/kg (Smyth); 0.9 ml/kg (Kimura).

Spirit of Chloroform. An alcoholic soln of chloroform contg 6% by vol of chloroform, corresponding to 10.5% by wt, and ~89% abs alcohol by vol. Has been used as a carminative. Colorless, clear liquid; chloroform odor. d ~0.85.

Caution: Potential symptoms of overexposure are dizziness, mental dullness, nausea and confusion; headache, fatigue; anesthesia; enlarged liver; direct contact may cause irritation to eyes and skin. *See NIOSH Pocket Guide to Chemical Hazards* (DHHS/NIOSH 97-140, 1997) p 64. This substance is reasonably anticipated to be a human carcinogen: *Report on Carcinogens, Eleventh Edition* (PB2005-104914, 2004) p III-54.

USE: In the manuf of fluorocarbon-22. As a solvent for fats, oils, rubber, alkaloids, waxes, gutta-percha, resins; as cleansing agent; in fire extinguishers to lower the freezing temp of carbon tetrachloride; in the rubber industry.

2142. Chlorogenic Acid. [327-97-9] [1*S*-(1α,3β,4α,5α)]-3-[[3-(3,4-Dihydroxyphenyl)-1-oxo-2-propenyl]oxy]-1,4,5-trihydroxycyclohexanecarboxylic acid; 1,3,4,5-tetrahydroxycyclohexanecarboxylic acid 3-(3,4-dihydroxycinnamate); 3-caffeoylquinic acid; 3-(3,4-dihydroxycinnamoyl)quinic acid. $C_{16}H_{18}O_9$; mol wt 354.31. C 54.24%, H 5.12%, O 40.64%. Important factor in plant metabolism. Isoln from green coffee beans: Freudenberg, *Ber.* **53**, 237 (1920). Chlorogenic acid and its isomers isochlorogenic acid and neochlorogenic acid occur also in fruit, leaves and other tissues of dicotyledenous plants: Sondheimer, *Arch. Pharm.* **293**, 721 (1960). Forms caffeic acid on hydrolysis: Fiedler, *Arzneim.-Forsch.* **4**, 41 (1954). Structure: Fischer, Dangschat, *Ber.* **65**, 1037 (1932); Barnes *et al., J. Am. Chem. Soc.* **72**, 4178 (1950); Corse *et al., Tetrahedron* **18**, 1207 (1962). Synthesis: Panizzi *et al., Gazz. Chim. Ital.* **86**, 913 (1956).

Hemihydrate. Needles from water. Becomes anhyd at 110°. mp 208°. $[\alpha]_D^{26}$ −35.2° (c = 2.8). pKa (27°) 2.66. R_f values: Fiedler, *loc. cit.* Soly in water at 25° about 4%, much more sol in hot water. Alkaline solns acquire an orange color. Freely sol in alcohol, acetone. Very slightly sol in ethyl acetate. Heating with dil HCl yields caffeic acid. Forms a black compd with iron, said to be responsible for the blackening of cut and cooked potatoes: *Chem. Ind. (London)* **1958**, 627.

3'-Methyl ether. 3-Feruloylquinic acid. $C_{17}H_{20}O_9$. Crystals from ethyl acetate + petr ether, mp 196-197°. $[\alpha]_D^{25}$ −42.8° (ethanol). uv max (ethanol): 325 nm (ε 19,200).

2143. Chlorogenin. [562-34-5] (3β,5α,6α,25*R*)-Spirostan-3,6-diol. $C_{27}H_{44}O_4$; mol wt 432.64. C 74.96%, H 10.25%, O 14.79%. Isoln from bulbs of the California soap plant, amole: *Chlorogalum pomeridianum* (DC.) Kunth, *Liliaceae:* Liang, Noller, *J. Am. Chem. Soc.* **57**, 525 (1935). Chlorogenin occurs in amole as a saponin which kills or stuns fish without rendering them inedible. Structure: Marker, Rohrmann, *ibid.* **61**, 947, 3479 (1939); Marker *et al., ibid.* **62**, 2537, 3006 (1940). On hydrogenation the 3β,6β-isomer (β-chlorogenin) is produced.

Needles from methanol, mp 273-276°. $[\alpha]_{546}^{24}$ −52° (chloroform or isopropanol).

2144. 1-Chlorohexane. [544-10-5] *n*-Hexyl chloride. C_6-$H_{13}Cl$; mol wt 120.62. C 59.74%, H 10.86%, Cl 29.39%. CH_3-$(CH_2)_4CH_2Cl$. Prepd from 1-hexanol by treatment with fuming HCl: Henry, *Chem. Zentralbl.* **1905, II**, 214; with excess $SOCl_2$ or with PCl_5 + $ZnCl_2$: Clark, Streight, *Trans. R. Soc. Can. Sect. 3* **23, III**, 77 (1929).

Mobile liquid. d_4^{20} 0.8780. bp_{760} 134°. n_D^{20} 1.4236 (Clark, Streight, *loc. cit.*); n_D^{20} 1.4195 (Mumford, Phillips, *J. Chem. Soc.* **1950**, 75). Insol in water. Refluxing with 10% aq NaOH decomposes 1-chlorohexane to 1-hexanol.

2145. α-Chlorohydrin. [96-24-2] 3-Chloro-1,2-propanediol; 3-chloro-1,2-dihydroxypropane; α-monochlorohydrin; β,β′-dihydroxyisopropyl chloride; glycerol α-monochlorohydrin; 3-chloropropylene glycol; Epibloc. $C_3H_7ClO_2$; mol wt 110.54. C 32.60%, H 6.38%, Cl 32.07%, O 28.95%. $CH_2ClCHOHCH_2OH$. Prepd from glycerol and HCl gas: Conant, Quayle, *Org. Synth.* **coll. vol. I,** 294 (1941). Toxicity study: C. H. Hine *et al., Arch. Ind. Health* **14**, 250 (1956).

Liquid. Sweetish taste. Tendency to turn straw color. d_4^{20} 1.3218. n_D^{20} 1.4831. bp_{760} 213° (dec); bp_{14} 114-120°; bp_{11} 115-117°. Sol in water, alcohol, ether. LD_{50} in mice, rats (g/kg): 0.16, 0.15 orally (Hine).

USE: To lower the freezing point of dynamite; in the manuf of dye intermediates. As rodent chemosterilant.

2146. Chloromethyl Methyl Ether. [107-30-2] Chloromethoxymethane; methyl chloromethyl ether; monochloromethyl ether; chlorodimethyl ether; CMME. C_2H_5ClO; mol wt 80.51. C 29.84%, H 6.26%, Cl 44.04%, O 19.87%. CH_3OCH_2Cl. Prepd by passing HCl through a mixture of formalin and methanol: C. S. Marvel, P. K. Porter, *Org. Synth.* **coll. vol. I,** 377 (1941). *See also Beilstein* **1**, 580 (1918) and supplements. Commercial product usually contaminated by *sym*-dichloromethyl ether, *q.v.* Review of carcinogenic risk: *IARC Monographs* **4**, 239-245 (1974).

Colorless liquid, bp 59°. d_4^{20} 1.0605. n_D^{20} 1.39737.

Caution: Potential symptoms of overexposure are irritation of eyes, skin and mucous membranes; pulmonary edema, pulmonary congestion and pneumonia; skin burns, necrosis; coughing, wheezing; blood stained sputum; weight loss; bronchial secretions. *See NIOSH Pocket Guide to Chemical Hazards* (DHHS/NIOSH 97-140, 1997) p 66. The technical grade is listed as a known human carcinogen: *Report on Carcinogens, Eleventh Edition* (PB2005-104914, 2004) p III-56.

USE: In synthesis of chloromethylated compounds, plastics and ion-exchange resins.

2147. 1-Chloro-2-methyl-1-propene. [513-37-1] α-Chloroisobutylene; β,β-dimethylvinyl chloride; isocrotyl chloride; 2-methyl-1-propenyl chloride. C_4H_7Cl; mol wt 90.55. C 53.06%, H 7.79%, Cl 39.15%. Prepn from isobutyraldehyde: Kirrmann, *Bull. Soc. Chim. Fr.* **1948**, 163; by isomerization of 3-chloro-2-methylpropene with 80% H_2SO_4: Backhurst *et al., J. Chem. Soc.* **1959**, 2742.

Liquid, bp 68.1°. d_4^{20} 0.9186. n_D^{20} 1.4221.

Caution: This substance is reasonably anticipated to be a human carcinogen: *Report on Carcinogens, Eleventh Edition* (PB2005-104914, 2004) p III-110.

USE: In organic syntheses; research chemical.

2148. 3-Chloro-2-methyl-1-propene. [563-47-3] γ-Chloroisobutylene; methallylchloride; β-methallyl chloride; β-methyl-

allylchloride. C_4H_7Cl; mol wt 90.55. C 53.06%, H 7.79%, Cl 39.15%. $ClCH_2(CH_3)CCH_2$. Prepn by chlorination of isobutylene: Burgin *et al., Ind. Eng. Chem.* **31**, 1413 (1939). Manuf: Carlson, **US 2494034**; Cherniavsky, Brown, **US 2612530**; Cheney *et al., US 2642464* (1950, 1952, 1953 all to Shell).

Liquid, bp 71-72°. d_4^{15} 0.9210, d_4^{20} 0.9165 (commercial grade d_{20}^{20} 0.926-0.930). n_D^{15} 1.4318, n_D^{20} 1.4274.

Caution: This substance is reasonably anticipated to be a human carcinogen: *Report on Carcinogens, Eleventh Edition* (PB2005-104914, 2004) p III-57.

USE: Insecticide, fumigant. Chemical intermediate in organic syntheses.

2149. 1-Chloronaphthalene. [90-13-1] α-Chloronaphthalene. $C_{10}H_7Cl$; mol wt 162.62. C 73.86%, H 4.34%, Cl 21.80%. Prepd by passing chlorine into boiling naphthalene with or without solvent such as chlorobenzene and with or without catalyst such as I_2: DeWitt, Ekeley, *Univ. Colo. Stud.* **18**, 119 (1931), *C.A.* **26**, 2974 (1932). From α-naphthylamine by diazotization and Sandmeyer CuCl reaction: von Auwers, Frühling, *Ann.* **422**, 194, 200, 202 (1921); Hampson, Weissberger, *J. Chem. Soc.* **1936**, 394.

Oily liquid. Volatile with steam. d_4^{20} 1.19382. mp −2.5°. bp_{760} 259.3°; bp_{400} 230.8°; bp_{200} 204.2°; bp_{100} 180.4°; bp_{60} 165.6°; bp_{40} 153.2°; bp_{20} 134.4°; bp_{10} 118.6°; bp_5 104.8°; $bp_{1.0}$ 80.6°. n_D^{20} 1.63321. Sol in benzene, petr ether, alcohol.

Compound with 2,4,6-trinitro-*m*-cresol. $C_{17}H_{12}ClN_3O_7$. mp 78°.

Styphnate. $C_{16}H_{10}ClN_3O_8$. Yellow needles from alcohol, mp 112°.

USE: As immersion liquid in the (microscopic) determn of the refractive index of crystals. Solvent for oils, fat, DDT.

2150. 2-Chloronaphthalene. [91-58-7] β-Chloronaphthalene. $C_{10}H_7Cl$; mol wt 162.62. C 73.86%, H 4.34%, Cl 21.80%. Prepd from β-naphthylamine by diazotization and Sandmeyer CuCl reaction: Scheid, *Ber.* **34**, 1813 (1901); van der Kam, *Rec. Trav. Chim.* **45**, 568 (1926); Hampson, Weissberger, *J. Chem. Soc.* **1936**, 394. By chlorination of gaseous naphthalene at 530° in the presence of iodine, ~50% of the product being 1-chloronaphthalene which is sepd by fractional freezing: Britton, Reed, **US 1917822** (1933).

Monoclinic plates, leaflets from dil alcohol. mp 59.5°. bp_{760} 256°; bp_{60} 161°; bp_{20} 132.6°; bp_{11} 119.7°. Volatile with steam. $n_D^{70.7}$ 1.60787. Sol in alcohol, ether, benzene, chloroform, carbon disulfide.

2151. Chloronitrobenzene. Nitrochlorobenzene. C_6H_4-$ClNO_2$; mol wt 157.55. C 45.74%, H 2.56%, Cl 22.50%, N 8.89%, O 20.31%. Prepn of *m*-isomer: W. W. Hartman, M. R. Brethen, *Org. Synth.* **coll. vol. I** (2nd ed., 1964) p 162.

m-**Chloronitrobenzene.** [121-73-3] 1-Chloro-3-nitrobenzene; *m*-nitrochlorobenzene. Pale-yellow orthorhombic prisms from alcohol. d_4^4 1.534. mp 46°. bp_{760} 236°; bp_{12} 117°. Insol in water. Sparingly sol in cold alcohol; freely sol in hot alcohol, chloroform, ether, carbon disulfide, glacial acetic acid.

o-**Chloronitrobenzene.** [88-73-3] Yellow crystals. d 1.305. mp 32-33°. bp 245-246°. Insol in water. Sol in alcohol, benzene, ether.

p-**Chloronitrobenzene.** [100-00-5] Yellow crystals. d 1.520. mp 82-84°. bp 242°. Flash pt 127°C. Insol in water. Sparingly sol in cold alcohol, freely in boiling alcohol, ether, carbon disulfide.

Caution: Absorbed by inhalation, skin penetration and ingestion. Potential symptoms of overexposure to *p*-isomer are anoxia; unpleasant taste; anemia; methemoglobinemia. Direct contact may cause allergic dermatitis. Potential occupational carcinogen. *See NIOSH Pocket Guide to Chemical Hazards* (DHHS/NIOSH 97-140, 1997) p 226; *Clinical Toxicology of Commercial Products*, R. E. Gosselin *et al.*, Eds. (Williams & Wilkins, Baltimore, 5th ed., 1984) Section II, p 214, Section III, p 31-36.

USE: In dye chemistry.

2152. Chlorophacinone. [3691-35-8] 2-[(4-Chlorophenyl)-phenylacetyl]-1*H*-indene-1,3(2*H*)-dione; 2-[(*p*-chlorophenyl)phenylacetyl]-1,3-indandione; LM-91; Caid; Drat; Liphadione; Quick; Raviac; Rozol. $C_{23}H_{15}ClO_3$; mol wt 374.82. C 73.70%, H 4.03%, Cl 9.46%, O 12.81%. Prepn: D. Molho *et al.*, US 3153612 (1964 to Lipha). HPLC determn in serum: M. G. Palazoglu *et al.*, *J. Agric. Food Chem.* **46**, 4260 (1998).

Light yellow silky needles from ethanol or acetone, mp 138°. Absorption max (acetone): 325 nm. Sol in organic solvents; very sparingly sol in water.

USE: Anticoagulant rodenticide.

2153. *p*-Chlorophenacyl Bromide. [536-38-9] 2-Bromo-1-(4-chlorophenyl)ethanone; 2-bromo-4'-chloroacetophenone; 4-chloro-ω-bromoacetophenone; α-bromo-*p*-chloroacetophenone. C_8H_6BrClO; mol wt 233.49. C 41.15%, H 2.59%, Br 34.22%, Cl 15.18%, O 6.85%. Prepn from bromoacetyl chloride, chlorobenzene, and $AlCl_3$: Collet, *Compt. Rend.* **125**, 718 (1897); by bromination of *p*-chloroacetophenone: *idem, Bull. Soc. Chim. Fr.* [3] **21**, 69 (1899). Toxicity study: Dat-Xuong *et al.*, *Med. Exp.* **11**(3), 137 (1964).

Needles, mp 96-96.5°. LD_{50} orally in mice: >2000 mg/kg (Dat-Xuong).

USE: In the prepn of quaternary salts of methenamine and of chlorophenol glyoximes.

2154. Chlorophenols. C_6H_5ClO; mol wt 128.56. C 56.05%, H 3.92%, Cl 27.58%, O 12.45%. Prepn of *o*-form: Holleman, Rinkes, *Rec. Trav. Chim.* **30**, 48 (1911); Huston, Neely, *J. Am. Chem. Soc.* **57**, 2176 (1935). *cis-trans* equilibria in *o*-halophenols: Baker, *ibid.* **80**, 3598 (1958). Prepn of *p*-form: Crawford, Willson, US 1910679 (1927 to Monsanto); Neu, *Ber.* **72**, 1505 (1939); Hodgson, Norris, *J. Chem. Soc.* **1949**, Suppl. 1, S181. Manuf: Britton, Keil, US 2725402 (1955 to Dow). Prepn of *m*-form: Acheson, Taylor, *J. Chem. Soc.* **1956**, 4727. Manuf: Stoesser, Gentry; Barnard, Meyer, US 2835707 and US 2852567 (both 1958 to Dow). Toxicity data: Deichmann, *Fed. Proc.* **2**, 76 (1943). Review of toxicology and human exposure: *Toxicological Profile for Chlorophenols* (PB99-166639, 1999) 260 pp.

***m*-Chlorophenol.** [108-43-0] 3-Chlorophenol. Needles, mp 33.5°. bp 214°. d_4^{45} 1.245, d_4^{78} 1.214. n_D^{40} 1.5565. Strong medicinal taste and odor. Dipole moment in benzene, 2.10D. Slightly sol in cold water; sol in alcohol, ether, caustic alkali solns. LD_{50} orally in rats: 0.57 g/kg (Deichmann).

***o*-Chlorophenol.** [95-57-8] 2-Chlorophenol. Liquid, bp 175°. mp 9.3°. d_4^{23} 1.2573. n_D^{25} 1.5565; *n* 1.5473. Strong medicinal taste and odor. Dipole moment in benzene, 1.33D. Freely sol in alcohol, ether, caustic alkali solns; slightly sol in water. LD_{50} orally in rats: 0.67 g/kg (Deichmann).

***p*-Chlorophenol.** [106-48-9] 4-Chlorophenol. Crystals with characteristic phenolic odor, mp 43.2-43.7°. bp 220°. d_4^{78} 1.2238. n_D^{55} 1.5419; n_D^{40} 1.5579. Dipole moment in benzene, 2.22D. Sparingly sol in water, liquid petrolatum; very sol in alcohol, glycerin, ether, chloroform, fixed and volatile oils: *U.S.P.* **XXI**, 1467. LD_{50} orally in rats: 0.67 g/kg (Deichmann).

Caution: Potential symptoms of overexposure are tremors, convulsions, dyspnea, coma. Direct contact may cause skin irritation. *See: Patty's Industrial Hygiene and Toxicology* Vol. **2A**, G. D. Clayton, F. E. Clayton, Eds. (Wiley-Interscience, New York, 3rd ed., 1981) pp 2612-2615.

USE: Biocide; disinfectant for home, hospital and farm.

THERAP CAT: Antiseptic.

2155. Chlorophyll. [1406-65-1] The green pigment of plants. Higher plants and green algae contain chlorophyll a and chlorophyll b in the approx ratio of 3:1. Chlorophyll c is found together with chlorophyll a in many types of marine algae: Jeffrey, *Biochem. J.* **86**, 313 (1963). Red algae *(Rhodophyta)* contain principally chlorophyll a and also chlorophyll d: Manning, Strain, *J. Biol. Chem.* **151**, 1 (1943). Isoln by chromatography: Tswett, *Ber. Dtsch. Bot. Ges.* **24**, 316, 385 (1906); Willstätter, Stoll, *Investigations on Chlorophyll* (transl by Schertz and Merz: Lancaster, 1928); Schertz, *Ind. Eng. Chem.* **30**, 1073 (1938); Fischer-Orth-Stern, *Die Chemie des Pyrrols* Vol. **II**, part 2 (Leipzig, 1940); Zechmeister, Cholnoky, *Principles and Practice of Chromatography* (New York, 1943). Industrial large-scale isoln processes: Judah *et al., Ind. Eng. Chem.* **46**, 2262 (1954). Structure: Fischer-Orth-Stern, *loc. cit.*; Ficken *et al., J. Chem. Soc.* **1956**, 2273. Total synthesis of chlorophyll a: Woodward *et al., J. Am. Chem. Soc.* **82**, 3800 (1960); *Angew. Chem.* **72**, 651 (1960); Strell *et al., ibid.* 169; Woodward, *Pure Appl. Chem.* **2**, 383 (1963). Abs config of chlorophylls a and b: Brockmann, *Ann.* **754**, 139 (1971); Brockmann, Bode, *Ann.* **1974** (7), 1017. ^{13}C-NMR study of chlorophyll a: S. Lötjönen, P. H. Hynninen, *Org. Magn. Reson.* **16**, 304 (1981); of chlorophyll b: N. Risch, H. Brockmann, *Tetrahedron Lett.* **24**, 173 (1983). Review of syntheses: Johnson, *Sci. Prog.* **49**, 77 (1961). Comprehensive reviews with bibliography: Stoll, Wiedemann, *Fortschr. Chem. Org. Naturst.* **1**, 159-254 (1938); *Fortschr. Chem. Forsch.* **2**, 538 (1952); *The Chlorophylls*, L. P. Vernon, G. R. Seely, Eds. (Academic Press, New York, 1966) 679 pp; Inhoffen *et al., Fortschr. Chem. Org. Naturst.* **26**, 284-298 (1968); Inhoffen, *Pure Appl. Chem.* **17**, 443-460 (1968).

	R_1	R_2	R_3
Chlorophyll a	CH_3	CH_2CH_3	X
Chlorophyll b	CHO	CH_2CH_3	X

Chlorophyll a. [479-61-8] $C_{55}H_{72}MgN_4O_5$; mol wt 893.49. R = CH_3. Sepn and purification: Anderson, Calvin, *Nature* **194**, 285 (1962). Waxy blue-black microcrystals, usually aggregates of thin, lancet-like leaflets, mp 117-120°. $[\alpha]_D^{20}$ −262° (acetone). Absorption max (ether): 660, 613, 577, 531, 498, 429, 409 nm. Freely sol in ether, ethanol, acetone, chloroform, carbon disulfide, benzene. Sparingly sol in cold methanol. Practically insol in petr ether. The alcoholic soln is blue-green with a deep-red fluorescence.

Chlorophyll b. [519-62-0] $C_{55}H_{70}MgN_4O_6$; mol wt 907.47. R = CHO. Waxy blue-black microcrystals. Sinters between 86° and 92°, becomes a viscous liquid at 120-130° and then begins to puff up in large bubbles. $[\alpha]_D^{20}$ −267° (acetone-methanol). Absorption max (ether): 642, 593, 565, 545, 453, 427 nm. Sparingly sol in petr ether, ligroin, cold methanol. Freely sol in abs alcohol, ether. The ether soln has a brilliant green color. Solns with other organic solvents are usually green to yellowish-green with red fluorescence.

Chlorophyll c. Structure: Dougherty *et al., J. Am. Chem. Soc.* **88**, 5037 (1966). Reddish-black hexagonal bipyramids or four-sided plates from dil ethanol. Absorption max (acetone): 628, 580, 442 nm ($E_{1cm}^{0.1\%}$ 15.8, 10.7, 115.9). Sol in methanol, ethanol, ethyl acetate; practically insol in ether, acetone.

Chlorophyll d. $C_{54}H_{70}MgN_4O_6$; mol wt 895.46. Chlorophyll a with the 9-vinyl group replaced by a formyl group: Holt, Morley, *Can. J. Chem.* **37**, 507 (1959); Holt, *Can. J. Bot.* **39**, 327 (1961). Absorption max (ether): 686, 445 nm. The chlorophyll of commerce is an intensely dark-green, aq, alc, or oil soln. Careful alkaline hydrolysis of chlorophyll opens the cyclopentanone ring and replaces the methyl and phytyl ester groups with Na or K; the resulting salts are called *chlorophyllins* and are water sol, e.g. sodium magnesium chlorophyllin, $C_{34}H_{31}N_4Na_3MgO_6$. Acid treatment of chlorophyll removes the Mg replacing it with H_2 which can be replaced with other metals, e.g. iron pheophytin, $C_{55}H_{72}$-FeN_4O_5, sol in oil. Comprehensive review with 89 refs: "Chlorophyll Derivatives, Their Chemistry, Commercial Preparation and Uses" by J. C. Kephart in *Econ. Bot.* **9**, 3-38 (1955). Exhaustive analysis and description of commercial chlorophyllin prepns: Strell *et al., Arzneim.-Forsch.* **5**, 640 (1955); **6**, 8 (1956). Trademarks: *Chloresium, Chlorofolin, Darotol, Ennds, Exodor-Grun, Nullo Chlorophyll, Stozzon-Chlorophyll.*

USE: To color soaps, oils, fats, waxes, confectionery, preserves, liquors, cosmetics, perfumes. Source of phytol. For dyeing leather. As sensitizer for color film. Has been used as antiknock agent in gasoline; as accelerator in the vulcanizing of rubber; in deodorizers.

THERAP CAT: Deodorant.

THERAP CAT (VET): Has been used orally to reduce odors, and topically to promote healing of skin lesions.

2156. Chloropicrin. [76-06-2] Trichloronitromethane; acquinite; nitrochloroform; Larvacide 100; Picfume. CCl_3NO_2; mol wt 164.38. C 7.31%, Cl 64.70%, N 8.52%, O 19.47%. First prepd in 1848 by Stenhouse from picric acid and bleach powder. Review of prepn, properties, physiological action, and uses: Jackson, *Chem. Rev.* **14**, 251 (1934). Manuf from nitromethane and alkaline hypochlorite: Wilhelm, **US 3106588** (1963).

Slightly oily liquid, intense odor; bp_{757} 112°. mp −64°; mp −69.2° (corr). d_4^{20} 1.6558, d_4^{25} 1.6483. n_D^{20} 1.4611, n_D^{25} 1.4596. Dipole moment in heptane or benzene, 1.80D. Practically insol in water. Soly in water (g/100 ml): 0.2272 (0°), 0.1621 (25°). Miscible with benzene, abs alc, carbon disulfide; sol in ether.

Caution: Potential symptoms of overexposure are irritation of eyes, skin, respiratory system; lacrimation; cough, pulmonary edema; nausea, vomiting. *See NIOSH Pocket Guide to Chemical Hazards* (DHHS/NIOSH 97-140, 1997) p 66.

USE: Disinfecting cereals and grains; in synthesis, esp in manuf of methyl violet; fumigant; soil insecticide; war gas.

2157. Chloroprednisone. [52080-57-6] (6α)-Chloro-17,21-dihydroxypregna-1,4-diene-3,11,20-trione; 6α-chloro-1,4-pregnadiene-17α,21-diol-3,11,20-trione; $C_{21}H_{25}ClO_5$; mol wt 392.87. C 64.20%, H 6.41%, Cl 9.02%, O 20.36%. Prepn: Batres *et al.*, **DE 1079042** (1960 to Syntex). Prepn of the 21-acetate by selenium dioxide dehydrogenation of 6α-chlorocortisone 21-acetate: Ringold *et al., J. Am. Chem. Soc.* **80**, 6464 (1958); Ringold, Rosenkranz, **US 2957895** (1960 to Syntex).

21-Acetate. [14066-79-6] Topilan. $C_{23}H_{27}ClO_6$; mol wt 434.91. Crystals from acetone + hexane, mp 217-219°. uv max (ethanol): 237 nm (log ε 4.19). $[\alpha]_D$ +144° (chloroform).

THERAP CAT: Glucocorticoid (topical).

2158. Chloroprocaine Hydrochloride. [3858-89-7] 4-Amino-2-chlorobenzoic acid 2-(diethylamino)ethyl ester monohydrochloride; 2-chloro-4-aminobenzoic acid diethylaminoethyl ester hydrochloride; Nesacaine. $C_{13}H_{20}Cl_2N_2O_2$; mol wt 307.22. C 50.82%, H 6.56%, Cl 23.08%, N 9.12%, O 10.42%. Description: Hädicke, *Pharm. Zentralhalle* **94**, 384 (1955).

Crystals, mp 176-178° (microstage). Bitter taste. Slowly sol in water. Soly in water at 20° about one gram in 22 ml. Aq solns are just acid to litmus and turn yellow on standing. Soly in 95% ethanol about one gram in 100 ml.

THERAP CAT: Anesthetic (local).

2159. β-Chloropropionic Acid. [107-94-8] 3-Chloropropanoic acid. $C_3H_5ClO_2$; mol wt 108.52. C 33.20%, H 4.64%, Cl 32.67%, O 29.49%. CH_2ClCH_2COOH. Prepd by the hydrolysis of ethylene cyanohydrin with hydrochloric acid; by the oxidation of β-chloropropionaldehyde or of trimethylene chlorohydrin by nitric acid: Moureu, Chaux, *Org. Synth.* **8**, 54 (1928); Powell, *ibid.* 58; Paal, Lobeck, *Ber.* **64**, 2142 (1931).

Leaflets from ligroin. Somewhat hygroscopic. mp 41°. bp_{765} 200°; bp_{35} 127°; bp_{25} 124°; bp_{12} 108°. pK (25°) 4.00. Freely sol in water, alc, chloroform, slightly less in ether.

Methyl ester. $C_4H_7ClO_2$. From β-chloropropionic acid with methanol and HCl or from acrylic acid chloride and methanol. d_4^0 1.198. bp 155-157°.

2160. β-Chloropropionitrile. [542-76-7] 3-Chloropropanenitrile; 3-chloropropanonitrile. C_3H_4ClN; mol wt 89.52. C 40.25%, H 4.50%, Cl 39.60%, N 15.65%. $ClCH_2CH_2CN$. Prepd from acrylonitrile and hydrogen chloride or bromide: Moureu, Clarke, *Bull. Soc. Chim. Fr.* [4] **27**, 905 (1920); Stewart, Clarke, *J. Am. Chem. Soc.* **69**, 714 (1947); Shirley, *Preparation of Organic Intermediates* (Wiley, New York, 1951) p 82.

Liquid. Acrid, characteristic odor. *Poisonous!* mp −51°. d_4^{25} 1.1363. bp_{760} 176° (dec); bp_{200} 132° (dec); bp_{50} 95.2°; bp_5 46.0°. Flash pt 168°F (75.5°C). n_D^{25} 1.4341. Begins to dec when heated above 130° evolving HCl. Absorbs strongly in the infrared. Transparent to uv above 220 nm. Soly in water at 25°: 4.5 g/100 ml. Soly of water in β-chloropropionitrile at 25°: 2.2 ml/100 g. Miscible with ethanol, ether, acetone, benzene, carbon tetrachloride. LD_{50} orally in mice, rats: 9, 100 mg/kg, Fassett in *Industrial Hygiene and Toxicology* vol. 2, F. A. Patty, Ed. (Interscience, New York, 2nd ed., 1962) pp 2025-2026.

Caution: Exposure by any route should be avoided. Somewhat less hazardous than acrylonitrile because of lower vapor pressure. Readily penetrates skin to produce systemic cyanide poisoning, death.

USE: In pharmaceutical and polymer synthesis. Combines the reactivity of a nitrile and an alkyl halide. Because of the cyano group the chlorine atom is more reactive than in ordinary alkyl halides.

2161. 6-Chloropurine. [87-42-3] $C_5H_3ClN_4$; mol wt 154.56. C 38.85%, H 1.96%, Cl 22.94%, N 36.25%. Prepd by the action of phosphorus oxychloride on hypoxanthine in N,N-dimethylaniline: Bendich *et al.*, *J. Am. Chem. Soc.* **76**, 6073 (1954). Antineoplastic activity *in vivo:* A. C. Sartorelli, B. A. Booth, *Experientia* **21**, 457 (1965).

Blunt needles from water, dec 175-177° (hot stage preheated to 170°). Also reported as not melted at 290°. uv max (pH 5.2): 265 nm (ε 9120); (pH 13): 274 nm (ε 8790). Soly in water: 0.5% at 20°, also reported as 1 g/182 ml at 24°. Sol in ether, dimethylformamide.

2162. Chloropyramine. [59-32-5] N-[(4-Chlorophenyl)-methyl]-N',N'-dimethyl-N-2-pyridinyl-1,2-ethanediamine; 2-[(p-chlorobenzyl)[2-(dimethylamino)ethyl]amino]pyridine; N-dimethylaminoethyl-N-p-chlorobenzyl-α-aminopyridine; N,N-dimethyl-N'-(p-chlorobenzyl)-N'-(2-pyridyl)ethylenediamine; halopyramine. $C_{16}H_{20}ClN_3$; mol wt 289.80. C 66.31%, H 6.96%, Cl 12.23%, N 14.50%. Prepn: Phillips, Cates, **US 2607778** (1952 to Merck & Co.); Howard, **US 2569314** (1951 to Am. Cyanamid); **CH 264754**; **CH 266234**; **CH 266235** (1950); **GB 651596** (1951) (all to Geigy).

Light yellow, viscous, oily liquid. Pungent odor. bp$_{0.2}$ 154-155°.
Hydrochloride. [6170-42-9] Synopen; Synpen. $C_{16}H_{20}$-ClN_3.HCl; mol wt 326.26. Crystals from acetone, mp 172-174°.
THERAP CAT: Antihistaminic.

2163. Chloroquine. [54-05-7] N^4-(7-Chloro-4-quinolinyl)-N^1,N^1-diethyl-1,4-pentanediamine; 7-chloro-4-(4-diethylamino-1-methylbutylamino)quinoline; SN-7618; RP-3377. $C_{18}H_{26}ClN_3$; mol wt 319.87. C 67.59%, H 8.19%, Cl 11.08%, N 13.14%. Prepd by the condensation of 4,7-dichloroquinoline with 1-diethylamino-4-aminopentane: **DE 683692** (1939); H. Andersag *et al.*, **US 2233970** (1941 to Winthrop); Surrey, Hammer, *J. Am. Chem. Soc.* **68**, 113 (1946). *Review:* Hahn in *Antibiotics* vol. **3**, J. W. Corcoran, F. E. Hahn, Eds. (Springer-Verlag, New York, 1975) pp 58-78. Comprehensive description: D. D. Hong, *Anal. Profiles Drug Subs.* **5**, 61-85 (1976). Comparative clinical trial with dapsone in rheumatoid arthritis: P. D. Fowler *et al.*, *Ann. Rheum. Dis.* **43**, 200 (1984); with penicillamine: T. Gibson *et al.*, *Br. J. Rheumatol.* **26**, 279 (1987).

mp 87°.
Diphosphate. [50-63-5] Arechin; Avloclor; Malaquin; Resochin. $C_{18}H_{26}ClN_3$.2H$_3$PO$_4$; mol wt 515.86. Bitter, colorless crystals. Dimorphic. One modification, mp 193-195°; the other, mp 215-218°. Freely sol in water; pH of 1% soln about 4.5; less sol at neutral and alkaline pH. Stable to heat in solns of pH 4.0 to 6.5. Practically insol in alcohol, benzene, chloroform, ether.

Sulfate. [132-60-5] Aralen; Nivaquine. $C_{18}H_{26}ClN_3$.H$_2$SO$_4$; mol wt 417.95.
THERAP CAT: Antimalarial; antiamebic; antirheumatic. Lupus erythematosus suppressant.

2164. *N*-Chlorosuccinimide. [128-09-6] 1-Chloro-2,5-pyrrolidinedione; succinchlorimide. $C_4H_4ClNO_2$; mol wt 133.53. C 35.98%, H 3.02%, Cl 26.55%, N 10.49%, O 23.96%. Prepn from succinimide: Hirst, Macbeth, *J. Chem. Soc.* **121**, 2169 (1922); Zimmer, Audrieth, *J. Am. Chem. Soc.* **76**, 3856 (1954). Crystal structure: Brown, *Acta Crystallogr.* **9**, 193 (1956); **14**, 711 (1961). Toxicity data: Stohlman, Smith, *Public Health Rep.* **59**, 541 (1944).

Orthorhombic crystals, mp 150-151°. Odor of chlorine. Acid to litmus (1:50 aq soln). One gram dissolves in about 70 ml water, 150 ml alcohol, 50 ml benzene. Sparingly sol in ether, chloroform, carbon tetrachloride. Liberates iodine from potassium iodide solns, and bromine from sodium bromide solns. MLD orally in rats: 2.7 g/kg (Stohlman, Smith).
USE: Chlorinating agent.

2165. Chlorosulfonic Acid. [7790-94-5] Sulfuric chlorohydrin; chlorosulfuric acid. $ClHO_3S$; mol wt 116.52. Cl 30.43%, H 0.87%, O 41.19%, S 27.52%. SO_2(OH)Cl. Prepd by the reaction of HCl gas with SO_3: Simon, Kratsch, *Z. Anorg. Allg. Chem.* **242**, 369 (1939); Briggs, **US 1442335** (1922 to General Chem.). Purification: Kaplar, Shechter, *Inorg. Synth.* **4**, 52 (1953). *Review:* H. O. Burrus in *Kirk-Othmer Encyclopedia of Chemical Technology* vol. **5** (Wiley-Interscience, New York, 3rd ed., 1979) pp 873-880.

Colorless or slightly yellow, very corrosive liquid, causes severe burns; fumes in air; pungent odor. d_{20}^{20} 1.76-1.77; d_4^0 1.784; d_4^{20} 1.753. mp $-80°$. bp$_{755}$ 151-152°; bp$_{19}$ 74-75°; bp$_{2-4}$ 60-64°. n_D^{14} 1.437. On dropping into water dec with explosive violence. *Keep tightly closed.* When used for the prepn of sulfate esters, the common solvent is pyridine. Other solvents are liquid sulfur dioxide and dichloroethane.
Caution: Highly irritating and corrosive to eyes, skin, mucous membranes.
USE: Manuf sulfone compds, saccharin. As chlorosulfonating and condensing agent in organic syntheses.

2166. Chlorothalonil. [1897-45-6] 2,4,5,6-Tetrachloro-1,3-benzenedicarbonitrile; tetrachloroisophthalonitrile; m-tetrachlorophthalodinitrile; 2,4,5,6-tetrachloro-1,3-dicyanobenzene; 1,3-dicyano-2,4,5,6-tetrachlorobenzene; chlorthalonil; DAC-2787; Daconil 2787; Bravo. $C_8Cl_4N_2$; mol wt 265.91. C 36.13%, Cl 53.33%, N 10.53%. Fungicidal properties first described by N. J. Turner *et al.*, *Contrib. Boyce Thompson Inst.* **22**, 303 (1964). Prepn: R. D. Battershell, H. Bluestone, **US 3290353** (1966 to Diamond Alkali); R. M. Bimber, **US 3652637** (1972 to Diamond Shamrock). Toxicity studies in mice: H. Yoshikawa, K. Kawai, *Ind. Health* **4**, 11 (1966). Review of carcinogenic risk: *IARC Monographs* **30**, 319-328 (1983).

Crystals. d_4^{25} 1.7. mp 250-251°. bp$_{760}$ 350°. Vapor press <0.01 at 40°. Practically insol in water (soly at room temp reported as 0.6 ppm). Soly in organic solvents at 25° (w/w): xylene 8%, cyclohexanone 3%, acetone 2%, kerosine <1.0%. LD$_{50}$ orally in rats: >10.0 g/kg (Turner).
USE: Fungicide, bactericide, nematocide. Agricultural and horticultural fungicide.

2167. Chlorothen. [148-65-2] *N*-[(5-Chloro-2-thienyl)-methyl]-*N'*,*N'*-dimethyl-*N*-2-pyridinyl-1,2-ethanediamine; 2-[(5-chloro-2-thenyl)(2-dimethylaminoethyl)amino]pyridine; *N*,*N*-dimethyl-*N'*-(2-pyridyl)-*N'*-(5-chloro-2-thenyl)ethylenediamine; *N*,*N*-dimethyl-*N'*-(α-pyridyl)-*N'*-(2-methyl-5-chlorothienyl)ethylenediamine; *N*-5-chloro-2-thienylmethyl-*N'*,*N'*-dimethyl-*N*-2-pyridylethylenediamine; chloropyrilene; chloromethapyrilene; chlorothenylpyramine. $C_{14}H_{18}ClN_3S$; mol wt 295.83. C 56.84%, H 6.13%, Cl 11.98%, N 14.20%, S 10.84%. Prepd by the condensation of 5-chloro-2-thenyl chloride and *N*,*N*-dimethyl-*N'*-(2-pyridyl)ethylenediamine in the presence of sodium or potassium amide: R. C. Clapp *et al.*, *J. Am. Chem. Soc.* **69**, 1549 (1947); L. P. Kyrides, US **2581869** (1952 to Monsanto). Toxicity data: J. C. Castillo *et al.*, *J. Pharmacol. Exp. Ther.* **96**, 388 (1949).

Liquid. $bp_{1.0}$ 155-156°. Strong base.
Hydrochloride. Thenclor. $C_{14}H_{18}ClN_3S.HCl$; mol wt 332.29. Crystals, mp 106-108°. Freely sol in water.
Citrate. [148-64-1] Tagathen. $C_{14}H_{18}ClN_3S.C_6H_8O_7$; mol wt 487.95. Crystals, mp 112-116°. On further heating gradually solidifies and remelts 125-140° (dec). uv max: 240 nm ($E_{1cm}^{1\%}$ 390-410). One gram dissolves in 35 ml water, in about 65 ml alc. Practically insol in ether, chloroform, benzene, pH of 1% aq soln 3.9 to 4.1. LD_{50} i.p. in mice: 105 mg/kg (Castillo).

THERAP CAT: Antihistaminic.

2168. Chlorothiazide. [58-94-6] 6-Chloro-2*H*-1,2,4-benzothiadiazine-7-sulfonamide 1,1-dioxide; 6-chloro-7-sulfamoyl-2*H*-1,2,4-benzothiadiazine 1,1-dioxide; 6-chloro-7-sulfamyl-1,2,4-benzothiadiazine 1,1-dioxide; Chlotride; Diuril; Saluric. $C_7H_6ClN_3O_4S_2$; mol wt 295.72. C 28.43%, H 2.05%, Cl 11.99%, N 14.21%, O 21.64%, S 21.69%. Prepn: F. C. Novello, US **2809194** (1957 to Merck & Co.); F. C. Novello, J. M. Sprague, *J. Am. Chem. Soc.* **79**, 2028 (1957). HPLC determn in urine: R. O. Fullinfaw *et al.*, *J. Chromatogr.* **415**, 347 (1987). Comprehensive description: H. G. Brittain, *Anal. Profiles Drug Subs.* **18**, 33-56 (1989).

Colorless needles from dil alc, mp 342.5-343°. pKa_1 6.85, pKa_2 9.45. Freely sol in DMSO, DMF; slightly sol in methanol, pyridine; very slightly sol in water. Practically insol in diethyl ether, chloroform, benzene. Soly (g/L): water (pH 4) 0; (pH 7) 0.65. Sol in alkaline aq solns with decompn upon standing or heating.
Sodium salt. [7085-44-1] 6-Chloro-7-sulfamoyl-2*H*-1,2,4-benzothiadiazin-2-ylsodium 1,1-dioxide. $C_7H_5ClN_3NaO_4S_2$; mol wt 317.71.

THERAP CAT: Diuretic; antihypertensive.
THERAP CAT (VET): Diuretic.

2169. Chlorothricin. [34707-92-1] $C_{50}H_{63}ClO_{16}$; mol wt 955.48. C 62.85%, H 6.65%, Cl 3.71%, O 26.79%. Macrolide antibiotic active against gram-positive bacteria. Isolated together with its dechloro analog from Tü 99, a strain of *Streptomyces antibioticus*: Keller-Schierlein *et al.*, *Helv. Chim. Acta* **52**, 127 (1969). Degradation products studies: Muntwyler *et al.*, *ibid.* **53**, 1544 (1970). Structure: Muntwyler, Keller-Schierlein, *ibid.* **55**, 2071 (1972). Non-competitive inhibitor of pyruvate carboxylase: P. W. Schindler, H. Zaehner, *Arch. Mikrobiol.* **82**, 66, (1972); P. W. Schindler, M. C. Scrutton, *ibid.* **55**, 543 (1975). Biosynthetic studies: O. Mascaretti *et al.*, *J. Nat. Prod.* **42**, 455 (1979); *eidem, Biochemistry* **20**, 919 (1981). Partial synthesis of the aglycone, *chlorothricolide*:

R. E. Ireland, W. J. Thompson, *J. Org. Chem.* **44**, 3041 (1979); R. E. Ireland *et al.*, *ibid.* **46**, 4863 (1981); W. R. Roush, S. E. Hall, *J. Am. Chem. Soc.* **103**, 5200 (1981). Alternate synthetic approach: R. E. Ireland, M. D. Varney, *J. Org. Chem.* **51**, 635 (1986). *Review:* Keller-Schierlein, *Fortschr. Chem. Org. Naturst.* **30**, 394-396 (1973); H. G. Floss, C.-J. Chang, *Antibiotics* **vol. IV**, J. W. Corcoran, Ed. (Springer-Verlag, New York, 1981) pp 193-214.

Colorless crystals from methylene chloride-methyl acetate, mp 206-207°. uv max (alc): 222, 260 nm (log ε 4.20, 3.81); (0.01*N* alc KOH): 221, 259 nm (log ε 4.09, 3.95). Dibasic acid; pK: 5.01, 7.91. (The above data applies to a 5:1 mixture with dechlorothricin, Muntwyler, Keller-Schierlein, *loc. cit.*). Slightly sol in water; readily sol in organic solvents of medium polarity.

2170. Chlorothymol. [89-68-9] 4-Chloro-5-methyl-2-(1-methylethyl)phenol; 6-chlorothymol; 4-chlorothymol; 1-methyl-3-hydroxy-4-isopropyl-6-chlorobenzene; 6-chloro-4-isopropyl-1-methyl-3-phenol. $C_{10}H_{13}ClO$; mol wt 184.66. C 65.04%, H 7.10%, Cl 19.20%, O 8.66%. Made by the action of sulfuryl chloride on thymol in CCl_4: Satriana *et al.*, *J. Am. Pharm. Assoc.* **39**, 135 (1950); H. Pahlicke, DE **905738** (1954 to Diwag), *C.A.* **52**, 16294i (1958). Antifungal properties: M. Iannarone, *Drug Stand.* **25**, 190 (1957).

Crystals. mp 62-64° (59-61° *N.F.* **XII**). One gram dissolves in about 1000 ml water, 0.5 ml alcohol, 2 ml benzene, 2 ml chloroform, 1.5 ml ether, about 10 ml petr ether; also sol in dil aq NaOH.

2171. Chlorotoluene. C_7H_7Cl; mol wt 126.58. C 66.42%, H 5.57%, Cl 28.01%. Prepn from diazotized toluidine: Neogi, Mitra, *J. Chem. Soc.* **1928**, 1332; Marvel, McElvain, *Org. Synth.* **coll. vol. I**, 170 (1941). Manuf of *o*- and *p*-isomers by catalytic chlorination of toluene: Di Bella, US **3000975** (1959 to Heyden Newport Chem.). Absorption spectrum of *m*- and *p*-isomers: Baly, *J. Chem. Soc.* **99**, 1704 (1911); of *m*- and *o*-isomers: Purvis, *ibid.* 1704. Metabolism of *o*-isomer by bacteria: P. A. Vandenbergh *et al.*, *Appl. Environ. Microbiol.* **42**, 737 (1981); by rats: G. B. Quistad *et al.*, *J. Agric. Food Chem.* **31**, 1158 (1983). Brief review: S. Gelfand in *Kirk-Othmer Encyclopedia of Chemical Technology* **vol. 5** (Wiley-Interscience, New York, 3rd ed., 1979) pp 819-827.

m-**Chlorotoluene.** [108-41-8] 1-Chloro-3-methylbenzene. Liquid, bp 161.75°. $d_4^{18.7}$ 1.0760. mp $-47.8°$. n_D^{20} 1.5218.

o-**Chlorotoluene.** [95-49-8] 1-Chloro-2-methylbenzene. Liquid, bp 158.97°. Vapor harmful. d_4^{20} 1.0826. mp $-35.59°$. n_D^{20} 1.5258. Volatile with steam. Slightly sol in water; freely sol in alcohol, benzene, chloroform, ether.

p-**Chlorotoluene.** [106-43-4] 1-Chloro-4-methylbenzene. Liquid, bp 162.4°. d_4^{20} 1.0697. mp 7.5°. n_D^{20} 1.5211. Slightly sol in water; sol in alcohol, benzene, chloroform, ether.

Caution: Potential symptoms of overexposure to *o*-chlorotoluene are irritation of eyes, skin, mucous membranes; dermatitis; drowsiness, incoordination, anesthesia; cough; liver and kidney injury. *See NIOSH Pocket Guide to Chemical Hazards* (DHHS/NIOSH 97-140, 1997) p 68.

USE: Solvent; dyestuff intermediate; in organic syntheses.

2172. Chlorotoluron. [15545-48-9] N'-(3-Chloro-4-methylphenyl)-*N,N*-dimethylurea; 3-(3-chloro-*p*-tolyl)-1,1-dimethylurea; Dicuran; Tolurex. $C_{10}H_{13}ClN_2O$; mol wt 212.68. C 56.47%, H 6.16%, Cl 16.67%, N 13.17%, O 7.52%. Photosynthesis inhibitor used to control grass weeds in cereals. Prepn: C. W. Todd, **US 2655445** (1952 to Du Pont); T. Mizuno *et al., Synth. Commun.* **9**, 1675 (2000). Degradation in soil and identification of metabolites: D. Gross *et al., Pestic. Biochem. Physiol.* **10**, 49 (1979). HPLC determn in technical products and formulations: W. Y. Yan *et al., Pestic. Sci.* **49**, 400 (1997). Movement in sandy soil: C. Zander *et al., J. Environ. Qual.* **28**, 1817 (1999). Field trial on grassy weeds in wheat: S. Singh, R. K. Malik *Indian J. Agron.* **39**, 23 (1994).

Crystals from toluene, mp 148.3°.

USE: Herbicide.

2173. Chlorotoxin. [163515-35-3] ClTx; Ctx. Small neurotoxic peptide (36 amino acids) isolated from the venom of the scorpion, *Leiurus quinquestriatus* characterized by 4 disulfide linkages. Specific blocker of small conductance chloride channels. Isoln, purification, and characterization: J. A. DeBin *et al., Am. J. Physiol.* **264**, C361 (1993). Solid phase synthesis: J. Najib *et al., 3rd Int. Symp. 1993 Innovation Perspect. Solid Phase Synth. Collect. Pap.* **1994**, 615. NMR and secondary structure: G. Lippens *et al., ibid.* 583; and solution structure: *eidem, Biochemistry* **34**, 13 (1995). Identification of chloride channel in gliomas: N. Ullrich *et al., Neuroscience* **83**, 1161 (1998); inhibition of glioma cell invasion: J. Deshane *et al., J. Biol. Chem.* **278**, 4135 (2003). Use in cell topography: G. Tobasnick, A. S. G. Curtis, *Eur. Cells Materials* **2**, 49 (2001).

M-C-M-P-C-F-T-T-D-H-Q-M-A-R-K-C-D-D-C-C-G-G-K-G-R-G-K-C-Y-G-Q-C-L-C-R-NH₂

USE: Biochemical probe for voltage-gated chloride channels.

2174. Chlorotrianisene. [569-57-3] 1,1′,1″-(1-Chloro-1-ethenyl-2-ylidene)tris[4-methoxybenzene]; chlorotris(*p*-methoxyphenyl)ethylene; tri-*p*-anisylchloroethylene; tris(*p*-methoxyphenyl)chloroethylene; Hormonisene; Merbentul; Tace. $C_{23}H_{21}ClO_3$; mol wt 380.86. C 72.53%, H 5.56%, Cl 9.31%, O 12.60%. Prepd by reacting tri-*p*-anisylethylene or tri-*p*-anisylethanol with Cl in an

inert solvent: Basford and I.C.I., **GB 561508** (1944). Synthesis from *p*-(*p*-anisoyl)anisole: Shelton, Van Campen, Jr., **US 2430891** (1947 to Merrell).

Crystals from methanol, mp 114-116°. Softens at 108°. uv max (chloroform): 310 nm, ($E_{1cm}^{1\%}$ 423); min 278 nm. Practically insol in water. Soly in alcohol: 0.28 g/100 ml; in ether: 3.6 g/100 ml. Also sol in glacial acetic acid, acetone, chloroform, carbon tetrachloride, benzene, vegetable oils.

THERAP CAT: Estrogen.

2175. Chloroxine. [773-76-2] 5,7-Dichloro-8-quinolinol; 5,7-dichloro-8-hydroxyquinoline; Capitrol. $C_9H_5Cl_2NO$; mol wt 214.05. C 50.50%, H 2.35%, Cl 33.13%, N 6.54%, O 7.47%. Prepd by chlorinating 8-quinolinol: Hebebrand, *Ber.* **21**, 2977 (1888), F. J. Welcher, *Organic Analytical Reagents* **vol. I** (Van Nostrand, 1947) pp 328-329.

Crystals from alc, mp 179-180°. Soluble in benzene, acetone; slightly sol in cold alcohol, acetic acid; readily sol in sodium and potassium hydroxides and in acids, forming yellow solns.

USE: Analytical reagent.

THERAP CAT: Antiseborrheic.

2176. Chloroxylenol. [88-04-0] 4-Chloro-3,5-dimethylphenol; *p*-chloro-*m*-xylenol; 4-chloro-3,5-xylenol; parachlorometaxylenol; 2-chloro-*m*-xylenol; 2-chloro-5-hydroxy-*m*-xylene; 2-chloro-5-hydroxy-1,3-dimethylbenzene; Benzytol; Dettol. C_8H_9ClO; mol wt 156.61. C 61.35%, H 5.79%, Cl 22.64%, O 10.22%. Prepd by treating 3,5-dimethylphenol with Cl_2 or SO_2Cl_2: Lesser, Gad, *Ber.* **56**, 974, 976 (1923); von Auwers *et al., Chem. Zentralbl.* **1924, II,** 2267, *C.A.* **19,** 2339 (1925); Gladden, Cocker, **US 2350677** (1944).

Crystals from benzene, mp 115.5°. Phenolic odor. Volatile with steam. bp 246°. One gram dissolves in 3 liters of water at 20°. More stable in hot water. Soluble in 1 part of 95% alcohol, ether, benzene, terpenes, fixed oils, in solns of alkali hydroxides.

USE: Antiseptic and germicide; for mildew prevention. Claimed to be about 60 times as potent as phenol.

THERAP CAT: Antibacterial; antiseptic (topical and urinary).

THERAP CAT (VET): Antiseptic (topical).

2177. Chlorozotocin. [54749-90-5] 2-[[[(2-Chloroethyl)-nitrosoamino]carbonyl]amino]-2-deoxy-D-glucose; 2-[3-(2-chloroethyl)-3-nitrosoureido]-2-deoxy-D-glucopyranose; 1-(2-chloroethyl)-1-nitroso-3-(D-glucos-2-yl)urea; DCNU; NSC-178248. C_9H_{16}-ClN_3O_7; mol wt 313.69. C 34.46%, H 5.14%, Cl 11.30%, N 13.40%, O 35.70%. Chloroethylnitrosourea derivative with antitumor activity. Similar to carmustine, lomustine, nimustine, ranimustine, *q.q.v;* 2-chloroethyl analog of streptozotocin, *q.v.* Synthesis: H. D. Burns *et al., Org. Prep. Proced. Int.* **6**, 259 (1974); T. P. Johnston *et al., J. Med. Chem.* **18**, 104 (1975). Pharmacology: T. Anderson *et al., Cancer Res.* **35**, 761 (1975); P. S. Schein *et al., Cancer Treat. Rep.* **60**, 801 (1976). Decomposition in aqueous media: J. A. Montgomery *et al., J. Med. Chem.* **18**, 568 (1975).

Ivory colored crystals, mp 147-148° (dec with the evolution of gas), (Burns, Heindel). Also reported as mp 140-141° (dec), (Johnston). Sol in water.

Caution: This substance is reasonably anticipated to be a human carcinogen: *Report on Carcinogens, Eleventh Edition* (PB2005-104914, 2004) p III-62.

THERAP CAT: Antineoplastic.

2178. Chlorphenesin. [104-29-0] 3-(4-Chlorophenoxy)-1,2-propanediol; *p*-chlorophenyl α-glyceryl ether; Adermykon; Mycil. $C_9H_{11}ClO_3$; mol wt 202.63. C 53.35%, H 5.47%, Cl 17.50%, O 23.69%. Prepd by condensing equimol amts of *p*-chlorophenol and glycidol in the presence of a tertiary amine or a quaternary ammonium salt as catalyst: Bradley, Forrest, **GB 628497** (1949 to British Drug Houses).

Crystals, mp 77-79°. Soly in water is less than 1%, may be increased by the addition of solubilizers such as ethylurea or propylene glycol: Berger *et al., US 2468423* (1949 to British Drug Houses).

THERAP CAT: Antifungal (topical).

2179. Chlorphenesin Carbamate. [886-74-8] 3-(4-Chlorophenoxy)-1,2-propanediol-1-carbamate; carbamic acid 3-(*p*-chlorophenoxy)-2-hydroxypropyl ester; 3-(*p*-chlorophenoxy)-2-hydroxypropyl carbamate; 1,2-propanediol-3-(*p*-chlorophenoxy)-1-carbamate; Maolate; Rinlaxer. $C_{10}H_{12}ClNO_4$; mol wt 245.66. C 48.89%, H 4.92%, Cl 14.43%, N 5.70%, O 26.05%. Prepn: Collins, Matthews, **US 3161567**; Parker, **US 3214336** (1964, 1965 both to Upjohn). Clinical evaluation of analgesic activity: L. J. Cass, W. S. Frederick, *J. New Drugs* **2**, 366 (1962).

Crystals from benzene + toluene, mp 89-91°. Readily sol in 95% ethanol, acetone, ethyl acetate; fairly readily sol in dioxane. Almost insol in cold water, benzene, cyclohexane. LD_{50} orally in rats: 748 mg/kg; i.v. in mice: 239 mg/kg (Cass, Frederick).

THERAP CAT: Muscle relaxant (skeletal).

THERAP CAT (VET): Muscle relaxant (skeletal).

2180. Chlorpheniramine. [132-22-9] γ-(4-Chlorophenyl)-*N,N*-dimethyl-2-pyridinepropanamine; 2-[*p*-chloro-α-(2-dimethylaminoethyl)benzyl]pyridine; 1-(*p*-chlorophenyl)-1-(2-pyridyl)-3-dimethylaminopropane; 1-(*p*-chlorophenyl)-1-(2-pyridyl)-3-*N,N*-dimethylpropylamine; 3-(*p*-chlorophenyl)-3-(2-pyridyl)-*N,N*-dimethylpropylamine; γ-(4-chlorophenyl)-γ-(2-pyridyl)propyldimethylamine; chlorprophenpyridamine; chlorphenamine; Haynon. C_{16}-

$H_{19}ClN_2$; mol wt 274.79. C 69.93%, H 6.97%, Cl 12.90%, N 10.19%. Synthesis: Sperber *et al.,* **US 2567245, US 2676964** (1951, 1954, both to Schering). Prepn of *d*-form: L. A. Walter, **US 3061517** (1962 to Schering). Solutions: Foley, Ilavsky, **US 2766174** (1956 to Schering). Pharmacology: F. E. Roth, W. M. Govier, *J. Pharmacol. Exp. Ther.* **124**, 347 (1958). Toxicity data: R. B. Smith *et al., Toxicol. Appl. Pharmacol.* **28**, 240 (1974). Comprehensive description: C. G. Eckhart, T. McCorkle, *Anal. Profiles Drug Subs.* **7**, 43-80 (1978).

Oily liquid, $bp_{1.0}$ 142°.

Maleate. [113-92-8] Allergisan; Chlor-Trimeton; Piriton; Teldrin. $C_{16}H_{19}ClN_2·C_4H_4O_4$; mol wt 390.86. Crystals, mp 130-135°. uv max (water): 261 nm (ε 5760). Soly in mg/ml at 25°: ethanol 330; chloroform 240; water 160; methanol 130. Slightly sol in benzene, ether. pH of a 2% aq soln about 5. LD_{50} orally in mice: 162 mg/kg (Smith).

d-Form. [25523-97-1] Dexchlorpheniramine; *d*-chlorpheniramine. Oily liquid. $[\alpha]_D^{25}$ +49.8° (c = 1 in DMF).

d-Form maleate. [2438-32-6] Phenamin; Polamin; Polaramine; Polaronil. Crystals from ethyl acetate, mp 113-115°. $[\alpha]_D^{25}$ +44.3° (c = 1 in dimethylformamide). pH of 1% soln 4-5.

THERAP CAT: Antihistaminic.

THERAP CAT (VET): Antihistaminic.

2181. Chlorphenoxamine. [77-38-3] 2-[1-(4-Chlorophenyl)-1-phenylethoxy]-*N,N*-dimethylethanamine; 2-[(*p*-chloro-α-methyl-α-phenylbenzyl)oxy]-*N,N*-dimethylethylamine; β-dimethylaminoethyl (*p*-chloro-α-methylbenzhydryl) ether; [1-(*p*-chlorophenyl)-1-phenyl]ethyl (β-dimethylaminoethyl) ether. $C_{18}H_{22}$-ClNO; mol wt 303.84. C 71.16%, H 7.30%, Cl 11.67%, N 4.61%, O 5.27%. Prepn: Arnold *et al., US 2785202* (1957 to Asta-Werke). Synthesis: G. Cahiez *et al., Tetrahedron Lett.* **29**, 3659 (1988). Pharmacology: *eidem, Arzneim.-Forsch.* **4**, 189 (1954); Brock *et al., ibid.* 262. Toxicity studies: Kerley *et al., Toxicol. Appl. Pharmacol.* **4**, 638 (1962). Metabolism: C. Koppel *et al., Arzneim.-Forsch.* **37**, 1062 (1987). GC-MS determn in urine: H. Maurer, K. Pfleger, *J. Chromatogr.* **428**, 43 (1988).

$bp_{0.05}$ 150-155°.

Hydrochloride. [562-09-4] Clorevan; Systral. $C_{18}H_{22}$-ClNO.HCl; mol wt 340.29. Needles, mp 128°. Soluble in water; aq solns are stable.

THERAP CAT: Antihistaminic.

2182. Chlorphentermine. [461-78-9] 4-Chloro-α,α-dimethylbenzeneethanamine; 4-chloro-α,α-dimethylphenethylamine; α,α-dimethyl-*p*-chlorophenethylamine; 1-(*p*-chlorophenyl)-2-methyl-2-propylamine; 1-(*p*-chlorophenyl)-2-methyl-2-aminopropane; clorfentermina; Lucofen; Teramine. $C_{10}H_{14}ClN$; mol wt 183.68. C 65.39%, H 7.68%, Cl 19.30%, N 7.63%. Prepn: Bachman *et al., J. Am. Chem. Soc.* **76**, 3972 (1954); Ferrari, *Farmaco Ed. Sci.* **15**, 337 (1960); **FR M1299** and **FR 1296132** (1962 to Simes), *C.A.* **58**, 4467e, 3352g (1963); **GB 906331** (1962 to Kefalas), *C.A.* **58**, 6654c (1963). Pharmacology: Jun *et al., Can. J. Pharm. Sci.* **4**, 27 (1969); Ciborska *et al., Acta Pol. Pharm.* **26**, 595 (1969); Moeller-Nielsen, Dubnick, *Proc. Int. Symp. Amphetamines Relat. Com-*

pounds 1969, E. Costa, Ed. (Raven Press, New York, 1970) pp 63-73.

Liquid. bp$_2$ 100-102°.

Hydrochloride. [151-06-4] Pre-Sate. C$_{10}$H$_{14}$ClN.HCl; mol wt 220.14. Crystals from alcohol + ether, mp 234°. Soly in water: >20%. pH of 1% aq soln ~5.5. LD$_{50}$ in mice (mg/kg): 270 orally; 267 s.c. (Ciborska).

Note: This is a controlled substance (stimulant): **21 CFR,** 1308.13.

THERAP CAT: Anorexic.

2183. Chlorproethazine. [84-01-5] 2-Chloro-*N,N*-diethyl-10*H*-phenothiazine-10-propanamine; 2-chloro-10-(3-diethylamino-propyl)phenothiazine; 3-chloro-10-(3-diethylaminopropyl)pheno-thiazine; RP-4909. C$_{19}$H$_{23}$ClN$_2$S; mol wt 346.92. C 65.78%, H 6.68%, Cl 10.22%, N 8.07%, S 9.24%. Prepn: Buisson *et al.,* **US 2769002** (1956 to Rhône-Poulenc).

Hydrochloride. [4611-02-3] Neuriplege. C$_{19}$H$_{23}$ClN$_2$S.HCl; mol wt 383.38. Crystals, mp 178°. (Free base bp$_1$ 225-240°). Sensitive to light. Soly in water about 1.0 g/60 ml, ethanol about 1.0 g/300 ml, chloroform 1.0 g/5 ml. Practically insol in acetone, ether, benzene. pH of 1% aq soln 4.8.

THERAP CAT: Topical analgesic.

2184. Chlorproguanil. [537-21-3] *N*-(3,4-Dichlorophen-yl)-*N'*-(1-methylethyl)imidodicarbonimidic diamide; 1-(3,4-dichlo-rophenyl)-5-isopropylbiguanide; *N^1*-3,4-dichlorophenyl-*N^5*-isopro-pylbiguanide; *N^1*-3,4-dichlorophenyl-*N^5*-isopropyldiguanide; M-5943. C$_{11}$H$_{15}$Cl$_2$N$_5$; mol wt 288.18. C 45.85%, H 5.25%, Cl 24.60%, N 24.30%. Method of prepn: Crowther *et al., J. Chem. Soc.* **1951,** 1780; Curd *et al.,* **US 2544827** (1951); Crowther *et al.,* **GB 667116** (1952) (both to ICI). Clinical trial with dapsone, *q.v.,* in drug-resistant malaria: T. Mutabingwa *et al., Lancet* **358,** 1218 (2001).

Hydrochloride. [15537-76-5] Lapudrine. C$_{11}$H$_{15}$Cl$_2$N$_5$.HCl; mol wt 324.64. Crystals, mp 246-247°. Soly in water: 1 g/100 ml. Solns may be boiled without dec.

THERAP CAT: Antimalarial.

2185. Chlorpromazine. [50-53-3] 2-Chloro-*N,N*-dimethyl-10*H*-phenothiazine-10-propanamine; 2-chloro-10-(3-dimethyl-aminopropyl)phenothiazine; 3-chloro-10-(3-dimethylaminopropyl)-phenothiazine; *N*-(3-dimethylaminopropyl)-3-chlorophenothiazine; 2601-A; HL-5746; RP-4560; SKF-2601-A. C$_{17}$H$_{19}$ClN$_2$S; mol wt 318.86. C 64.03%, H 6.01%, Cl 11.12%, N 8.79%, S 10.06%. Prepn: Charpentier *et al., Compt. Rend.* **235,** 59 (1952); Charpentier, **US 2645640** (1953 to Rhône-Poulenc). Effects of neuroleptics on dopamine receptors: N.-E. Anden *et al., Eur. J. Pharmacol.* **11,** 303 (1970). Toxicity study: E. I. Goldenthal, *Toxicol. Appl. Phar-macol.* **18,** 185 (1971). Review of analytical methods for determn in pharmaceutical prepns: L. F. S. Chagonda, J. S. Millership, *J. Pharm. Biomed. Anal.* **7,** 271-278 (1989). Brief historical review: G. Curzon, *Trends Pharmacol. Sci.* **11,** 61-63 (1990).

Oily liq. Amine odor. Alkaline reaction. bp$_{0.8}$ 200-205°.

Hydrochloride. [69-09-0] Ampliactil; Amplictil; Chloractil; Chlorazin; Contomin; Fenactil; Hibernal; Largactil; Plegomazin; Promacid; Promactil; Propaphenin; Prozin; Taroctyl; Thorazine; Wintermin. C$_{17}$H$_{19}$ClN$_2$S.HCl; mol wt 355.33. Crystals, dec 179-180° (capillary); 194-196° (microblock). uv curve: Neuhoff, Auterhoff, *Arch. Pharm.* **288,** 400 (1955). pH of 5% aq soln 4.0-5.5. One gram dissolves in 2.5 ml water. Sol in methanol, ethanol, chloroform. Practically insol in ether, benzene. Slightly acid to litmus. LD$_{50}$ orally in rats: 225 mg/kg (Goldenthal).

THERAP CAT: Antiemetic; antipsychotic.

THERAP CAT (VET): Antiemetic; tranquilizer.

2186. Chlorpropamide. [94-20-2] 4-Chloro-*N*-[(propyl-amino)carbonyl]benzenesulfonamide; 1-(*p*-chlorophenylsulfonyl)-3-propylurea; 1-(*p*-chlorobenzenesulfonyl)-3-propylurea; *N*-pro-pyl-*N'*-(*p*-chlorobenzenesulfonyl)urea; P-607; Adiaben; Asucrol; Catanil; Chloronase; Diabechlor; Diabenal; Diabetoral; Diabinese; Melitase; Millinese; Oradian; Stabinol. C$_{10}$H$_{13}$ClN$_2$O$_3$S; mol wt 276.74. C 43.40%, H 4.73%, Cl 12.81%, N 10.12%, O 17.34%, S 11.59%. Prepn: Marshall, Sigal, *J. Org. Chem.* **23,** 927 (1958); **GB 853555**; W. M. McLamore, **US 3349124** (1960, 1967 both to Pfizer); Bauer *et al., J. Org. Chem.* **31,** 3440 (1960). Pharmacology and metabolism: Khurana *et al., Indian J. Med. Res.* **55,** 1084 (1967); Brotherton *et al., Clin. Pharmacol. Ther.* **10,** 505 (1969); Madsen *et al., Eur. J. Pharmacol.* **13,** 374 (1971). Toxicity study: E. I. Gold-enthal, *Toxicol. Appl. Pharmacol.* **18,** 185 (1971).

Crystals from dil ethanol, mp 127-129°. uv max (0.01*N* HCl): 232.5 nm (ε 16500). Soly in water at pH 6: 2.2 mg/ml. Practically insol at pH 7.3. Sol in alc; moderately sol in chloroform; sparingly sol in ether, benzene. LD$_{50}$ i.p. in rats: 580 mg/kg (Goldenthal).

THERAP CAT: Antidiabetic.

2187. Chlorpropham. [101-21-3] (3-Chlorophenyl)car-bamic acid 1-methylethyl ester; *m*-chlorocarbanilic acid isopropyl ester; isopropyl-*m*-chlorocarbanilate; isopropyl *N*-(3-chlorophenyl)-carbamate; chloro-IPC; chloropropham; CIPC; Chlor-IFC; Furloe; Sprout-Nip. C$_{10}$H$_{12}$ClNO$_2$; mol wt 213.66. C 56.21%, H 5.66%, Cl 16.59%, N 6.56%, O 14.98%. Prepn: E. D. Witman, **US 2695225**; Strain, **US 2734911** (1954, 1956 both to Columbia-South-ern Chem.); Brockway, **US 2806051** (1957 to B. F. Goodrich). Toxicology: E. M. Boyd, E. Carsky, *Arch. Environ. Health* **19,** 621 (1969).

Solid, mp 40.7-41.1°. bp$_2$ 149°. n_D^{20} 1.5388. Commercial prod-uct is a liquid. Slightly sol in water; miscible with most oils and organic solvents. LD$_{50}$ orally in rats: 1.2 g/kg (Boyd, Carsky).

USE: Herbicide; plant growth regulator.

2188. Chlorprothixene. [113-59-7] (*Z*)-3-(2-Chloro-9*H*-thioxanthen-9-ylidene)-*N,N*-dimethyl-1-propanamine; (*Z*)-2-chlo-ro-*N,N*-dimethylthioxanthene-Δ^{9,γ}-propylamine; *cis*-2-chloro-*N,N*-dimethyl-3-thioxanthen-9-ylidenepropylamine; α-2-chloro-10-(3-dimethylaminopropylidene)thiaxanthene; N-714; Taractan; Tara-san; Truxal; Truxaletten. C$_{18}$H$_{18}$ClNS; mol wt 315.86. C

68.45%, H 5.74%, Cl 11.22%, N 4.43%, S 10.15%. Prepn: **GB 829763**; E. L. Engelhardt, **US 3046283** (1960, 1962 both to Merck & Co.). Structure-activity study: G. E. Bonvicino *et al., J. Org. Chem.* **26**, 2383 (1961). Comprehensive description: B. C. Rudy, B. Z. Senkowski, *Anal. Profiles Drug Subs.* **2**, 63-84 (1973). HPLC determn in serum: M. Bagli *et al., J. Chromatogr.* **B 657**, 141 (1994). Clinical pharmacokinetics: *idem et al., Arzneim.-Forsch.* **46**, 247 (1996).

Pale´yellow crystals, mp 97-98°. Practically insol in water; sol in alcohol, ether, chloroform. Incompatible with acids, alkalies, phenobarbital, thiopental sodium, mepazine.

Hydrochloride. [6469-93-8] $C_{18}H_{18}ClNS.HCl$. Crystals, mp 221°. Freely sol in water at pH 6 to 6.5.

THERAP CAT: Antipsychotic.

2189. Chlorpyrifos. [2921-88-2] Phosphorothioic acid *O,O*-diethyl *O*-(3,5,6-trichloro-2-pyridinyl) ester; *O,O*-diethyl *O*-3,5,6-trichloro-2-pyridyl phosphorothioate; chlorpyrifos-ethyl; Dowco 179; ENT-27311; Affront; Dursban; Empire; Lock-On; Lorsban; Pyrinex. $C_9H_{11}Cl_3NO_3PS$; mol wt 350.59. C 30.83%, H 3.16%, Cl 30.34%, N 4.00%, O 13.69%, P 8.83%, S 9.15%. Prepn: R. H. Rigterink, **FR 1360901**; *idem*, **US 3244586** (1964, 1966 both to Dow); R. H. Rigterink, E. E. Kenaga, *J. Agric. Food Chem.* **14**, 394 (1966). Activity: E. E. Kenaga *et al., J. Econ. Entomol.* **58**, 1043 (1965). Metabolism: G. N. Smith *et al., J. Agric. Food Chem.* **15**, 132 (1967); W. H. Gutenmann *et al., ibid.* **16**, 45 (1968). Toxicity study: Schafer, *Toxicol. Appl. Pharmacol.* **21**, 315 (1972). Review of environmental fate: K. D. Racke, *Rev. Environ. Contam. Toxicol.* **131**, 1-154 (1993); of toxicology and human exposure: *Toxicological Profile for Chlorpyrifos* (PB98-103088, 1997) 217 pp.

White granular crystals, mp 41-42°. Vapor pressure at 25°: 1.87 × 10⁻⁵ mm Hg. Soly at 25°: water 2 ppm; isooctane 79% w/w; methanol 43% w/w. Soly (g/100g): acetone 650, benzene 790, carbon disulfide 590, carbon tetrachloride 310, chloroform 630, diethyl ether 510, ethanol 63, ethyl acetate >200, isooctane 79, kerosene 60, methanol 45, methylene chloride 400, propylene glycol 4, toluene 150, 1,1,1-trichloroethane 400, triethylene glycol 5, xylene 140. Readily sol in other org solvents. uv max: 208, 230, 290 nm. LD_{50} orally in rats: 145 mg/kg (Schafer).

O,O-**Dimethyl analog.** [5598-13-0] Chlorpyrifos-methyl; Dowco 214; ENT-27520; Reldan. $C_7H_7Cl_3NO_3PS$; mol wt 322.53. Crystals, mp 45.5-46.5°. Vapor pressure at 25°: 4.22 × 10⁻⁵ mm Hg. Soly in water at 25°: 5 mg/l.

Caution: Potential symptoms of overexposure are wheezing, laryngeal spasms, salivation; bluish lips and skin; miosis, blurred vision; nausea, vomiting, abdominal cramps, diarrhea. *See NIOSH Pocket Guide to Chemical Hazards* (DHHS/NIOSH 97-140, 1997) p 70.

USE: Insecticide; acaricide.

THERAP CAT (VET): Ectoparasiticide.

2190. Chlorquinaldol. [72-80-0] 5,7-Dichloro-2-methyl-8-quinolinol; 5,7-dichloro-8-quinaldinol; 5,7-dichloro-8-hydroxyquinaldine; 5,7-dichloro-2-methyl-8-hydroxyquinoline; hydroxydichloroquinaldine; chloroquinaldol; Gynotherax; Sterosan; Steroxin. $C_{10}H_7Cl_2NO$; mol wt 228.07. C 52.66%, H 3.09%, Cl

31.09%, N 6.14%, O 7.02%. Prepd by chlorination of 8-hydroxyquinaldine with or without formic acid as solvent: Senn, **US 2411670** (1946 to Geigy).

Yellow needles from alc, mp 114-115° (slight decompn). Medicinal odor. uv max (ethanol): 316 nm ($A_{1cm}^{1\%}$ 170); min 280 nm. Practically insol in water. Soly (25°) in ethanol 1.0 g/100 ml of soln; chloroform 5.0 g; acetone 4.0 g; ether 3.0 g; 0.1N NaOH 1.4 g. Also sol in benzene, glacial acetic acid.

THERAP CAT: Antibacterial.

THERAP CAT (VET): Antibacterial; antifungal.

2191. Chlorsulfuron. [64902-72-3] 2-Chloro-*N*-[[(4-methoxy-6-methyl-1,3,5-triazin-2-yl)amino]carbonyl]benzenesulfonamide; DPX-4189; Glean; Telar. $C_{12}H_{12}ClN_5O_4S$; mol wt 357.77. C 40.29%, H 3.38%, Cl 9.91%, N 19.58%, O 17.89%, S 8.96%. Selective pre- and post-emergence herbicide. Prepn: G. Levitt, **DE 2715786**; *idem*, **US 4127405** (1977, 1978 both to du Pont). Activity: G. Levitt *et al., J. Agric. Food Chem.* **29**, 416 (1981). Mode of action: T. B. Ray, *Pestic. Biochem. Physiol.* **17**, 10 (1982).

Crystals from ether, mp 174-178°. Soly in water: 125 ppm. Moderately sol in methylene chloride; less sol in acetone, acetonitrile. Low soly in hydrocarbon solvents. LD_{50} in male, female rats (mg/kg): 5545, 6293 orally (Levitt).

USE: Herbicide.

2192. Chlortetracycline. [57-62-5] [4S-(4α,4aα,5aα,6β,-12aα)]-7-Chloro-4-dimethylamino-1,4,4a,5,5a,6,11,12a-octahydro-3,6,10,12,12a-pentahydroxy-6-methyl-1,11-dioxo-2-naphthacene-carboxamide; 7-chlorotetracycline; Acronize; Aureocina; Aureomycin; Biomitsin; Centreaureo; Chrysomykine; Orospray. $C_{22}H_{23}$-ClN_2O_8; mol wt 478.88. C 55.18%, H 4.84%, Cl 7.40%, N 5.85%, O 26.73%. Antibiotic substance isolated from the substrate of *Streptomyces aureofaciens:* Duggan, *Ann. N.Y. Acad. Sci.* **51**, 177 (1948); **US 2482055** (1949 to Am. Cyanamid); Broschard *et al., Science* **109**, 199 (1949). Structure: Stephens *et al., J. Am. Chem. Soc.* **74**, 4976 (1952); **76**, 3568 (1954). Crystal structure: Donohue *et al., ibid.* **85**, 851 (1963). Absolute configuration: Dobrynin *et al., Tetrahedron Lett.* **1962**, 901. Purification: Winterbottom *et al.,* **US 2899422** (1959 to Am. Cyanamid). Improved process: Miller *et al.;* Goodman, **US 2987449**; **US 3050446** (1961, 1962 to Am. Cyanamid). Toxicity: E. I. Goldenthal, *Toxicol. Appl. Pharmacol.* **18**, 185 (1971). Comprehensive description: G. Schwartzman *et al., Anal. Profiles Drug Subs.* **8**, 101-137 (1979).

Golden-yellow crystals, mp 168-169°. $[\alpha]_D^{23}$ −275.0° (methanol). uv max (0.1N HCl): 230, 262.5, 367.5 nm; (0.1N NaOH): 255, 285, 345 nm. Soly in water: 0.5-0.6 mg/ml. Very sol in aq solns above pH 8.5. Freely sol in the Cellosolves, dioxane, and

Carbitol. Slightly sol in methanol, ethanol, butanol, acetone, ethyl acetate, benzene. Practically insol in ether, petr ether.

Crystal salt. White powder. Insol in water. Marketed as suspension preserved with methyl and propyl *p*-hydroxybenzoate; stable and fully active for at least one year at room temps.

Hydrochloride. [64-72-2] Aureociclina; Isphamycin. $C_{22}H_{23}ClN_2O_8 \cdot HCl$; mol wt 515.34. Bitter, yellow rhomboid crystals. Dec above 210°. $[\alpha]_D^{23}$ −240°. Soly at about 28° (mg/ml): water 8.6; methanol 17.4; ethanol 1.7: Weiss *et al.*, *Antibiot. Chemother.* **7**, 374 (1957). Sol in solns of alkali hydroxides and carbonates. Practically insol in acetone, ether, chloroform, dioxane. pH of satd aq soln 2.8-2.9. LD_{50} orally in rats: 10300 mg/kg (Goldenthal).

THERAP CAT: Antibacterial; antiamebic.

THERAP CAT (VET): Antimicrobial.

2193. Chlorthalidone. [77-36-1] 2-Chloro-5-(2,3-dihydro-1-hydroxy-3-oxo-1*H*-isoindol-1-yl)benzenesulfonamide; 2-chloro-5-(1-hydroxy-3-oxo-1-isoindolinyl)benzenesulfonamide; 3-hydroxy-3-(4-chloro-3-sulfamylphenyl)phthalimidine; 2-chloro-5-(3-hydroxy-1-oxoisoindolin-3-yl)benzenesulfonamide; 1-oxo-3-(3-sulfamyl-4-chlorophenyl)-3-hydroxyisoindoline; 3-(4'-chloro-3'-sulfamoylphenyl)-3-hydroxyphthalimidine; 1-keto-3-(3'-sulfamyl-4'-chlorophenyl)-3-hydroxyisoindoline; chlorphthalidone; phthalamudine; phthalamodine; G-33182; Higroton; Hydro-long; Hygroton; Thalitone. $C_{14}H_{11}ClN_2O_4S$; mol wt 338.77. C 49.64%, H 3.27%, Cl 10.47%, N 8.27%, O 18.89%, S 9.47%. Prepn: Graf *et al.*, *Helv. Chim. Acta* **42**, 1085 (1959). Activity and side effects: Holtmeier *et al.*, *Med. Welt* **1967**, 1384; Zsoter *et al.*, *J. Pharmacol. Exp. Ther.* **180**, 723 (1972). Metabolism: Beisenherz *et al.*, *Arch. Int. Pharmacodyn. Ther.* **161**, 76 (1966). Comprehensive description: J. M. Singer *et al.*, *Anal. Profiles Drug Subs.* **14**, 1-36 (1985).

Crystals from 50% acetic acid, dec 224-226°. mp range may extend from 218 to 264° on slow heating. Can form a monohydrate. uv max (methanol): <220 nm. Soly in water: 12 mg/100 ml (20°); 27 mg/100 ml (37°); in 0.1*N* Na_2CO_3: 577 mg/100 ml (20°); 990 mg/100 ml (37°). More sol in aq solns of NaOH. Soluble in warm ethanol; slightly sol in ether.

THERAP CAT: Diuretic; antihypertensive.

THERAP CAT (VET): Diuretic.

2194. Chlorzoxazone. [95-25-0] 5-Chloro-2(3*H*)-benzoxazolone; 5-chloro-2-benzoxazolol; 5-chloro-2-hydroxybenzoxazole; 2-hydroxy-5-chlorobenzoxazole; 5-chlorbenzoxazolin-2-one; 5-chlorobenzoxazolidone; Paraflex; Biomioran; Solaxin. $C_7H_4ClNO_2$; mol wt 169.57. C 49.58%, H 2.38%, Cl 20.91%, N 8.26%, O 18.87%. Prepn from 2-amino-5-chlorobenzoxazole: Marsh, **US 2895877** (1959 to McNeil Labs.). LC determn in plasma: I. L. Honigsberg *et al.*, *J. Pharm. Sci.* **68**, 253 (1979). Fluorometric determn in tablets and biological fluids: J. T. Stewart, C. W. Chan, *ibid.* 910. Clinical studies: R. Herman, *Curr. Ther. Res.* **9**, 537 (1967); J. J. Scheiner, *ibid.* **19**, 51 (1976). Metabolism study: R. Twele, G. Spiteller, *Arzneim.-Forsch.* **32**, 759 (1982). Toxicity: G. Hofrichter *et al.*, *Arzneim.-Forsch.* **17**, 242 (1967). Review of clinical studies: J. K. Elenbaas, *Am. J. Hosp. Pharm.* **37**, 1313 (1980). Comprehensive description: J. T. Stewart, C. A. Janicki, *Anal. Profiles Drug Subs.* **16**, 119-144 (1987).

Crystals from acetone, mp 191-191.5°. Sparingly sol in water; sol in methanol, ethanol, isopropanol. Freely sol in aq solns of alkali hydroxides and ammonia. LD_{50} in mice (mg/kg): 3650

orally, 380 i.p. (suspensions); 440 orally, 183 i.p. (solns of Na salt) (Hofrichter).

THERAP CAT: Muscle relaxant (skeletal).

2195. Cholane. [548-98-1] $C_{24}H_{42}$; mol wt 330.59. C 87.19%, H 12.81%. Prepn from bisnorcholyl methyl ketone: Wieland *et al.*, *Z. Physiol. Chem.* **161**, 80, 109 (1926); from potassium cholanate: Kazuno *et al.*, *Proc. Jpn. Acad.* **28**, 416 (1952).

Stout prisms from alc, mp 90°; bp$_{0.001}$ 190°. Sparingly sol in methanol.

2196. Cholanic Acid. [25312-65-6] Cholan-24-oic acid; ursocholanic acid; 17β-(1-methyl-3-carboxypropyl)etiocholane. $C_{24}H_{40}O_2$; mol wt 360.57. C 79.94%, H 11.18%, O 8.87%. Steroidal acid probably formed by the dehydration and hydrogenation of certain bile acids commonly found in animals. Considered to be a chemical trademark certifying the prehistoric presence of some type of animal, *see* Seifert, *Pure Appl. Chem.* **34**, 633 (1973). This status as a natural product of exclusive animal origins now questioned by its isolation from the embryo of the jequirity bean, *Abrus precatorius, Leguminosae:* Mandava *et al.*, *Steroids* **23**, 357 (1974). Prepn from coprostane, cholic acid, lithocholic acid, desoxy- and chenodesoxycholic acid: Wieland, Weil, *Z. Physiol. Chem.* **80**, 287 (1912); Wieland, Boersch, *ibid.* **106**, 193 (1919); Windaus, Neukirchen, *Ber.* **52**, 1915 (1919); Wieland, Vocke, *Z. Physiol. Chem.* **191**, 69 (1930). From 3-ketocholanic acid diethyl thioacetal by hydrogenolysis: Bernstein, Dorfman, **US 2440660** (1948 to Am. Cyanamid). 5β-Cholanic acid differs from the thermodynamically more stable 5α-isomer, by being *cis* at the A/B steroid ring function rather than *trans*.

Needles from alc, mp 163-164°. $[\alpha]_D^{20}$ +21.7° (chloroform). Sol in chloroform, alcohol, acetic acid. Forms a molecular compd with allocholanic acid, mp 163.5°.

Methyl ester. $C_{25}H_{42}O_2$. mp 86-87°.

Ethyl ester. $C_{26}H_{44}O_2$. Needles from 80% alc, mp 93-94°; bp$_{12}$ 273°. $[\alpha]_D^{19}$ +21° (chloroform).

Note: The name cholanic acid was formerly applied to desoxybilianic acid, $C_{24}H_{36}O_7$.

USE: In chemotaxonomical classification.

2197. Cholanthrene. [479-23-2] 1,2-Dihydrobenz[*j*]aceanthrylene. $C_{20}H_{14}$; mol wt 254.33. C 94.45%, H 5.55%. Synthesis from 1-β-naphthylhydrindene: Cook *et al.*, *J. Chem. Soc.* **1935**, 667; from 4-indanyl-MgBr and 1-naphthoyl chloride: Fieser, Seligman, *J. Am. Chem. Soc.* **57**, 2174 (1935).

Faintly yellow plates from benzene + ether, mp 173°. Sublimes 210-215° at 0.2 mm Hg. Absorption max: Fieser, Hershberg, *J.*

Am. Chem. Soc. **60**, 940 (1938). Sol in benzene, xylene, toluene. Slightly sol in methanol. Insol in water. May be solubilized by aq solns of Na desoxycholate.

Molecular complex with 2,4,7-trinitrofluorenone. Olive green crystals, mp 245-246°: Orchin, Woolfolk, *J. Am. Chem. Soc.* **68**, 1727 (1946).

2198. Cholecystokinin. [9011-97-6] Pancreozymin; cholecystokinin-pancreozymin; CCK-PZ. Polypeptide hormone found in the mammalian gastrointestinal tract and brain. Stimulates pancreatic exocrine secretion and growth. May also play a role in appetite satiation, pain perception, and neuronal transmission. First shown to cause gallbladder contraction: Ivy, Oldberg, *Am. J. Physiol.* **86**, 599 (1928). Discovery of a substance, designated as pancreozymin, which promotes secretion of digestive enzymes by the pancreas: Harper, Raper, *J. Physiol. (London)* **102**, 115 (1943). Identity with pancreozymin: Jorpes *et al., Acta Chem. Scand.* **18**, 2408 (1964). The *C*-terminal pentapeptide has been shown to be identical to that of gastrin and caerulein: V. Mutt, J. E. Jorpes, *Eur. J. Biochem.* **6**, 156 (1968); *eidem, Biochem. J.* **125**, 57P (1971). Various biologically active, amino-truncated forms have been identified. Cholecystokinin consisting of 33 amino acids (CCK-33) is the predominant gastrointestinal form; CCK-39 and CCK-58 have also been identified. CCK-8 is the predominant CNS form. Identification of CCK in brain: J. J. Vanderhaeghen *et al., Nature* **257**, 604 (1975); G. J. Dockray, *ibid.* **264**, 568 (1976). Distribution and molecular heterogeneity: J. F. Rehfeld, *J. Biol. Chem.* **253**, 4022 (1978). Synthesis of the *C*-terminal dodecapeptide: M. A. Ondetti *et al., J. Am. Chem. Soc.* **92**, 195 (1970). Synthesis of the *N*-terminal hexapeptide of porcine CCK-33: Bodanszky *et al., J. Org. Chem.* **37**, 2303 (1972). Cloning and nucleotide sequence of the human cholecystokinin gene: Y. Takahashi *et al., Proc. Natl. Acad. Sci. USA* **82**, 1931 (1985). Total synthesis of porcine CCK-33: Y. Kurano, *Chem. Commun.* **1987**, 323; of human CCK-33: N. Fujii *et al., ibid.* **1988**, 324. Proposed role in suppression of food intake: M. A. Della-Fera, C. A. Baile, *Science* **206**, 471 (1979); C. J. Savory, M. J. Gentle, *Experientia* **36**, 1191 (1980); M. A. Della-Fera *et al., Science* **212**, 687 (1981); in regulation of hypothalamic peptides: S. Itoh *et al., Life Sci.* **25**, 1725 (1979); in modulation of catecholaminergic activity: K. Fuxe *et al., Eur. J. Pharmacol.* **67**, 329 (1980). There is also evidence that CCK acts as a specific antagonist of opiate analgesia: P. L. Faris *et al., Science* **219**, 310 (1983). *Reviews:* E. Straus, R. S. Yalow, *Fed. Proc.* **38**, 2320-2324 (1979); V. Mutt, *Biochem. Soc. Trans.* **8**, 11-14 (1980); *idem, Vitam. Horm.* **39**, 231-426 (1982). Review of physiology: G. J. Dockray, *Br. Med. Bull.* **38**, 253-258 (1982); of role in appetite satiation and pain perception: G. Stacher, *Psychoneuroendocrinology* **11**, 39-48 (1986). Symposium on neuronal CCK: *Ann. N.Y. Acad. Sci.* **448**, 1-697 (1985).

Lys–Ala–Pro–Ser–Gly–Arg–Met–Ser–Ile–Val–Lys–Asn–Leu–Gln–Asn–Leu–Asp
|
H₂NPhe–Asp–Met–Trp–Gly–Met–Tyr–Asp–Arg–Asp–Ser–Ile–Arg–His–Ser–Pro
|
SO₃H

Human CCK - 33

***C*-Terminal octapeptide** *see* Sincalide.

2199. (5α)-Cholestane. [481-21-0] C₂₇H₄₈; mol wt 372.67. C 87.02%, H 12.98%. The *trans*-decalin homolog of coprostane, *q.v.* Prepd from cholesteryl chloride: Diels, Linn, *Ber.* **41**, 548 (1908); Windaus, *Ber.* **50**, 136 (1917); Ruzicka *et al., Helv. Chim. Acta* **16**, 327 (1933). Crystal structure: Haner, Norton, *Acta Crystallogr.* **20**, 930 (1966).

Scales from ether + alcohol. mp 80°. [α]²⁰_D +24.4° or +30.2° (c = 2 in chloroform). n⁸⁸_D 1.4887. Freely sol in chloroform, ether, benzene, slightly in abs alcohol.

2200. Cholestanol. [80-97-7] (3β,5α)-Cholestan-3-ol; Dihydrocholesterol; 3β-hydroxycholestane; β-cholestanol. C₂₇H₄₈O; mol wt 388.67. C 83.44%, H 12.45%, O 4.12%. Occurs in human feces, in gallstones, in eggs. Prepn by reduction of cholesterol: Willstätter, Mayer, *Ber.* **41**, 2199 (1908); Ellis, Gardner, *Biochem. J.* **12**, 72 (1918). From coprostenone: Diels, Abderhalden, *Ber.* **39**, 884 (1906). *See also* Bruce, Ralls, *Org. Synth.* **coll. vol. II**, 191 (1943).

Monohydrate, scales from alc, mp 141.5-142°. [α]²²_D +24.2° (c = 1.3 in chloroform). One gram dissolves in about 100 ml alcohol, in 200 ml dry methanol. Freely sol in hot alc, ether, chloroform. Pptd by digitonin.

Methyl ether. C₂₈H₅₀O. Needles from acetone, mp 82.5-83°. [α]²⁰_D +20.0°.

Acetate. C₂₉H₅₀O₂. Prisms from ethyl acetate + methanol, mp 111°. [α]²⁰_D +13.3° (c = 2 in chloroform).

2201. Cholesterol. [57-88-5] (3β)-Cholest-5-en-3-ol; cholesterin. C₂₇H₄₆O; mol wt 386.65. C 83.87%, H 11.99%, O 4.14%. Principal sterol of the higher animals. Found in all body tissues, esp in the brain, spinal cord, and in animal fats or oils. Main constituent of gallstones. Prepd commercially from the spinal cord of cattle by petr ether extraction of the nonsaponifiable matter. Also produced from wool grease. Cholesterol from animal organs always contains cholestanol (dihydrocholesterol) and other satd sterols. Purification by repeated bromination: Schoenheimer, *J. Biol. Chem.* **105**, 355 (1934); Fieser, *Org. Synth.* **coll. vol. IV**, 195 (1963). Laboratory procedure for isoln from gallstones: L. F. Fieser, *Organic Experiments* (Heath, Boston, 3rd ed., 1964) p 70. Total synthesis: Keana, Johnson, *Steroids* **4**, 457 (1964). Reviews and bibliographies: Fieser, Fieser, *Steroids* (Reinhold, New York, Chapman & Hall, London, 1959); Lettré *et al., Ueber Sterine, Gallensäuren und verwandte Naturstoffe* (Stuttgart, 2nd ed., 1955); R. P. Cook, *Cholesterol (Chemistry, Biochemistry and Pathology)* (Academic Press, New York, 1958) 542 pp; J. T. Gwynne, J. F. Strauss, *Endocr. Rev.* **3**, 299-329 (1982).

Monohydrate, pearly leaflets or plates from dil alcohol. Becomes anhydr at 70-80°. When anhydr mp 148.5°. Has been sublimed as orthorhombic needles. bp₀.₅ 233°; bp₇₆₀ 360° (some decompn). d 1.03 (monohydrate); d¹⁹_19 1.052 (anhydr). [α]²⁰_D −31.5° (c = 2 in ether); [α]²⁰_D −39.5° (c = 2 in chloroform). Absorption spectrum: Heilbron *et al., J. Chem. Soc.* **1928**, 47. Practically insol in water (about 0.2 mg/100 ml H₂O). Slightly sol in alc (1.29% w/w at 20°), more sol in hot alc (100 g of satd 96% alcoholic soln contains 28 g at 80°). One gram dissolves in 2.8 ml ether, in 4.5 ml chloroform, in 1.5 ml pyridine. Also sol in benzene, petr ether, oils, fats. Soly in aq solns of bile salts: Rosin, *Z. Physiol. Chem.* **124**, 282 (1923). Solubilization: Gemant, *Life Sci.* **1**, 233 (June 1962). Is pptd by digitonin. Gives intense red color with rosaniline in chloroform soln.

Methyl ether. $C_{28}H_{48}O$. Crystals from acetone, mp 84°. $[\alpha]_D^{20}$ −45.8° (c = 1.2 in chloroform).

Acetate. $C_{29}H_{48}O_2$. Needles from acetone, mp 115-116°. $[\alpha]_D^{20}$ −47.4° (c = 2 in chloroform).

Benzoate. $C_{34}H_{50}O_2$. mp 145.5° (the melt becomes clear at 180°). $[\alpha]_D^{25}$ −13.7° (c = 0.9 in chloroform).

USE: Pharmaceutic aid (emulsifying agent).

2202. Cholestyramine Resin. [11041-12-6] Colestyramin; Dowex 1-X2-Cl; MK-135; Cholybar; Cuemid; Quantalan; Questran. A synthetic, strongly basic anion exchange resin contg quaternary ammonium functional groups which are attached to a styrene-divinylbenzene copolymer. Main constituent: Polystyrene trimethylbenzylammonium as Cl^- anion, also contains divinylbenzene. Avg polymeric mol wt $>10^6$; Cl^- content 14-17%. Effect of particle size on bile salt binding capacity: L. M. Hagerman *et al., Proc. Soc. Exp. Biol. Med.* **139**, 248 (1972). Review of pharmacology: H. R. Casdorph in *Lipid Pharmacology* Vol. **2**(2), R. Paoletti, C. J. Glueck, Eds. (Academic Press, New York, 1976) pp 222-256. Clinical evaluation in chlordecone detoxification: W. J. Cohn *et al., N. Engl. J. Med.* **298**, 243 (1978). Review of pharmacology and therapeutic efficacy: M. Ast, W. H. Frishman, *J. Clin. Pharmacol.* **30**, 99-106 (1990).

typified structure of main polymeric groups

White to buff-colored, hygroscopic, fine powder. Odorless or has not more than a slight amine-like odor. Insol in water, alcohol, benzene, chloroform, ether.

THERAP CAT: Antilipemic; ion-exchange resin (bile salts).

2203. Cholic Acid. [81-25-4] $(3\alpha,5\beta,7\alpha,12\alpha)$-3,7,12-Trihydroxycholan-24-oic acid; cholalic acid; 17β-(1-methyl-3-carboxypropyl)etiocholane-3α,7α,12α-triol; Colalin. $C_{24}H_{40}O_5$; mol wt 408.57. C 70.55%, H 9.87%, O 19.58%. Occurs in conjugation with glycine or taurine in bile of most vertebrates. Extraction from beef bile: Wieland, Siebert, *Z. Physiol. Chem.* **262**, 1 (1939); laboratory procedure: Gattermann-Wieland, *Praxis des Organischen Chemikers* (de Gruyter, Berlin, 40th ed., 1961) p 360. Structure and synthesis: Fieser, Fieser, *Steroids* (Reinhold, New York, 1959).

Monohydrate. Plates from dil acetic acid. Bitter taste with sweetish aftertaste. When anhyd, mp 198°. $[\alpha]_D^{20}$ +37° (c = 0.6 in alcohol). pK = 6.4. Not precipitated by digitonin. Soly at 15° in water 0.28 g/l; in alcohol 30.56 g/l; in ether 1.22 g/l; in chloroform 5.08 g/l; in benzene 0.36 g/l; in acetone 28.24 g/l; in glacial acetic acid 152.12 g/l. Sol in solns of alkali hydroxides or carbonates.

Methyl ester. $C_{25}H_{42}O_5$. Crystals from 95% alcohol + water, mp 155-156°.

Ethyl ester. $C_{26}H_{44}O_5$. Crystals from ethyl acetate + petr ether, mp 162-163°.

Sodium salt. Sodium cholate. $C_{24}H_{39}NaO_5$. Crystals. Soly in water at 15°: >568.9 g/l.

Caution: The names "sodium cholate" and "sodium choleate" are sometimes used for mixtures of bile salts. The term "sodium choleate" is to be preferred for bile salts, *see* Ox Bile Extract.

Note: The property of forming molecular compds is common to bile acids. For instance a blue molecular compd $(C_{24}H_{40}O_5I)_4$.-$KI.H_2O$, may be prepd by mixing an alcoholic soln of cholic acid and a soln of iodine in aq potassium iodide: Barger, Field, *J. Chem. Soc.* **101**, 1404 (1912).

THERAP CAT: Choleretic.

2204. Choline. [62-49-7] 2-Hydroxy-*N,N,N*-trimethylethanaminium; (β-hydroxyethyl)trimethylammonium; bilineurine. $[C_5H_{14}NO]^+$. Basic constituent of lecithin. Found in many plants and animal organs, *e.g.* bile, brain, yolk of eggs, hops, belladonna, strophanthus. Usually made synthetically from trimethylamine and ethylene chlorohydrin or ethylene oxide: Blackett, Soliday, **US 2774759** (1956 to Am. Cyanamid). *Review:* T. H. Jukes in *Kirk-Othmer Encyclopedia of Chemical Technology* vol. **6** (Wiley-Interscience, New York, 3rd ed., 1979) pp 19-28.

Hydroxide. Bursine; fagine; gossypine; luridine; sincaline; vidine. $C_5H_{15}NO_2$. Viscid, strongly alkaline liq, has been crystallized; absorbs CO_2 from the air. Very sol in water, alcohol. Insol in ether. *Keep tightly closed.*

2205. Choline Alfoscerate. [28319-77-9] 2-[[[(2*R*)-2,3-Dihydroxypropoxy]hydroxyphosphinyl]oxy]-*N,N,N*-trimethylethanaminium hydroxide inner salt; D-choline hydroxide 2,3-dihydroxypropyl hydrogen phosphate inner salt; L-α-glycerylphosphorylcholine; *sn*-glycero-3-phosphorylcholine; L-α-GPC; Brezal; Delecit; Gliatilin. $C_8H_{20}NO_6P$; mol wt 257.22. C 37.36%, H 7.84%, N 5.45%, O 37.32%, P 12.04%. Phospholipid; precursor in choline biosynthesis; intermediate in catabolic pathway of phosphatidylcholine. Isoln from bovine pancreas: G. Schmidt *et al., J. Biol. Chem.* **161**, 523 (1945). Synthesis: E. Baer, M. Kates, *J. Am. Chem. Soc.* **70**, 1394 (1948); and properties: N. H. Tattrie *et al., Biochem. Prep.* **6**, 16 (1958). HPLC determn: G. Abbiati *et al., J. Chromatogr.* **566**, 445 (1991). Metabolism and biodistribution: idem *et al., Eur. J. Drug Metab. Pharmacokinet.* **18**, 173 (1993). Clinical pharmacology: N. Canal *et al., Int. J. Clin. Pharmacol. Ther. Toxicol.* **29**, 103 (1991). Clinical pharmacokinetics: G. Gatti *et al., ibid.* **30**, 331 (1992). Clinical study in multi-infarct dementia: L. Frattola *et al., Curr. Ther. Res.* **49**, 683 (1991); in Alzheimer's type dementia: L. Parnetti *et al., Drugs Aging* **3**, 159 (1993).

White crystals, mp 142.5-143°, sinters at 141°. Extremely hygroscopic. Sol in water. $[\alpha]_{25}^D$ −2.7° (c = 2.7 in water, pH 2.5). $[\alpha]_{25}^D$ −2.8° (c = 2.6 in water, pH 5.8).

THERAP CAT: Nootropic.

2206. Choline Chloride. [67-48-1] 2-Hydroxy-*N,N,N*-trimethylethanaminium chloride; Biocolina; Hepacholine; Lipotril. $C_5H_{14}ClNO$; mol wt 139.62. C 43.01%, H 10.11%, Cl 25.39%, N 10.03%, O 11.46%. $[HOCH_2CH_2N^+(CH_3)_3]Cl^-$. Prepn: Klein, Kapp, **US 2623901** (1952 to Nopco Chem.). Polymorphism: Collin, *J. Am. Chem. Soc.* **79**, 6086 (1957). Enhancement of human serial learning: N. Sitaram *et al., Life Sci.* **22**, 1555 (1978); *eidem, Science* **201**, 274 (1978). Toxicity data: Hartung, Cornish, *Toxicol. Appl. Pharmacol.* **12**, 486 (1968).

Deliquesc crystals. Very sol in water or alcohol. The aq soln is practically neutral. *Keep tightly closed.* LD_{50} in rats (g/kg): 0.400 i.p.; 6.64 orally (Hartung, Cornish).

THERAP CAT: Lipotropic.

THERAP CAT (VET): Nutritional factor. Dietary source of choline (lipotropic factor) in poultry.

2207. Choline Dihydrogen Citrate. [77-91-8] (2-Hydroxyethyl)trimethylammonium citrate; Chothyn; Cirrocolina; Citracholine. $C_{11}H_{21}NO_8$; mol wt 295.29. C 44.74%, H 7.17%, N 4.74%, O 43.35%. [$HOCH_2CH_2N^+(CH_3)_3$][$C_6H_7O_7^-$]. Prepn: Klein *et al.,* **US 2870198** (1959).

Granules, mp 105-107.5°. Acrid taste. Freely sol in water; very slightly sol in alcohol. Practically insol in benzene, chloroform, ether. The pH of a 25% aq soln is 4.25. May be formulated with calcium citrate for better taste and easier tabletting.

THERAP CAT: Lipotropic.

THERAP CAT (VET): Dietary source of choline (lipotropic factor) in poultry.

2208. Choline Esterase. [9001-08-5] There are at least two choline esterases. **Acetylcholinesterase** is a "specific" choline esterase, hydrolyzing predominantly choline esters, and characterized by high concns in brain, nerve and red blood cells. The other type, called **butyrylcholinesterase,** is a nonspecific choline esterase ("pseudo" choline esterase), hydrolyzing other esters as well as choline esters, and found in blood serum, pancreas and liver, *cf.* Sumner and Somers, *Chemistry and Methods of Enzymes* (New York, 1947). Prepn from dog pancreas: Mendel, Mundell, *Biochem. J.* **37,** 64 (1943); from horse serum: Strelitz, *ibid.* **38,** 86 (1944). *Reviews:* Davies, Green, *Adv. Enzymol.* **20,** 283 (1958); Froede, Wilson, "Acetylcholinesterase" in *The Enzymes* **vol. 5,** P. D. Boyer, Ed. (Academic Press, N. Y., 3rd ed., 1971) pp 87-114.

Specific choline esterase develops its max activity at pH 7 and at low levels of acetylcholine (less than 2.5 mg %). Both enzymes are inhibited by very small quantities of physostigmine (eserine). Acetylcholinesterase is inhibited by phosphorus-containing insecticides and nerve gases.

2209. Choline Salicylate. [2016-36-6] 2-Hydroxy-*N,N,N*-trimethylethanaminium salt with 2-hydroxybenzoic acid (1:1); (2-hydroxyethyl)trimethylammonium salicylate; choline salicylic acid salt; salicylic acid choline salt; Actasal; Arthropan; Artrobione; Audax; Mundisal. $C_{12}H_{19}NO_4$; mol wt 241.28. C 59.73%, H 7.94%, N 5.81%, O 26.52%. Prepn from choline chloride and sodium salicylate: Broh-Kahn, *Int. Rec. Med.* **173,** 219 (Apr. 1960); *cf.* Johnson, **GB 8031** (1919); Broh-Kahn *et al.,* **US 3069321** (1962 to Labs. for Pharmaceut. Dev.). Variations of process: **BE 583513** (1960 to Mundipharma, AG).

Extremely hygroscopic solid, mp 49.5-50.0°. Very freely sol in water. Also sol in alcohol, acetone, other hydrophilic solvents. Practically insol in ether, petr ether, benzene, oils. Aq solns are stable, they contain the compd in the form of its dissociated choline and salicylate ions. pH of 10% aq soln 6.5. Aq solns are easily discolored by minute traces of iron. The addition of acid to aq solns immediately precipitates free salicylic acid, while choline base, readily recognized by its fishy odor, is liberated upon the addition of alkali.

THERAP CAT: Analgesic; antipyretic.

2210. Choline Theophyllinate. [4499-40-5] 2-Hydroxy-*N,N,N*-trimethylethanaminium salt with 3,7-dihydro-1,3-dimethyl-1*H*-purine-2,6-dione; theophylline cholinate; theophylline salt of choline; oxtriphylline; oxytrimethylline; Sabidal; Teokolin; Teofilcolina; Filoral; Cholinophylline; Choledyl; Theoxylline; Soliphylline. $C_{12}H_{21}N_5O_3$; mol wt 283.33. C 50.87%, H 7.47%, N 24.72%, O 16.94%. Prepn: Ladenburg *et al.,* **US 2776287** (1957 to Nepera Chem.).

White granules (contains about 60% of anhydr theophylline). One gram dissolves in 1 ml water.

Note: Also sold as Cholinophylline Magnesium Glycinate which contains 43% of anhydr theophylline.

THERAP CAT: Bronchodilator.

2211. Chondrillasterol. [481-17-4] (3β,5α,22*E*,24*R*)-Stigmasta-7,22-dien-3-ol. $C_{29}H_{48}O$; mol wt 412.69. C 84.40%, H 11.72%, O 3.88%. Stereoisomeric with α-spinasterol, *q.v.* Isolated from the green alga *Scenedesmus obliquus* (Turpin) Kuetz., *Scenedesmaceae:* Bergmann, Feeney, *J. Org. Chem.* **15,** 812 (1950). Synthesis: W. Sucrow *et al., Phytochemistry* **15,** 1533 (1976); M. Anastasia *et al., J. Chem. Soc. Perkin Trans. 1* **1981,** 2561.

Crystals from chloroform-methanol, mp 168-169°. $[\alpha]_D^{24}$ −2° (chloroform).

Acetate. $C_{31}H_{50}O_2$. Crystals from chloroform-methanol, mp 174.5-175.5°. $[\alpha]_D^{24}$ −0.7° (chloroform).

Benzoate. $C_{36}H_{52}O_2$. Crystals from dioxane, mp 194-195°. $[\alpha]_D^{24}$ +3.9° (chloroform).

2212. Chondrocurine. [477-58-7] 6,6′-Dimethoxy-2,2′-dimethyltubocuraran-7′,12′-diol; *d*-chondocurine; *d*-tubocurine. $C_{36}H_{38}N_2O_6$; mol wt 594.70. C 72.71%, H 6.44%, N 4.71%, O 16.14%. Isoln from *Chondodendron tomentosum* Ruiz & Pav., *Menispermaceae:* Wintersteiner, Dutcher, *Science* **97,** 467 (1943); King, *J. Chem. Soc.* **1948,** 1945; Bick, Clezy, *ibid.* **1960,** 2402; Boissier *et al., Lloydia* **28,** 191 (1965), *C.A.* **64,** 948b (1966). Structure: Dutcher, *J. Am. Chem. Soc.* **68,** 419 (1946); Hultin, *Acta Chem. Scand.* **15,** 1130 (1961). Configuration: Bick, Clezy, *J. Chem. Soc.* **1953,** 3893; Hultin, *Acta Chem. Scand.* **17,** 753 (1963). Revised structure: Everett *et al., Chem. Commun.* **1970,** 1020. ^{13}C-NMR: L. Koike *et al., J. Org. Chem.* **46,** 2385 (1981).

Slender needles from methanol, mp 232-234°; also reported as mp 218-220° (Boissier). $[\alpha]_D^{24}$ +200° (c = 0.5 in 0.1*N* HCl). $[\alpha]_D^{24}$ +105° (c = 0.9 in pyridine).

Sulfate tetrahydrate. $C_{36}H_{38}N_2O_6.H_2SO_4.4H_2O$. Rectangular plates from water. Contains 9.43% H_2O. After drying, mp 263-265° (dec). $[\alpha]_D^{24}$ +184° (c = 0.375 in methanol).

Methiodide. mp 270-275°.

Dimethiodide. $C_{38}H_{44}I_2N_2O_6$. Pale amorphous precipitate, mp 275° (dec). $[\alpha]_D^{24}$ +184° (c = 0.375 in methanol). uv max (water): 225, 280 nm (ε 62000, 7030).

USE: Methiodides have curarizing power.

2213. Chondrofoline. [31944-97-5] (1β)-6,6′,7′-Trimethoxy-2,2′-dimethyltubocuraran-12′-ol; (*R,R*)-7-*O*-methylbebeerine; 7-*O*-methylcurine. $C_{37}H_{40}N_2O_6$; mol wt 608.72. C 73.00%, H 6.62%, N 4.60%, O 15.77%. Alkaloid isolated from the leaves of *Chondrodendron platyphyllum* (A. St. Hil.) Miers, *Menispermaceae:* King, *J. Chem. Soc.* **1940,** 737. Structure, stereochemistry, NMR and mass spectrum: Baldas *et al., Chem. Commun.* **1971,** 132. ^{13}C-NMR: L. Koike *et al., J. Org. Chem.* **46,** 2385 (1981).

Solvated plates from methanol, mp about 135°. $[\alpha]_{5461}^{20}$ $-281°$ (0.1N HCl).

Nitrate hydrate. $C_{37}H_{40}N_2O_6 \cdot 2HNO_3 \cdot H_2O$. Needles from water, dec 225°.

2214. Chondroitin Sulfate. [9007-28-7] Chondroitinsulfuric acid; Chonsurid; Structum. Mol wt estimated at 50,000 depending on source and method of prepn: Schubert, *Fed. Proc.* **17**, 1099 (1958). High viscosity mucopolysaccharides (glycosaminoglycans) with N-acetylchondrosine as a repeating unit and with one sulfate group per disaccharide unit. These biological polymers act as the flexible connecting matrix between the tough protein filaments in cartilage to form a polymeric system similar to reinforced rubber. Chondroitin 4-sulfate and chondroitin 6-sulfate are the most abundant mucopolysaccharides in the body and occur both in skeletal and soft connective tissue. Isoln: Bray *et al., Biochem. J.* **38**, 142 (1944); Patat, Elias, *Z. Physiol. Chem.* **316**, 1 (1959); Kasavina *et al., SU 157466* (1962); Wheat, Davidson, *Biochem. Prep.* **10**, 52 (1963); Haneno, *JP 64 7650* (1964 to Yasushi Hano). Structure: Davidson, Meyer, *J. Am. Chem. Soc.* **77**, 4796 (1955). Absorption spectrum of A: Orr, *Biochim. Biophys. Acta* **14**, 173 (1954); of B + C: Mathews, *Nature* **181**, 421 (1958). Clinical trials in atherosclerosis: K. Nakazawa, K. Murata, *J. Int. Med. Res.* **6**, 217 (1978); *eidem, Z. Alternsforsch.* **34**, 153 (1979). *Reviews:* K. Meyer, "Chondroitin Sulfates" in *Polysaccharides in Biology*, Trans. 4th Conf. 1958, G. F. Springer, Ed. (Josiah Macy Jr. Foundn., New York, 1959) p 11; Muir, *Am. J. Med.* **47**, 673-690 (1969); Rodén, *Pure Appl. Chem.* **35**, 181-193 (1973). Review of clinical use in osteoarthritis: T. E. McAlindon *et al., J. Am. Med. Assoc.* **283**, 1469-1475 (2000). *See also* Chondrosine.

Chondroitin sulfate A　R = SO₃H　R' = H
Chondroitin sulfate C　R = H　R' = SO₃H

Chondroitin 4-sulfate. [24967-93-9] Chondroitin sulfate A; CSA; Atheroitin. $[\alpha]_D$ -28 to $-32°$.

Chondroitin 4-sulfate disodium salt. [39455-18-0] Condrosulf; Lacrypos.

Chondroitin 6-sulfate. [25322-46-7] Chondroitin sulfate C. $[\alpha]_D$ -12 to $-18°$.

Dermatan sulfate. [24967-94-0] Chondroitin sulfate B; β-heparin. Present in soft connective tissue and abundant in skin, arterial walls and heart valves. Differs from chondroitin sulfate A by containing iduronic acid in place of glucuronic acid, its epimer, at carbon atom 5. Pharmacodynamics: A. M. Traini *et al., J. Int. Med. Res.* **22**, 323 (1994). Clinical evaluation in deep vein thrombosis: B. P. Imbimbo *et al., Thromb. Haemostasis* **71**, 553 (1994). $[\alpha]_D$ -60 to $-70°$.

THERAP CAT: Chondroprotectant; in treatment of osteoarthritis.

2215. Chondrosine. [499-14-9] 2-Amino-2-deoxy-3-O-β-D-glucopyranurosyl-D-galactose; β-D-glucopyranosyluronic acid 2-deoxy-2-amino-D-galactose. $C_{12}H_{21}NO_{11}$; mol wt 355.30. C 40.57%, H 5.96%, N 3.94%, O 49.53%. Disaccharide unit of chondroitins 4-sulfate and 6-sulfate. Isoln: Hebting, *Biochem. Z.* **63**, 353 (1914); Levene, *J. Biol. Chem.* **140**, 267 (1941); Wolfrom *et*

al., *J. Am. Chem. Soc.* **74**, 1491 (1952); Davidson, Meyer, *ibid.* **76**, 5686 (1954). Structure: *eidem, ibid.* **77**, 4796 (1955). Synthesis: Takanashi *et al., ibid.* **84**, 3029 (1962). Chondrosine yields on acid hydrolysis chondrosamine (D-galactosamine, *q.v.*). Prepn and derivatives: Stacey, *J. Chem. Soc.* **1944**, 272; Wolfrom, Onodera, *J. Am. Chem. Soc.* **79**, 4737 (1957).

D-Glucuronic acid　　　Chondrosamine

Crystals from aq ethanol. $[\alpha]_D^{24}$ +40° (0.05 HCl). $[\alpha]_D^{20}$ +39° (water). Dec on heating.

Methyl ester hydrochloride. $C_{13}H_{24}ClNO_{11}$. Crystals from hot ethanol, mp 159-161°. $[\alpha]_D^{23}$ +42° (c = 2 in water).

2216. Chorionic Gonadotropin. Choriogonadotropin; CG. Glycoprotein hormone synthesized by chorionic tissue of the placenta; found in blood and urine during pregnancy. Maintains the function of the corpus luteum and stimulates ovarian steroid secretion in the early stages of gestation. Bioactivity closely resembles that of luteinizing hormone. Structurally similar to LH, FSH, and TSH, *q.q.v.*, all are dimers consisting of noncovalently linked α and β subunits. Within a species, the α-subunits of the four hormones are essentially identical, while the β-subunits, although exhibiting varying degrees of homology, are unique and believed to be responsible for the biological specificity of the individual hormones. Produced by trophoblastic cell neoplasms and used in the diagnosis and management of trophoblastic malignancies. Also produced by cancer cells of various histological types. Discovery in human pregnancy urine: S. Aschheim, B. Zondek, *Klin. Wochenschr.* **6**, 1322 (1927); in serum of pregnant mares: H. H. Cole, G. H. Hart, *Am. J. Physiol.* **93**, 57 (1930). Isoln of human CG: B. Zondek, S. Aschheim, *Klin. Wochenschr.* **7**, 831 (1928); S. Gurin *et al., J. Biol. Chem.* **128**, 525 (1939); P. A. Katzman *et al., ibid.* **148**, 501 (1943). Review of early literature: J. A. Loraine, *J. Reprod. Fertil.* **12**, 23-31 (1966). Purification and physicochemical properties: O. P. Bahl, *J. Biol. Chem.* **244**, 567 (1969). Isoln of α and β subunits: N. Swaminathan, O. P. Bahl, *Biochem. Biophys. Res. Commun.* **40**, 422 (1970); F. J. Morgan, R. E. Canfield, *Endocrinology* **88**, 1045 (1971). Amino acid sequence of α-subunit: R. Bellesario *et al., J. Biol. Chem.* **248**, 6796 (1973); of the β-subunit: R. B. Carlsen *et al., ibid.* **6810**; F. J. Morgan *et al., ibid.* **250**, 5247 (1975). Crystal structure: A. J. Lapthorn *et al., Nature* **369**, 438 (1994). Purification using HPLC: M. A. Chlenov *et al., J. Chromatogr.* **631**, 261 (1993). Comparison of gonadotropins of various species: J. G. Pierce, T. F. Parsons, *Annu. Rev. Biochem.* **50**, 465-495 (1981). Review of biosynthesis: R. O. Hussa, *Endocr. Rev.* **1**, 268-294 (1980). Diagnostic use as a tumor marker: L. A. Cole *et al., Cancer Res.* **48**, 1356 (1988); D. L. Blithe *et al., Trends Endocrinol. Metab.* **1**, 394 (1990). Secretion in normal, nonpregnant humans: W. D. Odell *et al., ibid.* **418**. Synthesis and expression by tumor cells: H. F. Acevedo *et al., Cancer* **76**, 1467 (1995). Review of clinical assay methods: R. J. Norman *et al., Ann. Clin. Biochem.* **27**, 183-194 (1990). Review of structure, secretion and bioactivity of equine CG: B. D. Murphy, S. D. Martinuk, *Endocr. Rev.* **12**, 27-44 (1991).

Human Chorionic Gonadotropin. [9002-61-3] HCG; pregnancy urine extract; urinary hCG; Choragon; Coriantin; Corulon; Endocorion; Physex; Predalon; Pregnesin; Pregnyl; Primogonyl; Profasi. Stable in dry form. Freely sol in water; sol in aq glycerol and glycols. Insol in alcohol, acetone, ether. pI 2.95. mol wt ~39500 Da. α subunit consists of 92 amino acids; β subunit, 145 amino acids. Total carbohydrate content: ~30% by wt.

Equine Chorionic Gonadotropin. [9002-70-4] Pregnant mare serum gonadotropin; PMSG; serum gonadotropin; Seragon; Serotropin. Sol in water, dil glycerol and glycols. pI 2.60-2.65. α subunit consists of 96 amino acids; β subunit, 149 amino acids. Total carbohydrate content: ~45% by wt.

Choriogonadotropin alfa. [177073-44-8] Chorionic gonadotropin (human α-subunit protein moiety reduced) complex with chorionic gonadotropin (human β-subunit protein moiety reduced); human chorionic gonadotropin, glycoform α; rhCG; Ovidrel; Ovitrelle. Recombinant human CG derived from genetically engineered Chinese hamster ovary cells. Clinical trial in assisted reproductive technology: P. Chang *et al.*, *Fertil. Steril.* **76**, 67 (2001).

THERAP CAT: Gonad-stimulating principle.

THERAP CAT (VET): Gonad-stimulating principle.

2217. Chorismic Acid. [617-12-9] (3*R-trans*)-3-[(1-Carboxyethenyl)oxy]-4-hydroxy-1,5-cyclohexadiene-1-carboxylic acid; 3-enolpyruvic ether of *trans*-3,4-dihydroxycyclohexa-1,5-diene carboxylic acid; α-(5-carboxy-1,2-dihydro-2-hydroxyphenoxy)-acrylic acid. $C_{10}H_{10}O_6$; mol wt 226.18. C 53.10%, H 4.46%, O 42.44%. The first branch point intermediate in the biosynthesis of aromatic amino acids via the shikimate pathway in bacteria, fungi, and higher plants; naturally occurring as the (−)-form. Its existence was predicted, then discovered during development of a mutant of *A. aerogenes:* M. I. Gibson *et al.*, *Nature* **195**, 1173 (1962); M. I. Gibson, F. Gibson, *Biochim. Biophys. Acta* **65**, 160 (1962). NMR and preliminary structure study: F. Gibson, M. Jackman, *Nature* **198**, 388 (1963). Isoln and metabolism study: M. Gibson, F. Gibson, *Biochem. J.* **90**, 248 (1964). Prepn and characterization of the barium salt: F. Gibson, *ibid.* 256. Structure, relative and abs config, prepn of the monohydrate: J. M. Edwards, L. M. Jackman, *Aust. J. Chem.* **18**, 1227 (1965). Total synthesis of racemic chorismic acid: D. A. McGowan, G. A. Berchtold, *J. Am. Chem. Soc.* **104**, 1153 (1982); B. Ganem *et al.*, *ibid.* 6787; improved synthesis: G. A. Berchtold *et al.*, *ibid.* **105**, 6265 (1983); short formal synthesis: G. H. Posner *et al.*, *J. Org. Chem.* **52**, 4836 (1987). Total synthesis of (−)-form: J. L. Pawlak, G. A. Berchtold, *ibid.* 1765. Potential use in development of herbicides: S. Stinson, *Chem. Eng. News* **60**, 31 (Dec. 6, 1982). Reviews of chorismic acid in biosynthesis of aromatic amino acids: F. Gibson, J. Pittard, *Bacteriol. Rev.* **32**, 465-492 (1968); R. J. Ife *et al.*, *J. Chem. Soc. Perkin Trans. 1* **1976**, 1776-1783; U. Weiss, J. M. Edwards, *The Biosynthesis of Organic Compounds* (Wiley, New York, 1980) pp 134-143. *See also* shikimic acid.

Crystals may be obtained but show marked tendency toward solvent retention, mp 105-108° (dec). $[\alpha]_D$ −274° (c = 0.16 in water).

Barium salt trihydrate. $C_{10}H_8BaO_6.3H_2O$. Unstable. uv max (aq soln): 272 nm (ε 2700).

Monohydrate. Colorless crystals from ethyl acetate + light petroleum, mp 148-149° (dec); from ether + light petroleum, mp 112° (dec); from ethyl acetate + carbon tetrachloride, mp 115° (dec). $[\alpha]_{5890}^{25}$ −295.5° (c = 0.2 in water). uv max (water): 275 nm (ε 2630).

(±)-Form. Crystals from ethyl acetate/hexane, mp 139.4-141° (dec).

2218. Chromafenozide. [143807-66-3] 3,4-Dihydro-5-methyl-2*H*-1-benzopyran-6-carboxylic acid 2-(3,5-dimethylbenzoyl)-2-(1,1-dimethylethyl)hydrazide; 2'-*tert*-butyl-5-methyl-2'-(3,5-xyloyl)chromane-6-carbohydrazide; ANS-118; Matric. $C_{24}H_{30}N_2O_3$; mol wt 394.51. C 73.07%, H 7.66%, N 7.10%, O 12.17%. Diacylhydrazine ecdysone mimetic for use in food crops. Prepn: M. Yanagi *et al.*, **EP 496342**; *eidem*, **US 5378726** (1992, 1995 both to Nippon Kayaku; Sankyo). Properties and biological activity: M. Yanagi *et al.*, *BCPC Conf. - Pests Dis.* **2000**, 27. Field trial against apple tortix: R. Ichinose *et al.*, *Annu. Rep. Sankyo Res. Lab.* **52**, 59 (2000). Mode of action: T. Toya *et al.*, *Biochem. Biophys. Res. Commun.* **292**, 1087 (2002). Series of articles on design, synthesis, and activity: Y. Sawada *et al.*, *Pest Manage. Sci.* **59**, 25-57 (2003). Review of development, environmental chemistry, safety, and toxicity: K. Tanaka *et al.*, *Annu. Rep. Sankyo Res. Lab.* **53**, 1-49 (2001).

White crystalline powder, mp 186.4°. Log P (octanol/water): 2.7 (22°). Vapor pressure at 25°: ≤4 × 10⁻⁹ Pa. Soly in water at 20°: 1.12 mg/l. Moderately sol in polar organic solvents. LD_{50} (mg/kg) orally in rats, mice: >5000; dermally in rabbits: >2000; LC_{50} (mg/l) in rats: >4.68 by inhalation; in carp, rainbow trout (96 hr): >47.25, >18.9 (Yanagi).

USE: Insecticide.

2219. Chromic Acetate. [1066-30-4] $C_6H_9CrO_6$; mol wt 229.13. C 31.45%, H 3.96%, Cr 22.69%, O 41.90%. $Cr(CH_3-COO)_3$. The commercial material, usually sold as a concd soln of the basic acetate, $Cr(OH)(C_2H_3O_2)_2$, contains Na acetate or Na_2SO_4 impurities. Industrial prepn: Stover; Drew, **US 2650239**; **US 2678328** (1953, 1954 both to Socony-Vacuum Oil). Prepn of hexahydrate: Hein, Herzog in *Handbook of Preparative Inorganic Chemistry* vol. 2, G. Brauer, Ed. (Academic Press, New York, 2nd ed., 1965) p 1371. Toxicity data: Cavalli, *Arch. Int. Pharmacodyn.* **62**, 330 (1939). *Review: ACS Monograph Series* **no. 132**, entitled "Chromium," vol. 1, M. J. Udy, Ed. (Reinhold, New York, 1956) pp 229-233.

Hydrate. Approx $Cr(C_2H_3O_2)_3.H_2O$, gray-green powder or violet plates. Slightly sol in water. Practically insol in alc. MLD in frogs, mice, rabbits (mg/kg): 6185, 2290, 1604 i.v. (Cavalli).

Hexahydrate. Hexaaquochromium triacetate. Blue-violet needles. Readily sol in water, with partial hydrolysis, giving a soln which is blue under the incident light and red under transmitted light; solvolyzed by alc.

Basic. $Cr(OH)(C_2H_3O_2)_2$. Violet cryst powder. Freely sol in water.

USE: As a mordant in dyeing; in tanning; in hardening photographic emulsions; to improve light stability and dye affinity of textiles and polymers; in catalyst for polymerization of olefins; as an oxidation catalyst.

2220. Chromic Bromide. [10031-25-1] Br_3Cr; mol wt 291.71. Br 82.17%, Cr 17.82%. $CrBr_3$. Prepd by passing Br_2 vapor over Cr powder at 1000°: Hein, Herzog, in *Handbook of Preparative Inorganic Chemistry* vol. 2, G. Brauer, Ed. (Academic Press, New York, 2nd ed., 1965) p 1341.

Black, lustrous, hexagonal crystals; green in transmitted and reddish in reflected light. Sol in cold water only upon addition of chromous salts; sol in boiling water.

Hexahydrate. At least two isomeric forms exist. *Dibromo-tetraaquochromium bromide dihydrate*, $[CrBr_2(H_2O)_4]Br.2H_2O$; green, deliquesc crystals; sol in water, alc. *Hexaaquochromium tribromide*, $[Cr(H_2O)_6]Br_3$; violet, deliquesc crystals; sol in water. Insol in alc. Both forms practically insol in ether.

USE: In catalysts for polymerization of olefins.

2221. Chromic Carbonate. [29689-14-3] $Cr_2O_3.xCO_2.-yH_2O$. A basic carbonate of indefinite composition, contg. 50-55% Cr. Obtained by pptg a chromic salt with a sol carbonate or bicarbonate.

Blue-green amorphous powder. Practically insol in water. Slightly sol in CO_2-contg water; sol in mineral acids.

USE: Prepn of chromic salts.

2222. Chromic Chloride. [10025-73-7] Cl_3Cr; mol wt 158.36. Cl 67.16%, Cr 32.83%. $CrCl_3$. Prepn: Heisig *et al.*, *Inorg. Synth.* **2**, 193 (1946); Pray, *ibid.* **5**, 153 (1953); Vavoulis *et al.*, *ibid.* **6**, 129 (1960); Hein, Herzog in *Handbook of Preparative Inorganic Chemistry* vol. 2, G. Brauer, Ed. (Academic Press, New York, 2nd ed., 1965) pp 1338-1340; prepn of hexahydrates: *eidem*, *ibid.*, pp 1348-1350. Toxicity data: Cavalli, *Arch. Int. Pharmacodyn.* **62**, 330 (1939).

Violet, lustrous, hexagonal, cryst scales. Greasy feel. mp 1152°; dissociates above 1300°. d^{25} 2.87. The rate of soln in water, acids, organic solvents is extremely slow. Addition of a trace of $CrCl_2$ or wetting agent aid in rapid soln in water, alcohol. Also exists in hygroscopic, sol, peach-blossom colored form. *Keep tightly closed.* MLD in frogs, mice, rabbits (mg/kg): 187, 801, 288 i.v. (Cavalli).

Hexahydrates. Several known isomers. *Dichlorotetraaquochromium chloride dihydrate,* [*trans*-[CrCl$_2$(H$_2$O)$_4$]Cl.2H$_2$O]; dark green salt, monoclinic crystals; d 1.849: Freeman, Dance, *Inorg. Chem.* **4,** 1555 (1965); Morosin, *Acta Crystallogr.* **21,** 280 (1966). *Hexaaquochromium trichloride,* [[Cr(H$_2$O)$_6$]Cl$_3$]; violet, rhombohedral hydrate. *Chloropentaaquochromium dichloride monohydrate,* [[CrCl(H$_2$O)$_5$]Cl$_2$.H$_2$O]; light green isomer. All are deliquesc in air. Sol in water; dil aq solns are violet, concd aq solns are green. pH of 0.2 molar aq soln 2.4. Sol in alcohol; slightly sol in acetone. Practically insol in ether. *Keep well closed.*

USE: In chromizing; manuf of Cr metal and compds; as catalyst for polymerization of olefins and other organic reactions; as textile mordant; in tanning; in corrosion inhibitors; as waterproofing agent.

2223. Chromic Fluoride. [7788-97-8] CrF$_3$; mol wt 108.99. Cr 47.71%, F 52.29%. Prepd by heating CrCl$_3$ in a current of HF: Kwasnik in *Handbook of Preparative Inorganic Chemistry* **vol. 1,** G. Brauer, Ed. (Academic Press, New York, 2nd ed., 1963) p. 257. Review of chromium halides: Fergusson in *Halogen Chemistry* **vol. 3,** V. Gutmann, Ed. (Academic Press, New York, 1967) pp 227-302.

Dark green needles, d 3.8. mp 1100°. Sublimes at 1100-1200°. Practically insol in water, alcohol. Sol in HCl with violet color.

Trihydrate. Triaquochromium trifluoride. Discussion of other hydrates or Werner complexes: *ACS Monograph Series* **no. 132,** entitled "Chromium," vol. 1, M. J. Udy, Ed. (Reinhold, New York, 1956) p 183. Green crystals from solns of Cr or Cr(OH)$_3$ in hydrofluoric acid. Sparingly sol in water.

USE: The hydrates in printing and dyeing woolens; coloring and hardening marble; mothproofing woolen fabrics; treating silk; polishing metals; halogenation catalyst.

2224. Chromic Formate. [27115-36-2] C$_3$H$_3$CrO$_6$; mol wt 187.05. C 19.26%, H 1.62%, Cr 27.80%, O 51.32%. Cr(HCOO)$_3$. Prepd from Cr(OH)$_3$ and formic acid: Akhmedli, Negretov, *J. Gen. Chem. USSR* **20,** 2045 (1950).

Hexahydrate. Fine green crystals or gray-green powder. Dec above 300°, evolving CO and CO$_2$. Sol in water; concd aq soln is blue under incident light, red under transmitted light; dil aq soln is green.

USE: In printing cotton in skeins; in leather tanning and waterproofing.

2225. Chromic Hydroxide. [1308-14-1] Chromium hydroxide; chromic oxide gel; chromic oxide, hydrous. CrH$_3$O$_3$; mol wt 103.02. Cr 50.47%, H 2.94%, O 46.59%. Cr(OH)$_3$. Occurs only as hydrates. Prepn: Ruthroff, *Inorg. Synth.* **2,** 190 (1946); Hein, Herzog in *Handbook of Preparative Inorganic Chemistry* **vol. 2,** G. Brauer, Ed. (Academic Press, New York, 2nd ed., 1965) pp 1345-1346.

Trihydrate. Cr(OH)$_3$.3H$_2$O. Or Cr$_2$O$_3$.9H$_2$O, blue-green powder. Practically insol in water. Sol in dil mineral acids when freshly prepd, giving blue or green soln; becomes insol in acids on aging. Cr(OH)$_3$.nH$_2$O, shining, vitrous, jet-black particles. Useful as catalyst in dehydrogenation of alcohols and paraffins, hydrogenation of olefins.

USE: As pigment; in tanning industry; as mordant; as catalyst for organic reactions.

2226. Chromic Nitrate. [13548-38-4] Nitric acid chromium(3+) salt; chromium(III) nitrate. CrN$_3$O$_9$; mol wt 238.01. Cr 21.85%, N 17.65%, O 60.50%. Cr(NO$_3$)$_3$. Prepn of anhydr salt from N$_2$O$_5$ and Cr(CO)$_6$: Addison, Chapma, *J. Chem. Soc.* **1964,** 539. Prepn of nonahydrate from Cr(OH)$_3$ and dil HNO$_3$ or by reducing CrO$_3$ in the presence of HNO$_3$: *ACS Monograph Series* **no. 132,** entitled "Chromium," vol. 1, M. J. Udy, Ed. (Reinhold, New York, 1956) pp 203-204. Toxicity study: Smyth *et al., Am. Ind. Hyg. Assoc. J.* **30,** 470 (1969).

Pale green, extremely deliquesc powder. Non-volatile. Dec above 60°. Sol in water, ethyl acetate, DMSO. Practically insol in benzene, CCl$_4$, CHCl$_3$. Reacts with ether, sometimes vigorously.

Nonahydrate. Deep violet, rhombic, monoclinic crystals. mp about 60°; dec above 100°. Sol in water, alcohol. Aq soln slowly

becomes green on heating and rapidly recovers the reddish-violet color on cooling. LD$_{50}$ orally in rats: 3.25 g/kg (Smyth).

USE: Prepn of Cr catalyst; in textile printing; corrosion inhibitor.

2227. Chromic Phosphate. [7789-04-0] CrO$_4$P; mol wt 146.97. Cr 35.38%, O 43.54%, P 21.07%. CrPO$_4$. Prepn: Ness *et al., J. Am. Chem. Soc.* **74,** 4685 (1952); Eickhoff, Kebrich, **US 2749214** (1956 to National Lead); Wegenknecht, **DE 1046597** (1958); **DE 1056104** (1959).

Gray-brown to black crystals of amorphous solid. Does not melt by 1800°. d$^{32.5}$ 2.94. Partially oxidizes to CrO$_3$ on heating in air. Practically insol in water, acetic acid, HCl, aqua regia.

Hemiheptahydrate. Arnaudon's green; Plessy's green. Blue-green powder. d 2.15. Practically insol in water. Sol in acids.

Hexahydrate. Violet crystals. Loses water gradually on heating, becoming anhydr after one hour at 800° or 3-4 hrs at 500°. d^{14} 2.121. Practically insol in water. Slightly sol in acetic acid solns; readily sol in mineral acids, alkalis, oxalic acid solns.

Radioactive Form. [24381-60-0] Phosphocol. Cr^{32}PO$_4$.

USE: Green pigment; in wash primers; in catalysts for dehydrogenation of hydrocarbons or polymerization of olefins.

THERAP CAT: Radioactive form as antineoplastic (radioactive agent).

2228. Chromic Potassium Oxalate. [14217-01-7] Tripotassium tris(ethanedioato)chromate(3−); tripotassium tris(oxalato)-chromate(3−); potassium trioxalatochromate(III); potassium chromic oxalate. C$_6$CrK$_3$O$_{12}$; mol wt 433.35. C 16.63%, Cr 12.00%, K 27.07%, O 44.30%. K$_3$[Cr(C$_2$O$_4$)$_3$]. Prepd by treatment of oxalic acid and K$_2$C$_2$O$_4$ with K$_2$Cr$_2$O$_7$: Bailar, Jr., Jones, *Inorg. Synth.* **1,** 37 (1939); Hein, Herzog in *Handbook of Preparative Inorganic Chemistry* **vol. 2,** G. Brauer, Ed. (Academic Press, New York, 2nd ed., 1965) p 1372.

Trihydrate. Potassium trioxalatotriaquochromate(III). Black-green, monoclinic scales with transparent blue edges. Freely sol in water; practically insol in alcohol.

USE: In tanning industry; dyeing chromate colors on wool.

2229. Chromic Potassium Sulfate. [10141-00-1] Potassium chromic sulfate; potassium disulfatochromate(III). CrKO$_8$S$_2$; mol wt 283.22. Cr 18.36%, K 13.80%, O 45.19%, S 22.64%. KCr(SO$_4$)$_2$. Dodecahydrate produced by reduction of K$_2$Cr$_2$O$_7$ with SO$_2$: Copson in *ACS Monograph Series* **no. 132,** entitled "Chromium," vol. 1, M. J. Udy, Ed. (Reinhold, New York, 1956) p 281; electrolytic manuf: Nishihara *et al., JP 60 2164 C.A.* **55,** 5200e (1961).

Dodecahydrate. Chrome alum. K[Cr(SO$_6$H$_4$)(H$_2$O)$_2$].6H$_2$-O: Duval, *Chim. Anal. (Paris)* **44,** 102 (1962); *C.A.* **57,** 9479d (1962). Large, violet-red to black, octahedral, cubic crystals; ruby-red under transmitted light. d^{25} 1.83. mp 89°; at 400° loses all its H$_2$O. Sol in 4 parts cold, 2 parts boiling water; practically insol in alcohol. The aq soln is violet when cold, green when hot. The violet color returns after a few weeks at room temp.

USE: Mordant for dyeing fabrics uniformly; tanning leather; printing calico; rendering glue and gum insol; manuf ink, other chromium salts; waterproofing fabrics; hardening photographic emulsions.

2230. Chromic Sulfate. [10101-53-8] Sulfuric acid chromium(3+) salt (3:2); chromium(III) sulfate. Cr$_2$O$_{12}$S$_3$; mol wt 392.18. Cr 26.52%, O 48.96%, S 24.53%. Cr$_2$(SO$_4$)$_3$. Prepn of anhydr salt by dehydration of hydrated forms: Rollinson, Bailar, Jr., *Inorg. Synth.* **2,** 197 (1946). Toxicity data: Cavalli, *Arch. Int. Pharmacodyn.* **62,** 330 (1939).

Peach-colored solid. d 3.012. Practically insol in water and acids. MLD in frogs, mice, rabbits (mg/kg): 37, 246.8, 215 i.v. (Cavalli).

Hydrates. Are known in both green and violet modifications, and have several degrees of hydration up to 18H$_2$O: Lukaszewski, Redfern, *Nature* **190,** 805 (1961); Udy in *Chromium* vol. 1, M. J. Udy, Ed., A.C.S. Monograph Series no. **132** (Reinhold, New York, 1956) pp 213-217, 288. The technical product comes in the form of a finely granular, dark-green flake or powder approximating the formula Cr$_2$(SO$_4$)$_3$.10H$_2$O. Readily sol in water. Almost insol in alc.

Basic chromic sulfates. Of the type Cr(OH)SO$_4$.nH$_2$O are of importance in the tanning industry: Udy, *loc. cit.* and pp 278-280,

305-308. Technical grades are available in two degrees of basicity, one-third and one-half, as finely granular dark-green flakes or powder contg about 25% Cr_2O_3. Readily sol in water.

USE: Insolubilization of gelatin; in catalyst prepn; as mordant in textile industry; in tanning of leather; in chrome plating; in manuf of Cr, CrO_3, and Cr alloys; to improve dispersibility of vinyl polymers in water; in manuf of green varnishes, paints, inks, glazes for porcelain.

2231. Chromium. [7440-47-3] Cr; at. wt 51.9961; at. no. 24; valences 1-6. Group VIB (6). Four naturally occurring isotopes: 50 (4.31%); 52 (83.76%); 53 (9.55%); 54 (2.38%). Artificial radioactive isotopes: 45-49; 51; 55-57; longest-lived isotope is ^{51}Cr ($T_{\frac{1}{2}}$ 27.704 days) prepd by (n,γ) reaction from ^{50}Cr. Abundance in earth's crust: 122 ppm. Isoln from *crocoite* ($PbCrO_4$): L. N. Vauquelin, *J. Mines* **6**, ser. 1, 737 (1787); *idem, Ann.* **70**, 70 (1809). Commercial sources obtained from chrome ore, *chromite* ($FeO.Cr_2O_3$). Reviews of chromium, its alloys and compds: *ACS Monograph Series* **no. 132**, entitled "Chromium," M. J. Udy, Ed. (Reinhold, New York, 1956) **vol. 1**, 433 pp; **vol. 2**, 402 pp; C. L. Rollinson, "Chromium, Molybdenum and Tungsten" in *Comprehensive Inorganic Chemistry* **vol. 3**, J. C. Bailar, Jr. *et al.*, Eds. (Pergamon Press, Oxford, 1973) pp 623-700; *Chemistry of the Elements*, N. N. Greenwood, A. Earnshaw, Eds. (Pergamon Press, New York, 1984) pp 1167-1210; J. H. Westbrook in *Kirk-Othmer Encyclopedia of Chemical Technology* **vol. 6** (Wiley-Interscience, New York, 4th ed., 1993) pp 228-263; B. J. Page, G. W. Loar, *ibid.* pp 263-311. Review of biological function of the Cr(III) ion as essential trace element: Mertz, *Physiol. Rev.* **49**, 163-239 (1969). Review of carcinogenic risk: *IARC Monographs* **2**, 100-125 (1973); *ibid.* **23**, 205-323 (1980); of metabolism and toxicity: M. D. Cohen *et al., Crit. Rev. Toxicol.* **23**, 255-281 (1993); of toxicology and human exposure: *Toxicological Profile for Chromium* (PB2000-108022, 2000) 461 pp. Books: *Chromium: Metabolism and Toxicity*, D. Burrows, Ed. (CRC Press, Boca Raton, 1983) 172 pp; *Chromium in the Natural and Human Environments*, J. O. Nriagu, E. Nieboer, Eds. (John Wiley & Sons, New York, 1988) 571 pp.

Steel-gray, lustrous metal; body-centered cubic structure; hard as corundum and less fusible than platinum. Takes a high polish. mp 1903 ±10°. bp 2642°. d^{20} 7.14. Heat capacity (25°): 5.58 cal/mol/deg C. Heat of fusion: 3.5 kcal/mol; heat of vaporization: 81.7 kcal/mol (at bp); heat of sublimation (25°): 94.8 kcal/mol (Rollinson). Also reported as mp 1875°. bp 2680°. d^{20} 7.19. Specific heat (25° C): 23.9 J/mol/deg K. Heat of fusion: 14.6 kJ/mol; heat of vaporization: 305 kJ/mol (at bp) (Westbrook). Resistant to common corroding agents, highly acid resistant. Reacts with dil HCl, H_2SO_4; not with HNO_3. Resists atmospheric attack at ambient temperatures.

Caution: Potential symptom of overexposure to chromium metal by inhalation is histologic fibrosis of the lungs. *See NIOSH Pocket Guide to Chemical Hazards* (DHHS/NIOSH 97-140, 1997) p 72. Chromic acid and chromate salts are irritating to exposed tissues. Toxic effects due to overexposure may include dermatitis, skin ulcers; nasal inflammation, perforation of nasal septum; cancer of the lungs, nasal cavity and paranasal sinus. *See Patty's Industrial Hygiene and Toxicology* **vol. 2C**, G. D. Clayton, F. E. Clayton, Eds. (John Wiley & Sons, New York, 4th ed., 1994) p 1973-1985. Chromium hexavalent compounds are listed as known human carcinogens: *Report on Carcinogens, Eleventh Edition* (PB2005-104914, 2004) p III-63.

USE: In manuf of chrome-steel or chrome-nickel-steel alloys (stainless steel), nonferrous alloys, heat resistant bricks for refractory furnaces. To greatly increase strength, hardness and resistance of metals to abrasion, corrosion and oxidation. For chrome plating of other metals; leather tanning; as pigment and mordant; wood preservative. Use of ^{51}Cr as diagnostic aid *see* sodium chromate(VI).

2232. Chromium Carbonyl. [13007-92-6] Chromium hexacarbonyl. C_6CrO_6; mol wt 220.06. C 32.75%, Cr 23.63%, O 43.62%. $Cr(CO)_6$. Prepn from Cr salts and CO in the presence of a Grignard reagent: Owen *et al., Inorg. Synth.* **3**, 156 (1950); in the presence of Mg and ether: Wender, **US 3012858** (1961 to Diamond Alkali); in the presence of Na and diglyme: Podall *et al., J. Am. Chem. Soc.* **83**, 2057 (1961); in the presence of Na and an aromatic hydrocarbon: Pruett, Wyman, **US 3053629** (1962 to Union Car-

bide); in the presence of I_2 and a nitrile: Wotiz, **US 3100687** (1963 to Diamond Alkali). Toxicity study: Strohmeier, *Z. Naturforsch.* **19b**, 540 (1964).

Orthorhombic, highly refractive crystals. Sublimes at room temp. Sinters at 90°; dec at 130°; explodes at 210°. Burns with a luminous flame. d^{18} 1.77. Vapor pressure (mm): 0.04 (0°); 1.0 (48°); 66.5 (100°). Almost insol in water, ethanol, methanol. Sol in ether, $CHCl_3$, other organic solvents. Solns or impure solid dec by light. LD_{50} i.v. in mice: 100 mg/kg (Strohmeier).

USE: In catalysts for olefin polymerization and isomerization; gasoline additive to increase octane number; prepn of chromous oxide, CrO.

2233. Chromium Dioxide. [12018-01-8] CrO_2; mol wt 83.99. Cr 61.91%, O 38.10%. Prepn: Wöhler, *Ann.* **111**, 117 (1859); Thamer *et al., J. Am. Chem. Soc.* **79**, 547 (1957); Swoboda *et al., J. Appl. Phys.* **32**, Suppl. no. 3, 374 (1961); Arthur; Arthur, Ingraham, **US 2959955**; **US 3117093** (1960, 1964 both to du Pont). *Reviews:* Hund, *Farbe Lack* **78**, 11-16 (1972); Rollinson in *Comprehensive Inorganic Chemistry* **vol 3**, J. C. Bailar, Jr. *et al.*, Eds. (Pergamon Press, Oxford, 1973) pp 689-690.

Black, ferromagnetic crystals; rutile structure. d 4.89. Metastable in air; various temperatures (250-500°) reported for decompn to Cr_2O_3.

USE: In magnetic recording tapes; as catalyst.

2234. Chromium(III) Oxide. [1308-38-9] Chromium oxide (Cr_2O_3); anadonis green; chrome green; chrome ocher; chrome oxide green; chromia; chromic oxide; chromium sesquioxide; green cinnabar; green oxide of chromium; green rouge; leaf green; oil green; ultramarine green; C.I. Pigment Green 17; C.I. 77288. Cr_2O_3; mol wt 151.99. Cr 68.42%, O 31.58%. Prepd by reaction of sodium dichromate or chromate with sulfur: Copson in *ACS Monograph Series* **no. 132**, entitled "Chromium," vol. 1, M. J. Udy, Ed. (Reinhold, New York, 1956) pp 277-278. *Review:* Wiesburg, *Paint Ind. Mag.* **71**(2), 11 (1956). *See also Colour Index* **vol. 4** (3rd ed., 1971) p 4662. Use as catalyst: R. Uma, J. C. Kuriacose, *Indian Chem. Manuf.* **8**, 11 (1970). Cytotoxic effects: V. Bianchi *et al., Toxicology* **17**, 219 (1980).

Light to dark green, fine, hexagonal crystals. mp about 2435°. bp about 3000°. d^{25} 5.22. Turns brown on heating but reverts to green color on cooling. Cryst Cr_2O_3 is extremely hard; will scratch quartz, topaz, zircon. Practically insol in water, alc, acetone. Slightly sol in acids, alkalies.

Caution: Trivalent chromium may cause skin irritation: S. Fregert, H. Rorsman, *Arch. Dermatol.* **90**, 4 (1964).

USE: In abrasives, refractory materials, electric semiconductors; as pigment, particularly in coloring glass; in alloys; printing fabrics and banknotes; as catalyst for organic and inorganic reactions.

2235. Chromium(VI) Oxide. [1333-82-0] Chromium oxide (CrO_3); chromic anhydride; chromium trioxide. CrO_3; mol wt 99.99. Cr 52.00%, O 48.00%. Produced commercially by the action of concd H_2SO_4 on a soln of chromate or dichromate: *Faith, Keyes & Clark's Industrial Chemicals*, F. A. Lowenheim, M. K. Moran, Eds. (Wiley-Interscience, New York, 4th ed., 1975) pp 270-274.

Dark red, deliquesc bipyramidal prismatic crystals, flakes or granular power. d 2.70. mp 197°. Dec at 250° to Cr_2O_3 and O_2. Very sol in water; sol in H_2SO_4. Powerful oxidizer; oxidizes alcohol and most other organic substances, sometimes with dangerous violence. Contact with combustible material may cause fire.

Caution: Potential symptoms of overexposure are respiratory system irritation, nasal septum perforation; liver and kidney damage; leukocytosis, leukopenia, monocytosis, eosinophilia; eye injury, conjunctivitis; skin ulcers, sensitization dermatitis. *See NIOSH Pocket Guide to Chemical Hazards* (DHHS/NIOSH 97-140, 1997) p 70. Chronic overexposure may lead to severe liver damage, CNS involvement and lung cancer. *See Clinical Toxicology of Commercial Products*, R. E. Gosselin *et al.*, Eds. (Williams & Wilkins, 5th ed., 1984) Section II, p 108. *See also Patty's Industrial Hygiene and Toxicology* **vol. 2C**, G. D. Clayton, F. E. Clayton, Eds. (Wiley-Interscience, New York, 4th ed., 1994) p 1973-1985. Chromium hexavalent compounds are listed as known human carcinogens: *Report on Carcinogens, Eleventh Edition* (PB2005-104914, 2004) p III-63.

USE: Chromium plating; copper stripping; aluminum anodizing; corrosion inhibitor; photography; purifying oil and acetylene; hardening microscopical prepns; oxidizing agent in organic chemistry.

THERAP CAT (VET): Has been used in solution as a topical antiseptic and astringent.

2236. Chromium Picolinate. [14639-25-9] Tris(2-pyridinecarboxylato-N^1,O^2)chromium; chromium tripicolinate; chromium(III) trispicolinate; Chromax. $C_{18}H_{12}CrN_3O_6$; mol wt 418.30. C 51.68%, H 2.89%, Cr 12.43%, N 10.05%, O 22.95%. Biologically active form of chromium. General prepn, chemical and biological properties: G. W. Evans, D. J. Pouchnik, *J. Inorg. Biochem.* **49**, 177 (1993). Clinical effect on insulin metabolism: G. W. Evans, *Int. J. Biosocial Med. Res.* **11**, 163 (1989). Clinical evaluation of lipid-lowering activity: R. I. Press *et al.*, *West. J. Med.* **152**, 41 (1990). Clinical pharmacokinetics: M. L. Gargas *et al.*, *Drug Metab. Dispos.* **22**, 522 (1994). Use as veterinary diet supplement: M. D. Lindemann *et al.*, *J. Anim. Sci.* **73**, 457 (1995). Review of clinical pharmacology: M. F. McCarty, *J. Appl. Nutr.* **43**, 58-66 (1991); *idem, J. Optim. Nutr.* **2**, 36-53 (1993); of safety studies: T. O. Berner *et al.*, *Food Chem. Toxicol.* **42**, 1029-1042 (2004).

Lipophilic. Soly: water (pH 7.0) 0.6 mM, chloroform 2.0 mM. uv max (water): 264 nm (a_M 15546 L mol^{-1}cm^{-1}).

THERAP CAT: Chromium supplement.

2237. Chromocarb. [4940-39-0] 4-Oxo-4H-1-benzopyran-2-carboxylic acid; 2-chromonecarboxylic acid; 4-oxo-4H-chromene-2-carboxylic acid; benzo-γ-pyronecarboxylic acid. $C_{10}H_6$-O_4; mol wt 190.15. C 63.16%, H 3.18%, O 33.66%. Prepn: S. Ruhemann, H. E. Stapleton, *J. Chem. Soc.* **77**, 1179 (1900); J. Schmutz *et al.*, *Helv. Chim. Acta* **34**, 767 (1951); G. Pifferi *et al.*, *J. Heterocycl. Chem.* **14**, 1257 (1977). Prepn of diethylamine salt: P. A. Tronche, **ZA 6807352**; *eidem*, **US 3816470** (1969, 1974 both to Ferlux). Pharmacology of diethylamine salt in animals: J. Couquelet *et al.*, *C.R. Seances Soc. Biol. Ses Fil.* **164**, 329 (1970); P. Conquet *et al.*, *ibid.* 800. Clinical comparison with dipyridamole effect on platelet function: A. Vittoria *et al.*, *Curr. Ther. Res.* **35**, 1033 (1984). Clinical trial in diabetes with vascular disease: N. Ciavarella *et al.*, *ibid.* **36**, 293 (1984). Bioavailability in humans: J.-M. Aiache *et al.*, *Biopharm. Drug Dispos.* **7**, 301 (1986).

Colorless needles from alcohol, mp 250-251° (dec) (Ruhemann, Stapleton); also reported as mp 255-256° (Pifferi). uv max: 230, 305 nm (ε 20220, 8075). Sol in alcohol, ammonia. Sparingly sol in water.

Diethylamine. [23915-80-2] Angiophtal; Campel; Fludarene. $C_{14}H_{17}NO_4$; mol wt 263.29. Microcrystalline powder from alcohol + acetone, mp 138°. Sol in water. LD$_{50}$ in mice: ~800 mg/kg i.v.; >5 g/kg orally (Tronche, 1974).

THERAP CAT: Diethylamine salt as capillary protectant.

2238. Chromomycin A$_3$. [7059-24-7] (1S)-1-C-[(2S,3S)-7-[[4-O-Acetyl-2,6-dideoxy-3-O-(2,6-dideoxy-4-O-methyl-α-D-*lyxo*-hexopyranosyl)-β-D-*lyxo*-hexopyranosyl]oxy]-3-[[O-4-O-acetyl-2,6-dideoxy-3-C-methyl-α-L-*arabino*-hexopyranosyl-(1 → 3)-O-2,6-

dideoxy-β-D-*arabino*-hexopyranosyl-(1 → 3)-2,6-dideoxy-β-D-*arabino*-hexopyranosyl]oxy]-1,2,3,4-tetrahydro-5,10-dihydroxy-6-methyl-4-oxo-2-anthracenyl]-5-deoxy-1-O-methyl-D-*threo*-2-pentulose; 3^D-O-(4-O-acetyl-2,6-dideoxy-3-C-methyl-α-L-*arabino*-hexopyranosyl)-7-methylolivomycin D; aburamycin B; toyomycin. $C_{57}H_{82}O_{26}$; mol wt 1183.25. C 57.86%, H 6.99%, O 35.16%. Major component of an antitumor antibiotic complex produced by *Streptomyces griseus*. Binds specifically to guanine-cytosine base pairs in DNA; does not intercalate. The aglycone, *chromomycinone*, is identical to that of plicamycin, *q.v.* Isoln of complex and antibacterial activity: M. Shibata *et al.*, *J. Antibiot.* **13B**, 1 (1960), *C.A.* **54**, 22835g (1960). Characterization: K. Mizuno, *J. Antibiot.* **16A**, 22 (1963). Structure: M. Miyamoto *et al.*, *Tetrahedron* **23**, 421 (1967). Abs config: N. Harada *et al.*, *J. Am. Chem. Soc.* **91**, 5896 (1969). Revised structure: J. Thiem, B. Meyer, *J. Chem. Soc. Perkin Trans. 2* **1979**, 1331. Pharmacology and toxicity: M. Slavik, S. K. Carter, *Adv. Pharmacol. Chemother.* **12**, 1 (1975). Fluorescence characteristics: R. H. Jensen, *J. Histochem. Cytochem.* **25**, 573 (1977). Use for analysis and identification of chromosomes: J. H. van de Sande *et al.*, *Science* **195**, 400 (1977); in high-speed chromosome sorting: J. W. Gray *et al.*, *ibid.* **238**, 323 (1987); in flow karyotyping: M. F. Bartholdi, *Pathobiology* **58**, 118 (1990). Review of staining methods: H. A. Crissman, R. A. Tobey, *Methods Cell Biol.* **33**, 97-103 (1990).

Yellow powder, dec. 185°. $[\alpha]_D^{23}$ −57° (ethanol). uv max (ethanol): 230, 281, 304, 318, 330, 412 nm (log ε 4.39, 4.72, 3.85, 3.92, 3.84, 4.07). Excitation max: ~445 nm. Emission max: ~575 nm. Sol in ethanol, ethyl acetate, DMSO, methanol. LD$_{50}$ in mice (mg/kg): 1.85 i.v. (Slavik, Carter). *Protect from light.*

USE: Fluorescent DNA stain in flow cytometry and karyotype analysis of chromosomes.

2239. Chromonar. [804-10-4] [[3-[2-(Diethylamino)ethyl]-4-methyl-2-oxo-2H-1-benzopyran-7-yl]oxy]acetic acid ethyl ester; 3-(β-diethylaminoethyl)-4-methyl-7-(carbethoxymethoxy)coumarin; 3-(β-diethylaminoethyl)-4-methyl-7-(carbethoxymethoxy)-2H-1-benzopyran-2-one; ethyl [[3-[2-(diethylamino)ethyl]-4-methyl-2-oxo-2H-1-benzopyran-7-yl]oxy]acetate; carbochromen; carbocromen. $C_{20}H_{27}NO_5$; mol wt 361.43. C 66.46%, H 7.53%, N 3.88%, O 22.13%. Prepn: **BE 621327**; Ritter *et al.*, **US 3282938** (1963, 1966 both to Casella Farbwerke Mainkur). Toxicity study: R. E. Nitz, E. Potzch, *Arzneim.-Forsch.* **13**, 243 (1963). Metabolic studies: Schraven *et al.*, *ibid.* **20**, 1905 (1970). Series of articles on pharmacology: *ibid.* **13**, 243-268 (1963); on distribution: *ibid.* **22**, 479-511 (1972).

Practically insol in water.

Hydrochloride. [655-35-6] Cassella 4489; Antiangor; Intenkordin; Intensain. $C_{20}H_{27}NO_5.HCl$; mol wt 397.89. Crystalline powder, mp 159-160°. Freely sol in water, alc, methylene chloride, chloroform. Sparingly sol in acetone, methyl ethyl ketone, benzene, ether. Aq solns show blue fluorescence. LD_{50} in mice (g/kg): 6.3 orally; 0.528 i.p.; 0.0355 i.v. (Nitz, Potzch).

THERAP CAT: Vasodilator (coronary).

2240. Chromotrope 2B. [548-80-1] 4,5-Dihydroxy-3-[(4-nitrophenyl)azo]-2,7-naphthalenedisulfonic acid disodium salt; C.I. Acid Red 176; *p*-nitrobenzeneazochromotropic acid sodium salt; C.I. 16575. $C_{16}H_9N_3Na_2O_{10}S_2$; mol wt 513.37. C 37.43%, H 1.77%, N 8.19%, Na 8.96%, O 31.17%, S 12.49%. Prepn from diazotized *p*-nitroaniline and chromotropic acid, see: *Colour Index* vol. 4 (3rd ed., 1971) p 4097.

Reddish-brown powder. Sol in water with a yellowish-red color. Insol in alcohol.

USE: As a dye; as a reagent for boric acid or borates.

2241. Chromotropic Acid. [148-25-4] 4,5-Dihydroxy-2,7-naphthalenedisulfonic acid; 1,8-dihydroxynaphthalene-3,6-disulfonic acid. $C_{10}H_8O_8S_2$; mol wt 320.30. C 37.50%, H 2.52%, O 39.96%, S 20.02%. Prepn from 4-chloro-5-hydroxy-2,7-naphthalenedisulfonic acid: **DE 147852** (1904 to BASF); alternate methods: *Frdl.* **3,** 460-466.

Dihydrate. White needles, soluble in water.

Disodium salt dihydrate. $C_{10}H_6Na_2O_8S_2.2H_2O$. White needles or leaflets. Very sol in water.

USE: Analytical reagent; intermediate for azo dyes.

2242. Chromous Acetate. [628-52-4] $C_4H_6CrO_4$; mol wt 170.08. C 28.25%, H 3.56%, Cr 30.57%, O 37.63%. $Cr(C_2H_3-O_2)_2$. Prepn of monohydrate: Balthis, Jr., Bailar, Jr., *Inorg. Synth.* **1,** 122 (1939); Hatfield, *ibid.* **3,** 148 (1950); Kranz, Witkowska, *ibid.* **6,** 144 (1960); Ocone, Block, *ibid.* **8,** 125 (1966). Toxicity study: H. F. Smyth *et al., Am. Ind. Hyg. Assoc. J.* **30,** 470 (1969).

Monohydrate. Deep red powder, or monoclinic crystals; composed of dimeric units. Easily oxidized, especially when moist, to chromic acetate. Loses H_2O when dried over P_2O_5 at 100°, changing color to brown. d 1.79. Slightly sol in cold water; readily sol in hot water; sol in and reacts with most acids; slightly sol in alcohol. Practically insoluble in ether. *Keep tightly closed.* LD_{50} orally in rats: 11.26 g/kg (Smyth).

USE: Prepn of other chromous salts; as O_2 absorber in gas analysis.

2243. Chromous Bromide. [10049-25-9] Br_2Cr; mol wt 211.80. Br 75.45%, Cr 24.55%. $CrBr_2$. Prepn: Hein, Herzog in *Handbook of Preparative Inorganic Chemistry* Vol. 2, G. Brauer, Ed. (Academic Press, New York, 2nd ed. 1965) p 1340. Review of chromium halides: Fergusson in *Halogen Chemistry* Vol. 3, V. Gutmann, Ed. (Academic Press, New York, 1967) pp 227-302.

White monoclinic crystals, becoming yellow when heated. mp 842°; d_4^{25} 4.236. Stable in dry air, oxidizes in moist air. Sol in water (exothermic) giving blue soln; sol in alcohol. *Keep well closed.*

USE: In chromizing.

2244. Chromous Chloride. [10049-05-5] Cl_2Cr; mol wt 122.90. Cl 57.69%, Cr 42.31%. $CrCl_2$. Prepn: Burg, *Inorg. Synth.* **3,** 150 (1950); Hein, Herzog, in *Handbook of Preparative*

Inorganic Chemistry Vol. 2, G. Brauer, Ed. (Academic Press, New York, 2nd ed. 1965) pp 1336-1338. Prepn of tetrahydrate: Balthis, Jr., Bailar, Jr., *Inorg. Synth.* **1,** 125 (1939); Holah, Fackler, *ibid.* **10,** 26 (1967). Toxicity study: H. F. Smyth *et al., Am. Ind. Hyg. Assoc. J.* **30,** 470 (1969).

Lustrous needles or fused, fibrous mass. mp 824°; d_4^{14} 2.751. Very hygroscopic; stable in dry air but oxidizes rapidly if moist. Powerful reducing agent. Soluble in water giving a blue soln. *Keep well closed.* LD_{50} orally in rats: 1.87 g/kg (Smyth).

Tetrahydrate. Tetraaquochromium dichloride. Bright blue, hygroscopic crystals. Above 38° changes to isomeric green modification. Loses $1H_2O$, forming trihydrate, at 51°. Absorbs O_2 even when dry, forming a greenish-black oxychloride. Sol in water. Almost insol in concd HCl. On standing in soln it is oxidized by the water with liberation of H_2. *Keep well closed.*

USE: In chromizing; in prepn of Cr metal; in catalysts for organic reactions; as O_2 absorbent; in analysis.

2245. Chromous Fluoride. [10049-10-2] CrF_2; mol wt 89.99. Cr 57.78%, F 42.22%. Prepd from $CrCl_2$ + HF: Poulenc, *Compt. Rend.* **116,** 254 (1893); Kwasnik in *Handbook of Preparative Inorganic Chemistry* Vol. 1, G. Brauer, Ed. (Academic Press, New York, 2nd ed., 1963) pp 256-257. Review of other preparative methods: Sturm, *Inorg. Chem.* **1,** 665-672 (1962).

Blue-green, monoclinic crystals with iridescent sheen. d 3.79. mp 894°. Sparingly sol in water; practically insol in alcohol; sol in boiling HCl; not attacked by hot dil H_2SO_4 or HNO_3. Changes to Cr_2O_3 when heated in air.

USE: In chromizing; in catalytic cracking of hydrocarbons; alkylation catalyst; in nuclear reactor fuels.

2246. Chromous Formate. [4493-37-2] $C_2H_2CrO_4$; mol wt 142.03. C 16.91%, H 1.42%, Cr 36.61%, O 45.06%. $Cr(HCOO)_2$. Prepd from $CrCl_2$ and Na formate: Lux, Illman, *Ber.* **91,** 2143 (1958); Earnshaw *et al., Proc. Chem. Soc. London* **1963,** 281. Prepn of blue and red anhydrous forms from hydrated formates: Herzog, Kalies, *Z. Chem.* **5,** 273 (1965).

Hemihydrate. Violet to blue crystals. Sol in water.

Monohydrate. Red needles. Sol in water to give blue soln.

Hemipentahydrate. Large, dark-red cubic crystals. Sol in water, alcohol, ether, acetone.

USE: In baths for Cr electroplating; in catalysts for organic reactions.

2247. Chromous Sulfate. [13825-86-0] CrO_4S; mol wt 148.06. Cr 35.12%, O 43.22%, S 21.66%. $CrSO_4$. Prepn of pentahydrate: Lux, Illman, *Ber.* **91,** 2143 (1958); Holah, Fackler, *Inorg. Synth.* **10,** 26 (1967). The common hydrated form, long considered to be the heptahydrate, has been reported to be the pentahydrate: Lux, Illman, *loc. cit.;* Lux *et al., Ber.* **97,** 503 (1964). Prepn of standard soln for use as an analytical reagent: Lingane, Pecsok, *Anal. Chem.* **20,** 425 (1948).

Pentahydrate. Blue crystals. Stable in air if dry. Sol in water; slightly sol in alcohol; practically insol in acetone. Soluble in dil, dec by concd H_2SO_4. Solns are rapidly oxidized by atmospheric oxygen.

USE: Analytical reagent; absorption of O_2 from gas mixtures; dehydrohalogenating and reducing agent.

2248. Chromyl Chloride. [14977-61-8] Dichlorodioxochromium; chromium dioxychloride. Cl_2CrO_2; mol wt 154.90. Cl 45.78%, Cr 33.57%, O 20.66%. CrO_2Cl_2. Prepn from CrO_3 + HCl: Sisler, *Inorg. Synth.* **2,** 205 (1946); Hein, Herzog in *Handbook of Preparative Inorganic Chemistry* Vol. 2, G. Brauer, Ed. (Academic Press, New York, 2nd ed., 1965) p 1384; and $AlCl_3$; Flesch, Svec, *J. Am. Chem. Soc.* **80,** 3189 (1958); from Cr_2O_3 and $TiCl_4$: Braos, Cohen, **US 3111380** (1963 to Natl. Distillers & Chem.). Review of chromium halides: Fergusson in *Halogen Chemistry* Vol. 3, V. Gutmann, Ed. (Academic Press, New York, 1967) pp 227-302.

Deep red liq; appears black under reflected light. Fumes in moist air. *Handle only in well-ventilated hood.* mp −96.5°; bp 117°; d_4^{25} 1.91. Slightly less viscous than water. Nonconductor of electricity. Strong oxidizing agent; *can react explosively with combustible organic and inorganic substances.* Hydrolyzes vigorously on contact with water. Reacts vigorously with liq or gaseous ammonia.

Sol in CCl_4, CS_2, benzene, nitrobenzene, $CHCl_3$, $POCl_3$. Its soln in CCl_4 is fairly stable. Liquid CrO_2Cl_2 is stable indefinitely in glass, aluminum, stainless steel containers if protected from light and moisture. CrO_2Cl_2 dissolves CrO_3, yielding a powerful oxidant.

Caution: Potential symptoms of overexposure are irritation of eyes, skin, upper respiratory system; eye, skin burns. *See NIOSH Pocket Guide to Chemical Hazards* (DHHS/NIOSH 97-140, 1997) p 72.

USE: Catalyst for polymerization of olefins; oxidation of hydrocarbons; in the Etard reaction for production of aldehydes and ketones; in the prepn of various coordination complexes of Cr.

2249. Chromyl Fluoride. [7788-96-7] Difluorodioxochromium; chromium oxyfluoride. CrF_2O_2; mol wt 121.99. Cr 42.62%, F 31.15%, O 26.23%. CrO_2F_2. Prepn of impure product from CrO_2Cl_2 and F_2: von Wartenberg, *Z. Anorg. Allg. Chem.* **247**, 140 (1941). Prepn from CrO_3 and SeF_4: Bartlett, Robinson, *J. Chem. Soc.* **1961**, 3549; from $K_2Cr_2O_7$ and HF or from Cr, KNO_3 and HF: Wiechert, *Z. Anorg. Allg. Chem.* **261**, 315 (1950). Review of earlier prepns and prepn from CrO_3 and ClF, COF_2, MoF_6 or WF_6: P. J. Green, G. L. Gard, *Inorg. Chem.* **16**, 1243 (1977). Review of chromium halides: Fergusson in *Halogen Chemistry* vol. 3, V. Gutmann, Ed. (Academic Press, New York, 1967) pp 227-302.

Red-violet to black rhombic or monoclinic crystals; described as a gas or a liq in earlier work with impure samples. Sublimation temp 29.6°; mp 31.6° (885 mm). *Extremely reactive;* etches glass, quartz. Ignites hydrocarbons such as methane or butane at elevated temps; mixtures burn with a bright flame producing fumes of Cr_2O_3 and CrF_3. Can be stored in a sealed aluminum phosphate glass tube or in a Kel-F tube. Stable indefinitely at room temp in the dark. Polymerizes slowly if exposed to visible, ultraviolet or infrared light to a gray-white solid, mp 200°.

USE: Fluorination catalyst; to increase olefin-polymer receptivity for dyes.

2250. Chrysanthemaxanthin. [27780-11-6] (3S,3'R,5R,-6'R,8S)-5,8-Epoxy-5,8-dihydro-β,ε-carotene-3,3'-diol. $C_{40}H_{56}O_3$; mol wt 584.87. C 82.14%, H 9.65%, O 8.21%. Carotenoid pigment. Occurs together with flavoxanthin, *q.v.*. Has same structural formula, mp, rotation, and absorption as flavoxanthin, but differs sterically. Can be separated chromatographically: in a zinc carbonate column the chrysanthemaxanthin zone locates itself below flavoxanthin and above lutein epoxide. Isoln from asters: Karrer, Jucker, *Helv. Chim. Acta* **26**, 626 (1943). Partial synthesis from lutein, *eidem, ibid.* **28**, 300 (1945). For absolute configuration see: H. Cadosch *et al., ibid.* **61**, 783 (1978).

Golden yellow leaflets, mp 184-185°, also reported as mp 178.5-180° (Codosch). $[\alpha]_D^{23}$ +104° ±5% (c = 1.833 mg/ml in chloroform). Absorption max (CHCl_3): 459, 430 nm. uv max (ethanol): 204, 251, 298, 311, 399, 422, 448 nm (ε 27300, 28800, 10000, 13100, 97700, 150400, 148500). Freely sol in chloroform, benzene, acetone. Less sol in methanol, ethanol. Almost insol in petr ether.

Note: Chrysanthemaxanthin has no vitamin A activity.

2251. Chrysanthemic Acid. [10453-89-1] 2,2-Dimethyl-3-(2-methyl-1-propenyl)cyclopropanecarboxylic acid; chrysanthemummonocarboxylic acid; chrysanthemumic acid. $C_{10}H_{16}O_2$; mol wt 168.23. C 71.39%, H 9.59%, O 19.02%. Occurs as esters in pyrethrum flowers, *see* Pyrethrin I and Cinerin I, *also* Allethrin (a synthetic product). Isoln and structure: Staudinger, Ruzicka, *Helv. Chim. Acta* **7**, 177, 201 (1924). Synthesis: Staudinger *et al., ibid.* 390; Campbell, Harper, *J. Chem. Soc.* **1945**, 283; M. J. Devos, A. Krief, *Tetrahedron Lett.* **1978**, 1845; **1979**, 1891; O. A. Nesmeyanova *et al., Synthesis* **1982**, 296. Asymmetric synthesis: T. Aratani *et al., ibid.* **1977**, 2599. Stereoselective synthesis of *dl-trans*-chrys-

anthemic acid: Mills *et al., Chem. Commun.* **1971**, 555; *eidem, J. Chem. Soc. Perkin Trans. 1* **1973**, 133; S. C. Welch, T. A. Valdes, *J. Org. Chem.* **42**, 2108 (1977); J. P. Genet *et al., Tetrahedron Lett.* **21**, 3183 (1980); of *dl-cis*-form: J. Mann, A. Thomas, *ibid.* **27**, 3533 (1986). Synthesis of (−)-*cis*- and (+)-*trans*-forms: Gopichand *et al., Indian J. Chem.* **13**, 433 (1975).

d-trans form

dl-cis-Form. [2935-23-1] Cubic prisms from ethyl acetate, mp 115-116°.

dl-trans-Form. [705-16-8] Long prisms, mp 54°. Very sol in ethyl acetate. Exhibits a marked negative heat of soln in ethyl acetate or in methanol.

l-trans-Form. [2259-14-5] Elongated prisms, mp 17-21°. $[\alpha]_D^{25}$ −14.01° (c = 1.535 in abs alc).

d-trans-Form. [4638-92-0] Elongated prisms, mp 17-21°. $[\alpha]_D^{25}$ +14.16° (c = 1.554 in abs alc).

2252. Chrysanthenone. [473-06-3] 2,7,7-Trimethylbicyclo[3.1.1]heptan-6-one; 2-pinen-7-one. $C_{10}H_{14}O$; mol wt 150.22. C 79.95%, H 9.39%, O 10.65%. A constituent of the essential oil of *Chrysanthemum indicium* L., also extracted from *C. sinense* Sabin, *Compositae.* Prepared by photochemical rearrangement of *l*- or d-verbenone, *q.v.*: Hurst, Whitham, *J. Chem. Soc.* **1960**, 2864; Erman, *J. Am. Chem. Soc.* **89**, 3828 (1967); Schuster, Widman, *Tetrahedron Lett.* **1971**, 3571. Structure: Kotake, Nonaka, *Ann.* **607**, 153 (1957); Blanchard, *Chem. Ind. (London)* **1958**, 293. Chemistry: Erman, *J. Am. Chem. Soc.* **91**, 779 (1969).

d-Form. Herbaceous odor. bp_{12} 88-89°. n_D^{22} 1.4720. $[\alpha]_D$ +37° (c = 2.1 in chloroform). uv max: 290 nm (ε 120). Insoluble in water; sol in alcohol.

2253. Chrysarobin. [491-59-8] Purified Goa powder; purified araroba. Improperly called *"medicinal chrysophanic acid"*. The name chrysarobin today has two meanings: (1) A commercial product consisting of 70-85% of different anthraquinone derivs extracted from Goa powder (Araroba); (2) A pure substance, (*1,8-dihydroxy-3-methyl-9-anthrone; 3-methyl-1,8,9-anthracenetriol*), reduction product of chrysophanic acid, *q.v.* This pure substance constitutes about 30% of commercial chrysarobin. Isoln of the commercial product from the wood of *Andira araroba* Aguiar [*Vouacapoua araroba* (Aguiar) Lyons], *Leguminosae:* Liebermann, Siedler, *Ann.* **212**, 29 (1882); Hesse; *ibid.* **309**, 53 (1899). Prepn of the pure substance by reduction of chrysophanic acid: Naylor, Gardner, *J. Am. Chem. Soc.* **53**, 4114 (1931).

Commercial product, brownish to orange-yellow, microcrystalline, odorless, tasteless powder. Irritating to mucous membranes; causes dangerous inflammation if it enters the eye. Very slightly sol in water; 1 g dissolves in 385 ml alcohol, 30 ml benzene, 15 ml chloroform, 160 ml ether, 180 ml carbon disulfide; also sol in fats. Dissolves in alkali hydroxides or in H_2SO_4 with a red color and is pptd from the H_2SO_4 soln by diluting with H_2O.

Pure substance. [491-58-7] $C_{15}H_{12}O_3$. Yellow needles from glacial acetic acid, mp 203.4-204°.

Caution: Ingestion may cause renal damage, severe gastroenteritis. Application to large areas of skin may cause renal irritation by percutaneous absorption. Inadvertent conjunctival contact frequently produces conjunctivitis. Allergic reaction of skin has been reported.

THERAP CAT: Has been used as antipsoriatic.

THERAP CAT (VET): Has been used in ringworm, and noninfectious diseases of the skin.

2254. 6-Chrysenamine. [2642-98-0] 6-Chrysenylamine; 6-aminochrysene; 6-chrysylamine; CP-1001; Chrysenex. $C_{18}H_{13}N$; mol wt 243.30. C 88.86%, H 5.39%, N 5.76%. Prepd by reduction of 6-nitrochrysene: Newman, Cathcart, *J. Org. Chem.* **5,** 620 (1940).

Leaflets from alc, mp 210-211°. Slightly sol in alcohol, benzene, ethyl acetate.

USE: In biochemical research to produce leukopenia.

2255. Chrysene. [218-01-9] 1,2-Benzphenanthrene. $C_{18}H_{12}$; mol wt 228.29. C 94.70%, H 5.30%. Occurs in coal tar, *q.v.* Is formed during distillation of coal, in very small amount during distillation or pyrolysis of many fats and oils. Isoln from coal tar: Liebermann, *Ann.* **158,** 299, 307 (1871). Purification by chromatography: Winterstein, Schön, *Z. Physiol. Chem.* **230,** 146 (1934); Winterstein *et al., ibid.* 158. Synthesis by heating H_2 and acetylene to 800°: Meyer, *Ber.* **45,** 1633 (1912). From cholesterol on heating with palladium charcoal or activated charcoal: Schmid, Zentner, *Monatsh. Chem.* **49,** 96 (1928). Review of toxicology and human exposure: *Toxicological Profile for Polycyclic Aromatic Hydrocarbons* (PB95-264370, 1995) 487 pp.

Orthorhombic bipyramidal plates from benzene. d_4^{20} 1.274. mp 254°. Sublimes easily *in vacuo.* bp 448°. Strong fluorescence under ultraviolet light. Absorption spectrum: Marchlewski, Moroz, *Bull. Soc. Chim. Fr.* [4] **33,** 1406 (1923). Slightly sol in alc, ether, carbon bisulfide, glacial acetic acid. At 25° one gram dissolves in 1300 ml abs alc, 480 ml toluene. About 5% is sol in toluene at 100°. Moderately sol in boiling benzene. Insol in water. Slightly sol in cold organic solvents, but fairly sol in these solvents when hot, including glacial acetic acid.

2256. Chrysin. [480-40-0] 5,7-Dihydroxy-2-phenyl-4*H*-1-benzopyran-4-one; 5,7-dihydroxyflavone; chrysidenon 1438. C_{15}-$H_{10}O_4$; mol wt 254.24. C 70.86%, H 3.96%, O 25.17%. From heartwood of *Pinus monticola* Dougl., *P. excelsa* Wall., and *P. aristata* Engelm., *Pinaceae:* Linstedt, *Acta Chem. Scand.* **3,** 1147, 1375 (1949); **4,** 55 (1950); from bark of *Dolichandrone falcata* Seem., *Bisnomiaceae:* Kincl, *Naturwissenschaften* **42,** 646 (1955). Synthesis: Seka, Prosche, *Monatsh. Chem.* **69,** 284 (1936); Hutchins, Wheeler, *J. Chem. Soc.* **1939,** 91; Teoule *et al., Bull. Soc. Chim. Fr.* **1961,** 546.

Light yellow prisms from methanol, mp 285°. uv max: 270, 329 nm (log ε 4.40, 3.90). Practically insol in water; sol in alkali hydroxide solns; slightly sol in alcohol, chloroform, ether.

Diacetoxychrysin. $C_{19}H_{14}O_6$. Crystals from ethanol, mp 194-195°.

Methylchrysin. Tectochrysin. $C_{16}H_{12}O_4$. It is present as such or in the form of a glucoside in buds of *Populus* spp., *Salicaceae.* Use of tectochrysin as diuretic: Perrault, US 3155579 (1964 to Laroche Navarron). Yellow needles, mp 163°. Sol in alcohol, benzene, chloroform.

2257. Chrysoidine. [532-82-1] 4-(Phenylazo)-1,3-benzenediamine monohydrochloride; 4-phenylazo-*m*-phenylenediamine hydrochloride; 2,4-diaminoazobenzene hydrochloride; chrysoidine orange; chrysoidine Y; C.I. 11270; C.I. Basic Orange 2. $C_{12}H_{13}ClN_4$; mol wt 248.71. C 57.95%, H 5.27%, Cl 14.25%, N 22.53%. Prepn: Hofmann, *Ber.* **10,** 213 (1877); Maximoff, US 2053095 (1935 to Azodal Co.). Prepn of salt: DE 562392 (1933 to Chem.-Pharm. Fabrik Hubold & Bartsch). *See also Colour Index* vol. 4 (3rd ed., 1971) p 4019; *H. J. Conn's Biological Stains,* R. D. Lillie, Ed. (Williams & Wilkins, Baltimore, 9th ed., 1977) p 87.

Reddish-brown crystalline powder, mp 118-118.5°. Solubility at 15°: water 5.5%; abs ethanol 4.75%; cellosolve 6.0%; anhydr ethylene glycol 9.5%; xylene 0.005%; slightly sol in acetone. Practically insol in benzene. Gives yellow soln in concd H_2SO_4, orange soln in dil H_2SO_4 and in HNO_3.

Citrate. [5909-04-6] 4-Phenylazo-*m*-phenylenediamine hydrochloride citrate; 2,4-diaminoazobenzene hydrochloride citrate; Azoangin; Azohel. $C_{12}H_{13}ClN_4 \cdot C_6H_8O_7$; mol wt 440.83. Sol in water (up to 4%), alcohol.

Free base. [495-54-5] C.I. Solvent Orange 3. $C_{12}H_{12}N_4$.

USE: Dyeing silk and cotton. Biological stain.

THERAP CAT: Citrate as antiseptic.

2258. Chrysophanic Acid. [481-74-3] 1,8-Dihydroxy-3-methyl-9,10-anthracenedione; 1,8-dihydroxy-3-methylanthraquinone; 3-methylchrysazin; chrysophanol. $C_{15}H_{10}O_4$; mol wt 254.24. C 70.86%, H 3.96%, O 25.17%. Occurs in the free state and as glucoside in cascara sagrada, senna and various species of *Rumex* and *Rheum* (rhubarb). Isoln from rhubarb root: Tutin, Clewer, *J. Chem. Soc.* **99,** 946 (1911); Siesto, Bartoli, *Farmaco Ed. Prat.* **12,** 517 (1957); Carelli, Giuliano, *ibid.* 184; from *Penicillium islandicum* Sopp.: Howard, Raistrick, *Biochem. J.* **46,** 49 (1950); from *Chaetonium affine* Corda: Arkley *et al., Croat. Chem. Acta* **29,** 141 (1957), *C.A.* **53,** 1287h (1959). Synthesis: Eder, Widmer, *Helv. Chim. Acta* **5,** 3 (1922); **6,** 419 (1923); Ayyangar *et al., J. Sci. Ind. Res.* **20B,** 493 (1961). Total synthesis: M. E. Jung, J. A. Lowe, *Chem. Commun.* **1978,** 95.

Hexagonal or monoclinic crystals from alcohol or benzene, mp 196°. Sublimes. Absorption max: 226, 256, 278, 288, 436 nm (ε × 10^{-3} 41, 28, 14, 14, 11.8). Practically insol in water. Slightly sol in cold, freely in boiling alc; sol in benzene, chloroform, ether, glacial acetic acid, acetone, solns of alkali hydrides, and in hot solns of alkali carbonates; very slightly sol in petr ether.

Glucoside. Chrysophanein; chrysophaniin. $C_{21}H_{20}O_9$. Fine yellow needles from alc, mp 248-249°. Slightly sol in hot water; sol in pyridine. Practically insol in cold water, chloroform, ether.

2259. Chymopapain. [9001-09-6] BAX-1526; Chymodiactin; Discase. Proteolytic enzyme which is the major component of the crude latex of *Carica papaya, Caricaceae.* A sulfhydryl enzyme similar to papain, *q.v.,* with respect to substrate specificities, but differing in electrophoretic mobility, stability and solubility. Original crystallization and partial characterization: Jansen, Balls, *J. Biol. Chem.* **137**, 459 (1941); *eidem*, US 2313875 (1943). Consists of four components, two of which have molecular wts of about 35,000 and have been isolated and studied. Chymopapain A: Erbata, Yasunobu, *J. Biol. Chem.* **237**, 1086 (1962); chymopapain B: Kunimitsu, Yasunobu, *Biochim. Biophys. Acta* **139**, 405 (1966); Isunoda, Yasunobu, *J. Biol. Chem.* **241**, 4610 (1966). Purification: Stern, US 3558433 (1971 to Baxter Labs.). Specificity studies: Ebata, Takahashi, *Biochim. Biophys. Acta* **118**, 201 (1966). *Reviews:* Kunimitsu, Yasunobu, *Methods Enzymol.* **19**, 244-252 (1970); Glazer, Smith, *The Enzymes* vol. III, P. D. Boyer, Ed. (Academic Press, New York, 3rd ed., 1971) pp 537-538. Review of use in herniated disk treatment: M. J. David, *J. Am. Med. Assoc.* **243**, 2043 (1980).

Powder, more sol in aq soln than papain. Extremely stable at pHs as low as 1.8 and sol in satd NaCl above pH 3. Most active at pHs 2.5 to 4.0. uv max (pH 7): 280 nm ($A_{1cm}^{1\%}$ 18.7 (A); 18.4 (B)). The ratio of milk-clotting to proteolytic activity is twice that of papain although the clotting capacities are the same.

USE: In meat tenderizer.

THERAP CAT: Proteolytic enzyme (used in chemonucleolysis).

2260. Chymotrypsins. Avazyme; Catarase; Chymetin; Chymolase; Kymo-trypure; Quimoral; Quimotrase; Zolyse. A group of major proteolytic enzymes in the pancreatic juice. Produced in the form of inactive chymotrypsinogen by the acinous cells of pancreas, and carried as such by the pancreatic juice into the duodenum where they are activated by trypsin. They split secondary amide or peptide bonds, carboxylic or phenolic ester bonds and even carbon-carbon bonds. Their main function is to hydrolyze peptide bonds during the intestinal digestion of proteins. Cattle pancreatic juice contains nearly equal quantities of two chymotrypsinogens: A which is cationic at pH 8 and B which is anionic. Chymotrypsinogen A is converted by trypsin into π-chymotrypsin. In the presence of large amounts of trypsin, π-chymotrypsin is degraded to δ-chymotrypsin. In the presence of small amounts of trypsin, π-chymotrypsin is autolyzed to α-chymotrypsin. After long standing α-chymotrypsin gives rise to β- and γ-chymotrypsin which differ from it in their crystal habits. Prepn of π- and δ-chymotrypsins: Bettelheim, Neurath, *J. Biol. Chem.* **212**, 241 (1955). Prepn of α-, β-, γ- and δ-chymotrypsins (and chymotrypsin B): Laskowski, *Methods Enzymol.* **2**, 8 (1955). Amino acid sequence of chymotrypsinogen A: Hartley, *Nature* **201**, 1284 (1964); Melorin *et al., Biochim. Biophys. Acta* **130**, 543 (1966); of chymotrypsinogen B: Hartley *et al., Nature* **207**, 1157 (1965); Smillie *et al., ibid.* **218**, 343 (1968). *Reviews:* Bender *et al., J. Polym. Sci.* **49**, 75 (1961); Desnuelle, *The Enzymes* vol. 4, P. D. Boyer *et al.,* Eds. (Academic Press, New York, 2nd ed., 1960) pp 93-118; Kraut; Blow; Hess, *ibid.* vol. 3 (3rd ed., 1971) pp 165, 185, 213.

α-Chymotrypsin. [9004-07-3] Alpha-Chymocutan; Chymotase (tabl.); Chymozym; Impral; Kimopsin; Kimoral. Arrangement of molecules in monoclinic crystal form: Blow *et al., J. Mol. Biol.* **8**, 65 (1964). Structure: Matthews *et al., Nature* **214**, 652 (1967); Blow *et al., ibid.* **221**, 337 (1969). *Review:* Niemann, *Science* **143**, 1287 (1964).

THERAP CAT: Enzyme (proteolytic).

THERAP CAT (VET): Topically for enzymatic debridement.

2261. Ciafos. [2636-26-2] Phosphorothioic acid *O*-(4-cyanophenyl) *O,O*-dimethyl ester; phosphorothioic acid *O,O*-dimethyl ester, *O*-ester with *p*-hydroxybenzonitrile; *O,O*-dimethyl *O*-(4-cyanophenyl) phosphorothioate; *O,O*-dimethyl *O*-(4-cyanophenyl) thionophosphate; cyanophos; Bay 34727; S-4084; Sumitomo S-4084; Cyanox. $C_9H_{10}NO_3PS$; mol wt 243.22. C 44.44%, H 4.14%, N 5.76%, O 19.73%, P 12.73%, S 13.18%. Prepn: Nishizawa, Mizutani, JP 62 18184; Kuramoto *et al.,* US 3150040 (1962, 1964 both to Sumitomo); Sakamoto, Nishizawa, *Agric. Biol. Chem.* **26**, 252 (1962); D. N. Bernhart, DE 2162344; *idem*, US 3792132 (1972, 1974 to Stauffer). Pharmacology and metabolism: H. Yamamoto *et al., Oyo Yakuri* **5**, 75 (1971), *C.A.* **76**, 68907a (1972); Wakimura, Miyamoto, *Agric. Biol. Chem.* **35**, 410 (1971). Evaluation as an insecticide: Nishiyawa *et al., ibid.* **25**, 597 (1961); Tamura *et al., ibid.* 773. Evaluation of neurotoxicity: H. Ohkawa *et al., Biochem. Pharmacol.* **29**, 2721 (1980).

Yellow to reddish-yellow transparent liquid. $bp_{0.09}$ 119-120° (dec). mp 14-15°. $n_D^{32.5}$ 1.5404. Very sol in methanol, ethanol, acetone, chloroform. Sparingly sol in *n*-hexane, kerosene; slightly sol in water. Rapidly dec under alkaline conditions and upon exposure to light, *Jpn. Med. Gaz.* **11**(7), 7 (1974). LD_{50} in mice (mg/kg): 1000 orally; 880 i.p. (Yamamoto).

Caution: Cholinesterase inhibitor.

USE: Insecticide.

2262. Cichoriin. [531-58-8] 7-(β-D-Glucopyranosyloxy)-6-hydroxy-2*H*-1-benzopyran-2-one; 6,7-dihydroxycoumarin-7-glucoside. $C_{15}H_{16}O_9$; mol wt 340.28. C 52.94%, H 4.74%, O 42.32%. Isomeric with esculin. In flowers of the chicory plant *(Cichorium intybus* L., *Compositae)*. Extraction procedure: Merz, *Arch. Pharm.* **270**, 476 (1932). Synthesis: Head, Robertson, *J. Chem. Soc.* **1939**, 1266; also Merz, *loc. cit.* *Review:* Sethna, Shah, *Chem. Rev.* **36**, 1 (1945).

Needles with $2H_2O$, mp 213-215° (after drying in desiccator). $[\alpha]_D^{18}$ −105° (c = 3 in 50% dioxane). Sol in hot water, alc, glacial acetic acid. Insol in ether, petr ether. Sol in dil alkalies with yellow color, but no fluorescence (difference from esculin). Absorption spectrum of soln: Merz, *loc. cit.*

2263. Ciclesonide. [126544-47-6] (11β,16α)-16,17-[[(*R*)-Cyclohexylmethylene]bis(oxy)]-11-hydroxy-21-(2-methyl-1-oxopropoxy)pregna-1,4-diene-3,20-dione; BY-9010; Alvesco. $C_{32}H_{44}$-O_7; mol wt 540.69. C 71.08%, H 8.20%, O 20.71%. Inhaled corticosteroid. Prodrug converted to the active metabolite, *ciclesonide-active principle*, in the lung. Prepn: J. Calatayud *et al.,* DE 4129535; *eidem*, US 5482934 (1992, 1996 both to Elmu). Pharmacokinetics and pharmacodynamics: S. Rohatagi *et al., J. Clin. Pharmacol.* **43**, 365 (2003). Clinical evaluation in asthma: D. A. Taylor *et al., Am. J. Respir. Crit. Care Med.* **160**, 237 (1999); in allergic rhinitis: B. M. W. Schmidt *et al., J. Clin. Pharmacol.* **39**, 1062 (1999). Review of clinical experience: G. Dent, *Curr. Opin. Invest. Drugs* **3**, 78-83 (2002).

THERAP CAT: Glucocorticoid.

2264. Cicletanine. [89943-82-8] 3-(4-Chlorophenyl)-1,3-dihydro-6-methylfuro[3,4-*c*]pyridin-7-ol; 1,3-dihydro-3-(4-chlorophenyl)-7-hydroxy-6-methylfuro[3,4-*c*]pyridine; cicletanide; cycletanide. $C_{14}H_{12}ClNO_2$; mol wt 261.70. C 64.25%, H 4.62%, Cl 13.55%, N 5.35%, O 12.23%. Furopyridine derivative with antihypertensive and diuretic properties. Prepn: A. Esanu, BE 891797; *idem*, US 4383998 (1982, 1983 both to Soc. Conseils Recher. Sci.). Studies on mechanism of action: P. Braquet *et al.,*

Lancet **1**, 1218 (1983); G. R. Elliott et al., Thromb. Res. **33**, 549 (1984). Cardiovascular pharmacology in dogs: R. Jouve et al., J. Cardiovasc. Pharmacol. **8**, 208 (1986). In vitro comparison of antihistaminic activity of isomers: P. Schoeffter et al., Eur. J. Pharmacol. **136**, 235 (1987). HPLC determn in biological fluids: G. Cuisinaud et al., J. Chromatogr. **341**, 97 (1985). Effect on human prostaglandin metabolism: P. Guinot, J. C. Frölich, Arzneim.-Forsch. **35**, 1714 (1985). Effect on potassium ion transport in hypertensive patients: R. Garay et al., J. Hypertens. **4**, Suppl. 5, S208 (1986). Pharmacokinetics in humans: J. M. Lize et al., Therapie **42**, 399 (1987).

Hydrochloride. [82747-56-6] BN-1270; Coverine; Justar; Secletan; Tenstaten. $C_{14}H_{12}ClNO_2.HCl$; mol wt 298.16. White crystals, mp 219-228°. Insol in water.

THERAP CAT: Antihypertensive.

2265. Ciclonicate. [53449-58-4] 3-Pyridinecarboxylic acid 3,3,5-trimethylcyclohexyl ester; trans-3,3,5-trimethylcyclohexyl nicotinate; cyclonicate; P-350; Bled. $C_{15}H_{21}NO_2$; mol wt 247.33. C 72.84%, H 8.56%, N 5.66%, O 12.94%. Deriv of nicotinic acid, q.v. Prepn: K. Matsuda et al., **DE 1910481** (1969 to Takeda), C.A. **72**, 12769g (1970); G. Massaroli, **DE 2406849** (1974 to Poli), C.A. **82**, 4129 (1975). Chromatographic study: G. Sekules et al., Boll. Chim. Farm. **119**, 521 (1980). Antilipolytic activity in rats: D. Faini et al., Farmaco Ed. Prat. **36**, 478 (1981). In vitro effect on lipolysis: F. Tessari et al., Farmaco Ed. Sci. **36**, 1029 (1981). Clinical study: C. Fossati, Gazz. Med. Ital. **139**, 43 (1980).

Liq, $bp_{0.6}$ 127-128°.

THERAP CAT: Vasodilator.

2266. Ciclopirox. [29342-05-0] 6-Cyclohexyl-1-hydroxy-4-methyl-2(1H)-pyridinone. $C_{12}H_{17}NO_2$; mol wt 207.27. C 69.54%, H 8.27%, N 6.76%, O 15.44%. Broad spectrum antimycotic agent with some antibacterial activity. Prepn: G. Lohaus, W. Dittmar, **ZA 6906039**; eidem, **US 3883545** (1970, 1975 both to Hoechst). In vitro study: eidem, Arzneim.-Forsch. **23**, 670 (1973). Series of articles on pharmacokinetics, pharmacology, teratology, toxicity studies: Oyo Yakuri **9**, 57-115 (1975), C.A. **83**, 53159d, 53538b, 53539c, 71844c, 90833q (1975). Series of articles on chemistry, mechanism of action, toxicology, clinical trials: Arzneim.-Forsch. **31**, 1309-1386 (1981). Toxicity data: H. G. Alpermann, E. Schutz, ibid. 1328. Review: S. G. Jue et al., Drugs **29**, 330-341 (1985). Review of clinical experience in seborrheic dermatitis: A. Starova, R. Aly, Expert Opin. Drug Saf. **4**, 235-239 (2005).

Solid, mp 144°.

Ethanolamine salt (1:1). [41621-49-2] Ciclopirox olamine; HOE-296; Batrafen; Brumixol; Ciclochem; Dafnegin; Loprox; Mi-

coxolamina; Mycoster. $C_{14}H_{24}N_2O_3$; mol wt 268.35. LD_{50} in mice, rats (mg/kg): 2898, 3290 orally (Alpermann, Schutz).

THERAP CAT: Antifungal.

2267. Cicutoxin. [505-75-9] (8E,10E,12E,14R)-8,10,12-Heptadecatriene-4,6-diyne-1,14-diol. $C_{17}H_{22}O_2$; mol wt 258.36. C 79.03%, H 8.58%, O 12.39%. Poisonous principle of the water hemlock (Cicuta virosa L., Umbelliferae); naturally occurring as the (−)-form. Isoln: Jacobson, J. Am. Chem. Soc. **37**, 916 (1915). Structure: Anet et al., J. Chem. Soc. **1953**, 309. Synthesis of (±)-form: Hill et al., ibid. **1955**, 1770. Antileukemic activity: T. Konoshima, K.-H. Lee, J. Nat. Prod. **49**, 1117 (1986). Simple analytical method: R. A. Smith, D. Lewis, Vet. Hum. Toxicol. **29**, 240 (1987).

Prisms from ether + petr ether, transformed in air and light to yellow oily resin. mp 54°. $[\alpha]_D^{15}$ −14.5° (c = 1.7 in ethanol). Sol in alc, chloroform, ether, hot water, alkali hydroxides. Practically insol in petr ether. Very toxic.

(±)-Form. Crystals from ether + petr ether, mp 67°. uv max (alc): 242, 252, 318.5, 335.5 nm ($\varepsilon \times 10^{-3}$ 14.6, 21.6, 50.6, 60.3).

2268. Cidofovir. [113852-37-2] [[(1S)-2-(4-Amino-2-oxo-1(2H)-pyrimidinyl)-1-(hydroxymethyl)ethoxy]methyl]phosphonic acid; (S)-1-[3-hydroxy-2-(phosphonylmethoxy)propyl]cytosine; (S)-HPMPC; GS-504; Vistide. $C_8H_{14}N_3O_6P$; mol wt 279.19. C 34.42%, H 5.05%, N 15.05%, O 34.38%, P 11.09%. DNA synthesis inhibitor. Prepn: A. Holy et al., **EP 253412**; eidem, **US 5142051** (1988, 1992 both to Ceskoslov. Akad. Ved; Rega Inst.); and activity vs cytomegalovirus: R. Snoeck et al., Antimicrob. Agents Chemother. **32**, 1839 (1988). Syntheses: J. J. Bronson et al., Nucleosides Nucleotides **9**, 745 (1990); P. R. Brodfuehrer et al., Tetrahedron Lett. **35**, 3243 (1994). Activity vs herpes simplex virus: G. Andrei et al., Eur. J. Clin. Microbiol. Infect. Dis. **11**, 143 (1992). Review of pharmacology and clinical studies: M. J. M. Hitchcock et al., Antiviral Chem. Chemother. **7**, 115-127 (1996). Review of clinical potential in poxvirus infections: E. De Clercq, Trends Pharmacol. Sci. **23**, 456-458 (2002).

Fluffy white powder, mp 260° (dec). $[\alpha]_D^{20}$ −97.3° (c = 0.80 in water). Monohydrate, uv max (pH 2): 279 nm (ε 13000).

THERAP CAT: Antiviral.

2269. Cifenline. [53267-01-9] 2-(2,2-Diphenylcyclopropyl)-4,5-dihydro-1H-imidazole; (±)-2-(2,2-diphenylcyclopropyl)-2-imidazoline; 1-(2-Δ²-imidazolinyl)-2,2-diphenylcyclopropane; cibenzoline; Ro-22-7796; UP-33-901. $C_{18}H_{18}N_2$; mol wt 262.35. C 82.41%, H 6.92%, N 10.68%. Prepn: **BE 807630**; J. C. Cognaco, **US 3903104** (1974, 1975 both to Hexachemie). Activity and tolerance: D. Herpin et al., Acta Cardiol. **36**, 131 (1981). Electrophysiological effects in man: J. F. Thizy et al., Lyon Med. **245**, 119 (1981). Clinical trial: D. Herpin et al., Curr. Ther. Res. **30**, 742 (1981).

Crystals from petr ether, mp 103-104°. LD_{100} in rats (mg/kg): 64 i.v. (Cognaco).

Succinate. [100678-32-8] Cibenol; Cipralan; Exacor. $C_{18}H_{18}$-$N_2.C_4H_6O_4$; mol wt 380.44. Crystals from ethanol + ether, mp 165°.

THERAP CAT: Antiarrhythmic.

2270. Ciguatoxins. CTX. Potent sodium channel activators found in a wide variety of fish, the toxins were ultimately traced to a dinoflagellate *Gambierdiscus spp.* Family of lipid soluble polyether toxins responsible for ciguatera food poisoning; structural variations are associated with the oceanic region from which the dinoflagellate originates. Isoln from eels: P. J. Scheuer *et al., Science* **155**, 1267 (1967). Purification from dinoflagellate: R. Bagnis *et al., Rev. Int. Oceanogr. Med.* **45-46**, 29 (1977). Structure: M. Murata *et al., J. Am. Chem. Soc.* **112**, 4380 (1990). Purification and characterization of 3 major forms CTX 1-3: R. J. Lewis *et al., Toxicon* **29**, 1115 (1991); absolute configuration: M. Satake *et al., J. Am. Chem. Soc.* **119**, 11325 (1997). Isoln and characterization of Pacific CTX: R. J. Lewis, A. Jones, *Toxicon* **35**, 159 (1997); of Caribbean CTX: J.-P. Vernoux, R. J. Lewis, *ibid.* **889**; of Indian CTX: B. Hamilton *et al., ibid.* **40**, 685 (2002). Effect on sodium channels: J.-N. Bidard *et al., J. Biol. Chem.* **259**, 8353 (1984); E. Benoit *et al., Neuroscience* **71**, 1121 (1996). Review of use as research tool: J. Molgo *et al., Methods Neurosci.* **8**, 149-164 (1992); of mechanism of action: C. Frelin *et al., ACS Symp. Ser.* **418**, 192-199 (1996); of neurobiological actions: C. Mattei *et al., J. Soc. Biol.* **193**, 329-344 (1999).

CIGUATOXIN 1

CTX-1. [11050-21-8] $C_{60}H_{86}O_{19}$; mol wt 1111.31. White solid. LD_{50} i.p. in mice: 0.25 μg/kg (Lewis 1991).

CTX-2. [142185-85-1] $C_{60}H_{86}O_{18}$; mol wt 1095.31. White amorphous solid. LD_{50} i.p. in mice: 2.3 μg/kg (Lewis 1991).

CTX-3. [139341-09-6] $C_{60}H_{86}O_{18}$; mol wt 1095.31. Total synthesis: M. Inoue, M. Hirama, *Synlett.* **2004**, 577. White amorphous solid. LD_{50} i.p. in mice: 0.9 μg/kg (Lewis 1991).

2271. Cilansetron. [120635-74-7] (10*R*)-5,6,9,10-Tetrahydro-10-[(2-methyl-1*H*-imidazol-1-yl)methyl]-4*H*-pyrido[3,2,1-jk]carbazol-11(8*H*)-one; *l*-10[(2-methyl-1*H*-imidazol-1-yl)methyl]-5,6,8,9,10,11-hexahydro-4*H*-pyrido[3,2,1-jk]carbazol-11-one; KC-9946. $C_{20}H_{21}N_3O$; mol wt 319.40. C 75.21%, H 6.63%, N 13.16%, O 5.01%. Serotonin 5-HT$_3$ receptor antagonist. Prepn: H. H. Haeck *et al., EP 297651; eidem, US 4939136* (1989, 1990 both to Duphar Int. Res.); I. van Wijngaarden *et al., J. Med. Chem.* **36**, 3693 (1993). Absolute configuration studies: P. G. Jones *et al., Acta Crystallogr.* **E59**, o38, o41 (2003). Pharmacology: A. Botella *et al., Fundam. Clin. Pharmacol.* **12**, 619 (1998). Mechanism of action study: K. Hillsley *et al., Neurosci. Lett.* **278**, 137 (2000). Clinical pharmacology: G. Stacher *et al., Br. J. Clin. Pharmacol.* **49**, 429 (2000). Review of development and therapeutic potential: *idem, Curr. Opin. Invest. Drugs* **2**, 1432-1436 (2001); of clinical experience: W. D. Chey, B. D. Cash, *Expert Opin. Invest. Drugs* **14**, 185-193 (2005).

Hydrochloride. [120635-72-5]; [209859-87-0] (monohydrate). Calmactin. $C_{20}H_{21}N_3O.HCl$; mol wt 355.86. Crystals, mp 226-228°. $[α]_D^5$ −5.0° (c = 1.8 in methanol).

THERAP CAT: In treatment of irritable bowel syndrome.

2272. Cilastatin. [82009-34-5] (2*Z*)-7-[[(2*R*)-2-Amino-2-carboxyethyl]thio]-2-[[[(1*S*)-2,2-dimethylcyclopropyl]carbonyl]-amino]-2-heptenoic acid; MK-791. $C_{16}H_{26}N_2O_5S$; mol wt 358.45. C 53.61%, H 7.31%, N 7.82%, O 22.32%, S 8.95%. Prevents renal metabolism of penem and carbapenem antibiotics by specific and reversible dehydropeptidase I inhibition. Synthesis and combination with thienamycins: D. W. Graham *et al., EP 48301;* H. Kropp *et al., EP 48025* (both 1982 to Merck & Co.), *C.A.* **97**, 145271b, 145270a (1982). Combination with penems: F. M. Kahan, H. Kropp, *EP 72014* (1983 to Merck & Co.), *C.A.* **99**, 70272h (1983). The articles cited below discuss the activity of cilastatin alone and in combination with imipenem, *q.v.* Dipeptidase inhibition, pharmacokinetics: S. R. Norrby *et al., Antimicrob. Agents Chemother.* **23**, 300 (1983). Stimulation of granulocyte function: H. Gnarpe *et al., ibid.* **25**, 179 (1984). HPLC determn in serum: C. M. Myers, J. L. Blumer, *ibid.* **26**, 78 (1984). Enhances intrathecal and ocular penetration of imipenem: A. W. Chow *et al., ibid.* **23**, 634 (1983) and K. R. Finlay *et al., Invest. Ophthalmol. Visual Sci.* **24**, 1147 (1983), respectively. In experimental meningitis: D. E. Washburn *et al., J. Antimicrob. Chemother.* **12**, 39 (1983). Series of articles on pharmacokinetics, safety and tolerance and efficacy of cilastatin/imipenem: *ibid.* **12**, Suppl. D, 1-155 (1983); *Infection* **14**, Suppl. 2, S111-S180 (1986).

Sodium salt. [81129-83-1] Cilastatin sodium. $C_{16}H_{25}N_2$-NaO$_5$S. Off-white to yellowish-white hygroscopic, amorphous solid. pKa$_1$ 2.0; pKa$_2$ 4.4; pKa$_3$ 9.2. Very sol in water, methanol.

THERAP CAT: Antibacterial adjunct (dipeptidase inhibitor).

2273. Cilazapril. [88768-40-5] (1*S*,9*S*)-9-[[(1*S*)-1-(Ethoxy-carbonyl)-3-phenylpropyl]amino]octahydro-10-oxo-6*H*-pyridazino[1,2-*a*][1,2]diazepine-1-carboxylic acid; (1*S*,9*S*)-9-[[(*S*)-1-carboxy-3-phenylpropyl]amino]octahydro-10-oxo-6*H*-pyridazino[1,2-*a*][1,2]diazepine-1-carboxylic acid 9-ethyl ester; Ro-31-2848; Dynorm. $C_{22}H_{31}N_3O_5$; mol wt 417.50. C 63.29%, H 7.48%, N 10.06%, O 19.16%. Angiotensin-converting enzyme (ACE) inhibitor; hydrolyzed *in vivo* to the active diacid metabolite. Prepn: M. R. Attwood *et al., DE 3317290; eidem, US 4512924* (1983, 1985 both to Hoffmann-La Roche); *eidem, J. Chem. Soc. Perkin Trans. 1* **1986**, 1011. HPLC determn in urine and pharmaceutical formulations: J. A. Prieto *et al., J. Chromatogr. B* **714**, 285 (1998). Pharmacology: I. L. Natoff *et al., J. Cardiovasc. Pharmacol.* **7**, 569 (1985). Review of clinical pharmacology: C. H. Kleinbloesem *et al., Am. J. Med.* **87**, Suppl. 6B, 45S-49S (1989). Review of clinical experience in hypertension: T. Szucs, *Drugs* **41**, Suppl. 1, 18-24 (1991); in chronic heart failure: L. Dössegger *et al., J. Cardiovasc. Pharmacol.* **24**, Suppl. 3, S38-S41 (1994); in combination with hydrochlorothiazide: R. C. Pordy, *Cardiology* **86**, 41-48 (1995).

Monohydrate. [92077-78-6] Inhibace; Initiss; Justor; Vascace. $C_{22}H_{31}N_3O_5 \cdot H_2O$; mol wt 435.51. White to off-white crystalline powder, mp 98° (dec). $[\alpha]_D^{20}$ −62.51° (c = 1% in ethanol). Soly in water (25°): 0.5 g/100 ml. pKa$_1$ 3.3; pKa$_2$ 6.4. Partition coefficient (octanol/pH 7.4 buffer, 22°): 0.8.

Diacid. [90139-06-3] Cilazaprilat; Ro-31-3113. $C_{20}H_{27}N_3O_5$; mol wt 389.45. Crystals from water, mp 242°. $[\alpha]_D^{20}$ −74.7° (c = 0.5 in 1M NaOH).

THERAP CAT: Antihypertensive.

2274. Ciliary Neurotrophic Factor. CNTF. Neurotrophic factor unrelated to the neurotrophins, *q.v.* Cytosolic peptide produced by Schwann cells in the peripheral nervous system and by astrocytes in the CNS; not expressed by target tissues. Promotes survival of a broad range of neurons and enhances differentiation of neurons and astrocytes. Initial identification as *in vitro* survival factor for chick ciliary neurons: R. Adler *et al., Science* **204,** 1434 (1979). Purification from chick eye: G. Barbin *et al., J. Neurochem.* **43,** 1468 (1984); from rat sciatic nerve: M. Manthorpe *et al., Brain Res.* **367,** 282 (1986). Molecular cloning of rat CNTF: K. A. Stöckli *et al., Nature* **342,** 920 (1989); of rabbit CNTF: L.-F. H. Lin *et al., Science* **246,** 1023 (1989); of human CNTF: A. Lam *et al., Gene* **102,** 271 (1991); A. Negro *et al., Eur. J. Biochem.* **201,** 289 (1991). Effect on motoneuron survival and proposed role as a "lesion factor" released in pathophysiological conditions: M. Sendtner *et al., J. Cell Sci.* **Suppl. 15,** 103 (1991). Review of bioactivity and structural relationship with hematopoietic cytokines: N. Y. Ip, G. D. Yancopoulos, *Prog. Growth Factor Res.* **4,** 139-155 (1992). Review of CNTF receptor: S. Davis, G. D. Yancopoulos, *Curr. Opin. Neurobiol.* **5,** 281-285 (1993). *Review:* M. Manthorpe *et al.* in *Neurotrophic Factors,* S. E. Loughlin, J. H. Fallon, Eds. (Academic Press, San Diego, 1993) pp 443-473.

Human CNTF. [133423-39-9] 200 Amino acid peptide. mol wt ~23,000 Da. pI ~6.0. Exhibits ~83% amino acid homology with rat CNTF; ~87% with rabbit CNTF.

2275. Cilnidipine. [132203-70-4] 1,4-Dihydro-2,6-dimethyl-4-(3-nitrophenyl)-3,5-pyridinedicarboxylic acid 2-methoxyethyl (2E)-3-phenyl-2-propenyl ester; (±)-(E)-cinnamyl 2-methoxyethyl 1,4-dihydro-2,6-dimethyl-4-(m-nitrophenyl)-3,5-pyridinedicarboxylate; FRC-8653; Atelec; Cinalong; Siscard. $C_{27}H_{28}N_2O_7$; mol wt 492.52. C 65.84%, H 5.73%, N 5.69%, O 22.74%. Dihydropyridine calcium channel blocker. Prepn: T. Kutsuma *et al.,* **EP 161877**; *eidem,* **US 4672068** (1985, 1987 both to Fujirebio). Pharmacology: K. Ikeda *et al., Oyo Yakuri* **44,** 433 (1992). Mechanism of action study: M. Hosono *et al., J. Pharmacobio-Dyn.* **15,** 547 (1992). LC-MS determn in plasma: K. Hatada *et al., J. Chromatogr.* **583,** 116 (1992). Clinical study: M. Ishii, *Jpn. Pharmacol. Ther.* **21,** 59 (1993). Acute toxicity study: S. Wada *et al., Yakuri to Chiryo* **20,** Suppl. 7, S1683 (1992), *C.A.* **118,** 32711 (1992).

Crystals from methanol, mp 115.5-116.6°. LD$_{50}$ in male, female mice, rats (mg/kg): ≥5000, ≥5000, ≥5000, 4412 orally; ≥5000 all species s.c.; 1845, 2353, 441, 426 i.p. (Wada).

THERAP CAT: Antihypertensive.

2276. Cilomilast. [153259-65-5] *cis*-4-Cyano-4-[3-(cyclopentyloxy)-4-methoxyphenyl]cyclohexanecarboxylic acid; SB-207499; Ariflo. $C_{20}H_{25}NO_4$; mol wt 343.42. C 69.95%, H 7.34%, N 4.08%, O 18.64%. Selective phosphodiesterase 4 (PDE4) inhibitor. Prepn: S. B. Christensen, **WO 9319749**; *idem,* **US 5552438** (1993, 1996 both to SmithKline Beecham); *idem et al., J. Med. Chem.* **41,** 821 (1998). Anti-inflammatory activity: M. S. Barnette *et al., J. Pharmacol. Exp. Ther.* **284,** 420 (1998); D. E. Griswold *et al., ibid.* 705. Pharmacology and therapeutic potential in asthma and chronic obstructive pulmonary disease (COPD): T. J. Torphy *et al., Pulm. Pharmacol. Ther.* **12,** 131-135 (1999). Clinical

pharmacokinetics and bioavailability: B. D. Zussman *et al., Pharmacotherapy* **21,** 653 (2001). Clinical trial in COPD: C. H. Compton *et al., Lancet* **358,** 265 (2001). Review of pharmacology and clinical experience: M. A. Giembycz, *Expert Opin. Invest. Drugs* **10,** 1361-1379 (2001).

White solid, mp 157°.

THERAP CAT: Antiasthmatic; in treatment of chronic obstructive pulmonary disease.

2277. Cilostazol. [73963-72-1] 6-[4-(1-Cyclohexyl-1H-tetrazol-5-yl)butoxy]-3,4-dihydro-2(1H)-quinolinone; 6-[4-(1-cyclohexyl-1H-tetrazol-5-yl)butoxy]-3,4-dihydrocarbostyril; 6-[4-(1-cyclohexyl-5-tetrazolyl)butoxy]-1,2,3,4-tetrahydro-2-oxoquinoline; OPC-13013; Pletal. $C_{20}H_{27}N_5O_2$; mol wt 369.46. C 65.02%, H 7.37%, N 18.96%, O 8.66%. Phosphodiesterase (PDE III) inhibitor; induces vasodilation and inhibits platelet aggregation. Prepn: **BE 878548**; T. Nishi, K. Nakagawa, **US 4277479** (1979, 1981 both to Otsuka); T. Nishi *et al., Chem. Pharm. Bull.* **31,** 1151 (1983). Physical properties: T. Shimizu *et al., Arzneim.-Forsch.* **35,** 1117 (1985). HPLC determn in plasma: H. Akiyama *et al., J. Chromatogr.* **338,** 456 (1985). Acute toxicity study: G. Nomura *et al., Iyakuhin Kenkyu* **16,** 1200 (1985), *C.A.* **104,** 102207f (1986). Clinical pharmacokinetics: A. Suri *et al., J. Clin. Pharmacol.* **38,** 144 (1998). Clinical evaluation to prevent stent thrombosis: S.-W. Park *et al., Am. J. Cardiol.* **84,** 511 (1999); to prevent restenosis after angioplasty: E. Tsuchikane *et al., Circulation* **100,** 21 (1999). Review of pharmacology and clinical efficacy in intermittent claudication: E. M. Sorkin, A. Markham, *Drugs Aging* **14,** 63-71 (1999).

Colorless needle-like crystals from methanol, mp 159.4-160.3°. uv max (methanol): 257 nm (ε 15200). Freely sol in acetic acid, chloroform, n-methyl-2-pyrrolidone, DMSO. Practically insol in ether, water, 0.1N HCl, 0.1N NaOH. LD$_{50}$ in mice, rats (mg/kg): >2000, >2000 i.p.; >5000, >5000 orally (Nomura).

THERAP CAT: Antithrombotic; in treatment of intermittent claudication.

2278. Cimaterol. [54239-37-1] 2-Amino-5-[1-hydroxy-2-[(1-methylethyl)amino]ethyl]benzonitrile; (±)-5-[1-hydroxy-2-(isopropylamino)ethyl]anthranilonitrile; 1-(4-amino-3-cyanophenyl)-2-isopropylaminoethanol; AB-A-663; CL-263780; AC-263780. $C_{12}H_{17}N_3O$; mol wt 219.28. C 65.73%, H 7.81%, N 19.16%, O 7.30%. β-Adrenergic agonist, related to clenbuterol and mabuterol, *q.q.v.* Prepn: G. Engelhardt *et al., DE 2261914* (1974 to Thomae). Pharmacology: G. Engelhardt, *Arzneim.-Forsch.* **34,** 1625 (1984). Effect on lipid metabolism in sheep: C. Y. Hu *et al., J. Anim. Sci.* **66,** 1393 (1988). Efficacy as a repartitioning agent in livestock: R. W. Jones *et al., ibid.* **61,** 905 (1985); D. H. Beermann *et al., ibid.* **62,** 370 (1986). *Review:* M. Lafontan *et al., Reprod. Nutr. Dev.* **28,** 61-84 (1988).

Crystals, mp 159-161°.

THERAP CAT (VET): Repartitioning agent.

2279. Cimetidine. [51481-61-9] N-Cyano-N'-methyl-N''-[2-[[(5-methyl-1H-imidazol-4-yl)methyl]thio]ethyl]guanidine; SKF-92334; Acibilin; Acinil; Cimal; Cimetag; Cimetum; Edalene; Dyspamet; Eureceptor; Gastromet; Peptol; Stomédine; Tagamet; Tametin; Tratul; Ulcedin; Ulcedine; Ulcerfen; Ulcimet; Ulcofalk; Ulcomedina; Ulcomet; Ulhys. $C_{10}H_{16}N_6S$; mol wt 252.34. C 47.60%, H 6.39%, N 33.30%, S 12.71%. Competitive histamine H_2-receptor antagonist which inhibits gastric acid secretion and reduces pepsin output. Prepn: G. J. Durant et al., **BE 804144**; eidem, **US 3950333** (1974, 1976 both to SK&F); P. Kairisalo, E. Honkanen, Arch. Pharm. **316**, 688 (1983). Chemistry, pharmacology and toxicology: R. W. Brimblecombe et al., J. Int. Med. Res. **3**, 86 (1975); eidem, Br. J. Pharmacol. **53**, 435p (1975). Use in combination with other drugs for cancer treatment: R. D. Thornes et al., Lancet **2**, 328 (1982); S. Borgström et al., N. Engl. J. Med. **307**, 1080 (1982); **308**, 591 (1983). Controlled clinical study in treatment of acute upper gastrointestinal tract bleeding: D. Barer et al., ibid. 1571; for prevention of recurrent duodenal ulcer: S. Sontag et al., ibid. **311**, 689 (1984). Immunoregulatory effect: J. L. Jorizzo et al., Ann. Intern. Med. **92**, 192 (1980); W. B. White, M. Ballow, N. Engl. J. Med. **312**, 198 (1985). Review of effect on endocrine secretion: C. Scarpignato, G. Bertaccini, Drugs Exp. Clin. Res. **5**(4-5), 129-140 (1979). Symposium on clinical efficacy, cytoprotection and antifibrinolytic effects: Scand. J. Gastroenterol. **21**, Suppl. 121, 1-62 (1986).

Crystals, mp 141-143°. Soly in water at 37°: 1.14%. Soly increased by dil HCl. LD_{50} in mice, rats (mg/kg): 2600, 5000 orally; 150, 106 i.v.; 470, 650 i.p. (Brimblecombe).

Hydrochloride. [70059-30-2] Aciloc; Biomag; Brumetidina; Notul. $C_{10}H_{16}N_6S$.HCl; mol wt 288.80.

THERAP CAT: Antiulcerative.

2280. Cimetropium Bromide. [51598-60-8] (1α,2β,4β,5α,-7β)-9-(Cyclopropylmethyl)-7-[(2S)-3-hydroxy-1-oxo-2-phenyl-propoxy]-9-methyl-3-oxa-9-azoniatricyclo[3.3.1.0^{2,4}]nonane bromide; 8-(cyclopropylmethyl)-6β,7β-epoxy-3α-hydroxy-1αH,5αH-tropanium bromide (−)-(S)-tropate; N-cyclopropylmethyl-scopolamine bromide; DA-3177; Alginor. $C_{21}H_{28}BrNO_4$; mol wt 438.36. C 57.54%, H 6.44%, Br 18.23%, N 3.20%, O 14.60%. Spasmolytic agent with affinity for intestinal muscarinic receptors. Prepn: S. Casadio, A. Donetti, **DE 2316728**; eidem, **US 3853886** (1973, 1974 both to De Angeli). Crystal and molecular structure: G. Giuseppetti et al., Farmaco Ed. Sci. **35**, 231 (1980). Molecular conformation in solution: A. Gallazzi et al., ibid. 913. Pharmacology: A. Schiavone et al., Arzneim.-Forsch. **35**, 796 (1985); C. Scarpignato, G. Bianchi Porro, Int. J. Clin. Pharmacol. Res. **5**, 467 (1985). Clinical trials in treatment of irritable bowel syndrome: G. Piai et al., Clin. Trials J. **23**, 6 (1986); A. Ferrari et al., Clin. Ther. **8**, 320 (1986).

Crystals from acetonitrile, mp 174°. $[α]_D^{20}$ −18.3° (c = 3).
THERAP CAT: Antispasmodic.

2281. Cimigenol. [3779-59-7] (3β,15α,16α,23R,24S)-16,23:16,24-Diepoxy-9,19-cyclolanostane-3,15,25-triol; cimicifugol. $C_{30}H_{48}O_5$; mol wt 488.70. C 73.73%, H 9.90%, O 16.37%. From the resin of Cimicifuga racemosa Nutt. (Actaea racemosa L.),

Ranunculaceae: Corsano, Spano, Atti Accad. Naz. Lincei Cl. Sci. Fis. Mat. Nat. Rend. **32**, 674 (1962), C.A. **58**, 11408e (1963). Structure: Corsano et al., Chem. Commun. **1965**, 185; Corsano, Piancatelli, Ric. Sci. **37**, 366 (1967); eidem, Gazz. Chim. Ital. **99**, 1140 (1969). Identity with cimicifugol: J. Pharm. Soc. Jpn. **87**, 1569 (1967).

Needles from methanol, mp 227.5-228.5°. $[α]_D$ +38° (c = 0.86 in chloroform).

Diacetate. $C_{34}H_{52}O_7$. Needles from hexane, mp 202-204°. $[α]_D$ +46.3° (c = 1.07 in chloroform).

Triacetate. $C_{36}H_{54}O_8$. Needles from hexane, mp 149.5-150.5°. $[α]_D$ +25.4° (chloroform).

2282. Cinacalcet. [226256-56-0] (αR)-α-Methyl-N-[3-[3-(trifluoromethyl)phenyl]propyl]-1-napthalenemethanamine; (R)-N-(3-(3-(trifluoromethyl)phenyl)propyl)-1-(1-naphtyl)ethylamine; AMG-073; KRN-1493. $C_{22}H_{22}F_3N$; mol wt 357.41. C 73.93%, H 6.20%, F 15.95%, N 3.92%. Calcimimetic. Prepn: B. C. Van Wagenen et al., **US 6211244** (2001 to NPS Pharmaceuticals). Review of pharmacology and mechanism of action: M. Wada, N. Nagano, Nephrol. Dial. Transplant. **18**, Suppl. 3, iii13-iii17 (2003); of clinical development: N. Franceschini et al., Expert Opin. Invest. Drugs **12**, 1413-1421 (2003). Clinical trial in secondary hyperparathyroidism: G. A. Block et al., N. Engl. J. Med. **350**, 1516 (2004).

Hydrochloride. [364782-34-3] Mimpara; Sensipar. $C_{22}H_{22}$-F_3N.HCl; mol wt 393.87. White to off-white, crystalline solid. Sol in methanol, 95% ethanol; slightly sol in water.

THERAP CAT: Antihyperparathyroid.

2283. Cinchomeronic Acid. [490-11-9] 3,4-Pyridine-dicarboxylic acid. $C_7H_5NO_4$; mol wt 167.12. C 50.31%, H 3.02%, N 8.38%, O 38.29%. Prepd in 42% yield by boiling quinine with nitric and fuming nitric acid: Ternájgo, Monatsh. Chem. **21**, 448 (1900); cf. Kirpal, ibid. **23**, 248 (1902); Kaas, ibid. 252; by selenium dioxide oxidation of isoquinoline: Mueller, **US 2436660** (1948 to Allied Chem.).

Crystals from acidulated water, mp 256°. On heating, a small portion sublimes without decompn. Strong acid. Sparingly sol in hot alc, ether, benzene. Insol in chloroform.

Disodium salt dihydrate. $C_7H_3NNa_2O_4.2H_2O$. Plates, moderately sol in water, alcohol.

Dimethyl ester. $C_9H_9NO_4$. Crystals, mp 141°.

2284. Cinchona. Calisaya bark; Peruvian bark; Cinchona bark; Jesuit's bark. Dried bark of stem or root of various species of Cinchona, fam. Rubiaceae, largely of C. officinalis L. (C. ledgeriana Moens) cultivated mostly in Java, of C. officinalis L. (C. calisaya Wedd.) from Bolivia, of C. officinalis L. and C. micrantha R. & P. from Peru, of C. pubescens Vahl. (C. succirubra Pav.) from Ecuador and C. pitayensis Wedd. from Colombia. Habit. South

America, cultivated mostly in Java, also in India. *Constit.* About 35 alkaloids; cinchotannic, quinic and quinovic acids; cinchona red; volatile oils. The alkaloid content varies according to the source of the bark. The cultivated bark contains 7-10% total alkaloids of which about 70% is quinine. *Cinchona succirubra* Pav. and some other varieties contain more cinchonidine and cinchonine and sometimes quinidine than the cultivated. The standardized method for the assay of cinchona, named "Brussels 1949" is published in the journal *De Belgische Chemische Industrie (Ind. Chim. Belge)* **15**, 328-338 (1950).

On heating a small portion of the bark in a test tube a characteristic purple vapor is evolved. Dil H_2SO_4 extracts have a blue fluorescence.

THERAP CAT: Antimalarial.

2285. Cinchonamine. [482-28-0] [1S-(1α,2α,4α,5β)]-2-(5-Ethenyl-1-azabicyclo[2.2.2]oct-2-yl)-1*H*-indole-3-ethanol; 3-(β-hydroxyethyl)-2-(5-vinyl-2-quinuclidyl)indole. $C_{19}H_{24}N_2O$; mol wt 296.41. C 76.99%, H 8.16%, N 9.45%, O 5.40%. From the bark of *Remijia purdieana* Wedd., *Rubiaceae:* Arnaud, *Compt. Rend.* **93**, 593 (1881); Hesse, *Ann.* **225**, 211 (1884). Prepn by reduction of quinamine with lithium aluminum hydride and structure: Goutarel *et al., Helv. Chim. Acta* **33**, 150 (1950). Synthesis: Chen *et al., C.A.* **53**, 7219e (1959). Total synthesis: G. Grethe *et al., Helv. Chim. Acta* **59**, 2271 (1976). Stereochemistry: Wenkert, Bringi, *J. Am. Chem. Soc.* **80**, 3484 (1958); Augustine, *Chem. Ind. (London)* **1959**, 1071; Sawa, Matsumura, *Tetrahedron* **26**, 2923 (1970). Biosynthetic studies: Battersby, Parry, *Chem. Commun.* **1971**, 31. Conversion of cinchona alkaloids of the quinoline series to those of the indole series: Ochiai *et al., C.A.* **59**, 14040h (1963).

Triboluminescent, orthorhombic prisms from methanol, mp 186°, also reported as mp 194°. $[\alpha]_D^{20}$ +123° (c = 0.66 in ethanol). pK in 80% methyl Cellosolve: 8.28. uv max (methanol): 223, 292 nm (log ε 4.60, 3.88). One gram dissolves in about 35 ml alcohol, 105 ml ether. Sol in benzene, chloroform, petr ether, CS_2; practically insol in water.

Hydrochloride monohydrate. $C_{19}H_{24}N_2O.HCl.H_2O$. Cubic crystals. One gram dissolves in 200 ml water. Sol in alc.

2286. Cinchonidine. [485-71-2] (8α,9R)-Cinchonan-9-ol; cinchovatine; α-quinidine. $C_{19}H_{22}N_2O$; mol wt 294.39. C 77.52%, H 7.53%, N 9.52%, O 5.43%. Occurs in most varieties of cinchona bark, especially in bark of *Cinchona pubescens* Vahl. (*C. succirubra* Pav.) and *C. pitayensis* Wedd., *Rubiaceae*. Isoln: Leers, *Ann.* **82**, 147 (1852). Structure: Rabe, *ibid.* **365**, 359 (1909). Stereoisomeric with cinchonine: Koenigs, *ibid.* **347**, 182 (1906). Configuration: Prelog, Zalán, *Helv. Chim. Acta* **27**, 535 (1944); Prelog, Häfliger, *ibid.* **33**, 2021 (1950); Roth, *Pharmazie* **16**, 257 (1961); Lyle, Keefer, *Tetrahedron* **23**, 3253 (1967). Biosynthetic studies: Battersby, Parry, *Chem. Commun.* **1971**, 31. Toxicity studies: C. C. Johnson, C. F. Poe, *Acta Pharmacol. Toxicol.* **4**, 265 (1948); E. W. Schafer, Jr. *et al., Ecotoxicol. Environ. Saf.* **6**, 149 (1982).

Orthorhombic plates, prisms from alcohol, mp 210°. $[\alpha]_D^{20}$ −109.2° (alc). uv absorption data: Kamath *et al., Indian J. Chem.* **6**, 510 (1968). Sol in alcohol and chloroform; moderately sol in ether. Practically insol in water. pK_1 5.80, pK_2 10.03. *Protect from light.* LD_{50} i.p. in rats: 206 mg/kg (Johnson, Poe). LD_{50} orally in quail: >316 mg/kg (Schafer).

Dihydrochloride. $C_{19}H_{22}N_2O.2HCl$. White or slightly yellow crystals or powder. Freely sol in water or alcohol. *Protect from light.*

Hydrochloride dihydrate. $C_{19}H_{22}N_2O.HCl.2H_2O$. Cryst powder; loses all of its H_2O at 120°. $[\alpha]_D^{20}$ −117.5° (water). Sol in 25 parts cold water, more sol in boiling water; sol in alcohol, chloroform, slightly in ether. The aq soln is practically neutral. *Protect from light.*

Sulfate trihydrate. $(C_{19}H_{22}N_2O)_2.H_2SO_4.3H_2O$. Silky, acicular crystals; efflorescent on exposure to air and darkens in light. mp when anhydr ~240° with decompn. One gram dissolves in 70 ml water, 20 ml hot water, 90 ml alcohol, 40 ml hot alc, 620 ml chloroform. Practically insol in ether. The aq soln is practically neutral. *Protect from light.*

Epicinchonidine. [550-54-9] (8α,9S)-Cinchonan-9-ol. mp 104°, $[\alpha]_D^{20}$ +63° (c = 0.804 in alc): Rabe *et al., Ann.* **492**, 253 (1932).

THERAP CAT: Antimalarial.

2287. Cinchonine. [118-10-5] (9S)-Cinchonan-9-ol. C_{19}-$H_{22}N_2O$; mol wt 294.39. C 77.52%, H 7.53%, N 9.52%, O 5.43%. Occurs in most varieties of cinchona bark, especially in bark of *Cinchona micrantha* R. & P., *Rubiaceae*. Isoln and structure: Rabe, *Ber.* **41**, 63 (1908). Stereoisomeric with cinchonidine: Koenigs, *Ann.* **347**, 182 (1906). Configuration: Prelog, Zalán, *Helv. Chim. Acta* **27**, 535 (1944); Prelog, Häfliger, *ibid.* **33**, 2021 (1950); Roth, *Pharmazie* **16**, 257 (1961); Lyle, Keefer, *Tetrahedron* **23**, 3253 (1967). Crystal and molecular structure: B. Oleksyn *et al., Acta Crystallogr.* **B35**, 440 (1979). Biosynthetic studies: Battersby, Parry, *Chem. Commun.* **1971**, 31. Toxicity study: C. C. Johnson, C. F. Poe, *Acta Pharmacol. Toxicol.* **4**, 265 (1949).

Prisms, needles from alcohol or ether. mp about 265°; begins to sublime at 220°. $[\alpha]_D$ +229° (alcohol). uv absorption data: Kamath *et al., Indian J. Chem.* **6**, 510 (1968). One gram dissolves in 60 ml alcohol, 25 ml boiling alcohol, 110 ml chloroform, 500 ml ether. Practically insol in water. pK_1 5.85, pK_2 9.92. *Protect from light.* LD_{50} i.p. in rats: 152 mg/kg (Johnson, Poe).

Dihydrochloride. $C_{19}H_{22}N_2O.2HCl$. White or faintly yellow crystals or crystalline powder. Freely sol in water or alcohol. *Protect from light.*

Hydrochloride dihydrate. $C_{19}H_{22}N_2O.HCl.2H_2O$. Fine crystals. mp when anhydr about 215° with dec. One gram dissolves in 20 ml water, 3.5 ml boiling water, 1.5 ml alcohol, 20 ml chloroform; slightly sol in ether. The aq soln is practically neutral. *Protect from light.*

Sulfate dihydrate. $(C_{19}H_{22}N_2O)_2.H_2SO_4.2H_2O$. Lustrous, very bitter crystals. mp when anhydr about 198°. One gram dissolves in 65 ml water, 30 ml hot water, 12.5 ml alc, 7 ml hot alc, 47 ml chloroform; slightly sol in ether. The aq soln is practically neutral.

Epicinchonine. [485-70-1] (9R)-Cinchonan-9-ol. mp 83°, $[\alpha]_D^{22}$ +120.3° (c = 0.806 in alc), Rabe *et al., Ann.* **492**, 253 (1932).

THERAP CAT: Antimalarial.

2288. Cinchophen. [132-60-5] 2-Phenyl-4-quinolinecarboxylic acid; 2-phenylcinchoninic acid; Atophan; Quinophan; Phenoquin; Agotan; Artam; Alutyl; Cinconal; Vantyl; Viophan; Atocin; Mylofanol; Rhematan; Rheumin; Tophol; Polyphlogin; Quinofen; Tophosan. $C_{16}H_{11}NO_2$; mol wt 249.26. C 77.10%, H 4.45%, N 5.62%, O 12.84%. Quinoline derivative formerly used in treatment of chronic gout: A. B. Gutman, *Arthritis Rheum.* **16**, 431 (1973). Prepd by heating pyruvic acid with aniline and benzaldehyde or with benzylidene aniline in abs alcohol: Doebner, Gieseke, *Ann.* **242**, 290 (1887). Also from acetophenone and isatinic acid in alcoholic KOH: Pfitzinger, *J. Prakt. Chem.* **38**, 582 (1882); **56**, 293 (1897). Cinchophen as ulcerogenic agent: T. P. Churchill, F. H. van Wagoner, *Arch. Pathol.* **13**, 850 (1932); N. Umeda *et al., Toxicol. Appl. Pharmacol.* **18**, 102 (1971); T. H. Stewart *et al., J. Pathol.* **131**, 363 (1980). Mitochondrial toxicity of cinchophen and derivatives: H. Vainio *et al., Biochem. Pharmacol.* **20**, 1589 (1971).

Needles, mp 213-216°. Stable to air, but turns yellow under the influence of light. Slightly bitter taste. Practically insol in water. One gram dissolves in about 400 ml chloroform, in about 100 ml ether and in about 120 ml alcohol.

Hydrochloride. [132-58-1] Chloroxyl. $C_{16}H_{11}NO_2 \cdot HCl$; mol wt 285.72. Yellow cryst powder, slightly bitter, astringent taste; mp about 223°. Practically insol in water. Slightly sol in alcohol; sol in chloroform, ether.

Allyl ester. [524-34-5] Allyl 2-phenylcinchoninate; Atoquinol. $C_{19}H_{15}NO_2$; mol wt 289.33. Prepn: Gams, **US 1336972** (1920). Long needles from alc, mp 30°. bp$_{15}$ 260°. Practically insol in water. Readily sol in alcohol, ether, acetone, oils. Tasteless.

USE: Experimentally to induce ulcers.

THERAP CAT: Formerly as analgesic.

2289. Cinchotoxine. [69-24-9] (3*R-cis*)-3-(3-Ethenyl-4-piperidinyl)-1-(4-quinolinyl)-1-propanone; 9-deoxy-9-oxo-1,8-secocinchonine; cinchonicine. $C_{19}H_{22}N_2O$; mol wt 294.39. C 77.52%, H 7.53%, N 9.52%, O 5.43%. A rearrangement product of cinchonine or cinchonidine obtained by boiling with acetic acid: Pasteur, *Compt. Rend.* **37**, 110 (1853). Miller, Rohde, *Ber.* **33**, 3214 (1900). Conversion to cinchonidinone and cinchonine: Rabe, *Ber.* **44**, 2088 (1911); **41**, 62 (1908). Prepn from cinchonine: Prostenik, Prelog, *Helv. Chim. Acta* **26**, 1965 (1943).

Bitter needles. mp 58-60°. $[\alpha]_D^{15}$ +47° in alcohol. Sparingly sol in water; sol in alcohol, ether, chloroform.

2290. Cinepazet. [23887-41-4] 4-[1-Oxo-3-(3,4,5-trimethoxyphenyl)-2-propenyl]-1-piperazineacetic acid ethyl ester; 4-(3,4,5-trimethoxycinnamoyl)-1-piperazineacetic acid ethyl ester; ethyl 4-3-(3,4,5-trimethoxycinnamoyl)-1-piperazineacetate; 4-(3′,4′,5′-trimethoxycinnamoyl)-1-(ethoxycarbonylmethyl)piperazine; cinepazic acid ethyl ester; ethyl cinepazate. $C_{20}H_{28}N_2O_6$; mol wt 392.45. C 61.21%, H 7.19%, N 7.14%, O 24.46%. Prepn: C. Fauran *et al.,* **GB 1168108**; *eidem,* **US 3590034** (1969, 1971 both to Delalande). Synthesis and structure-activity studies of the hydrochloride: Fauran, Turin, *Chim. Ther.* **4**, 290 (1969); Huguet *et al., ibid.* 293. Pharmacology and toxicology: Pourrias *et al., Ther-*

apie **26**, 845, 859 (1971). Metabolic data: Chasseaud *et al., Arzneim.-Forsch.* **22**, 2003 (1972).

Solid from isopropyl ether, mp 96°.

Hydrochloride. mp 200° (dec). LD$_{50}$ in mice (mg/kg): 300 i.v., 1300 orally (Fauran, 1969).

Maleate. [50679-07-7] MD-6753; Vascoril. $C_{20}H_{28}N_2O_6 \cdot C_4H_4O_4$; mol wt 508.52. Crystals, mp 130°.

THERAP CAT: Antianginal.

2291. Cinepazide. [23887-46-9] 1-[2-Oxo-2-(1-pyrrolidinyl)ethyl]-4-[1-oxo-3-(3,4,5-trimethoxyphenyl)-2-propenyl]-piperazine; 1-[(1-pyrrolidinylcarbonyl)methyl]-4-(3,4,5-trimethoxycinnamoyl)piperazine; 1-[4-[2-oxo-2-(1-pyrrolidinyl)ethyl]-1-piperazinyl]-3-(3,4,5-trimethoxyphenyl)-2-propen-1-one; 1-[4-[(3′,4′,5′-trimethoxycinnamoyl)-1-piperazinyl]acetyl]pyrrolidine. $C_{22}H_{31}N_3O_5$; mol wt 417.50. C 63.29%, H 7.48%, N 10.06%, O 19.16%. Prepn: **BE 730345**; C. P. Fauran *et al.,* **US 3634411** (1969, 1972 both to Delalande); C. P. Fauran, M. J. Turin, *Chim. Ther.* **4**, 290 (1969). Pharmacology: G. Huguet *et al., ibid.* 293; E. Marmo *et al., Farmaco Ed. Prat.* **28**, 132 (1973); B. M. Pourrias *et al., Therapie* **29**, 29, 43 (1974).

Maleate. [26328-04-1] MD-67350; Brendil; Vasodistal. $C_{22}H_{31}N_3O_5 \cdot C_4H_4O_4$; mol wt 533.57. Crystals from abs ethanol, mp 135°. LD$_{50}$ in mice, rats (mg/kg): 1000, 1310 orally; 617, 414 i.v. (Pourrias).

THERAP CAT: Vasodilator (peripheral).

2292. Cinerins. Active insecticidal constituents of pyrethrum flowers. Isoln: Ward, *Chem. Ind. (London)* **1953**, 586; Stephenson, *Pyrethrum Post* **5**, no. 4, 22 (1960); *C.A.* **55**, 13753g (1961). Structure: Schechter *et al., J. Am. Chem. Soc.* **71**, 3165 (1949); Godin *et al., J. Chem. Soc. C* **1966**, 332. Stereochemistry: Begley *et al., Chem. Commun.* **1972**, 1276. *Review:* Crombie, Elliott, *Fortschr. Chem. Org. Naturst.* **19**, 120-164 (1961). Review of toxicology and human exposure: *Toxicological Profile for Pyrethrins and Pyrethroids* (PB2004-100004, 2003) 332 pp.

Cinerin I   R = CH$_3$
Cinerin II   R = COOCH$_3$

Cinerin I. [25402-06-6] (1*R*,3*R*)-2,2-Dimethyl-3-(2-methyl-1-propenyl)cyclopropanecarboxylic acid (1*S*)-3-(2*Z*)-(2-butenyl)-2-methyl-4-oxo-2-cyclopenten-1-yl-ester. $C_{20}H_{28}O_3$; mol wt 316.43. Viscous liquid. Oxidizes rapidly and becomes inactive in presence of air. bp$_{0.008}$ 136-138°. n_D^{20} 1.5064. $[\alpha]_D^{20}$ −22° (hexane). uv max: 222 nm (ε 21400). Practically insol in water. Sol in alcohol, petr ether, kerosene, carbon tetrachloride, ethylene dichloride, nitromethane.

Cinerin II. [121-20-0] (1*R*,3*R*)-3-[(1*E*)-3-Methoxy-2-methyl-3-oxo-1-propenyl]-2,2-dimethylcyclopropanecarboxylic acid (1*S*)-3-(2*Z*)-(2-butenyl)-2-methyl-4-oxo-2-cyclopenten-1-yl ester. $C_{21}H_{28}O_5$; mol wt 360.44. Viscous liquid. Oxidizes rapidly and becomes inactive in presence of air. bp$_{0.001}$ 182-184°. n_D^{20} 1.5183. $[\alpha]_D^{16}$ +16° (isooctane). uv max: 229 nm (ε 28700). Practically insol in water. Sol in alcohol, petr ether (less sol than Cinerin I), kerosene, carbon tetrachloride, ethylene dichloride, nitromethane.

Caution: Direct skin contact and inhalation may cause allergic attacks in sensitive people. Potential symptoms of overexposure are severe dermatitis, asthma, vasomotor rhinitis, anaphylactic reactions; numbness of lips and tongue, sneezing, vomiting, diarrhea; headache, restlessness, tinnitis, incoordination, clonic convulsions, stupor, prostration; death due to respiratory paralysis. *See: Clinical Toxicology of Commercial Products*, R. E. Gosselin *et al.*, Eds. (Williams & Wilkins, Baltimore, 5th ed., 1984) Section III, pp 352-355.

USE: Insecticide.

2293. Cinidon-ethyl. [142891-20-1] (2*Z*)-2-Chloro-3-[2-chloro-5-(1,3,4,5,6,7-hexahydro-1,3-dioxo-2*H*-isoindol-2-yl)phenyl]-2-propenoic acid ethyl ester; ethyl (*Z*)-2-chloro-3-[2-chloro-5-(1,3-dioxo-4,5,6,7-tetrahydroisoindol-2-yl)phenyl]acrylate; BAS-615H; Bingo; Lotus; Orbit; Solar; Vega. $C_{19}H_{17}Cl_2NO_4$; mol wt 394.25. C 57.88%, H 4.35%, Cl 17.99%, N 3.55%, O 16.23%. Post-emergence herbicide which inhibits protoporphyrinogen oxidase. Prepn: P. Plath *et al.*, **DE 3603789**; *eidem*, **US 5062884** (1987, 1991 both to BASF). Biochemical mode of action: K. Grossman, H. Schiffer, *Pestic. Sci.* **55**, 687 (1999). Field trials in cereals: W. Nuyken *et al.*, *Brighton Crop Prot. Conf. - Weeds* **1999**, 81.

USE: Herbicide.

2294. Cinitapride. [66564-14-5] 4-Amino-*N*-[1-(3-cyclohexen-1-ylmethyl)-4-piperidinyl]-2-ethoxy-5-nitrobenzamide. $C_{21}H_{30}N_4O_4$; mol wt 402.49. C 62.67%, H 7.51%, N 13.92%, O 15.90%. Prepn: A. Vega-Noverola *et al.*, **DE 2751139** (1978 to Anphar); *eidem*, **US 5026858** (1991 to Walton). Pharmacology: R. Massingham *et al.*, *J. Auton. Pharmacol.* **5**, 41 (1985). Spectral determn in pharmaceutical preps: M. Blanco *et al.*, *J. Pharm. Sci.* **82**, 834 (1993). Clinical evaluation in functional dyspepsia, in comparison with metoclopramide, *q.v.*: F. Mora *et al.*, *Ann. Med. Interne* **10**, 323 (1993).

Tartrate. [96623-56-2] LAS-17177; Cidine.

THERAP CAT: Gastroprokinetic.

2295. Cinmethylin. [87818-31-3] *exo*-(±)-1-Methyl-4-(1-methylethyl)-2-[(2-methylphenyl)methoxy]-7-oxabicyclo[2.2.1]heptane; (±)-2-*exo*-(2-methylbenzyloxy)-1-methyl-4-isopropyl-7-oxabicyclo[2.2.1]heptane; SD-95481; Cinch. $C_{18}H_{26}O_2$; mol wt 274.40. C 78.79%, H 9.55%, O 11.66%. Pre-emergence grass herbicide. Member of the cineole eucalyptol, *q.v.*, family. Prepn: G. B. Payne *et al.*, **EP 81893** (1983 to Shell); *eidem*, **US 4670041** (1987 to Du Pont). Physical and chemical properties: B. T. Grayson *et al.*, *Pestic. Sci.* **21**, 143 (1987). Mechanism of action study:

M. H. El-Deek, F. D. Hess, *Weed Sci.* **34**, 684 (1986). Metabolism in rats: P. W. Lee *et al.*, *J. Agric. Food Chem.* **34**, 162 (1986). Mobility in soil: D. R. Wendt *et al.*, *Proc. South. Weed Sci. Soc.* **1987**, 391; and herbicidal activity: P. C. Lolas, A. Galopoulos, *Zizaniology* **1**, 221 (1985). Field studies in tobacco: P. C. Lolas, *Proc. Br. Crop Prot. Conf. - Weeds* **1985**, 841; in soybeans: P. C. Bhowmik, *Weed Sci.* **36**, 678 (1988).

Colorless liquid, bp 313 ±2°. d^{20} 1015 kg/m³. Viscosity (20°): 70-90 mPa. Vapor pressure (20°): 7.6 × 10⁻⁵ mm Hg. Moderately volatile. Partition coefficient (*n*-octanol/water): 6850. Miscible with most organic solvents. Slightly sol in water. Soly in water (20°): 63 ± 2 mg/l. LD$_{50}$ orally in rats: 4.5 g/kg; LD$_{50}$ dermally in rabbits: >2 g/kg (Lee).

USE: Herbicide.

2296. Cinnabarine. [146-90-7] 2-Amino-9-hydroxymethyl-3-oxo-3*H*-phenoxazine-1-carboxylic acid; 1-carboxy-2-amino-9-hydroxymethylphenoxazin-3-one; polystictine. $C_{14}H_{10}N_2O_5$; mol wt 286.24. C 58.74%, H 3.52%, N 9.79%, O 27.95%. Antibiotic substance produced by the fungus *Trametes cinnabarina* Jacq.: Gripenberg, *Acta Chem. Scand.* **5**, 590 (1951); from *Coriolus sanguineus* (Fr.) (*Polystictus cinnabarinus* Jacq.): Cavill *et al.*, *J. Chem. Soc.* **1953**, 525. Identity with polystictine: Gripenberg *et al.*, *Acta Chem. Scand.* **11**, 1485 (1957). Structure: Gripenberg, *ibid.* **12**, 603 (1958); **13**, 1305 (1959). Cavill *et al.*, *Tetrahedron* **5**, 275 (1959). Syntheses: Weinstein, Brattesani, *J. Heterocycl. Chem.* **4**, 151 (1967); Schäfer, Schlude, *Tetrahedron Lett.* **1968**, 2161.

Red needles, dec 320°. Absorption max: 234, 430, 455 nm (log ε 4.2, 4.0, 4.0). Soly in acetone: 0.04% (20°); in dioxane: 0.1% (100°). Practically insol in ethanol, chloroform and dimethyl sulfoxide. Sol in cold concd HCl.

O-Methyl ether. $C_{15}H_{12}N_2O_5$. Orange red prisms from ethyl acetate + petr ether, mp 200-202°.

2297. Cinnamaldehyde. [104-55-2] 3-Phenyl-2-propenal; cinnamic aldehyde; phenylacrolein; cinnamal. C_9H_8O; mol wt 132.16. C 81.79%, H 6.10%, O 12.11%. Found in Ceylon and Chinese cinnamon oils as the *trans*-form. Prepn by condensation of benzaldehyde and acetaldehyde: Peine, *Ber.* **17**, 2117 (1884); **JP 163097** (1944 to Ogawa Chem. Ind.); from 2-chloroallylbenzene: Bert, Dorier, *Compt. Rend.* **191**, 332 (1930); Bert, Annequin, *ibid.* **192**, 1315 (1931); by condensation of styrene with formylmethylaniline: **GB 504125** (1939 to I. G. Farben); by oxidation of cinnamyl alc: Holum, *J. Org. Chem.* **26**, 4814 (1961); Traynelis, Hergenrother, *J. Am. Chem. Soc.* **86**, 298 (1964). Isoln from wood-rotting fungus, *Stereum subpileatum* Berk. & Curt.: Birkinshaw *et al.*, *Biochem. J.* **66**, 188 (1957). Toxicity data: P. M. Jenner *et al.*, *Food Cosmet. Toxicol.* **2**, 327 (1964). Review of risk assessment as fragrance ingredient: D. Bickers *et al.*, *Food Chem. Toxicol.* **43**, 799-836 (2005); of toxicology: J. Cocchiara *et al.*, *ibid.* 867-923.

Yellowish oily liquid, strong odor of cinnamon. d_{25}^{25} 1.048-1.052. Volatile with steam. mp $-7.5°$. $bp_{1.0}$ 76.1°; bp_5 105.8°; bp_{10} 120.0°; bp_{20} 135.7°; bp_{40} 152.2°; bp_{60} 163.7°; bp_{100} 177.7°; bp_{200} 199.3°; bp_{400} 222.4°; bp_{760} 246.0° (some dec). n_D^{20} 1.618-1.623. Flash point, closed cup: >100°C. Dissolves in about 700 parts water, in about 7 vols of 60% alc. Misc with alcohol, ether, chloroform, oils. LD_{50} in rats (mg/kg): 2220 orally (Jenner).

USE: In the flavor and perfume industry.

2298. Cinnamedrine. [90-86-8] α-[1-[Methyl(3-phenyl-2-propenyl)amino]ethyl]benzenemethanol; N-cinnamylephedrine; α-[1-(N-cinnamyl-N-methylamino)ethyl]benzyl alcohol. $C_{19}H_{23}NO$; mol wt 281.39. C 81.10%, H 8.24%, N 4.98%, O 5.69%. Smooth muscle relaxant. Prepn: Stolz, Flaecher, US 1959392 (1934 to Winthrop Chem.); Welsh, Keenan, *J. Am. Pharm. Assoc. Sci. Ed.* **30**, 123 (1941).

dl-Hydrochloride. $C_{19}H_{23}NO\cdot HCl$. Bitter crystals from ethyl acetate + chloroform. mp 180-185° (base, mp 72-78°). Sol in about 80 parts water and 10 parts alc at 20°, more easily sol at higher temps; sol in 50 parts chloroform; sparingly sol in ether, benzene.

THERAP CAT: Antispasmodic.

2299. Cinnamic Acid. [621-82-9] 3-Phenyl-2-propenoic acid; β-phenylacrylic acid. $C_9H_8O_2$; mol wt 148.16. C 72.96%, H 5.44%, O 21.60%. Occurs as the *trans*-form in storax, balsam Peru or Tolu, oil of cinnamon, coca leaves. Isoln: Beilstein, Kuhlberg, *Ann.* **163**, 123 (1872); von Miller, *Ann.* **188**, 196 (1877). Synthesis (Perkin reaction) from benzaldehyde, acetic anhydride, and potassium acetate: *Org. React.* **I**, 248 (1942); from oxalyl bromide + styrene: Treibs *et al., Naturwissenschaften* **45**, 85 (1958); from acetylene + benzaldehyde: Herbetz, *Ber.* **92**, 541 (1959). Prepn of *cis*- and *trans*-isomers: Comte *et al., Compt. Rend.* **245**, 1144 (1957). Isoln from wood-rotting fungus, *Stereum subpileatum* Berk. & Curt.: Birkinshaw *et al., Biochem. J.* **66**, 188 (1957). Review of risk assessment as fragrance ingredient: D. Bickers *et al., Food Chem. Toxicol.* **43**, 799-836 (2005); of toxicology: C. S. Letizia *et al., ibid.* 925-943.

Monoclinic crystals, honey, floral odor, d_4^4 1.2475. mp 134°; bp_3 147°. Flash point, closed cup: >93.3°C. Distilling at 146° causes decarboxylation to styrene. pK (25°) 4.46. uv max (alc): 273 nm. One gram dissolves in about 2000 ml water at 25° (more sol in hot water), in 6 ml alc, 5 ml methanol, 12 ml chloroform. Freely sol in benzene, ether, acetone, glacial acetic acid, carbon disulfide, oils. The alkali salts are sol in water. LD_{50} (g/kg): 3.57 orally in rats; >5.0 dermally in rabbits (Letizia).

Methyl ester. [103-26-4] $C_{10}H_{10}O_2$. Crystals, odor fruity and balsamic, reminiscent of strawberries. mp 36°. d_0^{36} 1.042. bp 261.9°; bp_{15} 132.5-134°. n_D^{21} 1.5766. Freely sol in alcohol, ether. Practically insol in water. Clearly sol in 80% alc.

Ethyl ester. [103-36-6] Ethyl cinnamate; ethyl phenylacrylate. $C_{11}H_{12}O_2$. Almost colorless, oily liquid, fruity and balsamic odor, reminiscent of cinnamon with an amber note. d_{25}^{25} 1.045-1.048. d_4^{20} 1.049. bp 271°. mp 6-10°. n_D^{20} 1.559-1.561. Miscible with alcohol, ether. Insol in water. Soluble in 3 vols of 70% alc.

n-Butyl ester. [538-65-8] Butyl cinnamate; Eliminoxy. $C_{13}H_{16}O_2$; mol wt 204.26. Liquid, agreeable ethereal odor when pure. bp_{13} 145°. d_4^{18} 1.012. Very sparingly sol in water (<0.5%). Sol in 95% alc, ether, acetone, chloroform, benzene. Incompatible with alkalies; stable to light, air, and storage temps.

Anhydride. [538-56-7] Cinnamic anhydride. $C_{18}H_{14}O_3$. Crystals, mp 136°. Practically insol in water. Freely sol in warm benzene; slightly sol in alc.

USE: Fragrance and flavoring ingredient.

2300. Cinnamon. Ceylon cinnamon. Tropical evergreen tree, *Cinnamomum zeylanicum* Bl. (syn. *C. verum* Presl.), *Lauraceae*; cultivated for the aromatic bark which is widely used in cooking and in traditional medicine. Leaves and root bark are also used for their essential oil. *Habit.* Sri Lanka and southeast Asia. *Saigon cinnamon* is obtained from the bark of *C. loureirii* Nees. *Cassia*, also known as **Chinese cinnamon**, is often used as a substitute; obtained from the related species, *C. cassia* Presl. (syn. *C. aromaticum* Nees). *Constit.* Volatile oil (up to 4%), tannins, catechins, pre-anthocyanidins, resins, mucilage, gum, sugars, calcium oxalate, coumarins, and the insecticidal compounds, cinnzeylanin and cinnzeylanol. Comprehensive description: J. Thomas, P. P. Duethi in *Handbook of Herbs and Spices*, K. V. Peter, Ed., (CRC Press, Boca Raton, 2001) pp 143-153. Analysis of volatile constituents: U. M. Senanayake *et al., J. Agric. Food Chem.* **26**, 822 (1978). Authentication method: M. J. Cikalo *et al., J. Planar Chromatogr.* **5**, 135 (1992). Review of cinnamon: J. Barnes *et al., Herbal Medicines* (Pharmaceutical Press, London, 2nd Ed., 2002) pp 135-136; of cassia: *idem, ibid.* pp 112-113. *Review:* A. Y. Leung, S. Foster, *Encyclopedia of Common Natural Ingredients*, (Wiley-Interscience, Hoboken, 2nd Ed., 2003) pp 167-170.

Cinnamon bark oil. [8015-91-6] Oil of cinnamon, Ceylon. Volatile oil obtained by steam distillation from the dried inner bark of *C. zeylanicum. Constit.* Complex mixture of components chiefly, cinnamaldehyde (60-75%), cinnamyl acetate, eugenol, caryophyllene, linalool. Yellow liquid with a spicy burning taste and the characteristic odor of cinnamon. d_{25}^{25} 1.010-1.030. n_D^{20} 1.573-1.591. Rotation between $-2°$ and 0°. Sol in most fixed oils, propylene glycol, in 3 vols 70% alcohol. Insol in glycerin, mineral oil.

Cinnamon leaf oil. Oil of cinnamon leaf. Volatile oil obtained by steam distillation of the leaves and twigs of *C. zeylanicum. Constit.* Eugenol (80-88%), other components similar to bark oil. Light to dark brown liquid with spicy cinnamon-clove odor and taste. d_{25}^{25} 1.030-1.050. n_D^{20} 1.529-1.537. Rotation between $-2°$ and $+1°$. Sol in most fixed oils, propylene glycol, in 1.5 vols 70% alcohol. Sol with cloudiness in mineral oil. Insol in glycerin.

Cassia oil. [8007-80-5] Oil of cassia; oil of Chinese cinnamon. Volatile oil obtained by steam distillation from the leaves and twigs of *C. cassia. Constit.* Cinnamaldehyde (75-90%), salicylaldehyde, methylsalicylaldehyde, methyleugenol. Yellow or brown liquid with characteristic odor and taste. Darkens and thickens upon aging or exposure to air. d_{25}^{25} 1.045-1.063. n_D^{20} 1.602-1.614. Rotation between $-1°$ and $+1°$. Sol in glacial acetic acid, in 2 vols 70% alcohol.

USE: Used extensively as spice and flavoring in foods, beverages, pharmaceuticals. Ingredient in spice blends such as garam masala.

THERAP CAT: Carminative, antiseptic, astringent.

THERAP CAT (VET): Carminative.

2301. Cinnamoyl Chloride. [102-92-1] 3-Phenyl-2-propenoyl chloride. C_9H_7ClO; mol wt 166.60. C 64.88%, H 4.24%, Cl 21.28%, O 9.60%. $C_6H_5CH{=}CHCOCl$. Prepn by the action of oxalyl chloride on sodium cinnamate: Adams, Ulich, *J. Am. Chem. Soc.* **42**, 605 (1920).

Yellowish crystals. mp 35-36°; bp_{58} 170-171°; bp_{25} 154°; bp_{16} 147°; bp_2 101°; $d_4^{45.3}$ 1.1617; $n_D^{42.5}$ 1.614.

USE: Titrimetric determination of small amts of water.

2302. Cinnamyl Alcohol. [104-54-1] 3-Phenyl-2-propen-1-ol; cinnamic alcohol; styryl carbinol; γ-phenylallyl alcohol. $C_9H_{10}O$; mol wt 134.18. C 80.56%, H 7.51%, O 11.92%. The *trans*-form occurs (in the esterified form) in storax and in balsam Peru, cinnamon leaves, hyacinth oil. Obtained by the alkaline hydrolysis of storax. Prepd synthetically by reducing cinnamal diacetate with iron filings and acetic acid; from cinnamaldehyde by Meerwein-Ponndorf reduction with aluminum isopropoxide: Meerwein, Schmidt, *Ann.* **444**, 221 (1925). Review of risk assessment as fragrance ingredient: D. Bickers *et al., Food Chem. Toxicol.* **43**, 799-836 (2005); of toxicology: C. S. Letizia *et al., ibid.* 837-866.

Needles or cryst mass. Odor of hyacinth. mp 30°. d_{35}^{35} 1.0397. bp 258°. n_D^{20} 1.58190; n_D^{33} 1.57580. Flash point, closed cup: >93.3°C. When small amounts of impurities are present as in the natural article (cinnamyl alcohol from storax), it remains fluid at lower temps than the melting point. Minimum congealing points specified by the Essential Oil Assn are: 33.0° for cinnamic alcohol pure; 28.0° for cinnamic alcohol prime; 20.0° for cinnamic alcohol from storax. Is oxidized slowly on exposure to heat, light and air. Sol in water, glycerol. Clearly sol in 3 vols 50% alc. Freely sol in alc, ether, other common organic solvents. LD_{50} (g/kg): 2.0 orally in rats; >5.0 dermally in rabbits (Letizia).

USE: In perfumery; as deodorant in 12.5% soln in glycerol.

2303. Cinnamyl Anthranilate. [87-29-6] 2-Aminobenzoic acid 3-phenyl-2-propenyl ester; anthranilic acid cinnamyl ester; 3-phenyl-2-propenyl anthranilate; cinnamyl o-aminobenzoate. $C_{16}H_{15}NO_2$; mol wt 253.30. C 75.87%, H 5.97%, N 5.53%, O 12.63%. Synthetic imitation grape or cherry flavoring agent. Prepn: A. Seldner, *Am. Perfum. Essent. Oil Rev.* **54**, 295 (1949); R. P. Staiger, E. B. Miller, *J. Org. Chem.* **24**, 1214 (1959). Carcinogenicity studies: G. D. Stoner *et al.*, *Cancer Res.* **33**, 3069 (1973); *Fed. Regist.* **45**, 85832 (1980). Review: D. L. Opdyke, *Food Cosmet. Toxicol.* **13**, Suppl., 751-752 (1975).

(E)-form

Crystals, mp 61-61.5°.

USE: Flavoring agent in food; fragrance in soaps and perfumes.

2304. Cinnamyl Cinnamate. [122-69-0] 3-Phenyl-2-propenoic acid 3-phenyl-2-propenyl ester; cinnamic acid cinnamyl ester; cinnyl cinnamate; styracin. $C_{18}H_{16}O_2$; mol wt 264.32. C 81.79%, H 6.10%, O 12.11%. $C_6H_5CH{=}CHCOOCH_2{-}CH{=}CHC_6H_5$. From buds of *Populus balsamifer* L., *Salicaceae*: Goris, Canal, *Bull. Soc. Chim. Fr.* **3**, 1982 (1936); from *Lavanga scandens* Buch.-Ham., *Lavangalata*: Baslas, Deshapande, *J. Indian Chem. Soc.* **27**, 379 (1950). Synthesis of *trans*-cinnamyl *trans*-cinnamate: Klemm *et al.*, *Tetrahedron* **20**, 871 (1964).

trans-trans-Form. Needles from abs ethanol, mp 44°. uv max (95% ethanol): 216, 223 nm (log ε 3.45, 3.25). Practically insol in water. 1 g dissolves in 22 ml cold, 3 ml boiling alcohol, 3 ml ether.

2305. Cinnarizine. [298-57-7] 1-(Diphenylmethyl)-4-(3-phenyl-2-propenyl)piperazine; N-benzhydryl-N'-*trans*-cinnamylpiperazine; 1-cinnamyl-4-diphenylmethylpiperazine; 1-*trans*-cinnamyl-4-diphenylmethylpiperazine; 1-cinnamyl-4-benzhydrylpiperazine; 1-diphenylmethyl-4-*trans*-cinnamylpiperazine; cinnipirine; 516-MD; Aplactan; Aplexal; Apotomin; Artate; Carecin; Cerebolan; Cerepar; Cinaperazine; Cinazyn; Cinnacet; Cinnageron; Corathiem; Denapol; Dimitron; Eglen; Folcodal; Giganten; Glanil; Hilactan; Ixertol; Katoseran; Labyrin; Midronal; Mitronal; Olamin; Processine; Sedatromin; Sepan; Siptazin; Spaderizine; Stugeron; Stutgeron; Stutgin; Toliman. $C_{26}H_{28}N_2$; mol wt 368.51. C 84.74%, H 7.66%, N 7.60%. Calcium channel blocker with antiallergic and anti-vasoconstricting activity. Prepn: Janssen, **US 2882271** (1959, Janssen). Pharmacology: Van Nueten, Janssen, *Arch. Int. Pharmacodyn. Ther.* **204**, 37 (1973). Metabolism: Soudijn, van Wijngaarden, *Life Sci.* **7**, 231 (1968). Clinical study in treatment of intermittent claudication: J. H. Barber *et al.*, *Pharmatherapeutica* **2**, 401 (1980). Assessment of calcium antagonist effects: M. Spedding, *Arch. Pharmacol.* **318**, 234 (1982). HPLC determn in blood and plasma: M. Puttemans *et al.*, *J. Liq. Chromatogr.* **7**, 2237 (1984). Comparison of clinical pharmacokinetics with other antihistamines: D. M. Paton, D. R. Webster, *Clin. Pharmacol.* **10**, 477-497 (1985).

Hydrochloride. $C_{26}H_{28}N_2{\cdot}HCl$. mp 192° (dec). Soly in water: 2 mg/100 ml.

Mixture with vitamin B$_6$. Emesazine.

THERAP CAT: Antihistaminic. Vasodilator (peripheral, cerebral).

2306. Cinnoline. [253-66-7] 1,2-Benzodiazine; benzo[c]pyridazine; 1,2-diazanaphthalene; α-phenodiazine. $C_8H_6N_2$; mol wt 130.15. C 73.83%, H 4.65%, N 21.52%. First prepd by reduction of 4-chlorocinnoline: Busch, Rast, *Ber.* **30**, 521, 524 (1897). Synthesis from methyl anthranilate: Jacobs *et al.*, *J. Am. Chem. Soc.* **68**, 1310 (1946); from cinnoline-4-carboxylic acid: Morley, *J. Chem. Soc.* **1951**, 1971. Crystal and molecular structure: C. Huiszoon *et al.*, *Acta Crystallogr.* **33B**, 1867 (1977).

Pale yellow clusters of crystals from ligroin, mp 38°; also reported as mp 40-41° (Morley). Solvated needles from ether (contg 1 mol ether), mp 24-25°. bp$_{0.35}$ 114°. uv spectrum: Hearn *et al.*, *J. Chem. Soc.* **1951**, 3318. Geranium-like odor. *Poisonous!* Bitter taste resembling the taste of quinine. Must be kept under nitrogen. On exposure to air it has a tendency to liquefy and turn green. Strong base: *ibid.* **1949**, 1356. Freely sol in the usual solvents.

Hydrochloride. $C_8H_6N_2{\cdot}HCl$. Brownish needles from alcohol + ether, mp 156-160°. Volatilizes around 100° on slow heating. Freely sol in water, alcohol.

2307. Cinobufotalin. [1108-68-5] (3β,5β,15β,16β)-16-(Acetyloxy)-14,15-epoxy-3,5-dihydroxybufa-20,22-dienolide; 14,15β-epoxy-3β,5,16β-trihydroxy-5β-bufa-20,22-dienolide 16-acetate. $C_{26}H_{34}O_7$; mol wt 458.54. C 68.10%, H 7.47%, O 24.42%. Isolated from the Chinese drug Ch'an Su which is prepd from Chinese toads (*Bufo asiaticus* = *bufo gargarizans* Cantor). Isoln: Kotake, Kuwada, *C.A.* **31**, 7065² (1937); Ruckstubl, Meyer, *Helv. Chim. Acta* **40**, 1270 (1957). Structure: Bernoulli *et al.*, *ibid.* **45**, 240 (1962).

Octahedrons from acetone, mp 259-262°. $[\alpha]_D^{20}$ +11°. uv max: 295 nm (log ε 3.72).

2308. Cinolazepam. [75696-02-5] 7-Chloro-5-(2-fluorophenyl)-2,3-dihydro-3-hydroxy-2-oxo-1H-1,4-benzodiazepine-1-propanenitrile; 1-(2-cyanoethyl)-7-chloro-3-hydroxy-5-(2'-fluorophenyl)-1,3-dihydro-2H-1,4-benzodiazepin-2-one; OX-373; Gerodorm. $C_{18}H_{13}ClFN_3O_2$; mol wt 357.77. C 60.43%, H 3.66%, Cl 9.91%, F 5.31%, N 11.75%, O 8.94%. Prepn: L. H. Schlager, **DE 2950235**; *idem*, **US 4388313** (1980, 1983 both to Gerot). Benzodiazepine receptor affinity: W. Sieghart, A. Schuster, *Biochem. Pharmacol.* **33**, 4033 (1984). Polarographic and HPLC analyses:

H. Oelschläger *et al.*, *Arch. Pharm.* **325**, 65 (1992). Clinical pharmacokinetics: J. Grünberger *et al.*, *Adv. Ther.* **4**, 84 (1987). Clinical evaluation in insomnia: B. Saletu *et al.*, *Int. J. Clin. Pharmacol. Res.* **7**, 407 (1987).

Crystals from ethanol, mp 190-193°.

THERAP CAT: Sedative, hypnotic.

2309. Cinoxacin. [28657-80-9] 1-Ethyl-1,4-dihydro-4-oxo[1,3]dioxolo[4,5-*g*]cinnoline-3-carboxylic acid; 1-ethyl-6,7-methylenedioxy-4(1*H*)-oxocinnoline-3-carboxylic acid; compd 64716; Cinobac; Noxigram; Uronorm. $C_{12}H_{10}N_2O_5$; mol wt 262.22. C 54.96%, H 3.84%, N 10.68%, O 30.51%. Quinolone antibacterial; analog of oxolinic acid, *q.v.* Prepn: W. A. White, **DE 2005104**; *idem*, **US 3669965** (1970, 1972 both to Lilly). *In vitro* and *in vivo* study: W. E. Wick *et al.*, *Antimicrob. Agents Chemother.* **4**, 415 (1973). Pharmacology: J. J. Szwed *et al.*, *J. Antimicrob. Chemother.* **4**, 451 (1978); K. S. Israel *et al.*, *J. Clin. Pharmacol.* **18**, 491 (1978). Metabolism: R. L. Wolen *et al.* in *Stable Isotopes*, T. A. Baillie, Ed. (Univ. Park Press, Baltimore, 1978) pp 113-125. Clinical studies: S. Colleen *et al.*, *J. Antimicrob. Chemother.* **3**, 579 (1977); S. N. Rous, *J. Urol.* **120**, 196 (1978). Toxicity: I. Narama *et al.*, *Chemotherapy (Tokyo)* **28**, Suppl. 4, 406 (1980), *C.A.* **94**, 25007 (1981). Pharmacokinetics: M. Ohkawa *et al.*, *J. Antimicrob. Chemother.* **8**, 447 (1981); R. Barbhaiya *et al.*, *Antimicrob. Agents Chemother.* **21**, 472 (1982). *Review:* J. M. Scavone *et al.*, *Pharmacotherapy* **2**, 266-271 (1982). Review of pharmacology and therapeutic efficacy: T. S. Sisca *et al.*, *Drugs* **25**, 544-569 (1983).

Light tan crystals, mp 261-262° (dec). Sol in most polar organic solvents. LD_{50} in rats (mg/kg): 4160 orally; 900 i.v. (Narama).

Sodium salt. $C_{12}H_9N_2NaO_5$. White crystalline solid. Sol in aqueous solvents.

THERAP CAT: Antibacterial.

2310. Cinoxate. [104-28-9] 3-(4-Methoxyphenyl)-2-propenoic acid 2-ethoxyethyl ester; *p*-methoxycinnamic acid 2-ethoxyethyl ester; 2-ethoxyethyl *p*-methoxycinnamate; Give-Tan; Sun-Dare. $C_{14}H_{18}O_4$; mol wt 250.29. C 67.18%, H 7.25%, O 25.57%. Prepn: **GB 856411** (1960 to Givaudan).

(E)-form

Viscous liq; bp_2 184-187°. May have a slightly yellow tinge. Practically odorless. Solidifies below −25°. d_{25}^{25} 1.102. n_D^{20} 1.5670. Sapon no. 225.5. Practically insol in water (soly ~0.05%). Soly in glycerol 0.5%, in propylene glycol 5.0%. Miscible with alcohols, esters, vegetable oils.

THERAP CAT: Ultraviolet screen.

2311. Cinromide. [58473-74-8] (2*E*)-3-(3-Bromophenyl)-*N*-ethyl-2-propenamide; *trans*-3-bromo-*N*-ethylcinnamamide; BW-122U; Vumide. $C_{11}H_{12}BrNO$; mol wt 254.12. C 51.99%, H 4.76%, Br 31.44%, N 5.51%, O 6.30%. Cinnamic acid derivative with anti-epileptic activity. Prepn: E. M. Grivsky, **DE 2535599**; *idem*, **US 4041071** (1976, 1977 to Burroughs Wellcome). Pharmacology: F. E. Soroko *et al.*, *J. Pharm. Pharmacol.* **33**, 741 (1981); G. H. Fromm *et al.*, *Epilepsia* **24**, 394 (1983). Pharmacokinetics and metabolism: R. R. Maddox, B. B. Wannamaker, *Curr. Ther. Res.* **32**, 165 (1982). Mass spec determn in plasma and urine: R. J. Perchalski *et al.*, *Anal. Chem.* **54**, 1466 (1982). Controlled clinical trials: J. W. Allen *et al.*, *Epilepsia* **24**, 422 (1983); B. Spilker *et al.*, *Curr. Ther. Res.* **34**, 7 (1983).

Crystals from ethanol-water, mp 89-90°. LD_{50} in mice (mg/kg): 660 ±28 i.p.; 2277 ±250 orally (Soroko).

THERAP CAT: Anticonvulsant.

2312. Cintredekin Besudotox. [372075-36-0] Toxin hIL13-PE38QQR (plasmid phuIL13-Tx); IL-13PE38. Recombinant chimeric protein consisting of human interleukin 13 (IL-13) fused to a truncated form of *Pseudomonas* exotoxin A, PE38QQR; designed to target human epithelial carcinomas bearing the IL-13 receptor. Prepn: W. Debinski *et al.*, *J. Biol. Chem.* **270**, 16775 (1995); R. K. Puri *et al.*, **WO 9629417**; *idem*, **US 5919456** (1996, 1999 both to U.S. Dept. Health Human Serv.). Review of pharmacology: S. R. Husain, R. K. Puri, *J. Neuro-Oncol.* **65**, 37-48 (2003). Molecular mode of action study and gene expression profile: J. Han *et al.*, *ibid.* **72**, 35 (2005). Review of clinical experience in malignant glioma: N. G. Rainov, A. Söling, *Curr. Opin. Mol. Ther.* **7**, 170-181 (2005).

THERAP CAT: Antineoplastic.

2313. Ciprofibrate. [52214-84-3] 2-[4-(2,2-Dichlorocyclopropyl)phenoxy]-2-methylpropanoic acid; 2-[4-(2,2-dichlorocyclopropyl)phenoxy]isobutyric acid; Win-35833; Ciprol; Lipanor; Modalim. $C_{13}H_{14}Cl_2O_3$; mol wt 289.15. C 54.00%, H 4.88%, Cl 24.52%, O 16.60%. Hypolipemic agent, related structurally to clofibrate, *q.v.* Prepn: D. K. Phillips, **DE 2343606**; *idem*, **US 3948973** (1974, 1976 both to Sterling). Pharmacokinetics in animals and man: C. Davison *et al.*, *Drug Metab. Dispos.* **3**, 520 (1975). Inhibition of cholesterol biosynthesis in rats: A. Arnold *et al.*, *Atherosclerosis* **32**, 155 (1979). Blood levels, distribution, duration of action: J. Edelson *et al.*, *ibid.* **33**, 351 (1979). Metabolic effects: A. Arnold *et al.*, *J. Pharm. Sci.* **68**, 1557 (1979). Teratology study: H. Tuchman-Duplessis *et al.*, *Toxicology* **12**, 1 (1979).

Pale cream solid from hexane, mp 114-116°.

THERAP CAT: Antilipemic.

2314. Ciprofloxacin. [85721-33-1] 1-Cyclopropyl-6-fluoro-1,4-dihydro-4-oxo-7-(1-piperazinyl)-3-quinolinecarboxylic acid; Bay q 3939. $C_{17}H_{18}FN_3O_3$; mol wt 331.34. C 61.62%, H 5.48%, F 5.73%, N 12.68%, O 14.49%. Fluorinated quinolone antibacterial. Prepn: K. Grohe *et al.*, **DE 3142854**; *idem*, **US 4670444** (1983, 1987 both to Bayer AG); K. Grohe, H. Heitzer, *Ann.* **1987**, 29. Antibacterial spectrum *in vitro*: B. Watt, F. V. Brown, *J. Antimicrob. Chemother.* **17**, 605 (1986); C. M. Bassey *et al.*, *ibid.* 623. HPLC determn in biological fluids: W. Gau *et al.*, *J. Liq. Chromatogr.* **8**, 485 (1985). Pharmacokinetics: G. Hoffken *et al.*, *Antimicrob. Agents Chemother.* **27**, 375 (1985). Clinical trials: C. A. Ramirez *et al.*, *ibid.* **28**, 128 (1985); B. E. Scully *et al.*, *Lancet* **1**,

819 (1986). Symposia on antibacterial spectrum and clinical use: *Am. J. Med.* **82**, Suppl. 4A, 1-404 (1987); *J. Antimicrob. Chemother.* **26**, Suppl. F, 3-193 (1990). Review of clinical safety and efficacy in children: R. Kubin, *Infection* **21**, 413-421 (1993).

Dec 255-257°.

Monohydrochloride monohydrate. [86393-32-0] Bay o 9867; Baycip; Ciflox; Ciloxan; Cipro; Ciprobay; Ciproxan; Ciproxin; Flociprin; Septicide; Uniflox; Velmonit. C_{17}H_{18}FN_3O_3·HCl·H_2O; mol wt 385.82. Light yellow crystalline powder. mp 318-320°.

THERAP CAT: Antibacterial.

2315. Circulins. Polypeptide antibiotics related to polymyxins. Produced by *Bacillus circulans,* a microorganism found in soil and dust: Murray, Tetrault, *Proc. Soc. Am. Bact.* **1**, 20 (1948); McLeod, *J. Bacteriol.* **56**, 749 (1948); Murray *et al., ibid.* **57**, 305 (1949). Isoln yields circulins A and B, circulin A being the major component: Tetrault, **US 2676133** (1954 to Purdue Res. Found.). *Review:* Vogner, Studer, *Experientia* **22**, 345 (1966).

DAB = α,γ-diaminobutyric acid

Circulin A   R = (+)-6-methyloctanoyl
Circulin B   R = isooctanoyl

Circulin A. C_{53}H_{100}N_{16}O_{13}; mol wt 1169.46. Structure: Fujikawa *et al., Experientia* **21**, 307 (1965). Synthesis: Studer *et al., Helv. Chim. Acta* **49**, 974 (1966).

Sulfate. C_{53}H_{100}N_{16}O_{13}·2½H_2SO_4. Crystals or amorphous solid, dec 226-228°. $[\alpha]_D^{25}$ -61.6° (c = 1.25). Sol in water; less sol in the lower alcs. Practically insol in acetone and water-immiscible solvents.

Circulin B. C_{52}H_{98}N_{16}O_{13}; mol wt 1155.43. Structure: Hayashi *et al., Experientia* **24**, 656 (1968).

2316. Cisapride. [81098-60-4] *cis*-4-Amino-5-chloro-*N*-[1-[3-(4-fluorophenoxy)propyl]-3-methoxy-4-piperidinyl]-2-methoxybenzamide; *cis*-4-amino-5-chloro-*N*-[1-[3-(*p*-fluorophenoxy)propyl]-3-methoxy-4-piperidinyl]-*o*-anisamide. C_{23}H_{29}ClFN_3O_4; mol wt 465.95. C 59.29%, H 6.27%, Cl 7.61%, F 4.08%, N 9.02%, O 13.73%. Serotonin 5-HT_4 receptor agonist. Prepn: G. Van Daele, **EP 76530**; *idem,* **US 4962115** (1983, 1990 both to Janssen); and pharmacology: *idem et al., Drug Dev. Res.* **8**, 225 (1986). Pharmacokinetics: J. A. Barone *et al., Clin. Pharm.* **6**, 640 (1987). Review of pharmacology and therapeutic efficacy: L. R. Wiseman, D. Faulds, *Drugs* **47**, 116-152 (1994).

Monohydrate. R-51619; Acenalin; Alimix; Cipril; Prepulsid; Propulsid; Risamol. C_{23}H_{29}ClFN_3O_4·H_2O; mol wt 483.96. Crystals from 2-propanol, mp 109.8°. Sol in acetone. Sparingly sol in methanol. Practically insol in water.

THERAP CAT: Gastroprokinetic.

2317. Cisplatin. [15663-27-1] (*SP*-4-2)-Diamminedichloroplatinum; *cis*-diamminedichloroplatinum; *cis*-platinum II; *cis*-DDP; CACP; CPDC; DDP; NSC-119875; Briplatin; Cismaplat; Cisplatyl; Citoplatino; Lederplatin; Neoplatin; Platamine; Platinex; Platiblastin; Platinol; Platinoxan; Platistin; Platosin; Randa. Cl_2-H_6N_2Pt; mol wt 300.05. Cl 23.63%, H 2.02%, N 9.34%, Pt 65.02%. Prepn: M. Peyrone, *Ann.* **51**, 1 (1845); G. B. Kauffman, D. O. Cowan, *Inorg. Synth.* **7**, 239 (1963); S. C. Dhara, *Indian J. Chem.* **8**, 193 (1970). Originally known as **Peyrone's salt** or **Peyrone's chloride**, it was primarily of interest in the development of coordination theory. Early structural studies: R. Werner, *Z. Anorg. Chem.* **3**, 267 (1893); H. D. K. Drew *et al., J. Chem. Soc.* **1932**, 988. Discovery of anti-tumor activity: B. Rosenberg *et al., Nature* **205**, 698 (1965); **222**, 385 (1972). Use as neoplasm inhibitor: M. L. Tobe *et al.,* **DE 2318020** (1972 to Rustenburg Platinum Mines Ltd.), *C.A.* **80**, 55897e (1974); M. J. Cleare *et al.,* **DE 2329485** (1972 to Research Corp.), *C.A.* **81**, 21172v (1974). Mechanism of action: J. J. Roberts, J. M. Pascoe, *Nature* **235**, 282 (1972); A. Khan, J. M. Hill, *Transplant* **13**, 55 (1972); G. L. Cohen *et al., Science* **203**, 1014 (1979). X-ray structure of cisplatin-DNA adduct: S. E. Sherman *et al., Science* **230**, 412 (1985). Inhibition of *in vitro* DNA synthesis: A. L. Pinto, S. J. Lippard, *Proc. Natl. Acad. Sci. USA* **82**, 4616 (1985). Pharmacology: A. Sirica *et al., Proc. Am. Assoc. Cancer Res.* **12**, 4 (1971); C. L. Litterst *et al., Cancer Res.* **36**, 2340 (1976); N. P. Johnson *et al., Chem. Biol. Interact.* **23**, 267 (1978). Metabolism: R. C. Lange *et al., J. Nucl. Med.* **14**, 191 (1973). Clinical studies: J. J. Ochs *et al., Cancer Treat. Rep.* **62**, 239 (1978); H. M. Pinedo *et al., Eur. J. Cancer* **14**, 1149 (1978). Cisplatin has been shown to have trypanocidal effects: M. S. Wysor *et al., Science* **217**, 454 (1982). Toxicology: R. L. Dixon, *Proc. 7th Int. Congr. Chemother.* **Vol. 2** (University Park Press, Baltimore, 1972) pp 241-243; R. W. Fleishman *et al., Toxicol. Appl. Pharmacol.* **33**, 320 (1975). *Reviews:* D. D. Von Hoff, M. Rozencweig in *Advances in Pharmacology and Chemotherapy* vol. 16, S. Garattini *et al.,* Eds. (Academic Press, New York, 1979) pp 273-294; S. J. Lippard, *Science* **218**, 1075-1082 (1982). Review of carcinogenicity studies: *IARC Monographs* **26**, 154-161 (1981); of neurotoxicity: R. J. Cersosimo, *Cancer Treat. Rev.* **16**, 195-211 (1989). Comprehensive description: C. M. Riley, L. M. Sternson, *Anal. Profiles Drug Subs.* **14**, 77-105 (1985). Book: *Cisplatin, Current Status and New Developments,* A. W. Prestayko *et al.,* Eds. (Academic Press, New York, 1980) 527 pp.

Deep yellow solid, dec 270°. Soly in water 0.253 g/100 g at 25°; slowly changes to *trans*-form in aq soln. Insol in most common solvents. Sol in DMF. LD_{50} in guinea pigs: 9.7 mg/kg i.p. (Fleishman).

Caution: This substance is reasonably anticipated to be a human carcinogen: *Report on Carcinogens, Eleventh Edition* (PB2005-104914, 2004) p III-67.

THERAP CAT: Antineoplastic.

2318. Citalopram. [59729-33-8] 1-[3-(Dimethylamino)propyl]-1-(4-fluorophenyl)-1,3-dihydro-5-isobenzofurancarbonitrile; 1-[3-(dimethylamino)propyl]-1-(4-fluorophenyl)-5-phthalancarbonitrile; nitalapram; Lu-10-171. C_{20}H_{21}FN_2O; mol wt 324.39. C 74.05%, H 6.53%, F 5.86%, N 8.64%, O 4.93%. Selective serotonin reuptake inhibitor (SSRI). Prepn: K. P. Boegesoe, A. S. Toft, **DE 2657013**; *idem,* **US 4136193** (1977, 1979 both to Kefalas); A. J. Bigler *et al., Eur. J. Med. Chem. - Chim. Ther.* **12**, 289 (1977). Prepn of enantiomers: K. P. Boegesoe, J. Perregaard, **EP 347066**; *idem,* **US 4943590**, reissued as **US RE 34712** (1989, 1990, 1994 all to Lundbeck). Pharmacology: A. V. Christensen *et al., Eur. J. Pharmacol.* **41**, 153 (1977). HPLC determn in plasma and urine: E. Oyehaug *et al., J. Chromatogr.* **308**, 199 (1984). Comparative biotransformation of enantiomers: L. L. Von Moltke *et al., Drug Metab. Dispos.* **29**, 1102 (2001). Review of clinical pharmacokinetics: K. Brosen, C. A. Naranjo, *Eur. Neuropsychopharmacol.* **11**, 275-283 (2001). Review of clinical experience in depression: M. B. Keller, *J. Clin. Psychiatry* **61**, 896-908 (2000). Clinical trial of *S*-form in depression: W. J. Burke *et al., ibid.* **63**, 331 (2002).

bp$_{0.03}$ 175-181°.

Hydrobromide. [59729-32-7] Celexa; Cipramil; Elopram; Seropram. $C_{20}H_{21}FN_2O\cdot HBr$; mol wt 405.30. Crystals from isopropanol, mp 182-183°.

S-(+)-Form. [128196-01-0] Escitalopram. $[\alpha]_D$ +12.33° (c = 1 in methanol).

Escitalopram oxalate. [219861-08-2] Lu-26-054-0; Cipralex; Gaudium; Lexapro. $C_{20}H_{21}FN_2O\cdot C_2H_2O_4$; mol wt 414.43. Fine white to slightly yellow powder. Crystals from acetone, mp 147-148°. $[\alpha]_D$ +12.31° (c = 1 in methanol). Freely sol in methanol, DMSO; sol in isotonic saline; sparingly sol in water, ethanol; slightly sol in ethyl acetate. Insol in heptane.

THERAP CAT: Antidepressant.

2319. Citicoline. [987-78-0] Cytidine 5'-(trihydrogen diphosphate) P'-[2-(trimethylammonio)ethyl] ester inner salt; choline cytidine 5'-pyrophosphate (ester); cytidine diphosphate choline ester; CDP-choline; Difosfocin; Nicholin; Recognan; Rexort; Somazina. $C_{14}H_{26}N_4O_{11}P_2$; mol wt 488.32. C 34.43%, H 5.37%, N 11.47%, O 36.04%, P 12.69%. Naturally occurring nucleotide; intermediate in the major pathway of lecithin biosynthesis. Identification: E. P. Kennedy, S. B. Weiss, *J. Am. Chem. Soc.* **77**, 250 (1955). Crystallization from yeast extract: I. Lieberman *et al., Science* **124**, 81 (1956). Synthesis: E. P. Kennedy, *J. Biol. Chem.* **222**, 185 (1956); K. Kikugawa *et al., Chem. Pharm. Bull.* **19**, 1011, 2466 (1971). Molecular structure: M. A. Viswamitra *et al., Nature* **258**, 497 (1975). Series of articles on pharmacology and toxicology: *Arzneim.-Forsch.* **33**, 1009-1080 (1983). Acute toxicity: T. Grau *et al., ibid.* 1033. Clinical trial in ischemic stroke: W. M. Clark *et al., Neurology* **49**, 671 (1997). Review of biosynthesis, metabolism, pharmacology: G. B. Weiss, *Life Sci.* **56**, 637-660 (1995); and clinical experience: J. J. Secades, G. Frontera, *Methods Find. Exp. Clin. Pharmacol.* **17**, Suppl. B, 1-54 (1995).

Amorphous, somewhat hygroscopic powder. $[\alpha]_D^{25}$ +19.0° (c = 0.86 in H_2O). uv max (pH 1): 280 nm (ε 12800). Dissolves readily in water to form acidic soln. Practically insol in most organic solvents. pKa 4.4. LD$_{50}$ in mice, rats (mg/kg): 4600 ±335, 4150 ±370 i.v.; both species 8 g/kg orally (Grau).

Sodium salt. [33818-15-4] Acticolin; Brassel; Ceraxon; Neuroton; Sintoclar. $C_{14}H_{25}N_4NaO_{11}P_2$; mol wt 510.31. White, crystalline, spongy, hygrosopic powder, dec 250°. $[\alpha]_D^{20}$ +12.5° (c = 1.0 in H_2O). Sol in water. Practically insol in alcohol.

THERAP CAT: Neuroprotective. In treatment of ischemic stroke and head trauma.

2320. Citiolone. [1195-16-0] 2-Acetamido-4-mercaptobutyric acid γ-thiolactone; *N*-(tetrahydro-2-oxo-3-thienyl)-

acetamide; *N*-acetylhomocysteinethiolactone; α-acetamido-γ-thiobutyrolactone; AHCTL; BO-714; Citiolase. $C_6H_9NO_2S$; mol wt 159.21. C 45.26%, H 5.70%, N 8.80%, O 20.10%, S 20.14%. Prepn: Wagner *et al.,* **DE 1134683** (1962 to Degussa, vorm Roessler), *C.A.* **58**, 4648c (1963); Nakanishi *et al.,* **JP 62 16712** (1962 to Yoshitomi), *C.A.* **59**, 11660h (1963); Takayananagi *et al.,* **JP 64 3420**, *C.A.* **61**, 3193h (1964); Ogino, Yasui, **JP 65 1376**, *C.A.* **62**, 14822c (1965) (1964, 1965 both to Sumitomo). Chemistry: Benesch, Benesch, *J. Am. Chem. Soc.* **78**, 1597 (1956); Laliberté *et al., J. Chem. Soc.* **1963**, 2756. Pharmacology: E. -J. Kirnberger *et al., Arzneim.-Forsch.* **8**, 72 (1958); Varga *et al., ibid.* **13**, 1867 (1963).

Needles from toluene, mp 111.5-112.5°. uv max: 238 nm (ε 4400). LD$_{50}$ i.v. in mice: 1200 mg/kg (Kirnberger).

USE: Photographic antifogging agent: Dersch, **US 3068100** (1962); Weber, **DE 1164828** (1964 to Adox Fotowerke Schleussner GmbH), *C.A.* **60**, 14050f (1964); protector against radiation: Langendorff, Koch, *Strahlentherapie* **106**, 451 (1958); Braun *et al., ibid.* **108**, 262 (1959), *C.A.* **52**, 18841h (1958); **53**, 17325e (1959).

THERAP CAT: In treatment of hepatic disorders.

2321. Citraconic Acid. [498-23-7] (*Z*)-2-Methyl-2-butenedioic acid; methylmaleic acid. $C_5H_6O_4$; mol wt 130.10. C 46.16%, H 4.65%, O 49.19%. Obtained by carefully heating citric acid at about 175°. Production of citraconic anhydride from itaconic acid: Humphrey, **US 2966498** (1960 to Pfizer). Toxicity study: P. M. Jenner *et al., Food Cosmet. Toxicol.* **2**, 327 (1964).

Hygroscopic monoclinic crystals; characteristic odor. d 1.62. mp ~90° (dec). Freely sol in water, alc, ether, slightly in chloroform. Practically insol in benzene, petr ether. LD$_{50}$ in rats, mice (mg/kg): 1320, 2260 orally (Jenner).

2322. Citral. [5392-40-5] 3,7-Dimethyl-2,6-octadienal. $C_{10}H_{16}O$; mol wt 152.23. C 78.90%, H 10.59%, O 10.51%. Constituent of many commercial oils such as lemon grass, verbena, lemon, and orange. Citral from natural sources is a 2:1 mixture of two geometric isomers geranial and neral. Isoln from lemongrass: F. W. Semmler, *Ber.* **23**, 2965 (1890); F. D. Dodge, *Am. Chem. J.* **12**, 553 (1890). Separation of isomers: Y. R. Naves, *Bull. Soc. Chim. Fr.* **1952**, 521. IR determn in lemon and orange oils: P. L. Mahia *et al., Food Chem.* **46**, 193 (1993). Stability in food emulsions and beverages: E. J. Freeburg *et al., Perfum. Flavor.* **19**(4), 23 (1994). Review of toxicity: D. L. J. Opdyke, *Food Cosmet. Toxicol.* **17**, 259-266 (1979); of reaction chemistry: R. K. Baslas, B. Gupta, *Indian Perfum.* **32**, 266-272 (1988). Comprehensive reviews: J. L. Simonsen, *The Terpenes* vol. I, 83-100 (1947); P. Z. Bedoukian, *Perfumery and Flavoring Synthetics* (Allured Publishing Corporation, Wheaton, IL, 3rd ed., 1986) pp 106-117.

Geranial   Neral

Mobile pale yellow liquid having a strong lemon-like odor. d$_{25}^{25}$ 0.885-0.891. n_D^{20} 1.4860-1.4900. Flash point: 99.5°C (208°F). LD$_{50}$ orally in rats: 4.96 g/kg (Opdyke).

Geranial. [141-27-5] Trans-citral; citral a. Light oily liquid with strong lemon odor. bp$_{2.6}$ 92-93°. d$_4^{20}$ 0.8888. n_D^{20} 1.4898.

Practically insol in water. Miscible with alc, ether, benzyl benzoate, diethyl phthalate, glycerol, propylene glycol, mineral oil, essential oils.

Neral. [106-26-3] *cis*-Citral; citral b. Light oily liquid with a lemon odor not as intense but sweeter than gerianal. $bp_{2.6}$ 91-92°. d_4^{20} 0.8860. n_D^{20} 1.4869. Solubilities same as gerianal.

USE: In the synthesis of vitamin A, ionone and methylionone. As a flavor and in perfumery for its citrus effect.

2323. Citramalic Acid. [2306-22-1] 2-Hydroxy-2-methyl-butanedioic acid; 2-methylmalic acid; 2-hydroxy-2-methylsuccinic acid; α-hydroxypyrotartaric acid. $C_5H_8O_5$; mol wt 148.11. C 40.55%, H 5.44%, O 54.01%. Enzymatic synthesis: Barker, Blair, *Biochem. Prep.* **9**, 21 (1962). Chemical synthesis: Barker, *ibid.* 25; J. B. Wilkes, R. G. Wall, *J. Org. Chem.* **45**, 247 (1980). Stereoselective synthesis: E. G. J. Staring *et al., Rec. Trav. Chim.* **105**, 374 (1986).

dl-**Form.** Deliquescent monoclinic prisms from ethyl acetate + petr ether, mp 117°. Sublimes. Freely sol in water, acetone. Sol in ethyl acetate, ether. Practically insol in petr ether, benzene.

d-**Form.** Crystals, mp 112.2-112.8°. $[\alpha]_D^{22}$ +23.6° (c = 3 in H_2O).

l-**Form.** Crystals, mp 112-113°. $[\alpha]_D^{20}$ −23.4° (c = 3 in H_2O).

2324. β-Citraurin. [650-69-1] 3-Hydroxy-8'-apo-β,ψ-carotenal; citraurin. $C_{30}H_{40}O_2$; mol wt 432.64. C 83.28%, H 9.32%, O 7.40%. Carotenoid pigment found only in orange peel. Isoln by chromatography: Zechmeister, Tuzson, *Ber.* **69**, 1878 (1936); **70**, 1966 (1937). The peels from 100 kilos of oranges yield about 35 mg. Structure: Zechmeister, Tuzson, *loc. cit.;* Karrer, Solmssen, *Helv. Chim. Acta* **20**, 682 (1937); Karrer *et al., ibid.* 1020; Zechmeister, v. Cholnoky, *Ann.* **530**, 291 (1937); Karrer *et al., Helv. Chim. Acta* **21**, 445 (1938). Abs config: Bartlett *et al., J. Chem. Soc. C* **1969**, 2527. Synthesis: H. Pfander *et al., Helv. Chim. Acta* **63**, 1377 (1980).

Thin orange or yellow-colored plates from benzene + petr ether, mp 147°. Absorption max (benzene): 497, 467 nm. Freely sol in acetone, ethanol, ether, benzene, and carbon disulfide. Sparingly sol in petr ether.

2325. Citrazinic Acid. [99-11-6] 1,2-Dihydro-6-hydroxy-2-oxo-4-pyridinecarboxylic acid; 2,6-dihydroxyisonicotinic acid; 2,6-dihydroxy-4-pyridinecarboxylic acid. $C_6H_5NO_4$; mol wt 155.11. C 46.46%, H 3.25%, N 9.03%, O 41.26%. Prepn from citric acid with aq NH_3 at 140-160° under pressure: Bavley, Hamilton, US 2729647 (1956 to Pfizer). Purification: Bavley *et al.,* US 2738352 (1956 to Pfizer).

Yellowish powder with a greenish tinge; carbonizes above 300° without melting. Ultrapure material which is white or colorless, has been prepared. Almost insol in water; slightly sol in hot HCl; sol in alkali hydroxide or carbonate solns. Alkaline solns turn blue on standing.

2326. Citric Acid. [77-92-9] 2-Hydroxy-1,2,3-propanetricarboxylic acid; β-hydroxytricarballylic acid. $C_6H_8O_7$; mol wt 192.12. C 37.51%, H 4.20%, O 58.29%. Widely distributed in plants and in animal tissues and fluids. Produced by mycological fermentation on an industrial scale using crude sugar solns, such as molasses and strains of *Aspergillus niger: See* review by Von Loesecke, *Chem. Eng. News* **23**, 1952 (1945); Schweiger, US

2970084 (1961 to Miles Labs.); *Faith, Keyes & Clark's Industrial Chemicals*, F. A. Lowenheim, M. K. Moran, Eds. (Wiley-Interscience, New York, 4th ed., 1975) pp 275-279. Also extracted from citrus fruits (lemon juice contains 5 to 8%) and from pineapple waste. *Reviews:* Wilson, *Chem. Metall. Eng.* **29**, 787 (1923); Browne, *Ind. Eng. Chem.* **13**, 81 (1921); Warneford, Hardy, *ibid.* **17**, 1283 (1925); E. F. Bouchard, E. G. Merritt in *Kirk-Othmer Encyclopedia of Chemical Technology* vol. 6 (Wiley-Interscience, New York, 3rd ed., 1979) pp 150-179. Toxicity: C. M. Gruber, Jr., W. A. Halbeisen, *J. Pharmacol. Exp. Ther.* **94**, 65 (1948).

Anhydr form, mp 153°. Crystals are monoclinic holohedra and crystallize from hot concd aq soln. d 1.665. At 25°, pK_1 3.128; pK_2 4.761; pK_3 6.396, Bates, Pinching, *J. Am. Chem. Soc.* **71**, 1274 (1949). Soly in water: 54.0% w/w at 10°; 59.2% at 20°; 64.3% at 30°; 68.6% at 40°; 70.9% at 50°; 73.5% at 60°; 76.2% at 70°; 78.8% at 80°; 81.4% at 90°; 84.0% at 100°. LD_{50} in mice, rats (mmol/kg): 5.0, 4.6 i.p. (Gruber, Halbeisen).

Monohydrate. Orthorhombic crystals from cold aq solns. Pleasant, sour taste. d 1.542. Monohydrate crystals lose water of crystn in dry air or when heated at about 40 to 50°, slightly deliquescent in moist air. Softens at 75°. mp ~100°. pH of 0.1N soln = 2.2. Densities of aqueous soln (15°/15°): 10% = 1.0392; 20% = 1.0805; 30% = 1.1244; 40% = 1.1709; 50% = 1.2204; 60% = 1.2738. Soly in g/100 g satd soln: ether 2.17; chloroform 0.007; amyl alcohol 15.43; amyl acetate 5.98; ethyl acetate 5.28. Soly at 19° in g/100 g solvent: methanol 197; propanol 62.8.

Barium salt heptahydrate. Barium citrate. $C_{12}H_{10}Ba_3O_{14}$.-7H_2O. Powder. Loses all H_2O at 150°. Sol in 1750 parts water; freely sol in dil HCl or HNO_3; practically insol in alcohol.

Ethyl ester. Ethyl citrate; triethyl citrate. $C_{12}H_{20}O_7$. Bitter, oily liq. d^{20} 1.137. bp_{760} 294°; $bp_{1.0}$ 127°. Viscosity at 25°: 35.2 cP. Pour pt ~10°. n_D^{20} 1.4455. Soly: water ~6.9%; peanut oil 0.8%. Misc with alc, ether.

Disodium salt. [144-33-2] Disodium hydrogen citrate; sodium acid citrate; Alkacitron. $C_6H_6Na_2O_7$; mol wt 236.09. White powder, saline taste. One gram of sesquihydrate dissolves in slightly less than 2 ml water; pH of a 3% w/v soln in water: 4.9 to 5.2. LD_{50} in mice, rats (mmol/kg): 7.5, 7.3 i.p. (Gruber, Halbeisen).

Trisodium salt. *See* Sodium Citrate.

USE: Anticoagulant, generally in solution with glucose, to prevent the clotting of blood intended for transfusion. Acidulant in beverages, confectionery, effervescent salts, in pharmaceutical syrups, elixirs, in effervescent powders and tablets, to adjust the pH of foods and as synergistic antioxidant, in processing cheese. Used in beverages, jellies, jams, preserves and candy to provide tartness. In the manuf of alkyd resins; in esterified form as plasticizer, foam inhibitor. In the manuf of citric acid salts. As sequestering agent to remove trace metals. As mordant to brighten colors; in electroplating; in special inks; in analytical chemistry for determining citrate-soluble P_2O_5; as reagent for albumin, mucin, glucose, bile pigments.

2327. Citrinin. [518-75-2] (3R,4S)-4,6-Dihydro-8-hydroxy-3,4,5-trimethyl-6-oxo-3H-2-benzopyran-7-carboxylic acid; Antimycin. $C_{13}H_{14}O_5$; mol wt 250.25. C 62.39%, H 5.64%, O 31.97%. Antibiotic substance produced by a white spore aspergillus which has been placed under the species name *Aspergillus niveus* (Thorn and Raper). Also produced in small quantities by *Penicillium citrinum*: Hetherington, Raistrick, *Trans. R. Soc. London* **B220**, 269 (1931); Raistrick, Smith, *Chem. Ind. (London)* **60**, 828 (1941); Timonin, *Science* **96**, 494 (1942); Timonin, Rovatt, *Can. J. Public Health* **35**, 80 (1944). Identity with antimycin: Haese, *Arch. Pharm.* **296**, 227 (1963). Structure: Brown *et al., J. Chem. Soc.* **1949**, 867; Warren *et al., J. Am. Chem. Soc.* **79**, 3812 (1957); Kovac *et al., Nature* **190**, 1104 (1961). Synthesis: Cartwright *et al., J. Chem. Soc.* **1949**, 1563; J. A. Barber *et al., J. Chem. Soc. Perkin Trans. 1* **1986**, 2101. Stereochemistry: Cram, *J. Am. Chem. Soc.* **72**, 1001 (1950); Mehta, Whalley, *J. Chem. Soc.* **1963**, 3777; Mathieson, Whalley, *ibid.* **1964**, 4640. Physical characteristics and toxicity: Nagai *et al.*, *Chem. Zentralbl.* **1958**, 8088, *C.A.* **55**, 1914 (1961). Crystal and molecular structure: Rodig, *Chem. Commun.* **1971**, 1553. Biosynthesis: J. Barber *et al.*, *J. Chem. Soc. Perkin Trans. 1* **1981**, 2577; L. Colombo *et al.*, *ibid.* 2594. Physicochemical data: A. E. Pohland *et al.*, *Pure Appl. Chem.* **54**, 2219 (1982). Toxicology: A. M. Ambrose, F. De Eds, *J. Pharmacol. Exp. Ther.* **88**, 173 (1946). *Review:* Saito *et al.*, "Yellowed Rice Toxins" in *Microbial Toxins* vol. **VI**, A. Ciegler, S. Kadis, A. Ajl, Eds. (Academic Press, New York, 1971) pp 357-367.

Lemon-yellow needles from alcohol, dec 175°. $[\alpha]_D^{18}$ −37.4° (c = 1.15 in alc.). uv max: 250, 331 nm ($E_{1cm}^{1\%}$ 370, 418). Strong acid. Practically insol in water. Sol in alcohol, dioxane, dilute alkali. Solns change color with changes in pH, from lemon-yellow at pH 4.6 to cherry-red at pH 9.9. *Poisonous!* LD_{50} in mice, rats (mg/kg): 35, 67 i.p. (Ambrose, De Eds).

Methyl citrinin. $C_{14}H_{16}O_5$. Plates from benzene, dec 139°. $[\alpha]_D^{18}$ +217.1° (c = 0.38 in acetone). uv max: 260, 334 nm ($E_{1cm}^{1\%}$ 520, 151.6). Sol in hot alcohol; moderately sol in chloroform. Practically insol in petr ether.

Dihydrocitrinin. $C_{13}H_{16}O_5$. Prisms from benzene, dec 171°. $[\alpha]_D^{18}$ −18.8° (c = 4.148 in chloroform). uv max: 260, 330 nm ($E_{1cm}^{1\%}$ 400, 100). Sol in alcohol, acetone, chloroform; sparingly sol in benzene, petr ether.

2328. Citromycetin. [478-60-6] 8,9-Dihydroxy-2-methyl-4-oxo-4*H*,5*H*-pyrano[3,2-*c*][1]benzopyran-10-carboxylic acid; frequentic acid. $C_{14}H_{10}O_7$; mol wt 290.23. C 57.94%, H 3.47%, O 38.59%. Antibiotic substance produced by *Penicillium frequentans* Westling and *P. vesiculosum* Bainier and by *Citromyces* spp: Hetherington, Raistrick, *Philos. Trans. R. Soc. London Ser. B* **220**, 209 (1931); Grove, Brian, *Nature* **167**, 995 (1951). Structure: Robertson *et al.*, *J. Chem. Soc.* **1951**, 2013. Biosynthesis: Birch *et al.*, *ibid.* **1958**, 4576; Money, *Nature* **199**, 592 (1963). Total synthesis: M. Yamauchi *et al.*, *J. Chem. Soc. Perkin Trans. 1* **1987**, 395.

Dihydrate. Yellow crystals, effervescence at 155°, dec 290-300° (considerable antecedent blackening). Freely sol in ethanol; readily sol in aq sodium carbonate soln; sparingly sol in water, chloroform. Insol in benzene, hexane. Stable to acid and alkali at 100°.

2329. Citronellal. [106-23-0] 3,7-Dimethyl-6-octenal. $C_{10}H_{18}O$; mol wt 154.25. C 77.87%, H 11.76%, O 10.37%. Chief constituent of citronella oil; also found in many other volatile oils, such as lemon, lemon grass, melissa: Tiemann, *Ber.* **32**, 834 (1899); Spoon, *Chem. Weekbl.* **54**, 236 (1958). Structure: Naves, *Bull. Soc. Chim. Fr.* **1951**, 505; Eschinazi, *J. Org. Chem.* **26**, 3072 (1961).

Liquid. bp_1 47°. n_D^{20} 1.4460. $[\alpha]_D^{25}$ +11.50°. d 0.848-0.856. Soluble in alcohols; very slightly sol in water.

α-citronellal. [141-26-4] 3,7-Dimethyl-7-octenal; rhodinal. Liquid. $bp_{1.4}$ 51°. n_D^{20} 1.4410. $[\alpha]_D^{20}$ +9.75°.

USE: In soap perfumes; insect repellent.

2330. β-Citronellol. [106-22-9] 3,7-Dimethyl-6-octen-1-ol; 2,6-dimethyl-2-octen-8-ol; citronellol; cephrol. $C_{10}H_{20}O$; mol wt 156.27. C 76.86%, H 12.90%, O 10.24%. *l*-Form is a constituent of rose and geranium oils. *d*-Form occurs in Ceylon and Java citronella oils. History: J. L. Simonsen, L. N. Owen, *The Terpenes* vol. **I** (University Press, Cambridge, 2nd ed, 1947). Prepn of (±)-form: Adams, Garvey, *J. Am. Chem. Soc.* **48**, 477 (1926); Ofner *et al.*, *Helv. Chim. Acta* **42**, 2577 (1959). Prepn of (+)-form: Rienäcker, Ohloff, *Angew. Chem.* **73**, 240 (1961); Naves, Tullen, *Helv. Chim. Acta* **44**, 1867 (1961); Eschinazi, *J. Org. Chem.* **26**, 3072 (1961); Rienäcker, *Chimia* **27**, 97 (1973); C. G. Overberger, J. L. Weise, *J. Am. Chem. Soc.* **90**, 3525 (1968); T. Sato *et al.*, *Tetrahedron Lett.* **1980**, 3377. Prepn of (−)-form: Ohloff, *loc. cit.*; Rienäcker, *loc. cit.*; Shono *et al.*, *Tetrahedron Lett.* **1974**, 1295; K. Mori, T. Sugai, *Synthesis* **1982**, 752. Synthesis of (+) or (−)-form from isoprene: Hidai *et al.*, *Chem. Commun.* **1975**, 170. Stereospecific prepn via microbiological (*Saccharomyces cerevisiae*) reduction: P. Gramatica *et al.*, *Experientia* **38**, 775 (1982). Manuf: Woroch *et al.*; Bain; Webb, **US 2990422**; **US 3005845**; **US 3028431** (1961, 1961, 1962, all to Glidden); Eschinasi, **US 3052730** (1962 to Givaudan). Abs config of the (+)-form: Freudenberg, Hohmann, *Ann.* **584**, 54 (1953); Freudenberg, Lwowski, *ibid.* **587**, 213 (1954). NMR, HPLC determn of *R/S* enantiomer ratios: D. Valentine *et al.*, *J. Org. Chem.* **41**, 62 (1976). *See also* Rhodinol.

R-(+)-β-Citronellol

(+)-**Form.** Oily liquid, bp 224.5°, bp_{10} 108.4°, d_4^{20} 0.8550. n_D^{20} 1.4559. $[\alpha]_D^{20}$ +5.22°. Very slightly sol in water, miscible with with alcohol, ether.

(−)-**Form.** β-Rhodinol; Levocitrol. bp_{10} 108-109°. d_4^{18} 1.4576. $[\alpha]_D^{20}$ −4.76°.

(±)-**Form.** Dihydrogeraniol. $d_4^{23.5}$ 0.851. $n_D^{23.5}$ 1.454.

USE: In perfumery.

2331. Citrulline. [372-75-8] N^5-(Aminocarbonyl)-L-ornithine; δ-ureidonorvaline; α-amino-δ-ureidovaleric acid; N^δ-carbamylornithine. $C_6H_{13}N_3O_3$; mol wt 175.19. C 41.13%, H 7.48%, N 23.99%, O 27.40%. $H_2NCONH(CH_2)_3CH(NH_2)COOH$. An amino acid, first isolated from the juice of watermelon, *Citrullus vulgaris* Schrad., *Cucurbitaceae:* Wada, *Biochem. Z.* **224**, 420 (1930); isoln from casein: Wada, *ibid.* **257**, 1 (1933). Synthesis from ornithine through copper complexes: Kurtz, *J. Biol. Chem.* **122**, 477 (1938); by alkaline hydrolysis of arginine: Fox, *ibid.* **123**, 687 (1938); from cyclopentanone oxime: Fox *et al.*, *J. Org. Chem.* **6**, 410 (1941). Crystallization: Matsuda *et al.*, **JP 71 174** (1971 to Ajinomoto), *C.A.* **74**, 126056u (1971). Crystal and molecular structure: Naganathan, Venkatesan, *Acta Crystallogr.* **27B**, 1079 (1971); Ashida *et al.*, *ibid.* **28B**, 1367 (1972). Use in asthenia and hepatic insufficiency: **FR 2198739** (1974 to Hublot & Vallet), *C.A.* **82**, 144952c (1975). Clinical trial in treatment of lysinuric protein intolerance: J. Rajantie *et al.*, *J. Pediatr.* **97**, 927 (1980); T. O. Carpenter *et al.*, *N. Engl. J. Med.* **312**, 290 (1985).

Prisms from methanol + water, mp 222°. $[\alpha]_D^{20}$ +3.7° (c = 2). pK_1 2.43; pK_2 9.41. Sol in water. Insol in methanol, ethanol.

Hydrochloride. [34312-10-2] $C_6H_{13}N_3O_3 \cdot HCl$. Crystals, dec 185°. $[\alpha]_D^{22}$ +17.9° (c = 2).

Malate (salt). [54940-97-5] Stimol. $C_6H_{13}N_3O_3 \cdot C_4H_6O_5$; mol wt 309.27.

THERAP CAT: Treatment of asthenia.

2332. Citrullol. [1390-93-8] $C_{22}H_{38}O_4$; mol wt 366.53. C 72.09%, H 10.45%, O 17.46%. From fruit pulp of *Citrullus colo-*

cynthis Schrad., *Cucurbitaceae:* Power, Moore, *J. Chem. Soc.* **97**, 99 (1910); Power, Salway, *ibid.* **103**, 399, 1022 (1913); Khadem, Rahman, *Tetrahedron Lett.* **1962**, 1137.

Crystals, mp 282-283°. uv max: 242, 272, 282 nm (log ε 2.85, 2.68, 2.68). Sol in pyridine; practically insol in usual organic solvents.

Diacetate. $C_{26}H_{42}O_6$. Crystals, mp 162°.

2333. Citrus Red 2. [6358-53-8] 1-[(2,5-Dimethoxyphenyl)azo]-2-naphthalenol; C.I. Solvent Red 80; C.I. 12156. $C_{18}H_{16}N_2O_3$; mol wt 308.33. C 70.12%, H 5.23%, N 9.09%, O 15.57%. Prepn: H. W. Elley, H. W. Daudt, US 2224904 (1940 to Du Pont). Metabolism: J. L. Radomski, *J. Pharmacol. Exp. Ther.* **134**, 100 (1961); **136**, 378 (1962). Toxicology: M. Sharratt *et al., Food Cosmet. Toxicol.* **4**, 493 (1966). Review of carcinogenicity studies: *IARC Monographs* **8**, 101-106. *See also Colour Index* **vol. 4** (3rd ed., 1971) p 4033.

Crystals, mp 155-157°. Slightly sol in water; partially sol in ethanol and vegetable oils.

USE: To color orange skins.

2334. Civet. Zibeth. Unctuous secretion from receptacles between the anus and genitalia of both male and female civet cat. *Constit.* Civetone and similar compds.

Semi-solid, yellowish to brown unctuous substance; unpleasant, subacrid, bitter taste; fusible and burns without leaving much residue. Insol in water; partly sol in hot alcohol or in ether.

USE: As a fixative in perfumery.

2335. Civetone. [542-46-1] (Z)-9-Cycloheptadecen-1-one. $C_{17}H_{30}O$; mol wt 250.42. C 81.54%, H 12.07%, O 6.39%. 17-Membered macrocyclic musk, constituent of civet: Ruzicka, *Helv. Chim. Acta* **9**, 230 (1926); Ruzicka *et al., ibid.* **10**, 695 (1927). Occurs in nature as *cis*-form. Synthesis of *cis*-civetone: Stoll *et al., ibid.* **31**, 543 (1948); J. Tsuji, T. Mondai, *Tetrahedron Lett.* **1977**, 3285; E. Seoane *et al., J. Chem. Ind. (London)* **1978**, 165. Synthesis of *trans*-form: H. Hunsdiecker, *Ber.* **77**, 185 (1944); H. H. Mathur, S. C. Bhattacharyya, *J. Chem. Soc.* **1968**, 114. Crystal and molecular structure of *cis*-civetone: G. Bernardinelli, R. Gerdil, *Helv. Chim. Acta* **65**, 558 (1982).

(cis)-form

Crystals, mp 31-32°. Musky odor becoming pleasant in extreme dilns. d_4^{33} 0.917. bp_{742} 342°; bp_2 59°. $n_D^{33.4}$ 1.4830.

USE: In perfumery.

2336. Cizolirtine. [142155-43-9] *N,N*-Dimethyl-2-[(1-methyl-1*H*-pyrazol-5-yl)phenylmethoxy]ethanamine; 1-methyl-α-phenyl-*O*-(2-dimethylaminoethyl)-1*H*-pyrazole-5-methanol; E-3710. $C_{15}H_{21}N_3O$; mol wt 259.35. C 69.47%, H 8.16%, N 16.20%, O 6.17%. Antinociceptive agent that inhibits release of calcitonin gene related peptide and substance P, *q.v.*, from the spinal cord. Prepn: A. Colombo *et al., EP 289380; eidem, US 5017596* (1988, 1991 both to Esteve). Prepn of isomers: J. A. Hueso-Rodriguez *et al., Bioorg. Med. Chem. Lett.* **3**, 269 (1993). CE determn of chemical and enantiomeric purity: A. Gómez-Gomar *et al., J. Chromatogr. A* **950**, 257 (2002). Pharmacology: I. Al-

varez *et al., Methods Find. Exp. Clin. Pharmacol.* **22**, 211 (2000). Mechanism of action study: S. Ballet *et al., Neuropharmacology* **40**, 578 (2001). Clinical evaluation in chronic neuropathic pain: P. Shembalkar *et al., Curr. Med. Res. Opin.* **17**, 262 (2001); in renal colic: I. Pavlik *et al., Curr. Ther.* **26**, 1061 (2004). *Review:* N. Monck, *Curr. Opin. Invest. Drugs* **2**, 1269-1272 (2001).

Citrate. [142155-44-0] E-4018. $C_{15}H_{21}N_3O \cdot C_6H_8O_7$; mol wt 451.47.

THERAP CAT: Analgesic.

2337. Cladribine. [4291-63-8] 2-Chloro-2'-deoxyadenosine; 2-chloro-6-amino-9-(2-deoxy-β-D-*erythro*-pentofuranosyl)-purine; 2-chlorodeoxyadenosine; 2-CdA; CldAdo; NSC-105014-F; Leustatin. $C_{10}H_{12}ClN_5O_3$; mol wt 285.69. C 42.04%, H 4.23%, Cl 12.41%, N 24.51%, O 16.80%. Substituted purine nucleoside with antileukemic activity. Prepn as intermediate in synthesis of 2-deoxynucleosides: H. Venner, *Ber.* **93**, 140 (1960); M. Ikehara, H. Tada, *J. Am. Chem. Soc.* **85**, 2344 (1963); *eidem, ibid.* **87**, 606 (1965). Synthesis and biological activity: L. F. Christensen *et al., J. Med. Chem.* **15**, 735 (1972). Stereospecific synthesis: Z. Kazimierczuk *et al., J. Am. Chem. Soc.* **106**, 6379 (1984); R. K. Robins, G. R. Revankar, *EP 173059; eidem, US 4760137* (1986, 1988 both to Brigham Young Univ.). Specific toxicity to lymphocytes: D. A. Carson *et al., Proc. Natl. Acad. Sci. USA* **77**, 6865 (1980); *eidem, Blood* **62**, 737 (1983). Mechanism of action: S. Seto *et al., J. Clin. Invest.* **75**, 377 (1985). Clinical evaluation in chronic lymphocytic leukemia: L. D. Piro *et al., Blood* **72**, 1069 (1988); in hairy cell leukemia: *eidem, N. Engl. J. Med.* **322**, 1117 (1990).

Crystals from water, softens at 210-215°, solidifies and turns brown (Christensen). Also reported as crystals from ethanol, mp 220° (softens), resolidifies, turns brown and does not melt below 300° (Kazimierczuk). $[\alpha]_D^{25}$ −18.8° (c = 1 in DMF). uv max in 0.1N NaOH: 265 nm; in 0.1N HCl: 265 nm.

THERAP CAT: Antineoplastic.

2338. Clanobutin. [30544-61-7] 4-[(4-Chlorobenzoyl)(4-methoxyphenyl)amino]butanoic acid; 4-[p-chloro-*N*-(p-methoxyphenyl)benzamido]butyric acid; *N*-(p-chlorobenzoyl)-γ-(p-anisidino)butyric acid; Bykahepar. $C_{18}H_{18}ClNO_4$; mol wt 347.79. C 62.16%, H 5.22%, Cl 10.19%, N 4.03%, O 18.40%. Prepn: K. Klemm *et al., DE 1917036; eidem, US 3780095* (1971, 1973 both to Byk-Gulden). Series of articles on synthesis, physical and pharmacological properties: *Arzneim.-Forsch.* **29**, 1-15 (1979). *In vitro* biochemical study: H. Wolf *et al., Biochem. Pharmacol.* **29**, 1649 (1980). Effect on bile excretion in rats, dogs: P. Berchtold *et al., Arzneim.-Forsch.* **30**, 1878 (1980).

Cryst from ethyl acetate, mp 115-116°. pKa 5.04. Soly in water at 37°: 4.02×10^{-2} mol/l at pH 7. LD$_{50}$ in rats (mg/kg): >2000 orally; 570 i.v. (Klemm).

THERAP CAT: Choleretic.

THERAP CAT (VET): Choleretic; in treatment of piroplasmosis and anaplasmosis.

2339. Clarithromycin. [81103-11-9] 6-O-Methylerythromycin; A-56268; TE-031; Biaxin; Clarosip; Clathromycin; Cyllind; Klacid; Klaricid; Macladin; Naxy; Veclam; Zeclar. $C_{38}H_{69}NO_{13}$; mol wt 747.95. C 61.02%, H 9.30%, N 1.87%, O 27.81%. Semisynthetic macrolide antibiotic; derivative of erythromycin, q.v. Prepn: Y. Watanabe et al., **EP 41355**; eidem, **US 4331803** (1981, 1982 both to Taisho); and in vitro antibacterial activity: S. Morimoto et al., J. Antibiot. **37**, 187 (1984). In vitro and in vivo antibacterial activity: P. B. Fernandes et al., Antimicrob. Agents Chemother. **30**, 865 (1986). Comparative antibacterial spectrum in vitro: C. Benson et al., Eur. J. Clin. Microbiol. **6**, 173 (1987); H. M. Wexler, S. M. Finegold, ibid. 492. HPLC determn in biological fluids: D. Croteau et al., J. Chromatogr. **419**, 205 (1987); in plasma: H. Amini, A. Ahmadiani, J. Chromatogr. B **817**, 193 (2005). Acute toxicity study: S. Abe et al., Chemotherapy (Tokyo) **36**, Suppl. 3, 274 (1988). Symposium on pharmacology and comparative clinical studies: J. Antimicrob. Chemother. **27**, Suppl. A, 1-124 (1991). Comprehensive description: I. I. Salem, Anal. Profiles Drug Subs. Excip. **24**, 45-85, (1996).

Colorless needles from chloroform + diisopropyl ether (1:2), mp 217-220° (dec). Also reported as crystals from ethanol, mp 222-225° (Morimoto). uv max (CHCl$_3$): 288 nm (ε 27.9). uv max (CHCl$_3$): 240, 288 nm; (methanol): 211, 288 nm. [α]$_D^{20}$ −90.4° (c = 1 in CHCl$_3$). Stable at acidic pH. LD$_{50}$ in male, female mice, male, female rats (mg/kg): 2740, 2700, 3470, 2700 orally, 1030, 850, 669, 753 i.p., >5000 all s.c. (Abe).

THERAP CAT: Antibacterial.

2340. Clathrates. Compounds that are capable of trapping other substances within their own crystal lattices. The cavities of the host molecules are classified as cages, tunnels, or layered types, depending on the way they include guest molecules. The geometry of the cavities limits the guest molecules by size and shape, rather than by chemical similarity with the host molecules. Among common clathrates are *molecular sieves, cyclotriphosphazenes*, and *Dianin's compound*, as well as hydroquinone, cyclodextrins, and deoxycholic acid, q.q.v. *Cavitands* are organic hosts with enforced (rigid) cavities: D. J. Cram, Science **219**, 1177 (1983); R. C. Helgeson et al., Chem. Commun. **1983**, 101. Comprehensive book: Clathrate Compounds, V. M. Bhatnagar, Ed. (Chemical Pub. Co., New York, 1970) 244 pp. Reviews: D. D. MacNicol et al., Chem. Soc. Rev. **7**, 65-87 (1978); E. C. Makin, "Clathration" in Kirk-Othmer Encyclopedia of Chemical Technology **Vol. 6** (Wiley-Interscience, New York, 3rd ed., 1979) pp 178-189.

USE: As complexing agent; stabilizing agent. In analytical separations.

2341. Clavulanic Acid. [58001-44-8] [2R-(2α,3Z,5α)]-3-(2-Hydroxyethylidene)-7-oxo-4-oxa-1-azabicyclo[3.2.0]heptane-2-carboxylic acid; MM 14151. $C_8H_9NO_5$; mol wt 199.16. C 48.25%, H 4.55%, N 7.03%, O 40.17%. β-Lactamase inhibitor. Antibiotic produced by Streptomyces clavuligerus; first reported naturally occurring fused β-lactam containing oxygen. Isoln: M.

Cole et al., **DE 2517316** (1975 to Beecham), C.A. **84**, 72635t (1976); A. G. Brown et al., J. Antibiot. **29**, 668 (1976). Structure, x-ray crystallography: T. T. Howarth et al., Chem. Commun. **1976**, 266. Total synthesis of (±)-form: P. H. Bentley et al., ibid. **1977**, 748, 905; eidem, Tetrahedron Lett. **1979**, 1889. β-Lactamase inhibition and antibacterial spectrum: C. Reading, M. Cole, Antimicrob. Agents Chemother. **11**, 852 (1977). Mechanism of action: B. G. Spratt et al., ibid. **12**, 406 (1977). Antibacterial activity, pharmacology and clinical efficacy of combination with amoxicillin: A. P. Ball et al., Lancet **1**, 620 (1980); R. N. Brogden et al., Drugs **22**, 337-362 (1981). In vitro and in vivo synergism with ticarcillin: R. Sutherland et al., Am. J. Med. **79**, Suppl. 5B, 13 (1985).

Combination of potassium salt with amoxicillin trihydrate. Co-amoxiclav; Amoksiklav; Augmentin; Ciblor; Clavamox; Clavulin; Klavocin; Neo-Duplamox; Synulox.

Combination of potassium salt with ticarcillin disodium. [116876-37-0] Betabactyl; Timentin.

Methyl ester. $C_9H_{11}NO_5$. Oil. [α]$_D^{22}$ +38°.

p-Nitrobenzyl ester. $C_{15}H_{14}N_2O_7$. Monoclinic crystals, mp 117.5-118°.

THERAP CAT: Combination with β-lactam antibiotics as antibacterial.

THERAP CAT (VET): Combination with β-lactam antibiotics as antibacterial.

2342. Clazosentan. [180384-56-9] N-[6-(2-Hydroxyethoxy)-5-(2-methoxyphenoxy)-2-[2-(1H-tetrazol-5-yl)-4-pyridinyl]-4-pyrimidinyl]-5-methyl-2-pyridinesulfonamide; 5-methylpyridine-2-sulfonic acid 6-(2-hydroxyethoxy)-5-(2-methoxyphenoxy)-2-(2-1H-tetrazol-5-ylpyridin-4-yl)pyrimidin-4-ylamide. $C_{25}H_{23}N_9O_6$-S; mol wt 577.57. C 51.99%, H 4.01%, N 21.83%, O 16.62%, S 5.55%. Nonpeptide selective endothelin ET$_A$ receptor antagonist. Prepn: V. Breu et al., **WO 9619459**; eidem, **US 6004965** (1996, 1999 both to Hoffmann-La Roche). Pharmacology and receptor binding study: S. Roux et al., J. Pharmacol. Exp. Ther. **283**, 1110 (1997). Clinical pharmacology: T. J. L. Vuurmans et al., Hypertension **41**, 1253 (2003). Cerebrovascular characterization: H. Vatter et al., J. Neurosurg. **102**, 1101, 1108 (2005). Clinical effect on vasospasm following subarachnoid hemorrhage: P. Vajkoczy et al., ibid. **103**, 9 (2005). Review of development and therapeutic potential: D. Uhlmann, Curr. Opin. Invest. Drugs **7**, 272-281 (2006).

White substance from acetonitrile, mp 239-241°.

Disodium salt. [503271-02-1] AXV-034343; Ro-61-1790; VML-588. $C_{25}H_{21}N_9Na_2O_6S$; mol wt 621.54. pKa$_1$ 4.5; pKa$_2$ 3.3. Soly in water: 25% at physiol pH.

THERAP CAT: In treatment of cerebral vasospasm.

2343. Clazuril. [101831-36-1] 2-Chloro-α-(4-chlorophenyl)-4-(4,5-dihydro-3,5-dioxo-1,2,4-triazin-2(3H)-yl)benzeneacetonitrile; (±)-[2-chloro-4-(4,5-dihydro-3,5-dioxo-as-triazin-2(3H)-

yl)phenyl](*p*-chlorophenyl)acetonitrile; Appertex. $C_{17}H_{10}Cl_2N_4$-O_2; mol wt 373.19. C 54.71%, H 2.70%, Cl 19.00%, N 15.01%, O 8.57%. Prepn: G. M. Boeckx *et al.*, **EP 170316**; *eidem*, **US 4631278** (both 1986 to Janssen). Anticoccidial effect in pigeons: W. Coussement *et al.*, *Res. Vet. Sci.* **45**, 117 (1988).

mp 196.8°.
THERAP CAT (VET): Coccidiostat.

2344. Clebopride. [55905-53-8] 4-Amino-5-chloro-2-methoxy-*N*-[1-(phenylmethyl)-4-piperidinyl]benzamide; 4-amino-*N*-(1-benzyl-4-piperidyl)-5-chloro-*o*-anisamide; *N*-(1′-benzyl-4′-piperidyl)-2-methoxy-4-amino-5-chlorobenzamide. $C_{20}H_{24}ClN_3$-O_2; mol wt 373.88. C 64.25%, H 6.47%, Cl 9.48%, N 11.24%, O 8.56%. Dopamine receptor antagonist related to metoclopramide, *q.v.* Prepn: R. G. Spickett *et al.*, **DE 2513136**; A. V. Noverola *et al.*, **US 4138492** (1975, 1979 both to Anphar); J. Prieto *et al.*, *J. Pharm. Pharmacol.* **29**, 147 (1977). Pharmacological study: J. L. Masso, D. J. Roberts, *ibid.* **32**, 727 (1980). *In vitro* metabolism studies: G. Huizing *et al.*, *Xenobiotica* **10**, 211 (1980); G. Huizing, A. H. Beckett, *ibid.* 593. Pharmacokinetics: J. Segura *et al.*, *J. Pharm. Pharmacol.* **33**, 214 (1981). Comparative study of antiemetic and gastrointestinal effects: P. Berga *et al.*, *Arch. Farmacol. Toxicol.* **7**, 189 (1981). Efficacy in healing exptl ulcers: Y. Matsuo *et al.*, *Oyo Yakuri* **24**, 251 (1982); S. Okabe *et al.*, *ibid.* 261, *C.A.* **97**, 208081n, 208082p (1982). Determn in urine and plasma by radioimmunoassay: M. Yano *et al.*, *Chem. Pharm. Bull.* **32**, 1491 (1984). Clinical effect in postoperative nausea: D. F. Duarte *et al.*, *Clin. Ther.* **7**, 365 (1985).

Cryst from methanol, mp 194-195°.
Hydrochloride monohydrate. $C_{20}H_{24}ClN_3O_2$.HCl.H_2O. Cryst, mp 217-219°. Approx oral LD_{50} in male Swiss mice: >1000 mg/kg (Prieto).
Malate. [57645-91-7] Amicos; Clanzol; Clast; Cleboril; Cleprid; Motilex. $C_{20}H_{24}ClN_3O_2$.$C_4H_6O_5$; mol wt 507.96.
THERAP CAT: Antiemetic; antispasmodic.

2345. Clemastine. [15686-51-8] (2*R*)-2-[2-[(1*R*)-1-(4-Chlorophenyl)-1-phenylethoxy]ethyl]-1-methylpyrrolidine; (+)-2-[2-[(*p*-chloro-α-methyl-α-phenylbenzyl)oxy]ethyl]-1-methylpyrrolidine; 1-methyl-2-[2-(α-methyl-*p*-chlorobenzhydryloxy)ethyl]pyrrolidine; 1-methyl-2-[2-(methyl-*p*-chlorodiphenylmethyloxy)ethyl]pyrrolidine; meclastine. $C_{21}H_{26}ClNO$; mol wt 343.89. C 73.34%, H 7.62%, Cl 10.31%, N 4.07%, O 4.65%. Prepn: **GB 942152** (1963 to Sandoz). Synthesis and abs config: A. Ebnöther, H. P. Weber, *Helv. Chim. Acta* **59**, 2462 (1976). Pharmacology and toxicology of the hydrogen fumarate: Weidmann *et al.*, *Boll. Chim. Farm.* **106**, 467 (1967). HPLC determn in plasma: V. Horváth *et al.*, *J. Chromatogr. B* **816**, 153 (2005).

Free base, bp$_{0.02}$ 154°. n_D^{22} 1.5582. $[α]_D^{20}$ +33.6° (ethanol).

Hydrogen fumarate. [14976-57-9] HS-592; Aloginan; Alphamin; Anhistan; Fuluminol; Inbestan; Kinotomin; Lacretin; Lecasol; Maikohis; Mallermin-F; Marsthine; Masletine; Piloral; Reconin; Tavegil; Tavegyl; Tavist; Telgin-G; Trabest; Xolamin. $C_{25}H_{30}$-ClNO$_5$; mol wt 459.96. mp 177-178°. $[α]_D^{21}$ +16.9° (methanol). LD_{50} in mice, rats (mg/kg): 730, 3550 orally; 43, 82 i.v. (Weimann).
THERAP CAT: Antihistaminic.

2346. Clemizole. [442-52-4] 1-[(4-Chlorophenyl)methyl]-2-(1-pyrrolidinylmethyl)-1*H*-benzimidazole; 1-(*p*-chlorobenzyl)-2-(1-pyrrolidinylmethyl)benzimidazole; 1-(*p*-chlorobenzyl)-2-pyrrolidylmethylenebenzimidazole. $C_{19}H_{20}ClN_3$; mol wt 325.84. C 70.04%, H 6.19%, Cl 10.88%, N 12.90%. Prepn: D. Jerchel *et al.*, *Ann.* **575**, 162 (1952); **GB 703272**; M. Schenck, W. Heinz, **US 2689853** (both 1954 to Schering A.G.).

Crystals from dil alc, mp 167°.
Hydrochloride. [1163-36-6] Allercur. $C_{19}H_{20}ClN_3$.HCl; mol wt 362.30. White microscopic rods from butanol, mp 239-241°. Sol in water.
THERAP CAT: Antihistaminic.

2347. Clenbuterol. [37148-27-9] 4-Amino-3,5-dichloro-α-[[(1,1-dimethylethyl)amino]methyl]benzenemethanol; 4-amino-α-[(*tert*-butylamino)methyl]-3,5-dichlorobenzyl alcohol; NAB-365; Monores. $C_{12}H_{18}Cl_2N_2O$; mol wt 277.19. C 52.00%, H 6.55%, Cl 25.58%, N 10.11%, O 5.77%. Substituted phenylethanolamine with $β_2$ sympathomimetic activity. Prepn: J. Keck *et al.*, **ZA 6705692**; *eidem*, **US 3536712** (1968, 1970 both to Thomae); *eidem*, *Arzneim.-Forsch.* **22**, 861 (1972). Series of articles on pharmacology, reproductive toxicology, pharmacokinetics and metabolism: *ibid.* **26**, 1403-1419, 1427-1460 (1976). Toxicity: M. Ueberberg *et al.*, *ibid.* 1420. Clinical studies: M. Tschan *et al.*, *Eur. J. Clin. Pharmacol.* **15**, 159 (1979); C. Pasotti *et al.*, *Int. J. Clin. Pharmacol. Biopharm.* **17**, 176 (1979). Effect on weight gain in lambs: M. E. Nichols *et al.*, *1991 Animal Science Research Report* (Oklahoma Agric. Exp. Station, Oklahoma State University, 1991) 303.

Hydrochloride. [21898-19-1] NAB-365Cl; Spiropent; Ventipulmin. $C_{12}H_{18}Cl_2N_2O$.HCl; mol wt 313.65. Colorless microcrystalline powder from isopropyl alc, mp 174-175.5°. Very sol in water, methanol, ethanol, slightly sol in chloroform. Insol in benzene. LD_{50} in mice, rats, guinea pigs (mg/kg): 176, 315, 67.1 orally; 27.6, 35.3, 12.6 i.v. (Ueberberg).
THERAP CAT: Bronchodilator.
THERAP CAT (VET): Bronchodilator; tocolytic.

2348. Clentiazem. [96125-53-0] (2*S*,3*S*)-3-(Acetyloxy)-8-chloro-5-[2-(dimethylamino)ethyl]-2,3-dihydro-2-(4-methoxyphenyl)-1,5-benzothiazepin-4(5*H*)-one; (+)-(2*S*,3*S*)-8-chloro-5-[2-(dimethylamino)ethyl]-2,3-dihydro-3-hydroxy-2-(*p*-methoxyphenyl)-1,5-benzothiazepin-4(5*H*)-one acetate (ester). $C_{22}H_{25}ClN_2O_4S$; mol wt 448.96. C 58.85%, H 5.61%, Cl 7.90%, N 6.24%, O 14.25%, S 7.14%. Calcium channel blocker; 8-chloro derivative of diltiazem. Prepn: M. Takeda *et al.*, **EP 127882**; *eidem*, **US 4567175** (1984, 1986 both to Tanabe); H. Inoue *et al.*, *J. Med. Chem.* **34**, 675 (1991). Cardiovascular pharmacology: H. Narita *et al.*, *Arzneim.-Forsch.* **38**, 515 (1988). Clinical pharmacokinetics: A. K. Shah *et al.*, *J. Clin. Pharmacol.* **33**, 354 (1993). Clinical evaluation in hypertension: S. Kawakita *et al.*, *Clin. Cardiol.* **14**, 53 (1991).

Maleate. [96128-92-6] TA-3090; Logna. $C_{22}H_{25}ClN_2O_4 \cdot S.C_4H_4O_4$; mol wt 565.04. Crystals from ethanol, mp 160.5-161.5°. $[\alpha]_D^{20}$ +76.5° (c = 1 in methanol).

THERAP CAT: Antihypertensive.

2349. Clethodim. [99129-21-2] 2-[1-[[(3-Chloro-2-propen-yl)oxy]imino]propyl]-5-[2-(ethylthio)propyl]-3-hydroxy-2-cyclo-hexen-1-one; (±)-2-[(E)-1-[(E)-3-chloroallyloxyimino]propyl]-5-[2-(ethylthio)propyl]-3-hydroxycyclohex-2-enone; RE-45601; Prism; Select. $C_{17}H_{26}ClNO_3S$; mol wt 359.91. C 56.73%, H 7.28%, Cl 9.85%, N 3.89%, O 13.34%, S 8.91%. Systemic grami-nicide. Prepn: T. Luo, **BE 897413**; *idem*, **US 4440566** (1983, 1984 both to Chevron). Properties and biological profile: R. T. Kincade *et al.*, *Proc. Br. Crop Prot. Conf. - Weeds* **1987**, 49. Degradation studies: L. N. Falb *et al.*, *J. Agric. Food Chem.* **38**, 875 (1990). Persistence in soil and efficacy against grasses: A. Rahman *et al.*, *Proc. 41st N. Z. Weed Pest Control Conf.* **1988**, 39. Field trial against grasses: J. H. Hunter, *Weed Technol.* **9**, 432 (1995).

Clear amber liquid. Sol in most organic solvents. LD_{50} in male, female rats (mg/kg): 1630, 1360 orally; LC_{50} in trout: 56 mg/l; 8 day feeding in quail: > 6000 ppm (Kincade).

USE: Post-emergent herbicide.

2350. 1,6-Cleve's Acid. [119-79-9] 5-Amino-2-naphtha-lenesulfonic acid; 1-naphthylamine-6-sulfonic acid. $C_{10}H_9NO_3S$; mol wt 223.25. C 53.80%, H 4.06%, N 6.27%, O 21.50%, S 14.36%. Prepn: Erdmann, *Ann.* **275**, 262 (1893).

Crystals. Sol in 1000 parts water. Practically insol in alc, ether.

USE: In manuf of azo dyes.

2351. 1,7-Cleve's Acid. [119-28-8] 8-Amino-2-naphtha-lenesulfonic acid; 1-naphthylamine-7-sulfonic acid. $C_{10}H_9NO_3S$; mol wt 223.25. C 53.80%, H 4.06%, N 6.27%, O 21.50%, S 14.36%. Prepn: Erdmann, *Ann.* **275**, 262 (1893); Roos *et al.*, **US 2875243** (1959 to Bayer). Industrial synthesis: Nakahara *et al.*, *J. Synth. Org. Chem. Jpn.* **29**, 1129 (1971).

Needles or prisms from water contg $1H_2O$. Sol in 220 parts water; very slightly sol in alcohol, ether.

USE: In manuf of azo dyes.

2352. Clevidipine. [167221-71-8] 4-(2,3-Dichlorophenyl)-1,4-dihydro-2,6-dimethyl-3,5-pyridinedicarboxylic acid methyl (1-oxybutoxy)methyl ester; butyroxymethyl methyl 4-(2',3'-dichloro-phenyl)-2,6-dimethyl-1,4-dihydropyridine-3,5-dicarboxylate; Clevelox. $C_{21}H_{23}Cl_2NO_6$; mol wt 456.32. C 55.27%, H 5.08%, Cl 15.54%, N 3.07%, O 21.04%. Ultrashort-acting dihydropyridine calcium channel antagonist. Prepn: K. H. Andersson *et al.*, **WO 9512578**; *eidem*, **US 5856346** (1995, 1999 both to Astra). Improved prepn: A. Mattson *et al.*, **WO 0031035** (2000 to AstraZe-neca). Capillary GC/MS determn in whole blood: C. Fakt, H. Stenhoff, *J. Chromatogr. B* **723**, 211 (1999). Clinical pharmaco-kinetics: H. Ericsson *et al.*, *Br. J. Clin. Pharmacol.* **47**, 531 (1999); and pulmonary extraction during cardiopulmonary bypass: A. Vuylsteke *et al.*, *Br. J. Anaesth.* **85**, 683 (2000). Clinical evaluation in hypertension in postoperative cardiac surgical patients: N. Kiel-er-Jensen *et al.*, *Acta Anaesthesiol. Scand.* **44**, 186 (2000); J. M. Bailey *et al.*, *Anesthesiology* **96**, 1086 (2002). Review of pharma-cology and clinical development: M. Nordlander *et al.*, *Cardiovasc. Drug Rev.* **22**, 227-250 (2004).

Crystals from diisopropylether, mp 136.2-138.5°. Soly in water: 0.1 mg/ml.

THERAP CAT: Antihypertensive.

2353. Clevudine. [163252-36-6] 1-(2-Deoxy-2-fluoro-β-L-arabinofuranosyl)-5-methyl-2,4-(1H,3H)-pyrimidinedione; 1-(2-de-oxy-2-fluoro-β-L-arabinofuranosyl)thymine; 2'-fluoro-5-methyl-β-L-arabinofuranosyluridine; L-FMAU. $C_{10}H_{13}FN_2O_5$; mol wt 260.22. C 46.16%, H 5.04%, F 7.30%, N 10.77%, O 30.74%. Nucleoside analog; specific inhibitor of viral DNA synthesis. Prepn: C. K. Chu *et al.*, **WO 9520595**; *eidem*, **US 5587362** (1995, 1996 both to Univ. Georgia Res. Found.; Yale Univ.); T. Ma *et al.*, *J. Med. Chem.* **39**, 2835 (1996). Synthesis: M. L. Sznaidman *et al.*, *Nucleosides Nucleotides Nucleic Acids* **21**, 155 (2002). *In vitro* antiviral activity: C. K. Chu *et al.*, *Antimicrob. Agents Chemother.* **39**, 979 (1995). Pharmacokinetics: J. D. Wright *et al.*, *Pharm. Res.* **12**, 1350 (1995). Mechanism of action study: Y. Chong, C. K. Chu, *Bioorg. Med. Chem. Lett.* **12**, 3459 (2002). Clinical evaluation in chronic hepatitis B: P. Marcellin *et al.*, *Hepatology* **40**, 140 (2004). Review of preclinical pharmacol-ogy: C. K. Chu *et al.* in *Therapies for Viral Hepatitis*, R. F. Schinazi *et al.*, Eds. (Int. Med. Press, London, 1998) pp 303-312; of develop-ment and clinical experience: G. R. Painter *et al.* in *Frontiers in Viral Hepatitis*, R. F. Schinazi *et al.*, Eds. (Elsevier, New York, 2003) pp 281-300.

Crystals from methanol/chloroform, mp 184-185°. $[\alpha]_D^{25}$ $-111.77°$ (c = 0.23 in methanol). uv max in water: 265.0 (pH 2), 265.5 (pH 7), 265.5 nm (pH 11) (ε 9695, 9647, 7153). LD$_{50}$ in mice, rats (mg/kg): >5000, >3000 orally (Painter).

Triphosphate. [174625-00-4] L-FMAU-TP. $C_{10}H_{16}FN_2O_{14}$-P_3; mol wt 500.16.

THERAP CAT: Antiviral.

2354. Clidinium Bromide. [3485-62-9] 3-[(Hydroxydiphenylacetyl)oxy]-1-methyl-1-azoniabicyclo[2.2.2]octane bromide; 3-hydroxy-1-methylquinuclidinium bromide benzilate; 1-methyl-3-benziloyloxyquinuclidinium bromide; 3-benziloyloxy-1-azabicyclo[2.2.2]octane methobromide; Ro-2-3773; Quarzan. $C_{22}H_{26}$-BrNO$_3$; mol wt 432.35. C 61.12%, H 6.06%, Br 18.48%, N 3.24%, O 11.10%. Anticholinergic. Prepn: Sternbach, US 2648667 (1953 to Hoffmann-La Roche). Comprehensive description: B. C. Rudy, B. Z. Senkowski, *Anal. Profiles Drug Subs.* **2,** 145-161 (1973).

Crystals from methanol + acetone + ether, mp 240-241°.
THERAP CAT: Antispasmodic.

2355. Clinafloxacin. [105956-97-6] 7-(3-Amino-1-pyrrolidinyl)-8-chloro-1-cyclopropyl-6-fluoro-1,4-dihydro-4-oxo-3-quinolinecarboxylic acid. $C_{17}H_{17}ClFN_3O_3$; mol wt 365.79. C 55.82%, H 4.68%, Cl 9.69%, F 5.19%, N 11.49%, O 13.12%. Fluorinated quinolone antibacterial. Prepn: S. Suzue *et al.,* **EP 195316** (1986 to Kyorin). Antibacterial spectrum: M. S. Barrett *et al., Diagn. Microbiol. Infect. Dis.* **14,** 389 (1991); S. M. H. Qadri *et al., Chemotherapy (Basel)* **38,** 92 (1992).

Milk-white powder from chloroform-methanol-conc. aq. ammonia, mp 253-258° (dec).

Hydrochloride. [105956-99-8] AM-1091; CI-960; PD-127391. $C_{17}H_{17}ClFN_3O_3$·HCl; mol wt 402.25. Light yellow prisms from methanol, mp 263-265° (dec).

THERAP CAT: Antibacterial.

2356. Clindamycin. [18323-44-9] Methyl 7-chloro-6,7,8-trideoxy-6-[[[(2S,4R)-1-methyl-4-propyl-2-pyrrolidinyl]carbonyl]amino]-1-thio-L-*threo*-α-D-*galacto*-octopyranoside; 7(S)-chloro-7-deoxylincomycin; 7-deoxy-7(S)-chlorolincomycin; clinimycin (rescinded); U-21251. $C_{18}H_{33}ClN_2O_5S$; mol wt 424.98. C 50.87%, H 7.83%, Cl 8.34%, N 6.59%, O 18.82%, S 7.55%. Semi-synthetic antibiotic prepd from lincomycin, *q.v.* Prepn: Magerlein *et al., Antimicrob. Agents Chemother.* **1966,** 727. Manuf process: R. D. Birkenmeyer, **US 3475407** (1969 to Upjohn). Synthesis and structure: R. D. Birkenmeyer, F. Kagan, *J. Med. Chem.* **13,** 616 (1970). Stability studies: Oesterling, *J. Pharm. Sci.* **59,** 63 (1970). Activity studies: McGehee *et al., Am. J. Med. Sci.* **256,** 279 (1968); D. A. Leigh, *J. Antimicrob. Chemother.* **7**(suppl. A), 3 (1981). Toxicology: J. E. Gray *et al., Toxicol. Appl. Pharmacol.* **21,** 516 (1972). Comprehensive description of the hydrochloride: L. W. Brown, W. F. Beyer, *Anal. Profiles Drug Subs.* **10,** 75-91 (1981).

Yellow, amorphous solid. $[\alpha]_D$ +214° (chloroform).

Hydrochloride. [21462-39-5]; [58207-19-5] (monohydrate). Antirobe; Clinsol; Clintabs; Dalacin C; Sobelin. $C_{18}H_{33}ClN_2O_5$-S·HCl; mol wt 461.44. Various hydrated forms exist. White crystals from ethanol-ethyl acetate, mp 141-143° (anhydrous). $[\alpha]_D$ +144° (H$_2$O). pKa 7.6. Sol in water, pyridine, ethanol, DMF. LD$_{50}$ in mice (mg/kg): 245 i.v.; 361 i.p.; 2618 orally (Gray).

2-Dihydrogen phosphate. [24729-96-2] U-28508; Cleocin; Dalacin T; Klimicin; Zindaclin. $C_{18}H_{34}ClN_2O_8PS$; mol wt 504.96. Sol in water.

THERAP CAT: Antibacterial.

THERAP CAT (VET): Antibacterial.

2357. Clinofibrate. [30299-08-2] 2,2′-[Cyclohexylidenebis(4,1-phenyleneoxy)]bis[2-methylbutanoic acid]; 2,2′-(4,4′-cyclohexylidenediphenoxy)-2,2′-dimethyldibutyric acid; S-8527; Lipoclin. $C_{28}H_{36}O_6$; mol wt 468.58. C 71.77%, H 7.74%, O 20.49%. Anti-atherosclerosis agent, related structurally to clofibrate, *q.v.* Prepn: Y. Nakamura *et al.,* **DE 2017331**; *eidem,* **US 3716583** (1970, 1973 both to Sumitomo). Hypolipidemic activity: K. Toki *et al., Atherosclerosis* **18,** 101 (1973); K. Suzuki *et al., Jpn. J. Pharmacol.* **24,** 407 (1974), *C.A.* **82,** 25821z (1975). Effect on cholesterol and lipoprotein metabolism in rats: K. Suzuki, *Biochem. Pharmacol.* **25,** 325 (1976). General pharmacology: H. Nakatani *et al., Oyo Yakuri* **16,** 687 (1978), *C.A.* **90,** 145808 (1979).

Off-white powder, mp 143-146° (dec). Sol in methanol, ethanol, acetone, chloroform, glacial acetic acid. Slightly sol in CCl$_4$. Practically insol in water.

THERAP CAT: Antilipemic.

2358. Clinprost. [88931-51-5] (3aS,5R,6R,6aS)-1,3a,4,5,6,-6a-Hexahydro-5-hydroxy-6-(3-hydroxy-1-octenyl)-2-pentalenepentanoic acid methyl ester; isocarbacyclin methyl ester; TEI-9090; TTC-909. $C_{22}H_{36}O_4$; mol wt 364.52. C 72.49%, H 9.95%, O 17.56%. Chemically stable prostacyclin (PGI$_2$) analog. Prepn: S. Kurozumi, S. Ikegami, **WO 8402902**; *eidem,* **US 4736058** (1984, 1988 both to Teijin); M. Shibasaki *et al., Tetrahedron Lett.* **24,** 3493 (1983). Stereosynthesis: H. Park *et al., Bull. Korean Chem. Soc.* **14,** 86 (1993). Series of articles on pharmacology: *Arzneim.-Forsch.* **45,** 967-993 (1995). Clinical trial as lipid emulsion in peripheral vascular disorders: K. Esato, *Adv. Prostaglandin Thromboxane Leukotriene Res.* **23,** 405 (1995).

Colorless oil.

Free acid. [88911-35-7] Isocarbacyclin; 9(*O*)-methano-$\Delta^{6(9)}$-prostaglandin I$_1$; TEI-7165. $C_{21}H_{34}O_4$; mol wt 350.49. Solid, mp 73-79°. $[\alpha]_D^{25}$ +16° (c = 0.25 in MeOH).

THERAP CAT: Antithrombotic.

2359. Clobazam. [22316-47-8] 7-Chloro-1-methyl-5-phenyl-1*H*-1,5-benzodiazepine-2,4(3*H*,5*H*)-dione; 1-phenyl-5-chloro-1,2,4,5-tetrahydro-2,4-dioxo-3*H*-1,5-benzodiazepine; H-4723; HR-376; LM-2717; Frisium; Urbadan; Urbanyl. $C_{16}H_{13}$-ClN_2O_2; mol wt 300.74. C 63.90%, H 4.36%, Cl 11.79%, N 9.31%, O 10.64%. Benzodiazepine psychotherapeutic agent in which the nitrogens in the heterocyclic ring are in the 1,5- rather than in the more common 1,4-positions. Prepn: **BE 707667**; S. Rossi, **US 3984398** (1968, 1976 both to Roussel-UCLAF); S. Rossi *et al., Chim. Ind. (Milan)* **51**, 479 (1969); K. H. Weber *et al., Ann. 756,* 128 (1972). Toxicology: E. Schütz, *Br. J. Clin. Pharmacol.* **7**, 33S (1979). Review of pharmacology and therapeutic use in anxiety: R. N. Brogden *et al., Drugs* **20**, 161-178 (1980). Symposium on pharmacology: *Drug Dev. Res.* **1982**, Suppl. 1, 1-186. Metabolism: A. G. Borel, F. S. Abbott, *Drug Metab. Dispos.* **21**, 415 (1993). GC determn in serum: D. F. LeGatt, D. P. McIntosh, *Clin. Biochem.* **26**, 159 (1993). Clinical experience in refractory epilepsy: Canadian Clobazam Cooperative Group, *Epilepsia* **32**, 407 (1991). Review of pharmacology and clinical studies in epilepsy: S. D. Shorvon, "Clobazam" in *Antiepileptic Drugs*, R. H. Levy *et al.*, Eds. (Raven Press, New York, 3rd ed., 1989) pp 821-840.

Crystals from 50% ethanol, mp 166-168°.

Note: This is a controlled substance (depressant): **21 CFR,** 1308.14.

THERAP CAT: Anxiolytic; anticonvulsant.

2360. Clobenfurol. [3611-72-1] α-(4-Chlorophenyl)-2-benzofuranmethanol; 2-benzofuryl-*p*-chlorophenylcarbinol; Menacor. $C_{15}H_{11}ClO_2$; mol wt 258.70. C 69.64%, H 4.29%, Cl 13.70%, O 12.37%. Prepn: **BE 644176**; Ghelardoni, Russo, **GB 1160925** (1964, 1969 both to Menarini), *C.A.* **63**, 8319h (1965); **71**, 124212f (1969); Ghelardoni, Russo, *Boll. Chim. Farm.* **109**, 48 (1970). Pharmacology of the hemisuccinate deriv: Pisanti, Volterra, *Farmaco Ed. Sci.* **26**, 312 (1971).

White, odorless powder, mp 48-49°.

Hemisuccinate. $C_{19}H_{15}ClO_5$. mp 95-97° from petr ether. LD$_{50}$ in mice, rats (mg/kg): 321, 300 i.p. (Pisanti, Volterra).

THERAP CAT: Vasodilator (coronary).

2361. Clobenoside. [29899-95-4] Ethyl 5,6-bis-*O*-[(4-chlorophenyl)methyl]-3-*O*-propyl-D-glucofuranoside; ethyl 3-*O*-*n*-propyl-5,6-di-*O*-(4-chlorobenzyl)-D-glucofuranoside; ZY-15028; Arvigol; Floganol. $C_{25}H_{32}Cl_2O_6$; mol wt 499.42. C 60.12%, H 6.46%, Cl 14.20%, O 19.22%. Congener of tribenoside, *q.v.* Prepn: **NL 6812906**; A. Rossi, **US 3542761** (1969, 1970 both to Ciba). Pharmacology and bioavailability in cats: G. Hennings *et al., Arzneim.-Forsch.* **35**, 498 (1985). Effect on glycoprotein biosynthesis *in vitro:* W. Reutter, C. Bauer, *Adv. Enzyme Regul.* **24**, 405 (1985). Mechanism of action study: D. Araujo *et al., Arch. Int. Pharmacodyn.* **277**, 192 (1985).

Faintly yellowish oil, $[\alpha]_D^{20}$ −17 ±1° (c = 1 in chloroform). Poorly sol in water.

THERAP CAT: Vasoprotectant.

2362. Clobenzorex. [13364-32-4] (+)-*N*-[(2-Chlorophenyl)methyl]-α-methylbenzeneethanamine; (+)-*N*-(*o*-chlorobenzyl)-α-methylphenethylamine; *d*-*N*-(1-phenyl-2-propyl)-2-chlorobenzylamine. $C_{16}H_{18}ClN$; mol wt 259.77. C 73.98%, H 6.98%, Cl 13.65%, N 5.39%. Prepn and pharmacology: J. R. Boissier, R. Ratouis, **FR 1429306** (1966 to Soc. Ind. Fabric. Antibiot.), *C.A.* **66**, 46195h (1967); J. R. Boissier *et al., Ann. Pharm. Fr.* **24**, 57 (1966). Synthesis of labelled compound: J. Lintermans *et al., J. Labelled Compd.* **6**, 289 (1970). Metabolic studies: M. Thomasset *et al., Experientia* **26**, 692 (1970); B. Glasson *et al., Arzneim.-Forsch.* **21**, 1985 (1971).

bp$_{0.1}$ 132-134°.

Hydrochloride. [5843-53-8] Ba-7205; SD-271-12; Dinintel; Rexigen. $C_{16}H_{18}ClN.HCl$; mol wt 296.23. Crystals, mp 182-183° (isopropanol). $[\alpha]_D^{20}$ +26.3° (water). Sol in water, ethanol. Slightly sol in methanol, chloroform. LD$_{50}$ i.p. in mice: 103 mg/kg (Boissier *et al.*).

THERAP CAT: Anorexic.

2363. Clobetasol. [25122-41-2] (11β,16β)-21-Chloro-9-fluoro-11,17-dihydroxy-16-methylpregna-1,4-diene-3,20-dione. $C_{22}H_{28}ClFO_4$; mol wt 410.91. C 64.30%, H 6.87%, Cl 8.63%, F 4.62%, O 15.57%. Topical corticosteroid. Prepn: Elks *et al.*, **DE 1902340**; *eidem,* **US 3721687** (1969, 1973 both to Glaxo). Review of pharmacology and clinical efficacy in skin disorders: E. A. Olsen, R. C. Cornell, *J. Am. Acad. Dermatol.* **15**, 246-255 (1986).

17-Propionate. [25122-46-7] GR-2/925; Clobesol; Dermovate; Olux; Psorex; Temovate. $C_{25}H_{32}ClFO_5$; mol wt 466.97. White or almost white colorless, crystalline powder, mp 195.5-197°. $[\alpha]_D$ +103.8° (c = 1.04 in dioxane). uv max (ethanol): 237 nm (ε 15000). Insol in water.

THERAP CAT: Glucocorticoid; anti-inflammatory.

2364. Clobetasone. [54063-32-0] (16β)-21-Chloro-9-fluoro-17-hydroxy-16-methylpregna-1,4-diene-3,11,20-trione; 21-chloro-11-dehydrobetamethasone. $C_{22}H_{26}ClFO_4$; mol wt 408.89. C 64.62%, H 6.41%, Cl 8.67%, F 4.65%, O 15.65%. Prepn: Elks *et al.*, **DE 1902340**; *eidem,* **US 3721687** (1969, 1973, both to Glaxo). Activity: Munro, Wilson, *Br. Med. J.* **3**, 626 (1975). Radioimmunoassay: W. A. Webb, R. V. Brooks, *Acta Endocrinol. Suppl.* **212**, 203 (1977). Toxicology: J. Tamura *et al., J. Toxicol. Sci.* **5**, 45, 177 (1980). Comparative clinical studies: A. Lassus, *Curr. Med. Res. Opin.* **6**, 165 (1979); T. Fredriksson, K. Nordin, *ibid.* 322. Clinical evaluation of ophthalmic form: D. Lloyd-Jones *et al., Br. J. Oph-thalmol.* **65,** 641 (1981); L. A. Eilon, S. R. Walker, *ibid.* 644; K. R. Wilhelmus *et al., ibid.* 699.

17-Butyrate. [25122-57-0] GR-2/1214; Emovate; Eumovate. $C_{26}H_{32}ClFO_5$; mol wt 478.98. Crystals from methanol, mp 90-100°.

THERAP CAT: Glucocorticoid; anti-inflammatory.

2365. Clobutinol. [14860-49-2] 4-Chloro-α-[2-(dimethylamino)-1-methylethyl]-α-methylbenzeneethanol; *p*-chloro-α-[2-(dimethylamino)-1-methylethyl]-α-methylphenethyl alcohol; 2-(*p*-chlorobenzyl)-3-dimethylaminomethyl-2-butanol; 1-*p*-chlorophenyl-2,3-dimethyl-4-dimethylamino-2-butanol. $C_{14}H_{22}ClNO$; mol wt 255.78. C 65.74%, H 8.67%, Cl 13.86%, N 5.48%, O 6.26%. Prepn: **GB 898010**; Berg, **US 3121087** (1962, 1964 both to Thomae). Pharmacology: Engelhorn, *Arzneim.-Forsch.* **10,** 785 (1960). Metabolism: Beisenherz *et al., ibid.* **19,** 79 (1969).

bp_{12} 179-180°.
Hydrochloride. [1215-83-4] KAT-256; Biotertussin; Silomat. $C_{14}H_{22}ClNO.HCl$; mol wt 292.24. Minute crystals, mp 169-170°. Slightly bitter, acidic taste. Numbs the tongue. Sol in water. LD_{50} in mice (mg/kg): 600 orally; 130 i.p. (Engelhorn).

THERAP CAT: Antitussive.

2366. Clocapramine. [47739-98-0] 1'-[3-(3-Chloro-10,11-dihydro-5*H*-dibenz[*b,f*]azepin-5-yl)propyl][1,4'-bipiperidine]-4'-carboxamide; 3-chloro-5-[3-(4-piperidino-4-carbamoylpiperidino)-propyl]-10,11-dihydro-5*H*-dibenz[*b,f*]azepine; 3-chlorocarpyramine; clocarpramine; CCP. $C_{28}H_{37}ClN_4O$; mol wt 481.07. C 69.91%, H 7.75%, Cl 7.37%, N 11.65%, O 3.33%. Prepn: M. Nakanishi, C. Tashiro, **DE 1905765**; *eidem,* **US 3668210** (1969, 1972, both to Yoshitomi); M. Nakanishi *et al., J. Med. Chem.* **13,** 644 (1970). Pharmacology and toxicity: M. Nakanishi *et al., Arzneim.-Forsch.* **21,** 391 (1971). Effect on metabolism of serotonin and catecholamines: M. Nakanishi, M. Setoguchi, *ibid.* **23,** 806 (1973). Metabolism: M. Nakanishi *et al., J. Pharm. Soc. Jpn.* **91,** 1042 (1971). HPLC determn in plasma: K. Hikida *et al., Anal. Sci.* **6,** 367 (1990). *Review: Jpn. Med. Gaz.* **10**(7), 5 (1973).

Dihydrochloride monohydrate. [60789-62-0] Y-4153; Clofekton. $C_{28}H_{37}ClN_4O.2HCl.H_2O$; mol wt 572.01. White, bitter tasting, crystalline powder, mp 267°. Soly in water: <3.5 g/100 ml. Freely sol in glacial acetic acid. Practically insol in ether, acetone. LD_{50} in mice, rats (mg/kg): 160, 125 i.p.; 2550, 6800 orally (Nakanishi).

THERAP CAT: Antipsychotic.

2367. Clocinizine. [298-55-5] 1-[(4-Chlorophenyl)phenyl-methyl]-4-(3-phenyl-2-propenyl)piperazine; 1-(*p*-chloro-α-phenyl-benzyl)-4-cinnamylpiperazine; 1-cinnamyl-4-(4-chlorobenzhy-dryl)piperazine; cliocinizine. $C_{26}H_{27}ClN_2$; mol wt 402.96. C 77.50%, H 6.75%, Cl 8.80%, N 6.95%. Prepn: **GB 809760** (1959 to Janssen). HPLC determn in cough-cold preparations: G. Cavazzutti *et al., J. Liq. Chromatogr.* **18,** 227 (1995).

Hydrochloride. Crystals, mp 200-201°.
THERAP CAT: Antihistaminic.

2368. Cloconazole. [77175-51-0] 1-[1-[2-[(3-Chlorophen-yl)methoxy]phenyl]ethenyl]-1*H*-imidazole; 1-[1-[2-[(3-chloroben-zyl)oxy]phenyl]vinyl]-1*H*-imidazole; croconazole. $C_{18}H_{15}ClN_2O$; mol wt 310.78. C 69.56%, H 4.86%, Cl 11.41%, N 9.01%, O 5.15%. Antimycotic vinylimidazole. Prepn and antifungal properties: M. Ogata *et al.,* **BE 883665**; *eidem,* **US 4328348** (1980, 1982 both to Shionogi); *eidem, J. Med. Chem.* **26,** 768 (1983). Pharmacology: K. Yamamoto *et al., Oyo Yakuri* **27,** 533 (1984), *C.A.* **101,** 16881c (1984). Series of articles on metabolism in rats and rabbits: K. Mizojiri *et al., Iyakuhin Kenkyu* **16,** 177-206 (1985), *C.A.* **103,** 47788y; 47789z; 47790t (1985). Mechanism of action study: T. Hiratani, H. Yamaguchi, *Chemotherapy (Tokyo)* **33,** 579 (1985).

mp 72-73°. Sol in ethyl acetate.
Monohydrochloride. [77174-66-4] 710674-S; Pilzcin. C_{18}-$H_{15}ClN_2O.HCl$; mol wt 347.24. Crystals from ethyl acetate + acetonitrile, mp 148.5-150°. LD_{50} in rats (mg/kg): 7000 s.c.; 2500 orally (Ogata, 1983).

THERAP CAT: Antifungal (topical).

2369. Clocortolone. [4828-27-7] (6α,11β,16α)-9-Chloro-6-fluoro-11,21-dihydroxy-16-methylpregna-1,4-diene-3,20-dione; 9-chloro-6α-fluoro-16α-methyl-1,4-pregnadiene-11β,21-diol-3,20-di-one. $C_{22}H_{28}ClFO_4$; mol wt 410.91. C 64.30%, H 6.87%, Cl 8.63%, F 4.62%, O 15.57%. Prepn: **NL 6412708**; E. K. Kaspar, R. Philippson, **DE 2011559**; *eidem,* **US 3729495** (1965, 1971, 1973 all to Schering AG). Clinical trials: Wortmann, *Wien. Med. Wochenschr.* **122,** 701 (1972); Baumann, *Praxis* **61,** 536 (1972).

Crystals from methanol-methylene chloride, mp 254° (dec).
21-Acetate. [4258-85-9] SH-818. $C_{24}H_{30}ClFO_5$; mol wt 452.94. Crystals from methanol-methylene chloride, mp 252° (dec).

21-Pivalate. [34097-16-0] CL-68; SH-863; Cloderm; Purantix. $C_{27}H_{36}ClFO_5$; mol wt 495.02.
THERAP CAT: Glucocorticoid.

2370. Clodinafop-Propargyl. [105512-06-9] (2R)-2-[4-[(5-Chloro-3-fluoro-2-pyridinyl)oxy]phenoxy]propanoic acid 2-propynyl ester; 2-propynyl (R)-2-[4-(5-chloro-3-fluoro-2-pyridyl-oxy)phenoxy]propionate; CGA-184927; Topik. $C_{17}H_{13}ClFNO_4$; mol wt 349.74. C 58.38%, H 3.75%, Cl 10.14%, F 5.43%, N 4.00%, O 18.30%. Pyridyloxyphenoxy herbicide for use in cereal crops. Prepn: R. Schurter, **EP 248968**; R. Schurter, H. Rempfler, **US 4713109** (both 1987 to Ciba-Geigy). Description: J. Amrein et al., Brighton Crop Prot. Conf. - Weeds **1989**, 71-76. HPLC determn in soil and plant samples: S. Roy, S. B. Singh, J. Chromatogr. A **1065**, 199 (2005). Review of field trials with the crop safener, cloquintocet, q.v.: D. W. Cornes, ibid. 729-734; R. D. Welsh, Proc. 47th N. Z. Plant Prot. Conf. **1994**, 22-26.

Odorless, crystalline solid, mp 59.3°. $[\alpha]_D^{20}$ +45.4° (c = 2 in acetone). Vapor pressure (20°): 5.3×10^{-6} Pa. Soly in water (20°): 2.5 ppm. Sol in most organic solvents. LD_{50} in rats (mg/kg): 1829 orally; >2000 dermally. LC_{50} in rats (4 hr): >2325 mg/m³ by inhalation (Amrein).
USE: Herbicide.

2371. Clodronic Acid. [10596-23-3] (Dichloromethyl-ene)bisphosphonic acid; (dichloromethylene)diphosphonic acid; di-chloromethanediphosphonic acid; Cl_2MDP; DMDP. $CH_4Cl_2O_6P_2$; mol wt 244.89. C 4.90%, H 1.65%, Cl 28.95%, O 39.20%, P 25.30%. Bisphosphonate antiresorptive agent. Prepn and use as detergent additive: **BE 672205** (1966 to Procter and Gamble), C.A. **67**, 4040u (1967). Prepn: O. T. Quimby et al., J. Org. Chem. **32**, 4111 (1967). Effect on hydroxyapatite durapatite, q.v., crystal aggregation: N. M. Hansen et al., Biochim. Biophys. Acta **451**, 549 (1976); S. Bisaz et al., ibid. **617**, 291 (1993). Symposium on therapeutic efficacy in neoplastic bone disease: Bone **8**, Suppl. 1, S1-S86 (1987). Review of pharmacology and clinical efficacy in resorptive bone disease: G. L. Plosker, K. L. Goa, Drugs **47**, 945-982 (1994). Clinical reduction of new meta-stases in breast cancer: I. J. Diel et al., N. Engl. J. Med. **339**, 357 (1998).

mp 249-251°.
Disodium salt. [22560-50-5]; [88416-50-6] (tetrahydrate). Clodronate disodium; Bonefos; Clasteon; Clastoban; Difosfonal; Loron; Lytos; Mebonat; Ossiten; Ostac. $CH_2Cl_2Na_2O_6P_2$; mol wt 288.86. Occurs as the tetrahydrate.
THERAP CAT: Bone resorption inhibitor.

2372. Clofarabine. [123318-82-1] 2-Chloro-9-(2-deoxy-2-fluoro-β-D-arabinofuranosyl)-9H-purin-6-amine; 2-chloro-9-(2-de-oxy-2-fluoro-β-D-arabinofuranosyl)adenine; 2-chloro-2′-arabino-fluoro-2′-deoxyadenosine; Cl-F-ara-A; Clolar. $C_{10}H_{11}ClFN_5O_3$; mol wt 303.68. C 39.55%, H 3.65%, Cl 11.67%, F 6.26%, N 23.06%, O 15.81%. Second generation purine nucleoside analog; antimetabolite that inhibits DNA synthesis and resists deamination by adenosine deaminase. Prepn: K. A. Watanabe et al., **EP 219829**; eidem, **US 4918179** (1987, 1990 both to Sloan-Kettering Inst. Cancer Res.); J. A. Montgomery et al., J. Med. Chem. **35**, 397 (1992). Improved synthesis: W. E. Bauta et al., Org. Process Res. Dev. **8**, 889 (2004). Antineoplastic activity: W. R. Waud et al., Nucleosides Nucleotides Nucleic Acids **19**, 447 (2000). Clinical

pharmacology: H. M. Kantarjian et al,. J. Clin. Oncol. **21**, 1167 (2003). Clinical pharmacokinetics: V. Gandhi et al., Clin. Cancer Res. **9**, 6335 (2003). Clinical evaluation in acute leukemia: H. Kantarjian et al., Blood **102**, 2379 (2003); in pediatric patients: S. Jeha et al., ibid. **103**, 784 (2004). Review of development: A. Sternberg, Curr. Opin. Invest. Drugs **4**, 1479-1487 (2003); of mech-anism of action and clinical experience: S. Faderl et al., Cancer **103**, 1985-1995 (2005).

Crystals from water, mp 225-227° (Montgomery). Also reported as crystals from methanol, mp 237° (Bauta). uv max (water): 212, 263 nm (ε 22500, 15989).
THERAP CAT: Antineoplastic.

2373. Clofazimine. [2030-63-9] N,5-Bis(4-chlorophenyl)-3,5-dihydro-3-[(1-methylethyl)imino]-2-phenazinamine; 3-(p-chlo-roanilino)-10-(p-chlorophenyl)-2,10-dihydro-2-(isopropyl-imino)phenazine; 2-(4-chloroanilino)-3-isopropylimino-5-(4-chlo-rophenyl)-3,5-dihydrophenazine; 2-p-chloroanilino-5-p-chloro-phenyl-3,5-dihydro-3-isopropyliminophenazine; G-30320; B-663; Lampren(e). $C_{27}H_{22}Cl_2N_4$; mol wt 473.40. C 68.50%, H 4.68%, Cl 14.98%, N 11.83%. Prepn: V. C. Barry et al., **US 2948726** (1960 to Geigy); Barry et al., Nature **179**, 1013 (1957); Barry et al., J. Chem. Soc. **1958**, 859; Belton et al., Proc. R. Irish Acad. Sect. B **62**, 9 (1961), C.A. **58**, 4556d (1963). Activity studies: Vischer, Arzneim.-Forsch. **18**, 1529 (1968). HPLC determn in plasma: J. H. Peters et al., J. Chromatogr. **229**, 503 (1982). Toxicity data: Stenger et al., Arzneim.-Forsch. **20**, 794 (1970). Clinical studies: Mathies, ibid. 1838; Karat et al., Br. Med. J. **1**, 198 (1970). Review of clinical pharmacokinetics: M. R. Holdi-ness, Clin. Pharmacokinet. **16**, 74-85 (1989); of clinical use: J. C. Garrelts, DICP Ann. Pharmacother. **25**, 525-531 (1991). Compre-hensive description: V. K. Kapoor, Anal. Profiles Drug Subs. **18**, 91-120 (1989); C. M. O'Driscoll, O. I. Corrigan, Anal. Profiles Drug Subs. Excip. **21**, 75-108 (1992).

Dark-red crystals, mp 210-212°. uv max (0.01M methanolic HCl): 284, 486 nm (abs. ~1.30, ~0.64). pKa 8.37; also reported as 8.51. Sol in dil acetic acid, DMF. Sol in 15 parts of chloroform, 700 parts of ethanol, 1000 parts of ether. Practically insol in water. Log P (octanol/water): 7.48; (isooctane/pH 5.15 buffer) at 20°: 5.01; (n-octanol/pH 5.15 buffer) at 20°: 4.30; (n-octanol/pH 5.15 buffer) at 37°: 4.40; (n-octanol/pH 5.15 buffer) at 45°: 4.48; (n-octanol/pH 5.15 buffer) at 55°: 4.54. LD_{50} orally in mice, rats, and guinea pigs: >4 g/kg (Stenger).
THERAP CAT: Antibacterial (tuberculostatic, leprostatic).

2374. Clofenamide. [671-95-4] 4-Chloro-1,3-benzenedi-sulfonamide; 4-chloro-m-benzenedisulfonamide; 1-chlorobenzene-2,4-disulfonamide; chlorphenamide; monochlorphenamide; Salco; Saltron; Soluran; Aquedux; Haflutan. $C_6H_7ClN_2O_4S_2$; mol wt

270.71. C 26.62%, H 2.61%, Cl 13.10%, N 10.35%, O 23.64%, S 23.69%. Prepn: Olivier, *Rec. Trav. Chim.* **37**, 307 (1918); Davies, Wood, *J. Chem. Soc.* **1928**, 1125.

Needles, mp 206-207° (Davies), mp 217-219° (Olivier). Sol in hot alcohol, water; slightly sol in cold solvents.

THERAP CAT: Diuretic.

2375. Clofencet. [129025-54-3] 2-(4-Chlorophenyl)-3-ethyl-2,5-dihydro-5-oxo-4-pyridazinecarboxylic acid; MON-21200. C$_{13}$H$_{11}$ClN$_2$O$_3$; mol wt 278.69. C 56.03%, H 3.98%, Cl 12.72%, N 10.05%, O 17.22%. Hybridizing agent for wheat. Prepn: D. R. Patterson, **EP 49971**; *idem*, **US 4732603** (1982, 1988 both to Rohm & Haas). Improved prepn: J. D. Clark *et al., Org. Process Res. Dev.* **8**, 176 (2004). Sorption behavior in soils: I. G. Dubus *et al., Chemosphere* **45**, 767 (2001). Comprehensive description: *Clofencet Pesticide Fact Sheet* (U.S. EPA, Feb. 1997) 12 pp.

Technical grade: tan/yellow solid, mp 269° (dec). d^{20} 1.44. Soly (%w:v): distilled water >55.2, pH 5 >65.5, pH 7 >69.6, pH 9 >65.8; methanol 1.6; acetone <0.05; dichloromethane <0.04; toluene <0.04; ethyl acetate <0.05; *n*-hexane <0.06. Vapor pressure (25°): <10^{-7} mm Hg. pKa 2.83 (20°). Log P (octanol/water): −2.2 (25°). LD$_{50}$ in rats (mg/kg/day): 3306 orally; >5000 dermally (U.S. EPA).

Potassium salt. [82697-71-0] MON-21233; Genesis. C$_{13}$H$_{10}$-ClKN$_2$O$_3$; mol wt 316.78. LC$_{50}$ in rats (mg/l): >3.8 (U.S. EPA).

Sodium salt. [82697-16-3] C$_{13}$H$_{10}$ClN$_2$NaO$_3$; mol wt 300.67. mp 190-191°.

USE: Plant growth regulator.

2376. Clofentezine. [74115-24-5] 3,6-Bis(2-chlorophenyl)-1,2,4,5-tetrazine; bisclofentezin; NC-21314; Apollo. C$_{14}$H$_8$Cl$_2$N$_4$; mol wt 303.15. C 55.47%, H 2.66%, Cl 23.39%, N 18.48%. Contact acaricide active against eggs and early motile stages of phytophagous mites. Prepn: J. H. Parsons, **EP 5912**; *idem*, **US 4237127** (1979, 1980 both to Fisons). Physical properties, toxicity and bioactivity: K. M. G. Bryan *et al., Proc. Br. Crop Prot. Conf. - Pests Dis.* **1981**, 67. Field trial on apple trees: A. J. Read, *Proc. 36th N.Z. Weed Pest Control Conf.*, 261 (1983). *Review:* F. Rauch, *Def. Veg.* **39**, 11-17 (1985).

Magenta solid. Crystals from ethyl acetate, mp 179-182°. Soly: 50 g/l in chloroform; 2.5 g/l in benzene; <1 g/l in hexane; <1 mg/l in water. LD$_{50}$ in rats, mice (mg/kg): >3200 orally; LC$_{50}$ (96 hr) in rainbow trout: 100 mg/l (Bryan).

USE: Pesticide.

2377. Clofibrate. [637-07-0] 2-(4-Chlorophenoxy)-2-methylpropanoic acid ethyl ester; ethyl 2-(*p*-chlorophenoxy)-2-methylpropionate; ethyl *p*-chlorophenoxyisobutyrate; Amotril; Anparton; Apolan; Artevil; Ateculon; Ateriosan; Atheropront; Atromidin; Atromid-S; Bioscleran; Claripex; Clobren-SF; Clofinit; CPIB; Hyclorate; Liprinal; Neo-Atromid; Normet; Normolipol; Recolip; Regelan; Serotinex; Sklerolip; Skleromexe; Sklero-Tablinen; Xyduril. C$_{12}$H$_{15}$ClO$_3$; mol wt 242.70. C 59.39%, H 6.23%, Cl 14.61%, O

19.78%. Prepn: W. G. M. Jones *et al.*, **GB 860303**; *eidem*, **US 3262850** (1961, 1966 both to I.C.I.). Clinical trials in the primary prevention of ischaemic heart disease: *Br. Heart J.* **40**, 1069 (1978); *Lancet* **2**, 379 (1980). Toxicity data: G. Metz *et al., Arzneim.-Forsch.* **27**, 1173 (1977). Review of pharmacology: M. Chevais, *Therapie* **35**, 5-22 (1980); of metabolism: M. N. Cayen, *Rev. Drug Metab. Drug Interact.* **3**, 77-103 (1980); of toxicity studies: *IARC Monographs* **24**, 39-58 (1980). Comprehensive description: M. M. A. Hassan, A. A. Elazzouny, *Anal. Profiles Drug Subs.* **11**, 197-224 (1982).

Oil, bp$_{20}$ 148-150°. Practically insol in water. Misc with ethanol, acetone, chloroform, ether. LD$_{50}$ in mice, rats (g/kg): 1.28, 1.65 orally (Metz).

Mixture with androsterone. [8075-95-8] Atromid.

THERAP CAT: Antilipemic.

2378. Clofibric Acid. [882-09-7] 2-(4-Chlorophenoxy)-2-methylpropanoic acid; 2-(*p*-chlorophenoxy)-2-methylpropionic acid; α-(*p*-chlorophenoxy)isobutyric acid; chlorophibrinic acid; Arteriohom; Regulipid. C$_{10}$H$_{11}$ClO$_3$; mol wt 214.65. C 55.95%, H 5.17%, Cl 16.52%, O 22.36%. Prepn: Galimberti, Defranceschi, *Gazz. Chim. Ital.* **77**, 431 (1947); Gilman, Wilder, *J. Am. Chem. Soc.* **77**, 6644 (1955); Jones *et al.*, **GB 860303** (1961 to I.C.I.). Prepn and resolution of isomers: Witiak *et al., J. Med. Chem.* **11**, 1086 (1968). Activity thought to be due to its displacement of thyroxin and its inhibition of cholesterol biosynthesis. *See* Chang *et al., Biochem. Pharmacol.* **16**, 2053 (1967); Walsh *et al., Arch. Biochem. Biophys.* **130**, 7 (1969); Witiak *et al., J. Med. Chem.* **14**, 754 (1971). Metabolism: Almirante *et al., Boll. Chim. Farm.* **108**, 292 (1969).

Crystals from water or methanol, mp 118-119°.

Basic aluminum salt. [24818-79-9] Alufibrate; Atherolip; Atherolipin. C$_{20}$H$_{21}$AlCl$_2$O$_7$; mol wt 471.26.

Magnesium salt. [14613-30-0] Magnesium clofibrate; UR-112; Clomag. C$_{20}$H$_{20}$Cl$_2$MgO$_6$; mol wt 451.58. White powder, mp 326-328°. Soly in g/100 mg: water 4.5; abs ethanol 0.7; chloroform 0.02.

Pyridoxine salt. [29952-87-2] Pyridoxine *p*-chlorophenoxy-isobutyrate; Claresan. C$_{10}$H$_{11}$ClO$_3$.C$_8$H$_{11}$NO$_3$; mol wt 383.82. Prepn: Sarbach *et al.*, **DE 1915497** (1970 to Inst. Rech. Sci.), *C.A.* **74**, 13011g (1971).

Ethyl ester *see* Clofibrate.

Etofylline ester *see* Theofibrate.

THERAP CAT: Antilipemic.

2379. Cloflucarban. [369-77-7] *N*-(4-Chlorophenyl)-*N*′-[4-chloro-3-(trifluoromethyl)phenyl]urea; 4,4′-dichloro-3-(trifluoromethyl)carbanilide; Irgasan CF3. C$_{14}$H$_9$Cl$_2$F$_3$N$_2$O; mol wt 349.14. C 48.16%, H 2.60%, Cl 20.31%, F 16.32%, N 8.02%, O 4.58%. Prepn: Schetty *et al.*, **US 2745874** (1956 to Geigy); Sydor, **BE 617117** (1962 to Am. Cyanamid), compd included but not specifically described in abstract, *C.A.* **59**, 1542a (1963).

White crystalline solid, mp 214-215°. Insol in water; dissolves well in organic solvents.

THERAP CAT: Disinfectant.

2380. Clofoctol. [37693-01-9] 2-[(2,4-Dichlorophenyl)-methyl]-4-(1,1,3,3-tetramethylbutyl)phenol; α-(2,4-dichlorophenyl)-4-(1,1,3,3-tetramethylbutyl)-*o*-cresol; Gramplus; Octofene. $C_{21}H_{26}Cl_2O$; mol wt 365.34. C 69.04%, H 7.17%, Cl 19.41%, O 4.38%. Prepn: J. Debat, **US 3830852** (1974 to Inst. Recherches Chim. Biol. Appl.). Activity against gram positive and gram negative bacteria: A. Buogo, *Drugs Exp. Clin. Res.* **10,** 321 (1984). Pharmacokinetics in rats: M. Del Tacca *et al.* in *Recent Advances in Chemotherapy, Antimicrobial Section 3,* J. Ishigami, Ed. (University of Tokyo Press, 1985) pp 1927-28; in man: *eidem, J. Antimicrob. Chemother.* **19,** 679 (1987). Mechanism of action: J. Combe *et al., J. Pharmacol.* **11,** 411 (1980); F. Yablonsky, G. Simonet, *ibid.* **13,** 515 (1982). Clinical trials in respiratory infections: J. Vialatte, *Diagnostics* **207,** 65 (1978); in infectious bronchopulmonary diseases: R. Danesi, M. Del Tacca, *Int. J. Clin. Pharmacol. Res.* **5,** 175 (1985); in ear, nose and throat infections: P. L. Ghilardi, A. Casani, *Drugs Exp. Clin. Res.* **11,** 815 (1985).

Crystals from petr ether, mp 78°. LD_{50} orally in male rats: >4 g/kg (Debat).

THERAP CAT: Antibacterial.

2381. Clomazone. [81777-89-1] 2-[(2-Chlorophenyl)methyl]-4,4-dimethyl-3-isoxazolidinone; dimethazone; FMC-57020; Command. $C_{12}H_{14}ClNO_2$; mol wt 239.70. C 60.13%, H 5.89%, Cl 14.79%, N 5.84%, O 13.35%. Pre-emergence herbicide; inhibits biosynthesis of photosynthetic pigments in susceptible species. Prepn: J. H. Chang, **BE 889040**; *idem,* **US 4405357** (1982, 1983 both to FMC). Use on soybeans: M. P. Mascianica, *Proc. Annu. Meet. Northeast. Weed Sci. Soc.* **39,** 25 (1985); on white potatoes: C. C. Kupatt *et al., ibid.* 166. Fate in soil: T. L. Mervosh *et al., J. Agric. Food Chem.* **43,** 537 (1995). Review of properties and analytical methods: A. W. Chen in *Comprehensive Analytical Profiles of Important Pesticides,* J. Sherma, T. Cairns, Eds. (CRC Press, Boca Raton, 1993) pp 131-148.

Light brown viscous liquid, mp 25°. Vapor pressure at 25°: 1.4 × 10^{-6} mm Hg. d^{20} 1.19. Solv in water: 1100 ppm. Readily sol in chloroform, methanol, methylene chloride, heptane, acetonitrile, toluene, acetone, dioxane, xylene, hexane. LD_{50} in male rats, female rats, mallard duck-bobwhite quail (mg/kg): 2077, 1369, >2510 orally; in rabbits (mg/kg): >2000 dermally (Chen).

USE: Herbicide.

2382. Clomestrone. [4091-75-2] (16α)-16-Chloro-3-methoxyestra-1,3,5(10)-trien-17-one; 16α-chloroestrone 3-methyl ether; Arterolo; Atheran. $C_{19}H_{23}ClO_2$; mol wt 318.84. C 71.57%, H 7.27%, Cl 11.12%, O 10.04%. Prepn: Mueller *et al., J. Am. Chem. Soc.* **80,** 1769 (1958); Mueller, **US 2855411** (1958 to Searle); Ravizza, **CH 343396** (1959). Alternate route: Labs. Sobio, **FR 1350100** (1964).

Crystals from chloroform, mp 179-180°. $[\alpha]_D$ +161° (chloroform).

2383. Clometacin. [25803-14-9] 3-(4-Chlorobenzoyl)-6-methoxy-2-methyl-1*H*-indole-1-acetic acid; [2-methyl-3-(*p*-chlorobenzoyl)-6-methoxyindol-1-yl]acetic acid; clometazin; mindolic acid; R-3959; C-1656; Dupéran. $C_{19}H_{16}ClNO_4$; mol wt 357.79. C 63.78%, H 4.51%, Cl 9.91%, N 3.91%, O 17.89%. Prepn: Allais, Nomine, **DE 1901167** (1969 to Roussel-UCLAF), *C.A.* **72,** 43440x (1970).

White powder, mp 242°.

THERAP CAT: Analgesic.

2384. Clomethiazole. [533-45-9] 5-(2-Chloroethyl)-4-methylthiazole; 4-methyl-5-(β-chloroethyl)thiazole; chlorethiazol; chlormethiazole; S.C.T.Z.. C_6H_8ClNS; mol wt 161.65. C 44.58%, H 4.99%, Cl 21.93%, N 8.66%, S 19.84%. Prepd by condensation of thioformamide with chloroacetopropyl alcohol: Buchman, *J. Am. Chem. Soc.* **58,** 1803 (1936); by chlorination of 4-methyl-5-(β-ethoxyethyl)thiazole: Clarke, Gurin, *ibid.* **57,** 1876 (1935); by treating 5-(2-hydroxyethyl)-4-methylthiazole with thionyl chloride: Sawa, Ishida, *J. Pharm. Soc. Jpn.* **76,** 337 (1956); by H_2O_2 oxidation of 2-mercapto-4-methyl-5-(β-chloroethyl)thiazole: **CH 200248** (1938 to Hoffmann-La Roche). Prepn of methane and ethanedisulfonate: Charonnat *et al.,* **US 3031457** (1962).

Oily, viscous liquid. d_4^{25} 1.233. Characteristic disagreeable odor of thiazole compds. bp_7 92°.

Hydrochloride. [6001-74-7] $C_6H_8ClNS.HCl$. Crystals from abs ethanol + ether, mp 130°. Sol in water, alcohol.

Methanedisulfonate. $C_{13}H_{20}Cl_2N_2O_6S_4$. Crystals from methanol + ether, mp 120°.

Ethanedisulfonate. [1867-58-9] Distraneurin; Hemineurin; Heminevrin. $C_{14}H_{22}Cl_2N_2O_6S_4$; mol wt 513.50. Crystals from methanol + ether, mp 124°.

USE: Intermediate in some processes of vitamin B_1 manufacture.

THERAP CAT: Sedative, hypnotic, anticonvulsant.

2385. Clometocillin. [1926-49-4] (2*S*,5*R*,6*R*)-6-[[(3,4-Dichlorophenyl)methoxyacetyl]amino]-3,3-dimethyl-7-oxo-4-thia-1-azabicyclo[3.2.0]heptane-2-carboxylic acid; 3,4-dichloro-α-methoxybenzylpenicillin; 6-(α-methoxy-3,4-dichlorophenylacetamido)-penicillanic acid; clometacillin; clomethacillin; no. 356; penicillin 356. $C_{17}H_{18}Cl_2N_2O_5S$; mol wt 433.31. C 47.12%, H 4.19%, Cl 16.36%, N 6.46%, O 18.46%, S 7.40%. Semi-synthetic antibiotic related to penicillin. Prepn: Vanderhaeghe *et al., Antimicrob. Agents Chemother.* **1961,** 581; **US 3007920** (1961 to Recherche et Ind. Therap.). Activity studies: van Dijck *et al., Antibiot. Chemother.* **12,** 192 (1962).

Sodium salt. [54530-86-8] Rixapen. $C_{17}H_{17}Cl_2N_2NaO_5S$; mol wt 455.29. $[\alpha]_D$ +210-220°. Pure epimers were prepared by fractional crystn. First crop: Crystals, dec 232-235°. $[\alpha]_D^{20}$ +182° (water). Second crop: $[\alpha]_D^{20}$ +207°. Third crop: Crystals, dec 180-183°. $[\alpha]_D^{20}$ +261° (water). The free acid yields two diastereoisomers: $[\alpha]_D$ +177° and $[\alpha]_D$ +257°.

THERAP CAT: Antibacterial.

2386. Clomiphene. [911-45-5] 2-[4-(2-Chloro-1,2-diphen-ylethenyl)phenoxy]-*N*,*N*-diethylethanamine; 2-[*p*-(2-chloro-1,2-di-phenylvinyl)phenoxy]triethylamine; 2-[*p*-(β-chloro-α-phenyl-styryl)phenoxy]triethylamine; 1-[*p*-(β-diethylaminoethoxy)phen-yl]-1,2-diphenylchloroethylene; clomifene; chloramifene; MRL-41; WSM-5008. C$_{26}$H$_{28}$ClNO; mol wt 405.96. C 76.92%, H 6.95%, Cl 8.73%, N 3.45%, O 3.94%. Synthetic estrogen ago-nist-antagonist. Prepn: R. E. Allen *et al.*, US 2914563 (1959 to Merrell); F. P. Palopoli *et al.*, *J. Med. Chem.* **10**, 84 (1967). Ste-reochemistry of the geometric isomers: Ernst *et al.*, *J. Pharm. Sci.* **65**, 148 (1976). Induction of ovulation: R. B. Greenblatt, *Fertil. Steril.* **12**, 402 (1961). Clinical trial in anovulatory women: J. Garcia *et al.*, *ibid.* **28**, 707 (1977). Use in male infertility: P. J. Sorbie, R. Perez-Marrero, *J. Urol.* **131**, 425 (1984). HPLC determn of isomers in human plasma: C. L. Baustian, T. J. Mikkelson, *J. Pharm. Biomed. Anal.* **4**, 237 (1986). Review of development, pharmacology and clinical experience: R. P. Dickey, D. E. Holt-kamp, *Hum. Reprod. Update* **2**, 483-506 (1996).

Enclomiphene

Citrate. [50-41-9] Clomid; Clostilbegyt; Pergotime; Serofene; Serophene. C$_{26}$H$_{28}$ClNO.C$_6$H$_8$O$_7$; mol wt 598.08. Crystals, mp 116.5-118°. Slightly sol in water, chloroform; freely sol in meth-anol; sparingly sol in alcohol. Insol in ether.

***cis*-Form.** [15690-55-8] Zuclomiphene. Hydrochloride salt mp 156.5-158.0°. uv max (methanol): 230, 291 nm (ε 20500, 12700).

***trans*-Form.** [15690-57-0] Enclomiphene. Hydrochloride salt mp 149.0-150.5°. uv max (methanol): 239, 297 nm (ε 22100, 11600).

THERAP CAT: Gonad-stimulating principle.

2387. Clomipramine. [303-49-1] 3-Chloro-10,11-dihydro-*N*,*N*-dimethyl-5*H*-dibenz[*b*,*f*]azepine-5-propanamine; 3-chloro-5-[3-(dimethylamino)propyl]-10,11-dihydro-5*H*-dibenz[*b*,*f*]azepine; 5-(γ-dimethylaminopropyl)-3-chloroiminodibenzyl; chlorimipra-mine; G-34586. C$_{19}$H$_{23}$ClN$_2$; mol wt 314.85. C 72.48%, H 7.36%, Cl 11.26%, N 8.90%. Serotonin reuptake inhibitor. Prepn: P. N. Craig *et al.*, *J. Org. Chem.* **26**, 135 (1961); W. Schindler, H. Dietrich, **CH 371799**; *eidem*, **US 3467650** (1963, 1969 both to Geigy). Crystal and molecular structure of the hydrochloride: M. L. Post, A. S. Horn, *Acta Crystallogr.* **33B**, 2590 (1977). HPLC determn in serum: H. Weigmann *et al.*, *J. Chromatogr. B* **710**, 227 (1998). Veterinary trial in canine compulsive disorder: C. J. Hewson *et al.*, *J. Am. Vet. Med. Assoc.* **213**, 1760 (1998); in canine separation anxiety: S. Petit *et al.*, *Rev. Med. Vet.* **150**, 133 (1999). Review of pharmacology and clinical experience in obsessive-com-pulsive disorder and depression: M. D. Peters *et al.*, *Clin. Pharm.* **9**, 165-178 (1990).

bp$_{0.3}$ 160-170°.

Hydrochloride. [17321-77-6] Anafranil; Clomicalm. C$_{19}$H$_{23}$-ClN$_2$.HCl; mol wt 351.31. Crystals from acetone-ether/methanol-ether, mp 189-190° (Craig); also reported as crystals from acetone,

mp 191.5-192° (Schindler, Dietrich). Freely sol in water, methanol, methylene chloride. Practically insol in ethyl ether, hexane.

THERAP CAT: Antidepressant; antiobsessional agent.

THERAP CAT (VET): In treatment of canine separation anxiety.

2388. Clomocycline. [1181-54-0] 7-Chloro-4-(dimethyl-amino)-1,4,4a,5,5a,6,11,12a-octahydro-3,6,10,12,12a-pentahy-droxy-*N*-(hydroxymethyl)-6-methyl-1,11-dioxo-2-naphthacenecar-boxamide; chlormethylenecycline; *N*^{2}-(hydroxymethyl)chlortetra-cycline; *N*-methylol-7-chlortetracycline; Megaclor. C$_{23}$H$_{25}$ClN$_2$-O$_9$; mol wt 508.91. C 54.28%, H 4.95%, Cl 6.97%, N 5.50%, O 28.29%. Semi-synthetic broad spectrum antibiotic related to tetra-cycline, *q.v.* Prepn: Banci, Tubaro, *Boll. Chim. Farm.* **102**, 471 (1963); BE 628142 (1963 to AB Leo), *C.A.* **60**, 15805f (1964).

Yellow material. Dec 145-170°. Sensitive to light and air. pH of 2% aq soln 6.3-6.5. Sol in citrate-phosphate buffer, pH 6-8.

THERAP CAT: Antibacterial.

2389. Clonazepam. [1622-61-3] 5-(2-Chlorophenyl)-1,3-dihydro-7-nitro-2*H*-1,4-benzodiazepin-2-one; 7-nitro-5-(2-chloro-phenyl)-3*H*-1,4-benzodiazepin-2(1*H*)-one; Ro-5-4023; Clonopin; Iktorivil; Klonopin; Landsen; Rivotril. C$_{15}$H$_{10}$ClN$_3$O$_3$; mol wt 315.71. C 57.07%, H 3.19%, Cl 11.23%, N 13.31%, O 15.20%. Antiepileptic agent with anxiolytic and antimanic properties. Prepn: L. H. Sternbach *et al.*, *J. Med. Chem.* **6**, 261 (1963); O. Keller *et al.*, US 3121076 (1964 to Hoffmann-La Roche). Prepd but not claimed: J. Kariss, H. L. Newmark, US 3116203 (1963 to Hoffmann-La Roche). Alternate process: A. Focella, A. I. Ra-chlin, US 3335181 (1967 to Hoffmann-La Roche). Pharmacology: Guerrero-Figueroa *et al.*, *Curr. Ther. Res.* **11**, 40 (1969); Lechat *et al.*, *Therapie* **25**, 893 (1970); D'Armagnac *et al.*, *ibid.* **26**, 439 (1971). Toxicology: Blum *et al.*, *Arzneim.-Forsch.* **23**, 377 (1973). Determn of clonazepam and its main metabolites: S. Ebel, H. Schütz, *ibid.* **27**, 325 (1977). Clinical efficacy in acute mania: G. Chouinard, *Psychosomatics* **26**(12), Suppl., 7 (1985); in panic disorders and agitation: R. Fontaine, *ibid.* 13. Comprehen-sive description: W. C. Winslow, *Anal. Profiles Drug Subs.* **6**, 61-81 (1977).

White crystals from ethanol-methylene chloride, mp 236.5-238.5°. uv max (7.5% methanol in isopropanol): 248, 310 nm (ε 14500, 11600). Soly in mg/ml at 25°: acetone 31; chloroform 15; methanol 8.6; ether 0.7; benzene 0.5; water <0.1. pK$_1$ 1.5, pK$_2$ 10.5. LD$_{50}$ orally in mice: >4000 mg/kg (Blum).

Note: This is a controlled substance (depressant): **21 CFR,** 1308.14.

THERAP CAT: Anticonvulsant.

2390. Clonidine. [4205-90-7] *N*-(2,6-Dichlorophenyl)-4,5-dihydro-1*H*-imidazol-2-amine; 2-(2,6-dichloroanilino)-2-imidazo-line; 2,6-dichloro-*N*-2-imidazolidinylidenebenzenamine; 2-(2,6-di-chloroanilino)-1,3-diazacyclopentene-(2); 2-[(2,6-dichlorophenyl)-imino]-2-imidazoline. C$_9$H$_9$Cl$_2$N$_3$; mol wt 230.09. C 46.98%, H 3.94%, Cl 30.82%, N 18.26%. α$_2$-Adrenergic agonist. Prepn: Zeile *et al.*, US 3202660 (1965 to Boehringer, Ing.). Use in shaving soap formulations: *eidem,* **US 3190802** (1965 to Boehringer, Ing.). Pharmacology: Bolme, Fuxe, *Eur. J. Pharmacol.* **13,** 168 (1971). Revised structure: L. M. Jackman, T. Jen, *J. Am. Chem. Soc.* **97,** 2811 (1975). GC determn in plasma: P. O. Edlund, *J. Chromatogr.* **187,** 161 (1980). Preliminary studies on potential antidepressant activity: D. C. Jimerson *et al., Biol. Psychiatry* **15,** 45 (1980); J. B. Malick, *Prog. Clin. Biol. Res.* **71,** 165 (1981). Exptl use in drug rehabilitation: M. S. Gold, A. C. Pottash, *Ann. N.Y. Acad. Sci.* **362,** 191-202 (1981). Activity as α-adrenoceptor agonist: A. G. Roach *et al., J. Pharmacol. Exp. Ther.* **227,** 421 (1983). Symposium on cardiovascular and psychotropic pharmacology and clinical experience: *Central Blood Pressure Regulation: The Role of α2-Receptor Stimulation,* K. Hayduk, K. B. Bock, Eds. (Steinkopff Verlag, Darmstadt, 1983) 284 pp. Effects in acute smoking withdrawal syndrome: A. H. Glassman *et al., Science* **226,** 864 (1984); in alcoholism withdrawal: Z. Jraidi *et al., Therapie* **42,** 21 (1987). Clinical trial in Tourette's syndrome: J. F. Leckman *et al., Neurology* **35,** 343 (1985); in cigarette smoking cessation: R. Davison *et al., Clin. Pharmacol. Ther.* **44,** 265 (1988). Clinical trial for intractable cancer pain: J. C. Eisenach *et al., Pain* **61,** 391 (1995). *Reviews:* A. Walland in *Pharmacological and Biochemical Properties of Drug Substances* **vol. 1,** M. E. Goldberg, Ed. (Am. Pharm. Assoc., Washington, D.C., 1977) pp 67-107; H. Schmitt, *Handb. Exp. Pharmacol.* **39,** 299-396 (1977); M. C. Houston, *Prog. Cardiovasc. Dis.* **23,** 337-350 (1981). Comprehensive description: M. A. Abounassif *et al., Anal. Profiles Drug Subs. Excip.* **21,** 109-147 (1992).

Crystals, mp 130°.

Hydrochloride. [4205-91-8] ST-155; Catapres; Catapresan; Clonistada; Dixarit; Duraclon; Isoglaucon; Tenso-Timelets. C_9H_9-Cl_2N_3.HCl; mol wt 266.55. Crystals, mp 305°. Sol in abs. ethanol; slightly sol in chloroform. Practically insol in ether. One gram is sol in 6 mls water (60°C); about 13 mls water (20°C); about 5.8 mls methanol; about 25 mls ethanol; about 5000 mls chloroform. uv max (water): 213, 271, 302 nm (ε 8290.327, 713.074, 339.876). LD_{50} in mice, rats (mg/kg): 328, 270 orally; 18, 29 i.v. (Walland).

USE: In shaving soaps.

THERAP CAT: Antihypertensive; analgesic for neuropathic pain.

2391. Clonitrate. [2612-33-1] 3-Chloro-1,2-propanediol dinitrate; 3-chloropropyleneglycol dinitrate; dinitrochlorohydrin; D-ylate. $C_3H_5ClN_2O_6$; mol wt 200.53. C 17.97%, H 2.51%, Cl 17.68%, N 13.97%, O 47.87%. Prepn from 3-chloro-1,2-propanediol: Henry, *Ann.* **155,** 165 (1870).

$$CH_2ONO_2$$
$$|$$
$$CHONO_2$$
$$|$$
$$CH_2Cl$$

Slightly yellow liq, bp$_{760}$ 190-195° (some decompn); bp$_{15}$ 121-123°; bp$_{10}$ 117.5°. d^9 1.5112; d^{15} 1.5408. Sol in alc, acetone, chloroform; practically insol in water, acids.

THERAP CAT: Vasodilator (coronary).

2392. Clonixin. [17737-65-4] 2-[(3-Chloro-2-methylphenyl)amino]-3-pyridinecarboxylic acid; 2-(3-chloro-*o*-toluidino)-nicotinic acid; 2-(2-methyl-3-chloroanilino)nicotinic acid; 2-(3-chloro-2-methylanilino)nicotinic acid; clonixic acid; CBA-93626; Sch-10304. $C_{13}H_{11}ClN_2O_2$; mol wt 262.69. C 59.44%, H 4.22%, Cl 13.50%, N 10.66%, O 12.18%. Nonsteroidal anti-inflammatory agent. Prepn: M. H. Sherlock, N. Sperber, **BE 679271;** *eidem,* **US 3337570** (1965, 1967 both to Schering). Pharmacology: A. S. Watnick *et al., Arch. Int. Pharmacodyn.* **190,** 78 (1971). Metabolism in humans: B. Katchen *et al., J. Pharmacol. Exp. Ther.* **187,** 152 (1973). Clinical evaluation of analgesic activity: J. S. Finch, T. J. DeKornfeld, *J. Clin. Pharmacol.* **15,** 371 (1971). GC determn

in plasma: C. Giachetti *et al., J. High Resolut. Chromatogr.* **13,** 789 (1990). Toxicology studies: H. Tanaka *et al., Oyo Yakuri* **7,** 655 (1973), *C.A.* **80,** 44091m (1974).

Crystals from isopropyl acetate, mp 233-235°. Extremely bitter taste. LD_{50} in male mice, rats (mg/kg): 415, 335 orally; 198, 148 i.p.; 296, 325 s.c. (Tanaka).

Lysine salt. [55837-30-4] L-104; Clonix; Deltar; Dolalgial; Dorixina. $C_{13}H_{11}ClN_2O_2.C_6H_{14}N_2O_2$; mol wt 408.88.

THERAP CAT: Analgesic.

2393. Clopamide. [636-54-4] *rel*-3-(Aminosulfonyl)-4-chloro-*N*-[(2R,6S)-2,6-dimethyl-1-piperidinyl]benzamide; *cis*-1-(4-chloro-3-sulfamoylbenzamido)-2,6-dimethylpiperidine; *cis*-*N*-(2′,6′-dimethyl-1′-piperidyl)-3-sulfamoyl-4-chlorobenzamide; *cis*-4-chloro-*N*-(2′,6′-dimethyl-1′-piperidyl)-3-sulfamoylbenzamide; chlosudimeprimyl; DT-327; Adurix; Brinaldix. $C_{14}H_{20}ClN_3O_3S$; mol wt 345.84. C 48.62%, H 5.83%, Cl 10.25%, N 12.15%, O 13.88%, S 9.27%. Prepn (stereochemistry unspecified): **BE 610039;** E. Jucker, A. J. Lindenmann, **US 3459756** (1962, 1969 both to Sandoz). Prepn of *cis*- and *trans*-forms: *eidem, Helv. Chim. Acta* **45,** 2316 (1962). HPLC determn: R. T. Sane *et al., J. Chromatogr.* **356,** 468 (1986). Pharmacokinetics and diuretic effect in humans: J. J. McNeil *et al., Clin. Pharmacol. Ther.* **42,** 299 (1987). Clinical trial of combination with pindolol, *q.v.,* in essential hypertension: D. Crowder, E. G. M. Cameron, *Curr. Med. Res. Opin.* **6,** 342 (1979).

Mixture with pindolol. [71789-16-7] Viskaldix.

Hydrazine deriv. Crystals from methanol + diisopropyl ether, mp 244-246°.

THERAP CAT: Antihypertensive; diuretic.

2394. Clopenthixol. [982-24-1] 4-[3-(2-Chloro-9*H*-thioxanthen-9-ylidene)propyl]-1-piperazineethanol; 2-chloro-9-[3-[4-(2-hydroxyethyl)-1-piperazinyl]propylidene]thiaxanthene. C_{22}-$H_{25}ClN_2OS$; mol wt 400.96. C 65.90%, H 6.28%, Cl 8.84%, N 6.99%, O 3.99%, S 8.00%. Thioxanthene neuroleptic. Prepn (configuration not specified): **BE 585338;** P. V. Petersen *et al., US 3116291** (1960, 1963 both to Kefalas A/S). Prepn of the pharmacologically active *cis*-isomer: **BE 816855;** N. Lassen, **US 3996211** (1974, 1976 both to Kefalas A/S). Pharmacology: Cazzullo, Andreola, *Acta Neurol.* **20,** 162 (1965); Weissman, *Mod. Probl. Pharmacopsychiatry* **2,** 15 (1969); Moeller Nielsen, *ibid.* 23. Metabolism: Khan, *Acta Pharmacol. Toxicol.* **27,** 202 (1969). HPLC determn of isomers in serum: T. Aaes-Jorgensen, *J. Chromatogr.* **188,** 239 (1980). Series of articles on pharmacology and clinical studies: *Acta Psychiatr. Scand.* **64,** Suppl. 294, 1-77 (1981).

cis-isomer

Colorless syrup. Sparingly sol in ether. Readily sol in methanol.

Dihydrochloride. [633-59-0] AY-62021; N-746; Ciatyl; Sordenac; Sordinol. $C_{22}H_{25}ClN_2OS.2HCl$; mol wt 473.89. Crystals from ethanol, mp 250-260° (dec). Freely sol in water; sparingly sol in alcohol. Practically insol in other organic solvents. LD_{50} in male mice (mg/kg): 111 i.v. (Lassen).

cis(Z)-Form. [53772-83-1] α-Clopenthixol; zuclopenthixol. Crystals, mp 84-85°.

cis(Z)-Form dihydrochloride. [58045-23-1] Cisordinol; Clopixol. Crystals, mp 250-260° (dec). LD_{50} in male mice (mg/kg): 105 i.v. (Lassen).

THERAP CAT: Antipsychotic.

2395. Cloperastine. [3703-76-2] 1-[2-[(4-Chlorophenyl)-phenylmethoxy]ethyl]piperidine; 1-[2-[(p-chloro-α-phenylbenzyl)-oxy]ethyl]piperidine; p-chlorobenzhydryl 2-(1-piperidyl)ethyl ether. $C_{20}H_{24}ClNO$; mol wt 329.86. C 72.82%, H 7.33%, Cl 10.75%, N 4.25%, O 4.85%. Prepn: **GB 670622** (1952 to Parke, Davis); Fujie, *Yakugaku Zasshi* **81**, 693 (1961), *C.A.* **55**, 25848f (1961). Prepn of salts: **GB 1179945** (1970 to Yoshitomi Pharm.), *C.A.* **72**, 132549g (1970). Pharmacology: Takagi *et al., Yakugaku Zasshi* **85**, 550 (1965); **87**, 907 (1967), *C.A.* **63**, 8932f (1965); **67**, 107101u (1967). Metabolism: Kato, Furuta, *Oyo Yakuri* **5**, 735 (1972).

$bp_{0.06}$ 172-174°, $bp_{0.15}$ 178-180°.
Hydrochloride. [14984-68-0] Hustazol; Nitossil; Novotusil; Seki. $C_{20}H_{24}ClNO.HCl$; mol wt 366.32. Crystals, mp 147.9°.
Methiodide. $C_{20}H_{24}ClNO.CH_3I$. Crystals, mp 140°.
THERAP CAT: Antitussive.

2396. Clopidogrel. [113665-84-2] (αS)-α-(2-Chlorophenyl)-6,7-dihydrothieno[3,2-c]pyridine-5(4H)-acetic acid methyl ester; methyl (+)-(S)-α-(o-chlorophenyl)-6,7-dihydrothieno[3,2-c]pyridine-5(4H)-acetate; (+)-methyl-α-5-[4,5,6,7-tetrahydro[3,2-c]thienopyridyl]-(2-chlorophenyl)acetate; SR-25990. $C_{16}H_{16}ClNO_2S$; mol wt 321.82. C 59.71%, H 5.01%, Cl 11.02%, N 4.35%, O 9.94%, S 9.96%. Analog of ticlopidine, q.v.; inhibits ADP-induced platelet aggregation. Prepn (unspec. stereochem.): D. Aubert *et al.,* **EP 99802**; *eidem,* **US 4529596** (1984, 1985 both to Sanofi). Prepn of (+)-form: A. Badorc, D. Fréhel, **EP 281459**; *eidem,* **US 4847265** (1988, 1989 both to Sanofi). Clinical pharmacology and mechanism of action: D. C. B. Mills *et al., Arterioscler. Thromb.* **12**, 430 (1992). Clinical trial vs aspirin for prevention of atherothrombotic events: CAPRIE Steering Committee, *Lancet* **348**, 1329 (1996). Review of pharmacology and therapeutic potential: G. Feuerstein *et al., Expert Opin. Invest. Drugs* **4**, 425-430 (1995); of use in secondary prevention in stroke: H.-C. Diener *et al., Expert Opin. Pharmacother.* **6**, 755-764 (2005).

Colorless oil. $[\alpha]_D^{20}$ +51.52° (c = 1.61 in methanol).
Hydrogen sulfate. [135046-48-9] SR-25990C; Plavix. $C_{16}H_{16}ClNO_2S.H_2SO_4$; mol wt 419.90. White crystals, mp 184°. $[\alpha]_D^{20}$ +55.10° (c = 1.891 in methanol). Sol in water, methanol.
THERAP CAT: Antithrombotic.

2397. Clopidol. [2971-90-6] 3,5-Dichloro-2,6-dimethyl-4-pyridinol; meticlorpindol; clopindol; Coyden. $C_7H_7Cl_2NO$; mol wt 192.04. C 43.78%, H 3.67%, Cl 36.92%, N 7.29%, O 8.33%. Prepn: Stevenson, **US 3206358** (1965 to Dow). Metabolism studies in chickens: Smith, *Poult. Sci.* **48**, 420 (1969). Toxicity study: Plisek *et al., Vet. Spofa* **12**, 111 (1970), *C.A.* **74**, 138780p (1971).

Solid, mp >320°. Practically insol in water. LD_{50} orally in rats: 18 g/kg (Plisek).
Caution: Potential symptoms of overexposure are irritation of eyes, skin, nose, throat; cough. *See NIOSH Pocket Guide to Chemical Hazards* (DHHS/NIOSH 97-140, 1997) p 72.
THERAP CAT (VET): Coccidiostat.

2398. Cloprednol. [5251-34-3] (11β)-6-Chloro-11,17,21-trihydroxypregna-1,4,6-triene-3,20-dione; 6-chloro-$\Delta^{1,4,6}$-pregnatriene-11β,17α,21-triol-3,20-dione; RS-4691; Cloradryn; Novacort; Syntestan. $C_{21}H_{25}ClO_5$; mol wt 392.87. C 64.20%, H 6.41%, Cl 9.02%, O 20.36%. Prepn: H. J. Ringold, G. Rosenkranz, **FR 1271981** *C.A.* **58**, 1148a (1963); *eidem,* **US 3232965** (1962, 1966 both to Syntex). Metabolic effects: E. Ortega *et al., J. Clin. Pharmacol.* **16**, 122 (1976). Effects on hypothalamic-pituitary-adrenal axis function: *eidem, J. Int. Med. Res.* **4**, 326 (1976). Bioavailability in humans: E. Mroszczak *et al., J. Pharm. Sci.* **67**, 920 (1978). HPLC determn in plasma: C. Lee *et al., ibid.* **70**, 669 (1981).

Crystals from acetone/hexane.
THERAP CAT: Glucocorticoid.

2399. Cloprostenol. [40665-92-7] (5Z)-rel-7-[(1R,2R,3R,5S)-2-[(1E,3R)-4-(3-Chlorophenoxy)-3-hydroxy-1-butenyl]-3,5-dihydroxycyclopentyl]-5-heptenoic acid. $C_{22}H_{29}ClO_6$; mol wt 424.92. C 62.18%, H 6.88%, Cl 8.34%, O 22.59%. Aryloxymethyl analog of prostaglandin $F_{2\alpha}$, q.v. Prepn: J. Bowler, **DE 2223365** (1972 to ICI), *C.A.* **78**, 110692v (1973); D. Binder *et al., Prostaglandins* **6**, 87 (1974). Synthesis and biological activity: *eidem, ibid.* **15**, 773 (1978). Short synthesis: N. R. A. Beeley *et al., Tetrahedron* **37**, Suppl. 9, 411 (1981). Disposition in the rat and marmoset: G. R. Bourne *et al., Xenobiotica* **9**, 623 (1979). Effect on fertility in cows: N. Baishya *et al., Br. Vet. J.* **136**, 227 (1980); on superovulation, fertilization, egg transport in ewes: D. Whyman, R. W. Moore, *J. Reprod. Fertil.* **60**, 267 (1980).

Sodium salt. [55028-72-3] ICI-80996; Estrumate; Planate. $C_{22}H_{28}ClNaO_6$; mol wt 446.90.
THERAP CAT (VET): In treatment of infertility in sows, gilts. In synchronization of estrus.

2400. Clopyralid. [1702-17-6] 3,6-Dichloro-2-pyridinecarboxylic acid; 3,6-dichloropicolinic acid; 3,6-DCP; Dowco 290. $C_6H_3Cl_2NO_2$; mol wt 192.00. C 37.53%, H 1.57%, Cl 36.93%, N 7.30%, O 16.67%. Systemic post-emergence herbicide for use in food crops and mesquite. Prepn: H. Johnston, **BE 644105**; *idem,* **US 3317549** (1964, 1967 both to Dow). Alternate process: S. D. McGregor, **US 4087431** (1978 to Dow). Physicochemical properties, toxicity and herbicidal activity: J. G. Brown, S. D. Uprichard, *Proc. Br. Crop Prot. Conf. - Weeds* **1976,** 119. GLC determn: A. J. Pik, G. W. Hodgson, *J. Assoc. Off. Anal. Chem.* **59,** 264 (1976). Persistence in soil: A. J. Pik *et al., J. Agric. Food Chem.* **25,** 1054 (1977). Field trial in mesquite control: R. W. Bovey, R. E. Meyer, *Weed Sci.* **33,** 349 (1985).

White, odorless crystalline solid, mp 151-152°. Vapor pressure at 25°: 1.2×10^{-5} mm Hg. Soly at 25°: ~1000 ppm in water, >25% w/w in methanol, acetone, xylene. LD_{50} in male, female rats (mg/kg): >5000, 4300 orally; LC_{50} (96 hr) to rainbow trout: 103.5 mg/l (Brown, Uprichard).

Monoethanolamine salt. [57754-85-5] Dow Shield; Lontrel; Reclaim; Stinger; Transline. $C_6H_3Cl_2NO_2.C_2H_7NO$; mol wt 253.08.

USE: Herbicide.

2401. Cloquintocet-Mexyl. [99607-70-2] [(5-Chloro-8-quinolinyl)oxy]acetic acid 1-methylhexyl ester; CGA-185072. $C_{18}H_{22}ClNO_3$; mol wt 335.83. C 64.38%, H 6.60%, Cl 10.56%, N 4.17%, O 14.29%. Safening agent to protect crops from herbicidal injury. Prepn: A. Hubele, **EP 94349**; *idem,* **US 4902340** (1983, 1990 both to Ciba-Geigy). Description: J. Amrein *et al., Brighton Crop Prot. Conf. - Weeds* **1989,** 71-76. Effects on herbicide metabolism in cereals: K. Kreuz *et al., Z. Naturforsch.* **46C,** 901 (1991).

Odorless crystals, mp 69°. Vapor pressure (20°): 2.5×10^{-6} Pa. Soly in water (20°): 0.8 ppm. Sol in most organic solvents. LD_{50} in rats (mg/kg): >2000 orally; >2000 dermally. LC_{50} (4 hr) in rats: >935 mg/m³ by inhalation (Amrein).

Mixture with clodinafop-propargyl. Célio; Horizon.

USE: Herbicide safener.

2402. Cloranolol. [39563-28-5] 1-(2,5-Dichlorophenoxy)-3-[(1,1-dimethylethyl)amino]-2-propanol; 1-(*tert*-butylamino)-3-(2,5-dichlorophenoxy)-2-propanol. $C_{13}H_{19}Cl_2NO_2$; mol wt 292.20. C 53.44%, H 6.55%, Cl 24.27%, N 4.79%, O 10.95%. β-Adrenergic blocker. Prepn: G. Richter, **DE 2213044** (1972 to Res. Inst. Pharm. Chem. Hungary), *C.A.* **78,** 15780p (1973). Effect on plasma renin and blood pressure: I. Tenyi, *Curr. Ther. Res.* **21,** 823 (1977). Pharmacology: M. I. K. Fekete *et al., Arch. Int. Pharmacodyn.* **248,** 190 (1980). Electrophysiological characteristics: F. Solti, E. Czako, *Int. J. Clin. Pharmacol. Ther. Toxicol.* **18,** 229 (1980). Clinical-pharmacological evaluation: E. Török *et al., ibid.* 200. GC-MS determn in plasma: E. Tomori, E. Elekes, *J. Chromatogr.* **204,** 355 (1981). Multicenter clinical trial: E. Török *et al., Int. J. Clin. Pharmacol. Ther. Toxicol.* **23,** 650 (1985).

Crystals, mp 82-83°.

Hydrochloride. [54247-25-5] GYKI-41099; Tobanum. $C_{13}H_{19}Cl_2NO_2.HCl$; mol wt 328.66. Crystals, mp 210-212°.

THERAP CAT: Antiarrhythmic.

2403. Clorazepic Acid. [23887-31-2] 7-Chloro-2,3-dihydro-2-oxo-5-phenyl-1*H*-1,4-benzodiazepine-3-carboxylic acid. $C_{16}H_{11}ClN_2O_3$; mol wt 314.72. C 61.06%, H 3.52%, Cl 11.26%, N 8.90%, O 15.25%. Prepn: **NL 6507637**; J. Schmitt, **US 3516988**; reissued as **US RE 28315** (1965, 1970, 1975 all to Clin-Byla). Synthesis and activity of the dipotassium salt: J. Schmitt *et al., Chim. Ther.* **4,** 239 (1969). Solution chemistry: R. Raveux, M. Briot, *ibid.* 303. Metabolism: P. Gros, R. Raveux, *ibid.* 312. Toxicity data: M. Brunaud *et al., Arzneim.-Forsch.* **20,** 123 (1970). Series of articles on pharmacology and clinical use: *ibid,* 123-137. HPLC determn in plasma: P. Colin, G. Sirois, *J. Chromatogr.* **273,** 367 (1983). Clinical trial in anxiety: W. W. K. Zung, *J. Clin. Psychiatry* **48,** 13 (1987); in comparison with buspirone, *q.v.*: K. Rickels *et al., Arch. Gen. Psychiatry* **45,** 444 (1988). Comprehensive description: J. A. Raihle, V. E. Papendick, *Anal. Profiles Drug Subs.* **4,** 91-112 (1975).

Dipotassium salt. [57109-90-7] 7-Chloro-2,3-dihydro-2-oxo-5-phenyl-1*H*-1,4-benzodiazepine-3-carboxylic acid monopotassium salt compd with potassium hydroxide; clorazepate dipotassium; Abbott 35516; CB-4306; Belseren; Mendon; Tranxilène; Tranxilium; Transene; Tranxene. $C_{16}H_{10}ClKN_2O_3.KOH$; mol wt 408.92. White powder, freely sol in water. Very poorly sol in ethanol. Practically insol in ether, chloroform. Aq solns are alkaline to phenolphthalein. uv max (anhydrous product in water): 231, 311 nm (ε 33500, 2450). LD_{50} in mice (mg/kg): 700 orally; 290 i.p. LD_{50} orally in rats: >1000 mg/kg (Brunaud).

Monopotassium salt. [5991-71-9] CB-4311; Azene. $C_{16}H_{10}ClKN_2O_4$; mol wt 368.81.

Note: This is a controlled substance (depressant): **21 CFR,** 1308.14.

THERAP CAT: Anxiolytic.

2404. Clorexolone. [2127-01-7] 6-Chloro-2-cyclohexyl-2,3-dihydro-3-oxo-1*H*-isoindole-5-sulfonamide; 6-chloro-2-cyclohexyl-3-oxo-5-isoindolinesulfonamide; 5-chloro-2-cyclohexyl-1-oxo-6-sulfamoylisoindoline; 5-chloro-2-cyclohexyl-6-sulfamoylisoindolin-1-one; 5-chloro-2-cyclohexylphthalimidine-6-sulfonamide; M & B 8430; RP-12833; Flonatril; Nefrolan. $C_{14}H_{17}ClN_2O_3S$; mol wt 328.81. C 51.14%, H 5.21%, Cl 10.78%, N 8.52%, O 14.60%, S 9.75%. Prepn: **BE 620654**; G. E. Lee, W. R. Wragg, **US 3183243** (1963, 1965 both to May & Baker).

Prisms, mp 266-268°. Soly in water at 25°: 16 mg/l.

THERAP CAT: Diuretic.

2405. Cloricromen. [68206-94-0] [[8-Chloro-3-[2-(diethylamino)ethyl]-4-methyl-2-oxo-2*H*-1-benzopyran-7-yl]oxy]acetic acid ethyl ester; ethyl [[8-chloro-3-[2-(diethylamino)ethyl]-4-methyl-2-oxo-2*H*-1-benzopyran-7-yl]oxy]acetate; 8-monochloro-3-(β-diethylaminoethyl)-4-methyl-7-ethoxycarbonylmethoxycoumarin; 8-chlorocarbochromen; AD$_6$. $C_{20}H_{26}ClNO_5$; mol wt 395.88. C 60.68%, H 6.62%, Cl 8.96%, N 3.54%, O 20.21%. Derivative of coumarin, *q.v.* Prepn: F. della Valle, **BE 871315**; *idem,* **US 4452811** (1979, 1984 both to Fidia). *In vivo* studies of activity as coronary vasodilator: F. Aporti *et al., Pharmacol. Res. Commun.* **10,** 469 (1978); as inhibitor of platelet aggregation: M. Prosdocimi *et al., Thromb. Res.* **39**, 399 (1985). Pharmacology in human platelets: R. A. Travagli *et al., ibid.* **54**, 327 (1989). Mechanism of action: S. Porcellati *et al., Agents Actions* **29**, 364 (1990).

Crystals from ethyl acetate, mp 147-148°.

Hydrochloride. [74697-28-2] Cromocap; Proendotel. C_{20}-$H_{26}ClNO_5$·HCl; mol wt 432.34. mp 219-220°.

THERAP CAT: Antithrombotic; vasodilator (coronary).

2406. Clorindione. [1146-99-2] 2-(4-Chlorophenyl)-1*H*-indene-1,3(2*H*)-dione; 2-(*p*-chlorophenyl)-1,3-indandione; 2-(4-chlorophenyl)indan-1,3-dione; chlophenadione; G-25766; MG-2552; Indaliton. $C_{15}H_9ClO_2$; mol wt 256.68. C 70.19%, H 3.53%, Cl 13.81%, O 12.47%. Prepn: Cavallini *et al., Farmaco Ed. Sci.* **10**, 710 (1955); **GB 748251** (1956 to Geigy). Pharmacokinetics: Danek, Pogonowska-Wala, *Pol. J. Pharmacol. Pharm.* **25**, 307 (1973), *C.A.* **79**, 111540b (1973). Toxicity study: Fontaine *et al., Med. Pharmacol. Exp.* **17**, 497 (1967).

Dark red needles from alcohol, pale yellow needles from dil acetic acid, mp 145-146°. Practically insol in water. Sol in organic solvents except petr ether. LD_{50} orally in mice: 1220 mg/kg (Fontaine).

THERAP CAT: Anticoagulant.

2407. Clorophene. [120-32-1] 4-Chloro-2-(phenylmethyl)-phenol; 4-chloro-α-phenyl-*o*-cresol; 2-benzyl-4-chlorophenol; 5-chloro-2-hydroxydiphenylmethane; *o*-benzyl-*p*-chlorophenol; Septiphene; Santophen 1. $C_{13}H_{11}ClO$; mol wt 218.68. C 71.40%, H 5.07%, Cl 16.21%, O 7.32%. Prepn: Klarmann *et al., J. Am. Chem. Soc.* **54**, 3315 (1932); Klarmann, Gate, **US 1967825** (to Lehn & Fink); from Na or K phenoxide and benzyl chloride followed by chlorination of the resulting *o*-benzylphenol: Kaiser, **DE 703955** (1941 to Deutsche Hydrierwerke).

Crystals, mp 48.5°. $bp_{3.5}$ 160-162°. $d_{15.5}^{55}$ 1.186-1.190.

USE: In household, hospital and veterinary disinfectant preparations.

2408. Clorprenaline. [3811-25-4] 2-Chloro-α-[[(1-methylethyl)amino]methyl]benzenemethanol; *o*-chloro-α-(isopropylaminomethyl)benzyl alcohol; 1-(*o*-chlorophenyl)-2-isopropylaminoethanol; *N*-(β-*o*-chlorophenyl-β-hydroxyethyl)isopropylamine; isoprophenamine; isoprofenamine. $C_{11}H_{16}ClNO$; mol wt 213.70. C 61.82%, H 7.55%, Cl 16.59%, N 6.55%, O 7.49%. β-Adrenergic agonist. Prepn: Mills, **US 2816059** (1957 to Lilly); Nash, **US 2887509** (1959 to Lilly).

Hydrochloride monohydrate. [5588-22-7] Broncon; Clopinerin; Conselt; Fusca; Kalutein; Pentadoll; Restanolon. $C_{11}H_{16}$-$ClNO$·HCl·H_2O; mol wt 268.18. mp 163-164°.

THERAP CAT: Bronchodilator.

2409. Clorsulon. [60200-06-8] 4-Amino-6-(trichloroethenyl)-1,3-benzenedisulfonamide; 4-amino-6-(trichlorovinyl)-*m*-benzenedisulfonamide; MK-401; Curatrem. $C_8H_8Cl_3N_3O_4S_2$; mol wt 380.66. C 25.24%, H 2.12%, Cl 27.94%, N 11.04%, O 16.81%, S 16.85%. Benzenedisulfonamide with fasciolicidal activity. Prepn: H. H. Mrozik, **DE 2556122** (1976 to Merck & Co.), *C.A.* **85**, 94100n (1976); H. Mrozik *et al., J. Med. Chem.* **20**, 1225 (1977). GLC determn in biological fluids: W. J. A. Vanden Heuvel *et al., J. Agric. Food Chem.* **25**, 389 (1977). Efficacy against liver fluke, *Fasciola hepatica:* D. A. Ostlind *et al., Br. Vet. J.* **133**, 211 (1977); M. D. Schulman *et al., J. Parasitol.* **65**, 555 (1979). *In vitro* inhibition of glycolysis: M. D. Schulman, D. Valentino, *Exp. Parasitol.* **49**, 206 (1980). Mechanism of action: M. D. Schulman *et al., Mol. Biochem. Parasitol.* **5**, 133 (1982). Pharmacokinetics: *eidem, J. Parasitol.* **68**, 603 (1982).

Crystals from ether, mp 194-203°. Another crystal form from water, mp 203-205°. uv max (CH$_3$OH): 325, 267, 227 nm (ε 4530, 17395, 36310). LD_{50} in mice (mg/kg): 761 i.p.; >10,000 orally (Ostlind).

THERAP CAT (VET): Anthelmintic (Trematodes).

2410. Clortermine. [10389-73-8] 2-Chloro-α,α-dimethylbenzeneethanamine; *o*-chloro-α,α-dimethylphenethylamine; 1-(*o*-chlorophenyl)-2-methyl-2-propylamine; 1-(*o*-chlorophenyl)-2-methyl-2-aminopropane. $C_{10}H_{14}ClN$; mol wt 183.68. C 65.39%, H 7.68%, Cl 19.30%, N 7.63%. Prepn and use as anorexic agent: **BE 665244; GB 1066616**; Finocchio, Huebner, **US 3415937** (1965, 1967, 1968, all to Ciba). Toxicity data: E. I. Goldenthal, *Toxicol. Appl. Pharmacol.* **18**, 185 (1971).

bp_{16} 116-118°.

Hydrochloride. [10389-72-7] Su-10568; Voranil. $C_{10}H_{14}$-ClN·HCl; mol wt 220.14. Crystals from ethanol, mp 245-246°. LD_{50} orally in rats: 332 ±23 mg/kg (Goldenthal).

Note: This is a controlled substance (stimulant): **21 CFR**, 1308.13.

THERAP CAT: Anorexic.

2411. Closantel. [57808-65-8] *N*-[5-Chloro-4-[(4-chlorophenyl)cyanomethyl]-2-methylphenyl]-2-hydroxy-3,5-diiodobenzamide; R-31520; Flukiver; Seponver. $C_{22}H_{14}Cl_2I_2N_2O_2$; mol wt 663.07. C 39.85%, H 2.13%, Cl 10.69%, I 38.28%, N 4.22%, O 4.83%. Salicylanilide derivative. Prepn: M. A. C. Janssen, V. K. Sipido, **BE 839481**; *eidem,* **US 4005218** (1976, 1977 both to Janssen). Effectiveness against *Taenia pisiformis* in rabbits: R. A. F. Chevis *et al., Vet. Parasitol.* **7**, 333 (1980); against *Ancylostoma caninum:* J. Guerrero *et al., J. Parasitol.* **68**, 616 (1983); against *Fasciola hepatica* in sheep: B. E. Stromberg *et al., ibid.* **70**, 446 (1984). Prolonged effect on *Haemonchus contortus* in sheep: C. A. Hall *et al., Res. Vet. Sci.* **31**, 104 (1981). Acts by uncoupling oxidative phosphorylation: H. Van den Bossche *et al., Arch. Int. Physiol. Biochim.* **87**, 851 (1979); H. J. Kane *et al., Mol. Biochem. Parasitol.* **1**, 347 (1980).

Crystals from methanol, mp 217.8°.
THERAP CAT (VET): Anthelmintic.

2412. Clospirazine. [24527-27-3] 8-[3-(2-Chloro-10*H*-phenothiazin-10-yl)propyl]-1-thia-4,8-diazaspiro[4.5]decan-3-one; 8-[3-(2-chloro-10-phenothiazinyl)propyl]-3-oxo-1-thia-4,8-diazaspiro[4.5]decane; spiclomazine. $C_{22}H_{24}ClN_3OS_2$; mol wt 446.03. C 59.24%, H 5.42%, Cl 7.95%, N 9.42%, O 3.59%, S 14.38%. Prepn: Nakanishi *et al.*, **JP 69 23091**; **US 3574204** (1969, 1971 both to Yoshitomi). Pharmacological and metabolic studies: Nakanishi *et al., J. Pharm. Soc. Jpn.* **90**, 800, 808 (1970); Imamura *et al., ibid.* 813. *Review: Jpn. Med. Gaz.* **8**(11), 10 (1971).

mp 154-156° (acetone).
Hydrochloride. [27007-85-8] APY-606; Diceplon; Disepron. White to brownish, tasteless, odorless crystals or powder, mp 262-264° (dec). Sparingly sol in methanol; slightly sol in chloroform; very slightly sol in water. Decomposes slowly when exposed to light. LD_{50} in mice, rats (mg/kg): 3400, 2950 i.p.; >5490, >5490 s.c.; 3800, 4000 orally (Nakanishi, 1970).
THERAP CAT: Antipsychotic.

2413. Clostebol. [1093-58-9] (17β)-4-Chloro-17-hydroxy-androst-4-en-3-one; 4-chlorotestosterone. $C_{19}H_{27}ClO_2$; mol wt 322.87. C 70.68%, H 8.43%, Cl 10.98%, O 9.91%. Prepn: Camerino *et al., Farmaco Ed. Sci.* **11**, 586 (1956); *eidem, J. Am. Chem. Soc.* **78**, 3540 (1956); Ringold *et al., J. Org. Chem.* **21**, 1432 (1956); Camerino, **US 2953582** (1960 to Farmitalia); Julian, Printy, **US 2933510** (1960 to Julian Labs.). Clinical pharmacology of the acetate: Molinatti *et al., Folia Endocrinol.* **14**, 528 (1961); Krueskemper, Morgner, *Int. Z. Klin. Pharmakol. Ther. Toxikol.* **1**, 455 (1968).

Crystals from acetone + hexane, mp 188-190°. $[\alpha]_D^{20}$ +148° ($CHCl_3$). uv max (95% ethanol): 256 nm (log ε 4.13).
Acetate. [855-19-6] Macrobin; Steranabol. $C_{21}H_{29}ClO_3$; mol wt 364.91. Crystals from methanol, mp 228-230°. $[\alpha]_D$ +118 ±4° ($CHCl_3$). uv max: 255 nm (ε 13,300). Sol in ethanol.
Note: This is a controlled substance (anabolic steroid): **21 CFR**, 1308.13, as defined in 1300.01.
THERAP CAT: Anabolic.

2414. Clothianidin. [210880-92-5] [*C*(*E*)]-*N*-[(2-Chloro-5-thiazolyl)methyl]-*N'*-methyl-*N''*-nitroguanidine; (*E*)-1-(2-chloro-1,3-thiazol-5-ylmethyl)-3-methyl-2-nitroguanidine; TI-435; Arena; Poncho. $C_6H_8ClN_5O_2S$; mol wt 249.68. C 28.86%, H 3.23%, Cl

14.20%, N 28.05%, O 12.82%, S 12.84%. Neonicotinoid insecticide for use in food crops. Prepn: H. Uneme *et al.*, **EP 376279**; *eidem*, **US 5034404** (1990, 1991 both to Takeda); *eidem, Pestic. Sci.* **55**, 202 (1999). Synthesis: P. Maienfisch *et al., Tetrahedron Lett.* **41**, 7187 (2000). Insecticidal activity and physical properties: Y. Ohkawara *et al., Brighton Crop Prot. Conf. - Pests Dis.* **1**, 51 (2002). Field trials in sugar beets: R. H. Meredith *et al., ibid.* **2**, 691 (2002); and cereals: A. M. Dewar *et al., ibid.* 647. Ecotoxicological profile: R. Schmuck, J. Keppler, *Pflanzenschutz-Nachr. Bayer* **56**, 26 (2003). Metabolism studies: O. Klein, *ibid.* 75. Review of use in corn: W. Andersch, M. Schwarz, *ibid.* 147-172.

White crystalline powder, mp 176.8°. Vapor pressure (Pa): 1.3 × 10⁻¹⁰ (25°); 3.8 × 10⁻⁷ (20°). Soly (g/l) at 20°: water 0.327; at 25°: acetone 15.2, methanol 6.26, ethyl acetate 2.03, xylene 0.013. Log P (*n*-octanol/water) at 25°: 0.7. LD_{50} in rats (mg/kg): >5000 orally; >2000 dermally. LC_{50} in rats (mg/l): >6.1 inhalation. LC_{50} in bobwhite quail, mallard duck (ppm): >5200, >5200 (dietary). LC_{50} (96 hr) in rainbow trout, bluegill (mg/l): >100, >120 (Ohkawara).
USE: Insecticide.

2415. Clothiapine. [2058-52-8] 2-Chloro-11-(4-methyl-1-piperazinyl)dibenzo[*b,f*][1,4]thiazepine; Entumine; Etumine. C_{18}-$H_{18}ClN_3S$; mol wt 343.87. C 62.87%, H 5.28%, Cl 10.31%, N 12.22%, S 9.32%. Prepn: **FR CAM 51** (1964 to Dr. A. Wander), *C.A.* **61**, 8328h (1964).

Crystals from ether + petr ether, mp 118-120°.
THERAP CAT: Antipsychotic.

2416. Clotiazepam. [33671-46-4] 5-(2-Chlorophenyl)-7-ethyl-1,3-dihydro-1-methyl-2*H*-thieno[2,3-*e*]-1,4-diazepin-2-one; Y-6047; Clozan; Rise; Rize; Rizen; Tienor; Trecalmo; Veratran. $C_{16}H_{15}ClN_2OS$; mol wt 318.82. C 60.28%, H 4.74%, Cl 11.12%, N 8.79%, O 5.02%, S 10.06%. A thienodiazepine tranquilizer with biological activity similar to the benzodiazepines. Prepn: M. Nakanishi *et al.*, **DE 2107356**; *eidem*, **US 3849405** (1971, 1974 both to Yoshitomi); *eidem, J. Med. Chem.* **16**, 214 (1973). Pharmacology: *eidem, Arzneim.-Forsch.* **22**, 1905 (1972). Effects on biogenic amine metabolism: *eidem, ibid.* 1914. Metabolism: *eidem, Yakugaku Zasshi* **93**, 311 (1973), *C.A.* **79**, 13397r (1973). Clinical studies: S. Sieberns, *Fortschr. Med.* **97**, 1705 (1979).

Crystals from hexane, mp 105-106°. LD_{50} in mice (mg/kg): 440 i.p., 636 orally (Nakanishi).

Note: This is a controlled substance (depressant): **21 CFR,** 1308.14.

THERAP CAT: Anxiolytic.

2417. Clotrimazole. [23593-75-1] 1-[(2-Chlorophenyl)diphenylmethyl]-1*H*-imidazole; 1-(*o*-chloro-α,α-diphenylbenzyl)imidazole; 1-[α-(2-chlorophenyl)benzhydryl]imidazole; 1-[(*o*-chlorophenyl)diphenylmethyl]imidazole; diphenyl-(2-chlorophenyl)-1-imidazolylmethane; 1-(*o*-chlorotrityl)imidazole; FB-5097; Bay b 5097; Canesten; Canifug; Empecid; Gyne-Lotrimin; Lotrimin; Mono-Baycuten; Mycelex-G; Mycofug; Mycosporin; Pedisafe; Rimazole; Tibatin; Trimysten. $C_{22}H_{17}ClN_2$; mol wt 344.84. C 76.63%, H 4.97%, Cl 10.28%, N 8.12%. Prepn: K. H. Buechel *et al.*, **ZA 6805392**; *eidem*, **US 3705172** (1969, 1972 both to Bayer). Pharmacology: Plempel *et al.*, *Antimicrob. Agents Chemother.* **1969**, 271; *eidem, Dtsch. Med. Wochenschr.* **94**, 1356 (1969). Clinical findings: Oberste-Lehn *et al., ibid.* 1365. Series of articles on prepn, toxicology, pharmacokinetics, clinical studies: *Arzneim.-Forsch.* **22**, 1260-1272, 1276-1299 (1972). Toxicity: D. Tettenborn, *ibid.* 1276. Comprehensive description: J. G. Hoogerheide, B. E. Wyka, *Anal. Profiles Drug Subs.* **11**, 225-255 (1982).

Crystals, mp 147-149°. A weak base, slightly sol in water, benzene, toluene; sol in acetone, chloroform, ethyl acetate, DMF. Hydrolyzes rapidly upon heating in aq acids. LD_{50} in male mice, rats (mg/kg): 923, 708 orally (Tettenborn).

Hydrochloride. $C_{22}H_{17}ClN_2$·HCl. mp 159°.

THERAP CAT: Antifungal.

THERAP CAT (VET): Antifungal.

2418. Clove. Caryophyllus. Evergreen tree, *Syzygium aromaticum* (L.) Merr. et Perry, also known as *Eugenia caryophyllata* Thunb. and *Caryophyllus aromaticus* L., Myrtaceae. *Habit.* Southeast Asia; cultivated in tropical regions worldwide. Parts used are the dried buds (cloves) and the essential oil produced from them. *Constit.* 15-21% volatile oil, sterols, *e.g.* sitosterol, ~6% protein, ~61% carbohydrate, ~20% lipids. *Review*: A. Y. Leung, *Encyclopedia of Common Natural Ingredients Used in Food, Drugs and Cosmetics* (Wiley-Interscience, New York, 1980) pp 130-132.

Clove oil. Oil of clove. Volatile oil from dried flower buds. *Constit.* 60-90% eugenol, 2-27% eugenyl acetate, 5-12% β-caryophyllene, minor constituents such as methyl amyl ketone, methyl salicylate, benzaldehyde. Extraction procedures: A. A. Clifford *et al., J. Anal. Chem.* **364**, 635 (1999). Colorless to pale yellow liq, becoming darker and thicker with age. d_{25}^{25} 1.038-1.060. n_D^{20} 1.530. Insol in water. Sol in 2 vols 70% alcohol. *Keep well closed, cool and protected from light.*

USE: Flavoring agent in foods; fragrance component in dentifrices, soaps, lotions, perfumes; commercial source of eugenol. Pharmaceutic aid (flavor).

THERAP CAT: Carminative, counterirritant. Clove oil as analgesic (dental).

2419. Cloxacillin. [61-72-3] (2*S*,5*R*,6*R*)-6-[[[3-(2-Chlorophenyl)-5-methyl-4-isoxazolyl]carbonyl]amino]-3,3-dimethyl-7-oxo-4-thia-1-azabicyclo[3.2.0]heptane-2-carboxylic acid; [3-(*o*-chlorophenyl)-5-methyl-4-isoxazolyl]penicillin; [5-methyl-3-(*o*-chlorophenyl)-4-isoxazolyl]penicillin; 6-[3-(*o*-chlorophenyl)-5-methyl-4-isoxazolecarboxamido]penicillanic acid. $C_{19}H_{18}ClN_3O_5S$; mol wt 435.88. C 52.35%, H 4.16%, Cl 8.13%, N 9.64%, O 18.35%, S 7.36%. Semi-synthetic antibiotic related to penicillin; chlorinated deriv of oxacillin, *q.v.* Prepn: F. P. Doyle, J. H. C. Nayler, **US 2996501** (1961); F. P. Doyle *et al., J. Chem. Soc.* **1963**, 5838. Manuf: *Ind. Chem.* **39**, 513 (1963), *C.A.* **60**, 1543a (1964). Properties and pharmacology: J. H. C. Nayler *et al., Nature* **195**, 1264 (1962). Toxicity data: E. I. Goldenthal, *Toxicol. Appl. Pharmacol.* **18**, 185 (1971). Comprehensive description: D. L. Mays, *Anal. Profiles Drug Subs.* **4**, 113-136 (1975).

Sodium salt monohydrate. [7081-44-9]; [642-78-4] (anhydrous). Sodium cloxacillin; BRL-1621; Cloxapen; Cloxypen; Ekvacillin; Latocillin; Orbenin; Methocillin-S; Tegopen. $C_{19}H_{17}ClN_3NaO_5S$·H_2O; mol wt 475.88. Microcryst powder, dec 170°. $[\alpha]_D^{20}$ +163° (c = 1 in water). pH of 1% aq soln = 6.0-7.5. Sol in water, methanol, ethanol, pyridine, ethylene glycol. LD_{50} in rats, mice (mg/kg): 1630 ±112, 1280 ±50 i.p. (Goldenthal).

Benzathine salt. [23736-58-5] Dry Clox; Noroclox. $C_{54}H_{56}Cl_2N_8O_{10}S_2$; mol wt 1112.11.

THERAP CAT: Antibacterial.

THERAP CAT (VET): Antibacterial.

2420. Cloxazolam. [24166-13-0] 10-Chloro-11b-(2-chlorophenyl)-2,3,7,11b-tetrahydrooxazolo[3,2-*d*][1,4]benzodiazepin-6(5*H*)-one; 7-chloro-5-(2-chlorophenyl)tetrahydrooxazolo[5,4-*b*]-2,3,4,5-tetrahydro-1*H*-1,4-benzodiazepin-2-one; 10-chloro-11b-(2-chlorophenyl)-2,3,5,6,7,11b-hexahydrobenzo[6,7]-1,4-diazepino[5,4-*b*]oxazol-6-one; 10-chloro-11b-(2-chlorophenyl)-6-oxo-2,3,5,6,7,11b-hexahydrooxazolo[3,2-*d*][1,4]benzodiazepine; CS-370; Betavel; Enadel; Lubalix; Olcadil; Sepazon; Tolestan. $C_{17}H_{14}Cl_2N_2O_2$; mol wt 349.21. C 58.47%, H 4.04%, Cl 20.30%, N 8.02%, O 9.16%. Prepn: R. Tachikawa *et al.*, **DE 1812252** and **DE 1952201**; *eidem*, **US 3772371** and **US 3696094** (1969, 1970, 1973, 1972 all to Sankyo); T. Miyadera *et al., J. Med. Chem.* **14**, 520 (1971). Pharmacology: T. Kamioka *et al., Arzneim.-Forsch.* **22**, 884 (1972). Metabolism: Murata *et al., Chem. Pharm. Bull.* **21**, 404 (1973). Multicenter trials and complementary studies: K. A. Fischer-Cornelssen, *Arzneim.-Forsch.* **31**, 1757 (1981).

Crystals, mp 202-204° (dec). Freely sol in glacial acetic acid; sparingly sol in chloroform; slightly sol in acetone, dehydrated ethanol, ethyl acetate, benzene. Practically insol in water. LD_{50} in mice (g/kg): 3.3 orally; >2.0 i.p. (Kamioka).

Note: This is a controlled substance (depressant): **21 CFR,** 1308.14.

THERAP CAT: Anxiolytic.

2421. Cloxotestosterone. [53608-96-1] (17β)-17-(2,2,2-Trichloro-1-hydroxyethoxy)androst-4-en-3-one; testosterone 17-chloral hemiacetal. $C_{21}H_{29}Cl_3O_3$; mol wt 435.81. C 57.87%, H 6.71%, Cl 24.40%, O 11.01%. Prepn: P. Borrevang, **US 2933514** (1960 to Lövens Kemiske Fabrik); *idem, Acta Chem. Scand.* **16**, 883 (1962).

Crystals from ethyl acetate, mp 200-201°. uv max (ethanol): 241 nm (ε 16300).

Acetate. [13867-82-8] Caprosem. $C_{23}H_{31}Cl_3O_4$; mol wt 477.85. Crystals from ethyl acetate, mp 192-193°. uv max (ethanol): 241 nm (ε 16400).

THERAP CAT: Androgen.

2422. Cloxyquin. [130-16-5] 5-Chloro-8-quinolinol; 5-chloro-8-hydroxyquinoline; 5-chloro-8-oxychinolin; cloxiquine; Chlorisept. C_9H_6ClNO; mol wt 179.60. C 60.19%, H 3.37%, Cl 19.74%, N 7.80%, O 8.91%. Prepn: Bratz, Niementowski, *Ber.* **52**, 189 (1919); Weizmann, Bograchov, *J. Am. Chem. Soc.* **69**, 1222 (1947); Manske *et al.*, *Can. J. Res.* **27F**, 359 (1949). Crystal structure: T. Banerjee, N. N. Saha, *Acta Crystallogr.* **C42**, 1408 (1986).

Crystals from ethanol, mp 130°. Sparingly sol in cold, dil HCl.

Hydrochloride. $C_9H_6ClNO.HCl$. Yellow needles. mp 256-258°.

Acetate (ester). 5-Chloro-8-acetoxyquinoline. $C_{11}H_8ClNO_2$.

THERAP CAT: Antibacterial; antifungal.

2423. Clozapine. [5786-21-0] 8-Chloro-11-(4-methyl-1-piperazinyl)-5*H*-dibenzo[*b,e*][1,4]diazepine; HF-1854; Clozaril; Leponex. $C_{18}H_{19}ClN_4$; mol wt 326.82. C 66.15%, H 5.86%, Cl 10.85%, N 17.14%. Combined serotonin (5HT$_2$) and dopamine (D$_2$) receptor antagonist. Prepn: **FR 1334944** (1963 to Wander); Schmutz, Hunziker, **US 3539573** (1970); **NL 293201** (1965 to Wander), *C.A.* **64**, 8221a (1966); Hunziker *et al.*, *Helv. Chim. Acta* **50**, 1588 (1967). Structure-activity studies: Schmutz *et al.*, *Chim. Ther.* **2**, 424 (1967). Pharmacology: Stille *et al.*, *Farmaco Ed. Prat.* **26**, 603 (1971). Metabolism: Gauch, Michaelis, *ibid.* 667. Toxicology: Lindt *et al.*, *ibid.* 585. *Review:* A. C. Sayers, H. A. Amsler, in *Pharmacological and Biochemical Properties of Drug Substances* **vol. 1**, M. E. Goldberg, Ed. (Am. Pharm. Assoc., Washington, DC, 1977) pp 1-31. Review of pharmacology and clinical use: R. J. Baldessarini, F. R. Frankenburg, *N. Engl. J. Med.* **324**, 746-754 (1991). Comprehensive description: M. J. McLeish *et al.*, *Anal. Profiles Drug Subs. Excip.* **22**, 145-184 (1993). Overview of mechanism of action: H. Y. Meltzer, *J. Clin. Psychiatry* **55**, Suppl. B, 47-52 (1994). Clinical trial in suicide prevention in schizophrenia: H. Y. Meltzer *et al.*, *Arch. Gen. Psychiatry* **60**, 82 (2003). Review of safety and tolerability: J. Fitzsimons *et al.*, *Expert Opin. Drug Saf.* **4**, 731-744 (2005).

Yellow crystals from acetone-petr ether, mp 183-184°. Soly w/w at 25° (%): acetone >5; acetonitrile 1.9; chloroform >20; ethyl acetate >5; abs ethanol 4.0; water <0.01. pKa$_1$ 3.70; pKa$_2$ 7.60. Partition coefficient (octanol/water): 0.4 (pH 2); 600 (pH 7); 1000 (pH 7.4); 1500 (pH 8). uv max (ethanol): 215, 230, 261, 297 nm (ε 27400, 25800, 16800, 10500). LD$_{50}$ in mice, rats (mg/kg): 61, 58 i.v.; 199, 260 orally (Lindt).

THERAP CAT: Antipsychotic.

2424. Clupeine. [9007-31-2] Protamine found in herring (*Clupea pallasii*) sperm. Isoln from herring testes contg ripe sperm: Kossel, *The Protamines and Histones* (London, 1928); Rasmussen, *Z. Physiol. Chem.* **224**, 97 (1934); Felix, Mager, *ibid.* **249**, 111 (1937); Block *et al.*, *Proc. Soc. Exp. Biol. Med.* **70**, 494 (1949).

Separated into two main fractions, Y and Z, and fraction Y separated into Y$_I$ and Y$_{II}$: Ando, Sawada, *J. Biochem. (Tokyo)* **49**, 252 (1961). Chemical structure of fraction Z: Ando *et al.*, *Biochim. Biophys. Acta* **56**, 628 (1962); Felix, Hashimoto, *Z. Physiol. Chem.* **330**, 205 (1963). Complete amino acid sequence of Z component: Iwai *et al.*, *J. Biochem. (Tokyo)* **69**, 493 (1971); of Y$_{II}$ component: Suzuki, Ando, *ibid.* **72**, 1419 (1972); of Y$_I$ component: *eidem, ibid.* 1433. Solid-phase synthesis of clupeine Z: Yonezawa *et al.*, *C.A.* **79**, 19093k (1973).

White powder, strongly alkaline reaction. pKa 7.4-8.0; pKb 2.9-3.3.

Disulfate. White powder, $[\alpha]_D^{22}$ −85.49° (satd aq soln). One gram dissolves in 80 ml water at room temp. Freely sol in hot water, separates from the supersatd soln on cooling as a clear, colorless oil contg 50% H$_2$O, n_D^{20} 1.4435. Clupeine is split by protaminase, active trypsin and by chymotrypsin. Compds of clupeine with nucleic acids are described by Kossel, *loc. cit.*

2425. Cnicin. [24394-09-0] (3*R*)-(3a*R*,4*S*,6*E*,10*Z*,11a*R*)-3,4-Dihydroxy-2-methylenebutanoic acid 2,3,3a,4,5,8,9,11a-octahydro-10-(hydroxymethyl)-6-methyl-3-methylene-2-oxocyclodeca[*b*]furan-4-yl ester; (*Z,E*)-6α,8α,15-trihydroxygermacra-1(10),4,11(13)-trien-12-oic acid 12,6-lactone 8-(3,4-dihydroxy-2-methylenebutyrate); cynisin; centaurin. $C_{20}H_{26}O_7$; mol wt 378.42. C 63.48%, H 6.93%, O 29.60%. Bitter principle of *Cnicus benedictus* L., *Compositae*. Isolation and review: Korte, Bechmann, *Naturwissenschaften* **45**, 390 (1958). Structure: Suchy *et al.*, *Tetrahedron Letters* no. 10, 5 (1969); *Ber.* **93**, 2449 (1960). Revised structure: Samek *et al.*, *Tetrahedron Lett.* **1969**, 2931. Stereochemistry: Tori *et al.*, *J. Chem. Soc. B* **1971**, 1084.

Crystals, mp 143°. $[\alpha]_D^{20}$ +158° (c = 2.3 in ethanol). uv max: 220 nm (log ε 4.34). Slightly sol in water; freely sol in alcohol. Practically insol in ether.

2426. Coal Tar. Clinitar; Psorigel; T/Gel. A by-product in the destructive distillation of coal. *Constit.* Benzene, toluene, naphthalene, anthracene, xylene, and other aro-matic hydrocarbons; phenol, cresol, and other phenol bodies; ammonia, pyridine, and some other organic bases; thiophene. Monographs: *Coal Tar Data Book*, 2nd ed., 1965, compiled and published by The Coal Tar Res. Assoc., Gomersal (Leeds), England; H. G. Franck, G. Collin, *Steinkohlenteer* (Springer Verlag, Heidelberg-New York, 1968) 255 pp. Review of carcinogenic risk: *IARC Monographs* **35**, 83-159 (1985); of toxicology and human exposure: *Toxicological Profile for Wood Creosote, Coal Tar Creosote, Coal Tar, Coal Tar Pitch, and Coal Tar Pitch Volatiles* (PB2003-100136, 2002) 394 pp.

Almost black, thick liq or semisolid; characteristic odor. A small portion of coal tar dissolves in water; all or almost all dissolves in benzene or nitrobenzene; partly dissolves in alcohol, ether, chloroform, carbon disulfide, methanol, acetone, petr ether, or sodium hydroxide soln. Practically insol in water. Sol in 20 parts alcohol; miscible with abs alcohol, acetone, petrolatum, oils and fats.

Purified coal tar. Pixalbol. Light-yellow, thin, oily liq.

Caution: Coal tar and coal tar pitches are listed as known human carcinogens: *Report on Carcinogens, Eleventh Edition* (PB2005-104914, 2004) p III-68.

USE: Prodn of creosote, coal tar pitch, crude naphthalene and anthracene oils; as fuel for furnaces in steel industry.

THERAP CAT: Antieczematic (topical).

THERAP CAT (VET): Topically in skin disorders.

2427. Cobalt. [7440-48-4] Co; at. wt 58.933195; at. no. 27; valences 1, 2, 3; rarely 4, 5. Group VIII (9). One naturally occurring isotope: ^{59}Co; artificial, radioactive isotopes: 54-58; 60-64. Widely distributed in nature; abundance in earth's crust 0.001-

0.002%. Principle ores include *cobaltite* ($CoS_2.CoAs_2$), *linnaeite* (Co_3S_4), *smaltite* ($CoAs_2$) and erythrite ($3CoO.As_2O_5.8H_2O$). Metal first isolated in 1735 by Brandt. Reviews of prepn: Whittemore in *Rare Metals Handbook*, C. A. Hampel, Ed. (Reinhold, New York, 1956) pp 105-146; Houot, *Ann. Mines* **1969** (April), 9-36. Prepn of high purity metal: Ware in *Ultrapurification of Semiconductor Materials*, M. S. Brooks, J. K. Kennedy, Eds. (Macmillan, New York, 1962) pp 192-204. Cobalt appears to be essential to life. Plays an important part in animal nutrition; the absence of cobalt-contg vitamin B_{12} causes pernicious anemia. The reactor-produced ^{60}Co ($T_{1/2}$ 5.263 years; β^- 0.314 Mev; γ 1.173, 1.332 Mev) is a widely used source of radioactivity: Centre d'Information du Cobalt, *Cobalt Monograph* (Brussels, 1960) 515 pp. Comprehensive reviews of cobalt and its compds: *ACS Monograph Series* **no. 149**, entitled "Cobalt, Its Chemistry, Metallurgy and Uses," R. S. Young, Ed. (Reinhold, New York, 1960) 424 pp; Nicholls in *Comprehensive Inorganic Chemistry* **vol. 3**, J. C. Bailar, Jr. *et al*, Eds. (Pergamon Press, Oxford, 1973) pp 1053-1107; F. Planinsek, J. B. Newkirk in *Kirk-Othmer Encyclopedia of Chemical Technology* **vol. 6** (Wiley-Interscience, New York, 3rd ed., 1979) pp 481-494. Review of toxicology and human exposure: *Toxicological Profile for Cobalt* (PB2004-104398, 2004) 486 pp.

Gray, hard, magnetic, ductile, somewhat malleable metal. Exists in two allotropic forms. At room temp the hexagonal form is more stable than the cubic form; both forms can exist at room temperature. Stable in air or toward water at ordinary temp. d 8.92. mp 1493°. bp about 3100°. Brinell hardness: 125. Latent heat of fusion 62 cal/g, latent heat of vaporization 1500 cal/g. Specific heat (15-100°): 0.1056 cal/g/°C. Readily sol in dil HNO_3; very slowly attacked by HCl or cold H_2SO_4. The hydrated salts of cobalt are red, and the sol salts form red solns which become blue on adding concd HCl.

Caution: Potential symptoms of overexposure to metal, dust or fumes are coughing, dyspnea; wheezing and decreased pulmonary function; weight loss; dermatitis; diffuse nodular fibrosis; respiratory hypersensitivity; asthma. *See NIOSH Pocket Guide to Chemical Hazards* (DHHS/NIOSH 97-140, 1997) p 74.

USE: For alloys; manuf cobalt salts; in nuclear technology. Since ^{60}Co can be encapsulated compactly, it has replaced radium in exptl medicine and cancer research. Cobalt is also used in the cobalt bomb, a hydrogen bomb surrounded by a cobalt metal shell. When the nuclear explosion occurs ^{60}Co is formed from ^{59}Co by neutron capture. Considered a "dirty bomb" because of long half-life and intense β^- and γ radiation. Max permissible concentration of ^{60}Co in air: $10^{-7}\mu Ci/cc$, *Natl. Bur. Stand. Handb.* **69**, 31 (1959).

THERAP CAT: Trace mineral; ^{60}Co as radiation source (antineoplastic).

2428. Cobaltic Acetate. [917-69-1] $C_6H_9CoO_6$; mol wt 236.07. C 30.53%, H 3.84%, Co 24.96%, O 40.66%. $Co(C_2H_3O_2)_3$. Prepd by electrolytic oxidation of $Co(C_2H_3O_2)_2.4H_2O$ in glacial acetic acid contg 2% (v/v) water: Sharp, White, *J. Chem. Soc.* **1952**, 110; by oxidation of solns of cobaltous salts by alkaline persulfates in the presence of acetic acid: Peschanski, Wormser, *Compt. Rend.* **252**, 1607 (1961). Generally considered to be a hydroxo-bridged binuclear complex.

Dark-green, very hygroscopic powder or green octahedral crystals. Becomes black and dec on heating to 100°. Sol in water, acetic acid, alcohol, *n*-butanol; dec by mineral acids. Aq solns hydrolyze slowly at room temp, rapidly at 60-70°; reduced by light or $FeSO_4$.

USE: Catalyst for cumene hydroperoxide decompn.

2429. Cobaltic-Cobaltous Oxide. [1308-06-1] Cobalto-cobaltic oxide; cobaltosic oxide; tricobalt tetroxide. Co_3O_4; mol wt 240.80. Co 73.42% O 26.58%. Prepn: *Gmelins, Cobalt* (8th ed.) **58** (Part A), 231-235 (1932) and supplement, **202**, 491-496 (1961). *Review:* de Bie, Doyen, *Cobalt* **15**, 3-13; **16**, 3-15 (1962).

Black or grey octahedral crystals of cubic system. d 6.11. Commercial material is black and contains about 71% Co. Above 900° loses O_2 to form CoO; absorbs O_2 at lower temps but cryst structure is unchanged. Absorbs water but no definite hydrate has been identified. Readily reduced to Co metal by C, CO, or H_2. Practically insol in water. Sol in acids, alkalies.

USE: In enamels; in semiconductors; in grinding wheels.

2430. Cobaltic Fluoride. [10026-18-3] Cobalt trifluoride. CoF_3; mol wt 115.93. Co 50.84%, F 49.16%. Prepn from F_2, and CoF_2, $CoCl_2$, or Co_2O_3: Priest, *Inorg. Synth.* **3**, 175 (1950); Kwasnik in *Handbook of Preparative Inorganic Chemistry* **vol. 1**, G. Brauer, Ed. (Academic Press, New York, 2nd ed., 1963) p 268; from ClF_3 and $CoCl_2$: Rochow, Kukin, *J. Am. Chem. Soc.* **74**, 1615 (1952).

Minute, light brown, hexagonal crystals, d 3.88. Discolors rapidly on exposure to moist air. Reacts with water giving off O_2. Comparatively stable to heat, at 600° the fluorine pressure over the solid is less than 0.1 atm. Volatilizes in an F_2 stream at 600-700°. May be stored in hermetically sealed glass, quartz, or metal containers.

USE: Important fluorinating agent, particularly for complete fluorination of hydrocarbons by the Fowler process.

2431. Cobaltic Oxide Monohydrate. [12016-80-7] Cobalt hydroxide oxide; cobaltic hydroxide. $CoHO_2$; mol wt 91.94. Co 64.10%, H 1.10%, O 34.80%. CoO(OH). Alternate formula $Co_2O_3.H_2O$. Prepn: Glemser in *Handbook of Preparative Inorganic Chemistry* **vol 2**, G. Brauer, Ed. (Academic Press, New York, 2nd ed., 1965) pp 1520-1521; Schrader, Petzold, *Z. Anorg. Allg. Chem.* **353**, 186 (1967). Existence of anhydrous cobaltic oxide (Co_2O_3) has not been established: Pagel *et al.*, *J. Am. Chem. Soc.* **57**, 2552 (1935); Nicholls in *Comprehensive Inorganic Chemistry* **vol 3**, J. C. Bailar, Jr. *et al.*, Eds. (Pergamon Press, Oxford, 1973) p 1096. *See also* de Bie, Doyen, *Cobalt* **15**, 3 (1962). Structure: Schrader, Petzold, *loc. cit.*; Delaplane *et al.*, *J. Chem. Phys.* **50**, 1920 (1969).

Dark-brown to black powder; hexagonal crystal structure. Converted to Co_3O_4 on heating to 148-150° in a vacuum. Practically insol in water. Sol in HCl, evolving Cl_2; sol in HNO_3, H_2SO_4.

USE: Oxidation catalysts, in separation of cobalt from nickel.

2432. Cobaltic Potassium Nitrite. [13782-01-9] Hexakis(nitrito-*N*)cobaltate(3−) tripotassium; potassium hexanitrocobaltate(III); potassium cobaltinitrite; potassium nitrocobaltate(III); cobalt yellow; Fischer's yellow; C.I. Pigment Yellow 40; C.I. 77357. $CoK_3N_6O_{12}$; mol wt 452.26. Co 13.03%, K 25.94%, N 18.58%, O 42.45%. $K_3Co(NO_2)_6$. Incorrectly called *"Indian Yellow"*. Prepd by addition of KNO_2 to a solution of a Co salt: Salyer, Sweet, *Anal. Chem.* **32**, 548 (1962).

Sesquihydrate, yellow, octahedral, cubic crystals. Very slightly sol in water, dil acetic acid. Practically insol in alcohol; dec by mineral acids.

USE: As an oil- and water-color pigment; in painting on glass and porcelain; in coloring rubber; in separation of Co from Ni; in Co analysis.

2433. Cobaltous Acetate. [71-48-7] $C_4H_6CoO_4$; mol wt 177.02. C 27.14%, H 3.42%, Co 33.29%, O 36.15%. $Co(C_2H_3O_2)_2$. Prepd commercially from cobaltous hydroxide or carbonate and an excess of dil acetic acid: Morral in *Kirk-Othmer Encyclopedia of Chemical Technology* **vol. 5** (Interscience, New York, 2nd ed., 1964) p 737; prepn from powdered Co and acetic acid: Hahl, US 3133942 (1964 to BASF); prepn by oxidation of Co carbonyls in the presence of acetic acid: Gwynn *et al.*, US 3246024 (1966 to Gulf). *Review:* de Bie, Doyen, *Cobalt* **15**, 3-13; **16**, 3-15 (1962).

Light-pink crystals. Readily sol in water.

Tetrahydrate. Bis(acetato)tetraaquocobalt. Intense red, monoclinic, prismatic crystals. d 1.705. On heating becomes anhydrous by 140°. Sol in water, alcohols, dil acids, pentyl acetate. pH of 0.2 molar aq soln 6.8.

USE: Bleaching agent and drier for lacquers, varnishes; in anodizing; catalyst for oxidation and esterification; foam stabilizer for malt beverages.

2434. Cobaltous Arsenate. [7785-24-2] C.I. 77350. $As_2Co_3O_8$; mol wt 454.64. As 32.96%, Co 38.89%, O 28.15%. $Co_3(AsO_4)_2$. Octahydrate occurs in nature as *erythrite* or *cobalt bloom*. Prepn: *Gmelins, Cobalt* (8th ed.) **58**, (part A), 305 (1932) and supplement, 752 (1961); Charles-Messance *et al.*, *Bull. Soc. Chim. Fr.* **1962**, 574. *See Colour Index* **vol. 4** (3rd ed., 1971) p 4664.

Octahydrate, pink to blood-red, monoclinic, fine needles. On heating becomes anhydr by 400°. Dec by 1000° to $Co_6As_2O_{11}$. d 2.9-3.1. Practically insol in water. Sol in dil mineral acids, in NH_4OH.

USE: Painting on glass and porcelain.

2435. Cobaltous Bromide. [7789-43-7] Cobalt dibromide. Br_2Co; mol wt 218.74. Br 73.06%, Co 26.94%. $CoBr_2$. Prepn of hexahydrate from $CoCO_3$ and HBr: Clark, Buchner, *J. Am. Chem. Soc.* **44**, 230 (1922). Prepn of anhyd: *eidem, loc. cit.;* Watt *et al., ibid.* **77**, 2752 (1955); Wydeven, Gregory, *J. Phys. Chem.* **68**, 3249 (1964).

Bright green solid or lustrous green cryst leaflets. mp 678° (under HBr and N_2); d_4^{25} 4.909. Hygroscopic, forms hexahydrate in air. Readily sol in water, methanol, ethanol, acetone, methyl acetate.

Hexahydrate. Red to reddish-purple, deliquesc, prismatic crystals. mp 47-48°. d_4^{25} 2.46. Loses $4H_2O$ at 100° giving the purple dihydrate, and all H_2O by 130°. Sol in water giving red or blue soln depending on concn and temp, in methanol giving red soln, in ethanol, acetone, ether, methyl acetate giving blue solns. *Keep well closed.*

USE: Chiefly in hygrometers; also in catalysts for organic reactions.

2436. Cobaltous Carbonate. [513-79-1] $CCoO_3$; mol wt 118.94. C 10.10%, Co 49.55%, O 40.35%. $CoCO_3$. Occurs in nature as the mineral **cobalt spar** or **sphaerocobaltite.** Prepd by heating a soln of a cobaltous salt with Na_2CO_3: Schlessinger, *Inorg. Synth.* **6**, 189 (1963) where it is the starting material for the prepn of trinitrotriamminecobalt. *Review:* de Bie, Doyen, *Cobalt* **15**, 3-13; **16**, 3-15 (1962).

Red powder or rhombohedral crystals. d 4.13. Almost insol in water, alcohol, methyl acetate. Does not react with cold concd HNO_3 or HCl; when heated, dissolves with evolution of CO_2. Oxidized by air or weak oxidizing agents to cobaltic carbonate.

Hexahydrate. Pink to violet-red cryst needles. Pptd when excess CO_2 is present during prepn. On heating becomes anhydr by 140°. Stable in air.

Cobalt carbonate basic. Cobalt carbonate hydroxide. C_2-$H_6Co_5O_{12}$; mol wt 516.73. $Co_5(OH)_6(CO_3)_2$. Pale-red powder, usually containing some water. Practically insol in water; sol in dilute acids and ammonia.

USE: In ceramics; manuf of Co pigments; prepn of Co compds.

THERAP CAT (VET): Nutritional factor. Used in cobalt deficiency in ruminants.

2437. Cobaltous Chloride. [7646-79-9] Cobalt dichloride. Cl_2Co; mol wt 129.84. Cl 54.61%, Co 45.39%. $CoCl_2$. Prepn of anhydr from Co powder and Cl_2: Osthoff, West, *J. Am. Chem. Soc.* **76**, 4732 (1954); from the acetate and acetyl chloride: Watt *et al., ibid.* **77**, 2752 (1955); by dehydration of the hexahydrate with $SOCl_2$: Hecht, *Z. Anorg. Chem.* **254**, 51 (1947). Prepn of the hexahydrate by treating an aqueous soln of a cobaltous salt with HCl: *ACS Monograph Series* **no. 149**, entitled "Cobalt - Its Chemistry, Metallurgy, and Uses," R. S. Young, Ed. (Reinhold, New York, 1960) p 76. *Review:* de Bie, Doyen, *Cobalt* **15**, 3-13; **16**, 3-15 (1962). Toxicity studies: G. J. A. Speijers *et al., Food Chem. Toxicol.* **20**, 311 (1982); P. P. Singh, A. Y. Junnarkar, *Indian J. Pharmacol.* **23**, 153 (1991). Review of toxicology: B. Venugopal, T. D. Luckey, *Environ. Qual. Safety* Suppl. 1, 4-73 (1975).

Pale-blue hygroscopic leaflets; colorless in very thin layers; turns pink on exposure to moist air. mp 735°; bp 1049°; d_4^{25} 3.367. Dec 400° on long heating in air. Sublimes at 500° in HCl gas, forming iridescent, fluffy, colorless cryst. Sol in water, alcohols, acetone, ether, glycerol, pyridine. LD_{50} in mice, rats (mg/kg): 360.0, 171.0 orally; 92.6, 36.9 i.p.; 23.3, 4.3 i.v. (Singh, Junnarkar).

Hexahydrate. [7791-13-1] Monoclinic crystals. Structure is reported to be $[CoCl_2(H_2O)_4].2H_2O$: Mizuno *et al., J. Phys. Soc. Jpn.* **14**, 383 (1959), *C.A.* **53**, 14630i (1959). Pink to red, slightly deliquesc, monoclinic, prismatic crystals. mp 87°; d^{20} 1.924. On heating loses $4H_2O$ at 52-56° forming the dihydrate, violet or blue crystals, d_{25}^{25} 2.477, stable unless exposed directly to moisture. Loses another H_2O by 100°, giving monohydrate, violet, hygroscopic, amorphous solid or needles. Remaining H_2O lost at 120-140°. Sol in water, alcohols, acetone, ether, glycerol. pH of 0.2 molar aq soln 4.6. The aq soln is pink to red, but turns blue when heated or when HCl or H_2SO_4 is added. *Keep well closed.* LD_{50} orally in rats: 766 mg/kg (Speijers).

Caution: Large amounts of $CoCl_2$ depress erythrocyte production. May lead to death in children. Other effects include cuta-

neous flushing, chest pains, dermatitides, tinnitus, nausea and vomiting, nerve deafness, thyroid hyperplasia, myxedema, congestive heart failure. *See* E. Beutler *et al., Clinical Disorders of Iron Metabolism* (Grune & Stratton, New York, 1963) pp 175-178.

USE: Invisible ink; humidity and water indicator; in hygrometers; temp indicator in grinding; in electroplating; for painting on glass and porcelain; prepn of catalysts; fertilizer and feed additive; foam stabilizer in beer; as absorbent for military poison gas and ammonia; in manuf of vitamin B_{12}. Radioactive cobalt chloride, $^{57}CoCl_2$ (half-life 271.79 days, pure gamma emitter) used in Mössbauer effect (nuclear clock).

THERAP CAT: Hematinic.

THERAP CAT (VET): Nutritional factor. Used in cobalt deficiency in ruminants.

2438. Cobaltous Chromate(III). [12016-69-2] Chromium cobalt oxide (Cr_2CoO_4); cobalt chromite. $CoCr_2O_4$; mol wt 226.92. Co 25.97%, Cr 45.83%, O 28.20%. Prepn: *Gmelins, Cobalt* (8th ed.) **58**, (part A), 479 (1932) and supplement, 874-876 (1961).

Brilliant greenish-blue powder having a cubic spinel structure. Almost insol in concd HCl and HNO_3.

USE: Green pigment for ceramics.

2439. Cobaltous Cyanide. [542-84-7] Cobalt cyanide. C_2-CoN_2; mol wt 110.97. C 21.65%, Co 53.11%, N 25.24%. Prepn: Ray, Sahu, *J. Indian Chem. Soc.* **23**, 161 (1946); *Gmelins, Cobalt* (8th ed.) **58**, (part A), 364 (1932) and supplement, 712 (1961). Structure reported as $Co_3[Co(CN)_6]_2$: P. S. Poskozim *et al., J. Inorg. Nucl. Chem.* **35**, 687 (1973). Prepn and structure as $Co(CN)_2$: D. M. S. Mosha, D. Nicholls, *Inorg. Chim. Acta* **38**, 127 (1980).

Deep-blue, very hygroscopic powder. d_4^{25} 1.872.

Di- to trihydrate. Pink to reddish-brown powder or needles. Practically insol in water, acids, methyl acetate; sol in alkali cyanide solns.

USE: In cobalt catalysts.

2440. Cobaltous Fluoride. [10026-17-2] Cobalt difluoride. CoF_2; mol wt 96.93. Co 60.80%, F 39.20%. Prepd by the action of HF on anhydr $CoCl_2$: Kwasnik in *Handbook of Preparative Inorganic Chemistry* **vol. 1**, G. Brauer, Ed. (Academic Press, New York, 2nd ed., 1963) p 267; on $CoCO_3$: Clark, Buchner, *J. Am. Chem. Soc.* **44**, 230 (1922). on Co: Muetterties, Castle, *J. Inorg. Nucl. Chem.* **18**, 148 (1961).

Rosy-red tetragonal crystals. mp 1100-1200°, forming a red liq. Volatilizes at about 1400°. d 4.43. Sparingly sol in water; readily sol in warm mineral acids. Forms di-, tri-, and tetrahydrates, all sol in water; their aq solns are dec by boiling, forming the oxyfluoride $CoF_2.CoO.H_2O$.

USE: Catalyst for organic reactions.

2441. Cobaltous Formate. [544-18-3] $C_2H_2CoO_4$; mol wt 148.97. C 16.12%, H 1.35%, Co 39.56%, O 42.96%. $Co(HCOO)_2$. Prepn: *Gmelins, Cobalt* (8th ed.) **58** (part A), 350 (1932) and supplement, 702 (1961).

Dihydrate. Red, cryst powder. d^{22} 2.13. Sol in water; almost insol in alcohol. Becomes anhydr at 140°.

USE: In prepn of Co catalysts.

2442. Cobaltous Hydroxide. [21041-93-0] CoH_2O_2; mol wt 92.95. Co 63.40%, H 2.17%, O 34.43%. $Co(OH)_2$. Prepd from a solution of a cobaltous salt and an alkali hydroxide: Glemser in *Handbook of Preparative Inorganic Chemistry* **vol. 2**, G. Brauer, Ed. (Academic Press, New York, 2nd ed., 1965) p 1521; Weiser, Milligan, *J. Phys. Chem.* **36**, 722 (1932). *Review:* de Bie, Doyen, *Cobalt* **15**, 3-13; **16**, 3-15 (1962).

Blue-green or rose-red powder or microscopic rhombohedral crystals; red form is the more stable of the two. d_4^{15} 3.597. Easily oxidized by air or weak oxidizing agents to $Co(OH)_3$. Amphoteric. Loses water on heating, forming CoO at 168° *in vacuo.* Very slightly sol in water; readily sol in acids; practically insol in dil alkalies; sol in ammonia.

USE: Manuf of Co compds; drier for paints; in enhancing drying properties of lithographic printing inks; in storage battery electrode impregnating solns.

2443. Cobaltous Iodide. [15238-00-3] Cobalt diiodide. CoI_2; mol wt 312.74. Co 18.84%, I 81.16%. Prepn: Clark, Buchner, *J. Am. Chem. Soc.* **44**, 230 (1922); Chaigneau, *Bull. Soc. Chim. Fr.* **1957**, 886; Chaigneau, Chastagnier, *ibid.* **1958**, 1192; Glemser in *Handbook of Preparative Inorganic Chemistry* vol. **2**, G. Brauer, Ed. (Academic Press, New York, 2nd ed., 1965) p 1518.

The anhyd salt exists in two isomorphous forms. α-CoI_2: black, graphite-like solid. mp 515-520° (in high vacuum). d_4^{25} 5.584. Very hygroscopic, becomes blackish-green in air. Sol in water to give pink to red soln. β-CoI_2: ochre-yellow powder. Blackens at 400° and converts to α-form. d_4^4 5.45. Very hygroscopic; deliquesce in moist air forming green droplets. Sol in water to give colorless soln which becomes pink on heating.

Hexahydrate. Dark red hexagonal prisms. Loses H_2O on heating becoming anhyd by 130°. d 2.90. Loses I_2 on exposure to air and light. Sol in water to give soln which is red below 20°, olive green at 20 to 40°, and green at higher temps. Sol in ethanol (blue soln), ether (blue to green soln), chloroform (blue soln), acetone.

USE: Indicator for moisture and humidity; determination of water in organic solvents; catalyst for organic reactions.

2444. Cobaltous Nitrate. [10141-05-6] CoN_2O_6; mol wt 182.94. Co 32.21%, N 15.31%, O 52.47%. $Co(NO_3)_2$. Prepn: *Gmelins, Cobalt* (8th ed.) **58** (part A), 252-262 (1932) and supplement, 515-521 (1961); Weigel *et al., Bull. Soc. Chim. Fr.* **1964**, 836; Addison, Sutton, *J. Chem. Soc.* **1964**, 5553. Toxicity study: G. J. A. Speijers *et al., Food Chem. Toxicol.* **20**, 311 (1982). Review of toxicology: B. Venugopal, T. D. Luckey, *Environ. Qual. Safety* Suppl. 1, 4-73 (1975). *Review:* de Bie, Doyen, *Cobalt* **15**, 3-13; **16**, 3-15 (1962).

Pale red powder. Dec at 100-105°. d 2.49. Sol in water. LD in rabbits (mg/kg): 250 orally, 75 s.c. (Venugopal, Luckey).

Hexahydrate. [10026-22-9] Red, deliquesc, monoclinic crystals. mp ~55°. Red liq becomes green and dec to the oxide above 74°. d 1.88. Very sol in water, alcohol, most organic solvents. *Keep well closed in a cool place.* LD_{50} orally in rats: 691 mg/kg (Speijers).

USE: Manuf of cobalt pigments and invisible inks; decorating stoneware and porcelain; prepn of catalysts; production of vitamin B_{12} supplements.

2445. Cobaltous Oxalate. [814-89-1] C_2CoO_4; mol wt 146.95. C 16.35%, Co 40.10%, O 43.55%. CoC_2O_4. Prepn: Robin, *Bull. Soc. Chim. Fr.* **1953**, 1078; *Gmelins, Cobalt* (8th ed.) **58** (part A) p 355 (1932) and supplement, pp 704-706 (1961). *Review:* de Bie, Doyen, *Cobalt* **15**, 3-13; **16**, 3-15 (1962).

d_4^{25} 3.021. Readily absorbs moisture from air to form hydrates.

Dihydrate. Light pink microcryst powder or needles. Almost insol in water; slightly sol in acids; almost insol in aq oxalic acid; freely sol in aq ammonia. Dec on heating with aq KOH or Na_2CO_3 soln.

Tetrahydrate. Yellowish-pink amorphous powder. Effloresces on exposure to air. Loses water on heating to 100° giving the dihydrate. Very slightly sol in water; slightly sol in acids; readily sol in aq ammonia.

USE: Prepn of Co catalysts, Co metal powder for powder-metallurgical applications; stabilizer for HCN; temperature indicator.

2446. Cobaltous Oxide. [1307-96-6] CoO; mol wt 74.93. Co 78.65%, O 21.35%. Prepn: Amiel *et al., Compt. Rend.* **259**, 3512 (1964); Wilke, *Z. Anorg. Allg. Chem.* **330**, 164 (1964). Toxicity study: Smyth *et al., Am. Ind. Hyg. Assoc. J.* **30**, 470 (1969). *Review:* de Bie, Doyen, *Cobalt* **15**, 3-13; **16**, 3-15 (1962).

Powder, or cubic or hexagonal crystals. Color varies from olive green to red, depending on the particle size, but the commercial material is usually dark grey and contains about 76% Co. mp ~1935°. d 5.7 to 6.7, depending on method of prepn. Readily absorbs O_2 even at room temp. Practically insol in water. Sol in acids or alkalies. Easily reduced to Co by C or CO. Reacts at high temperatures with silica, alumina, zinc oxide to form pigments. LD_{50} orally in rats: 1.70 g/kg (Smyth).

Note: The commercial oxides are usually not definite chemical compds but mixtures of the cobalt oxides.

USE: In pigments for ceramics; glass coloring and decolorization; oxidation catalyst for drying oils, fast-drying paints and varnishes;

prepn of cobalt-metal catalysts, Co powder for binder in sintered tungsten carbide; in semiconductors.

2447. Cobaltous Phosphate. [13455-36-2] C.I. Pigment Violet 14; C.I. 77360. $Co_3O_8P_2$; mol wt 366.74. Co 48.21%, O 34.90%, P 16.89%. $Co_3(PO_4)_2$. Prepn from $CoCl_2$ and $(NH_4)_2$-HPO_4: Klement, Haselbeck, *Z. Anorg. Allg. Chem.* **334**, 27 (1964); from $Ca(H_2PO_4)_2$: Vickery, *US 2914380* (1959 to Horizons). *Review:* de Bie, Doyen, *Cobalt* **15**, 3-13; **16**, 3-15 (1962). *See also Colour Index* vol. **4** (3rd ed., 1971) p 4665.

Octahydrate. Pink to lavender amorph powder. d 2.77. Practically insol in water; sol in mineral acids.

USE: In ceramic pigments; in artists' colors, plastic resins.

2448. Cobaltous Sulfate. [10124-43-3] CoO_4S; mol wt 155.00. Co 38.02%, O 41.29%, S 20.69%. $CoSO_4$. Hexahydrate occurs in nature as the mineral *bieberite*. Prepn: Clark *et al., J. Am. Chem. Soc.* **42**, 2483 (1920); Hammel, *Ann. Chim.* **11**, 247 (1939); *Gmelins, Cobalt* (8th ed.) **58**, (part A) 324-336 (1932) and supplement, 628-647 (1961). *Review:* de Bie, Doyen, *Cobalt* **15**, 3-13; **16**, 3-15 (1962).

Red to lavender dimorphic, orthorhombic crystals. d_4^{25} 3.71. Stable to 708°. Dissolves slowly in boiling water.

Monohydrate. Rose-colored, monoclinic crystals. Structure reported to be $Co(H_2SO_5)$. d_4^{25} 3.08. Dissolves slowly in boiling water.

Heptahydrate. [10026-24-1] Pink to red monoclinic, prismatic crystals. On heating dehydrates to the hexahydrate (monoclinic, prismatic crystals) at 41.5°, and to the monohydrate at 71°. d_4^{25} 2.03. Sol in water; slightly sol in methanol, ethanol.

Caution: Cobaltous sulfate is reasonably anticipated to be a human carcinogen: *Report on Carcinogens* (PB2005-104914, 2004) p III-70.

USE: Usual source of water-soluble cobalt since it is the most economical and it shows less tendency to deliquesc or dehydrate than the chloride or nitrate. Used in storage batteries; in Co-electroplating baths; as drier for lithographic inks, varnishes; in ceramics, enamels, glazes to prevent discoloring; in Co pigments for decorating porcelain.

2449. Cobaltous Sulfide. [1317-42-6] CoS; mol wt 91.00. Co 64.76%, S 35.24%. Prepn: Glemser in *Handbook of Preparative Inorganic Chemistry* vol. **2**, G. Brauer, Ed. (Academic Press, New York, 2nd ed., 1965) p 1523.

Exists in two forms. α-CoS: black, amorphous powder. Forms Co(OH)S in air. Sol in HCl. β-CoS: grey powder or reddish-silver octahedral crystals. mp >1100°; d 5.45. Practically insol in water; sol in acids.

USE: Catalyst for hydrogenation or hydrodesulfurization.

2450. Cobaltous Thiocyanate. [3017-60-5] Cobaltous rhodanide; cobaltous sulfocyanate. $C_2CoN_2S_2$; mol wt 175.10. C 13.72%, Co 33.66%, N 16.00%, S 36.62%. $Co(SCN)_2$. Prepn: *Gmelins, Cobalt* (8th ed.) **58** (part A), 380 (1932) and supplement, 720-722 (1961); Schlessinger, *Inorganic Laboratory Preparations* (Chemical Publishing, New York, 1962) p 44.

Yellow-brown powder. Soluble in water to give a rose-colored soln; sol in ethanol, methanol, ether, acetone, $CHCl_3$ to give blue solns.

Trihydrate. Violet to violet-brown rhombic crystals; red in transmitted light. Sol in water to give blue soln which becomes pink on dilution; sol in ethanol, ether, acetone to give blue solns.

USE: As humidity indicator.

2451. Cobamamide. [13870-90-1] Co-(5'-deoxyadenosine-5') deriv of 3'-ester of cobinamide dihydrogen phosphate (ester) with 5,6-dimethyl-1-α-D-ribofuranosyl-1*H*-benzimidazole, inner salt; cobamamidum; coenzyme B_{12}; DBC; adenosyl-B_{12}; 5'-deoxyadenosyl-B_{12}; 5'-deoxyadenosylcobalamine; dibencozide; dibenzcozamide; dimebenzcozamide; 5,6-dimethylbenzimidazolylcobamide coenzyme; 5,6-dimethylbenzimidazolylcobamide 5'-deoxyadenosine; vitamin B_{12} coenzyme; Actimide; Ademide; Betarin; Calomide; Cobalion; Cobaltamin S; Cobanzyme; Cobazymase; Coenzile; Dolonevran; Enzicoba; Héraclène; Hi-Fresmin; Hycobal; Indusil; Ripresil; Sabalamin; Xobaline. $C_{72}H_{100}CoN_{18}O_{17}P$; mol wt 1579.58. C 54.75%, H 6.38%, Co 3.73%, N 15.96%, O 17.22%, P

1.96%. The coenzyme is the metabolically active form of vitamin B$_{12}$: Barker *et al., Proc. Natl. Acad. Sci. USA* **44**, 1093 (1958); Weissbach, Taylor, *Vitam. Horm.* **26**, 395 (1968). Isoln from a culture of *Propionibacterium shermanii:* Barker *et al., J. Biol. Chem.* **235**, 181, 480 (1960); *Biochem. Prep.* **10**, 27 (1964). Prepn of aquocobalamin and 2′,3′-*O*-isopropylidene-5′-*O*-*p*-tolylsulfonyl-adenosine: Hogenkamp, Pailes, *ibid.* **12**, 124 (1968); from treatment of a cobalamin-thiol complex: Murakami *et al., US 3461114* (1969 to Yamanouchi). The coenzyme differs from Vitamin B$_{12}$ by the presence of a 5′-deoxyadenosyl group in the axial ligand occupied by the cyanide in the vitamin. Structure: Lenhert, Hodgkin, *Nature* **192**, 937 (1961). The nucleoside is linked to the cobalt via the 5′-carbon atom of its deoxyribosyl moiety and the biological and chemical reactivity reside in this C to Co bond: Hogenkamp *et al., J. Biol. Chem.* **240**, 3641 (1965) and *Fed. Proc.* **25**, 1623 (1966). *Review:* Smith, *Vitamin B$_{12}$* (Methuen & Co., London, 3rd ed., 1965).

Yellow-orange six-faced crystals which become deep red upon exposure to air. Absorption max (H$_2$O): 260, 375, 522 nm (A × 10^{-6} 34.7, 10.9, 8.0 cm^2/mole). Soly in water (24°): 16.4 mmol. Solns of pH <3.5 are yellow, >3.5, red. Sol in ethanol, phenol. Practically insol in acetone, ether, dichloroethylene, dioxane. pKa 3.5. Stability studies: Collado, Nieto, *Ann. Pharm. Fr.* **27**, 427 (1969). Highly sensitive to light, to cyanide and moderately sensitive to acid. Solns are most stable at pH 6-7 stored in the dark. Heating of acid or alkaline solns produces slow inactivation.

THERAP CAT: Vitamin (hematopoietic).

THERAP CAT (VET): Vitamin (hematopoietic).

2452. Cobrotoxin. [12584-83-7] The main toxic protein in cobra venom. Crystallization and properties: Yang, *J. Biol. Chem.* **240**, 1616 (1965). Composed of a single peptide chain having 62 amino acid residues intramolecularly cross-linked by four disulfide bonds. Amino acid sequence: Yang *et al., Biochim. Biophys. Acta* **188**, 65 (1969). Complete structure: *eidem, ibid.* **214**, 355 (1970). Synthetic study: H. Aoyagi *et al., ibid.* **263**, 823 (1972). *Review:* C. C. Yang, "Biochemical Studies on the Toxic Nature of Snake Venom Cobrotoxin from Formosan Cobra Venom" in *Toxins of Animal and Plant Origin* **I**, A. de Vries, E. Kochva, Eds. (Gordon and Breach Science Publishers, New York, 1971) pp 205-236. *See also* A. T. Tu, *Venoms: Chemistry and Molecular Biology* (John Wiley and Sons, New York, 1977) pp 174-189.

2453. Coca. Erythroxylon; cuca; hayo; ipado. Dried leaves of *Erythroxylon coca* Lam., *Erythroxylaceae. Habit.* Bolivia, Brazil, Peru, cultivated in Java. *Constit.* 0.5-1% alkaloids in the South American, 1.5-2.5% in the Javanese leaves. In the former, the major alkaloid is cocaine; in the latter, there is very little cocaine, the alkaloids consisting chiefly of ecgonine derivatives such as benzoyl ecgonine, methyl ecgonine, etc. The Java leaves also contain small quantities of tropococaine which is apparently absent in the South American leaves. Other "cocaine" alkaloids present are truxillococaine, isatropylcocaine or cocamine, cocaicine.

Note: This is a controlled substance: **21 CFR**, 1308.12.

THERAP CAT: CNS stimulant.

2454. Cocaethylene. [529-38-4] [1*R*-(*exo,exo*)]-3-(Benzoyloxy)-8-methyl-8-azabicyclo[3.2.1]octane-2-carboxylic acid ethyl ester; ecgonine ethyl ester benzoate (ester); *O*-benzoyl-*l*-ecgonine ethyl ester; ethylbenzoylecgonine; Homocaine. C$_{18}$H$_{23}$NO$_4$; mol wt 317.38. C 68.12%, H 7.30%, N 4.41%, O 20.16%. Homolog of cocaine. Prepn: Merck, *Ber.* **18**, 2952 (1885); Einhorn, *ibid.* **21**, 47 (1888).

Prisms from alcohol, mp 109°. Almost insol in water. Sol in alcohol, ether.

THERAP CAT: Anesthetic (local).

2455. Cocaine. [50-36-2] [1*R*-(*exo,exo*)]-3-(Benzoyloxy)-8-methyl-8-azabicyclo[3.2.1]octane-2-carboxylic acid methyl ester; 3β-hydroxy-1α*H*,5α*H*-tropane-2β-carboxylic acid methyl ester benzoate; 2β-carbomethoxy-3β-benzoxytropane; ecgonine methyl ester benzoate; *l*-cocaine; β-cocaine; benzoylmethylecgonine. C$_{17}$H$_{21}$-NO$_4$; mol wt 303.35. C 67.31%, H 6.98%, N 4.62%, O 21.10%. From the leaves of *Erythroxylon coca* Lam. and other species of *Erythroxylon, Erythroxylaceae* or by synthesis. Extraction procedure: Squibb, *Pharm. J.* [3] **15**, 775, 796; **16**, 67 (1885); Emde in *Ullmanns Encyklopädie der technischen Chemie* Schwyzer, *Die Fabrikation pharmazeutischer und chemisch-technischer Produkte* (Berlin, 1931). Configuration: Findlay, *J. Am. Chem. Soc.* **76**, 2855 (1954); O. Kovacs *et al., Helv. Chim. Acta* **37**, 892 (1954). Synthesis: R. Willstätter *et al., Ann.* **434**, 111 (1923). Stereospecific synthesis of *dl*-form: J. J. Tufariello *et al., Tetrahedron Lett.* **1978**, 1733; *eidem, J. Am. Chem. Soc.* **101**, 2435 (1979). Biosynthesis: E. Leete, S. H. Kim, *J. Am. Chem. Soc.* **110**, 2976 (1988). Absorption spectrum: J. J. Dobbie, J. J. Fox, *J. Chem. Soc.* **103**, 1193 (1913); Fischer, *Arch. Exp. Pathol. Pharmakol.* **170**, 610 (1933). Toxicity: C. L. Rose *et al., J. Lab. Clin. Med.* **15**, 731 (1930). Vapor pressure studies: A. H. Lawrence *et al., Can. J. Chem.* **62**, 1886 (1984). Comprehensive description: F. J. Muhtadi, A. A. Al-Badr, *Anal. Profiles Drug Subs.* **15**, 151-231 (1986). Review of pharmacology and pharmacotherapies for abuse: M. Rocío *et al., Bioorg. Med. Chem.* **12**, 5019-5030 (2004).

Monoclinic tablets from alcohol, mp 98°. Volatile, esp above 90°, but the sublimate is not crystalline. bp$_{0.1}$ 187-188°. [α]$_D^{18}$ −35° (50% alcohol); [α]$_D^{20}$ −16° (c = 4 in chloroform). Aq solns are alkaline to litmus. pKa (15°) 8.61. pKb (15°) 5.59. One gram dissolves in 600 ml water, 270 ml water at 80°, 6.5 ml alcohol, 0.7 ml chloroform, 3.5 ml ether, 12 ml oil turpentine, 12 ml olive oil, 30-50 ml liquid petrolatum. Also sol in acetone, ethyl acetate, carbon disulfide. LD$_{50}$ i.v. in rats: 17.5 mg/kg (Rose).

Hydrochloride. [53-21-4] Cocaine muriate. $C_{17}H_{21}NO_4 \cdot$ HCl. Crystals, granules, or powder; saline, slightly bitter taste; numbs tongue and lips. mp ~195°. $[\alpha]_D$ −72° (c = 2 in aq soln pH 4.5). One gram dissolves in 0.4 ml water; 3.2 ml cold, 2 ml hot alcohol; 12.5 ml chloroform. Also sol in glycerol, acetone. Insol in ether or oils. Avoid heat in preparing soln as it decomposes. Preserve in well-closed, light-resistant containers.

Note: This is a controlled substance: **21 CFR,** 1308.12.

THERAP CAT: Anesthetic (local).

THERAP CAT (VET): Topical anesthetic (ophthalmic).

2456. Cocculus. Fish-berry; Indian berry; *Cocculus indicus*; oriental berry. Dried fruit of *Anamirta cocculus* (L.) Wight & Arn., *Menispermaceae. Habit.* East Indies, Malay Archipelago. *Constit.* Menispermine, paramenispermine, about 1% picrotoxin, picrotoxic acid, cocculine alkaloid, about 50% fat. *Poisonous!*

THERAP CAT: CNS and respiratory stimulant.

2457. Cochineal. The dried female insect, *Coccus cacti* L., enclosing the young larvae. *Habit.* Mexico, Central America; cultivated in West Indies, Canary Islands, Algiers, and Southern Spain. About 70,000 insects to 1 lb. *Constit.* About 10% carminic acid, about 2% coccerin (a wax), about 10% fat. The coloring matter, alkali carminate, is contained only in the fatty parts of the insect and in the yolk of the eggs, to the extent of 10-14%.

USE: Coloring food products and toilet preparations; the source of carmine and carminic acid for manuf red and pink inks and lakes.

2458. Cocillana. Dried bark of *Guarea rusbyi* (Britt.) Rusby, *Meliaceae. Habit.* Bolivia. *Constit.* Rusbyine, about 2.5% resins, about 2.5% fat, tannin.

THERAP CAT: Expectorant.

THERAP CAT (VET): Has been used as an expectorant.

2459. Coclaurine. [486-39-5] (1S)-1,2,3,4-Tetrahydro-1-[(4-hydroxyphenyl)methyl]-6-methoxy-7-isoquinolinol; 1-(*p*-hydroxybenzyl)-6-methoxy-7-hydroxy-1,2,3,4-tetrahydroisoquinoline; machiline. $C_{17}H_{19}NO_3$; mol wt 285.34. C 71.56%, H 6.71%, N 4.91%, O 16.82%. Isolated as the racemate from species of *Machilus (Lauraceae)* and *Cocculus (Menispermaceae).* First isoln from *C. laurifolius* D.C. believed to be of the *d*-form: Kondo, Kondo, *J. Pharm. Soc. Jpn.* No. **524,** 876 (1925), *C.A.* **20,** 604[7] (1926); *see also* Johns *et al., Aust. J. Chem.* **20,** 1729 (1967). Structure: Kondo, Kondo, *J. Pharm. Soc. Jpn.* **48,** 1156 (1928); Tomita, Kusuda, *ibid.* **72,** 280 (1952). Synthesis: Kratzl, Billek, *Monatsh. Chem.* **82,** 568 (1951); Finkelstein, *J. Am. Chem. Soc.* **73,** 550 (1951). Identity with machiline: Tomita *et al., J. Pharm. Soc. Jpn.* **83,** 218 (1963), *C.A.* **59,** 2874a (1963). Crystal structure and absolute configuration: Fridrichsons, Mathieson, *Tetrahedron* **24,** 5785 (1968).

Plates, tablets from alc, mp 220-221°. Sol in hot alc, hot acetone; slightly sol in water, alc, chloroform, ether, acetone; practically insol in benzene, petr ether.

Hydrochloride. $C_{17}H_{19}NO_3 \cdot$HCl. Crystals, mp 263-264°.

2460. Cocoa. A powder prepd from the roasted and cured kernels of ripe seeds of *Theobroma cacao* L. and other species of *Theobroma, Sterculiaceae.* For bibliography *see* Cacao Shell.

Brownish powder of chocolate odor and taste.

USE: In nutrient beverages; as flavoring.

2461. Coconut Oil. Copra oil. Expressed oil from kernels of *Cocos nucifera* L., *Palmae. Constit.* Trimyristin, trilaurin, tripalmitin, tristearin; also various other glycerides.

White, semisolid, lard-like fat; stable to air. Remains bland and edible for several years under ordinary storage conditions. d_4^0 0.903. mp 21-25°. n_D^{40} 1.4485-1.4495. Sapon. no. 255-258. Iodine no. 8-

9.5. Acid no. not over 6. Surface tension (20°): 33.4 dyn/cm; (80°): 28.4 dyn/cm. Practically insol in water, 95% alc, more sol in abs alc; very sol in chloroform, ether, carbon disulfide. Soly data: Rao, Arnold, *J. Am. Oil Chem. Soc.* **33,** 389 (1956).

USE: Manuf soap, edible fats, chocolate, candies; in baking instead of lard; in candles and night lights; in dyeing cotton; as an ointment base; in hair dressing; in massage.

2462. Codamine. [21040-59-5] (1S)-1-[(3,4-Dimethoxyphenyl)methyl]-1,2,3,4-tetrahydro-6-methoxy-2-methyl-7-isoquinolinol; 1,2,3,4-tetrahydro-6-methoxy-2-methyl-1-veratryl-7-isoquinolinol. $C_{20}H_{25}NO_4$; mol wt 343.42. C 69.95%, H 7.34%, N 4.08%, O 18.64%. Minor opium alkaloid. Constitutes about 0.003% of Turkish opium. Isoln: Hesse, *Ann.* **282,** 213 (1894). Structure: Späth, Epstein, *Ber.* **59B,** 2791 (1926). Synthesis: Schöpf, Thierfelder, *Ann.* **537,** 143 (1939); Billek, *Monatsh. Chem.* **87,** 106 (1956).

dl-**Form.** Large, six-sided prisms from ether, mp 127°. Very sol in alcohol, chloroform. Somewhat sol in boiling water. In soln codamine reacts strongly basic. The salts are bitter in taste, whereas the base is said to be tasteless.

2463. Codeine. [76-57-3] (5α,6α)-7,8-Didehydro-4,5-epoxy-3-methoxy-17-methylmorphinan-6-ol; methylmorphine; morphine monomethyl ether; morphine 3-methyl ether; Codicept. $C_{18}H_{21}NO_3$; mol wt 299.36. C 72.22%, H 7.07%, N 4.68%, O 16.03%. Present in opium from 0.7 to 2.5%, depending on the source, but mostly prepd by methylation of morphine, *q.v.* Discussion of structure and bibliography: Small, Lutz, "Chemistry of the Opium Alkaloids," in *U.S. Public Health Reports* **Suppl. No. 103** (Washington, 1932). Prepn of (+)-codeine and racemate: Goto, Yamamoto, *Proc. Jpn. Acad.* **30,** 769 (1954), *C.A.* **50,** 1052h (1956); of (−)-form: E. J. Bijsterveld, H. J. Sinnige, *Rec. Trav. Chim.* **95,** 24 (1976); H. C. Beyerman *et al., ibid.* **97,** 127 (1978). Manuf from morphine: W. R. Heumann, *Bull. Narc.* **X,** 15 (1958). Facile synthesis from thebaine, *q.v.:* W. G. Dauben *et al., J. Org. Chem.* **44,** 1567 (1979). Toxicity of the hydrochloride: Eddy, Sumwalt, *J. Pharmacol. Exp. Ther.* **67,** 127 (1939). Comprehensive description of codeine and codeine phosphate, *q.v.:* F. J. Muhtadi, M. M. A. Hassan, *Anal. Profiles Drug Subs.* **10,** 93-138 (1981).

Monohydrate. Orthorhombic sphenoidal rods or tablets (octahedra) from water or dil alcohol, mp 154-156° (after drying at 80°). Sublimes (when anhydr) at 140-145° under 1.5 mm pressure. Melts to oily drops when heated in an amount of water insufficient for complete soln, crystallizes on cooling. d_4^{20} 1.32. $[\alpha]_D^{15}$ −136° (c = 2 in alcohol), $[\alpha]_D^{15}$ −112° (c = 2 in chloroform). pK (15°) 6.05; pH of satd aq soln 9.8. One gram dissolves in 120 ml water, 60 ml water at 80°, 2 ml alcohol, 1.2 ml hot alcohol, 13 ml benzene, 18 ml ether, 0.5 ml chloroform; freely sol in amyl alcohol, methanol, dil acids. Almost insol in petr ether or in solns of alkali hydroxides.

Hydrochloride. [1422-07-7] $C_{18}H_{21}NO_3 \cdot$HCl. Dihydrate, small needles, mp ~280° with some decompn. $[\alpha]_D^{22}$ −108°. One gram dissolves in 20 ml water, 1 ml boiling water, 180 ml alcohol. pH about 5. LD_{50} s.c. in mice: 300 mg/kg (Eddy, Sumwalt).

Sulfate. [1420-53-7] $(C_{18}H_{21}NO_3)_2 \cdot H_2SO_4$; mol wt 696.81. C 62.05%, H 6.36%, N 4.02%, O 22.96%, S 4.60%. Trihydrate, crystals or cryst powder. One gram dissolves in 30 ml water, 6.5 ml water at 80°, 1300 ml alc. Insol in chloroform or ether. pH: 5.0. Store in airtight containers; protect from light.

Note: This is a controlled substance (opiate): **21 CFR,** 1308.12.

THERAP CAT: Analgesic (narcotic); antitussive.

THERAP CAT (VET): Analgesic (narcotic); antitussive.

2464.   Codeine Phosphate. [52-28-8] Galcodine. $C_{18}H_{24}$-NO_7P; mol wt 397.36. C 54.41%, H 6.09%, N 3.52%, O 28.18%, P 7.79%.

Hemihydrate. (U.S.P.), fine, white, needle-shaped crystals or cryst powder. Odorless; affected by light. Solns acid to litmus. Freely sol in water; very sol in hot water; slightly sol in alcohol; more sol in boiling alcohol.

Sesquihydrate. Very efflorescent, small crystals or cryst powder. One gram dissolves in 2.3 ml water, 0.5 ml water at 80°, 325 ml alcohol, 125 ml boiling alcohol, 4500 ml chloroform, 1875 ml ether. pH of a 2% aq soln: 4.6. *Keep well closed.*

Note: This is a controlled substance (opiate): **21 CFR,** 1308.12.

THERAP CAT: Analgesic (narcotic); antitussive.

THERAP CAT (VET): Analgesic (narcotic); antitussive.

2465.   Cod Liver Oil. Gaduol; Tunol. The partially destearinated fixed oil expressed from fresh livers of *Gadus morrhua* L., and other species of *Gadidae*. *Constit.* Most important are vitamins A and D, each gram containing at least 850 U.S.P. units vitamin A (255 μg) and at least 85 U.S.P. units vitamin D (2.125 μg); glycerides of palmitic, stearic, etc. acids ($\approx$19% saturated fatty acids; remainder unsaturated); cholesterol, batyl alcohol esters. Source of omega 3 fatty acid: N. Haagsma *et al., J. Am. Oil Chem. Soc.* **59**, 117 (1982). Brief description: D. Hilditch, P. Williams, *The Chemical Constitution of Natural Fats* (Wiley-Interscience, New York, 4th ed., 1964) p 43; *Bailey's Industrial Oil and Fat Products* **Vol. 1**, D. Swern (Wiley-Interscience, New York, 4th ed., 1979) pp 451-453.

Pale-yellow, thin liq; bland, slightly fishy taste and odor. Becomes yellow, acquires a somewhat disagreeable odor on exposure to air and light. d 0.918-0.927. n_D^{40} 1.4705-1.4745. Sapon no. 180-190. Iodine no. 145-180. Acid no. not over 1.2. Slightly sol in alcohol; freely sol in chloroform, ether, carbon disulfide, ethyl acetate, petr ether.

THERAP CAT: Vitamins A and D source.

THERAP CAT (VET): Source of vitamins A and D. Locally to promote healing.

2466.   Coenzyme A. [85-61-0] CoA. $C_{21}H_{36}N_7O_{16}P_3S$; mol wt 767.53. C 32.86%, H 4.73%, N 12.77%, O 33.35%, P 12.11%, S 4.18%. An essential cofactor in enzymatic acetyl transfer reactions. Synthesized in cells from pantothenate, ATP and cysteine. Found ubiquitously in mammalian cells. Isoln from animal sources: Lipmann *et al., J. Biol. Chem.* **167**, 869 (1947); **186**, 235 (1950). Many microorganisms contain large amounts of the coenzyme. Isoln from *Streptomyces fradiae:* Kaplan, Lipmann, *ibid.* **174**, 37 (1948). Purifications: De Vries *et al., J. Am. Chem. Soc.* **72**, 4838 (1950); Gregory *et al., ibid.* **74**, 854 (1952). Structure: Baddiley *et al., Nature* **171**, 76 (1953). Total synthesis: Moffatt, Khorana, *J. Am. Chem. Soc.* **81**, 1265 (1959); **83**, 663 (1961); Shimizu *et al., Chem. Pharm. Bull.* **13**, 1142 (1965). Reviews: Lipmann, *Bacteriol. Rev.* **17**, 1-16 (1953); Baddiley, *Adv. Enzymol.* **16**, 1 (1955); Jaenicke, Lynen in *The Enzymes* vol. 3, P. D. Boyer *et al.,* Eds. (Academic Press, New York, 2nd ed., 1960) pp 3-103. Review of metabolism: J. D. Robishaw, J. R. Neely, *Am. J. Physiol.* **248**, E1-E9 (1985); of clinical evaluations in hyperlipoproteinemia: A. Perin, G. Fraticelli, *Int. J. Tissue React.* **13**, 111-114 (1991); of biochemical role in cellular toxicity: E. P. Brass, *Chem. Biol. Interact.* **90**, 203-214 (1994).

White powder; characteristic thiol odor. May be dried *in vacuo* over phosphorus pentoxide at 34°. uv max: 259.5 nm (ε 16800). Fairly strong acid. pK 9.6 (thiol); pK 6.4 (secondary phosphate); pK 4.0 (adenine NH_3^+). Soluble in water. Practically insol in ethanol, ether, acetone. Pure dry coenzyme is best stored in evacuated ampuls at room temp. Readily oxidized by air to the catalytically inactive disulfide.

2467.   Coffee, Green. Coffee beans. Dry, unroasted seeds of *Coffea arabica* L., *Rubiaceae. Habit.* Tropical Africa, especially Abyssinia; cultivated in many tropical countries, *e.g.,* Java, West Indies, Brazil, etc. *Constit.* Caffeine 1-2%, coffee oil 10-15%, sucrose and other sugars about 8%, proteins about 11%, ash about 5%, chlorogenic and caffeic acids about 6%. Other constituents include cellulose, hemicelluloses, trigonelline, tannic acid, volatile oils. Monograph: M. Sivetz, H. E. Foote, *Coffee Processing Technology,* 2 vols (Avi Publ., 1963).

2468.   Coffee Oil. Coffee bean oil. A fatty oil found in coffee beans to the extent of about 15% (dry basis). Byproduct in the manufacture of instant coffees. Obtained in 2.7% yield by petr ether extraction of green Santos beans after previous dewaxing with tetrachloroethane: Schuette *et al., J. Am. Chem. Soc.* **56**, 2085 (1934). Coffee oil seems devoid of linolenic acid, however positive tests for linoleic (25.66%) and oleic (12.36%) acids were obtained.

Greenish-brown oil. Odor characteristic of green coffee beans. d_{25}^{25} 0.9653. n_D^{25} 1.4790. Iodine no. (Wijs) 100.72. Saponification no. 195.53; Reichert-Meissl no. 0.36. Saturated acids 33.60%. Unsaturated fatty acids 38.02%. Unsaponifiable matter 12.63%.

2469.   Coherin. [9044-70-6] A peptide factor present in the bovine neurohypophysis which may be involved in the normal physiological regulation of intestinal motility in mammals. Appears to stimulate the coordinated or "coherent" contraction of the intestine needed to keep food moving down the tract. Mol wt ~4000. Amino acid analysis (residue/mole): lysine 0.59; aspartic acid 3.9; threonine 0.11; serine 0.22; glutamic acid 4.0; proline 5.1; glycine 4.7; alanine 0.90; half-cystine 4.9; isoleucine 3.3; leucine 3.1; tyrosine 2.9; phenylalanine 0.88. Isoln from bovine posterior pituitary and preliminary data: Goodman, Hiatt, *Science* **178**, 419 (1972). Localization of formation site: I. Galasinska-Pomykol, M. Chilimoniuk, *Endokrynol. Pol.* **24**, 429 (1973), *C.A.* **81**, 102499j (1974). Effect on electrical rhythm of dog ileum *in vivo:* R. B. Hiatt *et al., Am. J. Dig. Dis.* **22**, 108 (1977). Effects on idiopathic delayed gastric emptying in humans: E. D. Davidson *et al., Am. J. Gastroenterol.* **74**, 419 (1980).

Relatively thermostable, losing only 10% of its activity when heated in a boiling water bath at pH 3 for 1 hour. Isoelectric point: pH 6.0.

2470.   Colchiceine. [477-27-0] *N*-[(7*S*)-5,6,7,9-Tetrahydro-10-hydroxy-1,2,3-trimethoxy-9-oxobenzo[*a*]heptalen-7-yl]acetamide; 7-acetamido-10-hydroxy-1,2,3-trimethoxy-6,7-dihydro-benzo[*a*]heptalen-9(5*H*)-one. $C_{21}H_{23}NO_6$; mol wt 385.41. C 65.44%, H 6.02%, N 3.63%, O 24.91%. Deriv of colchicine, *q.v.,* isolated from *Colchicum autumnale* L., *Liliaceae:* Santavy, Macák, *Collect. Czech. Chem. Commun.* **19**, 805 (1954). Toxicity data: B. Goldberg *et al., Cancer* **3**, 124 (1950). Structure and synthesis: Nakamura, *Chem. Pharm. Bull.* **10**, 299 (1962). Circular dichroism: J. Hrbek *et al., Collect. Czech. Chem. Commun.* **47**, 2258 (1982). Effect on antibody response induced *in vitro:* J. Sterzl *et al., Folia Microbiol.* **27**, 256 (1982).

Yellow crystals from dioxane + ether, mp 178-179°. $[\alpha]_D^{25}$ −255.1° (c = 1 in chloroform). uv max (95% ethanol): 351,

244 nm (log ε 4.28, 4.51). Slightly sol in water; freely sol in alcohol, chloroform. Almost insol in benzene, ether.

Ethyl ether. $C_{23}H_{27}NO_6$. Needles from ethyl acetate + ether, mp 135-139°. $[\alpha]_D^{25}$ −129.4° (c = 1 in chloroform). uv max (95% ethanol): 351, 243.5 nm (log ε 4.21, 4.45). LD_{50} i.p. in mice: 84 mg/kg (Goldberg).

2471. Colchicine. [64-86-8] N-[(7S)-5,6,7,9-Tetrahydro-1,-2,3,10-tetramethoxy-9-oxobenzo[a]heptalen-7-yl]acetamide. C_{22}-$H_{25}NO_6$; mol wt 399.44. C 66.15%, H 6.31%, N 3.51%, O 24.03%. A major alkaloid of *Colchicum autumnale* L., *Liliaceae*. Extraction procedure: Chemnitius, *J. Prakt. Chem.* [II] **118**, 29 (1928); F. E. Hamerslag, *Technology and Chemistry of Alkaloids* (New York, 1950) pp 66-80. Structure: Dewar, *Nature* **155**, 141 (1945); King *et al., Acta Crystallogr.* **5**, 437 (1952); Horowitz, Ullyot, *J. Am. Chem. Soc.* **74**, 487 (1952). Crystal structure: L. Lessinger, T. N. Margulis, *Acta Crystallogr.* **B34**, 578 (1978). Total synthesis: Schreiber *et al., Helv. Chim. Acta* **44**, 540 (1961); Van Tamelen *et al., Tetrahedron* **14**, 8 (1961); Nakamura, *Chem. Pharm. Bull.* **8**, 843 (1960); Sunagawa *et al., ibid.* **9**, 81 (1961); **10**, 281 (1962); Scott *et al., Tetrahedron* **21**, 3605 (1965); Woodward, *Harvey Lectures,* Ser. **59** (Academic Press, New York, 1965) p 31; Kotani *et al., Chem. Commun.* **1974**, 300; D. A. Evans *et al., J. Am. Chem. Soc.* **103**, 5813 (1981). Biosynthesis: Leete, *Tetrahedron Lett.* **1965**, 333; Battersby *et al., J. Chem. Soc.* **1964**, 4257; Hill, Unrau, *Can. J. Chem.* **43**, 709 (1965). Tubulin-binding activity: J. M. Andreu, S. N. Timasheff, *Proc. Natl. Acad. Sci. USA* **79**, 6753 (1982). Toxicity: S. J. Rosenbloom, F. C. Ferguson, *Toxicol. Appl. Pharmacol.* **13**, 50 (1968); R. P. Beliles, *ibid.* **23**, 537 (1972). Clinical evaluations in cirrhosis of the liver: M. M. Kaplan *et al., N. Engl. J. Med.* **315**, 1448 (1986); D. Kershenobich *et al., ibid.* **318**, 1709 (1988). Bibliography of early literature: Eigsti, *Lloydia* **10**, 65 (1947). Monograph: O. J. Eigsti, P. Dustin, Jr., *Colchicine in Agriculture, Medicine, Biology and Chemistry* (Iowa State College Press, Ames, Iowa, 1955). *Reviews:* Fleming, *Selected Organic Syntheses* (John Wiley, London, 1973) pp 183-207; G. Lagrue *et al., Ann. Med. Interne* **132**, 496-500 (1981); F. D. Malkinson, *Arch. Dermatol.* **118**, 453-457 (1982). Comprehensive description: D. K. Wyatt *et al., Anal. Profiles Drug Subs.* **10**, 139-182 (1981).

Pale yellow scales or powder, mp 142-150°. Darkens on exposure to light. Has been crystallized from ethyl acetate, pale yellow needles, mp 157°. $[\alpha]_D$ −429° (c = 1.72). $[\alpha]_D^{17}$ −121° (c = 0.9 in chloroform). pK at 20°: 12.35; pH of 0.5% soln: 5.9. uv max (95% ethanol): 350.5, 243 nm (log ε 4.22; 4.47). One gram dissolves in 22 ml water, 220 ml ether, 100 ml benzene; freely sol in alcohol or chloroform. Practically insol in petr ether. Forms two cryst compds with chloroform, B.CHCl₃ or B.2CHCl₃, which do not give up their chloroform unless heated between 60 and 70° for considerable time. LD_{50} in rats (mg/kg): 1.6 i.v. (Rosenbloom, Ferguson); in mice (mg/kg): 4.13 i.v. (Beliles).

USE: In research in plant genetics (for doubling chromosomes).

THERAP CAT: Gout suppressant. Treatment of Familial Mediterranean Fever.

THERAP CAT (VET): Has been used as an antineoplastic.

2472. Colchicum Corm. Meadow saffron; autumn crocus; wild saffron; meadow crocus. Dried corm of *Colchicum autumnale* L., *Liliaceae*. *Habit.* Central and Southern Europe, North Africa. *Constit.* 0.3-0.5% colchicine, colchicein, colchicoresin, starch, etc. Detn of colchicine in colchicine corm: Self, Corfield, *Q. J. Pharm. Pharmacol.* **5**, 347 (1932).

THERAP CAT: Gout suppressant.

2473. Colesevelam Hydrochloride. [182815-44-7] N,N,N-Trimethyl-6-(2-propenylamino)-1-hexanaminium chloride polymer with (chloromethyl)oxirane, 2-propen-1-amine and N-2-propenyl-1-decanamine, hydrochloride; GT-31-104; CholestaGel; Welchol. Bile acid sequestrant composed of a polyallylamine cross-linked with epichlorohydrin and alkylated with 1-bromodecane and 6-bromohexyltrimethylammonium bromide. Prepn: H. W. Mandeville, III, S. R. Holmes-Farley, **WO 9534585**; *eidem,* **US 5693675** (1995, 1997 both to GelTex); and bile acid binding: W. H. Mandeville *et al., Mater. Res. Soc. Symp. Proc.* **550**, 3 (1999). Absorption, distribution and excretion: D. P. Rosenbaum *et al., J. Pharm. Sci.* **86**, 591 (1997). Clinical trial in hypercholesterolemia: W. Insull, Jr. *et al., Mayo Clin. Proc.* **76**, 971 (2001). Review of pharmacology and clinical experience: M. A. Aldridge, M. K. Ito, *Ann. Pharmacother.* **35**, 898-907 (2001).

THERAP CAT: Antilipemic.

2474. Colestilan. [95522-45-5] 2-Methyl-1H-imidazole polymer with (chloromethyl)oxirane; 2-methylimidazole polymer with 1-chloro-2,3-epoxypropane; colestimide; MCI-196; Cholebine. $(C_4H_6N_2.C_3H_5ClO)n$. Bile acid sequestering anion exchange resin. Prepn: H. Toda, K. Kihara, **JP Kokai 59138228** (1984 to Mitsubishi Petrochem.); and bile acid binding activity: H. Toda *et al., J. Pharm. Sci.* **77**, 531 (1988). Series of articles on pharmacology and toxicology: *Jpn. Pharmacol. Ther.* **24**, Suppl. 4, 1-181 (1996). Clinical evaluation in type II hyperlipoproteinemia: Y. Homma *et al., Nutr. Metab. Cardiovasc. Dis.* **6**, 211 (1996); in hyperphosphatemia: S. Kurihara *et al., Nephrol. Dial. Transplant.* **20**, 424 (2005).

Odorless, tasteless, white powder. Ion exchange capacity: 4.9 mEq/g. Particle size: 44-149 μm.

THERAP CAT: Antilipemic.

2475. Colestipol. [26658-42-4] N-(2-Aminoethyl)-N'-[2-[(2-aminoethyl)amino]ethyl]-1,2-ethanediamine polymer with (chloromethyl)oxirane. A basic anion exchange resin described as a high molecular wt copolymer of diethylenetriamine and 1-chloro-2,3-epoxypropane (hydrochloride), with approx 1 out of 5 amine nitrogens protonated, for which no structural formula has been assigned and for which no specific mol wt information is available, due to the highly cross-linked and insoluble nature of the material. Prepn: Nelson, Van den Berg, **DE 1927336**; *eidem,* **US 3692895** (1969, 1971 to Upjohn); Lednicer, Peery, **DE 2053585**; *eidem,* **US 3803237** (1971, 1974 to Upjohn). Activity studies: Parkinson *et al., Atherosclerosis* **11**, 531 (1970); **17**, 167 (1973); Marmo *et al., G. Arterioscler.* **8**, 229 (1970); Goodman *et al., J. Clin. Invest.* **52**, 2646 (1973). Toxicology: Webster, Bollert, *Toxicol. Appl. Pharmacol.* **28**, 57 (1974). Review of pharmacology and therapeutic efficacy: R. C. Heel *et al., Drugs* **19**, 161-180 (1980).

Hydrochloride. [37296-80-3] U-26597A; Cholestabyl; Colestid; Lestid. Light yellow, hygroscopic resin. Insol in water. Swells when suspended in water or aqueous fluids. LD_{50} in rats (mg/kg): >4000 i.p.; >1000 orally (Webster, Bollert).

THERAP CAT: Antilipemic.

2476. Colforsin. [66575-29-9] (3R,4aR,5S,6S,6aS,10S,-10aR,10bS)-5-(Acetyloxy)-3-ethenyldodecahydro-6,10,10b-trihydroxy-3,4a,7,7,10a-pentamethyl-1H-naphtho[2,1-b]pyran-1-one; 7β-acetoxy-8,13-epoxy-1α,6β,9α-trihydroxylabd-14-en-11-one; forskolin; boforsin (obsolete); HL-362. $C_{22}H_{34}O_7$; mol wt 410.50. C 64.37%, H 8.35%, O 27.28%. Diterpene isolated from *Coleus forskohlii,* Briq. *Labiatae,* possessing vasodilating and cardiostimulatory properties. Isoln and characterization: S. V. Bhat *et al., Tetrahedron Lett.* **1977**, 1669; *eidem,* **DE 2557784**; *eidem,* **US 4088659** (1977, 1978 both to Hoechst). Synthesis by hydroxylation of 9-deoxyforskolin: N. J. Hrib, *Tetrahedron Lett.* **28**, 19 (1987); *see also* F. E. Ziegler *et al., J. Am. Chem. Soc.* **109**, 8115 (1987). Stereocontrolled synthesis of the 3-ring system: S. Hashimoto *et al., Chem. Commun.* **1987**, 24. Total synthesis of (±)-forskolin: S.

Hashimoto *et al., J. Am. Chem. Soc.* **110**, 3670 (1988); E. J. Corey *et al., ibid.* 3672. Positive inotropic and blood-pressure lowering activity: E. Lindner *et al., Arzneim.-Forsch.* **28**, 284 (1978). Activates adenylate cyclase: H. Metzger, E. Lindner, *ibid.* **31**, 1248 (1981). Binds to catalytic site of adenylate cyclase: T. Pfeuffer, H. Metzger, *FEBS Lett.* **146**, 369 (1982). Lowers intraocular pressure: J. Capriolli, M. Sears, *Lancet* **1**, 958 (1983). In treatment of glaucoma: *eidem,* US 4476140 (1984 to Yale University). *Reviews:* K. B. Seaman, J. W. Daly, *J. Cyclic Nucleotide Res.* **1981**, 201; K. B. Seaman, "Forskolin and Adenylate Cyclase: New Opportunities in Drug Design" in *Annu. Rep. Med. Chem.* **19**, D. M. Bailey, Ed. (Academic Press, New York, 1984) pp 293-302.

Colorless crystals from ethyl acetate/petr ether, mp 230-232°. uv max 210, 305 nm (ε 1000, 50). $[\alpha]_D^{25}$ $-26.19°$ (c = 1.68 in $CHCl_3$).

USE: In purification of adenylate cyclase.

2477. Colfosceril Palmitate. [63-89-8] (7*R*)-4-Hydroxy-*N,N,N*-trimethyl-10-oxo-7-[(1-oxohexadecyl)oxy]-3,5,9-trioxa-4-phosphapentacosan-1-aminium inner salt 4-oxide; L-α-dipalmitoyl lecithin; dipalmitoyl-L-α-glycerylphosphorylcholine; dipalmitoyl phosphatidylcholine; DPPC; Exosurf Neonatal. $C_{40}H_{80}NO_8P$; mol wt 734.04. C 65.45%, H 10.99%, N 1.91%, O 17.44%, P 4.22%. Major phospholipid constituent and primary surface tension lowering component of natural lung surfactant. Isoln from lung extracts: S. J. Thannhauser *et al., J. Biol. Chem.* **166**, 669 (1946); E. S. Brown, *Am. J. Physiol.* **207**, 402 (1964). Enantioselective synthesis: E. Baer, M. Kates, *J. Am. Chem. Soc.* **72**, 942 (1950). Clinical study in combination therapy for neonatal respiratory distress syndrome (RDS): C. J. Morley *et al., Lancet* **1**, 64 (1981). Diagnostic use as predictor of fetal lung maturity: A. Lohninger *et al., Clin. Chem.* **29**, 650 (1983). HPTLC determn in amniotic fluid: J. G. Alvarez *et al., J. Chromatogr. B* **665**, 79 (1995). Review of early literature: D. F. Tierney, *Am. J. Physiol.* **257**, L1-L12 (1989); of role in pulmonary function and clinical use: L. M. G. van Golde *et al., Physiol. Rev.* **68**, 374-455 (1988); of structure and function as surface active agent: B. A. Hills, *Br. J. Anaesth.* **65**, 13-29 (1990); of biosynthesis: H. P. Haagsman, L. M. G. van Golde, *Annu. Rev. Physiol.* **53**, 441-464 (1991).

Occurs as monohydrate, crystals from hot diisobutyl ketone, softens at 75-79°, mp 234-235°. $[\alpha]_D^{23}$ +6.6° (c = 4.2 in 1:1 chloroform-methanol). Readily sol in chloroform, hot diisobutyl ketone, hot dioxane. Readily emulsified in water. Soly at 22-23° (g/100 ml): ethanol 1.5, ether 0.02, acetone 0.02, pyridine 1.1, acetic acid 4.0, methanol 1.4.

THERAP CAT: Pulmonary surfactant. Diagnostic aid (fetal lung maturity).

2478. Colicins. Colicine. Antibiotic substances, or complexes of antibiotic substances, which are highly specific, are produced by certain strains of intestinal bacteria, and act upon other related strains: Fredericq, *Annu. Rev. Microbiol.* **11**, 7 (1957). Colicins produced by various strains may differ in many characteristics, the most conspicuous of which are activity spectra and the specificity of resistant mutants. They give the general reactions of proteins, are antigenic, and their activity is destroyed by proteolytic enzymes: Fredericq, *J. Theor. Biol.* **4**, 159 (1963). Production of colicin A: Barry *et al., Nature* **198**, 211 (1963); of colicin V:

Hutton, Goebel, *Proc. Natl. Acad. Sci. USA* **47**, 1498 (1961); of colicins E_4, N, P,V_2, V_3, V_4 and V_5: Hamon, Péron, *Ann. Inst. Pasteur* **107**, 44 (1964). Mechanism of action of colicins: Nomura, *Proc. Natl. Acad. Sci. USA* **52**, 1514 (1964). *Reviews: idem* in *Antibiotics* vol. 1, D. Gottlieb, P. D. Shaw, Eds. (Springer-Verlag, New York, 1967) pp 696-704; Wendt, *ibid.* vol. 3, J. W. Corcoran, F. E. Hahn, Eds. (1975) pp 588-605.

2479. Colistin. [1066-17-7] Polymyxin E. Cyclic polypeptide antibiotic produced by *Bacillus polymyxa* subsp. *colistinus.* Complex mixture of at least 30 components, primarily colistins A and B. Isoln from Japanese soil: Y. Koyama, JP 52 1546 (1952). Identification of colistins A, B and C: T. Suzuki *et al., J. Biochem. (Tokyo)* **54**, 25 (1963). Structure of colistin A: *eidem, ibid.* 173, 412. Identity of colistin A with polymyxin E_1: S. Wilkinson, L. A. Lowe, *J. Chem. Soc.* **1964**, 4107. Synthesis of colistin A: R. O. Studer *et al., Helv. Chim. Acta* **48**, 1371 (1965). Prepn of sodium sulfomethyl derivs and toxicity study: M. Barnett *et al., Br. J. Pharmacol. Chemother.* **23**, 552 (1964). Comparative pharmacology of sulfate and methansulfonate salts: A. A. Al-Khayyat, A. L. Aronson, *Chemotherapy (Basel)* **19**, 82 (1973). HPLC determn in medicated animal feeds: B. Cancho-Grande *et al., Chromatagraphia* **54**, 481 (2001); in human plasma: J. Li *et al., J. Chromatogr. B* **761**, 167 (2001). Review and comparison with polymyxin B, *q.v.*: J. Horton, G. A. Pankey, *Med. Clin. North Am.* **66**, 135-142 (1982); M. E. Evans *et al, Ann. Pharmacother.* **33**, 960-967 (1999). Review of clinical experience in cystic fibrosis: J. M. Littlewood *et al., Respir. Med.* **94**, 632 (2000); in treatment of multi-resistant bacterial infections: J. Li *et al., Int. J. Antimicrob. Ag.* **25**, 11-25 (2005).

Colistin A   R = (+)-6-methyloctanoyl
Colistin B   R = 6-methylheptanoyl

Colistin sodium methanesulfonate. [8068-28-8] Colistimethate sodium; Alficetin; Colimicina; Colimycine; Colomycin; Coly-Mycin M; Methacolimycin; Promixin. $C_{58}H_{105}N_{16}Na_5O_{28}S_5$; mol wt 1749.82. Prepd by treating colistin complex with formaldehyde and sodium bisulfite. Sol in water and stable in the dry form. LD_{50} i.v. in mice: >550 mg/kg (Barnett).

Sulfate. [1264-72-8] Belcomycine; Colomycin (tabl.).

Colistin A. [7722-44-3] Polymyxin E_1. $C_{53}H_{100}N_{16}O_{13}$; mol wt 1169.46. $[\alpha]_{5461}^{22}$ $-93.3°$ (2% acetic acid).

Colistin B. [7239-48-7] Polymyxin E_2. $C_{52}H_{98}N_{16}O_{13}$; mol wt 1155.43. $[\alpha]_{5461}^{22}$ $-94.5°$ (2% acetic acid).

THERAP CAT: Antibacterial.

THERAP CAT (VET): Antibacterial.

2480. Collagen. Ossein. Mol wt about 130,000. Polypeptide substance comprising one third of the total protein in mammalian organisms; main constituent of skin, connective tissue, and the organic substance of bones and teeth. Prepd from bones by dissolving the mineral part of the bones with phosphoric acid: Sciallano, FR 688104 (1929), *C.A.* **25**, 786 (1931). Isoln of sol collagens from corium tissue: Reizo, Sakata, *Kumamoto Med. J.* **13**, 27 (1960). Purification: Bloch, Oneson, US 2973302 (1961 to Ethicon). Commercial extraction process: Highberger, US 2979438 (1961 to United Shoe Machinery). Collagen production in the body is preceded by the formation of a much larger molecule, the biosynthetic precursor **procollagen**, which is degraded by specific enzymes to make collagen. Different types of collagens exist. They are all composed of molecules containing three polypeptide chains, α-chains, arranged in a triple helical conformation. The amino acid sequence of the α-chain is mostly a repeating structure with glycine in every third position and proline or 4-hydroxyproline frequently preceding the glycine residues. Slight differences in the primary structure (amino acid sequence) establish differences between types. Review of structural studies: Tanzer, *Science* **180**, 561-566 (1973); P. Bornstein, H. Sage, *Annu. Rev. Biochem.* **49**, 959 (1980). Collagen is differentiated from the accompanying fibrous proteins, elastin, and reticulin, *q.q.v.,* by (*1*) its content of proline, hydroxyproline and hydroxylysine, by (*2*) the absence of tryptophan and its low tyrosine and sulfur content, but particularly by (*3*) its high content of polar groups originating from the difunctional amino acids. The polar groups are responsible for the swelling properties leading eventually to dispersion of collagen in dil acid. Denaturation of collagen is the conversion of the rigidly coiled helix to a random coil called gelatin, *q.v.* Description of the native and denatured states of sol collagen: Boedtker, Doty, *J. Am. Chem. Soc.* **78**, 4267 (1956). Biosynthesized in fibroblastic cells. Review of biosynthesis: Bornstein, *Annu. Rev. Biochem.* **43**, 567-603 (1974). *Reviews:* Gross, *Sci. Am.* **204**, 121 (May 1961); Harrington, von Hippel, *Adv. Protein Chem.* **16**, 1-138 (1961); Grassmann *et al., Fortschr. Chem. Org. Naturst.* **23**, 195-314 (1965); P. Bornstein, W. Traub, "The Chemistry and Biology of Collagen" in *The Proteins* vol. **IV**, H. Neurath, R. L. Hill, Eds. (Academic Press, New York, 1979) pp 411-632; D. R. Eyre, *Science* **207**, 1315-1322 (1980); *Methods Enzymol.* **82**, 3-555 (1982). Summary of recent studies of the role of collagen in disease: *Chem. Eng. News* **60**, 32 (Jan. 25, 1982). Books: A. Veis, *The Macromolecular Chemistry of Gelatin* (Academic Press, New York, 1964) 433 pp; *Biochemistry of Collagen*, G. N. Ramachandran *et al.,* Eds. (Plenum, New York, 1976) 536 pp; P. P. Fietzek in *Collagen in Health and Disease*, M. I. V. Jayson, J. B. Weiss, Eds. (Churchill-Livingstone, New York, 1982).

USE: As fibers in sutures, in leather substitutes; as a gel in photographic emulsions, in coatings; in food casings.

2481. Collagenase. [9001-12-1] Clostridiopeptidase A; Iruxol; Santyl. Rare proteolytic enzyme capable of digesting native undenatured collagen, *q.v.,* found in certain *Clostridia* bacteria culture filtrates. Crude prepn from *C. histolyticum:* Mandl *et al., J. Clin. Invest.* **32**, 1323 (1953). Purified prepn: Keller, Mandl, *Arch. Biochem. Biophys.* **101**, 81 (1963). Also isolated from culture media of human wound tissue, skin, bone, leukocytes, gingiva, cornea, rheumatoid synovium; from involuting rat uterus and tadpole tailfin tissue. Sepn of fractions A and B having the respective mol wts 105,000 and 57,400: Harper *et al., Biochem. Biophys. Res. Commun.* **18**, 627 (1965). Amino acid composition: Mandl *et al., Biochemistry* **3**, 1737 (1964); Yoshida, Noda, *Biochim. Biophys. Acta* **105**, 562 (1965). Potential use in treatment of herniated discs: Sussman, *FR* **2008611** (1970 to Worthington Biochemical). Review of early studies: Mandl, *Adv. Enzymol.* **23**, 163-264 (1961). *Reviews: idem, Science* **169**, 1234-1238 (1970); Nordwig, *Adv. Enzymol. Relat. Areas Mol. Biol.* **34**, 155-205 (1971); Lazarus, *Br. J. Dermatol.* **86**, 193-199 (1972). Book: *Collagenase*, I. Mandl, Ed. (Gordon and Breach, N.Y., 1972) 215 pp.

USE: In investigation of the structure and biosynthesis of collagen; in dispersion of cells for tissue culture studies.

THERAP CAT: Debriding agent.

2482. Collinomycin. [27267-69-2] 6-[2-(4,9-Dihydro-8-hydroxy-5,7-dimethoxy-4,9-dioxonaphtho[2,3-*b*]furan-2-yl)ethyl]-7,8-dihydroxy-1-oxo-1*H*-2-benzopyran-3-carboxylic acid methyl ester; α-rubromycin. C$_{27}$H$_{20}$O$_{12}$; mol wt 536.44. C 60.45%, H 3.76%, O 35.79%. Antibiotic substance produced by *Streptomyces collinus:* Brockmann, Renneberg, *Naturwissenschaften* **40**, 166 (1953); *DE* **918162** (1954 to Bayer). Identity with α-rubromycin: Brockmann *et al., Tetrahedron Lett.* **1966**, 3525. Structure: Brockmann, Zeeck, *Ber.* **103**, 1709 (1970). Shows considerable *in vitro* activity against *Staph. aureus.*

Orange prisms from chloroform-methanol, mp 280-282°. Moderately sol in chloroform, acetone, dioxane; sparingly sol in ether, low-molecular alcohols. Practically insol in petr ether, water, aq sodium bicarbonate soln.

2483. Collinsonia. Stone-root; knob root; horse balm; richweed. Root of *Collinsonia canadensis* L., *Labiatae. Habit.* North America, from Ontario to Florida and west to Kansas. *Constit.* Resin, saponin, tannin, mucilage.

2484. Collodion. A soln of 4 g pyroxylin (chiefly nitrocellulose) in 100 ml of a mixture of 25 ml alcohol and 75 ml ether. Contains about 70% ether and 24% abs alc by vol.

Colorless, or slightly yellow, clear or slightly opalescent, syrupy liquid. Has the odor of ether. d$_{25}^{25}$ 0.765-0.775. Exposed in thin layers, it evaporates leaving a tough, colorless film. On the addition of water the pyroxylin ppts.

Flexible collodion. Mixture of simple collodion with 2% camphor and 3% castor oil (by wt). Yellow syrupy liquid; contains about 67% ether and about 22% abs alcohol by volume.

Styptic collodion. Mixture of flexible collodion with 18% tannic acid by wt. Contains about 61% ether and about 21% abs alcohol by volume.

Caution: Highly flammable! Keep tightly closed in a cool place and away from flame!

USE: Collodion in photography; manuf lacquers, patent and artificial leathers, artificial pearls; process engraving; in cements.

THERAP CAT: Collodion and flexible collodion as topical protectant; styptic collodion as hemostatic.

THERAP CAT (VET): Skin protectant.

2485. Colloidal Bismuth Subcitrate. [57644-54-9] CBS; De-Nol; De-Noltab; Duosol; Ulcerone. Cytoprotective, polymeric bismuth citrato complex; also known as *tripotassium dicitrato bismuthate.* General prepn of colloidal bismuth solution: L. Vanino, cited in *Mellor's* vol. **IX**, 598 (1929). Manufacturing processes: C. J. McLoughlin, R. B. Himstedt, *DE* **2501787**; P. J. H. Bos *et al., EP* **75992**; *eidem,* US **4801608** (1975, 1985, 1989 all to Gist-Brocades). Analytical study: D. R. Williams, *J. Inorg. Nucl. Chem.* **39**, 711 (1977). Crystal structure: E. Asato *et al., Chem. Lett.* **1992**, 1967. Pharmacology: J. Wieriks *et al., Scand. J. Gastroenterol.* **17**, Suppl. 80, 11 (1982). Modes of action: D. W. R. Hall, *ibid.* **24**, Suppl. 157, 3 (1989); S. P. Lee, *ibid.* **26**, Suppl. 185, 1 (1991). Pharmacokinetics and safety: L. Z. Benet *ibid.* 29. Symposia on pharmacology and clinical efficacy: *ibid.* **21**, Suppl. 122, 1-54 (1986); *Digestion* **37**, Suppl. 2, 1-64 (1987). Clinical trials in *Helicobacter pylori* associated gastritis and ulcer: T. Rokkas *et al., Gut* **29**, 1386 (1988); W. A. de Boer *et al., Am. J. Gastroenterol.* **89**, 1993 (1994).

White, amorphous powder. Sol in water, dil alkali, ammonia. Forms precipitate of bismuth oxychloride and bismuth citrate at pH <5.

THERAP CAT: Antiulcerative.

2486. Colocynth. Bitter apple; bitter cucumber; bitter gourd. Perennial trailing vine, *Citrullus colocynthis* Schrad., *Cucurbitaceae*, bearing round, yellow, bitter, poisonous fruit with numerous white or brownish seeds. The dried fruit pulp has been used in traditional medicine as a purgative. *Habit.* Semi-arid, tropical and subtropical regions of Asia and N. Africa. *Constit.* Colocynthin, *q.v.,* colocynthidin, cucurbitacins, citrullol, pectin, albuminoids, 1-3% fixed oil. Seeds contain fixed oil, protein, crude fiber. Constituents of seeds: W. N. Sawaya *et al., J. Agric. Food Chem.* **34**, 285 (1986). Review of constituents and medicinal uses: C. P. Khare, *Indian Herbal Remedies* (Springer-Verlag, Berlin, 2004) pp 148-149; J. Gruenwald *et al., PDR for Herbal Medicines* (Medical Economics, Montvale, 3rd Ed., 2004) pp 85-86.

Caution: Potential symptoms of overexposure by ingestion are vomiting, bloody diarrhea, colic and kidney irritation, convulsions, paralysis, death (Gruenwald).

2487. Colocynthin. [1398-78-3] 25-(Acetyloxy)-2-(β-D-glucopyranosyloxy)-16,20-dihydroxy-9-methyl-19-norlanosta-1,5,23-triene-3,11,22-trione; 2-*O*-β-D-glucopyranosylcucurbitacin E. C$_{38}$H$_{54}$O$_{13}$; mol wt 718.83. C 63.49%, H 7.57%, O 28.93%. Glucoside from fruit of *Citrullus colocynthis* Schrad., *Cucurbitaceae:* Walz, *Neues Jahrb. Pharm.* **9**, 16, 225 (1858); **16**, 10 (1861); Henke, *Arch. Pharm.* **221**, 200 (1883); Naylas, Chappel, *Pharm. J.*

25, 117 (1907); Lavie *et al., Acta Univ. Int. Contra Cancerum* **15**, 177 (1959); Khadem, Rahman, *Tetrahedron Lett.* **1962**, 1137. Other isolns: H. Ripperger, K. Seifert, *Tetrahedron* **31**, 1561 (1975); H. Ripperger, *ibid.* **32**, 1567 (1976). Structure: Khadem, Rahman, *J. Chem. Soc.* **1963**, 4991.

Yellow crystals, mp 158-160°. $[\alpha]_D$ +50° (c = 0.4 in ethanol). uv max: 234-236 nm (log ε 4.11). Sol in ethanol, acetone, chloroform; slightly sol in ether, water.

THERAP CAT: Cathartic.

2488. Colony Stimulating Factors. CSFs. Family of hematopoietic growth factors that regulate the production of myeloid cells. Glycoprotein hormones that stimulate cell proliferation, survival, differentiation commitment, and end-cell functional activity; important to the inflammatory and immune response. Cell types capable of producing one or more CSFs include monocytes, T-lymphocytes, endothelial cells, fibroblasts and skin epithelial cells. Originally identified by their ability to stimulate the *in vitro* growth of hematopoietic progenitor cells into colonies in semisolid media: D. H. Pluznick, L. Sachs, *J. Cell. Comp. Physiol.* **66**, 319 (1965); T. R. Bradley, D. Metcalf, *Aust. J. Exp. Biol. Med. Sci.* **44**, 287 (1966). Distinguished by the type(s) of progeny cells which result from stimulation by the specific factor, CSFs include: granulocyte-CSF (G-CSF), granulocyte-macrophage CSF (GM-CSF), macrophage-CSF (M-CSF) and multi-CSF or interleukin-3 (IL-3), *q.q.v.* G-CSF and M-CSF are thought to act on late progenitor cells already committed to their respective lineages. GM-CSF and IL-3 act on earlier, pluripotential progenitors. Potential clinical applications include the reduction of myelosuppression during cancer chemotherapy; augmentation of host defense in infection; and differentiation induction in hematological malignancies. Reviews: D. Metcalf, *Science* **229**, 16-22 (1985); S. C. Clark, R. Kamen, *ibid.* **236**, 1229-1237 (1987); J. D. Griffin, *Oncology* **2**, 15-21 (1988). Role in infectious disease: R. M. Rose, *Semin. Oncol.* **19**, 415-421 (1992). Reviews of biological effects and clinical potential: J. L. Gabrilove, *Cancer Chemother. Biol. Response Modif.* **10**, 492-506 (1988); J. E. Groopman *et al., N. Engl. J. Med.* **321**, 1449-1459 (1989); J. A. Hamilton, *Immunol. Today* **14**, 18-24 (1993).

2489. Colpormon. [1247-71-8] (16α)-3,16-Bis(acetyloxy)estra-1,3,5(10)-trien-17-one; 3,16α-dihydroxyestra-1,3,5(10)-trien-17-one diacetate; 16α-hydroxyestrone diacetate; 3,16α-diacetoxy-Δ^{1,3,5}-estratrien-17-one; Colpogynon. $C_{22}H_{26}O_5$; mol wt 370.44. C 71.33%, H 7.07%, O 21.60%. Prepn: Leeds *et al., J. Am. Chem. Soc.* **76**, 2943 (1954); **FR M1390** (1962 to Lab. Albert Rolland), *C.A.* **58**, 3484c (1963).

Crystals, mp 179-180°. $[\alpha]_D^{28}$ +122° (chloroform).

THERAP CAT: Estrogen.

2490. Coltsfoot. Coughwort. Dried leaves of *Tussilago farfara* L., *Compositae. Habit.* Northern Europe and Asia; naturalized in Northeastern U.S. *Constit.* Pectin, bitter glucoside, tannin, volatile oil, resin, saponin, caoutchouc.

2491. Colubrines. $C_{22}H_{24}N_2O_3$; mol wt 364.44. C 72.50%, H 6.64%, N 7.69%, O 13.17%. Minor alkaloids found in *Strychnos nux vomica L.;* naturally occurring in two chemically distinct forms, α and β. Isolation from mother liquor of commercial strychnine extraction: K. Warnat, *Helv. Chim. Acta* **14**, 997 (1931). Isolation and characterization from *S. nux vomica L.:* G. B. Marini-Bettolo *et al., J. Assoc. Off. Anal. Chem.* **51**, 185 (1968). Structure of α- and β-colubrine: S. P. Findlay, *J. Am. Chem. Soc.* **73**, 3008 (1951); of β-colubrine: P. Rosenmund, *Ber.* **95**, 2639 (1962); of α-colubrine: J. M. Culver, M. Sainsbury, *J. Chem. Res. Synop.* **1987**, 304. Synthesis from strychnine: P. Rosenmund, H. Franke, *Ber.* **97**, 1677 (1964). Determn by GLC: N. G. Bisset, P. Fouché, *J. Chromatogr.* **37**, 172 (1968); by HPLC: G. M. Iskander *et al., J. Liq. Chromatogr.* **5**, 1481 (1982). Chiroptical properties of β-colubrine: J. W. Snow, T. M. Hooker, Jr., *Can. J. Chem.* **56**, 1222 (1978).

α-Colubrine: $R_1 = OCH_3$ $R_2 = H$
β-Colubrine: $R_1 = H$ $R_2 = OCH_3$

α-Colubrine. [509-44-4] 3-Methoxystrychnidin-10-one; 11-methoxystrychnine. Pyramids from ethyl acetate, mp 189-193°. $[\alpha]_D^{20}$ −72.4° (c = 0.9 in alc). uv max (ethanol): 255, 297 nm (log ε 4.03, 3.77). Sol in alc, benzene, chloroform.

β-Colubrine. [509-36-4] 2-Methoxystrychnidin-10-one; 10-methoxystrychnine. Crystals from dil alcohol, mp 222°. Very bitter. $[\alpha]_D^{19}$ −107.7° (c = 2.5 in 80% alcohol). $[\alpha]_D^{21}$ −156° (c = 0.042 in chloroform). uv max (ethanol): 262, 297 nm (log ε 4.40, 3.80). Sol in alcohol, benzene, chloroform.

2492. Columbamine. [3621-36-1] 5,6-Dihydro-2-hydroxy-3,9,10-trimethoxydibenzo[a,g]quinolizinium; 7,8,13,13α-tetradehydro-2-hydroxy-3,9,10-trimethoxyberbinium. $[C_{20}H_{20}NO_4]^+$. Found in *Jatrorrhiza palmata* (DC.) Miers (*J. columba* Miers), *Menispermaceae:* Breslau, *Arch. Pharm.* **245**, 586 (1908); Späth, Burger, *Ber.* **59**, 1486 (1926); Reed, *Diss. Abstr.* **23**, 3638 (1963); from *Berberis lambertii* R. N. Parker, *Berberidaceae:* Chatterjee, Banerjee, *J. Indian Chem. Soc.* **30**, 705 (1953). Synthesis from berberine: Cava, Reed, *J. Org. Chem.* **32**, 1640 (1967).

The free base has not been described, but its quaternary salts are known.

Chloride hemipentahydrate. $C_{20}H_{20}ClNO_4 \cdot 2\frac{1}{2}H_2O$. Orange-yellow needles, mp 194°. Sol in water, alcohol.

Chloride tetrahydrate. $C_{20}H_{20}ClNO_4 \cdot 4H_2O$. Orange-yellow prisms, mp 184°.

Iodide. Orange-yellow needles, mp 224°. Sol in water, alcohol.

2493. Columbin. [546-97-4] 9-(3-Furanyl)decahydro-4-hydroxy-4a,10a-dimethyl-1,4-etheno-3*H*,7*H*-benzo[1,2-*c*:3,4-*c'*]dipyran-3,7-dione; 15,16-epoxy-1β,4,12-trihydroxy-5,9-dimethyl-17,18-dinor-8β*H*,9β*H*,10α-labda-2,13(16),14-triene-19,20-dioic acid 19,1:20,12-dilactone. $C_{20}H_{22}O_6$; mol wt 358.39. C 67.03%, H 6.19%, O 26.79%. Major bitter principle from the root of *Jatrorrhiza palmata* (DC.) Miers (*J. columba* Miers), *Menispermaceae.* Isoln: Wittstock, *Poggendorff's Ann.* **19**, 298 (1830). Structure: Barton, Elad, *J. Chem. Soc.* **1956,** 2090. Stereochemistry: Cava *et al., Tetrahedron Lett.* **1959,** 1; Overton *et al., J. Chem. Soc. C* **1966,** 1482; Cheung *et al., ibid. (B)* **1966,** 853.

Very bitter needles from methanol, mp 195°. $[\alpha]_D$ +52.5° (pyridine). uv max (ethanol): 209 nm (log ε 3.78). Practically insol in water. One gram dissolves in 30 ml acetone, 50 ml ethyl acetate, 75 ml methanol; sol also in chloroform, methylene chloride. Bitterness threshold 1:60,000. Easily isomerized to isocolumbin.

Isocolumbin. $C_{20}H_{22}O_6$; mol wt 358.39. Needles from methanol, dec 190°. $[\alpha]_D^{17}$ +0.17° (alk alc). uv max (alc): 209 nm (log ε 3.80).

2494. Combretastatins. A group of compounds isolated from the bark and stem wood of the South African bushwillow tree, *Combretum caffrum,* which inhibit tubulin polmerization. The most active are combretastatins A-2 and A-4. Used in folk medicine, extracts have shown antileukemic properties. Isoln: G. R. Pettit *et al., Can. J. Chem.* **60,** 1374 (1982); of A-2: G. R. Pettit, S. B. Singh, *ibid.* **65,** 2390 (1987); of A-4: *idem et al., Experientia* **45,** 209 (1989). Enantioselective synthesis: A. Ramacciotti *et al., Tetrahedron: Asymmetry* **7,** 1101 (1996). Mechanism of action study: C. M. Lin *et al., Biochemistry* **28,** 6984 (1989). Antineoplastic activity of A-4: A. A. E. El-Zayat *et al., Anti-Cancer Drugs* **4,** 19 (1993); inhibition of tumor vascularization: G. G. Dark *et al., Cancer Res.* **57,** 1829 (1997). Review of structure-activity of combretastatins, podophyllotoxin, *q.v.* and steganacin: D. L. Sackett, *Pharmacol. Ther.* **59,** 163-228 (1993).

Combretastatin   Combretastatin A-4

Combretastatin. [82855-09-2] (*R*)-3-Hydroxy-4-methoxy-α-(3,4,5-trimethoxyphenyl)benzeneethanol; (−)-combretastatin. $C_{18}H_{22}O_6$; mol wt 334.36. Needles from acetone-hexane, mp 130-131°. $[\alpha]_D^{26}$ −8.51° (c = 1.41 in chloroform). uv max (methanol): 212, 228 (shoulder), 279, 287 nm (shoulder) (log ε 4.33, 4.11, 3.47, 3.36). d 1.33.

Combretastatin A-4. [117048-59-6] (*Z*)-2-Methoxy-5-[2-(3,-4,5,-trimethoxyphenyl)ethenyl]phenol; 3,4,5-trimethoxy-3′-hydroxy-4′-methoxy-(*Z*)-stilbene; CS-A4. $C_{18}H_{20}O_5$; mol wt 316.35. Fine crystals from ethylacetate-hexane, mp 84.5-85.5°.

2495. Concanavalin A. [11028-71-0] ConA. The most extensively investigated member of the lectin family of plant proteins. Unlike most lectins, it lacks covalently bound carbohydrate and therefore is not a glycoprotein. Isolated from jack bean, *Canavalia ensiformis, Papilionatae:* J. B. Sumner, S. F. Howell, *J. Bacteriol.* **32,** 227 (1936). Its function in *C. ensiformis* is unknown, but it agglutinates a variety of somatic and germ line cells through specific interaction with saccharide-containing cell surface receptors and restores the growth pattern of virus-transformed fibroblasts in tissue culture to that of normal cells, *cf.* M. M. Burger, K. D. Noonan, *Nature* **228,** 512 (1970); G. M. Edelman, C. F. Millette,

Proc. Natl. Acad. Sci. USA **68,** 2436 (1971). Differential toxicity on normal and transformed cells *in vitro* and inhibition of tumor development *in vivo* have also been reported: J. Shoham *et al., Nature* **227,** 1244 (1970). The molecule consists of identical polypeptide subunits of mol wt about 27,000, existing as dimers in soln at pH <6 and as tetramers at physiologic pH. The proposed amino acid sequence contains 238 residues; con A has also been shown to have binding site for transition metal ions and calcium ions in addition to saccharide binding sites: G. M. Edelman *et al., Proc. Natl. Acad. Sci. USA* **69,** 2580 (1972). The transition ion, usually Mn^{+2} or Ca^{+2}, apparently stabilizes the formation of the specific saccharide binding site: M. Shoham *et al., Biochemistry* **12,** 1914 (1973). Circular dichroism-NMR study of metal binding sites: A. R. Palmer *et al., ibid.* **19,** 5063 (1980). Oligosaccharide binding study: A. Vanlands *et al., Eur. J. Biochem.* **103,** 307 (1980). Use of con A to study immunoregulation of human T cells: D. M. Dwyer, C. Johnson, *Clin. Exp. Immunol.* **46,** 237 (1981); E. L. Larson *et al., Immunobiology* **161,** 5 (1982). For general refs, *see* Lectins.

USE: As a reagent in analytical and preparative biochemistry; as a probe in studies of cell surface membrane dynamics and cell division.

2496. Condurangin. [1401-98-5] Kondurangin. Bitter principle from the bark of the Condurango vine, *Marsdenia condurango* Reichb. f., *Asclepiadaceae,* also known as *eagle vine, mataperro, condor vine. Habit.* Ecuador, Peru. Isoln: Korte, Korte, *Z. Naturforsch.* **10b,** 223 (1955); Zechner, Zölss, *Sci. Pharm.* **24,** 107 (1956). Separation of fractions: Cellarius, Zechner, *ibid.* **34,** 10 (1966). Proposed structure of the aglycone, *condurangogenin A:* Tschesche *et al., Tetrahedron* **21,** 1777, 1797 (1965); **23,** 1461 (1967).

Crystals from dil methanol, mp 186-188°. uv max (methanol): 277 nm. Soluble in chloroform, methanol; slightly sol in water. Practically insol in ether, petr ether. Bitterness threshold 1:20,000.

THERAP CAT: Astringent.

2497. Conessine. [546-06-5] (3β)-*N,N*-Dimethylcon-5-enin-3-amine; 3β-(dimethylamino)con-5-enine; neriine; roquessine; wrightine. $C_{24}H_{40}N_2$; mol wt 356.59. C 80.84%, H 11.31%, N 7.86%. Antiamebic, antifungal principle in Kurchi bark, the bark of *Holarrhena anti-dysenterica* Wall., *Apocynaceae,* native to India; also found in African species, such as *H. africana* A.DC.; *H. congolensis* Stapf; *H. wulfsbergii* Stapf, and *H. febrifuga* Klotzsch, *Apocynaceae.* Isoln: Haines, *Trans. Med. Soc. Bombay* **4,** 28 (1858); Warnecke, *Ber.* **19,** 60 (1886); Bertho, *Arch. Pharm.* **277,** 237 (1939); Siddiqui, Pillay, *J. Indian Chem. Soc.* **9,** 553 (1932). Structure: Haworth *et al., J. Chem. Soc.* **1953,** 1102; Haworth, McKenna, *Chem. Ind. (London)* **1957,** 1510; Bertho, Götz, *Ann.* **619,** 96 (1958). Discussion of structure in Fieser, Fieser, *Steroids* (New York, 1959), p 858. Synthesis from Δ⁵-pregnene-3β,20β-diol: Barton, Morgan, *Proc. Chem. Soc. London* **1961,** 206; *J. Chem. Soc.* **1962,** 622. Total synthesis: Marshall, Johnson, *J. Am. Chem. Soc.* **84,** 1485 (1962); Stork *et al., ibid.* 2018; Nagata *et al., Tetrahedron Lett.* **1963,** 869.

Leaflets or broad plates from acetone, mp 127-128.5°. $[\alpha]_D^{20}$ +25.3° (c = 0.7 in abs alc). Sparingly sol in water.

Dihydrochloride monohydrate. $C_{24}H_{40}N_2.2HCl.H_2O$. Crystals, sol in water, mp >340°. $[\alpha]_D^{20}$ +9.3° (c = 0.9 in H_2O).

Dihydrobromide. [5913-82-6] $C_{24}H_{40}N_2.2HBr$. Crystals, dec 340°. Very bitter taste. $[\alpha]_D^{20}$ +7.0° (c = 5 in H_2O). Sol in water. Slightly sol in 95% ethanol. Very slightly sol in ether. Practically insol in petr ether.

2498. Congo Red. [573-58-0] 3,3'-[[1,1'-Biphenyl]-4,4'-diylbis(azo)]bis[4-amino-1-naphthalenesulfonic acid] disodium salt; C.I. Direct Red 28; sodium diphenyldiazo-bis-α-naphthylaminesulfonate; C.I. 22120. $C_{32}H_{22}N_6Na_2O_6S_2$; mol wt 696.66. C 55.17%, H 3.18%, N 12.06%, Na 6.60%, O 13.78%, S 9.21%. Prepn: Böttiger, **DRP 28753** (1884); *Frdl.* **1**, 470; Whitehead, *Chem. Trade J.* **77**, 386 (1925); Kline, *J. Chem. Educ.* **15**, 129 (1938). Purification: Bedaux *et al., Pharm. Weekbl.* **98**, 189 (1963). *See also Colour Index* vol. 4 (3rd ed., 1971) p 4166; *H. J. Conn's Biological Stains*, R. D. Lillie, Ed. (Williams & Wilkins, Baltimore, 9th ed., 1977) p 148. Toxicity: Richardson, Dillon, *Am. J. Med. Sci.* **198**, 73 (1939). Clinical evaluation as diagnostic aid: E. Ouchi *et al., Tohoku J. Exp. Med.* **118**, Suppl., 191 (1976). Use in combination with Sirius red as histological stain: I. R. Hinds, *Lab. Med.* **16**, 366 (1985).

Brownish-red powder. Absorption max (pH 7.3): 488 nm ($E_{1cm}^{1\%}$ 595). Sol in water (yellowish-red) and in ethanol (orange); very slightly sol in acetone. Practically insol in ether. LD_{50} i.v. in rats: 190 mg/kg (Richardson, Dillon).

Congo Red Paper. Riegel's paper; Herzberg's paper. Paper charged with a 0.1% aq soln of Congo Red.

USE: As indicator, usually in 0.1% aq soln for estimating free mineral acids, particularly in presence of organic acids. pH: 3.0 blue-violet, 5.0 red. Detecting and estimating free HCl in gastric contents; detecting acidity of papers. As addition to culture media; reagent for bitter-almond water; dye; biological stain.

THERAP CAT: Diagnostic aid (amyloidosis).

2499. Congressane. [2292-79-7] Decahydro-3,5,1,7-[1,2,-3,4]butanetetraylnaphthalene; pentacyclo[7.3.1.1⁴,¹².0²,⁷.0⁶,¹¹]-tetradecane; diamantane. $C_{14}H_{20}$; mol wt 188.31. C 89.29%, H 10.71%. Isoln from petroleum: Hala *et al., Angew. Chem. Int. Ed.* **5**, 1045 (1966). Synthesis: Cupas *et al., J. Am. Chem. Soc.* **87**, 917 (1965); Gund *et al., J. Org. Chem.* **39**, 2979 (1974). Structure: Karle, Karle, *J. Am. Chem. Soc.* **87**, 918 (1965).

Crystals, mp 236-237°.
Note: Structure is congress emblem of the International Congress of Pure and Applied Chemistry.

2500. Conhydrine. [495-20-5] [R-(R^*,S^*)]-α-Ethyl-2-piperidinemethanol; 2-(α-hydroxypropyl)piperidine. $C_8H_{17}NO$; mol wt 143.23. C 67.08%, H 11.96%, N 9.78%, O 11.17%. From seeds of *Conium maculatum* L., *Umbelliferae.* Isoln: Späth, Adler, *Monatsh. Chem.* **63**, 127 (1933). Stereochemistry: Hill, *J. Am. Chem. Soc.* **80**, 1609 (1958); Sicher, Ticky, *Collect. Czech. Chem. Commun.* **23**, 2081 (1958).

Crystals from ether, mp 121°. bp 226°. [α]$_D$ +10°. Slightly sol in water; sol in alc, chloroform, ether.

2501. β-Coniceine. [538-90-9] 2-(1-Propenyl)piperidine; α-allylpiperidine. $C_8H_{15}N$; mol wt 125.21. C 76.74%, H 12.07%, N 11.19%. Prepn from conhydrine: Löffler, Friederick, *Ber.* **42**, 107 (1909); Löffler, Tschunke, *ibid.* 929.

dl-Form. Liquid, solidifies around 8°. bp 168°. d_4^{15} 0.8716. Sol in alcohol, ether; very slightly sol in water.
dl-Form hydrochloride. $C_8H_{15}N.HCl$. mp 206°. Sol in water.
d-Form. Needles, mp 39°. bp 168°. [α]$_D^{45}$ +50°. Sol in alcohol, ether; very slightly sol in water.
d-Form hydrochloride. mp 182°. Sol in water.
l-Form. Crystals, mp 40°. bp 168°. [α]$_D^{45}$ −50°. Sol in alcohol, ether; very slightly sol in water.
l-Form hydrochloride. mp 183°. Sol in water.

2502. γ-Coniceine. [1604-01-9] 2,3,4,5-Tetrahydro-6-propylpyridine; 2-n-propyl-3,4,5,6-tetrahydropyridine; 2-n-propyl-Δ¹-piperidine. $C_8H_{15}N$; mol wt 125.21. C 76.74%, H 12.07%, N 11.19%. Easily reduced to *dl*-coniine, *q.v.* From seeds of *Conium maculatum* L., *Umbelliferae:* Cromwell, *Biochem. J.* **64**, 259 (1956); Fairbairn, Challen, *ibid.* **72**, 556 (1959); Fairbairn, Sewal, *Phytochemistry* **1**, 38 (1961). Structure: Beyerman *et al., Rec. Trav. Chim.* **80**, 513 (1961). Synthesis: Lukes *et al., Collect. Czech. Chem. Commun.* **12**, 641 (1947); Cervinka, *Chem. Listy* **52**, 1145 (1958).

Alkaline liquid, mousy odor. bp 171°; bp$_{15}$ 63°. Volatile with steam. d_4^{15} 0.8753. n_D^{16} 1.4661. Slightly sol in water; freely sol in alcohol, chloroform, ether.

Hydrochloride. $C_8H_{15}N.HCl$. Hygroscopic crystals from ether, mp 143°.

2503. Coniferin. [531-29-3] 4-(3-Hydroxy-1-propenyl)-2-methoxyphenyl β-D-glucopyranoside; 4-hydroxy-3-methoxy-1-(γ-hydroxypropenyl)benzene-4-D-glucoside; abietin; laricin. $C_{16}H_{22}$-O_8; mol wt 342.34. C 56.13%, H 6.48%, O 37.39%. Principal glucoside of the conifers. Also in comfrey root, sugar beet, and asparagus. Extraction from the cambium layer of fir: Solntsev, *C.A.* **38**, 3780 (1944). Synthesis: Pauley, Feuerstein, *Ber.* **60**, 1031 (1927). Hydrolysis by emulsin yields coniferyl alcohol and D-glucose. Yields lignin-like material by enzymatic dehydrogenation and polymerization: Freudenberg *et al., Ber.* **85**, 641 (1952); Freudenberg, Rasenack, *Ber.* **86**, 756 (1953).

Dihydrate. Crystals from water. Anhydr after 4 hrs at 100°. Anhydr coniferin, mp 186°. [α]$_D^{20}$ −68° (c = 0.5). Absorption spectrum: Patterson, Hibbert, *J. Am. Chem. Soc.* **65**, 1862 (1943). One gram dissolves in 200 ml water, freely sol in boiling water; sol in pyridine; sparingly sol in alc. Practically insol in ether.

2504. Coniferyl Alcohol. [458-35-5] 4-(3-Hydroxy-1-propenyl)-2-methoxyphenol; 3-(4-hydroxy-3-methoxyphenyl)-2-propen-1-ol; 4-hydroxy-3-methoxycinnamic alcohol; γ-hydroxyisoeugenol. $C_{10}H_{12}O_3$; mol wt 180.20. C 66.65%, H 6.71%, O 26.64%. In benzoin, especially Siam benzoin, as coniferyl benzoate (up to 78%): Reinitzer, *Arch. Pharm.* **264**, 131 (1926). From coniferin by hydrolysis with emulsin. From ferula aldehyde (coniferyl aldehyde) by the action of fermenting yeast. Small amounts of coniferyl alcohol are found in brandy from beet molasses.

Consult the Name Index before using this section.

Prisms, mp 74°. Freely sol in ether; moderately sol in alc; almost insol in water; sol in alkalies. Polymerized by dil acids; converted to an amorphous gum. Absorption spectrum: Herzog, Hillmer, *Ber.* **64B**, 1288 (1931).

2505. Coniine. [458-88-8] (2*S*)-2-Propylpiperidine; cicutine; conicine. $C_8H_{17}N$; mol wt 127.23. C 75.52%, H 13.47%, N 11.01%. Toxic principle of poison hemlock, *Conium maculatum* L., *Umbelliferae*: Ladenburg, *Ber.* **19**, 439 (1886); Koller, *Monatsh. Chem.* **47**, 393 (1926). Occurs naturally as the (*S*)-(+)-isomer. Review of early literature: Marion in *The Alkaloids* **vol. I**, R. H. F. Manske, H. L. Holmes, Eds. (Academic Press, New York, 1950) pp 211-217. Isoln from the pitcher plant, *Sarracenia flava* and insect paralyzing properties: N. V. Mody *et al. Experientia* **32**, 829 (1976). Absolute configuration: J. C. Craig, S. K. Roy, *Tetrahedron* **21**, 401 (1965). Resolution of (±)-form: J. C. Craig, A. R. Pinder, *J. Org. Chem.* **36**, 3648 (1971). Synthesis of (*S*)-(+)-form: K. Aketa *et al., Chem. Pharm. Bull.* **24**, 621 (1976); of (*R*)-(−)-form: D. Lathbury, T. Gallagher, *Chem. Commun.* **1986**, 114; of (±)-form: T. Nagasaka *et al., Heterocycles* **27**, 1685 (1988). Enantiospecific synthesis of (+)- and (−)-forms: L. Guerrier *et al., J. Am. Chem. Soc.* **105**, 7754 (1983).

Colorless alkaline liquid, darkens and polymerizes on exposure to light and air. Mousy odor. mp $\sim -2°$. bp 166-166.5°; bp_{20} 65-66°. Volatile with steam. d_4^{20} 0.844-0.848. n_D^{23} 1.4505. $[\alpha]_D^{25}$ +8.4° (c = 4.0 in $CHCl_3$); $[\alpha]_D^{23}$ +14.6° (neat). pK 3.1. One ml dissolves in 90 ml water, less in hot water. The base dissolves about 25% water at room temp. Sol in alcohol, ether, acetone, benzene, amyl alcohol; slightly sol in chloroform.

Hydrobromide. [637-49-0] $C_8H_{17}N.HBr$. Prisms, mp 211°. One gram dissolves in 2 ml water, 3 ml alcohol; sol in chloroform, ether.

Hydrochloride. [555-92-0] $C_8H_{17}N.HCl$. Rhomboids, mp 221°. Freely sol in water, alcohol, chloroform.

(*R*)-(−)-Form. Liquid, bp_{756} 165°. $[\alpha]_D^{25}$ −8.1° (c = 4.0 in $CHCl_3$); $[\alpha]_D^{23}$ −14.2° (neat).

(±)-Form. bp 200-210°.

Caution: Potential symptoms of overexposure include drowsiness, paresthesias, weakness, ataxia, nausea, profuse salivation, and bradycardia followed by tachycardia. *See: Clinical Toxicology of Commercial Products,* R. E. Gosselin *et al.,* Eds. (Williams & Wilkins, Baltimore, 5th ed., 1984) Section II, pp 249-250.

2506. Conium Fruit. Hemlock; poison hemlock; spotted hemlock; poison parsley; spotted cowbane. Full-grown, but unripe, carefully dried fruit of *Conium maculatum* L., *Umbelliferae. Habit.* Europe, Asia, naturalized in U.S. *Constit.* 0.5-1.5% coniine, conhydrine, pseudoconhydrine, methylconiine, ethylpiperidine, coniic acid, volatile and fixed oil. Has antispasmodic activity.

2507. Conivaptan. [210101-16-9] *N*-[4-[(4,5-Dihydro-2-methylimidazo[4,5-*d*][1]benzazepin-6(1*H*)-yl)carbonyl]phenyl][1,1'-biphenyl]-2-carboxamide; 4'-[(2-methyl-1,4,5,6-tetrahydroimidazo[4,5-*d*][1]benzazepin-6-yl)carbonyl]-2-phenylbenzanilide. $C_{32}H_{26}N_4O_2$; mol wt 498.57. C 77.09%, H 5.26%, N 11.24%, O 6.42%. Nonpeptide, dual vasopressin V_{1a}/V_2 receptor antagonist. Prepn: A. Tanaka *et al.,* **WO 9503305**; *eidem,* **US 5723606** (1995, 1998 both to Yamanouchi); A. Matsuhisa *et al., Chem. Pharm. Bull.* **48**, 21 (2000). Pharmacology: Y. Yatsu *et al., Eur. J. Pharmacol.* **321**, 225 (1997). Binding specificity study: A. Tahara *et al., Peptides* **19**, 691 (1998). Clinical pharmacokinetics: M. Burnier *et al., Eur. J. Clin. Pharmacol.* **55**, 633 (1999). Clinical evaluation in advanced heart failure: J. E. Udelson *et al., Circulation* **104**, 2417 (2001). Review of clinical development: S. A. Doggrell, *Curr. Opin. Invest. Drugs* **6**, 317-326 (2005).

Hydrochloride. [168626-94-6] Cl-1025; YM-087; YM-35087; Vaprisol. $C_{32}H_{26}N_4O_2.HCl$; mol wt 535.04. Crystals, mp >250°.
THERAP CAT: In treatment of congestive heart failure.

2508. Conjugated Estrogens. [12126-59-9] Conjugated equine estrogens; CEE; Premarin. Complex mixture of natural estrogens obtained from equine urine or synthetically from estrone and equilin. Principal components are sodium estrone sulfate and sodium equilin sulfate; also known to contain 17α-dihydroequilin, 17α-estradiol, and 17β-dihydroequilin as sodium sulfate conjugates. Purification from urine of pregnant mares: R. W. Bates, H. Cohen, **US 2565115** (1951 to Squibb); E. T. Stiller, E. O'Keefe, **US 2720483** (1955 to Olin Mathieson). HPLC determn of major components in serum: S. Y. Su *et al., Biomed. Chromatogr.* **6**, 265 (1992). Review of pharmacokinetics and metabolism: B. R. Bhavnani, *Proc. Soc. Exp. Biol. Med.* **217**, 6-16 (1998); of pharmacology and neuroprotective effects: *idem, J. Steroid Biochem. Mol. Biol.* **85**, 473-482 (2003). Clinical assessment of efficacy and safety in combination with progestin in hormone replacement therapy: J. E. Rossouw *et al., J. Am. Med. Assoc.* **288**, 321 (2002); of conjugated estrogens alone: G. L. Anderson *et al., ibid.* **291**, 1701 (2004).

Caution: These substances are listed as known human carcinogens: *Report on Carcinogens, Eleventh Edition* (PB2005-104914, 2004) p III-115.

THERAP CAT: Estrogen.

2509. Connexins. Family of gap-junction structural proteins found in virtually all metazoans; the assembly of which permits rapid intercellular communication by ions, second messengers and small metabolites. Named as the species of origin Cx, where x is the predicted molecular mass in kDa, e.g. rat C43. These transmembrane proteins are characterized by 2 extracellular loops, 4 hydrophobic membrane regions and a cytoplasmic loop. Oligomerization into a hexamer forms a *connexon* or hemichannel which interacts across the extracellular gap with a corresponding connexon to complete the intercellular channel. Description of connexon structure and composition: D. L. D. Caspar *et al., J. Cell Biol.* **74**, 605, 629 (1977). Isolation of rat C32 via molecular cloning: D. L. Paul, *ibid.* **103**, 123 (1986). Tissue distribution: E. C. Beyer *et al., ibid.* **108**, 595 (1987). Review of early works on gap junction structure: P. N. T. Unwin, G. Zampighi, *Nature* **283**, 545-549 (1980); of molecular structure and biochemical characterization: E. C. Beyer *et al., J. Membr. Biol.* **116**, 187-194 (1990). Review of biosynthesis, function and turnover: D. W. Laird, *J. Bioenerg. Biomembr.* **28**, 311-318 (1996); of structure/activity: C. Peracchia, X. G. Wang, *Braz. J. Med. Biol. Res.* **30**, 577-590 (1997); of mutations in human genetic diseases: V. Krutovskikh, H. Yamasaki, *Mutat. Res.* **462**, 197-207 (2000). *Review:* D. A. Goodenough *et al., Annu. Rev. Biochem.* **65**, 475-502 (1996).

2510. Conotoxins. Ctx. Family of related peptide neurotoxins isolated from the venom of genus *Conus,* the marine cone snail. Wide variety of venoms are found, almost all of which are under 30 amino acids in length. The most common classes are ω-and δ-conotoxins which target voltage-gated calcium and sodium channels respectively; α-conotoxins which inhibit acetylcholine receptor; μ-conotoxins which block sodium channels. Review characterizing binding of ω-Ctx: E. Sher, F. Clementi, *Neuroscience* **42**, 301-307 (1991); and use: K. Takeda, J. J. Nordmann, *Methods Neurosci.* **8**, 202-222 (1992). Review of α-CTX isolation and binding: J. M. McIntosh, "α-*Conotoxins and Nicotinic Acetylcholine Receptors"*, in *Biochemical Aspects of Marine Pharmacology,* P. Lazarovici *et al.,* Eds. (Alaken Inc., Fort Collins, CO, 1996) pp 28-34. *Review:* B. M. Olivera *et al., ACS Symp. Ser.* **418**, 256-278 (1990).

USE: Biochemical probes for ion channels.

2511. Convallaria. Lily of the valley; May lily; Park lily; May blossom. Dried flowers of *Convallaria majalis* L., *Liliaceae.*

Habit. U.S., Europe, Northern Asia; cultivated in gardens. *Constit.* of dried flowers: Convallatoxin, convallarin, volatile oil; of dried rhizome and roots: Glycosides of convallamarin, convallatoxin, convallarin. Extraction and identification of glycosides: Tschesche, Seehofer, *Ber.* **87,** 1108 (1954); Erbring, Patt, *Arzneim.-Forsch.* **8,** 554 (1958).

Convallaria glycosides. Convacard; Convallan; Convallen; Convalyt; Convasid. An aqueous extract containing the total glycosides of Convallaria.

THERAP CAT: Cardiotonic.

THERAP CAT (VET): Has been used as a cardiotonic and diuretic.

2512.   Convallatoxin. [508-75-8] (3β,5β)-3-[(6-Deoxy-α-L-mannopyranosyl)oxy]-5,14-dihydroxy-19-oxocard-20(22)-enolide; strophanthidin α-L-rhamnoside; Convallaton; Corglykon; Korglykon. C$_{29}$H$_{42}$O$_{10}$; mol wt 550.64. C 63.26%, H 7.69%, O 29.06%. From blossoms of lily of the valley *(Convallaria majalis* L., *Liliaceae):* Karrer, *Helv. Chim. Acta* **12,** 506 (1929); from *Ornithogalum umbellatum* L., *Liliaceae:* Mrozik *et al., ibid.* **42,** 683 (1959); from *Antiaris toxicaria* Lesch, *Moraceae:* Juslen *et al., ibid.* **46,** 117 (1963). Structure: Tschesche, Haupt, *Ber.* **69,** 459 (1936); Fieser, Jacobsen, *J. Am. Chem. Soc.* **59,** 2335 (1937). Cleavage into L-rhamnose and strophanthidin: Reichstein, Katz, *Pharm. Acta Helv.* **18,** 521 (1943); *see also C.A.* **38,** 2046. Synthesis from strophanthidin and acetobromrhamnose: Reyle *et al., Helv. Chim. Acta* **33,** 1541 (1950); Haede *et al.,* **DE 1933090** (1971 to Hoechst). Toxicity study: W. Förster *et al., Arch. Int. Pharmacodyn.* **155,** 165 (1965).

Prisms from methanol + ether. mp 235-242°. [α]$_D^{22}$ −1.7 ± 3° (c = 0.65 in methanol); [α]$_D^{25}$ −9.4 ± 3° (c = 0.72 in dioxane). Sol in alcohol, acetone; slightly sol in chloroform, ethyl acetate, and water (1:2000). Practically insol in ether, petr ether. Gives Legal's reaction. LD$_{50}$ in mice, rats (mg/kg): 10.0 i.p., 16.0 i.v. (Förster).

Tri-O-acetyl-convallatoxin. C$_{35}$H$_{48}$O$_{13}$. Needles from acetone + ether, mp 215-238°. [α]$_D^{25}$ −5.5 ± 2° (c = 0.962 in chloroform).

THERAP CAT: Cardiotonic.

2513.   Convicine. [19286-37-4] 6-Amino-5-(β-D-glucopyranosyloxy)-2,4(1*H*,3*H*)-pyrimidinedione. C$_{10}$H$_{15}$N$_3$O$_8$; mol wt 305.24. C 39.35%, H 4.95%, N 13.77%, O 41.93%. From seeds of *Vicia sativa* L., *Leguminosae:* Ritthausen, *J. Prakt. Chem.* [2] **24,** 202 (1881); *Ber.* **29,** 894 (1896). Structure: Johnson, *J. Am. Chem. Soc.* **36,** 337 (1914); Fisher, Johnson, *ibid.* **54,** 2038 (1932); Bendick, Clements, *Biochim. Biophys. Acta* **12,** 462 (1953); Bien *et al., J. Chem. Soc. C* **1968,** 496. Synthesis: *eidem, J. Chem. Soc. Perkin Trans. 1* **1973,** 1089.

Leaflets from boiling water, dec without melting at 287°. uv max (pH 7): 245, 271 nm (log ε 3.43, 4.16). Sol in hot water, dil NaOH;

slightly sol in cold water, alcohol. Practically insol in chloroform, glacial acetic acid.

2514.   COP. [26591-04-8] 2-Methyl-2-propenoic acid oxiranylmethyl ester polymer with ethyl 2-propenoate; poly-(glycidyl methacrylate-co-ethyl acrylate); [P(GMA-co-EA)]; glycidyl methacrylate-ethyl acrylate polymer; COP Resist. (C$_7$H$_{10}$-O$_3$.C$_5$H$_8$O$_2$)$_x$. Negative electron resist. Prepn and characterization: L. F. Thompson *et al., Tech. Pap. Reg. Tech Conf. Soc. Plast. Eng.* **1973,** (Oct.) 127. Molecular parameters and lithographic performance: L. F. Thompson *et al., J. Vac. Sci. Technol.* **12,** 1280 (1975). Radiation chemistry: E. D. Feit *et al., ACS Org. Coat. Plast. Chem.* **35,** 287 (1975). Use as matrix for deep UV resist materials: C. Kutal, S. K. Weit, *J. Coat. Technol.* **62,** 63 (1990); S. K. Weit *et al., Chem. Mater.* **4,** 453 (1992).

USE: In photosensitive materials as polymer matrix. Photoresist.

2515.   Copaene. [3856-25-5] [1*R*-(1α,2α,6α,7α,8α)]-1,3-Dimethyl-8-(1-methylethyl)tricyclo[4.4.0.0^{2,7}]dec-3-ene; (1*R*,2*S*,6*S*,-7*S*,8*S*)-(−)-8-isopropyl-1,3-dimethyltricyclo[4.4.0.0^{2,7}]dec-3-ene; α-copaene. C$_{15}$H$_{24}$; mol wt 204.35. C 88.16%, H 11.84%. Tricyclic sesquiterpene occurring in African copaiba balsam oil; in the so-called supa oil from *Sindora supa* Merr. (*S. wallichii* F.-Vill.), *Leguminosae:* Henderson *et al., J. Chem. Soc.* **1926,** 3077. Also in the essential oil of *Phyllocladus trichomanoides* D. Don, *Podocarpaceae:* Briggs, Sutherland, *J. Org. Chem.* **13,** 1 (1948); from *Cyperus articulatus* Michx., *Cyperaceae:* Couchman *et al., Tetrahedron* **20,** 2037 (1964). Structural studies: Kapadia *et al., ibid.* **21,** 607 (1965). Absolute stereostructure: deMao *et al., ibid.* 619. Synthesis: Heathcock, *J. Am. Chem. Soc.* **88,** 4110 (1966); Heathcock *et al., ibid.* **89,** 4133 (1967); Corey, Watt, *ibid.* **95,** 2303 (1973). *Review:* J. Simonsen, D. H. R. Barton, *The Terpenes* vol. **III** (University Press, Cambridge, 1952) pp 88-91. *See also* Ylangene.

Oily liquid, bp 246-251°; bp$_{10}$ 119-120°; d$_{15}^{15}$ 0.9077; n$_D^{20}$ 1.4894. [α]$_D^{22}$ −6.3° (c = 1.20 in chloroform).

2516.   Copaiba. [8001-61-4] Balsam copaiba; balsam capivi; Jesuit's balsam. Oleoresin from trees of the genus, *Copaifera, Leguminosae,* particularly *C. reticulata* Ducke (Para balsam), *C. langsdorffii* Desf. (Maranhao balsam) and *C. guianensis* (Maracaibo balsam). Used in traditional medicine as an antiseptic, diuretic and anti-inflammatory. *Habit.* Tropical regions of South America and southern Africa. *Constit.* Varies among the species; volatile oil (20-90%); diterpene acids, such as kaurenoic, copalic, hardwickiic acids. Brief description: D. L. J. Opdyke, *Food Cosmet. Toxicol.* **14,** 687 (1976); of copaiba oil: *idem, ibid.* **11,** 1075 (1973). Chemical characterization of 3 species: V. Cascon, B. Gilbert, *Phytochemistry* **55,** 773 (2000). Volatile constituents of *C. langsdorffii:* N. V. Gramosa, E. R. Silveira, *J. Essent. Oil Res.* **17,** 130 (2005). Review of ethnobotany and uses: C. Plowden, *Econ. Bot.* **58,** 729-739 (2004).

Color, scent and viscosity varies widely ranging from pale yellow fluid to thick, brownish-yellow liquid; characteristic odor; unpleasant taste. Insol in water. Sol in benzene, chloroform, ether, oils, carbon disulfide, abs alcohol, petr ether, partly in 95% alcohol.

Volatile oil. [8013-97-6] Oil of copaiba. Obtained by steam distillation of the oleoresin. *Constit.* Highly variable, chiefly β-caryophyllene, β-bisabolene, α-copaene, α-humulene. Colorless or pale yellow liquid; slightly bitter and pungent taste. d$_{25}^{25}$ 0.880-0.907. bp 250-275°. Rotation −7 to −33°. n$_D^{20}$ 1.493-1.500. Sol in alcohol, most fixed oils, mineral oil. Insol in glycerin, propylene glycol. *Keep well closed, cool and protected from light.*

USE: In varnishes, paints, lacquer; for restoration of oil paintings. As frangrance or odor fixative in soaps, shampoo, lotions, perfumes.

2517.   Copal. [9000-14-0] Resin copal; gum copal; anime (soft copal); kaurie; cowrie. A resin found as a fossil in Zaire, or exuding from various species of *Trachylobium, Hymenaea courbaril* L., etc., *Leguminosae.* Occurs as hard or soft copals. *Habit.*

Zanzibar, Mozambique, also S. America, Australia, Philippine Islands and West Indies. *Constit.* Zanzibar copal contains 80% trachylolic acid, 4% isotrachylolic acid, 6% resene and volatile oil. Kaurie copal contains dammaric acid, dammaran and a resin.

Yellowish to yellowish-brown pieces of various sizes; conchoidal fracture; odorless and tasteless. Hard copals are almost insol in usual solvents; soft copals are partly sol in alcohol, chloroform or glacial acetic acid; both copals after having been fused are sol in oil turpentine and linseed oil.

USE: In varnishes and cements; as substitute for amber; manuf oil cloths and linoleum. In dentistry, for modeling compds and cavity varnishes.

2518. Coparaffinate. [8001-60-3] Isopar. A mixture of water-insol isoparaffinic acids partially neutralized with hydroxy-benzyldialiphatic amines. The water-insol isoparaffinic acids are obtained by oxidation of petroleum hydrocarbons by the passage of a current of oxygen under pressure at an elevated temp in the presence of a metal catalyst. The water-insol mono- and dicarboxylic acids with from 6 to 16 carbon atoms are separated and purified by fractional distillation. The hydroxybenzyldialiphatic amines are combined directly with the isoparaffinic acids or in suitable solvent.The latter is then removed by distillation: C. E. Earle, **US 2262720** (1941).

Dark-brown, viscous, oily liq. Odor of burnt petroleum. d 0.970-0.980. Immiscible with water. Freely sol in alc, volatile and fixed oils. Marketed as a 17% ointment, which also contains 4% titanium dioxide in an ointment base consisting of beeswax, cetyl alcohol, lanolin, and petrolatum.

THERAP CAT: Antifungal (topical).

2519. Copper. [7440-50-8] Cu; at. wt 63.546; at. no. 29; valences 1, 2. Group IB (11). Occurrence in the earth's crust: 70 ppm; also present in seawater: 0.001-0.02 ppm. Two naturally occurring isotopes: 63 (69.09%), 65 (30.91%); nine artificial isotopes: 58-62, 64, 66-68. One of the earliest known metals. Found in nature in its native state; also in combined form in several minerals including chalcopyrite, *q.v.*, ***chalcocite***, ***bornite***, (Cu$_5$-FeS$_4$), ***tetrahedrite*** (Cu$_{12}$Sb$_4$S$_{13}$), ***enargite*** (Cu$_3$AsS$_4$), ***antlerite*** (Cu$_3$H$_4$O$_8$S). Extraction from ores: Clark-Hawley, *Encyclopedia of Chemistry* (Reinhold, New York, 2nd ed., 1966) p 288. Metallurgy of copper and its alloys: *Metals Reference Book* **vols. 1, 2,** C. J. Smithells, Ed. (Butterworth's, London, 3rd ed., 1962). A trace element essential to many plants and animals. Occurs in biological complexes such as ***pheophytin*** (analog of chlorophyll), hemocyanin, tyrosinase and ceruloplasmin, *q.q.v.* Reviews of copper and copper compounds: *ACS Monograph Series* **no. 122,** entitled "Copper," A. Butts, Ed. (Reinhold, New York, 1954) 936 pp; Massey, "Copper" in *Comprehensive Inorganic Chemistry* vol. 3, J. C. Bailar, Jr. *et al.,* Eds. (Pergamon Press, Oxford, 1973) pp 1-78; W. M. Tuddenham, P. A. Dougall, *Kirk-Othmer Encyclopedia of Chemical Technology* vol. 6 (Wiley-Interscience, New York, 3rd ed., 1979) pp 819-869. Book: *Inflammatory Diseases and Copper,* J. R. J. Sorenson, Ed. (Humana Press, Clifton, NJ, 1982) 622 pp. Review of role in human diseases: G. J. Brewer, *Curr. Opin. Chem. Biol.* **7,** 207-212 (2003); of toxicology and human exposure: *Toxicological Profile for Copper* (PB2004-107333, 2004) 318 pp.

Reddish, lustrous, ductile, malleable metal; face-centered cubic structure; commercially available in the form of ingots, sheets, wire or powder. Becomes dull when exposed to air. In moist air gradually becomes coated with green basic carbonate. d 8.94. mp 1083°. bp 2595°. Mohs' hardness 3.0. Resistivity 1.673 microhm-cm. Heat of fusion 48.9 cal/g; heat of vaporization 1150 cal/g. Heat capacity at constant pressure (solid) 0.092 cal/g/°C (20°), (liq) 0.112 cal/g/°C. E^0 (aq) Cu$^+$/Cu +0.521 V; E^0 (aq) Cu^{2+}/Cu +0.337 V. Very slowly attacked by cold hydrochloric or dil sulfuric acid; readily by dil nitric acid, and by both hot concd H$_2$SO$_4$ and HBr. It is also attacked by acetic and other organic acids. Slowly sol in ammonia water. Water-soluble cupric salts yield with sodium hydroxide a bluish-green precipitate of cupric hydroxide which is changed to black cupric oxide on warming. Potassium ferrocyanide produces a brownish-red precipitate of copper ferrocyanide. Hydrogen sulfide produces in acid solns a black precipitate of cupric sulfide which is sol in soln of sodium cyanide. Aluminum, iron or zinc precipitate metallic copper from its solns.

Caution: Potential symptoms of overexposure to dusts and mists are irritation of eyes, nose, pharynx; nasal perforation; metallic taste; dermatitis. Potential symptoms of overexposure to fumes are irritation of eyes, upper respiratory system; metal fume fever (chills, muscle aches, nausea, fever; dry throat, cough, weakness, lassitude); metallic or sweet taste; discoloration of skin and hair. *See NIOSH Pocket Guide to Chemical Hazards* (DHHS/NIOSH 97-140, 1997) p 76.

USE: Manuf bronzes, brass, other copper alloys, electrical conductors, ammunition, copper salts, works of art.

2520. Copper Phthalocyanine. [147-14-8] (*SP*-4-1)-[29*H*,31*H*-Phthalocyaninato(2−)-$N^{29},N^{30},N^{31},N^{32}$]copper; C.I. Pigment Blue 15; C.I. 74160. C$_{32}$H$_{16}$CuN$_8$; mol wt 576.07. C 66.72%, H 2.80%, Cu 11.03%, N 19.45%. Discoverers: Dandridge *et al., Angew. Chem.* **68,** 133 (1956); Sanielevici *et al., Rec. Chim. (Bucharest)* **12,** 281 (1961); Raab, Hoernle, **GB 930150** (1963 to Bayer). Purification: Heinle, Mau, **DE 1167307** (1964 to G. Siegle); Sanielevici *et al.,* **BE 657307** (1965 to Romania, Ministry of Petroleum and Chemical Industry); H. Tomoda *et al., Chem. Lett.* **1980,** 1277. Properties: Dent, Linstead, *J. Chem. Soc.* **1934,** 1027; Easton, Smith, *J. Oil Colour Chem. Assoc.* **49,** 614 (1966). *See also Colour Index* vol. 4 (3rd ed., 1971) p 4618.

Bright blue microcrystals with purple lustre; sol in 98% H$_2$SO$_4$ from which it can be almost quantitatively pptd by dilution with water. Practically insol in water, alcohol, and hydrocarbons. Stable toward heat (crystalline and analytically pure sublimate obtained at about 580° in low pressure atmosphere of nitrogen or carbon dioxide), alkalies, dilute acids. Dec by hot nitric acid, or dilute acid permanganate to yield phthalimide. Exists in two forms: the thermodynamically less stable, redder α-form is a better pigment than the more stable greener β-form. In the presence of aromatic solvents, heat, high shear, etc., α-form is converted to β-form.

USE: In inks and paints. In polypropylene sutures.

2521. Copper(I) Thiophene-2-carboxylate. [68986-76-5] (2-Thiophenecarboxylato-$\kappa O^2,\kappa S^1$)copper; CuTC. C$_5$H$_3$CuO$_2$S; mol wt 190.69. C 31.49%, H 1.59%, Cu 33.32%, O 16.78%, S 16.82%. Copper(I) reagent; promotes modified Stille cross-coupling reactions and Ullman-type couplings. Prepn: G. D. Allred, L. S. Liebeskind, *J. Am. Chem. Soc.* **118,** 2748 (1996). Synthetic applications: S. Zhang *et al., J. Org. Chem.* **62,** 2312 (1997); I. Paterson, J. Man, *Tetrahedron Lett.* **38,** 695 (1997); C. Savarin *et al., Org. Lett.* **3,** 91, 2149 (2001); G. Borsato *et al., J. Org. Chem.* **67,** 7894 (2002); M. d'Augustin *et al., Angew. Chem. Int. Ed.* **44,** 1376 (2005). *Brief review*: A. Innitzer, *Synlett* **2005,** 2405-2406.

Tan, air-stable, non-hygroscopic powder.

USE: Mediator in intermolecular cross-coupling reactions, asymmetric 1,4-additions, and allylation reactions.

2522. Coprogen. [31418-71-0] C$_{35}$H$_{53}$FeN$_6$O$_{13}$; mol wt 821.67. C 51.16%, H 6.50%, Fe 6.80%, N 10.23%, O 25.31%. Iron-contg, growth-promoting complex. Isoln from *Penicillium* spp: Hesseltine *et al., J. Am. Chem. Soc.* **74,** 1362 (1952). Pidacks *et al., ibid.* **75,** 6064 (1953); Gaeumann, Vischer, **US 3297526** (1967 to Ciba). Isoln from *Aspergillaceae*: Zaehner *et al., Arch. Mikrobiol.* **45,** 119 (1963). Structure: Keller-Schierlein, Diekmann, *Helv. Chim. Acta* **53,** 2035 (1970).

Coprostane

Clusters of brick-red needles from ethanol. Absorption max (ethanol): 217, 250, 440 nm (log ε 4.46, 4.22, 3.47). Sol in water, methanol, ethanol (amorphous coprogen only), propanol, benzyl alcohol, Cellosolves. Practically insol in ether, ethyl acetate, chloroform, benzene, Cellosolve esters.

Desferricoprogen. Iron-free coprogen, may be obtained by treating an aq solution with 8-quinolinol yielding a light brown powder.

USE: Coprogen as growth-promoting agent in various organisms. Desferricoprogen to bring about excretion of iron.

2523. Coprostane. [481-20-9] 5β-Cholestane; pseudocholestane. $C_{27}H_{48}$; mol wt 372.67. C 87.02%, H 12.98%. The cis-decalin homolog of cholestane. Prepn: Wieland, Jacobi, Ber. **59**, 2064 (1926); Young et al., J. Am. Chem. Soc. **81**, 1452 (1959); Dart, Henbest, J. Chem. Soc. **1960**, 3563; Nickon, Bagli, J. Am. Chem. Soc. **83**, 1498 (1961); Caglioti, Grasselli, Chem. Ind. (London) **1964**, 153.

Needles from alcohol, mp 72°. $[α]_D^{11}$ +25.1° (c = 2 in CHCl₃). n_D^{88} 1.4884. Freely soluble in ether, chloroform; slightly in abs alcohol.

2524. Coprosterol. [360-68-9] (3β,5β)-Cholestan-3-ol; 3β-coprostanol; stercorin. $C_{27}H_{48}O$; mol wt 388.67. C 83.44%, H 12.45%, O 4.12%. Found in feces of man and of carnivorous animals: Bondzynski, Humnicki, Z. Physiol. Chem. **22**, 396 (1896); Wells et al., Arch. Biochem. Biophys. **57**, 437 (1955); Samuel et al., J. Chromatogr. **14**, 508 (1964). Prepn from coprostenone: Ruzicka et al., Helv. Chim. Acta **17**, 1407 (1934); Shoppee, Summers, J. Chem. Soc. **1950**, 687. From coprostenol: Schönheimer, Evans, J. Biol. Chem. **114**, 567 (1936); Ruzicka et al., Helv. Chim. Acta **21**, 498 (1938); Agashe, Summers, J. Chem. Soc. **1957**, 3107; Dart, Henbest, ibid. **1960**, 3563. Prepn from cholesterol: Rosenfeld, Gallagher, Steroids **4**, 515 (1964).

Needles from methanol, mp 101°. $[α]_D^{18}$ +28° (c = 1.8 in CHCl₃). Freely sol in ether, chloroform, benzene; slightly sol in methanol (one gram dissolves in 145 ml MeOH). Insol in water.

2525. Coptine. [1391-14-6] From root of Coptis trifolia Salisb., Ranunculaceae: Gross, Am. J. Pharm. **45**[4], 193 (1873); Mollett, Christensen, J. Am. Pharm. Assoc. **23**, 310 (1934); from C. teeta Wall.: Chatterjee et al., J. Indian Chem. Soc. **28**, 97 (1951); from C. chinensis Wils.: Schramm, Tang, Pharmazie **14**, 405 (1959).

Crystals. Practically insol in water, ammonia, alkali hydroxides; sol in hot alcohol, dil acids.

2526. Coptis. Goldthread. Dried plant of Coptis trifolia Salisb., Ranunculaceae. Habit. U.S., northern and middle Atlantic States; Canada. Constit. Berberine, coptine.

THERAP CAT: Bitter tonic.

2527. Coptisine. [3486-66-6] 6,7-Dihydrobis[1,3]benzodioxolo[5,6-a:4′,5′-g]quinolizinium; 7,8,13,13a-tetradehydro-2,3:9,10-bismethylenedioxyberbinium; bis[methylenedioxy]-protoberberine. $[C_{19}H_{14}NO_4]^+$. From root of Coptis japonica Makino, Ranunculaceae. Extraction procedure: Kitasato, C.A. **21**, 2700 (1927). Structure: Späth, Posega, Ber. **62**, 1029 (1929); cf. Huang-Minlon, Ber. **69**, 1744 (1936). Prepn from rhoeagenine-diol: Klásek et al., Tetrahedron Lett. **1968**, 4549.

Hydroxide. $C_{19}H_{15}NO_5$. Yellowish needles from alc, mp 218°. Absorption spectrum: Kitasato, Acta Phytochim. **3**, 175 (1927). Very slightly sol in water; sparingly in alcohol; sol in alkalies.

Chloride. Orange prisms, not melted at 300°.

Iodide. Yellow needles, dec above 280°.

Sulfate. Yellow crystals, insol in water and alcohol (enables separation from berberine and worenine).

2528. Cord Factor(s). [61512-20-7] Trehalose 6,6′-dimycolate; 6,6′-di-O-mycolyl-α,α-trehalose; (6-O-mycolyl-α-D-glucopyranosyl)-6-O-mycolyl-α-D-glucopyranoside. Naturally occurring 6,6′-diesters of trehalose and mycolic acids, β-hydroxy α-branched long chain acids produced by Mycobacteria, Nocardia, and Corynebacteria. 3 major classes identified which are based on the size of the acid and the producing strain: corynomycolic acids (C_{32}), nocardomycolic acids (C_{48}-C_{60}); mycobacteria mycolic acids (C_{60}-C_{90}). The formation of "cords" by tubercule bacilli was first described in 1884 by R. Koch. Isolation of the factor from Mycobacterium tuberculosis: H. Bloch, J. Exp. Med. **91**, 197 (1950). Structure: J. Asselineau, E. Lederer, Biochim. Biophys. Acta **17**, 161 (1955). Synthesis: J. Polonsky et al., Carbohydr. Res. **65**, 295 (1978); Y. Gama, Yakugaku **44**, 671 (1995). Antitumor activity: A. Bekierkunst et al., Science **174**, 1240 (1971); M. V. Pimm et al., Int. J. Cancer **24**, 780 (1979). Molecular packing and surface properties: R. Almog, C. A. Mannella, Biophys. J. **71**, 3311 (1996). Use as antigen in serodiagnosis of Mycobacterium avium-intracellulare complex: K. Enomoto et al., Microbiol. Immunol. **42**, 689 (1998); in tuberculosis: J. Pan et al., ibid. **43**, 863 (1999). Review of early literature: E. Lederer, Springer Semin. Immunopathol. **2**, 133-148 (1979). Review of classes of cord factors and their chemistry: idem, Microbiol. Ser. **15**, 361-378 (1984).

R = Mycolic acids

Consult the Name Index before using this section.

2529. Cordycepin. [73-03-0] 3'-Deoxyadenosine; 9-cordyceposidoadenine. $C_{10}H_{13}N_5O_3$; mol wt 251.24. C 47.81%, H 5.22%, N 27.88%, O 19.10%. First reported nucleoside antibiotic. Isoln from culture fluids of *Cordyceps militaris* (Linn.) Link: K. G. Cunningham *et al., J. Chem. Soc.* **1951,** 2299; N. M. Kredich, A. J. Guarino, *Biochim. Biophys. Acta* **41,** 363 (1960). Proposed structure: H. R. Bentley *et al., J. Chem. Soc.* **1951,** 2301. Identity with 3'-deoxyadenosine and revised structure: E. A. Kaczka *et al., Biochem. Biophys. Res. Commun.* **14,** 456 (1964). Biosynthesis: R. Suhadolnik *et al., J. Am. Chem. Soc.* **86,** 948 (1964). Synthesis: A. R. Todd, T. L. Ulbricht, *J. Chem. Soc.* **1960,** 3275; W. W. Lee *et al., J. Am. Chem. Soc.* **83,** 1906 (1961); E. Walton *et al., ibid.* **86,** 2952 (1964); Y. Ito *et al., ibid.* **103,** 6739 (1981). Cordycepin and cordycepin triphosphate have been used extensively in the study of messenger RNA transcription, *see* H. T. Shigeura, G. E. Boxer, *Biochem. Biophys. Res. Commun.* **17,** 758 (1964); S. Penman *et al., Proc. Natl. Acad. Sci. USA* **67,** 1878 (1970). *Reviews:* J. J. Fox. *et al.,* "Nucleoside Antibiotics" in *Prog. Nucleic Acid Res. Mol. Biol.* **5,** 258-262 (1966); A. J. Guarino, "Cordycepin" in *Antibiotics* **I,** D. Gottlieb, P. Shaw, Eds. (Springer-Verlag, New York, 1967) pp 468-480.

Needles from ethanol, *n*-butanol, *n*-propanol or water. mp 225-226°. $[\alpha]_D^{20}$ −47°. $[\alpha]_D^{27}$ −42°. uv max (ethanol): 260 nm (ε 14600). pH aq soln: 7.1.

Triphosphate. Cordycepin-5'-triphosphate; 3'-deoxy ATP; 3'-deoxyadenosine-5'-(tetrahydrogen triphosphate). $C_{10}H_{13}N_5O_{12}P_3$. Formation by conversion of 3'-deoxyadenosine in Ehrlich ascites tumor: H. Klenow, *Biochim. Biophys. Acta* **76,** 347 (1963). Metabolism in KB cells: H. Shigeura, S. Sampson, *ibid.* **138,** 26 (1967). Synthesis: J. J. Novak, F. Sorm, *Collect. Czech. Chem. Commun.* **38,** 113 (1973); M. Blandin, *J. Carbohyd. Nucl., Nucl.* **3**(5/6), 341 (1976). Inhibits the final step of RNA biosynthesis by termination of the ribonucleotide chain due to the absence of the 3'-hydroxyl group.

2530. Coriamyrtin. [2571-86-0] (1a*S*,1b*R*,2*S*,2'*R*,5*S*,6a*R*,-7a*R*,8*R*)-Hexahydro-1b-hydroxy-6a-methyl-8-(1-methylethenyl)-spiro[2,5-methano-7*H*-oxireno[3,4]cyclopent[1,2-*d*]oxepin-7,2'-oxiran]-3(2*H*)-one. $C_{15}H_{18}O_5$; mol wt 278.30. C 64.74%, H 6.52%, O 28.74%. Sesquiterpene of the picrotoxane group. Main toxic principle from leaves and fruit of *Coraria myrtifolia* L., *Coriariaceae:* M. J. Riban, *C.R. Hebd. Seances Acad. Sci.* **57,** 798 (1863) and *C. japonica* A. Gray, *Coriariaceae:* Kariyone, Sato, *J. Pharm. Soc. Jpn.* **50,** 106 (1930); Okuda, *Pharm. Bull.* **2,** 185 (1954). Series of articles on structure, absolute configuration, stereochemistry and derivatives: T. Okuda, T. Yoshida, *Chem. Pharm. Bull.* **9,** 379, 404 (1961); **15,** 1687, 1697 (1967). Structural relationship to tutin, *q.v.: eidem, Tetrahedron Lett.* **1965,** 439. Biosynthetic studies: M. Biollaz, D. Arigoni, *Chem. Commun.* **1969,** 633. Synthetic studies: K. Tanaka *et al., Chem. Pharm. Bull.* **31,** 1943, 1958, 1972 (1983). Pharmacology: E. E. Swanson, K. K. Chen, *J. Pharmacol. Exp. Ther.* **57,** 410 (1936). Structure-activity relationship: C. H. Jarboe *et al., J. Med. Chem.* **11,** 729 (1968).

Bitter, monoclinic prisms, mp 229-230°. $[\alpha]_D^{14}$ +79°. Slightly sol in water, cold alc; freely sol in hot alc, in ether. LD_{50} i.p. in mice: 3 mg/kg (Jarboe).

2531. Coriander. Annual plant, *Coriandrum sativum* L., *Umbelliferae,* with characteristic "bug-like" odor. *Habit.* Asia, Europe, North and South America. *Constit.* About 1% volatile oil; fixed oils, malic acid, tannin, mucilage. Medicinal parts are the dried ripe fruit and volatile oil. The leaf, known as **cilantro**, and whole or ground seeds are used in cooking. Description and medicinal uses: M. Wichtl, N. G. Bisset, *Herbal Drugs and Phytopharmaceuticals,* English Ed. (CRC Press, Boca Raton, 1994) pp 159-160. Production and constituents of seed oil: B. M. Smallfield *et al., J. Agric. Food Chem.* **49,** 118 (2001).

Volatile oil. [8008-52-4] Obtained by steam distillation of dried ripe fruit. *Constit.* Chiefly 60-70% linalool, α-pinene, γ-terpinene, limonene, camphor, geraniol and geranyl acetate. Colorless or pale yellow liquid. d_{25}^{25} 0.863-0.875. α_D^{25} +8 to +15°. n_D^{20} 1.4620-1.4720. Almost insol in water; sol in 3 vols 70% alcohol; more sol in stronger alcohol; very sol in chloroform, ether, glacial acetic acid.

USE: Flavoring in foods; component of spice blends such as curry powder.

THERAP CAT: Carminative.

2532. Cork. The bark of the cork oak tree, *Quercus suber* L., *Fagaceae* and to a lesser degree of *Quercus occidentalis* Gray, *Fagaceae,* indigenous to the African and European shores of the western Mediterranean. *Constit.* 35-60% suberin, 30-33% cellulose, 27-32% lignin; small amounts of cerin (a wax), fats, inorganic manganese compds, decacrylic acid. Suberin contains phellonic acid, suberic acid, phloionic acid, phloionolic acid, suberolcarboxylic acid, eicosadicarboxylic acid, stearic acid, cortic acid. Used to seal wine casks since antiquity: Theophrastus, *Historia Plantarum* **3,** 16 and 17. Plinius (major), *Historia Naturalis* **16,** 8, 13. *Reviews and monographs:* A. Klauber, *Monographie des Korkes* (Weber, Berlin, 1920); W. Herrmann, *Kork* in *Ullmanns Encyklopädie der technischen Chemie* **vol. 10,** (Urban & Schwarzenberg, Munich, 3rd ed., 1958) pp 634-637; G. B. Cooke, *Cork and the Cork Tree* (Pergamon Press, New York, 1961).

Pale tan, elastic mass. Floats on water. Specific gravity about 0.10 to 0.25 g/ml. Excellent insulator against heat and sound. Stable to heat up to about 100°. Unaffected by water, brine, dil acids, alcohols, bland oils. Attacked by concd mineral acids, strong alkali and ammonia, free halogens, hydrogen peroxide, ozone.

USE: Bottle stoppers, sound deadeners, heat insulators, life preservers, gaskets, linoleum manufacture, cork tile, bulletin boards, dart boards, inlays for shoes.

2533. Corn Oil. Maize oil; Maydol; Mazola. Obtained as a byproduct by wet milling the grain of *Zea mays* L., *Gramineae* for the manuf of corn starch, corn syrup, glucose, dextrins, etc.: E. W. Eckey, *Vegetable Fats and Oils* (Reinhold, New York, 1954). *Constit.* Glycerides of the following fatty acids: Myristic 0.1-1.7%, palmitic 8-12%, stearic 2.5-4.5%, hexadecenoic 0.2-1.6%, oleic 19-49%, linoleic 34-62%. Unsaponifiable fraction: 1-3% (γ-tocopherol 0.1%, the rest is mostly isomeric sitosterols and wax such as myricyl and ceryl alcohols). The crude oil may contain up to 2% phospholipids (vegetable lecithin, inositol esters). The following constants are for the refined product.

Yellow oil. Faint characteristic odor and taste. d_{25}^{25} 0.916-0.921. mp 18 to −10°. Titer 14-20°. Flash pt 610°F (321°C). Ignition pt 740°F (393°C). n_D^{25} 1.470-1.474; n_D^{40} 1.464-1.468. Acid value 2-6. Saponification value 187-196. Iodine value 109-133. Thiocyanogen value 71-77. Hydroxyl value 8-12. Reichert-Meissl value <0.5. Polenske value <0.5. Hehner value 92-96. Classed as a semidrying oil. On prolonged exposure to air it thickens and becomes rancid. Miscible with chloroform, ether, benzene, petr ether. Slightly sol in alc.

USE: As salad and cooking oil; in prepn of margarine. As pharmaceutic aid (solvent). Some use in the preparation of nonyellowing enamel paint.

2534. Corn Steep Liquor. Corn steep water. Cleaned corn grain is washed thoroughly and then steeped for 36 to 40 hours in approx twice its volume of water contg 0.2% SO_2 at a temp of 46-

50°C. As the steep water is drawn from the corn it contains between 6 and 9 lbs of solids per 100 lbs of water. The corn should be soft to the touch, but must not be slimy or smeary which occurs when steeped either too hot or too long. The steep liquor is then evaporated under 25 mm Hg pressure in a "Swenson" evaporator to what is called heavy steep liquor with a gravity of 16 to 20° Bé and contg 50-60% of solids. In this form it is sold to manufacturers of antibiotics who may have their own specifications as to age, gravity and SO₂ content. *See* Bowden, Peterson, *Arch. Biochem.* **9**, 387-399 (April 1946); Graefe, *Staerke* **4**, 275-282 (1952).

USE: In production of penicillin, *meso*-inositol; source of phytin.

2535. Cornus. Dogwood; flowering dogwood. Dried root bark of *Cornus florida* L., *Cornaceae*. *Habit*. Eastern U.S. and Ontario. *Constit*. Cornin Verbenalin, *q.v.*

THERAP CAT: Astringent bitter.

2536. Coronene. [191-07-1] $C_{24}H_{12}$; mol wt 300.35. C 95.97%, H 4.03%. Planar polycyclic aromatic hydrocarbon; found in almost pure form as the mineral *pendletonite*. Environmental pollutant produced as a byproduct of hydrocarbon combustion; impurity in natural carbon deposits. Possible source of infrared emission from interstellar matter. Prepn: R. Scholl, K. Meyer, *Ber.* **65**, 902 (1932); M. S. Newman, *J. Am. Chem. Soc.* **62**, 1683 (1940). Isoln from coal-hydrogenation oil: M. Orchin, J. Feldman, *J. Org. Chem.* **18**, 609 (1953). UV absorption spectrum: J. W. Patterson, *J. Am. Chem. Soc.* **64**, 1485 (1942). Photophysical properties: R. Katraro *et al., Chem. Phys.* **42**, 121 (1979); N. Nijegorodov *et al., Spectrochim. Acta A* **57**, 2673 (2001). Calorimetry study: Y. Nagano, *J. Chem. Thermodyn.* **32**, 973 (2000). Quantitative structure-property relationships for polycyclic aromatic hydrocarbons: M. M. C. Ferreira, *Chemosphere* **44**, 125 (2001). Thermodynamic properties: J. S. Chickos *et al., J. Chem. Thermodyn.* **34**, 1195 (2002).

mp 429-430° (Scholl, Meyer). Also reported as pale yellow needles from dilute benzene, mp 437-440° (Newman). bp 590.0°. d 1.39. Soly in water at 25°, log *S*: −3.85 g/m³.

USE: Ultraviolet phosphor for charge-coupled devices.

2537. Coroxon. [321-54-0] Phosphoric acid 3-chloro-4-methyl-2-oxo-2*H*-1-benzopyran-7-yl diethyl ester; 3-chloro-7-hydroxy-4-methylcoumarin diethyl phosphate; 3-chloro-4-methylumbelliferone diethyl phosphate; *O,O*-diethyl *O*-(3-chloro-4-methyl-7-coumarinyl) phosphate; *O,O*-diethyl *O*-7-(3-chloro-4-methylumbelliferone) phosphate; coumaphos oxygen analog; Coralox. $C_{14}H_{16}ClO_6P$; mol wt 346.70. C 48.50%, H 4.65%, Cl 10.23%, O 27.69%, P 8.93%. Metabolite of coumaphos, *q.v.* Prepn: Fusco *et al., US 2951851* (1960 to Montecatini); G. C. Amin, C. M. Christian, *Indian Chem. Manuf.* **12**, 22 (1974). Crystal and molecular structure: M. R. Gifkins, R. A. Jacobson, *J. Agric. Food Chem.* **24**, 232 (1976). Determn in eggs and milk: K. D. White *et al., J. Assoc. Off. Anal. Chem.* **66**, 1358 (1983). Ophthalmic cholinesterase inhibitor: M. Kadin, *Am. J. Ophthalmol.* **50**, 622 (1960).

Practically insol in water. Somewhat sol in acetone, chloroform, corn oil.

Mixture with phenothiazine. Coopex.

THERAP CAT (VET): Anthelmintic.

2538. Corticosterone. [50-22-6] (11β)-11,21-Dihydroxypregn-4-ene-3,20-dione; 4-pregnene-11β,21-diol-3,20-dione; Kendall's compound B; Reichstein's substance H; compd B. $C_{21}H_{30}$-O_4; mol wt 346.46. C 72.80%, H 8.73%, O 18.47%. Endogenous glucocorticoid; intermediate in the biosynthesis of aldosterone from progesterone. Isoln from adrenal cortex: Mason *et al., J. Biol. Chem.* **114**, 613 (1936); Reichstein, von Euw, *Helv. Chim. Acta* **21**, 1197 (1938); Jeanloz *et al., US 2676904* (1954 to Searle); from adrenal extract: Reichstein, *US 2166877* (1939 to Roche-Organon). Prepn from desoxycholic acid: Wallis, Chakravorty, *US 2341250* (1944 to Research Corp.); from 11-deoxycorticosterone: Zaffaroni, *US 2671752* (1954 to Syntex); from cortisone: Oliveto *et al., US 2927108* (1960 to Schering).

Trigonal plates from acetone, mp 180-182°. $[\alpha]_D^{15}$ +223° (c = 1.1 in alc). uv max: 240 nm. Insol in water. Sol in usual organic solvents. Upon moistening with concd H_2SO_4 it gives an orange-yellow soln which has a strong fluorescence.

21-Acetate. $C_{23}H_{32}O_5$. Clusters of needles from acetone + ether, mp 145°. $[\alpha]_D^{20}$ +195° (c = 0.62 in acetone).

2539. Cortisone. [53-06-5] 17,21-Dihydroxypregn-4-ene-3,11,20-trione; 17-hydroxy-11-dehydrocorticosterone; 11-dehydro-17-hydroxycorticosterone; Δ⁴-pregnene-17α,21-diol-3,11,20-trione; Kendall's compound E; Wintersteiner's compound F; Reichstein's substance Fa. $C_{21}H_{28}O_5$; mol wt 360.44. C 69.98%, H 7.83%, O 22.19%. Isoln from suprarenal glands: Pfiffner *et al., J. Biol. Chem.* **111**, 585 (1935); **116**, 291 (1936); Mason *et al., ibid.* **114**, 613 (1936); Reichstein, *Helv. Chim. Acta* **19**, 1107 (1936); Kuizenga, Cartland, *Endocrinology* **24**, 526 (1939). Synthesis of the monoacetate from desoxycholic acid: Sarett, *J. Biol. Chem.* **162**, 601 (1946). Further development of prepn methods: Meystre, Wettstein, *Experientia* **3**, 185 (1947); *Helv. Chim. Acta* **30**, 1037, 1256 (1947); Reichstein *et al., ibid.* **26**, 562, 705, 721 (1943); **27**, 821 (1944); Reichstein, *US 2403683* (1946); Kendall *et al., J. Biol. Chem.* **166**, 345 (1946); Gallagher, *US 2447325* (1948); Peterson, Murray, *J. Am. Chem. Soc.* **74**, 1871 (1952); Perlman, *ibid.* 2126; Sarett, *ibid.* **70**, 1454 (1948); **71**, 2443 (1949); Mattox, Kendall, *ibid.* **70**, 882 (1948). Stereospecific total synthesis: Sarett *et al., ibid.* **74**, 4974 (1952).

Rhombohedral platelets from 95% alcohol, mp 220-224° (some decompn) when heated in evac capillary. $[\alpha]_D^{25}$ +209° (c = 1.2 in 95% alcohol); $[\alpha]_{546}^{25}$ +269° (c = 0.125 in benzene); $[\alpha]_{546}^{25}$ +248° (c = 0.1 to 0.2 in alcohol). uv max: 237 nm (ε 1.4×10⁴) *see* Mason *et al., J. Biol. Chem.* **116**, 267 (1936); Wintersteiner, Pfiffner, *ibid.* 291. Fairly sol in cold methanol, ethanol, acetone; much less sol in ether, benzene, chloroform; slightly sol in water (28 mg/100 ml at 25°). The water soln is neutral. Gives orange-red soln with intense green fluorescence in concd H_2SO_4. Reduces Benedict's soln on heating.

21-Acetate. [50-04-4] Cortisone acetate; Cortistab; Cortisyl; Cortogen; Cortone. $C_{23}H_{30}O_6$; mol wt 402.48. Flat needles from acetone; clusters of radiating rods from chloroform. Becomes opaque at 70-100°, mp 235-238° with slight sintering at 230°. $[\alpha]_D^{25}$ +164° (c = 0.5 in acetone), $[\alpha]_D^{25}$ +208 to +217° (dioxane). uv max:

238 nm (ε 1.58×10⁴), *see* Sarett, *J. Biol. Chem.* **162**, 630 (1946). Soly at 25° in water: 2.2 mg/100 ml; in propylene glycol 44 mg/100 ml; in chloroform 182 mg/g. Reduces ammoniacal silver nitrate soln at room temp. Sol in sulfuric acid giving a yellow soln without fluorescence (difference from hydrocortisone acetate).

21-Cyclopentanepropionate. [509-00-2] $C_{29}H_{40}O_6$. Needles from diisopropyl ether, mp 158-161°. $[\alpha]_D^{20}$ +190° (chloroform). uv max (ethanol): 239 nm (ε 16350). Sol in ether, glycols, vegetable oils, especially sesame, peanut, and corn oils.

THERAP CAT: Glucocorticoid.

THERAP CAT (VET): Glucocorticoid, anti-inflammatory agent.

2540. Cortivazol. [1110-40-3] (11β,16α)-21-(Acetyloxy)-11,17-dihydroxy-6,16-dimethyl-2'-phenyl-2'*H*-pregna-2,4,6-trieno[3,2-*c*]pyrazol-20-one; 1,2,3,3a,3b,7,10,10a,10b,11,12,12a-dodecahydro-1,11-dihydroxy-2,5,10a,12a-tetramethyl-7-phenylcyclopenta[7,8]phenanthro[2,3-*c*]pyrazol-1-yl hydroxymethyl ketone acetate; 6,16α-dimethyl-11β,17α,21-trihydroxy-2'-phenyl[3,2-*c*]pyrazolo-4,6-pregnadien-20-one 21-acetate; MK-650; H-3625; Altim; Diaster; Dilaster. $C_{32}H_{38}N_2O_5$; mol wt 530.65. C 72.43%, H 7.22%, N 5.28%, O 15.08%. Prepn: Fried *et al.*, *J. Am. Chem. Soc.* **85**, 236 (1963); Tishler *et al.*, **US 3067194** and **US 3300483** (1962, 1967 to Merck & Co.).

Double mp 160-165° and 229-230°; $[\alpha]_D^{23}$ +14° (CHCl₃). uv max (methanol): 283, 315 nm (ε 15700, 19000).

THERAP CAT: Glucocorticoid.

2541. Cortol. [516-38-1] (3α,5β,11β,20S)-Pregnane-3,11,-17,20,21-pentol. $C_{21}H_{36}O_5$; mol wt 368.51. C 68.44%, H 9.85%, O 21.71%. Isolated from human urine after administration of hydrocortisone or ACTH: Fukushima *et al.*, *J. Biol. Chem.* **212**, 449 (1955).

α-**Cortol.** 5β-Pregnane-3α,11β,17,20α,21-pentol. Crystals from ethyl acetate, mp 250.5-254°. $[\alpha]_D^{26}$ +23.7° (ethanol).

α-**Cortol 3,20,21-triacetate.** $C_{27}H_{42}O_8$. Crystals from benzene + cyclohexane, mp 168-170°.

β-**Cortol.** 5β-Pregnane-3α,11β,17,20β,21-pentol. Crystals from methanol, mp 262-264.5°. $[\alpha]_D^{25}$ +33.3° (ethanol).

2542. Cortolone. [516-42-7] (3α,5β,20S)-3,17,20,21-Tetrahydroxypregnan-11-one; 3α,17α,20α,21-pregnanetetrol-11-one. $C_{21}H_{34}O_5$; mol wt 366.49. C 68.82%, H 9.35%, O 21.83%. Isolated from human urine after administration of cortisone, hydrocortisone or ACTH: D. K. Fukushima *et al.*, *J. Biol. Chem.* **212**, 449 (1955). Synthesis: L. H. Sarett, *J. Am. Chem. Soc.* **71**, 1169 (1949); A. H. Soloway *et al.*, *ibid.* **76**, 2941 (1954).

Crystals from acetone, mp 208-209°. $[\alpha]_D^{25}$ +44° (c = 0.5 in ethanol); also reported as $[\alpha]_D^{28}$ +34.2° (ethanol).

3,20,21-Triacetate. [2638-46-2] $C_{27}H_{40}O_8$. Crystals from methanol, mp 214-216° (Fukushima); also reported as mp 213-214° (Sarett). $[\alpha]_D^{28}$ +28° (ethanol); also reported as $[\alpha]_D^{25}$ +18° (c = 1 in acetone).

2543. Corydaldine. [493-49-2] 3,4-Dihydro-6,7-dimethoxy-1(2*H*)-isoquinolinone; 3,4-dihydro-6,7-dimethoxyisocarbostyril; 1,2,3,4-tetrahydro-6,7-dimethoxy-1(2*H*)-1-isoquinolone. $C_{11}H_{13}NO_3$; mol wt 207.23. C 63.75%, H 6.32%, N 6.76%, O 23.16%. Synthesis: Späth, Dobrowsky, *Ber.* **58**, 1274 (1925); Mohunta, Ray, *J. Chem. Soc.* **1934**, 1263; Wiesner *et al.*, *J. Am. Chem. Soc.* **77**, 675 (1955); Brossi *et al.*, *Helv. Chim. Acta* **43**, 1459 (1960); Mahuzier, Hamon, *Bull. Soc. Chim. Fr.* **1969**, 684.

Monoclinic prisms from water or alcohol, mp 175°. Sol in water, alcohol, ether, benzene, chloroform. Practically insol in petr ether.

2544. Corydaline. [518-69-4] (13S-*trans*)-5,8,13,13a-Tetrahydro-2,3,9,10-tetramethoxy-13-methyl-6*H*-dibenzo[*a,g*]quinolizine; 2,3,9,10-tetramethoxy-13α-methyl-13aβ-berbine; *d*-corydaline. $C_{22}H_{27}NO_4$; mol wt 369.45. C 71.52%, H 7.37%, N 3.79%, O 17.32%. Alkaloid isolated from many species of *Corydalis.* Discovery in *C. tuberosa*: Wackenroder, *Kustner's Arch.* **8**, 423 (1826), as cited in: C. Wehmer, *Die Pflanzenstoffe* **I** (G. Fischer, Jena, 1929) p 389. Isoln from *Corydalis aurea* Willd. and *C. solida* (L.) Swartz, *Fumariaceae*: Manske, *Can. J. Res.* **16B**, 81 (1938); *Can. J. Chem.* **34**, 1 (1956). Structure: von Bruchhausen, Stippler, *Arch. Pharm.* **265**, 152 (1927). Synthesis: Späth, Kruta, *Ber.* **62**, 1024 (1929); T. Kametani *et al.*, *J. Chem. Soc. Perkin Trans. 1* **1977**, 1151; M. Cushman, F. W. Dekon, *Tetrahedron* **1978**, 1435; Z. Kiparissides *et al.*, *Can. J. Chem.* **58**, 2770 (1980). Stereochemistry: Bersch, *Arch. Pharm.* **291**, 595 (1958); Jeffs, *Experientia* **21**, 690 (1965). Pharmacology: Berezhinskaya, *C.A.* **78**, 119087j (1973). Toxicity study: R. C. Anderson, K. K. Chen, *Fed. Proc.* **5**, 163 (1946).

Prisms from alc, mp 135°. $[\alpha]_D^{20}$ +311° (c = 0.8 in alc). uv max: 396 nm. Sol in chloroform; moderately sol in ether; sparingly sol in methanol, ethanol. Practically insol in water. LD₅₀ in mice (mg/kg): 135.5 ± 12.8 i.v. (Anderson, Chen).

Hydrochloride hydrate. $C_{22}H_{27}NO_4 \cdot HCl \cdot H_2O$. Four-sided columns, mp 230-240°.

dl-**Form.** mp 135°. Slightly sol in water.

dl-**Mesocorydaline.** mp 158°. The (13R-*cis*)-analog of corydaline. Slightly sol in water.

d-**Mesocorydaline.** Rhombic crystals, mp 152°. $[\alpha]_D^{20}$ +82° (c = 1.4); +180° (c = 3 in chloroform).

l-**Mesocorydaline.** Rhombic crystals, mp 152°. $[\alpha]_D^{20}$ −85° (c = 1.4); −181° (c = 3 in chloroform).

2545. Corydalis. Squirrel corn; turkey corn. Dried tuber of *Dicentra (Bicuculla) cucullaria* (L.) Bernh., or of *Dicentra canadensis* (DC.) Walp., *Fumariaceae. Habit.* Ontario to Kentucky and Missouri. *Constit.* Corydaline, bulbocapnine, isocorydine, corytuberine, corycavine, corybulbine, corydine, fumaric acid, acrid resin, protopine.

2546. Corydine. [476-69-7] (6aS)-5,6,6a,7-Tetrahydro-2,10,11-trimethoxy-6-methyl-4H-dibenzo[de,g]quinolin-1-ol; 2,10,11-trimethoxy-6aα-aporphin-1-ol; 1-hydroxy-2,10,11-trimethoxyaporphine. $C_{20}H_{23}NO_4$; mol wt 341.40. C 70.36%, H 6.79%, N 4.10%, O 18.75%. The methyl ether of corytuberine. Occurs in *Corydalis cava* (L.) Schweigg & Körte (*C. tuberosa* DC), *Fumariaceae*, in the dextrorotatory form. Isoln: Gadamer, Ziegenbein, *Arch. Pharm.* **240**, 94 (1902). Structure: Späth, Berger, *Ber.* **64**, 2038 (1931). Synthesis: Hey, Palluel, *J. Chem. Soc.* **1957**, 2926; Arumugam *et al., Ber.* **91**, 40 (1958); Jackson, Martin, *Chem. Commun.* **1965**, 142, 420; *eidem, J. Chem. Soc. C* **1966**, 2222. uv spectrum: Shamma, Yao, *J. Org. Chem.* **36**, 3253 (1971).

Tetragonal prisms from ether, mp 149°. $[\alpha]_D^{20}$ +204° (c = 1.6 in chloroform). Freely sol in chloroform, alcohol, ethyl acetate; moderately sol in ether.

dl-**Hydrochloride monohydrate.** $C_{20}H_{23}NO_4 \cdot HCl \cdot H_2O$. Crystals from ethanol + ether, sinters at 205°, dec 228°. Sparingly sol in water.

2547. Corynantheine. [18904-54-6] (16E)-16,17,18,19-Tetradehydro-17-methoxycorynan-16-carboxylic acid methyl ester; (E)-16,17,18,19-tetradehydro-17-methoxy-17,18-secoyohimban-16-carboxylic acid methyl ester. $C_{22}H_{26}N_2O_3$; mol wt 366.45. C 72.11%, H 7.15%, N 7.64%, O 13.10%. Isolated from *Corynanthe johimbe* K. Schum., and *Pseudocinchona africana* A. Cheval., *Rubiaceae:* Karrer *et al., Helv. Chim. Acta* **9**, 1059 (1926); **35**, 851 (1952). Structure: Janot *et al., ibid.* **34**, 1207 (1951). Stereochemistry: Van Tamelen *et al., J. Am. Chem. Soc.* **79**, 6426 (1957). Total synthesis of *dl*- form: Van Tamelen, Wright, *Tetrahedron Lett.* **1964**, 295; *eidem, J. Am. Chem. Soc.* **91**, 7349 (1969). Total synthesis of *d*-form: Autrey, Scullard, *ibid.* **90**, 4917 (1968).

Crystals: α-form mp 103-107°; β-form mp 165-166°. $[\alpha]_D$ +28° (c = 1 in methanol). uv max (methanol): 227, 280, 291 nm (log ε 4.64, 3.82, 3.80).

Hydrochloride. $C_{22}H_{26}N_2O_3 \cdot HCl$. Needles from alcohol + ether, mp 194-206°. Also reported as mp 176-179°. $[\alpha]_D^{20}$ +12° (water). Sol in alcohol, sparingly sol in water.

Dihydrocorynantheine. $C_{22}H_{28}N_2O_3$. Total synthesis of *dl*-form: Van Tamelen, Hester, *J. Am. Chem. Soc.* **81**, 3805 (1959); *eidem, ibid.* **91**, 7342 (1969). Plates from alcohol + water, mp 177-177.5°. $[\alpha]_D$ +28°.

Hydrochloride. $C_{22}H_{28}N_2O_3 \cdot HCl$. mp 212-213°. Also reported as crystals from 95% ethanol-ethyl acetate, mp 242.2-243.3° (dec) (sealed tube), Van Tamelen, Hester, *loc. cit.* (1969).

2548. Corynanthine. [483-10-5] (16β,17α)-17-Hydroxy-yohimban-16-carboxylic acid methyl ester; rauhimbine. $C_{21}H_{26}N_2O_3$; mol wt 354.44. C 71.16%, H 7.39%, N 7.90%, O 13.54%. From bark of *Pseudocinchona africana* Chev., *Corynanthe johimbe* K. Schum., *Rubiaceae* and *Rauwolfia serpentina* (L.) Benth., *Apocynaceae:* Raymond-Hamet, *Compt. Rend.* **212**, 305 (1941); Jorio, *Ann. Chim. Farm.* **1939**, 50, *C.A.* **33**, 9306⁹ (1939); Le Hir *et al., Ann. Pharm. Fr.* **11**, 546 (1953); Hofmann, *Helv. Chim. Acta* **37**, 314 (1954). Identity with rauhimbine: *idem, ibid.* 849. Structure and stereochemistry: Janot *et al., Bull. Soc. Chim. Fr.* **1952**, 1085; **1961**, 637.

Stout prisms from acetone, dec 225-226°. $[\alpha]_D^{19}$ −85° (c = 0.5 in pyridine). uv max (methanol): 226, 283, 290 nm (log ε 4.56, 3.87, 3.79). Practically insol in water or petr ether. Sol in 40 parts of boiling chloroform, in 60 parts of boiling benzene, in 20 parts of boiling ethyl acetate, in 5 parts of boiling alcohol.

O,N-**Dibutyrylcorynanthine hydrochloride.** Prepn: Reiser *et al., US 2975183* (1961 to Chemische Werke Albert). Crystals from benzene, mp 208-210°.

O,N-**Dipropionylcorynanthine hydrochloride.** Prepn: Reiser *et al., loc. cit.* Crystals from isopropanol, mp 236-237°.

2549. Corypalmine. [6018-40-2] 5,8,13,13a-Tetrahydro-2,9,10-trimethoxy-6H-dibenzo[a,g]quinolizin-3-ol; 2,9,10-trimethoxyberbin-3-ol; 3-hydroxy-2,9,10-trimethoxyberbine; tetrahydrojatrorrhizine. $C_{20}H_{23}NO_4$; mol wt 341.40. C 70.36%, H 6.79%, N 4.10%, O 18.75%. In *Corydalis cava* (L.) Schweigg & Körte (*C. tuberosa* D.C.) and other varieties of *Corydalis, Fumariaceae*. Synthesis of *dl*-corypalmine: Govindachari *et al., Ber.* **92**, 1654 (1959).

d-**Form.** Small crystals, mp 236°. $[\alpha]_D^{16}$ +280° (chloroform). Insol in water; sol in alcohol and chloroform: Späth *et al., Ber.* **56**, 878 (1923); **58**, 2133 (1925); **60**, 383 (1927).

l-**Form.** Crystals from chloroform-methanol, mp 246° (in vac): Manske, *Can. J. Res.* **20B**, 57 (1942); **21B**, 111 (1943).

dl-**Form.** Crystals from methanol, mp 207°.

2550. Corytuberine. [517-56-6] (6aS)-5,6,6a,7-Tetrahydro-2,10-dimethoxy-6-methyl-4H-dibenzo[de,g]quinoline-1,11-diol; 2,10-dimethoxy-6aα-aporphine-1,11-diol; 1,11-dihydroxy-2,10-dimethoxyaporphine. $C_{19}H_{21}NO_4$; mol wt 327.37. C 69.71%, H 6.47%, N 4.28%, O 19.55%. In *Corydalis cava* (L.) Schweigg & Körte (*C. tuberosa* (Andr.) Walp., *Fumariaceae.* Isoln: Späth, Berger, *Ber.* **64**, 2038 (1931); Manske, *Can. J. Res.* **10**, 521 (1934). Synthesis of (±)-form: Tomita, Kikkawa, **JP 58 6466** (1958 to Shionogi), *C.A.* **54**, 1584i (1960); T. Kametani, M. Ihara, *J. Chem. Soc. Perkin Trans. 1* **1980**, 629. Biosynthesis studies: Blaschke, *Biochem. Physiol. Alkaloide, Int. Symp., 4th,* K.

Mothes, Ed. (Akad.-Verlag, Berlin, 1972) pp 283-286. Biomimetric total synthesis: T. Kametani *et al.*, *Heterocycles* **5**, 175 (1976).

Pentahydrate. Leaflets, plates, turning gray on exposure to light. mp 240° dec (dry). uv max (methanol): 227, 272, 311.5 nm. Sol in alc, hot water; slightly sol in ether, chloroform, ethyl acetate. $[\alpha]_D^{20}$ +283° (alc). The dried crystals are hygroscopic and quickly attract 1 mol H_2O from the air.

Hydrochloride. $C_{19}H_{21}NO_4$·HCl. Crystals from alcohol-ether, dec above 250°; $[\alpha]_D^{20}$ +168°; sparingly sol in water.

Methyl ether see Corydine.

2551. Cosyntropin. [16960-16-0] α^{1-24}-Corticotropin; β^{1-24}-corticotropin; tetracosactide; Cortrosyn. $C_{136}H_{210}N_{40}O_{31}S$; mol wt 2933.44. C 55.68%, H 7.22%, N 19.10%, O 16.91%, S 1.09%. Synthetic polypeptide corresponding to the first 24 amino acids of ACTH, *q.v.* Identification of activity: R. G. Shepherd *et al.*, *J. Am. Chem. Soc.* **78**, 5067 (1956). Synthesis: H. Kappeler, R. Schwyzer, *Helv. Chim. Acta* **44**, 1136 (1961); *eidem, ibid.* **46**, 1550 (1963); solid-state synthesis: R. Matsueda *et al.*, *J. Am. Chem. Soc.* **97**, 2573 (1975). Assessment of hormone levels for adrenal function in cats: M. E. Peterson *et al.*, *Res. Vet. Sci.* **37**, 331 (1984); in dogs: L. A. Frank *et al.*, *Domest. Anim. Endocrinol.* **24**, 43 (2003). Review as diagnostic aid in assessment of secondary adrenal insufficiency: T. A. M. Abdu, R. N. Clayton, *Curr. Opin. Endocrinol. Diabetes* **7**, 116-121 (2000); in primary or secondary adrenal insufficiency: R. I. Dorin *et al.*, *Ann. Intern. Med.* **139**, 194-204, E205-E206 (2003).

Ser-Tyr-Ser-Met-Glu-His-Phe-Arg-Trp-Gly-Lys-Pro-Val-Gly
|
Lys
|
Pro-Tyr-Val-Lys-Val-Pro-Arg-Arg-Lys

Hexaacetate. [22633-88-1] α^{1-24}-Corticotropin hexaacetate (salt); Synacthen. $[\alpha]_D^{22}$ −88 ±2° (c = 0.511 in 1% acetic acid). uv max (0.1 *N* NaOH): 283, 289 nm (ε 8550, 8810).

THERAP CAT: Diagnostic aid (adrenal function).

THERAP CAT (VET): Diagnostic aid (adrenal function).

2552. Cotarnine. [82-54-2] 5,6,7,8-Tetrahydro-4-methoxy-6-methyl-1,3-dioxolo[4,5-*g*]isoquinolin-5-ol. $C_{12}H_{15}NO_4$; mol wt 237.25. C 60.75%, H 6.37%, N 5.90%, O 26.97%. Prepd by the oxidation of narcotine with dil nitric acid. Synthesis: Salway, *J. Chem. Soc.* **97**, 1208 (1910). Is tautomeric. Structure studies: Small, Lutz, "Chemistry of the Opium Alkaloids," Supplement No. 103, *U.S. Public Health Reports* (Washington, 1932) p 49; Schneider, Müller, *Ann.* **615**, 34 (1958). Absorption spectrum: Csokán, *Z. Anal. Chem.* **124**, 344 (1942).

Small needles from benzene, dec 132-133°. Sol in alcohol, chloroform, ether, benzene; slightly sol in water; sol in dil acids, in ammonia or sodium carbonate soln, but only slightly in potassium hydroxide soln. Aq or alcoholic solns are yellow.

Hydrochloride. [36647-02-6] Secalysat. $C_{12}H_{15}NO_4$·HCl; mol wt 273.71.

Chloride. [10018-19-6] 7,8-Dihydro-4-methoxy-6-methyl-1,3-dioxolo[4,5-*g*]isoquinolinium chloride; cotarnine chloride; cotarninium chloride; Stypticin. $C_{12}H_{14}ClNO_3$; mol wt 255.70. Dihy-

drate, light-yellow powder; deliquesc in moist air. Sol in about 1 part water, 4 parts alc. *Keep well closed.*

Phthalate. [6190-36-9] Styptol. $C_{32}H_{32}N_2O_{10}$; mol wt 604.60.

THERAP CAT: Hemostatic.

2553. Cotinine. [486-56-6] 1-Methyl-5-(3-pyridinyl)-2-pyrrolidinone; *N*-methyl-2-(3-pyridyl)-5-pyrrolidone. $C_{10}H_{12}N_2$-O; mol wt 176.22. C 68.16%, H 6.86%, N 15.90%, O 9.08%. Nicotine metabolite first described by Pinner, *Arch. Pharm.* **231**, 378 (1893). Isolated from autoxidized nicotine, nicotine treated with hydrogen peroxide, from nicotine irradiated with ultraviolet light: Frankenburg, Vaitekunas, *J. Am. Chem. Soc.* **79**, 149 (1957).

Viscous oil, bp$_6$ 210-211°. Absorption spectra: Frankenburg, Vaitekunas, *loc. cit.*

Fumarate. [5695-98-7] Scotine. $(C_{10}H_{12}N_2O)_2$·$C_4H_4O_4$; mol wt 468.50.

THERAP CAT: Antidepressant.

2554. Cotton-root Bark. Dried root-bark of one or more of the cultivated species of *Gossypium herbaceum* L. and of other species of *Gossypium, Malvaceae*. **Habit.** Asia (India, China, Arabia), Egypt, U.S., West Indies, S. America, Australia, Spain, etc. **Constit.** Yellow chromogen about 8% of a pale yellow resin, fixed oil, sugar.

THERAP CAT: Oxytocic.

2555. Cottonseed Oil. Fixed oil from seeds of cultivated varieties of *Gossypium herbaceum* L. or of other species of *Gossypium*.

Pale yellow, oily, practically odorless liq. d_{25}^{25} 0.915-0.921. Solidif 0° to −5°. n_D^{40} 1.4645-1.4655. Sapon no.: 190-198. Iodine no.: 105-114. Surface tension (20°) = 35.4 dyn/cm; (80°) = 31.3 dyn/cm. Slightly sol in alcohol; miscible with chloroform, ether, carbon disulfide, petr ether.

USE: Manuf soaps, oleomargarine, hydrogenated fats, lard substitute, glycerol, leather dressings, lubricants, cosmetics; emollient; also as salad and cooking oil; packing fish. Pharmaceutic aid (solvent).

THERAP CAT (VET): Pediculicide, acaricide, laxative, emollient.

2556. Coumachlor. [81-82-3] 3-[1-(4-Chlorophenyl)-3-oxobutyl]-4-hydroxy-2*H*-1-benzopyran-2-one; 3-(α-acetonyl-*p*-chlorobenzyl)-4-hydroxycoumarin; 3-(α-*p*-chlorophenyl-β-acetyl-ethyl)-4-hydroxycoumarin; G-21133. $C_{19}H_{15}ClO_4$; mol wt 342.77. C 66.58%, H 4.41%, Cl 10.34%, O 18.67%. Structural analog of warfarin. Prepn: F. Litvan, W. Stoll, US 2648682 (1953 to J. R. Geigy). Anticoagulant activity: M. Reiff, R. Weismann, *Acta Trop.* **8**, 97 (1951), *C.A.* **50**, 10976d (1956). Review of comparative toxicology: H. Wanntorp, *Acta Pharmacol. Toxicol.* **16**, Suppl. 2, 123 pp (1959).

Crystals, mp 169-171°. Sol in alc, acetone, chloroform. Slightly sol in benzene, ether. Practically insol in water. MLD in dog, swine (mg/kg): <5, <5 orally (Wanntorp).

Caution: Similar to warfarin, with delayed actions on prothrombin level and blood clotting, resulting in death by hemorrhage. *See Clinical Toxicology of Commercial Products*, R.E. Gosselin *et al.*, Eds. (Williams & Wilkins, Baltimore, 5th ed., 1984) Section II, pp 348.

USE: Rodenticide.

2557. Coumalic Acid. [500-05-0] 2-Oxo-1,2H-pyran-5-carboxylic acid; α-pyrone-5-carboxylic acid. $C_6H_4O_4$; mol wt 140.09. C 51.44%, H 2.88%, O 45.68%. Prepd by heating anhydr malic acid with oleum: v. Pechmann, *Ann.* **264**, 262, 272 (1891); Wiley, Smith, *Org. Synth.* **coll. vol. IV**, 201 (1963).

Bright yellow prisms from methanol, mp 205-210° (partial decompn). bp$_{120}$ 218°; sublimes partially. Sparingly sol in cold water. Dec by boiling water. Sol in alcohol, glacial acetic acid. Slightly sol in ether, acetone, ethyl acetate. Insol in chloroform, benzene, ligroin.

Methyl ester. $C_7H_6O_4$. Leaflets from ligroin, mp 73-74°. bp$_{60}$ 178-180°. bp$_{760}$ 250-260°.

Ethyl ester. $C_8H_8O_4$. Crystals, mp 36°. bp$_{760}$ 262-265°. Distills without decompn.

2558. Coumaphos. [56-72-4] Phosphorothioic acid O-(3-chloro-4-methyl-2-oxo-2H-1-benzopyran-7-yl) O,O-diethyl ester; 3-chloro-7-hydroxy-4-methylcoumarin O-ester with O,O-diethyl phosphorothioate; 3-chloro-4-methylumbelliferone O-ester with O,O-diethyl phosphorothioate; O,O-diethyl O-(3-chloro-4-methyl-7-coumarinyl) phosphorothioate; O,O-diethyl O-(3-chloro-4-methylumbelliferone) thiophosphate; coumafos; Bayer 21/199; Asuntol; Baymix; Co-ral; Meldane; Muscatox; Resitox. $C_{14}H_{16}ClO_5PS$; mol wt 362.77. C 46.35%, H 4.45%, Cl 9.77%, O 22.05%, P 8.54%, S 8.84%. Prepn: Schrader, **DE 881194**; **US 2748146** (1951, 1956 both to Bayer); Krueger *et al., J. Agric. Food Chem.* **7**, 183 (1959). Toxicity: T. B. Gaines, *Toxicol. Appl. Pharmacol.* **14**, 515 (1969).

Crystals, mp 91°. The commercial product may be slightly brownish. Practically insol in water. Somewhat sol in acetone, chloroform, corn oil. Stable in water. LD$_{50}$ in female, male rats (mg/kg): 16, 41 orally (Gaines).

USE: Insecticide, nematocide.

THERAP CAT (VET): Anthelmintic.

2559. Coumaran. [496-16-2] 2,3-Dihydrobenzofuran; cumaran; dihydrocoumarone. C_8H_8O; mol wt 120.15. C 79.97%, H 6.71%, O 13.32%. Synthesis: Bennett, Mahmoud Hafez, *J. Chem. Soc.* **1941**, 287; *cf.* Hurd, Hoffmann, *J. Org. Chem.* **5**, 212 (1940); Rindfusz, *J. Am. Chem. Soc.* **41**, 669 (1919); J. M. Bakke, H. M. Roholdt, *Acta Chem. Scand.* **B34**, 73 (1980).

Oily liq, bp 188-189°, bp$_{13}$ 74-75°. d$_4^{25}$ 1.058, n$_D^{20}$ 1.5426. Sol in alcohol, ether, chloroform, carbon disulfide.

2560. p-Coumaric Acid. [7400-08-0] 3-(4-Hydroxyphenyl)-2-propenoic acid; p-hydroxycinnamic acid; β-[4-hydroxyphenyl]acrylic acid. $C_9H_8O_3$; mol wt 164.16. C 65.85%, H 4.91%, O 29.24%. Isoln: Hlasiwetz, *Ann.* **136**, 31 (1865); Bamberger, *Monatsh. Chem.* **12**, 459 (1891). Prepn: Eigel, *Ber.* **20**, 2528 (1887); Konek, Pacsu, *Ber.* **51**, 856 (1918). uv data: Wheeler, Covarrubias, *J. Org. Chem.* **28**, 2015 (1963).

Needles, mp 210-213° (reported in early lit as 206°). Crystallizes in anhydrous form from conc hot aq soln, but as monohydrate from dil aq soln on slow cooling. Slightly sol in cold water; sol in hot water and alc, ether. Practically insol in benzene and ligroin. uv max (95% ethanol): 223, 286 nm (ε 14450, 19000).

2561. Coumarilic Acid. [496-41-3] 2-Benzofurancarboxylic acid; coumarone-2-carboxylic acid. $C_9H_6O_3$; mol wt 162.14. C 66.67%, H 3.73%, O 29.60%. Synthesis from coumarin: Fuson *et al., Org. Synth.* **coll. vol. III**, 209 (1955). *Review:* Sethna, Shah, *Chem. Rev.* **36**, 1 (1945).

Needles from water, bitter taste. mp 192-193°. bp 310-315° with slight decompn. Sol in boiling water, in alcohol; slightly sol in chloroform, carbon disulfide.

2562. Coumarin. [91-64-5] 2H-1-Benzopyran-2-one; 1,2-benzopyrone; *cis-o*-coumarinic acid lactone; cumarin; coumarinic anhydride; tonka bean camphor. $C_9H_6O_2$; mol wt 146.14. C 73.97%, H 4.14%, O 21.90%. In tonka beans, lavender oil, woodruff (*Asperula* species), in sweet clover (*Melilotus*). Crystal and molecular structure: *Chem. Commun. (Univ. Stockholm)* **1976**, 21. Toxicity: Jenner *et al., Food Cosmet. Toxicol.* **2**, 327 (1964). *Review:* Sethna, Shah, *Chem. Rev.* **36**, 1 (1945); W. C. Meuly in *Kirk-Othmer Encyclopedia of Chemical Technology* **vol. 7** (Wiley-Interscience, New York, 3rd ed., 1979) pp 196-206.

Orthorhombic, rectangular plates. Pleasant, fragrant odor resembling that of vanilla beans, burning taste. mp 68-70°. bp 297-299°. bp$_5$ 139°. One gram dissolves in 400 ml cold, 50 ml boiling water. Freely sol in alc, chloroform, ether, oils; also sol in alkali hydroxide solns. LD$_{50}$ orally in rats, guinea pigs: 680, 202 mg/kg (Jenner).

USE: Pharmaceutic aid (flavor).

2563. Coumarin-3-carboxylic Acid. [531-81-7] 2-Oxo-2H-1-benzopyran-3-carboxylic acid. $C_{10}H_6O_4$; mol wt 190.15. C 63.16%, H 3.18%, O 33.66%. By heating salicylaldehyde with malonic acid in glacial acetic acid. *Review:* Sethna, Shah, *Chem. Rev.* **36**, 1 (1945).

Needles from water, mp 188° (dec). Slightly sol in water; sol in alc, alkalies. Insol in ether, benzene, petr ether.

2564. Coumestrol. [479-13-0] 3,9-Dihydroxy-6H-benzofuro[3,2-c][1]benzopyran-6-one; 2-(2,4-dihydroxyphenyl)-6-hydroxy-3-benzofurancarboxylic acid δ-lactone; 7',6-dihydroxycoumarino(3',4',3,2)coumarone. $C_{15}H_8O_5$; mol wt 268.22. C 67.17%, H 3.01%, O 29.83%. An estrogenic factor occurring naturally in forage crops, esp in ladino clover (*Trifolium repens* L.), strawberry clover (*T. fragiferum* L.) and alfalfa (*Medicago sativa* L., *Leguminosae*). Isoln: Bickoff *et al., J. Agric. Food Chem.* **6**, 536 (1958); Bickoff, Booth, **US 2890116** (1959 to U.S.A.). Structure: Bickoff *et al., J. Am. Chem. Soc.* **80**, 3969 (1958). Synthesis: Emerson, Bickoff, *ibid.* 4381; **US 2884427** (1959 to U.S.A.); Jurd, *Tetrahedron Lett.* **1963**, 1151; Kappe, Brandner, *Z. Naturforsch.* **29B**, 292 (1974). Biosynthesis: Grisebach, Barz, *Chem. Ind. (London)* **1963**, 690.

Crystals, mp 385°. Sublimes at 325°; sublimes in high vacuum at about 175°. uv max (methanol): 208, 243, 343 nm. Exhibits bright blue fluorescence in neutral or acid soln, greenish-yellow fluorescence in strong alkali. Absorption and fluorescence spectra: O. S. Wolfbeis, K. Schaffner, *Photochem. Photobiol.* **32**, 143 (1980). Practically insol in water at acid and neutral pH, in petr ether. Sparingly sol in water at alkaline pH (pH 11-12); slightly sol in methanol, chloroform, ether; very slightly sol in carbon tetrachloride, benzene.

Diacetate. $C_{19}H_{12}O_7$. Crystals from acetic acid, mp 237°.

Dimethyl ether. $C_{17}H_{12}O_5$. Crystals from methanol, mp 198°.

2565. Coumingine. [26241-81-6] [2S-(2α,4aα,4bβ,7E,8β,8aα,10aβ)]-3-Hydroxy-3-methylbutanoic acid 7-[2-[2-(dimethylamino)ethoxy]-2-oxoethylidene]tetradecahydro-1,1,4a,8-tetramethyl-9-oxo-2-phenanthrenyl ester. $C_{29}H_{47}NO_6$; mol wt 505.69. C 68.88%, H 9.37%, N 2.77%, O 18.98%. Cardiotonic principle from the bark of *Erythrophleum couminga* Baillon, *Leguminosae*. Isoln: Ruzicka *et al.*, *Helv. Chim. Acta* **24**, 63 (1941). Structure: Ruzicka *et al.*, *ibid.* 1449.

Thin shiny needles from ether, mp 142°. $[\alpha]_D^{20}$ −70°. Sol in methanol, ethanol, acetone, acetic acid, benzene, chloroform. Practically insol in water, hexane, ether.

Hydrochloride. $C_{29}H_{47}NO_6 \cdot HCl$. Crystals from ethanol + ether, mp 195°. Sol in ethanol, water.

2566. Crabtree's Catalyst. [64536-78-3] [(1,2,5,6-η)-1,5-Cyclooctadiene](pyridine)(tricyclohexylphosphine)iridium(1+) hexafluorophosphate(1−); Felkin-Crabtree catalyst. $C_{31}H_{50}$-IrNP.F_6P; mol wt 804.89. C 46.26%, H 6.26%, Ir 23.88%, N 1.74%, P 7.70%, F 14.16%. Stereoselective organoiridium based catalyst used primarily for hydrogenation of the general formula [Ir(cod)L(py)]metal complex where cod is 1,5-cyclooctadiene, L is tertiary phosphine, py is pyridine. Prepn: R. H. Crabtree, G. E. Morris, *J. Organomet. Chem.* **135**, 395 (1977); R. H. Crabtree *et al.*, *ibid.* **141**, 205 (1977); R. H. Crabtree, S. M. Morehouse, *Inorg. Synth.* **24**, 173 (1986). Hydrogenation study: J. W. Suggs *et al.*, *Tetrahedron Lett.* **22**, 303 (1981); directing effects: J. M. Brown, S. A. Hall, *Tetrahedron* **41**, 4639 (1985); R. H. Crabtree, M. W. Davis, *J. Org. Chem.* **51**, 2655 (1986). Structure: M. S. Abbassioun *et al.*, *Acta Crystallogr.* **C45**, 331 (1989). Synthetic applications: M. Weck *et al.*, *J. Org. Chem.* **64**, 5463 (1999); J. M. Bueno *et al.*, *Tetrahedron Lett.* **41**, 4379 (2000).

Orange crystalline solid. d 1.67 g/cm³. Air stable. Sol in CH_2Cl_2, $CHCl_3$ and Me_2CO. Insol in alcohols, water, benzene, diethyl ether and hexane.

Tetrafluoroborate. [80409-82-1] $C_{31}H_{50}IrNP.BF_4$; mol wt 746.73.

USE: Catalyst for selective reduction of hindered carbon-carbon double bonds.

2567. Crataegus. Hawthorn; English hawthorn; haws; haw apple; aubépine. Berries, flowers, and leaves of *Crataegus oxyacantha* L., *Rosaceae*. Habit. All temperate zones, abundant in Europe, a garden escape in North America. Constit. Triterpene acids (oleanolic, ursolic, crataegolic); purines; anthocyanin type pigments and flavone deriv (pelargonin, quercitrin); choline; acetylcholine; trimethylamine; chlorogenic acid; caffeic acid; ascorbic acid; a growth hormone for caterpillars; a substance named RN 30/9: Hahn *et al.*, *Arzneim.-Forsch.* **10**, 825 (1960). Some commercial extracts are: *Curtacrat*; *Crataegus-Kreussler*; *Esbericard*. Review and bibliography: F. Berger, *Handbuch der Drogenkunde* **vol. 3** (Vienna, 1952) pp 202-211.

THERAP CAT: Cardiotonic, vasodilator (coronary).

2568. Creatine. [57-00-1] N-(Aminoiminomethyl)-N-methylglycine; N-amidinosarcosine; (α-methylguanido)acetic acid; N-methyl-N-guanylglycine; methylglycocyamine. $C_4H_9N_3O_2$; mol wt 131.13. C 36.64%, H 6.92%, N 32.04%, O 24.40%. Amino acid that participates in the transfer of high energy phosphate in muscle cells. Predominantly found in skeletal and cardiac muscle; occurring also in its phosphorylated form, *see* phosphocreatine. Produced by liver, pancreas and kidneys by the transfer of the guanidine moiety of arginine to glycine which is then methylated to give creatine. First identified in meat extracts by Chevreul in 1835; name derived from the Greek "kreas," meaning flesh. Synthesis by heating cyanamide with sarcosine: Strecker, *Jahresber. Chem.* **1868**, 686; *cf.* Volhard, *Z. Chem.* **5**, 318 (1869); Paulmann, *Arch. Pharm.* **232**, 638 (1894); Bergmann, Zervas, *Z. Physiol. Chem.* **173**, 80 (1928); King *J. Chem. Soc.* **1930**, 2374. Use in diagnosis of myocardial infarction: J. Delanghe *et al.*, *Ann. Clin. Biochem.* **25**, 383 (1988). HPLC determn in cardiac muscle: T. Teerlink *et al.*, *Anal. Biochem.* **214**, 278 (1993). Review of role in energy metabolism: S. P. Bessman, C. L. Carpenter, *Annu. Rev. Biochem.* **54**, 831-862 (1985). Review of efficacy and safety as nutritional supplement: A. S. Graham, R. C. Hatton, *J. Am. Pharm. Assoc.* **39**, 803-810 (1999); of effects of dietary supplementation on exercise performance: T. W. Demant, E. C. Rhodes, *Sports Med.* **28**, 49-60 (1999); A. Casey, P. L. Greenhaff, *Am. J. Clin. Nutr.* **72**, Suppl., 607S-617S (2000).

Monoclinic prisms from water as the monohydrate. Becomes anhyd at 100°; dec 303°. Neutral reaction to litmus. pKb (20°) 11.02. Adsorption on various chromatographic agents: Grettie, Williams, *J. Am. Chem. Soc.* **50**, 671 (1928). Absorption spectrum: Abderhalden, Haas, *Z. Physiol. Chem.* **164**, 7 (1927). One gram of the monohydrate dissolves in 75 ml water, in about 9 liters alcohol. Insol in ether.

2569. Creatinine. [60-27-5] 2-Amino-1,5-dihydro-1-methyl-4H-imidazol-4-one; 2-amino-1-methyl-4-imidazolidinone; 1-methylhydantoin-2-imide; 1-methylglycocyamidine. $C_4H_7N_3O$; mol wt 113.12. C 42.47%, H 6.24%, N 37.15%, O 14.14%. The end product of creatine catabolism. Normal constituent of urine; daily output about 25 mg/kg of body weight. Also found together with creatine in muscle tissues and blood. Occurs in all soils and in grain seeds and other vegetable matter. Has been found in certain fish and in crab meat extract. Isoln from urine: Maly, *Ann.* **159**, 279 (1871); Folin, *J. Biol. Chem.* **17**, 463 (1914); Benedict, *ibid.* **18**, 183 (1914). The isoln from urine is tedious, and creatinine is usually prepd from commercial creatine by treatment with HCl: Edgar, Hinegardner, *ibid.* **56**, 881 (1923); *Org. Synth.* **4**, 15 (1925).

Monoclinic plates. Leaflets from water. Dec about 300°. pKb (40°) 10.45. Sol in 12 parts water; slightly sol in alc. Practically insol in acetone, ether, chloroform.

2570. Creolin. [12751-04-1] Pearson's creolin. Prepd from refined coal-tar oils. Approx composition: Tar acids and oils 75-77%; emulsifying soaps 15-17%; water 8-10%.

Dark brown liquid, characteristic odor resembling that of phenol. Phenol coefficient (against *B. typhosus*) about 10. d 1.02-1.04. Forms stable milky emulsions when dil with much water. Miscible with a small amount of water; also miscible with alcohol, ether, chloroform.

USE: As a general industrial and household disinfectant and deodorant in 1-3% emulsion in water.

THERAP CAT (VET): Antiseptic, parasiticide. Do not use on cats.

2571. Creosol. [93-51-6] 2-Methoxy-4-methylphenol; 2-methoxy-*p*-cresol; 4-methylguaiacol; 3-methoxy-4-hydroxytoluene; 4-hydroxy-3-methoxy-1-methylbenzene. $C_8H_{10}O_2$; mol wt 138.16. C 69.55%, H 7.30%, O 23.16%. Occurs in beechwood tar. It is one of the active constituents of creosote. Obtained by the Clemmensen reduction of vanillin using amalgamated zinc and toluene as auxiliary solvent: Fletcher, Tarbell, *J. Am. Chem. Soc.* **65**, 1431 (1943); Schwarz, Hering, *Org. Synth.* **coll. vol. IV**, 203 (1963).

Colorless to yellowish, strongly refractive, aromatic liq. d_4^{25} 1.092. bp_{760} 220°; bp_{15} 105°; bp_4 79°. mp 5.5°. n_D^{25} 1.5353. Slightly sol in water; miscible with alcohol, benzene, chloroform, ether, glacial acetic acid.

Note: Not to be confused with cresol.

2572. Creosote, Coal Tar. [8001-58-9] Coal tar creosote. A distillate of coal tar produced by high temp carbonization of bituminous coal. *Constit.* Liq and solid aromatic hydrocarbons, tar acids (up to 3%) and tar bases. History and composition: Roche, *J. For. Prod. Res. Soc.* **2**, 75 (1952). Characterization by GLC: F. H. M. Nestler, *Anal. Chem.* **46**, 46 (1974). GC-MS analysis in treated railroad ties: W. Rotard, W. Mailahn, *ibid.* **59**, 65 (1987). Review of constituents, uses and carcinogenic risk: *IARC Monographs* **35**, 83-159 (1985); of toxicology and human exposure: *Toxicological Profile for Wood Creosote, Coal Tar Creosote, Coal Tar, Coal Tar Pitch, and Coal Tar Pitch Volatiles* (PB2003-100136, 2002) 394 pp.

Translucent brown to black, oily liq. Flammable. Characteristic sharp, penetrating smoky odor; burning caustic taste. Heavier than water. *Typical specification:* $d_{15.5}^{38.0}$ 1.06. Distillation ranges: Up to 210° not >5%; up to 235° not >25% nor <5%; up to 270° not <20%; up to 355° not >85% nor <60%. Flash pt 165°F (75°C); ignition temp 637°F (335°C). Practically insol in water.

Caution: Readily absorbed through GI tract and skin. Potential symptoms following oral overexposure are intense GI irritation and congestion. Symptoms of systemic poisoning include salivation, vomiting, respiratory difficulties, thready pulse, vertigo, headache, loss of pupillary reflexes, hypothermia, cyanosis and mild convulsions. Direct contact may cause skin, eye or mucous membrane irritation, burning and itching, erythema, papular and vesicular eruptions, keratoconjunctivitis. *See Patty's Industrial Hygiene and Toxicology* **Vol. 2B**, G. D. Clayton, F. E. Clayton, Eds. (John Wiley & Sons, Inc., New York, 4th ed., 1994) pp 1602-1605. Coal tar and coal tar pitches are listed as known human carcinogens: *Report on Carcinogens, Eleventh Edition* (PB2005-104914, 2004) p III-68.

USE: Wood preservative, disinfectant, insecticide.

THERAP CAT (VET): Has been used as an anthelmintic.

2573. Creosote, Wood. [8021-39-4] Wood creosote; beechwood creosote; Creasote. Liquid obtained from wood tars by dis-

tillation; composed chiefly of guaiacol and creosol, *q.q.v.* Analysis of constituents by GC-MS and HPLC: N. Ogata, T. Baba, *Res. Commun. Chem. Pathol. Pharmacol.* **66**, 411 (1989). Acute toxicity: T. Miyazato *et al., Oyo Yakuri* **21**, 899 (1981), *C.A.* **96**, 28311h (1982). Chronic toxicity and carcinogenicity studies: *eidem, ibid.* **28**, 909, 925 (1984), *C.A.* **102**, 41238b, 57380c (1985). *See also: Clinical Toxicology of Commercial Products*, R. E. Gosselin *et al.*, Eds. (Williams & Wilkins, Baltimore, 5th ed., 1984) Section II, p 192. Review of toxicology and human exposure: *Toxicological Profile for Wood Creosote, Coal Tar Creosote, Coal Tar, Coal Tar Pitch, and Coal Tar Pitch Volatiles* (PB2003-100136, 2002) 394 pp.

Almost colorless or yellowish, very refractive, oily liq; characteristic smoky odor; caustic, burning taste. d_{25}^{25} not below 1.076. Begins to boil at about 203° and at least 90% by vol distills between 203-220°. Does not solidify at −20°. Sol in 150-200 parts water, in glycerol, glacial acetic acid, fixed alkali hydroxide solns; miscible with alcohol, chloroform, ether, oils.

Benzoate. Yellowish liquid. Insol in water. Freely sol in alcohol or ether.

Carbonate. Colorless to yellowish, clear, viscid, oily liquid; odorless and tasteless or slight odor and taste of creosote. d_{25}^{25} not below 1.145. Insol in water. Freely sol in alcohol; sol in petr ether, fixed oils. Miscible with benzene, chloroform.

Oleate. Oleocreosote. Yellowish, oily liquid. d 0.950. Insol in water. Sol in benzene, chloroform, ether.

Phosphate. Phosote. Mixture of the phosphoric acid esters of creosote. Yellowish, almost odorless, viscid mass. d_{15}^{15} 1.19. bp 230-235° with decompn. Insol in water. Sol in alcohol.

Valerate. Eosote. Colorless to yellowish liquid. bp about 240°. Insol in water. Sol in alcohol, ether.

THERAP CAT: Antiseptic; expectorant.

THERAP CAT (VET): Antiseptic, parasiticide, deodorant; has been used as expectorant, gastric sedative and gastrointestinal antiseptic. Do not use in cats.

2574. Creosotic Acid. Mixture of the isomeric cresotic acids. White or reddish-white powder. Slightly sol in water; sol in alcohol, ether, alkali hydroxide solns.

USE: Disinfectant generally and in veterinary medicine in 1:500 aq or soap soln; manuf dyes and artificial tannin.

2575. Creslan®. Fiber X-54; Exlan. A copolymer of acrylonitrile possibly with acrylamide or a substituted acrylamide. *Ref:* R. W. Moncrieff, *Man-Made Fibres* (John Wiley, New York, 1963) p 483.

Off-white fiber. Specific gravity 1.17. Sticks at 210°. Shrinkage in boiling water, 1%. Sunlight has negligible effect. Resistance to acids: good except to mineral acids. Resistance to alkalies: fair to dilute, poor to concd. Good resistance to cleaning solvents. Superior to its forerunner, *fiber X-51*, in the ease with which it can be dyed.

USE: Recommended for those uses that acrylics generally fill. It is claimed that it can be durably pleated.

2576. *o*-Cresolphthalein. [596-27-0] 3,3-Bis(4-hydroxy-3-methylphenyl)-1(3*H*)-isobenzofuranone; 3,3′-dimethylphenolphthalein. $C_{22}H_{18}O_4$; mol wt 346.38. C 76.28%, H 5.24%, O 18.48%. Prepn: F. J. Welcher, *Organic Analytical Reagents* **vol. 4** (Van Nostrand, New York, 1948) p 482; Hubacher *et al., J. Am. Pharm. Assoc.* **42**, 23 (1953).

Crystals from alc, mp 223°. Slightly sol in water; sol in alcohol. pK 9.4.

USE: As indicator: pH range, 8.2 colorless, 9.8 red. Analytical reagent.

2577. Cresol Purple. [2303-01-7] 4,4′-(1,1-Dioxido-3*H*-2,1-benzoxathiol-3-ylidene)bis[3-methylphenol]; *m*-cresolsulfonphthalein. C$_{21}$H$_{18}$O$_5$S; mol wt 382.43. C 65.95%, H 4.74%, O 20.92%, S 8.38%. pH sensitive dye. Prepn: W. R. Orndorff, A. C. Purdy, *J. Am. Chem. Soc.* **48**, 2212 (1926). Solvent effects: J. Barbosa *et al.*, *Mikrochim. Acta* **106**, 327 (1992). Ionization and spectral properties: R. Casula *et al.*, *Talanta* **40**, 1781 (1993); M. C. Aragoni *et al.*, *ibid.* **42**, 1157 (1995). Titrimetric determn: K. Vytras *et al.*, *Analyst* **114**, 479 (1989). Use as pH indicator for emission of NO$_2$ in museum collections: J. Fenn, *Polym. Prepr.* **37**, 170 (1996); in wine: E. N. Gaiao *et al.*, *Analyst* **124**, 1727 (1999); in buffered solns: S. Paula *et al.*, *Biochemistry* **38**, 3025 (1999).

Slightly sol in ethanol; sol in ethanol denatured with 10% methanol. pH 1.2 red; pH 2.8 yellow; pH 7.4 yellow; pH 9.0 purple.
USE: Acid-base indicator.

2578. Cresol Red. [1733-12-6] 4,4′-(1,1-Dioxido-3*H*-2,1-benzoxathiol-3-ylidene)bis[2-methylphenol]; α-hydroxy-α,α-bis(4-hydroxy-*m*-tolyl)-*o*-toluenesulfonic acid γ-sultone; *o*-cresolsulfonphthalein. C$_{21}$H$_{18}$O$_5$S; mol wt 382.43. C 65.95%, H 4.74%, O 20.92%, S 8.38%. pH sensitive dye. Prepn: M. D. Sohon, *Am. Chem. J.* **20**, 257 (1898); and properties: H. A. Lubs, W. M. Clark, *J. Wash. Acad. Sci.* **6**, 481 (1916). Raman spectrum: K. Machida *et al.*, *J. Raman Spectrosc.* **8**, 172 (1979). Ionization and spectral properties: R. Casula *et al.*, *Talanta* **40**, 1781 (1993); M. C. Aragoni *et al.*, *ibid.* **42**, 1157 (1995). Protein dye binding stoichiometry: I. Molnár-Perl *et al.*, *Food Chem.* **35**, 69 (1990). Use in detection of alkaloids via ion-associates: Z. Skalican *et al.*, *Anal. Lett.* **28**, 1223 (1995); as pH indicator for emission of NO$_2$ in museum collections: J. Fenn, *Polym. Prepr.* **37**, 170 (1996); for archived photographic films: J. C. Harthan *et al.*, *Imaging Sci. J.* **45**, 81 (1997); for microbiological media: L. A. Actis *et al.*, *J. Microbiol. Methods* **39**, 79 (1999).

Reddish-brown cryst powder. Sol in alcohol. pH 0.2: red; pH 1.8 yellow; pH 7.2 yellow; pH 8.8 reddish-purple.
USE: Acid-base indicator.

2579. Cresols. [1319-77-3] Cresylic acid; cresylol; tricresol. C$_7$H$_8$O; mol wt 108.14. C 77.75%, H 7.46%, O 14.80%. Mixture of the three isomeric cresols, in which the *m*-isomer predominates. Obtained from coal tar: Paulsen, US **2998457** (1962 to Ashland Oil & Ref.). Usually contains a few per cent phenol. Prepn by sulfonation of toluene: Englund *et al.*, *Ind. Eng. Chem.* **45**, 189 (1953); by oxidation of toluene: Braunwarth, Winsted, US **2994722** (1961 to Pure Oil). Toxicity study: W. B. Deichmann, S. Witherup, *J. Pharmacol. Exp. Ther.* **80**, 233 (1944). Review of manuf processes: *Faith, Keyes & Clark's Industrial Chemicals*, F. A. Lowenheim, M. K. Moran, Eds. (Wiley-Interscience, New York,

4th ed., 1975) pp 285-293; of toxicology and human exposure: *Toxicological Profile for Cresols* (PB93-110732, 1992) 175 pp.

Colorless, yellowish, brownish-yellow or pinkish liq; phenolic odor; becomes darker with age and on exposure to light. *Poisonous!* d$_{25}^{25}$ 1.030-1.038. Not less than 90% by vol distills between 195-205°. Soluble in about 50 parts water; miscible with alcohol, benzene, ether, glycerol, petr ether; also sol in solns of fixed alkali hydroxides. A soln in water is neutral to bromocresol purple. *Protect from light.*

m-**Cresol.** [108-39-4] 3-Methylphenol. Obtained from coal tar: Maesawa, Kurakano, **JP 55 8929** (1955 to Osaka Gas), *C.A.* **52**, 1231d (1958); Macak, Rehak, *Brennst.-Chem.* **43**, 80 (1962). Prepn from toluene: Toland, US **2760991** (1956 to California Res. Corp.); by oxidation of *o*- or *p*-toluic acid: Kaeding *et al.*, *Ind. Eng. Chem.* **53**, 805 (1961). Colorless or yellowish liquid; phenolic odor. d$_4^{20}$ 1.034. bp 202°. mp 11-12°. Flash pt, closed cup: 187°F (86°C). n$_D^{20}$ 1.5398. Sol in about 40 parts water, in solns of fixed alkali hydroxides; miscible with alc, chloroform, ether. LD$_{50}$ orally in rats: 2.02 g/kg (Deichmann, Witherup).

o-**Cresol.** [95-48-7] 2-Methylphenol; *o*-cresylic acid; *o*-hydroxytoluene. Prepn from *m*-toluic acid: Toland, US **2766294** (1956 to California Res. Corp.); Barnard, Meyer, US **2852567** (1958 to Dow). Crystals or liq, becoming dark with age and exposure to air and light; phenolic odor. d$_4^{20}$ 1.047. bp 191-192°. mp 30°. Flash pt 81-83°C. n$_D^{20}$ 1.553. Sol in about 40 parts water, in solns of the fixed alkali hydroxides. Miscible with alcohol, chloroform, ether. *Protect from light.* LD$_{50}$ orally in rats: 1.35 g/kg (Deichmann, Witherup).

p-**Cresol.** [106-44-5] 4-Methylphenol. Obtained from coal tar. Laboratory prepn from *p*-toluenesulfonic acid by fusion with potassium hydroxide: W. W. Hartman, *Org. Synth.* **coll. vol. I**, 175 (2nd ed., 1941); from toluene: Braunwarth, US **3046305** (1962 to Pure Oil). Crystals. Phenolic odor. d$_4^{20}$ 1.0341. mp 35.5°. bp$_{760}$ 201.8°; bp$_{200}$ 179.4°; bp$_{100}$ 140.0°; bp$_{40}$ 117.7°; bp$_{20}$ 102.3°; bp$_{10}$ 88.6°; bp$_5$ 76.5°; bp$_{1.0}$ 53.0°. Flash pt (closed cup) 86°C (187°F). Volatile in steam. n$_D^{20}$ 1.5395. 100 ml water dissolves about 2.5 g at 50°, about 5 g at 100°. Sol in aq solns of alkali hydroxides, in the usual organic solvents. LD$_{50}$ orally in rats: 1.8 g/kg (Deichmann, Witherup).

Caution: Potential symptoms of overexposure to *o*-, *m*- or *p*-isomers are irritation of eyes, skin and mucous membranes; CNS effects; confusion, depression and respiratory failure; dyspnea, irregular rapid respiration and weak pulse; skin and eye burns; dermatitis; lung, liver, kidney and pancreas damage. *See* NIOSH *Pocket Guide to Chemical Hazards* (DHHS/NIOSH 97-140, 1997) p 78. Symptoms of intoxication are similar to those produced by phenol, *q.v.* Acute exposure may cause muscular weakness, gastroenteric disturbances, severe depression, collapse and death. Chronic exposure may cause digestive disturbances, liver and kidney damage, and skin eruptions. Cresol has a marked corrosive action on tissues, producing burns and dermatitis. *See Patty's Industrial Hygiene and Toxicology* **vol. 2A**, G. D. Clayton, F. E. Clayton, Eds. (Wiley-Interscience, New York, 3rd ed., 1981) pp 2597-2601.

USE: For making synthetic resins; in disinfectants and fumigants; as industrial solvent; *m*-cresol in photographic developers, explosives.

THERAP CAT: Disinfectant.

THERAP CAT (VET): Local antiseptic, parasiticide, disinfectant; has been used as an intestinal antiseptic.

2580. *m*-Cresotic Acid. [50-85-1] 2-Hydroxy-4-methylbenzoic acid; 2,4-cresotic acid; *m*-homosalicylic acid; *m*-cresotinic acid; 2-hydroxy-*p*-toluic acid; γ-cresotic acid. C$_8$H$_8$O$_3$; mol wt 152.15. C 63.15%, H 5.30%, O 31.55%. Prepn: Prelog *et al.*, *Helv. Chim. Acta* **30**, 675 (1947); Baine *et al.*, *J. Org. Chem.* **19**, 510 (1954); Hauptschein *et al.*, *J. Am. Chem. Soc.* **77**, 2284 (1955).

Crystals or leaflets, mp 177°; volatile with steam. Soly as of the *o*-acid.

Caution: Toxicity is similar to salicylic acid, *q.v.*

USE: In manuf of dyes.

2581. *o*-Cresotic Acid. [83-40-9] 2-Hydroxy-3-methyl-benzoic acid; 2,3-cresotic acid; *o*-homosalicylic acid; *o*-cresotinic acid; 2-hydroxy-*m*-toluic acid; 3-methylsalicylic acid. $C_8H_8O_3$; mol wt 152.15. C 63.15%, H 5.30%, O 31.55%. Prepn: Baine *et al., J. Org. Chem.* **19**, 510 (1954); Jones, *Chem. Ind. (London)* **1958**, 228; Blicke, McCarty, *J. Org. Chem.* **24**, 1061 (1959); Wessely *et al., Ber.* **93**, 2840 (1960).

White to slightly reddish, odorless cystals, mp 165-166°; volatile with steam. Slightly sol in cold, more sol in hot water; sol in chloroform, alcohol, ether, alkali hydroxides.

Caution: Toxicity is similar to salicylic acid.

USE: In manuf of dyes.

2582. *p*-Cresotic Acid. [89-56-5] 2-Hydroxy-5-methyl-benzoic acid; 2,5-cresotic acid; *p*-cresotic acid; 6-hydroxy-*m*-toluic acid. $C_8H_8O_3$; mol wt 152.15. C 63.15%, H 5.30%, O 31.55%. Prepn: Cameron *et al., J. Org. Chem.* **15**, 233 (1950); Baine *et al., ibid.* **19**, 510 (1954); Thomas *et al., J. Am. Chem. Soc.* **80**, 5864 (1958); Blicke, McCarty, *J. Org. Chem.* **24**, 1061 (1959).

White or slightly reddish, almost odorless crystals, mp 151°. Volatile with steam. Sublimes with partial decompn. Soly as of the *o*-acid.

Caution: Toxicity is similar to salicylic acid.

2583. *m*-Cresyl Acetate. [122-46-3] Acetic acid 3-methyl-phenyl ester; *m*-tolyl acetate; *m*-cresol acetic acid ester; acetic acid *m*-cresol ester; acetylmetacresol; metacresol acetate; Cresatin. $C_9H_{10}O_2$; mol wt 150.17. C 71.98%, H 6.71%, O 21.31%. Germicide with pain-relieving properties. Prepn: Claus, Hirsch, *J. Prakt. Chem.* [2] **39**, 62 (1889); Eijkman, *Chem. Weekbl.* **1**, 453 (1904); *see also* US **1031971** (1912 to N. Sulzberger). Purification: Lebeau-Janot, *Traité Pharm. Chim.* **II**, 882 (Paris, 1955). Use in dentistry: J. M. Gergely, P. M. DiFiore, *Gen. Dent.* **41**, 328 (1993).

Oily liq. Volatile with steam. Characteristic phenolic odor with a reminiscence of acetone. d_4^{26} 1.048. bp 212°; bp_{13} 99°. uv max (methanol): 262.5, 269.5 nm. Practically insol in water, glycerol.

Miscible with alc, ether, chloroform, petr ether, benzene. Soly in liq petrolatum about 5%. Also sol in cottonseed oil.

THERAP CAT: Antiseptic (topical).

THERAP CAT (VET): Antiseptic (topical).

2584. *o*-Cresyl Acetate. [533-18-6] Acetic acid 2-methyl-phenyl ester; acetic acid *o*-tolyl ester; *o*-cresol acetate; acetyl-*o*-cresol; *o*-cresylic acetate; *o*-tolyl acetate. $C_9H_{10}O_2$; mol wt 150.17. C 71.98%, H 6.71%, O 21.31%. $CH_3C_6H_4OCOCH_3$.

Liquid. bp ~208°. Almost insol in cold, sol in hot water; freely sol in usual organic solvents, in oils.

2585. *p*-Cresyl Phenylacetate. [101-94-0] Benzeneacetic acid 4-methylphenyl ester; *p*-tolyl phenylacetate. $C_{15}H_{14}O_2$; mol wt 226.27. C 79.62%, H 6.24%, O 14.14%. Synthetic organic ester in perfumery. Prepn: W. Autenrieth, G. Thomae, *Ber.* **57**, 423 (1924). Fragrance monograph: *Food Cosmet. Toxicol.* **13**, 775 (1975). Photochemistry study: C.-H. Tung, Y.-M. Ying, *J. Chem. Soc. Perkin Trans.* 2 **1997**, 1319. Synthesis using montmorillonite catalysts: C. R. Reddy *et al., J. Mol. Catal. A* **223**, 117 (2004). Environmentally benign synthesis of perfumery grade product: G. D. Yadav, S. V. Lande, *Org. Process Res. Dev.* **9**, 288 (2005).

Prisms from alcohol, mp 75-76°. Organoleptic character similar to honey, nuts, and butter. LD_{50} (g/kg): >5 orally in rats; >5 dermally in rabbits (*Food Cosmet. Toxicol.*).

USE: In jasmine, narcissus, hyacinth, lily, and jonquille perfume compositions; fixative; fragrance ingredient in soaps and household products.

2586. CRF. [9015-71-8] Corticotropin-releasing factor; CRH; corticoliberin(e); corticotropin-releasing hormone. Hypothalamic substance that stimulates secretion of ACTH, *q.v.* and β-endorphin from the pituitary. First direct evidence for its presence in hypothalami: R. Guillemin, B. Rosenberg, *Endocrinology* **57**, 599 (1955); M. Saffran, A. V. Schally, *Can. J. Biochem. Physiol.* **33**, 408 (1955). Purification and characterization of a 41-residue ovine hypothalamic CRF that is highly potent in stimulating secretion of corticotropin and β-endorphin-like immunoactivities: W. Vale *et al., Science* **213**, 1394 (1981). Primary structure: J. Spiess *et al., Proc. Natl. Acad. Sci. USA* **78**, 6517 (1981). When centrally administered, CRF activates the sympathetic nervous system and may therefore function as a key hormone in stress mobilization of the organism, *cf.* W. Vale *et al., loc. cit.;* M. Brown *et al., Life Sci.* **30**, 207 (1982). CRF also stimulates α-MSH secretion and cyclic AMP accumulation in rat pars intermedia cells: H. Meunier *et al., ibid.* **31**, 2129 (1982). A functional relationship between CRF and dynorphin-related opioid peptides has also been suggested: K. A. Roth *et al., Science* **219**, 189 (1983). *Reviews:* A. V. Schally *et al., Recent Prog. Horm. Res.* **24**, 497-588 (1968); R. Burgus, R. Guillemin, *Annu. Rev. Biochem.* **39**, 499-526 (1970); M. Saffran in *Hypothalamic Peptide Hormones and Pituitary Regulation,* J. C. Porter, Ed. (Plenum Press, New York, 1977) pp 225-235; W. Vale *et al.* in *The Role of Peptides in Neuronal Function,* J. L. Barker, J. G. Smith, Eds. (Dekker, New York, 1980) pp 432-454; several authors in *Polypeptide Hormones,* R. F. Beers, E. G. Bassett, Eds. (Raven Press, New York, 1980) pp 165-291; B. Lutz-Bucher *et al., J. Physiol.* **77**, 939-950 (1981); N. Yasuda *et al., Endocr. Rev.* **3**, 123-140 (1982); E. Stark, G. B. Makara in *Hormonally Active Brain Peptides: Structure and Function,* K. W. McKerns, V. Pantic, Eds. (Plenum Press, New York, 1982) pp 157-179.

Activity is destroyed by trypsin; unaffected by thioglycolate, pepsin, chymotrypsin.

2587. Crilanomer. [37291-07-9] Starch polymer with 2-propenenitrile; Super-Slurper; Clinagel; Intrasite. Hydrolyzed starch-polyacrylonitrile graft copolymers capable of absorbing 2000 times their initial weight of liquid. Prepn: L. A. Gugliemelli *et al., J. Appl. Polym. Sci.* **13**, 2007 (1969). Continuous production: Z. Reyes *et al., Ind. Eng. Chem. Process Des. Dev.* **12**, 62 (1973);

manufacturing process: M. O. Weaver *et al., Staerke* **29,** 413 (1977). Analysis: R. J. Dennenberg, T.P. Abbott, *J. Polym. Sci. Polym. Lett. Ed.* **14,** 693 (1976). Use in wound dressings: W. R. Spence, **US 4226232** (1980 to Spenco Med). Clinical evaluation in leg ulceration: M. Hornemann, G. Raptis, *Z. Hautkrankhr.* **62,** 41 (1987); B. Esch, G. Raptis, *ibid.* **64,** 1135 (1989). Brief description: H.-G. Elias, *Polym. News* **4,** 26 (1977).

Dry powder.

USE: In dressings for wounds. Absorption of liquids in products ranging from disposable diapers to seed coatings.

2588. Croceic Acid. [132-57-0] 7-Hydroxy-1-naphthalene-sulfonic acid; 2-naphthol-8-sulfonic acid; Bayer's acid. $C_{10}H_8O_4$-S; mol wt 224.23. C 53.56%, H 3.60%, O 28.54%, S 14.30%. Prepn: Nietzki, Zübelen, *Ber.* **22,** 453 (1889); Forster, Keyworth, *J. Soc. Chem. Ind. London* **46,** 26T (1927).

On evaporation of an aq soln, the free acid dec into sulfuric acid and β-naphthol. However, very concd solns of the acid can be obtained. The normal sodium salt is sol in water, and readily sol in alcohol, crystallizing with 2 mols of alcohol. *Ref:* Forster, Keyworth, *loc. cit.*

2589. Crocetin. [27876-94-4] 8,8′-Diapo-ψ,ψ-carotene-dioic acid; *trans*-crocetin. $C_{20}H_{24}O_4$; mol wt 328.40. C 73.15%, H 7.37%, O 19.49%. Carotenoid-dicarboxylic acid isolated from *Crocus sativus* L.; *C. albiflorus* var. *neapolitanus* Hort.; *C. luteus* Lam., *Iridaceae.* Extraction procedure and structure: Jucker, Karrer, *Carotinoide* (Basel, 1948) p 282.

Brick-red rhombs from acetic anhydride, mp 285°. Absorption max (pyridine): 464, 436, 411 nm. Sol in pyridine, in very dil NaOH solns. Very sparingly sol in water, and in the usual organic solvents except pyridine and similar organic bases. Forms a solid dipyridyl salt.

Dimethyl ester. $C_{22}H_{28}O_4$. Brick-red elongated leaflets, mp 222.5°. Total synthesis: Buchta, Andree, *Naturwissenschaften* **46,** 74 (1959).

Di-gentiobiose ester. [42553-65-1] Crocin. $C_{44}H_{64}O_{24}$; mol wt 976.96. One of the yellow-red pigments of saffron. Isoln and structure: Karrer, Salomon, *Helv. Chim. Acta* **10,** 397 (1927); **11,** 513, 711 (1928); Karrer *et al., ibid.* **12,** 985 (1929); **13,** 392 (1930); Kuhn, Winterstein, *Ber.* **67,** 344 (1934); Reichstein, *Angew. Chem.* **74,** 887 (1962). Hydrated brownish-red needles from methanol, mp 186° (effervescence). Absorption max (methanol): 464, 434 nm. Freely sol in hot water giving an orange-colored soln. Sparingly sol in abs alcohol, ether, other organic solvents.

2590. Cromolyn. [16110-51-3] 5,5′-[(2-Hydroxy-1,3-propanediyl)bis(oxy)]bis[4-oxo-4*H*-1-benzopyran-2-carboxylic acid]; 5,5′-[(2-hydroxytrimethylene)dioxy]bis(4-oxo-4*H*-1-benzopyran-2-carboxylic acid); 5,5′-(2-hydroxytrimethylenedioxy)bis(4-oxochromene-2-carboxylic acid); 1,3-bis(2-carboxychromon-5-yloxy)-2-hydroxypropane; 1,3-di(2-carboxy-4-oxochromen-5-yloxy)-propan-2-ol; cromoglycic acid. $C_{23}H_{16}O_{11}$; mol wt 468.37. C 58.98%, H 3.44%, O 37.58%. Chromone complex which blocks mast cell degranulation. Prepn: **NL 6603997**; C. Fitzmaurice, T. B. Lee, **US 3419578** (1966, 1968 both to Fisons). Metabolism: M. J. Ashton *et al., Toxicol. Appl. Pharmacol.* **26,** 319 (1973). Mechanism of action: T. C. Theoharides *et al., Science* **207,** 80 (1980); R. G. Alvarez *et al., Agents Actions* **11,** 94 (1981). Toxicology in primates: J. E. Beach *et al., Toxicol. Appl. Pharmacol.* **57,** 367 (1981). Clinical study in allergic conjunctivitis: G. A. Friday *et al., Am. J. Ophthalmol.* **95,** 169 (1983). Review of pharmacology

and clinical use: G. G. Shapiro, P. Konig, *Pharmacotherapy* **5,** 156-170 (1985). *Review:* J. S. G. Cox in *Pharmacological and Biochemical Properties of Drug Substances* vol. **1,** M. E. Goldberg, Ed. (Am. Pharm. Assoc., Washington, DC, 1977) pp 277-310; W. Storms, M. A. Kaliner, *J. Asthma* **42,** 79-89 (2005).

mp 241-242° (dec).

Monohydrate. Colorless crystals from ethanol + ether, mp 216-217° (dec).

Disodium salt. [15826-37-6] Cromolyn sodium; disodium cromoglycate; DSCG; FPL-670; Alloptrex; Allergocrom; Colimune; Cromabak; Cromadoses; Cromedil; Cromogen; Cromoptic; Duracroman; Gastrofrenal; Hay-Crom; Intal; Intercron; Lomudal; Lomupren; Lomusol; Multicrom; Nalcrom; Nalcron; Nasalcrom; Ophtacalm; Opticrom; Rynacrom; Vividrin. $C_{23}H_{14}Na_2O_{11}$; mol wt 512.33. Hygroscopic. Freely sol in water (100 mg/ml at 20°). Practically insol in chloroform and alcohol. LD_{50} in mice, rats (mg/kg): >8000 orally (Cox).

THERAP CAT: Antiasthmatic; antiallergic.

THERAP CAT (VET): Antiallergic.

2591. Cropropamide. [633-47-6] *N*-[1-[(Dimethylamino)-carbonyl]propyl]-*N*-propyl-2-butenamide; *N*-(1-dimethylcarbamoylpropyl)-*N*-propylcrotonamide; α-(*N*′-crotonyl-*N*′-propyl)-amino-*N,N*-dimethylbutyramide. $C_{13}H_{24}N_2O_2$; mol wt 240.34. C 64.97%, H 10.07%, N 11.66%, O 13.31%. Prepn: Martin, Gysin, **US 2447587** (1948 to Geigy).

Liquid, $bp_{0.25}$ 128-130°. Easily sol in water, ether.

Combination with crotethamide. [8015-51-8] Prethcamide; Micoren; Respirot.

THERAP CAT: Analgesic. Combination as respiratory stimulant.

2592. Croscarmellose Sodium. [74811-65-7] Ac-Di-Sol. Internally cross-linked form of carboxymethylcellulose sodium (NaCMC), *q.v.* Prepd by lowering pH of NaCMC in solution, then heating: *Technical Literature,* FMC Corp. Use as tablet disintegrant: D. Gissinger, A. Stamm, *Pharm. Ind.* **42,** 189 (1980); M. E. Sangalli *et al., Boll. Chim. Farm.* **128,** 242 (1989). Evaluation of drug-excipient interaction: R. G. Hollenbeck *et al., J. Pharm. Sci.* **72,** 325 (1983). Water sorption and thermal behavior: D. Faroongsarng, G. E. Peck, *Drug Dev. Ind. Pharm.* **20,** 779 (1994). Mechanism of action study: R. Thibert, B. C. Hancock, *J. Pharm. Sci.* **85,** 1255 (1996).

Free flowing, odorless, white powder. Bulk density (g/cc) 0.48. pH 5.0-7.0. Hydrophilic. Insol in water.

USE: Pharmaceutic aid (tablet disintegrant).

2593. Crotamine. [37196-57-9] One of the poisonous principles found in the venom of Brazilian rattlesnakes, *Crotalus terrificus crotaminicus* Goncalves, *Crotalidae.* A polypeptide having mol wt 10,000-15,000 and isoelectric point at pH 10.3. Purification and properties: Goncalves in *Venoms,* E. E. Buckley, N. Porges, Eds. (Publ. no. **44** of the Am. Assoc. Adv. Science, Washington, D.C., 1956) pp 261-274. Pharmacology: Moussatché *et al., ibid.* pp 275-279.

2594. Crotamiton. [483-63-6] *N*-Ethyl-*N*-(2-methylphenyl)-2-butenamide; *N*-ethyl-*o*-crotonotoluidide; crotonyl-*N*-ethyl-*o*-toluidine; Crotamitex; Eurax; Euraxil; Veteusan. $C_{13}H_{17}NO$; mol wt 203.28. C 76.81%, H 8.43%, N 6.89%, O 7.87%. Prepd by treating crotonic acid *o*-toluidide with diethyl sulfate: **CH 253472**; **CH 253473**; **GB 615137** (1949 to Geigy).

Yellowish oil, bp_{13} 153-155°. Sol in methanol, ethanol.
USE: Fungicide, insecticide.
THERAP CAT: Scabicide.
THERAP CAT (VET): Scabicide; antipruritic.

2595. Crotethamide. [6168-76-9] *N*-[1-[(Dimethylamino)-carbonyl]propyl]-*N*-ethyl-2-butenamide; *N*-(1-dimethylcarbamoyl-propyl)-*N*-ethylcrotonamide; α-(*N'*-crotonyl-*N'*-ethyl)amino-*N,N*-dimethylbutyramide. $C_{12}H_{22}N_2O_2$; mol wt 226.32. C 63.68%, H 9.80%, N 12.38%, O 14.14%. Prepn: Martin, Gysin, **US 2447587** (1948 to Geigy).

Liquid, $bp_{0.03}$ 132-134°. Easily sol in water, ether.
Combination with cropropamide *see* Cropropamide.
THERAP CAT: Analgesic; combination as respiratory stimulant.

2596. Crotonaldehyde. [4170-30-3] 2-Butenal; crotonic aldehyde; β-methylacrolein. C_4H_6O; mol wt 70.09. C 68.54%, H 8.63%, O 22.83%. $CH_3CH=CHCHO$. Commercial product is a 95:5 mixture of *trans:cis* isomers. Prepn: v. Auwers, Eisenlohr, *J. Prakt. Chem.* **82**, 115 (1910); Hibbert, *J. Am. Chem. Soc.* **37**, 1759 (1915). Alternate synthesis: J. Smidt *et al., Angew. Chem.* **71**, 176 (1959). Toxicity studies: H. F. Smyth, C. P. Carpenter, *J. Ind. Hyg. Toxicol.* **26**, 269 (1944). Review of use in commercial processes: O. Horn, *Ind. Eng. Chem.* **51**, 655-658 (1959). *Reviews:* J. E. Fernandez, T. W. G. Solomons, *Chem. Rev.* **62**, 485-502 (1962); W. Blau *et al., in Ullmann's Encyclopedia of Industrial Chemistry* vol. **A8** (VCH, Weinheim, 5th ed., 1987) pp 83-89. Review of carcinogenic potential: V. J. Feron *et al., Mutat. Res.* **259**, 363-385 (1991); of role in DNA adduct formation: S. S. Hecht *et al., Toxicology* **166**, 31-36 (2001).
Flammable liq. *Lacrimator!* mp −69°; bp 102.2°; d_{20}^{20} 0.853; $n_D^{17.3}$ 1.4384. Flash pt when anhydr: 13°C (55°F) (open cup). Explosive limits in air 2.95-15.5% v/v. Vapor density 2.41 (air = 1). Heat capacity: 0.7 cal/g/°C; heat of vaporization: 123 cal/g. Dimerizes under strong acid conditions, slowly oxidizes to crotonic acid. Soly in water (g/100 g) at 20°: 18.1; at 5°: 19.2. Soly of water in crotonaldehyde (g/100 g) at 20°: 9.5; at 5°: 8.0. LD_{50} orally in rats: 0.3 g/kg (Smyth, Carpenter).
Caution: Potential symptoms of overexposure is irritation of eyes and respiratory system. *See NIOSH Pocket Guide to Chemical Hazards* (DHHS/NIOSH 97-140, 1997) p 80.
USE: Manuf of butyl alcohol, butyraldehyde, methoxy-butyraldehyde, sorbic acid, maleic acid, crotonic acid, crotyl alcohol. In polymer chemistry: manuf of resins and polyvinyl acetals, solvent for polyvinyl chloride, rubber antioxidant, increases rubber strength with ketones. In prepn of insecticides and fertilizers. In production of flavors.

2597. Crotonic Acid. [107-93-7] (2*E*)-2-Butenoic acid; β-methylacrylic acid; α-crotonic acid; solid crotonic acid; *trans*-crotonic acid. $C_4H_6O_2$; mol wt 86.09. C 55.81%, H 7.02%, O 37.17%. Has been found in clay soil in Texas; formed during the dry distillation of wood. Obtained on a commercial scale exclusively by oxygen- or air-oxidation of crotonaldehyde: Kennedy, **US 2413235** (1946 to Shawinigan Chem.); Leupold, PB report 70249 (1942); Matthews, B.I.O.S. report 758 (1946). Laboratory procedure using alkaline silver oxide: Young, *J. Am. Chem. Soc.* **54**, 2498

(1932); from acetaldehyde and malonic acid in pyridine: v. Auwers, *Ann.* **432**, 46 (1923); Backer, Bloemen, *Rec. Trav. Chim.* **45**, 102 (1926); Florence, *Bull. Soc. Chim. Fr.* [4] **41**, 440 (1927); Letch, Linstead, *J. Chem. Soc.* **1932**, 454. Toxicity study: Smyth, Carpenter, *J. Ind. Hyg. Toxicol.* **26**, 269 (1944). *Review:* W. Blau *et al., in Ullmann's Encyclopedia of Industrial Chemistry* vol. **A8** (VCH, Weinheim, 5th ed., 1987) pp 83-89.

Monoclinic needles, prisms from water or ligroin. Corrosive and combustible solid. d_4^{15} 1.018; d_4^{80} 0.964. mp 71.6°. bp_{10} 80.0°; bp_{20} 93.0°; bp_{40} 107.8°; bp_{60} 116.7°; bp_{100} 128.0°; bp_{200} 146.0°; bp_{400} 165.5°; bp_{760} 185.0°. n_D^{80} 1.4228. pKa (25°) 4.817. Heat of combustion: 2.00 MJ/mol. Heat of fusion: 150.9 J/g. Soly in water (g/l) at 0°: 41.5; at 10°: 54.6; at 20°: 76.1; at 25°: 94; at 30°: 122; at 40°: 656. Soly in ethanol at 25°: 52.5% w/w; acetone: 53.0% w/w; toluene: 37.5% w/w. LD_{50} orally in rats: 1.0 g/kg (Smyth, Carpenter).
Methyl ester. $C_5H_8O_2$. Liq, bp 121°; d_4^{20} 0.9444; n_D^{20} 1.4242.
Ethyl ester. $C_6H_{10}O_2$. Liq, bp 138°; d_4^{20} 0.9175; n_D^{20} 1.4245.
Vinyl ester. $C_6H_8O_2$. Liq, bp 133°; d_4^{20} 0.9410; n_D^{20} 1.450.
USE: In the manuf of copolymers with vinyl acetate used in lacquers and paper sizing; in the manuf of softening agents for synthetic rubber. In medicinal chemistry, e.g., in the manuf of DL-threonine, vitamin A.

2598. Croton Oil. Fixed oil expressed from seeds of *Croton tiglium* L., *Euphorbiaceae*. *Constit.* Croton resin; glycerides of stearic, palmitic, myristic, lauric, tiglic, etc. acids; crotin; phorbol esters, *q.v. Review:* Hecker, Schmidt, *Fortschr. Chem. Org. Naturst.* **31**, 377 (1974).
Pale-yellow or brownish-yellow, rather viscid liq; slight disagreeable odor. *Poisonous!* d_{25}^{25} 0.935-0.950. n_D^{40} 1.470-1.473. Sapon no. 205-220. Iodine no. 102-118. Slightly sol in alcohol, increasing with age. Freely sol in chloroform, ether, oils, petr ether, carbon disulfide, glacial acetic acid. *Keep well closed and protected from light.*
Caution: Potential symptom of overexposure is hemorrhagic gastroenteritis. Direct contact may cause vesiculation, necrosis and sloughing of skin. *See Clinical Toxicology of Commercial Products,* R. E. Gosselin *et al.,* Eds. (William & Wilkins, Baltimore, 5th ed., 1984) Section II, p. 228.
USE: Has been used as an irritant and cocarcinogen in cancer research.
THERAP CAT: Cathartic, counterirritant.
THERAP CAT (VET): Formerly used as a counterirritant and a purgative.

2599. Crotoxin. [9007-40-3] Neurotoxin. One of the toxic principles isolated from rattlesnake venom: Slotta, Fraenkel-Conrat, *Ber.* **71**, 1076 (1938). A polypeptide complex of probably two components, one acidic and one basic, having mol wts of ~9000 and 12,000 resp. The subunits do not retain the toxicity of crotoxin but show synergistic action in combination: Hendon, Fraenkel-Conrat, *Proc. Natl. Acad. Sci. USA* **68**, 1560 (1971). Amino acid analyses and fractionation studies: Fraenkel-Conrat, Singer, *Arch. Biochem. Biophys.* **60**, 64 (1956); Rübsamen *et al., Arch. Pharmacol.* **270**, 274 (1971); Horst *et al., Biochem. Biophys. Res. Commun.* **46**, 1042 (1972). Review of early chemical studies: Fraenkel-Conrat, Singer, *Publ. Am. Assoc. Advan. Sci.* **44**, 259 (1956). *Monograph:* Behringwerk-Mitteilungen Sonderband, *Die Giftschlangen der Erde* (N. G. Elwert, Marburg, 1963) 464 pp. Pharmacology: Brazil, Excell, *J. Physiol. (London)* **212**, 34P (1970); Brazil *et al., ibid.* **234**, 63P (1973); Habermann *et al., Arch. Pharmacol.* **273**, 313 (1972). *See also* Crotamine.
Caution: When injected by snake bite, local pain, redness, hemorrhage and necrosis result. Systemic effects are dizziness, sensory and motor depression, collapse, shock. May be fatal. *Antidote:* Rattlesnake antivenin.

2600. Crotoxyphos. [7700-17-6] (*E*)-3-[(Dimethoxyphosphinyl)oxy]-2-butenoic acid 1-phenylethyl ester; 3-hydroxycrotonic acid α-methylbenzyl ester dimethyl phosphate; *O,O*-dimethyl *O*-[1-

methyl-2-(1-phenylcarbethoxy)vinyl] phosphate; dimethyl 2-(α-methylbenzyloxycarbonyl)-1-methylvinyl phosphate; ENT-24717; SD-4294; Ciodrin. $C_{14}H_{19}O_6P$; mol wt 314.27. C 53.50%, H 6.09%, O 30.55%, P 9.86%. Prepn: **GB 855238** (1960 to Bataafse Petroleum Maatschappij N.V.); Whetstone, Stiles, **US 2982686** (1961 to Shell). Activity: C. P. Weidenback, R. L. Younger, *J. Econ. Entomol.* **55**, 793 (1962). Metabolism and degradn: K. I. Beynon *et al., Residue Rev.* **47**, 55 (1973). Toxicity study: T. B. Gaines, *Toxicol. Appl. Pharmacol.* **14**, 515 (1969).

Light straw-colored liq, bp$_{0.03}$ 135°. n_D^{25} 1.4988. d^{25} 1.19. Vapor pressure at 20°: 1.4×10^{-5} mm Hg. Soly in water at room temp: 0.1%. Slightly sol in kerosine, saturated hydrocarbons. Sol in acetone, chloroform, ethanol, highly chlorinated hydrocarbons. LD$_{50}$ in female, male rats (mg/kg): 74, 110 orally (Gaines).

Caution: A cholinesterase inhibitor.

USE: Insecticide for external use on livestock.

2601. Crotyl Alcohol. [6117-91-5] 2-Buten-1-ol; crotonyl alcohol. C_4H_8O; mol wt 72.11. C 66.62%, H 11.18%, O 22.19%. $CH_3CH=CHCH_2OH$. Prepn by reduction of crotonaldehyde: Nystrom, Brown, *J. Am. Chem. Soc.* **69**, 1197 (1947); Olivier, Young, *ibid.* **81**, 5811 (1959); Smith, Holm, **US 2761883**; Finch, Furman, **US 2763696** (both 1956 to Shell); Foreman, **US 3109865** (1963 to Standard Oil Co., Ohio). Prepn of *cis*- and *trans*-forms: Hatch, Nesbitt, *J. Am. Chem. Soc.* **72**, 727 (1950); Hiskey *et al., J. Org. Chem.* **21**, 429 (1956); of *cis*-form only: Clarke, Crombie, *Chem. Ind. (London)* **1957**, 143. Toxicity study: H. F. Smyth *et al., Am. Ind. Hyg. Assoc. J.* **23**, 95 (1962).

Liquid, bp 122°. d$_4^{20}$ 0.8532. n_D^{20} 1.4285. Sol in 6 parts water; misc with alc. LD$_{50}$ orally in rats: 0.93 ml/kg (Smyth).

cis-**Form.** Liquid, bp 123.6°. mp −90.15°. d$_4^{20}$ 0.8662. n_D^{20} 1.4342.

trans-**Form.** Liquid, bp 121.2°. d$_4^{25}$ 0.8454. n_D^{20} 1.4289, n_D^{25} 1.4270.

2602. Crown Ethers. Crown compounds. Macrocyclic polyethers with the repeating unit $(-CH_2-CH_2-O-)_n$, where n is greater than 2. Crown compounds with other heteroatoms (N, S, P) are known. Prepd by C. J. Pedersen, *J. Am. Chem. Soc.* **89**, 2495, 7017 (1967). Described as "crown" ethers due to appearance of space-filling models and ability to "crown" cations. Proposed nomenclature lists non-ring substituents, number of atoms in ring, the class (crown), and the number of heteroatoms in the ring; e.g. dibenzo-18-crown-6. Bicyclic crowns are called *cryptates*. Crowns complex with cations and solubilize inorganic reagents in organic solvents. Selectivity results from the definite size of the crown cavity which admits only cations of corresponding ionic radii. The stability of complexes depends on the size of the cation and the size of the polyether ring. Chiral crowns are used in optical resolution of enantiomers. *Reviews:* D. J. Cram, J. M. Cram, *Science* **183**, 803-809 (1974); *eidem, Acc. Chem. Res.* **11**, 8-14 (1978); J. J. Christensen *et al., Chem. Rev.* **74**, 351-384 (1974); G. W. Gokel, H. D. Durst, *Synthesis* **1976**, 168-184; A. C. Knipe, *J. Chem. Educ.* **53**, 618-622 (1976); V. Prelog, *Pure Appl. Chem.* **50**, 893-904 (1978). Historical overview: C. J. Pedersen, *Science* **241**, 536-540 (1988).

Dibenzo-18-crown-6

18-Crown-6. 1,4,7,10,13,16-Hexaoxacyclooctadecane. $C_{12}H_{24}O_6$; mol wt 264.32. Prepn: G. W. Gokel *et al., Org. Synth.* **57**, 30 (1977). Crystals from acetonitrile, mp 38-39.5°.

Dibenzo-18-crown-6. 2,3,11,12-Dibenzo-1,4,7,10,13,16-hexaoxacyclooctadeca-2,11-diene. $C_{20}H_{24}O_6$; mol wt 360.40. The first crown ether discovered. Prepn: C. J. Pedersen, **US 3687978** (1972 to Du Pont). White crystals from acetone, mp 164°, bp$_{679}$ 380-384°.

Dicyclohexano-18-crown-6. Dicyclohexyl-18-crown-6. $C_{20}H_{36}O_6$; mol wt 372.50. Approx LD in rats (mg/kg): 300 orally (Pedersen, 1967).

Caution: Direct contact may cause eye and skin irritation (Pedersen, 1967).

USE: In organic synthesis as phase transfer reagents, catalysts and in sepn of enantiomers.

2603. CRP. [9007-41-4] C-Reactive Protein. Homogeneous acute phase protein, found in man and most other animals. Discovered as a result of its precipitation with C-polysaccharide (CPS) in sera of patients with infections and inflammatory disease: W. S. Tillet, T. Francis, *J. Exp. Med.* **52**, 561 (1930). Characterization as a protein and identification of its calcium ion requirement for interaction with CPS: T. J. Abernathy, O. T. Avery, *ibid.* **73**, 173 (1941). CRP is a trace serum protein consisting of single subunits of mol wt about 21,000. In serum and in the purified state, the subunits aggregate as cyclic pentamers having mol wts of 110,000-144,000. The concentrations of C-reactive protein increase up to 1000-fold in inflammatory conditions and in tissue necrosis. In addition, it can initiate reactions of agglutination, precipitation, and opsonization for phagocytosis and can activate the complement system. Other biological activities with platelets and lymphocytes have also been described, but the full biological functions of CRP have not yet been completely elucidated. Review of CRP and the acute phase response: H. Gewurz *et al., Adv. Intern. Med.* **27**, 345-372 (1982). Review of structure and function: M. B. Pepys, *Eur. J. Rheumatol. Inflammation* **5**, 386-397 (1982). Book: *Ann. N.Y. Acad. Sci.* **389**, entitled "C-Reactive Protein and the Plasma Protein Response to Tissue Injury", I. Kushner *et al.,* Eds. (1982) 482 pp.

2604. Crufomate. [299-86-5] Methylphosphoramidic acid 2-chloro-4-(1,1-dimethylethyl)phenyl methyl ester; methylphosphoramidic acid 4-*tert*-butyl-2-chlorophenyl methyl ester; 4-*tert*-butyl-2-chlorophenyl N-methyl O-methylphosphoramidate; Dowco 132; Montrel; Ruelene. $C_{12}H_{19}ClNO_3P$; mol wt 291.71. C 49.41%, H 6.57%, Cl 12.15%, N 4.80%, O 16.45%, P 10.62%. Prepn: Wasco *et al.,* **US 2929762** (1960 to Dow). Toxicity study: T. B. Gaines, *Toxicol. Appl. Pharmacol.* **14**, 515 (1969). Anthelmintic activity in dairy cattle: E. T. Lyons *et al., Am. J. Vet. Res.* **43**, 1072 (1982).

Crystals from petr ether, mp 60-60.5°. Relatively stable in aq dispersions at pH 7 or below. Commercial product is a yellow oil, bp$_{0.01}$ 117-118°. n_D^{20} 1.5142. Sol in acetone, benzene, carbon tetrachloride. Practically insol in water, light petroleum. LD$_{50}$ in male, female rats (mg/kg): 635, 460 orally (Gaines).

Caution: Potential symptoms of overexposure are irritation of eyes, skin, respiratory system; wheezing, dyspnea; blurred vision, lacrimation; sweating; abdominal cramps, diarrhea, nausea, anorexia. *See NIOSH Pocket Guide to Chemical Hazards* (DHHS/NIOSH 97-140, 1997) p 80.

USE: Insecticide.

THERAP CAT (VET): Anthelmintic.

2605. Cryofluorane. [76-14-2] 1,2-Dichloro-1,1,2,2-tetrafluoroethane; Freon 114; Frigen 114; Arcton 114. $C_2Cl_2F_4$; mol wt 170.92. C 14.05%, Cl 41.48%, F 44.46%. $ClCF_2CClF_2$. Prepn: Henne, *Org. React.* **2**, 49 (1944).

Colorless, practically odorless, noncorrosive, nonirritating, nonflammable gas. Faint, ether-like odor in high concentrations. d$_{liq}^0$

1.5312. mp −94°. bp$_{760}$ 4.1°. n_D^0 1.3092. Critical temp 145.7°; crit pressure 474 lb/sq in. abs. Practically insol in water. Sol in alcohol, ether. Absorbs less than 0.0025% water. Has little, if any, anesthetic or toxic effect on humans, but toxic substances may be formed on contact with a flame or hot metal surface.

Caution: Potential symptoms of overexposure are irritation of respiratory system; asphyxia; cardiac arrhythmias, cardiac arrest; direct contact with liquid may cause frostbite. *See NIOSH Pocket Guide to Chemical Hazards* (DHHS/NIOSH 97-140, 1997) p 102. *Note:* Consult latest Government regulations on use as aerosol propellant.

USE: Refrigerant, aerosol propellant.

2606. Cryolite. [15096-52-3] Kryolith; ice spar; sodium aluminum fluoride. AlF$_6$Na$_3$; mol wt 209.94. Al 12.85%, F 54.30%, Na 32.85%. 3NaF.AlF$_3$. A mineral named for its resemblance to ice; large deposits existed in Greenland and in the Urals. Synthetic cryolite is usually made from NaAlO$_2$, NaHCO$_3$ and NaF. *See* the review by Vogel, *Chem. Ztg.* **75**, 603 (1951).

Snow-white, semi-opaque masses, vitreous fracture. Monoclinic crystals with cubic habit, perfect cleavage (001) (110) (101). The natural form may be colored reddish or brown or even black, but loses this discoloration on heating. d 2.95. Mohs' hardness 2.5-3. Fuses fairly easily, mp 1000°. Sol in concd H$_2$SO$_4$. Dec by boiling with aq alkali hydroxides or aq calcium hydroxide.

Caution: Potential symptoms of overexposure are irritation of eyes and respiratory system; nausea, abdominal pain, diarrhea; salivation, thirst and sweating; stiff spine; dermatitis; calcification of ligaments of ribs and pelvis. *See NIOSH Pocket Guide to Chemical Hazards* (DHHS/NIOSH 97-140, 1997) p 280.

2607. Cryptophycins. Cytotoxic, cyclic depsipeptides isolated from blue-green algae *Nostoc* sp. Named for their antifungal activity against the genus *Cryptococcus* sp. The parent compound is cryptophycin-1; at least 21 other naturally-occurring cryptophycins have been isolated; many other analogs have been synthesized. Interacts with the *Vinca* alkaloid binding domain of tubulin. Isoln: C. F. Hirsch *et al.*, **GB 2220657**; *eidem*, **US 4946835** (both 1990 to Merck & Co.); R. E. Schwartz *et al.*, *J. Ind. Microbiol.* **5**, 113 (1990). Prepn: R. E. Moore *et al.*, **WO 9640184**; *eidem*, **US 6013626** (1996, 2000 both to Univ. of Hawaii and Wayne State Univ.). Structure determn: G. Trimurtulu *et al.*, *J. Am. Chem. Soc.* **116**, 4729 (1994); and stability and antitumor evaluation: *idem et al.*, *ibid.* **117**, 12030 (1995). Mechanism of action: C. D. Smith, X. Zhang, *J. Biol. Chem.* **271**, 6192 (1996); D. Panda *et al.*, *Proc. Natl. Acad. Sci. USA* **95**, 9313 (1998). Effect on tubulin ring structures: N. R. Watts, *et al.*, *Biochemistry* **41**, 12662 (2002). Review of syntheses: M. A. Tius, *Tetrahedron* **58**, 4343-4367 (2002); and anticancer activity: M. Eggen, G. I. Georg, *Med. Res. Rev.* **22**, 85-101 (2002).

Cryptophycin-1   R = H
Cryptophycin-52 R = CH$_3$

Cryptophycin-52. [186256-67-7] Cyclo[2,2-dimethyl-β-alanyl-(2S)-2-hydroxy-4-methylpentanoyl-(2E,5S,6S)-5-hydroxy-6-[(2R,3R)-3-phenyloxiranyl]-2-heptenoyl-3-chloro-o-methyl-D-tyrosyl]; LY-355703. C$_{36}$H$_{45}$ClN$_2$O$_8$; mol wt 669.20. C 64.61%, H 6.78%, Cl 5.30%, N 4.19%, O 19.13%. Synthetic cryptophycin analog under investigation for treatment of solid tumors. Enantioselective synthesis: A. K. Ghosh, L. Swanson, *J. Org. Chem.* **68**, 9823 (2003). Clinical evaluation in lung cancer: M. J. Edelman *et*

al., Lung Cancer **39**, 197 (2003); in platinum-resistant ovarian cancer: G. D'Agostino *et al.*, *Int. J. Gynecol. Cancer* **16**, 71 (2006). White solid. [α]$_D$ +19.9° (c = 0.5 in CHCl$_3$). uv max (methanol): 204, 218 nm (ε 35100, 20900).

Cryptophycin-1. [124689-65-2] Cyclo[(2R)-2-methyl-β-alanyl-(2S)-2-hydroxy-4-methylpentanoyl-(2E,5S,6S)-5-hydroxy-6-[(2R,3R)-3-phenyloxiranyl]-2-heptenoyl-3-chloro-o-methyl-D-tyrosyl]; cryptophycin A. C$_{35}$H$_{43}$ClN$_2$O$_8$; mol wt 655.18. C 64.16%, H 6.62%, Cl 5.41%, N 4.28%, O 19.54%. White or light colored glassy solid. [α]$_D$ +33.8° (c = 1.83 in methanol). uv max: 208, 218, 228, 280 nm (ε 42400, 33700, 23800, 2210). Sol in organic solvents.

2608. Cryptopine. [482-74-6] 4,6,7,13-Tetrahydro-9,10-dimethoxy-5-methylbenzo[e]-1,3-dioxolo[4,5-l][2]benzazecin-12(5H)-one; cryptocavine. C$_{21}$H$_{23}$NO$_5$; mol wt 369.41. C 68.28%, H 6.28%, N 3.79%, O 21.66%. Occurs in opium (0.003-0.03%). Has been found in *Corydalis sempervirens* (L.) Pers., and in *Dicentra* spp., *Fumariaceae:* Manske, *Can. J. Res.* **8**, 407 (1933); **7**, 265 (1932); **15B**, 274 (1937). Structure: Perkin, *Chem. Soc.* **115**, 713 (1919). Synthesis: Haworth, Perkin, *ibid.* **1926**, 1769. Crystal structure: S. R. Hall, F. R. Ahmed, *Acta Crystallogr.* **B24**, 346 (1968).

Crystallizes as six-sided prisms or plates from benzene, mp 220-221°. d 1.35. Almost insol in water and ether. Soluble in chloroform, acetic acid. One part dissolves in 455 parts alc or 80 parts boiling alc. Sparingly sol in most other organic solvents. May be crystallized from hot alc, benzene, petr ether, methyl ethyl ketone, isoamyl alcohol, acetophenone, pyridine, or an alcohol-pyridine mixture. The salts tend to oil out, but can be crystallized by warming, redissolving, and slow cooling.

2609. Cryptoxanthin. [472-70-8] (3R)-β,β-Caroten-3-ol; cryptoxanthol; caricaxanthin; hydroxy-β-carotene; β-caroten-3-ol; all-trans-cryptoxanthin. C$_{40}$H$_{56}$O; mol wt 552.87. C 86.90%, H 10.21%, O 2.89%. Carotenoid pigment with vitamin A activity, best isolated from petals and berries of *Physalis* species: Kuhn, Grundmann, *Ber.* **66**, 1746 (1933). Widely distributed, also was isolated from orange rind, *Carica papaya* L., *Caricaceae, Cucurbita pepo* L., *Cucurbitaceae, Zea mays* L., *Gramineae*, egg yolk, butter, bovine blood serum. Structure: Kuhn, Grundmann, *Ber.* **66**, 1746 (1933); Karrer, Schlientz, *Helv. Chim. Acta* **17**, 55 (1934); Cholnoky *et al.*, *Ann.* **616**, 207 (1958). Total synthesis: Isler *et al.*, *Helv. Chim. Acta* **40**, 456 (1957); Loeber *et al.*, *J. Chem. Soc. C* **1971**, 404.

all-*trans*-form

Red plates with metallic luster from ether + methanol. mp 158-159° (racemate); 169° (natural). Absorption max: 452, 480 nm (E$_{1cm}^{1\%}$ 2380, 2080). Freely sol in chloroform, benzene, pyridine, carbon disulfide. Less sol in ligroin, petr ether, alcohol, methanol.

Monoacetate. C$_{42}$H$_{58}$O$_2$. Deep red leaflets, mp 117.5°.

2610. Crystallins. Major water-soluble structural proteins found in fiber cells of vertebrate eye lenses; account for the transparency of the lens. Heterogeneous family composed of four groups α, β, γ, δ which have been separated on the basis of size, charge, immunological properties and source. α, β, δ crystallins occur in avian and reptilian lenses while α, β, γ crystallins occur in all other lenses. Several other minor forms have also been identified. Identification and isolation of α, β, γ: C. T. Mörner, Z.

Consult the Name Index before using this section.

Physiol. Chem. **18,** 61 (1894); of δ: M. Rabaey, *Exp. Eye Res.* **1,** 310 (1962). Review of early isolation procedures: A. Spector, *Invest. Ophthalmol.* **3,** 182-193 (1964). Structural studies of α: A. F. Van Dam, G. Ten Cates, *Biochim. Biophys. Acta* **121,** 183 (1966); H. A. Kramps *et al., Eur. J. Biochem.* **50,** 503 (1975); of β: H. P. C. Driessen *et al., ibid.* **121,** 83 (1981); G. Wistow *et al., FEBS Lett.* **133,** 9 (1981); of γ: T. Blundell *et al., Nature* **289,** 771 (1981); L. Summers *et al., Pept. Protein Rev.* **3,** 147 (1984); of δ: J. Horwitz, J. Piatigorsky, *Biochim. Biophys. Acta* **624,** 21 (1980); L. A. Williams *et al., ibid.* **708,** 49 (1982). Short-range spatial ordering is essential for lens transparency: M. Delaye, A. Tardieu, *Nature* **302,** 415 (1983). Photoinduced aggregation; implications for cataract formation: U. P. Andley *et al., Photochem. Photobiol.* **40,** 343 (1984); K. Mandal *et al., ibid.* **47,** 583 (1988); M. Kono *et al., ibid.* 593. Role of crystallin aging in cataract formation: R. J. Siezen *et al., Proc. Natl. Acad. Sci. USA* **82,** 1701 (1985); H. J. Hoenders, G. J. H. Bessems, *Lens Res.* **3,** 281 (1986). Evolution and expression of crystallin genes: J. Piatigorsky, *Cell* **38,** 620 (1984); W. W. de Jong, W. Hendriks, *J. Mol. Evol.* **24,** 121 (1986). *Reviews:* A. Spector, *Invest. Ophthalmol.* **4,** 579-591 (1965); W. W. de Jong, *Co-ord. Regul. Gene Expression - Proc. 2nd Int. Workshop,* R. M. Clayton, Ed. (Plenum Press, New York, 1986) pp 281-291; G. J. Wistow, J. Piatigorsky, *Annu. Rev. Biochem.* **57,** 479-504 (1988). Review of δ-crystallin: J. Piatigorsky, *Mol. Cell. Biochem.* **59,** 33-56 (1984). Book: *Molecular and Cellular Biology of the Eye Lens,* H. Bloemendal, Ed. (John Wiley & Sons, New York, 1981).

α-Crystallin. High molecular wt multimeric (35-50 subunits) polypeptide for which two major subunit forms exist αA_1, αA_2; M_r unit 20 kDa. Most acidic crystallin, pI 4.8-5.0.

β-Crystallin. Dioctamer for which several (6-7) subunit forms exist; M_r unit 23-25 kDa. pI 5.7-7.0.

γ-Crystallin. Monomer, M_r 20 kDa. pI 7.1-8.1.

δ-Crystallin. Tetramer for which two possible subunit forms exist; M_r (monomer) 48-50 kDa. pI 4.9-5.3.

2611. Cubane. [277-10-1] Pentacyclo[4.2.0.0^{2,5}.0^{3,8}.- 0^{4,7}]octane. C_8H_8; mol wt 104.15. C 92.26%, H 7.74%. Prepn from bromocyclopentadienone dimer: Eaton, Cole, *J. Am. Chem. Soc.* **86,** 3157 (1964). Structure: Fleischer, *ibid.* 3889.

Rhombic crystals from methanol followed by sublimation at just above room temperature and atmospheric pressure, mp 130-131° (sealed capillary). Thermally unstable. Dec at 200°.

2612. Cubeb. Tailed pepper; Java pepper. Dried, unripe, nearly full-grown fruit of *Piper cubeba* L.f., *Piperaceae. Habit.* Southern Asia, Java, Borneo, Sumatra; cultivated in W. Indies and Ceylon. Berries are globular, 4-5 mm in diameter; blackish-gray; intern. whitish and hollow; strong, spicy odor; aromatic, pungent taste. *Constit.* 10-18% volatile oil, cubebin, about 1% cubebic acid, resin, fat, wax. Review of constituents: N. B. Shankaracharya *et al., PAFAI J.* **17,** 33-39 (1995). Botanical description and medicinal uses: J. Gruenwald *et al., PDR for Herbal Medicines* (Medical Economics, Montvale, 2nd Ed., 2000) p 235.

Volatile oil. [8007-87-2] Obtained by steam distillation of the mature, unripe, sun-dried fruit. *Constit.* α- and β-cubebenes, co-paene, cubebol, δ-cadinene, humulenes. Description: D. L. J. Opdyke, *Food Cosmet. Toxicol.* **14,** Suppl., 729 (1976). Colorless or pale green to blue-green liquid. d_{25}^{25} 0.898-0.928. n_D^{20} 1.492-1.502. Sol in 10 vols 90% alcohol. Sol in most fixed oils, mineral oil. Insol in glycerin, propylene glycol.

USE: Fragrance and flavoring agent; as a spice in cooking.

THERAP CAT: Urinary antiseptic; expectorant.

2613. Cubebin. [18423-69-3] 3,4-Bis(1,3-benzodioxol-5-ylmethyl)tetrahydro-2-furanol; tetrahydro-3,4-dipiperonyl-2-furanol; 5-hydroxy-3,4-bis(3,4-methylenedioxybenzyl)tetrahydrofuran. $C_{20}H_{20}O_6$; mol wt 356.37. C 67.41%, H 5.66%, O 26.94%. From cubeb. Isoln: Capitaine, Soubeiran, *Ann.* **31,** 190 (1839). Structure: Haworth, Kelly, *Chem. Ind. (London)* **1936,** 901; Haen-

sel *et al., Arch. Pharm.* **300,** 559 (1967). Synthesis: Batterbee *et al., J. Chem. Soc. C* **1969,** 2470.

Slender prisms from methanol, mp 131-132°. $[\alpha]_D^{14}$ −17° (acetone). Practically insol in water. Sol in alcohol, chloroform, ether.

Note: "Cubebine" is the French designation for ethereal extract of cubeb.

2614. Cucurbitacins. A group of tetracyclic triterpenes, commonly referred to as "bitter principles of cucurbits", which have antineoplastic and anti-gibberellin activity. They are isolated from various spp of cucurbitaceous plants known since antiquity for their beneficial and toxic properties. The plants have been used as vermifuges, emetics, narcotics, and antimalarials and have been implicated in sporadic livestock poisoning in S. Africa. Seventeen cucurbitacins have been isolated, most from plants of the *Cucurbitaceae* family, but also from *Begoniaceae, Cruciferae, Datisceae, Euphorbiaceae,* and *Scrophulariaceae.* Cucurbitacins B and E are the most commonly identified. Isoln of cucurbitacins A, B, C, D, F: P. R. Enslin, *J. Sci. Food Agric.* **5,** 410 (1954); of G, H, J, K, L: *idem, ibid.* **8,** 673 (1957); of E and I: D. Lavie, S. J. Szinai, *J. Am. Chem. Soc.* **80,** 707 (1958). of O, P, Q and antitumor activity: S. Kupchan *et al., J. Org. Chem.* **35,** 2891 (1970). Structures of A, B, C, D, E, I: W. T. DeKock *et al., J. Chem. Soc.* **1963,** 3828; of B, D, F: D. Lavie *et al., Chem. Ind. (London)* **1959,** 951; of G, H: C. W. Holzapfel, P. R. Enslin, *J. S. Afr. Chem. Inst.* **17,** 142 (1964), *C.A.* **62,** 10467c (1965); of J, K, L: P. R. Enslin, K. B. Norton, *J. Chem. Soc.* **1964,** 529. Stereochemistry of B, D, E, F, I: D. Lavie *et al., J. Org. Chem.* **28,** 1790 (1963). ^{13}C-NMR study of cucurbitacins: V. V. Velde, D. Lavie, *Tetrahedron* **39,** 317 (1983). Use as plant growth regulators: J. Guha, S. P. Sen, *Nature New Biol.* **244,** 273 (1973). Toxicity studies: J. LeMen *et al., Chim. Ther.* **4,** 459 (1969); D. Albert *et al., Chim. Ther.* **5,** 205 (1970). *Reviews:* D. Lavie, E. Glotter, *Fortschr. Chem. Org. Naturst.* **29,** 308-357 (1971); J. Guha, S. P. Sen, *Plant Biochem. J.* **2,** 12-28 (1975); A. Shrotria, *Botanica* **26,** 28-31 (1976).

Cucurbitacin B. [6199-67-3] (2β,9β,10α,16α,23E)-25-(Acetyloxy)-2,16,20-trihydroxy-9-methyl-19-norlanosta-5,23-diene-3,11,22-trione; 1,2-dihydro-α-elaterin. $C_{32}H_{46}O_8$; mol wt 558.70. Crystals from abs ethanol, mp 184-186°. $[\alpha]_D^{25}$ +88° (c = 1.55 in ethanol). LD$_{10}$ orally in mice: 5 mg/kg (LeMen).

Cucurbitacin E. [18444-66-1] (9β,10α,16α,23E)-25-(Acetyloxy)-2,16,20-trihydroxy-9-methyl-19-norlanosta-1,5,23-triene-3,11,22-trione; α-elaterin. $C_{32}H_{44}O_8$; mol wt 556.69. White hexagonal plates from methanol, mp 232-233° (dec). $[\alpha]_D$ −59° (c = 0.7 in chloroform). uv max (chloroform): 234, 267 nm (ε 11700, 8350). LD$_{50}$ orally in mice: 340 mg/kg (Albert).

2615. Cudbear. Crottle. Common names for the lichen *Ochrolechia tartarea* L., *Lecanoraceae* and for the coloring matter from this and other lichens, especially *Lecanoraceae* and *Roccellaceae.* A source of litmus, *q.v.* Acids in lichens (e.g. lecanoric acid) hydrolyze to orcinol, *q.v.,* which, in the presence of ammonia can be oxidized to the dye orcein, *q.v.* The dyes **French Purple, Persio, Orchil,** and **Orseilles** derive from the salts of orcein: *Colour Index* **Vol. 3** (3rd ed., 1971) p 3241.

Purplish-red powder. Imparts fine purplish-red color to alcohol, acid and neutral liquids. The purple tinge may be covered by adding a few drops of burnt-sugar coloring.

USE: Color for syrups, elixirs etc.

2616. Cuelure. [3572-06-3] 4-[4-(Acetyloxy)phenyl]-2-butanone; 4-(*p*-hydroxyphenyl)-2-butanone acetate. $C_{12}H_{14}O_3$; mol wt 206.24. C 69.88%, H 6.84%, O 23.27%. Synthetic sex pheromone developed as a lure for melon flies, *Dacus cucurbitae* (Coq.); analog of raspberry ketone. Prepn and biological activity: M. Beroza *et al., Science* **131**, 1044 (1960); B. H. Alexander *et al., J. Agric. Food Chem.* **10**, 270 (1962). Extraction and GC-MS determn in soil: J. P. Alcantara-Licudine *et al., J. Chromatogr. Sci.* **34**, 238 (1996). Field studies in fruit fly eradication: R. T. Cunningham, L. F. Steiner, *J. Econ. Entomol.* **65**, 505 (1972). Acute toxicity study: M. Beroza *et al., Toxicol. Appl. Pharmacol.* **31**, 421 (1975).

Colorless to pale yellow liquid with a raspberry-like odor, bp$_{0.2}$ 123-124°. n_D^{25} 1.5061. d 1.099. Sol in alcohol, hydrocarbons, ether. Insol in water. LD$_{50}$ in rats (mg/kg): 3038 ±1266 orally; in rabbits (mg/kg): >2025 dermally; LC$_{50}$ (24 hr) in rainbow trout, bluegill sunfish (ppm): ≈21, 18 (Beroza).

USE: As attractant in melon fly traps.

2617. Cumene. [98-82-8] (1-Methylethyl)benzene; cumol; isopropylbenzene. C_9H_{12}; mol wt 120.19. C 89.94%, H 10.06%. Manuf: *Faith, Keyes & Clark's Industrial Chemicals,* F. A. Lowenheim, M. K. Moran, Eds. (Wiley-Interscience, New York, 4th ed., 1975) pp 294-297. Toxicity study: Smyth *et al., Arch. Ind. Hyg. Occup. Med.* **4**, 119 (1951). *Review:* D. J. Ward in *Kirk-Othmer Encyclopedia of Chemical Technology* **vol. 7** (Wiley-Interscience, New York, 3rd ed., 1979) pp 286-290.

Colorless liquid. d$_4^{20}$ 0.862. bp 152-153°. Flash pt, closed cup: 102°F (39°C). n_D^{20} 1.4914: Hirschler, Faulconer, *J. Am. Chem. Soc.* **68**, 210 (1946). Insol in water. Sol in alcohol and many other organic solvents. LD$_{50}$ orally in rats: 2.91 g/kg (Smyth).

Caution: Potential symptoms of overexposure are irritation of eyes, skin and mucous membranes; dermatitis; headache, narcosis, coma. *See NIOSH Pocket Guide to Chemical Hazards* (DHHS/NIOSH 97-140, 1997) p 80.

USE: In manuf of phenol, acetone, acetophenone, α-methylstyrene.

2618. Cumic Acid. [536-66-3] 4-(1-Methylethyl)benzoic acid; *p*-isopropylbenzoic acid; cuminic acid. $C_{10}H_{12}O_2$; mol wt 164.20. C 73.15%, H 7.37%, O 19.49%.

Triclinic crystals. d^4 1.162. mp 115-117°. Sparingly sol in water; sol in alcohol, ether; also sol in concd H_2SO_4 without decompn, and pptd unchanged by adding water.

2619. Cumic Alcohol. [536-60-7] 4-(1-Methylethyl)-benzenemethanol; cuminol; cuminyl alcohol; *p*-isopropylbenzyl alcohol. $C_{10}H_{14}O$; mol wt 150.22. C 79.95%, H 9.39%, O 10.65%. Found in caraway seed. Prepd by the reduction of cuminal; also by treating a suspension of cuminylmagnesium chloride in ether with dry oxygen.

Liquid; intense, persistent, caraway-like odor and burning, aromatic taste. d^{15} 0.981. bp 248.4°. n_D^{24} 1.522. Insol in water; miscible with alcohol, ether.

2620. Cumidine. [99-88-7] 4-(1-Methylethyl)benzenamine; 4-aminocumene; *p*-isopropylaniline; 4-amino-1-isopropylbenzene; β-(4-aminophenyl)propane. $C_9H_{13}N$; mol wt 135.21. C 79.95%, H 9.69%, N 10.36%. Prepn from aniline and isopropyl alcohol: Louis, *Ber.* **16**, 111 (1883); by nitration and subsequent reduction of cumene: Constam, Goldschmidt, *Ber.* **21**, 1157 (1898); Vavon, Callier, *Bull. Soc. Chim. Fr.* [4] **41**, 677 (1927).

Liquid. bp$_{745}$ 226-227°. d 0.9526. Insol in water.

Hydrochloride. $C_9H_{13}N.HCl$. Prisms from water or alc.

Sulfate. $C_9H_{13}N.\frac{1}{2}H_2SO_4$. Leaflets, mp 205°. Sol in hot water or alcohol, less sol in cold water, ether.

USE: In the determination of tungsten.

2621. Cuminaldehyde. [122-03-2] 4-(1-Methylethyl)-benzaldehyde; *p*-isopropylbenzaldehyde; cuminal; cumaldehyde. $C_{10}H_{12}O$; mol wt 148.20. C 81.04%, H 8.16%, O 10.80%. Constituent of eucalyptus, myrrh, cassia, cumin, and other essential oils; prepared synthetically from *p*-isopropylbenzoyl chloride. Alternate synthesis by formylation of isopropylbenzene under pressure: Crounse, *J. Am. Chem. Soc.* **71**, 1263 (1949). Toxicity study: P. M. Jenner *et al., Food Cosmet. Toxicol.* **2**, 327 (1964).

Colorless to yellowish, oily liq; strong persistent odor; acrid, burning taste. d^{20} 0.978. bp$_{760}$ 235-236°; bp$_{35}$ 131-135°. n_D^{20} 1.5301. Practically insol in water. Sol in alc, ether. LD$_{50}$ orally in rats: 1390 mg/kg (Jenner).

Thiosemicarbazone. [3811-20-9] SHCH-58. $C_{11}H_{15}N_3S$; mol wt 221.32. Prepn: P. P. T. Sah, T. C. Daniels, *Rec. Trav. Chim.* **69**, 1545 (1950); J. Bernstein *et al., J. Am. Chem. Soc.* **73**, 906 (1951). Stout platelets from methanol, mp 147°. Practically insol in water. Moderately sol in alc.

USE: In perfumery.

2622. Cupferron. [135-20-6] *N*-Hydroxy-*N*-nitrosobenzenamine ammonium salt; *N*-nitrosophenylhydroxylamine ammonium salt. $C_6H_9N_3O_2$; mol wt 155.15. C 46.45%, H 5.85%, N 27.08%, O 20.62%. Prepd from phenylhydroxylamine by treating with NaNO$_2$ at 0° in presence of HCl, filtering, dissolving in ether and treating with NH$_3$, or by treating an ether soln of phenylhydroxylamine with butyl or amyl nitrite and NH$_3$ in the cold: Marvel, Kamm, *Org. Synth.* **4**, 19 (1925).

Crystals, mp 163-164°. Freely sol in water or alc. *Keep in well-closed containers to which a piece of ammonium carbonate has been added.*

Caution: This substance is reasonably anticipated to be a human carcinogen: *Report on Carcinogens, Eleventh Edition* (PB2005-104914, 2004) p III-73.

USE: As a reagent for separating Sn from Zn, and Cu and Fe from other metals. Ppts iron quantitatively from strongly acid soln; as a quantitative reagent for vanadates with which it gives a dark-red ppt sol in alkali soln, and for Ti with which it forms a yellow ppt; also suitable for the colorimetric estimation of Al.

2623. Cupreine. [524-63-0] (8α,9R)-Cinchonan-6′,9-diol; hydroxycinchonidine; ultraquinine. $C_{19}H_{22}N_2O_2$; mol wt 310.39. C 73.52%, H 7.14%, N 9.03%, O 10.31%. In bark and seeds of *Remijia pedunculata* Flueck., *Rubiaceae*. Isoln: Howard, Hodgkin, *J. Chem. Soc.* **41**, 16 (1882). Separated from homoquinine by treatment with NaOH: Hesse, *Ann.* **230**, 55 (1885). Reduction to *hydrocupreine*: Giemsa, Halberkann, *Ber.* **51**, 1325 (1918). Conversion into cinchonidine: King, *J. Chem. Soc.* **1946**, 523.

Monoclinic plates from alcohol, mp 202°. $[\alpha]_D^{17}$ −176°, (methanol). pK_1 6.57. Sol in alcohol, NaOH soln, but not in NH_4OH. Sparingly sol in water, ether, chloroform, benzene, petr ether. The neutral salts give yellow aq solns; the acid salts remain colorless in aq soln.

Monomethyl ether *see* Quinine.

2624. Cupric Acetate. [142-71-2] Acetic acid copper (2+) salt. $C_4H_6CuO_4$; mol wt 181.63. C 26.45%, H 3.33%, Cu 34.99%, O 35.24%. $Cu(CH_3COO)_2$. Prepd by the action of acetic acid on CuO or $CuCO_3$: Winter *et al.*, in *Kirk-Othmer Encyclopedia of Chemical Technology* vol. 6 (Interscience, New York, 2nd ed., 1965) p 267. Toxicity study: H. F. Smyth *et al.*, *Am. Ind. Hyg. Assoc. J.* **30**, 470 (1969).

Monohydrate. Neutral verdigris. Dark green, monoclinic crystals; exists in dimeric units. mp 115°; dec at 240°; d 1.882. Sol in water, alcohol; slightly sol in ether, glycerol. LD_{50} orally in rats: 0.71 g/kg (Smyth).

Verdigris. [8007-61-2] C.I. Pigment Green 20; C.I. 77408. Prepn: *Colour Index* vol. 4 (3rd ed, 1971) p 4666. Commercial product is a mixture of *basic cupric acetate* salts with variable waters of hydration, resulting in blue to green powders. Slightly sol in water, ethanol; sol in dil acids, ammonia.

USE: Intermediate in manuf of Paris green, *q.v.*; as fungicide; as catalyst for organic reactions, including rubber aging; in textile dyeing; as pigment for ceramics.

2625. Cupric Acetoarsenite. [12002-03-8] (Acetato)trimetaarsenitodicopper; Paris green; copper acetate arsenite; emerald green; French green; imperial green; mineral green; Mitis green; parrot green; Schweinfurt green; Vienna green; C.I. Pigment Green 21; C.I. 77410. $C_4H_6As_6Cu_4O_{16}$; mol wt 1013.79. C 4.74%, H 0.60%, As 44.34%, Cu 25.07%, O 25.25%. $Cu(C_2H_3O_2)_2$·$3Cu(AsO_2)_2$. Usually contains some water. Prepn: Serciron, US 2159864 (1939); Krefft, US 2268123 (1944 to Chemical Marketing); Glemser, Sauer in *Handbook of Preparative Inorganic Chemistry* vol. 2, G. Brauer, Ed. (Academic Press, New York, 2nd ed., 1965) p 1027. *See also Colour Index* vol. 4 (3rd ed., 1971) p 4667. Toxicity study: T. B. Gaines, *Toxicol. Appl. Pharmacol.* **14**, 515 (1969).

Emerald green, crystalline powder. *Poisonous!* Stable to air, light. Practically insol in water. Dec on prolonged heating in water. Unstable in acids, bases, and toward H_2S. LD_{50} orally in female rats: 100 mg/kg (Gaines).

Caution: Toxicity primarily result of arsenic content. Gastric disturbance, tremors or muscular cramps, and peripheral neuritis. Local effects on the skin, mucous membranes and conjunctiva.

USE: Insecticide; wood preservative; as pigment, particularly for ships and submarines.

2626. Cupric Arsenite. [10290-12-7] Arsonic acid copper(2+) salt (1:1); arsenious acid copper(2+) salt (1:1); Scheele's green. Compound of variable composition. Usually considered to be $CuHAsO_3$; mol wt 187.46. Also reported as $Cu(AsO_2)_2$: Bhadraver, *Bull. Chem. Soc. Jpn.* **35**, 1770 (1962). Prepd by reaction of a cupric salt with an alkaline or ammoniacal arsenite: R. N. Kust in *Kirk-Othmer Encyclopedia of Chemical Technology* vol. 7 (Interscience, New York, 3rd ed., 1979) p 102. *See also: Colour Index* vol. 4 (3rd ed., 1971) p 4667.

Yellowish-green powder. *Poisonous!* Practically insol in water, alcohol. Sol in acids, ammonia.

USE: As pigment, wood preservative, insecticide, fungicide, rodenticide.

2627. Cupric Bisglycinate. [13479-54-4] Bis(glycinato-κN,κO)copper; cupric aminoacetate; glycocoll-copper; Copper Chelazome. $C_4H_8CuN_2O_4$; mol wt 211.66. C 22.70%, H 3.81%, Cu 30.02%, N 13.24%, O 30.24%. Prepn: J. Mauthner, W. Suida, *Monatsh. Chem.* **11**, 373 (1890); and characterization: H. Ley, Z. *Elektrochem.* **10**, 954 (1904); and isomerization study: K. Tomita, *Bull. Chem. Soc. Jpn.* **34**, 280 (1961). Thermodynamics of complex formation: K. P. Anderson *et al., Inorg. Chem.* **5**, 2106 (1966). Kinetics of complex formation: A. F. Pearlmutter, J. Stuehr, *J. Am. Chem. Soc.* **90**, 858 (1968). Clinical evaluation in maintenance of bone mineral density: J. Eaton-Evans *et al., J. Trace Elem. Exp. Med.* **9**, 87 (1996).

Monohydrate. Long, deep-blue, rhombic needles. Loses H_2O at 123°, chars at 213°, and dec with gas evolution at 228°. Sol in water; slightly sol in alcohol.

Dihydrate. Light blue, powdery crystals. Loses one H_2O at 103°, remaining H_2O at about 140°. Dec with gas evolution at about 225°. Sol in water.

THERAP CAT: Copper supplement.

THERAP CAT (VET): Nutritional factor. Given parenterally for copper deficiency in ruminants.

2628. Cupric Borate. [39290-85-2] A material of indefinite composition prepd by the reaction of a borax soln with $CuSO_4$: Barnard, Jr. in *ACS Monograph Series* **no. 122**, entitled "Copper," A. Butts, Ed. (Reinhold, New York, 1954) p 794.

Blue to blue-green solid. Extremely hard material.

Caution: Symptoms of acute toxicity include vomiting, diarrhea, tremors, convulsions, shock, dermatitis; renal, hepatic and CNS degeneration. Symptoms of chronic ingestion include skin disorders, kidney lesions.

USE: As ceramic color, pigment in oil paint; in dehydrogenation catalysis; as insulating and sealing medium for lead wires in lamps and mercury rectifiers, as fireproofing agent and preservative for wood; as fungicide, insecticide, parasiticide.

2629. Cupric Bromide. [7789-45-9] Br_2Cu; mol wt 223.35. Br 71.55%, Cu 28.45%. $CuBr_2$. Prepn: Watt *et al., J. Am. Chem. Soc.* **77**, 2752 (1955); Glemser, Sauer in *Handbook of Preparative Inorganic Chemistry* vol. 2, G. Brauer, Ed. (Academic Press, New York, 2nd ed., 1965) p 1009.

Almost black, iodine-like, deliquesc monoclinic crystals or cryst powder. mp 498°; bp 900°; d_4^{20} 4.710. Very sol in water; sol in alcohol, acetone, ammonia; practically insol in benzene, ether, concd H_2SO_4. *Keep well closed.*

USE: As intensifier in photography; as brominating agent in organic synthesis; as humidity indicator; as wood preservative; in solid-electrolyte battery; as stabilizer for acetylated polyformaldehyde.

2630. Cupric Butyrate. [540-16-9] $C_8H_{14}CuO_4$; mol wt 237.74. C 40.42%, H 5.94%, Cu 26.73%, O 26.92%. $Cu(CH_3-CH_2CH_2COO)_2$. Prepn from a cupric salt and butyric acid or Na butyrate: Graddon, *J. Inorg. Nucl. Chem.* **17**, 222 (1955); Martin,

Waterman, *J. Chem. Soc.* **1957**, 2545; from powdered Cu and butyric acid: Hahl, **US 3133942** (1964 to BASF).

Monohydrate. Large, dark green, monoclinic, hexagonal plates. Becomes dull and disintegrates after several days exposure to air. Sol in water, dioxane, benzene; slightly sol in chloroform, alcohol.
USE: In catalysts; in lubricants.

2631. Cupric Carbonate, Basic. [12069-69-1] Copper carbonate hydroxide; cupric subcarbonate; Bremen blue; Bremen green. $CH_2Cu_2O_5$; mol wt 221.12. C 5.43%, H 0.91%, Cu 57.48%, O 36.18%. $CuCO_3.Cu(OH)_2$. Occurs in nature as the mineral *malachite* (dark green monoclinic crystals). Prepd by adding $CuSO_4$ soln to Na_2CO_3 soln: Winter *et al.*, in *Kirk-Othmer Encyclopedia of Chemical Technology* **vol. 6** (Interscience, New York, 2nd ed., 1965) p 270. The commercial product usually contains 50-55% Cu.

Green to blue amorphous powder or dark-green monoclinic crystals. Practically insol in water, alcohol; sol in dil acids, ammonia.

Note: Another form of basic copper carbonate, $2CuCO_3.$-$Cu(OH)_2$, occurs in nature as the mineral *azurite* or *chessylite*. See also Burgundy Mixture.

USE: As seed treatment fungicide; in pyrotechnics; as paint and varnish pigment; in animal and poultry feeds; in sweetening of petrol sour crude stock; in manuf of other Cu salts.

THERAP CAT (VET): Nutritional factor. Used in copper deficiency in ruminants.

2632. Cupric Chlorate. [14721-21-2] Cl_2CuO_6; mol wt 230.45. Cl 30.77%, Cu 27.57%, O 41.66%. $Cu(ClO_3)_2$. Prepn: *Gmelins, Copper* (8th ed.) **60B**, 332-334 (1958).

Hexahydrate. Blue to green, deliquesc, octahedral crystals. mp 65°. Dec at 100°. Very sol in water, alcohol. *Keep well closed and out of contact with organic matter.*
USE: Mordant in dyeing and printing of textiles.

2633. Cupric Chloride. [7447-39-4] Cl_2Cu; mol wt 134.45. Cl 52.74%, Cu 47.26%. Prepn: Pray, *Inorg. Synth.* **5**, 153 (1957); *Gmelins, Copper* (8th ed.) **60B**, 253-295 (1958); Glemser, Sauer in *Handbook of Preparative Inorganic Chemistry* **vol. 2**, G. Brauer, Ed. (Academic Press, New York, 2nd ed., 1965) p 1008.

Yellow to brown, deliquesc, microcryst powder. Partially dec above 300° to CuCl + Cl_2. mp (extrapolated) 630°. mp of 498° usually reported for this compd is the melting pt of a mixture of $CuCl_2$ and CuCl. d_4^{25} 3.39. Forms the dihydrate in moist air. Sol in water, alc, acetone. *Keep well closed.*

Dihydrate. Green to blue powder or orthorhombic, bipyramidal crystals. Deliquesc in moist air, efflorescent in dry air. Water loss occurs from 70-200°: Bell, Coultard, *J. Chem. Soc. A* **1968**, 1417. mp ~100°; d 2.51. Freely sol in water, methanol, ethanol; moderately sol in acetone, ethyl acetate; slightly sol in ether. The aq soln is acid to litmus; pH of 0.2 molar soln 3.6.

Caution: Irritating to skin, mucous membranes.

USE: As catalyst for organic and inorganic reactions; in petroleum industry as deodorizing, desulfurizing, and purifying agent; as mordant for dyeing and printing textiles; as oxidizing agent for aniline dyestuffs; in indelible, invisible and laundry-marking inks; in metallurgy in wet process for recovering mercury from ores; in refining Cu, Ag, Au; in tinting-baths for Fe, Sn; in electrotyping baths for plating Cu on Al; in photography as a fixer, desensitizer and reagent; in producing color in pyrotechnic compositions; in manuf of acrylonitrile, fast black (melanin); in pigments for glass, ceramics; as feed-additive, wood preservative, disinfectant.

2634. Cupric Chromate(VI). [13548-42-0] Neutral cupric chromate. $CrCuO_4$; mol wt 179.54. Cr 28.96%, Cu 35.39%, O 35.65%. $CuCrO_4$. Prepn from $CuCO_3$, Na_2CrO_4 and CrO_3: Briggs, *J. Chem. Soc.* **1929**, 242; from CuO and CrO_3: Campbell, Lemaire, *Can. J. Res.* **25B**, 243 (1947); from $Cu(OH)_2$ and K_2Cr_2-O_7: Winter *et al.*, in *Kirk-Othmer Encyclopedia of Chemical Technology* **vol. 6** (Interscience, New York, 2nd ed., 1965) p 270.

Reddish-brown crystals. Gradually dec to $CuCr_2O_4$ above 400°. Practically insol in water; sol in acids.

Basic cupric chromates. Several cupric chromate-cupric hydroxide compounds are known. $CuCrO_4.Cu(OH)_2$ forms yellow, copper-red or chocolate-brown to lilac crystals; $CuCrO_4.2Cu(OH)_2$,

a light brown powder; $2CuCrO_4.3Cu(OH)_2$, yellow to yellowish-brown crystals. Prepn: Campbell, Lemaire, *loc. cit.*; Winter *et al.*, *loc. cit.* All are practically insol in water.

USE: In fungicides, seed protectants, and wood preservatives; as mordant in dyeing textiles; in protecting textiles against insects and microorganisms.

2635. Cupric Chromite. [12018-10-9] Cupric chromate(III). Cr_2CuO_4; mol wt 231.54. Cr 44.91%, Cu 27.44%, O 27.64%. $CuCr_2O_4$. Prepd by heating $CuCrO_4$ at 400°: Stroupe, *J. Am. Chem. Soc.* **71**, 569 (1949); or by decompn of $(NH_4)_2$-$Cu(CrO_4)_2.2NH_3$ at 700°: Whipple, Wold, *J. Inorg. Nucl. Chem.* **24**, 23 (1962).

Grayish-black to black tetragonal crystals. Dec to $CuCrO_2$ and CrO_3 above 900°. Practically insol in water, dil acids, concd HCl.

Copper-chromium oxide. A mixture of $CuCr_2O_4$ and CuO formed on decompn at temps below 400°, of orange copper ammonium chromate complex prepd from $Cu(NO_3)_2$, $Na_2Cr_2O_7$ and NH_4OH: Adkins *et al.*, *J. Am. Chem. Soc.* **72**, 2626 (1950); Wagner in *Handbook of Preparative Inorganic Chemistry* **vol. 2**, G. Brauer, Ed. (Academic Press, New York, 2nd ed., 1965) p 1672. Fine, brownish-black to black powder. Stable in atmospheric O_2 and moisture. Practically insol in water, dil acids.

USE: Selective hydrogenation catalysts.

2636. Cupric Citrate. [866-82-0] 2-Hydroxy-1,2,3-propanetricarboxylic acid copper (2+) salt (1:2); Cuprocitrol. C_6H_4-Cu_2O_7; mol wt 315.18. C 22.86%, H 1.28%, Cu 40.32%, O 35.53%. Prepd by the interaction of hot aq solns of $CuSO_4$ and Na citrate: *U.S.D.* 25th ed., p 1653.

Hemipentahydrate. Green or bluish-green, odorless, cryst powder. Loses its water at about 100°. Slightly sol in water; sol in ammonia, dil acids; slightly sol in cold, freely in hot solns of alkali citrates.

THERAP CAT: Astringent, antiseptic.

2637. Cupric Ferrocyanide. [13601-13-3] Hexakis(cyano-C)ferrate(4−) copper(2+) (1:2); hexacyanoferrate(4−) dicopper(2+); cupric hexacyanoferrate(II); Hatchett's brown; C.I. Pigment Brown 9. $C_6Cu_2FeN_6$; mol wt 339.04. C 21.26%, Cu 37.49%, Fe 16.47%, N 24.79%. $Cu_2Fe(CN)_6$. Prepd by addition of $K_4$$Fe(CN)_6$ to an aqueous soln of a sol cupric salt: Weiser *et al.*, *J. Phys. Chem.* **42**, 945 (1938); **46**, 99 (1942).

Reddish-brown powder or cubic crystals; ppts as a colloid or gel. Practically insol in water, dil acids, most organic solvents. Sol in NH_4OH, solns of alkali cyanides.

USE: As pigment; in photographic toning baths; to lower electric resistance of soil and electrode-to-soil contacts.

2638. Cupric Fluoride. [7789-19-7] CuF_2; mol wt 101.54. Cu 62.58%, F 37.42%. Prepd by fluorinating Cu or a Cu salt with F_2: von Wartenberg, *Z. Anorg. Allg. Chem.* **241**, 381 (1939); Jache, Cady, *J. Phys. Chem.* **56**, 1106 (1952); Haendler *et al.*, *J. Am. Chem. Soc.* **76**, 2178 (1954); Ritter, Smith, *J. Phys. Chem.* **70**, 805 (1966); **71**, 2036 (1971).

Monoclinic crystals; turns blue in moist air due to formation of dihydrate. mp ~785° (N_2 atm), 950° (HF atm); d 4.85. Soly in water (20°) 4.7 g/100 ml; hydrolyzed to CuFOH in hot water. May be stored in sealed glass ampuls.

Dihydrate. Blue monoclinic crystals. Dec above 130°. d_4^{25} 2.934. Slightly sol in cold water, hydrolyzed to oxyfluoride in hot water.

USE: Anhydr in cathodes in nonaq galvanic cells; high temperature fluorinating agent; dihydrate as flux in casting gray iron.

2639. Cupric Formate. [544-19-4] Tubercuprose. C_2H_2-CuO_4; mol wt 153.58. C 15.64%, H 1.31%, Cu 41.38%, O 41.67%. $Cu(HCOO)_2$. Prepd from cupric carbonate and formic acid: Martin, Waterman, *J. Chem. Soc.* **1959**, 1359.

Three forms of anhydrous compd exist: powder-blue, turquoise, or royal blue crystals. Sol in water. Practically insol in most organic solvents.

Dihydrate. Very pale blue, monoclinic needles. Loses $2H_2O$ on standing in air. Turquoise, anhydrous modification formed by dehydration at 100° *in vacuo* over phosphoric oxide. Sol in water.

Tetrahydrate. Large, light-blue, monoclinic, holohedral prisms. Powder-blue modification formed by dehydration over $CaCl_2$ under reduced press. Sol in water; very slightly sol in alc. Practically insol in most organic solvents.

USE: As antibacterial agent in the treatment of cellulose.

2640. Cupric Gluconate. [527-09-3] Bis(D-gluconato-$\kappa O^1,\kappa O^2$) copper; copper(II) gluconate. $C_{12}H_{22}CuO_{14}$; mol wt 453.84. C 31.76%, H 4.89%, Cu 14.00%, O 49.35%. $Cu[CH_2-OH(CHOH)_4CO_2]_2$. Prepd from gluconic acid and basic cupric carbonate: Suzuki *et al.*, *JP 63 2889* (1963 to Dainippon), *C.A.* **59**, 11264c (1963).

Hydrate. Light blue to bluish-green, odorless crystals or cryst powder. Astringent taste. Soly in water 30 g/100 ml at 25°; slightly sol in alc. Practically insol in most other organic solvents.

USE: Oral deodorant.

THERAP CAT: Copper supplement.

2641. Cupric Hexafluorosilicate. [12062-24-7] Cupric fluosilicate; cupric silicofluoride. CuF_6Si; mol wt 205.62. Cu 30.90%, F 55.44%, Si 13.66%. $CuSiF_6$. Prepn: Worthington, Haring, *Ind. Eng. Chem. Anal. Ed.* **3**, 7 (1931).

Tetrahydrate. Blue, monoclinic, efflorescent crystals. d 2.56: Clark *et al.*, *Can. J. Chem.* **47**, 3859 (1969). Readily sol in water. *Keep well closed.*

USE: Dyeing and hardening white marble; treating plant diseases.

2642. Cupric Hydroxide. [20427-59-2] Copper hydrate; hydrated cupric oxide. CuH_2O_2; mol wt 97.56. Cu 65.14%, H 2.07%, O 32.80%. $Cu(OH)_2$. Commercial prepn: Furness, **US 1800828** (1931 to Cellosilk); idem, **US RE 24324** (1957 to Copper Research); Rowe, **US 2536096** (1951 to Mountain Copper); laboratory prepn: Weiser *et al.*, *J. Am. Chem. Soc.* **64**, 503 (1942); Gauthier, *Bull. Soc. Chim. Fr.* **1960**, 353.

Blue to blue-green gel or light blue cryst powder. Stability is dependent on the method of prepn; may dec to black CuO on standing a few days or on heating. d 3.37. Practically insol in water. Sol in concd alkali when freshly pptd; sol in acids, NH_4OH.

USE: In manuf of rayon, battery electrodes, other Cu salts; as mordant in dyeing; as pigment; in fungicides, insecticides; as feed additive; in treating and staining paper; in prepn of Schweitzer's reagent; in catalysts.

2643. Cupric Nitrate. [3251-23-8] CuN_2O_6; mol wt 187.56. Cu 33.88%, N 14.94%, O 51.18%. $Cu(NO_3)_2$. Prepn: *Gmelins, Copper* (8th ed.) **60B**, 164-179 (1958); Addison, Hathaway, *J. Chem. Soc.* **1958**, 3099. Toxicity: H. F. Smyth *et al.*, *Am. Ind. Hyg. Assoc. J.* **30**, 470 (1969).

Large, blue-green, deliquesc, orthorhombic crystals. Sublimes at 150-225°. mp 255-256°. Sol in water, ethyl acetate, dioxane; dissolves in and reacts vigorously with ether. *Keep well closed.*

Trihydrate. Gerhardite. Blue, deliquesc, rhombic plates. mp 114.5°; d 2.05. Freely sol in water, alcohol. Practically insol in ethyl acetate. pH of 0.2 molar aq soln 4.0. *Keep well closed.* LD_{50} orally in rats: 0.94 g/kg (Smyth).

Hexahydrate. Blue, deliquesc prismatic crystals. Decomposes to trihydrate at 26.4°. d 2.07. Freely sol in water; sol in alc. *Keep well closed.*

Caution: Irritating to skin, mucous membranes.

USE: In light-sensitive reproductive papers; as ceramic color; as mordant and oxidizing agent in textile dyeing and printing; as reagent for burnishing iron, for giving a black "antique" finish to copper, for coloring zinc brown; in nickel-plating baths; in aluminum brighteners; in wood-preservatives, fungicides, herbicides; in pyrotechnic compositions; as catalyst component in solid rocket fuel; as nitrating agent for aromatic organosilicon compds; as catalyst for organic reactions.

2644. Cupric Oleate. [1120-44-1] 9-Octadecenoic acid copper salt. $C_{36}H_{66}CuO_4$; mol wt 626.45. C 69.02%, H 10.62%, Cu 10.14%, O 10.22%. $(C_{17}H_{33}COO)_2Cu$. Prepd from $CuSO_4$ and K oleate: Nelson, Pink, *J. Chem. Soc.* **1954**, 4412.

Blue to green solid. Practically insol in water. Slightly sol in alcohol; sol in ether.

Note: Ingredient of *Cuprex*, a hydrocarbon mixture used as a topical pediculicide.

USE: In antifouling compositions; as emulsifier and dispersing agent; as antioxidant in lubricating oils; as combustion-improver in fuel oils; as stabilizer for amide polymers; as catalyst.

2645. Cupric Oxalate. [814-91-5] Ethanedioic acid copper salt. C_2CuO_4; mol wt 151.57. C 15.85%, Cu 41.93%, O 42.22%. CuC_2O_4. Prepd by reaction of $CuSO_4$ with oxalic acid: David, *Bull. Soc. Chim. Fr.* **1960**, 719. Usually contains some water.

Blue-white powder. Loses any hydrated water by 200°; dec in air at 310° to CuO. Practically insol in water, alcohol, ether, acetic acid; sol in NH_4OH.

USE: As catalyst for organic reactions; as stabilizer for acetylated polyformaldehyde; in anticaries compositions; in seed treatments to repel birds and rodents.

2646. Cupric Oxide. [1317-38-0] Copper oxide (CuO); black copper oxide; C.I. 77403; C.I. Pigment Black 15; copper(II) oxide. CuO; mol wt 79.55. Cu 79.88%, O 20.11%. Occurs in nature as the mineral *tenorite*. Prepn: R. Ruer, J. Kuschmann, *Z. Anorg. Allg. Chem.* **154**, 69 (1926); O. Glemser, H. Sauer in *Handbook of Preparative Inorganic Chemistry* **vol. 2**, G. Brauer, Ed. (Academic Press, New York, 2nd ed., 1965) p 1012. Soly study: A. Hayward *et al.*, *Nature* **215**, 730 (1967). Bioavailability study: S. Aoyagi, D. H. Baker, *Poult. Sci.* **72**, 1075 (1993). Review of physical properties: E. Gmelin, *Indian J. Pure Appl. Phys.* **30**, 596-608 (1992); of use as a nutritional supplement: D. H. Baker, *J. Nutr.* **129**, 2278-2279 (1999).

Pure CuO (tenorite) is a steel-grey to black *p*-type semiconductor, mp ≈1330°. d ≈6.4. Insol in water. Slightly sol in alkalis; sol in acids and ammonia. Heat of formation (25°): −37.1 kcal/mol.

USE: As pigment in glass, ceramics, enamels, porcelain glazes, artificial gems; in mfr of rayon, other Cu compds; in sweetening petr gases; in galvanic electrodes; as flux in metallurgy; in correcting Cu deficiencies in soil; as optical-glass polishing agent; in antifouling paints, pyrotechnic compositions; as exciter in phosphor mixtures; as catalyst for organic reactions; in high temp superconductors.

THERAP CAT: Copper supplement.

THERAP CAT (VET): Copper supplement in ruminants.

2647. Cupric Perchlorate. [13770-18-8] Cl_2CuO_8; mol wt 262.45. Cl 27.02%, Cu 24.21%, O 48.77%. $Cu(ClO_4)_2$. Prepd from $Cu(NO_3)_2$ and perchloric acid or nitrosyl perchlorate: Caven, Bryce, *J. Chem. Soc.* **1934**, 514; Hathaway, Underhill, *ibid.* **1960**, 648; **1961**, 3091; Hathaway, *Proc. Chem. Soc. London* **1958**, 344.

Very pale green, hygroscopic crystals. Volatilizes on heating. Thermally stable to 130°; above 130° dec to a basic perchlorate. mp about 230-240°. Soluble in water, ether, dioxane, ethyl acetate. Practically insol in benzene, CCl_4, hexane.

Hexahydrate. Deep blue, monoclinic crystals. Freely sol in water, methanol, ethanol, acetic acid, acetic anhydride, acetone; slightly sol in ether, ethyl acetate.

USE: Analytical reagent: Kolb, *Ind. Eng. Chem. Anal. Ed.* **11**, 197 (1939); **16**, 38 (1944); Serjeant, *Nature* **186**, 963 (1960). Also in copper electrodeposition; in catalysts for combustion and propellants.

2648. Cupric Phosphate. [7798-23-4] $Cu_3O_8P_2$; mol wt 380.58. Cu 50.09%, O 33.63%, P 16.28%. $Cu_3(PO_4)_2$. Basic salts occur in nature as the minerals: *cornetite, dihydrite, libethenite, phosphorochalcite, pseudolibethenite, pseudomalachite, tagilite*. Prepn from $CuSO_4$ and $(NH_4)_2HPO_4$: Klement, Haselbeck, *Z. Anorg. Allg. Chem.* **334**, 27 (1964).

Trihydrate. Blue or olive orthorhombic crystals or blue to bluish-green powder. Dec on heating. Practically insol in cold water. Slightly sol in hot water; sol in acids, NH_4OH.

USE: Fungicide; catalyst for organic reactions, fertilizer; emulsifier; corrosion inhibitor for H_3PO_4; protectant for metal surfaces against oxidation.

2649. Cupric Salicylate. [16048-96-7] 2-Hydroxybenzoic acid copper salt. $C_{14}H_{10}CuO_6$; mol wt 337.77. C 49.78%, H 2.98%, Cu 18.81%, O 28.42%. $Cu[C_6H_4(OH)COO]_2$. Prepd from reaction of $CuSO_4$ with Na salicylate: Hanic, Michalov, *Acta Crystallogr.* **13**, 299 (1960); Inoue *et al.*, *Inorg. Chem.* **3**, 239 (1964).

Brown, blue-green or green powder. Absorbs water in moist air to form the tetrahydrate.

Tetrahydrate. Pale-blue needles or blue-green plates. Blue-green modification loses water on standing in air. Sol in water, alcohol, NH_4OH.

USE: In the separation of monoolefinic from di- or polyolefinic hydrocarbons.

2650. Cupric Selenate. [15123-69-0] CuO_4Se; mol wt 206.50. Cu 30.77%, O 30.99%, Se 38.24%. $CuSeO_4$. Prepd by the action of selenic acid on cupric carbonate: Klein, *Ann. Chim.* **14**, 263 (1940).

Pentahydrate. Light-blue triclinic crystals. Loses water above 80°, forming the monohydrate at 150-220° and becoming anhyd by 265°; dec to the selenite and basic selenite at ~480° and to CuO at ~700°. d 2.56. Sol in water; very slightly sol in acetone. Practically insol in alcohol.

USE: In coloring Cu or Cu alloys black.

2651. Cupric Selenide. [1317-41-5] CuSe; mol wt 142.51. Cu 44.59%, Se 55.41%. Occurs in nature as the mineral *klockmannite*. Prepd by reduction of cupric selenite with hydrazine: Benzing *et al., J. Am. Chem. Soc.* **80**, 2657 (1958); Kulifay, *J. Inorg. Nucl. Chem.* **25**, 75 (1965).

Blue-black to greenish-black prismatic needles or hexagonal plates. Dec at a dull red heat. d 6.0-6.6. Sol in HCl with H_2Se evolved, in H_2SO_4 with SO_2 evolved; oxidized to $CuSeO_3$ by HNO_3.

USE: Catalyst in Kjeldahl digestions; in semiconductors.

2652. Cupric Stearate. [660-60-6] Octadecanoic acid copper salt. $C_{36}H_{70}CuO_4$; mol wt 630.48. C 68.58%, H 11.19%, Cu 10.08%, O 10.15%. $(C_{17}H_{35}COO)_2Cu$. Prepd by metathesis of alcohol cupric acetate with an alcohol soln of stearic acid: Martin, Waterman, *J. Chem. Soc.* **1957**, 2545; Rai, Mehrotra, *J. Inorg. Nucl. Chem.* **21**, 311 (1961).

Pale-blue to blue-green amorphous powder. Considered to be dimeric. mp ~250°: Grant, *Can. J. Chem.* **42**, 951 (1964). Practically insol in water, methanol, ethanol, acetone, ether. Sol in pyridine, dioxane, acetic anhydride; sol in hot but practically insol in cold benzene, toluene, CCl_4, $CHCl_3$, ethyl acetate.

USE: In antifouling paints; in textile and wood preservatives; in rubber aging; as catalyst.

2653. Cupric Sulfate. [7758-98-7] Sulfuric acid copper (2+) salt (1:1); copper(II) sulfate. CuO_4S; mol wt 159.61. Cu 39.81%, O 40.10%, S 20.09%. $CuSO_4$. Occurs in nature as the mineral *hydrocyanite*. Commercial preparation of pentahydrate: *Faith, Keyes & Clark's Industrial Chemicals*, F. A. Lowenheim, M. K. Moran, Eds. (Wiley-Interscience, New York, 4th ed., 1975) pp 280-284; other prepns: *Gmelins, Copper* (8th ed.) **60B**, 491-560 (1958). Toxicity: Smyth *et al., Am. Ind. Hyg. Assoc. J.* **30**, 470 (1969).

Grayish-white to greenish-white rhombic crystals or amorphous powder. On heating dec above 560°. d 3.6. Hygroscopic. Sol in water. Practically insol in alcohol. *Keep tightly closed.*

Monohydrate. [10257-54-2] Dried cupric sulfate. Hygroscopic, almost white powder. Sol in water. Practically insol in alcohol. *Keep tightly closed.*

Pentahydrate. [7758-99-8] Bluestone; blue vitriol; Roman vitriol; Salzburg vitriol. Occurs in nature as the mineral *chalcanthite*. Large, blue or ultramarine, triclinic crystals or blue granules or light-blue powder. Slowly effloresces in air. Loses $2H_2O$ at 30°, 2 more H_2O at 110°; becomes anhyd by 250°. $d_4^{15.6}$ 2.286. Very sol in water; sol in methanol, glycerol; slightly sol in ethanol. pH of 0.2 molar aq soln 4.0. LD_{50} orally in rats: 960 mg/kg (Smyth).

Caution: A strong irritant. *See also* Copper.

USE: Anhyd salt for detecting and removing trace amounts of water from alcohols and other organic compds; as fungicide. Pentahydrate as agricultural fungicide, algicide, bactericide, herbicide; food and fertilizer additive; in insecticide mixtures; in manuf of other Cu salts; as mordant in textile dyeing; in prepn of azo dyes; in preserving hides; in tanning leather; in preserving wood; in electroplating solns; as battery electrolyte; in laundry and metal-marking inks; in petroleum refining; as flotation agent; pigment in paints, varnishes and other materials; in mordant baths for intensifying photographic negatives; in pyrotechnic compositions; in water-resistant adhesives for wood; in metal coloring and tinting baths; in antirusting compositions for radiator and heating systems; as reagent toner in photography and photoengraving; etc.

THERAP CAT: Antidote to phosphorus; antifungal (topical); copper supplement.

THERAP CAT (VET): Nutritional factor. Used in copper deficiency of ruminants. Has also been used as an anthelmintic, emetic, fungicide.

2654. Cupric Sulfate, Basic. [1332-14-5] Copper hydroxide sulfate; cupric subsulfate; Basi-Cop; Cuproxat. Salts of variable compositions of cupric sulfate and cupric hydroxide or oxide. Occurs in nature as the mineral *dolerophane*, $CuSO_4 \cdot CuO$. *Reviews:* Frear, *Chemistry of the Pesticides* (Van Nostrand, New York, 3rd ed., 1955) pp 316-323; *idem, Agricultural Chemistry* **vol. 2** (Van Nostrand, New York, 1951) pp 524-525; *Gmelins, Copper* (8th ed.) **60B**, 579-589 (1958). *See also* Burgundy Mixture.

Copper sulfate tribasic. $Cu_4H_6O_{10}S$; mol wt 452.29. Occurs in nature as the mineral *brochantite*; monohydrate as the mineral *langite*. Initial product formed during preparation of Bordeaux mixture, *q.v.*, from $CuSO_4$ and $Ca(OH)_2$: Frear, *loc. cit.* Also prepd from $CuSO_4$ and $Cu(OH)_2$: Denk, Leschhorn, *Z. Anorg. Allg. Chem.* **336**, 58 (1965). Very finely divided, light blue, gelatinous particles. Practically insol in water. Sol in plant and mineral acids, NH_4OH.

Copper sulfate dibasic. $Cu_3H_4O_8S$; mol wt 354.73. Occurs in nature as the mineral *antlerite*. Blue-green, rhombic, bipyramidal crystals. Practically insol in water.

USE: Fungicide for plants, seed treatment.

2655. Cupric Sulfide. [1317-40-4] CuS; mol wt 95.61. Cu 66.46%, S 33.54%. Occurs in nature as the mineral *covellite*, or *indigo copper* (blue, hexagonal or monoclinic crystals). Prepn: Glemser, Sauer in *Handbook of Preparative Inorganic Chemistry* **vol. 2**, G. Brauer, Ed. (Academic Press, New York, 2nd ed., 1965) p 1017.

Black powder. Stable in air when dry, oxidized to $CuSO_4$ by moist air. Practically insol in water, alcohol, dil acids, alkalies. Sol in KCN soln, NH_4OH, hot HNO_3.

USE: In antifouling paints; in prepn of mixed catalysts; in development of aniline black dye in textile printing.

2656. Cupric Tartrate. [815-82-7] (2*R*,3*R*)-2,3-Dihydroxybutanedioic acid copper (2+) salt (1:1). $C_4H_4CuO_6$; mol wt 211.62. C 22.70%, H 1.91%, Cu 30.03%, O 45.36%. Prepd by reaction of K tartrate with $Cu(NO_3)_2$: Kirschner, Kiesling, *J. Am. Chem. Soc.* **82**, 4174 (1960).

Trihydrate. Green to blue, odorless powder. Slightly sol in water; sol in acids, alkali solns.

USE: In baths for Cu electroplating.

2657. Cupric Tungstate(VI). [13587-35-4] Cupric wolframate. CuO_4W; mol wt 311.38. Cu 20.41%, O 20.55%, W 59.04%. $CuWO_4$. Prepn: Kosek *et al., Collect. Czech. Chem. Commun.* **24**, 2034 (1959).

Dihydrate. Light green powder. Becomes brown to greyish-yellow on heating, with loss of H_2O. Practically insol in water. Slightly sol in acetic acid; sol in NH_3, H_3PO_4; dec by mineral acids.

USE: In semiconductors, nuclear reactors; as catalyst for polyester formation.

2658. Cuprous Acetate. [598-54-9] Acetic acid copper(1+) salt. $C_2H_3CuO_2$; mol wt 122.59. C 19.59%, H 2.47%, Cu 51.84%, O 26.10%. CH_3COOCu. Obtained as a sublimate by heating cupric acetate *in vacuo* to temps above 220°: Angel, Harcourt, *J. Chem. Soc.* **81**, 1385 (1902); prepn from cuprous oxide and acetic acid-acetic anhydride: Shimizu, Mehler, *J. Am. Chem. Soc.* **74**, 4469 (1952). Crystal structure: T. Ogura *et al., J. Am. Chem. Soc.* **95**, 949 (1973).

Transparent, leafy crystals. Volatilizes on heating; dec on strong heating. Rapidly hydrolyzed by water with the formation of yellow Cu_2O.

2659. Cuprous Bromide. [7787-70-4] BrCu; mol wt 143.45. Br 55.70%, Cu 44.30%. CuBr. Prepn: Briggs, *J. Chem. Soc.* **127**, 496 (1925); Keller, Wycoff, *Inorg. Synth.* **2**, 3 (1946); Wagner, Wagner, *J. Chem. Phys.* **26**, 1597 (1957).

White powder or cubic crystals, (zinc blende structure); turns green to dark-blue on exposure to sunlight. mp 504°; bp 1345°;

d_4^{25} 4.72. Slightly sol in cold water, dec in hot water, HNO_3. Sol in HCl, HBr, NH_4OH with formation of complexes. Practically insol in acetone, concd H_2SO_4. *Keep tightly closed in a dark place.*

USE: As catalyst for organic reactions.

2660. Cuprous Chloride. [7758-89-6] Cu-lyt. ClCu; mol wt 99.00. Cl 35.81%, Cu 64.19%. CuCl. Occurs in nature as the mineral *nantokite* (colorless to grey cubic crystals). Prepn: Keller, Wycoff, *Inorg. Synth.* **2**, 1 (1946); Glemser, Sauer in *Handbook of Preparative Inorganic Chemistry* **vol. 2**, G. Brauer, Ed. (Academic Press, New York, 2nd ed., 1965) p 1005.

White cryst powder or cubic crystals (zinc-blende structure); stable to air and light if dry, but in presence of moisture turns green on exposure to air and blue to brown on exposure to light. mp 430°; d_4^{25} 4.14. Sparingly sol in water with partial decompn; practically insol in alcohol, acetone; sol in concd HCl, concd NH_4OH with formation of complexes. Solns oxidize rapidly in air. *Keep tightly closed and protected from light.*

USE: As catalyst for organic reactions; catalyst, decolorizer and desulfuring agent in petr industry; in denitration of cellulose; as condensing agent for soaps, fats and oils; in gas analysis to absorb carbon monoxide.

2661. Cuprous Cyanide. [544-92-3] Cupricin. CCuN; mol wt 89.56. C 13.41%, Cu 70.95%, N 15.64%. CuCN. Commercial prepns: Winter *et al.*, *Kirk-Othmer Encyclopedia of Chemical Technology* **vol. 6** (Interscience, New York, 2nd ed., 1965) p 271; laboratory prepns: Barber, *J. Chem. Soc.* **1943**, 79; Norberg, Jacobson, *Acta Chem. Scand.* **3**, 174 (1949); Vaughan, McCane, *J. Am. Chem. Soc.* **76**, 2504 (1954). Review of toxicology and human exposure: *Toxicological Profile for Cyanide* (PB98-101207, 1997) 291 pp.

White to cream-colored powder, colorless or dark green orthorhombic crystals, or dark red monoclinic crystals. *Poisonous!* mp 474°. Practically insol in water, alcohol, cold dil acids. Sol in NH_4OH; dec by HNO_3, boiling dil HCl. Sol in alkali cyanide solns because of formation of stable cyanocuprate(I) ions.

USE: In electroplating Cu or Fe; as insecticide, fungicide; as antifouling agent in marine paints; as polymerization catalyst.

2662. Cuprous Iodide. [7681-65-4] Hydro-Giene. CuI; mol wt 190.45. Cu 33.37%, I 66.63%. Occurs in nature as the mineral *marshite* (red-brown crystals). Prepn: Kaufman, Pinnel, *Inorg. Synth.* **6**, 3 (1960); Glemser, Sauer in *Handbook of Preparative Inorganic Chemistry* **vol 2**, G. Brauer, Ed. (Academic Press, New York, 2nd ed., 1965) p 1007.

Dense powder or cubic crystals (zinc-blende structure). Less photosensitive than CuBr or CuCl. mp 588-606°; bp ~1290°; d_4^{25} 5.63. Extremely insol in water; practically insol in dil acids, alcohol; sol in aq solns of NH_3, alkali cyanides, thiosulfates, iodides; dec by concd H_2SO_4 and HNO_3.

USE: As catalyst in organic reactions; as ice-nucleating chemical; as coating in cathode-ray tubes; as source of iodine in animal feeds; with HgI_2 as temp indicator; bactericide.

2663. Cuprous Mercuric Iodide. [13876-85-2] (T-4)-Dicopper(1+) tetraiodomercurate(2−); copper(I) iodomercurate(II); cuprous tetraiodomercurate(II); mercuric cuprous iodide. Cu_2HgI_4; mol wt 835.30. Cu 15.22%, Hg 24.01%, I 60.77%. Superionic, thermochromic material; exists in two temperature dependent forms; a structurally ordered low temperature β-form and the more random high temperature α-form. Prepn and structural studies: J. A. A. Ketelaar, *Z. Kristallogr.* **80**, 190 (1931). Prepn and phase diagram: M. Friesel *et al.*, *Physica Scripta* **35**, 34 (1987); J. Nölting *et al.*, *Ber. Bunsen-Ges. Phys. Chem.* **93**, 1335 (1989). Optical properties: H.-R. C. Jaw *et al.*, *Inorg. Chem.* **26**, 1387 (1987). Crystal structure and phase transition studies: L. Eriksson *et al.*, *Z. Kristallogr.* **197**, 235 (1991). High temperature powder neutron diffraction studies: S. Hull, D. A. Keen, *J. Phys. Condens. Matter* **13**, 5597 (2001). Use in holography: J. M. Yang, D. W. Sweeney, *Appl. Optics* **18**, 2398 (1979); in titrimetric applications: O. E. S. Godinho *et al.*, *Anal. Lett.* **17**, 135 (1984).

Deep-red, thermochromic cryst powder. Changes from scarlet to chocolate-brown at 67°. *Poison!* Practically insol in water, alcohol.

USE: For detecting overheating of machine bearings, etc. In pigments to prepare paints. Recording material for infrared holograms. Analytical reagent in titrimetric determn.

2664. Cuprous Oxide. [1317-39-1] Red copper oxide; C.I. 77402; yellow cuprocide; Cacobre; Cooper-Sandoz. Cu_2O; mol wt 143.09. Cu 88.82%, O 11.18%. Occurs in nature as the mineral *cuprite* (red to reddish-brown octahedral or cubic crystals). Prepd commercially by furnace reduction of mixtures of copper oxides with Cu: Drapeau, Johnson, US 2758014; US 2891842 (1956, 1959 both to Glidden); by decompn of copper ammonium carbonate: Rowe, US 2474497; Klein, US 2474533 (both 1949 to Lake Chemical); Rowe, US 2536096; Munn, US 2670273 (1951, 1954 both to Mountain Copper); by treatment of $Cu(OH)_2$ with SO_2: Rowe, US 2665192 (1954 to Mountain Chemical); or by electrolysis of an aq soln of NaCl between Cu electrodes: Arend, *Paint Technol.* **13**, 265 (1948). Laboratory prepns: Glemser, Sauer in *Handbook of Preparative Inorganic Chemistry* **vol. 2**, G. Brauer, Ed. (Academic Press, New York, 2nd ed., 1965) p 1011. Toxicity study: H. F. Smyth *et al.*, *Am. Ind. Hyg. Assoc. J.* **30**, 470 (1969).

Cubic crystals or microcrystalline powder. Color may be yellow, red, or brown depending on the method of prepn and the particle size. Stable in dry air; gradually oxidizes in moist air to CuO. mp 1232°; d_4^{25} 6.0. Practically insol in water. Sol in NH_4OH; in HCl forming CuCl which dissolves in excess HCl. With dil H_2SO_4 or dil HNO_3, the cupric salt is formed and half the copper is pptd as the metal. LD_{50} orally in rats: 0.47 g/kg (Smyth).

USE: Fungicide; antiseptic for fishnets; in antifouling paints for marine use; in photoelectric cells; as red pigment for glass, ceramic glazes; in brazing pastes; in rectifiers; as catalyst.

2665. Cuprous Potassium Cyanide. [13682-73-0] Potassium bis(cyano-*C*)cuprate(1−); potassium dicyanocuprate(I); potassio-cuprous cyanide; potassium cyanocuprate(I). C_2CuKN_2; mol wt 154.68. C 15.53%, Cu 41.08%, K 25.28%, N 18.11%. $KCu(CN)_2$. Prepd by evaporation of an aq soln of CuCN and KCN: Staritzky, Walker, *Anal. Chem.* **28**, 419 (1956).

Monoclinic, prismatic crystals. d 2.38. Practically insol in water; dec to CuCN by cold dil H_2SO_4 or heating in water; sol in DMSO.

USE: In electroplating copper and brass.

2666. Cuprous Selenide. [20405-64-5] Berzeline; selenkupfer. Cu_2Se; mol wt 206.05. Cu 61.68%, Se 38.32%. Occurs in nature as the mineral *berzelianite* which in addition to copper and selenium contains 4.73-8.50% silver, 0.35-0.54% iron, up to 0.38% thallium and traces of lead and magnesium. Prepd by reduction of an ammoniacal soln of a cupric salt and H_2SeO_3 with hydrazine: Benzing *et al.*, *J. Am. Chem. Soc.* **80**, 2657 (1958); Kulifay, *J. Inorg. Nucl. Chem.* **25**, 75 (1963); alternate methods: Glemser, Sauer in *Handbook of Preparative Inorganic Chemistry* **vol. 2**, G. Brauer, Ed. (Academic Press, New York, 2nd ed., 1965) p 1019.

Blue-black to black, tetragonal or cubic crystals with a metallic luster. mp 1113°. d_4^{21} 6.84. Sol in HCl with evolution of H_2Se, in H_2SO_4 with evolution of SO_2, in KCN soln; oxidized by HNO_3 to $CuSeO_3$.

USE: In semiconductors.

2667. Cuprous Sulfide. [22205-45-4] Cu_2S; mol wt 159.16. Cu 79.85%, S 20.15%. Occurs in nature as the mineral *chalcocite* also called *copper glance* (grey, black, green, blue, or violet rhombic crystals). Prepn: Glemser, Sauer in *Handbook of Preparative Inorganic Chemistry* **vol. 2**, G. Brauer, Ed. (Academic Press, New York, 2nd ed., 1965) p 1016.

Blue to grayish-black lustrous powder, granules, or orthorhombic crystals. mp ~1100°. d_4^{20} 5.6. On heating in the absence of air it forms Cu and CuS; in the presence of air it forms CuO, $CuSO_4$ and SO_2. Practically insol in water, acetic acid; very sparingly sol in HCl; dec by HNO_3, concd H_2SO_4. Partially sol in NH_4OH, readily in cyanide solns due to complex ion formation.

USE: In luminous paints; in electrodes for thermoelements; in preparation of $CuSO_4$; in solid-lubricant compositions; as catalyst.

2668. Cuprous Sulfite. [13982-53-1] Cu_2O_3S; mol wt 207.16. Cu 61.35%, O 23.17%, S 15.48%. Cu_2SO_3. Prepn and review: Dasent, Morrison, *J. Inorg. Nucl. Chem.* **26**, 1122 (1964).

Hemihydrate. Etard's salt. White to pale-yellow hexagonal crystals. Slightly sol in water; sol in HCl, NH_4OH, alkali solns. Practically insol in ether, alcohol.

Cupro-cupric sulfate. Chevreul's salt. $Cu_3O_6S_2$; mol wt 350.76. Dihydrate, red microcryst powder or prismatic crystals. Practically insol in water, alcohol. Sol in NH_4OH, HCl.

Rogojski's salt. Formerly considered to be $Cu_2SO_3 \cdot H_2O$; shown to be an equimolar mixture of Chevreul's salt and metallic copper (Dasent, Morrison, *loc. cit.*). Brick-red solid.

USE: As fungicide for grape vines; in dyeing polyacrylic fibers; polymerization catalyst. Chevreul's salt is a selective molluscicide.

2669. Cuprous Thiocyanate. [1111-67-7] Cuprous sulfocyanate; cuprous sulfocyanide. CCuNS; mol wt 121.63. C 9.87%, Cu 52.25%, N 11.52%, S 26.36%. CuSCN. Prepn: Demmerle *et al., Ind. Eng. Chem.* **42**, 2 (1950); Newman, *Analyst* **88**, 500 (1963).

White to yellow amorphous powder. d 2.85. Practically insol in water, dil acids, alc, acetone; sol in NH_4OH, ether, solns of alkali thiocyanates; dec by concd mineral acids.

USE: In marine antifouling paints; in primer compositions for explosives industry.

2670. Cuproxoline. [13007-93-7] Tetrahydrogen bis[8-hydroxy-5,7-quinolinedisulfonato(3−)-N^1,O^8]cuprate(4−) compd with *N*-ethylethanamine (1:4); 8-hydroxy-5,7-quinolinedisulfonic acid copper derivative compound with diethylamine; cupric bis[8-hydroxyquinoline di(diethylammonium sulfonate)]; copper DOS; Dicuprene; Cujec; Cuprimyl. $C_{34}H_{56}CuN_6O_{14}S_4$; mol wt 964.65. C 42.33%, H 5.85%, Cu 6.59%, N 8.71%, O 23.22%, S 13.30%. Clinical efficacy in treatment of arthritis: W. C. Kuzell *et al., Ann. Rheum. Dis.* **10**, 328 (1951). Veterinary use as parenteral copper supplement: I. J. Cunningham, *N. Z. Vet. J.* **7**, 15 (1959); N. F. Suttle, *Vet. Rec.* **109**, 304 (1981); G. J. Judson *et al., Aust. Vet. J.* **61**, 40 (1984). Review of use of organic copper complexes in treatment of rheumatoid and degenerative diseases: J. R. J. Sorenson, W. Hangarter, *Inflammation* **2**, 217-238 (1977). Review of veterinary use: W. M. Allen, C. B. Mallinson, *Vet. Rec.* **114**, 451-454 (1984).

Green platelets. Sol in water, giving a dark-green soln. A 10% aq soln is almost neutral and can be sterilized by autoclaving. LD_{50} i.m. in rats: 126 mg/kg (Kuzell).

THERAP CAT: Antirheumatic.

THERAP CAT (VET): Copper supplement.

2671. Curare. [8063-06-7] Ourari; urari; woorari; woorali; wourara. Rendering of an Indian name given to the unstandardized extracts derived mainly from the bark of various spp. of Strychnos and Chondodendron, prepared for use as arrow poisons by Indians in the Amazon and Orinoco valleys, and in the Guianas; the physiologically active principle of which is (+)-tubocurarine chloride, *q.v.* Three kinds of curare have appeared in commerce, distinguished by the kind of containers in which they were packed: **Tube cucare** or **bamboo curare, pot curare,** and **gourd curare** or **calabash curare.** Listing of members of the family *Menispermaceae*, botanical components of tube or bamboo curare and of pot curare: Krukoff, Moldenke, *Studies of American Menispermaceae, with special reference to species used in the preparation of arrow poisons in Brittonia* **3**, 1-74 (1938), also suppl. no. 1-5. (Note that the curare available for medical use under the name Intocostrin is a physiologically standardized extract from *Chondodendron tomentosum* R. & P., *Menispermaceae*). Listing of *Strychnos* spp. *Loganiaceae*, botanical components of calabash curare and of pot curare: Kruk-

off, Monachino, *The American Species of Strychnos* in *Brittonia* **4**, 248-322 (1942), also suppl. no. 1-6. Alkaloids from calabash curare and bark of *Strychnos* spp.: P. Karrer, *J. Pharm. Pharmacol.* **8**, 161-164 (1956); Schmid, Karrer, *Helv. Chim. Acta* **29**, 1853 (1946); **30**, 1162 (1947); Marino-Bettolo, *Festschrift Arthur Stoll* (Birkhäuser-Verlag, Basel 1957) pp 257-280. Review of history, chemistry, and use of arrow-poison curare: McIntyre, *Curare* (Chicago, 1947); Bovet *et al., Curare and Curare-like Agents* (Van Nostrand, Princeton, 1959).

Curare is sol in water and in dil alcohol. Stable aq solns (in ampuls) are standardized to contain 20 units per ml.

THERAP CAT: Neuromuscular blocking agent.

2672. C-Curarine I. [7168-64-1] $[C_{40}H_{44}N_4O]^{2+}$. Isoln from calabash-curare: Wieland, Pistor, *Ann.* **536**, 68 (1938); Karrer, Schmid, *Helv. Chim. Acta* **29**, 1853 (1946); Zürcher *et al., J. Am. Chem. Soc.* **80**, 1500 (1958). Structure: Nagyvàry *et al., Tetrahedron* **14**, 138 (1961); Grdinic *et al., J. Am. Chem. Soc.* **86**, 3357 (1964); Jones, Nowacki, *Chem. Commun.* **1972**, 805. Prepn of *C*-dihydrotoxiferine chloride: Bernauer *et al., Helv. Chim. Acta* **40**, 1999 (1957).

Dichloride. $C_{40}H_{44}Cl_2N_4O$. Needles from methanol + ether, mp >350°. $[\alpha]_D^{20}$ +73.6° (c = 1 in water). uv max (95% alc): 260, 296 nm (log ε 4.41, 4.07). Sol in water, alc; practically insol in ether, acetone.

2673. Curcumin. [458-37-7] (1E,6E)-1,7-Bis(4-hydroxy-3-methoxyphenyl)-1,6-heptadiene-3,5-dione; turmeric yellow; diferuloylmethane; C.I. 75300; C.I. Natural Yellow 3. $C_{21}H_{20}O_6$; mol wt 368.38. C 68.47%, H 5.47%, O 26.06%. Natural dyestuff from root of *Curcuma longa* L., *Zingiberaceae*. Isoln: Vogel, *Ann.* **44**, 297 (1842); Perkin, Phipps, *J. Chem. Soc.* (Trans.) **85, I,** 64 (1904); Rao, Shintre, *J. Soc. Chem. Ind.* **47**, 54T (1928). Synthesis: Lampe, *Ber.* **51**, 1347 (1918). Production: Stieglitz, Horn, **DE** 859145 (1952 to Hoechst). Biosynthesis studies: Roughley, Whiting, *Tetrahedron Lett.* **1971**, 3741. Chromatography: Srinivasan, *J. Pharm. Pharmacol.* **5**, 448 (1953). *See also: H. J. Conn's Biological Stains,* R. D. Lillie, Ed. (Williams & Wilkins, Baltimore, 9th ed., 1977) pp 474-476. Pharmacology and anti-inflammatory activity: Srimal, Dhawan, *ibid.* **25**, 447 (1973).

Orange-yellow, cryst powder, mp 183°. Insol in water, ether. Sol in alcohol, glacial acetic acid. Gives a brownish-red color with alkali; a light-yellow color with acids.

USE: For preparing curcuma paper, pH range 8-9. In the detection of boron.

2674. Curine. [436-05-5] (13aR,25aR)-2,3,13a,14,15,16,-25,25a-Octahydro-18,29-dimethoxy-1,14-dimethyl-13*H*-4,6:21,24-dietheno-8,12-metheno-1*H*-pyrido[3′,2′:14,15][1,11]dioxacycloeicosino[2,3,4-*ij*]isoquinoline-9,19-diol; (1β)-6,6′-dimethoxy-2,2′-

dimethyltubocuraran-7′,12′-diol; *l*-bebeerine. $C_{36}H_{38}N_2O_6$; mol wt 594.70. C 72.71%, H 6.44%, N 4.71%, O 16.14%. From tubocurare *(Chondodendron tomentosum* R. & P., *Menisperma-ceae):* Boehm, *Arch. Pharm.* **235**, 660 (1897); Späth *et al., Ber.* **61**, 1698 (1928). Structure: Späth, Kuffner, *Ber.* **67**, 55 (1934); Faltis *et al., Ber.* **69**, 1269 (1936); King, *J. Chem. Soc.* **1939**, 1157. Configuration: Bick, Clezy, *ibid.* **1953**, 3893; Hultin, *Acta Chem. Scand.* **17**, 753 (1963). Biosynthetic study: D. S. Bhakuni *et al., Tetrahedron* **43**, 3975 (1987). Ca^{2+} channel interactions: J. P. Felix *et al., Biochemistry* **31**, 11793 (1992).

Efflorescent crystals from methanol. mp 213°; mp 221° *in vacuo*; four sided prisms from benzene containing one mol benzene, mp 161°. $[\alpha]_D^{20} -328°$ (pyridine). Sol in benzene, chloroform, pyridine.

2675. Curium. [7440-51-9] Cm; at. no. 96; valence 3, 4. Man-made radioactive element. No stable nuclides; known isotopes (mass numbers): 238-251. Longest-lived known isotope: 247 (T$_{\frac{1}{2}}$ 1.56×10^7 years, rel. at. mass 247.0703, α-decay). Prepn of first isotope, ^{242}Cm (T$_{\frac{1}{2}}$ 162.9 days, α-decay), in 1944 by G. T. Seaborg *et al.* in *The Transuranium Elements,* G. T. Seaborg *et al.,* Eds. (McGraw-Hill, New York, 1949) pp 1554-1571. Prepn of metal: J. C. Wolfmann *et al., J. Am. Chem. Soc.* **73**, 493 (1951). Properties: Cunningham, Wallman, *J. Inorg. Nucl. Chem.* **26**, 271 (1964); Smith *et al., J. Chem. Phys.* **50**, 5066 (1969). *Reviews:* M. Haissinsky, J.-P. Adloff, *Radiochemical Survey of the Elements* (Elsevier, New York, 1965) pp 41-43; C. Keller, *The Chemistry of the Transuranium Elements* (Verlag Chemie, Weinheim, English Ed., 1971) pp 529-551; *Comprehensive Inorganic Chemistry* **vol 5**, J. C. Bailar, Jr. *et al.,* Eds. (Pergamon Press, Oxford, 1973) *passim; Handb. Exp. Pharmakol.* **36**, 689-928 (1973); P. G. Eller, R. A. Penneman in *The Chemistry of the Actinide Elements* **vol. 2**, J. J. Katz *et al.,* Eds. (Chapman and Hall, New York, 1986) pp 962-988.

Silvery, lusterous, malleable metal. Two allotropic modifications: double hexagonal close-packed α-form, d 13.51, transforms to β-form at ~1277°; face-centered cubic β-form, d 12.9, exists from ~1277° to mp. mp 1345°. bp (calc) 3110°. Metal dissolves rapidly in dilute acid solns; oxidizes rapidly in the presence of traces of oxygen. Pyrophoric when finely divided. Chemistry of trivalent state similar to that of trivalent lanthanides.

Caution: Radiation hazard; handling requires special equipment and shielding facilities (Katz *et al., loc. cit.* **vol. 2**, p 1128).

USE: ^{242}Cm and ^{244}Cm as power sources in radionuclide batteries for space and medical applications. ^{242}Cm as radioactive heat source. ^{248}Cm in accelerator studies to form superheavy elements.

2676. Curvularin. [10140-70-2] 4,5,6,7,8,9-Hexahydro-11,13-dihydroxy-4-methyl-2*H*-3-benzoxacyclododecin-2,10(1*H*)-dione. $C_{16}H_{20}O_5$; mol wt 292.33. C 65.74%, H 6.90%, O 27.37%. Mold metabolite from a species of *Convalaria:* Musgrave, *J. Chem. Soc.* **1956**, 4301; from *Penicillium steckii:* Fennell *et al., Chem. Ind. (London)* **1959**, 1382. Structure: Birch *et al., J. Chem. Soc.* **1959**, 3146. Synthesis: H. Gerlach, *Helv. Chim. Acta* **60**, 3039 (1977); of *dl-O,O*-dimethyl ether: Baker *et al., J. Chem. Soc. C* **1967**, 1913; T. Takahashi *et al., Tetrahedron Lett.* **21**, 3885 (1980); H. H. Wasserman, R. J. Gambale, *ibid.* **22**, 4849 (1981).

Plates from hot benzene + methanol, mp 206-206.5°. $[\alpha]_D^{18} -36.3°$ (c = 3.8 in ethanol). uv max (ethanol): 223, 272, 304.5 nm (ε 11300; 6350; 5100). Sol in ethanol, methanol, dioxane, acetone, pyridine, concd H_2SO_4; moderately sol in acetic acid, ether; sparingly sol in benzene, petr ether, chloroform, water. Gives yellow solns with aq ammonia, sodium carbonate, and sodium hydroxide. Alkaline solns darken rapidly in air, eventually becoming purple.

Dibenzoate. $C_{30}H_{28}O_7$. Needles from benzene + petr ether, mp 133-134°. $[\alpha]_D^{18} -10.8°$ (c = 1.9 in chloroform). uv max (ethanol): 236 nm (ε 36700).

O,O-**Dimethyl ether.** $C_{18}H_{24}O_5$. Short rods from aq ethanol, mp 72°. $[\alpha]_D^{18} -2.9°$ (c = 2.7 in chloroform). uv max (ethanol): 223, 267.5 nm (ε 10500; 5100).

2677. Cuscohygrine. [454-14-8] 1,3-Bis(1-methyl-2-pyrrolidinyl)-2-propanone; cuskhygrine; bellaradine. $C_{13}H_{24}N_2O$; mol wt 224.34. C 69.60%, H 10.78%, N 12.49%, O 7.13%. In coca leaves of various origin. Found in crude hygrine. Readily converted to hygrine by acids and bases. Isoln: Liebermann, *Ber.* **22**, 679 (1898); Liebermann, Cybulski, *ibid.* **28**, 578 (1895). Identity with bellaradine: Steinegger, Phokas, *Pharm. Acta Helv.* **30**, 441 (1955). Structure: Hess, Fink, *Ber.* **53**, 794 (1920); Sohl, Shriner, *J. Am. Chem. Soc.* **55**, 3828 (1933); Rapoport, Jorgensen, *J. Org. Chem.* **14**, 664 (1949). Synthesis: Späth, Tuppy, *Monatsh. Chem.* **79**, 119 (1948); Galinovsky *et al., ibid.* **82**, 551 (1951). Enzymatic synthesis: Tuppy, Faltaous, *ibid.* **91**, 167 (1960). Stereochemistry: Galinovsky, Zuber, *ibid.* **84**, 798 (1953). Biosynthesis: E. Leete, *Chem. Commun.* **1980**, 1170.

Oily liquid, bp$_{23}$ 169-170°; bp$_{14}$ 152°; bp$_2$ 118-125°. d$_4^{20}$ 0.9733. n$_D^{20}$ 1.4832. Miscible with water. Sol in alcohol, ether, benzene.

Hemiheptahydrate. Needles, mp 40°.

Hydrobromide. $C_{13}H_{24}N_2O.2HBr$. Prisms from alc, mp 234°.

2678. Cy 3. [146397-20-8] 1-[6-[(2,5-Dioxo-1-pyrrolidinyl)oxy]-6-oxohexyl]-2-[3-[1-[6-[(2,5-dioxo-1-pyrrolidinyl)oxy]-6-oxohexyl]-1,3-dihydro-3,3-dimethyl-5-sulfo-2*H*-indol-2-ylidene]-1-propenyl]-3,3-dimethyl-5-sulfo-3*H*-indolium inner salt. $C_{43}H_{50}$-$N_4O_{14}S_2$; mol wt 911.01. C 56.69%, H 5.53%, N 6.15%, O 24.59%, S 7.04%. One of a family of indocyanine dyes with high fluorescence. Conjugates easily to proteins and oligonucleotides for labelling. Prepn: A. S. Waggoner *et al.,* **DE 3912046**; *eidem,* **US 5268486** (1990, 1993 both to Carnegie-Mellon). Use with fiber optic biosensors: L. A. Tempelman *et al., Proc. SPIE Int. Soc. Opt. Eng.* **2293**, 139 (1994). Use with neuropeptides for detection of receptors: N. W. Bunnett *et al., Histochem. J.* **28**, 811 (1996); for detection of synaptic vesicle mobility: K. Kraszewski *et al., J. Neurosci.* **16**, 5905 (1996).

Potassium salt. Water soluble. Absorbance max: 552 nm; emission max: 565 nm; extinction coefficient >130,000 M^{-1}cm^{-1}.

USE: Fluorescent label.

2679. Cy 5. [146368-15-2] 1-[6-[-(2,5-Dioxo-1-pyrrolidinyl)oxy]-6-oxohexyl]-2-[5-[1-[6-[(2,5-dioxo-1-pyrrolidinyl)oxy]-6-oxohexyl]-1,3-dihydro-3,3-dimethyl-5-sulfo-2*H*-indol-2-ylidene]-1,3-pentadienyl]-3,3-dimethyl-5-sulfo-3*H*-indolium inner salt. $C_{45}H_{52}N_4O_{14}S_2$; mol wt 937.04. C 57.68%, H 5.59%, N 5.98%,

O 23.90%, S 6.84%. Indocyanine dye with high fluorescence which is easily coupled to proteins. Named CyX.Y where X is the number of bridge carbons and Y represents a unique dye structure. Prepn: A. S. Waggoner *et al.*, **DE 3912046**; *eidem*, **US 5268486** (1990, 1993 both to Carnegie-Mellon). Use with fiber optic biosensors: L. A. Tempelman *et al.*, *Proc. SPIE Int. Soc. Opt. Eng.* **2293**, 139 (1994); for antibody/antigen detection: R. M. Wadkins *et al.*, *ibid.* **2676**, 148 (1996). Use in resonance energy transfer: P. R. Selvin *et al*, *J. Am. Chem. Soc.* **116**, 6029 (1994).

Water soluble.

Potassium salt. Water soluble. Absorbance max 650 nm; emission max 667 nm (ε >200,000). Quantum yield 0.28.

Cy 5.5. [172777-84-5] Water soluble. Absorbance max 678 nm; emission max 703 nm (ε 250,000). Quantum yield 0.28.

USE: Fluorescent label.

2680. Cyacetacide. [140-87-4] Cyanoacetic acid hydrazide; malononitrile hydrazide; cyanoacetohydrazide; cyanazide; cyanizide; cyanacethydrazine; cyanacethydrazide; cyanoethydrazide; cyanacetylhydrazide; Dictyzide; Mackreazid; Armazal; Reacid; Reazide; Hidacian; Leandin; Neohydrazid; Dictycide. $C_3H_5N_3O$; mol wt 99.09. C 36.36%, H 5.09%, N 42.41%, O 16.15%. $NCCH_2CONHNH_2$. Prepd by boiling ethyl or methyl cyanoacetate with hydrazine hydrate in alc: Rothenburg, *Ber.* **27**, 687 (1894); Darapsky, Hillers, *J. Prakt. Chem.* **92**[2], 313 (1915); Klosa, *Arch. Pharm.* **288**, 453 (1955). Prepn of dosage forms: Muset, **US 2849369** (1958 to Labs OM).

Stout prisms from alc, mp 114.5-115° (evac tube). Rapidly dec by heat. Very slightly acid to litmus. Very sol in water. Sol in alcohol. Practically insol in ether. Aq solns become discolored after a few days and the pH becomes alkaline.

Hydrochloride. $C_3H_5N_3O.HCl$. Crystals, mp 145°. Freely sol in water. Acid reaction. Aq solns are more stable than those of the free hydrazide.

THERAP CAT: Antibacterial (tuberculostatic).

THERAP CAT (VET): Anthelmintic (lungworms).

2681. Cyadox. [65884-46-0] [(1,4-Dioxido-2-quinoxalinyl)methylene]hydrazide cyanoacetic acid; 2-formylquinoxaline-1,4-dioxide cyanoacetylhydrazone; $C_{12}H_9N_5O_3$; mol wt 271.23. C 53.14%, H 3.34%, N 25.82%, O 17.70%. Antimicrobial growth promoting feed additive for poultry, calves and pigs. Growth promoting effects in chickens: J. Broz, B. Sevcik, *Biol. Chem. Vyz. Zvirat* **13**, 357, 375 (1977). Prepn: J. Hebky *et al.*, **DE 2829580**; *eidem*, **US 4225604** (1979, 1980 both to Spofa). Adsorptive voltammetry determn in plasma: I. Sestáková, M. Kopanica, *Talanta* **35**, 816 (1988). LC determn in animal feeds and gastrointestinal samples: G. J. De Graaf, T. J. Spierenburg, *J. Chromatogr.* **447**, 244 (1988); in goat tissue: Y. Zhang *et al.*, *Anal. Sci.* **21**, 1495 (2005). Heat stability study: *idem et al.*, *J. Agric. Food Chem.* **53**, 9737 (2005). Subchronic toxicity study: G. Fang *et al.*, *Food Chem. Toxicol.* **44**, 36 (2006).

Yellow solid, mp 255-260°. *Light sensitive.*

THERAP CAT (VET): Growth promotant.

2682. Cyamelide. [462-02-2] 1,3,5-Trioxane-2,4,6-triimine; insoluble cyanuric acid. $C_3H_3N_3O_3$; mol wt 129.07. C

27.92%, H 2.34%, N 32.56%, O 37.19%. Formed by polymerization of cyanic acid (gaseous or liquid). Prepd by digesting equal parts of potassium cyanate and oxalic acid: Liebig, Wöhler, *Berzelius Jahresber.* **11**, 85. Crude cyamelide contains cyanuric acid which is removed by washing with water: Senier, Walsh, *J. Chem. Soc.* **81**, 290 (1902). Mechanism of polymerization: Werner, Fearon, *ibid.* **117**, 1358 (1920).

White amorphous powder. Practically insol in water. Insol in organic solvents. Slightly sol in ammonia water, in concd acids, in concd NaOH with salt formation.

2683. Cyamemazine. [3546-03-0] 10-[3-(Dimethylamino)-2-methylpropyl]-10*H*-phenothiazine-2-carbonitrile; 2-cyano-10-(3-dimethylamino-2-methylpropyl)phenothiazine; 10-(3-dimethylamino-2-methylpropyl)-3-cyanophenothiazine; cyamepromazine; RP-7204; TH-2602; Kyamepromazine; cyamepromazine; RP-7204; TH-2602; Kyamepromazine; Cianatil; Tercian. $C_{19}H_{21}N_3S$; mol wt 323.46. C 70.55%, H 6.54%, N 12.99%, S 9.91%. Prepn: Jacob, Robert, **US 2877224** (1959 to Rhône-Poulenc). Synthesis: Craig *et al.*, *J. Org. Chem.* **26**, 1138 (1961). Biotransformation studies: Robinson, *J. Pharm. Pharmacol.* **18**, 19 (1966). Chemistry: Kiger, Kiger, *Ann. Pharm. Fr.* **23**, 489 (1965).

Yellow oil, $bp_{0.2-0.5}$ 205-220°; also reported as yellow powder, mp 89-96° (Kiger). Practically insol in water. Sol in ethanol and in organic solvents.

Maleate. $C_{23}H_{25}N_3O_4S$. Pale yellow plates from methanol-ethanol, mp 196-197° (Craig).

THERAP CAT: Antipsychotic.

2684. Cyanamide. [420-04-2] Carbodiimide; hydrogen cyanamide; carbimide; cyanogenamide; amidocyanogen. CH_2N_2; mol wt 42.04. C 28.57%, H 4.80%, N 66.64%. $H_2NC≡N$. Prepd commercially by continuous carbonation of calcium cyanamide in water. *Ref.* "Cyanamide," Process Chemicals Dept., Am. Cyanamid (New York, 1959) p 19. Acute toxicity data: J. Doull *et al.*, *Survey of Compounds for Radiation Protection* (AD277689, USAF Radiation Lab., 1962) 124 p.

Deliquescent, orthorhombic, elongated, six-sided tablets from dimethyl phthalate. d_4^{20} 1.282. mp 45-46°. $bp_{0.5}$ 83°. Formn of dicyandiamide begins at 122°. Dipole moment in benzene at 20°: 3.8. Cryoscopic constant (water) 26.8-28.4. Sp ht 0.547 cal/g/°C between 0° and 39°. Heat of formation 14.05 kcal/mole (25°); heat of combustion −176.4 kcal/mole (25°); heat of fusion 2.1 kcal/mole. Heat of vaporization 16.4 kcal/mole. Soly (g/100 g soln) in water at 15°: 77.5, at 43°: 100; in butanol at 20°: 28.8, in methyl ethyl ketone: 50.5, in ethyl acetate: 42.4. Sol in alcohols, phenols, amines, ethers, ketones. Very sparingly sol in benzene, halogenated hydrocarbons. Practically insol in cyclohexane. Solid cyanamide should be stored in a cool, dry place. Polymerizes at 122°. Optimum pH for storage of solns is ~4. Attacks various metals. Solns can be stored in glass provided they are stabilized with phosphoric, acetic, sulfuric, or boric acid. LD_{50} i.p. in male mice: 200-300 mg/kg (Doull).

Note: Term "cyanamide" is also used to designate calcium cyanamide.

Caution: Potential symptoms of overexposure are irritation of eyes, skin, respiratory system; eye, skin burns; miosis, salivation, lacrimation, twitching; Antabuse-like effects. *See NIOSH Pocket Guide to Chemical Hazards* (DHHS/NIOSH 97-140, 1997) p 80.

2685. Cyanazine. [21725-46-2] 2-[[4-Chloro-6-(ethylamino)-1,3,5-triazin-2-yl]amino]-2-methylpropanenitrile; 2-[[4-chloro-6-(ethylamino)-s-triazin-2-yl]amino]-2-methylpropionitrile; SD-15418; WL-19805; DW-3418; Bladex; Fortrol. $C_9H_{13}ClN_6$; mol wt 240.69. C 44.91%, H 5.44%, Cl 14.73%, N 34.92%. Selective pre-emergence herbicide. Prepn: **GB 1132306**; W. Schwarze, **US 3505325** (1968, 1970 both to Degussa). Activity: T. Chapman *et al., Proc. 9th Br. Weed Control Conf.* **2**, 1018 (1968). Metabolism: J. V. Crayford, D. H. Hutson, *Pestic. Biochem. Physiol.* **2**, 295 (1975). Persistence in soil: J. T. Majka, T. L. Lavy, *Weed Sci.* **25**, 401 (1977).

White crystals, mp 167.5-169°. Vapor pressure at 20°: 1.6×10^{-9} mmHg. Soly in water at 25°: 171 mg/l. Soly at 25° (g/l): benzene 15, chloroform 210, ethanol 45, hexane 15. LD_{50} in rats, mice (mg/kg): 182, 380 orally (Chapman).

USE: Herbicide.

2686. Cyanic Acid. [420-05-3] Hydrogen cyanate. CHNO; mol wt 43.02. C 27.92%, H 2.34%, N 32.56%, O 37.19%. Best prepd in the laboratory by dry distillation of cyanuric acid: Linhard, *Z. Anorg. Allg. Chem.* **236**, 200 (1938). *See also* Isocyanic Acid.

$$HO-C\equiv N$$

Liquid. *Acrid odor, strong lacrimator and vesicant.* d_4^{20} 1.140; d_4^{-20} 1.156. mp $-86°$. bp_{760} 23.5°. Heat of formation -36.5 kcal/mol. Dipole moment 1.592. pK (20°) 3.66. Rapid heating of the liq may result in an explosion. Polymerizes on standing forming cyamelide and cyanuric acid. Sol in water with decompn to carbon dioxide and ammonia. Dil solns in ice water may be kept for several hours. Dil solns in ether, benzene, toluene can be kept for several weeks.

Caution: Highly irritating to eyes, skin, and mucous membranes. *See Clinical Toxicology of Commercial Products*, R. E. Gosselin *et al.,* Eds. (Williams & Wilkins, Baltimore, 5th ed., 1984) Section II, p 110.

USE: In formation of some cyanates.

2687. Cyanidin Chloride. [528-58-5] 2-(3,4-Dihydroxyphenyl)-3,5,7-trihydroxy-1-benzopyrylium chloride; 3,3′,4′,5,7-pentahydroxyflavylium chloride; 3,3′,4′,5,7-pentahydroxy-2-phenylbenzopyrylium chloride. $C_{15}H_{11}ClO_6$; mol wt 322.70. C 55.83%, H 3.44%, Cl 10.99%, O 29.75%. Prepd by acid hydrolysis of cyanin chloride: Willstätter, Everest, *Ann.* **401**, 189 (1913). Isoln from bananas: Simmonds, *Nature* **173**, 402 (1954). Prepn by reduction of quercetin: Bauer *et al., Chem. Ind. (London)* **1954**, 433; King, White, *J. Chem. Soc.* **1957**, 3901. Structure: Willstätter, Mallison, *Ann.* **408**, 147 (1915). Synthesis: Willstätter *et al., Ber.* **57**, 1938 (1924); Robertson, Robinson, *J. Chem. Soc.* **1928**, 1528. Biosynthesis: Fritsch *et al., Z. Naturforsch.* **26b**, 581 (1971). *See also* Bioflavonoids.

Metallic brownish-red needles (monohydrate) from dil alcoholic HCl. The anhydr compd does not melt below 300°. Absorption max (methanolic HCl): 535 nm. Freely sol in alcohol and in amyl alcohol giving a violet soln. Sol in sodium carbonate soln with blue color. Sparingly sol in dil HCl or H_2SO_4.

3-Glucoside. Chrysanthemin; asterin; kuromanin. $C_{21}H_{21}$-ClO_{11}. From winter aster (*Chrysanthemum indicum* L., Composi-

tae): Willstätter, Bolton, *Ann.* **412**, 136 (1917); from wild strawberries (*Fragaria vesca* L., *Rosaceae):* Sondheimer, Karash, *Nature* **178**, 648 (1956); from sweet cherries (*Prunus avium* L., *Rosaceae):* Li, Wagenknecht *ibid.* **182**, 657 (1958). Identity with asterin: Robinson, Willstätter, *Ber.* **61**, 2503 (1928). Structure and synthesis: Murakami *et al., J. Chem. Soc.* **1931**, 2665. Reddish-brown plates or prisms with a metallic shine from dil alcoholic HCl, dec 205° without melting. Absorption max (methanolic HCl): 525 nm. Sol in alc with strong fluorescence and in sodium carbonate with violet-blue color.

3-Rhamnoglucoside. Keracyanin; antirrhinin; sambucin; Meralop; Meralops. $C_{27}H_{31}ClO_{15}$; mol wt 630.98. From skin of sweet cherries (*Prunus avium* L,. *Rosaceae):* Willstätter, Zollinger, *Ann.* **412**, 164 (1917); from sour cherries (*Prunus cerasus* L., *Rosaceae*): Li, Wagenknecht, *J. Am. Chem. Soc.* **78**, 979 (1956). Structure: Robertson, Robinson, *J. Chem. Soc.* **1927**, 2196. Prepn by reduction of quercetin-3-rhamnoglucoside: Bauer *et al., Chem. Ind. (London)* **1954**, 433. Reduces time to adjust to darkness: F. Trimarchi *et al., Min. Oftalmol.* **18**, 143 (1977). Mechanism of action: F. Trimarchi *et al., Ann. Ottalmol. Clin. Ocul.* **105**, 111 (1979). Red needles from dil HCl or dark prisms from dil methanolic HCl. Absorption max (ethanolic HCl): 532, 333, 282 nm. Sol in hot water, alcohol.

3-Galactoside. Idaein; idein. $C_{21}H_{21}ClO_{11}$. From cranberries (*Vaccinium vitis idaea* L., *Ericaceae):* Willstätter, Mallison, *Ann.* **408**, 15 (1915); from Winesap apple (*Pyrus malus* Linn., *Rosaceae):* Duncan, Dustman, *J. Am. Chem. Soc.* **58**, 1511 (1936). Structure and synthesis: Grove, Robinson, *J. Chem. Soc.* **1931**, 2722. Red needles with bronze metallic luster from dil ethanolic HCl, dec 210-212°. Sol in water, ethanol, methanol, dil HCl. Practically insol in 7% HCl.

3,5-Diglucoside. Cyanin; shisonin A. $C_{27}H_{31}ClO_{16}$. From cornflower (*Centaurea cyanus* L., *Compositae):* Willstätter, Everest, *loc. cit.* Structure: Léon, Robinson, *J. Chem. Soc.* **1932**, 221. Synthesis: Robinson, Todd, *ibid.* 2488. Plates with a metallic luster from dil alcoholic HCl, mp 203-204°. $[\alpha]_D$ $-258°$ (in 0.05% HCl). Absorption max (methanolic HCl): 522 nm.

3-Sophoroside. Mecocyanin. $C_{27}H_{31}ClO_{16}$. From the flowers of *Papaver rhoeas* L., *Papaveraceae:* Willstätter, Weil, *Ann.* **412**, 231 (1917); from sour cherries: Li, Wagenknecht, *J. Am. Chem. Soc., loc. cit.* Structure: Harborne, *Experientia* **19**, 7 (1963); *Phytochemistry* **2**, 85 (1963). (Alternate structure: Grove *et al., J. Chem. Soc.* **1934**, 1608). Dark-red crystals from dil HCl + HOAc or dark-red needles from 2% alcoholic HCl. Absorption max (methanolic HCl): 523 nm. Sol in water. Pptd by glacial acetic acid or acetone.

THERAP CAT: 3-Rhamnoglucoside in treatment of night blindness.

2688. Cyanoacetamide. [107-91-5] Malonamide nitrile. $C_3H_4N_2O$; mol wt 84.08. C 42.85%, H 4.80%, N 33.32%, O 19.03%. $CNCH_2CONH_2$. Prepd by the action of aq or alcoholic ammonia on cyanoacetic ester: Hesse, *Am. Chem. J.* **18**, 724 (1896); Thole, Thorpe, *J. Chem. Soc.* **99**, 429 (1911); Ott, Löpmann, *Ber.* **55**, 1258 (1922); Corson *et al., Org. Synth.* **coll. vol. I** (2nd ed., 1941) p 179.

Needles from alc, mp 119.5°. One gram dissolves in 6.5 ml of cold water. Soly in 100 ml of 95% alc: 1.3 g at 0°; 3.1 g at 26°; 7.0 g at 44°; 14.0 g at 62°; 21.5 g at 71°.

USE: In organic syntheses (*e.g.,* starting material for vitamin B_6 synthesis).

2689. Cyanoacetic Acid. [372-09-8] Malonic mononitrile. $C_3H_3NO_2$; mol wt 85.06. C 42.36%, H 3.55%, N 16.47%, O 37.62%. $N\equiv CCH_2COOH$. Prepd from chloroacetic acid and NaCN: Ruggli, Businger, *Helv. Chim. Acta* **25**, 35 (1942); Lapworth, Baker, *Org. Synth.* **coll. vol. I**, 181 (1941); **GB 824640** (1959); Eaker, **US 2539238** (1951 to Monsanto).

Hygroscopic crystals, mp 66°; dec at 160° into CO_2 and acetonitrile. bp_{15} 108°. Sol in water, alcohol, ether, slightly in benzene, chloroform. *Keep well closed.*

USE: Synthesis of intermediates; manuf barbital.

2690. 1-Cyanobenzotriazole. [15328-32-2] 1H-Benzotriazole-1-carbonitrile. $C_7H_4N_4$; mol wt 144.13. C 58.33%, H 2.80%, N 38.87%. Cyanating agent. Prepn: M. E. Hermes, F. D. Marsh,

J. Am. Chem. Soc. **89**, 4760 (1967); T. V. Hughes *et al., J. Org. Chem.* **63**, 401 (1998). Electronic structure: P. Rademacher *et al., J. Mol. Struct.* **513**, 47 (1999). Use in cyanation: A. R. Katritzky *et al., Rev. Roum. Chim.* **36**, 573 (1991); T. V. Hughes, M. P. Cava, *J. Org. Chem.* **64**, 313 (1999); corrected: *ibid.* 2599.

[Chemical structure: benzotriazole with CN group]

Colorless needles, mp 73-75°. uv max (ethanol): 253, 293 nm (ε 6620, 3300).

USE: In chemical synthesis as a cyanating reagent.

2691. Cyanogen. [460-19-5] Ethanedinitrile; dicyan; oxalic acid dinitrile. C_2N_2; mol wt 52.03. C 46.17%, N 53.84%. N≡C—C≡N. Prepn by adding an aq soln of sodium or potassium cyanide to an aq soln of copper(II) sulfate or chloride: Janz, *Inorg. Synth.* **5**, 43 (1957); from HCN by the use of CuO: Fierce, Millikan, US 2841472 (1958 to Pure Oil); from HCN and NO_2: Fierce, Sander, *Ind. Eng. Chem.* **53**, 985 (1961). *Review:* Brotherton, Lynn, *Chem. Rev.* **59**, 841-883 (1959). Review of toxicology and human exposure: *Toxicological Profile for Cyanide* (PB98-101207, 1997) 291 pp.

Highly poisonous gas. Almond-like odor. Acrid and pungent when in lethal concns. Burns with pink flame having a bluish border. mp −27.9° (also reported as −34.4°). bp −21.17°. $d_4^{-21.17}$ 0.9537. Heat of vaporization (liquid) 5.778 kcal/mole. Above 500° polymerizes to insol paracyanogen $(CN)_n$. One vol of water dissolves about 4 vols of cyanogen gas. Also sol in alcohol, ether. Slowly hydrolyzed in aq soln giving oxalic acid and ammonia.

Caution: Potential symptoms of overexposure are irritation of eyes, nose, upper respiratory system; lacrimation; cherry red lips; tachypnea, hyperpnea, bradycardia; headache, vertigo, convulsions; dizziness, loss of appetite, weight loss. Direct contact with liquid may cause frostbite. *See NIOSH Pocket Guide to Chemical Hazards* (DHHS/NIOSH 97-140, 1997) p 82.

2692. Cyanogen Azide. [764-05-6] Carbon pernitride. CN_4; mol wt 68.04. C 17.65%, N 82.34%. Prepd by suspending NaN_3 in dry acetonitrile and distilling cyanogen chloride into the cooled suspension: Marsh, Hermes, *J. Am. Chem. Soc.* **86**, 4506 (1964); *see also Chem. Eng. News* **42**, 51 (Oct. 26, 1964); Marsh, US 3410658 (1968); Marsh, *J. Org. Chem.* **37**, 2966 (1972). Spectrum, structure, dipole moment: Costain, Kroto, *Can. J. Phys.* **50**, 1453 (1972); Almenningen *et al., Acta Chem. Scand.* **27**, 1531 (1973).

$^-N{=}N{=}^+N{-}C{\equiv}N$

Clear, colorless, oily liquid. *Caution: The pure azide detonates violently upon thermal, electrical or mechanical shock!* Can be handled relatively safely in solvents. Half-life of a 27% soln in acetonitrile is 15 days at room temp, more stable at lower temps.

USE: In organic synthesis. Has a versatility and scope of chemical reactivity that is very broad and useful, *e.g.* reacts with alkanes to give primary alkylcyanamides: Anastassiou *et al., J. Am. Chem. Soc.* **87**, 2296 (1965).

2693. Cyanogen Bromide. [506-68-3] Bromine cyanide. CBrN; mol wt 105.92. C 11.34%, Br 75.44%, N 13.22%. BrCN. Prepd from potassium or sodium cyanide and bromine: Hartman, Dreger, *Org. Synth.* **11**, 30 (1931). Industrial prepn from sodium bromide, sodium chlorate, and sodium cyanide in 30% H_2SO_4: Ewan, *Chem. Zentralbl.* **1907, I**, 591; Göpner, *ibid.* **1908, I**, 1807; Grignard, Crouzier, *Bull. Soc. Chim. Fr.* [4] **29**, 214 (1921). Brief review of synthetic applications: V. Kumar, *Synlett* **2005**, 1638-1639.

Crystalline solid; dec in the presence of moisture. *Vapors are highly irritating and very poisonous!* d_4^{20} 2.015. mp 52°. bp 61-62°. Freely sol in water, alcohol, ether. Aq solns of alkalies dec it to alkali cyanide and alkali bromide.

Caution: Toxic effects similar to those of hydrogen cyanide, *q.v.*

USE: Reagent for the synthesis of cyanamides.

2694. Cyanogen Chloride. [506-77-4] CClN; mol wt 61.47. C 19.54%, Cl 57.68%, N 22.79%. CNCl. Prepd by action of Cl on HCN. Review of toxicology and human exposure: *Toxicological Profile for Cyanide* (PB98-101207, 1997) 291 pp.

Liquid. *Vapors are highly irritant and very poisonous!* d 1.186. bp 13.8°. mp −6°. Sol in water, alc, ether.

Caution: Potential symptoms of overexposure are irritation of eyes, upper respiratory system; cough, delayed pulmonary edema; weakness, headache, giddiness, dizziness, confusion, nausea, vomiting; irregular heart beat; direct contact with liquid may cause skin irritation. *See NIOSH Pocket Guide to Chemical Hazards* (DHHS/NIOSH 97-140, 1997) p 82.

USE: In chemical synthesis. Military poison gas.

2695. Cyanogen Iodide. [506-78-5] Iodine cyanide. CIN; mol wt 152.92. C 7.85%, I 82.99%, N 9.16%. CNI. Prepd by the action of iodine on sodium cyanide: Bak, Hillebert, *Org. Synth.* **coll. vol. IV**, 207 (1963).

White needles; very pungent odor; acrid taste. *Very poisonous!* mp 146-147°. Sol in water, alcohol, ether, volatile oils.

Caution: Causes convulsions, paralysis, death from respiratory failure. Lacks inhalation hazard.

USE: Generally for destroying all lower forms of life. In taxidermy for preserving insects, butterflies, etc.

2696. 1-Cyanoimidazole. [36289-36-8] 1*H*-Imidazole-1-carbonitrile; *N*-cyanoimidazole. $C_4H_3N_3$; mol wt 93.09. C 51.61%, H 3.25%, N 45.14%. Coupling and cyanating agent. Prepn: H. Giesemann, *J. Prakt. Chem.* **4(1)**, 345 (1955); by thermolysis of tetrazolopyrazine: C. Wentrup, *Helv. Chim. Acta* **55**, 565 (1972); P. B. W. McCallum *et al., Aust. J. Chem.* **52**, 159 (1999). Use as a condensing agent: J. P. Ferris *et al., Nucleosides Nucleotides* **8**, 407 (1989); K. J. Luebke, P. B. Dervan, *J. Am. Chem. Soc.* **113**, 7447 (1991); as a cyanating agent: Y. Wu *et al., Org. Lett.* **2**, 795 (2000).

[Chemical structure: imidazole with N—CN]

White hygroscopic needles, mp 59.5-60.5°. bp_{760} 185-189°; bp_{27} 95°.

USE: In chemical synthesis as a cyanating agent; as condensing agent in DNA ligation.

2697. Cyanopsin. Photoreceptor protein found in the retinal cone cells of fresh water and migratory fish, lampreys, and certain amphibians; corresponds to the rod pigment, porphyropsin, *q.v.* Absorption maximum ~620 nm. Composed of the chromophore 11-*cis*-3-dehydroretinal, *q.v.*, bound to a photopsin, the specific protein component of cone cells (*see* Opsins). Proposed existence as a visual pigment and *in vitro* synthesis from 3-dehydroretinal and chicken photopsin: G. Wald, *Science* **118**, 505 (1953). Demonstration of natural occurrence by microspectrophotometry: P. Liebman, G. Entine, *Nature* **216**, 501 (1967). Methods for prepn and assay: R. Hubbard *et al., Methods Enzymol.* **18**, 615-653 (1971). Photochemistry and biological activity: G. Wald, *Science* **162**, 230 (1968). A trichromatic cone system utilizing 3-dehydroretinal as chromophore has been noted to occur in certain amphibians and fish. Three photochemically distinct pigments, corresponding to those of retinal-based color vision, have been identified: P. A. Liebman in *Handbook of Sensory Physiology* Vol. VII(1), H. J. A. Dartnall, Ed. (Springer-Verlag, New York, 1972) pp 481-528. A visual system is generally based on one type of chromophore combined with various opsins. However, pigments utilizing both types of chromophore have been found to co-exist in the retina of some of these species. Demonstration of paired-pigment cone systems: E. R. Loew, H. J. A. Dartnall, *Vision Res.* **11**, 551 (1976); A. T. C. Tsin *et al., ibid.* **21**, 943 (1981). Absorption spectrum: J. E. M. Mooij, T. J. T. P. van den Berg, *ibid.* 23 (1983).

2698. Cyanuric Acid. [108-80-5] 1,3,5-Triazine-2,4,6(1*H*,3*H*,5*H*)-trione; *sym*-triazinetriol; 2,4,6-trihydroxy-1,3,5-triazine; tricyanic acid; trihydroxycyanidine. $C_3H_3N_3O_3$; mol wt 129.07. C 27.92%, H 2.34%, N 32.56%, O 37.19%. Prepn: Schmidt, *J. Prakt. Chem.* [2] **5**, 41-52 (1872); Venable, Moore, *J. Am. Chem. Soc.* **39**, 1752 (1917). HPLC determn: P. Beilstein *et al., J. Agric. Food Chem.* **29**, 1132 (1981); in urine and pool water: T. V. Briggle *et al., J. Assoc. Off. Anal. Chem.* **64**, 1222 (1981). Review of prepn, properties and uses: E. M. Smolin, L. Rapoport, "s-Triazines and Derivatives" in *The Chemistry of Heterocyclic Compounds* **vol. 13**, A. Weissberger, Ed.(Interscience, New York, 1959) pp 17-48; of chemistry, toxicity and antibacterial activity as applied to swimming pools: E. Canelli, *Am. J. Public Health* **64**, 155-162 (1974); F. W. Linda, R. C. Hollenbach, *J. Environ. Health* **40**, 324-329 (1978); of toxicology: B. G. Hammond *et al., Environ. Health Perspect.* **69**, 287-292 (1986). *Review:* J. A. Wojtowicz in *Kirk-Othmer Encyclopedia of Chemical Technology* **vol. 7** (John Wiley & Sons, 4th ed., 1993) pp 834-851.

White crystalline solid; does not melt up to 330°, sublimes and dissociates to isocyanic acid at higher temps. pKa_1 6.88; pKa_2 11.40; pKa_3 13.5. uv max (0.1M HCl): 214 nm (log ε 3.38). uv max (0.1M phosphate buffer pH 7): 214 nm (log ε 4.00). uv max (0.1M NaOH) 213 nm (log ε 4.64). Slightly sol in common organic solvents such as acetone, benzene, diethyl ether, ethanol, hexane. Soly (%): DMF 7.2; DMSO 17.4. Soly in water (%): 0.2 at 25°; 2.6 at 90°; 10.0 at 150°. Soly in 96% H_2SO_4 (25°): 14.1%. Sol in hot alcohols, pyridine, concd HCl without decompn; in aq solns of NaOH and KOH. Insol in cold methanol, ether, acetone, benzene, chloroform. Forms dihydrate in aq soln; crystallizes as colorless monoclinic prisms that effloresce in dry air. d^{25} 1.75 (anhydr); d^{25} 1.66 (dihydrate). Predominant tautomeric form in solid state and soln is keto form, *isocyanuric acid*; in basic soln the enol form is more stable. LD_{50} orally in rats: >5.00 g/kg (Canelli).

USE: Convenient lab source of cyanic acid gas. In prepn of melamine, sponge rubber, herbicides, dyes, resin, antimicrobial agents. As stabilizer and disinfectant in swimming pool water.

2699. Cyanuric Chloride. [108-77-0] 2,4,6-Trichloro-1,3,5-triazine; trichloro-s-triazine. $C_3Cl_3N_3$; mol wt 184.41. C 19.54%, Cl 57.68%, N 22.79%. Versatile coupling agent for proteins and nucleic acids; reagent in synthetic organic chemistry. Prepn: A. Gautier, *Ann.* **141**, 122 (1867); H. Herlinger, *Angew. Chem.* **76**, 437 (1964). Structural studies: A. W. Hofmann, *Ber.* **19**, 2061 (1886); R. A. Pascal, Jr., D. M. Ho, *Tetrahedron Lett.* **33**, 4707 (1992); S. J. Maginn *et al., ibid.* **34**, 4349 (1993); V. Krishnakumar, R. Ramasamy, *Spectrochim. Acta A* **61**, 3112 (2005). Polarographic determn in air: V. Stará *et al., Anal. Chim. Acta* **147**, 371 (1983). Synthetic applications as a chlorinating reagent for alcohols: S. R. Sandler *et al., J. Org. Chem.* **35**, 3967 (1970); for carboxylic acids: K. Venkataraman, D. R. Wagle, *Tetrahedron Lett.* **20**, 3037 (1979); in macrocyclic lactonization: *eidem, ibid.* **21**, 1893 (1980); as a Beckmann rearrangement catalyst: Y. Furuya *et al., J. Am. Chem. Soc.* **127**, 11240 (2005); as a dehydrating agent: K. P. Haval *et al., Tetrahedron* **62**, 937 (2006). Use as a linking agent in molecular biology applications: H.-D. Hunger *et al., Anal. Biochem.* **156**, 286 (1986); *idem et al., ibid.* **165**, 45 (1987); R. A. Abuknesha *et al., J. Immunol. Methods* **306**, 211 (2005).

Crystals from ether, mp 146°. bp 198°. Crystal density: 1.93 g/cm³.

Caution: Eye irritant; avoid skin contact and inhalation (Hunger, 1986).

USE: Intermediate in the synthesis of active dyes, agricultural products, and drug substances. Reagent in organic synthesis. Coupling agent for nucleic acids and proteins; cyanuric chloride-activated paper is used in capillary and electroblotting applications, dot tests, and hybridization protocols.

2700. Cyazofamid. [120116-88-3] 4-Chloro-2-cyano-N,N-dimethyl-5-(4-methylphenyl)-1H-imidazole-1-sulfonamide; 4-chloro-2-cyano-N,N-dimethyl-5-p-tolylimidazole-1-sulfonamide; IKF-916; Ranman. $C_{13}H_{13}ClN_4O_2S$; mol wt 324.79. C 48.07%, H 4.03%, Cl 10.92%, N 17.25%, O 9.85%, S 9.87%. Imidazole fungicide for use on food crops; inhibits mitochondrial complex III at the Qi (ubiquinone-reducing) site. Prepn: R. Nasu *et al., AU* **8812883**; *eidem, US* **4995898** (1988, 1991 both to Ishihara Sangyo Kaisha). Mode of action study: S. Mitani *et al., Pestic. Biochem. Physiol.* **71**, 107 (2001). Review of properties and field performance: S. Mitani *et al., Brighton Crop Prot. Conf. - Pests Dis.* **1998**, 351-358; S. Mitani, *Agrochem. Jpn.* **78**, 17-20 (2001).

Odorless ivory powder, mp 152.7°. Log P (n-octanol/water): 3.2 (25°). Vapor pressure: <1.33 × 10⁻⁵ Pa. Soly in water at 20°: 0.121 µg/ml (pH 5). LD_{50} orally in mice, rats: >5000, >5000 mg/kg; dermally in rats: >2000 mg/kg. LC_{50} in rats: >5.5 mg/l by inhalation. LC_{50} (48 hr) in carp, rainbow trout: >69.6, >100 mg/l (Mitani).

USE: Agricultural fungicide.

2701. Cycasin. [14901-08-7] (Methyl-*ONN*-azoxy)methyl β-D-glucopyranoside; methylazoxymethanol β-D-glucoside; β-D-glucosyloxyazoxymethane. $C_8H_{16}N_2O_7$; mol wt 252.22. C 38.10%, H 6.39%, N 11.11%, O 44.40%. Toxic substance from seeds of *Cycas revoluta* Thumb. and *C. circinalis* L., *Cycadaceae* from Guam: Nishida *et al., Bull. Agric. Chem. Soc. Jpn.* **19**, 77 (1955), *C.A.* **50**, 13756g (1956); Riggs, *Chem. Ind. (London)* **1956**, 926; Matsumoto, Strong, *Arch. Biochem. Biophys.* **101**, 299 (1963). Biological effects, metabolism and mechanism of action of cycasin and its aglycone, *methylazoxymethanol:* Spatz, *Ann. N.Y. Acad. Sci.* **163**, 848 (1969). Structure: Korsch, Riggs, *Tetrahedron Lett.* **1964**, 523. Toxicology: Laqueur, Spatz, *Cancer Res.* **28**, 2262 (1968). Carcinogenicity and neurotoxicity studies: I. Hirono, *Fed. Proc.* **31**, 1493 (1972). Review of carcinogenicity studies: *IARC Monographs* **10**, 121-138 (1976).

Needles from water + acetone + ether, dec 154°. $[\alpha]_D^{18}$ −44° (c = 0.62). uv max (0.4M H_2SO_4): 217 nm. LD_{50} in rats, mice, hamsters, rabbits, guinea pigs (mg/kg): 562, 500, <250, ~30, <20 orally (Hirono).

Tetraacetate. $C_{16}H_{24}N_2O_{11}$. Plates from acetone + petr ether, mp 137°. $[\alpha]_D^{18}$ −27° (c = 0.98 in CHCl₃).

Caution: Cycasin has been listed as reasonably anticipated to be a carcinogen: *Fourth Annual Report on Carcinogens* (NTP 85-002, 1985) p 64; delisted because no U.S. residents exposed: *Fifth Annual Report on Carcinogens* (NTP 89-239, 1989) p 340.

2702. Cyclacillin. [3485-14-1] (2S,5R,6R)-6-[[(1-Amino-cyclohexyl)carbonyl]amino]-3,3-dimethyl-7-oxo-4-thia-1-azabicyclo[3.2.0]heptane-2-carboxylic acid; 6-(1-aminocyclohexanecarboxamido)penicillanic acid; (1-aminocyclohexyl)penicillin; ciclacillin; Wy-4508; Calthor; Citosarin; Cyclapen; Syngacillin; Ultracillin; Vastcillin; Vatracin; Vipicil; Wyvital. $C_{15}H_{23}N_3O_4S$; mol wt 341.43. C 52.77%, H 6.79%, N 12.31%, O 18.74%, S 9.39%. Semi-synthetic antibiotic related to penicillin. Prepn: Alburn *et al., US* **3194802**; C. A. Robinson, J. J. Nescio, *DE* **1800698**; *eidem, US* **3478018** (1965, 1969, 1969, all to Am. Home Prods.). Activity studies: Rosenman *et al., Antimicrob. Agents Chemother.* **1967**, 590; Hopper *et al., ibid.* 597; Yurchenco *et al., ibid.* 602; *Chemotherapy* **15**, 209 (1970). Metabolic studies: Poole, *J. Pharm. Sci.* **59**, 1255 (1970); Tucker *et al., Toxicol. Appl. Pharmacol.* **19**, 361

(1971). Physicochemical data: Alburn *et al.*, *Antimicrob. Agents Chemother.* **1967**, 586; Hou, Poole, *J. Pharm. Sci.* **58**, 1510 (1969); Poole, Bahal, *ibid.* **59**, 1265 (1970).

Crystals, mp 182-183° (anhydrate) (Hou, Poole); also reported as mp 156-158° (dec) (Alburn *et al.*). $[\alpha]_D^{25}$ +268° (water). pK_1, pK_2 in water: 2.68, 7.50; in 50% dioxane: 4.16, 7.04. Stable in acid. Soly at 38°: about 29 mg/ml.

THERAP CAT: Antibacterial.

2703. Cyclamic Acid. [100-88-9] Cyclohexylsulfamic acid; cyclohexanesulfamic acid; Hexamic Acid. $C_6H_{13}NO_3S$; mol wt 179.24. C 40.21%, H 7.31%, N 7.81%, O 26.78%, S 17.89%. Prepn: Audrieth, Sveda, US 2275125 (1942 to du Pont); *J. Org. Chem.* **9**, 89 (1944); Thompson, US 2800501 (1957 to du Pont); Shah, Bernsen, US 3361799 (1968 to Abbott). Prepn of the Na salt: Robinson, US 2383617 (1945 to du Pont). Other prepns and metabolism: *See* Calcium Cyclamate. Sweetness of the sodium salt discovered by Michael Sveda at the University of Illinois in 1937. Toxicity: Taylor *et al.*, *Food Cosmet. Toxicol.* **6**, 313 (1968). Review of long-term toxicity and carcinogenicity of sodium cyclamate in mice: Brantom *et al.*, *Food Cosmet. Toxicol.* **11**, 735 (1973).

Sweet-sour crystals. mp 169-170°. Fairly strong acid. Very sparingly soluble in water. Slowly hydrolyzed by hot water.

Sodium salt. Sodium cyclohexylsulfamate; cyclamate sodium; sodium cyclamate; Assugrin; Sucaryl Sodium; Sucrosa. C_6H_{12}-$NNaO_3S$; mol wt 201.22. Crystals. Pleasantly sweet to the taste. Freely sol in water. About 30 times as sweet as refined cane sugar. Sweetness is still easily perceptible at a dilution of 1:10,000 (sugar 1:140; saccharin 1:50,000). pH of 10% aq soln between 5.5 and 7.5. Practically insol in alcohol, ether, benzene, chloroform. LD_{50} orally in mice, rats: 17.0, 15.25 g/kg (Taylor).

Note: Consult latest Government regulations on use in food.

USE: Non-nutritive sweetener.

2704. Cyclandelate. [456-59-7] α-Hydroxybenzeneacetic acid 3,3,5-trimethylcyclohexyl ester; mandelic acid 3,3,5-trimethylcyclohexyl ester; 3,3,5-trimethylcyclohexyl mandelate; 3,5,5-trimethylcyclohexyl amygdalate; 3,3,5-trimethylcyclohexanol α-phenyl-α-hydroxyacetate; BS-572; Cyclergine; Cyclobral; Cyclolyt; Cyclomandol; Cyclospasmol; Natil; Novodil; Perebral; Spasmocyclon. $C_{17}H_{24}O_3$; mol wt 276.37. C 73.88%, H 8.75%, O 17.37%. Prepn: N. Brock *et al.*, *Arzneim.-Forsch.* **2**, 165 (1952); A. B. H. Funcke *et al.*, *ibid.* **3**, 503 (1953); van Sluis, *Chem. Prod.* **17**, 375 (1954); GB 707237; W. T. Nauta, US 2707193 (1954, 1955 both to Brocades-Stheeman). Purification: D. Flitter, US 3663597 (1972 to Am. Home Prods.). Pharmacokinetics: A. Orr, J. R. Whittier, *Int. J. Nucl. Med. Biol.* **1**, 205 (1974). GLC determn in human plasma: G. Andermann, M. Dietz, *J. Chromatogr.* **223**, 365 (1981). Clinical trial in chronic cerebrovascular disease: S. Bassi *et al.*, *Br. J. Clin. Pract.* **38**, 344 (1984). Review of efficacy as cerebral and peripheral vasodilator: C. B. Blakemore, *ibid.* **34**, Suppl., 3-9 (1984). Symposium on calcium modulation and clinical effects: *Drugs* **33**, Suppl. 2, 1-141 (1987). Comprehensive description: C. M. Shearer, *Anal. Profiles Drug Subs. Excip.* **21**, 149-168 (1992).

Crystals, mp 55.0-56.5°. bp_{14} 192-194°. uv max (ethanol): 269, 258, 251 nm (ε 1575, 2020, 1630). Very sol in chloroform, methanol; freely sol in acetonitrile, ethyl acetate, DMF, toluene. Insol in water.

THERAP CAT: Vasodilator (peripheral, cerebral).

2705. Cyclazocine. [3572-80-3] 3-(Cyclopropylmethyl)-1,-2,3,4,5,6-hexahydro-6,11-dimethyl-2,6-methano-3-benzazocin-8-ol; Win-20740; NSC-107429. $C_{18}H_{25}NO$; mol wt 271.40. C 79.66%, H 9.28%, N 5.16%, O 5.90%. Analgesic with mixed narcotic agonist-antagonist properties. Prepn: Archer, BE 611000 (1962 to Sterling Drug), *C.A.* **58**, 2439c (1963). Crystal structure: I. L. Karle *et al.*, *Acta Crystallogr.* **B25**, 1469 (1969). Supraspinal analgesic effects: S. Sasson, C. Kornetsky, *Life Sci.* **38**, 21 (1986). Evaluation in anorexia and motor disruption in rats: J. W. Henck *et al.*, *Pharmacol. Biochem. Behav.* **22**, 671 (1985). Determn by HPLC: I. Jane, A. McKinnon, *J. Chromatogr.* **323**, 191 (1985). Review of use in treatment of opiate addiction: M. J. Goldstein, *Int. J. Addict.* **15**, 939 (1980).

Crystals from methanol, mp 201-204°.

THERAP CAT: Narcotic antagonist.

2706. Cyclethrin. [97-11-0] 2,2-Dimethyl-3-(2-methyl-1-propenyl)cyclopropanecarboxylic acid 3-(2-cyclopenten-1-yl)-2-methyl-4-oxo-2-cyclopenten-1-yl ester; 3-(2-cyclopentenyl)-2-methyl-4-oxo-2-cyclopentenyl ester of chrysanthemummonocarboxylic acid; chrysanthemummonocarboxylic acid ester with 3-(2-cyclopenten-1-yl)-2-methyl-4-oxo-2-cyclopenten-1-ol. $C_{21}H_{28}O_3$; mol wt 328.45. C 76.79%, H 8.59%, O 14.61%. Prepn and insecticidal activity: H. L. Haynes *et al.*, *Contrib. Boyce Thompson Inst.* **18**, 1 (1954); H. R. Guest, H. A. Stansbury, US 2891888 (1959 to Union Carbide). Product is a mixture of isomers including four racemic forms or eight optical and geometric isomers which have not yet been isolated and evaluated. Toxicology: C. P. Carpenter *et al.*, *Arch. Ind. Hyg. Occup. Med.* **10**, 162 (1954).

Liquid. n_D^{30} 1.5120. d_{20}^{20} 1.033. LD_{50} orally in rats: 1.4-2.8 g/kg (Carpenter).

USE: Insecticide for flies, roaches, and grain pests.

2707. Cyclexedrine. [532-52-5] N,β-Dimethylcyclohexaneethanamine; cyclohexylisopropylmethylamine; 2-cyclohexyl-N-methylpropylamine; 1-cyclohexyl-1-methyl-2-methylaminoethane; ethylhexedrine; isopropylhexedrine. $C_{10}H_{21}N$; mol wt 155.28. C 77.35%, H 13.63%, N 9.02%. Prepn: DE 970480 (1958 to Knoll).

Hydrochloride. [64011-61-6] Eventin. $C_{10}H_{21}N\cdot HCl$; mol wt 191.74. Crystalline powder, bitter taste. mp 138-140°. Soluble in water, ethanol, chloroform; slightly sol in ether.

THERAP CAT: Sympathomimetic; anorexic.

2708. Cyclic AMP. [60-92-4] Adenosine cyclic 3′,5′-(hydrogen phosphate); adenosine 3′,5′-cyclic monophosphate; adenosine 3′,5′-cyclic phosphate; adenosine 3′,5′-monophosphate; adenosine 3′,5′-phosphate; cyclic adenosine 3′,5′-monophosphate; acrasin; 3′,5′-AMP; cAMP. $C_{10}H_{12}N_5O_6P$; mol wt 329.21. C 36.48%, H 3.67%, N 21.27%, O 29.16%, P 9.41%. Key intracellular regulator of a number of cellular processes; found in most animal cells, in bacteria, and in some higher plants. First isoln and identification: Rall et al., J. Biol. Chem. **224**, 463 (1957); Sutherland, Rall, ibid. **232**, 1077 (1958). Molecular structure and conformation: Cook et al., J. Am. Chem. Soc. **79**, 3607 (1957); Lipkin et al., ibid. **81**, 6198 (1959); Watenpaugh et al., Science **159**, 206 (1968). Syntheses: Smith et al., J. Am. Chem. Soc. **83**, 698 (1961); Borden, Smith, J. Org. Chem. **31**, 3247 (1966). Physical data: D. Lipkin et al., J. Am. Chem. Soc. **81**, 6075 (1959). Functions as a mediator of hormone-action for a variety of hormones such as epinephrine, glucagon and ACTH, q.q.v. Activates phosphorylation of proteins by protein kinases. Defined as a "second messenger" because of its response to hormones ("first messengers"). Converted from adenosine triphosphate (ATP) by the enzyme **adenylate cyclase**. Deactivated by **cyclic nucleotide phosphodiesterases** which convert it to 5′-adenylic acid. Reviews of biochemical model: Sutherland et al., J. Biol. Chem. **237**, 1220-1243 (1962); Robison et al., Annu. Rev. Biochem. **37**, 149 (1968); Jost, Rickenberg, ibid. **40**, 741 (1971); Sutherland, J. Am. Med. Assoc. **214**, 1281 (1970); Pastan, Perlman, Nature New Biol. **229**, 5 (1971); G. A. Robison et al., Eds., Ann. N.Y. Acad. Sci. **185**, (1971); Losert, Pharmazie **28**, 351 (1973). See also Cyclic GMP. Identity with acrasin from cellular slime molds (Dictyostelium species), where it acts as a "first" rather than a "second messenger": Konijn et al., Proc. Natl. Acad. Sci. USA **58**, 1152 (1967). Review of quantitative methods: Methods in Molecular Biology vol. 3, "Methods in Cyclic Nucleotide Research", Mark Chasin, Ed. (Marcel Dekker, New York, 1972). Books: G. A. Robison et al., Cyclic AMP (Academic Press, New York, 1971); Advan. Cyclic Nucleotide Res. vols. **1, 2, 3**, P. Greengard, G. A. Robison, Eds. (Raven Press, New York, 1972, 1973); Handb. Exp. Pharmacol. **58**, "Cyclic Nucleotides", Pt I: Biochemistry and Pt II: Physiology & Pharmacology, J. A. Nathanson, J. W. Kobabian, Eds. (Springer-Verlag, New York, 1982) 736 and 1000 pp resp.

Hydrate crystallizes from water as platelets with pearly luster, mp 219-220° (with gas evolution). $[\alpha]_D$ −51.3° (c = 0.67). uv max (pH 2): 256 nm (ε 14500); (pH 7): 258 nm (ε 14650). Heat stable; resistant to inactivation by acid or alkali. Found in concns of 10^{-7} to 10^{-6} moles/kg in living cells.

2709. Cyclic GMP. [7665-99-8] Guanosine cyclic 3′,5′-(hydrogen phosphate); cyclic guanosine 3′,5′-monophosphate; guanosine 3′,5′-cyclic monophosphate; guanosine 3′,5′-cyclic phosphate; guanosine 3′-monophosphate; 3′,5′-GMP; cGMP. $C_{10}H_{12}N_5O_7$-P; mol wt 345.21. C 34.79%, H 3.50%, N 20.29%, O 32.44%, P 8.97%. A cellular regulatory agent which has been described as a "second messenger". See Cyclic AMP. First synthesized because of the interest in cyclic nucleotides generated by cyclic AMP: Smith et al., J. Am. Chem. Soc. **83**, 698 (1961); Borden, Smith, J. Org. Chem. **31**, 3247 (1966). Has subsequently been found in animal and bacterial cells in concentrations of 10^{-8} to 10^{-6} moles/kg. First isoln from rat urine: Ashman et al., Biochem. Biophys. Res. Commun. **11**, 330 (1963). Structure and conformation: Chwang, Sundaralingam, Nature New Biol. **244**, 136 (1973). Proposed as an antagonist of cyclic AMP in bidirectional systems such as contraction-relaxation or glycogen synthesis-glycogen

breakdown. Cyclic GMP levels increase in response to a variety of hormones including acetylcholine, insulin and oxytocin. Formed by conversion of guanosine triphosphate by the enzyme **guanylate cyclase** and hydrolyzed by cyclic nucleotide phosphodiesterases. Found to activate specific protein kinases. Reviews of biochemical model: Goldberg et al., in Pharmacology and the Future of Man **vol. 5**, R. A. Maxwell, G. H. Acheson, Eds. (Karger, New York, 1973) pp 146-169; eidem in Advan. Cyclic Nucleotide Res. **vol. 3**, P. Greengard, G. A. Robison, Eds. (Raven Press, New York, 1973) pp 155-223; Kolata, Science **182**, 149-151 (1973); Nature **246**, 186 (1973); N. D. Goldberg, M. K. Haddox, Annu. Rev. Biochem. **46**, 823-896 (1977). Book: Handb. Exp. Pharmacol. **58**, entitled "Cyclic Nucleotides", Pt. I: Biochemistry and Pt. II: Physiology & Pharmacology, J. A. Nathanson, J. W. Kobabian, Eds. (Springer-Verlag, New York, 1982) 736 and 1000 pp resp.

Calcium salt. $C_{20}H_{22}CaN_{10}O_{14}P_2$. Decahydrate. uv max (pH 1): 256.5 nm (ε 11350); (pH 7): 254 nm (ε 12950); (pH 12): 262 nm (ε 12400).

2710. Cyclizine. [82-92-8] 1-Diphenylmethyl-4-methylpiperazine; N-benzhydryl-N′-methylpiperazine; N-methyl-N′-benzhydrylpiperazine; (N-benzhydryl)(N′-methyl)diethylenediamine; Compd 47-83; Wellcome prepn 47-83; Marzine; Marezine. C_{18}-$H_{22}N_2$; mol wt 266.38. C 81.16%, H 8.32%, N 10.52%. Prepn: R. Baltzly et al., J. Org. Chem. **14**, 775 (1949); eidem, US 2630435 (1953 to Burroughs Wellcome). Metabolism: R. Kuntzman et al., Ann. N.Y. Acad. Sci. **226**, 131 (1973). Physical properties and analysis: S. A. Benezra, Anal. Profiles Drug Subs. **6**, 83 (1977). Crystallographic study: V. Bertolasi et al., Acta Crystallogr. **B36**, 1975 (1980). HPLC determn: R. B. Walker, I. Kanfer, J. Chromatogr. B **672**, 172 (1995). Clinical antiemetic efficacy: G. Rowlands, W. J. Currie, Br. J. Clin. Pract. **30**, 197 (1976); W. N. Chestnutt et al., Eur. J. Anaesthesiol. **3**, 27 (1986).

Light-sensitive crystals from petr ether, mp 105.5-107.5°. uv max (0.1N HCl): 269, 263, 258, 225 (ε 540, 742, 694, 11300). Soly in g/ml at 25°: chloroform 1.1; ether 0.17; ethanol 0.17; in mg/ml: water <0.1.

Hydrochloride. [303-25-3] Valoid. $C_{18}H_{22}N_2$.HCl; mol wt 302.84. Crystals, moderately sol in water. Protect from light.

THERAP CAT: Antiemetic.

THERAP CAT (VET): Antiemetic.

2711. Cyclobarbital. [52-31-3] 5-(1-Cyclohexen-1-yl)-5-ethyl-2,4,6(1H,3H,5H)-pyrimidinetrione; 5-(1-cyclohexen-1-yl)-5-ethylbarbituric acid; cyclobarbitone; hexamal; tetrahydrophenobarbital; Cavonyl; Cyclodorm; Cyklodorm; Fanodormo; Irifan; Namuron; Palinum; Phanodorn; Phanodorm; Philodorm; Prälumin; Pro-Sonil; Sonaform. $C_{12}H_{16}N_2O_3$; mol wt 236.27. C 61.00%, H 6.83%, N 11.86%, O 20.31%. Prepn: **GB 231150** (1924 to Bayer); Schulemann, Meisenburg, **US 1690796** (1929 to

Winthrop); Eckstein, *Przem. Chem.* **9**, 390 (1953), *C.A.* **49**, 11668c (1955). Toxicity data: G. Hofrichter *et al., Arzneim.-Forsch.* **17**, 242 (1967).

Shiny crystals, insipid bitter taste, mp 171-174°. Very slightly sol in cold water, appreciably sol in boiling water. One gram dissolves in 5 ml alcohol, 20 ml ether. LD_{50} in mice, rats (mg/kg): 350, 290 i.p. (Hofrichter).

Calcium salt. [143-76-0] Hexemal calcium; Itridal; Koller-dormfix; Pronox. $C_{24}H_{30}CaN_4O_6$; mol wt 510.60. Minute crystals. Appreciably bitter taste. Slightly basic reaction. Soly in water about 1 part in 70 parts (w/w), in 95% alc about 1 part in 500 parts. Practically insol in ether, chloroform.

Note: This is a controlled substance (depressant): **21 CFR, 1308.13**.

THERAP CAT: Sedative, hypnotic.

THERAP CAT (VET): Has been used as an anesthetic and sedative.

2712. Cyclobendazole. [31431-43-3] [5-(Cyclopropyl-carbonyl)-1*H*-benzimidazol-2-yl]carbamic acid methyl ester; ciclo-bendazole; CC-2481; R-17147; Haptocil. $C_{13}H_{13}N_3O_3$; mol wt 259.26. C 60.22%, H 5.05%, N 16.21%, O 18.51%. Prepn: J. L. Van Gelder *et al.,* **DE 2029637**; *eidem,* **US 3657267** (1971, 1972 both to Janssen). Synthesis and anthelmintic activity: A. H. M. Raeymaekers *et al., Arzneim.-Forsch.* **28**, 586 (1978). Embryotoxic and antimitotic properties: P. Delatour, Y. Richard, *Therapie* **31**, 505 (1976). Pharmacokinetics: R. R. Brodie *et al., Arzneim.-Forsch.* **27**, 593 (1977). Biotransformation: B. C. Mayo *et al., Drug Metab. Dispos.* **6**, 518 (1978). Clinical evaluation: A. De-grémont, E. Stahel, *Schweiz. Med. Wochenschr.* **108**, 1430 (1978).

Crystals from acetic acid, mp 250.5°.

THERAP CAT: Anthelmintic (Nematodes).

2713. Cyclobenzaprine. [303-53-7] 3-(5*H*-Dibenzo[*a*,-*d*]cyclohepten-5-ylidene)-*N*,*N*-dimethyl-1-propanamine; *N*,*N*-di-methyl-5*H*-dibenzo[*a*,*d*]cyclohepten-Δ^{5,γ}-propylamine; 5-(3-dimethylaminopropylidene)dibenzo[*a*,*e*]cycloheptatriene; 1-(3-di-methylaminopropylidene)-2,3:6,7-dibenzo-4-suberene; prohepta-triene; MK-130; Ro-4-1577; RP-9715. $C_{20}H_{21}N$; mol wt 275.39. C 87.23%, H 7.69%, N 5.09%. Prepn: **GB 858187** (1961 to Hoffmann-La Roche); Villani *et al., J. Med. Pharm. Chem.* **5**, 373 (1962); Winthrop *et al., J. Org. Chem.* **27**, 230 (1962). Pharmacol-ogy: C. D. Barnes, W. L. Adams, *Neuropharmacology* **17**, 445 (1978); N. N. Share, *ibid.* 721; and toxicology: J. Metysova *et al., Arch. Int. Pharmacodyn. Ther.* **144**, 481 (1963). Metabolism: G. Belvedere *et al., Biomed. Mass Spectrom.* **1**, 329 (1974); H. B. Hucker *et al., Drug Metab. Dispos.* **6**, 184 (1978). Bioavailability: *eidem, J. Clin. Pharmacol.* **17**, 719 (1977). Clinical studies: J. V. Basmajian, *Arch. Phys. Med. Rehabil.* **5**, 58 (1978); B. R. Brown, J. Womble, *J. Am. Med. Assoc.* **240**, 1151 (1978). Comprehensive description: M. L. Cotton, G. R. B. Down, *Anal. Profiles Drug Subs.* **17**, 41-72 (1988).

bp$_1$ 175-180°. uv max: 224, 289 nm (log ε 4.57, 4.02), (Villani, *et al.*)

Hydrochloride. [6202-23-9] Flexeril; Flexiban. $C_{20}H_{21}$-N.HCl; mol wt 311.85. Use as muscle relaxant: N. N. Share, **FR 2100873** (1972 to Frosst), *C.A.* **78**, 47801n (1973). Crystals from isopropanol, mp 216-218°. Soly in water: >20 g/100 ml. Freely sol in water, methanol, ethanol; sparingly sol in isopropanol; slightly sol in chloroform, methylene chloride. Practically insol in hydrocarbons. uv max: 226, 295 nm (ε 52300, 12000). LD_{50} in mice (mg/kg): 35 i.v., 250 orally (Metysova).

THERAP CAT: Muscle relaxant (skeletal).

2714. Cyclobutane. [287-23-0] Tetramethylene. C_4H_8; mol wt 56.11. C 85.62%, H 14.37%. Prepd by hydrogenaton of cyclobutene in the presence of nickel at 100°: Willstätter, Bruce, *Ber.* **40**, 3988 (1907); *see also* Heisig, J. *Am. Chem. Soc.* **63**, 1698 (1941); by pyrolysis of ether, along with other products: Peytral, *Bull. Soc. Chim. Fr.* [4] **35**, 964 (1924). In 39% yield from cyclo-butanecarboxylic acid: Cason, Way, *J. Org. Chem.* **14**, 31 (1949), for the prepn of this acid *see* Heisig, Stodola, *Org. Synth.* **coll. vol. III**, 213 (1955).

Gas. Burns with a luminous flame. mp −80°. bp$_{741}$ 13.08°. d^0 0.7038; d^{-5} 0.7185. n_D^0 1.37520. Insol in water; freely sol in alcohol, acetone.

2715. Cyclobutyrol. [512-16-3] α-Ethyl-1-hydroxycyclo-hexaneacetic acid; 1-cyclohexanol-α-butyric acid; α-(1-hydroxy-cyclohexyl)butyric acid; 1-hydroxy-α-ethylcyclohexylacetic acid. $C_{10}H_{18}O_3$; mol wt 186.25. C 64.49%, H 9.74%, O 25.77%. Prepd by hydrolysis of the ethyl ester obtained by the Reformatski reac-tion: Kon, Naravanan, *J. Chem. Soc.* **1927**, 1536; Kandiah, Lin-stead, *ibid.* **1929**, 2150; J. G. Maillard *et al., Bull. Soc. Chim. Fr.* **1958**, 244; *eidem,* **DE 1094254**; *eidem,* **US 3065134** (1959, 1962 to Lab. Jacques Logeais). Activity studies: Roquet, Jousse, *Arch. Int. Pharmacodyn.* **125**, 172 (1960).

Colorless crystals from ether-petr ether, mp 81-82°. Formerly reported as viscous oil. $d_4^{18.8}$ 1.0010. bp$_{24}$ 164°; bp$_{16}$ 167-170°; $n_D^{18.8}$ 1.4680 (Kon, Naravanan, *loc. cit.*). Slightly sol in water, petr ether. Very sol in alcohols, acetone, dioxane, chloroform, ether. Completely sol in aq alkalies at pH 7.5-8.

Sodium salt. [1130-23-0] Bilimix; Bis-Bil; Colepan; Dimene; Epa-Bon; Hebucol; Maricolene; Tachicol; Tri-Bil; Tribilina. C_{10}-$H_{17}NaO_3$; mol wt 208.23. White crystalline, slightly hygroscopic powder, mp 299-300°.

THERAP CAT: Choleretic.

2716. Cyclobuxine D. [2241-90-9] (3β,5α,16α,20S)-14-Methyl-3,20-bis(methylamino)-4-methylene-9,19-cyclopregnan-16-ol; cyclobuxine. $C_{25}H_{42}N_2O$; mol wt 386.61. C 77.67%, H 10.95%, N 7.25%, O 4.14%. From *Buxus sempervirens* L., *Bux-aceae*: E. Schlittler *et al., Helv. Chim. Acta* **32**, 2209 (1949). Probably identical with Alkaloid A: Heusler, Schlittler, *ibid.* 2226. Structure: Brown, Kupchan, *J. Am. Chem. Soc.* **84**, 4590 (1962). Stereochemistry: *eidem, ibid.* **86**, 4424 (1964).

Crystals, dec 245-247°. $[\alpha]_D^{23}$ +98° (chloroform).

Dihydrobromide. $C_{25}H_{42}N_2O.2HBr$. Crystals, dec 288-292°.

N,N'-Dimethylcyclobuxine D. [4282-16-0] $C_{27}H_{46}N_2O$; mol wt 414.67. Crystals, dec 204-205°. $[\alpha]_D^{25}$ +99° (chloroform).

2717. Cyclocumarol. [518-20-7] 3,4-Dihydro-2-methoxy-2-methyl-4-phenyl-2H,5H-pyrano[3,2-c][1]benzopyran-5-one; 2-methyl-2-methoxy-4-phenyl-5-oxodihydropyrano[3,2-c][1]benzo-pyran; 3,4-(2'-methyl-2'-methoxy-4'-phenyl)dihydropyranocou-marin; 4-hydroxycoumarin anticoagulant no 63; BL-5; Cumopyran; Cumopyrin. $C_{20}H_{18}O_4$; mol wt 322.35. C 74.52%, H 5.63%, O 19.85%. Prepn: M. Ikawa et al., J. Am. Chem. Soc. **66**, 902 (1944); M. A. Stahmann, et al., US 2427579 (1947 to Wisconsin Alumni Res. Found.).

Crystals from ethanol, mp 166°. One gram dissolves in 100 ml water. Slightly sol in alcohol, vegetable oil.

THERAP CAT: Anticoagulant.

2718. Cyclodextrins. Cycloamyloses; cycloglucans; Schar-dinger dextrins. Naturally occurring clathrates, q.v. Obtained from the action of Bacillus macerans amylase on starch to form homoge-neous cyclic α-(1 → 4) linked D-glucopyranose units. α-, β- and γ-cyclodextrins are composed of six, seven and eight units, resp. Isoln of β-cyclodextrin: A. Villiers, Compt. Rend. **112**, 536 (1891); of α- and β-cyclodextrin: F. Schardinger, Z. Untersuch. Nahr. Genussm. **6**, 865 (1903); of γ-cyclodextrin: K. Freudenberg, R. Jacobi, Ann. **518**, 102 (1935). X-ray mol wt determn: D. French, R. E. Rundle, J. Am. Chem. Soc. **64**, 1651 (1942); D. French et al., ibid. **72**, 5150 (1950). Have hydrophobic cavities; form inclusion compds with organic substances, salts and halogens in the solid state or in aq solns. Model for enzyme action: I. Tabushi, Acc. Chem. Res. **15**, 66 (1982). Reviews: D. French, Adv. Carbo-hydr. Chem. **12**, 189-260 (1957); J. A. Thoma, L. Stewart, Starch: Chemistry and Technology vol. **1**, R. L. Whistler, E. F. Paschall, Eds. (Academic Press, New York, 1965) pp 209-249; F. Cramer, H. Hettler, Naturwissenschaften **154**, 625-632 (1967). Book: M. L. Bender, M. Komiyama, Cyclodextrin Chemistry (Springer-Verlag, New York, 1978) 96 pp.

α-Cyclodextrin

α-Cyclodextrin. Cyclohexaamylose. $C_{36}H_{60}O_{30}$; mol wt 972.84. Hexagonal plates or blade-shaped needles. $[\alpha]_D$ +150.5°.

β-Cyclodextrin. Cycloheptaamylose. $C_{42}H_{70}O_{35}$; mol wt 1134.98. Parallelogram shaped crystals. $[\alpha]_D$ +162.0°.

γ-Cyclodextrin. Cyclooctaamylose. $C_{48}H_{80}O_{40}$; mol wt 1297.12. Square plates or rectangular rods. $[\alpha]_D$ +177.4°.

USE: As complexing agent; in study of enzyme action.

2719. Cyclodrine. [52109-93-0] 1-Hydroxy-α-phenyl-cyclopentaneacetic acid 2-diethylaminoethyl ester; β-diethylamino-ethyl (1-hydroxycyclopentyl)phenylacetate; 2-phenyl-2-(1-hy-droxycyclopentyl)acetic acid β-(diethylamino)ethyl ester. $C_{19}H_{29}$-NO_3; mol wt 319.44. C 71.44%, H 9.15%, N 4.38%, O 15.03%. Anticholinergic. Prepn: Blicke, US 2922795 (1960 to Univ. of Michigan). Activity studies: Lands, Luduena, J. Pharmacol. Exp. Ther. **117**, 331 (1956); Karczman, Long, ibid. **123**, 230 (1958).

Hydrochloride. [78853-39-1] GT-92; Cyclopent. $C_{19}H_{29}$-$NO_3.HCl$; mol wt 355.90. Crystals from isopropanol-isopropyl ether, mp 133-135°.

THERAP CAT: Mydriatic.

2720. Cyclofenil. [2624-43-3] 4-[[4-(Acetyloxy)phenyl]cy-clohexylidenemethyl]phenol acetate; α-cyclohexylidene-α-(p-hy-droxyphenyl)-p-cresol diacetate; bis(p-acetoxyphenyl)cyclohexyli-denemethane; 4,4'-diacetoxybenzhydrylidenecyclohexane; F-6066; H-3452; ICI-48213; Fertodur; Neoclym; Ondogyne; Rehibin; Sa-nocrisin; Sexovid. $C_{23}H_{24}O_4$; mol wt 364.43. C 75.80%, H 6.64%, O 17.56%. Prepn: Miquel et al., J. Med. Chem. **6**, 774 (1963); Olsson et al., US 3287397 (1966). Pharmacology: Hira-matsu et al., Oyo Yakuri **6**, 1045 (1972), C.A. **78**, 131963z (1973).

Crystals from ethanol, mp 135-136°. uv max (ethanol): 247 nm (ε 17000).

Free diol. F-6060. $C_{19}H_{20}O_2$; mol wt 280.36. mp 235-236°.

THERAP CAT: Gonad-stimulating principle.

2721. Cycloguanil. [516-21-2] 1-(4-Chlorophenyl)-1,6-di-hydro-6,6-dimethyl-1,3,5-triazine-2,4-diamine; 4,6-diamino-1-(p-chlorophenyl)-1,2-dihydro-2,2-dimethyl-s-triazine; 2,4-diamino-1-p-chlorophenyl-1,6-dihydro-6,6-dimethyl-1,3,5-triazine; 1-p-chlo-rophenyl-2,4-diamino-6,6-dimethyl-1,6-dihydro-1,3,5-triazine; chlorazine (Russian); chlorguanide triazine; TCl; M-10580; D-20. $C_{11}H_{14}ClN_5$; mol wt 251.72. C 52.49%, H 5.61%, Cl 14.08%, N 27.82%. Metabolic product formed from the antimalarial drug chlorguanide: Carrington et al., Nature **168**, 1080 (1951). Prepn: Modest et al., J. Am. Chem. Soc. **74**, 855 (1952); Loo, ibid. **76**, 5096 (1954); Carrington et al., J. Chem. Soc. **1954**, 1017; Bami, J. Sci. Ind. Res. **14C**, 231 (1955); Modest, J. Org. Chem. **21**, 1 (1956); US 2900385 (1959 to Children's Cancer Res. Found.); Elslager, Worth, US 3074947 (1963 to Parke, Davis).

Prisms from chloroform + ether, mp 146°. uv max (water): 241 nm (log ε 4.11).

Hydrochloride. $C_{11}H_{14}ClN_5.HCl$. Prisms from water, mp 210-215°. uv max (water): 241 nm (log ε 4.12).

Dihydrochloride. $C_{11}H_{14}ClN_5.2HCl$. Crystals from acetone, mp 190-196°.

Pamoate. [609-78-9] Cycloguanil embonate; CI-501; Camolar. $(C_{11}H_{14}ClN_5)_2.C_{23}H_{16}O_6$; mol wt 891.80. Yellow crystals, mp 231-234°. Soly in water: 0.003%.

THERAP CAT: Antimalarial.

2722. Cycloheptanone. [502-42-1] Suberone; ketohepta-methylene; ketocycloheptane. $C_7H_{12}O$; mol wt 112.17. C 74.95%, H 10.78%, O 14.26%. Prepn from cyclohexanol with 1-(aminomethyl)cyclohexanol as the intermediate: Blicke *et al., J. Am. Chem. Soc.* **74,** 2924 (1952). Other methods: *Org. Synth.* **coll. vol. IV,** 221-228 (1963).

Liquid. d_4^{20} 0.9490. bp_{760} 179-181°. bp_{16} 66-70°. n_D^{20} 1.4608. Dipole moment 2.98. Practically insol in water. Freely sol in alcohol. Sol in ether.

Oxime. Suberoxime. $C_7H_{13}NO$. mp 23°, bp_{20} 152°.

2723. Cyclohexane. [110-82-7] Hexahydrobenzene; hexamethylene; hexanaphthene. C_6H_{12}; mol wt 84.16. C 85.63%, H 14.37%. Occurs in petr (0.5-1.0%). Obtained in the distillation of petr or by hydrogenation of benzene. In the distillation of petr the C_4-400°F boiling range naphthas are fractionated to obtain a C_5-200°F naphtha contg 10-14% cyclohexane which on superfractionation yields an 85% concentrate (which is sold as such); further purification necessitates isomerization of pentanes to cyclohexane, heat cracking for removing open chain hydrocarbons and sulfuric acid treatment to remove aromatic compds. The hydrogenation of benzene is done in the liq phase at 150° using Raney nickel catalyst and at least 10 atm H_2 pressure: Sabatier, *Ind. Eng. Chem.* **18,** 1005 (1926). Review and bibliography: Sachanen, *Chemical Constituents of Petroleum* (New York, 1945). Prepn of high purity cyclohexane: Seyer *et al., Ind. Eng. Chem.* **31,** 759 (1939). Cyclohexane can exist in two interconvertible conformations, the boat and the chair. In the chair form its 12 extracyclic bonds fall into two classes: six lie parallel to the main axis of symmetry and are designated "axial", while six extend radially outward at ±109.5° angles to the axis and are designated as "equatorial", Barton *et al., Nature* **172,** 1096 (1954); *Science* **119,** 49 (1954). Toxicity: Lazarew, *Arch. Exp. Pathol. Pharmakol.* **143,** 223 (1929). Physical properties and methods of purification: L. Scheflan, M. B. Jacobs, *The Handbook of Organic Solvents* (Van Nostrand, 1953) p 233; *Techniques of Chemistry* vol. II, entitled "Organic Solvents", J. D. Riddick, W. B. Bunger, Eds. (Wiley-Interscience, New York, 3rd ed., 1970) p 592. *Review:* M. L. Campbell in *Kirk-Othmer Encyclopedia of Chemical Technology* vol. 12 (Wiley-Interscience, New York, 3rd ed., 1980) pp 931-937.

boat   chair

Flammable liq. Solvent odor. Pungent when impure. d_4^{20} 0.7781; d_4^{80} 0.7206. mp 6.47°. bp_{760} 80.7°; bp_{400} 60.8°; bp_{200} 42.0°; bp_{100} 25.5°; bp_{60} 14.7°; bp_{40} 6.7°. n_D^{20} 1.4264. Flash pt, closed cup: 1°F (−18°C). Flammability limits in air 1.3-8.4% v/v. Soly in water at 23.5°C (w/w): 0.0052%. 100 ml of methanol dissolves 57 grams at 20°C; miscible with ethanol, ethyl ether, acetone, benzene, carbon tetrachloride. LC in mice: ~60-70 mg/l air (Lazarew).

Caution: Potential symptoms of overexposure are irritation of eyes, skin and respiratory system; drowsiness; dermatitis; narcosis, coma. *See NIOSH Pocket Guide to Chemical Hazards* (DHHS/-NIOSH 97-140, 1997) p 82.

USE: Solvent for lacquers and resins. Paint and varnish remover. In the extraction of essential oils. In analytical chemistry for mol wt determinations (cryoscopic constant 20.3). In the manuf of adipic acid, benzene, cyclohexyl chloride, nitrocyclohexane, cyclohexanol

and cyclohexanone. In the manuf of solid fuel for camp stoves. In fungicidal formulations (possesses slight fungicidal action). In the industrial recrystn of steroids.

2724. Cyclohexanecarboxylic Acid. [98-89-5] Hexahydro-benzoic acid. $C_7H_{12}O_2$; mol wt 128.17. C 65.60%, H 9.44%, O 24.97%. Prepn from anisic acid: Lumsden, *J. Chem. Soc.* **87,** 90 (1905); from 2-chlorocycloheptanone: Gutsche, *J. Am. Chem. Soc.* **71,** 3513 (1949); by carbonation of cyclohexylmagnesium chloride: Wagner, Moore, *ibid.* **72,** 974 (1950); from cyclohexane + KI + active Ni: Reppe *et al., Ann.* **582,** 38 (1953); by oxidation of cycloheptanone: Payne, Smith, *J. Org. Chem.* **22,** 1680 (1957); from cyclohexane + HCOOH or CO_2: McKursick *et al., J. Am. Chem. Soc.* **82,** 723 (1960); McKursick, *US 2940913* (1960 to du Pont).

Liquid. bp 232.5°; bp_{20} 131°; bp_8 110°; $bp_{<1}$ 63-67°. Crystal-lizes, on cooling, in monoclinic prisms, mp 29°. Odorless but when liq or in soln has a valerian odor. d_4^{15} 1.0480. n_D^{20} 1.4530. Soly in 100 g water at 15°: 0.201 g. Sol in most organic solvents.

Methyl ester. $C_8H_{14}O_2$. Fragrant liq, bp 183°. d_4^{15} 0.9954.

USE: Solubilizer for vulcanized rubber; clarifier for mineral oil; in insecticide formulations.

2725. Cyclohexanol. [108-93-0] Hexalin; hexahydrophe-nol. $C_6H_{12}O$; mol wt 100.16. C 71.95%, H 12.08%, O 15.97%. Obtained by oxidation of cyclohexane or hydrogenation of phenol: *Faith, Keyes & Clark's Industrial Chemicals,* F. A. Lowenheim, M. K. Moran, Eds. (Wiley-Interscience, New York, 4th ed., 1975) pp 304-309. Toxicity study: H. F. Smyth *et al., Am. Ind. Hyg. Assoc. J.* **23,** 95 (1962).

Hygroscopic crystals; camphor odor. d^{20} 0.962. mp 23-25°. bp 161°. Flash pt, closed cup: 154°F (68°C). n_D^{22} 1.465. At 20° soly in water: 3.6% (w/w); soly of water in cyclohexanol: 11% (w/w). Miscible with ethanol, ethyl acetate, linseed oil, petr solvents, aromatic hydrocarbons. LD_{50} orally in rats: 2.06 g/kg (Smyth).

Caution: Potential symptoms of overexposure are irritation of eyes, nose, throat and skin; narcosis. *See NIOSH Pocket Guide to Chemical Hazards* (DHHS/NIOSH 97-140, 1997) p 84.

USE: Solvent for alkyd resins, alcohol-sol phenolic resins, ethyl cellulose. Manuf celluloid; finishing textiles; insecticides.

2726. Cyclohexanone. [108-94-1] Ketohexamethylene; pimelic ketone; Hytrol O; Anone; Nadone. $C_6H_{10}O$; mol wt 98.14. C 73.43%, H 10.27%, O 16.30%. Obtained from cyclohexanol by catalytic dehydrogenation or by oxidation (which yields cyclohexanone and adipic acid) or from cyclohexane by oxidation (yielding cyclohexanone and cyclohexanol): *GB 310055* (1928 to Schering-Kahlbaum); *US 2223493; US 2223494; US 2285914* (1940, 1940, 1942 to Du Pont). Review of manuf processes: *Faith, Keyes & Clark's Industrial Chemicals,* F. A. Lowenheim, M. K. Moran, Eds. (Wiley-Interscience, New York, 4th ed., 1975) pp 304-309. Toxicity: Smyth *et al., Am. Ind. Hyg. Assoc. J.* **30,** 470 (1969).

Oily liq. Odor reminiscent of peppermint and acetone. d_4^{20} 0.9478; d_4^{25} 0.9421. mp −32.1°. bp_{760} 155.6°; bp_{400} 132.5°; bp_{200} 110.3°; bp_{100} 90.4°; bp_{60} 77.5°; bp_{40} 67.8°; bp_{20} 52.5°; bp_{10}

38.7°; bp$_5$ 26.4°; bp$_{1.0}$ 1.4°. n_D^{20} 1.4507. Flash pt closed cup: 147°F (63°C). Soly in water: 150 g/l at 10°; 50 g/l at 30°. Soly of water in cyclohexanone: 87 g/l at 20°. Sol in alcohol, ether and in other common organic solvents. LD$_{50}$ orally in rats: 1.62 ml/kg (Smyth).

2,4-Dinitrophenylhydrazone. Golden yellow needles, mp 160°. uv max (CHCl$_3$): 262 nm (ε 22500); (0.01N NaOH): 435 nm (ε 19000).

Caution: Potential symptoms of overexposure are irritation of eyes, skin and mucous membranes; headache; narcosis, coma; dermatitis. *See NIOSH Pocket Guide to Chemical Hazards* (DHHS/-NIOSH 97-140, 1997) p 84.

• USE: Solvent for cellulose acetate, nitrocellulose, natural resins, vinyl resins, crude rubber, waxes, fats, shellac, DDT. In the production of adipic acid for nylon. In the prepn of cyclohexanone resins. 2,4-Dinitrophenylhydrazone deriv as standard in elemental analysis.

2727. Cyclohexene. [110-83-8] 1,2,3,4-Tetrahydrobenzene. C$_6$H$_{10}$; mol wt 82.14. C 87.73%, H 12.27%. Occurs in coal tar. Prepd by dehydration of cyclohexanol at high temps over various catalysts. Lab prepn using H$_2$SO$_4$ as dehydrating agent: Coleman, Johnstone, *Org. Synth.* **5**, 33 (1925); Wagner, *J. Chem. Educ.* **10**, 113 (1933); by distn of cyclohexanol over silica gel or alumina: Hershberg, Ruhoff, *Org. Synth.* **17**, 25 (1937).

Liquid. d$_4^{20}$ 0.8098; d^{50} 0.7823; d^{100} 0.7355. mp −103.5°. bp$_{760}$ 83°. n_D^{20} 1.4465; n_D^{27} 1.4428. Absorption spectrum: Purvis, *Proc. Cambridge Philos. Soc.* **23**, 588 (1927); *Chem. Zentralbl.* **1927**, II, 379; *cf.* Hartley, Dobbie, *J. Chem. Soc.* **77**, 846 (1900).

Caution: Potential symptoms of overexposure are irritation of eyes, respiratory system and skin; drowsiness. *See NIOSH Pocket Guide to Chemical Hazards* (DHHS/NIOSH 97-140, 1997) p 84.

USE: Alkylation component. In the manuf of adipic acid, maleic acid, hexahydrobenzoic acid and aldehyde. To prepare butadiene in the laboratory. Has been suggested for the synthesis of maleic acid and as stabilizer for high octane gasoline.

2728. Cycloheximide. [66-81-9] 4-[(2R)-2-[(1S,3S,5S)-3,5-Dimethyl-2-oxocyclohexyl]-2-hydroxyethyl]-2,6-piperidinedione; 3-[2-(3,5-dimethyl-2-oxocyclohexyl)-2-hydroxyethyl]glutarimide; actidione; naramycin A; NSC-185; U-4527. C$_{15}$H$_{23}$NO$_4$; mol wt 281.35. C 64.03%, H 8.24%, N 4.98%, O 22.75%. Antibiotic substance isolated from the beers of streptomycin-producing strains of *Streptomyces griseus:* B. E. Leach *et al., J. Am. Chem. Soc.* **69**, 474 (1947); J. H. Ford, B. E. Leach, *ibid.* **70**, 1223 (1948); A. J. Whiffen *et al., US 2574519* (1951 to Upjohn). Production, assay and antibiotic activity: A. J. Whiffen, *J. Bacteriol.* **56**, 283 (1948). Improved production method: Kominek, *US 3915802; US 3915803* (both 1975 to Upjohn). Structure: E. C. Kornfeld *et al., J. Am. Chem. Soc.* **71**, 150 (1949). Absolute configuration: E. J. Eisenbraun *et al., ibid.* **80**, 1261 (1958); F. Johnson, N. A. Starkovsky, *Tetrahedron Lett.* **1962**, 1173; F. Johnson *et al., J. Am. Chem. Soc.* **87**, 4612 (1965). Synthesis of *dl-* and *l*-forms: F. Johnson *et al., ibid.* **88**, 149 (1966).

Plates from amyl acetate or water or 30% methanol, mp 119.5-121° (Whiffen, 1951); also reported as mp 115-116° (Johnson, 1966). [α]$_D^{29}$ −3.38° (c = 9.47 in methanol); [α]$_D^{25}$ +6.8° (c = 2 in H$_2$O). Soly at 2°: water 2.1 g/100 ml, amyl acetate 7 g/100 ml. Also sol in chloroform, ether, acetone, methanol, ethanol, other common organic solvents except satd hydrocarbons. Relatively

heat-stable, acid-stable, destroyed by boiling in aq soln at pH 7 for 1 hr, but shows no loss of activity after 15 min boiling. At pH 2 it is not destroyed by boiling for 1 hr. Rapidly inactivated at room temp by dil alkali with the formation of a volatile, fragrant ketone, 2,4-dimethylcyclohexanone. Extremely repellent to rats. LD$_{50}$ i.v. in mice: 150 mg/kg (Leach).

Acetate. C$_{17}$H$_{25}$NO$_5$. Glistening plates from methanol, mp 148-149°. [α]$_D^{25}$ +22° (c = 2.3 in methanol).

USE: Fungicide; plant growth regulator. As protein synthesis inhibitor.

2729. Cyclohexylamine. [108-91-8] Cyclohexanamine; aminocyclohexane; hexahydroaniline. C$_6$H$_{13}$N; mol wt 99.17. C 72.67%, H 13.21%, N 14.12%. Prepd by the catalytic hydrogenation of aniline at elevated temps and pressures. Fractionation of the crude reaction product yields cyclohexylamine, unchanged aniline, and a high-boiling residue contg N-phenylcyclohexylamine (cyclohexylaniline) and dicyclohexylamine. Review and bibliography: Carswell, Morrill, *Ind. Eng. Chem.* **29**, 1247 (1937). Toxicity data: H. F. Smyth *et al., Am. Ind. Hyg. Assoc. J.* **30**, 470 (1969).

Liquid. Strong, fishy, amine odor. d$_{25}^{25}$ 0.8647. mp −17.7°. bp$_{760}$ 134.5°; bp$_{500}$ 118.9°; bp$_{300}$ 102.5°; bp$_{100}$ 72.0°; bp$_{50}$ 56.0°; bp$_{30}$ 45.1°; bp$_{25}$ 41.3°; bp$_{20}$ 36.4°; bp$_{15}$ 30.5°. n_D^{25} 1.4565. Strong base. Completely misc with water and with common organic solvents, including alcohols, ethers, ketones, esters, aliphatic hydrocarbons, aromatic hydrocarbons and their chlorinated derivatives. On distillation with water, cyclohexylamine forms an azeotropic mixture contg 44.2% cyclohexylamine by weight, bp$_{760}$ 96.4°. Reacts with excess ammonia and zinc chloride at 350° to produce α-picoline: Nordt, *Conversion of Hexahydroaniline into Pyridine Bases,* Off. Pub. Bd., Report PB 704 (1941). LD$_{50}$ orally in rats: 0.71 ml/kg (Smyth).

Caution: Potential symptoms of overexposure are irritation of eyes, skin, mucous membranes, respiratory system; eye, skin burns; skin sensitization; cough, pulmonary edema; drowsiness, lightheadedness, dizziness; diarrhea, nausea, vomiting. *See NIOSH Pocket Guide to Chemical Hazards* (DHHS/NIOSH 97-140, 1997) p 84.

USE: In organic synthesis, manuf insecticides, plasticizers, corrosion inhibitors, rubber chemicals, dyestuffs, emulsifying agents, dry-cleaning soaps, acid gas absorbents.

2730. Cyclohexyl Bromide. [108-85-0] Bromocyclohexane. C$_6$H$_{11}$Br; mol wt 163.06. C 44.19%, H 6.80%, Br 49.00%. Liquid; penetrating odor. d$_{15}^{15}$ 1.329. bp 163-165°. n_D^{15} 1.4956. Insol in water. Sol in alcohol, etc.

2731. Cyclohexylcarbinol. [100-49-2] Cyclohexanemethanol; cyclohexanecarbinol; hydroxymethylcyclohexane; hexahydrobenzyl alcohol. C$_7$H$_{14}$O; mol wt 114.19. C 73.63%, H 12.36%, O 14.01%. Prepd from cyclohexylmagnesium bromide and formaldehyde in ether: Gilman, Catlin, *Org. Synth.* **coll. vol. I** (2nd ed., 1941) p 188; Hiers, Adams, *J. Am. Chem. Soc.* **48**, 2385 (1926); Marvel *et al., ibid.* **50**, 2810 (1928). For prepn of cyclohexylmagnesium bromide *see Org. Syn., loc. cit.;* Gilman, Zoellner, *J. Am. Chem. Soc.* **53**, 1945 (1931).

Liquid. Slight odor of camphor. d$_4^{25}$ 0.9215. bp$_{784}$ 184-186°; bp$_{23}$ 91-92°. n_D^{15} 1.4640. Sol in alc, ether.

Acetate. bp$_{740}$ 199-201°.

2732. Cyclohexyl Chloride. [542-18-7] Chlorocyclohexane. C$_6$H$_{11}$Cl; mol wt 118.60. C 60.76%, H 9.35%, Cl 29.89%

Colorless liquid; suffocating odor. d_4^{20} 1.000. mp $-44°$. bp 142°. n_D^{20} 1.4626. Insol in water. Sol in alcohol, etc.

2733. 2-Cyclohexyl-4,6-dinitrophenol. [131-89-5] 2,4-Dinitro-6-cyclohexylphenol; dinitro-*o*-cyclohexylphenol; DNOCHP; SN-46. $C_{12}H_{14}N_2O_5$; mol wt 266.25. C 54.13%, H 5.30%, N 10.52%, O 30.05%. Prepd from phenol, H_2SO_4, and cyclohexene or cyclohexanol: **GB 620026** (1949 to Pest Control); from *o*-cyclohexylphenol by nitration in chloroform: Baroni, Kleinan, *Monatsh. Chem.* **68**, 251 (1936).

Crystals, mp 106.5-107.5°. Soly in petr oils 2.5 to 6%. Sol in benzene, DMF; very slightly sol in water.

Sodium salt. 2-Cyclohexyl-4,6-dinitrophenate; Anobesina. $C_{12}H_{13}N_2NaO_5$; mol wt 288.23. Crystals, sol in water, alcohol.

USE: Insecticide, esp in control of citrus red mite.

2734. Cycloleucine. [52-52-8] 1-Aminocyclopentanecarboxylic acid; ACPC; CB-1639; NSC-1026. $C_6H_{11}NO_2$; mol wt 129.16. C 55.79%, H 8.58%, N 10.84%, O 24.77%. Synthetic amino acid thought to act as a valine antagonist. Prepn: Zelinsky, Stadnikoff, *Z. Physiol. Chem.* **75**, 350 (1911); Connors, Ross, *J. Chem. Soc.* **1960**, 2119; Cremlyn, *ibid.* **1962**, 3977; Sudo, Ichihara, *Bull. Chem. Soc. Jpn.* **36**, 34 (1963). Manuf: **NL 6607754** (1966 to Rohm & Haas), *C.A.* **67**, 73159b (1967). *Review:* R. B. Ross *et al.*, *J. Med. Pharm. Chem.* **3**, 1 (1961). Immunopharmacology: Rosenthale *et al.*, *J. Pharmacol. Exp. Ther.* **180**, 501 (1972); Brambilla *et al.*, *Cancer Chemother. Rep. Part 1* **56**, 579 (1972).

Crystals from ethanol-water, mp 330° (dec). Soly in water approx 5 g/100 ml. Forms stable metal salts.

Hydrochloride. [92398-48-6]; [66146-62-1] (monohydrate). Prismic crystals from water, mp 274° (dec). LD_{50} in mice, rats (mg/kg): 309, 290 orally; in rats (mg/kg): 340 i.v. (Ross).

USE: Biological testing material for immunosuppressive properties in mice; for amino acid transport studies.

2735. Cyclomethycaine. [139-62-8] 4-(Cyclohexyloxy)-benzoic acid 3-(2-methyl-1-piperidinyl)propyl ester; *p*-cyclohexyloxybenzoic acid ester of *N*-(3-hydroxypropyl)pipecoline; 3-(2-methylpiperidino)propyl *p*-cyclohexyloxybenzoate; Surfacaine; Surfathesin; Topocaine. $C_{22}H_{33}NO_3$; mol wt 359.50. C 73.50%, H 9.25%, N 3.90%, O 13.35%. Prepn: McElvain, Carney, *J. Am. Chem. Soc.* **68**, 2592 (1946), *eidem*, **US 2439818** (1948). Toxicity data: Schmidt *et al.*, *Toxicol. Appl. Pharmacol.* **1**, 454 (1959).

Hydrochloride. [537-61-1] $C_{22}H_{33}NO_3 \cdot HCl$. Crystals, dec 178-180°. Soly in water: slightly >1 g/100 ml.

Sulfate. $(C_{22}H_{33}NO_3)_2 \cdot H_2SO_4$. Crystals, mod sol in water.

THERAP CAT: Topical anesthetic.

THERAP CAT (VET): Surface anesthetic.

2736. Cyclonite. [121-82-4] Hexahydro-1,3,5-trinitro-1,3,5-triazine; cyclotrimethylenetrinitramine; *sym*-trimethylenetrinitramine; 1,3,5-trinitrohexahydro-*s*-triazine; hexogen; royal demolition explosive; RDX; T_4. $C_3H_6N_6O_6$; mol wt 222.12. C 16.22%, H 2.72%, N 37.84%, O 43.22%. Prepd by treating methenamine with fuming nitric acid: Henning, **DE 104280** (1899); Hale, *J. Am. Chem. Soc.* **47**, 2754 (1925). Two moles of cyclonite

can be obtained from one mole of methenamine, if ammonium nitrate and acetic anhydride are added: Bachmann, Sheehan, *ibid.* **71**, 1842 (1949). Manuf by nitrolysis of hexamethylenetetramine: Ruth, **US 3049543** (1962 to Olin Mathieson). Physical data relating to detonation, explosion, and blasting action: *ACS Monograph Series* **no. 139**, entitled "Science of High Explosives," M. A. Cook, Ed. (Reinhold, New York, 1958). Structure: Wood, *Proc. 4th Int. Meet. Mol. Spectrosc.* **2**, 955 (1962). Review of toxicology and human exposure: *Toxicological Profile for RDX* (PB95-264255, 1995) 145 pp.

Orthorhombic crystals from acetone, mp 205-206°. d_4^{20} 1.82. *Very explosive*. One gram dissolves in 25 ml acetone. Slightly sol in methanol, ether, ethyl acetate, glacial acetic acid. Practically insol in water, carbon tetrachloride, carbon disulfide.

Mixture with pentaerythritol tetranitrate. [52441-47-1] Semtex. Plastic explosive manufactured in two forms, *Semtex H* and *Semtex A*, which differ in the proportion of the two components RDX and pentaerythritol tetranitrate, *q.v.* Used in the destruction of PanAm Flight 103 in Dec. 1988 over Lockerbie, Scotland. Identification by MS: J. Yinon, *Can. Soc. Forensic Sci. J.* **21**, 46 (1988); by time of flight-MS: A. Marshall *et al.*, *Rapid Commun. Mass Spectrom.* **8**, 521 (1994). Description of incidents of illicit use: A. W. Feraday in *Adv. Anal. Detect. Explosives*, J. Yinon, Ed. (Kluwer Academic Publishers, Netherlands, 1993) pp 67-72. Analysis of Semtex H and A: J. R. Hobbs, *ibid.* pp. 409-427.

Caution: Potential symptoms of overexposure are irritation of eyes and skin; headache, irritability, fatigue, weakness, tremor, nausea, dizziness, vomiting, insomnia, convulsions. *See NIOSH Pocket Guide to Chemical Hazards* (DHHS/NIOSH 97-140, 1997) p 86.

USE: High explosive; rat poison.

2737. Cyclonium Iodide. [6577-41-9] 1-[(2-Cyclohexyl-2-phenyl-1,3-dioxolan-4-yl)methyl]-1-methylpiperidinium iodide; *N*-methyl-*N*-[(2-cyclohexyl-2-phenyl-1,3-dioxolan-4-yl)-methyl]-piperidinium iodide; 1-(2-phenyl-2-cyclohexyl-1,3-dioxolan-4-yl)-methyl-1-methylpiperidinium iodide; ciclonium iodide; oxapium iodide; SH-100; Esperan. $C_{22}H_{34}INO_2$; mol wt 471.42. C 56.05%, H 7.27%, I 26.92%, N 2.97%, O 6.79%. Prepn: M. Kimura *et al.,* **JP 66 6585** (1966 to Toyama), *C.A.* **65**, 7191 (1966); and separation of isomers: I. Saikawa, **JP 70 16475** (1970 to Toyama), *C.A.* **73**, 45355t. Stability studies: Shiuchi, Miyazaki, *Bunseki Kagaku* **18**, 455 (1969), *C.A.* **71**, 74097z (1969). Incompatibility studies: Kunita *et al.*, *Yakuzaigaku* **28**, 84 (1968), *C.A.* **69**, 99335x (1968). Anticholinergic activity and acute toxicity: J. Faff *et al.*, *Pol. J. Pharmacol. Pharm.* **30**, 493 (1978). *Review: Jpn. Med. Gaz.* **8**(9), 11 (1971).

α-Form. White crystals from monochlorobenzene or isopropyl alcohol, mp 195-197°. Insol in trichloroethylene.

β-Form. White crystals from monochlorobenzene, mp 150-152°. Sol in hot trichloroethylene. Both sol in methanol, ethanol, chloroform and tetrachlorethane. Hardly sol in benzene, toluene, xylene and water. LD_{50} i.p. in mice: 106 mg/kg (Faff).

THERAP CAT: Antispasmodic.

2738. Cyclooctyne. [1781-78-8] C_8H_{12}; mol wt 108.18. C 88.82%, H 11.18%. Highly strained, highly reactive cycloalkyne. Prepn: A. T. Blomquist, L. H. Liu, *J. Am. Chem. Soc.* **75**, 2153 (1953); G. Wittig, A. Krebs, *Ber.* **94**, 3260 (1961). Improved synthesis: L. Brandsma, H. D. Verkruijsse, *Synthesis* **1978**, 290.

Molecular structure: M. Traetteberg *et al., J. Mol. Struct.* **128**, 217 (1985). Review of synthetic applications: D. Heber *et al., Eur. J. Org. Chem.* **2005**, 4231-4247.

bp$_{740}$ 157.5-158°. bp$_{20}$ 50-55°. mp −34° to −32°. n_D^{20} 1.4876. d$_4^{20}$ 0.868.

USE: Building block in cycloaddition reactions.

2739. Cyclopentadiene. [542-92-7] 1,3-Cyclopentadiene. C$_5$H$_6$; mol wt 66.10. C 90.85%, H 9.15%. Obtained from the distillates produced in carbonization of coal, esp from the foreruns of coke-oven light oil: Ward, **US 2211038** (1940); process involving the liquefaction of coke-oven gas: Horclois, *Chim. Ind. (Paris)*, special issue April 1934, pp 357-363. Also obtained during the cracking of petr hydrocarbons: Tropsch *et al., Ind. Eng. Chem.* **30**, 169 (1938); *cf.* Dedussenko, *J. Gen. Chem. USSR* **7**, 1467 (1937); *Chem. Zentralbl.* **109, I,** 793 (1938). Synthesis by passing vaporized cyclopentane over activated alumina and oxides of molybdenum, chromium, or vanadium: Grosse *et al., Ind. Eng. Chem.* **32**, 309 (1940); **US 2157202; US 2157203; US 2157939.** Lab prepn by depolymerization of *dicyclopentadiene*: Moffett, *Org. Synth.* **coll. vol. IV,** 238 (1963). Toxicity study: Smyth *et al., Arch. Ind. Hyg. Occup. Med.* **10**, 61 (1954). *Review and discussion of structure:* Wilson, Wells, *Chem. Rev.* **34**, 1 (1944). *Review:* M. Fefer, A. B. Small in *Kirk-Othmer Encyclopedia of Chemical Technology* vol. 7 (Wiley-Interscience, New York, 3rd ed., 1979) pp 417-429.

Liquid. d$_4^0$ 0.8235; d$_4^{10}$ 0.8131; d$_4^{20}$ 0.8021; d$_4^{25}$ 0.7966; d$_4^{30}$ 0.7914. mp −85°. bp$_{760}$ 41.5-42.0°. n_D^{16} 1.44632. Absorption spectrum: Pickett *et al., J. Am. Chem. Soc.* **63**, 1073 (1941). Insol in water. Miscible with alc, ether, benzene, carbon tetrachloride. Sol in carbon disulfide, aniline, acetic acid, liquid petrolatum. Cyclopentadiene polymerizes to dicyclopentadiene on standing. Polymerization is accelerated by the presence of peroxides or trichloroacetic acid. The dimer is cryst, mp 32.5°, with a camphor-like odor, having the structure of a partially hydrogenated indene contg a bridged methylene group. It is a more convenient form in which to handle cyclopentadiene, and is easily depolymerized by distilling at atmospheric pressure. LD$_{50}$ of dimer orally in rats: 0.82 g/kg (Smyth).

Caution: Potential symptoms of overexposure are irritation of eyes and nose. *See NIOSH Pocket Guide to Chemical Hazards* (DHHS/NIOSH 97-140, 1997) p 86.

USE: Manuf resins; in organic synthesis as the diene in the Diels-Alder reaction producing sesquiterpenes, synthetic alkaloids, camphors.

2740. Cyclopentamine. [102-45-4] *N,α*-Dimethylcyclopentaneethanamine; *N,α*-dimethylcyclopentaneethylamine; 1-cyclopentyl-2-methylaminopropane; *β*-(methylamino)propylcyclopentane; cyclopentadrine; Sinos; Cyklosal; Cyclonarol; Clopane. C$_9$H$_{19}$N; mol wt 141.25. C 76.53%, H 13.56%, N 9.92%. Prepn: Rohrmann, **US 2520015** (1950 to Lilly).

Hydrochloride. [3459-06-1] C$_9$H$_{19}$N.HCl. Crystals, mp 113-115° (base bp$_{30}$ 83-86°, n_D^{25} 1.4500). Bitter taste. Freely sol in water.

THERAP CAT: Adrenergic (vasoconstrictor); nasal decongestant.

2741. Cyclopentane. [287-92-3] Pentamethylene. C$_5$H$_{10}$; mol wt 70.13. C 85.63%, H 14.37%. Occurs in petroleum. Found in petr ether fractions. Prepd by cracking cyclohexane in the presence of alumina at high temps and pressure: Haensel, Ipatieff, *Ind.*

Eng. Chem. **35**, 632 (1943); by reduction of cyclopentadiene: David *et al., Bull. Soc. Chim. Fr.* [5] **11**, 561 (1944). Toxicity data: Lazarew, *Arch. Exp. Pathol. Pharmakol.* **149**, 116 (1930).

Mobile, flammable liq. mp −94.4°. bp 49.3°. d$_4^{20}$ 0.7460. n_D^{20} 1.4068. Insol in water. Miscible with other hydrocarbon solvents, alcohol, ether. LC (2 hr in air) in mice: 110 mg/l (Lazarew).

Caution: Potential symptoms of overexposure are irritation of eyes, skin, nose and throat; lightheadedness, dizziness, euphoria, incoordination, nausea, vomiting, stupor; dry, cracking skin. *See NIOSH Pocket Guide to Chemical Hazards* (DHHS/NIOSH 97-140, 1997) p 86.

2742. Cyclopentanol. [96-41-3] Cyclopentyl alcohol; hydroxycyclopentane. C$_5$H$_{10}$O; mol wt 86.13. C 69.72%, H 11.70%, O 18.58%. Prepd by modified Meerwein-Pondorf-Verley reduction of cyclopentanone in the presence of aluminum isopropoxide and sodium hydroxide: Truett, Moulton, *J. Am. Chem. Soc.* **73**, 5913 (1951); by catalytic hydrogenation of pure cyclopentanone with copper chromite at 150° and 150 atm: Kögl, Ultée, *Rec. Trav. Chim.* **69**, 1576 (1950); by catalytic hydrogenation of cyclopentanone with platinum oxide and platinum black at 2-3 atm: Noller, Adams, *J. Am. Chem. Soc.* **48**, 1084 (1926); by hydration of cyclopentene in aq H$_2$SO$_4$: Hepp, **US 2414646** (1947 to Phillips Petr.); by reduction of cyclopentanone with LiAlH$_4$ in ether at room temp: Nystrom, Brown, *J. Am. Chem. Soc.* **69**, 1197 (1947).

Liquid, odor of amyl alcohol. d$_4^0$ 0.96253; d$_4^{15}$ 0.95078; d$_4^{20}$ 0.9488; d$_4^{30}$ 0.93908. mp −19°. bp 140.85°. Flash pt 124°F. n_D^{15} 1.45512; n_D^{20} 1.4520. Sparingly sol in water. Sol in ethanol.

2743. Cyclopentanone. [120-92-3] Ketocyclopentane; ketopentamethylene; adipic ketone. C$_5$H$_8$O; mol wt 84.12. C 71.39%, H 9.59%, O 19.02%. Prepd by heating adipic acid to 285-295° in the presence of barium hydroxide, distilling, extracting with ether and fractionating: Thorpe, Kon, *Org. Synth.* **coll. vol. I,** 192 (2nd ed., 1941).

Liquid. Agreeable odor, somewhat like peppermint. d$_4^{18}$ 0.9509. mp −58.2°. bp$_{760}$ 130.6°; bp$_{10}$ 23-24°. Flash pt 85°F. n_D^{20} 1.4366. Slightly sol in water. Miscible with alc, ether. Polymerizes easily, esp in presence of acids.

2744. 1,2-Cyclopentenophenanthrene. [482-66-6] C$_{17}$H$_{14}$; mol wt 218.29. C 93.54%, H 6.46%. Prepn: Ruzicka *et al., Helv. Chim. Acta* **16**, 838 (1933), *cf.* Kon, *J. Chem. Soc.* **1933**, 1081; Cook, Hewett, *Chem. Ind. (London)* **52**, 451 (1933); Hawthorne, Robinson, *J. Chem. Soc.* **1936**, 763; Bachmann, Kloetzel, *J. Am. Chem. Soc.* **59**, 2207 (1937).

Needles from alc or petr ether, mp 135-136°. Absorption spectrum: Mayneord, Roe, *Proc. Roy. Soc. London* **A152**, 299 (1935).

2745. Cyclopenthiazide. [742-20-1] 6-Chloro-3-(cyclopentylmethyl)-3,4-dihydro-2*H*-1,2,4-benzothiadiazine-7-sulfonamide 1,1-dioxide; 6-chloro-3-cyclopentylmethyl-3,4-dihydro-7-sulfamoyl-2H-1,2,4-benzothiadiazine 1,1-dioxide; 3-cyclopentyl-methyl-6-chloro-7-sulfamyl-3,4-dihydro-1,2,4-benzothiadiazine 1,1-dioxide; cyclomethiazide; tsiklometiazid; Su-8341; Navidrex; Salimid. $C_{13}H_{18}ClN_3O_4S_2$; mol wt 379.88. C 41.10%, H 4.78%, Cl 9.33%, N 11.06%, O 16.85%, S 16.88%. Prepn: Whitehead *et al., J. Org. Chem.* **26**, 2814 (1961); **BE 587225** (1960 to Ciba). Pharmacology: W. E. Barrett *et al., Arch. Int. Pharmacodyn.* **131**, 325 (1961).

Crystals from dil alc, mp 230°. LD_{50} in rats, mice (mg/kg): 141.8 ±24, 232.4 ±25 i.v. (Barrett).

THERAP CAT: Antihypertensive.

2746. Cyclopentolate. [512-15-2] α-(1-Hydroxycyclopentyl)benzeneacetic acid 2-(dimethylamino)ethyl ester; 1-hydroxy-α-phenylcyclopentaneacetic acid 2-(dimethylamino)ethyl ester; 2-dimethylaminoethyl 1-hydroxy-α-phenylcyclopentaneacetate; β-dimethylaminoethyl (1-hydroxycyclopentyl)phenylacetate; 2-phenyl-2-(1-hydroxycyclopentyl)ethanoic acid β-(dimethylamino)ethyl ester. $C_{17}H_{25}NO_3$; mol wt 291.39. C 70.07%, H 8.65%, N 4.81%, O 16.47%. Ophthalmic anticholinergic. Prepn: Treves, **US 2554511** (1951 to Schieffelin).

Hydrochloride. [5870-29-1] Ak-Pentolate; Alnide; Mydplegic; Cyclogyl; Mydrilate; Zyklolat. $C_{17}H_{25}NO_3 \cdot HCl$; mol wt 327.85. Crystals from ethyl acetate, mp 137-141°. pH of 1% aq soln: 5.0-5.4. Freely sol in water, alcohol. Practically insol in ether.

THERAP CAT: Mydriatic.

2747. Cyclophosphamide. [6055-19-2]; [50-18-0] (anhydrous). N,N-Bis(2-chloroethyl)tetrahydro-2H-1,3,2-oxazaphosphorin-2-amine 2-oxide monohydrate; 1-bis(2-chloroethyl)amino-1-oxo-2-aza-5-oxaphosphoridin monohydrate; bis(2-chloroethyl)phosphamide cyclic propanolamide ester monohydrate; N,N-bis(β-chloroethyl)-N',O-propylenephosphoric acid ester diamide monohydrate; cyclophosphane; cytophosphane; B-518; Cycloblastin; Cyclostin; Cytoxan; Endoxan; Procytox; Sendoxan. $C_7H_{15}Cl_2N_2O_2$-P.H_2O; mol wt 279.10. C 30.12%, H 6.14%, Cl 25.41%, N 10.04%, O 17.20%, P 11.10%. Oxazaphosphine cytostatic agent; supresses B-cell activity and antibody formation. Prepn: H. Arnold, F. Bourseaux, *Angew. Chem.* **70**, 539 (1958). Optical resolution study: T. Kawashima *et al., J. Org. Chem.* **43**, 1111 (1978). Toxicology: A. G. Wheeler *et al., Toxicol. Appl. Pharmacol.* **4**, 324 (1962). Book: D. L. Hill, *A Review of Cyclophosphamide* (Charles C Thomas, Springfield, 1975) 340 pp. Reviews of carcinogenicity studies: *IARC Monographs* **9**, 135-156 (1975); of field trials as defleecing agent for sheep: M. H. Fahmy, Y. Moride, *Anim. Breed. Abstr.* **52**, 7-19 (1984); of clinical toxicology: L. H. Fraiser *et al., Drugs* **42**, 781-795 (1991); of mechanism of action and clinical use: O. M. Colvin, *Curr. Pharmaceut. Design* **5**, 555-560 (1999); of analytical methods: M. Malet-Martino *et al., ibid.* 561-586; and metabolism: F. Baumann, R. Preiss, *J. Chromatogr. B* **764**, 173-192 (2001).

mp 41-45° (Arnold); also reported as mp 47-49° (Hill). Soly in water: 40 g/l. Sol in alcohol, benzene, ethylene glycol, chloro-

form, dioxane; sparingly sol in ether and acetone. LD_{50} orally in mice, rats: 350, 94 mg/kg (Wheeler). Also marketed as the anhydrous form: crystals from ether, mp 51.5-52.5°.

Caution: This substance is listed as a known human carcinogen: *Report on Carcinogens, Eleventh Edition* (PB2005-104914, 2004) p III-74.

USE: Defleecing agent for sheep.

THERAP CAT: Antineoplastic; immunosuppressant.

2748. Cyclopropane. [75-19-4] Trimethylene. C_3H_6; mol wt 42.08. C 85.63%, H 14.37%. Prepd by reduction of 1,2-dibromocyclopropane with zinc and alcohol: Lott, Christiansen, *J. Am. Pharm. Assoc.* **19**, 341 (1930); Schlatter, *J. Am. Chem. Soc.* **63**, 1733 (1941); from 1,3-dibromopropane with zinc and alcohol in absence of water: Ashdown *et al., ibid.* **58**, 850 (1936); by the action of sodium vapor on 1,3-dibromopropane: Bawn, Hunter, *Trans. Faraday Soc.* **34**, 608 (1938); from 1,3-dichloropropane heated with an excess of zinc dust, iodine and ethanol in 80% yield: Hass *et al., Ind. Eng. Chem.* **28**, 1178 (1936); from 1,3-dichloropropane with zinc in presence of sodium iodide: **US 2102556** (1937); *cf.* **US 2098239**; **GB 498225**; **US 2211787**; **US 2235679**; **US 2235762**; **US 2240513**; **US 2240514**; **US 2242235**. From ethylene by the reaction with methylene iodide and a zinc-copper couple in 29% yield: Simmons, Smith, *J. Am. Chem. Soc.* **80**, 5323 (1958); *Chem. Eng. News* **36**, 40 (Dec 8, 1958).

Flammable gas. Characteristic odor resembling that of petr ether. mp −127°. bp −33°. Liquefies at 4-6 atms. One liter of cyclopropane (at 1 atm, 0°) weighs 1.879 g. One vol of cyclopropane dissolves in about 2.7 vols of water at 15°. Freely sol in alcohol, ether. Sol in fixed oils. Concd H_2SO_4 absorbs the gas readily.

Caution: Mixture of cyclopropane with oxygen or air may explode when brought in contact with a flame or other causes of ignition. Explosive limits (% by vol in air), lower: 2.41; upper: 10.3. The explosibility is greater than that of other anesthetic-oxygen mixtures because of the comparatively larger amounts of oxygen that are compatible with cyclopropane anesthesia. Rich oxygen mixtures are therefore to be avoided.

THERAP CAT: Anesthetic (inhalation).

THERAP CAT (VET): Anesthetic (inhalation).

2749. Cyclopropyl Methyl Ether. [540-47-6] Methoxycyclopropane; cyprome ether. C_4H_8O; mol wt 72.11. C 66.62%, H 11.18%, O 22.19%. Prepd from 1,3-dibromo-2-methoxypropane by reduction with Zn: Olson *et al., J. Am. Chem. Soc.* **69**, 2454 (1947); *see also* Krantz, Jr. *et al., J. Pharmacol.* **69**, 207 (1940); Krantz, Jr., Drake, **US 2330979** (1944); Haller, **US 2424029** (1947).

Mobile, flammable liq. Odor similar to that of cyclopropane. d_4^{25} 0.786. mp −119°; bp 44.7°; n_D^{20} 1.3802. 100 ml of water dissolve 5.5 g of cyprome ether at 25°. Oil-water coefficient: 6.7 (ethyl ether = 4.5). Vapor press. at 26° (measured in nitrometer): 414 mm (ethyl ether = 555 mm). Explosive mixture, lower limit for air or oxygen: 2.0% v/v (ethyl ether vapor = 2.5 v/v).

Caution: Narcotic in high concns.

USE: Insecticide.

2750. Cyclorphan. [4163-15-9] 17-(Cyclopropylmethyl)-morphinan-3-ol; (−)-3-hydroxy-N-cyclopropylmethylmorphinan. $C_{20}H_{27}NO$; mol wt 297.43. C 80.76%, H 9.15%, N 4.71%, O 5.38%. Prepn: Gates, Montzka, *J. Med. Chem.* **7**, 127 (1964); Gates, **US 3285922** (1966 to Res. Corp.). Pharmacology: Harris *et al., Arch. Int. Pharmacodyn. Ther.* **165**, 112 (1967).

Crystals from ethyl acetate, mp 187.5-189°. $[\alpha]_D^{30}$ $-120°$ (c = 2.26). LD_{50} in mice, rats (mg/kg): 24, 23 i.v. (Gates, 1966).

2751. Cycloserine. [68-41-7] D-4-Amino-3-isoxazolidinone; D-4-amino-3-isoxazolidone; orientomycin; PA-94; 106-7; Closina; Farmiserina; Micoserina; Oxamycin; Seromycin. C_3H_6-N_2O_2; mol wt 102.09. C 35.29%, H 5.92%, N 27.44%, O 31.34%. Antibiotic substance produced by *Streptomyces garyphalus* sive *orchidaceus*: Kuehl, Jr., *et al.*, *J. Am. Chem. Soc.* **77**, 2344 (1955); Hidy *et al.*, *ibid.* 2345; Shull, Sardinas, *Antibiot. Chemother.* **5**, 398 (1955); Shull *et al.*, US 2773878 (1956 to Pfizer); Harned, US 2789983 (1957 to Commercial Solvents); GB 768007 (1957 to Commercial Solvents); *C.A.* **51**, 10847e (1957); US 3124590 (1964 to Commercial Solvents); Howe, US 2845433 (1958 to Merck & Co.). Synthesis: Stammer *et al.*, *J. Am. Chem. Soc.* **77**, 2346 (1955); Peck, US 2772280 (1956 to Merck & Co.); Plattner *et al.*, *Helv. Chim. Acta* **40**, 1531 (1957); Holly, Stammer, US 2840565 (1958 to Merck & Co.). Prepn of crystalline calcium and magnesium salts: Harris *et al.*, US 2832788 (1958 to Merck & Co.). HPLC determn in plasma and urine: D. G. Musson *et al.*, *J. Chromatogr.* **414**, 121 (1987). Comprehensive description: J. W. Lamb, *Anal. Profiles Drug Subs.* **1**, 53-64 (1972); H. A. El-Obeid, A. A. Al-Badr, *ibid.* **18**, 567-597 (1989).

Crystals, decomp 155-156°. $[\alpha]_D^{23}$ $+116°$ (c = 1.17); $[\alpha]_{546}^{25}$ $+137°$ (c = 5 in 2N NaOH). uv max: 226 nm ($E_{1cm}^{1\%}$ 402). Sol in water, slightly sol in methanol, propylene glycol. Aq solns have a pH around 6. Forms salts with acids and bases. Neutral or acid solns are unstable. Aq solns buffered to pH 10 with sodium carbonate can be stored without loss for one week at refrigerator temps.

THERAP CAT: Antibacterial (tuberculostatic).

2752. Cyclosporins. Group of nonpolar cyclic oligopeptides with immunosuppressant activity; produced by *Tolypocladium inflatum* Gams (formerly designated as *Trichoderma polysporum* [Link ex Pers.] Rifai) and other fungi imperfecti. Cyclosporins A through Z have been identified with A being the major component. Characterized by a C_9-amino acid, MeBmt, *q.v.*, cyclosporins bind to the cytosolic protein, cyclophilin, to form an active complex which inhibits the enzyme, calcineurin, a key component of T-cell activation. Isoln of A and C, structure of A: A. Rüegger *et al.*, *Helv. Chim. Acta* **59**, 1075 (1976); structure of C: R. Traber *et al.*, *ibid.* **60**, 1247 (1977). Production of A and C: E. Härri *et al.*, US 4117118 (1978 to Sandoz). Review of isoln, structure elucidation, synthesis and bioactivity: A. von Wartburg, R. Traber, *Prog. Med. Chem.* **25**, 1-33 (1988); of biosynthesis and mode of action: A. Lawen, *ibid.* **33**, 53-97 (1996). Review of role of calcineurin on bioactivity of cyclosporins: K. A. Jorgensen *et al.*, *Scand. J. Immunol.* **57**, 93-98 (2003). HPLC separation of components from fungal fermentation samples: J. Tuominen *et al.*, *Rapid Commun. Mass Spectrom.* **12**, 1085 (1998). HPLC-MS determn in blood: B. Vollenbroeker *et al.*, *Transplant. Proc.* **37**, 1741 (2005).

Cyclosporin A

Cyclosporin A. [59865-13-3] Cyclosporine; ciclosporin; 27-400; Atopica; Sandimmun(e); Neoral; Optimmune; Restasis. C_{62}-$H_{111}N_{11}O_{12}$; mol wt 1202.61. Comprehensive description: M. M. Hassan, M. A. Al-Yahya, *Anal. Profiles Drug Subs.* **16**, 145-206

(1987). Toxicological evaluation: B. Ryffel *et al.*, *Arch. Toxicol.* **53**, 107 (1983). Symposium on therapeutic use in dermatology: *J. Am. Acad. Dermatol.* **23**, part 2, 1241-1334 (1990). Review of use in canine skin diseases: E. Guaguere *et al.*, *Vet. Dermatol.* **15**, 61-74 (2004). Review of clinical experience in organ transplantation: C. J. Dunn *et al.*, *Drugs* **61**, 1957-2016 (2001); in treatment of dry eye: H. D. Perry, E. D. Donnenfeld, *Expert Opin. Pharmacother.* **5**, 2099-2107 (2004). White prismatic needles from acetone at $-15°$. mp 148-151°. $[\alpha]_D^{20}$ $-244°$ (c = 0.6 in chloroform); $[\alpha]_D^{20}$ $-189°$ (c = 0.5 in methanol). Sol in methanol, ethanol, acetone, ether, chloroform; slightly sol in water and saturated hydrocarbons. LD_{50} in mice, rats, rabbits (mg/kg): 107, 25, >10 i.v.; 2329, 1480, >1000 orally (Ryffel).

Cyclosporin B. [63775-95-1] Ala²-cyclosporine. $C_{61}H_{109}$-$N_{11}O_{12}$; mol wt 1188.58. Amorphous white powder, mp 149-152°. $[\alpha]_D^{20}$ $-238°$ (c = 0.62 in chloroform). $[\alpha]_D^{20}$ $-168°$ (c = 0.56 in methanol).

Cyclosporin C. [59787-61-0] Thr²-cyclosporine. $C_{62}H_{111}$-$N_{11}O_{13}$; mol wt 1218.61. Colorless prismatic needles from acetone at $-15°$. mp 152-155°. $[\alpha]_D^{20}$ $-255°$ (c = 0.5 in chloroform). $[\alpha]_D^{20}$ $-182°$ (c = 0.5 in methanol). Solubility similar to cyclosporin A.

Cyclosporin D. [63775-96-2] Val²-cyclosporine. $C_{63}H_{113}$-$N_{11}O_{12}$; mol wt 1216.64. Colorless prisms from acetone at $-15°$. mp 148-151°. $[\alpha]_D^{20}$ $-245°$ (c = 0.52 in $CHCl_3$). $[\alpha]_D^{20}$ $-211°$ (c = 0.51 in methanol).

Cyclosporin G. [74436-00-3] 7-L-Norvaline cyclosporin A; Nva²-cyclosporine. $C_{63}H_{113}N_{11}O_{12}$; mol wt 1216.64. Immunosuppressive profile: P. C. Hiestand *et al.*, *Transplant. Proc.* **17**, 1362 (1985); *eidem*, *Immunology* **55**, 249 (1985). Colorless, polyhedric crystals from ether + petroleum ether, mp 196-197°. $[\alpha]_D^{20}$ $-245°$ (c = 1.0 in chloroform). $[\alpha]_D^{20}$ $-191°$ (c = 1.04 in methanol).

Caution: Cyclosporin A is listed as a known human carcinogen: *Report on Carcinogens, Eleventh Edition* (PB2005-104914, 2004) p III-75.

THERAP CAT: Cyclosporin A as immunosuppressant.

THERAP CAT (VET): In the control of canine atopic dermatitis and immune-mediated dermatological diseases.

2753. Cyclotheonamides. Naturally occurring family of macrocyclic peptides that inhibit serine proteases such as thrombin, *q.v.* Isolated from the Japanese marine sponge *Theonella swinhoei*; the two major forms, A and B, contain a vinylogous tyrosine (V-Tyr) and an α-ketoarginine residues — amino acids which were previously unknown in nature. Isoln and initial structure of A and B: N. Fusetani *et al.*, *J. Am. Chem. Soc.* **112**, 7053 (1990). Reassignment of stereochemistry and total synthesis of B: M. Hagihara, S. L. Schreiber, *ibid.* **114**, 6570 (1992). Facile synthesis of B: H. M. M. Bastiaans *et al.*, *Tetrahedron Lett.* **36**, 5963 (1995). Isoln of C, D, E: Y. Nakao *et al.*, *Bioorg. Med. Chem.* **3**, 1115 (1995). Inhibition of thrombin and other serine proteases: S. D. Lewis *et al.*, *Thromb. Res.* **70**, 173 (1993). Molecular basis of inhibition and synthesis of A: B. E. Maryanoff *et al.*, *Proc. Natl. Acad. Sci. USA* **90**, 8048 (1993).

Cyclotheonamide A   R = H
Cyclotheonamide B   R = CH₃

Cyclotheonamide A. [129033-04-1] [*S*(*E*)]-3-[[4-Amino-5-(4-hydroxyphenyl)-1-oxo-2-pentenyl]amino]-*N*-formyl-L-alanyl-L-prolyl-*N*⁶-(aminoiminomethyl)-2-oxo-L-3,6-diaminohexanoyl-D-phenylalanine cyclic (4 → 1)-peptide; MS-1144. $C_{36}H_{45}N_9O_8$; mol wt 731.80. uv max (methanol): 278 nm (ε 1940). $[\alpha]_D^{23}$ −13° (c = 0.2 in methanol).

Cyclotheonamide B. [129033-05-2] $C_{37}H_{47}N_9O_8$; mol wt 745.82. $[\alpha]_D^{23}$ −13.5° (c = 0.2 in methanol).

2754. Cyclothiazide. [2259-96-3] 3-Bicyclo[2.2.1]hept-5-en-2-yl-6-chloro-3,4-dihydro-2*H*-1,2,4-benzothiadiazine-7-sulfonamide 1,1-dioxide; 6-chloro-3,4-dihydro-3-(2-norbornen-5-yl)-2*H*-1,2,4-benzothiadiazine-7-sulfonamide 1,1-dioxide; 6-chloro-3,4-dihydro-3-(2-norbornen-5-yl)-7-sulfamoyl-1,2,4-benzothiadiazine 1,1-dioxide; 6-chloro-3,4-dihydro-3-(2-norbornen-5-yl)-7-sulfamoyl-1,2,4-benzothiadiazine 1,1-dioxide; 6-chloro-3-(2-norbornen-5-yl)-7-sulfamyl-3,4-dihydro-1,2,4-benzothiadiazine 1,1-dioxide; Lilly 35483; Aquirel; Anhydron; Doburil; Fluidil. $C_{14}H_{16}ClN_3O_4S_2$; mol wt 389.88. C 43.13%, H 4.14%, Cl 9.09%, N 10.78%, O 16.41%, S 16.45%. Prepn: C. W. Whitehead *et al.*, *J. Org. Chem.* **26**, 2814 (1961); E. Müller, K. Hasspacher, **US 3275625** (1966 to Boehringer, Ing.). Comprehensive description: C. D. Wentling, *Anal. Profiles Drug Subs.* **1**, 65-77 (1972).

Crystals from dil alc, mp 234°.
THERAP CAT: Diuretic; antihypertensive.
THERAP CAT (VET): Diuretic.

2755. Cyclovalone. [579-23-7] 2,6-Divanillylidenecyclohexanone; 2,6-bis(4-hydroxy-3-methoxybenzylidene)cyclohexanone; divanillalcyclohexanone; Beveno; Divanil; Divanon (obsolete); DVC. $C_{22}H_{22}O_5$; mol wt 366.41. C 72.11%, H 6.05%, O 21.83%. Prepn: Vorländer, Koch, *Ber.* **62**, 534 (1929); Rumpel, **AT 180258** (1954 to Chem-Pharm. Fabrik Waldheim).

Crystals from acetic acid, mp 178-179°. Soluble in alcohol, water.
THERAP CAT: Choleretic, cholagogue.

2756. Cyfluthrin. [68359-37-5] 3-(2,2-Dichloroethenyl)-2,2-dimethylcyclopropanecarboxylic acid cyano(4-fluoro-3-phenoxyphenyl)methyl ester; (*R,S*)-α-cyano-4-fluoro-3-phenoxybenzyl-(1*R,S*)-*cis,trans*-3-(2,2-dichlorovinyl)-2,2-dimethylcyclopropanecarboxylate; cyfoxylate; FCR-1272; BAY FCR 1272; Baythroid; Renounce; Tempo. $C_{22}H_{18}Cl_2FNO_3$; mol wt 434.29. C 60.84%, H 4.18%, Cl 16.33%, F 4.37%, N 3.23%, O 11.05%. Synthetic pyrethroid insecticide. Commercial product is mixture of 8 isomers, the (1*R*)-isomers primarily responsible for the bioactivity. Prepn of racemic mixture: R. Fuchs *et al.*, **DE 2709264**; *eidem*, **US 4218469** (1978, 1980 both to Bayer AG). Prepn of stereoisomers: *eidem*, **EP 22970**; *eidem*, **US 4287208** (both 1981 to Bayer AG). Chiral phase HPLC separation of enantiomers: R. A. Chapman, *J. Chromatogr.* **258**, 175 (1983). Metabolism by cell suspension cultures: U. Preiss *et al.*, *Chemosphere* **13**, 861 (1984). Field evaluation against cotton insect pests: J. A. Durant, *J. Agric. Entomol.* **1**, 201 (1984). Review of chemistry, bioactivity and field studies: I. Hammann, R. Fuchs, *Pflanzenschutz-Nachr.* **34**, 121-151 (1981); of formulations and potential uses: W. Behrenz *et al.*, *ibid.* **36**, 127-176 (1983). Review of toxicology and human exposure: *Toxicological Profile for Pyrethrins and Pyrethroids* (PB2004-100004, 2003) 332 pp.

(1*R*,3*R*,α*R*)-form

Yellowish-brown oil, n_D^{23} 1.5511. Soly in water (20°): 1-2 × 10^{-6} g/l. LD_{50} in male, female rats, male, female mice (mg/kg): 500-800, 1200, 300, 600 orally in Lutrol (Behrenz). LC_{50} (96 hr) in rainbow trout: 0.0006 mg/l (Hammann).

(1*R*,3*R*,α*R*)-Form. [85649-12-3] Colorless oil. $[\alpha]_D^{20}$ −15.0° (c = 1.0 in CHCl₃).
(1*R*,3*R*,α*S*)-Form. [85649-15-6] Crystals, mp 50-52°. $[\alpha]_D^{20}$ +24.5° (c = 1.0 in CHCl₃).
(1*R*,3*S*,α*S*)-Form. [85649-19-0] Crystals from *m*-hexane mp 68-69°. $[\alpha]_D^{20}$ −2.1° (c = 1.0 in CHCl₃).
USE: Agricultural insecticide.

2757. Cyhalothrin. [68085-85-8] 3-(2-Chloro-3,3,3-trifluoro-1-propenyl)-2,2-dimethylcyclopropanecarboxylic acid cyano(3-phenoxyphenyl)methyl ester; Grenade. $C_{23}H_{19}ClF_3NO_3$; mol wt 449.85. C 61.41%, H 4.26%, Cl 7.88%, F 12.67%, N 3.11%, O 10.67%. Synthetic pyrethroid insecticide. Prepn: R. K. Huff, **DE 2802962**; *idem*, **US 4183948** (1977, 1980 both to ICI). Activity: P. D. Bently *et al.*, *Pestic. Sci.* **11**, 156 (1980); V. K. Stubbs *et al.*, *Aust. Vet. J.* **59**, 152 (1982). Review of toxicology and human exposure: *Toxicological Profile for Pyrethrins and Pyrethroids* (PB2004-100004, 2003) 332 pp.

(*Z*)-(1*S*)-*cis*-form

Commercial product exists as a mixture consisting of 95% *cis*-isomers.
USE: Insecticide; acaricide.

2758. λ-Cyhalothrin. [91465-08-6] (1*S*,3*S*)-*rel*-3-[(1*Z*)-2-Chloro-3,3,3-trifluoro-1-propenyl]-2,2-dimethylcyclopropanecarboxylic acid (*R*)-cyano(3-phenoxyphenyl)methyl ester; (±)-α-cyano-3-phenoxybenzyl 3-(2-chloro-3,3,3-trifluoroprop-1-enyl)-2,2-dimethylcyclopropane carboxylate; PP-321; Karate; Warrior. $C_{23}H_{19}ClF_3NO_3$; mol wt 449.85. C 61.41%, H 4.26%, Cl 7.88%, F 12.67%, N 3.11%, O 10.67%. Synthetic pyrethroid; 1:1 mixture of the *Z*-(1*R*,3*R*) *S*-ester isomers and *Z*-(1*S*,3*S*) *R*-ester isomers of cyhalothrin, *q.v.* Prepn: M. J. Robson, J. Crosby, **EP 106469**; J. Crosby, **US 4510098** (1984, 1985 both to ICI); M. J. Robson *et al.*, *Brighton Crop Prot. Conf. - Pests Dis.* **1984**, 853. Description of chemical properties and biological activities: A. R. Jutsum *et al.*, *ibid.* 421. Field trials for mosquito control: A. A. Weathersbee *et al.*, *J. Am. Mosq. Control Assoc.* **7**, 238 (1991); for sandfly control: D. A. Elnaiem *et al.*, *Med. Vet. Entomol.* **13**, 310 (1999). Effect on beneficial insects: J. S. White *et al.*, *Brighton Crop Prot. Conf. - Pests Dis.* **1990**, 969. Dissipation on soil: B. D. Hill, D. J. Inaba, *J. Agric. Food Chem.* **39**, 2282 (1991). Determination in natural waters: S. T. Hadfield *et al.*, *Pestic. Sci.* **34**, 207 (1992). Review of early field trials on horticultural crops: D. Wilson, J. Trevenna, *Brighton Crop Prot. Conf. - Pests Dis.* **1986**, 323.

Z-(1*S*,3*S*) *R*-form

Consult the Name Index before using this section.

White odorless solid, mp 49.2°. Vapor pressure at 20°: 2×10^{-10} kPa. Soly (mg/l): purified water 5×10^{-3}; buffered water 4×10^{-3}. Sol in common range of solvents at 21°C. LD_{50} (technical grade) in male, female rats (mg/kg): 79, 56 orally; 632, 696 dermally (Jutsum).

USE: Insecticide.

2759. Cyheptamide. [7199-29-3] 10,11-Dihydro-5H-dibenzo[a,d]cycloheptene-5-carboxamide; dibenzo[a,d][1,4]-cycloheptadiene-5-carboxamide; AY-8682. $C_{16}H_{15}NO$; mol wt 237.30. C 80.98%, H 6.37%, N 5.90%, O 6.74%. Prepn: M. A. Davis et al., FR 1355829 (1964 to Ayerst, McKenna & Harrison); M. A. Davis, S. O. Winthrop, US 3242212 (1966 to Am. Home Prods.). Prepn and anticonvulsant activity: M. A. Davis et al., J. Med. Chem. 7, 88 (1964). Physical characteristics: H. J. Doorenbos et al., Pharm. Weekbl. 104, 732 (1969). Pharmacology: A. B. H. Funcke et al., Arch. Int. Pharmacodyn. 187, 174 (1970). Toxicological studies: C. J. van Eeken et al., ibid. 188, 79 (1970). Metabolism in animals and man: M. Kraml et al., Biochem. Pharmacol. 20, 2327 (1971). Comparison of potency with other anticonvulsants: G. L. Jones et al., J. Pharm. Sci. 70, 618 (1981). Elucidation of structure by x-ray diffraction, mode of action: P. W. Codding et al., J. Med. Chem. 27, 649 (1984).

Long needles from acetonitrile, mp 193-194°. Sol in chloroform; sparingly sol in methanol, acetone; slightly sol in ethanol, ether. Practically insol in water. LD_{50} in mice (g/kg): 4.2-5.2 orally; 2.4-2.6 i.p. (Funcke).

2760. Cyhexatin. [13121-70-5] Tricyclohexylhydroxystannane; TCTH; tricyclohexylstannol; tricyclohexyltin hydroxide; ENT-27395; Dowco 213; Plictran. $C_{18}H_{34}OSn$; mol wt 385.17. C 56.13%, H 8.90%, O 4.15%, Sn 30.82%. Prepn: E. E. Kenaga, US 3264177 (1966 to Dow). Activity studies: W. E. Allison et al., J. Econ. Entomol. 61, 1254 (1968); L. R. Jeppson et al., ibid., 1502. Biochemical mode of action: S. Ahmad, C. O. Knowles, Comp. Gen. Pharmacol. 3, 125 (1972). Biodegradation: E. H. Blair, Environ. Qual. Saf. Suppl. 3, 406 (1975). Toxicity data: T. B. Gaines, R. E. Linder, Fundam. Appl. Toxicol. 7, 299 (1986). Acute toxicity studies in livestock: J. H. Johnson et al., Toxicol. Appl. Pharmacol. 31, 66 (1975).

Whitish crystalline powder, mp 195-198°. Insol in water. Slightly sol in most organic solvents. Degraded when exposed in thin layers to uv light. LD_{50} in adult male, female rats (mg/kg): 779, 826 orally (Gaines, Linder).

Caution: Potential symptoms of overexposure are irritation of eyes, skin, respiratory system; headache, vertigo; sore throat, cough; abdominal pain, vomiting; skin burns, pruritis. See NIOSH Pocket Guide to Chemical Hazards (DHHS/NIOSH 97-140, 1997) p 86.

USE: Acaricide.

2761. Cymarin. [508-77-0] 3β-[(2,6-Dideoxy-3-O-methyl-β-D-$ribo$-hexopyranosyl)oxy]-5β,14-dihydroxy-19-oxocard-20(22)-enolide; K-strophanthin-α; Alvonal MR. $C_{30}H_{44}O_9$; mol wt

548.66. C 65.67%, H 8.08%, O 26.24%. A glycoside of cymarose, the aglucon being strophanthidin. Isoln from Strophanthus kombé Oliv., Apocynaceae: Jacobs, Hoffmann, J. Biol. Chem. 67, 609 (1926); Stoll et al., Helv. Chim. Acta 20, 1484 (1937); from Adonis vernalis L., and A. chrysocyathus Hook., Ranunculaceae: Reichstein, Rosenmund, Pharm. Acta Helv. 15, 150 (1940); Pitra, Cekan, Collect. Czech. Chem. Commun. 26, 1551 (1961); Abubakirov, Yamatova, Zh. Obshch. Khim. 31, 2424 (1961); from Pentopetia androsaemifolia Decne., Asclepiadaceae: Wyss et al., Helv. Chim. Acta 43, 664 (1960); from Castilloa elastica Cerv., Moraceae: Adams, Wilkinson, J. Pharm. Pharmacol. 13, 279 (1961). Structure: Kochetkov et al., Dokl. Akad. Nauk SSSR 136, 613 (1961). Toxicity data: V. G. Vogel, E. Kluge, Arzneim.-Forsch. 11, 848 (1961).

Needles from methanol, mp 148°. $[\alpha]_D^{20}$ +39.2° (methanol); $[\alpha]_D^{22}$ +39.0° (c = 1.7 in chloroform). Sol in methanol, chloroform. Practically insol in water. LD_{50} i.v. in rats: 24.8 ± 1.8 mg/kg (Vogel, Kluge).

Sesquihydrate. Hexagonal plates from dil ethanol, mp 184-185°.

Monoacetylcymarin. $C_{32}H_{46}O_{10}$. Needles from dil methanol, mp 175-176°. $[\alpha]_D^{22}$ +45.1° (ethanol). Sol in chloroform. Practically insol in water.

THERAP CAT: Cardiotonic.

2762. Cymarose. [579-04-4] 2,6-Dideoxy-3-O-methyl-$ribo$-hexose; 3-methyldigitoxose. $C_7H_{14}O_4$; mol wt 162.18. C 51.84%, H 8.70%, O 39.46%. By hydrolysis of a number of cardiac glycosides from the Apocynaceae family. From Apocynum cannabinum L., A. androsaemifolium L., A. venetum L.: Windaus, Hermanns, Ber. 48, 979 (1915); Trabert, Arzneim.-Forsch. 10, 197 (1960); from Strophanthus kombé Oliv., Periploca graeca L.: Jacobs, Hoffmann, J. Biol. Chem. 67, 609 (1926); 79, 519 (1928); from S. emini Aschers & Pax: Lamb, Smith, J. Chem. Soc. 1936 442; also from Castilla elastica Cerv., Moraceae: Adams, Wilkinson, J. Pharm. Pharmacol. 13, 279 (1961). Structure: S. F. Dyke, The Carbohydrates (Interscience, New York, 1960) p 104. Synthesis: Bollinger, Ulrich, Helv. Chim. Acta 35, 93 (1952). Review: R. C. Elderfield, "The Carbohydrate Components of Cardiac Glycosides" in W. W. Pigman, M. L. Wolfrom, Advances in Carbohydrate Chemistry vol. I (Academic Press, New York, 1945) pp 147-173.

Prisms from ether + petr ether, mp 93-94°. $[\alpha]_D^{20}$ +54.7° (c = 3.2 in water after 24 hrs). Sol in water, alcohol, acetone; sparingly sol in ether, petr ether, chloroform, benzene. Reduces Fehling soln. Does not form an osazone.

2763. Cymene. [25155-15-1] Methyl(1-methylethyl)-benzene; isopropyltoluene; methylisopropylbenzene. $C_{10}H_{14}$; mol wt 134.22. C 89.49%, H 10.51%. Usually prepd by alkylation of toluene; m-, o- and p-isomers obtained: Allen, Yats, J. Am. Chem. Soc. 83, 2799 (1961). Purification and properties of the three isomers: Streiff et al., Anal. Chem. 27, 411 (1955). Separation of the three isomers by gas chromatography: Rihani, Froment, J. Chromatogr. 18, 150 (1965). Toxicity study: P. M. Jenner et al., Food Cosmet. Toxicol. 2, 327 (1964).

m-**Cymene.** [535-77-3] 1-Methyl-3-(1-methylethyl)benzene. Liquid, bp 175.14°. mp $-63.75°$. d_4^{20} 0.8610, d_4^{25} 0.8570. n_D^{20}

1.4930, n_D^{25} 1.4906. Practically insol in water. Miscible with alcohol, ether.

***o*-Cymene.** [527-84-8] 1-Methyl-2-(1-methylethyl)benzene. Liquid, bp 178.15°. mp −71.54°; also reported as −75.24° and −81.53° for two unstable solid forms (Streiff). d_4^{20} 0.8766, d_4^{25} 0.8726. n_D^{20} 1.5006, n_D^{25} 1.4982. Practically insol in water. Miscible with organic solvents.

***p*-Cymene.** [99-87-6] 1-Methyl-4-(1-methylethyl)benzene; Dolcymene. Occurs in a number of essential oils. Liquid, bp 177.10°. mp −67.94°. d_4^{20} 0.8573, d_4^{25} 0.8533. n_D^{20} 1.4909, n_D^{25} 1.4885. Flash pt, closed cup: 117°F (47°C). Practically insol in water. Misc with alcohol, ether. LD$_{50}$ orally in rats: 4750 mg/kg (Jenner).

2764. Cymiazole. [61676-87-7] 2,4-Dimethyl-*N*-(3-methyl-2(3*H*)-thiazolylidene)benzenamine; 2-(2′,4′-dimethylphenyl-imino)-3-methylthiazoline; *N*-(3-methyl-4-thiazolin-2-ylidene)-2,4-xylidine; xymiazole; CGA-50439; Tifatol. C$_{12}$H$_{14}$N$_2$S; mol wt 218.32. C 66.02%, H 6.46%, N 12.83%, S 14.69%. Prepn: D. Duerr, W. D. Traber, **DE 2619724** (1976 to Ciba-Geigy), *C.A.* **86**, 72627h (1977). Activity: R. M. Immler *et al., Proc. Br. Crop Prot. Conf. - Pests Dis.* **1977**, 383.

USE: Acaricide.

THERAP CAT (VET): Ectoparasiticide.

2765. Cymoxanil. [57966-95-7] 2-Cyano-*N*-[(ethylamino)carbonyl]-2-(methoxyimino)acetamide; 2-cyano-*N*-ethylcarbamoyl-2-methoxyiminoacetamide; 1-(2-cyano-2-methoxyiminoacetyl)-3-ethylurea; DPX-3217; Biozate; Curzate. C$_7$H$_{10}$N$_4$O$_3$; mol wt 198.18. C 42.42%, H 5.09%, N 28.27%, O 24.22%. Systemic fungicide primarily for potato blight. Prepn: S. H. Davidson, **US 3957847** (1976 to DuPont). Metabolism in plants: Y. Cohen, U. Gisi, *Crop Prot.* **12**, 284 (1993). *In vitro* sensitivity study: R. A. Hamlen, R. J. Power, *Pestic. Sci.* **53**, 101 (1998). GC determn in plants and food products: R. F. Holt, *ibid.* **10**, 455 (1979). Field trials in blight: M. Absi, *Proc. Br. Crop Prot. Conf. - Pests Dis.* **1979**, 311. Brief description: H. L. Klopping, C. J. Delp, *J. Agric. Food Chem.* **28**, 467 (1980).

Crystals from acetone, mp 160-161°. Soly in water approx. 1000 ppm. For 80% formulations, LD$_{50}$ orally in male rats: 1425 mg/kg; dermally in male rabbits: >3000 mg/kg. LC$_{50}$ orally in bobwhite quails, mallard ducks: 2847, >10000 ppm. LC$_{50}$ (96 hr) in bluegill sunfish, rainbow trout (ppm): 13.5, 18.7 (Klopping, Delp).

USE: Agricultural fungicide.

2766. Cynarin(e). [30964-13-7] [1*R*-(1α,3α,4α,5β)]-1,3-Bis[[3-(3,4-dihydroxyphenyl)-1-oxo-2-propenyl]oxy]-4,5-dihydroxycyclohexanecarboxylic acid; 1,3-dicaffeoylquinic acid; 1,5-dicaffeylquinic acid; 3,4-dihydroxycinnamic acid 1-carboxy-4,5-dihydroxy-1,3-cyclohexylene ester; caffeic acid 1-carboxy-4,5-dihydroxy-1,3-cyclohexylene ester; 1-carboxy-4,5-dihydroxy-1,3-cyclohexylenebis-(3,4-dihydroxycinnamate); quinic acid 1,5-dicaffeic ester; Cinarine; Listrocol; Plemocil. C$_{25}$H$_{24}$O$_{12}$; mol wt 516.45. C 58.14%, H 4.68%, O 37.18%. Active principle of artichoke, *Cynara scolymus* L., *Compositae:* L. Panizzi, M. L. Scarpati, *Gazz. Chim. Ital.* **84**, 792 (1954). Synthesis of originally proposed structure: L. Panizzi *et al., ibid.* 806; L. Panizzi *et al.,* **US 2863909**; US

3100224 (1958, 1963 both to Farmitalia); Alberti *et al.,* **US 2918477** (1959). Revised structure: L. Panizzi, M. L. Scarpati, *Gazz. Chim. Ital.* **95**, 71 (1965). NMR confirmation of structure: I. Horman *et al., J. Agric. Food Chem.* **32**, 538 (1984). HPLC determn in pharmaceutics: A. Bettero, *Boll. Chim. Farm.* **120**, 49 (1981). Inhibition of fatty acid mobilization: P. Dorigo, G. Fassina, *Pharmacol. Res. Commun.* **2**, 109 (1970). Reduction of cholesterol levels in rats: J. Wojcicki, *Drug Alcohol Depend.* **3**, 143 (1978). Clinical trial in hyperlipemic syndrome: M. Montini *et al., Arzneim.-Forsch.* **25**, 1311 (1975).

Crystals from dil acetic acid. Sweet taste. mp 225-227°. $[α]_D^{25}$ −59° (c = 2 in methanol). uv max (methanol): 326 nm (E$_{1cm}^{1\%}$ 616). Sparingly sol in cold, more in boiling water; sol in glacial acetic acid, alcohols.

THERAP CAT: Choleretic.

2767. Cypermethrin. [52315-07-8] 3-(2,2-Dichloroethenyl)-2,2-dimethylcyclopropanecarboxylic acid cyano(3-phenoxyphenyl)methyl ester; (±)-α-cyano-3-phenoxybenzyl-(±)-*cis,trans*-3-(2,2-dichlorovinyl)-2,2-dimethylcyclopropane carboxylate; NRDC-149; FMC-30980; PP-383; Ammo; Arrivo; Barricade; Basathrin; Cymbush; Cynoff; Demon; Flectron; Ripcord. C$_{22}$H$_{19}$Cl$_2$NO$_3$; mol wt 416.30. C 63.47%, H 4.60%, Cl 17.03%, N 3.36%, O 11.53%. Synthetic pyrethroid insecticide, usually exists as a mixture of cis and trans isomers. Prepn of racemic mixture: M. Elliot *et al.,* **DE 2326077**; *eidem,* **US 4024163** (1974, 1977 to NRDC). Activity: *eidem, Pestic. Sci.* **6**, 537 (1975); M. H. Breese, *ibid.* **8**, 264 (1977). Soil degradation: T. R. Roberts, M. E. Standen, *ibid.* 305; D. D. Kaufman *et al., J. Agric. Food Chem.* **29**, 239 (1981). Metabolism: T. Shono *et al., ibid.* **27**, 316 (1979); M. J. Crawford *et al., ibid.* **29**, 130 (1981). Analysis: A. Sapiets *et al., Anal. Methods Pestic. Plant Growth Regul.* **13**, 33-51 (1984). Repellent activity against flies on cattle: J. A. Shemanchuk, *Pestic. Sci.* **12**, 412 (1981); J. E. Hillerton *et al., Br. Vet. J.* **141**, 160 (1985). Acute toxicity study: F. Cantalamessa, *Arch. Toxicol.* **67**, 510 (1993). Review of toxicology and human exposure: *Toxicological Profile for Pyrethrins and Pyrethroids* (PB2004-100004, 2003) 332 pp.

Commercial product is a mixture of eight isomers. Viscous semisolid, mp 60-80°. Insol in water. Sol in methanol, acetone, xylene, methylene dichloride. LD$_{50}$ in 8 day old rats, adult male rats (mg/kg): 14.9, 250.0 orally (Cantalamessa).

USE: Insecticide.

THERAP CAT (VET): Ectoparasiticide.

2768. Cyphenothrin. [39515-40-7] 2,2-Dimethyl-3-(2-methyl-1-propenyl)cyclopropanecarboxylic acid cyano(3-phenoxyphenyl)methyl ester; (*RS*)-α-cyano-3-phenoxybenzyl (1*R*)-*cis,trans*-chrysanthemate; α-cyano-*m*-phenoxybenzyl 2,2-dimethyl-3-(2-methylpropenyl)cyclopropanecarboxylate; 3-phenoxy-α-cyanobenzylchrysanthemate; S-2703; S-2703 Forte; Gokilaht. C$_{24}$H$_{25}$-

NO_3; mol wt 375.46. C 76.77%, H 6.71%, N 3.73%, O 12.78%. Synthetic pyrethroid. Prepn: T. Matsuo *et al.*, **DE 2231312**; *eidem*, **US 3835176** (1973, 1974 to Sumitomo). Insecticidal activity: M. Elliot *et al.*, *Pestic. Sci.* **13**, 407 (1982); T. Matsunaga *et al.*, *Pesticide Chemistry: Human Welfare and the Environment* **2**, Miyamoto *et al.*, Eds (Pergamon Press, Oxford, 1983) pp 231-238; T. Itoh *et al.*, *J. Am. Mosq. Control Assoc.* **2**, 503 (1986). Mechanism of action: T. Narahashi, *Neurobehav. Toxicol. Teratol.* **4**, 753 (1982). Series of articles on stereoselective syntheses of labelled *cis* and *trans* forms: H. Kanamaru *et al.*, *Radioisotopes* **35**, 103, 109, 242 (1986).

Yellowish viscous liquid. d_{25}^{25} 1.083. Vapor pressure at 30°: 3.11×10^{-6} mm Hg. Viscosity at 30°: 808.8 cP.

Note: Commercial product is a mixture (35:65) of *cis* and *trans* forms.

USE: Insecticide.

2769. Cyprenorphine. [4406-22-8] (5α,7α)-17-(Cyclopropylmethyl)-4,5-epoxy-3-hydroxy-6-methoxy-α,α-dimethyl-6,14-ethenomorphinan-7-methanol; *N*-(cyclopropylmethyl)-7,8-dihydro-7α-(1-hydroxy-1-methylethyl)-*O*⁶-methyl-6,14-*endo*-ethenonormorphine; *N*-(cyclopropylmethyl)-6,14-*endo*-etheno-7α-(2-hydroxy-2-propyl)tetrahydronororipavine; *N*-(cyclopropylmethyl)-6,14-*endo*-ethenotetrahydronororipavine. $C_{26}H_{33}NO_4$; mol wt 423.54. C 73.73%, H 7.85%, N 3.31%, O 15.11%. Narcotic antagonist closely related to diprenorphine, *q.v.* Prepn (7α- or 7β-linkage unspecified): **BE 629070** (1963 to J. F. Macfarlan), *C.A.* **61**, 13364g (1964); K. W. Bentley, **US 3474101** (1969 to Reckitt & Sons); of 7α: K. W. Bentley, D. G. Hardy, *J. Am. Chem. Soc.* **89**, 3281 (1967). Activity in rats: K. W. Bentley *et al.*, *Nature* **206**, 102 (1965). Use in large animals: M. R. Jainudeen, *Vet. Rec.* **89**, 686 (1971); K. R. Presnell *et al.*, *J. Wildl. Dis.* **9**, 336 (1973). Binding to neuroleptic receptors: A. Czlonkowski *et al.*, *Life Sci.* **22**, 953 (1978). Determn by HPLC: I. Jane, A. McKinnon, *J. Chromatogr.* **323**, 191 (1985).

Prisms from methanol, mp 234° (7α- or 7β-linkage unspecified).

Hydrochloride. [16550-22-4] M-285. $C_{26}H_{33}NO_4 \cdot HCl$. Crystals from methanol, mp 248°.

Note: This is a controlled substance (opium derivative): **21 CFR**, 1308.11.

THERAP CAT (VET): Etorphine antagonist.

2770. Cypripedium. Lady's slipper; American valerian; nerve root; yellow moccasin flower; Noah's ark. Dried rhizome and roots of *Calypso bulbosa* (L.) Oakes (*Cypripedium bulbosum* L.), *Cypripedium pubescens* Willd., or of *Cypripedium parviflorum* Salisb., *Orchidaceae*. *Habit.* Nova Scotia south to Alabama, west to Nebraska and Missouri. *Constit.* Volatile oil, volatile acid, tannin, resins.

THERAP CAT: Sedative.

2771. Cyproconazole. [94361-06-5] α-(4-Chlorophenyl)-α-(1-cyclopropylethyl)-1*H*-1,2,4-triazole-1-ethanol; (2*RS*,3*RS*)-2-(4-chlorophenyl)-3-cyclopropyl-1-(1*H*-1,2,4-triazol-1-yl)butan-2-ol; SAN-619F; SN-108266; Alto; Atemi; Bonanza; Paindor; Sentinel. $C_{15}H_{18}ClN_3O$; mol wt 291.78. C 61.75%, H 6.22%, Cl 12.15%, N 14.40%, O 5.48%. Broad spectrum triazole antifungal; sterol demethylase inhibitor. Prepn: F. Schaub, **DE 3406993**; *idem*, **US 4664696** (1984, 1987 both to Sandoz). Mode of action: M. S. Fuller *et al.*, *Pestic. Biochem. Physiol.* **36**, 115 (1990). Synergism with herbicides: H. R. Kataria, U. Gisi, *Crop Prot.* **9**, 403 (1990). Field trials in winter wheat: J. P. Devey *et al.*, *Brighton Crop Prot. Conf. - Pests Dis.* **1990**, 801; in cereals in combination with prochloraz, *q.v.*: R. I. Harris *et al.*, *ibid.* 813. *Review:* U. Gisi *et al.*, *Proc. Br. Crop Prot. Conf. - Pests Dis.* **1986**, 33-40.

Colorless crystals from hexane/CH_2Cl_2, mp 103-105°. Soly at 25° (%w/w): water 0.0140 ±0.0004; acetone >23; ethanol >23; xylene 12; DMSO >18. Vapor pressure at 20°: 2.6×10^{-7} torr. LD_{50} in male and female rats (mg/kg): 1020, 1330 orally; in rats: 2000 dermally. LD_{50} in carp: 18.9 mg/l; in trout 7.2 mg/l; in bluegill sunfish 6.0 mg/l in water. LD_{50} in bobwhite quail (mg/kg): 150 orally; LD_{50} (8 day dietary) in bobwhite quail, mallard duck: 816, 1197 mg/kg (Gisi, 1986).

Combination with prochloraz. Sportak Delta; Tiptor; Epicure.

USE: Agricultural fungicide.

2772. Cyprodinil. [121552-61-2] 4-Cyclopropyl-6-methyl-*N*-phenyl-2-pyrimidinamine; *N*-(4-cyclopropyl-6-methylpyrimidin-2-yl)aniline; 2-phenylamino-4-methyl-6-cyclopropylpyrimidine; CGA-219417; Chorus; Unix; Vangard. $C_{14}H_{15}N_3$; mol wt 225.29. C 74.64%, H 6.71%, N 18.65%. Methionine biosynthesis inhibitor. Prepn: A. Hubele, **EP 310550**; *idem*, **US 5153200** (1989, 1992 both to Ciba-Geigy). Comprehensive description: U. J. Heye *et al.*, *Crop Prot.* **13**, 541-549 (1994). Mechanism of action: P. Masner *et al.*, *Pestic. Sci.* **42**, 163 (1994). Review of field trials: N. J. Leadbitter *et al.*, *Br. Crop Prot. Counc. Monogr.* **57**, 73-78 (1994).

White crystalline solid, mp 75.9°. vapor pressure (25°): 5.1×10^{-4} Pa (crystal modif. A); 4.7×10^{-4} Pa (crystal modif. B). Log P (*n*-octanol/water): 3.9 (pH 5.0); 4.0 (pH 7.0); 4.0 (pH 9.0). Soly in water at 25° (mg/l): 20 (pH 5.0); 13 (pH 7.0); 15 (pH 9.0). LD_{50} orally or dermally in rats: >2000 mg/kg (Heye).

USE: Agricultural fungicide.

2773. Cyproheptadine. [129-03-3] 4-(5*H*-Dibenzo[*a,d*]-cyclohepten-5-ylidene)-1-methylpiperidine; 1-methyl-4-(5*H*-dibenzo[*a,d*]cycloheptenylidene)piperidine; 5-(1-methylpiperidyl-idene)-4-5*H*-dibenzo[*a,d*]cycloheptene; 1-methyl-4-(5-dibenzo-[*a,e*]cycloheptatrienylidene)piperidine; Periactinol. $C_{21}H_{21}N$; mol wt 287.40. C 87.76%, H 7.36%, N 4.87%. Prepn: Engelhardt, **US 3014911** (1961 to Merck & Co.); Engelhardt *et al.*, *J. Med. Chem.* **8**, 829 (1965). Metabolism: C. C. Porter *et al.*, *Drug Metab. Dispos.* **3**, 189 (1975). Toxicity study: J. J. Loux *et al.*, *Arzneim.-Forsch.* **28**, 1644 (1978). Comprehensive description: H. Y. Aboul-Enein, A. A. Al-Badr, *Anal. Profiles Drug Subs.* **9**, 155-179 (1980).

Crystals from dil ethanol, mp 112.3-113.3°.

Hydrochloride sesquihydrate. [41354-29-4] Antegan; Ifrasarl; Nuran; Periactin; Vimicon; Cipractin; Peritol. $C_{21}H_{22}$-$ClN.1\frac{1}{2}H_2O$; mol wt 332.87. Crystals from abs ethanol + ether, dec 252.6-253.6°. uv max $(0.1N\ H_2SO_4)$: 224, 285 nm $(E_{1cm}^{1\%}$ 1656, 355). 1.0 g is sol in 1.5 ml methanol, 16 ml chloroform, 35 ml alc, 275 ml H_2O. Practically insol in ether. LD_{50} orally in mice: 74.2 mg/kg (Loux).

Hydrochloride monohydrate. [6032-06-0] Crystals, mp 214-216°. Soly in water: ~5 mg/ml.

THERAP CAT: Antihistaminic; antipruritic.

2774. Cyproterone. [2098-66-0] $(1\beta,2\beta)$-6-Chloro-1,2-dihydro-17-hydroxy-3'H-cyclopropa[1,2]pregna-1,4,6-triene-3,20-dione; 6-chloro-17-hydroxy-1α,2α-methylenepregna-4,6-diene-3,20-dione; 6-chloro-6-dehydro-17α-hydroxy-1,2α-methyleneprogesterone; 6-chloro-1,2α-methylene-4,6-pregnadien-17α-ol-3,20-dione; SH-881; SH-80881. $C_{22}H_{27}ClO_3$; mol wt 374.90. C 70.48%, H 7.26%, Cl 9.46%, O 12.80%. Prepn of free alcohol: Wiechert, Neumann, **DE 1189991** *C.A.* **63,** 1842e (1965); Wiechert, US **3234093** (1965, 1966 both to Schering AG). Biodynamics in man: Gerhards *et al., Arzneim.-Forsch.* **23,** 1550 (1973). The free alcohol is an anti-androgen; the acetate is both an anti-androgen and a progestogen. Effect on hormone secretion and on spermatogenesis in man: L. Moltz *et al., Contraception* **21,** 393 (1980). Review of pharmacology and clinical studies (acetate) on acne and hirsutism in women: J. Hammerstein *et al., J. Steroid Biochem.* **19,** 591 (1983).

Crystals from ethyl acetate, mp 237.5-240°.

Acetate. [427-51-0] CPA; SH-714; Androcur; Cyprostat. C_{24}-$H_{29}ClO_4$; mol wt 416.94. Crystals from diisopropyl ether, mp 200-201°. uv max (methanol): 281 nm (ε 17280).

Mixture of acetate with ethinyl estradiol. Diane 35; Dianette.

THERAP CAT: The acetate as antiandrogen; combination with estrogen in treatment of acne.

2775. Cyromazine. [66215-27-8] N-Cyclopropyl-1,3,5-triazine-2,4,6-triamine; 2-cyclopropylamino-4,6-diamino-s-triazine; CGA-72662; Larvadex; Neporex; Trigard; Vetrazin. $C_6H_{10}N_6$; mol wt 166.18. C 43.37%, H 6.07%, N 50.57%. Insect growth regulator. Prepn: H. U. Brechbuhler *et al.,* **DE 2736876**; *eidem,* US **4225598** (1978, 1980 to Ciba-Geigy). Activity: R. D. Hall, M. C. Foehse, *J. Econ. Entomol.* **73,** 564 (1980); R. J. Hart *et al., Aust. Vet. J.* **59,** 104 (1982).

Crystals, mp 219-222°.

USE: Insecticide.

THERAP CAT (VET): Ectoparasiticide.

2776. Cystamine. [51-85-2] 2,2'-Dithiobisethanamine; 2,2'-dithiobis[ethylamine]; β,β'-diaminodiethyl disulfide; bis[β-aminoethyl]disulfide; decarboxycystine. $C_4H_{12}N_2S_2$; mol wt 152.28. C 31.55%, H 7.94%, N 18.40%, S 42.11%. $(H_2NCH_2$-$CH_2)_2S_2$. Forms when cystine is distilled: Neuberg, Ascher, *Chem. Zentralbl.* **1907,** II, 1156. Prepd by H_2O_2 oxidation of H_2-NCH_2CH_2SH: Mills, Jr., Bogert, *J. Am. Chem. Soc.* **62,** 1173 (1940); Barnett, *J. Chem. Soc.* **1944,** 5.

Viscous oil. Cannot be distilled without decompn (even in high vacuum). Freely sol in water. Sol in alc.

Dihydrochloride. $C_4H_{12}N_2S_2.2HCl$. Needles from methanol, dec 203-214°. Sol in water.

2777. L-Cystathionine. [56-88-2] S-[(2R)-2-Amino-2-carboxyethyl]-L-homocysteine; L-2-amino-4-[(2-amino-2-carboxyethyl)thio]butyric acid. $C_7H_{14}N_2O_4S$; mol wt 222.26. C 37.83%, H 6.35%, N 12.60%, O 28.79%, S 14.43%. An amino acid whose homocysteine and serine moieties are both L in configuration. Intermediate in transsulfuration whereby the mammal transfers the sulfur of methionine via homocysteine to cysteine: Hope, *Proc. 4th Int. Congr. Biochem.* **13,** 63 (1960). Preparation: du Vigneaud *et al., J. Biol. Chem.* **143,** 59 (1942); Weiss, Stekol, *J. Am. Chem. Soc.* **73,** 2497 (1951); Schöberl, Täuber, *Ann.* **599,** 23 (1956). Isolation from human brain: Tallau *et al., J. Biol. Chem.* **230,** 707 (1958). Abs config: G. Jung *et al., Eur. J. Biochem.* **35,** 436 (1973); C.-S. Chen *et al., Biochim. Biophys. Acta* **538,** 534 (1978). *Review:* J. P. Greenstein, M. Winitz, *Chemistry of the Amino Acids* vol. 3 (John Wiley, N. Y., 1961) p 2682.

Crystals (rectangular parallelepipeds), dec 312° (darkening at 270°). $[\alpha]_D^{20}$ +23.7° (1N HCl).

2778. Cystatins. Protein superfamily of endogenous cysteine proteinase inhibitors. All inhibit papain-type peptidases, including serveral cathepsins. Widely distributed in animals, plants, and protozoa; at least 12 cystatins have been identified in humans. Type 1 (cystatins A and B), also known as *stefins*, are intracellular, single-chain peptides of ~100 residues with no disulfide bonds or carbohydrate. Type 2, comprising the largest group, are extracellular, secreted proteins, typically 120-125 residues with 2 disulfide bonds; broadly distributed and found in most body fluids. Type 3, known as kininogens, *q.v.,* are intravascular, multi-functional, glycosylated proteins of mol wt 60-120 kDa that also serve as kinin precursors. Discovery of a papain inhibitor in chicken egg white: K. Fossum, J. R. Whitaker, *Arch. Biochem. Biophys.* **125,** 367 (1968). Sequence homologies and evolutionary relationship: W. Müller-Esterl *et al., FEBS Lett.* **191,** 221 (1985). Review of physiological role in malignant progression and prognosis: J. Kos, T. T. Lah, *Oncol. Rep.* **5,** 1349-1361 (1998). *Reviews:* A. J. Barrett, *Biomed. Biochim. Acta* **45,** 1363-1374 (1986); M. Abrahamson *et al., Biochem. Soc. Symp.* **70,** 179-199 (2003).

Cystatin A. [107544-29-6] Stefin A; CPI-A; acidic cysteine proteinase inhibitor. Found primarily in epithelial cells and polymorphonuclear leukocytes; also occurs in amniotic fluid and tears. Purification from human epidermis: M. Järvinen, *J. Invest. Dermatol.* **72,** 114 (1978); from human granulocytes: J. Brzin *et al., Z. Phys. Chem.* **364,** 1475 (1983). Mature human form is a single chain, non-glycosylated peptide containing 98 amino acid residues; mol wt 11.0 kDa. Isoelectric point: 4.5-4.7.

Cystatin B. [99194-04-4] Stefin B; CPI-B; NCPI; neutral cysteine proteinase inhibitor. Broadly distributed in human cells and tissues; general cytosolic inhibitor to protect against leakage of lysosomal enzymes. Mutations in the cystatin B gene have been associated with progressive myoclonus epilepsy. Isoln from human spleen: M. Järvinen, A. Rinne, *Biochim. Biophys. Acta* **708**, 210 (1982); from human liver: G. D. J. Green *et al., Biochem. J.* **218**, 939 (1984). Review of role in Unverricht-Lundborg disease: A.-E. Lehesjoki, *EMBO J.* **22**, 3473-3478 (2003). Mature human form is a single chain, non-glycosylated peptide containing 98 amino acid residues; mol wt 11.2 kDa. Isoelectric point: 5.6-6.3.

Cystatin C. [91448-99-6] Post-γ-globulin; γ-CSF; γ-trace. Found ubiquitously in vertebrates; major extracellular cysteine peptidase inhibitor in mammals. Isoln from human CSF: J. Clausen, *Proc. Soc. Exp. Biol. Med.* **107**, 170 (1961); from urine of patients with renal dysfunction: E. A. Butler, F. V. Flynn, *J. Clin. Pathol.* **14**, 172 (1961). Identification as a cystatin: A. J. Barrett *et al., Biochem. Biophys. Res. Commun.* **120**, 631 (1984). Review of biochemistry and clinical role: M. Mussap, M. Plebani, *Crit. Rev. Clin. Lab. Sci.* **41**, 467-550 (2004); of efficacy as biomarker for glomerular filtration rate: G. Filler *et al., Clin. Biochem.* **38**, 1-8 (2005). Clinical evaluation to predict risk of cardiovascular events in elderly patients: M. G. Shlipak *et al., N. Engl. J. Med.* **352**, 2049 (2005). Mature human form is a single chain, non-glycosylated peptide containing 120 amino acid residues; mol wt 13.3 kDa. Isoelectric point: 9.3. Electrophoretic mobility: γ_3 (agarose gel electrophoresis at pH 8.6). $E_{1cm}^{1\%}$ 9.1 (280 nm). Conc in plasma of healthy adults: 0.8 to 1.2 mg/l.

THERAP CAT: Cystatin C as diagnostic aid (renal function).

2779. Cysteamine. [60-23-1] 2-Aminoethanethiol; mercaptamine; β-mercaptoethylamine; 2-aminoethyl mercaptan; thioethanolamine; decarboxycysteine; MEA; mercamine; L-1573; Becaptan; Lambratene (formerly). C_2H_7NS; mol wt 77.15. C 31.14%, H 9.15%, N 18.16%, S 41.56%. $HSCH_2CH_2NH_2$. A sulfhydryl compound with a variety of biological effects. Prepn: Gabriel, Leupold, *Ber.* **31**, 2837 (1898); Knorr, Rössler, *ibid.* **36**, 1281 (1903); Mills, Jr., Bogart, *J. Am. Chem. Soc.* **62**, 1173 (1940); Wenker, *ibid.* **57**, 2328 (1935); D. A. Shirley, *Preparation of Organic Intermediates* (Wiley, New York, 1951) p 189. Use in treatment of paracetamol (acetaminophen) poisoning: L. F. Prescott *et al., Lancet* **2**, 109 (1976); A. L. Harris, *Br. Med. J.* **284**, 825 (1982). Effects in nephropathic cystinosis: M. Yudkoff *et al., N. Engl. J. Med.* **304**, 141 (1981). Radioprotective effects: R. P. Bird, *Radiat. Res.* **72**, 290 (1980); C. J. Koch, R. L. Howell, *ibid.* **87**, 265 (1981). Cysteamine has been shown to be a duodenal ulcerogen in rats: H. Selye', S. Szabo, *Nature* **244**, 458 (1973); S. Szabo, *Am. J. Pathol.* **93**, 273 (1978); P. Kirkegaard *et al., Scand. J. Gastroenterol.* **15**, 621 (1980). *Review:* S. Szabo, *Lab. Invest.* **51**, 121 (1984). It has also been found to deplete somatostatin concentration: S. Szabo, S. Reichlein, *Endocrinology* **109**, 2255 (1981); S. M. Sagar *et al., J. Neurosci.* **2**, 225 (1982). In pituitary tissue, cysteamine is a potent depletor of prolactin concentrations *in vivo* and *in vitro*: W. J. Millard *et al., Science* **217**, 452 (1982). Toxicity studies: E. Beccari *et al., Arzneim.-Forsch.* **5**, 421 (1955); D. L. Klayman *et al., J. Med. Chem.* **12**, 510 (1969); P. K. Srivastava, L. Field, *ibid.* **18**, 798 (1975).

Crystals by sublimation *in vacuo*. Disagreeable odor. mp 97-98.5°. Oxidizes to cystamine on standing in air. Freely sol in water, alkaline reaction. LD_{50} in mice (mg/kg): 625 orally; 250 i.p. (Klayman); (Srivastava, Field).

Hydrochloride. $C_2H_7NS.HCl$. Crystals from alc, mp 70.2-70.7°. Sol in water, alcohol. LD_{50} (cg/kg): 23.19 i.p. in rats; 14.95 i.v. in rabbits (Beccari).

USE: Experimentally as a radioprotective agent and to produce acute and chronic duodenal ulcers in rats.

THERAP CAT: Antidote to acetaminophen.

2780. Cysteic Acid. [13100-82-8] 3-Sulfoalanine; α-amino-β-sulfopropionic acid. $C_3H_7NO_5S$; mol wt 169.16. C 21.30%, H 4.17%, N 8.28%, O 47.29%, S 18.96%. $HOOCCH(NH_2)CH_2$-SO_3H. Has been isolated from human hair oxidized with permanganate: Lissizin, *Z. Physiol. Chem.* **173**, 309 (1928). Occurs normally in the outer part of the sheep's fleece, where the wool is exposed to light and weather: Martin, Synge, *Adv. Protein Chem.* **2**,

3 (1945). Prepd from cystine or cysteine by oxidation with bromine in water: Friedmann, *Beitr. Chem. Physiol. Pathol.* **3**, 25, 38; Gortner, Hoffman, *J. Biol. Chem.* **72**, 435 (1927).

L-Form. Octahedra or needles from dil alc (also forms a monohydrate, prismatic needles). When anhydr, dec 260°. $[\alpha]_D^{20}$ +8.66° (1.85 g in 25 ml). pKa_1 (25°): 1.89; pKa_2 8.7; pKb about 12.7. Soluble in water. Insol in alcohol.

DL-Form. Crystals, dec 245°.

2781. Cysteine. [52-90-4] L-Cysteine; Cys; C; β-mercapto-alanine; (R)-2-amino-3-mercaptopropanoic acid; 2-amino-3-mercaptopropionic acid; α-amino-β-thiolpropionic acid; half-cystine; thioserine. $C_3H_7NO_2S$; mol wt 121.16. C 29.74%, H 5.82%, N 11.56%, O 26.41%, S 26.47%. A non-essential amino acid in human development. Readily oxides to form a dimeric amino acid, cystine, *q.v.*, in which the two Cys are linked via a disulfide bridge, a common structural feature in proteins. Early chemistry and biochemistry: *Amino Acids and Proteins*, D. M. Greenberg, Ed. (Charles C. Thomas, Springfield, IL, 1951) 950 pp., *passim*; J. P. Greenstein, M. Winitz, *Chemistry of the Amino Acids* vol 1-3 (John Wiley and Sons, Inc., New York, 1961) pp. 1879-1928, *passim*. Simple synthesis of racemic cysteine: V. J. Martens *et al., Angew. Chem. Int. Ed.* **20**, 668 (1981). Determn in proteins: J. G. Hoogerheide, C. M. Campbell, *Anal. Biochem.* **201**, 146 (1992); D. Atherton *et al., ibid.* **212**, 98 (1993). Review of biosynthesis: N. M. Kredich *et al., Ciba Found. Symp.* (Netherlands) **72**, 87-99 (1980). Review of transport in mammalian cells: S. Bannai, *Biochim. Biophys. Acta* **779**, 289-306 (1984). Review of effects on acrylonitrile toxicity: D. E. Nerland *et al., Drug Metab. Rev.* **20**, 233-246 (1989). Review of thermodynamics and kinetics: T. R. Ralph *et al., J. Electroanal. Chem.* **375**, 1-15 (1994); of electrosynthesis: *eidem, ibid.* 17-27. Review of role in chemo- and radio-protectant strategies: J. C. Roberts, *Amino Acids* **8**, 113-124 (1995).

Crystals. $[\alpha]_D^{25}$ +6.5° (5N HCl); $[\alpha]_D^{25}$ +13.0° (glacial acetic acid). pK_1 1.71; pK_2 8.33; pK_3 10.78. Absorption spectrum: Abderhalden, Rossner, *Z. Physiol. Chem.* **178**, 160 (1928). Freely sol in water, alcohol, acetic acid, ammonia water. Insol in ether, acetone, ethyl acetate, benzene, carbon disulfide, carbon tetrachloride. In neutral or slightly alkaline aq solns it is oxidized to cystine by air. More stable in acidic solns.

Hydrochloride. [52-89-1] $C_3H_7NO_2S.HCl$. Crystals, dec 175-178°. $[\alpha]_D^{25}$ +5.0° (5N HCl); $[\alpha]_D^{25}$ +10.0° (glacial acetic acid). Sol in water, alcohol, acetone; the aq soln is acid. *Keep tightly closed.* Decomposes and oxidizes slowly; hygroscopic.

USE: As dough conditioner.

THERAP CAT (VET): Has been used as a detoxicant.

2782. Cystine. [56-89-3] L-Cystine; [R-(R*,R*)]-3,3'-dithiobis[2-aminopropanoic acid]; dicysteine; β,β'-dithiodialanine; α-diamino-β-dithiolactic acid; β,β'-diamino-β,β'-dicarboxydiethyl disulfide; bis(β-amino-β-carboxyethyl) disulfide; Gelucystine. $C_6H_{12}N_2O_4S_2$; mol wt 240.30. C 29.99%, H 5.03%, N 11.66%, O 26.63%, S 26.69%. Non-essential amino acid for human development. Formed by the dimerization of two cysteines, *q.v.* through the sulfur. These disulfide bridges occur both within and between polypeptides; often found in extracellular proteins. First amino acid described in 1810 by Wollaston. Isoln from horn hydrolysate: K. A. H. Mörner, *Z. Physiol. Chem.* **28**, 595 (1899). Early chemistry and biochemistry: *Amino Acids and Proteins*, D. M. Greenberg, Ed. (Charles C. Thomas, Springfield, IL, 1951) 950 pp. *passim*; J. P. Greenstein, M. Winitz, *Chemistry of the Amino Acids* **vols 1-3** (John Wiley and Sons, Inc., New York, 1961) pp. 1879-1928, *passim*. Distribution in protein: R. C. Fahey *et al., J. Mol. Evol.* **10**, 155 (1977). Review of lysosomal transport including pathophysiology: W. Gahl in *Pathophysiol. Lysosomal Transp.*, J. G. Thoene, Ed. (CRC Press, Boca Raton, FL, 1992) pp 45-71. Review of thermodynamics and kinetics: T. R. Ralph *et al., J. Electroanal. Chem.* **375**, 1-15 (1994); of electrosynthesis: *eidem, ibid.* 17-27.

Hexagonal tablets from water, dec 260-261° (sealed tube). $[\alpha]_D^{20}$ −223.4° (1.0N HCl). pK$_1$ 1; pK$_2$ 2.1; pK$_3$ 8.02; pK$_4$ 8.71 at 35°. Soly in water (g/l) at 25°: 0.112; at 50°: 0.239; at 75°: 0.523; at 100°: 1.142. Quite sol in aq solns below pH 2 or above pH 8. Soly curves: Sano, *Biochem. Z.* **168,** 14 (1926). Insol in alc. Absorption spectrum: Marchlewski, Nowotonowna, *Bull. Soc. Chim. Fr.* [4] **39,** 163, 166 (1926).

D-Form. [349-46-2] Crystals. $[\alpha]_D^{20}$ +223° (1.0N HCl). Soly in water at 25°: 0.057 g/l.

DL-Form. [923-32-0] Crystals. Soly in water at 25°: 0.057 g/l.

***meso*-Form.** [6020-39-9] Crystals. Soly in water: 0.056 g/l.

2783.   L-Cystine *S,S*-Dioxide. [30452-69-8] 2-Amino-2-carboxyethyl 2-amino-2-carboxyethanethiosulfonate; L-cystine thiosulfonate; sacysyl-cysteine. C$_6$H$_{12}$N$_2$O$_6$S$_2$; mol wt 272.30. C 26.47%, H 4.44%, N 10.29%, O 35.25%, S 23.55%. Oxidation product of cystine. Prepn: G. Toennies, T. F. Lavine, *J. Biol. Chem.* **113,** 571 (1936); R. Emilozzi, L. Pichat, *Bull. Soc. Chim. Fr.* **1959,** 1887. Orignally thought to be a mixture of two isomers, cystine *S,S*-dioxide and ***cystine *S,S'*-dioxide***: G. E. Utzinger, *Experientia* **17,** 374 (1961). Elucidaton of structures: G. Axelson *et al., Spectrochim. Acta* **23A,** 2015 (1967); L. D. Setiawan *et al., Surf. Interface Anal.* **7,** 188 (1985). Use in determn of sulfite: T. Ubuka *et al., Anal. Biochem.* **126,** 273 (1982); *idem et al., ibid.* **140,** 449 (1984).

Solid, relatively unstable in aqueous solns; disproportionates to cystine and cysteine sulfinic acid.

USE: In detection of sulfites and thiosulfate.

2784.   Cytarabine. [147-94-4] 4-Amino-1-β-D-arabinofuranosyl-2(1H)-pyrimidinone; 1-β-D-arabinofuranosylcytosine; Ara-C; β-cytosine arabinoside; aracytidine; CHX-3311; U-19920; Alexan; Aracytine; Cytosar; Depocyte; Udicil. C$_9$H$_{13}$N$_3$O$_5$; mol wt 243.22. C 44.44%, H 5.39%, N 17.28%, O 32.89%. Nucleoside analog; converted by cellular kinases into the active metabolite, ***AraCTP.*** Prepn: J. H. Hunter, US 3116282 (1963 to Upjohn); T. Y. Shen *et al., J. Org. Chem.* **30,** 835 (1965). NMR soln structure of Ara-C within a DNA dodecamer: B. I. Schweitzer *et al., Biochemistry* **33,** 11460 (1994). Crystal structure of complex with human topoisomerase I: J. E. Chrencik *et al., J. Biol. Chem.* **278,** 12461 (2003). Clinical pharmacology and toxicology: R. C. Donehower *et al., Cancer Treat. Rep.* **70,** 1059 (1986). Symposium on clinical pharmacology, pharmacokinetics and efficacy in leukemia: *Scand. J. Haematol.* **36,** Suppl. 44, 1-74 (1986). Review of development of a high dose treatment for acute myeloid leukemia: R. L. Capizzi, *Invest. New Drugs* **14,** 249-256 (1996); of cellular metabolism and mechanism of action: S. Grant, *Adv. Cancer Res.* **72,** 197-233 (1998).

Crystals from ethanol, mp 212-213°. $[\alpha]_D^{24}$ +153° (c = 0.5 in water). uv max at pH 2: 281.0, 212.5 nm (ε 13171, 10230); at pH 12: 272.5 nm (ε 9259).

THERAP CAT: Antineoplastic.

2785.   Cythioate. [115-93-5] Phosphorothioic acid O-[4-(aminosulfonyl)phenyl] O,O-dimethyl ester; phosphorothioic acid O,O-dimethyl ester O-ester with p-hydroxybenzenesulfonamide; O,O-dimethyl O-p-sulfamoylphenylphosphorothioate; CL-26691; ENT-25640; Proban. C$_8$H$_{12}$NO$_5$PS$_2$; mol wt 297.29. C 32.32%, H 4.07%, N 4.71%, O 26.91%, P 10.42%, S 21.57%. Prepn: G. Berkelhammer, US 3005004 and R. I. Hewitt, G. Berkelhammer, US 3179560 (1961, 1965 to Am. Cyanamid). Pharmacodynamics: H. G. Smith, R. L. Goulding, *J. Econ. Entomol.* **63,** 1640 (1970). Efficacy as ectoparasiticide: C. P. Doval, I. Gupta, *Indian Vet. J.* **55,** 890 (1978); P. M. Bowen, N. J. Caldwell, *Vet. Med. Small Anim. Clin.* **77,** 79 (1982). Toxicity data: E. E. Kenaga, W. E. Allison, *Bull. Entomol. Soc. Am.* **15,** 85 (1969).

Crystals, mp 70-71°. n_D^{25} 1.5346. LD$_{50}$ orally in rats: 160 mg/kg (Kenaga, Allison).

USE: Insecticide.

THERAP CAT (VET): Ectoparasiticide.

2786.   Cytidine. [65-46-3] 4-Amino-1-β-D-ribofuranosyl-2-(1H)-pyrimidinone; cytosine riboside; 1-β-D-ribofuranosylcytosine. C$_9$H$_{13}$N$_3$O$_5$; mol wt 243.22. C 44.44%, H 5.39%, O 17.28%, O 32.89%. Constituent of nucleic acids. Isoln from yeast nucleic acid: Levene, Jacobs, *Ber.* **43,** 3154 (1910); Levene, La Forge, *ibid.* **45,** 608 (1912). Sepn from other nucleosides by ion-exchange chromatography: Cohn in Chargaff-Davidson, *The Nucleic Acids* **vol. I** (New York, 1955) p 211. Synthesis: Howard *et al., J. Chem. Soc.* **1947,** 1052. Crystal structure: Furberg *et al., Acta Crystallogr.* **18,** 313 (1965). *Review: Basic Principles in Nucleic Acid Chemistry* **vol. 1,** P. O. P. Ts'o, Ed. (Academic Press, New York, 1974) *passim.*

Long needles from 90% ethanol, dec 220-230°. $[\alpha]_D^{25}$ +31° (c = 0.7 in water). Freely sol in water, less sol in alcohol. pK (amino, cationic) 4.22; pK (sugar, anionic) 12.5. uv max (pH 8.2): 271 nm (ε 9100); (pH 2.2): 280 nm (ε 13400), Voet *et al., Biopolymers* **1,** 193 (1963).

Sulfate. (C$_9$H$_{13}$N$_3$O$_5$)$_2$.H$_2$SO$_4$. Long prismatic needles, mp 224-225° (dec with effervescence). $[\alpha]_{589}^{25}$ +34°; $[\alpha]_{546}^{25}$ +43°.

2787.   2'-Cytidylic Acid. [85-94-9] Cytidine-2'-monophosphate; cytidylic acid *a*; 2'-cytidinephosphoric acid; cytidine-2'-phosphate; 2'-cytosylic acid; 2'-CMP. C$_9$H$_{14}$N$_3$O$_8$P; mol wt 323.20. C 33.45%, H 4.37%, N 13.00%, O 39.60%, P 9.58%. Ribonuclease inhibitor. Prepn from yeast ribonucleic acid: Cohn, Carter, *J. Am. Chem. Soc.* **72,** 2606 (1950); Loring *et al., J. Biol. Chem.* **196,** 807 (1952); by phosphorylation of $N^6,O^{3'},O^{5'}$-tribenzoylcytidine: Rammler, Khorana, *J. Am. Chem. Soc.* **84,** 3112 (1962). Crystal structure and conformation of the trihydrate: Kartha *et al., Science* **179,** 495 (1973). *Reviews: See* Cytidine.

Crystals, dec 238-240°. $[\alpha]_D^{20}$ +20.7° (water); $[\alpha]_D^{25}$ −3° (aq NaOH adjusted to pH 10). uv max at pH 2: 278 nm (ε 12.7); at pH 12: 272 nm (ε 8.6). pKa$_1$ 0.8; pKa$_2$ 4.36; pKa$_3$ 6.17. Sparingly sol in water. Less sol than 3′-cytidylic acid.

2788. 3′-Cytidylic Acid. [84-52-6] Cytidine-3′-monophosphate; cytidylic acid b; 3′-cytidinephosphoric acid; cytidine-3′-phosphate; 3′-cytosylic acid; 3′-CMP. $C_9H_{14}N_3O_8P$; mol wt 323.20. C 33.45%, H 4.37%, N 13.00%, O 39.60%, P 9.58%. Ribonuclease inhibitor. Prepn from yeast ribonucleic acid: *see* refs under 2′-Cytidylic Acid. Prepn by pancreatic-ribonuclease-catalyzed ring opening of dicyclohexylguanidinium cytidine 2′,3′-cyclic phosphate: Lohrmann, Khorana, *J. Am. Chem. Soc.* **86**, 4188 (1964). X-ray analysis studies of orthorhombic form: Alver, Furberg, *Acta Chem. Scand.* **13**, 910 (1959); Sundaralingam, Jensen, *J. Mol. Biol.* **13**, 914 (1965); of monoclinic form: Bugg, Marsh, *ibid.* **25**, 67 (1967). *Reviews: See* Cytidine.

Crystals, dec 232-234°. $[\alpha]_D^{20}$ +49.4° (c = 1 in water). $[\alpha]_D^{25}$ +50.0° (c = 1 in aq NaOH adjusted to pH 10). uv max at pH 2: 279 nm (ε 13.0); at pH 12: 272 nm (ε 8.90). pKa$_1$ 0.8; pKa$_2$ 4.28; pKa$_3$ 6.0. Moderately sol in water; more sol than 2′-cytidylic acid.

2789. Cytisine. [485-35-8] *(1R)*-1,2,3,4,5,6-Hexahydro-1,5-methano-8H-pyrido-[1,2-a][1,5]diazocin-8-one; baptitoxine; sophorine; ulexine; Cytiton. $C_{11}H_{14}N_2O$; mol wt 190.24. C 69.45%, H 7.42%, N 14.73%, O 8.41%. Toxic principle in seed of *Laburnum anagyroides* Medik. and other *Leguminosae.* Extraction: Ing, *J. Chem. Soc.* **1931,** 2200; Späth, Galinovsky, *Ber.* **65,** 1526 (1932); **66,** 1338 (1933); Lecoq, *Bull. Soc. Chim. Fr.* **10,** 153 (1943). Structure: Ing, *J. Chem. Soc.* **1932,** 2778. Synthesis: Bohlmann *et al., Angew. Chem.* **67,** 708 (1955); Van Tamelen, Baran, *J. Am. Chem. Soc.* **77,** 4944 (1955). Absolute configuration: Okuda *et al., Chem. Ind. (London)* **1961,** 1751. Pharmacological properties: R. B. Barlow, L. J. McLeod, *Br. J. Pharmacol.* **35,** 161 (1969).

Orthorhombic prisms from acetone, mp 152-153°. Sublimes. bp$_2$ 218°. $[\alpha]_D^{17}$ −120°. pK$_1$ 6.11; pK$_2$ 13.08. Sol in 1.3 parts

water, 13 parts acetone, 1.3 parts methanol, 3.5 parts alcohol, 30 parts benzene, 10 parts ethyl acetate, 2.0 parts chloroform. Practically insol in petr ether. LD$_{50}$ in mice (mg/kg): 1.73 i.v.; 9.4 i.p.; 101 orally (Barlow, McLeod).

Hydrochloride. $C_{11}H_{14}N_2O.HCl.$ Deliquescent crystals, sol in water and alcohol. pH of 0.1 molar aq soln 4.3.

Nitrate monohydrate. $C_{11}H_{14}N_2O.HNO_3.H_2O.$ Needles or leaflets, $[\alpha]_D$ −81.5°. Sol in water, slightly sol in alcohol. Practically insol in ether.

2790. Cytochalasins. A class of mold metabolites exhibiting a number of unusual and varied effects on animal cells. More than twenty cytochalasins are known, isolated from several different mold spp. All are characterized by a highly substituted hydrogenated isoindole ring of known configuration to which is fused a macrocyclic ring. This ring may vary from 11 to 14 atoms in size and may be either a carbocycle or a lactone. Isoln and structure of cytochalasins A, B, C, D: Aldridge *et al., J. Chem. Soc. C* **1967,** 1667; *eidem, Chem. Commun.* **1967,** 26; of E and F: Aldridge *et al., ibid.* **1972,** 148. Revised structures of cytochalasins E and F: Aldridge *et al., ibid.* **1973,** 551; Büchi *et al., J. Am. Chem. Soc.* **95,** 5423 (1973). Isoln of H, also known as *paspaline-P* or *kodo-cytochalasin-1*: G. S. Pendse, *Experientia* **30,** 107 (1974). Structure of H: S. A Patwardhan *et al., Phytochemistry* **13,** 1985 (1974); M. A. Beno *et al., J. Am. Chem. Soc.* **99,** 4123 (1977); x-ray crystal and molecular structure: J. A. McMillan *et al., Chem. Commun.* **1977,** 105. Isoln of K, L, M from *Chalara microspora* and proposed structures: T. Fex, *Tetrahedron Lett.* **22,** 2703 (1981). Isoln of E and K from *Aspergillus clavatus* and proposed alternate structure of K: P. S. Steyn *et al., J. Chem. Soc. Perkin Trans. 1* **1982,** 541. Partial synthesis of A and B: S. Masamune *et al., J. Am. Chem. Soc.* **99,** 6756 (1977). Total synthesis of B: G. Stork *et al., ibid.* **100,** 7775 (1978). Major biological effects are the blockage of cytoplasmic cleavage by blocking formation of contractile microfilament structures, resulting in multinucleate cell formation, the reversible inhibition of cell movement, and the induction of nuclear extrusion: Carter, *Nature* **213,** 261 (1967); Krishan, *J. Cell Biol.* **54,** 657 (1972); E. D. Korn, *Physiol. Rev.* **62,** 703 (1982). Correlation between effects of cytochalasins on cellular structures and cellular events and those on actin *in vitro*: I. Yahara *et al., J. Cell Biol.* **92,** 69 (1982). Other reported effects include the inhibition of glucose transport, of thyroid secretion, of growth hormone release, of phagocytosis, and of platelet aggregation and clot contraction. *See* D. A. Hume *et al., Nature* **272,** 359 (1978). Nomenclature: M. Binder *et al., J. Chem. Soc. Perkin Trans. 1* **1973,** 1146. *Reviews:* M. Binder, C. Tamm, *Angew. Chem. Int. Ed.* **12,** 370 (1973); R. B. Herbert in *The Alkaloids* vol. 7, J. E. Saxton, Ed. (The Chemical Society, London, 1977) pp 29-30; W. G. Thilly *et al., Front. Biol.* **46,** 53-64 (1978); L. V. Domnina *et al., Proc. Natl. Acad. Sci. USA* **79,** 7754-7757 (1982); W. Siess *et al., ibid.* 7709-7713.

Cytochalasin B

Cytochalasin B. [14930-96-2] (7S,13E,16R,20R,21E)-7,20-Dihydroxy-16-methyl-10-phenyl-24-oxo[14]cytochalasa-6(12),13,21-triene-1,23-dione; (E,E)-16-benzyl-6,7,8,9,10,12a,13,14,15,15a,-16,17-dodecahydro-5,13-dihydroxy-9,15-dimethyl-14-methylene-2H-oxacyclotetradec[2,3-d]isoindole-2,18(5H)-dione; phomin. $C_{29}H_{37}NO_5$; mol wt 479.61. The most important and biologically studied of the cytochalasins. Formerly isolated from cultures of a *Phoma* sp. and called phomin: Rothweiler, Tamm, *Experientia* **22,** 750 (1966). Physicochemical data: A. E. Pohland *et al., Pure Appl. Chem.* **54,** 2219 (1982). Felted needles from acetone, mp 218-221°. Completely stable under normal conditions. Solutions in DMSO show no decrease in potency when stored at 4° for three years (Aldrich data sheet). Solubility (mg/ml at 24°): acetone 10.3; ethanol 35.4; DMSO 371; DMF 492. Insol in water.

USE: As tools in cytological research and in characterization of polymerization properties of actin, _q.v._

2791. Cytochrome _c_. [9007-43-6] Myohematin; hematin-protein; Cytorest. Electron transport protein found in the mitochondrial intermembrane space of all eukaryotes. Transfers electrons between complex III and complex IV of the respiratory chain. Synthesized in the cytosol as **apocytochrome _c_**, then transported across the mitochondrial outer membrane. Heme lyase covalently attaches the heme _c_ prosthetic group, a derivative of iron protoporphyrin IX, _q.v._ During apoptosis, cytochrome _c_ is released from the mitochondia and acts as a cofactor for caspase, _q.v._ activation. Human form consists of a single polypeptide chain of 104 amino acid residues with the heme group covalently attached through thioether linkages at cysteine residues 14 and 17. Isoln from muscle tissue: C. A. MacMunn, _Proc. R. Soc. London_ **39**, 248 (1886). Identification and absorption spectra of cellular pigments called cytochromes: D. Keilin, _Proc. R. Soc. London Ser. B_ **98**, 312 (1925). Redox function and isoln from baker's yeast: _idem, ibid._ **106**, 418 (1930). Absorption spectrum: M. Dixon _et al., ibid._ **109**, 29 (1931). Improved prepn from vertebrate and invertebrate sources: E. Margoliash, O. F. Walasek, _Methods Enzymol._ **10**, 339 (1967). Isoln and purification from plant sources: M. Richardson _et al., Phytochemistry_ **9**, 2271 (1970). Oxidation-reduction potentials: F. L. Rodkey, E. G. Ball, _J. Biol. Chem._ **182**, 17 (1950). First crystn from King penguin: G. Bodo, _Nature_ **176**, 829 (1955). Electron transport function in respiration: E. C. Slater, _Adv. Enzymol. Relat. Subj. Biochem._ **20**, 147 (1958). First elucidation of amino acid sequence was horse heart: E. Margoliash _et al., J. Biol. Chem._ **237**, 2148, 2151, 2161 (1962); of human heart: H. Matsubara, E. L. Smith, _ibid._ **238**, 2732 (1963). Crystal structure of horse heart and bonito cytochrome _c_: R. E. Dickerson _et al., J. Biol. Chem._ **246**, 1511 (1971). Structural properties of apo-, iron-free porphyrin, and native cytochrome _c_: W. R. Fisher _et al., J. Biol. Chem._ **248**, 3188 (1973). Discovery and characterization of apoptotic function: X. Liu _et al., Cell_ **86**, 147 (1996); H. Zou _et al., J. Biol. Chem._ **274**, 11549 (1999). Review of role in apoptosis: X. Jiang, X. Wang, _Annu. Rev. Biochem._ **73**, 87-106 (2004). _Reviews:_ R. Lemberg, J. W. Legge, _Hematin Compounds and Bile Pigments_ (Wiley, New York, 1949); E. Margoliash, A. Schejter, _Adv. Protein Chem._ **21**, 113-286 (1966); H. A. Harbury, R. H. L. Marks, in _Inorganic Biochemistry_ vol. 2, G. L. Eichhorn, Ed. (Elsevier, New York, 1973) pp 902-954. _Books: Structure and Function of Cytochromes_, K. Okunuki _et al._, Eds. (University Park Press, Baltimore, 1968) 742 pp; G. W. Pettigrew, G. R. Moore, _Cytochromes c: Biological Aspects_, (Springer-Verlag, Berlin, 1987) 282 pp.; G. R. Moore, G. W. Pettigrew, _Cytochromes c: Evolutionary, Structural and Physicochemical Aspects_, (Springer-Verlag, Berlin, 1990) 478 pp.; _Cytochrome c: A Multidisciplinary Approach_, R. A. Scott, A. G. Mauk, Eds. (University Science, Sausalito, 1996) 738 pp.

Red, basic, water soluble protein. Mol wt about 12500. pI: 10.65 (0°); 10.05 (20°). $E_0' = +0.254$ v (pH 1.75-7.8). Extinction ratio for sequences containing 1 tryptophan: $E_{550 \text{ red}}/E_{280 \text{ ox}} = 1.25$; for sequences containing two tryptophans: $E_{550 \text{ red}}/E_{280 \text{ ox}} = 1.04$-1.06. Reduced form, _Ferrocytochrome c_: absorption max 416, 520, 550 nm (ε_{416} 129.1, ε_{550} 29.5 mM); oxidized form, _Ferricytochrome c_: 279, 360, 410, 530 nm (ε_{410} 106.1 mM). Contains one heme per mole weight of 12,500.

2792. Cytochromes P$_{450}$. P$_{450}$. Hemoproteins involved in enzyme hydroxylation, demethylation, and _N_-oxidation; present in a number of mammalian tissues but in highest concentrations in adrenal and liver microsomes. Has also been found in insects, yeast, plants, and bacteria. Existence of mitochondrial P$_{450}$ first reported by Harding _et al., Biochim. Biophys. Acta_ **92**, 415 (1964). Extraction and purification: Mitani, Horie, _J. Biochem._ **65**, 269 (1969). Acts as a monooxygenase in catalyzing metabolic functions; influences the rate of drug metabolism. Name derived from the characteristic absorption at 450 nm. _Reviews:_ several authors in _Oxidases and Redox Systems_ vol. 2, King _et al._, Eds. (University Park Press, Baltimore, 1971); J. T. Groves, _Advances in Inorganic Biochemistry_ vol. 1, G. L. Eichhorn, L. G. Marzilla, Eds. (Elsevier/North-Holland, New York, 1979) pp 119-145; several authors in

Xenobiotica **12**, 671-800 (1982). _Books: Cytochromes P-450 & B5: Structure, Function & Interaction_, D. Y. Cooper _et al._, Eds. (Plenum, New York, 1975) 554 pp; _Cytochrome P-450_, R. Sato, T. Omura, Eds. (Academic Press, New York, 1978) 233 pp; _Biochemistry, Biophysics and Regulation of Cytochrome P-450_, J. A. Gustafsson _et al._, Eds. (Elsevier/North-Holland, New York, 1980) 626 pp.

2793. Cytohemin. [19554-22-4] (_SP_-5-13)-Chloro[(4_E_,-8_E_)-7-ethenyl-17-formyl-12-(1-hydroxy-5,9,13-trimethyl-4,8,12-tetradecatrienyl)-3,8,13-trimethyl-21_H_,23_H_-porphine-2,18-dipropanoato(4−)-$\kappa N^{21}, \kappa N^{22}, \kappa N^{23}, \kappa N^{24}$]ferrate(2−) dihydrogen; chloro[dihydrogen-3-formyl-8-(1-hydroxy-5,9,13-trimethyltetradecyl)-7,12,17-trimethyl-13-vinyl-2,18-porphinedipropionato(2−)]iron. $C_{49}H_{56}ClFeN_4O_6$; mol wt 888.29. C 66.25%, H 6.35%, Cl 3.99%, Fe 6.29%, N 6.31%, O 10.81%. Isoln from heart muscle: Warburg, Gewitz, _Z. Physiol. Chem._ **288**, 1 (1951); Lemberg, _Biochem. Z._ **338**, 97 (1963). Structure: M. Grassl _et al., ibid._ **337**, 35 (1963); **338**, 771 (1963). Side chain appears to be a mixture of saturated and unsaturated forms: R. Sayffert _et al., 3rd Proc. Colloq. Hemes Hemoproteins, 1966,_ 45-59. Unsaturated form drawn.

Amorphous powder.

2794. Cytolipin H. [4682-48-8] 1-_O_-(4-_O_-β-D-Galactopyranosyl-β-D-glucopyranosyl)ceramide; lactosylceramide; ceramide-β-lactoside; cerebronylsphingosylglucosidogalactoside; Galβ1 → 4Glcβ1 → 1cer. A glycosphingolipid containing lactose and a ceramide (_N_-acyl fatty acid deriv of a sphingosine). Fatty acid composition is variable but is primarily palmitic, behenic and lignoceric acids. First isolated from human epidermoid carcinoma cells, later found to be one of the major neutrophil glycolipids serving as a neutrophil-differentiation marker. Isoln: M. M. Rapport _et al., Cancer_ **12**, 438 (1959). Simplified prepn from ox spleen: M. M. Rapport _et al., J. Biol. Chem._ **237**, 1056 (1962). Structure elucidation: A. C. Schram _et al., Nature_ **197**, 1074 (1963). Synthesis: D. Shapiro, E. S. Rachaman, _ibid._ **201**, 878 (1964); K. C. Nicolaou _et al., J. Am. Chem. Soc._ **110**, 7910 (1988). Serological activity: M. M. Rapport, L. Graf, _Nature_ **201**, 879 (1964); and effect of fatty acid chain length: L. Graf, M. M. Rapport, _Chem. Phys. Lipids_ **13**, 367 (1974). Characterization and distribution of glycolipids in leukemic and nonleukemic blood cells: J. Hildebrand _et al., J. Lipid Res._ **12**, 361 (1971); in neutrophils: B. A. Macher, J. C. Klock, _J. Biol. Chem._ **255**, 2092 (1980). Role as neutrophil cell surface marker: F. W. Symington _et al., J. Immunol._ **134**, 2498 (1985). Intracellular localization: _eidem, J. Biol. Chem._ **262**, 11356 (1987). TLC determn: K. Ogawa _et al., J. Chromatogr._ **426**, 188 (1988). Clinical implications in inflammatory bowel disease: C. R. Stevens _et al., Gut_ **29**, 580 (1988). Review of structure, organization and role of glycolipids in the cell surface membrane: S. Hakomori, _Annu. Rev. Biochem._ **50**, 733-764 (1981).

Coral-like clusters from pyridine + acetone, mp 230-240° with sintering at 180-190°. $[\alpha]_D^{24} - 10.8°$ (c = 2 in pyridine). Practically insol in water, cold methanol, acetone, cold acetic acid, ether, acetonitrile. Soluble in pyridine, chloroform, hot methanol, hot acetic acid. Dissolves readily in chloroform + methanol mixtures of high chloroform content.

2795. Cytosine. [71-30-7] 4-Amino-2(1_H_)-pyrimidinone; 4-amino-2-oxo-1,2-dihydropyrimidine; 4-amino-2-pyrimidinol; 4-amino-2-hydroxypyrimidine. $C_4H_5N_3O$; mol wt 111.10. C 43.24%, H 4.54%, N 37.82%, O 14.40%. Widely distributed in nature; constituent of nucleic acids. Isoln by hydrolysis of thymus nucleic acids: Levene, Bass, *Nucleic Acids* (New York, 1931) p 57. Syntheses: Hilbert, Johnson, *J. Am. Chem. Soc.* **52,** 1152 (1930); Hilbert *et al., ibid.* **57,** 552 (1935); *cf.* Hunter, Hlynka, *Biochem. J.* **31,** 486 (1937); Ballweg, *Tetrahedron Lett.* **1968,** 2171; David, Lubineau, *Bull. Soc. Chim. Fr.* **1969,** 816. Synthesis from carbon dioxide and ammonia on kaolinite: G. R. Harvey *et al., Naturwissenschaften* **58,** 624 (1971). Exists in keto form. Structure: Barker, Marsh, *Acta Crystallogr.* **17,** 1581 (1964); of monohydrate: Jeffrey, Kinoshita, *ibid.* **16,** 20 (1963); R. J. McClure, B. M. Craven, *ibid.* **B29,** 1234 (1973). Tautomerism: Y. P. Wong, *J. Am. Chem. Soc.* **95,** 3511 (1973). *Review:* Ts'o, "Bases, Nucleosides and Nucleotides" in *Basic Principles in Nucleic Acid Chemistry* **vol. 1,** P. O. P. Ts'o, Ed. (Academic Press, New York, 1974) pp 453-584.

Monohydrate. Lustrous monoclinic or triclinic platelets from water. Anhydr at 100°; brown around 300°; dec 320-325°. uv max (pH 8.8): 196.5, 267 nm ($\varepsilon \times 10^{-3}$ 22.5, 6.1). pK_1 4.60; pK_2 12.16. One gram dissolves in 130 ml water. Slightly sol in alcohol, insol in ether. Gives red color when dissolved in soln of sodium hypochlorite to which a drop of NH_4OH is added. Forms salts with acids.

D

2796. 2,4-D. [94-75-7] (2,4-Dichlorophenoxy)acetic acid; Trinoxol. $C_8H_6Cl_2O_3$; mol wt 221.04. C 43.47%, H 2.74%, Cl 32.08%, O 21.71%. Prepd from 2,4-dichlorophenol and monochloroacetic acid in aq NaOH: Pokorny, *J. Am. Chem. Soc.* **63**, 1768 (1941); Foster, **GB 573476** (1945); by chlorination of molten phenoxyacetic acid: Manske, **US 2471575** (1949 to U.S. Rubber); from 2,4-dichlorophenol, sodium, and ethyl chloroacetate followed by hydrolysis of the ester: Haskelberg, *J. Org. Chem.* **12**, 426 (1947). Toxicology: V. K. Rowe, T. A. Hymas, *Am. J. Vet. Res.* **15**, 622 (1954); J. M. Way, *Residue Rev.* **26**, 37 (1969).

Crystals from benzene, mp 138°. $bp_{0.4}$ 160°. Almost insol in water. Sol in organic solvents. LD_{50} in mice, rats (mg/kg): 368, 375 orally (Rowe, Hymas).

Sodium salt. $C_8H_5Cl_2NaO_3$. Needles from alc, dec 215°. Soly in water: 3.5%.

Isopropyl ester. Esteron 44. $C_{11}H_{12}Cl_2O_3$; mol wt 263.12. Liquid, d_{25}^{25} 1.255-1.270. Solidifies at +5°. Sol in oil.

Butyl ester. Lironox; Weedone. $C_{12}H_{14}Cl_2O_3$; mol wt 277.14. Prepn: Nagel, **DE 1144288** (1963 to Bayer), *C.A.* **59**, 6315e (1963).

Amine salts. Sol in water. The following amines form useful salts: Dimethylamine, isopropylamine, triethylamine, diethanolamine, triethanolamine. These salts are much more sol than the sodium salt. A small amount of sequestering agent, such as ethylenediaminetetraacetic acid, is generally added to prevent complex formation in hard water.

Note: The name Hedonal was formerly a synonym for carbamic acid 1-methylbutyl ester.

Caution: Potential symptoms of overexposure to 2,4-D are weakness, stupor, hyporeflexia and muscle twitch; convulsions; dermatitis. *See NIOSH Pocket Guide to Chemical Hazards* (DHHS/NIOSH 97-140, 1997) p 88.

USE: Herbicide. To increase latex output of old rubber trees.

2797. Dabigatran. [211914-51-1] *N*-[[2-[[[4-(Aminoiminomethyl)phenyl]amino]methyl]-1-methyl-1*H*-benzimidazol-5-yl]carbonyl]-*N*-2-pyridinyl-β-alanine; 3-[[2-[(4-carbamimidoylphenylamino)methyl]-1-methyl-1*H*-benzoimidazole-5-carbonyl]-pyridin-2-ylamino]propionic acid; BIBR-953. $C_{25}H_{25}N_7O_3$; mol wt 471.51. C 63.68%, H 5.34%, N 20.79%, O 10.18%. Nonpeptide, direct thrombin inhibitor. Prepn and crystal structure of complex with thrombin: N. Hauel *et al.*, **WO 9837075**; *eidem*, **US 6087380** (1998, 2000 both to Boehringer, Ing.); *eidem*, *J. Med. Chem.* **45**, 1757 (2002). Review of pharmacology: D. Mungall, *Curr. Opin. Invest. Drugs* **3**, 905-907 (2002). Clinical pharmacokinetics: J. Stangier *et al.*, *J. Clin. Pharmacol.* **45**, 555 (2005). Clinical evaluations in joint replacement: B. I. Eriksson *et al.*, *J. Thromb. Haemostas.* **2**, 1573 (2004); *idem et al.*, *ibid.* **3**, 103 (2005).

White crystals, mp 276-277°. Log P (*n*-octanol/buffer, pH 7.4): −2.4.

Etexilate. [211915-06-9] *N*-[[2-[[[4-[[(Hexyloxy)carbonyl]-amino]iminomethyl]phenyl]amino]methyl]-1-methyl-1*H*-benzimidazol-5-yl]carbonyl]-*N*-2-pyridinyl-β-alanine ethyl ester; ethyl 3-[[[2-[[[4-[[(hexyloxy)carbonyl]amino]iminomethyl]phenyl]amino]methyl]-1-methyl-1*H*-benzimidazol-5-yl]carbonyl](pyridin-2-yl)amino]propanoate; BIBR-1048; Rendix. $C_{34}H_{41}N_7O_5$; mol wt 627.73. Colorless crystals, mp 128-129°. Log P (*n*-octanol/-buffer, pH 7.4): 2.6.

THERAP CAT: Antithrombotic.

2798. Dacarbazine. [4342-03-4] 5-(3,3-Dimethyl-1-triazenyl)-1*H*-imidazole-4-carboxamide; 5(or 4)-(dimethyltriazeno)-imidazole-4(or 5)-carboxamide; DIC; DTIC; NSC-45388; Dacatic; DTIC-Dome; Deticene. $C_6H_{10}N_6O$; mol wt 182.18. C 39.56%, H 5.53%, N 46.13%, O 8.78%. First synthesized in 1959 at the Southern Research Institute. Prepn: Shealy *et al.*, *J. Org. Chem.* **27**, 2150 (1962); Hano *et al.*, *Gann* **59**, 207 (1968), *C.A.* **69**, 42527g (1968). Antitumor activity: Shealy *et al.*, *Biochem. Pharmacol.* **11**, 674 (1962); Hano *et al.*, *Gann* **56**, 417 (1965), *C.A.* **63**, 18856g (1965). Mechanism of action studies: Saunders, Schultz, *Biochem. Pharmacol.* **19**, 911 (1970). Metabolism: Skibba *et al.*, *ibid.* 2043; Mizuno, Humphrey, *Cancer Chemother. Rep. Part 1* **56**, 465 (1972). *Review:* Carter, Friedman, *Eur. J. Cancer* **8**, 85-92 (1972), *see also* the series of articles on history, activity, mechanism of action and clinical studies: *Cancer Treat. Rep.* **60**, 123-214 (1976).

Ivory microcrystalline substance; explosive decomp 250-255°. Also reported as mp 205°, Hano *et al.*, *loc. cit.* (1965). uv max (0.1*N* HCl): 223 nm (7500); (pH 7): 237 nm (11200); both solns protected from light. Stable in neutral soln in absence of light.

Caution: This substance is reasonably anticipated to be a human carcinogen: *Report on Carcinogens, Eleventh Edition* (PB2005-104914, 2004) p III-76.

THERAP CAT: Antineoplastic.

2799. Daclizumab. [152923-56-3] Anti-(human interleukin 2 receptor) immunoglobulin G1 (human-mouse monoclonal clone 1H4 γ1-chain) disulfide with human-mouse monoclonal clone 1H4 light chain, dimer; humanized anti-Tac; HAT; dacliximab; Ro-24-7375; Zenapax. Humanized monoclonal antibody directed against the α-subunit (p55 alpha, CD25, or Tac subunit) of the human interleukin-2 receptor (IL-2Rα) that is expressed on the surface of activated T lymphocytes. Glycoprotein, mol wt ~150 kDa. DNA sequence is ~90% human origin and ~10% mouse origin. Prepn: C. Queen *et al.*, *Proc. Natl. Acad. Sci. USA* **86**, 10029 (1989). *See also:* C. L. Queen, H. E. Selick, **US 5530101** (1996 to Protein Design Labs). ELISA determn in serum: B. E. Fayer *et al.*, *J. Immunol. Methods* **186**, 47 (1995). Clinical trial in renal transplantation: B. Nashan *et al.*, *Transplantation* **67**, 110 (1999); in cardiac transplantation: A. Beniaminovitz *et al.*, *N. Engl. J. Med.* **342**, 613 (2000). Review of development: J. Hakimi *et al.* in *Antibody Therapeutics*, W. J. Harris, J. R. Adair, Eds. (CRC Press, Boca Raton, 1997) pp 277-300; of clinical efficacy in solid organ transplantation: A. M. Wiland, B. Philosophe, *Expert Opin. Biol. Ther.* **4**, 729-740 (2004).

THERAP CAT: Immunosuppressant.

2800. Dactinomycin. [50-76-0] Actinomycin D; actinomycin-[thr-val-pro-sar-meval]; meractinomycin; actinomycin A$_{IV}$; actinomycin IV; actinomycin C$_1$; actinomycin I$_1$; actinomycin X$_1$; NSC-3053; Cosmegen. $C_{62}H_{86}N_{12}O_{16}$; mol wt 1255.42. C 59.32%, H 6.90%, N 13.39%, O 20.39%. Antibiotic substance belonging to the actinomycin complex, produced by several *Streptomyces* spp. Historical background of actinomycins and chemistry, toxicology, pharmacology of actinomycin D: *Ann. N.Y. Acad. Sci.* **89**, 285-485 (1960). Isoln from broth cultures of *S. parvulus*: Manaker *et al.*, *Antibiot. Ann.* **1954/55**, 853. Structure: Bullock, Johnson, *J. Chem. Soc.* **1957**, 3280. Synthesis: Brockmann, Manegold, *Naturwissenschaften* **51**, 383 (1964); Brockmann, Lackner, *ibid.* 384, 435 (1964); Brockmann *et al.*, **DE 1172680** (1964 to Bayer); *eidem, Ber.* **101**, 1312 (1968); Meienhofer, *J. Am. Chem. Soc.* **92**, 3771 (1970); T. Tanaka *et al.*, *Bull. Chem. Soc. Jpn.* **53**, 1352 (1980); K. Nakajima *et al.*, *Pept. Chem.* **19**, 143-148 (1981). Conformation from NMR: Conti, DeSantis, *Nature* **227**, 1239 (1970); Lackner, *Ber.* **104**, 3653 (1971). Toxicity data: F. S. Philips *et al.*, *Ann. N.Y. Acad. Sci.* **89**, 348 (1960). Review and evaluation of studies of carcinogenic action in laboratory animals: *IARC Monographs* **12**, 29-41 (1976).

Trihydrate. Bright red, rhomboid prisms from abs alc, dec 241.5-243°. $[\alpha]_D^{28}$ −315° (c = 0.25 in methanol). Abs max (methanol): 244, 441 nm ($A_{1cm}^{1\%}$ 281, 206). Dil solns are very sensitive to light. Sol in alc, propylene glycol, water + glycol mixtures. LD_{50} orally in mice, rats: 13.0, 7.2 mg/kg (Philips).

THERAP CAT: Antineoplastic.

2801. Daidzein. [486-66-8] 7-Hydroxy-3-(4-hydroxyphenyl)-4H-1-benzopyran-4-one; 4′,7-dihydroxyisoflavone. $C_{15}H_{10}O_4$; mol wt 254.24. C 70.86%, H 3.96%, O 25.17%. The aglucon of daidzin, prepd by hydrolysis with HCl in methanol: Walz, Ann. **489,** 118 (1931). Isoln from red clover: Wong, J. Sci. Food Agric. **13,** 304 (1962); from the mold Micromonospora halophytica: Ganguly, Sarre, Chem. Ind. (London) **1970,** 201. Synthesis: Baker et al., J. Chem. Soc. **1933,** 274; Wessely et al., Ber. **66,** 685 (1933); Mahal et al., J. Chem. Soc. **1934,** 1769; Baker et al., ibid. **1953,** 1852; Farkas, Ber. **90,** 2940 (1957). Biosynthetic study: Grisebach, Zilg, Z. Naturforsch. **23b,** 494 (1968).

Pale-yellow prisms from dil alc, dec 315-323°. uv max: 250 nm (log ε 4.44). Sol in alcohol, ether.

7-Glucoside. Daidzin. $C_{21}H_{20}O_9$. Isoln from soybean meal (Soja hispida): Walz, loc. cit. Synthesis: Farkas, Várady, Ber. **92,** 819 (1959). Monohydrate, needles from water, dec 234-236°. $[\alpha]_D^{20}$ −36.4° (0.02N NaOH). Sol in water and aq alcohol.

2802. Dalapon. [75-99-0] 2,2-Dichloropropanoic acid; α,α-dichloropropionic acid. $C_3H_4Cl_2O_2$; mol wt 142.97. C 25.20%, H 2.82%, Cl 49.60%, O 22.38%. Selective systemic herbicide for control of annual and perennial grasses. Prepn: **GB 752761** (1956 to Dow); E. J. Kowolik, J. W. Fisher, **GB 892584** (1962 to British Celanese); of free acid and sodium salt: Smeykal, Pallutz, Chem. Tech. (Leipzig) **15** (11), 654 (1963), C.A. **60,** 6741c (1964). Acute toxicity: T. B. Gaines, R. E. Linder, Fundam. Appl. Toxicol. **7,** 299 (1986). Toxicity data for the sodium salt: G. W. Bailey, J. L. White, Residue Rev. **10,** 97 (1965). Quantitative NMR purity determn: R. J. Wells et al., J. Agric. Food Chem. **50,** 3366 (2002).

Liquid, bp$_{20}$ 98-99°. d^{20} 1.4014. n_D^{20} 1.4551. LD_{50} in male, female rats (mg/kg): 7126, 6936 orally (Gaines, Linder).

Sodium salt. [127-20-8] Basfapon; Dowpon; Radapon. C_3H_3-Cl_2NaO_2; mol wt 164.95. Crystals, dec 174-176°. Soly in water at 25°, 45 g/100 ml; aq solns hydrolyze above 70°. Corrosive to iron.

2-(2,4,5-Trichlorophenoxy)ethyl Ester. [136-25-4] Erbon; Baron; Novon. $C_{11}H_9Cl_5O_3$; mol wt 366.45. Prepn: H. F. Brust, H. O. Senkbeil, **US 2754324** (1956 to Dow). Crystals, mp 49-50°. bp$_{0.5}$ 161-164°. d$_4^{50}$ 1.55. Sol in acetone, alc, kerosene, xylene. Insol in water. LD_{50} orally in rats: 1120 mg/kg (Bailey, White).

Caution: Potential symptoms of dalapon overexposure are irritation of eyes, skin, upper respiratory system; eye and skin burns; lassitude, loss of appetite, diarrhea, vomiting, slowing of pulse; CNS

depression. See NIOSH Pocket Guide to Chemical Hazards (DHHS/NIOSH 97-140, 1997) p 100.

USE: Herbicide.

2803. Dalbavancin. [171500-79-1] 5,31-Dichloro-38-de-(methoxycarbonyl)-7-demethyl-19-deoxy-56-O-[2-deoxy-2-[(10-methyl-1-oxoundecyl)amino]-β-D-glucopyranuronosyl]-38-[[[3-(dimethylamino)propyl]amino]carbonyl]-42-O-α-D-mannopyrano-syl-N^{15}-methylristomycin A aglycone; BI-397; MDL-63397. C_{88}-$H_{100}Cl_2N_{10}O_{28}$; mol wt 1816.69. C 58.18%, H 5.55%, Cl 3.90%, N 7.71%, O 24.66%. Semisynthetic glycopeptide antibiotic derived from the natural glycopeptide, A-40926. Structurally related to teicoplanin, q.v. Prepn: A. Malabarba et al., J. Antibiot. **48,** 869 (1995). In vitro antibacterial activity: J. M. Streit et al., Diagn. Microbiol. Infect. Dis. **48,** 137 (2004). Clinical pharmacology: A. Leighton et al., Antimicrob. Agents Chemother. **48,** 940 (2004). Clinical evaluation in skin and soft-tissue infections: E. Seltzer et al., Clin. Infect. Dis. **37,** 1298 (2003); in catheter-related bloodstream infections: I. Raad et al., ibid. **40,** 374 (2005). Series of articles on development and antibacterial activity: J. Antimicrob. Chemother. **55,** Suppl. S2, ii5-ii35 (2005).

THERAP CAT: Antibacterial.

2804. Dalfopristin. [112362-50-2] (26R,27S)-26-[[2-(Di-ethylamino)ethyl]sulfonyl]-26,27-dihydrovirginiamycin M1; 26-(2-diethylaminoethyl)sulfonylpristinamycin IIB; RP-54476. C_{34}-$H_{50}N_4O_9S$; mol wt 690.85. C 59.11%, H 7.29%, N 8.11%, O 20.84%, S 4.64%. Semisynthetic polyunsaturated macrolactone type II streptogramin, q.v. Prepn: J.-C. Barriere et al., **EP 191662**; eidem, **US 4668669** (1986, 1987 both to Rhone-Poulenc). In vitro activity: H. C. Neu et al., J. Antimicrob. Chemother. **30,** Suppl. A, 83 (1992). HPLC determn in plasma: A. Le Liboux et al., J. Chromatogr. B **708,** 161 (1998)

White solid, mp ~150°.

Mixture with quinupristin. [126602-89-9] RP-59500; Synercid. Semisynthetic streptogramin comprised of two synergistic components in a defined 70:30 percent w/w mixture of dalfopristin and quinupristin, q.v., mesylate salts. HPLC determn for quality control: B. Vasselle et al., J. Pharm. Biomed. Anal. **19,** 641 (1999). In vitro activity in comparison with pristinamycin, q.v.: A. Lozniewski et al., Pathol. Biol. **48,** 463 (2000). Clinical trial in vancomycin resistant Enterococcus faecium (VREF) infection: R. C. Moellering et al., J. Antimicrob. Chemother. **44,** 251 (1999); in skin infections: R. L. Nichols *et al., ibid.* 263. *Review*: B. Pavan, *Curr. Opin. Invest. Drugs* **1**, 173-180 (2000).

THERAP CAT: Antibacterial.

2805. Dalteparin. Tedelparin. Low molecular weight fragment of heparin, *q.v.*, prepd by nitrous acid depolymerization of porcine mucosal heparin. Mean mol wt 4000-6000 daltons. Prepn: U. Lindahl *et al.,* **WO 8001383**; *eidem,* **US 4303651** (1980, 1981 both to Kabi AB). *See also: eidem, Proc. Natl. Acad. Sci. USA* **76**, 3198 (1979). Comparison of bioactivity with standard heparin: E. Holmer *et al., Thromb. Res.* **18**, 861 (1980). Clinical pharmacokinetics: G. Bratt *et al., ibid.* **42**, 613 (1986). Symposia on pharmacology and clinical efficacy: *Haemostasis* **16**, Suppl. 2, 1-71 (1986); *Semin. Thromb. Hemostasis* **16**, Suppl., 1-76 (1990). Clinical trial in unstable angina: W. Klein *et al., Circulation* **96**, 61 (1997); in unstable coronary artery disease: FRISC II Investigators, *Lancet* **354**, 701 (1999). *Review*: C. J. Dunn, E. M. Sorkin, *Drugs* **52**, 276-305 (1996).

Sodium salt. Kabi 2165; FR-860; Boxol; Fragmin.

THERAP CAT: Antithrombotic.

2806. Daltroban. [79094-20-5] 4-[2-[[(4-Chlorophenyl)-sulfonyl]amino]ethyl]benzeneacetic acid; [*p*-[2-(*p*-chlorobenzene-sulfonamido)ethyl]phenyl]acetic acid; BM-13505; SKF-96148. $C_{16}H_{16}ClNO_4S$; mol wt 353.82. C 54.31%, H 4.56%, Cl 10.02%, N 3.96%, O 18.09%, S 9.06%. Thromboxane A_2-receptor antagonist. Prepn: E. C. Witte *et al.,* **DE 3000377**; *eidem,* **US 4443477** (1981, 1984 both to Boehringer, Mann.). Receptor binding study: A. Yanagisawa *et al., Eur. J. Pharmacol.* **133**, 89 (1987). Pharmacological evaluations in animals: D. J. Lefer *et al., Arch. Int. Pharmacodyn.* **287**, 89 (1987); E. F. Smith, III, J. McDonald, *Pharmacology* **36**, 340 (1988); P. Löbel *et al., Biomed. Biochim. Acta* **47**, S 86 (1988). GC determn in biological fluids: V. Uebis, *J. Chromatogr.* **419**, 345 (1987).

THERAP CAT: Antithrombotic.

2807. Damar. [9000-16-2] Gum Damar; Dammar; resin Damar. Resinous exudate from a species of *Shorea, Dipterocarpaceae. Habit.* East Indies, Philippines. *Constit.* Volatile oil, resins, bitter substance.

Yellowish-white, roundish, or stalactite shaped, friable masses; semi-transparent, conchoidal fracture; varying degrees of hardness. d 1.04-1.12. mp ~120°. Insol in water. Sol in alcohol, chloroform, ether, carbon disulfide, oil rosemary; partly sol in oil turpentine.

USE: In plasters, varnishes, lacquers, etc. A soln of the purified material in chloroform or xylene is used for preserving animal and vegetable specimens for microscopy.

2808. Damascenine. [483-64-7] 3-Methoxy-2-(methylamino)benzoic acid methyl ester; 2-(methylamino)-*m*-anisic acid methyl ester; methyl 2-(methylamino)-3-methoxybenzoate; methyldamascenine; nigelline. $C_{10}H_{13}NO_3$; mol wt 195.22. C 61.52%, H 6.71%, N 7.17%, O 24.59%. Odoriferous principle of oil of Nigella from seeds of *Nigella damascena* L. and *Nigella arvensis* L., *Ranunculaceae.* Early syntheses: Ewins, *J. Chem. Soc.* **101**, 544 (1912); Kaufman, Rothlin, *Ber.* **49**, 578 (1916); Sornet, *Manuf. Chem.* **5**, 87 (1924); Keller, Schulze, *Arch. Pharm.* **263**, 481 (1925). Improved synthesis: Mutschler, *ibid.* **298**, 861 (1965); M. Thoinet *et al., Ann. Pharm. Fr.* **36**, 337 (1978). Toxicity study: Bekemeier *et al., Arch. Int. Pharmacodyn. Ther.* **168**, 199 (1967).

Prisms from abs. alc. Nutmeg-like odor, mp 27-29°. bp 270° (slight dec), bp_{10} 147°. Volatile with steam. Insol in water. Freely sol in alc, ether, chloroform, petr ether, oils.

Hydrochloride. Deliquesc prisms, mp 156°. (Hydrate, mp 122°). LD_{50} orally in mice: 1800 mg/kg (Bekemeier).

2809. β-Damascenone. [23726-93-4]; [23696-85-7] (stereo unspecified). (2*E*)-1-(2,6,6-Trimethyl-1,3-cyclohexadien-1-yl)-2-buten-1-one; *trans*-2,6,6-trimethyl-1-crotonylcyclohexa-1,3-diene; Doricenone. $C_{13}H_{18}O$; mol wt 190.28. C 82.06%, H 9.53%, O 8.41%. Terpenic ketone; odorant in fruits, vegetables, honey, wine and beer. Isoln from Bulgarian rose oil, *Rosa damascena* Mill., and synthesis: E. Demole *et al., Helv. Chim. Acta* **53**, 541 (1970). Synthetic studies: G. Büchi, H. Wüest, *ibid.* **54**, 1767 (1971); K. S. Ayyar *et al., J. Chem. Soc. Perkin Trans. 1* **1975**, 1727. Identification in grapes: T. E. Acree *et al., J. Agric. Food Chem.* **29**, 688 (1981); in tomato volatiles: R. G. Buttery *et al., Chem. Ind. (London)* **1988**, 238. Quantitative determn in foods: A. Sen *et al., J. Agric. Food Chem.* **39**, 757 (1991); in beers: F. Chevance *et al., ibid.* **50**, 3818 (2002). Reactivity in wine: M. A. Daniel *et al., ibid.* **52**, 8127 (2004).

Pale yellow to yellow liquid; powerful floral, fruity odor. $bp_{0.001}$ 57°. $bp_{0.08}$ 51°. bp_{13} 116-118°. d_4^{20} 0.942. n_D^{20} 1.5123. Flash pt (closed cup): >100°C. uv max (cyclohexane): 220, 253, 302 nm (ε 10000, 4120, 2270). uv max (ethanol): 228, 255, 310 nm (ε 12000, 500, 2000). Sol in ethanol (95°). Odor threshold in water: 0.02-0.09 ng/g.

USE: In perfumery.

2810. Daminozide. [1596-84-5] Butanedioic acid mono(2,-2-dimethylhydrazide); *N*-(dimethylamino)succinamic acid; succinic acid 2,2-dimethylhydrazide; B-9; B-995; Alar; B-Nine; Kylar. $C_6H_{12}N_2O_3$; mol wt 160.17. C 44.99%, H 7.55%, N 17.49%, O 29.97%. HOOCCH$_2$CH$_2$CONHN(CH$_3$)$_2$. Prepn: **BE 613799**, *C.A.* **57**, 10281d (1962); H. A. Hageman, W. L. Hubbard, **US 3257414** (1962, 1966 both to U.S. Rubber). Effect in controlling growth in apples: F. W. Southwick *et al., Proc. Am. Soc. Hortic. Sci.* **92**, 71 (1968); D. W. Greene *et al., Fruit Var. J.* **40**, 41 (1986). *In vitro* and *in vivo* mechanism of action studies: K. Ryugo, R. M. Sachs, *J. Am. Soc. Hortic. Sci.* **94**, 529 (1969). Hydrolysis to 1,1-dimethylhydrazine, *q.v.,* and determn in food products: W. H. Newsome, *J. Agric. Food Chem.* **28**, 319 (1980); M. K. Conditt, J. R. Baumgardner, *J. Assoc. Off. Anal. Chem.* **71**, 735 (1988). Discussion of toxicological evaluation: D. Campt, *EPA Journal* **13**, 32 (1987).

Crystals, mp 154-155°. Soly 10% in water, 2.5% in acetone, 5% in methanol.

USE: Plant growth regulator.

2811. Danaparoid. Mucoglucuronan. Low molecular weight heparinoid derived from hog intestinal mucosa. Mixture of glycosaminoglycans with a mean mol wt of 6000 Da (range 4000-10000 Da). Consists of heparan sulfate (~83%), dermatan sulfate (~12%) and chondroitin sulfate (~5%). Prepn: A. L. M. Saunders *et al.,* **EP 66908**; *eidem,* **US 4438108** (1982, 1984 both to Akzo). Pharmacology: D. G. Meuleman *et al., Thromb. Res.* **27**, 353 (1982). Determn in plasma: H. ten Cate *et al., Clin. Chem.* **30**, 860 (1984). Series of articles on pharmacology and clinical efficacy: *Haemostasis* **22**, 55-112 (1992). Clinical trial in deep venous thromboembolism: H. W. de Valk *et al., Ann. Intern. Med.* **123**, 1 (1995).

Sodium salt. Org-10172; Organan.

THERAP CAT: Antithrombotic.

2812. Danazol. [17230-88-5] (17α)-Pregna-2,4-dien-20-yno[2,3-*d*]isoxazol-17-ol; 1-ethynyl-2,3,3a,3b,4,5,10,10a,10b,11,-12,12a-dodecahydro-10a,12a-dimethyl-1*H*-cyclopenta[7,8]phenanthro[3,2-*d*]isoxazol-1-ol; 17α-ethynyl-17β-hydroxy-4-androsteno[2,3-*d*]isoxazole; Win-17757; Bonzol; Cyclomen; Danatrol;

Danocrine; Danol; Danoval; Ladogal; Winobanin. $C_{22}H_{27}NO_2$; mol wt 337.46. C 78.30%, H 8.06%, N 4.15%, O 9.48%. Anterior pituitary supressant. Anabolic steroid deriv of ethisterone, *q.v.*, with mild androgenic side effects (an impeded androgen). Prepn: **GB 905844** (1962 to Sterling Drug), *C.A.* **58**, 6895c (1963); Manson *et al., J. Med. Chem.* **6**, 1 (1963); Clinton, Manson, **US 3135743** (1964 to Sterling Drug). Activity studies: Sherins *et al., J. Clin. Endocrinol. Metab.* **32**, 522 (1971); Dmowski *et al., Fertil. Steril.* **22**, 9 (1971). Clinical studies in endometriosis and other endocrine disorders: R. B. Greenblatt *et al., ibid.* 102. Series of articles on pharmacology, pharmacokinetics and clinical use: *Drugs* **19**, 321-372 (1980). Use in idiopathic thrombocytopenic purpura: Y. S. Ahn *et al., N. Engl. J. Med.* **308**, 1396 (1983); in hemophilia: H. R. Gralnick *et al., ibid.* 1393.

Crystals from acetone, mp 224.4-226.8°. $[\alpha]_D^{25}$ +7.5° (ethanol); $[\alpha]_D^{25}$ +21.9° (chloroform). uv max (ethanol): 286 nm (ε 11300).

THERAP CAT: Antigonadotropin.

2813. Danofloxacin. [112398-08-0] 1-Cyclopropyl-6-fluoro-1,4-dihydro-7-[(1*S*,4*S*)-5-methyl-2,5-diazabicyclo[2.2.1]hept-2-yl]-4-oxo-3-quinolinecarboxylic acid. $C_{19}H_{20}FN_3O_3$; mol wt 357.38. C 63.85%, H 5.64%, F 5.32%, N 11.76%, O 13.43%. Fluorinated quinolone antibacterial. Prepn: M. R. Jefson, P. R. McGuirk, **EP 215650**; *eidem*, **US 4861779** (1987, 1989 both to Pfizer). *See also:* F. R. Busch *et al.*, **EP 342849** (1989 to Pfizer), *C.A.* **113**, 6177m (1990). Evaluation in treatment of pneumonia in cattle: W. T. R. Grimshaw *et al., Dtsch. Tieraerztl. Wochenschr.* **97**, 529 (1990); C. J. Giles *et al., Vet. Rec.* **128**, 296 (1991). Efficacy in treatment of *E. coli* diarrhoea in calves: S. J. Sunderland *et al., Res. Vet. Sci.* **74**, 171 (2003).

mp 268-272°.

Methanesulfonate. [119478-55-6] CP-76136-27; Advocin. $C_{19}H_{20}FN_3O_3 \cdot CH_3SO_3H$; mol wt 453.48.

THERAP CAT (VET): Antibacterial.

2814. Dansyl Chloride. [605-65-2] 5-(Dimethylamino)-1-naphthalenesulfonyl chloride. $C_{12}H_{12}ClNO_2S$; mol wt 269.75. C 53.43%, H 4.48%, Cl 13.14%, N 5.19%, O 11.86%, S 11.89%. Reagent for fluorescent labelling of amines, amino acids and proteins. Synthesis: G. Weber, *Biochem. J.* **51**, 155 (1952); A. Mendel, *J. Chem. Eng. Data* **15**, 340 (1970). In amino acid analysis: J. Airhart *et al., Anal. Biochem.* **53**, 132 (1973). In HPLC analysis of phenols: R. M. Cassidy, D. S. LeGay, *J. Chromatogr. Sci.* **12**, 85 (1974). In protein microassays: T. Kinoshita *et al., Anal. Biochem.* **66**, 104 (1975). In measurement of desquamation: R. Marks *et al., Br. J. Dermatol.* **111**, 265 (1984).

Yellow-orange crystals from hexane, mp 66.5-68°. Sol in acetone, pyridine, benzene, dioxane. Insol in water.

USE: In fluorescent labelling, column chromatography, HPLC.

2815. Danthron. [117-10-2] 1,8-Dihydroxy-9,10-anthracenedione; 1,8-dihydroxyanthraquinone; 1,8-Dihydroxyanthraquinone; chrysazin; dantron; Altan; Antrapurol; Diaquone; Istizin; Modane. $C_{14}H_8O_4$; mol wt 240.21. C 70.00%, H 3.36%, O 26.64%. Prepn: Fierz-David, Blangey, *Farbenchemie* (Vienna, 5th ed., 1943) pp 224-225; Kozlov, *Dokl. Akad. Nauk SSSR* **61**, 281 (1948). Clinical trial with poloxalkol in constipation: L. Mundow, *Br. J. Clin. Pract.* **29**, 95 (1975). Mutation study: J. P. Brown, R. J. Brown, *Mutat. Res.* **40**, 203 (1976). Toxicology: M. T. Case *et al., Drug Chem. Toxicol.* **1**, 89 (1977). Review of toxicity and carcinogenic risk: *IARC Monographs* **50**, 265-275 (1990).

Orange needles from alc, mp 193-197°. Sublimes. Absorption max: 430, 250 nm (log ε 4.35, 4.60). Almost insol in water (6.5 × 10^{-6} mols/l at 25°), in alcohol (1:2000). Moderately sol in ether (1:500), in chloroform; sol in 10 parts hot glacial acetic acid. Very slightly sol in aq solns of alkali hydroxides: about 0.8 g dissolves in 100 ml 0.5*N* NaOH. (Disodium salt is reported to have a water soly of 0.05%.) LD_{50} orally in mice: <7 g/kg (Case).

Caution: This substance is reasonably anticipated to be a human carcinogen: *Report on Carcinogens, Eleventh Edition* (PB2005-104914, 2004) p III-77.

USE: Important intermediate in the manuf of alizarin and indanthrene dyestuffs; forms insol Ca, Ba, Pb lakes. Antioxidant in synthetic lubricants; fungicide.

THERAP CAT: Cathartic.

THERAP CAT (VET): Purgative.

2816. Dantrolene. [7261-97-4] 1-[[[5-(4-Nitrophenyl)-2-furanyl]methylene]amino]-2,4-imidazolidinedione; 1-[[5-(*p*-nitrophenyl)furfurylidene]amino]hydantoin. $C_{14}H_{10}N_4O_5$; mol wt 314.25. C 53.51%, H 3.21%, N 17.83%, O 25.46%. Direct acting skeletal muscle relaxant; probably inhibits the release of calcium from the sarcoplasmic reticulum of skeletal muscle. Prepn: **NL 6612588**; Davis, Snyder, **US 3415821** (1967, 1968 both to Norwich Pharmacal); Snyder *et al., J. Med. Chem.* **10**, 807 (1967); Frimm *et al., Chem. Zvesti* **23**, 916 (1969). HPLC determn in plasma: M. Lalande *et al., J. Chromatogr.* **430**, 187 (1988). Toxicity data: K. O. Ellis *et al., J. Pharm. Sci.* **69**, 327 (1980). Review of pharmacology: G. G. Harrison, *Br. J. Anaesth.* **60**, 279 (1988); and therapeutic use: A. Ward *et al., Drugs* **32**, 130-168 (1986). Review of efficacy in malignant hyperthermia: R. Ben Abraham *et al., Q. J. Med.* **90**, 13-18 (1997).

Crystals from aqueous DMF, mp 279-280°.

Sodium salt hemiheptahydrate. [24868-20-0]; [14663-23-1] (anhydrous). F-440; Dantamacrin; Dantrium. $C_{14}H_9N_4Na-O_5 \cdot 3\frac{1}{2}H_2O$; mol wt 399.29. Orange powder. Slightly soluble in water; more sol in alkaline soln. LD_{50} (calculated as base) orally in mice: 1110 mg/kg (Ellis).

THERAP CAT: Muscle relaxant (skeletal); in treatment of malignant hyperthermia.

2817. Daphnetin. [486-35-1] 7,8-Dihydroxy-2*H*-1-benzopyran-2-one; 7,8-dihydroxycoumarin. $C_9H_6O_4$; mol wt 178.14. C 60.68%, H 3.39%, O 35.93%. The aglucon of daphnin. By boiling daphnin with dil mineral acids; by enzymatic hydrolysis of daphnin; by sublimation from daphnin; by synthesis: v. Pechmann,

Ber. **17**, 934 (1884); Gatterman, Köbner, *Ber.* **32**, 287 (1899); Baker, Savage, *J. Chem. Soc.* **1938**, 1602; Späth, Galinovsky, *Ber.* **70B**, 235 (1937); Sethna, Shah, *Chem. Rev.* **36**, 1 (1945).

Crystals from dil alc, mp 256° (dec). Sublimes. Sol in boiling water, hot dil alcohol, hot glacial acetic acid; very sparingly sol in ether, in carbon bisulfide, in chloroform, in benzene. Sol in alkali and alkali carbonate solns giving a yellow color. Aq solns give a green color with ferric chloride which turns red on addition of sodium carbonate.

2818. Daphnin. [486-55-5] 7-β-D-Glucopyranosyloxy-8-hydroxy-2*H*-1-benzopyran-2-one; 7,8-dihydroxycoumarin 7-β-D-glucoside; daphnetin 7-β-D-glucoside; 7-glucosido-8-hydroxycoumarin. $C_{15}H_{16}O_9$; mol wt 340.28. C 52.94%, H 4.74%, O 42.32%. In bark and flower of *Daphne* spp. Extraction from fresh bark of *D. mezereum* L., *Thymelaeaceae: Beilstein* **XXXI**, 248. Structure: Wessely, Sturm, *Ber.* **63**, 1299 (1930); Hattori, *Chem. Zentralbl.* **1930** II, 2138. Synthesis: Gandini, *Gazz. Chim. Ital.* **70**, 611 (1940), *C.A.* **35**, 1394 (1941).

Monohydrate, prisms from water. Anhydr after drying at 80-90° at 2 mm Hg. When anhydrous, dec 215° (Wessely, Sturm); dec 224° (Hattori); dec 229° (older data). Optical rotations of monohydrate: $[\alpha]_D^{22}$ −124° (15 mg in 4 ml MeOH); after 2 recrystns from water: $[\alpha]_D^{22}$ −115° (abs MeOH) (Wessely, Sturm); $[\alpha]_D^{15}$ −84.2° (MeOH) (Hattori). Sol in hot water, alcohol; sol in aq solns of alkalies and alkali carbonates with yellow color. Insol in ether. Hydrolyzed by dilute acid yielding 7,8-dihydroxycoumarin and D-glucose. Also split by emulsin.

2819. Daphnoline. [479-36-7] 6,6′-Dimethoxy-2-methyl-oxyacanthan-7,12′-diol; trilobamine. $C_{35}H_{36}N_2O_6$; mol wt 580.67. C 72.39%, H 6.25%, N 4.82%, O 16.53%. From bark of *Daphnandra micrantha* Benth., *Monimiaceae.* Isoln: Pyman, *J. Chem. Soc.* **105**, 1679 (1914). Identity with trilobamine: Bick *et al., ibid.* **1949**, 2767. Structure: Bick *et al., ibid.* **1960**, 4928.

Crystals from chloroform, mp 194-196°. $[\alpha]_D$ +459° (c = 0.3 in chloroform). uv max (methanol): 285 nm (log ε 3.9). Practically insol in water, ethyl acetate, acetone, ether, petr ether. Sparingly sol in methanol, ethanol, xylene, hot chloroform sol in dil acids, cold aq 5% sodium hydroxide.

Daphnandrine. [1183-76-2] 6,6′,12′-Trimethoxy-2-methyl-oxyacanthan-7-ol. $C_{36}H_{38}N_2O_6$. Needles from methanol, dec 270°. $[\alpha]_D^{16}$ +480° (c = 1.2 in chloroform). uv max (methanol): 284 nm (log ε 3.92). Practically insol in hot methanol, ethanol, acetone, ether, petr ether. Sparingly sol in hot methanol, ethanol, xylene, cold chloroform; sol in hot chloroform.

2820. Dapiprazole. [72822-12-9] 5,6,7,8-Tetrahydro-3-[2-[4-(2-methylphenyl)-1-piperazinyl]ethyl]-1,2,4-triazolo[4,3-*a*]pyridine; 5,6,7,8-tetrahydro-3-[2-(4-*o*-tolyl-1-piperazinyl)ethyl]-*s*-

triazolo[4,3-*a*]pyridine. $C_{19}H_{27}N_5$; mol wt 325.45. C 70.12%, H 8.36%, N 21.52%. α-Adrenergic blocker. Prepn: B. Silvestrini, L. Baiocchi, **DE 2915318**; *eidem,* **US 4252721** (1979, 1981 both to Angelini Francesco). Series of articles on general pharmacology: *Arzneim.-Forsch.* **32**, 674-681 (1982); and toxicity: B. Silvestrini *et al., ibid.* 668. Ocular pharmacokinetics in rabbits: P. Valeri *et al., Pharmacol. Res. Commun.* **18**, 1093 (1986). Topical effects in human eye: A. Reibaldi *et al., Acta Ther.* **10**, 381 (1984); C. Malpassi *et al., ibid.* **12**, 55 (1986). Clinical trial in reversal of mydriasis: R. W. Allinson *et al., Ann. Ophthalmol.* **22**, 131 (1990).

mp 158-160°.
Monohydrochloride. [72822-13-0] AF-2139; Glamidolo; Reversil; Rev-Eyes. $C_{19}H_{27}N_5$.HCl; mol wt 361.91. Crystals from absolute ethanol, mp 206-207°. LD_{50} in mice (mg/kg): 260 i.p. (Silvestrini).

THERAP CAT: Antiglaucoma; miotic.

2821. Dapoxetine. [119356-77-3] (α*S*)-*N,N*-Dimethyl-α-[2-(1-naphthalenyloxy)ethyl]benzenemethanamine; (+)-*N,N*-dimethyl-1-phenyl-3-(1-naphthalenyloxy)propanamine; LY-210448. $C_{21}H_{23}NO$; mol wt 305.41. C 82.59%, H 7.59%, N 4.59%, O 5.24%. Selective serotonin reuptake inhibitor (SSRI). Prepn: D. W. Robertson *et al.,* **EP 288188**; *eidem,* **US 5135947** (1988, 1992 both to Lilly). Chiral synthesis: W. J. Wheeler, D. D. O'Bannon, *J. Labelled Compd. Radiopharm.* **31**, 305 (1992). HPLC determn in plasma: C. L. Hamilton, J. D. Cornpropst, *J. Chromatogr.* **612**, 253 (1993). Review of pharmacology and clinical experience: B. Feret, *Formulary* **40**, 227-230 (2005).

Hydrochloride. [129938-20-1] $C_{21}H_{23}NO$.HCl; mol wt 341.87. White crystalline solid from hydrochloric acid and ethyl acetate. $[\alpha]_D$ +135.78° (c = 2.18 in methanol).

THERAP CAT: In treatment of premature ejaculation.

2822. Dapsone. [80-08-0] 4,4′-Sulfonylbisbenzeneamine; 4,4′-sulfonyldianiline; bis(4-aminophenyl)sulfone; 4,4′-diaminodiphenyl sulfone; DDS; diaphenylsulfone; DADPS; 1358F; Avlosulfon; Croysulfone; Diphenasone; Disulone; Dumitone; Eporal; Novophone; Sulfona-Mae; Sulphadione; Udolac. $C_{12}H_{12}N_2O_2S$; mol wt 248.30. C 58.05%, H 4.87%, N 11.28%, O 12.89%, S 12.91%. Prepn: **FR 829926** (1938 to I. G. Farbenind.), *C.A.* **33**, 1761 (1939); Buckles, *J. Chem. Educ.* **31**, 36 (1954); Ferry *et al., Org. Synth.* **coll. vol. III**, 239 (1955). Antibacterial action and metabolism: J. Francis, A. Spinks, *Br. J. Pharmacol.* **5**, 565 (1950). Mechanism of toxic action: Wu, DuBois, *Arch. Int. Pharmacodyn. Ther.* **183**, 36 (1970). Comprehensive description: C. E. Orzech *et al., Anal. Profiles Drug Subs.* **5**, 87-114 (1976). Review of pharmacology and therapeutic use: J. Uetrecht, *Clin. Dermatol.* **7**, 111-120 (1989). Clinical trial with chlorproguanil, *q.v.,* in drug-resistant malaria: T. Mutabingwa *et al., Lancet* **358**, 1218 (2001).

Crystals from 95% ethanol. mp 175-176° (also a higher melting form, mp 180.5°). pKb 13.0. Soluble in alcohol, methanol, acetone, dil hydrochloric acid. Practically insol in water.

USE: Hardening agent in the curing of epoxy resins.

THERAP CAT: Antibacterial (leprostatic); in treatment of dermatitis herpetiformis.

THERAP CAT (VET): Antibacterial; coccidostat.

2823. Daptomycin. [103060-53-3] LY-146032; Cidecin; Cubicin. $C_{72}H_{101}N_{17}O_{26}$; mol wt 1620.67. C 53.36%, H 6.28%, N 14.69%, O 25.67%. Cyclic lipopeptide antibiotic derived from a fermentation product of *Streptomyces roseosporus*; disrupts plasma membrane function in gram-positive bacteria. Prepn: B. J. Abbott *et al.*, **US 4537717** (1985 to Eli Lilly); M. Debono *et al.*, *J. Antibiot.* **41**, 1093 (1988). Mechanism of action study: N. E. Allen *et al.*, *Antimicrob. Agents Chemother.* **31**, 1093 (1987); and structure determn: D. Jung *et al.*, *Chem. Biol.* **11**, 949 (2004). Comparative *in vitro* antibacterial spectrum: I. A. Critchley *et al.*, *J. Antimicrob. Chemother.* **51**, 639 (2003). Clinical pharmacokinetics: J. R. Woodworth *et al.*, *Antimicrob. Agents Chemother.* **36**, 318 (1992). Clinical trial in skin infections: R. D. Arbeit *et al.*, *Clin. Infect. Dis.* **38**, 1673 (2004). Review of pharmacology and clinical evaluations: F. P. Tully *et al.*, *Expert Opin. Invest. Drugs* **8**, 1223-1238 (1999); L. P. Kotra *Curr. Opin. Anti-Infect. Invest. Drugs* **2**, 185-205 (2000).

uv max (ethanol): 220, 260 nm (ε 46500, 10000). LD_{50} i.v. in mice: 600 mg/kg (Debono).

THERAP CAT: Antibacterial.

2824. Darbepoetin Alfa. [209810-58-2] [30-Asparagine,32-threonine,87-valine,88-asparagine,90-threonine]erythropoietin (human); novel erythropoiesis stimulating protein; NESP; Aranesp. Hyperglycosylated analog of human erythropoietin, *q.v.*, produced by recombinant DNA technology. mol wt ~38 kDa. Engineered to contain 2 extra carbohydrate addition sites, leading to increased circulating half-life. Prepn: S. G. Elliott, T. E. Byrne, **WO 9505465** (1995 to Amgen). Review of development and pharmacology: I. C. Macdougall, *Semin. Nephrol.* **20**, 375-381 (2000); of clinical experience in treatment of anemia of kidney disease: A. R. Nissenson, *Am. J. Kidney Dis.* **38**, 1390-1397 (2001); of chemotherapy induced anemia: J. Vansteenkiste, I. Wauters, *Expert Opin. Pharmacother.* **6**, 429-440 (2005). Series of articles on clinical experience in cancer-related anemia: *Br. J. Cancer* **84**, Suppl. 1, 1-38 (2001).

THERAP CAT: Hematopoietic.

2825. Darifenacin. [133099-04-4] (3*S*)-1-[2-(2,3-Dihydro-5-benzofuranyl)ethyl]-α,α-diphenyl-3-pyrrolidineacetamide; 3-(*S*)-(−)-(1-carbamoyl-1,1-diphenylmethyl)-1-[2-(2,3-dihydrobenzofuran-5-yl)ethyl]pyrrolidine; (*S*)-2-[1-[2-(2,3,-dihydrobenzofuran-5-yl)ethyl]-3-pyrrolidinyl]-2,2-diphenylacetamide; UK-88525. $C_{28}H_{30}N_2O_2$; mol wt 426.55. C 78.84%, H 7.09%, N 6.57%, O 7.50%. Selective muscarinic M_3-receptor antagonist. Prepn: P. E. Cross, A. R. MacKenzie, **EP 388054**; *eidem*, **US 5096890** (1990, 1992 both to Pfizer). HPLC/MS determn in plasma: B. Kaye *et al.*, *Anal. Chem.* **68**, 1658 (1996). Binding profile for receptor subtypes: C. M. Smith, R. W. Wallis, *J. Recept. Signal Transduction Res.* **17**, 177 (1997); and pharmacology: R. M. Wallis, C. M. Napier, *Life Sci.* **64**, 395 (1999). Pharmacokinetics and metabolism: K. C. Beaumont *et al.*, *Xenobiotica* **28**, 63 (1998). Clinical trial in overactive bladder: F. Haab *et al.*, *Eur. Urol.* **45**, 420 (2004). Review of clinical experience: C. R. Chapple, *Expert Opin. Invest. Drugs* **13**, 1493-1500 (2004).

Foam or colorless glass. $[\alpha]_D^{25}$ −20.6° (c = 1.0 in methylene chloride). pKa (25°): 9.2.

Hydrobromide. [133099-07-7] Emselex; Enablex. $C_{28}H_{31}N_2O_2Br$. mp 229°. $[\alpha]_D^{25}$ −30.3° (c = 1.0 in methylene chloride). Soly at 37° (mg/ml): water 6.03.

THERAP CAT: Antispasmodic; in treatment of urinary incontinence.

2826. Darmstadtium. [54083-77-1] Element 110; ununnilium. Ds, Uun; at. no. 110. Group VIII (10). Transuranium element. No stable nuclides. Prepn and decay of isotopes [269]110 ($T_{1/2}$ ~170 μsec, α decay) by [208]Pb([62]Ni,n) and isotopes [271]110 ($T_{1/2}$ ~1.1 msec, α decay) and [271m]110 ($T_{1/2}$ ~56 msec, α decay) by [208]Pb([64]Ni,n): S. Hofmann *et al.*, *Z. Phys. A* **350**, 277 (1995). Production of isotope [273]110 ($T_{1/2}$ ~76 μsec, α decay) as a decay product of isotope [277]112: Y. A. Lazarev, *Phys. Rev. C* **54**, 620 (1996); of isotope [273]110 ($T_{1/2}$ ~118 msec, α decay): S. Hofmann *et al.*, *Z. Phys. A* **354**, 229 (1996). Review of production and properties: *idem, Rep. Prog. Phys.* **61**, 639-689 (1998).

2827. Darunavir. [206361-99-1] [(1*S*,2*R*)-3-[[(4-Aminophenyl)sulfonyl] (2-methylpropyl)amino]-2-hydroxy-1-(phenylmethyl)propyl]carbamic acid (3*R*,3a*S*,6a*R*)-hexahydrofuro[2,3-*b*]furan-3-yl ester; (1*S*,2*R*,3'*R*,3'a*S*,6'a*R*)-[3'-hexahydrofuro[2,3-*b*]furanyl]-[3-(4-aminobenzenesulfonyl)isobutylamino]-1-benzyl-2-hydroxypropyl]carbamate; TMC-114; UIC-94017. $C_{27}H_{37}N_3O_7S$; mol wt 547.66. C 59.21%, H 6.81%, N 7.67%, O 20.45%, S 5.85%. Second generation HIV-1 protease inhibitor; structurally similar to amprenavir, *q.v.* Prepn: A. K. Ghosh *et al.*, *Bioorg. Med. Chem. Lett.* **8**, 687 (1998); *idem et al.*, *J. Org. Chem.* **69**, 7822 (2004). *See also*: J. W. Erickson, S. V. Gulnik, **WO 9967417** (1999 to U.S. Dept. Health Human Serv.); J. W. Erickson *et al.*, **US 05158713** (2005 to Univ. Illinois). *In vitro* activity vs multidrug resistant HIV isolates: Y. Koh *et al.*, *Antimicrob. Agents Chemother.* **47**, 3123 (2003). Crystal structures of complex with protease variants: Y. Tie *et al.*, *J. Mol. Biol.* **338**, 341 (2004). Structure activity study and pharmacokinetic analysis: D. L. N. G. Surleraux *et al.*, *J. Med. Chem.* **48**, 1813 (2005). Review of pharmacology and clinical experience: A. C. Shurtleff, *Curr. Opin. Invest. Drugs* **5**, 879-886 (2004). Clinical evaluation of combination with ritonavir: K. Arastéh *et al.*, *AIDS* **19**, 943 (2005).

White amorphous solid, mp 74° (dec).

THERAP CAT: Antiviral.

2828. Darvan®. [9003-24-1] Vinylidene cyanide-vinyl acetate copolymer; Darlan; Travis. *Methylenemalononitrile copolymer with vinyl acetate* contg about equal parts of each component. Polymerization of vinylidene cyanide with vinyl acetate: Gilbert *et al.*, *J. Am. Chem. Soc.* **78**, 1669 (1956); Gilbert, Miller, **US 2615866** and Sayre, **US 2975158** (1952, 1961, both to B. F. Goodrich). *Review*: R. W. Moncrieff, *Man-Made Fibres* (John Wiley, New York, 4th ed., 1963) pp 488-494. Approximate structure:

A wool-like fiber, sp gr 1.18. Softens at about 175°. Flammability similar to cotton and viscose. Insol in acetone, methylene chloride. Good resistance to sunlight, clothes-moth and carpet-beetle attack, and mildew; moderate resistance to 10% H_2SO_4 at 100° for hrs, and to 0.5% caustic soda at 43° for 7 days. Shrinks about 1% when immersed in boiling water for 3 minutes. Difficult to dye. Relatively resistant to pilling.

USE: Knitted garments, pile coats, and in blends for tropical suitings and men's shirtings.

2829. Dasatinib. [302962-49-8] *N*-(2-Chloro-6-methylphenyl)-2-[[6-[4-(2-hydroxyethyl)-1-piperazinyl]-2-methyl-4-pyrimidinyl]amino]-5-thiazolecarboxamide; BMS-354825. $C_{22}H_{26}$- ClN_7O_2S; mol wt 488.01. C 54.15%, H 5.37%, Cl 7.26%, N 20.09%, O 6.56%, S 6.57%. Orally bioactive, ATP-competitive dual inhibitor of Src and Abl kinases. Prepn: J. Das *et al.*, **WO 0062778**; *eidem* **US 6596746** (2000, 2003 both to Bristol-Myers Squibb); and Src/Abl kinase inhibition study: L. J. Lombardo *et al.*, *J. Med. Chem.* **47**, 6658 (2004). *In vivo* evaluation vs imatinib-resistant mutants in chronic myeloid leukemia: N. P. Shah *et al.*, *Science* **305**, 399 (2004). Mechanism of action study: M. R. Burgess *et al.*, *Proc. Natl. Acad. Sci. USA* **102**, 3395 (2005). Review of therapeutic potential in chronic myeloid leukemia: T. O'Hare *et al.*, *Curr. Opin. Genet. Dev.* **16**, 92-99 (2006).

mp 279-280°.
THERAP CAT: Antineoplastic.

2830. Datiscetin. [480-15-9] 3,5,7-Trihydroxy-2-(2-hydroxyphenyl)-4*H*-1-benzopyran-4-one; 2′,3,5,7-tetrahydroxyflavone; 2′-hydroxycrysidenolon 1493. $C_{15}H_{10}O_6$; mol wt 286.24. C 62.94%, H 3.52%, O 33.54%. Cleavage product of datiscin: Stenhouse, *Ann.* **98**, 166 (1856). From roots of *Datisca cannabina* L., *Datiscaceae:* Marchlewski, *Biochem. Z.* **3**, 286 (1907). Structure: Leskiewicz, Marchlewski, *Ber.* **47**, 1599 (1914). Synthesis: Kalf, Robinson, *J. Chem. Soc.* **127**, 1968 (1925); Simpson, Wally, *ibid.* **1955**, 166.

Pale yellow needles from alc, mp 271°. uv max (96% alc): 264.0, 375.0 nm (log ε 4.265, 4.005). Sol in alcohol, ether, other organic solvents; practically insol in water. Sol in alkaline solns with yellow color.

2831. Daucol. [887-08-1] Octahydro-6,8a-dimethyl-3-(1-methylethyl)-1*H*-3a,6-epoxyazulen-7-ol; 2,3,4,5,6,7a,8,8a-octahydro-3-isopropyl-6,8a-dimethyl-1*H*-3a,6-epoxyazulen-7-ol. C_{15}-$H_{26}O_2$; mol wt 238.37. C 75.58%, H 10.99%, O 13.42%. From oil of carrot seeds, *Daucus carota* L., *Umbelliferae:* Richter, *Arch. Pharm.* **247**, 391 (1909). Structure: Sykora *et al.*, *Collect. Czech. Chem. Commun.* **26**, 788 (1961); Zalkow *et al.*, *J. Org. Chem.* **26**,

981 (1961). Stereochemistry: Levisalles, Rudler, *Bull. Soc. Chim. Fr.* **1964**, 2020; **1967**, 2059. Synthesis of (−)-form: DeBroissia *et al.*, *Chem. Commun.* **1972**, 855; *eidem, Bull. Soc. Chim. Fr.* **1972**, 4314.

(−)-Daucol

Crystals (from petr ether at −30°), mp 113-115°. bp₂ 124-132°. $[\alpha]_D^{20}$ −16.9° (c = 2.76 in ethanol).

2832. Daunorubicin. [20830-81-3] (8*S-cis*)-8-Acetyl-10-[(3-amino-2,3,6-trideoxy-α-L-*lyxo*-hexopyranosyl)oxy]-7,8,9,10-tetrahydro-6,8,11-trihydroxy-5,12-naphthacenedione; daunomycin; leukaemomycin C; rubidomycin; RP-13057; Cerubidin. $C_{27}H_{29}NO_{10}$; mol wt 527.52. C 61.47%, H 5.54%, N 2.66%, O 30.33%. Anthracycline antibiotic related to the rhodomycins, *q.v.* Isolated from fermentation broths of *Streptomyces peucetius:* G. Cassinelli, P. Orezzi, *G. Microbiol.* **11**, 167 (1963), *C.A.* **62**, 9482b (1965); A. Di Marco *et al.*, *Nature* **201**, 706 (1964); *eidem,* **BE 639897**; *eidem,* **US 4012284** (1964, 1977 both to Soc. Farmaceut. Italia); S. Pinnert *et al.*, **US 3997662** (1976 to Rhone-Poulenc). Daunorubicin is a glycoside formed by a tetracyclic aglycone, *daunomycinone*, ($C_{21}H_{18}O_8$) and an amino sugar, *daunosamine*, ($C_6H_{13}NO_3$), 3-amino-2,3,6-trideoxy-L-*lyxo*-hexose: F. Arcamone *et al.*, *J. Am. Chem. Soc.* **86**, 5334, 5335 (1964); R. H. Iwamoto *et al.*, *Tetrahedron Lett.* **1968**, 3891. Absolute stereochemistry: F. Arcamone *et al.*, *Gazz. Chim. Ital.* **100**, 949-989 (1970). Identity with rubidomycin: G. L. Tong *et al.*, *J. Pharm. Sci.* **56**, 1691 (1967). Synthesis of daunosamine: J. P. Marsh *et al.*, *Chem. Commun.* **1967**, 973; T. Yamaguchi, M. Kojimo, *Carbohydr. Res.* **59**, 343 (1977); P. M. Wovkulich, M. R. Uskokovic, *J. Am. Chem. Soc.* **103**, 3956 (1981); of daunomycinone: C. M. Wong *et al.*, *Can. J. Chem.* **51**, 466 (1973); J. S. Swenton, P. W. Reynolds, *J. Am. Chem. Soc.* **100**, 6188 (1978); K. Krohn, K. Tolkiehn, *Ber.* **112**, 3453 (1979); F. M. Hauser, S. Prasanna, *J. Am. Chem. Soc.* **103**, 6378 (1981). Total synthesis of daunorubicin: E. M. Acton *et al.*, *J. Med. Chem.* **17**, 659 (1974). Purification: E. Oppici *et al.*, **BE 898506**; *eidem,* **GB 2133005** (both 1984 to Farmitalia). Toxicity data: A. Di Marco *et al.*, *Cancer Chemother. Rep. Part 1* **53**, 33 (1969). Review of properties, biosynthesis, fermentation: R. J. White, R. M. Stroshane, *Drugs Pharm. Sci.* **22**, 569-594 (1984); of carcinogenic action in laboratory animals: *IARC Monographs* **10**, 145-152 (1976); of toxicology: R. J. Maral *et al.*, *Cancer Treat. Rep.* **65**, Suppl. 4, 9-18 (1981); of use in treatment of solid tumors: R. B. Weiss *et al.*, *ibid.* 25-28; of interactions with nucleic acids: S. Neidle, M. R. Sanderson, in *Molecular Aspects of Anti-cancer Drug Action*, S. Neidle, M. J. Waring, Eds. (Verlag-Chemie, Florida, 1983) pp 35-55; of mechanism of cytotoxicity: H. S. Schwartz, *ibid.* pp 93-125; of metabolism and clinical pharmacokinetics: C. E. Riggs, Jr., *Semin. Oncol.* **11**, Suppl. 3, 2-11 (1984). *Review:* A. DiMarco *et al.*, *Antibiotics* vol. 3, J. W. Corcoran, F. E. Hahn, Eds. (Springer Verlag, New York, 1975) pp 101-128.

Daunomycinone

Daunosamine

mp 208-209°. LD₅₀ in mice, rats (mg/kg): 20, 13 i.v.; 5, 8 i.p. (DiMarco, 1977).

Hydrochloride. [23541-50-6] Cérubidine; Daunoblastina; Ondena. $C_{27}H_{29}NO_{10}$·HCl; mol wt 563.98. Thin red needles, dec 188-190°. $[\alpha]_D^{20}$ +248 ±5° (c = 0.05-0.1 in methanol). Sol in water, methanol, aq alcohols. Practically insol in chloroform, ether, benzene. Color of aq soln changes from pink at acid pH to blue at alkaline pH. Absorption max (methanol): 234, 252, 290, 480, 495, and 532 nm ($E_{1cm}^{1\%}$ 665, 462, 153, 214, 218, and 112). LD_{50} in mice (mg/kg): 26 i.v. (DiMarco, 1969).

THERAP CAT: Antineoplastic.

2833. Dauricine. [524-17-4] 4-[[(1R)-1,2,3,4-Tetrahydro-6,7-dimethoxy-2-methyl-1-isoquinolinyl]methyl]-2-[4-[[(1R)-1,2,-3,4-tetrahydro-6,7-dimethoxy-2-methyl-1-isoquinolinyl]methyl]-phenoxy]phenol. $C_{38}H_{44}N_2O_6$; mol wt 624.77. C 73.05%, H 7.10% N 4.48%, O 15.37%. From *Menispermum dauricum* DC., and *M. canadense* L., *Menispermaceae:* Kondo, Narita, *J. Pharm. Soc. Japan* no. 542, 279 (1927); *C.A.* **21**, 2700 (1927); Manske, *Can. J. Res.* **21B**, 17 (1943). Structure: Kondo *et al., Ber.* **68**, 519 (1935); Kondo, Tomita, *Arch. Pharm.* **274**, 65 (1936); Inubushi, Niwa, *J. Pharm. Soc. Jpn.* **72**, 762 (1952); *C.A.* **47**, 6430e (1953). Total synthesis: Kametani, Fukumoto, *J. Chem. Soc.* **1965**, Suppl. 2, 6141.

Slightly yellow amorphous base, mp 115°. $[\alpha]_D^{11}$ −139° in methanol. Sol in alc, acetone, benzene; slightly sol in ether.

Dimethiodide. $C_{38}H_{44}N_2O_6$·2CH$_3$I. Needles, mp 204°. $[\alpha]_D^{20}$ −114°.

2834. Dazomet. [533-74-0] Tetrahydro-3,5-dimethyl-2H-1,3,5-thiadiazine-2-thione; 2-thio-3,5-dimethyltetrahydro-1,3,5-thiadiazine; 3,5-dimethyl-2-thionotetrahydro-1,3,5-thiadiazine; dimethylformocarbothialdine; DMTT; UCC 974; Crag 974; Mylone. $C_5H_{10}N_2S_2$; mol wt 162.28. C 37.01%, H 6.21%, N 17.26%, S 39.52%. Prepd by the action of carbon disulfide on trimethyl-trimethylenetriimine: Delépine, *Bull. Soc. Chim.* **15**, 891 (1897); from formaldehyde and methylammonium methyldithiocarbamate: Bodendorf, *J. Prakt. Chem.* **126**, 233 (1930); Ainley *et al., J. Chem. Soc.* **1944**, 147. Prepd commercially by the reaction of carbon disulfide, methylamine and caustic soda: *Chem. Week* **79**, no. 18, 82-83 (1956). Toxicology study: H. F. Smyth, Jr. *et al., Toxicol. Appl. Pharmacol.* **9**, 521 (1966).

Needles from benzene, mp 106-107°. Soluble in alc with decompn. Dec by water, dil acids. uv max (cyclohexane): 242, 289 nm (ε 7150, 9900). LD_{50} in rats, mice, guinea pigs, rabbits (g/kg): 0.32-0.62, 0.18, 0.16, 0.12 orally; in rats, rabbits, dogs (g/kg): 0.087, 0.127, 0.047-0.063 i.p.; in rabbits (g/kg): 7.1 dermally (Smyth).

USE: Soil fungicide, nematocide, weed killer; slimicide in paper making.

2835. 2,4-DB. [94-82-6] 4-(2,4-Dichlorophenoxy)butanoic acid; 4-(2,4-dichlorophenoxy)butyric acid; Butyrac; Legumex D. $C_{10}H_{10}Cl_2O_3$; mol wt 249.09. C 48.22%, H 4.05%, Cl 28.47%, O 19.27%. Selective post-emergence, translocated herbicide. First described as a plant growth regulator: M. E. Synerholm and P. W. Zimmerman, *Contrib. Boyce Thompson Inst.* **14**, 369 (1947).

Prepn: G. W. Kitchingman, A. C. Tucker, **GB 804565** and **GB 883255** (1958, 1961, both to ICI). Similar in activity to 2,4-D, *q.v.,* but more selective. Mechanism of selectivity studies: D. L. King, D. E. Bayer, *Proc. West. Soc. Weed Sci.* **25**, 37 (1972).

White crystals, mp 117-119°. Soly in water at 25°: 46 ppm. Sol in acetone, ethanol, diethyl ether. Slightly sol in benzene, toluene, kerosene.

Sodium salt. Embutox. $C_{10}H_9Cl_2NaO_3$; mol wt 271.07. Water soluble; hard water will show precipitate as the calcium and magnesium salts.

Dimethylamine salt. Butoxone. $C_{12}H_{17}Cl_2NO_3$; mol wt 294.17. Water sol; calcium and magnesium salts precipitate in hard water.

USE: Herbicide.

2836. DBHBT. [63147-28-4] Mercaptoacetic acid [3,5-bis(1,1-dimethylethyl)-4-hydroxyphenyl]methyl ester; 3,5-di-*tert*-butyl-4-hydroxybenzylthioglycollate. $C_{17}H_{26}O_3S$; mol wt 310.45. C 65.77%, H 8.44%, O 15.46%, S 10.33%. Thermal stabilizer. Prepn: K. S. Cottman, **US 4020042** (1977 to Goodyear); and stabilization of acrylonitrile-butadiene-styrene (ABS) terpolymer: E. G. Kolawole, J. B. Adeniyi, *Eur. Polym. J.* **18**, 469 (1982). Stabilization of polystyrene and poly(methyl methacylate): E. G. Kolawole, *J. Appl. Polym. Sci.* **27**, 3437 (1982); of Nigerian natural rubber: G. C. Ebi, E. G. Kolawole, *ibid.* **45**, 2239 (1992).

White crystals from benzene, mp 107.5-108.5° (Cottman); also reported as mp 110° (Kolawole, Adeniyi).

USE: Antioxidant.

2837. DBMC. [497-39-2] 2,4-Bis(1,1-dimethylethyl)-5-methylphenol; 4,6-di-*tert*-butyl-*m*-cresol; 3-methyl-4,6-di-*tert*-butylphenol. $C_{15}H_{24}O$; mol wt 220.35. C 81.76%, H 10.98%, O 7.26%. Prepn: Weinrich, *Ind. Eng. Chem.* **35**, 264 (1943).

Crystals, mp 62.1°. bp 282°, bp$_{100}$ 211°, bp$_{20}$ 167°. d_4^{80} 0.912. Practically insol in water, ethylene glycol; sol in alcohol, benzene, carbon tetrachloride, ether, acetone.

USE: Intermediate in the production of rubber chemicals modified phenolic resins, synthetic musks of the ambrette type.

2838. DCM. [51325-91-8] [2-[2-[4-(Dimethylamino)phenyl]ethenyl]-6-methyl-4H-pyran-4-ylidene]propanedinitrile; 4-dicyanomethylene-2-methyl-6-p-dimethylaminostyryl-4H-pyran. $C_{19}H_{17}N_3O$; mol wt 303.36. C 75.23%, H 5.65%, N 13.85%, O 5.27%. Laser dye characterized by a broad tuning range. Prepn: F. G. Webster, W. C. McColgin, **FR 2156723**; *eidem,* **US 3852683** (1973, 1974 both to Eastman Kodak); P. R. Hammond, *Opt. Commun.* **29**, 331 (1979). Fluorescence lifetime measurements of cis/-trans isomers: M. Meyer *et al., Chem. Phys. Lett.* **150**, 484 (1988). Photophysical properties and consequences for use: J.-C. Mialocq, M. Meyer, *Laser Chem.* **10**, 277 (1990). Transient spectra: S. A. Kovalenko *et al., Chem. Phys. Lett.* **258**, 445 (1996). Use in polyimide systems for electro-optic devices: S. Ermer *et al., Appl. Phys. Lett.* **61**, 2272 (1992); in chemical actinometers: J.-C. Mialocq *et al., J. Photochem. Photobiol. A* **69**, 351 (1993).

Dark brown plates from benzene, mp 210-212°.
USE: Laser dye.

2839. DCPA. [1861-32-1] 2,3,5,6-Tetrachloro-1,4-benzene-dicarboxylic acid dimethyl ester; 2,3,5,6-tetrachloroterephthalic acid dimethyl ester; dimethyl 2,3,5,6-tetrachloroterephthalate; chlorthal-methyl; Dacthal; Rid. $C_{10}H_6Cl_4O_4$; mol wt 331.96. C 36.18%, H 1.82%, Cl 42.72%, O 19.28%. Prepn: Lindemann, US 2923634 (1960 to Diamond Alkali). Toxicity data: G. W. Bailey, J. L. White, *Residue Rev.* **10**, 97 (1965).

Crystals from methanol, mp 155-156°. Solubility: <5% in water; >5% in acetone, cyclohexanone, xylene. LD_{50} orally in rats: >3000 mg/kg (Bailey, White).
USE: Pre-emergent herbicide.

2840. DDD (Analytical). [6088-51-3] 6,6'-Dithiobis-2-naphthalenol; 6,6'-dithiodi-2-naphthol; bis(6-hydroxy-2-naphthyl)disulfide; 2,2'-dihydroxy-6,6'-dinaphthyl disulfide; 6,6'-dithiobis(2-naphthol). $C_{20}H_{14}O_2S_2$; mol wt 350.45. C 68.54%, H 4.03%, O 9.13%, S 18.30%. Prepn: Zincke, Dereser, *Ber.* **51**, 352 (1918).

Leaflets, mp 221-222°.
Note: Not to be confused with the insecticide, *p,p'*-DDD [1,1-dichloro-2,2-bis(*p*-chlorophenyl)ethane].
USE: For determination of protein-bound sulfhydryl groups.

2841. DDT. [50-29-3] 1,1'-(2,2,2-Trichloroethylidene)-bis[4-chlorobenzene]; 1,1,1-trichloro-2,2-bis(*p*-chlorophenyl)-ethane; α,α-bis(*p*-chlorophenyl)-β,β,β-trichlorethane; dichloro-diphenyltrichloroethane; chlorophenothane; clofenotane; dico-phane; pentachlorin; *p,p'*-DDT; Gesapon; Gesarex; Gesarol. $C_{14}H_9Cl_5$; mol wt 354.49. C 47.43%, H 2.56%, Cl 50.01%. Poly-chlorinated nondegradable pesticide; has been used as an ectopar-asiticide. Prepn: Zeidler, *Ber.* **7**, 1180 (1874); P. Müller, US 2329074 (1944 to Geigy); Rueggeberg, Torrans, *Ind. Eng. Chem.* **38**, 211 (1946); Cook *et al.*, *ibid.* **39**, 868, 1683 (1947). Convenient lab procedures: Bailes, *J. Chem. Educ.* **22**, 122 (1945); Ginsburg, *Science* **108**, 339 (1948). Large scale production: Mosher *et al.*, *Ind. Eng. Chem.* **38**, 916 (1946). Chemical composition of techni-cal grade: H. L Haller *et al.*, *J. Am. Chem. Soc.* **67**, 1591 (1945). Activity: P. Müller, *Helv. Chim. Acta* **29**, 1560 (1946). Compre-hensive monograph (in English and German): *DDT*, P. Müller, Ed., 3 vols (Birkhäuser Verlag, Basel and Stuttgart, 1955). Toxicity data: Gaines, *Toxicol. Appl. Pharmacol.* **2**, 88 (1960); **14**, 515 (1969). Review of toxicology and human exposure: *Toxicological Profile for DDT, DDE, DDD* (PB2003-100137, 2002) 497 pp; of toxicology and environmental impact: V. Turusov *et al.*, *Environ. Health Perspect.* **110**, 125-128 (2002).

Biaxial elongated tablets, needles from 95% alc. mp 108.5-109°. uv max (95% alc): 236 nm. Vapor pressure at 20° = 1.5×10^{-7} mm Hg. Practically insol in water, dil acids, alkalies. Soly (g/100 ml): acetone 58; benzene 78; benzyl benzoate 42; carbon tetra-chloride 45; chlorobenzene 74; cyclohexanone 116; 95% alc 2; ethyl ether 28; gasoline 10; isopropanol 3; kerosene 8-10; morpholine 75; peanut oil 11; pine oil 10-16; tetralin 61; tributyl phosphate 50; freely sol in pyridine, dioxane. The soly in organic solvents in-creases sharply with a rise in temp. Resistant to destruction by light and oxidation. Its unusual stability has resulted in difficulties in residue removal from water, soil and foodstuffs. Should not be kept in iron containers and should not be mixed with iron and aluminum salts nor with alkaline substances. High storage temps should also be avoided. Setting point of technical grade: 88.6-91.4°. LD_{50} in male, female rats (mg/kg): 113, 118 orally (Gaines, 1960).
Caution: Poisoning may occur by ingestion or by absorption through skin or respiratory tract. Potential symptoms of overexpo-sure are numbness, paresthesias, malaise, headache, sore throat, fatigue, weakness, coarse tremors, convulsions and coma; death due to respiratory failure. *See Clinical Toxicology of Commercial Products,* R. E. Gosselin *et al.*, Eds. (Williams & Wilkins, Balti-more, 5th ed., 1984) Section III, pp 134-138. This substance is reasonably anticipated to be a human carcinogen: *Report on Car-cinogens, Eleventh Edition* (PB2005-104914, 2004) p III-89.
USE: Contact insecticide.

2842. Deaminooxytocin. [113-78-0] 1-(3-Mercaptopropa-noic acid)oxytocin; demoxytocin; desaminooxytocin; ODA-914; Sandopart. $C_{43}H_{65}N_{11}O_{12}S_2$; mol wt 992.17. C 52.05%, H 6.60%, N 15.53%, O 19.35%, S 6.46%. Highly potent analog of the posterior pituitary hormone oxytocin, *q.v.*, differing in structure at the 1 position where the free amino group in the half-cystine residue is replaced by hydrogen. Synthesis and biological activity: du Vigneaud *et al.*, *J. Biol. Chem.* **235**, P.C. 64 (1960); Hope *et al.*, *ibid.* **237**, 1563 (1962); Takashima *et al.*, *J. Am. Chem. Soc.* **90**, 1323 (1968). Isoln and purifn: Ferrier *et al.*, *J. Biol. Chem.* **240**, 4264 (1965). Structure-activity correlation: Jarvis, du Vigneaud, *Sci-ence* **143**, 545 (1964). Synthesis of D-isomer: G. Flouret, V. du Vigneaud, *J. Med. Chem.* **14**, 556 (1971). Crystal structure analy-sis: S. P. Wood *et al.*, *Science* **232**, 633 (1986). Pharmacology and comparison with oxytocin: Chan, du Vigneaud, *Endocrinology* **71**, 977 (1962). *Review: Adv. Exp. Med. Biol.* vol. 2, 53-104 (1968).

$CH_2—CH_2—\overset{O}{\overset{\|}{C}}—Tyr–Ile–Gln–Asn–Cys–Pro–Leu–GlyNH_2$

L-Isomer. White plate-like crystals from water, mp 179° (Fer-rier); 182-183° (Takashima). For amorphous powder; $[\alpha]_D^{20}$ −88.3° (Ferrier); $[\alpha]_D^{21}$ −107° (Hope); $[\alpha]_D^{25}$ −95.1° (Takashima); all (c = 0.5 in 1N acetic acid). Anhydrous form is very hygroscopic.
D-Isomer. White, fluffy powder, $[\alpha]_D^{20}$ +104° (c = 0.5 in 1N acetic acid).
THERAP CAT: Oxytocic.

2843. Deanol. [108-01-0] 2-(Dimethylamino)ethanol; β-di-methylaminoethyl alcohol; N,N-dimethyl-2-hydroxyethylamine. $C_4H_{11}NO$; mol wt 89.14. C 53.90%, H 12.44%, N 15.71%, O 17.95%. $(CH_3)_2NCH_2CH_2OH$. Prepd from equimolar amounts of ethylene oxide and dimethylamine: Knorr, *Ber.* **37**, 3508 (1904); Hanhart, Ingold, *J. Chem. Soc.* **1927**, 1012. Clinical trial in hyper-kinetic children: N. Coleman *et al.*, *Psychosomatics* **17**, 68 (1976); in involuntary movement disorders: D. E. Casey, *Dis. Nerv. Syst.* **38**, 7 (1977).
Liquid. d_4^{20} 0.8866. bp_{758} 135°. n_D^{20} 1.43. Miscible with water, alcohol, ether.
Aceglumate. [3342-61-8] Clérégil; Risatarun. $C_4H_{11}NO.C_7H_{11}NO_5$; mol wt 278.30. Prepn: **FR M2487** (1964 to Interco Fribourg), *C.A.* **61**, 12085c (1964). Sol in water.
Acetamidobenzoate. [3635-74-3] Deaner; Pabenol. $C_4H_{11}NO.C_9H_9NO_3$; mol wt 268.31. Prepn: **GB 879259** (1957 to Riker Labs); A. Lasslo *et al.*, *J. Am. Pharm. Assoc. Sci. Ed.* **48**, 345 (1959). Crystals from absolute ethanol + ethyl acetate, mp 159-161.5°. Sol in water.
Bitartrate. [5988-51-2] Liparon. $C_4H_{11}NO.C_4H_6O_6$; mol wt 239.22. Crystals, sol in water.

Hemisuccinate. Tonibral; Rischiaril. $C_4H_{11}NO.C_4H_6O_4$; mol wt 207.22. White, hygroscopic crystalline powder. Very soluble in water, ethanol; sparingly sol in chloroform, benzene.

THERAP CAT: CNS stimulant.

2844. Debrisoquin. [1131-64-2] 3,4-Dihydro-2($1H$)-isoquinolinecarboximidamide; 3,4-dihydro-2($1H$)-isoquinolinecarboxamidine; 2-amidino-1,2,3,4-tetrahydroisoquinoline; isocaramidine. $C_{10}H_{13}N_3$; mol wt 175.23. C 68.54%, H 7.48%, N 23.98%. Prepn of derivs: W. Wenner, **BE 629007**; *idem*, **US 3157573** (1963, 1964 both to Hoffmann-La Roche); *idem, J. Med. Chem.* **8**, 125 (1965). Pharmacology: Moe *et al., Curr. Ther. Res.* **6**, 299 (1964); Abrams *et al., J. New Drugs* **4**, 268 (1964). Possible mechanism of action: Medina *et al., Biochem. Pharmacol.* **18**, 891 (1969); Pocelinko *et al., Int. Z. Klin. Pharmakol. Ther. Toxikol.* **2**, 13 (1969). Toxicity study: E. I. Goldenthal, *Toxicol. Appl. Pharmacol.* **18**, 185 (1971).

Sulfate. [581-88-4] Ro-5-3307/1; Declinax; Tendor. $2(C_{10}H_{13}N_3).H_2SO_4$; mol wt 448.54. Crystals, mp 278-280°, 284-285° or 266-268° (H_2O), depending on humidity. Freely sol in water. LD_{50} in neonate, adult rats (mg/kg): 88 ±18, 1580 ±163 orally (Goldenthal).

THERAP CAT: Antihypertensive.

2845. Decaborane(14). [17702-41-9] Decaboron tetradecahydride. $B_{10}H_{14}$; mol wt 122.22. B 88.46%, H 11.55%. Prepd by the pyrolysis of diborane(6). Reviews of chemistry: Griffo, *Diss. Abstr.* **22**, 2976 (1962); Stanko *et al., Usp. Khim.* **34**(6), 1011-1039 (1965). Review of structure and properties: Campbell, Jr., in *Progress in Boron Chemistry* vol. 1, Steinberg, McCloskey, Eds. (Macmillan, New York, 1964) pp 173-188. Reviews of toxicity: Levinskas, "Toxicology of Boron Compounds" in *Boron, Metallo-Boron Compounds and Boranes*, R. M. Adams, Ed. (Interscience, New York, 1964) pp 693-737; E. Browning, *Toxicity of Industrial Metals* (Appleton-Century-Crofts, New York, 2nd ed., 1969) pp 92-97. General reviews: Stock, *Hydrides of Boron and Silicon* (Cornell Univ. Press, Ithaca, 1933) *passim;* Siegel, Mack, *J. Chem. Educ.* **34**, 314-317 (1957); Major, *Chem. Eng. Prog.* **54**(3), 49-54 (1958); Lipscomb, *Boron Hydrides* (Benjamin, New York, 1963) *passim;* Adams in *Boron, Metallo-Boron Compounds and Boranes loc. cit.,* pp 647-663; Hawthorn in *Adv. Inorg. Chem. Radiochem.* **5**, 307-345 (1963); Greenwood in *Comprehensive Inorganic Chemistry* vol. 1, J. C. Bailar, Jr. *et al.*, Eds. (Pergamon Press, Oxford, 1973) pp 818-837.

Orthorhombic crystals. mp 99.6-99.7°; bp 213°; bp_{19} 100°. d_4^{25} 0.94; d_4^{100} (liq) 0.78. Stable indefinitely at room temp; decomp slowly into B + H_2 at 300°. Heat of fusion: 7.8 kcal/mole; of sublimation: 18.33 kcal/mole; of vaporization: 11.6 kcal/mole. Slightly sol in cold water; hydrolyzes in hot water. Sol in ethyl acetate, 1-bromopropane, ethyl silicate, carbon disulfide, benzene, alcohol, acetic anhydride, acetic acid, ethyl borate, carbon tetrachloride. *Highly reactive.* Reacts with amides, acetone, butyraldehyde, acetonitrile at room temp. Decaborane mixtures with carbon tetrachloride are dangerously shock sensitive.

Caution: Potential symptoms of overexposure are dizziness, headache, nausea, lightheadedness and drowsiness; incoordination, local muscle spasms, tremor and convulsions; fatigue. *See NIOSH Pocket Guide to Chemical Hazards* (DHHS/NIOSH 97-140, 1997) p 88. See also *Patty's Industrial Hygiene and Toxicology* vol. 2B, G. D. Clayton, F. E. Clayton, Eds. (Wiley-Interscience, New York, 3rd ed., 1981) 2987-2990.

USE: In rocket propellants; as catalyst in olefin polymerization.

2846. Decalin®. [91-17-8] Decahydronaphthalene; perhydronaphthalene; bicyclo[4.4.0]decane; naphthalane; naphthane; DeKalin. $C_{10}H_{18}$; mol wt 138.25. C 86.88%, H 13.12%. Occurs in two forms: *cis* and *trans.* Hydrogenation of naphthalene in glacial acetic acid in the presence of platinum catalyst at 25° and 130 atm yields a mixture of 77% *cis*-Decalin and 23% *trans*-Dec-

alin. Hydrogenation of Tetralin under the same conditions yields almost only *cis*-Decalin: Baker, Schuetz, *J. Am. Chem. Soc.* **69**, 1250 (1947). Hydrogenation of $\Delta^{4a(8a)}$-octalin in ethanol in the presence of platinum yields *trans*-Decalin as the main component: Linstead *et al., J. Chem. Soc.* **1937**, 1136. Separation of *trans*- and *cis*-forms: Seyer, Walker, *J. Am. Chem. Soc.* **60**, 2125 (1938). Prepn of *trans*-Decalin from *cis*-Decalin: Zelinsky, *Ber.* **65**, 1299 (1932). Conformation studies: Barton, *J. Chem. Soc.* **1948**, 340; Moniz, Dixon, *J. Am. Chem. Soc.* **83**, 1671 (1961). Toxicity data: Smyth *et al., Arch. Ind. Hyg. Occup. Med.* **4**, 119 (1951).

trans   cis

Liquid. Slight odor resembling menthol. Pure Decalin does not smell of naphthalene. Volatile with steam. The commercial product may be practically all *trans*-Decalin, or a mixture contg up to 60% *cis*-Decalin. The commercial mixture has a flash pt (closed cup) of about 136°F (58°C). Autoignition temp 504°F. Insol in water. Very sol in alcohol, methanol, ether, chloroform. Miscible with propyl and isopropyl alcohol; miscible with most ketones and esters. LD_{50} orally in rats: 4.2 g/kg; LC (in air) in rats: 500 ppm (Smyth).

cis-Form. mp −43.26°. bp 195.7°; bp_9 67.0°. d_4^{20} 0.8963. n_D^{20} 1.48113.

trans-Form. mp −30.4°. bp 187.25°; bp_9 62.0°. d_4^{20} 0.8700. n_D^{20} 1.46968.

USE: Solvent for naphthalene, fats, resins, oils, waxes; used instead of turpentine in lacquers, shoe polishes, floor waxes. In motor fuel and lubricants. As patent fuel in stoves.

2847. Decamethonium Bromide. [541-22-0] N,N,N,N',N',N'-Hexamethyl-1,10-decanediaminium dibromide; decamethylenebis[trimethylammonium bromide]; C-10; Syncurine. $C_{16}H_{38}Br_2N_2$; mol wt 418.29. C 45.94%, H 9.16%, Br 38.21%, N 6.70%. $[(CH_3)_3N^+(CH_2)_{10}N^+(CH_3)_3].2Br^-$. Prepn: Blomquist *et al., J. Am. Chem. Soc.* **81**, 678 (1959).

Crystals from methanol + acetone, dec 268-270°. Freely sol in water, alcohol; very slightly sol in chloroform. Practically insol in ether. Aq solns are stable and may be sterilized by autoclaving.

THERAP CAT: Neuromuscular blocking agent.

2848. Decamethylcyclopentasiloxane. [541-02-6] D_5. $C_{10}H_{30}O_5Si_5$; mol wt 370.77. C 32.39%, H 8.16%, O 21.58%, Si 37.87%. Cyclic siloxane. Isolated from the hydrolysis product of dimethyldichlorosilane: W. Patnode, D. F. Wilcock, *J. Am. Chem. Soc.* **68**, 358 (1946). HPLC determn and GC-MS characterization of metabolites in urine: S. Varaprath *et al., Drug Metab. Dispos.* **31**, 206 (2003). Physicochemical properties: M. Palczewska-Tulinska, P. Oracz, *J. Chem. Eng. Data* **50**, 1711 (2005).

Colorless volatile liquid. mp −38°. bp_{760} 210°; bp_{20} 101°. d 0.9593. n_D^{20} 1.3982. Soly in water: 17 ppb. Vapor pressure (50°): 2 mm Hg.

USE: Intermediate in the mfr of high mol wt siloxane polymers. Carrier ingredient in personal care products; dry cleaning solvent.

2849. Decamethylene Glycol. [112-47-0] 1,10-Decanediol. $C_{10}H_{22}O_2$; mol wt 174.28. C 68.92%, H 12.72%, O 18.36%. $HO(CH_2)_{10}OH$. Prepd by the reduction of dimethyl or diethyl sebacate with sodium and ethyl alcohol: Bouveault, Blanc, *Compt. Rend.* **137**, 329 (1903); *Bull. Soc. Chim.* [3] **31**, 1205 (1904); **DE**

164294; *Frdl.* **8,** 1260 (1905); Chuit, *Helv. Chim. Acta* **9,** 264 (1926); Manske, *Org. Synth.* **14,** 20 (1934). By catalytic hydrogenation of sebacic esters: Folkers, Adkins, *J. Am. Chem. Soc.* **54,** 1146 (1932).

Needles from water or dil alcohol. mp 74°. bp$_{20}$ 192°; bp$_{11}$ 179°; bp$_8$ 170°. Freely sol in alcohol, warm ether; almost insol in petr ether and water.

Diethyl ether. 1,10-Diethoxydecane. $C_{14}H_{30}O_2$. d_0^0 0.850; bp 260°.

2850. Decamethyltetrasiloxane. [141-62-8] $C_{10}H_{30}O_3Si_4$; mol wt 310.69. C 38.66%, H 9.73%, O 15.45%, Si 36.16%. Prepn: Patnode, Wilcock, *J. Am. Chem. Soc.* **68,** 358 (1946).

$$(H_3C)_3Si-O-\underset{CH_3}{\overset{H_3C}{Si}}-O-\underset{CH_3}{\overset{H_3C}{Si}}-O-Si(CH_3)_3$$

Liquid. bp 194°. d 0.8536. n_D^{20} 1.3895. mp ~ −70°. Stable. Inert to most chemical reagents and rubber. Maintains about the same viscosity over a wide temp range. Sol in benzene and the lighter hydrocarbons; slightly sol in alc and heavy hydrocarbons.

USE: As a basis for silicone oils or fluids designed to withstand extremes of temp; as a foam suppressant in petr lubricating oil.

2851. Dechlorane® Plus. [13560-89-9] 1,2,3,4,7,8,9,10,- 13,13,14,14-Dodecachloro-1,4,4a,5,6,6a,7,10,10a,11,12,12a-dodec- ahydro-1,4:7,10-dimethanodibenzo[a,e]cyclooctene; bis(hexachlo- rocyclopentadieno)cyclooctane. $C_{18}H_{12}Cl_{12}$; mol wt 653.72. C 33.07%, H 1.85%, Cl 65.08%. Polychlorinated hydrocarbon. Prepn by Diels-Alder reaction between cyclooctadiene and hexa- chlorocyclopentadiene: K. Ziegler, H. Froitzheim-Kühlhorn, *Ann.* **589,** 157 (1954). Use as fire-retardant for plastics: E. V. Gouin- lock, Jr., *US* **3382204** (1965 to Hooker). Accumulation in juvenile Atlantic salmon: V. Zitko, *Chemosphere* **9,** 73 (1980). Brief re- view of fire retardant props: T. J. Machmer, *Life Prop. Protect., Fire Retard. Chem. Assoc., Semi-Annu. Meet.* **1977,** 156-174.

Colorless crystals, mp >325°. Soluble in *o*-dichlorobenzene.

USE: Fire retardant for plastics.

2852. Decimemide. [14817-09-5] 4-(Decyloxy)-3,5-di- methoxybenzamide; EGYT-1050; Denegyt. $C_{19}H_{31}NO_4$; mol wt 337.45. C 67.63%, H 9.26%, N 4.15%, O 18.97%. Prepn: **NL** **6605460**; E. Kasztreiner *et al.*, *US* **3432549** (1966, 1969 both to EGYT). Pharmacology: E. Kasztreiner, *Magy. Kem. Lapja* **27,** 370 (1972), *C.A.* **78,** 66697z (1973); I. Kiraly *et al.*, *Acta Physiol. Acad. Sci. Hung.* **47,** 200 (1976). Metabolism study: G. Molnar *et al.*, *Acta Pharm. Hung.* **48,** Suppl., 58 (1978). Toxicity data: E. Usdin, D. H. Efron, Eds., *Psychotropic Drugs and Related Compounds* (NIH, Washington, D. C., 2nd Ed., 1972) p 377.

Cryst from methanol, mp 121-122°. LD$_{50}$ in mice, rats (mg/kg): 2950, 1650 orally (Udsin, Efron).

THERAP CAT: Anticonvulsant.

2853. Decitabine. [2353-33-5] 4-Amino-1-(2-deoxy-β- *erythro*-pentofuranosyl)-1,3,5-triazin-2(1*H*)-one; 5-aza-2′-deoxycy- tidine; NSC-127716; Dacogen. $C_8H_{12}N_4O_4$; mol wt 228.21. C 42.10%, H 5.30%, N 24.55%, O 28.04%. Pyrimidine analog that inhibits DNA methylation and induces differentiation of leukemic cells. Prepn: J. Pliml, F. Sorm, *Collect. Czech. Chem. Commun.* **29,** 2576 (1964); A. Piskala, F. Sorm, in *Nucleic Acid Chemistry* Part 1 (Wiley, New York, 1978) pp 443-449. Improved synthesis: J. Ben-Hattar, J. Jiricny, *Nucleosides Nucleotides* **6,** 393 (1987). Chemical stability in soln: K.-T. Lin *et al.*, *J. Pharm. Sci.* **70,** 1228 (1981). HPLC determn in plasma: *eidem, J. Chromatogr.* **345,** 162 (1985). Clinical trial in chronic myelogenous leukemia: H. M. Kantarjian *et al.*, *Cancer* **98,** 522 (2003). Review of phar- macology and mechanism of action: R. L. Momparler, *Pharmacol. Ther.* **30,** 287-299 (1985); *idem et al.*, *Leukemia* **11,** Suppl. 1, 1-6 (1997); of clinical experience: B. T. Hennessy *et al.*, *Expert. Opin. Invest. Drugs* **12,** 1985-1993 (2003).

Crystals from methanol, mp 201-202° (dec). $[\alpha]_D^{22}$ +68.5° (30 min) → +57.8° (6 hr) (c = 0.5 in water). uv max (pH 7): 244 nm (log ε 3.86). LD$_{50}$ in mice (mg/kg): 190 i.p. (Momparler, 1985).

THERAP CAT: Antineoplastic.

2854. Decoquinate. [18507-89-6] 6-Decyloxy-7-ethoxy-4- hydroxy-3-quinolinecarboxylic acid ethyl ester; ethyl 6-(*n*-decyl- oxy)-7-ethoxy-4-hydroxyquinoline-3-carboxylate; M & B 15497; Deccox. $C_{24}H_{35}NO_5$; mol wt 417.54. C 69.04%, H 8.45%, N 3.35%, O 19.16%. Description of compd: Ball *et al.*, *Chem. Ind. (London)* **1968,** 56; **BE 698305** (1966 to May & Baker). Metabo- lism and residue studies: Craine *et al.*, *J. Agric. Food Chem.* **19,** 1228 (1971); Kouba *et al.*, *ibid.* 1234.

THERAP CAT (VET): Coccidiostat.

2855. *n*-Decyl Alcohol. [112-30-1] 1-Decanol; nonylcarbi- nol. $C_{10}H_{22}O$; mol wt 158.28. C 75.88%, H 14.01%, O 10.11%. $CH_3(CH_2)_8CH_2OH$. Prepn from caprinaldehyde: Krafft, *Ber.* **16,** 1717 (1883); from capric acid methyl ester: Bouveault, Blanc, *Bull. Soc. Chim.* [3] **31,** 674 (1904); from 1-chlorodecane: Schultz, *Ber.* **42,** 3611 (1909); from nonylmagnesium bromide and formaldehyde: Yohe, Adams, *J. Am. Chem. Soc.* **50,** 1507 (1928). Manuf: *Faith, Keyes & Clark's Industrial Chemicals,* F. A. Lowenheim, M. K. Moran, Eds. (Wiley-Interscience, New York, 4th ed., 1975) pp 310- 317.

Moderately viscous, strongly refractive liq. Solidifies forming rectangular plates or leaflets; mp 6.4°. bp$_{760}$ 232.9°; bp$_{15}$ 115-120°; bp$_8$ 109.5°. d_4^{20} 0.8297. n_D^{20} 1.43587. Insol in water. Sol in alcohol, ether.

USE: In the manuf of plasticizers, synthetic lubricants, petroleum additives, herbicides, surface active agents, solvents. Has moderate antifoaming capacity.

2856. Deet. [134-62-3] *N,N*-Diethyl-3-methylbenzamide; *N,N*-diethyl-*m*-toluamide; M-Det; *m*-DETA; ENT-20218; *m*-Del- phene; Detamide; Dieltamid; Flypel; Metadelphene; OFF!; Repel. $C_{12}H_{17}NO$; mol wt 191.27. C 75.35%, H 8.96%, N 7.32%, O 8.36%. Technical deet contains a minimum of 95% meta isomer; commercial formulations contain 11.27-100% deet by weight. Prepn from *m*-toluoyl chloride and diethylamine in benzene or ether: Maxim, *Bull. Soc. Chim. Romania* **11,** 29 (1929); *Chem. Zentralbl.* **1929,** II, 2324, *C.A.* **24,** 94 (1930); *Beilstein* **9,** II, 325; E. T. McCabe *et al.*, *J. Org. Chem.* **19,** 493 (1954). Repellent activity vs mosquitoes: I. H. Gilbert *et al., J. Econ. Entomol.* **48,** 741 (1955). Toxicity study: A. M. Ambrose *et al., Toxicol. Appl. Pharmacol.* **1,** 97 (1959). Metabolism: L. Blomquist, W. Thorsell, *Acta Pharmacol. Toxicol.* **41,** 235 (1977). Physical, chemical and toxicological properties and insect repellent efficacy: *Pesticide Registration Standard - Deet* (U.S. EPA 504/RS-81-004, Washington, D.C., 1980) 82 pp. HPLC determn including metabolites: J. M. Yeung, W. G. Taylor, *Drug Metab. Dispos.* **16,** 600 (1988). Comparative study of efficacy vs mosquitoes: M. S. Fradin, J. F. Day, *N. Engl. J. Med.* **347,** 13 (2002). Review of safety: T. G. Osimitz, R. H. Grothaus, *J. Am. Mosq. Control Assoc.* **11,** 274-278 (1995); and pharmacokinetics and formulation: H. Qiu *et al., ibid.* **14,** 12-27 (1998).

Nearly colorless to amberlike liquid, faint aromatic odor. $bp_{1.0}$ 111°. d^{25} 0.990-1.000. n_D^{25} 1.5206. Flash pt, open cup: 311°F (155°C). Partition coefficient (octane/water): 105. Vapor pressure at 25°: 1.67×10^{-3} mm Hg. Viscosity at 30°: 13.3 cP. Soly in water at 25°: 9.9 mg/ml. Practically insol in glycerin. Miscibile with ethanol, ether, isopropanol, chloroform, benzene, and carbon disulfide. Hygroscopic. Light sensitive. LD_{50} orally in male rats (ml/kg): 2.43; in female rats: 1.78; dermally in rabbits: ≥3.18. LC_{50} by inhalation in rats (mg/l): 5.95 (U.S. EPA).

Caution: Direct contact may cause eye irritation (U.S. EPA). *See also: Clinical Toxicology of Commercial Products,* R. E. Gosselin *et al.,* Eds. (Williams & Wilkins, Baltimore, 5th ed., 1984) Section II, p 346.

USE: Insect repellent.

2857. Defensins. [103220-14-0] A class of low molecular weight cationic peptides which have *in vitro* microbiocidal activity against various bacteria, fungi, and viruses, originally isolated from mammalian neutrophils. Possess similar arginine-rich, cysteine-rich structures of 29-35 amino acids with a conserved core of 8-11 residues. Characterized by six cysteines comprising 3 disulfide linkages. Abbreviated NP (neutrophil peptide) where NP is used for rabbit, HNP for human, GPNP for guinea pig etc.; defensins represent a major protein component of granulocytes. Initial identification studies: H. I. Zeya, J. K. Spitznagel, *Science* **142,** 1085 (1961); *eidem, J. Bacteriol.* **91,** 750 (1966). Isoln, antimicrobial activities and amino acid sequence of six NPs: M. E. Selsted *et al., Infect. Immun.* **45,** 150 (1984); M. E. Selsted *et al., J. Biol. Chem.* **260,** 4579 (1985); of three HNPs: T. Ganz *et al., J. Clin. Invest.* **76,** 1427 (1985); M. E. Selsted *et al., ibid.* 1436. Crystal structure of HNP-3: C. P. Hill *et al., Science* **251,** 1481 (1991). Direct inactivation of enveloped viruses: K. A. Daher *et al., J. Virol.* **60,** 1068 (1986). *In vitro* cytolysis of tumor cells: A. Lichtenstein *et al., Blood* **68,** 1407 (1986). Mechanism of cytolysis: *eidem, J. Immunol.* **140,** 2686 (1988). Identification and isoln of insect defensins from haemolymph of dipteran: J. A. Hoffmann, D. Hoffmann, *Res. Immunol.* **141,** 910 (1990). Structure determn of insect forms: P. Lepage *et al., Eur. J. Biochem.* **196,** 735 (1991). Review of insect forms: J. A. Hoffmann, C. Hetru, *Immunol. Today* **13,** 411-415 (1992). *Review:* B. L. Kagan *et al., Toxicology* **87,** 131-149 (1994); including insect forms: T. Ganz, R. I. Lehrer, *Pharmacol. Ther.* **66,** 191-205 (1995).

2858. Deferasirox. [201530-41-8] 4-[3,5-Bis(2-hydroxyphenyl)-1*H*-1,2,4-triazol-1-yl]benzoic acid; ICL-670; ICL-670A; CGP-72670; Exjade. $C_{21}H_{15}N_3O_4$; mol wt 373.36. C 67.56%, H 4.05%, N 11.25%, O 17.14%. Orally active tridentate iron chelator. Prepn: R. Lattmann, P. Acklin, **WO 9749395**; *eidem,* **US 6465504** (1997, 2002 both to Novartis); U. Heinz *et al., Angew. Chem. Int. Ed.* **38,** 2568 (1999). HPLC determn in plasma: M. C. Rouan *et al., J. Chromatogr. B* **755,** 203 (2001). Iron complex formation study: S. Steinhauser *et al., Eur. J. Inorg. Chem.* **2004,** 4177. Pharmacology: C. Hershko *et al., Blood* **97,** 1115 (2001). Clinical pharmacokinetics: R. Galanello *et al., J. Clin. Pharmacol.*

43, 565 (2003). Clinical trial in thalassemia: E. Nisbet-Brown *et al., Lancet* **361,** 1597 (2003). Review of structure activity: H. Nick *et al., Curr. Med. Chem.* **10,** 1065-1076 (2003); of preclinical and clinical experience: M. D. Cappellini, *Best Prac. Res. Clin. Haematol.* **18,** 289-298 (2005).

Crystals from ethanol, mp 264-265°. Soly in water at 25° (mg/ml): 0.4 (pH 7.40). pKa_1 4.57, pKa_2 8.71, pKa_3 10.56 (Nick). Also reported in H_2O/DMSO ($X_{DMSO} = 0.20$) as pKa_1 4.61, pKa_2 10.12, pKa_3 12.08 (Steinhauser). Partition coefficient (octanol/water): 6.3 (pH 7.40). uv max (H_2O/DMSO, pH < 2): 284 nm (ε 1.5×10^4).

THERAP CAT: Chelating agent (iron).

2859. Deferiprone. [30652-11-0] 3-Hydroxy-1,2-dimethyl-4(1*H*)-pyridinone; 1,2-dimethyl-3-hydroxypyrid-4-one; DMHP; L1; CP-20; Kelfer. $C_7H_9NO_2$; mol wt 139.15. C 60.42%, H 6.52%, N 10.07%, O 23.00%. Orally active chelator that promotes urinary iron excretion. Prepn: M. Yasue *et al., Yakugaku Zasshi* **90,** 1222 (1970), *C.A.* **74,** 23102b (1971); G. J. Kontoghiorghes *et al., Arzneim.-Forsch.* **37,** 1099 (1987). Iron binding studies: *idem, Inorg. Chim. Acta* **135,** 145 (1987). HPLC determn in serum and urine: B. Dresow *et al., J. Anal. Chem.* **352,** 562 (1995). Clinical pharmacokinetics: F. N. Al-Refaie *et al., Br. J. Haematol.* **89,** 403 (1995). Clinical studies in transfusional iron overload: *idem et al., ibid.* **91,** 224 (1995); N. F. Olivieri *et al., N. Engl. J. Med.* **332,** 918 (1995). Review of pharmacology and clinical experience: G. J. Kontoghiorghes, *Ann. N.Y. Acad. Sci.* **612,** 339-350 (1990); F. N. Al-Refaie, A. V. Hoffbrand, *Baill. Clin. Haematol.* **7,** 941-963 (1994); of toxicology: G. J. Kontoghiorghes, *Toxicol. Lett.* **80,** 1-18 (1995).

Needles from water, mp 266-268° (Yasue); also reported as mp 263-266° (Kontoghiorghes *et al.,* 1987). Very bitter taste. Soly at 37° (mg/ml): water ~20 (pH 7.40). pKa_1 3.3, pKa_2 9.7. uv max (phosphate buffer saline, pH 7.3): 460 nm (ε 3600). Hydrophilic chelator; forms red colored complexes with iron. LD_{50} i.p. in rats, mice: 650 mg/kg, 0.8-1.0 g/kg; i.g. in rats: 2.0-3.0 g/kg (Kontoghiorghes, 1995).

THERAP CAT: Chelating agent (iron and aluminum).

2860. Deferoxamine. [70-51-9] *N'*-[5-[[4-[[5-(Acetylhydroxyamino)pentyl]amino]-1,4-dioxobutyl]hydroxyamino]pentyl]-*N*-(5-aminopentyl)-*N*-hydroxybutanediamide; *N*-[5-[3-[(5-aminopentyl)hydroxycarbamoyl]propionamido]pentyl]-3-[[5-(*N*-hydroxyacetamido)pentyl]carbamoyl]propionohydroxamic acid; 1-amino-6,17-dihydroxy-7,10,18,21-tetraoxo-27-(*N*-acetylhydroxylamino)-6,11,17,22-tetraazaheptaeicosane; desferrioxamine B. $C_{25}H_{48}N_6O_8$; mol wt 560.68. C 53.55%, H 8.63%, N 14.99%, O 22.83%. Natural product forming iron complexes, isolated from *Streptomyces pilosus* Ettlinger *et al.* Prepn from ferrioxamine B and structure: H. Bickel *et al., Helv. Chim. Acta* **43,** 2129 (1960). Syntheses: V. Prelog, A. Walser, *ibid.* **45,** 631 (1962); **BE 609053**; E. Gaeumann *et al.,* **US 3471476** (1962, 1969 both to Ciba). Derivatives: H. Bickel *et al., Helv. Chim. Acta* **46,** 1385 (1963). Clinical efficacy in thallasemia major (Cooley's anemia): B. Modell *et al., Br. Med. J.* **284**, 1081 (1982). Treatment of hemodialysis-induced aluminum accumulation in brain: P. Ackril *et al, Lancet* **2**, 692 (1980); in bone: H. H. Malluche *et al., N. Engl. J. Med.* **311**, 140 (1984). Neurotoxicity study: N. F. Olivieri *et al., ibid.* **314**, 869 (1986). Review of clinical experience: R. Propper, D. Nathan, *Annu. Rev. Med.* **33**, 509-519 (1982).

Monohydrate. Crystals from dil alcohol, mp 138-140°. Sol in water at 20°: 1.2%.

Hydrochloride. [1950-39-6] Ba-29837. $C_{25}H_{48}N_6O_8 \cdot HCl$; mol wt 597.14. Crystals from slightly acidic methanol, mp 172-175°.

Methanesulfonate. [138-14-7] Desferrioxamine mesylate; DFOM; Desferal. $C_{25}H_{48}N_6O_8 \cdot CH_3SO_3H$; mol wt 656.79. Crystals from dil alcohol, mp 148-149°. Sol in water at 20°: >20%.

N-Acetyl derivative. *N*-Acetyldeferoxamine; *N*-acetyldesferrioxamine B. $C_{27}H_{50}N_6O_9$. Crystals from *n*-propanol, mp 180-182°.

Iron complex. Ferrioxamine B. $C_{25}H_{45}FeN_6O_8$. A natural microbial growth factor. Isoln: H. Bickel *et al., Helv. Chim. Acta* **43**, 2118 (1960); E. Gaeumann *et al.,* **US 3118823; US 3153621** (both 1964 to Ciba).

Note: Reviews on iron-containing metabolites with growth stimulating properties, *sideramines*, or with antibiotic properties, *sideromycins, ferrimycins*: H. Bickel *et al., Experientia* **16**, 129-133 (1960); V. Prelog, *Pure Appl. Chem.* **6**, 327-338 (1963); F. Knüsel, J. Nüesch, *Nature* **206**, 674-676 (1965); T. F. Emery, *Adv. Enzymol. Relat. Areas Mol. Biol.* **35**, 135-185 (1971); Knüsel, Zimmermann, in *Antibiotics* vol. 3, J. W. Corcoran, F. E. Hahn, Eds. (Springer-Verlag, New York, 1975) pp 653-667.

THERAP CAT: Parenteral chelating agent (iron and aluminum). Methanesulfonate as antidote to iron poisoning.

2861. Defibrotide. [83712-60-1] Fraction P; defibrinotide; Dasovas; Noravid; Prociclide. Sodium salt of polydeoxyribonucleotide extract from mammalian lung which stimulates fibrinolysis. mol wt 45,000-50,000 daltons. Prepn: A. Butti *et al.,* **DE 2154278**; *eidem,* **US 3899481** (1972, 1975 both to Crinos). Antithrombotic activity: R. Niada *et al., Thromb. Res.* **23**, 233 (1981). Pharmacokinetics and profibrinolytic activity in rabbits: R. Pescador *et al., ibid.* **30**, 1 (1983). Clinical trial as antithrombotic: S. Coccheri *et al., Int. J. Clin. Pharmacol. Res.* **2**, 227 (1982). Clinical evaluation in thrombotic microangiopathy: V. Bonomini *et al., Nephron* **40**, 195 (1985). Symposium on pharmacology and clinical efficacy: O. N. Ulutin, Ed., *Haemostasis* **16**, Suppl. 1, 1-68 (1986). Review of pharmacology and therapeutic use: K. J. Palmer, K. L. Goa, *Drugs* **45**, 259-294 (1993).

THERAP CAT: Antithrombotic.

2862. Deflazacort. [14484-47-0] (11β,16β)-21-(Acetyloxy)-11-hydroxy-2'-methyl-5'*H*-pregna-1,4-dieno[17,16-*d*]oxazole-3,20-dione; 11β,21-dihydroxy-2'-methyl-5'β*H*-pregna-1,4-dieno[17,16-*d*]oxazole-3,20-dione 2l-acetate; pregna-1,4-diene-11β,21-diol-3,20-dione[17α,16α-*d*]-2'-methyloxazoline 21-acetate; oxazacort; azacort; DL-458-IT; L-5458; Calcort; Deflan; Dezacor; Flantadin; Lantadin. $C_{25}H_{31}NO_6$; mol wt 441.52. C 68.01%, H 7.08%, N 3.17%, O 21.74%. Systemic corticosteroid; oxazoline derivative of prednisolone, *q.v.* Prepn: G. Nathansohn, G. Winters, **BE 679820**; *eidem,* **GB 1077393**; *eidem,* **US 3436389** (1966, 1967, 1969 all to Lepetit); G. Nathansohn *et al., J. Med. Chem.* **10**, 799 (1967). Pharmacology: P. Schiatti *et al., Arzneim.-Forsch.* **30**, 1543 (1980). Pharmacokinetics: A. Assandri *et al., Eur. J. Drug Metab. Pharmacokinet.* **5**, 207 (1980); *eidem, Adv. Exp. Med. Biol.* **171**, 9 (1984). Immunosuppressive activity in humans: B. H. Hahn *et al., J. Rheumatol.* **8**, 783 (1981). Effect on human mineral metabolism: T. J. Hahn *et al., Calcif. Tissue Int.* **31**, 109 (1980); on human glucose metabolism: P. Cavallo-Perin *et al., Eur. J. Clin. Pharmacol.* **26**, 357 (1984). Clinical comparison with prednisone, *q.v.,* in rheumatoid arthritis and lupus: B. Imbimbo *et al., Adv. Exp. Med. Biol.* **171**, 241 (1984).

Crystals from acetone-hexane, mp 255-256.5°. $[\alpha]_D$ +62.3° (c = 0.5 in chloroform). uv max (methanol): 241-242 nm ($E_{1cm}^{1\%}$ 352.5). LD_{50} orally in mice: 5200 mg/kg (Schiatti).

THERAP CAT: Anti-inflammatory; glucocorticoid.

2863. Deguelin. [522-17-8] (7a*S-cis*)-13,13a-Dihydro-9,10-dimethoxy-3,3-dimethyl-3*H*-bis[1]benzopyrano[3,4-*b*:6',5'-*e*]pyran-7(7a*H*)-one. $C_{23}H_{22}O_6$; mol wt 394.42. C 70.04%, H 5.62%, O 24.34%. From roots of *Tephrosia toxicaria* Pers., leaves of *Tephrosia vogelii* Hook f., *Leguminosae*, and from derris and cubé roots: H. L. Haller, F. B. LaForge, *J. Am. Chem. Soc.* **56**, 2415 (1934); E. Brierly, H. J. Smith, *J. Pharm. Pharmacol.* **20**, 840 (1968). Structure: Clark, *J. Am. Chem. Soc.* **54**, 3000 (1932). Stereoselective synthesis: P. B. Anzeveno, *J. Org. Chem.* **44**, 2578 (1979). Total synthesis of racemate: Fukami *et al., Agric. Biol. Chem.* **25**, 252 (1961); Omokawa, Yamashita, *ibid.* **38**, 1731 (1974). Stereochemical studies: Djerassi *et al., J. Chem. Soc.* **1961**, 1448.

Yellow oil, $[\alpha]_D^{27}$ −97.2° (c = 0.2 in benzene).

(±)-Form. Pale green crystals, mp 171°. Practically insol in water. Sol in alc.

Caution: Irritates skin. Inhalation may cause fatal pulmonary damage.

USE: Insecticide.

2864. DEHP. [117-81-7] 1,2-Benzenedicarboxylic acid bis(2-ethylhexyl) ester; bis(2-ethylhexyl) phthalate; di(2-ethylhexyl) phthalate; DOP; dioctyl phthalate; Octoil. $C_{24}H_{38}O_4$; mol wt 390.56. C 73.81%, H 9.81%, O 16.39%. Dialkyl phthalate ester plasticizer used to impart softness and flexiblilty to PVC products. Prepn: P. J. Garner, G. Watson, **US 2508911** (1950 to Shell). Effect on dynamic mechanical properties: D. L. Hertz, Jr., *Elastomerics* **116**, 20 (1984); interaction with PVC polymer: B. Garnaik, S. Sivaram, *Macromolecules* **29**, 185 (1996). HPLC determn in PVC packaging: M. F. Aignasse *et al., Int. J. Pharm.* **113**, 241 (1995). GC/MS determn in toys: R. Stringer *et al., Environ. Sci. Pollut. Res. Int.* **7**, 27 (2000). Evaluation of carcinogenic risk: J. Doull *et al., Regul. Toxicol. Pharmacol.* **29**, 327 (1999); of health effects: M. Fay *et al., Toxicol. Ind. Health* **15**, 651 (1999). *Review:* L. G. Krauskopf, *Plast. Compd.* **6**, 28-38 (1983). Review of environmental fate: C. A. Staples *et al., Chemosphere* **35**, 667-749 (1997); of aquatic toxicity: idem *et al., Environ. Toxicol. Chem.* **16**, 875 (1997); of toxicology and human exposure: *Toxicological Profile for Di(2-ethylhexyl)phthalate* (PB2003-100138, 2002) 337 pp.

Liquid, mp −47°. bp$_{5mm\ Hg}$ 231°. Flash point (closed cup): 206°C (403°F). d$_{20}^{20}$ 0.986. n$_D^{20}$ 1.486. Viscosity (cSt): 386 (0°); 22 (20°); 31 (37.8°); 5 (100°). Vapor pressure (mm Hg): (100°) 0.003; (200°) 1.20; (300°) 96.

Caution: Potential symptoms of overexposure are irritation of eyes and mucous membranes. *See NIOSH Pocket Guide to Chemical Hazards* (DHHS/NIOSH 97-140, 1997) p 118. This substance is reasonably anticipated to be a human carcinogen: *Report on Carcinogens, Eleventh Edition* (PB2005-104914, 2004) p III-123.

USE: As plasticizer in PVC applications and flexible vinyls.

2865. Dehydroacetic Acid. [520-45-6] 3-Acetyl-6-methyl-2*H*-pyran-2,4(3*H*)-dione; 2-acetyl-5-hydroxy-3-oxo-4-hexenoic acid δ-lactone; methylacetopyronone; DHA. $C_8H_8O_4$; mol wt 168.15. C 57.14%, H 4.80%, O 38.06%. Polymerization product of ketene: Steele *et al., J. Org. Chem.* **14**, 460 (1949). From ethyl acetoacetate: Arndt, *Org. Synth.* **coll. vol. III**, 231 (1955). Toxicity study: H. C. Spencer *et al., J. Pharmacol. Exp. Ther.* **99**, 57 (1950). Series of articles on toxicity studies, pharmacology, mechanism of action, absorption, distribution, renal action: *ibid.* 57-111.

White to cream crystalline powder, mp 109-111° (sublimes). bp 269.9°. Soly (w/w at 25°): in acetone 22%; benzene 18%; methanol 5%; carbon tetrachloride 3%; U.S.P. ethanol 3%; ether 5%; glycerol <0.1%, *n*-heptane 0.7%; olive oil 1.6%; propylene glycol 1.7%; water <0.1%. LD$_{50}$ orally in rats: 1000 mg/kg (Spencer).

Sodium salt hydrate. DHA-S. $C_8H_7NaO_4 \cdot H_2O$; mol wt 208.14. Tasteless white powder. Soly (w/w at 25°): in water 33%; propylene glycol 48%; olive oil <0.1%; methanol 14%; U.S.P. ethanol 1%; *n*-heptane <0.1%; glycerol 15%; ether <0.1%; carbon tetrachloride <0.1%; benzene <0.1%; acetone 0.2%. LD$_{50}$ orally in rats: 570 mg/kg (Spencer).

USE: In organic syntheses; as plasticizer, compatible with nitrocellulose, polystyrene, methacrylate, vinylite resins; as fungicide and bactericide; in antienzyme toothpastes; to reduce pickle bloating.

2866. Dehydroascorbic Acid. [490-83-5] L-*threo*-2,3-Hexodiulosonic acid γ-lactone. $C_6H_6O_6$; mol wt 174.11. C 41.39%, H 3.47%, O 55.14%. The reversibly oxidized form of ascorbic acid. Prepd by the action of benzoquinone on ascorbic acid: Ohle, Erlbach, *Ber.* **67**, 555 (1934); Moll, Wieters, *E. Merck's Jahresber.* **50**, 65 (1936); by the action of iodine: Herbert *et al., J. Chem. Soc.* **1933**, 1270; Kenyon, Munro, *ibid.* **1948**, 158; by oxidn with *peri*-naphthindan-2,3,4-trione hydrate: Moubasher, *J. Biol. Chem.* **176**, 533 (1948); *see also* Müller-Mulot, *Z. Physiol. Chem.* **351**, 52 (1970). Isomerization and formn of derivs: Egge, *Tetrahedron Lett.* **1969**, 801. Structure studies: Teichmann, Ziebarth, *Z. Prakt. Chem.* **33**, 124 (1966). Toxicity studies: Gaudiano *et al., Boll. Soc. Ital. Biol. Sper.* **43**, 674 (1967).

Fine needles, dec 225°. Sol in water at 60°. In soln the two carbonyl groups (in position 2 and 3) assume the hydrated form —C(OH)$_2$—C(OH)$_2$—. Practically neutral reaction. pKa: 3.90. [α]$_D^{20}$ +56°. Aq solns are much less stable than those of ascorbic acid. Detailed stability data: Bogdanski, Bogdanska, *Bull. Acad. Pol. Sci. Cl. 2* **3**, 41 (1955). *See also* Velisek *et al., Collect. Czech. Chem. Commun.* **37**, 1465 (1972). Undecomposed dehydroascorbic acid in soln is easily converted to ascorbic acid by reduction with sulfurous acid. Has same antiscorbutic activity in humans as ascorbic acid (upon oral ingestion).

2867. (3β)-7-Dehydrocholesterol. [434-16-2] Cholesta-5,7-dien-3-ol; provitamin D$_3$. $C_{27}H_{44}O$; mol wt 384.64. C 84.31%, H 11.53%, O 4.16%. Occurs in higher animals and in man. Isoln from the horned snail, *Buccinum undatum:* Windaus *et al., Z. Physiol. Chem.* **241**, 100 (1936); from pigskin: Windaus, Bock, *ibid.* **245**, 168 (1937); Boer *et al., Proc. K. Ned. Akad. Wet.* **39**, 622 (1936). Synthesis: Windaus *et al., Ann.* **520**, 98 (1935); Rosenberg, Tinker, **US 2215727**; Buisman *et al., Rec. Trav. Chim.* **66**, 83 (1947); P. N. Confalone *et al., J. Org. Chem.* **46**, 1030 (1981). Irradiation with ultraviolet light produces vitamin D$_3$; also lumisterol$_3$ and tachysterol$_3$: Windaus *et al., Ann.* **533**, 118 (1938).

Hydrated plates from ether-methanol. The water of crystn is held tenaciously: Schenck *et al., Ber.* **69**, 2705 (1936). When anhydr mp 150-151°. [α]$_D^{20}$ −113.6° (c = 1 in chloroform), Koch, Koch, *J. Biol. Chem.* **116**, 757 (1936); [α]$_D^{20}$ −127.1° in benzene (Boer). All provitamins D have the same uv maxima at 260, 270, 281, 293.5 nm. Insol in water, sol in the usual organic solvents.

Acetate. $C_{29}H_{46}O_2$. Crystals from methanol, mp 129-130°; [α]$_D^{20}$ −85.3° (c = 1.2 in benzene).

Benzoate. $C_{34}H_{48}O_2$. Plates from chloroform-acetone, mp 139-140°; [α]$_D^{20}$ −53.2° in chloroform.

2868. Dehydrocholic Acid. [81-23-2] (5β)-3,7,12-Trioxo-cholan-24-oic acid; 3,7,12-triketocholanic acid; Acolen; Bilidren; Cholagon; CholDgOn; Decholin; Dehychol; Deidrocolico Vita; Didrocolo; Erebile; Felacrinos; Procholon. $C_{24}H_{34}O_5$; mol wt 402.52. C 71.61%, H 8.51%, O 19.87%. Prepd from cholic acid by oxidation with CrO$_3$ in glacial acetic acid: Hammarsten in *Abderhalden's Handbuch der Biol. Arbeitsmethoden*, Abt. **I**, Teil 6, p 238 (1925); by using chlorine instead of CrO$_3$: Hinkley, Singleton, **US 2966499** (1960 to Merck & Co.).

Bitter crystals from acetone, mp 237°. [α]$_D^{20}$ +26° (c = 1.4 in alc). Soly at 15° (g/l): water 0.18; alcohol 3.3; ether 0.46; chloroform 9.04; benzene 1.04; acetone 7.76; ethyl acetate 7.4; glacial acetic acid 7.42.

Sodium salt. [145-41-5] Sodium dehydrocholate; Carachol; Dycholium; Suprachol. $C_{24}H_{33}NaO_5$; mol wt 424.51. Very sol in water. pH of aq soln about 9.0.

THERAP CAT: Choleretic.

2869. 11-Dehydrocorticosterone. [72-23-1] 21-Hydroxy-pregn-4-ene-3,11,20-trione; Δ^4-pregnen-21-ol-3,11,20-trione; 17-(1-keto-2-hydroxyethyl)-Δ^4-androsten-3,11-dione; Kendall's compound A. $C_{21}H_{28}O_4$; mol wt 344.44. C 73.23%, H 8.19%, O 18.58%. Found in adrenal cortex. 1000 lbs of beef glands yield 333 mg: Kendall, *Cold Spring Harbor Symp. Quant. Biol.* **5**, 299 (1937). Isoln procedure: Mason *et al., J. Biol. Chem.* **114**, 613 (1936); *see also* Kendall *et al., Proc. Staff Meet. Mayo Clin.* **12**, 136 (1937). Prepn from corticosterone 21-acetate: Reichstein, *Helv. Chim. Acta* **20**, 953 (1937); from desoxycholic acid: Lardon, Reichstein, *ibid.* **26**, 747 (1943); Gallagher, *Recent Progress in Hormone Research* (New York, 1946) p 83; from 3α-acetoxy-11-ketobisnorcholanic acid: Sarett, *J. Biol. Chem.* **162**, 601 (1946); *J. Am. Chem. Soc.* **68**, 2478 (1946); from 3α-acetyl-11-ketolithocholic acid methyl ester: Wettstein, Meystre, *Helv. Chim. Acta* **30,** 1262 (1947). Manuf: Wettstein, **US 2778776** (1957 to Ciba).

Large prisms from aq acetone, mp 178-180°. Can be distilled in high vacuum. $[\alpha]_{546}^{25}$ +299°, also given as +347° (c = 0.23 in benzene); $[\alpha]_D^{25}$ +258° (alc). Relatively good soly in benzene.
  Acetate. $C_{23}H_{30}O_5$. Needles from alc, mp 179-181°. $[\alpha]_{546}^{18}$ +285° (dioxane); $[\alpha]_D^{18}$ +233.7° (dioxane).

2870. Dehydroemetine. [4914-30-1] 2,3-Didehydro-6′,7′,-10,11-tetramethoxyemetan; 2,3-dehydroemetine; 2-dehydro-emetine. $C_{29}H_{38}N_2O_4$; mol wt 478.62. C 72.77%, H 8.00%, N 5.85%, O 13.37%. Synthetic analog of emetine, *q.v.;* the (−)-form is therapeutically active. Synthesis of racemic 2,3-dehydroemetine: Brossi *et al., Helv. Chim. Acta* **42,** 772 (1959). Stereospecific synthesis of (±)-form and (±)-*2,3-dehydroisoemetine,* the (1′β)-isomer: Clark *et al., J. Chem. Soc.* **1962,** 2479. Separation of the four possible isomers: Brossi, Burkhardt, *Experientia* **18,** 211 (1962). Absolute configuration and bioactivity of isomers: A. Brossi *et al., Helv. Chim. Acta* **45,** 2219 (1962). Prepn of pure (−)-form: A. Brossi, **BE 629898**; *eidem,* **US 3311633** (1963, 1967 both to Hoffmann-La Roche); N. Whittaker *J. Chem. Soc. C* **1969,** 94. Antiprotozoal activity *in vitro:* G. H. Al-Khateeb *et al., Chemotherapy (Basel)* **23,** 267 (1977). Review of use in amebiasis: G. Woolfe, *Prog. Drug Res.* **8,** 12 (1965).

Crystals from isopropyl ether, mp 94-96°. $[\alpha]_D$ −183°.
  (−)-Form dihydrobromide. $C_{29}H_{38}N_2O_4.2HBr$. Crystals, mp 243-245°. $[\alpha]_D$ −97° (methanol). uv max (alc): 282 nm (ε 7300).
  (+)-Form dihydrobromide. Crystals, mp 241-243°. $[\alpha]_D$ +95° (methanol). uv max (alc): 282 nm (ε 7350).
  (±)-Form dihydrochloride. [14358-43-1] Mebadin. $C_{29}H_{38}$-$N_2O_4.2HCl$; mol wt 551.54. Crystals from ethanol + ether, mp 235°.
  (±)-2,3-Dehydroisoemetine hydrochloride. Crystals from ethanol + ether, mp 220-225°.
  (−)-2,3-Dehydroisoemetine dihydrobromide. $C_{29}H_{38}N_2$-$O_4.2HBr$. Crystals, mp 257-260°. $[\alpha]_D$ −107° (methanol). uv max (alc): 285 nm (ε 7400).
  (+)-2,3-Dehydroisoemetine dihydrobromide. Crystals, mp 257-260°. $[\alpha]_D$ +109° (methanol). uv max (alc): 285 nm (ε 7450).
  THERAP CAT: Antiamebic.

2871. Dehydroepiandrosterone. [53-43-0] (3β)-3-Hydroxyandrost-5-en-17-one; prasterone; dehydroisoandrosterone; *trans*-dehydroandrosterone; Δ^5-androsten-3β-ol-17-one; DHEA. $C_{19}H_{28}O_2$; mol wt 288.42. C 79.12%, H 9.79%, O 11.09%. Major secretory steroidal product of the adrenal gland; secretion progressively declines with aging. May have estrogen- or androgen-like effects depending on the hormonal milieu. Intracellularly converted to androstenedione, *q.v.* Isoln from male urine: Butenandt, Tscherning, *Z. Physiol. Chem.* **229,** 167 (1934); Butenandt, Dannenbaum, *ibid.* 192. Prepn from cholesterol: Butenandt *et al., ibid.* **237,** 57 (1935); Ruzicka, Wettstein, *Helv. Chim. Acta* **18,** 986

(1935); Wallis, Fernholz, *J. Am. Chem. Soc.* **57,** 1379, 1504 (1935); Schoeller *et al., Naturwissenschaften* **23,** 337 (1935); from sitosterol: Oppenauer, *Nature* **135,** 1039 (1935). High yield prepn: H. Hosoda *et al., J. Org. Chem.* **38,** 4209 (1973). Metabolism study: P. Knapstein *et al. Acta Endocrinol.* **58,** 261 (1968). Toxicity study of the sulfate: M. Yahara *et al., J. Toxicol. Sci.* **2,** 161 (1977). Clinical evaluation in hormone replacement therapy: A. J. Morales *et al., J. Clin. Endocrinol. Metab.* **78,** 1360 (1994); in systemic lupus erythematosus: R. F. van Vollenhoven *et al., Arthritis Rheum.* **38,** 1826 (1995). Review of physiological importance: P. Ebeling, V. A. Koivisto, *Lancet* **343,** 1479-1481 (1994). Symposium on role in aging: *Ann. N.Y. Acad. Sci.* **774,** 1-350 (1995). Review of therapeutic potential: B. Allolio, W. Arlt, *Trends Endocrinol. Metab.* **13,** 288-294 (2002).

Dimorphous, needles, mp 140-141°; leaflets, mp 152-153°. $[\alpha]_D^{18}$ +10.9° (c = 0.4 in alc). Pptd by digitonin. Sol in benzene, alcohol, ether; sparingly sol in chloroform, petr ether.
  Sulfate. [651-48-9] DHEAS. $C_{19}H_{28}O_5S$; mol wt 368.49. Hydrophilic storage form that circulates in the blood.
  Sodium sulfate. [1099-87-2] Sodium dehydroepiandrosterone sulfate; Astenile; Mylis. $C_{19}H_{27}NaO_5S$; mol wt 390.47. White cryst powder, mp 154° (dec). Sol in methanol, slightly sol in water, abs ethanol. Practically insol in acetone, chloroform, benzene.
  THERAP CAT: In treatment of menopausal syndrome.

2872. Dehydroergosterol. [516-85-8] (3β,22E)-Ergosta-5,-7,9(11),22-tetraen-3-ol. $C_{28}H_{42}O$; mol wt 394.63. C 85.22%, H 10.73%, O 4.05%. Prepd from ergosterol: Windhaus, Linsert, *Ann.* **465,** 148 (1928); Callow, Rosenheim, *J. Chem. Soc.* **1933,** 387. From isopyrocalciferol: Windhaus, Dimroth, *Ber.* **70,** 376 (1937).

Solvated plates from alcohol, needles from ether. When dry, mp 146°. bp$_{0.5}$ 230°. $[\alpha]_D^{15}$ +149.2° (c = 1.9 in chloroform). Absorption spectrum: Morton, de Gouveia, *J. Chem. Soc.* **1934,** 916. One gram dissolves in 800 ml methanol. Freely sol in ether, chloroform, benzene.
  Acetate. $C_{30}H_{44}O_2$. mp 146°. $[\alpha]_D^{16}$ +204° (c = 1.1 in chloroform).
  Methyl ether. $C_{29}H_{44}O$. mp 106°. $[\alpha]_D^{20}$ +166° (c = 2 in chloroform).

2873. 3-Dehydroretinal. [472-87-7] 3,4-Didehydroretinal; (*all-E*)-3,7-dimethyl-9-(2,6,6-trimethyl-1,3-cyclohexadien-1-yl)-2,-4,6,8-nonatetraenal; *all-trans*-3,4-dehydroretinal; retinal 2; retinene 2; vitamin A$_2$ aldehyde. $C_{20}H_{26}O$; mol wt 282.42. C 85.06%, H 9.28%, O 5.67%. Carotenoid chromophore of porphyropsin and cyanopsin, *q.q.v.,* which are visual pigments of certain fish, crustaceans and amphibians. May also occur in combination with retinal, *q.v.,* in mixed visual systems. Isoln from retinas of fresh-water fish: G. Wald, *Nature* **139,** 1017 (1937). Recognition as vitamin A$_2$ aldehyde: R. A. Morton, *ibid.* **153,** 69 (1944). Prepn by the oxidation of vitamin A$_2$: G. Wald, *Biochim. Biophys. Acta* **4,** 215 (1950). Synthesis: K. R. Farrar *et al., J. Chem. Soc.* **1952,** 1414; of stereoisomers: U. Schwieter *et al., Helv. Chim. Acta* **45,** 517, 528, 541 (1962); R. S. H. Liu *et al., J. Am. Chem. Soc.* **99,** 8095 (1977).

HPLC separation: K. Tsukida *et al., J. Chromatogr.* **192,** 395 (1980); T. Suzuki, M. Makino-Tasaka, *Anal. Biochem.* **129,** 111 (1983). Biological activity: G. Wald, *J. Gen. Physiol.* **22,** 775 (1939); *idem, Fed. Proc.* **12,** 606 (1953). *Reviews:* G. Wald, *Science* **162,** 230-239 (1968); R. Hubbard *et al., Methods Enzymol.* **18,** 615-653 (1971). Book: *The Retinoids* Vol. 1-2, M. B. Sporn *et al.,* Eds. (Academic Press, New York, 1984).

All-*trans*

11-*cis* isomer

Orange-red prisms from pentane, mp 77-78°. uv max (ethanol): 401 nm ($E_{1cm}^{1\%}$ 1470).

11-*cis*-Isomer. [41470-05-7] Oil from petr ether-ether. uv max (ethanol): 393 nm ($E_{1cm}^{1\%}$ 882).

USE: As tool in biological energy transduction research.

2874. 3-Dehydroretinol. [79-80-1] 3,4-Didehydroretinol; (*all-E*)-3,7-dimethyl-9-(2,6,6-trimethyl-1,3-cyclohexadien-1-yl)-2,-4,6,8-nonatetraen-1-ol; *all-trans*-3-dehydroretinol; retinol$_2$; vitamin A$_2$. $C_{20}H_{28}O$; mol wt 284.44. C 84.45%, H 9.92%, O 5.62%. Naturally occurring retinoid originally discovered in livers of freshwater fish. Constitutes 20-25% of total retinoid content in human epidermis; levels are markedly elevated in patients with hyperproliferative dermatoses such as psoriasis. Discovery in freshwater fish: E. Lederer *et al., Nature* **140,** 233 (1937); J. R. Edisbury *et al., ibid.* 234. Isoln from pike liver oils: E. M. Shantz, *Science* **108,** 417 (1948). Structure and synthesis: K. R. Farrar *et al., J. Chem. Soc.* **1952,** 2657. Synthesis and characteristics of stereoisomers: U. Schwieter *et al., Helv. Chim. Acta* **45,** 517, 528, 541, 548 (1962). HPLC determn in fish oils: B. Stancher, F. Zonta, *J. Chromatogr.* **312,** 423 (1984). Identification in human skin: A. Vahlquist, *Experientia* **36,** 317 (1980). Comparative levels in psoriasis patients: O. Rollman, A. Vahlquist, *Arch. Dermatol. Res.* **278,** 17 (1985). Biosynthesis from retinol, *q.v.,* in cultured keratinocytes: O. Rollman *et al., Biochem. J.* **293,** 675 (1993).

Light yellow needles from petr ether, mp 63-65°. uv max (ethanol): 350 nm ($E_{1cm}^{1\%}$ 1455).

2875. 7-Dehydrositosterol. [521-04-0] (3β)-Stigmasta-5,7-dien-3-ol. $C_{29}H_{48}O$; mol wt 412.69. C 84.40%, H 11.72%, O 3.88%. From soy bean oil β-sitosterol: Wunderlich, *Z. Physiol. Chem.* **241,** 116 (1936). Starting with cholesterol: **US 2386635** (1945).

Platelets from alc, browns on contact with air, mp 144-145°. $[\alpha]_D^{21}$ −116° (c = 2 in chloroform). Sparingly sol in methanol, somewhat more in alcohol, freely sol in the other usual organic solvents. Insol in water.

Acetate. $C_{31}H_{50}O_2$. mp 151-152°. $[\alpha]_D^{21}$ −71° (c = 2 in chloroform).

2876. Delapril. [83435-66-9] *N*-[(1*S*)-1-(Ethoxycarbonyl)-3-phenylpropyl]-L-alanyl-*N*-(2,3-dihydro-1*H*-inden-2-yl)glycine; *N*-[*N*-[*(S)*-1-(ethoxycarbonyl)-3-phenylpropyl]-L-alanyl]-*N*-(indan-2-yl)glycine; ethyl *(S)*-2-[[(*S*)-1-[(carboxymethyl)-2-indanylcarbamoyl]ethyl]amino]-4-phenylbutyrate; alindapril; indalapril. C_{26}-$H_{32}N_2O_5$; mol wt 452.54. C 69.01%, H 7.13%, N 6.19%, O 17.68%. Angiotensin-converting enzyme (ACE) inhibitor. Prepn: Y. Oka *et al., EP 51391; idem, US 4385051* (1982, 1983 both to Takeda); J. T. Suh *et al., Eur. J. Med. Chem. - Chim. Ther.* **20,** 563 (1985); A. Miyake *et al., Chem. Pharm. Bull.* **34,** 2852 (1986). Pharmacology in animals: Y. Inada *et al., Jpn. J. Pharmacol.* **42,** 1 (1986); *eidem, ibid.,* 99. Pharmacology and metabolism in humans: T. Ogihara *et al., Curr. Ther. Res.* **41,** 809 (1987). Pharmacokinetics and evaluation in hypertension: H. Shionoiri *et al., Clin. Pharmacol. Ther.* **41,** 74 (1987).

Hydrochloride. [83435-67-0] CV-3317; REV-6000A; Adecut; Cupressin. $C_{26}H_{32}N_2O_5 \cdot HCl$; mol wt 489.00. Colorless plates from acetone + hydrochloric acid, mp 166-170° (dec). $[\alpha]_D^{22}$ +18.5° (c = 1 in methanol).

THERAP CAT: Antihypertensive.

2877. Delavirdine. [136817-59-9] 1-[3-[(1-Methylethyl)-amino]-2-pyridinyl]-4-[[5-[(methylsulfonyl)amino]-1*H*-indol-2-yl]carbonyl]piperazine; 1-(5-methanesulfonamido-1*H*-indol-2-ylcarbonyl)-4-[3-(1-methylethylamino)pyridinyl]piperazine; 1-[3-(iso-propylamino)-2-pyridyl]-4-[(5-methanesulfonamidoindol-2-yl)carbonyl]piperazine; U-90152. $C_{22}H_{28}N_6O_3S$; mol wt 456.56. C 57.88%, H 6.18%, N 18.41%, O 10.51%, S 7.02%. Bisheteroarylpiperazine non-nucleoside reverse transcriptase inhibitor of HIV-1. Prepn: D. L. Romero *et al., WO 9109849;* J. R. Palmer *et al., US 5563142* (1991, 1996 both to Upjohn). Structure-activity studies: D. L. Romero *et al., J. Med. Chem.* **36,** 1505 (1993). *In vitro* activity vs HIV-1: T. J. Dueweke *et al., Antimicrob. Agents Chemother.* **37,** 1127 (1993); P. J. Pagano, K.-T. Chong, *J. Infect. Dis.* **171,** 61 (1995). Enzyme kinetic studies: I. W. Althaus *et al., Biochem. Pharmacol.* **47,** 2017 (1994). NMR characterization of crystalline forms: P. Gao, *Pharm. Res.* **15,** 1425 (1998). HPLC determn in plasma: C.-L. Cheng *et al., J. Chromatogr. B* **769,** 297 (2002). Review of discovery and development: W. J. Adams *et al., in Pharm. Biotechnol.,* R. T. Borchardt *et al.,* Eds. (Plenum Press, New York, 1998) pp 285-312; of clinical use in HIV infection: L. J. Scott, C. M. Perry, *Drugs* **60,** 1411-1444 (2000).

Crystals from ethyl acetate + hexane, mp 226-228°. Aqueous soly at 23° (μg/ml): 2942 (pH 1.0); 295 (pH 2.0); 0.81 (pH 7.4). pKa$_1$ 4.56. pKa$_2$ 8.9. Log P (*n*-octanol/water): 2.84.

Methanesulfonate. [147221-93-0] Delavirdine mesylate; U-90152S; Rescriptor. $C_{22}H_{28}N_6O_3S \cdot CH_3SO_3H$; mol wt 552.67.

THERAP CAT: Antiviral.

2878. Delmadinone Acetate. [13698-49-2] 17-(Acetyloxy)-6-chloropregna-1,4,6-triene-3,20-dione; 6-chloro-17-hydroxypregna-1,4,6-triene-3,20-dione acetate; 1,6-bisdehydro-6-chloro-17α-acetoxyprogesterone; Δ¹-chlormadinone acetate; RS-1301; Delminal; Estrex; Tardastrex; Tarden; Zenadrex. $C_{23}H_{27}ClO_4$; mol wt 402.91. C 68.56%, H 6.75%, Cl 8.80%, O 15.88%. Prepn: Ringold *et al., J. Am. Chem. Soc.* **81**, 3485 (1959); **GB 890315** (1962 to Upjohn), *C.A.* **57**, 5996c (1962); **76**, 14813y (1972); Campbell, Babcock, **DE 1243682** (1967 to Upjohn), *C.A.* **67**, 100343r (1967). Activity studies: Dorfman, Kincl, *Steroids* **1**, 185 (1963); Weichert *et al., Arzneim.-Forsch.* **17**, 1103 (1967); Gerber *et al., J. Small Anim. Pract.* **14**, 151 (1973).

Crystals, mp 168-170°. [α]$_D$ −83° (chloroform). uv max (ethanol): 229, 258, 297 nm (log ε 4.00, 4.00, 4.03).

THERAP CAT: Progestogen.

THERAP CAT (VET): Progestogen.

2879. Delmopinol. [79874-76-3] 3-(4-Propylheptyl)-4-morpholineethanol. $C_{16}H_{33}NO_2$; mol wt 271.44. C 70.80%, H 12.25%, N 5.16%, O 11.79%. Surface-active agent that reduces dental plaque formation. Prepn: **BE 888052**; S. E. H. Hernestam *et al.*, **US 4636382** (1981, 1987 both to Ferrosan). Stereoselective HPLC determn in plasma: G. Egginger *et al., J. Chromatogr. A* **666**, 275 (1994). *In vitro* effect on bacterial cell walls: J. Rundegren *et al., Oral Microbiol. Immunol.* **10**, 102 (1995). Home usage trials of mouthwash: A. J. Elworthy *et al., J. Clin. Periodontol.* **22**, 527 (1995); N. Claydon *et al., ibid.* **23**, 220 (1996).

Hydrochloride. [98092-92-3] M-1650; Decapinol. $C_{16}H_{33}NO_2 \cdot HCl$; mol wt 307.90. mp 70-72°. pKa 7.1. Soly in water: >40%.

THERAP CAT: In treatment of gingivitis.

2880. Delphinidin. [528-53-0] 3,5,7-Trihydroxy-2-(3,4,5-trihydroxyphenyl)-1-benzopyrylium chloride; 3,3′,4′,5,5′,7-hexahydroxyflavylium chloride; 3,3′,4′,5,5′,7-hexahydroxy-2-phenylbenzopyrylium chloride; delphinidol. $C_{15}H_{11}ClO_7$; mol wt 338.70. C 53.19%, H 3.27%, Cl 10.47%, O 33.07%. The aglucone of delphinin: Willstätter, Mieg, *Ann.* **408**, 61 (1915); the aglucone of violanin: Willstätter, Weil, *ibid.* **412**, 178 (1917). Occurrence in plants: Acheson, *Can. J. Biochem. Physiol.* **37**, 1 (1959). Synthesis: Pratt, Robinson, *J. Chem. Soc.* **127**, 166 (1925); Bradley *et al., ibid.* **1930**, 793.

Chocolate-brown prisms or needles with metallic luster from 5% HCl. Crystallizes from water with 1, 2 or 4 mols H_2O. When anhydr does not melt below 350°. Absorption max (methanolic HCl): 544 nm. Sol in methanol, ethanol, ethyl acetate.

3-Glucoside. Myrtillin-a. $C_{21}H_{21}ClO_{12}$. From the whortleberry *(Vaccinium myrtillus* L., *Ericaceae):* Willstätter, Zollinger, *Ann.* **408**, 83 (1915); **412**, 195 (1916); from the pansy *(Viola tricolor* L., *Violaceae):* Karrer, de Meuron, *Helv. Chim. Acta* **16**, 292 (1933). Structure and synthesis: Reynolds, Robinson, *J. Chem. Soc.* **1934**, 1039. Deep purple crystals from dil HCl. Absorption max (methanolic HCl): 535 nm.

3,5-Diglucoside. 3,5-Bis(glucosyloxy)-3′,4′,5′,7-tetrahydroxyflavylium chloride; delphin; delphoside; hyacin. $C_{27}H_{31}ClO_{17}$. From flowers of *Salvia patens* Cav., *Labiatae,* structure and synthesis: Reynolds *et al., J. Chem. Soc.* **1934**, 1235; from flowers of *Verbena hybrida* Hart., *Verbenaceae:* Scott-Moncrieff, Sturgess, *Biochem. J.* **34**, 268 (1940); from grape skins: Bockian *et al., J. Agric. Food Chem.* **3**, 695 (1955). Identity with hyacin: Saito *et al., Proc. Jpn. Acad.* **36**, 340 (1960). Leaflets with bronze luster from dil HCl. Absorption max (methanolic HCl): 534 nm. Practically insol in cold water, alcohol, dil acids; sol in hot dil HCl.

Compound with glucose + hydroxybenzoic acid. Delphinin. $C_{41}H_{39}ClO_{21}$. From *Delphinium consolida* L., *Ranunculaceae:* Willstätter, Mieg, *loc. cit.* Dark red-brown plates or prisms from 3% HCl. dec 200-203°. Sol in water with decompn, dil alcohol, acetone, boiling alcohol.

Compound with glucose + rhamnose + *p*-hydroxycinnamic acid. Violanin. $C_{36}H_{37}ClO_{18}$. From flowers of *Viola tricolor* L., *Violaceae:* Karrer, de Meuron, Weil, *loc. cit.* Structure: Karrer, de Meuron, *loc. cit.* Bluish-violet plates with green metallic luster from methanolic HCl + ether. Sol in amyl alcohol, in 0.15-0.5% HCl; less sol in 1% HCl; slightly sol in water; practically insol in 5-12% HCl.

2881. Delphinine. [561-07-9] (1α,6α,14α,16β)-1,6,16-Trimethoxy-4-(methoxymethyl)-20-methylaconitane-8,13,14-triol 8-acetate 14-benzoate. $C_{33}H_{45}NO_9$; mol wt 599.71. C 66.09%, H 7.56%, N 2.34%, O 24.01%. A toxic alkaloid from seeds of *Delphinium staphisagria* L., *Ranunculaceae.* Isoln: Markwood, *J. Am. Pharm. Assoc.* **16**, 928 (1927). Purification: Schneider, *Arch. Pharm.* **283**, 243 (1950). Structure: Jacobs, Pelletier, *J. Am. Chem. Soc.* **78**, 3542 (1956); Wiesner *et al., Can. J. Chem.* **47**, 2734 (1969). Configuration: Wiesner *et al., Tetrahedron Lett.* **1959**, no. 3, 12; **1960**, no. 15, 23; Gilman, Marion, *ibid.* **1962**, 923; Birnbaum *et al., ibid.* **1971**, 867. Synthesis: Wiesner *et al., Can. J. Chem.* **50**, 1925 (1972).

Orthorhombic, six-sided plates from alc, mp 197.5-199°. [α]$_D^{20}$ +25° (ethanol). Practically insol in water. Sol in 25 parts alcohol, 20 parts chloroform, 10 parts ether.

Hydrochloride. $C_{33}H_{45}NO_9 \cdot HCl$. Crystals, dec 214°.

2882. Delsoline. [509-18-2] (1α,6β,14α,16β)-20-Ethyl-6,14,16-trimethoxy-4-(methoxymethyl)aconitane-1,7,8-triol. $C_{25}H_{41}NO_7$; mol wt 467.60. C 64.21%, H 8.84%, N 3.00%, O 23.95%. From seeds of *Dephinium consolida* L., *Ranunculaceae:* Markwood, *J. Am. Pharm. Assoc.* **13**, 696 (1924); Cionga, Iliescu, *Ber.* **74**, 1031 (1941); Marion, Edwards, *J. Am. Chem. Soc.* **69**, 2010 (1947). Structure: Anet *et al., Can. J. Chem.* **35**, 397 (1957); Skaric, Marion, *J. Am. Chem. Soc.* **80**, 4434 (1958); *eidem, Can. J. Chem.* **38**, 2433 (1960); **39**, 1579 (1961).

Delsoline R = CH₃
Delcosine R = H

Prisms from methanol, mp 213-216.5° (when immersed at 205°). $[\alpha]_D^{22}$ +53.4° (c = 2.04 in chloroform). Slightly sol in water, sol in alcohol or chloroform.

Delcosine. [545-56-2] $C_{24}H_{39}NO_7$; mol wt 453.57. Alkaloid also found in *D. consolida*. mp 203-204°, $[\alpha]_D^{25}$ +56.8° (c = 2.01 in chloroform). Quite sol in water.

USE: Glycosidal dyestuff.

2883. Deltamethrin. [52918-63-5] (1*R*,3*R*)-3-(2,2-Dibro-moethenyl)-2,2-dimethylcyclopropanecarboxylic acid (*S*)-cyano(3-phenoxyphenyl)methyl ester; (*S*)-α-cyano-3-phenoxybenzyl-(1*R*)-*cis*-3-(2,2-dibromovinyl)-2,2-dimethylcyclopropane carboxylate; decamethrin; esbecythrin; FMC-45498; NRDC-161; RU-22974; Butox; Decis; K-Othrine; Scalibor. $C_{22}H_{19}Br_2NO_3$; mol wt 505.20. C 52.30%, H 3.79%, Br 31.63%, N 2.77%, O 9.50%. Synthetic pyrethroid insecticide. Prepn of racemic mixture: M. Elliot *et al.*, DE 2439177 (1975 to NRDC), *C.A.* **83**, 73519z (1975); of decamethrin and isomers: *eidem, Pestic. Sci.* **9**, 105 (1978). Activity: *eidem, Nature* **248**, 710 (1974); *eidem, Pestic. Sci.* **9**, 112 (1978). Absolute configuration: J. D. Owen, *J. Chem. Soc. Perkin Trans. 1* **1975**, 1865. Photochemistry: L. O. Ruzo *et al., J. Agric. Food Chem.* **25**, 1385 (1977). Metabolism: *eidem, ibid.* **26**, 918 (1978). Toxicology: R. Kavlock *et al., J. Environ. Pathol. Toxicol.* **2**, 751 (1979). Pharmacological effects on central nervous system: P. H. Chanh *et al., Arzneim.-Forsch.* **34**, 175 (1984). Review of toxicology and human exposure: *Toxicological Profile for Pyrethrins and Pyrethroids* (PB2004-100004, 2003) 332 pp.

Crystals, mp 98-101°. Sol in ethanol, acetone, dioxane. Insol in water. LD₅₀ in female rats (mg/kg): 31 orally; 4 i.v. (Kavlock).

USE: Insecticide.

THERAP CAT (VET): Ectoparasiticide.

2884. Demanyl Phosphate. [6909-62-2] Mono[2-(dimeth-ylamino)ethyl]phosphoric acid ester; 2-dimethylaminoethanol dihy-drogen phosphate; phosphoryldimethylaminoethanol; phosphoryl-dimethylcolamine; phosphoryldimethylethanolamine; P-DMEA; Panclar. $C_4H_{12}NO_4P$; mol wt 169.12. C 28.41%, H 7.15%, N 8.28%, O 37.84%, P 18.31%. $(CH_3)_2NCH_2CH_2OPO_3H_2$. Prepn: Aron-Samuel *et al.*, FR 992802 (1951), *C.A.* **51**, 458e (1957); Cherbuliez, Rabinowitz, *Helv. Chim. Acta* **41**, 1168 (1958); GB 861463; US 3098072 (1961, 1963 to Ciba). The phosphate ester of a possible choline precursor. Has been isolated from a choline-requiring mutant of *Neurospora crassa*, strain 47904: Wolf, Nyc, *J. Biol. Chem.* **234**, 1068 (1959). Biosynthetic studies: Ansell, Choj-nacki, *Nature* **196**, 545 (1962); *eidem, Biochem. J.* **98**, 303 (1966).

Crystals, mp 175-176°.

Monohydrate. mp 78-81°.

THERAP CAT: Psychotonic.

2885. Demecarium Bromide. [56-94-0] 3,3′-[1,10-Decane-diylbis[(methylimino)carbonyloxy]]bis[*N*,*N*,*N*-trimethylbenz-enaminium]dibromide; (*m*-hydroxyphenyl)trimethylammonium bromide, decamethylenebis(methylcarbamate); *N*,*N*′-bis[3-trimeth-ylammoniumphenoxycarbonyl]-*N*,*N*′-dimethyldecamethylenedi-amine dibromide; decamethylenebis[*m*-dimethylaminophenyl *N*-methylcarbamate] dimethobromide; decamethylenebis[*N*-methyl-carbamic acid *m*-dimethylaminophenyl ester] bromomethylate;

BC-48; Tosmilen; Humorsol. $C_{32}H_{52}Br_2N_4O_4$; mol wt 716.59. C 53.63%, H 7.31%, Br 22.30%, N 7.82%, O 8.93%. Prepn: Schmid, US 2789981 (1957 to Oesterreichische Stickstoffwerke).

White, slightly hygroscopic powder, dec 162-167°. Freely sol in water, alc. Sparingly sol in acetone. Insol in ether. Aq solns are neutral, stable, and may be sterilized by heat.

THERAP CAT: Cholinergic (ophthalmic).

2886. Demeclocycline. [127-33-3] [4*S*-(4α,4aα,5aα,6β,-12aα)]-7-Chloro-4-(dimethylamino)-1,4,4a,5,5a,6,11,12a-octahy-dro-3,6,10,12,12a-pentahydroxy-1,11-dioxo-2-naphthacenecarbox-amide; 7-chloro-6-demethyltetracycline; demethylchlortetracycline (obsolete); RP-10192; Bioterciclin; Declomycin; Deganol; Leder-mycin; Periciclina. $C_{21}H_{21}ClN_2O_8$; mol wt 464.85. C 54.26%, H 4.55%, Cl 7.63%, N 6.03%, O 27.53%. Antibiotic related to tetra-cycline produced by *Streptomyces aureofaciens*. Prepn: McCor-mick *et al., J. Am. Chem. Soc.* **79**, 4561 (1957); US 2878289 (1959 to Am. Cyanamid). Improved fermentation processes: Szumski, US 3012946; Goodman, Matrishin, US 3019172; Goodman, US 3050446 (1961, 1962, 1962 all to Am. Cyanamid); FR 1344645 (1963 to Merck & Co.); Neidleman, US 3154476 (1964 to Olin Mathieson). Abs config: Dobrynin *et al., Tetrahedron Lett.* **1962**, 901. Toxicity data: E. I. Goldenthal, *Toxicol. Appl. Pharmacol.* **18**, 185 (1971).

Sesquihydrate. mp 174-178° (dec). $[\alpha]_D^{25}$ −258° (c = 0.5 in 0.1*N* H_2SO_4). Solubilities: Marsh, Weiss, *J. Assoc. Off. Anal. Chem.* **50**, 457 (1967).

Hydrochloride. [64-73-3] Clortetrin; Demetraciclina; Detra-vis; Meciclin; Mexocine. LD₅₀ orally in rats: 2372 mg/kg (Gold-enthal).

THERAP CAT: Antibacterial.

THERAP CAT (VET): Antibacterial.

2887. Demecolcine. [477-30-5] 6,7-Dihydro-1,2,3,10-tetra-methoxy-7-(methylamino)benzo[*a*]heptalen-9(5*H*)-one; *N*-deace-tyl-*N*-methylcolchicine; *N*-methyl-*N*-desacetylcolchicine; colcha-mine; Santavy's substance F; colcemid. $C_{21}H_{25}NO_5$; mol wt 371.43. C 67.91%, H 6.78%, N 3.77%, O 21.54%. Antitumor alkaloid; depolymerizes microtubules and inhibits spindle formation during metaphase. Isoln from *Colchicum autumnale* L., *Liliaceae*: Santavy, *Pharm. Acta Helv.* **25**, 248 (1950); Santavy, Reichstein, *Helv. Chim. Acta* **33**, 1606 (1950); Schlittler, Uffer, DE 936268 (1955 to Ciba), *C.A.* **53**, 1396 (1959). Structure: Santavy *et al., Helv. Chim. Acta* **36**, 1319 (1953). Synthesis: Uffer *et al., ibid.* **37**, 18 (1954); H. G. Capraro, A. Brossi, *ibid.* **62**, 965 (1979). Effect on the mitotic cycle: C. L. Rieder, R. E. Palazzo, *J. Cell Sci.* **102**, 387 (1992). Use in oocyte enucleation: E. Ibáñez *et al., Biol. Reprod.* **68**, 1249 (2003).

Pale yellow prisms from ethyl acetate + ether, mp 186°. $[\alpha]_D^{20}$ −129.0° (c = 1 in chloroform). uv max (alc): 245, 355 nm (log ε 4.55, 4.24). Basic reaction. Soluble in acidified water, in alcohol, ether, chloroform, benzene.

USE: Cell synchronization agent; for chromosome visualization; to induce oocyte enucleation for somatic cell cloning.

2888. Demegestone. [10116-22-0] 17-Methyl-19-norpregna-4,9-diene-3,20-dione; 17α-methyl-19-nor-$\Delta^{4,9}$-pregnadiene-3,20-dione; 17α-methyl-Δ^9-19-norprogesterone; R-2453; Lutionex. $C_{21}H_{28}O_2$; mol wt 312.45. C 80.72%, H 9.03%, O 10.24%. Prepn: **NL 6517141**; R. Joly *et al.*, **US 3547959** (1966, 1970 both to Roussel-UCLAF); L. Velluz *et al.*, *Tetrahedron Suppl.* **8**, part II, 495 (1966); R. Joly *et al.*, *Bull. Soc. Chim. Fr.* **1973**, 2694.

Crystals from ether, mp 106°. $[\alpha]_D$ −275° (c = 0.5 in ethanol). uv max (ethanol): 214, 302 nm (ε 6350, 21000).

THERAP CAT: Progestogen.

2889. Demeton. [8065-48-3] Phosphorothioic acid O,O-diethyl O-[2-(ethylthio)ethyl] ester mixture with O,O-diethyl S-[2-(ethylthio)ethyl]phosphorothioate; mercaptophos; Bayer 8169; E-1059; Systox. $C_8H_{19}O_3PS_2$; mol wt 258.34. C 37.19%, H 7.41%, O 18.58%, P 11.99%, S 24.82%. Cholinesterase inhibitor. Isomeric mixture consisting of demeton-O and demeton-S (O,O-diethyl O(and S)-ethylmercaptoethyl thiophosphates). Another name for demeton-S is *Isosystox*. Prepn: Schrader, **US 2571989** and **US 2597534** (1951, 1952 both to Bayer); Gardner, Heath, *Anal. Chem.* **25**, 1849 (1953). Toxicity study: T. B. Gaines, *Toxicol. Appl. Pharmacol.* **14**, 515 (1969).

Oily liq. Faint odor. bp_2 134°. Virtually insol in water. Sol in ethanol, propylene glycol, toluene and similar hydrocarbons. Absorbed by plants, rendering the foliage and plant fluids toxic to insects. LD_{50} in female, male rats (mg/kg): 2.5, 6.2 orally; 8.2, 14 dermally (Gaines).

Caution: Potential symptoms of overexposure are miosis, aching eyes, rhinorrhea and headache; chest tightening, wheezing, laryngeal spasms, salivation and cyanosis; anorexia, nausea, vomiting, abdominal cramps and diarrhea; local sweating; muscle fasciculation, weakness and paralysis; giddiness, confusion and ataxia; convulsions, coma; low blood pressure; cardiac irregularities; irritation of eyes and skin. *See NIOSH Pocket Guide to Chemical Hazards* (DHHS/NIOSH 97-140, 1997) p 90.

USE: Insecticide.

2890. Demexiptiline. [24701-51-7] 5H-Dibenzo[a,d]cyclohepten-5-one O-[2-(methylamino)ethyl]oxime. $C_{18}H_{18}N_2O$; mol wt 278.35. C 77.67%, H 6.52%, N 10.06%, O 5.75%. Prepn: S. Schütz *et al.*, **DE 1247302**; *eidem*, **US 3963778** (1967, 1976 both to Bayer). Synthesis and pharmacological properties: G.

Aichinger *et al.*, *Arzneim.-Forsch.* **19**, 838 (1969); S. Rossi *et al.*, *Farmaco Ed. Sci.* **24**, 685 (1969).

Colorless oil.

Hydrochloride. [18059-99-9] LM-2909; Deparon. $C_{18}H_{18}$-N_2O.HCl; mol wt 314.81. Crystals from isopropanol, mp 232-233°. LD_{50} in rats (mg/kg): 330 orally, 25 i.v. (Rossi).

THERAP CAT: Antidepressant.

2891. Denatonium Benzoate. [3734-33-6] N-[2-[(2,6-Dimethylphenyl)amino]-2-oxoethyl]-N,N-diethylbenzenemethanaminium benzoate; benzyldiethyl[(2,6-xylylcarbamoyl)methyl]ammonium benzoate; lignocaine benzyl benzoate; Bitrex. $C_{28}H_{34}N_2O_3$; mol wt 446.58. C 75.31%, H 7.67%, N 6.27%, O 10.75%. Prepn: J. E. Hay, **US 3080327** (1963 to T. & H. Smith Ltd.); *idem*, **US 3268575** (1966 to Edinburgh Pharm. Ind.). HPLC determn in rapeseed oil: C. E. Damon, B. C. Pettitt, Jr., *J. Chromatogr.* **195**, 243 (1980). Brief review of substance history and uses: H. A. S. Payne, *Chem. Ind. (London)* **22**, 721-723 (1988).

Crystals from isopropyl alcohol + ethyl acetate, mp 166-170°. Among the most bitter substances known to man. Soluble in water, alcohol; sparingly sol in acetone. Practically insol in ether.

USE: Pharmaceutic aid (alcohol denaturant; flavor). Added to toxic substances as a deterrent to accidental ingestion. Can replace brucine or quassin as denaturant for ethyl alcohol.

2892. Dendrotoxins. [74811-93-1] DTX. Family of low molecular weight (∼7K) proteins isolated from the venom of mamba snakes. Inhibits voltage-dependent potassium (K^+) channels at nanomolar ranges. Characterized by 3 conserved disulfide linkages in a 57-60 amino acid sequence. Isoln from *Dendroaspis angusticeps:* A. L. Harvey, E. Karlsson, *Arch. Pharmacol.* **312**, 1 (1980). K^+-channel blockade: J. V. Halliwell *et al.*, *Proc. Natl. Acad. Sci. USA* **83**, 493 (1986); relative potencies as blockers: D. G. Owen *et al.*, *Br. J. Pharmacol.* **120**, 1029 (1997). NMR and 2° structure of I: M.-F. Foray *et al.*, *Eur. J. Biochem.* **211**, 813 (1993). Syntheses and sequences: M. E. Byrnes *et al.*, *Protein Pept. Lett.* **1**, 239 (1995); H. Nishio *et al.*, *Pept. Chem.* **34**, 105 (1996). Structure-activity study of K: L. A. Smith *et al.*, *Biochemistry* **36**, 7690 (1997). Comparison of neurotoxic effects with apamin, *q.v.*: G. Lallement *et al.*, *Toxicology* **104**, 47 (1995). *Review:* A. L. Harvey, *Gen. Pharmacol.* **28**, 7-12 (1997).

USE: Biochemical tool for K^+ channels.

2893. Denileukin Diftitox. [173146-27-5] N-L-Methionyl-387-L-histidine-388-L-alanine-1-388-toxin (*Corynebacterium diphtheriae* strain C7) (388 → 2')-protein with 2-133-interleukin 2 (human clone pTIL2-21a); $DAB_{389}IL2$; LY-335348; Ontak. Recombinant fusion protein consisting of the catalytic and translocation domains of diphtheria toxin fused to interleukin 2, *q.v.* Immunotoxin that selectively targets eukaryotic cells expressing the interleukin 2 receptor. Prepn: D. Williams *et al.*, *J. Biol. Chem.* **265**, 11885 (1990). Clinical evaluation in cutaneous T cell lymphoma: M. Duvic *et al.*, *Am. J. Hematol.* **58**, 87 (1998). Review of development and clinical experience: F. M. Foss *et al.*, *Curr. Top. Microbiol. Immunol.* **234**, 63-81 (1998).

THERAP CAT: Antineoplastic.

2894. Denopamine. [71771-90-9] (αR)-α-[[[2-(3,4-Dimethoxyphenyl)ethyl]amino]methyl]-4-hydroxybenzenemethanol; (−)-

(R)-α-[[(3,4-dimethoxyphenethyl)amino]methyl]-p-hydroxybenzyl alcohol; (−)-(R)-1-(4-hydroxyphenyl)-2-(3,4-dimethoxyphenethyl-amino)ethanol; TA-064; Carguto; Kalgut. $C_{18}H_{23}NO_4$; mol wt 317.38. C 68.12%, H 7.30%, N 4.41%, O 20.16%. Selective β_1-adrenoceptor agonist with positive inotropic activity. Prepn: M. Ikezaki *et al.*, **BE 833731**; *eidem*, **US 4032575** (1976, 1977 both to Tanabe Seiyaku); N. Umino *et al.*, *Chem. Pharm. Bull.* **27**, 1479 (1979). Effect on carbohydrate and lipid metabolism in rats: M. Inamasu *et al.*, *Biochem. Pharmacol.* **33**, 2171 (1984). Cardiovascular pharmacology in animals: T. Nagao *et al.*, *Jpn. J. Pharmacol.* **35**, 415 (1984); in humans: M. Kino *et al.*, *Am. J. Cardiol.* **51**, 802 (1983). Metabolism in humans: T. Suzuki *et al.*, *Drug Metab. Dispos.* **11**, 377 (1983). GC-MS determn in human urine: *eidem*, *Chem. Pharm. Bull.* **33**, 2549 (1985). Binding affinity and selectivity: K. Naito *et al.*, *Jpn. J. Pharmacol.* **38**, 235 (1985). Clinical efficacy in congestive cardiomyopathy: J. Thormann *et al.*, *Am. Heart J.* **110**, 426 (1985). Series of articles on pharmacokinetics, metabolism and disposition in animals: *Arzneim.-Forsch.* **36**, 643-667 (1986).

l-**Form hydrochloride.** $C_{18}H_{23}NO_4 \cdot HCl$. Crystals from isopropanol, mp 138-139.5°. $[\alpha]_D^{25}$ −38.0° (c = 1 in methanol).
dl-**Form hydrochloride.** Crystals from isopropanol + isopropyl ether, mp 164-167°.
THERAP CAT: Cardiotonic.

2895. Denopterin. [22006-84-4] N-[4-[[1-(2-Amino-1,4-di-hydro-4-oxo-6-pteridinyl)ethyl]methylamino]benzoyl]-L-glutamic acid; 9,10-dimethylpteroylglutamic acid; N^{10},9-dimethylfolic acid; Dimetfol; $C_{21}H_{23}N_7O_6$; mol wt 469.45. C 53.73%, H 4.94%, N 20.89%, O 20.45%. Prepn: Hultquist *et al.*, *J. Am. Chem. Soc.* **71**, 619 (1949); Hultquist, Smith, **GB 667098** (1952 to Am. Cyanamid).

Yellow-orange microcrystals. uv max (0.1N NaOH): 253, 305, 365 nm; (0.1N HCl): 315 nm.
THERAP CAT: Antineoplastic.

2896. Denufosol. [211448-85-0] Uridine 5'-(pentahydrogen tetraphosphate) $P'''\rightarrow 5'$-ester with 2'-deoxycytidine; P^1-(uridine 5')-P^4-(2'-deoxycytidine 5')tetraphosphate; UP_4dC. $C_{18}H_{27}N_5O_{21}P_4$; mol wt 773.32. C 27.96%, H 3.52%, N 9.06%, O 43.45%, P 16.02%. Nucleotide $P2Y_2$ purinoceptor agonist. Prepn: W. Pendergast *et al.*, **WO 9834942**; *eidem*, **US 6348589** (1998, 2002 both to Inspire); and structure-activity study: S. R. Shaver *et al.*, *Purinergic Signal.* **1**, 183 (2005). Pharmacology: B. R. Yerxa *et al.*, *J. Pharmacol. Exp. Ther.* **302**, 871 (2002). Clinical evaluation in cystic fibrosis: R. Deterding *et al.*, *Pediatr. Pulmonol.* **39**, 339 (2005).

Tetrasodium salt. [318250-11-2] INS-37217. $C_{18}H_{23}N_5Na_4$-$O_{21}P_4$; mol wt 861.25.
THERAP CAT: In treatment of cystic fibrosis.

2897. Deoxo-Fluor®. [202289-38-1] (T-4)-Trifluoro[2-methoxy-N-(2-methoxyethyl)ethanaminato-κN]sulfur; bis(2-meth-oxyethyl)aminosulfur trifluoride. $C_6H_{14}F_3NO_2S$; mol wt 221.24. C 32.57%, H 6.38%, F 25.76%, N 6.33%, O 14.46%, S 14.49%. Broad-spectrum deoxofluorinating agent. Prepn: G. S. Lal *et al.*, **EP 908448**; *eidem* **US 6207860** (1999, 2001 both to Air Prods. Chem.); *idem et al.*, *Chem. Commun.* **1999**, 215; *idem et al.*, *J. Org. Chem.* **64**, 7048 (1999). Review of use in fluorination reactions of organic compds: R. P. Singh, J. M. Shreeve, *Synthesis* **2002**, 2561-2578.

Yellow liquid, colorless after distillation. bp_{10} 60°. Dec onset ~140°. d 1.2. Sol in hexane, ethers, halogenated organics, toluene.
Caution: Reacts violently with water to form HF.
USE: Versatile, thermally stable nucleophilic fluorinating reagent.

2898. 6-Deoxy-L-ascorbic Acid. [528-81-4] $C_6H_8O_5$; mol wt 160.12. C 45.01%, H 5.04%, O 49.96%. Prepn starting with 2,3-monoacetone-L-sorbomethylose: Müller, Reichstein, *Helv. Chim. Acta* **21**, 273 (1938). Alternative procedure: **CH 203549** and **CH 209587** (1939 and 1940, both to Hoffmann-La Roche).

Stout prisms from ethyl acetate, mp 168°. Sublimes at 10^{-3} mm and 160°. $[\alpha]_D^{22}$ +36.7° (0.1N HCl). Freely sol in water; sol in acetone, alcohol; sparingly sol in ethyl acetate. Practically insol in ether.

2899. Deoxycholic Acid. [83-44-3] (3α,5β,12α)-3,12-Dihy-droxy-5-cholan-24-oic acid; 17β-(1-methyl-3-carboxypropyl)-etiocholane-3α,12α-diol; desoxycholic acid. $C_{24}H_{40}O_4$; mol wt 392.57. C 73.43%, H 10.27%, O 16.30%. Lacks the C-7 hydroxy group of cholic acid. Occurs in bile of man, ox, sheep, dog, goat, and rabbit. Isoln: Wieland, Siebert, *Z. Physiol. Chem.* **262**, 1 (1939). From cholic acid: Sifferd, **US 2765316** (1956 to Armour). Structure and synthesis: L. F. Fieser, M. Fieser, *Steroids* (Reinhold, New York, 1959). Laboratory prepn from ox bile: Gattermann-Wieland, *Praxis des Organischen Chemikers* (de Gruyter, Berlin, 40th ed., 1961) p 361. Forms molecular coordination compds (so-called **choleic acids**) with many substances. Complexes wth fatty acids have been studies extensively: Sobotka, Goldberg, *Biochem. J.* **26**, 555 (1932); Sobotka, *Chem. Rev.* **15**, 362 (1934). Surface activity: *idem, Chemistry of the Steroids*, New York (1938).

Crystals from alc, mp 176-178°. Not precipitated by digitonin. $[\alpha]_D^{20}$ +55° (alc). pK 6.58. Soly at 15° in water 0.24 g/l; in alcohol 220.7 g/l; in ether 1.16 g/l; in chloroform 2.94 g/l; in benzene 0.12 g/l; in acetone 10.46 g/l; in glacial acetic acid 9.06 g/l. Sol in solns of alkali hydroxides or carbonates.

Sodium salt. Sodium deoxycholate. $C_{24}H_{39}NaO_4$. Soly in water at 15°: >333 g/l.

THERAP CAT: Choleretic.

2900. Deoxycorticosterone. [64-85-7] 21-Hydroxypregn-4-ene-3,20-dione; 4-pregnen-21-ol-3,20-dione; 21-hydroxy-progesterone; desoxycorticosterone; 11-deoxycorticosterone; cortexone; desoxycortone; Kendall's desoxy compound B; Reichstein's substance Q. $C_{21}H_{30}O_3$; mol wt 330.46. C 76.33%, H 9.15%, O 14.52%. Occurs in adrenal cortex: Reichstein, von Euw, *Helv. Chim. Acta* **21**, 1197 (1938); Steiger, Reichstein, *ibid.* **20**, 1164 (1937). Numerous prepns from other steroids: Schindler *et al.*, *ibid.* **24**, 371 (1941); Reichstein, **DE 875353** (1953 to Schering); Bockmühl *et al.*, **DE 871153** (1953 to Hoechst); Wettstein *et al.*, **US 2778776** (1957 to Ciba); **NL 89575** (1958 to Organon); Kaspar *et al.*, **DE 1028572** (1958 to Schering). Isoln from the prothoracal glands of the water beetle, *Dytiscus marginalis*: Schildknecht *et al.*, *Angew. Chem.* **78**, 392 (1966).

Plates from ether, mp 141-142°. $[\alpha]_D^{22}$ +178° (alc). uv max: 240 nm. Freely sol in alcohol, acetone.

Acetate *see* Deoxycorticosterone Acetate.

Tetraacetyl-β-D-glucoside. $C_{35}H_{48}O_{12}$. Clusters of needles from 50% alc, mp 176-176.5°. $[\alpha]_D^{24}$ +80° (c = 0.515 in chloroform). Believed to occur in nature in this glycosidic form: Johnson, *J. Am. Chem. Soc.* **63**, 3238 (1941).

THERAP CAT: Mineralocorticoid.

2901. Deoxycorticosterone Acetate. [56-47-3] 21-Acetyloxypregn-4-ene-3,20-dione; 21-hydroxypregn-4-ene-3,20-dione 21-acetate; 11-deoxycorticosterone acetate; cortexone acetate; desoxycorticosterone acetate; desoxycortone acetate; DCA; Cortate; Cortiron; Decosteron; Doca; Dorcostrin; Percorten; Syncortyl. $C_{23}H_{32}O_4$; mol wt 372.50. C 74.16%, H 8.66%, O 17.18%.

Orthorhombic needles from alcohol, stable in air, mp 154-160°. Sublimes in high vacuum. $[\alpha]_D^{20}$ +168 to +176° (dioxane). Slightly sol in alcohol, methanol, acetone, ether, dioxane, propylene glycol (10 mg/ml), vegetable oils. Practically insol in water.

THERAP CAT: Mineralocorticoid.

THERAP CAT (VET): Adrenocortical steroid, mineralocorticoid.

2902. Deoxydihydrostreptomycin. [26086-49-7] *O*-2-De-oxy-2-(methylamino)-α-L-glucopyranosyl-(1 → 2)-*O*-3,5-dideoxy-3-(hydroxymethyl)-α-L-arabinofuranosyl-(1 → 4)-*N,N'*-bis(amino-iminomethyl)-D-streptamine; dihydrodeoxystreptomycin; Desoxymycin; Mervastrept. $C_{21}H_{41}N_7O_{11}$; mol wt 567.59. C 44.44%, H 7.28%, N 17.27%, O 31.01%. Reduction product of streptomycin. Prepn and structure: Ikeda, *C.A.* **50**, 13765g (1956); Yabuta *et al.*, **US 2837510** (1958); Gailliot, Baget, **FR 1198042** (1959 to Rhône-Poulenc). TLC separation: H. Heding, *Acta Chem. Scand.* **24**, 3086 (1970). Comparative antibacterial activity of streptomycin analogs: H. Heding, O. Lützen, *J. Antibiot.* **25**, 287 (1972).

Needles, dec 190-195°. $[\alpha]_D^{20}$ −102.5° (water).

Sulfate. $[\alpha]_D^{20}$ −78° (c = 2).

THERAP CAT: Antibacterial (tuberculostatic).

2903. Deoxyepinephrine. [501-15-5] 4-[2-(Methylamino)-ethyl]-1,2-benzenediol; 4-[2-(methylamino)ethyl]pyrocatechol; 3,4-dihydroxyphenylethylamine; methyl[β-(3,4-dihydroxyphenyl)ethyl]amine; *N*-methyldopamine; epinine. $C_9H_{13}NO_2$; mol wt 167.21. C 64.65%, H 7.84%, N 8.38%, O 19.14%. Adrenergic and dopamine receptor agonist; active metabolite of ibopamine, *q.v.* Prepd by heating HCl and 1-keto-6,7-dimethoxy-2-methyltetrahydroisoquinoline obtained from laudanosine or papaverine: Pyman, *J. Chem. Soc.* **95**, 1266, 1610 (1909). Synthesis from veratrole: Kindler, Peschke, *Arch. Pharm.* **270**, 340 (1932); Kindler, Hesse, *ibid.* **271**, 439 (1933). From methylhomoveratrylamine: Buck, *J. Am. Chem. Soc.* **52**, 4119 (1930); Bretschneider, *Monatsh. Chem.* **76**, 335 (1947). Precursor in biosynthesis of epinephrine: W. F. Bridgers, S. Kaufman, *J. Biol. Chem.* **237**, 526 (1962). Cardiovascular pharmacology: I. Martínez-Mir *et al.*, *Gen. Pharmacol.* **31**, 75 (1998). Comparison with 3,4-dihydroxybenzylamine in catecholamine analysis: H. He *et al.*, *J. Chromatogr. B* **701**, 115 (1997).

Crystals, mp 188-189°.

Hydrochloride. $C_9H_{13}NO_2 \cdot HCl$. Crystals. Sol in water, alcohol. *Sensitive to light.*

USE: Internal standard in chromatographic analysis of catecholamines.

2904. 2-Deoxy-D-glucose. [154-17-6] 2-Deoxy-D-*arabino*-hexose; D-*arabino*-2-desoxyhexose; 2-deoxyglucose; 2-DG; Ba-2758. $C_6H_{12}O_5$; mol wt 164.16. C 43.90%, H 7.37%, O 48.73%. Antimetabolite of glucose, *q.v.*, with antiviral activity. Synthesis: M. Bergmann *et al.*, *Ber.* **55**, 158 (1922); **56**, 1052 (1923); J. C. Sowden, H. O. L. Fischer, *J. Am. Chem. Soc.* **69**, 1048 (1947); H. R. Bolliger, *Helv. Chim. Acta* **89** (1954); H. R. Bolliger, M. D. Schmid, *ibid.* 1597, 1671; H. R. Bolliger, "2-Deoxy-D-*arabino*-hexose (2-Deoxy-D-glucose)" in *Methods in Carbohydrate Chemistry* vol. I, R. L. Whistler, M. L. Wolfrom, Eds. (Academic Press, New York, 1962) pp 186-189. Inhibition of influenza virus multiplication: E. D. Kilbourne, *Nature* **183**, 271 (1959). Effects on herpes simplex virus: R. J. Courtney *et al.*, *Virology* **52**, 447 (1973). Mechanism of action studies: M. R. Steiner *et al.*, *Biochem. Biophys. Res. Commun.* **61**, 745 (1974); E. K. Ray *et al.*, *Virology* **58**, 118 (1978). Use in human genital herpes infections: H. A. Blough, R. L. Giuntoli, *J. Am. Med. Assoc.* **241**, 2798 (1979); L. Corey, K. K. Holmes, *ibid.* **243**, 29 (1980). Effect vs respiratory syncytial viral infections in calves: S. B. Mohanty *et al.*, *Am. J. Vet. Res.* **42**, 336 (1981).

Cryst from acetone or butanone, mp 142-144°. $[\alpha]_D^{17.5}$ +38.3° (35 min) → +45.9° (c = 0.52 in water); +22.8° (24 hrs) → +80.8° (c = 0.57 in pyridine).

α-Form. Cryst from isopropanol, mp 134-136°. $[\alpha]_D^{26}$ +156° → +103° (c = 0.9 in pyridine).

USE: Exptlly as an antiviral agent.

2905. 1-Deoxynojirimycin. [19130-96-2] (2R,3R,4R,5S)-2-(Hydroxymethyl)-3,4,5-piperidinetriol; D-5-amino-1,5-dideoxyglucopyranose; 1,5-dideoxy-1,5-imino-D-glucitol; (2R,3R,4R,5S)-2-hydroxymethyl-3,4,5-trihydroxypiperidine; moranoline; Bay m 5595; S-GI. $C_6H_{13}NO_4$; mol wt 163.17. C 44.17%, H 8.03%, N 8.58%, O 39.22%. α-Glucosidase inhibitor. Prepd by reduction of nojirimycin: S. Inouye et al., J. Antibiot. **19A,** 290 (1966); S. Inouye et al., Tetrahedron **23,** 2125 (1968). Isoln from mulberry, Morus spp. (Moraceae): M. Yagi et al., Nippon Nogei Kagaku Kaishi **50,** 571 (1976), C.A. **86,** 167851r (1977). Production by Bacillus subtilis DSM704: D. C. Stein et al., Appl. Environ. Microbiol. **48,** 280 (1984). Total synthesis: H. Setoi et al., Chem. Pharm. Bull. **34,** 2642 (1986); H. J. G. Broxterman et al., Rec. Trav. Chim. **106,** 571 (1987). HPLC determn: M. D. Cole et al., J. Chromatogr. **445,** 295 (1988). Inhibition of α-glucosidase: Y. Yoshikuni, Agric. Biol. Chem. **52,** 121 (1988). Antiviral activity: P. S. Sunkara et al., Biochem. Biophys. Res. Commun. **148,** 206 (1987). Inhibition of glycoprotein synthesis and secretion: N. Peyrieras et al., EMBO J. **2,** 823 (1983); V. Gross et al., Biochem. J. **236,** 853 (1986); M. Bollen et al., Biochem. Pharmacol. **37,** 905 (1988).

Prisms from water/ethanol, mp 195°. $[\alpha]_D^{21}$ +47° (c = 1.045 in water); $[\alpha]_D^{20}$ +46.7° (c = 0.2 in water); $[\alpha]_D^{20}$ +36° (c = 0.02 in water). pKa 6.6.

2906. Deoxyribonuclease I. [9003-98-9] Deoxyribonuclease (pancreatic); pancreatic dornase; pancreatic desoxyribonuclease; DNase I. Endonuclease enzyme that hydrolyzes DNA; produced by the mammalian pancreas. Variably glycosylated, single polypeptide chain with two disulfide bridges; multiple isoforms exist. The human form consists of 260 amino acid residues; mol wt ~37 kDa. Prepn from beef pancreas: M. Kunitz, Science **108,** 19 (1948); Baumgarten, Johnson, US 2801956; eidem, US 3042587 (1957, 1962 both to Merck & Co.). Properties of purified DNase I: Price et al., J. Biol. Chem. **244,** 917 (1969). Reviews of purification and characterization: M. Laskowski in The Enzymes vol. 4, P. D. Boyer, Ed. (Academic Press, New York, 3rd ed., 1971) pp 289-311; S. Moore, ibid. vol. 14 281-296 (1981); T.-H. Liao, Mol. Cell. Biochem. **34,** 15-22 (1981).

Bovine pancreatic deoxyribonuclease. Deanase; Dinase; Dornavac. Mixture of 4 isoforms. DNAse A is the most predominant. Contains 257 amino acid residues; mol wt 31 kDa. pI ~5.

Dornase alfa. [143831-71-4] Deoxyribonuclease (human clone 18-1 protein moiety); rhDNase I; Pulmozyme. Human DNase I produced in Chinese hamster ovary cells by recombinant DNA technology. Cloning and expression of human form and effect on sputum viscosity: S. Shak et al., Proc. Natl. Acad. Sci. USA **87,** 9188 (1990); S. Shak, WO 9007572 (1990 to Genentech). HPLC purification: J. Cacia et al., J. Chromatogr. **634,** 229 (1993). Clinical study in cystic fibrosis: H. J. Fuchs et al., N. Engl. J. Med. **331,** 637 (1994). Expert report on pharmacology and toxicology: J. D. Green, Hum. Exp. Toxicol. **13,** Suppl. 1, S1-S42 (1994).

THERAP CAT: Debriding agent. In treatment of cystic fibrosis and other pulmonary disease to reduce viscosity of sputum.

THERAP CAT (VET): Debriding agent.

2907. Deoxyribonucleic Acid. Desoxyribonucleic acid; DNA; thymus nucleic acid; Desoxiribon; Eucytol. Polynucleotide; essential component of chromosomes in cell nuclei. In its role as the carrier of genetic information, DNA must have two functions: be exactly reproducible in order to transmit its genetic information to future generations; contain information, in chemical code, to direct the development of the cell according to its inheritance. Reviews of biological function: Hotchkiss in The Nucleic Acids vol. 2, E. Chargaff, J. N. Davidson, Eds. (Academic Press, New York, 1955) pp 435-473; Crick, Nature **227,** 561 (1970); J. N. Davidson, The Biochemistry of Nucleic Acids (Academic Press, New York, 7th ed., 1972) pp 6-28. The purine and pyrimidine bases of the nucleosides are primarily adenine, guanine, cytosine and thymine; the sugar is D-2-deoxyribose, q.q.v. The nucleosides are linked together by phosphates in diester linkage from the 3'-hydroxyl of one sugar to the 5'-hydroxyl of the next. The repeating sugar-phosphate linkage forms the backbone of the single polynucleotide strand which is the primary structure of DNA. Chemical analyses of DNA from different species show that the purine content is equal to the pyrimidine content; adenine content equal to thymine; guanine equal to cytosine: Chargaff, Experientia **6,** 201 (1950); idem, Fed. Proc. **10,** 654 (1951). In the Watson-Crick model of its secondary structure (based on chemical analysis and x-ray studies), DNA consists of two polynucleotide chains forming right-handed helices coiled around the same axis with the sequence of atoms in the two sugar-phosphate backbones running in opposite direction. Two major families of right-handed helix were proposed. *A-DNA* and *B-DNA*, each having its own intrinsic restrictions on chain-folding and structure. B-DNA is believed to be the predominant form in biological systems. The purine and pyrimidine bases are inside the helical structure formed by the sugar phosphate backbones; those on one chain form hydrogen bonds to those on the other. Adenine in one chain is always bonded to thymine in the complementary chain by hydrogen bonds; similarly guanine is bonded to cytosine. The linear sequence of bases in one strand completely determines the sequence in the complementary strand. Thus each strand can serve as a template for the replication of the original DNA molecule: Watson, Crick, Nature **171,** 737, 964 (1953). X-ray studies: Wilkins et al., ibid. 738; Marvin et al., J. Mol. Biol. **3,** 547 (1961); Fuller et al., ibid. **12,** 60 (1965). DNA also acts as a template in the formation of ribonucleic acids, q.v., which play a fundamental role in the synthesis of proteins in the cell. Another form of DNA, termed *Z-DNA*, is also known. Its structure is an antiparallel double helix with Watson-Crick base pairing, but it is a left-handed helix with the ribose-phosphate backbone following a zig-zag course. Molecular structure, atomic resolution x-ray crystallographic analysis: A. H.-J. Wang et al., Nature **282,** 680 (1979). First identification of Z-DNA in material of biological origin: A. Nordheim et al., ibid. **294,** 417 (1981). Studies of B- and Z-DNA: D. J. Patel et al., Proc. Natl. Acad. Sci. USA **79,** 1413 (1982). Comparison of A-, B-, and Z-DNA: R. E. Dickerson et al., Science **216,** 475 (1982). Demonstration of Z-DNA immunoreactivity in rat tissues: G. Morgenegg et al., Nature **309,** 540 (1983).

2908. D-2-Deoxyribose. [533-67-5] 2-Deoxy-D-*erythro*-pentose; desoxyribose; D-2-deoxyarabinose; D-2-ribodesose; D-*erythro*-2-deoxypentose; thyminose. $C_5H_{10}O_4$; mol wt 134.13.

C 44.77%, H 7.51%, O 47.71%. Isoln from deoxyribonucleic acid by acidic hydrolysis of purine deoxyribonucleosides which have been isolated by ion-exchange resin chromatography: Laland, Overend, *Acta Chem. Scand.* **8,** 192 (1954). Synthesis: Felton, Freudenberg, *J. Am. Chem. Soc.* **57,** 1637 (1935); Deriaz *et al., J. Chem. Soc.* **1949,** 1879, 2836; Hough, *Chem. Ind. (London)* **1951,** 406; Sowden, *Biochem. Prep.* **5,** 75 (1957); I. Ziderman, E. Dimant, *J. Org. Chem.* **32,** 1267 (1967); J. R. Hauske, H. Rapoport, *ibid.* **44,** 2472 (1979); T. Harada, T. Mukaiyama, *Chem. Lett.* **1981,** 1109. *Review:* Overend, Stacey, in Chargaff-Davidson, *Nucleic Acids* **vol. 1,** E. Chargaff, N. J. Davidson, Eds. (Academic Press, New York, 1955) pp 1-80.

Crystals from isopropanol, mp 91°. Shows mutarotation. Final $[\alpha]_D^{22}$ −56.2° (H$_2$O). Sol in water, pyridine. Slightly sol in alc.

1,3,4-Triacetate. C$_{11}$H$_{16}$O$_7$. Needles from methanol, mp 98°. $[\alpha]_D^{23}$ −171.8° (c = 0.56 in chloroform): Allerton, Overend, *J. Chem. Soc.* **1951,** 1480.

3,4,5-Triacetate. Oily liq, bp$_{0.001}$ 105°. $[\alpha]_D^{21}$ +3.4° (c = 4.57 in pyridine): Zinner *et al., Ber.* **90,** 2696 (1957).

1,3,4-Tribenzoate. Small white nodules from ethanol, mp 127°. $[\alpha]_D^{23}$ −65° (c = 1.02 in chloroform) (Allerton, Overend). Probably a mixture of the two anomeric 2-deoxy-D-ribopyranose tribenzoates: Pedersen *et al., J. Am. Chem. Soc.* **82,** 3425 (1960).

3,4,5-Tribenzoate. Fine needles from ethyl acetate + petr ether, mp 118-119°. $[\alpha]_D^{18}$ −2.8° (c = 1.44 in pyridine) (Zinner).

2909. 2-Deoxystreptamine. [2037-48-1] 2-Deoxy-1,3-*myo*-inosadiamine; 1,3-diamino-4,5,6-trihydroxycyclohexane. C$_6$H$_{14}$N$_2$O$_3$; mol wt 162.19. C 44.43%, H 8.70%, N 17.27%, O 29.59%. Important component of several aminocyclitol antibiotics. Production by acid hydrolysis of neamine, *q.v.* and structure: F. A. Kuehl *et al., J. Am. Chem. Soc.* **73,** 881 (1952). Also obtained from hydrolysis products of kanamycins, paromomycins, gentamicins, *q.q.v.* and other aminoglycoside antibiotics. *See* K. L. Rinehart, *J. Infect. Dis.* **119,** 345 (1969); S. Hanessian, T. H. Haskell, *The Carbohydrates* **vol. IIA,** W. Pigman, D. Horton, Eds. (Academic Press, New York, 2nd ed., 1970) pp 159-172. Configuration: J. Daly *et al., J. Am. Chem. Soc.* **82,** 5928 (1960); H. E. Carter *et al., ibid.* **83,** 3723 (1961); R. U. Lemieux, R. J. Cushley, *Can. J. Chem.* **41,** 858 (1963). Synthesis: M. Nakajima *et al., Tetrahedron Lett.* **1964,** 967; T. Suami *et al., ibid.* **1967,** 2671; S. Ogawa *et al., J. Org. Chem.* **39,** 812 (1974); H. Prinzbach *et al., Angew. Chem. Int. Ed.* **14,** 225 (1975); S. Ogawa *et al., J. Org. Chem.* **42,** 3083 (1977). Review of syntheses: G. F. Busscher *et al., Chem. Rev.* **105,** 775-791 (2005).

Colorless crystals from ethanol, mp 225-228°.

Dihydrochloride. [14429-30-2] C$_6$H$_{14}$N$_2$O$_3$.2HCl. Crystals, mp 325° (dec), H. Hitomi *et al., Chem. Pharm. Bull.* **9,** 340 (1961).

2910. Deoxyuridine. [951-78-0] 2′-Deoxyuridine; 1-(2-deoxy-β-D-*erythro*-pentofuranosyl)uracil; 1-(2-deoxy-β-D-ribofurano-syl)uracil; uracil deoxyriboside. C$_9$H$_{12}$N$_2$O$_5$; mol wt 228.20. C 47.37%, H 5.30%, N 12.28%, O 35.06%. Prepn: Dekker, Todd, *Nature* **166,** 557 (1950); Brown *et al., J. Chem. Soc.* **1958,** 3035; Prystas *et al., Collect. Czech. Chem. Commun.* **28,** 3140 (1963); Smejkal *et al., ibid.* **31,** 291 (1966). Conformation: Rahman, Wilson, *Nature* **232,** 333 (1971).

Needles from abs alc or 95% alc, mp 163° (Dekker, Todd) and 167° (Brown *et al.*). $[\alpha]_D^{22}$ +50° (c = 1.1 in *N* NaOH).

α-Anomer. 1-(2-Deoxy-α-D-*erythro*-pentofuranosyl)uracil; 1-(2-deoxy-α-D-ribofuranosyl)uracil. Prepn: Prystas *et al., loc. cit.*

2911. Depreotide. [161982-62-3] Cyclo(L-homocysteinyl-*N*-methyl-L-phenylalanyl-L-tyrosyl-D-tryptophyl-L-lysyl-L-valyl), (1 → 1′)-thioether with 3-[(mercaptoacetyl)amino]-L-alanyl-L-lysyl-L-cysteinyl-L-lysinamide; cyclo-(*N*-Me)Phe-Tyr-(D-Trp)-Lys-Val-Hcy(CH$_2$CO-(β-Dap)-Lys-Cys-Lys-NH$_2$); cyclo.(*N*-CH$_3$)FYW$_D$-KV.Hcy(CH$_2$CO.(β-Dap)KCK.amide); P829. C$_{65}$H$_{96}$N$_{16}$O$_{12}$S$_2$; mol wt 1357.69. C 57.50%, H 7.13%, N 16.51%, O 14.14%, S 4.72%. Synthetic cyclic peptide of 10 amino acids; somatostatin analog designed to bind to somatostatin receptor-bearing tumors. ^{99m}Tc-Labeled complex functions as scintigraphic imaging agent. Prepn: R. T. Dean *et al.,* **WO 9500553** (1995 to Diatech); *eidem,* **US 6051206** (2000 to Diatide); D. A. Pearson *et al., J. Med. Chem.* **39,** 1361 (1996). Binding studies: I. Virgolini *et al., Cancer Res.* **58,** 1850 (1998). Clinical study in diagnosis of pulmonary nodules: J. Blum *et al., Chest* **117,** 1232 (2000).

^{99m}Tc-Labeled form. ^{99m}Tc-P829; NeoTect.

THERAP CAT: Diagnostic aid (radioactive imaging agent).

2912. Deptropine. [604-51-3] *endo*-3-[(10,11-Dihydro-5*H*-dibenzo[*a,d*]cyclohepten-5-yl)oxy]-8-methyl-8-azabicyclo[3.2.1]-octane; 3α-[(10,11-dihydro-5*H*-dibenzo[*a,d*]cyclohepten-5-yl)oxy]-1α*H*,5α*H*-tropane; dibenzheptropine. C$_{23}$H$_{27}$NO; mol wt 333.47. C 82.84%, H 8.16%, N 4.20%, O 4.80%. Prepn: Van der Stelt *et al., J. Med. Pharm. Chem.* **4,** 335 (1961). Pharmacology: Funcke *et al., Arch. Int. Pharmacodyn.* **148,** 135 (1964); Timmerman *et al., ibid.* **187,** 291 (1970). Metabolism: Hespe *et al., ibid.* **164,** 397 (1966).

Citrate. [2169-75-7] BS-6987; Brontine. C$_{23}$H$_{27}$NO.C$_6$H$_8$O$_7$; mol wt 525.59. LD$_{50}$ in mice (mg/kg): 32 i.v.; 300 orally (Timmerman).

Maleate. C$_{23}$H$_{27}$NO.C$_4$H$_4$O$_4$. Crystals from ethanol, acetone, ethyl acetate or chloroform, mp 133-136°.

THERAP CAT: Antihistaminic.

2913. Dequalinium Chloride. [522-51-0] 1,1'-(1,10-Decanediyl)bis-[4-amino-2-methylquinolinium chloride]; 1,1'-decamethylenebis[4-aminoquinaldinium chloride]; BAQD-10; decamine; dekamin; Decatylen; Dekadin; Dequadin Chloride; Dequafungan; Dequavet; Dequavagyn; Eriosept; Evazol; Grocreme; Labosept; Optipect; Phylletten; Polycidine; Sorot. $C_{30}H_{40}Cl_2N_4$; mol wt 527.57. C 68.30%, H 7.64%, Cl 13.44%, N 10.62%. Prepn: Taylor *et al.*, **GB 745956** (1956 to Allen & Hanburys), *C.A.* **50**, 16878e (1956); Austin *et al., J. Chem. Soc.* **1958**, 1489.

Crystals from ethanol, mp 326° (dec). Soly in water (25°): about one g/200 ml.

Ingredient of *Efisol, Gargilon, Gramipan, Hexalyse, Micrin.*
USE: Bacteriostat.
THERAP CAT: Antiseptic, disinfectant.
THERAP CAT (VET): Antimicrobial.

2914. Deracoxib. [169590-41-4] 4-[3-(Difluoromethyl)-5-(3-fluoro-4-methoxyphenyl)-1*H*-pyrazol-1-yl]benzenesulfonamide; SC-046; SC-59046; Deramaxx. $C_{17}H_{14}F_3N_3O_3S$; mol wt 397.37. C 51.38%, H 3.55%, F 14.34%, N 10.57%, O 12.08%, S 8.07%. Selective cyclooxygenase-2 (COX-2) inhibitor. Prepn: J. J. Talley *et al.,* **WO 9515316**; M. J. Graneto, **US 5521207** (1995, 1996 both to Searle); T. D. Penning *et al., J. Med. Chem.* **40**, 1347 (1997). Structure activity study: G. R. Desiraju *et al., Molecules* **5**, 945 (2000). Effect in experimental synovitis in dogs: D. L. Millis *et al, Vet. Ther.* **3**, 453 (2002); HPLC determn in plasma: S. K. Cox *et al., J. Chromatogr. B* **819**, 181 (2005).

Light tan solid, mp 159-161°.
THERAP CAT (VET): Anti-inflammatory; analgesic.

2915. Deramciclane. [120444-71-5] *N,N*-Dimethyl-2-[[(1*R*,2*S*,4*R*)-1,7,7-trimethyl-2-phenylbicyclo[2.2.1]hept-2-yl]oxy]-ethanamine; (−)-[1*R*,2*S*,4*R*]-2-(2-dimethylaminoethoxy)-2-phenyl-1,7,7-trimethylbicyclo[2.2.1]heptane. $C_{20}H_{31}NO$; mol wt 301.47. C 79.68%, H 10.36%, N 4.65%, O 5.31%. Serotonin (5-HT_2)-receptor antagonist. Prepn: **BE 886579**; Z. Budai *et al.,* **US 4342762** (1981, 1982 both to Egyt); L. Ladanyi *et al., Chirality* **11**, 689 (1999). LC/MS/MS determn in plasma: A. Tolokán *et al., J. Chromatogr. A* **896**, 279 (2000). Receptor binding profile and pharmacology: I. Gacsalyi *et al., Drug Dev. Res.* **40**, 333 (1997). Clinical pharmacokinetics and tolerability: H. Kanerva *et al., Int. J. Clin. Pharmacol. Ther.* **37**, 589 (1999). Clinical evaluation in generalized anxiety disorder: H. Naukkarinen *et al., Eur. Neuropsychopharmcol.* **15**, 617 (2005). Review: S. Koks, E. Vasar, *Curr. Opin. Invest. Drugs* **3**, 289-294 (2002).

Colorless oil. Log P (octanol/water): 5.9. Soly in water (25°): 0.0088 g/100 ml.
Fumarate. [120444-72-6] EGIS-3886. $C_{20}H_{31}NO.C_4H_4O_4$; mol wt 417.54. Crystals from DMF, mp 210-213°. $[\alpha]_{436}^{20}$ −88.0° ± 1 (c = 0.4 in DMSO). Log P (octanol/water): 1.41. pKa 9.61.
THERAP CAT: Anxiolytic.

2916. Derris Root. Tuba root; Deguelia root. The roots of plants belonging to the genus *Derris,* of which more than 80 species have been described. *Derris elliptica* (Wall.) Benth. and *D. malaccensis* Prain, *Leguminosae* are cultivated in British Malaya and the Dutch East Indies. Toxicity data: Haag *et al., Proc. Soc. Exp. Biol. Med.* **54**, 140 (1943).
LD_{50} orally in mice: 350 mg/kg (as the dry powdered root (Haag)).
USE: As insecticide; as a source of rotenone and rotenoid compds.

2917. Desaspidin BB. [114-43-2] 2-[[2,4-Dihydroxy-6-methoxy-3-(1-oxobutyl)phenyl]methyl]-3,5-dihydroxy-4,4-dimethyl-6-(1-oxobutyl)-2,5-cyclohexadien-1-one; 3'-[(5-butyryl-2,4-dihydroxy-3,3-dimethyl-6-oxo-1,4-cyclohexadien-1-yl)methyl]-2',6'-dihydroxy-4'-methoxybutyrophenone; desaspidin; rosapin. $C_{24}H_{30}O_8$; mol wt 446.49. C 64.56%, H 6.77%, O 28.67%. Isoln from the rhizome of *Dryopteris austriaca* (Jacq.) Wojnar, *Polypodiaceae:* Aebi *et al., Helv. Chim. Acta* **40**, 266 (1957); from *D. caucasica* (A. Br.) Fraser-Jenkins et Corley: Widén *et al., ibid.* **56**, 831 (1973). Structure: Aebi *et al., ibid.* **40**, 572 (1957). Toxicity study: Airaksinan *et al., Acta Pharmacol. Toxicol.* **25**, 33 (1967).

Crystals from ether + petr ether, mp 150-150.5°. uv max: 230, 274 nm (ε 23000, 16800) in cyclohexane. Freely sol in ether, benzene, acetone. Practically insol in methanol, ethanol, petr ether. LD_{50} orally in mice: 340 mg/kg (Airaksinan).

2918. Deserpidine. [131-01-1] (3β,16β,17α,18β,20α)-17-Methoxy-18-[(3,4,5-trimethoxybenzoyl)oxy]-3,20-yohimban-16-carboxylic acid methyl ester; 11-desmethoxyreserpine; canescine; recanescine; Harmonyl; Raunormine. $C_{32}H_{38}N_2O_8$; mol wt 578.65. C 66.42%, H 6.62%, N 4.84%, O 22.12%. Isoln from roots of *Rauwolfia canescens* L., *Apocynaceae:* A. Stoll, A. Hofmann, *J. Am. Chem. Soc.* **77**, 820 (1955); M. W. Klohs *et al., ibid.* 4084; N. Neuss *et al., ibid.* 4087; H. B. MacPhillamy *et al., ibid.* 4335; E. Schlittler *et al., Experientia* **11**, 64 (1955); **GB 791241** (1958 to Penick); **GB 809912**; P. R. Ulshafer, **US 2982769** (1959, 1961 both to Ciba). Stereochemistry: C. F. Huebner *et al., Experientia* **11**, 303 (1955); P. E. Aldrich *et al., J. Am. Chem. Soc.* **81**, 2481 (1959). Synthesis: L. Bláha *et al., Collect. Czech. Chem. Commun.* **25**, 237 (1960); **CA 678216** (1964 to Roussel-UCLAF).

Exists in three cryst forms from methanol: α-form, mp 228-232°; β-form, mp 230-232°; and γ-form, mp 138° and 226-232° with resolidification at 175°. $[\alpha]_D^{20}$ −163° (c = 0.5 in pyridine). pKa

6.68 in 40% methanol. uv max (ethanol): 218, 272, 290 nm (log ε 4.79, 4.26, 4.07).

Hydrochloride. [6033-69-8] $C_{32}H_{38}N_2O_8 \cdot HCl$. Thin rectangular plates from acetone, dec 253-256°.

Nitrate. $C_{32}H_{38}N_2O_8 \cdot HNO_3$. Crystals, dec 254-260°.

Oxalate. [119506-01-3] $C_{32}H_{38}N_2O_8 \cdot C_2H_2O_4$. Crystals, dec 239-243°.

10-Methoxy deriv. [865-04-3] 10-Methoxydeserpidine; methoserpidine; Decaserpyl. $C_{33}H_{40}N_2O_9$; mol wt 608.68.

THERAP CAT: Antihypertensive.

2919. Desflurane. [57041-67-5] 2-(Difluoromethoxy)-1,1,-1,2-tetrafluoroethane; (±)-2-difluoromethyl 1,2,2,2-tetrafluoroethyl ether; I-653; Suprane. $C_3H_2F_6O$; mol wt 168.04. C 21.44%, H 1.20%, F 67.84%, O 9.52%. $CHF_2OCHFCF_3$. Prepd but not claimed: J. P. Russell *et al.,* **US 3897502** (1975 to Airco). Prepn and use as anesthetic: R. C. Terrell, **US 4762856** (1988 to BOC). Series of articles on pharmacology and physical properties: E. I. Eger II *et al., Anesth. Analg.* **66,** 971-985 (1987); and toxicity studies: *eidem, ibid.* 1227, 1230. Series of articles on clinical pharmacology and kinetics: *Anesthesiology* **74,** 412-439; 479-498. *Review:* R. M. Jones, *Br. J. Anaesth.* **65,** 527-536 (1990).

Volatile liquid. Slight non-pungent odor. Nonflammable, soda lime stable. bp 23.5°. d 1.44. Vapor pressure (20°): 88.53 kPa. Vapor pressure (22-23°): ~700mm. Partition coefficient at 37° (blood/gas): 0.424 ±0.024; (saline/gas): 0.225 ±0.002; (oil/gas): 18.7 ±1.1.

THERAP CAT: Anesthetic (inhalation).

2920. Desipramine. [50-47-5] 10,11-Dihydro-*N*-methyl-5*H*-dibenz[*b,f*]azepine-5-propanamine; 10,11-dihydro-5-[3-(methylamino)propyl]-5*H*-dibenz[*b,f*]azepine; 5-(γ-methylaminopropyl)-iminodibenzyl; *N*-(3-methylaminopropyl)iminobenzyl; desmethylimipramine; norimipramine. $C_{18}H_{22}N_2$; mol wt 266.38. C 81.16%, H 8.32%, N 10.52%. Prepn: **GB 908788; BE 614616** (both 1962 to Geigy); J. H. Biel, C. I. Judd, **GB 980231** (1965 to Lakeside); *eidem*, **US 3454554** (1969 to Colgate Palmolive). Chemistry, pharmacology: E. Eriksoo, O. Rohte, *Arzneim.-Forsch.* **20,** 1561 (1970). Clinical response, plasma levels, pharmacokinetics: P. D. Hrdina, Y. D. Lapierre, *Prog. Neuro-Psychopharmacol.* **4,** 591 (1980). Mechanism of action study: S. A. Checkley *et al., Br. J. Psychiatry* **138,** 248 (1981). Efficacy in depression: W. Z. Potter *et al., Psychopharmacol. Bull.* **17,** 26 (1981); J. W. Stewart *et al., ibid.* 136. Teratological study: L. Aeppli, *Arzneim.-Forsch.* **19,** 1617 (1969). Carcinogenicity and mutagenicity study: H. Kubinski *et al., Mutat. Res.* **89,** 95 (1981). Has been found to be the most effective cmpds described for *in vitro* and *in vivo* reversal of chloroquine, *q.v.,* resistance in *Plasmodium falciparum:* A. J. Bitonti *et al., Science* **242,** 1301 (1988).

bp$_{0.02}$ 172-174°. uv max: 213, 252 nm (log ε 4.39, 3.93).

Hydrochloride. [58-28-6] G-35020; JB-8181; NSC-114901; Norpramin; Nortimil; Pertofran; Pertofrane; Petylyl. $C_{18}H_{22}N_2$. HCl; mol wt 302.84. Crystals from methanol ether, mp 215-216°. Sol in water. LD$_{50}$ in mice, rats (mg/kg): 500, 385 orally; 94, 48 i.p.; 420, 183 s.c. (Eriksoo, Rohte).

THERAP CAT: Antidepressant.

2921. Deslanoside. [17598-65-1] (3β,5β,12β)-3-[(*O*-β-D-Glucopyranosyl-(1 → 4)-*O*-2,6-dideoxy-β-D-*ribo*-hexopyranosyl-(1 → 4)-*O*-2,6-dideoxy-β-D-*ribo*-hexopyranosyl-(1 → 4)-2,6-dideoxy-β-D-*ribo*-hexopyranosyl)oxy]-12,14-dihydroxycard-20(22)-enolide; deacetyllanatoside C; desacetyldigilanide C; Cedilanide; Desace; Desaci. $C_{47}H_{74}O_{19}$; mol wt 943.08. C 59.86%, H 7.91%, O 32.23%. Cardiac glycoside. Isoln from leaves of *Digitalis lanata* Ehrh., *Scrophulariaceae:* Stoll, Kreis, *Helv. Chim. Acta* **16,** 1049, 1390 (1933). Prepn by alkaline degradation of lanatoside C: Kroszczynski *et al., Acta Pol. Pharm.* **21,** 357 (1964), *C.A.* **62,**

10292b (1965). Hemodynamic effects in heart failure: E. Ambrosioni *et al., Int. J. Clin. Pharmacol. Biopharm.* **17,** 416 (1979). Clinical pharmacokinetics: A. Marzo *et al., Farmaco Ed. Prat.* **37,** 28 (1982). Determn in blood and urine by HPLC/MS/MS: F. Guan *et al., Anal. Chem.* **71,** 4034 (1999).

β-D-glucose–(β-D-digitoxose)$_3$–O

Crystals from methanol, dec 265-268°. $[\alpha]_D^{20}$ +12° (c = 1.084 in 75% alc). One part dissolves in 5000 parts water, 200 parts methanol and 2500 parts ethanol; very slightly sol in chloroform. Practically insol in ether.

THERAP CAT: Cardiotonic.

2922. Desloratadine. [100643-71-8] 8-Chloro-6,11-dihydro-11-(4-piperidinylidene)-5*H*-benzo[5,6]cyclohepta[1,2-*b*]pyridine; descarboethoxyloratadine; Sch-34117; Clarinex. $C_{19}H_{19}$-ClN_2; mol wt 310.82. C 73.42%, H 6.16%, Cl 11.41%, N 9.01%. Nonsedating-type histamine H$_1$-receptor antagonist; active metabolite of loratadine, *q.v.* Also inhibits generation and release of inflammatory mediators from basophils and mast cells. Prepn: D. P. Schumacher *et al.,* **EP 208855;** F. J. Villani, J. K. Wong, **US 4659716** (both 1987 to Schering). GLC determn in plasma: R. Johnson *et al., J. Chromatogr. B* **657,** 125 (1994). Pharmacology: W. Kreutner *et al., Arzneim.-Forsch.* **50,** 345 (2000). Series of articles on clinical efficacy in rhinitis, asthma and urticaria: *Allergy* **56,** Suppl. 65, 1-32 (2001). Review of pharmacology, pharmacokinetics and clinical efficacy: R. S. Geha, E. O. Meltzer, *J. Allergy Clin. Immunol.* **107,** 751-762 (2001); D. K. Agrawal, *Expert Opin. Invest. Drugs* **10,** 547-560 (2001).

Crystals from hexane, mp 150-151°. Slightly sol in water; very sol in ethanol, propylene glycol.

THERAP CAT: Antihistaminic.

2923. Deslorelin. [57773-65-6] 6-D-Tryptophan-9-(*N*-ethyl-L-prolinamide)-10-deglycinamideluteinizing hormone-releasing factor (pig); [D-Trp^6,des-Gly^{10}]-LH-RH ethylamide; Somagard. $C_{64}H_{83}N_{17}O_{12}$; mol wt 1282.45. C 59.94%, H 6.52%, N 18.57%, O 14.97%. Synthetic nonapeptide agonist analog of LH-RH, *q.v.* Prepn: D. H. Coy *et al., J. Med. Chem.* **19,** 423 (1976); W. Kornreich *et al., Int. J. Pept. Protein Res.* **25,** 414 (1985). Pharmacology: K. Sundaram *et al., Life Sci.* **28,** 83 (1981). Pharmacokinetics and metabolism: B. Candas *et al., J. Clin. Endocrinol. Metab.* **70,** 1046 (1990). Clinical inhibition of spermatogenesis: R. Linde *et al., N. Engl. J. Med.* **305,** 663 (1981). Clinical trial in combination with flutamide, *q.v.,* for prostatic carcinoma: A. Dupont *et al., Eur. J. Cancer Clin. Oncol.* **24,** 659 (1988). Clinical evaluation in precocious puberty: P. K. Manasco *et al., J. Pediatr.* **115,** 105 (1989).

5-oxoPro–His–Trp–Ser–Tyr–D-Trp–Leu–Arg–ProNHCH$_2$CH$_3$

$[\alpha]_D^{24}$ −61° (c = 0.37 in 0.1*M* acetic acid).

THERAP CAT: Treatment of precocious puberty.

2924. Desmopressin. [16679-58-6] 1-(3-Mercaptopropanoic acid)-8-D-arginine vasopressin; 8-D-arginine-1-(3-mercaptopropanoic acid) vasopressin; 1-desamino-8-D-arginine vasopressin. $C_{46}H_{64}N_{14}O_{12}S_2$; mol wt 1069.22. C 51.67%, H 6.03%, N 18.34%, O 17.96%, S 6.00%. Synthetic analog of vasopressin, q.v., with antidiuretic activity and decreased pressor effects. Improves hemostasis by increasing plasma levels of von Willebrand factor, factor VIII and tissue plasminogen activator, q.q.v. Prepn: M. Zaoral et al., FR 1540536; eidem, US 3497491 (1968, 1970 both to Ceskoslovenska Akad. Ved). Syntheses: R. L. Huguenin, R. A. Boissonnas, Helv. Chim. Acta 49, 695 (1966); M. Zaoral et al., Collect. Czech. Chem. Commun. 32, 1250 (1967). Review of clinical experience in bleeding disorders: P. M. Mannucci, Blood 90, 2515-2521 (1997); in treatment of nocturnal enuresis: P. E. V. van Kerrebroeck, BJU Int. 89, 420-425 (2002); of mechanism of hemostatic effects: J. E. Kaufmann, U. M. Vischer, J. Thromb. Haemostasis 1, 682-689 (2003).

S–CH₂–CH₂–C–Tyr–Phe–Gln–Asn–Cys–Pro–D-Arg–GlyNH₂
  ‖
  O

$[\alpha]_D^{25}$ +85.5 ± 2° (calculated for the free peptide).
Monoacetate. [62288-83-9] Adiuretin SD; DDAVP; Desmospray; Minirin; Octim; Octostim; Presinex; Stimate. $C_{46}H_{64}N_{14}O_{12}S_2.C_2H_4O_2$; mol wt 1129.27. Occurs as the trihydrate.

THERAP CAT: Antidiuretic; hemostatic.

2925. Desmosterol. [313-04-2] 3β-Cholesta-5,24-dien-3-ol; 24-dehydrocholesterol; desmesterol. $C_{27}H_{44}O$; mol wt 384.64. C 84.31%, H 11.53%, O 4.16%. Has been isolated from chick embryos and the skin of rats: Stokes et al., J. Biol. Chem. 220, 415 (1956). From barnacles: Fagerlund, Idler, J. Am. Chem. Soc. 79, 6473 (1957); from red algae: Idler et al., Steroids 11, 465 (1968). Synthesis: Dasgupta et al., J. Org. Chem. 39, 1658 (1974); M. A. Apfel, ibid. 43, 2284 (1978). Stereospecific synthesis: M. Koreeda et al., ibid. 45, 1172 (1980); S. Takano et al., Chem. Commun. 1983, 760.

Platelets from methanol, mp 121.5°, also reported as 119-119.5°. $[\alpha]_D^{27}$ −41.0° (c = 1 in chloroform).

2926. Desogestrel. [54024-22-5] (17α)-13-Ethyl-11-methylene-18,19-dinorpregn-4-en-20-yn-17-ol; 17α-ethynyl-18-methyl-11-methylene-Δ⁴-estren-17β-ol; Org-2969; Cerazette. $C_{22}H_{30}O$; mol wt 310.47. C 85.11%, H 9.74%, O 5.15%. Progestogen with low androgenic potency. Prepn: A. J. van den Broek, DE 2361120; idem, US 3927046 (1974, 1975 both to Akzo); A. J. van den Broek et al., Rec. Trav. Chim. 94, 36 (1975). Biological effects: L. Viinikka et al., Acta Endocrinol. 83, 429 (1976). Endocrinological studies in animals: J. van der Vies, J. de Visser, Arzneim.-Forsch. 33, 231 (1983). Radioimmunoassay: L. Viinikka, J. Steroid Biochem. 9, 979 (1978). Metabolism, pharmacokinetics in humans: L. Viinikka et al., Eur. J. Clin. Pharmacol. 15, 349 (1979). Receptor binding study: E. W. Bergink et al., J. Steroid Biochem. 14, 175 (1981). Clinical trial in combination with ethinyl estradiol: M. J. Weijers, Clin. Ther. 4, 359 (1982); as progestogen-only contraceptive: T. Korver et al., Eur. J. Contracept. Reprod. Health Care 3, 169 (1998).

Crystals, mp 109-110°. $[\alpha]_D^{20}$ +55° (chloroform).
Mixture with ethinyl estradiol. [71138-35-7] Cyclosa; Desogen; Dicromil; Marvelon 150/30; Mercilon; Ortho-Cept; Oviol; Varnoline.

THERAP CAT: Progestogen. Alone or in combination with estrogen as oral contraceptive.

2927. Desomorphine. [427-00-9] 4,5a-Epoxy-17-methylmorphinan-3-ol; dihydrodesoxymorphine-D; Permonid. $C_{17}H_{21}$-NO_2; mol wt 271.35. C 75.25%, H 7.80%, N 5.16%, O 11.79%. Synthesis, physical data: L. F. Small et al., J. Am. Chem. Soc. 55, 3863 (1933).

Rectangular plates from acetone-water. Sublimes in high vacuum between 140° and 170°. Anhydr base, mp 189°. $[\alpha]_D^{28}$ −77° (c = 1.6 in methanol). Sol in acetone, ethyl acetate. Alcoholic solns darken and acquire a reddish color.
Hemihydrate. Crystals from ethyl acetate, mp 162-164°. $[\alpha]_D^{28}$ −79° (c = 1.08 in ethyl acetate).
Hydrochloride. $C_{17}H_{21}NO_2.HCl$. Crystals from alcohol, $[\alpha]_D^{27}$ −67° (c = 0.90). Very sol in water.
Hydrogen sulfate dihydrate. $(C_{17}H_{21}NO_2)_2.H_2SO_4.2H_2O$. Scales, plates from water, brown at 210°, unmelted at 230°. Sol in 40 parts water; freely sol in hot water. Soln is stable to boiling. $[\alpha]_D^{29}$ −60° (c = 1.43).
Note: This is a controlled substance (opium derivative): 21 CFR, 1308.11.

THERAP CAT: Analgesic (narcotic).

2928. Desonide. [638-94-8] (11β,16α)-11,21-Dihydroxy-16,17-[(1-methylethylidene)bis(oxy)]pregna-1,4-diene-3,20-dione; 11β,16α,17,21-tetrahydroxypregna-1,4-diene-3,20-dione cyclic 16,17-acetal with acetone; 16α-hydroxyprednisolone-16α,17-acetonide; 11β,21-dihydroxy-16α,17-isopropylidenedioxy-1,4-pregnadiene-3,20-dione; 16α-hydroxy-Δ¹-hydrocortisone-16α,17α-acetonide; 16α,17α-isopropylidenedioxyprednisolone; prednacinolone; D-2083; Locapred; Locatop; Sterax; Steroderm; Topifug; Tridesilon. $C_{24}H_{32}O_6$; mol wt 416.51. C 69.21%, H 7.74%, O 23.05%. Prepn and activity: Bernstein et al., J. Am. Chem. Soc. 81, 4573 (1959); Bernstein, Allen, US 2990401 (1961 to Am. Cyanamid); Lee et al. and Diassi, Principe, US 3536586 and US 3549498 (both 1970 to Squibb). Pharmacological and toxicological studies: Mascitelli-Coriandoli, Fraia, Arzneim.-Forsch. 20, 111 (1970); Phillips et al., Toxicol. Appl. Pharmacol. 20, 522 (1971). Structure-activity studies: Ringler et al., Proc. Soc. Exp. Biol. Med. 107, 451 (1961). Chemical and physical properties: Mantica et al., Arzneim.-Forsch. 20, 109 (1970).

Small plates or white to off-white odorless powder, mp 274-275° from methanol (Mantica); also reported as mp 263-266° from ethyl acetate-petr ether (Bernstein). $[\alpha]_D^{25}$ +123° (c = 0.5 in DMF). uv max: 242 nm ($E_{1cm}^{1\%}$ 356). LD_{50} in rats (mg/kg): 93 s.c. (Phillips).

THERAP CAT: Anti-inflammatory.

2929. Desosamine. [5779-39-5] 3,4,6-Trideoxy-3-(dimethylamino)-D-xylo-hexose; 4-dimethylaminotetrahydro-6-methylpyran-2,3-diol; picrocine. $C_8H_{17}NO_3$; mol wt 175.23. C

54.83%, H 9.78%, N 7.99%, O 27.39%. Sugar component of several macrolide antibiotics, such as the erythromycins. Isoln: Clark, *Antibiot. Chemother.* **3**, 663 (1953). Identity with picrocine: Brockmann *et al., Ber.* **87**, 856 (1954). Stereochemistry: Woo *et al., Tetrahedron Lett.* **1962**, 735. Configuration: Bolton *et al., Chem. Ind. (London)* **1962**, 1945; Foster *et al., J. Chem. Soc.* **1965**, 2318. Synthesis of DL-form: Korte *et al., Tetrahedron* **18**, 657 (1962); Newman, *Chem. Ind. (London)* **1963**, 372; *J. Org. Chem.* **29**, 1461 (1964). Stereospecific synthesis of the natural D-form: Richardson, *J. Chem. Soc.* **1964**, 5364; of the L-form: Baer, Chiu, *Can. J. Chem.* **52**, 122 (1974).

Crystals, mp 86-87°.

Hydrochloride. $C_8H_{17}NO_3 \cdot HCl$. Needles from ethanol + acetone, dec 191-193°. $[\alpha]_D^{20}$ +49.5° (c = 10.0); $[\alpha]_D^{20}$ +53.4° (c = 2.1 in ethanol).

2930. Desoximetasone. [382-67-2] (11β,16α)-9-Fluoro-11,21-dihydroxy-16-methylpregna-1,4-diene-3,20-dione; 9α-fluoro-16α-methyl-17-desoxyprednisolone; 9α-fluoro-16α-methyl-Δ¹-corticosterone; desoxymethasone; A-41-304; R-2113; HOE-304; Esperson; Stiedex LP; Topicort; Topisolon. $C_{22}H_{29}FO_4$; mol wt 376.46. C 70.19%, H 7.76%, F 5.05%, O 17.00%. Prepn: R. Joly *et al.*, **FR 1296544**; *eidem,* **US 3099654** (1962, 1963 to Roussel-UCLAF); **BE 614196**; Kieslich *et al.*, **US 3232839** (1962, 1966 to Schering AG); R. Joly *et al., Arzneim.-Forsch.* **24**, 1 (1974). Activity studies: Branceni *et al., Steroids* **6**, 451 (1965); Schröder *et al., Arzneim.-Forsch.* **24**, 3 (1974). NMR data: Lukacs *et al., C.R. Seances Acad. Sci. Ser. C* **274**, 1458 (1972). Review of pharmacology and therapeutic efficacy in dermatoses: R. C. Heel *et al., Drugs* **16**, 302-321 (1978).

Crystals from ethyl acetate, mp 217°. $[\alpha]_D$ +109° (chloroform). uv max: 238 nm (ε 15750). Sol in alcohol, acetone, chloroform, hot ethyl acetate; slightly sol in ether, benzene. Insol in water, dil aq acids and alkalies.

THERAP CAT: Anti-inflammatory; glucocorticoid.

2931. 6-Desoxy-D-glucosamine. [6018-53-7] 2-Amino-2,6-dideoxy-D-glucose; 6-deoxy-D-glucosamine; 2,6-didesoxy-2-amino-D-glucose. $C_6H_{13}NO_4$; mol wt 163.17. C 44.17%, H 8.03%, N 8.58%, O 39.22%. May be prepd by tosylation of the primary alcohol group of a suitable derivative of D-glucosamine, followed by acetylation and replacement of the tosyl group by iodine, and catalytic cleavage of the halide with Raney nickel in the presence of triethylamine: Morel, *Helv. Chim. Acta* **41**, 1501 (1958).

Hydrochloride. $C_6H_{13}NO_4 \cdot HCl$. Crystals from abs ethanol + ether, dec 172-173°. Shows mutarotation. Final value: $[\alpha]_D^{20}$ +55° (H_2O).

1,3,4-Tri-O-acetyl-N-acetyl-6-desoxy-β-D-glucosamine. $C_{14}H_{21}NO_8$; mol wt 331.32. Crystals from alc, mp 209-210°. $[\alpha]_D^{20}$ +17.5° (chloroform).

USE: In the investigation of amino acid metabolism.

2932. 11-Desoxy-17-hydroxycorticosterone. [152-58-9] 17,21-Dihydroxypregn-4-ene-3,20-dione; 17-hydroxydesoxycorticosterone; 4-pregnene-17α,21-diol-3,20-dione; 17-(1-keto-2-hydroxyethyl)-4-androsten-17α-ol-3-one; Reichstein's Substance S; 11-desoxycortisone; cortexolone. $C_{21}H_{30}O_4$; mol wt 346.46. C 72.80%, H 8.73%, O 18.47%. Isoln and partial synthesis: Reichstein, von Euw, *Helv. Chim. Acta* **21**, 1197 (1938); Reichstein, *ibid.* 1490; Reichstein, von Euw, *ibid.* **23**, 1258 (1940). Partial synthesis involving the chromic acid oxidation of 4-pregnene-17α,20,21-triol-3-one 21-monoacetate: Sarett, *J. Biol. Chem.* **162**, 627 (1946). Prepn from 3α-formoxy-17α-hydroxypregnan-20-one: Gallagher *et al., J. Am. Chem. Soc.* **71**, 3262 (1949); from 16,17-oxido-5-pregnen-3β-ol-20-one acetate: Julian *et al., ibid.* 3574; from 5-pregnen-3β-ol-20-one: Julian *et al., ibid.* **72**, 5145 (1950).

Fine, glistening plates from ether. mp 212.8-216.8°; gives no depression of melting point when mixed with cortisone. Very sparingly sol in water, ether. Sol in acetone, methanol, alcohol. Gives a carmine-red fluorescence reaction with concd H_2SO_4. Reduces ammoniacal silver nitrate soln at room temp. uv max: 242 nm ($E_{1cm}^{1\%}$ 500). Oxidation with chromic acid in glacial acetic acid yields 4-androstene-3,17-dione.

Acetate. $C_{23}H_{32}O_5$. mp 237.2-240.2° (sinters at 230°); $[\alpha]_D^{24}$ +116° (acetone); uv max (methanol): 242 nm ($E_{1cm}^{1\%}$ 448). When dissolved in concd sulfuric acid produces a typical scarlet color.

2933. Dess-Martin Periodinane. [87413-09-0] 1,1,1-Tris(acetyloxy)-1,1-dihydro-1,2-benziodoxol-3(1H)-one; triacetoxyperiodinane. $C_{13}H_{13}IO_8$; mol wt 424.14. C 36.81%, H 3.09%, I 29.92%, O 30.18%. Pentacoordinate organoiodine (periodinane); selectively oxidizes primary and secondary alcohols, aldehydes and ketones. Prepn: D. B. Dess, J. C. Martin, *J. Org. Chem.* **48**, 4155 (1983); R. E. Ireland, L. Liu, *ibid.* **58**, 2899 (1993). Structure and reaction conditions: D. B. Dess, J. C. Martin, *J. Am. Chem. Soc.* **113**, 7277 (1991); acceleration by water: S. D. Meyer, S. L. Schreiber, *J. Org. Chem.* **59**, 7549 (1994). Synthetic applications: N. E. Jenkins *et al., Synth. Commun.* **30**, 947 (2000); A. G. Myers *et al., Tetrahedron Lett.* **41**, 1359 (2000).

White crystalline solid, mp 134°. Sparingly sol in hexane or ether. Sol in chloroform, methylene chloride, acetonitrile and acetone.

USE: Oxidizing reagent.

2934. Desthiobiotin. [533-48-2] (4R-cis)-5-Methyl-2-oxo-4-imidazolidinehexanoic acid; 5-methyl-2-oxo-4-imidazolidinecaproic acid; ε-(4-methyl-5-imidazolidone-2)-caproic acid; 4-methyl-5-(ω-carboxyamyl)imidazolidone-2. $C_{10}H_{18}N_2O_3$; mol wt 214.26. C 56.06%, H 8.47%, N 13.07%, O 22.40%. Prepd from biotin by hydrogenolysis of the sulfide linkage: du Vigneaud *et al., J. Biol. Chem.* **146**, 475 (1942). Improved prepn procedure: Melville *et al., Science* **98**, 497 (1943). Synthesis: Melville, *J. Am. Chem. Soc.* **66**, 1422 (1944); Wood, du Vigneaud, *ibid.* **67**, 210 (1945); Duschinsky, Dolan, *ibid.* 2079; Bourquin *et al., Helv. Chim. Acta* **28**, 528 (1954).

Long needles from water. mp 156-158°. $[\alpha]_D^{21}$ +10.7° (c = 2). Sol in water.

Methyl ester. $C_{11}H_{20}N_2O_3$. Crystals from methanol. Can be sublimed at 10^{-5} mm and 100°. mp 69-70°. $[\alpha]_D^{28}$ +2.6° (c = 2 in chloroform). Readily sol in chloroform.

2935. Destomycin A. [14918-35-5] *O*-6-Amino-6-deoxy-L-*glycero*-D-*galacto*-heptopyranosylidene-(1 → 2-3)-*O*-β-D-talopyranosyl-(1 → 5)-2-deoxy-*N'*-methyl-D-streptamine; 5-*O*-[2,3-*O*-[6-(1-amino-2-hydroxyethyl)tetrahydro-3,4,5-trihydroxy-2*H*-pyran-2-ylidene]-β-D-talopyranosyl]-2-deoxy-*N*³-methyl-D-streptamine; Destonate 20. $C_{20}H_{37}N_3O_{13}$; mol wt 527.52. C 45.54%, H 7.07%, N 7.97%, O 39.43%. Aminoglycoside antibiotic, member of the orthosomycin family. Destomycins A, B and C are known; A is the major component. Isoln of A and B from culture broth of *Streptomyces rimofaciens:* S.-I. Kondo *et al., J. Antibiot.* **18A,** 38 (1965); of C: *eidem, ibid.* **28,** 83 (1975). Prepn: *eidem,* JP 67 7598 (1967 to Meiji Seika Kaisha). Structure of A: *eidem, J. Antibiot.* **19A,** 139 (1966); of A and B: *eidem, ibid.* **28,** 79 (1975). Stereochemical study: S. Horito *et al., Bull. Chem. Soc. Jpn.* **54,** 2147 (1981). Synthesis of destomycin C: J. Yoshimura *et al., Chem. Lett.* **1985,** 1335; J.-I. Tamura *et al., Carbohydr. Res.* **174,** 181 (1988). Anthelmintic activity in poultry: I. Sawada, *Kiseichugaku Zasshi* **21,** 45 (1972), *C.A.* **77,** 135668j (1972). HPLC determn in pork samples: K. Nakaya *et al., Shokuhin Eiseigaku Zasshi* **28,** 487 (1987), *C.A.* **109,** 5359c (1988).

White powder, mp 180-190° (dec). $[\alpha]_D^{22}$ +7° (c = 2). Freely sol in water, lower alcohols. Insol or poorly sol in most organic solvents. LD_{50} in mice (after 2-week observation) (mg/kg): 5-10 i.v.; 50-100 orally (Kondo, 1965).

THERAP CAT (VET): Broad spectrum antimicrobial; anthelmintic.

2936. Detaxtran. [9015-73-0] Dextran 2-(diethylamino)-ethyl ether; diethylaminoethyldextran; DEAE-dextran; basic dextran. Cationic derivative of dextran, *q.v.,* with antilipemic activity. Prepn: W. McKernan, C. R. Ricketts, *Chem. Ind. (London)* **1959,** 1490; E. Antonini *et al., G. Biochem.* **14,** 88 (1965); *C.A.* **63,** 4375h (1965). Effect on platelet aggregation: R. Brossmer, Th. Pflederer, *Naturwissenschaften* **53,** 464 (1966); A. Larcon *et al., Experientia* **28,** 1096 (1972). Use to lower hypercholesterolemia: T. M. Parkinson, US 3627872 (1971 to Upjohn); to reduce blood lipid levels: F. Kuzuya *et al.,* US 3851057 (1974 to Meito Sangyo). Clinical trial in hyperlipoproteinemia: F. Pupita, A. Barone, *Int. J. Clin. Pharmacol. Res.* **3,** 287 (1983).

Powder, soluble in water, saline.

Hydrochloride. [9064-91-9] Dexide; Pulsar.

THERAP CAT: Antilipemic.

2937. Detomidine. [76631-46-4] 4-[(2,3-Dimethylphenyl)-methyl]-1*H*-imidazole; 4-(2',3'-dimethylbenzyl)imidazole. $C_{12}H_{14}N_2$; mol wt 186.25. C 77.38%, H 7.58%, N 15.04%. α_2-Adrenoceptor agonist with sedative and analgesic activity. Prepn: A. J. Karjalayne, K. O. A. Kurkela, EP 24829; *eidem,* US 4443466 (1981, 1984 both to Farmos). Physical studies: E. Laine *et al., Acta Pharm. Suec.* **20,** 451 (1983). Crystal structure: L. H. J. Lajunen *et al., ibid.* **21,** 163 (1984). Pharmacology: R. Virtanen, L. Nyman, *Eur. J. Pharmacol.* **108,** 163 (1985); R. Virtanen, E. MacDonald, *ibid.* **115,** 277 (1985). Mechanism of action: *eidem, J. Vet. Pharmacol. Ther.* **8,** 30 (1985).

Crystals from acetone, mp 114-116°. LD_{50} i.v. in mice: 35 mg/kg (Karjalayne, Kurkela).

Hydrochloride. Domosedan. $C_{12}H_{14}N_2 \cdot HCl$; mol wt 222.71. Crystals, mp 160°. Converts reversibly to monohydrate at room temp, 80% humidity.

THERAP CAT (VET): Sedative.

2938. Detoxin Complex. DX.C. A group of selective antagonists of blasticidin S, *q.v.,* produced by *Streptomyces caespitosus* var. *detoxicus* 7072 GC₁. The complex counteracts the inhibitory action of blasticidin S (BS) against *Bacillus cereus* but not against *Piricularia oryzal,* the causative agent of rice blast disease. DX.C also depresses the phytotoxicity of BS to rice plants, and a combination of the two showed less eye irritation in animals than BS alone. Isoln, production, biological properties: H. Yonehara *et al., J. Antibiot.* **21,** 369 (1968); *eidem, Agric. Biol. Chem.* **37,** 2771 (1973). Separation of the complex yields eight groups of detoxins designated A through H, the major components being C and D: N. Otake *et al., J. Antibiot.* **21,** 371 (1968); *eidem, Agric. Biol. Chem.* **37,** 2777 (1973). Detoxin D₁, the major component of the D group, has been shown to have the highest specific activity. It is a unique depsipeptide containing the amino acid *detoxinine* (β,3-dihydroxy-2-pyrrolidinepropanoic acid). Structure of D₁: K. Kakenuma *et al., Tetrahedron Lett.* **1972,** 2509. ¹³C-NMR: T. Ogita *et al., Agric. Biol. Chem.* **42,** 2403 (1978). Structures of the minor components of the D group: N. Otake *et al., J. Antibiot.* **27,** 484 (1974). Structures of detoxins A₁, B₁, B₃, C₁, C₂, C₃, E₁: N. Otake *et al., Experientia* **37,** 926 (1981); T. Ogita *et al., Agric. Biol. Chem.* **45,** 2605 (1981). Effect of D on BS uptake in *B. cereus:* A. Shimazu *et al., Experientia* **37,** 365 (1981).

Detoxin D₁   R = CH(CH₃)CH₂CH₃
Detoxin C₁   R = CH₃

Light colored fine powder.

Detoxin D₁. [37878-19-6] *N*-(2-Methyl-1-oxobutyl)-L-phenylalanine (1*S*)-1-[(2*S*,3*R*)-3-(acetyloxy)-1-[(2*S*)-2-amino-3-methyl-1-oxobutyl]-2-pyrrolidinyl]-2-carboxyethyl ester. $C_{28}H_{41}N_3O_8$; mol wt 547.64. Fine crystalline powder, mp 156-158°. $[\alpha]_D^{25}$ −16° (c = 1 in methanol). uv max (methanol): 253, 258, 265, 268 nm ($E_{1cm}^{1\%}$ 3.1, 3.58, 2.77, 1.85). Amphoteric. pKa 4.0, 8.0.

Detoxin C₁. [74717-53-6] *N*-Acetyl-L-phenylalanine (1*S*)-1-[(2*S*,3*R*)-3-(acetyloxy)-1-[(2*S*)-2-amino-3-methyl-1-oxobutyl]-2-pyrrolidinyl]-2-carboxyethyl ester; detoxin C₀₁. $C_{25}H_{35}N_3O_8$; mol wt 505.56. Microneedles from water, mp 142-144°. Amphoteric. pKa 8.0, 3.9. $[\alpha]_D^{25}$ −23° (c = 1 in methanol). uv max (methanol): 248, 253, 259, 265, 269 nm ($E_{1cm}^{1\%}$ 3.7, 3.18, 2.65, 2.8, 1.85).

USE: In mixtures with blasticidin S, to decrease phytotoxicity to rice plants.

2939. Deuterium. [7782-39-0] Heavy hydrogen. ²H or D. Exists in the diatomic state, D_2; mol wt 4.028. Stable, non-radioactive isotope of hydrogen, *q.v.* Shows *ortho* and *para* isomerism. Prepd by electrolysis of heavy water, D_2O (obtained by the H_2S/H_2-O exchange process) or by fractional distillation of liq hydrogen: Urey *et al., Phys. Rev.* **39,** 164 (1932); Spevack, US 2787526 (1957 to USAEC). The hydrogen bomb contains lithium deuteride (LiD) as explosive and plutonium (Pu) as initiator. After detonation by Pu the following reaction sequence takes place (nuclear fusion): ⁶Li + D = 2⁴He; ⁶Li + n = ⁴He + T; ⁶Li + T = 2⁴He + n (n = neutrons, coming from Pu in the second reaction). Since the explosion does not start by itself, there is no critical mass and no limit to the size of the bomb. Use as chemical tracer: Wiberg, *Chem. Rev.* **55,** 713-743 (1955). Toxicology: J. F. Thomson, *Biological Effects of Deuterium* (Pergamon Press, 1964). *Review:* Mackay, Dove in *Comprehensive Inorganic Chemistry* vol. 1, J. C. Bailar, Jr. *et al.,*

Eds. (Pergamon Press, Oxford, 1973) pp 77-116; *Chemistry of the Elements*, N. N. Greenwood, A. Earnshaw, Eds. (Pergamon Press, New York, 1984) pp 38-74; J. J. Katz in *Kirk-Othmer Encyclopedia of Chemical Technology* **vol. 8** (Wiley-Interscience, New York, 4th ed., 1993) pp 1-17.

Colorless, odorless, flammable gas having properties similar to hydrogen. d (liq, 20.4 K) 0.169. bp $-249.49°$ (23.67 K). mp $-254.43°$ (18.73 K) at 128.5 mm (triple point). Crit temp $-234.75°$. Crit press. 16.432 atm. Flammable limits in air: 5-75%. Calculation of vapor press. from the triple point to the crit point: Friedman *et al., J. Am. Chem. Soc.* **73**, 1310 (1951).

Caution: Can act as an asphyxiant by displacing air. *See: Matheson Gas Data Book* (Matheson, 6th ed., Lyndhurst, NJ, 1980) pp 215-218.

USE: Used extensively in small amts as tracer in the establishment of rates and kinetics of chemical reactions.

2940. Deuterium Oxide. [7789-20-0] Heavy water; water-d_2. ^2H_2O. D_2O.

More associated than H_2O. mp 3.81°; triple point temp 3.82°. bp 101.42°. Critical temp 371.5°. d^{25} 1.1044. Temp of max density 11.23°; $d^{11.23}$ 1.1059. Sp heat of liq (4-25°) 1.028 cal/g/°C. Heat of fusion 1.501 kcal/mole: Long, Kemp, *J. Am. Chem. Soc.* **58**, 1829 (1936). Heat of evapn 9.917 kcal/mole. Dielectric const (25°): 78.06, Vidulich *et al., J. Phys. Chem.* **71**, 656 (1966). Dipole moment in benzene (25°) 1.78, in dioxane 1.87. The surface tension is very slightly smaller and the viscosity at 25° is 1.23 times as great as that of water. On mixing with water, heat is evolved. Reacts with hydrogen at 100° in the presence of 0.2 to $1N$ NaOH forming DOH + HD + OD⁻. Ionization const 1.95×10^{-15}: W. F. K. Wynne-Jones, *Trans. Faraday Soc.* **32**, 1397 (1936). pK (25°) 14.955 (molarity scale); 16.653 (mole fraction scale): A. K. Covington *et al., J. Phys. Chem.* **70**, 3820 (1966). *See also* Water.

USE: To study chemical reaction rates and mechanisms. The cross section of deuterium for the capture of thermal neutrons is very low which makes it useful, in the form of heavy water, as a neutron moderator in nuclear reactors. Produces a considerable decrease in neutron energy per collision.

2941. Devarda's Metal. [8049-11-4] Devarda's alloy. Consists of 50 parts Cu, 45 Al and 5 Zn.

Gray powder. Partly sol in HCl with residue of Cu.

USE: Reducing agent for determination of nitrogen in nitrates and nitrites.

2942. Devil's Claw. Herbaceous, perennial plant, *Harpagophyrum procumbens* DC, Pedaliaceae, used in African traditional medicine as a bitter tonic, febrifuge and analgesic. Medicinal formulations are prepared from the dried secondary tubers. *Habit.* Kalahari savannas of southern Africa and Namibia. *Constit.* Iridoid glucosides, primarily harpagoside (the pharmacologically active component), harpagide and procumbide; sugars such as stachyose, raffinose, sucrose; caffeic and cinnamic acids. HPLC determn of active component in commercial extracts: L. Guillerault *et al., J. Liq. Chromatogr.* **17**, 2951 (1994). Pharmacology: B. Baghdikian *et al., Planta Med.* **63**, 171 (1997). Clinical comparison with diacerein, *q.v.*, in osteoarthritis: P. Chantre *et al., Phytomedicine* **7**, 177 (2000). Reviews of medicinal uses: S. Chrubasik, E. Eisenberg, *Pain Clinic* **11**, 171-178 (1999); C. Hansen, *Dtsch. Apoth.* **140**, 85-89 (2000).

Dry extract. Arthrosetten; Arthrotabs; Doloteffin; Herbadon; Rivoltan.

THERAP CAT: Analgesic.

2943. Dexamethasone. [50-02-2] (11β,16α)-9-Fluoro-11,17,21-trihydroxy-16-methylpregna-1,4-diene-3,20-dione; 9α-fluoro-16α-methylprednisolone; 16α-methyl-9α-fluoro-1,4-pregnadiene-11β,17α,21-triol-3,20-dione; 16α-methyl-9α-fluoroprednisolone; 1-dehydro-16α-methyl-9α-fluorohydrocortisone; 16α-methyl-9α-fluoro-Δ¹-hydrocortisone; hexadecadrol; Aeroseb-Dex; Decadron; Dexacortal; Dexacortin; Dexamonozon; Dexapos; Dexasine; Dexasone; Fortecortin; Isopto-Dex; Loverine; Luxazone; Maxidex. $C_{22}H_{29}FO_5$; mol wt 392.46. C 67.33%, H 7.45%, F 4.84%, O 20.38%. Prepn: Arth *et al., J. Am. Chem. Soc.* **80**, 3161 (1958); Oliveto *et al., ibid.* 4431; Muller *et al., US 3007923* (1961 to Lab. Franc. Chimiother.); Arth *et al., DE 1113690* (1961 to Merck & Co.); *GB 869511* (to Upjohn). Pharmacology in guinea pigs: L. Zicha *et al., Arzneim.-Forsch.* **10**, 831 (1960). Clinical trial of anti-

emetic efficacy in chemotherapy-induced nausea: M. Markman *et al., N. Engl. J. Med.* **311**, 549 (1984); in combination with ondansetron, *q.v.:* F. Roila *et al., ibid.* **342**, 1554 (2000). Use as diagnostic aid in depression: B. J. Carroll *et al., Arch. Gen. Psychiatry* **38**, 15 (1981); P. P. Hubain *et al., Neuropsychobiology* **16**, 57 (1986); M. Ansseau *et al., ibid.* 68. Comprehensive description: E. M. Cohen, *Anal. Profiles Drug Subs.* **2**, 163-197 (1973). Reviews of diagnostic use in Cushing's syndrome: L. Crapo, *Metabolism* **28**, 955 (1979); in depression: L. Braddock, *Br. J. Psychiatry* **148**, 363 (1986).

Crystals from ether, mp 262-264°; mp 268-271° (Arth, 1961). $[α]_D^{25}$ +77.5° (dioxane). Soly in water (25°): 10 mg/100 ml. Sol in acetone, ethanol, chloroform.

21-Acetate. [1177-87-3] Decadronal; Decadron-LA; Dectancyl. $C_{24}H_{31}FO_6$; mol wt 434.50. Crystals, mp 215-221° (Arth, 1958); mp 229-231° (Oliveto); mp 238-240° (Arth, 1961). $[α]_D^{25}$ +73° (chloroform) (Arth, 1958); $[α]_D$ +77.6° (Oliveto). uv max: 239 nm (ε 14900).

21-Phosphate disodium salt. [2392-39-4] Dexamethasone 21-(dihydrogen phosphate) disodium salt; dexamethasone sodium phosphate; Ak-Dex; Dalalone; Desocort; Dexabene; Hexadrol; Oradexon; Orgadrone; SoluDecadron; Soldesam; Solupen N; Totocortin. $C_{22}H_{28}FNa_2O_8P$; mol wt 516.40. Used as an injectable form of dexamethasone. Prepn: Chemerda *et al., US 2939873* (1960 to Merck & Co.); Irmscher, *Chem. Ind. (London)* **1961**, 1035. Crystals, mp 233-235°. $[α]_D$ +57° (water). Also reported as $[α]_D^{25}$ +74 ±4° (calcd on water-free and alcohol-free basis, concn of 10 mg/ml): *USP XIX*, p 124. uv max (ethanol): 238-239 nm (ε 14000). Sol in water.

21-Isonicotinate. Dexamethasone 21-(4-pyridinecarboxylate); Auxisone. $C_{28}H_{32}FNO_6$; mol wt 497.56. Crystals, mp 250-252°. $[α]_D^{27}$ +183.5° (dioxane).

17,21-Dipropionate. THS-101; Methaderm. $C_{28}H_{37}FO_7$; mol wt 504.59.

THERAP CAT: Glucocorticoid; anti-inflammatory. Diagnostic aid (Cushing's syndrome, depression).

THERAP CAT (VET): Glucocorticoid; anti-inflammatory.

2944. Dexanabinol. [112924-45-5] (6aS,10aS)-3-(1,1-Dimethylheptyl)-6a,7,10,10a-tetrahydro-1-hydroxy-6,6-dimethyl-6H-dibenzo[b,d]pyran-9-methanol; (+)-(3S,4S)-7-hydroxy-Δ⁶-tetrahydrocannabinol-1,1-dimethylheptyl; (+)-11-OH-Δ⁸-THC-DMH; HU-211. $C_{25}H_{38}O_3$; mol wt 386.57. C 77.67%, H 9.91%, O 12.42%. NMDA antagonist. Nonpsychotropic derivative of tetrahydrocannabinol, *q.v.* Prepn: R. Mechoulam *et al., DE 3735990*; *eidem, US 4876276* (1988, 1989 both to Yissum Res. Dev. Co.); R. Mechoulam *et al., Tetrahedron: Asymmetry* **1**, 315 (1990). Cannabinoid receptor binding study: A. C. Howlett *et al., Neuropharmacology* **29**, 161 (1990). Inhibition of nuclear factor-κB (NF-κB): E. Jüttler *et al., Neuropharmacology* **47**, 580 (2004). Pharmacology: N. Eshhar *et al., Eur. J. Pharmacol.* **283**, 19 (1995). Clinical pharmacokinetics: M. E. Brewster *et al., Int. J. Clin. Pharmacol. Ther.* **35**, 361 (1995). Clinical evaluation in severe head injury: N. Knoller *et al., Crit. Care Med.* **30**, 548 (2002).

Crystals from pentane, mp 141-142°. $[α]_D$ +227° (CHCl₃).

THERAP CAT: Neuroprotective.

2945. Dexetimide. [21888-98-2] (3*S*)-3-Phenyl-1'-(phenyl-methyl)-[3,4'-bipiperidine]-2,6-dione; (*S*)-(+)-2-(1-benzyl-4-piperi-dyl)-2-phenylglutarimide; (+)-3-(1-benzyl-4-piperidyl)-3-phenyl-piperidine-2,6-dione; (+)-1-benzyl-4-(2,6-dioxo-3-phenyl-3-piperi-dyl)piperidine; dexbenzetimide; dexbenzetimide. $C_{23}H_{26}N_2O_2$; mol wt 362.46. C 76.21%, H 7.23%, N 7.73%, O 8.83%. The dextroenantiomer responsible for the pharmacological activity of racemic benzetimide, *q.v.* Resolution of isomers and comparative pharmacology: Janssen *et al., Arzneim.-Forsch.* **21**, 1365 (1971). Abs config studies: van Wijngaarden *et al., Life Sci.* **9**, part 1, 1289 (1970); Spek *et al., Nature* **232**, 575 (1971). Clinical trials: De Smedt *et al., J. Clin. Pharmacol.* **10**, 207 (1970).

Crystals, mp 181-183°. $[\alpha]_D^{20}$ +125° (chloroform).
Hydrochloride. [21888-96-0] R-16470; Tremblex. $C_{23}H_{26}$-N_2O_2.HCl; mol wt 398.93. Crystals, mp 270-275°. $[\alpha]_D^{20}$ +125° (methanol). LD_{50} i.v. in rats: 45 mg/kg (Janssen).
THERAP CAT: Antiparkinsonian.

2946. Dexmedetomidine. [113775-47-6] 4-[(1*S*)-1-(2,3-Di-methylphenyl)ethyl]-1*H*-imidazole; *d*-medetomidine; MPV-1440. $C_{13}H_{16}N_2$; mol wt 200.28. C 77.96%, H 8.05%, N 13.99%. α_2-Adrenergic agonist; (+)-isomer of medetomidine, *q.v.* Prepn: A. J. Karjalainen *et al., GB 2206880; eidem,* **US 4910214** (1989, 1990 both to Farmos). Physical properties: R. Rajala *et al., Eur. J. Pharm. Sci.* **1**, 219 (1994). Clinical pharmacokinetics: P. Talke *et al, Anesth. Analg.* **85**, 1136 (1997). Clinical evaluation as anesthetic adjunct: J. Jalonen *et al., Anesthesiology* **86**, 331 (1997). Review of pharmacology and clinical experience for sedation of patients in intensive care: N. Bhana *et al., Drugs* **59**, 263-270 (2000).

Hydrochloride. [145108-58-3] Precedex. $C_{13}H_{16}CN_2$.HCl; mol wt 248.75. White or almost white crystalline powder, mp 156.5-157.5°. d 1.17 g/cm^3. $[\alpha]$ +52.4° (c = 1 in water). pH of 1% soln in water: 4.3.
THERAP CAT: Sedative; analgesic.

2947. Dexpanthenol. [81-13-0] 2,4-Dihydroxy-*N*-(3-hy-droxypropyl)-3,3-dimethylbutanamide; D(+)-α,γ-dihydroxy-*N*-(3-hydroxypropyl)-β,β-dimethylbutyramide; pantothenylol; *N*-pan-toyl-3-propanolamine; pantothenol; pantothenyl alcohol; Alcopan-250; Intrapan; Pantenyl; Panthoderm; Motilyn; Bepanthen; Co-zyme; Ilopan; Urupan. $C_9H_{19}NO_4$; mol wt 205.25. C 52.67%, H 9.33%, N 6.82%, O 31.18%. Prepd by the addition of propanol-amine to optically active α,γ-dihydroxy-β,β-dimethylbutyrolactone: Schnider, *Jubilee Vol. Emil Barell* **1946**, 85; CH 227706 (1943); GB 582156 (1946); US 2413077 (1946 to Hoffmann-La Roche). Only the D(+)-form has vitamin activity.

Viscous, somewhat hygroscopic liq. Slightly bitter taste. d_{20}^{20} 1.2. $bp_{0.02}$ 118-120°. Easily dec on distn. $[\alpha]_D^{20}$ +29.5° (c = 5). n_D^{20} 1.497. Freely sol in water, alcohol, methanol. Slightly sol in ether. Natural pH about 9.5. Reasonably stable to usual steriliza-tion time and temp in aq solns adjusted to pH 3.0-4.0, but long heating causes racemization. Hydrolyzed by alkali and strong acid. Usually more stable than salts of pantothenic acid if pH can be adjusted between 3 and 5. For add'l stability data *see* Rubin, *J. Am. Pharm. Assoc. Sci. Ed.* **37**, 502 (1948). Aq solns can be stabilized with pantolactone: US 2898373 (1959).
***dl*-Form.** Panthenol.
THERAP CAT: Cholinergic; *dl*-form as vitamin.
THERAP CAT (VET): Nutritional factor. Dietary source of panto-thenic acid.

2948. Dextran. [9004-54-0] Gentran; Hemodex; Intradex; Promit. A term applied to polysaccharides produced by bacteria growing on a sucrose substrate, contg a backbone of D-glucose units linked predominantly α-D(1 → 6). Several organisms produce dex-trans but only *Leuconostoc mesenteroides* and *L. dextranicum (Lac-tobacteriaceae)* have been used commercially. Chemical and phys-ical properties of the dextrans vary with the methods of production. Native dextrans usually have high mol wt; lower mol wt clinical dextrans usually prepared by depolymerization of native dextrans or by synthesis. All dextrans are composed exclusively of α-D-gluco-pyranosyl units, differing only in degree of branching and chain length. Prepn: Tarr, Hibbert, *Can. J. Res.* **5**, 414 (1931); Novak, Stoycos, US 2841578 (1958 to Commonwealth Eng. of Ohio). Enzymic synthesis: Sugg, Hehre, *J. Immunol.* **43**, 119 (1942); Behrens, Ringpfeil, US 3044940 (1962 to Serum Werk Bernburg). The crude dextran may be isolated from the culture by precipitation with methanol. Continuous dialysis process: Shurter, US 2717853 (1955 to C.S.C.). Elimination of pyrogens: Levi, Lozinski, US 2762727 (1956 to Frosst). Method of producing clinical dextran: Novak, Witt, US 2972567 (1961). Structure studies: Fowler *et al., Can. J. Res.* **B15**, 486 (1937); Fairhead *et al., ibid.* **B16**, 151 (1938); Peat *et al., J. Am. Chem. Soc.* **1939**, 581; Goldstein, Whelan, *ibid.* **1962**, 170, 176. ^{13}C-NMR structure study: F. R. Seymour *et al., Carbo-hydr. Res.* **51**, 179 (1976). *Reviews:* Evans, Hibbert, *Adv. Carbo-hydr. Chem.* **2**, 204 (1946); Neely, *ibid.* **15**, 341 (1960); Ricketts, *Prog. Org. Chem.* **5**, 73 (1961); Murphy, Whistler, in *Industrial Gums,* R. L. Whistler, Ed. (Academic Press, New York, 2nd ed., 1973) pp 513-542.
Dextran 40. LMD; LMWD; LVD; Gentran 40; Rheomacrodex. Produced by action of *L. mesenteroides* on sucrose; average mol wt: 40,000.
Dextran 70. Gentran 70; Hyskon; Macrodex. Average mol wt: 70,000.
USE: In soft center confections, as a partial substitute for barley malt. Mixed ethers and esters of dextran can be used in lacquers.
THERAP CAT: Plasma volume expander; Dextran 40 also as blood flow adjuvant.
THERAP CAT (VET): Plasma extender.

2949. Dextranase. [9025-70-1] α-1,6-Glucan 6-glucanohy-drolase; EC 3.2.1.11. Enzyme which hydrolyzes the α-1 → 6 glu-cosidic linkages of the bacterial polysaccharide dextran. *Endodex-tranases* (dextranases which preferentially split glucosidic linkages remote from end groups) are secreted by various molds and a few bacteria. *Exodextranases* occur predominantly in mammalian tis-sues. Prepn: from *Penicillium lilacinum, P. funiculosum,* and *Ver-ticillium coccorum,* Nordström, Hultin, *Sven. Kem. Tidskr.* **60**, 283 (1948), *C.A.* **43**, 3050i (1949); from *Aspergillus,* Carlson, Carlson, *Science* **115**, 43 (1952), *eidem,* US 2709150 (1955 to Enzymatic Chemicals), *eidem,* US 2716084, and Novak, Stoycos, US 2841578 (1955 and 1958 both to Commonwealth Eng. of Ohio); from *P. lilacinum, P. funiculosum, P. verruculosum,* and *Spicaria violacea,* Tsuchiya *et al.,* US 2742399 and Corman, Tsuchiya, US 2776925 (1956 and 1957 both to U.S. Secy. Agr.); from *P. lilacinum,* Charles, Farrell, *Can. J. Microbiol.* **3**, 239 (1957); from *Lactobacillus bifidus,* Bailey, Clarke, *Biochem. J.* **72**, 49 (1959). Tested as dental caries-control agent in hamsters: Fitzgerald *et al., J. Am. Dent. Assoc.* **76**, 301 (1968). *Review:* E. H. Fischer, E. A. Stein, "Cleavage of *O*- and *S*-Glycosidic Bonds (Survey)" in *The Enzymes* vol. 4, P. D.

Boyer *et al.*, Eds. (Academic Press, New York, 2nd ed., 1960) pp 304-307.

USE: In prepn of dextran for clinical use; in dentifrices.

2950. Dextranomer. [56087-11-7] Dextran 2,3-dihydroxypropyl 2-hydroxy-1,3-propanediyl ethers; Debrisan; Debrisorb. Three-dimensional hydrophilic network of a dextran polymer, linked by cross-chains of epichlorohydrin, *q.v.*; it absorbs moisture and small molecules from suppurating wounds. Chronic tissue response to implantation: J. Falk, G. Tollerz, *Clin. Ther.* **1**(3), 185 (1977). Potential allergic contact sensitization in guinea pigs: G. Jonsson, *ibid.* **1**(4), 260 (1978). Efficacy in treatment of ulcers and wounds: J. Soul, *Br. J. Clin. Pract.* **32**, 172 (1978); P. N. Sawyer *et al.*, *Surgery* **85**, 201 (1979); S. Di Mascio, *Am. J. Nurs.* **79**, 684 (1979). *Review:* R. C. Heel *et al.*, *Drugs* **18**, 89-102 (1979).

Insol in all solvents; stable in water, salt solns and in alkaline and weakly acidic soln.

THERAP CAT: Vulnerary.

2951. Dextran Sulfate Sodium. [9011-18-1] Dextran sulfuric acid ester sodium salt; Asuro; Colyonal; Dexulate; Dextrarine; MDS. Heparin-like polysaccharide containing approx. 17% S with up to three sulfate groups per glucose molecule. Mol wt ranges from 4,000-500,000 Da; variations in mol wt are associated with differences in biological activity. Prepn, properties and anticoagulant activity: A. Grönwall *et al.*, *Upsala Laekarefoeren. Foerh.* **50**, 397 (1945); C. R. Ricketts, *Biochem. J.* **51**, 129 (1952). Evaluation of toxicity as a function of mol wt: K. W. Walton, *Br. J. Pharmacol.* **9**, 1 (1954); of carcinogenicity: I. Hirono *et al.*, *Cancer Lett.* **18**, 29 (1983). Use in serum HDL cholesterol determn: P. R. Finley *et al.*, *Clin. Chem.* **24**, 931 (1978); G. R. Warnick *et al.*, *ibid.* **28**, 1379 (1982). Antiscrapie effect: B. Ehlers, H. Diringer, *J. Gen. Virol.* **65**, 1325 (1984); R. H. Kimberlin, C. A. Walker, *Antimicrob. Agents Chemother.* **30**, 409 (1986). Anti-HIV-1 activity *in vitro*: H. Mitsuya *et al.*, *Science* **240**, 646 (1988); M. Baba *et al.*, *Proc. Natl. Acad. Sci. USA* **85**, 6132 (1988).

White powder from alcohol + ether. Freely sol in water. Activity about 17 international heparin units/mg. Aq solns must be buffered (*e.g.*, with sodium bicarbonate) to prevent dec during autoclaving.

USE: Clinical reagent (HDL cholesterol determn).

THERAP CAT: Anticoagulant.

2952. Dextri-Maltose®. [8006-91-5] Maltose and dextrins obtained by enzymic action of barley malt on corn flour.

Light, amorphous powder. Readily sol in water or milk. One leveled tablespoonful (8 grams) supplies 27 calories.

USE: As carbohydrate modifier for use with milk and milk products in infants' formulas.

2953. Dextrin. [9004-53-9] Pyrodextrin; torrefaction dextrin. $(C_6H_{10}O_5)_n.xH_2O$. Produced by the dry heating of unmodified starches. The term also includes products resulting from enzyme or acid-catalyzed hydrolysis of wet starch. *Review:* R. W. Satterthwaite, D. J. Iwinski, in *Industrial Gums*, R. L. Whistler, Ed. (Academic Press, New York, 2nd ed., 1973) pp 577-599.

British gum. Starch gum. Produced at high temp in the absence of acid. Dark brown color, odorous. High viscosity; very sol in

cold water. Does not reduce Fehling's soln; gives reddish-brown color with iodine.

Canary dextrin. Yellow dextrin. Hydrolyzed at high temp for long period of time in the presence of small amts of acid. Light brown to yellow color, slight odor. Low viscosity; very sol in cold water.

White dextrin. Hydrolyzed at low temp for short period of time in the presence of large amts of acid. White color, odorless. Slightly sol in cold water giving a red color with iodine. Very sol in hot water giving a blue color with iodine.

USE: Excipient for dry extracts and pills; for preparing emulsions and dry bandages; for thickening dye pastes and mordants used in printing fabrics in fast colors; sizing paper and fabrics; printing tapestries; preparing felt; manuf printer's inks, glues and mucilage; polishing cereals; in matches, fireworks, and explosives.

2954. Dextroamphetamine. [51-64-9] (αS)-α-Methylbenzeneethanamine; (+)-α-methylphenethylamine; *d*-amphetamine; (*S*)-1-phenyl-2-aminopropane; *d*-β-phenylisopropylamine; dexamphetamine. $C_9H_{13}N$; mol wt 135.21. C 79.95%, H 9.69%, N 10.36%. Prepn by resolution of amphetamine: Temmler, **GB 508757** (1939); Nabenhauer, **US 2276508** (1942 to SK&F); Magidson, Garkusha, *J. Gen. Chem. USSR* **11**, 339 (1941); from D-phenylalanine: D. B. Repke *et al.*, *J. Pharm. Sci.* **67**, 1167 (1978). Toxicity data: E. J. Warawa *et al.*, *J. Med. Chem.* **18**, 71 (1975). GC-MS determn in urine: V. A Tetlow, J. Merrill, *Ann. Clin. Biochem.* **33**, 50 (1996). Review of pharmacology: S. J. Chee, *Neurosci. Biobehav. Rev.* **16**, 481-496 (1992).

Sulfate. [51-63-8] Dexamin; Dexedrine; Dextrostat. White, odorless, crystalline powder with bitter taste. mp >300°. $[\alpha]_D^{20}$ +21.8° (c = 2). Freely sol in water (about 1:10); slightly sol in alcohol (about 1:800). Insol in ether. pH 5% aq soln: 5.0 to 6.0. LD_{50} orally in mice: 10 mg/kg (Warawa).

Tannate. [1407-85-8] Synatan; Synatan. Prepn: Cavallito, **US 2950309** (1960 to Irwin, Neisler and Co.).

Note: This is a controlled substance (stimulant): **21 CFR,** 1308.12.

THERAP CAT: CNS stimulant; anorexic.

2955. Dextromoramide. [357-56-2] 1-[(3*S*)-3-Methyl-4-(4-morpholinyl)-1-oxo-2,2-diphenylbutyl]pyrrolidine; (+)-1-(3-methyl-4-morpholino-2,2-diphenylbutyryl)pyrrolidine; 4-[2-methyl-4-oxo-3,3-diphenyl-4-(1-pyrrolidinyl)butyl]morpholine; *d*-2,2-diphenyl-3-methyl-4-morpholinobutyrylpyrrolidine; pyrrolamidol; R-875; SKF-5137; *d*-Moramid(e); Palfium; Palphium; Jetrium; Dimorlin. $C_{25}H_{32}N_2O_2$; mol wt 392.53. C 76.50%, H 8.22%, N 7.14%, O 8.15%. Synthesis: Janssen, *J. Am. Chem. Soc.* **78**, 3862 (1956); **GB 822055** (1959 to Janssen).

Crystals, mp 180-184°. $[\alpha]_D^{20}$ +25.5° (c = 5 in benzene). uv max (0.01*N* isopropanol-HCl): 254, 260, 264 nm. Practically insol in water. Soly in 0.1*N* HCl: 1:25 (w/v). Soly (g/100 ml) in ethanol 50; in methanol 40; in acetone 50; in ethyl acetate 40; in benzene 5; in chloroform 5. Sol in ether.

Bitartrate. $C_{25}H_{32}N_2O_2.C_4H_6O_6$. Minute crystals, bitter taste. Dec 189-192°. Soly (w/v) at 25°: Water 20%, chloroform 30%, methanol 40%, ethanol 100%, acetone 100%.

Note: This is a controlled substance (opiate): **21 CFR,** 1308.11.

THERAP CAT: Analgesic (narcotic).

2956. Dezocine. [53648-55-8] (5*R*,11*S*,13*S*)-13-Amino-5,-6,7,8,9,10,11,12-octahydro-5-methyl-5,11-methanobenzocyclodecen-3-ol; Wy-16225; Dalgan. $C_{16}H_{23}NO$; mol wt 245.36. C 78.32%, H 9.45%, N 5.71%, O 6.52%. Synthetic opiate agonist-antagonist. Prepn: M. E. Freed *et al.*, **DE 2159324** (1972 to Am. Home Products), *C.A.* **79**, 53094w (1973); *eidem, J. Med. Chem.* **16**, 595 (1973). Pharmacology: J. L. Malis *et al., J. Pharmacol. Exp. Ther.* **194**, 488 (1975). Metabolism: S. F. Sisenwine, C. O. Tio, *Drug Metab. Dispos.* **9**, 37 (1981). Pharmacokinetics: S. F. Sisenwine *et al., ibid.* **10**, 366 (1982). Clinical studies: W. Oosterlinck, A. Verbaeys, *Curr. Med. Res. Opin.* **6**, 472 (1980); J. W. Downing *et al., Br. J. Anaesth.* **53**, 59 (1981).

Hydrobromide salt. $C_{15}H_{23}NO.HBr$. Crystalline powder, mp 269-270°. pH (2% aq soln): 4.6. Soly in water: >20 mg/ml. LD_{50} in female mice, rats (mg/kg): 313, 232 orally; 129, 270 i.m. (Malis).

THERAP CAT: Analgesic (narcotic).

2957. DFDT. [475-26-3] 1,1'-(2,2,2-Trichloroethylidene)-bis[4-fluorobenzene]; 1,1,1-trichloro-2,2-bis(*p*-fluorophenyl)-ethane; difluorodiphenyltrichloroethane; fluorogesarol; HO-2474; Gix. $C_{14}H_9Cl_3F_2$; mol wt 321.58. C 52.29%, H 2.82%, Cl 33.07%, F 11.82%. Prepn: Sumerford, *J. Am. Pharm. Assoc.* **36**, 127 (1947); Cross, **US 2581174** (1952). Toxicity: Piekarski, Holz, *Arch. Exp. Pathol. Pharmakol.* **210**, 71 (1950).

Crystals from aq ethanol, mp 44-45°. Practically insol in water; very sol in oils, most organic solvents.

Caution: Effects similar to DDT [1,1,1-trichloro-2,2-bis(*p*-chlorophenyl)ethane], *q.v.*

USE: Contact insecticide.

2958. Dhurrin. [499-20-7] (αS)-α-(β-D-Glucopyranosyloxy)-4-hydroxybenzeneacetonitrile; *p*-hydroxymandelonitrile-β-D-glucoside; β-D-glucopyranosyloxy-L-*p*-hydroxymandelonitrile. $C_{14}H_{17}NO_7$; mol wt 311.29. C 54.02%, H 5.50%, N 4.50%, O 35.98%. From the fruit of young Egyptian plants of *Sorghum vulgare* Pers., *Gramineae:* Dunstan, Henry, *Chem. News* **85**, 301 (1902). Biosynthesis: Koukol *et al., J. Biol. Chem.* **237**, 3223 (1962). Absolute configuration: Towers *et al., Tetrahedron* **20**, 71 (1964). Allied to amygdalin, *q.v.* and the mandelonitrile glucosides.

Leaflets from water, prisms from alcohol, dec 200°. $[\alpha]_D^{20}$ −65° (alc). uv max: 228 nm (ε 13000). Sol in water, alcohol. Alkali labile.

Pentaacetate. $C_{24}H_{27}NO_{12}$. Needles from ethyl acetate + petr ether, mp 132-132.5°. $[\alpha]_D^{20}$ −50.5° (c = 0.24 in alc).

Caution: Yields HCN on hydrolysis.

2959. Diaboline. [509-40-0] 1-Acetyl-19,20-didehydro-17,18-epoxycuran-17-ol; *N*-acetyl-Wieland-Gumlich aldehyde. $C_{21}H_{24}N_2O_3$; mol wt 352.43. C 71.57%, H 6.86%, N 7.95%, O 13.62%. From *Strychnos diaboli* Sandw., *Loganiaceae:* King, *J. Chem. Soc.* **1949**, 955; Bader *et al., Helv. Chim. Acta* **36**, 1256 (1953); Casinovi *et al., Nature* **193**, 1178 (1962). Structure: Bat-

tersby, Hodson, *Proc. Chem. Soc. London* **1959**, 123. Synthesis: Deyrup *et al., Helv. Chim. Acta* **45**, 2266 (1962). ^{13}C-NMR study: E. Wenkert *et al., J. Org. Chem.* **43**, 1099 (1978).

Needles from ether, mp 187°. $[\alpha]_D^{22}$ +37.8° (c = 1.72 in chloroform). uv max (ethanol): 249 nm (log ε 4.06).

Hydrochloride monohydrate. $C_{21}H_{24}N_2O_3.HCl.H_2O$. Needles from alcohol + ethyl acetate, mp 300°. For anhydr, $[\alpha]_{5461}^{20}$ +184° (c = 0.57 in water).

2960. Diacerein. [13739-02-1] 4,5-Bis(acetyloxy)-9,10-dihydro-9,10-dioxo-2-anthracenecarboxylic acid; 9,10-dihydro-4,5-dihydroxy-9,10-dioxo-2-anthroic acid diacetate; 1,8-diacetoxy-3-carboxyanthraquinone; diacerhein; diacetylrhein; DAR; SF-277; Artrodar; Fisiodar. $C_{19}H_{12}O_8$; mol wt 368.29. C 61.96%, H 3.28%, O 34.75%. Diacetyl derivative of rhein, *q.v.* Demonstrates anti-arthritic activity without inhibiting prostaglandin synthesis. Prepn: A. Tschirch, K. Heuberger, *Arch. Pharm.* **240**, 596 (1902); V. K. Murty *et al., Tetrahedron* **23**, 515 (1967). Effect on prostaglandin release: P. Pomarelli *et al., Farmaco Ed. Sci.* **35**, 836 (1980). Inhibition of proteases: L. Raimondi *et al., Pharmacol. Res. Commun.* **14**, 103 (1982). Use in arthritis: C. A. Friedmann, **DE 2711493**; *idem,* **US 4244968** (1977, 1981 both to Proter). Preliminary clinical study in osteoarthritis: A. G. Kay *et al., Curr. Med. Res. Opin.* **6**, 548 (1980). Use in multiple sclerosis, amyotrophic lateral sclerosis: C. A. Friedmann, **US 4346103** (1982); *idem,* **JP Kokai 83 225015** (1983 to Proter), *C.A.* **100**, 144991e (1984). Clinical trial in osteoarthritis: S. Adami *et al., Clin. Ter.* **112**, 439 (1985).

Yellow plates from acetic acid, mp 217-218°.
THERAP CAT: Antiarthritic.

2961. Diacetin. [25395-31-7] 1,2,3-Propanetriol diacetate; glycerol diacetate; glyceryl diacetate. $C_7H_{12}O_5$; mol wt 176.17. C 47.72%, H 6.87%, O 45.41%. Commercial material is probably a mixture of glycerol 1,2- and 1,3-diacetates. Prepn of the 1,2- and 1,3-compounds: Wegscheider, Zmerzlikar, *Monatsh. Chem.* **34**, 1061 (1913); of the 1,2-compd: Golendeev, *J. Gen. Chem. USSR* **6**, 1841 (1936); of the 1,3-compd: Lagenbeck, Bollow, *Naturwissenschaften* **42**, 389 (1955).

Hygroscopic liquid, bp 259°. d_4^{16} 1.184. n_D^{20} 1.44. Sol in water, alc, ether, benzene; practically insol in CS_2.

dl-**1,2-Compd.** 1,2-Diacetin. bp_{12} 140-142°, bp_{40} 172-173.5°. d_4^{15} 1.1173.

1,3-Compd. 1,3-Diacetin. bp$_{40}$ 172-174°. d^{15} 1.179. n_D^{20} 1.4395.

USE: Technical grade as a plasticizer and softening agent, and as a solvent.

2962. Diacetonamine. [625-04-7] 4-Amino-4-methyl-2-pentanone. $C_6H_{13}NO$; mol wt 115.17. C 62.57%, H 11.38%, N 12.16%, O 13.89%. $CH_3COCH_2C(CH_3)_2NH_2$. Prepd from mesityl oxide with aq NH_3: Haeseler, *J. Am. Chem. Soc.* **47**, 1195 (1925); Orthner, *Ann.* **456**, 245 (1927); Haeseler, *Org. Synth.* **coll. vol. I** (2nd ed., 1941) p 196. From mesityl oxide with liquid ammonia: Smith, Adkins, *J. Am. Chem. Soc.* **60**, 408 (1938).

Liq, bp$_{0.2}$ 25°. Amine odor. Lighter than water. Strongly alkaline. Sol in water, but aq solns prepd in the cold become turbid on heating; miscible with alc, ether. Dec easily forming mesityl oxide and NH_3. Decompn is prone to take place in aq solns or during distillation.

Acid oxalate monohydrate. $C_6H_{13}NO.C_2H_2O_4.H_2O$. Spear-shaped crystals, mp 126-127°.

2963. Diacetone Acrylamide. [2873-97-4] *N*-(1,1-Dimethyl-3-oxobutyl)-2-propenamide; *N*-(1,1-dimethyl-3-oxobutyl)-acrylamide; *N*-[2-(2-methyl-4-oxopentyl)]acrylamide. $C_9H_{15}NO_2$; mol wt 169.22. C 63.88%, H 8.93%, N 8.28%, O 18.91%. Highly reactive vinyl monomer. Prepd by the reaction of acrylonitrile with acetone in presence of conc sulfuric acid: Coleman *et al., J. Polym. Sci.* **3A**, 1601 (1965); Coleman, **US 3277056** (1966 to Lubrizol). Toxicity data: K. Hashimoto *et al., Arch. Toxicol.* **47**, 179 (1981). *Review: idem, "N-Oxoalkylacrylamides" in Encyclopedia of Polymer Science and Technology* **vol. 15**, N. M. Bikales, Exec. Ed. (Wiley-Interscience, New York, 1971) pp 353-364.

White crystalline solid, mp 57-58°. bp$_{0.1-0.3}$ 93-100°; bp$_8$ 120°. Hygroscopic. Has long shelf life; shows no polymerization on prolonged storage. A 50% neutral water soln is stable at pH 7.5-7.7 for up to six months. Similar to acrylic esters in polymerization behavior. Forms high mol wt polymers in bulk, solution, or emulsion. Esp suitable for electropolymerization. LD$_{50}$ orally in mice: 7.7 mmol/kg (Hashimoto).

USE: In the manufacture of coatings, laminates, sealers, adhesives, lubricating oils.

2964. Diacetone Alcohol. [123-42-2] 4-Hydroxy-4-methyl-2-pentanone; Pyranton. $C_6H_{12}O_2$; mol wt 116.16. C 62.04%, H 10.41%, O 27.55%. $(CH_3)_2C(OH)CH_2COCH_3$. Prepd by the action of barium hydroxide or of calcium hydroxide on acetone: Conant, Tuttle, *Org. Synth.* **vol. 1**, p 45 (1921); **coll. vol. I**, 193; *cf.* Jacquemain, *Compt. Rend.* **196**, 1622 (1933). Industrial process using KOH and acetone: Schmitt, Disteldorf, **DE 1052970** (1959 to Hibernia). Toxicity study: Smyth, Carpenter, *J. Ind. Hyg. Toxicol.* **30**, 63 (1948).

Flammable liq; faint, pleasant odor. d$_4^{25}$ 0.9306 (0.940 for tech grades). bp$_{760}$ 167.9°. bp$_{100}$ 108.2°. bp$_{20}$ 72.0°. bp$_{10}$ 58.8°. bp$_{1.0}$ 22.0°. mp −44°; n_D^{20} 1.4232: Lantz, *J. Am. Chem. Soc.* **62**, 3260 (1940). Flash pt reagent grade: 66°C (151°F). Flash pt commercial grades: 8°C (48°F) (closed cup); 13°C (55°F) (open cup). Vapor density 4.00 (air = 1.00). Miscible with water, alcohol, ether, and other solvents. Is dec by prolonged exposure to alkalies and by distillation at atmospheric pressure. LD$_{50}$ orally in rats: 4.0 g/kg (Smyth).

Caution: Potential symptoms of overexposure are irritation of eyes, nose, throat and skin; corneal damage. *See NIOSH Pocket Guide to Chemical Hazards* (DHHS/NIOSH 97-140, 1997) p 90.

USE: Solvent for cellulose acetate, nitrocellulose, celluloid, fats, oils, waxes, resins. As a preservative in pharmaceutical prepns. In some antifreeze solns and in hydraulic fluids.

2965. Diacetoneglucose. [582-52-5] 1,2:5,6-Bis-*O*-(1-methylethylidene)-D-glucofuranose; 1,2:5,6-diisopropylidene-D-glucose; 1,2:5,6-diisopropylidene-D-glucofuranose. $C_{12}H_{20}O_6$; mol wt 260.28. C 55.37%, H 7.75%, O 36.88%. Prepd by shaking

glucose wih acetone contg 1% HCl: Fischer, Rund, *Ber.* **49**, 90, 93 (1916). Improved procedure (90% yield) using 85% H_3PO_4 and anhydr $ZnCl_2$ in a mechanically stirred suspension of glucose in acetone: Glen *et al., US 2715121* (1955 to Am. Home Prod.).

Needles from ether or petr ether. Bitter taste. mp 110-111°. Sublimes. $[\alpha]_D^{20}$ −18.5° (c = 5). Reduces Fehling's soln. One part dissolves in about 7 parts of boiling water and in about 200 parts of boiling petr ether. Freely sol in chloroform, alc, acetone, warm ether. Precipitated from aq soln by NaOH soln. Is not split by yeast or emulsin.

2966. Diacetyl. [431-03-8] 2,3-Butanedione; biacetyl; dimethyl diketone; dimethylglyoxal; 2,3-diketobutane. $C_4H_6O_2$; mol wt 86.09. C 55.81%, H 7.02%, O 37.17%. $CH_3COCOCH_3$. Found in bay and other oils; also in butter. Made from methyl ethyl ketone by converting to the isonitroso compd and then decomposing to diacetyl by hydrolysis with HCl; by special fermentation of glucose *via* methylacetylcarbinol: Suomalainen, Jännes, *Nature* **157**, 336 (1946). Toxicity study: P. M. Jenner *et al., Food Cosmet. Toxicol.* **2**, 327 (1964).

Yellowish-green liq; quinone odor; the vapors have a Cl-like odor. d$_{15}^{15}$ 0.990. bp 88°. n_D^{18} 1.3933. Sol in ~4 parts water; misc with alcohol, ether. LD$_{50}$ orally in rats: 1580 mg/kg (Jenner).

USE: Carrier of aroma of butter, vinegar, coffee, and other foods.

2967. Diacetyldihydromorphine. [509-71-7] (5α,6α)-4,5-Epoxy-17-methylmorphinan-3,6-diol diacetate (ester); dihydroheroin; paralaudin. $C_{21}H_{25}NO_5$; mol wt 371.43. C 67.91%, H 6.78%, N 3.77%, O 21.54%. Prepn from dihydromorphine: Eddy, Howes, *J. Pharmacol.* **53**, 430 (1935); Small, Mallonee, *J. Org. Chem.* **12**, 558-566 (1947); K. W. Bentley, *The Chemistry of the Morphine Alkaloids* (Oxford, 1954).

Needles, mp 165-167°. Slightly sol in water; sol in chloroform, alcohol, ether.

Hydrochloride. $C_{21}H_{25}NO_5.HCl$. Flakes, scales. mp 215-218°. $[\alpha]_D^{29}$ −59° (c = 1.2). Very sol in water.

2968. Diacetylmorphine. [561-27-3] (5α,6α)-7,8-Didehydro-4,5-epoxy-17-methylmorphinan-3,6-diol diacetate (ester); heroin; diamorphine; acetomorphine. $C_{21}H_{23}NO_5$; mol wt 369.41. C 68.28%, H 6.28%, N 3.79%, O 21.66%. Narcotic analgesic prepared from morphine and acetic anhydride: O. Hesse, *Ann.* **220**, 203 (1883); from morphine and acetyl chloride: Small, Lutz, *Chemistry of the Opium Alkaloids,* Supplement No. 103, Public Health Reports, Washington (1932); K. W. Bentley, *The Chemistry of the Morphine Alkaloids* (Oxford, 1954). Comparison with acetylmorphine: N. B. Eddy, H. A. Howes, *J. Pharmacol. Exp. Ther.* **53**, 430 (1935). Pharmacodynamics: J. G. Umans, C. E. Inturrisi, *ibid.* **218**, 409 (1981). Toxicity: *eidem, Eur. J. Pharmacol.* **85**, 317 (1982). Vapor pressure studies: A. H. Lawrence *et al., Can. J. Chem.* **42**, 1886 (1984). Comprehensive description: D. K. Wyatt, L. T. Grady, *Anal. Profiles Drug Subs.* **10**, 357-403 (1981).

Orthorhombic plates, tablets from ethyl acetate. mp 173°. bp$_{12}$ 272-274°. $[\alpha]_D^{25}$ −166° (c = 1.49 in methanol). One gram dissolves in 1.5 ml chloroform, 31 ml alcohol, 100 ml ether, 1700 ml water. Slightly sol in ammonia or sodium carbonate soln, sol in alkalies, dec by boiling with water. Turns pink and emits acetic odor on prolonged exposure to air. LD$_{50}$ i.v. in mice: 59 μmol/kg (Umans, Inturrisi).

Hydrochloride monohydrate. C$_{21}$H$_{23}$NO$_5$.HCl.H$_2$O. Fine crystals, mp 243-244°. $[\alpha]_D^{24}$ −156° (c = 1.044). Sol in 2 parts water, 11 parts alcohol. Insol in ether.

Methyl iodide. C$_{21}$H$_{23}$NO$_5$.CH$_3$I. Needles, mp 252°, $[\alpha]_D^{15}$ −107° (c = 0.896).

Note: "*China White*" has been used as a term for very pure Southeast Asian heroin. This term has also been erroneously used to refer to *3-methylfentanyl* and α-methylfentanyl, *q.v.*, which are potent derivs of fentanyl, *q.v.* See: S. Stinson, *Chem. Eng. News* **59**, 71 (Jan. 19, 1981).

Note: This is a controlled substance (opium derivative): **21 CFR**, 1308.11.

2969. Diafenthiuron. [80060-09-9] *N*-[2,6-Bis(1-methylethyl)-4-phenoxyphenyl]-*N*′-(1,1-dimethylethyl)thiourea; 1-*tert*-butyl-3-(2,6-diisopropyl-4-phenoxyphenyl)thiourea; CGA-106630; Pegasus; Polo. C$_{23}$H$_{32}$N$_2$OS; mol wt 384.58. C 71.83%, H 8.39%, N 7.28%, O 4.16%, S 8.34%. Thiourea proinsecticide that acts via its carbodiimide metabolite to inhibit mitochondrial ATPase. Prepn: J. Drabek, M. Böger, **FR 2465720**; *eidem*, **US 4939257** (1981, 1990 both to Ciba-Geigy). Properties and insecticidal activity: H. P. Streibert *et al., Brighton Crop Prot. Conf. - Pests Dis.* **1988**, 25. Field trials: H. P. Streibert, D. Kaeding, *ibid.* **1994**, 743. Mechanism of action studies: F. J. Ruder *et al., Pestic. Biochem. Physiol.* **41**, 207 (1991); E. Petroske, J. E. Casida, *ibid.* **53**, 60 (1995).

Colorless crystals, mp 149.6°. Vapor pressure: 1.8×10^{-8} Pa. Soly at 20° (g/100ml): water 0.00005; cyclohexanone 38; xylene 21; hexane 0.8. LD$_{50}$ in rats (mg/kg): 2068 orally; >2000 dermally; LC$_{50}$ (14 hr) in rats: 558 mg/m^3 by inhalation (Streibert, 1988).

USE: Insecticide.

2970. Diallate. [2303-16-4] Bis(1-methylethyl)carbamothioic acid *S*-(2,3-dichloro-2-propenyl) ester; diisopropylthiocarbamic acid *S*-2,3-dichloroallyl ester; *S*-2,3-dichloroallyl diisopropylthiocarbamate; DATC; CP-15336; Avadex. C$_{10}$H$_{17}$Cl$_2$NOS; mol wt 270.22. C 44.45%, H 6.34%, Cl 26.24%, N 5.18%, O 5.92%, S 11.87%. Prepn: **GB 882111**; M. W. Harman, J. J. D'Amico, **US 3330823** (1961, 1967 both to Monsanto). Toxicity data: Bailey, White, *Residue Rev.* **10**, 97 (1965). Mutagenicity studies: F. DeLorenzo *et al., Cancer Res.* **38**, 13 (1978); I. Schuphan *et al., Science* **205**, 1013 (1979). Herbicidal activity: R. Grover *et al., Weed Res.* **19**, 363 (1979). GLC determn in milk and plant tissue: L. W. Cook *et al., J. Assoc. Off. Anal. Chem.* **65**, 215 (1982). Review of carcinogenic risk: *IARC Monographs* **30**, 235-244 (1983).

Brown liquid, bp$_9$ 150°. Very slightly sol in water (40 ppm); sol in acetone, benzene, chloroform, ether, heptane. LD$_{50}$ orally in rats: 395 mg/kg (Bailey, White).

USE: Herbicide.

2971. Diallylamine. [124-02-7] *N*-2-Propenyl-2-propen-1-amine; di-2-propenylamine. C$_6$H$_{11}$N; mol wt 97.16. C 74.17%, H 11.41%, N 14.42%. (CH$_2$=CHCH$_2$)$_2$NH. Prepd from allylamine and allyl bromide: Ladenburg, *Ber.* **14**, 1879 (1881); from allylamine and allyl chloride: Liebermann, Hagen, *Ber.* **16**, 1641 (1883); from diallylcyanamide by refluxing with dil H$_2$SO$_4$: Vliet, *J. Am. Chem. Soc.* **46**, 1307 (1924); *Org. Synth.* **coll. vol. I** (2nd ed.,1941) p 201. Toxicity study: H. F. Smyth *et al., Am. Ind. Hyg. Assoc. J.* **23**, 95 (1962).

Liquid. bp 112°. LD$_{50}$ orally in rats: 0.65 g/kg (Smyth).

2972. Diallylcyanamide. [538-08-9] Di-2-propenylcyanamide; *N*-cyanodiallylamine. C$_7$H$_{10}$N$_2$; mol wt 122.17. C 68.82%, H 8.25%, N 22.93%. (CH$_2$=CHCH$_2$)$_2$NCN. Prepd by the action of allyl bromide on disodium cyanamide: Vliet, *J. Am. Chem. Soc.* **46**, 1307 (1924); *Org. Synth.* **coll. vol. I**, 203 (1941); North, **US 1659793** (1929).

Liquid. bp$_{90}$ 140-145°; bp$_{57}$ 128-133°; bp$_{18}$ 105-110°. Insol in water, sol in the usual organic solvents.

2973. Diallyl Trisulfide. [2050-87-5] Di-2-propenyl trisulfide; allyl trisulfide; DATS. C$_6$H$_{10}$S$_3$; mol wt 178.34. C 40.41%, H 5.65%, S 53.94%. (CH$_2$=CHCH$_2$)$_2$S. Component of the essential oil of garlic; formed by pyrolysis of diallyl disulfide. Major component of the Chinese traditional medicine, *allitridium*. Exhibits antifungal, antitumor and antioxidant activity. Isoln from garlic oil: F. W. Semmler, *Arch. Pharm.* **230**, 434 (1892); E. Block *et al., J. Am. Chem. Soc.* **110**, 7813 (1988). Synthesis: B. Milligan *et al., J. Chem. Soc.* **1961**, 4850; A. Banerji, G. P. Kalena, *Tetrahedron Lett.* **21**, 3003 (1980). Inhibitory effect on mammary tumor cells *in vitro*: S. G. Sundaram, J. A. Milner, *Cancer Lett.* **74**, 85 (1993). Mechanism of action study: X. Hu *et al., Arch. Biochem. Biophys.* **336**, 199 (1996). Antifungal activity: J. Shen *et al., Planta Med.* **62**, 415 (1996).

Oil. bp$_6$ 92°; bp$_{0.0008}$ 66-67°. n_D^{20} 1,5896.

2974. Diamfenetide. [36141-82-9] *N,N*′-[Oxybis(2,1-ethanediyloxy-4,1-phenylene)]bisacetamide; β,β′-oxybis[*p*-acetophenetidide]; β,β′-bis(4-acetamidophenyloxy)ethyl ether; diamphenethide; Coriban. C$_{20}$H$_{24}$N$_2$O$_5$; mol wt 372.41. C 64.50%, H 6.50%, N 7.52%, O 21.48%. Prepn: Harfenist, **DE 2143570** (1972), *C.A.* **77**, 19404w (1972). Activity: Dickerson *et al., Br. Vet. J.* **127**, xl (1971); Kingsbury, Rowlands, *ibid.* **128**, 235 (1972); Armour, Corba, *Vet. Rec.* **91**, 211 (1972). *Review:* Rowlands, *Pestic. Sci.* **4**, 883 (1973).

THERAP CAT (VET): Anthelmintic (Trematodes).

2975. Diamine Oxidase. [9001-53-0] Histaminase; benzylamine oxidase; histamine deaminase; histamine oxidase; DAO; EC 1.4.3.6. Copper containing enzyme present in various tissues, esp in the intestinal mucosa; catalyzes the oxidative deamination of histamine and other biogenic amines to form the corresponding aldehydes, ammonia and hydrogen peroxide. Rate-limiting enzyme in the terminal catabolism of polyamines that are essential for cell proliferation. Discovery of a histamine-inactivating enzyme in lung tissue: C. H. Best, *J. Physiol.* **67**, 256 (1929). Identification of activity on other diamines: E. A. Zeller, *Helv. Chim. Acta* **21**, 880

(1938). Extraction from hog kidneys: B. Swedin, *Acta Med. Scand.* **114**, 21 (1943). Improved purification: D. Wilflingseder, H. G. Schwelberger, *J. Chromatogr. B* **737**, 161 (2000). HPLC determn in plasma: P. A. Biondi *et al., J. Chromatogr.* **507**, 333 (1990). *Reviews:* F. Buffoni, *Pharmacol. Rev.* **18**, 1163-1199 (1966); M. C. J. Wolvekamp, R. W. F. de Bruin, *Dig. Dis.* **12**, 2-14 (1994). Review of role in polyamine metabolism: A. Sessa, A. Perin, *Agents Actions* **43**, 69-77 (1994); of role in cell growth and differentiation: P. Pietrangeli, B. Mondovi, *Neurotoxicology* **25**, 317-324 (2004).

2976. 2,4-Diaminoanisole. [615-05-4] 4-Methoxy-1,3-benzenediamine; 4-methoxy-*m*-phenylenediamine; 2,4-DAA; 4-MMPD; C.I. 76050; C.I. Oxidation Base 12. $C_7H_{10}N_2O$; mol wt 138.17. C 60.85%, H 7.29%, N 20.27%, O 11.58%. Prepd by reduction of 2,4-dinitroanisole with iron and acetic acid: **DE 258653** (1912 to BASF), *Frdl.* **11**, 392 (1912-14). Alternate prepn: K. Fries, *Ann.* **454**, 147 (1927). Prepn of hydrochloride: F. Kehrmann, *Ber.* **50**, 562 (1917). Mutagenicity studies: B. N. Ames *et al., Proc. Natl. Acad. Sci. USA* **72**, 2423 (1975); D. J. N. Hossack, J. C. Richardson, *Experientia* **33**, 377 (1977); W. G. H. Blijleven, *Mutat. Res.* **48**, 181 (1977). Toxicity studies: C. Burnett *et al., Food Cosmet. Toxicol.* **13**, 353 (1975); *eidem, J. Toxicol. Environ. Health* **1**, 1027 (1976); *eidem, ibid.* **2**, 657 (1977); G. K. Lloyd *et al., Food Cosmet. Toxicol.* **15**, 607 (1977).

Needles from ether, mp 67-68°. Darkens on exposure to light. LD_{50} of an aq soln containing 0.05% Na_2SO_3: 460 mg/kg orally in rats (Lloyd).

Sulfate. [39156-41-7] 4-MMPDS. $C_7H_{10}N_2O.H_2SO_4$. Off white to violet powder. Sol in water and ethanol. When heated to decomposition, it emits very toxic fumes of nitrogen oxides and sulfur oxides. LD_{50} in rats (mg/kg): 372 i.p.; >4000 orally (Burnett, 1977).

Caution: Potential symptoms of overexposure in exptl animals are skin irritation; thyroid and liver changes; teratogenic effects. See *NIOSH Pocket Guide to Chemical Hazards* (DHHS/NIOSH 97-140, 1997) p 90. 2,4-Diaminoanisole sulfate is reasonably anticipated to be a human carcinogen: *Report on Carcinogens, Eleventh Edition* (PB2005-104914, 2004) p III-78.

USE: In prepn of dyes, esp hair and fur dyes; intermediates in the production of C. I. Basic Brown 2; as corrosion inhibitor for steel.

2977. *p*-Diaminoazobenzene. [538-41-0] 4,4'-Azobisbenzenamine; 4,4'-azodianiline; *p*-azoaniline; 4,4'-diaminoazobenzene. $C_{12}H_{12}N_4$; mol wt 212.25. C 67.91%, H 5.70%, N 26.40%. Prepn: Witt, Kopetschini, *Ber.* **45**, 1136 (1912); Brode *et al., J. Am. Chem. Soc.* **77**, 2762 (1955). Lab procedure starting with *p*-aminoacetanilide; Santurri *et al., Org. Synth.* **40**, 18 (1960).

Golden-yellow needles, dec 238-241°. Absorption max (ethanol): 400 nm. Slightly soluble in water, benzene, petr ether; freely sol in alcohol.

2978. 3,5-Diaminobenzoic Acid. [535-87-5] $C_7H_8N_2O_2$; mol wt 152.15. C 55.26%, H 5.30%, N 18.41%, O 21.03%. Prepn from 3,5-dinitrobenzoic acid: Griess, *Ann.* **154**, 327 (1870).

Monohydrate. Needles. Loses its water of crystn at about 110°, mp 228°. Slightly sol in water; the aqueous soln dec on standing. Sol in alcohol or ether.

Ethyl ester. $C_9H_{12}N_2O_2$. Prisms from ether, mp 84°. Moderately sol in hot water. Sol in alcohol, benzene, other organic solvents.

USE: Detection and determination of nitrites.

2979. 4,4'-Diaminodiphenylamine. [537-65-5] *N*-(4-Aminophenyl)-1,4-benzenediamine; *p*-*p*'-diaminodiphenylamine. $C_{12}H_{13}N_3$; mol wt 199.25. C 72.34%, H 6.58%, N 21.09%. Prepn from *p*-phenylenediamine and aniline hydrochloride: Nietzki, *Ber.* **16**, 474 (1883); from *p*-aminoazobenzene: Barbier, Sisley, *Bull. Soc. Chim. Fr.* [3] **33**, 1232 (1905); by reducing bis(*p*-nitrophenyl)-nitroxide with tin chloride and hydrochloric acid: Wieland, Roth, *Ber.* **53**, 213, 226 (1920).

Leaflets from water, mp 158°. Oxidized to bromanil and bromonitromethane by bromine and concd nitric acid.

USE: Dyeing fur: **DE 367690; DE 371231**; manuf dyes. In the detection of hydrogen cyanide.

2980. *p,p*'-Diaminodiphenylmethane. [101-77-9] 4,4'-Methylenebis[benzenamine]; 4,4'-methylenedianiline. $C_{13}H_{14}N_2$; mol wt 198.26. C 78.75%, H 7.12%, N 14.13%. Prepn from aniline and formaldehyde: Scanlon, *J. Am. Chem. Soc.* **57**, 887 (1935); by hydrogenolysis of *p,p*'-diaminobenzophenone with $LiAlH_4$: Conover, Tarbell, *ibid.* **72**, 3586 (1950). Identified as causative agent in clinical outbreak of hepatoxicity called Epping Jaundice: H. Kopelman *et al., Br. Med. J.* **1**, 514 (1966); D. B. McGill, J. D. Motto, *N. Engl. J. Med.* **291**, 278 (1974). Review of toxicology and human exposure: *Toxicological Profile for Methylenedianiline* (PB99-102568, 1998) 194 pp.

Crystals from water or benzene. mp 91.5-92°. bp_{768} 398-399°; bp_{18} 257°; bp_{15} 249-253°; bp_9 232°. Slightly sol in cold water. Very sol in alcohol, benzene, ether.

Caution: Potential symptoms of overexposure by ingestion are jaundice, weakness, abdominal pain, nausea, vomiting, anorexia, fever, chills, hepatotoxicity (Kopelman). Direct contact may cause skin irritation (PB99-102568). This substance and its dihydrochloride are reasonably anticipated to be human carcinogens: *Report on Carcinogens, Eleventh Edition* (PB2005-104914, 2004) p III-169.

USE: As chemical intermediate in prodn of isocyanates and polyisocyantes for prepn of polyurethane foams, Spandex fibers; as curing agent for epoxy resins and urethane elastomers; in production of polyamides; in the determination of tungsten and sulfates; in prepn of azo dyes; as corrosion inhibitor.

2981. 2,4-Diamino-6-hydroxypyrimidine. [56-06-4] 2,6-Diamino-4(1*H*)-pyrimidinone. $C_4H_6N_4O$; mol wt 126.12. C 38.09%, H 4.80%, N 44.42%, O 12.69%. Prepn from guanidine hydrochloride and cyanoacetic ester: Traube, *Ber.* **33**, 1371 (1900).

Crystallizes from water as the monohydrate. When anhydrous, dec 286°.

USE: In the detection of nitrites and nitrates.

2982. 2,3-Diaminophenazine. [655-86-7] 2,3-Phenazinediamine. $C_{12}H_{10}N_4$; mol wt 210.23. C 68.56%, H 4.79%, N 26.65%. Prepn from o-phenylenediamine: Ullmann, Mauthner, *Ber.* **35**, 4304 (1902); Knoevenagel, *J. Prakt. Chem.* [2] **89**, 25 (1914); Richter *Ber.* **44**, 3469 (1911).

Brown to yellow needles. On careful heating sublimes forming yellow leaflets. mp 264°. Sol in alcohol, benzene. Yields 2-aminophenazine and small amounts of phenazine when heated with zinc dust.

USE: Detection of bismuth, cadmium, lead, copper, and mercury.

2983. 2,4-Diaminophenol. [95-86-3] $C_6H_8N_2O$; mol wt 124.14. C 58.05%, H 6.50%, N 22.57%, O 12.89%. Prepn by reduction of 2,4-dinitrophenol: Braude *et al., J. Chem. Soc.* **1954**, 3586; Neilson *et al., ibid.* **1962**, 371; from m-nitroaniline: Bean, **US 2525515** (1950 to Eastman Kodak).

Crystals, dec 78-80°. Somewhat sol in alcohol, acetone; sparingly sol in ether, chloroform, petr ether; readily sol in acids, alkalies.

Dihydrochloride. Acrol; Amidol. $C_6H_8N_2O.2HCl$; mol wt 197.06. Crystals, mp 205°. Soly in water at 15°: 27.5 g/100 ml. Slightly sol in alcohol.

USE: Dihydrochloride as photographic developer, in fur and hair dyeing, in test for formaldehyde and ammonia.

2984. 2,3-Diaminopropionic Acid. [515-94-6] 3-Amino-alanine; 2,3-diaminopropanoic acid; α,β-diaminopropionic acid. $C_3H_8N_2O_2$; mol wt 104.11. C 34.61%, H 7.75%, N 26.91%, O 30.74%. Prepd by treating 2,3-dibromopropionic acid with ammonia: Klebs, *Z. Physiol. Chem.* **19**, 314 (1894); Winterstein, Küng, *ibid.* **59**, 146 (1909); Neuberg, Silbermann, *Ber.* **37**, 341 (1904); Frankland, *J. Chem. Soc.* **97**, 1318 (1910); by treating 2-amino-3-chloropropionic acid with ammonia under pressure: Fisher *et al., Ber.* **40**, 3717 (1907); by the reduction of cyanooximoacetic acid esters: Godefroi, **US 2738363** (1956 to Parke, Davis). Configuration: Karrer *et al., Helv. Chim. Acta* **9**, 314 (1926). *See also* Bergmann, Grafe, *Z. Physiol. Chem.* **187**, 187 (1930).

DL-Form. Radially arranged cryst masses. Hygroscopic, also absorbs CO_2 from air. Begins to melt at 97°, completely liq at 110-120°. Sol in water, yielding alkaline solns. Practically insol in alcohol, ether.

Hydrochloride. $C_3H_8N_2O_2.HCl$. Needles or leaflets, mp 236-237°. One gram dissolves in 12 ml water, practically insol in alcohol.

Sulfate hemihydrate. $(C_3H_8N_2O_2)_2.H_2SO_4.\frac{1}{2}H_2O$. Six-sided leaflets from water, dec 233-234°. One gram dissolves in 31 ml water at 20°.

Methyl ester dihydrochloride. $C_4H_{10}N_2O_2.2HCl$. Crystals, dec 170°. Freely sol in water.

Ethyl ester dihydrochloride. $C_5H_{12}N_2O_2.2HCl$. Crystals, mp 164.5-165° (some decompn). Freely sol in water.

L-Form hydrochloride. $C_3H_8N_2O_2.HCl$. Needles from water, $[\alpha]_D^{20}$ +25.0° (c = 5 in 1.0N HCl).

D-Form hydrochloride. $C_3H_8N_2O_2.HCl$. Needles from water, $[\alpha]_D^{20}$ −25.3° (c = 5 in 1.0N HCl).

USE: The salts as growth inhibitors for microorganisms.

2985. 2,6-Diaminopurine. [1904-98-9] 1H-Purine-2,6-diamine; 2,6-diamino-9H-purine. $C_5H_6N_6$; mol wt 150.14. C 40.00%, H 4.03%, N 55.97%. Antagonist of naturally occurring purines: Hitchings, Elion in *Metabolic Inhibitors* vol. I, R. M. Hochster, J. H. Quastel, Eds. (Academic Press, New York, 1963) pp 216-232. Molecular and electronic structure: Veillard, Pullman, *J. Theor. Biol.* **4**, 37 (1963). First synthesized by Traube, *Ber.* **37**, 4547 (1904) by cyclization of 2,4,5,6-tetraaminopyrimidine. Prepn from guanidine carbonate in 70% yield and refs to earlier prepns: Taylor *et al., J. Am. Chem. Soc.* **81**, 2442 (1959).

Crystals from ethanol + water, mp 302°. uv max (pH 1.9): 241, 282 nm (log ε 3.98, 4.00).

2986. 3,4-Diaminopyridine. [54-96-6] 3,4-Pyridinediamine; 3,4-DAP. $C_5H_7N_3$; mol wt 109.13. C 55.03%, H 6.47%, N 38.50%. Potassium channel blocker; antagonizes non-depolarizing neuromuscular blockade. Prepn: O. Bremer, *Ann.* **518**, 274 (1935); J. W. Clark-Lewis, R. P. Singh, *J. Chem. Soc.* **1962**, 2379; J. B. Campbell *et al., J. Heterocycl. Chem.* **23**, 669 (1986). HPLC determn in serum: J. Leslie, C. T. Bever, *J. Chromatogr.* **496**, 214 (1989). Acute toxicity: P. Lechat *et al., Ann. Pharm. Fr.* **26**, 345 (1968). Effect on neuromuscular transmission: J. Molgo *et al., Eur. J. Pharmacol.* **61**, 25 (1980); R. H. Thomsen, D. F. Wilson, *J. Pharmacol. Exp. Ther.* **227**, 260 (1983). Evaluation in human botulism: A. P. Ball *et al., Q. J. Med.* **48**, 473 (1979). Clinical evaluations in myasthenic syndromes: K. M. McEvoy *et al., N. Engl. J. Med.* **321**, 1567 (1989); J. Palace *et al., J. Neurol. Neurosurg. Psychiatry* **54**, 1069 (1991); in multiple sclerosis: C. T. Bever, Jr. *et al., Ann. Neurol.* **27**, 421 (1990); *idem, ibid.* **36**, S118 (1994).

Needles from water, mp 220° (Clark-Lewis, Singh); also reported as white to beige crystals from water, mp 218-219° (Campbell). Readily sol in water, alcohol; slightly sol in ether. LD_{50} i.v. in mice: 13 mg/kg (Lechat).

USE: Intermediate in synthesis of heterocyclic compds.

2987. Diamond. [7782-40-3] A crystalline form of carbon. Mined as a mineral, principally in South Africa. (Non-commercial) synthesis from other carbon compds (e.g., lignin) by means of elevated temperatures (about 2700°) and pressures (about 800,000 lbs/sq inch): Desch, *Nature* **152**, 148 (1943); Neuhaus, *Angew. Chem.* **66**, 525 (1954); Hall, *Chem. Eng. News* **33**, 718 (1955); Bridgman, *Sci. Am.* **1955**, 46; Hall, *J. Chem. Educ.* **38**, 484 (1961); Bundy, *Ann. N.Y. Acad. Sci.* **105**, 951-982 (1964). Books: S. Tolansky, *History and Use of Diamond* (London, 1962) 166 pp; R. Berman, *Physical Properties of Diamond* (Oxford, 1965) 442 pp.

Face-centered cubic crystal lattice. Burns when heated with a hot enough flame (over 800°, oxygen torch). d_4^{25} 3.513. n_D^{20} 2.4173. Hardness = 10 (Mohs' scale). Sp heat at 100 K: 0.606 cal/g-atom/K. Entropy at 298.16 K: 0.5684 cal/g-atom/K. Band gap energy: 6.7 ev. Dielectric constant 5.7. Electron mobility: ~1800 cm²/v-sec. Hole mobility: 1200 cm²/v-sec. Can be pulverized in a steel mortar. Attacked by laboratory-type cleaning soln (potassium dichromate + concd H_2SO_4). In the jewelry trade the unit of weight for diamonds is one carat = 200 mg. *Ref: Wall Street J.* **164**, no. 36, p 10 (Aug 19, 1964).

USE: Jewelry. Polishing, grinding, cutting glass, bearings for delicate instruments; manuf dies for tungsten wire and similar hard wires; making styli for recorder heads, long-lasting phonograph needles. In semiconductor research.

2988. Diampromide. [552-25-0] N-[2-[Methyl(2-phenylethyl)amino]propyl]-N-phenylpropanamide; N-[2-(methylphenethylamino)propyl]propionanilide. $C_{21}H_{28}N_2O$; mol wt 324.46. C 77.74%, H 8.70%, N 8.63%, O 4.93%. Synthesis: Wright *et al.*, *J. Am. Chem. Soc.* **81**, 1518 (1959); **US 2944081** (1960 to American Cyanamid).

Liquid, $bp_{0.5}$ 174-178°. n_D^{26} 1.546.

Sulfate. $C_{21}H_{30}N_2O_5S$. Crystals from ethanol + ether, mp 110-111°.

Note: This is a controlled substance (opiate): **21 CFR**, 1308.11.

THERAP CAT: Analgesic (narcotic).

2989. Diamyl Sodium Sulfosuccinate. [922-80-5] Sulfobutanedioic acid 1,4-dipentyl ester sodium salt; sulfosuccinic acid dipentyl ester sodium salt; Aerosol AY; Alphasol AY. $C_{14}H_{25}$-NaO_7S; mol wt 360.40. C 46.66%, H 6.99%, Na 6.38%, O 31.08%, S 8.90%. The amyl or 1-methylbutyl diester of the monosodium salt of sulfosuccinic acid or a mixture of both. Wetting agent prepd by the action of the appropriate alcohols on maleic anhydride followed by addtion of sodium bisulfite: Jaeger, **US 2028091** and **US 2176423** (1936, 1939 to Am. Cyanamid).

Available as a mixture of white, hard pellets and powder. Soly in water at 25° = 392 g/liter; at 70° = 502 g/liter. Maximum concn of electrolyte soln in which 1% of the wetting agent is sol: 3% NaCl; 2-4% NH_4Cl (turbid); 3-6% $(NH_4)_2HPO_4$ (turbid); 4% $NaNO_3$ (slightly turbid); 15% Na_2SO_4 (very slightly turbid). Also sol in pine oil, oleic acid, acetone, hot kerosene, carbon tetrachloride, glycerol, hot olive oil; insol in liq petrolatum. Surface tension in water: 0.001% = 69.4 dyn/cm; 0.02% = 68.3 dyn/cm; 0.1% = 50.2 dyn/cm; 0.25% = 41.6 dyn/cm; 1% = 29.2 dyn/cm. Interfacial tension 1% in water *vs.* liquid petrolatum: 5 seconds = 7.55 dyn/cm; 30 seconds = 7.37 dyn/cm; 15 minutes = 7.03 dyn/cm. Interfacial tension 0.1% in water *vs.* liquid petrolatum: 5 seconds = 29.5 dyn/cm; 30 seconds = 28.6 dyn/cm; 15 minutes = 27.5 dyn/cm. Stable in acid and neutral solns, hydrolyzes in alkaline solns.

USE: As emulsifier in emulsion polymerization and as a wetting agent.

2990. 1,2-Dianilinoethane. [150-61-8] N,N'-Diphenyl-1,2-ethanediamine; N,N'-diphenylethylenediamine; N,N'-diphenyl-α,ω-diaminoethane; *sym*-diphenylethylenediamine. $C_{14}H_{16}N_2$; mol wt 212.29. C 79.21%, H 7.60%, N 13.20%. Prepd by heating aniline with dichloroethane: Büchi *et al.*, *Helv. Chim. Acta* **39**, 950 (1956); by heating aniline with dibromoethane: Wanzlick, Löchel, *Ber.* **86**, 1463 (1953).

Crystals from dil ethanol, mp 67.5°; (also reported as the monohydrate). bp_{12} 228-230°. Very sol in alc, ether.

USE: Identification of aldehydes; stabilizer for resins and rubber. Intermediate in the manufacture of antihistamines.

2991. Dianisidine. [119-90-4] 3,3'-Dimethoxy-[1,1'-biphenyl]-4,4'-diamine; 3,3'-dimethoxybenzidine; 3,3'-dimethoxy-

4,4'-diaminobiphenyl. $C_{14}H_{16}N_2O_2$; mol wt 244.29. C 68.83%, H 6.60%, N 11.47%, O 13.10%. Prepn: Meier, Böhler, *Ber.* **89**, 2301 (1956); Sogn, **US 2794047** (1957 to Allied Chem.). Manuf of stabilized product: Cashion, **US 2966519** (1960 to Allied Chem.). Review of carcinogenicity studies: *IARC Monographs* **4**, 41-47 (1974).

Crystals, becoming violet, mp 137-138°. Practically insol in water. Sol in alcohol, benzene, ether.

Caution: Potential symptom of overexposure by direct contact is skin irritation. *See NIOSH Pocket Guide to Chemical Hazards* (DHHS/NIOSH 97-140, 1997) p 90. 3,3'-Dimethoxybenzidine and dyes metabolized to 3,3'-dimethoxybenzidine are reasonably anticipated to be human carcinogens: *Report on Carcinogens, Eleventh Edition* (PB2005-104914, 2004) p III-104.

USE: Manuf of azo dyes and pigments.

2992. Diatrizoate Sodium. [737-31-5] 3,5-Bis(acetylamino)-2,4,6-triiodobenzoic acid sodium salt; 3,5-diacetamido-2,4,6-triiodobenzoic acid sodium salt; sodium 3,5-diacetamido-2,4,6-triiodobenzoate; urografic acid sodium salt; sodium amidotrizoate; sodium diatrizoate; Hypaque Sodium; Triognost. $C_{11}H_8I_3$-N_2NaO_4; mol wt 635.90. C 20.78%, H 1.27%, I 59.87%, N 4.41%, Na 3.62%, O 10.06%. Prepn of the acid: Larsen *et al.*, *J. Am. Chem. Soc.* **78**, 3210 (1956). Description: Langecker *et al.*, *Arch. Exp. Pathol. Pharmakol.* **222**, 584 (1954). Use in separation of leukocytes from whole blood: R. J. Perper *et al.*, *J. Lab. Clin. Med.* **72**, 842 (1968); L. P. Bignold, A. Ferrante, *J. Immunol. Methods* **96**, 29 (1987); J. R. Kalmar *et al.*, *ibid.* **110**, 275 (1988). Comprehensive description: H. H. Lerner, *Anal. Profiles Drug Subs.* **4**, 137-167 (1975).

Rhombic needles, slightly salty taste, mp 261-262° (dec). Soly in water at 20°: 60 g/100 ml. pH of a 50% aq soln 7.0 to 7.5. On chilling solns may become cloudy or form a precipitate which disappears at room temp. Solns may be sterilized by autoclaving. Should be protected from light. LD_{50} i.v. in rats: 14.7 g/kg (Langecker).

Free acid. Crystals from dil DMF, mp >300°.

Note: See also Meglumine Diatrizoate.

USE: Density gradient reagent for blood cell separation.

THERAP CAT: Diagnostic aid (radiopaque medium).

THERAP CAT (VET): Diagnostic aid (radiopaque medium).

2993. Diaveridine. [5355-16-8] 5-[(3,4-Dimethoxyphenyl)-methyl]-2,4-pyrimidinediamine; 2,4-diamino-5-veratrylpyrimidine; 2,4-diamino-5-(3',4'-dimethoxybenzyl)pyrimidine. $C_{13}H_{16}N_4O_2$; mol wt 260.29. C 59.99%, H 6.20%, N 21.52%, O 12.29%. Prepn: Falco *et al.*, *J. Am. Chem. Soc.* **73**, 3758 (1951). Hitchings, Falco, **US 2624732** (1953 to Burroughs Wellcome); Stenbuck *et al.*, *J. Org. Chem.* **28**, 1983 (1963); Hoffer, **US 3341541** (1967 to Hoffmann-La Roche); M. Hoffer *et al.*, *J. Med. Chem.* **14**, 462 (1971). Crystal structure: T. F. Koetzle, G. Williams, *Acta Crystallogr.* **B34**, 323 (1978).

Crystals, mp 233°.

Ingredient of *Darvisul* which also contains sulfaquinoxaline.

THERAP CAT (VET): Antiprotozoan (in combination with sulfa-quinoxaline).

2994. Diazepam. [439-14-5] 7-Chloro-1,3-dihydro-1-meth-yl-5-phenyl-2H-1,4-benzodiazepin-2-one; 7-chloro-1-methyl-5-phenyl-3H-1,4-benzodiazepin-2(1H)-one; methyl diazepinone; di-acepin; LA-III; Ro-5-2807; Wy-3467; NSC-77518; Apaurin; Bial-zepam; Calmpose; Ceregulart; Dialar; Diastat; Diazemuls; Eurosan; Faustan; Gewacalm; Lamra; Noan; Novazam; Paceum; Paxate; Re-lanium; Seduxen; Servizepam; Stesolid; Unisedil; Valiquid; Valium; Vival. $C_{16}H_{13}ClN_2O$; mol wt 284.74. C 67.49%, H 4.60%, Cl 12.45%, N 9.84%, O 5.62%. Prepn: L. H. Sternbach, E. Reeder, *J. Org. Chem.* **26**, 4936 (1961); E. Reeder, L. H. Sternbach, US 3371085 (1968 to Hoffmann-La Roche). Synthesis: M. Gates, *J. Org. Chem.* **45**, 1675 (1980); M. Ishikura *et al., ibid.* **47**, 2456 (1982). Binding study in rat brain: R. F. Squires, C. Braestrup, *Nature* **266**, 732 (1977). Comprehensive description: A. MacDonald *et al., Anal. Profiles Drug Subs.* **1**, 79-99 (1972). Review of clinical pharmacokinetics: M. Mandelli *et al., Clin. Pharmacokinet.* **3**, 72-91 (1978); and metabolism: L. Bertilsson *et al., Pharmacol. Ther.* **45**, 85-91 (1990). Review of clinical experience and dependency potential in anxiety: J. B. Murray, *J. Psychol.* **124**, 655-674 (1990); of use in seizure treatment: J. M. Pellock, *Drug Saf.* **27**, 383-392 (2004).

Colorless to light yellow crystalline compound. Prisms from ethanol, mp 131.5-134.5°. pKa 3.4. Sol in chloroform, DMF, benzene, acetone, alc. Practically insol in water.

Note: This is a controlled substance (depressant): **21 CFR,** 1308.14.

THERAP CAT: Anxiolytic; muscle relaxant (skeletal); anticonvul-sant.

2995. Diazinon. [333-41-5] Phosphorothioic acid O,O-di-ethyl O-[6-methyl-2-(1-methylethyl)-4-pyrimidinyl] ester; thio-phosphoric acid 2-isopropyl-4-methyl-6-pyrimidyl diethyl ester; O,O-diethyl O-2-isopropyl-4-methyl-6-pyrimidyl thiophosphate; diethyl 2-isopropyl-4-methyl-6-pyrimidyl thionophosphate; dim-pylate; G-24480; Antigal; Basudin; Diazol; HelfaCat; HelfaDog; Neocidol; Parasitex; Sarolex; Spectracide; Taberdog; Tabergat. $C_{12}H_{21}N_2O_3PS$; mol wt 304.35. C 47.36%, H 6.95%, N 9.20%, O 15.77%, P 10.18%, S 10.54%. Cholinesterase inhibitor. Prepn: Gysin, Margot, US 2754243 (1956 to Geigy). Insecticidal proper-ties: Gasser, *Z. Naturforsch.* **8b**, 225 (1953). Toxicity data: T. B. Gaines, *Toxicol. Appl. Pharmacol.* **14**, 515 (1969). Review of toxicology and human exposure: *Toxicological Profile for Diazinon* (PB97-121107, 1996) 245 pp.

Liquid. Faint ester-like odor. d_4^{20} 1.116-1.118. $bp_{0.002}$ 83-84°. n_D^{20} 1.4978-1.4981. Vapor pressure at 20°: 1.4×10^{-4}; at 40°: 1.1×10^{-3} (~5 times vapor pressure of parathion). Volatility at 20°: 2.4 mg/m³; at 40°: 17.6 mg/m³. Decomposes above 120°. Soly in water at 20°: 0.004%. Miscible with alcohol, ether, petr

ether, cyclohexane, benzene, and similar hydrocarbons. More sta-ble in alkaline formulations, then when at neutral or acid pH. LD_{50} in male, female rats (mg/kg): 250, 285 orally (Gaines).

Caution: Potential symptoms of overexposure are eye irritation; miosis, blurred vision; dizziness, confusion, weakness, convulsions; dyspnea; salivation, abdominal cramps, nausea, vomiting. *See NIOSH Pocket Guide to Chemical Hazards* (DHHS/NIOSH 97-140, 1997) p 92.

USE: Insecticide.

THERAP CAT (VET): Ectoparasiticide.

2996. Diaziquone. [57998-68-2] [2,5-Bis(1-aziridinyl)-3,6-dioxo-1,4-cyclohexadiene-1,4-diyl]biscarbamic acid diethyl ester; 2,5-bis(1-aziridinyl)-3,6-dioxo-1,4-cyclohexadiene-1,4-dicarbamic acid diethyl ester; 2,5-diaziridinyl-3,6-bis(ethoxycarbonylamino)-1,4-benzoquinone; aziridinylbenzoquinone; AZQ; CI-904; NSC-182986. $C_{16}H_{20}N_4O_6$; mol wt 364.35. C 52.74%, H 5.53%, N 15.38%, O 26.35%. Quinone-containing lipophilic alkylating agent. Prepn as intermediate in dyestuffs: S. Petersen *et al.,* US 2913453 (1959 to Schenley Ind.). Synthesis and antitumor activity: A. H. Khan, J. S. Driscoll, *J. Med. Chem.* **19**, 313 (1976); J. S. Driscoll *et al.,* US 4146622 (1979 to U.S. Gov't). *In vivo* antitumor studies: J. S. Driscoll *et al., J. Pharm. Sci.* **68**, 185 (1979). Intra-cerebral penetration and tissue distribution in humans: N. Savaraj *et al., J. Neuro-Oncol.* **1**, 15 (1983). LC determn: B. A. Allen *et al., J. Chromatogr.* **222**, 146 (1981). Pharmacokinetics: S. Zimm *et al., Cancer Res.* **44**, 1698 (1984). Clinical studies in treatment of CNS neoplasms: R. T. Eagan *et al., J. Neuro-Oncol.* **5**, 309 (1987); E. Tapazoglou *et al., Am. J. Clin. Oncol.* **11**, 474 (1988). *Review:* J. F. Bender *et al., Invest. New Drugs* **1**, 71-84 (1983).

Orange needles from ethanol, mp 230° (dec); also reported as yellowish-brown crystals from ethanol decomposing at temperatures above 250° (Petersen). uv max (methanol): 340 nm (log ε 4.17). Soly in water: 0.5 mg/ml. LD_{50} in mice (mg/m²): 30.9 i.v. (Bender).

THERAP CAT: Antineoplastic.

2997. Diazoacetic Ester. [623-73-4] Ethyl diazoacetate; ethyl diazoethanoate. $C_4H_6N_2O_2$; mol wt 114.10. C 42.11%, H 5.30%, N 24.55%, O 28.04%. $^-N{=}N^+{=}CHCOOC_2H_5$. Prepd by the action of sodium nitrite on glycine ethyl ester hydrochloride: Curtius *J. Prakt. Chem.* [2] **38**, 396 (1888); Silberrad, *J. Chem. Soc.* **81**, 600 (1902); Womack, Nelson, *Org. Synth.* **24**, 56 (1944).

Yellow oil. Pungent odor. Very volatile. Explosive. *Distilla-tion, even under reduced pressure, is dangerous.* mp −22°. $d_4^{17.6}$ 1.0852. bp_5 42°; bp_{12} 45°; bp_{88} 85-86°; bp_{720} 140-141°. $n_D^{17.6}$ 1.4588. Slightly sol in water. Neutral reaction. Volatile with steam, ether, and benzene vapors. Miscible with alcohol, benzene, ligroin, ether. Explodes on contact with concd H_2SO_4.

2998. Diazoaminobenzene. [136-35-6] 1,3-Diphenyl-1-tri-azene; anilinoazobenzene; benzeneazoaniline. $C_{12}H_{11}N_3$; mol wt 197.24. C 73.07%, H 5.62%, N 21.30%. Made by diazotizing aniline dissolved in HCl with $NaNO_2$ and then adding a concd soln of sodium acetate: Hartman, Dickey, *Org. Synth.* **coll. vol. II,** 163 (1943).

Golden-yellow, small crystals. mp 98°. *Explodes when heated to 150°.* Insol in water. Freely sol in benzene, ether, hot alc.

Caution: This substance is reasonably anticipated to be a human carcinogen: *Report on Carcinogens, Eleventh Edition* (PB2005-104914, 2004) p III-80.

2999. *p*-Diazobenzenesulfonic Acid. [305-80-6] 4-Sulfobenzenediazonium inner salt; DABS; diazotized sulfanilic acid ; Pauly's reagent; sulfanilic acid diazonium salt. $C_6H_4N_2O_3S$; mol wt 184.17. C 39.13%, H 2.19%, N 15.21%, O 26.06%, S 17.41%. Prepn by diazotization of sulfanilic acid: E. Fischer, *Ann.* **190,** 67 (1878); K. B. Whetsel *et al., J. Am. Chem. Soc.* **78,** 3360 (1956); G. Kaupp *et al., Chem. Eur. J.* **8,** 1395 (2002). Crystal structure.: C. Bugg *et al., Acta Crystallogr.* **17,** 767 (1964). Use as denaturant for membrane proteins: R. T. Giaquinta *et al., Arch. Biochem. Biophys.* **162,** 200 (1974); M.-J. Bouchet *et al., J. Med. Chem.* **30,** 2222 (1987); of protein components: S. K. Nishimoto *et al., Anal. Biochem.* **216,** 156 (1994). Determn of bilirubin: J. B. Landis, H. L. Pardue, *Clin. Chem.* **24,** 1690 (1978); P. Fossati *et al., ibid.* **35,** 173 (1989); of phenols: C. Baiocchi *et al., Anal. Lett.* **15,** 1539 (1982); M. C. Quintero *et al., Talanta* **36,** 717 (1989); of halides: M. Pandey *et al., Analyst* **123,** 2319 (1998); S. Gosain *et al., J. AOAC Int.* **82,** 167 (1999).

N≡N⁺—⟨benzene ring⟩—SO₃⁻

Solid. *Explodes* upon heating to mp 104°; shock sensitive (hammer and anvil test). Insol in water.

USE: Reagent for determination of phenols, bilirubin, halides and amines. Irreversible probe in membrane protein studies.

3000. Diazolidinyl Urea. [78491-02-8] *N*-[1,3-Bis(hydroxymethyl)-2,5-dioxo-4-imidazolidinyl]-*N*,*N* '-bis(hydroxymethyl)urea; *N*-(hydroxymethyl)-*N*-(1,3-dihydroxymethyl-2,5-dioxo-imidazolidinyl)-*N* '-(hydroxymethyl)urea; Germall II. $C_8H_{14}N_4O_7$; mol wt 278.22. C 34.54%, H 5.07%, N 20.14%, O 40.25%. Member of a family of heterocyclic substituted urea compounds with formaldehyde releasing activity. Prepn: P. A. Berke, W. E. Rosen, **WO 8100566**; *eidem,* **US 4271176** (both 1981 to Sutton). Chemistry, toxicity and antimicrobial activity: *eidem, Cosmet. Toiletries* **97,** 49 (1982). Determn in cosmetic products: R. J. Geise *et al., J. Soc. Cosmet. Chem.* **45,** 173 (1994). Review of use and safety assessment: *J. Am. Coll. Toxicol.* **9,** 229-245 (1990).

⟨chemical structure⟩

Fine, white, free-flowing powder. Sol in water as a 30% soln. Insol in fats. LD₅₀ orally in rats: 2.57 g/kg; dermally in rabbits: >2.0 g/kg (Berke, Rosen).

USE: Antimicrobial preservative in cosmetics and toiletries.

3001. Diazomethane. [334-88-3] Azimethylene. CH_2N_2; mol wt 42.04. C 28.57%, H 4.80%, N 66.64%. $CH_2=N^+=N^-$. Prepd from chloroform and hydrazine by reaction with potassium hydroxide: Staudinger, Kupfer, *Ber.* **45,** 501 (1912); McManus *et al., J. Org. Chem.* **33,** 4272 (1968); from KOH and nitrosomethylurea: Dessaux, Durand, *Bull. Soc. Chim. Fr.* **1963,** 41. These methods yield gaseous diazomethane. The following procedures yield ether solns of diazomethane. From *N*-nitroso-β-methylaminoisobutyl methyl ketone in ether and isopropanol by reaction with sodium isopropoxide or from the same ketone in ether by reaction with sodium cyclohexoxide: Redemann *et al., Org. Synth.* **25,** 28 (1945). By KOH saponification of nitrosomethylurea in ether: Arndt, *Org. Synth.* **coll. vol. II,** 165 (1943), or of nitrosomethylurethan in ether: von Pechmann, *Ber.* **27,** 1888 (1894); **28,** 855 (1895); Meerwein, Burneleit, *Ber.* **61,** 1845 (1928). In the laboratory diazomethane may be prepd most simply by the action of alkali on the commercially available *N*-methyl-*N*-nitroso-*N* '-nitroguanidine, *cf.* McKay, *J. Am. Chem. Soc.* **70,** 1974 (1948); McKay *et al., Can. J. Res.* **28,** 683 (1950); Fieser and Fieser, *Organic Chemistry* (Reinhold, New York, 3rd ed., 1956) p 176. Alternate intermediate: *p*-tolylsulfonylmethylnitrosamide ("Di-

azald" Aldrich Chemical Co.), *see* De Boer, Backer, *Org. Synth.* **coll. vol. IV,** 250 (1963).

Very toxic yellow gas. *Explosive!* Use safety screen. Insidious poison, a well-ventilated hood is absolutely necessary, avoid vapor. mp −145°; bp −23°. Undil liq and concd solns may explode violently, especially if impurities are present. Gaseous diazomethane may explode on heating to 100° or on rough glass surfaces. Ground glass apparatus and glass stirrers with glass sleeve bearings where grinding may occur, should not be used. Alkali metals also produce explosions with diazomethane. Sol in ether, dioxane. Such solns dec only slowly at low temps. Decompn is more rapid if alcohols or water are present. Copper powder causes active decompn with the evolution of nitrogen and the formation of insol white flakes of polymethylene $(CH_2)_x$. Solid calcium chloride or boiling stones have the same effect. This phenomenon appears to occur always during the action of diazomethane on solid substances.

Caution: Potential symptoms of overexposure are eye irritation; coughing, shortness of breath; headache; fatigue, flushing of skin, fever; chest pain, pulmonary edema, pneumonitis; asthma; direct contact with liquid may cause frostbite. *See NIOSH Pocket Guide to Chemical Hazards* (DHHS/NIOSH 97-140, 1997) p 92. May act as a respiratory sensitizer. *See Patty's Industrial Hygiene and Toxicology* **vol. 2A,** G. D. Clayton, F. E. Clayton, Eds. (Wiley-Interscience, New York, 3rd ed., 1981) pp 2784-2786.

USE: Powerful methylating agent for acidic compds such as carboxylic acids, phenols, enols. For syntheses with diazomethane *see* the reviews by Smith, *Chem. Rev.* **23,** 193 (1938); Eistert, *Z. Angew. Chem.* **54,** 99, 124 (1941) translated by Spangler in *Newer Methods of Preparative Organic Chemistry* (New York, 1948) p 513; J. S. Pizey, *Synthetic Reagents* **vol. 2** (John Wiley, New York, 1974) pp 65-142.

3002. 6-Diazo-5-oxo-L-norleucine. [157-03-9] DON. $C_6H_9N_3O_3$; mol wt 171.15. C 42.11%, H 5.30%, N 24.55%, O 28.04%. $N_2CHCOCH_2CH_2CH(NH_2)COOH$. Antitumor antibiotic produced by an unidentified species of *Streptomyces* from Peruvian soil: Dion *et al., J. Am. Chem. Soc.* **78,** 3075 (1956); Ehrlich *et al., Antibiot. Chemother.* **6,** 487 (1956). Several methods of synthesis: De Wald, Moore, *ibid.* **80,** 3941 (1958); *eidem,* **US 2965634** (1960 to Parke, Davis). *Review:* Pittillo, Hunt, *Antibiotics* **vol 1,** D. Gottlieb, P. D. Shaw, Eds. (Springer-Verlag, New York, 1967) pp 481-493.

Pale yellow crystals from dil ethanol, dec 145-155°. $[\alpha]_D^{26}$ +21° (c = 5.4). uv max (phosphate buffer): 244, 275 nm ($E_{1cm}^{1\%}$ 376, 683). Freely sol in water. The pH of aq solns should be maintained between 4.5 and 6.5. Also sol in aq solns of methanol, ethanol, acetone. Sparingly sol in absolute alcs.

3003. 5-Diazouracil. [2435-76-9] 5-Diazo-2,4(1*H*,3*H*)-pyrimidinedione; DU; 2,4-dioxo-5-diazopyrimidine; 5-diazo-2,4-dioxopyrimidine. $C_4H_2N_4O_2$; mol wt 138.08. C 34.79%, H 1.46%, N 40.58%, O 23.17%. Prepd by diazotization of 5-aminouracil: Johnson *et al., Ber.* **64,** 2629 (1931). Revised structure: Thurber, Townsend, *J. Heterocycl. Chem.* **9,** 629 (1972). Has significant activity against gram-positive and gram-negative bacteria *in vivo:* Hunt, Pittillo, *Appl. Microbiol.* **16,** 1792 (1968).

⟨chemical structure⟩

Crystals, conflagrates at 198°. The stout prisms obtained from ice water should be white, not yellow or red. Sensitive to light, temp and air. Best stored in evacuated, refrigerated ampuls. Acid reactions. IR spectrum: Band at 4.57 μ. Forms alcoholates, also a red monohydrate, $C_4H_4N_4O_3$, from which a potassium salt, $KC_4H_3N_4O_3$, is obtained which is slightly sol in water with neutral reaction.

USE: In cancer research.

3004. Diazoxide. [364-98-7] 7-Chloro-3-methyl-2*H*-1,2,4-benzothiadiazine 1,1-dioxide; 3-methyl-7-chloro-1,2,4-benzothiadiazine 1,1-dioxide; SRG-95213; Eudemine Injection; Proglicem;

Hyperstat; Hypertonalum; Mutabase; Proglycem. $C_8H_7ClN_2O_2S$; mol wt 230.67. C 41.66%, H 3.06%, Cl 15.37%, N 12.14%, O 13.87%, S 13.90%. Hypotensive agent that inhibits secretion of insulin from pancreatic beta cells. Prepn: A. A. Rubin *et al.*, *Science* **133**, 2067 (1961); J. G. Topliss *et al.*, **US 2986573**; *eidem*, **US 3345365** (1961, 1967 both to Schering); Raffa, Monzani, *Farmaco Ed. Sci.* **17**, 244 (1962). Crystal and molecular structure: G. Bandoli, M. Nicolini, *J. Cryst. Mol. Struct.* **7**, 229 (1978). Review of effect on insulin secretion: *Nutr. Rev.* **30**, 194-198 (1972); of pharmacology and efficacy in hypertension: J. Koch-Weser, *N. Engl. J. Med.* **294**, 1271-1274 (1976).

Crystals from dil alc, mp 330-331°. uv max (methanol): 268 nm (ε 11300). Sol in alcohol and alkaline solns. Insol in water.

THERAP CAT: Antihypoglycemic; antihypertensive.

3005. Dibekacin. [34493-98-6] *O*-3-Amino-3-deoxy-α-D-glucopyranosyl-(1 → 6)-*O*-[2,6-diamino-2,3,4,6-tetradeoxy-α-D-*erythro*-hexopyranosyl-(1 → 4)]-2-deoxy-D-streptamine; DKB; 3',4'-dideoxykanamycin B; debecacin. $C_{18}H_{37}N_5O_8$; mol wt 451.52. C 47.88%, H 8.26%, N 15.51%, O 28.35%. Semisynthetic analog of kanamycin, *q.v.*, effective against kanamycin-resistant bacteria. Prepn: Umezawa *et al.*, *J. Antibiot.* **24**, 485 (1971); *eidem*, *Bull. Chem. Soc. Jpn.* **45**, 3624 (1972); Umezawa *et al.*, **DE 2135191** (1972 to Microbiochem. Res. Found.). Improved synthesis: T. Yoneta *et al.*, *Bull. Chem. Soc. Jpn.* **52**, 1131 (1979). Antibacterial activity: A. G. Paradelis *et al.*, *Antimicrob. Agents Chemother.* **14**, 514 (1978). Metabolic studies: Shimizu, *Jpn. J. Antibiot.* **26**, 522 (1973). Toxicology: Koeda *et al.*, *ibid.* 221. Pharmacokinetics and acute toxicity: I. Komiya *et al.*, *J. Pharmacobio-Dyn.* **4**, 356 (1981). HPLC determn in serum: H. Kubo *et al.*, *Antimicrob. Agents Chemother.* **28**, 521 (1985). *Review:* P. Noone, *Drugs* **27**, 548-578 (1984).

$[\alpha]_D^{20}$ +132° (c = 0.65). LD_{50} in mice (mg/kg): 61.0-68.0 i.v., 373.0-380.0 i.m. (Komiya).

Sulfate. [58580-55-5] Débékacyl; Icacine; Orbicin; Panamicin; Panimycin; Tokocin. White or yellowish-white powder. Slightly bitter taste. Sol in water. Practically insol in ethanol, acetone, and other organic solvents.

THERAP CAT: Antibacterial.

3006. Dibenzalacetone. [538-58-9] 1,5-Diphenyl-1,4-pentadien-3-one; dibenzylidene acetone; distyryl ketone; $C_{17}H_{14}O$; mol wt 234.29. C 87.15%, H 6.02%, O 6.83%. $C_6H_5CH=CHCO-CH=CHC_6H_5$. Prepn from benzaldehyde + acetone: Conrad, Dolliver, *Org. Synth.* **12**, 22 (1939); Haslam, **US 2719863** (1955 to du Pont); Tokár *et al.*, *Acta Chim. Acad. Sci. Hung.* **19**, 83 (1959). Prepn of geometrical isomers: Dinwiddie *et al.*, *J. Org. Chem.* **27**, 327 (1962).

trans-trans-Form. Crystals from hot ethyl acetate, mp 110-111°. uv max: 330 nm (ε 34,300). Practically insol in water. Slightly sol in alc, ether; sol in acetone, chloroform.

cis-trans-Form. Light yellow needles from ethanol, mp 60°. uv max: 295 nm (ε 20,000).

cis-cis-Form. Yellow oil, $bp_{0.02}$ 130°. uv max: 287 nm (ε 11,000).

USE: In sun protection preparations.

3007. 1,2:5,6-Dibenzanthracene. [53-70-3] Dibenz[*a,h*]anthracene. $C_{22}H_{14}$; mol wt 278.35. C 94.93%, H 5.07%. From methyl dinaphthyl ketone: Clar, *Ber.* **62**, 350, 1378 (1929); Fieser, Dietz, *ibid.* 1827; Bachmann, *J. Org. Chem.* **1**, 347 (1937). Separation by chromatography: Winterstein, Schön, *Z. Physiol. Chem.* **230**, 146 (1934). Absorption spectrum: Mayneord, Roe, *Proc. Roy. Soc. London* **A152**, 299 (1935). *Review:* E. Clar, *Polycyclic Hydrocarbons* Vol. 1 & 2 (Academic Press, New York, 1964). Review of carcinogenic risk: *IARC Monographs* **3**, 178-196 (1973); of toxicology and human exposure: *Toxicological Profile for Polycyclic Aromatic Hydrocarbons* (PB95-264370, 1995) 487 pp.

Plates, leaflets from acetic acid. Crystals may be monoclinic or orthorhombic. Sublimes. mp 266°. Sol in petr ether, benzene, toluene, xylene, oils, other organic solvents; slightly sol in alcohol and ether. Insol in water.

Caution: This substance is reasonably anticipated to be a human carcinogen: *Report on Carcinogens, Eleventh Edition* (PB2005-104914, 2004) p III-220.

3008. Dibenzepin. [4498-32-2] 10-[2-(Dimethylamino)ethyl]-5,10-dihydro-5-methyl-11*H*-dibenzo[*b,e*][1,4]diazepin-11-one; 5-methyl-10β-dimethylaminoethyl-10,11-dihydro-11-oxodibenzo[*b,e*][1,4]diazepine; HF-1927. $C_{18}H_{21}N_3O$; mol wt 295.38. C 73.19%, H 7.17%, N 14.23%, O 5.42%. Prepn: F. Hunziker *et al.*, *Arzneim.-Forsch.* **13**, 324 (1963); **GB 961106**; J. Schmutz, F. Hunziker, **US 3312689** and **US 3419547** (1964, 1967, 1968 all to Wander). Metabolism: H. Lehner *et al.*, *Arzneim.-Forsch.* **17**, 185 (1967). Comprehensive description: A. Egli, W. R. Michaelis, *Anal. Profiles Drug Subs.* **9**, 181-206 (1980).

mp 116-117°. $bp_{0.01}$ 185°.

Hydrochloride. [315-80-0] Neodalit; Noveril. $C_{18}H_{21}N_3O\cdot$HCl; mol wt 331.84. Crystals, mp 238°. uv max (0.1*N* HCl): 204, 220 nm (log ε 4.530, 4.458). pKa 8.25. Sol in water, alcohol, chloroform. LD_{50} orally in mice: 215 mg/kg (Hunziker).

THERAP CAT: Antidepressant.

3009. Dibenzoylmethane. [120-46-7] 1,3-Diphenyl-1,3-propanedione; phenyl-α-hydroxystyryl ketone; ω-benzoylacetophenone; phenyl phenacyl ketone; γ-benzoylchalcone. $C_{15}H_{12}O_2$; mol wt 224.25. C 80.34%, H 5.39%, O 14.27%. $C_6H_5COCH_2-COC_6H_5$. Prepd by the action of sodium methylate on benzylideneacetophenone dibromide: Allen *et al.*, *Org. Synth.* **coll. vol. I** (2nd ed., 1941) p 205.

Orthorhombic plates, tablets from petr ether, mp 80°. bp_{18} 219-221°. 100 parts alc dissolve 4.43 parts at 19°. Sol in ether, chloroform, aq NaOH. Equilibrium mixtures in methanol, alcohol, and glacial acetic acid contain 96-98% of the enol form.

Monoxime. $C_{15}H_{13}NO_2$. Prepd by adding 4 mols hydroxylamine to 1 mol dibenzoylmethane in alcohol. Prisms from ether, mp 165°. Sparingly sol in cold alcohol.

3010. 2,3:6,7-Dibenzphenanthrene. [222-93-5] Pentaphene; dibenzo[*b,h*]phenanthrene; β,β'-dibenzphenanthrene; naphtho-2′,3′-1,2-anthracene. $C_{22}H_{14}$; mol wt 278.35. C 94.93%, H 5.07%. Prepn by pyrolysis of 1,2- or 1,4-di-*o*-toluylbenzene: Clar *et al.*, *Ber.* **62**, 947 (1924); Clar, John, *Ber.* **64**, 986 (1931); Winterstein, Schön, *Z. Physiol. Chem.* **230**, 146 (1934); from phthalic anhydride + *o*-tolylmagnesium bromide: Clar, Stewart, *J. Chem. Soc.* **1951**, 3215; from 2-benzoylbenzoic acid: Marsili, Isola, *Tetrahedron Lett.* **1965**, 3023; Franck, Zander, *Ber.* **99**, 396 (1966).

Yellowish-green needles or leaflets from xylene; mp 257°. Absorption max (alc): 423.5, 412, 399, 379, 356, 345, 329, 314.5, 302, 289.5, 257.5, 245 nm. Sol in benzene, xylene; sparingly sol in alcohol, ether. Solns exhibit blue fluorescence in daylight.

Dipicrate. $C_{22}H_{14}\cdot 2C_6H_3N_3O_7$. Orange needles, mp 184°.

3011. Dibenzylamine. [103-49-1] *N*-(Phenylmethyl)benzenemethanamine. $C_{14}H_{15}N$; mol wt 197.28. C 85.23%, H 7.66%, N 7.10%. $C_6H_5CH_2NHCH_2C_6H_5$. Prepd by the action of alcoholic ammonia on benzyl chloride: Mason, *J. Chem. Soc.* **63**, 1312 (1893).

Oil; ammoniacal odor. bp 300° with partial decompn. Practically insol in water; sol in alcohol or ether.

USE: Detection of cobalt, cyanate and iron.

3012. Dibenzyl Chlorophosphonate. [538-37-4] Phosphorochloridic acid bisphenylmethyl ester; benzyl phosphorochloridate; dibenzylchlorophosphate; DBPCl; dibenzylphosphoryl chloride. $C_{14}H_{14}ClO_3P$; mol wt 296.69. C 56.68%, H 4.76%, Cl 11.95%, O 16.18%, P 10.44%. Prepd by adding sulfuryl chloride to dibenzyl phosphite at 17-19° in CCl_4 diluent: Atherton *et al.*, *J. Chem. Soc.* **1948**, 1106; by adding chlorine to dibenzyl phosphite in CCl_4 at below 0°: Atherton *et al.*, US 2490573 (1949 to Hoffmann-La Roche).

Thick oil, dec on standing or distillation. Identified by its reaction with ammonia or amines to form corresponding dibenzyl aminophosphonates.

USE: In solns with inert solvents such as chloroform, carbon tetrachloride, benzene and ether for the phosphorylation of nucleosides and amino acids.

3013. Dibenzyl Disulfide. [150-60-7] Bis(phenylmethyl) disulfide; benzyl disulfide; α-(benzyldithio)toluene; di(phenylmethyl)disulfide. $C_{14}H_{14}S_2$; mol wt 246.39. C 68.25%, H 5.73%, S 26.03%. $C_6H_5CH_2SSCH_2C_6H_5$. Prepd by the reaction of benzyl chloride with sodium disulfide or polysulfide: Blanksma, *Rec. Trav. Chim.* **20**, 137 (1901); Moran, Crandall, US 2113092 (1938); Wojcik, US 2185007 (1939).

Leaflets from alcohol, mp 71-72°. Another modification mp 69-70°. Dec >270°. Practically insol in water. Sol in ether, benzene, hot methanol, hot ethanol.

USE: Antioxidant in rubber compounding, stabilizer for petr fractions, additive to silicone oils. The soly in oils is increased by the presence of benzyl alcohol.

3014. Dibenzyl Phosphite. [17176-77-1] Phosphonic acid bis(phenylmethyl) ester; dibenzyl hydrogen phosphite; benzyl phosphite. $C_{14}H_{15}O_3P$; mol wt 262.24. C 64.12%, H 5.77%, O 18.30%, P 11.81%. $(HO)P(OCH_2C_6H_5)_2$. Prepd by adding dropwise a mixture of dimethylaniline and benzyl alc to a soln of phosphorus trichloride in benzene: Atherton *et al.*, *J. Chem. Soc.* **1945**, 382; US 2490573 (1949 to Hoffmann-La Roche).

Liquid. mp 0 to 5°. $bp_{0.1}$ 160-164°; (decompn); $bp_{0.01}$ 110-120°; also reported as $bp_{0.001}$ 120-130°. n_D^{18} 1.5521.

USE: In preparation of *N*-phosphorylated amines.

3015. Diborane(6). [19287-45-7] Boroethane; diboron hexahydride. B_2H_6; mol wt 27.67. B 78.14%, H 21.86%. Review of methods of prepn: Adams in *Borax to Boranes, Advances Chem. Ser.* **No. 32** (American Chemical Society, 1961) pp 60-68. Review of structure and properties: Campell, Jr. in *Progress in Boron Chemistry* vol. 1, Steinberg, McCloskey, Eds. (Macmillan, New York, 1964) pp 167-184. Reviews of reaction chemistry: Schenker, *Angew. Chem.* **73**, 81-107 (1961); Long in *Adv. Inorg. Chem. Radiochem.* **16**, 201-296 (1974). Review of toxicity: *see* Decaborane(14). General reviews: Stock, *Hydrides of Boron and Silicon* (Cornell Univ. Press, Ithaca, 1933), *passim;* Siegel, Mack, *J. Chem. Educ.* **34**, 314-317 (1957); Major, *Chem. Eng. Prog.* **54**(3), 49-54 (1958); Mikhailov, *Usp. Khim.* **31**, 417-451 (1962); *Russian Chem. Rev.* (Eng. Ed.) **31**, 224-235 (1962); Adams, *Boron, Metallo-Boron Compounds and Boranes* (Interscience, New York, 1964) pp 555-605; Lipscomb, *Boron Hydrides* (Benjamin, New York, 1963) *passim;* Long, *Prog. Inorg. Chem.* **15**, 1-99 (1972); Greenwood in *Comprehensive Inorganic Chemistry* vol. **1**, J. C. Bailar, Jr., *et al.*, Eds. (Pergamon Press, Oxford, 1973) pp 763-783.

Colorless, flammable gas; repulsive, sickly-sweet odor. mp −165°; bp −92.5°. d^{-112} 0.447; $d^{-29.6}$ 0.33; $d^{15.0}$ 0.210. Critical temp 16.7°; critical press. 39.5 atm; Cp at 25°: 13.60 cal/mole/°C. Dec at red heat to B + H_2, at lower temps to H_2 and other boron hydrides. Spontaneous ignition temp in air about 40-50°; presence of contaminants may lower the temp limit so that ignition or detonation of diborane(6)-air mixtures may occur at or below room temp. Hydrolyzes in water to H_2 + H_3BO_3. Sol in CS_2. Reacts with NH_3 to form diborane diammoniate; reacts slowly with Br_2 and explosively with Cl_2 to form boron halides; reacts with hydrocarbons or organoboron compds to give alkyl- or arylboron compds; reacts with metal alkyls to form metal borohydrides; reacts with strong electron pair donors to form borane adduct compds.

Caution: Potential symptoms of overexposure are tightening of chest, precordial pain, shortness of breath, nonproductive cough and nausea; headache, lightheadedness, vertigo, chills, fever, fatigue, weakness, tremor and muscle fasciculation. *See* NIOSH *Pocket Guide to Chemical Hazards* (DHHS/NIOSH 97-140, 1997) p 92. *See also Patty's Industrial Hygiene and Toxicology* vol. **2B**, G. D. Clayton, F. E. Clayton, Eds. (Wiley-Interscience, New York, 3rd ed., 1981) pp 2987, 2990-2992.

USE: As catalyst for olefin polymerization; as rubber vulcanizer; as reducing agent; as flame-speed accelerator; in rocket propellants; in intermediate in prepn of the boron hydrides; in conversion of olefins to trialkylboranes and primary alcohols; as a doping gas.

3016. Diboron Tetrachloride. [13701-67-2] Tetrachlorodiborane(4); boron chloride. B_2Cl_4; mol wt 163.43. B 13.23%, Cl 86.77%. Prepd by passing gaseous boron trichloride through flow discharge between mercury or copper electrodes: Urry *et al.*, *J. Am. Chem. Soc.* **76**, 5293 (1954); Wartik *et al.*, *Inorg. Synth.* **10**, 118 (1967); by passing boron trichloride vapor over boron monoxide at 200°: McCloskey *et al.*, *J. Am. Chem. Soc.* **83**, 4750 (1961). Infrared and Raman spectra: Linevsky *et al.*, *J. Am. Chem. Soc.* **75**, 3287 (1953). Review of boron halides: Massey, *Adv. Inorg. Chem. Radiochem.* **10**, 1-152 (1967).

Liquid, ignites in air. mp −92.6°. bp_1 −63.5°; bp_{45} 0°; bp (calc) 65.5°.

3017. Dibromantin. [77-48-5] 1,3-Dibromo-5,5-dimethyl-2,4-imidazolidinedione; 1,3-dibromo-5,5-dimethylhydantoin; DBH; DBDMH. $C_5H_6Br_2N_2O_2$; mol wt 285.92. C 21.00%, H 2.12%, Br 55.89%, N 9.80%, O 11.19%. Stable, efficient, and economic bromination reagent; alternative to bromine or NBS, *q.q.v.* Prepn: O. O. Orazi, J. Meseri, *An. Asoc. Quim. Argent.* **38**, 5 (1950); I. Markish, O. Arrad, *Ind. Eng. Chem. Res.* **34**, 2125 (1995). Analytical applications in determn of iodide, iodine values, propylthiouracil, and selenium sulfide: M. Hilp, S. Senjuk, *J. Pharm. Biomed. Anal.* **25**, 363 (2001); *idem, ibid.* **28**, 81, 303, 337 (2002). Use in aromatic bromination reactions: H. Eguchi *et al.*, *Bull. Chem. Soc. Jpn.* **67**, 1918 (1994); X. Herault *et al.*, *Org. Prep. Proced. Int.* **27**, 652 (1995); C. Chassaing *et al.*, *Tetrahedron Lett.* **38**, 4415 (1997); in oxidation of thiols: A. Khazaei *et al.*, *Synthesis* **2004**, 2959.

Review of bromination chemistry: R. A. Reed, *Chem. Prod.* **23**, 299-302 (1960); A. Alam, *Synlett* **2005**, 2403-2404.

Yellow to buff colored solid, mp ~190° (dec).

USE: Brominating agent. Analytical reagent for determn of iodide and organic iodine, and for identification tests.

3018. 9,10-Dibromoanthracene. [523-27-3] $C_{14}H_8Br_2$; mol wt 336.02. C 50.04%, H 2.40%, Br 47.56%. Made by brominating a suspension of anthracene in CCl_4: Heilbron, Heaton, *Org. Synth.* **3**, 41 (1923).

Yellow needles from xylene, mp 226°. Sublimes. Absorption max: Conrad-Billroth, *Z. Phys. Chem. (Leipzig)* **33B**, 133 (1936). Insol in water; slightly sol in alcohol, ether, cold benzene; sol in hot benzene, hot toluene. Oxidation gives anthraquinone.

Addn compd with *sym*-trinitrobenzene. $C_{20}H_{11}Br_2N_3O_6$. mp 179°.

3019. *p*-Dibromobenzene. [106-37-6] $C_6H_4Br_2$; mol wt 235.90. C 30.55%, H 1.71%, Br 67.74%. Prepn from diazotized *p*-bromoaniline: Fry, Grote, *J. Am. Chem. Soc.* **48**, 710 (1926); by catalytic bromination of bromobenzene: Ferguson *et al.*, *ibid.* **76**, 1250 (1954).

Crystals, mp 87.31°. bp 220.40°. $d^{99.6}$ 0.9641. $n_D^{99.3}$ 1.5743. Practically insol in water; sol in about 70 parts alcohol; sol in benzene, chloroform; very sol in ether.

3020. Dibromochloropropane. [96-12-8] 1,2-Dibromo-3-chloropropane; 3-chloro-1,2-dibromopropane; DBCP; OS-1897; Fumazone; Nemafume; Nemagon. $C_3H_5Br_2Cl$; mol wt 236.33. C 15.25%, H 2.13%, Br 67.62%, Cl 15.00%. $ClCH_2CHBrCH_2Br$. Prepn: Darmstädter, *Ann.* **152**, 320 (1869). Activity: C. W. McBeth, G. B. Bergeson, *Plant Dis. Rep.* **39**, 223 (1955). Toxicity study: T. R. Torkelson *et al.*, *Toxicol. Appl. Pharmacol.* **3**, 545 (1961). Carcinogenicity studies: W. A. Olsen *et al.*, *J. Natl. Cancer Inst.* **51**, 1993 (1973); E. K. Weisburger, *Environ. Health Perspect.* **21**, 7 (1977). Mutagenicity study: H. S. Rosenkranz, *Bull. Environ. Contam. Toxicol.* **14**, 8 (1975). Review of toxicology and human exposure: *Toxicological Profile for 1,2-Dibromo-3-chloropropane* (PB93-110906, 1992) 164 pp.

Brown liq; pungent odor. bp 196°; bp_{16} 78°; $bp_{0.8}$ 21°. d^{14} 2.093. n_D^{14} 1.553. Vapor press at 21°: 0.8 mm Hg. Slightly sol in water; misc with oils, dichloropropane, isopropyl alcohol. LD_{50} in rats, mice (g/kg): 0.17, 0.26 orally (Torkelson).

Caution: Potential symptoms of overexposure are drowsiness; nausea, vomiting; irritation of eyes, nose, throat and skin; pulmonary edema; liver and kidney injury; sterility. *See NIOSH Pocket Guide to Chemical Hazards* (DHHS/NIOSH 97-140, 1997) p 92. *See also Clinical Toxicology of Commercial Products*, R. E. Gosselin *et al.*, Eds. (Williams & Wilkins, Baltimore, 5th ed., 1984) Section II, pp 167-168. This substance is reasonably anticipated to be a human carcinogen: *Report on Carcinogens, Eleventh Edition* (PB2005-104914, 2004) p III-81.

USE: Soil fumigant; nematocide; intermediate in organic synthesis.

3021. 1,2-Dibromo-2,4-dicyanobutane. [35691-65-7] 2-Bromo-2-(bromomethyl)pentanedinitrile; 2-bromo-2-(bromomethyl)glutaronitrile; Tektamer 38. $C_6H_6Br_2N_2$; mol wt 265.93. C 27.10%, H 2.27%, Br 60.09%, N 10.53%. Prepn: N. Grier, S. J. Lederer, **DE 2164723**; *eidem*, **US 3833731** (1972, 1974 to Merck & Co.).

Crystals from ethanol, mp 51.2-52.5°. Mildly pungent odor. Very sol in DMF, acetone, chloroform, ethyl acetate, benzene. Sol in methanol, ethanol, ether. Insol in water.

USE: Preservative for latex paints, adhesives, latex emulsions, dispersed pigments, joint cements, metal working fluids.

3022. 4′,5′-Dibromofluorescein. [596-03-2] 4′,5′-Dibromo-3′,6′-dihydroxyspiro[isobenzofuran-1(3*H*),9′-[9*H*]xanthen]-3-one; 4,5-dibromo-3,6-fluorandiol; D & C Orange No. 5; C.I. Solvent Red 72; C.I. 45370:1. $C_{20}H_{10}Br_2O_5$; mol wt 490.10. C 49.01%, H 2.06%, Br 32.61%, O 16.32%. Prepn from fluorescein, *q.v.*: A. Baeyer, *Ann.* **183**, 1 (1876); M. A. Phillips, *J. Chem. Soc.* **1932**, 724. Metabolism: J. M. Webb *et al.*, *J. Pharmacol. Exp. Ther.* **137**, 141 (1962). *See also: Colour Index* **vol. 4** (3rd ed., 1971) p 4425.

Red plates, mp 285°. Slightly sol in water (orange with faint yellow fluorescence); sol in ethanol (orange with greenish-yellow fluorescence) and in acetone (pink with yellow fluorescence). Red-yellow soln in conc H_2SO_4, turning yellow-brown with orange ppt on dilution. Absorption spectra: R. C. Gibbs, C. V. Shapiro, *J. Am. Chem. Soc.* **51**, 1769 (1929).

Disodium salt. C.I. Acid Orange 11. $C_{20}H_8Br_2Na_2O_5$.

USE: D & C Orange No. 5 permitted for use in lipsticks, mouthwashes and dentifrices: *Fed. Regist.* **47**, 49632 (1982).

3023. 3,5-Dibromo-4-hydroxybenzenesulfonic Acid. [4232-99-9] 2,6-Dibromophenol-4-sulfonic acid; *p*-hydroxy-3,5-dibromobenzenesulfonic acid. $C_6H_4Br_2O_4S$; mol wt 331.97. C 21.71%, H 1.21%, Br 48.14%, O 19.28%, S 9.66%. Prepn: Senhofer, *Ann.* **156**, 103 (1870); Armstrong, Brown, *J. Chem. Soc.* **25**, 858 (1872). Prepn of the sodium salt: Cannell, *J. Am. Chem. Soc.* **79**, 2927 (1957).

Rectangular platelets. Freely sol in water, alcohol; less sol in ether.

Sodium salt dihydrate. Dibromol. $C_6H_3Br_2NaO_4S.2H_2O$; mol wt 389.98. Needles. Freely sol in hot water, less sol in cold water.

THERAP CAT: Disinfectant.

3024. Dibromopropamidine. [496-00-4] 4,4′-[1,3-Propanediylbis(oxy)]bis(3-bromobenzenecarboximidamide); 4,4′-(trimethylenedioxy)bis(3-bromobenzamidine); 2′,2″-dibromo-4′,4″-diamidino-1,3-diphenoxypropane. $C_{17}H_{18}Br_2N_4O_2$; mol wt 470.16. C 43.43%, H 3.86%, Br 33.99%, N 11.92%, O 6.81%. Prepn: S. S. Berg, G. Newbery, **GB 598911** (1948 to May & Baker); *eidem, J. Chem. Soc.* **1949**, 642. Antibacterial activity: R. Wien *et al.*,

Lancet **254,** 711 (1948); A. D. Russell, J. R. Furr, *Int. J. Pharm.* **34,** 115 (1986). Mode of action: W. Woodside, *Microbios* **8,** 23 (1973). Clinical use in *Acanthamoeba* keratitis: J. J. Wiens, W. B. Jackson, *Can. J. Ophthalmol.* **23,** 107 (1988). HPLC determn in cosmetics: B. Wyhowski de Bukanski, M. O. Masse, *Int. J. Cosmet. Sci.* **6,** 283 (1984).

Isethionate. [614-87-9] Brolene Ointment; Brulidine. C_{21}-$H_{30}Br_2N_4O_{10}S_2$; mol wt 722.42. Prismatic needles from ethanol, mp 226°. Freely sol in water. One gram dissolves in 2 ml of water at 20°, in 60 g of 95% alcohol at 20°. Sol in glycerol. Practically insol in ether, chloroform, fixed oils, liquid petrolatum. Aq solns are very slightly acidic. Solns may be sterilized by heating at 100° for 30 min, but they should not be stored for more than a few days, and then only in neutral glass containers since some hydrolysis occurs with the formation of sparingly sol urea derivs. *Incompat.* with chlorides, sulfates, and many organic anions, all of which form sparingly sol salts.

USE: Preservative in cosmetics.

THERAP CAT: Antiseptic; antiamebic.

THERAP CAT (VET): Antiseptic, antimicrobial.

3025. 2,3-Dibromopropene. [513-31-5] 2,3-Dibromopropylene; 2-bromoallyl bromide; α-bromoallyl bromide; α-epidibromohydrin. $C_3H_4Br_2$; mol wt 199.87. C 18.03%, H 2.02%, Br 79.96%. $BrCH_2CBr\!=\!CH_2$. Prepd by the action of sodium hydroxide on 1,2,3-tribromopropane: Lespieau, Bourguel, *Org. Synth.* **5,** 49 (1925); *cf.* Tapley, Giesy, *J. Am. Pharm. Assoc.* **15,** 173 (1926).

Liquid. d_4^{20} 1.9336. bp_{760} 140-143°; bp_{75} 75-76°; bp_{18} 42-43°. n_D^{20} 1.5157. May be distilled under atmospheric pressure with very slight decompn, but becomes highly colored on standing in glass-stoppered bottle.

3026. 2,6-Dibromoquinone-4-chlorimide. [537-45-1] 2,6-Dibromo-4-(chloroimino)-2,5-cyclohexadien-1-one; 2,6-dibromo-*N*-chloro-*p*-benzoquinoneimine; 2,6-dibromo-*N*-chloroquinonimine; BQC reagent. $C_6H_2Br_2ClNO$; mol wt 299.35. C 24.07%, H 0.67%, Br 53.39%, Cl 11.84%, N 4.68%, O 5.34%. Prepn: Hartman *et al., Org. Synth.* **coll. vol. II,** 175 (1943).

Yellow prisms from alc or glacial acetic acid, mp 83°. Sol in about 17,000 parts water; moderately sol in hot alc, hot glacial acetic acid. Gives a blue color with alk phenol soln.

USE: As a reagent for phenol and phosphatases: Ljunggren, *Proc. 13th Int. Dairy Congr.* **3,** 1319 (1953).

3027. 3,5-Dibromosalicylaldehyde. [90-59-5] 3,5-Dibromo-2-hydroxybenzaldehyde. $C_7H_4Br_2O_2$; mol wt 279.91. C 30.04%, H 1.44%, Br 57.09%, O 11.43%. Prepd by bromination of salicylaldehyde in glacial acetic acid with cooling: Wentworth, Brady, *J. Chem. Soc.* **117,** 1043 (1920); Brewster, *J. Am. Chem. Soc.* **46,** 2464 (1924); by bromination in the presence of sodium acetate in glacial acetic acid at 50°: Lindemann, Forth, *Ann.* **435,** 223 (1924).

Pale yellow prisms, mp 86°. Sublimes forming leaflets and needles. Volatile with steam. Sparingly sol in water. Aq solns are yellow. Readily sol in ether, benzene, chloroform, hot petr ether, alcohol, glacial acetic acid.

3028. 3,5-Dibromosalicylic Acid. [3147-55-5] 3,5-Dibromo-2-hydroxybenzoic acid. $C_7H_4Br_2O_3$; mol wt 295.91. C 28.41%, H 1.36%, Br 54.01%, O 16.22%. Prepd from salicylic acid and Br_2: Earle, Jackson, *J. Am. Chem. Soc.* **28,** 111 (1906); Robertson, *J. Chem. Soc.* **82,** 1481 (1902); and HOBr: Leulier, Pinet, *Bull. Soc. Chim. Fr.* [4] **41,** 1362 (1927).

Needles, mp 223°. Sparingly sol in H_2O; sol in alc, ether.

3029. 2,3-Dibromosuccinic Acid. [526-78-3] 2,3-Dibromobutanedioic acid; α,α′-dibromosuccinic acid; *sym*-dibromosuccinic acid. $C_4H_4Br_2O_4$; mol wt 275.88. C 17.41%, H 1.46%, Br 57.93%, O 23.20%. Prepn of *dl*-form by bromination of maleic acid: McKenzie, *J. Chem. Soc.* **101,** 1196 (1912); Young *et al., J. Am. Chem. Soc.* **61,** 1640 (1939); of *meso*-form by bromination of fumaric acid: *eidem, ibid.;* Rhinesmith, *Org. Synth.* **coll. vol. II,** 177 (1943). Resolution of *dl*-form: McKenzie, *loc. cit.*

dl-**Form.** *threo*-2,3-Dibromosuccinic acid. Crystals, mp 167°. Very sol in cold water.

d-**Form.** Crystalline powder from ethyl acetate + CCl_4, mp 157-158°. $[\alpha]_D^{18}$ +64.4° (c = 5 in water), +135.8° (c = 5 in alc), +147.8° (c = 5 in ethyl acetate).

l-**Form.** Needles from benzene, decomp 157-158°. $[\alpha]_D^{13}$ −148.0° (c = 5.8 in ethyl acetate). Very sol in cold water; sol in ethyl acetate, acetone, methanol, ethanol; sparingly sol in chloroform, petr ether, CCl_4.

meso-**Form.** *erythro*-2,3-Dibromosuccinic acid. Cryst from water, dec 255-256°, also reported as mp 270-273°. Sol in 50 parts cold water, more sol in hot water; sol in alcohol, ether; sparingly sol in chloroform.

3030. 3,5-Dibromo-L-tyrosine. [300-38-9] β-(3,5-dibromo-4-hydroxyphenyl)alanine; Biotiren; Bromotiren. $C_9H_9Br_2$-NO_3; mol wt 338.98. C 31.89%, H 2.68%, Br 47.14%, N 4.13%, O 14.16%. Obtained upon saponification of gorgonin, a substance isolated from coral *(Primnoa lepadifera)* stems: Mörner, *Z. Physiol. Chem.* **88,** 139, 152 (1913). Prepd by the action of bromine vapor on tyrosine: Gorup-Besanez, *Ann.* **125,** 281 (1863). By treating tyrosine in aq HBr with Br: Aloy, Rabaut, *Bull. Soc. Chim. Fr.* [4] **3,** 392 (1908); Zeynek, *Z. Physiol. Chem.* **114,** 275 (1921). Clinical evaluation in thyroid function: A. Isidori, *Int. J. Clin. Pharmacol. Biopharm.* **16,** 180 (1978).

L-Form dihydrate. Efflorescent needles, plates (orthorhombic) from water. When anhydr, dec 245°. $[\alpha]_D^{20}$ +1.3° (c = 5 in 4% HCl). pK_1 2.17; pK_2 6.45; pK_3 7.60. One gram dissolves in 250 ml water at 25°, in 30 ml at boiling temp. Slightly sol in alcohol; insol in ether. Freely sol in alkalies and in dil mineral acids. Forms HBr and HCl salts; stable in boiling water.

DL-Form. Efflorescent prisms, platelets from water probably contg 1 mol water of crystn. Dec at about 245°. Aq solns are acid to litmus. Behaves as a monobasic acid when titrated with

NaOH and phenolphthalein. One gram dissolves in about 590 ml water at 20°.

THERAP CAT: Thyroid inhibitor.

3031. Dibucaine. [85-79-0] 2-Butoxy-*N*-[2-(diethylamino)-ethyl]-4-quinolinecarboxamide; 2-butoxy-*N*-(2-diethylaminoethyl)-cinchoninamide; cinchocaine. $C_{20}H_{29}N_3O_2$; mol wt 343.46. C 69.94%, H 8.51%, N 12.23%, O 9.32%. Prepn: Miescher, **US 1825623** (1931 to Ciba). Comprehensive description: G. R. Padmanabhan, *Anal. Profiles Drug Subs.* **12**, 105-134 (1983). Spectrometric determn in pharmaceutical formulations: N. T. Abdel-Ghani *et al.*, *Farmaco* **60**, 419 (2005).

White to off-white powder; slight characteristic odor. mp 64°.
Hydrochloride. [61-12-1] Nupercainal. $C_{20}H_{29}N_3O_2$.HCl; mol wt 379.92. Hygroscopic crystals. Dec 90-98°. uv max (1*N* HCl): 247, 320 nm (ε 24700, 8810). Sol in 0.5 part water; freely sol in alcohol, acetone, chloroform; slightly sol in benzene, ethyl acetate and toluene (on warming); insol in ether and in oils. The aq soln, about 1 in 20, is faintly alkaline to litmus.

THERAP CAT: Anesthetic (local).

3032. *n*-Dibutylamine. [111-92-2] *N*-Butyl-1-butanamine. $C_8H_{19}N$; mol wt 129.24. C 74.35%, H 14.82%, N 10.84%. (C_4-$H_9)_2$NH. Prepn from butyl bromide and ammonia with separation of the mono-, di-, and tributylamines formed: Werner, *J. Chem. Soc.* **115**, 1010 (1919). Manuf: Engel, Hoog, **US 2574693** (1951 to Shell); Davies *et al.*, **US 2609394** (1952 to I.C.I.); Lemon, Myerly, **US 3022349** (1962 to Union Carbide); Brois, Rutkowski, **US 3147310** (1964 to Esso). Toxicity study: H. F. Smyth *et al.*, *Arch. Ind. Hyg. Occup. Med.* **10**, 61 (1954).
Liquid, bp 159-160°. mp −60° to −59°. d_4^{20} 0.7601. n_D^{20} 1.4177. Flash pt, open cup: 135°F (57°C). Sol in water, alc. LD_{50} orally in rats: 550 mg/kg (Smyth).

3033. Di-*tert*-butyl Ether. [6163-66-2] 2,2′-Oxybis[2-methylpropane]. $C_8H_{18}O$; mol wt 130.23. C 73.78%, H 13.93%, O 12.29%. $[(CH_3)_3C]_2O$. Prepn: R. J. Moore, G. J. O'Donnell, **GB 652809** (1951 to Bataafsche Petrol.); *C.A.* **46**, 1023d (1952). Synthesis from *t*-butyl chloride and silver carbonate: J. Erickson, W. M. Ashton, *J. Am. Chem. Soc.* **63**, 1769 (1941); from *t*-butyl perbenzoates and Grignard reagents: S. O. Lawesson, N. C. Yang, *ibid.* **81**, 4230 (1959); by alkylation of *t*-butyl alcohol with trimethylcarbenium fluoroantimonate: G. A. Olah *et al.*, *Synthesis* **1975**, 315; from lithium *tert*-butoxide with aromatic sulfonyl chlorides: H. Masada *et al.*, *Tetrahedron Lett.* **1979**, 1315.
Clear liquid with camphorous odor. bp 106.5-107.0°. n_D^{20} 1.3949; d_4^{20} 0.7658. Decomposes in the presence of acids.

USE: Gasoline additive.

3034. Di-*tert*-butyl Malonate. [541-16-2] Propanedioic acid bis(1,1-dimethylethyl) ester; malonic acid di-*tert*-butyl ester. $C_{11}H_{20}O_4$; mol wt 216.27. C 61.09%, H 9.32%, O 29.59%. $(CH_3)_3COOCCH_2COOC(CH_3)_3$. Prepd from malonic acid, liq isobutylene and sulfuric acid: McCloskey *et al.*, *Org. Synth.* **34**, 26 (1954).
Liquid. mp −6.1 to −5.9°. bp_{31} 112-115°; bp_{10} 93°; bp_1 65-67°. n_D^{20} 1.4184; $n_D^{24.2}$ 1.4161; n_D^{25} 1.4158-1.4161.

USE: In the prepn of ketones.

3035. Dibutyl Phthalate. [84-74-2] 1,2-Benzenedicarboxylic acid dibutyl ester; *n*-butyl phthalate; phthalic acid dibutyl ester; DBP. $C_{16}H_{22}O_4$; mol wt 278.34. C 69.04%, H 7.97%, O 22.99%. Prepn: Farrar, Wienkauff, *Chem. Ind. (London)* **1962**, 2144. Manuf: Bruno, **US 2628249** (1953 to Pittsburgh Coke & Chemical). Toxicity study: C. C. Smith, *Arch. Ind. Hyg. Occup. Med.* **7**, 310 (1953). Review of toxicology and human exposure: *Toxico-*

logical Profile for Di-n-butyl phthalate (PB2001-109104, 2001) 225 pp.

Oily liquid. bp 340°. d^{20} 1.0459 and 1.0465, Kemppinen, Gokeen, *J. Phys. Chem.* **60**, 126 (1956). n_D^{20} 1.4900. Flash pt, open cup: 340°F (171°C). Sol in about 2500 parts water; very sol in alcohol, ether, acetone, benzene.
Caution: Potential symptoms of overexposure are irritation of eyes, upper respiratory system and stomach. *See NIOSH Pocket Guide to Chemical Hazards* (DHHS/NIOSH 97-140, 1997) p 94.

USE: Plasticizer; solvent for oil-soluble dyes, insecticides and other organics; antifoam agent; textile fiber lubricant; fragrance fixative; insect repellent.

3036. 2,6-Di-*tert*-butylpyridine. [585-48-8] 2,6-Bis(1,1-dimethylethyl)pyridine. $C_{13}H_{21}N$; mol wt 191.31. C 81.62%, H 11.06%, N 7.32%. Prepd by reacting *tert*-butyllithium with 2-*tert*-butylpyridine: Brown, Kanner, *J. Am. Chem. Soc.* **75**, 3865 (1953); **US 2780626** (1957 to Research Corp.).

Liquid, mp 2.2°. bp_{23} 100-101°. n_D^{20} 1.5733. pKa 3.58. The base neutralizes HCl but does not react with alkyl halides or boron trifluoride. Undergoes nuclear sulfonation with sulfur trioxide forming a sulfonic acid, $C_{13}H_{21}NSO_3$, mp 310° (decompn).
Chloroaurate. $C_{13}H_{22}NAuCl_4$. mp 184.2-184.5°.

USE: Has been proposed as an additive for lubricating oil, gasoline and for stabilizing Cl-containing polymers.

3037. Di-*tert*-butyl Succinate. [926-26-1] Butanedioic acid bis(1,1-dimethylethyl) ester; succinic acid di-*tert*-butyl ester. C_{12}-$H_{22}O_4$; mol wt 230.30. C 62.58%, H 9.63%, O 27.79%. $(CH_3)_3$-$COOCCH_2CH_2COOC(CH_3)_3$. Prepd from succinic acid, liq isobutylene, and sulfuric acid in dioxane: McCloskey *et al.*, *Org. Synth.* **coll. vol. IV**, 263 (1963).
Liquid, mp 36-37°. bp_9 109-110°; bp_7 105-107°.

USE: In Stobbe condensation of ketones.

3038. Dibutyltin Dilaurate. [77-58-7] Dibutylbis[(1-oxododecyl)oxy]stannane; dibutylbis(lauroyloxy)tin; Butynorate; Davainex; Tinostat. $C_{32}H_{64}O_4Sn$; mol wt 631.56. C 60.86%, H 10.21%, O 10.13%, Sn 18.80%. $(C_4H_9)_2Sn[OOC(CH_2)_{10}CH_3]_2$. Prepn: Sheverdina *et al.*, *Khim. Prom.* **1962** (10), 707, *C.A.* **59**, 8776f (1963); **FR 1320473** (1963 to Noury & van der Lande), *C.A.* **59**, 8789b (1963), corresp to **GB 975369**. Compd claimed but not described: Eberly, **US 2560034** (1951 to Firestone).
Soft crystals or yellow liq, mp 22-24° (Sheverdina). n_D^{20} 1.4683, (**FR 1320473**). Practically insol in water, methanol. Soluble in petr ether, benzene, acetone, carbon tetrachloride, ether, organic esters.

USE: Stabilizer for polyvinyl chloride resins. Catalyst for curing certain silicones.

THERAP CAT (VET): Anthelmintic (vs. chicken tapeworms).

3039. Di-*tert*-butyl Tricarbonate. [24424-95-1] Tricarbonic acid bis(1,1-dimethylethyl)ester. $C_{11}H_{18}O_7$; mol wt 262.26. C 50.38%, H 6.92%, O 42.70%. Mild reagent which converts most primary amines quantitatively into their corresponding isocyanate. Prepn: C. S. Dean, D. S. Tarbell, *Chem. Commun.* **1969**, 728; B. M. Pope *et al.*, *Org. Synth.* **57**, 45 (1977). Kinetic study: *eidem, J. Org. Chem.* **43**, 2410 (1978). Use in prepn of isocyanates: H. W. I. Peerlings, E. W. Meijer, *Tetrahedron Lett.* **40**, 1021 (1999); of polyurethanes: R. V. Versteegen *et al.*, *Angew. Chem. Int. Ed.* **38**, 2917 (1999).

(H₃C)₃CO—C(=O)—O—C(=O)—O—C(=O)—OC(CH₃)₃

Crystalline solid, mp 64-65° (Dean); also reported as colorless prisms, mp 62-63° (Pope).

USE: In synthesis of polyurethanes.

3040. Dicamba. [1918-00-9] 3,6-Dichloro-2-methoxy-benzoic acid; 3,6-dichloro-*o*-anisic acid; 2-methoxy-3,6-dichloro-benzoic acid; dianat; Velsicol 58-CS-11; Banvel; Clarity. C_8H_6-Cl_2O_3; mol wt 221.04. C 43.47%, H 2.74%, Cl 32.08%, O 21.71%. Sometimes misnamed *methoxydichlorobenzoate*. Prepn: S. B. Richter, **US 3013054** (1961 to Velsicol). Metabolism: D. D. Oehler, G. W. Ivie, *J. Agric. Food Chem.* **28**, 685 (1980). Toxicity: Bailey, White, *Residue Rev.* **10**, 97 (1965).

Crystals from pentane, mp 114-116°. Vapor pressure at 100°: 3.75×10^{-3} mm Hg. Sol in ethanol and acetone. Very slightly sol in water. LD_{50} orally in rats: 1040 mg/kg (Bailey, White).

USE: Herbicide.

3041. Dicentrine. [517-66-8] 6,7,7a,8-Tetrahydro-10,11-di-methoxy-7-methyl-5*H*-benzo[*g*]-1,3-benzodioxolo[6,5,4-*de*]quino-line; 9,10-dimethoxy-1,2-(methylenedioxy)aporphine; 1,2-methyl-enedioxy-9,10-dimethoxyaporphine. $C_{20}H_{21}NO_4$; mol wt 339.39. C 70.78%, H 6.24%, N 4.13%, O 18.86%. *d*-Form prevalent in nature. Found in *Dicentra pusilla* Sieb. & Zucc., *Fumariaceae* and several other *Dicentra* species. Related to actinodaphnine, and laurotetanine, *q.q.v.* Isoln: Y. Asahina, *Arch. Pharm.* **247**, 201 (1909). Isoln of *l*-form from *Duguetia* A. St. Hil., *Annonaceae*: Casagrande, Ferrari, *Farmaco Ed. Sci.* **25**, 442 (1970). Synthesis of *dl*-form: Haworth *et al.*, *J. Chem. Soc.* **127**, 2018 (1925); Cava *et al.*, *Tetrahedron* **29**, 2245 (1973). Resolution of isomers: Haworth *et al.*, *J. Chem. Soc.* **129**, 29 (1926).

d-Dicentrine

dl-Form. Prisms from methanol, mp 178-179°. Freely sol in chloroform, ethyl acetate, acetone, benzene, hot alcohol. Moderately sol in ether, cold alcohol. Absorption max: Girardet, *J. Chem. Soc.* **1931**, 2630.

d-Form. Long prisms from ether. mp 169°. $[\alpha]_D^{17}$ +64.1° (c = 1.433 in chloroform). Freely sol in alcohol, ethyl acetate, benzene.

l-Form. Long prisms from ether. mp 169°. $[\alpha]_D^{17}$ −63.5° (c = 1.70 in chloroform).

dl-Hydrochloride. $C_{20}H_{21}NO_4 \cdot HCl$. Small needles from water, dec 263-265°.

dl-Methiodide monohydrate. $C_{20}H_{21}NO_4 \cdot CH_3I \cdot H_2O$. Plates, mp 228-229°.

3042. Dichlobenil. [1194-65-6] 2,6-Dichlorobenzonitrile; H-133; Niagara 5006; Casoron. $C_7H_3Cl_2N$; mol wt 172.01. C 48.88%, H 1.76%, Cl 41.22%, N 8.14%. Prepn: Reich, *Bull. Soc. Chim. Fr.* [4] **21**, 217 (1917); Norris, Klemka, *J. Am. Chem. Soc.* **62**, 1432 (1940); Chang *et al.*, *C.A.* **53**, 6134d (1959); Koopman, *Rec. Trav. Chim.* **80**, 1075 (1961); Hackmann, ten Haken **GB 861899**; Higson, **GB 862937** (both 1961 to Shell). Use as herbicide: Koopman, Daams, **US 3027248** (1962 to N. A. Phillips). Fate in crops, soil and animals: Beynon, Wright, *Residue Rev.* **43**, 23 (1972);

Veroop, *ibid.* 55. Toxicity data: G. W. Bailey, J. L. White, *ibid.* **10**, 97 (1965).

Crystals from petr ether, mp 144-145°. Soly in water at 25°: 25 ppm; at 20°: 18 ppm. Vapor pressure at 20°: 3×10^{-6} mm Hg; at 25°: 5×10^{-4} mm. Absorption spectrum see Koopman, *loc. cit.* LD_{50} in rats, mice (mg/kg): 2710, 6800 orally (Bailey, White).

USE: Herbicide.

3043. Dichlofenthion. [97-17-6] Phosphorothioic acid *O*-2,4-dichlorophenyl *O,O*-diethyl ester; *O*-2,4-dichlorophenyl *O,O*-diethyl phosphorothioate; *O,O*-diethyl *O*-2,4-dichlorophenyl phos-phorothioate; VC-13 Nemacide. $C_{10}H_{13}Cl_2O_3PS$; mol wt 315.15. C 38.11%, H 4.16%, Cl 22.50%, O 15.23%, P 9.83%, S 10.17%. Cholinesterase inhibitor. Prepd from *O,O*-diethyl phosphoro-chloridothioate, 2,4-dichlorophenol and NaOH: Smithey, Jr., **US 3004054** (1960 to Virginia-Carolina Chemical). Toxicity data: T. B. Gaines, R. E. Linder, *Fundam. Appl. Toxicol.* **7**, 299 (1986).

Liquid, $bp_{0.1}$ 164-169°. n_D^{25} 1.5291. d_{20} 1.300. Slightly sol in water; miscible with most organic solvents. LD_{50} in male, female rats (mg/kg): 185, 172 orally; 576, 355 dermally (Gaines, Linder).

USE: Nematocide, insecticide.

3044. Dichlofluanid. [1085-98-9] 1,1-Dichloro-*N*-[(di-methylamino)sulfonyl]-1-fluoro-*N*-phenylmethanesulfenamide; *N*-[(dichlorofluoromethyl)thio]-*N* ',*N* '-dimethyl-*N*-phenylsulfamide; Bayer 47531; KUE 13032c; Elvaron; Euparen(e). $C_9H_{11}Cl_2FN_2$-O_2S_2; mol wt 333.23. C 32.44%, H 3.33%, Cl 21.28%, F 5.70%, N 8.41%, O 9.60%, S 19.24%. Prepn: E. Klauke *et al.*, **BE 609868**; *eidem*, **US 3285929** and **US 3341403** (1962, 1966, 1967 to Bayer). Antifungal activity: E. Kuhle *et al.*, *Angew. Chem.* **76**, 807 (1964); F. Grewe, *Phytiatr.-Phytopharm.* **17**, 47 (1968). UV degradation: T. Clark, D. Watkins, *Pestic. Sci.* **9**, 225 (1978). GC determn in plants and beverages: R. Brennecke, *Pflanzenschutz-Nachr.* **41**, 137 (1988).

White powder, mp 105.0-105.6°. Vapor press at 20°: 1×10^{-6} mm Hg. Insol in water. Sol in acetone, methanol, xylene. Soly at 20° (g/1000 ml): water 0.0013; dichloromethane >200; *n*-hexane 2-5; 2-propanol 10-20; toluene 100-200. Light sensitive; decomp by strong alkaline media. LD_{50} in rats, guinea pigs, rabbits (mg/kg): 1.000 orally in all species (Grewe).

USE: Fungicide.

3045. Dichlone. [117-80-6] 2,3-Dichloro-1,4-naphthalene-dione; 2,3-dichloro-1,4-naphthoquinone; USR-604; Phygon; Phy-gon Paste; Phygon XL. $C_{10}H_4Cl_2O_2$; mol wt 227.04. C 52.90%, H 1.78%, Cl 31.23%, O 14.09%. Prepd by chlorination of 1,4-naphthoquinone: Bertheim, *Ber.* **34**, 1554 (1901); Brass, Köhler, *Ber.* **55**, 2554 (1922); Sjöstrand, **US 2975196** (1961 to Svenska Oljeslageri Aktiebolaget); by oxidation of 2,3-dichloro-5,8-dihy-dro-1,4-naphthohydroquinone: Gaertner, **US 2750427** (1956 to Monsanto); by oxidation of 2,3-dichloro-*p*-benzoquinone: Grinev *et al.*, *Zh. Obshch. Khim.* **29**, 90 (1959). Toxicity data: G. W.

Bailey, J. L. White, *Residue Rev.* **10**, 97 (1965). *Review:* Ter Horst, *Ind. Eng. Chem.* **35**, 1255 (1943).

Golden yellow needles or leaflets from alc, mp 193°. Sublimes. Practically insol in water (soly about 1 part in 10 million parts H_2O). Soly in xylene and *o*-dichlorobenzene about 4%. Moderately sol in acetone, ether, benzene, dioxane. LD_{50} orally in rats: 1300 mg/kg (Bailey, White).

Caution: Irritating to skin, mucous membranes; CNS depressant: *Clinical Toxicology of Commercial Products*, R. E. Gosselin *et al.*, Eds. (Williams & Wilkins, Baltimore, 5th ed., 1984) Section II, p 318.

USE: Fungicide for agriculture and textiles; herbicide.

3046. Dichloralphenazone. [480-30-8] 1,2-Dihydro-1,5-dimethyl-2-phenyl-3*H*-pyrazol-3-one compd with 2,2,2-trichloro-1,1-ethanediol(1:2); dichloralantipyrine; Bonadorm; Dormwell; Welldorm. $C_{15}H_{18}Cl_6N_2O_5$; mol wt 519.03. C 34.71%, H 3.50%, Cl 40.98%, N 5.40%, O 15.41%. $[CCl_3CH(OH)_2]_2.C_{11}H_{12}N_2O$. Prepn: Pfeiffer, Seidel, *Z. Physiol. Chem.* **178**, 97 (1928). GLC determn in pharmaceutical formulation: F. M. Plakogiannis, A. M. Saad, *J. Pharm. Sci.* **66**, 604 (1977). Clinical trial of combination with isometheptene and acetaminophen, *q.q.v.*, in treatment of migraine: S. Diamond, *Headache* **15**, 282 (1976).

Small prismatic needles from water, mp 68°.

Note: This is a controlled substance (depressant): **21 CFR,** 1308.14.

THERAP CAT: Sedative, hypnotic.

3047. Dichloramine T. [473-34-7] *N,N*-Dichloro-4-methylbenzenesulfonamide; *N,N*-dichloro-*p*-toluenesulfonamide; *p*-toluenesulfonic acid dichloramide. $C_7H_7Cl_2NO_2S$; mol wt 240.11. C 35.02%, H 2.94%, Cl 29.53%, N 5.83%, O 13.33%, S 13.35%. Prepn from *p*-toluenesulfonic acid: Soper, *J. Chem. Soc.* **125**, 1899 (1924); van Andel, **US 2495489** (1950 to Shell).

Prisms from chloroform + petr ether, mp 83°. Strong chlorine odor; dec on exposure to air with loss of chlorine. mp about 80°. Almost insol in water, dec by alcohol when warmed; one gram dissolves in about 1 ml benzene, 1 ml chloroform, 2.5 ml carbon tetrachloride; sol in eucalyptol, chlorinated paraffin hydrocarbons, glacial acetic acid; slightly sol in petr ether. *Keep well closed and protected from light.*

USE: Germicide.

THERAP CAT: Antibacterial.

3048. Dichlorisone. [7008-26-6] (11β)-9,11-Dichloro-17,21-dihydroxypregna-1,4-diene-3,20-dione; 9α,11β-dichloro-1,4-pregnadiene-17α,21-diol-3,20-dione; 9α,11β-dichloro analog of prednisolone; Diloderm; Disoderm. $C_{21}H_{26}Cl_2O_4$; mol wt 413.33. C 61.02%, H 6.34%, Cl 17.15%, O 15.48%. Prepn: Robinson *et al.*, *J. Am. Chem. Soc.* **81**, 2191 (1959); Gould *et al.*, **US 2894963** (1959 to Schering).

Crystals from acetone, dec 238-241°. $[\alpha]_D^{20}$ +134° (pyridine). uv max (methanol): 237 nm (ε 15400).

21-Acetate. [79-61-8] Astroderm. $C_{23}H_{28}Cl_2O_5$; mol wt 455.37. Crystals from acetone, dec 246-253°. $[\alpha]_D^{25}$ +162° (dioxane). uv max (methanol): 237 nm (ε 15000).

THERAP CAT: Antipruritic (topical).

3049. Dichlormid. [37764-25-3] 2,2-Dichloro-*N,N*-di-2-propenylacetamide; *N,N*-diallyl-2,2-dichloroacetamide; R-25788. $C_8H_{11}Cl_2NO$; mol wt 208.09. C 46.18%, H 5.33%, Cl 34.07%, N 6.73%, O 7.69%. Increases corn tolerance to thiocarbamate and chloroacetanilide herbicides. Field and growth room trials in protection of corn from herbicide injury: F. Y. Chang *et al.*, *Can. J. Plant Sci.* **52**, 707 (1972); *eidem, Weed Res.* **13**, 399 (1973). Effects on uptake and metabolism of EPTC, *q.v.*: *eidem, J. Agric. Food Chem.* **22**, 245 (1974). Prepn and use in combination with thiocarbamate herbicides: F. M. Pallos *et al.*, **US 4021224** (1977 to Stauffer). Synergistic activity with herbicides that affect photosynthesis: C. Fedtke, R. H. Strang, *Z. Naturforsch.* **45c**, 565 (1990). Effects on lipid biosynthesis in maize: I. Cs. Barta, *ibid.* **46c**, 926 (1991); in barley and wild oats: A. Baldwin *et al.*, *J. Exp. Bot.* **54**, 1289 (2003). Environmental tolerances: *Fed. Regist.* **65**, 16143 (2000). Photodegradation study: A. W. Abu-Qare, H. J. Duncan, *Chemosphere* **46**, 1183 (2002).

$bp_{0.4 kPa}$ 96°. n_D^{30} 1.4990. LD_{50} orally in rats: 2146 mg/kg (*Fed. Regist.*).

Combination with acetochlor. [144115-48-0] Surpass; Top-Notch.

USE: Herbicide safener.

3050. Dichloroacetic Acid. [79-43-6] Bichloracetic acid; dichlorethanoic acid; DCA. $C_2H_2Cl_2O_2$; mol wt 128.94. C 18.63%, H 1.56%, Cl 54.99%, O 24.82%. $CHCl_2COOH$. Transformation of chloral to dichloroacetic acid: Wallach, *Ann.* **173**, 288 (1874); Frantzen, Fikentscher, *ibid.* **623**, 68 (1959); Rosenblum *et al.*, *Chem. Ind. (London)* **1960**, 718. Toxicity: Smyth *et al.*, *Arch. Ind. Hyg. Occup. Med.* **4**, 119 (1951); P. W. Stacpoole *et al.*, *N. Engl. J. Med.* **300**, 372 (1979); J. L. Cicmanec *et al.*, *Fundam. Appl. Toxicol.* **17**, 376 (1991). Mutagenicity studies: V. Herbert *et al.*, *Am. J. Clin. Nutr.* **33**, 1179 (1980). Use in treatment of lactic acidosis: P. W. Stacpoole *et al.*, *N. Engl. J. Med.* **309**, 390 (1983).

Liquid; pungent odor. d_4^{20} 1.563. bp 193-194°. Apparently occurs in two cryst forms, mp 9.7° and −4°. n_D^{22} 1.4659. Miscible with water, alc, ether. LD_{50} orally in rats: 2.82 g/kg (Smyth).

Ethyl ester. $C_4H_6Cl_2O_2$. Liquid, bp 158.3-158.7°. d_4^{20} 1.282. n_D^{20} 1.4386. Slightly sol in water; miscible with alcohol, ether.

THERAP CAT: Caustic; keratolytic; topical astringent.

3051. 1,1-Dichloroacetone. [513-88-2] 1,1-Dichloro-2-propanone; α,α-dichloroacetone; *uns*-dichloroacetone; dichloromethyl methyl ketone. $C_3H_4Cl_2O$; mol wt 126.97. C 28.38%, H 3.18%, Cl 55.84%, O 12.60%. $CH_3COCHCl_2$. Prepn: Borsche, Fittig, *Ann.* **133**, 113 (1865).

Oily liq. d_{15}^{18} 1.305. bp 120°. Slightly sol in water; sol in alcohol; miscible with ether. Boiling with Na_2CO_3 gives acrylic acid.

3052. 1,3-Dichloroacetone. [534-07-6] 1,3-Dichloro-2-propanone; α,γ-dichloroacetone; *sym*-dichloroacetone; bis(chloromethyl) ketone. $C_3H_4Cl_2O$; mol wt 126.97. C 28.38%, H 3.18%, Cl 55.84%, O 12.60%. $CH_2ClCOCH_2Cl$. Prepd by the oxidation of dichlorohydrin with sodium dichromate: Conant, Quayle, *Org. Synth.* **2**, 13 (1922).

Plates, needles on distillation. mp 45°. bp 173°. d_4^{46} 1.3826. n_D^{46} 1.47144. Sol in water, very sol in alc, ether.

Caution: Lacrimator, vesicant.

3053. 2,2-Dichloroacetyl Chloride. [79-36-7] Dichloroethanoyl chloride. C_2HCl_3O; mol wt 147.39. C 16.30%, H

0.68%, Cl 72.16%, O 10.86%. $Cl_2CHCOCl$. Prepd from pentachloroethane: Ott, **DE 362748** (1922 to Weiler ter Meer); from chloroform and carbon monoxide in presence of aluminum chloride at high pressure (21% yield): Frank *et al., Ind. Eng. Chem.* **41**, 2061 (1949). Toxicity study: Smyth *et al., Arch. Ind. Hyg. Occup. Med.* **4**, 119 (1951).

Liquid. Fumes in air; acrid, penetrating odor. d_4^{16} 1.5315. bp_{760} 107-108°; bp_{739} 106-107°. n_D^{16} 1.4638. Dec upon contact with water, alcohol. Miscible with ether. LD_{50} orally in rats: 2.46 g/kg (Smyth).

Caution: Irritating to eyes, mucous membranes.

3054.   3,4-Dichloroaniline. [95-76-1] 3,4-Dichlorobenzeneamine. $C_6H_5Cl_2N$; mol wt 162.02. C 44.48%, H 3.11%, Cl 43.76%, N 8.65%. Prepd by chlorination of *p*-chloroaniline with $AlCl_3$—HCl: Suthers *et al., J. Org. Chem.* **27**, 447 (1962). Manuf by catalytic reduction of 3,4-dichloro-1-nitrobenzene: Dietzler, Keil, **US 3067253** (1962 to Dow).

Crystals, mp 71-72°. bp 272°. Practically insol in water. Very sol in alcohol, ether; slightly sol in benzene.

3055.   *m*-Dichlorobenzene. [541-73-1] 1,3-Dichlorobenzene. $C_6H_4Cl_2$; mol wt 147.00. C 49.02%, H 2.74%, Cl 48.24%. Prepn by Sandmeyer procedure from the appropriate chloroaniline, and, along with *o*- and *p*-dichlorobenzenes, by chlorination of chlorobenzene: Engelsma *et al., Rec. Trav. Chim.* **76**, 325 (1957). Separation of mixture contg *m*-, *o*-, and *p*-dichlorobenzenes by distillation and crystn: Mueller, Wolz, **FR 1374863** (1964 to Bayer), *C.A.* **62**, 4936e (1965); **GB 999845**. Physical properties: *Rev. Environ. Contam. Toxicol.* **106**, 51 (1988).

Liquid, bp 173°. mp −24.76°. d_4^{20} 1.2884, d_4^{25} 1.2828. n_D^{20} 1.5459. Log P (olive oil:water) 3.69. Vapor pressure (39°) 5 mm Hg. Soly in water 1.23 mg/L. Sol in alcohol, ether.

3056.   *o*-Dichlorobenzene. [95-50-1] 1,2-Dichlorobenzene; orthodichlorobenzene. $C_6H_4Cl_2$; mol wt 147.00. C 49.02%, H 2.74%, Cl 48.24%. Prepn and separation from *m*- and *p*-dichlorobenzenes, *see m*-isomer above. Manuf: *Faith, Keyes & Clark's Industrial Chemicals*, F. A. Lowenheim, M. K. Moran, Eds. (Wiley-Interscience, New York, 4th ed., 1975) pp 258-265. Review of toxicology: *Rev. Environ. Contam. Toxicol.* **106**, 51-68 (1988).

Liquid, bp 180.5°. mp −17.03°. d_4^{20} 1.3059, d_4^{25} 1.3003. n_D^{20} 1.5515, n_D^{25} 1.5491. Flash pt, closed cup: 151°F (66°C). Vapor pressure (25°) 1.56 mm Hg. Log P (olive oil:water) 3.65. Soly in water 145 mg/L. Miscible with alc, ether, benzene.

Caution: Potential symptoms of overexposure are irritation of nose and eyes; liver and kidney damage; skin blisters. *See NIOSH Pocket Guide to Chemical Hazards* (DHHS/NIOSH 97-140, 1997) p 96. Exposure to high concentrations may result in CNS depression. *See Patty's Industrial Hygiene and Toxicology* vol. 2B, G. D. Clayton, F. E. Clayton, Eds. (Wiley-Interscience, New York, 3rd ed., 1981) pp 3611-3617.

USE: Solvent for waxes, gums, resins, tars, rubbers, oils, asphalts; insecticide for termites and locust borers; fumigant; deodorizer; removing sulfur from illuminating gas; as degreasing agent for metals, leather, wool; as ingredient of metal polishes; as heat transfer medium; as intermediate in the manuf of dyes.

3057.   *p*-Dichlorobenzene. [106-46-7] Paracide; PDB; Paradichlorobenzene; Para-zene; Di-chloricide; Paramoth. $C_6H_4Cl_2$;

mol wt 147.00. C 49.02%, H 2.74%, Cl 48.24%. Prepn and separation from *m*- and *o*-dichlorobenzene, *see m*-dichlorobenzene. Crystal structure of triclinic form (*β*-modification): Housty, Clastre, *Acta Crystallogr.* **10**, 695 (1957); of monoclinic form (*α*-modification) and transformation to triclinic form: Panatoni *et al., Gazz. Chim. Ital.* **93**, 813 (1963). Manuf: *Faith, Keyes & Clark's Industrial Chemicals*, F. A. Lowenheim, M. K. Moran, Eds. (Wiley-Interscience, New Yok, 4th ed., 1975) pp 258-265. Toxicity study: T. B. Gaines, R. E. Linder, *Fundam. Appl. Toxicol.* **7**, 299 (1986). Review of toxicology: *Rev. Environ. Contam. Toxicol.* **106**, 51-68 (1988); and human exposure: *Toxicological Profile for 1,4-Dichlorobenzene* (PB99-121972, 1998) 300 pp.

Volatile crystals with a characteristic penetrating odor. Sublimes at ordinary temps. mp 53.5° (*α*-modification), 54° (*β*-modification). bp 174.12°. n_D^{60} 1.5285. Flash pt (closed cup) 150°F. Log P (olive oil/water) 3.65. Vapor pressure (25°) = 0.4 mm Hg. d^{20} 1.46. Practically insol in water. Sol in alcohol, ether, benzene, chloroform, carbon disulfide. Non-corrosive; non-staining. LD_{50} in male, female rats (mg/kg): 3863, 3790 orally; >6000, >6000 dermally (Gaines, Linder).

Caution: Potential symptoms of overexposure are eye irritation, periorbital swelling; profuse rhinitis; headache; anorexia, nausea and vomiting; weight loss, jaundice and cirrhosis. *See NIOSH Pocket Guide to Chemical Hazards* (DHHS/NIOSH 97-140, 1997) p 96. Direct contact with fumes or solid may cause skin irritation. *See Patty's Industrial Hygiene and Toxicology* vol. 2B, G. D. Clayton, F. E. Clayton, Eds. (Wiley-Interscience, New York, 3rd ed., 1981) pp 3617-3626. This substance is reasonably anticipated to be a human carcinogen: *Report on Carcinogens, Eleventh Edition* (PB2005-104914, 2004) p III-85.

USE: Insecticidal fumigant. For domestic use against clothes moths; as space deodorant in room deodorizers, toilet bowl blocks and diaper pail deodorizers. Intermediate in production of plastics for electronic components.

3058.   2,2′-Dichlorobenzidine. [84-68-4] 2,2′-Dichloro[1,1′-biphenyl]-4,4′-diamine. $C_{12}H_{10}Cl_2N_2$; mol wt 253.13. C 56.94%, H 3.98%, Cl 28.01%, N 11.07%. Prepn from *m*-chloronitrobenzene: Laubenheimer, *Ber.* **8**, 1625 (1875); Cain, May, *J. Chem. Soc.* **97**, 723 (1910).

Needles from water or prisms from alc, mp 165°. Almost insol in water; moderately sol in alc; readily sol in ether.

Hydrochloride. $C_{12}H_{10}Cl_2N_2$.2HCl. Leaflets from water, moderately sol in water.

USE: Manuf azo dyes.

3059.   3,3′-Dichlorobenzidine. [91-94-1] 3,3-Dichloro-(1,1′-biphenyl)-4,4′-diamine; 3,3′-dichloro-4,4′-biphenyldiamine; DCB. $C_{12}H_{10}Cl_2N_2$; mol wt 253.13. C 56.94%, H 3.98%, Cl 28.01%, N 11.07%. Prepn from *o*-chloronitrobenzene: Cohn, *Ber.* **33**, 3552 (1900). Review of carcinogenicity studies: *IARC Monographs* **4**, 49-55 (1974); of bioactivation and toxicity: M. M. Iba, *Drug Metab. Rev.* **21**, 377-400 (1990).

Needles from alc or benzene, mp 132-133°. Almost insol in water. Readily sol in alc, benzene, glacial acetic acid.

Dihydrochloride. [612-83-9] $C_{12}H_{10}Cl_2N_2$.2HCl. Needles. Slightly sol in water, readily sol in alc.

Caution: Potential symptoms of overexposure are skin sensitization; dermatitis; headache, dizziness; caustic burns; frequent urination, dysuria; hematuria; GI upsets; upper respiratory infection. *See NIOSH Pocket Guide to Chemical Hazards* (DHHS/NIOSH 97-140, 1997) p 96. 3,3′-Dichlorobenzidine and its dihydrochloride are reasonably anticipated to be human carcinogens: *Report on Carcinogens, Eleventh Edition* (PB2005-104914, 2004) p III-87.

USE: Manuf azo dyes and pigments; as an intermediate for the Benzidine Yellow pigments. As curing agent for isocyanate polymers and solid urethane plastics.

3060. Dichlorobenzyl Alcohol. [1777-82-8] 2,4-Dichlorobenzenemethanol; Dybenal. $C_7H_6Cl_2O$; mol wt 177.03. C 47.49%, H 3.42%, Cl 40.05%, O 9.04%. Prepn: Van de Lande, *Rec. Trav. Chim.* **51**, 98 (1932); Metayer, Dat-Xuong, *Bull. Soc. Chim. Fr.* **1954**, 615.

Crystals, mp 59.5°.
THERAP CAT: Antiseptic.

3061. 1,1-Dichloro-2,2-bis(p-chlorophenyl)ethane. [72-54-8] 1,1'-(2,2-Dichloroethylidene)bis[4-chlorobenzene]; tetrachlorodiphenylethane; TDE; dichlorodiphenyldichloroethane; DDD; *p,p'*-DDD; *p,p'*-TDE; Rhothane. $C_{14}H_{10}Cl_4$; mol wt 320.04. C 52.54%, H 3.15%, Cl 44.31%. Non-degradable pesticide; a component of technical grade DDT, *q.v.* Prepd by condensing dichloroacetaldehyde with chlorobenzene: Haller *et al., J. Am. Chem. Soc.* **67**, 1596, 1600 (1945). Toxicity study: T. B. Gaines, *Toxicol. Appl. Pharmacol.* **14**, 515 (1969). Review of toxicology and human exposure: *Toxicological Profile for DDT, DDE, DDD* (PB2003-100137, 2002) 497 pp.

Crystals, mp 109-110°. The chemical properties and solys are similar to those of DDT. LD_{50} orally in rats: >4000 mg/kg (Gaines).
Caution: Potential symptoms of overexposure are similar to DDT.
USE: Insecticide.

3062. Dichloro(2-chlorovinyl)arsine. [541-25-3] (2-Chloroethenyl)arsonous dichloride; 2-chlorovinyldichloroarsine; chlorovinylarsine dichloride; Lewisite. $C_2H_2AsCl_3$; mol wt 207.32. C 11.59%, H 0.97%, As 36.14%, Cl 51.30%. ClCH=CHAsCl$_2$. Vesicant used as chemical weapon. Prepn: S. J. Green, T. S. Price, *J. Chem. Soc.* **119**, 448 (1921); W. L. Lewis, G. A. Perkins, *Ind. Eng. Chem.* **15**, 290 (1923). Review of military experience: G. N. Jarman in *Adv. Chem. Ser.* **23**, entitled "Metal-Organic Compounds," M. Sittig, Ed. (ACS, Washington DC, 1959) pp 328-337. Determn of degradation products in soil: B. A. Tomkins *et al., J. Chromatogr. A* **909**, 13 (2001); in urine: J. V. Wooten *et al., J. Chromatogr. B* **772**, 147 (2002). Review of chemistry, toxicology and biological effects: M. Goldman, J. C. Dacre, *Rev. Environ. Contam. Toxicol.* **110**, 75-115 (1989).

Colorless, slightly oily liquid; darkens with time becoming violet-black or green. Faint odor of geranium. *Vesicant.* $bp_{12.5}$ 76-77°; bp_{26} 93°; bp_{760} 190°. d_4^{20} 1.888. Sol in the common organic solvents. Insol in water, dil mineral acids. Absorbed by rubber, paint, varnish and porous materials. Rapidly hydrolyzed in aqueous medium. LD_{50} in rats (mg/kg): 50 orally; in rats, rabbits (mg/kg): 24, 6 dermally; 1, 2 s.c. (Goldman, Dacre).
Caution: Vapors are extremely toxic. Contact with skin may produce immediate, persistent stinging, followed by erythema and blistering; irritating to eyes; inhalation of 0.50 mg/l for 5 min is considered lethal in humans (Goldman, Dacre). *Antidote:* Dimercaprol, *q.v.*
USE: Chemical warfare agent.

3063. 2,3-Dichloro-5,6-dicyanobenzoquinone. [84-58-2] 4,5-Dichloro-3,6-dioxo-1,4-cyclohexadiene-1,2-dicarbonitrile;

DDQ. $C_8Cl_2N_2O_2$; mol wt 227.00. C 42.33%, Cl 31.24%, N 12.34%, O 14.10%. Prepn: Thiele, Günther, *Ann.* **349**, 45 (1906); Walker, Waugh, *J. Org. Chem.* **30**, 3240 (1965).

Yellow to orange crystals, mp 213.5-215°. Dec in water. Sol in benzene, dioxane, acetic acid. Slightly sol in chloroform, methylene chloride.
USE: Oxidizing agent, especially in steroid synthesis.

3064. Dichlorodifluoromethane. [75-71-8] Difluorodichloromethane; Arcton 12; Freon 12; Frigen 12; Genetron 12; Halon; Isotron 2. CCl_2F_2; mol wt 120.91. C 9.93%, Cl 58.64%, F 31.43%. Prepn: Henne, *Org. React.* **2**, 49 (1944); Swarts, *Chem. Zentralbl.* **1907, II**, 581. Manuf: *Faith, Keyes & Clark's Industrial Chemicals,* F. A. Lowenheim, M. K. Moran, Eds. (Wiley-Interscience, New York, 4th ed., 1975) pp 325-330.

Colorless, practically odorless, noncorrosive, nonirritating, nonflammable gas. Faint, ether-like odor in high concentrations. Stable up to 550°. $d_{liq}^{-29.8}$ 1.486. mp $-158°$. bp_{760} $-29.8°$; bp_{2atm} $-12.2°$; bp_{5atm} 16.1°; bp_{10atm} 42.4°; bp_{20atm} 74.0°; bp_{30atm} 95.6°. Critical temp 111.5°; critical pressure 39.6 atm (582 lb/sq inch). Dipole moment 0.51. Insol in water. Sol in alcohol, ether. Absorbs less than 0.0025% water. Has little, if any, anesthetic or toxic action, but toxic substances may be formed on contact with a flame or hot metal surface.
Caution: Potential symptoms of overexposure are dizziness, tremors, asphyxia, unconsciousness, cardiac arrhythmias and cardiac arrest; direct contact with liquid may cause frostbite. *See NIOSH Pocket Guide to Chemical Hazards* (DHHS/NIOSH 97-140, 1997) p 96. *Note:* Consult latest Government regulations on use as aerosol propellant.
USE: Refrigerant, aerosol propellant.

3065. 1,3-Dichloro-5,5-dimethylhydantoin. [118-52-5] 1,3-Dichloro-5,5-dimethyl-2,4-imidazolidinedione; Dactin; Halane. $C_5H_6Cl_2N_2O_2$; mol wt 197.02. C 30.48%, H 3.07%, Cl 35.99%, N 14.22%, O 16.24%. Prepd by passing chlorine through an aq soln of 5,5-dimethylhydantoin: Biltz, Slotta, *J. Prakt. Chem.* **113**, 248 (1926); Orazi, Orio, *An. Asoc. Quim. Argent.* **41**, 153 (1953), *C.A.* **48**, 13634 (1954). Structure: Bogaert-Verhoogen, Martin, *Bull. Soc. Chim. Belg.* **58**, 567 (1949). Purification by dissolving in concd H_2SO_4 and diluting with ice-water: Lorenz, US 2828308 (1958 to Purex).

Four-sided, pointed prisms from chloroform, d_{20}^{20} 1.5. mp 132°. Sublimes at 100°. Turns brown and conflagrates at 212° (after melting at 132°). The dry crystals [combined available chlorine 77.6% (theory)] may be stored without much loss of available chlorine. After 14 weeks at 60° the loss was 1.5% Cl compared with a loss of 37.5% suffered by 70% calcium hypochlorite. On contact with water and esp hot water hypochlorous acid is liberated. At pH 9 nitrogen chloride is formed. Soly in water at 25° 0.21%; at 60° 0.60%. pH of aq soln about 4.4. Freely sol in chlorinated and highly polar solvents at 25°: Chloroform 14%, methylene chloride 30.0%, carbon tetrachloride 12.5%, ethylene dichloride 32.0%, *sym*-tetrachlorethane 17.0%, benzene 9.2%.
Caution: Potential symptoms of overexposure are irritation of eyes, mucous membranes and respiratory system. *See NIOSH Pocket Guide to Chemical Hazards* (DHHS/NIOSH 97-140, 1997) p 98.

USE: Chlorinating agent, disinfectant, industrial deodorant. In water treatment. Active ingredient of powder laundry bleaches such as Sage's Dry Bleach, Colgate's Pruf. Intermediate for amino acids, drugs, insecticides. Stabilizer for vinyl chloride polymers. Polymerization catalyst.

3066. *sym*-Dichloroethyl Ether. [111-44-4] 1,1'-Oxybis[2-chloroethane]; bis(2-chloroethyl) ether; β,β'-dichloroethyl ether; DCEE; Chlorex. $C_4H_8Cl_2O$; mol wt 143.01. C 33.59%, H 5.64%, Cl 49.58%, O 11.19%. [ClCH₂CH₂]₂O. Prepn: O. Kamm, J. H. Waldo, *J. Am. Chem. Soc.* **43**, 2223 (1921). Toxicity: H. F. Smyth, Jr., C. P. Carpenter, *J. Ind. Hyg. Toxicol.* **30**, 66 (1948). Evaluation of carcinogenic risk: *IARC Monographs* **9**, 117 (1975). Review of toxicology and human exposure: *Toxicological Profile for Bis(2-chloroethyl)ether* (PB90-168683, 1989) 83 pp.

Colorless, clear liq; pungent odor. Vapor harmful. d_{20}^{20} 1.22. bp 178°. mp −50°. n_D^{20} 1.457. Flash pt, closed cup: 145°F (63°C), Buckman Laboratories, IC literature; also reported as 131°F (55°C), *Ind. Eng. Chem.* **32**, 880 (1940). Insol in water. Sol in most organic solvents. It dissolves oils, fats, greases, etc. LD_{50} orally in rats: 75 mg/kg (Smyth, Carpenter).

Caution: Potential symptoms of overexposure are lacrimation; irritation of nose, throat and respiratory system; coughing; nausea, vomiting. Potential occupational carcinogen. *See NIOSH Pocket Guide to Chemical Hazards* (DHHS/NIOSH 97-140, 1997) p 98.

USE: Reagent for organic synthesis; solvent. Has been used as a scouring agent for textiles; as soil fumigant.

3067. 4′,5′-Dichlorofluorescein. [2320-96-9] 4′,5′-Di-chloro-3′,6′-dihydroxyspiro[isobenzofuran-1(3H),9′-[9H]xanthen]-3-one; D & C Orange no. 8; 4,5-dichloro-3,6-fluorandiol. $C_{20}H_{10}$-Cl_2O_5; mol wt 401.20. C 59.87%, H 2.51%, Cl 17.67%, O 19.94%. Prepd by condensation of 2-chlororesorcinol with phthalic anhydride: *Colour Index* **vol. 4** (3rd ed., 1971) p 4424.

Orange powder, insol in water and in dil acids. Sol in alcohol and in dil alkali yielding solns which are orange with a greenish-yellow fluorescence. Slightly sol in glycerol and the glycols. Practically insol in oils, fats and waxes. If a soln of the dye in strong alkali is heated, a violet color is produced.

Disodium salt. C.I. Solvent Orange 32; C.I. 45365. $C_{20}H_8Cl_2$-Na_2O_5.

Note: Structure depicted as the open tautomer.

3068. 2,6-Dichloroindophenol Sodium. [620-45-1] 2,6-Di-chloro-4-[(4-hydroxyphenyl)imino]-2,5-cyclohexadien-1-one sodium salt; sodium 2,6-dichloroindophenol; sodium 2,6-dichloro-N-(p-hydroxyphenyl)-p-benzoquinone imine; 2,6-dichloro-1,4-benzo-quinone-4-(4-hydroxyanil) sodium; 2,6-dichlorophenol-indophenol sodium; Tillman's reagent. $C_{12}H_6Cl_2NNaO_2$; mol wt 290.08. C 49.69%, H 2.08%, Cl 24.44%, N 4.83%, Na 7.93%, O 11.03%. Prepd from 2,6-dichloro-p-quinone-4-chlorimide and phenol in alkaline soln: Gibbs *et al.*, *Public Health Rep.* **40**, 650 (1925); Till-mans *et al.*, *Z. Unters. Lebensm.* **56**, 273 (1932).

Dark green powder. May contain up to 2 mols H_2O. Freely sol in water, alc. The aq soln is deep blue, changed to red by acids. It liberates iodine from KI in acid solns.

USE: Analytical reagent in the determination of ascorbic acid (vitamin C) which reduces the dye to a colorless hydroxy compd.

3069. *sym*-Dichloromethyl Ether. [542-88-1] Oxybis[chloromethane]; bis(chloromethyl) ether; BCME. $C_2H_4Cl_2O$; mol wt 114.96. C 20.90%, H 3.51%, Cl 61.68%, O 13.92%. (CH₂Cl)₂O. Review of carcinogenic risk: *IARC Monographs* **4**, 231-238 (1974); of toxicology and human exposure: *Toxicological Profile for Bis (Chloromethyl) Ether* (PB90-168691, 1989) 77 pp.

Colorless liquid; suffocating odor. d_4^{20} 1.315. bp 106°. n_D^{20} 1.4346. Unstable in moist air; dec by water into HCl and formaldehyde.

Caution: Potential symptoms of overexposure are irritation of eyes, skin, mucous membranes and respiratory system; pulmonary congestion, edema; corneal damage, necrosis; decreased pulmonary function, coughing, dyspnea and wheezing; blood stained sputum, bronchial secretions. *See NIOSH Pocket Guide to Chemical Hazards* (DHHS/NIOSH 97-140, 1997) p 64. This substance is listed as a known human carcinogen: *Report on Carcinogens, Eleventh Edition* (PB2005-104914, 2004) p III-56.

USE: Manuf of plastics and ion exchange resins.

3070. 4,5-Dichloro-2-octyl-3-isothiazolone. [64359-81-5] 4,5-dichloro-2-octyl-3(2H)-isothiazolone; 2-n-octyl-4,5-dichloro-1-isothiazolin-3-one; 4,5-dichloro-2-n-octyl-4-isothiazolin-3-one; DCOI; C-9211; RH-5287; Sea-Nine. $C_{11}H_{17}Cl_2NOS$; mol wt 282.23. C 46.81%, H 6.07%, Cl 25.12%, N 4.96%, O 5.67%, S 11.36%. Prepn: E. D. Weiler *et al.*, *J. Heterocycl. Chem.* **14**, 627 (1977). Physical properties and ecological risk assessment: W. D. Shade *et al.*, *ASTM Spec. Tech. Publ.* **STP 1216**, 381 (1993). HPLC analysis and persistence in seawater and sediment: A. Jacobson *et al.*, *ACS Symp. Ser.* **522**, 127 (1993). *Review:* G. L. Willingham, A. H. Jacobson, *ibid.* **640**, 224-233 (1996).

Crystals from hexane, mp 44-46°. Technical product is reported as tan-to-brown waxy solid with pungent aromatic odor, mp 40-41°. d^{25} 1.28 g/ml. Vapor pressure (25°): 7.4 × 10^{-6} mm Hg. Log P (octanol/water): 2.85 (Willingham, Jacobson); also reported as 4.5 (Shade). Miscible in most organic solvents. Soly (ppm): 6.5 in deionized water; 4.7 in synthetic seawater. LC_{50} (96 hr) in bluegill sunfish, adult bay mussel, fiddler crab: 14, 850, 1312 ppb (Willingham, Jacobson).

USE: Marine antifoulant.

3071. Dichlorophen. [97-23-4] 2,2′-Methylenebis[4-chloro-phenol]; 2,2′-dihydroxy-5,5′-dichlorodiphenylmethane; 5,5′-di-chloro-2,2′-dihydroxydiphenylmethane; bis[5-chloro-2-hydroxy-phenyl]methane; di[5-chloro-2-hydroxyphenyl]methane; dichloro-phene; G-4; Anthiphen; Dicestal; Didroxane; Di-phenthane-70; Parabis; Plath-Lyse; Preventol G-D; Wespuril. $C_{13}H_{10}Cl_2O_2$; mol wt 269.12. C 58.02%, H 3.75%, Cl 26.35%, O 11.89%. Prepn by adding a CH_2O yielding reagent, e.g. aq HCHO, to p-chlorophenol: Gump, Luthy, **US 2334408** (1944 to Burton T. Bush). Acute toxicity: T. B. Gaines, R. E. Linder, *Fundam. Appl. Toxicol.* **7**, 299 (1986).

Crystals from toluene, mp 177-178°. Practically insol in water. Sparingly sol in toluene. One gram dissolves in 1 g of 95% ethanol, in less than 1 g of ether. Also sol in methanol, isopropyl ether, petr ether. Sol (with decompn) in alkaline aq solns. LD_{50} in adult male, female rats (mg/kg): 1506, 1683 orally (Gaines, Linder).

USE: Agricultural fungicide; antimicrobial; germicide in soaps, shampoos, etc.

THERAP CAT: Anthelmintic (Cestodes).

THERAP CAT (VET): Anthelmintic, antiprotozoan, fungicide.

3072. 2,4-Dichlorophenol. [120-83-2] $C_6H_4Cl_2O$; mol wt 163.00. C 44.21%, H 2.47%, Cl 43.50%, O 9.82%. Key intermediate in synthesis of the herbicide 2,4-D, *q.v.* Prepn by chlorination of phenol: M. Kohn, S. Sussmann, *Monatsh. Chem.* **46**, 575 (1926); B. O. Pray, D. N. Sukow, US 2759981 (1956 to Columbia-Southern Chem. Corp.); by chlorination of *o*- or *p*-chlorophenol: L. G. Groves *et al., J. Chem. Soc.* **1929**, 512; from 2,4-dinitrophenol: A. Ghosh, *J. Indian Chem. Soc.* **28**, 155 (1951). ^{1}H NMR study: J. B. Rowbotham, T. Schaefer, *Can. J. Chem.* **52**, 3037 (1974). Review of toxicology and human exposure: *Toxicological Profile for Chlorophenols* (PB99-166639, 1999) 260 pp.

Needle-like crystals, with strong medicinal taste and odor. mp 45°. bp 209-211°. Volatile with steam. Sol in CCl_4.

USE: Biocide; intermediate in production of herbicides.

3073. 2,6-Dichlorophenol. [87-65-0] $C_6H_4Cl_2O$; mol wt 163.00. C 44.21%, H 2.47%, Cl 43.50%, O 9.82%. Synthesis from ethyl 3,5-dichloro-4-hydroxybenzoate: D. S. Tarbell *et al., Org. Synth.* **coll. vol. III**, 267. Crystal structure: C. Bavoux, P. Michel, *Acta Crystallogr.* **30B**, 2043 (1974). Isoln and identification as sex pheromone of lone star tick: R. S. Berger, *Science* **177**, 704 (1972).

White crystals from petr ether, mp 64.5-65.5°.

3074. 1,3-Dichloro-2-propanol. [96-23-1] α-Dichlorohydrin; *sym*-glycerol dichlorohydrin; glycerol α,γ-dichlorohydrin; *sym*-dichloroisopropyl alcohol. $C_3H_6Cl_2O$; mol wt 128.99. C 27.93%, H 4.69%, Cl 54.97%, O 12.40%. $CH_2ClCHOHCH_2Cl$. Prepd from glycerol, acetic acid and HCl gas: Conant, Quayle, *Org. Synth.* **2**, 29 (1922); **coll. vol. I** (2nd ed.) p 292. Toxicity study: Smyth *et al., Am. Ind. Hyg. Assoc. J.* **23**, 95 (1962).

Liquid. Ethereal odor. d_4^{17} 1.3506. mp −4°. bp_{760} 174.3°; bp_{100} 114.8°; bp_{40} 93°; bp_{20} 78°; bp_5 52°; $bp_{1.0}$ 28°. n_D^{17} 1.480245. Sol in 10 parts water; miscible with alcohol, ether. LD_{50} orally in rats: 110 mg/kg, Smyth *et al., Am. Ind. Hyg. Assoc. J.* **23**, 95 (1962).

USE: Solvent for hard resins and nitrocellulose; manuf photographic and Zapon lacquer; cement for celluloid; binder for water colors.

3075. 1,3-Dichloropropene. [542-75-6] α,γ-Dichloropropylene; 1,3-dichloropropylene; γ-chloroallyl chloride; 1,3-D; Curfew; Telone II. $C_3H_4Cl_2$; mol wt 110.97. C 32.47%, H 3.63%, Cl 63.90%. $ClCH_2CH{=}CHCl$. Prepd from 1,2,3-trichloropropane with NaOH: Friedel, Silva, *Compt. Rend.* **75**, 81 (1872); Reboul, *Ann. Chim.* [3] **60**, 37 (1860); from 3-chloro-2-propen-1-ol with PCl_3: Kirrmann *et al., Bull. Soc. Chim. Fr.* [5] **1**, 860 (1934); from acrolein with PCl_5: van Romburgh, *ibid.* [2] **36**, 549 (1881); from 3,3-dichloropropene by isomerization with conc HCl: *idem, ibid.* The usual industrial prepn is from 1,3-dichloro-2-propanol by dehydration with $POCl_3$ or with P_2O_5 in benzene: Hurd, Webb, *J. Am. Chem. Soc.* **58**, 2191 (1936). Prepn of stereoisomers: L. F. Hatch, A. C. Moore, *ibid.* **66**, 285 (1944). Configuration: H. A. Smith, W. H. King, *ibid.* **70**, 3528 (1948); L. F. Hatch, R. H. Perry, *ibid.* **71**, 3262 (1949). Persistence in soil: I. J. Thomason, M. V. McKenry, *Hilgardia* **42**, 393 (1974). GC determn of isomers in rat

blood: P. E. Kastl, E. A. Hermann, *J. Chromatogr.* **265**, 277 (1983). Toxicity study: T. R. Torkelson, F. Oyen, *Am. Ind. Hyg. Assoc. J.* **38**, 217 (1977). Review of toxicology and human exposure: *Toxicological Profile for 1,3-Dichloropropene* (PB93-110765, 1992) 151 pp.

Liquid with chloroform odor. d^{25} 1.220. bp 108°. n_D^{22} 1.4735. Technical product is mixture of *cis*- and *trans*-isomers. LD_{50} (92% technical product) in male, female rats (mg/kg): 713, 470 orally (10% soln in corn oil); in rabbits (mg/kg): 504 dermally (Torkelson, Oyen).

cis-**Form.** [10061-01-5] bp 104.3°. d_4^{20} 1.224. n_4^{20} 1.4682.

trans-**Form.** [10061-02-6] bp 112.0°. d_4^{20} 1.217. n_4^{20} 1.4730.

Caution: Potential symptoms of overexposure are irritation of skin, eyes, and respiratory system; eye and skin burns; lacrimation; headache, dizziness, coma; gasping, refusal to breathe, cough, substernal pain; possible liver, kidney and heart injury. *See NIOSH Pocket Guide to Chemical Hazards* (DHHS/NIOSH 97-140, 1997) p 100; *Clinical Toxicology of Commercial Products*, R. E. Gosselin *et al.,* Eds. (Williams & Wilkins, Baltimore, 5th Ed., 1984) Section III, pp 141-142. The technical grade is reasonably anticipated to be a human carcinogen: *Report on Carcinogens, Eleventh Edition* (PB2005-104914, 2004) p III-93.

USE: Soil fumigant; nematocide. In manuf of pesticides.

3076. Dichloroxylenol. [133-53-9] 2,4-Dichloro-3,5-dimethylphenol; 2,4-dichloro-3,5-xylenol; DCMX. $C_8H_8Cl_2O$; mol wt 191.05. C 50.29%, H 4.22%, Cl 37.11%, O 8.37%. Prepn: Lesser, Gad, *Ber.* **56**, 963 (1923); Jones, *J. Chem. Soc.* **1941**, 267; Gemmell, *Manuf. Chem.* **23**, 63 (1952).

Crystals from petr ether, mp 95-96°. Sublimes. Volatile with steam. Soly in water: one part in 5000. Soly at 15° in 100 parts of solvent: benzene, 14; toluene, 15; acetone, 73; diethyl ketone, 59; petr ether, 4; chloroform, 25; CCl_4, 10.

USE: Bacteriostat in soaps; mold inhibitor, preservative.

3077. Dichlorphenamide. [120-97-8] 4,5-Dichloro-1,3-benzenedisulfonamide; 1,3-disulfamyl-4,5-dichlorobenzene; 4,5-dichloro-1,3-disulfamoylbenzene; Antidrasi; Daranide; Oratrol. $C_6H_6Cl_2N_2O_4S_2$; mol wt 305.16. C 23.62%, H 1.98%, Cl 23.24%, N 9.18%, O 20.97%, S 21.02%. Prepn: Schultz, US 2835702 (1958 to Merck & Co.).

Needles from DMSO + water, mp 239-241° (patent, mp 228.5-229°). Practically insol in water. Sol in alkaline solns.

THERAP CAT: Carbonic anhydrase inhibitor.

3078. Dichlorprop. [120-36-5] 2-(2,4-Dichlorophenoxy)propanoic acid; (±)2-(2,4-dichlorophenoxy)propionic acid; 2,4-DP; dichloroprop; Dicopur DP; Polymore. $C_9H_8Cl_2O_3$; mol wt 235.06. C 45.99%, H 3.43%, Cl 30.17%, O 20.42%. Selective pre- and post-emergent herbicide. Exists in two optically active forms; only the (+)-isomer shows biological activity. First prepd and described as a plant growth regulator: M. E. Synerholm, P. W. Zimmerman, *Contrib. Boyce Thompson Inst.* **14**, 91 (1945). Commercial prepn: H. A. Stevenson, R. F. Brookes, GB 822199 (1959 to Boots). Resoln of enantiomers and biological activity: S. T. Collins, F. E. Smith: *J. Sci. Food Agric.* **3**, 248 (1952). Field studies and toxicology: W. O. G. Nuyken *et al., Meded. Fac. Landbouwwet. Rijksuniv. Gent* **52**, 1139 (1987). Enantiomeric effects on degradation: A.W. Garrison *et al., Environ. Sci. Technol.* **30**,

2449 (1996). GC/MS determn in soil: T. Heberer, H.-J. Stan, *J. AOAC Int.* **79**, 1428 (1996).

Colorless crystals, mp 117-118°. Soly in water at 20°: 350 ppm. Readily sol in organic solvents. Corrosive to metals in the presence of water.

(**R**)-(+)-**Form.** [15165-67-0] Dichlorprop-P; Duplosan DP. Colorless needles from benzene, mp 124°. $[\alpha]_D^{21}$ +26.6° (c = 1.23 in ethanol).

USE: Herbicide.

3079. Dichlorvos. [62-73-7] Phosphoric acid 2,2-dichloroethenyl dimethyl ester; phosphoric acid 2,2-dichlorovinyl dimethyl ester; *O,O*-dimethyl *O*-(2,2-dichlorovinyl) phosphate; dichlorophos; dichlorovos; DDVP; SD-1750; Atgard; Dedevap; Divipan; Doom; Nuvan; Task; Vapona. $C_4H_7Cl_2O_4P$; mol wt 220.98. C 21.74%, H 3.19%, Cl 32.09%, O 28.96%, P 14.02%. Cholinesterase inhibitor. Prepn: Whetstone, Harman, US 2956073 (1960 to Shell). Toxicity: T. B. Gaines, *Toxicol. Appl. Pharmacol.* **14**, 515 (1969). Review of carcinogenicity studies: M. D. Reuber, *Clin. Toxicol.* **18**, 47-84 (1981); of toxicology and human exposure: *Toxicological Profile for Dichlorvos* (PB98-101124, 1997) 248 pp.

Liquid. Practically non-flammable. d_4^{25} 1.415. bp_{20} 140°; $bp_{1.0}$ 84°; $bp_{0.5}$ 72°; $bp_{0.01}$ 30°. n_D^{25} 1.451. Vapor pressure at 20°: 1.2 × 10^{-2} mm Hg. Misc with alcohol and most non-polar solvents. Soly in water: about 1 g/100 ml; in glycerol: about 0.5 g/100 ml. LD_{50} orally in male, female rats: 80, 56 mg/kg (Gaines).

Caution: Potential symptoms of overexposure are miosis, aching eyes; rhinorrhea; headache; chest tightening, wheezing, laryngeal spasms and salivation; cyanosis; anorexia, nausea, vomiting and diarrhea; sweating; muscle fasciculation, paralysis, giddiness and ataxia; convulsions; low blood pressure, cardiac irregularities; irritation of eyes and skin. See *NIOSH Pocket Guide to Chemical Hazards* (DHHS/NIOSH 97-140, 1997) p 102.

USE: Insecticide.

THERAP CAT (VET): Anthelmintic, insecticide.

3080. Diclazuril. [101831-37-2] 2,6-Dichloro-α-(4-chlorophenyl)-4-(4,5-dihydro-3,5-dioxo-1,2,4-triazin-2(3*H*)-yl)benzeneacetonitrile; (*p*-chlorophenyl)[2,6-dichloro-4-(4,5-dihydro-3,5-dioxo-*as*-triazin-2(3*H*)-yl)phenyl]acetonitrile; R-64433; Clinacox. $C_{17}H_9Cl_3N_4O_2$; mol wt 407.64. C 50.09%, H 2.23%, Cl 26.09%, N 13.74%, O 7.85%. Nucleotide analog with broad-spectrum anticoccidial activity. Prepn: G. M. Boeckx *et al.*, EP 170316; *eidem*, US 4631278 (both 1986 to Janssen). Mechanism of action studies: L. Maes *et al.*, *J. Parasitol.* **74**, 931 (1988); A. Verheyen *et al.*, ibid. 939. Efficacy against *Eimeria* species in turkeys: O. Vanparijs *et al.*, *Avian Dis.* **33**, 479 (1989); in chickens: O. Vanparijs *et al.*, *Poult. Sci.* **69**, 60 (1990). Preliminary evaluation in coccidial enteritis in AIDS patients: K. Kayembe *et al.*, *Lancet* **1**, 1397 (1989).

mp 290.5°.

THERAP CAT (VET): Coccidiostat.

3081. Diclofenac. [15307-86-5] 2-[(2,6-Dichlorophenyl)-amino]benzeneacetic acid; [*o*-(2,6-dichloroanilino)phenyl]acetic acid; Motifene. $C_{14}H_{11}Cl_2NO_2$; mol wt 296.15. C 56.78%, H 3.74%, Cl 23.94%, N 4.73%, O 10.80%. Prepn: NL 6604752; A. Sallmann, R. Pfister, US 3558690 (1966, 1971 both to Geigy). Pharmacology: Renaud, Lecompte, *Thromb. Diath. Haemorrh.* **24**, 577 (1970), *C.A.* **74**, 86215m (1971); Krupp *et al.*, *Experientia* **29**, 450 (1973). HPLC determn in plasma and urine: J. Godbillon *et al.*, *J. Chromatogr.* **338**, 151 (1985). Symposium on pharmacology and clinical experience: *Semin. Arthritis Rheum.* **15**, Suppl. 1, 57-110 (1985); on pharmacology, efficacy and safety: *Am. J. Med.* **80**, Suppl. 4B, 1-87 (1986). Comprehensive description: C. M. Adeyeye, P-K. Li, *Anal. Profiles Drug Subs.* **19**, 123-144 (1990). Review of clinical trials in actinic keratosis: D. C. Peters, R. H. Foster, *Drugs Aging* **14**, 313-319 (1999).

Crystals from ether-petr ether, mp 156-158°.

Diethylammonium salt. [78213-16-8] Voltarol. $C_{14}H_{11}Cl_2$-$NO_2 \cdot C_4H_{11}N$; mol wt 369.29.

Sodium salt. [15307-79-6] GP-45840; Allvoran; Benfofen; Dealgic; Deflamat; Delphinac; Dicloflex; Diclomax; Diclophlogont; Dicloreum; Duravolten; Ecofenac; Effekton; Lexobene; Neriodin; Novapirina; Primofenac; Prophenatin; Rewodina; Rhumalgan; Voldal; Voltaren; Xenid. $C_{14}H_{10}Cl_2NNaO_2$; mol wt 318.13. Crystals from water, mp 283-285°. uv max (methanol) 283 nm (ε 1.05 × 10^5); (phosphate buffer, pH 7.2) 276 nm (ε 1.01 × 10^5). Soly at 25°C (mg/ml): deionized water (pH 5.2) >9; methanol >24; acetone 6; acetonitrile <1; cyclohexane <1; HCl (pH 1.1) <1; phosphate buffer (pH 7.2) 6. pKa 4. Partition coefficient (*N*-octanol/aq. buffer): 13.4. LD_{50} in mice, rats (mg/kg): ~390, 150 orally (Krupp).

Potassium salt. [15307-81-0] CGP-45840B; Cataflam. C_{14}-$H_{10}Cl_2KNO_2$; mol wt 334.24.

THERAP CAT: Anti-inflammatory.

3082. Diclofop-methyl. [51338-27-3] 2-[4-(2,4-Dichlorophenoxy)phenoxy]propanoic acid methyl ester; methyl 2-[4-(2,4-dichlorophenoxy)phenoxy]propionate; HOE-23408; Hoelon; Hoegrass; Illoxan. $C_{16}H_{14}Cl_2O_4$; mol wt 341.19. C 56.32%, H 4.14%, Cl 20.78%, O 18.76%. Selective post-emergence herbicide. Prepn: W. Becker *et al.*, DE 2223894; *eidem*, US 3954442 (1973, 1976 to Hoechst). Soil degradn: A. E. Smith, *J. Agric. Food Chem.* **25**, 893 (1977); **27**, 1145 (1979).

mp 39-41°. $bp_{0.1}$ 175-177°. Soly in water: 0.3 mg/100 ml. Soly (g/100 ml): acetone 249; ethanol 11; xylene 253.

USE: Herbicide.

3083. Diclosulam. [145701-21-9] *N*-(2,6-Dichlorophenyl)-5-ethoxy-7-fluoro[1,2,4]triazolo[1,5-*c*]pyrimidine-2-sulfonamide; XDE-564; Strongarm. $C_{13}H_{10}Cl_2FN_5O_3S$; mol wt 406.22. C 38.44%, H 2.48%, Cl 17.46%, F 4.68%, N 17.24%, O 11.82%, S 7.89%. Pre-emergent, soil-applied herbicide for broadleaf weed control in peanuts and soybeans. Prepn: J. C. Van Heertum *et al.*, EP 343752; *eidem*, US 5163995 (1989, 1992 both to DowElanco). Field study in peanuts: W. A. Bailey *et al.*, *Weed Technol.* **13**, 450, 771 (1999); W. J. Grichar *et al.*, *Peanut Sci.* **26**, 23 (1999). Field trial in soybeans: D. R. Shaw *et al.*, *Weed Technol.* **13**, 791 (1999).

Consult the Name Index before using this section.

mp 234-237°.
USE: Herbicide.

3084. Dicloxacillin. [3116-76-5] (2*S*,5*R*,6*R*)-6-[[[3-(2,6-Dichlorophenyl)-5-methyl-4-isoxazolyl]carbonyl]amino]-3,3-dimethyl-7-oxo-4-thia-1-azabicyclo[3.2.0]heptane-2-carboxylic acid; 6-[3-(2,6-dichlorophenyl)-5-methyl-4-isoxazolecarboxamido]-penicillanic acid; 3-(2,6-dichlorophenyl)-5-methyl-4-isoxazolylpenicillin; BRL-1702; Maclicine. $C_{19}H_{17}Cl_2N_3O_5S$; mol wt 470.33. C 48.52%, H 3.64%, Cl 15.08%, N 8.93%, O 17.01%, S 6.82%. Semi-synthetic antibiotic related to penicillin. Prepn: J. H. C. Naylor, **GB 978299**; *eidem,* **US 3239507** (1965, 1969 to Beecham). Toxicity data: C. Gloxhuber *et al., Arzneim.-Forsch.* **15,** 322 (1965). Series of articles on chemistry, pharmacology and toxicology: *ibid.* 322-348; Matsuzaki, *Jpn. J. Antibiot.* **21,** 274, 284 (1968), *C.A.* **70,** 95267z, 95265x (1969).

Sodium salt monohydrate. [13412-64-1] Sodium dicloxacillin monohydrate; P-1011; Brispen; Dichlor-Stapenor; Diclocil; Dycill; Dynapen; Noxaben; Pathocil; Pen-Sint; Syntarpen; Veracillin. C_{19}-$H_{16}Cl_2N_3NaO_5S.H_2O$; mol wt 510.32. Crystals, dec 222-225°. $[\alpha]_D^{20}$ +127.2° (water). Sol in water, methanol; less sol in butanol; slightly sol in acetone and the usual organic solvents. LD_{50} in mice (g/kg): 0.9 i.v.; in rats (g/kg): 0.63 i.p.; >5 orally (Gloxhuber).

THERAP CAT: Antibacterial.

THERAP CAT (VET): Antibacterial.

3085. Dicobalt Octacarbonyl. [10210-68-1] Di-μ-carbonylhexacarbonyldicobalt; octacarbonyldicobalt; cobalt tetracarbonyl; cobalt octacarbonyl. $C_8Co_2O_8$; mol wt 341.95. C 28.10%, Co 34.47%, O 37.43%. $Co_2(CO)_8$. Prepn: Mond *et al., J. Chem. Soc.* **97,** 798 (1910); Gilmont, Blanchard, *Inorg. Synth.* **2,** 238 (1946); Wender *et al., ibid.* **5,** 190 (1957); Chini *et al., Chim. Ind. (Milan)* **55,** 120 (1973). Crystal structure: Sumner *et al., Acta Crystallogr.* **17,** 732 (1964). Two isomeric forms exist in soln: Noack, *Spectrochim. Acta* **19,** 1925 (1963); Bor, *ibid.* 2065; Noack, *Helv. Chim. Acta* **47,** 1064, 1555 (1964). Toxicity studies: Kincaid *et al., Arch. Ind. Hyg. Occup. Med.* **10,** 210 (1954); Brief *et al., Arch. Environ. Health* **23,** 373 (1971); Kalekin, *C.A.* **78,** 67751z (1973); Spiridonova, Shabalina, *Gig. Sanit.* **1973,** 73, *C.A.* **78,** 119835b (1973). Reviews of prepn, properties and chemistry of cobalt carbonyls: I. Wender *et al., Bull. U.S. Bur. Mines* **600,** 83 pp (1960); *Organic Syntheses via Metal Carbonyls* vol. 1, I. Wender, P. Pino, Eds. (Interscience, New York, 1968) *passim;* Chalk, Harrod, "Catalysis by Cobalt Carbonyls" in *Adv. Organomet. Chem.* **6,** 119-170 (1968); Nicholls in *Comprehensive Inorganic Chemistry* vol. 3, J. C. Bailar, Jr. *et al.,* Eds. (Pergamon Press, Oxford, 1973) pp 1059-1064.

Orange platelets obtained by vacuum sublimation. d 1.87. mp 51°; dec above 52°. Stable in atm of H_2 and CO; dec on exposure to air. Insol in water. Sol in organic solvents such as ether, alcohol, CS_2, naphtha. Slowly attacked by HCl, H_2SO_4, more rapidly by HNO_3, Br_2. LD_{50} in mice, rats (mg/kg): 377.7, 753.8 by gavage (Spiridonova, Shabalina).

Cobalt carbonyl hydride. Cobalt hydrocarbonyl; tetracarbonylhydridocobalt; tetracarbonylhydrocobalt. C_4HCoO_4; mol wt 171.98. Unstable catalytic intermediate; active species in some reactions catalyzed by $Co_2(CO)_8$. Yellow, toxic, foul-smelling liquid. mp −26°. Dec at room temp to $Co_2(CO)_8$. Sparingly

sol in water (3×10^{-3} moles/l); behaves as a strong acid. Readily oxidized in air.

Caution: Potential symptoms of overexposure are irritation of eyes, skin, mucous membranes; cough, decreased pulmonary function, wheezing, dyspnea. *See NIOSH Pocket Guide to Chemical Hazards* (DHHS/NIOSH 97-140, 1997) p 74.

USE: Catalyst for hydroformylation, hydrogenation, hydrosilation, isomerization, carboxylation, carbonylation and polymerization reactions.

3086. Dicofol. [115-32-2] 4-Chloro-α-(4-chlorophenyl)-α-(trichloromethyl)benzenemethanol; 4,4′-dichloro-α-(trichloromethyl)benzhydrol; 1,1-bis(*p*-chlorophenyl)-2,2,2-trichloroethanol; di(*p*-chlorophenyl)trichloromethylcarbinol; DTMC; ENT-23648; FW-293; Acarin; Kelthane; Mitigan. $C_{14}H_9Cl_5O$; mol wt 370.49. C 45.39%, H 2.45%, Cl 47.85%, O 4.32%. Prepn: Wilson, Craig, **US 2812280**; Wilson, Wolffe, **US 2812362** (both 1957 to Rohm & Haas); Bergmann, Kaluszyner, *J. Org. Chem.* **23,** 1306 (1958); **GB 831421** (1960 to Metal & Thermit Corp.). Miticidal activity: J. S. Baker, F. B. Maughan, *J. Econ. Entomol.* **49,** 458 (1956). Toxicology: R. B. Smith *et al., Toxicol. Appl. Pharmacol.* **1,** 119 (1959). Metabolism: J. R. Brown *et al., ibid.* **15,** 30 (1969); K. Tabata *et al., Appl. Entomol. Zool.* **14,** 490 (1979). Review of carcinogenic risk: *IARC Monographs* **30,** 87-101 (1983).

Crystals from petr ether, mp 77-78°. uv max (ethanol): 226, 258, 266, 276 nm (4.43, 2.82, 2.85, 2.60). Practically insol in water. Sol in most aliphatic and aromatic solvents. LD_{50} in rats (mg/kg): 1495 orally; 1150 i.p. (Brown).

USE: Acaricide.

3087. Dicrotophos. [141-66-2] Phosphoric acid 3-(dimethylamino)-1-methyl-3-oxo-1-propenyl dimethyl ester; phosphoric acid dimethyl ester, ester with *cis*-3-hydroxy-*N,N*-dimethylcrotonamide; 3-(dimethoxyphosphinyloxy)-*N,N*-dimethyl-*cis*-crotonamide; dimethyl 2-dimethylcarbamoyl-1-methylvinyl phosphate; dimethyl 1-dimethylcarbamoyl-1-propen-2-yl phosphate; C-709; ENT-24482; SD-3562; Bidrin. $C_8H_{16}NO_5P$; mol wt 237.19. C 40.51%, H 6.80%, N 5.91%, O 33.73%, P 13.06%. Cholinesterase inhibitor. Prepn of diethyl ester: Whetstone, Stiles, **US 2802855** (1957 to Shell). Activity: R. A. Corey, *J. Econ. Entomol.* **58,** 112 (1965). Metabolism and degradn: R. I. Beynon *et al., Residue Rev.* **47,** 55 (1973). Toxicity data: T. B. Gaines, *Toxicol. Appl. Pharmacol.* **14,** 515 (1969).

Liquid, commercial grade is brown. bp_{760} 400°. d_{15}^{15} 1.216. n_D^{23} 1.468. Misc with water, ethanol, xylene; somewhat sol in kerosene. Dec at 90° after 7 days; at 75° after 31 days. LD_{50} in female, male rats (mg/kg): 16, 21 orally; 42, 43 dermally (Gaines).

Caution: Potential symptoms of overexposure are headache, nausea, dizziness, anxiety, restlessness, muscle twitching, weakness, tremor, incoordination, vomiting, abdominal cramps, diarrhea; salivation, sweating, lacrimation, rhinitis; anorexia, malaise. *See NIOSH Pocket Guide to Chemical Hazards* (DHHS/NIOSH 97-140, 1997) p 102.

USE: Insecticide.

3088. Dicryl. [2164-09-2] *N*-(3,4-Dichlorophenyl)-2-methyl-2-propenamide; 3′,4′-dichloro-2-methylacrylanilide; *N*-(3,4-dichlorophenyl)methacrylamide; chloranocryl; Niagara 4556. C_{10}-H_9Cl_2NO; mol wt 230.09. C 52.20%, H 3.94%, Cl 30.82%, N 6.09%, O 6.95%. Post-emergence herbicide. Prepn from 3,4-dichloroaniline with methacryloyl chloride in the presence of triethylamine. Prepd but not claimed: Thompson, **US 3169850** (1965).

Toxicity study: G. W. Bailey, J. L. White, *Residue Rev.* **10**, 97 (1965).

Crystals from ethanol + petr ether, mp 128°. Practically insol in water. Soluble in acetone, alcohol, isophorone, dimethyl sulfoxide. LD$_{50}$ orally in rats: 3160 mg/kg (Bailey, White).

USE: Herbicide.

3089. Dictamnine. [484-29-7] 4-Methoxyfuro[2,3-*b*]quinoline; dictamine. C$_{12}$H$_9$NO$_2$; mol wt 199.21. C 72.35%, H 4.55%, N 7.03%, O 16.06%. Alkaloid from root of *Dictamnus albus* Linn., *Skimmia repens* Nakai, *Aegle marmelos* Correa, *Zanthoxylum alatum* Roxb., *Rutaceae:* Thoms, *Ber.* **33**, 68 (1923); Asahina *et al.*, *ibid.* **63**, 2045 (1930); Chatterjee, Roy, *J. Indian Chem. Soc.* **36**, 267 (1959); Deb *et al., ibid.* **39**, 493 (1962). Structure: M. F. Brundon, N. J. McCorkindale, *Chem. Ind. (London)* **1956**, 1091. Synthesis: Tuppy, Bohm, *Angew. Chem.* **68**, 388 (1956); M. Sato *et al., Chem. Pharm. Bull.* **35**, 1319 (1987).

Prisms from alcohol, ethyl acetate, benzene + ethyl acetate, mp 133°. Sol in hot alcohol, chloroform; slightly sol in ether. Practically insol in water.

Hydrochloride. C$_{12}$H$_9$NO$_2$.HCl. Needles from alcohol, dec 170°.

3090. Dicumarol. [66-76-2] 3,3′-Methylenebis[4-hydroxy-2*H*-1-benzopyran-2-one]; 3,3′-methylenebis[4-hydroxycoumarin]; bishydroxycoumarin (rescinded); Dicoumarol; Dicoumarin; Dicumol; Melitoxin. C$_{19}$H$_{12}$O$_6$; mol wt 336.29. C 67.86%, H 3.60%, O 28.55%. Originally isolated from spoiled sweet clover (improperly cured Melilotus hay): Link *et al., J. Biol. Chem.* **138**, 21, 513, 529 (1941); **142**, 941 (1942); now prepd synthetically by the action of formaldehyde on 4-hydroxycoumarin (obtained as the Na derivative by the action of sodium metal on methyl acetylsalicylate): Link, *Fed. Proc.* **4**, 176 (1945), and patents (The Wisconsin Alumni Res. Found.). Toxicity data: Rose *et al., Proc. Soc. Exp. Biol. Med.* **50**, 228 (1942).

Minute crystals. Slight pleasant odor. Has a slightly bitter taste. mp 287-293°. Sol in aq alkaline solns, in pyridine and similar organic bases. Slightly sol in benzene and chloroform. Practically insol in water, alcohol, ether. LD$_{50}$ orally in rats: 541.6 mg/kg (Rose).

THERAP CAT: Anticoagulant.

3091. Dicyanine. [52260-69-2] 1-Ethyl-2-[3-(1-ethyl-2-methyl-4(1*H*)-quinolinylidene)-1-propenyl]-4-methylquinolinium iodide; 1-ethyl-2-[3-(1-ethyl-4(1*H*)-quinaldylidene)propenyl]-lepidinium iodide; 1-ethyl-2-[3-(1-ethyl-2-methyl-4(1*H*)-quinolylidene)propenyl]-4-methylquinolinium iodide; 2′,4-dimethyl-1,1′-diethyl-2,4′-carbocyanine iodide. C$_{27}$H$_{29}$IN$_2$; mol wt 508.44. C 63.78%, H 5.75%, I 24.96%, N 5.51%. Prepn by J. A. Aeschlimann as reported by Mills, Odams, *J. Chem. Soc.* **125**, 1913 (1924). See also *Beilstein* 2nd suppl. **vol. 23**, p 284. Has photoconductive properties that increase sharply with a rise in temp and is classed as an O$_2$-photoconductor: Meier, *Z. Phys. Chem. (Leipzig)* **208**, 325 (1958). Gives a color reaction with magnesium ions: Babenko, *Zh. Anal. Khim.* **13**, 496 (1958).

Olive-green crystals with metallic sheen from methanol. Crystals are usually solvated. Drying at 110° expels methanol of crystn. Decomp 244-252°. Absorption max (methanol): 603.5, 655.5 nm (A$_{1cm}^{1\%}$ 63, 218). Soly in methanol: about 2%. Methanol solns appear deep blue when viewed under incident daylight. Soly in water about 0.2%. Aq solns are dichroic and may appear brownish green. Also sol in abs ethanol (0.5%), in ethylene glycol (1.5%), and in Cellosolve (2.0%). Practically insol in benzene, xylene.

USE: In color photography (sensitizer for extreme reds). Diagnostic stain for cytodiagnosis of ruptured fetal membranes.

3092. Dicyanodiamide. [461-58-5] Cyanoguanidine. C$_2$H$_4$N$_4$; mol wt 84.08. C 28.57%, H 4.80%, N 66.64%. Prepared by controlled polymerization of cyanamide in water in the presence of ammonia, alkaline earth hydroxides, or other suitable bases: Grube, Nitsche, *Z. Angew. Chem.* **27**, 368 (1914); Pinck, Hetherington, *Ind. Eng. Chem.* **27**, 834 (1935); Pinck, *Inorg. Synth.* **3**, 43 (1950).

Monoclinic prismatic crystals from water or alcohol, mp 209.5°. d$_4^{25}$ 1.400. Eutectic with cyanamide at 35.6° (15% dicyanodiamide). Specific heat 0.456 at 0-204°. Neutral reaction. Soly in water at 13°: 2.26%, more sol in hot water. Solns above 80° dec slowly, yielding ammonia. Soly in abs ethanol at 13°: 1.26%; in ether: 0.01%. Insol in benzene, chloroform. Sol in liq ammonia.

USE: In the plastics industry (manuf of melamine). In the pharmaceutical industry (barbiturates, guanidine derivs).

3093. Dicyanodiamidine Sulfate. [591-01-5] (Aminoiminomethyl)urea sulfate (2:1); biuretamidine sulfate; carbamylguanidine sulfate; guanylurea sulfate. C$_4$H$_{14}$N$_8$O$_6$S; mol wt 302.27. C 15.89%, H 4.67%, N 37.07%, O 31.76%, S 10.61%. Prepd by heating dicyanodiamide with H$_2$SO$_4$ and H$_2$O.

Dihydrate. White needles. At 110° loses its water. Sol in about 20 parts cold, 3 parts boiling water; slightly sol in alc.

USE: For detecting and determining Ni and its separation from Co and other metals.

3094. 9-Dicyanomethylene-2,4,7-trinitrofluorene. [1172-02-7] (2,4,7-trinitro-9*H*-fluoren-9-ylidene)propanedinitrile; DTF. C$_{16}$H$_5$N$_5$O$_6$; mol wt 363.24. C 52.90%, H 1.39%, N 19.28%, O 26.43%. Prepn from 2,4,7-trinitrofluorenone: Mukherjee, Levasseur, *J. Org. Chem.* **30**, 644 (1965).

Yellow crystals from acetonitrile, mp 266-268°. uv max (dichloromethane): 365 nm (log ε 4.38).

USE: Forms charge-transfer complexes with aromatic hydrocarbons and amines.

3095. Dicyclohexylamine. [101-83-7] *N*-Cyclohexylcyclohexanamine; dodecahydrodiphenylamine. $C_{12}H_{23}N$; mol wt 181.32. C 79.49%, H 12.79%, N 7.72%. Prepn by hydrogenation of equimolar amounts of cyclohexanone and cyclohexylamine: C. F. Winans, H. Adkins, *J. Org. Chem.* **54**, 306 (1932); R. M. Robinson, W. C. Braaten, US 3154580 (1964 to Abbott). Forms crystalline derivatives with *N*-protected amino acids: E. Klieger *et al.*, *Ann.* **640**, 157 (1961). *Review:* T. S. Carswell, H. L. Morrill, *Ind. Eng. Chem.* **29**, 1265 (1937).

Liquid. Faint fishy odor. d_{25}^{25} 0.9104. mp −0.1°. pKa 10.4. bp$_{760}$ 255.8°; bp$_{300}$ 214.5°; bp$_{200}$ 199.0°; bp$_{100}$ 174.4°; bp$_{50}$ 154.3°; bp$_{25}$ 135.4°; bp$_{11}$ 121°; bp$_{4}$ 99.3°; bp$_{1.0}$ 83°. n_D^{25} 1.4823. Flash pt: 110°C. Strong base. Sparingly sol in water; sol in the usual organic solvents. Miscible with cyclohexylamine. Readily forms adducts with solvents.

Caution: A skin irritant and possible sensitizer.

USE: Industrial solvent; corrosion inhibitor.

3096. Dicyclohexylcarbodiimide. [538-75-0] *N,N′*-Methanetetraylbiscyclohexanamine; carbodicyclohexylimide; DCC; DCCI. $C_{13}H_{22}N_2$; mol wt 206.33. C 75.67%, H 10.75%, N 13.58%. Coupling agent in peptide synthesis: Sheehan, Hess, *J. Am. Chem. Soc.* **77**, 1067 (1955); Khorana, *Chem. Ind. (London)* **1955**, 1087. Prepn: Schmidt *et al.*, *Ber.* **71**, 1933 (1938); Schmidt, Schnegg, US 2656383 (1953 to Bayer); Stevens *et al.*, *J. Org. Chem.* **32**, 2895 (1967); Bestmann *et al.*, *Ann.* **718**, 24 (1968).

Cryst mass, mp 35-36°. bp$_{11}$ 154-156°; bp$_{0.5}$ 98-100°.

Caution: Contact allergen.

USE: In the synthesis of peptides.

3097. Dicyclomine. [77-19-0] [1,1′-Bicyclohexyl]-1-carboxylic acid 2-(diethylamino)ethyl ester; β-diethylaminoethyl 1-cyclohexylcyclohexanecarboxylate; bis(cyclohexyl)carboxylic acid diethylaminoethyl ester; dicycloverin. $C_{19}H_{35}NO_2$; mol wt 309.49. C 73.74%, H 11.40%, N 4.53%, O 10.34%. Anticholinergic; binds to muscarinic M_1 receptors. Prepn: C. H. Tilford *et al.*, *J. Am. Chem. Soc.* **69**, 2903 (1947); M. G. Van Campen, C. H. Tilford, US 2474796 (1949 to Merrell). Receptor binding study: H. Kilbinger, A. Stein, *Br. J. Pharmacol.* **94**, 1270 (1988). Capillary GC determn in plasma: B. J. Walker *et al.*, *J. Chromatogr.* **416**, 150 (1987). Clinical trial in functional abdominal pain: M. G. Grillage *et al.*, *Br. J. Clin. Pract.* **44**, 176 (1990).

Hydrochloride. [67-92-5] Bentyl; Bentylol; Merbentyl; Wyovin. $C_{19}H_{35}NO_2 \cdot HCl$; mol wt 345.95. Crystals from butanone, mp 164-166°. Bitter taste. Sol in water; freely sol in alcohol, chloroform; very slightly sol in ether.

THERAP CAT: Antispasmodic.

3098. Didanosine. [69655-05-6] 2′,3′-Dideoxyinosine; dideoxyinosine; ddI; ddIno; BMY-40900; NSC-612049; Videx. $C_{10}H_{12}N_4O_3$; mol wt 236.23. C 50.84%, H 5.12%, N 23.72%, O 20.32%. Hypoxanthine nucleoside with antiviral activity; metabolic product of dideoxyadenosine, *q.v.* Enzymatic prepn from

dideoxyadenosine: W. Plunkett, S. S. Cohen, *Cancer Res.* **35**, 1547 (1975). Synthesis: G. W. Koszalka, T. A. Krenitsky, **EP 206497** (1986 to Wellcome Found.); R. R. Webb *et al.*, *Nucleosides Nucleotides* **7**, 147 (1988). *In vitro* inhibition of HIV-I: H. Mitsuya, S. Broder, *Proc. Natl. Acad. Sci. USA* **83**, 1911 (1986); of HIV-II: D. D. Richman, *Antimicrob. Agents Chemother.* **31**, 1879 (1987). Antiretroviral spectrum *in vitro:* J. E. Dahlberg *et al.*, *Proc. Natl. Acad. Sci. USA* **84**, 2469 (1987). Cellular pharmacol in cloned human T-cells: G. Ahluwalia *et al.*, *Biochem. Pharmacol.* **36**, 3797 (1987). HPLC determn in human plasma: G. Ray, E. Murrill, *Anal. Lett.* **20**, 1815 (1987). Clinical evaluations in AIDS: J. S. Lambert *et al.*, *N. Engl. J. Med.* **322**, 1333 (1990); T. P. Cooley *et al.*, *ibid.* 1340. Comprehensive description: M. N. Nassar *et al.*, *Anal. Profiles Drug Subs. Excip.* **22**, 185-227 (1993).

White solid, mp 160-163°. Soly at 23° (mg/ml): acetone <1; acetonitrile <1; *t*-butanol <1; chloroform <1; dimethylacetamide 45; DMSO 200; ethanol 1; ethyl acetate <1; hexane <1; methanol 6; methylene chloride <1; polyethylene glycol-300 1; 1-propanol <1; 2-propanol <1; propylene glycol 8. pKa 9.12 ±0.02. Partition coefficient (1-octanol/0.05*M* phosphate buffer pH 7) 0.068 ±0.005. $[\alpha]_D^{25}$ −26.3° (c = 10 in water). uv max 240 nm (pH 2); 254 nm (pH 12).

THERAP CAT: Antiviral.

3099. Didecyldimethylammonium Chloride. [7173-51-5] *N*-Decyl-*N,N*-dimethyl-1-decanaminium chloride; dimethyldidecylammonium chloride; Bardac 2250/2280; BTC-1010; Dodigen 1881; Querton 210CL. $C_{22}H_{48}ClN$; mol wt 362.08. C 72.98%, H 13.36%, Cl 9.79%, N 3.87%. Quaternary alkyl ammonium compound with fungicidal and bactericidal activity. Prepn: A. W. Ralston *et al.*, *J. Org. Chem.* **13**, 186 (1948). Conductivity of aqueous soln: *eidem*, *J. Am. Chem. Soc.* **70**, 977 (1948). Mothproofing agent: A. M. Schwartz, C. A. Rader, US 3746767 (1971 to USDA). In carpet dyeing: F. F. Bartsch, R. Feigin, US 3758269 (1971 to Sybron). Germicidal activity: R. J. Wright, DE 2810998; *eidem*, US 4272395 (1978, 1981 both to Unilever). Ion-pair extracting agent in carbapenem isoln: J. D. Hood *et al.*, *J. Antibiot.* **32**, 295 (1979). In froth-flotation recovery of metals: V. Petrovich, US 4225428 (1980). Eliminates ice-nucleating effect of bacteria in plants: E. A. Youngman, R. C. Schnell, EP 37593; *eidem*, US 4311517 (1981, 1982 both to Shell). Breaks oil-in-water emulsions created during oil-spill recovery procedures: J. Newcombe, US 4374734 (1983 to Cities Service). Fungidal wood preservative: A. F. Preston: *J. Am. Oil Chem. Soc.* **60**, 567 (1983).

Extremely hygroscopic. Sol in acetone, extremely sol in benzene. Insol in hexane.

Caution: Causes eye damage and skin irritation. Harmful if swallowed.

USE: General purpose disinfectant, sanitizer; mildew preventative in commercial laundries; water treatment in cooling towers and oil field flood waters; wood preservative.

3100. Didemnins. Biologically active depsipeptides extracted from a Caribbean tunicate (sea squirt) family *Didemnidae*, genus *Trididemnum*. First marine natural product to enter clinical trials as antineoplastic. The three components, didemnins A, B and C are basic compds with antiviral, antitumor activity. Didemnin A is the most abundant, whereas didemnin B is generally the most active. Isoln and bioactivity: K. L. Rinehart, Jr. *et al.*,

Science **212**, 933 (1981). Extraction and purification: K. L. Rinehart, Jr., **EP 48149**; *idem*, **US 4493796** (1982, 1985 both to Univ. Illinois). Structure determn: K. L. Rinehart, Jr. *et al., J. Am. Chem. Soc.* **103**, 1857 (1981). Revised structure and total synthesis: K. L. Rinehart, Jr. *et al., ibid.* **109**, 6846 (1987). *See also:* U. Schmidt *et al., Tetrahedron Lett.* **29**, 3057 (1988); *eidem, ibid.* 4407. Crystal structure of B: M. B. Hossain *et al., Proc. Natl. Acad. Sci. USA* **85**, 4118 (1988). Efficient total synthesis of A and B: Y. Hamada *et al., J. Am. Chem. Soc.* **111**, 669 (1989). Mechanism of action study: L. H. Li *et al., Cancer Lett.* **23**, 279 (1984). *In vitro* and *in vivo* immunosuppressive activity of B: D. W. Montgomery, C. F. Zukowski, *Transplantation* **40**, 49 (1985). HPLC determn in biological fluids: J. N. Hartshorn *et al., J. Liq. Chromatogr.* **9**, 1489 (1986). Clinical pharmacology, pharmacokinetics: F. A. Dorr *et al., Eur. J. Cancer Clin. Oncol.* **24**, 1699 (1988). Review of bioactivity of A and B: K. L. Rinehart, Jr. *et al., Fed. Proc.* **42**, 87-90 (1983); of activity and toxicology of B: H. G. Chun *et al., Invest. New Drugs* **4**, 279-284 (1986); of biological activity, structure and synthesis: W.-R. Li, M. M. Joullie, *Stud. Nat. Prod. Chem.* **10**, 241-302 (1992).

Didemnin A. [77327-04-9] $C_{49}H_{78}N_6O_{12}$; mol wt 943.18. Greenish-white solid. Sol in methanol, ethanol, dioxane, chloroform. Insol in water.

Didemnin B. [77327-05-0] NSC-325319. $C_{57}H_{89}N_7O_{15}$; mol wt 1112.35. Yellow-white amorphous solid. Sol in methanol, ethanol, dioxane, ethyl acetate, chloroform. Insol in water.

Didemnin C. [77327-06-1] $C_{52}H_{82}N_6O_{14}$; mol wt 1015.24. Oil. Sol in methanol, ethanol, isopropanol, dioxane, ethyl acetate and chloroform. Sparingly sol in toluene. Insol in water.

3101. Dideoxyadenosine. [4097-22-7] 2′,3′-Dideoxyadenosine; 6-amino-9-(2′,3′-dideoxy-β-D-*glycero*-pentofuranosyl)purine; DDA; ddAdo. $C_{10}H_{13}N_5O_2$; mol wt 235.24. C 51.06%, H 5.57%, N 29.77%, O 13.60%. Purine nucleoside analog with antiviral (retrovirus) activity. Prepn: M. J. Robins, R. K. Robins, *J. Am. Chem. Soc.* **86**, 3585 (1964); G. L. Tong *et al., J. Org. Chem.* **30**, 2854 (1965); J. R. McCarthy *et al., J. Am. Chem. Soc.* **88**, 1549 (1966). *In vitro* inhibition of bacterial DNA synthesis: L. Toji, S. S. Cohen, *Proc. Natl. Acad. Sci. USA* **63**, 871 (1969). Antibacterial activity in mice: G. Beskid *et al., Antimicrob. Agents Chemother.* **19**, 424 (1981). Inhibition of *in vitro* infectivity of HIV-1 virus: H. Mitsuya, S. Broder, *Proc. Natl. Acad. Sci. USA* **83**, 1911 (1986). HPLC determn in biological fluids: P. A. Blau *et al., J. Chromatogr.* **420**, 1 (1987). Metabolism by cloned human T-cells: D. A. Cooney *et al., Biochem. Pharmacol.* **36**, 1765 (1987).

Crystals from ethanol, mp 184-186°. $[\alpha]_D^{25}$ −25.2° (c = 1.01 in water). uv max in methanol: 259.5 nm (ε 14800).

THERAP CAT: Antiviral.

3102. DIDS. [53005-05-3] 2,2′-(1,2-Ethenediyl)bis[5-isothiocyanatobenzenesulfonic acid]; 4,4′-diisothiocyanato-2,2′-stilbenedisulfonic acid. $C_{16}H_{10}N_2O_6S_4$; mol wt 454.52. C 42.28%, H 2.22%, N 6.16%, O 21.12%, S 28.22%. Classic inhibitor of ion transport across biological membranes. Prepn: Z. I. Cabantchik, A. Rothstein, *J. Membr. Biol.* **10**, 311 (1972); of tritated form: S. Ship *et al., ibid.* **33**, 311 (1977). Inhibition of chloride transport: T. Janas *et al., Am. J. Physiol.* **257**, C601 (1989); J.-A. Kim *et al., Biochem. Biophys. Res. Commun.* **309**, 291 (2003); of non-selective cation conductance: A. Diakov *et al., Pflugers Arch. Eur. J. Physiol.* **442**, 700 (2001). Effects of ionic strength and pH on membrane penetration: V. A. Tverdislov *et al., Colloids Surfaces B* **5**, 205 (1995). Mechanism of inhibition in erythrocytes: J. M. Salhany, *Blood Cells Mol. Dis.* **27**, 901 (2001); of cardiac ryanodine receptor: A. P. Hill, R. Sitsapesan, *Biophys. J.* **82**, 3037 (2002).

White crystalline solid. uv max: 340 nm (ε 16000).

USE: Ion channel inhibitor; especially of anion transport.

3103. Dieldrin. [60-57-1] (1aα,2β,2aα,3β,6β,6aα,7β,7aα)-3,4,5,6,9,9-Hexachloro-1a,2,2a,3,6,6a,7,7a-octahydro-2,7:3,6-dimethanonaphth[2,3-b]oxirene; 1,2,3,4,10,10-hexachloro-6,7-epoxy-1,4,4a,5,6,7,8,8a-octahydro-*endo,exo*-1,4:5,8-dimethanonaphthalene; insecticide no. 497; HEOD; ENT-16225; compd 497; Octalox. $C_{12}H_8Cl_6O$; mol wt 380.91. C 37.84%, H 2.12%, Cl 55.84%, O 4.20%. Stereoisomer of endrin, *q.v.* Activity: C. W. Kearns *et al., J. Econ. Entomol.* **42**, 127 (1949). Prepn from aldrin, *q.v.*: Soloway, **US 2676131** (1954 to Shell); Payne, Smith, **US 2776301** (1957 to Shell). Synthesis: Korte, Rechmeier, *Ann.* **656**, 131 (1962). Metabolism: M. K. Baldwin *et al., Chem. Ind. (London)* **1970**, 595; C. T. Bedford, D. H. Hutson, *ibid.* **1976**, 440. Toxicity data: Gaines, *Toxicol. Appl. Pharmacol.* **14**, 515 (1969). Review of toxicology and human exposure: *Toxicological Profile for Aldrin/Dieldrin* (PB2003-100134, 2002) 354 pp.

Crystals, mp 176-177°. Vapor press at 20°: 3.1×10^{-6} mm Hg. Practically insol in water. Moderately sol in common organic solvents except aliphatic petr solvents and methyl alcohol. Stable in org and inorg alkalies and acids commonly used in agriculture. Affected by strong mineral acids. LD_{50} orally in rats: 46 mg/kg (Gaines).

Caution: Absorbed through skin, respiratory mucosa and GI tract. Potential symptoms of overexposure are malaise, headache, nausea, vomiting, dizziness, sweating, tremors, myoclonic limb jerks; clonic and tonic convulsions, coma, respiratory failure; leukocytosis, increased blood pressure, tachycardia, arrhythmia, metabolic acidosis, fever. Potential occupational carcinogen. *See*

NIOSH Pocket Guide to Chemical Hazards (DHHS/NIOSH 97-140, 1997) p 104; *Clinical Toxicology of Commercial Products*, R. E. Gosselin *et al.*, Eds. (Williams & Wilkins, Baltimore, 5th ed., 1984) Section III, pp 143-146.

USE: Formerly as insecticide.

3104. Dienestrol. [84-17-3] 4,4'-(1,2-Diethylidene-1,2-ethanediyl)bisphenol; 4,4'-(diethylideneethylene)diphenol; 3,4-bis(*p*-hydroxyphenyl)-2,4-hexadiene; 4,4'-dihydroxy-γ,δ-diphenyl-β,δ-hexadiene; di(*p*-oxyphenyl)-2,4-hexadiene; dienoestrol; estrodienol; Cycladiene; Dienol; Dinovex; DV; Estroral; Gynefollin; Hormofemin; Oestrasid; Oestrodiene; Oestroral; Restrol; Retalon; Synestrol. $C_{18}H_{18}O_2$; mol wt 266.33. C 81.17%, H 6.81%, O 12.01%. Synthesis: Dodds *et al.*, *Proc. Roy. Soc.* **127B**, 162 (1939); Hobday, Short, *J. Chem. Soc.* **1943**, 609; Short, Hobday, US 2464203 (1949 to Boots); Adler, US 2465505 (1949 to Hoffmann-La Roche). Configuration: Koch, *Nature* **161**, 309 (1948); Lane, Spialter, *J. Am. Chem. Soc.* **73**, 4408 (1951).

(trans-trans)-form

Minute needles from dil alcohol, mp 227-228°. Sublimes at 130° and 1 mm Hg. The sublimate mp 231-234°. Freely sol in alcohol, methanol, ether, acetone, propylene glycol; sol in chloroform, aq solns of alkali hydroxides; sol in vegetable oils after warming, but crystallizes out on standing. Practically insol in water, dil acids.

Diacetate. [84-19-5] Lipamone; Retalon-Oral. $C_{22}H_{22}O_4$; mol wt 350.41. Prisms from alc, mp 119-120°.

THERAP CAT: Estrogen.

THERAP CAT (VET): Estrogenic hormone therapy.

3105. Dienochlor. [2227-17-0] 1,1',2,2',3,3',4,4',5,5'-Decachlorobi-2,4-cyclopentadien-1-yl; bis(pentachloro-2,4-cyclopentadien-1-yl); decachlor; HRS-16; Pentac. $C_{10}Cl_{10}$; mol wt 474.64. C 25.30%, Cl 74.69%. Acaricide to control mites on ornamental plants. Prepn from hexachlorocyclopentadiene, characterization: E. T. McBee *et al.*, *J. Am. Chem. Soc.* **77**, 4375 (1955). Prepn and rubber vulcanizing props: E. C. Ladd, US 2732409 (1956 to U.S. Rubber). Prepn and insecticidal props: J. T. Rucker, US 2934470 (1960 to Hooker). Effectiveness as miticide: W. W. Allen *et al.*, *J. Econ. Entomol.* **57**, 187 (1964). Crystal structure: G. Smith *et al.*, *J. Chem. Soc. Perkin Trans.* 2 **1976**, 796. Photodegradation: G. B. Quistad, K. M. Mulholland, *J. Agric. Food Chem.* **31**, 621 (1983). Effect on oogenesis of Mexican bean beetle: P. R. Hughes, M. A. Penton, *J. Econ. Entomol.* **76**, 1156 (1983).

Yellow prisms from petr ether, mp 121.5-122°. uv max: 330 nm (ε 2950). Stable to alkali.

USE: Miticide.

3106. Dienogest. [65928-58-7] (17α)-17-Hydroxy-3-oxo-19-norpregna-4,9-diene-21-nitrile; 17α-cyanomethyl-17β-hydroxy-13β-methylgona-4,9-dien-3-one; 17α-cyanomethyl-17β-hydroxy-4,9-estradien-3-one; dienogestril; STS-557; Endometrion. $C_{20}H_{25}$-NO_2; mol wt 311.42. C 77.14%, H 8.09%, N 4.50%, O 10.28%. Derivative of 19-nortestosterone. Prepn: K. Ponsold *et al.*, DE 2718872; *eidem*, US 4167517 (1977, 1979 both to VEB Jenapharm); M. Hübner *et al.*, *Arzneim.-Forsch.* **30**, 401 (1980). Structure-activity study: M Hübner, K. Ponsold, *Exp. Clin. Endocrinol.* **81**, 109 (1983). Evaluation of combination with estrogen as oral contraceptive: J. Spona *et al.*, *Contraception* **56**, 185 (1997); as hormone

replacement therapy: T. Gräser *et al.*, *Maturitas* **35**, 253 (2000). Review of pharmacology and clinical experience: R. H. Foster, M. I. Wilde, *Drugs* **56**, 825-833 (1998).

Needles from ethyl acetate + acetonitrile, mp 209-214°. $[\alpha]_D^{25}$ -290° (c = 0.5 in pyridine).

Mixture with ethinyl estradiol. [170475-05-5] Certostat; Valette.

THERAP CAT: Progestogen. In combination with estrogen as oral contraceptive.

3107. Diethanolamine. [111-42-2] 2,2'-Iminobisethanol; 2,2'-iminodiethanol; diethylolamine; bis(hydroxyethyl)amine; 2,2'-dihydroxydiethylamine. $C_4H_{11}NO_2$; mol wt 105.14. C 45.69%, H 10.55%, N 13.32%, O 30.43%. $(HOCH_2CH_2)_2NH$. Produced along with mono- and triethanolamine by ammonolysis of ethylene oxide. *See refs under* Ethanolamine. Toxicity study: H. F. Smyth *et al.*, *J. Ind. Hyg. Toxicol.* **23**, 259 (1941).

Deliquescent prisms, mp 28°. Usually offered as a viscous liquid. Mild ammoniacal odor. d_4^{30} 1.0881; d_4^{60} 1.0693. One U.S. gallon weighs 9.09 lbs at 30°. Viscosity at 30°: 351.9 cP; at 60°: 53.85 cP. bp_{760} 268.8°; bp_{150} 217°; $bp_{0.01}$ 20°. Strong base: pH of 0.1N aq soln: 11.0. n_D^{30} 1.4753. Dipole moment 2.81. Flash pt 300°F. Miscible with water, methanol, acetone. Soly at 25° in benzene: 4.2%, in ether: 0.8%, in carbon tetrachloride: <0.1%, in *n*-heptane: <0.1%. LD_{50} orally in rats: 12.76 g/kg (Smyth).

Caution: Potential symptoms of overexposure are irritation of eyes, skin, nose and throat; eye and skin burns, corneal necrosis; lacrimation, cough, sneezing. *See NIOSH Pocket Guide to Chemical Hazards* (DHHS/NIOSH 97-140, 1997) p 104.

USE: To scrub gases as indicated under ethanolamine. Diethanolamine can be used with cracking gases and coal or oil gases which contain carbonyl sulfide that would react with monoethanolamine. As rubber chemicals intermediate. In the manuf of surface active agents used in textile specialties, herbicides, petr demulsifiers. As emulsifier and dispersing agent in various agricultural chemicals, cosmetics, and pharmaceuticals. In the production of lubricants for the textile industry. As humectant and softening agent. In organic syntheses.

3108. Diethazine. [60-91-3] *N,N*-Diethyl-10*H*-phenothiazine-10-ethanamine; 10-(2-diethylaminoethyl)phenothiazine; *N*-(diethylaminoethyl)thiodiphenylamine; *N*-(2'-diethylaminoethyl)-dibenzoparathiazine; RP-2987; Deparkin; Dinezin; Dolisina; Eazaminum; Ethylemin; Parkazin. $C_{18}H_{22}N_2S$; mol wt 298.45. C 72.44%, H 7.43%, N 9.39%, S 10.74%. Anticholinergic. Prepd by reacting 10-phenothiazineethyl chloride with diethylamine in presence of copper powder or by reacting diethylaminoethyl chloride with phenothiazine: Charpentier, *Compt. Rend.* **225**, 306 (1947); Huttrer, *Enzymologia* **12**, 293 (1948); Charpentier, US 2530451 (1950 to Rhône-Poulenc); Berg, Ashley, US 2607773 (1952 to Rhône-Poulenc). Toxicity study: Bovet *et al.*, *Therapie* **2**, 115 (1947).

Oily liquid. bp_{4-5} 195-208°; $bp_{0.4-0.5}$ 167-175°.

Hydrochloride. [341-70-8] Antipar; Aparkazin; Diparcol; Latibon; Thiantan; Thiontan. $C_{18}H_{22}N_2S$·HCl; mol wt 334.91. Crystals, mp 184-186°. Burning taste, producing a temporary numbness of the tongue. One part dissolves in about 5 parts water, 6 parts ethanol, 5 parts chloroform. Practically insol in ether. pH of 10% aq soln 5.0-5.3. LD_{50} orally in mice: 450 mg/kg (Bovet).

THERAP CAT: Antiparkinsonian.

3109. Diethofencarb. [87130-20-9] (3,4-Diethoxyphenyl)-carbamic acid 1-methylethyl ester; isopropyl 3,4-diethoxy-carbanilate; isopropyl N-(3,4-diethoxyphenyl)carbamate; S-165; S-1605; S-32165; Powmil. $C_{14}H_{21}NO_4$; mol wt 267.32. C 62.90%, H 7.92%, N 5.24%, O 23.94%. Prepn: H. Noguchi et al., **EP 78663**; eidem, **US 4608385** (1983, 1986 both to Sumitomo). In vitro and greenhouse antifungal activities: M. L. Gullino et al., Tagungsber. Akad. Landwirtschaftswiss. **253**, 165 (1987); M. L. Gullino, A. Garibaldi, Meded. Fac. Landbouwwet. Rijksuniv. Gent **52**, 895 (1987). Structure-activity study: J. Takahashi et al., J. Chromatogr. **436**, 316 (1988). Mechanism of action study: M. Fujimura et al., ACS Symp. Ser. **421**, 224-236 (1990). Metabolism in rats: K. Shiba et al., J. Pestic. Sci. **15**, 395 (1990). Review: M. Fujimura et al., Jpn. Pestic. Inf. **57**, 7-11 (1990).

Crystalline solid, mp 101.3°. Vapor pressure at 20°: 6.3 × 10^{-5}, at 25°: 1.1 × 10^{-4} mm Hg. Soluble in most organic solvents. Soly at 25 ±2° in water: 26.6 ±0.3 mg/l. LD_{50} in male and female rats (mg/kg): >5000, >5000 orally; >5000, >5000 dermally. LC_{50} (48 hrs) in carp: 13.5 mg/l; (3 hrs) in Daphnia pulex: >10 mg/l (Fujimura, review).

USE: Agricultural fungicide.

3110. Diethylacetic Acid. [88-09-5] 2-Ethylbutanoic acid. $C_6H_{12}O_2$; mol wt 116.16. C 62.04%, H 10.41%, O 27.55%. (CH_3-$CH_2)_2$CHCOOH.

Colorless liq; odor somewhat resembling that of caproic acid. d_4^{18} 0.920. bp 194-195°, also stated as 190°. mp ~ −15°. n_D^{10} 1.4179. Slightly sol in water; freely sol in alcohol or ether.

3111. Diethylamine. [109-89-7] N-Ethylethanamine. C_4-$H_{11}N$; mol wt 73.14. C 65.69%, H 15.16%, N 19.15%. Prepn from ethyl iodide and NH_3 with separation of mono-, di-, and triethyl-amines formed: Watt, Otto, J. Am. Chem. Soc. **69**, 836 (1947). Manuf from ethanol and NH_3, obtained along with mono- and triethylamines: Davies et al., **US 2609394** (1952 to ICI); Lemon, Myerly, **US 3022349** (1962 to Union Carbide). Toxicity data: Smyth et al., Arch. Ind. Hyg. Occup. Med. **4**, 119 (1951).

Flammable, strongly alkaline liq, bp 55.5°. mp −50°. d_4^{20} 0.7074. n_D^{20} 1.3864. Flash pt <20°F. Forms a hydrate, $B_2.H_2O$, mp −19°. Miscible with water, alc. It is usually supplied as a soln. Keep well closed. LD_{50} orally in rats: 540 mg/kg (Smyth).

Hydrochloride. $C_4H_{11}N.HCl$. Crystals from alcohol + ether, mp 226°. Hygroscopic. bp 320-330°. d_4^{21} 1.048. Sol in water, alcohol, chloroform. Practically insol in ether.

Caution: Potential symptoms of overexposure are eye, skin and respiratory system irritation. See NIOSH Pocket Guide to Chemical Hazards (DHHS/NIOSH 97-140, 1997) p 106. See also Patty's Industrial Hygiene and Toxicology vol. 2B, G. D. Clayton, F. E. Clayton, Eds. (Wiley-Interscience, New York, 3rd ed., 1981) p 3149.

USE: In the rubber and petroleum industry; in flotation agents; in resins; dyes, pharmaceuticals.

3112. 2-Diethylaminoethanol. [100-37-8] β-Diethylami-noethyl alcohol; 2-hydroxytriethylamine. $C_6H_{15}NO$; mol wt 117.19. C 61.49%, H 12.90%, N 11.95%, O 13.65%. Prepd by the action of ethylene chlorohydrin on diethylamine: Ladenburg, Ber. **14**, 1878 (1881); Soderman, Johnson, J. Am. Chem. Soc. **47**, 1394 (1925); Hartman, Org. Synth. coll. vol. II, 183 (1943); by the action of ethylene oxide on diethylamine: Horne, Shriner, J. Am. Chem. Soc. **54**, 2928 (1932); Headlee et al., ibid. **55**, 1066 (1933).

Liquid. d^{25} 0.8800. bp_{760} 163°; bp_{80} 100°; bp_{10} 55°. n_D^{25} 1.4389. Sol in water, alcohol, ether, benzene.

p-Nitrophenylurethan. Crystals, mp 59-60°.

Caution: Potential symptoms of overexposure are nausea, vomiting; irritation of respiratory system, skin and eyes. See NIOSH Pocket Guide to Chemical Hazards (DHHS/NIOSH 97-140, 1997) p 106.

3113. Diethylaminosulfur Trifluoride. [38078-09-0] (T-4)-(N-Ethylethanaminato)trifluorosulfur; DAST. $C_4H_{10}F_3NS$; mol wt 161.19. C 29.81%, H 6.25%, F 35.36%, N 8.69%, S 19.89%. Versatile fluorinating agent. Prepn: S. P. von Halasz, O. Glemser, Ber. **103**, 594 (1970); and fluorination of aldehydes and alcohols: W. J. Middleton, J. Org. Chem. **40**, 574 (1975). Thermal decompn study: P. A. Messina et al., J. Fluorine Chem. **42**, 137 (1989). Brief review of chemistry: K. A. Jolliffe, Aust. J. Chem. **54**, 75 (2001). Review of applications in nucleophilic fluorination reactions: M. Hudlicky, Org. React. **25**, 513-637 (1988); R. P. Singh, J. M. Shreeve, Synthesis **2002**, 2561-2578.

Pale yellow liquid, bp_{10} 46-47°; bp_{12} 43-44°. n_D^{20} 1.4125. d 1.22-1.23. Reacts violently with water.

Caution: Thermally unstable. Undergoes explosion or detonation when heated to >90° (Jolliffe).

USE: Nucleophilic fluorinating reagent.

3114. Diethylaniline. [91-66-7] N,N-Diethylbenzenamine. $C_{10}H_{15}N$; mol wt 149.23. C 80.48%, H 10.13%, N 9.39%. Prepd by ethylation of aniline: Whitman, **US 2501556** (1950 to du Pont); Voltz, J. Org. Chem. **22**, 48 (1957); Closson et al., ibid. **22**, 646 (1957); Horyna, Cerny, Collect. Czech. Chem. Commun. **21**, 906 (1956); from bromobenzene, sodium amide + diethylamine: Bunnett, Brotherton, J. Org. Chem. **22**, 832 (1957).

Colorless to yellow liq. d_4^{25} 0.9302. bp 215-216°; bp_3 62-66°. mp −38°. n_D^{24} 1.5394. Volatile with steam. uv max (isooctane): 303, 259 nm (ε × 10^{-3} 2.37, 16.7). Slightly sol in alcohol, chloroform, ether. One gram dissolves in 70 ml water at 12°.

USE: As dyestuff intermediate, in organic syntheses.

3115. N,N-Diethylbenzhydrylamine. [519-72-2] N,N-Di-ethyl-α-phenylbenzenemethanamine; diethylaminodiphenylmeth-ane. $C_{17}H_{21}N$; mol wt 239.36. C 85.30%, H 8.84%, N 5.85%. Prepd by addn of an excess of phenylmagnesium bromide to N,N-diethylformamide and treating the reaction mixture with ammonium chloride: Maxim, Mavrodineanu, Bull. Soc. Chim. Fr. [5] **3**, 1084 (1936). Proposed as an antihistaminic: Capraro, C.A. **41**, 6989 (1947).

Viscous liquid, bp_{17} 170°. Solidifies on deep cooling, then mp 56° (Maxim, Mavrodineanu); mp 58-59° [Sommelet, *Compt. Rend.* **175**, 1149 (1922)]; mp 61° [Titov, *C.A.* **43**, 4217 (1949)].

USE: In the detection of nitrates.

3116. Diethylcarbamazine. [90-89-1] *N,N*-Diethyl-4-methyl-1-piperazinecarboxamide; 1-diethylcarbamoyl-4-methylpiperazine; carbamazine; 1-diethylcarbamyl-4-methylpiperazine; 84L; RP-3799; Carbilazine; Caricide; Cypip; Ethodryl; Notézine; Spatonin. $C_{10}H_{21}N_3O$; mol wt 199.29. C 60.27%, H 10.62%, N 21.08%, O 8.03%. Prepn: Kushner *et al.*, *J. Org. Chem.* **13**, 151 (1948); Kushner, Brancone, US 2467893; US 2467895 (1949 to Am. Cyanamid). Pharmacology and toxicology: Harned *et al.*, *Ann. N.Y. Acad. Sci.* **50**, 141 (1948). GC determn in blood: S. Nene *et al.*, *J. Chromatogr.* **308**, 334 (1984). Mode of action: J.-Y. Cesbron *et al.*, *Nature* **325**, 533 (1987). Review of pharmacology, mechanisms of action and clinical uses: C. D. MacKenzie, M. A. Kron, *Trop. Dis. Bull.* **82**(10), R1-R37 (1985).

Crystals, mp 47-49°. bp_3 108.5-111°.

Hydrochloride. $C_{10}H_{21}N_3O.HCl$. Crystals from acetone, mp 156.5-157°. Very sol in water; sol in chloroform, dioxane.

Citrate. [1642-54-2] Banocide; Dec; Dirocide; Filaribits; Filazine; Franocide; Hetrazan; Loxuran; Longicid. $C_{10}H_{21}N_3O.C_6H_8$-O_7; mol wt 391.42. Crystals, mp 141-143°. Freely sol in water (>75% at 20°). Sparingly sol in cold alc; freely sol in hot alc. Practically insol in benzene, acetone, ether, chloroform. LD_{50} orally in rats: 1.38 g/kg (Harned).

Phosphate. Ditrazin. Crystals, freely sol in water.

THERAP CAT: Anthelmintic (Nematodes).

THERAP CAT (VET): Citrate as an anthelmintic.

3117. N,N'-Diethylcarbanilide. [85-98-3] *N,N'*-Diethyl-*N,N'*-diphenylurea; *sym*-diethyldiphenylurea; centralite I; ethyl centralite. $C_{17}H_{20}N_2O$; mol wt 268.35. C 76.09%, H 7.51%, N 10.44%, O 5.96%. $C_2H_5(C_6H_5)NCON(C_6H_5)C_2H_5$. Prepn from ethylaniline and phosgene: Michler, *Ber.* **9**, 712 (1876). Alternate synthesis: N. R. Ayyangar *et al.*, *Chem. Ind. (London)* **1988**, 599.

Crystals from alc, mp 79°. Insol in water.

USE: As stabilizer of smokeless explosives.

3118. Diethyl Carbitol®. [112-36-7] 1,1'-Oxybis(2-ethoxy)ethane; diethylene glycol diethyl ether. $C_8H_{18}O_3$; mol wt 162.23. C 59.23%, H 11.18%, O 29.59%. $(C_2H_5OCH_2CH_2)_2O$. Toxicity data: H. F. Smyth *et al.*, *J. Ind. Hyg. Toxicol.* **23**, 259 (1941).

Liquid. d_4^{20} 0.907. bp 188°. Very sol in water, alcohol, and other organic solvents. LD_{50} orally in rats: 4.97 g/kg (Smyth).

USE: Solvent; high boiling reaction medium.

3119. Diethylene Glycol. [111-46-6] 2,2'-Oxybisethanol; 2,2'-oxydiethanol. $C_4H_{10}O_3$; mol wt 106.12. C 45.27%, H 9.50%, O 45.23%. Manuf from ethylene oxide and glycol: *Faith, Keyes & Clark's Industrial Chemicals*, F. A. Lowenheim, M. K. Moran, Eds. (Wiley-Interscience, New York, 4th ed., 1975) pp 397-402. Toxicity study: H. F. Smyth *et al.*, *J. Ind. Hyg. Toxicol.* **23**, 259 (1941).

Colorless, hygroscopic, practically odorless liq; sharply sweetish taste. d_{20}^{20} 1.118. Solidifies at −10.45° (when pure). mp −6.5°. bp 244-245°. n_D^{20} 1.4475. Flash pt, open cup: 290°F (143°C). Misc with water, alc, ether, acetone, ethylene glycol. Practically insol in benzene, carbon tetrachloride. LD_{50} in rats, guinea pigs (g/kg): 20.76, 13.21 orally (Smyth).

Caution: Symptoms on ingestion similar to ethylene glycol, *q.v.* Fatal poisoning resulted from its use as a solvent in an elixir. *See* E. Browning, *Toxicity and Metabolism of Industrial Solvents* (Elsevier, New York, 1965) pp 624-628, 686-690; *Patty's Industrial Hygiene and Toxicology* vol. 2C, G. D. Clayton, F. E. Clayton, Eds. (Wiley-Interscience, New York, 3rd ed., 1982) pp 3832-3838.

USE: In antifreeze soln for sprinkler systems, water seals for gas tanks, etc. (water with 40% diethylene glycol freezes at −18°; with 50% at −28°); as lubricating and finishing agent for wool, worsted, cotton, rayon, and silk; as solvent for vat dyes; in composition corks, glues, gelatin, casein, and pastes to prevent drying out.

3120. Diethylene Glycol Monolaurate. [141-20-8] Dodecanoic acid 2-(2-hydroxyethoxy)ethyl ester; diethylene glycol laurate; diglycol laurate; Glaurin. $C_{16}H_{32}O_4$; mol wt 288.42. C 66.63%, H 11.18%, O 22.19%. Prepared by controlled esterification of diethylene glycol with lauric acid.

Oily liq. d_4^{25} 0.9572; d_{20}^{20} 0.963-0.968. mp 17-18°. bp ~270° (some dec). May be heated to 250° without decompn. Practically insol in water. Sol in methanol, ethanol, benzene, toluene, chlorinated hydrocarbons, acetone, ethyl acetate, cottonseed oil. Slightly sol in petr naphtha.

USE: Dispersing agent, emulsifier, plasticizer.

3121. Diethyl Ketone. [96-22-0] 3-Pentanone; dimethylacetone; propione; methacetone. $C_5H_{10}O$; mol wt 86.13. C 69.72%, H 11.70%, O 18.58%. $CH_3CH_2COCH_2CH_3$. Liquid, acetone odor. d_4^{19} 0.816. bp 101.5°. mp −42°. n_D^{25} 1.3905. Sol in about 25 parts water; miscible with alcohol, ether. LD_{50} orally in rats: 2.1 g/kg, Smyth *et al.*, *Arch. Ind. Hyg. Occup. Med.* **10**, 61 (1954).

3122. Diethylmagnesium. [557-18-6] Magnesium diethyl. $C_4H_{10}Mg$; mol wt 82.43. C 58.28%, H 12.23%, Mg 29.49%. $Mg(C_2H_5)_2$. Prepd by the action of magnesium metal on mercury diethyl in ether: Schlenk, Jr., *Ber.* **64**, 734, 736 (1931).

Solvated crystals from ether, $MgEt_2.Et_2O$, plates, rods. mp 0°. Liquid at room temp. Spontaneously flammable in air. Violent explosion on contact with water. Loses its ether of crystn on heating *in vacuo*. Not volatile in high vac up to 250° when decompn sets in. Sol in ether. Dec by alc and ammonia. Will glow and catch fire even in CO_2. Must be handled in high vac, or under dry nitrogen or hydrogen.

3123. Diethyl Maleate. [141-05-9] (2Z)-2-Butenedioic acid, diethyl ester; maleic acid, diethyl ester; ethyl maleate. C_8-$H_{12}O_4$; mol wt 172.18. C 55.81%, H 7.02%, O 37.17%. Prepn from maleic acid and ethanol: V. M. Mitchovitch, *Bull. Soc. Chim. Fr.* **4**, 1667 (1937). Physical properties: G. H. Jeffrey, A. I. Vogel, *J. Chem. Soc.* **1948**, 658. Copolymerization with styrene: F. M. Lewis *et al.*, *J. Am. Chem. Soc.* **70**, 1519, 1529 (1948). In Diels-Alder reactions: N. L. Bauld *et al.*, *Tetrahedron Lett.* **1972**, 2443. In Michael additions: G. Arsenault *et al.*, *Chem. Commun.* **1983**, 437. Conjugation with glutathione, *q.v.*: E. Boyland, L. F. Chasseaud, *Biochem. J.* **104**, 95 (1967); *eidem, ibid.* **109**, 651 (1968). Toxicity: H. F. Smyth *et al.*, *J. Ind. Hyg. Toxicol.* **31**, 60 (1949).

Oil, bp_{758} 219.5°. d_4^{20} 1.0674. n_D^{20} 1.4402. Insol in water. Soluble in ethanol, ether. LD_{50} orally in rats: 0.30 g/kg (Smyth).

USE: In organic synthesis.

3124. Diethylmalonic Acid. [510-20-3] Diethylpropanedioic acid; 3,3-pentanedicarboxylic acid. $C_7H_{12}O_4$; mol wt 160.17. C 52.49%, H 7.55%, O 39.96%. Prepn: Daimler, *Ann.* **249**, 173 (1888); Speck, *J. Am. Chem. Soc.* **74**, 2876 (1952). Spectral studies: J. L. Delarbre *et al.*, *J. Raman Spectrosc.* **16**, 11 (1985). Crystal structure: A. Dubourg *et al.*, *Acta Crystallogr.* **C44**, 1987 (1988).

Crystals, mp 127°. Dec at 170-180° with liberation of CO_2 and formation of diethylacetic acid. Very sol in water; freely sol in alcohol, ether, slightly in chloroform.

3125. Diethyl Oxalate. [95-92-1] Ethanedioic acid diethyl ester; ethyl oxalate; diethyl ethanedioate; oxalic acid diethyl ester. $C_6H_{10}O_4$; mol wt 146.14. C 49.31%, H 6.90%, O 43.79%. C_2-$H_5OOCCOOC_2H_5$. Prepn: Clarke, Davis, *Org. Synth.* **coll. vol. I,** 256 (2nd ed., 1941); Kenyon, *ibid.* 261.

Liquid. d_4^{20} 1.0785. mp −40.6°; bp_{760} 185.7°; bp_{100} 130.8°; bp_{20} 96.8°; $bp_{1.0}$ 47°. n_D^{20} 1.41011. Flash pt, open cup: 168°F (75°C). Sparingly sol in water which dec it gradually; miscible with alcohol, ether, and other usual org solvents.

USE: Manuf phenobarbital, ethylbenzyl malonate, triethylamine, and similar chemicals, plastics, dyestuff intermediates. Solvent for cellulose esters, perfumes.

3126. N,N-Diethylphenylacetamide. [2431-96-1] *N,N*-Di-ethylbenzeneacetamide; DEPA. $C_{12}H_{17}NO$; mol wt 191.27. C 75.35%, H 8.96%, N 7.32%, O 8.36%. Substituted amide with broad spectrum repellent activity. Prepn: G. Hausknecht, *Ber.* **22,** 324 (1889); R. Mukherjee, *J. Chem. Soc. D* **1971,** 1113; and structure-activity relationship studies: M. V. S. Suryanarayana *et al., J. Pharm. Sci.* **80,** 1055 (1991). Comparative studies with deet and dimethyl phthalate, *q.q.v.,* vs mosquitoes, black flies and land leeches: S. Kumar *et al., Indian J. Med. Res.* **80,** 541 (1984); vs bedbugs: *idem et al., ibid.* **102,** 20 (1995); vs rat flea: K. K. Mathur *et al., ibid.* **83,** 466 (1986); vs sandflies: M. Kalyanasundaram *et al., Med. Vet. Entomol.* **8,** 68 (1994). Comparison with deet and dibutyl phthalate, *q.q.v.,* in prevention of scrub typhus: R. Tilak *et al., Indian J. Med. Res.* **113,** 98 (2001). GC determn in urine: S. S. Rao *et al., J. Chromatogr. B* **493,** 210 (1989). Toxicity and metabolism studies: *idem. et al., Toxicology* **58,** 81 (1989); *idem et al., Toxicol. Lett.* **45,** 67 (1989). Development of polysiloxane based slow release formulations and efficacy vs mosquitoes : D. C. Gupta *et al., J. Polym. Mater.* **17,** 215 (2000). *Review*: S. S. Rao, K. M. Rao, *J. Med. Entomol.* **28,** 303-306 (1991).

Liquid, $bp_{0.3}$ 120-122°. Log P (methanol/water): 2.40. Vapor pressure at 30°: 0.1043 cm Hg. LD_{50} in guinea pigs, rats, rabbits, mice (g/kg): 7, 3-4, 3.5, ∼2 dermally (Rao, 1991).

USE: Insect repellent.

3127. Diethylpropion. [90-84-6] 2-(Diethylamino)-1-phenyl-1-propanone; 2-diethylaminopropiophenone; α-benzoyltriethylamine; amfepramone. $C_{13}H_{19}NO$; mol wt 205.30. C 76.05%, H 9.33%, N 6.82%, O 7.79%. Prepn: Hyde *et al., J. Am. Chem. Soc.* **50,** 2287 (1928); Schutte, **US 3001910** (1961 to Temmler-Werke). Pharmacology: Cahen *et al., Therapie* **17,** 373-412 (1962). Clinical trial in obesity: R. Abramson *et al., J. Clin. Psychiatry* **41,** 234 (1980).

Hydrochloride. [134-80-5] Anorex; Dobesin; Moderatan; Prefamone; Regenon; Tenuate; Tepanil. $C_{13}H_{19}NO.HCl$; mol wt 241.76. Crystals, dec 168°.

Note: This is a controlled substance (stimulant): **21 CFR,** 1308.14.

THERAP CAT: Anorexic.

3128. Diethylsilane. [542-91-6] $C_4H_{12}Si$; mol wt 88.22. C 54.46%, H 13.71%, Si 31.84%. $(C_2H_5)_2SiH_2$. Prepd from ethylene and silane: Hurd, **US 2537763** (1951); Fritz, *Z. Naturforsch.* **7b,** 207 (1952); White, Rochow, *J. Am. Chem. Soc.* **76,** 3897 (1954); Clasen, *Angew. Chem.* **70,** 180 (1958).

Liquid. Stable to air when pure. bp_{741} 56°; d_4^{20} 0.6843; n_D^{20} 1.3921. Quickly oxidized by Ag_2O and HgO. Oxidation can be slowed by soln in petr ether or by cooling to −80°.

3129. Diethylstilbestrol. [56-53-1] 4,4'-[(*1E*)-1,2-Diethyl-1,2-ethenediyl]bisphenol; *(E)*-α,α'-diethyl-4,4'-stilbenediol; *(E)*-3,4-bis(4-hydroxyphenyl)-3-hexene; 4,4'-dihydroxy-α,β-diethylstilbene; stilbestrol; stilboestrol; DES; Apstil; Cyren A; Distilbène; Stilbetin. $C_{18}H_{20}O_2$; mol wt 268.35. C 80.56%, H 7.51%, O 11.92%. Synthetic, nonsteroidal estrogen. Prepn: E. C. Dodds *et al., Nature* **141,** 247 (1938); *eidem, Proc. R. Soc. London Ser. B* **127,** 140 (1939). Prepn of ethers: E. E. Reid, E. Wilson, *J. Am. Chem. Soc.* **64,** 1625 (1942). Review of early literature: U. V. Solmssen, *Chem. Rev.* **37,** 481-598 (1945). HPLC determn in plasma and urine: A. T. Rhys Williams *et al., J. Chromatogr.* **235,** 461 (1982). Clinical trial in breast cancer: A. C. Carter *et al., J. Am. Med. Assoc.* **237,** 2079 (1977); in prostate cancer: C. J. Nickel. A. Morales, *Can. J. Surg.* **26,** 434 (1983). Review of metabolism: M. Metzler, *Crit. Rev. Biochem.* **10,** 171-212 (1981). Review of toxicology and use as a growth promotant in livestock: K. E. McMartin *et al., J. Environ. Pathol. Toxicol.* **1,** 279-313 (1978). Book: *Developmental Effects of Diethylstilbestrol (DES) in Pregnancy,* A. L. Herbst, H. A. Bern, Eds. (Thieme-Verlag, New York, 1981) 203 pp. Comprehensive description: A. A. Al-Badr, A. G. Mekkawi, *Anal. Profiles Drug Subs.* **19,** 145-192 (1990).

Small plates from benzene, mp 169-172°. uv max (0.1*N* NaOH): 259 nm ($E_{1cm}^{1\%}$ 764). Almost insol in water. Sol in alcohol, ether, chloroform, fatty oils, dil hydroxides.

Diphosphate *see* Fosfestrol.

Dipropionate. [130-80-3] Cyren B; Dibestil. $C_{24}H_{28}O_4$; mol wt 380.48. Plates from methanol, mp 104°. Sol in organic solvents and in vegetable oils.

Dimethyl ether *see* Dimestrol.

Monomethyl ether. [18839-90-2] 4-[(*1E*)-1-Ethyl-2-(4-methoxyphenyl)-1-butenyl]phenol; mestilbol. $C_{19}H_{22}O_2$; mol wt 282.38. Crystals from benzene + petr ether, mp 116-117.5°.

Caution: Diethylstilbestrol is listed as a known human carcinogen: *Report on Carcinogens, Eleventh Edition* (PB2005-104914, 2004) p III-98.

THERAP CAT: Antineoplastic (hormonal).

3130. Diethyl Sulfate. [64-67-5] Sulfuric acid diethyl ester. $C_4H_{10}O_4S$; mol wt 154.18. C 31.16%, H 6.54%, O 41.51%, S 20.80%. $(C_2H_5)_2SO_4$. Prepd from ethanol + sulfuric acid; by absorption of ethylene in sulfuric acid; from diethyl ether and fuming sulfuric acid. Review of prepn and uses: R. Page, J. A. John in *Ethylene and its Industrial Derivatives* S. A. Miller, Ed. (Benn, London, 1969) pp 774-787. Toxicity data: H. F. Smyth *et al., J. Ind. Hyg. Toxicol.* **31,** 60 (1949). Review of carcinogenicity studies: *IARC Monographs* **4,** 277-281 (1974). *Reviews*: C. M. Suter, *The Organic Chemistry of Sulfur* (John Wiley, 1944) pp 62-65; E. E. Gilbert, *Sulfonation and Related Reactions* (Interscience, New York, 1965).

Colorless, oily liquid; peppermint odor. *Poisonous!* Darkens with age. bp 209.5° with decompn; bp_{15} 96°; bp_5 75°. mp −25°. d_4^{23} 1.1774. n_D^{20} 1.40037, A. I. Vogel, D. M. Cowan, *J. Chem. Soc.* **1943,** 16. Flash pt: 220°F. Vapor density (air = 1) 5.31. Vapor pressure at 47° = 1 mm. Practically insol in water, gradually dec by it. Rapidly dec by hot water into monoethyl sulfate and alcohol. Miscible with alcohol, ether. LD_{50} orally in rats: 0.88 g/kg (Smyth).

Caution: This substance is reasonably anticipated to be a human carcinogen: *Report on Carcinogens, Eleventh Edition* (PB2005-104914, 2004) p III-97.

USE: Chiefly as an ethylating agent; as an accelerator in the sulfation of ethylene; in some sulfonations.

3131. Diethylzinc. [557-20-0] Zinc diethyl. $C_4H_{10}Zn$; mol wt 123.53. C 38.89%, H 8.16%, Zn 52.95%. $Zn(C_2H_5)_2$. Prepd by the interaction of zinc and ethyl iodide: Simonowitch, *Chem. Zentralbl.* **1899**, I, 1066; Lachmann, *Am. Chem. J.* **24**, 32 (1900); Dennis, Hance, *J. Am. Chem. Soc.* **47**, 370 (1925); from zinc and ethyl bromide, ethyl iodide: C. R. Noller, *Org. Synth.* **coll. vol. II**, 184. Used in synthesis of cyclopropanes: J. Furukawa *et al., Tetrahedron* **24**, 53 (1968); *eidem, Tetrahedron Lett.* **1968**, 3495; in synthesis of ketocarbenes: L. T. Scott, W. D. Cotton, *J. Am. Chem. Soc.* **95**, 2708 (1973); in ring expansion of arenes: S. Miyano, H. Hashimoto, *Chem. Commun.* **1973**, 216; in preservation of papers: J. C. Williams, G. B. Kelly Jr., **US 3969549** (1976 to U.S.A.); *eidem* in *Adv. Chem. Ser.* **193**, entitled "Preservation of Paper and Textiles of Historic and Artistic Value 2," J. C. Williams, Ed. (ACS, Washington DC, 1981) pp 109-117.

Mobile liq. Stable in sealed tube and carbon dioxide. d_4^{20} 1.2065; d_4^8 1.245; mp $-28°$; bp_{760} 118°; bp_{30} 27°; n_{Ha}^{20} 1.4936. *Ignites in air*, burns with a blue flame, giving off a peculiar, garlic-like odor. Miscible with ether, petr ether, benzene, other hydrocarbons.

USE: In organic synthesis; in preservation on archival papers.

3132. Difemerine. [80387-96-8] α-Hydroxy-α-phenylbenzeneacetic acid 2-(dimethylamino)-2-methylpropyl ester; 2-(dimethylamino)-1,1-dimethylethyl benzilate. $C_{20}H_{25}NO_3$; mol wt 327.42. C 73.37%, H 7.70%, N 4.28%, O 14.66%. Anticholinergic. Prepn: S. G. Kuznetsov, A. G. El'tsov, *Zh. Obshch. Khim.* **32**, 511 (1962), *C.A.* **58**, 470d (1963); C. Hoffmann, **FR M3406** (1965 to Labs. U.P.S.A.), *C.A.* **63**, 13163ab (1965). Toxicity: S. N. Golikov, S. G. Kuznetsov, *C.A.* **61**, 8790b (1964). Comparison of side effects with those of atropine: L. Moser, P. V. Lundt, *Med. Welt* **31**, 1795 (1980). Crystal structure: A. Carpy *et al., Acta Crystallogr.* **B35**, 882 (1979).

Solid, mp 78-78.3°.
Hydrochloride. [70280-88-5] Luostyl. $C_{20}H_{25}NO_3 \cdot HCl$; mol wt 363.88. Crystals from isopropanol, mp 182°.
THERAP CAT: Antispasmodic.

3133. Difenacoum. [56073-07-5] 3-(3-[1,1'-Biphenyl]-4-yl-1,2,3,4-tetrahydro-1-naphthalenyl)-4-hydroxy-2*H*-1-benzopyran-2-one; 3-[3-(biphenyl-4-yl)-1,2,3,4-tetrahydro-1-naphthyl]-4-hydroxycoumarin; 3-(3-*p*-biphenyl-1,2,3,4-tetrahydronaphth-1-yl)-4-hydroxycoumarin; Neosorexa; Ratak. $C_{31}H_{24}O_3$; mol wt 444.52. C 83.76%, H 5.44%, O 10.80%. Second generation anticoagulant rodenticide. Prepn: M. R. Hadler, R. S. Shadbolt, **DE 2424806**; *idem*, **US 3957824** (1975, 1976 both to Ward Blenkinsop); R. S. Shadbolt *et al., J. Chem. Soc. Perkin Trans. 1* **1976**, 1190. Comprehensive description: J. O. Bull, *Proc. Vertebr. Pest Conf.* **7**, 72 (1976). HPLC determn of rat blood and liver: M. J. Kelly *et al., J. Chromatogr.* **620**, 105 (1993); of residue levels in rats: H. Atterby *et al., Environ. Toxicol. Chem.* **24**, 318 (2005). Field and laboratory studies against the house mouse: F. P. Rowe *et al., J. Hyg. Camb.* **87**, 171 (1981). Pharmacokinetics and pharmacodynamics in rabbits: A. M. Breckenridge *et al., Br. J. Pharmacol.* **84**, 81 (1985). Pharmacological variation between rodent sexes: M. J. Winn *et al., J. Pharm. Pharmacol.* **39**, 219 (1987).

Crystals from ethyl acetate, mp 215-217°. LD_{50} orally in Wistar male, female rats (mg/kg): 1.8, 2.5; in male rabbits: 2.0 mg/kg; in dogs: 50 mg/kg; in cats: 100 mg/kg (Bull).
USE: Pesticide.

3134. Difenamizole. [20170-20-1] 2-(Dimethylamino)-*N*-(1,3-diphenyl-1*H*-pyrazol-5-yl)propanamide; 1,3-diphenyl-5-(2-dimethylaminopropionamido)pyrazole; AP-14; Pasalin. $C_{20}H_{22}N_4$-O; mol wt 334.41. C 71.83%, H 6.63%, N 16.75%, O 4.78%. Prepn: Kameyama, Niwa, **JP 68 6621** (1968 to Takeda), *C.A.* **69**, 106704x (1968). Physicochemical properties and stability: Uda, Yashiki, *Takeda Kenkyusho* **29**, 42 (1970), *C.A.* **73**, 28847n (1970). Pharmacology: Fukuda *et al., ibid.* **30**, 389 (1971); Saji *et al., ibid.* 406; Nagawa *et al., ibid.* 427, *C.A.* **76**, 108025v, 108021r, 108023t (1972), resp. Toxicity studies: Tanaka *et al., Oyo Yakuri* **6**, 279 (1972). Mechanism of action studies: Yasuhara *et al., ibid.* 313. Acute toxicity: M. Hayashi *et al., Gifu Daigaku Igakubu Kiyo* **20**, 360 (1972), *C.A.* **78**, 92505e (1973). *Review: Jpn. Med. Gaz.* **10**(11), 12 (1973).

White to pale yellow, odorless powder, mp 123-128°. Also reported as mp 120-122°. Freely sol in acetone, chloroform, benzene. Practically insol in water. Stable to heat, humidity and sunlight for 3 months. LD_{50} in mice (mg/kg): 103 i.v.; 186 i.p.; 525 s.c.; 560 orally (Hayashi).
THERAP CAT: Analgesic, anti-inflammatory.

3135. Difenoconazole. [119446-68-3] 1-[[2-[2-Chloro-4-(4-chlorophenoxy)phenyl]-4-methyl-1,3-dioxolan-2-yl]methyl]-1*H*-1,2,4-triazole; *cis,trans*-3-chloro-4-[4-methyl-2-(1*H*-1,2,4-triazol-1-ylmethyl)-1,3-dioxolan-2-yl]phenyl 4-chlorophenyl ether; CGA-169374; Dividend; Plandom; Score; Spectro. $C_{19}H_{17}Cl_2N_3$-O_3; mol wt 406.26. C 56.17%, H 4.22%, Cl 17.45%, N 10.34%, O 11.81%. Ergosterol biosynthesis inhibitor. Prepn: A. Hubele, P. Riebli, **GB 2098607** (1982 to Ciba-Geigy). Properties and antifungal activity: W. Ruess *et al., Brighton Crop Prot. Conf. - Pests Dis.* **1988**, 543. Field studies: A. J. Leadbeater *et al., ibid.* 917; A. B. Bassi, Jr. *et al., Br. Crop Prot. Counc. Monogr.* **57**, 91 (1994). Uptake and translocation in crops: H. Dahmen, T. Staub, *Plant Dis.* **76**, 523 (1992).

White crystalline solid, mp 76°. Vapor pressure (20°): 1.2×10^{-7} Pa. Soly (20°): 5 mg/l in water. Very soluble in most organic solvents. LD_{50} in rats (mg/kg): 1453 orally; in rabbits: >2010 dermally (Ruess).
USE: Agricultural fungicide.

3136. Difenoxin. [28782-42-5] 1-(3-Cyano-3,3-diphenylpropyl)-4-phenyl-4-piperidinecarboxylic acid; 1-(3-cyano-3,3-diphenylpropyl)-4-phenylisonipecotic acid; difenoxilic acid; difenoxylic acid; McN-JR-15403-11; Lyspafen. $C_{28}H_{28}N_2O_2$; mol wt 424.53. C 79.22%, H 6.65%, N 6.60%, O 7.54%. Active metabolite of diphenoxylate, *q.v.*, from which it may be prepared by hydrolysis of the ethyl ester: W. Soudijn, I. van Wijngaarden, **DE**

1953342; *eidem*, **US 3646207** (1970, 1972 to Janssen). Series of articles on pharmacology, toxicology, metabolism: *Arzneim.-Forsch.* **22**, 513-531 (1972). Toxicity data: Niemegeers *et al., ibid.* 516.

Hydrochloride. R-15403. $C_{28}H_{28}N_2O_2$.HCl; mol wt 461.00. White amorphous power, mp 290°. Very slightly sol in water (0.023%); sparingly sol in chloroform, tetrahydrofuran, dimethylacetamide, DMSO. Stable, can be stored for several years under normal conditions; not hygroscopic; not affected by light. LD_{50} orally in rats: 149 mg/kg (Niemegeers).

Note: This is a controlled substance (opiate): **21 CFR**, 1308.11.
THERAP CAT: Antiperistaltic; antidiarrheal.

3137. Difenpiramide. [51484-40-3] *N*-2-Pyridinyl-[1,1'-biphenyl]-4-acetamide; diphenpyramide; Z-876; Difenax. $C_{19}H_{16}$-N_2O; mol wt 288.34. C 79.14%, H 5.59%, N 9.72%, O 5.55%. Prepn: F. Tenconi, R. M. Tagliabue, **DE 2325309** to Zambeletti; L. Molteni *et al.*, **US 3868380** (1975). Pharmacological properties: S. Caliari *et al., Arzneim.-Forsch.* **27**, 2086 (1977). Physicochemical profile: A. Trebbi, G. Filippi, *Boll. Chim. Farm.* **118**, 729 (1979). Therapeutic use: C. Ortolani *et al., Clin. Ter.* **89**, 391 (1979).

Crystals, mp 122-124°. LD_{50} in male mice, rats (mg/kg): 2590, 2075 orally; 1421, 1396 i.p. (Caliari).
THERAP CAT: Anti-inflammatory.

3138. Difenzoquat. [49866-87-7] 1,2-Dimethyl-3,5-diphenyl-1*H*-pyrazolium. $[C_{17}H_{17}N_2]^+$. Post-emergence herbicide for food crops; also effective vs mildew. Prepn of salts: B. Walworth, E. Klingsberg, **DE 2260485**; *eidem*, **US 3882142** (1973, 1975 both to Am. Cyanamid); B. Cross *et al., J. Heterocycl. Chem.* **17**, 905 (1980). Physical properties and herbicidal activity: N. E. Shafer, *Proc. 12th Br. Weed Control Conf.* **1974**, 831. Effect vs mildew: R. J. Winfield *et al., Proc. Br. Crop Prot. Conf. - Pests Dis.* **1977**, 57. HPLC determn in commercial formulations: C. Barry, R. K. Pike, *J. Assoc. Off. Anal. Chem.* **63**, 64 (1980); in water: M. C. Carneiro *et al., J. Chromatogr. A* **669**, 217 (1994).

Methyl sulfate. [43222-48-6] AC-84777; CL-84777; Avenge; Finaven. $C_{17}H_{17}N_2$.CH_3O_4S; mol wt 360.43. Crystals from acetone, mp 146-148° (Cross). Soly in water (25°): ~70%. Relatively insol in non-polar solvents. LD_{50} (technical grade) orally in rats: 470 mg/kg; dermally in rabbits: 3540 mg/kg (Shafer).
USE: Herbicide; agricultural fungicide.

3139. Difethialone. [104653-34-1] 3-[3-(4'-Bromo[1,1'-biphenyl]-4-yl)-1,2,3,4-tetrahydro-1-naphthalenyl]-4-hydroxy-2*H*-1-benzothiopyran-2-one; LM-2219; Generation; Hombre. $C_{31}H_{23}$-BrO_2S; mol wt 539.48. C 69.02%, H 4.30%, Br 14.81%, O 5.93%, S 5.94%. Second generation anticoagulant rodenticide; member of the hydroxy-4-benzothiopyranone family. Prepn: J.-J. Berthelon, **FR 2562893**; *idem*, **US 4585786** (1985, 1986 both to Lipha). HPLC determn of residue levels in rats: D. A. Goldade *et al., J. Agric. Food Chem.* **46**, 504 (1998). Use against warfarin-resistant rodents: K. Nahas *et al., Anal. Rech. Vét.* **20**, 159 (1989). Toxicity in rodents and non-target species: J. C. Lechevin, R. M. Poche, *Proc. Vetebr. Pest Conf.* **13**, 59 (1988); S. Moran, *Crop Prot.* **12**, 501 (1993). Laboratory and field studies: C. Sheikher, P. Sood, *Indian J. Agric. Sci.* **70**, 312 (2000). Use in conjunction with compounds to improve bait acceptance: H. Kaur, V. R. Parshad, *Int. Pest Control* **46**, 88 (2004).

Prepd as a variable proportion of the (1*RS*,3*RS*) and (1*RS*,3*SR*) racemates, mp 203-227°. LD_{50} orally in male, female rats, mice (mg/kg): 0.62, 0.42, 0.52, 0.43 (non-resistant); 0.27, 0.39, 0.46, 0.52 (warfarin resistant). LD_{50} in hare: 0.75 mg/kg. LC_{50} in mallard duck, bobwhite quail (ppm): 1.94, 0.56. LD_{50} at 48 hrs in daphnia magna, bluegill sunfish, rainbow trout (μg/l): 4.4, 110, 67 (Lechevin).
USE: Pesticide.

3140. Diflorasone. [2557-49-5] (6α,11β,16β)-6,9-Difluoro-11,17,21-trihydroxy-16-methylpregna-1,4-diene-3,20-dione; 6α,9α-difluoro-16β-methyl-$\Delta^{1,4}$-pregnadiene-11β,17α,21-triol-3,20-dione; 6α,9α-difluoro-16β-methylprednisolone. $C_{22}H_{28}F_2O_5$; mol wt 410.45. C 64.38%, H 6.88%, F 9.26%, O 19.49%. The 16β-analog of flumethasone, *q.v.* Prepn of free alcohol and 21-acetate: **GB 881334** (1961 to Pfizer), *C.A.* **56**, 15586c (1962); **GB 898293**; F. H. Lincoln *et al.*, **US 3557158** (1962, 1971 both to Upjohn); **GB 912015** (1962 to Merck & Co.). Prepn of the 17,21-diacetate: D. E. Ayer *et al.*, **DE 2308731**; *eidem*, **US 3980778** (1973, 1976 both to Upjohn). Proposed mechanism of action: S. Hammarstrom *et al., Science* **197**, 994 (1977). Pharmacology: S. Wickrema *et al., J. Invest. Dermatol.* **71**, 372 (1978). Clinical study: S. M. Bluefarb *et al., J. Int. Med. Res.* **4**, 454 (1976).

Diacetate. [33564-31-7] U-34865; Dermaflor; Diacort; Florone; Maxiflor; Psorcon; Soriflor. $C_{26}H_{32}F_2O_7$; mol wt 494.52. Crystals from ethyl acetate-Skellysolve C and acetone-methanol, mp 221-223° (dec). uv max (alc): 238 nm (ε 17250). $[\alpha]_D$ +61° (chloroform).
THERAP CAT: Anti-inflammatory (topical); glucocorticoid.

3141. Difloxacin. [98106-17-3] 6-Fluoro-1-(4-fluorophenyl)-1,4-dihydro-7-(4-methyl-1-piperazinyl)-4-oxo-3-quinolinecarboxylic acid. $C_{21}H_{19}F_2N_3O_3$; mol wt 399.39. C 63.15%, H

4.80%, F 9.51%, N 10.52%, O 12.02%. Fluoroquinolone antibacterial structurally related to norfloxacin, *q.v.* Prepn: D. T. W. Chu, **EP 131839**; *idem,* **US 4730000** (1985, 1988 both to Abbott); D. T. W. Chu *et al., J. Med. Chem.* **28**, 1558 (1985); H. Narita *et al.,* **JP Kokai 85 237069** (1985 to Toyama). Antibacterial spectrum *in vitro:* J. M. Stamm *et al., Antimicrob. Agents Chemother.* **29**, 193 (1986); *in vivo:* P. B. Fernandes *et al., ibid.* 201. Activity vs anaerobic bacteria: *eidem, J. Antimicrob. Chemother.* **18**, 693 (1986). HPLC determn in biological fluids: G. R. Granneman, L. T. Sennello, *J. Chromatogr.* **413**, 199 (1987). Pharmacokinetics in humans: G. R. Granneman *et al., Antimicrob. Agents Chemother.* **30**, 689 (1986).

Monohydrochloride. [91296-86-5] Abbott 56619; A-56619; Dicural. $C_{21}H_{19}F_2N_3O_3 \cdot HCl$; mol wt 435.85. Crystals, mp >275°.

THERAP CAT (VET): Antibacterial.

3142. Diflubenzuron. [35367-38-5] *N*-[[(4-Chlorophenyl)-amino]carbonyl]-2,6-difluorobenzamide; 1-(4-chlorophenyl)-3-(2,6-difluorobenzoyl)urea; difluron; DU-112307; PH-60-40; TH-6040; ENT-29054; OMS-1804; Dimilin; Duphacid; Micromite. $C_{14}H_9ClF_2N_2O_2$; mol wt 310.68. C 54.12%, H 2.92%, Cl 11.41%, F 12.23%, N 9.02%, O 10.30%. Substituted benzoylphenylurea, inhibits chitin deposition in insect cuticle. Prepn: K. Wellinga, R. Mulder, **DE 2123236**; *eidem,* **US 3748356** (1971, 1973 both to Philips). Insecticidal activity: K. Wellinga *et al., J. Agric. Food Chem.* **21**, 993 (1973); R. Mulder, M. J. Gijswijt, *Pestic. Sci.* **4**, 737 (1973). Mode of action: E. Hunter, J. F. V. Vincent, *Experientia* **30**, 1432 (1974); S. M. Meola, R. T. Mayer, *Science* **207**, 985 (1980). Field trials against locusts and grasshoppers: A. Bouaichi *et al., Crop Prot.* **13**, 53, 60 (1994). Brief review: J. L. Marx, *Science* **197**, 1170-1172 (1977). Review of activity, environmental fate, mode of action: A. Verloop, C. D. Ferrell, *ACS Symp. Ser.* **37**, 237-270 (1977); of chemistry and analyses: B. Rabenort *et al., Anal. Methods Pestic. Plant Growth Regul.* **10**, 57-72 (1978).

White to yellowish brown crystalline solid, mp 210-230° (technical grade); mp 239° (pure compd). Soly in water ≈0.2 ppm at 20°. Moderate to good soly in polar to very polar solvents; e.g. acetone 0.65 gm/100 ml at 20°. Partition coefficient (dichloromethane): 50 (pH 5.6); (1-octanol/water): ~5000. LD_{50} in mice, rats (formulation with 50% kaolin) (g/kg): 4.64, >10 orally (Mulder, Gijswijt).

USE: Insecticide.

3143. Diflucortolone. [2607-06-9] (6α, 11β, 16α)-6,9-Difluoro-11,21-dihydroxy-16-methylpregna-1,4-diene-3,20-dione; 6α,9α-difluoro-16α-methyl-1,4-pregnadiene-11β,21-diol-3,20-dione; 6α,9α-difluoro-16α-methyl-1-dehydrocorticosterone. $C_{22}H_{28}$-F_2O_4; mol wt 394.45. C 66.99%, H 7.15%, F 9.63%, O 16.22%. The 9α-fluoro deriv of fluocortolone, *q.v.* Prepn: **BE 639708**; K. Kieslich *et al.,* **US 3426128** (1964, 1969, both to Schering AG); *eidem, Arzneim.-Forsch.* **26**, 1462 (1976). Toxicity: P. Gunzel *et al., ibid.* 1476. Series of articles on pharmacology, toxicity, metabolism and clinical studies: *ibid.* **26**, 1463-1513 (1976).

Crystals from ethyl acetate-ether, mp 240-244°. uv max: 237 nm (ε 16600) (Kieslich, 1969). Also reported as mp 248-249°. $[\alpha]_D^{22}$ +111° (methanol) (Kieslich, 1976).

21-Valerate. [59198-70-8] Neribas; Neriforte; Nerisona; Nerisone; Temetex; Texmeten. $C_{27}H_{36}F_2O_5$; mol wt 478.57. Crystals, mp 195-195.5°. $[\alpha]_D^{22}$ +100.8° (dioxane). Approx LD_{50} in mice, rats: >4, 3.1 g/kg orally; 180, 13 mg/kg s.c.; 450, 98 mg/kg i.p. (Gunzel).

THERAP CAT: Anti-inflammatory.

3144. Diflufenican. [83164-33-4] *N*-(2,4-Difluorophenyl)-2-[3-(trifluoromethyl)phenoxy]-3-pyridinecarboxamide; *N*-(2,4-difluorophenyl)-2-(3-trifluoromethylphenoxy)nicotinamide; 2',4'-difluoro-2-(α,α,α-trifluoro-*m*-tolyloxy)nicotinanilide; M & B 38544; Fenican. $C_{19}H_{11}F_5N_2O_2$; mol wt 394.29. C 57.88%, H 2.81%, F 24.09%, N 7.10%, O 8.12%. Pre and post emergence foliar absorbed herbicide for winter weed control in cereal crops; carotenoid biosynthesis inhibitor. Prepn: M. C. Cramp *et al.,* **EP 53011**; *eidem,* **US 4618366** (1981, 1986 both to May & Baker). Description of physical properties, toxicity and activity: M. C. Cramp *et al., Proc. Br. Crop Prot. Conf. - Weeds* **1985**, 23. Mode of action: G. Britton *et al., ibid.* **1987**, 1015. GC determn in runoff and soil: L. Patty, C. Guyot, *Bull. Environ. Contam. Toxicol.* **55**, 802 (1995). Degradation and persistence in soil: E. Conte *et al., J. Agric. Food Chem.* **46**, 4766 (1998).

White crystalline solid, without odor, from toluene, mp 161-162°. Soly at 20°: acetone 10%; acetophenone 5%; aromasol H 1%; cyclohexane 1%; DMF 10%; ethylcellosolve 1%; isophorone 3.5%; kerosene 1%; xylene 2%; water 0.05 mg/l. Vapor pressure at 25°: 4.25 × 10^{-6} Pa. LD_{50} in mice, rats (mg/kg): >1000, >2000 orally; in rats (mg/kg): >2000 dermally (Cramp).

USE: Herbicide.

3145. Diflufenzopyr. [109293-97-2] 2-[1-[[[(3,5-Difluorophenyl)amino]carbonyl]hydrazono]ethyl]-3-pyridinecarboxylic acid; 2-[1-[4-(3,5-difluorophenyl)semicarbazono]ethyl]nicotinic acid; SAN-835H. $C_{15}H_{12}F_2N_4O_3$; mol wt 334.28. C 53.90%, H 3.62%, F 11.37%, N 16.76%, O 14.36%. Auxin transport inhibitor. Prepn: R. J. Anderson, M. M. Leippe, **JP Kokai 62 45570**; *eidem et al.,* **US 5098466** (1987, 1992 both to Sandoz). Synergy with auxin type herbicides: R. G. Lym, K. M. Christianson, *Proc. West. Soc. Weed Sci.* **51**, 59 (1998). Field trial of combination with dicamba in corn: P. H. Sikkema *et al., Weed Technol.* **13**, 283 (1999). Review of physical properties, mode of action, and activity: S. Bowe *et al., Brighton Crop Prot. Conf. - Weeds* **1999**, 35-40.

Off-white solid, mp 155° (Bowe); also reported as 186° (Anderson). Soly in water: 63 mg/l. Vapor pressure at 20°: $<1.3 \times 10^{-5}$ Pa. Log P (octanol/water, pH 7): 0.3. LD_{50} in rats (mg/kg): >5000 orally; >5000 dermally; LC_{50} in rats (mg/l): 2.93 by inhalation; LC_{50} in rainbow trout, bluegill sunfish (mg/l): 106, 135 (Bowe).

Mixture with dicamba. [211050-90-7] BAS-662; SAN-1269H; Distinct.

USE: Herbicide.

3146. Diflunisal. [22494-42-4] 2',4'-Difluoro-4-hydroxy-[1,1'-biphenyl]-3-carboxylic acid; 2',4'-difluoro-4-hydroxy-3-biphenylcarboxylic acid; 2',4'-difluoro-4-hydroxy-[1',1-diphenyl]-3-carboxylic acid; 2-(hydroxy)-5-(2,4-difluorophenyl)benzoic acid; 5-(2,4-difluorophenyl)salicylic acid; MK-647; Adomal; Difludol; Dolisal; Dolobid; Dolobis; Flovacil; Fluniget; Fluodonil; Flustar. $C_{13}H_8F_2O_3$; mol wt 250.20. C 62.41%, H 3.22%, F 15.19%, O 19.18%. Prepn: W. V. Ruyle et al., ZA 6701021; eidem, FR 1522570; eidem, US 3714226 (1968, 1968, 1973, all to Merck & Co.); J. Hannah et al., J. Med. Chem. 21, 1093 (1978). Metabolism: P. J. DeSchepper et al., Br. J. Clin. Pharmacol. 4, 645P (1977). Clinical studies: J. A. Wojtulewski et al., Curr. Med. Res. Opin. 5, 562 (1978); J. A. Hicklin, ibid. 572; in sickle cell anemia: E. A. Oyewo, Clin. Trials J. 24, 249 (1987). Review of chemistry, pharmacology, clinical pharmacology: S. L. Steelman et al., ibid. 506-514. Comprehensive description: M. Cotton, R. A. Hux, Anal. Profiles Drug Subs. 14, 491-526 (1985). Review: Br. J. Clin. Pharmacol. 4, Suppl. 1, 1S-52S (1977); C. A. Winter et al., in Pharmacological and Biochemical Properties of Drug Substances vol. 3, M. E. Goldberg, Ed. (Am. Pharm. Assoc., Washington, DC, 1981) pp 291-323. Comprehensive review of pharmacological properties and therapeutic use in pain: R. N. Brogden et al., Drugs 19, 84-106 (1980); Pharmacotherapy 3, no. 2, pt. 2, 1S-82S (1983).

Crystals from toluene, mp 210-211°. Sparingly sol in water. LD_{50} orally in female mice: 439 mg/kg (Stone).

THERAP CAT: Analgesic; anti-inflammatory.

3147. 2,4-Difluoroaniline. [367-25-9] 2,4-Difluorobenzenamine. $C_6H_5F_2N$; mol wt 129.11. C 55.82%, H 3.90%, F 29.43%, N 10.85%. Prepn: Swarts, Rec. Trav. Chim. 35, 164 (1916); Kutepov, Rozanova, Zh. Obshch. Khim. 27, 2848 (1957), C.A. 52, 8067 (1958); Nad et al., C.A. 53, 14976i (1959).

mp −7.5°. bp$_{753}$ 169.5°. n_D^{25} 1.5043. Specific gravity at 25°: 10.72 lb/gal. Flash pt 158°F (70°C).

USE: In organic syntheses.

3148. p-Difluorobenzene. [540-36-3] $C_6H_4F_2$; mol wt 114.09. C 63.16%, H 3.53%, F 33.30%. Prepd by diazotizing p-fluoroaniline in hydrofluoric acid and heating the diazonium salt to 120°: Swarts, Chem. Zentralbl. 1913, II, 760.

Liquid, pungent, aromatic odor. mp −23.7°. bp 88.82°. d^{20} 1.17006. $n_D^{18.9}$ 1.44219.

3149. 4,4'-Difluorodiphenyl. [398-23-2] 4,4'-Difluoro-1,1'-biphenyl. $C_{12}H_8F_2$; mol wt 190.19. C 75.78%, H 4.24%, F

19.98%. NMR spectrum: T. K. Halstead et al., J. Chem. Soc. Faraday Trans. 2 1981, 1817.

Crystalline powder; aromatic odor. d 1.04. mp 92-95°. bp 254-255°. Insol in water. Freely sol in alc, chloroform, ether, oils.

3150. Difluoroiodotoluene. [371-11-9] Difluoro(4-methylphenyl)iodine; 4-iodotoluene difluoride; p-tolyliododifluoride. $C_7H_7F_2I$; mol wt 256.03. C 32.84%, H 2.76%, F 14.84%, I 49.57%. Hypervalent iodine(III) difluoride reagent used to transfer of fluorine to organic substrates. Prepn: R. F. Weinland, W. Stille, Ann. 328, 132 (1903); W. Bockemüller, Ber. 64, 522 (1931); and spectral studies: D. Naumann, G. Rüther, J. Fluorine Chem. 15, 213 (1980). Improved prepn: M. Sawaguchi et al., Synthesis 2002, 1802. Synthetic applications in fluorination reactions: W. B. Motherwell et al., J. Chem. Soc. Perkin Trans. 1 2002, 2809; M. A. Arrica, T. Wirth, Eur. J. Org. Chem. 2005, 395.

White needles from hexane, mp 98° (Sawaguchi). Also reported as white solid, mp 110° (dec) (Motherwell). Easily sol in chloroform; sparingly sol in petroleum ether, 40% hydrofluoric acid.

USE: Fluorinating agent.

3151. Difluoromethane. [75-10-5] HFC-32; methylene difluoride; R-32; Genetron 32. CH_2F_2; mol wt 52.02. C 23.09%, H 3.88%, F 73.04%. Hydrofluorocarbon refrigerant with zero ozone-depletion potential. Prepn: A. L. Henne et al., J. Am. Chem. Soc. 59, 1400 (1937). Structural studies: L. O. Brockway, J. Phys. Chem. 41, 185, 747 (1937); W. C. Hamilton, K. Hedberg, J. Am. Chem. Soc. 75, 5529 (1952). Microwave spectrum: D. R. Lide, Jr., ibid. 74, 3548 (1952). UV absorption spectrum: P. Wagner, A. B. F. Duncan, ibid. 77, 2609 (1955). Thermodynamic properties: P. F. Malbrunot et al., J. Chem. Eng. Data 13, 16 (1968); D. R. Defibaugh et al., ibid. 39, 333 (1994). Viscosity study: M. Takahashi et al., ibid. 40, 900 (1995). Toxicology and metabolism in rats: M. K. Ellis et al., Fundam. Appl. Toxicol. 31, 243 (1996).

Colorless gas, bp −51.6°. mp −136°. d^0 (liq) 1.052. d^{25} (liq) 0.961. Critical temp 78.4°; critical press 57.54 atm; critical d 0.430. Dipole moment 1.98 D.

USE: Refrigerant.

3152. Difluprednate. [23674-86-4] (6α,11β)-21-(Acetyloxy)-6,9-difluoro-11-hydroxy-17-(1-oxobutoxy)pregna-1,4-diene-3,20-dione; 6α,9-difluoro-11β,17,21-trihydroxypregna-1,4-diene-3,20-dione 21-acetate 17-butyrate; 6α,9α-difluoroprednisolone-21-acetate-17-butyrate; CM-9155; W-6309; Epitopic; Myser. $C_{27}H_{34}F_2O_7$; mol wt 508.55. C 63.77%, H 6.74%, F 7.47%, O 22.02%. Prepn: A. Ercoli, R. Gardi, ZA 6803686; A. Ercoli et al., US 3780177 (1968, 1973 both to Warner-Lambert). Anti-inflammatory properties: G. Di Pasquale et al., Steroids 16, 663, 679 (1970); R. Gardi et al., J. Med. Chem. 15, 556 (1972). Pharmacological study: J. Navarro et al., Arzneim.-Forsch. 28, 2302 (1978). Vasoconstrictive activity in man: A. Barbier et al., Therapie 33, 607 (1978). Bioavailability study: C. Lafille et al., Dermatologica 159, 277 (1979).

Crystals from methylene chloride/ether/petr ether, mp 191-194°. $[\alpha]_D^{22}$ +31.7° (c = 0.5 in dioxane). uv max (ethanol): 237-238 nm ($E_{1cm}^{1\%}$ 320).

THERAP CAT: Anti-inflammatory.

3153. Digallic Acid. [536-08-3] 3,4-Dihydroxy-5-[(3,4,5-trihydroxybenzoyl)oxy]benzoic acid; gallic acid 5,6-dihydroxy-3-carboxyphenyl ester; 4,5-dihydroxybenzoic acid monogallate; gallic acid 3-monogallate; *m*-digallic acid; *m*-galloylgallic acid. $C_{14}H_{10}O_9$; mol wt 322.22. C 52.18%, H 3.13%, O 44.69%. Isoln from Aleppo gallotannin and Chinese gallotannin: Nierenstein, *Ber.* **43**, 628 (1910). Synthesis: Fischer, Freudenberg, *Ber.* **46**, 1128 (1913). Structure: Nierenstein *et al., J. Am. Chem. Soc.* **47**, 846 (1925). Determn by HPLC: P. Delahaye, M. Verzele, *J. Chromatogr.* **265**, 363 (1983); in tannic acids: M. Verzele *et al., Bull. Soc. Chim. Belg.* **92**, 181 (1983). Role in corrosion inhibition: A. M. Beccaria, E. D. Mor, *Br. Corrosion J.* **11**, 156 (1976).

Hydrated needles from alc + water, anhydr at 110°; dec 280°. Sol in 1900 parts water at 25°; in 50-60 parts boiling water; sol in methanol, ethanol, acetone; sparingly sol in ether, glacial acetic acid. Upon addn of KCN to an aq soln a transitory pink color appears, which returns on shaking.

Note: In pharmaceutical literature the name digallic acid is frequently confused with tannic acid.

3154. Digalogenin. [6877-35-6] (3β,5α,15β,25R)-Spirostan-3,15-diol. $C_{27}H_{44}O_4$; mol wt 432.64. C 74.96%, H 10.25%, O 14.79%. Aglycon of digalonin. Isoln from saponin mixture and partial synthesis from digitogenin: Tschesche, Wulff, *Ber.* **94**, 2019 (1961).

Crystals from methanol, mp 218.5-220.5°. $[\alpha]_D^{21}$ −75° (CHCl₃). IR spectrum: Tschesche, Wulff *loc. cit.* Sol in chloroform.

3155. Diginatigenin. [559-57-9] (3β,5β,12β,16β)-3,12,14,-16-Tetrahydroxycard-20(22)-enolide; 12-hydroxygitoxigenin; 16-hydroxydigoxigenin. $C_{23}H_{34}O_6$; mol wt 406.51. C 67.96%, H 8.43%, O 23.61%. Aglycone of diginatin from *Digitalis lanata* Ehrk., *Scrophulariaceae:* Murphy, *J. Am. Pharm. Assoc. Sci. Ed.* **44**, 719 (1955). Aglycone of lanatoside D: Angliker *et al., Ann.* **607**, 131 (1957). Obtained by microbiological conversion of gitoxigenin: Tamm, Gubler, *Helv. Chim. Acta* **41**, 1762 (1958); Okado *et al., Chem. Pharm. Bull.* **8**, 530 (1960). Structure: Linde *et al., Helv. Chim. Acta* **42**, 2040 (1959); Okado *et al., Chem. Pharm. Bull.* **8**, 535 (1960).

Needles from water, mp 157°. $[\alpha]_D^{20}$ +34° (methanol). Absorption max (ethanol): 318 nm (log ε 4.18); (98% w/w H_2SO_4): 230, 310, 390, 490 nm ($E_{1cm}^{1\%}$ 160, 130, 210, 85).

3156. Diginatin. [52589-12-5] (3β,5β,12β,16β)-3-[(*O*-2,6-Dideoxy-β-D-*ribo*-hexopyranosyl-(1 → 4)-*O*-2,6-dideoxy-β-D-*ribo*-hexopyranosyl-(1 → 4)-2,6-dideoxy-β-D-*ribo*-hexopyranosyl)oxy]-12,14,16-trihydroxy-card-20(22)-enolide. $C_{41}H_{64}O_{15}$; mol wt 796.94. C 61.79%, H 8.09%, O 30.11%. Cardiac glycoside from *Digitalis lanata* Ehrk., *Scrophulariaceae:* Murphy, *J. Am. Pharm. Assoc. Sci. Ed.* **44**, 719 (1955); Angliker *et al., Ann.* **607**, 131 (1957); von Wartburg *et al., Experientia* **14**, 439 (1958). Acid hydrolysis yields 1 mol diginatigenin + 3 mols D-digitoxose. The sugar residue is attached to the hydroxyl group at C-3 of the aglycon.

Prisms from acetone, mp 251-253°. Somewhat hygroscopic. $[\alpha]_D^{20}$ +20.5 ±2°; $[\alpha]_{546}^{20}$ +26.3 ±2° (c = 0.6 in methanol). Absorption max (98% w/w H_2SO_4): 230, 310, 390, 480, 560 nm ($E_{1cm}^{1\%}$ 185, 175, 315, 230, 120). Sol in alcohol, dil alcohol, dioxane; slightly sol in acetone. One part sol in 1000 parts water and in 2000 parts chloroform at 25°.

Acetyldiginatin-α. $C_{43}H_{66}O_{16}$. Flat plates from methanol + chloroform+ ether, mp 199-202°. $[\alpha]_D^{20}$ +30.1° (c = 0.6 in pyridine). uv max: 218 nm (log ε 4.1).

3157. Diginin. [467-53-8] (3β,12α,14β,17α,20S)-3-[(2,6-Dideoxy-3-*O*-methyl-D-lyxohexopyranosyl)oxy]-12,20-epoxy-pregn-5-ene-11,15-dione; 3β-(diginosyloxy)-12α,20α-epoxy-14β,17α-pregn-5-ene-11,15-dione. $C_{28}H_{40}O_7$; mol wt 488.61. C 68.83%, H 8.25%, O 22.92%. Isoln from leaves of *Digitalis purpurea* L., *Scrophulariaceae:* Karrer in *E. Barell Festschrift* (1936) p 238; *Chem. Zentralbl.* **1936**, II, 2727. Isoln: Shoppee, Reichstein, *Helv. Chim. Acta* **23**, 975 (1940); Shoppee, *ibid.* **27**, 426 (1944). Structure: Shoppee *et al., J. Chem. Soc.* **1962**, 3610; Tschesche, Brügmann, *Tetrahedron* **20**, 1469 (1964). Mild hydrolysis yields **diginigenin** and **diginose.** Attempted partial synthesis of diginigenin: Tschesche, Schwinum, *Ber.* **100**, 464 (1967); Tschesche, Müller-Albrecht, *Ber.* **103**, 350 (1970).

Stout prisms from dil alc. Indistinct melting range: 155-183°. $[\alpha]_D^{14}$ −223° (c = 2.3 in chloroform). uv max (ethanol) 309 nm (log ε 1.94). Freely sol in chloroform; slightly sol in ether, acetone, ethyl acetate, carbon tetrachloride. Practically insol in water. Positive Legal's test. The Keller reaction produces a brilliant yellow band with diginigenin.

3158. Digitalin. [752-61-4] (3β,5β,16β)-3-[(6-Deoxy-4-*O*-β-D-glucopyranosyl-3-*O*-methyl-β-D-galactopyranosyl)oxy]-14,16-dihydroxycard-20(22)-enolide; digitalinum verum; digitalinum true; Schmiedeberg's digitalin; Diginorgin. $C_{36}H_{56}O_{14}$; mol wt 712.82. C 60.66%, H 7.92%, O 31.42%. Obtained from seeds of *Digitalis purpurea* L., *Scrophulariaceae*, and from roots of *Adenium honghel* A. DC., *Apocynaceae:* Schmiedeberg, *Arch. Exp. Pathol. Pharmakol.* **3**, 16 (1874); Windaus, Haack, *Ber.* **62**, 475 (1929); Hunger, Reichstein, *Helv. Chim. Acta* **33**, 76 (1950); Sasakawa, *J. Pharm. Soc. Jpn.* **74**, 474 (1954); Miyatake *et al., Pharm. Bull.* **5**, 157 (1957).

Crystals from methanol + ether and methanol + water, mp 240-243°. $[\alpha]_D^{20}$ −1.1° (c = 0.894 in methanol). Slightly sol in water, chloroform or ether; sol in alcohol.

16-Acetyldigitalinum verum. $C_{38}H_{58}O_{15}$. Prepn: Miyatake *et al.*, US 3023147 (1962). Amorphous powder. Freely sol in water, alcohol, acetone. Practically insol in benzene, ether. uv max: 217 nm (log ε 4.16). $[\alpha]_D^{26}$ −21.1° (methanol).

THERAP CAT: Cardiotonic.

3159. Digitalis. Foxglove; fairy gloves; purple foxglove. Dried leaves of *Digitalis purpurea* L., *Scrophulariaceae*. Habit. Southern and central Europe, cultivated in the U.S. *Constit*. Digitoxin (0.2-0.4%), digitonin, digitalin, antirhinic acid, digitalosmin, digitoflavone, inositol, pectin. One U.S.P. digitalis unit represents the potency of 0.1 g of the U.S.P. Digitalis Reference Standard. Toxicology: A. P. Somlyo, *Am. J. Cardiol.* **5**, 523 (1960). Review of mechanism of action and clinical use: T. W. Smith, *N. Engl. J. Med.* **318**, 358-365 (1988). Book: C. Fisch, B. Surawicz, *Digitalis* (Grune & Stratton, New York, 1969) 244 pp.

Caution: Potential symptoms of overexposure are anorexia, nausea, salivation, vomiting, diarrhea, headache, drowsiness, disorientation, delirium, hallucinations; death may result. *See Clinical Toxicology of Commercial Products*, R. E. Gosselin *et al.*, Eds. (Williams & Wilkins, Baltimore, 4th ed., 1976) Section III, pp 124-133.

THERAP CAT: Cardiotonic.

THERAP CAT (VET): Cardiotonic.

3160. Digitogenin. [511-34-2] (2α,3β,5α,15β,25R)-Spirostan-2,3,15-triol. $C_{27}H_{44}O_5$; mol wt 448.64. C 72.28%, H 9.89%, O 17.83%. The aglycon of digitonin: Tschesche, *Ber.* **68**, 1090 (1935); Tschesche, Hagedorn, *Ber.* **69**, 797 (1936). Structure and stereochemistry: Marker *et al.*, *J. Am. Chem. Soc.* **64**, 1843 (1942); Meystre *et al.*, *Helv. Chim. Acta* **38**, 381 (1955). Klass *et al.*, *J. Am. Chem. Soc.* **77**, 3829 (1955); and IR spectra: Djerassi *et al.*, *ibid.* **78**, 3166 (1956).

Needles from alc, dec 296°. $[\alpha]_D^{19}$ −81° (c = 1.4 in chloroform). Practically insol in water. Sol in 30 parts chloroform, 35 parts boiling alc, 100 parts alc at 20°.

2,3-Diacetate. Crystals from methanol-chloroform, mp 241.5-242°. $[\alpha]_D$ −104°.

Triacetate. Minute needles from ether, mp 190°.

3161. Digitonin. [11024-24-1] Digitin. $C_{56}H_{92}O_{29}$; mol wt 1229.31. C 54.71%, H 7.54%, O 37.74%. Obtained from the

seeds of *Digitalis purpurea* L., *Scrophulariaceae*. Extraction procedure: Gisvold, *J. Am. Pharm. Assoc.* **23**, 664 (1934). Purification of commercial digitonin and its separation into two fractions: G. Ruhenstroth-Bauer, P. M. Breitenfeld, *Z. Physiol. Chem.* **302**, 111 (1955). Structure: Tschesche, Wulff, *Tetrahedron* **19**, 1213 (1963). Use as clinical reagent: H. H. Leffler, *Am. J. Clin. Pathol.* **31**, 310 (1959).

Crystals from alc, sinters 225°. Indistinct mp 235-240°. $[\alpha]_D^{20}$ −54° (0.45 g in 15.8 ml methanol). One gram dissolves in 57 ml abs alc, in 220 ml 95% alc. Practically insol in water, forming a soapy suspension. Also practically insol in chloroform, ether.

USE: Clinical reagent (cholesterol determination).

3162. Digitoxigenin. [143-62-4] (3β,5β)-3,14-Dihydroxycard-20(22)-enolide; $Δ^{20:22}$-3,14,21-trihydroxynorcholenic acid lactone; cerberigenin; echujetin; evonogenin; Thevetigenin. $C_{23}H_{34}O_4$; mol wt 374.51. C 73.76%, H 9.15%, O 17.09%. The aglycon of digitoxin, thevetin, cerberin, echujin, evomonosid. Prepn by refluxing digitoxin in a mixture of water + alcohol + HCl: Cloetta, *Arch. Exp. Pathol. Pharmakol.* **88**, 113 (1920); Stoll, Kreiss, *Helv. Chim. Acta* **17**, 592 (1934). Structure: Jacobs, Hoffmann, *J. Biol. Chem.* **67**, 333 (1926); Jacobs, Gustus, *ibid.* **78**, 573; **79**, 533 (1928); **82**, 402 (1929); Jacobs, Elderfield, *ibid.* **108**, 497 (1935); Elderfield, *Chem. Rev.* **17**, 187 (1935). Stereochemistry: Meyer, *Helv. Chim. Acta* **30**, 1976 (1947). Synthesis: Danieli *et al.*, *Tetrahedron* **22**, 3189 (1966); W. Fritsch *et al.*, *Ann.* **1974**, 621; S. F. Donovan *et al.*, *Tetrahedron Lett.* **1979**, 3287; R. Marinibettolo *et al.*, *Can. J. Chem.* **59**, 1403 (1981); T. Milkova *et al.*, *Tetrahedron Lett.* **23**, 413 (1982). Biosynthesis from neriifolin, *q.v.*: A. Cruz *et al.*, *J. Org. Chem.* **42**, 3580 (1977).

Stout prisms from 40% alc, mp 253°. $[\alpha]_D^{17}$ +19.1° (c = 1.36 in methanol). Sol in alc, chloroform, acetone; slightly sol in ethyl acetate; very sparingly sol in ether, water.

3-Acetyldigitoxigenin. $C_{25}H_{36}O_5$. Hexagonal plates from acetone + ether, mp 222-227°. $[\alpha]_D^{17}$ +21.4° (c = 1.02 in chloroform).

3163. Digitoxin. [71-63-6] (3β,5β)-3-[(O-2,6-Dideoxy-β-D-*ribo*-hexopyranosyl-(1 → 4)-O-2,6-dideoxy-β-D-*ribo*-hexopyranosyl-(1 → 4)-2,6-dideoxy-β-D-*ribo*-hexopyranosyl)oxy]-14-hydroxycard-20(22)-enolide; digitalin, crystalline; digitophyllin; Carditoxin; Coramedan; Cristapurat; Crystodigin; Digicor; Digilong; Digimerck; Digimed; Digipural; Ditaven; Lanatoxin; Myodigin; Purodigin; Purpurid; Tardigal. $C_{41}H_{64}O_{13}$; mol wt 764.94. C 64.38%, H 8.43%, O 27.19%. Secondary glycoside from *Digitalis purpurea* L., *Scrophulariaceae*. Extracted from the dried leaves with 50% alc. Extraction procedure: Cloetta, *Arch. Exp. Pathol.*

Pharmakol. **112,** 261 (1926). Purification: Windaus, Freese, *Ber.* **58,** 2503 (1925). Ten kilo leaves yield about 6 grams pure digitoxin. Identity with digitophyllin: Cloetta, *Arch. Exp. Pathol. Pharmakol.* **88,** 113 (1920). Structure: *See* reviews by Elderfield in *Chem. Rev.* **17,** 187 (1935), and Stoll, *The Cardiac Glycosides* (London, 1937); also Shoppee in *Annu. Rev. Biochem.* **11,** 103 (1942). Acid hydrolysis yields 1 mol digitoxigenin + 3 mol digitoxose. The sugar residue is attached to the hydroxyl group at C-3 of the aglycon. Structure of the sugar moiety: Lichti *et al., Helv. Chim. Acta* **45,** 868 (1962). Digitoxin U.S.P. is either pure digitoxin or a mixture of cardioactive glycosides obtained from *Digitalis purpurea* and consisting chiefly of digitoxin. The potency of digitoxin U.S.P. corresp to the potency of an equal wt of U.S.P. Digitoxin Reference Standard. A deviation of 20% is permitted. The physical characteristics given below are those of the pure compd. Toxicity data: Foerster *et al., Arch. Int. Pharmacodyn. Ther.* **159,** 1 (1966). Comprehensive description: I. M. Jakovljevic, *Anal. Profiles Drug Subs.* **3,** 149-172 (1974).

Very small elongated, rectangular plates from dil alc. May contain ½ or 1 mol H_2O or EtOH which is given up at 118° *in vacuo.* When anhydrous, mp 256-257°. $[\alpha]_D^{20}$ +4.8° (c = 1.2 in dioxane). One gram dissolves in about 40 ml chloroform, about 60 ml alcohol, about 400 ml ethyl acetate. Also sol in acetone, amyl alcohol, pyridine, sparingly sol in ether, petr ether, water (1 g/100 liter at 20°). LD_{50} in guinea pigs, cats (mg/kg): 60.0, 0.18 orally (Foerster).

Acetyl derivatives *see* Acetyldigitoxins.

THERAP CAT: Cardiotonic.

THERAP CAT (VET): Cardiotonic.

3164. Digitoxose. [527-52-6] 2,6-Dideoxy-D-*ribo*-hexose; 2-desoxy-D-altromethylose; 2,6-didesoxy-D-allose. $C_6H_{12}O_4$; mol wt 148.16. C 48.64%, H 8.16%, O 43.19%. Obtained by mild acid hydrolysis of the glycosides digitoxin, gitoxin and digoxin: Cloetta, *Arch. Exp. Pathol. Pharmakol.* **88,** 113 (1920); **112,** 261 (1926); Windaus, Stein, *Ber.* **61,** 2436 (1928); Kraft, *Arch. Pharm.* **250,** 118 (1912); Mannich *et al., ibid.* **268,** 453 (1930); Smith, *J. Chem. Soc.* **1930,** 508; **1931,** 23. Configuration: Micheel, *Ber.* **63,** 347 (1930). Structure: S. F. Dyke, *The Carbohydrates* (Interscience, New York, 1960) p 104. Synthesis: Gut, Prins, *Helv. Chim. Acta* **30,** 1223 (1947); Bolliger, Ulrich, *ibid.* **35,** 93 (1952). Stereochemical study: S. Tsukamoto *et al., J. Chem. Soc. Perkin Trans. 1* **1988,** 2621. *Review:* R. C. Elderfield in W. W. Pigman, M. L. Wolfrom, *Advances in Carbohydrate Chemistry* vol. **I** (Academic Press, New York, 1945) pp 159-164.

Crystals from methanol + ether, from ethyl acetate or from acetone + ether, mp 112°. $[\alpha]_D^{17}$ +46.3° (in water); $[\alpha]_D^{20}$ +39.1° (in methanol); $[\alpha]_D^{18}$ +27.9° → +43.3° (after 24 hrs in pyridine). Freely sol in water; sol in acetone, ethanol. Practically insol in ether.

3165. Diglyme. [111-96-6] 1,1'-Oxybis[2-methoxyethane]; bis(2-methoxyethyl) ether; diethylene glycol dimethyl ether. $C_6H_{14}O_3$; mol wt 134.17. C 53.71%, H 10.52%, O 35.77%. $(CH_3-OCH_2CH_2)_2O$. Prepn: Cretcher, Pittenger, *J. Am. Chem. Soc.* **47,** 163 (1925); Gallaugher, Hibbert, *ibid.* **58,** 813 (1936).

Liquid, bp_{760} 162°; bp_{200} 116°; bp_{35} 75°; bp_3 20°. d_{20}^{20} 0.9451. mp −68°. Flash pt (open cup) 158°F (70°C). n_D^{20} 1.4097. Miscible with water, alcohol, ether, hydrocarbon solvents.

USE: Solvent; reaction medium for Grignard and similar syntheses.

3166. Digoxigenin. [1672-46-4] (3β,5β,12β)-3,12,14-Trihydroxycard-20(22)-enolide; $\Delta^{20:22}$-3β,12β,14,21-tetrahydroxynorcholenic acid lactone; lanadigenin. $C_{23}H_{34}O_5$; mol wt 390.51. C 70.74%, H 8.78%, O 20.49%. The aglycon of digoxin. By hydrolysis of digoxin: Smith, *J. Chem. Soc.* **1930,** 508. From *Digitalis orientalis* L. and *D. lanata* Ehrh., *Scrophulariaceae:* Mannick, Schneider, *Arch. Pharm.* **279,** 223 (1941); Pataki *et al., Helv. Chim. Acta* **36,** 1295 (1953). Structure: Meyer, Reichstein, *Expe-*

rientia **9,** 253 (1953); Cardwell, Smith, *ibid.* 367; *eidem, J. Chem. Soc.* **1954,** 2012. Synthesis: P. Welzel, H. Stein, *Tetrahedron Lett.* **22,** 3385 (1981).

Dihydrate. Prismatic rods from dil alc. Anhydr as stout prisms from ethyl acetate, mp 222°. $[\alpha]_{546}^{20}$ +27.0° (c = 1.77 in methanol). Although it is a 3β-alcohol, it is not precipitated by digitonin (Pataki).

3,12-Diacetyldigoxigenin. Prisms from dil methanol, mp 222-223°. $[\alpha]_{546}^{20}$ +61.3° (c = 2 in methanol).

3167. Digoxin. [20830-75-5] (3β,5β,12β)-3-[(*O*-2,6-Dideoxy-β-D-*ribo*-hexopyranosyl-(1 → 4)-*O*-2,6-dideoxy-β-D-*ribo*-hexopyranosyl-(1 → 4)-2,6-dideoxy-β-D-*ribo*-hexopyranosyl)oxy]-12,14-dihydroxycard-20(22)-enolide; Digacin; Dilanacin; Eudigox; Lanicor; Lanoxin; Lanoxicaps; Lenoxin; Neo-Dioxanin; Rougoxin. $C_{41}H_{64}O_{14}$; mol wt 780.94. C 63.06%, H 8.26%, O 28.68%. Secondary glycoside from *Digitalis lanata* Ehrh., or *D. orientalis* Lam., *Scrophulariaceae:* S. Smith, *J. Chem. Soc.* **1930,** 508; Stoll, *The Cardiac Glycosides* (London, 1937); M. M. Dhar *et al.,* **IN 62497** (1958 to Council Sci. Indust. Res.), *C.A.* **53,** 653b (1959). *See also* ref under Digoxigenin. Acid hydrolysis of digoxin yields 1 mol digoxigenin + 3 mols digitoxose. The sugar residue is attached to the hydroxyl group at C-3 of the aglycon. Clinical pharmacokinetics: J. K. Aronson, *Clin. Pharmacokinet.* **5,** 137 (1980). Comprehensive description: P. R. B. Foss, S. A. Benezra, *Anal. Profiles Drug Subs.* **9,** 207-243 (1980).

Radially arranged, four- and five-sided triclinic plates from dil alcohol or dil pyridine, decomp 230-265°. $[\alpha]_{Hg}^{25}$ +13.4 to 13.8° (c = 10 in pyridine). uv max (ethanol): 220 nm (ε 12800). Sol in dil alcohol, pyridine, or mixt of chloroform and alcohol. Almost insol in ether, acetone, ethyl acetate, chloroform, water. More sol in hot 80% alcohol than gitoxin.

β-Methyldigoxin. [30685-43-9] Medigoxin; metildigoxin; 4'''-*O*-methyldigoxin; 3β,12β,14β-trihydroxy-5β-card-20(22)-enolide-3-(4'''-*O*-methyltridigitoxoside); Cardiolan; Lanirapid; Lanitop. $C_{42}H_{66}O_{14}$; mol wt 794.97. Obtained by the *O*-methylation of digoxin: F. Kaiser *et al.,* **ZA 6806079;** *eidem,* **US 3538078** (1969, 1970 both to Boehringer, Mann.). Pharmacology and toxicity studies: W. Schaumann, R. Wegerle, *Arzneim.-Forsch.* **21,** 225 (1971); H. Czerwek *et al., ibid.* 231. Crystals, mp 227-231°. LD_{50} in rats, mice (mg/kg): 4.8, 4.9 i.v.; 6.2, 4.8 i.p.; 8.3, 7.8 orally (Czerwek).

α-Acetyldigoxin. [5511-98-8] Lanatilin; Sandolanid. $C_{43}H_{66}O_{15}$; mol wt 822.98. Obtained by enzymatic hydrolysis of digilanide. Prisms from methanol + chloroform, dec 225°. $[\alpha]_D^{20}$ +18.9° (pyridine). Very sparingly sol in ethyl acetate.

β-Acetyldigoxin. [5355-48-6] Kardiamed; Longdigox; Novodigal; Stillacor. Needles from alcohol + chloroform, dec 240°. $[\alpha]_D^{20}$ +30.4° (c = 1.2 in alc). More sol in ethyl acetate than the α-form.

THERAP CAT: Cardiotonic.

THERAP CAT (VET): Cardiotonic.

3168. Dihexyverine. [561-77-3] [1,1'-Bicyclohexyl]-1-carboxylic acid 2-(1-piperidinyl)ethyl ester; 1-cyclohexylcyclohexanecarboxylic acid β-piperidinoethyl ester; dicyclohexylacetic acid 2-piperidinoethyl ester; dihexiverine. $C_{20}H_{35}NO_2$; mol wt 321.50. C 74.72%, H 10.97%, N 4.36%, O 9.95%. Anticholinergic. Prepn: Kopp, Tchoubar, *Bull. Soc. Chim. Fr.* **1952,** 84. Pharmacology: Buchel *et al., Arch. Sci. Physiol.* **16,** 57 (1962); **21,** 537 (1967); Guyonneau, *Med. Exp.* **6,** 245 (1962).

Hydrochloride. [5588-25-0] JL-1078; Metaspas; Diverine; Olimplex; Seclin; Dispas; Neospasmina; Spasmodex; Spasmalex.

$C_{20}H_{35}NO_2 \cdot HCl$; mol wt 357.96. Crystals, mp 175° (copper block). mp 200° (capillary). LD_{50} i.p. in mice: 212 mg/kg (Buchel).

THERAP CAT: Antispasmodic.

3169. Dihydralazine. [484-23-1] 2,3-Dihydro-1,4-phthalazinedione dihydrazone; 1,4-dihydrazinophthalazine. $C_8H_{10}N_6$; mol wt 190.21. C 50.52%, H 5.30%, N 44.18%. Vasodilator. Prepn: J. Druey, US 2484785 (1949 to Ciba); J. Druey, B. H. Ringier, *Helv. Chim. Acta* **34**, 195 (1951); Zerweck, Kunze, US 2786839 (1957 to Cassella Farbw.). Pharmacology: P. A. Van Zwieten, *Arzneim.-Forsch.* **18**, 79 (1968). Mechanism of action: I. W. Reimann *et al.*, *Clin. Sci.* **61**, 319s (1981); *eidem, Clin. Exp. Pharmacol. Physiol.* **12**, 79 (1985). Cerebrovascular effects in rats: L. M. Auer *et al.*, *Acta Med. Scand.* **Suppl. 678**, 73 (1983); D. I. Barry *et al.*, *Stroke* **15**, 102 (1984). Hemodynamic responses in man: G. G. Belz, *Clin. Pharmacol. Ther.* **37**, 48 (1985). Clinical studies: A. Salvadeo *et al.*, *Int. J. Clin. Pharmacol. Ther. Toxicol.* **19**, 372 (1981); P. I. Salmela *et al.*, *Ann. Clin. Res.* **13**, 433 (1981). Toxicity data: G. Steiner *et al.*, *J. Med. Chem.* **24**, 59 (1981).

Orange needles from water, dec about 180°. LD_{50} i.p. in rats: 1084 μmol/kg (Steiner).
Sulfate. [7327-87-9] Pressunic. $C_8H_{10}N_6 \cdot H_2SO_4$; mol wt 288.28. Needles, dec 233°.
Sulfate hemipentahydrate. Depressan; Dihyzin; Nepresol; Népressol.
Methanesulfonate. Dihydralazine mesylate; Nepresol Inject. $C_8H_{10}N_6 \cdot CH_3SO_3H$; mol wt 286.31.
THERAP CAT: Antihypertensive.

3170. Dihydroactinidiolide. [15356-74-8] 5,6,7,7a-Tetrahydro-4,4,7a-trimethyl-2(4H)-benzofuranone; 2-oxo-4,4,7a-trimethyl-2,4,5,6,6,7a-hexahydrobenzofuran; (2,6,6-trimethyl-2-hydroxycyclohexylidene)acetic acid lactone. $C_{11}H_{16}O_2$; mol wt 180.24. C 73.30%, H 8.95%, O 17.75%. Found in many plant sources including tea and tobacco. (−)-Form is naturally occurring. Produced by photo-oxidation of carotenoid flavor compounds. Pheromone component for queen recognition in red fire ants. Isoln from black tea aroma: J. Bricout *et al.*, *Helv. Chim. Acta* **50**, 1517 (1967); from *Actinidia polygama* Miq. and structure determn: T. Sakan *et al.*, *Tetrahedron Lett.* **8**, 1623 (1967); from tobacco and synthesis: W. C. Bailey, Jr. *et al.*, *J. Org. Chem.* **33**, 2819 (1968). Synthesis: S. Isoe *et al.*, *Tetrahedron Lett.* **9**, 5561 (1968); by photo-oxidation of β-carotene: *eidem, ibid.* **10**, 279 (1969). Abs config study: *eidem, ibid.* **13**, 2517 (1972). Prepn of enantiomers: K. Mori, Y. Nakazono, *Tetrahedron* **42**, 283 (1986). Improved prepns: G. V. Subbaraju *et al.*, *Tetrahedron Lett.* **32**, 4871 (1991); A. Bosser *et al.*, *Biotechnol. Prog.* **11**, 689 (1995). Prepn of (R)-form: S. Yao *et al.*, *J. Org. Chem.* **63**, 118 (1998). Germination inhibition in wheat grains: T. Kato *et al.*, *J. Agric. Food Chem.* **51**, 2161 (2003).

(R)-Form

Tan oil, bp_{800} 108-109°. mp 42-43°. Fruity aroma. uv max: 241 nm (ε 10000).
(R)-Form. [17092-92-1] mp 70-71°. $[\alpha]_D^{24}$ −121.0° (c = 1.05 in $CHCl_3$).
(S)-Form. [81800-41-1] mp 67-68°. $[\alpha]_D^{23}$ +120.9° (c = 1.00 in $CHCl_3$).
USE: Flavor ingredient; inhibitor of seed germination.

3171. Dihydrocodeine. [125-28-0] (5α,6α)-4,5-Epoxy-3-methoxy-17-methylmorphinan-6-ol; 6-hydroxy-3-methoxy-N-methyl-4,5-epoxymorphinan; dihydroneopine; drocode; Codhydrine; Dehacodin; DF 118; DH-codeine; Didrate; Dihydrin; Hydrocodin; Nadeine; Novicodin; Paracodin; Parzone; Rapacodin. $C_{18}H_{23}NO_3$; mol wt 301.38. C 71.73%, H 7.69%, N 4.65%, O 15.93%. Prepd by reduction of codeine or neopine: Skita, Franck, *Ber.* **44**, 2862 (1911); Wieland, Koralek, *Ann.* **433**, 269 (1923); Stein, *Pharmazie* **10**, 180 (1955).

Crystals from methanol + water, mp 112-113°; bp_{15} 248°.
Bitartrate (acid tartrate). Fortuss; DHC; Dico. $C_{18}H_{23}NO_3 \cdot C_4H_6O_6$; mol wt 451.47. Crystals from methanol, contains 66.8% dihydrocodeine when completely anhyd. mp 192-193° (Stein). The commercial medicinal grade usually melts at 186-190°. $[\alpha]_D^{25}$ −72 to −75° (c = 1 in H_2O). One gram dissolves in 4.5 ml water. Sparingly sol in alcohol. Insol in ether.
Note: This is a controlled substance (opiate): **21 CFR**, 1308.12.
THERAP CAT: Analgesic (narcotic). Antitussive.

3172. Dihydrocodeinone Enol Acetate. [466-90-0] (5α)-6,7-Didehydro-4,5-epoxy-3-methoxy-17-methylmorphinan-6-ol acetate (ester); demethyldihydrothebaine acetate (ester); acetyldemethyldihydrothebaine; acetyldihydrocodeinone; thebacon. $C_{20}H_{23}NO_4$; mol wt 341.40. C 70.36%, H 6.79%, N 4.10%, O 18.75%. Prepn by refluxing dihydrocodeinone with acetic anhydride and anhyd sodium acetate: Small *et al.*, *J. Org. Chem.* **3**, 204 (1938).

Needles from methanol, mp 154°. Practically insol in water. Soluble in most organic solvents.
Hydrochloride. [20236-82-2] Acedicon. $C_{20}H_{23}NO_4 \cdot HCl$; mol wt 377.86. Crystals, mp 132-135° (dec). Very sol in water. Stable in boiling water.
Note: This is a controlled substance (opium derivative): **21 CFR**, 1308.11.
THERAP CAT: Analgesic (narcotic). Antitussive.

3173. Dihydroequilin. [3563-27-7] (17β)-Estra-1,3,5(10),-7-tetraene-3,17-diol. $C_{18}H_{22}O_2$; mol wt 270.37. C 79.96%, H 8.20%, O 11.84%. Occurs in the 17α- and 17β-forms. Prepn of β-form by reduction of equilin with sodium in alc: David, *Acta Brev. Nederland* **4**, 63 (1934); Serini *et al.*, US 2221340 (1940 to Schering). Isoln of β-form from pregnant mares' urine: Gaudry, Glen, *Ind. Chim. Belge* **Suppl. 2**, 435 (1959). Prepn of α-form by reduction of equilin with aluminum isopropoxide: Carol *et al.*, *J. Biol. Chem.* **185**, 267 (1950). Isoln of α-form from pregnant mares' urine: Glen *et al.*, *Nature* **177**, 753 (1956). α-Form was formerly called β-dihydroequilin and vice versa: Banes *et al.*, *J. Biol. Chem.* **187**, 557 (1950).

Consult the Name Index before using this section.

β-Form

Crystals from actone, mp 174.5-174.6°. $[\alpha]_D^{20}$ +220° (dioxane).
17α-Form. [651-55-8] Plates from 30% ethanol, mp 205.5-205.6°. $[\alpha]_D^{20}$ +213° (ethanol).

3174. Dihydroergotamine. [511-12-6] 9,10-Dihydro-12′-hydroxy-2′-methyl-5′-(phenylmethyl)ergotaman-3′,6′,18-trione. $C_{33}H_{37}N_5O_5$; mol wt 583.68. C 67.91%, H 6.39%, N 12.00%, O 13.71%. α-Adrenergic blocker with selective venoconstrictor properties. Also binds to serotonin 5HT₁-receptors. Prepn from ergotamine: Stoll, Hofmann, *Helv. Chim. Acta* **26**, 2070 (1943). Clinical pharmacology: H. de Marées *et al., Eur. J. Clin. Pharmacol.* **30**, 685 (1986). Neurotransmitter receptor binding study: B. G. McCarthy, S. J. Peroutka, *Headache* **29**, 420 (1989). Clinical trials in migraine: P. Winner *et al., ibid.* **33**, 471 (1993); D. Ziegler *et al., Neurology* **44**, 447 (1994).
Strongly refractive prisms from dil acetone, contg 2 mols acetone and 2 mols water of crystn. mp 239°. $[\alpha]_D^{20}$ −64°; $[\alpha]_{546}^{20}$ −79° (c = 0.5 in pyridine). Insol in water. Sparingly sol in methanol, ethanol, chloroform, benzene.
Tartrate. Divegal. $(C_{33}H_{37}N_5O_5)_2 \cdot C_4H_6O_6$; mol wt 1317.44. Six-sided plates from methanol, dec 210-215°.
Methanesulfonate. [6190-39-2] Dihydroergotamine mesylate; Agit; Angionorm; Dergotamine; DET MS; D.H.E. 45; Diergo; Dihydergot; Dirgotarl; Endophleban; Ergomimet; Ergont; Ergotonin; Ikaran; Migranal; Orstanorm; Séglor; Tonopres; Verladyn. $C_{33}H_{37}N_5O_5 \cdot CH_3SO_3H$; mol wt 679.78. Large prisms from 95% alc. mp 230-235°. Moderately sol in water.
THERAP CAT: Antimigraine.

3175. Dihydro-β-erythroidine. [23255-54-1] (3β)-1,6-Didehydro-14,17-dihydro-3-methoxy-16(15H)-oxaerythrinan-15-one; 12,13-didehydro-2,7,13,14-tetrahydro-α-erythroidine. $C_{16}H_{21}$-NO_3; mol wt 275.34. C 69.79%, H 7.69%, N 5.09%, O 17.43%. The more active of the two isomers that constitute the principal alkaloidal fraction of seeds from several *Erythrina* spp. In contrast to curare, *q.v.*, it retains its ability to block neuromuscular transmission even when administered orally: K. Unna, J. G. Greslin, *J. Pharmacol.* **80**, 53 (1944); K. Unna *et al., ibid.* 39. Prepd by catalytic hydrogenation of β-erythroidine or a salt of β-erythroidine: Folkers, Koniuszy, US 2370651 (1945 to Merck & Co.). Structure: Boekelheide *et al., J. Am. Chem. Soc.* **75**, 2550 (1953). Configuration: Hanson, *Proc. Chem. Soc. London* **1963**, 52.

Crystals from anhydr ethyl ether, dec 85-86°. $[\alpha]_D^{25}$ +102.5°. Soluble in ethanol. Alkaline hydrolysis yields sodium dihydro-β-erythroidinate.
Hydrochloride. Crystals from abs ethanol, mp 238°. $[\alpha]_D^{25}$ +124.7°.
Hydrobromide. Crystals from abs ethanol or abs ethanol + abs ether, dec 242°. Bitter taste. $[\alpha]_D^{25}$ +106-107.5°. Soly in water 0.8 g/ml; in ethanol 0.5 g/100 ml.

3176. Dihydroisocodeine. [795-38-0] (5α,6β)-4,5-Epoxy-3-methoxy-17-methylmorphinan-6-ol; DHIC. $C_{18}H_{23}NO_3$; mol wt 301.38. C 71.73%, H 7.69%, N 4.65%, O 15.93%. Differs from dihydrocodeine only by the spatial arrangement of the —CHOH— group. Prepn by catalytic reduction of isocodeine: Speyer, Krauss, *Ann.* **432**, 233 (1923); Lutz, Small, *J. Am. Chem.*

Soc. **54**, 4724 (1932); Rapoport, Payne, *J. Org. Chem.* **15**, 1097 (1950); by epimerization of dihydrocodeine: Baizer, US 2774762 (1956 to N.Y. Quinine and Chem. Works).
Prisms from ethanol, mp 199-200°.
Acid tartrate. $C_{18}H_{23}NO_3 \cdot C_4H_6O_6$. Crystals, mp 192°, $[\alpha]_D^{29}$ −65.3°.
Acid tartrate trihydrate. $C_{18}H_{23}NO_3 \cdot C_4H_6O_6 \cdot 3H_2O$. Crystals from water, mp about 180°. $[\alpha]_D^{26}$ −62.4° (c = 1.94). Soly at 24° = 4.5 g/100 ml H_2O.
Methiodide. $C_{18}H_{23}NO_3 \cdot CH_3I$. Crystals from ethanol, dec 269-272°.

3177. Dihydromorphine. [509-60-4] (5α,6α)-4,5-Epoxy-17-methylmorphinan-3,6-diol. $C_{17}H_{21}NO_3$; mol wt 287.35. C 71.06%, H 7.37%, N 4.87%, O 16.70%. Prepd by hydrogenation of morphine or opium; by demethylation of tetrahydrothebaine; from dihydrocodeine. *Ref:* Small, Lutz, "Chemistry of the Opium Alkaloids" in *U.S. Public Health Reports* **Suppl. No. 103** (Washington, 1932); Eddy, Reid *J. Pharmacol.* **52**, 468 (1934); K. W. Bentley, *The Chemistry of the Morphine Alkaloids* (Oxford, 1954).

Monohydrate. Prisms from chloroform, mp (dry) 157° (dec). Insoluble in water. Sol in acetone, alcohol, chloroform, dil acids.
Hydrochloride. Paramorphan; paramorfan. $C_{17}H_{21}NO_3 \cdot HCl$. Prismatic crystals, unmelted at 280° *in vacuo.* $[\alpha]_D^{25}$ −112° (c = 1.6). Very sol in water; sparingly sol in abs alcohol.
Hydriodide. $C_{17}H_{21}NO_3 \cdot HI$. Crystals, soften at 270°. mp 275°.
Note: This is a controlled substance (opium derivative): **21 CFR**, 1308.11.
THERAP CAT: Analgesic (narcotic).

3178. Dihydroresorcinol. [504-02-9] 1,3-Cyclohexanedione; hydroresorcinol. $C_6H_8O_2$; mol wt 112.13. C 64.27%, H 7.19%, O 28.54%.

Crystals, mp about 105° with decompn. Sol in water, alcohol, chloroform, acetone, boiling benzene; slightly sol in ether, carbon disulfide, petr ether.

3179. Dihydrostreptomycin. [128-46-1] O-2-Deoxy-2-(methylamino)-α-L-glucopyranosyl-(1 → 2)-O-5-deoxy-3-C-(hydroxymethyl)-α-L-lyxofuranosyl-(1 → 4)-N,N′-bis(aminoiminomethyl)-D-streptamine; DHSM; DST; Abiocine; Vibriomycin. C_{21}-$H_{41}N_7O_{12}$; mol wt 583.59. C 43.22%, H 7.08%, N 16.80%, O 32.90%. Semi-synthetic antibiotic prepd by reduction of streptomycin: Bartz *et al., J. Am. Chem. Soc.* **68**, 2163 (1946); Fried, Wintersteiner, *ibid.* **69**, 79 (1947); Peck, US 2498574 (1950 to Merck & Co.); Carboni, Regna, US 2522858 (1950 to Pfizer); Levy, US 2663685 (1953 to Schenley); Dolliver, Semenoff, US 2717236 (1955 to Olin Mathieson); Kaplan, US 2790792 (1957 to Bristol); Sokol, Popino, US 2784181 (1957 to Cyanamid); Jurist, US 2945850 (1960 to Olin Mathieson). Isoln from fermentation broth of *Streptomyces humidus:* Nakazawa *et al.,* and Tatsuoka *et al.,* US 2931756 and US 2950277 (both 1960 to Takeda). Crystn of free base (obtained from the sulfate): Rhodehamel *et al., Science* **111**, 233 (1950). Crystn of the hydrochloride: Wolf *et al., ibid.* **109**, 515 (1949); Wolf, US 2590139; US 2594245 (both 1952 to Merck & Co.). Crystn of the sulfate: Solomons, Regna, *Science* **109**, 515 (1949); Wolf *et al., ibid.* 515; Wolf, US 2590140; US 2590141 (both

1952 to Merck & Co.); R. B. Peet, **US 2640054** (1953 to Heyden Chem.); Katz, **US 2744892** (1956 to Schenley). Total synthesis: Umezawa *et al., J. Am. Chem. Soc.* **96**, 920 (1974); *eidem, Bull. Chem. Soc. Jpn.* **48**, 563 (1975); T. Yamasaki *et al., J. Antibiot.* **31**, 1233 (1978).

Hydrate. Crystals from aq acetone. Chars at 240°, turning black up to 300° without melting.

Trihydrochloride. [6533-54-6] $C_{21}H_{41}N_7O_{12}$.3HCl. Amorphous solid, dec 190-195°, or crystals from methanol. Soly in methanol at 25°: 45 mg/ml for crystalline form; >1 g/ml for amorphous form. Crystals contain methanol of crystn which is lost on heating at 100°C. $[\alpha]_D^{25}$ −95° (1% soln).

Sesquisulfate. [5490-27-7] Didromycine; Double-mycin; Sol-Mycin; Streptomagma. $(C_{21}H_{41}N_7O_{12})_2$.3$H_2SO_4$; mol wt 1461.42. Amorphous solid; crystalline form from water + (methanol, methyl ethyl ketone, or other low boiling solvent). Crystals, dec 255-265°, also reported as dec 250°. $[\alpha]_D^{25}$ −88.5° (1% soln). Crystals show very little hygroscopicity in contrast to amorphous form. Both forms are very sol in water. Solubility in 50% methanol + water: 0.8 mg/ml for crystals; 100 mg/ml for amorphous form. Soly at 28° (mg/ml): >20 in water; 0.35 in methanol; 0.10 in ethanol: Weiss *et al., Antibiot. Chemother.* **7**, 374 (1957). Each milligram contains 800 micrograms of dihydrostreptomycin base on a potency basis.

Pantothenate. [3563-84-6] Didrothenat; Pantostrep. $C_{21}H_{41}$-N_7O_{12}.$C_9H_{17}NO_5$; mol wt 802.82.

THERAP CAT: Antibacterial (tuberculostatic).

THERAP CAT (VET): Antibacterial.

3180. Dihydrotachysterol. [67-96-9] $(3\beta,5E,7E,10\alpha,22E)$-9,10-Secoergosta-5,7,22-trien-3-ol; dichystrolum; anti-tetany substance 10; AT 10; Antitanil; Calcamine; Dygratyl; Dihydral; Hytakerol; Parterol; Tachyrol. $C_{28}H_{46}O$; mol wt 398.66. C 84.36%, H 11.63%, O 4.01%. Prepn by reduction of tachysterol: Windaus *et al., Ann.* **499**, 198 (1932); v. Werder, **US 2228491** (1941 to Winthrop), *cf. Z. Physiol. Chem.* **260**, 119 (1939). Activity similar to parathyroid extract.

Needles from 90% methanol, mp 125-127°. $[\alpha]_D^{22}$ +97.5° (chloroform). uv max: 242, 251, 261 nm ($E_{1cm}^{1\%}$ 870, 1010, 650). Insol in water. Easily sol in organic solvents.

THERAP CAT: Calcium regulator.

3181. Dihydrothebaine. [561-25-1] (5α)-6,7-Didehydro-4,5-epoxy-3,6-dimethoxy-17-methylmorphinan. $C_{19}H_{23}NO_3$; mol wt 313.39. C 72.82%, H 7.40%, N 4.47%, O 15.32%. Prepd by reduction of thebaine: Small *et al., J. Am. Chem. Soc.* **58**, 1457 (1936); K. W. Bentley, *The Chemistry of the Morphine Alkaloids* (Oxford, 1954) p 204.

Prisms from ethyl acetate, mp 162-163°. $[\alpha]_D^{20}$ −267° (c = 1.02 in benzene). Sol in alcohol, benzene, ethyl acetate. Insol in water, alkalies.

Methyl iodide. $C_{20}H_{23}NO_4$.CH_3I. Rods from alc, mp 257°.

3182. Dihydroxyacetone. [96-26-4] 1,3-Dihydroxy-2-propanone; 1,3-dihydroxydimethyl ketone; Protosol; Ketochromin. $C_3H_6O_3$; mol wt 90.08. C 40.00%, H 6.71%, O 53.28%. HOCH$_2$-COCH$_2$OH. Produced from glycerol by *Acetobacter* sp. under aerobic conditions: Bernhauer, Schoen, *Z. Physiol. Chem.* **177**, 107 (1928); Rutten, *Rec. Trav. Chim.* **70**, 449 (1951); Bousfield *et al., J. Inst. Brew.* **53**, 258 (1947); **US 2948658** (1960 to Baxter). *Review: Chem. Eng. News* **38**, 62 (Feb. 22, 1960), 54 (Aug. 15, 1960).

Cryst powder; fairly hygroscopic; characteristic odor; sweet, cooling taste. mp about 75-80°. The normal form is a dimer, slowly sol in 1 part water, 15 parts alcohol. When freshly prepd reverts rapidly to monomer in soln. The monomer is very sol in water, alcohol, ether, acetone.

USE: Artificial tanning agent; active ingredient in *Man-Tan*; *Oxatone*; *Tanorama*; *Q.T. (Quick Tan)*; *Tan Tone*; *Magic Tan*. Formulations: Barmak, *Am. Perfum.*, March 1960, p 57; Andreadis, Miklean, **US 2949403** (1960).

3183. Dihydroxyaluminum Aminoacetate. [13682-92-3] (Glycinato-*N*,*O*)dihydroxyaluminum; dihydroxy(glycinato)aluminum; aluminum aminoacetate (basic); aluminum dihydroxyaminoacetate; aluminum glycinate; glycine, aluminum salt; Ada; Alamine; Alubasine; Alzinox; Aspogen; Dimothyn; Doraxamin; Elcosal; Robalate. $C_2H_6AlNO_4$; mol wt 135.05. C 17.79%, H 4.48%, Al 19.98%, N 10.37%, O 47.39%. NH$_2$CH$_2$COOAl(OH)$_2$. Prepd by adding a soln of aluminum isopropoxide in isopropanol to an aq soln of glycine: Krantz *et al., J. Pharmacol.* **82**, 247 (1944).

Very fine powder. Bland taste. Insol in water. Mixes easily with water forming suspensions which do not separate readily. At 25° the pH of the aq suspension (1 in 25) is 7.4. One gram consumes 200 ml of 0.1N HCl under conditions of the pharmacopoeial test for aluminum hydroxide gel.

THERAP CAT: Antacid.

3184. Dihydroxyaluminum Sodium Carbonate. [539-68-4] [Carbonato(1−)-*O*]dihydroxyaluminum monosodium salt; aluminum sodium carbonate hydroxide; Kompensan; Minicid. CH$_2$-AlNaO$_5$; mol wt 143.99. C 8.34%, H 1.40%, Al 18.74%, Na 15.97%, O 55.56%. (HO)$_2$AlOCO$_2$Na. Prepd by the reaction between an aluminum alkoxide and NaHCO$_3$ in water: Grote, **US 2783179** (1957 to Chattanooga Medicine).

Amorphous powder or poorly formed crystals. May contain 10 to 11% H$_2$O. d 2.144. pH of water suspension: 9.7. Acid consuming power: 230 ml 0.1N HCl/gram.

THERAP CAT: Antacid.

3185. Dihydroxymaleic Acid. [526-84-1] (Z)-2,3-Dihydroxy-2-butenedioic acid; 1,2-dihydroxyethylenedicarboxylic acid.

$C_4H_4O_6$; mol wt 148.07. C 32.45%, H 2.72%, O 64.83%. Prepn from tartaric acid: Fenton, *J. Chem. Soc.* **87**, 811 (1905); Nef, *Ann.* **357**, 291 (1907).

Plates from water, usually crystallizes as the dihydrate. The anhyd acid dec 155° without melting. Slightly sol in cold water, ether, acetic acid; more sol in alcohol. Aq solns are unstable.

USE: In the detection of fluorides and of titanium. Has been proposed as antioxidant for frozen foods.

3186. 9,10-Dihydroxystearic Acid. [120-87-6] 9,10-Dihydroxyoctadecanoic acid. $C_{18}H_{36}O_4$; mol wt 316.48. C 68.31%, H 11.47%, O 20.22%. $CH_3(CH_2)_7CH(OH)CH(OH)(CH_2)_7COOH$.

White, odorless, tasteless, lustrous crystals; fatty feel. mp 132-136°. Insol in water. Sol in hot alc or acetone, slightly in ether.

USE: Manuf cosmetic and toilet preparations.

3187. Dihydroxytartaric Acid. [76-30-2] Tetrahydroxybutanedioic acid; diketosuccinic acid. $C_4H_6O_8$; mol wt 182.09. C 26.38%, H 3.32%, O 70.29%. $HOOCC(OH)_2C(OH)_2COOH$.

White, cryst powder. mp ~114-115° with decompn. Very sol in water; the aq soln dec on heating.

USE: As a reagent for the determination of sodium.

3188. 2,4-Diiodoaniline. [533-70-0] 2,4-Diiodobenzenamine. $C_6H_5I_2N$; mol wt 344.92. C 20.89%, H 1.46%, I 73.58%, N 4.06%.

Brown crystals. d 2.75. mp 95-96°. Slightly sol in cold water, moderately in hot water or in alcohol; freely sol in chloroform, ether, acetone, carbon disulfide, boiling alc.

3189. 4',5'-Diiodofluorescein. [38577-97-8] 3',6'-Dihydroxy-4',5'-diiodospiro[isobenzofuran-1(3H),9'-[9H]xanthen]-3-one; hydroxydiiodo-o-carboxyphenylfluorone; D & C Orange No. 10; C.I. Solvent Red 73; C.I. 45425:1. $C_{20}H_{10}I_2O_5$; mol wt 584.10. C 41.13%, H 1.73%, I 43.45%, O 13.70%. Prepd by reaction of fluorescein with I_2 and HIO_4 or ICl in alkali: *Colour Index* vol. 4 (3rd ed., 1971) p 4427.

Orange-red powder. Slightly sol in water; sol in alcohol, in alkali hydroxide solns.

Sodium salt. Erythrosine Extra Yellowish; D & C Orange No. 11; C.I. Acid Red 95; C.I. 45425. $C_{20}H_8I_2Na_2O_5$.

Note: Structure depicted as the open tautomer.

USE: As an adsorption indicator in the determn of iodides in the presence of chlorides and bromides. The salts in dyeing and printing cotton, in printing half-silk, in dyeing jute, straw, etc.

3190. 3,5-Diiodosalicylic Acid. [133-91-5] 2-Hydroxy-3,5-diiodobenzoic acid. $C_7H_4I_2O_3$; mol wt 389.91. C 21.56%, H 1.03%, I 65.09%, O 12.31%. Prepn from salicylic acid and ICl: Woollett, Johnson, *Org. Synth.* **coll. vol. II**, 343 (1943); and iodine + H_2O_2: Jurd, *Aust. J. Sci. Res.* **3A**, 587 (1950).

Colorless, odorless needles or slightly yellow cryst powder. Sweetish, bitter taste. mp 235-236° dec. Sol in 5200 parts water at 25°; freely sol in alcohol, ether and most other organic solvents. Practically insol in $CHCl_3$, benzene.

Bismuth salt. Bijosal. Pollano, *Minerva Med.* **1930 I**, 786; *C.A.* **24**, 4854[7] (1930).

Ethyl ester. Ethyl 3,5-diiodosalicylate. $C_9H_8I_2O_3$. Crystals, mp 133°. Practically insol in H_2O. Sol in alc, ether, benzene.

USE: As I_2 source in foods; in animal feeds as growth promotant.

3191. 3,5-Diiodothyronine. [534-51-0] *O*-(4-Hydroxyphenyl)-3,5-diiodotyrosine; 3-[4-(*p*-hydroxyphenoxy)-3,5-diiodophenyl]alanine. $C_{15}H_{13}I_2NO_4$; mol wt 525.08. C 34.31%, H 2.50%, I 48.34%, N 2.67%, O 12.19%. Prepn of DL-form: Harington, McCartney, *Biochem. J.* **21**, 852 (1927); Borrows *et al.*, *J. Chem. Soc.* **1949**, Suppl. Issue No. 1, S199, S204; Siedel *et al.*, **US 2894977** (1959 to Hoechst). Prepn of L(+)-form: Harington, *Biochem. J.* **22**, 1429 (1928); Chambers *et al.*, *J. Chem. Soc.* **1949**, 3424; Hillmann, **US 2886592** (1959); as the hydrochloride: Anthony, **US 2950315** (1960 to Baxter); Meltzer, **US 3102136** (1963 to Warner-Lambert). Prepn of D(−)-form: Harington, *loc. cit.*; Elks, Waller, *J. Chem. Soc.* **1952**, 2366.

DL-Form. Plates, dec 256-257°.

L(+)-Form. Crystals, dec 256°. $[\alpha]_D^{22}$ +26° (c = 1.06 in a 1:2 mixture of 1N HCl + alcohol).

L(+)-Form hydrochloride. Crystals, mp 235-240°.

D(−)-Form. Crystals, dec 256° (Harington), 265° (Elks, Waller). $[\alpha]_D^{20}$ −27.1° (c = 1 in 1N alc HCl:alc, 1:2 by vol).

USE: An intermediate in manuf of thyroxine.

3192. 3,5-Diiodotyrosine. [66-02-4] 3,5-Diiodo-4-hydroxy-β-phenylalanine; iodogorgoic acid; Agontan. $C_9H_9I_2NO_3$; mol wt 432.98. C 24.97%, H 2.10%, I 58.62%, N 3.23%, O 11.09%. Found in the skeletal proteins of corals, sponges, and other marine organisms. Isoln from *Gorgonia cavollini* as the DL acid: Drechsel, *Z. Biol.* **33**, 99; *Jahresber. Tierchemie* **1896**, 574; Henze, *Z. Physiol. Chem.* **38**, 71 (1903); isoln from the common sponge: Wheeler, Mendel, *J. Biol. Chem.* **7**, 1 (1909-10); Low, *J. Mar. Res.* **10**, 239 (1951); from marine algae: Coulson, *Chem. Ind. (London)* **1953**, 997; prepn from L- or DL-tyrosine: Henze, *Z. Physiol. Chem.* **51**, 67 (1907); Borrows *et al.*, *J. Chem. Soc.* **1949**, Suppl. Issue no. 1, S185; Jurd, *J. Am. Chem. Soc.* **77**, 5747 (1955); Boyle, Zlatkis, **US 2835700** (1958 to Basic, Inc.).

L-Form. Bunches of needles from water or 70% alcohol, dec 213°. $[\alpha]_D^{20}$ +2.89° (0.246 g in 5 g 4% HCl); $[\alpha]_D^{20}$ +2.27° (0.227 g in 5 g 25% NH_3). pK_1 2.12; pK_2 6.48; pK_3 7.82. Soly in water (g/l): at 0° = 0.204; at 25° = 0.617; at 50° = 1.862; at 75° = 5.62; at 100° = 17.00. On boiling with dil alc the crystals swell, and after prolonged boiling a gelatinous precipitate is formed.

DL-Form. Double wedge crystals from 70% alc, rectangular plates from water. Dec about 200°. Soly in water (g/l): at 0° = 0.149; at 25° = 0.340; at 50° = 0.773. On cooling a boiled hydroalcoholic soln, no gelatinous precip is formed.

THERAP CAT: Thyroid inhibitor.

3193. Diisoamylamine. [544-00-3] 3-Methyl-*N*-(3-methylbutyl)-1-butanamine; isodiamylamine. $C_{10}H_{23}N$; mol wt 157.30. C 76.36%, H 14.74%, N 8.90%. $(CH_3)_2CHCH_2CH_2NHCH_2CH_2-CH(CH_3)_2$.

Liquid. d_4^{20} 0.767. bp 188°. mp −44°. n_D^{21} 1.4229. Slightly sol in water; sol in alcohol, chloroform, ether.

Hydrochloride. $C_{10}H_{23}N \cdot HCl$. Vitreous mass, mp 276°. Freely sol in water, alcohol, ether.

Caution: Irritating to skin, mucous membranes. Has pressor effect.

3194. Diisobutyl Sodium Sulfosuccinate. [127-39-9] Sulfosuccinic acid diisobutyl ester *S*-sodium salt; Aerosol IB; Alphasol IB. $C_{12}H_{21}NaO_7S$; mol wt 332.35. C 43.37%, H 6.37%, Na 6.92%, O 33.70%, S 9.65%. The isobutyl or butyl or 1-methylpropyl diester of the monosodium salt of sulfosuccinic acid or a mixture of all three esters. Wetting agent prepd by the action of the appropriate alcohols on maleic anhydride followed by addition of sodium bisulfite: Jaeger, **US 2028091**; **US 2176423**; **GB 446568**; **FR 776495**.

The mixture of the three esters is available as a white, powder-like, easily grindable material. Soly in water at 25°: 760 g/l; at 60°: 804 g/l. Maximum concn of electrolyte soln in which 1% of the wetting agent is sol: 20% NaCl; 20% NH_4Cl; 30% $NaNO_3$; 20% Na_2SO_4. Also sol in glycerol, pine oil, oleic acid. Insol in acetone, kerosene, liq petrolatum, carbon tetrachloride, 2B ethanol, benzene, olive oil. Surface tension (dynes/cm) in water: 0.001% = 72.2; 0.1% = 67.5; 0.5% = 53.4; 1% = 49.1. Interfacial tension 1% in water *vs.* liq petrolatum: 10 seconds = 32.5 dynes/cm; 30 seconds = 32.3 dynes/cm; 15 minutes = 31.2 dynes/cm. Stable in acid and neutral solns; hydrolyzes in alkaline solns.

Caution: Irritating to eyes, mucous membranes.

USE: Wetting agent.

3195. Diisopropanolamine. [110-97-4] 1,1′-Iminobis-2-propanol; bis(2-hydroxypropyl)amine; DIPA. $C_6H_{15}NO_2$; mol wt 133.19. C 54.11%, H 11.35%, N 10.52%, O 24.02%. Secondary alkanolamine. Prepn: J. N. Wickert, **US 1988225** (1935 to Carbide & Carbon Chem.). Densities, viscosities, diffusivities: H. Hikita *et al., J. Chem. Eng. Jpn.* **14**, 411 (1981). Absorption and mass transfer study: P. M. M. Blauwhoff, W. P. M. Van Swaaij, *ACS Symp. Ser.* **196**, 377 (1982). Safety assessment and use: K. H. Beyer *et al., J. Am. Coll. Toxicol.* **6**, 53 (1987). Review of use in 'Sulfinol' process: K. E. Zarker, *Fert. Sci. Technol. Ser.* **2**, 219-232 (1974); in gas purification: K. F. Butwell *et al., Hydrocarbon Process. Int. Ed.* **61**, 109-116 (1982).

White, waxy solid, mp 32-42°. bp 249°. Freezing pt 107°F. Flash point (open cup) 255°F (127°C). Critical density 0.31 g/cc. d_{20}^{45} 0.9890. n^{60} 1.4450-1.4550. pH of 5% aq soln: 11.5. Completely miscible with water and alcohol, slightly sol in toluene. Insol in hydrocarbons.

USE: Emulsifying and neutralizing agent in cosmetics. Removal of H_2S and CO_2 from natural and industrial gases. Antimicrobial agent in cutting fluids.

3196. Diisopropylamine. [108-18-9] *N*-(1-Methylethyl)-2-propanamine. $C_6H_{15}N$; mol wt 101.19. C 71.22%, H 14.94%, N 13.84%. $[(CH_3)_2CH]_2NH$. Prepn: A. Siersch, *Ann.* **148**, 263 (1868); M. Van der Zande, *Rec. Trav. Chim.* **8**, 202 (1889). Enthalpy of formation: M. A. V. Ribeiro da Silva *et al., J. Chem. Thermodyn.* **29**, 1025 (1997). Toxicity study: H. F. Smyth *et al., Arch. Ind. Hyg. Occup. Med.* **10**, 61 (1954). Safety assessment: *J. Am. Coll. Toxicol.* **14**, 182-192 (1995).

Liquid; characteristic odor; strongly alkaline. d^{22} 0.722. bp 84°. Flash pt, open cup: 21°F (−6°C). Sol in water, alc. LD_{50} orally in rats: 0.77 g/kg (Smyth).

Lithium salt. [4111-54-0] LDA; lithiodiisopropylamine; lithium diisopropylamide. Strong nucleophile. Crystal structure: N. D. R. Barnett *et al. J. Am. Chem. Soc.* **113**, 8187 (1991). Use as nucleophile: Y. Tanaka *et al., Bull. Chem. Soc. Jpn.* **60**, 788 (1987);

S. Saito *et al., J. Am. Chem. Soc.* **119**, 611 (1997). Review of chemistry: *Reagents for Organic Synthesis* vol. 8, M. Fieser, Ed. (Wiley-Interscience, New York, 1980) pp 292-299. Powder, melts with decompn. Air and moisture sensitive.

Caution: Potential symptoms of overexposure are irritation of eyes, skin and respiratory system; nausea, vomiting; headache; visual disturbance. *See NIOSH Pocket Guide to Chemical Hazards* (DHHS/NIOSH 97-140, 1997) p 110.

USE: pH adjuster in colognes and toilet waters. In organic synthesis, particularly, the lithium salt.

3197. Diisopropylamine Dichloroacetate. [660-27-5] Dichloroacetic acid compd with *N*-(1-methylethyl)-2-propanamine (1:1); dichloroacetic acid diisopropylammonium salt; diisopropyl-ammonium dichloroacetate; diisopropylamine dichloroethanoate; DADA; DIPA-DCA; DIEDI; IS-401; Disotat; Kalodil; Oxypangam. $C_8H_{17}Cl_2NO_2$; mol wt 230.13. C 41.75%, H 7.45%, Cl 30.81%, N 6.09%, O 13.90%. Prepn: **GB 862248** (1961 to Italseber). Pharmacology: V. A. E. Kraushaar *et al., Arzneim.-Forsch.* **13**, 109 (1963). Ames mutagenicity test: M. D. Gelernt, V. Herbert, *Nutr. Cancer* **3**, 129 (1982). Pharmacokinetics and TLC determn in racehorses: J.-M. Yang *et al., Gen. Pharmacol.* **19**, 683 (1988). Review of pharmacology: P. W. Stacpoole, *J. Clin. Pharmacol. J. New Drugs* **9**, 282-291 (1969).

Crystals, mp 119-121°. Soly in water: >50%. LD_{50} orally in mice: 1700 mg/kg (Kraushaar).

THERAP CAT: Vasodilator, hypotensive.

3198. Diisopropyl Paraoxon. [3254-66-8] Bis(1-methylethyl)phosphoric acid 4-nitrophenyl ester; diisopropyl *p*-nitrophenyl phosphate; Mioticol; Propicol. $C_{12}H_{18}NO_6P$; mol wt 303.25. C 47.53%, H 5.98%, N 4.62%, O 31.66%, P 10.21%. Prepn: **GB 687596** (1953 to Albright & Wilson).

THERAP CAT: Cholinergic (ophthalmic).

3199. Dikegulac. [18467-77-1] 2,3:4,6-Bis-*O*-(methylethylidene)-α-L-*xylo*-2-hexulofuranosonic acid; α-2,3:4,6-di-*O*-isopropylidene-L-*xylo*-hexulofuranosonic acid; di-*O*-isopropylidene-2-keto-L-gulonic acid; diacetone-2-ketogulonic acid; diacetone-2-oxo-L-gulonic acid; oxogulonic acid diacetonide. $C_{12}H_{18}O_7$; mol wt 274.27. C 52.55%, H 6.61%, O 40.83%. Intermediate in the manuf of ascorbic acid, *q.v.* Manufacturing process: G. M. Jaffe, E. J. Pleven, **DE 2123621**; *eidem,* **US 3832355** (1970, 1974 both to Hoffmann-La Roche). Use as a plant growth regulator: W. Szkrybalo, **DE 2339239**; *eidem,* **US 4337080** (1974, 1982 both to Hoffmann-La Roche); P. Bocian *et al., Nature* **258**, 142 (1975). Physicochemical properties, toxicity and growth retardant effect: W. H. de Silva *et al., Proc. Br. Crop Prot. Conf. - Weeds* **1976**, 349. Activity: S. S. Purohit, *Comp. Physiol. Ecol.* **4**, 264 (1979); **6**, 261 (1981).

Sodium salt. Dikegulac-sodium; Ro-7-6145; Atrinal. $C_{12}H_{17}$-NaO_7; mol wt 296.25. Powder, mp >300°. Vapor pressure at 25°: $<10^{-10}$ mm Hg. Soly at 20° (g/l): water 590; methanol 390; ethanol 230; chloroform 60; acetone <10; hexane <10; cyclohexanone <10. LD_{50} in mice, male, female rats (mg/kg): 19500, 31000, 18000 orally; LC_{50} (96 hr) in bluegill sunfish, rainbow trout (ppm): >10000, >5000 (de Silva).

USE: Plant growth regulator; herbicide.

3200. Dilazep. [35898-87-4] 3,4,5-Trimethoxybenzoic acid (tetrahydro-1H-1,4-diazepine-1,4(5H)-diyl)di-3,1-propanediyl ester; 3,4,5-trimethoxybenzoic acid diester with tetrahydro-1H-1,4-diazepine-1,4(5H)-dipropanol; 1,4-bis[3-(3,4,5-trimethoxybenzoyloxy)propyl]perhydro-1,4-diazepine; N,N'-bis[3-(3,4,5-trimethoxybenzoyloxy)propyl]homopiperazine; N,N'-(bis-ω-hydroxypropyl)-homopiperazine 3,4,5-trimethoxybenzoate (diester). $C_{31}H_{44}N_2$-O_{10}; mol wt 604.69. C 61.57%, H 7.33%, N 4.63%, O 26.46%. Prepn: GB 1107470; H. Arnold et al., US 3532685 (1968, 1970 both to Asta-Werke). Series of articles on pharmacology and metabolism: Arzneim.-Forsch. **22**, 639-666 (1972). Toxicology: H. H. Abel et al., ibid. 667. Clinical results: Messerich, Med. Welt **1972**, 563.

Dihydrochloride. [20153-98-4] Asta C 4898; Comelian; Cormelian; Labitan. $C_{31}H_{44}N_2O_{10}$.2HCl; mol wt 677.61. Crystals from ethanol, mp 194-198° (monohydrate). LD_{50} in male mice, male rats (mg/kg): 26.6, 19.1 i.v.; 161, 90.1 i.p.; 3740, >2150 orally (Abel).

THERAP CAT: Vasodilator (coronary).

3201. Diloxanide. [579-38-4] 2,2-Dichloro-N-(4-hydroxyphenyl)-N-methylacetamide; 2,2-dichloro-4'-hydroxy-N-methylacetanilide; N-dichloroacet-4-hydroxy-N-methylanilide; 4-hydroxy-N-methyldichloroacetanilide; Entamide. $C_9H_9Cl_2NO_2$; mol wt 234.08. C 46.18%, H 3.88%, Cl 30.29%, N 5.98%, O 13.67%. Prepn: P. Oxley et al., US 2912438 (1959 to Boots Pure Drug). Spectrophotometric determn in 2-component tablet formulation: S. M. Galal et al., J. Pharm. Belg. **46**, 315 (1991). Clinical trial of combination with metronidazole, q.v., in amoebiasis and giardiasis: H. Qureshi et al., J. Int. Med. Res. **25**, 167 (1997). Review of clinical experience: J. B. McAuley et al., Clin. Infect. Dis. **15**, 464-468 (1992).

Crystals from ethyl acetate, mp 175°.
Furoate. [3736-81-0] Diloxanide 2-furoic acid ester; Furamide.

THERAP CAT: Antiamebic.

3202. Diltiazem. [42399-41-7] (2S-cis)-3-(Acetyloxy)-5-[2-(dimethylamino)ethyl]-2,3-dihydro-2-(4-methoxyphenyl)-1,5-benzothiazepin-4(5H)-one; (+)-cis-5-[2-(dimethylamino)ethyl]-2,3-dihydro-3-hydroxy-2-(p-methoxyphenyl)-1,5-benzothiazepin-4(5H)-one acetate (ester). $C_{22}H_{26}N_2O_4S$; mol wt 414.52. C 63.74%, H 6.32%, N 6.76%, O 15.44%, S 7.74%. Calcium channel blocker with vasodilating activity. Prepn (unspec stereochem): H. Kugita et al., DE 1805714; eidem, US 3562257 (1969, 1971 both to Tanabe Seiyaku); eidem, Chem. Pharm. Bull. **19**, 54 (1971). Resolution of optical isomers: H. Inoue et al., Yakugaku Zasshi **93**, 729 (1973), C.A. **79**, 66331w (1974). Stereospecific synthesis: K. Igarashi, T. Honma, DE 3415035; eidem, US 4552695 (1984, 1985 both to Shionogi). Structure-activity studies: Sato et al., Arzneim.-Forsch. **21**, 1338 (1971); T. Nagao et al., Chem. Pharm. Bull. **21**, 92 (1973). Pharmacology and toxicity: eidem, Jpn. J. Pharmacol. **22**, 467 (1972). Metabolism: Meshi et al., Chem.

Pharm. Bull. **19**, 1546 (1971). Review of synthesis and pharmacology: H. Inoue, T. Nagao, Chron. Drug Discovery **3**, 207-238 (1993). Comprehensive description: D. J. Mazzo et al., Anal. Profiles Drug Subs. Excip. **23**, 53-98 (1994). Review of pharmacology and efficacy in angina: M. Chaffman, R. N. Brogden, Drugs **29**, 387-454 (1985); in hypertension: M. R. Weir, J. Clin. Pharmacol. **35**, 220-232 (1995). Comparative clinical trial in prevention of complications of hypertension: L. Hansson et al., Lancet **356**, 359 (2000).

Hydrochloride. [33286-22-5] CRD-401; Adizem; Altiazem; Angizem; Cardizem; Deltazen; Dilacor XR; Diladel; Dilpral; Dilrene; Dilzem; Dilzene; Masdil; Tiazac; Tildiem; Zilden. $C_{22}H_{26}$-N_2O_4S.HCl; mol wt 450.98. Fine needles from ethanol-isopropanol, mp 207.5-212°. Odorless, with a bitter taste. $[\alpha]_D^{24}$ +98.3 ± 1.4° (c = 1.002 in methanol). Freely sol in water, methanol, chloroform, formic acid; slightly sol in abs ethanol. Practically insol in benzene. Insol in ether. LD_{50} in male, female mice, male, female rats (mg/kg): 61, 58, 38, 39 i.v.; 260, 280, 520, 550 s.c.; 740, 640, 560, 610 orally (Nagao, 1972).

THERAP CAT: Antianginal; antihypertensive; antiarrhythmic (class IV).

3203. Dimecrotic Acid. [7706-67-4] 3-(2,4-Dimethoxyphenyl)-2-butenoic acid; 2,4-dimethoxy-β-methylcinnamic acid; 3-(2,4-dimethoxyphenyl)crotonic acid. $C_{12}H_{14}O_4$; mol wt 222.24. C 64.85%, H 6.35%, O 28.80%. Prepn: DE 1915023 (1969 to Unicler), C.A. **72**, 66630y (1970). TLC determn in pharmaceutics: M.-F. Etcheverry et al., Sci. Tech. Pharm. **7**, 51 (1978).

mp 149°.
Magnesium salt. [54283-65-7] Fisiobil; Hepadial. $C_{24}H_{26}$-MgO_8; mol wt 466.76. mp 135°. LD_{50} in mice, rats (mg/kg): 1.3, 1.0 i.p. (DE 1915023).

THERAP CAT: Choleretic.

3204. Dimefline. [1165-48-6] 8-[(Dimethylamino)methyl]-7-methoxy-3-methyl-2-phenyl-4H-1-benzopyran-4-one; 8-[(dimethylamino)methyl]-7-methoxy-3-methylflavone; 8-dimethylaminomethyl-7-methoxy-3-methyl-2-phenylchromone. $C_{20}H_{21}NO_3$; mol wt 323.39. C 74.28%, H 6.55%, N 4.33%, O 14.84%. Prepn: Da Re et al., Arzneim.-Forsch. **10**, 800 (1960); GB 882537; P. Da Re, US 3147258 (1961, 1964 both to Recordati). Pharmacology: Setnikar et al., J. Pharmacol. Exp. Ther. **128**, 176 (1960); eidem, J. Med. Pharm. Chem. **3**, 471 (1961).

Hydrochloride. [2740-04-7] Rec-7-0267; Remeflin. $C_{20}H_{21}$-$NO_3 \cdot HCl$; mol wt 359.85. Crystals from alcohol + ether, dec 213-214°.

THERAP CAT: Respiratory stimulant.

3205. Dimefox. [115-26-4] Tetramethylphosphorodiamidic fluoride; tetramethyldiamidophosphoric fluoride; bis(dimethyl-amido)phosphoryl fluoride; fluophosphoric acid di(dimethylamide); bisdimethylaminofluorophosphine oxide; bis(dimethylamido)-fluorophosphate; Pestox XIV. $C_4H_{12}FN_2OP$; mol wt 154.12. C 31.17%, H 7.85%, F 12.33%, N 18.18%, O 10.38%, P 20.10%. Prepd by fluorination of bis(dimethylamido)phosphoryl chloride: Schrader, *Angew. Chem. Suppl.* **62**, 18 (1951); *BIOS Final Report No. 714* (1947); Holmsted, *Acta Physiol. Scand. Suppl.* **90**, 33 (1951); Heap, Saunders, *J. Chem. Soc.* **1948**, 1313; **GB 692446** (1953); McCombie *et al.*, **US 2489917** (1949). Toxicity data: A. J. Okinaka *et al.*, *J. Pharmacol. Exp. Ther.* **112**, 231 (1954). *Review:* Kilby, *Chem. Ind. (London)* **1953**, 856.

Liquid. Fishy odor. d_4^{20} 1.1151. $bp_{4.0}$ 67°; bp_{15} 86°. n_D^{20} 1.4267. Freely sol in water, ether, benzene. Aq solns are stable. LD_{50} in rats (mg/kg): 5.0 i.p.; 7.5 orally (Okinaka).

Caution: A highly toxic cholinesterase inhibitor. Symptoms similar to parathion, *q.v.*: *Clinical Toxicology of Commercial Products*, R. E. Gosselin *et al.*, Eds. (Williams & Wilkins, Baltimore, 5th ed., 1984) Section II, p 299.

USE: Insecticide; acaricide.

3206. Dimemorfan. [36309-01-0] $(9\alpha,13\alpha,14\alpha)$-3,17-Di-methylmorphinan; *d*-3-methyl-*N*-methylmorphinan; AT-17. C_{18}-$H_{25}N$; mol wt 255.40. C 84.65%, H 9.87%, N 5.48%. Prepn: Murakami *et al.*, **DE 2128607**; *eidem*, **US 3786054** (1971, 1974 both to Yamanouchi); *eidem*, *Chem. Pharm. Bull.* **20**, 1706 (1972). Pharmacology: Ida, Fujii, *Oyo Yakuri* **6**, 1207 (1972); Y. Kasé *et al.*, *Arzneim.-Forsch.* **26**, 353 (1976).

Pale yellow oil, $bp_{0.3}$ 130-136°; or white crystals from acetone, mp 90-93°.

Phosphate. [36304-84-4] Astomin. $C_{18}H_{25}N \cdot H_3PO_4$; mol wt 353.39. White to yellowish-white, odorless, bitter crystals, mp 267-269°. $[\alpha]_D^{23}$ +25.7° (c = 0.5 in methanol). Freely sol in glacial acetic acid; sparingly sol in water, methanol. Practically insol in ethanol, acetone, chloroform, benzene, ether. LD_{50} in mice (mg/kg): 223 s.c.; 475 orally (Kasé).

THERAP CAT: Antitussive.

3207. Dimenhydrinate. [523-87-5] 8-Chloro-3,7-dihydro-1,3-dimethyl-1*H*-purine-2,6-dione compd with 2-(diphenylmeth-oxy)-*N,N*-dimethylethanamine (1:1); 2-(benzhydryloxy)-*N,N*-di-methylethylamine 8-chlorotheophyllinate; β-dimethylaminoethyl benzhydryl ether 1,3-dimethyl-8-chloroxanthine; diphenhydramine 8-chlorotheophyllinate; *N,N*-dimethyl-2-diphenylmethoxyethyl-amine 8-chlorotheophyllinate; *O*-benzhydryldimethylaminoethanol 8-chlorotheophyllinate; chloranautine; Amosyt; Anautine; Andra-mine; Antemin; Diamarin; Dimate; Dramamine; Dramarin; Dram-ocen; Dramyl; Emedyl; Emes; Epha; Gravol; Menhydrinate; Travel-Gum; Travelin; Travelmin; Vomex A; Xamamina; Faston. $C_{24}H_{28}$-ClN_5O_3; mol wt 469.96. C 61.34%, H 6.01%, Cl 7.54%, N 14.90%, O 10.21%. Prepn: Cusic, *Science* **109**, 574 (1949); Cusic, **US 2499058** and **US 2534813** (1950 to Searle).

Crystals, mp 102-107°. Freely sol in alcohol, chloroform. Soluble in benzene. Soly in water: about 3 mg/ml. Almost insol in ether. A satd aq soln has a pH between 6.8 and 7.3.

THERAP CAT: Antiemetic.

THERAP CAT (VET): Has been used as an antiemetic.

3208. Dimenoxadol. [509-78-4] α-Ethoxy-α-phenylben-zeneacetic acid 2-(dimethylamino)ethyl ester; ethoxydiphenylacetic acid 2-dimethylaminoethyl ester; α,α-diphenyl-α-ethoxyacetic acid β-dimethylaminoethyl ester; 2-dimethylaminoethyl ethoxydiphen-ylacetate; Lokarin. $C_{20}H_{25}NO_3$; mol wt 327.42. C 73.37%, H 7.70%, N 4.28%, O 14.66%. Prepd by the reaction of diphenyl-ethoxyacetic acid with dimethylchloroethylamine in the presence of isopropanol: Klosa, *Arch. Pharm.* **288**, 42 (1955). Improved prepn: C. N. Yakhontov *et al.*, *Pharm. Chem. J.* **8**, 189 (1974). HPLC determn: I. Jane, A. McKinnon, *J. Chromatogr.* **323**, 191 (1985).

Hydrochloride. $C_{20}H_{25}NO_3 \cdot HCl$. Long needles, mp 170-172°. Sol in water and alcohols; only slightly sol in chloroform and acetone. Insol in ether, ethyl acetate, benzene. pH (2% aq soln) 4.0-5.5. LD_{50} i.v. in rats: 66 mg/kg (Yakhontov).

Note: This is a controlled substance (opiate): **21 CFR**, 1308.11.

THERAP CAT: Analgesic (narcotic).

3209. Dimercaprol. [59-52-9] 2,3-Dimercapto-1-propanol; 1,2-dithioglycerol; British anti-lewisite; BAL; Dicaptol; Sulfactin. $C_3H_8OS_2$; mol wt 124.23. C 29.00%, H 6.49%, O 12.88%, S 51.62%. Developed as an antidote to the vesicant warfare agent, dichloro(2-chlorovinyl)arsine, *q.v.*, also known as Lewisite. Inhib-its the toxic action of arsenic on pyruvate dehydrogenase. Discov-ery and development: R. A. Peters *et al.*, *Nature* **156**, 616 (1945); L. L. Waters, C. Stock, *Science* **102**, 601 (1945). Prepn by hydro-genation of hydroxypropylene trisulfide: W. J. Peppel, F. K. Sig-naigo, **US 2402665** (1946 to DuPont). Stereospecific synthesis: A. K. M. Anisuzzaman, L. N. Owen, *J. Chem. Soc. C* **1967**, 1021. GC/MS determn in plasma: C. E. Byers *et al.*, *J. Anal. Toxicol.* **28**, 384 (2004). Toxicity study: P. Zvirblis, R. I. Ellin, *Toxicol. Appl. Pharmacol.* **36**, 297 (1976). Review of discovery, biochemistry and clinical applications: J. A. Vilensky, K. Redman, *Ann. Emerg. Med.* **41**, 378-383 (2003).

Viscous oily liq. Pungent offensive odor of mercaptans. d_4^{25} 1.2385. n_D^{25} 1.5720. $bp_{0.0001}$ 68-69°. Vapor pressure at 80°: 1.9 mm Hg; at 140°: 40 mm Hg. Soly in water: 8.7 g/100 g. Sol in vegetable oils. LD_{50} i.m. in rats: 86.7 mg/kg (Zvirblis, Ellin).

THERAP CAT: Antidote (heavy metal poisoning).

THERAP CAT (VET): Antidote (heavy metal poisoning).

3210. 2,3-Dimercapto-1-propanesulfonic Acid. [74-61-3] 2,3-Dithiolpropanesulfonic acid. $C_3H_8O_3S_3$; mol wt 188.29. C 19.14%, H 4.28%, O 25.49%, S 51.09%. $HSCH_2CH(SH)CH_2$-SO_3H. Chelating agent related to BAL dimercaprol, *q.v.* Prepn:

N. S. Johary, L. N. Owen, *J. Chem. Soc.* **1955**, 1307; V. E. Petrun'-kin, *Ukr. Khim. Zh.* **22**, 603 (1956), *C.A.* **51**, 5692h (1957). Distribution and excretion in rats: B. Gabard, *Arch. Toxicol.* **39**, 289 (1978). Metabolism study: B. Gabard, R. Walser, *J. Toxicol. Environ. Health* **5**, 759 (1979). Use in removal of internally deposited gold: B. Gabard, *Br. J. Pharmacol.* **68**, 607 (1980). Protection of mice vs lethal effects of sodium arsenite: H. V. Aposhian *et al., Toxicol. Appl. Pharmacol.* **61**, 385 (1981). Pharmacokinetics in dogs: P. Wiedemann *et al., Biopharm. Drug Dispos.* **3**, 267 (1982). Anti-lewisite activity and stability: H. V. Aposhian *et al., Life Sci.* **31**, 2149 (1982). Toxicological studies: F. Planas-Bohne *et al., Arzneim.-Forsch.* **30**, 1291 (1980).

Sodium salt. [4076-02-2] DMPS; unitiol; Dimaval. C_3H_7-NaO_3S_3; mol wt 210.27. Leaflets, mp 235°. LD_{50} i.p. in mice: 5.22 mmol/kg (Aposhian, 1981).

THERAP CAT: Antidote (heavy metal poisoning).

3211. Dimestrol. [130-79-0] 1,1'-[(1E)-1,2-Diethyl-1,2-ethenediyl]bis[4-methoxybenzene]; (E)-α,α'-diethyl-4,4'-dimethoxystilbene; stilbestrol dimethyl ether; (E)-3,4-bis(p-methoxyphenyl)-3-hexene; (E)-3,4-dianisyl-3-hexene. $C_{20}H_{24}O_2$; mol wt 296.40. C 81.04%, H 8.16%, O 10.80%. Nonsteroidal synthetic estrogen; dimethyl ether of diethylstilbestrol, *q.v.* Prepn: Dodds *et al., Nature* **142**, 211, 247 (1938); Reid, Wilson, *J. Am. Chem. Soc.* **64**, 1625 (1942); Sisido, Nozaki, *J. Am. Chem. Soc.* **70**, 777 (1948). Improved stereospecific prepn: T. Hiyama, H. Nozaki, *Bull. Chem. Soc. Jpn.* **46**, 2248 (1973). Crystal structure: G. Ruban, P. Luger, *Acta Crystallogr.* **B31**, 2658 (1975). Biological activities: Y. Inamori *et al., Chem. Pharm. Bull.* **33**, 4478 (1985). Review and bibliography: Solmssen, *Chem. Rev.* **37**, 481 (1945).

Crystals from petr ether, mp 124°. Less sol than the monomethyl ether, mestilbol. Practically insol in water. Sol in alcohol; freely sol in acetone, ether; also sol in dil aq or alcoholic solns of alkali hydroxides and in vegetable oils.

3212. Dimetacrine. [4757-55-5] N,N,9,9-Tetramethyl-10(9H)-acridinepropanamine; 10-[3-(dimethylamino)propyl]-9,9-dimethylacridan; 5,5-dimethyl-10-dimethylaminopropylacridan; dimethacrine. $C_{20}H_{26}N_2$; mol wt 294.43. C 81.59%, H 8.90%, N 9.51%. Prepn: Holm, *GB 933875* (1963 to Kefalas), *C.A.* **60**, 510a (1964); Molnar, Wagner-Jauregg, *Helv. Chim. Acta* **48**, 1782 (1965); *FR 1438357* (1966 to Siegfried), *C.A.* **66**, 10856k (1967). Pharmacology and metabolism: Schatz *et al., Arzneim.-Forsch.* **18**, 862 (1968); Ishitani *et al., Jpn. J. Pharmacol.* **20**, 432 (1970).

Free base, bp_1 200°.
Hydrochloride. $C_{20}H_{26}N_2$.HCl. Crystals from abs alc + acetone, mp 151-154°.
Tartrate. [3759-07-7] SD-709; Istonil.
THERAP CAT: Antidepressant.

3213. Dimethadione. [695-53-4] 5,5-Dimethyl-2,4-oxazolidinedione; DMO; AC-1198; BAX-1400Z; NSC-30152; Eupractone. $C_5H_7NO_3$; mol wt 129.11. C 46.51%, H 5.46%, N 10.85%, O 37.18%. Active metabolite of trimethadione, *q.v.* Prepn: F. Urech, *Ber.* **13**, 485 (1880); R. W. Stoughton, *J. Am. Chem. Soc.* **63**, 2376 (1941). Anticonvulsant activity: C. D. Withrow *et al., J. Pharmacol. Exp. Ther.* **161**, 335 (1968); in comparison

with trimethadione: H. Ferngren, *Acta Pharmacol. Toxicol.* **26**, 177 (1968). Use in measurement of intracellular pH and cellular pH gradients: S. Addanki *et al., J. Biol. Chem.* **243**, 2337 (1968); V. Ehrhardt, *Biochim. Biophys. Acta* **775**, 182 (1984); J. B. Arnold *et al., J. Cereb. Blood Flow Metab.* **5**, 369 (1985). GLC determn: W. Gazdzik, W. Kmiotek, *J. Chromatogr.* **378**, 482 (1986); LC determn in serum: E. Tanaka, S. Misawa, *J. Chromatogr.* **413**, 376 (1987).

Crystals, mp 76-77°. Weak organic acid, pKa (37°) 6.13. LD_{50} i.v. in mice: 450 mg/kg (Stoughton).
USE: *In vivo* measurement of intracellular pH.
THERAP CAT: Anticonvulsant.

3214. Dimethenamid. [87674-68-8] 2-Chloro-N-(2,4-dimethyl-3-thienyl)-N-(2-methoxy-1-methylethyl)acetamide; SAN-582H; Frontier; Guardsman. $C_{12}H_{18}ClNO_2S$; mol wt 275.79. C 52.26%, H 6.58%, Cl 12.86%, N 5.08%, O 11.60%, S 11.63%. Preemergence herbicide for use in food crops. Prepn: K. Seckinger *et al., GB 2114566*; eidem, *US 4666502* (1983, 1987 both to Sandoz). Bioactivity of stereoisomers: M. Couderchet *et al., Pestic. Sci.* **50**, 221 (1997). Comprehensive description: J. Harr *et al., Proc. Br. Crop Prot. Conf. - Weeds* **1991**, 87-92. Review of field trials and persistence in soil: A. Rahman, T. K. James, *Proc. 45th N. Z. Plant Prot. Conf.* **1992**, 84-88.

Yellowish-brown, viscous liquid. Odorless to weak tar-like odor. Mixture of 4 stereoisomers (1RS,aRS). $bp_{26.7 Pa}$ 127°. Vapor pressure (25°): 36.7 mPa. d^{25} 1.187. Soly (25°): water 1174 mg/l; heptane 28.2 g/100 g; isooctane 22.0 g/100 g; ether, kerosene, ethanol >50%. LD_{50} in rats (mg/kg): 1570 orally; >2000 dermally; LC_{50} in bluegill sunfish, rainbow trout (mg/l): 6.4, 2.6 (Harr).
Dimethenamid P. [163515-14-8] DMTA-P; BAS-656H; Outlook. Consists of the 1S,aRS isomers. Prepn: K. Seckinger *et al., US 5457085* (1995 to Sandoz). Review of properties and activity: T. Guillet *et al., Phytoma* **546**, 50-53 (2002). Faintly yellow viscous liquid. $[\alpha]_D^{23}$ +3.5° (c = 1.102 in CH_3OH). $bp_{9.3 Pa}$ 122.6°. d^{20} 1.195. Vapor pressure (25°): 2.5×10^{-3} Pa. Soly in water (25°): 1449 mg/l. LD_{50} in rats (mg/kg): 429 orally; >2000 dermally. LC_{50} (96 hr) in rainbow trout (mg/l): 6.3 (Guillet).
USE: Herbicide.

3215. Dimethicone. [9006-65-9] Dimethyl polysiloxane; dimeticon; polydimethylsiloxane; α-(trimethylsilyl)-ω-methylpoly[oxy(dimethylsilylene)]. Silicone oil consisting of a mixture of fully methylated linear siloxane polymers end-blocked with trimethylsiloxy units. Prepn of homologous liquid methyl siloxane polymers: J. F. Hyde, *US 2441098* (1948 to Corning Glass). Dimethicone mixed with silicon dioxide is known as simethicone. Clinical evaluation of simethicone in functional upper GI disease: J. E. Bernstein, A. M. Kasich, *J. Clin. Pharmacol.* **14**, 617 (1974). Stability of simethicone + antacid mixtures in pharmaceutical preparations: J. A. Rider, *Curr. Ther. Res.* **52**, 681 (1992). Review of use of dimethicones in skin and hair products: A. Disapio, P. Fridd, *Int. J. Cosmet. Sci.* **10**, 75-89 (1988). Review of medical use in soft-tissue augmentation: V. J. Selmanowitz, N. Orentreich, *J. Dermatol. Surg. Oncol.* **3**, 597-611 (1977); D. M. Duffy, *Adv. Dermatol.* **5**, 93-109 (1990). *See also:* Silicones.

Clear colorless liquids. Viscosity increases with degree of polymerization. Immiscible with water, alcohol. Miscible with chloroform, ether.

Mixture with silicon dioxide. [8050-81-5] Simethicone; activated dimethicone; Antifoam A; Baros; Colicon; Endo-Paractol; Gas-X; Infacol; Lefax; Mylicon; Phasil; Phazyme; sab simplex; Silain. Average number of dimethylsiloxane units is 200 to 350. mol wt 14000-21000. Gray, translucent, viscous liquid. Insol in water, alcohol.

Dimethicone 350. Specific polydimethylsiloxane characterized by the following properties. Viscosity (25°): 350 cSt. d 0.965-0.973. n_D^{25} 1.4013-1.4053.

USE: Oleaginous ointment base, skin protectant, antifoaming agent; prosthetic aid (soft tissue).

THERAP CAT: Antiflatulent.

THERAP CAT (VET): Antibloating agent.

3216. Dimethindene. [5636-83-9] N,N-Dimethyl-3-[1-(2-pyridinyl)ethyl]-1H-indene-2-ethanamine; 2-[1-[2-[2-(dimethyl-amino)ethyl]inden-3-yl]ethyl]pyridine; 3-[α-(2′-pyridyl)ethyl]-2-(β-dimethylaminoethyl)indene; dimethpyrindene. $C_{20}H_{24}N_2$; mol wt 292.42. C 82.15%, H 8.27%, N 9.58%. Synthesis: Huebner *et al., J. Am. Chem. Soc.* **82,** 2077 (1960); Huebner, US **2970149** (1961 to Ciba). Pharmacology: W. E. Barrett *et al., Toxicol. Appl. Pharmacol.* **3,** 534 (1961).

Maleate. [3614-69-5] Fenistil. $C_{20}H_{24}N_2.C_4H_4O_4$; mol wt 408.49. Crystals, mp 159-161°. LD_{50} in rats (mg/kg): 26.8 i.v.; 618.2 orally (Barrett).

THERAP CAT: Antihistaminic.

3217. Dimethirimol. [5221-53-4] 5-Butyl-2-(dimethylamino)-6-methyl-4(1H)-pyrimidinone; 5-butyl-2-(dimethylamino)-6-methyl-4-pyrimidinol; 2-dimethylamino-4-methyl-5-n-butyl-6-hydroxypyrimidine; PP-675; Milcurb. $C_{11}H_{19}N_3O$; mol wt 209.29. C 63.13%, H 9.15%, N 20.08%, O 7.64%. Prepn: B. K. Snell *et al., ZA* **6701373**; *eidem, US* **3980781** (1968, 1976 both to ICI). Systemic fungicidal activity: R. S. Elias, *Nature* **219,** 1160 (1968); K. J. Bent, *Ann. Appl. Biol.* **66,** 103 (1970). Metabolism and mode of action: A. Calderbank, *Acta Phytopathol.* **6,** 355 (1971). Metabolism: H. Bratt *et al., Food Cosmet. Toxicol.* **10,** 489 (1972).

Needles from ethanol, mp 102°. Vapor pressure at 30°: 1.1 × 10^{-5} mm Hg. uv max (methanol): 229, 304 nm (ε 15500, 7700). Soly in (g/l) at 25°: water 1.2; acetone 45; chloroform 1200; ethanol 65; xylene 360. LD_{50} in female rats (mg/kg): 200-400 i.p., >4000 orally (Elias).

USE: Fungicide.

3218. Dimethisoquin. [86-80-6] 2-[(3-Butyl-1-isoquinolin-yl)oxy]-N,N-dimethylethanamine; 3-butyl-1-[2-(dimethylamino)-ethoxy]isoquinoline; 1-(β-dimethylaminoethoxy)-3-n-butylisoquin-oline; quinisocaine. $C_{17}H_{24}N_2O$; mol wt 272.39. C 74.96%, H 8.88%, N 10.28%, O 5.87%. Prepn: Wilson *et al., J. Am. Chem. Soc.* **71,** 937 (1949); Anderson *et al., J. Am. Pharm. Assoc. Sci. Ed.* **41,** 643 (1952); Ullyot, US **2612503** (1952 to SK & F). Clinical studies: Robinson: *South. Med. J.* **50,** 367 (1957). Toxicity study: Fellows, Macko, *J. Pharmacol. Exp. Ther.* **103,** 306 (1951).

Liquid, bp₃ 155-157°. n_D^{20} 1.5486.

Hydrochloride. [2773-92-4] Haenal; Isochinol. $C_{17}H_{24}N_2$-O.HCl; mol wt 308.85. Crystals, sol in water, alcohol, chloroform. Practically insol in ether. pH of 1% aq soln: ~4.2. LD_{50} i.p. in rats: 45-50 mg/kg (Fellows, Macko).

THERAP CAT: Anesthetic (topical).

THERAP CAT (VET): Anesthetic (topical).

3219. Dimethisterone. [79-64-1] (6α,17β)-17-Hydroxy-6-methyl-17-(1-propynyl)androst-4-en-3-one; 6α-methyl-17-(1-pro-pynyl)testosterone; 6α,21-dimethyl-17β-hydroxy-17α-pregn-4-en-20-yn-3-one; 6α,21-dimethylethisterone; 17α-ethynyl-6α,21-di-methyltestosterone; 17α-ethynyl-17-hydroxy-6α,21-dimethyl-androst-4-en-3-one; Secrosteron (obsolete). $C_{23}H_{32}O_2$; mol wt 340.50. C 81.13%, H 9.47%, O 9.40%. Orally active progestogen; formerly used in combinations as oral contraceptive. Prepn: S. P. Barton *et al., J. Chem. Soc.* **1959,** 1957; *eidem, US* **2939819** (1960 to Brit. Drug Houses). Structure-activity study: G. K. Suchowsky, G. Baldratti, *J. Endocrinol.* **30,** 159 (1964). Evaluation of risk for endometrial cancer: N. S. Weiss *et al., N. Engl. J. Med.* **302,** 551 (1980). Review of carcinogenicity studies: *IARC Monographs* **21,** 377-385 (1979).

Crystals, mp 102°. $[\alpha]_D^{20}$ +10° (c = 1 in chloroform). uv max (isopropanol): 240 nm ($E_{1cm}^{1\%}$ 450). Practically insol in water. Sol in ethanol; slightly sol in acetone, chloroform.

Mixture with ethinyl estradiol. [8015-19-8] Oracon (obsolete).

THERAP CAT: Progestogen.

3220. Dimethoate. [60-51-5] Phosphorodithioic acid O,O-dimethyl S-[2-(methylamino)-2-oxoethyl] ester; phosphorodithioic acid O,O-dimethyl ester, ester with 2-mercapto-N-methylacetamide; O,O-dimethyl S-methylcarbamoylmethyl phosphorodithioate; American Cyanamid 12880; Cygon; Fostion MM; Perfekthion; Rogor; Roxion. $C_5H_{12}NO_3PS_2$; mol wt 229.26. C 26.19%, H 5.28%, N 6.11%, O 20.94%, P 13.51%, S 27.97%. Prepn: Cassaday *et al.,* Young, US **2494283** and US **2996531** (1950, 1961, both to Am. Cyanamid); GB **791824** (1958 to Montecatini), *C.A.* **52,** 18222 (1958). Toxicity data: E. W. Schafer, *Toxicol. Appl. Pharmacol.* **21,** 315 (1972). Teratogenicity study: K. D. Courtney *et al., J. Environ. Sci. Health* **B20,** 373 (1985).

Crystals, mp 52-52.5°. d^{65} 1.277. n_D^{65} 1.5334. Burns readily on contact with flame. Very slightly sol in water. Freely sol in most organic solvents, except saturated hydrocarbons. Stable in aq soln; hydrolyzed by aq alkali. LD_{50} orally in rats: 250 mg/kg (Schafer).

Caution: Cholinesterase inhibitor: *Clinical Toxicology of Commercial Products,* R. E. Gosselin *et al.,* Eds. (Williams & Wilkins, Baltimore, 5th ed., 1984) Section II, p 297.

USE: Systemic and contact insecticide.

3221. Dimethocaine. [94-15-5] 3-(Diethylamino)-2,2-dimethyl-1-propanol p-aminobenzoate; 3-diethylamino-2,2-dimethylpropyl p-aminobenzoate; 1-aminobenzoyl-2,2-dimethyl-3-diethylaminopropanol; p-aminobenzoate of diethylaminoneopentyl alcohol; Larocaine. $C_{16}H_{26}N_2O_2$; mol wt 278.39. C 69.03%, H 9.41%, N 10.06%, O 11.49%. Prepn: Mannich, Wilder, *Ber.* **65**, 378 (1932); C. Mannich, **US 1889678** (1932). Pharmacology: O. Gebner *et al., Arch. Exp. Pathol. Pharmakol.* **168**, 447 (1932); and toxicology review: A. D. Hirschfelder, R. N. Bieter, *Physiol. Rev.* **12**, 190-282 (1932).

Hydrochloride. [553-63-9] $C_{16}H_{26}N_2O_2 \cdot HCl$. Minute crystals or powder, sometimes fine leaflets. Bitter taste. mp 196-197°. One part dissolves in 3 parts water at 20°, more sol in hot water. One part dissolves also in 10 parts of cold alcohol, in 5 parts of boiling alcohol. Practically insol in ether, oils, fats. Aq solns are slightly acid to litmus, and may be sterilized by heating at 105° for 10 minutes. MLD in mice, rabbits (g/kg): 0.30, 0.15 s.c.; 0.04, 0.015 i.v. (Hirschfelder, Bieter).

THERAP CAT: Anesthetic (local).

3222. Dimethomorph. [110488-70-5] 4-[3-(4-Chlorophenyl)-3-(3,4-dimethoxyphenyl)-1-oxo-2-propenyl]morpholine; 3-(4-chlorophenyl)-3-(3,4-dimethoxyphenyl) acrylic acid morpholide; CME-151; Acrobat; Forum. $C_{21}H_{22}ClNO_4$; mol wt 387.86. C 65.03%, H 5.72%, Cl 9.14%, N 3.61%, O 16.50%. Antifungal cinnamic acid derivative; comprised of a mixture of *E*- and *Z*-isomers. Process for prepn: J. Curtze, **EP 294907**; *idem*, **US 4933449** (1988, 1990 both to Shell Int.). Comprehensive description: G. Albert *et al., Brighton Crop Prot. Conf. - Pests Dis.* **1988**, 17-24. Mechanism of action study: P. J. Kuhn *et al., Mycol. Res.* **95**, 333 (1991). Efficacy vs downy mildew of grapevines: T. Wicks, B. Hall, *Plant Dis.* **74**, 114 (1990). Toxicological evaluation: G. E. Veenstra, D. E. Owen, *Arch. Toxicol.* **1992**, Suppl 15, 113.

Z-isomer

Colorless, odorless, crystalline solid. mp 127-148°. Soly (g/l) at 25°: water <0.05, acetone 50, toluene 20, methanol 20, dichloromethane 500. LD_{50} in rats (mg/kg): 321 i.p.; 3900 orally; >5000 dermally; LC_{50} (4-hr inhalation): >4.2 mg/ml (Veenstra, Owen).

USE: Agricultural fungicide.

3223. Dimethoxane. [828-00-2] 2,6-Dimethyl-1,3-dioxan-4-ol acetate; 6-acetoxy-2,4-dimethyl-*m*-dioxane; 2,6-dimethyl-*m*-dioxan-4-yl acetate; acetomethoxane; Dioxin (obsolete); Giv-Gard DXN; $C_8H_{14}O_4$; mol wt 174.19. C 55.16%, H 8.10%, O 36.74%. Prepn: C. S. Marvel *et al., J. Org. Chem.* **4**, 252 (1939); Späth *et al., Ber.* **76**, 57 (1943). Description: *Am. Perfum. Cosmet.* **77**, no. 12, 32-34 (1962), *C.A.* **58**, 8848c (1963).

Liquid, bp$_6$ 74-75°. n_D^{20} 1.4310; d_4^{20} 1.0655. Mustard-like odor. Miscible with water, many organic solvents.

USE: Preservative for cutting oils, resin emulsions, water-based paints, cosmetics, inks. Effective range of concn: 0.03-0.1%. Gasoline additive: Chafetz *et al.,* **US 3036904** (1962 to Texaco).

3224. 1,2-Dimethoxyethane. [110-71-4] Ethylene glycol dimethyl ether; monoglyme; α,β-dimethoxyethane; glyme; Dimethyl Cellosolve. $C_4H_{10}O_2$; mol wt 90.12. C 53.31%, H 11.18%, O 35.51%. $CH_3OCH_2CH_2OCH_3$. Prepd from ethylene glycol monomethyl ether, methyl sulfate and metallic sodium: Kranzfelder, Vogt, *J. Am. Chem. Soc.* **60**, 1714 (1938); from ethylene glycol monomethyl ether, methyl chloride and sodium: Capinjola, *ibid.* **67**, 1615 (1945); from chloromethyl methyl ether in the presence of sodium by Wurtz reaction: Geist, Mason, *ibid.* **76**, 3728 (1954). Series of articles on toxicology: *Environ. Health Perspect.* **57**, 1-275 (1984).

Liquid. Sharp ethereal odor. d_4^{15} 0.86877; d_4^{20} 0.86285; d_4^{33} 0.8602; d_{20}^{20} 0.8692. mp −58° (also reported as mp −71°). bp$_{760}$ 82-83°; bp$_{61.2}$ 20°; bp$_{50}$ 16°; bp$_{10}$ −14°. n_D^{24} 1.3739; n_D^{20} 1.3813. Flash pt 4.5°C (40°F). Miscible with water, alcohol. Sol in hydrocarbon solvents.

USE: Solvent, to facilitate the formation of alkali metal-hydrocarbon adducts; in the Reformatsky reaction with methyl γ-bromocrotonate.

3225. 2,6-Dimethoxyquinone. [530-55-2] 2,6-Dimethoxy-2,5-cyclohexadiene-1,4-dione; 2,6-dimethoxybenzoquinone. $C_8H_8O_4$; mol wt 168.15. C 57.14%, H 4.80%, O 38.06%. Obtained from pyrogallol-1,3-dimethyl ether-2-acetate upon oxidation with potassium dichromate: Hofmann, *Ber.* **11**, 337 (1878); or by heating with nitric acid in alc soln: Graebe, Hess, *Ann.* **340**, 237 (1905); by treating pyrogallol trimethyl ether with nitric acid: Will, *Ber.* **21**, 608 (1888); from syringa acid: Graebe, Martz, *ibid.* 221; from sinapic acid: Gadamer, *Ber.* **30**, 2333 (1897); from antiarole by oxidation with ferric chloride: Baker, *J. Chem. Soc.* **1928**, 1029.

Monoclinic golden-yellow prisms from acetic acid, mp 256°. Sublimes easily. Volatile with steam. Slightly sol in hot water, in ether, in alcohol; freely sol in hot glacial acetic acid and in alkaline solns.

3226. Dimethylacetal. [534-15-6] 1,1-Dimethoxyethane; acetaldehyde dimethyl acetal; ethylidene dimethyl ether. $C_4H_{10}O_2$; mol wt 90.12. C 53.31%, H 11.18%, O 35.51%. $CH_3CH(OCH_3)_2$. Prepn from acetaldehyde and methanol: Meadows, Darwent, *Can. J. Chem.* **30**, 501 (1952); Frevel, Hedelund, **US 2691684** (1954 to Dow). Toxicity study: H. F. Smyth *et al., J. Ind. Hyg. Toxicol.* **31**, 60 (1949).

Liquid, bp 64.5°. d_4^{20} 0.8516. n_D^{20} 1.3665. Miscible with water, alcohol, chloroform, ether. LD_{50} orally in rats: 6.5 g/kg; LC (in air) in rats: 16000 ppm (Smyth).

USE: As Mering's mixture which is 2 vol dimethylacetal and 1 vol chloroform.

3227. N,N-Dimethylacetamide. [127-19-5] Acetic acid dimethylamide; DMAC. C_4H_9NO; mol wt 87.12. C 55.15%, H 10.41%, N 16.08%, O 18.36%. $CH_3CON(CH_3)_2$. Prepn from tris(dimethylamido)phosphate and acetic anhydride: Dye, **US 2667510** (1954 to Chemstrand); from acetic anhydride and dimethylformamide: Coppinger, *J. Am. Chem. Soc.* **76**, 1372 (1954). Toxicity study: W. Bartsch *et al., Arzneim.-Forsch.* **26**, 1581 (1976).

Liquid. d_4^{25} 0.9366; d_4^{20} 0.9429; d_4^0 0.9599. bp$_{760}$ 163-165°; bp$_{80}$ 96°; bp$_{33}$ 85-87°; bp$_{26}$ 74-74.5°; bp$_{15}$ 66-67°; bp$_{12}$ 62-63°. n_D^{20} 1.4373; also reported as n_D^{20} 1.4230; n_D^{25} 1.4358. Flash pt 66°C (151°F). Miscible with water and most organic solvents. LD_{50} orally in rats: 5.4 ml/kg (Bartsch).

Caution: Potential symptoms of overexposure are jaundice, liver damage; depression, lethargy, hallucinations and delusions; skin irritation. *See NIOSH Pocket Guide to Chemical Hazards* (DHHS/-NIOSH 97-140, 1997) p 110.

USE: Solvent for many organic reactions and in industrial applications.

3228. Dimethylamine. [124-40-3] *N*-Methylmethanamine. C_2H_7N; mol wt 45.08. C 53.29%, H 15.65%, N 31.07%. $(CH_3)_2$-NH. Prepn from methanol + ammonia: Smith, **US 2456599** (1948 to Commercial Solvents); Serban, *Rev. Chim. (Bucharest)* **14,** 451 (1963), *C.A.* **60,** 5097b (1964); by catalytic hydrogenation of nitrosodimethylamine: Livering, Maury, **GB 797483** (1958 to Hercules Powder). Toxicity studies: R. Hazard *et al., Arch. Int. Pharmacodyn.* **112,** 36 (1957); W. H. Steinhagen *et al., Am. Ind. Hyg. Assoc. J.* **43,** 411 (1982).

A gas at ordinary temp; characteristic odor. d_4^0 (liq) 0.680. bp 7°, mp −96°. Very sol in water forming a very strong alkaline soln; sol in alcohol or ether. Has been marketed in compressed liq form in tubes or as a 33% aq soln.

Hydrochloride. [506-59-2] $C_2H_7N.HCl$. Deliquesc leaflets, mp 171°. Very sol in water; sol in alcohol, chloroform. Practically insol in ether. *Keep well closed.* LD_{50} in mice (g/kg): 1.21 i.v., 2.00 s.c. (Hazard). LC_{50} in mice (ppm): 7650 (48 hr), 4725 (14 day); in rats (ppm): 4540 (6 hr) (Steinhagen).

Caution: Potential symptoms of overexposure are irritation of nose and throat; sneezing, coughing and dyspnea; pulmonary edema; conjunctivitis; dermatitis; direct contact with liquid may cause frostbite. *See NIOSH Pocket Guide to Chemical Hazards* (DHHS/NIOSH 97-140, 1997) p 110.

USE: As accelerator in vulcanizing rubber, tanning, manuf detergent soaps, or attracting boll weevils to exterminate them. As reagent for Mg.

3229. *p*-Dimethylaminoazobenzene. [60-11-7] *N,N*-Dimethyl-4-(phenylazo)benzenamine; butter yellow; methyl yellow; C.I. Solvent Yellow 2; C.I. 11020. $C_{14}H_{15}N_3$; mol wt 225.29. C 74.64%, H 6.71%, N 18.65%. Prepn: *Colour Index* vol. 4 (3rd ed., 1971) p 4014. Review of carcinogenic risk: *IARC Monographs* **8,** 125-146 (1975).

Yellow cryst leaflets, mp 114-117°. Insol in water. Sol in alc, benzene, $CHCl_3$, ether, petr ether, mineral acids, oils.

Caution: Potential symptoms of overexposure are enlarged liver; hepatic and renal dysfunction; contact dermatitis; coughing, wheezing, difficulty breathing; bloody sputum; bronchial secretions; frequent urination, hematuria and dysuria. *See NIOSH Pocket Guide to Chemical Hazards* (DHHS/NIOSH 97-140, 1997) p 110. This substance is reasonably anticipated to be a human carcinogen: *Report on Carcinogens, Eleventh Edition* (PB2005-104914, 2004) p III-103.

USE: For determination of free HCl in gastric juice; spot test identification of peroxidized fats; pH indicator (red 2,9, yellow 4.0).

3230. *p*-Dimethylaminobenzaldehyde. [100-10-7] 4-Dimethylaminobenzenecarbonal; Ehrlich's reagent. $C_9H_{11}NO$; mol wt 149.19. C 72.46%, H 7.43%, N 9.39%, O 10.72%. Prepd by formylation of dimethylaniline with dimethylformamide: Campaigne, Archer, *Org. Synth.* **coll. vol. IV,** 331 (1963).

Small granular crystals or leaflets from alcohol + water. Unless extremely pure, the crystals are lemon-colored and may turn pink on exposure to light. mp 74°. bp_{17} 176-177°. Slightly sol in water; sol in alcohol, ether, chloroform, acetic acid, many other organic solvents.

Hydrochloride. Crystals, mp 109°.

USE: Manuf dyes; reagent for arsphenamine, anthranilic acid, antipyrine, indole, skatole, indican, tryptophan, albumin, ergot al-kaloids, colon bacteria, typhoid coli; for differentiating between serum eruptions and true scarlet fever.

3231. *p*-Dimethylaminobenzalrhodanine. [536-17-4] 5-[[4-(Dimethylamino)phenyl]methylene]-2-thioxo-4-thiazolidinone; 5-[*p*-(dimethylamino)benzylidene]rhodanine. $C_{12}H_{12}N_2OS_2$; mol wt 264.37. C 54.52%, H 4.58%, N 10.60%, O 6.05%, S 24.26%. Prepn: Mackie, Misra, *J. Chem. Soc.* **1954,** 3919.

Deep red needles from xylene, dec 270°, also reported as dec 246°. Sintering ~260° and melting ~280°. Practically insol in water. Very slightly sol in chloroform, ether, benzene; slightly sol in boiling alc; moderately sol in acetone; sol in strong acids with a yellow color.

USE: As 0.03% soln in acetone for detection of silver, mercury, copper, gold, platinum and palladium ions.

3232. 4-(Dimethylamino)benzoic Acid. [619-84-1] C_9H_{11}-NO_2; mol wt 165.19. C 65.44%, H 6.71%, N 8.48%, O 19.37%. Prepn: Willstätter, Kahn, *Ber.* **37,** 411 (1904); Morton, Stevens, *J. Am. Chem. Soc.* **53,** 4028, 4031 (1931); Gilman, Banner, *ibid.* **62,** 344 (1940); Bowman, Stroud, *J. Chem. Soc.* **1950,** 1342. Use of esters as sunscreening agents: Kreps, Ohlsson, **US 3403207** (1968); Worthington, **GB 1162337** and **FR 1566396** (both 1969 to Van Dyk).

Crystals from water, mp 242.5-243.5°. Soluble in alcohol, HCl and KOH solns, sparingly sol in ether. Practically insol in acetic acid. pKa 6.027; pKb 11.488.

3-Methylbutyl ester. [21245-01-2] Padimate A; Escalol 506. $C_{14}H_{21}NO_2$; mol wt 235.32.

2-Ethylhexyl ester. [21245-02-3] Padimate O; Escalol 507; Sundown. $C_{17}H_{27}NO_2$; mol wt 277.40.

Glyceryl ester *see* Glyceryl *p*-Aminobenzoate.

THERAP CAT: Esters as ultraviolet screen.

3233. *p*-Dimethylaminobenzophenone. [530-44-9] [4-(Dimethylamino)phenyl]phenylmethanone. $C_{15}H_{15}NO$; mol wt 225.29. C 79.97%, H 6.71%, N 6.22%, O 7.10%. *p*-$(CH_3)_2N$-$C_6H_4COC_6H_5$. Prepd from benzanilide, dimethylaniline, and phosphorus oxychloride: **DE 41751** *Frdl.* **1,** 44 (1887); Meisenheimer *et al., Ann.* **423,** 84 (1921); Hurd, Webb, *Org. Synth.* **7,** 24 (1927).

Leaflets from alc, mp 92-93°. Insol in water. Slightly sol in cold alcohol; freely sol in hot alcohol and in ether. Very weak base, sol in concd mineral acids from which it is precipitated by water.

syn-**Oxime.** $C_{15}H_{16}N_2O$. Prisms from H_2O + alc, mp 163°.

anti-**Oxime.** mp 176°.

3234. *N,N*-Dimethylaniline. [121-69-7] *N,N*-Dimethylbenzenamine; dimethylphenylamine. $C_8H_{11}N$; mol wt 121.18. C 79.29%, H 9.15%, N 11.56%. Made by heating aniline, methyl alcohol, and H_2SO_4 under pressure, the sulfate formed being converted by NaOH to the free base. Toxicity data: H. F. Smyth *et al., Am. Ind. Hyg. Assoc. J.* **23,** 95 (1962).

Oily liq. *Poisonous!* d_4^{20} 0.956. bp 192-194°. mp 2°. Flash pt 61°C. n_D^{20} 1.5582. Insol in water. Freely sol in alcohol, chloroform, ether. LD_{50} orally in rats: 1.41 ml/kg (Smyth).

Caution: Potential symptoms of overexposure are anoxia, cyanosis, weakness, dizziness and ataxia; methemoglobinemia. *See NIOSH Pocket Guide to Chemical Hazards* (DHHS/NIOSH 97-140, 1997) p 112.

USE: Solvent; manuf vanillin, Michler's ketone, methyl violet and other dyes. As reagent for methanol, methyl furfural, H_2O_2, nitrate, alcohol, formaldehyde.

3235. 9,10-Dimethyl-1,2-benzanthracene. [57-97-6] 7,12-Dimethylbenz[*a*]anthracene; 1,4-dimethyl-2,3-benzphenanthrene. $C_{20}H_{16}$; mol wt 256.34. C 93.71%, H 6.29%. Synthesis from *o*-(α-methyl-α-1-naphthyl)toluic acid: Newman, *J. Am. Chem. Soc.* **60**, 1141 (1938). From 9,10-dimethyl-9,10-dihydroxy-9,10-dihydro-1,2-benzanthracene: Bachmann, Chemerda, *J. Am. Chem. Soc.* **60**, 1023 (1938). From 9,10-dimethyl-9,10-dimethoxy-9,10-dihydro-1,2-benzanthracene: *eidem, ibid.* **61**, 2358 (1939). From 9-methyl-1,2-benzanthracen-10-one by a Reformatsky reaction: Mikhailov, Chernova *J. Gen. Chem. USSR* **9**, 2171 (1939), *C.A.* **34**, 4068 (1940).

Plates, leaflets from acetone-alc, faint greenish-yellow tinge. mp 122-123°. Maximum fluorescence at 440 nm: *C.A.* **38**, 1276 (1944). Freely sol in benzene; moderately sol in acetone; slightly sol in alcohol. Insol in water. May be solubilized in water by purines such as caffeine, tetramethyluric acid. The nucleosides, adenosine, and guanosine also show a solvent action.

3236. 5,6-Dimethylbenzimidazole. [582-60-5] $C_9H_{10}N_2$; mol wt 146.19. C 73.94%, H 6.89%, N 19.16%. Obtained by acid hydrolysis of vitamin B_{12}: Brink, Folkers, *J. Am. Chem. Soc.* **71**, 2951 (1949); **72**, 4442 (1950). Synthesis by refluxing 4,5-diamino-1,2-dimethylbenzene and formic acid in 4*N* HCl: Hobrecker, *Ber.* **5**, 921 (1872); Phillips, *J. Chem. Soc.* **1928**, 2393.

Crystals from ether, mp 205-206°. Sublimes at 140° and 3 mm. uv max (95% ethanol acidified with HCl to be 0.01*N*): 274.5, 284 nm. Alkaline to litmus. Soluble in water, chloroform, ether; freely sol in dil acids.

3237. *p*,α-Dimethylbenzyl Alcohol. [536-50-5] α,4-Dimethylbenzenemethanol; *p*-tolylmethylcarbinol; methyl-*p*-tolylcarbinol; 4-(α-hydroxyethyl)toluene; 4-methyl-α-phenethyl alcohol; 1-*p*-tolyl-1-ethanol. $C_9H_{12}O$; mol wt 136.19. C 79.37%, H 8.88%, O 11.75%. Constituent of the essential oil from *Curcuma longa* L., *Zingiberaceae* and related plants: Dieterle, Kaiser, *Arch. Pharm.* **271**, 337 (1933). Prepd from *p*-tolylmagnesium bromide and acetaldehyde in ether: v. Auwers, Kolligs, *Ber.* **55**, 42 (1922); Eisenlohr, Schulz, *Ber.* **57**, 1816 (1924); from 4-methylacetophenone: Gastaldi, Cherchi, *Gazz. Chim. Ital.* **45**, II, 274 (1915).

Viscous liq. Odor somewhat like that of menthol. The natural product is probably levorotatory. Constants for the synthetic *dl*-form: $d_4^{15.5}$ 0.9668. bp_{756} 219°; bp_{14} 134°; bp_{11} 115-116°. Very sparingly sol in water. Miscible with abs alcohol, ether. Also sol in isopropanol, liq petrolatum.

Phenylurethan. $C_{16}H_{17}NO_2$. Crystals, mp 97.5°.

3238. 2,3-Dimethyl-1,3-butadiene. [513-81-5] Diisopropenyl; β,γ-dimethyl-Δ-α,γ-butadiene. C_6H_{10}; mol wt 82.14. C

87.73%, H 12.27%. Occurs in the 66-70° fraction of Puertollano shale oil. Prepd by slow distillation of anhydr pinacol in the presence of hydrobromic acid: Allen, Bell, *Org. Synth.* **coll. vol. III**, 312; by rapid distillation of anhydr pinacol over alumina at 420-470°: Newton, Coburn, *ibid.* 313.

Liquid. d_{20}^{20} 0.7273; d_4^{20} 0.7267; d_4^{25} 0.7222. mp −76°. bp_{769} 69.2°; bp_{760} 68.8°. n_D^{25} 1.4362.

USE: In the manuf of synthetic rubber and polymers.

3239. Dimethylcadmium. [506-82-1] Cadmium dimethyl. C_2H_6Cd; mol wt 142.48. C 16.86%, H 4.24%, Cd 78.90%. $Cd(CH_3)_2$. Prepn from a Grignard reagent and a cadmium halide: Krause, *Ber.* **50**, 1813 (1917); Gilman, Nelson, *Rec. Trav. Chim.* **55**, 518 (1936); Anderson, Taylor, *J. Phys. Chem.* **56**, 161 (1952).

Liquid. Disagreeable odor. May be kept in a sealed tube. mp −4.5°; bp_{758} 105.5°; $d_4^{17.9}$ 1.9846; n_D 1.5488. Dec with explosive violence when heated above 150°. Catches fire when dropped on filter paper and produces dense clouds of first white, then brown cadmium oxide smoke. When thrown into water, it sinks to the bottom in large drops, which dec in a series of sudden explosive jerks, with crack-ling sounds. Sol in hydrocarbons.

USE: In organic synthesis; as polymerization catalyst.

3240. Dimethyl Carbate. [39589-98-5] (*endo,endo*)-Bicyclo[2.2.1]hept-5-ene-2,3-dicarboxylic acid dimethyl ester; *cis*-3,6-*endo*-methylene-Δ^4-tetrahydrophthalic acid dimethyl ester; *cis*-5-norbornene-2,3-dicarboxylic acid dimethyl ester; dimalone. $C_{11}H_{14}O_4$; mol wt 210.23. C 62.84%, H 6.71%, O 30.44%. Prepd by a Diels-Alder condensation of cyclopentadiene and maleic anhydride, followed by esterification of resulting anhydride: Bode, *Ber.* **70**, 1167 (1937); Morgan *et al., J. Am. Chem. Soc.* **66**, 404 (1944). Toxicology studies: J. H. Draize *et al., J. Pharmacol. Exp. Ther.* **93**, 26 (1948).

Crystals, mp 38° when very pure. The usual product is a viscous, syrupy liquid. $bp_{12.5}$ 137°; bp_9 130°; $bp_{1.5}$ 115°. d_4^{21} 1.164. n_D^{20} 1.4852. Practically insol in water. Soluble in the usual organic solvents. Solubility in kerosene and mineral oils ~6%. LD_{50} in mice, rats (ml/kg): 1.4, 1.0 orally; in rats (ml/kg): 10.0 dermally (Draize).

Caution: Can cause CNS excitation followed by depression.

USE: Insect repellent.

3241. Dimethyl Carbonate. [616-38-6] Carbonic acid dimethyl ester; methyl carbonate. $C_3H_6O_3$; mol wt 90.08. C 40.00%, H 6.71%, O 53.28%. Prepn: B. Röse, *Ann.* **205**, 227 (1880); V. Grignard *et al., Ann. Chim. (Paris)* **9**, 229 (1920). Review of mfr and characteristics as a fuel additive: M. A. Pacheco, C. L. Marshall, *Energy Fuels* **11**, 2-29 (1997); of synthesis and chemical reactions: Y. Ono, *Appl. Catal. A* **155**, 133-166 (1997); of production and eco-friendly applications: D. Delledonne *et al., ibid.* **221**, 241-251 (2001); and chemistry: P. Tundo, M. Selva, *Acc. Chem. Res.* **35**, 706-716 (2002).

Liquid. *Flammable.* d_4^{20} 1.07. mp 4.6°. bp 90.3°. Viscosity (20°): 0.625 cP. Flash pt, open cup: 71.1°F (21.7°C). Heat of vaporization: 88.2 kcal/kg. Soly in H_2O: 13.9 g/100g. Miscible with alc, ethers, esters, ketones. Dielectric constant at 25°: 3.087.

Dipole moment: 0.91. LD$_{50}$ in rats (g/kg): 13.8 orally; 2.5 dermally. LC$_{50}$ (4 hr) in rats (mg/l): 140 by inhalation (Ono).

USE: Environmentally benign substitute for dimethyl sulfate, *q.v.*, and methyl halides in methylation reactions and for phosgene, *q.v.*, in methylcarbonylation reactions.

3242. 5,5-Dimethyl-1,3-cyclohexanedione. [126-81-8] 1,1-Dimethyl-3,5-diketocyclohexane; 1,1-dimethyl-3,5-cyclohexandione; dimethyldihydroresorcinol; dimedone; methone. C$_8$H$_{12}$O$_2$; mol wt 140.18. C 68.54%, H 8.63%, O 22.83%. Prepd from mesityl oxide and diethyl malonate: Shriner, Todd, *Org. Synth.* **coll. vol. II**, 200 (1943).

Needles from water, prisms from alcohol + ether. Dec 148-150°. Slightly volatile with steam (50 ml of a distillate contained 0.016 g). The dry crystals may be stored in a brown bottle for several years at room temp. Aq solns oxidize on exposure to air and light or upon prolonged storage in the dark. 100 ml of a satd aq soln contains 0.401 g at 19°; 0.416 g at 25°; 1.185 g at 50°; 3.020 g at 80°; 3.837 g at 90°. Monobasic acid in water. pK (25°): 5.15. Dipole moment 3.46. Also sol in methanol, ethanol, chloroform, benzene, acetic acid, and in 50% ethanol-water mixture.

USE: For the separation and identification of aldehydes. Gives insol condensation products with aldehydes, but not with ketones. The use of piperidine as a catalyst is recommended.

3243. N,N-Dimethylformamide. [68-12-2] DMF; DMFA. C$_3$H$_7$NO; mol wt 73.09. C 49.30%, H 9.65%, N 19.16%, O 21.89%. HCON(CH$_3$)$_2$. Prepd from dimethylamine and formic acid: Mitchell, Reid, *J. Am. Chem. Soc.* **53**, 1879 (1931); Brown, *J. Appl. Chem.* **1**, Suppl. Issue no. 2, S159 (1951); Campbell, **US 3015674** (1962 to Commercial Solvents); Surman, **US 3072725** (1963 to du Pont); from dimethylamine + HCN: Benneville *et al.*, *J. Org. Chem.* **21**, 772 (1956); from HCN + methanol: Fukuoka, Kominami, *Chem. Tech.* **1972** (Nov.), 640. Toxicity study: W. Bartsch *et al.*, *Arzneim.-Forsch.* **26**, 1581 (1976). Reviews of chemical uses: R. S. Kittila, *Dimethylformamide Chemical Uses* (du Pont, Wilmington, 1967) 264 pp and Suppl. (1973) 148 pp; J. S. Pizey, *Synthetic Reagents* **Vol. 1** (John Wiley, New York, 1974) pp 4-99; C. L. Eberling in *Kirk-Othmer Encyclopedia of Chemical Technology* **vol. 11** (Wiley-Interscience, New York, 3rd ed., 1980) pp 263-268. Review of carcinogenic risk: *IARC Monographs* **47**, 171-197 (1989).

Colorless to very slightly yellow liquid. Faint amine odor. mp −61°. bp$_{760}$ 153°; bp$_{39}$ 76°; bp$_{3.7}$ 25°. d$_4^2$ 0.9445. n$_D^{25}$ 1.42803. Flash pt, open cup: 153°F (67°C). Misc with water and most common organic solvents. pH of 0.5 molar soln in H$_2$O = 6.7. LD$_{50}$ in mice, rats (ml/kg): 6.8, 7.6 orally; 6.2, 4.7 i.p. (Bartsch).

Caution: Potential symptoms of overexposure are irritation of eyes, skin and respiratory system; nausea, vomiting and colic; liver damage, hepatomegaly; high blood pressure; facial flush; dermatitis. *See NIOSH Pocket Guide to Chemical Hazards* (DHHS/NIOSH 97-140, 1997) p 114.

USE: Solvent for liqs and gases. In the synthesis of organic compounds. Solvent for Orlon and similar polyacrylic fibers. Wherever a solvent with a slow rate of evaporation is required. Has been termed the universal organic solvent.

3244. N,N-Dimethylglycine. [1118-68-9] (Dimethylamino)acetic acid; *N*-methylsarcosine; DMG. C$_4$H$_9$NO$_2$; mol wt 103.12. C 46.59%, H 8.80%, N 13.58%, O 31.03%. (CH$_3$)$_2$-NCH$_2$COOH. Prepn: H. T. Clarke *et al.*, *J. Am. Chem. Soc.* **55**, 4571 (1933); D. E. Pearson, J. D. Bruton, *ibid.* **73**, 864 (1951). Mutagenicity study: N. Colman *et al.*, *Proc. Soc. Exp. Biol. Med.* **164**, 9 (1980). Constituent of some products sold in the U.S. as "pangamic acid".

Hygroscopic crystals, mp 157-160°.

Hydrochloride. C$_4$H$_9$NO$_2$.HCl. mp 189-190°. Sol in alc, water. Insol in chloroform, acetone.

3245. N,N-Dimethylglycine Hydrazide Hydrochloride. [539-64-0] Girard's reagent D. C$_4$H$_{12}$ClN$_3$O; mol wt 153.61. C 31.28%, H 7.87%, Cl 23.08%, N 27.36%, O 10.42%. (CH$_3$)$_2$-NCH$_2$CONHNH$_2$.HCl. Prepd from *N,N*-dimethylglycine ethyl ester and hydrazine hydrate in abs alc: Viscontini, Meier, *Helv. Chim. Acta* **33**, 1773 (1950).

Crystals from alc, mp 181°.

Dihydrochloride. C$_4$H$_{11}$N$_3$O.2HCl. mp 214.5°.

USE: Reagent for aldehydes and ketones.

3246. Dimethylglyoxime. [95-45-4] 2,3-Butanedionedioxime; diacetyldioxime; Chugaev's reagent. C$_4$H$_8$N$_2$O$_2$; mol wt 116.12. C 41.37%, H 6.94%, N 24.12%, O 27.56%. Prepn: Semon, Damerell, *Org. Synth.* **coll. vol. II**, 204 (1943). Manuf: Kamlet, **US 2732404** (1956 to National Distillers Product Corp.). Crystal structure: *Anal. Chem.* **21**, 1428 (1949); Merritt, Lanterman, *Acta Crystallogr.* **5**, 811 (1952).

Triclinic crystals from alc + water, mp 238-240°, also reported as melting 242° and 246°. Practically insol in water. Sol in alc, ether, pyridine, acetone.

USE: Detection and determination of Ni and its separation from Co and many other metals. Forms a scarlet red ppt with Ni even in dil solns. Separation of Pd from Sn, Au, Rh, and Ir, also to detect Bi with which it forms a bright yellow color and ppt.

3247. 1,1-Dimethylhydrazine. [57-14-7] *unsym*-Dimethylhydrazine; *asym*-dimethylhydrazine; *N,N*-dimethylhydrazine; UDMH; Dimazine. C$_2$H$_8$N$_2$; mol wt 60.10. C 39.97%, H 13.42%, N 46.61%. (CH$_3$)$_2$NNH$_2$. Prepd industrially by the reaction of dimethylamine and chloramine; by reduction of nitrosodimethylamine (obtained by treating a dimethylamine salt with sodium nitrite): Hatt, *Org. Synth.* **coll. vol. II**, 211 (1943). Toxicity studies: Witkin, *Arch. Ind. Health* **13**, 34 (1956); Cornish, Hartung, *Toxicol. Appl. Pharmacol.* **15**, 62 (1969). Review of carcinogenic risk: *IARC Monographs* **4**, 137-143 (1974); of toxicology and human exposure: *Toxicological Profile for Hydrazines* (PB98-101025, 1997) 224 pp.

Flammable. Hygroscopic, mobile liquid. Fumes in air and gradually turns yellow. Characteristic ammonia-like fishy odor of aliphatic hydrazines. d$_4^{22}$ 0.791; d$_{25}^{25}$ 0.782. mp −58°. bp$_{760}$ 63.9°. n$_D^{22.3}$ 1.40753. Miscible with water with evolution of heat. Also miscible with alcohol, ether, dimethylformamide, hydrocarbons. LD$_{50}$ in mice, rats (mg/kg): 265, 122 orally; 250, 119 i.v. (Witkin).

Hydrochloride. C$_2$H$_8$N$_2$.HCl. Hygroscopic crystals from abs ethanol, mp 83°. Sol in water, ethanol. Practically insol in ether.

Caution: Potential symptoms of overexposure are irritation of eyes and skin; choking, chest pain and dyspnea; lethargy; nausea; anoxia; convulsions; liver injury. *See NIOSH Pocket Guide to Chemical Hazards* (DHHS/NIOSH 97-140, 1997) p 114. *See also Patty's Industrial Hygiene and Toxicology* **vol. 2A**, G. D. Clayton, F. E. Clayton, Eds. (Wiley-Interscience, New York, 3rd ed., 1981) pp 2801-2803. 1,1-Dimethylhydrazine is reasonably anticipated to be a human carcinogen: *Report on Carcinogens, Eleventh Edition* (PB2005-104914, 2004) p III-107.

USE: Base in rocket fuel formulations.

3248. 1,2-Dimethylhydrazine. [540-73-8] *N,N'*-Dimethylhydrazine; *sym*-dimethylhydrazine; SDMH. C$_2$H$_8$N$_2$; mol wt 60.10. C 39.97%, H 13.42%, N 46.61%. CH$_3$NHNHCH$_3$. Prepn from dibenzoylhydrazine: Folpmers, *Rec. Trav. Chim.* **34**, 34 (1915); Hatt, *Org. Synth.* **coll. vol. II**, 208 (1943). Electrosynthesis from nitromethane: Iversen, *Ber.* **104**, 2195 (1971). Toxicity study: Witkin, *Arch. Ind. Health* **13**, 34, (1956). Review of carcinogenic risk: *IARC Monographs* **4**, 145-150 (1974); and of toxicology and human exposure: *Toxicological Profile for Hydrazines* (PB98-101025, 1997) 224 pp.

Flammable, hygroscopic, mobile liquid. Fumes in air and gradually turns yellow. *Corrosive to skin!* Characteristic ammoniacal odor of aliphatic hydrazines. d$_4^{20}$ 0.8274. bp$_{753}$ 81°. n$_D^{20}$ 1.4209. Miscible with water with much evolution of heat. Also miscible with alcohol, ether, dimethylformamide, hydrocarbons. LD_{50} in mice, rats (mg/kg): 36, 160 orally; 29, 175 i.v. (Witkin).

Dihydrochloride. $C_2H_8N_2 \cdot 2HCl$. Extremely hygroscopic prisms, dec 168°. Freely sol in water, ethanol.

Caution: For toxic symptoms *see* 1,1-Dimethylhydrazine.

3249. 1,3-Dimethyl-2-imidazolidinone. [80-73-9] *N,N'*-Dimethylethyleneurea; DMI. $C_5H_{10}N_2O$; mol wt 114.15. C 52.61%, H 8.83%, N 24.54%, O 14.02%. Aprotic basic solvent. Prepn: W. R. Boon, *J. Chem. Soc.* **1947**, 307; M. W. Farlow, **US 2422400** (1947 to du Pont); E. V. Dehmlow, Y. R. Rao, *Synth. Commun.* **18**, 487 (1988). Prepn and pharmacological activity: E. J. Lien, W. D. Kumler, *J. Med. Chem.* **11**, 214 (1968). Prepn and spectral properties: H. Kohn *et al., J. Org. Chem.* **42**, 941 (1977). Evaluation as replacement solvent for HMPA, q.v.: C.-C. Lo, P.-M. Chao, *J. Chem. Ecol.* **16**, 3245 (1990).

mp 8.2° (Dehmlow, Rao); also reported as mp below −4° (Lo, Chao). bp_{754} 220°. bp_{17} 106-108°. bp_2 67-68°. n_D^{20} 1.4720. d^{25} 1.0519 g/ml. Dipole moment (dioxane, benzene): 4.09 ± 0.01 D, 4.05 ± 0.01 D. Dielectric constant (25°): 37.6. Viscosity (25°): 1.944 cP. Soly in toluene: >5%. LD_{50} i.p. in mice: 2840 mg/kg (Lien).

USE: As substitute solvent for HMPA in organic synthesis.

3250. Dimethylmercury. [593-74-8] Mercury, dimethyl; methyl mercury. C_2H_6Hg; mol wt 230.66. C 10.41%, H 2.62%, Hg 86.96%. $(CH_3)_2Hg$. Environmental contaminant found together with **monomethyl mercury** compounds in fish and birds. Prepns: Buckton, *Ann.* **108**, 103 (1858); **109**, 219 (1859); Jones, Werner, *J. Am. Chem. Soc.* **40**, 1257 (1918); Gilman, Brown, *ibid.* **52**, 3314 (1930); Wade, **US 3636020** (1972 to Ventron); H. H. Sisler *et al., J. Org. Chem.* **45**, 1329 (1980). Synthesized in bottom sediments: Jensen, Jernelöv, *Nature* **223**, 753 (1969). Physical properties: Wilde, *J. Chem. Soc.* **1949**, 72. Formation and degradation studies: Bertilsson, Neujahr, *Biochemistry* **10**, 2805 (1971); DeSimone *et al., Biochim. Biophys. Acta* **304**, 851 (1973); Spangler *et al., Science* **180**, 192 (1973); *eidem, Appl. Microbiol.* **25**, 488 (1973). Neurotoxicity studies: Dales, *Am. J. Med.* **53**, 219 (1972); Skerfving, *Food Cosmet. Toxicol.* **10**, 545 (1972); Kojima, Fujita, *Toxicology* **1**, 43 (1973).

Colorless, volatile, toxic liquid; easily inflammable. bp_{740} 92°. d^{20} 3.1874. n_D^{20} 1.5452. Easily sol in ether, alc. Insol in H_2O.

USE: As inorganic reagent.

3251. Dimethyl(methylene)ammonium Iodide. [33797-51-2] *N*-Methyl-*N*-methylenemethanaminium iodide; Eschenmoser's salt. C_3H_8IN; mol wt 185.01. C 19.48%, H 4.36%, I 68.59%, N 7.57%. $H_2C{=}N(CH_3)_2I$. Mannich type intermediate originally developed to introduce methyl groups into corrin chromophore. Prepn from trimethylamine and diiodomethane: J. Schreiber *et al., Angew. Chem. Int. Ed.* **10**, 330 (1971); from *N,N,N',N'*-tetramethylmethylenediamine: T. A. Bryson *et al., J. Org. Chem.* **45**, 524 (1980). Used in prepn of Mannich bases: J. Hooz, J. N. Bridson, *J. Am. Chem. Soc.* **95**, 602 (1973). In functionalization of indoles: A. P. Kozikowski, H. Isida, *Heterocycles* **14**, 55 (1980). In prepn of α-methylene carbonyls: J. L. Roberts *et al., Tetrahedron Lett.* **1977**, 1621; of terminal olefins: *eidem, ibid.* 1299.

Colorless crystals from tetrahydrothiophene dioxide, dec ∼240°. Sublimes at 120° at 0.05 torr.

USE: In organic synthesis.

3252. *N,N*-Dimethyl-1-naphthylamine. [86-56-6] *N,N*-Dimethyl-1-naphthalenamine; 1-dimethylaminonaphthalene. $C_{12}H_{13}N$; mol wt 171.24. C 84.17%, H 7.65%, N 8.18%. Prepn by heating in a closed tube 1-naphthylamine and methyl iodide in methyl alcohol: Landshoff, *Ber.* **11**, 643 (1878); by heating 1-naphthylamine with dimethyl sulfate in sodium hydroxide in presence of pyridine: Germuth, *J. Am. Chem. Soc.* **51**, 1556 (1929). Use: F. G. Germuth, *Ind. Eng. Chem. Anal. Ed.* **1**, 28 (1929).

Oil; aromatic odor. bp_{711} 274.5°, bp_{90} 193°, bp_{69} 184.5°, bp_{13} 139-140°; d_4^4 1.0522, d_{15}^{15} 1.0446, d_{25}^{25} 1.0391; n_D^{20} 1.622. Readily sol in alcohol or ether.

USE: Detection and determination of nitrites.

3253. Dimethylolpropionic Acid. [4767-03-7] 3-Hydroxy-2-(hydroxymethyl)-2-methylpropanoic acid; 2,2-bis(hydroxymethyl)propionic acid; dihydroxypivalic acid; DMPA. $C_5H_{10}O_4$; mol wt 134.13. C 44.77%, H 7.51%, O 47.71%. Prepn: H. Koch, T. Zerner, *Monatsh. Chem.* **22**, 447, 450 (1891); K. E. Wilzbach *et al., J. Am. Chem. Soc.* **70**, 4069 (1948); R. Riemschneider *et al., Monatsh. Chem.* **88**, 1099 (1957); H. Vieregge, J. F. Arens, *Rec. Trav. Chim.* **78**, 921 (1959).

Free-flowing granular powder, mp 181-185°. Sol in water, methanol. Slightly sol in acetone. Insol in benzene.

USE: In prepn of water-sol alkyl resins.

3254. Dimethyl-*p*-phenylenediamine. [99-98-9] *N,N*-Dimethyl-1,4-benzenediamine; *p*-aminodimethylaniline. $C_8H_{12}N_2$; mol wt 136.19. C 70.55%, H 8.88%, N 20.57%. Prepn from *p*-nitrosodimethylaniline which is obtained from dimethylaniline: Gattermann-Wieland, *Praxis des Organischen Chemikers* (de Gruyter, Berlin, 40th ed., 1961) p 273. By reduction of methyl orange: A. I. Vogel, *Practical Organic Chemistry* (Longmans, London, 3rd ed., 1959) p 624.

Reddish-violet crystals. mp 53°, also stated as 41°. bp 262°. Sol in water, alcohol, chloroform, ether. *Keep tightly closed and protected from light.*

Dihydrochloride. $C_8H_{12}N_2 \cdot 2HCl$. White to grayish-white, hygroscopic crystalline powder. Freely sol in water; sol in alcohol.

USE: Dihydrochloride in microscopy and in tests for acetone, uric acid, thallic salts, oxydases, lignin, ozone, H_2O_2, H_2S, Br.

3255. Dimethyl Phthalate. [131-11-3] 1,2-Benzenedicarboxylic acid dimethyl ester; phthalic acid dimethyl ester; methyl phthalate; dimethyl 1,2-benzenedicarboxylate; DMP; Palatinol M; Fermine; Avolin; Mipax. $C_{10}H_{10}O_4$; mol wt 194.18. C 61.85%, H 5.19%, O 32.96%. Prepd industrially from phthalic anhydride and methanol: *Faith, Keyes & Clark's Industrial Chemicals*, F. A. Lowenheim, M. K. Moran, Eds. (Wiley-Interscience, New York, 4th ed., 1975) pp 318-324. Metabolite of *Gibberella fujikuroi:* Cross *et al., J. Chem. Soc.* **1963**, 2937. Toxicity data: J. H. Draize *et al., J. Pharmacol. Exp. Ther.* **93**, 26 (1948).

Oily liq. Slight aromatic odor. $d_{15.6}^{15.6}$ 1.196; d_{20}^{20} 1.1940; d_{25}^{25} 1.189. One gallon weighs 9.93 lbs. Flash pt 295°F (146°C). mp 5.5° (the commercial product freezes around 0°). bp_{760} 283.7°; bp_{400} 257.8°; bp_{200} 232.7°; bp_{100} 210.0°; bp_{60} 194.0°; bp_{40} 182.8°; bp_{20} 164.0°; bp_{10} 147.6°; bp_5 131.8°; $bp_{1.0}$ 100.3°. Vapor pressure at 20° <0.0l mm. The vapor is heavy, d = 6.69 (air = 1). n_D^{20} 1.5168.

Viscosity at 25° = 17.2 cP. Heat of vaporization: 93.1 g-cal/g; heat of combustion: 119.7 kg-cal/mole. uv max (ethanol): 277 nm ($E_{1cm}^{1\%}$ 57.7). Miscible with alcohol, ether, chloroform. Practically insol in water (0.43 g/100 ml), petr ether, and other paraffin hydrocarbons. Soly in mineral oil at 20°: 0.34 g/100 g. LD_{50} in mice, rats, guinea pigs (ml/kg): 7.2, 6.9, 2.4 orally (Draize).

Caution: Potential symptoms of overexposure are irritation of eyes, upper respiratory system; stomach pain. *See NIOSH Pocket Guide to Chemical Hazards* (DHHS/NIOSH 97-140, 1997) p 114.

USE: Solvent and plasticizer for cellulose acetate and cellulose acetate-butyrate compositions. Insect repellent for personal protection against biting insects.

3256. Dimethyl Sulfate. [77-78-1] Sulfuric acid dimethyl ester; DMS. $C_2H_6O_4S$; mol wt 126.13. C 19.04%, H 4.79%, O 50.74%, S 25.42%. $(CH_3)_2SO_4$. Prepn by distillation of a mixture of oleum and methanol: Guyot, Simon, *Compt. Rend.* **169,** 796 (1919). Technical production from dimethyl ether and SO_3: *BIOS Final Report* No. 986, p 176. *Review:* C. M. Suter, *The Organic Chemistry of Sulfur* (John Wiley, New York, 1944) p 49-61. Use as methylating agent: L. Fieser, M. Fieser, *Reagents for Organic Synthesis* (John Wiley, New York, 1967) pp 293-295. Toxicity data: Smyth *et al., Arch. Ind. Hyg. Occup. Med.* **4,** 119 (1951). Review of toxicology: E. Browning, *Toxicity and Metabolism of Industrial Solvents* (Elsevier, New York, 1965) pp 713-721; of carcinogenicity studies: *IARC Monographs* **4,** 271-276 (1974); of mutagenicity studies: G. R. Hoffmann, *Mutat. Res.* **75,** 63-129 (1980).

Colorless oily liq. *Poisonous. Corrosive.* bp ~188° (with dec); bp_{15} 76°. mp −27°. d_4^{20} 1.3322. n_D^{20} 1.3874. Flash pt 182°F (83°C). Soly in water 2.8 g/100 ml at 18°. Hydrolysis is rapid at or above this temp. Vapor density 4.35. Sol in ether, dioxane, acetone, aromatic hydrocarbons. Sparingly sol in carbon disulfide, aliphatic hydrocarbons. LD_{50} orally in rats: 440 mg/kg (Smyth).

Caution: Vapors and liquid can be absorbed through the skin or respiratory tract, causing local and systemic toxicity. Potential symptoms of overexposure are irritation of eyes and nose; conjunctivitis; eye and skin burns; headache; giddiness; delerium; photophobia; periorbital edema; dysphonia, aphonia, dysphagia; cough, chest pain; dyspnea; cyanosis; vomiting; diarrhea, dysuria; analgesia; fever; albuminuria, hematuria. *See NIOSH Pocket Guide to Chemical Hazards* (DHHS/NIOSH 97-140, 1997) p 116; P. Grandjean, "Skin Penetration: Hazardous Chemicals at Work" (Taylor & Francis, New York, 1990) pp 173-174. This substance is reasonably anticipated to be a human carcinogen: *Report on Carcinogens, Eleventh Edition* (PB2005-104914, 2004) p III-109.

USE: Methylating agent in the manuf of many organic chemicals. War gas.

3257. 2,4-Dimethylsulfolane. [1003-78-7] Tetrahydro-2,4-dimethylthiophene 1,1-dioxide; 2,4-dimethylthiacyclopentane 1,1-dioxide; 2,4-dimethyltetramethylene sulfone; 2,4-dimethylcyclotetramethylene sulfone. $C_6H_{12}O_2S$; mol wt 148.22. C 48.62%, H 8.16%, O 21.59%, S 21.63%. Prepd by catalytic hydrogenation of 2,4-dimethyl-3-sulfolene: Morris, Melchior, **US 2451298** (1948 to Shell).

Colorless to yellow liquid. d_4^{20} 1.1362. n_D^{20} 1.4733. bp_5 123.3°; bp 280-281° (some decompn). Miscible with lower aromatic hydrocarbons; partially miscible with naphthenes, olefins, paraffins. Limited miscibility with water.

USE: Solvent for liquid-liquid and vapor-liquid extraction processes.

3258. Dimethyl Sulfone. [67-71-0] Sulfonylbismethane; $DMSO_2$; methyl sulfone; methylsulfonylmethane. $C_2H_6O_2S$; mol wt 94.13. C 25.52%, H 6.42%, O 33.99%, S 34.06%. CH_3SO_2-CH_3. Has been found in primitive plants such as *Equisetum arvense* L., *Equisetaceae* and in the adrenal cortex of cattle: Pfiffner, North,

J. Biol. Chem. **134,** 781 (1940). Easily prepd by oxidation of dimethyl sulfide: Douglas, *J. Am. Chem. Soc.* **68,** 1072 (1946); McAllan *et al., ibid.* **73,** 3627 (1951).

Crystals, mp 109°. bp_{760} 238°. Sublimes at 13 mm and 90° to 100°. Infrared absorption (solid) 7600-8700 nm. Dipole moment 4.44 (vapor). Freely sol in water, methanol, ethanol, acetone. Sparingly sol in ether.

USE: High temp solvent for many inorganic and organic substances.

3259. Dimethyl Sulfoxide. [67-68-5] Sulfinylbismethane; methyl sulfoxide; DMSO; SQ-9453; Deltan; Dolicur; Domoso; Kemsol; Rheumabene; Rimso-50. C_2H_6OS; mol wt 78.13. C 30.75%, H 7.74%, O 20.48%, S 41.04%. $(CH_3)_2SO$. Dipolar, aprotic solvent. Attributed with a wide range of bioactivities including analgesic, anti-inflammatory and cryoprotective properties. Prepn: A. Saytzeff, *Ann.* **144,** 148 (1867). Usually obtained as a by-product of paper manufacture: M. D. Robbins, *Chem. Eng.* **68,** 100 (June 26, 1961). Toxicity data: W. Bartsch *et al., Arzneim.-Forsch.* **26,** 1581 (1976). Review of properties and use in organic chemistry: D. Martin *et al., Angew. Chem. Int. Ed.* **6,** 318-334 (1967). Reviews of pharmacology and toxicology: S. W. Jacob, D. C. Wood, *Arzneim.-Forsch.* **17,** 1553-1560 (1967); N. A. David, *Annu. Rev. Pharmacol.* **12,** 353-374 (1972); of clinical experience: *Ann. N.Y. Acad. Sci.* **411,** entitled "Biological Actions and Medical Applications of Dimethyl Sulfoxide", J. C. de la Torre, Ed. (1983) 402 pp; B. N. Swanson, *Rev. Clin. Basic Pharmacol.* **5,** 1-33 (1985); of use in rheumatic disorders: J. M. Trice, R. S. Pinals, *Semin. Arthritis Rheum.* **15,** 45-60 (1985). Review of veterinary uses: C. F. Brayton, *Cornell Vet.* **76,** 61-90 (1986).

Very hygroscopic liquid. Practically no odor or color. Slightly bitter with sweet after-taste. d_4^{20} 1.100. mp 18.55°. bp_{760} 189°; bp_{16} 79.83°; bp_{12} 72.5°. Flash pt, open cup: 203°F (95°C). n_D^{20} 1.4783. Viscosity (20°): 2.47 cP. Specific heat (25°): 0.4698 cal/g. Dielectric constant: 45. Sol in water, ethanol, acetone, ether, benzene, chloroform. LD_{50} orally in rats: 17.9 ml/kg (Bartsch).

Caution: Rapidly absorbed through skin and mucous membranes; enhances dermal absorption of many other chemicals. Repeated topical application may result in mild, erythamatous, scaling dermatitis. Corneal opacities have been produced in exptl animals. *See Clinical Toxicology of Commercial Products,* R. E. Gosselin *et al.,* Eds. (Williams & Wilkins, Baltimore, 5th ed., 1984) Section II, p 407.

USE: Solvent for many organic compds including fats, carbohydrates, dyes, resins, and polymers. In organic reactions. As antifreeze or hydraulic fluid when mixed with water. To cryopreserve and store cultured cells.

THERAP CAT: In treatment of interstitial cystitis and scleroderma.

THERAP CAT (VET): Topically to reduce swelling due to trauma.

3260. Dimethylthiambutene. [524-84-5] *N,N*-Dimethyl-4,4-di-2-thienyl-3-buten-2-amine; *N,N,*1-trimethyl-3,3-di-2-thienyl-allylamine; 3-dimethylamino-1,1-bis(2-thienyl)-1-butene; 3-dimethylamino-1,1-di(2'-thienyl)but-1-ene; 338C48; NIH-4542; Ohton; Aminobutene; Dimethibutin; Kobaton; Takaton. $C_{14}H_{17}NS_2$; mol wt 263.42. C 63.83%, H 6.50%, N 5.32%, S 24.35%. Prepn: Grignard reaction of ethyl β-dimethylaminobutyrate with 2-thienyllithium and dehydration of the resulting 3-dimethylamino-1,1-di-2-thienylbutanol with HCl: Adamson, *J. Chem. Soc.* **1950,** 885; **US 2561899** (1951 to Burroughs Wellcome); **GB 657301** (1951 to Wellcome Foundation). Toxicity data: Y. Kase *et al., Chem. Pharm. Bull.* **7,** 372 (1959).

Viscous, dark brown or yellow oil, $bp_{0.05}$ 123-125°; bp_3 157-158°. Sol in chloroform, ether. LD_{50} in mice (mg/10 kg): 1.21 s.c.; in dogs (mg/kg): 20.3 i.v. (Kase).

Hydrochloride. $C_{14}H_{18}ClNS_2$. May be recrystallized from mixt of ethyl acetate and ethanol, mp 168-169°. Sol in water, chloroform. LD_{50} in mice (mg/10 kg): 1.37 s.c.; in dogs (mg/kg): 20.3 i.v. (Kase).

Note: This is a controlled substance (opiate): **21 CFR,** 1308.11.

THERAP CAT: Analgesic (narcotic).

3261.   N,N'-Dimethylthiourea. [534-13-4] Dimethylthio-carbamide. $C_3H_8N_2S$; mol wt 104.17. C 34.59%, H 7.74%, N 26.89%, S 30.78%. $CH_3NHCSNHCH_3$.

Colorless, exceedingly deliquesc crystals. mp 60-62°. Very sol in water, alcohol, acetone; sparingly sol in benzene, ether, carbon disulfide, very slightly in petr ether. *Keep tightly closed.*

3262.   N,N-Dimethyltryptamine. [61-50-7] N,N-Dimethyl-1H-indole-3-ethanamine; 3-[2-(dimethylamino)ethyl]indole; DMT. $C_{12}H_{16}N_2$; mol wt 188.27. C 76.55%, H 8.57%, N 14.88%. Occurs naturally in plants with hallucinogenic properties. Isoln from the leaves of *Prestonia amazonica* (Benth.) Macbride (*Haemadictyon amazonicum* Spruce & Benth.), *Apocynaceae:* Hockstein, Paradies, *J. Am. Chem. Soc.* **79,** 5735 (1957). Metabolism: St. Szára, *Experientia* **12,** 441 (1956); B. R. Sitaram *et al., Biochem. Pharmacol.* **36,** 1509 (1987). Relationship between hallucinogenic activity and electronic configuration: Snyder, Merril, *Proc. Natl. Acad. Sci. USA* **54,** 258 (1965). Synthesis: I. Fleming, M. Woolias, *J. Chem. Soc. Perkin Trans. 1* **1979,** 829. Differential interaction with serotonin receptor subtypes: A. V. Deliganis *et al., Biochem. Pharmacol.* **41,** 1739 (1991). Fluorometric detection: O. Jules *et al., Anal. Chim. Acta* **169,** 355 (1985). Review of biosynthesis, metabolism and bioactivity: S. A. Barker *et al., Int. Rev. Neurobiol.* **22,** 83-110 (1981).

Crystals, mp 44.6-46.8°; also reported as plates from ethanol and light petroleum, mp 46° (Fleming, Woolias). bp 60-80°. pKa 8.68 (ethanol-water). Freely sol in dil acetic and dil mineral acids.

Methiodide. mp 216-217°.

Note: This is a controlled substance (hallucinogen): **21 CFR,** 1308.11.

3263.   Dimethylzinc. [544-97-8] Zinc dimethyl. C_2H_6Zn; mol wt 95.48. C 25.16%, H 6.33%, Zn 68.51%. $Zn(CH_3)_2$. Prepd by the interaction of zinc and methyl iodide: Simonowitch, *Chem. Zentralbl.* **1899, I,** 1066; Bamford *et al., J. Chem. Soc.* **1946,** 468.

Mobile liquid. Stable in sealed tube and under CO_2. $d_4^{10.5}$ 1.386; mp $-40°$; bp 46°. *Ignites in air,* burns with a blue flame, giving off a peculiar, garlic-like odor. Very slow oxidation with traces of air produces methylzinc methylate, CH_3ZnOCH_3. Sol in ether, miscible with hydrocarbons.

3264.   Dimetofrine. [22950-29-4] 4-Hydroxy-3,5-dimethoxy-α-[(methylamino)methyl]benzenemethanol; 1-(3,5-dimethoxy-4-hydroxyphenyl)-2-(methylamino)ethanol; dimethophrine; dimetrophine. $C_{11}H_{17}NO_4$; mol wt 227.26. C 58.14%, H 7.54%, N 6.16%, O 28.16%. Selective α_1-adrenergic receptor agonist. Prepn: **GB 1145637;** M. Giani *et al.,* **US 3646144** (1969, 1972 both to Zambeletti). Pharmacology: Scrollini *et al., Atti Accad. Med. Lomb.* **25,** 193, 203 (1970), *C.A.* **76,** 54270a, 54425e (1972). Pharmacokinetics and metabolism: P. Boselli *et al., Arzneim.-Forsch.* **26,** 2038 (1976); M. S. Benedetti *et al., ibid.* **27,** 158 (1977). TLC determn: G. Musumarra *et al., J. Chromatogr.* **350,** 151 (1985). Double blind clinical evaluations: V. Baldrighi *et al., Curr. Med. Res. Opin.* **9,** 78 (1984); U. Marini *et al., ibid.* 265.

mp 178° (dec). pK 9.71.

Hydrochloride. [22775-12-8] Pressamina. $C_{11}H_{17}NO_4.HCl$; mol wt 263.72. mp 171-173°.

THERAP CAT: Antihypotensive.

3265.   Dimetridazole. [551-92-8] 1,2-Dimethyl-5-nitro-1H-imidazole; RP-8595; Emtryl; Unizole. $C_5H_7N_3O_2$; mol wt 141.13. C 42.55%, H 5.00%, N 29.77%, O 22.67%. Prepn: Bhagwat, Pyman, *J. Chem. Soc.* **127,** 1832 (1925).

Needles from water, mp 138-139°. Freely sol in alcohol; sparingly sol in cold water, ether.

Hydrochloride. $C_5H_7N_3O_2.HCl$. Prisms from dil HCl, mp 195°. Freely sol in water, alcohol; sparingly sol in acetone. Also used as the dihydrogen phosphate, freely sol in water.

THERAP CAT (VET): Antiprotozoal (Histomonas).

3266.   Diminazene Aceturate. [908-54-3] N-Acetylglycine compd with 4,4'-(1-triazene-1,3-diyl)bis(benzenecarboximidamide) (2:1); N-acetylglycine compd with 4,4'-(diazoamino)dibenzamidine; diminazene diaceturate; 4,4'-(diazoamino)dibenzamidine diaceturate; 1,3-bis(p-amidinophenyl)triazene bis(N-acetylglycinate); 1,3-bis[4-guanylphenyl]triazene diaceturate; 4,4'-diamidinodiazoaminobenzene diaceturate; p,p'-diguanyldiazoaminobenzene diaceturate; Berenil. $C_{22}H_{29}N_9O_6$; mol wt 515.52. C 51.26%, H 5.67%, N 24.45%, O 18.62%. Prepn: Brodersen *et al.,* **US 2838485** (1958 to Hoechst); Stavrovskaya, Drusvyatskaya, *C.A.* **59,** 15199a (1963). Mode of action: Festy *et al., C.R. Seances Acad. Sci. Ser. D* **271,** 730 (1970). Chemotherapeutic characteristics: Schmulevich *et al., Veterinariya (Moscow)* **38,** 23 (1961), *C.A.* **56,** 13512b (1962). *Review:* Newton in *Antibiotics* vol. 3, J. W. Corcoran, F. E. Hahn, Eds. (Springer-Verlag, New York, 1975) pp 34-47.

Yellow solid, dec 217°. Sol in 14 parts water (20°); slightly sol in alcohol; very slightly sol in ether, chloroform.

THERAP CAT (VET): Antiprotozoal (Trypanosoma, Babesia).

3267.   β,β'-Dinaphthylamine. [532-18-3] N-2-Naphthalenyl-2-naphthalenamine; $C_{20}H_{15}N$; mol wt 269.34. C 89.19%, H 5.61%, N 5.20%. Prepn from β-naphthol: Merz, Weith, *Ber.* **13,** 1300 (1880), Benz, *Ber.* **16,** 15 (1883); from β-naphthylamine: Klopsch, *Ber.* **18,** 1586 (1885); Liebermann, Jacobson, *Ann.* **211,** 43 (1882).

Glistening silvery leaves from benzene, mp 170.5°. Slightly sol in boiling alc; readily sol in boiling glacial acetic acid.

USE: Detection of nitrites, nitrates, and chlorates: Sa, *An. Farm. Bioquim.* **5,** 111 (1934), *C.A.* **30,** 6672 (1936).

3268.   Diniconazole. [83657-24-3] (βE)-β-[(2,4-Dichlorophenyl)methylene]-α-(1,1-dimethylethyl)-1H-1,2,4-triazole-1-ethanol; (E)-1-(2,4-dichlorophenyl)-4,4-dimethyl-2-(1,2,4-triazol-1-yl)-1-penten-3-ol; S-3308-10; S-3308L; XE-779L; Ortho Spotless; Spotless; Sumi-8. $C_{15}H_{17}Cl_2N_3O$; mol wt 326.22. C 55.23%, H 5.25%, Cl 21.74%, N 12.88%, O 4.90%. Prepn: Y. Funaki *et al.,* **DE 3010560;** *eidem,* **US 4554007;** resolution of enantiomers: Y. Funaki *et al.,* **EP 54431;** *eidem,* **US 4435203** (1980, 1985, 1982, 1984 all to Sumitomo). Metabolism of racemate in rats: N. Isobe *et al., Nippon Noyaku Gakkaishi* **10**, 475 (1985), *C.A.* **104**, 103703b (1986); of enantiomers: *eidem, ibid.* **12**, 421 (1987), *C.A.* **108**, 1715x (1988). Mechanism of sterol inhibition: Y. Yoshida *et al., Biochem. Biophys. Res. Commun.* **137**, 513 (1986); T. Katagi, *J. Agric. Food Chem.* **36**, 344 (1988). Fungicidal activity of the (−)-form and plant growth regulating activity of the (+)-form: C. S. Kvien *et al., J. Plant Growth Regul.* **6**, 233 (1987); D. J. Daigle *et al., Proc. 14th Ann. Mtg. Plant Growth Regul. Soc. Am. 1987*, p 108. Field trials as foliar fungicide: A. R. Biggs, J. Warner, *Can. J. Plant Pathol.* **9**, 41 (1987); A. K. Hagan *et al., J. Environ. Hort.* **6**, 67 (1988); against soil-borne diseases: A. S. Csinos *et al., Appl. Agric. Res.* **2**, 113 (1987). Comprehensive description: H. Takano, *Jpn. Pestic. Inf.* **49**, 18 (1986).

Crystals from isopropanol, mp 148-149°. Vapor pressure at 20°: 2.2 × 10⁻⁵ mm Hg. Soly at 25° (% v/w): water 4.01; at 23°: acetone 9.5; methanol 9.5; xylene 1.4. Stable to heat, sunlight and moisture. LD₅₀ in male, female rats (mg/kg): 639, 474 orally; >5000, >5000 dermally (Takano).

(−)-**Form.** [83657-18-5] Crystals from carbon tetrachloride/*n*-hexane, mp 160-161°. [α]²⁴_D −31.7° (c = 1 in CHCl₃).

(+)-**Form.** [83657-19-6] Crystals from carbon tetrachloride/*n*-hexane, mp 160-161°. [α]²⁴_D +26° (c = 1 in CHCl₃).

USE: Agricultural fungicide.

3269. Dinitolmide. [148-01-6] 2-Methyl-3,5-dinitrobenzamide; 3,5-dinitro-*o*-toluamide; 3,5-dinitro-2-methylbenzamide; Zoalene; Zoamix. C₈H₇N₃O₅; mol wt 225.16. C 42.67%, H 3.13%, N 18.66%, O 35.53%. Prepn: McGookin *et al., J. Soc. Chem. Ind.* **59**, 92 (1940); Harris *et al.*, US 2937204 (1960 to Dow). Activity studies: Peterson, *Poult. Sci.* **39**, 739 (1960); Joyner, *Res. Vet. Sci.* **1**, 363 (1960). Metabolism: Smith *et al., J. Agric. Food Chem.* **11**, 253 (1963); Smith, *Anal. Biochem.* **7**, 461 (1964).

Crystals from dil alc, mp 181°.
Caution: Potential symptom of overexposure by direct contact is eczema. *See NIOSH Pocket Guide to Chemical Hazards* (DHHS/NIOSH 97-140, 1997) p 116.
THERAP CAT (VET): Coccidiostat.

3270. 2,4-Dinitroaniline. [97-02-9] 2,4-Dinitrobenzenamine. C₆H₅N₃O₄; mol wt 183.12. C 39.35%, H 2.75%, N 22.95%, O 34.95%. Prepn: Wells, Allen, *Org. Synth. coll. vol.* **II**, 221 (1943). Liquid chromatographic determn: A. L. Scher, *J. Assoc. Off. Anal. Chem.* **68**, 474 (1985). Metabolism and disposition in rats: H. B. Matthews *et al., Xenobiotica* **16**, 1 (1986). Toxicity study: E. G. Feldmann, W. O. Foye, *J. Am. Pharm. Assoc. Sci. Ed.* **48**, 419 (1959).

Yellow needles from dil acetone, greenish-yellow plates from alcohol. mp 187.5-188°. pKa 18.46. Practically insol in cold water. Very sparingly sol in boiling water. 5.8 parts dissolve in 1000 parts of 88% alc at 18°; one part dissolves in 132.6 parts of 95% alc at 21°.
Caution: May be irritating to skin, mucous membranes.
USE: In prepn of azo dyes.

3271. 2,6-Dinitroaniline. [606-22-4] 2,6-Dinitrobenzenamine. C₆H₅N₃O₄; mol wt 183.12. C 39.35%, H 2.75%, N 22.95%, O 34.95%. Synthesis starting with chlorobenzene, fuming sulfuric acid, and potassium nitrate: Schultz, *Org. Synth.* **coll. vol. IV**, 364 (1963).

Light orange needles from alc, mp 139-140°. Soly in 95% ethanol about 0.4 g/100 ml. Also sol in ether, hot benzene. Practically insol in water, petr ether. Dipole moment: 1.9.

3272. 2,4-Dinitrobenzaldehyde. [528-75-6] C₇H₄N₂O₅; mol wt 196.12. C 42.87%, H 2.06%, N 14.28%, O 40.79%. Prepn: *p*-Nitrosodimethylaniline hydrochloride, obtained by reacting dimethylaniline and sodium nitrite, is condensed with 2,4-dinitrotoluene in the presence of sodium carbonate. The product, dinitrobenzylidene-*p*-aminodimethylaniline is split under steam agitation with HCl: Bennett, Bell, *Org. Synth.* **coll. vol. II**, 223 (1943).

Yellow to light brown crystals, mp 72°. bp₁₀₋₂₀ 190-210°. Freely sol in alc, ether, benzene, slightly sol in petr ether, water.
USE: In prepn of Schiff bases.

3273. Dinitrobenzene. C₆H₄N₂O₄; mol wt 168.11. C 42.87%, H 2.40%, N 16.66%, O 38.07%. Commercial product usually consists of a mixture of the *m*, *o* and *p* isomers. Toxicity study: T. E. Cody *et al., J. Toxicol. Environ. Health* **7**, 829 (1981). Review of toxicology and human exposure: *Toxicological Profile for 1,3-Dinitrobenzene and 1,3,5-Trinitrobenzene* (PB95-264289, 1995) 178 pp.

m-**Dinitrobenzene.** [99-65-0] 1,3-Dinitrobenzene. Yellowish crystals. mp 89-90°. bp 300-303°. Volatile with steam. One gram dissolves in 2000 ml cold water, 320 ml boiling water, 37 ml alc, 20 ml boiling alcohol; freely sol in benzene, chloroform, ethyl acetate. LD₅₀ in male, female rats (mg/kg): 91, 81 orally (Cody).

o-**Dinitrobenzene.** [528-29-0] 1,2-Dinitrobenzene. White crystals. d 1.57. mp 118°. bp 319°. Volatile with steam. One gram dissolves in 6600 ml cold water, 2700 ml boiling water, about 60 ml alc, 3 ml boiling alc, 20 ml benzene; freely sol in chloroform, ethyl acetate.

p-**Dinitrobenzene.** [100-25-4] 1,4-Dinitrobenzene. White crystals; sublimable. d 1.63. mp 173-174°. bp 299°. Volatile with steam. One gram dissolves in 12,500 ml cold water, 555 ml boiling water, 300 ml alcohol; sparingly soluble in benzene, chloroform, ethyl acetate.
Caution: Potential symptoms of overexposure include methemoglobinemia, headache, nausea, dizziness, general malaise (*See Toxicological Profile*); anoxia, cyanosis; visual disturbances, central

scotomas; bad taste, burning mouth, dry throat, thirst; yellowing hair, eyes, skin; anemia; liver damage. *See NIOSH Pocket Guide to Chemical Hazards* (DHHS/NIOSH 97-140, 1997) p. 116-119.

USE: Manuf of dyes, dye intermediates, explosives, plastics.

3274. 2,4-Dinitrobenzenesulfenyl Chloride. [528-76-7] $C_6H_3ClN_2O_4S$; mol wt 234.62. C 30.72%, H 1.29%, Cl 15.11%, N 11.94%, O 27.28%, S 13.67%. Prepd from bis(2,4-dinitrophenyl)disulfide and chlorine in ethylene bromide: Kharasch *et al., J. Am. Chem. Soc.* **69**, 1612 (1947); **72**, 1796 (1950); *J. Chem. Educ.* **33**, 585 (1956); from 2,4-dinitrothiophenol and chlorine in benzene: Perold, Snyman, *J. Am. Chem. Soc.* **73**, 2379 (1951); from 2,4-dinitrophenylbenzyl sulfide and sulfuryl chloride in ethylene chloride: Kharasch, Langford, *Org. Synth.* **44**, 47 (1964). *Review:* Kharasch, *Organic Sulfur Compounds* **vol. 1** (Pergamon Press, New York, 1961) pp 375-396.

Yellow crystals from carbon tetrachloride, mp 96°. Sol in glacial acetic acid, methylene chloride, ethylene chloride, trichlorethylene, benzene, xylene. Somewhat less sol in carbon tetrachloride. Insol in ether. Reacts with alc (even in the cold) to produce ethyl 2,4-dinitrobenzenesulfenate.

USE: Analytical reagent for the characterization of organic compds: Kharasch, *J. Chem. Ed.* **33**. 585 (1956); Langford, Lawson, *ibid.* **34**, 510 (1957).

3275. 3,4-Dinitrobenzoic Acid. [528-45-0] $C_7H_4N_2O_6$; mol wt 212.12. C 39.64%, H 1.90%, N 13.21%, O 45.26%. Prepd by treating 3-nitro-4-aminotoluene with Caro's acid and oxidizing the 3-nitro-4-nitrosotoluene with potassium dichromate: Langley, *Org. Synth.* **22**, 47 (1942); by oxidation of 3,4-dinitrotoluene: Goldstein, Voegeli, *Helv. Chim. Acta* **26**, 475 (1943).

Crystals from water + alc. Bitter taste. mp 166°; (mp 165.5-166.5°, Goldstein). 0.673 g dissolves in 100 parts water at 25°. Freely sol in alc, ether and hot water. Sublimes.

USE: In quantitative sugar analysis.

3276. 3,5-Dinitrobenzoic Acid. [99-34-3] $C_7H_4N_2O_6$; mol wt 212.12. C 39.64%, H 1.90%, N 13.21%, O 45.26%. Prepd by nitration of benzoic acid with fuming nitric acid: Brewster *et al., Org. Synth.* **22**, 48 (1942); Saunders *et al., Biochem. J.* **36**, 368 (1942). Purification: Jensen *et al., Chem. Weekbl.* **43**, 731 (1947), *C.A.* **42**, 2307d (1948).

Monoclinic prismatic crystals from alc. mp 205-207°, (mp 206.5-207.2° purified). One gram dissolves in 53 parts of boiling water; much less sol in cold water. Very sol in alc and glacial acetic acid; sparingly sol in ether, carbon disulfide and benzene. Sublimes.

USE: Identification of alcohols, alkyl halides; chromatographic determination of the essential oil constituents.

3277. 3,5-Dinitrobenzoyl Chloride. [99-33-2] $C_7H_3ClN_2O_5$; mol wt 230.56. C 36.47%, H 1.31%, Cl 15.38%, N 12.15%, O

34.70%. Prepd from 3,5-dinitrobenzoic acid and PCl_5 at 120-130°: Saunders *et al., Biochem. J.* **36**, 368 (1942).

Needles from light petr (bp 40-60°), mp 69.5°. bp_{10-12} 196°.
Caution: A strong irritant.

USE: Identification of amino acids; characterization of the alcohol part of acetals and ketals without prior hydrolysis and separation of the alcohol.

3278. 4,4'-Dinitrocarbanilide. [587-90-6] *N,N'*-Bis(4-nitrophenyl)urea; DNC; 4,4'-dinitrodiphenylurea. $C_{13}H_{10}N_4O_5$; mol wt 302.24. C 51.66%, H 3.33%, N 18.54%, O 26.47%. Prepd by heating 4-nitroaniline and diphenyl carbonate for 3 hrs at 200°: Vittenet, *Bull. Soc. Chim. Fr.* [3] **21**, 149 (1899); by nitration of diphenylurea with 68.28% HNO_3 in concd H_2SO_4 at 0°: Kogan, Kutepov, *J. Gen. Chem. USSR* **21**, 1297 (1951), *C.A.* **46**, 2003d (1952); by the action of dil HNO_3 on diphenylurea at up to 100°: *eidem*, **SU** 78379 (1949), *C.A.* **48**, 7056i (1954).

Yellow needles from alc, mp 312° (dec). Sublimes above 310°. Moderately sol in boiling nitrobenzene; sparingly sol in boiling alc, somewhat more sol in a mixture of glacial acetic acid and nitric acid. Practically insol in acetone, chloroform, benzene, dioxane, acetic acid, ether and linseed oil. Solubilities in g/100 ml solvent at 25°: water 2×10^{-6}; ethanol 0.007; ethyl acetate 0.015; petr ether 0.0; xylene <0.01; methyl Cellosolve 0.1; dimethyl acetamide 0.14; dimethyl sulfoxide 0.47.

3279. Dinitrocresol. [534-52-1] 2-Methyl-4,6-dinitrophenol; 4,6-dinitro-*o*-cresol; 3,5-dinitro-2-hydroxytoluene; 3,5-dinitro-*o*-cresol; DN; DNC; DNOC; Antinonnin; Detal; Dinitrol; Elgetol; K III; K IV; Ditrosol; Prokarbol; Effusan; Lipan; Selinon; Sinox; Dekrysil. $C_7H_6N_2O_5$; mol wt 198.13. C 42.43%, H 3.05%, N 14.14%, O 40.38%. Prepd by sulfonation of *o*-cresol followed by controlled nitration: Noelting, de Salis, *Ber.* **14**, 987 (1881); Bovini, *Chem. Zentralbl.* **1928**, II, 112; Bures, *C.A.* **22**, 63 (1928); Datta, Varma, *J. Indian Chem. Soc.* **4**, 321 (1927); Monti, Cianetti, *Gazz. Chim. Ital.* **67**, 628 (1937). Acute toxicity data: R. Ben-Dyke *et al., World Rev. Pest Control* **9**, 119-127 (1970). Review of toxicology and human exposure: *Toxicological Profile for Dinitrocresols* (PB95-264321, 1995) 204 pp.

Yellow prisms from alc, mp 87.5°. Moderately volatile with steam. Sparingly sol in water; readily sol in alkaline aq solns, in ether, acetone, alcohol (about 10%); sparingly sol in petr ether. LD_{50} in rats (mg/kg): 25-40 orally, 200-600 dermally (Ben-Dyke).

Sodium salt. $C_7H_5N_2O_5Na$. Red powder. Hydrate, yellow needles very freely sol in water.

Caution: Potential symptoms of overexposure to dinitrocresol are a sense of well being; headache, fever, lassitude, profuse sweating, excessive thirst, tachycardia, hyperpnea, coughing, shortness of breath and coma. *See NIOSH Pocket Guide to Chemical Hazards* (DHHS/NIOSH 97-140, 1997) p 118. *See also Clinical Toxicology of Commercial Products*, R. E. Gosselin *et al.,* Eds. (Williams & Wilkins, Baltimore, 5th ed., 1984) Section II, p 196.

USE: Selective herbicide, insecticide (ovicidal spray for dormant fruit trees).

3280.　2,4-Dinitrophenol. [51-28-5] α-Dinitrophenol; Aldifen. $C_6H_4N_2O_5$; mol wt 184.11. C 39.14%, H 2.19%, N 15.22%, O 43.45%. Prepd by the action of NaOH on 1-chloro-2,4-dinitrobenzene. Crystal and molecular structure: F. Iwasaki, Y. Kawano, *Acta Crystallogr.* **33B**, 2455 (1977). Toxicity data: E. W. Schafer, *Toxicol. Appl. Pharmacol.* **21**, 315 (1972). Review of toxicology and human exposure: *Toxicological Profile for Dinitrophenols* (PB95-264339, 1995) 262 pp.

Yellowish to yellow orthorhombic crystals. d 1.683. mp 112-114°. Sublimes when carefully heated. Volatile with steam. Very sparingly sol in cold water; soly in water (g/100 g of satd soln): at 54.5° = 0.137; at 75.8° = 0.301; at 87.4° = 0.587; at 96.2° = 1.22. Soly at 15° (g/100 g soln): Ethyl acetate 15.55; acetone 35.90; chloroform 5.39; pyridine 20.08; carbon tetrachloride 0.423; toluene 6.36. Sol in alcohol, benzene, aq alkaline solns. Forms crystalline sodium salt which is sol in water. LD_{50} orally in rats: 30 mg/kg (Schafer).

Caution: Rapidly absorbed through GI tract, respiratory tract and intact skin. Potential symptoms of overexposure are marked fatigue, tremendous thirst, profuse sweating, flushing of face; nausea, vomiting, abdominal pain, diarrhea; restlessness, anxiety, excitement; rise in body temperature; tachycardia, hyperpnea, dyspnea, cyanosis, muscle cramps; kidney and liver injury. *See Clinical Toxicology of Commercial Products,* R. E. Gosselin *et al.,* Eds. (Williams & Wilkins, Baltimore, 5th ed., 1984) Section III, pp 156-159.

USE: Manuf dyes, diaminophenol, wood preservative, insecticide; also as indicator. pH range: 2.6 colorless, 4.4 yellow. Reagent for the detection of potassium and ammonium ions.

3281.　2,5-Dinitrophenol. [329-71-5] Review of toxicology and human exposure: *Toxicological Profile for Dinitrophenols* (PB95-264339, 1995) 262 pp.

Yellow crystals. mp 108°; also stated as 104°. Slightly sol in water or cold alcohol; sol in hot alcohol, ether, fixed alkali hydroxides.

USE: Manuf dyes and organic chemicals, as indicator. pH range: 4.0 colorless, 5.4 yellow.

3282.　2,6-Dinitrophenol. [573-56-8] Review of toxicology and human exposure: *Toxicological Profile for Dinitrophenols* (PB95-264339, 1995) 262 pp.

Light yellow crystals. mp 63-64°. Slightly sol in cold water or cold alc; freely sol in chloroform, ether, boiling alc, fixed alkali hydroxide solns.

USE: Manuf dyes and organic chemicals; as indicator. pH range: 2.0 colorless, 4.0 yellow.

3283.　2,4-Dinitrophenylhydrazine. [119-26-6] $C_6H_6N_4$-O_4; mol wt 198.14. C 36.37%, H 3.05%, N 28.28%, O 32.30%. $C_6H_3(NO_2)_2NHNH_2$.

Red, cryst powder. mp ~200°. Slightly sol in water or alcohol; sol in moderately dil inorganic acids; readily sol in diglyme.

USE: For the determination of aldehydes and ketones.

3284.　2,4-Dinitroresorcinol. [519-44-8] 2,4-Dinitro-1,3-benzenediol. $C_6H_4N_2O_6$; mol wt 200.11. C 36.01%, H 2.01%, N 14.00%, O 47.97%.

Yellow crystals, mp 146-148°. Explodes when strongly heated. Sublimes partially undec. Very slightly sol in water or cold alcohol; sol in solns of fixed alkali hydroxides.

USE: For dyeing fabrics mordanted with iron a green color. As a reagent for Co (brown-red ppt) and for Fe (olive-green color).

3285.　Dinobuton. [973-21-7] Carbonic acid 1-methylethyl 2-(1-methylpropyl)-4,6-dinitrophenyl ester; carbonic acid 2-*sec*-butyl-4,6-dinitrophenyl isopropyl ester; 2-*sec*-butyl-4,6-dinitrophenyl isopropyl carbonate; dinitro-*sec*-butylphenyl isopropyl carbonate; isopropyl 2,4-dinitro-6-*sec*-butylphenyl carbonate; Acrex; Dessin; Sytasol. $C_{14}H_{18}N_2O_7$; mol wt 326.30. C 51.53%, H 5.56%, N 8.59%, O 34.32%. Prepn: Pianka, Polton, US **3234082**; US **3234260** (both 1966 to Murphy Chem.). Metabolism studies: Bandal, Casida, *J. Agric. Food Chem.* **20**, 1235 (1972). Toxicity study: T. B. Gaines, *Toxicol. Appl. Pharmacol.* **14**, 515 (1969).

Crystals from methanol or petr ether, mp 56-57°. LD_{50} in male, female rats (mg/kg): 59, 71 orally (Gaines).

USE: Miticide.

3286.　Dinocap. [39300-45-3] DNOCP; CR-1639; ENT-24727; Karathane. $C_{18}H_{24}N_2O_6$; mol wt 364.39. C 59.33%, H 6.64%, N 7.69%, O 26.34%. Originally thought to be 2-(1-methylheptyl)-4,6-dinitrophenyl butenoate, it is actually a mixture of 2(or 4)-octyl-4,6(or 2,6)-dinitrophenyl butenoate in which the octyl is a mixture of 1-methylheptyl, 1-ethylhexyl, and 1-propylpentyl. Prepn: W. F. Hester *et al.,* US **2526660** (1950 to Rohm & Haas). Fungicidal activity and chemical constitution: A. H. M. Kirby *et al., Ann. Appl. Biol.* **57**, 211 (1966); R. J. W. Byrde *et al., ibid.* 223. Mitocidal activity: N. D. Rishi, A. Q. Rather, *J. Entomol. Res.* **7**, 39 (1983). Degradation in soil: W. Mittelstaedt, F. Fuhr, *J. Agric. Food Chem.* **32**, 1151 (1984). Persistence on crops: B. D. Ripley *et al., Can. J. Plant Sci.* **65**, 229 (1985). HPLC residue analysis in crops: D. Liang *et al., J. Chromatogr.* **387**, 385 (1987). Acute and chronic toxicity: P. S. Larson *et al., Arch. Int. Pharmacodyn. Ther.* **119**, 31 (1959). Evaluation of developmental toxicity in rodents of technical grade and selected isomers: L. E. Gray, Jr. *et al., Teratog. Carcinog. Mutagen.* **6**, 33 (1986); J. M. Rogers *et al., ibid.* **7**, 341 (1987).

$R = $ —CH(CH$_2$)$_5$CH$_3$　or　—CH(CH$_2$)$_4$CH$_3$　or　—CH(CH$_2$)$_3$CH$_3$
　　　　　|　　　　　　　　　　　　|　　　　　　　　　　　　|
　　　　CH$_3$　　　　　　　　　CH$_2$CH$_3$　　　　　　(CH$_2$)$_2$CH$_3$

Dark brown liquid. bp$_{0.05}$ 138-140°. Incompatible with oil, oil based sprays, and lime-sulfur mixtures. LD_{50} in male rats (mg/kg): 23 i.v.; 980 orally (Larson).

Caution: Skin irritant. *See Clinical Toxicology of Commercial Products,* R. E. Gosselin *et al.,* Eds. (Williams & Wilkins, Baltimore, 5th ed., 1984) Section II, p 197.

USE: Acaricide; fungicide.

3287.　Dinoseb. [88-85-7] 2-(1-Methylpropyl)-4,6-dinitrophenol; 2-*sec*-butyl-4,6-dinitrophenol; DNBP; ENT-1122; WSX-8365; Chemox PE; Dow General; Premerge; Subitex; Caldon; Basanite. $C_{10}H_{12}N_2O_5$; mol wt 240.21. C 50.00%, H 5.04%, N 11.66%, O 33.30%. Prepn: L. E. Mills, B. L. Fayerweather, US **2192197** (1940 to Dow). Activity: A. S. Crafts, *Science* **101**, 417 (1945). Metabolism: S. K. Bandal, J. E. Casida, *J. Agric. Food Chem.* **20**, 1235 (1972); K. Ingebrigtsen, A. Froeslie, *Acta Pharmacol. Toxicol.* **46**, 326 (1980). Toxicology: R. G. Bough *et al., Toxicol. Appl. Pharmacol.* **7**, 353 (1965); T. B. Gaines, R. E. Linder, *Fundam. Appl. Toxicol.* **7**, 299 (1986).

Orange-brown viscous liquid, mp 38-42°. pKa 4.62. Sol in most organic solvents. LD_{50} in adult male, female rats (mg/kg): 27, 28 orally (Gaines, Linder).

Acetate. [2813-95-8] HOE-2904; Aretit; Ivosit. $C_{12}H_{14}N_2O_6$; mol wt 282.25. Brown oil, vinegar-like odor, mp 26-27°. Vapor press at 20°: 6×10^{-4} mm Hg. Sol in aromatics.

Ammonium salt. [6365-83-9] Chemox Selective; Dow Selective; Sinox W. $C_{10}H_{15}N_3O_5$; mol wt 257.24.

Triethanolamine salt. [6420-47-9] DN-289; Chemox DN; Gebutox. $C_{16}H_{27}N_3O_8$; mol wt 389.40.

USE: Herbicide; insecticide; miticide.

3288. Dinosterol. [58670-63-6] $(3\beta,4\alpha,5\alpha,22E)$-4,23-Dimethylergost-22-en-3-ol; 4α-methyl-$5\alpha(H)$-Δ^{22}-23,24-dimethylcholesten-3β-ol; Black Sea sterol. $C_{30}H_{52}O$; mol wt 428.73. C 84.04%, H 12.23%, O 3.73%. Biogenetically important marine sterol isolated from the toxic dinoflagellate, *Gonyaulax tamarensis*. Isoln and structure determn: Y. Shimizu *et al., J. Am. Chem. Soc.* **98,** 1059 (1976). Stereochemistry: J. Finer *et al., J. Org. Chem.* **43,** 1990 (1978). Identity with the Black Sea sterol: J. J. Boon *et al., Nature* **277,** 125 (1979). Stereospecific synthesis: A. Y. L. Shu, C. Djerassi, *Tetrahedron Lett.* **22,** 4627 (1981).

Needles from methanol-chloroform, mp 220-222° (Shimizu). Also reported as mp 211-214° (Shu, Djerassi). $[\alpha]_D^{20}$ −2.2° (in $CHCl_3$).

3289. Dinotefuran. [165252-70-0] *N*-Methyl-*N'*-nitro-*N''*-[(tetrahydro-3-furanyl)methyl]guanidine; 1-methyl-2-nitro-3-[(3-tetrahydrofuryl)methyl]guanidine; MTI-446; Starkle. $C_7H_{14}N_4O_3$; mol wt 202.21. C 41.58%, H 6.98%, N 27.71%, O 23.74%. Neonicotinoid insecticide. Prepn: K. Kodaka *et al., EP 649845; eidem, US 5434181* (both 1995 to Mitsui Toatsu); T. Wakita *et al., Pest Manage. Sci.* **59,** 1016 (2003). Comprehensive description: *eidem, Brighton Crop Prot. Conf. - Pests Dis.* **1998,** 21-26. Efficacy vs mosquitoes: V. Corbel *et al., J. Med. Entomol.* **41,** 712 (2004).

White solid from isopropyl ether, mp 94.5-101.5°. Relative density 1.33. Soly in purified water (20°): 54.3 ± 1.3 g/l. Log P (octanol/water): −0.664 (pH 7). LD_{50} in male, female mice, male, female rats (mg/kg): 2450, 2275, 2804, 2000 orally; in rats (mg/kg): >2000 dermally. LC_{50} in carp, rainbow trout, crayfish, daphnia (ppm): >1000 (96 hr), >40 (48 hr), 5-10 (48 hr), 1000 (48 hr) (Kodaka).

USE: Insecticide.

3290. DINP. [28553-12-0] 1,2-Benzenedicarboxylic acid diisononyl ester; diisononyl phthalate. $C_{26}H_{42}O_4$; mol wt 418.61.

C 74.60%, H 10.11%, O 15.29%. Dialkyl phthalate ester plasticizer used to impart softness and flexiblilty to PVC products. Prepn: P. J. Garner, G. Watson, *US 2508911* (1950 to Shell). Effects on behavior and properties of PVC: S. V. Patel, M. Gilbert, *Plast. Rubber Process. Appl.* **6,** 321 (1986); *eidem, ibid.* **8,** 215 (1987). Effects of temperature on viscosity and density: L. D. Lorenzi *et al., J. Chem. Eng. Data* **43,** 183 (1998). GC/MS determn in toys: R. Stringer *et al., Environ. Sci. Pollut. Res. Int.* **7,** 27 (2000). *Review:* L. G. Krauskopf, *Plast. Compd.* **6,** 28-38 (1983). Review of environmental fate: C. A. Staples *et al., Chemosphere* **35,** 667-749 (1997). Review of health effects and risk assessment: C. F. Wilkinson, J. C. Lamb, *Regul. Toxicol. Pharmacol.* **30,** 140-155 (1999); and environmental fate and toxicology: U. S. Gill *et al., Rev. Environ. Contam. Toxicol.* **172,** 87-127 (2001).

Liquid mp −48°. $bp_{5\ mm\ Hg}$ 252°. Flash point (closed cup): 213°C (415°F). d_{20}^{20} 0.972. n_D^{20} 1.486. Viscosity (cSt): 500 (0°); 102 (20°); 37 (37.8°); 6 (100°). Vapor pressure (mm Hg): (100°) 0.0018; (200°) 0.50; (300°) 40. Partition coefficient (octanol/water): 9.37.

USE: General purpose plasticizers for PVC applications and flexible vinyls.

3291. Diopterin. [6807-82-5] *N*-[*N*-[4-[[(2-Amino-1,4-dihydro-4-oxo-6-pteridinyl)methyl]amino]benzoyl]-L-α-glutamyl]-L-glutamic acid; pteroyl-α-glutamylglutamic acid; pteroyldiglutamic acid; PDGA. $C_{24}H_{26}N_8O_9$; mol wt 570.51. C 50.53%, H 4.59%, N 19.64%, O 25.24%. Folic acid analog. Synthesis: Mowat *et al., J. Am. Chem. Soc.* **70,** 1096 (1948); Hutchings, and Geraci, *US 2500825* and *US 2501168* (both 1950 to Am. Cyanamid); Geraci, *US 2766240* (1956 to Aries Labs.).

Precipitate from hot water. Sol in dil NaOH solns.

3292. Dioscin. [19057-60-4] (25R)-Spirost-5-en-3β-yl *O*-6-deoxy-α-L-mannopyranosyl-(1 → 2)-*O*-[6-deoxy-α-L-mannopyranosyl-(1 → 4)]-β-D-glucopyranoside; diosgenin bis-α-L-rhamnopyranosyl-(1 → 2 and 1 → 4)-β-D-glucopyranoside. $C_{45}H_{72}O_{16}$; mol wt 869.04. C 62.19%, H 8.35%, O 29.46%. From *Dioscorea tokoro* Mal., *Dioscoreaceae*. Isoln: Tsukamoto *et al., Pharm. Bull.* **4,** 35 (1956); Heitz, *Compt. Rend.* **248,** 283 (1958). Structure: Kawasaki, Yamauchi, *Chem. Pharm. Bull.* **10,** 703 (1962).

Crystals, decomp 275-277°. $[\alpha]_D^{13}$ −115° (c = 0.373 in ethanol).

3293. Dioscorea. Wild yam; colic root; rheumatism root. Dried rhizome of *Dioscorea villosa* L., *Dioscoreaceae*. *Habit.* North America. *Constit.* Saponin, acrid resin. Account of the nature, origins, cultivation and utilization of the useful members of the *Dioscoreaceae*: D. G. Coursey, *Yams* (London, Longmans, 1967) 230 pp. *See also* Yam, Mexican.

3294. Dioscorine. [3329-91-7] [1*R*-(1α,4α,5α)]-2,4'-Dimethylspiro[2-azabicyclo[2.2.2]octane-5,2'-[2*H*]pyran]-6'(3'*H*)-one. $C_{13}H_{19}NO_2$; mol wt 221.30. C 70.56%, H 8.65%, N 6.33%, O 14.46%. Found in the tubers of *Dioscorea hirsuta* Blume and *D. hispida* Dennst., *Dioscoreaceae*: H. W. Schutte, *Chem. Zentralbl.* **68, II,** 130 (1897); M. K. Gorter, *Rec. Trav. Chim.* **30,** 161 (1911); A. R. Pinder, *Nature* **168,** 1090 (1951); *idem, J. Chem. Soc.* **1952,** 2236. Structure: W. A. M. Davies *et al., Chem. Ind. (London)* **1961,** 1410; *eidem, Tetrahedron* **18,** 405 (1962); Morris, A. R. Pinder, *J. Chem. Soc.* **1963,** 1841. Synthesis: Page, A. R. Pinder, *ibid.* **1964,** 4811. Absolute configuration: A. F. Beecham *et al., Tetrahedron Lett.* **1969,** 3745. Biosynthetic studies: E. Leete, A. R. Pinder, *Chem. Commun.* **1971,** 1499; E. Leete, *J. Am. Chem. Soc.* **99,** 648 (1977). Pharmacology: A. R. Pinder, *J. Chem. Soc.* **1953,** 1826. Evaluation of toxic components: J. Webster *et al., J. Agric. Food Chem.* **32,** 1087 (1984).

Greenish-yellow prisms from ether, mp 54-55°. $[\alpha]_D^{18}$ −35.0° (c = 3.4 in chloroform). uv max (methanol): 215 nm (ε 10160). Distills unchanged *in vacuo*. Sol in water, alcohol, acetone, chloroform; slightly sol in ether, benzene, petr ether.

Hydrochloride. $C_{13}H_{19}NO_2 \cdot HCl$. Needles from alcohol + ether, dec 210-211°.

3295. Diosgenin. [512-04-9] (3β,25*R*)-Spirost-5-en-3-ol; nitogenin. $C_{27}H_{42}O_3$; mol wt 414.62. C 78.21%, H 10.21%, O 11.58%. Aglycone of saponin dioscin. From *Dioscorea tokoro* Makino, *Dioscoreaceae*: Tsukamoto, *J. Pharm. Soc. Jpn.* **56,** 135 (1936); from rhizomes of *Trillium erectum* L., *Liliaceae* and *D. villosa* L., *Dioscoreaceae*: Marker *et al., J. Am. Chem. Soc.* **62,** 2542 (1940). Plant sources for diosgenin: Marker *et al., ibid.* **65,** 1199 (1943); Wall *et al., J. Am. Pharm. Assoc. Sci. Ed.* **46,** 653 (1957). Identity with nitogenin: Marker *et al., J. Am. Chem. Soc.* **65,** 1248 (1943). Structure: Marker *et al., ibid.* **62,** 2525 (1940). Configuration at C_{25}: James, *J. Chem. Soc.* **1955,** 637. Synthesis: Mazur *et al., J. Am. Chem. Soc.* **82,** 5889 (1960); Kessar *et al., Tetrahedron Lett.* **1966,** 4319. Obtained commercially from *Dioscorea composita* Hemsl. and *D. terpinapensis* Uline (see under Barbasco). Isoln from barbasco varieties: Julian, US 3019220 (1962 to Julian Labs.).

Crystals from acetone, mp 204-207°. $[\alpha]_D^{25}$ −129° (c = 1.4 in CHCl$_3$). Sol in the usual organic solvents, in acetic acid.

Acetate. $C_{29}H_{44}O_4$. Crystals from acetic acid, mp 198°. $[\alpha]_D^{20}$ −119° (pyridine).

USE: Can be converted to pregnenolone and progesterone: Marker *et al., J. Am. Chem. Soc.* **69,** 2167 (1947).

3296. Diosmetin. [520-34-3] 5,7-Dihydroxy-2-(3-hydroxy-4-methoxyphenyl)-4*H*-1-benzopyran-4-one; 3',5,7-trihydroxy-4'-methoxyflavone; cyanidenon-4'-methyl ether 1479; luteolin-4'-methyl ether. $C_{16}H_{12}O_6$; mol wt 300.26. C 64.00%, H 4.03%, O 31.97%. Aglycone of diosmin, *q.v.* Prepn from diosmin isolated from various plant sources: O. A. Oesterle, G. Wander, *Helv. Chim. Acta* **8,** 519 (1925); isoln from lemons *(Citrus limon* Linn., *Rutaceae)*: R. M. Horowitz, *J. Org. Chem.* **21,** 1184 (1956). Synthesis and structural elucidation: G. Zemplén, R. Bognár, *Ber.* **76,** 452 (1943). Synthesis: A. Lovecy *et al., J. Chem. Soc.* **1930,** 817; N. B. Lorette *et al., J. Org. Chem.* **16,** 930 (1951); J. H. Looker, M. J. Holm, *ibid.* **24,** 1019 (1959). HPLC determn in biological fluids: D. Baylocq *et al., Ann. Pharm. Fr.* **41,** 115 (1983).

Hemimethanolate. $C_{16}H_{12}O_6 \cdot \frac{1}{2}CH_3OH$. Yellow needles from alcohol/ethyl acetate, sinters at 248°. mp 253-254°. Also reported as small yellow needles from methanol, mp 258-259° (Horowitz). uv max: 345, 268, 253 nm (log ε 4.32, 4.25, 4.28).

Triacetate. $C_{22}H_{18}O_9$. Colorless needles from methanol, mp 195-196°.

3297. Diosmin. [520-27-4] 7-[[6-*O*-(6-Deoxy-α-L-mannopyranosyl)-β-D-glucopyranosyl]oxy]-5-hydroxy-2-(3-hydroxy-4-methoxyphenyl)-4*H*-1-benzopyran-4-one; 3',5,7-trihydroxy-4'-methoxyflavone-7-rutinoside; 5-hydroxy-2-(3-hydroxy-4-methoxyphenyl)-7-(*O*⁶-α-L-rhamnopyranosyl-β-D-glucopyranosyloxy)-chromen-4-one; 5-hydroxy-2-(3-hydroxy-4-methoxyphenyl)-7-β-rutinosyloxy-4*H*-chromen-4-one; diosmetin 7-β-rutinoside; barosmin; buchu resin; Diosmil; Diosven; Diovenor; Flebosmil; Flebosten; Hemerven; Insuven; Litosmil; Tovene; Varinon; Ven-Detrex; Venosmine. $C_{28}H_{32}O_{15}$; mol wt 608.54. C 55.26%, H 5.30%, O 39.44%. Naturally occurring flavonic glycoside; rhamnoglycoside of diosmetin, *q.v.* Isolation from various plant sources: O. A. Oesterle, G. Wander, *Helv. Chim. Acta* **8,** 519 (1925). Elucidation of structure: G. Zemplén, R. Bognár, *Ber.* **76,** 452 (1943). Prepn from hesperidin, *q.v.: eidem, ibid.;* N. B. Lorette *et al., J. Org. Chem.* **16,** 930 (1951). Isoln from lemon peel *(Citrus limon* Linn. *Rutaceae)*: R. M. Horowitz, *J. Org. Chem.* **21,** 1184 (1956); from *Zanthoxylum avicennae, Rutaceae:* H. R. Arthur *et al., J. Chem. Soc.* **1956,** 632; H. R. Arthur *et al., ibid.* **1959,** 4007; from flowers of *Sophora microphylla* Ait. *Leguminosae:* L. H. Briggs *et al., ibid.* **1960,** 1955. Toxicology studies: H. Heusser, W. Osswald, *Arch. Farmacol. Toxicol.* **3,** 33 (1977). NMR spectrum: J. L. Nieto, A. M. Gutierrez, *Spectrosc. Lett.* **19,** 427 (1986). Mechanism of action: C. Boudet, L. Peyrin, *Arch. Int. Pharmacodyn.* **283,** 312 (1986). Pharmacology: J. R. Caseley-Smith, J. R. Caseley-Smith, *Agents Actions* **17,** 1 (1985); M. Damon *et al., Arzneim.-Forsch.* **37,** 1149 (1987). HPLC determn in biological fluids: D. Baylocq *et al., Ann. Pharm. Fr.* **41,** 115 (1983). Clinical study in post-phlebitic ulcers: M. C. Nguyen, K. Morere, *Gaz. Med.* **92,** 71 (1985); in acute hemorrhoids: A. Tajana *et al., Minerva Med.* **79,** 387 (1988). Clinical trial in chronic venous insufficiency: R. Laurent *et al., Int. Angiol.* **7,** Suppl. 2, 39 (1988).

Monohydrate. $C_{28}H_{32}O_{15} \cdot H_2O$. mp 275-277° (dec) (Zemplén). Also reported as fine needles from aq pyridine or aq DMF, mp 283° (dec) (Briggs). uv max (ethanol): 255, 268, 345 nm (log ε 4.28, 4.25, 4.30). Practically insol in water, alcohol.

Flavonoid extract. Daflon; Flebopex; Flebotropin.
THERAP CAT: Capillary protectant.

3298. Diosphenol. [490-03-9] 2-Hydroxy-3-methyl-6-(1-methylethyl)-2-cyclohexen-1-one; 1-methyl-4-isopropyl-1-cyclohexen-2-ol-3-one; 2-hydroxypiperitone; 1-p-menthen-2-ol-3-one; Buchu camphor; Barosma camphor. $C_{10}H_{16}O_2$; mol wt 168.23. C 71.39%, H 9.59%, O 19.02%. The crystalline portion of an oil obtained from Buchu leaves which come from various species of *Barosma,* such as *B. betulina* Bartl. & Wendl., *B. serratifolia* (Curt.) Willd. and *B. crenulata* (L.) Hook., *Rutaceae:* Flückiger, *Pharm. J.* **11,** 174, 219 (1880); Spica, *Gazz. Chim. Ital.* **15,** 195 (1885); Shimoyama, *Arch. Pharm.* **226,** 403 (1888); Kondakov *et al., J. Prakt. Chem.* [II] **54,** 433 (1896); [II] **63,** 49 (1901). Structure: Semmler, McKenzie, *Ber.* **39,** 1160 (1906).

Crystals, mp 83°. Sublimes. bp$_{760}$ 233° (dec); bp$_{10}$ 109°. d$_4^{99.2}$ 0.9542. n$_D^{99.8}$ 1.4607. Absorption spectrum: Lowry, Lishmund, *J. Chem. Soc.* **1935,** 1313; Gillan *et al., ibid.* **1941,** 62. Sparingly sol in water; moderately sol in alcohol; sol in ether, chloroform, carbon disulfide.

3299. Dioxadrol. [6495-46-1] 2-(2,2-Diphenyl-1,3-dioxolan-4-yl)piperidine; 2,2-diphenyl-4-(2-piperidyl)-1,3-dioxolane. $C_{20}H_{23}NO_2$; mol wt 309.40. C 77.64%, H 7.49%, N 4.53%, O 10.34%. Prepn of *dl*-forms and resolution of α-racemates: Hardie, Halverstadt, **BE 613262; US 3262938** (1962, 1966 both to Cutter Labs.); W. R. Hardie *et al., J. Med. Chem.* **9,** 127 (1966).

Oily liquid.
Hydrochloride. [3666-69-1] Rydar. $C_{20}H_{23}NO_2$.HCl; mol wt 345.86. Crystals from methanol, mp 256-260°. LD$_{50}$ orally in mice: 240 mg/kg (Hardie).
d-Form hydrochloride. [1162-15-8] Dexoxadrol hydrochloride; Relane. Crystals, dec 254°. [α]$_D^{20}$ +34° (c = 2 in methanol). LD$_{50}$ orally in mice: 340 mg/kg (Hardie).
l-Form hydrochloride. Levoxadrol hydrochloride; Levoxan. Crystals, mp 248-254°. [α]$_D^{20}$ −34.5° (c = 2 in methanol). LD$_{50}$ orally in mice: 230 mg/kg (Hardie).
THERAP CAT: Base as antidepressant; *d*-form hydrochloride as stimulant (central), analgesic; *l*-form hydrochloride as anesthetic (local), relaxant (smooth muscle).

3300. Dioxane. [123-91-1] 1,4-Diethylene dioxide. C_4H_8-O_2; mol wt 88.11. C 54.53%, H 9.15%, O 36.32%. Prepd by distilling ethylene glycol with dil H_2SO_4. Monograph: W. Stumpf, *Chemie und Anwendungen des 1,4-Dioxans* (Verlag Chemie, 1956). Toxicity data: E. P. Laug *et al., J. Ind. Hyg. Toxicol.* **21,** 173 (1939). Carcinogenicity studies: M. F. Argus *et al., J. Natl. Cancer Inst.* **35,** 949 (1965); R. J. Kociba *et al., Toxicol. Appl. Pharmacol.* **30,** 275 (1974).

Flammable liq; faint pleasant odor. Vapor harmful. d$_4^{20}$ 1.0329. mp 11.80°. bp$_{760}$ 101.1°; bp$_{400}$ 81.8°; bp$_{200}$ 62.3°; bp$_{100}$ 45.1°; bp$_{60}$ 33.8°; bp$_{40}$ 25.2°; bp$_{20}$ 12°. Cryoscopic constant 4.83. Trouton constant 21.90. Heat of combustion: 581 kcal/mol. Heat of fusion: 2.98 kcal/mol. Specific heat at 20° = 0.0370 kcal/mol/°C. Viscosity (25°): 0.0120 P. Crit temp 312°. Crit press 50.7 atm. Flash pt 5-18°C. n$_D^{20}$ 1.4175. Dipole moment: zero. Azeotropic mixture with water: 81.6% dioxane, bp 87.8°. Azeotropic mixture with ethanol: 9.3% dioxane, bp 78.1°. Sol in water and the usual organic solvents. Tends to form explosive peroxides, especially when anhydr. LD$_{50}$ in mice, rats (ml/kg): 5.7, 5.2 orally (Laug).
Caution: Potential symptoms of overexposure are drowsiness, headache; nausea, vomiting; irritation of eyes, skin, nose and throat; liver damage; kidney failure. *See NIOSH Pocket Guide to Chemical Hazards* (DHHS/NIOSH 97-140, 1997) p 120. This substance is reasonably anticipated to be a human carcinogen: *Report on Carcinogens, Eleventh Edition* (PB2005-104914, 2004) p III-110.
USE: Stabilizer in chlorinated solvents. Solvent for cellulose acetate, ethyl cellulose, benzyl cellulose, resins, oils, waxes, oil and spirit-sol dyes, and many other organic as well as some inorganic compds.

3301. Dioxathion. [78-34-2] Phosphorodithioic acid *S,S'*-1,4-dioxane-2,3-diyl *O,O,O',O'*-tetraethyl ester; 2,3-p-dioxanedithiol *S,S*-bis(*O,O*-diethyl phosphorodithioate); AC-528; ENT-22879; Hercules 528; Delnav; Navadel. $C_{12}H_{26}O_6P_2S_4$; mol wt 456.54. C 31.57%, H 5.74%, O 21.03%, P 13.57%, S 28.09%. Prepn: Diveley, Lohr, **US 2725328;** Speck, **US 2815350** (1955, 1957 both to Hercules); Diveley *et al., J. Am. Chem. Soc.* **81,** 139 (1959). Toxicity study: T. B. Gaines, *Toxicol. Appl. Pharmacol.* **14,** 515 (1969).

Tan liquid, d$_4^{26}$ 1.257. mp −20°. n$_D^{20}$ 1.5420. Practically insol in water. Partly sol in hexane. Hydrolyzed by alkali and by heating. LD$_{50}$ in female, male rats (mg/kg): 23, 43 orally; 63, 235 dermally (Gaines).
Caution: Potential symptoms of overexposure are eye, skin irritation; headache, giddiness, vertigo, weakness; rhinorrhea, chest tightness; miosis; nausea, vomiting, abdominal cramps, diarrhea, salivation; muscle fasciculations; confusion, drowsiness. *See NIOSH Pocket Guide to Chemical Hazards* (DHHS/NIOSH 97-140, 1997) p 120.
USE: Insecticide; acaricide.

3302. Dioxethedrine. [497-75-6] 4-[2-(Ethylamino)-1-hydroxypropyl]-1,2-benzenediol; *N*-ethyl-3,4-dihydroxynorephedrine; α-(1-ethylaminoethyl)protocatechuyl alcohol; 2-ethylamino-1-(3',4'-dihydroxyphenyl)-1-propanol; 1-(3',4'-dihydroxyphenyl)-2-ethylamino-1-propanol; C-247. $C_{11}H_{17}NO_3$; mol wt 211.26. C 62.54%, H 8.11%, N 6.63%, O 22.72%. β-Adrenergic agonist. Prepd by catalytic hydrogenation of the corresponding aminoketone: Lespagnol, Cuingnet, *Ann. Pharm. Fr.* **18,** 445 (1960). Only one of the two possible isomers, believed to be the "erythro" form, was isolated.

Hydrochloride. $C_{11}H_{17}NO_3$.HCl. Crystals from methanol + ether, mp 212-214°.
One of the ingredients of *Bexol.*
THERAP CAT: Bronchodilator.

3303. Dioxybenzone. [131-53-3] (2-Hydroxy-4-methoxyphenyl)(2-hydroxyphenyl)methanone; 2,2'-dihydroxy-4-methoxybenzophenone; 4-methoxy-2,2'-dihydroxybenzophenone; benzophenone-8; Cyasorb UV 24 (obsolete); Spectra-Sorb UV 24. $C_{14}H_{12}O_4$; mol wt 244.24. C 68.85%, H 4.95%, O 26.20%. Prepn: Hardy *et al.*, US 2853521 (1958 to Am. Cyanamid).

Yellow powder, mp 68°. Soly in g/100 ml at 25°: ethanol 21.8; isopropanol 17; propylene glycol 6.2; ethylene glycol 3.0; *n*-hexane 1.5.

THERAP CAT: Ultraviolet screen.

3304. 2,5-Di-*tert*-pentylhydroquinone. [79-74-3] 2,5-Bis(1,1-dimethylpropyl)-1,4-benzenediol; 2,5-di-*tert*-amylhydroquinone; 2,5-bis(1,1-dimethylpropyl)hydroquinone; Santovar A. $C_{16}H_{26}O_2$; mol wt 250.38. C 76.75%, H 10.47%, O 12.78%. Prepn: Erickson, GB 596461 (1948 to Mathieson Alkali Works).

Crystals, mp 179.4-180.4°.

USE: As a staining protector in rubber.

3305. Diphacinone. [82-66-6] 2-(Diphenylacetyl)-1*H*-indene-1,3(2*H*)-dione; 2-diphenylacetyl-1,3-diketohydrindene; 2-diphenylacetyl-1,3-indandione; diphenadione; U-1363; Diphacin; Ditrac; Ramik. $C_{23}H_{16}O_3$; mol wt 340.37. C 81.16%, H 4.74%, O 14.10%. Anticoagulant; inhibits vitamin K-dependent synthesis of factors II, VII and X. Prepn: D. G. Thomas, US 2672483 (1954 to Upjohn). Anticoagulant effects in rodents: J. T. Correll *et al.*, *Proc. Soc. Exp. Biol. Med.* **80**, 139 (1952). Metabolism in rats and mice: C. C. Yu *et al.*, *Drug Metab. Dispos.* **10**, 645 (1982). LC/MS determn in commercial rodenticides: M. Z. Mesmer, R. A. Flurer, *J. Chromatogr. A* **891**, 249 (2000).

Pale yellow crystals from ethanol, mp 146-147°. Practically insol in water. Slightly sol in benzene, hot ethanol. Sol in acetone, acetic acid. LD$_{50}$ orally (mg/kg): 3 in rats; 340 in mice; 35 in rabbits (Correll).

USE: Rodenticide.

3306. Diphemanil Methylsulfate. [62-97-5] 4-(Diphenylmethylene)-1,1-dimethylpiperidinium methyl sulfate; *p*-(α-phenylbenzylidene)-1,1-dimethylpiperidinium methylsulfate; *N*,*N*-dimethyl-4-piperidylidene-1,1-diphenylmethane methylsulfate; Prantal. $C_{21}H_{27}NO_4S$; mol wt 389.51. C 64.75%, H 6.99%, N 3.60%, O 16.43%, S 8.23%. Anticholinergic. Prepn: N. Sperber *et al.*, *J. Am. Chem. Soc.* **73**, 5010 (1951); N. Sperber *et al.*, US 2739968 (1956 to Schering). Pharmacological properties and toxicity data: S. Margolin *et al.*, *Proc. Soc. Exp. Biol. Med.* **78**, 576 (1951). Clinical evaluation in treatment of gustatory sweating: O. Laccourreye *et al.*, *Laryngoscope* **100**, 1651 (1990). Clinical pharmacokinetics: A. M. Vidal *et al.*, *Eur. J. Clin. Pharmacol.* **42**, 689 (1992).

Crystals, mp 194-195°. Soluble in water. LD$_{50}$ in rats, mice, guinea pigs (mg/kg): 1107, 64, 404 orally (Margolin).

THERAP CAT: In treatment of hyperhidrosis.

3307. Diphenamid. [957-51-7] *N*,*N*-Dimethyl-α-phenylbenzeneacetamide; *N*,*N*-dimethyl-2,2-diphenylacetamide; *N*,*N*-dimethyl-α,α-diphenyl acetamide; 2,2-diphenyl-*N*,*N*-dimethylacetamide; L-34314; Dymid; Enide. $C_{16}H_{17}NO$; mol wt 239.31. C 80.30%, H 7.16%, N 5.85%, O 6.69%. Selective pre-emergence herbicide. Prepn: Cheney *et al.*, *J. Org. Chem.* **17**, 770 (1952). Toxicity study: G. W. Bailey, J. L. White, *Residue Rev.* **10**, 97 (1965).

Crystals from ethyl acetate, mp 134.5-135.5°. Soluble in water, acetone, dimethylformamide, xylene, phenyl Cellosolve. LD$_{50}$ orally in rats: 700 mg/kg (Bailey, White).

USE: Herbicide.

3308. Diphencyprone. [886-38-4] 2,3-Diphenyl-2-cyclopropen-1-one; 1,2-diphenylcyclopropenone; DPC. $C_{15}H_{10}O$; mol wt 206.24. C 87.35%, H 4.89%, O 7.76%. Contact allergen, possibly the smallest neutral aromatic specie. Prepn: R. Breslow *et al.*, *J. Am. Chem. Soc.* **81**, 247 (1959). Crystal structure: H. L. Ammon, *ibid.* **95**, 7093 (1973). Strain energy: A. Greenberg *et al.*, *ibid.* **105**, 6855 (1983). Mechanism of photodissociation: Y. Hirata, N. Mataga, *Chem. Phys. Lett.* **193**, 287 (1992). Report as contact sensitizer: B. M. Hausen, J. Stute, *Chem. Ind.* **1980**, 699. Clinical evaluation in alopecia totalis: B. Monk, *Clin. Exp. Dermatol.* **14**, 154 (1989); of children with alopecia areata: S. MacDonald Hull *et al.*, *Br. J. Dermatol.* **125**, 164 (1991). Review of clinical efficacy: E. Hoting, A. Boehm, *ibid.* **127**, 625-629 (1992).

Crystallizes as monohydrate from cyclohexane, mp 87-90°. d 1.202 g/cm³. uv max (CH₃CN): 297, 282, 226, 220 nm (log ε 4.3, 4.25, 4.13, 4.16). mp (anhydrous): 118-120°.

THERAP CAT: Antialopecia agent.

3309. Diphenhydramine. [58-73-1] 2-Diphenylmethoxy-*N*,*N*-dimethylethanamine; 2-(benzhydryloxy)-*N*,*N*-dimethylethylamine; β-dimethylaminoethyl benzhydryl ether; *O*-benzhydryldimethylaminoethanol; β-dimethylaminoethanol diphenylmethyl ether; α-(2-dimethylaminoethoxy)diphenylmethane; benzhydramine. $C_{17}H_{21}NO$; mol wt 255.35. C 79.96%, H 8.29%, N 5.49%, O 6.27%. Prepn: G. Rieveschl, Jr., US 2421714 (1947 to Parke, Davis); *see also* H. Martin *et al.*, US 2397799 (1946 to Geigy). Toxicology study: O. M. Gruhzit, R. A. Fisken, *J. Pharmacol. Exp. Ther.* **89**, 227 (1947). Comprehensive description of the hydrochloride: I. J. Holcomb, S. A. Fusari, *Anal. Profiles Drug Subs.* **3**, 173-232 (1974). Clinical pharmacokinetics: J. M. Scavone *et al.*, *J. Clin. Pharmacol.* **38**, 603 (1998). Clinical trial in insomnia: K. Rickels *et al.*, *ibid.* **23**, 235 (1983).

bp$_{2.0}$ 150-165°.

Hydrochloride. [147-24-0] Allergina; Benadryl; Benocten; Dibondrin; Dolestan; Halbmond; Noctomin; Nytol; Sedopretten; Sekundal-D; Sominex; Unisom Sleepgels. $C_{17}H_{21}NO.HCl$; mol wt 291.82. Crystals from abs alcohol + ether, mp 166-170°. Bitter taste. Slowly darkens on exposure to light. Stable under ordinary conditions. One gram dissolves in 1 ml water, 2 ml alcohol, 2 ml chloroform, 50 ml acetone. Very slightly sol in benzene, ether. pH of 1% aq soln about 5.5. The aq soln forms a pink precipitate with satd Reinecke's salt soln. LD$_{50}$ orally in rats: 500 mg/kg (Gruhzit, Fisken).

THERAP CAT: Antihistaminic; sedative, hypnotic.

THERAP CAT (VET): Antihistaminic. Also in motion sickness.

3310. Diphenic Acid. [482-05-3] [1,1'-Biphenyl]-2,2'-dicarboxylic acid; o,o'-bibenzoic acid. $C_{14}H_{10}O_4$; mol wt 242.23. C 69.42%, H 4.16%, O 26.42%. Prepd from diazotized anthranilic acid by treatment with a cuproammonia-sulfite reducing agent: Vorländer, Meyer, *Ann.* **320,** 122 (1902); Atkinson, Lawler, *Org. Synth.* **coll. vol. I** (2nd ed, 1941) p 222. By chromic acid oxidation of phenanthrenequinone: Roberts, Johnson, *J. Am. Chem. Soc.* **47,** 1399 (1925). By heating potassium o-bromobenzoate with copper powder: Hurtley, *J. Chem. Soc.* **1929,** 1870.

Monoclinic prismatic rods upon slow cooling from water, leaflets from hot water, needles by careful sublimation. mp 228-229°. The satd aq soln is 0.0052N at 25°; soluble in the usual organic solvents.

Dimethyl ester. $C_{16}H_{14}O_4$. Monoclinic prismatic plates, tablets from methanol, mp 73.5°; bp$_{14}$ 204-206°.

Diethyl ester. $C_{18}H_{18}O_4$. Cubes from alcoholic HCl, mp 42°.

3311. Diphenidol. [972-02-1] α,α-Diphenyl-1-piperidinebutanol; 1,1-diphenyl-4-piperidino-1-butanol; diphenyl-[3-(1-piperidyl)propyl]carbinol; defenidol; SKF-478. $C_{21}H_{27}NO$; mol wt 309.45. C 81.51%, H 8.79%, N 4.53%, O 5.17%. Prepn: Miescher, Marxer, **US 2411664** (1946 to Ciba); Barrett, Wilkinson, **GB 683950** (1952 to Wellcome Foundation), *C.A.* **48,** 2112e (1954). Structure-activity studies: Gautier *et al., Med. Pharmacol. Exp.* **13,** 325 (1965). Clinical studies: Cutt *et al., Aerosp. Med.* **39,** 682 (1968); Benson, *ibid.* **40,** 589 (1969). Acute toxicity: E. I. Goldenthal, *Toxicol. Appl. Pharmacol.* **18,** 185 (1971).

Needles from petr ether, mp 104-105°. LD$_{50}$ s.c. in rats: 50 mg/kg (Goldenthal).

Hydrochloride. [3254-89-5] SKF-478-A; Ansmin; Cefadol; Celmidol; Difenidolin; Maniol; Mecalmin; Pineroro; Satanolon; Tenesdol; Vontrol; Wansar. $C_{21}H_{27}NO.HCl$; mol wt 345.91. Crystals from chloroform + ethyl acetate, mp 212-214°. Freely sol in methanol; sol in water, chloroform. Practically insol in ether, benzene, petr ether.

THERAP CAT: Antiemetic.

3312. Diphenolic Acid. [126-00-1] 4-Hydroxy-γ-(4-hydroxyphenyl)-γ-methylbenzenebutanoic acid; 4,4-bis[4'-hydroxyphenyl]pentanoic acid; γ,γ-bis-(p-hydroxyphenyl)valeric acid; DPA. $C_{17}H_{18}O_4$; mol wt 286.32. C 71.31%, H 6.34%, O 22.35%. Prepd by condensing 2.25-4.0 moles of phenol with one mole of levulinic acid in the presence of HCl: **GB 768206** (1957 to S. C. Johnson & Son); from one mole of phenol, 0.5 mole levulinic acid and HCl, H_2SO_4 or H_3PO_4: Bader, Kantowicz, *J. Am. Chem. Soc.* **76,** 4465 (1954); Bader, **US 2933520** (1960 to S. C. Johnson & Son).

Crystals from hot water. Higher melting modification, mp 171-172°. Appreciably sol in hot water; sol in acetone, acetic acid, ethanol, isopropanol, methyl ethyl ketone.

USE: Intermediate for surface coatings, lubricating oil additives, cosmetics, surfactants, plasticizers, textile chemicals.

3313. Diphenoxylate. [915-30-0] 1-(3-Cyano-3,3-diphenylpropyl)-4-phenyl-4-piperidinecarboxylic acid ethyl ester; 1-(3-cyano-3,3-diphenylpropyl)-4-phenylisonipecotic acid ethyl ester; ethyl 1-(3-cyano-3,3-diphenylpropyl)-4-phenyl-4-piperidinecarboxylate; ethyl 1-(3-cyano-3,3-diphenylpropyl)-4-phenylisonipecotate; 2,2-diphenyl-4-(4-carbethoxy-4-phenylpiperidino)butyronitrile; R-1132. $C_{30}H_{32}N_2O_2$; mol wt 452.59. C 79.61%, H 7.13%, N 6.19%, O 7.07%. Prepn: Janssen, **US 2898340** (1959). Pharmacokinetics and metabolism: Karim *et al., J. Pharmacol. Exp. Ther.* **177,** 546 (1971); *Clin. Pharmacol. Ther.* **13,** 407 (1972). See *also* Difenoxin, the active metabolite of diphenoxylate. Comprehensive description: D. D. Hung, *Anal. Profiles Drug Subs.* **7,** 149-169 (1978).

Hydrochloride. [3810-80-8] $C_{30}H_{32}N_2O_2.HCl$. Crystals, mp 220.5-222°. uv max (methanol): 252, 258, 264 nm. Soly in mg/ml at 25°: acetic acid 500; DMF 500; chloroform 360; methanol >50; ethanol 3; water 0.8; hexane 0.5.

Mixture of hydrochloride with atropine sulfate. Lomotil; Diarsed; Reasec.

Note: This is a controlled substance (opiate): **21 CFR,** 1308.12.

THERAP CAT: Antiperistaltic; antidiarrheal.

3314. Diphenyl. [92-52-4] 1,1'-Biphenyl; bibenzene; phenylbenzene. $C_{12}H_{10}$; mol wt 154.21. C 93.46%, H 6.54%. Toxicity data: Deichmann *et al., J. Ind. Hyg. Toxicol.* **29,** 1 (1947). *Review:* W. C. Weaver *et al.,* in *Kirk-Othmer Encyclopedia of Chemical Technology* vol. 7 (Wiley-Interscience, New York, 3rd ed., 1979) pp 782-793.

Colorless leaflets; pleasant, peculiar odor. d 1.041. mp 69-71°. bp 254-255°. n_D^{77} 1.588. Insol in water. Sol in alc, ether. LD$_{50}$ orally in rats: 3280 mg/kg (Deichmann).

Caution: Potential symptoms of overexposure are irritation of throat and eyes; headache, nausea, fatigue and numb limbs; liver damage. *See NIOSH Pocket Guide to Chemical Hazards* (DHHS/-NIOSH 97-140, 1997) p 120.

USE: As heat transfer agent; fungistat for oranges (applied to inside of shipping container or wrappers); in organic syntheses.

3315. Diphenylacetamide. [519-87-5] Acetyldiphenylamine. $C_{14}H_{13}NO$; mol wt 211.26. C 79.59%, H 6.20%, N 6.63%, O 7.57%. $CH_3CON(C_6H_5)_2$.

White, cryst powder. mp 103°. Sublimes without decomposition. Slightly sol in water; sol in alcohol, ether.

3316. Diphenylacetic Acid. [117-34-0] α-Phenylbenzeneacetic acid; diphenylmethane-α-carboxylic acid. $C_{14}H_{12}O_2$; mol wt 212.24. C 79.23%, H 5.70%, O 15.08%. $(C_6H_5)_2CHCOOH$. Prepd by the reduction of benzilic acid with hydriodic acid and red phosphorus: C. S. Marvel *et al., Org. Synth.* **coll. vol. I,** 224 (2nd ed., 1941). Ecologically and economically improved synthesis from benzilic acid: P. Strazzolini *et al., Synth. Commun.* **17,** 1919 (1987). Toxicity study: G. W. Bailey, J. L. White, *Residue Rev.* **10,** 97 (1965).

Small plates from alcohol, needles from water, mp 148°. Sublimes. Sol in hot water, alcohol, ether, chloroform.

Methyl ester. $C_{15}H_{14}O_2$. Crystals from dil alcohol, mp 60°.
Ethyl ester. $C_{16}H_{16}O_2$. Crystals from alcohol, mp 58°. bp_{15} 178°.
Amide. $C_{14}H_{13}NO$. mp 167-168°.
Nitrile. Diphenylacetonitrile; α-cyanodiphenylmethane; diphenatrile; Dipan. $C_{14}H_{11}N$; mol wt 193.24. mp 76°. bp_{12} 181°. Sol in alcohol, ether, propylene glycol. LD_{50} orally in rats: 3500 mg/kg (Bailey, White).
Chloride. $C_{14}H_{11}ClO$. Crystals from petr ether, mp 57°; bp_{15} 178°. Very sol in benzene. Sol in hot ligroin, in hot isopropyl ether.
Anhydride. $C_{28}H_{22}O_3$. mp 98°; bp_{15} 220°.
USE: Nitrile as herbicide.

3317. Diphenylamine. [122-39-4] *N*-Phenylbenzeneamine. $C_{12}H_{11}N$; mol wt 169.22. C 85.17%, H 6.55%, N 8.28%. C_6H_5-NHC_6H_5. Prepd by heating aniline with aniline hydrochloride.

Crystals; floral odor. d 1.16. mp 53-54°. bp 302°. Flash pt 153°C. Discolors in light. One gram dissolves in 2.2 ml alcohol, 4.5 ml propyl alcohol; freely sol in benzene, ether, glacial acetic acid, carbon disulfide. Insol in water. Forms salts with strong acids. *Keep protected from light.*

Hydrochloride. $C_{12}H_{11}N.HCl$. Crystals, turn blue in air. Freely sol in water, alcohol.
Sulfate. $C_{12}H_{11}N.H_2SO_4$. White to yellowish powder, mp 123-125°. Practically insol in water. Sol in alc, in H_2SO_4.

Caution: Potential symptoms of overexposure to diphenylamine are irritation of eyes, skin, mucous membranes; eczema; tachycardia, hypertension; cough, sneezing; methemoglobinemia; increased blood pressure and heart rate; proteinuria, hematuria, bladder injury. *See NIOSH Pocket Guide to Chemical Hazards* (DHHS/NIOSH 97-140, 1997) p 120.

USE: Manuf dyes; stabilizing nitrocellulose explosives and celluloid. In anal. chem for the detection of NO_3, ClO_3 and other oxidizing substances with which, in the presence of H_2SO_4, it gives a deep-blue color.

THERAP CAT (VET): Topically in antiscrewworm mixtures. In tests for nitrate or nitrite poisoning.

3318. Diphenylamine-2,2'-dicarboxylic Acid. [579-92-0] 2,2'-Iminobis[benzoic acid]. $C_{14}H_{11}NO_4$; mol wt 257.24. C 65.37%, H 4.31%, N 5.44%, O 24.88%. Prepn from the alkali salts of anthranilic acid and of 2-chlorobenzoic acid in presence of copper: Ullmann, *Ann.* **355,** 352 (1907).

Yellow crystals from alcohol, mp 296-297° (dec). Insoluble in water. Very slightly sol in alcohol, ether, chloroform, glacial acetic acid.

USE: Instead of diphenylamine in reactions with oxidizing agents. May be used as an oxidation-reduction indicator in strongly acid solns.

3319. *N,N'*-Diphenylbenzidine. [531-91-9] *N,N'*-Diphenyl-[1,1'-biphenyl]-4,4'-diamine. $C_{24}H_{20}N_2$; mol wt 336.43. C 85.68%, H 5.99%, N 8.33%.

Leaflets or plates, mp 242°. Insol in water. Freely sol in boiling toluene or ethyl acetate, slightly in alc, acetone. Is more sensitive to oxidizing substances than diphenylamine. *Keep protected from light.*

USE: *See* diphenylamine.

3320. 1,4-Diphenyl-1,3-butadiene. [886-65-7] 1,1'-(1,3-Butadiene-1,4-diyl)bisbenzene; distyryl; bistyryl; 1,4-diphenyl-erythrene. $C_{16}H_{14}$; mol wt 206.28. C 93.16%, H 6.84%. C_6H_5-$CH=CHCH=CHC_6H_5$. Prepd by the condensation of phenylacetic acid and cinnamic aldehyde: Kuhn, Winterstein, *Helv. Chim. Acta* **11,** 103 (1928); Corson, *Org. Synth.* **16,** 28 (1936). This method yields the *trans,trans*-form.

cis,cis-**Form.** Leaflets, needles, mp 70.5°. Changes to the *trans,trans*-form under the influence of light. $d_4^{100.6}$ 0.9697. $n_{H\alpha}^{100.6}$ 1.61831; $n_{H\beta}^{100.6}$ 1.66748; $n_{He}^{100.6}$ 1.63473. Soluble in ether, chloroform, benzene, petr ether, hot glacial acetic acid, slightly sol in alcohol.

cis,trans-**Form.** Obtained only in the absence of light. Oily liquid or crystals, mp 88°. $bp_{0.1}$ 133-135°. d_4^{22} 0.9974. $n_{H\alpha}^{22.2}$ 1.59679; $n_{H\beta}^{22.2}$ 1.62830; $n_{He}^{22.2}$ 1.60532.

trans,trans-**Form.** Crystals, mp 149.7°. bp_{720} 350°. Soluble in alcohol; sparingly sol in ether.

3321. *sym*-Diphenylcarbazide. [140-22-7] 2,2'-Diphenyl-carbonic dihydrazide. $C_{13}H_{14}N_4O$; mol wt 242.28. C 64.45%, H 5.82%, N 23.12%, O 6.60%. $C_6H_5NHNHCONHNHC_6H_5$.

White, cryst powder, gradually becomes pink. mp 168-171°. Very slightly sol in water; sol in hot alcohol, acetone, glacial acetic acid. *Keep protected from light.*

USE: As indicator in titrating Fe; for the colorimetric determination of Cr, detection of Cd, Hg, Mg, aldehydes, emetine.

3322. Diphenylcarbazone. [538-62-5] Phenyldiazenecarboxylic acid 2-phenylhydrazide. $C_{13}H_{12}N_4O$; mol wt 240.26. C 64.99%, H 5.03%, N 23.32%, O 6.66%. $C_6H_5N=NCONHNH-C_6H_5$.

Orange-red needles. mp about 157° with decompn. Insol in water. Sol in alcohol, chloroform, benzene.

USE: As a sensitive reagent for Hg, with which it gives a blue color.

3323. 1,1-Diphenylethene. [530-48-3] 1,1'-Ethenylidene-bis[benzene]; *unsym*-diphenylethylene; α,α-diphenylethylene; α-methylene-diphenylmethane. $C_{14}H_{12}$; mol wt 180.25. C 93.29%, H 6.71%. $(C_6H_5)_2C=CH_2$. Prepd by the action of phenylmagnesium bromide on ethyl acetate in ether, followed by treatment of the reaction product with ammonium chloride soln: Allen, Converse, *Org. Synth.* **coll. vol. I** (2nd ed., 1941) p 226. Absorption spectrum: Lardy, *J. Chim. Phys.* **21,** 361 (1924).

Liquid, mp 8.2°. d_4^{20} 1.0232. bp_{760} 277.0°; bp_{400} 249.8°; bp_{200} 222.8°; bp_{100} 198.6°; bp_{60} 183.4°; bp_{40} 170.8°; bp_{20} 151.8°; bp_{10} 135.0°; bp_5 119.6°; $bp_{1.0}$ 87.4°. n_D^{20} 1.60849.

3324. 1,3-Diphenylguanidine. [102-06-7] *N,N'*-Diphenyl-guanidine; *sym*-diphenylguanidine; Melaniline; Vulkazit. $C_{13}H_{13}$-N_3; mol wt 211.26. C 73.91%, H 6.20%, N 19.89%. Prepn: Naunton, *J. Soc. Chem. Ind. London* **45,** 376T (1926); Macholdt-Erdniss, *Ber.* **91,** 1992 (1958); Ferris, Schutz, *J. Org. Chem.* **28,** 71 (1963). Pharmacology: P. Valade *et al., C.R. Seances Soc. Biol. Ses Fil.* **143,** 815 (1949).

Crystals from ether, mp 150°. Dec at about 170°. d 1.13. Sparingly sol in water; sol in alcohol, chloroform, hot benzene, hot toluene; readily sol in dil mineral acids. Aq soln is strongly alkaline. MLD s.c. in guinea pigs: 200 mg/kg; i.v. in dogs: 25 mg/kg (Valade).

Phthalate. Guantal. $C_{34}H_{32}N_6O_4$; mol wt 588.66. Obtained as the hemihydrate, blue-white to light gray powder. mp 178°. d_4^{25} 1.20. Sol in alcohol. Practically insol in benzene, gasoline.

USE: Recommended as a primary material for standardizing acids. Free base and phthalate as accelerators for vulcanization of rubber.

3325. 1,1-Diphenylhydrazine. [530-50-7] $C_{12}H_{12}N_2$; mol wt 184.24. C 78.23%, H 6.56%, N 15.20%. $(C_6H_5)_2NNH_2$.

Yellow crystals. d 1.19. mp 34.5°; also reported as mp 44°. bp_{40} 220°. Insol in water. Freely sol in alc, ether.

Hydrochloride. $C_{12}H_{12}N_2$.HCl. White to grayish white, crystalline powder. Slightly sol in water; freely sol in alc.

USE: Hydrochloride as reagent for arabinose and lactose.

3326. Diphenylketene. [525-06-4] Diphenylethenone. $C_{14}H_{10}O$; mol wt 194.23. C 86.57%, H 5.19%, O 8.24%. $(C_6H_5)_2C{=}C{=}O$. Prepd from benzil monohydrazone: Smith, Hoehn, *Org. Synth.* **coll. vol. III**, 356 (1955).

Reddish-yellow liquid. Best stored under nitrogen. The addition of hydroquinone helps to retard polymerization. Solidifies in refrigerator. $d_4^{13.7}$ 1.1107. bp_{760} 265-270° (dec); bp_{12} 146°; $bp_{3.5}$ 119-121°. Should be distilled under reduced pressure (3 to 5 mm) in an atm of nitrogen. $n_D^{14.1}$ 1.615. Dipole moment in benzene at 25° = −1.9.

3327. Diphenylmagnesium. [555-54-4] Magnesium diphenyl. $C_{12}H_{10}Mg$; mol wt 178.51. C 80.74%, H 5.65%, Mg 13.62%. $Mg(C_6H_5)_2$. Prepd by the action of magnesium on mercury diphenyl: Schlenk, Jr., *Ber.* **64**, 736 (1931); Gilman, Brown, *Rec. Trav. Chim.* **49**, 202 (1930).

Solvated, feathery crystals from ether. Loses its ether *in vacuo* at around 37°. Dec 280°, dissociating into magnesium and diphenyl. Extremely reactive; catches fire in moist, although not in dry, air. Violently dec by water. The etherate is sol in benzene, but the dry compd is not.

3328. Diphenylmethane. [101-81-5] 1,1'-Methylenebis-[benzene]; benzylbenzene; ditan. $C_{13}H_{12}$; mol wt 168.23. C 92.81%, H 7.19%. $(C_6H_5)_2CH_2$. Prepd from methylene chloride and benzene with aluminum chloride as catalyst: Friedel, Crafts, *Bull. Soc. Chim.* [2] **41**, 324 (1884); from benzyl chloride and benzene: Hartman, Phillips, *Org. Synth.* **14**, 34 (1934); L. F. Fieser, *Experiments in Organic Chemistry* (Boston, 3rd ed., 1955) p 157.

Orthorhombic needles. Odor of oranges. d_4^{10} 1.3421 (solid). mp 25.9°. d_4^{26} 1.0008 (liq). bp_{760} 264.5°; bp_{400} 237.5°; bp_{200} 210.7°; bp_{100} 186.3°; bp_{60} 170.2°; bp_{40} 157.8°; bp_{20} 139.8°; bp_{10} 122.8°; bp_5 107.4°; $bp_{1.0}$ 76.0°. n_D^{20} 1.57683. Absorption spectrum in hexane: Castille, *Bull. Soc. Chim. Belg.* **36**, 296; *Chem. Zentralbl.* **1927**, I, 1126; in alcohol: Ondorff, *J. Am. Chem. Soc.* **49**, 1541 (1927). Freely sol in alcohol, ether, chloroform, hexane, benzene. Insol in liq ammonia.

3329. N,N'-Diphenyl-p-phenylenediamine. [74-31-7] N,N-Diphenyl-1,4-benzenediamine; 1,4-dianilinobenzene; DPPD. $C_{18}H_{16}N_2$; mol wt 260.33. C 83.05%, H 6.19%, N 10.76%. Prepd by condensing hydroquinone or p-aminophenol with aniline: Calm, *Ber.* **16**, 2805 (1883); Clemens, Magoffin, US 2503712 (1950 to Kodak). Purification: Pecherer, US 2833824 (1958 to Hoffmann-La Roche).

Colorless leaflets from alcohol. Commercial grades are greenish-brown. d 1.20. mp 150-151° (uncorr., Pecherer). $bp_{0.5}$ 220-225°. Sol in monochlorobenzene, benzene, DMF, ether, chloroform, acetone, ethyl acetate, isopropyl acetate, glacial acetic acid. Slightly sol in alcohol. Almost insol in petr ether, water.

USE: Polymerization inhibitor. Antioxidant for rubber, petr oils, feedstuffs.

THERAP CAT (VET): Antioxidant for feedstuffs.

3330. 1,1-Diphenyl-2-picrylhydrazyl (Free Radical). [1898-66-4] 2,2-Diphenyl-1-(2,4,6-trinitrophenyl)hydrazyl; DPPH. Prepn: Goldschmidt, Renn, *Ber.* **55B**, 628 (1922); Lyons, Watson, *J. Polym. Sci.* **18**, 141 (1955); Arbuzov, Valitova, *Zh. Obshch. Khim.* **27**, 2354 (1957). Structure: Poirier *et al.*, *J. Org. Chem.* **17**, 1437 (1952).

Large, dark violet prisms from benzene + petr ether, mp 127-129° (dec). mp also reported as 132-133°.

USE: Analytical reagent for reducing substances: Schenck *et al.*, *Tetrahedron Lett.* **1967**, 193.

3331. Diphenylpyraline. [147-20-6] 4-(Diphenylmethoxy)-1-methylpiperidine; diphenylpyrilene; 4-benzhydryloxy-N-methylpiperidine; 1-methyl-4-piperidyl benzhydryl ether; 1-methyl-4-hydroxypiperidine benzhydryl ether; P-253. $C_{19}H_{23}NO$; mol wt 281.39. C 81.10%, H 8.24%, N 4.98%, O 5.69%. Prepn: L. H. Knox, R. Kapp, US 2479843 (1949 to Nopco). Pharmacokinetics: G. Graham, A. G. Bolt, *J. Pharmacokinet. Biopharm.* **2**, 191 (1974). Clinical trial in allergic rhinitis: H. Puhakka *et al.*, *J. Int. Med. Res.* **5**, 37 (1977). GC determn in blood and urine: H. Hattori *et al.*, *J. Chromatogr.* **581**, 213 (1992).

Hydrochloride. [132-18-3] Dayfen; Diafen; Hispril; Histryl; Histyn; Kolton; Lergoban; Lergobine. $C_{19}H_{23}NO$.HCl; mol wt 317.85. Crystals from isopropanol + ether, mp 206°. Sol in water, ethanol, isopropanol. Practically insol in ether, benzene.

Hydrobromide. [5807-87-4] $C_{19}H_{23}NO$.HBr. Prepn: R. F. Phillips, US 2595405 (1952 to Merck & Co.). Crystals, mp 201-202°. Soluble in water, ethanol.

8-Chlorotheophyllinate. [606-90-6] Piprinhydrinate; diphenylpyraline theoclate; Mepedyl. $C_{19}H_{23}NO.C_7H_7ClN_4O_2$; mol wt 496.00. Prepn: W. A. Schuler, DE 934890 (1955 to Promonta), *C.A.* **52**, 20065i (1958). White to off-white crystalline powder, mp 174-176°. Sparingly sol in water. Freely sol in alcohol.

THERAP CAT: Antihistaminic.

3332. Diphenyl Sulfone. [127-63-9] 1,1'-Sulfonylbisbenzene; phenyl sulfone; sulfobenzide. $C_{12}H_{10}O_2S$; mol wt 218.27. C 66.03%, H 4.62%, O 14.66%, S 14.69%. $(C_6H_5)_2SO_2$. Prepd by sulfonation of benzene with sulfuric acid; formed as a by-product on production of benzenesulfonic acid and benzenesulfonyl chloride.

White monoclinic prisms or leaflets, mp 128-129°. bp 378-379°. Insoluble in cold water. Slightly sol in boiling water; sol in hot alcohol, in benzene. LD_{50} orally in rats: >2 g/kg, *Residue Rev.* **36**, 240 (1971).

USE: Ovicide; acaricide.

3333. sym-Diphenylthiourea. [102-08-9] *N,N'*-Diphenyl-thiourea; thiocarbanilide; sulfocarbanilide. $C_{13}H_{12}N_2S$; mol wt 228.31. C 68.39%, H 5.30%, N 12.27%, S 14.04%. C_6H_5-NHCSNHC$_6$H$_5$. Prepn from aniline and carbon disulfide: Fry, *J. Am. Chem. Soc.* **35**, 1539 (1913); Stasse, US 2435295 (1948 to Allied Chem. & Dye); from potassium ethylxanthate and aniline: Aravindakshan *et al., Indian J. Chem.* **1**(9), 395 (1963). Physical properties and toxicity data: P. J. Hanzlik, A. Irvine, *J. Pharmacol. Exp. Ther.* **17**, 349 (1921).

White crystalline solid, mp 153-154°. d 1.32. Distinct bitter taste. Practically insol in water. Sol in alcohol, ether, chloroform. MLD orally in rabbits: 1.5 g/kg (Hanzlik, Irvine).

USE: Vulcanizing accelerator; sulfur dyes.

3334. Diphosgene. [503-38-8] Carbonochloridic acid trichloromethyl ester; chloroformic acid trichloromethyl ester; trichloromethylchloroformate; trichloromethylcarbonochloridate. C_2Cl_4-O_2; mol wt 197.83. C 12.14%, Cl 71.68%, O 16.17%. ClCOOCCl$_3$. Used in synthesis as substitute for phosgene, *q.v.* Prepn by photochlorination of methyl formate: W. Hentschel, *J. Prakt. Chem.* **36**, 209 (1887); F. Grignard *et al., C.R. Hebd. Seances Acad. Sci.* **169**, 1074 (1919); *eidem, ibid.* 1143; by photochlorination of methyl chloroformate: A. Kling *et al., ibid.* 1046; K. Kurita, Y. Iwakura, *Org. Synth.* **59**, 195 (1980). Effect on air-blood barrier in rabbits, toxicity: E. Klika, A. Mysliveckova, *Folia Morphol. (Prague)* **19**, 5 (1971), *C.A.* **75**, 3433c (1971). Use in synthesis of isocyanides: G. Skorna, J. Ugi, *Angew. Chem. Int. Ed.* **16**, 259 (1977).

Suffocating liquid. bp 128°. bp$_{50}$ 49°. d$_{15}$ 1.664. n_D^{22} 1.45664. Stable at room temp, decomposes to phosgene at ~300°C. LC$_{100}$ in rabbits (10-20 minutes exposure to vapor): 0.9 mg/l air (Klika, Mysliveckova).

USE: In organic synthesis; as war gas.

3335. Dipicrylamine. [131-73-7] 2,4,6-Trinitro-*N*-(2,4,6-trinitrophenyl)benzenamine; 2,4,6,2',4',6'-hexanitrodiphenylamine. $C_{12}H_5N_7O_{12}$; mol wt 439.21. C 32.82%, H 1.15%, N 22.32%, O 43.71%. *Ref:* Winkel, Maas, *Angew. Chem.* **49**, 827 (1936).

Yellow prisms. Has a tendency to explode. mp about 238° with dec. Insol in water, acetone, alcohol or ether. Sol in alkalies, glacial acetic acid.

USE: Reagent for gravimetric determination of potassium.

3336. Dipin. [738-99-8] 1,4-Bis[bis(1-aziridinyl)phosphin-yl]piperazine; 1,4-piperazinediylbis[bis(1-aziridinyl)phosphine oxide]; piperazine-1,4-bis(*N,N'*-diethylenephosphonediamide); tetraethyleneimidopiperazine-*N,N'*-diphosphoric acid. $C_{12}H_{24}N_6O_2P_2$; mol wt 346.31. C 41.62%, H 6.99%, N 24.27%, O 9.24%, P 17.89%. Alkylating agent; exptl antineoplastic. Prepn: Kropacheva *et al., Zh. Obshch. Khim.* **30**, 3584 (1960), *C.A.* **55**, 18695c (1961). Spectrophotometric determn: L. Kh. Kartashova, E. M. Salomatin, *Farmatsiya (Moscow)* **33**, 72 (1983), *C.A.* **102**, 119736j (1985). Metabolism in rats: V. V. Chistyakov *et al., Khim. Farm. Zh.* **21**, 398 (1987), *C.A.* **107**, 146734s (1987).

Crystals, mp 187°.

3337. Dipipanone. [467-83-4] 4,4-Diphenyl-6-(1-piperidinyl)-3-heptanone; *dl*-4,4-diphenyl-6-piperidinoheptan-3-one; 6-piperidino-4,4-diphenylheptan-3-one; 2-(1-piperidino)-4,4-diphenyl-5-heptanone; phenylpiperone; 378C48; Hoechst 10805; Piperidyl

Amidone; Pamedon(e); Fenpidon; Pipadone. $C_{24}H_{31}NO$; mol wt 349.51. C 82.47%, H 8.94%, N 4.01%, O 4.58%. Prepn: Ofner, Walton, *J. Chem. Soc.* **1950**, 2158; GB 654975 (1951 to Wellcome Foundation). Variations of the synthesis using phenyllithium as condensing agent: Kazuhiko, Kubota, *Kumamoto Med. J.* **12**, 304-307 (1960).

Hydrochloride. [856-87-1] $C_{24}H_{31}NO.HCl$. Minute prisms from wet alcohol-ether, mp 123-126°. Also reported as mp 126-127°.

Hydrobromide. $C_{24}H_{31}NO.HBr$. Crystals from water, mp 103-106°.

Note: This is a controlled substance (opiate): 21 CFR, 1308.11.

THERAP CAT: Analgesic (narcotic).

3338. Dipivefrin. [52365-63-6] 2,2-Dimethylpropanoic acid 4-[1-hydroxy-2-(methylamino)ethyl]-1,2-phenylene ester; (±)-3,4-dihydroxy-α-[(methylamino)methyl]benzyl alcohol 3,4-dipivalate; 1-(3',4'-dipivaloyloxyphenyl)-2-methylamino-1-ethanol; dipivalyl epinephrine; DPE. $C_{19}H_{29}NO_5$; mol wt 351.44. C 64.93%, H 8.32%, N 3.99%, O 22.76%. Dipivalyl ester of epinephrine, *q.v.* Prepn: D. Henschler *et al., DE 2152058; eidem, US 4085270 (1973, 1978 both to Klinge); A. Hussain, J. E. Truelove, DE 2343657; eidem, US 3809714 and US 3839584 (all 1974 to Interx). *In vitro* study: A. H. Neufeld, E. D. Page, *Invest. Ophthalmol. Visual Sci.* **16**, 1118 (1977). Pharmacology: B. C. Wang *et al., J. Pharmacol. Exp. Ther.* **203**, 442 (1977). Effects on intraocular pressure in dogs: R. M. Gwin *et al., Am. J. Vet. Res.* **39**, 83 (1978). Metabolism: I. Abramovsky, J. S. Mindel, *Arch. Ophthalmol.* **97**, 1937 (1979). Clinical study: M. A. Kass *et al., ibid.* 1865. General pharmacology, toxicology and clinical experience in glaucoma: D. A. McClure, *ACS Symp. Ser.* **14**, 224-235 (1975). Comprehensive description: G. M. Wall, T. Y. Fan, *Anal. Profiles Drug Subs. Excip.* **22**, 229-262 (1993).

Crystals from ether, mp 146-147°.

Hydrochloride. [64019-93-8] Diopine; d Epifrin; Diphemin; Pivalephrine; Propine. $C_{19}H_{29}NO_5.HCl$; mol wt 387.90. Crystals from ethyl acetate, mp 158-159°. Sol in water and ethanol. pKa 8.40.

THERAP CAT: Adrenergic (ophthalmic); antiglaucoma.

3339. Diploicin. [527-93-5] 2,4,7,9-Tetrachloro-3-hydroxy-8-methoxy-1,6-dimethyl-11*H*-dibenzo[*b,e*][1,4]dioxepin-11-one; 3,5-dichloro-6-[(3,5-dichloro-6-hydroxy-4-methoxy-*o*-tolyl)oxy]-4,2-cresotic acid ε-lactone; 5,6'-dimethyl-2',3-dihydroxy-4'-methoxy-2,3',4,5'-tetrachloro-6-carboxydiphenyl ether 2',6-lactone. $C_{16}H_{10}Cl_4O_5$; mol wt 424.06. C 45.32%, H 2.38%, Cl 33.44%, O 18.86%. Antibiotic isolated from the lichen *Buellia canescens* (Dicks.) De Not. [*Diploicia canescens* (Dicks.) Massal.], *Lecideaceae*: Zopf, *Ann.* **336**, 58 (1904); Nolan, *Sci. Proc. R. Dublin Soc.* **21**, 67 (1934); Nolan *et al., Chem. Ind. (London)* **1935**, 577; Barry, *Nature* **158**, 131 (1946). Structure: Nolan *et al., Sci. Proc. R. Dublin Soc.* **24**, 319 (1948). Synthesis: Ollis, *ibid.* **27**, 161 (1956); Brown *et al., Proc. Chem. Soc. London* **1960**, 393; Hendrickson, Ramsay, *Chem. Commun.* **1968**, 1101; Hendrickson *et al., J. Am. Chem. Soc.* **94**, 6834 (1972); P. D. Djura *et al., J. Chem. Soc. Perkin Trans. 1* **1976**, 147.

White needles from methanol, mp 233-234°. uv max: 270 nm (log ε 3.79).

Acetate. $C_{18}H_{12}Cl_4O_6$. mp 234-235°.

3340. Diprenorphine. [14357-78-9] (5α,7α)-17-(Cyclopropylmethyl)-4,5-epoxy-18,19-dihydro-3-hydroxy-6-methoxy-α,α-dimethyl-6,14-ethenomorphinan-7-methanol; 21-cyclopropyl-6,7,8,-14-tetrahydro-7α-(1-hydroxy-1-methylethyl)-6,14-endo-ethanooripavine; N-(cyclopropylmethyl)-19-methylnororvinol; M-5050; RX-5050M. $C_{26}H_{35}NO_4$; mol wt 425.56. C 73.38%, H 8.29%, N 3.29%, O 15.04%. Closely related to cyprenorphine, q.v. Prepn: K. W. Bentley, D. G. Hardy, *J. Am. Chem. Soc.* **89**, 3281 (1967). Activity in rats: G. F. Blane, *J. Pharm. Pharmacol.* **19**, 367 (1967); G. F. Blane, D. Dugdall, *ibid.* **20**, 547 (1968). Use as etorphine antagonist in dogs: M. Grange *et al., Rev. Med. Vet.* **124**, 899 (1973); in large animals: B. T. Alford *et al., J. Am. Vet. Med. Assoc.* **164**, 702 (1974). Binding to opiate receptors: C. B. Pert *et al., Life Sci.* **16**, 1849 (1975); J. Pearson *et al., ibid.* **26**, 1047 (1980); to μ opiate receptors: J. J. Frost *et al., ibid.* **38**, 1597 (1986). Treatment of experimental stroke in cats: D. S. Baskin *et al., Neuropeptides* **5**, 307 (1985); *eidem, J. Neurosurg.* **64**, 99 (1986). Determn by HPLC: I. Jane, A. McKinnon, *J. Chromatogr.* **323**, 191 (1985). Toxicity data: N. S. Duggett *et al., Toxicol. Appl. Pharmacol.* **31**, 141 (1977).

Crystals from methanol, mp 185°.

Hydrochloride. Revivon. $C_{26}H_{35}NO_4 \cdot HCl$; mol wt 462.02. LD$_{50}$ s.c. in mice: 316.0 ± 28 mg/kg (Duggett).

THERAP CAT (VET): Narcotic antagonist.

3341. Dipropalin. [1918-08-7] 4-Methyl-2,6-dinitro-N,N-dipropylbenzenamine; 2,6-dinitro-N,N-dipropyl-p-toluidine; N,N-dipropyl-2,6-dinitro-4-methylaniline; 2,6-dinitro-N,N-dipropyl-4-methylaniline; 3,5-dinitro-4-dipropylaminotoluene; L-35355. $C_{13}H_{19}N_3O_4$; mol wt 281.31. C 55.50%, H 6.81%, N 14.94%, O 22.75%. Prepd from 2,6-dinitro-p-cresol, p-toluenesulfonate and dipropylamine: Hantzsch, *Ber.* **43**, 1662 (1910).

Yellow crystals, mp 80°.

USE: Herbicide.

3342. Dipropetryn. [4147-51-7] 6-(Ethylthio)-N,N'-bis(1-methylethyl)-1,3,5-triazine-2,4-diamine; 2-(ethylthio)-4,6-bis(isopropylamino)-s-triazine; GS-16068. $C_{11}H_{21}N_5S$; mol wt 255.38. C 51.73%, H 8.29%, N 27.42%, S 12.56%. Pre-emergence herbicide. Prepn: **NL 6414460**; H. Yamamoto, T. Namekawa, **US 3326912** (1965, 1967 both to Nippon Kayaku). Absorption and translocation in plants: E. Basler *et al., Weed Sci.* **26**, 358 (1978).

Powder, mp 104-106°. Vapor pressure at 20°: 7.3×10^{-7} mm Hg. Soly in water at 20°: 16 mg/l. Soluble in organic solvents.

USE: Herbicide.

3343. n-Dipropylamine. [142-84-7] N-Propyl-1-propanamine. $C_6H_{15}N$; mol wt 101.19. C 71.22%, H 14.94%, N 13.84%. $(CH_3CH_2CH_2)_2NH$.

Colorless liq; odor of ammonia. d_4^{20} 0.738. bp 110°. mp −63°. n_D^{20} 1.40455. Freely sol in water or alcohol. Forms a hydrate with H_2O. LD$_{50}$ orally in rats: 0.93 g/kg, H. F. Smyth *et al., Am. Ind. Hyg. Assoc. J.* **23**, 95 (1962).

3344. Dipropylene Glycol Monomethyl Ether. [34590-94-8] 1(or 2)-(2-Methoxymethylethoxy)propanol; DPGME; DPM; Arcosolv DPM; Dowanol DPM; Poly-Solv DPM. $C_7H_{16}O_3$; mol wt 148.20. C 56.73%, H 10.88%, O 32.39%. Commercial product, prepd from propylene oxide and methanol, may consist of as many as four structural isomers. Prepn of major isomer, *1-(2-methoxy-1-methylethoxy)-2-propanol*, depicted below: A. R. Sexton, E. C. Britton, *J. Am. Chem. Soc.* **75**, 4357 (1953). GC determn in urine: B. Hubner *et al., Fresenius J. Anal. Chem.* **342**, 746 (1992). Toxicity studies: H. F. Smyth, Jr. *et al., Am. Ind. Hyg. Assoc. J.* **23**, 95 (1962); T. D. Landry, B. L. Yano, *Fundam. Appl. Toxicol.* **4**, 612 (1984). Review of toxicology: *Patty's Industrial Hygiene and Toxicology* vol. **2D**, G. D. Clayton, F. E. Clayton, Eds. (Wiley-Interscience, New York, 4th ed., 1994) pp 2882-2886; G. Johansson, *NEG and NIOSH Basis for an Occupational Health Standard: Propylene Glycol Ethers and Their Acetates* (PB91-220749, 1991) 47 pp.

Colorless liquid. bp$_{760}$ 189.6°. fp −80°. d_4^{25} 0.948. n_D^{25} 1.419. Flash pt, open cup: 185°F. Vapor pressure at 25°: 0.41 mm Hg. Misc with water, benzene. LD$_{50}$ orally in rats, dermally in rabbits: 5.66, 10.0 (ml/kg) (Smyth).

Caution: Potential symptoms of overexposure are irritation of eyes, nose, throat; weakness, lightheadedness, headache. *See NIOSH Pocket Guide to Chemical Hazards* (DHHS/NIOSH 97-140, 1997) p 122.

USE: As solvent for automotive fluids, cleaners, dyes, coatings, inks, waxes, adhesives, agricultural products, insect repellents, and cosmetics; chemical intermediate.

3345. Dipropyl Ketone. [123-19-3] 4-Heptanone; butyrone. $C_7H_{14}O$; mol wt 114.19. C 73.63%, H 12.36%, O 14.01%. $CH_3CH_2CH_2COCH_2CH_2CH_3$. Made by passing butyric acid over precipitated $CaCO_3$ at 450°.

Colorless, very refractive liquid; penetrating odor; burning taste. d_4^{15} 0.821. bp 144°. mp −32.6°. n_D^{22} 1.4073. Insol in water; miscible with alcohol, ether.

Caution: Potential symptoms of overexposure are irritation of eyes, skin; CNS depression, dizziness, somnolence, decreased breathing. *See NIOSH Pocket Guide to Chemical Hazards* (DHHS/-NIOSH 97-140, 1997) p 122.

3346. Dipyridamole. [58-32-2] 2,2',2'',2'''-[(4,8-Di-1-piperidinylpyrimido[5,4-d]pyrimidine-2,6-diyl)dinitrilo]tetrakis-ethanol; 2,6-bis(diethanolamino)-4,8-dipiperidinopyrimido-[5,4-d]-pyrimidine; NSC-515776; RA-8; Anginal; Cardoxin; Cleridium; Coridil; Coronarine; Curantyl; Dipyridan; Gulliostin; Natyl; Peridamol; Persantine; Piroan; Prandiol; Protangix. $C_{24}H_{40}N_8O_4$; mol wt 504.63. C 57.12%, H 7.99%, N 22.21%, O 12.68%. Phosphodiesterase inhibitor that reduces platelet aggregation; also acts as a coronary vasodilator. Prepn: **GB 807826**; F. G. Fischer, *et al.*, **US 3031450** (1959, 1962 both to Thomae). Activity studies: Saraf, Seth, *Indian J. Physiol. Pharmacol.* **15**, 135 (1971). Toxicological study: F. Takenaka *et al., Arzneim.-Forsch.* **22**, 892 (1972). Symposium on pharmacology and clinical experience as antithrombotic: *Thromb. Res.* **60**, Suppl. 12, 1-99 (1990). Review of use as pharmacological stress agent in echocardiography: M. B. Buchalter *et al., Postgrad. Med. J.* **66**, 531-535 (1990); in ^{201}Tl cardiac imaging: S. G. Beer *et al., Am. J. Cardiol.* **67**, Suppl., 18D-26D (1991).

Deep yellow needles from ethyl acetate, mp 163°. Bitter taste. Slightly sol in H_2O; sol in dil acid having a pH of 3.3 or below; very sol in methanol, ethanol, chloroform; not too sol in acetone, benzene, ethyl acetate. Solns are yellow and show strong blue-green fluorescence. LD_{50} in rats: 8.4 g/kg orally; 208 mg/kg i.v. (Takenaka).

Combination with aspirin. Aggrenox. Review of pharmacology and clinical efficacy in secondary prevention of stroke: P. S. Hervey, K. L. Goa, *Drugs* **58**, 469-475 (1999).

THERAP CAT: Antithrombotic; diagnostic aid (cardiac stress testing).

3347.   α,α'-Dipyridyl. [366-18-7] 2,2'-Bipyridine; 2,2'-dipyridyl; CI-588. $C_{10}H_8N_2$; mol wt 156.18. C 76.90%, H 5.16%, N 17.94%. Prepn from pyridine: Smith, *J. Am. Chem. Soc.* **46**, 414 (1924). Manuf: Freeman, Ghosh, **US 2962502** (1960 to I.C.I.). Absorption spectrum: P. Krumholz, *J. Am. Chem. Soc.* **73**, 3487 (1951). Pharmacologic study: Bass *et al., J. Pharmacol. Exp. Ther.* **152**, 104 (1966). Toxicity data: R. W. Grady *et al., ibid.* **196**, 478 (1976).

Crystals from dil alcohol, mp 69.7°. bp 272-273°. Sol in about 200 parts water; very sol in alcohol, ether, benzene, chloroform, petr ether. LD_{50} i.p. in mice: 200 mg/kg (Grady).

USE: As a reagent for the determination of iron.

3348.   γ,γ'-Dipyridyl. [553-26-4] 4,4'-Bipyridine; 4,4'-dipyridyl. $C_{10}H_8N_2$; mol wt 156.18. C 76.90%, H 5.16%, N 17.94%. Prepn: Dimroth, Frister, *Ber.* **55**, 3695 (1922); Smith, *J. Am. Chem. Soc.* **46**, 414 (1924).

Dihydrate. Bitter needles from water, mp 73°. Anhydr form, mp 111-112°. bp_{760} 304.8°. Freely sol in alc, benzene, chloroform, ether; slightly sol in water. Absorption spectrum: Krumholz, *J. Am. Chem. Soc.* **73**, 3487 (1951).

Dihydrochloride. $C_{10}H_8N_2.2HCl$. Prisms from water. Soluble in water; practically insol in ether.

3349.   Dipyrocetyl. [486-79-3] 2,3-Bis(acetyloxy)benzoic acid; *o*-pyrocatechuic acid diacetate; diacetylpyrocatechol-3-carboxylic acid; 2,3-diacetoxybenzoic acid; Movirene; Artromialgina. $C_{11}H_{10}O_6$; mol wt 238.19. C 55.47%, H 4.23%, O 40.30%. Prepn: Rietz, **US 1140716** (1914); Simokoriyama, *Bull. Chem. Soc. Jpn.* **16**, 284 (1941).

mp 148-150° (Rietz); mp 146-170° (Simokoriyama). Sol in organic solvents. Practically insol in water.

THERAP CAT: Analgesic, antipyretic.

3350.   Dipyrone. [5907-38-0] [(2,3-Dihydro-1,5-dimethyl-3-oxo-2-phenyl-1*H*-pyrazol-4-yl)methylamino]methanesulfonic acid sodium salt monohydrate; (antipyrinylmethylamino)methanesulfonic acid sodium salt; 1-phenyl-2,3-dimethyl-5-pyrazolone-4-methylaminomethanesulfonate sodium; noraminopyrine methanesulfonate sodium; 4-methylamino-1,5-dimethyl-2-phenyl-3-pyrazolone sodium methanesulfonate; sodium methylaminoantipyrine methanesulfonate; methylmelubrin; methampyrone; metamizol; analgin; sulpyrin; Alginodia; Algocalmin; Bonpyrin; Conmel; Divarine; Dolazon; D-Pron; Dya-Tron; Espyre; Farmolisina; Feverall; Fevonil; Keypyrone; Metilon; Minalgin; Narone; Nartate; Nevralgina; Nolotil; Novacid; Novaldin; Novalgin; Novemina; Novil; Paralgin; Pyralgin; Pyril; Pyrilgin; Pyrojec; Tega-Pyrone; Unagen. $C_{13}H_{16}N_3NaO_4S.H_2O$; mol wt 351.35. C 44.44%, H 5.16%, N 11.96%, Na 6.54%, O 22.77%, S 9.13%. Prepd by methylating the amino group of sulfamipyrine, then treating with formaldehyde sodium bisulfite soln: **DE 254711**; **DE 259503**; **DE 259577** (all 1911 to Hoechst).

Minute crystals from alc. Sol in water (1 g/1.5 ml), methanol. Less sol in ethanol. Practically insol in ether, acetone, benzene, chloroform. Aq solns are neutral; may acquire a yellow discoloration without apparent potency loss.

Magnesium salt. [6150-97-6] Magnopyrol. $C_{26}H_{32}MgN_6O_8S_2$; mol wt 645.00.

THERAP CAT: Analgesic; antipyretic.

THERAP CAT (VET): Analgesic; antispasmodic.

3351.   Diquafosol. [59985-21-6] Uridine 5'-(pentahydrogen tetraphosphate) $P''' \rightarrow 5'$-ester with uridine; P^1,P^4-diuridine 5'-tetraphosphate; UP$_4$U. $C_{18}H_{26}N_4O_{23}P_4$; mol wt 790.31. C 27.36%, H 3.32%, N 7.09%, O 46.56%, P 15.68%. Uridine nucleotide analog. P2Y$_2$ purinoceptor agonist; stimulates mucin secretion from goblet cells. Prepn: M. J. Stutts, III *et al.*, **WO 9640059** (1996 to Univ. North Carolina at Chapel Hill); and receptor activity: W. Pendergast *et al., Bioorg. Med. Chem. Lett.* **11**, 157 (2001). Ocular pharmacology: T. Fujihara *et al., J. Ocul. Pharmacol. Ther.* **18**, 363 (2002). Review of development and therapeutic potential: J. Fischbarg, *Curr. Opin. Invest. Drugs* **4**, 1377-1383 (2003); K. K. Nichols *et al., Expert Opin. Invest. Drugs* **13**, 47-54 (2004). Clinical trial in dry eye disease: J. Tauber *et al., Cornea* **23**, 784 (2004).

Tetrasodium salt. [211427-08-6] INS-365. $C_{18}H_{22}N_4Na_4$-$O_{23}P_4$; mol wt 878.23.

THERAP CAT: In treatment of dry eye disease.

3352. Diquat Dibromide. [85-00-7] 6,7-Dihydrodipyr-ido[1,2-*a*:2',1'-*c*]pyrazinediium dibromide; 1,1'-ethylene-2,2'-dipyridylium dibromide; FB/2; Reglone. $C_{12}H_{12}Br_2N_2$; mol wt 344.05. C 41.89%, H 3.52%, Br 46.45%, N 8.14%. Prepn: Fielden *et al.*, **US 2823987** (1958 to ICI). Herbicidal properties: Brian *et al.*, *Nature* **181**, 446 (1958). Environmental fate and toxicity: Simsiman *et al.*, *Residue Rev.* **62**, 131-174 (1976). Acute toxicity study: T. B. Gaines, R. E. Linder, *Fundam. Appl. Toxicol.* **7**, 299 (1986). *Review:* Akhavein, Linscott, *ibid.* **23**, 97-145 (1968).

Monohydrate. [6385-62-2] Pale yellow crystals from water, mp <320° (dec). Also reported as mp 335-340°. uv max: 308.31 nm (ε 18000). Soly in water at 20°: 70%. Insoluble in organic solvents. Slightly sol in alcohol. Stable in acid or neutral soln. LD_{50} in male, female rats (mg/kg): 147, 121 orally; in male rats (mg/kg): 433 dermally (Gaines, Linder).

Caution: Potential symptoms of overexposure are irritation of eyes, skin, mucous membranes, respiratory system; rhinorrhea, epistaxis; skin burns; nausea, vomiting, diarrhea, malaise; kidney and liver injury; cough, chest pain, dyspnea, pulmonary edema; tremor, convulsions; delayed wound healing. See *NIOSH Pocket Guide to Chemical Hazards* (DHHS/NIOSH 97-140, 1997) p 122.

USE: Contact herbicide used also to produce desiccation and defoliation.

3353. 1,3-Di-6-quinolylurea. [532-05-8] *N,N'*-Di-6-quino-linylurea; *sym*-di-(6-quinolyl)urea; bis(6-quinolyl)urea; 6,6'-diquinolylurea; Babesan. $C_{19}H_{14}N_4O$; mol wt 314.34. C 72.60%, H 4.49%, N 17.82%, O 5.09%. Synthesis starting with 6-aminoquinoline: Schönhöfer, Henecka, **DE 583207** (1933 to I. G. Farben); Haskelberg, *J. Org. Chem.* **12**, 434 (1947); Reuter, *Aust. Chem. Inst. J. Proc.* **16**, 164 (1949).

Crystals from pyridine, mp 262°. Sol in dil acid.

Bismethosulfate. 6,6'-Ureylenebis[1,1'-dimethylquinolinium] sulfate; quinuronium sulfate; 6,6'-ureylenebis(1-methylquino-linium)bis(methosulfate); dimethyl quinolyl methylsulfate urea; SN-5870; Acaprin; Zothelone; Baburan; Pirevan; Pyroplasmin; Atral. $C_{23}H_{26}N_4O_9S_2$; mol wt 566.60. Yellow crystals from methanol, dec 237°. Freely sol in water.

THERAP CAT (VET): Antiprotozoal (*Babesia*).

3354. Dirithromycin. [62013-04-1] (1*R*,2*R*,3*R*,6*R*,7*S*,8*S*,-9*R*,10*R*,12*R*,13*S*,15*R*,17*S*)-7-[(2,6-Dideoxy-3-*C*-methyl-3-*O*-meth-yl-α-L-*ribo*-hexopyranosyl)oxy]-3-ethyl-2,10-dihydroxy-15-[(2-methoxyethoxy)methyl]-2,6,8,10,12,17-hexamethyl-9-[[3,4,6-tri-deoxy-3-(dimethylamino)-β-D-*xylo*-hexopyranosyl]oxy]-4,16-di-oxa-14-azabicyclo[11.3.1]heptadecan-5-one; [9*S*(*R*)]-9-deoxo-11-deoxy-9,11-[imino[2-(2-methoxyethoxy)ethylidene]oxy]erythro-mycin; LY-237216; AS-E 136; Dynabac; Noriclan; Nortron; Valodin. $C_{42}H_{78}N_2O_{14}$; mol wt 835.07. C 60.41%, H 9.41%, N 3.35%, O 26.82%. Semi-synthetic derivative of erythromycin, *q.v.* Prepn: **BE 840431** (1976 to Thomae); R. Maier *et al.*, **US 4048306** (1977 to Boehringer, Ing.). Synthesis, ^{1}H- and ^{13}C-NMR, and antimicrobial evaluation: F. T. Counter *et al.*, *Antimicrob. Agents Chemother.* **35**, 1116 (1991). X-ray structure determn: P. Luger, R. Maier, *J. Cryst. Mol. Struct.* **9**, 329 (1979). HPLC determn in plasma: G. W. Whitaker, T. D. Lindstrom, *J. Liq. Chromatogr.* **11**, 3011 (1988). Symposium on antibacterial activity, pharmacology, and clinical experience: *J. Antimicrob. Chemother.* **31**, Suppl. C, 1-185 (1993).

Crystals from ethanol/water, mp 186-189° (dec) (Counter). pKa 9.0 in 66% aq dimethyl fluoride. LD_{50} in mice (g/kg): >1 s.c.; >1 orally (Maier).

THERAP CAT: Antibacterial.

3355. Discodermolide. [127943-53-7] (3*R*,4*S*,5*R*,6*S*)-6-[(2*S*,3*Z*,5*S*,6*S*,7*S*,8*Z*,11*S*,12*R*,13*S*,14*S*,15*S*,16*Z*)-14-[(Aminocarbon-yl)oxy]-2,6,12-trihydroxy-5,7,9,11,13,15-hexamethyl-3,8,16,18-nonadecatetraenyl]tetrahydro-4-hydroxy-3,5-dimethyl-2*H*-pyran-2-one; YM-19020. $C_{33}H_{55}NO_8$; mol wt 593.79. C 66.75%, H 9.34%, N 2.36%, O 21.56%. Polyhydroxylated lactone isolated from the marine sponge, *Discodermia dissoluta*. Naturally occur-ring (+)-form stabilizes microtubles and inhibits cell proliferation with the same mechanism as paclitaxel, *q.v.* Isoln and structure determn: S. P. Gunasekera *et al.*, *J. Org. Chem.* **55**, 4912 (1990); correction: *ibid.* **56**, 1346 (1991). Total synthesis: D. T. Hung *et al.*, *J. Am. Chem. Soc.* **118**, 11054 (1996). Review of total synthe-ses: I. Paterson, G. J. Florence, *Eur. J. Org. Chem.* **2003**, 2193-2208. Series of articles on industrial-scale synthesis: S. J. Mickel *et al.*, *Org. Process Res. Dev.* **8**, 92-130 (2004). NMR soln structure determn: A. B. Smith, III *et al.*, *Org. Lett.* **3**, 695 (2001). Mech-anism of action: D. T. Hung *et al.*, *Chem. Biol.* **3**, 287 (1996); E. ter Haar *et al.*, *Biochemistry* **35**, 243 (1996). Synergistic activity with paclitaxel in cancer cells: S. Honore *et al.*, *Cancer Res.* **64**, 4957 (2004).

Monoclinic white crystals, mp 115-116°. uv max (methanol): 210, 226, 235 nm (ε 35400, 19500, 12500). $[\alpha]_D^{20}$ +14.0° (c = 0.6 in methanol); monohydrate: $[\alpha]_D$ +20.1° (c = 1 in methanol).

USE: Reagent for mitotic studies.

3356. Disilane. [1590-87-0] Disilicoethane; disilicon hexa-hydride; silicoethane; disilicane. H_6Si_2; mol wt 62.22. H 9.72%, Si 90.28%. Si_2H_6. Obtained by separation of mixed silanes prepd from magnesium silicide and hydrochloric acid: Moissan, Smiles, *Compt. Rend.* **134**, 569, 1549 (1902); Stock, Somiesky, *Ber.* **49**, 111 (1916); **54B**, 524 (1921); **56B**, 247 (1923); Culbertson, **US 2551571** (1951 to Union Carbide); prepd by conversion of silane to higher silanes in an ozonizer type electric discharge: Spanier, MacDiar-mid, *Inorg. Chem.* **1**, 432 (1962).

Gas; repulsive odor. d_4^{-25} 0.686. mp −132.5°. bp −14.5°. Dec 300°. Ignites spontaneously in air. Slowly dec in water.

Explodes on contact with sulfur hexafluoride; reacts vigorously with carbon tetrachloride and chloroform. Sol in carbon disulfide, ethyl alcohol, benzene, and ethyl silicate. Potassium hydroxide liberates hydrogen.

Caution: A powerful irritant.

3357. Disodium Phenyl Phosphate. [3279-54-7] C_6H_5-Na_2O_4P; mol wt 218.05. C 33.05%, H 2.31%, Na 21.09%, O 29.35%, P 14.20%. $C_6H_5PO_4Na_2$.

White, cryst powder. Freely sol in water, sparingly in alcohol; insol in acetone or ether.

USE: Reagent in the testing of milk for proper pasteurization and for the presence of unpasteurized milk.

3358. Disofenin. [65717-97-7] *N*-[2-[[2,6-Bis(1-methylethyl)phenyl]amino]2-oxoethyl]-*N*-(carboxymethyl)glycine; [[[(2,6-diisopropylphenyl)carbamoyl]methyl]imino]diacetic acid; (2,6-di-isopropylacetanilido)iminodiacetic acid; *N*-(carboxymethyl)-*N*-[2-(2,6-diisopropylphenyl)amino]-2-oxoethylglycine; DISIDA. C_{18}-$H_{26}N_2O_5$; mol wt 350.41. C 61.70%, H 7.48%, N 7.99%, O 22.83%. Iminodiacetic acid analog. Prepn of acid and ^{99m}Tc-complex: M. de Schrijver, **DE 2723605**; *idem,* **US 4316883** (1977, 1982 both to Solco Basel). High yield synthesis of acid: M. P. Best *et al., Aust. J. Chem.* **35,** 2371 (1982). Biodistribution: G. Subramanian *et al., Nuklearmedizin Suppl.* **16,** 136 (1978). Chromatographic determn of radiochemical purity: A. M. Zimmer *et al., Eur. J. Nucl. Med.* **7,** 88 (1982). Chemical and biological properties: B. Zmbova *et al., Appl. Radiat. Isot.* **38,** 35 (1987). Pharmacokinetics: I. A. Fraser *et al., Eur. J. Nucl. Med.* **14,** 431 (1988); J. E. Love *et al., ibid.* 436. Clinical evaluation as hepatobiliary imaging agent: R. C. Stadalnik *et al., Radiology* **140,** 797 (1981).

White crystals, mp 196-198° (Zmbova). Also reported as crystals from water, mp 191-192.5° (Best); and as mp 166-175° (de Schrijver). Insol in water.

^{99m}**Tc complex.** ^{99m}Tc diisopropyl IDA; ^{99m}Tc-DISIDA; Hepatolite. Distribution coefficient (ethylene dichloride/water): 0.0086.

THERAP CAT: ^{99m}Tc-complex as diagnostic aid (radioactive imaging agent).

3359. Disophenol. [305-85-1] 2,6-Diiodo-4-nitrophenol; DNP; Ancylol. $C_6H_3I_2NO_3$; mol wt 390.90. C 18.44%, H 0.77%, I 64.93%, N 3.58%, O 12.28%. Prepd by iodination of *p*-nitrophenol with iodine/potassium iodide soln in aq ammonia: Datta, Prosad, *J. Am. Chem. Soc.* **39,** 446 (1917). As an anthelmintic: Thorson *et al.,* **US 3081224** (1963 to Am. Cyanamid). Toxicity studies: J. A. Kaiser, *Toxicol. Appl. Pharmacol.* **6,** 232 (1964); Fowler, *Br. Vet. J.* **127,** 304 (1971). Comparative field trial in sheep: C. A. Hall *et al., Res. Vet. Sci.* **31,** 104 (1981).

Light yellow, feathery crystals from glacial acetic acid, mp 157°. Freely sol in alcohol, very sparingly sol in water. LD_{50} in rats, mice (mg/kg): 170, 212 orally; 105, 88 i.v.; 105, 107 i.p.; 122, 110 s.c. (Kaiser).

THERAP CAT (VET): Anthelmintic (hookworm).

3360. Disopyramide. [3737-09-5] α-[2-[Bis(1-methylethyl)amino]ethyl]-α-phenyl-2-pyridineacetamide; α-[2-(diisopropylamino)ethyl]-α-phenyl-2-pyridineacetamide; 4-(diisopropylamino)-2-phenyl-2-(2-pyridyl)butyramide; H-3292; SC-7031; Dicorantil; Isorythm; Lispine; Ritmodan; Rythmodan. $C_{21}H_{29}N_3O$; mol wt 339.47. C 74.30%, H 8.61%, N 12.38%, O 4.71%. Prepn: Cusic, Sause, **BE 617730** *C.A.* **58,** 12522e (1963) and **US 3225054** (1962 and 1965, both to Searle). Synthesis and biological activity: Adelstein, *J. Med. Chem.* **16,** 309 (1973). Pharmacology: *J. Am. Med. Assoc.* **213,** 697 (1970); Mathur, *Am. Heart J.* **84,** 764 (1972); B. Befeler, R. Lazzara, *Heart Lung* **9,** 475 (1980). Conformation-activity study: J. L. Czeisler, R. M. El-Rashidy, *J. Pharm. Sci.* **74,** 750 (1985). Toxicity: P. C. Ruenitz, C. M. Mokler, *J. Med. Chem.* **22,** 1142 (1979). *Reviews:* R. R. Dean *et al.,* in *Pharmacological and Biochemical Properties of Drug Substances* **vol. 2,** M. E. Goldberg, Ed. (Am. Pharm. Assoc., Washington, DC, 1979) pp 165-185; E. H. Taylor, A. A. Pappas, *Ann. Clin. Lab. Sci.* **16,** 289-295 (1986).

Crystals from hexane, mp 94.5-95.0°. pKa 10.2; also reported as 10.45. Soly in water: 1 mg/ml. Partition coefficient (chloroform/water): 3.1 (pH 7.2). LD_{50} i.p. in mice: 517 μmol/kg (Ruenitz, Mokler).

Phosphate. [22059-60-5] SC-13957; Dirythmin SA; Diso-Duriles; Norpace; Rythmodul. $C_{21}H_{29}N_3O.H_3PO_4$; mol wt 437.47. Freely sol in water.

THERAP CAT: Antiarrhythmic (class IA).

3361. Disparlure. [29804-22-6] (*cis*-form); [54910-51-9] (2S-*cis*-form). (2S-*cis*)-2-Decyl-3-(5-methylhexyl)oxirane; *cis*-7,8-epoxy-2-methyloctadecane; ENT-34886; Disrupt. $C_{19}H_{38}O$; mol wt 282.50. C 80.78%, H 13.56%, O 5.66%. Potent sex pheromone of the gypsy moth *Lymantria dispar* (formerly *Porthetria dispar*). Isoln and characterization: B. A. Bierl *et al., Science* **170,** 87 (1970); *eidem, J. Econ. Entomol.* **65,** 659 (1972). Synthesis: S. Iwaki *et al., J. Am. Chem. Soc.* **96,** 7842 (1974); D. G. Farnum *et al., Tetrahedron Lett.* **1977,** 4009; K. Mori *et al., Tetrahedron* **35,** 833 (1979); B. E. Rossiter *et al., J. Am. Chem. Soc.* **103,** 464 (1981); K. Mori, T. Ebata, *Tetrahedron Lett.* **22,** 4281 (1981). Synthesis of (±)-form: K. Eiter, *Angew. Chem. Int. Ed.* **11,** 60 (1972); *idem,* **DE 2145454**; *idem,* **US 3975409** (1973, 1976 both to Bayer); H. J. Bestmann *et al., Ber.* **109,** 3375 (1976). Activity of (+)- and (±)-forms: R. T. Cardé, R. P. Webster, *J. Chem. Ecol.* **5,** 935 (1979). Acute toxicity study: M. Beroza *et al., Toxicol. Appl. Pharmacol.* **31,** 421 (1975).

Viscous colorless oil, bp$_{0.25}$ 146-148°. $[\alpha]_D^{23}$ +0.8 ±0.2° (c = 10 in CCl_4). n_D^{23} 1.4450. LD_{50} in rats (mg/kg): >34600 orally; in rabbits (mg/kg): >2025 dermally; LC_{50} (24 hr) in rainbow trout, bluegill sunfish (ppm): >100, >100 (Beroza).

USE: Insect attractant.

3362. Distigmine Bromide. [15876-67-2] 3,3′-[1,6-Hexanediylbis[(methylimino)carbonyl]oxy]bis[1-methylpyridinium]dibromide; 3-hydroxy-1-methylpyridinium bromide hexamethylenebis[methylcarbamate]; hexamethylenebis[methylcarbamic acid] ester of 3-hydroxy-1-methylpyridinium bromide; hexamethylenebis[*N*-methylcarbamic acid ester bromomethylate]; hexamethylenebis[*N*-methylcarbaminoyl-1-methyl-3-hydroxypyridinium bromide]; hexamarium; BC-51; Ubretid. $C_{22}H_{32}Br_2N_4O_4$; mol wt 576.32. C 45.85%, H 5.60%, Br 27.73%, N 9.72%, O 11.10%. Prepn: Schmid, **US 2789981** (1957 to Oesterr. Stickstoffwerke).

Pharmacology: Hertting *et al., Arzneim.-Forsch.* **18**, 479 (1968); Hohenegger, Lindner, *Wien. Klin. Wochenschr.* **81**, 823 (1969). Stability studies: Suzuki, Tanimura, *Yakugaku Zasshi* **90**, 762 (1970).

Crystals, dec 149°.
THERAP CAT: Cholinesterase inhibitor.

3363. Disufenton. [168021-77-0] 4-[[(1,1-Dimethylethyl)-oxidoimino]methyl]-1,3-benzenedisulfonic acid; 2,4-disulfonyl-α-phenyl-*tert*-butylnitrone. $C_{11}H_{15}NO_7S_2$; mol wt 337.37. C 39.16%, H 4.48%, N 4.15%, O 33.20%, S 19.01%. Nitrone-based spin trapping agent; derivative of PBN, *q.v.* Prepn: J. M. Carney, **WO 9517876**; *idem,* **US 5488145** (1995, 1996 both to Oklahoma Med. Res. Found.). Pharmacology: S. Kuroda *et al., J. Cereb. Blood Flow Metab.* **19**, 778 (1999). Comparative radical trapping study: K. R. Maples *et al., Free Radical Res.* **34**, 417 (2001). Clinical pharmacokinetics: K. R. Lees *et al., Stroke* **32**, 675 (2001). Clinical trial in acute ischemic stroke: *idem et al., N. Engl. J. Med.* **354**, 588 (2006). Reviews of pharmacology and therapeutic potential: P. A. Lapchak, *Curr. Opin. Invest. Drugs* **3**, 1758-1762 (2002); P. A. Lapchak, D. M. Araujo, *CNS Drug Rev.* **9**, 253-262 (2003).

White powder. Soly (g/ml): water >1.
Sodium salt. [168021-79-2] Disodium 4-[(*tert*-butylimino)-methyl]benzene-1,3-disulfonate *N*-oxide; ARL-16556; CPI-22; CXY-059; NXY-059; Cerovive. $C_{11}H_{13}NNa_2O_7S_2$; mol wt 381.33.
THERAP CAT: Neuroprotective.

3364. Disulfiram. [97-77-8] Tetraethylthioperoxydicarbonic diamide; bis(diethylthiocarbamoyl) disulfide; tetraethylthiuram disulfide; bis(diethylthiocarbamyl) disulfide; teturamin; TTD; Antabuse; Esperal; Etabus. $C_{10}H_{20}N_2S_4$; mol wt 296.54. C 40.50%, H 6.80%, N 9.45%, S 43.25%. Prepn: Bailey, **US 1796977** (1931 to Roessler and Hasslacher); Adams, Newser, **US 1782111** (1931 to Naugatuck); *cf.* Cummings, Simmons, *Ind. Eng. Chem.* **20**, 1173 (1928). Toxicity study: Child, Cramp, *Acta Pharmacol. Toxicol.* **8**, 305 (1952). Comprehensive description: N. G. Nash, R. D. Daley, *Anal. Profiles Drug Subs.* **4**, 168-191 (1975).

Crystals, mp 70°. d 1.30. Practically insol in water (0.02 g/100 ml). Sol in alcohol (3.82 g/100 ml), in ether (7.14 g/100 ml), also sol in acetone, benzene, chloroform, carbon disulfide. LD₅₀ orally in rats: 8.6 g/kg (Child, Cramp).
Caution: Potential symptoms of overexposure are irritation of eyes, skin, respiratory system; sensitization dermatitis; lassitude, fatigue, tremor, restlessness, headache, dizziness; metallic taste; peripheral neuropathy; liver damage. Ingestion of alcohol after disulfiram administration causes intense vasodilation and flushing of face and neck, restlessness, anxiety; tachycardia and tachypnea; headache, nausea, vomiting, hyperpnea, chest pains, sweating, pallor, hypotension. *See NIOSH Pocket Guide to Chemical Hazards* (DHHS/NIOSH 97-140, 1997) p 122; *Clinical Toxicology of Com-*

mercial Products, R. E. Gosselin *et al.,* Eds. (Williams & Wilkins, Baltimore, 5th ed., 1984) Section III, pp 159-163, 383-386.
USE: Rubber accelerator; vulcanizer; seed disinfectant; fungicide.
THERAP CAT: Alcohol deterrent.

3365. Disulfoton. [298-04-4] Phosphorodithioic acid *O,O*-diethyl *S*-[2-(ethylthio)ethyl] ester; *O,O*-diethyl-*S*-ethylmercapto-ethyl dithiophosphate; thiodemeton; dithiodemeton; Bay 19639; ENT-23347; Di-Syston. $C_8H_{19}O_2PS_3$; mol wt 274.40. C 35.02%, H 6.98%, O 11.66%, P 11.29%, S 35.06%. Homolog of phorate, *q.v.* Prepn: Schrader, Lorenz, **US 2759010**; **GB 797307** (1956, 1958 both to Bayer). Toxicity study: T. B. Gaines, *Toxicol. Appl. Pharmacol.* **14**, 515 (1969). Review of toxicology and human exposure: *Toxicological Profile for Disulfoton* (PB95-264347, 1995) 239 pp.

Colorless oil, bp₀.₀₁ 108°, bp₁.₅ 132-133°. d₄²⁰ 1.144. n_D²⁰ 1.5348. Vapor pressure at 20°: 1.8×10^{-4} mm Hg. Insol in water. LD₅₀ in female, male rats (mg/kg): 2.3, 6.8 orally; 6, 15 dermally (Gaines).
Caution: Potential symptoms of overexposure are irritation of eyes, skin; nausea, vomiting, abdominal cramps, diarrhea, salivation; headache, giddiness, vertigo, weakness; rhinorrhea, chest tightness; blurred vision, miosis; cardiac irregularity; muscle fasciculation; dyspnea; eye and skin burns. *See NIOSH Pocket Guide to Chemical Hazards* (DHHS/NIOSH 97-140, 1997) p 124.
USE: Insecticide.

3366. Dita Bark. Alstonia cortex; Australian fever bark. The dried bark of *Alstonia scholaris* (L.) R. Br. and of *A. constricta* F. Muell., *Apocynaceae. Habit.* India, Ceylon, Philippine Islands, Australia. *Constit.* The alkaloids echitamine, echitenine, alsonine, porphyrine; echicerin—a non-nitrogenous substance; echitin, alstonidine and echitin.

3367. Ditazol. [18471-20-0] 2,2′-[(4,5-Diphenyl-2-oxazol-yl)imino]bisethanol; *N*-(4,5-diphenyloxazol-2-yl)diethanolamine; 2-[bis(β-hydroxyethyl)amino]-4,5-diphenyloxazole; 2,2′-dihy-droxy-*N*-(4,5-diphenyloxazol-2-yl)diethylamine; diethamphenazol; S-222; Ageroplas. $C_{19}H_{20}N_2O_3$; mol wt 324.37. C 70.35%, H 6.21%, N 8.64%, O 14.80%. Prepn: Marchetti *et al., J. Med. Chem.* **11**, 1092 (1968); **FR 1538009**; E. Marchetti, **US 3557135** (1968, 1971 to Ist. Farmacol. Serono). Series of articles on pharmacology and toxicology: L. Caprino *et al., Arzneim.-Forsch.* **23**, 1272-1291 (1973). Metabolism: Marchetti *et al., ibid.* 1291.

Monohydrate. Crystals from ethyl ether-petr ether, mp 96-98°. LD₅₀ in mice, rats (mg/kg): 9621, 11380 orally; 3390, 7770 i.p. (Caprino).
THERAP CAT: Anti-inflammatory.

3368. Dithianon. [3347-22-6] 5,10-Dihydro-5,10-dioxo-naphtho[2,3-*b*]-1,4-dithiin-2,3-dicarbonitrile; 1,4-dithiaanthraqui-none-2,3-dicarbonitrile; 2,3-dicyano-1,4-dithiaanthraquinone; IT-931; MV-119A; Delan. $C_{14}H_4N_2O_2S_2$; mol wt 296.32. C 56.75%, H 1.36%, N 9.45%, O 10.80%, S 21.64%. Prepn: van Schoor *et al.,* **US 2976296** (1961 to E. Merck). Properties and field trials: J. Berker *et al., Proc. 2nd Br. Insectic. Fungic. Conf.* **1963**, 351. LC determn in technical formulations: A. R. Hanks, *J. AOAC Int.* **78**, 1131 (1995). Environmental fate: M. Ueoka *et al., Chemo-*

sphere **35**, 2915 (1997). *Review:* E. Amadori, W. Heupt, *Anal. Methods Pestic. Plant Growth Regul.* **10**, 181-187 (1978).

Brown odorless crystals, mp 225°. d^{18} 1.55. Practically insol in water. Sol in dioxane, chlorobenzene, chloroform. LD_{50} orally in rats, guinea pigs: 638, 110 mg/kg (Amadori, Heupt).

USE: Fungicide.

3369. Dithiazanine Iodide. [514-73-8] 3-Ethyl-2-[5-(3-ethyl-2(3*H*)-benzothiazolylidene)-1,3-pentadienyl]benzothiazolium iodide; 3,3′-diethylthiadicarbocyanine iodide; Abminthic; Anelmid; Anguifugan; Delvex; Dejo; Déselmine; Dilombrin; Dizan; Nectocyd; Partel; Telmicid; Telmid. $C_{23}H_{23}IN_2S_2$; mol wt 518.48. C 53.28%, H 4.47%, I 24.48%, N 5.40%, S 12.37%. Prepn from 1-methylbenzothiazole ethiodide and β-(ethylmercapto)acrolein diethyl acetal: Kendall, Edwards, **US 2412815** (1946 to Ilford).

Green needles from methanol, dec 248°. Practically insol in water. Can be solubilized with polyvinylpyrrolidone: **CA 676636** (1963 to GAF).

USE: Sensitizer for photographic emulsions.

THERAP CAT: Anthelmintic (Nematodes).

THERAP CAT (VET): Anthelmintic.

3370. 2,2′-Dithiobis[benzothiazole]. [120-78-5] MBTS; 2,2′-dibenzothiazyl disulfide; benzothiazyl disulfide; dibenzthiazyl disulfide; mercaptobenzthiazyl ether; Thiofide. $C_{14}H_8N_2S_4$; mol wt 332.49. C 50.57%, H 2.43%, N 8.43%, S 38.58%. Formed by oxidation of 2-mercaptobenzothiazole.

Pale yellow needles from benzene. d 1.50. mp 180°; also reported as mp 186°; the commercial product, mp 168° min. Insoluble in water. Solubility at 25° (g/100 ml): in alcohol <0.2; in acetone <0.5; in benzene <0.5; in carbon tetrachloride <0.2 (somewhat more in chloroform); in ether <0.2; in naphtha <0.5.

USE: As accelerator in the rubber industry.

3371. 2,4-Dithiobiuret. [541-53-7] Thioimidodicarbonic diamide. $C_2H_5N_3S_2$; mol wt 135.21. C 17.77%, H 3.73%, N 31.08%, S 47.43%. $NH_2CSNHCSNH_2$. Prepd by the interaction of dicyandiamide and hydrogen sulfide in inert solvents under pressure: Sperry, **US 2371112** (1945 to Am. Cyanamid). *Review:* Kurzer, *Chem. Rev.* **56**, 138-144, 179-181 (1956).

Monoclinic or triclinic crystals. *Poisonous when ingested!* Apparent bulk density 1.522 g/ml at 30°. Dec 181°. uv max: 225, 280 nm (log ε 2.0, 2.2). Solubility at 27° = 0.27 g/100 ml water; 2.2 g/100 g ethanol; 16 g/100 g acetone; about 34 g/100 g Cellosolve. Solubility in boiling water about 8.0%. pH of satd aq soln at 30° = 5.8. Soluble in alkalies with formation of water-soluble salts. Solubility in 1% NaOH = 3.6 g/100 g soln; in 5% NaOH = 16 g/100 g; in 10% NaOH = 29 g/100 g.

Caution: Limited animal expts suggest high toxicity due to respiratory paralysis.

USE: Plasticizer, rubber accelerator, intermediate in resin manuf, in making insecticides and rodenticides. Can be used to delay the wilting of flowers.

3372. 4,4′-Dithiodimorpholine. [103-34-4] 4,4′-Dithiobis[morpholine]; morpholine *N,N*′-disulfide; dimorpholine *N,N*′-disulfide. $C_8H_{16}N_2O_2S_2$; mol wt 236.35. C 40.65%, H 6.82%, N 11.85%, O 13.54%, S 27.13%. Prepn: Blake, *J. Am. Chem. Soc.* **65**, 1267 (1943); *idem*, **US 2343524** (1944 to Monsanto); Harman, **US 2766236** and **GB 774570** (1956, 1957, both to Monsanto). Lambrech *et al.*, **US 2902402** (1959 to Pfizer).

Crystals, mp 124-125°.

USE: As staining protector in rubber; in vulcanization of rubber. As fungicide: Ladd, **US 2429097** (1949 to U.S. Rubber).

3373. 3,3-Dithiodipyridine Dihydrochloride. [538-45-4] 3,3′-Dithiobis[pyridine] dihydrochloride; 3,3-dipyridyl disulfide dihydrochloride. $C_{10}H_{10}Cl_2N_2S_2$; mol wt 293.24. C 40.96%, H 3.44%, Cl 24.18%, N 9.55%, S 21.87%. Prepd from 3-pyridinesulfonyl chloride and Na_2SO_3: Gibbs, Penny, **GB 582638** (1946).

Crystals from abs alc, mp 183°. Sol in water.

3374. Dithiopyr. [97886-45-8] 2-(Difluoromethyl)-4-(2-methylpropyl)-6-(trifluoromethyl)-3,5-pyridinedicarbothioic acid *S,S*-dimethyl ester; *S,S*-dimethyl 2-(difluoromethyl)-4-isobutyl-6-trifluoromethyl-3,5-pyridinedicarbothioate; MON-15100; MON-7200; Dimension. $C_{15}H_{16}F_5NO_2S_2$; mol wt 401.42. C 44.88%, H 4.02%, F 23.66%, N 3.49%, O 7.97%, S 15.98%. Selective herbicide for weed control in turfgrass and selected crops. Prepn: L. F. Lee, **EP 133612**; *idem*, **US 4692184** (1985, 1987 both to Monsanto). Herbicidal properties: M. Fujiyama, S. Yamane, *Shokubutsu no Kagaku Chosetsu* **24**, 49 (1989), *C.A.* **111**, 227154n (1989).

Colorless, crystalline solid with faint odor, mp 65°. vapor pressure at 25°: 4×10^{-6} mm Hg. Soly in water (20°): 1.38 ppm. LD_{50} orally in rats: >5000 mg/kg (Fujiyama, Yamane).

USE: Herbicide.

3375. Dithiosalicylic Acid. [527-89-9] 2-Hydroxybenzenecarbodithioic acid. $C_7H_6OS_2$; mol wt 170.25. C 49.38%, H 3.55%, O 9.40%, S 37.67%. Prepn from salicylaldehyde and ammonium polysulfide: Bruni, Levi, *Atti Accad. Naz. Lincei* **32**, (i), 5 (1923), *C.A.* **18**, 2694 (1924); *Beilstein* 2nd suppl. **vol. 10**, 78.

Orange-yellow needles, mp 48-50°. Moderately sol in water; sol in alcohol, ether, benzene, methanol.

3376. 1,4-Dithiothreitol. [3483-12-3] (2*R*,3*R*)-*rel*-1,4-Dimercapto-2,3-butanediol; Cleland's reagent; *threo*-2,3-dihydroxy-1,4-dithiolbutane. $C_4H_{10}O_2S_2$; mol wt 154.25. C 31.15%, H 6.53%, O 20.74%, S 41.58%. $HSCH_2(CHOH)_2CH_2SH$. Prepn: Evans *et al., J. Chem. Soc.* **1949**, 253.

Slightly hygroscopic needles from ether, mp 42-43°. Can be sublimed at 37° and 0.005 mm press; bp_2 125-130°. Redox potential: -0.33 volts at pH 7. Freely sol in water, ethanol, acetone, ethyl acetate, chloroform, ether.

USE: Protective agent for SH groups: Cleland, *Biochemistry* **3**, 480 (1964), *see also* "Cleland's Reagent" a detailed brochure and bibliography published by Calbiochem, Los Angeles.

3377. Dithizone. [60-10-6] Phenyldiazenecarbothioic acid 2-phenylhydrazide; (phenylazo)thioformic acid 2-phenylhydrazide; diphenylthiocarbazone. $C_{13}H_{12}N_4S$; mol wt 256.33. C 60.91%, H 4.72%, N 21.86%, S 12.51%. $C_6H_5N{=}NCSNHNHC_6H_5$. Prepn: E. Fischer, E. Besthorn, *Ann.* **212**, 316 (1882). Use as an analytical reagent: A. Stock, E. Pohland, *Angew. Chem.* **39**, 791 (1926); H. Fischer, *ibid.* **46**, 442 (1933); **50**, 919 (1937); *Organic Reagents for Metals* (Hopkins & Williams, 1934). Crystal structure: M. Laing, *J. Chem. Soc. Perkin Trans. 2* **1977**, 1248. Conformation in soln: A. T. Hutton, H. M. Irving, *Chem. Commun.* **1981**, 735. Monograph: *Analytical Sciences Monograph No. 5* entitled "Dithizone", H. M. Irving, Ed. (Chemical Society, London, 1977) 112 pp. *Review: idem, Crit. Rev. Anal. Chem.* **8**, 321-405 (1980).

Bluish-black cryst powder, mp 168° (dec). Insol in water. Sparingly sol in alc, freely in carbon tetrachloride, chloroform. Solns are not stable, but may be preserved by a layer of aq SO_2.

Caution: Has caused glycosuria and ocular injury in exptl animals.

USE: Sensitive reagent for several heavy metals, Co, Cu, Pb, and Hg; esp for the estimation of minute amounts of Pb.

3378. Ditiocarb Sodium. [148-18-5] Diethylcarbamodithioic acid sodium salt; diethyldithiocarbamic acid sodium salt; diethyldithiocarbamate sodium; dithiocarb; DTC; DDC; DEDC; DDTC; DeDTC; Imuthiol. $C_5H_{10}NNaS_2$; mol wt 171.26. C 35.07%, H 5.89%, N 8.18%, Na 13.42%, S 37.45%. $(C_2H_5)_2NCS_2Na$. Chelating agent with strong affinity for Hg, Cu, Ni and Zn. Also active as T-cell specific immunostimulant. Prepn: A. M. Clifford, J. G. Lichty, *J. Am. Chem. Soc.* **54**, 1163 (1932); A. L. Klebanskii, L. P. Fomina, *Zh. Obshch. Khim.* **30**, 794 (1960). Absorption spectrum: H. P. Koch, *J. Chem. Soc.* **1949**, 401. Inhibition of superoxide dismutase in mice: R. E. Heikkila *et al., J. Biol. Chem.* **251**, 2182 (1976); of cisplatin nephrotoxicity in rats: R. F. Borch *et al., Proc. Natl. Acad. Sci. USA* **77**, 5441 (1980). Clinical use in acute nickel carbonyl poisoning: F. W. Sunderman, F. W. Sunderman Jr., *Am. J. Med. Sci.* **236**, 26 (1958); F. W. Sunderman, *Ann. Clin. Lab. Sci.* **9**, 1 (1979); in acute cadmium poisoning: G. R. Gale *et al., ibid.* **11**, 476 (1981) and **13**, 207 (1983). Specific effects on T-cell regulation: A. Pompidou *et al., Int. J. Immunopharmacol.* **7**, 561 (1985). Clinical evaluation in T-cell deficient diseases: E. Lemarie *et al., Methods Find. Exp. Clin. Pharmacol.* **8**, 51 (1986); in AIDS-related complex: A. Pompidou *et al., Comp. Immunol. Microbiol. Infect. Dis.* **9**, 263 (1986). Review of pharmacology, toxicity and clinical uses: G. Renoux, *J. Pharmacol.* **13**, Suppl. 1, 95-134 (1982); of immunopharmacology and use in cancer immunotherapy: G. Renoux *et al., Adv. Exp. Med. Biol.* **166**, 223-239 (1983).

Trihydrate. $C_5H_{10}NNaS_2.3H_2O$. Thin, irregular plate-like crystals from acetone, mp 94-102°. Also reported as 90-92° (Sunderman, Sunderman). Freely sol in water; sol in ethanol, methanol, acetone. Insol in ether, benzene. The aq soln is alkaline to litmus and phenolphthalein and slowly dec. (pH of 10% aq soln is 11.6 at room temp). The addition of an acid to the aq soln produces a white turbidity due to the liberation of carbon disulfide. uv max (ethanol): 257, 290 nm (ε 1200, 13000). LD_{50} orally in rats, mice: 2830, 1870 mg/kg; i.v. in mice: >1000 mg/kg (Renoux, 1982).

USE: For colorimetric determination of small quantities of copper and for its separation from other metals.

THERAP CAT: Immunomodulator. Chelating agent (copper); Wilson's Disease treatment. Antidote (nickel, cadmium poisoning).

3379. 1,1-Di-*p*-tolylethane. [530-45-0] 1,1′-Ethylidenebis[4-methylbenzene]; α,α-di-*p*-tolylethane; *asym*-di-*p*-tolylethane; 4,4′-α-trimethyldiphenylmethane. $C_{16}H_{18}$; mol wt 210.31. C 91.38%, H 8.63%. Prepd by passing acetylene into a mixture of toluene and concd H_2SO_4 in presence of mercuric sulfate: Reichert, Nieuwland, *Org. Synth.* **IV**, 23 (1925).

Oily, highly refractive liquid. Aromatic odor. d_4^{20} 0.974. Not solid at $-20°$. bp 295-300°; bp_{12} 155-157°. Soluble in acetic acid.

3380. 1,2-Di-*p*-tolylethane. [538-39-6] 1,1′-(1,2-Ethanediyl)bis[4-methylbenzene]; α,β-di-*p*-tolylethane; *sym*-di-*p*-tolylethane; 4,4′-dimethyldibenzyl. $C_{16}H_{18}$; mol wt 210.31. C 91.38%, H 8.63%. Prepd by passing *p*-xylene vapor over red hot platinum wires: Meyer, Hofmann, *Monatsh. Chem.* **37**, 690 (1916).

Leaflets from methanol; plates from ligroin. mp 82°; bp_{730} 296-298°; bp_{18} 178°. Sol in benzene, moderately sol in alcohol, petr ether.

3381. *p*-Ditolylmercury. [537-64-4] Bis(4-methylphenyl)mercury. $C_{14}H_{14}Hg$; mol wt 382.85. C 43.92%, H 3.69%, Hg 52.39%. $(CH_3C_6H_4)_2Hg$. Prepd by the action of sodium iodide on *p*-tolylmercuric chloride in ethanol: Whitmore *et al., Org. Synth.* **3**, 65 (1923); by boiling *p*-bromotoluene with sodium amalgam in xylene in the presence of ethyl acetate as a catalyst: Dreher, Otto, *Ann.* **154**, 171 (1870); LaCoste, Michaelis, *ibid.* **201**, 246 (1880); *Compt. Rend.* **68**, 1298 (1869).

Needles from xylene. mp 238°. Insol in water. Slightly sol in cold alcohol; sol in hot benzene, xylene, chloroform, carbon disulfide.

3382. Diuron. [330-54-1] *N*′-(3,4-Dichlorophenyl)-*N*,*N*-dimethylurea; 1,1-dimethyl-3-(3,4-dichlorophenyl)urea; Diurex; Karmex; Urox D. $C_9H_{10}Cl_2N_2O$; mol wt 233.09. C 46.38%, H 4.32%, Cl 30.42%, N 12.02%, O 6.86%. Prepn: Jones, US **2768971** (1956 to I.C.I.). Toxicity data: E. M. Boyd, V. Krupa, *J. Agric. Food Chem.* **18**, 1104 (1970). Review of environmental impact: S. Giacomazzi, N. Cochet, *Chemosphere* **56**, 1021-1032 (2004).

Crystals, mp 158-159°. Soly in water at 25°: 42 ppm. Very low soly in hydrocarbon solvents. Vapor pressure at 50°: 3.1×10^{-6} mm Hg. Partition coefficient (octanol/water): 2.6. LD_{50} orally in rats: 1690 mg/kg (Boyd, Krupa).

Caution: Potential symptoms of overexposure are irritation of eyes, skin, nose, throat. Potential symptoms of overexposure in exptl animals are anemia, methemoglobinemia. *See NIOSH Pocket Guide to Chemical Hazards* (DHHS/NIOSH 97-140, 1997) p 124.

USE: Pre-emergent herbicide.

3383. Divicine. [32267-39-3] 2,6-Diamino-1,6-dihydro-4,5-pyrimidinedione; 2,6-diamino-4,5-pyrimidinediol; 2,6-diamine-5-hydroxy-4(3*H*)-pyrimidinone; 2,4-diamino-5,6-dihydroxypyrimidine. $C_4H_6N_4O_2$; mol wt 142.12. C 33.80%, H 4.26%, N 39.42%, O 22.52%. From vicine by heating with dil H_2SO_4: Ritthausen, *Ber.* **29**, 2108 (1896); Levene, Senior, *J. Biol. Chem.* **25**, 607 (1916). Structure: Bendich, Clements, *Biochim. Biophys. Acta* **12**, 462 (1953). Synthesis: Davall, Laney, *J. Chem. Soc.* **1956**, 2124; Chesterfield *et al., ibid.* **1964**, 1001.

Brownish needles, dec above 280°. One gram dissolves in 100 ml boiling water, in about 350 ml cold water. Soluble in 10% KOH.

Diacetate. $C_8H_{10}N_4O_4$. Crystals from water, dec 309-312°.

3384. Dixanthogen. [502-55-6] Thioperoxydicarbonic acid diethyl ester; dithiobis[thioformic acid] O,O-diethyl ester; O,O-diethyl dithiobis[thioformate]; bisethylxanthogen; diethyl xanthogenate; ethylxanthic disulfide; preparation K; EXD; Auligen; Aulinogen; Bexide; Herbisan; Lenisarin. $C_6H_{10}O_2S_4$; mol wt 242.40. C 29.73%, H 4.16%, O 13.20%, S 52.91%. Prepn: Losse, Wottgen, *J. Prakt. Chem.* **13**, 260 (1961). Metabolic studies: Gutenmann, Lisk, *J. Agric. Food Chem.* **19**, 200 (1971). Toxicity: G. W. Bailey, J. L. White, *Residue Rev.* **10**, 97 (1965).

Yellow needles, mp 28-32°. Onion-like odor. Soly in alcohol: 2 g/100 ml. Freely sol in benzene, ether, petr ether, oils. Almost insol in water. LD_{50} orally in rats: 480 mg/kg (Bailey, White).

USE: Insecticide formulations; herbicide.

THERAP CAT: Ectoparasiticide.

3385. Dixyrazine. [2470-73-7] 2-[2-[4-[2-Methyl-3-(10H-phenothiazin-10-yl)propyl]-1-piperazinyl]ethoxy]ethanol; 10-[2-methyl-3-(4-hydroxyethoxyethyl-1-piperazinyl)propyl]phenothiazine; 1-[2-(2-hydroxyethoxy)ethyl]-4-[2-methyl-3-(10-phenothiazinyl)propyl]piperazine; UCB-3412; Esucos; Roscal. $C_{24}H_{33}N_3$-O_2S; mol wt 427.60. C 67.41%, H 7.78%, N 9.83%, O 7.48%, S 7.50%. Prepn: H. Morren, **GB 861420** (1961). Partition properties: B.-A. Persson, *Acta Pharm. Suec.* **5**, 335 (1968). GC-MS determn in blood: G. Brante *et al., Eur. J. Clin. Pharmacol.* **20**, 307 (1981). Clinical pharmacokinetics: H. Liedholm *et al., Drug-Nutr. Interact.* **3**, 87 (1985). Clinical trial in postoperative nausea and vomiting: E. Kokinsky *et al., Acta Anaesthesiol. Scand.* **43**, 191 (1999); A. Johansson *et al., ibid.* **44**, 1093 (2000); as topical anesthetic for cataract surgery: E. Monestam *et al., J. Cataract Refract. Surg.* **27**, 445 (2001). Review of clinical chemistry and early clinical studies: T. Fokstuen, *Int. J. Neuropsychiat.* **340**, 294-299 (1965).

pKa₁: 7.8; pKa₂: 3.65.

Dihydrochloride. [60539-20-0] $C_{24}H_{33}N_3O_2S.2HCl$. Crystals from isopropanol, mp 192°.

THERAP CAT: Antipsychotic; antiemetic; anesthetic (local).

3386. Dizocilpine. [77086-21-6] 10,11-Dihydro-5-methyl-5H-dibenzo[a,d]cyclohepten-5,10-imine; (+)-5-methyl-10,11-dihydro-5H-dibenzo[a,d]cyclohepten-5,10-imine. $C_{16}H_{15}N$; mol wt 221.30. C 86.84%, H 6.83%, N 6.33%. Non-competitive NMDA, *q.v.*, receptor antagonist. Prepn of racemate: M. E. Christy *et al., J. Org. Chem.* **44**, 3117 (1979); T. R. Lamanec *et al., ibid.* **53**, 1768 (1988); and of enantiomers: **BE 882361**; P. Anderson *et al.,* **US 4399141** (1980, 1983 both to Merck & Co.). Series of papers on pharmacological activities: B. V. Clineschmidt *et al., Drug Dev. Res.* **2**, 123-163 (1982). NMDA receptor binding studies: E. H. F. Wong *et al., Proc. Natl. Acad. Sci. USA* **83**, 7104

(1986); A. C. Foster, E. H. F. Wong, *Br. J. Pharmacol.* **91**, 403 (1987); J. E. Huettner, B. P. Bean, *Proc. Natl. Acad. Sci. USA* **85**, 1307 (1988). Metabolism in animals: H. B. Hucker *et al., Drug Metab. Dispos.* **11**, 54 (1983). Pharmacokinetics: A. S. Troupin *et al., Curr. Probl. Epilepsy* **4**, 191 (1986). Protective effects against excitotoxic amino acid-induced neuronal degeneration: G. N. Woodruff *et al., Neuropharmacology* **26**, 903 (1987); A. C. Foster *et al., Neurosci. Lett.* **76**, 307 (1987); A. C. Foster *et al., J. Neurosci.* **8**, 4745 (1988); specifically in ischemia: R. Gill *et al., Neuroscience* **25**, 847 (1988); E. Ozyurt *et al., J. Cereb. Blood Flow Metab.* **8**, 138 (1988). Anticonvulsant activity in models of epilepsy: K. Sato *et al., Brain Res.* **463**, 12 (1988); M. E. Gilbert, *ibid.* **90**. Clinical evaluation in attention deficit disorder: F. W. Reimherr *et al., Psychopharmacol. Bull.* **22**, 237 (1986).

White solid from cyclohexane, mp 68.5-69°. $[\alpha]_{589}^{20}$ +161.4° (c = 0.038 g/2 ml ethanol).

Maleate. [77086-22-7] MK-801. $C_{16}H_{15}N.C_4H_4O_4$; mol wt 337.37. Crystalline solid, mp 208.5-210°. $[\alpha]_D^{20}$ +114° (c = 0.0128 g/2 ml ethanol).

(−)-Form. [77086-19-2] White solid from cyclohexane, mp 68.5-69.5°. $[\alpha]_{589}$ −160.8° (c = 0.032 g/2 ml ethanol).

USE: Biochemical probe for NMDA receptors.

3387. Djenkolic Acid. [498-59-9] S,S'-Methylenebis-L-cysteine; 3,3′-(methylenedithio)dialanine; 3,3′-methylenedithiobis(2-aminopropanoic acid); L-cysteine thioacetal of formaldehyde. C_7-$H_{14}N_2O_4S_2$; mol wt 254.33. C 33.06%, H 5.55%, N 11.01%, O 25.16%, S 25.22%. $CH_2[SCH_2CH(NH_2)COOH]_2$. An amino acid isolated from the djenkol bean (*Pithecolobium lobatum* Benth., *Leguminosae*): van Veen, Hyman, *Rec. Trav. Chim.* **54**, 493 (1935). Synthesis from 1 mol formaldehyde and 2 mols L-cysteine in strong HCl solution: Armstrong, du Vigneaud, *J. Biol. Chem.* **168**, 373 (1947); *cf.* du Vigneaud, Patterson, *ibid.* **114**, 633 (1936); Middlebrook, Phillips, *Biochem. J.* **41**, 218 (1947). Synthesis of homologs: Frankel, Gertner, *J. Chem. Soc.* **1960**, 898.

Rosettes of needles of various lengths. Gradually dec between 300 and 350°. $[\alpha]_D^{20.5}$ −65.0° (1.0N HCl); $[\alpha]_D^{25}$ −47.5° (c = 2 in 1.0N HCl). Very sparingly sol in cold water. Soly in boiling water about 1 in 200. Readily sol in aq solns of alkalies or acids.

Monohydrochloride. $C_7H_{14}N_2O_4S_2.HCl$. Slender prisms, dec 250-300°. Sol in water.

Dibenzoyldjenkolic acid. $C_{21}H_{22}N_2O_6S_2$. Crystals, mp 87.5-89°.

3388. DMAN. [20734-58-1] N,N,N',N'-Tetramethyl-1,8-naphthalenediamine; 1,8-bis(dimethylamino)naphthalene; proton sponge. $C_{14}H_{18}N_2$; mol wt 214.31. C 78.46%, H 8.47%, N 13.07%. Prototype of a class of neutral aromatic diamines with exceptionally high basicity known as proton sponges. Prepn: W. G. Brown, N. J. Letang, *J. Am. Chem. Soc.* **63**, 358 (1941); and basicity study: R. W. Alder *et al., J. Chem. Soc. Chem. Commun.* **1968**, 723. X-ray crystal structure: H. Einspahr *et al., Acta Crystallogr.* **B29**, 1611 (1973). Proton transfer studies: F. Hibbert, *J. Chem. Soc. Perkin Trans. 2* **1974**, 1862. Ab initio structural studies: J. A. Platts *et al., J. Org. Chem.* **59**, 4647 (1994); and fluorescence spectroscopy: A. Szemik-Hojniak *et al., J. Am. Chem. Soc.* **120**, 4840 (1998). Charge distribution: P. R. Mallinson *et al., ibid.* **121**, 4640 (1999). ^{13}C NMR study of hydrogen bonding: M. Pietrzak *et al., ibid.* **123**, 4338 (2001). Catalytic activity: I. Rodriguez *et al., J. Catal.* **183**, 14 (1999). Review of chemistry: H. A. Staab, T. Saupe, *Angew. Chem. Int. Ed.* **27**, 865-879 (1988); R. W. Alder, *Chem. Rev.* **89**, 1215-1223 (1989).

bp$_4$ 144-145°. mp 47-48°. d 1.12. Absorption max: 335 nm (log ε 3.96). pKa 12.1.

USE: Very strong base in organic synthesis and catalysis.

3389. DMAP. [1122-58-3] *N,N*-Dimethyl-4-pyridinamine; 4-(dimethylamino)pyridine. C$_7$H$_{10}$N$_2$; mol wt 122.17. C 68.82%, H 8.25%, N 22.93%. Basic nucleophilic catalyst. Prepn: E. Koenigs *et al., Ber.* **58**, 2571 (1925). Fluorescence spectra: S. Mishina *et al., J. Photochem. Photobiol. A* **141**, 153 (2001). Use in Baylis-Hillman chemistry: K. Y. Lee *et al., Bull. Korean Chem. Soc.* **23**, 659 (2002); in olefin hydroxylations: Q. Yao, *Org. Lett.* **4**, 2197 (2002); in regioselective acylations: T. Kurahashi *et al., Tetrahedron* **58**, 8669 (2002). Review of early literature and use in acylation chemistry: G. Höfle *et al., Angew. Chem. Int. Ed.* **17**, 569-583 (1978); U. Ragnarsson, L. Grehn, *Acc. Chem. Res.* **31**, 494-501 (1998); and of alkylation: E. F. V. Scriven, *Chem. Soc. Rev.* **12**, 129-161 (1983). Brief description and synthetic uses: A. Hassner, "4-(Dimethylamino)pyridine" in *Encyclopedia of Reagents for Organic Synthesis* **3**, L. A. Paquette, Ed. (John Wiley & Sons, New York, 1995) pp 2022-2023.

Colorless crystalline solid, mp 112-113°. pKa (20°): 9.70. Dipole moment (25°): 4.31 (benzene). Very sol in methanol, ethyl acetate, chloroform, methylene chloride, 1,2-dichloroethane, acetone and acetic acid; less sol in cold hexane, cyclohexane and water.

USE: In a wide variety of organic syntheses as a catalyst.

3390. DMC. [125376-11-6] 2-Chloro-4,5-dihydro-1,3-dimethyl-1*H*-imidazolium chloride; 2-chloro-1,3-dimethylimidazolinium chloride. C$_5$H$_8$Cl$_2$N$_2$; mol wt 167.04. C 35.95%, H 4.83%, Cl 42.45%, N 16.77%. Dehydrating agent under nearly neutral conditions. For prepn, *see:* H.-B. König *et al., US 3959258* (1976 to Bayer). NMR spectrum: H.-O. Kalinowski, H. Kessler, *Org. Magn. Reson.* **6**, 305 (1974). Series of articles on properties, dehydration and other reaction types: T. Isobe, T. Ishikawa, *J. Org. Chem.* **64**, 5832, 6984, 6989 (1999). Use as a dehydrating reagent: M. Node *et al., Tetrahedron Lett.* **39**, 6331 (1998).

Colorless and odorless prisms, mp 95-100°. Soly at room temperature (mL solvent/g DMC): acetic acid <1; water <1; methanol <1; ethanol <1; isopropanol <2; *n*-butanol <3; CHCl$_3$ <1; CCl$_4$ >50; *n*-hexane >50; THF >50; DMF 6.

USE: In organic syntheses for numerous reactions types such as condensations, chlorinations.

3391. DMMP. [756-79-6] Methylphosphonic acid dimethyl ester; dimethyl methylphosphonate. C$_3$H$_9$O$_3$P; mol wt 124.08. C 29.04%, H 7.31%, O 38.68%, P 24.96%. Testing chemical to simulate nerve agents such as sarin, *q.v.* Prepn: T. Milobedzki, K. Szulgin, *Chem. Zentralbl.* **89**, 914 (1918); by photolysis: M. Nakamura *et al., J. Chem. Soc. Perkin Trans. 1* **1994**, 141. Photodestruction: L. J. Radziemski, Jr., *J. Environ. Sci. Health* **B16**, 337 (1981). Raman spectroscopic determn: N. Taranenko *et al., J. Raman Spectrosc.* **27**, 379 (1996). Use as simulant in compd destruction study: M. G. Nickelsen *et al., J. Adv. Oxid. Technol.* **3**, 43 (1998). Use as cell volume probe: J. E. Raftos *et al., Biochim. Biophys. Acta* **968**, 160 (1988); J. A. Barry *et al., Biochemistry* **32**, 4665 (1993). Description of use as flame retardant: E. D. Weil in *Kirk-Othmer Encyclopedia of Chemical Technology* **vol. 10** (John Wiley, New York, 4th ed., 1993) pp 976-998. Review of toxicology: J. C. Rowland *et al., Health Advisory for Dimethyl Methylphosphonate (DMMP)* (PB 93-117018, 1993) 86 pp.

Colorless liquid, mp <50°. bp$_{754}$ 181°. d 1.145. Vapor pressure: (20°) <0.1 torr; (25°) 2.4 torr; (65°) 20 torr. pKa (20°) in water: 2.37. Sol in water. Miscible in alcohol, ether, benzene, acetone, carbon tetrachloride. Insol in heavy mineral oil. n 1.411. Log P (octanol/water): −1.88. LD$_{50}$ in rats, mice (mg/kg): 10190, >6810 orally (Rowland).

USE: NMR probe for cell volume. Flame retardant. Simulant for nerve agents.

3392. DMPA. [299-85-4] (1-Methylethyl)phosphoramidothioic acid *O*-(2,4-dichlorophenyl) *O*-methyl ester; isopropylphosphoramidothioic acid *O*-2,4-(dichlorophenyl) *O*-methyl ester; *O*-(2,4-dichlorophenyl) *O*-methyl isopropylphosphoramidothioate; K-22023; Dow 1329; ENT-25647; OMS-115; Dowco 118; Zytron. C$_{10}$H$_{14}$Cl$_2$NO$_2$PS; mol wt 314.17. C 38.23%, H 4.49%, Cl 22.57%, N 4.46%, O 10.19%, P 9.86%, S 10.21%. Prepn: Blair *et al., J. Agric. Food Chem.* **11**, 237 (1963). Synthesis of the optical isomers: Seiber, Tolkmith, *Tetrahedron* **25**, 381 (1969). Use as a herbicide: Leasure, *US 3074790* (1963 to Dow); as a plant growth regulator: Holmsen, *Weed Sci.* **17**, 187 (1969). Neurotoxicity in chickens: B. M. Francis *et al., J. Environ. Sci. Health* **B15**, 313 (1980). Toxicity study: E. W. Schafer, *Toxicol. Appl. Pharmacol.* **21**, 315 (1972).

Solid, mp 51.4°. Vapor pressure at 150°: 2 mm. Slightly sol in water (5 ppm); freely sol in acetone, benzene, carbon tetrachloride. LD$_{50}$ orally in rats: 270-360 mg/kg (Schafer).

USE: Herbicide; plant growth regulator.

3393. DMPO. [3317-61-1] 3,4-Dihydro-2,2-dimethyl-2*H*-pyrrole 1-oxide; 5,5-dimethyl-1-pyrroline 1-oxide. C$_6$H$_{11}$NO; mol wt 113.16. C 63.68%, H 9.80%, N 12.38%, O 14.14%. Nitrone spin trap. Prepn: R. Bonnett *et al., J. Chem. Soc.* **1959**, 2094; D. L. Haire *et al., J. Org. Chem.* **51**, 4298 (1986); and purification: E. G. Janzen *et al., Chem. Biol. Interact.* **70**, 167 (1989). uv absorption: L. S. Kaminsky, M. Lamchen, *J. Chem. Soc.* **1968**, 1085. Use as spin trap in biological systems: A. I. Cederbaum, G. Cohen, *Arch. Biochem. Biophys.* **204**, 397 (1980); A. S. W. Li *et al., Biochem. Biophys. Res. Commun.* **146**, 1191 (1987); for neutrophil activation studies: B. E. Britigan, D. R. Hamill, *Arch. Biochem. Biophys.* **275**, 72 (1989); *eidem, Free Radical Biol. Med.* **8**, 459 (1990); in reperfusion injury: C. M. Arroyo *et al., FEBS Lett.* **221**, 101 (1987); A. Tosaki, P. Braquet, *Am. Heart J.* **120**, 819 (1990). Use in HPLC quantitation of oxygen free radicals *in vivo*: P. S. Rao *et al., Chromatographia* **30**, 19 (1990).

Nitrone as white crystalline solid. Very hygroscopic. Turns yellow with time even at −20°C sealed under vacuum and protected from light. uv max in cyclohexane: 246 nm (ε 9000); ethanol: 234 nm (ε 7700); water: 226 nm (ε 8600); *N*-hydrochloric acid: 226 nm (ε 7000); ether: 246 nm.

USE: Spin trap agent for biological systems.

3394. Dobesilate Calcium. [20123-80-2] 2,5-Dihydroxybenzenesulfonic acid calcium salt; calcium dobesilate; hydroquinone calcium sulfonate; Dexium; Doxium. C$_{12}$H$_{10}$CaO$_{10}$S$_2$; mol wt 418.41. C 34.45%, H 2.41%, Ca 9.58%, O 38.24%, S 15.33%. Prepn: *ES 335945* (1967 to Labs. Esteve), *C.A.* **69**, 106253z (1968); *FR M6163*; A. Esteve-Subirana, *US 3509207* (1968, 1970 both to Labs. OM). Clinical trials: Berson, *Praxis* **59**, 1305 (1970); **61**, 52 (1972). Metabolism: A. Benakis *et al., Therapie* **29**, 211 (1974).

White, powdery crystals from water, mp >300° (dec). Color deepens to pink upon exposure to air. Very soluble in water and alcohol. Practically insol in ether, benzene, chloroform. LD_{50} in mice: 700 mg/kg (Esteve-Subirana).

THERAP CAT: Vasotropic.

3395. Dobutamine. [34368-04-2] 4-[2-[[3-(4-Hydroxyphenyl)-1-methylpropyl]amino]ethyl]-1,2-benzenediol; (±)-4-[2-[[3-(p-hydroxyphenyl)-1-methylpropyl]amino]ethyl]pyrocatechol; 3,4-dihydroxy-N-[3-(4-hydroxyphenyl)-1-methylpropyl]-β-phenylethylamine; Compound 81929. $C_{18}H_{23}NO_3$; mol wt 301.38. C 71.73%, H 7.69%, N 4.65%, O 15.93%. $β_1$-Adrenergic agonist; derivative of dopamine, q.v. Prepn: R. R. Tuttle, J. Mills, **DE 2317710**; eidem, **US 3987200** (1973, 1976 to Lilly). Pharmacology: R. Weber, R. R. Tuttle in *Pharmacological and Biochemical Properties of Drug Substances* vol. 1, M. E. Goldberg, Ed. (Am. Pharm. Assoc., Washington, DC, 1977) pp 109-124; E. H. Sonnenblick et al., *N. Engl. J. Med.* **300**, 17 (1979). Comprehensive description: R. H. Bishara, H. B. Long, *Anal. Profiles Drug Subs.* **8**, 139-158 (1979).

Hydrochloride. [49745-95-1] Inotrex (obsolete); Dobutrex. $C_{18}H_{23}NO_3 \cdot HCl$; mol wt 337.84. Crystals, mp 184-186°. uv max (methanol): 281, 223 nm (ε 4768, 14400). pKa 9.45. Rapidly oxidized at pH 11-13. LD_{50} i.v. in mice: ~73 mg/kg (Weber, Tuttle).

THERAP CAT: Cardiotonic.

3396. Docarpamine. [74639-40-0] 4-[2-[[(2S)-2-(Acetylamino)-4-(methylthio)-1-oxobutyl]amino]ethyl]-1,2-phenylene diethyl ester; (−)-(S)-2-acetamido-N-(3,4-dihydroxyphenethyl)-4-(methylthio)butyramide bis(ethylcarbonate) (ester); N-(N-acetyl-L-methionyl)-O,O-bis(ethoxycarbonyl)dopamine; N-(N-acetyl-L-methionyl)-3,4-diethoxycarboxyphenethylamine; TA-870; Tanadopa. $C_{21}H_{30}N_2O_8S$; mol wt 470.54. C 53.60%, H 6.43%, N 5.95%, O 27.20%, S 6.81%. Dopamine prodrug. Prepn: T. Kiguchi et al., **EP 7441**; eidem, **US 4228183** (both 1980 to Tanabe Seiyaku). Pharmacology: I. Yamaguchi et al., *J. Cardiovasc. Pharmacol.* **13**, 879 (1989). Mechanism of action: S. Nishiyama et al., ibid. **14**, 175 (1989). Pharmacokinetics: M. Yoshikawa et al., *Drug Metab. Dispos.* **16**, 754 (1988). Metabolism in humans: eidem, ibid. **18**, 212 (1990). HPLC determn in biological fluids: eidem, *Biomed. Chromatogr.* **4**, 181 (1990). Review: S. Nishiyama et al., *Cardiovasc. Drug Rev.* **10**, 101-116 (1992).

Crystals form ethyl acetate/n-hexane, mp 85-90°. $[α]_D^{20}$ −15.6° (c = 2 in methanol). Also reported as crystalline powder, mp 105-108° (Nishiyama, 1992). Slightly sol in water, readily sol in ethanol. LD_{50} in male, female rats (mg/kg): 1000-1400, ~1000 s.c.; in rats, dogs (mg/kg): >2000 orally (Nishiyama, 1992).

THERAP CAT: Cardiotonic.

3397. Docetaxel. [114977-28-5] (αR,βS)-β-[[(1,1-Dimethylethoxy)carbonyl]amino]-α-hydroxybenzenepropanoic acid (2aR,-4S,4aS,6R,9S,11S,12S,12aR,12bS)-12b-(acetyloxy)-12-(benzoyloxy)-2a,3,4,4a,5,6,9,10,11,12,12a,12b-dodecahydro-4,6,11-trihydroxy-4a,8,13,13-tetramethyl-5-oxo-7,11-methano-1H-cyclodeca[3,4]benz[1,2-b]oxet-9-yl ester; N-debenzoyl-N-(tert-butoxycarbonyl)-10-deacetyltaxol; NSC-628503; RP-56976; Taxotere. $C_{43}H_{53}NO_{14}$; mol wt 807.88. C 63.93%, H 6.61%, N 1.73%, O 27.73%. Semisynthetic derivative of paclitaxel, q.v., prepd using a natural precursor, **10-deacetylbaccatin III**, extracted from the needles of the European yew tree, *Taxus baccata* L., *Taxaceae*. Antimitotic agent that promotes the assembly of microtubules and inhibits their depolymerization to free tubulin. Prepn: M. Colin et al., **EP 253738**; eidem, **US 4814470** (1988, 1989 both to Rhône-Poulenc Sante); L. Mangatal et al., *Tetrahedron* **45**, 4177 (1989). Synthesis of the side chain: J.-N. Denis et al., *J. Org. Chem.* **56**, 6939 (1991). Structure-activity study: F. Guéritte-Voegelein et al., *J. Med. Chem.* **34**, 992 (1991). Cytotoxic activity and mechanism of action: I. Ringel, S. B. Horwitz, *J. Natl. Cancer Inst.* **83**, 288 (1991). *In vivo* antitumor activity: M.-C. Bissery et al., *Cancer Res.* **51**, 4845 (1991). HPLC determn: J. C. Vergniol et al., *J. Chromatogr.* **582**, 273 (1992). Clinical pharmacokinetics and toxicology: J.-M. Extra et al., *Cancer Res.* **53**, 1037 (1993). Clinical trials in prostate cancer: I. F. Tannock et al., *N. Engl. J. Med.* **351**, 1502 (2004); D. P. Petrylak et al., ibid. 1513. Symposium on clinical experience: *Semin. Oncol.* **27**, Suppl. 3, 1-29 (2000). Review of mechanism of action and combination therapies: R. S. Herbst, F. R. Khuri, *Cancer Treat. Rev.* **29**, 407-415 (2003); of clinical studies in non-small cell lung cancer: A. M. Davies et al., *Expert Opin. Pharmacother.* **4**, 553-565 (2003).

mp 232°. $[α]_D$ −36° (c = 0.74 in ethanol). uv max: 230, 275, 283 nm (ε 14800, 1730, 1670).

THERAP CAT: Antineoplastic.

3398. Docosahexaenoic Acid. [6217-54-5] (4Z,7Z,10Z,-13Z,16Z,19Z)-4,7,10,13,16,19-Docosahexaenoic acid; cervonic acid; doconexent; DHA. $C_{22}H_{32}O_2$; mol wt 328.49. C 80.44%, H 9.82%, O 9.74%. Omega-3 fatty acid found in marine fish oils and in many phospholipids. Major structural component of excitable membranes of the retina and brain; synthesized in the liver from α-linolenic acid, q.v. Isoln from oil of *Sardina ocellata* J. and structure: J. M. Whitcutt, *Biochem. J.* **67**, 60 (1957). Improved isoln from cod liver oil: S. W. Wright et al., *J. Org. Chem.* **52**, 4399 (1987). Effect on brain and behavioral development: P. E. Wainwright, *Neurosci. Biobehav. Rev.* **16**, 193 (1992). Review of uptake and metabolism by retinal cells: N. G. Bazan, E. B. Rodriguez de Turco, *J. Ocul. Pharmacol.* **10**, 591-603 (1994). Review of clinical studies in infant formula supplementation: M. Makrides et al., *Lipids* **31**, 115-119 (1996).

Clear, faintly yellow oil, mp −44.7 to −44.5°. n_D^{26} 1.5017.

USE: Nutritional supplement.

3399. n-Docosanol. [661-19-8] 1-Docosanol; behenic alcohol; behenyl alcohol; docosyl alcohol; Abreva; Lidakol. $C_{22}H_{46}O$;

mol wt 326.60. C 80.90%, H 14.20%, O 4.90%. $H_3C(CH_2)_{21}OH$. Naturally occurring alcohol; active principal of Pygeum africanum extract, *q.v.*, that has been used to treat benign prostatic hypertrophy (BPH). Prepn: R. Willstätter, E. W. Mayer, *Ber.* **41**, 1475 (1908); P. A. Levene, F. A. Taylor, *J. Biol. Chem.* **59**, 905 (1924). Surface thermodynamic properties: S. Pathak, S. S. Katti, *J. Chem. Eng. Data* **14**, 359 (1969). GC-MS determn in Pygeum africanum extract: N. Pierini *et al.*, *Boll. Chim. Farm.* **121**, 27 (1982). Antiviral activity: D. H Katz *et al.*, *Ann. N.Y. Acad. Sci.* **724**, 472 (1994). Study of mechanism of action in BPH: J. Müntzing *et al.*, *Invest. Urol.* **17**, 176 (1979); vs herpes simplex virus: L. E. Pope *et al.*, *Antiviral Res.* **40**, 85 (1998). Clinical evaluation in recurrent herpes labialis: L. Habbema *et al.*, *Acta Derm. Venereol.* **76**, 479 (1996). mp 70.5-71.5°. bp_{22mm} 180°. d^{75} 0.8063 g/ml; d^{85} 0.7986 g/ml; d^{95} 0.7911 g/ml. Surface tension (dyne/cm): 21.82 (75°); 21.17 (85°); 20.53 (95°). n^{75} 1.4360.

THERAP CAT: Antiviral (topical).

3400. Docusate Calcium. [128-49-4] Sulfobutanedioic acid 1,4-bis(2-ethylhexyl)ester calcium salt; bis[2-ethylhexyl]calcium sulfosuccinate; calcium dioctyl sulfosuccinate; dioctyl calcium sulfosuccinate; Surfak. $C_{40}H_{74}CaO_{14}S_2$; mol wt 883.22. C 54.40%, H 8.44%, Ca 4.54%, O 25.36%, S 7.26%. Prepd from dioctyl sodium sulfosuccinate dissolved in isopropanol and from calcium chloride dissolved in methanol: Klotz, US 3035973 (1962 to Lloyd Brothers).

White precipitate. Sol in mineral and vegetable oils, liq polyethylene glycol. Practically insol in glycerol. Claimed to have greater surface-active wetting properties than the sodium salt.

Ingredient of *Doxidan* which also contains phenolphthalein.

THERAP CAT: Stool softener.

3401. Docusate Sodium. [577-11-7] Sulfobutanedioic acid 1,4-bis(2-ethylhexyl) ester sodium salt; sulfosuccinic acid 1,4-bis(2-ethylhexyl) ester *S*-sodium salt; bis(2-ethylhexyl)sodium sulfosuccinate; dioctyl sodium sulfosuccinate; sodium dioctyl sulfosuccinate; DSS; Aerosol OT; Colace; Comfolax; Coprola; Dioctylal; Dioctyl; Diotilan; Disonate; Doxinate; Doxol; Dulcivac; Jamylène; Molatoc; Molcer; Nevax; Regutol; Soliwax; Velmol; Waxsol; Yal. $C_{20}H_{37}NaO_7S$; mol wt 444.56. C 54.03%, H 8.39%, Na 5.17%, O 25.19%, S 7.21%. Prepn: Jaeger, US 2028091; US 2176423 (1936, 1939, both to Am. Cyanamid). Structure and wetting power: Caryl, *Ind. Eng. Chem.* **33**, 731 (1941). Comprehensive description: S. Ahuja, J. Cohen, *Anal. Profiles Drug Subs.* **2**, 199-219 (1973); **12**, 713-720 (1983). For structure see Docusate calcium.

Available as wax-like solid, usually in rolls of tissue-thin material; also as 50-75% solns in various solvents. Soly in water (g/l): 15 (25°), 23 (40°), 30 (50°), 55 (70°). Sol in CCl₄, petr ether, naphtha, xylene, dibutyl phthalate, liq petrolatum, acetone, alcohol, vegetable oils. Very sol in water + alcohol, water + water-miscible organic solvents. Stable in acid and neutral solns; hydrolyzes in alkaline solns.

Note: Ingredient of the laxative *Peri-Colace* which also contains casanthranol.

Docusate potassium. [7491-09-0] Rectalad. $C_{20}H_{37}KO_7S$; mol wt 460.67.

USE: Sodium salt as pharmaceutic aid (surfactant); as wetting agent in industrial, pharmaceutical, cosmetic and food applications; dispersing and solubilizing agent in foods; adjuvant in tablet formation.

THERAP CAT: Stool softener.

THERAP CAT (VET): Stool softener.

3402. Dodecahedrane. [4493-23-6] Hexadecahydro-5,2,1-6,3,4-[2,3]butanediyl[1,4]diylidenedipentaleno[2,1,6-*cde*:2′,1′,6′-*gha*]pentalene; pentagonal dodecahedrane. $C_{20}H_{20}$; mol wt 260.37.

C 92.26%, H 7.74%. Classical uniform convex polyhedrane. Theoretical studies: O. Ermer, *Angew. Chem. Int. Ed.* **16**, 411 (1977); R. L. Disch, J. M. Schulman, *J. Am. Chem. Soc.* **103**, 3297 (1981). Review of synthetic studies: P. E. Eaton, *Tetrahedron* **35**, 2189-2223 (1979). Total synthesis: R. J. Ternansky *et al.*, *J. Am. Chem. Soc.* **104**, 4503 (1982).

Crystals from benzene, mp >450°.

3403. Dodecamethylcyclohexasiloxane. [540-97-6] $C_{12}H_{36}O_6Si_6$; mol wt 444.92. C 32.39%, H 8.16%, O 21.58%, Si 37.87%. Isolated from the hydrolysis product of dimethyldichlorosilane: Patnode, Wilcock, *J. Am. Chem. Soc.* **68**, 358 (1946).

Oily liquid. mp −3°. bp 245°. bp_{20} 128°. d 0.9762. n_D^{20} 1.4015.

3404. Dodecamethylpentasiloxane. [141-63-9] $C_{12}H_{36}O_4Si_5$; mol wt 384.84. C 37.45%, H 9.43%, O 16.63%, Si 36.49%. Prepn: Patnode, Wilcock, *J. Am. Chem. Soc.* **68**, 358 (1946).

Liquid. bp_{710} 229°. d 0.8755. n_D^{20} 1.3925. mp ~−80°. Stable. Inert to most chemical reagents and rubber. Maintains about the same viscosity over a wide temperature range. Sol in benzene and the lighter hydrocarbons; slightly sol in alcohol and the heavy hydrocarbons.

USE: As a basis for silicone oils or fluids designed to withstand extremes of temperature; as a foam suppressant in petr lubricating oil.

3405. 1-Dodecanol. [112-53-8] Dodecyl alcohol; lauryl alcohol. $C_{12}H_{26}O$; mol wt 186.33. C 77.35%, H 14.06%, O 8.59%. $CH_3(CH_2)_{11}OH$. Prepd by the reduction of esters of lauric acid with sodium and abs alcohol: Levene, Allen, *J. Biol. Chem.* **27**, 443 (1916); Ford, Marvel, *Org. Synth.* **10**, 62 (1930), or by high pressure hydrogenation of the esters using copper chromite catalyst: Adkins, Folkers, *J. Am. Chem. Soc.* **53**, 1095 (1931).

Leaflets from dil alc, mp 24°. d_4^{24} 0.8309 (liq); d_4^{40} 0.8201; d_4^{99} 0.7781. bp_{760} 259°; bp_{400} 235.7°; bp_{200} 213°; bp_{100} 192°; bp_{60} 177.8°; bp_{40} 167.2°; bp_{20} 150°; bp_{10} 134.7°; bp_5 120.2°; $bp_{1.0}$ 91.0°. Insol in water; sol in alcohol and ether.

Phenylurethan. $C_{19}H_{31}NO_2$. Needles from dilute methanol, mp 84°.

USE: Manuf of sulfuric acid esters which are used as wetting agents.

3406. [S-(all-E)]-3-(1,3,5,7,9-Dodecapentaenyloxy)-1,2-propanediol. [91423-46-0] Fecapentaene 12. $C_{15}H_{22}O_3$; mol wt 250.33. C 71.97%, H 8.86%, O 19.17%. A potent mutagen detected in human feces: W. R. Bruce *et al.*, *Cold Spring Harbor Conf. Cell Proliferation* **3**, 1641 (1977). Isoln and characterization: T. D. Wilkins *et al.*, *Am. J. Clin. Nutr.* **33**, 2513 (1980). Structure: N. Hirai *et al.*, *J. Am. Chem. Soc.* **104**, 6149 (1982). Implicated in human colon cancer: *Chem. Eng. News* **60**, 22 (Sept. 27, 1982); T. H. Maugh, *Science* **218**, 363 (1982).

Unstable, decomp rapidly in presence of air or acid. uv max: 325, 345, 365 nm. Sol in chloroform, benzene, ether. Insol in water.

3407. Dodemorph. [1593-77-7] 4-Cyclododecyl-2,6-dimethylmorpholine. $C_{18}H_{35}NO$; mol wt 281.48. C 76.81%, H 12.53%, N 4.98%, O 5.68%. Prepn: W. Sanne *et al.*, **BE 614214**; *eidem*, **US 3686399** (1962, 1972 both to BASF); K.-H. König *et al.*, *Angew. Chem. Int. Ed.* **4**, 336 (1965). Activity: J. Kradel, E. H. Pommer, *Proc. 4th Br. Insectic. Fungic. Conf.* **1967**, 170. Toxicity data: D. Marchand, G. Serra, *Def. Veg.* **27**, 144 (1973), *C.A.* **79**, 133569v (1973).

Oil, bp$_{1.5}$ 161-162°. n_D^{25} 1.4907.
Acetate. Cyclomorph; BAS-238F; Meltatox; Milban. $C_{18}H_{35}$-$NO.C_2H_4O_2$; mol wt 341.53. Yellow liquid, d 0.93. Misc with water. LD_{50} i.p. in mice: 100 mg/kg (Marchand, Serra).
USE: Fungicide.

3408. Dodine. [2439-10-3] Dodecylguanidine monoacetate; AC-5223; Carpene; Melprex. $C_{15}H_{33}N_3O_2$; mol wt 287.44. C 62.68%, H 11.57%, N 14.62%, O 11.13%. Prepn: B. Puetzer, **US 2213474** (1940 to Winthrop Chem. Co.). Degradation study: M. C. Goldberg, R. L. Wershaw, *Prepr. Pap. Natl. Meet., Div. Water, Air Waste Chem., Am. Chem. Soc.* **5**, 53 (1965). Mechanism of action: E. Somers, R. J. Pring, *Ann. Appl. Biol.* **58**, 457 (1966). Toxicology: G. J. Levinskas *et al.*, *Toxicol. Appl. Pharmacol.* **3**, 127 (1961); to aquatic organisms: A. Hourdakis *et al.*, *Fresenius Environ. Bull.* **4**, 679 (1995). Determn by titration in formulations: N. R. Pasarela, *J. Assoc. Off. Anal. Chem.* **52**, 1292 (1969); by GLC in fruit: J. Hajslová *et al.*, *J. Chromatogr.* **348**, 437 (1985). Field trial on apple trees: R. G. Ross *et al.*, *Can. J. Plant Sci.* **49**, 655 (1969).

Slightly waxy solid, mp 132-135°. Sol in ethanol, water. Insol in most organic solvents. LC_{50} in harlequin fish: 0.6 mg/l (Hourdakis).
Caution: Strong solns irritating to skin, mucous membranes. Ingestion causes vomiting, diarrhea.
USE: Agricultural fungicide.

3409. Dofetilide. [115256-11-6] *N*-[4-[2-[Methyl[2-[4-[(methylsulfonyl)amino]phenoxy]ethyl]amino]ethyl]phenyl]-methanesulfonamide; 1-(4-methanesulfonamidophenoxy)-2-[*N*-(4-methanesulfonamidophenethyl)-*N*-methylamino]ethane; UK-68798; Tikosyn. $C_{19}H_{27}N_3O_5S_2$; mol wt 441.56. C 51.68%, H 6.16%, N 9.52%, O 18.12%, S 14.52%. Potassium channel blocker. Prepn: J. E. Arrowsmith *et al.*, **EP 245997**; P. E. Cross *et al.*, **US 4959366** (1987, 1990 both to Pfizer); *idem et al.*, *J. Med. Chem.* **33**, 1151 (1990). HPLC determn in urine: D. K. Walker *et al.*, *J. Chromatogr.* **568**, 475 (1991). Mechanism of action study: D. Carmeliet, *J. Pharmacol. Exp. Ther.* **262**, 809 (1992). Review of pharmacology and pharmacokinetics: H. S. Rasmussen *et al.*, *ibid.* **20**, Suppl. 2, S96-S105 (1992). Clinical trial in atrial fibrillation and flutter: B. L. Norgaard *et al.*, *Am. Heart J.* **137**, 1062 (1999); in congestive heart failure: C. Torp-Pedersen *et al.*, *N. Engl. J. Med.* **341**, 857 (1999).

Crystals from ethyl acetate/methanol (10:1), mp 147-149° (Cross); from hexane/ethyl acetate, mp 151-152° (Arrowsmith). Also reported as white crystalline solid, mp 161° (Rasmussen). pKa 7.0, 9.0, 9.6. Distribution coefficient (pH 7.4): 0.96. Sol in 0.1*M* NaOH, acetone, 0.1*M* HCl; very slightly sol in water, propan-2-ol.
THERAP CAT: Antiarrhythmic (class III).

3410. Doisynolic Acid. [109784-48-7] 1-Ethyl-1,2,3,4,4a,-9,10,10a-octahydro-7-hydroxy-2-methyl-2-phenanthrenecarboxylic acid; 3-hydroxy-16,17-secoestra-1,3,5(10)-trien-17-oic acid. C_{18}-$H_{24}O_3$; mol wt 288.38. C 74.97%, H 8.39%, O 16.64%. Prepd by alkali fusion of estrone: MacCorquodale *et al.*, *J. Biol. Chem.* **99**, 327 (1933); **101**, 753 (1933); Heer, Miescher, *Helv. Chim. Acta* **28**, 156 (1945). Sixteen isomers are possible. If the hydrogen atom at position 4a is α- and the hydrogen atom at position 10a is β-, the acid belongs to the A series. If the hydrogen at 4a is β- and the hydrogen at 10a is α-, the acid belongs to the B series. If both hydrogens are α-, the acid belongs to the C series. If both hydrogens are β-, the acid belongs to the D series: Miescher, *Chem. Rev.* **43**, 367 (1948). If the hydrogen atom at position 1 and the methyl group at position 2 have either the α,α- or β,β-orientation, the acid is designated *cis;* if they are α,β- the acid is designated *trans:* L. F. Fieser, M. Fieser, *Steroids* (Reinhold, New York, 1959) pp 487-495. Synthesis of *dl-cis* and *dl-trans* of the A series and *dl-cis* of the B series: Anner, Miescher, *Helv. Chim. Acta* **29**, 1889 (1946); **30**, 1422 (1947). Synthesis of *dl-cis* of the C series: Jilck, Protiva, *Collect. Czech. Chem. Commun.* **23**, 692 (1958). Stereochemistry of *d-cis*-form: Iriarte, Crabbe, *Chem. Commun.* **1972**, 1110. *Reviews:* Shoppee, *Annu. Rep. Prog. Chem.* **44**, 190 (1948); Miescher in *Recent Progress in Hormone Research* **vol. 3**, G. Pincus Ed. (Academic Press, New York, 1948) pp 47-69.

B-type acid

dl-cis **Acid of the A series.** Crystals from methanol, mp 181-182°. Appears to have the highest estrogenic potency.
dl-trans **Acid of the A series.** Plates from methanol, mp 175-177°.
dl-cis **Acid of the B series.** Crystals from methanol, mp 212-214°.
dl-cis **Acid of the C series.** Crystals from methanol, mp 113-117°.

3411. Dolasetron. [115956-12-2] 1*H*-Indole-3-carboxylic acid (2α,6α,8α,9$\alpha\beta$)-octahydro-3-oxo-2,6-methano-2*H*-quinolizin-8-yl ester; *endo*-hexahydro-8-(3-indolylcarbonyloxy)-2,6-methano-2*H*-quinolizin-3(4*H*)-one; MDL-73147. $C_{19}H_{20}N_2O_3$; mol wt 324.37. C 70.35%, H 6.21%, N 8.64%, O 14.80%. Bridged pseudopelletierine derivative; specific serotonin (5HT$_3$) receptor antagonist. Prepn: M. W. Gittos, **EP 266730**; *idem et al.*, **US 4906755** (1988, 1990 both to Merrell Dow). Binding study: P. H. Boeijinga *et al.*, *Eur. J. Pharmacol.* **219**, 9 (1992). Pharmacology: R. C. Miller *et al.*, *Drug Dev. Res.* **28**, 87 (1993). Clinical pharmacokinetics: H. Boxenbaum *et al.*, *Biopharm. Drug Dispos.* **13**, 693 (1992); *eidem, ibid.* **14**, 131 (1993). GC-MS and LC determn in plasma: T. A. Gillespie *et al.*, *J. Pharm. Biomed. Anal.* **11**, 955 (1993). Clinical trial in emetogenic chemotherapy: A. A. Fauser *et al.*, *Eur. J. Cancer* **32A**, 1523 (1996); for prevention of postoperative nausea: S. G. Graczyk *et al.*, *Anesth. Analg.* **84**, 325 (1997).

Methanesulfonate. [115956-13-3] Dolasetron mesylate; MDL-73147EF; Anzemet. $C_{19}H_{20}N_2O_3.CH_3SO_3H$; mol wt 420.48. Crystalline solid, mp 278°.

THERAP CAT: Antiemetic.

3412. DOM. [15588-95-1] 2,5-Dimethoxy-α,4-dimethylbenzeneethanamine; 2,5-dimethoxy-α,4-dimethylphenethylamine; 1-(2,5-dimethoxy-4-methylphenyl)-2-aminopropane; ($\pm$)-2,5-dimethoxy-4-methylamphetamine; STP. $C_{12}H_{19}NO_2$; mol wt 209.28. C 68.87%, H 9.15%, N 6.69%, O 15.29%. Psychedelic compound of "hippie" culture. Prepn: A. T. Shulgin, **US 3547999** (1970 to Dow). Pharmacology: B. T. Ho *et al., J. Med. Chem.* **13**, 26 (1970). Clinical pharmacology: S. H. Snyder *et al., Am. J. Psychiatry* **125**, 357 (1968). Mechanism of action: R. A. Glennon, *Neuropsychopharmacology* **3**, 509 (1990); C. S. Aulakh *et al., J. Pharmacol. Exp. Ther.* **271**, 143 (1994). Abuse potential: P. B. Silverman, B. T. Ho, *Psychopharmacology* **68**, 209 (1980); D. Fiorella *et al., ibid.* **119**, 239 (1995). Activity comparison of enantiomers: F. Benington *et al., Nature* **242**, 185 (1973); sepn and determn of enantiomers by HPLC: J. Goto *et al., J. Liq. Chromatogr.* **2**, 1179 (1979). Analysis by TLC: I. Ojanperä *et al., J. Planar Chromatogr. Mod. TLC* **4**, 373 (1991). Brief description including prepn: A. Shulgin, A. Shulgin, *Pihkal* (Transform Press, Berkeley CA, 1991) pp 637-642.

mp 60.5-61°.
Hydrochloride. [15589-00-1] $C_{12}H_{19}NO_2.HCl$. White crystals from isopropanol/ether, mp 189-189.5°. LD_{50} i.p. in mice: 89 $\pm$4.2 mg/kg (Ho).

Note: This is a controlled substance (hallucinogen): **21 CFR,** 1308.11.

3413. Domesticine. [476-71-1] (6a*S*)-5,6,6a,7-Tetrahydro-2-methoxy-6-methyl-4*H*-benzo[*de*][1,3]benzodioxolo[5,6-*g*]quinolin-1-ol; 2-methoxy-9,10-(methylenedioxy)-6aα-aporphin-1-ol; 1-hydroxy-2-methoxy-9,10-methylenedioxyaporphine. $C_{19}H_{19}NO_4$; mol wt 325.36. C 70.14%, H 5.89%, N 4.30%, O 19.67%. In *Nandina domestica* Thunb., *Berberidaceae.* Isoln: Kitasato, Shishido, *Ann.* **527**, 176 (1937). Syntheses: Govindachari *et al., Indian J. Chem.* **7**, 841 (1969); Kessar *et al., ibid.* **8**, 468 (1970); Kametani *et al., J. Chem. Soc. C* **1971**, 2446, 2712; *eidem, Chem. Pharm. Bull.* **21**, 766 (1973); Horii *et al., ibid.* **22**, 583 (1974); Hoshino *et al., ibid.* **23**, 2048 (1975).

From methanol + water, mp 115-116°; from abs methanol or benzene, mp 84-85°; dried at 60° over P_2O_5, mp 152-153°. Easily oxidized in air. uv max (ethanol): 221, 283, 310 nm (log ε 4.56, 4.01, 4.17). Very sol in chloroform, sol in hot alc, ethyl acetate, acetic acid, alkalies; slightly sol in ether. Practically insol in water.
Methyl ether. Nantenine; domestine; epidicentrine. mp 139°. $[\alpha]_D^{18}$ +102° (c = 0.528 in chloroform).
dl-**Form.** Needles from methanol, mp 185-186° (dec).

3414. Domiodol. [61869-07-6] 2-(Iodomethyl)-1,3-dioxolane-4-methanol; 4-hydroxymethyl-2-iodomethyl-1,3-dioxolane; MG-13608; Mucolitico. $C_5H_9IO_3$; mol wt 244.03. C 24.61%, H 3.72%, I 52.00%, O 19.67%. Organic iodide mixture of *cis* and *trans* isomers. Prepn: M. Carissimi *et al.,* **DE 2610704**; *eidem,* **US 4085223** (1976, 1978 both to Maggioni). Prepn, expectorant and mucolytic activities: G. Cantarelli *et al., Farmaco Ed. Prat.* **34**, 393 (1979). Pharmacology, toxicity: K. Kogi *et al., Arzneim.-Forsch.* **33**, 1281 (1983). Separation of isomers and comparison of their pharmacological activity: M. Riva *et al., ibid.* 1091. Metabolism and tissue distribution in rats: T. Ohtsuki *et al., Farmaco Ed. Prat.* **39**, 291 (1984). Comparative study with *S*-carboxymethylcysteine, *q.v.,* in chronic obstructive lung disease: L. Casali *et al., Int. J. Clin. Pharmacol. Ther. Toxicol.* **20**, 554 (1982).

LD_{50} in male, female mice (mg/kg): 79, 89 i.p.; 140, 145 orally (Riva).
cis-**Form.** $bp_{0.2}$ 106-108°. LD_{50} orally in male mice: 135 mg/kg (Riva).
trans-**Form.** $bp_{0.2}$ 114-116°. LD_{50} orally in male mice: 150 mg/kg (Riva).

THERAP CAT: Mucolytic.

3415. Domiphen Bromide. [538-71-6] *N,N*-Dimethyl-*N*-(2-phenoxyethyl)-1-dodecanaminium bromide; dodecyldimethyl(2-phenoxyethyl)ammonium bromide; (β-phenoxyethyl)dimethyldodecylammonium bromide; PDDB; phenododecinium bromide; NSC-39415; Bradosol; Oradol; Modicare; Neo-Bradoral. $C_{22}H_{40}BrNO$; mol wt 414.46. C 63.75%, H 9.73%, Br 19.28%, N 3.38%, O 3.86%. Prepd by heating phenoxyethyldimethylamine with dodecyl bromide: Hartmann, Bosshard, **US 2581336** (1952 to Ciba).

Crystals, mild characteristic odor, bitter taste, mp 112-113°. Freely sol in water (100 g/100 ml), much less sol at low temps. Sol in ethanol, acetone, ethyl acetate, chloroform; very slightly sol in benzene. Aq solns are clear, colorless, and foam profusely on shaking. pH of 10% soln: 6.42; of 1% commercial product at 25°: 5.5; of 0.1%: 6.8. Surface tension values at 25° (by the capillary rise method) range from 26.75 dynes/cm (10% soln) to 22.08 dynes/cm (0.1% soln). Incompatible with soap.

THERAP CAT: Anti-infective (topical).

3416. Domitroban. [112966-96-8] (5*Z*)-7-[(1*R*,2*S*,3*S*,4*S*)-3-[(Phenylsulfonyl)amino]bicyclo[2.2.1]hept-2-yl]-5-heptenoic acid; (+)-(5*Z*)-7-[3-*endo*-[(phenylsulfonyl)amino]bicyclo[2.2.1]hept-2-*exo*-yl]-5-heptenoic acid; (+)-S-145. $C_{20}H_{27}NO_4S$; mol wt 377.50. C 63.63%, H 7.21%, N 3.71%, O 16.95%, S 8.49%. Thromboxane A_2-receptor antagonist. Prepn of ($\pm$)-form: F. Watanabe *et al.,* **EP 226346**; *eidem,* **US 4861913** (1987, 1989 both to Shionogi); and isomers: M. Narisada *et al., J. Med. Chem.* **31**, 1847 (1988). Prepn of (+)-form: M. J. Martinelli, *J. Org. Chem.* **55**, 5065 (1990); M. Ohtani *et al., ibid.* **56**, 2122 (1991). Pharmacology: A. Arimura *et al., Int. Arch. Allergy Immunol.* **98**, 239 (1992). GC determn in plasma: J. Okamoto *et al., J. Chromatogr.* **583**, 45 (1992); in urine: *eidem, ibid.* 53. Clinical pharmacokinetics: A. Fujimura *et al., J. Clin. Pharmacol.* **36**, 409 (1996). Clinical evaluation in asthma: M. Fujimura *et al.*, *Pulm. Pharmacol.* **8**, 251 (1995).

Colorless crystals from toluene + hexane, mp 60-62°. uv max (ethanol): 225 nm (ε 5270). $[\alpha]_{589}$ +28.7° (c = 1.00 in methanol).

Calcium salt. [132747-47-8] S-1452; Anboxan. $C_{40}H_{52}$-$CaN_2O_8S_2$; mol wt 793.06. Prepd as the dihydrate. Colorless pillars, mp >300° (dec). $[\alpha]_D^{26}$ +19.0 ±0.6° (c = 1.010 in methanol).

(±)-Form. [115266-92-7] S-145. Colorless plates from ether + *n*-hexane, mp 85-86°.

THERAP CAT: Antiasthmatic.

3417. Domoic Acid. [14277-97-5] (2*S*,3*S*,4*S*)-2-Carboxy-4-[(1*Z*,3*E*,5*R*)-5-carboxy-1-methyl-1,3-hexadienyl]-3-pyrrolidine-acetic acid. $C_{15}H_{21}NO_6$; mol wt 311.33. C 57.87%, H 6.80%, N 4.50%, O 30.83%. Excitatory amino acid isolated from the red alga *Chondria armata* Okamura, *Rhodomelaceae*, known in Japanese as "domoi". Structural analog of kainic acid, *q.v.* Shown to be responsible for amnesic shellfish poisoning associated with ingestion of certain cultured blue mussels. Isoln: T. Takemoto, K. Daigo, *Chem. Pharm. Bull.* **6**, 578 (1958); *eidem*, *Arch. Pharm.* **293**, 627 (1960). Series of articles on isoln, structure, and anthelminthic activity: K. Daigo, *Yakugaku Zasshi* **79**, 350-364 (1959), *C.A.* **53**, 14218 (1959). Structural studies: T. Takemoto *et al.*, *ibid.* **86**, 874 (1966), *C.A.* **66**, 28604m (1967). Total synthesis and revised structure: Y. Ohfune, M. Tomita, *J. Am. Chem. Soc.* **104**, 3511 (1982). Neuroexcitatory activity: T. J. Biscoe *et al.*, *Nature* **255**, 166 (1975); R. Zaczek, J. T. Coyle, *Neuropharmacology* **21**, 15 (1982). Effect on kainate receptor activation: G. Debonnel *et al.*, *Can. J. Physiol. Pharmacol.* **67**, 29, 904 (1989). Identification in toxic mussel extracts: J. L. C. Wright *et al.*, *Can. J. Chem.* **67**, 481 (1989). LC determn in shellfish products: J. F. Lawrence *et al.*, *J. Chromatogr.* **462**, 349, 419 (1989). *Reviews*: M. A. Quilliam, J. L. C. Wright, *Anal. Chem.* **61**, 1053A-1059A (1989); J. Clayden *et al.*, *Tetrahedron* **61**, 5713-5724 (2005).

Dihydrate. mp 217° (dec). $[\alpha]_D^{12}$ −109.6° (c = 1.314 in water). uv max: 242 nm (log ε 4.24). pKa in water: 2.10, 3.72, 4.93, 9.82. Sol in water, acetic acid. Insol in methanol, ethanol, chloroform, acetone, benzene.

3418. Domperidone. [57808-66-9] 5-Chloro-1-[1-[3-(2,3-dihydro-2-oxo-1*H*-benzimidazol-1-yl)propyl]-4-piperidinyl]-1,3-dihydro-2*H*-benzimidazol-2-one; 5-chloro-1-[1-[3-(2-oxo-1-benzimidazolinyl)propyl]-4-piperidyl]-2-benzimidazolinone; R-33812; Euciton; Evoxin; Gastronorm; Mod; Motilium; Nauzelin; Peridon; Peridys. $C_{22}H_{24}ClN_5O_2$; mol wt 425.91. C 62.04%, H 5.68%, Cl 8.32%, N 16.44%, O 7.51%. A novel *in vitro* dopamine antagonist with antinauseant properties. Prepn: J. Vandenberk *et al.*, *DE* **2632870**; *eidem*, *US* **4066772** (1977, 1978 both to Janssen). Pharmacology: C. Ennis *et al.*, *J. Pharm. Pharmacol.* **31**, Suppl., 14P (1979). Gastrokinetic properties: J. M. Van Neuten *et al.*, *Life Sci.* **23**, 453 (1978). ³H-domperidone studies: M. P. Martres *et al.*, *ibid.* 1781; M. Baudry *et al.*, *Arch. Pharmacol.* **308**, 231 (1979). Clinical studies: A. J. Reyntjens *et al.*, *Arzneim.-Forsch.* **28**, 1194 (1978); D. B. Wilson, J. W. Dundee, *Anaesthesia* **34**, 765 (1979). Review of pharmacology, pharmacokinetics and therapeutic efficacy: R. N. Brogden *et al.*, *Drugs* **24**, 360-400 (1982).

Crystals from DMF/water, mp 242.5°.
THERAP CAT: Antiemetic.

3419. Donepezil. [120014-06-4] 2,3-Dihydro-5,6-dimethoxy-2-[[1-(phenylmethyl)-4-piperidinyl]methyl]-1*H*-inden-1-one; 5,6-dimethoxy-2-[[1-(phenylmethyl)-4-piperidinyl]methyl]-2,3-dihydro-1*H*-inden-1-one; 1-benzyl-4-[(5,6-dimethoxy-1-indanon-2-yl)methyl]piperidine. $C_{24}H_{29}NO_3$; mol wt 379.49. C 75.96%, H 7.70%, N 3.69%, O 12.65%. Acetylcholinesterase inhibitor. Prepn: H. Sugimoto *et al.*, **EP 296560**, *eidem*, **US 4895841** (1988, 1990 both to Eisai). Synthesis: Y. Iimura *et al.*, *J. Labelled Compd. Radiopharm.* **27**, 835 (1989). Resolution of enantiomers: J. Haginaka, C. Seyama, *J. Chromatogr. B* **577**, 95 (1992). Clinical pharmacokinetics: A. Ohnishi *et al.*, *J. Clin. Pharmacol.* **33**, 1086 (1993). Clinical trials in Alzheimer's disease: R. C. Mohs *et al.*, *Neurology* **57**, 481 (2001); B. Winblad *et al.*, *ibid.* 489. Review of pharmacology and clinical experience in cognitive disorders: G. C. Román, S. J. Rogers, *Expert Opin. Pharmacother.* **5**, 161-180 (2004).

Hydrochloride. [120011-70-3] E-2020; Aricept. $C_{24}H_{29}$-NO_3.HCl; mol wt 415.95. Crystals from methanol/IPE, mp 211-212° (dec).

THERAP CAT: Nootropic.

3420. Dopa. 3-Hydroxytyrosine; 3-(3,4-dihydroxyphenyl)-alanine; β-(3,4-dihydroxyphenyl)-α-alanine; 2-amino-3-(3,4-dihydroxyphenyl)propanoic acid. $C_9H_{11}NO_4$; mol wt 197.19. C 54.82%, H 5.62%, N 7.10%, O 32.45%. An amino acid found in seedlings, pods and beans of *Vicia faba* L. (broad beans) *Stizolobium deeringianum* L. (velvet beans) *Leguminosae:* Torquati, *Arch. farm. sper.* **15**, 213, 308 (1913), *C.A.* **7**, 2774 (1913); Sealock, *Biochemical Preparations* vol. **1**, 25 (1949). Absolute configuration: Guggenheim, *Z. Physiol. Chem.* **88**, 276 (1913). Prepn of DL-, D-, and L-dopa: Yamada *et al.*, *Chem. Pharm. Bull.* **10**, 693 (1962).

DL-Form. [63-84-3] Prisms from water or from aq $NaHSO_3$ soln, dec 270-272°. Soly in water: 144 mg/40 ml. Readily sol in dil acids and alkalies; slightly sol in benzene, carbon disulfide. Practically insol in abs alcohol, ether, glacial acetic acid, petr ether, chloroform. Oxidizes readily.

D-Form. [5796-17-0] Needles from water, dec 276-278°. $[\alpha]_D^{11}$ +13.0° (c = 5.27 in 1*N* HCl). Soly in water: 66 mg/40 ml.

L-Form see Levodopa.

3421. Dopamine. [51-61-6] 4-(2-Aminoethyl)-1,2-benzenediol; 4-(2-aminoethyl)pyrocatechol; 3-hydroxytyramine; 3,4-dihydroxyphenethylamine; α-(3,4-dihydroxyphenyl)-β-aminoethane. $C_8H_{11}NO_2$; mol wt 153.18. C 62.73%, H 7.24%, N 9.14%, O 20.89%. Endogenous catecholamine with α and β-adrenergic activity. Isoln from *Hermidium alipes* (S. Watson) *Nyctaginaceae:* Buelow, Gisvold, *J. Am. Pharm. Assoc.* **33**, 270 (1944). Prepn from aminotyramine: Waser, Sommer, *Helv. Chim. Acta* **6**, 61 (1923). From homoveratrylamine: Schöpf, Bayeler, *Ann.* **513**,

196 (1934); Hahn, Stiehl, *Ber.* **69**, 2640 (1936). Comprehensive description of the hydrochloride: J. E. Carter *et al., Anal. Profiles Drug Subs.* **11**, 257-272 (1982). Review of pharmacology and clinical efficacy in oliguria: J. F. Dasta, M. G. Kirby, *Pharmacotherapy* **6**, 304 (1986).

Free base, stout prisms, highly sensitive to oxygen; discolors quickly.

Hydrochloride. [62-31-7] ASL-279; Cardiosteril; Dopastat; Dynatra; Inovan; Inotropin. $C_8H_{11}NO_2.HCl$; mol wt 189.64. Rosettes of needles from water, dec 241°; may be recrystallized from methanol + ether. Freely sol in water; sol in methanol, in hot 95% ethanol; in aq solns of alkali hydroxides. Practically insol in ether, petr ether, chloroform, benzene, toluene.

Hydrobromide. $C_8H_{11}NO_2.HBr$. Crystals, dec 210-214°.

THERAP CAT: Cardiotonic; antihypotensive.

3422. Dopan. [520-09-2] 5-[Bis(2-chloroethyl)amino]-6-methyl-2,4(1*H,3H*)-pyrimidinedione; 5-[bis(2-chloroethyl)amino]-6-methyluracil; 6-methyl-5-[bis(2-chloroethyl)amino]uracil; 4-methyl-5-[bis(β-chloroethyl)amino]uracil; 2,6-dihydroxy-4-methyl-5-bis[2-chloroethyl]aminopyrimidine; Elderfield pyrimidine mustard; NSC-23436. $C_9H_{13}Cl_2N_3O_2$; mol wt 266.12. C 40.62%, H 4.92%, Cl 26.64%, N 15.79%, O 12.02%. Description: Larionova, Platonova, *Vopr. Onkol.* **1**, no. 5, 36 (1955); *C.A.* **51**, 6862 (1957). Prepn: Nemets *et al.*, **SU 116912** (1959), *C.A.* **53**, 17438i (1959). Outline of synthesis of the demethyl compd: Petering, Lyttle, *Chem. Eng. News* **36**, 47 (Sept. 22, 1958). Monograph: L. F. Larionov, *Cancer Chemotherapy* (Pergamon Press, New York, 1965).

Snow-white crystals, dec 178-179°. Practically insol in cold water, acetone and benzene. Slightly sol in alc.

USE: In anticancer research: Louis, *J. Chronic Dis.* **15**, 273-281 (March 1962).

3423. Dopastin. [37134-80-8] (2*E*)-*N*-[(2*S*)-2-(Hydroxynitrosoamino)-3-methylbutyl]-2-butenamide; *N*-(2-nitrosohydroxylamino-3-methylbutyl)crotonamide. $C_9H_{17}N_3O_3$; mol wt 215.25. C 50.22%, H 7.96%, N 19.52%, O 22.30%. Dopamine β-hydroxylase inhibitor isolated from a culture filtrate of a bacterium of the *Pseudomonas* genus. Prodn, isoln and characterization: Iinuma *et al., Agric. Biol. Chem.* **38**, 2093 (1974). Structure and synthesis: Iinuma *et al., ibid.* 2099. Biochemical and biological studies: Iinuma *et al., ibid.* 2107.

Crystals from acetone + *n*-hexane or from ethyl ether, mp 116-119°. Monobasic acid, pKa 5.1. $[\alpha]_D^{21}$ −246° (c = 0.5 in alcohol). uv max (0.01*N* HCl): 215 nm (ε 20900).

Copper salt. $C_9H_{16}N_3O_3.\frac{1}{2}Cu$. Dark blue needles from ethanol, mp 142-144°.

3424. Dopexamine. [86197-47-9] 4-[2-[[6-[(2-Phenylethyl)amino]hexyl]amino]ethyl]-1,2-benzenediol; 4-[2-[6-(phenethylamino)hexyl]amino]ethyl]pyrocatechol; FPL-60278. $C_{22}H_{32}N_2$-O_2; mol wt 356.50. C 74.12%, H 9.05%, N 7.86%, O 8.98%. Dopamine receptor and β_2-adrenoreceptor agonist. Prepn: J. B. Farmer *et al., EP 72061* (1983 to Fisons). Unlike dopamine, dopex-

amine has little or no activity at the α- and β_1-adrenoceptors: R. A. Brown *et al., Br. J. Pharmacol.* **85**, 599 (1985). Cardiovascular activity in dogs: *eidem, ibid.* 609. Hemodynamic effects in chronic congestive heart failure: J. R. Dawson *et al., Br. Heart J.* **54**, 313 (1985); G. Svensson *et al., Eur. Heart J.* **7**, 697 (1986). Human renovascular effects: F. Magrini *et al., Eur. J. Clin. Pharmacol.* **32**, 1 (1987). Symposium on pharmacology and clinical efficacy: *Am. J. Cardiol.* **62**, Suppl., 1C-88C (1988).

Dihydrochloride. [86484-91-5] Dopexamine hydrochloride; FPL-60278AR; Dopacard. $C_{22}H_{32}N_2O_2.2HCl$; mol wt 429.42.

Dihydrobromide. $C_{22}H_{32}N_2O_2.2HBr$. Crystals from ethanol, mp 227-228°.

THERAP CAT: Cardiotonic.

3425. Doramectin. [117704-25-3] 25-Cyclohexyl-5-*O*-demethyl-25-de(1-methylpropyl)avermectin A$_{1a}$; 25-cyclohexyl-avermectin B$_1$; UK-67994; Dectomax. $C_{50}H_{74}O_{14}$; mol wt 899.11. C 66.79%, H 8.30%, O 24.91%. Mutational biosynthetic antiparasitic antibiotic structurally related to the avermectins, *q.v.* Isoln: S. P. Gibson *et al., EP 214731; eidem, US 5089480* (1987, 1992 both to Pfizer). Mutational biosynthesis: C. J. Dutton *et al., J. Antibiot.* **44**, 357 (1991). Pharmacokinetics and efficacy in cattle: *Vet. Parasitol.* **49**, 1-119 (1993). Clinical evaluation as prophylactic in canine spirocercosis: E. Lavy *et al., Res. Vet. Sci.* **75**, 217 (2003).

mp 116-119°.

THERAP CAT (VET): Antiparasitic.

3426. Dorzolamide. [120279-96-1] (4*S*,6*S*)-4-(Ethylamino)-5,6-dihydro-6-methyl-4*H*-thieno[2,3-*b*]thiopyran-2-sulfonamide 7,7-dioxide. $C_{10}H_{16}N_2O_4S_3$; mol wt 324.44. C 37.02%, H 4.97%, N 8.63%, O 19.73%, S 29.65%. Carbonic anhydrase inhibitor. Prepn: J. J. Baldwin *et al., EP 296879; eidem, US 4797413* (1988, 1989 both to Merck & Co.). Mechanism of action study: R.-F. Wang *et al., Arch. Ophthalmol.* **109**, 1297 (1991). HPLC determn in plasma and urine: B. K. Matuszewski, M. L. Constanzer, *Chirality* **4**, 515 (1992). Clinical evaluations in glaucoma and ocular hypertension: E. A. Lippa *et al., Ophthalmology* **98**, 308 (1991); E. A. Lippa *et al., Arch. Ophthalmol.* **110**, 495 (1992).

Hydrochloride. [130693-82-2] MK-507; Trusopt. $C_{10}H_{16}N_2$-$O_4S_3.HCl$; mol wt 360.90. mp 283-285°. $[\alpha]_D^{24}$ −8.34° (c = 1 in methanol). Sol in water.

THERAP CAT: Antiglaucoma agent.

3427. Dosmalfate. [122312-55-4] [μ_7-[7-[[6-O-[6-Deoxy-2,3,4-tri-O-(sulfo-κO)-α-L-mannopyranosyl]-2,3,4-tri-O-(sulfo-κO)-β-D-glucopyranosyl]oxy]-5-hydroxy-2-[4-methoxy-3-[(sulfo-κO)oxy]pheny]-4H-1-benzopyran-4-onato(7−)]]tetradeca-μ-hydroxyheneicosahydroxytetradecaaluminum; flavalfate; F-3616; Diotul. $C_{28}H_{60}Al_{14}O_{71}S_7$; mol wt 2134.93. C 15.75%, H 2.83%, Al 17.69%, O 53.21%, S 10.51%. Diosmin, $q.v.$, heptakis (hydrogen sulfate) aluminum complex. Prepn: A. Orjales-Venero, R. Mosquera-Pestana, **EP 558435**; $eidem$, **US 5296469** (1993, 1994 both to FAES). $In~vivo$ protective effect in exptl colitis: I. Villegas $et~al.$, $Eur.~J.~Pharmacol.$ **460**, 209 (2003). Series of articles on pharmacology, toxicity and clinical studies as gastroprotectant and anti-ulcerative: $Drugs~Today$ **36** (Suppl. A), 25-85 (2000).

R = $SO_3[Al_2(OH)_5]$

Yellow solid.
THERAP CAT: Gastroprotectant.

3428. Dotarizine. [84625-59-2] 1-(Diphenylmethyl)-4-[3-(2-phenyl-1,3-dioxolan-2-yl)propyl]piperazine; FI-6026. $C_{29}H_{34}N_2O_2$; mol wt 442.59. C 78.70%, H 7.74%, N 6.33%, O 7.23%. Mixed calcium channel blocker and serotonin (5-HT$_2$) receptor antagonist. Prepn: R. Foguet $et~al.$, **EP 97340**; $eidem$, **US 4883797** (1984, 1989 both to Ferrer); S. Gubert $et~al.$, $Arzneim.$-$Forsch.$ **37**, 1103 (1987). Clinical pharmacokinetics and tolerability: M. Farré $et~al.$, $Methods~Find.~Exp.~Clin.~Pharmacol.$ **19**, 343 (1997). Cerebrovascular study in goats: G. Torregrosa $et~al.$, $Arzneim.$-$Forsch.$ **49**, 668 (1999); in rabbits: N. Kuridze $et~al.$, $J.~Neurol.~Sci.$ **175**, 13 (2000). Mechanism of blockade: A. Ruiz-Nuno $et~al.$, $Eur.~J.~Pharmacol.$ **411**, 289 (2001).

White crystalline solid from methanol, mp 100-101° (Gubert); also reported as 93-97° (Foguet).
THERAP CAT: Antimigraine.

3429. Dothiepin. [113-53-1] 3-Dibenzo[b,e]thiepin-11(6H)-ylidene-N,N-dimethyl-1-propanamine; N,N-dimethyl-dibenzo[b,e]thiepin-$\Delta^{11(6H).\gamma}$-propylamine; 11-(3-dimethylamino-propylidene)-6,11-dihydrodibenzo[b,e]thiepin; dosulepin. $C_{19}H_{21}NS$; mol wt 295.44. C 77.24%, H 7.16%, N 4.74%, S 10.85%. Tricyclic antidepressant. Prepn: M. Protiva $et~al.$, $Experientia$ **18**, 326 (1962); **BE 618591**; M. Protiva $et~al.$, **US 3527766** (1962, 1970 both to SPOFA); M. Rajsner, M. Protiva, $Cesk.~Farm.$ **11**, 404 (1962), $C.A.$ **59**, 2772g (1963). Synthesis of isomers: M. Rajsner $et~al.$, $Collect.~Czech.~Chem.~Commun.$ **34**, 1963 (1969). Pharmacology: J. Metysova $et~al.$, $Arzneim.$-$Forsch.$ **13**, 1039 (1963). Clinical pharmacokinetics and metabolism: K. P. Maguire $et~al.$, $Br.~J.~Clin.~Pharmacol.$ **12**, 405 (1981). HPLC determn in plasma: P. J. Taylor $et~al.$, $J.~Chromatogr.$ **581**, 152 (1992). Review of clinical experience in depression: S. Donovan $et~al.$, $Prog.~Neuro$-$Psychopharmacol.~Biol.~Psychiatry$ **18**, 1143-1162 (1994).

bp$_{0.05}$ 171-172°. mp 55-57°.
Hydrochloride. [897-15-4] Prothiaden. $C_{19}H_{21}NS.HCl$; mol wt 331.90. Crystals from ethanol-ether, mp 218-221°. uv max (methanol): 232, 260, 309 nm (log ε 4.41, 3.97, 3.53).
THERAP CAT: Antidepressant.

3430. Dowicide 9®. [13347-42-7] 4-Chloro-2-cyclopentyl-phenol. $C_{11}H_{13}ClO$; mol wt 196.67. C 67.18%, H 6.66%, Cl 18.03%, O 8.14%. Prepn: **DE 615448** (1935 to Hoffmann-La Roche), $C.A.$ **29**, 6248^1 (1935); Pajeau, Begue, $Bull.~Soc.~Chim.~Fr.$ **1962**, 1923. Bactericidal properties: **NL 6513777**; Lorah, **US 3323988** (1966, 1967 both to Dow).

bp$_{18}$ 181-185°; bp$_{11}$ 160-162°.
USE: Germicide.

3431. Doxacurium Chloride. [106819-53-8] (1R,1'S,2S,-2'R)-rel-2,2'-[(1,4-Dioxo-1,4-butanediyl)bis(oxy-3,1-propane-diyl)]bis[1,2,3,4-tetrahydro-6,7,8-trimethoxy-2-methyl-1-[(3,4,5-trimethoxyphenyl)methyl]isoquinolinium] dichloride; (1R,2S;1S,-2R)-1,2,3,4-tetrahydro-2-(3-hydroxypropyl)-6,7,8-trimethoxy-2-methyl-1-(3,4,5-trimethoxybenzyl)isoquinolinium chloride succinate (2:1); $trans,trans$-2,2'-[dimethylenebis(carbonyloxytrimeth-ylene)]bis[1,2,3,4-tetrahydro-6,7,8-trimethoxy-2-methyl-1-(3,4,5-trimethoxybenzyl)isoquinolinium] dichloride; BW-A938U; Nuromax. $C_{56}H_{78}Cl_2N_2O_{16}$; mol wt 1106.13. C 60.81%, H 7.11%, Cl 6.41%, N 2.53%, O 23.14%. Benzylisoquinolinium, competitive neuromuscular blocker. Prepn: H. A. El-Sayad $et~al.$, **EP 54309** (1982 to Wellcome Found.); $eidem$, **US 4701460** (1987 to Burroughs Wellcome). Clinical pharmacology: S. J. Basta $et~al.$, $Anesthesiology$ **69**, 478 (1988). Clinical evaluation during anesthesia: R. P. F. Scott, J. Norman, $Br.~J.~Anaesth.$ **62**, 373 (1989).

Amorphous solid. Sol in water.
THERAP CAT: Neuromuscular blocking agent.

3432. Doxapram. [309-29-5] 1-Ethyl-4-[2-(4-morpholin-yl)ethyl]-3,3-diphenyl-2-pyrrolidinone. $C_{24}H_{30}N_2O_2$; mol wt 378.51. C 76.16%, H 7.99%, N 7.40%, O 8.45%. Prepn: C. D. Lunsford, A. D. Cale, **BE 613734**; $eidem$, **US 3192206** (1962, 1965 both to A. H. Robins); Lunsford $et~al.$, $J.~Med.~Chem.$ **7**, 302 (1964). Clinical comparison with mepixanon in chronic bronchopulmonary disease: M. Parziale $et~al.$, $G.~Ital.~Mal.~Torace$ **38**, 323 (1984). Toxicity data: E. I. Goldenthal, $Toxicol.~Appl.~Pharmacol.$ **18**, 185 (1971).

Hydrochloride monohydrate. [7081-53-0] AHR-619; Dopram; Doxapril; Stimulexin. $C_{24}H_{30}N_2O_2.HCl.H_2O$; mol wt 432.98. Crystals from isopropyl ether, mp 217-219°. Bitter taste. Sol in water; sparingly sol in alc, slightly sol in chloroform. LD_{50} orally in rats: 261 mg/kg (Goldenthal).

Benzoate. $C_{31}H_{36}N_2O_4$. Crystals, mp 123-124°.

THERAP CAT: Respiratory stimulant.

THERAP CAT (VET): Respiratory stimulant.

3433. Doxazosin. [74191-85-8] 1-(4-Amino-6,7-dimethoxy-2-quinazolinyl)-4-[(2,3-dihydro-1,4-benzodioxin-2-yl)carbonyl]piperazine; 4-amino-2-[4-(1,4-benzodioxan-2-carbonyl)-piperazin-1-yl]-6,7-dimethoxyquinazoline; UK-33274. $C_{23}H_{25}N_5O_5$; mol wt 451.48. C 61.19%, H 5.58%, N 15.51%, O 17.72%. Selective α_1-adrenergic blocker related to prazosin, q.v. Prepn: S. F. Campbell, **DE 2847623**; idem, **US 4188390** (1979, 1980 both to Pfizer). Cardiovascular pharmacology: P. B. Timmermans et al., Arch. Int. Pharmacodyn. Ther. **245**, 218 (1980). HPLC determn in plasma: M. G. Cowlishaw, J. R. Sharman, J. Chromatogr. **344**, 403 (1985). Clinical pharmacokinetics: H. L. Elliott et al., Br. J. Clin. Pharmacol. **13**, 699 (1982). Symposia on pharmacology and clinical efficacy in hypertension: Br. J. Clin. Pharmacol. **21**, Suppl. 1, 1S-92S (1986); Am. J. Cardiol. **59**, 1G-104G (1987). Review of clinical trials in benign prostatic hypertrophy: C. G. Roehrborn, R. L. Siegel, Urology **48**, 406-415 (1996).

Hydrochloride. $C_{23}H_{25}N_5O_5.HCl$. Crystals, mp 289-290°.

Methanesulfonate. [77883-43-3] Doxazosin mesylate; UK-33274-27; Alfadil; Alfamedin; Benur; Cardenalin; Cardular; Cardura; Carduran; Diblocin; Doxamax; Zoxan. $C_{23}H_{25}N_5O_5.CH_3$-SO_3H; mol wt 547.58.

THERAP CAT: Antihypertensive; in treatment of benign prostatic hypertrophy.

3434. Doxefazepam. [40762-15-0] 7-Chloro-5-(2-fluorophenyl)-1,3-dihydro-3-hydroxy-1-(2-hydroxyethyl)-2H-1,4-benzodiazepin-2-one; N-1-hydroxyethyl-3-hydroxyflurazepam; SAS-643; Doxans. $C_{17}H_{14}ClFN_2O_3$; mol wt 348.76. C 58.55%, H 4.05%, Cl 10.17%, F 5.45%, N 8.03%, O 13.76%. Prepn: G. F. Tamagnone et al., Arzneim.-Forsch. **25**, 720 (1975); eidem, J. Pharm. Pharmacol. **26**, 566 (1974); F. De Marchi, G. F. Tamagnone, **DE 2338058** (1974 to Schiapparelli), C.A. **80**, 121016v (1974). Comparison with flurazepam, q.v., and pharmacology, toxicity studies: M. Babbini et al., Arzneim.-Forsch. **25**, 1294 (1975). Structure-activity studies: eidem, Pharmacol. Res. Commun. **7**, 337 (1975). GC determn in blood and tissue: F. Marcucci et al., J. Chromatogr. **198**, 180 (1980); in plasma, urine: S. Mardente et al., Ther. Drug Monit. **3**, 351 (1981). Quantitative EEG, behavioral effects: W. G. Sanita et al., ibid. 341. Effect on sleep: G. Rodriguez et al., Neuropsychobiology **11**, 133 (1984).

Crystals from methylene chloride/petr ether, mp 138-140°. LD_{50} in rats, mice (mg/kg): 2550, >1500 orally; 586, 774 i.p. (Babbini).

THERAP CAT: Sedative, hypnotic.

3435. Doxepin. [1668-19-5] 3-Dibenz[b,e]oxepin-11(6H)-ylidene-N,N-dimethyl-1-propanamine; N,N-dimethyldibenz[b,e]-oxepin-$\Delta^{11(6H)}$,γ-propylamine; 11-(3-dimethylaminopropylidene)-6,11-dihydrodibenz[b,e]oxepin; P-3693A. $C_{19}H_{21}NO$; mol wt 279.38. C 81.68%, H 7.58%, N 5.01%, O 5.73%. Prepn of mixture of cis- and trans-isomers: K. Stach, F. Bickelhaupt, Monatsh. Chem. **93**, 896 (1962); F. Bickelhaupt et al., ibid. **95**, 485 (1964); **NL 6407758**; K. Stach, **US 3438981** (1965, 1969 both to Boehringer Mann.); and separation and activity of isomers: B. M. Bloom, J. R. Tretter, **BE 641498**; eidem, **US 3420851** (1964, 1969 both to Pfizer). Pharmacology: A. Ribbentrop, W. Schaumann, Arzneim.-Forsch. **15**, 863 (1965). Metabolism in animals: D. C. Hobbs, Biochem. Pharmacol. **18**, 1941 (1969). Determn in plasma by GC/MS: T. P. Davis et al., J. Chromatogr. **273**, 436 (1983); by HPLC: T. Emm, L. J. Lesko, ibid. **419**, 445 (1987). Clinical study in depression: K. Rickels et al., Arch. Gen. Psychiatry **42**, 134 (1985). Comparative clinical trial with cimetidine, q.v., in treatment of ulcer: R. K. Shrivastava et al., Clin. Ther. **7**, 181 (1985). Review of pharmacology and therapeutic efficacy: R. M. Pinder et al., Drugs **13**, 161 (1977).

Oily liq consisting of a mixture of cis- and trans-isomers. $bp_{0.03}$ 154-157°, $bp_{0.2}$ 260-270°. LD_{50} in mice, rats (mg/kg): 26, 16 i.v.; 79, 182 i.p.; 135, 147 orally (Ribbentrop, Schaumann).

Hydrochloride. [1229-29-4] Adapin; Aponal; Curatin; Quitaxon; Sinequan. $C_{19}H_{21}NO.HCl$; mol wt 315.84. Crystals, mp 184-186°, 188-189°.

Maleate. Crystals, mp 161-164°, 168-169°.

trans-Form hydrochloride. [3607-18-9] mp 192-193°.

cis-Form hydrochloride. [25127-31-5] Cidoxepin hydrochloride; P-4599. Crystals, mp 209-210.5°.

THERAP CAT: Antidepressant.

THERAP CAT (VET): Antipruritic.

3436. Doxercalciferol. [54573-75-0] (1α,3β,5Z,7E,22E)-9,10-Secoergosta-5,7,10(19),22-tetraene-1,3-diol; 1α-hydroxyvitamin D_2; 1-hydroxyergocalciferol; Hectorol. $C_{28}H_{44}O_2$; mol wt 412.65. C 81.50%, H 10.75%, O 7.75%. Synthetic vitamin D prohormone. Prepn: H.-Y. P. Lam et al., Science **186**, 1038 (1974); eidem, Steroids **30**, 671 (1977); H. E. Paaren et al., J. Org. Chem. **45**, 3253 (1980). Comparative activity and toxicity: G. Sjöden et al., Proc. Soc. Exp. Biol. Med. **178**, 432 (1985). Metabolism to bioactive form: J. C. Knutson et al., Endocrinology **136**, 4749 (1995). Pharmacology: J. W. Coburn et al., Nephrol. Dial. Transplant. **11**, Suppl. 3, 153 (1996). Clinical trial for suppression of secondary hyperparathyroidism in hemodialysis: J. M. Frazao et al., ibid. **13**, Suppl. 3, 68 (1998).

Crystals, mp 138-140°. uv max (ethanol): 265 nm (ε 18300). LD_{50} orally in rats: 3.5-6.5 mg/kg (Sjöden).

THERAP CAT: Antihyperparathyroid.

3437. Doxifluridine. [3094-09-5] 5'-Deoxy-5-fluoro-uridine; 1-(β-D-5'-deoxyribofuranosyl)-5-fluorouracil; 5'-DFUR; 5'-dFUrd; Ro-21-9738; Flutron; Furtulon. $C_9H_{11}FN_2O_5$; mol wt 246.19. C 43.91%, H 4.50%, F 7.72%, N 11.38%, O 32.49%. Fluorinated pyrimidine nucleoside with cytostatic activity. Prepn: A. F. Cook, **US 4071680** (1978 to Hoffmann-La Roche); H. Hrebabecky, J. Beranek, *Nucleic Acids Res.* **5**, 1029 (1978); A. F. Cook *et al., J. Med. Chem.* **22**, 1330 (1979). Stereospecific synthesis: J. Kiss *et al., Helv. Chim. Acta* **65**, 1522 (1982). Mechanism of action studies: H.-R. Hartmann, A. Matter, *Cancer Res.* **42**, 2412 (1982); R. D. Armstrong *et al., Cancer Chemother. Pharmacol.* **11**, 102 (1983). Kinetics and metabolism in humans: J.-P. Sommadossi *et al., Cancer Res.* **43**, 930 (1983). Clinical trials in colorectal carcinoma: R. Abele *et al., J. Clin. Oncol.* **1**, 750 (1983); S. D. Fossa *et al., Cancer Chemother. Pharmacol.* **15**, 161 (1985). Series of articles on animal toxicology: *Yakuri to Chiryo* **13**, Suppl. 2, 221-430 (1985); acute toxicity: M. Shimizu *et al., ibid.* **209**, *C.A.* **104**, 14673z-14678e (1986). Evaluation of neurotoxicity in humans: M. S. Heier, S. D. Fossa, *Acta Neurol. Scand.* **73**, 449 (1986).

Crystals from ethyl acetate, mp 189-190° (Cook). Also reported as crystals from 2-propanol, mp 186-188° (Hrebabecky, Beranek); needles from methanol + ethyl acetate, mp 192-193° (Kiss). pKa 7.4. $[\alpha]_D^{25}$ +18.4° (c = 0.419 in water). uv max (in methanol): 268-269 nm (ε 8550). LD_{50} (14 day) in mice or rats (mg/kg): >1000 i.v.: >2000 s.c.; in male, female mice, male, female rats (mg/kg): >5000, >5000, 3471, 3390 orally (Shimizu).

THERAP CAT: Antineoplastic.

3438. Doxofylline. [69975-86-6] 7-(1,3-Dioxolan-2-yl-methyl)-3,7-dihydro-1,3-dimethyl-1*H*-purine-2,6-dione; 7-(1,3-di-oxolan-2-ylmethyl)theophylline; 2-(7'-theophyllinemethyl)-1,3-di-oxolane; doxophylline; dioxyfilline; ABC-12/3; Ansimar; Maxivent; Ventax. $C_{11}H_{14}N_4O_4$; mol wt 266.25. C 49.62%, H 5.30%, N 21.04%, O 24.04%. Prepn: U. Avico *et al., Farmaco Ed. Sci.* **17**, 73 (1962). Use as bronchodilator: **BE 868556**; J. S. Franzone, T. Tamietto, **US 4187308** (1978, 1980 to Istituto Biologico Chemioterapico ABC). Pharmacology: J. S. Franzone *et al., Farmaco Ed. Sci.* **36**, 201 (1981). Pharmacodynamics and toxicity in rats: J. S. Franzone *et al., ibid.* 220. HPLC determn in pharmaceutical compositions: C. Badini *et al., Farmaco Ed. Prat.* **37**, 320 (1982). Clinical trial in obstructive pneumopathy: C. Bucca *et al., Int. J. Clin. Pharmacol. Res.* **11**, Suppl 1, 101 (1982).

Crystals, mp 144-145.5°. Sol in water, acetone, ethyl acetate, benzene, chloroform, dioxane, hot methanol or hot ethanol. Practically insol in ethyl ether or petr ether. LD_{50} in mice (mg/kg): 841 orally; 215.6 i.v.; in rats: 1022.4 orally, 445 i.p. (Franzone).

THERAP CAT: Bronchodilator.

3439. Doxorubicin. [23214-92-8] (8*S*,10*S*)-10-[(3-Amino-2,3,6-trideoxy-α-L-*lyxo*-hexopyranosyl)oxy]-7,8,9,10-tetrahydro-6,8,11-trihydroxy-8-(hydroxyacetyl)-1-methoxy-5,12-naphthacene-dione; 14-hydroxydaunomycin; NSC-123127; FI-106. $C_{27}H_{29}$-NO_{11}; mol wt 543.52. C 59.66%, H 5.38%, N 2.58%, O 32.38%.

Anthracycline antibiotic; interferes with topoisomerase II function. Isoln from *Streptomyces peucetius* var *caesius*: F. Arcamone *et al.,* **ZA 6802378**; *eidem,* **US 3590028** (1968, 1971 both to Farmitalia); *eidem, Biotechnol. Bioeng.* **11**, 1101 (1969). Structural studies: F. Arcamone *et al., Tetrahedron Lett.* **10**, 1007 (1969). Synthesis from daunomycin, *q.v.: eidem, Chim. Ind. (Milan)* **51**, 834 (1969). Biochemical comparison with daunomycin: Wang *et al., Proc. Am. Assoc. Cancer Res.* **12**, No. 62, 77 (1971). In acid environment doxorubicin breaks up into **adriamycinone** and **daunosamine**: A. Di Marco *et al., Cancer Chemother. Rep. Part 1* **53**, 33 (1969). Pharmacokinetic and chemotherapeutic studies: E. Arena *et al., Arzneim.-Forsch.* **21**, 1258 (1971). LC/MS/MS determn of doxorubicin and metabolites: R. D. Arnold *et al., J. Chromatogr. B* **808**, 141 (2004). Toxicity study: C. Bertazzoli *et al., Experientia* **26**, 389 (1970). Comprehensive description: A. Vigevani, M. J. Williamson, *Anal. Profiles Drug Subs.* **9**, 245-274 (1980). Book: *Doxorubicin,* F. Arcamone, Ed. (Academic Press, New York, 1981) 369 pp. Review of clinical development: R. H. Blum, S. K. Carter, *Ann. Intern. Med.* **80**, 249-259 (1974); of efficacy in cancer therapy: H. L. Davis, T. E. Davis, *Cancer Treat. Rep.* **63**, 809-815 (1979); of clinical pharmacokinetics: P. A. J. Speth *et al., Clin. Pharmacokinet.* **15**, 15-31 (1988); of mechanism of cardiotoxicity: R. D. Olson, P. S. Mushlin, *FASEB J.* **4**, 3076-3086 (1990); of mechanism of action: G. Aubel-Sadron, D. Londos-Gagliardi, *Biochimie* **66**, 333-352 (1984); D. A. Gewirtz, *Biochem. Pharmacol.* **57**, 727-741 (1999); of liposomal formulations: D. N. Waterhouse *et al., Drug Saf.* **24**, 903-920 (2001).

Adriamycinone

Daunosamine

Hydrochloride. [25316-40-9] Adriacin; Adriablastina; Adriamycin. $C_{27}H_{29}NO_{11}$·HCl; mol wt 579.98. Red crystalline solid, mp 205° (dec). $[\alpha]_D^{20}$ +248±2° (c = 0.1 in methanol). Absorption max (methanol): 233, 253, 290, 477, 495, 530 nm (ε 38150, 25500, 8400, 13050, 13000, 7200). Apparent partition coefficient (1-octanol/Tris buffer pH 7.0): 0.52. Readily sol in water, normal saline, methanol, acetonitrile, THF. Practically insol in acetone, benzene, chloroform, ethyl ether and petr ether. Aq solns are yellow-orange at acid pHs, orange-red at neutral pHs and violet-blue at pH >9. LD_{50} i.v. in mice: 21.1 mg/kg (Bertazzoli, 1970).

Liposomal complex of the citrate. [111266-55-8] (doxorubicin citrate). Myocet. Doxorubicin citrate encapsulated in liposome carriers composed of egg phosphatidylcholine and cholesterol. Review of development and clinical efficacy in breast cancer: G. Batist *et al., Expert Opin. Pharmacother.* **3**, 1739-1751 (2002).

Liposomal complex of the hydrochloride. Caelyx; Doxil. Doxorubicin HCl encapsulated in liposome carriers composed of *N*-(carbonyl-methoxypolyethylene glycol 2000)-1,2-distearoyl-*sn*-glycero-3-phosphoethanolamine sodium salt, fully hydrogenated soy phosphatidylcholine, and cholesterol. Review of pharmacology and toxicology: P. K. Working, A. D. Dayan, *Hum. Exp. Toxicol.* **15**, 752-785 (1996); of clinical experience in solid and hematological malignancies and AIDS-related Kaposi's sarcoma: M. Sharpe *et al., Drugs* **62**, 2089-2126 (2002); of pharmacokinetics: A. Gabizon *et al., Clin. Pharmacokinet.* **42**, 419-436 (2003). LD_{50} in mice: 38.3±7.2 mg/kg (Working, Dayan).

Caution: Doxorubicin hydrochloride is reasonably anticipated to be a human carcinogen: *Report on Carcinogens, Eleventh Edition* (PB2005-104914, 2004) p III-8.

THERAP CAT: Antineoplastic.

3440. Doxycycline. [17086-28-1] (monohydrate); [564-25-0] (anhydrous). [4*S*-(4α,4aα,5α,5aα,6α,12aα)]-4-(Dimethylamino)-1,4,4a,5,5a,6,11,12a-octahydro-3,5,10,12,12a-pentahydroxy-6-methyl-1,11-dioxo-2-naphthacenecarboxamide monohydrate; α-6-

deoxy-5-hydroxytetracycline monohydrate; α-6-deoxyoxytetracy-cline monohydrate; 5-hydroxy-α-6-deoxytetracycline monohydrate; GS-3065; Doxirobe; Supracyclin. $C_{22}H_{24}N_2O_8.H_2O$; mol wt 462.45. C 57.14%, H 5.67%, N 6.06%, O 31.14%. Prepn of family of 6-deoxytetracyclines: C. R. Stephens *et al., J. Am. Chem. Soc.* **80,** 5324 (1958). *See also:* McCormick, Jensen, **US 3019260** (1962 to Am. Cyanamid). Prepn, separation and configuration of 6α- and 6β-epimers: M. S. von Wittenau *et al., J. Am. Chem. Soc.* **84,** 2645 (1962); C. R. Stephens *et al., ibid.* **85,** 2643 (1963). Prepn of 6α-deoxyoxytetracycline: R. K. Blackwood *et al.,* **US 3200149** (1965 to Pfizer). ^{1}H-NMR study: M. S. von Wittenau, R. K. Blackwood, *J. Org. Chem.* **31,** 613 (1966). Biological properties: English, *Proc. Soc. Exp. Biol. Med.* **122,** 1107 (1966). Pharmacology: Fabre, *Chemotherapia* **11,** 73 (1966); Gibaldi, *ibid.* **12,** 265 (1967). Toxicity of hyclate: Goldenthal, *Toxicol. Appl. Pharmacol.* **18,** 185 (1971). Clinical trial in prophylaxis of leptospirosis: E. T. Takafuji *et al., N. Engl. J. Med.* **310,** 497 (1984). Clinical trial in periodontitis: A. M. Polson *et al., J. Periodontol.* **68,** 110, 119 (1997). *Review:* C. Edwards in *Pharmacological and Biochemical Properties of Drug Substances* vol. 2, M. E. Goldberg, Ed. (Am. Pharm. Assoc., Washington, DC, 1979) pp 305-332.

Hydrochloride hemiethanolate hemihydrate. [24390-14-5] Doxycycline hyclate; Atridox; Azudoxat; Bassado; Clinofug; Diocimex; Doryx; Doxicrisol; Doxylar; Duradoxal; Granudoxy; Mespafin; Retens; Ronaxan; Spanor; Tetradox; Unacil; Vibramycin; Vibra-Tabs; Vibraveineuse; Vibravenös; Zadorin. $C_{22}H_{25}ClN_2O_8.\frac{1}{2}C_2H_6O.\frac{1}{2}H_2O$; mol wt 512.94. Light yellow, crystalline powder from ethanol + HCl. Chars without melting at about 201°. $[\alpha]_D^{25} -110°$ (c = 1 in 0.01N methanolic HCl). uv max (0.01N methanolic HCl): 267, 351 nm (log ε 4.24, 4.12). Sol in water. The alcohol and water of crystallization are lost by drying at 100° under reduced pressure. More active biologically than the corresponding 6β-epimer hydrochloride (Wittenau, 1962). LD50 i.p. in rats: 262 mg/kg (Goldenthal).

THERAP CAT: Antibacterial.
THERAP CAT (VET): Antibacterial.

3441. Doxylamine. [469-21-6] *N,N*-Dimethyl-2-[1-phenyl-1-(2-pyridinyl)ethoxy]ethanamine; 2-[α-(2-dimethylaminoethoxy)-α-methylbenzyl]pyridine; phenyl-2-pyridylmethyl-β-*N,N*-dimethylaminoethyl ether; 2-dimethylaminoethoxyphenylmethyl-2-picoline. $C_{17}H_{22}N_2O$; mol wt 270.37. C 75.52%, H 8.20%, N 10.36%, O 5.92%. Prepn: C. H. Tilford *et al., J. Am. Chem. Soc.* **70,** 4001 (1948); N. Sperber *et al., ibid.* **71,** 887 (1949). Pharmacology: B. B. Brown, H. Werner, *J. Lab. Clin. Med.* **33,** 325 (1948). GC determn: H. C. Thompson *et al., J. Chromatogr. Sci.* **20,** 373 (1982). Chronic toxicity study: C. D. Jackson, B. Blackwell, *J. Am. Coll. Toxicol.* **12,** 1 (1993). Review of properties and pharmacology: T. J. Haley, *Dangerous Prop. Ind. Mater. Rep.* **2,** 17-20 (1982). Clinical evaluation as hypnotic: P. Sjöqvist, L. Lasagna, *Clin. Pharmacol. Ther.* **8,** 48 (1967); as antihistaminic for use in colds: R. Eccles *et al., J. Pharm. Pharmacol.* **47,** 990 (1995).

Liquid, bp0.5 137-141°. Sol in acids. Slightly volatile, darkens on exposure to light.
Succinate. [562-10-7] Gittalun; Hoggar; Mereprine; Sedaplus; Unisom. $C_{17}H_{22}N_2O.C_4H_6O_4$; mol wt 388.46. Crystals, mp 100-

104°, sol in water. One gram dissolves in 1 ml water, 2 ml alcohol, 2 ml chloroform. Slightly sol in benzene and ether. pH (1% aq soln): 4.9 to 5.1. LD50 in mice, rabbits (mg/kg): 470, 250 orally; 62, 49 i.v.; in mice, male rats, female rats (mg/kg): 460, 440, 445 s.c. (Brown, Werner).

Combination with pyridoxine hydrochloride. Bendectin; Diclectin. Has been used for nausea of pregnancy. Some formulations also contained dicyclomine, *q.v.* Review of therapeutic use and the issue of teratogenicity: L. J. Sheffield, R. Batagol, *Med. J. Aust.* **143,** 143-147 (1985); R. L. Brent, *Reprod. Toxicol.* **9,** 337-349 (1995).

THERAP CAT: Antihistaminic; sedative, hypnotic.
THERAP CAT (VET): Antihistaminic.

3442. DPQ. [129075-73-6] 3,4-Dihydro-5-[4-(1-piperidin-yl)butoxy]-1(2*H*)-isoquinolinone. $C_{18}H_{26}N_2O_2$; mol wt 302.41. C 71.49%, H 8.67%, N 9.26%, O 10.58%. Competitive inhibitor of poly (ADP-ribose)polymerase (PARP). Prepn: M. J. Suto *et al.,* **EP 355720**; *eidem,* **US 5177075** (1990, 1993 both to Warner-Lambert). Use and effects as inhibitor: M. J. L. Eliasson *et al., Nat. Med.* **3,** 1089 (1997); K. Takahashi *et al., Brain Res.* **829,** 46 (1999).

Crystals from water, mp 107-109°. Water soluble.
USE: Reagent for inhibition of PARP.

3443. Dragon's Blood. A resinous secretion found on the fruits of *Daemonorops propinquus* Becc., *D. draco* Blume, and probably other species of *Daemonorops, Palmae* (Rattan palms). *Habit.* Sumatra, Borneo, India. *Constit.* About 55% of a red resin contg about 12-15% of bright-yellow, amorphous dracoresene; 2-3% white amorphous dracoalban. Isoln of the main coloring matter, dracorubin: Brockmann, Haase, *Ber.* **69,** 1950 (1936). Chemical studies of resin pigments: Olaniyi *et al., J. Chem. Soc. Perkin Trans. 1* **1973,** 179.

Red sticks, pieces, or cakes; vitreous fracture; makes a bright-crimson powder; odorless and almost tasteless. mp ~120° with sublimation of some benzoic acid. Insol in water; sol in alcohol.

USE: For coloring lacquers and varnishes; occasionally for coloring plasters; in photoengraving on zinc to protect metal parts against etching.

3444. Drimenin. [2326-89-8] [5a*S*-(5aα,9aβ,9bα)]-5,5a,6,-7,8,9,9a,9b-Octahydro-6,6,9a-trimethylnaphtho[1,2-*c*]furan-1(3*H*)-one. $C_{15}H_{22}O_2$; mol wt 234.33. C 76.88%, H 9.46%, O 13.66%. From bark of *Drimys winteri* Forst., *Magnoliaceae:* Appel, Dohr, *Scientia* **25,** 137 (1958); *C.A.* **54,** 4663f (1960). Structure and stereochemistry: Appel *et al., J. Chem. Soc.* **1960,** 4685. Synthesis: Wenkert, Strike, *J. Am. Chem. Soc.* **86,** 2044 (1964); Yamagawa, *et al., Synthesis* **1970,** 257; M. Jallali-Naini *et al., Tetrahedron Lett.* **22,** 2995 (1981).

Crystals from methanol and sublimed at 110°/0.1 mm, mp 133°. $[\alpha]_D -42°$ (c = 0.76 in benzene); $[\alpha]_D^{25} -35.8°$ (chloroform). Soluble in organic solvents; practically insol in water, acids, bases.

3445. Drofenine. [1679-76-1] α-Cyclohexylbenzeneacetic acid 2-(diethylamino)ethyl ester; α-phenylcyclohexaneacetic acid

2-(diethylamino)ethyl ester; 2-diethylaminoethyl α-phenylcyclo-hexaneacetate; hexahydroadiphenine. $C_{20}H_{31}NO_2$; mol wt 317.47. C 75.67%, H 9.84%, N 4.41%, O 10.08%. Prepn: Miescher, Hoffman, US 2265184; US 2265185 (both 1941 to Ciba). Pharmacology and toxicity: Fleisch *et al., Arzneim.-Forsch.* **11**, 1119 (1961).

bp$_{0.15}$ 158°.

Hydrochloride. [548-66-3] $C_{20}H_{31}NO_2$.HCl; mol wt 353.93. Crystals from alc + petr ether, mp 145-147°. Freely sol in water; very sparingly sol in alc, ether. A 5% aq soln is neutral to litmus. LD$_{50}$ i.v. in mice: 65.6 mg/kg (Fleisch).

THERAP CAT: Antispasmodic.

3446. Droloxifene. [82413-20-5] 3-[(1E)-1-[4-[2-(Dimeth-ylamino)ethoxy]phenyl]-2-phenyl-1-butenyl]phenol; (E)-α-[p-[2-(dimethylamino)ethoxy]phenyl]-α'-ethyl-3-stilbenol; (E)-1-[4'-(2-dimethylaminoethoxy)phenyl]-1-(3-hydroxyphenyl)-2-phenylbut-1-ene; 3-hydroxytamoxifen. $C_{26}H_{29}NO_2$; mol wt 387.51. C 80.59%, H 7.54%, N 3.61%, O 8.26%. Estrogen-receptor antago-nist. Prepn: H. Schickaneder *et al.*, **EP 54168**; *eidem*, **US 5047431** (1982, 1991 both to Klinge); P. C. Ruenitz *et al., J. Med. Chem.* **25**, 1056 (1982). Symposium on pharmacology and clinical studies: *Am. J. Clin. Oncol.* **14**, Suppl. 2, S1-S63 (1991). Clinical trial in breast cancer: P. F. Bruning, *Eur. J. Cancer* **28A**, 1404 (1992).

Colorless crystals from ether, mp 162-163° (Schickaneder); also reported as white crystals from benzene-hexane, mp 160-162° (Rue-nitz).

Citrate. [97752-20-0] K-21060E; FK-435. $C_{26}H_{29}NO_2.C_6H_8O_7$; mol wt 579.64. Slightly sol in water, methanol, ethanol. Insol in chloroform.

THERAP CAT: Antineoplastic (hormonal).

3447. Drometrizole. [2440-22-4] 2-(2H-Benzotriazol-2-yl)-4-methylphenol; 2-(2H-benzotriazol-2-yl)-p-cresol; 2-(2'-hy-droxy-5'-methylphenyl)benzotriazole; Tinuvin P. $C_{13}H_{11}N_3O$; mol wt 225.25. C 69.32%, H 4.92%, N 18.65%, O 7.10%. Prepn: Heller *et al.*, **US 3004896**; **US 3189615** (1961, 1965 to Geigy). Stabilization mechanism in acrylonitrile-butadiene-styrene (ABS) latex: J. B. Adeniyi, *J. Polym. Mater.* **3**, 25 (1986). HPLC determn in plastic: B. Niklasson, B. Björkner, *Contact Dermatitis* **21**, 330 (1989). Review of uses: Dunn, Fogg, *J. Appl. Polym. Sci.* **2**, 367 (1959); of toxicology and cosmetic use: CTFA, *J. Am. Coll. Tox-icol.* **5**, 455-470 (1986).

Minute crystals, mp 131-133°. bp$_{10}$ 225°. Sol in ethyl acetate, acetone, caprolactam solns, dioctylphthalate, oleyl alcohol, hot pet-

rolatum. Stable to conditions and chemicals used in polymerization or compounding of plastics.

USE: An ultraviolet light absorber for stabilizing plastics and other organic materials against discoloration and deterioration.

THERAP CAT: Ultraviolet screen.

3448. Dromostanolone. [58-19-5] (2α,5α,17β)-17-Hy-droxy-2-methyl-androstan-3-one; 17β-hydroxy-2α-methyl-5α-an-drostan-3-one; 2α-methylandrostan-17β-ol-3-one; 2α-methyl-dihydrotestosterone; drostanolone. $C_{20}H_{32}O_2$; mol wt 304.47. C 78.90%, H 10.59%, O 10.51%. Synthetic estrogen antagonist. Prepn: H. J. Ringold *et al., J. Am. Chem. Soc.* **81**, 427 (1959); H. J. Ringold, G. Rosenkranz, **US 3118915** (1964 to Syntex). GC-MS determn of urinary metabolites: D. DeBoer *et al., J. Steroid Bio-chem. Mol. Biol.* **42**, 411 (1992).

Crystals from acetone/hexane, mp 149-153°. [α]$_D$ +32° (etha-nol).

Propionate. [521-12-0] NSC-12198; Drolban; Emdisterone; Masterid; Masteril; Masterone; Permastril. $C_{23}H_{36}O_3$; mol wt 360.53. Crystals from hexane, mp 126-130°. [α]$_D$ +24°.

Note: This is a controlled substance (anabolic steroid): **21 CFR**, 1308.13, as defined in 1300.01.

THERAP CAT: Antineoplastic.

3449. Dronedarone. [141626-36-0] N-[2-Butyl-3-[4-[3-(di-butylamino)propoxy]benzoyl]-5-benzofuranyl]methanesulfona-mide; N,N-dibutyl-3-[4-[(2-butyl-5-methylsulfonamido)benzo-furan-3-ylcarbonyl]phenoxy]propylamine; SR-33589. $C_{31}H_{44}N_2O_5S$; mol wt 556.76. C 66.87%, H 7.97%, N 5.03%, O 14.37%, S 5.76%. Noniodinated analog of amiodarone, *q.v.* Prepn: J. Gubin *et al.*, **EP 471609**; *eidem*, **US 5223510** (1992, 1993 both to Sanofi). Hemodynamic and antiadrenergic effects in dogs: L. Djandjighian *et al., J. Cardiovasc. Pharmacol.* **36**, 376 (2000). Electrophysiological effects in canine heart: A. Varró *et al., Br. J. Pharmacol.* **133**, 625 (2001). Clinical pharmacokinetics and inter-action with metoprolol, *q.v.*: T. Damy *et al., Fundam. Clin. Phar-macol.* **18**, 113 (2004). Clinical evaluation in atrial fibrillation: P. Touboul *et al., Eur. Heart J.* **24**, 1481 (2003).

Crystals from hexane, mp 65.3°.

Hydrochloride. [141625-93-6] SR-33589B. $C_{31}H_{45}ClN_2O_5S$; mol wt 593.22. Colorless solid from acetone, mp 143°.

THERAP CAT: Antiarrhythmic (class III).

3450. Droperidol. [548-73-2] 1-[1-[4-(4-Fluorophenyl)-4-oxobutyl]-1,2,3,6-tetrahydro-4-pyridinyl]-1,3-dihydro-2H-benzimi-dazol-2-one; 1-[1-[3-(p-fluorobenzoyl)propyl]-1,2,3,6-tetrahydro-4-pyridyl]-2-benzimidazolinone; 1-[1-[4-(p-fluorophenyl)-4-oxo-butyl]-1,2,3,6-tetrahydro-4-pyridyl]-2-benzimidazolinone; R-4749; Dehydrobenzperidol; Dridol; Droleptan; Inapsine. $C_{22}H_{22}FN_3O_2$; mol wt 379.43. C 69.64%, H 5.84%, F 5.01%, N 11.07%, O 8.43%.

Prepn: P. A. J. Janssen, J. F. Gardocki, US 3161645 (1964 to Janssen). Pharmacology and toxicity: J. Yelnosky *et al., Toxicol. Appl. Pharmacol.* **6**, 37 (1964). Comprehensive description: C. A. Janicki, R. K. Gilpin, *Anal. Profiles Drug Subs.* **7**, 171-192 (1978).

Hydrate. Crystals, mp 145-146.5°. uv max (9:1, 0.1*M* HCl:methanol): 245, 280 nm (ε 15600, 7500). Soly at 25° (g/100 ml): chloroform 40; DMF 17; benzene 0.55; methanol 0.41; ethanol 0.34; ether 0.24; 0.1*M* HCl 0.15; water <0.001. pKa 7.64. Heat and light sensitive. LD$_{50}$ in mice (mg/kg): 125 s.c.; 43 i.v. (Yelnosky).
Note: Ingredient of **Thalamonal, Innovar.**
THERAP CAT: Antipsychotic.
THERAP CAT (VET): Tranquilizer.

3451. Droprenilamine. [57653-27-7] *N*-(2-Cyclohexyl-1-methylethyl)-γ-phenylbenzenepropanamine; (±)-*N*-(3,3-diphenyl-propyl)-α-methylcyclohexaneethylamine; droprenylamine. C$_{24}$-H$_{33}$N; mol wt 335.53. C 85.91%, H 9.91%, N 4.17%. Vasodilator with antiarrhythmic and hypotensive activity. Prepn: M. Carissimi *et al.,* DE 2521113 (1976 to Maggioni), *C.A.* **84**, 164388t (1976). Synthesis and pharmacological study: G. Carenini *et al., Arzneim.-Forsch.* **26**, 2127 (1976). Hemodynamic and metabolic effects: R. J. Marshall, J. R. Parratt, *Br. J. Pharmacol.* **59**, 311 (1977). Clinical evaluation: F. Rengo *et al., G. Ital. Cardiol.* **10**, 473 (1980).

Hydrochloride. [59182-63-7] MG-8926; Valcor. C$_{24}$H$_{33}$-N.HCl; mol wt 371.99. Crystals from isopropanol, mp 175-176°. LD$_{50}$ in mice (mg/kg): 2850 orally; 68 i.p. (Carenini).
THERAP CAT: Vasodilator (coronary).

3452. Dropropizine. [17692-31-8] 3-(4-Phenyl-1-pipera-zinyl)-1,2-propanediol; 1-phenyl-4-(2,3-dihydroxypropyl)-piperazine; 1-(2,3-dihydroxypropyl)-4-phenylpiperazine; 1-phenyl-4-(2,3-dihydroxypropyl)diethylenediamine; UCB-1967; Ribex. C$_{13}$H$_{20}$N$_2$O$_2$; mol wt 236.31. C 66.07%, H 8.53%, N 11.85%, O 13.54%. Cough suppressive phenylpiperazine derivative. Prepn: H. G. Morren, BE 601394; *eidem,* US 3163649 (1961, 1964 to UCB); H. Howell *et al., J. Org. Chem.* **27**, 1709 (1962); J. Bourdais, *Bull. Soc. Chim. Fr.* **1968**, 3246. Prepn of enantiomers: M. Borsa *et al.,* EP 147847; *eidem,* US 4699911 (1985, 1987 both to Dompé). LC-MS-MS determn in plasma: Y. Tang *et al., J. Chromatogr. B* **819**, 185 (2005). Pharmacology: K. Cartwright, J. L. Paterson, *J. Pharm. Pharmacol.* **23**, Suppl., 247S (1971). Controlled clinical trials: G. C. Moreo *et al., Gazz. Med. Ital.* **140**, 409 (1981); A. Ravetta, M. Ravetta, *ibid.* **141**, 531 (1982). Chronic oral toxicity: P. R. B. Noel, *Arzneim.-Forsch.* **19**, 1246 (1969).

Crystals from benzene, mp 105° (Morren); also reported as mp 108° (Bourdais). LD$_{50}$ in rats (mg/kg): 200 i.v., 750 orally (Morren).
S-Form. [99291-24-8] Levodropropizine; Danka; Levotuss; Rapitux. White solid from acetone, mp 98-100°. [α]$_D^{25}$ −10° (c = 1.0 in ethanol). LD$_{50}$ in mice, rats (mg/kg): 1287.2, 886.6 orally; 408.0, 401.3 i.p. (Borsa).
R-Form. Crystals from acetone, mp 104-105°. [α]$_D^{25}$ +9.7° (c = 1.0 in ethanol). LD$_{50}$ in mice, rats (mg/kg): 871.7, 721.3 orally; 319.2, 363.4 i.p. (Borsa).
THERAP CAT: Antitussive.

3453. Drosera. Common sundew; round-leafed sundew; youthwort. Air-dried, flowering plant, *Drosera rotundifolia* L., frequently mixed with closely allied species *D. anglica* Hudson and *D. longifolia* L., *Droseraceae. Habit.* Europe, Asia, North America, south to Florida. *Constit.* Malic and citric acids, resin, tannin.

3454. Drospirenone. [67392-87-4] (2'S,6R,7R,8R,9S,10R,-13S,14S,15S,16S)-1,3',4',6,7,8,9,10,11,12,13,14,15,16,20,21-Hexa-decahydro-10,13-dimethylspiro[17*H*-dicyclopropa[6,7:15,16]-cyclopenta[a]phenanthrene-17,2'(5'H)-furan]-3,5'(2H)-dione; 6β,-7β,15β,16β-dimethylene-3-oxo-4-androstene-[17(β-1')-spiro-5']-perhydrofuran-2'-one; 6β,7β,15β,16β-dimethylen-3-oxo-17α-pregn-4-ene-21,17-carbolactone; dihydrospirorenone; ZK-30595. C$_{24}$H$_{30}$O$_3$; mol wt 366.49. C 78.65%, H 8.25%, O 13.10%. Synthetic progestogen exhibiting antimineralocorticoid and antian-drogenic activity. Prepn: R. Wiechert *et al.,* DE 2652761; *eidem,* US 4129564 (both 1978 to Schering AG); D. Bittler *et al., Angew. Chem.* **94**, 718 (1982). HPLC determn in human plasma: W. Krause, U. Jakobs, *J. Chromatogr.* **230**, 37 (1982). Pharmacolog-ical profile: P. Muhn *et al., Contraception* **51**, 99 (1995). Review of synthesis: H. Laurent *et al., J. Steroid Biochem.* **19**, 771-776 (1983); of pharmacology and clinical experience: W. Oelkers, *Mol. Cell. Endocrinol.* **217**, 255-261 (2004).

mp 201.3°. [α]$_D^{22}$ −182° (c = 0.5 in chloroform). uv (methanol): 265 nm (ε 19000).
Mixture with ethinyl estradiol. Angeliq; Yasmin. Clinical trial as oral contraceptive: K. S. Parsey, A. Pong, *Contraception* **61**, 105 (2000); in treatment of menopausal symptoms: R. Schür-mann *et al., Climacteric* **7**, 189 (2004).
THERAP CAT: Progestogen. In combination with estrogen as oral contaceptive and in treatment of menopausal symptoms.

3455. Drotaverine. [14009-24-6] 1-[(3,4-Diethoxyphenyl)-methylene]-6,7-diethoxy-1,2,3,4-tetrahydroisoquinoline; 1-(3,4-di-ethoxybenzylidene)-6,7diethoxy-1,2,3,4-tetrahydroisoquinoline; isodihydroperparine. C$_{24}$H$_{31}$NO$_4$; mol wt 397.51. C 72.52%, H 7.86%, N 3.52%, O 16.10%. Analogue of papaverine, *q.v.* Prepn: BE 621917 (1962 to Chinoin), *C.A.* **59**, 8713g (1963). Synthesis: E. Koltai *et al., J. Labelled Compd. Radiopharm.* **16**, 351 (1979). Crystal structure: Z. Böcksei *et al., Acta Crystallogr.* **C51**, 1587 (1995). Absorption study: P. Szentmiklosi, S. Marton, *Pharmazie* **38**, 611 (1983). Platelet aggregation and hemorrheological effects: Z. Kapui *et al., Thromb. Res.* **66**, 693 (1992). Clinical pharmaco-kinetics and bioavailability: O. O. Bolaji *et al., Eur. J. Drug Metab. Pharmacokinet.* **21**, 217 (1996). HPLC determn in biological flu-ids: *eidem, J. Chromatogr.* **622**, 93 (1993). Clinical evaluation: D. Vecsey, *Ther. Hung.* **32**, 127 (1984). Clinical effects on fetal development: A. E. Czeizel, M. Rockenbauer, *Prenatal Neonat. Med.* **1**, 137 (1996).

Acephyllinate. [61954-97-0] Drotaverine theophylline-7-acetic acid; 6,7,3',4'-tetraethoxy-1-benzyl-3,4-dihydroisoquinoline xanthine-7-acetate; DRA; Depogen. $C_{24}H_{31}NO_4 \cdot C_9H_{10}N_4O_4$; mol wt 635.71. Exists as monohydrate.

Hydrochloride. [985-12-6] No-Spa. Pale yellow crystals from ethanol, mp 197-200° (uncorr).

THERAP CAT: Antispasmodic.

3456. Drotebanol. [3176-03-2] (6β)-3,4-Dimethoxy-17-methylmorphinan-6,14-diol; 6β,14-dihydroxy-3,4-dimethoxy-N-methylmorphinan; 14-hydroxydihydro-6β-thebainol 4-methyl ether; dihydro-14-hydroxy-4-O-methyl-6β-thebainol; dihydro-14-hydroxy-6β-thebainol 4-methyl ether; oxymethebanol; Metebanyl. $C_{19}H_{27}NO_4$; mol wt 333.42. C 68.44%, H 8.16%, N 4.20%, O 19.19%. Prepn from thebaine: **JP 64 26726** (1964 to Sankyo), C.A. **62**, 11869b (1965). Metabolism: H. Shindo *et al., Yakugaku Zasshi* **90**, 36 (1970), C.A. **72**, 88520q (1970). Pharmacology: S. Kobayashi *et al., Arzneim.-Forsch.* **20**, 43 (1970). Dependence potential in rhesus monkeys: T. Yanagita *et al., Bull. Narc.* **29**, 33 (1977).

Minute crystals, very slightly hygroscopic, slightly bitter taste. mp 165.5-166.5°. Slightly sol in water. Freely sol in ethanol, chloroform. Sol in acetone, benzene, toluene. Very slightly sol in ether. LD_{50} in mice (mg/kg): 1300 orally, 1150 s.c., 91 i.v. (Kobayashi).

Note: This is a controlled substance (opium derivative): **21 CFR**, 1308.11.

THERAP CAT: Antitussive.

3457. Droxidopa. [23651-95-8] *threo*-β,3-Dihydroxy-L-tyrosine; L-*threo*-3-(3,4-dihydroxyphenyl)serine; (−)-(2S,3R)-2-amino-3-hydroxy-3-(3,4-dihydroxyphenyl)propionic acid; *threo*-dopaserine; L-*threo*-DOPS; L-DOPS; SM-5688; Dops. $C_9H_{11}NO_5$; mol wt 213.19. C 50.70%, H 5.20%, N 6.57%, O 37.52%. Synthetic amino acid precursor of norepinephrine, *q.v.* Prepn of racemate: K. W. Rosenmund, H. Dornsaft, *Ber.* **52B**, 1734 (1919). Separation and resolution of diastereomers: B. Hegedüs *et al., Helv. Chim. Acta* **58**, 147 (1975); B. Hegedüs, A. Krasso, **US 3920728** (1975 to Hoffmann-La Roche). Improved process for production: N. Ohashi *et al.,* **US 4319040** (1982 to Sumitomo). Pharmacology of stereoisomers: G. Bartholini *et al. J. Pharmacol. Exp. Ther.* **193**, 523 (1975). Clinical pharmacology of L-*threo*-form and clinical evaluation in familial amyloid polyneuropathy (FAP): T. Suzuki *et al., Eur. J. Clin. Pharmacol.* **17**, 429 (1980). Reversed-phase chromatography determn in plasma and urine: F. Boomsma *et al., J. Chromatogr.* **427**, 219 (1988). Pharmacokinetics in FAP: T. Suzuki *et al., Eur. J. Clin. Pharmacol.* **23**, 463 (1982); in parkinsonism: T. Suzuki *et al., Neurology* **34**, 1446 (1984). Metabolism to norepinephrine: T. Suzuki *et al., Life Sci.* **36**, 435 (1985). Clinical studies in Parkinson's disease: N. Ogawa *et al., J. Med.* **16**, 525 (1985); H. Narabayashi *et al., Adv. Neurol.* **45**, 593 (1986).

Crystals from ethanol and ether, mp 232-235° (dec). $[\alpha]_D^{20} -39°$ (c = 1 in 1N aq HCl). Also cited as crystals from water and L-ascorbic acid, mp 229-232° (dec) (Ohashi). $[\alpha]_D^{20} -42.0°$ (c = 1 in 1N aq HCl).

THERAP CAT: Antiparkinsonian.

3458. DSIP. [62568-57-4] Delta sleep-inducing peptide (rabbit); delta sleep peptide; delta sleep factor. $C_{35}H_{48}N_{10}O_{15}$; mol wt 848.81. C 49.53%, H 5.70%, N 16.50%, O 28.27%. A nonapeptide that shows enhancement and induction of delta (slow-wave) and spindle EEG patterns. Its occurrence was suspected during dialysis of cerebral venous blood of rabbits during sleep induced by electrical stimulation of the thalamus: M. Monnier, L. Hösli, *Science* **146**, 796 (1964). Initial isoln: *eidem, Pfluegers Arch.* **282**, 60 (1965). Isoln, characterization: G. A. Schoenenberger *et al., Experientia* **28**, 919 (1972). Amino acid sequence, synthesis of DSIP and analogs: G. A. Schoenenberger, M. Monnier, *Proc. Natl. Acad. Sci. USA* **74**, 1282 (1977). Solid phase synthesis: Y. P. Shvachkin *et al., Zh. Obshch. Khim.* **51**, 719 (1981), C.A. **95**, 43644s (1981). Rapid liquid phase synthesis: S. Nozaki, I. Muramatsu, *Bull. Chem. Soc. Jpn.* **55**, 2165 (1982). HPLC separation: M. Dizaroglu *et al., J. Chromatogr.* **237**, 417 (1982). Effect on human sleep: D. Schneider-Helmert *et al., Lancet* **1**, 1256 (1981); *eidem, Int. J. Clin. Pharmacol. Ther. Toxicol.* **19**, 341 (1981); D. Schneider-Helmert, G. A. Schoenenberger, *Experientia* **37**, 913 (1981).

Trp–Ala–Gly–Gly–Asp–Ala–Ser–Gly–Glu

3459. DSPA. Vampire bat salivary plasminogen activator; BatPA; v-PA. Plasminogen activator naturally occurring in the saliva of the vampire bat, *Desmodus rotundus*. Four isoforms have been identified. All are single chain peptides that are structurally homologous to human tissue plasminogen activator, *q.v.* DSPA-α1 and -α2 are comprised of 477 amino acid residues containing 4 distinct domains; isoforms β and γ are smaller, truncated versions. DSPA-α1 and -α2 bind to fibrin; all isoforms require fibrin as a cofactor for plasminogen activation: Isoln: C. Hawkey, *Nature* **211**, 434 (1966). Cloning, characterization and structure: S. J. Gardell *et al., J. Biol. Chem.* **264**, 17947 (1989). Identification of isoforms: J. Krätzschmar *et al., Gene* **105**, 229 (1991). Review of purification, properties and activity: S. J. Gardell, P. A. Friedman, *Methods Enzymol.* **223**, 233-249 (1993). Study of structural mechanism of catalytic activity: M. Renatus *et al., Biochemistry* **36**, 13483 (1997).

Desmoteplase. [145137-38-8] Plasminogen activator (Desmodus rotundus isoform α1 protein moiety reduced); rDSPA alpha 1. DSPA-α1 produced by recombinant technology; mol wt 55-58 kDa. Prepn: B. Baldus *et al.,* **WO 9009438**; *eidem,* **US 6008019** (1990, 1999 both to Schering AG); T. Petri *et al., J. Biotechnol.* **39**, 75 (1995). CE/MS method for pharmaceutical formulations: J. A. Chakel *et al., J. Chromatogr. B* **689**, 215 (1997). Pharmacology: W.-D. Schleuning, *Haemostasis* **31**, 118 (2001). Clinical evaluation in acute ischemic stroke: W. Hacke *et al., Stroke* **36**, 66 (2005). *Review:* T. Debens, *Curr. Opin. Mol. Ther.* **6**, 567-575 (2004).

THERAP CAT: Thrombolytic.

3460. DTAF. [51306-35-5] 5-[(4,6-Dichloro-1,3,5-triazin-2-yl)amino]-3',6'-dihydroxyspiro[isobenzofuran-1(3H),9'-[9H]xanthen]-3-one; 5-(4,6-dichlorotriazinyl)aminofluorescein. $C_{23}H_{12}Cl_2N_4O_5$; mol wt 495.27. C 55.78%, H 2.44%, Cl 14.32%, N 11.31%, O 16.15%. Fluorochrome labelling agent related to fluorescein, *q.v.* Prepn: V. E. Barskii *et al., Izv. Akad. Nauk Ser. Biol.* **1968**, 744, C.A. **70**, 79127 (1969); and use as label: D. Blakeslee, M. G. Baines, *J. Immunol. Methods* **13**, 305 (1976). Practical comparison with FITC, *q.v.,* for labelling: S. P. D. Lalljie, P. Sandra, *Chromatographia* **40**, 519 (1995). Use as label for carbohydrates and proteins: R. Schumann, D. Rentsch, *Mar. Ecol. Prog.*

Ser. **163,** 77 (1998); for poloxamers, *q.v.*: F. Ahmed *et al., Langmuir* **17,** 537 (2001). Ultrasensitive chromatographic/fluorescent determn of amino acid herbicides: M. Molina, M. Silva, *Electrophoresis* **23,** 1096 (2002).

Bright yellow powder. Very stable when dry; hydrolyzes in alkaline solutions (pH 9.0). Absorption max: 492 nm; emission max: 513 nm (c = 5 × 10^{-7} M in 0.1 *M* sodium borate).

USE: Fluorescent reagent for conjugation of fluorescein to proteins, carbohydrates and selected polymers.

3461. DTBP. [110-05-4] Bis(1,1-Dimethylethyl) peroxide; di-*tert*-butyl peroxide. $C_8H_{18}O_2$; mol wt 146.23. C 65.71%, H 12.41%, O 21.88%. $(CH_3)_3COOC(CH_3)_3$.
Flammable liq; d_4^{20} 0.7940; mp −40°; bp_{284} 80°; n_D^{20} 1.3890. Flash pt (Tag open cup) 65°F (18°C). Soluble in organic solvents, in most resin monomers and in partial polymers. Soly in water about 0.01%.

USE: As polymerization catalyst.

3462. Dubnium. [53850-35-4] Element 105; hahnium; nielsbohrium; unnilpentium. Db, Ha, Ns, Unp; at. no. 105. Group VB(5). No stable nuclides. Prepn of α-emitting ^{260}105 isotope ($T_{1/2}$ 1.6±0.3 sec) by ^{249}Cf (^{15}N,4n): A. Ghiorso *et al., Phys. Rev. Lett.* **24,** 1498 (1970). Prepn of ^{261}105 isotope (decay by spontaneous fission, $T_{1/2}$ 1.8 ±0.6 sec) by ^{243}Am (^{22}Ne,4n): G. N. Flerov *et al., At. Energ.* **29,** 243 (1970); *eidem, Nucl. Phys. A* **160,** 181 (1971); *eidem, Proc. Int. Conf. Heavy Ion Phys.* **1971** pp 125-143, *C.A.* **80,** 139758y (1974). Prepn of α-emitting isotopes ^{261}105 ($T_{1/2}$ 1.7 sec) by ^{249}Bk (^{16}O,4n) or by ^{250}Cf (^{15}N,4n); ^{262}105 ($T_{1/2}$ 40.0 ±10 sec, longest-lived known isotope, rel. at. mass 262.1144) by ^{249}Bk(^{18}O,5n): A. Ghiorso *et al., Phys. Rev.* **C4,** 1850 (1971); and revised $T_{1/2}$ 34.1 ±4.6 sec for ^{262}105: C. E. Bemis, Jr. *et al., Phys. Rev. Lett.* **39,** 1246 (1977). Discussion of conflicting claims of discovery: Holcomb, *Science* **168,** 810 (1970); G. N. Flerov, *ibid.* **170,** 15 (1970); A. Ghiorso, *ibid.* **171,** 127 (1971). Solution chemistry: K. E. Gregorich *et al., Radiochim. Acta* **43,** 223 (1988); M. K. Gober *et al., ibid.* **57,** 77 (1992); and identification of ^{263}105 isotope ($T_{1/2}$ 27 sec, α-emitter) by ^{249}Bk(^{18}O,4n): M. Schädel *et al., ibid.* 85. Reviews of history, prepn and properties: C. Keller, *The Chemistry of the Transuranium Elements* (Verlag Chemie, Weinheim, English Ed., 1971) pp 619-622; Silva, "Trans-Curium Elements" in *MTP Int. Rev. Sci.: Inorg. Chem., Ser. One* **vol. 8,** A. G. Maddock, Ed. (University Park Press, Baltimore, 1972) pp 71-105; R. J. Silva in *The Chemistry of the Actinide Elements* **vol. 2,** J. J. Katz *et al.,* Eds. (Chapman and Hall, New York, 1986) pp 1106-1109; E. K. Hyde *et al., Radiochim. Acta* **42,** 57-102 (1987); Transfermium Working Group, *Pure Appl. Chem.* **65,** 1757-1814 (1993). Review of chemistry: D. C. Hoffman, *Proc. Robert A. Welch Found. Conf. on Chem. Res., XXXIV, Fifty Years with Transuranium Elements* (Houston, Texas, 1990) pp 255-276.

3463. Dulcamara. Bittersweet; woody nightshade; scarlet berry. Dried stems of *Solanum dulcamara* L., *Solanaceae*. *Habit.* Europe, Western Asia, Northern Africa, natural in U.S. *Constit.* Solaniceine (about 1%), dulcamarin, dulcamaric and dulcamaretic acids.

3464. Dulcin. [150-69-6] (4-Ethoxyphenyl)urea; *p*-phenetolcarbamide; *p*-phenetylurea; Sucrol; Valzin. $C_9H_{12}N_2O_2$; mol wt 180.20. C 59.99%, H 6.71%, N 15.55%, O 17.76%. Made by treating *p*-phenetidine with phosgene and then with ammonia:

Berlinerblau, *J. Prakt. Chem.* **30,** 103 (1883); from *p*-phenetidine and urea: Kurzer, *Org. Synth.* **coll. vol. IV,** 52 (1963).

Lustrous needles. Very sweet taste, about 250 times as sweet as cane sugar. mp 173-174°. Sol in 800 parts cold water, 50 parts boiling water, 25 parts alcohol.

USE: Non-nutritive sweetener.

3465. Duloxetine. [116539-59-4] (γS)-*N*-Methyl-γ-(1-naphthalenyloxy)-2-thiophenepropanamine; (+)-(*S*)-*N*-methyl-γ-(1-naphthyloxy)-2-thiophenepropylamine; (+)-*N*-methyl-3-(1-naphthalenyloxy)-3-(2-thienyl)propanamine; LY-248686. $C_{18}H_{19}NOS$; mol wt 297.41. C 72.69%, H 6.44%, N 4.71%, O 5.38%, S 10.78%. Dual serotonin and norepinephrine reuptake inhibitor (SNRI). Prepn: D. W. Robertson *et al.,* **EP 273658;** *eidem,* **US 5023269** (1988, 1991 both to Lilly); and abs config: J. Deeter *et al., Tetrahedron Lett.* **31,** 7101 (1990). Improved process: R. A. Berglund, **US 5362886** (1994 to Lilly). Pharmacology: D. T. Wong *et al., Neuropsychopharmacology* **8,** 23 (1993). Neurochemical effects *in vivo*: R. W. Fuller *et al., J. Pharmacol. Exp. Ther.* **269,** 132 (1994). Determn of chiral purity: E. C. Rickard, R. J. Bopp, *J. Chromatogr. A* **680,** 609 (1994). Clinical pharmacokinetics: A. Sharma *et al., J. Clin. Pharmacol.* **40,** 161 (2000). Clinical trial in stress incontinence: P. A. Norton *et al., Am. J. Obstet. Gynecol.* **187,** 40 (2002); in depression: M. J. Detke *et al., J. Psychiatr. Res.* **36,** 383 (2002).

Hydrochloride. [136434-34-9] Ariclaim; Cymbalta; Yentreve. $C_{18}H_{19}NOS.HCl$. White solid. pKa in DMF-water (66:34): 9.6.

THERAP CAT: Antidepressant; in treatment of stress urinary incontinence.

3466. DuPHOS. Series of chiral bis(phospholane) compounds with C_2 symmetry used as rhodium complexes for catalysis. Prepn: M. J. Burk, *J. Am. Chem. Soc.* **113,** 8518 (1991); and configuration: *idem et al., ibid.* **115,** 10125 (1993). Use in asymmetric synthesis of warfarin: A. Robinson *et al, Tetrahedron Lett.* **37,** 8321 (1996); hydrogena-tions of β-(acylamino)acrylates: G. Zhu *et al., J. Org. Chem.* **64,** 6907 (1999).

(R,R)-Ethyl DuPHOS

(R,R)-**Me-DuPHOS.** [147253-67-6] [2R-[1(2′*R**,5′*R**),2α,-5β]]-1,1′-(1,2-Phenylene)bis[2,5-dimethylphospholane]. $C_{18}H_{28}$-P_2; mol wt 306.36.

(S,S)-**Me-DuPHOS.** [136735-95-0] (*S,S*)-1,2-Bis(2,5-dimethylphospholano)benzene. $C_{18}H_{28}P_2$; mol wt 306.36. Colorless crystals from methanol, mp 79-81°. $[α]_D^{25}$ +476± 5° (c = 1 in hexane).

(R,R)-Et-DuPHOS. [136705-64-1] (2R,2'R,5R,5'R)-1,1'-(1,2-Phenylene)bis[2,5-diethylphospholane]. $C_{22}H_{36}P_2$; mol wt 362.47. Colorless oil. $[\alpha]_D^{25}$ −265° (c = 1 in hexane). $bp_{0.045}$ 138-145°.

USE: Catalyst for asymmetric hydrogenations.

3467. Durapatite. [1306-06-5] Hydroxylapatite; calcium phosphate hydroxide; calcium orthophosphate basic; hydroxyapatite; Alveograf; Ossopan; Periograf. $3Ca_3(PO_4)_2 \cdot Ca(OH)_2$ or $Ca_{10}(PO_4)_6(OH)_2$. Also considered as pentacalcium monohydroxyorthophosphate $Ca_5(OH)(PO_4)_3$. Calcd as $Ca_{10}H_2O_{26}P_6$; Ca 39.89%, H 0.20%, O 41.41%, P 18.50%. Occurs as a mineral in phosphate rock. Constitutes the mineral portion of bone. Prepn from $Ca(NO_3)_2$ and KH_2PO_4: Warington, *J. Chem. Soc.* **26**, 983 (1873); Rathje, *Ber.* **74**, 342 (1941); Hayek in *Handbook of Preparative Inorganic Chemistry*, G. Brauer, Ed. (Academic Press, 2nd ed., 1963) p 545; from calcium phosphate, dibasic: Perloff, Posner, *Inorg. Synth.* **6**, 16 (1960); from $Ca(NO_3)_2 \cdot 4H_2O$ and $(NH_4)_3PO_4$ plus NH_4OH: Hayek, Newesely, *ibid.* **7**, 63 (1963). Formation and structure of synthetic bone hydroxyapatites: A. S. Posner *et al., Prog. Cryst. Growth Charact.* **3**, 3 (1980).

Hexagonal needles arranged in rosettes. Dec above 1100°. Practically insol in water, even when freshly prepd. Crystallographic data: a_0 9.425; C_0 6.935; C_0/a_0 0.736.

USE: Prosthetic aid (artificial bone and teeth).

THERAP CAT: Calcium supplement; phosphorus supplement.

3468. Durene. [95-93-2] 1,2,4,5-Tetramethylbenzene; Durol. $C_{10}H_{14}$; mol wt 134.22. C 89.49%, H 10.51%. Occurs in coal tar. Usually prepd from xylene and methyl chloride in the presence of $AlCl_3$: Smith, *Org. Synth.* **vol. 10**, 32 (1930); *cf.* Smith, Dobrovolny, *J. Am. Chem. Soc.* **48**, 1413 (1926).

Scales with camphor-like odor from alcohol. d_4^{81} 0.84. mp 80°. bp 191-193°. Sublimes and is volatile with steam. Insol in water; freely sol in alcohol, ether, benzene.

3469. Durohydroquinone. [527-18-4] 2,3,5,6-Tetramethyl-1,4-benzenediol; tetramethyl-*p*-hydroquinone; dihydroxydurene. $C_{10}H_{14}O_2$; mol wt 166.22. C 72.26%, H 8.49%, O 19.25%. For prepn *see* refs under Duroquinone.

Needles from alcohol. mp 233°. Begins to sinter at 220°. Sparingly sol in ether. Treatment with ferric chloride yields duroquinone.

Diacetyldurohydroquinone. Needles from alc, mp 207°.

3470. Duroquinone. [527-17-3] 2,3,5,6-Tetramethyl-2,5-cyclohexadiene-1,4-dione; tetramethyl-*p*-benzoquinone. $C_{10}H_{12}O_2$; mol wt 164.20. C 73.15%, H 7.37%, O 19.49%. Prepn by reduction of dinitrodurene: Smith, *Org. Synth.* **vol. 10**, 40 (1930); Smith, Dobrovolny, *J. Am. Chem. Soc.* **48**, 1420 (1926); by condensation of 2,3-diketopentane with itself in presence of alkalies: von Pechmann, *Ber.* **21**, 1420 (1888); by the action of alkalies on 3,3-dichloropentan-2-one: Faworsky, *J. Prakt. Chem.* [2] **51**, 538 (1895).

Yellow needles from alc, mp 111-112°. Sublimes. Volatile with steam. Insol in water; sol in alcohol, benzene, ether, hot petr ether.

3471. Dutasteride. [164656-23-9] (4aR,4bS,6aS,7S,9aS,9bS,11aR)-N-[2,5-Bis(trifluoromethyl)phenyl]-2,4a,4b,5,6,6a,7,8,-9,9a,9b,10,11,11a-tetradecahydro-4a,6a-dimethyl-2-oxo-1H-indeno[5,4-f]quinoline-7-carboxamide; 17β-N-[2,5-Bis(trifluoromethyl)phenyl]carbamoyl-4-aza-5α-androst-1-en-3-one; GG-745; GI-198745; Avodart; Avolve. $C_{27}H_{30}F_6N_2O_2$; mol wt 528.53. C 61.36%, H 5.72%, F 21.57%, N 5.30%, O 6.05%. Dual inhibitor of 5α-reductase isoenzymes types 1 and 2; structurally related to finasteride, *q.v.* Prepn: K. W. Batchelor, S. V. Frye, **WO 9507927** (1995 to Glaxo). Structure-activity study: R. K. Bakshi *et al., J. Med. Chem.* **38**, 3189 (1995). Clinical pharmacokinetics: P. O. Gisleskog *et al., Br. J. Clin. Pharmacol.* **47**, 53 (1999). Clinical trial in benign prostatic hyperplasia: C. G. Roehrborn *et al., Urology* **60**, 434 (2002). Review of discovery and development: S. V. Frye *et al., Pharm. Biotechnol.* **11**, 393-422 (1998); of clinical experience: B. Djavan *et al., Expert Opin. Pharmacother.* **6**, 311-317 (2005).

White crystalline solid, mp 245-245.5°.

THERAP CAT: In treatment of benign prostatic hyperplasia.

3472. Duthaler-Hafner Reagent. [132068-98-5] Chloro-(η^5-2,4-cyclopentadien-1-yl)[(4R,5R)-2,2-dimethyl-$\alpha,\alpha,\alpha',\alpha'$-tetraphenyl-1,3-dioxolane-4,5-dimethanolato(2−)-$\kappa O^4,\kappa O^5$]titanium. $C_{36}H_{33}ClO_4Ti$; mol wt 612.96. C 70.54%, H 5.43%, Cl 5.78%, O 10.44%, Ti 7.81%. Enantioselective allyl-transfer reagent. Prepn: R. O. Duthaler *et al., Pure Appl. Chem.* **62**, 631 (1990). As reagent in prepn of titanium transmetallation complexes: A. Hafner *et al., J. Am. Chem. Soc.* **114**, 2321 (1992). Use in aldol reactions: R. C. Cambie *et al., Aust. J. Chem.* **46**, 583 (1993); in asymmetric allylation: A. Fürstner, K. Langemann, *J. Am. Chem. Soc.* **119**, 9130 (1997). Review of prepn, structure and use: R. O. Duthaler *et al.*, in *Proc. 3rd Symp. Org. Synth. Organomet. 1990*, K. H. Doetz, R. W. Hoffmann Eds. (Vieweg, Braunschweig, Germany, 1991) pp 285-309.

mp 209-213°. $[\alpha]_D^{20}$ −246° (c = 1 in $CHCl_3$). Moisture sensitive, store under nitrogen. *Corrosive*.

(S,S)-Form. [140462-73-3] mp 209-213°. $[\alpha]_D^{20}$ +246° (c = 1 in $CHCl_3$). Moisture sensitive, store under nitrogen. *Corrosive*.

USE: Transmetallation of allyl-Grignard or allyl-Li compounds.

3473. Dyclonine. [586-60-7] 1-(4-Butoxyphenyl)-3-(1-piperidinyl)-1-propanone; 3-piperidino-4'-butoxypropiophenone; β-piperidinoethyl-4-butoxyphenyl ketone; 4-butoxy-β-piperidinopropiophenone; 4-*n*-butoxy-β-(1-piperidyl)propiophenone; 4-butoxyphenyl piperidineethyl ketone; 2-(1-piperidyl)ethyl *p*-butoxyphenyl ketone. $C_{18}H_{27}NO_2$; mol wt 289.41. C 74.70%, H 9.40%, N 4.84%, O 11.06%. Prepd from *p*-butoxyacetophenone by condensation with formaldehyde and piperidine hydrochloride: Pofft, *Chem. Tech. (Berlin)* **4**, 241 (1952), *C.A.* **47**, 10531 (1953).

Hydrochloride. [536-43-6] Dyclone; Tanaclone. $C_{18}H_{27}$-NO_2.HCl; mol wt 325.87. Crystals, mp 175-176°. Sol in water, alc, acetone. Phenol coefficient 3.6.

THERAP CAT: Anesthetic (local).

3474. Dydrogesterone. [152-62-5] (9β,10α)-Pregna-4,6-diene-3,20-dione; 10α-pregna-4,6-diene-3,20-dione; 6-dehydro-*retro*-progesterone; 10α-isopregnenone; Dufaston; Duphaston; Gynorest; Prodel; Retrone. $C_{21}H_{28}O_2$; mol wt 312.45. C 80.72%, H 9.03%, O 10.24%. Prepn: Westerhof, Reerink, *Rec. Trav. Chim.* **79**, 771 (1960); Rappoldt, Westerhof, *ibid.* **80**, 43 (1961).

Crystals from acetone + hexane, mp 169-170°. $[\alpha]_D^{25}$ −484.5° (chloroform). uv max: 286.5 nm (ε 26400).

THERAP CAT: Progestogen.

3475. Dymanthine. [124-28-7] *N,N*-Dimethyl-1-octadecanamine; *N,N*-dimethyloctadecylamine; dimantine. $C_{20}H_{43}N$; mol wt 297.56. C 80.73%, H 14.57%, N 4.71%. $CH_3(CH_2)_{17}$-$N(CH_3)_2$. Prepd from octadecylamine and formaldehyde: Reck *et al., J. Org. Chem.* **12**, 517 (1947).

mp 22.89°.

Hydrochloride. [1613-17-8] GS-1339; NSC-5547; Thelmesan. $C_{20}H_{43}N$.HCl; mol wt 334.02.

THERAP CAT: Anthelmintic (Nematodes).

THERAP CAT (VET): Anthelmintic (Nematodes).

3476. Dynamin. GTPase mechanoenzyme which plays an essential role in membrane budding and vesicle trafficking. Various isoforms which are tissue or function specific co-exist. Homotetramer which self-assembles into ring and spirals which form collars at the fission point. Isolation from bovine brain: H. S. Shpetner, R. B. Vallee, *Cell* **59**, 421, (1989). Model for mechanism of membrane fission: M. M. Kozlov, *Biophys. J.* **77**, 604 (1999). Review of function and nomenclature: R. Urrutia *et al., Proc. Natl. Acad. Sci. USA* **94**, 377-384 (1997); of functions: M. A. McNiven *et al., Trends Biochem. Sci.* **25**, 115-120 (2000). Review of structure and assembly: J. E. Hinshaw, *Curr. Opin. Struct. Biol.* **9**, 260-267 (1999). Review of functional diversity and related dynamin-like proteins: A. M. van der Bliek, *Trends Cell Biol.* **9**, 96-102 (1999).

3477. Dynel. Staple fiber copolymer of 60% vinyl chloride and 40% acrylonitrile wet spun from acetone, stretched hot as much as 1300% and then annealed by heat treatment: E. E. Stout, *Introduction to Textiles* (John Wiley, New York, 1960) pp 198-201; R. W. Moncrieff, *Man-Made Fibres* (John Wiley, New York, 1963) pp 411-420; Kennedy, "Modacrylic Fibers" in *Encyclopedia of Polymer Science and Technology* vol. **8**, N. M. Bikales, Ed. (Interscience, New York, 1968) pp 812-839.

Light cream fiber which can be bleached nearly white. Specific gravity 1.31. Tenacity ranges from 2.0 to 3.5 g/denier. Elongation is 30-40%; hygroscopicity is 0.4% under standard conditions. Has extremely good chemical resistance. Acetone is the best solvent; cyclohexanone and dimethylformamide also have some solvent action. Acetic anhydride, acetaldehyde, aniline, ethylene dichloride, and methyl ethyl ketone all plasticize or swell dynel. Resistant to clothes moths' larvae, to carpet beetles, and to mildew and fungus. Will burn in a flame, but if the flame is removed it is self-extinguishing. Resistant to water and non-felting and non-shrinking below the boil. Hot water delusters dynel. Must be ironed with the lowest iron setting and a dry cotton cover over the fabric. May be heat-set in permanent pleats. Can be dyed readily and may be solution-dyed. Resistant to perspiration and to salt-water deterioration.

USE: In apparel and household furnishings; simulated fur coats; chemically resistant clothing. In making wigs and doll hair; the hair can be washed, combed, set, and in some instances, redyed.

3478. Dynorphin. [74913-18-1] Extremely potent, widely distributed neuropeptide that has 17 amino acid residues and contains leu⁵-enkephalin as its NH_2-terminal sequence. Its name is derived from "dynamis", the Greek word for power, and endorphin, the name applied to the group of opioid peptides to which it belongs. Initially isolated from porcine pituitaries and termed *slow-reversing endorphin*: L. I. Lowney *et al., Life Sci.* **24**, 2377 (1979). Purification, description of properties and amino acid sequence of the first 13 residues: A. Goldstein *et al., Proc. Natl. Acad. Sci. USA* **76**, 6666 (1979). Complete amino acid sequence of the heptadecapeptide from porcine pituitary: *eidem, ibid.* **78**, 7219 (1981). Isoln from porcine duodenum and identity with pituitary dynorphin: S. Tachibana *et al., Nature* **295**, 339 (1982). Synthesis of porcine dynorphin$_{1-13}$: M. Wakimasu *et al., Chem. Pharm. Bull.* **29**, 2592 (1981). Soln conformation: R. Maroun, W. L. Mattice, *Biochem. Biophys. Res. Commun.* **103**, 442 (1981). Radioimmunoassay: V. E. Ghazarossian *et al., Life Sci.* **27**, 75 (1980). Comparison of distribution of dynorphin and enkephalin systems in brain: S. J. Watson *et al., Science* **218**, 1134 (1982). Behavioral effects of dynorphin$_{1-13}$ in mice and rats: J. M. Walker *et al., Peptides* **1**, 341 (1980); H. Zwiers *et al., Life Sci.* **28**, 2545 (1981). Opiate activity and receptor selectivity: M. Wuester *et al., Neurosci. Lett.* **20**, 79 (1980); C. Chavkin, A. Goldstein *Nature* **291**, 591 (1981). In the guinea pig ileum bioassay it has been shown to be 700 times more potent than leu⁵-enkephalin and its agonist effects are 1/13th as sensitive to naloxone antagonism: *eidem, Proc. Natl. Acad. Sci. USA* **78**, 6543 (1981). Dynorphin$_{1-13}$ has been proposed as the specific endogenous ligand of the *kappa* opioid receptor (*cf.* endorphins): C. Chavkin *et al., Science* **215**, 413 (1982). It has also been suggested that dynorphin$_{1-8}$ or dynorphin$_{1-9}$ may be transmitters or modulators at the kappa binding site and dynorphins 1-13 and 1-17 may act at a distance from the release site: A. D. Corbett *et al., Nature* **299**, 79 (1982). A possible regulatory role of dynorphin on morphine and β-endorphin-induced analgesia has been proposed: F. Tulunay *et al., J. Pharmacol. Exp. Ther.* **219**, 296 (1981); E. C. Petrie *et al., Peptides* **3**, 41 (1982). Several non-opiate effects have also been described: J. M. Walker *et al., Science* **218**, 1136 (1982); R. Przewlocki *et al., ibid.* **219**, 71 (1983).

Tyr–Gly–Gly–Phe–Leu–Arg–Arg–Ile–Arg–Pro–Lys–Leu–Lys–Trp–Asp–Asn–Gln

Porcine Dynorphin

Dynorphin$_{1-13}$. 1-13-Dynorphin (pig). $C_{75}H_{126}N_{24}O_{15}$; mol wt 1603.95. $[\alpha]_D^{23}$ −62.9° (c = 0.5 in 1% acetic acid).

3479. Dyphylline. [479-18-5] 7-(2,3-Dihydroxypropyl)-3,7-dihydro-1,3-dimethyl-1*H*-purine-2,6-dione; 7-(2,3-dihydroxypropyl)theophylline; (1,2-dihydroxy-3-propyl)theophylline; glyphylline; glyfyllin; diprophylline; AFI-phyllin; Astmamasit; Asthmolysin; Astrophyllin; Circair; Coronarin; Cor-Theophyllin; Dilor; Hiphyllin; Hyphylline; Lufyllin; Neostenovasan; Neothylline; Neotilina; Neo-Vasophylline; Neutrafil; Neutraphylline; Prophyllen; Silbephylline; Solufilin; Solufyllin; Theal ampules; Thefylan. C_{10}-$H_{14}N_4O_4$; mol wt 254.24. C 47.24%, H 5.55%, N 22.04%, O 25.17%. Prepn: Jones, Maney, US 2575344 (1951 to State Univ. of Iowa); Roth, *Arch. Pharm.* **292**, 234 (1959). Toxicity data: R. A. Al'tshuler, *Med. Prom. SSSR* **16**, 57 (1962), *C.A.* **61**, 6230g (1964).

Extremely bitter crystals from alcohol, mp 158°. uv max (0.001% in H_2O): 273 nm ($A_{1cm}^{1\%}$ 361). Freely sol in water; one gram dissolves in 3 ml H_2O at 25°. Soly (g/100 ml): alc 2; chloroform 1. pH (1% aq soln) 6.6 to 7.3. LD_{50} in mice (mg/kg): 3400 orally; 1430 s.c. (Al'tshuler).

THERAP CAT: Bronchodilator.

3480. Dypnone. [495-45-4] 1,3-Diphenyl-2-buten-1-one; β-methylchalcone. $C_{16}H_{14}O$; mol wt 222.28. C 86.45%, H 6.35%, O 7.20%. Prepd by self-condensation of acetophenone in the presence of aluminum *tert*-butoxide: Adkins, Cox, *J. Am. Chem. Soc.* **60**, 1151 (1938); W. Wayne, H. Adkins, *Org. Synth.* **coll. vol. III**, 367 (1955). Use as sunscreen: *Ind. Eng. Chem.* **46**, 15A (July 1954). Toxicity study: H. F. Smyth *et al., J. Ind. Hyg. Toxicol.* **31**, 60 (1949).

Liquid. d_4^{15} 1.1080. n_D^{20} 1.6343. bp_{760} 340-345° (partial decompn); bp_{22} 225°; $bp_{1.0}$ 150-155°. Insol in water. Sol in alcohol, ether. LD_{50} orally in rats: 3.6 g/kg (Smyth).

USE: Sunscreen.

3481. Dysidiolide. [182136-94-3] (5*R*)-5-Hydroxy-4-[(1*R*)-1-hydroxy-2-[(1*R*,2*R*,5*S*,8a*S*)-1,2,3,5,6,7,8,8a-octahydro-1,2,5-trimethyl-5-(4-methyl-4-pentenyl)-1-naphthalenyl]ethyl]-2(5*H*)-furanone; (−)-dysidiolide. $C_{25}H_{38}O_4$; mol wt 402.57. C 74.59%, H 9.51%, O 15.90%. Sesterterpene γ-hydroxybutenolide with a unique carbon skeleton isolated from the marine sponge *Dysidea etheria* de Laubenfels. First naturally occurring inhibitor of the protein phosphatase, cdc25; the inhibition of which blocks cell division. Isolation, activity and crystal structure: S. P. Gunasekera *et al., J. Am. Chem. Soc.* **118**, 8759 (1996). Enantioselective synthesis: E. J. Corey, B. E. Roberts, *ibid.* **119**, 12425 (1997). Total synthesis of racemate and preliminary biological activity: S. R. Magnuson *et al., ibid.* **120**, 1615 (1998).

Colorless crystals from CH_3OH/CH_2Cl_2, mp 186-187°. $[\alpha]_D^{24}$ −11.1° (c = 0.6 in CH_2Cl_2/CH_3OH, 1:1).

3482. Dysprosium. [7429-91-6] Dy; at. wt 162.500; at. no. 66; valences 2, 3, 4. A lanthanide; belongs to the yttrium group of rare earth metals. Naturally occurring isotopes (mass numbers): 156 (0.06%); 158 (0.10%); 160 (2.34%); 161 (18.9%); 162 (25.5%); 163 (24.9%); 164 (28.2%); known artificial radioactive isotopes: 145-155; 157; 159; 165-167. Abundance in earth's crust: ~4.5 ppm. Occurs in gadolinite, xenotime, samarskite and other rare

earth minerals. Discovered in 1886 by Lecoq de Boisbaudran. Sepn: Urbain, *Compt. Rend.* **139**, 736 (1904); **141**, 521 (1905); **142**, 785 (1906); Spedding *et al., J. Am. Chem. Soc.* **69**, 2812 (1947); **76**, 2557 (1954). Prepn of salt: Engle, Balke, *ibid.* **39**, 53 (1917); prepn of a Dy-Al alloy: Schumacher, Harris, *ibid.* **48**, 3108 (1926). Toxicity studies: Bruce *et al., Toxicol. Appl. Pharmacol.* **5**, 750 (1962); Haley *et al., ibid.* **8**, 37 (1966). Reviews of prepn, properties and compds: *The Rare Earths,* F. H. Spedding, A. H. Daane, Eds. (Krieger, Huntington, N.Y., 1971, reprint of 1961 ed.) 641 pp; Hulet, Bode, "Separation Chemistry of the Lanthanides and Transplutonium Actinides" in *MTP Int. Rev. Sci.: Inorg. Chem., Ser. One* **vol. 7**, K. W. Bagnall, Ed. (Univ. Park Press, Baltimore, 1972) pp 1-45; Moeller, "The Lanthanides" in *Comprehensive Inorganic Chemistry* **vol. 4**, J. C. Bailar, Jr. *et al.,* Eds. (Pergamon Press, Oxford, 1973) pp 1-101; F. H. Spedding in *Kirk-Othmer Encyclopedia of Chemical Technology* **vol. 19** (John Wiley & Sons, New York, 3rd ed., 1982) pp 833-854; *Chemistry of the Elements*, N. N. Greenwood, A. Earnshaw, Eds. (Pergamon Press, New York, 1984) pp 1423-1449. Brief review of properties: G. T. Seaborg, *Radiochim. Acta* **61**, 115-122 (1993).

Silver metal; tarnishes in moist air. Hexagonal close-packed crystals. d 8.5500. mp 1412°. bp 2567°. Heat of fusion: 10.782 kJ/mol. Heat of sublimation (25°): 290.4 kJ/mol. Forms greenish-yellow salts.

Oxide. Dysprosia. Dy_2O_3. White substance. Prepd by heating the oxalate or sulfate. d^{27} 7.81.

Hydroxide. $Dy(OH)_3$. A gelatinous precipitate. Prepd by adding ammonia to an aq soln of a dysprosium salt; forms a blue colloidal soln.

Chloride. $DyCl_3$. Obtained by passing S_2Cl_2 over heated dysprosia. A hexahydrate is formed from the aq soln. The anhyd chloride, yellow shining crystals, d 3.67; mp 680°. LD_{50} in mice: 585 mg/kg i.p.; 7.65 g/kg orally (Haley).

Sulfate. $Dy_2(SO_4)_3$. Octahydrate, yellow crystals. Prepd by dissolving the oxide in sulfuric acid and precipitating with alcohol; stable in air at 110°, dehydrated at 360°.

Nitrate. $Dy(NO_3)_3$. Pentahydrate, melts at 88.6° in its water of crystn. Sol in water. LD_{50} (hexahydrate) in rats: 295 mg/kg i.p.; 3.1 g/kg orally (Bruce).

USE: Oxide used in control rods of some nuclear power reactors.

3483. Dystrophin. Protein product of the human Duchenne muscular dystrophy (DMD) gene. Mol wt approx 400,000 daltons. Present in very small amounts in normal muscle (approx 0.002% of total muscle protein) but either absent or abnormal in muscular dystrophy patients. Thought to be an intracellular structural component of the plasma membrane system in normal muscle fibers. Complete cloning of DMD cDNA: M. Koenig *et al., Cell* **50**, 509 (1987). Isoln of dystrophin from mouse and human muscle tissue: E. P. Hoffman *et al., ibid.* **51**, 919 (1987). Subcellular localization studies: E. P. Hoffman *et al., Nature* **330**, 754 (1987); C. M. Knudson *et al., J. Biol. Chem.* **263**, 8480 (1988); E. E. Zubrzycka-Gaarn *et al., Nature* **333**, 466 (1988); S. C. Watkins *et al., ibid.* 863. Amino acid sequence and structural similarity to α-actinin and to the cytoskeletal protein, spectrin: M. Koenig *et al., Cell* **53**, 219 (1988). Characterization of DMD gene expression in normal and diseased human muscle: M. Oronzi Scott *et al., Science* **239**, 1418 (1988); in animal muscle and brain: U. Nudel *et al., Nature* **331**, 635 (1988). Differentiation of muscle and brain DMD mRNA: U. Nudel *et al., ibid.* **337**, 76 (1989). Correlation of clinical phenotype with dystrophin abnormalities: E. P. Hoffman *et al., N. Engl. J. Med.* **318**, 1363 (1988). Use of dystrophin cDNA for prenatal diagnosis and carrier detection in muscular dystrophy: B. T. Darras *et al., Am. J. Med. Genet.* **29**, 713 (1988).

E

tathione peroxidase mimic: H. Sies, *Free Radical Biol. Med.* **14**, 313-323 (1993).

3484. Ebastine. [90729-43-4] 1-[4-(1,1-Dimethylethyl)-phenyl]-4-[4-(diphenylmethoxy)-1-piperidinyl]-1-butanone; 4'-*tert*-butyl-4-[4-(diphenylmethoxy)piperidino]butyrophenone; 4-diphen-ylmethoxy-1-[3-(4-*tert*-butylbenzoyl)propyl]piperidine; LAS-W-090; Ebastel; Estivan; Evastel; Kestin; Kestine. $C_{32}H_{39}NO_2$; mol wt 469.66. C 81.83%, H 8.37%, N 2.98%, O 6.81%. Nonsedating type histamine H_1-receptor antagonist. Prepn: J. M. P. Soto *et al.*, **EP 134124**; *eidem*, **US 4550116** (both 1985 to Fordonal). Metabo-lized *in vivo* to *carebastine*, its active carboxylic acid metabolite. Clinical pharmacology, pharmacokinetics: J. Vincent *et al.*, *Br. J. Clin. Pharmacol.* **26**, 497 (1988). Effect on psychomotor perform-ance: J. Vincent *et al.*, *ibid.* 503.

Fumarate. $C_{32}H_{39}NO_2 \cdot C_4H_4O_4$. Crystals from ethanol, mp 197-198°.

THERAP CAT: Antihistaminic.

3485. Ebrotidine. [100981-43-9] [*N*(*E*)]-*N*-[[[2-[[[2-[(Am-inoiminomethyl)amino]-4-thiazolyl]methyl]thio]ethyl]amino]meth-ylene]-4-bromobenzenesulfonamide; (*E*)-*N*-*p*-bromobenzenesulfo-nyl-*N*′-[2-[[[2-[(aminoiminomethyl)amino]-4-thiazolyl]methyl]-thio]ethyl]formamidine; *p*-bromo-*N*-[(*E*)-[[2-[[[2-[(diaminomethyl-ene)amino]-4-thiazolyl]methyl]thio]ethyl]amino]methylene]ben-zenesulfonamide; FI-3542; Ebrocit; Ebrodin; Ulsanic. $C_{14}H_{17}$-$BrN_6O_2S_3$; mol wt 477.42. C 35.22%, H 3.59%, Br 16.74%, N 17.60%, O 6.70%, S 20.15%. Histamine H_2-receptor antagonist. Prepn: R. Foguet *et al.*, **EP 159012**; *eidem*, **US 4728655** (1985, 1988 both to Ferrer); L. Anglada *et al.*, *Eur. J. Med. Chem.* **23**, 97 (1988). Clinical pharmacology: S. J. Konturek *et al.*, *Scand. J. Gastroenterol.* **27**, 438 (1992); M. Maczka *et al.*, *J. Physiol. Phar-macol.* **43**, 139 (1992). Clinical evaluation in gastroesophageal reflux disease: E. Sito *et al.*, *ibid.* **44**, 259 (1993). HPLC determn in urine and metabolism study: E. Rozman *et al.*, *J. Pharm. Sci.* **83**, 252 (1994).

Crystals from ethyl acetate. mp 142.5-146°.

THERAP CAT: Antiulcerative.

3486. Ebselen. [60940-34-3] 2-Phenyl-1,2-benzisoselena-zol-3(2*H*)-one; PZ-51. $C_{13}H_9NOSe$; mol wt 274.18. C 56.95%, H 3.31%, N 5.11%, O 5.84%, Se 28.80%. Seleno-organic which shows antioxidant effects through glutathione peroxidase-like ac-tion. Prepn: R. Lesser, R. Weiss, *Ber.* **57**, 1077 (1924); R. Weber, M. Renson, *Bull. Soc. Chim. Fr.* **1976**, 1124; L. Engman, A. Hall-berg, *J. Org. Chem.* **54**, 2964 (1989). One-step synthesis: J. Op-penheimer, L. A. Silks, III, *J. Labelled Compd. Radiopharm.* **38**, 281 (1996). HPLC determn in plasma: R. Terlinden *et al.*, *J. Chroma-togr.* **430**, 438 (1988). Clinical trial as neuroprotectant in ischemic stroke: T. Yamaguchi *et al.*, *Stroke* **29**, 12 (1998); A. Ogawa *et al.*, *Cerebrovasc. Dis.* **9**, 112 (1999). Review of pharmacology: M. J. Parnham *et al.*, **32**, 4-9 (1991); and of biochemical interactions: T. Schewe, *Gen. Pharmacol.* **26**, 1153-1169 (1995). Review as glu-

Crystals from ethanol, mp 180-181°.

3487. Eburnamonine. [474-00-0] Eburnamenin-14(15*H*)-one; (+)-*cis*-eburnamonine. $C_{19}H_{22}N_2O$; mol wt 294.39. C 77.52%, H 7.53%, N 9.52%, O 5.43%. One of the *Vinca* alkaloids, naturally occurring as the (+)- and (±)-forms. Isoln of the (+)-form from *Hunteria eburnea* Pinchon, *Apocynaceae:* M. F. Bartlett *et al.*, *Compt. Rend.* **249**, 1259 (1959); of the (±)-form from *Vinca minor* L., *Apocynaceae:* J. Mokry *et al.*, *Experientia* **17**, 354 (1961). The (−)-form is obtained by acid hydrolysis of vincamine, *q.v.:* J. Trajanek *et al.*, *Tetrahedron Lett.* **1961**, 702; O. Clauder *et al.*, *ibid.* **1962**, 1147; *eidem*, **HU 151295** (1964 to Gedeon Richter), *C.A.* **60**, 14558e (1964). Structure and synthesis of the (±)-form: M. F. Bartlett, W. I. Taylor, *Tetrahedron Lett.* **20**, 20 (1959); *eidem*, *J. Am. Chem. Soc.* **82**, 5941 (1960); E. Wenkert, B. Wickberg, *ibid.* **87**, 1580 (1965). Short synthesis of the (±)-form: E. Wenkert *et al.*, *ibid.* **100**, 4893 (1978); high yield total synthesis: J. L. Her-mann *et al.*, *ibid.* **101**, 1540 (1979); T. Imanishi *et al.*, *Chem. Pharm. Bull.* **30**, 1521 (1982). Synthesis of the (−)-form: D. Cartier *et al.*, *Bull. Soc. Chim. Fr.* **1976**, 1961. Structural and biogenetic relation-ship to vincamine: J. Mokry *et al.*, *Tetrahedron Lett.* **1962**, 433. Pharmacology of the (−)-form: P. Lacroix *et al.*, *Arzneim.-Forsch.* **29**, 1094 (1979). Series of articles on the pharmacodynamics, metabolism, and therapeutic use of the (−)-form: *Eur. Neurol.* **17**, Suppl. 1, 1-172 (1978). *Reviews:* W. I. Taylor in *The Alkaloids* vol. 8, R. H. F. Manske, Ed. (Academic Press, New York, 1965) pp 253-259; *idem, ibid.* **vol. 11**, pp 108-110 (1968).

Cryst, mp 174°. $[\alpha]_D^{25}$ +89° (chloroform). uv max: 241, 268, 296, 302 nm (ε 19800, 10200, 4800, 4800).

(±)-**Form.** [2580-88-3] (±)-Eburnamenin-14(15H)-one; vin-canorine. Crystals from methanol, mp 201-202.5°. uv max (eth-anol): 227, 287, 294 nm (log ε 4.49, 3.89, 3.87).

(−)-**Form.** [4880-88-0] (3α,16α)-Eburnamenin-14(15*H*)-one; 16-oxoeburnane; vincamone; CH-846; Cervoxan. Solid, mp 168-170°; also reported as mp 177-178° (Cartier). $[\alpha]_D^{25}$ −102° (chlo-roform) (Clauder); $[\alpha]_D$ −100° (c = 0.783 in chloroform) (Cartier). uv max: 205, 240, 265, 290, 300 nm (log ε 4.28, 4.16, 3.90, 3.59, 3.57).

(−)-**Form phosphate.** [94134-60-8] Eburnal.

THERAP CAT: The (−)-form as vasodilator.

3488. Ecabapide. [104775-36-2] 3-[[2-[[2-(3,4-Dimeth-oxyphenyl)ethyl]amino]-2-oxoethyl]amino]-*N*-methylbenzamide; *m*-[[[(3,4-dimethoxyphenethyl)carbamoyl]methyl]amino]-*N*-meth-ylbenzamide; ecabamide; DQ-2511. $C_{20}H_{25}N_3O_4$; mol wt 371.43. C 64.67%, H 6.78%, N 11.31%, O 17.23%. α_2-Adrenoceptor ago-nist; reduces vagally-induced gastric acid secretion. Prepn: T. Miki *et al.*, **EP 185368**; *eidem*, **US 4985595** (1986, 1991 both to Daiichi); T. Hosokami *et al.*, *Chem. Pharm. Bull.* **40**, 2712 (1992). Pharmacology: K. Yokotani *et al.*, *Jpn. J. Pharmacol.* **48**, 299 (1988); M. Hirohashi *et al.*, *Arzneim.-Forsch.* **43**, 569 (1993). Efficacy in exptl ulcers: M Asano *et al.*, *ibid.* **40**, 276 (1990). Metabolism studies: Y. Fujimaki *et al.*, *Xenobiotica* **25**, 501 (1995).

Colorless needles from methanol/diethyl ether, mp 93-96.5°; recrystallized as colorless prisms from abs methanol, mp 133-134.5°. Soly (mg/ml) in water: 5.31 at 25°, 8.55 at 37°.

THERAP CAT: Antiulcerative.

3489. Ecabet. [33159-27-2] (1R,4aS,10aR)-1,2,3,4,4a,9,-10,10a-Octahydro-1,4a-dimethyl-7-(1-methylethyl)-6-sulfo-1-phenanthrenecarboxylic acid; dehydro-6-sulfoabietic acid; 12-sulfo-dehydroabietic acid. $C_{20}H_{28}O_5S$; mol wt 380.50. C 63.13%, H 7.42%, O 21.02%, S 8.43%. Prepn: L. F. Fieser, W. P. Campbell, *J. Am. Chem. Soc.* **60**, 2631 (1938); H. Wada *et al., Chem. Pharm. Bull.* **33**, 1472 (1985). Metabolism in animals: Y. Ito *et al., J. Pharmacobio-Dyn.* **14**, 533 (1991). Efficacy in healing expt ulcers in rats: Y. Onoda *et al., Arzneim.-Forsch.* **41**, 546 (1991). Gastroprotective effects in rats in comparison with sucralfate, *q.v.*: M. Kinoshita *et al., Dig. Dis. Sci.* **40**, 661 (1995). Bactericidal activity against *Helicobacter pylori*: K. Shibata *et al., Antimicrob. Agents Chemother.* **39**, 1295 (1995).

As the hemihydrate, $[\alpha]_D^{25}$ +72.4° (c = 2.5 in alcohol).
  Sodium salt. [86408-72-2] TA-2711; Gastron. $C_{20}H_{27}NaO_5$-S; mol wt 402.48. Occurs as pentahydrate, mp >300°. $[\alpha]_D^{20}$ +59.4° (c = 0.5).

THERAP CAT: Antiulcerative.

3490. Ecamsule. [92761-26-7] 3,3'-(1,4-Phenylenedimethylidyne)bis[7,7-dimethyl-2-oxo-bicyclo[2.2.1]heptane-1-methanesulfonic acid]; terephthalylidene-3,3'-dicamphor-10,10'-disulfonic acid; Mexoryl SX. $C_{28}H_{34}O_8S_2$; mol wt 562.69. C 59.77%, H 6.09%, O 22.75%, S 11.40%. Broad spectrum UVA absorber with some UVB absorption. Prepn: G. Lang *et al.,* **DE 3321679**; *eidem,* **US 4585597** (1983, 1986 both to L'Oreal). Evaluation of photomutagenicity: S.W. Dean *et al., Mutagenesis* **7**, 179 (1992). Evaluation of photoprotection: A. Fourtanier *et al., Photochem. Photobiol.* **55**, 549 (1992); R. D. Ley, A. Fourtanier, *ibid.* **65**, 1007 (1997).

Solid, mp 255° (dec). uv max (ethanol): 345 nm (ε 47000 $M^{-1}cm^{-1}$); uv max (water): 342 nm (ε 42300).

THERAP CAT: Ultraviolet screen.

3491. Ecdysteroids. Polyhydroxylated steroids formerly known as ecdysones. Originally identified as insect molting hormones controlling the pupation of insects. Later shown to be involved in many complex developmental processes in metamorphosis, differentiation and reproduction. Ecdysteroids have been detected in invertebrate species of several phylla belonging to the Protostomia and in some plant species. The terms *zooecdysteroids* and *phytoecdysteroids* are used to distinguish ecdysteroids isolated

from animal species from those of plant origin. Nomenclature: T. W. Goodwin *et al., Nature* **272**, 122 (1978). The two major ecdysteroids isolated are ecdysone and 20-hydroxyecdysone. Configuration: M. Koreeda *et al., J. Am. Chem. Soc.* **93**, 4084 (1971). Chromosomal action: M. Ashburner, *Nature* **285**, 435 (1980). GC and HPLC determn: R. P. Evershed *et al., J. Chromatogr.* **390**, 357 (1987). *Reviews:* Kilby, *Discovery* **18**, 13 (1957); P. Karlson, *Angew. Chem. Int. Ed.* **2**, 175-182 (1963); K. Nakanishi, *Pure Appl. Chem.* **25**, 167-195 (1971); M. Koreeda, B. A. Teicher, *Anal. Biochem. Insects* **1977**, 207-240; P. Karlson, *Dev. Endocrinol.* **7**, 1-11 (1980). *Book: Ecdysone: From Chemistry to Mode of Action,* J. Koolman, Ed. (Thieme, New York, 1989) 482 pp.

| | Ecdysone | R = H, R' = ---CH₃ |
| | 20-Hydroxyecdysone | R = OH, R' = ◄CH₃ |

Ecdysone. [3604-87-3] (2β,3β,5β,22R)-2,3,14,22,25-Pentahydroxycholest-7-en-6-one; α-ecdysone. $C_{27}H_{44}O_6$; mol wt 464.63. Secreted by ecdysial tissues, then transformed to more active compound, 20-hydroxyecdysone. First isoln from silkworm moths, *Bombyx mori:* A. Butenandt, P. Karlson, *Z. Naturforsch.* **9b**, 389 (1954). Isoln from rhizomes of *Polypodium vulgare* L.: G. Heinrich, H. Hoffmeister, *Experientia* **23**, 995 (1967); from bracken fern, *Pteridinium aquilinum:* J. N. Kaplanis *et al., Science* **157**, 1436 (1967). Structure: P. Karlson *et al., Ber.* **98**, 2394 (1965). Configuration: R. Huber, W. Hoppe, *ibid.* 2403. Synthesis: U. Kerb *et al., Helv. Chim. Acta* **49**, 1601 (1966); J. B. Siddall *et al., J. Am. Chem. Soc.* **88**, 379, 862 (1966); H. Mori *et al., Chem. Pharm. Bull.* **16**, 563 (1968). mp 238-239°. $[\alpha]_{578}^{20}$ +62°. uv max: 243 nm (ε 11600).

20-Hydroxyecdysone. [5289-74-7] (2β,3β,5β,22R,)-2,3,14,-20,22,25-Hexahydroxycholest-7-en-6-one; β-ecdysone; ecdysterone; crustecdysone; isoinokosterone; polypodine A. $C_{27}H_{44}O_7$; mol wt 480.63. Most widely occurring ecdysteroid in both plant and animal species. Isoln from *B. mori:* P. Hocks, R. Wiechert, *Tetrahedron Lett.* **1966**, 2989; from seawater crayfish, *Jasus lalandei:* F. Hampshire, D. H. S. Horn, *Chem. Commun.* **1966**, 37. Isolns from plant sources, *Achyranthes fauriei:* T. Takemoto *et al., Yakugaku Zasshi* **87**, 325 (1967); *P. elatus:* M. N. Galbraith, D. H. S. Horn, *Chem. Commun.* **1966**, 905; *P. vulgare:* J. Jizba *et al., Tetrahedron Lett.* **1967**, 1689. Isoln from parasitic helminths: H. H. Rees, J. G. Mercer, *Adv. Invertebr. Reprod.* **4**, 173 (1986). Configuration: Dammeier, Hoppe, *Ber.* **104**, 1660 (1971). Synthesis: G. Hüppi, J. B. Siddall, *J. Am. Chem. Soc.* **89**, 6790 (1967); U. Kerb *et al., Tetrahedron Lett.* **1968**, 4277; H. Mori, K. Shibata, *Chem. Pharm. Bull.* **17**, 1970 (1969). Total synthesis: T. Kametani *et al., Tetrahedron Lett.* **21**, 4855 (1980). From methanol-ethyl acetate, mp 240-242°. uv max: 243 nm (ε 10300). Unstable in alkaline soln.

3492. Ecgonidine. [484-93-5] (1R)-8-Methyl-8-azabicyclo[3.2.1]oct-2-ene-2-carboxylic acid; 2-tropidinecarboxylic acid; anhydroecgonin. $C_9H_{13}NO_2$; mol wt 167.21. C 64.65%, H 7.84%, N 8.38%, O 19.14%. Prepn from ecgonine and structure: Findlay, *J. Am. Chem. Soc.* **75**, 1033 (1953). Prepn and formation of *l*-form: de Jong, *Rec. Trav. Chim.* **42**, 980 (1923), **66**, 99 (1947). Synthesis of *dl*-form: Grundmann, Ottmann, *Ann.* **605**, 24 (1957); **US 2783235** (1957 to Olin Mathieson).

***dl*-Form.** Crystals from alcohol + ether, dec 235-236°. Soluble in water; sparingly sol in alcohol.

***l*-Form.** Crystals from abs alcohol, mp 235°. $[\alpha]_D^{14}$ −84.6° (c = 1.7).

THERAP CAT: Anesthetic (topical).

3493. Ecgonine. [481-37-8] [1*R*-(*exo,exo*)]-3-Hydroxy-8-methyl-8-azabicyclo[3.2.1]octane-2-carboxylic acid; 3β-hydroxy-1α*H*,5α*H*-tropane-2β-carboxylic acid. $C_9H_{15}NO_3$; mol wt 185.22. C 58.36%, H 8.16%, N 7.56%, O 25.91%. The principal part of the cocaine molecule; naturally occurring as the *l*-form. Obtained by hydrolysis of cocaine: Willstätter *et al., Ann.* **434**, 111 (1923); Bell, Archer, *J. Am. Chem. Soc.* **82**, 4642 (1960). From coca leaves: de Jong, *Rec. Trav. Chim.* **59**, 687 (1940). Structure: Gadamer, John, *Arch. Pharm.* **259**, 227 (1921). Stereochemistry: Fodor, *Nature* **170**, 278 (1952); Fodor, Kovács, *J. Chem. Soc.* **1953**, 724. Synthesis: Willstätter, Bommer, *Ann.* **422**, 15 (1920). *Review:* Stoll, Jucker, *Angew. Chem.* **66**, 376 (1954).

***l*-Form monohydrate.** [5796-30-5] Triboluminescent, monoclinic prisms from alc, mp 198° (anhydr, dec 205°). $[\alpha]_D^{15}$ −45° (c = 5). Neutral to litmus. pKa 11.11; pKb 11.22. One gram dissolves in 5 ml water, 67 ml alc, 20 ml methanol, 75 ml ethyl acetate. Sparingly sol in acetone, ether, benzene, chloroform, petr ether.

Hydrochloride. [5796-31-6] $C_9H_{15}NO_3 \cdot HCl$. Triclinic plates from water, mp 246°. $[\alpha]_D^{15}$ −59° (c = 10). Sol in water; slightly in alc.

***dl*-Form trihydrate.** Plates from 90% alcohol, mp 93-118° (anhydr dec 212°).

Note: This is a controlled substance: **21 CFR**, 1308.12.

THERAP CAT: Anesthetic (topical).

3494. Echinacea. Purple coneflower. Perennial plant of the family *Compositae (Asteraceae). Habit.* North American plains and southeast U.S.; cultivated in Europe. Widely used in traditional medicine as an immunostimulant. Medicinal formulations are prepared from the roots and aerial parts of three species: *E. angustifolia* DC, *E. pallida* (Nutt.) Nutt. or *E. purpurea* (L.) Moench. *Constit.* Alkamides such as **echinacein**, caffeic acid esters such as **echinacoside**, polysaccharides, volatile oil. Isoln of constituents from *E. augustifolia* DC: A. Stoll *et al., Helv. Chim. Acta* **33**, 1877 (1950); M. Jacobson, *Science* **120**, 1028 (1954). Analysis of alkamides: X. He *et al., J. Chromatogr. A* **815**, 205 (1998); of volatile components: G. Mazza, T. Cottrell, *J. Agric. Food Chem.* **47**, 3081 (1999). Review of clinical trials in treatment of upper respiratory infection: B. Barrett *et al., J. Fam. Pract.* **48**, 628-635 (1999); of use in Native American medicine: A. T. Borchers *et al., Am. J. Clin. Nutr.* **72**, 339-347 (2000).

THERAP CAT: In treatment of respiratory infections.

3495. Echinenone. [432-68-8] β,β-Caroten-4-one; 4-oxo-β-carotene; 4-keto-β-carotene; aphanin; myoxanthin. $C_{40}H_{54}O$; mol wt 550.86. C 87.21%, H 9.88%, O 2.90%. Carotenoid pigment occurring in algae. Isoln from *Aphanizomenon flos-aqua:* Tischer, *Z. Physiol. Chem.* **251**, 109 (1938); **260**, 257 (1939); from *Paracentrotus lividus:* Lederer, *Compt. Rend.* **201**, 300 (1935); from *Oscillatoria rubrescens:* Heilbron, Lythgoe, *J. Chem. Soc.* **1936**, 1376. Structure: Goodwin, Taha, *Biochem. J.* **47**, 244 (1950); **48**, 513 (1951); Goodwin, *ibid.* **63**, 481 (1956); Ganguly *et al., Arch. Biochem. Biophys.* **60**, 345 (1956). Synthesis: Akhtar, Weedon, *J. Chem. Soc.* **1958**, 3986; **1959**, 4058.

Orange-red crystals from benzene + methanol, mp 178-180°. Absorption max (chloroform): 472-478 nm. Freely sol in carbon disulfide, chloroform, benzene. Slightly sol in pyridine, ether. Practically insol in methanol. Provitamin A activity 54% of that of all-*trans*-β-carotene.

Oxime. $C_{40}H_{55}NO$. Red crystals from benzene, mp 208°. Absorption max (chloroform): 464-468 nm.

3496. Echinochrome A. [517-82-8] 2-Ethyl-3,5,6,7,8-pentahydroxy-1,4-naphthalenedione; 2-ethyl-3,5,6,7,8-pentahydroxy-1,4-naphthoquinone. $C_{12}H_{10}O_7$; mol wt 266.20. C 54.14%, H 3.79%, O 42.07%. The red pigment of the eggs of the sea urchin (*Arbacia pustulosa*). Isoln and structure: Kuhn, Wallenfels, *Ber.* **72**, 1407 (1939). Synthesis from 2-ethyl-1,3,4-trimethoxybenzene and dibenzoyloxymaleic anhydride: Wallenfels, Gauhe, *Ber.* **76**, 325 (1943).

Deep-red needles from dioxane-water, mp 220° (some decompn). Sublimes at 10^{-4} mm at 120°. Absorption max (chloroform): 533, 497, 462 nm. Very sparingly sol in cold water, yet more than sufficiently sol for chemotaxic effects. Readily sol in carbon disulfide, ether, chloroform, benzene, concd H_2SO_4.

3497. Echinomycin. [512-64-1] Quinomycin A. $C_{51}H_{64}N_{12}O_{12}S_2$; mol wt 1101.26. C 55.62%, H 5.86%, N 15.26%, O 17.43%, S 5.82%. A *"quinoxaline antibiotic"* similar to the triostins, *q.v.:* Kuroya, Ishida, *J. Antibiot.* **14A**, 324 (1961). Powerful, selective inhibitor of nucleic acid synthesis *in vitro*. Produced by *Streptomyces echinatus* from soil of Cuanza (Angola): Corbaz *et al., Helv. Chim. Acta* **40**, 199 (1957). Structure: Keller-Schierlein *et al., ibid.* **42**, 305 (1959). Revised structure: Dell *et al., J. Am. Chem. Soc.* **97**, 2497 (1975); D. G. Martin *et al., J. Antibiot.* **28**, 332 (1975). Identity with quinomycin A: Katagiri, Sugiura, *Antimicrob. Agents Chemother.* **1961**, 162. Biosynthesis: Arif *et al., Indian J. Biochem.* **7**, 193 (1970). Isoln and properties of the other quinomycins: Yoshida, Katagiri, *J. Antibiot.* **14A**, 330 (1961); Otsuka, Shoji, *ibid.* **19A**, 128 (1966); *eidem, Tetrahedron* **23**, 1535 (1967). Conformation in soln: H. T. Cheung *et al., J. Am. Chem. Soc.* **100**, 46 (1978). Review of chemistry and biochemistry of echinomycin: M. J. Waring in *Antibiotics* **vol. 5**(pt. 2), F. E. Hahn, Ed. (Springer-Verlag, New York, 1979) pp 173-194.

Slightly hygroscopic crystals, mp 217-218°. $[\alpha]_D^{20}$ −310° (c = 0.86 in chloroform). uv max (methanol): 243, 320 nm ($E_{1cm}^{1\%}$ 622, 100). Has lipophile solubilities. Easily sol in chloroform, dioxane. Insol in water, petr ether, hexane.

3498. Echinopsine. [83-54-5] 1-Methyl-4(1*H*)-quinolinone; 1-methyl-4(1*H*)-quinolone; 1,4-dihydro-1-methyl-4-oxoquinoline; *N*-methyl-4-quinolone. $C_{10}H_9NO$; mol wt 159.18. C 75.45%, H 5.70%, N 8.80%, O 10.05%. Isoln from *Echinops ritro* L. and other spp of *Echinops, Compositae:* Greshoff, *Rec. Trav. Chim.* **19**, 360 (1900); Ban'kovskii *et al., Dokl. Akad. Nauk SSSR* **148**, 1073 (1963). Structure: Späth, Kolbe, *Monatsh. Chem.* **43**, 469 (1923). Synthesis: Kondo, Ikawa, *J. Pharm. Soc. Jpn.* **51**, 702 (1931); Allison *et al., J. Chem. Soc.* **1954**, 403; King, Abramo, *J. Org. Chem.* **23**, 1609 (1958); Kamiya, *Chem. Pharm. Bull.* **10**, 669 (1962). Simple synthesis: J. R. Merchant, V. Shankaranarayan, *Chem. Ind. (London)* **1979**, 320. Pharmacology: A. D. Turova *et al., Pharmacol. Toxicol.* **20**, 236 (1957).

Needles from benzene, mp 152°. One gram dissolves in about 60 ml water, 6 ml boiling water. Soluble in alcohol, chloroform, hot benzene; slightly sol in ether. LD$_{100}$ s.c. in mice: 600 mg/kg (Turova).

Hydrochloride. $C_{10}H_9NO.HCl$. Crystals, mp 185-186°.

3499. Echinuline. [1859-87-6] (3*S-cis*)-3-[[2-(1,1-Dimethyl-2-propenyl)-5,7-bis(3-methyl-2-butenyl)-1*H*-indol-3-yl]methyl]-6-methyl-2,5-piperazinedione. $C_{29}H_{39}N_3O_2$; mol wt 461.64. C 75.45%, H 8.52%, N 9.10%, O 6.93%. From the dry mycelia of *Aspergillus echinulatus.* Quilico, Panizzi, *Ber.* **76**, 348 (1943). Structure: Casnati *et al., Gazz. Chim. Ital.* **92**, 105 (1962); Romanet *et al., Bull. Soc. Chim. Fr.* **1963**, 1048. Absolute configuration: Nakashima, Slater, *Tetrahedron Lett.* **1967**, 4433; **1971**, 2649. Synthetic studies: Houghton, Saxton, *J. Chem. Soc. C* **1969**, 595, 1003; Takamatsu *et al., Tetrahedron Lett.* **1971**, 4661. Total synthesis of optically active *cis* isomer: *eidem, ibid.* 4665; S. Inoue *et al., J. Pharm. Soc. Jpn.* **97**, 558 (1977). Epimerization of echinuline with triethylamine in ethanol gives the *trans* isomer, *epi-echinuline,* Westley *et al., Anal. Chem.* **40**, 1888 (1968).

Needles from butanol, mp 242-243°. $[\alpha]_D^{20}$ −26.0° (chloroform). uv max (ethanol): 230, 279, 286 nm (log ε 4.60, 3.98, 3.96). Sol in glacial acetic acid, chloroform, pyridine, dioxane; less sol in warm alcohol, warm butanol; slightly sol in benzene, ether, petr ether, carbon tetrachloride, acetone, cold alcohol.

3500. Echitamine. [6871-44-9] (3β,16*R*)-3,17-Dihydroxy-16-(methoxycarbonyl)-4-methyl-2,4(1*H*)-cyclo-3,4-secoakuammilanium; ditaine. $[C_{22}H_{29}N_2O_4]$+. From the bark of *Alstonia scholaris* (L.) R.Br., *A. congensis* Engl., *Apocynaceae; A. neriifolia:* Hesse, *Ann.* **203**, 150 (1880); Goodson, Henry, *J. Chem. Soc.* **127**, 1640 (1925); Goodson, *ibid.* **1932**, 2626; Chakravarti *et al., Bull. Calcutta Sch. Trop. Med.* **16**, 81 (1968); *C.A.* **71**, 3529f (1969); Roy, Chatterjee, *J. Indian Chem. Soc.* **45**, 21 (1968). Structure: Hamilton *et al., Proc. Chem. Soc. London* **1961**, 63; *J. Chem. Soc.* **1962**, 5061. Abs config: Manohar, Ramaseshan, *Tetrahedron Lett.* **1961**, 814. Synthetic studies: Fritz, Fischer, *Tetrahedron* **20**, 1737 (1964); Dolby, Esfandiari, *J. Org. Chem.* **37**, 43 (1972). *Review:* Govindachari, *J. Indian Chem. Soc.* **45**, 945-957 (1968).

Hydroxide. $C_{22}H_{30}N_2O_5$. White crystals, mp 206°. $[\alpha]_D^{20}$ −29° (alcohol). Sol in water, alcohol, chloroform, ether.

Chloride. $C_{22}H_{29}O_4N_2^+Cl^-$. Long needles from water, mp 295°. $[\alpha]_D^{15}$ −58°. uv max (ethanol): 235, 295 nm (log ε 3.93, 3.55).

3501. Echothiophate Iodide. [513-10-0] 2-[(Diethoxyphosphinyl)thio]-*N,N,N*-trimethylethanaminium iodide; (2-mercaptoethyl)trimethylammonium iodide *O,O*-diethyl phosphorothioate; diethoxyphosphinylthiocholine iodide; 2-diethoxyphosphinylthioethyltrimethylammonium iodide; *O,O*-diethyl *S*-(2-trimethylammoniumethyl)phosphorothioate iodide; *S*-β-dimethylaminoethyl-*O,O*-diethylthionophosphate methiodide; ecothiopate iodide; 217-MI; Phospholine Iodide. $C_9H_{23}INO_3PS$; mol wt 383.23. C 28.21%, H 6.05%, I 33.11%, N 3.65%, O 12.52%, P 8.08%, S 8.37%. Prepn: Tammelin, *Acta Chem. Scand.* **11**, 1340 (1957); Fitch, *US 2911430* (1959 to Campbell Pharmaceuticals). Comprehensive description: R. D. Daley, *Anal. Profiles Drug Subs.* **3**, 233-251 (1974).

Crystals, mp 138° (Tammelin); mp 124-124.5° (Fitch). Sol in water, alcohol, chloroform.

THERAP CAT: Cholinergic (ophthalmic).

3502. Econazole. [27220-47-9] 1-[2-[(4-Chlorophenyl)methoxy]-2-(2,4-dichlorophenyl)ethyl]-1*H*-imidazole; 1-[2,4-dichloro-β-[(*p*-chlorobenzyl)oxy]phenethyl]imidazole; SQ-13050. $C_{18}H_{15}Cl_3N_2O$; mol wt 381.68. C 56.64%, H 3.96%, Cl 27.87%, N 7.34%, O 4.19%. Prepn: Godefroi *et al., J. Med. Chem.* **12**, 784 (1969); Godefroi, Heeres, *DE 1940388; eidem, US 3717655* (1970, 1973 both to Janssen). Biological and toxicological properties: Thienpont *et al., Arzneim.-Forsch.* **25**, 224 (1975). Review of antifungal activity and therapeutic efficacy: R. C. Heel *et al., Drugs* **16**, 177-201 (1978). Comprehensive description: A. M. Dyas, H. Delargy, *Anal. Profiles Drug Subs. Excip.* **23**, 125-152 (1994).

mp 86.8°.

Nitrate. [24169-02-6] R-14827; Epi-Pevaryl; Gyno-Pevaryl; Ifenec; Micofugal; Micogin; Palavale; Pargin; Pevaryl; Spectazole. $C_{18}H_{15}Cl_3N_2O.HNO_3$; mol wt 444.70. White, odorless crystals from a mixture of 2-propanol, methanol and diisopropyl ether, mp 162°. uv max (methanol): 202, 225 nm. uv max (methanol): 265, 271, 280 nm ($A_{1cm}^{1\%}$ 9.4, 9.7, 4.9). Soly at 20° (g/100 ml): water <0.1; ethanol (96%) 2.0; acetone 1.5. LD$_{50}$ in mice, rats (mg/kg): 462.7, 667.7 orally (Thienpont).

THERAP CAT: Antifungal.

3503. Ecteinascidins. Family of tetrahydroisoquinoline alkaloids with antitumor activity isolated from the Caribbean tunicate, *Ecteinascidin turbinata.* Ecteinascidin 743 is the most abundant; bends DNA toward the major groove by selectively alkylating guanine from the minor groove. Prepn: K. L. Rinehart, T. G. Holt, **WO 8707610**; *eidem,* **US 5089273** (1987, 1992 both to Univ. Illinois); and structures: K. L. Rinehart *et al., J. Org. Chem.* **55**, 4512 (1990); R. Sakai *et al., Proc. Natl. Acad. Sci. USA* **89**, 11456 (1992). Crystal structures: Y. Guan *et al., J. Biomol. Struct. Dyn.* **10**, 793 (1993). Biosynthetic studies: R. G. Kerr, N. F. Miranda, *J. Nat. Prod.* **58**, 1618 (1995).

Trabectedin

Trabectedin. [114899-77-3] (1'*R*,6*R*,6a*R*,7*R*,13*S*,14*S*,16*R*)-5-(Acetyloxy)-3',4',6,6a,7,13,14,16-octahydro-6',8,14-trihydroxy-7',9-dimethoxy-4,10,23-trimethylspiro[6,16-(epithiopropanoxymethano)-7,13-imino-12*H*-1,3-dioxolo[7,8]isoquino[3,2-*b*][3]-benzazocine-20,1'(2'*H*)-isoquinolin]-19-one; ecteinascidin 743; ET-743; Yondelis. C$_{39}$H$_{43}$N$_3$O$_{11}$S; mol wt 761.84. Enantioselective total synthesis: E. J. Corey *et al., J. Am. Chem. Soc.* **118**, 9202 (1996). *In vitro* antitumor activity: E. Isbicka *et al., Ann. Oncol.* **9**, 981 (1998). HPLC determn in plasma: H. Rosing *et al., J. Chromatogr. B* **710**, 183 (1998). Clinical pharmacokinetics: C. van Kesteren *et al., Clin. Cancer Res.* **6**, 4725 (2000). Review of mechanism of action: G. J. Aune *et al., Anti-Cancer Drugs* **13**, 545-555 (2002); of clinical development: C. van Kesteren *et al., ibid.* **14**, 487-502 (2003); of metabolism and hepatotoxicity: J. H. Beumer *et al., Pharmacol. Res.* **51**, 391-398 (2005). [α]$_D^{25}$ +114° (c = 0.1 in methanol).

THERAP CAT: Antineoplastic.

3504. ECTEOLA-Cellulose. [9015-13-8] Cellulose-ECTEOLA. Anion-exchange material prepd from cellulose, epichlorohydrin, and triethanolamine: Peterson, Sober, *J. Am. Chem. Soc.* **78**, 751 (1956); Veder, *J. Chromatogr.* **10**, 507 (1963).

3505. Ectoine. [96702-03-3] (4*S*)-1,4,5,6-Tetrahydro-2-methyl-4-pyrimidinecarboxylic acid; ectoin; RonaCare Ectoin. C$_6$-H$_{10}$N$_2$O$_2$; mol wt 142.16. C 50.69%, H 7.09%, N 19.71%, O 22.51%. Naturally occurring cyclic amino acid. Organic osmolyte; synthesized by microorganisms to maintain osmotic equilibrium in saline environments and to protect enzymes and whole cells from denaturation. Isoln from the halophilic, phototrophic bacterium, *Ectothiorhodospira halochloris*, and characterization as a compatible solute: E. A. Galinski *et al., Eur. J. Biochem.* **149**, 135 (1985). Biosynthesis: P. Peters *et al., FEMS Microbiol. Lett.* **71**, 157 (1990). Calorimetric analysis of biosynthesis efficiency: T. Maskow, W. Babel, *Biochim. Biophys. Acta* **1527**, 4 (2001). Chromatographic determn: V. Riis *et al., Anal. Bioanal. Chem.* **377**, 203 (2003). Osmoprotection in *E. coli*: M. Jebbar *et al., J. Bacteriol.* **174**, 5027 (1992). Mechanism of osmoprotection study: *idem et al., ibid.* **187**, 1293 (2005). Enzyme stabilization study: K. Lippert, E. A. Galinski, *Appl. Microbiol. Biotechnol.* **37**, 61 (1992). *In vitro* prevention of UVA-induced skin damage: J. Buenger, H. Driller, *Skin Pharmacol. Physiol.* **17**, 232 (2004). Inhibition of β-amyloid peptide aggregation and neurotoxicity: M. Kanapathipillai *et al., FEBS Lett.* **579**, 4775 (2005).

Crystals from water-free methanol. mp ~280°. [α]$_D^{20}$ +140° (c = 1.0 in methanol). Soly at 4°: 6 mol/kg water. Non-ionic character at physiological pH.

USE: Stabilizer in biotechnological processes; protects the taste of food during dehydration; moisturizer in cosmetics; protects skin against photoaging and formation of sunburn cells.

3506. Eculizumab. [219685-50-4] Anti-(human complement C5α-chain)(human-mouse monoclonal 5G1.1 heavy chain)immunoglobulin, disulfide with human-mouse monoclonal 5G1.1 light chain, dimer; h5G1.1 Fab; h5G1.1VHC + h5G1.1VLC. Humanized monoclonal antibody directed against complement component C5; designed to prevent activation of complement-mediated inflammation and tissue injury. Prepn: M. J. Evans *et al.,* **WO 9529697**; *eidem,* **US 6355245** (1995, 2002 both to Alexion); and experiment inhibition study: T. C. Thomas *et al., Mol. Immunol.* **33**, 1389 (1996). Clinical evaluation in paroxysmal nocturnal hemoglobinuria: P. Hillmen *et al., N. Engl. J. Med.* **350**, 552 (2004); A. Hill *et al., Blood* **106**, 2559 (2005). Review of development and therapeutic potential: M. Kaplan, *Curr. Opin. Invest. Drugs* **3**, 1017-1023 (2002).

THERAP CAT: Anti-inflammatory.

3507. Edatrexate. [80576-83-6] *N*-[4-[1-[(2,4-Diamino-6-pteridinyl)methyl]propyl]benzoyl]-L-glutamic acid; 10-ethyl-10-deazaaminopterin; 10-EdAM; 10-EDAAM; CGP-30694. C$_{22}$H$_{25}$-N$_7$O$_5$; mol wt 467.48. C 56.52%, H 5.39%, N 20.97%, O 17.11%. Dihydrofolate reductase inhibitor. Prepn: F. M. Sirotnak, J. I. DeGraw, **FR 2464956** (1981 to SRI International); J. I. DeGraw, Jr., F. M. Sirotnak, **US 4369319** (1983). Synthesis: J. I. DeGraw *et al., J. Med. Chem.* **25**, 1227 (1982); and resolution of diastereomers: *eidem, ibid.* **29**, 1056 (1986). HPLC determn: J. J. Kinahan *et al., Anal. Biochem.* **150**, 203 (1985); O. Van Tellingen *et al., J. Chromatogr.* **529**, 135 (1990). Pharmacology and toxicology: M. P. Fanucchi *et al., Cancer Res.* **47**, 2334 (1987). Clinical evaluation in non-small cell lung cancer: J. S. Lee *et al, Invest. New Drugs* **8**, 299 (1990). Review of pharmacology and antitumor activity: F. M. Sirotnak *et al., NCI Monogr.* **5**, 127-131 (1987).

Prepd as 1.75 H$_2$O, uv max (pH 13): 255, 370 nm (ε 30731, 7582).

THERAP CAT: Antineoplastic.

3508. EDDS. [186459-75-6] *N,N'*-1,2-Ethanediylbisaspartic acid; ethylenediamine *N,N'*-disuccinic acid. C$_{10}$H$_{16}$N$_2$O$_8$; mol wt 292.24. C 41.10%, H 5.52%, N 9.59%, O 43.80%. Hexadentate chelating agent with 2 chiral centers; structural isomer of EDTA, *q.v. S,S*-form is naturally occurring and biodegradable. Prepn: M. Barbier *et al., Ann.* **668**, 132 (1963). *See also:* C. Kezerian, W. M. Ramsey, **US 3158635** (1964 to Stauffer). Synthesis and metal chelating behavior of *S,S*-form: J. A. Neal, N. J. Rose, *Inorg. Chem.* **7**, 2405 (1968); of isomers: M. Orama *et al., J. Chem. Soc. Dalton Trans.* **2002**, 4644. Bacterial production of *S,S*-form: R. Takahashi *et al., Biosci. Biotech. Biochem.* **63**, 1269 (1999). Crystal structure of *S,S*-form: F. E. Scarbrough, D. Voet, *Acta Crystallogr.* **B32**, 2715 (1976). Biodegradation analysis of isomers: R. Takahashi *et al., Biosci. Biotech. Biochem.* **61**, 1957 (1997); of *S,S*-form: P. C. Vandevivere *et al., Environ. Sci. Technol.* **35**, 1765 (2001). HPLC determn of *S,S*-form: S. Tandy *et al., J. Chromatogr. A* **1077**, 37 (2005). Study of use in radiochemical decontamination: P. W. Jones, D. R. Williams, *Appl. Radiat. Isot.* **54**, 587 (2001); in heavy metal phytoextraction from soil: H. Grcman *et al., J. Environ. Qual.* **32**, 500 (2003); E. Meers *et al., Chemosphere* **58**, 1011 (2005).

S,S-EDDS

Crystals from methanol, mp 128-132° (Barbier). Also reported as mp 220-222° (Kezerian, Ramsey). Slightly sol in water. Insol in ethanol, acetone, benzene, and most organic solvents. Acid dissociation constants (25°, 0.1 M KNO$_3$): pK$_1$ 2.4; pK$_2$ 3.9; pK$_3$ 6.8; pK$_4$ 9.8.

S,S-Form. [20846-91-7] Crystal density: 1.44 g/cm^3.

USE: Chelating agent in detergents, electroless plating, rust removal, photography, and soil remediation.

3509. Edestin. [9007-57-2] Globular protein originally obtained from hemp seed *(Cannabis sativa):* Osborne, *Am. Chem. J.* **14,** 662 (1892); Stockwell *et al., Proc. Seed Protein Conf.* **1963,** 56, *C.A.* **60,** 3090d (1964). Approx mol wt 300,000. Since the passage of the Marihuana Tax Act in the U.S.A. commercial hemp seed must be heat-treated to destroy its narcotic properties, a process which also destroys the edestin. Very closely related proteins may be obtained from seeds of *Cucurbita pepo* L. (pumpkin), *C. moschata* Duchesne, and *C. maxima* Duchesne (squash), *Citrullus vulgaris* Schrader (watermelon), *Cucumis melo* L. (cantaloupe), and *Cucumis sativus* L., *Cucurbitaceae* (cucumber). Isoln from *Cucurbita pepo:* Vickery *et al., Biochem. Prep.* **2,** 5 (1952). Extraction from hemp seed, prepn of crystalline form and x-ray data: J. Drenth, E. W. Wiebenga, *Rec. Trav. Chim.* **74,** 813 (1955). The amino acid compositions of these globulins are slightly different from hemp seed globulin and from each other: Smith *et al., J. Biol. Chem.* **164,** 159 (1946); Smith, Greene, *ibid.* **167,** 833 (1947); **172,** 111 (1948). Structure studies: Hall, *ibid.* **185,** 45 (1959); Cleemann, Kratky, *Z. Naturforsch.* **15b,** 526 (1960); Dlouhá *et al., Collect. Czech. Chem. Commun.* **28,** 2779 (1963); **29,** 1835 (1964). Electron microscopy and optical diffraction: A. M. H. Schepman *et al., Biochim. Biophys. Acta* **271,** 279 (1972). Electron spin resonance studies: L. J. Dimmey, W. Gordy, *Proc. Natl. Acad. Sci. USA* **77,** 343 (1980).

Octahedral crystals. Completely sol to a clear soln in 10% salt soln. Sol in dil mineral acids. Forms a water-soluble hydrochloride.

3510. Edifenphos. [17109-49-8] Phosphorodithioic acid *O*-ethyl *S,S*-diphenyl ester; *O*-ethyl *S,S*-diphenyl phosphorodithioate; EDDP; ediphenphos; Bayer 78418; Hinosan. C$_{14}$H$_{15}$O$_2$PS$_2$; mol wt 310.37. C 54.18%, H 4.87%, O 10.31%, P 9.98%, S 20.66%. Prepn: **NL 6611860**; G. Schrader *et al., US 3499951* (1967, 1970 both to Bayer). Degradn in soil: C. Tomizawa *et al., J. Environ. Sci. Health* **B11,** 231 (1976). Metabolism: I. Ueyama *et al., Agric. Biol. Chem.* **42,** 885 (1978). Mechanism of action: O. Kodama *et al., ibid.* **44,** 1015 (1980). Toxicology: T. S. Chen *et al., Toxicol. Appl. Pharmacol.* **23,** 519 (1972).

Clear yellow to light-brown liquid, bp$_{0.01}$ 154°. d$_4^{20}$ 1.23; n$_D^{22}$ 1.61. Practically insol in water. Sol in acetone, xylene. LD$_{50}$ in female, male rats (mg/kg): 25.5, 66.5 i.p. (Chen).

USE: Fungicide.

3511. Edifoligide Sodium. [328538-04-1] DNA d(*P*-Thio)- (C-T-A-G-A-T-T-T-C-C-C-G-C-G) complex with DNA d(*P*-thio)- (G-A-T-C-C-G-C-G-G-G-A-A-A-T)(1:1) hexacosasodium salt; E2F Decoy; E2FD; CGT-003; Double stranded oligodeoxynucleotide designed to bind and inactivate the cell-cycle transcription factor E2F. Transcription factor decoy used in *ex vivo* gene suppression therapy to prevent vein graft failure following coronary artery and peripheral artery bypass surgery. Description of sequence and use as decoy: V. J. Dzau *et al.,* **WO 9511687**; *eidem,* **US 02052333** (1995, 2002). Binding inhibition study in vascular smooth muscle: R. Morishita *et al., Proc. Natl. Acad. Sci. USA* **92,** 5855 (1995); in glomerular mesangial cells: N. Tomita *et al., Am. J. Physiol.* **275,** F278 (1998). Pharmacology: A. Ehsan *et al., J. Thorac. Cardiovasc. Surg.* **121,** 714 (2001). Clinical evaluation in vascular bypass: M. J. Mann *et al., Lancet* **354,** 1493 (1999). Review of mechanism of action: M. J. Mann, *Antisense Nucl. Acid Drug Dev.* **8,** 171-176 (1998).

THERAP CAT: Gene suppression therapy to prevent vein graft atherosclerosis.

3512. Edotecarin. [174402-32-5] 12-β-D-Glucopyranosyl-12,13-dihydro-2,10-dihydroxy-6-[[2-hydroxy-1-(hydroxymethyl)-ethyl]amino]-5*H*-indolo[2,3-*a*]pyrrolo[3,4-*c*]carbazole-5,7(6*H*)-dione; ED-749; J-107088; PF-804950; PHA-782615. C$_{29}$H$_{28}$N$_4$O$_{11}$; mol wt 608.55. C 57.24%, H 4.64%, N 9.21%, O 28.92%. Topoisomerase I inhibitor that induces single strand DNA cleavage. Prepn: K. Kojiri *et al.,* **EP 760375**; *eidem,* **US 5922860** (1997, 1999 both to Banyu Pharm.); M. Ohkubo *et al., Bioorg. Med. Chem. Lett.* **9,** 3307 (1999). Synthesis: A. Akao *et al., Tetrahedron* **57,** 8917 (2001). Mechanism of action study: T. Yoshinari *et al., Cancer Res.* **59,** 4271 (1999). *In vivo* antitumor activity: H. Arakawa *et al., Jpn. J. Cancer Res.* **90,** 1163 (1999). LC/MS/MS determn in plasma: A. Q. Wang *et al., Rapid Commun. Mass Spectrom.* **16,** 975 (2002). Review of development: W. A. Denny, *IDrugs* **7,** 173-177 (2004); and clinical experience: M. W. Saif, R. B. Diasio, *Clin. Colorectal Cancer* **5,** 27-36 (2005).

Orange solid, mp 330° (dec). [α]$_D^{23}$ +117° (c = 0.8 in 1:1 acetonitrile/water).

THERAP CAT: Antineoplastic.

3513. Edotreotide. [204318-14-9] *N*-[[4,7,10-Tris(carboxymethyl)-1,4,7,10-tetraazacyclododec-1-yl]acetyl]-D-phenylalanyl-L-cysteinyl-L-tyrosyl-D-tryptophyl-L-lysyl-L-threonyl-*N*-[(1*R*,2*R*)-2-hydroxy-1-(hydroxymethyl)propyl]-L-cysteinamide cyclic(2 → 7)-disulfide; (DOTA D-Phe^1,Tyr^3)octreotide; DOTATOC; SMT-487. C$_{65}$H$_{92}$N$_{14}$O$_{18}$S$_2$; mol wt 1421.64. C 54.92%, H 6.52%, N 13.79%, O 20.26%, S 4.51%. Octapeptide analog of somatostatin, *q.v.* Designed for targeted radiotherapy vs somatostatin receptor-expressing tumors. Prepn: R. Albert *et al.,* **EP 714911**; *eidem,* **US 6183721** (1996, 2001 both to Novartis); *idem, et al., Bioorg. Med. Chem. Lett.* **8,** 1207 (1998). Solution-phase synthesis: M. Schottelius *et al., Tetrahedron Lett.* **44,** 2393 (2003). *In vivo* antineoplastic activity: B. Stolz *et al., Eur. J. Nucl. Med.* **25,** 668 (1998). Receptor binding study: J. C. Reubi *et al., ibid.* **27,** 273 (2000). Clinical pharmacokinetics: F. Jamar *et al., Eur. J. Nucl. Med. Mol. Imaging* **30,** 510 (2003). Clinical evaluation in neuroendocrine tumors: C. Waldherr *et al., J. Nucl. Med.* **43,** 610 (2002).

Prepd as acetate. [α]$_{22}^D$ −14.75° (c = 0.52 in 95% acetic acid).

^{90}Y chelate. [322407-70-5] ^{90}Y-SMT-487; OctreoTher.

THERAP CAT: ^{90}Y chelate as antineoplastic.

3514. Edoxudine. [15176-29-1] 2′-Deoxy-5-ethyluridine; 5-ethyl-2′-deoxyuridine; 5-ethyl-3-(2′-deoxyribosyl)uracil; EDU;

EUDR; ORF-15817; Aedurid; Edurid. $C_{11}H_{16}N_2O_5$; mol wt 256.26. C 51.56%, H 6.29%, N 10.93%, O 31.22%. Substituted uracil with anti-herpes activity. Prepn and properties: K. K. Gauri, **GB 1170565**; *eidem*, **US 3553192** (1968, 1971 both to Robugen). Synthesis via organopalladium intermediates: D. E. Bergstrom, J. L. Ruth, *J. Am. Chem. Soc.* **98**, 1587 (1976); D. E. Bergstrom, M. K. Ogawa, *ibid.* **100**, 8106 (1978). Physical properties: M. Swierkowski, D. Shugar, *J. Med. Chem.* **12**, 533 (1969). Antiviral activity: E. De Clercq, D. Shugar, *Biochem. Pharmacol.* **24**, 1073 (1975). Preferential inhibition of herpes simplex virus type 2: C.-Z. Teh, S. L. Sacks, *Antimicrob. Agents Chemother.* **23**, 637 (1983). Synergistic effect with interferon-β, *q.v.*, on herpes simplex virus: C. Janz, R. Wigand, *Arch. Virol.* **73**, 135 (1982). Inhibitory effect on growth of murine leukemia cells: J. Balzarini *et al.*, *Invest. New Drugs* **2**, 35 (1984).

Long clear needles from acetone, mp 152-153°. uv max: 267 nm (ε 9610) at pH 2, 267 nm (ε 7280) at pH 1. pKa: 9.98.

THERAP CAT: Antiviral (herpes simplex).

3515. Edrecolomab. [156586-89-9] Anti-(human colon cancer tumor-associated antigen) immunoglobulin G2a (mouse monoclonal 17-1aγ_{2a}-chain) disulfide with mouse monoclonal 17-1A light chain, dimer; 17-1A antibody; Panorex. Murine monoclonal IgG2a antibody directed against the cell surface glycoprotein CO17-1A, a human tumor associated antigen expressed on malignant and normal epithelial cells. Prepn: M. Herlyn *et al.*, *Proc. Natl. Acad. Sci. USA* **76**, 1438 (1979). Pharmacology: D. Herlyn, H. Koprowski, *ibid.* **79**, 4761 (1982). Clinical studies in colorectal cancer: G. Riethmüller *et al.*, *Lancet* **343**, 1177 (1994); *eidem*, *J. Clin. Oncol.* **16**, 1788 (1998). Review of prepn and pharmacology: A. H. Ross *et al.*, *Immunol. Ser.* **43**, 107-122 (1989); and clinical experience: J. C. Adkins, C. M. Spencer, *Drugs* **56**, 619-626 (1998).

THERAP CAT: Antineoplastic.

3516. Edrophonium Chloride. [116-38-1] *N*-Ethyl-3-hydroxy-*N*,*N*-dimethylbenzenaminium chloride; ethyl(*m*-hydroxyphenyl)dimethylammonium chloride; (3-hydroxyphenyl)dimethylethylammonium chloride; 3-hydroxy-*N*,*N*-dimethyl-*N*-ethylanilinium chloride; Antirex; Enlon; Reversol; Tensilon. $C_{10}H_{16}ClNO$; mol wt 201.69. C 59.55%, H 8.00%, Cl 17.58%, N 6.94%, O 7.93%. Cholinesterase inhibitor. Prepn: J. A. Aeschlimann, A. Stempel, **US 2647924** (1953 to Hoffmann-La Roche). LC determn in biological fluids: M. G. M. DeRuyter *et al.*, *J. Chromatogr.* **183**, 193 (1980). Clinical evaluation in reversal of neuromuscular blockade: D. M. Fisher *et al.*, *Anesthesiology* **61**, 428 (1984). Clinical study in supraventricular tachycardia: J. D. Cantwell *et al.*, *Arch. Int. Med.* **130**, 221 (1972). Diagnostic use in myasthenia gravis: I. M. Williams *et al.*, *Clin. Exp. Neurol.* **22**, 1 (1986); in esophageal chest pain: C. A. Lee *et al.*, *Dig. Dis. Sci.* **32**, 682 (1987).

Crystals from isopropanol, dec 162-163°. pH of 1% aq soln 4-5. Very sol in water; freely sol in alcohol. Insol in chloroform, ether.

Edrophonium Bromide. Edrophone bromide; Ro-2-3198. $C_{10}H_{16}BrNO$; mol wt 246.14. Crystals from ethanol + ether, dec 151-152°. Bitter taste. Sol in water (more than 10%). Moderately sol in alcohol. Practically insol in ether. Solns are stable.

THERAP CAT: Cholinergic; antidote to curare; diagnostic aid (myasthenia gravis).

3517. EDTA. [60-00-4] *N*,*N*'-1,2-Ethanediylbis[*N*-(carboxymethyl)glycine]; ethylenebis(iminodiacetic acid); (ethylenedinitrilo)tetraacetic acid; ethylenediaminetetraacetic acid; edathamil; edetic acid; Versene Acid. $C_{10}H_{16}N_2O_8$; mol wt 292.24. C 41.10%, H 5.52%, N 9.59%, O 43.80%. Powerful chelating agent; forms stable complexes with most metal ions. Prepn: F. Münz, **US 2130505** (1938 to General Aniline); R. Smith *et al.*, *J. Org. Chem.* **14**, 355 (1949). Prepn of α- and β-form of crystals: R. B. Le Blanc, H. L. Spell, *J. Phys. Chem.* **64**, 949 (1960). Efficacy in animal models of cadmium toxicity: L. R. Cantilena, Jr., C. D. Klaassen, *Toxicol. Appl. Pharmacol.* **53**, 510 (1980). Lead mobilization by calcium and zinc salts: C. F. Brownie, A. L. Aronson, *ibid.* **75**, 167 (1984). Determn in pharmaceutical formulations and foods: A. A. Krokidis *et al.*, *Anal. Chim. Acta* **535**, 57 (2005). Clinical evaluation in calcific band keratopathy: D. M. Najjar *et al.*, *Am. J. Ophthalmol.* **137**, 1056 (2004). Review of laboratory uses: W. C. Broad, *Am. Lab.* **3**, 47-51 (1971); of toxicology: K. Heindorff *et al.*, *Mutat. Res.* **115**, 149-173 (1983); of use in personal care products: J. R. Hart, *Cosmet. Toiletries* **98**, 54-58 (1983); of determn methods: M. Sillanpää, M.-L. Sihvonen, *Talanta* **44**, 1487-1497 (1997); of properties and analysis methods: F. Belal, A. A. Al-Badr, *Anal. Profiles Drug Subs. Excip.* **29**, 57-104 (2002); of safety and efficacy in chelation therapy in atherosclerosis: M. T. Grier, D. G. Meyers, *Ann. Pharmacother.* **27**, 1504-1509 (1993); E. Ernst, *Am. Heart J.* **140**, 139-141 (2000). Safety assessment: *Int. J. Toxicol.* **21**, (Suppl. 2), 95-142 (2002).

White, crystalline powder, mp 240-241° (dec). Soly in water at 20°: 0.2 g/100 g. The free acid tends to decarboxylate when heated to temps of 150°. Stable on storage and on boiling in aq soln.

Calcium disodium salt. [62-33-9] [[*N*,*N*'-1,2-Ethanediylbis[*N*-(carboxymethyl)glycinato]](4−)-*N*,*N*',*O*,*O*',*O*^{N},*O*^{N}']calciate(2−)-disodium; edetate calcium disodium; Antallin; Calcium Disodium Versenate; Ledclair; Mosatil; Sormetal. $C_{10}H_{12}CaN_2Na_2O_8$; mol wt 374.27. Prepn: Astakhov, Kiseleva, *Zh. Obshch. Khim.* **20**, 1780 (1950), *C.A.* **45**, 2409 (1951). Tetrahydrate, powder. Sol in water: at 30° a 0.1*M* soln can be prepd (pH ~7). Practically insol in organic solvents.

Cobalt salt. [36499-65-7] Dicobalt edetate; Kelocyanor. $C_{10}H_{12}Co_2N_2O_8$; mol wt 406.08.

Disodium salt. [139-33-3] Edetate disodium; tetracemate disodium; Chelaplex III; Chelatran; Endrate disodium; Titriplex III; Versene Na$_2$. $C_{10}H_{14}N_2Na_2O_8$; mol wt 336.21. Dihydrate: crystals, mp 252° (dec). pH about 5.3. Soly in water at 20°: 10.8 g/100 ml.

Tetrasodium salt. [64-02-8] Edetate sodium; tetracemate tetrasodium; tetracemin; Endrate Tetrasodium; Versene 100; Sequestrene; Trilon B; Nullapon; Complexone; Distol 8; Calsol; Syntes 12a; Nervanaid B. $C_{10}H_{12}N_2Na_4O_8$; mol wt 380.17. Powder, mp 300° (dec). Apparent density: 6.9 lb/gallon. Sol in water: about 103 g/100 ml. pH of 1% soln 11.3. Less sol in alcohol than the potassium salt.

Trisodium salt. [150-38-9] Edetate trisodium; Limclair; Versene-9. $C_{10}H_{13}N_2Na_3O_8$; mol wt 358.19. Monohydrate: crystals from water, mp >300°. More sol in water than the corresp disodium salt or free acid. pH of 1% aq soln 9.3.

USE: Preservative and color retention agent in foods, flavoring agent. As antioxidant in foods. Pharmaceutic aid (chelating agent); anticoagulant for blood collection. Chelating agent in personal care products, in pulp and paper industry, in laboratory titrimetric analysis of metals and solubilization of metal compds.

THERAP CAT: Chelating agent (metal); dicobalt edetate as antidote (cyanide).

THERAP CAT (VET): In treatment of lead and heavy metal poisoning of farm animals.

3518. EEDQ. [16357-59-8] 2-Ethoxy-1(2H)-quinolinecarboxylic acid ethyl ester; N-carbethoxy-2-ethoxy-1,2-dihydroquinoline; N-ethoxycarbonyl-2-ethoxy-1,2-dihydroquinoline; BC-681. $C_{14}H_{17}NO_3$; mol wt 247.29. C 68.00%, H 6.93%, N 5.66%, O 19.41%. Coupling agent used in the synthesis of peptides: Belleau, Malek, J. Am. Chem. Soc. **90**, 1651 (1968); Yajima, Kawatani, Chem. Pharm. Bull. **19**, 1905 (1971); Sipos, Gaston, Synthesis **1971**, 321. Preparation: Weinberg, US 3389142 and US 3452140 (1968, 1969, to Bristol-Myers). Has CNS depressant activity: Belleau, J. Am. Chem. Soc. **90**, 823 (1968). Pharmacological studies: Martel et al., Can. J. Physiol. Pharmacol. **47**, 909 (1969); Chang et al., Pharmacol. Res. Commun. **2**, 63 (1970); Weissman, Muren, J. Med. Chem. **14**, 49 (1971).

mp 56-57°. bp$_{0.1}$ 125-128°.
USE: In the synthesis of peptides.

3519. Efalizumab. [214745-43-4] Anti-(human CD11a (antigen)) immunoglobulin G1 (human-mouse monoclonal hu1124 γ$_1$-chain) disulfide with human-mouse monoclonal hu1124 light chain, dimer; hu1124; Raptiva; Xanelim. Humanized monoclonal IgG1 antibody directed against the CD11a subunit of lymphocyte function-associated antigen-1 (LFA-1). Inhibits lymphocyte activation, migration and adhesion to endothelial cells. Prepn: P. M. Jardieu, L. G. Presta, **WO 9823761**; eidem, **US 6037454** (1998, 2000 both to Genentech); W. A. Werther et al., J. Immunol. **157**, 4986 (1996). Clinical pharmacokinetics: R. J. Bauer et al., J. Pharmacokinet. Biopharm. **27**, 397 (1999). Clinical study in psoriasis: M. Lebwohl et al., N. Engl. J. Med. **349**, 2004 (2003). Review of pharmacology and therapeutic potential: R. L. Dedrick et al., Transplant Immunol. **9**, 181-186 (2002); J. C. Cather et al., Expert Opin. Biol. Ther. **3**, 361-370 (2003); of use in chronic psoriasis: J. C. Cather, A. Menter, Expert Opin. Biol. Ther. **5**, 393-403 (2005).
THERAP CAT: Antipsoriatic; immunosuppressant.

3520. Efaproxiral. [131179-95-8] 2-[4-[2-[(3,5-Dimethylphenyl)amino]-2-oxoethyl]phenoxy]-2-methylpropanoic acid; 2-4-[[(3,5-dimethylanilino)carbonyl]methyl]phenoxy-2-methylpropionic acid; RSR-13. $C_{20}H_{23}NO_4$; mol wt 341.40. C 70.36%, H 6.79%, N 4.10%, O 18.75%. Allosteric modifier of hemoglobin (Hb). Binds in the central water cavity of the Hb molecule causing a conformational change such that bound oxygen is released more readily. Prepd not claimed: D. J. Abraham et al., **US 5049695** (1991 to Center Innovative Technol.); eidem., J. Med. Chem. **34**, 752 (1991). Oxygen binding affinities and mechanism of action: D. J. Abraham et al., Biochemistry **31**, 9141 (1992). Effect on myocardial oxygen concentration: P. S. Pagel et al., J. Pharmacol. Exp. Ther. **285**, 1 (1998). Antimetastatic effects: B. A. Teicher et al., Cancer Chemother. Pharmacol. **42**, 24 (1998). Clinical pharmacokinetics and pharmacodynamics: L. Kleinberg et al., J. Clin. Oncol. **17**, 2593 (1999). Clinical evaluation in brain tumor therapy: eidem, ibid. **20**, 3149 (2002).

mp 85°.
THERAP CAT: Antineoplastic adjunct (radiosensitizer).

3521. Efavirenz. [154598-52-4] (4S)-6-Chloro-4-(cyclopropylethynyl)-1,4-dihydro-4-(trifluoromethyl)-2H-3,1-benzoxazin-2-one; DMP-266; Stocrin; Sustiva. $C_{14}H_9ClF_3NO_2$; mol wt 315.67. C 53.27%, H 2.87%, Cl 11.23%, F 18.06%, N 4.44%, O 10.14%. Nonnucleoside HIV-1 reverse transcriptase inhibitor. Prepn: S. D. Young et al., **EP 582455**; eidem, **US 5519021**

(1994, 1996 both to Merck & Co.). Pharmacology: S. D. Young et al., Antimicrob. Agents Chemother. **39**, 2602 (1995). Enantioselective synthesis: A. S. Thompson et al., Tetrahedron Lett. **36**, 8937 (1995). Total synthesis and resolution of enantiomers: L. A. Radesca et al., Synth. Commun. **27**, 4373 (1997). Ionization behavior: S. R. Rabel et al., Pharm. Dev. Technol. **1**, 91 (1996). Clinical trial as component of combination therapy in HIV-1 infection in adults: S. Staszewski et al., N. Engl. J. Med. **341**, 1865 (1999); in children: S. E. Starr et al., ibid. 1874. Review of clinical experience: C. Fortin, V. Joly, Expert Rev. Anti Infect. Ther. **2**, 671-684 (2004).

Crystals from toluene:heptane, mp 139-141°. $[\alpha]_D^{20}$ −84.7° (c = 0.005 g/ml in CH$_3$Cl). $[\alpha]_D^{25}$ −94.1° (c = 0.300 in methanol). pKa 10.2.
THERAP CAT: Antiviral.

3522. Eflornithine. [67037-37-0] 2-(Difluoromethyl)-DL-ornithine; α-difluoromethylornithine; DFMO; RMI-71782. C_6H_{12}-$F_2N_2O_2$; mol wt 182.17. C 39.56%, H 6.64%, F 20.86%, N 15.38%, O 17.57%. Irreversible inhibitor of ornithine decarboxylase, an enzyme involved in polyamine biosynthesis. Prepn: B. W. Metcalf et al., J. Am. Chem. Soc. **100**, 2551 (1978); P. Bey et al., J. Org. Chem. **44**, 2732 (1979). Effect on polyamine biosynthesis in trypanosomes: C. J. Bacchi et al., Science **210**, 332 (1980). Clinical pharmacokinetics: K. D. Haegele et al., Clin. Pharmacol. Ther. **30**, 210 (1981). Reviews of clinical experience in Pneumocystis carinii pneumonia: J. Sahai, A. J. Berry, Pharmacotherapy **9**, 29-33 (1989); in cancer chemotherapy: F. L. Meyskens, Jr., E. W. Gerner, Clin. Cancer Res. **5**, 945-951 (1999); in trypanosomiasis: C. Burri, R. Brun, Parasitol. Res. **90**, S49-S52 (2003). Review of topical use in hirsutism: J. A. Barman Balfour, K. McClellen, Am. J. Clin. Dermatol. **2**, 197-201 (2001).

Hydrochloride monohydrate. [96020-91-6] Ornidyl; Vaniqa. $C_6H_{12}F_2N_2O_2 \cdot HCl \cdot H_2O$; mol wt 236.64. Crystals from ethanol/-water, mp 183°. Freely sol in water; sparingly sol in ethanol.
THERAP CAT: Antineoplastic; antipneumocystic; antiprotozoal (Trypanosoma). In treatment of hirsutism.

3523. Efloxate. [119-41-5] [(4-Oxo-2-phenyl-4H-1-benzopyran-7-yl)oxy]acetic acid ethyl ester; 7-flavone ethyl hydroxyacetate; ethyl flavon-7-yloxyacetate; ethyl 7-flavonoxyacetate; 7-flavonoxyacetic acid ethyl ester; oxyflavil; Re-1-0185; Recordil. $C_{19}H_{16}O_5$; mol wt 324.33. C 70.36%, H 4.97%, O 24.67%. Prepn: P. Da Re et al., Farmaco Ed. Sci. **13**, 561 (1958); **GB 803372** and **GB 824547** (1958, 1959 both to Recordati); P. Da Re, A. Colleoni, Ann. Chim. (Rome) **49**, 1632 (1959).

Crystals from 50% ethanol, mp 123-124°. Soluble in the usual organic solvents; slightly sol in water. LD$_{50}$ i.p. in rats: 3200 mg/kg (Da Re).
THERAP CAT: Vasodilator (coronary).

3524. Efonidipine. [111011-63-3] 5-(5,5-Dimethyl-1,3,2-dioxaphosphorinan-2-yl)-1,4-dihydro-2,6-dimethyl-4-(3-nitrophenyl)-3-pyridinecarboxylic acid 2-[phenyl(phenylmethyl)amino]ethyl ester, P-oxide; 2-(N-benzylanilino)ethyl(±)-1,4-dihydro-2,6-dimethyl-4-(m-nitrophenyl)-5-phosphononicotinate, cyclic 2,2-dimethyltrimethylene ester. $C_{34}H_{38}N_3O_7P$; mol wt 631.66. C 64.65%, H 6.06%, N 6.65%, O 17.73%, P 4.90%. Dihydropyridine calcium channel blocker. Prepn: K. Seto et al., **WO 8704439**; idem et al., **US 4885284** (1987, 1989 both to Nissan); and crystal structure: R. Sakoda et al., Chem. Pharm. Bull. **40**, 2362 (1992). Stereoselective synthesis of enantiomers and crystal structure of (S)-form: idem et al., ibid. 2377. Pharmacology: C. Shudo et al., J. Pharm. Pharmacol. **45**, 525 (1993). Mechanism of action study: T. Yamashita et al., Jpn. J. Pharmacol. **57**, 337 (1991). Clinical study: T. Saito et al., Curr. Ther. Res. **52**, 113 (1992).

Crystals from ethyl acetate, mp 169-170° (Sakoda); also reported as mp 155-156° (Seto).

Hydrochloride. [111011-53-1] $C_{34}H_{38}N_3O_7P\cdot HCl$. LD_{50} in mice (mg/kg): >600 orally (Seto).

Hydrochloride ethanol. [111011-76-8] NZ-105; Landel. $C_{34}H_{38}N_3O_7P\cdot C_2H_5OH\cdot HCl$; mol wt 714.18. Yellow crystals from aq ethanol, mp 151° (dec).

(S)- or (R)-Form. Pale yellow crystals from ethanol, mp 190-192°. $[\alpha]_D^{25}$ + or −7.0° resp (c = 0.50 in chloroform).

THERAP CAT: Antihypertensive.

3525. Efrotomycin. [56592-32-6] 31-O-[6-Deoxy-4-O-(6-deoxy-2,4-di-O-methyl-α-L-mannopyranosyl)-3-O-methyl-β-D-allopyranosyl]-1-methylmocimycin; 31-O-[6-deoxy-4-O-(6-deoxy-2,4-di-O-methylhexopyranosyl)-3-O-methylhexopyranosyl]-1-methylmocimycin; FR-02A; MK-621; Producil. $C_{59}H_{88}N_2O_{20}$; mol wt 1145.33. C 61.87%, H 7.74%, N 2.45%, O 27.94%. Antibiotic produced by Streptomyces lactamdurans NRRL 3802: R. G. Wax, W. M. Maiese, **DE 2450813** (1975 to Merck & Co.), C.A. **83**, 145755y (1975); R. G. Wax et al., J. Antibiot. **29**, 670 (1976). In vitro and in vivo activity: B. M. Frost et al., ibid. 1083; 32, 626 (1979). Production and growth promoting activity: W. M. Maiese, R. G. Wax, **US 4024251** (1977 to Merck & Co.). Synergism with bottromycin, q.v.: B. M. Frost et al., J. Antibiot. **32**, 1046 (1979). Structure: R. S. Dewey et al., ibid. **38**, 1691 (1985). Stereospecific total synthesis: R. E. Dolle, K. C. Nicolaou, J. Am. Chem. Soc. **107**, 1691, 1695 (1985). HPLC determn in feeds: J. D. Strong, Analyst **111**, 853 (1986). Effect on gain and feed efficiency in swine: A. G. Foster et al., J. Anim. Sci. **65**, 877 (1987).

Pale yellow solid. uv max (pH 7): 232, 327 nm ($E_{1cm}^{1\%}$ 464, 216). LD_{50} in mice (g/kg): >4 orally; >2 s.c. (Frost).

THERAP CAT (VET): Growth stimulant.

3526. EGCG. [989-51-5] 3,4,5-Trihydroxybenzoic acid, (2R,3R)-3,4-dihydro-5,7-dihydroxy-2-(3,4,5-trihydroxyphenyl)-2H-1-benzopyran-3-yl ester; (−)-epigallocatechin 3-O-gallate;

(−)-epigallocatechol gallate. $C_{22}H_{18}O_{11}$; mol wt 458.37. C 57.65%, H 3.96%, O 38.40%. Polyphenolic constituent of tea; inhibits tumor promotion. Initial identification and isoln from green tea: M. Tsujimura, Bull. Agric. Chem. Soc. Jpn. **6**, 70 (1930); C.A. **25**, 3637 (1931); and crystallization: L. Vuataz et al., J. Chromatogr. **2**, 173 (1959). Oxidation during tea fermentation: P. Coggon et al., J. Agric. Food Chem. **21**, 727 (1973). HPLC/MS extraction from black tea: R. G. Bailey et al., J. Sci. Food Agric. **66**, 203 (1994). HPLC determn in plasma and urine: M.-J. Lee et al., Cancer Epidemiol. Biomarkers Prev. **4**, 393 (1995). Antitumor promoting activity: S. Yoshizawa et al., Phytother. Res. **1**, 44 (1987); T. Yamane et al., Cancer Res. **55**, 2081 (1995). Inhibition of metastasis in mice: S. Taniguchi et al., Cancer Lett. **65**, 51 (1992). Modulation of endocrine systems and food intake: Y.-H. Kao, et al., Endocrinology **141**, 980 (2000).

White crystals from water, mp 218°. $[\alpha]_D$ −185 ±2°(ethanol). uv max (ethanol): 275 nm (ε 11500).

3527. EGF-Urogastrone. EGF-URO. Related polypeptides that are both potent stimulators of cellular proliferation and inhibitors of gastric acid secretion. *Urogastrone* was originally detected as an antisecretory agent during experiments on human urine: J. S. Gray et al., Science **89**, 489 (1939); M. H. F. Friedman et al., Proc. Soc. Exp. Biol. Med. **41**, 509 (1935). Isoln: J. S. Gray et al., Endocrinology **30**, 129 (1942); R. A. Gregory, J. Physiol. **129**, 528 (1955). Improved procedures led to the isoln and amino acid sequence determn of two polypeptides, *β-urogastrone* and *γ-urogastrone*: H. Gregory, Nature **257**, 325 (1975). These two peptides contain 3 disulfide bonds and consist of 53 and 52 amino acid residues, respectively. The only difference between them is the absence of a C-terminal arginine residue in the γ-peptide. *Epidermal growth factor*, or *EGF*, was isolated from submaxillary glands of male mice after first being detected during purification of a nerve growth promoting protein: S. Cohen, Proc. Natl. Acad. Sci. USA **46**, 302 (1960); idem, J. Biol. Chem. **237**, 1555 (1962). The primary structure of mouse EGF (mEGF) was found to be a 53 amino acid polypeptide containing 3 disulfide bonds: C. R. Savage et al., ibid. **247**, 7612 (1972); **248**, 7669 (1973). Sequence of an mEGF cDNA clone that predicts the synthesis of EGF as a large protein precursor of 1,168 amino acids: A. Gray et al., Nature **303**, 722 (1983). mEGF causes premature eye opening and stimulation of epithelial cell tissue growth when injected daily into newborn mice: S. Cohen, loc. cit. (1962); S. Cohen, J. M. Taylor, Recent Prog. Horm. Res. **30**, 533 (1974). The structural similarities between EGF and urogastrone led to experiments that established the gastric acid-inhibitory activity of mEGF and the proliferative activity of urogastrone, thus showing that both polypeptides have the same intrinsic biological activities, cf. H. Gregory, loc. cit. It has also been shown that both mEGF and urogastrone can share the same receptor sites in human tissue with almost equal affinities: M. D. Hollenberg, H. Gregory, Life Sci. **20**, 267 (1976). Human EGF has been isolated from urine: S. Cohen, G. Carpenter, Proc. Natl. Acad. Sci. USA **72**, 1317 (1975). The similarity of its amino acid composition and physicochemical properties to urogastrone has suggested the identity of these polypeptides. Although the mouse and human polypeptides are chemically distinct (16 differences in amino acid sequence), their identical intrinsic biological activities and their ability to share receptor sites with similar affinities has led to the use of the combined term EGF-urogastrone. *Reviews:* S. Cohen,

R. Savage, *Recent Prog. Horm. Res.* **30,** 551-574 (1974); M. D. Hollenberg, *Vitam. Horm.* **37,** 69-110 (1979); D. Gospodarowicz, *Annu. Rev. Physiol.* **43,** 251-263 (1981); P. Walker, *J. Endocrinol. Invest.* **5,** 183-196 (1982); M. Das, *Int. Rev. Cytol.* **78,** 233-256 (1982).

Mouse EGF-URO. Mol wt 6041. uv max: 280 nm ($E_{1cm}^{1\%}$ 30.9). Isoelectric pt 4.60. Heat stable and non-dialyzable. Biological activity stable in boiling water but destroyed by heating in dil acid or alkali. Incubation with chymotrypsin or a bacterial protease also destroys biological activity.

Human EGF-URO. Anthelone; anthelone U; uroanthelone; uroenterone. Mol wt 6201. Isoelectric pt 4.5. Very sol in water. Sol in methanol, ethylene gycol.

3528. Egg Oil. Oil of egg yolk. Obtained from fresh egg yolks by extraction with ethylene dichloride. Contains fatty glycerides, cholesterol, lecithin. The glyceride fraction is a mixture of the glycerides of satd and unsatd fatty acids. Palmitic, stearic, oleic, linoleic and clupanodonic acids have been isolated from both the glyceride and lecithin fractions. Preparation: Levin, Lerman, *J. Am. Oil Chem. Soc.* **28,** 441 (1951); **US 2503312** (to Vio-Bin Corp.).

Dark oil. d 0.95. n_D^{20} 1.4790. Sol in the common organic solvents. Miscible with other oils. Insol in water, but disperses readily when shaken with it to form emulsions.

USE: In the formulation of hydrophilic ointment bases for medicinal ointments and cosmetic creams: Bandelin, Tuschhoff, *J. Am. Pharm. Assoc. Pract. Pharm. Ed.* **14,** 106, 120 (1953); *Schimmel-Briefs,* no. 235 (Oct. 1954).

3529. EGTA. [67-42-5] 3,12-Bis(carboxymethyl)-6,9-dioxa-3,12-diazatetradecanedioic acid; [ethylenebis(oxyethylenenitrilo)]tetraacetic acid; ethylene glycol bis(β-aminoethylether)-*N*,-*N*,*N*′,*N*′-tetraacetic acid. $C_{14}H_{24}N_2O_{10}$; mol wt 380.35. C 44.21%, H 6.36%, N 7.37%, O 42.06%. Chelating agent. Prepn: H. Schläpfer, J. Bindler, **US 2709178** (1955 to Geigy). Toxicology: J. E. Wynn *et al., Toxicol. Appl. Pharmacol.* **16,** 807 (1970). Thermal properties: M. F. G. Esteban *et al., Thermochim. Acta* **62,** 267 (1983). Cathodic-stripping determn: M. Ciszkowska, Z. Stojek, *Talanta* **33,** 817 (1986). Use in calcium measurements: J. D. Johnson *et al., Am. J. Physiol.* **272,** C1437 (1997); in heavy metal remobilization from river sediment: K.-C. Yu *et al., Toxicol. Environ. Chem.* **58,** 85 (1997). Review of regulation of Ca^{+2} concentration in biological systems: S. Robertson, J. D. Potter, *Methods Pharmacol.* **5,** 63-75 (1984).

Disodium salt. [26082-78-0] $C_{14}H_{22}N_2Na_2O_{10}$; mol wt 424.31. LD$_{50}$ orally in rats: 3.96±0.50 g/kg (Wynn).

USE: Chelator for heavy metals. Reagent for maintaining calcium concentrations.

3530. Eicosamethylnonasiloxane. [2652-13-3] $C_{20}H_{60}O_8$-Si$_9$; mol wt 681.46. C 35.25%, H 8.87%, O 18.78%, Si 37.09%. Prepd by the reaction of hexamethyldisiloxane with octamethylcyclotetrasiloxane and sulfuric acid; by varying the proportions of these reactants, other methylpolysiloxanes of a desired average molecular weight may be prepd: Patnode, Wilcock, *J. Am. Chem. Soc.* **68,** 362 (1946).

Liquid. bp$_{4.9}$ 173°. d 0.918. n_D^{20} 1.3980. Stable. Inert to most chemical reagents and rubber. Maintains about the same viscosity over a wide temp range. Sol in benzene and the lighter hydrocarbons; slightly sol in alc and the heavy hydrocarbons.

USE: As a basis for silicone oils or fluids designed to withstand extremes of temp; as a foam suppressant in petr lubricating oil.

3531. Eicosapentaenoic Acid. [10417-94-4] (5Z,8Z,11Z,-14Z,17Z)-5,8,11,14,17-Eicosapentaenoic acid; (*all-Z*)-5,8,11,14,-17-eicosapentaenoic acid; *all-cis*-fatty acid 20:5 omega-3; EPA; icosapent. $C_{20}H_{30}O_2$; mol wt 302.45. C 79.42%, H 10.00%, O 10.58%. Important polyunsaturated fatty acid of the marine food chain that serves as a precursor for the prostaglandin-3 and thromboxane-3 families. It differs from arachidonic acid, *q.v.* (the eicosatetraenoic acid that is a precursor for the prostaglandin and thromboxane-2 families) by the extra double bond between the third and fourth carbons from the "methyl end" of the molecule. Isoln from cod liver oil: E. Klenk, D. Eberhagen, *Z. Physiol. Chem.* **307,** 42 (1957). Enzymatic conversion to prostaglandin E$_3$: S. Bergström *et al., J. Biol. Chem.* **239,** PC 4006 (1964). Review on role of platelets in thrombosis: K. C. Srivastava *et al., Biochem. Exp. Biol.* **16,** 317 (1980). Effects on prostacyclin-like material in human umbilical vasculature: J. Dyerberg, K. A. Jorgensen, *Artery* **8,** 12 (1980). A possible relationship between diets rich in EPA in marine oils and low rates of ischemic heart disease has been proposed: H. O. Bang *et al., Am. J. Clin. Nutr.* **33,** 2657 (1980); J. Dyerberg, *Philos. Trans. R. Soc. London Ser. B* **294,** 373 (1981). Clinical evaluation of lipid lowering effect: Y. Nagakawa *et al., Atherosclerosis* **47,** 71 (1983); of use in rheumatoid arthritis: J. M. Kremer *et al., Ann. Intern. Med.* **106,** 497 (1987); of use in Raynaud's phenomenon: R. A. DiGiacomo *et al., Am. J. Med.* **86,** 158 (1989).

Colorless oil. n_D^{20} 1.49865.

Ethyl ester. [86227-47-6] Epadel. $C_{22}H_{34}O_2$; mol wt 330.50.

THERAP CAT: Antilipemic.

3532. Einsteinium. [7429-92-7] Es; at. no. 99; valence 3, 2. Man-made radioactive element. No stable nuclides; known isotopes (mass numbers): 243-256. Longest-lived known isotope: 252 (T$_{½}$ 472 days, α-emitter, rel. at. mass 252.0830). ^{253}Es (T$_{½}$ 20.47 days, α-emitter) originally discovered in debris from a thermonuclear test explosion in Nov. 1952. Reviews of discovery: A. Ghiorso *et al., Phys. Rev.* **99,** 1048-1049 (1955); A. Ghiorso, G. T. Seaborg, *Sci. Am.* **195** (6), 67-80 (1956). Prepn of isotopes: A. Chetham-Strode, Jr., L. W. Holm, *Phys. Rev.* **104,** 1314 (1956); B. G. Harvey *et al., ibid.* 1315; G. T. Seaborg, *J. Chem. Educ.* **36,** 38 (1959). *Reviews:* C. Keller, *The Chemistry of the Transuranium Elements* (Verlag Chemie, Weinheim, English Ed., 1971) pp 583-589, Silva, "Trans-Curium Elements" in *MTP Int. Rev. Sci.: Inorg. Chem., Ser. One* vol. 8, A. G. Maddock, Ed. (University Park Press, Baltimore, 1972) pp 71-105; *Comprehensive Inorganic Chemistry* vol. 5, J. C. Bailar, Jr. *et al.,* Eds. (Pergamon Press, Oxford, 1973) *passim; Handb. Exp. Pharmakol.* **36,** 689-928 (1973); E. K. Hulet in *The Chemistry of the Actinide Elements* vol. 2, J. J. Katz *et al.,* Eds. (Chapman and Hall, New York, 1986) pp 1071-1085; *The Elements Beyond Uranium,* G. T. Seaborg, W. D. Loveland, Eds. (John Wiley & Sons, Inc., New York, 1990) pp 28-38.

Metal; two crystalline forms: double hexagonal close-packed α-form exists below 860°; face-centered cubic β-form, d 8.84. mp 860 ±50°.

Caution: Radiation hazard; handling requires special equipment and shielding facilities (Katz *et al., loc. cit.* vol. 2, p. 1128).

3533. Elaidic Acid. [112-79-8] (*E*)-9-Octadecenoic acid. $C_{18}H_{34}O_2$; mol wt 282.46. C 76.54%, H 12.13%, O 11.33%. Stereoisomer of oleic acid, *q.v.* Prepd by the action of HNO$_2$ on oleic acid. ^{13}C-NMR: J. G. Batchelor *et al., J. Org. Chem.* **39,** 1698 (1974).

White leaflets. d^{79} 0.851. mp 44-45°; also stated as 51°. bp$_{100}$ 288°; bp$_{15}$ 234°. n_D^{100} 1.4308.

3534. Elaiomycin. [23315-05-1] 4-Methoxy-3-(1-octenyl-*ONN*-azoxy)-2-butanol; (2*S*,3*S*)-4-methoxy-3-(1'-*cis*-octenyl-*cis*-azoxy)-2-butanol; D-*threo*-4-methoxy-3-(1-octenylazoxy)-2-butanol. $C_{13}H_{26}N_2O_3$; mol wt 258.36. C 60.43%, H 10.14%, N 10.84%, O 18.58%. Antibiotic substance produced by *Streptomyces hepaticus:* Haskell *et al., Antibiot. Chemother.* **4**, 141 (1954); Ehrlich *et al., ibid.* 338; Anderson *et al., ibid.* **6**, 100 (1956). Inhibits the growth of *Mycobacterium tuberculosis* var. *hominis in vitro:* Karlson, *ibid.* **12**, 446 (1962). Reported to have carcinogenic activity: Schoental, *Nature* **221**, 765 (1969). Structure: Stevens *et al., J. Am. Chem. Soc.* **78**, 3229 (1956); **80**, 6088 (1958). Configuration: Stevens *et al., ibid.* **81**, 1435 (1959); McGahren, Kunstmann, *ibid.* **92**, 1587 (1970). Total synthesis: R. A. Moss, M. Matsuo, *ibid.* **99**, 1643 (1977). Biosynthesis: R. J. Parry *et al., ibid.* **104**, 339 (1982).

Pale yellow oil. Stable to air. $[\alpha]_D^{26}$ +38.4° (c = 2.8 in abs ethanol). n_D^{25} 1.4798. uv max: 237.5 nm ($E_{1cm}^{1\%}$ 428). Sparingly sol in water; sol in practically all of the common organic solvents. Stable in neutral or slightly acidic aq solns. Dec into a yellow product when dissolved in 0.1*N* NaOH.

Acetate. $C_{15}H_{28}N_2O_4$. Oily liquid, $bp_{0.5}$ 84-90°. $[\alpha]_D^{27}$ +25.3° (c = 3 in alc). uv max (alc): 237.5 nm (ε 11000).

3535. Elastase. Serine proteases produced by many differnt cell types, named for its ability to break down the connective tissue protein elastin. Active site is a catalytic triad of residues Ser-195, His-57, and Asp-102. Hydrolyzes proteins at *N*-terminal peptide bonds of small aliphatic residues. First isolated from pancreatic extracts: J. Balo, I. Banga, *Biochem. J.* **46**, 384 (1950). Amino acid sequence comparison of mammalian elastases: T. Tani *et al., J. Biol. Chem.* **263**, 1231 (1988). Review and comparison of porcine pancreatic and human neutrophil elastase: W. Bode *et al., Biochemistry* **28**, 1951-1963 (1989). Review of role in atherosclerosis: L. Robert *et al., Atherosclerosis* **140**, 281-295 (1998); of role in pulmonary hypertension: M. Rabinovitch, *Chest* **114**, Suppl., 213S-224S (1998).

Pancreatic elastase. Elaszym. Stored as an inactive zymogen in the pancreas; secreted into intestines where it is activated by trypsin and participates in digestion. Mol wt about 25,000. Porcine form is a single polypeptide chain of 240 amino acid residues and four disulfide bridges. Purification and characterization: U. J. Lewis *et al., J. Biol. Chem.* **222**, 705 (1956); M. A. Naughton, F. Sanger, *Biochem. J.* **78**, 156 (1961). Primary structure: D. M. Shotton, B. S. Hartley, *Nature* **225**, 802 (1970); *eidem, Biochem. J.* **131**, 643 (1973). Crystal structure: H. C. Watson *et al., Nature* **225**, 806 (1970); D. M. Shotton, H. C. Watson, *ibid.* 811; E. Meyer *et al., Acta Crystallogr.* **B44**, 26 (1988). Review of diagnostic uses: R. Dominici, C. Franzini, *Clin. Chem. Lab. Med.* **40**, 325-332 (2002). White, lyophilized powder of slightly yellowish shade. pI 9.5 ±0.5. Maximum protease activity pH 8.1-8.8.

Neutrophil elastase. Leukocyte elastase; polymorphonuclear elastase; granulocyte elastase. Degrades extracellular matrix proteins including elastin, collagen (types I-IV), fibronectin, laminin, and proteoglycans. Necessary for migration of neutrophils through connective tissue. Defends against infectious bacteria by degrading bacterial structural proteins. Human form is a glycoprotein single peptide chain of 218 amino acid residues and four disulfide bridges. Mol wt about 33,000. Identification of elastolytic activity in polymorphonuclear leukocytes: A. Janoff, J. Scherer, *J. Exp. Med.* **128**, 1137 (1968). Isoln and characterization: A. Janoff, *Lab. Invest.* **29**, 458 (1973); K. Ohlsson, I. Olsson, *Eur. J. Biochem.* **42**, 519 (1974); R. J. Baugh, J. Travis, *Biochemistry* **15**, 836 (1976). Primary structure: S. Sinha *et al., Proc. Natl. Acad. Sci. USA* **84**, 2228 (1987). Crystal structure: H. R. Williams *et al., J. Biol. Chem.* **262**, 17178 (1987). Review of role in emphysema: A. Janoff, *Am. Rev. Respir. Dis.* **132**, 417-433 (1985); of role in acute lung injury: K. Kawabata *et al., Eur. J. Pharmacol.* **451**, 1-10 (2002). Maximum protease activity pH 7.5-9. pI 10-11.

3536. Elastin. Elastic, load-bearing protein fibers of animal connective tissue, particularly the ligaments of the vertebrae and the walls of the large arteries. Elastin is an insoluble, highly cross-linked hydrophobic protein, rich in nonpolar amino acid residues, such as valine, leucine, isoleucine, and phenylalanine. On the average, about every third residue is glycine and about every ninth residue is a prolyl residue. Unlike collagen, *q.v.*, which is rich in hydroxyproline, elastin contains only modest amounts. At least two types of elastin are distinguishable: type I elastin isolated from *liga-mentum nuchae*, aorta or skin and type II elastin isolated from cartilage. The most ready source of high purity elastin is the *ligamentum nuchae* of the larger ruminants: Partridge *et al., Biochem. J.* **61**, 11 (1955). Amino acid composition studies: Petruska, Sandberg, *Biochem. Biophys. Res. Commun.* **33**, 222 (1968). Its elastic properties are brought about by a cross-linked structure. Identification of new cross-linking amino acids in elastin: Partridge *et al., Biochem. J.* **93**, 30C (1964); Franzblau *et al., Biochem. Biophys. Res. Commun.* **21**, 575 (1965); Starcher *et al., Biochemistry* **6**, 2425 (1967). Molecular model: Gray *et al., Nature* **246**, 461 (1973). *Review:* Partridge, *Adv. Protein Chem.* **17**, 227-302 (1962); C. Franzblau, "Elastin" in *Comprehensive Biochemistry* vol. **26c**, M. Florkin, E. H. Stotz, Eds. (Elsevier, New York, 1971) pp 659-712; Ross, Bornstein, *Sci. Am.* **224**, 44 (June, 1971). Book (in English): I. Banga, *Structure and Function of Elastin and Collagen* (Akademiai Kiado, Budapest, 1967). Series of articles on structure, biosynthesis, and immunology: *Methods Enzymol.* **82**, 559-765 (1982).

Purified elastin has a pale yellow color and a bluish fluorescence in uv light. Resists acid and alkaline hydrolysis. Practically insol in a wide range of hydrogen-bond-breaking solvents at temps up to 100° and swells, but does not dissolve, in phenolic solvents. It appears practically impossible to bring elastin into soln except by hydrolytic reagents capable of rupturing peptide bonds. Elastin is one of only a few polymeric substances which, in the presence of water, exist in a form with rubber-like extensibility and low modulus of elasticity. Enzymes which dissolve fibers of the insol protein elastin undamaged and free from contamination are called elastases.

3537. Elcatonin. [60731-46-6] 1-Butanoic acid 1,7-dicarbacalcitonin (eel); 1,4,7,10,13,16-hexaazacyclotricosane cyclic peptide deriv; [aminosuberic acid 1,7]-eel calcitonin; [ASU^{1,7}]-ECT; carbocalcitonin; HC-58; Calcinil; Elcitonin; Turbocalcin. $C_{148}H_{244}N_{42}O_{47}$; mol wt 3363.77. C 52.84%, H 7.31%, N 17.49%, O 22.36%. Synthetic analog of eel calcitonin in which the 1 and 7 cystine residues have been modified to deaminosuberic acid. Inhibits osteoclast bone resorption and induces uptake of calcium from body fluids. Prepn: S. Sakakibara *et al., DE 2616399; eidem, US 4086221* (1976, 1978 both to Toyo Jozo); T. Morikawa *et al., Experientia* **32**, 1104 (1976). Structural characterization: P. L. Mauri *et al. Rapid Commun. Mass Spectrom.* **11**, 1292 (1997). Immunoassay determn in plasma: M. Takeyama *et al. Biol. Pharm. Bull.* **18**, 900 (1995); HPLC determn in pharmaceutical prepn: K. Maekawa *et al. Iyakuhin Kenkyu* **32**, 465 (2001). Mechanistic study: M. Ikegame *et al., J. Bone Miner. Res.* **9**, 25 (1994). Clinical pharmacology: T. Ishioka, *Pharmatherapeutica* **1**, 625 (1977); in Paget's disease patients: A. Caniggia *et al., Minerva Med.* **74**, 993 (1983). Clinical trial in osteoporosis: Italian Osteoporosis Network, *Curr. Ther. Res.* **45**, 502 (1989); in combination with alfacalcidol, *q.v.*: T. Fujita *et al. J. Bone Miner. Metab.* **15**, 223 (1997).

THERAP CAT: Calcium regulator. Treatment of Paget's disease.

3538. Elcometrine. [7759-35-5] 17-(Acetyloxy)-16-methylene-19-norpregn-4-ene-3,20-dione; 16-methylene-17α-hydroxy-19-nor-4-pregnene-3,20-dione 17-acetate; 16-methylene-17α-acetoxy-19-norpregn-4-ene-3,20-dione; ST-1435; Nestorone. $C_{23}H_{30}$-

O$_4$; mol wt 370.48. C 74.56%, H 8.16%, O 17.27%. Synthetic, non-orally active progestin. Prepn: V. Schwarz *et al., Tetrahedron Lett.* **1967**, 1925; *eidem, Collect. Czech. Chem. Commun.* **33**, 4337 (1968). Pharmacology: N. Kumar *et al., Steroids* **65**, 629 (2000). Clinical pharmacokinetics: G. Noé *et al., Contraception* **48**, 548 (1993). Metabolism: O. Heikinheimo *et al., ibid.* **50**, 275 (1994). Clinical trial of subdermal implant: S. Diaz *et al., ibid.* **51**, 33 (1995). Clinical trial of vaginal rings delivery system: I. Sivin *et al., ibid.* **69**, 137 (2004); *idem et al., ibid.* **71**, 122 (2005).

Crystals from methanol, mp 178-179°. $[\alpha]_D^{21}$ −105° (c = 1.2 in chloroform). uv max (methanol): 240 nm (log ε 4.21).

THERAP CAT: Progestogen; contraceptive (implantable).

3539. Eledoisin. [69-25-0] C$_{54}$H$_{85}$N$_{13}$O$_{15}$S; mol wt 1188.40. C 54.58%, H 7.21%, N 15.32%, O 20.19%, S 2.70%. A hendecapeptide from the posterior salivary glands of eledone spp (small octopus spp): Anastasi, Erspamer, *Br. J. Pharmacol.* **19**, 326 (1962); *eidem, Experientia* **18**, 58 (1962). Synthesis: Sandrin, Boissonnas, *ibid.* 59; *eidem, Helv. Chim. Acta* **47**, 1294 (1964); Lubke *et al., Ann.* **679**, 195 (1964); **GB 984810** (1965 to Farmitalia); solid-phase synthesis: P. G. Pietta *et al., J. Org. Chem.* **39**, 44 (1974). Its physiologic action resembles that of the other tachykinins, substance P and physalaemin, *q.q.v.* Stimulates extravascular smooth muscle, acts as a potent vasodilator and hypotensive agent; in certain species causes salivation, and increases capillary permeability. Pharmacology: Erspamer, Erspamer, *Br. J. Pharmacol.* **19**, 337 (1962); Sicuteri *et al., Experientia* **19**, 44 (1963); G. Bertaccini, *Pharmacol. Rev.* **28**, 127 (1976). *Review:* Erdös, *Adv. Pharmacol.* **4**, 64-72 (1966).

5-oxoPro–Pro–Ser–Lys–Asp–Ala–Phe–Ile–Gly–Leu–MetNH$_2$

Sesquihydrate. Powder, dec 230°. $[\alpha]_D^{22}$ −44° (c = 1 in 95% acetic acid). Slowly loses activity when incubated in blood.

Trifluoroacetate. [10129-92-7] Eloisin. C$_{54}$H$_{85}$N$_{13}$O$_{15}$S.C$_2$-HF$_3$O$_2$; mol wt 1302.42.

THERAP CAT: Hypotensive; stimulator of lacrimal secretion.

3540. Element 112. [54084-26-3] Ununbium. Uub; at. no. 112. Group IIb (12). Transuranium element. No stable nuclides. Prepn and decay of isotope ^{277}112 (T$_{1/2}$ ~240 μsec, α decay) by ^{208}Pb(^{70}Zn,n): S. Hoffmann *et al., Z. Phys. A* **354**, 229 (1996); of isotope ^{283}112 (T$_{1/2}$ ~81 sec, decay by SF) by ^{238}U(^{48}Ca,3n): Y. T. Oganessian *et al., Eur. Phys. J. A* **5**, 63 (1999). Observation of ^{281}112 as decay product of isotope ^{285}114 (T$_{1/2}$ ~890$_{-450}^{+1300}$ μsec, α decay): V. Ninov *et al., Phys. Rev. Lett.* **83**, 1104 (1999). Synthesis and decay chains: S. Hofmann *et al, Eur. Phys. J. A* **14**, 147 (2002); Y. T. Oganessian *et al., ibid.* **19**, 3 (2004). Review of production and properties: S. Hofmann, *Rep. Prog. Phys.* **61**, 639-689 (1998).

3541. Element 114. [54085-16-4] Ununquadium. Uuq; at. no. 114. Group IVa (14). Transuranium element. No stable nuclides. Prepn and decay of isotope ^{287}114 (T$_{1/2}$ 1.32 sec, α decay) by ^{242}Pu(^{48}Ca,3n): Y. T. Oganessian *et al., Nature* **400**, 242 (1999); of isotope ^{289}114 (T$_{1/2}$ 30.4 sec, α decay) by ^{244}Pu(^{48}Ca,3n): *eidem, Phys. Rev. Lett.* **83**, 3154 (1999). Observation of isotope ^{285}114 (T$_{1/2}$ 580 $_{-280}^{+870}$ μsec, α decay) as decay product of ^{293}118: V. Ninov *et al., ibid.* 1104. Review of production and properties: G. Münzenberg, *Proc. 7th Int. Conf. Clustering Aspects, Nucl. Struct. Dyn.* **2000**, 377-385. Historical review: Y. T. Oganessian *et al., Sci. Am.* **282**, 63-67 (2000).

3542. Element 116. [54100-71-9] Ununhexium. Uuh; at. no. 116. Group VIa (16). Transuranium element. No stable nuclides. Production of isotope ^{289}116 (T$_{1/2}$ 600 $_{-300}^{+860}$ μsec, α decay) as decay product of isotope ^{293}118: V. Ninov *et al., Phys. Rev. Lett.* **83**, 1104 (1999).

3543. Elenolide. [24582-91-0] (4S)-4-[(1E)-1-Formyl-1-propenyl]-3,4-dihydro-2-oxo-2H-pyran-5-carboxylic acid methyl ester. C$_{11}$H$_{12}$O$_5$; mol wt 224.21. C 58.93%, H 5.39%, O 35.68%. Hypotensive lactone from fruits, bark and leaves of the olive tree, *Olea europaea* L., *Oleaceae:* Veer *et al., Rec. Trav. Chim.* **76**, 839 (1957); **GB 789427** (1958 to Organon); **US 3033877** (1962 to Organon). Structure: Panizzi *et al., Gazz. Chim. Ital.* **90**, 1464 (1960); Beyerman *et al., Bull. Soc. Chim. Fr.* **1961**, 1812. Synthesis from secologanin: L. F. Tietze, H. C. Uzar, *Angew. Chem. Int. Ed.* **18**, 539 (1979).

Needles from hot alc, mp 155.5°. $[\alpha]_D^{20}$ +369° (chloroform). uv max (ethanol): 225, 317 nm (log ε 4.29, 1.75).

3544. Eletriptan. [143322-58-1] 3-[[(2R)-1-Methyl-2-pyrrolidinyl]methyl]-5-[2-(phenylsulfonyl)ethyl]-1H-indole; 5-[2-(benzenesulfonyl)ethyl]-3-(1-methylpyrrolidin-2(R)-ylmethyl)-1H-indole; UK-116044. C$_{22}$H$_{26}$N$_2$O$_2$S; mol wt 382.52. C 69.08%, H 6.85%, N 7.32%, O 8.37%, S 8.38%. Serotonin 5-HT$_{1B/1D}$ receptor agonist. Prepn: J. E. Macor, M. J. Wythes, **WO 9206973**; *eidem,* **US 5545644** (1992, 1996 both to Pfizer). Pharmacology: E. Willems *et al., Arch. Pharmacol.* **358**, 212 (1998). Affinity and specificity of receptor binding: C. Napier *et al., Eur. J. Pharmacol.* **368**, 259 (1999). Clinical trial in comparison with sumatriptan, *q.v.*: P. J. Goadsby *et al., Neurology* **54**, 156 (2000). Review of pharmacokinetics, and clinical efficacy: A. Bardsley-Elliot, S. Noble, *CNS Drugs* **12**, 325-333 (1999).

Hydrobromide. [177834-92-3] Relpax. C$_{22}$H$_{26}$N$_2$O$_2$S.HBr; mol wt 463.43. White to light pale colored powder. Readily sol in water.

THERAP CAT: Antimigraine.

3545. Eleutherobin. [174545-76-7] [(4R,4aS,5Z,7R,10S,-11S,12aR)-3,4,4a,7,10,11,12,12a-Octahydro-7-methoxy-1,10-dimethyl-4-(1-methylethyl)-11-[[(2E)-3-(1-methyl-1H-imidazol-4-yl)-1-oxo-2-propenyl]oxy]-7,10-epoxybenzocyclodecen-6-yl]methyl-β-D-arabinopyranoside 2-acetate. C$_{35}$H$_{48}$N$_2$O$_{10}$; mol wt 656.76. C 64.01%, H 7.37%, N 4.27%, O 24.36%. Cytotoxic glycosylated diterpene isolated from the marine soft coral, *Eleutherobia* sp. Enhances tubulin polymerization and stablization of microtubules similar to paclitaxel, *q.v.* Isoln and structure determn: W. H. Fenical *et al.,* **US 5473057** (1995 to Univ. Calif.). Induction of tubulin polymerization and mode of action: B. H. Long *et al., Cancer Res.* **58**, 1111 (1998). Total synthesis: K. C. Nicolaou *et al., J. Am. Chem. Soc.* **120**, 8674 (1998); X. T. Chen *et al., ibid.* **121**, 6563 (1999). Solid-state and solution conformations: B. Cinel *et al., Tetrahedron Lett.* **41**, 2811 (2000). Structure-activity: I. Ojima *et al., Proc. Natl. Acad. Sci. USA* **96**, 4256 (1999). Brief review: T. Lindel, *Angew. Chem. Int. Ed.* **37**, 774-776 (1998).

White non-crystalline solid. $[\alpha]_D^{25}$ −49.3°. (c = 3 in methanol). uv max (methanol): 290 nm (log ε 3.824).

USE: Biological reagent for tubulin and microtubulin studies.

3546. Elgodipine. [119413-55-7] 4-(1,3-Benzodioxol-4-yl)-1,4-dihydro-2,6-dimethyl-3,5-pyridinedicarboxylic acid 2-[[(4-fluorophenyl)methyl]methylamino]ethyl 1-methylethyl ester; 2-[(p-fluorobenzyl)methylamino]ethyl (±)- 1,4-dihydro-2,6-dimethyl-4-[2,3-(methylenedioxy)phenyl]-3,5-pyridinedicarboxylate. $C_{29}H_{33}FN_2O_6$; mol wt 524.58. C 66.40%, H 6.34%, F 3.62%, N 5.34%, O 18.30%. Dihydropyridine calcium channel blocker. Prepn: C. F. Torija, J. A. Galiano Ramos, **EP 302980**; *eidem*, **US 4952592** (1989, 1990 both to Inst. Invest. Desarr. Quimicobiol.). *In vitro* and *in vivo* cardiovascular effects: J. Tamargo *et al., Arzneim.-Forsch.* **41,** 895 (1991). Hemodynamic profile: C. Drieu la Rochelle *et al., Br. J. Pharmacol.* **111,** 49 (1994). Clinical evaluation in coronary artery disease: H. Suryapranata *et al., Am. J. Cardiol.* **69,** 1171 (1992). Clinical evaluation in chronic stable angina: D. U. Acharya *et al., Eur. Heart J.* **15,** 665 (1994).

Hydrochloride. [121489-04-1] IQB-875. $C_{29}H_{33}FN_2O_6 \cdot$ HCl; mol wt 561.04. Crystals from acetone, mp 194-195°. LD_{50} i.p. in mice: 30-40 mg/kg (Torija, Galiano Ramos).

THERAP CAT: Antianginal.

3547. Ellagic Acid. [476-66-4] 2,3,7,8-Tetrahydroxy[1]-benzopyrano[5,4,3-cde][1]benzopyran-5,10-dione; 4,4′,5,5′,6,6′-hexahydroxydiphenic acid 2,6,2′,6′-dilactone; benzoaric acid; Lagistase. $C_{14}H_6O_8$; mol wt 302.19. C 55.64%, H 2.00%, O 42.36%. Occurs free or combined in galls. Isoln from the kino of *Eucalyptus maculata* Hook and *E. hemipholia* F. Muell., *Myrtaceae*: Gell *et al., Aust. J. Chem.* **11,** 372 (1958); Hills, Carle, *ibid.* **16,** 147 (1963). Prepd by sodium persulfate oxidation of gallic acid or by acid hydrolysis of crude tannin from walnuts: Perkin, Nierenstein, *J. Chem. Soc.* **87,** 1412 (1905); Jurd, *J. Am. Chem. Soc.* **78,** 3445 (1956); **79,** 6043 (1957). Purification: **FR 1478523** (1967 to Prod. Chim. Celluloses Rey), *C.A.* **68,** 78267r (1968). Physicochemical properties: Press, Hardcastle, *J. Appl. Chem.* **19,** 247 (1969). Pharmacology: Bhargava *et al., J. Pharm. Sci.* **57,** 1728 (1968). Ellagic acid is a potent antagonist of the mutagenicity of bay-region diol epoxides of several aromatic hydrocarbons. Inhibition of the mutagenicity of the ultimate carcinogenic metabolite of benzo[a]-pyrene: A. W. Wood *et al., Proc. Natl. Acad. Sci. USA* **79,** 5513 (1982). Study of the reaction between this metabolite and ellagic acid: J. M. Sayer *et al., J. Am. Chem. Soc.* **104,** 5562 (1982). Brief discussion of ellagic acid as a prototype of a new class of cancer-preventing drugs: J. Fox, *Chem. Eng. News* **60,** 26 (Oct. 25, 1982).

Cream colored needles from pyridine, mp >360°. uv max (ethanol): 366, 255 nm (log ε 3.93, 4.60). Slightly sol in water or alcohol; sol in alkalies, in pyridine. Practically insol in ether.

Tetraacetate. $C_{22}H_{14}O_{12}$. Needles from acetic anhydride, mp 340°.

THERAP CAT: Hemostatic.

3548. Ellipticine. [519-23-3] 5,11-Dimethyl-6H-pyrido[4,-3-b]carbazole. $C_{17}H_{14}N_2$; mol wt 246.31. C 82.90%, H 5.73%, N 11.37%. Antitumor alkaloid isolated from *Ochrosia elliptica* Labill., *O. sandwicensis* A. DC., *O. viellardii, O. silvatica, Apocynaceae*: Goodwin *et al., J. Am. Chem. Soc.* **81,** 1903 (1959); Kan Fan *et al., Phytochemistry* **9,** 1351 (1970); Cosson, Schmid, *ibid.* 1353. Structure and synthesis: Woodward *et al., J. Am. Chem. Soc.* **81,** 4434 (1959). Syntheses: J. Bergman, R. Carlsson, *Tetrahedron Lett.* **1977,** 4663; D. A. Taylor *et al., J. Chem. Res. Miniprint* **1979,** 4801; S. Kano *et al., J. Org. Chem.* **46,** 2979 (1981); R. Besselievre, H. P. Husson, *Tetrahedron* **37,** 241 (1981). Regioselective synthesis: T.-L. Ho, S.-Y. Hsieh, *Helv. Chim. Acta* **89,** 111 (2006). Toxicity study: Rakieten *et al., U.S. Gov. Res. Dev. Rep.* **67,** 38 (1967), *C.A.* **68,** 20827g (1968). Review of syntheses: M. Sainsbury, *Synthesis* **1977,** 437-448; R. Barone, M. Chanon, *Heterocycles* **16,** 1357-1365 (1981). Review of antineoplastic activity: K. W. Kohn *et al., Antibiotics* **vol. 5** (pt. 2), F. E. Hahn, Ed. (Springer-Verlag, New York, 1979) pp 195-213.

Bright yellow needles from ethyl acetate, mp 311-315° (dec). uv max: 239, 277, 286, 294, 332, 382, 400 nm (log ε 4.23, 4.61, 4.76, 4.74, 3.65, 3.61, 3.53). LD_{50} in mice (mg/kg): 19.5-22.4 i.v.; 178-204 orally (Rakieten).

3549. Elliptinium Acetate. [58337-35-2] 9-Hydroxy-2,5,11-trimethyl-6H-pyrido[4,3-b]carbazolium acetate (salt); 9-hydroxy-2-methylellipticinium acetate; HME; NSC-264137; Celiptium. $C_{20}H_{20}N_2O_3$; mol wt 336.38. C 71.41%, H 5.99%, N 8.33%, O 14.27%. Deriv of ellipticine, *q.v.*, with anticancer activity. Prepn: J. LePecq *et al.*, **DE 2618223**; J. B. LePecq, C. Paoletti, **US 4310667** (1976, 1982 both to Agence Nat. Valorisation Recher.). Activity vs L 1210 mouse leukemia: *eidem, C.R. Seances Acad. Sci. Ser. D* **281,** 1365 (1975). HPLC determn: G. Muzard, J. B. LePecq, *J. Chromatogr.* **169,** 446 (1979). Metabolism, disposition: N. Van-Bac *et al., Cancer Treat. Rep.* **64,** 879 (1980). Antitumor activity, pharmacology, toxicity study: C. Paoletti *et al., Recent Results Cancer Res.* **74,** 107 (1980). Use in treatment of breast cancers: J. Rouesse *et al., Bull. Cancer* **68,** 437 (1981). Cytochemical and autoradiographic study: N. Sales, E. Puvion, *Eur. J. Cancer Clin. Oncol.* **18,** 291 (1982).

THERAP CAT: Antineoplastic.

3550. Elliptone. [478-10-4] 12,12a-Dihydro-8,9-dimeth-oxy[1]benzopyrano[3,4-*b*]furo[2,3-*h*][1]benzopyran-6(6a*H*)-one; derride. $C_{20}H_{16}O_6$; mol wt 352.34. C 68.18%, H 4.58%, O 27.25%. Found in derris resins of low rotenone content. Isoln of naturally occurring (−)-form from *Derris elliptica* (Wall.) Benth., *Leguminosae:* Buckley, *J. Soc. Chem. Ind.* **55**, 285T (1936); Harper, *Chem. Ind. (London)* **57**, 1059 (1938); **58**, 292 (1939); *J. Chem. Soc.* **1939**, 1099; *see also* Meyer, Koolhaas, *Rec. Trav. Chim.* **58**, 207 (1939). Structure: Harper, *J. Chem. Soc.* **1939**, 1424; **1942**, 593. Comparison with similar substances: Seiferle, Frear, *Ind. Eng. Chem.* **40**, 683 (1948). Total synthesis of (±)-form: Fukami *et al., Agric. Biol. Chem.* **29**, 82 (1965), *C.A.* **62**, 13115e (1963). Synthesis of (−)-form from rotenone, *q.v.:* P. B. Anzeveno, *J. Heterocycl. Chem.* **16**, 1643 (1979).

Needles from ethanol, mp 160° (Harper), also reported as mp 177-178° (Anzeveno). $[\alpha]_D^{20}$ −18° (benzene); $[\alpha]_D^{20}$ +55° (acetone).

3551. Ellman's Reagent. [69-78-3] 3,3′-Dithiobis[6-nitro-benzoic acid]; 5,5′-dithiobis[2-nitrobenzoic acid]; DTNB. $C_{14}H_8$-$N_2O_8S_2$; mol wt 396.35. C 42.42%, H 2.03%, N 7.07%, O 32.29%, S 16.18%. Reacts with thiols to produce the yellow dianion of 5-thio-2-nitrobenzoic acid (TNB). Prepn: G. L. Ellman, *Arch. Biochem. Biophys.* **82**, 70 (1959); and spectral properties: P. W. Riddles *et al., Anal. Biochem.* **94**, 75 (1979). Structure determn: E. Shefter, T. I. Kalman, *J. Chem. Soc. Chem. Commun.* **1969**, 1027. Reaction stoichiometry with protein disulfide groups: R. J. Ackerman, J. F. Robyt, *Anal. Biochem.* **50**, 656 (1972). Use in HPLC determn of alkylthiols: K. Kuwata *et al., Anal. Chem.* **54**, 1082 (1982). Molar absorption coefficients for TNB: P. Eyer *et al., Anal. Biochem.* **312**, 224 (2003).

Yellow crystals from DMF or glacial acetic acid, mp 237-238° (dec) (Ellman); also reported as pale yellow needles from ethanol, mp 239.7-240.3° (dec) (Riddles). d 1.67. Sol in water (pH 8). Absorption max (pH 7.27, 25°): 324 nm (ε 17780).

Ellman's anion. [77874-90-9] 5-Mercapto-2-nitrobenzoic acid ion (2−); 5-thio-2-nitrobenzoate anion; TNB^{2-}. $C_7H_3NO_4S$; mol wt 197.17. Absorption max (0.1 M phosphate buffer, pH 7.4): 412 nm (ε 14.15×10^3 at 25°, 13.8×10^3 at 37°).

USE: Chromogenic reagent for determn of thiols, covalent modification of protein thiols, kinetic assays of cholinesterase and other enzyme activities.

3552. Eltoprazine. [98224-03-4] 1-(2,3-Dihydro-1,4-benzodioxin-5-yl)piperazine; 1-(1,4-benzodioxan-5-yl)piperazine. $C_{12}H_{16}N_2O_2$; mol wt 220.27. C 65.43%, H 7.32%, N 12.72%, O 14.53%. Selective serotonin $5HT_1$ agonist; psychotropic agent with antiaggressive activity. Prepn: J. Hartog *et al., EP 138280; idem et al., EP 189612* (1985, 1986 both to Duphar). Prepd (not claimed): *idem et al., US 4833142* (1989 to Duphar). Crystal structure: M. L. Verdonk *et al., Acta Crystallogr.* **C48**, 2271 (1992). Series of articles on pharmacology, receptor binding and mechanism of action: *Drug Metab. Drug Interact.* **8**, 1-186 (1990). Pharmacokinetics: M. H. de Vries *et al., Eur. J. Clin. Pharmacol.* **41**, 485 (1991). Clinical evaluation in self-injury: W. M. A. Verhoeven *et al., Lancet* **340**, 1037 (1992); in violent psychiatric patients: J. Tiihonen *et al., ibid.* **341**, 307 (1993).

Hydrochloride. [98206-09-8] DU-28853. $C_{12}H_{16}N_2O_2 \cdot HCl$; mol wt 256.73. Crystals from ethanol, mp 256-258°. Soly in water: 19 g/100 ml.

THERAP CAT: Serenic.

3553. Elymoclavine. [548-43-6] 8,9-Didehydro-6-methyl-ergoline-8-methanol. $C_{16}H_{18}N_2O$; mol wt 254.33. C 75.56%, H 7.13%, N 11.01%, O 6.29%. An ergot alkaloid obtained from cultures of fungi parasitic on *Elymus mollis* Trin.: Abe *et al., US 2835675* (1958). Found in fungi parasitic on *Pennisetum typhoideum* Rich.: Stoll *et al., Helv. Chim. Acta* **37**, 1815 (1954). Structure and stereochemistry: Schreier, *Helv. Chim. Acta* **41**, 1984 (1958). Biosyntheses utilizing *Claviceps* cultures: Naidoo *et al., Chem. Commun.* **1970**, 472; Ogunlana *et al., ibid.* 775; Seiler *et al., ibid.* 1394; Cavender, Anderson, *Biochim. Biophys. Acta* **208**, 345 (1970).

Monoclinic prisms from methanol, 248-252° (dec). $[\alpha]_D^{20}$ −59° (c = 0.1 in ethanol) (Abe); $[\alpha]_D^{20}$ −152° (c = 0.9 in pyridine) (Stoll). uv max: 227, 283, 293 nm (log ε 4.31, 3.84, 3.76). Fairly sol in water with alkaline reaction. Sol in pyridine; very slightly sol in organic solvents.

3554. Emamectin. [137335-79-6]; [121124-29-6] (major component); [121424-52-0] (minor component). (4″*R*)-5-*O*-de-methyl-4″-deoxy-4″-(methylamino)avermectin A_{1a} and (4″*R*)-5-*O*-demethyl-25-de(1-methylpropyl)-4″-deoxy-4″-(methylamino)-25-(1-methylethyl)avermectin A_{1a} (9:1). Mixture of semi-synthetic avermectins, *q.v.,* consisting (9:1) of *4″-epi-(methylamino)-4″-deoxyavermectin B_{1a}*, ($C_{49}H_{75}NO_{13}$) and *4″-epi-(methylamino)-4″-deoxyavermectin B_{1b}*, ($C_{48}H_{73}NO_{13}$). Prepn: H. Mrozik, *US 4874749* (1989 to Merck & Co.); and insecticidal activity: H. Mrozik *et al., Experientia* **45**, 315 (1989). Synthesis: R. J. Cvetovich *et al., J. Org. Chem.* **59**, 7704 (1994). Avian toxicity studies: A. C. Chukwudebe *et al., Environ. Toxicol. Chem.* **17**, 1118 (1998). *Review:* M. H. Fisher, *ACS Symp. Ser.* **524**, 169-182 (1993); H. Mrozik, *ibid.* **551**, 54-73 (1994).

Component B_{1a} R = CH_2CH_3
Component B_{1b} R = CH_3

LC$_{50}$ (48 hr) in *Daphnia magna*: 2.9 μg/l; LC$_{50}$ in rainbow trout, bluegill sunfish (mg/l) at 24 hrs: >1.0, 0.75; at 48 hrs: >1.0, 0.45; at 96 hrs: 0.67, 0.24 (Mrozik, **US 4874749**).

Benzoate. [137512-74-8] 4″-Deoxy-4″-*epi*-N-methylamino-avermectin B$_1$ benzoate; MK-244; Affirm; Proclaim; Slice. Exists as the anhydrous and various hydrated forms having different crystal morphologies. Amt of water is nonstoichiometric. 1.1% form is an off white crystalline powder, mp 141-146°. [α]$_D$ −6.9° (c = 0.5% in methanol). uv max (10% methanol in water by volume): 244 nm (A$_1^{1\%}$ = 327 corr). log P (*n*-octanol/aq phosphate): 3.0 (pH 5.1); 5.0 (pH 7.0). pKa 4.2; 7.6. Soly 0.32 mg/ml at pH 5 (aq); 0.024 mg/ml at pH 7 (aq). Freely sol in chloroform and methanol. Insol in hexane. LD$_{50}$ in mallard ducks, northern bobwhite quail (mg/kg): 76, 264 orally (Chukwudebe).

USE: Insecticide.

3555. Embelin. [550-24-3] 2,5-Dihydroxy-3-undecyl-2,5-cyclohexadiene-1,4-dione; 2,5-dihydroxy-3-undecyl-*p*-benzoquinone; "Embelic acid". C$_{17}$H$_{26}$O$_4$; mol wt 294.39. C 69.36%, H 8.90%, O 21.74%. From fruit of *Embelia ribes* Burm., *Myrsinaceae*. Isoln: Heffter, Feuerstein, *Arch. Pharm.* **238**, 15 (1900). Structure and synthesis: Fieser, Chamberlin, *J. Am. Chem. Soc.* **70**, 71 (1948).

Glistening orange plates from alcohol, benzene or acetic acid, mp 142-143°. Soluble in the usual hot organic solvents or in alkali hydroxide solns; very slightly sol in petr ether. Practically insol in water.

Diammonium salt. Ammonium embelate. C$_{17}$H$_{34}$N$_2$O$_4$. Grayish-violet powder. Sol in water, dil alcohol.

Caution: Handle with care; irritates mucous membranes and may cause prolonged and violent sneezing!

Disemicarbazone. C$_{19}$H$_{32}$N$_6$O$_4$. Pale-brown needles from dil alcohol, dec 236°.

Dioxime. C$_{17}$H$_{28}$N$_2$O$_4$. Pale-yellow needles from acetic acid, mp 278°.

THERAP CAT: Ammonium embelate as an anthelmintic (Cestodes).

3556. Embramine. [3565-72-8] 2-[1-(4-Bromophenyl)-1-phenylethoxy]-*N,N*-dimethylethanamine; 2-[(*p*-bromo-α-methyl-α-phenylbenzyl)oxy]-*N,N*-dimethylethylamine; [2-(1-*p*-bromophenyl-1-phenylethoxy)ethyl]dimethylamine; 2-[1-(4-bromodiphenyl)eth-oxy]-*N,N*-dimethylethylamine; *p*-bromo-α-methylbenzhydryl 2-dimethylaminoethyl ether; 1-(*p*-bromophenyl)-1-phenyl-1-(2-dimethylaminoethoxy)ethane; β-dimethylaminoethyl *p*-bromo-α-methylbenzhydryl ether. C$_{18}$H$_{22}$BrNO; mol wt 348.28. C 62.07%, H 6.37%, Br 22.94%, N 4.02%, O 4.59%. Prepn: L. Novak, M. Protiva, *Collect. Czech. Chem. Commun.* **24**, 3966 (1959); M. Protiva, L. Novak, **DE 1240877** (1967 to SPOFA), *C.A.* **67**, 73338j (1967).

bp$_{0.3}$ 135-140°. bp$_1$ 163-170°.

Hydrochloride. [13977-28-1] Mebrophenhydramine; Bromadryl; Mebryl. C$_{18}$H$_{22}$BrNO.HCl; mol wt 384.74. Crystals from acetone + ether, mp 150-152°. LD$_{50}$ in mice (mg/kg): 80 i.v.; 330 orally (Protiva, Novak).

THERAP CAT: Antihistaminic.

3557. Emedastine. [87233-61-2] 1-(2-Ethoxyethyl)-2-(hexahydro-4-methyl-1*H*-1,4-diazepin-1-yl)-1*H*-benzimidazole; 1-

[2-(ethoxy)ethyl]-2-(4-methyl-1-homopiperazinyl)benzimidazole. C$_{17}$H$_{26}$N$_4$O; mol wt 302.41. C 67.52%, H 8.67%, N 18.53%, O 5.29%. Histamine H$_1$-receptor antagonist. Prepn: R. Iemura *et al.*, **EP 79545**; *eidem*, **US 4430343** (1983, 1984 both to Kanebo); *eidem, J. Med. Chem.* **29**, 1178 (1986). GC determn in plasma: T. Hamada *et al., Chem. Pharm. Bull.* **34**, 1168 (1986). Series of articles on pharmacology: *Arzneim.-Forsch.* **34**, 801-818 (1984). Toxicity data: T. Fukuda *et al., ibid.* 801.

Difumarate. [87233-62-3] KB-2413; LY-188695; Emadine. C$_{17}$H$_{26}$N$_4$O.2C$_4$H$_4$O$_4$; mol wt 534.56. Crystals from ethanol, mp 148-151°. LD$_{50}$ orally in guinea pigs: 744 mg/kg (Fukuda).

THERAP CAT: Antihistaminic.

3558. Emepronium Bromide. [3614-30-0] *N*-Ethyl-*N,N,α*-trimethyl-γ-phenylbenzenepropanaminium bromide; ethyldimethyl(1-methyl-3,3-diphenylpropyl)ammonium bromide; ethyl(3,3-diphenyl-1-methylpropyl)dimethylammonium bromide; (1-methyl-3,3-diphenylpropyl)dimethylethylammonium bromide; Cetiprin; Restenacht; Ripirin; Uro-Ripirin. C$_{20}$H$_{28}$BrN; mol wt 362.35. C 66.29%, H 7.79%, Br 22.05%, N 3.87%. Prepn: Carlsson, **SE 136606** (1952 to Aktiebolaget Recip.), *C.A.* **48**, 729a (1954).

Crystals, mp 204°.

THERAP CAT: Antispasmodic. In treatment of urinary incontinence.

3559. Emetine. [483-18-1] 6′,7′,10,11-Tetramethoxy-emetan; cephaeline methyl ether. C$_{29}$H$_{40}$N$_2$O$_4$; mol wt 480.64. C 72.47%, H 8.39%, N 5.83%, O 13.32%. Principal alkaloid of ipecac, the ground roots of *Uragoga ipecacuanha* (Brot.) Baill. *Rubiaceae*; occurs naturally as (−)-form. Extraction procedures: E. Merck, *BIOS Final Report* **No. 766** (1947); F. E. Hamerslag, *Technology and Chemistry of Alkaloids* (New York, 1950) chapter XI; Stoll, Jucker in *Ullmanns Encyklopädie der technischen Chemie* **3**, Aufl., Bd. III (München-Berlin, 1953) p 231; *Beilstein* 2nd suppl. **vol. 23**, 449. Structure: Robinson, *Nature* **162**, 524 (1948); Janot, *Bull. Soc. Chim. Fr.* **1949**, 185. Stereochemistry: Battersby, *Chem. Ind. (London)* **1958**, 1324; Battersby, Garrett, *J. Chem. Soc.* **1959**, 3512; Van Tamelen *et al., J. Am. Chem. Soc.* **81**, 6214 (1959). Total synthesis: Evstigneeva *et al., Proc. Acad. Sci. USSR* **75**, 539 (1950); Van Tamelen *et al., J. Am. Chem. Soc.* **91**, 7359 (1969); T. Kametani *et al., J. Chem. Soc. Perkin Trans. 1* **1979**, 1211. Alternate syntheses: Burgstahler, Bithos, *J. Am. Chem. Soc.* **82**, 5446 (1960); Openshaw, Whittaker, *J. Chem. Soc.* **1963**, 1461; S. Takano *et al., J. Org. Chem.* **43**, 4169 (1978); T. Fujii, S. Yoshifuji, *Tetrahedron* **36**, 1539 (1980). *See also* Clark *et al.*, **US 3102118** (1963 to Glaxo). Review of syntheses: M. Shamma, *The Isoquinoline Alkaloids* (Academic Press, New York, 1972) pp 426-457. Toxicity: Radomski *et al., J. Pharmacol. Exp. Ther.* **104**, 421 (1952); of dihydrochloride: Child *et al., J. Pharm. Pharmacol.* **16**, 65 (1964). *General review:* Grollman, Jarkovsky, in *Antibiotics* **Vol. 3**, J. W. Corcoran, F. E. Hahn, Eds. (Springer-Verlag, New York, 1975) pp 420-435. Comprehensive description: L. V. Feyns, L. T. Grady, *Anal. Profiles Drug Subs.* **10**, 289-335 (1981).

White, amorphous powder. mp 74°. Turns yellow on exposure to light and heat. $[\alpha]_D^{20}$ −50° (c = 2 in CHCl$_3$). Strong alkaline reaction. pK$_1$ 5.77; pK$_2$ 6.64. Freely sol in methanol, ethanol, acetone, ethyl acetate, ether, chloroform. Sparingly sol in water, petr ether. Moderately sol in dil ammonium hydroxide, but sparingly in solns of KOH and NaOH. Absorption spectrum: Bayard, *Chem. Zentralbl.* **1943,** **II,** 305. LD$_{50}$ i.p. in rats: 12.1 mg/kg (Radomski).

Dihydrochloride. [316-42-7] Emetine hydrochloride; Hemometina. C$_{29}$H$_{40}$N$_2$O$_4$.2HCl; mol wt 553.56. Contains water of crystallization varying from 3 to 8 H$_2$O. Clusters of needles after drying at 105°, mp 235-255° (dec). $[\alpha]_D$ +11° (c = 1) to $[\alpha]_D$ +21° (c = 8), calculated for the anhydrous salt. One gram of the hydrated salt dissolves in about 7 ml water. pH of aq soln (1 g in 50 ml) 5.6. Sol in alcohol. Solid and solutions turn yellow on exposure to light or heat. LD$_{50}$ (calculated as base) in mice (mg/kg): 32 s.c.; 30 orally (Child).

Emetamine. [483-19-2] 1′,2′,3′,4′-Tetrahydro-6′,7′,10,11-tetramethoxyemetan; tetradehydroemetine. C$_{29}$H$_{36}$N$_2$O$_4$. Occurs in small amounts in ipecac. Isoln: Pyman, *J. Chem. Soc.* **111,** 419 (1917). Structure: Battersby *et al., J. Chem. Soc.* **1959,** 1744. Synthesis: *eidem, J. Chem. Soc.* **1961,** 3899. Crystals from ether, mp 142-143°. uv max (ethanol): 236, 283 nm (log ε 4.85, 3.86).

THERAP CAT: Antiamebic.

THERAP CAT (VET): Hydrochloride has been used as an antiamebic and in lung worm infection.

3560. Emodepside. [155030-63-0] Cyclo[(αR)-α-hydroxy-4-(4-morpholinyl)benzenepropanoyl-*N*-methyl-L-leucyl-(2*R*)-2-hydroxypropanoyl-*N*-methyl-L-leucyl-(αR)-α-hydroxy-4-(4-morpholinyl)benzenepropanoyl-*N*-methyl-L-leucyl-(2*R*)-2-hydroxypropanoyl-*N*-methyl-L-leucyl]; Bay-44-4400; PF-1022-221. C$_{60}$H$_{90}$N$_6$O$_{14}$; mol wt 1119.39. C 64.38%, H 8.10%, N 7.51%, O 20.01%. Cyclic octadepsipeptide that binds to presynaptic latrophilin receptors in nematodes. Semisynthetic derivative of PF1022A, a fungal metabolite of *Mycelia sterilia.* Prepn: H. Nishiyama *et al.,* **WO 9319053**; *eidem,* **US 5514773** (1993, 1996 both to Fujisawa). *In vivo* anthelmintic activity: A Harder, G. von Samson-Himmelstjerna, *Parasitol. Res.* **87,** 924 (2001); H. Zahner *et al., Int. J. Parasitol.* **31,** 1515 (2001). Review of mechanism of action studies: A. Harder *et al., Parasitol. Res.* S1-S10 (2005).

White to yellowish powder. Soly in water: 8.1 mg/l (pH 4); 5.2 mg/l (pH 7), 6.1 mg/l (pH 10). Log P (octanol/water): 4.9 (pH 7).

Combination with praziquantel. Profender. Series of articles on therapeutic use in cats, reptiles and rodents: *Parasitol. Res.* **97,** S33-S69 (2005).

THERAP CAT (VET): Anthelmintic (Nematodes and Cestodes).

3561. Emodin. [518-82-1] 1,3,8-Trihydroxy-6-methyl-9,10-anthracenedione; 1,3,8-trihydroxy-6-methylanthraquinone; 4,5,7-trihydroxy-2-methylanthraquinone; frangula emodin; rheum emodin; archin; frangulic acid. C$_{15}$H$_{10}$O$_5$; mol wt 270.24. C 66.67%, H 3.73%, O 29.60%. Occurs mostly as the rhamnoside (*see* Frangulin) in rhubarb root, in alder buckthorn (*Rhamnus frangula* L.*),* in *Cascara sagrada (Rhamnus purshiana* DC.*, Rhamnaceae),* also in *Rumex* and in other *Polygonaceae.* Isoln from rhubarb root: Tutin, Clewer, *J. Chem. Soc.* **99,** 946 (1911); Carelli, Giuliano, *Farmaco Ed. Prat.* **12,** 184 (1957); from bark of alder buckthorn: Bridel, Charaux, *Bull. Soc. Chim. Biol.* **15,** 648 (1933). Identity with archin: Chaudhry *et al., J. Sci. Ind. Res.* **9B,** No. 6, 142 (1950), *C.A.* **44,** 9396h (1950). Synthesis from 3,5-dinitrophthalic anhydride and *m*-cresol: Elder, Widmer, *Helv. Chim. Acta* **6,** 966 (1923); from 2-methylanthraquinone: Ayyangar *et al., J. Sci. Ind. Res.* **20B,** 493 (1961), *C.A.* **57,** 8514b (1962).

Orange needles from alc or by sublimation at 12 mm. mp 256-257°. Absorption max (ethanol): 222, 252, 265, 289, 437 nm (log ε 4.55, 4.26, 4.27, 4.34, 4.10). Practically insol in water; sol in alc, aq alkali hydroxide solns (cherry-red color), Na$_2$CO$_3$ and NH$_3$ solns. Soly at 25° (g/100 ml of satd soln): ether 0.140; chloroform 0.071; carbon tetrachloride 0.010; carbon bisulfide 0.009; benzene 0.041.

3-Methyl ether. 1,8-Dihydroxy-3-methoxy-6-methylanthraquinone; rheochrysidin. C$_{16}$H$_{12}$O$_5$. Brick-red, monoclinic needles, mp 207°. Occurs naturally as *physcione* or *parietin.*

See also Aloe emodin.

Trimethyl ether. C$_{18}$H$_{16}$O$_5$. Pale yellow needles, mp 225°.

THERAP CAT: Cathartic.

3562. Emorfazone. [38957-41-4] 4-Ethoxy-2-methyl-5-(4-morpholinyl)-3(2*H*)-pyridazinone; M-73101; Nandron; Pentoyl. C$_{11}$H$_{17}$N$_3$O$_3$; mol wt 239.27. C 55.22%, H 7.16%, N 17.56%, O 20.06%. Prepn: K. Satoda *et al.,* **JP 72 24030** (1972 to Morishita), *C.A.* **77,** 164732f (1972); M. Takaya *et al., J. Med. Chem.* **22,** 53 (1979). Metabolism studies: T. Hayashi *et al., Chem. Pharm. Bull.* **26,** 3124 (1978); **27,** 317 (1979). General pharmacological study: M. Sato *et al., Nippon Yakurigaku Zasshi* **75,** 291 (1979), *C.A.* **91,** 117292 (1979). Mechanism of action studies: M. Sato, A. Yamaguchi, *Arzneim.-Forsch.* **32,** 379 (1982). Antigenicity study: M. Sato *et al., Oyo Yakuri* **18,** 65 (1979), *C.A.* **92,** 104391 (1980). Toxicity studies: *eidem, ibid.* **16,** 1011 (1978), *C.A.* **90,** 197741 (1979); C. Onodera *et al., J. Toxicol. Sci.* **4,** 229 (1979); K. Shimpo *et al., ibid.* 255.

Cryst from methanol/isopropyl ether, mp 89-91°. LD$_{50}$ i.p. in mice: 700 mg/kg (Takaya).

THERAP CAT: Anti-inflammatory; analgesic.

3563. EMPA. [1832-53-7] Methylphosphonic acid monoethyl ester; ethyl methylphosphonate. C$_3$H$_9$O$_3$P; mol wt 124.08. C 29.04%, H 7.31%, O 38.68%, P 24.96%. Degradation product of the chemical warfare agent, VX, *q.v.* Prepn as sodium salt: V. S. Abramov, M. N. Morozova, *J. Gen. Chem. USSR* **22,** 315 (1952). Capillary electrophoretic determn in soils: A.-E. F. Nassar *et al., Anal. Chem.* **71,** 1285 (1999). Determn in human urine samples after exposure to VX: M. Minami *et al., J. Toxicol. Sci.* **23,** Suppl. II 250 (1998).

USE: Marker for the detection of VX.

3564. EMPTA. [18005-40-8] Methylphosphonothioic acid *O*-ethyl ester. $C_3H_9O_2PS$; mol wt 140.14. C 25.71%, H 6.47%, O 22.83%, P 22.10%, S 22.88%. Degradation product and precursor of VX, inhibits cholinesterase. Prepn: M. I. Kabachnik *et al., Dokl. Akad. Nauk SSSR* **104**, 861 (1955), *C.A.* **50**, 11240a (1956); F. W. Hoffmann *et al., J. Am. Chem. Soc.* **81**, 148 (1959). Structure: H. Christol *et al., C.R. Seances Acad. Sci. Ser. C* **265**, 1511 (1967). NMR: M. Mikolajczyk *et al., J. Am. Chem. Soc.* **100**, 7003 (1978). Mass spec.: E. R. J. Wils, *Fresenius J. Anal. Chem.* **338**, 22 (1990). Ionspray-MS determn in water: R. Kostiainen *et al., J. Chromatogr.* **634**, 113 (1993).

Yellowish oil, $bp_{0.22mm}$ 63°. n_D^{25} 1.4912. d_4^{25} 1.1735.
USE: Precursor to chemical warfare agents.

3565. Emtricitabine. [143491-57-0] 4-Amino-5-fluoro-1-[(2*R*,5*S*)-2-(hydroxymethyl)-1,3-oxathiolan-5-yl]-2(1*H*)-pyrimidinone; (−)-*cis*-4-amino-5-fluoro-1-(2-hydroxymethyl-1,3-oxathiolan-5-yl)-(1*H*)-pyrimidin-2-one; (−)-(2*R*,5*S*)-5-fluoro-1-[2-(hydroxymethyl)-1,3-oxathiolan-5-yl]cytosine; (−)-β-2′,3′-dideoxy-5-fluoro-3′-thiacytidine; (−)-FTC; 524W91; BW-524W91; Coviracil; Emtriva. $C_8H_{10}FN_3O_3S$; mol wt 247.25. C 38.86%, H 4.08%, F 7.68%, N 16.99%, O 19.41%, S 12.97%. Reverse transcriptase inhibitor; nucleoside analog structurally related to lamivudine, *q.v.* Prepn: D. C. Liotta *et al.,* **WO 9214743** (1992 to Emory University); G. Dionne, **US 5538975** (1996 to BioChem Pharma, Inc.); L. S. Jeong *et al., J. Med. Chem.* **36**, 181 (1993). Absolute configuration: P. van Roey *et al., Antiviral Chem. Chemother.* **4**, 369 (1993). HPLC-NMR determn of urinary metabolites: J. P. Shockcor *et al., Xenobiotica* **26**, 189 (1996). Comparative efficacy of enantiomers vs HIV: R. F. Schinazi *et al., Antimicrob. Agents Chemother.* **36**, 2423 (1992). Pharmacokinetics: L. W. Frick *et al., ibid.* **38**, 2722 (1994). Mechanism of action study: J. Y. Feng *et al., FASEB J.* **13**, 1511 (1999). Clinical study in combination with didanosine and efavirenz: J.-M. Molina *et al., J. Infect. Dis.* **182**, 599 (2000). *Review:* P. Cahn, *Expert Opin. Invest. Drugs* **13**, 55-68 (2004).

White solid from ether and methanol, mp 136-140°. $[\alpha]_D^{25}$ −133.60° (c = 0.23 in MeOH). uv max (water): 287.8 nm (pH 2); 280.0 nm (pH 7); 279.8 nm (pH 11) (ε 14210, 11090, 11810).
THERAP CAT: Antiviral.

3566. Emylcamate. [78-28-4] 3-Methyl-3-pentanol carbamate; 1-ethyl-1-methylpropyl carbamate; diethyl methyl carbinol urethan; 3-methyl-3-pentyl carbamate; methyl diethyl carbinol urethan; *tert*-hexanol carbamate; Kabi 925; JD-91; Nuncital; Restetal; Statran; Striatran. $C_7H_{15}NO_2$; mol wt 145.20. C 57.90%, H 10.41%, N 9.65%, O 22.04%. Prepn: **DE 245491** (1912 to Chinifabr. Zimmer); **DE 254472** (1912 to E. Merck); Melander, Hanshoff, **US 2972564** (1961 to Kabi).

Needles from 30% ethanol, mp 56-58.5°. $bp_{1.0}$ 35°; $bp_{0.7}$ 24°. Slight odor of camphor. Soly in water: 4.0 mg/ml. Freely sol in alcohol, ether, benzene, glycol ethers.
THERAP CAT: Anxiolytic.

3567. Enalapril. [75847-73-3] *N*-[(1*S*)-1-(Ethoxycarbonyl)-3-phenylpropyl]-L-alanyl-L-proline; 1-[*N*-[(*S*)-1-carboxy-3-phenylpropyl]-L-alanyl]-L-proline 1′-ethyl ester. $C_{20}H_{28}N_2O_5$; mol wt 376.45. C 63.81%, H 7.50%, N 7.44%, O 21.25%. Angiotensin-converting enzyme (ACE) inhibitor; de-esterified *in vivo* to its active diacid metabolite, enalaprilat, *q.v.* Prepn: A. A. Patchett *et al., Nature* **288**, 280 (1980); *eidem,* **EP 12401**; E. E. Harris *et al.,* **US 4374829** (1980, 1983 both to Merck & Co.). Pharmacology: D. M. Gross *et al., J. Pharmacol. Exp. Ther.* **216**, 552 (1981); C. S. Sweet *et al., ibid.* 558. Bioavailability and metabolism: E. H. Ulm, *Drug Metab. Rev.* **14**, 99 (1983). Comprehensive description: D. P. Ip, G. S. Brenner, *Anal. Profiles Drug Subs.* **16**, 207-243 (1987). Clinical trial in congestive heart failure: Consensus Trial Study Group, *N. Engl. J. Med.* **316**, 1429 (1987). Review of clinical experience in hypertension: H. J. Gomez *et al., J. Cardiovasc. Pharmacol.* **15**, Suppl. 3, S26-S29 (1990); of clinical pharmacokinetics: R. J. MacFadyen *et al., Clin. Pharmacokinet.* **25**, 274-282 (1993); of combination with hydrochlorothiazide: P. L. Malini, *Adv. Ther.* **10**, 253-262 (1993).

Maleate. [76095-16-4] MK-421; Amprace; Cardiovet; Enacard; Enapren; Glioten; Hipoartel; Innovace; Pres; Renitec; Reniten; Renivace; Vasotec; Xanef. $C_{20}H_{28}N_2O_5 \cdot C_4H_4O_4$; mol wt 492.52. White to off-white crystalline powder, mp 143-144.5°. Soly (g/ml): water 0.025; alcohol 0.08; methanol 0.20. $[\alpha]_D^{25}$ −42.2° (c = 1 in methanol). pH (1% water) 2.6. pKa_1 3.0; pKa_2 (25°) 5.4.
Mixture of maleate with hydrochlorothiazide. Acesistem; Co-Renitec; Enaloc; Innozide; Lotrial D; Renacor; Vaseretic; Vasoretic; Xynertec.

THERAP CAT: Antihypertensive.
THERAP CAT (VET): In treatment of heart failure in dogs.

3568. Enalaprilat. [76420-72-9] *N*-[(1*S*)-1-Carboxy-3-phenylpropyl]-L-alanyl-L-proline dihydrate; enalaprilic acid; MK-422; Vasotec IV. $C_{18}H_{24}N_2O_5 \cdot 2H_2O$; mol wt 384.42. C 56.24%, H 7.34%, N 7.29%, O 29.13%. Nonsulfhydryl dipeptide angiotensin converting enzyme (ACE) inhibitor. Prepn: A. A. Patchett *et al., Nature* **288**, 280 (1980); *eidem,* **EP 12401**; E. E. Harris *et al.,* **US 4374829** (1980, 1983 both to Merck & Co.). Active metabolite of enalapril, *q.v.:* D. J. Tocco *et al., Drug Metab. Dispos.* **10**, 15 (1982). Pharmacology: D. M. Gross *et al., J. Pharmacol. Exp. Ther.* **216**, 552 (1981); M. A. Nelson *et al., Clin. Exp. Pharmacol. Physiol.* **Suppl. 7**, 87 (1982); T. A. Unger *et al., Biochem. Pharmacol.* **31**, 3063 (1982). Bioavailability: M. L. Cohen *et al., J. Pharmacol. Exp. Ther.* **226**, 192 (1983). Kinetics of enzyme inhibition: C. H. Reynolds, *Biochem. Pharmacol.* **33**, 1273 (1984). Pharmacokinetics: K. S. Pang *et al., Drug Metab. Dispos.* **12**, 309 (1984). Acute hemodynamic effects in essential hypertension: A. C. Simon *et al., Clin. Pharm. Ther.* **43**, 49 (1988). Clinical evaluation in severe and malignant hypertension: D. J. DiPette *et al., ibid.* **38**, 199 (1985).

Needles from H_2O, mp 148-151°. $[\alpha]_D$ −67.0° (0.1*M* HCl).
THERAP CAT: Antihypertensive.

3569. Enanthotoxin. [20311-78-8] (2*E*,8*E*,10*E*)-2,8,10-Heptadecatriene-4,6-diyne-1,14-diol; oenanthotoxin. $C_{17}H_{22}O_2$; mol wt 258.36. C 79.03%, H 8.58%, O 12.39%. The poisonous principle of *Oenanthe crocata* L., *Umbelliferae*, the hemlock water dropwort, a toxic plant known since 1746 and believed to be the most poisonous plant in England. Isoln: Clarke *et al.*, *J. Pharm. Pharmacol.* **1**, 377 (1949). Structure studies: Anet *et al.*, *Chem. Ind. (London)* **1952**, 757; *J. Chem. Soc.* **1953**, 309. Synthesis of DL-form: Bohlmann, Viehe, *Ber.* **88**, 1245 (1955). Fluorimetric determn: B. Del Castillo *et al.*, *Ital. J. Biochem.* **29**, 233 (1980). Blocking of sodium current and intramembrane charge movement: J. M. Dubois, M. F. Schneider, *Nature* **289**, 685 (1981); *eidem*, *Toxicon* **20**, 49 (1982). Toxicity study: M. P. Martinez-Honduvilla *et al.*, *Arch. Farmacol. Toxicol.* **7**, 197 (1981).

Large prisms (natural) or star-shaped crystals (synthetic). Unstable, dec by light and air to brown insol resin. mp 87° (natural), 68° (synthetic). $[\alpha]_D^{15}$ +30.5° (c = 2.0 in methanol). uv max: 213, 252, 267, 281, 296, 315.5, 337.5 ($\varepsilon \times 10^{-3}$ 17.5, 33, 29, 17.5, 30.5, 40, 29). Practically insol in water, petr ether, alkalies, dil mineral acids. Readily sol in chloroform, ethanol, methanol, ether, benzene. Average LD i.p. in mice: 0.83 mg/kg (Clarke). LD_{50} i.p. in rats: 2.94 mg/kg (Martinez-Honduvilla).

Caution: Very toxic. May cause convulsions, death.

3570. Encainide. [66778-36-7] 4-Methoxy-*N*-[2-[2-(1-methyl-2-piperidinyl)ethyl]phenyl]benzamide; (±)-2'-[2-(1-methyl-2-piperidyl)ethyl]-*p*-anisanilide; 4-methoxy-2'-[2-(1-methyl-2-piperidyl)ethyl]benzanilide. $C_{22}H_{28}N_2O_2$; mol wt 352.47. C 74.97%, H 8.01%, N 7.95%, O 9.08%. Anti-arrhythmic benzanilide derivative. Prepn: S. J. Dykstra, J. L. Minielli, **DE 2210154** (1972 to Bristol-Myers), *C.A.* **78**, 4138j (1973); *eidem*, **US 3931195** (1976 to Mead Johnson); S. J. Dykstra *et al.*, *J. Med. Chem.* **16**, 1015 (1973). Anti-arrhythmic pharmacology in animals: J. E. Byrne *et al.*, *J. Pharmacol. Exp. Ther.* **200**, 147 (1977). Clinical pharmacology and efficacy in chronic ventricular arrhythmia: D. M. Roden *et al.*, *N. Engl. J. Med.* **302**, 877 (1980). Electrophysiology and effects on cardiac conduction: M. Sami *et al.*, *Am. J. Cardiol.* **44**, 526 (1979). Hemodynamic effects: M. Sami *et al.*, *ibid.* **52**, 507 (1983). Adverse effects: R. A. Winkle *et al.*, *Am. Heart J.* **102**, 857 (1981). Comparison with other Class I anti-arrhythmic agents: A. Pottage, *Am. J. Cardiol.* **52**, 24C (1983). Series of articles on pharmacology, pharmacokinetics, metabolism, clinical safety and efficacy: *ibid.* **58**(5), 1C-116C (1986). Review: L. B. Mitchell, R. A. Winkle in *New Drugs Annual: Cardiovascular Drugs* **vol. 1**, A. Scriabine, Ed. (Raven Press, New York, 1983) pp 93-107.

Hydrochloride. [66794-74-9] MJ-9067; Enkaid. $C_{22}H_{28}N_2O_2 \cdot HCl$; mol wt 388.93. Crystals, mp 131.5-132.5°. Freely sol in water; slightly sol in ethanol. Insol in heptane. LD_{50} in mice, dogs (mg/kg): 86, 43 orally; 16, 17 i.v. (Mitchell, Winkle).

THERAP CAT: Antiarrhythmic (class IC).

3571. Endiandric Acids. A group of novel polycyclic compounds isolated from leaves of the 'Dorrigo Plum', *Endiandra introrsa* C. T. White, *Lauraceae,* a large tree occurring in rain forests of Australia. Although they have a number of asymmetric centers, endiandric acids occur in nature in racemic rather than enantiomeric forms. This fact led to a proposed hypothesis for the "biogenesis" of these compounds in nature from achiral precursors by a series of non-enzymatic electrocyclizations called the "endiandric acid cascade". Isoln from *E. introrsa* leaves (obtained in 1958) and structure of endiandric acid A: W. M. Bandaranayake *et al.*, *Chem.*

Commun. **1980**, 162. Postulated electrocyclic reactions, prediction of endiandric acid D as a natural product: *eidem, ibid.* 902. X-ray crystallographic structural elucidation of A and detailed report of isoln: *eidem, Aust. J. Chem.* **34**, 1655 (1981). Isoln and structure of endiandric acid B: *eidem, ibid.* **35**, 557 (1982); of C: *eidem, ibid.* 567. Stereocontrolled total synthesis of A and B, description of "endiandric acid cascade": K. C. Nicolaou *et al.*, *J. Am. Chem. Soc.* **104**, 5555 (1982). Stereocontrolled total synthesis of endiandric acids C-G: *eidem, ibid.* 5557. Synthesis of precursors and thermal studies: *eidem, ibid.* 5558, 5560.

Endiandric acid A
R = CH_2COOH

Endiandric acid C

Endiandric acid B
R = COOH

Endiandric Acid A. [74591-03-0] (1*R*,1a*R*,2a*R*,5*S*,5a*S*,7a*S*,-7b*R*,7c*R*)-*rel*-1a,2,2a,5,5a,7a,7b,7c-Octahydro-5-phenyl-1*H*-cyclobut[*bc*]acenaphthylene-1-acetic acid; 2-(6'-phenyltetracyclo[5,4,2,-$0^{3,13},0^{10,12}$]trideca-4',8'-dien-11'-yl)acetic acid. $C_{21}H_{22}O_2$; mol wt 306.40. Rods from aq ethanol, mp 147-149°. uv max (95% ethanol): 242, 255, 261, 268, 286 nm (log ε 2.19, 2.36, 2.45, 2.32, 1.45). pKa 5.1, 5.0. Gives a yellow color with tetranitromethane.

Endiandric Acid B. [76060-33-8] (2*E*)-*rel*-4-[(1*R*,1a*R*,2a*R*,-5*S*,5a*S*,7a*S*,7b*R*,7c*R*)-1a,2,2a,5,5a,7a,7b,7c-Octahydro-5-phenyl-1*H*-cyclobut[*bc*]acenaphthylen-1-yl]-2-butenoic acid; (*E*)-4-(6'-phenyltetracyclo[5,4,2,$0^{3,13},0^{10,12}$]trideca-4',8'-dien-11'-yl)but-2-enoic acid. $C_{23}H_{24}O_2$; mol wt 332.44. Rosettes from aq ethanol and chloroform/ petr ether, mp 163-165°. uv max (95% ethanol): 252, 258, 262, 265, 269 nm (log ε 3.11, 3.08, 3.07, 3.01, 2.97).

Endiandric Acid C. [76060-34-9] (1*R*,1a*R*,3*S*,3a*R*,6*S*,6a*S*,-6b*R*,7*S*)-*rel*-1,1a,2,3,3a,6,6a,6b-Octahydro-1-[(2*E*,4*E*)-5-phenyl-2,-4-pentadienyl]-3,6-methanocyclobut[*cd*]indene-7-carboxylic acid; 4-[(*E*,*E*)-5'-phenylpenta-2',4'-dien-1'-yl]tetracyclo[5,4,0,0^{2,5},0^{3,9}]-undec-10-ene-8-carboxylic acid. $C_{23}H_{24}O_2$; mol wt 332.44. Cryst from ethanol and methanol, mp 125-132° (variable and with dec). uv max (95% ethanol): 222, 228, 236, 280, 288 nm (log ε 4.10, 4.05, 3.89, 4.51, 4.53).

3572. Endorphins. Generic name derived from the term "endogenous morphine" and applied to a group of neuropeptides that are endogenous ligands of the opiate receptors. They are found in brain, pituitary gland and peripheral tissues of all vertebrates; the effects of endorphins on cells resemble those of opiates such as morphine. Their existence was postulated as a result of the discovery of stereospecific binding sites for narcotic analgesics in animal brain, *cf.* A. Goldstein *et al.*, *Proc. Natl. Acad. Sci. USA* **68**, 1742 (1971); C. B. Pert, S. H. Snyder, *Science* **179**, 1011 (1973); E. J. Simon *et al.*, *Proc. Natl. Acad. Sci. USA* **70**, 1947 (1973). Three types of stereochemically related opiate receptors have been postulated, *mu, delta, kappa*: W. R. Martin *et al.*, *J. Pharmacol. Exp. Ther.* **197**, 517 (1976); P. E. Gilbert, W. R. Martin, *ibid.* **198**, 66 (1976); J. A. H. Lord *et al.*, *Nature* **267**, 495 (1977). Of the endorphin group of peptides, several important members are known: α-, β- and γ-endorphins (β-endorphin being the most potent), α-neo-endorphin, β-neo-endorphin, dynorphin, *q.v.*, and met-enkephalin and leu-enkephalin, two naturally occurring pentapeptides belonging to the endorphin class. The amino acid sequences of α-, β- and γ-endorphins are contained within the sequence 61-91 of β-lipotropin, and in each, the amino terminal pentapeptide sequence is that of met-enkephalin. Dynorphin and α- and β-neo-endorphins have common terminal leu-enkephalin sequences. Initial isoln of active oligopeptide: L. Terenius, A. Wahlstrom, *Acta Pharmacol. Toxicol.* **35**, Suppl. 1, 55 (1974); J. Hughes, *Brain Res.* **88**, 295 (1975).

Isoln, characterization and synthesis of two active pentapeptides (*enkephalins*): J. Hughes *et al.*, *Life Sci.* **16**, 1753 (1975); G. W. Pasternak *et al., ibid.* 1765; J. Hughes *et al., Nature* **258**, 577 (1975); J. D. Bower *et al., J. Chem. Soc. Perkin Trans. 1* **1976**, 2488. Isoln and properties of β-endorphin from bovine pituitary: H. Teschemacher *et al., Life Sci.* **16**, 1771 (1975); B. M. Cox *et al., ibid.* 1777. Identity of β-endorphin with carboxy terminal amino acid sequence (61-91) of β-lipotropin: C. H. Li, D. Chang, *Proc. Natl. Acad. Sci. USA* **73**, 1145 (1976); B. M. Cox *et al., ibid.* 1821. Production of biologically active β-endorphin via expression of cloned gene sequences by *E. coli:* J. Shine *et al., Nature* **285**, 456 (1980). For a review of isoln, amino acid sequences, and synthesis of β-endorphins from various species, *see Hormonal Proteins and Peptides* vol. **X**, entitled "β-Endorphin", C. H. Li, Ed. (Academic Press, New York, 1981) pp 2-30. Isoln and structure of *α-endorphin* or *LPH (61-76)*: R. Guillemin *et al., C.R. Seances Acad. Sci. Ser. D* **282**, 783 (1976); isoln, structure, synthesis of α- and *γ-endorphin* or *LPH (61-77)*: N. Ling *et al., Proc. Natl. Acad. Sci. USA* **73**, 3942 (1976). High yield synthesis of met[5]-enkephalin: B. J. Dhotre *et al., J. Indian Chem. Soc.* **55**, 1128 (1978). Rapid synthesis of leu[5]-enkephalin: E. Vilkas *et al., Int. J. Pept. Protein Res.* **15**, 29 (1980). Isoln of *α-neo-endorphin*: K. Kagawa *et al., Biochem. Biophys. Res. Commun.* **86**, 153 (1979). Amino acid sequence: *eidem, ibid.* **99**, 871 (1981). Isoln, purification, amino acid sequence of *β-neoendorphin*: N. Minamino *et al., ibid.* 864. Metabolism and physiological effects of endorphins: H. W. Kosterlitz, J. Hughes, *Life Sci.* **17**, 91 (1975); L.-F. Tseng *et al., Proc. Natl. Acad. Sci. USA* **73**, 4187 (1976). Although the physiological role of the endorphins has not been completely elucidated, they are known to block inhibitory pathways in the vertebrate CNS and their possible effects on pain perception, addictive states, and psychiatric disorders have been investigated: D. T. Krieger, A. S. Liotta, *Science* **205**, 366 (1979); R. A. Nicoll *et al., Nature* **287**, 22 (1980). Studies have also suggested that endorphins may be involved in gluco-regulation: M. Feldman *et al., N. Engl. J. Med.* **308**, 350 (1983). *Reviews:* A. Goldstein, *Science* **193**, 1081-1086 (1976); *idem, Harvey Lect.* **79**, 291-314 (1979); R. A. North, *Life Sci.* **24**, 1527-1546 (1979); C. R. Beddell *et al., Prog. Med. Chem.* **17**, 1-39 (1980); several authors in *Adv. Biochem. Pharmacol.* **22**, 145-642 (1980); M. S. Gold *et al., Med. Res. Rev.* **2**, 211-246 (1982); S. Zakarian, D. G. Smyth, *Biochem. J.* **202**, 561-571 (1982). Books: *Opiates and Endogenous Opioid Peptides*, H. W. Kosterlitz, Ed. (Elsevier, New York, 1976) 466 pp; *Endorphins: Proceedings*, L. Graf *et al., Eds.* (Elsevier, New York, 1979) 471 pp; *Endorphins and Opiate Antagonists in Psychiatric Research*, N. Shah, A. G. Donald, Eds. (Plenum, New York, 1982) 425 pp.

```
      61
 –Tyr–Gly–Gly–Phe–Met–Thr–Ser–Glu–Lys–Ser–Gln–Thr–Pro–Leu–Val
                                                        |
                                                       Thr
                                                        |
                                                       Leu
                                                        |
      91
 HO–Glu–Gly–Lys–Lys–Tyr–Ala–Asn–Lys–Ile–Ile–Ala–Asn–Lys–Phe
```

Human β-Endorphin

β-Endorphin. β-Lipotropin C-fragment; β-lipotropin (61-91); LPH (61-91).

Met[5]-Enkephalin. Methionine[5]-enkephalin; met[5]-E; L-tyrosylglycylglycyl-L-phenylalanyl-L-methionine; LPH (61-55). $C_{27}H_{35}N_5O_7S$; mol wt 573.66. Needles from hot methanol, mp 196-198°. $[\alpha]_{589}^{22}$ −21.9° (c = 1 in DMF); +14° (c = 1 in *N* HCl).

Leu[5]-Enkephalin. Leucine[5]-enkephalin; leu[5]-E; L-tyrosylglycylglycyl-L-phenylalanyl-L-leucine. $C_{28}H_{37}N_5O_7$; mol wt 555.62. White crystalline solid, mp 206° (dec). $[\alpha]_{589}^{22}$ −23.4° (c = 1 in DMF); +18.3° (c = 1 in *N* HCl).

3573. Endostatin. [187888-07-9] Endogenous inhibitor of angiogenesis and tumor growth. mol wt ~20 kDa. C-terminal fragment of collagen XVIII, a collagen-like peptide localized around blood vessels. Released by the action of tumor-produced proteases on the collagen molecule. Isoln from murine hemangioendothelioma: M. S. O'Reilly *et al., Cell* **88**, 277 (1997); from human plasma: L. Ständker *et al., FEBS Lett.* **420**, 129 (1997). Crystal structure: E. Hohenester *et al., EMBO J.* **17**, 1656 (1998). Antitumor activity in mice: T. Boehm *et al., Nature* **390**, 404 (1997).

3574. Endosulfan. [115-29-7] 6,7,8,9,10,10-Hexachloro-1,5,5a,6,9,9a-hexahydro-6,9-methano-2,4,3-benzodioxathiepin 3-oxide; 1,4,5,6,7,7-hexachloro-5-norbornene-2,3-dimethanol cyclic sulfite; 1,2,3,4,7,7-hexachlorobicyclo[2.2.1]-2-heptene-5,6-bisoxymethylene sulfite; chlorthiepin; Malix; Thiodan; Thionex. $C_9H_6Cl_6O_3S$; mol wt 406.93. C 26.56%, H 1.49%, Cl 52.27%, O 11.80%, S 7.88%. Prepd by reaction of hexachlorocyclopentadiene with *cis*-butene-1,4-diol to form the bicyclic dialcohol, followed by esterification and cyclization with $SOCl_2$: Geering, Nelson, **US 2983732** (1961 to Hooker). Configuration studies: Reimschneider, Wuscherpfenning, *Z. Naturforsch.* **17b**, 585 (1962); Forman *et al., J. Org. Chem.* **30**, 169 (1965). Toxicity study: T. B. Gaines, *Toxicol. Appl. Pharmacol.* **14**, 515 (1969). Review of toxicology and human exposure: *Toxicological Profile for Endosulfan* (PB2000-108023, 2000) 323 pp.

Commercial product brown crystals. mp 70-100° (pure mp 106°). Practically insol in water. Sol in most organic solvents. Stable toward dil mineral acids; hydrolyzed rapidly by alkalies. Commercial product is a mixture of α-isomer, mp 108-110°, and β-isomer, mp 208-210°. LD_{50} orally in male, female rats: 43, 18 mg/kg (Gaines).

Caution: Potential symptoms of overexposure are skin irritation; nausea, confusion, agitation, flushing, dry mouth, tremors, convulsions, headache. *See NIOSH Pocket Guide to Chemical Hazards* (DHHS/NIOSH 97-140, 1997) p 126.

USE: Insecticide.

3575. Endothall. [145-73-3] 7-Oxabicyclo[2.2.1]heptane-2,3-dicarboxylic acid; 3,6-endoxohexahydrophthalic acid; endothal. $C_8H_{10}O_5$; mol wt 186.16. C 51.61%, H 5.41%, O 42.97%. Prepn: Olin, **US 2550494** (1951 to Sharples Chemicals). Of the three possible isomers, the *exo-cis* form has the greatest biological activity. Fate in the environment and toxicity: Simsiman *et al., Residue Rev.* **62**, 131-174 (1976); T. B. Gaines, R. E. Linder, *Fundam. Appl. Toxicol.* **7**, 299 (1986).

Solubility of the acid in g/100 g at 20°: water 10; acetone 7; benzene 0.01; methanol 28. Converted to the anhydride at 90°. LD_{50} in adult male, female rats (mg/kg): 57, 46 orally (Gaines, Linder).

Dipotassium salt. Aquathol; Aquathol K. $C_8H_8K_2O_5$; mol wt 262.34.

Caution: May be very irritating to skin, eyes, mucous membranes. Ingestion may cause severe G.I. inflammation with erosion. *See Clinical Toxicology of Commercial Products*, R. E. Gosselin *et al.*, Eds. (Williams & Wilkins, Baltimore, 5th ed., 1984) Section II, p 342.

USE: Herbicide; defoliant.

3576. Endothelin. [117399-94-7] Endothelin-1; ET-1. Potent vasoconstrictor peptide produced by mammalian vascular endothelial cells; present in low concentrations in normal serum. Composed of 21 amino acid residues; mol wt ~2500 Da. Isoln, characterization and cloning of porcine endothelin: M. Yanagisawa *et al., Nature* **332**, 411 (1988). Structural identity of porcine and human endothelin: Y. Itoh *et al., FEBS Lett.* **231**, 440 (1988). Structural similarity with the snake venom toxins, *sarafotoxins S6*: C. Y. Lee, V. A. Chiappinelli, *Nature* **335**, 303 (1988); C. Takasaki *et al., ibid.* 303. Identification in serum by radioimmunoassay: K. Ando *et al., FEBS Lett.* **245**, 164 (1989). Two additional isoforms, known as **endothelin-2** and **endothelin-3**, have been identified. Structures and comparative pharmacology of human endothelin isopeptides: A. Inoue *et al., Proc. Natl. Acad. Sci. USA* **86**, 2863 (1989). Mechanism of action study: Y. Hirata *et al., Biochem. Biophys. Res. Commun.* **154**, 868 (1988). Possible role in acute renal failure: J. D. Firth *et al., Lancet* **2**, 1179 (1988). *In vivo* effects on pulmonary and systemic hemodynamics: H. L. Lippton *et al., J. Appl. Physiol.* **66**, 1008 (1989). *Review:* T. Masaki, *J. Cardiovasc. Pharmacol.* **13**, Suppl. 5, S1-S4 (1989).

C–S–C–S–S–L–M–D–K–E–C–V–Y–F–C– H–L–D–I–I–W

3577. Endralazine. [39715-02-1] 6-Benzoyl-5,6,7,8-tetrahydropyrido[4,3-*c*]pyridazin-3(2*H*)-one hydrazone; 6-benzoyl-3-hydrazino-5,6,7,8-tetrahydropyrido[4,3-*c*]pyridazine. $C_{14}H_{15}N_5O$; mol wt 269.30. C 62.44%, H 5.61%, N 26.01%, O 5.94%. Prepn: E. Schenker, **DE 2221808**; *idem*, **US 3838125** (1972, 1974 both to Sandoz); E. Schenker, R. Salzmann, *Arzneim.-Forsch.* **29**, 1835 (1979). Pharmacology: R. Salzmann *et al., ibid.* 1843. Hemodynamic study: H. U. Lehmann *et al., Z. Cardiol.* **66**, 203 (1977). HPLC determn in human plasma: P. A. Reece *et al., J. Chromatogr.* **225**, 151 (1981). Clinical pharmacology: F. C. Reubi, *Eur. J. Clin. Pharmacol.* **13**, 185 (1978). Clinical study in hypertension: H. U. Lehmann *et al., Med. Welt* **29**, 1007 (1978).

Crystals from acetonitrile/water, mp 220-223° (dec).
Methanesulfonate. [65322-72-7] Endralazine mesylate; BQ 22-708; Miretilan. $C_{14}H_{15}N_5O.CH_3SO_3H$; mol wt 365.41. Cryst, mp 185-188° (dec).
THERAP CAT: Antihypertensive.

3578. Endrin. [72-20-8] (1a*R*,2*R*,2a*R*,3*R*,6*S*,6a*S*,7*S*,7a*S*)-*rel*-3,4,5,6,9,9-Hexachloro-1a,2,2a,3,6,6a,7,7a-octahydro-2,7:3,6-dimethanonaphth[2,3-*b*]oxirene; 1,2,3,4,10,10-hexachloro-6,7-epoxy-1,4,4a,5,6,7,8,8a-octahydro-*endo,endo*-1,4:5,8-dimethanonaphthalene; mendrin; nendrin; hexadrin; experimental insecticide no. 269; compd 269; ENT-17251. $C_{12}H_8Cl_6O$; mol wt 380.91. C 37.84%, H 2.12%, Cl 55.84%, O 4.20%. Stereoisomer of dieldrin, *q.v.* Prepn from isodrin: H. Bluestone, **US 2676132** (1954 to Shell); Marks, **US 2899446** (1959 to Velsicol). Metabolism: M. K. Baldwin *et al., Pestic. Sci.* **7**, 575 (1976). Carcinogenicity studies: M. D. Rueber, *Sci. Total Environ.* **12**, 101 (1979). Toxicity study: T. B. Gaines, *Toxicol. Appl. Pharmacol.* **14**, 515 (1969). Review of toxicology and human exposure: *Toxicological Profile for Endrin* (PB97-121040, 1996) 227 pp.

Crystals, dec 245°. Vapor pressure at 25°: 2×10^{-7} mm Hg. Soly in g/100 ml solvent at 25°: acetone 17, benzene 13.8, carbon tetrachloride 3.3, hexane 7.1, xylene 18.3. LD_{50} in female, male rats (mg/kg): 7.5, 18 orally (Gaines).
Caution: Potential symptoms of overexposure are epileptiform convulsions; stupor, headache and dizziness; abdominal discomfort, nausea and vomiting; insomnia; aggressiveness, confusion; lethargy, weakness; anorexia. *See NIOSH Pocket Guide to Chemical Hazards* (DHHS/NIOSH 97-140, 1997) p 126.
USE: Formerly as insecticide.

3579. Enduracidin. [11115-82-5] Enramycin. Cyclodepsipeptide antibiotic produced by *Streptomyces fungicidicus*, strain no. B5477, from a soil sample collected in Nishinomiya,

Hyogo Prefecture, Japan: Higashide *et al., J. Antibiot.* **21**, 126 (1968). Originally thought to be a single compound. Isoln and characterization: Asai *et al., ibid.* 138; **FR 1514139**; **GB 1163270** (1968, 1969 to Takeda). Manufacturing process: **JP Kokai 82 79896** (1982 to Takeda), *C.A.* **97**, 108525s (1982). Separation into two components, enduracidins A and B: Hori *et al., Chem. Pharm. Bull.* **21**, 1171 (1973). The two components are each composed of seventeen amino acids, sixteen of which form a macrocyclic peptide lactone, and only differ by one methylene group in their fatty acid moieties. Structural studies: Hori *et al., ibid.* 1175. Final structure: Iwasaki *et al., ibid.* 1184. Antibacterial activity: Goto *et al., J. Antibiot.* **21**, 119 (1968); Tsuchiya *et al., ibid.* 147; M. Kawakami *et al., ibid.* **24**, 583 (1971). Toxicology: H. Yokotani *et al., Takeda Kenkyusho Nempo* **28**, 76 (1969), *C.A.* **72**, 77300s (1970).
Monohydrochloride. Enradin. Yellowish powder, dec 234-238°. Slightly sol in water, methanol. Practically insol in acetone, ethanol, chloroform, benzene. LD_{50} in mice and rats (mg/kg): >10000 orally; >5000 i.m.; >5000 s.c. (Yokotani).
Enduracidin A hydrochloride. [33368-20-6] $C_{107}H_{138}Cl_2$-$N_{26}O_{31}$.HCl; mol wt 2391.76. mp 240-245°. $[\alpha]_D^{23}$ +92° (c = 0.5 in DMF). uv max (0.1*N* HCl): 231, 272 nm.
Enduracidin B hydrochloride. [34765-98-5] $C_{108}H_{140}Cl_2$-$N_{26}O_{31}$.HCl; mol wt 2405.79. mp 238-241°. $[\alpha]_D^{23}$ +92° (c = 0.5 in DMF). uv max (0.1*N* HCl): 231, 272 nm.
THERAP CAT: Antibacterial.

3580. Enfenamic Acid. [23049-93-6] 2-[(2-Phenylethyl)amino]benzoic acid; *N*-phenethyl anthranilic acid; RH-8; Tromaril. $C_{15}H_{15}NO_2$; mol wt 241.29. C 74.67%, H 6.27%, N 5.80%, O 13.26%. Nonsteroidal anti-inflammatory, antipyretic, analgesic. Prepn: S. R. Hashim *et al.*, **IN 103066** and **IN 114805** (both 1974 to Council Sci. Ind. Res.). Chemistry and pharmacology: P. Sisoda *et al., Proc. Symp. CNS Drugs* (Council of Scientific and Industrial Research, New Delhi, 1966) pp 238-248. Antithrombotic activity in rheumatoid arthritis and myocardial infarction: S. R. Manikeri *et al., Indian J. Med. Res.* **71**, 438 (1980). Natriuretic activity: N. Kshirsagar *et al., Br. J. Clin. Pharmacol.* **9**, 530 (1980). Clinical trial in nephrotic syndrome: *eidem, Indian J. Med. Res.* **70**, 801 (1979); as postpartum analgesic: S. Tandon *et al., Indian Med. Gaz.* **116**, 182 (1982).

Crystals, mp 116-117°. Insol in water. LD_{50} in mice (mg/kg): 575 i.p., >2000 orally (Sisoda).
THERAP CAT: Anti-inflammatory; analgesic.

3581. Enflurane. [13838-16-9] 2-Chloro-1-(difluoromethoxy)-1,1,2-trifluoroethane; 2-chloro-1,1,2-trifluoroethyl difluoromethyl ether; methylflurether; compd 347; NSC-115944; Alyrane; Efrane; Ethrane. $C_3H_2ClF_5O$; mol wt 184.49. C 19.53%, H 1.09%, Cl 19.22%, F 51.49%, O 8.67%. CHF_2OCF_2CHClF. Prepn by fluorination of the corresp dichloromethyl ether: R. C. Terrell, **GB 1138406**; *idem*, **US 3469011**; **US 3527813** (1969, 1969, 1970 all to Air Reduction). Synthesis and anesthetic properties: R. C. Terrell *et al., J. Med. Chem.* **14**, 517 (1971); **15**, 604 (1972). Enantiomeric resolution: J. Meinwald *et al., Science* **251**, 560 (1991).
Stable, volatile, non-flammable liq. bp 56.5°. n_D^{20} 1.3025. d_{25}^{25} 1.5167. Does not degrade in the presence of alkali or light. Miscible with other organic liquids incl. fats and oils.
Caution: Potential symptoms of overexposure are eye irritation; CNS depression, analgesia, anesthesia, seizures, respiratory depression. *See NIOSH Pocket Guide to Chemical Hazards* (DHHS/NIOSH 97-140, 1997) p 128.
THERAP CAT: Anesthetic (inhalation).

3582. Enfuvirtide. [159519-65-0] Pentafuside; DP-178; T-20; Fuzeon. $C_{204}H_{301}N_{51}O_{64}$; mol wt 4491.88. C 54.55%, H 6.75%, N 15.90%, O 22.80%. HIV fusion inhibitor. Synthetic, 36 amino acid peptide corresponding to a region of gp41, the transmembrane subunit of the HIV-1 envelope protein. Prepn and biological activity: D. P. Bolognesi *et al.*, **WO 9428920**; *eidem, US*

5464933 (1994, 1995 both to Duke Univ.); C. T. Wild *et al.*, *Proc. Natl. Acad. Sci. USA* **91**, 9770 (1994). Mechanism of action study: R. A. Furuta *et al.*, *Nat. Struct. Biol.* **5**, 276 (1998). Clinical pharmacokinetics: J. M. Kilby *et al.*, *AIDS Res. Hum. Retroviruses* **18**, 685 (2002). Review of development: N. Press *et al.*, *Curr. Opin. Anti-Infect. Invest. Drugs* **1**, 171-178 (1999); of clinical evaluations: A. Pozniak, *J. HIV Ther.* **6**, 91-94 (2001).

THERAP CAT: Antiviral.

3583. Enilconazole. [35554-44-0] 1-[2-(2,4-Dichlorophenyl)-2-(2-propenyloxy)ethyl]-1*H*-imidazole; (±)-1-[β-(allyloxy)-2,4-dichlorophenethyl]imidazole; imazalil; R-23979; Clinafarm; Imaverol. $C_{14}H_{14}Cl_2N_2O$; mol wt 297.18. C 56.58%, H 4.75%, Cl 23.86%, N 9.43%, O 5.38%. Broad spectrum antimycotic with agricultural and veterinary applications. Prepn: E. F. Godefroi, J. L. Schuermans, DE 2063857; *eidem*, US 3658813 (1971, 1972 both to Janssen). Efficacy vs citrus decay: P. R. Harding, *Plant Dis. Rep.* **60**, 643 (1976); S. Ben-Yehoshua *et al.*, *Pestic. Sci.* **12**, 485 (1981). Biological and toxicological properties: D. Thienpont *et al.*, *Arzneim.-Forsch.* **31**, 309 (1981). Residue analysis in treated grapefruit: E. R. Stein *et al.*, *J. Environ. Sci. Health* **B16**, 427 (1981).

Solidified oil. Slightly sol in organic solvents; poorly sol in water.

USE: As a disinfectant for stable and kennel equipment; exptly as an agricultural fungicide.

THERAP CAT: Antifungal.

THERAP CAT (VET): Antifungal.

3584. Eniluracil. [59989-18-3] 5-Ethynyl-2,4(1*H*,3*H*)-pyrimidinedione; 5-ethynyluracil; 5-EU; 776C85. $C_6H_4N_2O_2$; mol wt 136.11. C 52.95%, H 2.96%, N 20.58%, O 23.51%. Irreversible inhibitor of dihydropyrimidine dehydrogenase, the rate-determining enzyme in catabolism of 5-fluorouracil, *q.v.* Prepn: J. Perman *et al.*, *Tetrahedron Lett.* **1976**, 2427; P. J. Barr *et al.*, *Nucleic Acids Res.* **3**, 2845 (1976). Large scale synthesis: N. G. Kundu, S. A. Schmitz, *J. Heterocycl. Chem.* **19**, 463 (1982). Crystal structure determn: M. Sacchetti *et al.*, *J. Pharm. Sci.* **90**, 1049 (2001). Mechanism-based inactivation of dihydropyrimidine dehydrogenase: D. J. T. Porter *et al.*, *J. Biol. Chem.* **267**, 5236 (1992). Prolongs plasma concentration of 5-fluorouracil: D. P. Baccanari *et al.*, *Proc. Natl. Acad. Sci. USA* **90**, 11064 (1993). Clinical safety and efficacy: R. A. Humerickhouse *et al.*, *Clin. Cancer Res.* **5**, 291 (1999). Clinical study with 5-fluorouracil in advanced pancreatic cancer: M. L. Rothenberg *et al.*, *Ann. Oncol.* **13**, 1576 (2002); in metastatic/advanced colorectal cancer: R. L. Schilsky *et al.*, *J. Clin. Oncol.* **20**, 1519 (2002). Review of clinical development: J. A. Hohneker, *Oncology* **12**, 52-56 (1998).

Cream colored solid from methanol-water, mp 320° (dec). d 1.527. uv max (methanol): 284, 225 nm (ε 9450, 10330).

THERAP CAT: Antineoplastic adjunct (chemomodulator).

3585. Enniatins. Ionophore antibiotics produced by the fungus *Fusarium orthoceras* var. *enniatum* and other *Fusaria*: Gaumann *et al.*, *Experientia* **3**, 202 (1947); Plattner, Nager, *ibid.* 325; Plattner *et al.*, *Helv. Chim. Acta* **31**, 594 (1948). They are cyclic depsihexapeptides related structurally to valinomycin, *q.v.* Enniatins A, B, and C are known; A and B are obtained from natural

sources and C is a synthetic homolog. Structure and synthesis of enniatin A: Quitt *et al.*, *ibid.* **46**, 1715 (1963); **47**, 166 (1964); of enniatin B: Plattner *et al.*, *ibid.* **46**, 927 (1963); Shemyakin *et al.*, *Tetrahedron Lett.* **1963**, 885. Conformation of enniatin B: Ovchinnikov *et al.*, *Biochem. Biophys. Res. Commun.* **37**, 668 (1969). Synthesis of C: *eidem*, *Izv. Akad. Nauk SSSR Ser. Khim.* **1964**, 1912, *C.A.* **62**, 28246b (1965). Enniatins are able to form "sandwich" complexes with cations, a factor used to explain their ability to induce permeability in biological membranes to the complexed ion, *cf.* V. T. Ivanov, *Ann. N.Y. Acad. Sci.* **264**, 221 (1975). *Review*: Y. A. Ovchinnikov, V. T. Ivanov, "The Cyclic Peptides: Structure, Conformation, and Function" in *The Proteins* vol. **V**, H. Neurath, R. L. Hill, Eds. (Academic Press, New York, 3rd ed., 1982) pp 365-373, 516-529.

Enniatin A	R = CH(CH₃)CH₂CH₃
Enniatin B	R = CH(CH₃)₂
Enniatin C	R = CH₂CH(CH₃)₂

Enniatin A. $C_{36}H_{63}N_3O_9$; mol wt 681.90. Long needles from ethanol + water, mp 122-122.5°. Very slowly sublimes at 10^{-4} mm and 127-128° (oil bath temp). $[\alpha]_D^{18}$ −91.9° (c = 0.926 in chloroform). Sol in ether, benzene, ethyl acetate; sparingly sol in water. Solns are stable to heat, inactivated by alkali.

Enniatin B. $C_{33}H_{57}N_3O_9$; mol wt 639.82. Crystals from petr ether, mp 175-175.5°. $[\alpha]_D^{20}$ −107.9° (c = 0.63 in chloroform). Very sol in organic solvents; slightly sol in petr ether. Practically insol in water.

Enniatin C. $C_{36}H_{63}N_3O_9$; mol wt 681.90. Crystals, mp 160-161°. $[\alpha]_D^{23}$ −24°.

3586. Enocitabine. [55726-47-1] *N*-(1-β-D-Arabinofuranosyl-1,2-dihydro-2-oxo-4-pyrimidinyl)docosanamide; *N*(4)-behenoyl-1-β-D-arabinofuranosylcytosine; behenoylcytosine arabinoside; BH-AC; NSC-239336; Sunrabin. $C_{31}H_{55}N_3O_6$; mol wt 565.78. C 65.81%, H 9.80%, N 7.43%, O 16.97%. Deriv of cytarabine, *q.v.* Prepn: T. Ishida *et al.*, DE 2426304; *eidem*, US 3991045 (1975, 1976 both to Asahi); M. Akiyama *et al.*, *Chem. Pharm. Bull.* **26**, 981 (1978). Antitumor activity: M. Aoshima *et al.*, *Cancer Res.* **36**, 2726 (1976); *eidem*, *ibid.* **37**, 2481 (1977). Distribution, excretion: M. Fukama *et al.*, *Gan to Kagaku Ryoho* **7**, 2109 (1980), *C.A.* **95**, 35186 (1981). Effect and mode of action: T. Kataoka, Y. Sakurai, *Recent Results Cancer Res.* **70**, 147 (1980). Pharmacological and clinical studies: K. Yamada *et al.*, *ibid.* 219.

Crystals from DMSO, mp 141-142°. $[\alpha]_D$ +70° (c = 1 in THF, 22°). uv max (isopropyl alcohol): 216, 248, 303 nm (ε 16400, 15200, 8200).

THERAP CAT: Antineoplastic.

3587. Enoxacin. [74011-58-8] 1-Ethyl-6-fluoro-1,4-dihydro-4-oxo-7-(1-piperazinyl)-1,8-naphthyridine-3-carboxylic acid; AT-2266; CI-919; PD-107779; Comprecin; Flumark. $C_{15}H_{17}FN_4$-O_3; mol wt 320.32. C 56.24%, H 5.35%, F 5.93%, N 17.49%, O 14.98%. Fluorinated quinolone antibacterial; nalidixic acid analog. Prepn and antibacterial activity: J. Matsumoto *et al.*, **EP 9425**; *eidem*, **US 4352803**; *eidem*, **US 4359578** (1980, 1982, 1982 all to Dainippon and Roger Bellon); J. Matsumoto *et al.*, *J. Med. Chem.* **27,** 292 (1984). HPLC determn in plasma, urine: T. B. Vree *et al.*, *J. Chromatogr.* **343,** 449 (1985). *In vitro* comparison with other quinolones and azaquinolones: S. Selwyn, M. Bakhtiar, *Drugs Exp. Clin. Res.* **10,** 653 (1984). Pharmacokinetics, therapeutic efficacy: K. G. Naber *et al.*, *Infection* **13,** 219 (1985). Efficacy in treatment of urinary tract infections: R. R. Bailey, B. A. Peddie, *N. Z. Med. J.* **98,** 286 (1985). Toxicology studies: H. Senda *et al.*, *Chemotherapy (Tokyo)* **32,** Suppl. 3, 192 (1984). Series of articles on activity, pharmacology, metabolism, early clinical studies: *ibid.* 1-1093; *J. Antimicrob. Chemother.* **14,** Suppl. C, 1-96 (1984); on activity, pharmacokinetics, clinical safety and efficacy: *Infection* **14,** Suppl. 3, S183-S220 (1986).

Crystals from ethanol/methylene chloride, mp 220-224°. LD_{50} in male, female mice, male, female rats (mg/kg): 327, 391, 236, 294 i.v.; 1237, 1320, >2000, >2000 s.c.; all >5000 orally (Senda).

Sesquihydrate. [84294-96-2] Bactidan; Enoxen; Enoxor; Gyramid. $C_{15}H_{17}FN_4O_3.1\frac{1}{2}H_2O$; mol wt 329.33.

THERAP CAT: Antibacterial.

3588. Enoxaparin. Low molecular weight fragment of heparin, *q.v.*, prepd by depolymerization of a benzylic ester of porcine mucosal heparin. The majority of components present a 2-*O*-sulfo-α-L-*threo*-hex-4-enopyranuronic acid structure at the non-reducing end and a 2-*N*,6-*O*-disulfo-D-glucosamine structure at the reducing end of the chain. Average mol wt ~4500 daltons. Prepn: J. Mardiguian, **EP 40144** (1981 to Pharmindustrie), *C.A.* **96,** 218191s (1982). Determn in human plasma: L. Bara *et al.*, *Haemostasis* **17,** 127 (1987). Symposium on pharmacology and clinical efficacy: *ibid.* **16,** 69-188 (1986). Review of pharmacology and use in prevention and treatment of deep venous thrombosis: M. M. Buckley, E. M. Sorkin, *Drugs* **44,** 465-497 (1992); in unstable angina: S. Noble, C. M. Spencer, *ibid.* **56,** 259-272 (1998).

Sodium salt. PK-10169; RP-54563; Clexane; Lovenox.

THERAP CAT: Antithrombotic.

3589. Enoximone. [77671-31-9] 1,3-Dihydro-4-methyl-5-[4-(methylthio)benzoyl]-2*H*-imidazol-2-one; 4-methyl-5-[*p*-(methylthio)benzoyl]-4-imidazolin-2-one; fenoximone; MDL-17043; RMI-17043; Perfane; Perfan. $C_{12}H_{12}N_2O_2S$; mol wt 248.30. C 58.05%, H 4.87%, N 11.28%, O 12.89%, S 12.91%. Selective phosphodiesterase inhibitor with vasodilating and positive inotropic activity. Prepn: **BE 883856** (1980 to Richardson-Merrell); R. A. Schnettler *et al.*, **US 4405635** (1983 to Merrell-Dow); *eidem, J. Med. Chem.* **25,** 1477 (1982). Cardiovascular pharmacology in animals: R. C. Dage *et al.*, *J. Cardiovasc. Pharmacol.* **4,** 500 (1982); L. E. Roebel *et al.*, *ibid.* 721. *In vitro* mechanism of action studies: T. Kariya *et al.*, *ibid.* 509; H. S. Ahn *et al.*, *Biochem. Pharmacol.* **35,** 1113 (1986). Acute hemodynamic effects in congestive heart failure: B. F. Uretsky *et al.*, *Circulation* **67,** 823 (1983). HPLC determn in plasma: K. Y. Chan *et al.*, *J. Chromatogr.* **272,** 396 (1983). Pharmacokinetics in humans: R. G. Alken *et al.*, *Clin. Pharmacol. Ther.* **36,** 209 (1984). Symposium on pharmacology and clinical efficacy in congestive heart failure: *Am. J. Cardiol.* **60,** 1C-90C (1987).

Crystals from isopropanol + water, mp 255-258° (dec).

THERAP CAT: Cardiotonic.

3590. Enoxolone. [471-53-4] (3β,20β)-3-Hydroxy-11-oxo-olean-12-en-29-oic acid; 3β-hydroxy-11-oxoolean-12-en-30-oic acid; glycyrrhetic acid; 18β-glycyrrhetinic acid; uralenic acid; Arthrodont; Biosone; P.O. 12. $C_{30}H_{46}O_4$; mol wt 470.68. C 76.55%, H 9.85%, O 13.60%. From glycyrrhizic acid, *q.v.* Structure: Ruzicka *et al.*, *Helv. Chim. Acta* **26,** 2143, 2278 (1943). Stereochemistry: Beaton, Spring, *J. Chem. Soc.* **1955,** 3126. Prepn from shredded licorice root: Mer, *Am. Perfum. Aromat.* **74**(6), 39 (1959). Manuf: **GB 833184** (1960 to Carlo Erba). Identity with uralenic acid: Belous *et al.*, *Zh. Obshch. Khim.* **35,** 401 (1965). Metabolism: Parke *et al.*, *J. Pharm. Pharmacol.* **15,** 500 (1963). Mechanism of action: Helbing, Berntsen, *Pharm. Weekbl.* **100,** 1438 (1965).

Needles from alcohol + petr ether, mp 296°. $[\alpha]_D^{21}$ +86° (alc); $[\alpha]_D^{20}$ +145.5° (dioxane); $[\alpha]_D^{20}$ +163° (chloroform). Freely sol in chloroform, dioxane. Soluble in alcohol, pyridine, acetic acid. Practically insol in petr ether.

18α-Hydrogen Form. Platelets from dil alcohol, mp 335°. $[\alpha]_D^{20}$ +140° (alcohol); $[\alpha]_D$ +98° (c = 0.1 in chloroform). Sol in alcohol, dioxane, chloroform.

THERAP CAT: Anti-inflammatory (topical).

3591. Enprostil. [73121-56-9] *rel*-7-[(1*R*,2*R*,3*R*)-3-Hydroxy-2-[(1*E*,3*R*)-3-hydroxy-4-phenoxy-1-butenyl]-5-oxocyclopentyl]-4,5-heptadienoic acid methyl ester; (*dl*)-9-keto-11α,15α-dihydroxy-16-phenoxy-17,18,19,20-tetranorprosta-4,5,13-*trans*-trienoic acid methyl ester; RS-84135; Camleed; Gardrin(e). $C_{23}H_{28}$-O_6; mol wt 400.46. C 68.98%, H 7.05%, O 23.97%. Prostaglandin E_2 derivative with antisecretory activity. Prepn: A. R. Van Horn *et al.*, **US 4178457** (1979 to Syntex). Pharmacokinetics: D. R. Stanski *et al.*, *Clin. Pharmacol. Ther.* **31,** 273 (1982). Cytoprotective effect against aspirin-induced gastromucosal injury in humans: M. M. Cohen *et al.*, *Gastroenterology* **88,** 382 (1985). Clinical comparison with cimetidine of antisecretory and antigastrin activity in duodenal ulcer: V. Mahachai *et al.*, *ibid.* **89,** 555 (1985); of efficacy in ulcer healing: L. Carling *et al.*, *Scand. J. Gastroenterol.* **22,** 325 (1987). Series of articles on pharmacology, clinical efficacy and safety: *Am. J. Med.* **81,** Suppl. 2A, 1-88 (1986).

White to off-white waxy solid. Softens at 30°, liquid at 46°. Very slightly sol in water. Sol in alcohol, propylene glycol, propylene carbonate. uv max (methanol): 220, 265, 271, 277 nm (log ε 4.01, 3.14, 3.24, 3.16).

THERAP CAT: Antiulcerative.

3592. Enrofloxacin. [93106-60-6] 1-Cyclopropyl-7-(4-ethyl-1-piperazinyl)-6-fluoro-1,4-dihydro-4-oxo-3-quinolinecarboxylic acid; CFPQ; Bay Vp 2674; Baytril. $C_{19}H_{22}FN_3O_3$; mol wt 359.39. C 63.50%, H 6.17%, F 5.29%, N 11.69%, O 13.36%. Fluorinated quinolone antibacterial. Prepn: K. Grohe et al., **DE 3142854**; eidem, **US 4670444** (1983, 1987 both to Bayer AG); K. Grohe, H. Heitzer, Ann. **1987**, 29. Use as plant fungicide: K. Grohe et al., **US 4563459** (1986 to Bayer AG). Pharmacokinetics in calves: J. N. Davidson et al., Proc. West. Pharmacol. Soc. **29**, 129 (1986); in chickens: G. M. Conzelman et al., ibid. **30**, 393 (1987). Spectrofluorometric determn of residues in poultry tissues: T. B. Waggoner, M. C. Bowman, J. Assoc. Off. Anal. Chem. **70**, 813 (1987). Toxicology and physical properties: P. Altreuther, Vet. Med. Rev. **2**, 87 (1987). Series of articles on pharmacology, in vitro antibacterial activity and field trials: ibid. 90-140.

Pale yellow crystals, mp 219-221°. Slightly sol in water at pH 7. LD_{50} in male, female mice (mg/kg): >5000, 4336 orally; ~200, ~200 i.v.; in male rats, male rabbits (mg/kg): >5000, 500-800 orally (Altreuther).

THERAP CAT (VET): Antibacterial.

3593. Ensulizole. [27503-81-7] 2-Phenyl-1H-benzimidazole-5-sulfonic acid; phenylbenzimidazole sulfonic acid; Eusolex 232; Neo Heliopan Hydro; Parsol HS. $C_{13}H_{10}N_2O_3S$; mol wt 274.30. C 56.92%, H 3.67%, N 10.21%, O 17.50%, S 11.69%. UV-B filter in sunscreens and cosmetics. Synergistic increase in SPF occurs in combination with oil-soluble UV absorbers. Prepn: V. G. Sayapin et al., Khim. Geterotsikl. Soedin. **5**, 681 (1970), C.A. **73**, 45409p (1970). See also: U. Heywang et al., **US 5473079** (1995 to Merck Patent GmbH). DNA photosensitization study: C. Stevenson, R. J. H. Davies, Chem. Res. Toxicol. **12**, 38 (1999). Photochemical studies: J. J. Inbaraj et al., Photochem. Photobiol. **75**, 107 (2002). Fluorometric determn in urine: M. T. Vidal et al., Talanta **59**, 591 (2003). Complexation with cyclodextrins: S. Scalia et al., Eur. J. Pharm. Sci. **22**, 241 (2004).

mp 410° (dec). Absorption max (phosphate buffer, pH 7.4): 300 nm. Soly in water: ~0.03%.

Sodium salt. [5997-53-5] $C_{13}H_9N_2NaO_3S$; mol wt 296.28. Soly: water >30%; 1,2-propylene glycol >20%.

THERAP CAT: Ultraviolet screen.

3594. Entacapone. [130929-57-6] (2E)-2-Cyano-3-(3,4-dihydroxy-5-nitrophenyl)-N,N-diethyl-2-propenamide; (E)-α-cyano-N,N-diethyl-3,4-dihydroxy-5-nitrocinnamamide; (E)-2-cyano-N,N-diethyl-3-(3,4-dihydroxy-5-nitrophenyl)acrylamide; OR-611; Comtan; Comtess. $C_{14}H_{15}N_3O_5$; mol wt 305.29. C 55.08%, H 4.95%, N 13.76%, O 26.20%. Peripherally acting inhibitor of catechol-O-methyl transferase (COMT), an enzyme involved in the metabolism of catecholamine neurotransmitters and related drugs. Prepn (stereochemistry unspecified): R. J. Bäckström et al., **DE 3740383**; eidem, **US 5446194** (1988, 1995 both to Orion). Prepn of (E)-isomer: A. K. Pippuri et al., **EP 426468**; eidem, **US 5135950** (1991, 1992 both to Orion). Pharmacology: E. Nissinen et al., Arch. Pharmacol. **346**, 262 (1992). LC determn in plasma and urine: M. Karlsson, T. Wikberg, J. Pharm. Biomed. Anal. **10**, 593 (1992).

Identification of metabolites: T. Wikberg et al., Eur. J. Drug Metab. Pharmacokinet. **18**, 359 (1993). Clinical pharmacokinetics: T. Keränen et al., Eur. J. Clin. Pharmacol. **46**, 151 (1994). Clinical effect on levodopa bioavailability in Parkinson's disease: H. M. Routtinen, U. K. Rinne, J. Neurol. Neurosurg. Psychiatry **60**, 36 (1996).

Crystals from acetic acid + HCl, mp 162-163°. pKa ~4.5.

THERAP CAT: Antiparkinsonian.

3595. Entecavir. [142217-69-4] 2-Amino-1,9-dihydro-9-[(1S,3R,4S)-4-hydroxy-3-(hydroxymethyl)-2-methylenecyclopentyl]-6H-purin-6-one. $C_{12}H_{15}N_5O_3$; mol wt 277.28. C 51.98%, H 5.45%, N 25.26%, O 17.31%. Deoxyguanine nucleoside analog; inhibits hepatitis B virus (HBV) DNA polymerase. Prepn: R. Zahler, W. A. Slusarchyk, **EP 481754**; eidem, **US 5206244** (1992, 1993 both to Squibb); G. S. Bisacchi et al., Bioorg. Med. Chem. Lett. **7**, 127 (1997). In vitro antiviral activity: S. F. Innaimo et al, Antimicrob. Agents Chemother. **41**, 1444 (1997). Review of pharmacology and clinical experience: P. Honkoop, R. A. de Man, Expert Opin. Invest. Drugs **12**, 683-688 (2003); T. Shaw, S. Locarnini, Expert Rev. Anti Infect. Ther. **2**, 853-871 (2004). Clinical comparisons with lamivudine in chronic hepatitis B: T.-T. Chang et al., N. Engl. J. Med. **354**, 1001 (2006); C.-L. Lai et al., ibid. 1011.

Monohydrate. [209216-23-9] BMS-200475; SQ-200475; Baraclude. $C_{12}H_{15}N_5O_3 \cdot H_2O$; mol wt 295.29. White to off-white powder, mp >220°. $[\alpha]_D$ +35.0° (c = 0.38 in water). Soly in water: 2.4 mg/ml. pH of saturated soln in water is 7.9 at 25°±0.5°.

THERAP CAT: Antiviral.

3596. Enterobactin. [28384-96-5] N,N',N''-(2,6,10-Trioxo-1,5,9-trioxacyclododecane-3,7,11-triyl)tris[2,3-dihydroxy]benzamide; N,N',N''-(2,6,10-trioxo-1,5,9-trioxacyclododecane-3,7,11-triyl)tris-o-pyrocatechuamide; enterochelin. $C_{30}H_{27}N_3O_{15}$; mol wt 669.55. C 53.82%, H 4.06%, N 6.28%, O 35.84%. Physiologically active macrocyclic iron sequestering agent of the phenolate type, involved in microbial transport and metabolism of iron; it is overproduced by E. coli and related enteric bacteria under low-iron stress. Isoln from culture medium of Salmonella typhimurium LT2 and structure: J. R. Pollack, J. B. Neilands, Biochem. Biophys. Res. Commun. **38**, 989 (1970); also produced by Escherichia coli and Aerobacter aerogenes: I. G. O'Brien, F. Gibson, Biochim. Biophys. Acta **215**, 393 (1970). Conformation: M. Leinás et al., Biochemistry **12**, 3836 (1973). Total synthesis: E. J. Corey, S. Bhattacharyya, Tetrahedron Lett. **1977**, 3919. Synthesis of enterobactin and enantioenterobactin: W. H. Rastetter et al., J. Org. Chem. **45**, 5011 (1980); **46**, 3579 (1981). Biosynthetic study: J. R. Pollack et al., J. Bacteriol. **104**, 635 (1970). Stability constants and electrochemical behavior of ferric enterobactin: K. N. Raymond, J. Am. Chem. Soc. **101**, 6097 (1979). Kinetics and mechanism of iron removal from transferrin: C. J. Carrano et al., ibid. 5401. Review: J. B. Neilands in Inorg. Biochem. **1**, G. Eichorn, Ed. (Elsevier, New York, 1973) pp 167-202; idem, Bioinorg. Chem. **II**, K. N. Raymond, Ed. (A.C.S., Washington, 1977) pp 3-33.

Crystals from ethanol/water, mp 202-203°. $[\alpha]_D^{25}$ +7.40° (ethanol). uv max (ethyl acetate): 316 nm (ε 9390). Sol in acetone, dioxane, dimethyl sulfoxide, methanol. Practically insol in water, soly increases at pH 7 to 8. Neutral on paper electrophoresis at pH 5. Displays bright blue fluorescence under uv light.

Ferric enterobactin. $[C_{30}H_{21}FeN_3O_{15}]^{3-}$. Anionic complex of enterobactin. uv max: 495 nm (ε 5600).

USE: As a growth-promoting agent in various organisms.

3597. Enterogastrone. [9007-67-4] Anthelone E; enteroanthelone; Duosan; Ileogastrone. An inhibitor of gastric secretion, apparently different from urogastrone. Obtained from extracts of the intestinal mucosa of mammals: Gray, Ivy, *Cold Spring Harbor Symp. Quant. Biol.* **5,** 405 (1937); Ivy, Greengard, US 2477541 (1949 to Research Corp.). Comparison with urogastrone: Friedman, *Vitam. Horm.* **9,** 313 (1951); Gregory, *J. Physiol.* **129,** 528 (1955).

Amorphous buff-colored powder. Freely sol in water.

THERAP CAT: Gastric secretion inhibitor.

3598. Enterolactone. [78473-71-9] (3*R*,4*R*)-*rel*-Dihydro-3,4-bis[(3-hydroxyphenyl)methyl]-2(3*H*)-furanone; *trans*-(±)-2,3-bis(3'-hydroxybenzyl)-γ-butyrolactone; HPMF; HBBL; compd 180/442. $C_{18}H_{18}O_4$; mol wt 298.33. C 72.47%, H 6.08%, O 21.45%. Phenolic compound having 2,3-dibenzylbutane skeleton. First lignan, *q.v.*, found in animal species. Determn in female urine from humans, vervet monkeys and characterization: S. R. Stitch *et al., Nature* **287,** 738 (1980); K. D. R. Setchell *et al., ibid.* 740. Structure determn by GC-MS: *eidem, Biochem. J.* **197,** 447 (1981); *eidem, Biomed. Mass Spectrom.* **10,** 227 (1983). ^{1}H-NMR, X-ray crystal structure: G. Cooley *et al., J. Chem. Soc. Perkin Trans. 1* **1984,** 489. Synthesis: M. B. Groen, J. Leemhuis, *Tetrahedron Lett.* **21,** 5043 (1980); G. Cooley *et al., ibid.* **22,** 349 (1981); A. Pelter *et al., ibid.* 1549; P. A. Ganeshpure, R. Stevenson, *Chem. Ind. (London)* **1981,** 778; A. Pelter *et al., J. Chem. Soc. Perkin Trans. 1* **1983,** 643. Lignan excretion peaks during luteal phase of menstrual cycle: K. D. R. Setchell *et al., J. Steroid Biochem.* **12,** 375 (1980). Excretion as glucuronide conjugate: M. Axelson, K. D. R. Setchell, *FEBS Lett.* **122,** 49 (1980). Biosynthesis by intestinal bacteria: *eidem, ibid.* **123,** 337 (1981). Effect of diet on lignan excretion: H. Aldercreutz *et al., Med. Biol.* **59,** 337 (1981).

Gum, mp 141-143°. uv max (ethanol): 227, 261 nm (log ε 4.66, 4.64).

3599. Entprol. [102-60-3] 1,1',1'',1'''-(1,2-Ethanediyldinitrilo)tetrakis[2-propanol]; 1,1',1'',1'''-(ethylenedinitrilo)tetra-2-propanol; *N,N,N',N'*-tetrakis(2-hydroxypropyl)ethylenediamine; Quad-rol. $C_{14}H_{32}N_2O_4$; mol wt 292.41. C 57.50%, H 11.03%, N 9.58%, O 21.89%. $[CH_3CH(OH)CH_2]_2NCH_2CH_2N[CH_2CH(OH)CH_3]_2$. Prepd by the action of propylene oxide on ethylenediamine: Lundsted, Schulz, US 2697118 (1954 to Wyandotte).

Viscous liq. bp$_{1.0}$ 190°. Miscible with water. Sol in methanol, ethanol, toluene, ethylene glycol, perchloroethylene.

USE: Cross-linking agent and catalyst in the manuf of urethan foams; in epoxy resin curing; as complexing agent, humectant, emulsifier, plasticizer.

3600. Enviomycin. [33103-22-9] Tuberactinomycin N; (*R*)-1-[(3*R*,4*R*)-4-hydroxy-3,6-diaminohexanoic acid]-6-[L-2-(2-amino-1,4,5,6-tetrahydro-4-pyrimidinyl)glycine]viomycin. $C_{25}H_{43}N_{13}$-O_{10}; mol wt 685.69. C 43.79%, H 6.32%, N 26.56%, O 23.33%. Polypeptide antibiotic produced by a mutant of *Streptomyces griseoverticillatus* var. *tuberacticus*. Isoln and characterization: T. Ando *et al., J. Antibiot.* **24,** 680 (1971); A. Nagata *et al.,* in *Advan. Antimicrob. Antineopl. Chemother.* **vol. 1/2,** M. Hejzlar *et al.,* Eds. (University Park Press, Baltimore, 1972) pp 1039-1041. Prepn: J. Abe *et al.,* DE 2133181; *eidem,* US 3892732 (1972, 1975 both to Toyo Brewing Co., Ltd.). Structural studies: H. Yoshioka *et al., Tetrahedron Lett.* **1971,** 2043; T. Wakamiya, T. Shiba, *J. Antibiot.* **28,** 292 (1975). Pharmacology: H. Hamakawa *et al., Oyo Yakuri* **8,** 817 (1974), *C.A.* **82,** 51530y (1975). Metabolism: T. Shimizu *et al., Jpn. J. Antibiot.* **27,** 279 (1974). Total synthesis: T. Shiba *et al., J. Antibiot.* **32,** 1078 (1979).

Hydrochloride. $C_{25}H_{43}N_{13}O_{10}$.3HCl. White crystalline powder, mp >245° (dec). $[\alpha]_D^{21}$ −19.1°. uv max (water, 0.1*N* HCl): 268 nm (E$_{1cm}^{1\%}$ 342); uv max (0.1*N* NaOH): 288 nm (E$_{1cm}^{1\%}$ 215). Very sol in water, slightly sol in methanol, ethanol. Insol in common organic solvents.

Sulfate. Tuberactin. $C_{50}H_{92}N_{26}O_{32}S_3$; mol wt 1665.62. White crystalline powder. Very sol in water, slightly sol in usual organic solvents. LD$_{50}$ in mice, rats (mg/kg): 485, 680 i.v. (Hamakawa).

THERAP CAT: Antibacterial (tuberculostatic).

3601. Enviroxime. [72301-79-2] 6-[(Hydroxyimino)phenylmethyl]-1-[(1-methylethyl)sulfonyl]-1*H*-benzimidazol-2-amine; (*E*)-2-amino-6-benzoyl-1-(isopropylsulfonyl)benzimidazole oxime; *anti*-2-amino-1-(isopropylsulfonyl)-6-(α-hydroxyiminobenzyl)-benzimidazole; LY-122772. $C_{17}H_{18}N_4O_3S$; mol wt 358.41. C 56.97%, H 5.06%, N 15.63%, O 13.39%, S 8.95%. Benzimidazole deriv that inhibits rhinovirus multiplication. Prepn: C. J. Paget *et al.,* DE 2638551; *eidem,* US 4118742 (1977, 1978 both to Lilly). Synthesis and sepn of *syn* and *anti* isomers: J. H. Wikel *et al., J. Med. Chem.* **23,** 368 (1980). Inhibition of rhinovirus replication in organ culture: D. C. De Long, S. E. Reed, *J. Infect. Dis.* **141,** 87 (1980). Metabolic studies: J. F. Quay *et al., Fed. Proc.* **39,** 3079 (1980); C. J. Parli *et al., ibid.* 214. Activity vs rhinovirus infection in man: R. J. Phillpotts *et al., Lancet* **1,** 1342 (1981). Prophylactic activity: F. G. Haden, J. M. Gwaltney, *Antimicrob. Agents Chemother.* **21,** 892 (1982).

Cryst from acetonitrile, mp 198-199°. uv max (methanol): 218, 290 nm (ε 45600, 27100).

(Z)-isomer. Zinviroxime. Cryst from methanol, mp 182-183°. uv max (methanol): 254, 285 nm (ε 20800, 13200).

3602. Eosine I Bluish. [548-24-3] 4′,5′-Dibromo-3′,6′-dihydroxy-2′,7′-dinitrospiro[isobenzofuran-1(3H),9′-[9H]xanthen]-3-one disodium salt; 4′,5′-dibromo-2′,7′-dinitrofluorescein disodium salt; hydroxydibromodinitro-o-carboxyphenylfluorone sodium; C.I. Acid Red 91; C.I. 45400. $C_{20}H_6Br_2N_2Na_2O_9$; mol wt 624.06. C 38.49%, H 0.97%, Br 25.61%, N 4.49%, Na 7.37%, O 23.07%. Prepd by nitration of 4′,5′-dibromofluorescein: *Colour Index* vol. 4 (3rd ed., 1971) p 4427.

Red powder. Freely sol in water with green fluorescence; sol in alc.

USE: Dyeing wool, cotton, and paper. In histology as a stain for epithelia, muscular fibers, nuclei, etc.

3603. Eosine Yellowish —(YS). [17372-87-1] 2′,4′,5′,7′-Tetrabromo-3′,6′-dihydroxyspiro[isobenzofuran-1(3H),9′-[9H]xanthen]-3-one disodium salt; 2′,4′,5′,7′-tetrabromofluorescein; bromoeosine; tetrabromofluorescein sol; bromofluoresceic acid; eosin; eosine; eosin Y; D & C Red No. 22; C.I. Acid Red 87; C.I. 45380. $C_{20}H_6Br_4Na_2O_5$; mol wt 691.85. C 34.72%, H 0.87%, Br 46.20%, Na 6.65%, O 11.56%. Xanthene dye capable of photodynamic generation of singlet oxygen. Prepd by bromination of fluorescein: *Colour Index* vol. 4 (3rd ed., 1971) p 4426. Photodynamic injury to leaf tissue and inhibition of photosynthesis: J. P. Knox, A. D. Dodge, *Planta* 164, 22; 30 (1985). *Review: H. J. Conn's Biological Stains*, R. D. Lillie, Ed. (Williams & Wilkins, Baltimore, 9th ed., 1977), pp 342-344.

Red crystals with bluish tinge, or brownish-red powder. Freely sol in water, less in alcohol. Insol in ether. The concd aq soln is deep brownish-red, the dilute (1:500) soln is yellowish-red with greenish fluorescence; the alcoholic soln exhibits a strong green fluorescence.

Free acid. Eosine acid; D & C Red No. 21; C.I. Solvent Red 43; C.I. 45380:2. $C_{20}H_8Br_4O_5$. Bright yellowish red. Sol in acetone, ethanol. Insol in mineral oil, toluene.

USE: In microbiological differential media. Colorant in drugs and cosmetics such as lipstick and nail-polish; dyeing wool, silk and paper; in red inks; as biological stain.

3604. Eotaxin. Chemoattractant protein that is highly selective for eosinophils. Member of the family of proinflammatory substances known as CC (or β-) chemokines. Purification and proposed role in allergic asthma: D. A. Griffiths-Johnson *et al., Biochem. Biophys. Res. Commun.* 197, 1167 (1993); P. J. Jose *et al., J. Exp. Med.* 179, 881 (1994). Cloning of guinea pig eotaxin: *idem et al., Biochem. Biophys. Res. Commun.* 205, 788 (1994); of human eotaxin: P. D. Ponath *et al., J. Clin. Invest.* 97, 604 (1996). Cloning of the eosinophil eotaxin receptor (CKR-3): B. L. Daugherty *et al., J. Exp. Med.* 183, 2349 (1996); P. D. Ponath *et al., ibid.* 2437. Discussion of role in allergic inflammation: H. Kita, G. J. Gleich, *ibid.* 2421-2426.

3605. Epalrestat. [82159-09-9] (5Z)-5-[(2E)-2-Methyl-3-phenyl-2-propenylidene]-4-oxo-2-thioxo-3-thiazolidineacetic acid; 5-[(E,E)-β-methylcinnamylidene]-4-oxo-2-thioxo-3-thiazolidineacetic acid; 3-carboxymethyl-5-(2-methylcinnamylidene)rhodanine; ONO-2235; Kinedak; Sorbistat. $C_{15}H_{13}NO_3S_2$; mol wt 319.40. C 56.41%, H 4.10%, N 4.39%, O 15.03%, S 20.08%. Aldose reductase inhibitor. Prepn: T. Tadao *et al., EP 47109; eidem, US 4464382* (1982, 1984 both to Ono Pharmaceutical). Inhibitory effect on aldose reductase *in vitro*: H. Terashima *et al., J. Pharmacol. Exp. Ther.* 229, 226 (1983). Effect on motor nerve conduction and sorbitol levels in diabetic rats: R. Kikkawa *et al., Diabetologia* 24, 290 (1983). Effect in rats on peripheral nerve dysfunction: *eidem, Metabolism* 33, 212 (1984); on retinal microangiopathy: K. Kojima *et al., Jpn. J. Ophthalmol.* 29, 99 (1985).

Crystals from ethanol-water, mp 210-217°.
N-Methyl-D-glucamine salt. $C_{22}H_{30}N_2O_8S_2$. Crystals from methanol, mp 163-165°.
THERAP CAT: Treatment of diabetic neuropathy.

3606. Eperisone. [64840-90-0] 1-(4-Ethylphenyl)-2-methyl-3-(1-piperidinyl)-1-propanone; 4′-ethyl-2-methyl-3-piperidinopropiophenone. $C_{17}H_{25}NO$; mol wt 259.39. C 78.72%, H 9.71%, N 5.40%, O 6.17%. Spasmolytic agent related structurally to tolperisone, *q.v.* Prepn: E. Morita *et al., DE 2458638*; E. Morita, T. Kanai, *US 4181803* (1975, 1980 both to Eisai). Pharmacological study: K. Tanaka *et al., Nippon Yakurigaku Zasshi* 77, 511 (1981), *C.A.* 95, 35471t (1981). Absorption, distribution, excretion in rats and guinea pigs: T. Fujita *et al., Oyo Yakuri* 21, 835 (1981), *C.A.* 96, 28193w (1982). Toxicity study: H. Miyagawa *et al., ibid.* 939, *C.A.* 96, 79722a (1982).

Hydrochloride. [56839-43-1] EMPP; E-646; Mional; Myonal. $C_{17}H_{25}NO.HCl$; mol wt 295.85. Needles from isopropanol, mp 170-172°. LD_{50} in male S.D. rats, Wistar rats, mice (mg/kg): 1300, 1850, 1024 orally (Miyagawa).
THERAP CAT: Muscle relaxant (skeletal).

3607. Ephedra. Ma Huang. Stems and leaves of *Ephedra equisetina* Bunge, *Ephedraceae, E. sinica* Stapf. and other *Ephedra* species. *Habit.* China, India, Europe. *Constit.* 0.75-1% ephedrine, pseudoephedrine, norpseudoephedrine, N-methylephedrine, *q.q.v.*, (+)-N-methylpseudoephedrine, (−)-norephedrine. Used in traditional Chinese medicine as a diaphoretic, stimulant, and antiasthmatic. Brief description: V. E. Tyler in *The Honest Herbal* (Pharmaceutical Products Press, New York, 3rd ed., 1993) pp 119-121. Pharmacology of psychoactive alkaloids: P. Kalix, *J. Ethnopharmacol.* 32, 201 (1991). GC determn of alkaloids in Ma Huang preparations: J. M. Betz *et al., J. AOAC Int.* 80, 303 (1997). Review of cardiovascular and CNS effects of weight-loss supplements containing ephedra: C. A. Haller, N. L. Benowitz, *N. Engl. J. Med.* 343, 1833-1838 (2000). Review of clinical experience: S. R. Mehendale *et al., Am. J. Chin. Med.* 32, 1-10 (2004).

Morman Tea. Brigham tea; teamsters' tea; popotillo; whorehouse tea. Fresh or dried stems of *Ephedra nevadensis* Wats., *Ephedraceae,* a North American species, generally considered to be alkaloid free. Used by early American settlers as a remedy for venereal disease, colds and kidney disorders. Brief description: V. E. Tyler, *loc. cit.,* 215-216.

3608. Ephedrine. [299-42-3] (αR)-α-[(1S)-1-(Methylamino)ethyl]benzenemethanol; (1R,2S)-2-methylamino-1-phenylpropan-1-ol; L-*erythro*-2-(methylamino)-1-phenylpropan-1-ol; *l*-ephedrine. $C_{10}H_{15}NO$; mol wt 165.23. C 72.69%, H 9.15%, N

8.48%, O 9.68%. α- and β-Adrenergic agonist. Occurs in plants of the genus *Ephedra* (Ephedraceae) known in traditional medicine as Ma Huang. Isoln from *E. vulgaris:* Nagai, *Chem. Zentralbl.* **59**, 130 (1888). Syntheses: E. Späth, R. Göhring, *Monatsh. Chem.* **41**, 319 (1920); R. H. F. Manske, T. B. Johnson, *J. Am. Chem. Soc.* **51**, 580, 1906 (1929). Stereochemistry: K. Freudenberg *et al., ibid.* **54**, 234 (1932); K. Freudenberg, F. Nikolai, *Ann.* **510**, 223 (1934). Properties of crystalline forms: E. E. Moore, D. L. Tabern, *J. Am. Pharm. Assoc.* **24**, 211 (1935). Symposium on sympathomimetic agents: *Ind. Eng. Chem.* **37**, 116-148 (1945). Toxicity: M. D. Fairchild, G. A. Alles, *J. Pharmacol. Exp. Ther.* **158**, 135 (1967). Electrophoretic determn in urine: M. Chicharro *et al., J. Chromatogr.* **622**, 103 (1993). HPLC determn in Ma Huang: B. J. Gurley *et al., J. Pharm. Sci.* **87**, 1547 (1998). Clinical pharmacokinetics of botanical ephedrine: *eidem, Ther. Drug Monit.* **20**, 439 (1998). Review of use as bronchodilator: M. M. Weinberger, *Pediatr. Clin. North Am.* **22**, 121-127 (1975).

Waxy solid, crystals or granules. Gradually dec on exposure to light. Anhyd material is hygroscopic, mp 38.1°. Also occurs as the hemihydrate, mp 40°. bp$_{745}$ 260°. Sol in water, alcohol, chloroform, ether. *Keep well closed in a cool place.*

Hydrochloride. [50-98-6] Caniphedrin. $C_{10}H_{15}NO.HCl$; mol wt 201.69. Fine, white, odorless crystals or powder, affected by light, mp 217-220°. $[\alpha]_D^{25}$ −33 to −35.5° (c = 5). Freely sol in water; sol in alcohol. Practically insol in ether.

Sulfate. [134-72-5] Isofedrol. $(C_{10}H_{15}NO)_2.H_2SO_4$; mol wt 428.54. Fine, white, odorless crystals or powder. Darkens on exposure to light. mp 245° (dec). $[\alpha]_D^{25}$ −30 to −32.5° (c = 5). Freely sol in water; sparingly sol in alcohol.

dl-**Form.** [90-81-3] Racemic ephedrine; racephedrine. Crystals from chloroform-petr ether, mp 75°. Sol in water, alcohol, ether, chloroform, etc.

dl-**Form hydrochloride.** [134-71-4] Racephedrine hydrochloride. Crystals from alcohol-acetone, mp 189°. One gram dissolves in 4 ml water, in about 40 ml of 95% alc at 20°. Practically insol in ether. pH about 6.

(+)-***threo*-Form** see Pseudoephedrine.

THERAP CAT: Bronchodilator.

THERAP CAT (VET): Bronchodilator; in treatment of urinary incontinence.

3609. Epiandrosterone. [481-29-8] (3β,5α)-3-Hydroxyandrostan-17-one; 3β-hydroxy-17-androstanone; isoandrosterone; 3β-androstanol-17-one; 3β-hydroxyetioallocholan-17-one. $C_{19}H_{30}O_2$; mol wt 290.44. C 78.57%, H 10.41%, O 11.02%. Present in normal human urine as a minor constituent, it is a less active androgen than androsterone. Synthesis: Cardwell *et al., J. Chem. Soc.* **1953**, 361; Johnson *et al., J. Am. Chem. Soc.* **75**, 2275 (1953); Johnson *et al., ibid.* **78**, 6331 (1956). *Review:* R. I. Dorfman, R. A. Shipley, *Androgens* (Wiley, New York, 1956).

dl-**Form.** Crystals, mp 161-162°. Gives off a musk-like odor when hot.

d-**Form.** Crystals from ethyl acetate + petr ether, mp 174.5°. $[\alpha]_D^{20}$ +88° (in methanol). Precipitated by digitonin. Practically insol in water. Soluble in organic solvents.

Acetate. $C_{21}H_{32}O_3$. Stout prisms, mp 103-104°. $[\alpha]_D^{18}$ +68.5° (chloroform).

Benzoate. $C_{26}H_{34}O_3$. Crystals, mp 210-212°.

3610. Epibatidine. [140111-52-0] (1R,2R,4S)-2-(6-Chloro-3-pyridinyl)-7-azabicyclo[2.2.1]heptane. $C_{11}H_{13}ClN_2$; mol wt 208.69. C 63.31%, H 6.28%, Cl 16.99%, N 13.42%. First naturally occurring non-opioid, organochlorine, alkaloid analgesic; isolated from skin of the Ecuadoran poison frog, *Epipedobates tricolor.* Isoln and structural determn: T. F. Spande *et al., J. Am. Chem. Soc.* **114**, 3475 (1992). First natural product identified which contains the 7-azabicyclo[2.2.1]heptane ring system. Synthesis of (±)-form: C. A. Broka, *Tetrahedron Lett.* **1993**, 3251.

Basic, relatively polar, colorless oil. uv max (methanol): 217 nm, shoulder 250-280 nm.

3611. Epichlorohydrin. [106-89-8] Chloromethyloxirane; *dl*-α-epichlorohydrin; 1-chloro-2,3-epoxypropane; γ-chloropropylene oxide. C_3H_5ClO; mol wt 92.52. C 38.95%, H 5.45%, Cl 38.32%, O 17.29%. Prepn: H. T. Clarke, W. W. Hartman, *Org. Synth.* **coll. vol. I**, 233 (2nd ed., 1941); G. Braun, *ibid.* **coll. vol. II**, 256 (1943). Manuf: *Faith, Keyes & Clark's Industrial Chemicals*, F. A. Lowenheim, M. K. Moran, Eds. (Wiley-Interscience, New York, 4th ed., 1975) pp 335-338. Toxicity data: H. F. Smyth, C. P. Carpenter, *J. Ind. Hyg. Toxicol.* **30**, 63 (1948).

Liquid. d_4^{20} 1.1812; d_4^{25} 1.1750; d_4^{50} 1.1436; d_4^{75} 1.1101. bp$_{760}$ 117.9°; bp$_{400}$ 98.0°; bp$_{200}$ 79.3°; bp$_{100}$ 62.0°; bp$_{40}$ 42.0°; bp$_{10}$ 16.6°; bp$_{1.0}$ −16.5°. mp −25.6°. $n_D^{11.6}$ 1.44195; n_D^{16} 1.43969; n_D^{25} 1.43585. Flash pt, open cup: 105°F (40°C). Insol in water. Misc with alcohol, ether, chloroform, trichloroethylene, carbon tetrachloride; immiscible with petr hydrocarbons. LD$_{50}$ orally in rats: 0.09 g/kg (Smyth, Carpenter).

Caution: Potential symptoms of overexposure are nausea, vomiting; abdominal pain; respiratory distress, coughing; cyanosis; irritation of eyes and skin with deep pain; reproductive effects. *See NIOSH Pocket Guide to Chemical Hazards* (DHHS/NIOSH 97-140, 1997) p 128. *See also Patty's Industrial Hygiene and Toxicology* **vol. 2A**, G. D. Clayton, F. E. Clayton, Eds. (Wiley-Interscience, New York, 3rd ed., 1981) pp 2242-2247. This substance is reasonably anticipated to be a human carcinogen: *Report on Carcinogens, Eleventh Edition* (PB2005-104914, 2004) p III-113.

USE: Solvent for natural and synthetic resins, gums, cellulose esters and ethers, paints, varnishes, nail enamels and lacquers, cement for Celluloid. As stabilizer.

3612. Epicholestanol. [516-95-0] (3α,5α)-Cholestan-3-ol; 3α-hydroxycholestane; ε-cholestanol. $C_{27}H_{48}O$; mol wt 388.67. C 83.44%, H 12.45%, O 4.12%. The 3α-hydroxy epimer of cholestanol. Prepn from cholestanone: Ruzicka, *Helv. Chim. Acta* **17**, 1407 (1934); *cf.* Marker, *et al., J. Am. Chem. Soc.* **57**, 2359 (1935); Barnett *et al., J. Chem. Soc.* **1940**, 1390.

Needles from alcohol, mp 185-186°. $[\alpha]_D^{20}$ +34° (c = 1.7 in chloroform). Less sol than cholestanol. Not precipitated by digitonin.

Acetate. $C_{29}H_{50}O_2$. mp 95.5-96°. Crystals from methanol.

Benzoate. $C_{34}H_{52}O_2$. mp 102-103°. $[\alpha]_{546}$ +27.2° in chloroform.

3613. Epicholesterol. [474-77-1] (3α)-Cholest-5-en-3-ol. $C_{27}H_{46}O$; mol wt 386.65. C 83.87%, H 11.99%, O 4.14%. The 3α-hydroxy epimer of cholesterol. Prepd from 8-oxocholesteryl chloride or from cholest-5-en-3-one or by passing O_2 into a soln of cholesteryl Mg chloride: Ruzicka, Goldberg, *Helv. Chim. Acta* **19**, 1407 (1936); Marker, *et al., J. Am. Chem. Soc.* **58**, 481 (1936); Marker, **US 2117355** (1938); Barnett *et al., J. Chem. Soc.* **1940**, 1390.

Crystals from alcohol, mp 141.5°. $[\alpha]_D^{30}$ −35° (c = 1 in alcohol). Not precipited by digitonin.

Acetate. $C_{29}H_{48}O_2$. Crystals from methanol, mp 85°.

3614. Epicillin. [26774-90-3] (2S,5R,6R)-6-[[(2R)-Amino-1,4-cyclohexadien-1-ylacetyl]amino]-3,3-dimethyl-7-oxo-4-thia-1-azabicyclo[3.2.0]heptane-2-carboxylic acid; 6-[D-α-amino-2-(1,4-cyclohexadien-1-yl)acetamido]penicillanic acid; D-α-amino-(1,4-cyclohexadien-1-yl)methylpenicillin; SQ-11302; Dexacilina; Dexacillin; Spectacillin. $C_{16}H_{21}N_3O_4S$; mol wt 351.42. C 54.68%, H 6.02%, N 11.96%, O 18.21%, S 9.12%. Semi-synthetic antibiotic related to penicillin. Prepn: Weisenborn *et al.,* **US 3485819** (1969 to Squibb); Dolfini *et al., J. Med. Chem.* **14**, 117 (1971). Activity studies: Basch *et al., Infect. Immun.* **4**, 44 (1971); Gadebusch *et al., ibid.* 50. Clinical trials: Woodruff *et al., N. Y. State J. Med.* **71**, 1087 (1971); Beck *et al., Curr. Ther. Res.* **13**, 530 (1971); Reyes, *ibid.* 602; Landa, *ibid.* 654.

Crystals, dec 202° (hemihydrate).
THERAP CAT: Antibacterial.

3615. Epicocconone. [371163-96-1] (6S,9aS)-5,6-Dihydro-6-(hydroxymethyl)-3-[(1Z,4E,6E,8E)-1-hydroxy-3-oxo-1,4,6,8-decatetraenyl]-9a-methyl-2H-furo[3,2-g][2]benzopyran-2,9(9aH)-dione; Deep Purple; Lightning Fast. $C_{23}H_{22}O_7$; mol wt 410.42. C 67.31%, H 5.40%, O 27.29%. Fluorescent natural product isolated from the fungus *Epicoccum nigrum*. Reacts reversibly with primary amines to produce a highly fluorescent enamine. Prepn: P. J. L. Bell, P. Karuso, **WO 0181351** (2001 to Maquarie Res. Ltd.); *eidem,* **US 030157518** (2003). Isoln, characterization, and fluorescence applications: *eidem, J. Am. Chem. Soc.* **125**, 9304 (2003). Protein gel staining characteristics: J. A. Mackintosh *et al., Proteomics* **3**, 2273 (2003). Photostability study: G. B. Smejkal *et al., Electrophoresis* **25**, 2511 (2004). Mechanism of protein staining: D. R. Coghlan *et al., Org. Lett.* **7**, 2401 (2005).

Orange solid. $[\alpha]_D^{25}$ +110° (c = 0.009 in acetonitrile). Absorption max (methanol): 432, 555 nm (ε 10000, 4000). Absorption max (acetonitrile): 209, 290(sh), 317, 441 nm (ε 6000, 3000, 3000, 10000).

USE: Biodegradable fluorescent stain for detection of proteins in 1D and 2D gel electrophoresis.

3616. 16-Epiestriol. [547-81-9] (16β,17β)-Estra-1,3,5(10)-triene-3,16,17-triol; $\Delta^{1,3,5}$-estratriene-3,16β,17β-triol; 16-epioestriol; Actriol. $C_{18}H_{24}O_3$; mol wt 288.38. C 74.97%, H 8.39%, O 16.64%. Isoln from urine of pregnant women: Marrian, Bauld, *Biochem. J.* **59**, 136 (1955); Watson, Marrian, *ibid.* **63**, 64 (1956). From human placenta: Diczfalusy, Halla, *Acta Endocrinol.* **27**, 303 (1958). Prepn by reduction of 3,16β-diacetoxy-1,3,5(10)-estratrien-17-one: Biggerstaff, Gallagher, *J. Org. Chem.* **22**, 1220 (1957).

Crystals from methanol + benzene, mp 289-291°. $[\alpha]_D^{15}$ +76° (c = 0.297 in ethanol).

Epiestriol-3-allyl ether. Prepn: Huffman, **US 3002009** (1961 to Lasdon Found). Crystals, mp 156-156.5°.

3617. Epimedii Herba. Yinyanghuo. Chinese herbal medicine made from the dried aerial parts of *Epimedium* sp. (*Berberidaceae*). Used as a tonic and in the treatment of rheumatic disease and hypertension. Principal constituents are prenylflavone glycosides such as icariin, epimedosides, sagittatosides, and baohuosides. Isoln of icariin from *E. macranthum*: S. Akai, *J. Pharm. Soc. Jpn.* **55**, 537 (1935), *C.A.* **29**, 5850 (1935). Revised structure: Y. Tokuoka *et al., Yakugaku Zasshi* **95**, 825 (1975), *C.A.* **83**, 111072r (1975). HPLC determn of constituents: M. Mizuno *et al., Chem. Pharm. Bull.* **36**, 3487 (1988); Y. Ito *et al., J. Chromatogr.* **456**, 392 (1988). Immunoregulatory effects of icariin *in vitro:* W. He *et al., Arzneim.-Forsch.* **45**, 910 (1995). Review: W. Tang, G. Eisenbrand in *Chinese Drugs of Plant Origin* (Springer-Verlag, Berlin, 1992) pp 491-498.

Icariin. [489-32-7] 3-[(6-Deoxy-α-L-mannopyranosyl)oxy]-7-(β-D-glucopyranosyloxy)-5-hydroxy-2-(4-methoxyphenyl)-8-(3-methyl-2-butenyl)-4H-1-benzopyran-4-one; 4'-O-methyl-8-γ,γ-dimethylallylkaempferol-3-rhamnoside-7-glucoside. $C_{33}H_{40}O_{15}$; mol wt 676.66. Sesquihydrate, mp 231.5°. $[\alpha]_D^{15}$ −87.09° (in pyridine). Sol in pyridine. Insol in water, alcohol, chloroform, acetone, methanol, ethyl acetate.

3618. Epinastine. [80012-43-7] 9,13b-Dihydro-1H-dibenz-[c,f]imidazo[1,5-a]azepin-3-amine; 3-amino-9,13b-dihydro-1H-dibenz[c,f]imidazo[1,5-a]azepine; WAL-801. $C_{16}H_{15}N_3$; mol wt 249.31. C 77.08%, H 6.06%, N 16.85%. Tetracyclic, non-sedating histamine H_1 receptor antagonist. Prepn: G. Walther *et al.,* **GB 2071095**; *eidem,* **US 4313931** (1981, 1982 both to Boehringer, Ing.); and receptor binding studies: *idem et al., Arzneim.-Forsch.* **40**, 440 (1990). Pharmacology: A. Fügner *et al., ibid.* **38**, 1446 (1988). Clinical evaluation: W. S. Adamus *et al., ibid.* **37**, 569 (1987). Mechanism of action: K. Tasaka *et al., Oyo Yakuri* **39**, 365 (1990). Toxicology: J. Nishikawa *et al., ibid.* **42**, 151 (1991).

Crystals from acetonitrile, mp 205-208°. log P_a (octanol/ aqueous buffer, pH 7.4, 20°) −0.70. pKa 11.2.

Hydrobromide. [127786-29-2] Crystals from methanol/ethyl actate, mp 284-286°.

Hydrochloride. [108929-04-0] WAL-801CL; Alesion; Azusaleon; Elestat; Flurinol; Relestat; Talerc. $C_{16}H_{15}N_3$.HCl; mol wt 285.77. Crystals from methanol/ether, mp 273-275°. Freely sol in water. LD_{50} in male, female rats (mg/kg): 314, 192 orally; 17, 22 i.v. (Nishikawa).

THERAP CAT: Antihistaminic.

3619. Epinephrine. [51-43-4] 4-[(1R)-1-Hydroxy-2-(methylamino)ethyl]-1,2-benzenediol; (−)-3,4-dihydroxy-α-[(methylamino)methyl]benzyl alcohol; l-1-(3,4-dihydroxyphenyl)-2-(methylamino)ethanol; l-3,4-dihydroxy-1-[1-hydroxy-2-(methylamino)ethyl]benzene; l-methylaminoethanolcatechol; adrenaline; levorenin; Anapen; EpiPen; Primatene Mist; Sus-phrine. $C_9H_{13}NO_3$; mol wt 183.20. C 59.00%, H 7.15%, N 7.65%, O 26.20%. Endogenous catcholamine with combined α- and β-agonist activity. Principal sympathomimetic hormone produced by the adrenal medulla. Isoln from animal adrenal glands: Takamine, *J. Soc. Chem. Ind.* **20**, 746 (1901); Aldrich, *Am. J. Physiol.* **5**, 457 (1901). Synthesis of *dl*-form: Stolz, *Ber.* **37**, 4149 (1904); Payne, *Ind. Chem.* **37**, 523 (1961). Historic review of syntheses: Loewe, *Arzneim.-Forsch.* **4**, 583 (1954). Resolution of *dl*-form: Flächer, *Z. Physiol. Chem.* **58**, 189 (1908). Configuration: Pratesi *et al., J. Chem. Soc.* **1958**, 2069. Acute toxicity: A. M. Lands *et al., J. Pharmacol. Exp. Ther.* **90**, 110 (1947). HPLC determn in plasma and urine: C. R. Benedict, *J. Chromatogr.* **385**, 369 (1987). Comprehensive description: D. H. Szulczewski, W.-H. Hong, *Anal. Profiles Drug Subs.* **7**, 193-229 (1978). Physiologic review: Malmejac, *Physiol. Rev.* **44**, 186 (1964). Review of biosynthesis: L. A. Pohorecky, R. J. Wurtman, *Pharmacol. Rev.* **23**, 1-35 (1971); of pharmacology and clinical use in cardiopulmonary resuscitation: N. A. Paradis, E. M. Koscove, *Ann. Emerg. Med.* **19**, 1288-1301 (1990); P. Hebert *et al., J. Emerg. Med.* **9**, 487-495 (1991). Review of use in anaphylaxis: A. P. C. McLean-Tooke *et al., Br. Med. J.* **327**, 1332-1335 (2003).

Minute crystals, gradually browning on exposure to light and air. mp 211-212°. mp ~215° (dec) when rapidly heated. $[\alpha]_D^{25}$ −50.0° to −53.5° (in 0.6N HCl). Very slightly sol in water, alc. Readily sol in aq solns of mineral acids, NaOH, and KOH. Insol in aq solns of ammonia and of the alkali carbonates. Insol in chloroform, ether, acetone, oils. LD_{50} i.p. in mice: 4 mg/kg (Lands).

Hydrochloride. [55-31-2] Adrenalin; Epifrin; Glaucon; Suprarenin. $C_9H_{13}NO_3$.HCl; mol wt 219.67.

d-Bitartrate. [51-42-3] Asthmahaler; Medihaler-Epi. $C_9H_{13}NO_3.C_4H_6O_6$; mol wt 333.29. Crystals, mp 147-154° (some dec). Darkens slowly on exposure to air and light. One gram dissolves in about 3 ml water. Slightly sol in alc.

***dl*-Form.** [329-65-7] Racepinephrine. Sparingly sol in water, alcohol.

***dl*-Form hydrochloride.** [329-63-5] Vaponefrin. Crystals from alcohol, mp 157°. Readily sol in water; sparingly sol in abs alc.

THERAP CAT: Bronchodilator; cardiostimulant; mydriatic; antiglaucoma.

THERAP CAT (VET): Vasoconstrictor; cardiostimulant.

3620. Epiquinidine. [572-59-8] (9R)-6'-Methoxycinchonan-9-ol. $C_{20}H_{24}N_2O_2$; mol wt 324.42. C 74.04%, H 7.46%, N 8.63%, O 9.86%. Occurs in cinchona bark. Isoln from quinoidine:

Dirscherl, Thron, *Ann.* **521**, 48 (1938). By epimerization of quinine or quinidine: Rabe, Höter, *J. Prakt. Chem.* **154**, 66 (1940). Stereochemistry: Prelog, Zalán, *Helv. Chim. Acta* **27**, 535, 545 (1944); Prelog, Häfliger, *ibid.* **33**, 2021 (1950); Roth, *Pharmazie* **16**, 257 (1961). Synthesis: Grethe *et al., Helv. Chim. Acta* **55**, 1044 (1972); Gutzwiller, Uskokovic, *ibid.* **56**, 1494 (1973).

Lustrous leaflets from ether, mp 111-113°. $[\alpha]_D^{25}$ +107.8° (c = 1.02 in ethanol). Freely sol in alcohol; moderately sol in ether. Shows more blue fluorescence in H_2SO_4 than quinidine or quinine. Forms a double sulfate with epiquinine.

Dihydrochloride. $C_{20}H_{24}N_2O_2$.2HCl. Crystals from alc, dec 195-196°. $[\alpha]_D^{20}$ +46° (c = 0.8 in 99% alc).

Neutral dibenzoyl-*d*-tartrate. $(C_{20}H_{24}N_2O_2)_2.C_{18}H_{14}O_8$. Crystals from alcohol or acetone, dec 166-167°. $[\alpha]_D^{21}$ +3.7° (4:1 alcohol + chloroform).

3621. Epiquinine. [572-60-1] (8α,9S)-6'-Methoxycinchonan-9-ol. $C_{20}H_{24}N_2O_2$; mol wt 324.42. C 74.04%, H 7.46%, N 8.63%, O 9.86%. For refs see Epiquinidine.

Viscous oil, $[\alpha]_D^{22}$ +43° (c = 0.95 in 99% alc). Freely sol in organic solvents. Shows more blue fluorescence in H_2SO_4 than quinine. Forms a double sulfate with epiquinidine.

Dihydrochloride. $C_{20}H_{24}N_2O_2$.2HCl. Crystals from acetone, dec 196°. $[\alpha]_D^{20}$ +33° (c = 0.8 in 99% alc).

Neutral dibenzoyl-*d*-tartrate. $(C_{20}H_{24}N_2O_2)_2.C_{18}H_{14}O_8$. Crystals from acetone, dec 159°, $[\alpha]_D^{25}$ −24.3° (c = 0.93 in ethanol).

3622. Epirizole. [18694-40-1] 4-Methoxy-2-(5-methoxy-3-methyl-1H-pyrazol-1-yl)-6-methylpyrimidine; 2-(3-methyl-5-methoxy-1-pyrazolyl)-4-methoxy-6-methylpyrimidine; 2-(3-methoxy-5-methylpyrazol-2-yl)-4-methoxy-6-methylpyrimidine; 1-(4-methoxy-6-methyl-2-pyrimidinyl)-3-methyl-5-methoxypyrazole; mepirizole; DA-398; Mebron. $C_{11}H_{14}N_4O_2$; mol wt 234.25. C 56.40%, H 6.02%, N 23.92%, O 13.66%. Prepn: Naito *et al.,* ZA **6704936** (1968 to Daiichi Seiyaku), *C.A.* **70**, 57876q (1969); Naito *et al., Chem. Pharm. Bull.* **17**, 1467 (1969). Pharmacology and metabolism: Oshima *et al., ibid.* 1492; Takabatake *et al., ibid.* **18**, 1900 (1970). Toxicity data: H. Ogura *et al., J. Med. Chem.* **15**, 923 (1972).

Minute, white or cream-colored crystals from isopropyl ether, mp 90-92°. Characteristic odor, bitter taste. Sparingly sol in water. Sol in dil acids; freely sol in ethanol, benzene, dichloroethane. Also sol in ether, acetone. LD_{50} orally in mice: 820 mg/kg (Ogura).

THERAP CAT: Analgesic, antipyretic, anti-inflammatory.

3623. Epirubicin. [56420-45-2] (8S,10S)-10-[(3-Amino-2,3,6-trideoxy-α-L-*arabino*-hexopyranosyl)oxy]-7,8,9,10-tetrahydro-6,8,11-trihydroxy-8-(hydroxyacetyl)-1-methoxy-5,12-naphthacenedione; 3-glycoloyl-1,2,3,4,6,11-hexahydro-3,5,12-trihydroxy-10-methoxy-6,11-dioxo-1-naphthacenyl-3-amino-2,3,6-tridioxy-α-L-arabino-hexopyranoside; 4′-epidoxorubicin; 4′-epiadriamycin; pidorubicin; 4′-epi-DX; IMI-28. $C_{27}H_{29}NO_{11}$; mol wt 543.52. C 59.66%, H 5.38%, N 2.58%, O 32.38%. Analog of the anthracycline antibiotic doxorubicin, q.v., differing only in the position of the C-4 hydroxy group of the sugar moiety. Prepn: F. Arcamone *et al.*, **DE 2510866**; *eidem*, **US 4058519** (1975, 1977 both to Soc. Farmaceut. Italia); *eidem, J. Med. Chem.* **18**, 703 (1975); S. Penco, *Process Biochem.* **15**(5), 12 (1980). Purification: E. Oppici *et al.*, **BE 898506**; *eidem*, **GB 2133005** (both 1984 to Farmitalia Carlo Erba). Comparison with doxorubicin of *in vitro* activity: A. Di Marco *et al.*, *Cancer Res.* **36**, 1962 (1976). Tissue distribution: C. Italia *et al.*, *Br. J. Cancer* **47**, 545 (1983); F. Arcamone *et al.*, *Cancer Chemother. Pharmacol.* **12**, 157 (1984). HPLC determn in biological fluids: P. E. Deesen, B. Leyland-Jones, *Drug Metab. Dispos.* **12**, 9 (1984); G. Cassinelli *et al.*, *ibid.* 506. Clinical trials in solid tumors: K. Kolaric *et al.*, *J. Cancer Res. Clin. Oncol.* **106**, 148 (1983). Review of activity in experimental tumors: A. Goldin *et al.*, *Invest. New Drugs* **3**, 3-21 (1985). Review of pharmacology and clinical efficacy: F. Ganzina, *Cancer Treat. Rev.* **10**, 1-22 (1983); R. J. Cersosimo, W. K. Hong, *J. Clin. Oncol.* **4**, 425-439 (1986); P. Hurteloup, F. Ganzina, *Drugs Exp. Clin. Res.* **13**, 233-246 (1986). Review of epirubicin and other anthracycline antineoplastics: R. B. Weiss *et al.*, *Cancer Chemother. Pharmacol.* **18**, 185-97 (1986).

Hydrochloride. [56390-09-1] Ellence; Farmorubicina. C_{27}-$H_{29}NO_{11}$.HCl; mol wt 579.98. Red-orange crystals, mp 185° (dec). $[α]_D^{20}$ +274° (c = 0.01 in methanol). Solution should be protected from sunlight.

THERAP CAT: Antineoplastic.

3624. Epitiostanol. [2363-58-8] (2α,3α,5α,17β)-2,3-Epithioandrostan-17-ol; 10275-S; Thiodrol. $C_{19}H_{30}OS$; mol wt 306.51. C 74.45%, H 9.87%, O 5.22%, S 10.46%. Episulfide deriv of androstane, q.v. Prepn: **GB 977599**; T. Komeno, **US 3230215** (1964, 1966 both to Shionogi); K. Takeda *et al.*, *Tetrahedron* **1965**, 329; P. D. Klimstra *et al.*, *J. Med. Chem.* **9**, 693 (1966). Antitumor effect in mice: A. Matsuzawa, T. Yamamoto, *Cancer Res.* **37**, 4408 (1977). Teratogenicity study: T. Minesita *et al.*, *Oyo Yakuri* **7**, 723 (1973), *C.A.* **80**, 116474p (1974). Toxicity study: *eidem, ibid.* 805, *C.A.* **80**, 66865u (1974). Use in treatment of breast cancer: M. Fujimoro *et al.*, *Cancer* **31**, 789 (1973).

Crystals from acetone, mp 127-128°. $[α]_D^{27.5}$ +24.4° (c = 1.054 in chloroform). uv max (alcohol): 262 nm. LD_{50} in mice, rats (mg/kg): 1, 5 i.p. (Minesita, p 805).

THERAP CAT: Antineoplastic.

3625. Eplerenone. [107724-20-9] (7α,11α,17α)-9,11-Epoxy-17-hydroxy-3-oxopregn-4-ene-7,21-dicarboxylic acid γ-lactone methyl ester; 9α,11-epoxy-7α-(methoxycarbonyl)-3-oxo-17α-pregn-4-ene-21,17-carbolactone; 9α,11α-epoxy-7α-methoxycarbonyl-20-spirox-4-ene-3,21-dione; epoxymexrenone; CGP-30083; SC-66110; Inspra. $C_{24}H_{30}O_6$; mol wt 414.49. C 69.54%, H 7.30%, O 23.16%. Selective aldosterone receptor antagonist (SARA); structurally similar to spironolactone, q.v. Prepn: J. Grob, J. Kalvoda, **EP 122232**; *eidem*, **US 4559332** (1984, 1985 both to Ciba-Geigy); J. Grob *et al.*, *Helv. Chim. Acta* **80**, 566 (1997). Pharmacology and receptor binding studies: M. de Gasparo *et al.*, *J. Pharmacol. Exp. Ther.* **240**, 650 (1987). Clinical pharmacokinetics: W. R. Ravis *et al.*, *J. Clin. Pharmacol.* **45**, 810 (2005). Clinical trial in congestive heart failure after myocardial infarction: B. Pitt *et al.*, *N. Engl. J. Med.* **348**, 1309 (2003); in hypertension vs losartan: M. H. Weinberger *et al.*, *Am. Heart J.* **150**, 426 (2005). Review of pharmacology and clinical experience: J. A. Delyani *et al.*, *Cardiovasc. Drug Rev.* **19**, 185-200 (2001); E. Burgess, *Expert Opin. Pharmacother.* **5**, 2573-2581 (2004).

Crystals from methylene chloride + isopropanol, mp 240-242°. $[α]_D$ +5° (c = 0.437 in chloroform). uv max: 240 nm (ε 16800). Partition coefficient (octanol/water): 7.1 (pH 7.0). Sol in dichloromethane, acetonitrile; slightly sol in ethanol; sparingly sol in methyl ethyl ketone, methanol; very slightly sol in water.

THERAP CAT: Antihypertensive. In treatment of congestive heart failure.

3626. EPN. [2104-64-5] Phenylphosphonothioic acid O-ethyl O-(4-nitrophenyl) ester; ethyl p-nitrophenyl benzenethiophosphonate; O-ethyl O-p-nitrophenyl phenylphosphonothioate. C_{14}-$H_{14}NO_4PS$; mol wt 323.30. C 52.01%, H 4.36%, N 4.33%, O 19.80%, P 9.58%, S 9.92%. Cholinesterase inhibitor. Prepn: A. G. Jelinek, **US 2503390** (1950 to du Pont). Manufacturing process: N. Shindo *et al.*, **US 3327026** (1967 to Nissan). Insecticidal activity: R. L. McGarr, A. J. Chapman, *J. Econ. Entomol.* **59**, 1529 (1966); D. A. Wolfenbarger *et al.*, *ibid.* **63**, 1568 (1970). Determn by HPLC: J. M. Lasker *et al.*, *Anal. Biochem.* **109**, 369 (1980); X.-D. Ding, I. S. Krull, *J. Agric. Food Chem.* **32**, 622 (1984). Inhibition of acetylcholinesterase: O. Awad *et al.*, *Arzneim.-Forsch.* **22**, 1035 (1972); O. M. E. Awad, *Enzyme* **32**, 193 (1984). Metabolism in animals: R. L. Chrzanowski, A. G. Jelinek, *J. Agric. Food Chem.* **29**, 580 (1981). Toxicological study: H. C. Hodge *et al.*, *J. Pharmacol. Exp. Ther.* **112**, 29 (1954). Teratogenic evaluation in mice: K. D. Courtney *et al.*, *J. Environ. Sci. Health* **20B**, 373 (1985). Study of delayed neurotoxicity: B. M. Francis, *Bull. Environ. Contam. Toxicol.* **38**, 283 (1987). Toxicity data: T. B. Gaines, *Toxicol. Appl. Pharmacol.* **2**, 88 (1960).

Light yellow oil, aromatic odor. d^{25} 1.268. n_D^{25} 1.6021. Practically insol in water. Miscible with benzene, toluene, xylene, acetone, isopropanol, methanol. LD_{50} in female, male rats (mg/kg): 7.7, 36 orally; 25, 230 dermal (Gaines).

Caution: Potential symptoms of overexposure are miosis, lacrimation; rhinorrhea; headache; tight chest, wheezing and laryngeal spasm; salivation; cyanosis; anorexia, nausea, abdominal cramps and diarrhea; paralysis, convulsions; low blood pressure; cardiac irregularities; irritation of skin and eyes. *See NIOSH Pocket Guide to Chemical Hazards* (DHHS/NIOSH 97-140, 1997) p 128. *See also Clinical Toxicology of Commercial Products*, R. E. Gosselin *et al.*, Eds. (Williams & Wilkins, Baltimore, 5th ed., 1984) Section II, p 294.

USE: Insecticide; acaricide.

3627. Epostane. [80471-63-2] (4α,5α,17β)-4,5-Epoxy-3,17-dihydroxy-4,17-dimethylandrost-2-ene-2-carbonitrile; (2α,4α,5α,17β)-4,5-epoxy-17-hydroxy-4,17-dimethyl-3-oxoandrostane-2-carbonitrile; Win-32729. $C_{22}H_{31}NO_3$; mol wt 357.49. C 73.91%, H 8.74%, N 3.92%, O 13.43%. 3β-Hydroxysteroid dehydrogenase inhibitor; derivative of trilostane, *q.v.* Prepn as ketone tautomer: R. G. Christiansen, DE **2855091**; *idem,* US **4160027** (both 1979 to Sterling). Pharmacology and interceptive activity: J. E. Creange *et al., Contraception* **24**, 289 (1981); R. G. Christiansen *et al., J. Med. Chem.* **27**, 928 (1984). Clinical pharmacology: Z. M. Van der Spuy *et al., Clin. Endocrinol.* **19**, 521 (1983); N. S. Pattison *et al., Fertil. Steril.* **42**, 875 (1984). Clinical evaluation as abortifacient: L. Birgerson *et al., Contraception* **35**, 111 (1987); M. J. Crooij *et al., N. Engl. J. Med.* **319**, 813 (1988). Comparative clinical study with mifepristone, *q.v.*, as abortifacient: L. Birgerson, V. Odlind, *Fertil. Steril.* **48**, 565 (1987). Induction of labor in swine: P. A. Martin *et al., J. Anim. Sci.* **64**, 497 (1987); in sheep: M. Silver, *Vet. Rec.* **120**, 299 (1987). Regulation of ovulation in sheep: R. Webb, *J. Reprod. Fertil.* **79**, 231 (1987). Abortifacient efficacy in dogs: D. M. Keister *et al., Theriogenology* **30**, 497 (1988).

Crystals, mp 191-194° from DMF/H_2O. $[\alpha]_D^{25}$ +67.4° (c = 1 in pyridine).

THERAP CAT: Interceptive.

THERAP CAT (VET): Interceptive, labor inducer.

3628. Epothilones. Microtubule stabilizing 16-membered macrolides which mimic the biological effects of paclitaxel, *q.v.*, while retaining multidrug-resistant activity. Structurally lacking the taxane ring. Isoln of A and B from the myxobacterium *Sorangium cellulosum:* G. Höfle *et al.,* DE **4138042**, (1993 to Ges. Biotech. Forsch.), *C.A.* **120**, 52841 (1994). Purification of A and B, and mechanism of action: D. M. Bollag *et al., Cancer Res.* **55**, 2325 (1995). Total synthesis of A: A. Balog *et al., Angew. Chem. Int. Ed.* **35**, 2801 (1996); of B and D: D.-S. Su *et al., ibid.* **36**, 757 (1997). Crystal structure of A and B, and conformation in soln: G. Höfle *et al., ibid.* **35**, 1567 (1996). Isoln and structural studies of 39 natural epothilone variants: I. H. Hardt *et al., J. Nat. Prod.* **64**, 847 (2001). Isoln and crystallization of D: R. L. Arslanian *et al., ibid.* **65**, 570 (2002). Effects of A and B on microtubule proteins in comparison with paclitaxel: R. J. Kowalski *et al., J. Biol. Chem.* **272**, 2534 (1997). Review of properties and clinical potential: D. M. Bollag, *Expert. Opin. Invest. Drugs* **6**, 867-873 (1997); of biology, chemistry and therapeutic potential: K. C. Nicolaou *et al., Angew. Chem. Int. Ed.* **37**, 2014-2045 (1998); *idem et al., Chem. Commun.* **2001**, 1523-1535.

Epothilone A   R = H
Epothilone B   R = CH_3

Epothilone D

Epothilone A. [152044-53-6] (1S,3S,7S,10R,11S,12S,16R)-7,11-Dihydroxy-8,8,10,12-tetramethyl-3-[(1E)-1-methyl-2-(2-methyl-4-thiazolyl)ethenyl]-4,17-dioxabicyclo[14.1.0]heptadecane-5,9-dione. $C_{26}H_{39}NO_6S$; mol wt 493.66. Colorless crystals from ethyl acetate/toluene, mp 95°. Soly at 20° (g/l): water 0.7. uv max (methanol): 211, 249 nm (ε 17800, 12500). $[\alpha]_D^{21}$ −47.1° (c = 1.0 in methanol).

Epothilone B. [152044-54-7] Patupilone; EPO-906. $C_{27}H_{41}NO_6S$; mol wt 507.68. Colorless crystals from ethyl acetate, mp 93-94°. uv max (methanol): 211, 249 nm (ε 18600, 14100). $[\alpha]_D^{21}$ −35° (c = 0.7 in methanol).

Epothilone D. [189453-10-9] (4S,7R,8S,9S,13Z,16S)-4,8-Dihydroxy-5,5,7,9,13-pentamethyl-16-[(1E)-1-methyl-2-(2-methyl-4-thiazolyl)ethenyl]oxacyclohexadec-13-ene-2,6-dione; desoxyepothilone B; KOS-862. $C_{27}H_{41}NO_5S$; mol wt 491.68. Colorless crystals from ethanol + water, mp 120-121° (Arslanian). Also reported as colorless amorphous solid. $[\alpha]_D^{22}$ −61.3° (c = 2.5 in methanol). uv max (methanol): 210, 248 nm (ε 18400, 13200) (Hardt).

3629. Epoxiconazole. [133855-98-8]; [106325-08-0] (undefined). *rel*-1-[[(2R,3S)-3-(2-Chlorophenyl)-2-(4-fluorophenyl)-oxiranyl]methyl]-1H-1,2,4-triazole; (2RS,3RS)-1-[3-(2-chlorophenyl)-2,3-epoxy-2-(4-fluorophenyl)-propyl]-1H-1,2,4-triazole; BAS-480-F; Opus. $C_{17}H_{13}ClFN_3O$; mol wt 329.76. C 61.92%, H 3.97%, Cl 10.75%, F 5.76%, N 12.74%, O 4.85%. Ergosterol biosynthesis inhibitor. Prepn: S. Karbach *et al.,* EP **196038**; *ei-dem,* US **4906652** (1986, 1990 both to BASF). Properties and field trials: E. Ammermann *et al., Brighton Crop Prot. Conf. - Pests Dis.* **1990**, 407; R. Saur *et al., ibid.* 831. Mode of action: A. Akers *et al., ibid.* 837. Use in combination with fenpropimorph, *q.v.*: R. Saur *et al., Gesunde Pflanz.* **46**, 61 (1994). Brief review: A. Floquet, N. Martin, *Phytoma* **449**, 54-57 (1993).

Crystals from diisopropyl ether, mp 136.2°. Soly at 20° (g/100 ml): water 6.63×10^{-4}, acetone 18, dichloromethane 14, *n*-heptane <0.1. Partition coefficient (*n*-octanol/ water at pH 7) 3.44. LD_{50} in rats (mg/kg): >5000 orally, >2000 dermally; LC_{50} in rats (4 hr): >5.3 mg/l (dust aerosol) (Ammermann).

USE: Agricultural fungicide.

3630. Epoxomicin. [134381-21-8] *N*-Acetyl-*N*-methyl-L-isoleucyl-L-isoleucyl-*N*-[(1*S*)-3-methyl-1[[(2*R*)-2-methyloxiranyl]-carbonyl]butyl]-L-threoninamide; BU-4061T. $C_{28}H_{50}N_4O_7$; mol wt 554.72. C 60.63%, H 9.09%, N 10.10%, O 20.19%. *α',β'*-epoxyketone peptide which specifically inhibits proteasome activity. Isoln from actinomycetes: M. Konishi *et al.,* **EP 411660**; *eidem,* **US 5071957** (both 1991 to Bristol-Myers); and characterization: M. Hanada *et al., J. Antibiot.* **45,** 1746 (1992). Total synthesis: N. Sin *et al., Bioorg. Med. Chem. Lett.* **9,** 2283 (1999). Proteasome selectivity and antiinflammatory activity: L. Meng *et al., Proc. Natl. Acad. Sci. USA* **96,** 10403 (1999). Crystal structure and mechanism of selectivity: M. Groll *et al., J. Am. Chem. Soc.* **122,** 1237 (2000). Use as inhibitor to modulate antigen presentation: K. Schwarz *et al., J. Immunol.* **164,** 6147 (2000).

Colorless powder, mp 107-109°. $[\alpha]_D^{24.5}$ −66.1 ± 0.4° (c = 0.5 in MeOH). Readily sol in methanol, methylene chloride and ethyl acetate. Practically insol in water.

USE: In studies of proteasome biology.

3631. Epratuzumab. [205923-57-5]; [501423-23-0] (^{90}Y-labeled form). Anti-(human CD22 (antigen)) immunoglobulin G1 (human-mouse monoclonal IMMU-hLL2 γ-chain) disulfide with human-mouse monoclonal IMMU-hLL2 κ-chain dimer; hLL2; AMG-412; IMMU-hLL2; LymphoCide. Humanized monoclonal antibody directed against CD22, a transmembrane sialoglycoprotein expressed on the surface of B-cell malignancies. Prepn: S.-O. Leung, H. Hansen, **WO 9604925**; *eidem,* **US 5789554** (1996, 1998 both to Immunomedics); *idem et al., Mol. Immunol.* **32,** 1413 (1995). Characterization and binding study: J. Carnahan *et al., Clin. Cancer Res.* **9,** Suppl., 3982s (2003). Clinical pharmacokinetics and evaluation in non-Hodgkin's lymphoma: J. P. Leonard *et al., Clin. Cancer Res.* **10,** 5327 (2004). Review of clinical development: A. B. Siegel *et al., Semin. Oncol.* **30,** 457-464 (2003). ^{90}**Y Epratuzumab Tetraxetan.** [501423-25-2] ^{90}Y-DOTA-hLL2. Prepn and biodistribution studies: S. V. Govindan *et al., Bioconj. Chem.* **9,** 773 (1998); G. L. Griffiths *et al., J. Nucl. Med.* **44,** 77 (2003). Clinical pharmacokinetics and efficacy: R. M. Sharkey *et al., ibid.* 2000. Clinical evaluation in non-Hodgkin's lymphoma: O. Lindén *et al., Clin. Cancer Res.* **11,** 5215 (2005).

THERAP CAT: Antineoplastic. ^{90}Y-labeled form in radioimmunotherapy.

3632. Eprazinone. [10402-90-1] 3-[4-(2-Ethoxy-2-phenylethyl)-1-piperazinyl]-2-methyl-1-phenyl-1-propanone; 3-[4-(β-ethoxyphenethyl)-1-piperazinyl]-2-methylpropiophenone. $C_{24}H_{32}N_2$-O_2; mol wt 380.52. C 75.75%, H 8.48%, N 7.36%, O 8.41%. Prepn of the dihydrochloride: R. Y. Mauvernay, **NL 6602581**; *idem,* **US 3448192** (1966, 1969 both to Riom). Pharmacodynamics: J. Vacher *et al., Arch. Int. Pharmacodyn. Ther.* **165,** 1 (1967). Pharmacological study: Y. Kase *et al., Nippon Yakurigaku Zasshi* **73,** 605 (1977), *C.A.* **88,** 15657 (1978). Efficacy: W. Spitzer, *Fortschr. Med.* **98,** 871 (1980). Metabolism: P. Toffel-Nadolny, W. Gielsdorf, *Arzneim.-Forsch.* **31,** 719 (1981).

Dihydrochloride. [10402-53-6] 746-CE; Eftapan; Mucitux. $C_{24}H_{32}N_2O_2$·2HCl; mol wt 453.44. White, bitter-tasting crystalline powder, mp 201° (Toffel-Nadolny, Gielsdorf); also reported as

crystals from methanol, mp 160° (Mauvernay). LD_{50} in mice (mg/kg): 729 orally, 38 i.v. (Vacher).

THERAP CAT: Antitussive.

3633. Eprinomectin. [123997-26-2] (4"*R*)-4"-(Acetylamino)-4"-deoxyavermectin B₁; MK-397; Eprinex. Mixture of semisynthetic avermectins, *q.v.*; containing 90% or more of component B$_{1a}$ and 10% or less of component B$_{1b}$. Prepn: H. H. Mrozik, **US 4427663** (1984 to Merck & Co.). Synthesis: R. J. Cvetovich *et al., J. Org. Chem.* **59,** 7704 (1994) and biological activity: T. K. Jones *et al., J. Agric. Food Chem.* **42,** 1786 (1994). Mechanism of action study: J. P. Arena *et al., J. Parasitol.* **81,** 286 (1995).

Component B₁ₐ, R = C₂H₅
Component B₁ᵦ, R = CH₃

Crystalline solid, mp 163.3-165.7°. LD_{50} orally in mice: 24 mg/kg (Jones).

Component B$_{1a}$. [133305-88-1] (4"*R*)-4"-(Acetylamino)-5-*O*-demethyl-4"-deoxyavermectin A$_{1a}$; $C_{50}H_{75}NO_{14}$; mol wt 914.13.

Component B$_{1b}$. [133305-89-2] (4"*R*)-4"-(Acetylamino)-5-*O*-demethyl-25-de(1-methylpropyl)-4"-deoxy-25-(1-methylethyl)-avermectin A$_{1a}$; $C_{49}H_{73}NO_{14}$; mol wt 900.10.

THERAP CAT (VET): Antiparasitic.

3634. Episteride. [119169-78-7] (17β)-17-[[(1,1-Dimethylethyl)amino]carbonyl]androsta-3,5-diene-3-carboxylic acid; 17β-(*N-tert*-butylcarboxamido)androsta-3,5-diene-3-carboxylic acid; SKF-105657. $C_{25}H_{37}NO_3$; mol wt 399.57. C 75.15%, H 9.33%, N 3.51%, O 12.01%. 5α-Reductase inhibitor. Prepn and *in vitro* activity: D. A. Holt *et al.,* **EP 289327**; *eidem,* **US 4910226** and **US 5017568** (1988, 1990, 1991 all to SmithKline Beecham); D. A. Holt *et al., J. Med. Chem.* **33,** 943 (1990). Pharmacology: J. C. Lamb *et al., Endocrinology* **130,** 685 (1992). Antitumor effects in rats: J. C. Lamb *et al., Prostate* **21,** 15 (1992). Mechanism of action study: M. A. Levy *et al., Biochemistry* **29,** 2815 (1990). HPLC determn in human plasma: V. K. Boppana *et al., J. Chromatogr.* **631,** 251 (1993).

White crystals from ethyl acetate, mp 242-249°. pK 4.8.

THERAP CAT: Treatment of benign prostatic hypertrophy.

3635. Eprosartan. [133040-01-4] (*αE*)-α-[[2-Butyl-1-[(4-carboxyphenyl)methyl]-1*H*-imidazol-5-yl]methylene]-2-thiophenepropanoic acid; (*E*)-3-[2-butyl-1-[(4-carboxyphenyl)methyl]-imidazol-5-yl]-2-(2-thienylmethyl)-2-propenoic acid; SKF-108566. C_{23}-$H_{24}N_2O_4S$; mol wt 424.51. C 65.07%, H 5.70%, N 6.60%, O 15.08%, S 7.55%. Prototype of the imidazoleacrylic acid angiotensin II receptor antagonists. Prepn: J. A. Finkelstein *et al.,* **EP 403159** (1990 to SmithKline Beecman); *eidem,* **US 5185351** (1993 to SmithKline Beecham); J. Weinstock *et al., J. Med. Chem.* **34,**

1514 (1991); R. M. Keenan *et al.*, *ibid.* **36**, 1880 (1993). Pharmacology: R. M. Edwards *et al.*, *J. Pharmacol. Exp. Ther.* **260**, 175 (1992). Receptor binding study: H. T. Schambye *et al.*, *Mol. Pharmacol.* **47**, 425 (1995). Clinical pharmacokinetics: D. Tenero *et al.*, *Biopharm. Drug Dispos.* **19**, 351 (1998). Clinical trial in hypertension: W. J. Elliott *et al.*, *J. Hum. Hypertens.* **13**, 413 (1999). Review of clinical experience: L. Ruilope, B. Jäger, *Expert Opin. Pharmacother.* **4**, 107-114 (2003).

Crystals from methanol, mp 260-261°.
Monomethanesulfonate. [144143-96-4] Eprosartan mesylate; SKF-108566J; Teveten. $C_{23}H_{24}N_2O_4S.CH_3SO_3H$; mol wt 520.62. White to off-white crystalline powder, mp 248-250°. Insol in water. Freely sol in ethanol.
THERAP CAT: Antihypertensive.

3636. Eprozinol. [32665-36-4] 4-(2-Methoxy-2-phenylethyl)-α-phenyl-1-piperazinepropanol; 1-(2-methoxy-2-phenylethyl)-4-(3-hydroxy-3-phenylpropyl)piperazine. $C_{22}H_{30}N_2O_2$; mol wt 354.49. C 74.54%, H 8.53%, N 7.90%, O 9.03%. Prepn: Saunders, **GB 1188505** (1970); to R. Y. Mauvernay, N. Busch, **US 3705244** (1972). Pharmacology: Duchene-Marullaz *et al.*, *Therapie* **26**, 155 (1971). Clinical studies: Sors, Dutarte, *ibid.* 163.

Dihydrochloride. [27588-43-8] Alecor; Brovel; Eupnéron. $C_{22}H_{30}N_2O_2.2HCl$; mol wt 427.41. White crystalline powder, mp 164°. Sol in water and alcohol. LD_{50} orally in mice: 500 mg/kg (Mauvernay, Busch).
THERAP CAT: Bronchodilator.

3637. Epsiprantel. [98123-83-2] 2-(Cyclohexylcarbonyl)-2,3,6,7,8,12b-hexahydropyrazino[2,1-*a*][2]benzazepin-4(1*H*)-one; 2-cyclohexylcarbonyl-4-oxo-1,2,3,4,6,7,12b-octahydropyrazino[2,1-*a*][2]benzazepine; BRL-38705; Cestex. $C_{20}H_{26}N_2O_2$; mol wt 326.43. C 73.59%, H 8.03%, N 8.58%, O 9.80%. Anthelmintic structurally related to praziquantel, *q.v.* Prepn: R. J. Dorgan, R. L. Elliott, *eidem*, **EP 134984**; *eidem*, **US 4661489** (1985, 1987 both to Beecham); M. D. Brewer *et al.*, *J. Med. Chem.* **32**, 2058 (1989). Veterinary trials in dogs: R. M. Corwin *et al.*, *Am. J. Vet. Res.* **50**, 1076 (1989); in cats and dogs: B. R. Manger, M. D. Brewer, *Br. Vet. J.* **145**, 384 (1989).

White crystals from chloroform/petr ether, mp 189-190°.
THERAP CAT (VET): Anthelmintic (Cestodes).

3638. Eptastigmine. [101246-68-8] (3a*S*,8a*R*)-1,2,3,3a,8,8a-Hexahydro-1,3a,8-trimethylpyrrolo[2,3-*b*]indol-5-yl heptylcarbamic acid ester; *N*-demethyl-*N*-heptylphysostigmine; heptylphysostigmine; heptylstigmine. $C_{21}H_{33}N_3O_2$; mol wt 359.51. C 70.16%, H 9.25%, N 11.69%, O 8.90%. Cholinesterase inhibitor; analog of physostigmine, *q.v.* Prepn: M. Pomponi *et al.*, **EP 154864**; M. Brufani *et al.*, **US 4831155** (1985, 1989 both to Consiglio Naz. Ricerche). Prepn of tartrate: P. G. Pagella *et al.*, **EP 298202** (1989 to Mediolanum Farm. and Consiglio Naz. Ricerche). Prepn and pharmacology: M. Marta *et al.*, *Life Sci.* **43**, 1921 (1988). Anticholinesterase activity: P. De Sarno *et al.*, *Neurobiochem. Res.* **14**, 971 (1989). Clinical cholinesterase inhibition: L. K. Unni *et al.*, *Eur. J. Clin. Pharmacol.* **41**, 83 (1991).

Crystals from heptane, mp 60-64°; also reported as 58-62° (Marta). uv max (methanol): 303, 253 nm (ε 3300, 14200).
Tartrate. [121652-76-4] MF-201. $C_{21}H_{33}N_3O_2.C_4H_6O_6$; mol wt 509.59. Microcrystalline powder, mp 122-123°. Soly in water 70%. LD_{50} i.p. in mice: 35 mg/kg (De Sarno).
THERAP CAT: Cholinergic.

3639. Eptazocine. [72522-13-5] (1*S*)-2,3,4,5,6,7-Hexahydro-1,4-dimethyl-1,6-methano-1*H*-4-benzazonin-10-ol; (1*S*)-1,4-dimethyl-10-hydroxy-2,3,4,5,6,7-hexahydro-1,6-methano-1*H*-4-benzazonine; ST-2121; Sedapain. $C_{15}H_{21}NO$; mol wt 231.33. C 77.88%, H 9.15%, N 6.05%, O 6.92%. Opioid agonist-antagonist analgesic, related to pentazocine, *q.v.* Prepn: M. Ikeda *et al.*, **DE 2422309**; *eidem*, **US 4008219** (1974, 1977 both to Nihon Iyakuhin Kogyo). Chromatographic study: I. Hayashi *et al.*, *Iyakuhin Kenkyu* **12**, 442 (1981), *C.A.* **95**, 220196v (1981). Series of articles on pharmacological activities: *Nippon Yakurigaku Zasshi* **78**, 599-645 (1981), *C.A.* **96**, 62879, 79732, 79733 (1982). Opioid receptor binding study: T. Nabeshima *et al.*, *Res. Commun. Chem. Pathol. Pharmacol.* **48**, 173 (1985).

Hydrobromide. $C_{15}H_{22}BrNO$. Crystals, mp 207-210°.
THERAP CAT: Analgesic (narcotic).

3640. EPTC. [759-94-4] Dipropylcarbamothioic acid *S*-ethyl ester; dipropylthiocarbamic acid *S*-ethyl ester; *S*-ethyl dipropylthiocarbamate; R-1608; FDA-1541; Eptam. $C_9H_{19}NOS$; mol wt 189.32. C 57.10%, H 10.12%, N 7.40%, O 8.45%, S 16.94%. Selective pre-planting herbicide. Prepn: **GB 808753**; H. Tilles, J. Antognini, **US 2913327** (both 1959 to Stauffer). Activity: J. Antognini *et al.*, *Proc. Northeast. States Weed Control Conf.* **1957**, 3. Metabolism: V. Y. Ong, S. C. Fang, *Toxicol. Appl. Pharmacol.* **17**, 418 (1970); J. P. Hubbell, J. E. Casida, *J. Agric. Food Chem.* **25**, 404 (1977).

Liquid, bp_{20} 127°. d^{30} 0.9546; n_D^{30} 1.4750. Vapor pressure at 35°: 3.4×10^{-2} mm Hg. Soly in water at 20°: 365 mg/l. Miscible with benzene, alc, toluene, xylene. LD_{50} orally in rats: 1631 mg/kg (Antognini).
USE: Herbicide.

3641. Eptifibatide. [188627-80-7] N^6-(Aminoiminomethyl)-N^2-(3-mercapto-1-oxopropyl)-L-lysylglycyl-L-α-aspartyl-L-tryptophyl-L-prolyl-L-cysteinamide, cyclic (1 → 6)-disulfide; Integrilin. $C_{35}H_{49}N_{11}O_9S_2$; mol wt 831.96. C 50.53%, H 5.94%, N 18.52%, O 17.31%, S 7.71%. Fibrinogen receptor antagonist. Specifically inhibits fibrinogen binding to the platelet integrin GPIIb-IIIa which prevents platelet aggregation and subsequent clot formation. Synthetic, disulfide-linked cyclic heptapeptide based on **barbourin**, a specific GPIIb-IIIa antagonist isolated from venom of the southeastern pigmy rattlesnake, *Sistrurus m. barbouri*. Contains the Lys-Gly-Asp (KGD) amino acid sequence, a modification of the Arg-Gly-Asp (RGD) recognition site which appears to confer specificity: R. M. Scarborough *et al., J. Biol. Chem.* **266**, 9359 (1991). Design and structure-activity study of integrin antagonists: *eidem, ibid.* **268**, 1066 (1993). Prepn: R. M. Scarborough *et al.,* **US 5686570** (1997 to COR Therapeutics). Pharmacology: F. A. Nicolini *et al., Circulation* **89**, 1802 (1994); K. Uthoff *et al., ibid.* **90**, pt 2, II-269 (1994). Clinical trial in patients undergoing percutaneous cardiovascular intervention: IMPACT-II Investigators, *Lancet* **349**, 1422 (1997). Clinical trial in acute coronary syndromes: PURSUIT Trial Investigators, *N. Engl. J. Med.* **339**, 436 (1998).

THERAP CAT: Antithrombotic.

3642. Equilenin. [517-09-9] 3-Hydroxyestra-1,3,5,7,9-pentaen-17-one; 11,12,13,14,15,16-hexahydro-3-hydroxy-13-methyl-17H-cyclopenta[a]phenanthren-17-one; 1,3,5:10,6,8-estrapentaen-3-ol-17-one. $C_{18}H_{18}O_2$; mol wt 266.33. C 81.17%, H 6.81%, O 12.01%. Estrogenic steroidal hormone isolated from urine of pregnant mares: Girard *et al., Compt. Rend.* **195**, 981 (1932). Occurs naturally in the *d*-form. Not found in human urine. Component of Conjugated Estrogenic Hormones, *q.v.* Isoln by chromatography: Duschinsky, Lederer, *Bull. Soc. Chim. Biol.* **17**, 1534 (1935). Total synthesis: Bachmann *et al., J. Am. Chem. Soc.* **61**, 974 (1939); **62**, 824 (1940); Johnson *et al., ibid.* **67**, 2274 (1945); **69**, 2942 (1947); **72**, 505 (1950); Hughes, Smith, *Chem. Ind. (London)* **1960**, 1022; Bailey *et al., Chem. Commun.* **1967**, 1253; Stein *et al., Tetrahedron* **26**, 1917 (1970). Synthesis from estrone: Corbellini *et al., Farmaco Ed. Sci.* **19**, 913 (1964); O. N. Minailova *et al., Zh. Obshch. Khim.* **49**, 2633 (1979); A. R. Daniewski, T. Kowalczyk-Przewloka, *Tetrahedron Lett.* **1982**, 2411. Review of synthetic studies: Taub, "Naturally Occurring Aromatic Steroids" in *The Total Synthesis of Natural Products* vol. 2, J. ApSimon, Ed. (John Wiley & Sons, New York, 1973) pp 642-663.

Needles from dil alc, mp 258-259°. Sublimes at 170-180° at 0.01 mm Hg. $[\alpha]_D^{16}$ +87° (12.8 mg made up to 1.8 ml in dioxane). uv max (ethanol): 231, 270, 282, 292, 325, 340 nm. Soly/100 ml alcohol 0.63 (18°); 2.5 g (boiling).

Acetate. $C_{20}H_{20}O_3$. mp 156-157°.

Benzoate. $C_{25}H_{22}O_3$. mp 222-223° (vac).

Methyl ether. $C_{19}H_{20}O_2$. Needles from alc, mp 197-198°; mp 193-194° (vac).

THERAP CAT: Estrogen.

3643. Equilin. [474-86-2] 3-Hydroxyestra-1,3,5(10),7-tetraen-17-one; 1,3,5,7-estratetraen-3-ol-17-one. $C_{18}H_{20}O_2$; mol wt 268.35. C 80.56%, H 7.51%, O 11.92%. Steroidal hormone isolated from urine of pregnant mares: Girard *et al., Compt. Rend.* **195**, 981 (1932); Cartland, Meyer, *J. Biol. Chem.* **112**, 9 (1935/6). Structure: Serini, Logemann, *Ber.* **71**, 186 (1938); Pearlman, Wintersteiner, *J. Biol. Chem.* **130**, 35 (1939). Separation from estrone: Serini, Logemann, **US 2221340** (1941 to Schering). Synthesis: Zderic *et al., J. Am. Chem. Soc.* **80**, 2596 (1958); Bagli *et al., Tetrahedron Lett.* **1964**, 387; Stein *et al., ibid.* **1966**, 5015; *eidem, Tetrahedron* **26**, 1917 (1970). Prepn from testosterone by bacterial fermentation: Bowers *et al.,* **US 3067212** (1962 to Syntex). Prepn

by conversion of equilenin: Bailey *et al., Chem. Commun.* **1967**, 1253; Marshall, Deghenghi, *Can. J. Chem.* **47**, 3127 (1969). Component of Conjugated Estrogenic Hormones, *q.v.* Review of synthetic studies: Taub, "Naturally Occurring Aromatic Steroids" in *The Total Synthesis of Natural Products* **vol. 2**, J. ApSimon, Ed. (John Wiley & Sons, New York, 1973) pp 664-670.

Orthorhombic sphenoidal plates from ethyl acetate, mp 238-240°. $[\alpha]_D^{25}$ +308° (c = 2 in dioxane); $[\alpha]_D^{25}$ +325° (c = 2 in alc). uv max: 283-285 nm. Soluble in alcohol, dioxane, acetone, ethyl acetate, in other organic solvents; sparingly sol in water.

Benzoate. $C_{25}H_{24}O_3$. mp 196-197°.

Methyl ether. $C_{19}H_{22}O_2$. Needles from alc, mp 161-162°.

THERAP CAT: Estrogen.

3644. Equol. [531-95-3] 3,4-Dihydro-3-(4-hydroxyphenyl)-2H-1-benzopyran-7-ol; 4′,7-isoflavandiol; 4′,7-dihydroxyisoflavan; 7-hydroxy-3-(4′-hydroxyphenyl)chroman. $C_{15}H_{14}O_3$; mol wt 242.27. C 74.36%, H 5.82%, O 19.81%. Isoln from mare's urine: G. F. Marrian, G. A. D. Haslewood, *Biochem. J.* **26**, 1226 (1932); from human urine: M. Axelson *et al., ibid.* **201**, 353 (1982). Physical description: *eidem, ibid.* **29**, 1586 (1935); F. Wessely *et al., Monatsh. Chem.* **71**, 215 (1938). Structure: F. Wessely, F. Prillinger, *Ber.* **72B**, 629 (1939); E. L. Anderson, G. F. Marrian, *J. Biol. Chem.* **127**, 649 (1939). Abs config: H. Suginome, *Bull. Chem. Soc. Jpn.* **39**, 409 (1966). Prepn of (±)-form: J. A. Lamberton *et al., Aust. J. Chem.* **31**, 455 (1978).

Crystals from aq ethanol, mp 189-190.5°. $[\alpha]_D$ −21.5°.

3645. Erabutoxins. Neurotoxic principles isolated from venom of the sea-snake, *Laticauda semifasciata* (in Japanese, *erabu-umihebi)*. Their action on post-synaptic membrane blocks neuromuscular transmission. Separation and crystn of erabutoxins A and B: Tamiya, Arai, *Biochem. J.* **99**, 624 (1966). Structures are single polypeptide chains containing 62 amino acid residues with four S-S bridges, **erabutoxin A** differing from **erabutoxin B** only in the amino acid residue at position 26: Sato, Tamiya, *ibid.* **122**, 453 (1971); Endo *et al., ibid.* 463. Isoln and structure of the minor component, **erabutoxin C**: Tamiya, Abe, *ibid.* **130**, 547 (1972). Corrected amino acid sequences: N. Maeda, N. Tamiya, *Biochem. J.* **167**, 289 (1977). Three-dimensional structure of B, description of active site: B. W. Low, *Adv. Cytopharmacol.* **3**, 141 (1979). Molecular conformation: M. R. Kimball *et al., Biochem. Biophys. Res. Commun.* **88**, 950 (1979); F. Inagaki *et al., Eur. J. Biochem.* **109**, 129 (1980). Raman spectra: T. Takamatsu *et al., Biochim. Biophys. Acta* **622**, 189 (1980). Immunological studies: A. Tatsuya *et al., Toxicon* **17**, 571 (1979), *C.A.* **92**, 141459t (1980). Effect on transmission in autonomic ganglia: V. A. Chiappinelli *et al., Brain Res.* **211**, 107 (1981).

LD_{50} in mice, rats (g/g): 0.15, 0.07 i.m. (Tamiya, Arai).

3646. Erbium. [7440-52-0] Er; at. wt 167.26; at. no. 68; valence 3. Rare earth metal of the yttrium group; member of the lanthanide series. Naturally occurring isotopes (mass numbers): 162 (0.14%); 164 (1.61%); 166 (33.6%); 167 (22.95%); 168 (26.8%); 170 (14.9%). Known artificial radioactive isotopes: 147; 148; 150-161; 163; 165; 169; 171-173. Abundance in earth's crust: 2.47-3.5 ppm. Occurs in small quantities in all the rare earth minerals; main sources: xenotime, fergusonite, gadolinite, euxenite, polycrase, blomstrandine. Discovery: Mosander, *Skand. Naturför. Förh.* **3**, 387 (1842); *Philos. Mag.* [3] **23**, 241 (1843). Separation of oxide: James, *J. Am. Chem. Soc.* **32**, 517 (1910); **34**, 757 (1912); Hofmann, Burger, *Ber.* **41**, 308 (1908); Prandtl, *Z. Anorg. Chem.* **198**, 157 (1931). Sepn by ion-exchange: Spedding *et al.*, *J. Am. Chem. Soc.* **69**, 2812 (1947); **76**, 2557 (1954). Prepn of the metal: Klemm, Bommer, *Z. Anorg. Chem.* **213**, 138 (1937). Prepn of chloride, bromide: Jantsch *et al.*, *Z. Anorg. Chem.* **207**, 353 (1932). Radioactivity induced by neutron bombardment: Sugden, *Nature* **135**, 469 (1935); McLennan, Rann, *ibid.* **136**, 831 (1935). Spectrum: Eder, *Ber. Wien. Akad.* [2a] **124**, 790 (1915); deGramont, *Compt. Rend.* **171**, 1106 (1920); Mott, McDonald, *Trans. R. Soc. Can. Sect. 3* **21**, 230 (1927). Natural isotopic composition: Hayden *et al.*, *Phys. Rev.* **77**, 299 (1950). Toxicity study: Haley, *J. Pharm. Sci.* **54**, 663 (1965). Reviews of prepn, properties and compds: *The Rare Earths*, F. H. Spedding, A. H. Daane, Eds. (Krieger, Huntington, N.Y., 1971, reprint of 1961 ed.) 641 pp; Hulet, Bode, "Separation Chemistry of the Lanthanides and Transplutonium Actinides" in *MTP Int. Rev. Sci.: Inorg. Chem., Ser. One* **vol. 7**, K. W. Bagnall, Ed. (University Park Press, Baltimore, 1972) pp 1-45; Moeller, "The Lanthanides" in *Comprehensive Inorganic Chemistry* **vol. 4**, J. C. Bailar Jr. *et al.*, Eds. (Pergamon Press, Oxford, 1973) pp 1-101; F. H. Spedding in *Kirk-Othmer Encyclopedia of Chemical Technology* **vol. 19** (John Wiley & Sons, New York, 3rd ed., 1982) pp 833-854; *Chemistry of the Elements*, N. N. Greenwood, A. Earnshaw, Eds. (Pergamon Press, New York, 1984) pp 1423-1449. Brief review of properties: G. T. Seaborg, *Radiochim. Acta* **61**, 115-122 (1993).

Dark-gray metallic powder; hexagonal close-packed crystal lattice. d 9.066. mp 1529°. bp 2868°. Heat of fusion: 19.90 kJ/mol. Heat of sublimation (25°): 317.10 kJ/mol. E°(aq) Er^{3+}/Er −230 V (calc). Similar to the other rare earth metals, possesses two reduction potentials 1.770 and 1.875 volts (ref to the normal calomel electrode), Noddack, Brukl, *Angew. Chem.* **50**, 362 (1937).

Oxide. Erbia. Er_2O_3. Pinkish powder changing into cubic crystals on heating at 1300°; d 8.64; sp heat 0.065; prepd by igniting the oxalate or basic nitrate. Readily sol in acids. Soly in water: 1.28×10^{-5} g-mol/l at 29°.

Hydroxide. $Er(OH)_3$. Pale pink gelatinous ppt. Prepd by action of alkali hydroxide on a soln of erbium nitrate.

Chloride. $ErCl_3$. Hexahydrate, deliquesc crystals. Sol in water; slightly sol in alcohol. Dehydrated by heating in a stream of hydrogen chloride. Anhydr form is pinkish powder, d 4.1. LD_{50} in mice (mg/kg): 535 i.p.; 6.2 orally (Haley).

Bromide. $ErBr_3$. Nonahydrate, deliquesc rose crystals.

Nitrate. $Er(NO_3)_3$. Pentahydrate, reddish, deliquesc crystalline solid. Loses 4 mols of water on heating to 130°. LD_{50} of hexahydrate in female rats (mg/kg): 230 i.p.; 35.8 i.v. (Haley).

3647. Erdosteine. [84611-23-4] [[2-Oxo-2-[(tetrahydro-2-oxo-3-thienyl)amino]ethyl]thio]acetic acid; (±)-[[[(tetrahydro-2-oxo-3-thienyl)carbamoyl]methyl]thio]acetic acid; DL-S-[2-[N-3-(2-oxotetrahydrothienyl)acetamido]]thioglycolic acid; *N*-(carboxymethylthioacetyl)homocysteine thiolactone; dithiosteine; RV-144; Secresolv. $C_8H_{11}NO_4S_2$; mol wt 249.31. C 38.54%, H 4.45%, N 5.62%, O 25.67%, S 25.72%. Homocysteine thiolactone derivative with mucomodulating activity. Prepn: J. Gonella, **EP 61386**; *idem*, **US 4411909** (1982, 1983 both to Refarmed); M. Gobetti *et al.*, *Farmaco Ed. Sci.* **41**, 69 (1986). Clinical trial in bronchitis: G. Ricevuti *et al.*, *Thorax* **43**, 585 (1988). Clinical effect on α_1-antitrypsin levels in cigarette smokers: M. Vagliasindi, G. B. Fregnan, *Int. J. Clin. Pharmacol. Ther. Toxicol.* **27**, 238 (1989).

Crystals from ethanol, mp 156-158°. pKa 3.71. LD_{50} in mice and rats (g/kg): >10 orally; >3.5 i.v. (Gonella).

THERAP CAT: Mucolytic.

3648. Ergocornine. [564-36-3] (5′α)-12′-Hydroxy-2′,5′-bis(1-methylethyl)ergotaman-3′,6′,18-trione. $C_{31}H_{39}N_5O_5$; mol

wt 561.67. C 66.29%, H 7.00%, N 12.47%, O 14.24%. Natural ergot alkaloid derived from lysergic acid; component of ergotoxine, *q.v.* Isoln from ergot: Stoll, Hofmann, *Helv. Chim. Acta* **26**, 1570 (1943). Structure: Stoll *et al.*, *ibid.* **34**, 1544 (1951). Separation and purification: Stoll, Hofmann, **US 2447214** (1948 to Sandoz). Synthesis: Stadler *et al.*, *Helv. Chim. Acta* **52**, 1969 (1969). Determn in ergot by capillary electrophoresis: K. Frach, G. Blaschke, *J. Chromatogr. A* **808**, 247 (1998).

Solvated, polyhedra from methanol, dec 181° (contains 1 mole methanol). $[\alpha]_D^{20}$ −110° (pyridine); −175° (chloroform). uv max (methanol): 311 nm (log ε 3.91). Soluble in acetone, chloroform, ethyl acetate; slightly sol in ethyl and methyl alcohol. Nearly insol in water.

8α-Epimer. [564-37-4] Ergocorninine. Prisms from alc, dec 228°. $[\alpha]_D^{20}$ +409° (chloroform). uv max (methanol): 240.5, 312.5 (log ε 4.31, 3.92). Soluble in 15 parts boiling ethanol, 25 parts boiling methanol, 30 parts boiling benzene, 30 parts boiling ethyl acetate; freely sol in acetone, chloroform. Practically insol in water.

3649. Ergocristine. [511-08-0] (5′α)-12′-Hydroxy-2′-(1-methylethyl)-5′-(phenylmethyl)ergotaman-3′,6′,18-trione. $C_{35}H_{39}N_5O_5$; mol wt 609.71. C 68.95%, H 6.45%, N 11.49%, O 13.12%. Natural ergot alkaloid derived from lysergic acid; a member of the ergotoxine group. Isoln from ergot: Stoll, Burckhardt, *Z. Physiol. Chem.* **250**, 1 (1937); Stoll, Hofmann, *Helv. Chim. Acta* **26**, 1570 (1943). Structure: Stoll *et al.*, *ibid.* **34**, 1544 (1951). Separation and purification: Stoll, Hofmann, **US 2447214** (1948 to Sandoz). Synthesis: Stadler *et al.*, *Helv. Chim. Acta* **52**, 1549 (1969).

Orthorhombic crystals with $2C_6H_6$ from benzene. mp 155-157° (dec) (solvent-free base). $[\alpha]_D^{20}$ −183° (chloroform). Very sol in ethyl and methyl alcohol, acetone, chloroform, ethyl acetate. Slightly sol in ether. Practically insol in water, petr ether.

Phosphate. [6424-36-8] Crystals, dec 195°.

Ethanesulfonate. [6055-56-7] Crystals, dec 207°.

8α-isomer. [511-07-9] Ergocristinine. Crystallizes solvent-free, unlike ergocristine which tends to retain the solvent of crystn. Long prisms from abs alc, mp 226° (dec). $[\alpha]_D^{20}$ +366° (c = 0.68 in chloroform); +471° (c = 0.35 in pyridine). uv max (methanol/methylene chloride): 313 nm (log ε 3.96). Much less sol than ergocristine. Does not seem to form salts.

3650. Ergocryptine. Ergokryptine. $C_{32}H_{41}N_5O_5$; mol wt 575.70. C 66.76%, H 7.18%, N 12.16%, O 13.90%. Two closely related isomers of the ergotoxine group which differ in the peptide portion of the molecule; α-ergocryptine yielding L-leucine upon hydrolysis, β-ergocryptine yielding L-isoleucine. The ergocryptine discussed in the literature prior to 1967 is now referred to as α-ergocryptine. Isoln from ergot: Stoll, Hofmann, *Helv. Chim. Acta* **26**, 1570 (1943). Structure: Stoll *et al., ibid.* **34**, 1544 (1951). Separation and purification: Stoll, Hofmann, **US 2447214** (1948 to Sandoz). Separation of β-ergocryptine from α-ergocryptine: Schlientz *et al., Experientia* **23**, 991 (1967); *see also eidem, Pharm. Acta Helv.* **43**, 497 (1968). Synthesis of α- and β-ergocryptine: Stadler *et al., Helv. Chim. Acta* **52**, 1549 (1969).

α-Ergocryptine R = CH₂CH(CH₃)₂
β-Ergocryptine R = CH(CH₃)CH₂CH₃

α**-Ergocryptine.** [511-09-1] (5′α)-12′-Hydroxy-2′-(1-methylethyl)-5′-(2-methylpropyl)ergotaman-3′,6′,18-trione. Solvated prisms from acetone, benzene, methanol. With MeOH of crystn, mp 212° (dec). $[\alpha]_D^{20}$ −120° (pyridine); −198° (chloroform). uv max (methanol): 241, 312.5 nm (log ε 4.31, 3.95). Freely sol in alcohol, chlorofom. Almost insol in water.

β**-Ergocryptine.** [20315-46-2] [5′α(S)]-12′-Hydroxy-2′-(1-methylethyl)-5′-(1-methylpropyl)ergotaman-3′,6′,18-trione. Rectangular plates from benzene, mp 173° (dec). $[\alpha]_D^{20}$ −98° (c = 0.5 in pyridine); −179° (c = 0.5 in chloroform). uv max (methanol): 312 (log ε 3.93).

THERAP CAT: *See* Ergot.

3651. Ergocryptinine. [511-10-4] Ergokryptinine. $C_{32}H_{41}N_5O_5$; mol wt 575.70. C 66.76%, H 7.18%, N 12.16%, O 13.90%. Alkaloid pair isomeric with α- and β-ergocryptine, resp., but differing by an α-configuration at C-8. The literature prior to 1967 refers to α-ergocryptinine as ergocryptinine. Isolation, structure, separation and purification *see* ergocryptine. Production: Abe *et al.,* **US 2835675** (1958). Prepn of β-ergocryptinine from β-ergocryptine: Schlientz *et al., Experientia* **23**, 991 (1967). Synthesis of α- and β-ergocryptinin: Stadler *et al., Helv. Chim. Acta* **52**, 1549 (1969).

α**-Ergocryptinine.** 12′-Hydroxy-2′-(1-methylethyl)-5′α-(2-methylpropyl)-8α-ergotaman-3′,6′,18-trione. Crystallizes solvent-free, unlike ergocryptine which tends to retain the solvent of crystn. Fine needles from methanol, dec 240-242°. $[\alpha]_D^{20}$ +408° (chloroform); +485° (c = 0.5 in pyridine). uv max (methanol): 241.5, 312.5 nm (log ε 4.30, 3.94). Sol in 20 parts boiling ethanol, 50 parts boiling methanol; freely sol in acetone, chloroform; almost insol in water. Does not seem to form salts.

β**-Ergocryptinine.** Colorless needles from methylene chloride-methanol, mp 217-218° (dec). $[\alpha]_D^{20}$ +421° (chloroform); +497° (pyridine). uv max (methanol): 240.5, 312 nm (log ε 4.31, 3.94). Differs from the α-isomer by the 1-methylpropyl group at the 5′-position.

3652. Ergoflavin. [3101-51-7] (1S,1′S,3S,3′S,4S,4′S,4aS,-4′aS,9aR,9′aR)-1,1′,3,3′,4,4′,9a,9′a-Octahydro-4,4′,8,8′,9a,9′a-hexahydroxy-3,3′-dimethyl-[7,7′-bi-1,4a-(epoxymethano)-4aH-xanthene]-9,9′,11,11′(2H,2′H)-tetrone; ergochrome CC(2,2′). $C_{30}H_{26}O_{14}$; mol wt 610.52. C 59.02%, H 4.29%, O 36.69%. Principal pigment from ergot: Freeborn, *Pharm. J.* **88**, 568 (1912); Eglinton *et al., J. Chem. Soc.* **1958**, 1833. Structure: McPhail *et al., ibid.* **1966**, *Sect. B*, 18. Review of ergoflavin and other ergochromes: Franck, Flasch in *Fortschr. Chem. Org. Naturst.* **30**, 151-206 (1973).

Yellow needles from methanol, decomp 350°. $[\alpha]_D^{21}$ +37.5° (c = 1.236 in acetone). uv max: 240, 260, 381 nm ($E_{1cm}^{1\%}$ 350, 346, 130). Sol in acetone, pyridine; moderately sol in methanol, alcohol, ethyl acetate, dioxane; sparingly sol in ether, benzene. Practically insol in 2N aq $NaHCO_3$.

Hexaacetate. $C_{42}H_{38}O_{20}$. Prisms from chloroform + petr ether, dec 248-249°. $[\alpha]_D^{20}$ +61.2° (c = 0.62 in dioxane). uv max: 340, 338 nm ($E_{1cm}^{1\%}$ 343, 61).

3653. Ergoloid Mesylates. [8067-24-1] Dihydroergotoxine monomethanesulfonate (salt); co-dergocrine mesylate; CCK-179; Circanol; Coristin; Dacoren; DCCK; Decril; Dulcion; Ergodesit; Ergohydrin; Ergoplus; Hydergine; Lysergin; Novofluen; Orphol; Pérénan; Progeril; Redergin; Sponsin; Trigot. Hydrogenated ergot alkaloids, specifically an equiproportional mixture of dihydroergocornine methanesulfonate, dihydroergocristine methanesulfonate and α- and β-dihydroergocryptine methanesulfonate in the ratio of 1.5-2.5:1. Neuropharmacological investigations: D. M. Loew *et al., Postgrad. Med. J.* **52**, Suppl. 1, 40 (1976).

Dihydroergocornine R = CH(CH₃)₂
Dihydroergocristine R = CH₂C₆H₅
Dihydro-α-ergocryptine R = CH₂CH(CH₃)₂
Dihydro-β-ergocryptine R = CH(CH₃)CH₂CH₃

Dihydroergocristine methanesulfonate. [24730-10-7] Decme; Defluina; Enirant; Insibrin; Nehydrin; Simactil; Unergol. $C_{36}H_{45}N_5O_8S$; mol wt 707.84.

THERAP CAT: α-Adrenergic blocker (treatment of impaired mental function in the elderly).

3654. Ergometrinine. [479-00-5] [8α(S)]-9,10-Didehydro-N-(2-hydroxy-1-methylethyl)-6-methylgolinecarboxamide; D-lysergic acid D-propanolamide; ergonovinine. $C_{19}H_{23}N_3O_2$; mol wt 325.40. C 70.13%, H 7.12%, N 12.91%, O 9.83%. An alkaloid isomeric with ergonovine, *q.v.* Ergometrinine and ergonovine can be interconverted by simple chemical procedures: Smith, Timmis, *J. Chem. Soc.* **1936**, 1166. Chromatographic determn in cereal grains: G. H. Ware *et al., J. Assoc. Off. Anal. Chem.* **69**, 697 (1986). Stout prisms from acetone, dec 196°. $[\alpha]_D^{20}$ +416° (c = 0.45 in chloroform). pK 7.3. Freely sol in pyridine, moderately in chloroform; slightly sol in alcohol, acetone. Nearly insol in water.

Hydrobromide monohydrate. $C_{19}H_{24}BrN_3O_2 \cdot H_2O$. Needles from aq acetone + ether, dec 190°.

Hydrochloride monohydrate. $C_{19}H_{24}ClN_3O_2 \cdot H_2O$. Needles, dec 175-180°.

Mononitrate. $C_{19}H_{24}N_4O_5$. Stout prisms from aq MeOH + ether, dec 235°. $[\alpha]_D^{20}$ +282° (c = 1).

Perchlorate. $C_{19}H_{24}ClN_3O_6$. Needles, dec 225° (brown at 210°).

3655. Ergonovine. [60-79-7] [8β(S)]-9,10-Didehydro-N-(2-hydroxy-1-methylethyl)-6-methylergoline-8-carboxamide; N-[α-

(hydroxymethyl)ethyl]-D-lysergamide; D-lysergic acid L-2-propanolamide; ergometrine; Ergobasine; Ergotocine; Ergostetrine; Ergotrate; Ergoklinine; Syntometrine. $C_{19}H_{23}N_3O_2$; mol wt 325.40. C 70.13%, H 7.12%, N 12.91%, O 9.83%. From some ergots: A. Stoll *et al.*, **US 2809920** (1957 to Saul & Co.). Prepn from D-lysergic acid and L(+)-2-amino-1-propanol: A. Stoll, A. Hofmann, *Helv. Chim. Acta* **26**, 944 (1943); Pioch, **US 2736728** (1956 to Lilly); Patelli, Bernardi, **US 3141887** (1964 to Farmitalia). Structure: A. Stoll *et al., Helv. Chim. Acta* **34**, 1544 (1951). Total synthesis: E. C. Kornfeld *et al., J. Am. Chem. Soc.* **78**, 3087 (1956). Metabolism: Slaytor, Wright, *J. Med. Pharm. Chem.* **5**, 483 (1962). Comprehensive description of the maleate: V. D. Reif, *Anal. Profiles Drug Subs.* **11**, 273-312 (1982). Toxicity data: R. P. Beliles, *Toxicol. Appl. Pharmacol.* **23**, 537 (1972). Clinical use in diagnosis of angina: L. A. DiCarlo, Jr. *et al., Am. J. Cardiol.* **54**, 744 (1984); R. Nordlander, R. Orinius, *Acta Med. Scand.* **221**, 47 (1987).

Tetrahedra from ethyl acetate, fine needles from benzene. Tends to form solvated crystals, mp 162°. $[\alpha]_D^{20}$ +90° (in water). pK 6.8. Freely sol in lower alcohols, ethyl acetate, acetone; more sol in water than the other principal alkaloids of ergot; slightly sol in chloroform.

Hydrochloride. $C_{19}H_{23}N_3O_2$.HCl. Needles from ethyl alcohol, dec 246°. $[\alpha]_D^{25}$ +63° (c = 0.9). More sol in water than the hydrobromide.

Maleate. [129-51-1] Cornocentin; Ergotrate Maleate; Ermetrine. $C_{19}H_{23}N_3O_2.C_4H_4O_4$; mol wt 441.48. Crystals, dec 167°. $[\alpha]_D^{25}$ +48 to +57°. One gram dissolves in 36 ml water, 120 ml alcohol. Nearly insol in ether and chloroform. LD$_{50}$ i.v. in mice: 8.26 mg/kg (Beliles).

Tartrate hydrate. Basergin; Neofemergen. $(C_{19}H_{23}N_3O_2)_2.-C_4H_6O_6.H_2O$; mol wt 818.91. Crystals, slightly sol in water.

Hydracrylate. Ergotrate-H. $C_{41}H_{52}N_6O_7$; mol wt 740.89.

THERAP CAT: Oxytocic.

THERAP CAT (VET): Oxytocic.

3656. Ergosine. [561-94-4] 12'-Hydroxy-2'-methyl-5'α-(2-methylpropyl)ergotaman-3',6',18-trione. $C_{30}H_{37}N_5O_5$; mol wt 547.65. C 65.79%, H 6.81%, N 12.79%, O 14.61%. Isoln of ergosine and ergosinine from ergot: Smith, Timmis, *J. Chem. Soc.* **1937**, 396. Structure: Stoll *et al., Helv. Chim. Acta* **34**, 1544 (1951). Stereochemistry: Stoll *et al., ibid.* **37**, 2039 (1954). Total synthesis of ergosine and ergosinine: Stadler *et al., ibid.* **47**, 1911 (1964).

Prisms from ethyl acetate, dec 228°. $[\alpha]_D^{20}$ −161° (chloroform). Sol in chloroform; fairly sol in methanol, acetone; sparingly sol in ethyl acetate, benzene.

8α-Isomer. Ergosinine; ergoclavinine. $C_{30}H_{37}N_5O_5$. Prisms from 90% alcohol, aq acetone, benzene or ethyl acetate, dec 228°. Also reported as colorless needles, mp 190-191° (dec), Stadler *et al., loc. cit.* $[\alpha]_D^{20}$ +420° (chloroform); $[\alpha]_D^{20}$ +380° (acetone). Very readily sol in chloroform; readily sol in acetone; less sol in ethyl acetate; sparingly sol in benzene; very sparingly sol in methyl alcohol; almost insol in water.

Note: **Ergoclavine** is an equimolar mixture of ergosine and ergosinine.

3657. Ergostane. [511-20-6] 5α-Ergostane. $C_{28}H_{50}$; mol wt 386.70. C 86.97%, H 13.03%. Prepn from allocholanic acid: Fernholz, *Ber.* **69**, 1792 (1938).

Scales, plates from ether + methanol, mp 85°. $[\alpha]_D^{20}$ +17° (c = 2 in chloroform).

3658. Ergostanol. [6538-02-9] (3β,5α)-Ergostan-3-ol. $C_{28}H_{50}O$; mol wt 402.70. C 83.51%, H 12.51%, O 3.97%. Prepn by hydrogenation of ergosta-14,22-dien-7-one: Chen, *Ber.* **70**, 1432 (1937).

Crystals, mp 144-145°. $[\alpha]_D^{20}$ +15.9° (c = 1.8 in chloroform). Is precipitated by digitonin.

Acetate. $C_{30}H_{52}O_2$. mp 145°. $[\alpha]_D^{20}$ +6.0° (c = 1.8 in chloroform).

Benzoate. $C_{35}H_{54}O_2$. mp 163-165°.

3659. Ergosterol. [57-87-4] (3β,22E)-Ergosta-5,7,22-trien-3-ol; ergosta-5:6,7:8,22:23-trien-3-ol; ergosterin. $C_{28}H_{44}O$; mol wt 396.65. C 84.78%, H 11.18%, O 4.03%. Most important of the provitamins D. Usually obtained from yeast which synthesizes it from simple sugars such as glucose. Damp yeast yields about 2.5% ergosterol, the variety of the yeast being very important. Isoln procedure: Green *et al.*, **US 3006932** (1961 to Vitamins Ltd.). When irradiated with uv light, ergosterol develops powerful vitamin D$_2$, *q.v.*, activity. Askew *et al.*, in England and Windaus and collaborators in Germany isolated the antirachitic vitamin D$_2$. The main irradiation products of ergsterol are lumisterol → tachysterol → vitamin D$_2$. Structure: Chuang, *Ann.* **500**, 270 (1933). Oxidation products: Fuerst, *Arch. Pharm.* **300**, 144 (1967).

Small hydrated plates from alcohol, in hydrated needles from ether. The best crystallized form contains 1½ mol H_2O, mp 168°: Bills, Honeywell, *J. Biol. Chem.* **80**, 15 (1928). Complete removal of water is almost impossible and results in an amorphous mass, melting range 166-183°. $bp_{0.01}$ 250°. $[\alpha]_D^{20}$ −135° (c = 1.2 in $CHCl_3$ calcd as anhydr). $[\alpha]_{546}^{20}$ −171° ($CHCl_3$). uv max (ethanol): 262, 271, 282, 293 nm, Hogness *et al., ibid.* **120**, 239 (1937). Practically insol in water. One gram dissolves in 660 ml alcohol, in 45 ml boiling alcohol, in 70 ml ether, in 39 ml boiling ether, in 31 ml chloroform. Precipitated by digitonin. Affected by light and air, turns yellow. Oxygen forms peroxides and hydrogen may form polyhydro compds.

Acetate. $C_{30}H_{46}O_2$. mp 179°, clear at 181°.

Benzoate. $C_{35}H_{48}O_2$. Plates or needles, mp 169-171°. $[\alpha]_D^{23}$ −71° (c = 1.1 in $CHCl_3$), $[\alpha]_{546}$ −88° ($CHCl_3$).

22,23-Dihydro analog. 22,23-Dihydroergosterol. $C_{28}H_{46}O$. Prepn: A. Windhaus, R. Langer, *Ann.* **508**, 105 (1934); D. H. R. Barton *et al., J. Chem. Soc. Perkin Trans. 1* **1976**, 821; D. J. Curry *et al., ibid.* **1977**, 822. uv irradiation gives vitamin D_4, *q.v.* Solvated needles from ethyl acetate + methanol, mp 152-153° (dried). $[\alpha]_D^{19}$ −109° ($CHCl_3$) (Windhaus); also reported as needles from chloroform-methanol, mp 128-130°. $[\alpha]_D^{19}$ −121° (c = 0.1). uv max: 262, 272, 282, 294 nm (ε 8000, 11200, 11800, 6800) (Barton).

22,23-Dihydro analog acetate. $C_{30}H_{48}O_2$. mp 157-158°. $[\alpha]_D^{17}$ −75° (c = 2.1 in $CHCl_3$).

THERAP CAT: Vitamin (antirachitic).

3660. Ergot. Secale cornutum; spurred rye. Dried sclerotia of the fungus *Claviceps purpurea* (Fries) Tul., *Hypocreaceae*, parasitic on rye plants. *Habit*. Europe; cultivated in Spain, Germany, and France. Four main classes of ergot alkaloids can be distinguished: clavine alkaloids, lysergic acids, lysergic acid amides and ergot peptide alkaloids. There are ten ergot peptide alkaloids which are ergotamine, ergosine, ergocristine, ergocryptine, ergocornine, ergotaminine, ergosinine, ergocristinine, ergocryptinine, and ergocorninine, the last five alkaloids being isomers of the first five. These alkaloids are typified by a structure consisting of lysergic acid, dimethylpyruvic acid, proline, and phenylalanine joined in amide linkages. In 1943 A. Stoll and A. Hofmann, *Helv. Chim. Acta* **26**, 1570 (1943) made it clear that the ergotoxine reported by G. Barger and F. H. Carr, *J. Chem. Soc.* **91**, 377 (1907) and by F. Kraft, *Arch. Pharm.* **244**, 336 (1906) was but a mixture of ergocristine, ergocryptine, and ergocornine, and that the ergotinine, first reported by C. Tanret, *Compt. Rend.* **81**, 891 (1875), was also a mixture consisting of ergocristinine, ergocryptinine, and ergocorninine. Other constituents of ergot are ergonovine, ergometrinine, ergoclavine, elymoclavine, trimethylamine, putrescine, cadaverine, agmatine, histamine, tyramine, histidine, tyrosine, valine, leucine, betaine, choline, acetylcholine, ergothioneine, 15-30% fatty oil, ergosterol, mannitol, lactic acid, and succinic acid. Production of ergocryptinine and elymoclavine by cultures of fungi parasitic on *Elymus mollis* Trin: Abe *et al., US 2835675*. Production of ergot alkaloids by saprophytic cultures: Adams, *US 3117917* (1964 to Miles Labs.). Ergot alkaloid fermentation: W. J. Kelleher, *Adv. Appl. Microbiol.* vol. **11**, 211 (1969). Biosynthesis of ergot alkaloids: H. G. Floss, *Tetrahedron* **32**, 873 (1976). *Reviews:* Gröger in *Microbial Toxins* vol. VIII, S. Kadis *et al.,* Eds. (Academic Press, New York, 1972) pp 321-373; Stadler, Stütz, "The Ergot Alkaloids" in *The Alkaloids* vol. **15**, R. H. F. Manske, Ed. (Academic Press, New York, 1975) pp 1-40. Books: F. J. Bove, *The Story of Ergot* (Karger, Basel, 1970) 297 pp; *Handb. Exp. Pharmacol.* **49** entitled "Ergot Alkaloids and Related Compounds", B. Berde, H. O. Schild, Eds. (Springer-Verlag, New York, 1978) 1003 pp.

Caution: Potential symptoms of overexposure are CNS stimulation, nausea, vomiting, weakness, tremors, excitement, confusion, convulsions, tachycardia, mydriasis, peripheral vasoconstriction progressing to gangrene. *See Clinical Toxicology of Commercial Products*, R. E. Gosselin *et al.,* Eds. (Williams & Wilkins, Baltimore, 5th ed., 1984) Section II, pp 218-219.

THERAP CAT: Vasoconstrictor (specific in migraine).

THERAP CAT (VET): Has been used as an oxytocic.

3661. Ergotamine. [113-15-5] (5′α)-12′-Hydroxy-2′-methyl-(phenylmethyl)ergotaman-3′,6′,18-trione. $C_{33}H_{35}N_5O_5$; mol wt 581.66. C 68.14%, H 6.07%, N 12.04%, O 13.75%. Vasoconstrictor found in ergot of Central Europe. Extraction procedure: Stoll,

Helv. Chim. Acta **28**, 1283 (1945). Pharmacology: E. Rothlin, *Schweiz. Med. Wochenschr.* **76**, 1254 (1946). Structure: Stoll *et al., ibid.* **34**, 1544 (1951). Total synthesis: Hofmann *et al., Experientia* **17**, 206 (1961). Stereochemistry: Hofmann *et al., ibid.* **46**, 2306 (1963). Comprehensive description: B. Kreilgard, *Anal. Profiles Drug Subs.* **6**, 113-159 (1977). LC determn in tablets: U. R. Cieri, *J. Assoc. Off. Anal. Chem.* **70**, 538 (1987); GC/MS determn in plasma: N. Feng *et al., J. Chromatogr.* **575**, 289 (1992). Bioavailablity and efficacy in migraine: V. Ala-Hurula, *Headache* **22**, 167 (1982). Review of clinical pharmacokinetics and treatment of headache: V. L. Perrin, *Clin. Pharmacokinet.* **10**, 334-352 (1985). Review of teratogenic risk: G. V. Raymond, *Teratology* **51**, 344-347 (1995).

Elongated prisms from benzene. Very hygroscopic. Darkens and dec on exposure to air, heat and light. Dec 212-214°. $[\alpha]_D^{20}$ −160° (chloroform). Sol in about 70 parts methanol, 150 parts acetone, 300 parts alcohol; freely sol in chloroform, pyridine, glacial acetic acid; moderately sol in ethyl acetate; slightly in benzene. Almost insol in water, petr ether. LD_{50} in mice, rats, rabbits (mg/kg): 62, 80, 3 i.v.; in cats: 11 s.c. (Rothlin).

Hydrochloride. $C_{33}H_{35}N_5O_5$.HCl. Rectangular plates from 90% alc, mp 212° (dec). Sol in water-alcohol mixtures; sparingly in water or alcohol.

Tartrate. [379-79-3] Ergomar; Ergostat; Gynergen; Lingraine. $(C_{33}H_{35}N_5O_5)_2 \cdot C_4H_6O_6$; mol wt 1313.41. Solvated crystals, e.g. the dimethanolate, heavy rhombic plates from methanol, mp 203° (dec). $[\alpha]_D^{25}$ −125 to −155° (c = 0.4 in chloroform). One gram dissolves in 500 ml water or 500 ml alc. *Protect from light and heat.*

THERAP CAT: Antimigraine.

THERAP CAT (VET): Tartrate has been used as an oxytocic.

3662. Ergotaminine. [639-81-6] 12′-Hydroxy-2′-methyl-5′α-(phenylmethyl)-8α-ergotaman-3′,6′,18-trione. $C_{33}H_{35}N_5O_5$; mol wt 581.66. C 68.14%, H 6.07%, N 12.04%, O 13.75%. An alkaloid isomeric with ergotamine, *q.v.* Isoln from ergot: Stoll, *Helv. Chim. Acta* **28**, 1283 (1945); Stoll *et al., US 2809920* (1957 to Saul & Co.); Tabor, Vining, *Can. J. Microbiol.* **3**, 55 (1957).

Crystallizes solvent-free, unlike ergotamine which tends to retain the solvent of crystn. Thin rhombic plates from methanol, dec 241-243°. $[\alpha]_D^{20}$ +369° (c = 0.5 in chloroform). Much less sol than ergotamine; sol in about 1000 parts boiling alcohol, 1500 parts boiling methanol; fairly sol in chloroform, pyridine, glacial acetic acid. Does not seem to form salts.

3663. Ergothioneine. [497-30-3] (αS)-α-Carboxy-2,3-dihydro-*N,N,N*-trimethyl-2-thioxo-1*H*-imidazole-4-ethanaminium inner salt; [1-carboxy-2-[2-mercaptoimidazol-4-yl]ethyl]trimethylammonium hydroxide inner salt; L(+)-ergothioneine; thioneine; thiolhistidine-betaine; thiasine; sympectothion. $C_9H_{15}N_3O_2S$; mol wt 229.30. C 47.14%, H 6.59%, N 18.33%, O 13.95%, S 13.98%. First discovered in the sclerotia of the ergot fungus, *Claviceps purpurea*, by Tanret, *J. Pharm. Chim.* **30**, 145 (1909). Has since been found to occur in blood, semen and various mammalian tissues, principally liver and kidneys. Biosynthesis from histidine by *Claviceps purpurea* cultures: Heath, Wildy, *Nature* **179**, 196 (1957); also produced by *Neurospora crassa*: Melville *et al., Fed. Proc.* **15**, 314 (1956). Chemical synthesis: Heath *et al., J. Chem. Soc.* **1951**, 2215. Occurrence in the *Linulus polyphemus* L. (king crab): Ackermann, List, *Z. Physiol. Chem.* **313**, 30 (1958). *Review:* Melville, *Vitam. Horm.* **17**, 155 (1959).

Dihydrate. Needles or leaflets from dil ethanol, dec 256-257°. $[\alpha]_D^{20}$ +116.5°; $[\alpha]_D^{27}$ +115° (H_2O). uv max (water): 258 nm (ε 16000). One gram dissolves in 5 ml at 25°, much more sol in hot water. Slightly sol in hot methanol, hot ethanol, acetone. Practically insol in ether, chloroform, benzene.

3664. Ergotinine. [8006-08-4] A 1:1:1 mixture of ergocornine, ergocristinine, and ergocryptinine. Isomeric with the ergotoxine mixture, *q.v.* First reported by Tanret, *Compt. Rend.* **81,** 891 (1875). Resolution into three alkaloids: Stoll, Hofmann, *Helv. Chim. Acta* **26,** 1570 (1943).

Crystallizes solvent-free, unlike ergotoxine which tends to retain the solvent of crystn. Long prisms from acetone. mp 229° with decompn. $[\alpha]_D^{20}$ +365° (c = 0.35 in chloroform). Very sol in chloroform. Sol in 25 parts acetone, 420 parts alcohol, 1000 parts abs ether.

3665. Ergotoxine. [8006-25-5] Ecboline. A mixture of ergocornine, ergocristine, and ergocryptine, *q.q.v.*, with oxytocic activity. *See also* the isomeric ergotinine mixture. Prepn: Barger, Carr, *J. Chem. Soc.* **91,** 337 (1907); Smith, Timmis, *ibid.* **1930,** 1390; Kofler, *Arch. Pharm.* **275,** 455 (1937); Stoll, Hofmann, *Helv. Chim. Acta* **26,** 1570 (1943); Pitra, Sapara, *Cesk. Farm.* **5,** 585 (1956), *C.A.* **51,** 8369f (1957). Toxicity data: H. Kreitmair, *Arch. Exp. Pathol. Pharmakol.* **176,** 171 (1934).

Orthorhombic crystals with $2C_6H_6$ from benzene. The solvent of crystn is given up only after long drying and heating in high vacuum. mp ~190° (dec) (solvent-free base). $[\alpha]_D^{20}$ −197° (chloroform). Very sol in ethyl and methyl alcohol, acetone, chloroform, ethyl acetate; slightly sol in ether. Almost insol in water, petr ether. LD in mice (mg/kg): 0.107 s.c.; 0.032 i.v. (Kreitmair).

Ergotoxine phosphate. Clusters of needles, dec 187°. Sol in 320 parts water, 15 parts boiling alcohol.

Ergotoxine ethanesulfonate. Acicular crystals, dec 209°. Sol in methanol; slightly in alcohol. Almost insol in water. Solid and solns are sensitive to light and air.

3666. Erigeron. Fleabane; horseweed. Leaves and tops of *Conyza canadensis* (L.) Cron. (*Erigeron canadensis* L.), *Compositae.* Habit. Northern and central U.S. Constit. Volatile oil, tannin, gallic acid.

3667. Eriochrome® Black T. [1787-61-7] 3-Hydroxy-4-[(1-hydroxy-2-naphthalenyl)azo]-7-nitro-1-naphthalenesulfonic acid monosodium salt; C.I. Mordant Black 11; C.I. 14645. C_{20}-$H_{12}N_3NaO_7S$; mol wt 461.38. C 52.06%, H 2.62%, N 9.11%, Na 4.98%, O 24.27%, S 6.95%. Prepn: Hagenbach, **US 790363** (1904 to Geigy); *Colour Index* **vol. 4** (3rd ed., 1971) p 4067.

Brownish-black powder with a faint metallic sheen. Sol in hot water giving a reddish-brown soln when cold. Violet-brown precipitate with excess HCl. Deep blue, then red in aq soln of NaOH. Sol in concd H_2SO_4 giving a blackish-blue soln which yields a brown precipitate on dilution.

USE: To dye wool from an acid bath reddish-black, which can be converted to blue-black by afterchroming. As indicator in the determination of the total calcium and magnesium content of water.

3668. Eriodictyol. [552-58-9] 2-(3,4-Dihydroxyphenyl)-2,3-dihydro-5,7-dihydroxy-4*H*-1-benzopyran-4-one; 3′,4′,5,7-tetrahydroxyflavanone. $C_{15}H_{12}O_6$; mol wt 288.25. C 62.50%, H 4.20%, O 33.30%. Isoln from *Eriodictyon californicum* (H. & A.) Greene, *Hydrophyllaceae:* Geissman, *J. Am. Chem. Soc.* **62,**

3258 (1940); from lemon: Mager, *Z. Physiol. Chem.* **274,** 109 (1942); Horowitz, *J. Am. Chem. Soc.* **79,** 6561 (1957); **US 2857318** (1958 to U.S. Dept. Agr.). Structure and synthesis: Reichel *et al., Ann.* **550,** 146 (1942); Zemplén *et al., Ber.* **76B,** 1112 (1943); Pew, *J. Org. Chem.* **27,** 2935 (1962). Synthesis: G. Wurm, U. Geres, *Arch. Pharm.* **315,** 183 (1982). *See also* Bioflavanoids.

Needles with 1½ H_2O from dil alc, dec 257° (rapid heating). After drying in vacuo at 100° for 6 hours, dec 267°. uv max (alc): 290, 326 nm (log ε 2.54, 2.16). Sparingly sol in boiling water, hot alcohol, ether, glacial acetic acid; sol in dil alkalies.

7-L-Rhamnoside. Eriodictin. $C_{21}H_{22}O_{10}$. Isoln from citrin: Bruckner, Szent-Györgyi, *Nature* **138,** 1057 (1936). Structure: Mager, *loc. cit.* Crystals from ethyl acetate, dec 184-186°. $[\alpha]_D^{20}$ −51.5° (in pyridine). Sol in water, acetone, alcohol; practically insol in ether.

3669. Eriodictyon. Yerba santa; consumptive's weed; bear's weed; mountain balm; gum plant. Dried leaves of *Eriodictyon californicum* (H. & A.) Greene, *Hydrophyllaceae.* Habit. U.S. (California). Constit. Volatile oil, eriodictyol, homoeriodictyol, chrysoeriodictyol, xanthoeriodictyol, eriodonol, eriodictyonic acid, ericolin, resin.

USE: Pharmaceutic aid (flavor).

3670. Eritadenine. [23918-98-1] ($\alpha R,\beta R$)-6-Amino-α,β-dihydroxy-9*H*-purine-9-butanoic acid; 2(*R*),3(*R*)-dihydroxy-4-(9-adenyl)butyric acid; 4-(6-amino-9*H*-purin-9-yl)-4-deoxy-D-erythronic acid; lentinacin; lentysine. $C_9H_{11}N_5O_4$; mol wt 253.21. C 42.69%, H 4.38%, N 27.66%, O 25.27%. Hypocholesterolemic principle isolated from the Shiitake mushroom, *Lentinus edodes* Sing. Isoln, activity and structure: I. Chibata *et al., Experientia* **25,** 1237 (1969). Synthesis: T. Kamiya *et al., J. Heterocycl. Chem.* **9,** 359 (1972). GC/MS determn in mushroom extracts: G. Vitányi *et al., Rapid Commun. Mass Spectrom.* **12,** 120 (1998). Effect on phospholipid metabolism: K. Sugiyama *et al., J. Nutr.* **125,** 2134 (1995); on linoleic acid metabolism: *idem et al., Lipids* **32,** 859 (1997).

Crystals from 10% acetic acid, mp 278-279° (dec). $[\alpha]_D$ +51.4° (c = 1.6 in 0.1*N* NaOH). uv max (water): 261.5 nm (ε 14508).

Sodium salt. $C_9H_{10}N_5NaO_4$. Crystals from 50% ethanol, mp 275° (dec). $[\alpha]_D^{20}$ +45.5° (c = 1 in H_2O). IR, NMR: Chibata, *loc. cit.*

3671. Eritoran. [185955-34-8] 3-*O*-Decyl-2-deoxy-6-*O*-[2-deoxy-3-*O*-[(3*R*)-3-methoxydecyl]-6-*O*-methyl-2-[[(11*Z*)-1-oxo-11-octadecenyl]amino]-4-*O*-phosphono-β-D-glucopyranosyl]-2-[[(1,3-dioxotetradecyl)amino]-α-D-glucopyranose 1-(dihydrogen phosphate). $C_{66}H_{126}N_2O_{19}P_2$; mol wt 1313.66. C 60.34%, H 9.67%, N 2.13%, O 23.14%, P 4.72%. Toll-like receptor 4 (TLR4) antagonist. Synthetic analog of the lipid A component of endotoxin, a major constituent of the outer membrane of Gram negative bacteria. Prepn: W. J. Christ *et al.,* **WO 9639411;** *eidem,* **US 5750664** (1996, 1998 both to Eisai). Pharmacology: M. Mullarkey *et al., J. Pharmacol. Exp. Ther.* **304,** 1093 (2003). Clinical pharmacokinetics: Y. N. Wong *et al., J. Clin. Pharmacol.* **43,** 735 (2003); and lipid distribution profile: D. P. Rossignol *et al., Anti-*

microb. Agents Chemother. **48**, 3233 (2004). Clinical evaluation in experimental endotoxemia: M. Lynn *et al., J. Pharmacol. Exp. Ther.* **308**, 175 (2004). Review of pharmacology and clinical experience: D. P. Rossignol, M. Lynn, *Curr. Opin. Invest. Drugs* **6**, 496-502 (2005).

Tetrasodium salt. [185954-98-7] E-5564; B-1287. $C_{66}H_{122}$-$N_2Na_4O_{19}P_2$; mol wt 1401.58.

THERAP CAT: In treatment of severe sepsis.

3672. Erlotinib. [183321-74-6] *N*-(3-Ethynylphenyl)-6,7-bis(2-methoxyethoxy)-4-quinazolinamine. $C_{22}H_{23}N_3O_4$; mol wt 393.44. C 67.16%, H 5.89%, N 10.68%, O 16.27%. Selective epidermal growth factor receptor (EGFR)-tyrosine kinase inhibitor. Prepn: R. C. Schnur, L. D. Arnold, **WO 9630347**; *eidem,* **US 5747498** (1996, 1998 both to Pfizer). Mechanism of action study: J. D. Moyer *et al., Cancer Res.* **57**, 4838 (1997). Enzyme inhibition and antitumor activity: V. A. Pollack *et al., J. Pharmacol. Exp. Ther.* **291**, 739 (1999). HPLC determn in plasma: E. R. Lepper *et al., J. Chromatogr. B* **796**, 181 (2003). Clinical pharmacokinetics: M. Hidalgo *et al., J. Clin. Oncol.* **19**, 3267 (2001). Clinical evaluation in non-small-cell lung cancer: R. Pérez-Soler *et al., J. Clin. Oncol.* **22**, 3238 (2004). Review of pharmacology and clinical development: T. E. Kim, J. R. Murren, *Curr. Opin. Invest. Drugs* **3**, 1385-1395 (2002); and use in non-small cell lung cancer: F. H. Blackhall *et al., Expert Opin. Pharmacother.* **6**, 995-1002 (2005).

Hydrochloride. [183319-69-9] CP-358774; OSI-774; Tarceva. $C_{22}H_{23}N_3O_4$.HCl; mol wt 429.90. mp 228-230°. pKa (25°): 5.42. Soly in water (pH ~2): ~0.4 mg/ml. Slightly sol in methanol. Practically insol in acetonitrile, acetone, ethyl acetate, hexane.

THERAP CAT: Antineoplastic.

3673. Ertapenem. [153832-46-3] [4*R*,5*S*,6*S*]-3-[[(3*S*,5*S*)-5-[[(3-Carboxyphenyl)amino]carbonyl]-3-pyrrolidinyl]thio]-6-[(1*R*)-1-hydroxyethyl]-4-methyl-7-oxo-1-azabicyclo[3.2.0]hept-2-ene-2-

carboxylic acid; (1*R*,5*S*,6*S*,8*R*,2′*S*,4′*S*)-2-(2-(3-carboxyphenylcarbamoyl)pyrrolidin-4-ylthio)-6-(1-hydroxyethyl)-1-methylcarbapenem-3-carboxylic acid; ZD-443. $C_{22}H_{25}N_3O_7S$; mol wt 475.51. C 55.57%, H 5.30%, N 8.84%, O 23.55%, S 6.74%. Group 1 carbapenem antibiotic. Prepn: M. J. Betts *et al.,* **WO 9315078**; *eidem,* **US 5478820** (1993, 1995 both to Zeneca). Large-scale synthesis: J. M. Williams *et al., J. Org. Chem.* **70**, 7479 (2005). Pharmacokinetics in primates: J. G. Sundelof *et al., Antimicrob. Agents Chemother.* **41**, 1743 (1997). *In vivo* efficacy and pharmacokinetics: C. J. Gill *et al., ibid.* **42**, 1996 (1998). *In vitro* efficacy and β-lactamase stability: J. Kohler *et al., ibid.* **43**, 1170 (1999). HPLC determn in plasma and urine: D. G. Musson *et al., J. Chromatogr. B* **720**, 99 (1998); of residual crystallization solvents: T. K. Natishan, Y. Wu, *ibid. A* **800**, 275 (1998). Series of articles on pharmacology and clinical experience in complicated community-acquired infections: *J. Antimicrob. Chemother.* **53**, Suppl. S2, ii1-ii86 (2004).

Sodium salt. [153832-38-3] MK-826; Invanz. $C_{22}H_{24}N_3$-NaO_7S; mol wt 497.50. White to off-white hygroscopic, weakly crystalline powder. Sol in water, 0.9% sodium chloride soln. Practically insol in ethanol; insol in isopropyl acetate, THF.

THERAP CAT: Antibacterial.

3674. Erucic Acid. [112-86-7] (*Z*)-13-Docosenoic acid; Δ^{13}-*cis*-docosenoic acid. $C_{22}H_{42}O_2$; mol wt 338.57. C 78.04%, H 12.50%, O 9.45%. A monoethenoid acid found in the seed fats of *Cruciferae* and *Tropaeolaceae*. It constitutes 40 to 50% of the total fatty acids of rapeseed, mustard and wallflower seed, and it represents up to 80% of fatty acids of nasturtium seeds, *cf.* K. S. Markley, *Fatty Acids* Part I (Interscience, New York, 2nd ed., 1960) p 138-139. Prepn of a crude product by alkaline hydrolysis of rapeseed oil: Noller, Talbot, *Org. Synth.* **coll. vol. II**, 258 (1943). A purer product is obtained by the method of Dorée and Pepper, *J. Chem. Soc.* **1942**, 477, which involves a fractional precipitation and crystallization. Prepn of a pure product by acid soap crystallization: Chobanov *et al., Chem. Ind. (London)* **1965**, 606. Synthesis: Bowman, *J. Chem. Soc.* **1950**, 177, 325; Bounds *et al., ibid.* **1953**, 2393. Treatment with nitric acid yields the *trans* isomer, brassidic acid, *q.v.*: Dorée, Pepper, *loc. cit.* Brief review: E. Lower, *Manuf. Chem.* **56**(6), 61-63 (1985).

Needles from alcohol, mp 33.8°. Iodine value 74.98; neutralization value 165.72. d_4^{55} 0.860. bp_{760} 381.5° (decompn); bp_{400} 358.8°; bp_{100} 314.4°; bp_{60} 300.2°; bp_{20} 270.6°; bp_5 239.7°; $bp_{1.0}$ 206.7°. n_D^{45} 1.4534; $n_D^{}$ 1.44794. Insol in water. About 175 g dissolve in 100 ml ethanol and about 160 g dissolve in 100 ml methanol. Very sol in ether.

3675. Erythritol. [149-32-6] (2*R*,3*S*)-*rel*-1,2,3,4-Butanetetrol; *meso*-erythritol; tetrahydroxybutane; erythrol; erythrite; anti-erythrite; erythroglucin; phycite. $C_4H_{10}O_4$; mol wt 122.12. C 39.34%, H 8.25%, O 52.41%. All natural bulk sweetener found in various fruits and fermented foods; 60 to 70% as sweet as sucrose. Isoln from algae, lichens, grasses: Bamberger, Landsiedl, *Monatsh. Chem.* **21**, 571 (1900); Hesse, *J. Prakt. Chem.* **92**, 425 (1915); Hofmann, *Ber.* **7**, 508 (1874). Prepn by *Aspergillus niger*: Yuill, *Nature* **162**, 652 (1948); by *Penicillium herquei*: Galarraga *et al., Biochem. J.* **61**, 456 (1955); from 2-butene-1,4-diol: Reppe, Schnabel, **DE 734025** (1943 to I. G. Farbenind.); from periodate-oxidized starch: Jeanes, Hudson, *J. Org. Chem.* **20**, 1565 (1955). Structure: Shimada, *Acta Crystallogr.* **11**, 748 (1958). Review of metabolism, toxicology and clinical safety studies: I. C. Munro *et al., Food Chem. Toxicol.* **36**, 1139-1174 (1998); of use in beverage industry: P. de Cock, C.-L. Bechert, *Pure Appl. Chem.* **74**, 1281-1289 (2002).

CH₂OH

$$\begin{array}{c} CH_2OH \\ | \\ HC-OH \\ | \\ HC-OH \\ | \\ CH_2OH \end{array}$$

Tetragonal prisms, mp 121.5°. About twice as sweet as sucrose. bp 329-331°. Very sol in water (satd soln contains about 61% w/w); sol in pyridine (satd soln contains 2.5% w/w); slightly sol in alcohol. Practically insol in ether. pKa (18°): 13.903. LD_{50} in male, female rats (g/kg): 6.6, 9.6 i.v.; >16, >16 s.c.; 13.1, 13.5 orally (Munro).

USE: Non-nutritive sweetener in beverages.

3676. Erythritol Anhydride. [564-00-1] $(2R,2'S)$-rel-2,2'-Bioxirane; meso-1,2:3,4-diepoxybutane; butadiene diepoxide; butadiene dioxide; butanedione; Bioxiran. $C_4H_6O_2$; mol wt 86.09. C 55.81%, H 7.02%, O 37.17%. Prepn from erythrityl chlorohydrin: Przybytek, *Ber.* **17**, 1091 (1884); by refluxing 1,4-dichloro-2,3-butanediol in tetrahydrofuran with NaOH: Reppe, *Ann.* **596**, 141 (1955); meso-form from 1,4-dihydroxy-2-butene or from 3,4-epoxy-1-butene and dl-form from 1,4-dibromo-2-butene: Beech, *J. Chem. Soc.* **1951**, 2483. Use to prevent microbial spoilage: H. D. Michener, J. C. Lewis, US 2934439 (1960 to U.S. Secy of Agr.). Toxicity data: H. F. Smyth et al., *Arch. Ind. Hyg. Occup. Med.* **10**, 61 (1954).

Liquid. d_4^{18} 1.113. bp 138°; bp_{23} 50-51°. meso-form, bp_{761} 140-142°. mp −19°. Compd with piperidine, mp 106° (Beech). Misc with water which hydrolyzes it to erythritol. LD_{50} orally in rats: 0.078 g/kg (Smyth).

Caution: This substance is reasonably anticipated to be a human carcinogen: *Report on Carcinogens, Eleventh Edition* (PB2005-104914, 2004) p III-94.

USE: Curing polymers; crosslinking textile fibers.

3677. Erythrityl Tetranitrate. [7297-25-8] $(2R,3S)$-rel-1,2,3,4-Butanetetroltetranitrate; erythritol tetranitrate; erythrol tetranitrate; tetranitrol; tetranitrin; nitroerythrite; Cardilate; Cardiloid. $C_4H_6N_4O_{12}$; mol wt 302.11. C 15.90%, H 2.00%, N 18.55%, O 63.55%. Made by nitration of erythritol.

Leaflets from alcohol, mp 61°. Sol in alcohol, ether, glycerol. Insol in water. Reduces Fehling's soln. Explodes on percussion. Its use in pharmaceutical preparations is only in admixture with carbohydrate substances such as lactose. Sold in tablet form only. Such tablets are nonexplosive.

THERAP CAT: Vasodilator (coronary).

THERAP CAT (VET): Vasodilator.

3678. Erythrocentaurin. [50276-98-7] 3,4-Dihydro-1-oxo-1H-2-benzopyran-5-carboxaldehyde; 5-formyl-3,4-dihydroisocoumarin; 5-formyl-3,4-dihydro-1H-2-benzopyran-1-one. $C_{10}H_8$-O_3; mol wt 176.17. C 68.18%, H 4.58%, O 27.25%. From *Centaurium umbellatum* Gilib., (*Erythraea centaurium* Pers.), Gentianaceae or *Swertia japonica* (Maxim.) Makino, Gentianaceae. By hydrolysis of swertiamarin and erytaurin with emulsin. Isoln: Kariyone, Matsushima, *J. Pharm. Soc. Jpn.* **47**, 25 (1927). Structure: Kubota, Tomita, *Chem. Ind. (London)* **1958**, 230; Kubota et al., *Tetrahedron Lett.* **1961**, 223. Synthesis: Wenkert et al., *J. Org. Chem.* **29**, 2534 (1964).

Long needles, mp 140-141°. Turns red on exposure to sunlight. uv max: 223, 290 nm (log ε 4.30, 3.13).

THERAP CAT: Bitter tonic.

3679. α-Erythroidine. [466-80-8] $(3\beta,12\beta)$-1,2,6,7-Tetradehydro-12,17-dihydro-3-methoxy-16(15H)-oxaerythrinan-15-one. $C_{16}H_{19}NO_3$; mol wt 273.33. C 70.31%, H 7.01%, N 5.12%, O 17.56%. Isoln from *Erythrina* spp, *Leguminosae:* Folkers, Major, US 2373952 (1945 to Merck & Co.); Boekelheide, Grundon, *J. Am. Chem. Soc.* **75**, 2563 (1953). Structure: Godfrey et al., *ibid.* **77**, 3342 (1955). Absolute configuration: Hill, Shearer, *J. Org. Chem.* **27**, 921 (1962); Wenzinger, Boekelheide, *Proc. Chem. Soc. London* **1963**, 53. Conversion of α- to β-erythroidine: Boekelheide, Morrison, *J. Am. Chem. Soc.* **80**, 3905 (1958). Biosynthesis studies: Leete, Ahmad, *ibid.* **88**, 4722 (1966).

Needles from pentane, mp 58-60°. $[\alpha]_D^{27}$ +136° (c = 0.5 in water). Unstable on exposure to air.

Hydrochloride. $C_{16}H_{20}ClNO_3$. Prisms from ethanol, dec 226-228°. $[\alpha]_D^{32}$ +118° (c = 0.5 in water). uv max (ethanol): 224 nm (log ε 4.55).

Methiodide. $C_{17}H_{22}INO_3$. Yellow prisms from ethanol, mp 219-220°.

3680. β-Erythroidine. [466-81-9] (3β)-1,2,6,7-Tetradehydro-14,17-dihydro-3-methoxy-16(15H)-oxaerythrinan-15-one; 12,13-didehydro-13,14-dihydro-α-erythroidine. $C_{16}H_{19}NO_3$; mol wt 273.33. C 70.31%, H 7.01%, N 5.12%, O 17.56%. Skeletal muscle relaxant. Isolated from the seeds and other plant parts of *Erythrina* spp., *Leguminosae:* Folkers, Major, *J. Am. Chem. Soc.* **59**, 1580 (1937); eidem, US 2373952; US 2385266; US 2407713 (1945 and 1946 to Merck & Co.). Structural studies: Koniuszy, Folkers, *J. Am. Chem. Soc.* **72**, 5519 (1950); Boekelheide et al., *ibid.* **75**, 2550 (1953). Absolute configuration: Wenzinger, Boekelheide, *Proc. Chem. Soc. London* **1963**, 53; eidem, *J. Org. Chem.* **29**, 1307 (1964). Toxicity data: F. M. Berger, R. P. Schwartz, *J. Pharmacol. Exp. Ther.* **93**, 362 (1948). *Review:* Boekelheide, *Rec. Chem. Prog.* **16**, 227-239 (1955).

Crystals from abs ethanol, mp 99.5-100°. $[\alpha]_D^{25}$ +88.8°. Sol in water, benzene, chloroform, methanol, ethanol; moderately sol in diethyl ether. Reacts with NaOH to form sodium erythroidinate. LD_{50} i.p. in mice: 24.0 mg/kg (Berger, Schwartz).

Hydrochloride. $C_{16}H_{19}NO_3$.HCl. Small needles from abs ethanol, mp 232° (dec). $[\alpha]_D^{25}$ +10°. Unstable in air and light. Bitter taste. Sol in water, benzene, chloroform, methanol, ethanol; moderately sol in diethyl ether. *Incompat.* with oxidizing agents, alkaline solns, and akaloidal reagents.

Hydrochloride hemihydrate. $C_{16}H_{19}NO_3$.HCl.½H_2O. Small needles from abs ethanol, mp 229.5-230° (dec). $[\alpha]_D$ +95°. Has curare-like action which is antagonized by prostigmine.

Hydrobromide. $C_{16}H_{19}NO_3$.HBr. Crystals from abs ethanol, mp 222.5°. $[\alpha]_D^{25}$ +111.2°.

Hydriodide. $C_{16}H_{19}NO_3$.HI. Crystals from abs ethanol, mp 206°. $[\alpha]_D^{25}$ +108.1°.

Methiodide. $C_{16}H_{19}NO_3$.CH₃I. White prisms from alcohol, mp 211°.

3681. Erythromycin. [114-07-8] E-Base; E-Mycin; Erythromycin A; Aknemycin; Aknin; Emgel; Ery-Derm; Erymax; Ery-Tab; Erythromid; ERYC; Erycen; Erycin; Erycinum; Ermysin;

Gallimycin; Ilotycin; Inderm; PCE; Retcin; Staticin; Stiemycin. $C_{37}H_{67}NO_{13}$; mol wt 733.93. C 60.55%, H 9.20%, N 1.91%, O 28.34%. Antibiotic substance produced by a strain of *Streptomyces erythreus* (Waksman) Waksman & Henrici, found in a soil sample from the Philippine Archipelago. Isoln: McGuire *et al.*, *Antibiot. Chemother.* **2**, 281 (1952); Bunch, McGuire, US 2653899 (1953 to Lilly); Clark, Jr., US 2823203 (1958 to Abbott). Properties: Flynn *et al.*, *J. Am. Chem. Soc.* **76**, 3121 (1954). Solubility data: Weiss *et al.*, *Antibiot. Chemother.* **7**, 374 (1957). Structure: Wiley *et al.*, *J. Am. Chem. Soc.* **79**, 6062 (1957). Configuration: Hofheinz, Grisebach, *Ber.* **96**, 2867 (1963); Harris *et al.*, *Tetrahedron Lett.* **1965**, 679. There are three erythromycins produced during fermentation, designated A, B, and C; A is the major and most important component. Erythromycins A and B contain the same sugar moieties, desosamine, *q.v.*, and cladinose (3-*O*-methylmycarose). They differ in position 12 of the aglycone, erythronolide, A having an hydroxyl substituent. Component C contains desosamine and the same aglycone present in A but differs by the presence of mycarose, *q.v.*, instead of cladinose. Structure of B: P. F. Wiley *et al.*, *J. Am. Chem. Soc.* **79**, 6070 (1957); of C: *eidem, ibid.* 6074. Synthesis of the aglycone, erythronolide B: E. J. Corey *et al., ibid.* **100**, 4618, 4620 (1978); of erythronolide A: *eidem, ibid.* **101**, 7131 (1979). Asymmetric total synthesis of erythromycin A: R. B. Woodward *et al., ibid.* **103**, 3215 (1981). NMR spectrum of A: D. J. Ager, C. K. Sood, *Magn. Reson. Chem.* **25**, 948 (1987). HPLC determn in plasma: W. Xiao *et al., J. Chromatogr. B* **817**, 153 (2005). Biosynthesis: Martin, Goldstein, *Prog. Antimicrob. Anticancer Chemother., Proc. 6th Int. Congr. Chemother.* **II**, 1112 (1970); Martin *et al., Tetrahedron* **31**, 1985 (1975). Cloning and expression of clustered biosynthetic genes: R. Stanzak *et al., Biotechnology* **4**, 229 (1986). *Reviews:* T. J. Perun in *Drug Action and Drug Resistance in Bacteria* **I**, S. Mitsuhashi, Ed. (University Park Press, Baltimore, 1977) pp 123-152; Oleinick in *Antibiotics* vol. 3, J. W. Corcoran, F. E. Hahn, Eds. (Springer-Verlag, New York, 1975) pp 396-419; *Infection* **10**, Suppl. 2, S61-S118 (1982). Comprehensive description: W. L. Koch, *Anal. Profiles Drug Subs.* **8**, 159-177 (1979).

Erythromycin A

Hydrated crystals from water, mp 135-140°, resolidifies with second mp 190-193°. Melting point taken after drying at 56° and 8 mm. $[\alpha]_D^{25}$ −78° (c = 1.99 in ethanol). uv max (pH 6.3): 280 nm (ε 50). pKa_1 8.8. Basic reaction. Readily forms salts with acids. Soly in water: ~2 mg/ml. Freely sol in alcohols, acetone, chloroform, acetonitrile, ethyl acetate. Moderately sol in ether, ethylene dichloride, amyl acetate.

Ethylsuccinate. [41342-53-4] Anamycin; Arpimycin; E.E.S.; Eritrocina; Eryliquid; Eryped; Erythroped; Esinol; Monomycin; Paediathrocin; Pediamycin; Refkas. $C_{43}H_{75}NO_{16}$; mol wt 862.05. Prepn: GB 830846; R. K. Clark, US 2967129 (1960, 1961 both to Abbott). Hydrated crystals from acetone + water, mp 109-110°. $[\alpha]_D$ −42.5°.

THERAP CAT: Antibacterial.
THERAP CAT (VET): Antibacterial.

3682. Erythromycin Acistrate. [96128-89-1] Erythromycin 2'-acetate octadecanoate (salt); octadecanoic acid compd with erythromycin 2'-acetate; 2'-acetylerythromycin stearate; Erasis. $C_{57}H_{105}NO_{16}$; mol wt 1060.44. C 64.56%, H 9.98%, N 1.32%, O 24.14%. $C_{39}H_{69}NO_{14}\cdot CH_3(CH_2)_{16}COOH$. Ester prodrug of erythromycin, *q.v.* Prepn: M. L. A. Marvola *et al.*, BE 901411;

E. J. Honkanen *et al.*, US 4599326 (1985, 1986 both to Orionyhtymä Oy). Pharmacology, toxicity and clinical studies: *J. Antimicrob. Chemother.* **21**, Suppl D, 1-122 (1988). For structure see Erythromycin.

THERAP CAT: Antibacterial.

3683. Erythromycin Estolate. [3521-62-8] Erythromycin 2'-propanoate dodecyl sulfate (salt); erythromycin propionate lauryl sulfate; lauryl sulfate salt of the propionic acid ester of erythromycin; propionylerythromycin lauryl sulfate; Eritroger; Eromycin; Ilosone; Lauromicina; Neo-Erycinum; PELS; Roxomicina; Stellamicina; Eriscel; Estomicina; Eupragin; Marcoeritrex; Togiren. $C_{52}H_{97}NO_{18}S$; mol wt 1056.39. C 59.12%, H 9.26%, N 1.33%, O 27.26%, S 3.04%. $C_{40}H_{71}NO_{14}\cdot CH_3(CH_2)_{11}OSO_3H$. Prepn from propionyl erythromycin: Stephens *et al., J. Am. Pharm. Assoc.* **48**, 620 (1959); Bray, Stephens, US 3000874 (1961 to Lilly). Toxicity: E. I. Goldenthal, *Toxicol. Appl. Pharmacol.* **18**, 185 (1971). Comprehensive description: J. M. Mann, *Anal. Profiles Drug Subs.* **1**, 101-117 (1972). For structure see Erythromycin.

Long needles, mp 135-140° (dec). pKa 6.9. Soly in water: 0.024 mg/ml; sol in alcohol, acetone, chloroform. LD_{50} orally in rats: >5000 mg/kg (Goldenthal).

THERAP CAT: Antibacterial.

3684. Erythromycin Glucoheptonate. [23067-13-2] D-*glycero*-D-*gulo*-Heptonic acid compd with erythromycin (1:1); erythromycin glucoheptonic acid salt; erythromycin gluceptate; Ilotycin Gluceptate. $C_{44}H_{81}NO_{21}$; mol wt 960.11. C 55.04%, H 8.50%, N 1.46%, O 34.99%. $C_{37}H_{67}NO_{13}\cdot C_7H_{14}O_8$. Semi-synthetic macrolide antibiotic. Prepn: Shepler, US 2852429 (1958 to Lilly).

Crystals, mp 95-140°. Freely sol in water, alcohol, dioxane, acetone, propylene glycol. Practically insol in ether, carbon tetrachloride, toluene, benzene. 2% aq solns are levorotatory and have a pH of 6.0 to 7.5.

THERAP CAT: Antibacterial.

3685. Erythromycin Lactobionate. [3847-29-8] 4-*O*-β-D-Galactopyranosyl-D-gluconic acid compd with erythromycin (1:1); Erythrocin Lactobionate. Semi-synthetic macrolide antibiotic prepd from erythromycin base and lactobiono-δ-lactone in wateracetone: Hoffhine, US 2761859 (1956 to Abbott); alternate prepn and antibacterial activity: S. K. Dutta, K. S. Basu, US 4137397 (1979 to Jadavpur Univ.). Pharmacokinetics: R. L. Parsons *et al., J. Int. Med. Res.* **8**, suppl. 2, 15 (1980).

White, amorphous powder, mp 145-150°. Soly in water about 200 mg/ml. Freely sol in alcohol; slightly sol in ether. pH of a 2% aq soln 6.0-7.5. A 5% stock soln can be prepd with water or glucose soln but not with NaCl isotonic soln, because NaCl at this concn precipitates erythromycin base. Lower concns of inorganic salts are compatible.

THERAP CAT: Antibacterial.
THERAP CAT (VET): Antibacterial.

3686. Erythromycin Propionate. [134-36-1] Erythromycin 2'-propanoate; propionylerythromycin; monopropionylerythromycin; Propiocine. $C_{40}H_{71}NO_{14}$; mol wt 789.99. C 60.81%, H 9.06%, N 1.77%, O 28.35%. Semi-synthetic macrolide antibiotic. Prepn: V. C. Stephens, US 2993833 (1961 to Lilly); V. C. Stephens, J. W. Conine, *Antibiot. Annu.* **1958-59**, 346. Pharmacology and toxicology: C. Lee *et al., ibid.* 354. Clinical studies: R. S. Griffith, *ibid.* 364; D. M. Perry *et al., ibid.* 375. Clinical pharmacokinetics: M. Ducci *et al., Int. J. Clin. Pharmacol. Ther. Toxicol.* **19**, 494 (1981). HPLC determn in plasma: W. Xiao *et al., J. Chromatogr. B* **817**, 153 (2005).

Monohydrate. Crystals from acetone + water, mp 122-126°. $[\alpha]_D^{25}$ −81.6° (acetone). pKa: 6.9. Very slightly sol in water. Readily sol in methanol, ethanol, acetone, ethyl acetate, DMF. LD_{50} in mice, rats (g/kg): 2.87, >5.0 orally; >5.0, >5.0 s.c. (Lee).

THERAP CAT: Antibacterial.

3687. Erythromycin Stearate. [643-22-1] Erythromycin octadecanoate (salt); Abboticine; Bristamycin; Dowmycin E; Erypar; Eryprim; Erythro S; Erythrocin; Ethril; Ethryn; Gallimycin; Meberyt; Pantomicina; Pfizer-E; Wemid. $C_{55}H_{103}NO_{15}$; mol wt 1018.40. C 64.87%, H 10.19%, N 1.38%, O 23.57%. Semi-synthetic macrolide antibiotic. Prepn: O. F. Walasek, US 2881163 (1959 to Abbott). Bioavailability: A.-S. Malmborg, *J. Antimicrob.*

Chemother. **5,** 591 (1979). Pharmacokinetics and tolerance: D. C. Shanson *et al., ibid.* **14,** 157 (1984). Clinical efficacy in respiratory tract infections: J. P. Butler *et al., Chemotherapy (Basel)* **25,** 367 (1979); in acute otitis media: C. Rosen *et al., Acta Otolaryngol. (Stockholm)* **Suppl. 407,** 23 (1984). Prepn of erythromycin stearate (ester): Booth, Murray, **US 2862921** (1958 to Upjohn).

Crystals. Slightly bitter taste. Slightly sol in alc, ether, chloroform. Practically insol in water.

THERAP CAT: Antibacterial.

THERAP CAT (VET): Antibacterial.

3688. Erythropoietin. [11096-26-7] Erythropoiesis stimulating factor; hemopoietine; ESF; Ep; Epo. Glycoprotein hormone which stimulates red blood cell formation in higher organisms: P. Carnot, C. Deflandre, *Compt. Rend.* **143,** 384 (1906). Single chain, 165 amino acid polypeptide containing approx 40% carbohydrate. Produced in response to hypoxia, primarily in the kidneys and to a lesser extent in the liver. Occurs normally in low concentrations in plasma; elevated levels in urine and plasma under conditions of anemic or hypoxic stress. Isoln from sheep plasma: W. F. White *et al., Recent Prog. Horm. Res.* **16,** 219 (1960); from human urine: J. Espada, A. Gutnisky, *Biochem. Med.* **3,** 475 (1970). Purification from human urine: T. Miyake *et al., J. Biol. Chem.* **252,** 5558 (1977). Amino acid sequence: P.-H. Lai *et al., J. Biol. Chem.* **261,** 3116 (1986). Biogenesis and control of production: J. W. Fisher, *Proc. Soc. Exp. Biol. Med.* **173,** 289 (1983). Production by recombinant DNA technology in *E. coli:* S. Lee-Huang, *Proc. Natl. Acad. Sci. USA* **81,** 2708 (1984); in mammalian cells: K. Jacobs *et al., Nature* **313,** 806 (1985); F.-K. Lin *et al., Proc. Natl. Acad. Sci. USA* **82,** 7580 (1985). Review of chemistry, pharmacology and clinical efficacy of recombinant human Epo (*rHuEpo*): K. K. Flaharty *et al., Clin. Pharm.* **8,** 769-782 (1989). Review of clinical screening methods and abuse potential in sports: G. Lippi, G. Guidi, *Clin. Chem. Lab. Med.* **38,** 13-19 (2000). Review of clinical experience: K.-U. Eckardt, *Nephrol. Dial. Transplant.* **16,** 1745-1749 (2001); D. H. Henry, *Expert Opin. Pharmacother.* **6,** 295-310 (2005).

Epoetin alfa. [113427-24-0] Epogen; Eprex; Erypo; Procrit. Human Epo produced by recombinant technology. Contains 165 amino acids; mol wt 30.4 kDa.

Epoetin beta. [122312-54-3] Epogin; Recormon. Human Epo produced by recombinant technology. Contains 165 amino acids; mol wt ~30 kDa.

THERAP CAT: Hematopoietic.

3689. Erythropterin. [7449-03-8] 3-(2-Amino-4,5,6,8-tetrahydro-4,6-dioxo-7(3H)-pteridinylidene)-2-oxopropanoic acid; 2-amino-3,4,5,6-tetrahydro-4,6-dioxo-7-pteridinepyruvic acid. $C_9H_7N_5O_5$; mol wt 265.18. C 40.76%, H 2.66%, N 26.41%, O 30.17%. Pigment responsible for the red, orange and yellow color spots on the wings of butterflies. Has been detected also in the integument of other insects. Isoln: C. Schöpf, E. Becker, *Ann.* **524,** 49 (1936). Structure: R. Tschesche, H. Ende, *Ber.* **91,** 2074 (1958). Revised structure: W. Pfleiderer, *ibid.* **95,** 2195 (1962). Synthesis: M. Viscontini, H. Stierlin, *Helv. Chim. Acta* **46,** 51 (1963). Correlation to body coloration: E. J. Pfeiler, Jr., *J. Res. Lepid.* **7,** 183 (1968); C. Melber, G. H. Schmidt, *Comp. Biochem. Physiol.* **116A,** 17 (1997). Quantification: *eidem, ibid.* **101B,** 115 (1992); Y. Bel *et al., Arch. Insect Biochem. Physiol.* **34,** 83 (1997).

As the monohydrate, red microcrystals. Abs max (pH 1.0): 450 nm (log ε 4.02). Orange fluorescence from 254-365 nm.

3690. D-Erythrose. [583-50-6] (2R,3R)-2,3,4-Trihydroxybutanal. $C_4H_8O_4$; mol wt 120.10. C 40.00%, H 6.71%, O 53.29%. From calcium D-arabonate by oxidation with H_2O_2: Ruff, *Ber.* **32,** 3674 (1899); **33,** 1799 (1900). From D-glucose:

Perlin, *Methods Carbohydr. Chem.* **1** (Academic Press, New York, 1962) p 64. Synthesis of DL-erythrose: Sonogashira, Nakagawa, *Bull. Chem. Soc. Jpn.* **45,** 2616 (1972).

Syrup. Shows mutarotation. $[\alpha]_D^{20}$ +1° → −14.5° (3 days, c = 11). Sol in water. Slowly reduces cold Fehling's soln. Sodium amalgam reduces it to natural, inactive erythritol. No aldehyde reaction with benzenesulfhydroxamic acid. Not fermented by yeast.

Phenylosazone. $C_{16}H_{18}N_4O_2$. mp 164°.

3691. L-Erythrose. [533-49-3] (2S,3S)-2,3,4-Trihydroxybutanal. $C_4H_8O_4$; mol wt 120.10. C 40.00%, H 6.71%, O 53.29%. From calcium L-arabonate by oxidation with H_2O_2: Ruff, Meusser, *Ber.* **34,** 1365 (1901). From L-arabinose oxime: Wohl, *Ber.* **32,** 3667 (1899). From L-arabonamide by treatment with alkaline NaOCl: Weerman, *Rec. Trav. Chim.* **37,** 35 (1918).

Syrup. Sweet taste. Shows mutarotation. $[\alpha]_D^{24}$ +11.5° (8 min) → +15.2° (120 min) → +30.5° (final, c = 3): Felton, Freudenberg, *J. Am. Chem. Soc.* **57,** 1640 (1935). Soluble in water. Heating with HCl yields lactic acid. Oxidation with Br converts it to L-erythronic acid. Reduces Fehling's soln slowly in the cold. Not fermented by yeast.

Phenylosazone. $C_{16}H_{18}N_4O_2$. mp 164°.

3692. D-Erythrose 4-Phosphate. [585-18-2] (2R,3R)-2,3-Dihydroxy-4-(phosphonooxy)butanal; 4-D-erythrosephosphoric acid. $C_4H_9O_7P$; mol wt 200.08. C 24.01%, H 4.53%, O 55.98%, P 15.48%. Occurs in minute amounts in muscle flesh of all animals. Important natural intermediate in the Embden-Meyerhof scheme of alcoholic fermentation and glycolysis. Prepn by chemical synthesis: Ballou *et al., J. Am. Chem. Soc.* **77,** 2658, 5967 (1955). Outline: *Chem. Eng. News* **34,** 2506 (1956).

Obtained in aq soln only. Shows no observable optical rotation. Is condensed with phosphoenolpyruvate by a cell-free extract from an *E. coli* mutant to give a 90% yield. Best stored and transported as the cyclohexylammonium salt of 4-phosphoryl-D-erythrose dimethyl acetal from which it can be prepared readily when needed.

3693. Erythrosine. [16423-68-0] 3′,6′-Dihydroxy-2′,4′,5′,-7′-tetraiodospiro[isobenzofuran-1(3H),9′-[9H]xanthen]-3-one disodium salt; 2′,4′,5′,7′-tetraiodofluorescein disodium salt; erythrosine BS; erythrosine B; FD & C Red No. 3; C.I. Food Red 14; C.I. Acid Red 51; C.I. 45430. $C_{20}H_6I_4Na_2O_5$; mol wt 879.86. C 27.30%, H 0.69%, I 57.69%, Na 5.23%, O 9.09%. Prepn: Gilliard *et al.,* **DE 108838** (1899); *Frdl.* **5,** 215; Gomberg, Tabern, *J. Ind. Eng. Chem.* **14,** 1115 (1922); Dolinsky, Jones, *J. Assoc. Off. Agric. Chem.* **34,** 114 (1951); *Colour Index* vol. 4 (3rd ed., 1971) p 4428. Structure: Holmes, Scanlan, *J. Am. Chem. Soc.* **49,** 1594 (1927). HPLC determn: F. E. Lancaster, J. F. Lawrence, *J. Chromatogr.* **388,** 248 (1987). Acute toxicity: K. R. Butterworth *et al., Food*

Cosmet. Toxicol. **14,** 525 (1976); S. L. Yankell et al., J. Periodontol. **48,** 228 (1977). Carcinogenicity studies in rodents: J. F. Borzelleca et al., Food Chem. Toxicol. **25,** 723, 735 (1987).

Brown powder. Absorption max (water): 524 nm; in 95% alcohol: 531 nm. Soluble in water to cherry-red soln; sol in alcohol. HCl added to an aq soln produces a yellowish-brown ppt. Sodium hydroxide produces a red ppt sol in an excess of the reagent. LD_{50} in male, female mice, male, female rats (g/kg): 0.40, 0.32, 0.34, 0.37 i.p.; 6.7, 6.9, 7.4, 6.8 orally (Butterworth). Also reported as LD_{50} in mice, rats (mg/kg): 2558, 2891 orally (Yankell).

Note: Consult latest governmental regulations on use in food, drugs and cosmetics.

USE: Biological stain; color additive.

3694. L-Erythrulose. [533-50-6] (3S)-1,3,4-Trihydroxy-2-butanone; L-glycero-tetrulose. $C_4H_8O_4$; mol wt 120.10. C 40.00%, H 6.71%, O 53.29%. Prepn by bacterial oxidation of meso-erythritol: Müller et al., Helv. Chim. Acta **20,** 1468 (1937); Whistler, Underköfler, J. Am. Chem. Soc. **60,** 2507 (1937). Synthesis from D-fructose: Gorin et al., J. Chem. Soc. **1955,** 2699.

Syrup. $[\alpha]_D^{18}$ +11.4° (c = 2.4 in water). Very sensitive to alkali. Soluble in water, abs alc.

Phenylosazone. $C_{16}H_{18}N_4O_2$. Crystals from aq ethanol, mp 162°. $[\alpha]_D$ +32° (10 min) → 0° (24 hr, constant) (c = 0.75 in pyridine + ethanol, 3:2 v/v).

3695. Esaprazole. [64204-55-3] N-Cyclohexyl-1-piperazineacetamide; 1-piperazinyl-4-methylenecarbonylcyclohexylamine; N-(1-piperazinylacetyl)cyclohexylamine; N-[(N-cyclohexylcarbamoyl)methyl]piperazine; hexaprazol(e); exaprazole; C-63; Prazol. $C_{12}H_{23}N_3O$; mol wt 225.33. C 63.96%, H 10.29%, N 18.65%, O 7.10%. Prepn: C. Corvi-Mora, **DE 2702537;** idem, **US 4123530** (1977, 1978 both to Camillo Corvi). Metabolism in animals and man: P. Ventura et al., Farmaco Ed. Prat. **39,** 190 (1984). Cytoprotective activity: B. Lumachi, R. Scuri, Drugs Exp. Clin. Res. **11,** 693 (1985); and pharmacology: R. Scuri et al., Boll. Chim. Farm. **123,** 425 (1983). Pharmacology: G. Coruzzi et al., Farmaco Ed. Prat. **40,** 313 (1985); G. Coruzzi et al., ibid. 324. Antisecretory activity in humans: L. Erembourg et al., Int. J. Clin. Pharmacol. Res. **7,** 95 (1987). HPLC determn in biological fluids: M. A. Girometta et al., J. Chromatogr. **383,** 85 (1986). Clinical trial in comparison with cimetidine: L. Capurso et al., Clin. Trials J. **23,** 293 (1986).

Residue, mp 111-112°. $bp_{0.5}$ 190°. LD_{50} in mice (mg/kg): 1974 orally; 271 i.v.; in rats (mg/kg): 3900 orally (Corvi-Mora).

Hydrochloride. CO-1063. $C_{12}H_{23}N_3O \cdot HCl$; mol wt 261.79.

THERAP CAT: Antiulcerative.

3696. Escin. [6805-41-0] Aescin; Reparil. A mixture of saponins occurring in the seed of the horse chestnut tree, Aesculus hippocastanum L., Hippocastanaceae: Winterstein, Z. Physiol.

Chem. **199,** 25 (1931); Steiner, Holtzem in Paech-Tracey, Moderne Methoden der Pflanzenanalyse III (Springer-Verlag, 1955) p 117. Isoln by chromatography and purification: Fiedler, Arzneim.-Forsch. **4,** 213 (1953); using ion-exchange resins: Erbring et al., **US 3238190** (1966 to Madaus). Previously thought to be built up from the aglycon escigenin, glucuronic acid, glucose and xylose: Jermstadt, Waaler, Pharm. Acta Helv. **28,** 265 (1953); Patt, Winkler, Arzneim.-Forsch. **10,** 273 (1960); Tschesche et al., Ann. **669,** 171 (1963). Structural studies indicate that the two major glycosides in the mixture are built up from the aglycon, *protoescigenin,* which is acylated at C-22 by acetic acid, and from the sugar moiety, glucuronic acid and two D-glucose molecules. The two aglycons differ only at the C-21 position which is acylated by either angelic acid or tiglic acid, q.q.v. Structure and stereochemistry: Wulff, Tschesche, Tetrahedron **25,** 415 (1969); Wagner et al., Arzneim.-Forsch. **20,** 205 (1970); eidem, Z. Physiol. Chem. **351,** 1133 (1970). Early work identified two forms, *α-escin* and *β-escin*: Wagner, Basse, ibid. **320,** 27 (1960). Identity of *prosaponin B* with β-escin: Voigtlander, Rosenberg, Arzneim.-Forsch. **13,** 385 (1963). β-Escin is the natural form and can be converted to α-escin: Wagner, Schlemmer, **US 3450691** (1969 to Klinge); Wagner et al., Arzneimittel-Forsch., loc. cit. Pharmacology: H. Hampel et al., ibid. **20,** 209 (1970); Lang, Mennicke, ibid. **22,** 1928 (1972). Review: Tschesche, Wulff in Fortschr. Chem. Org. Naturst. **30,** 461-606 (1973). Review of pharmacology and clinical experience: C. R. Sirtori, Pharmacolog. Res. **44,** 183-193 (2001).

R = Tiglic acid or Angelic acid

Major glycosides of Escin

α-Escin. [66795-86-6] Amorphous powder, mp 225-227°. $[\alpha]_D^{25}$ −13.5° (c = 5 in methanol). Very sol in water. Hemolytic index: 1:20,000. LD_{50} in mice, rats, guinea pigs (mg/kg): 3.2, 5.4, 15.2 i.v.; 320, 720, 475 orally (Hampel).

Sodium salt. mp 251-252°.

β-Escin. [11072-93-8] Flogencyl. Leaflets from dil ethanol, mp 222-223°. $[\alpha]_D^{27}$ −23.7° (c = 5 in methanol). Practically insol in water. Hemolytic index: 1:40,000. LD_{50} in mice, rats, guinea pigs (mg/kg): 1.4, 2.0, 7.2 i.v.; 134, 400, 188 orally (Hampel).

THERAP CAT: In treatment of peripheral vascular disorders.

3697. Esculetin. [305-01-1] 6,7-Dihydroxy-2H-1-benzopyran-2-one; 6,7-dihydroxycoumarin; cichorigenin. $C_9H_6O_4$; mol wt 178.14. C 60.68%, H 3.39%, O 35.93%. The aglucon of esculin and of cichoriin. By hydrolysis of esculin or of cichoriin: Merz, Arch. Pharm. **270,** 486 (1932). By synthesis: Gattermann, Köbner, Ber. **32,** 288 (1899); Bert, Compt. Rend. **214,** 230 (1942). Review: Sethna, Shah, Chem. Rev. **36,** 1 (1945).

Prisms from glacial acetic acid; leaflets by vacuum sublimation. mp 268-270°. Soluble in dil alkalies with blue fluorescence; moderately sol in hot alcohol and in glacial acetic acid; almost insol in ether, in boiling water.

USE: In filters for absorption of ultraviolet light.

3698. Esculin. [531-75-9] 6-(β-D-Glucopyranosyloxy)-7-hydroxy-2*H*-1-benzopyran-2-one; 6,7-dihydroxycoumarin 6-glucoside; esculoside; bicolorin; enallachrome; polychrome; Escosyl. $C_{15}H_{16}O_9$; mol wt 340.28. C 52.94%, H 4.74%, O 42.32%. In leaves and bark of horse chestnut tree *Aesculus hippocastanum* L., *Hippocastanaceae.* Extraction procedure: Tumann, *Chem. Zentralbl.* **1916**, I, 1277. Synthesis: Merz, Hagemann, *Naturwissenschaften* **29**, 650 (1941); *eidem, Arch. Pharm.* **282**, 79 (1944); Amiard, Nominé, *Bull. Soc. Chim. Fr.* **1948**, 476. Use in bile-esculin test for identification of group D streptococci: C. Chuard, L. B. Reller, *J. Clin. Microbiol.* **36**, 1135 (1998).

Sesquihydrate. Needles from hot water, mp 204-206°. One gram dissolves in 580 ml water, 13 ml boiling water. Sol in hot alcohol, methanol, pyridine, ethyl acetate, acetic acid. Aq solns show blue fluorescence above pH 5.8. $[\alpha]_D^{18} -78.4°$ (c = 2.5 in 50% dioxane). Absorption spectrum: Merz, *Arch. Pharm.* **270**, 482 (1932); Goodwin, Pollock, *Arch. Biochem. Biophys.* **49**, 1 (1954). Has vitamin P activity.

Pentaacetate dihydrate. Needles from methanol, mp 163-164°.

4-Methylesculin. $C_{16}H_{18}O_9$. Prepn: Velluz, Amiard, *Bull. Soc. Chim. Fr.* **1948**, 1109.

USE: Reagent for microbiological identification test.

3699. Eseridine. [25573-43-7] (4a*S-cis*)-2,3,4,4a,9,9a-Hexahydro-2,4a,9-trimethyl-1,2-oxazino[6,5-*b*]indol-6-ol methylcarbamate ester; physostigmine aminoxide; eserine aminoxide; eserine oxide. $C_{15}H_{21}N_3O_3$; mol wt 291.35. C 61.84%, H 7.27%, N 14.42%, O 16.47%. From Calabar bean *(Physostigma venenosum* Balf., *Leguminosae):* Polonovski, Nitzberg, *Bull. Soc. Chim. Fr.* [5] **17**, 244 (1915); **21**, 191 (1917). Structure: Stedman, Barger, *J. Chem. Soc.* **127**, 247 (1925). Revised structure: Hootele, *Tetrahedron Lett.* **1969**, 2713. Stereochemistry: Robinson, Moorcroft, *J. Chem. Soc. C* **1970**, 2077. Total synthesis of racemate: K. Shishido *et al., Chem. Commun.* **1986**, 904.

Rectangular prisms from ether, mp 129°. $[\alpha]_D^{15} -175°$ (alc). Weak base, just alkaline to litmus; does not form crystn salts with mineral acids. Almost insol in water. Sol in alc, chloroform, benzene, ether, petr ether, acetone, dil acids.

Salicylate. [5995-96-0] Génésérine 3. $C_{22}H_{27}N_3O_6$; mol wt 429.47.

THERAP CAT: Cholinergic.

3700. Esmolol. [81147-92-4] 4-[2-Hydroxy-3-[(1-methylethyl)amino]propoxy]benzenepropanoic acid methyl ester; (±)-methyl 3-[4-[2-hydroxy-3-(isopropylamino)propoxy]phenyl]propionate; methyl *p*-[2-hydroxy-3-(isopropylamino)propoxy]hydrocinnamate. $C_{16}H_{25}NO_4$; mol wt 295.37. C 65.06%, H 8.53%, N 4.74%, O 21.67%. Cardioselective β-adrenergic blocker. Prepn: E. I. Carlsson *et al.,* **EP 41491** (1982 to A.B. Hässle), *C.A.* **96**, 122391f (1982); P. W. Erhardt *et al.,* **EP 53435**; *idem,* **US 4593119** (1982, 1986 both to Am. Hosp. Supply); P. W. Erhardt *et al., J. Med. Chem.* **25**, 1408 (1982). Pharmacology: R. J. Gorczynski *et al., J. Cardiovasc. Pharmacol.* **5**, 668 (1983); *eidem, ibid.* **6**, 1548 (1984).

Pharmacokinetics: A. Yacobi *et al., J. Pharm. Sci.* **72**, 711 (1983). GC-MS determn in blood: C. Y. Sum, A. Yacobi, *ibid.* **73**, 1177 (1984). Clinical studies of effect in supraventricular tachycardia: G. Klein *et al., Int. J. Clin. Pharmacol. Ther. Toxicol.* **22**, 112 (1984); R. J. Gray *et al., J. Am. Coll. Cardiol.* **5**, 1451 (1985). Symposium on pharmacology and clinical efficacy: *Am. J. Cardiol.* **56**(11), 1F-62F (1985). Review of pharmacology and clinical efficacy: P. Benfield, E. M. Sorkin, *Drugs* **33**, 392-412 (1987).

Oil, gradually forming crystalline rosettes at room temp, mp 48-50°.

Hydrochloride. [81161-17-3] ASL-8052; Brevibloc. $C_{16}H_{25}$-NO_4.HCl; mol wt 331.83. Crystals from methanol-ether, mp 85-86°.

THERAP CAT: Antiarrhythmic.

3701. Esparto Wax. Spanish grass wax; halfa wax. A wax derived from a tall, tough grass of the Mediterranean region (S. Europe and N. Africa and Libya). The grass is shipped to Scotland, where it is dewaxed and made into fine paper. The wax is a by-product. Two species of grass are cultivated for their excellent cellulose content: *Stipa tenacissima* L. *(Macrochloa tenacissima* (L.) Kunth.), *Graminaceae* and *Lygeum spartum* L., *Graminaceae.* Constit. Esparto wax consists of 15-17% free wax acids, 20-22% alcohols and hydrocarbons, 63-65% esters. The principal hydrocarbon is hentriacontane ($C_{31}H_{64}$, mp 68°). The acids include cerotic, montanic, myricinic ($C_{30}H_{60}O_2$, mp 68°), lacceric ($C_{32}H_{64}$-O_2, mp 70.5°) and hydroxy acids: A. H. Warth, *Chemistry and Technology of Waxes* (Reinhold, New York, 1947) p 139. Extraction of wax from grass: **DD 74703** (1970). TLC identification: H. Schmidt, *Am. Cosmet. Perfum.* **87**, 35 (1972).

Hard, tough wax. d_4^{25} 0.9887. mp 78.1°. Solidifies at 68.8°. Acid value 23.9. Saponification value 69.8. Soly in ethanol (25°): 0.244 g/100 ml; in ethylene chloride (37°): 1.48 g/100 ml.

USE: Substitute or extender for carnauba wax, *q.v.* Blends well with other waxes. Emulsifies easily and imparts smoothness to polishes. Preferred in the manufacture of carbon papers.

3702. Estazolam. [29975-16-4] 8-Chloro-6-phenyl-4*H*-[1,-2,4]triazolo[4,3-*a*][1,4]benzodiazepine; 8-chloro-6-phenyl-4*H-s*-triazolo[4,3-*a*][1,4]benzodiazepine; D-40TA; Cannoc; Esilgan; Eurodin; Julodin; Nemurel; Nuctalon; ProSom; Somnatrol. $C_{16}H_{11}$-ClN_4; mol wt 294.74. C 65.20%, H 3.76%, Cl 12.03%, N 19.01%. Prepn: J. B. Hester, **DE 2012190**; *idem,* **US 3701782** (1970, 1972 to Upjohn); Meguro, Kuwada, *Tetrahedron Lett.* **1970**, 4039; *eidem,* **DE 1955349** (1971 to Toyama), *C.A.* **74**, 88078t (1971); Tawada *et al.,* **DE 2114441** (1971 to Takeda), *C.A.* **76**, 34320p (1972); Hester *et al., J. Med. Chem.* **14**, 1078 (1971). Structure-activity studies: R. Nakajima *et al., Jpn. J. Pharmacol.* **21**, 489 (1971). Pharmacology: *eidem, ibid.* 497; *eidem, Takeda Kenkyushoho* **31**, 349 (1972), *C.A.* **78**, 24138m (1972). Toxicity: Yokotani *et al., ibid.* **32**, 152 (1973), *C.A.* **79**, 133006j (1973). Metabolism: Tanayama *et al., Xenobiotica* **4**, 33-64 (1974); *see also ibid.* 229, 441. Molecular structure studies: Kamiya *et al., Chem. Pharm. Bull.* **21**, 1520 (1973).

Crystals from ethyl acetate-Skellysolve B hexanes, mp 228-229°. LD_{50} orally in male mice, rats and rabbits: 740, 3200, 300 mg/kg (Yokotani).

Note: This is a controlled substance (depressant): **21 CFR, 1308.14.**

THERAP CAT: Sedative, hypnotic.

3703. Estradiol. [50-28-2] (17β)-Estra-1,3,5(10)-triene-3,17-diol; β-estradiol; *cis*-estradiol; 3,17-epidihydroxyestratriene; dihydrofollicular hormone; dihydrofolliculin; dihydroxyestrin; dihydrotheelin; Climara; Estrace; Estraderm; Estradot; Estring; Estrofem; Estrogel; Evorel; Menostar; Systen; Vivelle; Vivelle-Dot; Zumenon. $C_{18}H_{24}O_2$; mol wt 272.38. C 79.37%, H 8.88%, O 11.75%. Potent mammalian estrogenic hormone produced by the ovary. Triggers the production of gonadotropins leading to ovulation. Isoln from follicular fluid of sow ovaries: D. W. MacCorquodale *et al., J. Biol. Chem.* **115**, 435 (1936). Has also been isolated from urine of pregnant women and mares. Prepn from estrone: A. Butenandt, C. Georgens, *Z. Physiol. Chem.* **248**, 129 (1937); F. Hildebrandt *et al.,* US 2096744 (1938 to Schering); from cholesterol: H. H. Inhoffen, G. Zühlsdorff, *Ber.* **74**, 1914 (1941). Total syntheses: U. Eder *et al., Ber.* **109**, 2948 (1976); W. Oppolzer, D. A. Roberts, *Helv. Chim. Acta* **63**, 1703 (1980). Pharmacology: R. W. Lievertz, *Am. J. Obstet. Gynecol.* **156**, 1289 (1987). HPLC determn in plasma and urine: W. Slikker *et al.,J. Chromatogr.* **224**, 205 (1981). Pharmacokinetics: W. Kuhnz *et al., Arzneim.-Forsch.* **43**, 966 (1993). Clinical evaluation in osteoporosis: J. W. W. Studd *et al., Br. J. Obstet. Gynaecol.* **101**, 787 (1994). Comprehensive description: E. G. Salole, *Anal. Profiles Drug Subs.* **15**, 283-318 (1986). Physiologic review: H. G. Burger, *Int. J. Gynaecol. Obstet.* **1989**, Suppl. 1, 5-9. Review of clinical safety and efficacy in estrogen replacement therapy: A. Cheang *et al., Drug Saf.* **9**, 365-379 (1993); H. L. Judd, *J. Reprod. Med.* **39**, 343-352 (1994).

White crystalline powder. Prisms from 80% alc, stable in air, mp 173-179°. [α]$_D^{25}$ +76 to +83° (dioxane). uv max: 225, 280 nm. Precipitated by digitonin. Practically insol in water. Freely sol in alcohol; sol in acetone, dioxane, other organic solvents; solns of fixed alkali hydroxides; sparingly sol in vegetable oils. 1 mg = 10,000 international units.

Hemihydrate. [35380-71-3] Estroclim; Menorest; Vagifem. $C_{18}H_{24}O_2 \cdot \frac{1}{2}H_2O$; mol wt 281.39.

3-Acetate. [4245-41-4] Femring; Femtrace. $C_{20}H_{26}O_3$; mol wt 314.42.

3-Benzoate. [50-50-0] Estradiol benzoate; Agofollin; Duralease; Ovahormon; Progynon B. $C_{25}H_{28}O_3$; mol wt 376.49. Crystals from alc, mp 191-196°. Stable in air. [α]$_D^{25}$ +58 to +63° (c = 2 in dioxane). Sol in alc, acetone, dioxane; slightly sol in ether, vegetable oils.

17β-Cyclopentanepropanoate. [313-06-4] Estradiol cypionate; ECP. $C_{26}H_{36}O_3$; mol wt 396.56. Prepn: Ott, US 2611773 (1952 to Upjohn). Crystals from benzene + petr ether, mp 151-152°. [α]$_D^{25}$ +45° (chloroform). Sol in ether, methanol, benzene, chloroform, peanut oil, cottonseed oil, corn oil, sesame oil.

Dipropionate. [113-38-2] Ovahormon Depot. $C_{24}H_{32}O_4$; mol wt 384.51. Prepn: K. Miescher, C. Scholz, US 2205627 (1940 to Ciba). mp 104-105°.

17-Heptanoate. [4956-37-0] Estradiol enanthate; SQ-16150. $C_{25}H_{36}O_3$; mol wt 384.55. Prepn: Gauthier *et al., Ann. Pharm. Fr.* **16**, 757 (1958). Crystals from diisopropyl ether, mp 94-96°.

17-Valerate. [979-32-8] Climaval; Delestrogen; Pelanin Depot; Progynon Depot; Progynova. $C_{23}H_{32}O_3$; mol wt 356.50. Prepn: K. Miescher, C. Scholz, US 2233025 (1941 to Ciba). Comprehensive description: K. Florey, *Anal. Profiles Drug Subs.* **4**, 192-208 (1975). Crystals, mp 144-145°.

Caution: These substances are listed as known human carcinogens: *Report on Carcinogens, Eleventh Edition* (PB2005-104914, 2004) p III-115.

THERAP CAT: Estrogen.
THERAP CAT (VET): Estrogen.

3704. α-Estradiol. [57-91-0] (17α)-Estra-1,3,5(10)-triene-3,17-diol; 1,3,5-estratriene-3,17α-diol; 3,17-dihydroxyestratriene. $C_{18}H_{24}O_2$; mol wt 272.38. C 79.37%, H 8.88%, O 11.75%. Has been isolated from pregnancy urine of mares. Prepn from β-estradiol by inversion of the hydroxyl group at C-17 after tosylation: Allais, Hoffmann, US 2835681 (1958).

Needles with ½H_2O from 80% alcohol, mp 220-223°. [α]$_D^{20}$ +53 to +56° (c = 0.9 in dioxane). Not precipitated by digitonin (in 80% alcoholic soln). Soluble in alcohol, acetone, aq alkalies. One gram dissolves in more than 100 ml of boiling benzene. Slightly sol in ether, chloroform. Insol in water, aq dil acids.

Diacetate. $C_{22}H_{28}O_4$. mp 140-142°.

3-Benzoate. $C_{25}H_{28}O_3$. mp 156-157°; also reported as polymorphous: I, mp 63°; II, mp 153°; III, mp 158°.

3705. Estragole. [140-67-0] 1-Methoxy-4-(2-propenyl)-benzene; *p*-allylanisole; chavicol methyl ether; esdragol. $C_{10}H_{12}$-O; mol wt 148.20. C 81.04%, H 8.16%, O 10.80%. Main constituent of ***tarragon oil*** (*estragon oil*), the oil from *Artemisia dracunculus* L., *Compositae* (esdragon) where it occurs to an extent of 60-75%: Grimaux, *Bull. Soc. Chim.* [3] **11**, 34 (1894); Daufresne, *ibid.* [4] **3**, 333 (1908). Occurs also in pine oil and in American turpentine oil. Prepn: Tiffeneau, *Compt. Rend.* **139**, 482 (1904); Verley, **DE 154654**; D. Wigfield, K. Taymaz, *Tetrahedron Lett.* **1973**, 4841; P. Gramatica *et al., Gazz. Chim. Ital.* **104**, 629 (1974). Toxicity study: P. M. Jenner *et al., Food Cosmet. Toxicol.* **2**, 327 (1964).

Liquid. d_4^{21} 0.9645. bp_{764} 216°; bp_{25} 108-114°; bp_{12} 95-96°. $n_D^{17.5}$ 1.5230. Sol in alcohol, chloroform. Forms azeotropic mixtures with water. LD_{50} in rats, mice (mg/kg): 1820, 1250 orally (Jenner).

USE: In perfumes and as flavor in foods and liqueurs.

3706. Estramustine. [2998-57-4] (17β)-Estra-1,3,5(10)-triene-3,17-diol 3-[bis(2-chloroethyl)carbamate]; estradiol 3-bis(2-chloroethyl)carbamate; estra-1,3,5(10)triene-3,17β-diol 3-[*N,N*-bis(2-chloroethyl)carbamate]; Ro-21-8837. $C_{23}H_{31}Cl_2NO_3$; mol wt 440.40. C 62.73%, H 7.09%, Cl 16.10%, N 3.18%, O 10.90%. Carbamate ester linking estradiol to nor-nitrogen mustard; depolymerizes microtubules by binding to microtubule associated proteins (MAPs). Prepn: **BE 646319**; Fex *et al.,* US 3299104 (1963, 1967 to AB Leo); Niculescu-Duvaz *et al., J. Med. Chem.* **10**, 172 (1967). Clinical results: Anderes, *Praxis* **60**, 1375 (1971); Muntzing, Nilsson, *Z. Krebsforsch. Klin. Onkol.* **77**, 166 (1972). Review of mechanism of action: K. D. Tew, M. E. Stearns, *Pharmacol. Ther.* **43**, 299-319 (1989); of pharmacokinetics and pharmacodynamics: A. T. Bergenheim, R. Henriksson, *Clin. Pharmacokinet.* **34**, 163-172 (1998).

Crystals from benzene-petr ether, mp 104-105°. $[\alpha]_D^{20}$ +50° (in dioxane). uv max (alcohol): 270.7, 276.5 nm.

17-Phosphate. Estracyt. $C_{23}H_{32}Cl_2NO_6P$; mol wt 520.38. mp 155° (dec). $[\alpha]_D^{20}$ +30° (dioxane). Sol in aqueous and alkali solns.

17-(Dihydrogenphosphate) disodium salt monohydrate. [52205-73-9] (anhydrous). Emcyt. $C_{23}H_{30}Cl_2NNa_2O_6P.H_2O$; mol wt 582.36. Off-white powder; readily sol in water.

THERAP CAT: Antineoplastic.

3707.   Estriol. [50-27-1] (16α,17β)-Estra-1,3,5(10)-triene-3,16,17-triol; 1,3,5-estratriene-3β,16α,17β-triol; 3,16α,17β-trihydroxy-Δ^{1,3,5}-estratriene; 16α-hydroxyestradiol; follicular hormone hydrate; oestriol; trihydroxyestrin; Colpogyn; Destriol; Gynäsan; Hormomed; Klimax E; Oekolp; Ortho-Gynest; Ovesterin; Ovestin; Ovo-Vinces; Theelol; Trophicreme; Tridestrin; Triovex. $C_{18}H_{24}O_3$; mol wt 288.38. C 74.97%, H 8.39%, O 16.64%. A metabolite of, and considerably less potent than the hormone estradiol, q.v. It is usually the predominant estrogenic metabolite found in urine. During pregnancy the placenta produces relatively large amounts of estriol. Isoln from human pregnancy urine: Marrian, *Biochem. J.* **23**, 1090, 1233 (1929); probably occurs as a glucuronide: Cohen, Marrian, *ibid.* **29**, 1577 (1935). Isoln from human placenta: Collip, *Br. Med. J.* **II**, 1080 (1930); Collip et al., *Endocrinology* **18**, 71 (1934). Also obtained from plant sources. Isoln from pussywillows: Skarzynski, *Nature* **131**, 766 (1933). Structure: Huffman, Lott, *J. Am. Chem. Soc.* **69**, 1835 (1947). Crystal and molecular structure: Cooper et al., *Acta Crystallogr.* **25B**, 814 (1969). Soly studies: Ruchelman, Howe, *J. Chromatogr. Sci.* **7**, 340 (1969). Partial synthesis: Huffman, *J. Biol. Chem.* **169**, 167 (1947). Syntheses: Huffman, Lott, *J. Am. Chem. Soc.* **71**, 719 (1949); Leeds et al., *ibid.* **76**, 2943 (1954).

Very small, monoclinic crystals from dil alc. d 1.27. mp 282°. During heating on the microscope heating stage, rearrangement of the crystal structure takes place at 270° and 275° (rate of heating, 4°/min, Kofler microscope heating stage). $[\alpha]_D^{25}$ +58° ±5° (0.04 g in 1 ml dioxane). uv max: 280 nm. Precipitated by digitonin. Practically insol in water. Sol in alcohol, dioxane, chloroform, ether, vegetable oils; freely sol in pyridine, in solns of fixed alkali hydroxides.

Triacetate. $C_{24}H_{30}O_6$. Crystals from 90% alc. mp 126°.

16,17-Bis(sodium hemisuccinate). [113-22-4] Estriol succinate; Orgastyptin; Stiptanon; Synapause. $C_{26}H_{30}Na_2O_9$; mol wt 532.49. Prepn: GB 879014 (1960 to Organon).

THERAP CAT: Estrogen.

THERAP CAT (VET): Estrogenic hormone therapy.

3708.   Estrone. [53-16-7] 3-Hydroxyestra-1,3,5(10)-trien-17-one; 1,3,5-estratrien-3-ol-17-one; oestrone; folliculin; follicular hormone; tokokin; thelykinin; ketohydroxyestrin; Hiestrone; Menformon; Glandubolin; Cristallovar; Destrone; Endofolliculina; Estrol; Femidyn; Folikrin; Kolpon; Crinovaryl; Folisan; Disynformon; Hormovarine; Oestroperos; Wynestron; Thelestrin; Kestrone; Estrusol; Estrugenone; Femestrone Inj; Folipex; Follestrine; Follidrin (tablets); Follicunodis; Hormofollin; Oestrin; Ovifollin; Perlatan; Ketodestrin; Theelin. $C_{18}H_{22}O_2$; mol wt 270.37. C 79.96%, H 8.20%, O 11.84%. A metabolite of 17β-estradiol, q.v., possessing considerably less biological activity; isolated as d-form. Occurs in pregnancy urine of women and mares, in follicular liquor of many animals, in human placenta, in urine of bulls and stallions, in palm-kernel oil. Isoln: Butenandt, *Naturwissenschaften* **17**, 879 (1929); Doisy et al., *Am. J. Physiol.* **90**, 329 (1929). Also isolated from moghat roots and date palm pollen grains: Amin et al., *Phytochemistry* **8**, 295 (1969). Manuf: E. A. Doisy et al., US 1967350, US 1967351 (1934 both to St. Louis University); Joly et al., FR 1305992 (1962 to Roussel-Uclaf). Synthesis of a stereoisomer of estrone: W. E. Bachmann et al., *J. Am. Chem. Soc.* **64**, 974 (1942).

Total synthesis of natural estrone: G. Anner, K. Miescher, *Helv. Chim. Acta* **31**, 2173 (1948); **32**, 1957 (1949); **33**, 1379 (1950); W. S. Johnson et al., *J. Am. Chem. Soc.* **72**, 1426 (1950); **74**, 2832 (1952); I. V. Torgov et al., *Dokl. Akad. Nauk SSSR* **135**, 73 (1960), *C.A.* **55**, 11462f (1961). Stereochemistry of estrone isomers: W. S. Johnson et al., *J. Am. Chem. Soc.* **80**, 661 (1958). Review of estrone syntheses: L. F. Fieser, M. Fieser, *Steroids* (Reinhold, New York, 1959) pp 495-502; T. B. Windholz, M. Windholz, *Angew. Chem. Int. Ed.* **3**, 353 (1964); Taub, "Naturally Occurring Aromatic Steroids" in *The Total Synthesis of Natural Products* vol. 2, J. ApSimon, Ed. (John Wiley & Sons, New York, 1973) pp 670-725. Recent syntheses: P. A. Bartlett, W. S. Johnson, *J. Am. Chem. Soc.* **95**, 7501 (1973); S. Danishefsky, P. Cain, *ibid.* **98**, 4975 (1976); T. Kametani et al., *ibid.* **99**, 3461 (1977); P. A. Grieco et al., *J. Org. Chem.* **45**, 2247 (1980). Comprehensive description: D. Both, *Anal. Profiles Drug Subs.* **12**, 135-189 (1983).

Crystals from acetone, mp 254.5-256°. $[\alpha]_D^{22}$ +152° (c = 0.995 in CHCl$_3$). uv max (p-dioxane): 282, 296 nm (ε 2300, 2130); (conc H$_2$SO$_4$): 300, 450 nm; (0.1M NaOH): 239, 293 nm. Exists in three cryst phases, one monoclinic, the other two orthorhombic. Pptd by digitonin. Soly in water (25°): 0.003 g/100 ml. One gram of estrone dissolves in 250 ml of 96% alcohol at 15°, in 50 ml of boiling alcohol; in 50 ml acetone at 15°, in 110 ml chloroform at 15°, in 145 ml boiling benzene. Sol in dioxane, pyridine, fixed alkali hydroxide solns; slightly sol in ether, vegetable oils.

Acetate. [901-93-9] Hogival. $C_{20}H_{24}O_3$; mol wt 312.40. Crystals from alcohol, mp 125-127°.

Propionate. [975-64-4] $C_{21}H_{26}O_3$. mp 134-135°, US 2156599.

Sulfate. [481-97-0] Conjugol. Price, US 2917522 (1959 to Davis).

Sulfate piperazine salt. [7280-37-7] Estropipate; piperazine estrone sulfate; Harmogen; Ogen; Sulestrex Piperazine. $C_{22}H_{32}$-N_2O_5S; mol wt 436.56. Comprehensive description: Z. L. Chang, *Anal. Profiles Drug Subs.* **5**, 375-402 (1976). Cryst powder, melts at 190° to a liquid which resolidifies and then decomp at 245°. $[\alpha]_D^{25}$ +87.8° (c = 1 in 0.4% NaOH). uv max (0.04% NaOH): 275, 268 nm (ε 838, 851).

dl-Form. [19973-76-3] Crystals from acetone, mp 251-254°.

Methyl ether. [1091-94-7] $C_{19}H_{24}O_2$. Synthesis: T. A. Bryson, C. J. Reichel, *Tetrahedron Lett.* **21**, 2381 (1980). dl-Form, crystals from acetone + methanol, mp 143.2-144.2°. d-Form, crystals from methanol, mp 164-165°.

Caution: These substances are listed as known human carcinogens: *Report on Carcinogens, Eleventh Edition* (PB2005-104914, 2004) p III-115.

USE: In the prepn of commercial 19-norsteroids.

THERAP CAT: Estrogen.

THERAP CAT (VET): Estrogen.

3709.   Etafedrine. [7681-79-0] α-[1-(Ethylmethylamino)-ethyl]benzenemethanol; l-N-ethylephedrine; l-α-[1-(ethylmethylamino)ethyl]benzyl alcohol; 2-methylethylamino-1-phenyl-1-propanol; Menetryl; Novedrin. $C_{12}H_{19}NO$; mol wt 193.29. C 74.57%, H 9.91%, N 7.25%, O 8.28%. β-Adrenergic agonist. Prepn: Skita, Keil, *Ber.* **63**, 34 (1930); Ueda et al., *Pharm. Bull.* **3**, 465 (1955).

Hydrochloride. [5591-29-7] Nethamine. $C_{12}H_{19}NO.HCl$; mol wt 229.75. Crystals from acetone + alcohol, mp 183-184°.

One gram dissolves in 1.5 ml water, 8.0 ml alcohol. Aq solns are very stable.

THERAP CAT: Bronchodilator.

3710. Etafenone. [90-54-0] 1-[2-[2-(Diethylamino)ethoxy]phenyl]-3-phenyl-1-propanone; 2'-[2-(diethylamino)ethoxy]-3-phenylpropiophenone; o-diethylaminoethoxy-β-phenylpropiophenone; 2'-(β-diethylaminoethoxy)-3-phenylpropiophenone; β-phenyl-o-(diethylaminoethoxy)propiophenone; LG-11457. $C_{21}H_{27}$-NO_2; mol wt 325.44. C 77.50%, H 8.36%, N 4.30%, O 9.83%. Prepn: G. DiPaco, S. C. Tauro, *Ann. Chim. (Rome)* **48**, 1215 (1958); *eidem,* **DE 1265758** (1968 to Guidotti), *C.A.* **69**, 58950a (1968). Toxicity data: H.-J. Hapke, W. Sterner, *Arzneim.-Forsch.* **19**, 1664 (1969). Series of articles on pharmacology, toxicology, metabolism: *ibid.* 1664-1681.

Liquid, bp_{30} 264-268°.
Hydrochloride. Hetaphenone; Asamedol; Baxacor; Corodilan; Dialicor; Pagano-Cor; Relicor. $C_{21}H_{27}NO_2 \cdot HCl$; mol wt 361.91. Crystals, mp 129-130°. LD_{50} in rats (mg/kg): 716 orally; 20.8 i.v. (Hapke, Sterne).

THERAP CAT: Vasodilator (coronary).

3711. Etamiphyllin. [314-35-2] 7-[2-(Diethylamino)ethyl]-3,7-dihydro-1,3-dimethyl-1H-purine-2,6-dione; 7-(2-diethylaminoethyl)theophylline; 7-(2-diethylaminoethyl)-1,3-dimethylxanthine; 1,3-dimethyl-7-(2-diethylaminoethyl)xanthine; dietamiphylline; etamiphylline. $C_{13}H_{21}N_5O_2$; mol wt 279.34. C 55.90%, H 7.58%, N 25.07%, O 11.46%. Prepn: Quevauviller *et al., Bull. Soc. Chim. Biol.* **31**, 532 (1946); Moussalli *et al.,* **GB 669070** (1952); Klosa, *Arch. Pharm.* **288**, 301 (1955). Toxicity data on combinations: Baettig, *Arzneim.-Forsch.* **21**, 354 (1971). Pharmacokinetics, metabolism, and urinary determn in camels: M. Elghazali *et al., J. Vet. Pharmacol. Ther.* **25**, 43 (2002); GC/MS and LC/MS determn in greyhound urine: M. C. Dumasia, P. Teale, *J. Pharm. Biomed. Anal.* **36**, 1085 (2005).

Waxy solid, mp 75°. Very sol in water, acetone; slightly sol in ethanol, ether.
Hydrochloride. [17140-68-0] Solufilina. $C_{13}H_{21}N_5O_2 \cdot HCl$. Crystals, mp 239-241°. Very sol in water, forms stable neutral soln.
Camphorsulfonate. [19326-29-5] Etamiphylline camsylate; Millophyline. $C_{23}H_{37}N_5O_6S$; mol wt 511.63. Crystals, mp 174°.

THERAP CAT: Bronchodilator.
THERAP CAT (VET): Bronchodilator.

3712. Etanercept. [185243-69-0] 1-235-Tumor necrosis factor receptor (human) fusion protein with 236-467-immunoglobulin G1 (human γ1-chain Fc fragment); human tumor necrosis factor receptor p75 Fc fusion protein; TNFR:Fc; Enbrel. Recombinant protein consisting of the human soluble TNF receptor p75 linked to the Fc portion of human immunoglobulin G_1. Dimerizes via the cysteine residues in the Fc fragment to form an immunoglobulin-like structure. Inhibits the biological effects of tumor necrosis factor, *q.v.* Description of prepn and medicinal use: C. A. Smith, C. A. Jacobs, **WO 9406476**; *eidem,* **US 5605690** (1994, 1997 both to Immunex). Clinical pharmacokinetics: H. Lee *et al., Clin. Pharmacol. Ther.* **73**, 348 (2003). Clinical trial as monotherapy in plaque psoriasis: C. L. Leonardi *et al., N. Engl. J. Med.* **349**, 2014 (2003). Review of clinical experience in rheumatoid and psoriatic arthritis: B. Goffe, J. C. Cather, *J. Am. Acad. Dermatol.* **49**, S105-

S111 (2003); S. Nanda, J. M. Bathon, *Expert Opin. Pharmacother.* **5**, 1175-1186 (2004).

THERAP CAT: Anti-inflammatory; antipsoriatic.

3713. Etanidazole. [22668-01-5] N-(2-Hydroxyethyl)-2-nitro-1H-imidazole-1-acetamide; DUP-453; NSC-301467; SR-2508; Radinyl. $C_7H_{10}N_4O_4$; mol wt 214.18. C 39.25%, H 4.71%, N 26.16%, O 29.88%. Oxygen-mimetic which renders hypoxic cells sensitive to chemo- and radiotherapy. Prepn: A. G. Beaman *et al., Antimicrob. Agents Chemother.* **1967**, 520. *See also:* W. W. Lee *et al.,* **US 4371540** (1983 to U.S. Sec'y Health Human Serv.). Pharmacology: J. M. Brown *et al., Int. J. Radiat. Oncol. Biol. Phys.* **7**, 695 (1981). HPLC determn in biological materials: R. Ward, P. Workman, *J. Chromatogr.* **420**, 223 (1987). Clinical pharmacokinetics and efficacy in radiation therapy: T. H. Wasserman *et al., Radiother. Oncol.* **20**, Suppl. 1, 129 (1991). Evaluation in combination with alkylating agents: L. N. Shulman *et al., Int. J. Radiat. Oncol. Biol. Phys.* **29**, 545 (1994).

Crystals from ethanol, mp 162-163° (Beaman); also reported as white powder from ethyl acetate + methanol, mp 164.5-165° (Lee). Partition coefficient (octanol/water): 0.046. uv max (isopropanol): 313 nm (ε 7800). Soly in isotonic saline: 200 mg/ml.

THERAP CAT: Antineoplastic adjunct (radiosensitizer).

3714. Etaqualone. [7432-25-9] 3-(2-Ethylphenyl)-2-methyl-4(3H)-quinazolinone; 2-methyl-3-(o-ethylphenyl)-4-quinazolone; ethinazone; Aolan. $C_{17}H_{16}N_2O$; mol wt 264.32. C 77.25%, H 6.10%, N 10.60%, O 6.05%. Prepd by condensation of N-acetylanthranilic acid and 2-ethylaniline with $POCl_3$: **BE 615282** (1962 to P. Beiersdorf AG), *C.A.* **58**, 13971ef (1963). Structure-activity studies: Parmar *et al., J. Med. Chem.* **12**, 138 (1969).

mp 81°.
Hydrochloride. $C_{17}H_{16}N_2O \cdot HCl$. mp 247°.
THERAP CAT: Sedative, hypnotic.

3715. Eterobarb. [27511-99-5] 5-Ethyl-1,3-bis(methoxymethyl)-5-phenyl-2,4,6(1H,3H,5H)-pyrimidinetrione; 5-ethyl-1,3-bis(methoxymethyl)-5-phenylbarbituric acid; N,N'-dimethoxymethylphenobarbital; eterobarbital; Ex-12-095; Antilon. $C_{16}H_{20}$-N_2O_5; mol wt 320.34. C 59.99%, H 6.29%, N 8.74%, O 24.97%. Alkoxymethyl deriv of phenobarbital, *q.v.,* reported to have little or no hypnotic activity. Prepn: C. M. Samour, J. A. Vita, **DE 1939987**; J. A. Vita, **US 3595862** (1970, 1971 both to Kendall); C. M. Samour *et al., J. Med. Chem.* **14**, 187 (1971); J. Gal, *J. Pharm. Sci.* **68**, 1562 (1979). Spectrophotographic and polarographic analysis: M. Romer *et al., Anal. Chim. Acta* **88**, 261 (1977). Pharmacologic study: J. A. Vida, M. L. Hasker, *J. Med. Chem.* **16**, 602 (1973). Metabolism: M. A. Goldberg *et al., Ann. Neurol.* **5**, 121 (1979). Efficacy in febrile convulsions: R. M. Julien, G. G. Fowler, *Neuropharmacology* **16**, 719 (1977).

Crystals from ethanol, mp 116-118°. LD_{50} in mice: 470 mg/kg orally (Vida, Hooker).

Note: This is a controlled substance (depressant): **21 CFR, 1308.13.**

THERAP CAT: Anticonvulsant.

3716. Ethacridine. [442-16-0] 7-Ethoxy-3,9-acridinediamine; 6,9-diamino-2-ethoxyacridine; 2,5-diamino-7-ethoxyacridine; 2-ethoxy-6,9-diaminoacridine; etakridin. $C_{15}H_{15}N_3O$; mol wt 253.30. C 71.13%, H 5.97%, N 16.59%, O 6.32%. Prepn: **DE 364033; DE 364037; DE 393411; DE 395683** (1922); *Frdl.* **14**, 804, 807-812; A. Albert, W. Gledhill, *J. Soc. Chem. Ind.* **61**, 159 (1942). Toxicity: S. D. Rubbo, *Br. J. Exp. Pathol.* **28**, 1 (1947); N. J. Joshi *et al., Indian J. Exp. Biol.* **16**, 1038 (1978). Pharmacokinetics: T. J. Rising *et al., Arzneim.-Forsch.* **27**, 872 (1977). Use in protein analysis: R. H. Yue *et al., Thromb. Diath. Haemorrh.* **31**, 439 (1974); F. Franek, *Methods Enzymol.* **121**, 631-638 (1986); in serological detection of *Brucella sp.:* J. D. Huber, P. Nicoletti, *Am. J. Vet. Res.* **47**, 1529 (1986). Clinical evaluation in diarrhea: N. Madanagopalan *et al., Curr. Ther. Res.* **18**, 546 (1975); R. Raedsch *et al., Klin. Wochenschr.* **69**, 863 (1991); as an abortifacient: S. Gardo, M. Nagy, *Arch. Gynecol. Obstet.* **247**, 39 (1990).

Orange-yellow crystals from 50% alc. mp 226°.

Lactate monohydrate. [6402-23-9] Acrinol; Rimaon; Rivanol; Vucine; Acrolactine; Ethodin; Metifex. $C_{15}H_{15}N_3O.C_3H_6O_3.H_2O$; mol wt 361.39. Light yellow crystals from 90% alcohol + ether. Darkens at 200°, mp 235°. Slowly sol in 15 parts water; sol in 9 parts boiling water; in 110 parts alcohol at 22°, in 100 parts boiling alcohol. Solns are yellow, fluorescent and stable to boiling. LD_{50} s.c. in mice: 0.12 g/kg (Rubbo).

USE: Reagent in serological testing and protein chemistry.

THERAP CAT: Antiseptic. Abortifacient.

3717. Ethacrynic Acid. [58-54-8] [2,3-Dichloro-4-(2-methylene-1-oxobutyl)phenoxy]acetic acid; [2,3-dichloro-4-(2-methylenebutyryl)phenoxy]acetic acid; [4-(methylenebutyryl)-2,3-dichlorophenoxy]acetic acid; MK-595; Crinuryl; Edecril; Edecrin; Hydromedin; Reomax; Taladren; Uregit. $C_{13}H_{12}Cl_2O_4$; mol wt 303.14. C 51.51%, H 3.99%, Cl 23.39%, O 21.11%. Prepn: Schultz *et al., J. Med. Pharm. Chem.* **5**, 660 (1962); E. M. Schultz, J. M. Sprague, **BE 612755** C.A. **59**, 12712b (1963); *eidem,* **US 3255241** (1962, 1966 both to Merck & Co.). Pharmacology: Beyer *et al., J. Pharmacol. Exp. Ther.* **147**, 1 (1965). Crystal structure: J. Lamotte *et al., Acta Crystallogr.* **B34**, 2636 (1978). Toxicity study: Peck *et al., Fed. Proc.* **23**, 438 (1964). *Reviews:* Kim *et al., Am. J. Cardiol.* **27**, 407-415 (1971); H. E. Williamson, *J. Clin. Pharmacol.* **17**, 663-672 (1977).

Crystals, mp 121-122° (corr). pKa' 3.50. Sparingly sol in water, aq acids; sol in chloroform. LD_{50} in mice (mg/kg): 176 i.v.; 627 orally (Peck).

Sodium salt. [6500-81-8] Ethacrynate sodium; Sodium Edecrin. $C_{13}H_{11}Cl_2NaO_4$; mol wt 325.12. uv max (water): 225 nm (ε 15287). Soly in water at 25°: up to 9%. Solns at pH 7 at 25° stable for short periods of time. Stability decreased with an increase in pH, temperature and time.

THERAP CAT: Diuretic.

THERAP CAT (VET): Diuretic.

3718. Ethadione. [520-77-4] 3-Ethyl-5,5-dimethyl-2,4-oxazolidinedione; 3-ethyl-5,5-dimethyl-2,4-diketooxazolidine; Petidiol; Didione; Petidion; Epinyl; Etydion; Petisan; Neo-Absentol.

$C_7H_{11}NO_3$; mol wt 157.17. C 53.49%, H 7.05%, N 8.91%, O 30.54%. Prepn: Davis, Hook, **GB 626971** (1949 to Brit. Schering Res. Labs.).

Flat, vitreous prisms from ether, mp 76-77°.

THERAP CAT: Anticonvulsant.

3719. Ethalfluralin. [55283-68-6] N-Ethyl-N-(2-methyl-2-propenyl)-2,6-dinitro-4-(trifluoromethyl)benzenamine; N-ethyl-N-α,α,α-trifluoro-N-(2-methylallyl)-2,6-dinitro-p-toluidine; N-ethyl-N-methallyl-4-trifluoromethyl-2,6-dinitroaniline; EL-161; Sonalen; Sonalan. $C_{13}H_{14}F_3N_3O_4$; mol wt 333.26. C 46.85%, H 4.23%, F 17.10%, N 12.61%, O 19.20%. Selective, pre-emergent herbicide. Prepn: H. D. Porter, **DE 2511897**; *idem,* **GB 1505249** (1975, 1978 both to Eli Lilly). Activity: G. Skylakakis *et al., Proc. 12th Br. Weed Control Conf.* **2**, 795 (1974). Review of chemistry and analytical methods: E. W. Day, "Ethalfluralin" in *Analytical Methods for Pesticides and Plant Growth Regulators* **Vol. 10**, G. Zweig, J. Sherma, Eds. (Academic Press, New York, 1978) pp 341-352. Persistence in soil: B. J. Hayden, A. E. Smith, *Bull. Environ. Contam. Toxicol.* **25**, 508 (1983).

Yellow crystals from petr ether, mp 54-57°. Readily sol in acetone, acetonitrile, benzene, chloroform, hexane, methanol, xylene. Soly in water (25°): 0.3 ppm. uv max (methanol): 374, 267 nm. Vapor pressure (25°): 8.2×10^{-5} torr. LD_{50} in mice, rats (g/kg): >10 orally; LC_{50} in bluegill sunfish, rainbow trout, goldfish (ppb): 22, 37, 260 (Day).

USE: Pre-emergent herbicide.

3720. Ethambutol. [74-55-5] 2,2'-(1,2-Ethanediyldiimino)-bis-1-butanol; (+)-2,2'-(ethylenediimino)di-1-butanol; d-N,N'-bis(1-hydroxymethylpropyl)ethylenediamine; EMB. $C_{10}H_{24}N_2O_2$; mol wt 204.31. C 58.79%, H 11.84%, N 13.71%, O 15.66%. Prepn: Wilkinson *et al., J. Am. Chem. Soc.* **83**, 2212 (1961); *eidem, J. Med. Chem.* **5**, 835 (1962). Pharmacology: Kulig *et al., Diss. Pharm. Pharmacol.* **23**, 463 (1971), *C.A.* **76**, 81239d (1972). Comprehensive description: C. S. Lee, L. Z. Benet, *Anal. Profiles Drug Subs.* **7**, 231-249 (1978). Mechanism of action: W. H. Beggs in *Antibiotics* **vol. 5**(pt. 1), F. E. Hahn, Ed. (Springer-Verlag, New York, 1979) pp 43-66.

mp 87.5-88.8°. $[\alpha]_D^{25}$ +13.7° (c = 2 in water). Sol in chloroform, methylene chloride; less sol in benzene; sparingly sol in water.

Dihydrochloride. [1070-11-7] Dexambutol; Ebutol; Etibi; Etapiam; Myambutol; Mycobutol; Sural; Tibutol. $C_{10}H_{24}N_2O_2.2HCl$; mol wt 277.23. mp 198.5-200.3°; also reported as mp 201.8-202.6°. $[\alpha]_D^{25}$ +7.6° (c = 2 in water). Sol in water, DMSO; sparingly sol in ethanol; difficultly sol in acetone, chloroform.

Mixture with isoniazid methane sulfonate. [41663-50-7] (+)-2,2-(Ethylenediimino)dibutanol diisoniazide methanesulfonate; isobutol; Isoetam. Prepn: C. Ferrer-Salat *et al.,* **BE 753862; US 3718655** (1971, 1973 both to Lab. Ferrer). White powder, crystallizes as needles, mp 121-122° (dec). Sol in water, methanol, N,N-dimethylformamide. Insol in ethanol, ethyl ether, chloroform. uv max: 265 nm. $[\alpha]_D^{20}$ +3° (c = 5% in water). LD$_{50}$ in mice (g/kg): 2.800 orally; 2.210 i.p. (Ferrer-Salat).

THERAP CAT: Antibacterial (tuberculostatic).

3721. Ethamivan. [304-84-7] N,N-Diethyl-4-hydroxy-3-methoxybenzamide; N,N-diethylvanillamide; vanillic acid diethylamide; vanillic diethylamide; Vandid; Cardiovanil; Emivan. $C_{12}H_{17}NO_3$; mol wt 223.27. C 64.55%, H 7.67%, N 6.27%, O 21.50%. Prepd by dissolving vanillic acid O-acyl amide in NaOH and neutralizing with CO_2 or acid: Kratzl, Kvasnicka, *Monatsh. Chem.* **83**, 18 (1952); by refluxing a mixture of vanillic acid, P_2O_5 and powdered glass in xylene and treating with K_2CO_3: *eidem*, **US 2641612** (1953 to Oesterr. Stickstoffwerke). Toxicity study: Caujolle *et al.*, *Compt. Rend.* **243**, 609 (1956).

Needles from ligroin, mp 95-95.5°. LD$_{50}$ i.p. in rats: 28 mg/kg (Caujolle).

THERAP CAT: CNS stimulant; respiratory stimulant.

3722. Ethamsylate. [2624-44-4] 2,5-Dihydroxybenzenesulfonic acid compd with N-ethylethanamine; diethylammonium 2,5-dihydroxybenzenesulfonate; 1-hydroxy-4-oxo-2,5-cyclohexadiene-1-sulfonic acid compd with diethylamine; diethylammonium cyclohexadien-4-ol-1-one-4-sulfonate; cyclonamine; etamsylate; MD-141; E-141; Aglumin; Altodor; Biosinon; Dicynene; Dicynone. $C_{10}H_{17}NO_5S$; mol wt 263.31. C 45.61%, H 6.51%, N 5.32%, O 30.38%, S 12.18%. Prepn: **GB 895709** (1962 to Labs. OM); **ES 279303** (1962 to Labs. Esteve), *C.A.* **60**, 1652g (1964). Pharmacology: Demars, *Med. Exp.* **4**, 173 (1961); Huguet *et al.*, *Therapie* **24**, 429 (1969). Toxicity: Esteve *et al.*, *Therapie* **15**, 110 (1960).

Crystals from ethanol, mp 125°. LD$_{50}$ i.v. in mice, rats: 800, 1350 mg/kg (Esteve).

THERAP CAT: Hemostatic.

3723. Ethane. [74-84-0] Bimethyl; dimethyl; methylmethane; ethyl hydride. C_2H_6; mol wt 30.07. C 79.88%, H 20.11%. CH_3CH_3. Constituent of natural gas (about 9%). Can be recovered from the gases produced during the distillation of crude petroleum. *Review:* Smith, Hanson, *Oil Gas J.* **44**, no. 10, 119 (1945).

Colorless, odorless gas. *Flammable asphyxiant.* Burns with a faintly luminous flame. d_4^0 1.0493 (air = 1) or 1.3562 g/l. d_4^0 liq 0.446. mp −172°. bp −88°. Crit temp 32°; crit press. 48.2 atm. Heat of combustion: 1727 Btu/cu ft at 25° (one pound of CH_3CH_3 yields 20,420 Btu [net] at 15.56°). Flammable limits in air: 3.2 to 12.5% by vol. Ignition temp (in air): 530°. Soly in water at 20°: 4.7 ml/100 ml H_2O; in alc at 4°: 46 ml/100 ml alc.

Caution: Narcotic in high concns. A simple asphyxiant.

USE: In the manuf of chlorinated derivs; as refrigerant in some two-stage refrigeration systems where relatively low temps are produced; as fuel gas (so called "bottled gas" or "suburban propane" contains about 90% propane, 5% ethane, and 5% butane).

3724. 1,2-Ethanedisulfonic Acid. [110-04-3] 1,2-Ethylenedisulfonic acid. $C_2H_6O_6S_2$; mol wt 190.20. C 12.63%, H 3.18%, O 50.47%, S 33.72%. $HO_3SCH_2CH_2SO_3H$. Preparation of disodium salt from 1,2-dibromoethane and sodium sulfite: McElvain *et al.*, *J. Am. Chem. Soc.* **67**, 1578 (1945); Ohba *et al.*, **US 3022172** (1962 to Fuji Photo Film). Free acid obtained by conversion of disodium salt to barium salt followed by liberation with H_2SO_4: McElvain *et al.*, *loc. cit.* Review of prepns: Suter, *Organic Chemistry of Sulfur* (Wiley, New York, 1944) p 166; Gilbert, *Sulfonation and Related Reactions* (Interscience, New York, 1965).

Dihydrate. Crystals from acetic acid + acetic anhydride, mp 111-112°. Heating at 145° and 1 mm for 6 hours gives anhydr

compd, mp 172-174°. Somewhat soluble in anhydr ether, very sol in dioxane.

Sodium salt dihydrate. $C_2H_4Na_2O_6S_2.2H_2O$. Monoclinic prisms. Not very readily sol in water. Practically insol in alcohol.

USE: Base in hypnotics, sedatives.

3725. 1,2-Ethanedithiol. [540-63-6] Dithioethyleneglycol; ethylenedimercaptan. $C_2H_6S_2$; mol wt 94.20. C 25.50%, H 6.42%, S 68.08%. $HSCH_2CH_2SH$. Prepd by reacting ethanol, thiourea and ethylene dibromide and subsequent alkaline hydrolysis of the ethylenediisothiuronium bromide: Speciale, *Org. Synth.* **30**, 35 (1950), modified procedure: Grogan *et al.*, *J. Org. Chem.* **20**, 50 (1955).

Liquid. $d^{23.5}$ 1.123. bp$_{760}$ 146°; bp$_{150}$ 76-81°; bp$_{46}$ 63°; bp$_{24}$ 51-52°. n_D^{20} 1.5589. Freely sol in alcohol and in alkalies.

Caution: Vapors of ethanedithiol may cause severe headache and nausea.

3726. Ethanethiol. [75-08-1] Ethyl mercaptan; mercaptoethane; ethyl sulfhydrate; thioethyl alcohol. C_2H_6S; mol wt 62.13. C 38.66%, H 9.73%, S 51.61%. CH_3CH_2SH. Found in urine of rabbits after ingestion of cabbage. Is formed in vinous fermentation. Occurs in illuminating gas, in "sour" natural gas of W. Texas; in petroleum distillates from which it may be separated by chemical or physical methods: Thompson *et al.*, *Anal. Chem.* **27**, 175 (1955). Prepn from sodium ethylsulfate and KSH: Klason, *Ber.* **20**, 3407 (1887); catalytically from ethanol and hydrogen sulfide: Kramer, Reid, *J. Am. Chem. Soc.* **43**, 880 (1921). Review on occurrence, prepn, properties and reactions: E. Emmet Reid, *Organic Chemistry of Bivalent Sulfur* vol. I, 15-261 (Chemical Publishing Co., New York, 1958).

Liquid; penetrating leek-like odor: minimum detectable concn = 1 part in 50 billion parts of air. d_4^0 0.8617; d_4^{25} 0.83147. bp 34.7-35.04°; bp$_{400}$ 17.7°; bp$_{200}$ 1.5°; bp$_{100}$ −13.0°; bp$_{10}$ −50.2°; bp$_1$ −76.1°. mp −147.97 to −144.4°. n_D^{20} 1.431; n_D^{25} 1.420. Crit temp 225.5°. Crit pressure 54.2 atm. Explosive limits 2.8 and 18.2% by vol of vapor. Min ignition temp in air 299°, in oxygen 261°. Entropy at 25°: 70.77 cal/deg/mole. Heat capacity at 25°: 17.37 cal/deg/mole. Surface tension at 2°: 23.63 dynes/cm; at 16.7°: 21.62 dynes/cm. Viscosity at 20°: 0.003155 g/cm sec. Azeotrope with n-pentane (51% ethanethiol) bp 30.46°; with ether (40% ethanethiol) bp 31.50°. Soly in water at 20°: 6.76 g/l or 0.112 moles/l. Sol in alcohol, ether. *Keep tightly closed and in a cool place.*

Octadecahydrate. Needles. Practically insol in water, ethanethiol.

Sodium salt. C_2H_5NaS. Hydrolyzes instantly in water.

Caution: Potential symptoms of overexposure to ethanethiol are headache, nausea and irritation of mucous membranes. See *NIOSH Pocket Guide to Chemical Hazards* (DHHS/NIOSH 97-140, 1997) p 140.

USE: Odorant for natural gas; intermediate and starting material in manuf of plastics, insecticides, antioxidants.

3727. Ethanolamine. [141-43-5] 2-Aminoethanol; monoethanolamine; β-aminoethyl alcohol; 2-hydroxyethylamine; β-hydroxyethylamine; ethylolamine; colamine. C_2H_7NO; mol wt 61.08. C 39.33%, H 11.55%, N 22.93%, O 26.19%. $HOCH_2CH_2-NH_2$. Prepd on a large scale by ammonolysis of ethylene oxide: Knorr, *Ber.* **30**, 909 (1897); **FR 650574** (1928 to I. G. Farben); Reid, Lewis, **US 1904013** (1933 to Carbide & Carbon); Schwoegler, Olin, **US 2373199** (1945 to Sharples). Also from nitromethane and formaldehyde: *Ullmanns Encyklopädie der technischen Chemie* **3**, 102 (3rd ed., 1953). Manuf: *Faith, Keyes & Clark's Industrial Chemicals*, F. A. Lowenheim, M. K. Moran, Eds. (Wiley-Interscience, New York, 4th ed., 1975) pp 339-344. Toxicity: H. F. Smyth *et al.*, *J. Ind. Hyg. Toxicol.* **23**, 259 (1941).

Viscous, hygroscopic liq. Ammoniacal odor. Absorbs CO_2. d_4^{25} 1.0117; d_4^{40} 0.9998; d_4^{60} 0.9844. One gallon weighs 8.45 lbs in the U.S.A. Viscosity at 25°: 18.95 cP; at 60°: 5.03 cP. mp 10.3°. bp$_{760}$ 170.8°; bp$_{12}$ 70-72°. Strong base. pKa at 25°: 9.4. pH of 25% aq soln: 12.1; of 0.1N aq soln: 12.05. n_D^{20} 1.4539. Dipole moment 2.27. Flash pt 195°F. Misc with water, methanol, acetone. Soly at 25°: benzene 1.4%; ether 2.1%; carbon tetrachloride 0.2%; n-heptane <0.1%. LD$_{50}$ orally in rats: 10.20 g/kg (Smyth).

Hydrochloride. $C_2H_7NO.HCl$. Deliquesc crystals from alc, mp 75-77°.

Oleate. [2272-11-9] Antivariz; Esclerosina; Ethamolin. C_2H_7-$NO.C_{18}H_{34}O_2$; mol wt 343.54. Use as a sclerosing agent: S. E. Hedberg et al., Am. J. Surg. **143**, 426 (1982).

Caution: Potential symptoms of overexposure to ethanolamine are irritation of eyes, skin, respiratory system; lethargy. *See NIOSH Pocket Guide to Chemical Hazards* (DHHS/NIOSH 97-140, 1997) p 128.

USE: To remove CO_2 and H_2S from natural gas and other gases; in the synthesis of surface active agents; in polishes, hair waving solns, in emulsifiers; as softening agent for hides; dispersing agent for agricultural chemicals. Is reacted with other substances to form an accelerator in the manuf of antibiotics. Pharmaceutic aid (surfactant).

THERAP CAT: Oleate as sclerosing agent.

3728. Ethaverine. [486-47-5] 1-[(3,4-Diethoxyphenyl)-methyl]-6,7-diethoxyisoquinoline; 6,7-diethoxy-1-(3,4-diethoxy-benzyl)isoquinoline; ethylpapaverine; Dyscural. $C_{24}H_{29}NO_4$; mol wt 395.49. C 72.89%, H 7.39%, N 3.54%, O 16.18%. Tetraethyl homolog of papaverine. Synthesis: Wolf, **US 1962224** (1934).

Crystals from alcohol + ether, mp 99-101°. Insol in water. Readily sol in hot alc; slightly in ether and chloroform.

Hydrochloride. [985-13-7] Barbonin; Circubid; Diquinol; Ethabid; Isovex; Laverin; Perparin; Perperine. $C_{24}H_{29}NO_4.HCl$; mol wt 431.95. Prepn of stable solns: Hereld, **US 2971888** (1961). Crystals from abs alc, mp 186-188° (dec). One gram dissolves in about 40 ml water. pH of 1% soln 3.6; of 0.1% soln 4.6.

Acid oxalate. $C_{24}H_{29}NO_4.(COOH)_2$. Crystals from alc, soluble in hot water.

Salt with 7-iodo-8-hydroxyquinoline-5-sulfonic acid. Prepn: **HU 106906** (1931); v. Issekutz et al., Arch. Exp. Pathol. Pharmakol. **164**, 158 (1932).

THERAP CAT: Antispasmodic.

3729. Ethchlorvynol. [113-18-8] 1-Chloro-3-ethyl-1-penten-4-yl-3-ol; 5-chloro-3-ethylpent-1-yn-4-en-3-ol; ethyl β-chlorovinyl ethynyl carbinol; ethclorvynol; Placidyl; Arvynol; Serenesil; Roeridorm; Normoson. C_7H_9ClO; mol wt 144.60. C 58.14%, H 6.27%, Cl 24.52%, O 11.06%. Prepn: W. M. McLamore et al., J. Org. Chem. **20**, 109 (1955); Bavley, McLamore, **US 2746900** (1956 to Pfizer). Pharmacological studies: S. Y. P'an et al., J. Pharmacol. Exp. Ther. **114**, 326 (1955). Pharmacodynamics: Y. C. Martin, Biochem. Pharmacol. **16**, 2041 (1967). Evaluation as hypnotic: J. W. Middleton et al., Curr. Ther. Res. **8**, 391 (1966); J. H. Pattison et al., J. Am. Geriatr. Soc. **20**, 398 (1972). Study of metabolites: J. P. Horwitz et al., Drug Metab. Dispos. **8**, 77 (1980).

Liquid, pungent aromatic odor. Slowly darkens on exposure to light and air. d_4^{25} 1.065-1.070 (also reported as d_4^{20} 1.070). bp_{760} 173-174° (also reported as bp_{760} 181°); $bp_{0.1}$ 28.5-30°. n_D^{25} 1.4675-1.4800. Immiscible with water; miscible with most organic solvents. LD_{50} in mice (mg/kg): 290 orally; 240 s.c. (P'an).

Note: This is a controlled substance (depressant): **21 CFR,** 1308.14.

THERAP CAT: Sedative; hypnotic.

3730. 3-Ethenylpyridine. [1121-55-7] β-vinylpyridine; 3-EP. C_7H_7N; mol wt 105.14. C 79.96%, H 6.71%, N 13.32%. Combustion product of nicotine found in mainstream and sidestream smoke from cigarettes and cigars. Prepn: H. A. Iddles et al., J. Am. Chem. Soc. **59**, 1945 (1937). Electronic spectra: R. Abu-Eittah et al., Int. J. Quantum Chem. **39**, 211 (1991). Toxicology: K. D. Brunnemann et al., Cancer Lett. **65**, 107 (1992). Use as tracer for environmental tobacco smoke exposure: M. W. Ogden, Anal. Commun. **33**, 197 (1996); J. M. Daisey et al., J. Exposure Anal. Environ. Epidemiol. **8**, 313 (1998). Rapid chromatographic determn in indoor environments: G. Bertoni et al., Chromatographia **43**, 296 (1996).

Light-yellow liquid. Polymerizes at room temperatures. Sol in ether, partially sol in alcohol and very slightly sol in water. uv max (cyclohexane): 278, 239 nm (ε 3320, 3920 L/mol cm); uv max (methanol): 279, 238 nm (ε 3322, 3930 L/mol cm).

USE: Tracer compound for environmental tobacco smoke.

3731. Ethenzamide. [938-73-8] 2-Ethoxybenzamide; eth-benzamide; 2-ethoxybenzenecarbonamide; salicylamide o-ethyl ether; Lucamide; Protopyrin; Trancalgyl. $C_9H_{11}NO_2$; mol wt 165.19. C 65.44%, H 6.71%, N 8.48%, O 19.37%. Prepn: **GB 656746** (1951 to H. Lundbeck); Shapiro et al., J. Am. Chem. Soc. **81**, 3728 (1959); Bryk, Osowski, **PL 47822** (1961 to Polfa), C.A. **61**, 5573f (1964). Metabolism: Davison et al., J. Pharmacol. Exp. Ther. **136**, 226 (1962). Toxicity data: Starmer et al., Toxicol. Appl. Pharmacol. **19**, 20 (1971).

Crystals from ethyl acetate + hexane, mp 132-134°. LD_{50} orally in mice: 1160 mg/kg (Starmer).

THERAP CAT: Analgesic.

3732. Ethephon. [16672-87-0] (2-Chloroethyl)phosphonic acid; 2-chloroethanephosphonic acid; CEPA; camposan; Cerone; Ethrel; Prep. $C_2H_6ClO_3P$; mol wt 144.49. C 16.62%, H 4.19%, Cl 24.54%, O 33.22%, P 21.44%. $ClCH_2CH_2PO(OH)_2$. Ethylene-releasing agent used to control growth and ripening of fruit crops. Prepn: Kabachnik, Rossiiskaya, Izv. Akad. Nauk SSSR Otd. Khim. Nauk **1946**, 403-410, C.A. **42**, 7242e (1948); Beilstein **EIII 4**, 1780. Toxicity data: G. Hennighausen et al., Pharmazie **32**, 181 (1977). Review of use in viticulture: E. Szyjewicz et al., Am. J. Enol. Vitic. **35**, 117-123 (1984).

Very hygroscopic needles from benzene (must be dried over P_2O_5). mp 74-75°. Freely sol in water, methanol, acetone, ethylene glycol, propylene glycol. Slightly sol in benzene, toluene. Practically insol in petr ether. Aq solns are stable below pH 3.5. Above pH 3.5 hydrolysis begins with the release of free ethylene. LD_{50} orally in mice: 2850 mg/kg (Hennighausen).

Caution: Spray formulations are quite acidic, about pH 1.0. May be irritating to exposed skin and eyes, or if inhaled.

USE: Plant growth regulator.

3733. Ethinamate. [126-52-3] 1-Ethynylcyclohexanol carbamate; carbamic acid 1-ethynylcyclohexyl ester; ethynylcyclohexyl carbamate; Valamin; Valmid; Valmidate. $C_9H_{13}NO_2$; mol wt 167.21. C 64.65%, H 7.84%, N 8.38%, O 19.14%. Prepn: Junkmann, Pfeiffer, **US 2816910** (1957 to Schering, AG).

Needles from cyclohexane, mp 96-98°. bp_3 118-122°. Shows no optical activity. $n_D^{21.5}$ 1.4441 (20% in propylene glycol). Soly at 25° in water 0.25%, ethanol 35.0%, hexane 2.0%, sesame oil 0.7%,

1,2-propylene glycol 22%. Stable in N H_2SO_4 at 30°, but dec at 40° and in 0.02N acid at 60°. In 0.01N NaOH, CO_2 is split off at 30°. Lowers the surface tension in satd aq soln at 22° by 21%. Partition coefficient (oil/water): 1.48.

Note: This is a controlled substance (depressant): **21 CFR,** 1308.14. The trademark Valamin was used formerly to indicate a brand of *tert*-amyl isovalerate.

THERAP CAT: Sedative; hypnotic.

3734. Ethinyl Estradiol. [57-63-6] (17α)-19-Norpregna-1,3,5(10)-trien-20-yne-3,17-diol; 17α-ethynyl-1,3,5(10)-estratriene-3,17β-diol; 17-ethinylestradiol; ethynylestradiol; Estinyl; Feminone; Lynoral; Orestralyn; Primogyn C; Progynon C. $C_{20}H_{24}O_2$; mol wt 296.40. C 81.04%, H 8.16%, O 10.80%. Synthetic steroid with high oral estrogenic potency: Inhoffen, Hohlweg, *Naturwissenschaften* **26,** 96 (1938). Prepn from estrone: Inhoffen *et al., Ber.* **71,** 1024 (1938). *See also* **DE 702063; GB 516444; US 2243887; US 2251939; US 2265976; US 2267257.** Properties: Petit, Muller, *Bull. Soc. Chim. Fr.* **1951,** 121; L. Ehmann, A. Wettstein, *Pharm. Acta Helv.* **25,** 297 (1950). NMR: Hampel, Kraemer, *Ber.* **98,** 3255 (1965). Toxicity: E. I. Goldenthal, *Toxicol. Appl. Pharmacol.* **18,** 185 (1971). Randomized double-blind clinical studies: S. Koetsawang *et al., Contraception* **25,** 231 (1982); A. Sheth *et al., ibid.* 243. Clinical evaluation in gonadal dysgenesis: L. Cuttler *et al., J. Clin. Endocrinol. Metab.* **60,** 1087 (1985). General review: K. W. Thompson, *J. Clin. Pharmacol.* **8,** 1088-1098 (1948). Review of metabolism and pharmacokinetics: K. Fotherby, *Methods Find. Exp. Clin. Pharmacol.* **4,** 133-141 (1982); of carcinogenicity studies: *IARC Monographs* **21,** 233-255 (1979); *ibid.* Suppl. 4, 186-188 (1982).

Hemihydrate. Fine needles from methanol + water, mp 141-146°, $[\alpha]_D^{25}$ 0 ± 1° (dioxane). Dehydrates after melting and further heating, mp 182-184°. $[\alpha]_D^{24}$ +3.5 ± 0.5° (c = 2 in dioxane); −29.5 ± 1° (c = 2 in pyridine). uv max (ethanol): 281 nm (ε 2040 ± 60). Practically insol in water. Soly: 1 part in 6 of ethanol, 1 in 4 of ether, 1 in 5 of acetone, 1 in 4 of dioxane, and 1 in 20 of chloroform. Sol in vegetable oils, and in solns of fixed alkali hydroxides. LD_{50} in rats, mice (mg/kg): 2952, 1737 orally (Goldenthal).

3-Acetate. $C_{22}H_{26}O_3$. Crystals, mp 152-153°. $[\alpha]_D^{20}$ +3° (chloroform).

3-Benzoate. $C_{27}H_{28}O_3$. Needles from methanol, mp 200-202°.

Note: Also used in combination with chlormadinone acetate, desogestrel, ethynodiol, gestodene, lynestrenol, norethindrone or norgestrel, *q.q.v.* Has been used in combination with dimethisterone, medroxyprogesterone, or megestrol acetate, *q.q.v.*

Caution: These substances are listed as known human carcinogens: *Report on Carcinogens, Eleventh Edition* (PB2005-104914, 2004) p III-115.

THERAP CAT: Estrogen. In combination with progestogen as oral contraceptive.

THERAP CAT (VET): Estrogen.

3735. Ethiodized Oil. [8008-53-5] Ethyl ester of iodinated fatty acid of poppyseed oil; Ethiodol. Contains 37% organically bound iodine. Ref: Hom *et al., J. Am. Pharm. Assoc. Sci. Ed.* **46,** 254 (1957). Use in lymphography: R. M. Paxton *et al., Br. Med. J.* **I,** 120 (1975).

Amber-colored oil, extremely fluid, sp gr 1.28. Soluble in acetone, chloroform, ether, hexane. Insol in water.

THERAP CAT: Diagnostic aid (radiopaque medium). Antineoplastic when part of the iodine is ^{131}I.

3736. Ethion. [563-12-2] Phosphorodithioic acid S,S'-methylene O,O,O',O'-tetraethyl ester; ethyl methylene phosphorodithioate; O,O,O',O'-tetraethyl S,S'-methylenediphosphorodithioate; bis[S-(diethoxyphosphinothioyl)mercapto]methane; diethion; ENT-24105; FMC-1240; Niagara 1240; Commando; Rhodocide;

Tafethion. $C_9H_{22}O_4P_2S_4$; mol wt 384.48. C 28.11%, H 5.77%, O 16.65%, P 16.11%, S 33.36%. Cholinesterase inhibitor. Prepn: Willard, Henahan, **US 2873228; US 3014058** (1959, 1961 both to FMC). Toxicity study: T. B. Gaines, *Toxicol. Appl. Pharmacol.* **14,** 515 (1969). Review of toxicology and human exposure: *Toxicological Profile for Ethion* (PB2000-108024, 2000) 218 pp.

Liquid, mp −13 to −12°. d_4^{20} 1.220. n_D^{20} 1.5490. Vapor pressure: 1.5×10^{-6} mm Hg. Sol in xylene, methylated naphthalene, chloroform, acetone and kerosene + 1% methyl ethyl ketone or benzene; slightly sol in water. LD_{50} in female, male rats (mg/kg): 27, 65 orally; 62, 245 dermally (Gaines).

Caution: Potential symptoms of overexposure are eye, skin irritation; nausea, vomiting, abdominal cramps, diarrhea, salivation; headache, giddiness, vertigo, weakness; rhinorrhea, chest tightness; blurred vision, miosis; cardiac irregularities; muscle fasciculations; dyspnea. *See NIOSH Pocket Guide to Chemical Hazards* (DHHS/NIOSH 97-140, 1997) p 130.

USE: Insecticide; acaricide.

THERAP CAT (VET): Ectoparasiticide.

3737. Ethionamide. [536-33-4] 2-Ethyl-4-pyridinecarbothioamide; 2-ethylthioisonicotinamide; 3-ethylisothionicotinamide; 2-ethylisothionicotinamide; 2-ethyl-4-thiocarbamoylpyridine; α-ethylisonicotinoylthioamide; amidazine; ethioniamide; Bayer 5312; 1314-Th; Nisotin; Trescatyl; Aetina; Ethimide; Iridocin; Tio-Mid. $C_8H_{10}N_2S$; mol wt 166.24. C 57.80%, H 6.06%, N 16.85%, S 19.29%. Prepn: Libermann *et al., Compt. Rend.* **242,** 2409 (1956); *Bull. Soc. Chim. Fr.* **1958,** 687; **GB 800250** (1958 to Chimie et Atomistique). Mechanism of action study: K. Johnsson *et al., J. Am. Chem. Soc.* **117,** 5009 (1995).

Minute yellow crystals from ethanol, dec 164-166°. Very sparingly sol in water, ether. Sparingly sol in methanol, ethanol, propylene glycol. Sol in hot acetone, dichloroethane. Freely sol in pyridine.

THERAP CAT: Antibacterial (tuberculostatic).

3738. Ethionine. [13073-35-3] S-Ethyl-L-homocysteine; 2-amino-4-(ethylthio)butyric acid; α-amino-γ-(ethylmercapto)butyric acid; homocysteine S-ethyl ether. $C_6H_{13}NO_2S$; mol wt 163.24. C 44.15%, H 8.03%, N 8.58%, O 19.60%, S 19.64%. $CH_3CH_2SCH_2$-$CH_2CH(NH_2)COOH$. Prepn from ethanethiol and acrolein, purification via Zn salt: Norton, **US 2840587** (1958 to Dow). Prepn of DL-form and L-form: Armstrong, Lewis, *J. Org. Chem.* **16,** 749 (1951). Resolution of D- and L-isomers: Greenstein *et al., J. Biol. Chem.* **204,** 307 (1953). *Review:* E. Farber, "Ethionine Carcinogenesis" in A. Haddow, S. Weinhouse, *Advan. Cancer Res.* **vol. 7** (Academic Press, New York, 1963) pp 383-474.

Crystals, dec 272-274°. $[\alpha]_D^{24}$ +25.1°. Also reported as $[\alpha]_D^{23}$ +20.1° (1N HCl) (Armstrong, Lewis).

DL-Form. [67-21-0] Crystals, dec 257-260°. Also reported as dec 272-284° (Armstrong, Lewis).

3739. Ethiprole. [181587-01-9] 5-Amino-1-[2,6-dichloro-4-(trifluoromethyl)phenyl]-4-(ethylsulfinyl)-1H-pyrazole-3-carbonitrile; 5-amino-3-cyano-1-(2,6-dichloro-4-trifluoromethylphenyl)-4-ethylsulfinylpyrazole; RPA-107382; Curbix; Kirappu. $C_{13}H_9$-$Cl_2F_3N_4OS$; mol wt 397.20. C 39.31%, H 2.28%, Cl 17.85%, F 14.35%, N 14.11%, O 4.03%, S 8.07%. Insecticidal phenylpyrazole; analog of fipronil, *q.v.* Prepn: C. L. Haas *et al.,* **WO 9722593** (1997 to Rhone-Poulenc Agrochimie). Field trial vs stored-grain insects: F. H. Arthur, *J. Econ. Entomol.* **95,** 1314 (2002). Photochemistry, metabolism and GABAergic action compared with fipronil: P. Caboni *et al., J. Agric. Food Chem.* **51**, 7055 (2003).

mp ~174°. LD$_{50}$ in house flies (24 hr topical): 0.50 ±0.03 μg/g (Caboni).

USE: Insecticide for chewing and sucking insects.

3740. Ethirimol. [23947-60-6] 5-Butyl-2-(ethylamino)-6-methyl-4(1*H*)-pyrimidinone; 2-ethylamino-4-methyl-5-*n*-butyl-6-hydroxypyrimidine; PP-149; Milstem; Milgo; Milcurb Super. C$_{11}$-H$_{19}$N$_3$O; mol wt 209.29. C 63.13%, H 9.15%, N 20.08%, O 7.64%. Prepn: B. K. Snell *et al.,* **ZA 6701373**; *eidem,* **US 3980781** (1968, 1976 both to ICI). Systemic fungicidal activity: R. M. Bebbington, *Chem. Ind. (London)* **1969**, 1512; K. J. Bent, *Ann. Appl. Biol.* **66**, 103 (1970). Metabolism and mode of action: A. Calderbank, *Acta Phytopathol.* **6**, 355 (1971).

Crystalline solid, mp 159-160°. Vapor pressure at 25°: 2 × 10^{-6} mm Hg. Soly in water at 25°: 200 mg/l. Sol in chloroform, trichloroethylene, aq solns of strong acids and bases. Slightly sol in ethanol; sparingly sol in acetone. LD$_{50}$ orally in rats: 4000 mg/kg (Bebbington).

USE: Fungicide.

3741. Ethisterone. [434-03-7] 17α-Hydroxypregn-4-en-20-yn-3-one; 17α-ethynyltestosterone; 17α-ethynyl-17β-hydroxy-4-androsten-3-one; 17α-ethinyl-4-androsten-17β-ol-3-one; anhydrohydroxyprogesterone; pregneninolone. C$_{21}$-H$_{28}$O$_2$; mol wt 312.45. C 80.72%, H 9.03%, O 10.24%. Synthetic progestogen; metabolite of danazol, *q.v.*; intermediate in the synthesis of spironolactone, *q.v.* Prepn: Inhoffen *et al., Ber.* **71**, 1024 (1938). Crystal structure and photostability study: J. Reisch *et al., Monatsh. Chem.* **124**, 1169 (1993). GC/MS characterization as a metabolite of danazol: J. Y. Kim *et al., J. Vet. Pharmacol. Ther.* **24**, 147 (2001). HPLC/CD determn of isomers: D. Szegvári *et al., Anal. Bioanal. Chem.* **375**, 713 (2003).

Crystals from ethyl acetate, mp 269-275°. Sublimes in high vacuum at 190-195°. [α]$_D^{23}$ +23.8° (dioxane); [α]$_D^{25}$ −32.0° (pyridine). Crystal density: 1.220 g/cm^3. uv max (methanol): 241 nm (E$_{1cm}^{1\%}$ 513). Practically insol in water. Slightly sol in alcohol, acetone, ether, chloroform, vegetable oils.

3742. Ethofumesate. [26225-79-6] 2-Ethoxy-2,3-dihydro-3,3-dimethyl-5-benzofuranol methanesulfonate; NC-8438; Nortron; Tramat. C$_{13}$H$_{18}$O$_5$S; mol wt 286.34. C 54.53%, H 6.34%, O 27.94%, S 11.20%. Prepn: P. S. Gates *et al.,* **US 3689507** (1972 to Fisons). Biological properties and use: R. K. Pfeiffer, *3rd Symp. New Herbic.* **1969**, 1. Toxicity data: *Anal. Ref. Standards Suppl. Data* (PB85-143766, 1984) p 55. Field studies in grass: G. E. Coats, J. V. Krans, *Weed Sci.* **34**, 930 (1986); B. J. Johnson *et al,*

HortScience **24**, 102 (1989). HPLC determn in plant, soil, water: M. A. Alawi, *Anal. Lett.* **23**, 1695 (1990).

White crystalline solid, mp 70-72°. Vapor pressure at 25°: 8.6×10^{-7} mbar. Soly in water at 25°: 110 ppm. Relatively stable in water. LD$_{50}$ orally in rats: 1130 mg/kg (PB85-143766).

USE: Herbicide.

3743. Ethoheptazine. [77-15-6] Hexahydro-1-methyl-4-phenyl-1*H*-azepine-4-carboxylic acid ethyl ester; 4-carbethoxy-1-methyl-4-phenylhexamethylenimine; 4-carbethoxy-1-methyl-4-phenylazacycloheptane; ethyl heptazine; Wy-401. C$_{16}$H$_{23}$NO$_2$; mol wt 261.36. C 73.53%, H 8.87%, N 5.36%, O 12.24%. Prepd in several steps from 2-phenyl-4-dimethylaminobutyronitrile as a starting material, the final step being the hydrolysis and esterification of 1-methyl-4-phenyl-4-cyanoazacycloheptane: Diamond *et al., J. Org. Chem.* **22**, 399 (1957); Diamond, Bruce, **US 2666050** (1954 to Am. Home Prod.).

Liquid. d$_4^{26}$ 1.038. bp$_1$ 133-134°; bp$_{0.5}$ 127-129°; bp$_{0.3}$ 128-130°. n$_D^{26}$ 1.5210; n$_D^{28}$ 1.5220.

Hydrochloride. C$_{16}$H$_{23}$NO$_2$.HCl. Recrystallized from ethyl acetate + ether, mp 151-153°.

Citrate. [6700-56-7] Zactane. C$_{16}$H$_{23}$NO$_2$.C$_6$H$_8$O$_7$; mol wt 453.48.

Methobromide. C$_{16}$H$_{23}$NO$_2$.CH$_3$Br. Crystals from ether, mp 215-217°.

THERAP CAT: Analgesic.

3744. Ethohexadiol. [94-96-2] 2-Ethyl-1,3-hexanediol; 2-ethyl-3-propyl-1,3-propanediol; octylene glycol; 6-12. C$_8$H$_{18}$O$_2$; mol wt 146.23. C 65.71%, H 12.41%, O 21.88%. Prepn: Kulpinsky, Nord, *J. Org. Chem.* **8**, 256 (1943); B. G. Wilkes, **US 2407205** (1946 to Carbide & Carbon Chemicals). Activity: P. Granett, H. L. Haynes, *J. Econ. Entomol.* **38**, 671 (1945); W. V. King, *ibid.* **44**, 339 (1951); B. V. Travis, C. N. Smith, *ibid.* 428. As an additive in mosquito repellant: W. G. Reifenrath, L. C. Rutledge, *J. Pharm. Sci.* **72**, 169 (1983). Toxicity study: B. Ballantyne *et al., Vet. Hum. Toxicol.* **27**, 491 (1985).

Colorless, odorless, slightly viscous liq. d$_{20}^{20}$ 0.9422. d$_4^{22}$ 0.9325. bp$_{760}$ 244.2°; bp$_{50}$ 163°; bp$_{10}$ 129°; bp$_3$ 102°; bp$_{0.5}$ 94-96°. n$_D^{22}$ 1.4530. Flash pt 260°F. Vapor pressure at 20° <0.01 mm. Abs viscosity: 271 cP. Soly in water 0.6% w/w; soly of water in 2-ethyl-1,3-hexanediol 10.8% w/w; sol in ethanol, isopropanol, propylene glycol, castor oil. LD$_{50}$ in male, female rats (ml/kg): 9.85, 4.92 orally (Ballantyne).

Caution: Little or no skin absorption; ingestion causes CNS depression. *See: Clinical Toxicology of Commercial Products,* R. E. Gosselin *et al.,* Eds. (Williams & Wilkins, Baltimore, 5th ed., 1984) Section II, pp 347.

USE: Insect repellent.

3745. Ethopabate. [59-06-3] 4-Acetamido-2-ethoxybenzoic acid methyl ester; methyl 4-acetamido-2-ethoxybenzoate;

2-ethoxy-4-acetamidobenzoic acid methyl ester; ethyl pabate. C_{12}-$H_{15}NO_4$; mol wt 237.25. C 60.75%, H 6.37%, N 5.90%, O 26.97%. Prepn: Grimme, Schmitz, *Ber.* **87**, 179 (1954); E. F. Rogers, R. L. Clark, **BE 613166**; *eidem*, **US 3211610** (1962, 1965 both to Merck & Co.); **FR 1407055**; M. L. Thominet, **US 3357978** (1965, 1967 both to Soc. d'Etudes Sci. Ind. de l'Ile-de-France). Anticoccidial activity studies: Rogers *et al.*, *Proc. Soc. Exp. Biol. Med.* **117**, 488 (1964). Metabolism in chickens: Buhs *et al.*, *J. Pharmacol. Exp. Ther.* **154**, 357 (1966).

White to pinkish-white, practically odorless crystals from methanol and water, mp 148-149°. uv max (methanol): 298, 267 nm ($A_{1cm}^{1\%}$ 805, 365). Sol in methanol, ethanol, acetone, acetonitrile. Sparingly sol in isopropanol, *p*-dioxane, ethyl acetate, methylene chloride; very slightly sol in water and isooctane.

Mixture with amprolium. Amprol Plus.

THERAP CAT (VET): Mixture as coccidiostat.

3746. Ethoprop. [13194-48-4] Phosphorodithioic acid *O*-ethyl *S,S*-dipropyl ester; *O*-ethyl *S,S*-dipropylphosphorodithioate; ethoprophos; VC9-104; Mocap. $C_8H_{19}O_2PS_2$; mol wt 242.34. C 39.65%, H 7.90%, O 13.20%, P 12.78%, S 26.46%. Prepn: L. E. Goyette, **US 3112244** (1963 to Virginia-Carolina Chem. Corp.); J. H. Wilson, Jr., **US 3268393** (1966 to Mobil). Activity: C. R. Harris, J. L. Hitchon, *J. Econ. Entomol.* **63**, 2 (1970). Metabolism: Z. M. Iqbal, R. E. Menzer, *Biochem. Pharmacol.* **21**, 1569 (1972). Soil degradation: J. H. Smelt *et al.*, *Pestic. Sci.* **8**, 147 (1977).

Pale yellow oil, $bp_{0.2}$ 86-91°. d_4^{20} 1.094. Vapor press. at 26°: 3.5×10^{-4} mm Hg. Soly in water: 750 mg/l. Sol in most organic solvents.

USE: Insecticide; nematocide.

3747. Ethopropazine. [522-00-9] *N,N*-Diethyl-α-methyl-10*H*-phenothiazine-10-ethanamine; 10-(2-diethylaminopropyl)-phenothiazine; 10-(2-diethylamino-2-methylethyl)phenothiazine; 2-diethylamino-1-propyl-*N*-dibenzoparathiazine; phenopropazine; profenamine; RP-3356; W-483; Isothazine; Isothiazine; Parkin. $C_{19}H_{24}N_2S$; mol wt 312.47. C 73.03%, H 7.74%, N 8.97%, S 10.26%. Anticholinergic. Prepd from Grignard complexes of diethylaminopropyl halide and phenothiazine: S. S. Berg, J. N. Ashley, **US 2607773** (1952 to Rhône-Poulenc). Pharmacology: M. E. Farquharson, R. G. Johnston, *Br. J. Pharmacol.* **14**, 559 (1959). Pharmacokinetics: M. Maboudian-Esfahani, D. R. Brocks, *Biopharm. Drug Dispos.* **20**, 159 (1999). HPLC determn in plasma: *eidem*, *J. Chromatogr. B* **715**, 417 (1998).

Crystals, mp 53-55°. Usually obtained as an oil because of contamination with 10-(2-diethylamino-1-methylethyl)phenothiazine.

Hydrochloride. [1094-08-2] Dibutil; Lysivane; Pardisol; Parphezein; Parphezin; Parsidol; Parsitan; Parsotil; Rodipal. $C_{19}H_{24}$-$N_2S\cdot HCl$; mol wt 348.93. Crystals from ethylene dichloride, mp

223-225° (some decompn). Lower melting points reported are caused by admixture with 10-(2-diethylamino-1-methylethyl)-phenothiazine-HCl which melts at 166-168°. One gram dissolves in 400 ml water at 20°, in 20 ml water at 40°. Sol in ethanol, chloroform. Soly in abs ethanol at 25° = 1.0 g/30 ml. Sparingly sol in acetone. Practically insol in ether, benzene. pH of a 5% aq soln is about 5.8. LD_{50} s.c. in mice: 670 mg/kg (Farquharson, Johnston).

THERAP CAT: Antiparkinsonian.

3748. Ethosuximide. [77-67-8] 3-Ethyl-3-methyl-2,5-pyrrolidinedione; 2-ethyl-2-methylsuccinimide; α-ethyl-α-methylsuccinimide; 3-methyl-3-ethylpyrrolidine-2,5-dione; Atysmal; Capitus; Emeside; Epileo Petitmal; Ethymal; Mesentol; Pemal; Petinimid; Petinimid; Petnidan; Pyknolepsinum; Simatin; Succimal; Suxilep; Suximal; Suxinutin; Zarontin. $C_7H_{11}NO_2$; mol wt 141.17. C 59.56%, H 7.85%, N 9.92%, O 22.67%. Prepn: Najer *et al.*, *Bull. Soc. Chim. Fr.* **3**, 1119 (1966). Comparative clinical trial with valproic acid in epilepsy: S. Sato *et al.*, *Neurology* **32**, 157 (1982). Brief review: S. J. Wallace, *Neurol. Clin.* **4**, 601 (1986).

Crystals from acetone + ether, mp 64-65°. Freely sol in water. LD_{50} in mice (g/kg): 1.65 i.p.; 1.75 orally (Najer).

THERAP CAT: Anticonvulsant.

3749. Ethotoin. [86-35-1] 3-Ethyl-5-phenyl-2,4-imidazolidinedione; 3-ethyl-5-phenylhydantoin; 1-ethyl-2,5-dioxo-4-phenyl-imidazolidine; Peganone. $C_{11}H_{12}N_2O_2$; mol wt 204.23. C 64.69%, H 5.92%, N 13.72%, O 15.67%. Prepd by heating the potassium salt of 5-phenylhydantoin with ethyl bromide in alc at 100° in a sealed tube: Pinner, *Ber.* **21**, 2320 (1888). Use as anticonvulsant: W. J. Close, **US 2793157** (1957 to Abbott Labs.). Metabolism: Dudley *et al.*, *J. Pharmacol. Exp. Ther.* **175**, 27 (1970).

Stout prisms from water, mp 94°. Sparingly sol in cold water, more sol in hot water. Freely sol in alcohol, ether, benzene, dil aq solns of alkali hydroxides.

THERAP CAT: Anticonvulsant.

3750. 2-Ethoxyethanol. [110-80-5] Ethylene glycol monoethyl ether; Cellosolve; Oxitol. $C_4H_{10}O_2$; mol wt 90.12. C 53.31%, H 11.18%, O 35.51%. $HOCH_2CH_2OC_2H_5$. Manuf from ethylene oxide and ethanol: *Faith, Keyes & Clark's Industrial Chemicals*, F. A. Lowenheim, M. K. Moran, Eds. (Wiley-Interscience, New York, 4th ed., 1975) pp 403-407. Toxicity data: H. F. Smyth *et al.*, *J. Ind. Hyg. Toxicol.* **23**, 259 (1941). Series of articles on toxicology: *Environ. Health Perspect.* **57**, 1-275 (1984).

Colorless, practically odorless liq. d_{20}^{20} 0.931. bp 135°. mp −70°. Flash pt, closed cup: 112°F (44°C); open cup: 120°F (49°C). n_D^{25} 1.406. Misc with water, alc, ether, acetone, liq esters. It dissolves many oils, resins, waxes, etc. LD_{50} orally in rats: 3 g/kg (Smyth).

Caution: Potential symptoms of overexposure in exptl animals are irritation of eyes, respiratory system; blood changes; liver, kidney, lung damage; reproductive, teratogenic effects. *See* NIOSH Pocket Guide to Chemical Hazards (DHHS/NIOSH 97-140, 1997) p 130. *See also Patty's Industrial Hygiene and Toxicology* vol. 2D, G. D. Clayton, F. E. Clayton, Eds. (Wiley-Interscience, New York, 4th ed., 1994) pp 2765, 2777-2785.

USE: Solvent for nitrocellulose, lacquers and dopes; in varnish removers, cleansing solns, dye baths; finishing leather with water pigments and dye solns; increasing stability of emulsions.

3751. 2-Ethoxyethyl Acetate. [111-15-9] 2-Ethoxyethanol acetate; cellosolve acetate; ethylene glycol monoethyl ether acetate. $C_6H_{12}O_3$; mol wt 132.16. C 54.53%, H 9.15%, O 36.32%. C_2-$H_5OCH_2CH_2OOCCH_3$. Toxicity data: Smyth *et al., J. Ind. Hyg. Toxicol.* **23,** 259 (1941). Series of articles on toxicology: *Environ. Health Perspect.* **57,** 1-275 (1984).

Colorless liq, pleasant odor. d_{20}^{20} 0.975. bp 156°. Flash pt, open cup: 134°F (56°C). Sol in about 6 parts water. LD_{50} orally in rats: 5.1 g/kg (Smyth).

Caution: Potential symptoms of overexposure are vomiting; kidney damage; paralysis. Direct contact may cause irritation of eyes and nose. *See NIOSH Pocket Guide to Chemical Hazards* (DHHS/NIOSH 97-140, 1997) p 130. *See also Patty's Industrial Hygiene and Toxicology* vol. **2D,** G. D. Clayton, F. E. Clayton, Eds. (Wiley-Interscience, New York, 4th ed., 1994) pp 2921-2925.

USE: Automobile lacquers to retard evaporation and impart high gloss.

3752. 2-Ethoxynaphthalene. [93-18-5] Ethyl β-naphthyl ether; ethyl β-naphtholate; nerolin "new"; β-naphthyl ethyl ether; Bromelia. $C_{12}H_{12}O$; mol wt 172.22. C 83.69%, H 7.02%, O 9.29%. Prepd by heating β-naphthol with potassium ethyl sulfate, or with alcohol and H_2SO_4: Yokoyama *et al., Yakugaku Zasshi* **78,** 123 (1958); *C.A.* **52,** 10986c (1958); from β-naphthol + *p*-toluenesulfonyl chloride + ethyl alcohol: Drakowzal, Klamann, *Monatsh. Chem.* **82,** 588 (1951); from β-naphthol + H_2SO_4 + ethyl acetate: Patai, Bentov, *J. Am. Chem. Soc.* **74,** 6118 (1952); from β-naphthol + triethylphosphate + *p*-toluenesulfonic acid: Bell, **US 2683748** (1954 to Eastman Kodak).

Lustrous crystals, mp 37-38°. bp 28.2°. $n_D^{47.3}$ 1.5932. d_{20}^{20} 1.0640. Practically insol in water. Sol in alcohol, chloroform, ether, carbon disulfide, toluene, petr ether.

USE: In perfumery.

3753. Ethoxyquin. [91-53-2] 6-Ethoxy-1,2-dihydro-2,2,4-trimethylquinoline; 1,2-dihydro-6-ethoxy-2,2,4-trimethylquinoline; EMQ; Santoflex; Santoquin. $C_{14}H_{19}NO$; mol wt 217.31. C 77.38%, H 8.81%, N 6.45%, O 7.36%. Prepn: Knoevenagel, *Ber.* **54,** 1722 (1921); Baird *et al.,* **GB 505113** (1939 to ICI); C. C. Tung, *Tetrahedron* **19,** 1685 (1963). Structure: Cliffe, *J. Chem. Soc.* **1933,** 1327. Metabolism: R. H. Wilson *et al., Agric. Food Chem.* **7,** 206 (1959); J. U. Skaare, E. Solheim, *Xenobiotica* **9,** 649 (1979). Toxicity data: V. I. Piul'skaya *et al., C.A.* **90,** 4601c (1979).

Yellow liquid. bp_2 123-125°. n_D^{25} 1.569-1.672. d_{25}^{25} 1.029-1.031. LD_{50} orally in rats, mice: 1920, 1730 mg/kg (Piul'skaya).

USE: Antioxidant in feed and food; antidegradation agent for rubber.

3754. Ethoxysulfuron. [126801-58-9] [[(4,6-Dimethoxy-2-pyrimidinyl)amino]carbonyl]sulfamic acid 2-ethoxyphenyl ester; 3-(4,6-dimethoxypyrimidin-2-yl)-1-(2-ethoxyphenoxysulfonylurea); HOE-095404. $C_{15}H_{18}N_4O_7S$; mol wt 398.39. C 45.22%, H 4.55%, N 14.06%, O 28.11%, S 8.05%. Post-emergence herbicide for use in grains and sugarcane; inhibits the enzyme, acetohydroxyacid synthase. Prepn: H. Kehne *et al.,* **EP 342569**; *eidem,* **US 5104443** (1989, 1992 both to Hoechst). Comprehensive description: E. Hacker *et al., Brighton Crop Prot. Conf. - Weeds* **1995,** 73. Mode of selective action: H. Köcher, G. Dickerhof, *ibid.* 249. Field study in summer rice: M. K. Bhowmick, R. K. Ghosh, *Adv. Plant Sci.* **15,** 499 (2002).

Crystals from diethyl ether, mp 145-147°. Vapor pressure (20°): 6.6×10^{-5} Pa. Partition coefficient (octanol/water) at 20°: 773 (pH 3); 1.01 (pH 7); 0.06 (pH 9). Soly in water at 20° (ppm): 26 (pH 5); 1353 (pH 7); 9628 (pH 9). LD_{50} in rats (mg/kg): >3270 orally; >4000 dermally (Hacker).

USE: Herbicide.

3755. Ethoxzolamide. [452-35-7] 6-Ethoxy-2-benzothiazolesulfonamide; ethoxyzolamide; Ethamide; Glaucotensil. C_9-$H_{10}N_2O_3S_2$; mol wt 258.32. C 41.85%, H 3.90%, N 10.84%, O 18.58%, S 24.83%. Carbonic anhydrase inhibitor. Prepn: **GB 795174**; J. Korman, **US 2868800** (1958, 1959 both to Upjohn).

Crystals from ethyl acetate + Skellysolve B, mp 188-190.5°.

THERAP CAT: Diuretic.

THERAP CAT (VET): Diuretic.

3756. Ethybenztropine. [524-83-4] (3-*endo*)-3-(Diphenylmethoxy)-8-ethyl-8-azabicyclo[3.2.1]octane; 3α-(diphenylmethoxy)-8-ethyl-1α*H*,5α*H*-nortropane; *N*-ethylnortropine benzhydryl ether; tropethydrylin; *N*-ethyl-8-aza-3-bicyclo[3.2.1]octyl benzhydryl ether; *N*-ethylbenztropine; ethylbenzatropine; etybenzatropine. $C_{22}H_{27}NO$; mol wt 321.46. C 82.20%, H 8.47%, N 4.36%, O 4.98%. Anticholinergic. Prepn: **GB 804837** (1958 to Sandoz); Boehringer *et al.,* **GB 824875** (1959 to Boehringer, Ing.).

Hydrochloride. [26598-44-7] Ponalide. $C_{22}H_{27}NO \cdot HCl$; mol wt 357.92. Crystals from acetone, mp 190-191°.

Hydrobromide. [24815-25-6] $C_{22}H_{27}NO \cdot HBr$; mol wt 402.37. Crystals from methanol + ether, mp 226-228°.

THERAP CAT: Antiparkinsonian.

3757. Ethyl Acetate. [141-78-6] Acetic acid ethyl ester; acetic ether; vinegar naphtha. $C_4H_8O_2$; mol wt 88.11. C 54.53%, H 9.15%, O 36.32%. $CH_3COOC_2H_5$. Obtained by the slow distillation of a mixture of acetic acid, ethyl alc, and sulfuric acid: Alheritiere, Mercier, **US 2787636** (1957 to Usines de Melle); *Faith, Keyes & Clark's Industrial Chemicals,* F. A. Lowenheim, M. K. Moran, Eds. (Wiley-Interscience, New York, 4th ed., 1975) pp 350-354. Toxicity: H. F. Smyth *et al., Am. Ind. Hyg. Assoc. J.* **23,** 95 (1962).

Clear, volatile, flammable liq; characteristic fruity odor; pleasant taste when diluted. Slowly dec by moisture, then acquires an acid reaction. Absorbs water (up to 3.3% w/w). d_4^{20} 0.902; d_{25}^{25} 0.898. bp 77°. mp −83°. Ignition temp 800°F. Explosive limits (% vol in air): 2.2 to 11.5. n_D^{20} 1.3719. Vapor density 3.04 (air = 1). One ml dissolves in 10 ml water at 25°; more sol at lower and less sol at higher temps. Misc with alc, acetone, chloroform, ether. Azeotropic mixture with water (6.1% w/w) bp 70.4°. Azeotropic mixture with water (7.8% w/w) and alc (9.0% w/w) bp 70.3°. *Keep tightly*

Consult the Name Index before using this section.

closed in a cool place and away from fire. LD$_{50}$ orally in rats: 11.3 ml/kg (Smyth).

Caution: Potential symptoms of overexposure are irritation of eyes, skin, nose and throat; narcosis; dermatitis. *See NIOSH Pocket Guide to Chemical Hazards* (DHHS/NIOSH 97-140, 1997) p 130.

USE: Pharmaceutic aid (flavor); artificial fruit essences; solvent for nitrocellulose, varnishes, lacquers, and aeroplane dopes; manuf smokeless powder, artificial leather, photographic films and plates, artificial silk, perfumes; cleaning textiles, etc.

3758. Ethyl Acetoacetate. [141-97-9] 3-Oxobutanoic acid ethyl ester; acetoacetic acid ethyl ester; acetoacetic ester; ethyl 3-oxobutanoate. $C_6H_{10}O_3$; mol wt 130.14. C 55.37%, H 7.75%, O 36.88%. $CH_3COCH_2COOC_2H_5$. Only the equilibrium mixture of the keto and enol forms is described here. Prepd from ethyl acetate by the action of sodium, sodium ethoxide, sodamide, or calcium: Inglis, Roberts, *Org. Synth.* **coll. vol. I,** 235 (2nd ed., 1941); Hansley, Schott, **US 2843623** (1958 to Natl. Distillers); Scheibler, *Ann.* **565,** 176 (1949); Gattermann-Wieland, *Praxis des Organischen Chemikers* (de Gruyter, Berlin, 40th ed., 1961) p 218. Discussion of keto-enol tautomerism: Ward, *J. Chem. Educ.* **39,** 95 (1962). Toxicity study: H. F. Smyth *et al., J. Ind. Hyg. Toxicol.* **31,** 60 (1949).

Liq. Agreeable odor. d_4^{10} 1.0357; d_4^{17} 1.0288; d_4^{25} 1.0213; d_4^{54} 0.9924; d_4^{75} 0.9703. mp −45°. bp$_{760}$ 180.8°; bp$_{400}$ 158.2°; bp$_{200}$ 138.0°; bp$_{60}$ 106°; bp$_{20}$ 81.1°; bp$_5$ 54.0°; bp$_{1.0}$ 28.5°. n_D^{20} 1.41937. Absorption spectrum: Morton, Rosney, *J. Chem. Soc.* **1926,** 711. Flash pt, closed cup: 184°F. Sol in about 35 parts water; misc with the usual organic solvents. LD$_{50}$ orally in rats: 3.98 g/kg (Smyth).

Caution: Moderately irritating to skin, mucous membranes.

3759. Ethyl Acrylate. [140-88-5] 2-Propenoic acid ethyl ester; acrylic acid ethyl ester. $C_5H_8O_2$; mol wt 100.12. C 59.98%, H 8.05%, O 31.96%. CH_2=CHCOOCH$_2$CH$_3$. Prepd from ethylene chlorohydrin or acrylonitrile, ethanol, and sulfuric acid; also by an oxo reaction from acetylene, carbon monoxide, and ethanol in the presence of suitable catalysts. *See* the refs under Methyl Acrylate.

Monomer. Liquid, acrid, penetrating odor, retained by clothing. *Lacrimator.* d_4^{20} 0.9405. fp below −72°. bp$_{760}$ 99.4°; bp$_{39.2}$ 20° (polymerizes on distn). n_D^{20} 1.404. Specific heat at −60°: 0.442 cal/g/°C. Heat of vaporization 8.27 kcal/mol; heat of combustion 655.49 kcal/mol. Flash pt, open cup: 60°F (15°C). Vapor density 3.45 (air = 1). Soly in water at 20°: 2 g/100 ml. Soly of water in ethyl acrylate at 20°: 1.5 g/100 g. Sol in alcohol, ether. Azeotropes: 45.0% water = bp 81°; 56.8% ethanol = bp 76°. Easily polymerizes on standing; polymerization process speeded up by heat, light, and peroxides. If pure, the monomer can be stored below +10° without incurring polymerization.

Polymer. Transparent, elastic substance. Practically no odor. Little adhesive power. Resists the usual solvents.

Caution: Potential symptoms of overexposure to the monomer are irritation of eyes, respiratory system and skin. *See NIOSH Pocket Guide to Chemical Hazards* (DHHS/NIOSH 97-140, 1997) p 132. *See also Patty's Industrial Hygiene and Toxicology* vol. 2A, G. D. Clayton, F. E. Clayton, Eds. (Wiley-Interscience, New York, 3rd ed., 1981) p 2292-2296. This substance was formerly listed as reasonably anticipated to be a human carcinogen: *Eighth Report on Carcinogens* (PB99-128746, 1998) p III-627; delisted because the relevant data are not sufficient to meet the current criteria for this listing: *Ninth Report on Carcinogens* (PB2000-107509, 2000) p B-2.

USE: The monomer in the manuf of water emulsion paint vehicles; in production of emulsion-based polymers used in textile and paper coatings, leather finish resins and adhesives. Imparts flexibility to hard films.

3760. Ethyl Alcohol. [64-17-5] Ethanol; absolute alcohol; anhydrous alcohol; dehydrated alcohol; ethyl hydrate; ethyl hydroxide. C_2H_6O; mol wt 46.07. C 52.14%, H 13.13%, O 34.73%. C_2H_5OH. Manuf: by fermentation of starch, sugar, and other carbohydrates; from ethylene, acetylene, sulfite waste liquors, and synthesis gas (CO + H); by hydrolysis of ethyl sulfate, and oxidation of methane. Toxicity: G. S. Wiberg *et al., Toxicol. Appl. Pharmacol.* **16,** 718 (1970). Embryotoxicity in mammals: N. A. Brown *et al., Science* **206,** 573 (1979). Possible mechanism for actions of ethanol on the brain: G. Aston-Jones *et al., Nature* **296,** 857 (1982).

Ethanol-induced chromosomal abnormalities in mice: M. H. Kaufman, *ibid.* **302,** 258 (1983). Disruption of reproductive function in female primates following alcohol self-administration: N. K. Mello *et al., Science* **221,** 677 (1983). Review of metabolism and toxicity: C. S. Lieber in *Reviews in Biochemical Toxicology* vol. **5,** E. Hodgson *et al.,* Eds. (Elsevier, New York, 1983) pp 267-312; of pharmacology: L. Pohorecky, J. Brick, *Pharmacol. Ther.* **36,** 335-427 (1988); of hepatotoxicity: C. S. Lieber, L. M. DeCarli, *J. Hepatol.* **12,** 394-401 (1991). General reviews: P. Baud, "Ethyl Alcohol Industry" in Grignard, *Traité de Chimie Organique* vol. **5** (Masson, 1937) pp 841-975; Zabel, *Chem. Ind.* (now *Chem. Week*) **64,** 212 (1949); *Faith, Keyes & Clark's Industrial Chemicals,* F. A. Lowenheim, M. K. Moran, Eds. (Wiley-Interscience, New York, 4th ed., 1975) pp 355-364; P. D. Sherman, P. R. Kavasmaneck, "Ethanol" in *Kirk-Othmer Encyclopedia of Chemical Technology* vol. **9** (Interscience, New York, 3rd ed., 1980) pp 338-380.

Clear, colorless, very mobile, flammable liquid; pleasant odor; burning taste. Absorbs water rapidly from air. d_4^{20} 0.789. bp 78.5°. mp −114.1°. n_D^{20} 1.361. Flash pt, closed cup: 13°C. Miscible with water and with many organic liquids. *Keep tightly closed, cool, and away from flame!* LD$_{50}$ in young, old rats (g/kg): 10.6, 7.06 orally (Wiberg). The terms *95% alcohol* and *alcohol* (when used alone) refer to a binary azeotrope having a distillate composition of 95.57% ethyl alcohol (by wt) and bp 78.15°. *Alcohol, USP* is specified as containing not less than 92.3% and not more than 93.8% by weight, corresponding to not less than 94.9% and not more than 96.0% by vol of C_2H_5OH at 15.56°. d_{25}^{25} 0.810; d 0.816 at 15.56° (60°F). *Diluted alcohol,* prepd from equal vols 95% alcohol and water, contains about 41.5% by wt or about 48.9% by vol of C_2H_5OH. d_{25}^{25} 0.931; d 0.936 at 15.56° (60°F). *See U.S.P.* **XXI,** 22, 1530 (1985).

Caution: Potential symptoms of overexposure are irritation of eyes, skin, nose; headache, nausea, vomiting, drowsiness, fatigue; narcosis; cough; flushing, rapid pulse, sweating; mental excitement or depression; impaired perception, incoordination, stupor, coma; liver damage; anemia; reproductive and teratogenic effects. *See NIOSH Pocket Guide to Chemical Hazards* (DHHS/NIOSH 97-140, 1997) p 132; *Clinical Toxicology of Commercial Products,* R. E. Gosselin *et al.,* Eds. (Williams & Wilkins, Baltimore, 5th ed., 1984) Section III, pp 166-171.

USE: Most ethyl alcohol is used in alcoholic beverages in suitable dilutions. Other uses are as solvent in laboratory and industry, in the manufacture of denatured alcohol, pharmaceuticals (rubbing compds, lotions, tonics, colognes), in perfumery, in organic synthesis. Octane booster in gasoline. Pharmaceutical aid (solvent).

THERAP CAT: Antiseptic.

THERAP CAT (VET): Antiseptic. To destroy nerve tissue. Solvent and dehydrating agent.

3761. Ethyl Alcohol, Denatured. Denatured alcohol. Ethyl alcohol to which has been added some substance or substances which, while allowing the use of the alcohol in the most varied industries and arts, renders it entirely unfit for consumption as a beverage. The most commonly used denaturants, either alone or in combination, are the following: Methanol, camphor, Aldehol, amyl alcohol, gasoline, isopropanol, terpineol, benzene, castor oil, acetone, nicotine, aniline dyes, ether, cadmium iodide, pyridine bases, sulfuric acid, kerosene, diethyl phthalate. *Formula 1* is 5 gallons approved wood alcohol added to 100 gal of 95% ethanol. *Formula 2B* is 0.5 gal benzene added to 100 gal of 95% ethanol. Similarly *formula 3A* contains 5 gal commercial methanol, *formula 6B* contains 0.5 gal pyridine bases, *formula 12A* 5 gal benzene, *formula 13A* 10 gal ethyl ether, *formula 19* 4 gal methyl isobutyl ketone and 1 gal kerosene, *formula 20* 5 gal crude chloroform, *formula 23A* 10 gal acetone, *formula 28* 10 gal benzene, *formula 28A* 1 gal gasoline, *formula 30* 10 gal methanol, *formula 32* 5 gal ethyl ether, *formula 33* 30 lbs methyl violet, *formula 35A* 5 gal ethyl acetate, *formula 39C* 1 gal diethyl phthalate; *formula 44* contains 20 gal *n*-butanol. Additional permissible formulas are given in *Appendix to Regulations No. 3, Formulae for Completely and Specially Denatured Alcohol,* published by the U.S. Treasury Dept., Bureau of Industrial Alcohol. Reprinted in N. A. Lange, *Handbook of Chemistry.*

Caution: Denaturants, particularly methanol, may modify and increase toxic symptoms caused by ingestion and exposure to fumes.

3762. Ethylamine. [75-04-7] Ethanamine; monoethyl-amine; aminoethane. C_2H_7N; mol wt 45.08. C 53.29%, H 15.65%, N 31.07%. $C_2H_5NH_2$. Prepn from ethyliodide + liq ammonia: Watt, Otto, *J. Am. Chem. Soc.* **69**, 836 (1947); from ethanol + ammonia: Davies *et al.,* **US 2609394** (1952 to ICI); Lemon, Myerly, **US 3022349** (1962 to Union Carbide). Toxicity study: H. F. Smyth *et al., Arch. Ind. Hyg. Occup. Med.* **10**, 61 (1954).

Flammable, liq; ammonia odor; strong alkaline reaction. d_{15}^{15} 0.689. bp 16.6°. Solidif −80°. Miscible with water, alcohol, ether. *Keep tightly closed and in cold place.* LD_{50} orally in rats: 0.40 g/kg (Smyth).

Hydrochloride. [557-66-4] $C_2H_7N.HCl$. Crystals from ethanol + water, mp 110°. d 1.22. Soluble in 0.4 part water; freely sol in alcohol; slightly sol in chloroform or acetone. Practically insol in ether. *Keep well closed.*

Hydriodide. [506-58-1] $C_2H_7N.HI$. Hygroscopic crystals, mp 188°. d 2.10. Freely sol in water or alcohol. Practically insol in chloroform, ether. *Keep well closed and protected from light.*

Oleate. [39664-27-2] Ethanamine (Z)-9-octadecenoate; Etalate. $C_2H_7N.C_{18}H_{34}O_2$; mol wt 327.55. Commercial prepn is a 5% soln with 2% benzyl alcohol as anodyne.

Caution: Potential symptoms of overexposure are irritation of eyes, skin and respiratory system; skin burns; dermatitis. *See NIOSH Pocket Guide to Chemical Hazards* (DHHS/NIOSH 97-140, 1997) p 132.

USE: In resin chemistry; stabilizer for rubber latex; intermediate for dyestuffs, medicinals; in oil refining; in organic syntheses.

THERAP CAT: Oleate as a sclerosing agent.

3763. N-Ethylamphetamine. [457-87-4] N-Ethyl-α-methylbenzeneethanamine; N-ethyl-α-methylphenethylamine; N-ethyl-ω-phenylisopropylamine; 2-ethylamino-1-phenylpropane. $C_{11}H_{17}$-N; mol wt 163.26. C 80.92%, H 10.50%, N 8.58%. Prepn: Keil, Dobke, **DE 767263** (1952 to Theodor H. Temmler); Leonard *et al., J. Am. Chem. Soc.* **80**, 4858 (1958). Separation of isomers: **GB 814339** (1959 to Sterling Drug).

bp$_{14}$ 104.5-106°. n_D^{25} 1.4986.

Hydrochloride. [1858-47-5] MG-19973; Apetinil-Depo. C_{11}-$H_{17}N.HCl$; mol wt 199.72.

d-Form hydrochloride. $C_{11}H_{17}N.HCl$. mp 154-156°. $[\alpha]_D^{15}$ +17.2° (c = 2 in water).

l-Form hydrochloride. $C_{11}H_{17}N.HCl$. mp 155-156°. $[\alpha]_D^{25}$ −17.3° (c = 2 in water).

Note: This is a controlled substance (stimulant): **21 CFR,** 1308.11.

THERAP CAT: Anorexic.

3764. Ethylaniline. [103-69-5] N-Ethylbenzenamine; ethylphenylamine. $C_8H_{11}N$; mol wt 121.18. C 79.29%, H 9.15%, N 11.56%. Produced by heating aniline hydrochloride and alcohol at 180°. Toxicology: M. Sziza, L. Podhragyai, *Arch. Gewerbepathol. Gewerbehyg.* **15**, 447 (1957).

Very refractive liquid; rapidly becomes brown on exposure to light and air. Aniline-like odor. d_{25}^{25} 0.958. Solidifies below 80°. bp 204.5°. mp −63.5°. n_D^{20} 1.5559. Insol in water. Miscible with alc, ether and many other organic solvents. *Keep well closed and protected from light.* LD_{50} in rats (g/kg): 0.18 i.p., 0.28 orally, 4.7 s.c. (Sziza, Podhragyai).

3765. Ethylbenzene. [100-41-4] C_8H_{10}; mol wt 106.17. C 90.50%, H 9.49%. $C_6H_5C_2H_5$. Prepn from acetophenone: Clem-

mensen, *Ber.* **46**, 1838 (1913); Gattermann-Wieland, *Praxis des Organischen Chemikers* (de Gruyter, Berlin, 40th ed., 1961) p 332; by Huang-Minlon modification of Wolff-Kishner reduction: A. I. Vogel, *Practical Organic Chemistry* (Longmans, 3rd ed., 1959) p 516. Physical properties: L. C. Gibbons *et al., J. Am. Chem. Soc.* **68**, 1130 (1946). Manuf: *Faith, Keyes & Clark's Industrial Chemicals,* F. A. Lowenheim, M. K. Moran, Eds. (Wiley-Interscience, New York, 4th ed., 1975) pp 365-370. Toxicity study: H. F. Smyth *et al., Am. Ind. Hyg. Assoc. J.* **23**, 95 (1962). Review of toxicity and human exposure: *Toxicological Profile for Ethylbenzene* (PB99-166647, 1999) 280 pp.

Colorless liquid. *Flammable.* d_{25}^{25} 0.866. bp 136.25°. mp −95.01°. n_D^{25} 1.4932. Flash pt, closed cup: 64°F (18°C). Practically insol in water. Misc with the usual organic solvents. LD_{50} orally in rats: 5.46 g/kg (Smyth).

Caution: Potential symptoms of overexposure are irritation of eyes, skin and mucous membranes; headache; dermatitis; narcosis, coma. *See NIOSH Pocket Guide to Chemical Hazards* (DHHS/-NIOSH 97-140, 1997) p 132.

USE: For conversion to styrene monomer; as resin solvent.

3766. Ethyl Benzoate. [93-89-0] Benzoic acid ethyl ester. $C_9H_{10}O_2$; mol wt 150.17. C 71.98%, H 6.71%, O 21.31%. C_6-$H_5COOC_2H_5$.

Colorless, clear, refractive liq; aromatic odor; vapors cause cough. d_{25}^{25} 1.050. bp 211-213°. mp −34°. n_D^{20} 1.506. Almost insol in water; miscible with alcohol, chloroform, ether, petr ether. LD_{50} orally in rats: 6.48 g/kg, Smyth *et al., Arch. Ind. Hyg. Occup. Med.* **10**, 61 (1954).

USE: In perfumery under the name *Essence de Niobe*; in manuf of *Peau d'Espagne*; artificial fruit essence.

3767. Ethyl Benzoylacetate. [94-02-0] β-Oxobenzenepropanoic acid ethyl ester. $C_{11}H_{12}O_3$; mol wt 192.21. C 68.74%, H 6.29%, O 24.97%. $C_6H_5COCH_2COOC_2H_5$.

Liquid; pleasant odor; becomes yellow on exposure to air and light. d^{15} 1.122. bp 265-270° with decompn. Volatile with steam. n_D^{20} 1.5338. Insol in water; miscible with alcohol, ether. *Keep protected from air and light.*

3768. α-Ethylbenzyl Alcohol. [93-54-9] α-Ethylbenzenemethanol; ω-ethylbenzyl alcohol; 1-phenyl-1-propanol; 1-phenylpropyl alcohol; ethyl phenyl carbinol; α-hydroxypropylbenzene; SH-261; Ejibil; Livonal; Phenycholon; Phenicol; Phenychol; Felicur; Felitrope. $C_9H_{12}O$; mol wt 136.19. C 79.37%, H 8.88%, O 11.75%. Prepd from benzaldehyde or from ethyl phenyl ketone: Norris, Cortese, *J. Am. Chem. Soc.* **49**, 2640 (1927). Toxicity study: O. Linét *et al., Arzneim.-Forsch.* **12**, 347 (1962).

Oily liquid. Weak, ester-like odor. Sweetish, slightly irritating taste. bp$_{760}$ 219°; bp$_{15}$ 107°; bp$_3$ 78°. d_4^{25} 0.9915. n_D^{23} 1.5169. uv max (methanol): 250, 260 nm (ε 173, 114). Misc with methanol, ethanol, ether, benzene, toluene, olive oil. LD_{50} orally in rats: 1.6 ml/kg (Linét).

USE: As heat transfer medium; in perfumery.

THERAP CAT: Choleretic.

3769. Ethylbenzylaniline. [92-59-1] N-Ethyl-N-phenylbenzenemethanamine; N-ethyl-N-phenylbenzylamine. $C_{15}H_{17}N$; mol wt 211.30. C 85.26%, H 8.11%, N 6.63%. Prepn: Martin, MacQueen, **US 1887772** (1933 to Dow); Burgstahler, *J. Am. Chem. Soc.* **73**, 3021 (1951).

Consult the Name Index before using this section.

Light yellow, oily liq. d_4^{19} 1.034. bp$_{710}$ 287° with slight decompn; bp$_{14}$ 170-180°. n_D^{23} 1.5938. Practically insol in water. One ml dissolves in 5.5 ml alcohol; sol in the usual organic solvents.

USE: Manuf dyes; in organic syntheses.

3770. Ethyl Biscoumacetate. [548-00-5] 4-Hydroxy-α-(4-hydroxy-2-oxo-2H-1-benzopyran-3-yl)-2-oxo-2H-1-benzopyran-3-acetic acid ethyl ester; bis(4-hydroxy-2-oxo-2H-1-benzopyran-3-yl)acetic acid ethyl ester; ethyl bis(4-hydroxycoumarinyl)acetate; ethyldicoumarol acetate; bis-3,3'-(4-hydroxycoumarinyl)acetic acid ethyl ester; 3,3'-carboxymethylene bis(4-hydroxycoumarin)ethyl ester; ethyl 4,4'-dihydroxydicoumarinyl-3,3'-acetate; B.O.E.A.; Dicumacyl; Pelentan; Stabilene; Tromexan. $C_{22}H_{16}O_8$; mol wt 408.36. C 64.71%, H 3.95%, O 31.34%. Prepn: Rosicky, *Cas. Lek. Cesk.* **83**, 1200 (1944); US 2482510; US 2482511; US 2482512 (all 1949 to Spojené farm. zovody); Stahmann *et al., J. Am. Chem. Soc.* **65**, 2285 *sqq* (1943). Toxicity study: C. M. Gruber *et al., Fed. Proc.* **10**, 303 (1951).

Crystals, dimorphous, mp 177-182° and mp 154-157°. Bitter, persistent taste. Practically insol in water. Sol in 20 parts acetone, also sol in benzene. Slightly sol in alcohol, ether. LD$_{50}$ in mice, rats (g/kg): 0.88, 0.26 orally; 0.32, 1.1 i.p. (Gruber).

THERAP CAT: Anticoagulant.

3771. Ethyl Bromide. [74-96-4] Bromoethane; monobromoethane; bromic ether; hydrobromic ether. C_2H_5Br; mol wt 108.97. C 22.04%, H 4.62%, Br 73.33%. CH_3CH_2Br. Made by distilling from a mixture of HBr, ethyl alcohol and H_2SO_4: Kamm, Marvel, *Org. Synth.* **coll. vol. I**, 29 (1941). By phosphorus and bromine method: Goshorn *et al., ibid.* 36. Absorption spectrum: Hantzsch, *Ber.* **58**, 619 (1925). Physical properties: Mumford, Phillips, *J. Chem. Soc.* **1950**, 75. Toxicity data: E. H. Vernot *et al., Toxicol. Appl. Pharmacol.* **42**, 417 (1977).

Colorless, flammable, volatile liq; ethereal odor; burning taste; becomes yellowish on exposure to air and light. Vapor harmful. d_4^{20} 1.4612; d_4^{25} 1.4515. bp 38.2°. mp −119°. n_D^{20} 1.4242. Soly in water (g/100 g) at 0°: 1.067; 10°: 0.965; 20°: 0.914; 30°: 0.896; miscible with alcohol, ether, chloroform and with other organic solvents. Explosive limits (% by vol in air), lower 6.75, upper 11.25. Autoignition temp 952°F (511°C). LC$_{50}$ rats, mice (ppm): 27000, 16200 (Vernot).

Caution: Potential symptoms of overexposure are irritation of eyes, respiratory system and skin; CNS depression; pulmonary edema; liver and kidney disease; cardiac arrhythmias; cardiac arrest. *See NIOSH Pocket Guide to Chemical Hazards* (DHHS/NIOSH 97-140, 1997) p 134.

USE: Ethylating agent in organic synthesis; as refrigerant. Formerly used as a topical and inhalation anesthetic.

3772. Ethyl α-Bromopropionate. [535-11-5] 2-Bromopropanoic acid ethyl ester. $C_5H_9BrO_2$; mol wt 181.03. C 33.17%, H 5.01%, Br 44.14%, O 17.68%. $CH_3CHBrCOOC_2H_5$.

Liquid; sharp, pungent odor; becomes yellow on exposure to light. d_{20}^{20} 1.447. bp 159-160°; also stated as 160-165°. n_D^{20} 1.4469. Insol in water; miscible with alcohol, ether. *Protect from light.*

3773. Ethyl Butylacetylaminopropionate. [52304-36-6] N-Acetyl-N-butyl-β-alanine ethyl ester; 3-(N-butyl-N-acetyl)-aminopropionic acid ethyl ester; ethyl-3-(N-n-butyl-N-acetyl)aminopropionate; insect repellent 3535; IR 3535. $C_{11}H_{21}NO_3$; mol wt 215.29. C 61.37%, H 9.83%, N 6.51%, O 22.29%. N-Disubstituted derivative of β-alanine, *q.v.* Prepd (not claimed): M. Klier *et al.,* DE 2246433; *eidem,* US 4127672 (1974, 1978 both to Beiersdorf). Prepn, toxicity and insect repellency studies: M. Klier, F. Kuhlow, *J. Soc. Cosmetic Chem.* **27**, 141 (1976). Chemical, phys-

ical and toxicological properties: *WHO Interim Specification for IR 3535* (WHO/IS/TC/667/2001) 15 pp. Lab and field tests of efficacy vs mosquitoes: U. Thavara *et al., J. Am. Mosq. Control Assoc.* **17**, 190 (2001); and comparison to other repellents: D. R. Barnard *et al., J. Med. Entomol.* **39**, 895 (2002); M. S. Fradin, J. F. Day, *N. Engl. J. Med.* **347**, 13 (2002). HPLC determn in topical gel formulation: S. C. Marselos, H. A. Archontaki, *J. Chromatogr. A* **946**, 295 (2002). Assessment of efficiency of repellent formulations: R. Milutinovic *et al., SOFW-J.* **128**, 14 (2002). Review of repellency spectrum vs target pests: F. Marchio, *ibid.* **122**, 478-485 (1996).

Colorless to slightly yellowish, almost odorless liquid. mp <−20°. bp$_{0.2}$ 108-110°. bp$_{0.5}$ 126-127°. n_D^{20} 1.452-1.455. Flash point: 318°F (159°C). Log P (octanol/water): 1.7 (23°). Vapor pressure at 20°: 0.15 Pa. Soly at 20°: water 70 ±3 g/l (non-buffered). Sol in *n*-heptane, dichloromethane, ethyl acetate, *p*-xylene, acetone, methanol. LD$_{50}$ in rats (mg/kg): >5000 orally; LC$_{50}$ in rats (mg/l): >5.1 by inhalation (WHO).

USE: Insect repellent.

3774. Ethyl *tert*-Butyl Ether. [637-92-3] 2-Ethoxy-2-methylpropane; *tert*-butyl ethyl ether; ethyl *tert*-butyl oxide; 1,1-dimethylethyl ethyl ether; ethyl 1,1-dimethylethyl ether; ETBE. $C_6H_{14}O$; mol wt 102.17. C 70.53%, H 13.81%, O 15.66%. $(CH_3)_3$-C(OCH$_2$CH$_3$). Prepn J. U. Nef, *Ann.* **309**, 126 (1899). Synthesis: J. F. Norris, G. W. Rigby, *J. Am. Chem. Soc.* **54**, 2088 (1932). Physical properties: T. W. Evans, K. R. Edlund, *Ind. Eng. Chem.* **28**, 1186 (1936). Thermal decomposition: N. J. Daly, C. Wentrup, *Aust. J. Chem.* **21**, 1535 (1968). Brief review focusing on use as gasoline additive: M. Iborra *et al., Chemtech* **18**, 120-122 (1988).

fp −94.0°. bp$_{760}$ 72.8° (Evans, Edlund). Also reported as bp$_{760}$ 73.1° (Norris, Rigby). n_D^{25} 1.3728. n_D^{20} 1.3760. d_4^{15} 0.7456; d_4^{20} 0.7404; d_4^{25} 0.7353, d_4^{30} 0.7300. Vapor pressure at 25°: 130 mm Hg. Heat vaporization: 74.3 cal/g. Specific heat (liquid) at 25°: 0.51 cal/g/°C. Surface tension at 24°: 19.8 dynes/cm. Soly in water (20°): 1.2 g/100 g soln. Soly of water in compound (20°): 0.5 g/100 g soln.

USE: Gasoline additive.

3775. Ethyl Butyrate. [105-54-4] Butanoic acid ethyl ester; butyric acid ethyl ester; ethyl *n*-butyrate. $C_6H_{12}O_2$; mol wt 116.16. C 62.04%, H 10.41%, O 27.55%. $CH_3CH_2CH_2COOC_2H_5$. Toxicity data: P. M. Jenner *et al., Food Cosmet. Toxicol.* **2**, 327 (1964).

Colorless liq; pineapple odor. d_4^{20} 0.879. bp 120-121°. mp −93°. n_D^{20} 1.400. Flash pt, closed cup: 78°F (25°C); open cup: 85°F (29°C). Sol in about 150 parts water; misc with alcohol, ether. LD$_{50}$ orally in rats: 13,050 mg/kg (Jenner).

USE: Manuf artificial rum; perfumery; the alcoholic soln constitutes the so-called *"pineapple oil".*

3776. Ethyl Caprate. [110-38-3] Decanoic acid ethyl ester; ethyl decanoate. $C_{12}H_{24}O_2$; mol wt 200.32. C 71.95%, H 12.08%, O 15.97%. $CH_3(CH_2)_8COOC_2H_5$.

Colorless liq. d^{20} 0.862. bp 243-245°. Insoluble in water; miscible with alcohol, chloroform, ether.

USE: Manuf wine bouquets, cognac essence.

3777. Ethyl Caproate. [123-66-0] Hexanoic acid ethyl ester; ethyl hexanoate. $C_8H_{16}O_2$; mol wt 144.21. C 66.63%, H 11.18%, O 22.19%. $CH_3(CH_2)_4COOC_2H_5$.

Colorless to yellowish liquid; pleasant odor. d^{20} 0.873. bp 166-167°. Insol in water; miscible with alcohol, ether.

USE: Manuf artificial fruit flavors.

3778. Ethyl Caprylate. [106-32-1] Octanoic acid ethyl ester; ethyl octanoate; ethyl octylate. $C_{10}H_{20}O_2$; mol wt 172.26. C 69.72%, H 11.70%, O 18.58%. $CH_3(CH_2)_6COOC_2H_5$.

Colorless, clear, very mobile liquid; pleasant, pineapple odor. d^{17} 0.878. bp 207-209°. Insol in water; misc with alc, ether. LD$_{50}$

orally in rats: 25,960 mg/kg, P. M. Jenner *et al., Food Cosmet. Toxicol.* **2**, 327 (1964).

USE: Manuf fruit ethers; constit of enanthic, cocoic, and cognac ethers.

3779. Ethyl β-Carboline-3-carboxylate. [74214-62-3] 9*H*-Pyrido[3,4-*b*]indole-3-carboxylic acid ethyl ester; ethyl norharman-carboxylate; β-CCE. $C_{14}H_{12}N_2O_2$; mol wt 240.26. C 69.99%, H 5.03%, N 11.66%, O 13.32%. Deriv of **β-carboline** that is a potent displacer of ^{3}H-diazepam from brain benzodiazepine receptors. Isoln from human urine and brain and binding site study: C. Braestrup *et al., Proc. Natl. Acad. Sci. USA* **77**, 2288 (1980). Initially thought to be an endogenous ligand for benzodiazepine receptors in mammalian CNS, it is now believed to be formed during isoln and extraction procedures, R. F. Squires in *GABA and Benzodiazepine Receptors*, E. Costa *et al.*, Eds. (Raven Press, New York, 1980) pp 129-138; M. Nielson *et al., J. Neurochem.* **36**, 276 (1981). Synthesis and psychotropic activity: **JP Kokai 81 43283** (to Schering AG), *C.A.* **95**, 115508a (1981); U. Eder *et al.*, **EP 30254** (1981 to A/S Ferrosan; Schering AG). β-CCE has been shown to lower seizure threshold and to reverse the sedative effect of flurazepam, *q.v.:* P. J. Cowen *et al., Nature* **290**, 54 (1981). Neurochemical and pharmacological actions of β-CCE and other β-carbolines: M. Cain *et al., J. Med. Chem.* **25**, 1081 (1982). Anxiogenic and convulsant properties: L. Prado de Carvalho *et al., Nature* **301**, 64 (1983).

mp 229-233°. uv max (pH 7): 215, 242, 279 nm.

3-Hydroxymethyl-β-carboline. [65474-79-5] 9*H*-Pyrido[3,4-*b*]indole-3-methanol; 3-HMC. $C_{12}H_{10}N_2O$; mol wt 198.22. Prepn: F. Hamaguchi, S. Ohki, *Heterocycles* **8**, 383 (1977); M. Cain *et al., loc. cit.* Antagonism of anticonvulsant and anxiolytic actions of diazepam: P. Skolnick *et al., Eur. J. Pharmacol.* **68**, 381 (1980). Crystals, mp 225-228°.

USE: As tools for studying benzodiazepine receptors.

3780. Ethyl Carbonate. [105-58-8] Carbonic acid diethyl ester; diethyl carbonate; Eufin. $C_5H_{10}O_3$; mol wt 118.13. C 50.84%, H 8.53%, O 40.63%. $(C_2H_5O)_2C$=O. Prepn: Palomaa *et al., Ber.* **72**, 319 (1939). Manuf: Mador, Blackham, **US 3114762** (1963 to Natl. Distillers & Chem.).

Liquid, bp 126°. Pleasant ethereal odor, mp −43°. Flash pt, closed cup: 77°F (25°C). d_4^{20} 0.9764. n_D^{20} 1.3843. Practically insol in water; miscible with alcohol, ether.

USE: Solvent for nitrocellulose; manuf radio tubes; fixing rare earths to cathode elements.

3781. Ethyl Cellulose. [9004-57-3] Cellulose ethyl ether; Ethocel. Prepd from wood pulp or chemical cotton by treatment with alkali and ethylation of the alkali cellulose with ethyl chloride. Review and bibliography: E. Ott, *Cellulose and Cellulose Derivatives* (New York, 2nd ed., 1955).

White granules. Soly is dependent upon the degree of substitution. Commercial ethyl cellulose has an ethoxy content of 43-50%. A 47% product softens at 140° and is sol in ethyl acetate, ethylene dichloride, benzene, toluene, xylene, butyl acetate, acetone, methanol, ethanol, butanol, carbon tetrachloride. To avoid brittleness, ethyl cellulose formulations usually include an antioxidant such as hydroquinone monobenzyl ether, 4-hexylpyrocatechol, or diphenylamine.

USE: In the manuf of plastics and lacquers. Pharmaceutic aid (tablet binder).

3782. Ethyl Chloride. [75-00-3] Chloroethane; monochlorethane; chlorethyl; aethylis chloridum; ether chloratus; ether hydrochloric; ether muriatic; Kelene; Chelen; Anodynon; Chloryl Anesthetic; Narcotile. C_2H_5Cl; mol wt 64.51. C 37.24%, H 7.81%, Cl 54.96%. Prepd by the action of chlorine on ethylene in the presence of HCl and light: **US 2393509** (1946); by the action of chlorine on

ethylene in the presence of the chlorides of copper, iron, antimony, and calcium: **DE 298931**; Bähr, Zieber, *Angew. Chem.* **1930**, 233, 286; by heating alcohol, HCl and ZnCl₂: **US 2396639** (1946). Review of mfg processes: *Faith, Keyes & Clark's Industrial Chemicals*, F. A. Lowenheim, M. K. Moran, Eds. (Wiley-Interscience, New York, 4th ed., 1975) pp 371-375; of toxicology and human exposure: *Toxicological Profile for Chloroethane* (PB99-121956, 1998) 186 pp.

Flammable gas at ordinary temp and pressure. Characteristic ethereal odor; burning taste. At low temps or under increased pressure, ethyl chloride is a mobile, very volatile liquid. Keep away from heat, sparks, and open flame. Keep container closed, out of sun, and away from heat. Use with adequate ventilation. Carbon dioxide is recommended for extinguishing ethyl chloride fires. d_4^0 0.9214. Vapor density: 2.22 (air = 1.00). mp −138.7°. bp_{760} 12.3°. When ethyl chloride is liberated at ordinary room temp from its sealed container (usually a tube with automatic closure) it vaporizes at once. $bp_{2\ atm}$ 32.5°; $bp_{10\ atm}$ 92.6°; $bp_{30\ atm}$ 149.5°; $bp_{50\ atm}$ 180.5°. Crit temp = 187.2°; crit press = 52.0 atm. Soly in water: 0.574 g/100 ml at 20°; in alcohol: 48.3 grams/100 ml. Miscible with ether. Ethyl chloride burns with a smoky, greenish flame, producing hydrogen chloride. Flash pt: −50°C (−58°F) (closed cup); −43°C (−45°F) (open cup). Explosive limits (% by vol in air): lower 3.6; upper 14.8.

Caution: Potential symptoms of overexposure are incoordination, inebriation; abdominal cramps; cardiac arrhythmias, cardiac arrest; liver and kidney damage. *See NIOSH Pocket Guide to Chemical Hazards* (DHHS/NIOSH 97-140, 1997) p 134.

USE: Refrigerant, solvent, alkylating agent, starting point in the manuf of tetraethyl lead: **US 1907701** (1933).

THERAP CAT: Anesthetic (topical).

THERAP CAT (VET): Anesthetic (topical).

3783. Ethyl Chloroacetate. [105-39-5] Chloroacetic acid ethyl ester. $C_4H_7ClO_2$; mol wt 122.55. C 39.20%, H 5.76%, Cl 28.93%, O 26.11%. $CH_2ClCOOC_2H_5$. Prepn: Vogel, *J. Chem. Soc.* **1948**, 644.

Liquid; pungent odor. *Vapors irritate the eyes.* d_4^{20} 1.1498. mp −26°. bp 144-146°. Flash pt 54°C. n_D^{20} 1.4227. Insol in water; miscible with alcohol, ether.

3784. Ethyl Chloroformate. [541-41-3] Carbonochloridic acid ethyl ester; chloroformic acid ethyl ester; ethyl chlorocarbonate. $C_3H_5ClO_2$; mol wt 108.52. C 33.20%, H 4.64%, Cl 32.67%, O 29.49%. $ClCOOC_2H_5$. Prepn from phosgene and alc: Dumas, *Ann.* **10**, 277 (1834).

Corrosive, flammable liquid. Flash pt slightly below 61°F. bp 95°. d_4^{20} 1.1403. n_D^{20} 1.3947. Practically insol and gradually decomp by water; miscible with alcohol, benzene, chloroform, ether.

Caution: Vapors strongly irritate eyes, mucous membranes, and skin.

3785. Ethyl α-Chloropropionate. [535-13-7] 2-Chloropropanoic acid ethyl ester. $C_5H_9ClO_2$; mol wt 136.58. C 43.97%, H 6.64%, Cl 25.96%, O 23.43%. $CH_3CHClCOOC_2H_5$.

Liq; pleasant odor. d_4^{20} 1.087. bp 147-148°. n_D^{20} 1.4185. Insol in water; miscible with alcohol, ether.

3786. Ethyl Cyanoacetate. [105-56-6] Cyanoacetic acid ethyl ester; cyanoacetic ester; ethyl cyanoethanoate; malonic acid ethyl ester nitrile. $C_5H_7NO_2$; mol wt 113.11. C 53.09%, H 6.24%, N 12.38%, O 28.29%. $CNCH_2COOC_2H_5$. Made by the interaction of sodium cyanide and chloroacetic acid and subsequent esterification of the cyanoacetic acid formed: Kohler, Allen, *Org. Synth.* **3**, 53 (1923); Inglis, *ibid.* **8**, 74 (1928).

Liquid. Slight, pleasant odor. d_4^{25} 1.0560; d_4^{50} 1.0306; d_4^{70} 1.0110. mp −22°. bp_{760} 206.0°; bp_{100} 152.8°; bp_{40} 133.8°; bp_{20} 119.8°; bp_{10} 106.0°; bp_5 93.5°; $bp_{1.0}$ 67.8°. $n_D^{20.5}$ 1.41793. Insol in water. Miscible with alcohol, ether; sol in ammonia water, aq solns of alkalies.

3787. Ethyl Cyanoacrylate. [7085-85-0] 2-Cyano-2-propenoic acid ethyl ester; ECA; ethyl α-cyanoacrylate; ethyl 2-cyanoacrylate; Krazy Glue. $C_6H_7NO_2$; mol wt 125.13. C 57.59%, H 5.64%, N 11.19%, O 25.57%. Main constituent of **super glue**; polymerizes rapidly in various media including water. Preparative methods: A. E. Ardis, **US 2467927** (1949 to B. F. Goodrich); C. H.

McKeever, **US 2912454** (1959 to Rohm & Haas). Prepn, polymerization and degradation: F. Leonard *et al., J. Appl. Polym. Sci.* **10**, 259 (1966). Bioadhesive and histotoxic properties: B. J. Zumpano *et al., Surg. Neurol.* **18**, 452 (1982). Prepn and drug delivery applications of polymer nanoparticles: G. Cavallaro *et al., Int. J. Pharm.* **111**, 31 (1994). *In vitro* and *in vivo* studies in sclerotherapy: J.-C. Lin *et al., J. Biomed. Mater. Res.* **53**, 799 (2000). Review of chemistry and toxicology: R. Cary, *Concise Int. Chem. Assess. Doc. No. 36* (WHO, Geneva, 2001) 33 pp.

Clear, colorless liquid; strong, acrid odor; bp 54-56° (0.21-0.40 kPa); mp −20 to −25°. d^{20} 1.040. n_D^{20} 1.4391. Surface tension: 34.32 dynes/cm. Vapor pressure at 25°: <0.27 kPa. Sol in methyl ethyl ketone, toluene, acetone, DMF, nitromethane.

Polymer. [25067-30-5] Poly(ethyl 2-cyanoacrylate); PECA.

USE: In adhesives; in mfr of plastics, electronics, scientific instruments, jewelry, sports equip; in cable joining, manicuring, dentistry, mortuaries, fingerprint development. Polymer nanoparticles as pharmaceutic aid for controlled release drug delivery.

3788. Ethyl Dibunate. [5560-69-0] 3,6-Bis(1,1-dimethylethyl)-1-naphthalenesulfonic acid ethyl ester; 3,6-di-*tert*-butyl-1-naphthalenesulfonic acid ethyl ester; ethyl 3,6-di-*tert*-butyl-1-naphthalenesulfonate; 2,7-di-*tert*-butylnaphthalene-4-sulfonic acid ethyl ester; ethyl 2,7-di-*tert*-butylnaphthalene-4-sulfonate; dibunate ethyl; NDR-304; Neodyne. $C_{20}H_{28}O_3S$; mol wt 348.50. C 68.93%, H 8.10%, O 13.77%, S 9.20%. Prepn: Menard *et al., Can. J. Chem.* **39**, 729 (1961). Pharmacology: Shemano, *Arch. Int. Pharmacodyn. Ther.* **165**, 410 (1967). Clinical trial in chronic cough: H. Sevelius, J. P. Colmore, *Clin. Pharmacol. Ther.* **8**, 381 (1967).

Crystals from ethanol, mp 138-139°.
THERAP CAT: Antitussive.

3789. Ethyl Diethylmalonate. [77-25-8] Diethylpropanedioic acid diethyl ester. $C_{11}H_{20}O_4$; mol wt 216.27. C 61.09%, H 9.32%, O 29.59%. $C_2H_5COOC(C_2H_5)_2COOC_2H_5$. Produced by the action of sodium ethylate and ethylbromide on diethyl malonate.

Liquid. d 0.985-0.990. bp 228-230°. n_D^{20} 1.424. Insol in water; miscible with alcohol, ether.

USE: Manuf barbiturates.

3790. Ethyldimethyl-9-octadecenylammonium Bromide. [6458-13-5] *N*-Ethyl-*N,N*-dimethyl-9-octadecen-1-aminium bromide; Onyxide. $C_{22}H_{46}BrN$; mol wt 404.51. C 65.32%, H 11.46%, Br 19.75%, N 3.46%. Prepn: Du Bois, **US 2519747** (1950 to Onyx Oil & Chem.).

USE: A cationic surface active agent. Used in the control of algae. Sold as a 75% concentrate in isopropanol or propylene glycol.

3791. Ethylene. [74-85-1] Ethene; elayl; olefiant gas. C_2H_4; mol wt 28.05. C 85.64%, H 14.37%. $CH_2{=}CH_2$. Plant hormone; occurs in ripening fruit, in illuminating gas (up to 4%). Prepd by decompn of petr gases or by dehydration of alcohol. Lab prepn from alc: Gattermann-Wieland, *Praxis des Organischen Chemikers* (de Gruyter, Berlin, 40th ed, 1961) p 98; F. A. Wunder,

E. I. Leupold, *Angew. Chem. Int. Ed.* **19**, 126 (1980). Biosynthesis from 1-aminocyclopropane-1-carboxylic acid: D. Adams, S. F. Yang, *Proc. Natl. Acad. Sci. USA* **76**, 170 (1979). Proposed mechanism of biosynthesis: M. C. Pirrung, *J. Am. Chem. Soc.* **105**, 7207 (1983). Toxicity data: Flury, *Arch. Exp. Pathol. Pharmakol.* **138**, 65 (1928). Comprehensive monograph: S. A. Miller, *Ethylene and its Industrial Derivatives* (Ernest Benn Ltd., London, 1969) 1321 pp. Review of ethylene in biological systems: Spencer, *Fortschr. Chem. Org. Naturst.* **27**, 31-80 (1969); of manuf: *Faith, Keyes & Clark's Industrial Chemicals,* F. A. Lowenheim, M. K. Moran, Eds. (Wiley-Interscience, New York, 4th ed., 1975) pp 376-384; of carcinogenic risk: *IARC Monographs* **60**, 45-71 (1994). *Review:* K. M. Sundaram *et al.,* in *Kirk-Othmer Encyclopedia of Chemical Technology* **vol. 9** (Wiley-Interscience, New York, 4th ed., 1994) pp 877-915.

Colorless, flammable gas with faint sweet odor. Burns with a luminous flame. Solidif −181° forming monoclinic prisms. mp −169.4°, bp_{700} −102.4°. Vapor density 0.978 (air = 1.00). One liter of ethylene gas at 760 mm and 0° weighs 1.260 g. $bp_{2\,atm}$ −90.8°; $bp_{10\,atm}$ −52.8°; $bp_{30\,atm}$ −14.2°; $bp_{50\,atm}$ 8.9°. $d_4^{6.5}$ (liquid): 0.30342. Critical temp +9.6°; crit press. 50.7 atm. One volume of ethylene gas dissolves in about 4 vols of water at 0°, in about 9 vols of water at 25°, in 0.5 vol alcohol at 25°, in about 0.05 vol ether at 15.5°. Sol in acetone, benzene. Explosive limits (% vol in air), lower: 3.02; upper: 34. Autoignition temp: 1009°F (+543°C). LC for mice in air: 950,000 ppm (Flury).

Caution: Can act as a simple asphyxiant due to oxygen displacement. Exposure to high concns may cause CNS depression, unconsciousness. *See Patty's Industrial Hygiene and Toxicology* **vol. 2B,** G. D. Clayton, F. E. Clayton, Eds. (John Wiley & Sons, New York, 4th ed., 1994) p 1241-1244.

USE: Oxyethylene welding and cutting metals; manuf alcohol, mustard gas, and many other organics. Manuf ethylene oxide (for plastics), "Polythene", polystyrene and other plastics. Plant growth regulator; used commercially to accelerate the ripening of various fruits.

THERAP CAT: Anesthetic (inhalation).

THERAP CAT (VET): Has been used as inhalation anesthetic.

3792. Ethylene Bromohydrin. [540-51-2] 2-Bromoethanol; β-bromoethyl alcohol; glycol bromohydrin. C_2H_5BrO; mol wt 124.96. C 19.22%, H 4.03%, Br 63.94%, O 12.80%. $BrCH_2CH_2OH$. Prepd by the action of hydrobromic acid on ethylene oxide: Thayer *et al., Org. Synth.* **6**, 12 (1926).

Hygroscopic liq. d_4^0 1.7902; d_4^{15} 1.7696; d_4^{20} 1.7629; d_4^{25} 1.7560; d_4^{30} 1.7494. bp_{750} 149-150° (decompn); bp_{20} 56-57°; bp_{13} 48.5°. n_D^{20} 1.49361. Miscible with water; sol in the usual organic solvents, except petr ether. Hydrolysis of aq solns is accelerated by heat, acids, alkalies. Aq solns have a sweet, burning taste.

Caution: Ethylene bromohydrin vapors are an irritant to the eyes and the mucosa.

3793. Ethylene Chlorohydrin. [107-07-3] 2-Chloroethanol; 2-chloroethyl alcohol; glycol chlorohydrin. C_2H_5ClO; mol wt 80.51. C 29.84%, H 6.26%, Cl 44.04%, O 19.87%. $ClCH_2{-}CH_2OH$. Made from ethylene by action of a hypochlorite. Toxicity data: H. F. Smyth *et al., J. Ind. Hyg. Toxicol.* **23**, 259 (1941). *Review:* G. H. Riesser in *Kirk-Othmer Encyclopedia of Chemical Technology* **vol. 5** (Wiley-Interscience, New York, 3rd ed., 1979) pp 848-864.

Colorless liq. *Poisonous!* d_4^{20} 1.197. bp 128-130°. mp −67°. n_D^{20} 1.4419. Flash pt, open cup: 105°F (40°C). Miscible with water, alcohol. LD_{50} orally in rats: 0.095 g/kg (Smyth).

Caution: Potential symptoms of overexposure are irritation of mucous membranes; nausea, vomiting; vertigo, incoordination; numbness; visual disturbance; headache; thirst; delirium; low blood pressure; collapse, shock and coma; liver and kidney damage. *See NIOSH Pocket Guide to Chemical Hazards* (DHHS/NIOSH 97-140, 1997) p 134. *See also Patty's Industrial Hygiene and Toxicology* **vol. 2C,** G. D. Clayton, F. E. Clayton, Eds. (Wiley-Interscience, New York, 4th ed., 1982) pp 4675-4684.

USE: Solvent; manuf insecticides; treating sweet potatoes before planting.

3794. Ethylene Cyanohydrin. [109-78-4] 3-Hydroxypropanenitrile; hydracrylonitrile; glycol cyanohydrin; β-hydroxypropionitrile. C_3H_5NO; mol wt 71.08. C 50.69%, H 7.09%, N 19.71%, O 22.51%. $HOCH_2CH_2CN$. Prepd by the interaction of ethylene chlorohydrin and alkali cyanide: E. C. Kendall, B. McKenzie, *Org. Synth.* **coll. vol. I,** 256 (2nd ed., 1941). Toxicity study: H. F. Smyth, C. P. Carpenter, *J. Ind. Hyg. Toxicol.* **26,** 269 (1944).

Liquid. d_4^{25} 1.0404. mp $-46°$. bp_{760} 228° (slight dec); bp_{200} 178°; bp_{100} 157.7°; bp_{60} 144.7°; bp_{40} 134.1°; bp_{20} 117.9°; bp_{10} 102°; bp_5 87.8°; $bp_{1.0}$ 58.7°. n_D^{25} 1.4241. Miscible with water, acetone, methyl ethyl ketone, ethyl alcohol. Slightly sol in ether (2.3% w/w at 15°). Insol in benzene, petr ether, carbon disulfide, carbon tetrachloride. LD_{50} orally in rats: 10.0 g/kg (Smyth, Carpenter).

USE: Solvent for some cellulose esters and many inorganic salts.

3795. Ethylenediamine. [107-15-3] 1,2-Ethanediamine; 1,2-diaminoethane. $C_2H_8N_2$; mol wt 60.10. C 39.97%, H 13.42%, N 46.61%. $H_2NCH_2CH_2NH_2$. Manuf from ethylene dichloride and ammonia: *Faith, Keyes & Clark's Industrial Chemicals,* F. A. Lowenheim, M. K. Moran, Eds. (Wiley-Interscience, New York, 4th ed., 1975) pp 385-388. Toxicity: H. F. Smyth *et al., J. Ind. Hyg. Toxicol.* **23,** 259 (1941).

Colorless, clear, thick liq; ammonia odor. d_4^{25} 0.898. bp 116-117°. mp 8.5°. n_D^{26} 1.4540. Flash pt, closed cup: 110°F (43°C). Volatile with steam. Freely sol in water forming a hydrate, also in alcohol; slightly sol in ether; sol in benzene unless insufficiently dried: S. G. Boas-Traube *et al., Nature* **162,** 960 (1948). *Note:* Strongly alkaline and may readily absorb CO_2 from air to form a nonvolatile carbonate. Protect against undue exposure to the atmosphere. LD_{50} orally in rats: 1.16 g/kg (Smyth).

Monohydrate. mp 10°; bp 118°.

Dihydrochloride. $C_2H_8N_2.2HCl$. Crystals. Sublimes without melting. Freely sol in water. Practically insol in alcohol. Aq soln is practically neutral.

Caution: Potential symptoms of overexposure to ethylenediamine are irritation of nose, respiratory system; sensitization dermatitis; asthma; liver and kidney damage. *See NIOSH Pocket Guide to Chemical Hazards* (DHHS/NIOSH 97-140, 1997) p 136.

USE: Solvent for casein, albumin, shellac, and sulfur; emulsifier; stabilizing rubber latex; as inhibitor in antifreeze solns; in textile lubricants. Pharmaceutic aid (aminophylline injection stabilizer).

THERAP CAT (VET): Dihydrochloride has been used as a urinary acidifier.

3796. Ethylene Dibromide. [106-93-4] 1,2-Dibromoethane; *sym*-dibromoethane; ethylene bromide; EDB; Dowfume W 85. $C_2H_4Br_2$; mol wt 187.86. C 12.79%, H 2.15%, Br 85.07%. $BrCH_2CH_2Br$. Made from ethylene and bromine; also from acetylene and HBr. Manuf: *Faith, Keyes & Clark's Industrial Chemicals,* F. A. Lowenheim, M. K. Moran, Eds. (Wiley-Interscience, New York, 4th ed., 1975) pp 389-391. Toxicity data: G. W. Fischer *et al., J. Prakt. Chem.* **320,** 133 (1978). Carcinogenicity studies: W. A. Olson *et al., J. Natl. Cancer Inst.* **51,** 1993 (1973); *Clin. Toxicol.* **14,** 473 (1979). History of controversial use as a fumigant: J. Walsh, *Science* **215,** 1592 (1982). Review of toxicology and human exposure: *Toxicological Profile for 1,2-Dibromoethane* (PB93-110740, 1992) 173 pp.

Heavy liquid; chloroform odor. d_{25}^{25} 2.172. bp 131-132°. mp 9°. n_D^{20} 1.5379. Vapor pressure at 25°: 11 mm Hg. Sol in about 250 parts water; misc with alcohol, ether. *Protect from light.* LD_{50} i.p. in mice: 220 mg/kg (Fischer).

Caution: Potential symptoms of overexposure are irritation of skin, respiratory system and eyes; dermatitis with vesiculation; liver, heart, spleen, kidney damage; reproductive effects. *See NIOSH Pocket Guide to Chemical Hazards* (DHHS/NIOSH 97-140, 1997) p 136. *See also Patty's Industrial Hygiene and Toxicology* **vol. 2B,** G. D. Clayton, F. E. Clayton, Eds. (Wiley-Interscience, New York, 3rd ed., 1981) p 3497-3502. This substance is reasonably anticipated to be a human carcinogen: *Report on Carcinogens, Eleventh Edition* (PB2005-104914, 2004) p III-82.

USE: Soil and grain fumigant; as lead scavenger in anti-knock gasolines.

3797. Ethylene Dichloride. [107-06-2] 1,2-Dichloroethane; *sym*-dichloroethane; ethylene chloride; EDC; Dutch liquid; Brocide. $C_2H_4Cl_2$; mol wt 98.96. C 24.27%, H 4.07%, Cl 71.65%. $ClCH_2CH_2Cl$. Made from ethylene and chlorine; also from ace-

tylene and HCl: *Beilstein* **I,** 84 (1918). Manuf: *Faith, Keyes & Clark's Industrial Chemicals,* F. A. Lowenheim, M. K. Moran, Eds. (Wiley-Interscience, New York, 4th ed., 1975) pp 392-396. Toxicity data: Smyth *et al., Am. Ind. Hyg. Assoc. J.* **30,** 470 (1969). Review of carcinogenic risk: *IARC Monographs* **20,** 429-444 (1979); of toxicology and human exposure: *Toxicological Profile for 1,2-Dichloroethane* (PB2001-109103, 2001) 297 pp.

Heavy liq; burns with smoky flame; pleasant odor; sweet taste. d_4^{20} 1.2569. bp 83-84°. mp $\sim -40°$. Flash pt, closed cup: 56°F (13°C); open cup: 65°F (18°C). n_D^{20} 1.4443. Sol in about 120 parts water; misc with alcohol, chloroform, ether. LD_{50} orally in rats: 770 mg/kg (Smyth).

Caution: Potential symptoms of overexposure are CNS depression; nausea, vomiting; dermatitis; irritation of eyes, corneal opacity; liver, kidney, cardiovascular system damage. *See NIOSH Pocket Guide to Chemical Hazards* (DHHS/NIOSH 97-140, 1997) p 136. *See also Clinical Toxicology of Commercial Products,* R. E. Gosselin *et al.,* Eds. (Williams & Wilkins, Baltimore, 5th ed., 1984) Section II, pp 163-164. This substance is reasonably anticipated to be a human carcinogen: *Report on Carcinogens, Eleventh Edition* (PB2005-104914, 2004) p III-90.

USE: Manuf of vinyl chloride, acetyl cellulose; solvent for fats, oils, waxes, gums, resins, and particularly for rubber. Has been used as insect and soil fumigant.

3798. Ethylene Glycol. [107-21-1] 1,2-Ethanediol. $C_2H_6-O_2$; mol wt 62.07. C 38.70%, H 9.74%, O 51.55%. $HOCH_2CH_2-OH$. Prepd on a large scale by the hydration of ethylene oxide. Flowsheets: *Ullmanns Encyklopädie der technischen Chemie* **vol. 3** (3rd ed., 1953) p 137; M. Sittig, *Organic Chemical Process Encyclopedia* (Noyes Dev. Corp., Park Ridge, N.J., 1967) p 265. Manuf from ethylene and oxygen: *Faith, Keyes & Clark's Industrial Chemicals,* F. A. Lowenheim, M. K. Moran, Eds. (Wiley-Interscience, New York, 4th ed., 1975) pp 397-402. Toxicity studies: Smyth *et al., J. Ind. Hyg. Toxicol.* **23,** 259 (1941); Bornmann, *Arzneim.-Forsch.* **4,** 643 (1954). Monograph: G. O. Curme, F. Johnston, *Glycols* (Reinhold, New York, 1952). GC/MS determn in plasma: C. Giachetti *et al., Biomed. Environ. Mass Spectrom.* **18,** 592 (1989). Review of toxicology and human exposure: *Toxicological Profile for Ethylene Glycol and Propylene Glycol* (PB98-101108, 1997) 250 pp.

Slightly viscous liq. Sweet taste. *Poisonous! Do not swallow!* Considerably hygroscopic: Absorbs twice its weight of water at 100% relative humidity. d_4^0 1.1274. d_4^{10} 1.1204. d_4^{20} 1.1135. d_4^{30} 1.1065. One gallon weighs 9.3 lbs. Flash pt, open cup: 240°F (115°C). mp $-13°$. bp_{760} 197.6°; bp_{97} 140°; bp_{18} 100°; $bp_{3.0}$ 70°; $bp_{0.06}$ 20°. n_D^{15} 1.43312; n_D^{25} 1.43063. Viscosity (cP): 26 (15°); 21 (20°); 17.3 (25°). Dielectric constant at 20° and 150 meters wavelength: 38.66 esu. Dipole moment 2.20. Spec heat (20°): 0.561 cal/g/°C. Heat of formation -108.1 kcal/mol. Heat of fusion 44.7 cal/g. Heat of vaporization 191 cal/g. Heat of soln -6.5 cal/g of soln at 17° when 37 parts are mixed with 63 parts H_2O (w/w). Parachor 148.9 (theory 152.2). Surface tension at 20° = 48.4 dynes/cm. Miscible with water, lower aliphatic alcohols, glycerol, acetic acid, acetone and similar ketones, aldehydes, pyridine and similar coal tar bases. Slightly sol in ether (1:200). Practically insol in benzene and its homologs, chlorinated hydrocarbons, petr ether, oils. Density and freezing point of ethylene glycol-water mixtures: 10.15% ethylene glycol by wt d_{20}^{20} 1.013, fp $-3.5°$; 20.44% ethylene glycol d_{20}^{20} 1.027, fp $-8°$; 29.88% ethylene glycol d_{20}^{20} 1.040, fp $-15°$; 40.23% ethylene glycol d_{20}^{20} 1.054, fp $-24°$; 50.18% ethylene glycol d_{20}^{20} 1.067, fp $-36°$; 58.37% ethylene glycol d_{20}^{20} 1.0770, fp $-48°$. LD_{50} in rats, guinea pigs (g/kg): 8.54, 6.61 orally (Smyth); in mice (ml/kg): 13.79 orally (Bornmann).

Caution: Potential symptoms of overexposure by ingestion are nausea, vomiting, abdominal pain, weakness; dizziness, stupor, convulsions, CNS depression. Direct contact may cause irritation of eyes, nose, skin; skin sensitization. *See NIOSH Pocket Guide to Chemical Hazards* (DHHS/NIOSH 97-140, 1997) p 136. *See also Patty's Industrial Hygiene and Toxicology* **vol. 2F,** G. D. Clayton, F. E. Clayton, Eds. (Wiley-Interscience, New York, 4th ed., 1994) pp 4645-4657.

USE: Antifreeze in cooling and heating systems. In hydraulic brake fluids and de-icing solutions. Industrial humectant. Ingredient of electrolytic condensers (where it serves as solvent for boric acid and borates). Solvent in the paint and plastics industries. In the formulation of printers' inks, stamp pad inks, ball-point pen ink. Softening agent for cellophane. Stabilizer for soybean foam used to extinguish oil and gasoline fires. In the synthesis of safety explosives, glyoxal, unsatd ester type alkyd resins, plasticizers, elastomers, synthetic fibers (Terylene, Dacron), and synthetic waxes. To create artificial smoke and mist for theatrical uses.

3799. Ethylene Glycol Diacetate. [111-55-7] 1,2-Ethanediol diacetate; glycol diacetate; ethylene diacetate. $C_6H_{10}O_4$; mol wt 146.14. C 49.31%, H 6.90%, O 43.79%. $CH_3COOCH_2CH_2$-OOCCH$_3$. Prepn from glacial acetic acid and potassium acetate: Henry, *Bull. Soc. Chim.* [3] **17**, 207 (1897); Gattermann-Wieland, *Praxis des Organischen Chemikers* (de Gruyter, Berlin, 40th ed., 1961) p 107; from synthesis gas via homogeneous ruthenium catalysis: J. F. Knifton, *Chem. Commun.* **1981**, 188. Toxicity study: Smyth *et al., J. Ind. Hyg. Toxicol.* **23**, 259 (1941).

Liquid. d 1.104. bp 190-191°. mp −31°. n_D^{20} 1.415. Flash pt, open cup: 205°F (96°C). Sol in 7 parts water; miscible with alc, ether. LD_{50} orally in rats: 6.86 g/kg (Smyth).

USE: Solvent for oils, cellulose esters, explosives, etc.

3800. Ethylene Glycol Dinitrate. [628-96-6] 1,2-Ethanediol dinitrate; glycol dinitrate; nitroglycol; EGDN. $C_2H_4N_2O_6$; mol wt 152.06. C 15.80%, H 2.65%, N 18.42%, O 63.13%. O_2-NOCH$_2$CH$_2$ONO$_2$. Explosive. Prepn: L. Henry, *Ann. Chim. (Paris)* **4**, 253 (1872); P. Golding *et al., Tetrahedron* **49**, 7037 (1993). Determn in blood by GC: M. H. Litchfield, *Analyst* **93**, 653 (1968); in explosion debris by HPLC: R. J. Prime, J. Krebs, *Can. Soc. Forensic Sci. J.* **13**, 27 (1980); in vapor phase by ion mobility spectrometry: A. H. Lawrence, P. Neudorfl, *Anal. Chem.* **60**, 104 (1988). Measurement of vapor pressure: P. A. Pella, *J. Chem. Thermodyn.* **9**, 301 (1977). Adsorption kinetics: D. O. Henderson *et al., Appl. Spectrosc.* **47**, 528 (1993). Brief description of properties: *Am. Ind. Hyg. Assoc. J.* **27**, 574-577 (1966); V. Lindner in *Kirk-Othmer Encyclopedia of Chemical Technology* vol. **10**, (John Wiley & Sons, New York, 4th ed., 1993) pp 4, 21-26.

Colorless, odorless liquid with sweetish taste, mp −22.8°. d 1.490 g/cm³. n_D^{20} 1.395. Insol in water, very sol in alcohol and ether. *Combustible and Explosive!*

Caution: Potential symptoms of overexposure are throbbing headache; dizziness; nausea; vomiting; abdominal pain; hypotension; flushing; palpitations; methemoglobinemia; delirium; CNS depression. Direct contact may cause skin irritation. *See NIOSH Pocket Guide to Chemical Hazards* (DHHS/NIOSH 97-140, 1997) p 138.

USE: Explosive for mining and fuel industries. Additive to dynamite. Detection of hidden bombs by analysis of ambient air for EGDN.

3801. Ethylene Glycol Monoacetate. [542-59-6] 1,2-Ethanediol monoacetate; glycol-monoacetin. $C_4H_8O_3$; mol wt 104.10. C 46.15%, H 7.75%, O 46.11%. $CH_3COOCH_2CH_2OH$.

Liquid. d 1.108. bp 182°. Miscible with water, alcohol. LD_{50} orally in rats: 8.25 g/kg, Smyth *et al., J. Ind. Hyg. Toxicol.* **23**, 259 (1941).

3802. Ethylene Oxide. [75-21-8] Oxirane; Anprolene. C_2H_4O; mol wt 44.05. C 54.53%, H 9.15%, O 36.32%. Prepd from ethylene chlorohydrin and KOH: A. Wurtz, *Ann.* **110**, 125 (1859). Manuf by catalytic oxidation of ethylene: T. E. Lefort, *US 1998878* (1935 to Société Française de Catalyse Généralisée) reissued as *US RE 20370* (1937 to Carbide and Carbon). Physical props: W. H. Perkin, *J. Chem. Soc.* **63**, 488 (1893). Leukemia in workers exposed to ethylene oxide: C. Hogstedt *et al., J. Am. Med. Assoc.* **241**, 1132 (1979). Hazards and handling: L. G. Hess, V. V. Tilton, *Ind. Eng. Chem.* **42**, 1251 (1950). Genotoxicity: E. Agurell *et al., Mutat. Res.* **250**, 229 (1991). Review of toxicology and human exposure: *Toxicological Profile for Ethylene Oxide* (PB91-180554, 1990) 115 pp; of carcinogenic risk: *IARC Monographs* **60**, 73-159 (1994). *Review:* H. C. Schultze in *Glycols,* G. O. Curme, Jr., Ed. (Reinhold, New York, 1952) pp 74-113; J. P. Dever *et al.,* in *Kirk-Othmer Encyclopedia of Chemical Technology* vol. **9** (John Wiley & Sons, New York, 4th ed., 1994) pp 915-959.

Colorless, flammable gas at ordinary room temp and pressure; liquid below 12°. *Explosive!* bp 10.7°. d_4^4 0.891, d_7^7 0.887, d_{10}^{10} 0.882. mp −111°. n_D^7 1.3597. Sol in water, alcohol, ether.

Caution: Potential symptoms of overexposure are irritation of eyes, skin, nose and throat; peculiar taste; headache; nausea, vomiting and diarrhea; dyspnea, cyanosis and pulmonary edema; drowsiness, incoordination; EKG abnormalities; reproductive effects; direct contact with liquid or high vapor concentrations may cause burns to eyes and skin; direct contact with liquid may cause frostbite. *See NIOSH Pocket Guide to Chemical Hazards* (DHHS/NIOSH 97-140, 1997) p 138. This substance is listed as a known human carcinogen: *Report on Carcinogens, Eleventh Edition* (PB2005-104914, 2004) p III-118.

USE: Fumigant for foodstuffs and textiles; to sterilize surgical instruments; agricultural fungicide. In organic syntheses, esp in the production of ethylene glycol. Starting material for the manuf of acrylonitrile and nonionic surfactants.

3803. Ethylene Thiourea. [96-45-7] 2-Imidazolidinethione; imidazoline-2-thiol; 2-mercaptoimidazoline; ETU; Akrochem ETU-22; NA-22; Robac 22; Sanceller 22; Vulkacit NPV/C. $C_3H_6N_2S$; mol wt 102.16. C 35.27%, H 5.92%, N 27.42%, S 31.39%. Degradation product of ethylenebisdithiocarbamate fungicides such as mancozeb, maneb, zineb, *q.q.v.* Prepn: C. F. H. Allen *et al., Org. Synth.* **coll. vol. III**, 394 (1955); G. Matolcsy, *Ber.* **101**, 522 (1968). Identification as decomposition product: R A. Ludwig *et al., Can. J. Bot.* **32**, 48 (1954); G. Czegledi-Janko, *J. Chromatogr.* **31**, 89 (1967). Determn in various foods by GLC: W. H. Newsome, *J. Agric. Food Chem.* **20**, 967 (1972); by GLC, HPLC: J. H. Onley *et al., J. Assoc. Off. Anal. Chem.* **60**, 1105 (1977); J. H. Onley, *ibid.* 1111. Review of determn methods: P. Bottomley *et al., Residue Rev.* **95**, 45-89 (1985). Metabolism in mice: K. Savolainen, H. Pyysalo, *J. Agric. Food Chem.* **27**, 1177 (1979); in cats and rats: F. Iverson, *Toxicol. Appl. Pharmacol.* **52**, 16 (1980). Aquatic toxicity data: C. J. Van Leeuwen, *Aquat. Toxicol.* **7**, 145 (1985). Goitrogenic activity: S. L. Graham, W. H. Hansen, *Bull. Environ. Contam. Toxicol.* **7**, 19 (1972); D. M. Smith, *Br. J. Ind. Med.* **41**, 362 (1984). Use in rubber industry as crosslinking agent: J. T. Oetzel, *Rubber World* **172**, 55 (1975); C. Hepburn, M. S. Mahdi, *Kautsch. Gummi Kunstst.* **39**, 629 (1986). Review of toxicology: L. Fishbein, *J. Toxicol. Environ. Health* **1**, 713-756 (1976); of genotoxicity studies: K. L. Dearfield, *Mutat. Res.* **317**, 111-132 (1994).

Needles, prisms from alc or amyl alc. mp 203-204°. Soly in 100 ml water: 2 g at 30°, 9 g at 60°, 44 g at 90°. Moderately sol in methanol, ethanol, ethylene glycol, and pyridine. Insol in acetone, ether, chloroform, benzene, ligroin. LD_{50} orally in rats: 1832 mg/kg (Graham, Hansen).

Caution: Potential symptom of overexposure is eye irritation. *See NIOSH Pocket Guide to Chemical Hazards* (DHHS/NIOSH 97-140, 1997) p 138. This substance is reasonably anticipated to be a human carcinogen: *Report on Carcinogens, Eleventh Edition* (PB2005-104914, 2004) p III-122.

USE: Accelerator in synthetic rubber production.

3804. Ethylenimine. [151-56-4] Aziridine; azacyclopropane; dimethylenimine. C_2H_5N; mol wt 43.07. C 55.77%, H 11.70%, N 32.52%. Prepd by treating 2-chloroethylamine hydrochloride with NaOH: Wystrach *et al., J. Am. Chem. Soc.* **77**, 5915 (1955); **78**, 1263 (1956); from β-aminoethylsulfuric acid by reaction with NaOH: Allen *et al., Org. Synth.* **coll. vol. IV**, 433 (1963). Acute toxicity: H. F. Smyth *et al., J. Ind. Hyg. Toxicol.* **23**, 259 (1941). Toxicology: Weightman, Hoyle, *J. Am. Med. Assoc.* **189**, 543 (1964). Review of carcinogenicity studies: *IARC Monographs* **9**, 37 (1975).

Liquid. Intense odor of ammonia. *Poisonous! Handle in hood only!* Strongly alkaline. Polymerizes easily. d_4^{24} 0.8321. mp $-73.96°$. bp$_{760}$ 56-57°. n_D^{25} 1.412. Vapor press. (20°) 160 mm Hg. Miscible with water. Sol in alc. Can be stored for some time over a few pellets of sodium hydroxide. LD$_{50}$ orally in rats: 15 mg/kg (Smyth).

Caution: Potential symptoms of overexposure are nausea, vomiting; headache, dizziness; pulmonary edema; liver and kidney damage; eye burns; skin sensitization; irritation of eyes, skin, nose and throat. Potential occupational carcinogen. *See NIOSH Pocket Guide to Chemical Hazards* (DHHS/NIOSH 97-140, 1997) p 138.

USE: In the manuf of triethylenemelamine.

3805. Ethylestrenol. [965-90-2] (17α)-19-Norpregn-4-en-17-ol; 17α-ethylestr-4-en-17β-ol; 17α-ethyl-17β-hydroxy-4-estrene; 17β-hydroxy-17α-ethyl-19-nor-4-androstene; Orabolin; Durabolin-O; Orgaboral; Maxibolin; Orgabolin (obsolete). C$_{20}$H$_{32}$O; mol wt 288.47. C 83.27%, H 11.18%, O 5.55%. Prepn: de Winter *et al., Chem. Ind. (London)* **1959,** 905; Szpilfogel, de Winter, US 2878267 (1959 to Organon).

Crystals, mp 76-78°. [α]$_D$ +31° (chloroform).

Note: This is a controlled substance (anabolic steroid): **21 CFR,** 1308.13, as defined in 1300.01.

THERAP CAT: Anabolic.

3806. Ethyl Ether. [60-29-7] 1,1'-Oxybisethane; ethoxyethane; ether; diethyl ether; ethyl oxide; diethyl oxide; sulfuric ether; anesthetic ether. C$_4$H$_{10}$O; mol wt 74.12. C 64.82%, H 13.60%, O 21.59%. C$_2$H$_5$OC$_2$H$_5$. Produced on a large scale by dehydration of ethanol or by hydration of ethylene, both processes being carried out in the presence of sulfuric acid. Review of mfg processes: Himmler in *Ullmanns Encyklopädie der technischen Chemie* **vol. 5** (1954) pp 777-782; D. E. Keeley in *Kirk-Othmer Encyclopedia of Chemical Technology* **vol. 9** (Wiley-Interscience, New York, 3rd ed., 1980) pp 381-393.

Mobile, very volatile, highly flammable liq. *Explosive!* Vapor heavier than air. Characteristic, sweetish, pungent odor, more agreeable than chloroform. Burning taste. Tends to form explosive peroxides under the influence of air and light, esp when evaporation to dryness is attempted. Peroxides may be removed from ether by shaking with 5% aq ferrous sulfate soln. Addition of naphthols, polyphenols, aromatic amines, and aminophenols has been proposed for the stabilization of ethyl ether. d_4^0 0.7364; d_4^{10} 0.7249; d_4^{20} 0.7134; d_4^{30} 0.7019. Vapor density 2.55 (air = 1.0). mp $-116.3°$ (stable crystals); mp $-123.3°$ (metastable crystals). bp$_{760}$ 34.6°; bp$_{400}$ 17.9°; bp$_{200}$ 2.2°; bp$_{100}$ $-11.5°$; bp$_{10}$ $-48.1°$; bp$_{1.0}$ $-74.3°$. Satd vapor press. at 0°: 184.9 mm; at 10°: 290.8 mm; at 20°: 439.8 mm; at 50°: 1276 mm; at 70°: 2304 mm. Critical temp 192.7°; crit press. 35.6 atm. Flash pt, closed cup: $-49°$F $(-45°$C). Air-ether mixtures containing more than 1.85 volume-% of ether vapor, are explosive hazards. Autoignition temp 180-190°. n_D^{15} 1.35555. Dielectric constant at 26.9° and 85.8 kilocycles = 4.197; good insulator. When shaken under absolutely dry conditions ether can generate static electricity to start a fire. Surface tension at 20°: 17.06 dynes/cm. Viscosity at 20°: 0.2448 cP. Heat of vaporization at 30°: 89.80 cal/g. Produces considerable coldness on quick evaporation. Heat of formation -907 cal/g; heat of combustion -8.807 kcal/g. Ether is slightly sol in water and water is slightly sol in ether. A satd water soln contains 8.43% (w/w) of ether at 15° and 6.05% (w/w) at 25°. Ether satd with water contains 1.2% H$_2$O at 20°. Soly in water increased by HCl. Sol in concd hydrochloric acid. May explode when brought in contact with anhydr nitric acid. Miscible with lower aliphatic alcohols, benzene, chloroform, petr ether, other fat solvents, many oils. Azeotrope with water (1.3%), bp 34.2°.

Caution: Potential symptoms of overexposure are dizziness; drowsiness; headache, excitedness and narcosis; nausea, vomiting; irritation of eyes, upper respiratory system and skin. *See NIOSH Pocket Guide to Chemical Hazards* (DHHS/NIOSH 97-140, 1997) p 140.

USE: Solvent for waxes, fats, oils, perfumes, alkaloids, gums. Excellent solvent for nitrocellulose when mixed with alc. Important reagent in organic syntheses, esp in Grignard and Wurtz type reactions. Easily removable extractant of active principles (hormones, etc.) from plant and animal tissues. In the manuf of gun powder. As primer for gasoline engines.

THERAP CAT: Anesthetic (inhalation).

THERAP CAT (VET): Anesthetic (inhalation). Has been used orally in colic, subcutaneously as a stimulant.

3807. Ethyl Formate. [109-94-4] Formic acid ethyl ester. C$_3$H$_6$O$_2$; mol wt 74.08. C 48.64%, H 8.16%, O 43.19%. HCOOC$_2$H$_5$. Toxicity data: H. F. Smyth *et al., Arch. Ind. Hyg. Occup. Med.* **10,** 61 (1954).

Mobile, flammable liq. d^{20} 0.917. bp 53-54°. mp $-80°$. Flash pt, closed cup: $-4°$F $(-20°$C). n_D^{20} 1.3597. Sol in about 10 parts water with gradual decompn into free acid and alcohol; miscible with alcohol, ether. *Keep tightly closed and preferably in contact with calcium chloride.* LD$_{50}$ orally in rats: 4.29 g/kg (Smyth).

Caution: Potential symptoms of overexposure are irritation of eyes and upper respiratory system. *See NIOSH Pocket Guide to Chemical Hazards* (DHHS/NIOSH 97-140, 1997) p 140.

USE: As flavor for lemonades and essences; for manuf artificial rum and arrac; also as a solvent for nitrocellulose; as fungicide and larvicide for tobacco, cereals, dried fruits, etc.; in organic synthesis.

3808. 2-Ethyl-1-hexanol. [104-76-7] 2-Ethylhexyl alcohol. C$_8$H$_{18}$O; mol wt 130.23. C 73.78%, H 13.93%, O 12.29%. Manuf from butyraldehyde: *Faith, Keyes & Clark's Industrial Chemicals,* F. A. Lowenheim, M. K. Moran, Eds. (Wiley-Interscience, New York, 4th ed., 1975) pp 413-417. Toxicity study: H. F. Smyth *et al., Am. Ind. Hyg. Assoc. J.* **30,** 470 (1969).

Colorless liq. d_{20}^{20} 0.8344. bp 184-185°. n_D^{20} 1.4300. Flash pt 81°C. Soluble in about 720 parts water, in many organic solvents. It dissolves about 2.5% its weight of water at 25°. LD$_{50}$ orally in rats: 12.46 ml/kg (Smyth).

USE: Mercerizing textiles; as a solvent for dyes, resins, oils; also claimed to possess antifoaming properties.

3809. Ethylhexyl Triazone. [88122-99-0] 4,4',4''-(1,3,5-Triazine-2,4,6-triyltriimino)trisbenzoic acid tris(2-ethylhexyl) ester; octyl triazone; 2,4,6-trianilino-p-(carbo-2'-ethylhexyl-1'-oxy)-1,3,5-triazine; Uvinul T 150. C$_{48}$H$_{66}$N$_6$O$_6$; mol wt 823.07. C 70.04%, H 8.08%, N 10.21%, O 11.66%. Substituted s-triazine; uv absorber in cosmetic sunscreen products. Prepn: U. Hoppe *et al., EP 87098; eidem,* US 4617390 (1983, 1986 both to BASF). HPLC determn in cosmetic products: L. Gagliardi *et al., Anal. Lett.* **23,** 2123 (1990). Photochemical study: L. Douarre *et al., J. Photochem. Photobiol. A* **96,** 71 (1996).

Crystals from gasoline, mp 128°. uv max (ethanol): 218.7, 313.3 nm ($E_{1cm}^{1\%}$ 456, 1585). Readily sol in polar cosmetic oils.

THERAP CAT: Ultraviolet screen.

3810. Ethylidene Chloride. [75-34-3] 1,1-Dichloroethane. $C_2H_4Cl_2$; mol wt 98.96. C 24.27%, H 4.07%, Cl 71.65%. CH_3-$CHCl_2$. Prepd by the action of PCl_5 on acetaldehyde. Review of toxicology and human exposure: *Toxicological Profile for 1,1-Dichloroethane* (PB91-180539, 1990) 115 pp.

Chemical intermediate. Oily liquid; odor and taste as of chloroform. d_4^{20} 1.1757; d_4^{25} 1.1680. bp 57.3°: Mumford, Phillips, *J. Chem. Soc.* **1950**, 75. mp ~ −98°. n_D^{20} 1.4167. Sol in about 200 parts water; miscible with alcohol.

Caution: Potential symptoms of overexposure are CNS depression; skin irritation; lung, liver and kidney damage. *See NIOSH Pocket Guide to Chemical Hazards* (DHHS/NIOSH 97-140, 1997) p 98.

USE: Solvent for paint, varnishes; degreaser. Has been used as a surgical anesthetic.

3811. Ethylidene Diacetate. [542-10-9] 1,1-Ethanediol diacetate; 1,1-diacetoxyethane. $C_6H_{10}O_4$; mol wt 146.14. C 49.31%, H 6.90%, O 43.79%. $(CH_3COO)_2CHCH_3$. Made by heating acetaldehyde and acetic anhydride. Control of fungal and bacterial growth in crops and animal feedstuffs: D. L. Kensler *et al.*, US 3931412 and US 4012526 (1976 and 1977 to Chevron).

Liq; sharp, fruity odor. d_4^{12} 1.061. bp 167-169°. Slightly sol in water; miscible with alcohol. With NaOH it yields acetaldehyde.

USE: Agricultural fungicide.

3812. Ethylidene Dicoumarol. [1821-16-5] 3,3′-Ethylidenebis[4-hydroxy-2*H*-1-benzopyran-2-one]; 3,3′-ethylidenebis(4-hydroxycoumarin); 3,3-ethylidenebis(4-oxycoumarin); Pertrombon. $C_{20}H_{14}O_6$; mol wt 350.32. C 68.57%, H 4.03%, O 27.40%. Prepn: Jansen, Jensen, *Z. Phys. Chem.* **277**, 66 (1943); Sullivan *et al.*, *J. Am. Chem. Soc.* **66**, 2288 (1943); Stahmann *et al.*, *ibid.* **67**, 900 (1944); AT 196874 (1958 to Spofa), *C.A.* **52**, 10212d (1958); Fucik, CS 85918 (1957), *C.A.* **52**, 2930d (1958).

Crystals from ethanol + dioxane, mp 178°.
Dibenzoate. $C_{34}H_{22}O_8$. mp 209-210°.

THERAP CAT: Anticoagulant.

3813. Ethyl Iodide. [75-03-6] Iodoethane. C_2H_5I; mol wt 155.97. C 15.40%, H 3.23%, I 81.36%. CH_3CH_2I. Made by the action of iodine on alcohol in the presence of red phosphorus. Ethyl iodide contains about 98% CH_3CH_2I and about 2% alcohol.

Heavy, clear, very refractive liquid; ethereal odor. When freshly prepared it is colorless, but soon becomes red (on exposure to light and air) due to liberation of iodine. Silver leaf prevents or greatly retards decompn. d_{20}^{20} 1.950. bp 72°. mp −108°. n_D^{15} 1.5168. Sol in 250 parts water with gradual decompn; miscible with alcohol and most organic solvents. *Keep dry and cool, tightly closed, protected from light.*

3814. Ethyl Isobutyrate. [97-62-1] 2-Methylpropanoic acid ethyl ester. $C_6H_{12}O_2$; mol wt 116.16. C 62.04%, H 10.41%, O 27.55%. $(CH_3)_2CHCOOC_2H_5$.

Liquid; aromatic, fruity odor. d_{20}^{20} 0.870. bp 110-111°. mp −88°. n_D^{20} 1.3903. Slightly sol in water; miscible with alcohol, ether.

USE: Manuf flavoring compds and essences.

3815. Ethyl Isothiocyanate. [542-85-8] Isothiocyanatoethane; ethyl mustard oil. C_3H_5NS; mol wt 87.14. C 41.35%, H 5.78%, N 16.07%, S 36.80%. C_2H_5NCS. Obtained by the action of mercuric chloride on the product of the reaction of carbon disulfide with ethylamine.

Colorless to yellowish liq; pungent odor. d_4^{18} 1.003. bp 130-132°. mp −6°. n_D^{18} 1.5142. Insol in water. Miscible with alcohol, ether.

Caution: Vapors irritate the eyes; blister the skin.

USE: Military poison gas.

3816. Ethyl Isovalerate. [108-64-5] 3-Methylbutanoic acid ethyl ester. $C_7H_{14}O_2$; mol wt 130.18. C 64.58%, H 10.84%, O 24.58%. $(CH_3)_2CHCH_2COOC_2H_5$.

Colorless, oily liq; apple odor. d_{20}^{20} 0.868. bp 135°. mp −99°. n_D^{20} 1.4009. Sol in about 350 parts water; miscible with alcohol, benzene, ether.

USE: In alc soln for flavoring confectionery and beverages.

3817. Ethyl Lactate. [97-64-3] 2-Hydroxypropanoic acid ethyl ester; ethyl α-hydroxypropionate. $C_5H_{10}O_3$; mol wt 118.13. C 50.84%, H 8.53%, O 40.63%. $CH_3CHOHCOOC_2H_5$.

Colorless liquid; characteristic odor. d_4^{14} 1.042. bp 154°. $[\alpha]_D^{14}$ −10°. Flash pt, closed cup: 117°F (47°C). Miscible with water (with partial decompn), alcohol, ether. *Keep well closed.*

USE: As solvent for nitrocellulose and cellulose acetate.

3818. Ethyl Laurate. [106-33-2] Dodecanoic acid ethyl ester. $C_{14}H_{28}O_2$; mol wt 228.37. C 73.63%, H 12.36%, O 14.01%. $CH_3(CH_2)_{10}COOC_2H_5$.

Oil. d_{19}^{19} 0.867. mp −10°. bp 269°; bp_{25} 163°. n_D 1.4321. Insol in water. Very sol in alcohol, ether.

3819. Ethyl Levulinate. [539-88-8] 4-Oxopentanoic acid ethyl ester. $C_7H_{12}O_3$; mol wt 144.17. C 58.32%, H 8.39%, O 33.29%. $CH_3COCH_2CH_2COOC_2H_5$.

Liquid. d_{20}^{20} 1.012. bp 205-206°. n_D^{20} 1.4229. Freely sol in water; miscible with alcohol.

3820. Ethyl Linoleate. [544-35-4] (Z,Z)-9,12-Octadecadienoic acid ethyl ester; mandenol. $C_{20}H_{36}O_2$; mol wt 308.50. C 77.87%, H 11.76%, O 10.37%. Prepn from sunflower seed oil: McCutcheon, *Org. Synth.* **coll. vol. III**, 526 (1955); see also Parker *et al.*, *Biochem. Prep.* **4**, 88 (1955).

Colorless oil. More stable to air oxidation than linoleic acid. $d_4^{15.5}$ 0.8846; d^{20} 0.8919. bp_6 193°; $bp_{2.5}$ 175°; $bp_{0.001}$ 133°. n_D^{20} 1.46753; n_D^{48} 1.4489. Iodine value 162.5. Miscible with dimethylformamide, fat solvents, oils.

USE: In the vitamin industry.

3821. Ethyl Loflazepate. [29177-84-2] 7-Chloro-5-(2-fluorophenyl)-2,3-dihydro-2-oxo-1*H*-1,4-benzodiazepine-3-carboxylic acid ethyl ester; ethyl 7-chloro-5-(*o*-fluorophenyl)-2,3-dihydro-2-oxo-1*H*-1,4-benzodiazepine-3-carboxylate; CM-6912; Meilax; Victan. $C_{18}H_{14}ClFN_2O_3$; mol wt 360.77. C 59.93%, H 3.91%, Cl 9.83%, F 5.27%, N 7.76%, O 13.30%. Benzodiazepine tranquilizer. Prepn: J. Hellerbach *et al.*, DE 2001276; *eidem*, US 3657223 (1970, 1972 both to Hoffmann-La Roche). Analysis in plasma and urine: W. Cantreels, J. R. Jeanniot, *Biomed. Mass Spectrom.* **7**, 565 (1980). GC analysis of metabolites: J. P. Cano, *J. Chromatogr.* **226**, 413 (1981). Toxicologic evaluation: G. Mozue *et al.*, *Int. J. Clin. Pharmacol. Ther. Toxicol.* **19**, 453 (1981).

Crystals from ether, mp 193-194°.

Note: This is a controlled substance (depressant): **21 CFR**, 1308.14.

THERAP CAT: Anxiolytic.

3822. *N*-Ethylmaleimide. [128-53-0] 1-Ethyl-1*H*-pyrrole-2,5-dione. $C_6H_7NO_2$; mol wt 125.13. C 57.59%, H 5.64%, N

11.19%, O 25.57%. Prepd by heating *N*-ethylmaleamic acid in paraffin: Marrian, *J. Chem. Soc.* **1949**, 1515.

Crystals, mp 45°. Lacrimator when liquid.
Caution: Strong irritant.
USE: In cancer research (possible antimitotic activity.)

3823. Ethyl Malonate. [105-53-3] Propanedioic acid diethyl ester; diethyl malonate; malonic ester. $C_7H_{12}O_4$; mol wt 160.17. C 52.49%, H 7.55%, O 39.96%. $C_2H_5OOCCH_2COOC_2H_5$. Prepd from chloroacetic acid and sodium cyanide followed by esterification with ethanol and H_2SO_4: L. Gattermann, T. Wieland, *Praxis des Organischen Chemikers* (de Gruyter, Berlin, 40th ed., 1961) pp 220-221.

Liquid. Slightly aromatic, pleasant odor. d 1.055. bp 198-199°; bp_{20} 95°. mp −50°. n_D^{20} 1.4143. One gram dissolves in about 50 ml of water. Miscible with alcohol, ether.
USE: Manuf of barbiturates.

3824. Ethyl Maltol. [4940-11-8] 2-Ethyl-3-hydroxy-4*H*-pyran-4-one; 2-ethylpyromeconic acid; Veltol-Plus. $C_7H_8O_3$; mol wt 140.14. C 59.99%, H 5.75%, O 34.25%. Synthetic analog of maltol, *q.v.* Prepn: C. R. Stephens, Jr. *et al.,* **BE 651427**; C. R. Stephens, Jr., R. P. Allingham, **US 3376317** (1965, 1968 both to Pfizer). Synthesis: I. Ichimoto, C. Tatsumi, *Agric. Biol. Chem.* **34**, 961 (1970). Toxicity studies: E. J. Gralla *et al., Toxicol. Appl. Pharmacol.* **15**, 604 (1969). GC determn in apple juice: S. W. Gunner *et al., J. AOAC Int.* **51**, 959 (1968). Solid phase microextraction and microwave assisted extraction fom food products: Y. Wang *et al., J. High Resolut. Chromatogr.* **20**, 213 (1997). Metabolism in dogs: H. H. Rennhard, *J. Agric. Food Chem.* **19**, 152 (1971). Crystal structures of polymorphs: S. D. Brown *et al., Acta Crystallogr.* **C51**, 1335 (1995). Review of use as a food additive: D. T. LeBlanc, H. A. Akers, *Food Technol.* **43**, 78-84 (1989).

Crystals from chloroform, mp 89-90° (Ichimoto). Also reported as crystals from water, mp 89-92° (Gunner). Cotton candy, caramel-like odor. uv max (methanol): 278 nm (ε 8200). LD_{50} orally in male mice, male rats, female rats, chicks (mg/kg): 780, 1150, 1200, 1270 (Gralla).
USE: Flavor and fragrance enhancer in foods, esp baked goods, beverages, and synthetic berry and citrus flavorings; minimizes undesirable flavors in tobacco products, cough syrup, vitamins, cosmetics, and saccharin-containing products.

3825. Ethyl Menthane Carboxamide. [39711-79-0] *N*-Ethyl-5-methyl-2-(1-methylethyl)cyclohexanecarboxamide; *N*-ethyl-4-menthane-3-carboxamide; WS3. $C_{13}H_{25}NO$; mol wt 211.34. C 73.88%, H 11.92%, N 6.63%, O 7.57%. Prepn: **NL 7201523**; H. R. Watson *et al.,* **US 4193936** (1972, 1980 both to Wilkinson Sword). Structure-activity study: H. R. Watson *et al., J. Soc. Cosmet. Chem.* **29**, 185 (1978). Brief review: M. A. Parrish, *Manuf. Chem.* **58**, 31-32 (February, 1987).

White to nearly white powder, mp 88°. $[\alpha]_D$ −49 to −54°. Insol in water. Sol in most organic solvents. Average oral cooling threshold: 0.2 μg. LD_{50} in mice, rats (g/kg): 5.3, 2.9 orally (Parrish).
USE: Physiological coolant in foods, beverages, toiletries, cosmetics and pharmaceuticals.

3826. Ethylmercuric Chloride. [107-27-7] Chloroethylmercury; Granosan. C_2H_5ClHg; mol wt 265.10. C 9.06%, H 1.90%, Cl 13.37%, Hg 75.67%. CH_3CH_2HgCl. Prepd from ethylmercuric bromide by treating with methanolic KOH, filtering and neutralizing with HCl: Slotta, Jacobi, *J. Prakt. Chem.* [2] **120**, 249 (1929). Prepn from $HgCl_2$ and tetraethyl lead: Whelen in *Adv. Chem. Ser.* **23**, entitled "Metal-Organic Compounds," M. Sittig, Ed. (ACS, Washington DC, 1960) pp 82-86. For the prepn of the bromide from ethylmagnesium bromide and mercuric bromide *see* Slotta, Jacobi, *loc. cit.,* Marvel *et al., J. Am. Chem. Soc.* **47**, 3009 (1925). *Review:* Krause, von Grosse, *Die Chemie der Metallorganischen Verbindungen* (Berlin, 1937).

White, silvery leaflets from ethanol, mp 192°. Sublimes easily. Solubility in water at 18° = 1.4 × 10^{-4} g/100 ml, at 100° = 2.5 × 10^{-4} g/100 ml; in ethanol at 18° = 0.75 g/100 g; at 78° = 3.5 g/100 g; in chloroform at 18° = 2.6 g/100 g. Slightly sol in ether.
Note: A close analog, ***chloro-(2-methoxyethyl)mercury***, *Cere-san Wet*, is also used as seed fungicide. *Caution:* Highly toxic. Causes skin burns; is absorbed through the skin. Chronic exposure has caused permanent injury to brain.
USE: Applied at 2% strength (soln or mixed with solids) as a fungicide for treating seeds.

3827. Ethyl Methanesulfonate. [62-50-0] Methanesulfonic acid ethyl ester; ethyl methanesulfonic acid; ethyl mesylate; EMS; NSC-26805. $C_3H_8O_3S$; mol wt 124.16. C 29.02%, H 6.49%, O 38.66%, S 25.83%. $CH_3SO_2OCH_2CH_3$. Prepn: O. C. Billeter, *Ber.* **38**, 2015 (1905). Mutagenicity studies: T. Alderson, *Nature* **207**, 164 (1965); J. B. Jenkins, *Mutat. Res.* **4**, 90 (1967); A. P. Schalet, *ibid.* **49**, 313 (1978). Review of carcinogenicity studies: *IARC Monographs* **7**, 245-252 (1974). Review of comparative mutagenicity of EMS and methyl methanesulfonate, *q.v.*: S. Kondo, *Environ. Sci. Res.* **24**, 743-785 (1981).

Liquid, bp_{761} 213-213.5°; bp_{10} 85-86°. d_4^{22} 1.1452.
Caution: This substance is reasonably anticipated to be a human carcinogen: *Report on Carcinogens, Eleventh Edition* (PB2005-104914, 2004) p III-124.
USE: Exptlly as mutagen, teratogen and brain carcinogen.

3828. Ethyl Methyl Ether. [540-67-0] Methoxyethane; methyl ethyl ether. C_3H_8O; mol wt 60.10. C 59.95%, H 13.42%, O 26.62%. $C_2H_5OCH_3$.
Liquid. d_0^0 0.725. bp 10.8°. Sol in water; miscible with alcohol, ether.

3829. Ethylmethylthiambutene. [441-61-2] *N*-Ethyl-*N*-methyl-4,4-di-2-thienyl-3-buten-2-amine; *N*-ethyl-*N*,1-dimethyl-3,3-di-2-thienyl-2-propenamine; *N*-ethyl-*N*,1-dimethyl-3,3-di-2-thienylallylamine; 3-ethylmethylamino-1,1-di(2'-thienyl)but-1-ene; ethylmethiambutene; IC50; NIH-5145; Emethibutin. $C_{15}H_{19}NS_2$; mol wt 277.45. C 64.93%, H 6.90%, N 5.05%, S 23.11%. Prepn: Adamson, **US 2561899** (1951 to Burroughs Wellcome). Toxicology: N. B. Eddy, D. Leimbach, *J. Pharmacol. Exp. Ther.* **107**, 385 (1953).

$bp_{0.01}$ 110-113°; bp_{18} 75-76°.
Hydrochloride. $C_{15}H_{19}NS_2.HCl$. Crystals, mp 137-138°. LD_{50} in mice (mg/kg): 192 orally; 88 s.c. (Eddy, Leimbach).
Note: This is a controlled substance (opiate): **21 CFR**, 1308.11.
THERAP CAT: Analgesic (narcotic).

3830. Ethylmorphine. [76-58-4] 7,8-Didehydro-4,5-epoxy-3-ethoxy-17-methylmorphinan-6-ol. $C_{19}H_{23}NO_3$; mol wt

313.39. C 72.82%, H 7.40%, N 4.47%, O 15.32%. Prepd by ethylation of morphine: Baizer, Ellner, *J. Am. Pharm. Assoc.* **39**, 581 (1950); Gorecki, *Ann. Pharm. (Poznan)* **7**, 21 (1969). Toxicity data: M. Aurousseau, J. Navarro, *Ann. Pharm. Fr.* **15**, 640 (1957).

Crystals from ethanol, mp 199-201°.

Hydrochloride dihydrate. [6746-59-4] Codethyline. $C_{19}H_{23}$-$NO_3.HCl.2H_2O$; mol wt 385.88. White to faintly yellow crystalline powder, mp about 123° (dec); anhydrous form, mp about 170° (dec). One gram dissolves in 10 ml water and in 25 ml alcohol; slightly sol in chloroform, ether. LD_{50} in mice: 264.6 mg/kg s.c.; 0.771 g/kg orally (Aurousseau, Navarro).

Methiodide. [6696-59-9] Ethyl-*N*-methylmorphinium iodide; Trachyl. $C_{19}H_{23}NO_3.CH_3I$; mol wt 455.33.

Note: This is a controlled substance (opiate): **21 CFR**, 1308.12.

THERAP CAT: Analgesic (narcotic); antitussive.

THERAP CAT (VET): Analgesic (narcotic); antitussive; mydriatic.

3831. Ethyl Nitrite. [109-95-5] Nitrous acid ethyl ester; nitrous ether. $C_2H_5NO_2$; mol wt 75.07. C 32.00%, H 6.71%, N 18.66%, O 42.63%. C_2H_5ONO. Prepd by the action of sodium nitrite on a mixture of alcohol and H_2SO_4 in the cold. The article of commerce contains 90-95% ethyl nitrite, the remainder is chiefly alcohol as preservative. Laboratory generation of ethyl nitrite gas by placing 20 liters of 90% ethanol in a suitable vessel, diluting with 200 liters of water, and while stirring, adding to the dil alc 18.3 kg of nitrosyl chloride at the rate of 2.25 kg per hour; *see also* Chase, **US 2615896** (1952).

Colorless or yellowish, clear, flammable, exceedingly volatile liq. Characteristic odor; burning, sweetish taste. d_{15}^{15} 0.90. bp 17°. Slightly sol in water and dec by it; miscible with alcohol, ether. On keeping, it gradually dec, becoming acid and oxides of nitrogen form. Decompn is hastened by air, light, and moisture. *Keep tightly closed, in a cool place, protected from light.*

Spirit of Ethyl Nitrite. Spirit of nitrous ether; sweet spirit of niter. An alcoholic soln containing 3.5-4.5% ethyl nitrite. Pale yellow or faintly greenish-yellow, clear, mobile, volatile, flammable liquid; ethereal, pungent odor; sharp, burning taste. The ethyl nitrite evaporates rapidly; dec on exposure to air; dec in light. d not above 0.823 at 25°. Miscible with water and alcohol. *Keep tightly closed, protected from light, in a cool place, remote from fire.*

Caution: May cause methemoglobinemia and hypotension and, in high concns, narcosis.

THERAP CAT: Has been used as diaphoretic.

3832. Ethyl Nitrobenzoate. $C_9H_9NO_4$; mol wt 195.17. C 55.39%, H 4.65%, N 7.18%, O 32.79%.

Colorless crystals. Insol in water. Freely sol in alc, ether.

o-Ester. mp 30°. bp₁₈ 173°.

m-Ester. mp 47°. bp about 298°.

p-Ester. mp 57°.

3833. N-Ethyl-N-nitrosourea. [759-73-9] *N*-Nitroso-*N*-ethylurea; ENU. $C_3H_7N_3O_2$; mol wt 117.11. C 30.77%, H 6.02%, N 35.88%, O 27.32%. $C_2H_5N(NO)CONH_2$. Potent mouse mutagen. Prepn: E. A. Werner, *J. Chem. Soc.* **115**, 1093 (1919); F. Arndt, H. Scholz, *Angew. Chem.* **46**, 47 (1933). Carcinogenicity studies: M. F. Rajewsky, R. Goth, *Mol. Base Malig., Sel. Pap. Int. Symp.* **1976**, 2. Mutagenicity studies: W. L. Russell *et al., Proc. Natl. Acad. Sci. USA* **16**, 5818 (1979). Toxicity studies: H. Druckrey *et al., Nature* **210**, 1378 (1966).

Pale buff-yellow, hexagonal plates, mp 103-104°. LD_{50} i.v. in rats: 240 mg/kg (Druckrey).

Caution: This substance is reasonably anticipated to be a human carcinogen: *Report on Carcinogens, Eleventh Edition* (PB2005-104914, 2004) p III-201.

USE: Exptlly as mutagen; ethylating agent.

3834. Ethylnorepinephrine. [536-24-3] 4-(2-Amino-1-hydroxybutyl)-1,2-benzenediol; α-(1-aminopropyl)-3,4-dihydroxybenzyl alcohol; α-(1-aminopropyl)protocatechuyl alcohol; 1-(3,4-dihydroxyphenyl)-2-aminobutanol; 1-(3,4-dihydroxyphenyl)-1-hydroxy-2-aminobutane; ethylnoradrenaline; ethylnorsuprarenin; E.N.E.; E.N.S.. $C_{10}H_{15}NO_3$; mol wt 197.23. C 60.90%, H 7.67%, N 7.10%, O 24.34%. Prepd by catalytic hydrogenolysis of α-benzhydrylamino-3,4-dibenzyloxybutyrophenone-HCl: Suter, Ruddy, *J. Am. Chem. Soc.* **66**, 747 (1944); **US 2431285** (1947 to Winthrop-Stearns).

Hydrochloride. [3198-07-0] Bronkephrine. $C_{10}H_{15}NO_3$.-HCl; mol wt 233.69. Crystals, dec 199-200°. Soluble in water. Marketed as an 0.2% aq soln.

THERAP CAT: Bronchodilator.

3835. Ethyl Oenanthate. [106-30-9] Heptanoic acid ethyl ester; ethyl heptanoate; ethyl *n*-heptoate; oenanthic ether; cognac oil, synthetic; oil of grapes; aether oenanthicus; oleum vitis viniferae. $C_9H_{18}O_2$; mol wt 158.24. C 68.31%, H 11.47%, O 20.22%. $CH_3(CH_2)_5COOC_2H_5$. Obtained commercially either by esterification of heptanoic acid, yielding a high-grade product; or by the direct esterification of coconut oil yielding a mixture of the ethyl esters of lauric, myristic, palmitic, and other higher fatty acids plus ethyl and isoamyl alcohol. For some flavoring applications the latter product is more desirable. Prepn: Rogers, *J. Am. Pharm. Assoc. Sci. Ed.* **12**, 503 (1923). Toxicity: P. M. Jenner *et al., Food Cosmet. Toxicol.* **2**, 327 (1964).

Pure ester, liquid. Fruity, wine-like odor and taste with burning aftertaste. d_4^{15} 0.8723; d_4^{25} 0.8630. bp₇₆₀ 189°; bp₃₅ 95°; bp₈ 68°. Viscosity at 25°: 0.0111 g/cm/sec. Insol in water. Misc with alcohol, ether, chloroform. Forms an azeotrope with water, the azeotropic mixture boils at 98.5° and contains 72% w/w of ethyl oenanthate. LD_{50} orally in rats: >34640 mg/kg (Jenner).

Note: Artificial Ethyl Oenanthate, also known as *artificial cognac essence* or *oil of wine*, is a mixture of amyl and ethyl caprates with ethyl and isoamyl butyrates and caprylates.

USE: In the manuf of liqueurs. Plays an important part in the formulation of raspberry, gooseberry, grape, cherry, apricot, currant, bourbon, and other artificial essences.

3836. Ethyl Oxalacetate. [108-56-5] Oxobutanedioic acid diethyl ester; diethyl oxalacetate; oxaloacetic ester. $C_8H_{12}O_5$; mol wt 188.18. C 51.06%, H 6.43%, O 42.51%. $C_2H_5OOCCH_2$-$COCOOC_2H_5$. Obtained by the action of sodium on a mixture of ethyl oxalate and ethyl acetate.

Oily liquid. d_4^{20} 1.131. bp₂₄ 132°. $n_D^{16.6}$ 1.45614. Insol in water. Miscible with alc, benzene, ether. Dec when boiled at ordinary pressure. With water it gradually dec into alc and acetic and oxalic acids.

Semicarbazone. Crystals, mp 162°.

3837. Ethylparaben. [120-47-8] 4-Hydroxybenzoic acid ethyl ester; ethyl *p*-hydroxybenzoate; Nipagin A; Ethyl Parasept; Solbrol A. $C_9H_{10}O_3$; mol wt 166.17. C 65.05%, H 6.07%, O 28.88%. Prepd by esterification of *p*-hydroxybenzoic acid: Cavill, Vincent, *J. Soc. Chem. Ind. London* **66**, 175 (1947).

Crystals, mp 116°. bp 297-298° (decomp). Freely sol in alcohol, ether. Soly in water at 20°: 0.070% w/w; at 25°: 0.075% w/w.

USE: Preservative for pharmaceuticals.

3838. Ethyl Pelargonate. [123-29-5] Nonanoic acid ethyl ester; ethyl nonanoate; wine ether. $C_{11}H_{22}O_2$; mol wt 186.29. C

70.92%, H 11.90%, O 17.18%. $CH_3(CH_2)_7COOC_2H_5$. Toxicity data: P. M. Jenner *et al., Food Cosmet. Toxicol.* **2**, 327 (1964).

Liquid. d_4^{18} 0.866. bp ~220°. mp −44°. Insol in water. Misc with alc, ether. LD_{50} orally in rats: >43,000 mg/kg (Jenner). Marketed product is an alcoholic soln of various essences in form of a yellowish liq, d ~0.823. Used in production of cognac-like beverages; 1 part ethyl pelargonate and 20 parts alcohol constitute one kind of artificial "Cognac Essence".

3839. 2-Ethylphenol. [90-00-6] Phlorol; *o*-ethylphenol. $C_8H_{10}O$; mol wt 122.16. C 78.66%, H 8.25%, O 13.10%. Prepn: W. Suida, S. Plohn, *Monatsh. Chem.* **1**, 175 (1880). Purification and properties: D. P. Biddiscombe *et al., J. Chem. Soc.* **1963**, 5764. Colorimetric determn of isomeric purities in reagent grade chemicals: I. M. Jakovljevic, R. H. Bishara, *J. Chromatogr.* **192**, 425 (1980). Thermolytic reactions: P. Zhou, B. L. Crynes, *Ind. Eng. Chem. Process Des. Dev.* **25**, 898 (1986). Decomposition and oxidation of aqueous solns: C. J. Martino, P. E. Savage, *Ind. Eng. Chem. Res.* **38**, 1775 (1999).

Colorless liq; phenol odor. Cooling the liq to −30° gives a metastable cryst form, mp about −28°; when kept for 24-48 hrs, this changes to the stable cryst form, mp −3.4°. fp −3.31 ± 0.01° for repurified sample. bp$_{760}$ 204.52°. d_{20} 1.01885 ± 0.00001; d_{25} 1.01459; d_{30} 1.01033 ± 0.00001 (g/ml). Practically insol in water. Freely sol in alcohol, benzene, glacial acetic acid.

USE: Starting material and intermediate for pharmaceutical and agricultural chemicals.

3840. Ethyl Phenylacetate. [101-97-3] Benzeneacetic acid ethyl ester; α-toluic acid ethyl ester. $C_{10}H_{12}O_2$; mol wt 164.20. C 73.15%, H 7.37%, O 19.49%. $C_6H_5CH_2COOC_2H_5$. Prepd by heating benzyl cyanide with alcohol and H_2SO_4: Adams, Thal, *Org. Synth.* **2**, 27 (1922).

Liquid. Pleasant odor. d_4^{20} 1.0333. bp$_{760}$ 226°; bp$_{32}$ 135°; bp$_{20}$ 121°. $n_D^{18.5}$ 1.49921. Absorption spectrum: Baly, Collie, *J. Chem. Soc.* **87**, 1344 (1905); Baly, Tryhorn, *ibid.* **107**, 1063 (1915).

USE: In perfumery.

3841. Ethyl Phosphorochloridite. [589-57-1] Phosphorochloridous acid diethyl ester; diethylchlorophosphinate; diethylchlorophosphonate; diethylphosphorous acid chloride; ethyl chlorophosphite. $C_4H_{10}ClO_2P$; mol wt 156.55. C 30.69%, H 6.44%, Cl 22.65%, O 20.44%, P 19.79%. $(C_2H_5O)_2PCl$. Prepd by passing chlorine into diethylphosphorous acid in ligroin contg Na wire: Arbusow, Arbusow, *Ber.* **65**, 195 (1932); by heating triethyl phosphite and phosphorus trichloride; or by adding phosphorus trichloride to a soln of ethanol and diethylaniline in ether: Cook *et al., J. Chem. Soc.* **1949**, 2021.

Liquid. Characteristic odor of acid chlorides. Fumes in moist air; reacts violently with water. d_4^{20} 1.0816; d_0^0 1.0962; d_0^{20} 1.0747. bp$_{760}$ 153-155°; (also reported as bp$_{760}$ 143-148°); bp$_{30}$ 63-65°; bp$_{15}$ 45-53°; bp$_{10}$ 37-38°. n_D^{20} 1.4350.

USE: In peptide synthesis.

3842. 3-Ethyl-4-picoline. [529-21-5] 3-Ethyl-4-methylpyridine; β-collidine; 3-ethyl-γ-picoline; β-ethyl-γ-methylpyridine. $C_8H_{11}N$; mol wt 121.18. C 79.29%, H 9.15%, N 11.56%. Prepd from 2,6-dichloro-3-ethyl-4-methylpyridine by reduction with HI and red phosphorus: Ruzicka, Fornasir, *Helv. Chim. Acta* **2**, 338 (1919); from 3-acetyl-1,4-dimethyl-1,2,5,6-tetrahydropyridine: Prelog, Komzak, *Ber.* **74**, 1705 (1941); from γ-methylnicotinic acid: Rabe, Jantzen, *Ber.* **54**, 925 (1921); from β-ethylpyridine: Koenigs, Hoffmann, *Ber.* **58**, 194 (1925); from crotonaldehyde and ammonia: Tschitschibabin, Oparina, *Ber.* **60**, 1877 (1927).

Liquid, aromatic odor. d_4^{17} 0.9286. bp$_{753}$ 195-196°; bp$_{23}$ 88-90°; bp$_{12}$ 76°. Volatile with steam. Sparingly sol in water. Soluble in alcohol, ether, chloroform, dil acids.

Hydrochloride. $C_8H_{11}N.HCl$. Hygroscopic platelets, sol in water.

3843. 4-Ethyl-2-picoline. [536-88-5] 4-Ethyl-2-methylpyridine; α-methyl-γ-ethylpyridine; 4-ethyl-α-picoline; α-collidine. $C_8H_{11}N$; mol wt 121.18. C 79.29%, H 9.15%, N 11.56%. Prepd from 2-picoline and acetic anhydride in the presence of zinc dust: H. Maier-Bode, J. Altpeter, *Das Pyridin und Seine Derivate* (Halle, 1934) p 54; **DE 390333**.

Liquid. d_4^0 0.9291; d_4^{16} 0.9268. bp$_{751}$ 179°. Volatile with steam. Sol in alcohol, ether, benzene, dil acids. Sparingly sol in water.

3844. 5-Ethyl-2-picoline. [104-90-5] 5-Ethyl-2-methylpyridine; aldehyde-collidine; aldehydine; 2-methyl-5-ethylpyridine; 5-ethyl-α-picoline; 3-ethyl-6-methylpyridine. $C_8H_{11}N$; mol wt 121.18. C 79.29%, H 9.15%, N 11.56%. Prepd by heating acetaldehyde ammonia in a double vol of abs alc: Ador, Bayer, *Ann.* **155**, 297 (1870); by heating ammonia water and paraldehyde in presence of ammonium acetate: Dürkopf, Schlaugk, *Ber.* **21**, 294 (1888); **DE 347820**; **DE 349184**; **DE 349267**; H. Maier-Bode, J. Altpeter, *Das Pyridin und Seine Derivate* (Halle, 1934) p 56; Frank *et al., J. Am. Chem. Soc.* **68**, 1368 (1946); Dunn, **US 2717897** (1955 to UCC); R. L. Frank *et al., Org. Synth.* coll. vol. IV, 451 (1963). Continuous process: Takeba *et al.*, **US 2935513** (1960 to Takeda).

Liquid. Aromatic odor. d_4^{23} 0.9184. bp$_{747}$ 177.8°; bp$_{20}$ 74-75°; bp$_{17}$ 65-66°. n_D^{20} 1.4971. Volatile with steam. Practically insol in water. Sol in alcohol, ether, benzene, dil acids, concd H_2SO_4.

Hydrochloride. $C_8H_{11}N.HCl$. Hygroscopic needles, freely sol in water.

3845. 1-Ethyl-3-piperidinol. [13444-24-1] 1-Ethyl-3-hydroxypiperidine. $C_7H_{15}NO$; mol wt 129.20. C 65.07%, H 11.70%, N 10.84%, O 12.38%. Prepn: Biel *et al., J. Am. Chem. Soc.* **74**, 1485 (1952); Biel, **US 2802007** (1957 to Lakeside).

Liquid. bp$_{15}$ 93-95°. n_D^{14} 1.4777.

3846. Ethyl Propiolate. [623-47-2] 2-Propynoic acid ethyl ester; ethyl acetylenecarboxylate. $C_5H_6O_2$; mol wt 98.10. C 61.22%, H 6.16%, O 32.62%. Michael acceptor in organic synthesis. Prepn: W. H. Perkin, Jr., J. L. Simonsen, *J. Chem. Soc.* **1907**, 816. IR spectrum and rotational isomerism study: S. W. Charles *et al., J. Mol. Struct.* **26**, 249 (1975). Use in photochemical addition reactions: G. Büchi, S. H. Feairheller, *J. Org. Chem.* **34**, 609 (1969); in Michael addition reactions: A. Hong, J. M. Friedman, *Synth. Commun.* **27**, 2971 (1997); in halo aldol reactions with aldehydes: D. Chen *et al., Eur. J. Org. Chem.* **2004**, 3330. Review of use as a peptide coupling reagent: B. Iorga, J.-M. Campagne, *Synlett* **2004**, 1826-1828.

Distills at 119° (745 mm); also reported as bp 122° (Büchi, Feairheller). d_4^4 0.9788. d_{15}^{15} 0.9676. d_{25}^{25} 0.9583.

USE: In organic synthesis; peptide coupling reagent.

3847. Ethyl Propionate. [105-37-3] Propanoic acid ethyl ester. $C_5H_{10}O_2$; mol wt 102.13. C 58.80%, H 9.87%, O 31.33%. $CH_3CH_2COOC_2H_5$.

Colorless liquid; fruity odor. d_4^{20} 0.891. bp 99°. mp −73°. n_D^{20} 1.3844. Flash pt, closed cup: 12°C. Sol in about 60 parts water; miscible with alcohol, ether.

3848. 3-Ethylpyridine. [536-78-7] "β-Lutidine". C_7H_9N; mol wt 107.15. C 78.46%, H 8.47%, N 13.07%.

Colorless to brownish liquid. d^{23} 0.940. bp 162-165°. n_D^{22} 1.5021. Slightly sol in water; freely sol in alcohol, or ether.

3849. 4-Ethylpyridine. [536-75-4] γ-Ethylpyridine. C_7-H_9N; mol wt 107.15. C 78.46%, H 8.47%, N 13.07%. Found in California petr: Hackmann *et al., Rec. Trav. Chim.* **62**, 229 (1943). Best prepd from pyridine by treatment with acetic anhydride and zinc: Dohrn, Horsters, **DE 390333** (1924 to Schering); Wibaut, Arens, *Rec. Trav. Chim.* **60**, 119 (1941); Frank, Smith, *Org. Synth.* **27**, 38 (1947). Using iron powder: Tenenbaum, Fand, **US 2712019** (1955 to Nepera Chem.).

Liquid. Obnoxious odor. Turns brown if not very pure. d_4^{22} 0.9404. bp_{750} 169.6-170.0°. n_D^{18} 1.5029. Sparingly sol in water; sol in alcohol, ether.

Caution: Symptoms similar to pyridine, *q.v.*

3850. Ethyl Salicylate. [118-61-6] 2-Hydroxybenzoic acid ethyl ester; salicylic acid ethyl ester; salicylic ether; sal ethyl. C_9-$H_{10}O_3$; mol wt 166.17. C 65.05%, H 6.07%, O 28.88%.

Clear, very refractive liquid; pleasant odor resembling that of methyl salicylate. Becomes yellowish-brown on long exposure to air and light. d_4^{20} 1.131. bp 231-234°. mp 1°. n_D^{20} 1.5226. Slightly sol in water; miscible with alc, ether. *Protect from light.*

USE: Manuf artificial perfumes.

THERAP CAT (VET): Has been used as a counterirritant.

3851. Ethyl Silicate. [78-10-4] Silicic acid tetraethyl ester; tetraethyl silicate. $C_8H_{20}O_4Si$; mol wt 208.33. C 46.12%, H 9.68%, O 30.72%, Si 13.48%. $Si(OC_2H_5)_4$. Prepn from abs alcohol and silicon tetrachloride: J. J. Ebelmen, *Ann.* **57**, 319 (1846); A. W. Dearing, E. E. Reid, *J. Am. Chem. Soc.* **50**, 3058 (1928); G. Sumrell, E. E. Ham, *ibid.* **78**, 5573 (1956). Toxicological studies: H. F. Smyth, J. Seaton, *J. Ind. Hyg. Toxicol.* **22**, 288 (1940); V. H. Rowe *et al., ibid.* **30**, 332 (1948). *Review:* H. D. Cogan, C. A. Setterstrom, *Ind. Eng. Chem.* **39**, 1364 (1947).

Colorless, flammable liquid. mp −77°. bp 165-166°. Flash point 125°F (52°C). d_4^{20} 0.933; n_D^{25} 1.3818. Viscosity: 0.6 cP. Practically insol in water, and slowly dec by it. Miscible with alcohol.

Caution: Potential symptoms of overexposure are irritation of eyes and nose. *See NIOSH Pocket Guide to Chemical Hazards* (DHHS/NIOSH 97-140, 1997) p 142.

USE: In weatherproofing and hardening stone, arresting decay and disintegration; manuf weatherproof and acidproof mortars and cements. In the "lost wax" process for casting of high-melting alloys.

3852. Ethylstibamine. [1338-98-3] Bayer 693; Neostibosan; Stibamine; Astaril. A complex of *p*-aminobenzenestibonic acid (present largely as a tetramer), *p*-acetylaminobenzenestibonic acid (present largely as a dimer), antimonic acid and diethylamine in the approx molar ratio of 1:2:1:3. Contains 41 to 44% organic pentavalent antimony (the acetyl content is between 6 and 7%). The manuf requires special care since the compd is both a colloid and a molecular addition compd and slight variations affect its toxicity greatly: Schmidt, *Angew. Chem.* **43**, 963 (1930); **US 1988632**, *C.A.* **29**, 1586 (1935).

Light-yellow to yellowish-brown powder. Freely sol in water forming neutral, colloidal solns. The pH of a 5% soln is between 6.5 and 7.6. A 25% soln is approx isotonic. Solns for injection should be prepd immediately before use with sterile distilled water, as they are unstable on heating or standing.

THERAP CAT: Antiprotozoal (Leishmania).

3853. Ethyl Sulfate. [540-82-9] Sulfuric acid monoethyl ester; ethyl hydrogen sulfate; ethylsulfuric acid; sulfethylic acid; sulfovinic acid. $C_2H_6O_4S$; mol wt 126.13. C 19.04%, H 4.79%, O 50.74%, S 25.42%. $C_2H_5OSO_2OH$. Prepn: Hamid *et al., J. Chem. Soc.* **129**, 1098 (1926); Atwood, **US 2683731** (1954 to Natl. Petro-Chemicals). *Review:* C. M. Suter, *The Organic Chemistry of Sulfur* (John Wiley, 1944) p 23-27.

Corrosive.

Barium salt. Barium ethyl sulfate. $C_4H_{10}BaO_8S_2$. Dihydrate, lustrous leaflets. Freely soluble in water; slightly sol in alcohol. Not pptd by H_2SO_4 or sulfates.

Calcium salt. Calcium ethyl sulfate; calcium sulfovinate. C_4-$H_{10}CaO_8S_2$. Dihydrate, crystals. Soluble in water, alcohol.

See also Diethyl Sulfate.

USE: Intermediate in the manuf of ethanol from ethylene.

3854. Ethyl Sulfide. [352-93-2] 1,1′-Thiobisethane; diethyl sulfide; thioethyl ether. $C_4H_{10}S$; mol wt 90.19. C 53.27%, H 11.18%, S 35.55%. $(C_2H_5)_2S$. Made by distillation of sodium ethyl sulfate with a soln of K_2S.

Liquid; ethereal odor. d_4^{20} 0.837. bp 92°. n_D^{20} 1.44233. Insol in water; miscible with alcohol, ether.

USE: Solvent for anhydr mineral salts; in plating baths for coating metals with gold or silver.

3855. Ethyl Tartrate. [87-91-2] (2R,3R)-2,3-Dihydroxybutanedioic acid diethyl ester; diethyl tartrate. $C_8H_{14}O_6$; mol wt 206.19. C 46.60%, H 6.84%, O 46.56%. $C_2H_5OOCCH(OH)$-$CH(OH)COOC_2H_5$.

Colorless, thick, oily liquid. d_4^{20} 1.204. bp 280°; bp_{11} 150°. mp 17°. $[\alpha]_D^{20}$ +7.5°. n_D^{20} 1.4476. Slightly sol in water; miscible with alcohol or ether.

3856. Ethyl Tartrate, Acid. [608-89-9] (2R,3R)-2,3-Dihydroxybutanedioic acid monoethyl ester; monoethyl tartrate. C_6H_{10}-O_6; mol wt 178.14. C 40.45%, H 5.66%, O 53.89%. HOOC-$CH(OH)CH(OH)COOC_2H_5$.

Colorless, very hygroscopic crystals. Sweet taste. mp 90°. Sol in water, alcohol; insol in ether. *Keep well closed.*

USE: Printing with Indol Blue and Crystal Fast Blue on fustian, etc.

3857. 2-(Ethylthio)ethanol. [110-77-0] β-Hydroxydiethyl sulfide. $C_4H_{10}OS$; mol wt 106.19. C 45.24%, H 9.49%, O 15.07%, S 30.20%. $CH_3CH_2SCH_2CH_2OH$. Prepn from 2-chloroethanol and ethyl mercaptan: Demuth, Meyer, *Ann.* **240**, 310 (1887); Steinkopf *et al., Ber.* **53**, 1010 (1920); from 2-thioethanol and diethyl sulfate: Bergmann, *J. Am. Chem. Soc.* **74**, 829 (1952).

Liquid. d_{20}^{20} 1.015-1.025. bp_{760} 184.5°; bp_{28} 99°. Soluble in ether, other organic solvents.

USE: Intermediate for pesticides, lubricating and cutting oil additives, flotation agents, plasticizers.

3858. Ethyl p-Toluenesulfonate. [80-40-0] 4-Methylbenzenesulfonic acid ethyl ester. $C_9H_{12}O_3S$; mol wt 200.25. C 53.98%, H 6.04%, O 23.97%, S 16.01%. $CH_3C_6H_4SO_3C_2H_5$.

Monoclinic crystals. d 1.17. mp 33°. bp_{15} 173°.

USE: For ethylation.

3859. Ethyl Vanillin. [121-32-4] 3-Ethoxy-4-hydroxybenzaldehyde; ethylprotocatechuic aldehyde; bourbonal; ethylprotal; vanillal; Ethavan; Ethovan. $C_9H_{10}O_3$; mol wt 166.17. C 65.05%, H 6.07%, O 28.88%.

Colorless flakes possessing a finer and more intense vanilla odor and taste than vanillin. mp 77-78°. Sparingly sol in water; sol in alc, ether, glycerol, propylene glycol. Soly in 95% alc about 1 g/2 ml. LD_{50} orally in rats: >2000 mg/kg, P. M. Jenner *et al.*, *Food Cosmet. Toxicol.* **2**, 327 (1964).

USE: In flavoring and perfumery.

3860. Ethynodiol. [1231-93-2] (3β,17α)-19-Norpregn-4-en-20-yne-3,17-diol; 17α-ethynyl-19-norandrost-4-ene-3β,17β-diol; 17α-ethynyl-4-estrene-3β,17β-diol; ED. $C_{20}H_{28}O_2$; mol wt 300.44. C 79.95%, H 9.39%, O 10.65%. Prepn: F. B. Colton, US 2843609 (1958 to Searle). Prepn of the 3-acetate, 17-acetate, and diacetate: P. D. Klimstra, US 3176013 (1965 to Searle); *see also* F. Sondheimer, Y. Klibansky, *Tetrahedron* **5**, 15 (1959). Pharmacokinetics and metabolism: C. J. Lewis *et al.*, *Xenobiotica* **10**, 705 (1980). Comparative clinical study in oral contraceptives: M. H. Briggs, *J. Reprod. Med.* **28**, Suppl. 1, 92 (1983). Review of carcinogenicity studies: *IARC Monographs* **21**, 387-398 (1979). Comprehensive description: E. P. K. Lau, J. L. Sutter, *Anal. Profiles Drug Subs.* **3**, 253-279 (1974).

Diacetate. [297-76-7] 3β,17β-Diacetoxy-17α-ethynyl-4-estrene; SC-11800; Femulen; Luteonorm; Luto-Metrodiol; Metrodiol. $C_{24}H_{32}O_4$; mol wt 384.51. Crystals from methanol + water, mp ~126-127°. $[\alpha]_D$ −72.5° (chloroform).

Diacetate mixture with mestranol. Luteolas; Metrulen; Ovaras; Ovulen.

Diacetate mixture with ethinyl estradiol. Conova; Demulen; Miniluteolas.

THERAP CAT: Progestogen; in combination with estrogen as oral contraceptive.

3861. Ethynylbenzene. [536-74-3] Phenylacetylene. C_8H_6; mol wt 102.13. C 94.08%, H 5.92%. $C_6H_5C\equiv CH$. Prepd by dropping β-bromostyrene on molten potassium hydroxide and distilling: Hessler, *Org. Synth.* **2**, 67 (1922).

Liquid. d_4^{20} 0.9300. mp −44.8°. bp_{760} 142.4°; bp_{90} 75°; bp_{15} 39°. n_D^{20} 1.5489. Insol in water; miscible with alcohol, ether, other organic solvents.

3862. Etidocaine. [36637-18-0] N-(2,6-Dimethylphenyl)-2-(ethylpropylamino)butanamide; 2-(ethylpropylamino)-2',6'-butyroxylidide. $C_{17}H_{28}N_2O$; mol wt 276.42. C 73.87%, H 10.21%, N 10.13%, O 5.79%. Prepn: H. J. F. Adams *et al.*, DE 2162744; *eidem*, US 3812147 (1972, 1974 both to Astra). Activity and toxicity studies: *eidem, J. Pharm. Sci.* **61**, 1829 (1972).

Hydrochloride. [36637-19-1] W-19053; Duranest. $C_{17}H_{28}$-N_2O·HCl; mol wt 312.88. Crystals from abs ethanol-ether and

isopropanol-isopropylether, mp 203-203.5°. LD_{50} in female mice (mg/kg): 6.7 i.v.; 99 s.c. (Adams, 1972).

THERAP CAT: Anesthetic (local).

3863. Etidronic Acid. [2809-21-4] (1-Hydroxyethylidene)-bisphosphonic acid; (1-hydroxyethylidene)diphosphonic acid; ethane-1-hydroxy-1,1-diphosphonic acid; Dequest 2010; Fostex P. C_2-$H_8O_7P_2$; mol wt 206.03. C 11.66%, H 3.91%, O 54.36%, P 30.07%. Bisphosphonate antiresorptive agent. Prepn: H. von Baeyer, K. A. Hofmann, *Ber.* **30**, 1973 (1897); and characterization of the acid and disodium salt: F. Kasparek, *Monatsh. Chem.* **99**, 2016 (1968); B. Blaser *et al., Z. Anorg. Allg. Chem.* **381**, 247 (1971). Use as detergent builder: F. L. Diehl, US 3159581 (1964 to Proctor & Gamble). Determn in pharmaceutical formulations: E. W. Tsai *et al., J. Pharm. Biomed. Anal.* **11**, 513 (1993). Symposium on clinical efficacy in malignancy-related hypercalcemia: *Am. J. Med.* **82**, Suppl 2A, 1-78 (1987). Review of pharmacology and therapeutic efficacy in resorptive bone disease: C. J. Dunn *et al., Drugs Aging* **5**, 446-474 (1994); of clinical safety and efficacy in osteoporosis: T. P. van Staa *et al., Pharmacotherapy* **18**, 1121-1128 (1998).

Crystallizes from water as the monohydrate. pK_1 1.35 ±0.08; pK_2 2.87 ±0.01; pK_3 7.03 ±0.01; pK_4 11.3. Very sol in water (69% at 20° C). Insol in acetic acid.

Disodium salt. [7414-83-7] Disodium dihydrogen (1-hydroxyethylidene)bis[phosphonate]; etidronate disodium; Didronel; Diphos; Etidron. $C_2H_6Na_2O_7P_2$; mol wt 249.99. Crystallizes from water as the di- or tetrahydrate.

USE: Sequestering and chelating agent; scale and corrosion inhibitor.

THERAP CAT: Bone resorption inhibitor.

3864. Etifoxine. [21715-46-8] 6-Chloro-N-ethyl-4-methyl-4-phenyl-4H-3,1-benzoxazin-2-amine; 6-chloro-2-(ethylamino)-4-methyl-4-phenyl-4H-3,1-benzoxazine; HOE-36801. $C_{17}H_{17}ClN_2$-O; mol wt 300.78. C 67.88%, H 5.70%, Cl 11.79%, N 9.31%, O 5.32%. Psychotropic agent with anxiolytic and anticonvulsant activity. Prepn: FR M7358; H. Kuch *et al.*, US 3725404 (1969, 1973 both to Hoechst); I. Hoffmann *et al., Arzneim.-Forsch.* **20**, 975 (1970). Exptl psychopharmacological study: J. R. Boissier *et al., Therapie* **27**, 325 (1972). Analysis of EEG effects: D. Bente *et al., Arzneim.-Forsch.* **25**, 944 (1975). Evaluation of psychotropic effect: R. Corsico *et al., Psychopharmacologia* **45**, 301 (1976).

Colorless crystals from petr ether, mp 90-92°. uv max (ethanol): 273 nm (ε 21200). LD_{50} orally in mice: 12 g/kg (Hoffmann).

Hydrochloride. [56776-32-0] Stresam. $C_{17}H_{17}ClN_2O$·HCl; mol wt 337.24. Crystals, mp 150-151°.

THERAP CAT: Anxiolytic.

3865. Etilefrin. [709-55-7] α-[(Ethylamino)methyl]-3-hydroxybenzenemethanol; α-[(ethylamino)methyl]-m-hydroxybenzyl alcohol; m-hydroxy-α-(ethylaminomethyl)benzyl alcohol; α-(m-hydroxyphenyl)-β-(ethylamino)ethanol; ethylphenylephrine; etiladrianol. $C_{10}H_{15}NO_2$; mol wt 181.23. C 66.27%, H 8.34%, N 7.73%, O 17.66%. Sympathomimetic amine. Prepn: T. Goto, *J. Pharm. Soc. Jpn.* **74**, 318 (1954), *C.A.* **49**, 3960 (1955); ES 273595 (1962 to Labs. Fher S.A.), *C.A.* **60**, 1649e (1964). Clinical pharmacology: A. J. Coleman *et al., Eur. J. Clin. Pharmacol.* **8**, 41 (1975). Clinical pharmacokinetics and disposition: J. H. Hengstmann *et al., ibid.* **9**, 179 (1975). HPLC determn in plasma: K. Kojima *et al., J. Chromatogr.* **525**, 210 (1990). Clinical trial in arterial hypotension: T. Taivainen, *Acta Anaesthesiol. Scand.* **35**, 164 (1991); in neurocardiogenic syncope: F. Ammirati *et al., Am. J. Cardiol.* **86**, 472 (2000).

Crystals, mp 147-148°.

Hydrochloride. [534-87-2] Cardanat; Circupon; Effontil; Effortil; Efortil; Kertasin; Thomasin. $C_{10}H_{15}NO_2$.HCl; mol wt 217.69. Crystals, mp 121°. Bitter taste. Freely sol in water; sol in alcohol. Practically insol in chloroform.

THERAP CAT: Antihypotensive.

THERAP CAT (VET): Antihypotensive.

3866. Etiocholane. [438-23-3] (5β)-Androstane; 5-epiandrostane. $C_{19}H_{32}$; mol wt 260.46. C 87.62%, H 12.38%. Parent compd of alkyl substituted etiocholanes, such as pregnane, cholane, coprostane. Prepd from etiocholane-17-one semicarbazone: Butenandt, Dannenbaum, *Z. Physiol. Chem.* **229**, 192 (1934).

Needles from acetone, mp 78-80°.

3867. Etiocholanic Acid. [438-08-4] (5β,17β)-Androstane-17-carboxylic acid; aetiocholanic acid; etianic acid; etiocholane-17β-carboxylic acid. $C_{20}H_{32}O_2$; mol wt 304.47. C 78.90%, H 10.59%, O 10.51%. Prepn: Wieland *et al., Z. Physiol. Chem.* **161**, 80 (1926); Jacobs, Elderfield, *J. Biol. Chem.* **108**, 497 (1935); Tschesche, *Ber.* **68**, 9 (1935); Steiger, Reichstein, *Helv. Chim. Acta* **21**, 841 (1938).

Needles from glacial acetic acid; elongated leaflets from acetic acid. Sublimes at 0.002 mm press. and 160° bath temp, mp 228-229°. Insol in water; sol in pentane.

Methyl ester. $C_{21}H_{34}O_2$. Needles from methanol, mp 99-101°.

Note: The stem name "etianic acid" was proposed by the Subcommittee on Steroid Nomenclature of the National Research Council as a replacement for "etiocholanic acid" in order to avoid the use of the same name for parent hydrocarbons of different carbon content: *J. Am. Chem. Soc.* **74**, 2817 (1952).

3868. Etiocobalamin. [27792-36-5] Cobinamide dicyanide; vitamin B_{12p}; Factor B. $C_{50}H_{72}CoN_{13}O_8$; mol wt 1042.12. C 57.63%, H 6.96%, Co 5.66%, N 17.47%, O 12.28%. Vitamin B_{12} factor obtained by removal of the nucleotide from cyanocobalamin by acid hydrolysis. Isoln from calf feces: Ford, Porter, *Biochem. J.* **51**, V (1952). Prepn by acid hydrolysis: Gant *et al., ibid.* **56**, XXXIV (1954); Friedrich, Bernhauer, *Angew. Chem.* **65**, 627 (1953). Prepn from factor V_{1a} and D(−)-1-amino-2-propanol: Bernhauer *et al., Helv. Chim. Acta* **43**, 696 (1960); Bernhauer, US 3072674 (1963 to Hoffmann-La Roche).

Note: The term etiocobalamin is used by some authors to designate any cobalamin lacking the nucleotide group present in vitamin B_{12}.

3869. Etioporphyrin. [26608-34-4] 2,7,12,18-Tetraethyl-3,8,13,17-tetramethyl-21H,23H-porphine; 1,3,5,8-tetramethyl-2,4,-6,7-tetraethylporphine; etioporphyrin III; mesoetioporphyrin. $C_{32}H_{38}N_4$; mol wt 478.67. C 80.29%, H 8.00%, N 11.70%. Occurs in Bavarian oil shale, crude petr, ozokerite, amber, cannel coal and other hard varieties of bituminous coal: Treibs, *Ann.* **510**, 60 (1934); **517**, 184 (1935); *Angew. Chem.* **49**, 682 (1936). Prepd by decarboxylation of mesoporphyrin IX: Fischer, Treibs, *Ann.* **466**, 191, 206 (1928). Synthesis: Fischer, Stangler, *Ann.* **462**, 265 (1928); Johnson *et al., J. Chem. Soc.* **1959**, 3416. Structure: Abraham *et al., ibid.* **1961**, 3468. *Review:* Rimington, Kennedy, in M. Florkin, H. S. Mason, *Comparative Biochemistry* (Academic Press, New York, 1962) pp 557-614.

Long prismatic needles or butterflies from pyridine or from chloroform-petr ether, mp 360-363°. pKa 18. Absorption max: 246, 269, 396, 497, 532, 566, 620, 645 nm (log ε 3.90, 3.89, 5.22, 4.13, 3.99, 3.81, 3.65, 2.62).

Copper salt. $C_{32}H_{36}N_4Cu$. Red needles from pyridine-acetic acid.

Magnesium salt. $C_{32}H_{36}N_4Mg$. Crystals from methanol.

3870. Etiprednol Dicloacetate. [199331-40-3] (11β,17α)-17-[(Dichloroacetyl)oxy]-11-hydroxy-3-oxoandrosta-1,4-diene-17-carboxylic acid ethyl ester; ethyl 17α-dichloroacetoxy-11β-hydroxyandrosta-1,4-diene-3-one-17-carboxylate; BNP-166; Cronaze; Respicort. $C_{24}H_{30}Cl_2O_6$; mol wt 485.40. C 59.39%, H 6.23%, Cl 14.61%, O 19.78%. A so-called "soft" corticosteroid; designed to undergo predictable metabolism to an inactive compound. Prepn: N. S. Bodor, M. K. Baumeister, **WO 9742214**; *eidem*, **US 5981517** (1997, 1999 both to Soft Drugs, Inc.); A. Csanádi *et al., Pharmazie* **59**, 349 (2004). Toxicology and safety in animals: A. Miklós *et al., ibid.* **57**, 142 (2002). Pharmacology in animal model of asthma: I. Kurucz *et al., J. Pharmacol. Exp. Ther.* **307**, 83 (2003).

White crystalline powder from ethyl acetate, mp 201-202.5°.
THERAP CAT: Glucocorticoid; in treatment of Crohn's disease.

3871. Etiproston. [59619-81-7] (5Z)-7-[(1R,2R,3R,5S)-3,5-Dihydroxy-2-[(1E)-2-[2-(phenoxymethyl)-1,3-dioxolan-2-yl]-ethenyl]cyclopentyl]-5-heptenoic acid; (5Z,13E)-(8R,9S,11R,12R)-9,11-dihydroxy-15,15-ethylenedioxy-16-phenoxy-17,18,19,20-tetranorprostadienoic acid; 15-deoxy-15,15-ethylenedioxy-16-phenoxy-17,18,19,20-tetranorprostaglandin $F_{2\alpha}$; Prostavet; Vetiprost. $C_{24}H_{32}O_7$; mol wt 432.51. C 66.65%, H 7.46%, O 25.89%. Prostaglandin $F_{2\alpha}$ analog with estrus cycle synchronizing activity. Prepn: W. Skuballa *et al.*, **DE 2434133**; *eidem*, **US 4088775** (1976, 1978 both to Schering AG); and biological activity: W. Skuballa *et al.*, *J. Med. Chem.* **21**, 443 (1978).

Colorless oil.
THERAP CAT (VET): Luteolytic.

3872. Etiroxate. [17365-01-4] O-(4-Hydroxy-3,5-diiodophenyl)-3,5-diiodo-α-methyl-DL-tyrosine ethyl ester; DL-α-methylthyroxine ethyl ester; CG-635. $C_{18}H_{17}I_4NO_4$; mol wt 818.95. C 26.40%, H 2.09%, I 61.98%, N 1.71%, O 7.81%. Deriv of thyroxine, *q.v.* Prepn: **NL 6614150**; H. Kummer, R. Beckmann, **US 3930017** (1967, 1975 both to Grünenthal). Animal studies: R. Beckmann, *Arzneim.-Forsch.* **29**, 499 (1979). Effect on iodine metabolism in man: D. Emrich, *ibid.* **27**, 422 (1977). Use in hyperlipoproteinemia: H. Banz, F. P. Gall, *Fortschr. Med.* **97**, 1942 (1979); *eidem*, *Med. Klin.* **75**, 51 (1980).

Cryst from ethanol, mp 156-157°.
Hydrochloride. [55327-22-5] Skleronorm. $C_{18}H_{17}I_4NO_4$·HCl; mol wt 855.41.
THERAP CAT: Antilipemic.

3873. Etizolam. [40054-69-1] 4-(2-Chlorophenyl)-2-ethyl-9-methyl-6H-thieno[3,2-f][1,2,4]triazolo[4,3-a][1,4]diazepine; 1-methyl-6-o-chlorophenyl-8-ethyl-4H-s-triazolo[3,4-c]thieno[2,3-e]-1,4-diazepine; Y-7131; Depas. $C_{17}H_{15}ClN_4S$; mol wt 342.85. C 59.55%, H 4.41%, Cl 10.34%, N 16.34%, S 9.35%. Prepn: M. Nakanishi *et al.*, **DE 2229845**; *eidem*, **US 3904641** (1972, 1973 both to Yoshitomi). Pharmacology and toxicity studies: T. Tsumagari *et al.*, *Arzneim.-Forsch.* **28**, 1158 (1978). Effect on monoamine metabolism in brain: M. Setoguchi *et al.*, *ibid.* 1165; on rage responses in cats: T. Fukuda, T. Tsumagari, *Jpn. J. Pharmacol.* **33**, 885 (1983).

Crystals from toluene, mp 147-148°. LD_{50} in male, female rats, male, female mice (mg/kg): 3619, 3509, 4358, 4258 orally; 865, 825, 830, 783 i.p.; >5000 s.c. (Tsumagari).
THERAP CAT: Anxiolytic.

3874. Etodolac. [41340-25-4] 1,8-Diethyl-1,3,4,9-tetrahydropyrano[3,4-b]indole-1-acetic acid; etodolic acid; AY-24236; Etogesic; Lodine; Tedolan; Ultradol. $C_{17}H_{21}NO_3$; mol wt 287.35. C 71.06%, H 7.37%, N 4.87%, O 16.70%. Prepn: C. A. Demerson *et al.*, **DE 2301525** (1973 to Ayerst); *eidem*, **US 3939178** (1976 to Am. Home Products); *eidem*, *J. Med. Chem.* **19**, 391 (1976). Review of synthesis, pharmacology, metabolism and efficacy: L. G. Humber, *Med. Res. Rev.* **7**, 1-28 (1987). HPLC determn of enantiomers in plasma and urine: F. Jamali *et al.*, *J. Pharm. Sci.* **77**, 963 (1988). Veterinary trial for osteoarthritis in dogs: S. C. Budsberg *et al.*, *J. Am. Vet. Med. Assoc.* **214**, 206 (1999). Clinical trial for lumbar disc herniation: M. Hatori, S. Kokubun, *Curr. Med. Res. Opin.* **15**, 193 (1999). Review of pharmacology and therapeutic efficacy: J. A. Balfour, M. M.-T. Buckley, *Drugs* **42**, 274-299 (1991); of clinical pharmacokinetics: D. R. Brocks, F. Jamali, *Clin Pharmacokinet.* **26**, 259-274 (1994).

Crystals from hexane/chloroform, mp 145-148°. pKa 4.65. Insol in water. Sol in alcohols, chloroform, DMSO, aqueous polyethylene glycol.
THERAP CAT: Anti-inflammatory; analgesic.
THERAP CAT (VET): Anti-inflammatory; analgesic.

3875. Etofenamate. [30544-47-9] 2-[[3-(Trifluoromethyl)phenyl]amino]benzoic acid 2-(2-hydroxyethoxy)ethyl ester; N-(α,-α,α-trifluoro-m-tolyl)anthranilic acid 2-(2-hydroxyethoxy)ethyl ester; B-577; TV-485; Bayrogel; Glasel; Rheumon gel; Traumon Gel. $C_{18}H_{18}F_3NO_4$; mol wt 369.34. C 58.53%, H 4.91%, N 3.79%, O 17.33%. Percutaneously active antiphlogistic agent. Prepn: K. H. Boltze *et al.*, **DE 1939112**; *eidem*, **US 3692818** (1971, 1972 both to Troponwerke). Series of articles on chemistry, analysis, biochemistry, pharmacology, toxicology, and clinical studies: *Arzneim.-Forsch.* **27**, 1300-1363 (1977). Toxicity: H. Jacobi *et al.*, *ibid.* 1333. Metabolism and GC determn: *ibid.* **31**, 9-21 (1981).

Pale yellow viscous oil, thermolabile at 180°. $bp_{.001}$ 130-135°. uv max (methanol): 286 ($E_{1cm}^{1\%}$ 423). n_D^{25} 1.564. Sol in lower alcohols, ethyl acetate, acetone, chloroform, ether, benzene. Soly in water at 22°: 0.16 mg/100 ml. LD_{50} in male, female rats (mg/kg): 292, 470 orally; 140, 226 i.v.; 373, 397 i.p.; 643, 568 s.c. (Jacobi).
THERAP CAT: Anti-inflammatory.

3876. Etofenprox. [80844-07-1] 1-[[2-(4-Ethoxyphenyl)-2-methylpropoxy]methyl]-3-phenoxybenzene; 2-(4-ethoxyphenyl)-2-

methylpropyl-3-phenoxybenzyl ether; ethofenprox; ethoproxyfen; MTI-500; OMS-3002; Vectron. $C_{25}H_{28}O_3$; mol wt 376.49. C 79.75%, H 7.50%, O 12.75%. Non-ester pyrethroid insecticide. Prepn: K. Nakatani *et al.*, **FR 2481695**; *eidem*, **US 4397864** (1981, 1983 both to Mitsui Toatsu); T. K. Kim *et al.*, *Bull. Korean Chem. Soc.* **8**, 128 (1987). Fluorometric determn in potable water sources: M. Nakamura *et al.*, *Fresenius J. Anal. Chem.* **367**, 658 (2000). Field trial vs leafhoppers and planthoppers: N. V. Krishnaiah, M. B. Kalode, *Crop Prot.* **12**, 532 (1993); vs malarial vectors: S. Nalim *et al.*, *Southeast Asian J. Trop. Med. Public Health* **28**, 851 (1997). Review of physical properties and field trials: T. Tanaka, *Agrochem. Jpn.* **1999**, no. 74, 13-15.

White crystalline solid, mp 36.4-38.0°. Vapor pressure (100°): 2.4×10^{-4} mm Hg. Soly in water (25°): <1 ppb. $n_D^{20.2}$ 1.5732. LD_{50} in rats, mice (mg/kg): >2880, >107200 orally; >2140, >2140 dermally (Tanaka).

USE: Insecticide.

3877. Etofibrate. [31637-97-5] 3-Pyridinecarboxylic acid 2-[2-(4-chlorophenoxy)-2-methyl-1-oxopropoxy]ethyl ester; nicotinic acid 2-hydroxyethyl ester 2-(*p*-chlorophenoxy)-2-methylpropionate (ester); ethylene glycol 1-[2-(*p*-chlorophenoxy)-2-methylpropionate]-2-nicotinate; α-[(*p*-chlorophenoxy)isobutyroyl]-β-(nicotinoyl)glycol; ethofibrate; Lipo-Merz. $C_{18}H_{18}ClNO_5$; mol wt 363.79. C 59.43%, H 4.99%, Cl 9.75%, N 3.85%, O 21.99%. Glycol diester of nicotinic and clofibric acids, *q.q.v.* Prepn: A. Scherm, D. Peteri, **DE 1941217**; *eidem*, **US 3723446** (1971, 1973 both to Merz). Lipid lowering effects in rats: W. Sterner, A. Schultz, *Arzneim.-Forsch.* **24**, 1990 (1974). Metabolism: H. Oelschläger *et al.*, *ibid.* **30**, 984 (1980). *In vitro* effect on human platelet function: M. P. Ortega *et al.*, *Thromb. Res.* **19**, 409 (1980). HPLC determn in plasma: E. R. Garrett, M. R. Gardner, *J. Pharm. Sci.* **71**, 14 (1982). Bioavailability and pharmacokinetics in humans: K. I. Johnson *et al.*, *Arzneim.-Forsch.* **34**, 1785 (1984). Review of pharmacology and comparison with other hypolipidemic agents: R. Paoletti *et al.*, *Am. J. Cardiol.* **52**, Suppl B, 21B-27B (1983).

Crystalline powder, mp 100°.

THERAP CAT: Antilipemic.

3878. Etofylline. [519-37-9] 3,7-Dihydro-7-(2-hydroxyethyl)-1,3-dimethyl-1*H*-purine-2,6-dione; 7-(2-hydroxyethyl)theophylline; oxyethyltheophylline; Oxytheonyl; Oxphylline; Phyllocormin N. $C_9H_{12}N_4O_3$; mol wt 224.22. C 48.21%, H 5.39%, N 24.99%, O 21.41%. Obtained by the action of glycol monochlorohydrin upon theophylline in an alkaline medium: Lespagnol *et al.*, *Bull. Soc. Pharm. Lille* **1948**, no. 2, p 18; Roth, *Arch. Pharm.* **292**, 234 (1959); Fabbrini, Cencioni, *Farmaco Ed. Sci.* **17**, 660 (1962).

Crystals from abs ethanol, mp 158°. Freely sol in water. Moderately sol in alcohol. pH of a 5% aq soln 6.5-7.0. Solns may be sterilized by heating. Pharmacological action as of theophylline.

THERAP CAT: Bronchodilator.

3879. Etofylline Nicotinate. [13425-39-3] 3-Pyridinecarboxylic acid 2-(1,2,3,6-tetrahydro-1,3-dimethyl-2,6-dioxo-7*H*-purin-7-yl)ethyl ester; nicotinic acid ester with 7-(2-hydroxyethyl)theophylline; 7-(2-hydroxyethyl)theophylline nicotinate; Hesotanol; Hesotin. $C_{15}H_{15}N_5O_4$; mol wt 329.31. C 54.71%, H 4.59%, N 21.27%, O 19.43%. Prepn: Pongratz, Zirm, *Monatsh. Chem.* **88**, 330 (1957). Pharmacology: Fischbach, Haas, *Arzneim.-Forsch.* **17**, 313 (1967).

Fine dendritic needles from abs alcohol, mp 151-152°. Hydrated crystals from water. One gram dissolves in 50 ml boiling water; moderately sol in alcohol.

THERAP CAT: Vasodilator.

3880. Etoglucid. [1954-28-5] 2,2'-(2,5,8,11-Tetraoxadodecane-1,12-diyl)bisoxirane; 1,2:15,16-diepoxy-4,7,10,13-tetraoxahexadecane; 1,2-bis[2-(2,3-epoxypropoxy)ethoxy]ethane; triethylene glycol diglycidyl ether; TDE; ethoglucid; ICI-32865; Epodyl. $C_{12}H_{22}O_6$; mol wt 262.30. C 54.95%, H 8.45%, O 36.60%. Prepn: Greenshields *et al.*, **GB 901876** (1962 to ICI); Blyakhman, *Zh. Org. Khim.* **3**, 1423 (1967), *C.A.* **68**, 59384k (1968); X.-P. Gu *et al.*, *Synthesis* **1985**, 649. Pharmacology and metabolism: Duncan, Snow, *Biochem. J.* **82**, 8P (1962); James, Solheim, *Xenobiotica* **1**, 43 (1971). Clinical evaluation in bladder tumors: M. R. G. Robinson *et al.*, *J. Urol.* **118**, 972 (1977); J. Flamm, F. Grof, *Urologe* **B27**, 26 (1987).

Colorless liquid, mp −15 to −11°. $bp_{0.005}$ 140°; $bp_{0.1}$ 133-149°; bp_2 195-197°. d^{20} 1.1312. n_D^{20} 1.4584.

THERAP CAT: Antineoplastic.

3881. Etomidate. [33125-97-2] 1-[(1*R*)-1-Phenylethyl]-1*H*-imidazole-5-carboxylic acid ethyl ester; (*R*)-(+)-1-(α-methylbenzyl)imidazole-5-carboxylic acid ethyl ester; R-16659; Amidate; Hypnomidate. $C_{14}H_{16}N_2O_2$; mol wt 244.29. C 68.83%, H 6.60%, N 11.47%, O 13.10%. Prepn of the (±)-form: **BE 662474**; E. F. Godefroi, C. A. M. van der Eijcken, **US 3354173** (1965, 1967 both to Janssen); E. F. Godefroi *et al.*, *J. Med. Chem.* **8**, 220 (1965). Prepn of the (*R*)-(+)-form: L. F. C. Roevens *et al.*, **DE 2609573**; *eidem*, **US 3991072** (both 1976 to Janssen). Metabolism: E. Goetz, *Anaesthesist* **23**, 331 (1974). Pharmacokinetics: M. J. Van Hamme *et al.*, *Anesthesiology* **49**, 274 (1978). Pharmacology: P. A. J. Janssen *et al.*, *Arch. Int. Pharmacodyn. Ther.* **214**, 92 (1975). Clinical study: R. J. Fragen, N. Caldwell, *Anesthesiology* **50**, 242 (1979). Comprehensive description: Z. L. Chang, J. B. Martin, *Anal. Profiles Drug Subs.* **12**, 191-214 (1983).

Crystals from diisopropyl ether, mp 67°. $[\alpha]_D^{20}$ +66° (c = 1 in ethanol). uv max (isopropanol): 240 nm (ε 12200). Soly in water at 25°: 0.0045 mg/100 ml. Sol in chloroform, methanol, ethanol, propylene glycol, acetone. LD_{50} in mice, rats (mg/kg): 29.5, 14.8-24.3 i.v. (Janssen).

THERAP CAT: Hypnotic.

3882. Etomidoline. [21590-92-1] 2-Ethyl-2,3-dihydro-3-[[4-[2-(1-piperidinyl)ethoxy]phenyl]amino]-1*H*-isoindol-1-one; 2-ethyl-3-(β-piperidino-*p*-phenetidino)phthalimidine; K-2680; Smedolin. $C_{23}H_{29}N_3O_2$; mol wt 379.50. C 72.79%, H 7.70%, N 11.07%, O 8.43%. Anticholinergic antispasmodic. Prepn: N. Giraldi, V. Mariotti, **ZA 6705704**; *eidem*, **US 3624206** (1968, 1971 both to Erba). Quantitative evaluation in humans: G. Sacchetti *et al., Farmaco Ed. Prat.* **27**, 708 (1972). Spasmolytic properties: M. Takeda, *Oyo Yakuri* **7**, 903 (1973), *C.A.* **80**, 66678 (1974). Pharmacology: M. Takeda *et al., ibid.* 1073, *C.A.* **81**, 33285 (1974); T. Mukai *et al., Jpn. J. Pharmacol.* **31**, 147 (1981), *C.A.* **95**, 18068 (1981).

Crystals from ligroin, mp 106-107°. LD$_{50}$ in mice (mg/kg): 176 orally; 44.8 i.v. (Giraldi, Mariotti, 1971).

THERAP CAT: Antispasmodic.

3883. Etonitazene. [911-65-9] 2-[(4-Ethoxyphenyl)methyl]-*N,N*-diethyl-5-nitro-1*H*-benzimidazole-1-ethanamine; 1-[(2-diethylamino)ethyl]-2-(*p*-ethoxybenzyl)-5-nitrobenzimidazole; 2-*p*-ethoxybenzyl-1-(2-diethylaminoethyl)-5-nitrobenzimidazole. $C_{22}H_{28}N_4O_3$; mol wt 396.48. C 66.65%, H 7.12%, N 14.13%, O 12.11%. Prepn: Hunger *et al., Experientia* **13**, 400 (1957); Hoffmann *et al.*, **US 2935514** (1960 to Ciba). Crystal structure: C. Humblet *et al., Acta Crystallogr.* **B34**, 3828 (1978). Binds selectively to mu-opioid receptors: M. S. Moolten *et al., Life Sci.* **52**, PL199 (1993).

Hydrochloride. $C_{22}H_{28}N_4O_3 \cdot HCl$. mp 162-164°.
Note: This is a controlled substance (opiate): **21 CFR**, 1308.11.
THERAP CAT: Analgesic (narcotic).

3884. Etonogestrel. [54048-10-1] (17α)-13-Ethyl-17-hydroxy-11-methylene-18,19-dinorpregn-4-en-20-yn-3-one; 17-ethynyl-17β-hydroxy-18-methyl-11-methyleneestr-4-en-3-one; 3-ketodesogestrel; 3-oxodesogestrel; Org-3236; Implanon. $C_{22}H_{28}O_2$; mol wt 324.46. C 81.44%, H 8.70%, O 9.86%. Biologically active metabolite of desogestrel, *q.v.* Prepn: H. Hofmeister *et al.*, **EP 51762**; *eidem*, **US 4371529** (1982, 1983 both to Schering AG); H. Gao *et al., Steroids* **62**, 398 (1997). Series of articles on clinical experience: *Contraception* **58**, Suppl. 1, 75S-115S (1998). Clinical safety and efficacy: H. B. Croxatto *et al., Hum. Reprod.* **14**, 976 (1999). Review of clinical studies: J. E. Edwards, A. Moore, *Br. J. Fam. Plann.* **24**, 3-16 (1999).

mp 199-201°. [α]$_D$ +87.6°.
THERAP CAT: Progestogen; implantable contraceptive.

3885. Etoperidone. [52942-31-1] 2-[3-[4-(3-Chlorophenyl)-1-piperazinyl]propyl]-4,5-diethyl-2,4-dihydro-3*H*-1,2,4-triazol-3-one. $C_{19}H_{28}ClN_5O$; mol wt 377.91. C 60.39%, H 7.47%, Cl 9.38%, N 18.53%, O 4.23%. Psychotropic drug related structurally to trazodone, *q.v.* Prepn: G. Palazzo, **DE 2351739**; *idem*, **US 3857845** (both 1974 to Angelini). Pharmacology and acute toxicity: R. Lisciani *et al., Arzneim.-Forsch.* **28**, 417 (1978); M. T. Ramacci *et al., ibid.* **29**, 294 (1979). Clinical evaluation: P. Bertoletti, *G. Clin. Med.* **58**, 393 (1977). Teratology study: S. Barcellona *et al., Toxicology* **8**, 87 (1977). Acute cardiovascular toxicity study: R. Lisciani *et al., ibid.* **10**, 151 (1978).

Liq, bp$_{0.5}$ 230°.

Hydrochloride. [57775-22-1] AF-1191; ST-1191; Axiomin; Depracer; Etoran; Staff; Tropene. $C_{19}H_{28}ClN_5O \cdot HCl$; mol wt 414.37. Crystals from isopropanol, mp 197-198°. pH (2% aq soln): 4.1 ± 0.2. Sol in water, alc; slightly sol in chloroform. Practically insol in acetone, benzene, ether. LD$_{50}$ in mice, rats (mg/kg): 580, 720 orally; 72, 62 i.v.; 135, 120 i.p. (Lisciani).

THERAP CAT: Antidepressant.

3886. Etoposide. [33419-42-0] 9-[(4,6-*O*-Ethylidene-β-D-glucopyranosyl)oxy]-5,8,8a,9-tetrahydro-5-(4-hydroxy-3,5-dimethoxyphenyl)furo[3′,4′:6,7]naphtho[2,3-*d*]-1,3-dioxol-6(5a*H*)-one; 4′-demethylepipodophyllotoxin 9-[4,6-*O*-ethylidene-β-D-glucopyranoside]; EPEG; NSC-141540; VP-16-213; Lastet; Vepesid. $C_{29}H_{32}O_{13}$; mol wt 588.56. C 59.18%, H 5.48%, O 35.34%. DNA topoisomerase II inhibitor. Semi-synthetic deriv of podophyllotoxin, related structurally to teniposide, *q.q.v.* Prepn: C. Keller-Juslén *et al.*, **US 3524844** (1970 to Sandoz); *idem et al., J. Med. Chem.* **14**, 936 (1971). Teratogenicity and cytogenicity study: S. M. Sieber *et al., Teratology* **18**, 31 (1978). Review of pharmacokinetics and assay methods: P. I. Clark, M. L. Slevin, *Clin. Pharmacokinet.* **12**, 223-252 (1987). Comprehensive description: J. J. M. Holthuis *et al., Anal. Profiles Drug Subs.* **18**, 121-151 (1989). Review of pharmacology and clinical experience: J. D. Hainsworth, F. A. Greco, *Ann. Oncol.* **6**, 325-341 (1995); S. Joel, *Cancer Treat. Rev.* **22**, 179-221 (1996).

Crystals from methanol, mp 236-251°. [α]$_D^{20}$ −110.5° (c = 0.6 in chloroform). uv max (abs methanol): 283 nm (ε 4245). pKa 9.8. Very sol in methanol, chloroform; slightly sol in ethanol; sparingly sol in water.

Phosphate. [117091-64-2] BMY-40481; Etopophos. $C_{29}H_{33}O_{16}P$; mol wt 668.54. Review: A. H. I. Witterland *et al., Pharm. World Sci.* **18**, 163-170 (1996). Sol in water. Practically insol in organic solvents.

THERAP CAT: Antineoplastic.

3887. Etoricoxib. [202409-33-4] 5-Chloro-6′-methyl-3-[4-(methylsulfonyl)phenyl]-2,3′-bipyridine; 5-chloro-3-(4-methylsulfonyl)phenyl-2-(2-methyl-5-pyridinyl)pyridine; MK-663; MK-0663; Arcoxia. $C_{18}H_{15}ClN_2O_2S$; mol wt 358.84. C 60.25%, H 4.21%, Cl 9.88%, N 7.81%, O 8.92%, S 8.94%. Selective cyclooxygenase-2 (COX-2) inhibitor. Prepn: D. Dube *et al.*, **WO**

9803484; *eidem,* **US 5861419** (1998, 1999 both to Merck Frosst); R. W. Friesen *et al., Bioorg. Med. Chem. Lett.* **8**, 2777 (1998). Practical synthesis: I. W. Davies *et al., J. Org. Chem.* **65**, 8415 (2000). HPLC determn in urine and plasma: C. Z. Matthews *et al., J. Chromatogr. B* **751**, 237 (2001). Pharmacology: D. Riendeau *et al., J. Pharmacol. Exp. Ther.* **296**, 558 (2001); A. Dallob *et al., J. Clin. Pharmacol.* **43**, 573 (2003). Clinical comparison with indomethacin in acute gouty arthritis: H. R. Schumacher, Jr. *et al., Br. Med. J.* **324**, 1488 (2002). Clinical trial in rheumatoid arthritis: A. K. Matsumoto *et al., J. Rheumatol.* **29**, 1623 (2002); in osteoarthritis: S. P. Curtis *et al., BMC Musculoskel. Disord.* **6**, 58 (2005); in ankylosing spondylitis: D. van der Heijde *et al., Arthritis Rheum.* **52**, 1205 (2005). Gastrointestinal safety profile in inflammatory bowel diseases: Y. El Miedany *et al., Am. J. Gastroenterol.* **101**, 311 (2006). Review of pharmacology and clinical development: P. Patrignani *et al., Expert Opin. Pharmacother.* **4**, 265-284 (2003).

White solid, mp 127-128°. pKa 4.5. uv max (acetonitrile-phosphate buffer): 238, 280 nm.

THERAP CAT: Anti-inflammatory; analgesic.

3888. Etorphine. [14521-96-1] [5α,7α(*R*)]-4,5-Epoxy-3-hydroxy-6-methoxy-α,17-dimethyl-α-propyl-6,14-ethenomorphinan-7-methanol; tetrahydro-7α-(1-hydroxy-1-methylbutyl)-6,14-*endo*-ethenooripavine; 7,8-dihydro-7α-[1(*R*)-hydroxy-1-methylbutyl]-*O⁶*-methyl-6,14-*endo*-ethenomorphine; 7α-[1(*R*)-hydroxy-1-methylbutyl]-6,14-*endo*-ethenotetrahydrooripavine; 19-propylorvinol; tetrahydro-7α-(2-hydroxy-2-pentyl)-6,14-*endo*-ethenooripavine. $C_{25}H_{33}NO_4$; mol wt 411.53. C 72.96%, H 8.08%, N 3.40%, O 15.55%. Narcotic analgesic. Prepn: **BE 618392**; K. W. Bentley, **GB 937214** (1962, 1963 both to J. F. MacFarlan); and structure: K. W. Bentley, D. G. Hardy, *Proc. Chem. Soc. London* **1963**, 220. Improved prepn: W. R. Hydro, **US 3763167** (1973 to U.S. Army). Determn by HPLC: I. Jane, A. McKinnon, *J. Chromatogr.* **323**, 19 (1985). Analgesic activity: G. F. Blane, *J. Pharm. Pharmacol.* **19**, 367 (1967). Pharmacology: Lister, *ibid.* **16**, 364 (1964). Use as tranquilizer in dogs: J. L. Crooks *et al., Vet. Rec.* **87**, 498 (1970); M. Grange *et al., Rev. Med. Vet.* **124**, 899 (1973); in large animals: A. M. Harthoorn, *J. Am. Vet. Med. Assoc.* **149**, 875 (1966); B. T. Alford *et al., ibid.* **164**, 702 (1974).

White crystals from aqueous ethoxyethanol, mp 214-217°. (7β-isomer, melts at 280°).

Hydrochloride. M-99. $C_{25}H_{33}NO_4$.HCl; mol wt 447.99. mp 266-267°. (7β-isomer hydrochloride, dec at 290°).

Hydrochloride in combination with acepromazine. Immobilon.

3-Acetate. Acetorphine; *O³*-acetyl-7,8-dihydro-7α-[1(*R*)-hydroxy-1-methylbutyl]-*O⁶*-methyl-6,14-*endo*-ethenomorphine; 3-*O*-acetyl-7α-[1(*R*)-hydroxy-1-methylbutyl]-6,14-*endo*-ethenotetrahydrooripavine; 3-*O*-acetyl-17-propylorvinol. $C_{27}H_{35}NO_5$. Crystals from methanol, mp 195°.

3-Acetate hydrochloride. M-183. $C_{27}H_{35}NO_5$.HCl; mol wt 490.03. mp 206°.

Note: Acetorphine and etorphine are controlled substances (opium derivatives): **21 CFR**, 1308.11. Etorphine hydrochloride is a controlled substance (opiate): **21 CFR**, 1308.12.

Caution: Use with extreme care; very small amounts may bring about respiratory paralysis and death: D. W. Upson, *Upson's Handbook of Clinical Veterinary Pharmacology* (VM Publishing, Bonner Springs, 1980) pp 380-381.

THERAP CAT (VET): Used to immobilize large animals.

3889. Etoxadrol. [28189-85-7] (2*S*)-2-[(2*S*,4*S*)]-2-(2-Ethyl-2-phenyl-1,3-dioxolan-4-yl)piperidine; (+)-2-(2-Ethyl-2-phenyl-1,3-dioxolan-4-yl)piperidine; 2-ethyl-2-phenyl-4-(2-piperidyl)-1,3-dioxolane. $C_{16}H_{23}NO_2$; mol wt 261.36. C 73.53%, H 8.87%, N 5.36%, O 12.24%. Prepn of *dl*-form: Hardie *et al., J. Med. Chem.* **9**, 127 (1966); Hardie, Halverstadt, **US 3262938** (1966 to Cutter Labs). Resolution of the α-racemates: Allen *et al.,* **DE 2001616** (1970 to Cutter Labs), *C.A.* **74**, 13129b (1971). Pharmacological studies: Traber *et al., J. Pharmacol. Exp. Ther.* **175**, 395 (1970); Hidalgo *et al., Anesth. Analg.* **50**, 231 (1971); Kelly *et al., ibid.* 262.

(+)-Hydrochloride. [23239-37-4] CL-1848C; Thoxan. $C_{16}H_{23}NO_2$.HCl; mol wt 297.82. Crystals from isopropanol, mp 221.5-222°. $[\alpha]_D^{25}$ +16.63°.

THERAP CAT: Anesthetic (intravenous).

3890. Etoxazole. [153233-91-1] 2-(2,6-Difluorophenyl)-4-[4-(1,1-dimethylethyl)-2-ethoxyphenyl]-4,5-dihydrooxazole; 4-(4-*tert*-butyl-2-ethoxyphenyl)-2-(2,6-difluorophenyl)-4,5-dihydrooxazole; 2-(2,6-difluorophenyl)-4-(2-ethoxy-4-*tert*-butylphenyl)-2-oxazoline; YI-5301; Baroque; TetraSan; Zeal. $C_{21}H_{23}F_2NO_2$; mol wt 359.41. C 70.18%, H 6.45%, F 10.57%, N 3.90%, O 8.90%. Insect growth regulator; molting inhibitor for control of mites and aphids on fruits, vegetables and ornamentals. Prepn: J. Suzuki *et al.,* **WO 9322297**; *eidem,* **US 5478855** (1993, 1995 both to Yashima); and ovicidal and insecticidal activity: *idem et al., J. Pestic. Sci.* **26**, 215 (2001). Comprehensive description: T. Ishida *et al., Brighton Crop Prot. Conf. - Pests Dis.* **1994**, 37-44. Efficacy as a tick control agent: Y. Tamura *et al., Med. Entomol. Zool.* **55**, 303 (2004).

Colorless crystals from hexane, mp 101-102°. Vapor pressure (25°): 2.18×10^{-6} Pa. Log P (octanol/water): 5.59 at 25°. Soly at 20° (g/l solvent): water 75.4×10^{-6}; methanol 100; acetone 450; THF 850; *n*-hexane 15. LD_{50} in rats (mg/kg): >5000 orally; >2000 dermally. LC_{50} (96 hr) in Japanese carp: 0.89 mg/l (Ishida).

USE: Acaricide.

3891. Etozolin. [73-09-6] [3-Methyl-4-oxo-5-(1-piperidinyl)-2-thiazolidinylidene]acetic acid ethyl ester; 2-carbethoxymethylene-3-methyl-5-piperidino-4-thiazolidone; 3-methyl-4-oxo-5-piperidino-$\Delta^{2,\alpha}$-thiazolidineacetic acid ethyl ester; Gö-687; W-2900A; Elkapin. $C_{13}H_{20}N_2O_3S$; mol wt 284.37. C 54.91%, H 7.09%, N 9.85%, O 16.88%, S 11.28%. A member of a new class of heterocyclic compounds, the 2-methylenethiazolidones; a diuretic with choleretic properties. Prepn: Satzinger, *Ann.* **665**, 150 (1963); **US 3072653** (1963 to Warner-Lambert). Pharmacology: O. Heidenreich *et al., Arzneim.-Forsch.* **14**, 1242 (1964). Series of articles on activity, metabolism and toxicology: G. Satzinger *et al., ibid.* **27**, 1742-1817 (1977); M. Herrmann *et al., ibid.* 1745.

Crystals from methanol, mp 140°. uv max (methanol): 283, 243 nm (log ε 4.32, 4.0). LD$_{50}$ in male mice, rats (mg/kg): 1210, 1575 i.p.; in male, female mice, rats (mg/kg): 8670, 9360, 11040, 10250 orally (Herrmann).

Hydrochloride. C$_{13}$H$_{20}$N$_2$O$_3$S.HCl. Crystals, mp 158-159°.
Free acid. Ozolinone; Gödecke 3282. C$_{11}$H$_{16}$N$_2$O$_3$S.
THERAP CAT: Diuretic.

3892. Etretinate. [54350-48-0] (*all-E*)-9-(4-Methoxy-2,3,6-trimethylphenyl)-3,7-dimethyl-2,4,6,8-nonatetraenoic acid ethyl ester; Ro-10-9359; Tegison; Tigason. C$_{23}$H$_{30}$O$_3$; mol wt 354.48. C 77.93%, H 8.53%, O 13.54%. Aromatic analog of retinoic acid, *q.v.* Prepn: W. Bollag *et al., DE 2414619; eidem,* **US 4105681** and **US 4215215** (1974, 1978, 1980 all to Hoffmann-La Roche). Effects on skin metabolism: W. P. Raab, B. M. Gmeiner, *Arch. Dermatol. Res.* **256,** 247 (1976). Toxicity study in organ culture: D. R. Bard, I. Lasnitzki, *Br. J. Cancer* **35,** 110 (1977). Pharmacokinetics: R. Haenni, *Dermatologica* **157,** Suppl, 5 (1978). Mutation study: H. J. Juhl *et al., Mutat. Res.* **58,** 317 (1978). HPLC determn in plasma: R. Haenni *et al., J. Chromatogr.* **162,** 615 (1979). Toxicology, carcinogenicity and teratogenicity study: J. J. Kamm, *J. Am. Acad. Dermatol.* **6,** 652 (1982). Clinical evaluation in psoriatic arthritis: M. L. Ciompi *et al., Int. J. Tissue React.* **10,** 25 (1988). *Review:* H. Mayer *et al., Experientia* **34,** 1105-1119 (1978). Review of pharmacology and therapeutic efficacy: A. Ward *et al., Drugs* **26,** 9-43 (1983); of clinical pharmacology: A. Vahlquist, O. Rollman, *Dermatologica* **175,** Suppl. 1, 20-27 (1987). Book: *The Retinoids* Vol. **1-2,** M. B. Sporn *et al.,* Eds. (Academic Press, New York, 1984).

Crystals, mp 104-105°. LD$_{50}$ in mice (1 day): >4000 mg/kg i.p. (Bollag). LD$_{50}$ (20 day) in mice, rats (mg/kg): 1176, >2000 i.p.; >2000, >4000 orally (Kamm).

Free acid *see* Acitretin.
THERAP CAT: Antipsoriatic.

3893. Etrimfos. [38260-54-7] *O*-(6-Ethoxy-2-ethyl-4-pyrimidinyl)phosphorothioic acid *O,O*-dimethyl ester; *O,O*-dimethyl *O*-(2-ethyl-4-ethoxypyrimidinyl)-6-thionophosphate; SAN-197; Ekamet; Satisfar. C$_{10}$H$_{17}$N$_2$O$_4$PS; mol wt 292.29. C 41.09%, H 5.86%, N 9.58%, O 21.90%, P 10.60%, S 10.97%. Organophosphorous insecticide with stomach and contact activity against pests of fruit and vegetable crops. Prepn: K. Milzner, F. Reisser, **DE 2209554;** *eidem,* **US 3862188** (1972, 1975 both to Sandoz). Physical properties and activity: H. J. Knutti, F. Reisser, *Proc. 8th Br. Insectic. Fungic. Conf.* **2,** 675 (1975). Residue analysis and toxicity study: M. C. Bowman *et al., J. Agric. Food Chem.* **26,** 35 (1978). Metabolism in plants: M. Akram *et al., ibid.* 925. Field studies of formulations: D. A. Collins, D. A. Cook, *Crop Prot.* **17,** 521 (1998). Review of analytical methods: J. C. Karapally *et al., Anal. Methods Pestic. Plant Growth Regul.* **11,** 125-138 (1980).

Colorless oil, slight characteristic odor. mp −3.35°. d 1.195; n_D^{20} 1.5068. Vapor pressure at 20°: 6.5 × 10^{-5} mm Hg. Soly in

water at 23-24°: 40 ppm. Miscible with ethanol, dimethyl sulfoxide, ethyl acetate, acetone, ether, chloroform, xylene, hexane. LD$_{50}$ in male rats (mg/kg): 1800, 437 orally; LC$_{50}$ in carp (mg/l): 13.6 (48 hr); 13.3 (96 hr) (Knutti).
USE: Agricultural insecticide.

3894. β-Eucaine. [500-34-5] 2,2,6-Trimethyl-4-piperidinol benzoate (ester); α-4-benzoyloxy-2,2,6-trimethylpiperidine; α-vinyldiacetonalkamine benzoate; benzamine; betacaine; eucaine B. C$_{15}$H$_{21}$NO$_2$; mol wt 247.33. C 72.84%, H 8.56%, N 5.66%, O 12.94%. Prepn from lower melting form (α-form) of 2,2,6-trimethyl-4-piperidinol and benzoyl chloride: Harries, *Ann.* **417,** 107, *see* p 175 (1918). Stereochemistry: King, *J. Chem. Soc.* **125,** 41 (1924); Stenlake, *J. Pharm. Pharmacol.* **6,** 164 (1954). Configuration: Perks, Russell, *ibid.* **19,** 318 (1966). Toxicity data: Hirschfelder, *Physiol. Rev.* **12,** 262 (1932).

Crystals from petr ether, mp 70-71° (corr). MLD in frogs, rabbits (mg/kg): 1300, 400-500 s.c.; in rats, cats (mg/kg): 15-25, 10.0-12.5 i.v.; in guinea pigs (mg/kg): 310 s.c., 180 i.p., 30 i.v. (Hirschfelder).

Hydrochloride. Crystals from water, mp 277-279° (corr). pKa 9.4. One gram dissolves in 30 ml water, 35 ml alcohol, 6 ml chloroform; more sol in boiling water or boiling alcohol. Aq soln is neutral to litmus.
d-Form. Crystals from petr ether, mp 57-58° (corr).
d-Form hydrochloride. [α]$_D$ +11.5° (water).
l-Form. Crystals from petr ether, mp 57-58° (corr).
l-Form hydrochloride. Crystals, mp 244-245° (corr). [α]$_D$ −11.3° (water).

THERAP CAT: Anesthetic (local).
THERAP CAT (VET): Has been used as a local anesthetic.

3895. Eucalyptol. [470-82-6] 1,3,3-Trimethyl-2-oxabicyclo[2.2.2]octane; 1,8-epoxy-*p*-menthane; cineole; cajeputol. C$_{10}$H$_{18}$O; mol wt 154.25. C 77.87%, H 11.76%, O 10.37%. The chief constituent of oil of eucalyptus: Cloez, *Ann.* **154,** 372 (1870); Berry, *Australas. J. Pharm.* **1929,** 203; from wormwood oil: Wallach, Brass, *Ann.* **225,** 291 (1884). Identity with cajeputol: Wallach, *ibid.* 314. Identity with cineole: Wallach, *ibid.* 314. Identity with cineole: Jahns, *Ber.* **17,** 2941 (1884). Structure: Wallach, *Ann.* **291,** 342 (1896). Biosynthesis: Birch *et al., Tetrahedron Letters,* no. 3, 1 (1959). Activity: Jori *et al., Eur. J. Pharmacol.* **9,** 362 (1970). Cockroach repellent activity: T. H. Maugh, *Science* **218,** 278 (1982).

Colorless liquid; camphor-like odor; spicy, cooling taste. d$_{25}^{25}$ 0.921-0.923. bp 176-177°. mp 1.5°. n_D^{20} 1.455-1.460. Flash pt, closed cup: 118°F (48°C). Practically insol in water; miscible with alcohol, chloroform, ether, glacial acetic acid, oils.
USE: Pharmaceutic aid (flavor).

3896. Eucalyptus. Genus of evergreen trees of the Family *Myrtaceae,* having aromatic blue-grey leaves that yield a characteristic essential oil. *Habit.* Australia, cultivated in subtropical regions of Europe, Africa, Asia and U.S. More than 700 species are known; the Australian blue-gum, *Eucalyptus globulus* Labill., is the most predominant and said to be richest in essential oil. *Constit.* 0.5-3.5% volatile oil, resins, tannins, polyphenolic acids, and flavonoids such as quercetin, rutin, eucalyptin. Review of botany, cultivation and uses: M. Forrest, *Biologist* **47,** 139-142 (2000); of pharmacology and medicinal uses: A. Y. Leung, S. Foster, *Encyclopedia of Common Natural Ingredients,* (Wiley-Interscience, Hoboken, 2nd

Ed., 2003) pp 232-234; J. Gruenwald *et al.*, *PDR for Herbal Medicines* (Medical Economics, Montvale, 3rd Ed., 2004) pp 293-297.

Volatile oil. [8000-48-4] Oil of eucalyptus. Obtained by steam distillation from fresh leaves of *E. globulus*. *Constit.* 70-80% Eucalyptol (1,8-cineole), α-pinene, *d*-limonene, *p*-cymene, α-phellandrene, 1-α-terpineol. Description: E. Guenther, *The Essential Oils* vol. **4** (van Nostrand, New York, 1950) pp 437-525. Colorless to pale yellow liquid; characteristic camphoraceous odor; pungent, spicy, cooling taste. d_{25}^{25} 0.905-0.925. n_D^{20} 1.458-1.470. Almost insol in water; sol in 5 vols 70% alcohol. *Keep well closed, cool and protected from light.*

USE: Wood for timber, pulp, fuel, charcoal; cut foliage in floral arrangements. Oil as fragrance component in soaps, creams, lotions and as flavoring agent in pharmaceuticals, toothpastes, mouthwashes.

THERAP CAT: Oil as expectorant, antiseptic, externally for rheumatism.

3897. Eucatropine. [100-91-4] α-Hydroxybenzeneacetic acid 1,2,2,6-tetramethyl-4-piperidinyl ester; mandelic acid β-1,2,2,-6-tetramethyl-4-piperidyl ester; β-4-hydroxy-1,2,2,6-tetramethyl-piperidine mandelic acid ester; *N*-methyl-β-vinyldiacetonalkamine mandelate; β-4-mandeloyloxy-1,2,2,6-tetramethylpiperidine; β-1,-2,2,6-tetramethyl-4-piperidinol mandelate; Euphthalmine. $C_{17}H_{25}NO_3$; mol wt 291.39. C 70.07%, H 8.65%, N 4.81%, O 16.47%. Anticholinergic. Prepn from higher melting form (β-form) of 1,2,-2,6-tetramethyl-4-piperidinol and mandelic acid: Harries, *Ann.* **296**, 328 (1897); Kipping, *J. Chem. Soc.* **123**, 3115 (1923). Description: Harries, *Ber.* **31**, 665 (1898).

dl-**Form.** Prisms from petr ether sinters at 108°, mp 113°. Practically insol in cold water, more sol in hot water; readily sol in organic solvents other than petr ether.

dl-**Form hydrochloride.** Crystals from alcohol + ether, sinters at 181°, mp 183-184°. Very sol in water; sol in alcohol (1 g dissolves in 2 ml boiling alcohol), in chloroform. Practically insol in ether. Aq solns are neutral to litmus.

THERAP CAT: Mydriatic.

3898. Eugenol. [97-53-0] 2-Methoxy-4-(2-propenyl)-phenol; 4-allyl-2-methoxyphenol; allylguaiacol; eugenic acid; caryophyllic acid. $C_{10}H_{12}O_2$; mol wt 164.20. C 73.15%, H 7.37%, O 19.49%. Obtained from many natural sources: *Beilstein* vol. **6**, 961. Prepn: Claisen, *Ann.* **418**, 113 (1919); from oil of cloves: Waterman, Priester, *Rec. Trav. Chim.* **48**, 1272 (1929). Toxicity study: E. C. Hagan *et al.*, *Toxicol. Appl. Pharmacol.* **7**, 18 (1965).

Colorless or pale yellow liquid, bp 255°. Darkens and thickens on exposure to air. Odor of cloves; spicy, pungent taste. mp −9.2 to −9.1°. d_4^{20} 1.0664. n_D^{20} 1.5410. Practically insol in water. Misc with alcohol, chloroform, ether, oils. One ml dissolves in 2 ml 70% alcohol; sol in glacial acetic acid, in aq fixed alkali hydroxide solns. Ferric chloride, potassium permanganate. LD_{50} in rats, mice (mg/kg): 2680, 3000 orally (Hagan).

Benzoate. *O*-Benzoyleugenol. $C_{17}H_{16}O_3$. Crystals, mp 69-70°. bp 360°. Freely sol in benzene, chloroform, ether, hot alcohol. Practically insol in water.

USE: In perfumery instead of oil of cloves; manuf vanillin. As insect attractant.

THERAP CAT: Analgesic (dental).

3899. Euonymus. Wahoo; Indian arrow wood; bitter ash; burning bush; strawberry tree; spindle tree. Dried root bark of *Evonymus atropurpureus* Jacq., *Celastraceae*. *Habit.* U.S., Ontario to Florida east of Mississippi. *Constit.* Euonymol —an alcohol; euonysterol, atropurpurin, asparagine, citrullol, dulcite; malic, citric and tartaric acids.

THERAP CAT: Cathartic, diuretic.

3900. Euparin. [532-48-9] 1-[6-Hydroxy-2-(1-methylethenyl)-5-benzofuranyl]ethanone; 6-hydroxy-2-isopropenyl-5-benzo-furanyl methyl ketone; 5-acetyl-6-hydroxy-2-isopropenylbenzofuran. $C_{13}H_{12}O_3$; mol wt 216.23. C 72.21%, H 5.59%, O 22.20%. From roots of *Eupatorium purpureum* L., *E. cannabinum* L., *Compositae:* Kamthong, Robertson, *J. Chem. Soc.* **1939**, 925; Jermanowska, *C.A.* **48**, 5848h (1954). Structure: Kamthong, Robertson, *J. Chem. Soc.* **1939**, 933. Synthesis: Ramachandran *et al.*, *J. Org. Chem.* **28**, 2744 (1963). *Review:* Gizycki, *Pharmazie* **6**, 686 (1951).

Yellow needles from alcohol, mp 121-122°. uv max (ethanol): 263, 358 nm (ε 34400, 5900). Sol in alcohol, benzene, chloroform, ether. Practically insol in water, alkali.

Acetate. $C_{15}H_{14}O_4$. Prisms from petr ether, mp 80°.

O-**Methyl deriv.** *O*-Methyleuparin; 2-isopropenyl-6-methoxy-5-benzofuranyl methyl ketone. $C_{14}H_{14}O_3$. Needles from dil alcohol, mp 76-77°. Sol in the usual organic solvents.

3901. Eupatorin. [855-96-9] 5-Hydroxy-2-(3-hydroxy-4-methoxyphenyl)-6,7-dimethoxy-4*H*-1-benzopyran-4-one; 3′,5-di-hydroxy-4′,6,7-trimethoxyflavone. $C_{18}H_{16}O_7$; mol wt 344.32. C 62.79%, H 4.68%, O 32.53%. Isoln from *Eupatorium semiserratum* DC., *Compositae* and structure: Kupchan *et al.*, *J. Pharm. Sci.* **54**, 929 (1965).

Crystals from dioxane + water, mp 196-198°. uv max (alcohol): 243, 254, 274, 342 nm (ε 17400, 19300, 19800, 27700).

3902. Eupatorium. Boneset; thoroughwort. Flowering tops and dried leaves of *Eupatorium perfoliatum* L., *Compositae*. *Habit.* Canada to Florida and west to Texas and Nebraska. *Constit.* Eupatorin, volatile oil, resin, tannin, sugar, inulin, wax.

3903. Euphorbia. Pill-bearing spurge; snake-weed; cat's hair; Queensland asthma weed; flowery-headed spurge. Dried herb of *Euphorbia hirta* L. or *E. pilulifera* L., *Euphorbiaceae*. *Habit.* Queensland (Australia), India, widely distributed in tropical countries. *Constit.* Several resins, an unstable glucoside.

3904. Europium. [7440-53-1] Eu; at. wt 151.964; at. no. 63; valences 2, 3. A lanthanide; belongs to cerium group of rare earth metals. Naturally occurring isotopes (mass numbers): 151 (47.8%); 153 (52.2%); known artificial radioactive isotopes: 138-150; 152; 154-160. Abundance in earth's crust: 1.06-2.1 ppm. Commercially important sources are the rare earth minerals monazite and bastnaesite; also found in gadolinite. Has been detected spectroscopically in the sun and in certain stars. Discovered and prepd as the oxide: Demarçay, *Compt. Rend.* **122**, 728 (1896); **130**, 1019, 1469 (1900); **132**, 1484 (1901). Separation: Spedding *et al.*, *J. Am. Chem. Soc.* **76**, 2557 (1954); by paper chromatography: Lederer, *Nature* **176**, 462 (1953). Toxicity study: Haley, *J. Pharm. Sci.* **54**, 663 (1965). Reviews of prepn, properties and compds: *The Rare Earths*, F. H. Spedding, A. H. Daane, Eds. (Krieger, Huntington, N.Y., 1971, reprint of 1961 ed.) 641 pp; S. P. Sinha, *Europium*

(Springer, New York, 1967) 164 pp; Hulet, Bode, "Separation Chemistry of the Lanthanides and Transplutonium Actinides" in *MTP Int. Rev. Sci.: Inorg. Chem., Ser. One* **vol. 7,** K. W. Bagnall, Ed. (University Park Press, Baltimore, 1972) pp 1-45; Moeller, "The Lanthanides" in *Comprehensive Inorganic Chemistry* **vol. 4,** J. C. Bailar, Jr. *et al.,* Eds. (Pergamon Press, Oxford, 1973) pp 1-101; F. H. Spedding in *Kirk-Othmer Encyclopedia of Chemical Technology* **vol. 19** (John Wiley & Sons, New York, 3rd ed., 1982) pp 833-854; *Chemistry of the Elements,* N. N. Greenwood, A. Earnshaw, Eds. (Pergamon Press, New York, 1984) pp 1423-1449. Brief review of properties: G. T. Seaborg, *Radiochim. Acta* **61,** 115-122 (1993).

Body-centered cubic crystal lattice; d 5.244; mp 826°. bp 1429°. Heat of fusion: 9.221 kJ/mol. Heat of sublimation (25°): 144.7 kJ/mol. Sol in liq ammonia. Shows two reduction potentials −0.710 and −2.510 v. (referred to a normal calomel electrode): Noddack, Brukl, *Angew. Chem.* **50,** 362 (1937); gives two definite series of salts, in one the metal is divalent, and in the other it is trivalent.

Sesquioxide. Europia. Eu_2O_3. Pink powder, d 7.42, prepd by heating the hydroxide, nitrate, oxalate or sulfate at 1600°. The oxide of the divalent metal is prepd by reduction of the sesquioxide at elevated temp.

Hydroxide. $Eu(OH)_3$. Prepd by adding ammonia or an alkali hydroxide to a soln of an europic salt.

Europic chloride. $EuCl_3$. Greenish-yellow needles; mp 623° in nitrogen (in a closed tube), d^{35} 4.471, prepd by passing sulfur chloride over the heated oxide at 200-500°. LD_{50} of trichloride in mice: 550 mg/kg i.p.; 5 g/kg orally (Haley).

Europous chloride. $EuCl_2$. Prepd by reduction of $EuCl_3$ with hydrogen at 600°. White amorphous powder, sol in water.

Europic sulfate. $Eu_2(SO_4)_3$. Octahydrate, a pinkish cryst solid, prepd by dissolving the oxide in sulfuric acid. Soly in water: 2.56 parts per 100 parts at 20°, 1.93 parts per 100 parts at 40°. On heating at 375° yields the anhydr sulfate.

Europic nitrate. $Eu(NO_3)_3$. Hexahydrate, mp 85° in its water of crystallization (sealed tube). LD_{50} in rats (mg/kg): 210 i.p.; >5000 orally (Haley).

Europous sulfate. $EuSO_4$. Colorless crystals. Insol in water and in dil acids. Prepd by electrolytic reduction of europic salts.

USE: The salts in cathode ray tube coatings for color television receivers. Eu has a very high cross-section for the capture of thermal neutrons which is of value in the construction of electric atomic power stations. Organic derivs as shift reagents in NMR spectroscopy: C. C. Hinckley, *J. Am. Chem. Soc.* **91,** 5160 (1969); R. E. Sievers, *Nuclear Magnetic Resonance Shift Reagents* (Academic Press, New York, 1973).

3905. Evan's Blue. [314-13-6] 6,6′-[(3,3′-Dimethyl[1,1′-biphenyl]-4,4′-diyl)bis(azo)]bis[4-amino-5-hydroxy-1,3-naphthalenedisulfonic acid] tetrasodium salt; C.I. Direct Blue 53; 4,4′-bis[7-(1-amino-8-hydroxy-2,4-disulfo)naphthylazo]-3,3′-bitolyl tetrasodium salt; C.I. 23860; T-1824; Azovan Blue. $C_{34}H_{24}N_6Na_4O_{14}S_4$; mol wt 960.81. C 42.50%, H 2.52%, N 8.75%, Na 9.57%, O 23.31%, S 13.35%. Prepd by coupling 1 mol of diazotized *o*-tolidine with 2 mols of Chicago acid (1-amino-8-naphthol-2,4-disulfonic acid): **DE 35341; DE 38802** *Frdl.* **1,** 469, 488 (1877-1887); **DE 3949; DE 57327; DE 75469** *Frdl.* **3,** 685, 687, 690 (1890-1894); Hartwell, Fieser, *Org. Synth.* **coll. vol. II,** 145 (1943). Diagnostic use: M. H. Nielsen, N. C. Nielsen, *Scand. J. Clin. Lab. Invest.* **14,** 605 (1962); O. Linderkamp *et al., Eur. J. Pediatr.* **125,** 135 (1977).

Blue crystals with bronze to green luster. Sol in water, alcohol, acids, alkalies. Indicator changing color near pH 10. Destroyed by strong oxidizing and reducing agents and precipitated from soln by strong concns of neutral salts. Rather stable in aq soln, and may be autoclaved at 15 lbs pressure for 30 min. Dye made up in physiological saline should not be autoclaved.

THERAP CAT: Diagnostic aid (blood volume determination).

3906. Evening Primrose Oil. EPO. Seed oil of the evening primrose, *Oenothera biennis* L., *Onagraceae,* which contains approx 72% linoleic acid and approx 9% γ-linolenic acid, *q.q.v.,* as the two main constituents. Unique among vegetable oils because of its high content of γ-linolenic acid. Effect on prostaglandin biosynthesis in rats: B. A. Schölkens *et al., Prostaglandins Leukotrienes Med.* **8,** 273 (1982). Clinical studies in atopic eczema: C. R. Lovell *et al., Lancet* **1,** 278 (1981); S. Wright, J. L. Burton, *ibid.* **2,** 1120 (1982); P. L. Biagi *et al., Drugs Exp. Clin. Res.* **14,** 285 (1988). Ingredient in cosmetics for aging skin: J. P. Marty, **DE 3447618** (1985 to Roussel-UCLAF), *C.A.* **103,** 146984r (1985). Brief review including discussion of uses: A. J. Barber, *Pharm. J.* **240,** 723-725 (1988).

Clear, golden yellow oil. d_{15} 0.9283. n_D^{25} 1.4782. Sapon. no. 287.8. Iodine no. 154.8.

Note: Evening primrose oil products include **Efamol, Efamast, Epogam**.

USE: Dietary supplement.

THERAP CAT: In treatment of atopic eczema and mastaglia.

3907. Everolimus. [159351-69-6] 42-*O*-(2-Hydroxyethyl)-rapamycin; 40-*O*-(2-hydroxyethyl)rapamycin; RAD-001; SDZ RAD; Certican. $C_{53}H_{83}NO_{14}$; mol wt 958.22. C 66.43%, H 8.73%, N 1.46%, O 23.38%. Macrolide immunosuppressant; derivative of rapamycin, *q.v.* Inhibits cytokine-mediated lymphocyte proliferation. Prepn: S. Cottens, R. Sedrani, **WO 9409010;** *eidem,* **US 5665772** (1994, 1997 both to Sandoz). Pharmacology: W. Schuler *et al., Transplantation* **64,** 36 (1997). Whole blood determn by LC/MS: N. Brignol *et al., Rapid Commun. Mass Spectrom.* **15,** 898 (2001); by HPLC: S. Baldelli *et al., J. Chromatogr. B* **816,** 99 (2005). Clinical pharmacokinetics in combination with cyclosporine: J. M. Kovarik *et al., Clin. Pharmacol. Ther.* **69,** 48 (2001). Clinical study in prevention of cardiac-allograft vasculopathy: H. J. Eisen *et al., N. Engl. J. Med.* **349,** 847 (2003). *Review:* F. J. Dumont *et al., Curr. Opin. Invest. Drugs* **2,** 1220-1234 (2001); B. Nashan, *Ther. Drug Monit.* **24,** 53-58 (2002).

THERAP CAT: Immunosuppressant.

3908. Evodiamine. [518-17-2] 8,13,13b,14-Tetrahydro-14-methylindolo[2′,3′:3,4]pyrido[2,1-*b*]quinazolin-5(7*H*)-one. $C_{19}H_{17}N_3O$; mol wt 303.36. C 75.23%, H 5.65%, N 13.85%, O 5.27%. From *Evodia rutaecarpa* Hook. & Thoms and bark of *Zanthoxylum rhetsa* DC., *Rutaceae:* Y. Asahina, K. Kashiwaki, *J. Pharm. Soc. Jpn.* **1915,** 1293, *C.A.* **10,** 607 (1916); Gopinath *et al., Tetrahedron* **8,** 293 (1960). Structure: Y. Asahina *J. Pharm. Soc. Jpn.* **1924,** 1; Ohta, *J. Pharm. Soc. Jpn.* **65,** 15 (1945), *C.A.* **45,** 5697 (1951). Synthesis: Asahina, Ohta, *Ber.* **61B,** 319 (1928); T. Kametani *et al., J. Am. Chem. Soc.* **98,** 6186 (1976); *eidem, Heterocycles* **4,** 23 (1976). Biosynthesis: M. Yamazaki *et al., Tetrahedron Lett.* **1966,** 3221; **1967,** 3317. Mass spec.: J. Tamas *et al., Acta Chim. Acad. Sci. Hung.* **89,** 85 (1976).

Yellow plates from alc, mp 278°. $[\alpha]_D^{15}$ +352° (acetone); $[\alpha]_D$ +440° (chloroform). uv max (acetonitrile): 272, 280, 291, 335 nm (log ε 4.06, 4.02, 3.90, 3.30). Sol in acetone; slightly sol in alcohol, ether, chloroform. Practically insol in water, petr ether, benzene. Does not seem to form salts.

3909. Exalamide. [53370-90-4] 2-(Hexyloxy)benzamide; HBA; Hyperan. $C_{13}H_{19}NO_2$; mol wt 221.30. C 70.56%, H 8.65%, N 6.33%, O 14.46%. Deriv of salicylamide, q.v. Prepn: E. M. Bevin et al., J. Pharm. Pharmacol. **4**, 872 (1952); F. J. MacRae, D. E. Seymour, **GB 726786** (1955 to Herts Pharm.), C.A. **50**, 5751i (1956); L. V. Coates et al., J. Pharm. Pharmacol. **9**, 855 (1957). Metabolism: Y. Kanaiwa et al., Yakugaku Zasshi **95**, 411 (1975), C.A. **83**, 71428v (1975). General pharmacologic effects: R. Inoki et al., Oyo Yakuri **10**, 165 (1975), C.A. **88**, 115369 (1976). Comparative study of antifungal efficacy vs clinical isolates: T. Kusunoki, S. Harada, J. Dermatol. **11**, 227 (1984).

Cryst from ethanol, mp 71°. Sol in methanol, acetone, chloroform, benzene. Slightly sol in ether. Practically insol in water.

THERAP CAT: Antifungal (topical).

3910. Exaltolide®. [106-02-5] Oxacyclohexadecan-2-one; 15-hydroxypentadecanoic acid ε-lactone. $C_{15}H_{28}O_2$; mol wt 240.38. C 74.95%, H 11.74%, O 13.31%. Musk compd responsible for the pleasant odor of angelica root oil. Synthesis: Ruzicka, Stoll, Helv. Chim. Acta **11**, 1159 (1928); Carnduff et al., Chem. Ind. (London) **1960**, 559; Dhenkne et al., J. Chem. Soc. **1962**, 2348; Mathur, Bhattacharya, ibid. **1963**, 3505; Becker, Ohloff, Helv. Chim. Acta **54**, 2889 (1971). Alternate syntheses: T. Mukaiyama et al., Chem. Lett. **1977**, 441; K. Narasaka et al., ibid. 763; W. H. Kruizinga, R. M. Kellogg, Chem. Commun. **1979**, 286.

Thick oil. Odor of amber and musk. $bp_{0.25}$ 110°; bp_{15} 176°. d_4^{20} 0.9549. n_D^{20} 1.4708. When sublimed in vacuum, needles, mp 32°. Sol in alc.

USE: As a fixative in perfumery.

3911. Exametazime. [105613-48-7] (2E,2'E,3R,3'R)-rel-3,3'-[(2,2-Dimethyl-1,3-propanediyl)diimino]bis-2-butanone dioxime; (RR,SS)-4,8-diaza-3,6,6,9-tetramethylundecane-2,10-dione bisoxime; (±)-(3RS,3'RS)-3,3'-[(2,2-dimethyltrimethylene)diimino]di-2-butanone dioxime; d,l-hexamethylpropyleneamine oxime; d,l-HM-PAO; hexametazine; Ceretec. $C_{13}H_{28}N_4O_2$; mol wt 272.39. C 57.32%, H 10.36%, N 20.57%, O 11.75%. Propyleneamine oxime derivative that forms a neutral, lipophilic complex with ^{99m}Tc which diffuses across cellular membranes, including the blood brain barrier. Used in regional cerebral blood flow imaging. Prepn: L. R. Canning et al., **EP 194843**; eidem, **US 4789736** (1986, 1988 both to Amersham). Prepn and radiopharmacology of ^{99m}Tc

complex: D. P. Nowotnik et al., Nucl. Med. Commun. **6**, 499 (1985); R. D. Neirinckx et al., J. Nucl. Med. **28**, 191 (1987). Clinical comparison of isomers: P. F. Sharp et al., ibid. **27**, 171 (1986). Biodistribution in humans: K. Nakamura et al., Eur. J. Nucl. Med. **15**, 100 (1989). Clinical evaluation in single photon emission tomography (SPECT) of meningiomas: S. Nakano et al., J. Nucl. Med. **30**, 1101 (1989). ^{99m}Tc radiolabeling of human platelets: H. J. Danpure, S. Osman, Nucl. Med. Commun. **9**, 267 (1988); of human leukocytes: H. J. Danpure et al., ibid. 465. Clinical study of labeled leukocytes for imaging inflammatory lesions: J. H. Reynolds, Clin. Radiol. **42**, 195 (1990). Series of articles on basic and clinical studies: J. Cereb. Blood Flow Metab. **8**, S1-S126 (1988).

Crystals from ethyl acetate, mp 128-130°.

THERAP CAT: ^{99m}Tc complex as diagnostic aid (radioactive imaging agent).

3912. Exatecan. [171335-80-1] (1S,9S)-1-Amino-9-ethyl-5-fluoro-1,2,3,9,12,15-hexahydro-9-hydroxy-4-methyl-10H,13H-benzo[de]pyrano[3',4':6,7]indolizino[1,2-b]quinoline-10,13-dione; DX-8951. $C_{24}H_{22}FN_3O_4$; mol wt 435.45. C 66.20%, H 5.09%, F 4.36%, N 9.65%, O 14.70%. Topoisomerase I inhibitor; synthetic analogue of camptothecin, q.v. Prepn: H. Terasawa et al., **EP 495432** (1992 to Daiichi); of mesylate: S. Kamihara et al., **EP 737686**; eidem, **US 6552197** (1996, 2003 both to Daiichi). HPLC determn in mouse plasma: T. Oguma et al., Biol. Pharm. Bull. **24**, 176 (2001). Clinical pharmacokinetics and evaluation in advanced leukemia: F. J. Giles et al., Clin. Cancer Res. **8**, 2134 (2002); in advanced solid malignancies: M. A. Garrison et al., ibid. **9**, 2527 (2003); in breast cancer: F. J. Esteva et al., Cancer **98**, 900 (2003); in gastric cancer: J. A. Ajani et al., Invest. New Drugs **23**, 479 (2005).

Methanesulfonate dihydrate. [197720-53-9]; [169869-90-3] (anhydrous). Exatecan mesylate; DX-8951f. $C_{24}H_{22}FN_3O_4.CH_4O_3S.2H_2O$; mol wt 567.58. mp 245-255° (dec). Sol in water.

THERAP CAT: Antineoplastic.

3913. Exemestane. [107868-30-4] 6-Methyleneandrosta-1,4-diene-3,17-dione; FCE-24304; Aromasin. $C_{20}H_{24}O_2$; mol wt 296.40. C 81.04%, H 8.16%, O 10.80%. Irreversible aromatase inhibitor. Prepn: E. Di Salle et al., **DE 3622841**; F. Buzzetti et al., **US 4808616** (1987, 1989 both to Farmitalia Carlo Erba). Pharmacology: D. Giudici et al., J. Steroid Biochem. **30**, 391 (1988). HPLC determn in plasma: M. Breda et al., J. Chromatogr. **620**, 225 (1993). Clinical pharmacology: T. R. J. Evans et al., Cancer Res. **52**, 5933 (1992). Review of clinical experience in primary and secondary therapy for breast cancer: J. M. Dixon, Expert Rev. Anticancer Ther. **2**, 267-275 (2002). Clinical trial in sequential therapy following tamoxifen in breast cancer: R. C. Coombes et al., N. Engl. J. Med. **350**, 1081 (2004).

White to slightly yellow crystalline powder. mp 188-191°. uv max: 247 nm (ε 13750). Freely sol in DMF; sol in methanol. Practically insol in water.

THERAP CAT: Antineoplastic (hormonal).

3914. Exendins. Bioactive peptides isolated from the venom of *Heloderma suspectum* Helodermatidae (Gila monster) and *H. horridum* (Mexican beaded lizard). Carboxy-amidated peptides containing 39 amino acid residues; differ only at positions 2 and 3. Interact with mammalian receptors for glucagon like peptide-1 (GLP-1), a physiological regulator of insulin secretion, and exhibit similar activities. Structurally related peptides known as *helospectin* and *helodermin* have also been isolated from venom of these species and were considered exendins-1 and -2 but differ in bioactivity. Review of isoln, structure and activity: J. Eng, *Mt. Sinai J. Med.* **59,** 147-149 (1992); J.-P. Raufman, *Regul. Pept.* **61,** 1-18 (1996).

Exendin-3. [130391-54-7] Isoln from *H. horridum:* J. Eng *et al., J. Biol. Chem.* **265,** 20259 (1990).

Exendin-4. [141732-76-5] Exenatide; AC-2993; LY-2148568; Byetta. Isoln from *H. suspectum:* J. Eng *et al., J. Biol. Chem.* **267,** 7402 (1992). GLP-1 receptor binding study: R. Göke *et al., J. Biol. Chem.* **268,** 19650 (1993). Use as probe for human GLP-1 receptor: G. G. Chicchi *et al., Peptides* **18,** 319 (1997). Review of pharmacology: L. L. Nielsen *et al., Regul. Pept.* **117,** 77-88 (2004). Clinical trial in type 2 diabetes: J. B. Buse *et al., Diabetes Care* **27,** 2628 (2004). Review of pharmacology and clinical experience: G. M. Bray, *Am. J. Health-Syst. Pharm.* **63,** 411-418 (2006).

Exendin(9-39). [133514-43-9] 9-39-Exendin 3 (Helodermahorridum); 9-39-exendin 4; exendin (9-39) amide. Amino truncated fragment; specific antagonist of GLP-1 receptor. Prepn from exendin 3: J.-P. Raufman *et al., J. Biol. Chem.* **266,** 2897 (1991). Use as GLP-1 antagonist for *in vivo* studies: F. Kolligs *et al., Diabetes* **44,** 16 (1995).

USE: Biological probe.

THERAP CAT: Antidiabetic.

3915. Exifone. [52479-85-3] (2,3,4-Trihydroxyphenyl)(3,-4,5-trihydroxyphenyl)methanone; 2,3,3′,4,4′,5′-hexahydroxybenzophenone; 4-galloylpyrogallol; Adlone. $C_{13}H_{10}O_7$; mol wt 278.21. C 56.12%, H 3.62%, O 40.26%. Cognition enhancing agent. Prepn: H. Bleuler, A. G. Perkin, *J. Chem. Soc.* **109,** 529 (1916); *see also* DE 49149 (1889 to BASF). Prepd but not claimed: J. M. Gazave *et al.*, DE 2501443; *eidem*, US 4015017 (1975, 1977 both to Pharmascience). Pharmacology: R. D. Porsolt *et al., Arzneim.-Forsch.* **37,** 388 (1987). Animal studies in memory improvement: R. D. Porsolt *et al., Pharmacol. Biochem. Behav.* **27,** 253 (1987); in antagonism of benzodiazepine-induced amnesia: R. D. Porsolt *et al., Psychopharmacology* **95,** 291 (1988). Clinical evaluation in senile dementia: F. Piette *et al., Rev. Geriatr.* **11,** 375 (1986); in Parkinson's disease: H. Allain *et al., Fundam. Clin. Pharmacol.* **2,** 1 (1988).

Crystals from aqueous solution, mp 270° (Gazave); also reported as faintly yellow needles from water, mp 272-273° (Bleuler, Perkin). LD_{50} in rats (g/kg): 0.355 i.p.; 1.425 orally (Gazave).

THERAP CAT: Nootropic.

3916. Exisulind. [59973-80-7] (1Z)-5-Fluoro-2-methyl-1-[[4-(methylsulfonyl)phenyl]methylene]-1*H*-indene-3-acetic acid; *cis*-5-fluoro-2-methyl-1-(*p*-methylsulfonylbenzylidene)-3-acetic acid; sulindac sulfone; FGN-1; Aptosyn. $C_{20}H_{17}FO_4S$; mol wt 372.41. C 64.50%, H 4.60%, F 5.10%, O 17.18%, S 8.61%. Sulfone metabolite of sulindac, *q.v.*; induces apoptosis of cancer cells. Identification as metabolite: H. B. Hucker *et al., Drug Metab. Dispos.* **1,** 721 (1973). Prepn: H. Jones *et al., J. Carbohydr. Nucleosides Nucleotides* **3,** 369 (1974). Antiproliferative effect vs colon cancer cells: L. J. Hixson *et al., Cancer Epidemiol. Biomarkers Prev.* **3,** 433 (1994). HPLC determn in serum: M. Siluveru, J. T. Stewart, *J. Chromatogr. B* **673,** 91 (1995); and clinical pharmacokinetics: G. F. Ray *et al., J. Pharm. Biomed. Anal.* **14,** 213 (1995). Review of mechanism of action studies: D. J. Ahnen, *Eur. J. Surg. Suppl.* **582,** 111-114 (1998).

mp 194-196°. $[\alpha]_D$ −62° (c = 1 in $CHCl_3$).

THERAP CAT: In treatment of colorectal polyps.

3917. Exosurf®. [99732-49-7] (7*R*)-4-Hydroxy-*N,N,N*-trimethyl-10-oxo-7-[(1-oxohexadecyl)oxy]-3,5,9-trioxa-4-phosphapentacosan-1-aminium, inner salt, 4-oxide mixture with formaldehyde polymer with oxirane and 4-(1,1,3,3-tetramethylbutyl)phenol and 1-hexadecanol; Surfexo. $C_{40}H_{80}NO_8P.C_{16}H_{34}O.(C_{14}H_{22}$-O.C$_2H_4$O.CH$_2$O)$_x$. Protein-free synthetic lung surfactant composed of a 13.5:1.5:1 mixture of colfosceril palmitate, cetyl alcohol and tyloxapol, *q.q.v.* Prepn: J. A. Clements, US 5110806 (1992 to Univ. of Calif.). Pharmacology: D. J. Durand *et al., J. Pediatr.* **107,** 775 (1985); W. H. Tooley *et al., Am. Rev. Respir. Dis.* **136,** 651 (1987). Clinical trial in neonatal respiratory distress syndrome (RDS): W. Long *et al., J. Pediatr.* **118,** 595 (1991). Symposium on pulmonary mechanics and clinical use in RDS: *ibid.* **120,** Suppl., S1-S50 (1992). Review of pharmacodynamics, clinical efficacy and tolerance: K. L. Dechant, D. Faulds, *Drugs* **42,** 877-894 (1991); of metabolism: R. L. DeAngelis, J. W. Findlay, *Clin. Perinatol.* **20,** 697-710 (1993).

THERAP CAT: Pulmonary surfactant.

3918. Ezetimibe. [163222-33-1] (3*R*,4*S*)-1-(4-Fluorophenyl)-3-[(3*S*)-3-(4-fluorophenyl)-3-hydroxypropyl]-4-(4-hydroxyphenyl)-2-azetidinone; Sch-58235; Ezetrol; Zetia. $C_{24}H_{21}F_2NO_3$; mol wt 409.43. C 70.40%, H 5.17%, F 9.28%, N 3.42%, O 11.72%. Cholesterol absorption inhibitor. Prepn: S. B. Rosenblum *et al.*, WO 9508532; *eidem*, US 5767115 (1995, 1998 both to Schering); *idem et al., J. Med. Chem.* **41,** 973 (1998). Enantioselective synthesis: G. Wu *et al., J. Org. Chem.* **64,** 3714 (1999). Activity in animals: M. van Heek *et al., J. Pharmacol. Exp. Ther.* **283,** 157 (1997). Metabolism and distribution: *eidem, Br. J. Pharmacol.* **129,** 1748 (2000). Review of pharmacology and clinical studies: H. Bays, *Expert Opin. Invest. Drugs* **11,** 1587-1604 (2002).

White solid, mp 164-166°. $[\alpha]_D^{22}$ −33.9° (c = 3 in methanol).

THERAP CAT: Antilipemic.

F

3919. Factor V. [9001-24-5] Blood-coagulation factor V; proaccelerin; labile factor; accelerator globulin; Ac-globulin. Mol wt above 300,000. Participates in the later stages of blood coagulation. Activated by factor X, *q.v.*, and along with Ca^{2+} and phospholipid forms a complex which converts prothrombin to thrombin, *q.q.v.* Accelerates the interaction of prothrombin, thromboplastin and Ca^{2+} ions: Ware, Seegers, *Fed. Proc.* **7**, 131 (1948). Thrombin produces serum Ac-globulin, **accelerin**, a far more potent accelerator, from plasma Ac-globulin, apparently by catalytic action: Ware *et al., Science* **106**, 618 (1947); Rapaport *et al., Blood* **21**, 221 (1963). Purification: Ware, Seegers, *J. Biol. Chem.* **172**, 699 (1948); Blombäck, Blombäck, *Nature* **198**, 886 (1963). Role in the scheme of blood coagulation: Pavlovsky in *Fibrinogen and Fibrin Turnover of Clotting Factors*, R. B. Hunter *et al.*, Eds. (Schattauer-Verlag, Stuttgart, 1963) pp 443-454. Proaccelerin deficiency is characterized by prolonged Quick's prothrombin time, and cephalin time, abnormal thromboplastin generation test, abnormal prothrombin consumption, and prolonged whole blood clotting time: Owren in *Thrombolytic Activity and Related Phenomena*, I. S. Wright *et al.*, Eds. (Schattauer-Verlag, Stuttgart, 1961) pp 387-391. *Review:* R. W. Colman, *Prog. Hemostasis Thromb.* **3**, 109-143 (1976). Purification, stability, amino acid composition, physical properties of bovine and human factor V: R. W. Colman, R. M. Weinberg, *Methods Enzymol.* **45B**, 107-122 (1976).

3920. Factor VII. [9001-25-6] Blood-coagulation factor VII; proconvertin; co-thromboplastin; serum prothrombin conversion accelerator; SPCA. Enzyme which, in conjunction with tissue factor and Ca^{2+} ions initiates the activation of factor X, *q.v.* Isoln from human plasma or serum: Fantt, Osborn, *Thromb. Diath. Haemorrh.* **8**, 286 (1962); from bovine plasma: J. Jesty, Y. Nemerson, *J. Biol. Chem.* **249**, 509 (1974). Separation from factor X by DEAE cellulose: Hougie, Bunting, in *New Blood Clotting Factors*, I. S. Wright *et al.*, Eds. (Schattauer-Verlag, Stuttgart, 1960) pp 40-42. Purification and structure of bovine factor VII: J. Jesty, Y. Nemerson, *J. Biol. Chem.* **249**, 509 (1974); R. Radcliffe, Y. Nemerson, *ibid.* **250**, 388 (1975); *eidem, Methods Enzymol.* **45B**, 49 (1976). Its deficiency results in retarded prothrombin conversion and an elevated one-stage prothrombin time: Alexander in *Thrombolytic Activity and Related Phenomena*, I. S. Wright *et al.*, Eds. (Schattauer-Verlag, Stuttgart, 1961) pp 392-402. Factor VII deficiency is associated with severe liver disease, vitamin K deficiency and broad spectrum antibiotic therapy, or may follow anticoagulant coumarin therapy.

3921. Factor VIII. [9001-27-8] Blood-coagulation factor VIII; antihemophilic globulin; antihemophilic factor A; AHG; Alphanate; Hemofil-M; Humate-P; Koate-HP; Monoclate-P; Nordiocto; Profilate. Crucial, nonenzymatic cofactor in the intrinsic coagulation pathway leading to the localized generation of thrombin. Deficiency results in the bleeding disorder known as hemophilia A or classical hemophilia. Factor VIII is an X-linked gene product synthesized by hepatocytes. Mature, single chain protein contains 2332 amino acid residues; mol wt 265 kDa. Released into the circulation as a set of heterodimers that rapidly interact with von Willebrand factor to form a stable, noncovalent complex; present at extremely low concn in plasma. Converted by thrombin into a heterotrimer (factor VIIIa) that accelerates the activation of factor X by factor IXa. Inactivated by protein C. Identification in plasma: T. Addis, *J. Pathol. Bacteriol.* **15**, 427 (1911). Role in hemostasis: A. J. Patek, Jr., F. H. L.Taylor, *J. Clin. Invest.* **16**, 113 (1937). Isoln and characterization of human factor VIII: E. J. Hershgold *et al., J. Lab. Clin. Med.* **77**, 185 (1971). Purification and properties of bovine: G. A. Vehar, E. W. Davie, *Biochemistry* **19**, 401 (1980). Characterization of the human factor VIII gene: J. Gitschier *et al., Nature* **312**, 326 (1984). Series of articles on cloning, expression, and structure: *ibid.* 330-347. Review of bioregulation: R. J. Kaufman, *Annu. Rev. Med.* **43**, 325-339 (1992). Review of production methods and clinical use in treatment of factor VIII deficiency: J. C. Gill, *Semin. Thromb. Hemostasis* **19**, 1-12 (1993). Review of biosynthesis, structure and function: P. Lollar, *Adv. Exp. Med. Biol.* **386**, 3-17 (1995); P. J. Lenting *et al., Blood* **92**, 3983-3996 (1998).

Kogenate. [169149-90-0] Recombinant human factor VIII produced in baby hamster kidney cells. Review of manufacturing process: H.-D. Hörlein, *Prog. Biotechnol.* **9**, 731-734 (1994). Clinical trial in treatment of hemophilia: E. Aygören-Pürsün *et al., Thromb. Haemostasis* **78**, 1352 (1997).

Recombinate. Recombinant human factor VIII produced in Chinese hamster ovary cells. Review of manufacturing process: E. Gomperts *et al., Transfus. Med. Rev.* **6**, 247-251 (1992). Clinical trial in treatment of hemophilia: G. C. White II *et al., Thromb. Haemostasis* **77**, 660 (1997).

THERAP CAT: Antihemophilic factor (human).

3922. Factor IX. [9001-28-9] Blood-coagulation factor IX; Christmas factor; PTC; plasma thromboplastin component; antihemophilic factor B; autoprothrombin II. A plasma and serum glycoprotein that participates in the middle phases of blood coagulation. Activated by factor XI and Ca^{2+}. Interacts then with factor VIII, Ca^{2+}, and phospholipid to form the complex which converts factor X into factor X_a. Isoln and characterization of bovine factor IX: K. Fujikawa *et al., Biochemistry* **12**, 4938 (1973); K. Fujikawa, E. W. Davie, *Methods Enzymol.* **45B**, 74 (1976). Deficiency results in a congenital bleeding disorder known as Christmas disease or hemophilia B. *Review:* Macfarlane in *Thrombolytic Activity and Related Phenomena*, I. S. Wright *et al.*, Eds. (Schattauer-Verlag, Stuttgart, 1961) pp 408-415; B. N. Bouma, J. A. Van Mourik, *Haemostasis: Biochemistry, Physiology & Pathology*, D. Ogston, B. Bennett, Eds. (Wiley-Interscience, New York, 1977) pp 56-77.

Factor IX complex (human). Konyne; Profilnine; Proplex T. A mixture of human factors II, VII, IX, and X.

Factor IX (human). AlphaNine; Mononine.

THERAP CAT: Hemostatic.

3923. Factor X. [9001-29-0] Blood-coagulation factor X; Stuart-Prower factor; Stuart factor; Prower factor. Enzyme which is activated by a complex of factors IX, VIII, calcium ions and phospholipid, or by factor VII and tissue factor in the intrinsic and extrinsic pathways of blood coagulation resp. Non-physiological activators are trypsin and a specific protein from Russel's viper venom: *see* Fujikawa *et al., Biochemistry* **11**, 4892 (1972). Active factor X apparently acts upon factor V, *q.v.* in the presence of calcium ions and lipid to form a complex which activates the conversion of prothrombin to thrombin. Present in both plasma and serum because neither increases nor decreases during clotting. Presumably synthesized in the liver because level is reduced with coumarin drugs and in liver disease. Isoln and characterization of bovine factor X: *eidem., ibid.* 4882. Factor X_a is a serine protease which, in the presence of factor V, Ca^{2+} ions and phospholipids, activates prothrombin. Severe deficiency causes hemorrhagic state resembling hemophilia. Mild deficiency may result in easy bruising. In severe cases deep muscular and joint hemorrhages occur. Improved purification and bibliography of earlier isoln procedures: Bajaj, Mann, *J. Biol. Chem.* **248**, 7729 (1973). Comparison of the molecular forms generated by the different methods of activation: Radcliffe, Barton, *ibid.* 6788. *Review:* Graham, Hougie in *Thrombolytic Activity and Related Phenomena*, I. S. Wright *et al.*, Eds. (Schattauer-Verlag, Stuttgart, 1961) pp 416-420; C. M. Jackson, *Thromb. Diath. Haemorrh. Suppl.* **57**, 197-216 (1974). Reviews on prepn, physical properties and function in the coagulation process: K. Fujikawa, E. W. Davie, *Methods Enzymol.* **45B**, 89 (1976); J. Jesty, Y. Nemerson, *ibid.* p 95.

Stable at room temperature for several days. Adsorbed by $BaSO_4$, $Al(OH)_3$, $Ca_3(PO_4)_2$, Seitz filters, bentonite and DEAE cellulose. At 56° is destroyed rapidly, in serum, less rapidly as citrate eluate. At 65° is destroyed rapidly in any form. Stable between pH 6.1-9.0. Soluble in water. Precipitates from water between pH 8-4. Isoelec pt pH 4.3.

3924. Factor XI. [9013-55-2] Blood-coagulation factor XI; PTA; plasma thromboplastin antecedent. Participates in the initial phases of blood coagulation. In normal plasma, factor XI is present in a precursor form and is converted to an active form, factor XI_a, which in turn activates factor IX to factor IX_a in the presence of Ca^{2+} ions: Ratnoff, Davie, *Biochemistry* **1**, 677 (1962); Schiffman *et al., Blood* **22**, 733 (1963); K. Fujikawa *et al., Biochemistry* **13**, 4508 (1974). Deficiency is characterized by the moderate bleeding symptoms of hemophilia C; by pathological clotting and recalcification times, impaired prothrombin consumption, and delayed thromboplastin formation: Duckert, Soulier in *New Blood Clotting Factors*, I. S. Wright *et al.*, Eds. (Schattauer-Verlag, Stuttgart, 1960) pp 145-147, 123-131. Review on bovine factor XI: T. Koide, *Methods Enzymol.* **45B**, 65-73 (1976).

3925. Factor XII. [9001-30-3] Blood-coagulation factor XII; Hageman factor; HF. Mol wt about 82,000. An enzyme which circulates in zymogen form in blood and when activated initiates the first of a series of events in coagulation of blood plasma. Enzymatic nature of blood coagulation is described by the "cascade" theory in which clotting factors interact with one another in a stepwise manner, one acting as an enzyme, the other as substrate, in a sequence of reactions leading to the formation of thrombin, *q.v.*: Davie, Ratnoff, *Science* **145**, 1310 (1964); MacFarlane, *Nature* **202**, 498 (1964). Factor XII initiates clotting when blood or plasma comes into contact with glass, collagen, or surface-active agents. Once activated, it interacts with factor XI, *q.v.*, to convert it to an enzyme. Factor XII is a sialoglycoprotein with esterase activity. Its activation by glass may be viewed as a dynamic alteration of the tertiary structure of the protein moiety: Schoenmakers *et al., Biochim. Biophys. Acta* **101**, 166 (1965). Isoln of human and rabbit factor XII in zymogen form: C. G. Cochrane, K. D. Wuepper, *J. Exp. Med.* **134**, 986 (1971); H. Saito *et al., Circ. Res.* **34**, 641 (1974). Highly purified Hageman factor undergoes a change in physical properties during activation: Donaldson, Ratnoff, *Science* **150**, 754 (1965). Factor XII deficiency is termed the Hageman trait. Unlike deficiencies in all other clotting factors, persons with Hageman trait do not show significant bleeding tendencies. *Reviews:* Ratnoff in *New Blood Clotting Factors*, I. S. Wright *et al.*, Eds. (Schattauer-Verlag, Stuttgart, 1960) pp 116-122; Ratnoff *et al.*, in *Thrombolytic Activity and Related Phenomena*, I. S. Wright *et al.*, Eds. (Schattauer-Verlag, Stuttgart, 1961) pp 364-378; several authors in *Recent Advances in Blood Coagulation*, L. Poller, Ed. (J. & A. Churchill, London, 1969); J. Spragg, K. F. Austen, *Compr. Immunol.* **3**, 125-143 (1977); J. H. Griffin, C. G. Cochrane, *Methods Enzymol.* **45B**, 56-65 (1976).

Sedimentation coefficient, $s^{\circ}_{20,\omega} = 7.08$. Diffusion constant, $D^{\circ}_{20,\omega} = 7.14 \times 10^{-7}$ cm²/sec. uv max at pH 7: 280 nm ($E^{1\%}_{1cm}$ 12.0). Isoelectric pt pH 8.0.

3926. Factor XIII. [9013-56-3] Blood-coagulation factor XIII; fibrin-stabilizing factor; FSF; fibrinase; Laki-Lorand factor; LLF; Fibrogammin. Plasma enzyme precursor which, when activated by thrombin in the presence of Ca^{2+}, converts soluble fibrin, *q.v.* gel to a tough insoluble clot: Laki, Lorand, *Science* **108**, 280 (1948); Lorand, *Nature* **166**, 694 (1950). During the terminal stage of blood-clotting, factor XIII catalyzes the formation of cross-links in the fibrin gel by eliminating NH_3 in the transamidation reaction in which the ε-amino group of lysine from a fibrin molecule forms a peptide linkage with a glutaminyl residue from a nearby fibrin monomer: Lorand *et al., Biochem. Biophys. Res. Commun.* **25**, 629 (1966); Fuller, Doolittle, *ibid.* 694. Trypsin, papain, and reptilase also activate factor XIII: Lorand *et al., ibid.* **31**, 222 (1968). Structure contains two each of two types of soluble proteinaceous subunits called the α and β chains; mol wt of subunits each about 80,000: Schwartz *et al., J. Biol. Chem.* **248**, 1395 (1973). Amino acid sequence studies: Holbrook *et al., Biochem. J.* **135**, 901 (1973). Clinical studies: Cucuianu *et al., Thromb. Diath. Haemorrh.* **30**, 480 (1973). *Review:* L. Lorand, *Ann. N.Y. Acad. Sci.* **202**, 6-30 (1972); A. G. Loewy, *ibid.* 41-58; C. G. Curtis, L. Lorand, *Haemostasis: Biochemistry, Physiology & Pathology*, D. Ogston, B. Bennett, Eds. (Wiley-Interscience, New York, 1977) pp 186-201; *eidem, Methods Enzymol.* **45B**, 177-191 (1976).

uv max: 280 nm ($E^{1\%}$ 13.8). Retains activity in plasma kept at 0°; inactivated in a few days at room temperature. Activity destroyed if serum heated at 60° for 10 min. Does not dialyse out from plasma. Inactivated by *Echis coloratus* venom. Pretreatment with compounds containing an SH-group, such as cysteine, reduced glutathione, DL-penicillamine, or mercapto-1-propanol prevents inactivation as well as restores activity after venom treatment.

THERAP CAT: Antihemorrhagic.

3927. Fadrozole. [102676-47-1] 4-(5,6,7,8-Tetrahydroimidazo[1,5-a]pyridin-5-yl)benzonitrile; 5-p-cyanophenyl-5,6,7,8-tetrahydroimidazo[1,5-a]pyridine. $C_{14}H_{13}N_3$; mol wt 223.27. C 75.31%, H 5.87%, N 18.82%. Aromatase inhibitor. Prepn: L. J.

Browne, **EP 165904**; *idem,* **US 4617307** (1985, 1986 both to Ciba-Geigy); L. J. Browne *et al., J. Med. Chem.* **34**, 725 (1991). Effects on estrogen biosynthesis: R. E. Steele *et al., Steroids* **50**, 147 (1987). Pharmacology: K. Schieweck *et al., Cancer Res.* **48**, 834 (1988). GC/MS determn in plasma and urine: R. Ackermann, G. Kaiser, *Biomed. Environ. Mass Spectrom.* **18**, 558 (1989). Pharmacokinetics: G. M. Kochak *et al., J. Clin. Endocrinol. Metab.* **71**, 1349 (1990). Clinical evaluation in metastatic breast cancer: J. I. Raats *et al., J. Clin. Oncol.* **10**, 111 (1992).

mp 117-118°.

Hydrochloride. [102676-31-3] CGS-16949A; Afema. $C_{14}H_{13}N_3 \cdot HCl$; mol wt 259.73. Crystals from 2-propanol, mp 231-233°. Sol in water.

THERAP CAT: Antineoplastic.

3928. Fagarine. [524-15-2] 4,8-Dimethoxyfuro[2,3-b]quinoline; γ-fagarine; 8-methoxydictamnine. $C_{13}H_{11}NO_3$; mol wt 229.23. C 68.11%, H 4.84%, N 6.11%, O 20.94%. Antiarrhythmic principle in *Fagara coco* (Gill.) Engl., *Rutaceae*. Isoln: Deulofeu *et al., J. Am. Chem. Soc.* **64**, 2326 (1942); Briggs, Cambi, *Tetrahedron* **2**, 256 (1958). Structure: Berinzaghi *et al., J. Org. Chem.* **10**, 181 (1945). Synthesis: Grundon, McCorkindale, *Chem. Ind. (London)* **1956**, 1091.

Prisms from alcohol, mp 142°. uv max: 238, 332, 370 nm (log ε 4.76, 3.88, 3.89). Sol in chloroform, benzene, ether; slightly sol in water, petr ether.

Hydrochloride. $C_{13}H_{12}ClNO_3$. Needles from chloroform + ether, mp 158-159°.

3929. Famciclovir. [104227-87-4] 2-[2-(2-Amino-9H-purin-9-yl)ethyl]-1,3-propanediol diacetate (ester); 9-[4-acetoxy-3-(acetoxymethyl)but-1-yl]-2-aminopurine; FCV; BRL-42810; Oravir; Famvir. $C_{14}H_{19}N_5O_4$; mol wt 321.33. C 52.33%, H 5.96%, N 21.79%, O 19.92%. Prodrug of penciclovir, *q.v.* Prepn: M. R. Harnden, R. L. Jarvest, **AU 85 47560**; *eidem,* **US 5246937** (1986, 1993 both to Beecham); M. R. Harnden *et al., J. Med. Chem.* **32**, 1738 (1989). HPLC determn in plasma and urine: J. R. McMeekin *et al., Anal. Proc.* **29**, 178 (1992). Review of metabolism and mode of action: R. A. Vere Hodge, *Antiviral Chem. Chemother.* **4**, 67-84 (1993). Series of articles on pharmacology and pharmacokinetics: *ibid.* Suppl. 1, 37-68 (1993). Review of clinical efficacy in herpes zoster and genital herpes: R. Circelli *et al., Antiviral Res.* **29**, 141-151 (1996).

White shiny plates from ethyl acetate-hexane, mp 102-104°. uv max (methanol): 222, 244, 309 nm (ε 27500, 4890, 7160). Sol in water (25°): >25% w/v initially; rapidly ppts as sparingly sol monohydrate (2-3% w/v). Freely sol in acetone, methanol; sparingly sol in ethanol, isopropanol.

THERAP CAT: Antiviral.

3930. Famotidine. [76824-35-6] 3-[[[2-[(Aminoiminomethyl)amino]-4-thiazolyl]methyl]thio]-N-(aminosulfonyl)-propanimidamide; [1-amino-3-[[[2-[(diaminomethylene)amino]-4-thiazolyl]methyl]thio]propylidene]sulfamide; N-sulfamoyl-3-[(2-guanidinothiazol-4-yl)methylthio]propionamide; YM-11170; MK-208; Amfamox; Fadul; Famodil; Famosan; Famoxal; Ganor; Gaster; Gastridin; Gastropen; Lecedil; Motiax; Muclox; Pepcid; Pepcidac; Pepcidine; Pepdine; Pepdul; Peptan; Ulfamid. $C_8H_{15}N_7O_2S_3$; mol wt 337.45. C 28.47%, H 4.48%, N 29.06%, O 9.48%, S 28.51%. Histamine H_2-receptor antagonist. Prepn, NMR and mass spectral data: H. Yasufumi *et al.*, **BE 882071**; *eidem*, **US 4283408**; **JP Kokai 81 55383**, *C.A.* **95**, 203930n (1980, 1981, 1981 all to Yamanouchi). Inhibition of gastric acid and pepsin secretion in rats: M. Takeda *et al.*, *Arzneim.-Forsch.* **32**, 734 (1982); in man: M. Miwa *et al.*, *Int. J. Clin. Pharmacol. Ther. Toxicol.* **22**, 214 (1984). Effect on disposition of antipyrine in liver: Ch. Staiger *et al.*, *Arzneim.-Forsch.* **34**, 1041 (1984). Chromatographic determn in plasma and urine: W. C. Vincek *et al.*, *J. Chromatogr.* **338**, 438 (1985). Pharmacokinetics: T. Takabatke *et al.*, *Eur. J. Clin. Pharmacol.* **28**, 327 (1985). Clinical trial in Zollinger-Ellison syndrome: J. M. Howard *et al.*, *Gastroenterology* **88**, 1026 (1985). Symposia on pharmacology and clinical efficacy: *Am. J. Med.* **81**, Suppl. 4B, 1-64 (1986); *Scand. J. Gastroenterol.* **22**, Suppl. 134, 1-62 (1987).

mp 163-164°. Soly at 20° (%, w/v): 80 in DMF; 50 in acetic acid; 0.3 in methanol; 0.1 in water; <0.01 in ethanol, ethyl acetate, chloroform. LD_{50} i.v. in mice: 244.4 mg/kg (Yasufumi).

THERAP CAT: Antiulcerative.

3931. Famoxadone. [131807-57-3] 5-Methyl-5-(4-phenoxyphenyl)-3-(phenylamino)-2,4-oxazolidinedione; 3-anilino-5-methyl-5-(4-phenoxyphenyl)-1,3-oxazolidine-2,4-dione; DPX-JE874; Famoxate. $C_{22}H_{18}N_2O_4$; mol wt 374.39. C 70.58%, H 4.85%, N 7.48%, O 17.09%. Inhibits electron transport via blockage of ubiquinol:cytochrome c oxidoreductase. Prepd not claimed: D. Geffken, D. R. Rayner, **US 4957933** (1990 to DuPont). Biological activity and field trials: M. M. Joshi, J. A. Sternberg, *Proc. Br. Crop Prot. Conf. - Pests Dis.* **1996**, 21. Mode of action: B. B. Jordan *et al.*, *Pestic. Sci.* **55**, 105 (1999). Environmental fate: K. M. Jernberg, P. W. Lee, *ibid.* 587. Metabolic fate in plants and animals: P. W. Lee *et al.*, *ibid.* 589. Review of synthesis and structure-activity relationship: J. A. Sternberg *et al.*, *ACS Symp. Ser.* **686**, 216-227 (1998).

mp 140.3-141.8°. Log P (*n*-octanol/water): 4.65 (pH 7). Soly in water: 52 μg/L. LD_{50} in rats (mg/kg): >5000 orally; >2000 dermally (Joshi, Sternberg).

USE: Agricultural fungicide.

3932. Famphur. [52-85-7] Phosphorothioic acid O-[4-[(dimethylamino)sulfonyl]phenyl] O,O-dimethyl ester; phosphorothioic acid O,O-dimethyl ester, O-ester with p-hydroxy-N,N-dimethylbenzenesulfonamide; O,O-dimethyl-O,p-(dimethylsulfamoyl)-phenyl phosphorothioate; p-hydroxy-N,N-dimethylbenzenesulfonamide ester with phosphorothioic acid O,O-dimethyl ester; famophos; American Cyanamid 38023; ENT-25644; Warbex. $C_{10}H_{16}NO_5PS_2$; mol wt 325.34. C 36.92%, H 4.96%, N 4.31%, O 24.59%, P 9.52%, S 19.71%. Prepn: Berkelhammer, **US 3005004** (1961 to Am. Cyanamid). Metabolism: P. E. Gatterdam *et al.*, *J. Agric. Food Chem.* **15**, 845 (1967). Toxicology: E. W. Schafer, *Toxicol. Appl. Pharmacol.* **21**, 315 (1972); W. D. Black *et al.*, *ibid.* **50**, 167 (1979).

Crystals, mp 52.5-53.5°. LD_{50} orally in rats: 35 mg/kg (Schafer).

Caution: Cholinesterase inhibitor. *See* Parathion.

USE: Insecticide.

THERAP CAT (VET): Insecticide (grubicide).

3933. Fampridine. [504-24-5] 4-Pyridinamine; 4-aminopyridine; γ-aminopyridine; 4-pyridylamine; 4-AP; EL-970. $C_5H_6N_2$; mol wt 94.11. C 63.81%, H 6.43%, N 29.77%. Potassium channel blocker. Prepn: A. Kirpal, *Monatsh. Chem.* **23**, 244 (1902); R. Camps, *Arch. Pharm.* **240**, 345 (1902); C. R. Hauser, G. A. Reynolds, *J. Org. Chem.* **15**, 1224 (1950). Prolongs action potential in demyelinated nerve fibers: R. M. Sherratt *et al.*, *Nature* **283**, 570 (1980). HPLC determn in serum: A. van der Horst *et al.*, *J. Chromatogr.* **574**, 166 (1992). Neurophysiology and clinical efficacy in multiple sclerosis: H. A. M. van Diemen *et al.*, *J. Neurol. Sci.* **116**, 220 (1993). Clinical evaluation: C. H. Polman *et al.*, *Arch. Neurol.* **51**, 1136 (1994). Review of pharmacology and efficacy of aminopyridines in MS: C. T. Bever, Jr., *Ann. Neurol.* **36**, S118-S121 (1994).

Crystals from $CHCl_3$, mp 158-159°. Sol in water, alcohol; slightly sol in benzene, ether; very slightly sol in ligroin.

THERAP CAT: In treatment of multiple sclerosis.

3934. Fantofarone. [114432-13-2] 3,4-Dimethoxy-N-methyl-N-[3-[4-[[2-(1-methylethyl)-1-indolizinyl]sulfonyl]phenoxy]propyl]benzeneethanamine; 2-isopropyl-1-[4-[3-[N-methyl-N-(3,4-dimethoxy-β-phenethyl)amino]propyloxy]benzenesulfonyl]-indolizine; SR-33557. $C_{31}H_{38}N_2O_5S$; mol wt 550.71. C 67.61%, H 6.95%, N 5.09%, O 14.53%, S 5.82%. Indolizinsulfone calcium channel blocker. Prepn: J. Gubin *et al.*, **EP 235111**; J. Gubin *et al.*, **US 4957925** (1987, 1990 both to Sanofi); *eidem*, *J. Med. Chem.* **35**, 981 (1992). Binding studies: A. Schmid *et al.*, *Mol. Pharmacol.* **35**, 766 (1989); B. A. Kenny *et al.*, *Br. J. Pharmacol.* **108**, 93 (1993). X-ray structure and electronic properties: V. J. Gibon *et al.*, *Eur. J. Med. Chem.* **27**, 485 (1992). Pharmacokinetics: E. Bellissant *et al.*, *Eur. J. Clin. Pharmacol.* **41**, 329 (1991). Review of pharmacology and clinical evaluations: P. Chatelain *et al.*, *Cardiovasc. Drug Rev.* **9**, 123-146 (1991).

Monoclinic colorless sheets from diisopropyl ether/ $CHCl_2$, mp 82-83°. d_z 1.21 g/cm³. Sol in all organic solvents, in water at 0.06%. pKa 8.34 ± 0.05.

THERAP CAT: Antihypertensive.

3935. α-Farnesene. [502-61-4] 3,7,11-Trimethyl-1,3,6,10-dodecatetraene; 2,6,10-trimethyl-2,6,9,11-dodecatetraene; farnesene. $C_{15}H_{24}$; mol wt 204.35. C 88.16%, H 11.84%. Isoln of (E,E)-form from natural coating of apples: Huelin, Murray, *Nature* **210**, 1260 (1966); Murray, *Aust. J. Chem.* **22**, 197 (1969); from Dufour's gland in ants: Cavill *et al.*, *Tetrahedron Lett.* **1967**, 2201. Isoln of (Z,E)-form from oil of perilla: T. Sakai, Y. Hirose, *Bull.*

Chem. Soc. Jpn. **42,** 3615 (1969). Oxidation products of farnesene are believed to cause scald, a serious storage disorder of apples. Four possible geometric isomers. Synthetic studies: Ruzicka, *Helv. Chim. Acta* **6,** 490, 501 (1923); Ruzicka, Capato, *ibid.* **8,** 267 (1925). Configuration of *(E,E)*-form confirmed by synthesis from *trans*-β-farnesene: Brieger *et al., J. Org. Chem.* **34,** 3789 (1969). Stereospecific synthesis of *(E,Z)*- and *(Z,Z)*-isomers: Anet, *Aust. J. Chem.* **23,** 2101 (1970). Synthesis of *(E,E)*-form: Tanaka *et al., J. Am. Chem. Soc.* **97,** 3252 (1975). *(E,E)*- and *(Z,E)*-forms are components of aphid alarm pheromones: J. A. Pickett, D. C. Griffiths, *J. Chem. Ecol.* **6,** 349 (1980); of the trail pheromone of red imported fire ants: R. K. Vandermeer *et al., Tetrahedron Lett.* **22,** 1651 (1981).

(E,E)- α-Farnesene

Thin oil. bp_{12} about 125°. d_4^{20} 0.8410. n_D^{20} 1.4836. Practically insol in water. Misc with hydrocarbon solvents. uv max of *(E,E)*-form (alc): 233 nm (ε 27,000); of *(Z,E)*-form (alc): 238 nm (ε 11300).

3936. β-Farnesene. [18794-84-8] 7,11-Dimethyl-3-methylene-1,6,10-dodecatriene. $C_{15}H_{24}$; mol wt 204.35. C 88.16%, H 11.84%. The naturally occurring *trans* form or *(E)*-isomer is a constituent of various essential oils, *see* F. Sorm *et al., Collect. Czech. Chem. Commun.* **14,** 699 (1949); **15,** 626 (1951); also an alarm pheromone of several aphid species: Bowers *et al., Science* **177,** 1121 (1972); Edwards *et al., Nature* **241,** 126 (1973); W. S. Bowers *et al., J. Insect Physiol.* **23,** 697 (1977). Isoln from leaves of wild potato, *Solanum berthaultii* Hawkes, *Solanaceae:* R. W. Gibson, J. A. Pickett, *Nature* **302,** 608 (1983). Prepd by dehydration of farnesol: Bhati, *Perfum. Essent. Oil Rec.* **54,** 376 (1963); Brieger, *J. Org. Chem.* **32,** 3720 (1967); alternate syntheses: Tanaka *et al., J. Am. Chem. Soc.* **97,** 3252 (1975); S. Akutagawa *et al., Chem. Lett.* **1976,** 485; O. P. Vig *et al., Indian J. Chem. Sect. B* **18,** 33 (1979). Synthesis of *(Z)*-isomer: Anet, *Aust. J. Chem.* **23,** 2101 (1970); O. P. Vig *et al., J. Indian Chem. Soc.* **47,** 999 (1970); *eidem, Indian J. Chem.* **13,** 1244 (1975).

(E)- β-Farnesene

(E)-**Form.** Oil, bp 124°. d_4^{20} 0.8310. n_D^{20} 1.4870. uv max (hexane): 224 nm (ε 14000).

(Z)-**Form.** Oil, bp_{3-4} 95-107°. n_D^{32} 1.4780. uv max (hexane): 224 nm (ε 17300).

3937. Farnesol. [4602-84-0] 3,7,11-Trimethyl-2,6,10-dodecatrien-1-ol. $C_{15}H_{26}O$; mol wt 222.37. C 81.02%, H 11.79%, O 7.19%. Found in oils of citronella, neroli, cyclamen, lemon grass, tuberose, rose, musk, balsam Peru, and tolu. Isoln: Elge, *Chem. Ztg.* **34,** 857 (1910); **37,** 1422 (1913); Kerschbaum, *Ber.* **46,** 1732 (1913); Naves, *Helv. Chim. Acta* **32,** 1798, 2181 (1949); LaFace, *ibid.* **33,** 249 (1950). Synthesis: Ruzicka, *ibid.* **6,** 492 (1923); Ruzicka, Firmenich, *ibid.* **22,** 392 (1939); Nazarov *et al., Zh. Obshch. Khim.* **28,** 1444 (1958); Shvarts, Petrov, *ibid.* **30,** 3598 (1960); Popjak *et al., J. Biol. Chem.* **237,** 56 (1962). Four possible stereoisomers. Stereochemistry: Bates *et al., Chem. Ind. (London)* **1961,** 1907; *J. Org. Chem.* **28,** 1086 (1963). *trans-trans*-Farnesol is the only stereoisomer present in many essential oils but occurs mixed with *cis-trans*-farnesol in petitgrain oil and several other oils: Naves, *Compt. Rend.* **251,** 900 (1960). Stereospecific synthesis of *trans-trans*-farnesol: Corey *et al., J. Am. Chem. Soc.* **92,** 6637 (1970).

***trans-trans*-Farnesol.** Liquid. $bp_{0.35}$ 111°. n_D^{25} 1.4872. uv max: 192-196 nm (ε 28,500).

Commercial farnesol. $bp_{0.2}$ 110-113°. d_4^{20} 0.8871. n_D^{20} 1.4870.

USE: In perfumery, to emphasize the odor of sweet floral perfumes, such as lilac and cyclamen.

3938. Faropenem. [106560-14-9] (5R,6S)-6-[(1R)-1-Hydroxyethyl]-7-oxo-3-[(2R)-tetrahydro-2-furanyl]-4-thia-1-azabicyclo-[3.2.0]hept-2-ene-2-carboxylic acid; fropenem; (5R,6S,8R,2′R)-2-(2′-tetrahydrofuryl)-6-hydroxyethylpenem-3-carboxylate. $C_{12}H_{15}$NO$_5$S; mol wt 285.32. C 50.51%, H 5.30%, N 4.91%, O 28.04%, S 11.24%. Orally active, β-lactamase stable, penem antibiotic. Prepn: M. Ishiguro *et al.,* **EP 199446;** *eidem,* **US 4997829** (1986, 1991 both to Suntory); *eidem, J. Antibiot.* **41,** 1685 (1988). Pharmacokinetics: A. Tsuji *et al., Drug Metab. Dispos.* **18,** 245 (1990). *In vitro* antimicrobial spectrum: J. M. Woodcock *et al., J. Antimicrob. Chemother.* **39,** 35 (1997). β-Lactamase stability: A. Dalhoff *et al., Chemotherapy (Basel)* **49,** 229 (2003). HPLC determn in plasma: R. V. S. Nirogi *et al., Arzneim.-Forsch.* **55,** 762 (2005). Clinical trial in urinary tract infections: S. Arakawa *et al., Nishinihon J. Urol.* **56,** 300 (1994); in bacterial sinusitis: R. Siegert *et al., Eur. Arch. Otorhinolaryngol.* **260,** 186 (2003).

Sodium salt. [122547-49-3] Furopenem; ALP-201; SUN-5555; SY-5555; WY-49605; Farom. $C_{12}H_{15}$NNaO$_5$S; mol wt 308.31. $[\alpha]_D^{22}$ +60° (c = 0.10).

Daloxate. [141702-36-5] (5R,6S)-6-[(1R)-1-Hydroxyethyl]-7-oxo-3-[(2R)-tetrahydro-2-furanyl]-4-thia-1-azabicyclo[3.2.0]hept-2-ene-2-carboxylic acid (5-methyl-2-oxo-1,3-dioxol-4-yl)methyl ester; faropenem medoxomil; Bay-56-6854; SUN-208; Orapem. $C_{17}H_{19}$NO$_8$S; mol wt 397.40. Prepn: H. Iwata *et al.,* **WO 9203442;** *eidem,* **US 5830889** (1992, 1998 both to Suntory). Pale yellow crystals.

THERAP CAT: Antibacterial (antibiotics).

3939. Fasciculins. [86697-68-9] FAS. Group of low molecular wt (~6750 Da) toxic peptides isolated from the venom of green mamba snakes. Allosterically inhibits ($K_i \simeq 10^{-10}M$) most synaptic acetylcholinesterases (AChE). Cationic peptides characterized by 4 disulphide bridges. Isoln from *Dendroaspis angusticeps*: D. Rodriguez-Ithurralde *et al., Neurochem. Int.* **5,** 267 (1983). X-ray crystallography: M. H. le Du *et al., J. Biol. Chem.* **267,** 22112 (1992). Inhibition of AChE: P. Fossier *et al., Cell. Mol. Neurobiol.* **6,** 221 (1986). Allosteric control of inhibition: Z. Radic *et al., J. Biol. Chem.* **270,** 20391 (1995). Amino acid sequence and structure-activity study: C. Cervenansky *et al., Toxicon* **34,** 718 (1996). Review of neuropharmacology: F. Dajas *et al., Methods Neurosci.* **8,** 258-270 (1992).

USE: Research tool.

3940. Fasidotril. [135038-57-2] N-[(2S)-3-(Acetylthio)-2-(1,3-benzodioxol-5-ylmethyl)-1-oxopropyl]-L-alanine phenylmethyl ester; N-[(S)-α-(mercaptomethyl)-3,4-(methylenedioxy)-hydrocinnamoyl]-L-alanine, benzyl ester acetate (ester); aladotril; altriopril; BP-1137. $C_{23}H_{25}$NO$_6$S; mol wt 443.51. C 62.29%, H 5.68%, N 3.16%, O 21.64%, S 7.23%. Vasopeptidase inhibitor (VPI) exhibiting characteristic dual metalloprotease inhibition of neutral endopeptidase (NEP) and angiotensin converting enzyme (ACE). Prepn: J.-C. Plaquevent *et al.,* **EP 419327;** *eidem,* **US 5670531** (1991, 1997 both to Soc. Civile Bioprojet). Absolute configuration: V. Grosset *et al., Tetrahedron: Asymmetry* **14,** 2335 (2003). Enzyme inhibition activity: C. Gros *et al., Proc. Natl. Acad. Sci. USA* **88,** 4210 (1991). Preclinical and clinical pharmacology: S. Laurent *et al., Hypertension* **35,** 1148 (2000). Review of design and pharmacology: J. Bralet *et al., Cardiovasc. Drug Rev.* **18,** 1-24 (2000); of therapeutic potential: F. Ozdener, V. Ozdemir, *Curr. Opin. Invest. Drugs* **4,** 1113-1119 (2003).

mp 104°. $[\alpha]_D^{25}$ −50.6° (c = 1.35 in methanol). Also reported as white to yellowish microcrystalline powder, mp 108° (Bralet). Sol in acetone, chloroform, dimethylformamide. Nearly insol in water.

Diacid. [135038-59-4] Alatrioprilat; fasidotrilat. $C_{14}H_{17}NO_5$-S; mol wt 311.35. Biologically active metabolite. $[\alpha]_D^{25}$ +12.9° (c = 1.3 in methanol).

THERAP CAT: Antihypertensive.

3941. Fast Green FCF. [2353-45-9] *N*-Ethyl-*N*-[4-[[4-[eth-yl[(3-sulfophenyl)methyl]amino]phenyl](4-hydroxy-2-sulfophen-yl)methylene]-2,5-cyclohexadien-1-ylidene]-3-sulfobenzenemeth-anaminium inner salt disodium salt; FD & C Green No. 3; C.I. Food Green 3; C.I. 42053. $C_{37}H_{34}N_2Na_2O_{10}S_3$; mol wt 808.85. C 54.94%, H 4.24%, N 3.46%, Na 5.68%, O 19.78%, S 11.89%. Prepn: H. Johnson, P. Staub, *Ind. Eng. Chem.* **19**, 497 (1927). Toxicity studies: F. C. Lu, A. Lavalle, *Can. Pharm. J.* **97**, 30 (1964); W. H. Hansen *et al., Food Cosmet. Toxicol.* **4**, 389 (1966). Review of carcinogenicity studies: *IARC Monographs* **16**, 187-197 (1978). *See also: Colour Index* **vol. 4** (3rd ed., 1971) p 4383.

Dark green powder or granules with a metallic lustre. Absorption max: 628 nm. Very sol in water; sol in ethanol. Dull orange soln in conc H_2SO_4, changing to dull green on dilution. Orange soln in conc HCl or conc HNO_3. Bright blue soln in 10% aq NaOH. LD_{50} orally in rats: >2 g/kg (Lu, Lavalle).

USE: Biological stain. Color additive in food, drugs and cosmetics.

3942. Fasudil. [103745-39-7] Hexahydro-1-(5-isoquinolin-ylsulfonyl)-1*H*-1,4-diazepine; *N*-(5-isoquinolinesulfonyl)-1,4-per-hydrodiazepine; 1-(5-isoquinolinesulfonyl)homopiperazine. C_{14}-$H_{17}N_3O_2S$; mol wt 291.37. C 57.71%, H 5.88%, N 14.42%, O 10.98%, S 11.00%. Intracellular calcium antagonist. Prepn: H. Hidaka, T. Sone, **EP 187371**; *eidem*, **US 4678783** (1986, 1987 both to Asahi); A. Morikawa *et al., Chem. Pharm. Bull.* **40**, 770 (1992). Pharmacology: T. Asano *et al., Br. J. Pharmacol.* **98**, 1091 (1989). Mechanism of action: *idem et al., J. Pharmacol. Exp. Ther.* **241**, 1033 (1987). Clinical trials: M. Shibuya *et al., J. Neurosurg.* **76**, 571 (1992). Acute toxicity: H. Koga *et al., Yakuri to Chiryo* **20**, S1433 (1992), *C.A.* **117**, 226005b (1992). Review of pharmacology and clinical evaluation: M. Shirotani *et al., Cardiovasc. Drug Rev.* **10**, 333-357 (1992).

Hydrochloride. [105628-07-7] AT-877; HA-1077; Eril. C_{14}-$H_{17}N_3O_2S.HCl$; mol wt 327.83. Crystals from water, mp 220.5°. Also reported as white crystalline powder, mp 219.3° (Shirotani). Sol in water up to $2 \times 10^{-2}M$ at pH 5.0-7.0. LD_{50} in mice, rats (mg/kg): 67.5, 59.9 i.v.; 124.5, 123.2 s.c.; 273.9, 335.0 orally (Koga).

THERAP CAT: Vasodilator (cerebral).

3943. Fazadinium Bromide. [49564-56-9] 1,1′-Azobis[3-methyl-2-phenylimidazo[1,2-*a*]pyridinium] dibromide; AH-8165; Fazadon. $C_{28}H_{24}Br_2N_6$; mol wt 604.34. C 55.65%, H 4.00%, Br 26.44%, N 13.91%. A short-acting curarimimetic with rapid onset. Prepn: D. Jack, E. E. Glover, **DE 2127355**; *eidem*, **US 3773746** (1971, 1973 both to Allen & Hanburys); E. E. Glover, M. Yorke, *J. Chem. Soc. C* **1971**, 3280. Pharmacology: L. Bolger *et al., Nature* **238**, 354 (1972); and toxicity data: P. Bellani *et al., Farmaco Ed. Sci.* **39**, 846 (1984). Clinical pharmacokinetics: T. Busi *et al., Minerva Anestesiol.* **49**, 485 (1983). Clinical use: G. Minutella, G. Bongiovanni, *ibid.* 301; A. Lusini *et al., ibid.* 393.

Dihydrate. Yellow crystals from water, mp 215-219° (softens at 196°). Also reported as yellow solid from methanol/ethyl acetate, mp 218-220°. uv max (H_2O): 285, 297 nm (log ε 4.04, 4.34). LD_{50} i.v. in rats: 1.5 μM/k (Bellani).

THERAP CAT: Neuromuscular blocking agent.

3944. Febantel. [58306-30-2] [[2-[(Methoxyacetyl)amino]-4-(phenylthio)phenyl]carbonimidoyl]biscarbamic acid dimethyl ester; dimethyl [[2-(2-methoxyacetamido)-4-(phenylthio)phenyl]-imidocarbonyl]dicarbamate; Bay Vh 5757; Bay h 5757; Rintal. $C_{20}H_{22}N_4O_6S$; mol wt 446.48. C 53.80%, H 4.97%, N 12.55%, O 21.50%, S 7.18%. Prepn: H. Koelling *et al.*, **DE 2423679**; *eidem*, **US 3993682** (1975, 1976 both to Bayer). Anthelmintic efficacy: H. Wollweber *et al., Arzneim.-Forsch.* **28**, 2193 (1977); H. Thomas, *Res. Vet. Sci.* **25**, 290 (1978). Safety evaluation in horses: J. A. Shmidl, *Vet. Med. Small Anim. Clin.* **73**, 775 (1978).

Crystals, mp 129-130°.

THERAP CAT (VET): Anthelmintic.

3945. Febarbamate. [13246-02-1] 1-[2-[(Aminocarbonyl)-oxy]-3-butoxypropyl]-5-ethyl-5-phenyl-2,4,6(1*H*,3*H*,5*H*)-pyrimi-dinetrione; 1-(3-butoxy-2-hydroxypropyl)-5-ethyl-5-phenylbar-bituric acid carbamate; 1-(3-butoxy-2-carbamoyloxypropyl)-5-phenyl-5-ethylbarbituric acid; Gö-560; G-Tril; Tymium. $C_{20}H_{27}$-N_3O_6; mol wt 405.44. C 59.25%, H 6.71%, N 10.36%, O 23.68%. Prepn: P. Gold-Aubert, E. Gysin, *Helv. Chim. Acta* **44**, 105 (1961); P. Gold-Aubert, **US 3075983** (1963 to Sapos). Pharmacology: E. Frommel *et al., Helv. Physiol. Pharmacol. Acta* **19**, 241 (1961). Metabolism in rats: J. Vachta, P. Gold-Aubert, *Eur. J. Drug Metab. Pharmacokinet.* **7**, 147 (1982); in man: J. Vachta *et al., ibid.* **8**, 297 (1983).

Syrup; could not be crystallized, dec ~196°. Sol in alcohol, dioxane. Insol in water. LD_{50} orally in mice: 1065 mg/kg (Frommel).

THERAP CAT: Sedative, hypnotic.

3946. Febrifugine. [24159-07-8] (2*S-trans*)-3-[3-(3-Hydroxy-2-piperidinyl)-2-oxopropyl]-4(3*H*)-quinazolinone; 3-[3-(3-hydroxy-2-piperidyl)acetonyl]-4(3*H*)-quinazolinone; 3-[β-keto-γ-(3-hydroxy-2-piperidyl)propyl]-4-quinazolone; β-dichroine. $C_{16}H_{19}N_3O_3$; mol wt 301.34. C 63.77%, H 6.36%, N 13.94%, O 15.93%. Isolated from the *Dichroa febrifuga* Louv., *Saxifragaceae* and from the common hydrangea: Koepfli *et al., J. Am. Chem. Soc.* **71**, 1048 (1949). Identity with β-dichroine: Fu, Yang, *C.A.* **43**, 1530a (1949). Structure: Koepfli *et al., J. Am. Chem. Soc.* **72**, 3323 (1950). Synthesis: Baker *et al., J. Org. Chem.* **17**, 132 (1952); **18**, 178 (1953); Koepfli *et al.*, US 2504847 (1950 to U.S. Gov't); Baker, Querry, US 2651632 (1953 to Am. Cyanamid). Config: Hill, Edwards, *Chem. Ind. (London)* **1962**, 858. Revised stereochemistry: Barringer *et al., J. Org. Chem.* **38**, 1937 (1973).

Dimorphic crystals: needles from ethanol, mp 139-140°; from chloroform, mp 154-156°. $[α]_D^{25}$ +6° (c = 0.5 in chloroform); $[α]_D^{25}$ +28° (c = 0.5 in ethanol). Freely sol in methanol + chloroform, water + ethanol; slightly sol in water, ethanol, acetone, chloroform. Practically insol in ether, benzene, petr ether. LD_{50} orally in white mice: 2.5-3.0 mg/kg (Koepfli, 1949).

Dihydrochloride monohydrate. Crystals from 90% ethanol, mp 220-222°. $[α]_D^{25}$ +12.8° (c = 0.8).

THERAP CAT (VET): Coccidiostat.

3947. Febuprol. [3102-00-9] 1-Butoxy-3-phenoxy-2-propanol; H-33; K-10033; Valbil. $C_{13}H_{20}O_3$; mol wt 224.30. C 69.61%, H 8.99%, O 21.40%. Prepn: W. F. Minor *et al., J. Am. Chem. Soc.* **76**, 2993 (1954). Prepn and use as choleretic: H. Hoffmann *et al.*, DE 2120396; *eidem*, US 3839587 (1972, 1974 both to Klinge). Pharmacology: G. Hofrichter *et al., Arzneim.-Forsch.* **24**, 111 (1974). Pharmacokinetics, metabolism: K. Rehm *et al., ibid.* **26**, 813 (1976). Spasmolytic action: R. Eisenburger, *ibid.* **27**, 1429 (1977). Clinical studies: C. Wolf *et al., Muench. Med. Wochenschr.* **118**, 1285 (1976); W. E. Scholing, W. Weinert, *ibid.* **120**, 143 (1978); U. Ritter, H. J. Kyrein, *Arzneim.-Forsch.* **33**, 891 (1983).

Colorless oil, bp_{11} 165°; $bp_{1.0}$ 125-132°. n_D^{20} 1.5004. d_4^{20} 1.027. LD_{50} in mice, rats (mg/kg): 3050, 2370 orally; 436, 400 i.p. (Hofrichter).

THERAP CAT: Choleretic.

3948. Febuxostat. [144060-53-7] 2-[3-Cyano-4-(2-methylpropoxy)phenyl]-4-methyl-5-thiazolecarboxylic acid; 2-(3-cyano-4-isobutyloxyphenyl)-4-methyl-5-thiazolecarboxylic acid; TEI-6720; TMX-67. $C_{16}H_{16}N_2O_3S$; mol wt 316.37. C 60.74%, H 5.10%, N 8.85%, O 15.17%, S 10.14%. Xanthine oxidase/xanthine dehydrogenase inhibitor. Prepn: S. Kondo *et al.*, EP 513379; *eidem*, US 5614520 (1992, 1997 both to Teijin). Synthesis: M. Hasegawa, *Heterocycles* **47**, 857 (1998). Mechanism of action and

crystal structure study: K. Okamoto *et al., J. Biol. Chem.* **278**, 1848 (2003). Pharmacology: Y. Osada *et al., Eur. J. Pharmacol.* **241**, 183 (1993). Clinical pharmacokinetics: M. D. Mayer *et al., Am. J. Therap.* **12**, 22 (2005). Clinical evaluation in hyperuricemia and gout: M. A. Becker *et al., N. Engl. J. Med.* **353**, 2450 (2005). Review of clinical development: B. Tomlinson, *Curr. Opin. Invest. Drugs* **6**, 1168-1178 (2005).

Crystals from ethanol, mp 238-239° (dec). Also reported as crystals from acetone, mp 201-202° (Hasegawa).

THERAP CAT: Treatment of hyperuricemia and chronic gout.

3949. Fedotozine. [123618-00-8] (α*R*)-α-Ethyl-*N,N*-dimethyl-α-[[(3,4,5-trimethoxyphenyl)methoxy]methyl]benzenemethanamine; (+)-(*R*)-α-ethyl-*N,N*-dimethyl-α-[[(3,4,5-trimethoxybenzyl)oxy]methyl]benzylamine; (+)-(1*R*)-1-phenyl-1-[(3,4,5-trimethoxy)benzyloxymethyl]-*N,N*-dimethyl-*n*-propylamine. $C_{22}H_{31}NO_4$; mol wt 373.49. C 70.75%, H 8.37%, N 3.75%, O 17.14%. Peripheral kappa opioid receptor agonist. Prepn of racemate: NL 80 03601; D. R. Torossian *et al.*, US 4301163 (both 1981 to Soc. Ind. Prod. Synth.); of isomers: G. G. Aubard *et al.*, EP 384088; *eidem*, US 5245080 (1990, 1993 both to Jouveinal). Mechanism of action and pharmacokinetics in dogs: N. Pascaud *et al., J. Pharm. Pharmacol.* **42**, 546 (1990). Clinical trial in nonulcer dyspepsia: B. Fraitag *et al., Dig. Dis. Sci.* **39**, 1072 (1994).

Pale yellow, viscous oil. $[α]_D$ +16.5° (c = 6 in ethanol).

D(−)-Tartrate. [133267-27-3] JO-1196. $C_{22}H_{31}NO_4 \cdot C_4H_6O_6$; mol wt 523.57. Crystals from ethanol, mp 147°. $[α]_D^{25}$ +14.5° (c = 5 in HCl).

THERAP CAT: Gastroprokinetic.

3950. Felbamate. [25451-15-4] 2-Phenyl-1,3-propanediol dicarbamate; carbamic acid 2-phenyltrimethylene ester; ADD-03055; W-554; Felbamyl; Felbatol; Taloxa. $C_{11}H_{14}N_2O_4$; mol wt 238.24. C 55.46%, H 5.92%, N 11.76%, O 26.86%. Antiepileptic, structurally similar to meprobamate, *q.v.* Prepn: F. M. Berger, B. J. Ludwig, US 2884444 (1959 to Carter); B. J. Ludwig *et al., J. Med. Chem.* **12**, 462 (1969). Use in treatment of epileptic seizures: R. D. Sofia, US 4978680 (1990 to Carter-Walace). HPLC determn in plasma: R. P. Remmel *et al., Ther. Drug Monit.* **12**, 90 (1990). Pharmacology: E. A. Swinyard *et al., Epilepsia* **27**, 27 (1986). Metabolism in animals: J. T. Yang *et al., Drug Metab. Dispos.* **19**, 1126 (1991). Penetration of blood brain barrier: E. M. Cornford *et al., Epilepsia* **33**, 944 (1992). Clinical pharmacokinetics: A. J. Wilensky *et al., ibid.* **26**, 602 (1985). Clinical trial in refractory partial seizures: E. Faught *et al., Neurology* **43**, 688 (1993). Efficacy in childhood epileptic encephalopathy (Lennox-Gastaut syndrome): F. J. Ritter *et al., N. Engl. J. Med.* **328**, 29 (1993). Review of pharmacology, toxicology and clinical evaluation: R. D. Sofia *et al., Epilepsy Res.* Suppl. 3, 103-108 (1991).

White, odorless powder, mp 151-152°. Sparingly sol in water, methanol, ethanol, acetone and chloroform; freely sol in DMSO, 1-methyl-2-pyrrolidinone and DMF. LD_{50} i.p. in mice: 4000 mg/kg (Ludwig *et al.*).

THERAP CAT: Anticonvulsant.

3951. Felbinac. [5728-52-9] (1,1'-Biphenyl)-4-acetic acid; 4-biphenylacetic acid; 4-carboxymethylbiphenyl; BPAA; LY-61017; L-141; LJC-10141; Napageln; Traxam. $C_{14}H_{12}O_2$; mol wt 212.24. C 79.23%, H 5.70%, O 15.08%. One of the metabolites of fenbufen, *q.v.* Prepn: E. Schwenk, D. Papa, *J. Org. Chem.* **11**, 798 (1946). Improved prepn: G. R. Malone, A. I. Meyers, *ibid.* **39**, 618 (1974). Pharmacology: A. E. Sloboda, A. C. Osterberg, *Inflammation* **1**, 415 (1976). Mode of action study in ocular inflammation: E. L. Tolman *et al., Invest. Ophthalmol.* **15**, 1005 (1976). HPLC determn in serum: J. S. Fleitman *et al., J. Chromatogr.* **228**, 372 (1982).

White needles from ethyl ether, mp 164-165°. LD_{50} orally in rats: 164 mg/kg (Sloboda, Osterberg).

Ethyl ester. [14062-23-8] LM-001; Daitec. $C_{16}H_{16}O_2$; mol wt 240.30.

THERAP CAT: Anti-inflammatory, analgesic.

3952. Felinine. [471-09-0] S-(3-Hydroxy-1,1-dimethylpropyl)-L-cysteine; L-3-[(3-hydroxy-1,1-dimethylpropyl)thio]alanine; (−)-felinine. $C_8H_{17}NO_3S$; mol wt 207.29. C 46.35%, H 8.27%, N 6.76%, O 23.16%, S 15.47%. HOOCCH(NH$_2$)CH$_2$SC(CH$_3$)$_2$-CH$_2$CH$_2$OH. Sulfur containing amino acid; occurs as L-(−)-form in cat urine. Isoln: R. G. Westall, *Biochem. J.* **55**, 244 (1953). Synthesis of (±)-felinine: S. Trippett, *J. Chem. Soc.* **1957**, 1929; of (−)-felinine: H. Eggerer, *Ann.* **657**, 212 (1962); A. Schöberl *et al., Ber.* **101**, 373 (1968).

Needles from water + acetone, dec 177°. $[\alpha]_D^{25}$ −11.5° (c = 2.81 in water). Sol in water, ethanol. Practically insol in acetone, ethyl acetate, ether.

(±)-Felinine. Crystals from aq ethanol, dec 181°.

3953. Felodipine. [72509-76-3] 4-(2,3-Dichlorophenyl)-1,4-dihydro-2,6-dimethyl-3,5-pyridinedicarboxylic acid ethyl methyl ester; H-154/82; Agon; Feloday; Flodil; Hydac; Munobal; Plendil; Prevex; Splendil. $C_{18}H_{19}Cl_2NO_4$; mol wt 384.25. C 56.26%, H 4.98%, Cl 18.45%, N 3.65%, O 16.66%. Dihydropyridine calcium channel blocker marketed as the racemate. Prepn: P. B. Berntsson *et al., EP 7293; eidem, US 4264611* (1980, 1981 both to AB Hassle). Conformation: P. B. Berntsson, R. E. Carter, *Acta Pharm. Suec.* **18**, 221 (1981). Interaction with calmodulin, *q.v.*: S. L. Boström *et al., Nature* **292**, 777 (1981). Diuretic-natriuretic properties: G. F. Dibona *et al., Clin. Res.* **30**, 571A (1982). Hemodynamic effects in coronary patients: P. Decoster *et al., Eur. J. Clin. Invest.* **12**, 43 (1982). Enantioselective determn in plasma: P. A. Soons *et al., J. Chromatogr.* **528**, 343 (1990); HPLC-MS-MS determn in plasma: L. H. Miglioranca *et al., J. Chromatogr. B* **814**, 217 (2005). Pharmacokinetics and pharmacodynamics: B. Edgar *et al., Biopharm. Drug Dispos.* **8**, 235 (1987). Pharmacokinetics, vascular selectivity, effects on hypertension, hemodynamics and renal function: *Drugs* **29**, Suppl. 2, 1-212 (1985).

Crystals from isopropyl ether, mp 145°.
THERAP CAT: Antihypertensive; antianginal.

3954. Felypressin. [56-59-7] Vasopressin 2-(L-phenylalanine)-8-L-lysine; 2-(phenylalanine)-8-lysine vasopressin; Phe^2-

Lys^8-vasopressin; Phe^2-Phe^2-Lys^8-oxytocin; PLV-2; Octapressin. $C_{46}H_{65}N_{13}O_{11}S_2$; mol wt 1040.22. C 53.11%, H 6.30%, N 17.50%, O 16.92%, S 6.17%. Prepn: Boissonnas, Guttmann, *Helv. Chim. Acta* **43**, 190 (1960); Meienhofer, du Vigneaud, *J. Am. Chem. Soc.* **82**, 6336 (1960); **GB 928607**; R. Boissonnas, S. Guttmann, **US 3232923** (1963, 1966, both to Sandoz).

THERAP CAT: Vasoconstrictor.

3955. Femoxetine. [59859-58-4] (3R,4S)-3-[(4-Methoxyphenoxy)methyl]-1-methyl-4-phenylpiperidine; (+)-*trans*-1-methyl-3-[*p*-(methoxy)phenoxymethyl]-4-phenylpiperidine. $C_{20}H_{25}$-NO$_2$; mol wt 311.42. C 77.14%, H 8.09%, N 4.50%, O 10.28%. Serotonin uptake inhibitor. Prepn: J. A. Christensen, R. F. Squires, **BE 810310**; *eidem*, **US 3912743** (1974, 1975 both to A/S Ferrosan). Neuropharmacology: J. B. Lassen *et al., Psychopharmacologia* **42**, 21 (1975). Pharmacology and toxicity: *eidem, Eur. J. Pharmacol.* **32**, 108 (1975). GC determn in body fluids: E. Bechgaard, J. Lund, *J. Chromatogr.* **133**, 147 (1977). Metabolism: H. Larsson, J. Lund, *Acta Pharmacol. Toxicol.* **48**, 424 (1981). Bioavailability and pharmacokinetics: H. Mengel *et al., Arzneim.-Forsch.* **33**, 462 (1983). Double-blind clinical trials in treatment of migraine: P. G. Andersson, E. N. Petersen, *Acta Neurol. Scand.* **64**, 280 (1981); in treatment of endogenous depression: L.-E. Dahl *et al., Acta Psychiatr. Scand.* **66**, 9 (1982); P. N. Reebye *et al., Pharmacopsychiatria* **15**, 164 (1982).

Hydrochloride. [56222-04-9] FG-4963; Malexil. $C_{20}H_{25}$-NO$_2$.HCl; mol wt 347.88. LD_{50} in female, male mice (mg/kg): 48, 45 i.v.; 941, 723 s.c.; 1408, 1687 orally (Lassen).

THERAP CAT: Antidepressant.

3956. Fenamidone. [161326-34-7] (5S)-3,5-Dihydro-5-methyl-2-(methylthio)-5-phenyl-3-(phenylamino)-4H-imidazol-4-one; (S)-1-anilino-4-methyl-2-methylthio-4-phenylimidazolin-5-one; RPA-407213; Reason. $C_{17}H_{17}N_3OS$; mol wt 311.40. C 65.57%, H 5.50%, N 13.49%, O 5.14%, S 10.30%. Systemic, broad spectrum fungicide; mitochondrial electron transport inhibitor. Prepn: G. Lacroix *et al., EP 551048; eidem, US 6002016* (1993, 1999 both to Rhone-Poulenc). Physical and biological properties: R. T. Mercer *et al., Brighton Crop Prot. Conf. - Pests Dis.* **1998**, 319. Greenhouse studies: M. P. Latrose *et al., ibid.* 863. Field trials: G. DeWever *et al., Meded. Fac. Landbouwwet. Univ. Gent* **65**, 807 (2000).

White woolly powder, mp 137°. d 1.285. Soly in water (20°): 7.8 mg/l. Log P (octanol/water): 2.8 (20°). Vapor pressure (25°): 3.4×10^{-7} Pa. LD_{50} in male, female rats (mg/kg): >5000, 2028 orally; in rats (mg/kg): >2000 dermally. LC_{50} in bobwhite quail, mallard duck (mg/kg): >5200, >5200 dietary (Mercer).

USE: Fungicide.

3957. Fenamiphos. [22224-92-6] (1-Methylethyl)phosphoramidic acid ethyl 3-methyl-4-(methylthio)phenyl ester; isopropylphosphoramidic acid ethyl 4-(methylthio)-*m*-tolyl ester; ethyl 4-

(methylthio)-m-tolyl isopropylphosphoramidate; ethyl 3-methyl-4-(methylthio)phenyl (1-methylethyl)phosphoramidate; phenamiphos; Bay 68138; SRA-3886; B-68138; Bayer 68138; Nemacur. $C_{13}H_{22}NO_3PS$; mol wt 303.36. C 51.47%, H 7.31%, N 4.62%, O 15.82%, P 10.21%, S 10.57%. Systemic broad spectrum nematocide with anticholinesterase activity. Prepn: H. Kayser, G. Schrader, **US 2978479** (1961 to Bayer). Nematocidal activity: W. M. Zeck, *Pflanzenschutz-Nachr.* **24**, 114 (1971). Mode of action: B. Homeyer, K. Wagner, *Nematologica* **27**, 215 (1981). Effect on biological and chemical activity in soil: S. P. Mathur *et al., J. Environ. Sci. Health* **B15**, 61 (1980); D. J. Ross, T. W. Speir, *Soil Biol. Biochem.* **17**, 123 (1985). GC determn: M. J. Brown, *J. Agric. Food Chem.* **29**, 1129 (1981). Residual toxicity: D. C. Read, *J. Econ. Entomol.* **69**, 429 (1976). Acute toxicity: E. F. Hill, M. B. Camardese, *Ecotoxicol. Environ. Saf.* **8**, 551 (1984); E. W. Schafer, Jr., W. A. Bowles, Jr., *Arch. Environ. Contam. Toxicol.* **14**, 111 (1985). Solubility data: B. T. Bowman, W. W. Sans, *J. Environ. Sci. Health* **B18**, 221 (1983). *Review:* B. Homeyer, *Pflanzenschutz-Nachr.* **24**, 48-67 (1971). Review of metabolism and biochemical properties, efficacy: T. B. Waggoner, A. M. Khasawinah, *Residue Rev.* **53**, 79-97 (1974).

Crystals, mp 49°. Soly in water: 329 μg/ml. LD$_{50}$ orally in rats (mg/kg): 10-25 (Waggoner, Khasawinah). LD$_{50}$ orally in birds (mg/kg): 2.4 (Hill, Camardese).

Caution: Potential symptoms of overexposure are nausea, vomiting, abdominal cramps, diarrhea, salivation; headache, giddiness, vertigo, weakness; rhinorrhea, chest tightness; blurred vision, miosis; cardiac irregularities; muscle fasciculations; dyspnea. *See NIOSH Pocket Guide to Chemical Hazards* (DHHS/NIOSH 97-140, 1997) p 142.

USE: Nematocide.

3958. Fenarimol. [60168-88-9] α-(2-Chlorophenyl)-α-(4-chlorophenyl)-5-pyrimidinemethanol; 2,4′-dichloro-α-(pyrimidin-5-yl)benzhydryl alcohol; EL-222; Rubigan. $C_{17}H_{12}Cl_2N_2O$; mol wt 331.20. C 61.65%, H 3.65%, Cl 21.41%, N 8.46%, O 4.83%. Prophylactic and curative leaf fungicide; inhibits ergosterol biosynthesis. Prepn: **NL 6806106**; H. M. Taylor *et al.,* **US 3818009** (1968, 1974 both to Lilly). Improved prepn: *eidem,* **US 3869456**; use as fungicide: *eidem,* **US 3887708** (both 1975 to Lilly). Mode of action, efficacy against various fungi: H. Buchenauer, *Proc. Br. Crop Prot. Conf. - Pests Dis.* **1977**, 699. Absorption by leaf tissue, local systemic activity: I. F. Brown, H. R. Hall, *ibid.* **1981**(2), 573. In control of apple scab: J. M. Olivier, J. Guillaumes, *Monogr. Br. Crop Prot. Counc.* **31**, 485 (1985). Post-infection efficacy: A. L. O'Leary, T. B. Sutton, *Phytopathology* **76**, 119 (1986). Brief review: J.-M. Beraud *et al., Def. Veg.* **34**, 17 (1980).

White odorless crystals, mp 117-119°. Practically insol in water (13.7 ppm at pH 7). Sol in most organic solvents. Vapor pressure at 25° <10^{-7} millibar. LD$_{50}$ in mice, rats (mg/kg): 4500, 2500 orally (Beraud).

USE: Plant fungicide.

3959. Fenazaquin. [120928-09-8] 4-[2-[4-(1,1-Dimethylethyl)phenyl]ethoxy]quinazoline; 4-[2-[4-(*tert*-butyl)phenyl]-ethoxy]quinazoline; 4-*tert*-butylphenethyl quinazolin-4-yl ether; DE-436; EL-436; Magister. $C_{20}H_{22}N_2O$; mol wt 306.40. C 78.40%, H 7.24%, N 9.14%, O 5.22%. Acaricidal quinazoline;

inhibits Complex I of the mitochondrial electron transport chain. Prepn: B. A. Dreikorn *et al.,* **EP 326329** (1989 to Lilly); *idem et al.,* **US 5411963** (1995 to DowElanco). Mechanism of action study: E. Wood *et al., Pestic. Biochem. Physiol.* **54**, 135 (1996). Photodecomposition study: J. Bhattacharyya *et al., J. Agric. Food Chem.* **51**, 4013 (2003). GC determn in environmental and crop samples: A. R. Gambie, J. M. Perkins, *Brighton Crop Prot. Conf. - Pests Dis.* **1992**, 895. Field trials vs spider mites on ornamentals: R. T. Pollak *et al., ibid.* 1181. Comprehensive description: C. Longhurst *et al., ibid.* 51-58.

White to tan solid, mp 70-71° (Dreikorn); also reported as mp 77.5-80.0° (Gambie). Vapor pressure at 25°: 1.6×10^{-4} Pa. Log P at 25° (octanol/water): 5.51. Soly (g/ml): hexane 0.033-0.05; dichloromethane 70.6; acetone 0.4-0.5; acetonitrile 0.33-0.50; water 0.0001. Molar extinction coefficient at 262.2 nm: 1.24×10^4 (pH 7.83). LD$_{50}$ orally in rats, mice (mg/kg): 134, 1480; dermally in rabbits (mg/kg): >5000. LC$_{50}$ (96 hr) in bluegill, trout (μg/l): 34.1, 3.8 (Longhurst).

USE: Acaricide and insecticide.

3960. Fenbendazole. [43210-67-9] [5-(Phenylthio)-1*H*-benzimidazol-2-yl]carbamic acid methyl ester; 5-(phenylthio)-2-benzimidazolecarbamic acid methyl ester; methyl 5-(phenylthio)-2-benzimidazolecarbamate; HOE-881v; Panacur. $C_{15}H_{13}N_3O_2S$; mol wt 299.35. C 60.18%, H 4.38%, N 14.04%, O 10.69%, S 10.71%. Prepn: H. Loewe *et al.,* **DE 2164690**; *eidem,* **US 3954791** (1973, 1976 both to Hoechst); C. Baeder *et al., Experientia* **30**, 753 (1974). Efficacy vs gastrointestinal nematodes in swine: Enigk *et al., Dtsch. Tieraerztl. Wochenschr.* **81**, 177 (1974).

Light brownish-gray, odorless, tasteless crystalline powder, mp 233° (dec). Insol in water; insol or only very slightly sol in the usual solvents. Freely sol in DMSO.

THERAP CAT (VET): Anthelmintic (Nematodes).

3961. Fenbenicillin. [1926-48-3] (2*S*,5*R*,6*R*)-3,3-Dimethyl-7-oxo-6-[(phenoxyphenylacetyl)amino]-4-thia-1-azabicyclo[3.2.0]-heptane-2-carboxylic acid; 3,3-dimethyl-7-oxo-6-(2-phenoxy-2-phenylacetamido)-4-thia-1-azabicyclo[3.2.0]heptane-2-carboxylate; α-phenoxybenzylpenicillin; 6-(α-phenoxyphenylacetamido)-penicillanic acid; 6-(α-phenoxy-α-phenylacetamido)penicillanate; phenbenicillin. $C_{22}H_{22}N_2O_5S$; mol wt 426.49. C 61.96%, H 5.20%, N 6.57%, O 18.76%, S 7.52%. Semi-synthetic antibiotic related to penicillin. Prepn: **GB 877120** (1961 to Beecham). Bacteriological and pharmacological properties: Rollo, Burley, *Br. Med. J.* **I**, 76 (1962).

Potassium salt. [1177-30-6] Penspek (formerly). $C_{22}H_{21}$-KN_2O_5S; mol wt 464.58. Powder, mp 88-95°, dec 120-125°. Readily sol in water. LD$_{50}$ in mice (mg/kg): 225 i.v.; 520 i.p.; 3000 orally (Rollo, Burley).

THERAP CAT: Antibacterial.

3962. Fenbuconazole. [114369-43-6] α-[2-(4-Chlorophenyl)ethyl]-α-phenyl-1H-1,2,4-triazole-1-propanenitrile; (R,S)-4-(4-chlorophenyl)-2-phenyl-2-[(1H-1,2,4-triazol-1-yl)methyl]butyronitrile; fenethanil; RH-7592; Enable; Govern; Indar. C₁₉H₁₇ClN₄; mol wt 336.82. C 67.75%, H 5.09%, Cl 10.53%, N 16.63%. Systemic triazole antifungal for food and ornamental crops. Prepn: S. H. Shaber et al., DE 3721786; idem, US 5087635 (1988, 1992 both to Rohm & Haas). Comprehensive description: D. Driant et al., Brighton Crop Prot. Conf. - Pests Dis. 1988, 33-40. Field trials vs Botrytis infection in roses: Y. Elad et al., Crop Prot. 12, 69 (1993); vs root rot in barley: P. J. Cotterill, ibid. 273.

White crystalline solid, mp 124-126°. vapor pressure (20°): 0.37 × 10⁻⁷ torr. Soly in water (25°): 0.2 ppm. Sol in common organic solvents. Insol in aliphatic hydrocarbons. LD₅₀ in rats (mg/kg): >2000 orally; >5000 dermally (Driant).
USE: Agricultural fungicide.

3963. Fenbufen. [36330-85-5] γ-Oxo-[1,1'-biphenyl]-4-butanoic acid; 3-(4-biphenylylcarbonyl)propionic acid; β-p-phenylbenzoylpropionic acid; diphenyl-4-γ-oxo-γ-butyric acid; 4-(4-biphenylyl)-4-oxobutyric acid; CL-82204; Bufemid; Cinopal; Cinopol; Lederfen. C₁₆H₁₄O₃; mol wt 254.28. C 75.57%, H 5.55%, O 18.88%. Prepn: FR 798941 (1936 to I. G. Farbenind.), C.A. 30, 7729⁴ (1936); D. H. Hey, R. Wilkinson, J. Chem. Soc. 1940, 1030; cf. M. Weizmann et al., Chem. Ind. (London) 1940, 402; W. Reppe et al., Ann. 596, 223 (1955); A. S. Tomcufcik et al., DE 2147111; eidem, US 3784701 (1972, 1974 to Am. Cyanamid. Series of articles on chemistry, pharmacology, reproductive toxicology and clinical experience: Arzneim.-Forsch. 30, 695-720, 725-746 (1980). Toxicity: H. F. Bolte et al., ibid. 721. Review of pharmacology and therapeutic use: R. N. Brogden et al., Drugs 21, 1-22 (1981).

Crystals from ethanol, mp 185-187°. LD₅₀ in various strains of mice, rats (mg/kg): 795-1673, 200-720 orally; 506-811, 265-575 i.p. (Bolte).
THERAP CAT: Anti-inflammatory.

3964. Fenbutatin Oxide. [13356-08-6] Hexakis(2-methyl-2-phenylpropyl)distannoxane; di[tri-(2-methyl-2-phenylpropyl)tin]-oxide; hexakis(β,β-dimethylphenethyl)distannoxane; SD-14114; Torque; Vendex. C₆₀H₇₈OSn₂; mol wt 1052.68. C 68.46%, H 7.47%, O 1.52%, Sn 22.55%. Selective organotin miticide. Prepn: DE 2225666; C. A. Horne Jr., US 3657451 (1971, 1972 both to Shell Oil Co.). General description and analysis: G. Zweig, J. Sherma, Anal. Methods Pestic. Plant Growth Regul. 10, 139 (1978). HPLC/MS determn in fruits and vegetables: K. A. Barnes et al., Rapid Commun. Mass Spectrom. 11, 159 (1997). Suppression of citrus rust mite: V. French, J. Rio Grande Val. Hortic. Soc. 35, 121 (1982).

White crystalline powder, mp 145°. Soly at 23° (g/l): acetone 6; octanol 33; xylene 53; benzene 143; dichloromethane 377; methylene chloride 380. Soly in water: <5 µg/l. Converts to the hydroxide in the presence of water. Nontoxic to bees, toxic to fish. LD₅₀ in rats, rabbits (mg/kg): >2000 orally; >2000 percutaneously (Zweig).
USE: Acaricide.

3965. Fenbutrazate. [4378-36-3] α-Ethylbenzeneacetic acid 2-(3-methyl-2-phenyl-4-morpholinyl)ethyl ester; 2-phenylbutyric acid 2-(3-methyl-2-phenylmorpholino)ethyl ester; 2-(3-methyl-2-phenylmorpholino)ethyl 2-phenylbutyrate; phenbutrazate. C₂₃H₂₉NO₃; mol wt 367.48. C 75.17%, H 7.95%, N 3.81%, O 13.06%. Prepn: H. Siemer, O. Hengen, US 3018222 (1962 to Ravensberg). Physical properties and pharmacology: O. Hengen, H. Siemer, Arzneim.-Forsch. 5, 526 (1955).

Honey colored, viscous oil, bp₀.₀₅ 235-240°. Sol in methanol with neutral reaction.
Hydrochloride. [6474-85-7] R-381. C₂₃H₂₉NO₃.HCl; mol wt 403.94. Crystals, mp 154°. Slightly sol in water; sol in ethanol, acetone. Practically insol in ether, benzene. LD₅₀ in mice (mg/kg): 3200 orally; 2800 s.c. (Hengen, Seimer).
Hydrochloride mixture with phenmetrazine theoclate. [8004-38-4] Cafilon; Filon.
THERAP CAT: Anorexic.

3966. Fencamfamine. [1209-98-9] N-Ethyl-3-phenylbicyclo[2.2.1]heptan-2-amine; N-ethyl-3-phenyl-2-norbornanamine; 2-ethylamino-3-phenylnorcamphane; 2-phenyl-3-ethylamino-norbornane; 2-ethylamino-3-phenylnorbornane; 2-ethylamino-3-phenylbicyclo[2.2.1]heptane; Euvitol. C₁₅H₂₁N; mol wt 215.33. C 83.67%, H 9.83%, N 6.50%. Prepd from 3-amino-2-phenyl-norbornane and acetaldehyde followed by hydrogenation in the presence of PtO₂: Thesing et al., DE 1110159 (1961 to E. Merck), C.A. 56, 2352g (1962). Pharmacology: R. Hotovy et al., Arzneim.-Forsch. 11, 20 (1961).

bp₀.₁ 128-131°.
Hydrochloride. [2240-14-4] H-610. C₁₅H₂₁N.HCl; mol wt 251.79. Principal ingredient of Reactivan which also contains vitamins B₁, B₆, B₁₂ and C. Crystals from acetone, mp 192°. Freely sol in water, ethanol, methanol, chloroform; slightly sol in benzene. Practically insol in ether. LD₅₀ in mice, rats (mg/kg): 135.0, 113.0 orally; 85.5, 68.5 s.c.; 15.7, 23.5 i.v. (Hotovy).
Note: This is a controlled substance (stimulant): 21 CFR, 1308.14.
THERAP CAT: CNS stimulant.

3967. Fencamine. [28947-50-4] 3,7-Dihydro-1,3,7-trimethyl-8-[[2-[methyl(1-methyl-2-phenylethyl)amino]ethyl]amino]-1H-purine-2,6-dione; 8-[[2-[methyl(α-methylphenethyl)amino]ethyl]amino]caffeine; 8-[2-[N,α-dimethyl-β-phenyl)ethylamino]-1,3,7-trimethyl-2,6-dioxopurine; N¹-(1,3,7-trimethyl-2,6-dioxopurin-8-yl)-N²-(1-methyl)phenethyl-N²-methylethylenediamine; N-8-caffeyl-N'-methyl-N'-(α-methylphenethyl)ethylenediamine; phencamine; ST-374. C₂₀H₂₈N₆O₂; mol wt 384.48. C 62.48%, H 7.34%, N 21.86%, O 8.32%. Prepn: ES 347509; ES 352077 (both 1969 to Labs. Miquel); Pitarch et al., Quim. Ind. (Madrid) 17, 71 (1971). Pharmacology: eidem, ibid. 76. Colorimetric and TLC determn in urine: J. Mallol et al., Arzneim.-Forsch. 24, 1301 (1974). Toxicity data: E. Usdin, D. H. Efron, Psychotropic Drugs *and Related Compounds* (National Institute of Mental Health, Rockville, MD, 2nd ed., 1972) p 229. Clinical trial in depression: P. G. Quiros e Isla, *Rev. Clin. Esp.* **119**, 437 (1970).

Crystals from methanol, mp 150-152°.

Hydrochloride. [63918-50-3] Altimina; Sicoclor. $C_{20}H_{28}N_6$-O_2.HCl; mol wt 420.94. Slightly hygroscopic, bitter crystals, decomp 278-279°. uv max (water): 296 nm ($E_{1cm}^{1\%}$ 398). Sol in water; slightly sol in many organic solvents. LD_{50} in rats, mice (mg/kg): 93, 82 i.p.; 508, 418 orally (Usdin, Efron).

THERAP CAT: Analeptic.

3968. *d*-Fenchone. [4695-62-9] (1*S*)-1,3,3-Trimethylbicyclo[2.2.1]heptan-2-one; *d*-1,3,3-trimethyl-2-norbornanone; *d*-1,3,3-trimethyl-2-norcamphanone. $C_{10}H_{16}O$; mol wt 152.23. C 78.90%, H 10.59%, O 10.51%. Occurs in fennel oil and in the essential oil of *Lavandula stoechas* L., *Labiatae*. Isoln: Wallach, *Ann.* **263**, 129 (1891); **353**, 209 (1907); **369**, 63 (1909); Shavrygin, *J. Appl. Chem. USSR* **12**, 1201 (1939). Total synthesis: Boyle *et al., Chem. Commun.* **1971**, 395; G. Buchbauer, H. C. Rohner, *Ann.* **1981**, 2093. Toxicity study: P. M. Jenner *et al., Food Cosmet. Toxicol.* **2**, 327 (1964). *Review:* Simonsen, *The Terpenes* vol. II (Cambridge, 2nd ed., 1949) pp 560-580; D. L. J. Opdyke, *Food Cosmet. Toxicol.* **14**, Suppl., 769-771 (1976).

Oily liq. Camphor-like odor. d_4^{18} 0.948. mp 6.1°. bp_{760} 193.5°; bp_{100} 122°; bp_{20} 82°; bp_{15} 66°. $[\alpha]_D^{20}$ +66.9°. n_D^{18} 1.4636. Practically insol in water (pH of satd soln 6.82). Very sol in abs alcohol, ether. LD_{50} orally in rats: 6.16 g/kg (Jenner).

USE: As flavor in foods; in perfumes.

THERAP CAT: Counterirritant.

3969. **Fenclozic Acid.** [17969-20-9] 2-(4-Chlorophenyl)-4-thiazoleacetic acid; 2-(*p*-chlorophenyl)thiazol-4-ylacetic acid; acidum fenclozicum; ICI-54450; Myalex. $C_{11}H_8ClNO_2S$; mol wt 253.70. C 52.08%, H 3.18%, Cl 13.97%, N 5.52%, O 12.61%, S 12.64%. Prepn: W. Hepworth, G. J. Stacey, **NL 6614130**; *eidem,* **US 3538107** (1967, 1970 both to ICI); Aries, **FR 1561433** (1969), *C.A.* **72**, 43654y (1970). Pharmacology: W. Hepworth *et al., Nature* **221**, 582 (1969); Newbould, *Br. J. Pharmacol.* **35**, 487 (1969). Metabolic studies: Foulkes, *J. Pharmacol. Exp. Ther.* **172**, 115, 449 (1970). Clinical evaluation: Chalmers *et al., Ann. Rheum. Dis.* **28**, 590, 595 (1969).

Colorless crystalline solid from ethyl acetate, mp 155-156°. Soluble in most organic solvents; sparingly sol in water. LD_{50} in rats, mice (mg/kg): 850, 1000 orally; 250, 300 i.v. (Hepworth).

THERAP CAT: Anti-inflammatory.

3970. **Fendiline.** [13042-18-7] γ-Phenyl-*N*-(1-phenylethyl)-benzenepropanamine; *N*-(3,3-diphenylpropyl)-α-methylbenzylamine; *N*-(1-phenylethyl)-3,3-diphenylpropylamine. $C_{23}H_{25}N$; mol wt 315.45. C 87.57%, H 7.99%, N 4.44%. Calcium blocking agent. Prepn: **BE 621300**; Harsányi *et al.,* **US 3262977** (1962, 1966 both to Chinoin); *eidem, J. Med. Chem.* **7**, 623 (1964); Klosa,

J. Prakt. Chem. **34**, 312 (1966). Prepn and studies of the labelled compound: Volford, Harsányi, *J. Labelled Compd.* **9**, 219 (1973). Structure-activity studies: Leszkovszky *et al., Acta Physiol. Acad. Sci. Hung.* **29**, 283 (1966). Pharmacologic properties: W. R. Kukovetz *et al., Arzneim.-Forsch.* **26**, 1321 (1976); A. Fleckenstein *et al., ibid.* **27**, 562 (1977). Pharmacokinetics and tolerance: R. Weyhenmeyer *et al., ibid.* **37**, 58 (1987). Use in ischemic heart disease: Z. Antaloczy, I. Preda, *Ther. Hung.* **27**, 71 (1979). Assessment of Ca^{2+}-antagonist effects: M. Spedding, *Arch. Pharmacol.* **318**, 234 (1982).

$bp_{0.3}$ 206-210°.

Hydrochloride. [13636-18-5] HK-137; Cordan; Fendilar; Sensit. $C_{23}H_{25}N$.HCl; mol wt 351.91. Almost white or slightly pink powder, mp 204-205°. Very slightly sol in water; easily sol in methanol, ethanol, chloroform. LD_{50} in mice (mg/kg): 14.5 i.v.; 950 orally (Harsányi).

THERAP CAT: Vasodilator (coronary).

3971. **Fendosal.** [53597-27-6] 5-(4,5-Dihydro-2-phenyl-3*H*-benz[*e*]indol-3-yl)-2-hydroxybenzoic acid; 5-(4,5-dihydro-2-phenyl-3*H*-benz[*e*]indol-3-yl)salicylic acid; 3-(3-carboxy-4-hydroxyphenyl)-2-phenyl-4,5-dihydro-3*H*-benz[*e*]indole; HP-129; P-71-0129; Alnovin. $C_{25}H_{19}NO_3$; mol wt 381.42. C 78.72%, H 5.02%, N 3.67%, O 12.58%. Prepn: R. C. Allen, B. Anderson, **DE 2407671**; *eidem,* **US 3878225** (1974, 1975 both to Hoechst); V. B. Anderson *et al., J. Med. Chem.* **19**, 318 (1976). Pharmacology: H. B. Lassman *et al., Agents Actions* **8**, 209 (1978). Clinical study: S. S. Bloomfield *et al., Clin. Pharmacol. Ther.* **23**, 390 (1978).

Crystals from acetic acid, mp 223-225° (dec). LD_{50} in mice, rats, rabbits (mg/kg): 740, 450, 560 orally; in mice (mg/kg): 510 i.p. (Lassman).

THERAP CAT: Anti-inflammatory.

3972. **Fenethylline.** [3736-08-1] 3,7-Dihydro-1,3-dimethyl-7-[2-[(1-methyl-2-phenylethyl)amino]ethyl]-1*H*-purine-2,6-dione; 7-[2-[(α-methylphenethyl)amino]ethyl]theophylline; 7-[β-(α-methyl-β-phenylethylamino)ethyl]theophylline; 7-(phenylisopropylaminoethyl)theophylline; 7-(3-phenyl-2-propylaminoethyl)-theophylline; theophyllineethylamphetamine. $C_{18}H_{23}N_5O_2$; mol wt 341.41. C 63.32%, H 6.79%, N 20.51%, O 9.37%. Prepn from 7-(β-chloroethyl)theophylline and amphetamine: Kholstaedt, Klinger, **DE 1123329** (1962 to Degussa), *C.A.* **57**, 5933c (1962). Metabolism in man: T. Ellison *et al., Eur. J. Pharmacol.* **13**, 123 (1970).

Hydrochloride. [1892-80-4] H-814; Captagon. $C_{18}H_{23}N_5$-O_2.HCl; mol wt 377.87. Crystals, two different modifications, mp 227-229° and mp 237-239°.

d-Form hydrochloride. Crystals, mp 246-247°.

l-Form hydrochloride. Crystals, mp 246-247°.

Note: This is a controlled substance (stimulant): **21 CFR,** 1308.11.

THERAP CAT: CNS stimulant.

3973. Fenfluramine. [458-24-2] *N*-Ethyl-α-methyl-3-(tri-fluoromethyl)benzeneethanamine; *N*-ethyl-α-methyl-*m*-(trifluoro-methyl)phenethylamine; 2-ethylamino-1-(3-trifluoromethylphenyl)-propane; S-768. $C_{12}H_{16}F_3N$; mol wt 231.26. C 62.32%, H 6.97%, F 24.65%, N 6.06%. Prepn: L. G. Beregi *et al.*, **FR M1658**; *eidem*, **US 3198833** (1963, 1965 both to Sci. Union et Cie Soc. Franc. Recherche Méd.). Prepn of optical isomers: *eidem*, **US 3198834** (1965 to Sci. Union et Cie Soc. Franc. Recherche Med.). Pharma-cology: *Presse Med.* **71,** 181 (1963). Pharmacology and toxicity of isomers and racemate: J. C. Le Douarec *et al., Arch. Int. Pharma-codyn. Ther.* **161,** 206 (1966). Pharmacokinetics: S. Caccia *et al., Eur. J. Clin. Pharmacol.* **29,** 221 (1985). Clinical trial of dextro-fenfluramine in refractory obesity: N. Finer *et al., Curr. Ther. Res.* **38,** 847 (1985). Comprehensive review: Pinder *et al., Drugs* **10,** 241-323 (1975).

bp$_{12}$ 108-112°. LD$_{50}$ i.p. in mice: 144 mg/kg (**US 3198833**).

Hydrochloride. [404-82-0] Acino; Adipomin; Obedrex; Pesos; Ponderal; Ponderax; Ponderex; Pondimin; Rotondin. $C_{12}H_{16}F_3$-N.HCl; mol wt 267.72. Crystals from ethanol + ether, mp 166°.

d-Form. [3239-44-9] Dexfenfluramine; dextrofenfluramine. $[\alpha]_D^{25}$ +9.5° (c = 8 in ethanol). LD$_{50}$ orally in rats: 114.6 mg/kg (Le Douarec).

d-Form hydrochloride. [3239-45-0] Adifax; Glypolix; Iso-meride; Redux. Crystals from ethyl acetate, mp 160-161°.

l-Form. [37577-24-5] $[\alpha]_D^{25}$ −9.6° (c = 8 in ethanol). LD$_{50}$ orally in rats: 195 mg/kg (Le Douarec).

l-Form hydrochloride. [3616-78-2] Crystals from ethyl ace-tate, mp 160-161°.

Note: This is a controlled substance: **21 CFR,** 1308.14.

THERAP CAT: Anorexic.

3974. Fenhexamid. [126833-17-8] *N*-(2,3-Dichloro-4-hy-droxyphenyl)-1-methylcyclohexanecarboxamide; 1-methyl-cyclo-hexanecarboxylic acid (2,3-dichloro-4-hydroxy-phenyl)-amide; KBR-2738; Decree; Elevate. $C_{14}H_{17}Cl_2NO_2$; mol wt 302.20. C 55.64%, H 5.67%, Cl 23.46%, N 4.63%, O 10.59%. Hydroxy-anilide fungicide. Prepn: B.-W. Krüger *et al.,* **EP 339418**; *eidem*, **US 5059623** (1989, 1991 both to Bayer). Review of properties and activities: H.-J. Rosslenbroich *et al., Brighton Crop Prot. Conf. - Pests Dis.* **1998,** 327-334; of field trials on fruit crops: N. M. Adam, P. A. Birch, *ibid.,* 849-856.

mp 141°. Soly in water at 20°: 20 mg/l (pH 5-7). Vapor pressure at 20°: 4×10^{-7} Pa (extrapolated). Log P (*n*-octanol/-water) at 20°: 3.51 (pH 7). LD$_{50}$ in rats (mg/kg): >5000 orally; >5000 dermally (24 hr). LC$_{50}$ (4hr) in rats (mg/m^3): >5057 by inhalation. (Rosslenbroich).

USE: Fungicide.

3975. Fenipentol. [583-03-9] α-Butylbenzenemethanol; α-butylbenzyl alcohol; phenylbutylcarbinol; 1-phenyl-1-hydroxy-pentane; phenylpentanol; PC 1; Ph BC; Pancoral. $C_{11}H_{16}O$; mol wt 164.24. C 80.44%, H 9.82%, O 9.74%. Synthesis: Fourneau, Puyal, *An. Soc. Esp. Fis. Quim.* **18,** 323 (1920); Adams, Vander Werf, *J. Am. Chem. Soc.* **72,** 4368 (1950); Protiva *et al., Chem. Listy* **46,** 37 (1952). Prepn of the drug: Scheffler, Engelhorn, **GB 915815**; *eidem*, **US 3084100** (both 1963 to Thomae). Pharmacology: En-gelhorn, *Arzneim.-Forsch.* **10,** 255 (1960); Beck, Bierwisch, *ibid.* **20,** 693 (1970). Metabolism: Koss *et al., ibid.* **14,** 195 (1964).

Colorless or slightly yellow liquid. bp$_{12}$ 123-124°. n_D^{20} 1.5112. Miscible with organic liquids. Practically insol in water.

THERAP CAT: Choleretic. Also used in treatment of mild chronic pancreatitis.

3976. Fenitrothion. [122-14-5] Phosphorothioic acid *O,O*-dimethyl *O*-(3-methyl-4-nitrophenyl) ester; *O,O*-dimethyl *O*-4-ni-tro-*m*-tolyl phosphorothioate; *O,O*-dimethyl *O*-(3-methyl-4-nitro-phenyl) phosphorothioate; *O,O*-dimethyl *O*-4-nitro-*m*-tolyl thio-phosphate; MEP; metathion; Bayer 41831; Bayer S 5660; ENT-25715; OMS-45; AC-47300; Accothion; Cyten; Cyfen; Folithion; Sumithion. $C_9H_{12}NO_5PS$; mol wt 277.23. C 38.99%, H 4.36%, N 5.05%, O 28.86%, P 11.17%, S 11.57%. Prepn: **BE 594669** (1960 to Sumitomo); **BE 596091** (1960 to Bayer). Activity: Y. Nishi-zawa *et al., Agric. Biol. Chem.* **25,** 605 (1961). Toxicity study: G. Schrader, *Angew. Chem.* **73,** 331 (1961).

Yellow oil. bp$_{0.05}$ 118°. n_D^{25} 1.5528. d$_4^{25}$ 1.3227. Vapor press at 20°: 6×10^{-6} mm Hg. uv max: 269.5 nm (ε 6756). Practically insol in water. Low soly in aliphatic hydrocarbons; sol in most organic solvents. LD$_{50}$ orally in rats: 250 mg/kg (Schrader).

Caution: Cholinesterase inhibitor.

USE: Insecticide.

3977. Fennel. Large fennel; sweet fennel. Dried, ripe fruit of cultivated varieties of *Foeniculum vulgare* Mill., *Umbelliferae. Habit.* Southern Europe, Western Asia, widely cultivated. *Constit.* 2-6% volatile oil, fixed oil, protein, organic acids and flavonoids. Clinical trial of fennel oil emulsion in infantile colic: I. Alexan-drovich *et al., Alt. Ther. Health Med.* **9,** 58 (2003). Review: F. S. D'Amelio, Sr., *Botanicals* (CRC Press, Boca Raton, 1999) pp 105-106.

Volatile oil. [8006-84-6] Oil of fennel. *Constit.* 50-70% *trans*-anethole, up to 20% (+)-fenchone, methylchavicol, anisaldehyde, terpenoids including α-pinene, limonene, α-phellandrene. Color-less or pale yellow liquid with characteristic odor of fennel. d$_{25}^{25}$ 0.953-0.973. α_D^{25} +12 to +24°. n_D^{20} 1.532-1.543. Slightly sol in water; sol in 1 vol 90% or in 8 vols 80% alcohol; very sol in chloroform, ether. *Keep well closed, cool and protected from light.*

USE: Flavoring agent in foods and pharmaceuticals. Used in eye washes and in facial steams to soothe and clean skin.

THERAP CAT: Carminative.

3978. Fenofibrate. [49562-28-9] 2-[4-(4-Chlorobenzoyl)-phenoxy]-2-methylpropanoic acid 1-methylethyl ester; isopropyl [4′-(*p*-chlorobenzoyl)-2-phenoxy-2-methyl]propionate; procetofen; procetofene; LF-178; Ankebin; Elasterin; Fenobrate; Fenotard; Li-panthyl; Lipantil; Lipidil; Lipoclar; Lipofene; Liposit; Lipsin; No-lipax; Procetoken; Protolipan; Secalip; Tricor. $C_{20}H_{21}ClO_4$; mol wt 360.83. C 66.57%, H 5.87%, Cl 9.83%, O 17.74%. Prepn: A. Mieville, **DE 2250327** (1973 to Orchimed), *C.A.* **79,** 53029 (1973), addn to **DE 2003430**; *eidem*, **US 4058552** (1970, 1977 both to Orchimed). Series of articles on synthesis, metabolism, pharmacology and clinical trials: *Arzneim.-Forsch.* **26**, 885-909 (1976). Toxicity data: R. Sornay *et al., ibid.* 885. GC-MS of major metabolite in humans: L. F. Elsom *et al., J. Chromatogr.* **123**, 463 (1976). Efficacy in hyperlipidemias: H. B. Stähelin *et al., Praxis* **68**, 24 (1979). Effect on human biliary lipids: E. M. Grandjean *et al., Schweiz. Med. Wochenschr.* **109**, 601 (1979). Mechanism of action: W. Wülfert *et al., Artery* **9**, 120 (1981).

Crystals from isopropanol, mp 80-81°. Practically insol in water. Slightly sol in methanol, ethanol. Sol in acetone, ether, benzene, chloroform. LD_{50} in mice: 1600 mg/kg orally (Sornay).

THERAP CAT: Antilipemic.

3979. Fenoldopam. [67227-56-9] 6-Chloro-2,3,4,5-tetrahydro-1-(4-hydroxyphenyl)-1*H*-3-benzazepine-7,8-diol; 6-chloro-7,8-dihydroxy-1-*p*-hydroxyphenyl-2,3,4,5-tetrahydro-1*H*-3-benzazepine; SKF-82526. $C_{16}H_{16}ClNO_3$; mol wt 305.76. C 62.85%, H 5.27%, Cl 11.60%, N 4.58%, O 15.70%. Dopamine D_1-receptor agonist. Prepn: J. Weinstock, *DE 2751258; idem, US 4197297* (1978, 1980 both to SmithKline); J. Weinstock *et al., J. Med. Chem.* **23**, 973 (1980). HPLC determn in urine and plasma: V. K. Boppana *et al., J. Chromatogr.* **317**, 463 (1984). Clinical pharmacology: R. M. Stote *et al., Clin. Pharmacol. Ther.* **34**, 309 (1983); R. M. Carey *et al., J. Clin. Invest.* **74**, 2198 (1984). Hemodynamic effects in hypertension: H. O. Ventura *et al., Circulation* **69**, 1142 (1984); M. P. Caruana *et al., Br. J. Clin. Pharmacol.* **24**, 721 (1987). Clinical evaluation in congestive heart failure: G. S. Francis *et al., Am. Heart J.* **116**, 473 (1988).

Hydrobromide. $C_{16}H_{16}ClNO_3$.HBr. mp 277° (dec).
Methanesulfonate. [67227-57-0] Fenoldopam mesylate; SKF-82526-J; Corlopam. $C_{16}H_{16}ClNO_3$.CH_3SO_3H; mol wt 401.86. mp 274° (dec).

THERAP CAT: Antihypertensive.

3980. Fenoprofen. [31879-05-7] α-Methyl-3-phenoxybenzeneacetic acid; (±)-*m*-phenoxyhydratropic acid; α-*dl*-2-(3-phenoxyphenyl)propionic acid; Lilly 53838. $C_{15}H_{14}O_3$; mol wt 242.27. C 74.36%, H 5.82% O 19.81%. Prepn: W. S. Marshall, *FR 2015728; eidem, US 3600437* (1970, 1971 both to Lilly). Pharmacology: Rubin *et al., J. Pharm. Sci.* **60**, 1797 (1971); **61**, 800 (1972); Herrmann, *Proc. Soc. Exp. Biol. Med.* **139**, 548 (1972). Metabolism: Rubin *et al., J. Pharmacol. Exp. Ther.* **183**, 449 (1972). Toxicology: J. L. Emmerson *et al., Toxicol. Appl. Pharmacol.* **25**, 444 (1973). Comprehensive description: C. K. Ward, R. E. Schirmer, *Anal. Profiles Drug Subs.* **6**, 161-182 (1977). *Review:* R. N. Brogden *et al., Drugs* **13**, 241-265 (1977); R. Nickander *et al.,* in *Pharmacological and Biochemical Properties of Drug Substances* vol. 1, M. E. Goldberg, Ed. (Am. Pharm. Assoc., Washington, DC, 1977) pp 183-213.

Viscous oil, $bp_{0.11}$ 168-171°. n_D^{25} 1.5742. pKa 7.3.
Calcium salt dihydrate. [53746-45-5] Lilly 69323; Fenopron; Fepron; Feprona; Nalfon; Nalgesic; Progesic. $C_{30}H_{26}CaO_6$.$2H_2O$; mol wt 558.63. White crystalline powder. Soly in mg/ml at 37°: *n*-hexanol 11; methanol 8; water 2.5; chloroform 0.01. pKa 4.5. Aq solns sensitive to intense uv light. LD_{50} orally in mice: 800 mg/kg (Emmerson).

THERAP CAT: Anti-inflammatory; analgesic.

3981. Fenoterol. [13392-18-2] 5-[1-Hydroxy-2-[[2-(4-hydroxyphenyl)-1-methylethyl]amino]ethyl]-1,3-benzenediol; 3,5-dihydroxy-α-[[(*p*-hydroxy-α-methylphenethyl)amino]methyl]benzyl alcohol; 1-(3,5-dihydroxyphenyl)-1-hydroxy-2-[(4-hydroxyphenyl)isopropylamino]ethane; 1-(*p*-hydroxyphenyl)-2-[[β-hydroxy-β-(3′,5′-dihydroxyphenyl)ethyl]aminopropane; TH-1165. $C_{17}H_{21}$-NO_4; mol wt 303.35. C 67.31%, H 6.98%, N 4.62%, O 21.10%. $β_2$-Adrenergic agonist. Prepn and sepn of stereoisomers: **BE 640433**; Zelle *et al.,* **US 3341593** (1962, 1967 to Boehringer, Ing.). Pharmacology: Schuster, Baum, *Arzneim.-Forsch.* **19**, 1905 (1969); O'Donnell, *Eur. J. Pharmacol.* **12**, 35 (1970). Toxicity: E. I. Goldenthal, *Toxicol. Appl. Pharmacol.* **18**, 185 (1971). Metabolism in mice: S. Kojima *et al., Arzneim.-Forsch.* **30**, 959 (1980). HPLC determn in plasma: S. Kramer, G. Blaschke, *J. Chromatogr. B* **751**, 169 (2001). Clinical evaluation: Tweel, *Ann. Allergy* **29**, 142 (1971); Rebuck, Saunders, *Med. J. Aust.* **1**, 225 (1972). Comparison with ritodrine in preterm labor: J. Gerris *et al., Eur. J. Clin. Pharmacol.* **18**, 443 (1980). Review of pharmacology and therapeutic efficacy: R. C. Heel *et al., Drugs* **15**, 3-32 (1978); N. Svedmyr, *Pharmacotherapy* **5**, 109-126 (1985).

Hydrobromide. [1944-12-3] TH-1165a; Airum; Berotec; Dosberotec; Partusisten. $C_{17}H_{21}NO_4$.HBr; mol wt 384.26. Crystals from methanol-ether, mp 222-223°. LD_{50} in mice (mg/kg): 1100 s.c.; 1990 orally (Goldenthal).
Hydrochloride. [1944-10-1] $C_{17}H_{21}NO_4$.HCl. mp 183° (acetonitrile-ether).

THERAP CAT: Bronchodilator; tocolytic.

3982. Fenoverine. [37561-27-6] 10-[[4-(1,3-Benzodioxol-5-ylmethyl)-1-piperazinyl]acetyl]-10*H*-phenothiazine; 10-[4-(3,4-dioxymethylenebenzyl)-1-piperazinylacetyl]phenothiazine; 10-[(4-piperonyl-1-piperazinyl)acetyl]phenothiazine; Spasmopriv. C_{26}-$H_{25}N_3O_3S$; mol wt 459.56. C 67.95%, H 5.48%, N 9.14%, O 10.44%, S 6.98%. Piperonylpiperazine derivative with spasmolytic activity. Prepn: A. Buzas, R. Pierre, **FR 2092639** (1972), *C.A.* **77**, 140143p (1972). Pharmacology, clinical studies in gastrointestinal disorders, dysmenorrhea: R. Pierre, R. Roustan, *Med. Interne* **15**, 49 (1980). In treatment of colon dysfunction: Claudon, *Rev. Fr. Gastro-Enterol.* **198**, 31 (1984).

Crystals from isopropyl ether, mp 141-142°. LD_{50} in mice (g/kg): ~1.50 orally, ~2.50 i.p. (Buzas, Pierre).

THERAP CAT: Antispasmodic.

3983. Fenoxanil. [115852-48-7] *N*-(1-Cyano-1,2-dimethylpropyl)-2-(2,4-dichlorophenoxy)propanamide; AC-382042; NNF-9425; Achieve. $C_{15}H_{18}Cl_2N_2O_2$; mol wt 329.22. C 54.72%, H 5.51%, Cl 21.54%, N 8.51%, O 9.72%. Melanin biosynthesis inhibitor for control of rice blast fungus. Commercial product consists of a mixture of 4 isomers: 85% (*R,RS*) and 15% (*S,RS*). Prepn (stereochem unspec): W. Buck, E. Raddatz, **EP 262393** (1987 to Shell). Review of properties and field trials: E. Sieverding *et al., Brighton Crop Prot. Conf. - Pests Dis.* **1998**, 359-366.

Off white, odorless solid, mp 69.0-71.5°. d^{20} 1.22 g/cm³. Partition coefficient (*n*-octanol/water): 3390 ±133 (25°). Soly in water (20°): 30.7 ±0.3 × 10^{-3} g/l. Sol in most organic solvents. Vapor pressure (25°): 0.21 ±0.021 × 10^{-4} Pa. LD_{50} orally in mice, male rats, female rats (mg/kg): >5000, >5000, 4211 (Sieverding).

USE: Agricultural fungicide.

3984. Fenoxaprop-ethyl. [66441-23-4] 2-[4-[(6-Chloro-2-benzoxazolyl)oxy]phenoxy]propanoic acid ethyl ester; HOE-33171. $C_{18}H_{16}ClNO_5$; mol wt 361.78. C 59.76%, H 4.46%, Cl 9.80%, N 3.87%, O 22.11%. Selective postemergent herbicide to control grassy weeds in broadleaved crops and established turfgrass. Prepn: **BE 858618**; R. Handte *et al.*, **US 4130413** (both 1978 to Hoechst). Metabolism in soybeans: O. Wink *et al., J. Agric. Food Chem.* **32**, 187 (1984). Persistence in soil: A. E. Smith, *ibid.* **33**, 483 (1985). Field trials in agricultural crops: G. W. Selleck *et al., Proc. 36th N. Z. Weed Pest Control Conf.* 265 (1983); in turfgrass: P. H. Dernoeden, J. D. Fry, *Proc. Annu. Meet. Northeast. Weed Sci. Soc.* **39**, 282 (1985). Brief description: J. Bieringer *et al., Proc. Br. Crop Prot. Conf. - Weeds* **1982**, 11-17.

(*R*)-Form

mp 84-85°. bp 200° at 100 Pa. Vapor pressure at 20°: 0.19×10^{-5} Pa. Soly at 20° (%): >0.5 in hexane; >1 in cyclohexane, ethanol, 1-octanol; >20 in ethyl acetate; >30 in toluene; >50 in acetone. Soly in water at 25°: 0.9 mg/l. LD_{50} in male, female rats (mg/kg): 2357, 2500 orally; 739, 864 i.p. (Bieringer).

(*R*)-**Form.** [71283-80-2] Fenoxaprop-P-ethyl; HOE-46360; Acclaim; Furore Super; Puma; Ricestar; Whip. Comprehensive description: H. P. Huff *et al., Brighton Crop Prot. Conf. - Weeds* **1989**, 717-722. LD_{50} in male, female rats (mg/kg): 3040, 2090 orally; >2000, >2000 dermally (Huff).

USE: Postemergent herbicide.

3985. Fenoxazoline. [4846-91-7] 4,5-Dihydro-2-[[2-(1-methylethyl)phenoxy]methyl]-1*H*-imidazole; 2-[(*o*-cumenyloxy)-methyl]-2-imidazoline; 2-(*o*-isopropylphenoxymethyl)-2-imidazoline; phenoxazoline. $C_{13}H_{18}N_2O$; mol wt 218.29. C 71.53%, H 8.31%, N 12.83%, O 7.33%. Preparation: **FR 1365971** (1964 to Lab. Dausse and Soc. BMC). Use as sympathomimetic agent: Giudicelli, **US 3198703** (1965 to Lab. Dausse).

Hydrochloride. [21370-21-8] Aturgyl; Snup. $C_{13}H_{18}N_2O$.HCl; mol wt 254.76. Crystals, mp 174°. Sol in water, ethanol.
THERAP CAT: Sympathomimetic.

3986. Fenoxedil. [54063-40-0] 2-(4-Butoxyphenoxy)-*N*-(2,5-diethoxyphenyl)-*N*-[2-(diethylamino)ethyl]acetamide; 2-(*p*-butoxyphenyl)-*N*-[2-(diethylamino)ethyl]-2′,5′-diethoxyacetanilide.

$C_{28}H_{42}N_2O_5$; mol wt 486.64. C 69.11%, H 8.70%, N 5.76%, O 16.44%. Prepn: **DE 1964712**; Thuillier, Geffroy, **US 3818021** (1970, 1974 both to CERPHA).

Hydrochloride. [27471-60-9] Suplexedil. $C_{28}H_{42}N_2O_5$.HCl; mol wt 523.10. mp 140°. LD_{50} in mice (mg/kg): 750 orally, 17 i.v. (Thuillier, Geffroy).
THERAP CAT: Vasodilator.

3987. Fenoxycarb. [72490-01-8] [2-(4-Phenoxyphenoxy)-ethyl]carbamic acid ethyl ester; ethyl [2-(4-phenoxyphenoxy)ethyl]-carbamate; ABG-6215; Ro-13-5223; Comply; Insegar. $C_{17}H_{19}-NO_4$; mol wt 301.34. C 67.76%, H 6.36%, N 4.65%, O 21.24%. Insect growth regulator. Prepn: U. Fischer *et al.*, **EP 4334**; eidem, **US 4215139** (1979, 1980 both to Hoffmann-La Roche). Insecticidal properties: S. Dorn *et al., Z. Pflanzenkrankh. Pflanzenschutz* **88**, 269 (1981). Field trials, persistence in water, and bioaccumulation in fish: C. H. Schaefer *et al., J. Econ. Entomol.* **80**, 126 (1987).

Crystals from petr ether, mp 53-54°. Soly in water (23°): 5.76 ppm. LD_{50} in rats (mg/kg): 9220 i.p.; 16800 orally (Dorn).
USE: Insecticide.

3988. Fenozolone. [15302-16-6] 2-(Ethylamino)-5-phenyl-4(5*H*)-oxazolone; 2-ethylamino-4-oxo-5-phenyl-Δ²-oxazoline; 5-phenyl-2-(ethylimino)-4-oxazolidone; 5-phenyl-2-ethylamino-4-oxazolinone; LD-3394; Ordinator. $C_{11}H_{12}N_2O_2$; mol wt 204.23. C 64.69%, H 5.92%, N 13.72%, O 15.67%. Prepn: Najer, Giudicelli, *Bull. Soc. Chim. Fr.* **1961**, 1231; **BE 613985** and **DE 1297108** (1962, 1969 both to Dausse), *C.A.* **57**, 13761a (1962); **71**, 70586k (1969). Exists predominantly in the tautomeric ethylamino-oxazolinone form: Najer *et al., Compt. Rend.* **254**, 2173 (1962). Activity studies: Giudicelli *et al., ibid.* 2862.

Crystals from benzene, mp 148°. Stable in alkaline, unstable in acid soln. uv max (alcohol): 221 nm (log ε 4.42). LD_{50} in white mice (g/kg): 0.425 orally; 0.175 i.p. (**BE 613985**).
THERAP CAT: CNS stimulant.

3989. Fenpiclonil. [74738-17-3] 4-(2,3-Dichlorophenyl)-1*H*-pyrrole-3-carbonitrile; 3-(2,3-dichlorophenyl)-4-cyanopyrrole; 4-cyano-3-(2,3-dichlorophenyl)pyrrole; CGA-142705; Beret; Galbas; Gambit. $C_{11}H_6Cl_2N_2$; mol wt 237.08. C 55.73%, H 2.55%, Cl 29.91%, N 11.82%. Phenylpyrrole fungicide for seed treatment; structurally related to pyrrolnitrin, *q.v.* Prepd (not claimed): K. Ohkuma *et al.*, **GB 2024824**; eidem, **US 4229465** (both 1980 to Nippon Soda). Process: P. Martin, **EP 174910**; idem, **US 4812580** (1986, 1989 both to Ciba-Geigy). Comprehensive description: D. Nevill *et al., Brighton Crop Prot. Conf. - Pests Dis.* **1988**, 65-72. Field trials in potatoes: A. J. Leadbeater, W. W. Kirk, *ibid.* **1992**, 657. Mechanism of action study: A. B. K. Jespers, M. A. De Waard, *Pestic. Biochem. Physiol.* **49**, 53 (1994).

Colorless, odorless crystals, mp 152.9°. Soly in water (20°): 2 ppm. Log P (*n*-octanol/water): 4.3. LD_{50} in rats, mice, rabbits (mg/kg): >5000 orally. LD_{50} dermally in rats: >2000 mg/kg. LC_{50} (4 hr) in rats: >1502 mg/m^3 by inhalation (Nevill).

USE: Agricultural fungicide.

3990. Fenpiverinium Bromide. [125-60-0] 1-(4-Amino-4-oxo-3,3-diphenylbutyl)-1-methylpiperidinium bromide; 1-(3-carbamoyl-3,3-diphenylpropyl)-1-methylpiperidinium bromide; α,α-diphenyl-1-piperidinebutyramide methobromide; α,α-diphenyl-γ-piperidylbutyramide methobromide; 2,2-diphenyl-2-(2-piperidinoethyl)acetamide methyl bromide; (diphenylpiperidinoethyl)acetamide methyl bromide; fenpipramide methobromide; Hoechst 12494; Resantin. $C_{22}H_{29}BrN_2O$; mol wt 417.38. C 63.31%, H 7.00%, Br 19.14%, N 6.71%, O 3.83%. Anticholinergic. Prepn: **GB 708859** (1954 to Hoechst); Moffett, Aspergren, *J. Am. Chem. Soc.* **79**, 4451 (1957). Clinical trial in combination with pitofenone and diclofenac: K. B. Golhar, R. L. Gupta, *J. Indian Med. Assoc.* **97**, 398 (1999).

Crystals, mp 177.5-178.5°. Dimorphic crystals from isopropanol + ethyl acetate, mp 216-216.5°. Freely sol in water (water soln is neutral).

THERAP CAT: Antispasmodic.

3991. Fenpropathrin. [39515-41-8] 2,2,3,3-Tetramethylcyclopropane carboxylic acid cyano(3-phenoxyphenyl)methyl ester; α-cyano-3-phenoxybenzyl 2,2,3,3-tetramethylcyclopropanecarboxylate; fenpropanate; S-3206; SD-41706; WL-41706; Danitol; Meothrin; Rody. $C_{22}H_{23}NO_3$; mol wt 349.42. C 75.62%, H 6.63%, N 4.01%, O 13.74%. Synthetic pyrethroid insecticide with repellant and contact activity. Prepn: T. Matsuo *et al., DE* **2231312**; *eidem, US* **3835176** (1973, 1974 to Sumitomo). Commercial product is mixture of stereoisomers, the (*S*)-isomer primarily responsible for the bioactivity. Separation of enantiomers by chiral phase HPLC: R. A. Chapman, *J. Chromatogr.* **258**, 175 (1983). Pesticidal activity: M. H. Breese, *Pestic. Sci.* **8**, 264 (1977). Metabolism: M. J. Crawford, D. H. Hutson, *ibid.* 579. Degradn in soil: T. R. Roberts, M. E. Standen, *ibid.* 600; R. A. Chapman, *Bull. Environ. Contam. Toxicol.* **26**, 513 (1981). Fish toxicity: J. R. Coats, *ibid.* **23**, 250 (1979). Mammalian toxicity study: R. D. Verschoyle, W. N. Aldridge, *Arch. Toxicol.* **45**, 325 (1980). Review of toxicology and human exposure: *Toxicological Profile for Pyrethrins and Pyrethroids* (PB2004-100004, 2003) 332 pp.

Pale yellow oil, n_D^{26} 1.5283. LC_{50} (24 hr) in rainbow trout: 76.7 ppb (Coats). LD_{50} in rats (mg/kg): 2.5 i.v. (Verschoyle); in male, female rats (mg/kg): 24-36, 18-24 orally (Crawford).

USE: Insecticide, acaricide.

3992. Fenpropidin. [67306-00-7] 1-[3-[4-(1,1-Dimethylethyl)phenyl]-2-methylpropyl]piperidine; (*RS*)-1-[3-(4-*tert*-butylphenyl)-2-methylpropyl]piperidine; Tern. $C_{19}H_{31}N$; mol wt 273.46. C 83.45%, H 11.43%, N 5.12%. Piperidine fungicide active against powdery mildews of grain. Prepn: **BE 861002**; A. Pfiffner, **US 4241058** (1978, 1980 both to Hoffmann-La Roche). Improved process: N. Goetz, L. Hupfer, **EP 17893**; *eidem,* **US 4283534** (1980, 1981 both to BASF). Structure-activity relationships: W. Himmele, E.-H. Pommer, *Angew. Chem. Int. Ed.* **19**, 184 (1980). Inhibition of ergosterol biosynthesis: R. I. Baloch *et al., Phytochemistry* **23**, 2219 (1984).

Oil, $bp_{0.2}$ 117°; $bp_{0.045}$ 125°; also reported as $bp_{0.032}$ 104°.

USE: Agricultural fungicide.

3993. Fenpropimorph. [67306-03-0] 4-[3-[4-(1,1-Dimethylethyl)phenyl]-2-methylpropyl]-2,6-dimethylmorpholine; BAS-42100F; Ro-14-3169/000; Corbel; Mistral. $C_{20}H_{33}NO$; mol wt 303.48. C 79.15%, H 10.96%, N 4.62%, O 5.27%. Systemic fungicide for control of powdery mildew, rust in cereal crops. Prepn, fungicidal activity: W. Himmele *et al., DE* **2656747** (1978 to BASF), *C.A.* **89**, 109522k (1978). Synthesis using an ionic liquid solvent: S. A. Forsyth *et al., Org. Process Res. Dev.* **10**, 94 (2006). Field trials in control of cereal diseases: J. C. Atkin *et al., Proc. Br. Crop Prot. Conf. - Pests Dis.* **1981**, 307. Inhibition of ergosterol biosynthesis: R. I. Baloch *et al., Phytochemistry* **23**, 2219 (1984). Structure-activity relationships of 3-phenylpropylamines: W. Himmele, E.-H. Pommer, *Angew. Chem. Int. Ed.* **19**, 184 (1980); of substituted morpholines: E.-H. Pommer, *Pestic. Sci.* **15**, 285 (1984). Brief review: K. Bohnen *et al., Proc. Br. Crop Prot. Conf. - Pests Dis.* **1979**, 541-548.

cis-(−)-S-form

Liquid, $bp_{0.05}$ 120°. Soly in water: 1 gm/l; sol in most organic solvents. Vapor pressure at 20°: 2.5 × 10^{-5} mm Hg. LD_{50} in male, female rats (mg/kg): 3650, 3420 orally; 4200, 4380 dermally; in male, female mice (mg/kg): 1180, 1270 i.p. (Bohnen).

cis-**Form.** [67564-91-4] (±)-*cis*-4-[3-(4-*tert*-Butylphenyl)-2-methylpropyl]-2,6-dimethylmorpholine.

USE: Systemic fungicide.

3994. Fenproporex. [15686-61-0] 3-[(1-Methyl-2-phenylethyl)amino]propanenitrile; (±)-3-[(α-methylphenethyl)amino]propionitrile; (±)-*N*-2-cyanoethylamphetamine. $C_{12}H_{16}N_2$; mol wt 188.27. C 76.55%, H 8.57%, N 14.88%. Deriv of amphetamine, *q.v.* Prepn: **FR M4364**; P. Pohrbach, J. Blum, **US 3485924** (1966, 1969 both to Bottu). Pharmacological studies: B. M. Beecham *et al., J. Pharm. Pharmacol.* **23**, 140 (1971); A. H. Beckett *et al., ibid.* **24**, 194 (1972). Peripheral effects in human and rat adipose tissue: M. Dubost *et al., Br. J. Pharmacol.* **58**, 436P (1976). Chromatographic identification of amphetamine in urine of patients treated with fenproporex: R. B. Sznelvar, *Eur. J. Toxicol. Environ. Hyg.* **8**, 5 (1975). Clinical trial: G. Hertel, W. Fallot-Burghardt, *Fortschr. Med.* **96**, 2380 (1978).

Liquid, bp_2 126-127°.

Hydrochloride. [18305-29-8] Gacilin; Solvolip. $C_{12}H_{16}N_2 \cdot$HCl; mol wt 224.73. White, cryst, odorless powder from abs ethanol, mp 146°. Bitter taste. Sol in water, 95% ethanol.

Note: This is a controlled substance (stimulant): **21 CFR,** 1308.14.

THERAP CAT: Anorexic.

3995. **Fenprostalene.** [69381-94-8] (4S)-rel-7-[(1R,2R,3R,-5S)-3,5-Dihydroxy-2-[(1E,3R)-3-hydroxy-4-phenoxy-1-butenyl]-cyclopentyl]-4,5-heptadienoic acid methyl ester; (±)-9α,11α,15α-trihydroxy-16-phenoxy-17,18,19,20-tetranorprosta-4,5,13-*trans*-trienoic acid methyl ester; RS-84043; Bovilene; Porcilene; Synchrocept B. $C_{23}H_{30}O_6$; mol wt 402.48. C 68.64%, H 7.51%, O 23.85%. Synthetic analog of prostaglandin $F_{2\alpha}$, related structurally to prostalene, *q.v.* Prepn: J. M. Muchowski, J. H. Fried, **US 3985791**; A. R. Van Horn *et al.*, **US 4178457** (1976, 1979 both to Syntex). Effect on pregnancy in beagles: B. Vickery, G. McRae, *Biol. Reprod.* **22,** 438 (1980). Duration of action study: B. H. Vickery *et al.*, *Prostaglandins Med.* **5,** 93 (1980).

uv max (methanol): 220, 265, 271, 278 nm (log ε 3.99, 3.11, 3.23, 3.16).

THERAP CAT (VET): Luteolytic.

3996. **Fenpyroximate.** [134098-61-6] 4-[[[(E)-[(1,3-Dimethyl-5-phenoxy-1H-pyrazol-4-yl)methylene]amino]oxy]-methyl]benzoic acid 1,1-dimethylethyl ester; *tert*-butyl (E)-α-(1,3-dimethyl-5-phenoxypyrazol-4-ylmethyleneaminooxy)-*p*-toluate; NNI-850; HOE-555-02A; Sequel. $C_{24}H_{27}N_3O_4$; mol wt 421.49. C 68.39%, H 6.46%, N 9.97%, O 15.18%. Phenoxypyrazole based acaricide. Chemical, biological properties and field evaluation: T. Konno *et al.*, *Proc. Br. Crop Prot. Conf. - Pests Dis.* **1990,** 71. Mode of action: K. Motoba *et al.*, *Pestic. Biochem. Physiol.* **43,** 37 (1992). Control of spider mites: M. Van de Veire, D. Degheele, *Meded. Fac. Landbouwwet. Univ. Gent* **57,** 925 (1992). Metabolism in rats: H. Nishizawa *et al.*, *J. Pestic. Sci.* **18,** 59 (1993). Soil degradation: Y. Izawa *et al., ibid.* 67.

White crystalline powder, mp 101.1-102.4°. Vapor pressure at 25°: 5.6×10^{-8} mm Hg. Soly at 20° (g/l): water 0.015×10^{-3}; at 25°: methanol 15; *n*-hexane 4; xylene 175. Log P (octanol/water) at 20°: 5.01. LD_{50} in male, female rats (mg/kg): 480, 245 orally; >2000, >2000 dermally. LC_{50} (48hr) in carp: 6.1 µg/l; LC_{50} (3hr) in *daphnia pulex*: 85 µg/l (Konno).

USE: Acaricide.

3997. **Fenquizone.** [20287-37-0] 7-Chloro-1,2,3,4-tetrahydro-4-oxo-2-phenyl-6-quinazolinesulfonamide; 7-chloro-2-phenyl-6-sulfamyl-1,2,3,4-tetrahydro-4-quinazolinone; MG-13054. $C_{14}H_{12}ClN_3O_3S$; mol wt 337.78. C 49.78%, H 3.58%, Cl 10.50%, N 12.44%, O 14.21%, S 9.49%. Thiazide-like diuretic with saluretic and hypocalciuric activity. Prepn: M. G. Biressi *et al.*, *Farmaco Ed. Sci.* **24,** 199 (1969). Prepn of potassium salt: M. Carissimi, F. Ravenna, **BE 799087** (1973 to Maggioni); *eidem*, **US 3870720** (1975). Gas-liquid chromatography: A. Marzo *et al., J. Chromatogr.* **272,** 95 (1983). Metabolism in dogs: D. Ceriani *et al.*, *Farmaco Ed. Sci.* **31,** 379 (1976). Human pharmacokinetics: G. C. Maggi *et al.*, *Arzneim.-Forsch.* **35,** 994 (1985). Site of action: C. Ferrando *et al.*, *J. Pharm. Pharmacol.* **33,** 219 (1981). Clinical trials: O. Biadi *et al., Drugs Exp. Clin. Res.* 7, 763 (1981); N. Glorioso *et al.*, *Curr. Ther. Res.* **35,** 483 (1984); A. Cupisti *et al., ibid.* **38,** 293 (1985).

mp >310°. Insol in water.

Monopotassium salt. [52246-40-9] Idrolone. $C_{14}H_{12}ClKN_3O_3S$; mol wt 376.88. White crystalline powder. Sol in water. pH ~9.9 (1% aqueous soln).

THERAP CAT: Diuretic.

3998. **Fenretinide.** [65646-68-6] N-(4-Hydroxyphenyl)-retinamide; 4-HPR; *all-trans*-N-4'-hydroxyretinanilide; 4-(*all-trans*-retinoyl)aminophenol; McN-R-1967. $C_{26}H_{33}NO_2$; mol wt 391.55. C 79.75%, H 8.49%, N 3.58%, O 8.17%. Synthetic analog of vitamin A, *q.v.* Prepn: R. J. Gander, J. A. Gurney, **BE 847942**; *eidem*, **US 4190594** (1977, 1980 both to J & J); and pharmacology: R. C. Moon *et al.*, *Cancer Res.* **39,** 1339 (1979). Large scale prepn and physical properties: Y. F. Shealy *et al., J. Pharm. Sci.* **73,** 745 (1984). Clinical efficacy and safety in bladder cancer: A. Decensi *et al., Eur. J. Cancer Prev.* **3,** 377 (1994). Review of pharmacology and clinical evaluation in breast cancer prevention: *idem et al., Oncol. Rep.* **1,** 817-824 (1994); M. A. Cobleigh, *Leukemia* **8,** Suppl. 3, s59-s63 (1994); and oral leukoplakia: A. Costa *et al., Cancer Res.* **54,** Suppl., 2032s-2037s (1994).

Crystallizes in several polymorphic or solvated forms. Crystals from ethanol/water, mp 173-175° (Shealy). Crystals from chloroform/hexanes, mp 162-163°; solvated form obtained by slow crystallization from methanol, mp 178-181° (Moon). uv max (chloroform): 370 nm (ε 44500). uv max (methanol): 362 nm (47900).

THERAP CAT: Antineoplastic.

3999. **Fenspiride.** [5053-06-5] 8-(2-Phenylethyl)-1-oxa-3,8-diazaspiro[4.5]decan-2-one; decaspiride; DESP. $C_{15}H_{20}N_2O_2$; mol wt 260.33. C 69.20%, H 7.74%, N 10.76%, O 12.29%. α-Adrenergic blocker. Prepn: **NL 6504602**; Regnier *et al.*, **US 3399192** (1965 and 1968, both to Sci. Union et Cie-Soc. Franc. Recherche Méd.). Pharmacology: LeDouarec *et al.*, *Arzneim.-Forsch.* **19,** 1263 (1969); Duhault *et al., ibid.* **22,** 1947 (1972).

Hydrochloride. [5053-08-7] NAT-333; NDR-5998A; Decaspir; Fluiden; Pneumorel; Respiride; Tegencia; Viarespan. $C_{15}H_{20}N_2O_2$·HCl; mol wt 296.79. Crystals decomp 232-233°. Soluble in water. LD_{50} i.v. in mice: 106 mg/kg; orally in rats: 437 mg/kg (LeDouarec).

THERAP CAT: Bronchodilator.

4000. **Fensulfothion.** [115-90-2] Phosphorothioic acid O,O-diethyl O-[4-(methylsulfinyl)phenyl] ester; O,O-diethyl O-[*p*-(methylsulfinyl)phenyl] phosphorothioate; DMSP; Bay 25141; Dasanit; Terracur P. $C_{11}H_{17}O_4PS_2$; mol wt 308.35. C 42.85%, H 5.56%, O 20.75%, P 10.05%, S 20.80%. Organophosphate cholinesterase inhibitor. Prepn: Homeyer, Schrader, **BE 666012** (1965 to Bayer), *C.A.* **64,** 20555f (1966). Acute toxicity and anticholinesterase activity: K. P. DuBois, F. Kinoshita, *Toxicol. Appl. Pharmacol.* **6**, 78 (1964).

Liquid. bp$_{0.01}$ 138-141°. LD$_{50}$ in male, female rats (mg/kg): 5.5, 1.5 i.p.; 10.5, 2.2 orally; 30.0, 3.5 dermally; in male, female mice (mg/kg): 10.5, 7.0 i.p.; in male guinea pigs (mg/kg): 5.4 i.p., 9.0 orally (DuBois, Kinoshita).

Caution: Potential symptoms of overexposure are skin irritation; nausea, vomiting, abdominal cramps, diarrhea, salivation; headache, giddiness, vertigo, weakness; rhinorrhea, chest tightness; blurred vision, miosis; cardiac irregularities; muscle fasciculations; dyspnea. *See NIOSH Pocket Guide to Chemical Hazards* (DHHS/‑NIOSH 97-140, 1997) p 142.

USE: Nematocide, insecticide.

4001. Fentanyl. [437-38-7] *N*-Phenyl-*N*-[1-(2-phenylethyl)-4-piperidinyl]propanamide; *N*-(1-phenethyl-4-piperidyl)propionanilide; *N*-(1-phenethyl-4-piperidinyl)-*N*-phenylpropionamide; phentanyl; R-4263; Duragesic; Durogesic. C$_{22}$H$_{28}$N$_2$O; mol wt 336.47. C 78.53%, H 8.39%, N 8.33%, O 4.76%. Prepn: P. A. J. Janssen, **FR 1344366**; *idem*, **US 3164600** (1963, 1965 both to Janssen). Pharmacology: J. F. Gardocki, J. Yelnosky, *Toxicol. Appl. Pharmacol.* **6**, 48 (1964); R. Hess *et al., J. Pharmacol. Exp. Ther.* **179**, 474 (1971). Effects on cerebral circulation and metabolism in rats: C. Carlsson *et al., Anesthesiology* **57**, 375 (1982). Clinical studies: E. A. Welchew, J. A. Thornton, *Anaesthesia* **37**, 309 (1982); M. J. Stephens *et al., Med. J. Aust.* **1**, 419 (1982). Review of clinical experience with transdermal formulation: R. B. R. Muijsers, A. J. Wagstaff, *Drugs* **61**, 2289-2307 (2001).

Crystals, mp 83-84°. Partition coefficient (*n*-octanol/water): 860. pKa 8.4.

Citrate. [990-73-8] Actiq; Fentanest; Leptanal; Sublimaze. C$_{22}$H$_{28}$N$_2$O.C$_6$H$_8$O$_7$; mol wt 528.59. Crystalline powder, mp 149-151°. Bitter taste. One gram dissolves in about 40 ml water. Sol in methanol; sparingly sol in chloroform. LD$_{50}$ in mice (mg/kg): 11.2 i.v.; 62 s.c. (Gardocki, Yelnosky).

Note: This is a controlled substance (opiate): **21 CFR**, 1308.12.

THERAP CAT: Analgesic (narcotic).

THERAP CAT (VET): Analgesic; tranquilizer.

4002. Fenthion. [55-38-9] Phosphorothioic acid *O,O*-dimethyl *O*-[3-methyl-4-(methylthio)phenyl] ester; *O,O*-dimethyl *O*-(4-methylmercapto-3-methylphenyl) thionophosphate; *O,O*-dimethyl *O*-(3-methyl-4-methylthiophenyl) thiophosphate; *O,O*-dimethyl *O*-(4-methylthio-3-methylphenyl) thiophosphate; *O,O*-dimethyl *O*-[4-(methylthio)-*m*-tolyl] phosphorothioate; 4-methylmercapto-3-methylphenyl dimethyl thiophosphate; Bayer 29493; ENT-25540; S-1752; Baycid; Baytex; Entex (obsolete); Lebaycid; Mercaptophos; Queletox; Talodex; Tiguvon. C$_{10}$H$_{15}$O$_3$PS$_2$; mol wt 278.33. C 43.15%, H 5.43%, O 17.25%, P 11.13%, S 23.04%. Cholinesterase inhibitor. Prepn: Schrader, *Die Entwicklung neuer insektizider Phosphorsäure-Ester* (Verlag Chemie, 3rd ed., 1963) pp 298-313; Schlegk, Schrader, **DE 1116656** *C.A.* **56**, 14170g (1962); and **US 3042703** (1961 and 1962, both to Bayer); Nishizawa, Mizutani, **JP 64 15130** (1964 to Sumitomo), *C.A.* **61**, 16016h (1964).

Properties: Jung, *Bull. WHO* **21**, 215 (1959); Schrader, *loc. cit.* Toxicity: Gaines, *Toxicol. Appl. Pharmacol.* **2**, 88 (1960).

Liquid, slight odor of garlic. bp$_{0.01}$ 87°. Commercial product, bp$_{0.01}$ 105°. d$_4^{20}$ 1.250. n$_D^{20}$ 1.5698. Vapor pressure at 20°: 3×10^{-5} mm Hg. Thermally stable up to 210°; resistant to alkalies up to pH 9. Readily sol in methanol, ethanol, ether, acetone and many other organic solvents, esp chlorinated hydrocarbons. Practically insol in water (55 mg/l). LD$_{50}$ in male, female rats (mg/kg): 215, 245 orally (Gaines).

Caution: Potential symptoms of overexposure are nausea, vomiting, abdominal cramps, diarrhea, salivation; headache, giddiness, vertigo, weakness; rhinorrhea, chest tightness; blurred vision, miosis; cardiac irregularities; muscle fasciculations; dyspnea. *See NIOSH Pocket Guide to Chemical Hazards* (DHHS/NIOSH 97-140, 1997) p 144.

USE: Insecticide; acaricide.

THERAP CAT (VET): Ectoparasiticide.

4003. Fentiazac. [18046-21-4] 4-(4-Chlorophenyl)-2-phenyl-5-thiazoleacetic acid; BR-700; CH-800; Donorest; Flogene; Norvedan. C$_{17}$H$_{12}$ClNO$_2$S; mol wt 329.80. C 61.91%, H 3.67%, Cl 10.75%, N 4.25%, O 9.70%, S 9.72%. Prepn: K. Brown, **GB 1145884**; *idem*, **US 3476766** (both 1969 to Wyeth). Anti-inflammatory activity: K. Brown *et al., Nature* **219**, 164 (1968). Crystallographic study: R. Destro, *Acta Crystallogr.* **B34**, 959 (1978). Absorption: G. Zanolo *et al., Boll. Chim. Farm.* **119**, 209 (1980). Metabolism: S. Fumero *et al., Arzneim.-Forsch.* **30**, 1253 (1980). Pharmacokinetics in humans: M. Quattrini *et al., ibid.* **31**, 1046 (1981). Toxicity study: D. A. Shriver *et al., Toxicol. Appl. Pharmacol.* **42**, 75 (1977). Review of exptl and clinical pharmacology: E. Marmo, *Curr. Med. Res. Opin.* **6**, 53-63 (1979).

Colorless needles from benzene, mp 161-162°. LD$_{50}$ in rats, mice (mg/kg): 661, 692 orally (Marmo).

THERAP CAT: Anti-inflammatory.

4004. Fenticlor. [97-24-5] 2,2'-Thiobis[4-chlorophenol]; bis[2-hydroxy-5-chlorophenyl]sulfide; 2,2'-dihydroxy-5,5'-dichlorodiphenyl sulfide; S-7; Novex. C$_{12}$H$_8$Cl$_2$O$_2$S; mol wt 287.16. C 50.19%, H 2.81%, Cl 24.69%, O 11.14%, S 11.17%. Prepn by chlorination of bis[2-hydroxyphenyl]sulfide: Muth, **DE 568944** (1931 to I. G. Farben); Dunning *et al., J. Am. Chem. Soc.* **53**, 3466 (1931).

Fine needles from toluene, mp 175°. Sol in aq solns of NaOH, in alcohol, in hot benzene.

Note: Novex is also a trade name for a thermoplastic resin.

USE: Fungicide; esp used against *Monosporium apiospermum:* Reifferscheid, Seeliger, *Dtsch. Med. Wochenschr.* **80**, 1841, 1850 (1955).

THERAP CAT: Anti-infective.

4005. Fenticonazole. [72479-26-6] 1-[2-(2,4-Dichloro-phenyl)-2-[[4-(phenylthio)phenyl]methoxy]ethyl]-1*H*-imidazole; 1-[2,4-dichloro-β-[[*p*-(phenylthio)benzyl]oxy]phenethyl]imidazole; 1-(2,4-dichlorophenyl)-2-(*N*-imidazolyl)ethyl-4-phenylthiobenzyl ether; 2,4-dichloro-4'-phenylthio-(*N*-imidazolylmethyl)dibenzyl ether. $C_{24}H_{20}Cl_2N_2OS$; mol wt 455.40. C 63.30%, H 4.43%, Cl 15.57%, N 6.15%, O 3.51%, S 7.04%. Broad spectrum antimycotic; also active as antibacterial. Prepn: D. Nardi *et al.*, **DE 2917244**; *eidem*, **US 4221803** (1979, 1980 both to Recordati); *eidem, Arzneim.-Forsch.* **31**, 2123 (1981). Series of articles on physico-chemical properties, *in vitro* and *in vivo* antibacterial and antifungal activity, pharmacology and toxicology: *ibid.* 2127-2154. Toxicity data: G. Graziani *et al., ibid.* 2145. Preliminary clinical comparison with miconazole in vaginal candidiasis: A. Gastaldi, *Curr. Ther. Res.* **38**, 489 (1985). Comparative clinical trials in dermatomycoses: A. Finzi *et al., Mykosen* **29**, 41 (1986); E. M. Kokoschka *et al., ibid.* 45.

Mononitrate. [73151-29-8] Rec-15-1476; Falvin; Fentiderm; Fentigyn; Lomexin. $C_{24}H_{20}Cl_2NS.HNO_3$; mol wt 488.41. Odorless, white crystalline powder, mp 136°. uv max (methanol): 252 nm (ε 13894). Soly at 20° (mg/ml): water <0.1; ethyl ether <0.1; ethanol 30; methanol 100; chloroform 300; DMF 600. pKa 6.54. LD_{50} in mice, male rats, female rats (mg/kg): 1191, 440, 309 i.p.; all >3000 orally (Graziani).

THERAP CAT: Antifungal (topical).

4006. Fentonium Bromide. [5868-06-4] [3(*S*)-*endo*]-8-(2-[1,1'-Biphenyl]-4-yl-2-oxoethyl)-3-(3-hydroxy-1-oxo-2-phenyl-propoxy)-8-methyl-8-azoniabicyclo[3.2.1]octane bromide; 3α-hydroxy-8-(*p*-phenylphenacyl)-1α*H*,5α*H*-tropanium bromide (−)-tropate; *N*-(4-phenylphenacyl)-1-hyoscyaminium bromide; phentonium bromide; FA-402; Z-326; Ketoscilium; Ulcesium. $C_{31}H_{34}$-$BrNO_4$; mol wt 564.51. C 65.96%, H 6.07%, Br 14.15%, N 2.48%, O 11.34%. Anticholinergic. Prepn: U. Teotino, D. Della Bella, **GB 1026640**; *eidem*, **US 3356682** (1966, 1967 both to Whitefin Holding); Teotino *et al., Chim. Ther.* **3**, 453 (1968). Human pharmacology: Azzollini *et al., Curr. Ther. Res.* **12**, 734 (1970). Clinical studies: Alberto *et al., Minerva Med.* **62**, 852 (1971).

Crystals, mp 203-205° (dec). $[\alpha]_D^{23}$ −5.68° (c = 5 in DMF). Also reported as mp 193-194°. $[\alpha]_D^{25}$ −4.7° (c = 5 in DMF). LD_{50} in mice (mg/kg): 12.1 i.v.; >400 s.c. and orally (Teotino, Della Bella).

THERAP CAT: Antispasmodic.

4007. Fentrazamide. [158237-07-1] 4-(2-Chlorophenyl)-*N*-cyclohexyl-*N*-ethyl-4,5-dihydro-5-oxo-1*H*-tetrazole-1-carboxamide; 1-(2-chlorophenyl)-4-(*N*-cyclohexyl-*N*-ethylcarbamoyl)-5(4*H*)-tetrazolinone; BAY-YRC-2388; NBA-061; YRC-2388; Lecs. $C_{16}H_{20}ClN_5O_2$; mol wt 349.82. C 54.93%, H 5.76%, Cl 10.13%, N 20.02%, O 9.15%. Tetrazolinone herbicide for use in rice. Prepn: T. Goto *et al.*, **EP 612735**; *eidem*, **US 5362704** (both 1994 to Nihon Bayer). Mode of action study: C. Fedtke *et al.*,

Pestic. Sci. **55**, 566 (1999). Field trial in combination with propanil on seeded rice: H. Fürsch, *Brighton Crop Prot. Conf. - Weeds* **1999**, 99. Comprehensive review: Y. Yasui *et al., ibid.* **1997**, 67-72. Series of articles on properties, metabolism, and field trials: *Pflanzenschutz-Nachr. Bayer (Engl. Ed.)* **54**, 5-142 (2001).

Colorless crystals, mp 79°. d^{20} 1.30. Soly at 20° (g/l): pure water 0.0025; tap water (pH 4, 7, 9) 0.0023; *n*-heptane 20; 2-propanol 32; acetone >250; xylene >250. Vapor pressure at 20° (hPa): 5×10^{-10}; at 25°: 1×10^{-9}. Log P (octanol/water): 3.60 at 20°. LD_{50} in rats (mg/kg): >5000 orally, >5000 dermally. LC_{50} in rats (mg/m³): >5000 by inhalation. LC_{50} (48 hr) in carp, rainbow trout (mg/l): 3.2, 3.4 (Yasui).

USE: Herbicide.

4008. Fenugreek. Greek Hay. *Trigonella foenumgraecum* L., *Leguminosae*, an annual herb, cultivated in Southern Europe, Northern Africa and India for its seeds which are used in making curry. The seeds contain the alkaloid trigonelline and the steroidal sapogenin, diosgenin, *q.q.v.*: Fazli, Hardman, *Trop. Sci.* **10**, 66-78 (1968).

USE: Has been used in making imitation maple syrup and for culinary spices other than curry, flavoring agent.

THERAP CAT (VET): Emollient.

4009. Fenuron. [101-42-8] *N*,*N*-Dimethyl-*N*-phenylurea; *N*-phenyl-*N* ′,*N* ′-dimethylurea; Dybar. $C_9H_{12}N_2O$; mol wt 164.20. C 65.83%, H 7.37%, N 17.06%, O 9.74%. C_6H_5NHCON-$(CH_3)_2$. Prepn: Crosby, Niemann, *J. Am. Chem. Soc.* **76**, 4458 (1954); Gilbert, Sorma, **US 2729677** (1956 to Allied Chem.); Jones, **US 2768971** (1956 to ICI); Applegath *et al.*, **US 2857430** (1958 to Monsanto). Prepn of trichloroacetate: Gilbert *et al.*, **US 2782112** (1957 to Allied Chem.). Toxicity data: G. W. Bailey, J. L. White, *Residue Rev.* **10**, 97 (1965).

Crystals, mp 131-133°. Sparingly sol in water (0.29% at 24°); in hydrocarbons. LD_{50} orally in rats: 7500 mg/kg (Bailey, White).

Trichloroacetate. Fenuron TCA; Urab. $C_{10}H_{14}Cl_3N_2O_3$; mol wt 316.59. mp 65-68°. Esp effective in woody plant control.

Caution: If hydrolyzed to aniline can cause methemoglobinemia: *Clinical Toxicology of Commercial Products*, R. E. Gosselin *et al.*, Eds. (Williams & Wilkins, Baltimore, 5th ed., 1984) Section II, p 331.

USE: Herbicide.

4010. Fenvalerate. [51630-58-1] 4-Chloro-α-(1-methylethyl)benzeneacetic acid cyano(3-phenoxyphenyl)methyl ester; α-cyano-3-phenoxybenzyl α-(4-chlorophenyl)isovalerate; cyano(3-phenoxyphenyl)methyl 4-chloro-α-(1-methylethyl)benzeneacetate; α-cyano-3-phenoxybenzyl-2-(4-chlorophenyl)-3-methylbutyrate; phenvalerate; S-5602; SD-43775; WL-43775; Belmark; Pydrin; Pyridin; Sumicidin; Tirade. $C_{25}H_{22}ClNO_3$; mol wt 419.90. C 71.51%, H 5.28%, Cl 8.44%, N 3.34%, O 11.43%. Synthetic pyrethroid insecticide without the usual cyclopropane ring. Prepn: **DE 2335347**; K. Fujimoto *et al.*, **US 3996244** (1974, 1976, both to Sumitomo); D. A. Wood, **DE 2651341**; *idem*, **US 4061664** (1977, both to Shell). Has two chiral centers giving four possible optical isomers; prepn and comparative insecticidal activity of isomers: M. Hirano *et al.*, **DE 2737297**; *eidem*, **US 4503071** (1978, 1985 both to Sumitomo). Absolute configuration of most active isomer, esfenvalerate: K. Aketa *et al., Agric. Biol. Chem.* **42**, 895 (1978). GC separation of isomers: G. R. Cayley, B. W. Simpson, *J. Chromatogr.* **356**, 123 (1986); determn of esfenvalerate in technical prepn: S. Sakaue *et al., Agric. Biol. Chem.* **51**, 1671 (1987). Comprehensive description of activity and physical properties of esfenvalerate: H. Oo'uchi, *Jpn. Pestic. Inf.* **1985**, 21-24. Comparative soil metabolism of isomers: P.W. Lee *et al., J. Agric. Food Chem.* **35**, 384 (1987). Review of toxicology and human exposure: *Toxicological Profile for Pyrethrins and Pyrethroids* (PB2004-100004, 2003) 332 pp.

Clear yellow viscous liquid at 23°. d^{23} 1.17. n_D^{20} 1.5533. Vapor press at 25° = 1.1×10^{-8} mm Hg. Soly at 20° (g/l): acetone, >450; chloroform, >450; methanol, >450; hexane, 77. Insol in water. More stable in acidic soln than in alk soln. Dec gradually between 150-300°. No significant breakdown after 100 hrs at 75°. LD_{50} orally in rats: 451 mg/kg (DMSO); >3200 mg/kg (aqueous suspension), Shell Technical Data Bulletin. Highly toxic to fish and bees.

(S,S)-Isomer. [66230-04-4] Esfenvalerate; Aα; OMS-3023; S-1844; S-5602α; Sumi-alpha. White crystalline solid, mp 59-60.2°. $[\alpha]_D^{25}$ $-15.0°$ (c = 2.0 in CH_3OH). d_{23}^{23} 1.163. Vapor pressure at 20°: 2.63×10^{-7} mm Hg; at 25°: 5.00×10^{-7} mm Hg. Soly (1%): acetonitrile >60, chloroform >60, DMF >60, DMSO >60, ethyl acetate >60, acetone >60, ethyl cellosolve 40-50, n-hexane 1-5, kerosene <1, methanol 7-10, α-methylnaphthalene 50-60, xylene >60.

Caution: Eye, skin irritant.

USE: Insecticide.

THERAP CAT (VET): Ectoparasiticide.

4011. Fepradinol. [63075-47-8] α-[[(2-Hydroxy-1,1-dimethylethyl)amino]methyl]benzenemethanol; 1-phenyl-2-(α,α-dimethylethanolamino)ethanol. $C_{12}H_{19}NO_2$; mol wt 209.28. C 68.87%, H 9.15%, N 6.69%, O 15.29%. Prepn: E. Biekert, J. Sonnenbichler, *Ber.* **95**, 1451 (1962); G. Staibano, C. Protto, *Farmaco Ed. Sci.* **27**, 929 (1972); G. Staibano, **BE 774629** (1972 to Gentili). Pharmacology: J. M. Masso *et al., J. Pharm. Pharmacol.* **45**, 959 (1993). Mechanism of action study: *eidem, Arzneim.-Forsch.* **44**, 68 (1994). Clinical trial: C. Bestit *et al., Curr. Ther. Res.* **45**, 53 (1989).

White cryst from ethanol, mp 142-143°; also reported as mp 140-142° (Staibano). Cryst from benzene, mp 139° (Biekert). uv max (0.1N HCl): 250.5, 256.4, 262.0 nm (log ε 2.17, 2.28, 2.25).

Hydrochloride. Dalgen; Flexidol. $C_{12}H_{19}NO_2 \cdot HCl$; mol wt 245.75.

THERAP CAT: Anti-inflammatory.

4012. Feprazone. [30748-29-9] 4-(3-Methyl-2-butenyl)-1,2-diphenyl-3,5-pyrazolidinedione; 4-prenyl-1,2-diphenyl-3,5-pyrazolidinedione; 4-prenyl-1,2-diphenyl-3,5-dioxopyrazolidine; 4-(β-isoamylenyl)-1,2-diphenyl-3,5-pyrazolidinedione; 4-(2-isopentenyl)-1,2-diphenyl-3,5-pyrazolidinedione; phenylprenazone; prenazone; DA-2370; Analud; Methrazone; Zepelin. $C_{20}H_{20}N_2O_2$; mol wt 320.39. C 74.98%, H 6.29%, N 8.74%, O 9.99%. Nonsteroidal anti-inflammatory drug. Prepn: S. Casadio, G. Pala, **DE 2031238**; *eidem,* **US 3703528** (1971, 1972 both to Ist. De Angeli); Casadio *et al., Arzneim.-Forsch.* **22**, 171 (1972). Series of articles on physical-chemical data, pharmacology, toxicology and clinical studies: *ibid.* 174-281. Toxicity data: C. Bianchi, G. Bonardi, *ibid.* 196.

Fine, white odorless and tasteless crystalline powder, mp 156.5° (ethanol). Very sol in acetone, chloroform, DMF; sparingly sol in acetonitrile, benzene, 10% NaOH. Slightly sol in ether, methanol, ethanol, cyclohexane. Practically insol in 10% HCl, 10% acetic acid, water. uv max (ethanol): 246 nm (log ε 4.19); (pH 9-12 buffer): 264 nm (log ε 4.322-4.326). pKa 5.09 ± 0.07. LD_{50} in male mice, rats (mg/kg): 408.8, 386.4 i.p.; 1067, >2000 orally (Bianchi, Bonardi).

THERAP CAT: Anti-inflammatory.

4013. Ferbam. [14484-64-1] Tris(dimethylcarbamodithioato-S,S')iron; tris(dimethyldithiocarbamato)iron; dimethyldithiocarbamic acid iron salt; ferric dimethyldithiocarbamate; Carbamate; Ferbeck; Fermate; Ferradow; Karbam Black. $C_9H_{18}FeN_3S_6$; mol wt 416.49. C 25.95%, H 4.36%, Fe 13.41%, N 10.09%, S 46.19%. $[(CH_3)_2NCS_2]_3Fe$. Prepd from Na dimethyldithiocarbamate and a soln of a ferric salt: Tisdale, Williams, **US 1972961** (1934 to du Pont). Toxicity data: H. C. Hodge *et al., J. Am. Pharm. Assoc.* **41**, 662 (1952).

Black solid. mp >180° (dec). Solubility in water 120 ppm, pH of soln 5.0; sol in acetone, chloroform, pyridine, acetonitrile. Tends to decompose on prolonged storage or exposure to heat and moisture. LD_{50} in male mice, rats (mg/kg): 3000, 2700 i.p. (Hodge).

Caution: Potential symptoms of overexposure are irritation of eyes and respiratory tract; dermatitis; GI disturbance. *See NIOSH Pocket Guide to Chemical Hazards* (DHHS/NIOSH 97-140, 1997) p 144. *See also Clinical Toxicology of Commercial Products,* R. E. Gosselin *et al.,* Eds. (Williams & Wilkins, Baltimore, 5th ed., 1984) Section II, p 311.

USE: Fungicide.

4014. Fermium. [7440-72-4] Fm; at. no. 100; valence 3, 2. Man-made, radioactive element. No stable nuclides; known isotopes (mass numbers): 242-259. Longest-lived known isotope: 257 ($T_{1/2}$ 101 days, α-emitter, rel. at. mass 257.0951), produced by neutron bombardment of plutonium (or other elements with higher at. no.). ^{255}Fm ($T_{1/2}$ 20.07 hrs, α-emitter) originally discovered in debris from a thermonuclear test explosion in Nov. 1952. Reviews of discovery: A. Ghiorso *et al., Phys. Rev.* **99**, 1048-1049 (1955); A. Ghiorso, G. T. Seaborg, *Sci. Am.* **195**(6), 67-80 (1956). *Reviews:* G. T. Seaborg, *J. Chem. Educ.* **36**, 38-44 (1959); C. Keller, *The Chemistry of the Transuranium Elements* (Verlag Chemie, Weinheim, English Ed., 1971) pp 591-594; Silva, "Trans-Curium Elements" in *MTP Int. Rev. Sci.: Inorg. Chem., Ser. One* vol. 8, A. G. Maddock, Ed. (University Park Press, Baltimore, 1972) pp 71-105; *Comprehensive Inorganic Chemistry* vol. 5, J. C. Bailar, Jr. *et al.,* Eds. (Pergamon Press, Oxford, 1973) *passim; Handb. Exp. Pharmakol.* **36**, 689-738 (1973); R. J. Silva in *The Chemistry of the Actinide Elements* vol. 2, J. J. Katz *et al.,* Eds. (Chapman and Hall, New York, 1986) pp 1086-1092; *The Elements Beyond Uranium,* G. T. Seaborg, W. D. Loveland, Eds. (John Wiley & Sons, Inc., New York, 1990) pp 28-38.

Caution: Radiation hazard; handling requires special equipment and shielding facilities (Katz *et al., loc. cit.* **vol. 2**, p. 1128).

4015. Ferredoxins. A group of electron transfer factors found in plants and bacteria, which are non-heme iron-sulfur proteins and which play an important role in photosynthesis, nitrogen and carbon dioxide fixation, and respiration. They are generally classified by the presence of either 2 or 4 iron atom clusters and an equivalent amount of inorganic or "acid-labile" sulfide bonded to the peptide chain through 4 cysteine sulfhydryl groups. The two-iron ferredoxins are found primarly in plants and blue-green algae and are sometimes referred to as chloroplast or "plant type" ferredoxins; the four-iron ferredoxins are predominant in bacteria. Mol wts of chloroplast ferredoxins are about 12,000; those of bacterial ferredoxins range from about 6,000 to 24,000. Isoln from *Clostridium pasteurianum:* L. E. Mortenson *et al., Biochem. Biophys. Res. Commun.* **7**, 448 (1962). Prepn of bacterial ferredoxins: L. E. Mortenson, **US 3344130** (1960 to duPont). The amino acid sequence of several bacterial and chloroplast ferredoxins has been elucidated. Amino acid sequence of ferredoxin from *Clostridium pasteurianum:* Tanaka *et al., Biochem. Biophys. Res. Commun.* **16**, 422 (1964); *eidem, Biochemistry* **5**, 1666 (1966); from spinach: Matsubara, Sasaki, *J. Biol. Chem.* **243**, 1732 (1968). Synthesis of peptide chain of *C. pasteurianum* ferredoxins: Bayer *et al., Tetra-*

hedron **24,** 4853 (1968); Trakatellis, Schwartz, *Proc. Natl. Acad. Sci. USA* **63,** 436 (1969). *Reviews:* Buchanan, *Struct. Bonding* **1,** 109 (1966); Malkin, Rabinowitz, *Annu. Rev. Biochem.* **36,** 113 (1967); Arnon, *Naturwissenschaften* **56,** 295 (1969); Buchanan, Arnon, *Adv. Enzymol.* **33,** 119 (1970); W. Lovenberg, "Ferredoxin and Rubredoxin" in *Microbial Iron Metabolism,* J. B. Neilands, Ed. (Academic Press, New York, 1974) pp 161-182; D. C. Yoch, R. P. Carithers, *Microbiol. Rev.* **43,** 384-421 (1979).

Absorption max of bacterial ferredoxins: 280, 385-400 nm; of plant ferredoxins: 280, 325, 420, 463 nm. All show negative oxidation-reduction potentials near that of the hydrogen electrode: −0.390 V *(C. pasteurianum);* −0.420 V (spinach): Tagawa, Arnon, *Biochim. Biophys. Acta* **153,** 602 (1968). Autoxidizable. Acidification, as well as treatment with iron-chelating agents or mercurials, results in evolution of H_2S and loss of the visible absorption.

4016. Ferric Acetate, Basic. [10450-55-2] Bis(acetato-κO)hydroxyiron; basic iron(III) acetate. $C_4H_7FeO_5$; mol wt 190.94. C 25.16%, H 3.70%, Fe 29.25%, O 41.90%. $Fe(OH)(CH_3-COO)_2$. Prepd by heating ferric acetate soln: Casey, Doyle in *Kirk-Othmer Encyclopedia of Chemical Technology* **vol. 12** (Interscience, New York, 2nd ed., 1967) p 24.

Brownish-red scales or amorphous powder; faint acetic odor. Practically insol in water; sol in alcohol, acids. *Protect from light.*

USE: In the textile industry as a mordant in dyeing and printing, and for the weighting of silk and felt; as wood preservative; in leather dyes.

4017. Ferric Ammonium Citrate. [1185-57-5] 2-Hydroxy-1,2,3-propanetricarboxylic acid ammonium iron (3+) salt; ammonium ferric citrate; iron(III) ammonium citrate; FerriSeltz. Compounds of NH_3, iron, and citric acid of undetermined formula and structure. Prepn: H. J. Kruse, H. C. Mounce, US 2644828 (1953 to Mallinckrodt). ESR characterization of green and brown forms: R. A. Uphaus, M. I. Blake, *Naturwissenschaften* **68,** 270 (1981). Decomposition study: G. A. M. Hussein, *Powder Technol.* **80,** 265 (1994). Use in prevention of anemia in pigs: B. G. Harmon *et al., J. Anim. Sci.* **26,** 1051 (1967). Bioavailability: N. P. Wong *et al., Nutr. Rep. Int.* **29,** 135 (1984). Clinical evaluation in iron deficiency anemia: M. Taniguchi *et al., J. Nutr. Sci. Vitaminol.* **37,** 161 (1991); of use as an MRI contrast agent: S. Hirohashi *et al., Magn. Reson. Imaging* **12,** 837 (1994).

Two forms exist. The brown hydrated form exists as garnet-red transparent scales or granules, or brownish-yellow powder, and contains ∼9% NH_3, 16.5-18.5% Fe, and ∼65% hydrated citric acid. The green hydrated form exists as green transparent, deliquesc scales, granules, or powder, and contains ∼7.5% NH_3, 14.5-16% Fe, and ∼75% hydrated citric acid. Very sol in water. Insol in alcohol. Reduced to ferrous salt by light. *Keep well closed and protected from light.*

USE: For blueprints; in photography.

THERAP CAT: Hematinic.

THERAP CAT (VET): In iron deficiency anemia.

4018. Ferric Bromide. [10031-26-2] Br_3Fe; mol wt 295.56. Br 81.10%, Fe 18.89%. $FeBr_3$. Prepn from Fe and Br_2: Gregory, Thackrey, *J. Am. Chem. Soc.* **72,** 3176 (1950); Gregory, *ibid.* **73,** 472 (1951); from $Fe_2(SO_4)_3$ and LiBr: Lieser, Elias, *Z. Anorg. Allg. Chem.* **216,** 208 (1962).

Dark-red or black hexagonal, rhombic plates. Very hygroscopic. Loses some Br_2 on exposure to air and light. Sol in water, alcohol, ether, acetic acid; slightly sol in liq NH_3; aq soln dec to $FeBr_2 + Br_2$ on boiling. *Keep cool, well-closed and protected from light.*

Caution: Irritant.

USE: Catalyst for organic reactions, particularly in bromination of aromatic compds.

4019. Ferric Chloride. [7705-08-0] Flores martis. Cl_3Fe; mol wt 162.20. Cl 65.57%, Fe 34.43%. $FeCl_3$. Occurs in nature as the mineral *molysite.* Prepn: Tarr, *Inorg. Synth.* **3,** 191 (1950); Pray, *ibid.* **5,** 153 (1957); Epperson *et al., ibid.* **7,** 163 (1963); Lieser, Elias, *Z. Anorg. Allg. Chem.* **316,** 208 (1962); Attwood, Shelton, *J. Inorg. Nucl. Chem.* **26,** 1758 (1964); Bardawil *et al., Inorg. Chem.* **3,** 149 (1964). Acute toxicity: C. S. Hosking, *Aust. Paediatr. J.* **6,** 92 (1970). Use as clinical reagent: L. Cassidei *et al., Clin. Chim. Acta* **90,** 121 (1978).

Hexagonal, dark leaflets or plates. Red by transmitted light, green by reflected light; sometimes appears brownish-black. Very hygroscopic. Melts and volatilizes about 300°; bp ∼316°; d^{25} 2.90. Vapor density measurements show that it is dimeric at about 400° but monomeric above 750°. Dissociates at high temps to $FeCl_2$ and Cl_2. Readily absorbs water in air to form the hexahydrate. Readily sol in water, alcohol, ether, acetone; slightly sol in CS_2. Practically insol in ethyl acetate. *Keep well closed.*

Hexahydrate. Brownish-yellow or orange monoclinic crystals. d 1.82. Structure: *trans*-$[FeCl_2(H_2O)_4]Cl.2H_2O$: Lind, *J. Chem. Phys.* **47,** 990 (1967). Usually slight odor of HCl; very hygroscopic. mp ∼37°. Readily sol in water, alcohol, acetone, ether; pH of 0.1 molar aq soln 2.0. *Keep well closed.* LD_{50} i.v. in mice: 0.049 mg Fe/g (Hosking).

Caution: Potential symptoms of overexposure are irritation of eyes, skin, mucous membranes; abdominal pain, diarrhea, vomiting; possible liver damage. *See NIOSH Pocket Guide to Chemical Hazards* (DHHS/NIOSH 97-140, 1997) p 174.

USE: In photoengraving; photography; manuf of other Fe salts, pigments, ink; as catalyst in organic reactions; purifying factory effluents and deodorizing sewage; chlorination of Ag and Cu ores; as mordant in dyeing and printing textiles; oxidizing agent in dye manuf. Clinical reagent (amino acids in urine, esp in phenylketonuria).

THERAP CAT: Hexahydrate as astringent, styptic.

THERAP CAT (VET): Styptic, astringent.

4020. Ferric Chromate(VI). [10294-52-7] Chromic acid iron(3+) salt (3:2); C.I. Pigment Yellow 45; C.I. 77505; Siderin yellow. $Cr_3Fe_2O_{12}$; mol wt 459.67. Cr 33.93%, Fe 24.30%, O 41.77%. $Fe_2(CrO_4)_3$. Preparation: Boericke, Bangert, *Bur. Mines Rep. Invest.* **3813,** 19 pp (1945), *C.A.* **39,** 5164[7] (1945).

Yellow powder. Practically insol in water. Sol in HCl.

USE: Pigment for ceramics, glass and enamels.

4021. Ferric Citrate. [2338-05-8] (undefined); [28633-45-6] (undefined iron(III) salt); [3522-50-7] (1:1 iron(III) citrate salt). 2-Hydroxy-1,2,3-propanetricarboxylic acid iron salt. A combination of iron and citric acid of indefinite composition. Prepn: Belloni, *Gazz. Chim. Ital.* **50, II,** 159 (1920). Complex formation study: R. C. Warner, I. Weber, *J. Am. Chem. Soc.* **75,** 5086 (1953). Polymerization studies: T. G. Spiro *et al., ibid.* **89,** 5555, 5559 (1967). Role in iron uptake in plants: H. F. Bienfait, M. R. Scheffers, *Plant Soil* **143,** 141 (1992). Tumorigenicity study in mice: K. Inai *et al., Food Chem. Toxicol.* **32,** 493 (1994). Clinical evaluation in hyperphosphataemia: W.-C. Yang *et al., Nephrol. Dial. Transplant.* **17,** 265 (2002).

Garnet-red, transparent scales or pale-brown powder. Slowly but completely sol in cold water, readily sol in hot water, but diminishing in soly with age. Practically insol in alc.

THERAP CAT: Hematinic.

THERAP CAT (VET): In iron deficiency.

4022. Ferric Fluoride. [7783-50-8] F_3Fe; mol wt 112.84. F 50.51%, Fe 49.49%. FeF_3. Prepn from $FeCl_3$ and HF: Kwasnik in *Handbook of Preparative Inorganic Chemistry* **vol. 1,** G. Brauer, Ed. (Academic Press, New York, 2nd ed., 1963) p 266; Shinn *et al., Inorg. Chem.* **5,** 1927 (1966); from Fe_2O_3 or Fe_2S_3 and SF_4: Oppegard *et al., J. Am. Chem. Soc.* **82,** 3835 (1960); from $FeCl_3$ and CH_3CHF_2: Natta *et al.,* GB 995186 (1965 to Montecatini).

Green hexagonal crystals. Sublimes >1000°. d 3.87. Very slightly sol in water; freely sol in dil HF; practically insol in alcohol, ether, benzene. Soly in liq HF: 0.008 g/100 g HF, Jache, Cady, *J. Phys. Chem.* **56,** 1106 (1952).

USE: As catalyst in organic reactions.

4023. Ferric Formate. [555-76-0] $C_3H_3FeO_6$; mol wt 190.90. C 18.87%, H 1.58%, Fe 29.25%, O 50.29%. $Fe(HCOO)_3$. Prepn: Weinland, Reihlin, *Ber.* **46,** 3144 (1913); Starke, *J. Inorg. Nucl. Chem.* **25,** 823 (1963). May contain 1 or 2 H_2O.

Red or yellow microcryst powder. Readily hydrolyzed to basic formates. Sol in water; very slightly sol in alcohol. *Protect from light.*

USE: Preservation of silage.

4024. Ferrichromes. Growth-promoting iron chelates. Ferrichrome and ferrichrome A first isolated from the rust fungus, *Ustilago sphaerogena:* Neilands, *J. Am. Chem. Soc.* **74,** 4846

(1952); Garibaldi, Neilands, *ibid.* **77**, 2429 (1955). Ferrichrome and four related compounds, *ferrichrysin, ferricrocin, ferrirubin* and *ferrirhodin* have also been isolated from *Aspergillaceae* and from *Penicillium resticulosum:* Zähner *et al., Arch. Mikrobiol.* **45**, 119 (1963); Keller-Schierlein, Deer, *Helv. Chim. Acta* **46**, 1907 (1963); Keller-Schierlein, *ibid.,* 1920. Ferrichromes are cyclic hexapeptides containing three small, neutral amino acids and three derivatives of δ-N-hydroxy-L-ornithine [HONH(CH$_2$)$_3$CH(NH$_2$)-COOH]. Structure: Rogers, Neilands, *Biochemistry* **3**, 1850 (1964). Crystal and molecular structure of ferrichrome A: Zalkin *et al., J. Am. Chem. Soc.* **88**, 1810 (1966). Synthesis of ferrichrome: Keller-Schierlein, Maurer, *Helv. Chim. Acta* **52**, 603 (1969); Isowa *et al., Bull. Chem. Soc. Jpn.* **47**, 215 (1974). Reviews of ferrichromes and other hydroxamic acids: Neilands, *Struct. Bonding* **1**, 59-108 (1966); Emery, *Adv. Enzymol. Relat. Areas Mol. Biol.* **35**, 135-185 (1971); J. B. Neilands, *Bioinorg. Chem.* **II**, K. N. Raymond, Ed. (A.C.S., Washington, 1977), pp 3-32.

Ferrichrome	R = CH$_3$	R' = H
Ferrichrome A	R = *trans*-HOOCCH$_2$(CH$_3$)C=CH	R' = CH$_2$OH

Ferrichrome. C$_{27}$H$_{42}$FeN$_9$O$_{12}$; mol wt 740.52. Long, yellow needles from anhydr methanol, shrink and blacken at 240-242° without melting. $[\alpha]_D$ +300° (c = 0.04). Absorption max (methanol): 425 nm (E$_{1cm}^{1\%}$ 39.4). Sol in water and hot methanol; sparingly sol in ethanol, acetone, ether, chloroform.

Ferrichrome A. C$_{41}$H$_{58}$FeN$_9$O$_{20}$; mol wt 1052.79. Crystals from water. Absorption max (0.1*M* phosphate buffer; pH 7): 440 nm (E$_{1cm}^{1\%}$ 33.8). Very sol in methanol, ethanol, propanol; slightly sol in hot water. Practically insol in acetone, petr ether, ether, chloroform.

4025. Ferric Hydroxide. [20344-49-4] Ferric hydroxide oxide; hydrated ferric oxide. FeHO$_2$; mol wt 88.85. Fe 62.85%, H 1.13%, O 36.01%. FeO(OH). Occurs in nature as the minerals *goethite* [α-FeO(OH)], *lepidocrocite* [γ-FeO(OH)], and *limonite* [FeO(OH).nH$_2$O]. Other known allomorphic forms: β-FeO(OH); δ-FeO(OH). The hydroxide Fe(OH)$_3$ is not known. Prepn: Lux in *Handbook of Preparative Inorganic Chemistry* **vol 2**, G. Brauer, Ed. (Academic Press, New York, 2nd ed., 1965) p 1499. Crystal structure of α-FeO(OH): Sampson, *Acta Crystallogr.* **25B**, 1683 (1969). *Review:* Bernal *et al., Clay Miner. Bull.* **4**, 15-30 (1959).

Red to brown powder or crystals. Loses H$_2$O to form Fe$_2$O$_3$. d 3.4-3.9. Practically insol in water, alcohol. Sol in mineral acids.

USE: In purifying water; as absorbent in chemical processing; as pigment; as catalyst.

4026. Ferric Hypophosphite. [7783-84-8] FeH$_6$O$_6$P$_3$; mol wt 250.81. Fe 22.27%, H 2.41%, O 38.27%, P 37.05%. Fe(H$_2$-PO$_2$)$_3$. Prepn: *U.S.D.* 25th ed, p 573.

White or grayish-white powder. Odorless, tasteless. Sol in 2300 parts cold water, 1200 parts boiling water; more sol in water in presence of H$_3$PO$_2$; sol in warm concd solns of alkali citrates. *Protect from light.* Should not be heated or triturated with chlorates, nitrates, and other oxidizing agents.

USE: Formerly as dietary supplement for phosphorus.

4027. Ferric Nitrate. [10421-48-4] FeN$_3$O$_9$; mol wt 241.86. Fe 23.09%, N 17.37%, O 59.54%. Fe(NO$_3$)$_3$. Prepn: *Gmelins, Iron* (8th ed.) **59**, part B, 161-172 (1932). Toxicity study: H. F. Smyth *et al., Am. Ind. Hyg. Assoc. J.* **30**, 470 (1969).

Nonahydrate. Pale-violet to grayish-white, somewhat deliquesc crystals. mp 47°. Dec below 100°. d^{21} 1.68. Freely sol in water, alcohol, acetone; slightly sol in cold concd HNO$_3$. LD$_{50}$ orally in rats: 3.25 g/kg (Smyth).

Caution: Potential symptoms of overexposure are irritation of eyes, skin, mucous membranes; abdominal pain, diarrhea, vomiting; liver damage. *See NIOSH Pocket Guide to Chemical Hazards* (DHHS/NIOSH 97-140, 1997) p 174.

USE: As mordant in dyeing, weighting silks, tanning; as reagent in analytical chemistry; as corrosion inhibitor.

4028. Ferric Oxide. [1309-37-1] Ferric sesquioxide; jeweler's rouge. Fe$_2$O$_3$; mol wt 159.69. Fe 69.94%, O 30.06%. α-Form occurs in nature as the mineral *hematite*. γ-Form occurs in nature as the mineral *maghemite*; prepd by dehydration of α-FeO(OH): Giovanoli, Brütsch, *Chimia* **28**, 188 (1974). Prepn of a third allomorphic form, ε-Fe$_2$O$_3$: Schrader, Büttner, *Z. Anorg. Allg. Chem.* **320**, 220 (1963); Trautman, Forestier, *Compt. Rend.* **261**, 4423 (1965). Color and appearance of Fe$_2$O$_3$ are dependent upon the size and shape of the particles and the amount of combined water. Preparation and properties: *Gmelins, Iron* (8th ed.) **59**, part B, 63-94 (1932); Baudisch, Hartung, *Inorg. Synth.* **1**, 185 (1939); *Ullmanns Encyklopädie der technischen Chemie* **vol. 6**, 421-423 (1955); Bernal *et al., Clay Miner. Bull.* **4**, 15-30 (1959). Toxicology: L. T. Fairhall, *Industrial Toxicology* (Hafner, New York, 2nd ed., 1969) pp 64-66.

Note: The composition of the substance called δ-Fe$_2$O$_3$ is actually FeO(OH) (Bernal *et al.*).

Caution: Potential symptoms of overexposure to dust and fumes are benign pneumoconiosis with x-ray shadows indistinguishable from fibrotic pneumoconiosis. *See NIOSH Pocket Guide to Chemical Hazards* (DHHS/NIOSH 97-140, 1997) p 172.

USE: As pigment for rubber, paints, paper, linoleum, ceramics, glass; in paint for ironwork, ship hulls; as polishing agent for glass, precious metals, diamonds; in electrical resistors and semiconductors; in magnets, magnetic tapes; as catalyst; colloidal solns as stain for polysaccharides.

4029. Ferric Phosphate. [10045-86-0] FeO$_4$P; mol wt 150.82. Fe 37.03%, O 42.43%, P 20.54%. FePO$_4$. Occurs in nature as the minerals: *beraunite, cacoxenite, dufrenite, koninckite, phosphosiderite, strengite.* Prepn from Fe(H$_2$PO$_4$)$_3$: Remy, Boulle, *Compt. Rend.* **253**, 2699 (1961); from Fe(CO)$_5$ and H$_3$PO$_4$: Cate *et al., Soil Sci.* **88**(3), 130 (1959); from phosphate rock: Vickery, **US 2914380** (1959 to Horizons Inc.); from mill scale and H$_3$PO$_4$: Alexander, Mathes, **US 3070421** (1962 to Chemetron).

Dihydrate. White, grayish-white, or light pink, orthorhombic or monoclinic crystals or amorphous powder. Loses water above 140°. d 2.87. Practically insol in water. Slowly sol in HNO$_3$; readily sol in HCl.

USE: As food and feed supplement, particularly in bread enrichment; as fertilizer.

4030. Ferric Pyrophosphate. [10058-44-3] Diphosphoric acid iron(3+) salt (3:4); Ferro Angelini. Fe$_4$O$_{21}$P$_6$; mol wt 745.21. Fe 29.98%, O 45.09%, P 24.94%. Fe$_4$(P$_2$O$_7$)$_3$. Prepn: *Gmelins, Iron* (8th ed.) **59**, part B, 777 (1932); H. M. Knight, J. T. Kelly, **US 3014784** (1962 to American Oil). Magnetic structural study: W. M. Reiff, C. C. Torardi, *Hyperfine Interact.* **53**, 403 (1990). Bioavailability: H. Tsuchita *et al., J. Agric. Food Chem.* **39**, 316 (1991). Clinical evaluation in hemodialysis: A. Gupta *et al., Kidney Int.* **55**, 1891 (1999).

Nonahydrate. [10049-18-0] Yellowish-white powder. Practically insol in water or acetic acid. Sol in mineral acids.

USE: As catalyst; in fireproofing of synthetic fibers; in corrosion-preventing pigments.

THERAP CAT: Hematinic.

4031. Ferric Sodium Edetate. [15708-41-5] (*OC*-6-21)-[[N,N'-1,2-Ethanediylbis[N-[(carboxy-κO)methyl]glycinato-κN,-κO]](4−)]-ferrate(1−) sodium; sodium [(ethylenedinitrilo)tetraacetato]ferrate(1−); (ethylenedinitrilo)tetraacetic acid sodium salt iron complex; ferric monosodium ethylenediaminetetraacetate;

edetic acid sodium iron salt; sodium iron edetate; sodium feredetate; Ferrostrane; Ferrostrene; Sybron. $C_{10}H_{12}FeN_2NaO_8$; mol wt 367.05. C 32.72%, H 3.30%, Fe 15.21%, N 7.63%, Na 6.26%, O 34.87%. Prepd from disodium ethylenediaminetetraacetic acid and ferric nitrate: Sawyer, McKinnie, *J. Am. Chem. Soc.* **82**, 4191 (1960).

Crystals from water + ethanol.
THERAP CAT: Hematinic.

4032. Ferric Sulfate. [10028-22-5] Ferric persulfate; ferric sesquisulfate; ferric tersulfate. $Fe_2O_{12}S_3$; mol wt 399.88. Fe 27.93%, O 48.01%, S 24.06%. $Fe_2(SO_4)_3$. Prepn: *Gmelins, Iron* (8th ed.) **59**, part B, 439-462 (1932).

Grayish-white powder, or rhombic or rhombohedral crystals. Very hygroscopic. Commercial product usually contains about 20% water and is yellowish in color. d^{18} 3.097. Slowly sol in water, rapidly sol in the presence of a trace of $FeSO_4$; sparingly sol in alcohol; practically insol in acetone, ethyl acetate. Hydrolyzed slowly in aq soln. *Keep well closed and protected from light.*

Caution: Potential symptoms of overexposure are irritation of eyes, skin, mucous membranes; abdominal pain, diarrhea, vomiting; liver damage. *See NIOSH Pocket Guide to Chemical Hazards* (DHHS/NIOSH 97-140, 1997) p 174.

USE: In preparation of iron alums, other iron salts and pigments; as coagulant in water purification and sewage treatment; in etching aluminum; in pickling stainless steel and copper; as mordant in textile dyeing and calico printing; in soil conditioners; as polymerization catalyst.

4033. Ferric Tannate. Ferric gallotannate. Variable composition. Contains 8-10% Fe, 70-80% tannin.

Bluish-black powder. Insol in water; sol in dil mineral acids.
USE: In inks.

4034. Ferric Thiocyanate. [4119-52-2] Ferric sulfocyanate; ferric sulfocyanide. $C_3FeN_3S_3$; mol wt 230.09. C 15.66%, Fe 24.27%, N 18.26%, S 41.81%. $Fe(SCN)_3$. Prepn: *Gmelins, Iron* (8th ed.) part B, 747-761 (1932).

Sesquihydrate. Red, deliquesc crystals. Dec on heating. Sol in water, alcohol, ether, acetone, pyridine, ethyl acetate. Practically insol in $CHCl_3$, CCl_4, CS_2, toluene. *Keep well closed.*

USE: Analytical reagent.

4035. Ferrite. [1317-54-0] Ferrospinel. A crystalline, usually man-made material, having a spinel structure and consisting essentially of ferric oxide and at least one other metallic oxide which is usually, although not always, divalent in nature. When molded into compressed bodies, the material is characterized by high magnetic permeability. Typified composition: Fe_2O_3 67-70%; ZnO 10-10.5%; MnO_2 20-22.5%; CuO 0.1-10%; Co_3O_4 0.1%. Ferrites are prepd by ceramic techniques. The oxides or carbonates are milled in steel ball mills, and the mixture of very fine particles is dried and prefired in order to obtain a homogeneous end product: Hilpert, *Ber.* **42**, 2248 (1909). Prepn: J. O. Simpkiss, US 2723238; R. L. Harvey, US 2723239 (both 1955 to RCA). Prepn of single crystals: Rooymans, *Colloq. Int. Cent. Nat. Rech. Sci.* **No. 205**, 151 (1972). Books: Snoek, *New Developments in Ferromagnetic Materials* (Elsevier, New York, 1947); Smit, Wijn, *Ferrites* (John Wiley, New York, 1959); Soohov, *Theory and Applications of Ferrites* (Prentice Hall, 1960); Standley, *Oxide Magnetic Materials* (Clarendon Press, Oxford, 1962); *Ferrites, Proc. Int. Conf.*, Y. Hoshino *et al.*, Eds. (University Park Press, Baltimore, 1971) 671 pp; E. E. Riches, *Ferrites, A Review of Materials and Applications* (Mills and Boon, London, 1972) 88 pp. Reviews with bibliographies: Gorter, *Proc. IRE* **43**, 1945-1973 (1955); Fresh, "Methods of Preparation and Crystal Chemistry of Ferrites," *ibid.* **44**, 1303-1311 (1956); Brailsford, *Magnetic Materials* (John Wiley, New York, 3rd ed., 1960) pp 160-181; Hogen, *Sci. Am.* **202**, 92-104 (1960); Economos in *Kirk-Othmer Encyclopedia of Chemical Technology* vol. 8 (Interscience, New York, 2nd ed., 1965) pp 881-901; Gray, "Oxide

Spinels" in *High Temperature Oxides*, Part IV, A. M. Alper, Ed. (Academic Press, New York, 1971) pp 77-107.

Note: The term "ferrites" has been expanded to mean any oxidic magnetic material.

USE: Magnetic cores for inductors and transformers; microwave devices; information storage; electromechanical transducers: E. E. Riches, *loc. cit.;* Brockman, *Ceram. Ind.* **99**, 24 (1972).

4036. Ferritin. [9007-73-2] Ferrofolin; Ferrol; Ferrosprint; Ferrostar; Sanifer; Sideros; Unifer. Major iron storage protein; widely distributed in the plant and animal kingdoms. Consists of a 24-subunit protein shell surrounding a crystalline hydrous ferric oxide core. The core may contain up to 4500 Fe^{3+} ions. The protein shell, *apoferritin*, has a mol wt of ~445,000. Isoln and crystallization of horse spleen ferritin: V. Laufberger, *Bull. Soc. Chim. Biol.* **19**, 1575 (1937); S. Granick, *J. Biol. Chem.* **146**, 451 (1942). X-ray structural study of apoferritin: P. M. Harrison, *J. Mol. Biol.* **6**, 404 (1963). Review of properties and role in iron metabolism: S. Granick, *Chem. Rev.* **38**, 379-403 (1946); of structure, biosynthesis and function: R. R. Crichton, *N. Engl. J. Med.* **284**, 1413-1422 (1971); P. M. Harrison, T. G. Hoy, "Ferritin" in *Inorganic Biochemistry* vol. 1, G. L. Eichhorn, Ed. (Elsevier, New York, 1973) pp 253-279; H. N. Munro, M. C. Linder, *Physiol. Rev.* **58**, 317-396 (1978); of applications in clinical medicine: J. W. Halliday, L. W. Powell, *Prog. Hematol.* **11**, 229-266 (1979); of biology: M. Worwood, *Blood Rev.* **4**, 259-269 (1990); of structure and role in iron mineralization: N. D. Chasteen, P. M. Harrison, *J. Struct. Biol.* **126**, 182-194 (1999); of *mitochondrial ferritin*: J. Drysdale *et al., Blood Cells Mol. Dis.* **29**, 376-383 (2002); of role in dietary iron supplementation: E. C. Theil, *Annu. Rev. Nutr.* **24**, 327-343 (2004).

Red-brown, water-soluble protein. Forms cubic and orthorhombic crystals.

USE: Tool for the study of protein synthesis and regulatory mechanisms.

THERAP CAT: Hematinic.

4037. Ferrocene. [102-54-5] Dicyclopentadienyliron; bis-cyclopentadienyliron. $C_{10}H_{10}Fe$; mol wt 186.03. C 64.56%, H 5.42%, Fe 30.02%. Prepn: Kealy, Pauson, *Nature* **168**, 1039 (1951); Pauson, US 2680756 (1954 to Du Pont); Miller *et al., J. Chem. Soc.* **1952**, 632; Anzilotti, Weinmayr, US 2791597 (1957 to Du Pont). Other prepn: Pruett, Morehouse in *Adv. Chem. Ser.* **23**, entitled "Metal-Organic Compounds," M. Sittig, Ed. (ACS, Washington DC, 1959) pp 368-371; Wilkinson, *Org. Synth.* coll. vol. IV, 473 (1963); Cordes, FR 1341880 (1963 to BASF), *C.A.* **60**, 6873a (1964). Structure studies: Wilkinson *et al., J. Am. Chem. Soc.* **74**, 2125 (1952); Seibold, Sutton, *J. Chem. Phys.* **23**, 1967 (1955). Synthesis of a helical ferrocene: T. J. Katz, J. Pesti, *J. Am. Chem. Soc.* **104**, 346 (1982). *Reviews:* Rausch *et al., J. Chem. Educ.* **34**, 268-272 (1957); M. Rosenblum, *Chemistry of the Iron Group Metallocenes* (John Wiley, New York, 1965) 241 pp; Bruce, *Organomet. Chem. Rev. Sect. B* **10**, 75-122 (1972); B. W. Rockett, G. Marr, *J. Organomet. Chem.* **211**, 215-278 (1981).

Orange needles from methanol or ethanol; odor of camphor. mp 173-174°. Sublimes above 100°. Volatile in steam. Practically insol in water, 10% NaOH, and concd boiling HCl. Sol in alcohol, ether, benzene. Dissolves in dil nitric and concd sulfuric acids forming a deep red soln with blue fluorescence. The molecule is diamagnetic and the dipole moment is effectively zero.

Caution: Potential symptoms of overexposure are irritation of eyes, skin and respiratory system. *See NIOSH Pocket Guide to Chemical Hazards* (DHHS/NIOSH 97-140, 1997) p 104.

USE: Antiknock additive for gasoline; catalyst.

4038. Ferrocholinate. [1336-80-7] 2-Hydroxy-*N,N,N*-trimethylethanaminium (*OC*-6-44)-triaqua[2-(hydroxy-*κO*)-1,2,3-propanetricarboxylato(4−)-*κO¹,κO²*]ferrate(1−); [hydrogen citrato(3−)]triaquoiron, choline salt; iron choline citrate complex. C_{11}-$H_{24}FeNO_{11}$; mol wt 402.15. C 32.85%, H 6.02%, Fe 13.89%, N 3.48%, O 43.76%. Chelate prepd by interaction of equimolar quantities of choline dihydrogen citrate and freshly prepd $Fe(OH)_3$ or $FeCO_3$: F. J. Bandelin, **US 2575611** (1951 to Flint Eaton); by treatment of a freshly prepd solution of ferric citrate with an equimolar amount of choline: J. K. Chakrabarti, S. P. Sen, *Chem. Ind. (London)* **1961**, 1407. Pediatric use in anemia: J. Rose, *Clin. Med.* **69**, 1601 (1962). Clinical evaluation in iron deficient infants: J. C. Lee, *J. Catholic Med. Coll.* **30**, 479 (1977). Pharmaceutical prepn, characteristics and applications: G. N. Bookwalter *et al., J. Food Sci.* **38**, 618 (1973). Bioavailability in pigs: E. R. Miller *et al., J. Anim. Sci.* **52**, 783 (1981). Brief review in anemia: P. P. Gerbino, K. J. Tietze, *Am. J. Pharm.* **155**, 49-62 (1983).

Greenish-brown, reddish-brown or brown amorphous solid with glistening surface upon fracture. Freely sol in water, yielding stable solns; sol in acids, alkalies. One gram of pharmaceutical grade is equivalent to 120 mg of elemental iron and 360 mg of choline base.
Note: Was sold commerically under the names **Chel-Iron, Ferrolip, Chelafer.** Ferrocholinate is also used for other combinations of iron, choline and citric acid.
THERAP CAT: Formerly as a hematinic.

4039.   Ferroglycine Sulfate. [17169-60-7] (*T*-4)-Hydrogen (glycinato-*κN,κO*) [sulfato(2−)-*κO,κO′*]-ferrate(1−); ferrous aminoacetosulfate; iron sulfate-glycine complex; Ferrocontin; Plesmet; Ferrosanol. $C_2H_5FeNO_6S$; mol wt 226.97. C 10.58%, H 2.22%, Fe 24.60%, N 6.17%, O 42.29%, S 14.13%. Chelate of ferrous sulfate and glycine, *q.q.v.* Prepn: W. Rummell, **US 2877253** (1959 to Schwarz Arzneimittelfabrik). Tolerability study: J. Pomeranze, R. J. Gadek, *N. Engl. J. Med.* **257**, 73 (1957). Use in iron fortification of salt: S. Ranganathan *et al., Food Chem.* **57**, 311 (1996). Clinical evaluation in iron deficiency anemia vs ferrous fumarate, *q.v.*: A. Aronstam, D. L. Aston, *Pharmatherapeutica* **3**, 263 (1982).

THERAP CAT: Hematinic.

4040.   Ferrosoferric Oxide. [1317-61-9] Ferric ferrous oxide; triiron tetraoxide; black iron oxide; magnetic iron oxide; Ethiops iron. Fe_3O_4; mol wt 231.53. Fe 72.36%, O 27.64%. Occurs in nature as the mineral *magnetite* (red-black lumps). Prepn: *Gmelins, Iron* (8th ed) part B, 36-62 (1932); *Ullmanns Encyklopädie der technischen Chemie* vol. **6**, 420 (1955). *Review:* Robl, *Angew. Chem.* **70**, 367 (1958).
Black cubes or amorphous powder. mp 1538°; d 5.2. Oxidized to Fe_2O_3 on heating in air. Practically insol in water. Sol in acids.
USE: Pigment in paints, linoleum, ceramic glazes; in coloring glass; as a polishing compd; in the textile industry; in cathodes; as catalyst.

4041.   Ferrous Bisglycinate. [20150-34-9] Bis(glycinato-*κN,κO*) iron; bisglycino-iron(II) chelate; Ferrochel. $C_4H_8FeN_2O_4$; mol wt 203.96. C 23.56%, H 3.95%, Fe 27.38%, N 13.73%, O 31.38%. Nutritionally functional, totally reacted, metal amino acid chelate. Prepn: B. W. Fitzsimmons *et al., Inorg. Chim. Acta* **106**, 109 (1985). Clinical evaluation of tolerability vs ferrous sulfate: M. Coplin *et al., Clin. Ther.* **13**, 606 (1991); of iron bioavailability: M. Layrisse *et al., J. Nutr.* **130**, 2195 (2000). Clinical study in iron deficiency anemia in infants: O. Pineda, H. D. Ashmead, *Nutrition*

17, 381 (2001); in children: L. H. S. Miglioranza *et al., ibid.* **19**, 419 (2003). Toxicity study: R. B. Jeppsen, J. F. Borzelleca, *Food Chem. Toxicol.* **37**, 723 (1999). *Reviews:* M. R. Motyka, *Agro-Food-Ind. Hi-Tech* **12**, 6-8, 14-16 (2001).

Off-white solid. LD_{50} orally in rats: 560 mg iron/kg (Jeppsen).
THERAP CAT: Hematinic.

4042.   Ferrous Bromide. [7789-46-0] Br_2Fe; mol wt 215.65. Br 74.11%, Fe 25.90%. $FeBr_2$. Prepn: Baxter, *Z. Anorg. Chem.* **38**, 236 (1904); Baxter *et al., ibid.* **70**, 333 (1911); Schimmel, *Ber.* **62**, 963 (1929); Kühnl, Ernst, *Z. Anorg. Allg. Chem.* **317**, 84 (1962).
Light yellow to dark brown hygroscopic crystals. mp 684°. d_4^{25} 4.63. Very sol in water and alcohol. *Keep tightly closed.*
Hexahydrate. Pale green to bluish-green rhombic prisms. Forms tetrahydrate at 49°; dihydrate at 83°. Rapidly oxidized in moist air. *Keep tightly closed.*
USE: Polymerization catalyst.

4043.   Ferrous Chloride. [7758-94-3] Cl_2Fe; mol wt 126.75. Cl 55.94%, Fe 44.06%. $FeCl_2$. Occurs in nature as the mineral *lawrencite*. Preparation: Kovacic, Brace, *Inorg. Synth.* **6**, 172 (1960); Kühnl, Ernst, *Z. Anorg. Allg. Chem.* **317**, 84 (1962). Prepn of dihydrate: Gayer, Woontner, *Inorg. Synth.* **5**, 179 (1957).
White rhombohedral crystals; may sometimes have a green tint. Very hygroscopic. mp 674°; bp 1023°; d^{25} 3.16. Can be sublimed in a stream of HCl at about 700°. Forms $FeCl_3$ and Fe_2O_3 on heating in air. Freely sol in water, alc, acetone; slightly sol in benzene; practically insol in ether.
Dihydrate. White monoclinic crystals with pale green tint. Loses 1 H_2O at 120°: Gayer, Woontner, *loc. cit.;* also reported to lose 1 H_2O at 150-160°: Schafer, *Z. Anorg. Allg. Chem.* **258**, 69 (1949). Sol in water.
Tetrahydrate. Pale green to blue-green, monoclinic crystals or cryst powder. Loses $2H_2O$ at about 105-115°: Schafer, *loc. cit.* d 1.93. Sol in water, alcohol. The technical product may not be completely sol without the addn of acid. Aq solns are readily oxidized.
Caution: Potential symptoms of overexposure are irritation of eyes, skin, mucous membranes; abdominal pain, diarrhea, vomiting; possible liver damage. *See NIOSH Pocket Guide to Chemical Hazards* (DHHS/NIOSH 97-140, 1997) p 174.
USE: In metallurgy; as reducing agent; in pharmaceutical prepns; as mordant in dyeing.

4044.   Ferrous Citrate. [23383-11-1] Several forms of this salt are known. Prepn from citric acid and Fe powder: Oroshnik, Haffcke, **US 2904573** (1959 to Ortho); and ferrous salts: Carlson, **US 3091626** (1963 to Scherer).
Monohydrate. Monoferrous acid citrate monohydrate. Powder. Practically insol in water, alcohol, acetone.
Decahydrate. Triferrous dicitrate decahydrate. Very slightly colored powder or white crystals. Very stable to air oxidation. If H_2O is removed by vacuum desiccation, the dehydrated ferrous salt rapidly oxidizes to a ferric salt. Practically insol in water, acetone.
THERAP CAT: Hematinic.

4045.   Ferrous Fluoride. [7789-28-8] F_2Fe; mol wt 93.84. F 40.49%, Fe 59.51%. FeF_2. Prepn from $FeCl_2$ and HF gas: Kwasnik in *Handbook of Preparative Inorganic Chemistry*, G. Brauer, Ed. (Academic Press, New York, 2nd ed., 1963) p 266; from Fe powder and liq HF: Muetterties, Castle, *J. Inorg. Nucl. Chem.* **18**, 148 (1961).
Tetragonal crystals (rutile type) or powder. Sublimes at about 1100°. d 4.09. Sparingly sol in water; more sol in dil HF. Practically insol in alcohol, ether, benzene.
USE: As catalyst in organic reactions.

4046.   Ferrous Fumarate. [141-01-5] (*2E*)-2-Butenedioic acid iron(2+) salt (1:1); Erco-Fer; Ferronat; Ferrotemp; Fersaday;

Fersamal; Fumafer; Fumiron; Galfer; Heferol; Ircon; Meterfer; Palafer; Toleron; Tolferain. $C_4H_2FeO_4$; mol wt 169.90. C 28.28%, H 1.19%, Fe 32.87%, O 37.67%. Carboxyl groups in the fumarate act as bidentate ligands; overall structure is polymeric. Prepn: H. C. Bertsch, J. F. Lemp, US 2848366 (1958 to Mallinckrodt); and structural studies: C. P. Prabhakaran, C. C. Patel, *Indian J. Chem.* **7**, 266 (1969). Animal toxicity and human studies in treatment of anemia: M. C. Berenbaum *et al., Blood* **15**, 540 (1960). Pharmacokinetics in rats: F. Ryszka *et al., Boll. Chim. Farm.* **137**, 178 (1998). Clinical evaluation in dietary iron fortification: R. F. Hurrell *et al., Br. J. Nutr.* **65**, 271 (1991); with ascorbic acid, *q.v.*, in anemia in infants: S. Zlotkin *et al., Am. J. Clin. Nutr.* **74**, 791 (2001).

$$\text{Fe}^{++} \quad \begin{array}{c} ^-OOC \\ \\ H \end{array} \diagdown C=C \diagup \begin{array}{c} H \\ \\ COO^- \end{array}$$

Reddish-orange to reddish-brown, granular powder. d^{25} 2.435. Odorless; almost tasteless. Practically insol in water and common organic solvents including styrene and α-methylstyrene. LD_{50} in mice, rats (mg Fe/kg): 630, 580 orally (Berenbaum).

THERAP CAT: Hematinic.

4047. Ferrous Gluconate. [299-29-6] Bis(D-gluconato-O^1,O^2)-iron; Fergon; Ferlucon; Ferronicum; Iromon; Irox; Nionate. $C_{12}H_{22}FeO_{14}$; mol wt 446.14. C 32.31%, H 4.97%, Fe 12.52%, O 50.21%. Fe[HOCH$_2$(CHOH)$_4$CO$_2$]$_2$. Prepd from Ba gluconate and $FeSO_4$. Prepn of isotonic solns: Hammarlund, *Pharm. Acta Helv.* **35**, 593 (1960). Toxicity study: Hoppe *et al., Am. J. Med. Sci.* **230**, 491 (1955).

Dihydrate. Yellowish-gray or pale greenish-yellow powder. Slight odor of caramel. Acid to litmus. Sol in water. Practically insol in alcohol. Aq solns are stabilized by the addition of glucose. Extensive stability studies on aq solns: Johnson, Thomas, *J. Pharm. Pharmacol.* **6**, 1037 (1954). LD_{50} in mice: 114 mg/kg i.v.; 3.7 g/kg orally (Hoppe).

USE: As coloring and flavoring in foods.

THERAP CAT: Hematinic.

4048. Ferrous Hydroxide. [18624-44-7] FeH_2O_2; mol wt 89.86. Fe 62.15%, H 2.24%, O 35.61%. Fe(OH)$_2$. Prepn: Rihl, Fricke, Z. *Anorg. Allg. Chem.* **251**, 406 (1943); Leussing, Kolthoff, *J. Am. Chem. Soc.* **75**, 2476 (1953). Oxidation products: Feitknecht, Keller, Z. *Anorg. Chem.* **262**, 61 (1950); Mayne, *J. Chem. Soc.* **1953**, 129; Shipko, Douglas, *J. Phys. Chem.* **60**, 1519 (1956).

White, amorphous powder or white to pale green hexagonal crystals. Oxidized on exposure to air; may ignite spontaneously on exposure to air if finely divided. Practically insol in water. More sol in solns of NH_4 salts; sol in concd NaOH soln.

4049. Ferrous Iodide. [7783-86-0] FeI_2; mol wt 309.65. Fe 18.03%, I 81.97%. Prepn: Chaigneau, *Bull. Soc. Chim. Fr.* **1957**, 886; Lieser, Elias, Z. *Anorg. Allg. Chem.* **316**, 208 (1962); Lux in *Handbook of Preparative Inorganic Chemistry* **vol. 2**, G. Brauer, Ed. (Academic Press, New York, 2nd ed., 1965) p 1495.

Large, thin, red-violet crystals or black leaflets. Very hygroscopic. Sol in water, alcohol, ether; aq soln is readily oxidized by air. *Keep tightly closed and protected from light.*

USE: As catalyst for organic reactions.

4050. Ferrous Lactate. [5905-52-2] $C_6H_{10}FeO_6$; mol wt 233.99. C 30.80%, H 4.31%, Fe 23.87%, O 41.03%. Fe(C$_3$H$_5$O$_3$)$_2$. Prepn: *Gmelins, Iron* (8th ed.) **59**, part B, p 532 (1932). Prepn of isotonic solns: Hammarlund, *Pharm. Acta Helv.* **35**, 593 (1960). Toxicity study: T. H. Eickholt, W. F. White, *J. Pharm. Sci.* **54**, 1211 (1965). Review of toxicology: B. Venugopal, T. D. Luckey, *Environ. Qual. Safety* Suppl. 1, 4-73 (1975).

LD_{50} orally in mice: 147 $\pm$30 mg/kg (Eickholt, White).

Trihydrate. [6047-24-1] Greenish-white powder or cryst masses. Slight characteristic odor; mild, sweet and ferruginous taste. Sol in water; freely sol in alkali citrates forming a green soln. Almost insol in alc. On exposure to air it becomes darker and incompletely sol. *Keep well closed and protected from light.* LD in rabbits (mg/kg): 578 s.c., 287 i.v. (Venugopal, Luckey).

USE: Food coloring.

THERAP CAT: Hematinic.

4051. Ferrous Oxalate. [516-03-0] Ferrox. C_2FeO_4; mol wt 143.86. C 16.70%, Fe 38.82%, O 44.49%. FeC$_2$O$_4$. Prepn of dihydrate: *Gmelins, Iron* (8th ed.) **59**, part B, 532-533 (1932); prepn of anhydr salt: Waterman, Vivian, *J. Org. Chem.* **14**, 289 (1949).

Dihydrate. Pale yellow, odorless, cryst powder. d 2.28. Dec at 150-160° on heating in air. Slightly sol in water; sol in dil mineral acids.

USE: As a photographic developer for silver bromide-gelatin plates; to impart a greenish-brown tint to optical glass (sunglasses, windshields, railroad car windows), for decorative glassware; pigment for plastics, paints, lacquers.

4052. Ferrous Oxide. [1345-25-1] FeO; mol wt 71.84. Fe 77.74%, O 22.27%. Prepn: Lux in *Handbook of Preparative Inorganic Chemistry* **vol. 2**, G. Brauer, Ed. (Academic Press, New York, 2nd ed., 1965) p 1497.

Jet-black powder. mp 1360°; d 5.7. Easily oxidized by air. It is a strong base and readily absorbs CO$_2$. Practically insol in water and alkalies. Readily sol in acids.

USE: In manuf of green, heat-absorbing glass; in steel manuf; in enamels; as catalyst.

4053. Ferrous Phosphate. [14940-41-1] Fe$_3$O$_8$P$_2$; mol wt 357.48. Fe 46.87%, O 35.80%, P 17.33%. Fe$_3$(PO$_4$)$_2$. Prepn of octahydrate: *Gmelins, Iron* (8th ed.) **59**, part B, 771 (1932). Due to unavoidable oxidation, the article of commerce contains basic ferric phosphate.

Octahydrate. Grayish-blue powder or monoclinic crystals. d 2.58. Practically insol in water. Sol in mineral acids. *Keep well closed and protected from light.*

USE: In ceramics, as catalyst.

4054. Ferrous Phosphide. [1310-43-6] Iron phosphide; iron hemiphosphide; diiron phosphide. Fe$_2$P; mol wt 142.66. Fe 78.29%, P 21.71%. Prepn from Fe and red P: Rundqvist, Jellinek, *Acta Chem. Scand.* **13**, 425 (1959); Cadeville, Meyer, *Compt. Rend.* **252**, 1124 (1961).

Gray, hexagonal needles or blue-gray powder. d 6.85. Ferromagnetic. Insol in water, dil acid, dil alkali. Reacts with hot mineral acids.

4055. Ferrous Selenide. [1310-32-3] FeSe; mol wt 134.81. Fe 41.42%, Se 58.57%. Prepn from the elements: Gronvold, Westrum, *Acta Chem. Scand.* **13**, 241 (1959).

Black mass with metallic luster. Stable in air. Dec when heated in O$_2$. d 6.78. Practically insol in water. Sol in HCl with the evolution of H$_2$Se.

USE: In electrical semiconductors.

4056. Ferrous Succinate. [10030-90-7] Cerevon; Ferromyn. $C_4H_4FeO_4$; mol wt 171.92. C 27.94%, H 2.35%, Fe 32.48%, O 37.23%. Fe^{2+}(OOCCH$_2$CH$_2$COO)$^{2-}$. Prepn: Franke, *Ann.* **491**, 30 (1931).

Tetrahydrate. Sparingly sol in water. Also obtained as a dihydrate.

THERAP CAT: Hematinic.

4057. Ferrous Sulfate. [7720-78-7] FeO$_4$S; mol wt 151.91. Fe 36.76%, O 42.13%, S 21.11%. FeSO$_4$. Hydrates occur in nature as the minerals: *melanterite, siderotil, szomolnikite, tauriscite*. Heptahydrate prepd commercially by the action of H$_2$SO$_4$ on Fe: *Faith, Keyes & Clark's Industrial Chemicals*, F. A. Lowenheim, M. K. Moran, Eds. (Wiley-Interscience, New York, 4th ed., 1975) pp 418-421. Crystal structure of heptahydrate: Baur, *Acta Crystallogr.* **17**, 1167 (1964). Acute toxicity: Hoppe *et al., Am. J. Med. Sci.* **230**, 491 (1955).

Monohydrate. [17375-41-6] Dried ferrous sulfate; exsiccated ferrous sulfate; Feromax; Feroritard; Ferro-Gradumet; Fespan; Tetucur. White to yellow cryst powder. Loses H$_2$O at about 300°. Dec at higher temps. Sol in water.

Heptahydrate. [7782-63-0] Copperas; green vitriol; iron vitriol; Feosol; Feospan; Fesofor; Fero-Gradumet; Fer-in-Sol; Haemofort; Ironate; Mol-Iron; Presfersul; Sulferrous. Blue-green, monoclinic, odorless crystals or granules. Efflorescent in dry air; oxidizes in moist air forming a brown coating of basic ferric sulfate. Forms tetrahydrate at 56.6° and monohydrate at 65°. d 1.897. Sol in water. Practically insol in alcohol. Aq solns are oxidized slowly by air when cold, rapidly when hot; rate of oxidation increased by addn of alkali or exposure to light. LD_{50} in mice: 65 mg/kg i.v.; 1.52 g/kg orally (Hoppe).

Caution: Potential symptoms of overexposure are irritation of eyes, skin, mucous membranes; GI disturbances, abdominal pain, vomiting, diarrhea; dehydration; shock, pallor, cyanosis, coldness; rapid, weak pulse; low blood pressure; rapid, shallow respirations; drowsiness; hyporeflexia; dilated pupils; coma; liver damage. *See NIOSH Pocket Guide to Chemical Hazards* (DHHS/NIOSH 97-140, 1997) p 174; *Clinical Toxicology of Commercial Products*, R. E. Gosselin *et al.*, Eds. (Williams & Wilkins, Baltimore, 5th ed., 1984) Sect. III, pp 179-185.

USE: In manufacture of Fe, Fe compds, other sulfates; in Fe electroplating baths; in fertilizer; as food and feed supplement; in radiation dosimeters; as reducing agent in chemical processes; as wood preservative; as weed-killer; in prevention of chlorosis in plants; in other pesticides; in writing ink; in process engraving and lithography; as dye for leather; in etching aluminum; in water treatment; in qualitative analysis ("brown ring" test for nitrates); as polymerization catalyst.

THERAP CAT: Hematinic.

THERAP CAT (VET): In iron deficiency. Astringent.

4058. Ferrous Sulfide. [1317-37-9] Iron sulfuret. FeS; mol wt 87.91. Fe 63.53%, S 36.47%. Occurs in nature as the minerals: *magnetkies, pyrrhotine, troillite*. Usually prepd from the elements: Lux in *Handbook of Preparative Inorganic Chemistry* vol 2, G. Brauer, Ed. (Academic Press, New York, 2nd ed., 1965) p 1502. The commercial product is ~75-80% FeS.

Colorless hexagonal crystals when pure; usually gray to brownish-black lumps, rods or granular powder. mp 1194°; d 4.84. Trimorphic with transition points at 135° and 325°. Oxidized by moist air to S and Fe_3O_4. Practically insol in water. Soluble in acids with the evolution of H_2S.

USE: As a laboratory source of H_2S; in the ceramic industry; as a paint pigment; in anodes; in lubricant coatings.

4059. Ferrous Thiocyanate. [6010-09-9] Ferrous sulfocyanate; ferrous sulfocyanide. $C_2FeN_2S_2$; mol wt 172.01. C 13.97%, Fe 32.47%, N 16.29%, S 37.28%. $Fe(SCN)_2$. Prepn: *Gmelins, Iron* (8th ed) **59**, part B, 743-747 (1932); O'Brien, *Chem. Eng. News* **33**, 2008 (1955).

Trihydrate, pale green monoclinic prisms. Rapidly oxidized on exposure to air; dec by heat. Freely sol in water, alcohol, ether. *Keep tightly closed and protected from light.*

USE: Indicator for peroxides in organic solns.

4060. Fertilysin. [1477-57-2] *N,N'*-1,8-Octanediylbis[2,2-dichloroacetamide]; *N,N'*-octamethylenebis(2,2-dichloroacetamide); *N,N'*-bis(dichloroacetyl)-1,8-octamethylenediamine; Win-18446. $C_{12}H_{20}Cl_4N_2O_2$; mol wt 366.11. C 39.37%, H 5.51%, Cl 38.73%, N 7.65%, O 8.74%. $Cl_2CHCONH(CH_2)_8NHOC-CHCl_2$. Inhibits spermatogenesis without affecting production of gonadotropins in male laboratory animals. Prepn and biological activity: Surrey, Mayer, *J. Med. Pharm. Chem.* **3**, 419 (1961); Surrey, **US 3143566** (1964 to Sterling Drug). Assessment of antifertility activity in rats: S. Nag, J. J. Ghosh, *J. Steroid Biochem.* **11**(1B), 681 (1979). Teratological study: P. Taleporos *et al.*, *Teratology* **18**, 5 (1978). Toxicology study: F. Coulston *et al.*, *Toxicol. Appl. Pharmacol.* **2**, 715 (1960).

Crystals, mp 122.4-123.6°. LD_{50} orally in mice: >16000 mg/kg (Coulston).

4061. Fertirelin. [38234-21-8] 9-(*N*-Ethyl-L-prolinamide)-1-9-luteinizing hormone-releasing factor (swine); 9-(*N*-ethyl-L-prolinamide)-10-deglycinamide-luteinizing hormone-releasing factor (pig); Des-Gly[10]-NH$_2$-LH-RH-ethylamide; TAP-031. $C_{55}H_{76}N_{16}O_{12}$; mol wt 1153.29. C 57.28%, H 6.64%, N 19.43%, O 16.65%. Synthetic nonapeptide analog of LH-RH, *q.v.* Prepn: M. Fujino *et al.*, **DE 2321174**; *eidem*, **US 3853837** (1973, 1974 both to Takeda); S. Shinagawa, M. Fujino, *Chem. Pharm. Bull.* **23**, 229 (1975); *see also:* M. Fujino *et al.*, *Biochem. Biophys. Res. Commun.* **49**, 863 (1972). Enzyme immunoassay in bovine plasma: J. Okada, S. Kondo, *ibid.* **33**, 4464 (1985). HPLC determn of bulk drugs and formulations: P. A. Hartman, J. D. Stodola, *J. Chromatogr.* **444**,

177 (1988). Field trial in bovine cystic ovarian disease: T. Nakao *et al.*, *Jpn. J. Vet. Sci.* **45**, 269 (1983); to induce ovulation for insemination of dairy cows: T. Nakao *et al.*, *Theriogenology* **20**, 111 (1983); K. Yamada *et al.*, *Anim. Reprod. Sci.* **74**, 27 (2002).

5-oxoPro–His–Trp–Ser–Tyr–Gly–Leu–Arg–ProNHCH$_2$CH$_3$

Acetate. [66002-66-2] U-69689E; Conceral; Ovalyse. C_{55}-$H_{76}N_{16}O_{12}$·$C_2H_4O_2$; mol wt 1213.34. Pentahydrate as white, fluffy powder, $[\alpha]_D^{25}$ −53.6° (c = 0.5 in 5% acetic acid).

THERAP CAT (VET): Gonad stimulating principle.

4062. Ferulic Acid. [1135-24-6] 3-(4-Hydroxy-3-methoxyphenyl)-2-propenoic acid; 4-hydroxy-3-methoxycinnamic acid; 3-methoxy-4-hydroxycinnamic acid; caffeic acid 3-methyl ether. $C_{10}H_{10}O_4$; mol wt 194.18. C 61.85%, H 5.19%, O 32.96%. Widely distributed in small amounts in plants. Isoln from *Ferula foetida* Reg. *Umbelliferae:* H. Hlasiwetz, L. Barth, *Ann.* **138**, 61 (1866); from *Pinus laricio* Poir. *Abietineae:* M. Bamberger, *Monatsh. Chem.* **12**, 441 (1891); *see also Beilstein* **10**, 436 (1927) and supplements. Prepd by the interaction of vanillin, malonic acid and piperidine in pyridine for 3 weeks, then precipitating with HCl: Vorsatz, *J. Prakt. Chem.* **145**, 265 (1936); Pearl, Beyer, *J. Org. Chem.* **16**, 216 (1951). Sepn of *cis* and *trans* isomers: Comte *et al.*, *Compt. Rend.* **245**, 1144 (1957). ^{13}C NMR study: C. J. Kelley *et al.*, *J. Org. Chem.* **41**, 449 (1976). Discovery as a component of cell walls in wheat and barley: M. G. Smart, T. P. O'Brien, *Aust. J. Plant Physiol.* **6**, 485 (1979). Use as food preservative: T. Tsuchiya, M. Takasawa, **JP Kokai 75 18621** (1975 to Kyokuto Shibosan), *C.A.* **83**, 7602v (1975).

trans - Ferulic Acid

cis-**Form.** Yellow oil. uv max (alcohol): 316 nm.

trans-**Form.** Orthorhombic needles from water, mp 174°. uv max (alcohol): 236, 322 nm. Sol in hot water, alcohol, ethyl aetate. Moderately sol in ether. Sparingly sol in petr ether, benzene. Forms a sodium salt.

USE: Food preservative.

4063. Ferumoxides. [119683-68-0] AMI-25; Feridex; Endorem. Active ingredient of colloidal super paramagnetic iron oxide (SPIO) consisting of nonstoichiometric magnetite cores coated with dextran. Designed for use as hepatic MRI contrast agent. Prepn: E. V. Groman, L. Josephson, **WO 8800060**; *eidem*, **US 4770183** (both 1988 to Advanced Magnetics). Pharmacokinetics: S. Majumdar *et al.*, *Invest. Radiol.* **25**, 771 (1990). Physical and chemical properties: C. W. Jung, P. Jacobs, *Magn. Reson. Imaging* **13**, 661 (1995). Surface properties: C. W. Jung, *ibid.* 675. Clinical studies in hepatic imaging: T. J. Vogl *et al.*, *Radiology* **198**, 881 (1996); E. Senéterre *et al.*, *ibid.* **200**, 785 (1996). Series of articles on toxicology: *Jpn. Pharmacol. Ther.* **22**, 57-141 (1994). Review of physicochemical characteristics and clinical applications: O. Clement *et al.*, *Top. Magn. Reson. Imaging* **9**, 167-182 (1998).

Aqueous suspension, black to reddish-brown liquid. Osmolality: ~340 mOsm/kg. d 1.04.

THERAP CAT: Diagnostic aid (MRI contrast agent).

4064. Ferumoxsil. [171544-35-7] AMI-121; GastroMARK; Lumiren. Active ingredient of colloidal super paramagnetic iron oxide (SPIO) consisting of nonstoichiometric magnetite cores coated with siloxane ($FeO_x[C_3H_{13}N_2SiO_2]_y$); designed for use as negative MRI contrast agent. Prepn: M. S. Chagnon *et al.*, **EP 125995**, R. A. Whitehead *et al.*, **US 4554088** (1984, 1985 both to Advanced Magnetics). Physical and chemical properties: C. W. Jung, P. Jacobs, *Magn. Reson. Imaging* **13**, 661 (1995). Surface properties: C. W. Jung, *ibid.* 675. Clinical study in lower abdominal imaging: R. C. H. Heusler *et al.*, *J. Magn. Reson. Imaging* **4**,

385 (1995); A. D'Arienzo *et al.*, *Am. J. Gastroenterol.* **95**, 720 (2000).

Aqueous suspension, turbid, slightly viscous, dark brown to orange-brown liquid. Osmolality: 250 mOsm/kg. d 1.01.

THERAP CAT: Diagnostic aid (MRI contrast agent).

4065. Ferumoxtran 10. [189047-99-2] AMI-227; BMS-180549; Code-7227; Combidex; Sinerem. Ultrasmall superparamagnetic iron oxide (USPIO) magnetite nanoparticles covered with low molecular weight dextran T-10; designed for use as an MRI imaging agent to detect metastatic cancer in lymph nodes. Prepn: E. V. Groman *et al.*, *WO* **8800060**; S. Palmacci, L. Josephson, *US* **5262176** (1988, 1993 both to Advanced Magnetics). Physical and chemical properties: C. W. Jung, P. Jacobs, *Magn. Reson. Imaging* **13**, 661 (1995); surface properties: C. W. Jung, *ibid.* 675. Biodistribution study: H. H. Bengele *et al.*, *ibid.* **12**, 433 (1994). Clinical studies of diagnostic use: Y. Anai *et al.*, *Radiology* **228**, 777 (2003); A. G. Rockall *et al.*, *J. Clin. Oncol.* **23**, 2813 (2005). Review of clinical experience: M. G. Harisinghani *et al.*, *RadioGraphics* **24**, 867-878 (2004); of pharmacology and preclinical studies: P. Bourrinet *et al.*, *Invest. Radiol.* **41**, 313 2006.

Diameter of iron oxide core: 4.3-6.0 nm; of coated particle: 17-21 nm.

THERAP CAT: Diagnostic aid (MRI contrast agent).

4066. Fervenulin. [483-57-8] 6,8-Dimethylpyrimido[5,4-*e*]-1,2,4-triazine-5,7-(6*H*,8*H*)-dione; 6,8-dimethyl-5,7-dioxo-5,6,7,-8-tetrahydropyrimido[5,4-*e*]-*as*-triazine; 1,3-dimethylazalumazine; planomycin. $C_7H_7N_5O_2$; mol wt 193.16. C 43.53%, H 3.65%, N 36.26%, O 16.57%. Antibiotic from culture filtrates of *Streptomyces fervens:* Eble *et al.*, *Antibiot. Annu.* **1959-1960**, 227. Structure: Daves *et al.*, *J. Org. Chem.* **26**, 5256 (1961). Synthesis: Pfleiderer, Schündehütte, *Ann.* **615**, 42 (1958); Daves *et al.*, *J. Am. Chem. Soc.* **84**, 1724 (1962); Yoneda, Nagamatsu, *Bull. Chem. Soc. Jpn.* **48**, 2884 (1975); Taylor, Sowinski, *J. Org. Chem.* **40**, 2321 (1975); S. Senda *et al.*, *J. Am. Chem. Soc.* **99**, 7358 (1977).

Yellow orthorhombic crystals, mp 178-179°. uv max (ethanol): 238, 275, 340 nm (ε 18,500, 1600, 4200). Sol in practically all of the common organic solvents; sol in cold water to about 2 mg/ml; in hot water to about 40 mg/ml. Practically insol in hydrocarbons. Labile to alkali; stable to acid.

4-Oxide. $C_7H_7N_5O_3$. Synthesis: M. Ichiba *et al.*, *J. Heterocycl. Chem.* **14**, 175 (1977); K. Senga *et al.*, *Heterocycles* **6**, 273 (1977); synthesis and conversion to fervenulin: M. Ichiba *et al.*, *J. Org. Chem.* **43**, 469 (1978). Crystals from alc, mp 179-180°. uv max (alc): 240, 304 nm (log ε 4.10, 3.21).

4067. Feverfew. Featherfew; featherfoil; midsummer daisy. *Tanacetum parthenium* (L.) Sch. Bip., (formerly *Chrysanthemum parthenium* (L.) Bernh.) *Compositae;* a perennial, strongly aromatic herb found in Britain and the Balkan peninsula. Used medicinally since the Middle Ages as a febrifuge. Constituents include sesquiterpene lactones such as parthenolide, *q.v.:* P. J. Hylands, D. M. Hylands in *Development of Drugs and Modern Medicines*, J. W. Gorrod *et al.*, Eds. (Ellis Horwood, Chichester, 1986) pp 100-104. Inhibition of prostaglandin biosynthesis by feverfew extract: H. O. J. Collier *et al.*, *Lancet* **2**, 922 (1980). Effect on human platelet phospholipase: A. N. Makheja, J. M. Bailey, *ibid.* 1054 (1981); *eidem*, *Prostaglandins Leukotrienes Med.* **8**, 653 (1982); J. K. Thakkar *et al.*, *Biochim. Biophys. Acta* **750**, 134 (1983). Inhibition of platelet secretory activity: S. Heptinstall *et al.*, *Lancet* **1**, 1071 (1985); S. Heptinstall *et al.*, *J. Pharm. Pharmacol.* **39**, 459 (1987). Structure and anti-secretory activity study: W. A. Groenewegen *et al.*, *ibid.* **38**, 709 (1986). Clinical trials in migraine using freeze dried feverfew leaves: E. S. Johnson *et al.*, *Br. Med. J.* **291**, 569 (1985). Use of oil extract in migraine: E. S. Johnson *et al.*, *US* **4758433** (1988 to R. P. Scherer). *Review:* M. I. Berry, *Pharm. J.* **232**, 611-614 (1984). Brief review of activity and possible side effects: C. A. Baldwin *et al.*, *ibid.* **239**, 237-238 (1987).

4068. Fexofenadine. [83799-24-0] α,α-Dimethyl-4-[1-hydroxy-4-[4-(hydroxydiphenylmethyl)-1-piperidinyl]butyl]-benzeneacetic acid; carboxyterfenadine; terfenadine carboxylate; MDL-16455. $C_{32}H_{39}NO_4$; mol wt 501.66. C 76.61%, H 7.84%, N 2.79%, O 12.76%. Nonsedating-type histamine H_1-receptor antagonist. Prepn: A.A. Carr *et al.*, **DE 3007498**; *eidem*, **US 4254129** (1980, 1981 both to Richardson-Merrell). Identification as active metabolite of terfenadine, *q.v.*: D. A. Garteiz *et al.*, *Arzneim.-Forsch.* **32**, 1185 (1982). Synthesis: S. H. Kawai *et al.*, *J. Org. Chem.* **59**, 2620 (1994). HPLC separation from terfenadine: K. Y. Chan *et al.*, *J. Chromatogr.* **571**, 291 (1991); determn in biological fluids: A. Terhechte, G. Blaschke, *ibid. A* **694**, 219 (1995). Effects on cardiac K^+ channels: D. Rampe *et al.*, *Mol. Pharmacol.* **44**, 1240 (1993). Comparative analysis of cardiotoxic potential: J. A. Hey *et al.*, *Arzneim.-Forsch.* **46**, 153 (1996). Clinical pharmacology in children: F. E. R. Simons *et al.*, *J. Allergy Clin. Immunol.* **98**, 1062 (1996).

Crystals from methanol-butanone, mp 195-197° (Carr); also reported as white crystals from methanol, mp 142-143° (Kawai).

Hydrochloride. [153439-40-8] Allegra; Telfast. $C_{32}H_{39}$-NO_4.HCl; mol wt 538.12.

THERAP CAT: Antihistaminic.

4069. Fialuridine. [69123-98-4] 1-(2-Deoxy-2-fluoro-β-D-arabinofuranosyl)-5-iodo-2,4(1*H*,3*H*)-pyrimidinedione; 1-(2-deoxy-2-fluoro-β-D-arabinofuranosyl)-5-iodouracil; 5-iodo-2'-fluoroarauracil; FIAU. $C_9H_{10}FIN_2O_5$; mol wt 372.09. C 29.05%, H 2.71%, F 5.11%, I 34.11%, N 7.53%, O 21.50%. Exptl antiviral agent; nucleoside analog with antihepatitis B activity. Prepn: K. A. Watanabe *et al.*, *J. Med. Chem.* **22**, 21 (1979). Antiviral activity: J. M. Colacino, C. Lopez, *Antimicrob. Agents Chemother.* **24**, 505 (1983); K. A. Staschke *et al.*, *Antiviral Res.* **23**, 45 (1994). Clinical pharmacokinetics: R. R. Bowsher *et al.*, *Antimicrob. Agents Chemother.* **38**, 2134 (1994). Report of trial suspension: S. R. Ahmed, *Lancet* **342**, 166 (1993). Evaluation of mechanism of hepatotoxicity: L. Cui *et al.*, *J. Clin. Invest.* **95**, 555 (1995). Clinical toxicological profile: W. Stevenson *et al.*, *Transplant. Proc.* **27**, 1219 (1995).

Crystals from ethanol, mp 216-217°.

4070. Fibrin. [9001-31-4] Fibrin monomer is fibrinogen from which one or two peptides have been removed by means of thrombin: Laki, Chandrasekhar, *Nature* **197**, 1267 (1963). The term fibrin is usually applied to polymerized fibrin monomer. Terminal clotting takes place in four steps: (1) fibrinogen hydrolyzes under the influence of thrombin into fibrin and fibrinopeptide fragments; (2) fibrin forms soft clots which can be readily dispersed; (3) thrombin activates fibrin-stabilizing factor, *q.v.*, an enzyme precursor, present in blood plasma; (4) fibrin in the networks cross-links under the influence of the activated FSF to give the final hard clots: *Chem. Eng. News* **43**, no. 32, 38 (1965); O. D. Ratnoff, B. Bennett, *Science* **179**, 1291 (1973). Fibrin occurs in two principal forms, *fibrin-i,* "insoluble" fibrin, differing from *fibrin-s,* "soluble" fibrin, by urea solubility as well as other characteristics. Fibrin-i is formed through the reaction of a fibrinogen-like plasma protein, FSF, which in the presence of Ca^{2+} converts what would otherwise be a "soluble" weakly bonded gel into a covalently bonded, insol clot: Rosenberg, Carman, *Nature* **204,** 994 (1964). Chemical studies of crosslinking segments: Chen, Doolittle, *Proc. Natl. Acad. Sci. USA* **66,** 472 (1970); *eidem, Biochemistry* **10,** 4486 (1971); Doolittle *et al., Biochem. Biophys. Res. Commun.* **44,** 94 (1971). *Reviews:* W. H. Seegers, *Prothrombin* (Harvard University Press, 1962) 728 pp; Laki, Gladner, *Physiol. Rev.* **44,** 127 (1964); Lorand, *Fed. Proc.* **24,** no. 4, part 1, 784 (1965); A. L. Copley, *Thromb. Res.* **14,** 249 (1979). Review of chemistry: several authors, *Thromb. Diath. Haemorrh. Suppl.* **39** (1970).

4071. Fibrinogen. [9001-32-5] Factor I; Parenogen. A plasma glycoprotein belonging structurally to the keratin-myosin group. Synthesized and secreted by hepatic parenchymal cells. Present to the extent of 0.3-0.4 g/100 ml in human plasma. Essential to the clotting of blood. Its synthesis is greatly increased during acute inflammatory challenge. The fibrinogen molecule consists of three peptide chains, α (A), β (B), and γ (C), crosslinked by several disulfide bonds. The mol wt of about 400,000 represents a dimeric form of the molecule. Thrombin releases fibrinopeptides A and B from the *N*-terminal ends of the α and β chains of fibrinogen in the formation of fibrin during coagulation. Because fibrinogen is less sol than other plasma proteins it is readily separated by precipitation with sodium chloride: Florkin, *J. Biol. Chem.* **87,** 629 (1930); or with ammonium sulfate: Nanninga, *Arch. Neerl. Physiol.* **28,** 241 (1946). Prepn from human plasma: Edsall *et al., J. Am. Chem. Soc.* **69,** 2731 (1947). Purification: Cama *et al., Naturwissenschaften* **48,** 574 (1961). End group determination: Lorand, Middlebrook, *Science* **118,** 515 (1953). Structure studies: Schauenstein, Hochenegger, *Z. Naturforsch.* **8b,** 473 (1953); Edsall, *J. Polym. Sci.* **12,** 253 (1954). *Reviews:* Seegers, *Physiol. Rev.* **34,** 711 (1954); Lorand, *Fed. Proc.* **24,** no. 4, part 1, 784 (1965); several authors, *Thromb. Diath. Haemorrh. Suppl.* **39** (1970); A. L. Copley, *Thromb. Res.* **14,** 249 (1979). Fibrinogen has been shown to be the receptor for the endogenous lectin (agglutinin) secreted by activated platelets: T. K. Gartner *et al., Nature* **289,** 688 (1981). Review of biosynthesis: G. M. Fuller, D. G. Ritchie, *Ann. N.Y. Acad. Sci.* **389,** 308-322 (1982).

Sparingly sol in water. Aq solns are viscous. Isoelectric point 5.5. Readily denatured by heating to 56° or higher, and by chemical agents such as salicylaldehyde, naphthoquinone sulfonates, ninhydrin, and alloxan. Small amounts of papain will clot fibrinogen, but larger amounts will digest the clot.

THERAP CAT: Coagulant (clotting factor).

4072. Fibroblast Growth Factor. [62031-54-3] FGF. Growth stimulatory factor originally isolated from bovine brain and pituitary and found to stimulate DNA synthesis in cultured fibroblast cells. Isoln: D. Gospodarowicz, *Nature* **249,** 123 (1974). Mitogenic effect on cultured cell lines and induction of amphibian limb regeneration *in vivo:* D. Gospodarowicz *et al., Adv. Metab. Disord.* **8,** 301 (1975). Two closely related forms have been identified, known as basic (**bFGF**) and acidic (**aFGF**) fibroblast growth factors, having a total amino acid sequence homology of 55%. Both induce the proliferation and differentiation of a wide variety of cell types, including corneal and vascular endothelial cells, myoblasts, chondrocytes, osteoblasts and glial cells. FGF has neurotrophic and angiogenic activity and may play an important role in the wound healing process. Purification of bFGF from pituitary: D. Gospodarowicz, *J. Biol. Chem.* **250,** 2515 (1975); from brain: D. Gospodarowicz *et al., ibid.* **253,** 3736 (1978). Identification of aFGF from bovine brain: K. A. Thomas *et al., ibid.* **255,** 5517 (1980). Comparison of fibroblast growth factors: S. K. Lemmon *et al., J. Cell Biol.* **95,** 162 (1982). Purification and characterization of aFGF: K. A. Thomas *et al., Proc. Natl. Acad. Sci. USA* **81,** 357 (1984). Identity of bFGF from brain and pituitary: D. Gospodarowicz *et al., ibid.* 6963. Amino acid sequence of bFGF: F. Esch *et al., ibid.* **82,** 6507 (1985); of aFGF: G. Gimenez-Gallego *et al., Science* **230,** 1385 (1985); F. Esch *et al., Biochem. Biophys. Res. Commun.* **133,** 554 (1985). Possible identity of aFGF with *endothelial cell growth factor* (**ECGF**) and *eye-derived growth factor-II* (**EDGF-II**): A. B. Schreiber *et al., J. Cell Biol.*

101, 1623 (1985); of bFGF with *macrophage-derived growth factor* (**MDGF**): A. Baird *et al., Biochem. Biophys. Res. Commun.* **126,** 358 (1985); of FGFs with *retina-derived endothelial cell growth factors*: A. Baird *et al., Biochemistry* **24,** 7855 (1985). Cloning of cDNA for bovine bFGF: J. A. Abraham *et al., Science* **233,** 545 (1986); for human bFGF: T. Kurokawa *et al., FEBS Lett.* **213,** 189 (1987); M. Iwane *et al., Biochem. Biophys. Res. Commun.* **146,** 470 (1987). Expression of a chemically synthesized gene for bioactive bovine aFGF: D. L. Linemeyer *et al., Biotechnology* **5,** 960 (1987). Receptor binding study: G. Neufeld, D. Gospodarowicz: *J. Biol. Chem.* **261,** 5631 (1986). FGF-like factors have been isolated from several human tumor cell lines: R. R. Lobb *et al., Biochem. Biophys. Res. Commun.* **139,** 861 (1986); M. Klagsbrun *et al., Proc. Natl. Acad. Sci. USA* **83,** 2448 (1986); D. Moscatelli *et al., J. Cell. Physiol.* **129,** 273 (1986). FGF has also been shown to be structurally homologous to the protein products of several oncogenes: C. Dickson, G. Peters, *Nature* **326,** 833 (1987); M. Taira *et al., Proc. Natl. Acad. Sci. USA* **84,** 2980 (1987); P. Delli Bovi *et al., Cell* **50,** 729 (1987). Review of tissue distribution and bioactivity of bFGF: A. Baird *et al., Recent Prog. Horm. Res.* **42,** 143-205 (1986). Review of structural characterization and biological functions: D. Gospodarowicz *et al., Endocr. Rev.* **8,** 95-114 (1987). Potential role in the control of pituitary and gonad development: D. Gospodarowicz, N. Ferrara, *J. Steroid Biochem.* **32,** 183-191 (1989). *Reviews:* K. A. Thomas, G. Gimenez-Gallego, *Trends Biochem. Sci.* **11,** 81-84 (1986); D. Gospodarowicz *et al., Mol. Cell. Endocrinol.* **46,** 187-204 (1986); K. A. Thomas, *FASEB J.* **1,** 434-440 (1987).

Acidic fibroblast growth factor. [106096-92-8] pI 5-7. Exists in 2 microheterogeneous forms: *aFGF-1,* a 140 amino acid peptide, mol wt 15,900 daltons, and *aFGF-2,* an amino truncated form lacking 6 amino terminal residues, mol wt 15,200 daltons.

Basic fibroblast growth factor. [106096-93-9] pI 9.6. 146 amino acid peptide, mol wt ~16,000 daltons. Also exists as an amino truncated form, *des 1-15 bFGF,* lacking the first 15 amino acid residues.

4073. Fibroin. [9007-76-5] Protein filaments produced by members of the phylum *Arthropoda,* particularly by certain species belonging to the classes *Insecta* (insects) and *Arachnida* (spiders, etc.). Fibroin is the main protein of silk and is secreted by the insect in its silk glands together with *sericin,* the second silk protein, in aq soln and converted into silk by a process called "spinning." Organization of amino acid sequences in silk fibroin of *Bombyx mori* and general review of silk proteins: F. Lucas, K. M. Rudall in *Comprehensive Biochemistry* vol. 26B, M. Florkin, E. M. Stotz, Eds. (Elsevier, New York, 1968) pp 475-558. *See also* P. M. Lizardi, *Cell* **18,** 581 (1979); L. P. Gage, R. F. Manning, *J. Biol. Chem.* **255,** 9444 (1980). Chemical and crystalline structures: B. Lotz, F. Colonna Cesari, *Biochimie* **61,** 205 (1979).

Pale yellow mass resembling silk. Insol in water, alcohol, ether, dil alkalies. Sol in concd alkalies, concd mineral acids and in ammoniacal nickel oxide soln.

4074. Fibrolase. [116036-70-5] Fibrinolytic enzyme isolated from the venom of the southern copperhead snake, *Agkistrodon contortrix contortrix.* Single chain, zinc metalloproteinase which preferentially cleaves the Aα chain of fibrinogen and fibrin. Several isoforms have been identified; the longest form has 203 amino acid residues with mol wt of 23 kDa. Isoln: N. B. Egen *et al., Toxicon* **25,** 1189 (1987); and effect on human coagulation system: A. D. Retzios, F. S. Markland, Jr., *Thromb. Res.* **52,** 541 (1988). Amino acid sequence: A. Randoph *et al., Protein Sci.* **1,** 590 (1992). Resolution of isoforms: S. L. Loayza *et al., J. Chromatogr. B* **662,** 227 (1994). Three-dimensional structure: M. B. Bolger *et al., AAPS Pharmsci.* **3,** E16 (2001). Review and comparison with other snake venom fibrinolytic enzymes: S. Swenson, F. S. Markland, Jr., *Toxicon* **45,** 1021-1039 (2005).

pI ~6.8.

4075. Fibronectins. α_2-SB glycoproteins; α_2-opsonins; CIG; CSP; CAF; GAP A; LETS; Zeta protein. High mol wt multifunctional glycoproteins, found on cell surfaces, in body fluids (especially plasma), in soft connective tissue matrices, and in most basement membranes. Although fibronectins apparently function as adhesive ligand-like molecules, the full range of their biological activities and relationships are still being elucidated. Their importance in cell adhesion, oncogenic transformation, reticuloendothelial system function, embryonic differentiation, phagocytosis, hemostasis, and chemotaxis is being studied. Discovered as a result of isoln of a partially purified fraction of human plasma and initially termed "cold-insoluble globulin" or CIG: P. R. Morrison et al., J. Am. Chem. Soc. **70**, 3103 (1948). Subsequent studies described various proteins or factors, named according to sources or biological activities, that are now designated as fibronectins. At least two types are known to exist, termed plasma and cellular fibronectin, respectively. Both forms contain subunits of mol wt >200,000, joined by disulfide bonds. They are similar in amino acid compositions, carbohydrate structures and secondary and tertiary structures; they cannot be distinguished in biological activity in assays of cell interactions with substrates or in opsonic activity for macrophages. They differ in their effects on cell morphology, on alignment of transformed cells and on hemagglutination; they also have differences in solubility and in the number of subunits linked by disulfide bonds. Monoclonal antibody studies have indicated that the two forms are distinct: B. T. Atherton, R. O. Hynes, Cell **25**, 133 (1981); K. D. Noonan et al., J. Supramol. Struct. Cell. Biochem. **5**, Suppl, 302 (1981). Regulation of fibronectin biosynthesis: D. R. Senger et al., Am. J. Physiol. **245**, 144 (1983). Structure-function relationships: T. Vartio, A. Vaheri, Trends Biochem. Sci. **8**, 442 (1983). Role in cellular adhesion, spreading and cytoskeletal organization: I. Virtanen et al., Nature **298**, 660 (1982); in phagocytosis: L. Van de Water et al., Science **220**, 201 (1983); in wound healing: G. R. Martin et al., "Regulation of Tissue Structure and Repair by Collagen and Fibronectin" in The Surgical Wound, P. Dineen, C. Hildrick-Smith, Eds. (Lea & Febiger, Philadelphia, 1981) pp 110-122. Use in treatment of corneal trophic ulcer therapy: T. Nishida et al., Arch. Ophthalmol. **101**, 1046 (1983). Review of role in cellular adhesion: S. K. Akiyama et al., J. Supramol. Struct. Cell. Biochem. **16**, 345-358 (1981); role in inflammation: D. F. Mosher et al., Adv. Inflammation Res. **2**, 187-207 (1981); C. Bianco, Ann. N.Y. Acad. Sci. **408**, 602-609 (1983); actvity in various disease states: S. K. Akiyama, K. M. Yamada, "Fibronectin in Disease" in Monographs in Pathology **No. 24**, N. Kaufman, Ed., entitled "Connective Tissue Diseases", B. M. Wagner et al., Eds. (Williams & Wilkins, Baltimore, 1983). General Reviews: E. Pearlstein et al., Mol. Cell. Biochem. **29**, 103-128 (1980); M. W. Mosesson, D. L. Amrani, Blood **56**, 145-158 (1980); E. Ruoslahti, J. Oral Pathol. **10**, 3-13 (1981); R. O. Hynes, K. M. Yamada, J. Cell Biol. **95**, 369-377 (1982); R. O. Hynes, Sci. Am. **254**, 42-51 (1986).

4076. Fichtelite. [2221-95-6] [1S-(1α,4aα,4bβ,7β,8aα,-10aβ)]-Tetradecahydro-1,4a-dimethyl-7-(1-methylethyl)phenanthrene; 18-norabietane. $C_{19}H_{34}$; mol wt 262.47. C 86.94%, H 13.06%. From decayed wood of conifers: Bromeis, Ann. Pharm. **37**, 304 (1841). Structure: L. Ruzicka, E. Waldmann, Helv. Chim. Acta **18**, 611 (1935); Crowfoot, J. Chem. Soc. **1938**, 1241. Stereochemistry: Burgstahler, Marx, Tetrahedron Lett. **1964**, 3333. Synthesis from abietic acid: Jensen, Johnson, J. Org. Chem. **32**, 2045 (1967); Burgstahler, Marx, ibid. **34**, 1562 (1969). Synthesis of dl-form: Johnson et al., J. Am. Chem. Soc. **88**, 3859 (1966); **90**, 5872 (1968); D. F. Taber, S. A. Saleh, ibid. **102**, 5085 (1980).

Crystals from methanol, mp 45-46°. bp$_{43}$ 235-236°. d_4^{22} 0.9380. n_D^{20} 1.5052. $[\alpha]_D$ +19°.

4077. Ficin. [9001-33-6] Ficus proteinase; Ficus protease; Debricin; Higueroxyl Delabarre. A proteolytic enzyme of est. mol wt 23,800-25,500 which requires a free sulfhydryl group for activity and as such is a member of a group which includes papain and bromelain, q.q.v. Occurs in the latex of tropical trees of the genus

Ficus subgenus Pharmacosyce, Moraceae (Oje trees). The commercial product is a concentrate prepd by filtering and drying the latex of Ficus glabrata H. B. & K., Moraceae. First crystallized from fresh fig latex: Walti, J. Am. Chem. Soc. **60**, 493 (1938). Characterization: Cohen, Nature **182**, 659 (1958); Englund et al., Biochemistry **7**, 163 (1968). Purification: Gibian, Bratfisch, US 2950227 (1960 to Schering AG). Amino acid composition: Wong, Liener, Biochem. Biophys. Res. Commun. **17**, 470 (1964); Metrione et al., Arch. Biochem. Biophys. **122**, 137 (1967); Husain, Lowe, Biochem. J. **117**, 333 (1970). Pharmacodynamics: H. Heisto, M. K. Fagerhol, Transfusion **19**, 545 (1979); A. Perkash et al., ibid. **20**, 301 (1980). Toxicology: H. Molitor et al., J. Pharmacol. Exp. Ther. **71**, 20 (1941). Reviews: Liener, Friedenson, Methods Enzymol. **19**, 260-273 (1970); Glazer, Smith, The Enzymes **vol. III**, P. D. Boyer, Ed. (Academic Press, New York, 3rd ed., 1971) pp 538-542.

Buff to cream-colored hygroscopic powder. Acrid odor, growing stronger with age. Bulky, approx 3 ml/g, not free-flowing. Appears dry, even with 15% H_2O present. Not completely sol in water, 2-10% insol material. The sol portion of 1 g dissolves in 3 ml H_2O. pH (2% soln): 4.1. Insol in usual organic solvents. Loses about 10-20% activity when stored 1-3 yrs at ordinary temp and atm conditions. Aq solns inactivated at 100°, solid partially inactivated within a few hours. Solns relatively stable between pH 4-8.5; incompatible with iron, copper, aluminum. Gelatin, coagulated egg white, casein, meat and most protein-like material hydrolyzed in aq ficin solns. Ficin is 10-20 times as active as papain in regard to milk clotting; 4-10 times as active, in general. LD$_{50}$ orally in rats, mice: ~10 g/kg; in rabbits, guinea pigs: ~5 g/kg (Molitor).

Note: The name ficin is currently used to describe both the crude dried latex from different species of the genus Ficus, as well as the enzyme itself.

Caution: Handle ficin carefully because of its tissue-dissolving properties. Can cause irritation to skin, eyes, mucous membranes. Large doses by mouth cause purging.

USE: Protein digestant. In the brewing industry as a chill proofing agent in beer. In the cheese industry as a substitute for rennet in the coagulation of milk. In the meat industry as a meat tenderizer and as an agent for removing casings from formed sausage. In the leather industry for the bating of leather. In the textile industry for shrinkproofing wool, for removing gelatin from sized thread, and mixed with amylases and maltases as a spot remover. In the prepn of peptones. For solubilizing protein material in spent grains. Also used in the determination of the Rh factor. Speeds 10 times the agglutination of human blood cells by the Rh factor when in contact with the anti-Rh serum.

THERAP CAT (VET): Has been used as a trichuricide.

4078. Fidarestat. [136087-85-9]; [105300-43-4] (unspecified). (2S,4S)-6-Fluoro-2,3-dihydro-2′,5′-dioxospiro[4H-1-benzopyran-4,4′-imidazolidine]-2-carboxamide; (2S,4S)-6-fluoro-2′,5′-dioxospiro[chroman-4,4′-imidazolidine]-2-carboxamide; SNK-860. $C_{12}H_{10}FN_3O_4$; mol wt 279.22. C 51.62%, H 3.61%, F 6.80%, N 15.05%, O 22.92%. Aldose reductase inhibitor for treatment of diabetic complications. Prepn (stereo unspec): M. Kurono, et al., EP 193415; eidem, US 4740517 (1986, 1988 both to Sanwa). Prepn of isomers: T. Yamaguchi et al., Arzneim.-Forsch. **44**, 344 (1994). Pharmacological profile: K. Mizuno et al. in Current Concepts of Aldose Reductase and Its Inhibitions, N. Sakamoto et al., Eds. (Elsevier, Amsterdam, 1990) pp 89-96. Configuration and crystal structure of complex with aldose reductase: M. Oka et al., J. Med. Chem. **43**, 2479 (2000). Clinical efficacy in diabetic peripheral neuropathy: N. Hotta et al., Diabetes Care **24**, 1776 (2001). Clinical suppression of sorbitol accumulation in erythrocytes of diabetic patients: T. Asano et al., J. Diabetes Complications **16**, 133 (2002); eidem, ibid. **18**, 336 (2004). Review of clinical development: N. Giannoukakis, Curr. Opin. Invest. Drugs **4**, 1233-1239 (2003).

Crystals from methanol, mp 290-300° (dec). $[\alpha]_D^{27}$ +168° (c = 1.0 in methanol). LD$_{50}$ in rats, dogs (mg/kg): >2000 orally (Yamaguchi).

THERAP CAT: Treatment of diabetic neuropathy.

4079. Filicinic Acid. [2065-00-1] 3,5-Dihydroxy-4,4-dimethyl-2,5-cyclohexadien-1-one; 1,1-dimethylcyclohexane-2,4,6-trione; *gem*-dimethylphloroglucinol; filicinsäure (German). $C_8H_{10}O_3$; mol wt 154.16. C 62.33%, H 6.54%, O 31.14%. Isolated from male fern and by hydrolytic decompn of filixic acid or aspidin: Boehm, *Ann.* **302,** 171 (1898); **329,** 321 (1903). Synthesis: Robertson, Sandrock, *J. Chem. Soc.* **1933,** 1617; Angus *et al., Chem. Ind. (London)* **1954,** 546; Inagaki *et al., J. Pharm. Soc. Jpn.* **76,** 1258 (1956); Hoefer, Riedl, *Angew. Chem.* **74,** 501 (1962); *eidem, Ann.* **656,** 127 (1962).

Prisms from water or benzene, mp 214-215° (dec). pK 5.8. Practically insol in water, petr ether. Sol in 70 parts boiling water, 10 parts boiling alcohol; sparingly sol in ether, benzene, glacial acetic acid. Reduces Tollen's reagent.

3,5-Diacetylfilicinic acid. $C_{12}H_{14}O_5$. Crystals from methanol, mp 65-66°. pK 5.0. Sol in cold methanol, benzene, ether; slightly sol in hot water.

4080. Filipin. [11078-21-0] Filimarisin; U-5956; NSC-3364; Polyene antibiotic complex containing at least eight pentaene compounds, which has been resolved into three pure components, filipin II, III (major), and IV, which differ in the number of hydroxyl groups present (8, 9, 9, resp.) and filipin I, a mixture of at least 5 components. Described as a single entity in the earlier literature. Initial isolation from *Streptomyces filipenensis* in Philippine soil: Whitfield *et al., J. Am. Chem. Soc.* **77,** 4799 (1955). Early structural work: Dhar *et al., Proc. Chem. Soc. London* **1960,** 310; Djerassi *et al., Tetrahedron Lett.* **1961,** 383; Golding, Rickards, *ibid.* **1964,** 2615; Dhar *et al., J. Chem. Soc.* **1964,** 842; Ceder, Ryhage, *Acta Chem. Scand.* **18,** 588 (1964). Separation of filipin complex into components: Bergy, Eble, *J. Antibiot.* **23,** 414 (1970); *see also* Rickards *et al., ibid.* 603. Mechanism of action: R. W. Holz in *Antibiotics* **vol. 5,** pt. 2, F. E. Hahn, Ed. (Springer-Verlag, New York, 1979) pp 313-340. Filipin also interacts specifically with 3β-hydroxysterols (e.g. cholesterol): P. M. Elias *et al., J. Histochem. Cytochem.* **27,** 1247 (1979); *see also* N. J. Severs, H. J. Simons, *Nature* **303,** 637 (1983).

Filipin III

Yellow, feathery needles from chloroform, mp 195-205°. Sensitive to air. $[\alpha]_D^{22}$ -148.3° (c = 0.89 in methanol). uv max (methanol): 322, 338, 355 nm ($E_{1cm}^{1\%}$ 910, 1360, 1330). Freely sol in DMF, pyridine. Also sol in 95% ethanol, methanol, butanol, isopropanol, glacial acetic acid, ether. Practically insol in water, chloroform.

Filipin III. [480-49-9] 4,6,8,10,12,14,16,27-Octahydroxy-3-(1-hydroxyhexyl)-17,28-dimethyloxacyclooctacosa-17,19,21,23,-25-pentaen-2-one; 15-deoxylagosin. $C_{35}H_{58}O_{11}$; mol wt 654.83. Isomeric with filipin IV. Crystals from propanol, mp 163-180° (Bergy, Eble). $[\alpha]_D^{25}$ -245° (c = 0.8 in DMF). uv max (methanol): 243, 308, 321, 337, 354 nm ($E_{1cm}^{1\%}$ 62, 413, 851, 1368, 1343).

USE: Produces arthritis rapidly in rabbits: Pras, Weissman, *Drug Trade News,* July 4, 1966, p 40; as a sterol probe in freeze-fracture cytochemistry.

THERAP CAT: Antifungal.

4081. Filixic Acids. Filicin; filicic acid; Filixsäure (German). Natural filixic acid from male fern, *Dryopteris filix-mas,* is a mixture of six homologues, the 3 main components (BBB, PBB, PBP) of which are obtained by recrystallization from ethyl acetate. When raw filixic acid is purified by treatments with methanol but without recrystns from ethyl acetate, a product is obtained which seems to contain 3 additional homologues with an analogous composition but with acetyl groups in the side chain. Isoln: Luck, *Ann.* **54,** 119 (1845); Boehm, *ibid.* **318,** 253 (1901). Structure studies: Riedl, *Ann.* **585,** 32 (1954); Chan, Hassal, *Experientia* **13,** 349 (1957). Structure of the three main filixic acids: Penttilä, Sundman, *Acta Chem. Scand.* **17,** 191 (1963).

BBB	$R_1 = R_2 = C_3H_7$	
PBB	$R_1 = C_2H_5$	$R_2 = C_3H_7$
PBP	$R_1 = R_2 = C_2H_5$	

Natural filixic acid, pale-yellow plates from ethyl acetate, mp 184-185°. uv max: 228, 288 nm (ε 41000, 29000). Practically insol in water, methanol, acetone. Sol in chloroform, benzene, warm ethyl acetate, acetic acid; slightly sol in ether.

BBB. [4482-83-1] $C_{36}H_{44}O_{12}$; mol wt 668.73. Crystals from ethyl acetate, mp 172-174°.

PBB. [49582-09-4] $C_{35}H_{42}O_{12}$; mol wt 654.70. Crystals from ethyl acetate, mp 184-186°.

PBP. [51005-85-7] $C_{34}H_{40}O_{12}$; mol wt 640.67. Crystals from ethyl acetate, mp 192-194°.

THERAP CAT (VET): Has been used as an anthelmintic.

4082. Finasteride. [98319-26-7] (5α,17β)-N-(1,1-Dimethylethyl)-3-oxo-4-azaandrost-1-ene-17-carboxamide; 17β-(N-*tert*-butylcarbamoyl)-4-aza-5α-androst-1-en-3-one; MK-906; Chibro-Proscar; Finastid; Propecia; Proscar; Prostide. $C_{23}H_{36}N_2O_2$; mol wt 372.54. C 74.15%, H 9.74%, N 7.52%, O 8.59%. Inhibitor of 5α-reductase, the enzyme which converts testosterone to the more potent androgen, 5α-dihydrotestosterone. Prepn: G. H. Rasmusson, G. F. Reynolds, *EP 155096; eidem,* **US 4760071** (1985, 1988 both to Merck & Co.); G. H. Rasmusson *et al., J. Med. Chem.* **29,** 2298 (1986); A. Bhattacharya *et al., J. Am. Chem. Soc.* **110,** 3318 (1988). HPLC determn in plasma and urine: J. R. Carlin *et al., J. Chromatogr.* **427,** 79 (1988). Review of pharmacology and clinical uses: S. L. Sudduth, M. J. Koronkowski, *Pharmacotherapy* **13,** 309-329 (1993). Clinical trials in benign prostatic hyperplasia: J. L. Tenover *et al., Clin. Ther.* **19,** 243 (1997); J. D. McConnell *et al., N. Engl. J. Med.* **338,** 557 (1998); in male pattern hair loss: K. D. Kaufman *et al., J. Am. Acad. Dermatol.* **39,** 578 (1998).

White to off-white crystalline solid, mp ~257° (dried to anhydrous under N$_2$). Also reported as mp 252-254° (Rasmusson, 1988). $[\alpha]_{405}$ -59° (c = 1 in methanol). Freely sol in chloroform, DMSO, ethanol, methanol, *n*-propanol; sparingly sol in propylene glycol, polyethylene glycol 400; very slightly sol in 0.1N HCl, 0.1N NaOH, water.

THERAP CAT: Treatment of benign prostatic hypertrophy. Anti-alopecia agent.

4083. Fingolimod. [162359-55-9] 2-Amino-2-[2-(4-octyl-phenyl)ethyl]-1,3-propanediol. $C_{19}H_{33}NO_2$; mol wt 307.47. C 74.22%, H 10.82%, N 4.56%, O 10.41%. Immunomodulator evoking a reversible redistribution of lymphocytes from the circulation to secondary lymphatic tissue; synthetic analog of *myriocin (ISP-1)*, a fungal metabolite used in traditional Chinese herbal medicine. Prepn: T. Fujita *et al.*, **WO 9408943**; *eidem*, **US 5604229** (1994, 1997 both to Yoshitomi); K. Adachi *et al.*, *Bioorg. Med. Chem. Lett.* **5**, 853 (1995); M. Kiuchi *et al.*, *J. Med. Chem.* **43**, 2946 (2000). Efficient synthesis: P. Durand *et al.*, *Synthesis* **2000**, 505. Clinical pharmacokinetics: B. D. Kahan *et al.*, *Transplantation* **76**, 1079 (2003). Clinical evaluation in renal transplant: H. Tedesco-Silva *et al.*, *ibid.* **77**, 1826 (2004). Review of immunopharmacology: P. Troncoso, B. D. Kahan, *Clin. Biochem.* **31**, 369-373 (1998); of mechanism of action: V. Brinkmann, K. R. Lynch, *Curr. Opin. Immunol.* **14**, 569-575 (2002); and pharmacology: T. T. Aki, B. D. Kahan, *Exp. Opin. Biol. Ther.* **3**, 665-681 (2003); of development and therapeutic potential: F. J. Dumont, *IDrugs* **8**, 236-253 (2005).

Crystals from ethyl acetate, mp 103-105°.

Hydrochloride. [162359-56-0] FTY-720. $C_{19}H_{33}NO_2$.HCl; mol wt 343.93. Crystals from ethanol, mp 118-120°. Also reported as white solid from ethyl alcohol + ethyl acetate, mp 107-108° (Kiuchi). Sol in water, ethanol. LD_{50} orally in rats: 300-600 mg/kg (Troncoso).

THERAP CAT: Immunosuppressant.

4084. Fipexide. [34161-24-5] 1-(1,3-Benzodioxol-5-yl-methyl)-4-[(4-chlorophenoxy)acetyl]piperazine; 1-[(p-chlorophenoxy)acetyl]-4-piperonylpiperazine; 1-[2-(4-chlorophenoxy)acetyl]-4-(3,4-methylenedioxybenzyl)piperazine. $C_{20}H_{21}ClN_2O_4$; mol wt 388.84. C 61.78%, H 5.44%, Cl 9.12%, N 7.20%, O 16.46%. Prepn of hydrochloride: A. Buzas, R. Pierre, **FR M7524** (1970 to Lab Bouchard), *C.A.* **75**, 112865r (1971). Manufacturing process: G. P. Gardini *et al.*, **US 4225714** (1980 to Farmaceutici Geymon.). Improved prepn: G. P. Gardini *et al.*, *Synth. Commun.* **12**, 887 (1982). Determn by TLC: G. Musumarra *et al.*, *J. Chromatogr.* **350**, 151 (1985). Toxicology and pharmacology: G. David *et al.*, *Acta Ther.* **11**, 387 (1985). Clinical trial in the elderly: B. Bompani, G. Scali, *Curr. Med. Res. Opin.* **10**, 99 (1986).

Hydrochloride. [34161-23-4] BP-662; Attentil; Vigilor. $C_{20}H_{21}ClN_2O_4$.HCl; mol wt 425.31. Crystals from ethanol, mp 230-232°. LD_{50} in Swiss mice, Sprague-Dawley rats, Wistar rats (mg/kg): 4150, 4482, 7000 orally; 499, 537, 450 i.p. (David).

THERAP CAT: Nootropic.

4085. Fipronil. [120068-37-3] 5-Amino-1-[2,6-dichloro-4-(trifluoromethyl)phenyl]-4-[(trifluoromethyl)sulfinyl]-1H-pyrazole-3-carbonitrile; 5-amino-3-cyano-1-(2,6-dichloro-4-trifluoromethyl-phenyl)-4-trifluoromethylsulfinylpyrazole; (±)-5-amino-1-(2,6-di-chloro-α,α,α-trifluoro-p-tolyl)-4-trifluoromethylsulfinylpyrazole-3-carbonitrile; MB-46030; Frontline; Termidor. $C_{12}H_4Cl_2F_6N_4OS$; mol wt 437.15. C 32.97%, H 0.92%, Cl 16.22%, F 26.08%, N 12.82%, O 3.66%, S 7.34%. GABA-gated chloride channel blocker. Prototype of the phenylpyrazole insecticides known as *fiproles*. Prepn: I. G. Buntain *et al.*, **EP 295117** (1988 to May & Baker); L. R. Hatton *et al.*, **US 5232940** (1993). Mechanism of action study: L. M. Cole *et al.*, *Pestic. Biochem. Physiol.* **46**, 47

(1993). Comprehensive description: F. Colliot *et al.*, *Brighton Crop Prot. Conf. - Pests Dis.* **1992**, 29-34.

White solid, mp 200.5-201°. Vapor pressure (20°): 2.8×10^{-9} mm Hg. Log P (*n*-octanol/water): 4.0. Soly: water 2 mg/l; acetone >50%; corn oil >10,000 mg/l. LD_{50} in rats (mg/kg):100 orally; >2000 dermally (Colliot); in mice (mg/kg): 32 i.p. (Cole).

USE: Pesticide.

THERAP CAT (VET): Ectoparasiticide.

4086. Firefly Luciferin. [2591-17-5] (4S)-4,5-Dihydro-2-(6-hydroxy-2-benzothiazolyl)-4-thiazolecarboxylic acid; 2-(6-hy-droxybenzothiazol-2-yl)-2-thiazoline-4-carboxylic acid; D-(−)-lu-ciferin. $C_{11}H_8N_2O_3S_2$; mol wt 280.32. C 47.13%, H 2.88%, N 9.99%, O 17.12%, S 22.88%. Light emission in the American firefly, *Photinus pyralis,* has been shown to involve the interaction of magnesium ion, oxygen, ATP, the enzyme luciferase, and the oxidizable substrate luciferin. Isoln from fireflies (yield from 15,000 active fireflies about 9 mg): Bitler, McElroy, *Arch. Biochem. Biophys.* **72**, 358 (1957); from Japanese firefly *(Luciola cruciata)*: Kishi *et al.*, *Tetrahedron Lett.* **1968**, 2847. Structure and synthesis: E. H. White *et al.*, *J. Am. Chem. Soc.* **83**, 2402 (1961); **85**, 337 (1963); *J. Org. Chem.* **30**, 2344 (1965); S. Seto *et al.*, *Bull. Chem. Soc. Jpn.* **36**, 331 (1963). Configuration: G. E. Blank *et al.*, *Biochem. Biophys. Res. Commun.* **42**, 583 (1971). Measurement of ATP: D. M. Karl, O. Holm-Hansen, *Anal. Biochem.* **75**, 100 (1976). *Review:* L. J. Bowie, *Methods Enzymol.* **57**, 15 (1978).

Pale yellow needles from methanol, dec 189.5-190°. Recrystallizes with difficulty and sublimes with decomposition and decarboxylation. $[\alpha]_D^{22}$ −36° (c = 1.2 in DMF). uv max (H_2O): 268, 327 nm (log ε 3.88, 4.27). Slightly sol in water at pH 6.5. Sol in alkaline aq solns, methanol, acetone, ethyl acetate, DMF. Aqueous solns are sensitive to extremes in pH, esp. in presence of light and oxygen. Racemization occurs rapidly in some solvents. Should be stored for extended periods dry, under nitrogen atmosphere in light-tight containers.

USE: In the assay of ATP.

4087. Firocoxib. [189954-96-9] 3-(Cyclopropylmethoxy)-5,5-dimethyl-4-[4-(methylsulfonyl)phenyl]-2(5H)-furanone; ML-1785713; Previcox. $C_{17}H_{20}O_5S$; mol wt 336.40. C 60.70%, H 5.99%, O 23.78%, S 9.53%. Selective cyclooxygenase-2 (COX-2) inhibitor. Prepn: M. Belley *et al.*, **WO 9714691**; *eidem* **US 5981576** (1997, 1999 both to Merck Frosst). Pharmacokinetics and therapeutic efficacy in inflammatory synovitis in dogs: M. E. McCann *et al.*, *Am. J. Vet. Res.* **65**, 503 (2004).

THERAP CAT (VET): Anti-inflammatory; analgesic.

4088. Fisetin. [528-48-3] 2-(3,4-Dihydroxyphenyl)-3,7-di-hydroxy-4H-1-benzopyran-4-one; 3,3′,4′,7-tetrahydroxyflavone; 5-

desoxyquercetin; fisidenolon 1521; C.I. 75620; C.I. Natural Brown 1. $C_{15}H_{10}O_6$; mol wt 286.24. C 62.94%, H 3.52%, O 33.54%. Flavanoid present in the bark and stems of a variety of trees. Isolation from *Rhus cotinus* L. Anacardiaceae, Venetian Sumach: Chevreul, *Lecons Chim. Appl. a la Teint.* **2**, 169 (1833) [*cf.* J. Schmid, *Ber.* **19**, 1734 (1886)]; from heartwood of *Acacia* spp, *Leguminosae:* Roux *et al., Biochem. J.* **78**, 834 (1961). Structure: Seshadri, *Annu. Rev. Biochem.* **20**, 492 (1951). Synthesis: St. Kostanecki *et al., Ber.* **37**, 784 (1904); J. Allan, R. Robinson, *J. Chem. Soc.* **129**, 2334 (1926). Inhibition of aflatoxin cytotoxicity: A. G. Schwartz, W. R. Rate, *J. Environ. Pathol. Toxicol.* **2**, 1021 (1979). Mutagenicity studies: J. P. Brown *et al., Biochem. Soc. Trans.* **5**, 1489 (1977); *idem*, P. S. Dietrich, *Mutat. Res.* **66**, 223 (1979). TLC determn: D. Heimler, *J. Chromatogr.* **366**, 407 (1986).

Yellow needles from dil alc, dec 330°. uv max (ethanol): 252, 320, 360 nm (log $E^{1\%}_{1cm}$ 2.62, 2.51, 2.73). Sol in alcohol, acetone, acetic acid, solns of fixed alkali hydroxides. Practically insol in water, ether, benzene, chloroform and petr ether.

4089. FITC. [27072-45-3] (isomeric mixture); [3326-32-7] (5-isothiocyanate); [18861-78-4] (6-isothiocyanate). 3′,6′-Dihydroxy-5(or 6)-isothiocyanatospiro[isobenzofuran-1(3*H*),9′-[9*H*]-xanthen]-3-one; fluorescein isothiocyanate. $C_{21}H_{11}NO_5S$; mol wt 389.38. C 64.78%, H 2.85%, N 3.60%, O 20.54%, S 8.23%. Isomeric mixture of the 5- and 6-isothiocyanates; structural analog of the fluorochrome, fluorescein, *q.v.* Prepn: A. H. Coons *et al., J. Immunol.* **45**, 159 (1942); J. L. Riggs *et al., J. Am. Pathol.* **34**, 1081 (1958). Determn of purity of commerical product: R. M. McKinney *et al., Anal. Biochem.* **7**, 74 (1964); of properites and binding stoichiometry: A. Jobbágy, G. M. Jobbágy, *J. Immunol. Methods* **2**, 159, 169 (1972). Quantitative determn of bound FITC: H. G. de Bruin *et al., Vox Sang.* **45**, 373 (1983). Use as a pH probe: E. Lanz *et al., J. Fluorescence* **7**, 317 (1997); and evaluation of protonation kinetics: J. Widengren *et al., Chem. Phys.* **249**, 259 (1999). Immunofluorescent dye for microscopy: A. Entwistle, M. Noble, *J. Microsc.* **168**, 219 (1992). Label for amino acids: K. Muramoto *et al., Meth. Protein Seq. Anal.* **1993**, 29; F. Dang, Y. Chen, *Sci. China B* **42**, 663 (1999). Detection of anionic detergents: H.-W. Gao, D.-Y. Zhou, *Bull. Korean Chem. Soc.* **23**, 29 (2002).

Orange solid, dec upon heating.

USE: Fluorescent indicator and probe for biologic systems. Dye for sewage monitoring.

4090. Flavaspidic Acid. [114-42-1] 3,5-Dihydroxy-4,4-dimethyl-2-(1-oxobutyl)-6-[[2,4,6-trihydroxy-3-methyl-5-(1-oxobutyl)phenyl]methyl]-2,5-cyclohexadien-1-one; 3′-[(5-butyryl-2,4-dihydroxy-3,3-dimethyl-6-oxo-1,4-cyclohexadien-1-yl)methyl]-5′-methylphlorobutyrophenone; polystichocitrin; Toxifren. $C_{24}H_{30}$-O_8; mol wt 446.49. C 64.56%, H 6.77%, O 28.67%. Isolated from the rhizomes of male fern: Boehm, *Ann.* **318**, 253 (1901); **329**, 310 (1903). Structure and synthesis: McGookin *et al., J.*

Chem. Soc. **1953**, 1828; Riedl, *Ann.* **585**, 32 (1954); Aebi, *Helv. Chim. Acta* **39**, 153 (1956). Crystal structure of α- and β-forms: Erämetsä, Penttilä, *Acta Chem. Scand.* **24**, 3335 (1970). Toxicity study: Airaksinen *et al., Acta Pharmacol. Toxicol.* **25**, 33 (1967).

α-Form. Orthorhombic crystals from methanol or ethanol, mp 92°; solidifies again at 110° and melts again at 156°. LD_{50} orally in mice: 690 mg/kg (Airaksinen).

β-Form. Monoclinic crystals from benzene, xylene or acetic acid, mp 156°.

4091. Flavine-Adenine Dinucleotide. [146-14-5] Riboflavine 5′-(trihydrogen diphosphate) 5′ → 5′-ester with adenosine; adenosine 5′-(trihydrogen diphosphate) 5′ → 5′-ester with riboflavine; FAD; riboflavine 5′-adenosine diphosphate; isoalloxazine-adenine dinucleotide; Fademin; Flamitajin; Flanin F; Flavitan. $C_{27}H_{33}N_9$-$O_{15}P_2$; mol wt 785.55. C 41.28%, H 4.23%, N 16.05%, O 30.55%, P 7.89%. The prosthetic group of certain flavoproteins including D-amino acid oxidase, glucose oxidase, glycine oxidase, fumaric hydrogenase, histaminase, and xanthine oxidase. Isoln from yeast: Warburg *et al., Biochem. Z.* **297**, 417 (1938). Structure and isoln from liver, kidneys, hearts, muscles: Warburg, Christian, *ibid.* **298**, 150 (1938); isoln from the mycelium of *Eremothecium ashbyii:* Yagi, Tada, *Biochem. Prep.* **7**, 51 (1959); Masuda *et al.,* US 2973305 (1961 to Takeda). Synthesis: Christie *et al., J. Chem. Soc.* **1954**, 46; Huennekens, Kilgour, *J. Am. Chem. Soc.* **77**, 6716 (1955); DeLuca, Kaplan, *J. Biol. Chem.* **223**, 569 (1956); Moffatt, Khorana, *J. Am. Chem. Soc.* **80**, 3756 (1958). *Review:* A. Holmgren, *Experientia* **36** (Suppl), 149-180 (1980). Review of FAD and other flavin coenzymes: Beinert, *The Enzymes* vol. 2, P. D. Boyer *et al.,* Eds. (Academic Press, New York, 2nd ed., 1960) pp 339-416; *see also* vol. **XIII Part B** (Academic Press, New York, 3rd ed., 1975), several authors.

Barium salt. $C_{27}H_{31}BaN_9O_{15}P_2$. Small yellow spheres clustered like grapes. Absorption max: 366, 445 nm. The absorption curve is practically identical with that of riboflavine. There is some stronger absorption between 450 and 510 nm resulting in aq solns which are more reddish and less green than those of riboflavine. The appearance of a strong greenish fluorescence indicates decomposition and loss of catalytic activity.

4092. Flavone. [525-82-6] 2-Phenyl-4*H*-1-benzopyran-4-one; 2-phenylchromone; 2-phenyl-γ-benzopyrone; 2-phenyl-1,4-benzopyrone. $C_{15}H_{10}O_2$; mol wt 222.24. C 81.07%, H 4.54%, O 14.40%. Prepn: Feuerstein, Kostanecki, *Ber.* **31**, 1757 (1898);

Kostanecki, Tambor, *Ber.* **33**, 330 (1900); Kostanecki, Szabranski, *Ber.* **37**, 2634 (1904); Ruhemann, *Ber.* **46**, 2192 (1913); Bogert, Marcus, *J. Am. Chem. Soc.* **41**, 89 (1919). Isoln from *Primula malacoides*, Franch., *Primulaceae* and biological properties: Weller *et al., Antibiot. Chemother.* **3**, 603 (1953). Syntheses: Wheeler, *Org. Synth.* **coll. vol. IV**, 478 (1963); Y. Ashihara *et al., Bull. Chem. Soc. Jpn.* **50**, 3298 (1977); A. Banerji, N. C. Goomer, *Synthesis* **1980**, 874.

Crystals from petr ether, mp 99-100°. Practically insol in water. Sol in most organic solvents. Absorption max: 350, 405 nm.

4093. Flavopereirine. [486-18-0] 3-Ethyl-12*H*-indolo[2,3-a]quinolizin-5-ium inner salt; melinonine G. $C_{17}H_{14}N_2$; mol wt 246.31. C 82.90%, H 5.73%, N 11.37%. From *Strychnos melinoniana* Baillon., *Loganiaceae*: Bächli *et al., Helv. Chim. Acta* **40**, 1167 (1957); from *Geissospermum vellosii* Baillon., *Apocynaceae*: Rapoport *et al., J. Am. Chem. Soc.* **80**, 1601 (1958). Bertho *et al., Ber.* **91**, 2581 (1958). Structure: Bejar *et al., Compt. Rend.* **244**, 2066 (1957). Synthesis: Le Hir *et al., Bull. Soc. Chim. Fr.* **1958**, 551; Prasad, Swan, *J. Chem. Soc.* **1958**, 2024; G. W. Gribble, D. A. Johnson, *Tetrahedron Lett.* **28**, 5259 (1987); of perchlorate: J. Ninomiyo *et al., Heterocycles* **9**, 1527 (1978).

Orange crystals from acetone, mp 233-235°. uv max (ethanol): 230, 238, 248, 294, 351, 390 nm (log ε 4.40, 4.43, 4.39, 4.14, 4.25, 4.14).
Perchlorate. $C_{17}H_{15}ClN_2O_4$. Crystals from methanol, mp 307-308°. uv max (0.015*N* HCl-ethanol): 238, 294, 350, 389 nm (log ε 4.57, 4.22, 4.31, 4.21).

4094. Flavopiridol. [146426-40-6] *rel*-(−)-2-(2-Chlorophenyl)-5,7-dihydroxy-8-[(3*R*,4*S*)-3-hydroxy-1-methyl-4-piperidinyl]-4*H*-1-benzopyran-4-one; *cis*-(−)-2-(2-chlorophenyl)-5,7-dihydroxy-8-[4′-(3′-hydroxy-1′-methyl)-piperidinyl]-4H-1-benzopyran-4-one. $C_{21}H_{20}ClNO_5$; mol wt 401.84. C 62.77%, H 5.02%, Cl 8.82%, N 3.49%, O 19.91%. Flavone inhibitor of cyclin-dependent kinases; the (−)-cis form induces apoptosis in certain tumor cells. Prepn: S. L. Kattige *et al., EP 241003; eidem, US 4900727* (1987, 1990 both to Hoechst). Properties and formulation study: R.-M. Dannenfelser *et al., PDA J. Pharm. Sci. Technol.* **50**, 356 (1996). Mode of action study: S. Brüsselbach *et al., Int. J. Cancer* **77**, 146 (1998). Clinical evaluation in refractory cancers: A. M. Senderowicz *et al., J. Clin. Oncol.* **16**, 2986 (1998). Clinical pharmacokinetics: J. P. Thomas *et al., Cancer Chemother. Pharmacol.* **50**, 465 (2002). Review of chemistry, pharmacology, and antitumor spectrum: H. H. Sedlacek *et al., Int. J. Oncol.* **9**, 1143-1168 (1996).

Hydrochloride. [131740-09-5] L-86-8275; HMR-1275; NSC-649890. $C_{21}H_{20}ClNO_5 \cdot HCl$; mol wt 438.30. mp 169.5 ± 0.5° (Dannenfelser). Also reported as yellow powder, mp 188° containing 4.73-6.2% water of crystallization (Sedlacek). pKa 5.68 ± 0.06. $[\alpha]_D^{24}$ −1.73 to −3.9°. Soly (mg/ml): water, D5W, and normal saline all <5 at pH 4. Soly (mg/ml): ethanol 10.1; PEG 400 >73.8; propylene glycol >88.1; M-pyrol very much greater than 103.0; τ-butyrolactone very much greater than 105.5.
THERAP CAT: Antineoplastic.

4095. Flavoxanthin. [512-29-8] (3*S*,3′*R*,5*R*,6′*R*,8*R*)-5,8-Epoxy-5,8-dihydro-β,ε-carotene-3,3′-diol. $C_{40}H_{56}O_3$; mol wt 584.87. C 82.14%, H 9.65%, O 8.21%. Carotenoid pigment; stereoisomer of chrysanthemaxanthin, *q.v.* Often found in plants, but in minute amounts only and never as a principal pigment. Isoln from *Ranunculus acris* L., *Ranunculaceae*: Kuhn, Brockmann, *Z. Physiol. Chem.* **213**, 192 (1932). Structure: Karrer, Rutschmann, *Helv. Chim. Acta* **25**, 1144 (1942). Partial synthesis: Karrer, Jucker, *ibid.* **28**, 300 (1945). Absolute configuration: H. Cadosch *et al., ibid.* **61**, 783 (1978).

Golden-yellow aggregates of prisms, mp 184°. Absorption max (chloroform): 430, 459 nm. $[\alpha]_{Cd}^{20}$ +190° (c = 0.04 in benzene). Freely sol in chloroform, benzene, acetone; less sol in methanol, ethanol. Almost insol in petr ether.

4096. Flavoxate. [15301-69-6] 3-Methyl-4-oxo-2-phenyl-4*H*-1-benzopyran-8-carboxylic acid 2-(1-piperidinyl)ethyl ester; 3-methylflavone-8-carboxylic acid β-piperidinoethyl ester; 2-piperidinoethyl 3-methyl-4-oxo-2-phenyl-4*H*-1-benzopyran-8-carboxylate; 2-piperidinoethyl 3-methylflavone-8-carboxylate. $C_{24}H_{25}NO_4$; mol wt 391.46. C 73.64%, H 6.44%, N 3.58%, O 16.35%. Smooth muscle relaxant. Prepn of the hydrochloride: P. Da Re *et al., J. Med. Pharm. Chem.* **2**, 263 (1960); P. Da Re, *US 2921070* and *US 3350411* (1960 to Recordati and 1967 to Seceph). Pharmacological studies: I. Setnikar *et al., J. Pharmacol. Exp. Ther.* **130**, 356 (1960). Mechanism of action: P. Cazzulani *et al., Arch. Int. Pharmacodyn.* **274**, 189 (1985). Pharmacokinetics in rats: I. Setnikar *et al., Arzneim.-Forsch.* **25**, 1916 (1975); in man: M. Bertoli *et al., Pharmacol. Res. Commun.* **8**, 417 (1976). *In vivo* activity: C. Pietra, P. Cazzulani, *Farmaco Ed. Prat.* **41**, 267 (1986). Determn in tissues: A. Cova, I. Setnikar, *Arzneim.-Forsch.* **25**, 1707 (1975). Clinical evaluations: D. V. Bradley, R. J. Cazort, *J. Clin. Pharmacol.* **10**, 65 (1970); A. Zanollo, F. Catanzaro, *Urol. Int.* **35**, 176 (1980). Clinical comparison with phenazopyridine: S. Gould, *Urology* **5**, 612 (1975). Short review: R. Ruffmann, A. Sartini, *Drugs Exp. Clin. Res.* **13**, 57 (1987).

Crystals, pK 7.3. Soly in water at 37°: 0.001% (w/v). Sol in ethanol and chloroform. LD$_{50}$ in rats (mg/kg): 1110 orally; 20.8 i.v. (Setnikar, 1975).
Hydrochloride. [3717-88-2] DW-61; Rec-7-0040; Bladderon; Genurin; Patricin; Spasuret; Urispas. $C_{24}H_{25}NO_4 \cdot HCl$; mol wt 427.92. Crystals from ethanol + ether, mp 232-234°. LD$_{50}$ i.v. in rats: 27.4 mg/kg (Cazzulani).
Succinate. [28782-19-6] $C_{24}H_{25}NO_4 \cdot C_4H_6O_4$. Soly in water at 37°: 33.7% (w/v).
THERAP CAT: Antispasmodic; in treatment of urinary incontinence.

4097. Flazasulfuron. [104040-78-0] *N*-[[(4,6-Dimethoxy-2-pyrimidinyl)amino]carbonyl]-3-(trifluoromethyl)-2-pyridinesulfonamide; 1-(4,6-dimethoxypyrimidin-2-yl)-3-(3-trifluoromethyl-2-

pyridylsulfonyl)urea; OK-1166; SL-160; Katana; Shibagen. C_{13}-$H_{12}F_3N_5O_5S$; mol wt 407.33. C 38.33%, H 2.97%, F 13.99%, N 17.19%, O 19.64%, S 7.87%. Sulfonylurea herbicide. Prepn: F. Kimura *et al.*, **EP 184385**; *eidem*, **US 4744814** (1986, 1988 both to Ishihara Sangyo Kaisha); T. Haga *et al.*, *ACS Symp. Ser.* **443**, 107 (1991). Description of properties and biological activity: B. Hashizume, *Jpn. Pestic. Inf.* **57**, 27 (1990). Field trial for control of ragwort: T. K. James *et al.*, *Proc. 50th N. Z. Plant Prot. Conf.* **1997**, 447. Weed control management in grapevines: P. Bourdrez, J.-M. Béraud, *Phytoma* **521**, 66 (1999).

Odorless, white crystalline solid, mp 164-166°. Soly at 20° (w/w%): acetone 1.2%; toluene 0.06%; at 25° (w/v%): acetic acid 0.67%. Soly in water: 4.1 ppm (pH 1). Vapor pressure: 3.1×10^{-8} mm Hg. pKa (24°): 4.6. Log P (octanol/water): 1.08.LD_{50} mice, rats (mg/kg): >5000, >5000 orally; in rats (mg/kg): >2000 dermally (Hashizume).

USE: Herbicide.

4098. Flecainide. [54143-55-4] *N*-(2-Piperidinylmethyl)-2,5-bis(2,2,2-trifluoroethoxy)benzamide. $C_{17}H_{20}F_6N_2O_3$; mol wt 414.34. C 49.28%, H 4.87%, F 27.51%, N 6.76%, O 11.58%. Prepn: E. H. Banitt, W. R. Brown, **US 3900481** (1975 to Riker); of the acetate: *eidem*, **US 4005209** (1977 to Riker); E. H. Banitt *et al.*, *J. Med. Chem.* **20**, 821 (1977). Preliminary pharmacological study: J. R. Schmid *et al.*, *Fed. Proc.* **34**, 775 (1975). *In vitro* electrophysiological study: A. B. Hodess *et al.*, *J. Cardiovasc. Pharmacol.* **1**, 427 (1979). Antiarrhythmic effects: P. Somani, *Clin. Pharmacol. Ther.* **27**, 464 (1980). Use in acute exptl myocardial infarction: H. Gülker *et al.*, *Z. Cardiol.* **70**, 124 (1981). Clinical study in ventricular arrhythmias: J. L. Anderson *et al.*, *N. Engl. J. Med.* **305**, 473 (1981). Determn of acetate in human plasma by spectrophotofluorometry: S. F. Chang *et al.*, *Arzneim.-Forsch.* **33**, 251 (1983). Review of pharmacology and clinical efficacy: D. M. Roden, R. L. Woosley, *N. Engl. J. Med.* **315**, 36-41 (1986). Symposium on clinical experience: *Am. J. Cardiol.* **62**, Suppl., 1D-67D (1988). Comprehensive description: S. Alessi-Severini *et al.*, *Anal. Profiles Drug Subs. Excip.* **21**, 169-195 (1992).

uv max (ethanol): 205, 230, 300 nm ($E_{1cm}^{1\%}$ 521, 219, 59).

Monoacetate. [54143-56-5] R-818; Almarytm; Apocard; Ecrinal; Flécaine; Tambocor. $C_{17}H_{20}F_6N_2O_3 \cdot C_2H_4O_2$; mol wt 474.39. White granular solid from isopropyl alcohol/isopropyl ether, mp 145-147°. Soly at 37° (mg/ml): water 48.4, alcohol 300.

THERAP CAT: Antiarrhythmic (class IC).

4099. Fleroxacin. [79660-72-3] 6,8-Difluoro-1-(2-fluoroethyl)-1,4-dihydro-7-(4-methyl-1-piperazinyl)-4-oxo-3-quinolinecarboxylic acid; AM-833; Ro-23-6240; Megalocin; Megalone; Quinodis. $C_{17}H_{18}F_3N_3O_3$; mol wt 369.34. C 55.28%, H 4.91%, F 15.43%, N 11.38%, O 13.00%. Prepn: **BE 887574**; T. Irikura *et al.*, **US 4398029** (1981, 1983 both to Kyorin). Antibacterial spectrum *in vitro* and *in vivo*: K. Hirai *et al.*, *Antimicrob. Agents Chemother.* **29**, 1059 (1986). *In vitro* activity vs anaerobic bacteria: J. Wüst, U. Hardegger, *Eur. J. Clin. Microbiol.* **6**, 688 (1987). HPLC determn in biological fluids: H. Kusajima *et al.*, *J. Chromatogr.* **381**, 137 (1986). Pharmacokinetics and bioavailability: E. Weidekamm *et al.*, *Antimicrob. Agents Chemother.* **31**, 1909 (1987). Preliminary clinical evaluation in gonorrhea: J. B. J. Boerema *et al.*, *J. Antimicrob. Chemother.* **21**, 140 (1988).

Hydrochloride. $C_{17}H_{18}F_3N_3O_3 \cdot HCl$. Crystals from water, mp 269-271° (dec).

THERAP CAT: Antibacterial.

4100. Flesinoxan. [98206-10-1] *N*-[2-[4-[(2*R*)-2,3-Dihydro-2-(hydroxymethyl)-1,4-benzodioxin-5-yl]-1-piperazinyl]ethyl]-4-fluorobenzamide; (+)-(*S*)-*p*-fluoro-*N*-[2-[4-[2-(hydroxymethyl)-1,4-benzodioxan-5-yl]-1-piperazinyl]ethyl]benzamide. $C_{22}H_{26}$-FN_3O_4; mol wt 415.46. C 63.60%, H 6.31%, F 4.57%, N 10.11%, O 15.40%. Serotonin (5-HT_{1A})-receptor agonist; phenylpiperazine derivative. Prepn: J. Hartog *et al.*, **EP 138280**; *eidem*, **US 4833142** (1985, 1989 both to Duphar). Synthesis and resolution of enantiomers: M. D. Ennis, N. B. Ghazal, *Tetrahedron Lett.* **33**, 6287 (1992). GC determn in plasma and urine: M. P. van Berkel *et al.*, *Methodol. Surv. Biochem. Anal.* **18**, 209 (1988). Pharmacology: J. Schipper *et al.*, *Hum. Psychopharmacol.* **6**, S53 (1991). Clinical evaluation in depression: P. Grof *et al.*, *Int. Clin. Psychopharmacol.* **8**, 167 (1993).

$[\alpha]_D$ +26° (c = 1 in methanol).

Hydrochloride. [98205-89-1] DU-29373. $C_{22}H_{26}FN_3O_4 \cdot$HCl; mol wt 451.92. mp 184.5-185.5°. Also reported as crystals from ethanol/ether, mp 183.0-184.0° (Ennis). $[\alpha]_D$ +25° (c = 1 in methanol). Freely sol in water; sparingly sol in ethanol.

THERAP CAT: Anxiolytic.

4101. Flindersine. [523-64-8] 2,6-Dihydro-2,2-dimethyl-5*H*-pyrano[3,2-*c*]quinolin-5-one; 2,2'-dimethyl-α-pyrano(5',6',3,4)-2(1*H*)-quinolone. $C_{14}H_{13}NO_2$; mol wt 227.26. C 73.99%, H 5.77%, N 6.16%, O 14.08%. From wood of *Flindersia australis* R. Br., *Rutaceae*: Matthes, Schreiber, *Ber. Dtsch. Pharm. Ges.* **24**, 385 (1914). Structure: Brown *et al.*, *Aust. J. Chem.* **7**, 348 (1954). Synthesis: *eidem, ibid.* **9**, 277 (1956); Piozzi *et al.*, *Gazz. Chim. Ital.* **99**, 711 (1969); Bowman *et al.*, *Chem. Commun.* **1970**, 666; Huffman, Hsu, *Tetrahedron Lett.* **1972**, 141.

Crystals from methanol, dec 185-186°. uv max (methanol): 235, 333, 350, 365 nm (log ε 4.42, 4.00, 4.10, 3.93). Sol in alc, benzene, chloroform, glacial acetic acid, paraffin, fatty oils, alkali hydroxides, slightly sol in petr ether. Practically insol in water.

N-Methylflindersine. $C_{15}H_{15}NO_2$. Crystals from petr ether, mp 84°.

Dihydroflindersine. $C_{14}H_{15}NO_2$. Hexagons from ethyl acetate, mp 229°. uv max (methanol): 225, 272, 283, 312 nm (log ε 4.44, 3.94, 3.96, 3.93).

4102. Flocoumafen. [90035-08-8] 4-Hydroxy-3-[1,2,3,4-tetrahydro-3-[4-[[4-(trifluoromethyl)phenyl]methoxy]phenyl]-1-naphthalenyl]-2*H*-1-benzopyran-2-one; 4-hydroxy-3-[1,2,3,4-tetrahydro-3-[4-(4-trifluoromethylbenzyloxy)phenyl]-1-naphthyl]; WL-

108366; Storm. $C_{33}H_{25}F_3O_4$; mol wt 542.54. C 73.06%, H 4.64%, F 10.51%, O 11.80%. Second generation anticoagulant rodenticide. Prepn: I. D. Entwistle, P. Boehm, **EP 98629**; *eidem,* **US 4520007** (1983, 1985 both to Shell). Synthesis and separation of isomers: O. S. Park, B. S. Jang, *Arch. Pharmacal Res.* **18,** 277 (1995). HPLC determn in liver tissue: A. Jones, *Bull. Environ. Contam. Toxicol.* **56,** 8 (1996). Absorption and distribution in rats: K. R. Huckle *et al., Pestic. Sci.* **25,** 297 (1989). Efficacy against seven rodent species: J. E. Gill, *Int. Biodeterior. Biodegrad.* **30,** 65 (1992). Review of physical properties, mode of action, and field trials: D. J. Bowler *et al., Proc. Br. Crop Prot. Conf. - Pests Dis.* **1984,** 397.

White powder. Soly in water: 1.1 mg/l. Soly in acetone, alcohol, chloroform, dichloromethane: >10 g/l. Vapor pressure at 25°: approx 1×10^{-13} mm Hg. LD$_{50}$ in rats, mice, rabbits (mg/kg): 0.25, 0.8, 0.2 orally (Bowler).

USE: Rodenticide.

4103. Floctafenine. [23779-99-9] 2-[[8-(Trifluoromethyl)-4-quinolinyl]amino]benzoic acid 2,3-dihydroxypropyl ester; *N*-[8-(trifluoromethyl)-4-quinolyl]anthranilic acid 2,3-dihydroxypropyl ester; 4-[*o*-(2′,3′-dihydroxypropyloxycarbonyl)phenyl]amino-8-trifluoromethylquinoline; 8-trifluoromethyl-7-deschloroglafenine; R-4318; RU-15750; Idalon; Idarac; Novodolan. $C_{20}H_{17}F_3N_2O_4$; mol wt 406.36. C 59.11%, H 4.22%, F 14.03%, N 6.89%, O 15.75%. Prepn: A. Allais, J. Meier, **DE 1815467**; *eidem,* **US 3644368** (1969, 1972, both to Roussel-UCLAF); G. Mouzin *et al., Synthesis* **1980,** 54. Analgesic activity: Allais *et al., Chim. Ther.* **8,** 154 (1973); M. Peterfalvi *et al., Arch. Int. Pharmacodyn. Ther.* **216,** 97 (1975). Clinical investigation: Stenport, *Curr. Ther. Res.* **18,** 303 (1975). Toxicology: R. Glomot *et al., Toxicol. Appl. Pharmacol.* **36,** 173 (1976). Metabolism: R. K. Lynn *et al., J. Clin. Pharmacol.* **19,** 20 (1979).

Crystals from methanol, mp 179-180°. Sol in alcohol, acetone; very slightly sol in ether, chloroform, methylene chloride. Insol in water. LD$_{50}$ in male mice, rats (mg/kg): 3400, 960 orally; 180, 160 i.v. (Glomot).

THERAP CAT: Analgesic.

4104. Flomoxef. [99665-00-6] (6*R-cis*)-7-[[[(Difluoromethyl)thio]acetyl]amino]-3-[[[1-(2-hydroxyethyl)-1*H*-tetrazol-5-yl]thio]methyl]-7-methoxy-8-oxo-5-oxa-1-azabicyclo[4.2.0]oct-2-ene-2-carboxylic acid; 7-β-difluoromethylthioacetamido-7α-methoxy-3-[[1-(2-hydroxyethyl)-1*H*-tetrazol-5-yl]thiomethyl]-1-oxa-3-cephem-4-carboxylic acid. $C_{15}H_{18}F_2N_6O_7S_2$; mol wt 496.47. C 36.29%, H 3.65%, F 7.65%, N 16.93%, O 22.56%, S 12.92%. Semi-synthetic oxacephalosporin antibiotic. Prepn: T. Tsuji *et al., BE 898541; eidem,* **US 4532233** (1984, 1985 both to Shionogi); *eidem, J. Antibiot.* **38,** 466 (1985). *In vitro* activity and β-lactamase stability: H. C. Neu, N.-X. Chin, *Antimicrob. Agents Chemother.* **30,** 638 (1986).

Crystals from acetone + methylene chloride, mp 82.5-87.5°.
Sodium salt. [92823-03-5] 6315-S; Flumarin. $C_{15}H_{17}F_2N_6$-NaO$_7$S$_2$; mol wt 518.45.

THERAP CAT: Antibacterial.

4105. Flonicamid. [158062-67-0] *N*-(Cyanomethyl)-4-(trifluoromethyl)-3-pyridinecarboxamide; *N*-(cyanomethyl)-4-(trifluoromethyl)nicotinamide; F-1785; IKI-220; Aria; Urara. $C_9H_6F_3N_3$-O; mol wt 229.16. C 47.17%, H 2.64%, F 24.87%, N 18.34%, O 6.98%. Selective systemic aphicide. Prepn: T. Toki *et al.,* **EP 580374;** *eidem,* **US 5360806** (both 1994 to Ishihara Sangyo Kaisha). Comprehensive description: M. Morita *et al., BCPC Conf. - Pests Dis.* **2000,** 59-65. Field performance in cotton: H. G. Hancock, *Proc. Beltwide Cotton Conf.* **2004,** 1629.

Odorless, white crystalline powder, mp 157.5°. Vapor pressure (20°): 9.43×10^{-7} Pa. Log P (octanol/water): 0.30. Soly in water (20°): 5.2 g/l. LD$_{50}$ in male, female rats (mg/kg): 884, 1768 orally; in rats (mg/kg): >5000 dermally; in rats (mg/m^3): >4900 by inhalation. LC$_{50}$ in carp, rainbow trout (mg/l): >100, >91.9 (Morita).

USE: Insecticide.

4106. Flopropione. [2295-58-1] 1-(2,4,6-Trihydroxyphenyl)-1-propanone; 2′,4′,6-trihydroxypropiophenone; phloropropiophenone; RP-13907; Argobyl; Cospanon; Flopion; Gallepronin; Gasstenon; Labroda; Labrodax; Pasmus; Profenon; Spamorin; Spasmoril; Supanate; Supazlun. $C_9H_{10}O_4$; mol wt 182.17. C 59.34%, H 5.53%, O 35.13%. Prepn: Shinoda, *J. Pharm. Soc. Jpn.* **1927,** 111; Canter *et al., J. Chem. Soc.* **1931,** 1245; Howells, Little, *J. Am. Chem. Soc.* **54,** 2451 (1932).

Monohydrate. Needles from water. Anhydr compd, mp 175-176°. Sol in ethanol, ether, ethyl acetate, hot water; very slightly sol in cold water.

THERAP CAT: Antispasmodic.

4107. Florantyrone. [519-95-9] γ-Oxo-8-fluoranthenebutanoic acid; β-(8-fluoranthoyl)propionic acid; Zanchol. $C_{20}H_{14}O_3$; mol wt 302.32. C 79.46%, H 4.67%, O 15.88%. Prepn: R. R. Burtner, **US 2773091** (1956 to Searle). *See also:* O. E. Fancher, **US 2560425** (1951 to Miles Labs).

Lemon yellow crystals from acetic acid, mp ~208°. Soluble in methanol, ethanol, aq solns of sodium carbonate.

THERAP CAT: Choleretic.

4108. Florasulam. [145701-23-1] *N*-(2,6-Difluorophenyl)-8-fluoro-5-methoxy-[1,2,4]triazolo[1,5-*c*]pyrimidine-2-sulfonamide; 2′,6′,8-trifluoro-5-methoxy-*s*-triazolo[1,5-*c*]pyrimidine-2-sulfonanilide; Boxer; Nikos; Primus. $C_{12}H_8F_3N_5O_3S$; mol wt 359.28. C 40.12%, H 2.24%, F 15.86%, N 19.49%, O 13.36%, S 8.92%. Triazolopyrimidine herbicide for use in cereals. Acetolactate synthase (ALS) inhibitor. Prepn: J. C. Van Heertum *et al.*, **WO 8911782** (1989 to Dow); *eidem*, **US 5163995** (1992 to Dow-Elanco). Comprehensive description: A. R. Thompson *et al.*, *Brighton Crop Prot. Conf. - Weeds* **1999**, 73-80. Review of field trials: A. D. Bailey *et al., ibid.* 205-209. Photolytic degradation in soil and water: M. S. Krieger *et al., J. Agric. Food Chem.* **48**, 3710 (2000).

mp 220-221° (dec) (Van Heertum); also reported as 193.5-230.5° (Thompson). pKa: 4.54. Partition coefficient (octanol/water): 0.06G (pH 7.0). Vapor pressure (25°): 1×10^{-5} Pa. Soly in water (20°): 6.36 g/l (pH 7.0). LD_{50} in rat, quail (mg/kg): >6000, 1046 orally; percutaneously in rabbit: >2000 mg/kg. LC_{50} in rainbow trout, bluegill (96 hr): >96, >98 mg/l (Thompson).

USE: Herbicide.

4109. Florfenicol. [73231-34-2] 2,2-Dichloro-*N*-[(1*S*,2*R*)-1-(fluoromethyl)-2-hydroxy-2-[4-(methylsulfonyl)phenyl]ethyl]-acetamide; D-*(threo)*-1-*p*-methylsulfonylphenyl-2-amino-3-fluoro-1-propanol; fluorothiamphenicol; Sch-25298; Aquafen; Aquaflor; Florocol; Nuflor. $C_{12}H_{14}Cl_2FNO_4S$; mol wt 358.21. C 40.24%, H 3.94%, Cl 19.79%, F 5.30%, N 3.91%, O 17.87%, S 8.95%. Fluorinated derivative of thiamphenicol, *q.v.* Inhibits bacterial protein synthesis by binding to ribosome 50S and 70S subunits. Prepn: T. Nagabhushan, **EP 14437**; **US 4235692** (both 1980 to Schering); D. P. Schumacher *et al., J. Org. Chem.* **55**, 5291 (1990). Improved prepn: G. Wu *et al., ibid.* **62**, 2996 (1997). HPLC determn in fish plasma: C. Vue *et al., J. Chromatogr. B* **780**, 111 (2002). *In vitro* antibacterial activity: H. C. Neu, K. P. Fu, *Antimicrob. Agents Chemother.* **18**, 311 (1980); V. P. Syriopoulou *et al., ibid.* **19**, 294 (1981); vs bovine and porcine respiratory disease isolates: S. J. Shin *et al., Vet. Microbiol.* **106**, 73 (2005). Pharmacokinetics in veal calves: K. J. Varma *et al., J. Vet. Pharmacol. Ther.* **9**, 412 (1986); in sheep: J. Shen *et al., ibid.* **27**, 163 (2004). Therapeutic effect on pseudotuberculosis in yellowtail tuna: N. Yasunaga, S. Yasumoto, *Fish Pathol.* **23**, 1 (1988).

Crystals from 2-propanol/H_2O, mp 152-154°. $[\alpha]^{26}$ +17.9° (DMF). Sol in water.

THERAP CAT (VET): Antibacterial.

4110. Flosequinan. [76568-02-0] 7-Fluoro-1-methyl-3-(methylsulfinyl)-4(1*H*)-quinolinone; flosequinon; BTS-49465; Manoplax. $C_{11}H_{10}FNO_2S$; mol wt 239.27. C 55.22%, H 4.21%, F 7.94%, N 5.85%, O 13.37%, S 13.40%. Mixed arterial and venous vasodilator. Prepn: R. V. Davies *et al.*, **DE 3011994**; *eidem*, **US 4302460** (1980, 1981 both to Boots). Pharmacology: J. G. Smith, G. T. Kinasewitz, *J. Cardiovasc. Pharmacol.* **8**, 878 (1986); M. F. Sim *et al., Br. J. Pharmacol.* **94**, 371 (1988). HPLC determn in plasma, serum and urine: M. B. Slegowski *et al., J.*

Chromatogr. **425**, 227 (1988). Pharmacokinetics and hemodynamics in humans: A. J. Cowley *et al., J. Hypertens.* **2**, Suppl. 3, 547 (1984); R. D. Wynne *et al., Eur. J. Clin. Pharmacol.* **28**, 659 (1985). Preliminary evaluation in hypertension: A. J. Cowley *et al., ibid.* **33**, 203 (1987); in congestive heart failure: P. D. Kessler, M. Packer, *Am. Heart J.* **113**, 137 (1987); P. D. Kessler *et al., J. Cardiovasc. Pharmacol.* **12**, 6 (1988). Clinical study in chronic heart failure: A. J. Cowley *et al., Br. Med. J.* **297**, 169 (1988).

Crystals, mp 226-228°.

THERAP CAT: Antihypertensive.

4111. Floxacillin. [5250-39-5] (2*S*,5*R*,6*R*)-6-[[[3-(2-Chloro-6-fluorophenyl)-5-methyl-4-isoxazolyl]carbonyl]amino]-3,3-dimethyl-7-oxo-4-thia-1-azabicyclo[3.2.0]heptane-2-carboxylic acid; 3-(2-chloro-6-fluorophenyl)-5-methyl-4-isoxazolylpenicillin; 6-[3-(2-chloro-6-fluorophenyl)-5-methyl-4-isoxazolecarboxamido]-penicillanic acid; flucloxacillin; BRL-2039. $C_{19}H_{17}ClFN_3O_5S$; mol wt 453.87. C 50.28%, H 3.78%, Cl 7.81%, F 4.19%, N 9.26%, O 17.63%, S 7.06%. Semi-synthetic antibiotic active against penicillin-resistant staphylococci. Halogen-substituted derivative of oxacillin, *q.v.* Prepn: **ZA 6304323** (1964 to Beecham); Nayler, **GB 978299**; *idem*, **US 3239507** (1964, 1966 both to Beecham). Pharmacology and toxicity: R. Sutherland *et al., Br. Med. J.* **4**, 460 (1970). Clinical studies: Harding *et al., Clin. Trials J.* **7**, 368 (1970); Qureshi *et al., ibid.* 375.

Sodium monohydrate. [34214-51-2] Abboflox; Culpen; Floxapen; Ladropen; Stafoxil; Staphlipen; Staphylex. $C_{19}H_{16}ClFN_3$-$NaO_5S.H_2O$; mol wt 493.87. Freely sol in water. LD_{50} in mice (g/kg): 2.2 s.c., 3.8 orally (Sutherland).

THERAP CAT: Antibacterial.

4112. Floxuridine. [50-91-9] 2′-Deoxy-5-fluorouridine; 1-(2-deoxy-β-D-ribofuranosyl)-5-fluorouracil; 5-fluoro-2′-deoxy-β-uridine; NSC-27640; FUDR. $C_9H_{11}FN_2O_5$; mol wt 246.19. C 43.91%, H 4.50%, F 7.72%, N 11.38%, O 32.49%. Prepn: Hoffer *et al., J. Am. Chem. Soc.* **81**, 4112 (1959); Heidelberger, Duschinsky, **US 2885396** (1959); Duschinsky *et al.*, **US 2970139** (1961); Hoffer, **US 2949451**; **US 3041335** (1960, 1962 both to Hoffmann-La Roche). Structure: Lemieux, Hoffer, *Can. J. Chem.* **39**, 110 (1961). Crystal and molecular structure: Harris, *Diss. Abstr.* **24**, 4425 (1964); Harris, McIntyre, *Biophys. J.* **4**, 203 (1964). Conformation of furanose ring in molecule: Sundaralingam, *J. Am. Chem. Soc.* **87**, 599 (1965).

Crystals from butyl acetate, mp 150-151° (Hoffer, 1959); also reported as mp 145° (**US 3041335**). $[\alpha]_D$ +37° (water), +48.6°

Consult the Name Index before using this section.

(DMF). uv max (pH 7.2): 268 nm (ε 7570); (pH 14): 270 nm (ε 6480).

α-Anomer. 1-(2-Deoxy-α-D-*erythro*-pentofuranosyl)-5-fluorouracil. Crystals from butyl acetate, mp 150-151°. $[\alpha]_D^{25}$ −21° (c = 2 in water).

THERAP CAT: Antiviral; antineoplastic.

4113. Fluacizine. [30223-48-4] 10-[3-(Diethylamino)-1-oxopropyl]-2-(trifluoromethyl)-10*H*-phenothiazine; 10-(*N*,*N*-diethyl-β-alanyl)-2-(trifluoromethyl)phenothiazine; fluoracisine; fluoracizine; ftoracizine; Phtorazisin. $C_{20}H_{21}F_3N_2OS$; mol wt 394.45. C 60.90%, H 5.37%, F 14.45%, N 7.10%, O 4.06%, S 8.13%. Phenothiazine derivative with psychotropic activity. Prepn: Y. I. Vikhlyaev *et al.,* **SU 360342** (1972), *C.A.* **78,** 97683w (1973); of hydrochloride: S. V. Zhuravlev *et al.,* **GB 1191800** (1970), *C.A.* **73,** 25493h (1970); Y. I. Vikhlyaev *et al.,* **FR 2035748** (1971), *C.A.* **75,** 140872j (1971); *eidem,* **DE 1805659** (1979), *C.A.* **75,** 49101w (1971). Use as antidepressant: *eidem,* **SU 356992** (1972), *C.A.* **78,** 75888q (1973) (all to Inst. Pharmacol. Chemother., Acad. Med. Sci., USSR). Mass spectrum: S. Morosawa *et al., Org. Mass Spectrom.* **17,** 309 (1982). Effect on drug metabolism: V. Avakumov *et al., Biochem. Pharmacol.* **27,** 2177 (1978). Pharmacokinetics in animals, man: V. P. Zherdev *et al., Farmakol. Toksikol. (Moscow)* **45,** 83 (1982).

Hydrochloride. Fluoracyzine; toracizin. $C_{20}H_{21}F_3N_2OS\cdot HCl$. White cryst powder, mp 163-165°. Sol in water, warm alcohols.

THERAP CAT: Antidepressant.

4114. Fluanisone. [1480-19-9] 1-(4-Fluorophenyl)-4-[4-(2-methoxyphenyl)-1-piperazinyl]-1-butanone; 4′-fluoro-4-[4-(*o*-methoxyphenyl)-1-piperazinyl]butyrophenone; haloanisone; R-2028; Sedalande. $C_{21}H_{25}FN_2O_2$; mol wt 356.43. C 70.76%, H 7.07%, F 5.33%, N 7.86%, O 8.98%. Prepn: Janssen, **US 2997472** (1961). Determn in human plasma: M. P. Quaglio, A. M. Bellini, *Farmaco Ed. Prat.* **36,** 204 (1981). Comparison between biochemical and behavioral effects: G. B. Fregnan, R. Porta, *Arzneim.-Forsch.* **31,** 70 (1981). Toxicity study: C. Cascio *et al., Farmaco Ed. Sci.* **35,** 605 (1980).

Crystals, mp 67.5-68.5°. Sol in chloroform; sparingly sol in methanol; slightly sol in ether. Practically insol in water. LD_{50} i.p. in mice: 200 mg/kg (Cascio).

Hydrochloride. mp 205-205.5°.

THERAP CAT: Antipsychotic.

4115. Fluazacort. [19888-56-3] (11β,16β)-21-(Acetyloxy)-9-fluoro-11-hydroxy-2′-methyl-5′*H*-pregna-1,4-dieno[17,16-*d*]oxazole-3,20-dione; 9-fluoro-11β,21-dihydroxy-2′-methyl-5′β*H*-pregna-1,4-dieno[17,16-*d*]oxazole-3,20-dione 21-acetate; L-6400; Azacortid. $C_{25}H_{30}FNO_6$; mol wt 459.51. C 65.35%, H 6.58%, F 4.13%, N 3.05%, O 20.89%. Prepn of the 21-hydroxy compound: G. Nathansohn *et al., J. Med. Chem.* **10,** 799 (1967); of the 21-hydroxy and fluazacort: *eidem,* **GB 1119082**; *eidem,* **US 3461119** (1968, 1969 to Lepetit); *eidem, Steroids* **13,** 383 (1969). Pharmacological and physico-chemical properties: *eidem, ibid.* 365. Per-

cutaneous absorption: J. D. Lewis *et al., Arzneim.-Forsch.* **25,** 1646 (1975).

Crystals from ethanol, mp 252-255°. $[\alpha]_D$ +54.8° (c = 0.5 in CHCl₃). uv max (methanol): 238-240 nm ($E_{1cm}^{1\%}$ 330).

THERAP CAT: Anti-inflammatory.

4116. Fluazifop-butyl. [69806-50-4] 2-[4-[[5-(trifluoromethyl)-2-pyridinyl]oxy]phenoxy]propanoic acid butyl ester; butyl 2-[4-(5-trifluoromethyl-2-pyridyloxy)phenoxy]propionate; PP-009; TF-1169; Fusilade. $C_{19}H_{20}F_3NO_4$; mol wt 383.36. C 59.53%, H 5.26%, F 14.87%, N 3.65%, O 16.69%. Selective post-emergence herbicide. Prepn: R. Nishiyama *et al.,* **DE 2812571** (1979 to Ishihara Sangyo Kaisha), *C.A.* **90,** 152017g (1979). Activity: R. E. Plowman *et al., Proc. Br. Crop Prot. Conf. - Weeds* **1980,** 29; J. R. Finney, P. B. Sutton, *ibid.* 429.

bp₀.₀₅ 167°.

USE: Herbicide.

4117. Fluazinam. [79622-59-6] 3-Chloro-*N*-[3-chloro-2,6-dinitro-4-(trifluoromethyl)phenyl]-5-(trifluoromethyl)-2-pyridinamine; 3-chloro-*N*-(3-chloro-5-trifluoromethyl-2-pyridinyl)-α,α,α-trifluoro-2,6-dinitro-*p*-toluidine; *N*-(3-chloro-5-trifluoromethyl-2-pyridyl)-2,6-dinitro-3-chloro-4-trifluoromethylaniline; IKF-1216; ICIA-192; PP-192; Frowncide; Shirlan. $C_{13}H_4Cl_2F_6N_4O_4$; mol wt 465.09. C 33.57%, H 0.87%, Cl 15.25%, F 24.51%, N 12.05%, O 13.76%. Blight fungicide with uncoupling activity on oxidative phosphorylation. Prepn: R. Nishiyama *et al.,* **EP 31257**; *eidem,* **US 4331670** (1981, 1982 both to Ishihara Sangyo Kaisha). Mechanism of action study: Z. Guo *et al., Biochim. Biophys. Acta* **1056,** 89 (1991). Field trials in bulbs: B. P. Anema *et al., Meded. Fac. Landbouwwet. Rijksuniv. Gent* **53,** 635 (1988); in potatoes: B. P. Anema *et al., Brighton Crop Prot. Conf. - Pests Dis.* **1992,** 663.

mp 100-102°. pKa 7.11.

USE: Agricultural fungicide.

4118. Flubendazole. [31430-15-6] [5-(4-Fluorobenzoyl)-1*H*-benzimidazol-2-yl]carbamic acid methyl ester; 5-(*p*-fluorobenzoyl)-2-benzimidazolecarbamic acid methyl ester; R-17889; Flubenol; Flumoxal; Fluvermal. $C_{16}H_{12}FN_3O_3$; mol wt 313.28. C 61.34%, H 3.86%, F 6.06%, N 13.41%, O 15.32%. Fluoro analog of mebendazole, *q.v.* Prepn: J. L. H. Van Gelder *et al.,* **DE 2029637**; *eidem,* **US 3657267** (1971, 1972 both to Janssen); A. H. M. Raeymaekers *et al., Arzneim.-Forsch.* **28,** 586 (1978). Pharmacological, biological properties: D. Thienpont *et al., ibid.* 605. Anthelmintic activity in rats: O. Vanparijs *et al., Vet. Parasitol.* **5,** 237 (1979); in pigs: E. Telléz-Giron *et al., Am. J. Trop. Med. Hyg.* **30,** 135 (1981).

Crystals, mp 260°. LD_{50} in mice, rats, guinea pigs (mg/kg): >2560 orally (Thienpont).

THERAP CAT (VET): Anthelmintic.

4119. Flucarbazone. [145026-88-6] 4,5-Dihydro-3-methoxy-4-methyl-5-oxo-N-[[2-(trifluoromethoxy)phenyl]sulfonyl]-1H-1,2,4-triazole-1-carboxamide. $C_{12}H_{11}F_3N_4O_6S$; mol wt 396.30. C 36.37%, H 2.80%, F 14.38%, N 14.14%, O 24.22%, S 8.09%. Acetolactate synthase inhibitor for control of weeds in wheat. Prepn: K.-H. Müller *et al.,* **EP 507171**; *eidem,* **US 5534486** (1992, 1996 both to Bayer). Comprehensive description: H. J. Santel *et al., Brighton Crop Prot. Conf. - Weeds* 1999, 23-28. Field trials in wheat: K. J. Kirkland *et al., Weed Technol.* **15**, 48 (2001).

Sodium salt. [181274-17-9] BAY MKH 6562; MKH 6562; SJO 0498; Everest. $C_{12}H_{10}F_3N_4NaO_6S$; mol wt 418.28. Colorless, odorless crystalline powder, mp 200° (dec). Vapor pressure (20°): $<1 \times 10^{-9}$ Pa. d 1.59. pKa 1.9. Soly in water (20°): 44 g/l (pH 4-9). Log P (octanol/water): -0.89 (pH 4); -1.85 (pH 7); -1.89 (pH 9). LD_{50} in rats (mg/kg): >5000 orally; >5000 dermally. LD_{50} by inhalation in rats: >5.13 mg/l. LC_{50} in bluegill sunfish, rainbow trout: >99.3, >96.7 mg/l.

USE: Herbicide.

4120. Fluchloralin. [33245-39-5] N-(2-Chloroethyl)-2,6-dinitro-N-propyl-4-(trifluoromethyl)benzenamine; N-(2-chloroethyl)-α,α,α-trifluoro-2,6-dinitro-N-propyl-p-toluidine; BAS-392H; Basalin. $C_{12}H_{13}ClF_3N_3O_4$; mol wt 355.70. C 40.52%, H 3.68%, Cl 9.97%, F 16.02%, N 11.81%, O 17.99%. Soil incorporated, pre-planting herbicide. Prepn: K. H. Karl, K. Kiehs, **DE 2161879** (1973 to BASF), *C.A.* **79**, 65990y (1973). Photochemistry: G. P. Nilles, M. J. Zabik, *J. Agric. Food Chem.* **22**, 684 (1974). Degradn and metabolism in soil: S. Otto, *Environ. Qual. Saf. Suppl.* **3**, 277 (1975).

Orange-yellow cryst solid, mp 42-43°. Soly in water: 10 ppm. USE: Herbicide.

4121. Flucloronide. [3693-39-8] (6α,11β,16α)-9,11-Dichloro-6-fluoro-21-hydroxy-16,17-[(1-methylethylidene)bis(oxy)]-pregna-1,4-diene-3,20-dione; 9,11β-dichloro-6α-fluoro-16α,17,21-trihydroxypregna-1,4-dien-3,20-dione cyclic 16,17-acetal with acetone; 9α,11β-dichloro-6α-fluoro-21-hydroxy-16α,17α-(isopropylidenedioxy)pregna-1,4-diene-3,20-dione; 6α-fluoro-9α,11β-dichloro-1,4-pregnadiene-16α,17,21-triol-3,20-dione 16,17-acetonide; fluclorolone acetonide; RS-2252; Topilar. $C_{24}H_{29}Cl_2FO_5$; mol wt 487.39. C 59.14%, H 6.00%, Cl 14.55%, F 3.90%, O 16.41%. Prepn: Bowers, **US 3201391** (1965 to Syntex). Activity studies: Dorfman *et al., Acta Endocrinol.* **49**, 262 (1965); several authors in *Br. J. Dermatol.* **82**, suppl. 6, 53-98 (1970). Clinical studies: several authors in *Clin. Trials J.* **8**, 35-63 (1971).

THERAP CAT: Glucocorticoid.

4122. Fluconazole. [86386-73-4] α-(2,4-Difluorophenyl)-α-(1H-1,2,4-triazol-1-ylmethyl)-1H-1,2,4-triazole-1-ethanol; 2,4-difluoro-α,α-bis(1H-1,2,4-triazol-1-ylmethyl)benzyl alcohol; 2-(2,4-difluorophenyl)-1,3-bis(1H-1,2,4-triazol-1-yl)propan-2-ol; UK-49858; Biozolene; Diflucan; Elazor; Triflucan. $C_{13}H_{12}F_2N_6O$; mol wt 306.27. C 50.98%, H 3.95%, F 12.41%, N 27.44%, O 5.22%. Orally active bistriazole antifungal agent. Prepn: K. Richardson, **GB 2099818**; *idem,* **US 4404216** (1982, 1983 both to Pfizer). Antifungal activity *in vivo:* K. Richardson *et al., Antimicrob. Agents Chemother.* **27**, 832 (1985); and *in vitro:* T. E. Rogers, J. N. Galgiani, *ibid.* **30**, 418 (1986). Pharmacokinetics: M. J. Humphrey *et al., ibid.* **28**, 648 (1985). GC determn in human plasma and urine: P. R. Wood, M. H. Tarbit, *J. Chromatogr.* **383**, 179 (1986). Evaluation as maintenance therapy for cryptococcal meningitis in AIDS patients: S. A. Bozzette *et al., N. Engl. J. Med.* **324**, 580 (1991). Symposium on mode of action, toxicology, animal models and clinical studies: *International Telesymposium on Recent Trends in the Discovery, Development and Evaluation of Antifungal Agents* **Section 2**, R. A. Fromtling, Ed. (J. R. Prous Science Publ., Barcelona, 1987) pp 77-174. Infection prophylaxis in bone marrow transplantation patients: M. L. MacMillan *et al., Am. J. Med.* **112**, 369 (2002).

Crystals from ethyl acetate/hexane, mp 138-140°.
Dihydrogen phosphate ester. [194798-83-9] Fosfluconazole; 2-(2,4-difluorophenyl)-1,3-bis(1H-1,2,4-triazol-1-yl)propyl dihydrogen phosphate; Prodif. $C_{13}H_{13}F_2N_6O_4P$; mol wt 386.25. Prepn: C. W. Murtiashaw *et al., WO 9728169*; S. Green *et al.,* **US 6790957** (1997, 2004 both to Pfizer). Review of discovery and commercial process development: A. Bentley *et al., Org. Process Res. Dev.* **6**, 109-112 (2002). Water-soluble prodrug. White powder, mp 223-224°.

THERAP CAT: Antifungal.

4123. Flucycloxuron. [113036-88-7]; [94050-52-9] (E-isomer); [94050-53-0] (Z-isomer). N-[[[4-[[[[(4-Chlorophenyl)cyclopropylmethylene]amino]oxy]methyl]phenyl]amino]carbonyl]-2,6-difluorobenzamide; 1-[α-(4-chloro-α-cyclopropylbenzylideneaminooxy)-p-tolyl]-3-(2,6-difluorobenzoyl)urea; DU-319722; PH-70-23; UBI-A1335; Andalin. $C_{25}H_{20}ClF_2N_3O_3$; mol wt 483.89. C 62.05%, H 4.17%, Cl 7.33%, F 7.85%, N 8.68%, O 9.92%. Insect growth regulator which interferes with chitin biosynthesis. Prepn: M. S. Brouwer, A. C. Grosscurt, **EP 117320**; *eidem,* **US 4550202** (1984, 1985 both to Duphar). Comprehensive description: P. Scheltes *et al., Brighton Crop Prot. Conf. - Pests Dis.* **1988**, 559. Mechanism of action and insecticidal activity: A. C. Grosscurt *et al., Pestic. Sci.* **22**, 51 (1988). Determn in fruit and soil samples: J. van Zijtveld *et al., J. Chromatogr.* **600**, 211 (1992).

Odorless crystalline powder. Product consists of 50-80% E-isomer and 50-20% Z-isomer. Data given for ~70:30 E:Z mixture. mp 143.6°. vapor pressure (20°): <4.4 mPa. Soly (20°): water

<1μg/l; xylene 0.2 g/l; cyclohexane 3.3 g/l; ethanol 3.9 g/l. LC$_{50}$ (4 hr) in rats: 3.3 mg/l; LC$_{50}$ (96 hr) in rainbow trout, bluegill sunfish: >100 mg/l; LD$_{50}$ in rats (mg/kg): >5000 orally; >2000 dermally (Scheltes).

E-isomer

USE: Insecticide.

4124. Flucythrinate. [70124-77-5] 4-(Difluoromethoxy)-α-(1-methylethyl)benzeneacetic acid cyano(3-phenoxyphenyl)methyl ester; (±)-cyano-(3-phenoxyphenyl)methyl (+)-4-(difluoromethoxy)-α-(1-methylethyl)benzeneacetate; AC-222705; Cybolt; Guardian; Payoff; Stock Guard. C$_{26}$H$_{23}$F$_2$NO$_4$; mol wt 451.46. C 69.17%, H 5.14%, F 8.42%, N 3.10%, O 14.18%. Synthetic pyrethroid insecticide with contact and stomach poison activity. Prepn: G. Berkelhammer, V. Kameswaran, **DE 2757066**; *eidem*, **US 4199595** (1977, 1980 both to Am. Cyanamid). Activity: A. F. Saad *et al.*, *Proc. Br. Crop Prot. Conf. - Pests Dis.* **1981**, 381; K. Wettstein, *ibid.* 563. Efficacy in cattle fly control: S. M. Taylor *et al.*, *Vet. Rec.* **116**, 566 (1985). Review of toxicology and human exposure: *Toxicological Profile for Pyrethrins and Pyrethroids* (PB2004-100004, 2003) 332 pp.

Viscous liquid. Sol in acetone, xylene, 2-propanol.
USE: Insecticide.
THERAP CAT (VET): Ectoparasiticide.

4125. Flucytosine. [2022-85-7] 4-Amino-5-fluoro-2(1*H*)-pyrimidinone; 5-fluorocytosine; 5-FC; Ro-2-9915; Alcobon; Ancobon; Ancotil. C$_4$H$_4$FN$_3$O; mol wt 129.09. C 37.22%, H 3.12%, F 14.72%, N 32.55%, O 12.39%. Prepn: Duschinsky *et al.*, *J. Am. Chem. Soc.* **79**, 4559 (1957); Heidelberger, Duschinsky, **US 2802005** (1957); Duschinsky, Heidelberger, **US 2945038** and Duschinsky, **US 3040026** (1960, 1962 both to Hoffmann-La Roche); Undheim, Gacek, *Acta Chem. Scand.* **23**, 294 (1969). Patents as a fungicide: Berger, Duschinsky, **BE 628615** and **US 3368938** (1963, 1968 both to Hoffmann-La Roche). Activity studies: Grunberg *et al.*, *Antimicrob. Agents Chemother.* **1963**, 566; Shadomy *et al.*, *ibid.* **1968**, 452; Grunberg *et al.*, in *5th Int. Congr. Chemother.*, *Proc.* **vol. IV**, K. Spitzy, Ed. (Verlag Wiener Med. Akad., 1967, Austria) p 69. Metabolic studies: Koechlin *et al.*, *Biochem. Pharmacol.* **15**, 435 (1966). Clinical results: Utz *et al.*, *Antimicrob. Agents Chemother.* **1968**, 344; Warner *et al.*, *ibid.* **1970**, 473. Comprehensive description: E. H. Waysek, J. H. Johnson, *Anal. Profiles Drug Subs.* **5**, 115-138 (1976).

Odorless, white crystalline solid, mp 295-297° (dec). uv max (0.1*N* HCl): 285 nm (ε 8900). Soly in water: 1.5 g/100 ml at 25°C. pKa$_1$: 3.26. LD$_{50}$ in mice (mg/kg): >2000 orally and s.c.; 1190 i.p.; 500 i.v. (Grunberg, 1963).
THERAP CAT: Antifungal.

4126. Fludarabine. [21679-14-1] 9-β-D-Arabinofuranosyl-2-fluoro-9*H*-purin-6-amine; 9-β-D-arabinofuranosyl-2-fluoroadenine; 2-fluorovidarabine; 2-fluoro-9-β-D-arabinofuranosyladenine; 2-F-araA; NSC-118218; NSC-118218-H. C$_{10}$H$_{12}$FN$_5$O$_4$; mol wt 285.23. C 42.11%, H 4.24%, F 6.66%, N 24.55%, O 22.44%. Adenosine deaminase-resistant purine nucleoside antimetabolite. Prepn and *in vitro* cytotoxicity: J. A. Montgomery, K. Hewson, *J. Med. Chem.* **12**, 498 (1969). Improved prepn: J. A. Montgomery *et al.*, *J. Heterocycl. Chem.* **16**, 157 (1979); J. A. Montgomery, **US 4210745** (1980 to U.S. Dept. Health, Education and Welfare). Inhibition of DNA synthesis and *in vivo* antileukemic activity: R. W. Brockman *et al.*, *Biochem. Pharmacol.* **26**, 2193 (1977). Metabolized to 5′-monophosphate: R. W. Brockman *et al.*, *Cancer Res.* **40**, 3610 (1980). HPLC determn in human leukemia cells: V. Gandhi *et al.*, *J. Chromatogr.* **413**, 293 (1987). Prepn of 5′-monophosphate: J. A. Montgomery, A. T. Shortnacy, **US 4357324** (1982 to U.S. Dept. of Health and Human Services). Pharmacokinetics in humans: M. R. Hersh *et al.*, *Cancer Chemother. Pharmacol.* **17**, 277 (1986). Evaluation of therapeutic efficacy and CNS toxicity in acute refractory leukemia: R. P. Warrell, Jr., E. Berman, *J. Clin. Oncol.* **4**, 74 (1986); H. G. Chun *et al.*, *Cancer Treat. Rep.* **70**, 1225 (1986). Series of articles on pharmacology and therapeutic use: *Semin. Oncol.* **17**, Suppl. 8, 1-78 (1990).

Crystals from ethanol + water, mp 260°. [α]$_D^{25}$ +17 ±2.5° (c = 0.1 in ethanol). uv max (pH 1, pH 7, pH 13): 262, 261, 262 nm (ε × 10^{-3} 13.2, 14.8, 15.0). Sparingly sol in water, organic solvents.
5′-Monophosphate. [75607-67-9] 2-F-ara-AMP; NSC-328002; NSC-312887; Fludara. C$_{10}$H$_{13}$FN$_5$O$_7$P; mol wt 365.21. Sol in water.
THERAP CAT: Phosphate as antineoplastic.

4127. Fludeoxyglucose F^{18}. [105851-17-0] 2-Deoxy-2-(fluoro-^{18}F)-α-D-glucopyranose; 2-[^{18}F]fluoro-2-deoxy-D-glucose; ^{18}FDG. C$_6$H$_{11}$^{18}FO$_5$. Radioactive glucose analog used clinically to evaluate glucose metabolism by PET. Prepn: T. Ido *et al.*, *J. Labelled Compd. Radiopharm.* **14**, 175 (1978). Review of syntheses: T. J. Tewson, *Nucl. Med. Biol.* **16**, 533-551 (1989). Biodistribution: B. M. Gallagher *et al.*, *J. Nucl. Med.* **19**, 1154 (1978). Cerebral glucose measurement in man: M. Reivich *et al.*, *Circ. Res.* **44**, 127 (1979). Clinical evaluation of metabolic imaging in myocardium: R. J. Gropler *et al.*, *J. Nucl. Med.* **31**, 1749 (1990); in tumors: J. Okada *et al.*, *ibid.* **33**, 325 (1992); N. Y. Tse *et al.*, *Ann. Surg.* **216**, 27 (1992). Reviews of imaging in cerebrovascular disease: K. Herholz, W. D. Heiss, *Semin. Neurol.* **9**, 293-300 (1989); Alzheimer's disease: J. M. Hoffman *et al.*, *Eur. Neurol.* **29**, Suppl. 3, 16-24 (1989); brain tumors: R. E. Coleman *et al.*, *J. Nucl. Med.* **32**, 616-622 (1991); pancreatic cancer: M. Zimny, U. Buell, *Ann. Oncol.* **10**, Suppl. 4, S28-S32 (1999).

THERAP CAT: Diagnostic aid (radioactive imaging agent).

4128. Fludiazepam. [3900-31-0] 7-Chloro-5-(2-fluorophenyl)-1,3-dihydro-1-methyl-2*H*-1,4-benzodiazepin-2-one; ID-540; Ro-5-3438; Erispan. C$_{16}$H$_{12}$ClFN$_2$O; mol wt 302.73. C 63.48%, H 4.00%, Cl 11.71%, F 6.28%, N 9.25%, O 5.29%.

Fluorinated analog of diazepam, *q.v.* Prepn: E. Reeder *et al.,* **DE 1136709**; E. Reeder, L. H. Sternbach, **US 3371085** (1962, 1968 both to Hoffmann-LaRoche); L. H. Sternbach *et al., J. Org. Chem.* **27,** 3788 (1962). Synthesis and pharmacology: Y. Asami *et al., Arzneim.-Forsch.* **24,** 1563 (1974). Pharmacodynamics: M. Nakamura, H. Fukushima, *J. Pharm. Pharmacol.* **30,** 56, 254 (1978); T. Tsuchiya, H. Fukushima, *Eur. J. Pharmacol.* **48,** 421 (1978). Anxiolytic vs sedative properties: M. Babbini *et al., Life Sci.* **25,** 15 (1979).

Colorless prisms from *n*-hexane/isopropanol, mp 88-92°, (Asami); also reported as mp 69-72° (Sternbach). LD_{50} in mice (mg/kg): 910 orally; 360 i.p.; 1150 s.c. (Asami).

Note: This is a controlled substance (depressant): **21 CFR,** 1308.14.

THERAP CAT: Anxiolytic.

4129. Fludioxonil. [131341-86-1] 4-(2,2-Difluoro-1,3-benzodioxol-4-yl)-1*H*-pyrrole-3-carbonitrile; 3-(2,2-difluorobenzodioxol-4-yl)-4-cyanopyrrole; CGA-173506; Celest; Maxim; Medallion. $C_{12}H_6F_2N_2O_2$; mol wt 248.19. C 58.07%, H 2.44%, F 15.31%, N 11.29%, O 12.89%. Nonsystemic phenylpyrrole fungicide structurally related to pyrrolnitrin, *q.v.* Prepn: R. Nyfeler, J. Ehrenfreund, **EP 206999**; *eidem,* **US 4705800** (1986, 1987 both to Ciba-Geigy). Comprehensive description: K. Gehmann *et al., Brighton Crop Prot. Conf. - Pests Dis.* **1990,** 399-406. Review of field trials as seed treatment: E. Koch, A. J. Leadbeater, *ibid.* **1992,** 1137-1146.

Colorless, odorless crystals, mp 199.4°. Soly in water (20°): 1.53 ppm. log P (*n*-octanol/water): 2.6. LD_{50} in rats (mg/kg): >2000 orally; >2000 dermally; LC_{50} (4 hr) in rats: >2600 mg/m³ (Gehmann).

USE: Agricultural fungicide.

4130. Fludrocortisone. [127-31-1] (11β)-9-Fluoro-11,17,-21-trihydroxypregn-4-ene-3,20-dione; 9α-fluorohydrocortisone; 9α-fluoro-17-hydroxycorticosterone; 9α-fluorocortisol; fluodrocortisone; fluohydrisone; fluohydrocortisone; Astonin H. $C_{21}H_{29}FO_5$; mol wt 380.45. C 66.30%, H 7.68%, F 4.99%, O 21.03%. Prepn: J. Fried, E. F. Sabo, *J. Am. Chem. Soc.* **76,** 1455 (1954); **GB 792224**; J. Fried, **US 2852511** (both 1958 to Olin Mathieson). Series of articles on pharmacology and metabolism: *Arzneim.-Forsch.* **21,** 1103-1158 (1971). Comprehensive description of the acetate: K. Florey, *Anal. Profiles Drug Subs.* **3** 281-306 (1974).

Crystals, dec 260-262°. $[\alpha]_D^{23}$ +139° (c = 0.55 in 95% ethanol). uv max (ethanol): 239 nm (ε 17600). Soly in water: 0.14 mg/ml.

21-Acetate. [514-36-3] Florinef. $C_{23}H_{31}FO_6$; mol wt 422.49. Crystals, polymorphic, mp 233-234° (occasionally mp 205-208°, resolidifying on further heating, then mp 226-228°). Crystallizing procedure: R. P. Graber, C. S. Snoddy, **US 2957013** (1960 to Merck & Co.). $[\alpha]_D^{23}$ +123° (c = 0.64 in chloroform). uv max (ethanol): 238 nm (ε 16800). Soly (mg/ml): water 0.04; acetone 56; alc 20; chloroform 20; ether 4.

THERAP CAT: Mineralocorticoid.

THERAP CAT (VET): Mineralocorticoid.

4131. Flufenacet. [142459-58-3] *N*-(4-Fluorophenyl)-*N*-(1-methylethyl)-2-[[5-(trifluoromethyl)-1,3,4-thiadiazol-2-yl]oxy]-acetamide; *N*-isopropyl-(5-trifluoromethyl-1,3,4-thiadiazol-2-yl)-(4′-fluorooxyacetanilide); BAY FOE-5043; FOE-5043; Define. $C_{14}H_{13}F_4N_3O_2S$; mol wt 363.33. C 46.28%, H 3.61%, F 20.92%, N 11.57%, O 8.81%, S 8.83%. Oxyacetamide herbicide. Prepn: H. Förster *et al.,* **DE 3821600**; *eidem,* **US 4968342** (1989, 1990 both to Bayer). Ecotoxicological profile: T. Hall, *Pflanzenschutz-Nachr. Bayer (Engl. Ed.)* **50,** 187 (1997). Series of articles on chemical and biological properties, determn and field trials: *ibid.* 105-236. Review of properties and grass control in crops: R. Deege *et al., Brighton Crop Prot. Conf. - Weeds* **1995,** 43.

White to tan solid, mp 75-77°. Does not dissociate. Soly in water at 25° (mg/l): 56 pH 4; 56 pH 7; 54 pH 9. Log P (octanol/water): 3.2. Vapor pressure at 20°: 9.0×10^{-5} Pa. LD_{50} in rats (mg/kg): 589-1617 orally; >2000 dermally. LD_{50} orally in mice, bobwhite quail, mallard duck: 1331-1756, 1608, >2000 mg/kg. LC_{50} in sunfish, rainbow trout, sheepshead minnow: 2.1-2.4, 3.5-5.8, 3.3 mg/l (Hall).

USE: Pre-emergent herbicide.

4132. Flufenamic Acid. [530-78-9] 2-[[3-(Trifluoromethyl)phenyl]amino]benzoic acid; *N*-(α,α,α-trifluoro-*m*-tolyl)anthranilic acid; 3′-trifluoromethyldiphenylamine-2-carboxylic acid; CI-440; INF-1837; Achless; Ansatin; Arlef; Fullsafe; Meralen; Paraflu; Parlef; Ristogen; Sastridex; Surika; Tecramine. $C_{14}H_{10}F_3NO_2$; mol wt 281.23. C 59.79%, H 3.58%, F 20.27%, N 4.98%, O 11.38%. Prepn from *m*-aminobenzotrifluoride and *o*-iodobenzoic acid: Wilkinson, Finar, *J. Chem. Soc.* **1948,** 32. Pharmacology: Winder *et al., Arthritis Rheum.* **6,** 36 (1963); **12,** 472 (1969). Antiviral activity: Inglot, *J. Gen. Virol.* **4,** 203 (1969). Toxicity data: Zoni *et al., Farmaco Ed. Sci.* **26,** 191 (1971). Comprehensive description: E. Abignente, P. deCaprariis, *Anal. Profiles Drug Subs.* **11,** 313-346 (1982).

Pale yellow needles from 50% alc, mp 125°. LD_{50} in mice: 715 mg/kg orally (Zoni).

Aluminum salt. [61891-34-7] Aluminum flufenamate; Alfenamin; Opyrin. $C_{42}H_{27}AlF_9N_3O_6$; mol wt 867.65.

Butyl ester. [67330-25-0] Fenazol; Combec. $C_{18}H_{18}F_3NO_2$; mol wt 337.34.

THERAP CAT: Anti-inflammatory; analgesic.

4133. Flufenoxuron. [101463-69-8] *N*-[[[4-[2-chloro-4-(trifluoromethyl)phenoxy]-2-fluorophenyl]amino]carbonyl]-2,6-difluorobenzamide; 1-[4-(2-chloro-α,α,α-trifluoro-*p*-tolyloxy)-2-fluorophenyl]-3-(2,6-difluorobenzoyl)urea; *N*-(2,6-difluorobenzoyl)-*N*′-[2-fluoro-4-[2-chloro-4-(trifluoromethyl)phenoxy]phenylurea]; WL115110; DPX EY-059; Cascade. $C_{21}H_{11}ClF_6N_2O_3$; mol wt 488.77. C 51.60%, H 2.27%, Cl 7.25%, F 23.32%, N 5.73%, O 9.82%. Acylurea insecticide which inhibits chitin synthesis. Prepn: M. Anderson, **AU 8540924** (1985 to Shell); *idem,* **US**

4698365 (1987 to Du Pont). HPLC determn in grapes and wine: G. E. Miliadis *et al., J. Chromatogr. A* **835**, 113 (1999). Metabolism in caterpillars: B. S. Clarke, P. J. Jewess, *Pestic. Sci.* **28**, 357 (1990). Inhibition of chitin synthesis: *eidem, ibid.* 377. Field trial against German cockroach: B. L. Reid *et al., J. Econ. Entomol.* **48**, 1194 (1992). Review of physical properties and field trials: M. Anderson *et al., Proc. Br. Crop Prot. Conf. - Pests Dis.* **1986**, 89-96.

Colorless, odorless, crystals, mp 169-172° (dec). Soly (g/l) at 25°: water 4×10^{-6}, acetone 82, xylene 6, dichloromethane 24. LD_{50} in rats (mg/kg): >3000 orally; >2000 percutaneously (Anderson).

USE: Insecticide; acaricide.

4134. Fluindione. [957-56-2] 2-(4-Fluorophenyl)-1*H*-indene-1,3(2*H*)-dione; 2-(*p*-fluorophenyl)-1,3-indandione; LM-123; Previscan. $C_{15}H_9FO_2$; mol wt 240.23. C 75.00%, H 3.78%, F 7.91%, O 13.32%. Prepn: Geiger *et al.,* **DE 1130439** (1962 to USV), *C.A.* **57**, 12403a (1962); Molho, Boschetti, **FR 1369396** and **FR M 6913** (1964, 1969 to LIPHA), *C.A.* **62**, 3988g (1965); **74**, 141378u (1971). Alternate syntheses: Shapiro *et al., J. Org. Chem.* **26**, 3580 (1961); Hrnciar, Kovalcik, *Chem. Zvesti* **16**, 200 (1962). Activity and toxicity data: Fontaine *et al., Med. Pharmacol. Exp.* **17**, 497 (1967).

Crystals from acetic acid, mp 120°. LD_{50} orally in mice: 240 mg/kg (Fontaine).

THERAP CAT: Anticoagulant.

4135. Flumazenil. [78755-81-4] 8-Fluoro-5,6-dihydro-5-methyl-6-oxo-4*H*-imidazo[1,5-*a*][1,4]benzodiazepine-3-carboxylic acid ethyl ester; ethyl-8-fluoro-5,6-dihydro-5-methyl-6-oxo-4*H*-imidazo[1,5-*a*][1,4]benzodiazepine-3-carboxylate; flumazepil; Ro-15-1788; Anexate; Lanexat; Mazicon; Romazicon. $C_{15}H_{14}FN_3O_3$; mol wt 303.29. C 59.40%, H 4.65%, F 6.26%, N 13.85%, O 15.83%. Imidazodiazepine which selectively blocks the central effects of classic benzodiazepines. Prepn: W. Haefely *et al.,* **EP 27214**; M. Gerecke *et al.,* **US 4316839** (1981, 1982 both to Hoffmann-La Roche). Specific inhibition of benzodiazepine-receptor binding: W. Hunkeler *et al., Nature* **290**, 514 (1981). Electrophysiological study in animals: P. Pole *et al., Arch. Pharmacol.* **316**, 317 (1981). Antagonist, agonist and inverse agonist properties: S. E. File *et al., Psychopharmacology* **89**, 113 (1986). HPLC determn in human plasma: U. Timm, M. Zell, *Arzneim.-Forsch.* **33**, 358 (1983). Clinical reversal of benzodiazepine-induced sedation: A. Darragh *et al., Lancet* **2**, 8 (1981); *eidem, ibid.* 1042; B. Ricou *et al., Br. J. Anaesth.* **58**, 1005 (1986). Clinical evaluation in drug overdose: G. F. O'Sullivan *et al., Clin. Pharmacol. Ther.* **42**, 254 (1987).

Crystals from alcohol, mp 201-203°. LD_{50} in mice, rats (mg/kg): 4000, 1360 i.p.; 4300, 6000 orally (Hunkeler).

THERAP CAT: Benzodiazepine antagonist.

4136. Flumecinol. [56430-99-0] α-Ethyl-α-phenyl-3-(trifluoromethyl)benzenemethanol; α-ethyl-3-(trifluoromethyl)-benzhydrol; RGH-3332; Zixoryn; Zyxorin. $C_{16}H_{15}F_3O$; mol wt 280.28. C 68.56%, H 5.39%, F 20.34%, O 5.71%. Hepatic microsomal enzyme inducer. Prepn: E. Toth *et al.,* **DE 2438399**; *eidem,* **US 4039589** (1975, 1977 both to Gedeon-Richter). GC determn in biological fluids: I. Klebovich, L. Vereczkey, *J. Chromatogr.* **221**, 403 (1980). Toxicity study: M. Ledniczky *et al., Arzneim.-Forsch.* **28**, 669 (1978). Series of articles on metabolism, CNS effects, enzyme induction, pharmacological properties: *ibid.* 663-679.

Oil, $bp_{0.03}$ 106-108°. uv max (ethanol): 259, 265, 271 nm. LD_{50} orally in adult rats: 2235 mg/kg (Ledniczky).

THERAP CAT: Enzyme inducer (hepatic).

4137. Flumequine. [42835-25-6] 9-Fluoro-6,7-dihydro-5-methyl-1-oxo-1*H*,5*H*-benzo[*ij*]quinolizine-2-carboxylic acid; R-802; Apurone; Fantacin. $C_{14}H_{12}FNO_3$; mol wt 261.25. C 64.36%, H 4.63%, F 7.27%, N 5.36%, O 18.37%. Fluorinated quinolone antibacterial. Prepn: J. F. Gerster, **DE 2264163**; *idem,* **US 3896131** (1973, 1975 both to Riker). *In vitro* study: G. Stilwell *et al., Antimicrob. Agents Chemother.* **7**, 483 (1975). Bioevaluation: S. R. Rohlfing *et al., J. Antimicrob. Chemother.* **3**, 615 (1977). Activity vs *E. coli:* D. Greenwood, *Antimicrob. Agents Chemother.* **13**, 479 (1978).

White microcrystalline powder, mp 253-255°. Sol in alkaline solns and alcohol. Insol in water.

THERAP CAT: Antibacterial.

THERAP CAT (VET): Antibacterial.

4138. Flumethasone. [2135-17-3] (6α,11β,16α)-6,9-Difluoro-11,17,21-trihydroxy-16-methylpregna-1,4-diene-3,20-dione; 6α,9α-difluoro-16α-methylprednisolone; 6α-fluorodexamethasone; Aniprime; Cortexilar; Flucort; Methagon. $C_{22}H_{28}F_2O_5$; mol wt 410.45. C 64.38%, H 6.88%, F 9.26%, O 19.49%. Prepn: **GB 902292**; F. H. Lincoln *et al.,* **US 3499016** (1962, 1970 both to Upjohn). Prepn of the 21-acetate: J. A. Edwards *et al., J. Am. Chem. Soc.* **81**, 3156 (1959); **82**, 2318 (1960).

21-Acetate. $C_{24}H_{30}F_2O_6$. Crystals from acetone + hexane, mp 260-264°. $[\alpha]_D$ +91°. uv max (ethanol): 237 nm (log ε 4.16).
21-Pivalate. [2002-29-1] Locacorten; Locorten; Lorinden. $C_{27}H_{36}F_2O_6$; mol wt 494.57.

THERAP CAT: Glucocorticoid; anti-inflammatory.

THERAP CAT (VET): Glucocorticoid.

4139. Flumethiazide. [148-56-1] 6-(Trifluoromethyl)-2*H*-1,2,4-benzothiadiazine-7-sulfonamide 1,1-dioxide; 6-trifluoromethyl-7-sulfamoyl-4*H*-1,2,4-benzothiadiazine 1,1-dioxide; 6-trifluoromethyl-7-sulfamyl-1,2,4-benzothiadiazine 1,1-dioxide; trifluoro-methylthiazide; Ademol; Fludemil. $C_8H_6F_3N_3O_4S_2$; mol wt 329.28. C 29.18%, H 1.84%, F 17.31%, N 12.76%, O 19.44%, S 19.48%. Synthesis: Holdrege *et al., J. Am. Chem. Soc.* **81**, 4807 (1959); Yale *et al., ibid.* **82**, 2042 (1960); US 3040042 (1962 to Olin Mathieson); GB 861809 (1961 to SK&F).

Crystals, dec 305.4-307.8°. uv max: 278 nm ($E_{1cm}^{1\%}$ 335) (50% diglyme + 50% 0.1N HCl). Sparingly sol in water (50 mg/ml in boiling water with decompn); sol in methanol, ethanol, DMF. Practically insol in ethyl acetate, methyl ethyl ketone, benzene, toluene. Unstable in alkaline soln (conversion to precursor α,α,α-trifluoro-3-amino-4,6-disulfamoyltoluene).

THERAP CAT: Carbonic anhydrase inhibitor.

4140. Flumethrin. [69770-45-2] 3-[2-Chloro-2-(4-chlorophenyl)ethenyl]-2,2-dimethylcyclopropanecarboxylic acid cyano(4-fluoro-3-phenoxyphenyl)methyl ester; 3'-phenoxy-4'-fluoro-α-cyanobenzyl 2,2-dimethyl-3-[2-(4-chlorophenyl)-2-chlorovinyl]-cyclopropane carboxylate; Bayticol; Bayvarol. $C_{28}H_{22}Cl_2FNO_3$; mol wt 510.38. C 65.89%, H 4.34%, Cl 13.89%, F 3.72%, N 2.74%, O 9.40%. Synthetic pyrethroid insecticide. Prepn: R. Fuchs *et al.,* DE 2730515; *eidem,* US 4276306 (1979, 1981 both to Bayer). Series of articles on laboratory evaluation, efficacy and toxicology: *Vet. Med. Rev.* **2**, 115-139, 158-177 (1982).

Oil, n_D^{25} 1.5831.

USE: Insecticide; acaricide.

THERAP CAT (VET): Ectoparasiticide.

4141. Flumetsulam. [98967-40-9] N-(2,6-Difluorophenyl)-5-methyl[1,2,4]triazolo-[1,5-a]pyrimidine-2-sulfonamide; DE-498; Broadstrike; Python. $C_{12}H_9F_2N_5O_2S$; mol wt 325.29. C 44.31%, H 2.79%, F 11.68%, N 21.53%, O 9.84%, S 9.86%. Selective inhibitor of acetolactate synthase, a key enzyme in branched chain amino acid biosynthesis. Prepn: W. A. Kleschick *et al.,* EP 142152 (1985 to Dow). Improved process: L. H. McKendry, US 4910306 (1990 to Dow). Synthesis, toxicity and herbicidal activity: W. A. Kleschick *et al., J. Agric. Food Chem.* **40**, 1083 (1992). Degradation in soil: R. G. Lehmann *et al., Weed Res.* **33**, 187 (1993). Metabolism in wheat, corn and barley: D. S. Frear *et al., Pestic. Biochem. Physiol.* **45**, 178 (1993).

White powder, mp 250-251°. pKa 4.6. Partition coefficient (octanol/water): 0.21. Vapor pressure (25°): 3.7 × 10⁻¹³ Pa. Soly in water (g/l): 0.049 (pH 2.5); 5.65 (pH 7). LD$_{50}$ in rats (mg/kg): >5000 orally; in rabbits (mg/kg): >2000 dermally (Kleschick, 1992).

USE: Herbicide.

4142. Flumiclorac. [87547-04-4] [2-Chloro-4-fluoro-5-(1,-3,4,5,6,7-hexahydro-1,3-dioxo-2H-isoindol-2-yl)phenoxy]acetic acid; 2-chloro-4-fluoro-5-[(3,4,5,6-tetrahydro)phthalimido]phenoxyacetic acid; [2-chloro-5-(cyclohex-1-ene-1,2-dicarboximido)-4-fluorophenoxy]acetic acid. $C_{16}H_{13}ClFNO_5$; mol wt 353.73. C 54.33%, H 3.70%, Cl 10.02%, F 5.37%, N 3.96%, O 22.62%. Postemergent herbicide for use in food crops. Prepn: E. Nagano *et al.,* EP 83055; *eidem,* US 4770695 (1983, 1988 both to Sumitomo). Comprehensive description: K. Kamoshita *et al.,* in *Pest Management in Soybean,* L. G. Copping *et al.,* Eds. (Elsevier, London, 1992) pp 317-324.

Pentyl ester. [87546-18-7] V-23031; S-23031; Resource. C_{21}-$H_{23}ClFNO_5$; mol wt 423.86. mp 88.87-90.13°. Vapor pressure (22.4°): <1.0 × 10⁻⁷ mm Hg. d²⁰ 1.3316. Soly (25°): methanol 47.8 g/l; hexane 3.28 g/l; acetone 590 g/l; acetonitrile 589 g/l; water 0.189 mg/l. LD$_{50}$ in rats (mg/kg): >5000 orally; >2000 dermally (Kamoshita).

USE: Herbicide.

4143. Flumioxazin. [103361-09-7] 2-[7-Fluoro-3,4-dihydro-3-oxo-4-(2-propynyl)-2H-1,4-benzoxazin-6-yl]-4,5,6,7-tetrahydro-1H-isoindole-1,3(2H)-dione; N-(7-fluoro-3,4-dihydro-3-oxo-4-prop-2-ynyl-2H-1,4-benzoxazin-6-yl)cyclohex-1-ene-1,2-dicarboximide; S-53482; V-53482; Sumisoya; Valor. $C_{19}H_{15}FN_2O_4$; mol wt 354.33. C 64.40%, H 4.27%, F 5.36%, N 7.91%, O 18.06%. Selective postemergence herbicide that inhibits protoporphyrinogen oxidase. Prepn: E. Nagano *et al.,* EP 170191; *eidem,* US 4640707 (1986, 1987 both to Sumitomo). Field study in peanut: S. D. Askew *et al., Weed Technol.* **13**, 594 (1999). Metabolism in rat: Y. Tomigahara *et al., J. Agric. Food Chem.* **47**, 305, 2429 (1999). Review of physical properties, mode of action, and field trials: R. Yoshida *et al., Brighton Crop Prot. Conf. - Weeds* **1991**, 69-75.

Yellowish brown, odorless, powder, mp 201.83-203.83°. Soly in water at 25°: 1.79 mg/l. Sol in common organic solvents. Vapor pressure at 22°: 2.41 × 10⁻⁶ mmHg. d²⁰ 1.5132 g/ml. LD$_{50}$ in rats (mg/kg): >5000 orally; >2000 dermally. LC$_{50}$ (4 hr) in rats (mg/m³): >3930 by inhalation. LC$_{50}$ (96 hr) in bluegill, rainbow trout (mg/l): >21, 2.3 (Yoshida).

USE: Herbicide.

4144. Flunarizine. [52468-60-7] (E)-1-[Bis(4-fluorophenyl)methyl]-4-(3-phenyl-2-propenyl)piperazine; (E)-1-[bis(p-fluorophenyl)-methyl]-4-cinnamylpiperazine; 1-cinnamyl-4-(di-p-fluorobenzhydryl)piperazine. $C_{26}H_{26}F_2N_2$; mol wt 404.49. C 77.20%, H 6.48%, F 9.39%, N 6.93%. Calcium channel blocker; fluorinated deriv of cinnarizine, *q.v.* Prepn: P. A. J. Janssen, DE 1929330 and FR 2014487; *idem,* US 3773939 (1970, 1970, 1973, all to Janssen). Pharmacology: L. K. Desmedt *et al., Arzneim.-Forsch.* **25**, 1408 (1975); T. Godfraind, *Eur. J. Pharmacol.* **53**, 273 (1979). Clinical studies: J. Schetz *et al., Curr. Ther. Res.* **23**, 131 (1978); G. Rudofsky *et al., Angiology* **30**, 479 (1979). Rheological effects in humans: J. D. Cree *et al., ibid.* 505. Mechanism of calcium blocking activity: T. Godfraind, *Fed. Proc.* **40**, 2866 (1981). Clinical study in retinal vasculopathy: P. Nihard, *Angiology* **33**, 37 (1982). Clinical trial in chronic cerebrovascular disorders: A. Agnoli *et al., Int. J. Clin. Pharmacol. Res.* **8**, 189 (1988). Series of articles on absorption, distribution, excretion and metabolism: *Arzneim.-*

Forsch. **33**, 1135-1151 (1983). Review of pharmacology, toxicology and clinical studies: B. Holmes *et al., Drugs* **27**, 6 (1984).

Dihydrochloride. [30484-77-6] Dinaplex; Flugeral; Flunagen; Flunarl; Fluxarten; Gradient; Issium; Mondus; Sibelium. $C_{26}H_{26}$-$F_2N_2.2HCl$; mol wt 477.42. Crystals from a mixture of 2-propanol/ethanol, mp 251.5°.

THERAP CAT: Vasodilator (cerebral and peripheral).

4145. Flunisolide. [3385-03-3] (6α,11β,16α)-6-Fluoro-11,21-dihydroxy-16,17-[(1-methylethylidene)bis(oxy)]pregna-1,4-diene-3,20-dione; 6α-fluoro-11β,16α,17,21-tetrahydroxypregna-1,4-diene-3,20-dione cyclic 16,17-acetal with acetone; 6α-fluoro-11β,21-dihydroxy-16α,17-isopropylidenedioxy-Δ^{1,4}-pregnadiene-3,20-dione; RS-3999; Aerobid; Bronalide; Lunis; Nasalide; Rhinalar; Synaclyn; Syntaris. $C_{24}H_{31}FO_6$; mol wt 434.50. C 66.34%, H 7.19%, F 4.37%, O 22.09%. Synthetic fluorinated corticosteroid related to prednisolone, *q.v.* Prepn using *S. roseochromogenes*: **GB 933867** (1963 to Am. Cyanamid), *C.A.* **60**, 3070f (1964). Prepn using *Cunninghamella blakesleeana* 8688b: H. J. Ringold, G. Rosenkranz, **US 3124571**; H. J. Ringold *et al.*, **US 3126375** (both 1964 to Syntex). Metabolism: N. I. Chu *et al., Drug Metab. Dispos.* **7**, 81 (1979). Use in rhinitis: J. N. Sahay *et al., Clin. Allergy* **9**, 17 (1979); J. K. Sarsfield, G. E. Thomson, *Br. Med. J.* **2**, 95 (1979). Use in bronchial asthma: D. R. Webb *et al., Ann. Allergy* **42**, 80 (1979). Clinical study in chronic asthma: R. G. Slavin *et al., J. Allergy Clin. Immunol.* **66**, 379 (1980). Review of pharmacology and therapeutic efficacy: G. E. Pakes *et al., Drugs* **19**, 397-411 (1980); of clinical studies with HFA formulation: S. Shafazand, G. Colice, *Expert Opin. Pharmacother.* **5**, 1163-1173 (2004).

21-Acetate. [4533-89-5] RS-1320. $C_{26}H_{33}FO_7$; mol wt 476.53.

THERAP CAT: Glucocorticoid; antiasthmatic.

4146. Flunitrazepam. [1622-62-4] 5-(2-Fluorophenyl)-1,3-dihydro-1-methyl-7-nitro-2*H*-1,4-benzodiazepin-2-one; 1-methyl-7-nitro-5-(2-fluorophenyl)-3*H*-1,4-benzodiazepin-2(1*H*)-one; Ro 5-4200; Narcozep; Rohypnol; Roipnol. $C_{16}H_{12}FN_3O_3$; mol wt 313.28. C 61.34%, H 3.86%, F 6.06%, N 13.41%, O 15.32%. Prepn: L. H. Sternbach *et al., J. Med. Chem.* **6**, 261 (1963); J. Kariss, H. L. Newmark, **US 3116203** and **US 3123529**; O. Keller *et al.*, **US 3203990** (1963, 1964, 1965 all to Hoffmann-La Roche). Industrial prepn and purifn: J. M. Autin, **FR 2529203** (1983 to Fabre), *C.A.* **100**, 191913r (1984). Pharmacology and clinical studies: E. Eidelberg *et al., Neurology* **5**, 223 (1965); Schuler *et al., Psychopharmacologia* **27**, 123 (1972); J. M. Monti, H. Altier, *ibid.* **32**, 343 (1973); Schallek *et al., Arch. Int. Pharmacodyn. Ther.* **206**, 161 (1973); Kaplan *et al., J. Pharm. Sci.* **63**, 527 (1974). Review of pharmacology and therapeutic use: M. A. K. Mattila, H. M. Larni, *Drugs* **20**, 353-374 (1980).

Pale yellow needles from methylene chloride-hexane, mp 166-167°. Also reported as crystals from acetonitrile and methanol, mp 170-172°.

Note: This is a controlled substance (depressant): **21 CFR**, 1308.14.

THERAP CAT: Hypnotic.

4147. Flunixin. [38677-85-9] 2-[[2-Methyl-3-(trifluoromethyl)phenyl]amino]-3-pyridinecarboxylic acid; 2-(2-methyl-3-trifluoromethylanilino)nicotinic acid; 2-(α³,α³,α³-trifluoro-2,3-xylidino)nicotinic acid; Sch-14714. $C_{14}H_{11}F_3N_2O_2$; mol wt 296.24. C 56.76%, H 3.74%, F 19.24%, N 9.46%, O 10.80%. Cyclooxygenase inhibitor. Prepn: M. H. Sherlock, N. Sperber, **BE 679271**; *eidem*, **US 3337570** (1966, 1967 both to Schering). Prepn of the acid and meglumine salt: M. H. Sherlock, **BE 812772**; *idem*, **US 3839344** (both 1974 to Schering). Pharmacodynamics in horses: M. M. Hardee, J. N. Moore, *Res. Vet. Sci.* **40**, 152 (1986); and pharmacokinetics: L. R. Soma *et al., J. Vet. Pharmacol. Ther.* **15**, 292 (1992). GC determn in urine: M. Johansson, E. -L. Anlér, *J. Chromatogr.* **427**, 55 (1988). Clinical evaluation in horses: J. W. Houdeshell, P. W. Hennessey, *J. Equine Med. Surg.* **1**, 57 (1977). Experimental use in food-producing animals: M. Kopcha, A. S. Ahl, *J. Am. Vet. Med. Assoc.* **194**, 45 (1989). Comparative toxicological study in horses: C. G. MacAllister *et al., ibid.* **202**, 71 (1993).

Crystals from acetone/hexane, mp 226-228°. pKa' 5.82.

Meglumine salt. [42461-84-7] Banamine; Binixin; Finadyne. $C_{14}H_{11}F_3N_2O_2.C_7H_{17}NO_5$; mol wt 491.46. Colorless cryst from ethanol/ether, mp 135-137°. Crystals from acetonitrile, mp 136-139°. Sol in water.

THERAP CAT (VET): Anti-inflammatory; analgesic; antipyretic.

4148. Flunoxaprofen. [66934-18-7] (α*S*)-2-(4-Fluorophenyl)-α-methyl-5-benzoxazoleacetic acid; RV-12424; Priaxim. C_{16}-$H_{12}FNO_3$; mol wt 285.27. C 67.36%, H 4.24%, F 6.66%, N 4.91%, O 16.83%. Nonsteroidal anti-inflammatory. Prepn of racemate: D. Evans *et al.*, **DE 2324443**; *eidem*, **US 3912748** (1973, 1975 both to Lilly). Prepn of racemate and anti-inflammatory activity: D. W. Dunwell *et al., J. Med. Chem.* **18**, 53-58 (1975). Improved process for prepn of racemate and enantiomers: F. Mauri, R. Signorini, **BE 877887**; *eidem*, **US 4304918** (1979, 1981 both to Ravizza); R. Signorini, A. Verga, **DE 3325672** (1984 to Ravizza). HPLC determn of enantiomers in body fluids: S. Pedrazzini *et al., J. Chromatogr.* **415**, 214 (1987). Prophylactic and therapeutic treatment of asthma and other immediate hypersensitivity diseases: W. Dawson, **US 4416892** (1983 to Lilly).

Crystals from acetone-water or acetic acid, mp 162-164°. $[\alpha]_D^{20}$ +50° (c = 2% in DMF). LD_{50} orally in mice: ~1200 mg/kg (Dunwell).

THERAP CAT: Anti-inflammatory.

4149. Fluoboric Acid. [16872-11-0] Hydrogen tetrafluoroborate; borofluoric acid; hydrofluoboric acid. BF₄H; mol wt 87.81. B 12.31%, F 86.54%, H 1.15%. HBF₄. Prepd from H₃BO₃ + HF: Fichter, Thiele, *Z. Anorg. Allg. Chem.* **67**, 302 (1910); Mathers *et al.*, *J. Am. Chem. Soc.* **37**, 1516 (1915); Funk, Binder, *Z. Anorg. Allg. Chem.* **155**, 327; **159**, 121 (1926); Sheintsis, *J. Appl. Chem. USSR* **13**, 1101 (1940); Wamser, Christian, *J. Am. Chem. Soc.* **70**, 1209 (1948); Kwasnik in *Handbook of Preparative Inorganic Chemistry* **vol. 1**, G. Brauer, Ed. (Academic Press, New York, 2nd ed., 1963) pp 221-222. For other methods of prepn *see* H. S. Booth, D. R. Martin, *Boron Trifluoride and Its Derivatives* (New York, 1949). *Review:* Sharp, *Adv. Fluorine Chem.* **1**, 68-128 (1960).

Liquid. *Poisonous!* bp 130° (decompn). Miscible with water, alcohol. Strong acid. n_D^{20} of a 20% aq soln 1.3284. Heat of formn 388.5 kcal. Undergoes limited hydrolysis in water to form hydroxyfluoborate ions; major product is BF_3OH^-. Pure HBF₄ may be stored in glass vessels at room temps. Forms cryst salts with metals. The heavy metal salts and LiBF₄ and NaBF₄ are very sol in water. *See* Potassium Tetrafluoborate about color phenomena appearing in concd solns of fluoboric acid.

Caution: Strong caustic action on skin, mucous membranes. Irritating to eyes, respiratory tract. Plating solns contg fluoborates are considered toxic.

USE: As catalyst for preparing acetals, esterifying cellulose; to clean metal surfaces before welding; to brighten aluminum; as a solute in electrolytes for plating metals such as chromium, iron, nickel, copper, silver, zinc, cadmium, indium, tin, and lead (has a high throwing power). Reagent for sodium in the presence of magnesium and potassium ions; for making stabilized diazo salts (diazonium and tetrazonium fluoborates). An 0.1 to 0.5% soln retards fermentation: Homeyer, *Pharm. Ztg.* **34**, 761 (1889).

4150. Fluocinolone Acetonide. [67-73-2] (6α,11β,16α)-6,9-Difluoro-11,21-dihydroxy-16,17-[(1-methylethylidene)-bis(oxy)]-pregna-1,4-diene-3,20-dione; 6α,9α-difluoro-11β,16α,17,-21-tetrahydroxypregna-1,4-diene-3,20-dione cyclic 16,17-acetal with acetone; 6α,9α-difluoro-16α-hydroxyprednisolone 16,17-acetonide; 6α,9α-difluoro-16α,17α-isopropylidenedioxy-1,4-pregnadiene-3,20-dione; Coriphate; Cortiplastol; Dermalar; Fluonid; Fluovitef; Fluvean; Fluzon; Jellin; Localyn; Synalar; Synamol; Synandone; Synemol; Synotic; Synsac. C₂₄H₃₀F₂O₆; mol wt 452.49. C 63.70%, H 6.68%, F 8.40%, O 21.22%. Prepn: J. S. Mills *et al.*, *J. Am. Chem. Soc.* **82**, 3399 (1960); J. S. Mills, A. Bowers, **US 3014938**; H. J. Ringold *et al.*, **US 3126375** (1961, 1964 both to Syntex). IR spectrum: Sammul *et al.*, *J. Assoc. Off. Agric. Chem.* **47**, 952 (1964).

Crystals from acetone + hexane, mp 265-266°. [α]_D +95° (chloroform). uv max: 238 nm (log ε 4.21).

THERAP CAT: Glucocorticoid; anti-inflammatory.

THERAP CAT (VET): Adrenocortical steroid (topical use).

4151. Fluocinonide. [356-12-7] (6α,11β,16α)-21-(Acetyloxy)-6,9-difluoro-11-hydroxy-16,17-[(1-methylethylidene)-bis(oxy)]pregna-1,4-diene-3,20-dione; 6α,9-difluoro-11β,16α,17,-21-tetrahydroxypregna-1,4-diene-3,20-dione, cyclic 16,17-acetal with acetone, 21-acetate; 21-acetoxy-6α,9α-difluoro-11β-hydroxy-16α,17α-isopropylidenedioxy-1,4-pregnadiene-3,20-dione; 16α,17α-isopropylidene-6α-fluorotriamcinolone 21-acetate; fluocinolide (obsolete); fluocinolide acetate (obsolete); fluocinolone acetonide acetate; Biscosal; Dermaplus; Lidex; Metosyn; Synalate (rescinded); Straderm; Topsym; Topsymin; Topsyne; Topsyn. C₂₆H₃₂-F₂O₇; mol wt 494.52. C 63.15%, H 6.52%, F 7.68%, O 22.65%. Prepn: **GB 916996** (1963 to Olin Mathieson), *C.A.* **59**, 1716b (1963); H. J. Ringold, G. Rosenkranz, **US 3124571**; H. J. Ringold

et al., **US 3126375** (both 1964 to Syntex); J. Fried, **US 3197469** (1965 to Pharm. Res. Prod.). NMR: A. D. Cross, P. W. Landis, *J. Am. Chem. Soc.* **86**, 4005 (1964).

Crystals from methanol. mp 308-311°. [α]_D +83° (chloroform). uv max: 237 nm (log ε 4.18).

THERAP CAT: Anti-inflammatory; glucocorticoid.

4152. Fluocortin Butyl. [41767-29-7] (6α,11β,16α)-6-Fluoro-11-hydroxy-16-methyl-3,20-dioxopregna-1,4-dien-21-oic acid butyl ester; butyl 6α-fluoro-11β-hydroxy-16α-methyl-3,20-dioxopregna-1,4-dien-21-oate; SH K 203; Varlane; Vaspit. C₂₆H₃₅-FO₅; mol wt 446.55. C 69.93%, H 7.90%, F 4.25%, O 17.91%. The butyl ester deriv of fluocortolone, *q.v.*, in humans. Prepn: H. Laurent *et al.*, **DE 2150268**, **DE 2150270**; *eidem*, **US 3824260** (1973, 1973, 1974, all to Schering AG); H. Laurent *et al.*, *Angew. Chem.* **87**, 70 (1975). Description of this new corticoid structure type, the pregnan-21-oic esters, their activity and methods for synthesis: H. Laurent *et al.*, *J. Steroid Biochem.* **6**, 185 (1975). Toxicity data: P. Günzel *et al.*, *Arzneim.-Forsch.* **27**, 2217 (1977). Series of articles on synthesis, pharmacology and clinical trials: *ibid.* 2185-2246.

Crystals from acetone/hexane, mp 195.1°. [α]_D^{25} +136° (c = 0.5 in chloroform). uv max (methanol): 242 nm (ε 16800). Soluble in chloroform, ethanol; poorly sol in ethyl ether. Insol in water. LD₅₀ in mice, rats (g/kg): >4 orally and s.c. (Günzel).

THERAP CAT: Anti-inflammatory.

4153. Fluocortolone. [152-97-6] (6α,11β,16α)-6-Fluoro-11,21-dihydroxy-16-methylpregna-1,4-diene-3,20-dione; 6α-fluoro-16α-methyl-1-dehydrocorticosterone; 6α-fluoro-16α-methyl-Δ¹,⁴-pregnadiene-11β,21-diol-3,20-dione; Ultralan oral. C₂₂H₂₉-FO₄; mol wt 376.46. C 70.19%, H 7.76%, F 5.05%, O 17.00%. Prepn: **BE 614196**; Kieslich *et al.*, **US 3232839** (1962, 1966 to Schering AG); Doménico *et al.*, *Arzneim.-Forsch.* **15**, 46 (1965); Kieslich *et al.*, *Ann.* **726**, 168 (1969). Pharmacology: Doménico *et al.*, *loc. cit*; Gillich *et al.*, *Int. Z. Klin. Pharmakol. Ther. Toxikol.* **1**, 197 (1968); Von Schoening *et al.*, *Klin. Wochenschr.* **48**, 1448 (1970). Metabolism: Gerhards *et al.*, *Acta Endocrinol.* **68**, 98 (1971). Clinical studies: Breuer *et al.*, *Arzneim.-Forsch.* **15**, 50 (1965).

Crystals, mp 188-190.5°. Soly (mg/l): 295 in water (37°); 120 in ethanol (20°); 440 in toluene (20°). [α]$_D^{20}$ +100° (dioxane). uv max (methanol): 242 nm (ε 16300).

21-Acetate. C$_{24}$H$_{31}$FO$_5$. Crystals, mp 237-239°. uv max (methanol): 240 nm (ε 15860).

21-Hexanoate. [303-40-2] Fluocortolone 21-caproate; SH-770; Ficoid; Ultralanum. C$_{28}$H$_{39}$FO$_5$; mol wt 474.60. Crystals, mp 242-245°. [α]$_D^{20}$ +98.5° (dioxane). uv max (methanol): 242 nm (ε 16200). Soly (mg/l): 7.8 in water (37°); 450 in ethanol (20°); 440 in toluene (20°).

21-Pivalate. Fluocortolone trimethylacetate. C$_{22}$H$_{37}$FO$_5$. Crystals, mp 187°. Almost insol in water. Sol in chloroform, methanol. Slightly sol in ether.

THERAP CAT: Glucocorticoid.

4154. Fluometuron. [2164-17-2] N,N-Dimethyl-N'-[3-(tri-fluoromethyl)phenyl]urea; 1,1-dimethyl-3-(α,α,α-trifluoro-m-tolyl)-urea; N-(3-trifluoromethylphenyl)-N',N'-dimethylurea; Ciba 2059; Cotoran; Cottonex. C$_{10}$H$_{11}$F$_3$N$_2$O; mol wt 232.20. C 51.73%, H 4.77%, F 24.55%, N 12.06%, O 6.89%. Made by the reaction of dimethylamine on 3-trifluoromethylphenyl isocyanate: Abel, Chem. Ind. (London) **1957**, 1106. Herbicidal preparations: Martin, Aebi, US 3134665 (1964 to Ciba). Toxicity data: R. Ben-Dyke et al., World Rev. Pest Control **9**, 119 (1970). Review of carcinogenic risk: IARC Monographs **30**, 245-253 (1983).

Crystals, mp 163-164.5°. Soly in water at 25°: 80 ppm; sol in acetone, ethanol, isopropanol, DMF and other organic solvents. LD$_{50}$ in rats (mg/kg): 8900 orally; in rabbits (mg/kg): >10,000 dermally (Ben-Dyke).

USE: Herbicide.

4155. 9H-Fluorene. [86-73-7] o-Biphenylenemethane; di-phenylenemethane; 2,2'-methylenebiphenyl. C$_{13}$H$_{10}$; mol wt 166.22. C 93.94%, H 6.06%. Occurs in coal tar, q.v. (about 1.6%). Isoln: Kruber, Ber. **70**, 1556 (1937). Also found in coke-oven tar: Weiss, Downs, Ind. Eng. Chem. **15**, 1022 (1923). From acetylene and hydrogen in red-hot tube: Meyer, Ber. **45**, 1609 (1912); Meyer, Taeger, Ber. **53**, 1261 (1921). From charcoal by boiling with fuming HNO$_3$: Dimroth, Kerkovins, Ann. **399**, 120 (1913). From 2,2'-dibromodiphenylmethane on boiling with hydrazine hydrate in presence of Pd: Busch, Weber, J. Prakt. Chem. [2] **146**, 47 (1936). Reactions: Rieveschl Jr., Ray, Chem. Rev. **23**, 287 (1938). Review of toxicology and human exposure: Toxicological Profile for Polycyclic Aromatic Hydrocarbons (PB95-264370, 1995) 487 pp.

Dazzling white leaflets or flakes from alc. d 1.202. Sublimes easily in high vacuum. mp 116-117°. bp 295°. Absorption spectrum: Mayneord, Roe, Proc. Roy. Soc. London **A158**, 634 (1937). Freely sol in glacial acetic acid; sol in carbon disulfide, ether, benzene, hot alcohol. Soly data: Mortimer, J. Am. Chem. Soc. **45**, 633 (1923).

4156. 9H-Fluorene-2,7-diamine. [525-64-4] 2,7-Diamino-fluorene. C$_{13}$H$_{12}$N$_2$; mol wt 196.25. C 79.56%, H 6.16%, N 14.27%. Prepd by nitrating fluorene and reducing the 2,7-dinitro-fluorene formed with tin and hydrochloric acid: Schmidt, Hinderer, Ber. **64**, 1793 (1931).

Needles from water, mp 165°. Slightly sol in cold water, more sol in hot water. Readily sol in alc.

Hydrochloride. C$_{13}$H$_{12}$N$_2$.HCl. Crystals, readily sol in hot water.

USE: Detection of bromide, chloride, nitrate, persulfate, cadmium, copper, cobalt, zinc.

4157. N-2-Fluorenylacetamide. [53-96-3] N-9H-Fluoren-2-ylacetamide; 2-acetylaminofluorene; AAF; 2-FAA. C$_{15}$H$_{13}$NO; mol wt 223.27. C 80.69%, H 5.87%, N 6.27%, O 7.17%. Synthesis: Hayashi, Nakayama, J. Soc. Chem. Ind. Jpn. [Suppl] **36**, 127B (1933). Carcinogenicity studies: R. H. Wilson et al., Cancer Res. **1**, 595 (1941). Toxicity studies: Haley et al., Proc. Soc. Exp. Biol. Med. **143**, 1117 (1973); **146**, 648 (1974).

Crystals from alcohol + water, mp 194°. uv max: 285 nm. Insol in water. Sol in alcohols, glycols, fat solvents.

Caution: Potential symptoms of overexposure are reduced function of liver, kidneys, bladder and pancreas. See NIOSH Pocket Guide to Chemical Hazards (DHHS/NIOSH 97-140, 1997) p 4. This substance is reasonably anticipated to be a human carcinogen: Report on Carcinogens, Eleventh Edition (PB2005-104914, 2004) p III-3.

USE: As a positive control to study the carcinogenicity and mutagenicity of aromatic amines.

4158. Fluorescamine. [38183-12-9] 4-Phenylspiro[furan-2(3H),1'(3'H)-isobenzofuran]-3,3'-dione; 4-phenylspiro[furan-2(3H),1'-phthalan]-3,3'-dione; Ro-20-7234; Fluram. C$_{17}$H$_{10}$O$_4$; mol wt 278.26. C 73.38%, H 3.62%, O 23.00%. Non-fluorescent reagent that reacts readily with primary amines to form highly fluorescent compds: S. Udenfriend et al., Science **178**, 871 (1972). Prepn: M. Weigele et al., J. Am. Chem. Soc. **94**, 5927 (1972); eidem, J. Org. Chem. **41**, 388 (1976). Use as fluorometric reagent: W. Leimgruber, M. Weigele, DE 2350179; eidem, US 3830629 (both 1974 to Hoffmann-La Roche). Review of analytical uses: C. Y. Lai, Methods Enzymol. **47**, 236-243 (1977); S. Stein, Peptides in Neurobiology, H. Gainer, Ed. (Plenum, New York, 1977) pp 9-37; S. Udenfriend, Pharmacology **19**, 223-227 (1979).

mp 154-155°. uv max (ether): 235, 276, 284, 306 nm (ε 25900, 3950, 4100, 3800).

USE: Analytical reagent.

4159. Fluorescein. [2321-07-5] 3',6'-Dihydroxyspiro[iso-benzofuran-1(3H),9'-[9H]xanthen]-3-one; 9-(o-carboxyphenyl)-6-hydroxy-3H-xanthen-3-one; 3',6'-dihydroxyfluoran; 3',6'-fluorandiol; 9-(o-carboxyphenyl)-6-hydroxy-3-isoxanthenone; resorci-nolphthalein; D & C Yellow no. 7; C.I. Solvent Yellow 94; C.I. 45350:1. C$_{20}$H$_{12}$O$_5$; mol wt 332.31. C 72.29%, H 3.64%, O 24.07%. Prepd by heating phthalic anhydride with resorcinol: Fischer, Bollmann, J. Prakt. Chem. **104**, 123 (1922); McKenna, Sowa, J. Am. Chem. Soc. **60**, 124 (1938). Structure: Ramart-Lucas, Compt. Rend. **205**, 864 (1937); Nagase et al., J. Pharm. Soc. Jpn. **73**, 1033, 1039 (1953). Review of synthesis, properties and histological use: R. F. Steiner, H. Edelhoch, Chem. Rev. **62**, 457 (1962). Use as label in immunoassays: E. F. Ullman et al., J. Biol. Chem. **251**, 4172 (1976); Y. Suzuki et al., Jpn. J. Exp. Med. **49**, 179 (1979). Toxicity studies in fish: L. L. Marking, Prog. Fish Cult. **31**, 139 (1969). Toxicity data: S. L. Yankell, J. J. Loux, J. Perio-dontol. **48**, 228 (1977). See also: Colour Index vol. 4 (3rd ed., 1971) p 4424; H. J. Conn's Biological Stains, R. D. Lillie, Ed. (Williams & Wilkins, Baltimore, 9th ed., 1977) p 337.

Yellowish-red to red powder. mp 314-316° in sealed tube, with decompn. Insol in water, benzene, chloroform, ether. Sol in hot alcohol or glacial acetic acid; also sol in alkali hydroxides or carbonates with a bright green fluorescence appearing red by transmitted light. Absorption max: 493.5, 460 nm.

Disodium salt. [518-47-8] Soluble fluorescein; resorcinol phthalein sodium; uranin(e); uranine yellow; D & C yellow No. 8; C.I. Acid Yellow 73; C.I. 45350; Ak-Fluor; Fluorescite; Fluorets; Fluor-i-strip; Ful-Glo; Funduscein; Irescein. $C_{20}H_{10}Na_2O_5$; mol wt 376.27. Hygroscopic orange-red powder. Freely sol in water with yellowish-red color and intense yellowish-green fluorescence perceptible down to a dil of 0.02 ppm under uv light. The fluorescence disappears when the soln is made acid, and reappears when the soln is again made neutral or alkaline. Absorption max (water): 493.5 nm. Slightly sol in alc. LD_{50} in mice, rats (mg/kg): 4738, 6721 orally (Yankel, Loux).

USE: In examining subterranean waters. Serves to ascertain source of springs, connections between streams and sea, determining approx vol of water delivered by a spring, detecting source of contamination of drinking water, infiltration of soil with waste waters of factories. In externally applied drugs and cosmetics. Analytical reagent (protein label). Clinical reagent (immunohistological stain, immunofluorescent label).

THERAP CAT: Diagnostic aid (corneal trauma indicator), ophthalmic angiography, contact lens fitting.

THERAP CAT (VET): Diagnostic aid (corneal lesions, intraocular inflammation).

4160. Fluorescin. [518-44-5] 2-(3,6-Dihydroxy-9*H*-xanthen-9-yl)benzoic acid; resorcinolphthalin. $C_{20}H_{14}O_5$; mol wt 334.32. C 71.85%, H 4.22%, O 23.93%. Obtained by heating fluorescein with NaOH and zinc dust. Formation by *Pseudomonas aeruginosa*: King *et al.*, *Can. J. Res.* **26C**, 514 (1948); Totter, Moseley, *J. Bacteriol.* **65**, 45 (1953).

Bright yellow powder, mp 125-127°. Readily oxidizes to fluorescein. Practically insol in water. Sol in alkali hydroxides or carbonates, alcohol, ether. *Keep well closed.*

USE: Reagent for oxidases, peroxidases.

4161. Fluoresone. [2924-67-6] 1-(Ethylsulfonyl)-4-fluorobenzene; ethyl *p*-fluorophenyl sulfone; *p*-fluorophenyl ethyl sulfone; Bripadon; Caducid. $C_8H_9FO_2S$; mol wt 188.22. C 51.05%, H 4.82%, F 10.09%, O 17.00%, S 17.04%. Prepn: G. Thuillier *et al.*, *Compt. Rend.* **248**, 2492 (1959); P. Rumpf, G. Thuillier, **FR M399**; *eidem*, **US 3084101** (1962, 1963 both to Centre Nat. Recher. Scient.); A. A. Mignot, P. Rumpf, *Bull. Soc. Chim. Fr.* **1968**, 435. Pharmacology: J. Thuillier *et al.*, *Proc. 3rd Meet Coll. Int. Neuro-Psychopharmacol.* **1964**, 317-326 (Publ. 1964). Clinical evaluation: H. Akimoto, S. Taen, *ibid.* 326. Gas chromatography: E. Marozzi *et al.*, *Farmaco Ed. Prat.* **31**, 180 (1976).

Crystals, mp 41°. LD_{50} orally in mice: 2.5 g/kg (G. Thuillier); also reported as 850 mg/kg (J. Thuillier); 542 mg/kg (Akimoto, Taen).

THERAP CAT: Anticonvulsant; analgesic; anxiolytic.

4162. Fluorine. [7782-41-4] F; at. wt 18.9984032; at. no. 9; valence 1. A halogen, Group VIIA (17). Does not occur as elemental state, F_2, in nature. Occurrence in earth's crust 0.065% by wt. Naturally occurring isotope (mass number): 19 (100%). Know artificial radioactive isotopes; 15-17, 18 (longest-lived known isotope, $T_{1/2}$ 109.77 min, β^+ emitter), 20-27. Primary commercial source is fluorite, or fluorspar; other important sources are cryolite, and fluorapatite. Discovered in 1771 by Scheele. Isolated in 1886 by electrolyzing a soln of potassium fluoride in anhyd hydrogen fluoride at −23°, using platinum-iridium electrodes: H. Moissan, *Compt. Rend.* **102**, 1543 (1886); **103**, 202, 256. Toxicity data: Keplinger, Suissa, *Am. Ind. Hyg. Assoc. J.* **29**, 10 (1968). *Reviews:* Finger, "Fluorine Resources and Fluorine Utilization" in *Advances in Fluorine Chemistry* vol. 2, M. Stacey *et al.*, Eds. (Butterworths, London, 1961) pp 35-54; A. J. Rudge, *The Manufacture and Use of Fluorine and its Compounds* (Oxford University Press, 1962); T. A. O'Donnell, "Fluorine" in *Comprehensive Inorganic Chemistry* vol. 2, J. C. Bailar, Jr. *et al.*, Eds. (Pergamon Press, Oxford, 1973) pp 1009-1106; G. Shia in *Kirk-Othmer Encyclopedia of Chemical Technology* vol. 11 (Wiley-Interscience, New York, 4th ed., 1994) pp 241-267. Review of toxicology and human exposure: *Toxicological Profile for Fluorides, Hydrogen Fluoride and Fluorine* (PB2004-100002, 2003) 404 pp. Book: *Fluorine: The First Hundred Years (1886-1986)*, R. E. Banks *et al.*, Eds. (Elsevier Sequoia, Laussanne, 1986) 404 pp.

Pale yellow, diatomic gas with sharp penetrating odor. mp −219.61° (53.54 K); bp −188.13° (85.02 K); d (liq, −188.13°) 1.5127; vapor pressure data: Hu *et al.*, *J. Am. Chem. Soc.* **75**, 5642 (1953); White *et al.*, *ibid.* **76**, 2584 (1954). Crit temp: −129°; crit pressure: 55 atm. Most chemically reactive element; most powerful oxidizing agent, higher oxidation potential than ozone; most electronegative element; E° (calc) ½F/F⁻ 2.9 V. F-F bond weaker than Cl-Cl and Br-Br bonds; enthalpy of dissociation: 37.7 kcal. Reacts vigorously with most oxidizable substances at room temp, frequently with ignition. Combines directly or indirectly, to form fluorides with all the elements except helium, neon and argon. Dec water, giving hydrofluoric acid, HF, oxygen fluoride, OF_2, hydrogen peroxide, oxygen and ozone. Reacts with nitric acid, forming the explosive gas, fluorine nitrate, NO_3F; with sulfuric acid, giving fluorosulfuric acid, $HFSO_3$. Yields the metal fluorides, water, oxygen and oxygen fluoride when made to react with metal hydroxides in the cold. Reacts violently with organic compds, usually with disintegration of the molecule. Under controlled conditions, however, hydrocarbon vapors may be fluorinated with elemental fluorine. Solid fluorine explodes when brought in contact with liquid hydrogen. Under ordinary conditions it does not react directly with oxygen, nor does it react with oxides of sodium, potassium or calcium. LC_{50} (1 hr) inhalation by rats, mice, guinea pigs: 185, 150, 170 ppm (by vol) (Keplinger, Suissa).

Caution: Potential symptoms of overexposure are irritation of eyes, nose and respiratory system; laryngeal spasms, bronchial spasms; pulmonary edema; eye and skin burns. See *NIOSH Pocket Guide to Chemical Hazards* (DHHS/NIOSH 97-140, 1997) p 146. Chronic ingestion of high concentrations from water supply can cause mottled enamel of teeth and osteosclerosis. See *Clinical Toxicology of Commercial Products*, R. E. Gosselin *et al.*, Eds. (Williams & Wilkins, Baltimore, 5th ed., 1984) Section III, pp 185-193.

USE: In manuf of UF_6 for nuclear power generation, of SF_6 for dielectrics, of fluorinating and metal fluoride compounds.

4163. Fluorine Dioxide. [7783-44-0] Oxygen fluoride $((O_2)F_2)$; dioxygen difluoride. F_2O_2; mol wt 70.00. F 54.28%, O 45.71%. Prepd from O_2 and F_2: Ruff, Menzel, *Z. Anorg. Allg. Chem.* **211**, 204 (1933); **217**, 85 (1934); Goetschel *et al.*, *J. Am. Chem. Soc.* **91**, 4702 (1969). Chemical behavior: Streng, *ibid.* **85**, 130 (1963). *Review:* Kemmitt, Sharp, *Adv. Fluorine Chem.* **4**, 214-215 (1965).

Thermally unstable gas at room temp; begins to dec into fluorine and oxygen at −100°. Pale yellow solid or yellow liq at low temp. mp −154°C (119 K). Early prepns, described as brown gas, red liq and orange solid (mp −163.5°), probably contained other fluorine-oxygen compounds as impurities: Goetschel *et al., loc. cit.* Strong oxidizing and fluorinating agent.

4164. Fluorine Monoxide. [7783-41-7] Oxygen fluoride; fluorine oxide. F_2O; mol wt 54.00. F 70.36%, O 29.63%. Prepd by passing fluorine slowly through an aq NaOH soln: Yost, *Inorg. Synth.* **1,** 109 (1939); Schnizlein *et al., J. Phys. Chem.* **56,** 233 (1952). Toxicity data: Darmer *et al., Am. Ind. Hyg. Assoc. J.* **33,** 661 (1972). *Review:* Kemmitt, Sharp, *Adv. Fluorine Chem.* **4,** 213-314 (1965).

Colorless gas. Yellowish-brown when liq. Peculiar smell. Does not attack glass in the cold. Corrodes mercury. Reacts very slowly with water. The gas may be kept over water unchanged for a month. d (liq; −224°) 1.90. mp −223.8°. bp −145.3°. Trouton constant 20.65. Soly in water (0°) 6.8 ml gas/100 ml H_2O. LC_{50} (1 hr) inhalation by rats, mice: 2.6, 1.5 ppm (Darmer).

Caution: Potential symptoms of overexposure are headache; eyes, skin, respiratory system irritation; pulmonary edema; direct contact with gas under pressure may cause eye and skin burns. *See NIOSH Pocket Guide to Chemical Hazards* (DHHS/NIOSH 97-140, 1997) p 238.

4165. Fluorine Nitrate. [7789-26-6] Nitroxy fluoride; nitrogen trioxyfluoride; nitryl hypofluorite. FNO_3; mol wt 81.00. F 23.45%, N 17.29%, O 59.26%. $FONO_2$. Prepd by the action of fluorine on nitric acid: Cady, *J. Am. Chem. Soc.* **56,** 2635 (1934); Ruff, Kwasnik, *Angew. Chem.* **48,** 238 (1935); Kwasnik in *Handbook of Preparative Inorganic Chemistry* **vol. 1,** G. Brauer, Ed. (Academic Press, New York, 2nd ed., 1963) pp 187-189. *Reviews:* Kemmitt, Sharp, *Adv. Fluorine Chem.* **4,** 216-218 (1965); Woolf, *ibid.* **5,** 1-30 (1965); Schmutzler, *Angew. Chem. Int. Ed.* **7,** 440-455 (1968).

Colorless gas. Moldy, acrid odor. mp −175°. bp −45.9°. d (liq at bp) 1.507. $d^{-193.2}$ (solid) 1.951. Trouton const 20.8. The liq explodes on slight percussion. Hydrolyzed by water to OF_2, O_2, HF and HNO_3. Sol in acetone. Conflagrates on contact with alcohol, ether, aniline. May be stored in vacuum-sealed glass ampuls cooled by liq oxygen. Powerful oxidizing agent.

USE: Oxidizing agent in rocket propellants.

4166. Fluoroacetamide. [640-19-7] Fluoroacetic acid amide; monofluoroacetamide; 1081; Fluorakil 100; Fussol. C_2H_4FNO; mol wt 77.06. C 31.17%, H 5.23%, F 24.65%, N 18.18%, O 20.76%. CH_2FCONH_2. Numerous syntheses, e.g. from fluoroacetyl chloride and NH_3: Truce, *J. Am. Chem. Soc.* **70,** 2828 (1948). Mode of action study and toxicity data: F. Matsumura, R. D. O'Brien, *Biochem. Pharmacol.* **12,** 1201 (1963).

Crystals. Sublimes on heating. Freely sol in water; sol in acetone; sparingly sol in chloroform. LD_{50} i.p. in mice: 85 mg/kg (Matsumura, O'Brien).

USE: Rodenticide. Insecticide proposed mainly for use on fruits to combat scale insects, aphids, and mites.

4167. Fluoroacetic Acid. [144-49-0] Fluoroethanoic acid; gifblaar poison. $C_2H_3FO_2$; mol wt 78.04. C 30.78%, H 3.87%, F 24.34%, O 41.00%. CH_2FCOOH. Tricarboxylic acid cycle inhibitor. Toxic constituent of the poisonous South African plant, gifblaar, *Dichapetalum cymosum* (Hook.) Engl. (*Chailletia cymosa* Hook.), *Dichapetalaceae;* also contained in other poisonous plant species. Prepn: F. Swarts, *Bull. Soc. Chim.* [3] **15,** 1134 (1896); Gryszkiewicz-Trochimowski *et al., Rec. Trav. Chim.* **66,** 419 (1947). Review and biochemical aspects: Peters, *Endeavour* **13,** 147 (1954); Peters *et al., Biochem. J.* **77,** 17 (1960). Review of toxicity: Gribble, *J. Chem. Educ.* **50,** 460-462 (1973); and properties: A. J. Elliott in *Kirk-Othmer Encyclopedia of Chemical Technology* **vol. 11** (Wiley-Interscience, New York, 4th ed., 1994) pp 544-550.

Crystals. Burns with a green flame. mp 33°. bp 165°.

Sodium salt. [62-74-8] Sodium fluoroacetate; compound 1080; Fratol. $C_2H_2FNaO_2$; mol wt 100.02. Hygroscopic white solid. mp 200-202° (dec when heated above mp). Soly at 25° (g/100g): water 111, methanol 5, ethanol 1.4, acetone 0.04, carbon tetrachloride 0.004.

Methyl ester. [453-18-9] $C_3H_5FO_2$. Liq, odor of ethyl acetate. d_4^{15} 1.1613. bp 104.5°. Sol in water; slightly sol in petr ether.

Ethyl ester. [459-72-3] $C_4H_7FO_2$. Liq, odor of ethyl acetate. $d^{20.5}$ 1.0926. bp_{758} 121.6°. $n_D^{20.5}$ 1.3767. Sol in water.

Caution: Potential symptoms of overexposure to sodium fluoroacetate are vomiting; apprehension, auditory halucinations; facial paresthesia; twitching facial muscles; pulsus alternans, ectopic heartbeat, tachycardia, ventricular fibrillation; pulmonary edema; nystagmus; convulsions; liver, kidney damage. See *NIOSH Pocket Guide to Chemical Hazards* (DHHS/NIOSH 97-140, 1997) p 282; *Clinical Toxicology of Commercial Products,* R. E. Gosselin *et al.,* Eds. (Williams & Wilkins, Baltimore, 5th ed., 1984) Section III, pp 193-196.

USE: Sodium salt as water-soluble rodenticide.

4168. 3-Fluoro-D-alanine. [35455-20-0] *S*-2-Amino-3-fluoropropanoic acid; FA. $C_3H_6FNO_2$; mol wt 107.08. C 33.65%, H 5.65%, F 17.74%, N 13.08%, O 29.88%. Synthesis by *C*-photofluorination of D-alanine or by resolution of the DL-form: J. Kollonitsch, F. M. Kahan; J. Kollonitsch, **DE 2136067; DE 2229245** *C.A.* **76,** 100053p (1972); **78,** 72586d (1973); *idem,* **US 3839170** (1972, 1972, 1974 all to Merck & Co.). The 2-deuterated analog has also been prepared. Antibacterial activity: J. Kollonitsch *et al., Nature* **243,** 346 (1973).

Crystals from water, dec 168°. $[\alpha]_D^{20}$ −10° (c = 3 in 1*N* HCl). Stable at acid pH; less stable at pH >8.

4169. *p*-Fluoroaniline. [371-40-4] 4-Fluorobenzenamine. C_6H_6FN; mol wt 111.12. C 64.85%, H 5.44%, F 17.10%, N 12.61%. Prepd by reduction of 1-fluoro-4-nitrobenzene by Raney nickel: Benington *et al., J. Org. Chem.* **18,** 1508 (1953); Finger *et al., J. Am. Chem. Soc.* **81,** 98 (1959); by sulfurated sodium borohydride: Lalancette, Brindle, *Can. J. Chem.* **49,** 2990 (1971).

Liquid. d_4^{20} 1.1725; d_4^{25} 1.1690. mp −1.9°. bp 188°, bp_{20} 86°. n_D^{20} 1.51954. Heat of combustion 780.4 kcal/mol. Very slightly sol in water.

USE: Intermediate in the manuf of herbicides and plant growth regulators.

4170. Fluorobenzene. [462-06-6] C_6H_5F; mol wt 96.10. C 74.99%, H 5.24%, F 19.77%. Obtained by warming benzenediazonium chloride with concd HF. Solubility value: P. M. Gross *et al., J. Am. Chem. Soc.* **55,** 650 (1933). Pressure, vol, temp constants: Douslin *et al., J. Am. Chem. Soc.* **80,** 2031 (1958).

Liquid; benzene odor. d_4^{20} 1.024. bp_{760} 84.73°; $bp_{13\ atm}$ 200°; $bp_{38\ atm}$ 275°. mp −40°. n_D^{20} 1.4677. Miscible with alcohol, ether. Sol (30°C): 1.54 g/1000 g water.

4171. *p*-Fluorobenzoic Acid. [456-22-4] $C_7H_5FO_2$; mol wt 140.11. C 60.01%, H 3.60%, F 13.56%, O 22.84%. Prepd by treating *p*-carbethoxybenzenediazonium chloride with fluoboric acid, followed by thermal decompn of the resulting *p*-carbethoxybenzenediazonium fluoborate and by hydrolysis of the ensuing ethyl ester of *p*-fluorobenzoic acid: Schiemann, Winkelmüller, *Org. Synth.* **13,** 52 (1933).

Monoclinic prisms from water. Peculiar sweet taste. mp 182.6°. Sparingly sol in cold water; freely sol in hot water. Soly in water at 32°: 1.1 g/l. Water solns evaporate without leaving a residue. Sol in alc, ether. pK (25°): 3.85.

Ethyl ester. $C_9H_9FO_2$. Crystals, mp 26°. bp 210°.

4172. 1-Fluoro-2,4-dinitrobenzene. [70-34-8] 2,4-Dinitro-1-fluorobenzene; DNFB; FDNB; Sanger's reagent. $C_6H_3FN_2O_4$; mol wt 186.10. C 38.72%, H 1.62%, F 10.21%, N 15.05%, O 34.39%. Prepn: A. F. Holleman, J. W. Beekman, *Rec. Trav. Chim.* **23,** 225 (1904); Cook, Saunders, *Biochem. J.* **41,** 558

(1947). Use in peptide analysis: Sanger, *Biochem. J.* **39**, 507 (1945); **40**, 261 (1946); **45**, 563 (1949); Porter, Sanger, *ibid.* **42**, 287 (1948). Tumor promoting activity: F. G. Bock *et al., Cancer Res.* **29**, 179 (1969). Mutagenicity study: D. R. Jagannath *et al., Mutat. Res.* **78**, 91 (1980). Review of uses: *Reagents for Organic Synthesis*, L. F. Fieser, M. Fieser, Eds. (Wiley, New York, 1967) pp 321-322.

Pale yellow crystals from ether, mp 26°. bp$_{2.0}$ 137°. Sol in benzene, ether, propylene glycol.

Caution: Vesicant. For proper handling see: J. S. Thompson, O. P. Edmunds, *Ann. Occup. Hyg.* **23**, 27 (1980).

USE: Reagent for labeling a terminal amino acid group; in modified Wohl degradations of aldoses. As hapten.

4173. Fluoroform. [75-46-7] Trifluoromethane. CHF$_3$; mol wt 70.01. C 17.16%, H 1.44%, F 81.41%. Prepd from CHCl$_3$ and HF: Meslans, *Compt. Rend.* **110**, 717 (1890); Valentiner, **US 643835** (1900); Ruff, *Ber.* **69**, 299 (1936); Whallay, *J. Soc. Chem. Ind. London* **66**, 429 (1947); Kwasnik in *Handbook of Preparative Inorganic Chemistry* **vol. 1**, G. Brauer, Ed. (Academic Press, New York, 2nd ed., 1963) pp 204-205. Early industrial prepn: Pearlson in *Fluorine Chemistry* **vol. I**, J. H. Simons, Ed. (Academic Press, New York, 1950) p 467.

Colorless, odorless gas. Stable up to 1150°. Chemically very inert. d (solid) 1.935. d (liq; −100°) 1.52. mp −160°. bp −84.4°. Critical temp 33°, critical pressure 47 atm, critical density 0.516. May be stored over water. Practically non-toxic: N. V. Sidgwick, *The Chemical Elements and Their Compounds* **vol. II** (Oxford, 1950) p 1130.

Caution: May be slightly irritating to respiratory tract, and, in high concns, narcotic.

USE: Refrigerant for low temps.

4174. Fluoromethane. [593-53-3] Methyl fluoride. CH$_3$F; mol wt 34.03. C 35.29%, H 8.89%, F 55.83%. Prepn in 82% yield by heating fluorosulfonic acid methyl ester with KF: Zappel, Jonas, **DE 1131197** (1962 to Bayer).

Gas. Agreeable ether-like odor. Burns with evolution of HF, the flame being about as colorless as that of alc: Dumas, Peligot, *Ann.* **15**, 59 (1835). d (liq; −78°) 0.8774. d (gas) 1.1951 (air = 1); d (gas) 1.0813 (oxygen = 1). Dipole moment 1.81. Molecular volume: 22.03. Van der Waals constants: 0.00923; 0.002350. Critical temp 44.9°; crit press. 62.0 atm. Dielectric constant (for wavelengths below 10^4 cm) = 1.00948. mp −141.8°. bp$_{872}$ −75.7°; bp$_{760}$ −78.2°. bp$_{143}$ −103.7°. One hundred vols of water dissolve 166 vols of the gas at 15°. Freely sol in alcohol, ether.

Caution: Narcotic in high concns.

4175. Fluorometholone. [426-13-1] (6α,11β)-9-Fluoro-11,17-dihydroxy-6-methylpregna-1,4-diene-3,20-dione; 21-desoxy-9α-fluoro-6α-methylprednisolone; 21-desoxy-6α-methyl-9α-fluoroprednisolone; fluormetholon; Delmeson; Efflumidex; Fluaton; Flumetholon; Fluor-Op; FML. C$_{22}$H$_{29}$FO$_4$; mol wt 376.46. C 70.19%, H 7.76%, F 5.05%, O 17.00%. Prepn: F. H. Lincoln *et al.*, **US 2867637** (1959 to Upjohn). Prepn of acetate and other esters: B. J. Magerlein *et al.*, **US 3038914** (1962 to Upjohn). Pharmacology of acetate: A. Kupferman *et al., Arch. Ophthalmol.* **100**, 640 (1982). HPLC determn: H. Tokunaga *et al., Chem. Pharm. Bull.* **32**, 4012 (1984). Clinical evaluation in ocular inflammation: H. M. Leibowitz *et al., Ann. Ophthalmol.* **16**, 1110 (1984).

Crystals from acetone, mp 292-303°.

17-Acetate. [3801-06-7] Eflone. C$_{24}$H$_{31}$FO$_5$. Crystals from ethyl acetate + hexanes, mp 230-232°. [α]$_D$ +28° (chloroform).

THERAP CAT: Glucocorticoid; anti-inflammatory.

4176. 5-Fluoroorotic Acid. [703-95-7] 5-Fluoro-1,2,3,6-tetrahydro-2,6-dioxo-4-pyrimidinecarboxylic acid; 5-fluoroorotate; 5-fluoro-6-carboxyuracil; 5-FOA; ENT-26398; NSC-31712; Ro-2-9945; WR-152520. C$_5$H$_3$FN$_2$O$_4$; mol wt 174.09. C 34.50%, H 1.74%, F 10.91%, N 16.09%, O 36.76%. Pyrimidine precursor; selectively toxic to yeast cells that synthesize the enzyme orotidine-5′-P decarboxylase. Prepn: R. Duschinsky *et al., J. Am. Chem. Soc.* **79**, 4559 (1957); R. Duschinsky, C. Heidelberger, **US 2948725** (1960). Improved synthesis: D. H. R. Barton *et al., J. Chem. Soc. Perkin Trans. 1* **1974**, 2095; and mass spectrum: S. N. Alam *et al., Acta Pharm. Suec.* **12**, 375 (1975). Antitumor activity: C. Heidelberger *et al., Nature* **179**, 663 (1957). Inhibition of RNA synthesis: C. T. Garrett *et al., Arch. Biochem. Biophys.* **155**, 342 (1973). Clinical evaluation of antimycotic activity: K. Nikolova *et al., Methods Find. Exp. Clin. Pharmacol.* **9**, 85 (1987). Review of *in vitro* use in the positive selection of genetically transformed yeast cells: J. D. Boeke *et al., Methods Enzymol.* **154**, 164-175 (1987).

Monohydrate. Crystals, mp 255° (dec) (Duschinsky, 1957); also reported as 258-259° (Barton). Partially sol in water. uv max (0.1*N* HCl): 284-285 nm (ε 7100). LD$_{50}$ i.p. in male mice: 300 mg/kg (Nikolova).

USE: Research tool in molecular genetics.

4177. *p*-Fluorophenylacetic Acid. [405-50-5] 4-Fluorobenzeneacetic acid. C$_8$H$_7$FO$_2$; mol wt 154.14. C 62.34%, H 4.58%, F 12.33%, O 20.76%. Prepd by treating *p*-fluorobenzyl cyanide with sulfuric acid: Olah *et al., J. Org. Chem.* **22**, 879 (1957).

Crystals from chloroform, mp 86°. bp$_2$ 164°.

β-Dimethylaminoethyl ester HCl. Crystals, mp 103°.

USE: Intermediate in the manuf of fluorinated anesthetics.

4178. Fluorosalan. [4776-06-1] 3,5-Dibromo-2-hydroxy-*N*-[3-(trifluoromethyl)phenyl]benzamide; 3,5-dibromo-α,α,α-trifluoro-*m*-salicylotoluidide; 3,5-dibromo-3′-trifluoromethyl-salicylanilide; Fluorophene. C$_{14}$H$_8$Br$_2$F$_3$NO$_2$; mol wt 439.02. C 38.30%, H 1.84%, Br 36.40%, F 12.98%, N 3.19%, O 7.29%. Prepn: Stecker, **US 3041236** (1962).

THERAP CAT: Disinfectant.

4179. Fluorosulfonic Acid. [7789-21-1] Fluorosulfuric acid; fluosulfonic acid. FHO$_3$S; mol wt 100.07. F 18.99%, H 1.01%, O 47.96%, S 32.04%. HSO$_3$F. Prepn: Thorpe, Kirman, *J. Chem. Soc.* **61**, 921 (1892); Meyer, Schramm, *Z. Anorg. Allg. Chem.* **206**, 25 (1932); Kwasnik in *Handbook of Preparative Inorganic Chemistry* **vol. 1**, G. Brauer, Ed. (Academic Press, New York, 2nd ed., 1963) pp 177-178. Reviews of properties and chemistry: Gillespie, *Acc. Chem. Res.* **1**, 202-209 (1968); Thompson, "Fluorosulfuric Acid" in *Inorganic Sulfur Chemistry,* G. Nickless, Ed. (Elsevier, New York, 1968) pp 587-606; Jache in *Adv. Inorg. Chem. Radiochem.* **16,** 177-200 (1974).

Colorless liquid; fumes in moist air. d_4^{18} 1.740; d_4^{25} 1.726. mp $-89°$. bp_{760} 163°; bp_{120} 110.0°; bp_{19} 77.0°. Stable to 900°. Considerably more acidic than 100% H_2SO_4. Does not attack glass when anhydr and pure. Violent reaction with water although it is incompletely and reversibly hydrolyzed. Reddish-brown color with acetone. Forms stable salts which are little hydrolyzed by water and which may be recrystallized from water.

Methyl ester *see* Methyl Fluorosulfonate.

Caution: May be highly irritating to skin, mucous membranes.

USE: Fluorinating agent. Catalyst in alkylation, acylation, polymerization and condensation reactions; in hydrofluorination of olefins; in production of substituted pyridines. In production of petroleum products. *See* Thompson, *loc. cit.* **Magic Acid,** a 1:1 HSO_3F-SbF_5 soln, is used in the study of stable solns of alkyl- and arylcarbonium ions: Olah, *Science* **168,** 1298 (1970).

4180. Fluorotoluene. Fluoromethylbenzene. C_7H_7F; mol wt 110.13. C 76.34%, H 6.41%, F 17.25%. Prepn of *o-, m-, p-*isomers: A. F. Holleman, J. W. Beekman, *Rec. Trav. Chim.* **23,** 225 (1904); A. F. Holleman, *ibid.* **25,** 330 (1906); E. D. Bergmann, S. Berkovic, *J. Org. Chem.* **26,** 919 (1961).

Colorless liquids. Insol in water. Miscible with alc, ether.

*o-***Fluorotoluene.** [95-52-3] 1-Fluoro-2-methylbenzene. d^{13} 1.004. mp $\sim-80°$. bp 114°. n_D^{20} 1.4704.

*m-***Fluorotoluene.** [352-70-5] d^{13} 0.997. mp $-111°$. bp 116°. n_D^{20} 1.4691.

*p-***Fluorotoluene.** [352-32-9] Odor of oil of bitter almonds. d^{16} 1.001. bp 116°. n_D^{20} 1.470.

4181. Fluorouracil. [51-21-8] 5-Fluoro-2,4(1*H*,3*H*)-pyrimidinedione; 2,4-dioxo-5-fluoropyrimidine; 5-FU; Ro-2-9757; NSC-19893; Adrucil; Arumel; Efudex; Efudix; Fluril; Fluracil; Fluoroplex; Fluroblastin; Fluro Uracil; Timazin. $C_4H_3FN_2O_2$; mol wt 130.08. C 36.93%, H 2.32%, F 14.61%, N 21.54%, O 24.60%. Prepn: Duschinsky *et al., J. Am. Chem. Soc.* **79,** 4559 (1957); Heidelberger, Duschinsky, US 2802005 (1957); US 2885396 (1959); Barton *et al., J. Org. Chem.* **37,** 329 (1972); O. Miyashita *et al., Chem. Pharm. Bull.* **29,** 3181 (1981). Pharmacokinetics: W. Sadee, C. G. Wong, *Clin. Pharmacokinet.* **2,** 437 (1977). Site of action: F. Maley, G. F. Maley, *FEBS Symp.* **57,** 21 (1979). Comprehensive description: B. C. Rudy, B. Z. Senkowski, *Anal. Profiles Drug Subs.* **2,** 221-244 (1973); S. M. Bayomi, A. A. Al-Badr, *ibid.* **18,** 599-639 (1989). Review of clinical trials: R. M. Hansen, *Cancer Invest.* **9,** 637-642 (1991).

Crystals from water or methanol-ether, dec 282-283°. Sublimes (0.1 mm) 190-200°. uv max (0.1*N* HCl): 265-266 nm (ε 7070).

Sodium salt. Effluderm.

THERAP CAT: Antineoplastic.

4182. Fluosilicic Acid. [16961-83-4] Hydrogen hexafluorosilicate; hexafluosilicic acid; hydrosilicofluoric acid; hydrofluosilicic acid; silicofluoric acid; fluorosilicic acid. F_6H_2Si; mol wt 144.09. F 79.11%, H 1.40%, Si 19.49%. H_2SiF_6. Prepd from HF + SiO_2; also prepd by the action of water on SiF_4; by the action of H_2SO_4 on $BaSiF_6$: Hempel, *Ber.* **18,** 1438 (1885); Baur, Glaessner, *Ber.* **36,** 4215 (1903); Söll, *FIAT-Review* **23,** 257 (1946); Kwasnik in *Handbook of Preparative Inorganic Chemistry* **vol. 1,** G. Brauer, Ed. (Academic Press, New York, 2nd ed., 1963) p 214-

215; Lange in *Fluorine Chemistry* **vol. I,** J. H. Simon, Ed. (New York, 1950) p 129. Commercial grades of fluosilicic acid soln are obtained as a by-product in the superphosphate industry. *Review:* Colton, *J. Chem. Educ.* **35,** 562-563 (1958).

Liquid, when anhyd dissociates almost instantly into SiF_4 and HF. Marketed as aq soln only. A 60-70% soln solidifies around 19°, forming a cryst dihydrate. May be distilled without decompn only as a 13.3% aq soln. Fairly strong acid. Sour, pungent odor. $d_{17.5}^{17.5}$ 5% soln: 1.0407; 10%: 1.0834; 15%: 1.1281; 20%: 1.1748; 25%: 1.2235; 30%: 1.2742; 34%: 1.3162. The more concd solns (but not the anhydr liq) can be stored in glass, although some etching will take place around the surface. Usually stored in iron containers.

Caution: Severe corrosive effect on skin, mucous membranes.

USE: A 1-2% soln is used widely for sterilizing equipment in brewing and bottling establishments. Other concns are used in the electrolytic refining of lead, in electroplating, for hardening cement, crumbling lime or brick work, for the removal of lime from hides during the tanning process, to remove molds, as preservative for timber.

4183. Fluosol DA. [75216-20-5] Biologically inert fluorocarbon emulsion of perfluorodecalin and perfluorotripropylamine that performs the oxygen-carrying function of red blood cells. Has a particle size of 0.05 to 0.25μ and is stable at room temperature for years. Can be administered regardless of blood type; does not carry hepatitis or other infectious diseases. Prepn: K. Yokoyama *et al.,* **DE 2630586;** *eidem,* **US 4252827** (1977, 1981 to Green Cross). Hemodynamic and oxygen transport effects: K. K. Tremper *et al., Crit. Care Med.* **8,** 738 (1980). Clinical studies: H. Ohyanagi *et al., Clin. Ther.* **2,** 306 (1979); T. Suyama *et al., Prog. Clin. Biol. Res.* **55,** 609 (1981); T. Mitsuno *et al., Ann. Surg.* **195,** 60 (1982). *Review: Int. Congr. Ser. - Excerpta Med.* **486,** 1-471 (1979). Review of use as red cell substitute: K. C. Lowe, *Comp. Biochem. Physiol.* **87A,** 825-838 (1987).

20% Emulsion, *FDA-20.* Viscosity at 37°: 2.3 cP. pH 7.4.

Perfluorodecalin. [306-94-5] Octadecafluorodecahydronaphthalene; perflunafene; FDC. $C_{10}F_{18}$; mol wt 462.08. Prepn: E. T. McBee, L. D. Bechtol, *Ind. Eng. Chem.* **39,** 380 (1947). mp -10 to $-7°$. bp 140°. d_4^{20} 1.9456. n_D^{20} 1.3118. Vapor pressure at 37°: 12.7 mm Hg.

Perfluorotripropylamine. [338-83-0] 1,1,2,2,3,3,3-Heptafluoro-*N,N*-bis(heptafluoropropyl)-1-propanamine; heneicosafluorotripropylamine; perfluamine; FTPA. $C_9F_{21}N$; mol wt 521.07. Prepn: R. N. Haszeldine, *J. Chem. Soc.* **1951,** 102. bp 129.5-130.5°. d_4^{25} 1.822. n_D^{25} 1.279. Vapor press. at 37°: 20.0 mm Hg.

THERAP CAT: Blood substitute.

4184. Fluoxastrobin. [361377-29-9] (1*E*)-[2-[[6-(2-Chlorophenoxy)-5-fluoro-4-pyrimidinyl]oxy]phenyl](5,6-dihydro-1,4,2-dioxazin-3-yl)methanone *O*-methyloxime; HEC-5725; Fandango. $C_{21}H_{16}ClFN_4O_5$; mol wt 458.83. C 54.97%, H 3.51%, Cl 7.73%, F 4.14%, N 12.21%, O 17.43%. Leaf-systemic broad-spectrum fungicide for use in cereal and food crops; member of methoxyimidodihydro-dioxazines. Prepn (stereochem. unspecified): U. Heinemann *et al.,* **DE 19602095;** *eidem,* **US 6103717** (1997, 2000 both to Bayer). Comprehensive description: S. Dutzmann *et al., BCPC Conf. - Pests Dis.* **2002,** 365. Field trial in winter wheat seeds: I. Haeuser-Hahn *et al., BCPC Int. Cong. - Crop Sci. Tech.* **2003,** 801. Series of articles on chemistry, biology, determn, and environmental fate: *Pflanzenschutz-Nachr. Bayer (Engl. Ed.)* **57,** 299-449 (2004). Ecotoxicology: P. Breuer, *ibid.* 319.

White crystals with slight characteristic odor, mp 103-108°. bp 497° (est.). d_4^{20} 1.422. Log P (octanol/water): 2.86 (20°). Vapor pressure at 20° (extrapolated): 6×10^{-10} Pa. Soly at 20° (g/l): *n*-heptane 0.04; 2-propanol 6.7; xylene 38.1; dichloromethane >250;

in water (mg/l): 2.56 (unbuffered); 2.43 (pH 4); 2.29 (pH 7); 2.27 (pH 9). LD_{50} in rats, bobwhite quail (mg/kg): >2500, >2000 orally; LC_{50} (96 hr) rainbow trout, bluegill sunfish, carp (mg/l): 0.44, 0.97, 0.57 (Breuer).

USE: Agricultural fungicide.

4185. Fluoxetine. [54910-89-3] *N*-Methyl-γ-[4-(trifluoromethyl)phenoxy]benzenepropanamine; (±)-*N*-methyl-3-phenyl-3-[(α,α,α-trifluoro-*p*-tolyl)oxy]propylamine; *dl*-*N*-methyl-3-(*p*-trifluoromethylphenoxy)-3-phenylpropylamine. $C_{17}H_{18}F_3NO$; mol wt 309.33. C 66.01%, H 5.87%, F 18.43%, N 4.53%, O 5.17%. Selective serotonin reuptake inhibitor (SSRI). Prepn: B. B. Malloy, K. K. Schmiegel, **DE 2500110**; *eidem*, **US 4314081** (1975, 1982 both to Lilly). Pharmacology: D. T. Wong *et al., Life Sci.* **15,** 471 (1974). GC determn in plasma: J. F. Nash *et al., Clin. Chem.* **28,** 2100 (1982). Series of articles on clinical pharmacology and therapeutic efficacy in depression: *J. Clin. Psychiatry* **46,** Suppl. 3(2), 2-67 (1985). Toxicity data: P. Stark *et al., ibid.* 7. Clinical trial in bulimia nervosa: D. J. Goldstein *et al., Br. J. Psychiatry* **166,** 660 (1995); in obsessive-compulsive disorder: J. J. Lopez-Ibor, Jr. *et al., Eur. Neuropsychopharmacol.* **6,** 111 (1996). Veterinary trial in canine aggression: N. H. Dodman *et al., J. Am. Vet. Med. Assoc.* **209,** 1585 (1996). Comprehensive description: D. S. Risley, R. J. Bopp, *Anal. Profiles Drug Subs.* **19,** 193-219 (1990). Review of clinical experience: P. E. Stokes, A. Holtz, *Clin. Ther.* **19,** 1135-1250 (1997); in premenstrual dysphoric disorder: S. Romano *et al., Clin. Ther.* **21,** 615 (1999).

Hydrochloride. [59333-67-4] LY-110140; Adofen; Fluctin; Fluoxeren; Fontex; Foxetin; Lovan; Prozac; Reneuron; Sarafem. $C_{17}H_{18}F_3NO·HCl$; mol wt 345.79. White to off-white crystalline solid. mp 158.4-158.9°. Soly (mg/ml): methanol, ethanol >100; acetone, acetonitrile, chloroform 33-100; dichloromethane 5-10; ethyl acetate 2-2.5; toluene, cyclohexane, hexane 0.5-0.67. Maximum soly in water: 14 mg/ml. uv max (methanol) 227, 264, 268, 275 nm ($E_{1cm}^{1\%}$ 372.0, 29.2, 29.3, 21.5). LD_{50} in mice, rats (mg/kg): 248, 452 orally (Stark).

Oxalate. $C_{19}H_{18}F_3NO_5$. Crystals from ethyl acetate-methanol, mp 179-182° (dec).

THERAP CAT: Antidepressant; antiobessional; antibulimic.

4186. Fluoxymesterone. [76-43-7] (11β,17β)-9-Fluoro-11,17-dihydroxy-17-methylandrost-4-en-3-one; 11β,17β-dihydroxy-9α-fluoro-17α-methyl-4-androsten-3-one; 9α-fluoro-11β-hydroxy-17α-methyltestosterone; Halotestin. $C_{20}H_{29}FO_3$; mol wt 336.44. C 71.40%, H 8.69%, F 5.65%, O 14.27%. Prepn: Herr *et al., J. Am. Chem. Soc.* **78,** 501 (1956). *cf.* Herr, **US 2813881** (1957 to Upjohn). Comprehensive description: J. Kirschbaum, *Anal. Profiles Drug Subs.* **7,** 251-275 (1978).

Crystals, dec 270°. [α]$_D$ +109° (ethanol). uv max (ethanol): 240 nm (ε 16700). Sol in pyridine; slightly sol in acetone, chloroform; sparingly sol in methanol. Practically insol in water, ether, benzene, hexanes.

Note: This is a controlled substance (anabolic steroid): **21 CFR,** 1308.13, as defined in 1300.01.

THERAP CAT: Androgen.

4187. Flupentixol. [2709-56-0] 4-[3-[2-(Trifluoromethyl)-9*H*-thioxanthen-9-ylidene]propyl]-1-piperazineethanol; 2-trifluoro-

methyl-9-[3-[4-(β-hydroxyethyl)-1-piperazinyl]propylidene]thioxanthene; flupenthixol; N-7009; LC-44. $C_{23}H_{25}F_3N_2OS$; mol wt 434.52. C 63.58%, H 5.80%, F 13.12%, N 6.45%, O 3.68%, S 7.38%. Neuroleptic agent related structurally to thiothixene, *q.v.* Prepn: P. N. Craig, C. L. Zirkle, **US 3282930** (1966 to SKF). Prepn of *cis*- and *trans*-forms: **GB 925538** (1963 to SKF); P. V. Petersen, T. Ammitzboll, **US 3681346** (1972 to Kefalas). Metabolism of decanoate: A. Jorgensen *et al., Acta Pharmacol. Toxicol.* **29,** 339 (1971). α-Flupentixol, the *cis*-isomer, shows greater pharmacological activity than β-flupentixol, the *trans*-isomer: I. Moller Nielsen *et al., Acta Pharmacol. Toxicol.* **33,** 353 (1973). X-ray crystallography of isomers: M. L. Post *et al., Nature* **256,** 342 (1975).

cis-form

Dihydrochloride. [2413-38-9] Emergil; Fluanxol; Siplarol; Metamin. $C_{23}H_{25}F_3N_2OS·2HCl$; mol wt 507.44.

Decanoate. [30909-51-4] Lu-5-110; Depixol; Fluanxol Dépôt; Viscoleo.

THERAP CAT: Antipsychotic.

4188. Fluperolone Acetate. [2119-75-7] [11β,17α,17(*S*)]-17-[2-(Acetyloxy)-1-oxopropyl]-9-fluoro-11,17-dihydroxyandrosta-1,4-dien-3-one; 9-fluoro-11β,17α-dihydroxy-17(*S*)-lactoylandrosta-1,4-dien-3-one 17β-acetate; 9α-fluoro-11β,17α,21-trihydroxy-21-methylpregna-1,4-diene-3,20-dione 21-acetate; 17β-[2-acetoxypropionyl]-9α-fluoro-11β,17-dihydroxyandrosta-1,4-dien-3-one; 21-methyl-9α-fluoroprednisolone acetate; P-1742; ALAcortril; Methral. $C_{24}H_{31}FO_6$; mol wt 434.50. C 66.34%, H 7.19%, F 4.37%, O 22.09%. Prepn: E. J. Agnello *et al., Experientia* **16,** 357 (1960); *eidem, J. Org. Chem.* **28,** 1531 (1963); E. J. Agnello, G. D. Laubach, **US 3234095** (1966 to Pfizer). Activity studies: Child *et al., Arch. Dermatol.* **97,** 407 (1968).

Crystals, mp 251-253°. [α]$_D$ +87°. uv max: 239 nm (ε 15350).

THERAP CAT: Glucocorticoid; anti-inflammatory.

4189. Fluphenazine. [69-23-8] 4-[3-[2-(Trifluoromethyl)-10*H*-phenothiazin-10-yl]propyl]-1-piperazineethanol; 1-(2-hydroxyethyl)-4-[3-(trifluoromethyl-10-phenothiazinyl)propyl]piperazine; 10-[3'-[4''-(β-hydroxyethyl)-1''-piperazinyl]propyl]-3-trifluoromethylphenothiazine; 2-(trifluoromethyl)-10-[3-[1-(β-hydroxyethyl)-4-piperazinyl]propyl]phenothiazine; S-94; SQ-4918. $C_{22}H_{26}F_3N_3OS$; mol wt 437.52. C 60.39%, H 5.99%, F 13.03%, N 9.60%, O 3.66%, S 7.33%. Prepn: H. L. Yale, F. Sowinski, *J. Am. Chem. Soc.* **82,** 2039 (1960); **GB 829246**; G. E. Ullyot, **US 3058979** (1960, 1962 both to SKF); **GB 833474** (1960 to Scherico), *C.A.* **54,** 21143e (1960); E. L. Anderson *et al., Arzneim.-Forsch.* **12,** 937 (1962); H. L. Yale, R. C. Merrill, **US 3194733** (1965 to Olin Mathieson). Metabolism: J. Dreyfuss, A. J. Cohen, *J. Pharm. Sci.* **60,** 826 (1971). Comprehensive description of the enanthate ester: K. Florey, *Anal. Profiles Drug Subs.* **2,** 245-262 (1973); of the dihydrochloride: *idem, ibid.* 263-294; of the decanoate ester: G. Clarke, *ibid.* **9,** 275-294 (1980).

Dark brown viscous oil, $bp_{0.5}$ 268-274°; $bp_{0.3}$ 250-252°.

Dihydrochloride. [146-56-5] Anatensol; Dapotum; Lyogen; Moditen; Omca; Pacinol; Permitil; Prolixin; Siqualone; Tensofin; Valamina. $C_{22}H_{26}F_3N_3OS.2HCl$; mol wt 510.44. Crystals from abs ethanol, mp 235-237°. Also reported as mp 224.5-226°.

Decanoate. [5002-47-1] SQ-10733; QD-10733; Modecate. $C_{32}H_{44}F_3N_3O_2S$; mol wt 591.77. Pale yellow-orange, viscous liquid. Slowly crystallizes at room temp. mp 30-32°. Very sol in chloroform, ether, cyclohexane, methanol, ethanol. Insol in water.

Enanthate. [2746-81-8] SQ-16144. $C_{29}H_{38}F_3N_3O_2S$; mol wt 549.69. Pale yellow to yellow-orange viscous liquid or oily solid.

THERAP CAT: Antipsychotic.

4190. Flupirtine. [56995-20-1] [2-Amino-6-[[(4-fluoro-phenyl)methyl]amino]-3-pyridinyl]carbamic acid ethyl ester; 2-amino-6-[(p-fluorobenzyl)amino]-3-pyridinecarbamic acid ethyl ester; D-9998. $C_{15}H_{17}FN_4O_2$; mol wt 304.32. C 59.20%, H 5.63%, F 6.24%, N 18.41%, O 10.51%. Substituted pyridine with central analgesic properties. Prepn: K. Thiele, W. von Bebenburg, **ZA 6902364** (1970 to Degussa); W. von Bebenburg et al., Chem. Ztg. **103**, 387 (1979); eidem, ibid. **105**, 217 (1981). Prepn of maleate: W. von Bebenburg, S. Pauluhn, **BE 890331**; eidem, **US 4481205** (1980, 1984 both to Degussa). Comparison of pharmacology with other analgesics: V. Jakovlev et al., Arzneim.-Forsch. **35**, 30 (1985). Pharmacokinetic studies: K. Obermeier et al., ibid. 60. Effect on driving ability: B. Biehl, ibid. 77. Clinical trials in treatment of cancer pain: W. Scheef, D. Wolf-Gruber, ibid. 75. Efficacy in treatment of pain after hysterectomy: R. A. Moore et al., Br. J. Anaesth. **55**, 429 (1983). Symposium on pharmacology and clinical efficacy: Postgrad. Med. J. **63**, Suppl. 3, 1-113 (1987).

Crystals from isopropanol, mp 115-116°. 5% ethanol soln is colorless, turns green on exposure to air for 20 hours. LD_{50} orally in mice, rats: 617, 1660 mg/kg (Jakovlev).

Hydrochloride. $C_{15}H_{17}FN_4O_2.HCl$. Crystals from water, mp 214-215°. When prepd industrially contains intensely blue by-product.

Maleate. [75507-68-5] Katadolon. $C_{15}H_{17}FN_4O_2.C_4H_4O_4$; mol wt 420.39. Colorless crystals from isopropanol, mp 175.5-176°. Formed as mixture of two crystalline forms A and B; mixtures containing 60-90% A are preferred.

THERAP CAT: Analgesic.

4191. Fluprednidene Acetate. [1255-35-2] (11β)-21-(Ace-tyloxy)-9-fluoro-11,17-dihydroxy-16-methylenepregna-1,4-diene-3,20-dione; 9α-fluoro-11β,17,21-trihydroxy-16-methylenepregna-1,4-diene-3,20-dione 21-acetate; 9α-fluoro-16-methylene-$\Delta^{1,4}$-pregnadiene-11β,17,21-triol-3,20-dione 21-acetate; 16-methylene-9α-fluoroprednisolone 21-acetate; 9α-fluoro-16-methyleneprednisolone 21-acetate; fluprednylidene 21-acetate; StL-1106; Etacortin; Decoderm. $C_{24}H_{29}FO_6$; mol wt 432.48. C 66.65%, H 6.76%, F 4.39%, O 22.20%. Prepn: Taub et al., J. Org. Chem. **25**, 2258 (1960); **29**, 3486 (1964); v. Werder et al., Arzneim.-Forsch. **18**, 7 (1968); Wendler, Taub; Taub, Wendler; Taub et al.; Wendler et al., **US 3065239**;

US **3068224**; US **3068226** and US **3136760** (1960 and 1964 to Merck & Co.).

Crystals, mp 231-234°. $[\alpha]_D$ +43° ($CHCl_3$); $[\alpha]_D$ +32° (dioxane) (v. Werder). uv max (methanol): 238 nm (ε 15700).

THERAP CAT: Anti-inflammatory (topical).

4192. Fluprednisolone. [53-34-9] (6α,11β)-6-Fluoro-11,17,21-trihydroxypregna-1,4-diene-3,20-dione; 6α-fluoropredni-solone; 6α-fluoro-1,4-pregnadiene-11β,17α,21-triol-3,20-dione; 6α-fluoro-1-dehydrohydrocortisone; U-7800; NSC-47439; Etadrol. $C_{21}H_{27}FO_5$; mol wt 378.43. C 66.65%, H 7.19%, F 5.02%, O 21.14%. Prepn: Hogg, Spero, **US 2841600** (1958 to Upjohn); Batres et al., **DE 1079042** (1960 to Syntex); Lettré, Hotz, **DE 1088953** (1960 to Bayer).

Crystals, mp 208-213°. $[\alpha]_D$ +92°.

21-Acetate. $C_{23}H_{29}FO_6$. Crystals, mp 235-238°.

THERAP CAT: Glucocorticoid; anti-inflammatory.

THERAP CAT (VET): Anti-inflammatory.

4193. Fluproquazone. [40507-23-1] 4-(4-Fluorophenyl)-7-methyl-1-(1-methylethyl)-2(1H)-quinazolinone; 1-isopropyl-7-methyl-4-(p-fluorophenyl)-2(1H)-quinazolinone; RF-46-790; Tormosyl. $C_{18}H_{17}FN_2O$; mol wt 296.34. C 72.95%, H 5.78%, F 6.41%, N 9.45%, O 5.40%. Fluoro analog of proquazone, q.v. Prepn: G. E. Hardtmann et al., **DE 2230393** (1973 to Sandoz), C.A. **78**, 111363a (1973); G. E. Hardtmann, **US 3937705** (1976 to Sandoz). Analgesic effect: U. Herrmann et al., Clin. Pharmacol. Ther. **27**, 379 (1980); B. von Graffenried, E. Nuesch, Br. J. Clin. Pharmacol. **10**, Suppl. 2, 225 (1980). Series of articles on pharmacology, metabolism, analysis, clinical studies, toxicology: Arzneim.-Forsch. **31**, 871-940 (1981). Toxicity: G. Rüttimann et al., Arzneim.-Forsch. **31**, 882 (1981).

Crystals, mp 172-174°. LD_{50} in mice, rats, rabbits (mg/kg): >5000, >3000, 742 orally (Rüttimann).

THERAP CAT: Analgesic.

4194. **Fluprostenol.** [40666-16-8] (5Z)-rel-7-[(1R,2R,3R,-5S)-3,5-Dihydroxy-2-[(1E,3R)-3-hydroxy-4-[3-(trifluoromethyl)-phenoxy]-1-butenyl]cyclopentyl]-5-heptenoic acid; ICI-81008; Equimate. $C_{23}H_{29}F_3O_6$; mol wt 458.47. C 60.25%, H 6.38%, F 12.43%, O 20.94%. Potent luteolytic agent related to prostaglandin $F_{2\alpha}$, q.v.: Dukes, Walpole, Nature **250**, 330 (1974). Prepn: Binder et al., Prostaglandins **6**, 87 (1974). Induction of estrus and luteolysis in mares: Cooper, Farr, Vet. Rec. **94**, 161 (1974); Berwyn-Jones, Irvine, N. Z. Vet. J. **22**, 107 (1974).

Sodium salt. [55028-71-2] ICI-80008. $C_{23}H_{28}F_3NaO_6$; mol wt 480.45.

THERAP CAT (VET): Treatment of infertility in mares.

4195. **Flupyrsulfuron-methyl.** [144740-53-4] 2-[[[[(4,6-Dimethoxy-2-pyrimidinyl)amino]carbonyl]amino]sulfonyl]-6-(trifluoromethyl)-3-pyridinecarboxylic acid methyl ester; methyl 2-[(4,6-dimethoxypyrimidin-2-ylcarbamoyl)sulfamoyl]-6-(trifluoromethyl)nicotinate. $C_{15}H_{14}F_3N_5O_7S$; mol wt 465.36. C 38.71%, H 3.03%, F 12.25%, N 15.05%, O 24.07%, S 6.89%. Sulfonylurea postemergent herbicide which inhibits acetolactate synthetase. Prepn: T. A. Andrea, P. H. T. Liang, **EP 502740**; eidem, **US 5393734** (1992, 1995 both to Du Pont). Description of chemical and biological activities: S. R. Teaney et al., Brighton Crop Prot. Conf. - Weeds **1995**, 49. Metabolism and selectivity: M. K. Koeppe et al., Pestic. Biochem. Physiol. **59**, 105 (1998). LC determn in soil and water: C. R. Powley, P. A. de Bernard, J. Agric. Food Chem. **46**, 514 (1998). Environmental fate: S. K. Singles et al., Pestic. Sci. **55**, 288 (1999).

Solid, mp 130-137°.
Sodium salt. [144740-54-5] DPX-KE459; Lexus; Millenium. $C_{15}H_{13}F_3N_5NaO_7S$; mol wt 487.34. Solid, mp 172-173°. Most stable in aqueous solutions, pH 5-7; stable in most organic solvents including methanol, acetonitrile, acetone, ethyl acetate and methylene chloride. Soly in water at 25° (ppm): 62.7 (pH 5); 603 (pH 7). pKa: 4.9. LD_{50} in rats, Japanese quail, mallard duck (mg/kg): >5000, >2250, >2250 orally; in rabbits (mg/kg): >2000 dermally. LC_{50} (96hr) in rainbow trout, carp (mg/l): 470, 820; LC_{50} in rats (mg/l): >5.8 by inhalation (Teaney).
USE: Herbicide.

4196. **Fluquinconazole.** [136426-54-5] 3-(2,4-Dichlorophenyl)-6-fluoro-2-(1H-1,2,4-triazol-1-yl)-4(3H)-quinazolinone; SN-597265; Castellan; Jockey; Vista. $C_{16}H_8Cl_2FN_5O$; mol wt 376.17. C 51.09%, H 2.14%, Cl 18.85%, F 5.05%, N 18.62%, O 4.25%. Prepn: D. E. Green, A. Percival, **EP 183458**; eidem, **US 4731106** (1985, 1988 both to Schering Agrochem). Chemical and biological properties: P. E. Russell et al., Brighton Crop Prot. Conf. - Pests Dis. **1992**, 411. Fungicidal activity: G. Schnabel, L. Parisi, Acta Hortic. **466**, 83 (1998). Efficacy against root disease, Take-all, in seed treatment: M. Wenz et al., Brighton Crop Prot. Conf. - Pests Dis. **1998**, 907; in various crop stages: A. M. Löchel et al., ibid. 89.

Review of residue analysis: R. Hänel et al., Nachrichtenbl. Dtsch. Pflanzenschutzdienst **50**, 118 -126 (1998).

Off-white particulate, mp 191.5-193°. Soly at 20° (g/l): water 0.001; acetone 44; xylene 10; ethanol 3; DMSO 150. Log P (octanol/water): 3.4. Vapor pressure (20°): 6.4×10^{-9} Pa. LD_{50} in male, female mice, male, female rats (mg/kg): 325, 180, 112, 112 orally; in male, female rats (mg/kg): 2679, 625 dermally (Russell).
USE: Agricultural fungicide primarily for cereal crops.

4197. **Flurandrenolide.** [1524-88-5] (6α,11β,16α)-6-Fluoro-11,21-dihydroxy-16,17-[(1-methylethylidene)bis(oxy)]pregn-4-ene-3,20-dione; 6α-fluoro-11β,16α,17,21-tetrahydroxypregn-4-ene-3,20-dione cyclic 16,17-acetal with acetone; 6α-fluoro-16α,17α-isopropylidenedioxy-4-pregnene-11β,21-diol-3,20-dione; 6α-fluoro-11β,16α,17,21-tetrahydroxyprogesterone cyclic 16,17-acetal with acetone; fludroxycortide; flurandrenolone; flurandrenolone; flurandrenolone acetonide; Cordran; Drenison; Drocort; Sermaka. $C_{24}H_{33}FO_6$; mol wt 436.51. C 66.04%, H 7.62%, F 4.35%, O 21.99%. Prepn: H. J. Ringold et al., **DE 1131213**; eidem, **US 3126375** (1962, 1964 both to Syntex). HPLC determn in pharmaceutical cream: R. Pearlman et al., Int. J. Pharm. **18**, 53 (1984); in urine: E. Neufeld et al., J. Chromatogr. B **718**, 273 (1998). Clinical trial in psoriasis: G. G. Krueger et al., J. Am. Acad. Dermatol. **38**, 186 (1998).

Crystals from acetone + hexane, mp 247-255°. $[\alpha]_D$ +140-150° (CHCl_3). uv max: 236 nm (log ε 4.17).
THERAP CAT: Glucocorticoid; antipsoriatic.

4198. **Flurazepam.** [17617-23-1] 7-Chloro-1-[2-(diethylamino)ethyl]-5-(2-fluorophenyl)-1,3-dihydro-2H-1,4-benzodiazepin-2-one; Felmane; Noctosom; Stauroderm. $C_{21}H_{23}ClFN_3O$; mol wt 387.88. C 65.03%, H 5.98%, Cl 9.14%, F 4.90%, N 10.83%, O 4.12%. Prepn: G. A. Archer et al., **BE 629005** C.A. **60**, 15896f (1964); **NL 6401335** C.A. **62**, 5289a (1965); G. A. Archer et al., **US 3299053** (1963, 1964, 1967 all to Hoffmann-La Roche). Manuf process: R. Fryer, L. H. Sternbach, **US 3567710** (1971 to Hoffmann-La Roche). Synthesis: S. Inaba et al., Chem. Pharm. Bull. **19**, 263 (1971). Structure-activity studies: L. H. Sternbach et al., J. Med. Chem. **8**, 815 (1965); Armagnac et al., Therapie **26**, 439 (1971). Metabolism: Schwartz et al., J. Med. Chem. **11**, 770 (1968); eidem, J. Pharm. Sci. **59**, 1800 (1970). Pharmacology: L. O. Randall et al., Arch. Int. Pharmacodyn. Ther. **178**, 216 (1969). Toxicology: H. C. Rosenberg, Pharmacol. Biochem. Behav. **13**, 415 (1980). GC determn in plasma: Z. Salama et al., Arzneim.-Forsch. **38**, 400 (1988). Comprehensive description: B. C. Rudy, B. Z. Senkowski, Anal. Profiles Drug Subs. **3**, 307-331 (1974).

White rods from ether-petr ether, mp 77-82°.
Dihydrochloride. [1172-18-5] Flurazepam hydrochloride; Ro-5-6901; Benozil; Dalmadorm; Dalmane; Dalmate; Dormodor; Feli-

son; Insumin; Lunipax; Somlan. $C_{21}H_{23}ClFN_3O.2HCl$; mol wt 460.80. Pale yellow crystals from methanol + ether, mp 190-220°. LD_{50} in mice (mg/kg): 290 i.p.; 870 orally; 84 i.v. (Randall).

Note: This is a controlled substance (depressant): **21 CFR,** 1308.14.

THERAP CAT: Sedative, hypnotic.

4199. Flurbiprofen. [5104-49-4] 2-Fluoro-α-methyl[1,1'-biphenyl]-4-acetic acid; 2-(2-fluoro-4-biphenylyl)propionic acid; 3-fluoro-4-phenylhydratropic acid; BTS-18322; U-27182; Adfeed; Ansaid; Antadys; Cebutid; Froben; Flurofen; Ocufen; Stayban; Zepolas. $C_{15}H_{13}FO_2$; mol wt 244.26. C 73.76%, H 5.36%, F 7.78%, O 13.10%. Prepn: **FR M5737**; Adams *et al.,* **US 3755427** (1968, 1973 both to Boots Co., Ltd.). Pharmacology: Chalmers *et al., Ann. Rheum. Dis.* **31,** 319 (1972); *ibid.* **32,** 58 (1973); Glenn *et al., Agents Actions* **3,** 210 (1973); Nishizawa *et al., Thromb. Res.* **3,** 577 (1973). HPLC determn in urine and plasma: J. M. Hutzler *et al., J. Chromatogr. B* **749,** 119 (2000). Symposium on pharmacokinetics and clinical efficacy in pain management: *Am. J. Med.* **80,** Suppl. 3A, 1-157 (1986).

Crystals from petr ether, mp 110-111°. Slightly sol in water (pH 7.0); readily sol in most polar solvents.

THERAP CAT: Anti-inflammatory; analgesic.

4200. Flurogestone Acetate. [2529-45-5] (11β)-17-(Acetyloxy)-9-fluoro-11-hydroxypregn-4-ene-3,20-dione; 9-fluoro-11β,17-dihydroxypregn-4-ene-3,20-dione-17-acetate; 17α-acetoxy-9α-fluoro-11β-hydroxyprogesterone; 9-fluoro-11β,17-dihydroxyprogesterone 17-acetate; flugestone acetate; SC-9880; Chronogest; Cronolone; Synchronate. $C_{23}H_{31}FO_5$; mol wt 406.49. C 67.96%, H 7.69%, F 4.67%, O 19.68%. Prepn: Bergstrom *et al., J. Am. Chem. Soc.* **81,** 4432 (1959); Bergstrom, Dodson; Bergstrom, Nicholson, **US 2892851**; **US 2963498** (1959, 1960 to Searle).

Crystals from benzene + petr ether, or ethyl acetate + petr ether, mp 266-269°. [α]$_D$ +77.6° (in chloroform). uv max (methanol): 238 nm (ε 17500).

Component of *Syncro-Mate.*

THERAP CAT: Progestogen.

THERAP CAT (VET): Progestogen. Estrus regulation.

4201. Flurothyl. [333-36-8] 1,1'-Oxybis[2,2,2-trifluoroethane]; bis(2,2,2-trifluoroethyl) ether; hexafluorodiethyl ether; bis(trifluoroethyl) ether; Indoklon. $C_4H_4F_6O$; mol wt 182.06. C

26.39%, H 2.21%, F 62.61%, O 8.79%. $CF_3CH_2OCH_2CF_3$. Prepn: **GB 814493** (1959 to Pennsalt Chem.); **GB 889282** (1962 to Air Reduction). Toxicology in animals: A. Cherkin, *Psychopharmacologia* **15,** 404 (1969). Review of pharmacology: L. Arce, *Psychosomatics* **11,** 358-360 (1970); of clinical trials in psychiatric convulsant therapy: J. G. Small, I. F. Small, *Semin. Psychiatry* **4,** 13-26 (1972).

Colorless, mobile liq, mild ethereal, pleasant odor. d_4^{20} 1.41. bp 63.9°. Practically insol in water. Sol in alcohol.

THERAP CAT: CNS stimulant.

4202. Fluroxene. [406-90-6] (2,2,2-Trifluoroethoxy)-ethene; 2,2,2-trifluoroethyl vinyl ether; Fluoromar (formerly). $C_4H_5F_3O$; mol wt 126.08. C 38.11%, H 4.00%, F 45.21%, O 12.69%. $CF_3CH_2OCH=CH_2$. First clinical fluorinated inhalation anesthetic agent. Prepd (not claimed): J. G. Shukys, **US 2830007**; P. W. Townsend, **US 2870218** (1958, 1959 to Air Reduction). Anesthetic action: J. C. Krantz, Jr. *et al., J. Pharmacol. Exp. Ther.* **108,** 488 (1953). Review of metabolism and toxicity: V. Fiserova-Bergerova, *Environ. Health Perspect.* **21,** 225-230 (1977); L. S. Kaminsky, J. M. Fraser, *Crit. Rev. Toxicol.* **19,** 87-112 (1988).

Liquid. bp$_{751}$ 42.5°. n_D^{20} 3.3192. d_4^{20} 1.135. *Potentially explosive.*

Caution: Potential symptoms of overexposure are eye irritation; CNS depression, analgesia, anesthesia, seizures, respiratory depression. *See NIOSH Pocket Guide to Chemical Hazards* (DHHS/-NIOSH 97-140, 1997) p 146.

THERAP CAT: Formerly as anesthetic (inhalation).

4203. Fluroxypyr. [69377-81-7] [(4-Amino-3,5-dichloro-6-fluoro-2-pyridinyl)oxy]acetic acid. $C_7H_5Cl_2FN_2O_3$; mol wt 255.03. C 32.97%, H 1.98%, Cl 27.80%, F 7.45%, N 10.98%, O 18.82%. Auxin-type herbicide for use in cereals. Prepn: S. D. McGregor, **US 3761486** (1973 to Dow). Description: J. A. Paul *et al., Proc. Br. Crop Prot. Conf. - Weeds* **1985,** 939. Field trials in grassland: A. R. Thompson, *ibid.* **1987,** 735. Mode of action: G. E. Sanders, K. E. Pallet, *Ann. Appl. Biol.* **111,** 385 (1987). HPLC determn: R. G. Lehmann, J. R. Miller, *J. Chromatogr.* **485,** 581 (1989). Persistence in soil: L. F. Bergström *et al., Pestic. Sci.* **29,** 405 (1990). Uptake and metabolism in weeds: R. L. MacDonald *et al., Weed Res.* **34,** 333 (1994).

White crystalline solid, mp 232-233°. Vapor pressure (25°): 9.42×10^{-7} mm Hg. Soly at 20° (g/l): water 0.091; acetone 41.6. LD_{50} orally in rats: 2405 mg/kg; i.p. in male, female rats: 458, 519 mg/kg; percutaneous in rabbits >5000 mg/kg (Paul).

1-Methylheptyl ester. [81406-37-3] Fluroxypyr-meptyl; Dowco 433; Spotlight; Starane; Vista; WideMatch S. $C_{15}H_{21}Cl_2FN_2O_3$; mol wt 367.24.

USE: Herbicide.

4204. Flurprimidol. [56425-91-3] α-(1-Methylethyl)-α-[4-(trifluoromethoxy)phenyl]-5-pyrimidinemethanol; α-isopropyl-α-[p-(trifluoromethoxy)phenyl]-5-pyrimidinemethanol; Compd 72500; EL-500; Cutless. $C_{15}H_{15}F_3N_2O_2$; mol wt 312.29. C 57.69%, H 4.84%, F 18.25%, N 8.97%, O 10.25%. Growth regulator for use on established turfgrass. Prepn: R. L. Benefiel, **BE 815245** (1974 to Lilly), *C.A.* **83,** 97354t (1975); R. L. Benefiel, E. V. Krumkalns, **US 3967949**, **US 4002628** (1976, 1977 both to Lilly). Growth retardant properties, effect on turfgrass: L. G. Thompson, *Proc. West. Soc. Weed Sci.* **35,** 113 (1982). Effect on Kentucky bluegrass, comparison with other growth retardants: T. L. Watschke, *Proc. Annu. Meet. Northeast. Weed Sci. Soc.* **35,** 322 (1981); N. E. Christians, *J. Am. Soc. Hortic. Sci.* **110,** 765 (1985). Long term study of effect on bluegrass-fescue turf: P. H. Dernoeden, *Agron. J.* **76,** 807 (1984). Efficacy in dwarfing southern pine seedlings: R. C. Hare, *Can. J. For. Res.* **14,** 123 (1984).

Non-volatile white crystals, mp 94-96°. Sol in acetone, ethanol, methanol, DMSO, diethyl ether. LD_{50} dermally in rabbits: >2000 mg/kg (Thompson).

USE: Growth retardant for grasses.

4205. Flurtamone. [96525-23-4] 5-(Methylamino)-2-phenyl-4-[3-(trifluoromethyl)phenyl]-3(2H)-furanone; 5-methylamino-2-phenyl-4-(α,α,α-trifluoro-m-tolyl)furan-3(2H)-one; RE-40885; Baccara. $C_{18}H_{14}F_3NO_2$; mol wt 333.30. C 64.86%, H 4.23%, F 17.10%, N 4.20%, O 9.60%. Bleaching herbicide; inhibits carotenoid biosynthesis. Prepn: C. E. Ward, **DE 3422346**; idem, **US 4568376** (1984, 1986 both to Chevron). LC determn in soil: T. C. Mueller et al., J. Assoc. Off. Anal. Chem. **73**, 298 (1990). Mode of action study: G. Sandmann et al., Plant Physiol. **94**, 476 (1990). Persistence in soil: T. C. Mueller et al., Weed Sci. **38**, 411 (1990). Crystal structure: G. Pèpe et al., Acta Crystallogr. **C52**, 1514 (1996). Review of physical properties, mode of action, and field trials: D. D. Rogers et al., Proc. Br. Crop Prot. Conf. - Weeds **1987**, 69-75.

Ivory powder, mp 152-155°; also reported as colorless monoclinic crystals. d 1.38 mg/m³. Soly in water at 20°: 35 mg/l; in ethanol at 25°: 9.92 g/g solvent. Sol in acetone, methanol, methylene chloride. Slightly sol in isopropanol. LD_{50} in rats (mg/kg): 500 orally; in rabbits (mg/kg): 500 dermally (Rogers).

USE: Herbicide.

4206. Flusilazole. [85509-19-9] 1-[[Bis(4-fluorophenyl)-methylsilyl]methyl]-1H-1,2,4-triazole; bis(4-fluorophenyl)methyl(1H-1,2,4-triazol-1-ylmethyl)silane; fluzilazol; DPX-H6573; Nustar; Olymp; Punch. $C_{16}H_{15}F_2N_3Si$; mol wt 315.39. C 60.93%, H 4.79%, F 12.05%, N 13.32%, Si 8.91%. Sterol-inhibiting, broad spectrum foliar fungicide. Prepn: W. K. Moberg, **EP 68813**; idem, **US 4510136** (1983, 1985 both to Du Pont); W. K. Moberg et al., Pest. Sci. Biotech., Proc. 6th Int. Congr. Pest. Chem., 57 (1987). Field performance, physical properties and toxicity: T. M. Fort, W. K. Moberg, Proc. Br. Crop Prot. Conf. - Pests Dis. **1984**, 413. Field trials against apple scab: A. R. Biggs, J. Warner, Can. J. Plant Pathol. **9**, 41 (1987); and mildew: A. A. J. Swait et al., Tests Agrochem. Cultiv. **8**, 42 (1987).

Crystalline solid, mp 55°. Soly: >2 g/ml in many organic solvents. LD_{50} in male, female rats (mg/kg): 1110, 674 orally; in rabbits >2000 dermally (Fort, Moberg).

USE: Agricultural fungicide.

4207. Fluspirilene. [1841-19-6] 8-[4,4-Bis(4-fluorophenyl)butyl]-1-phenyl-1,3,8-triazaspiro[4.5]decan-4-one; R-6128; Imap; Redeptin. $C_{29}H_{31}F_2N_3O$; mol wt 475.57. C 73.24%, H 6.57%, F 7.99%, N 8.84%, O 3.36%. Prepn: **BE 633914**; P. A. J. Janssen, **US 3238216** (1963, 1966 both to Janssen). HPLC determn: A. H. Hikal, H. I. Al-Shoura, J. Liq. Chromatogr. **5**, 2205 (1982). Metabolism in rat: J. P. P. Heykants, Life Sci. **8**, Part I, 1029 (1969). Pharmacology: P. A. J. Janssen et al., Arzneim.-

Forsch. **20**, 1689 (1970). Calcium channel blocking activity: R. J. Gould et al., Proc. Natl. Acad. Sci. USA **80**, 5122 (1983); J. P. Galizzi et al., ibid. **83**, 7513 (1986). Clinical trials in schizophrenia: H. Immich et al., Arzneim.-Forsch. **20**, 1699 (1970); G. Chouinard et al., J. Clin. Psychopharmacol. **6**, 21 (1986).

White to yellowish amorphous or crystalline solid, mp 187.5-190°. Soly in water: 0.015-0.020 mg/ml. LD_{50} i.m. in rats: 146 ±14 mg/kg (Janssen).

THERAP CAT: Antipsychotic.

4208. Flutamide. [13311-84-7] 2-Methyl-N-[4-nitro-3-(trifluoromethyl)phenyl]propanamide; α,α,α-trifluoro-2-methyl-4'-nitro-m-propionotoluidide; 4'-nitro-3'-trifluoromethylisobutyranilide; niftolid; Sch-13521; Drogenil; Eulexin; Euflex; Flucinom; Flutamin; Fugerel. $C_{11}H_{11}F_3N_2O_3$; mol wt 276.21. C 47.83%, H 4.01%, F 20.63%, N 10.14%, O 17.38%. Prepn: Baker et al., J. Med. Chem. **10**, 93 (1967); Neri, Topliss, **DE 2130450** (1972 to Sherico), C.A. **78**, 58091g (1973); Gold, **DE 2261293**; idem, **US 3847988** (1973, 1974 both to Schering). Activity studies: Neri et al., Endocrinology **91**, 427 (1972); Peets et al., ibid. **94**, 532 (1974); B. A. Gladue, L. G. Clemens, Endocrinology **106**, 1917 (1980). Effect in prostatic cancer: P. C. Sogani, W. F. Whitmore, J. Urol. **122**, 640 (1979). Clinical evaluation in pancreatic cancer: B. A. Greenway, Br. Med. J. **316**, 1935 (1998).

Crystals from benzene, mp 111.5-112.5°.

THERAP CAT: Antiandrogen; antineoplastic (hormonal).

THERAP CAT (VET): Antiandrogen.

4209. Flutazolam. [27060-91-9] 10-Chloro-11b-(2-fluorophenyl)-2,3,7,11b-tetrahydro-7-(2-hydroxyethyl)oxazolo[3,2-d][1,-4]benzodiazepin-6(5H)-one; MS-4101; Ro-7-6102; Coreminal. $C_{19}H_{18}ClFN_2O_3$; mol wt 376.81. C 60.56%, H 4.81%, Cl 9.41%, F 5.04%, N 7.43%, O 12.74%. Tricyclic benzodiazepine deriv. Prepn: **BE 765253**; M. E. Derieg et al., **US 3905956** (1971, 1975 both to Hoffmann-La Roche). Physicochemical properties: A. Ito et al., Iyakuhin Kenkyu **9**, 787 (1978), C.A. **89**, 169013e (1979). Psychopharmacological profile: T. Mitsushima, S. Ueki, Folia Pharmacol. Jpn. **74**, 959 (1978), C.A. **90**, 180083u (1979). Toxicological studies: K. Ishimura et al., Oyo Yakuri **15**, 1081 (1978); eidem, ibid. **16**, 693 (1978), C.A. **90**, 16379z, 145909p (1979).

White prisms from toluene, mp 142-147°. pKa 5.40. Freely sol in chloroform, ethanol. Moderately sol in acetone, benzene, methanol. Practically insol in water.

THERAP CAT: Anxiolytic.

4210. Fluthiacet-methyl. [117337-19-6] [[2-Chloro-4-fluoro-5-[(tetrahydro-3-oxo-1*H*,3*H*-[1,3,4]thiadiazolo[3,4-*a*]pyridazin-1-ylidene)amino]phenyl]thio]acetic acid methyl ester; 9-(4-chloro-2-fluoro-5-methoxycarbonylmethylthiophenylimino)-8-thia-1,6-diazabicyclo-[4.3.0]nonane-7-one; KIH-9201; CGA-248757; Action. C₁₅H₁₅ClFN₃O₃S₂; mol wt 403.88. C 44.61%, H 3.74%, Cl 8.78%, F 4.70%, N 10.40%, O 11.88%, S 15.88%. Selective, post-emergence, isourazole herbicide which upon conversion to the urazole inhibits protoporphyrinogen oxidase. Prepn: M. Yamaguchi *et al.*, **EP 273417**; *eidem*, **US 4906279** (1988, 1990 both to Kumiai Chem. Ind.; Ihara Chem. Ind.). Description of physical properties, toxicity, and activity: T. Miyazawa *et al.*, *Brighton Crop Prot. Conf. - Weeds* **1993**, 23. Conversion to active metabolite and mode of action study: T. Shimizu *et al.*, *Plant Cell Physiol.* **36,** 625 (1995). Field study as harvest-aid for cotton: R. G. Lemon *et al.*, *Proc. Beltwide Cotton Conf.* **1999,** 605.

White powder, mp 104.6°. Soly in water at 29°: 0.64 mg/l. Vapor pressure: 9.2×10^{-6} Pa. Log P (octanol/water): 3.55. LD₅₀ in rats (mg/kg): >5000 orally; >2000 dermally (Miyazawa).

USE: Herbicide.

4211. Fluticasone Propionate. [80474-14-2] (6α,11β,16α,-17α)-6,9-Difluoro-11-hydroxy-16-methyl-3-oxo-17-(1-oxopropoxy)androsta-1,4-diene-17-carbothioic acid *S*-(fluoromethyl) ester; *S*-fluoromethyl 6α,9α-difluoro-11β-hydroxy-16α-methyl-17α-propionyloxy-3-oxoandrosta-1,4-diene-17β-carbothioate; CCI-18781; Cutivate; Flixonase; Flixotide; Flonase; Flovent; Flunase. C₂₅H₃₁F₃O₅S; mol wt 500.57. C 59.99%, H 6.24%, F 11.39%, O 15.98%, S 6.41%. Derivative of flumethasone, *q.v.* Prepn: **NL 81 00707**; G. H. Phillipps *et al.*, **US 4335121** (1981, 1982 both to Glaxo). Series of articles on structure-activity, pharmacology and clinical studies: *Respir. Med.* **84,** Suppl. A, 19-35 (1990). Clinical trials in allergic rhinitis: E. O. Meltzer *et al.*, *J. Allergy Clin. Immunol.* **86,** 221 (1990). Evaluation in untreated celiac disease: H. C. Mitchison *et al.*, *Gut* **32,** 260 (1991). Clinical trials in COPD: P. L. Paggiaro *et al.*, *Lancet* **351,** 773 (1998); P. S. Burge *et al.*, *Br. Med. J.* **320,** 1297 (2000). Clinical comparison with zafirlukast, *q.v.*, in persistant asthma: J. H. Brabson *et al.*, *Am. J. Med.* **113,** 15 (2002).

Crystals, mp 272-273° (dec). $[\alpha]_D$ +30° (c = 0.35). Practically insol in water. Freely sol in DMSO, DMF; slightly sol in methanol, 95% ethanol.

THERAP CAT: Antiallergic; antiasthmatic; anti-inflammatory.

4212. Flutolanil. [66332-96-5] *N*-[3-(1-Methylethoxy)-phenyl]-2-(trifluoromethyl)benzamide; *o*-trifluoromethyl-*m'*-isopropoxybenzoic anilide; α,α,α-trifluoro-3'-isopropoxy-*o*-toluanilide; NNF-136; Prostar; Moncut. C₁₇H₁₆F₃NO₂; mol wt 323.31. C 63.15%, H 4.99%, F 17.63%, N 4.33%, O 9.90%. Systemic benzanilide fungicide. Prepn: K. Yabutani *et al.*, **DE 2731522**; *eidem*,

US 4093743 (both 1978 to Nihon Nohyaku). Properties and biological activity: F. Araki, K. Yabutani, *Proc. Br. Crop Prot. Conf. - Pests Dis.* **1981,** 3; F. Araki, *Jpn. Pestic. Inf.* **47,** 23 (1985). Mode of action: K. Motoba *et al.*, *Agric. Biol. Chem.* **52,** 1445 (1988). Degradation study: M. Uchida *et al.*, *J. Pestic. Sci.* **8,** 529 (1983). Control of rice sheath blight: H. Mochizuki *et al.*, *ibid.* **12,** 29 (1987); of fungal diversity on peanuts: R. E. Baird *et al.*, *Phytoprotection* **76,** 101 (1995).

Odorless, white, crystalline solid. mp 108° (Araki, Yabutani), also reported as mp 104-105° (Araki, 1985). Stable in acid and alkaline solutions. Soly at 20° (g/l): water 0.0096; chloroform 341; methanol 480; benzene 131; xylene 29. Vapor pressure at 20°: 1.33×10^{-5} mm Hg. LD₅₀ in male and female rats, male and female mice (mg/kg): >10,000, >10,000 orally; in male and female rats (mg/kg): >5000 dermally (Araki).

USE: Agricultural fungicide.

4213. Flutoprazepam. [25967-29-7] 7-Chloro-1-(cyclopropylmethyl)-5-(2-fluorophenyl)-1,3-dihydro-2*H*-1,4-benzodiazepin-2-one; KB-509; ID-1937; Restar; Restas. C₁₉H₁₆ClFN₂O; mol wt 342.79. C 66.57%, H 4.70%, Cl 10.34%, F 5.54%, N 8.17%, O 4.67%. Benzodiazepine derivative. Prepn: H. Yamamoto *et al.*, **GB 1253368**; *eidem*, **US 3925364** (1971, 1975 both to Sumitomo). New process: T. Okamoto *et al.*, **DE 2151540**; *eidem*, **US 3832344** (1972, 1974 both to Sumitomo). Stability and degradation mechanism in aqueous solns: K. Akimoto *et al.*, *Int. J. Pharm.* **3,** 109 (1979). Pharmacokinetics and metabolism: A. Kozaki *et al.*, *Yakugaku Zasshi* **102,** 1177 (1982), *C.A.* **98,** 119080q (1983). Pharmacology of flutoprazepam and metabolites: K. Oki *et al.*, *Arch. Int. Pharmacodyn. Ther.* **269,** 180 (1984). Acute toxicity study: H. Takebe *et al.*, *Oyo Yakuri* **20,** 1055 (1980), *C.A.* **95,** 73630b (1981).

Crystals, mp 118-122°. LD₅₀ in male, female mice, rats (mg/kg): 2640, 2430, 13760, 10060 orally; 2400, 2110, 2460, 2230 i.p.; >5000 s.c. all species (Takebe).

THERAP CAT: Anxiolytic.

4214. Flutriafol. [76674-21-0] α-(2-Fluorophenyl)-α-(4-fluorophenyl)-1*H*-1,2,4-triazole-1-ethanol; (RS)-2,4'-difluoro-α-(1*H*-1,2,4-triazol-1-ylmethyl)benzhydryl alcohol; flutriafen; R-152450; PP-450; Impact. C₁₆H₁₃F₂N₃O; mol wt 301.29. C 63.78%, H 4.35%, F 12.61%, N 13.95%, O 5.31%. Prepn: K. P. Parry *et al.*, **EP 15756** (1980 to ICI). Activity, physical properties, and toxicology: A. M. Skidmore *et al.*, *Proc. 10th Int. Congr. Plant Prot.* **1,** 368 (1983). Mode of action: B. C. Baldwin *et al.*, *Meded. Fac. Landbouwwet. Rijksuniv. Gent* **49,** 303 (1984). Field trials: P. J. Northwood *et al.*, *Proc. 10th Int. Congr. Plant Prot.* **3,** 930 (1983); J. S. Brown, *Crop Prot.* **6,** 157 (1987).

White crystalline solid, mp 130°. Vapor pressure at 20°: 3.00×10^{-9} mm Hg. Soly at 20° (g/l): acetone 190; dichloromethane 150; hexane 0.30; methanol 69; xylene 12; water (pH 7.0) 0.13. LD$_{50}$ male, female rats (mg/kg): 1140, 1480 orally; rats, rabbits: >1000, >2000 percutaneously (Skidmore).

USE: Agricultural fungicide.

4215. Flutrimazole. [119006-77-8] 1-[(2-Fluorophenyl)(4-fluorophenyl)phenylmethyl]-1H-imidazole; 1-[o-fluoro-α-(p-fluorophenyl)-α-phenylbenzyl]imidazole; UR-4056; Micetal. C$_{22}$H$_{16}$F$_2$N$_2$; mol wt 346.37. C 76.29%, H 4.66%, F 10.97%, N 8.09%. Prepn: J. Bartroli, M. Anguita, EP 352352; eidem, US 5149707 (1990, 1992 both to Uriach). Series of articles on synthesis, antifungal activity, pharmacokinetics: Arzneim.-Forsch. 42, 832-863 (1992). Toxicity study: M. L. Vericat et al., ibid. 841. Clinical trial in dermatomycoses: O. Binet et al., Mycoses 37, 455 (1994).

Crystals from acetonitrile, mp 164-167°. Also reported as white solid, mp 161-163°. LD$_{50}$ in male, female mice, male, female rats (mg/kg): >1000, >1000, 808, 1214 orally; >2000, >2000, 1079, 1446 i.p. (Vericat).

THERAP CAT: Antifungal (topical).

4216. Flutropium Bromide. [63516-07-4] (endo,syn)-8-(2-Fluoroethyl)-3-[(hydroxydiphenylacetyl)oxy]-8-methyl-8-azoniabicyclo[3.2.1]octane bromide; (8r)-3α-benziloyloxy-8-(2-fluoroethyl)-8-methyl-8-azoniabicyclo[3.2.1]octane bromide; (8r)-8-(2-fluoroethyl)-3α-hydroxy-1αH,5αH-tropanium bromide benzilate; N-β-fluoroethylnortropine benzilate methobromide; benzilic acid N-β-fluoroethylnortropine ester methobromide; Ba-598Br; Flubron. C$_{24}$H$_{29}$BrFNO$_3$; mol wt 478.39. C 60.26%, H 6.11%, Br 16.70%, F 3.97%, N 2.93%, O 10.03%. Anticholinergic agent. Prepn: R. Banholzer et al., DE 2540633; eidem, US 4042700 (both 1977 to Boehringer, Ing.). Synthesis: R. Banholzer et al., Arzneim.-Forsch. 36, 1161 (1986). Molecular and crystal structure: G. Kiel, ibid. 1166. Pharmacology in animals: S. Yanaura et al., Jpn. J. Pharmacol. 33, 971 (1983); R. Bauer, A. Fügner, Arzneim.-Forsch. 36, 1348 (1986). Pharmacodynamics: K. Yoshimura et al., Iyakuhin Kenkyu 18, 240 (1987), C.A. 107, 17197v (1987).

White crystals from acetonitrile, mp 192-193° (dec); from ethanol-acetone, mp 198-199° (dec). LD$_{50}$ in male, female mice, male, female rats (mg/kg): 12.5, 11.0, 16.4, 18.4 i.v.; 760, 810, 830, 740 orally (Bauer, Fügner).

THERAP CAT: Bronchodilator.

4217. Fluvalinate. [69409-94-5] N-[2-Chloro-4-(trifluoromethyl)phenyl]-DL-valine cyano(3-phenoxyphenyl)methyl ester; ZR-3210; Mavrik. C$_{26}$H$_{22}$ClF$_3$N$_2$O$_3$; mol wt 502.91. C 62.09%, H 4.41%, Cl 7.05%, F 11.33%, N 5.57%, O 9.54%. Synthetic pyrethroid insecticide without the usual cyclopropane ring. Prepn: C. A. Henrick, B. A. Garcia, DE 2812169 (1978 to Zoecon), C.A. 90, 122072d (1970). Activity: C. A. Henrick et al.,

Pestic. Sci. 11, 224 (1980). Review of toxicology and human exposure: Toxicological Profile for Pyrethrins and Pyrethroids (PB2004-100004, 2003) 332 pp.

Yellow-amber liquid. Vapor press. at 25°: 1×10^{-7} mm Hg. Soly in water: 2.0 ppb. Sol in organic solvents.

USE: Insecticide.

4218. Fluvastatin. [93957-54-1] (3R,5S,6E)-rel-7-[3-(4-Fluorophenyl)-1-(1-methylethyl)-1H-indol-2-yl]-3,5-dihydroxy-6-heptenoic acid; ($\pm$)-(3R*,5S*,6E)-7-[3-(p-fluorophenyl)-1-isopropylindol-2-yl]-3,5-dihydroxy-6-heptenoate. C$_{24}$H$_{26}$FNO$_4$; mol wt 411.47. C 70.06%, H 6.37%, F 4.62%, N 3.40%, O 15.55%. Synthetic HMG-CoA reductase inhibitor. Prepn: F. G. Kathawala, WO 8402131; idem, US 4739073 (1984, 1988 both to Sandoz). Clinical pharmacology: J. Yuan et al., Atherosclerosis 87, 147 (1991). Clinical pharmacokinetics: F. L. S. Tse et al., J. Clin. Pharmacol. 32, 630 (1992). Metabolism in humans: J. G. Dain et al., Drug Metab. Dispos. 21, 567 (1993). HPLC determn in plasma: G. Kalafsky et al., J. Chromatogr. 614, 307 (1993). Clinical study in familial hypercholesterolaemia: E. Leitersdorf et al., Eur. J. Clin. Pharmacol. 45, 513 (1993); in prevention of cardiac events following percutaneous coronary intervention: P. W. J. Serruys et al., J. Am. Med. Assoc. 287, 3215 (2002). Review of pharmacology and therapeutic use: R. I. Levy et al., Circulation 87, Suppl. III, III-45–III-53 (1993).

Sodium salt. [93957-55-2] Fluindostatin; XU 62-320; Lescol; Lipaxan; Primexin. C$_{24}$H$_{25}$FNNaO$_4$; mol wt 433.45. mp 194-197°.

THERAP CAT: Antilipemic.

4219. Fluvoxamine. [54739-18-3] (E)-5-Methoxy-1-[4-(trifluoromethyl)phenyl]-1-pentanone O-(2-aminoethyl)oxime; 5-methoxy-4'-(trifluoromethyl)valerophenone (E)-O-(2-aminoethyl)-oxime. C$_{15}$H$_{21}$F$_3$N$_2$O$_2$; mol wt 318.33. C 56.60%, H 6.65%, F 17.90%, N 8.80%, O 10.05%. Selective serotonin reuptake inhibitor (SSRI). Prepn: NL 7503310; H. B. A. Welle, V. Claassen, US 4085225 (1975, 1978 both to Philips-Duphar). Inhibition of 5-HT uptake: V. Claassen et al., Br. J. Pharmacol. 60, 505 (1977). HPLC determn in plasma: G. J. De Jong, J. Chromatogr. 183, 203 (1980). Series of articles on pharmacology, pharmacokinetics and clinical trials in depression: Br. J. Clin. Pharmacol. 15, Suppl. 3, 347S-450S (1983). Clinical trial in obsessive-compulsive disorder: L. M. Koran et al., J. Clin. Psychopharmacol. 16, 121 (1996). Review of clinical experience in depression: M. R. Ware, J. Clin. Psychiatry 58, Suppl. 5, 15-23 (1997).

Maleate. [61718-82-9] DU-23000; MK-264; Dumirox; Faverin; Fevarin; Floxyfral; Luvox; Maveral. C$_{15}$H$_{21}$F$_3$N$_2$O$_2$.C$_4$H$_4$-

O_4; mol wt 434.41. Crystals from acetonitrile, mp 120-121.5°. Freely sol in ethanol, chloroform; sparingly sol in water. Practically insol in diethyl ether.

THERAP CAT: Antidepressant; antiobsessional.

4220. FM1-43. [149838-22-2] 4-[2-[4-(Dibutylamino)-phenyl]ethenyl]-1-[3-(triethylammonio)propyl]pyridinium dibromide; Neurodye GH1-43; SynaptoGreen. $C_{30}H_{49}Br_2N_3$; mol wt 611.54. C 58.92%, H 8.08%, Br 26.13%, N 6.87%. Green fluorescent styryl dye that binds to but is not translocated through biological membranes. Prepn and optical activity of *p*-aminostyrylpyridium probes: L. M. Loew *et al., Biochemistry* **17**, 4065 (1978); A. Grinvald *et al., Biophys. J.* **39**, 301 (1982). Optical analysis of synaptic vesicle recycling: W. J. Betz, G. S. Bewick, *Science* **255**, 200 (1992); W. J. Betz *et al., J. Neurosci.* **12**, 363 (1992); *eidem, Curr. Opin. Neurobiol.* **6**, 365 (1996). Interaction with lipid membranes: U. Schote, J. Seelig, *Biochim. Biophys. Acta* **1415**, 135 (1998); with background quenching: A. R. Kay *et al., Neuron* **24**, 809 (1999); J. L. Pyle *et al., ibid.* 803. Use in membrane recycling study: T. J. Diefenbach *et al., J. Neurosci.* **19**, 9436 (1999). Review of use and mechanism of action: M. A. Cousin, P. J. Robinson, *J. Neurochem.* **73**, 2227-2239 (1999).

Red-orange solid. Amphiphilic. Sol in water, DMSO. Practically nonfluorescent in aqueous solutions, becoming fluorescent upon membrane binding. Abs max (methanol): 510 nm (ε 56000). Emission max: 626 nm.

USE: Biological probe for membrane dynamics.

4221. Folic Acid. [59-30-3] *N*-[4-[[(2-Amino-1,4-dihydro-4-oxo-6-pteridinyl)methyl]amino]benzoyl]-L-glutamic acid; *N*-[*p*-[[(2-amino-4-hydroxy-6-pteridinyl)methyl]amino]benzoyl]glutamic acid; pteroylglutamic acid; *N*-(*p*-[2-amino-4-hydroxypyrimido-[4,5-*b*]pyrazin-6-yl)methylamino]benzoyl)glutamic acid; PGA; liver *Lactobacillus casei* factor; vitamin Bc; vitamin M; folsäure; Folacin; Foldine; Foliamin; Folicet; Folipac; Folettes; Folsan; Folvite; Incafolic; Millafol. $C_{19}H_{19}N_7O_6$; mol wt 441.40. C 51.70%, H 4.34%, N 22.21%, O 21.75%. Hematopoietic vitamin present, free or combined with one or more additional molecules of L(+)-glutamic acid, in liver, kidney, mushrooms, spinach, yeast, green leaves, grasses: Mitchell *et al., J. Am. Chem. Soc.* **63**, 2284 (1941). Isoln: Pfiffner *et al., ibid.* **69**, 1476 (1947); Stokstad *et al., ibid.* **70**, 3 (1948). Structure: Mowat *et al., ibid.* 14. Crystal structure: D. Mastropaolo *et al., Science* **210**, 334 (1980). History of the different folic acid factors: *Ann. N.Y. Acad. Sci.* **48**, 255-350 (1946). *See also* reviews by Subbarow *et al.* in *Vitam. Horm.* **3**, 237-296 (1945); Pfiffner, Hogan, *ibid.* **4**, 1-13 (1946). Several syntheses, *see* reviews by Gates, *Chem. Rev.* **41**, 63-95 (1947); Hutchings, Mowat, *Vitam. Horm.* **6**, 1-25 (1948); Sletzinger *et al., J. Am. Chem. Soc.* **77**, 6365 (1955); **US 2786056**; **US 2816109**; **US 2821527**; **US 2821528** (all 1958 to Merck & Co.); Sadao Kawanishi, **US 2956057** (1960 to Kongo Kagaku Kabushiki Kaisha). Alternate syntheses: Bieri, Viscontini, *Helv. Chim. Acta* **56**, 2905 (1973); E. Khalifa *et al., ibid.* **59**, 242 (1976). Comprehensive reviews: Jaenicki, Kutzbach, *Fortschr. Chem. Org. Naturst.* **21**, 183-274 (1963); Marchetti, *Acta Vitaminol. Enzymol.* **25**, 41-64 (1971); F. J. Al-Shammary *et al., Anal. Profiles Drug Subs.* **19**, 221-259 (1990). Review of role in prevention of neural tube defects: G. J. Locksmith, P. Duff, *Obstet. Gynecol.* **91**, 1027-1034 (1998).

Yellowish-orange crystals. Extremely thin platelets (elongated at two ends) from hot water, no mp. Darkens and chars from about 250°. $[\alpha]_D^{25}$ +23° (c = 0.5 in 0.1*N* NaOH). uv max (pH 13): 256, 283, 368 nm (log ε 4.43, 4.40, 3.96). Very slightly sol in cold water (0.0016 mg/ml at 25°), sol to about 1% in boiling water. Slightly sol in methanol, appreciably less sol in ethanol and butanol. Insol in acetone, chloroform, ether, benzene. Relatively sol in acetic acid, phenol, pyridine, solns of alkali hydroxides and carbonates. Sol in hot dil HCl and H_2SO_4. Injectable solns are prepd by dissolving folic acid in normal sodium bicarbonate soln (which should be sterilized by filtration) or by preparing solns of the sodium or methylglucamine salt. A suspension of 1 g folic acid in 10 ml water has a pH of 4.0-4.8. Aq solns prepd with sodium bicarbonate have a pH between 6.5 and 6.8.

THERAP CAT: Vitamin (hematopoietic).

THERAP CAT (VET): Nutritional factor (dietary requirement in poultry).

4222. Folinic Acid. [58-05-9] *N*-[4-[[(2-Amino-5-formyl-1,4,5,6,7,8-hexahydro-4-oxo-6-pteridinyl)methyl]amino]benzoyl]-L-glutamic acid; *N*-[*p*-[[(2-amino-5-formyl-5,6,7,8-tetrahydro-4-hydroxy-6-pteridinyl)methyl]amino]benzoyl]glutamic acid; 5-formyl-5,6,7,8-tetrahydropteroyl-L-glutamic acid; 5-formyl-5,6,7,8-tetrahydrofolic acid; CF; citrovorum factor; leucovorin. $C_{20}H_{23}N_7O_7$; mol wt 473.44. C 50.74%, H 4.90%, N 20.71%, O 23.66%. Intermediate product of the metabolism of folic acid; the active form into which that acid is converted in the body, ascorbic acid being a necessary factor in the conversion process. First reported as the *Leuconostoc citrovorum* 8081 growth factor: H. E. Sauberlich, C. A. Baumann, *J. Biol. Chem.* **176**, 165 (1948). Isoln from houseflies: S. Miller, A. S. Perry, *Life Sci.* **4**, 1573 (1965). Prepn: J. A. Brockman, Jr., *et al., J. Am. Chem. Soc.* **72**, 4325 (1950); E. Khalifa *et al., Helv. Chim. Acta* **63**, 2554 (1980). Isomers: D. B. Cosulich *et al., J. Am. Chem. Soc.* **74**, 4215 (1952). Structure: May *et al., ibid.* **73**, 3067 (1951); Pohland *et al., ibid.* 3247. Manuf: Shive, **US 2741608** (1956 to Res. Corp.). Stereoselective synthesis: J. Owens, *et al., J. Chem. Soc. Perkin Trans. 1* **7**, 871 (1993). Used as an antidote to folic acid antagonists such as methotrexate, *q.v.,* which block the conversion of folic acid into folinic acid. Review of clinical combination therapy with methotrexate: J. R. Bertino *et al., Ann. N.Y. Acad. Sci.* **186**, 486-495 (1971). Pharmacokinetics: P. F. Nixon, *Clin. Exp. Pharmacol. Physiol.* **Suppl. 5**, 35 (1979). Comprehensive description: L. O. Pont *et al., Anal. Profiles Drug Subs.* **8**, 315-350 (1979). Review of clinical synergy with fluorouracil in cancer: R. J. DeLap, *Yale J. Biol. Med.* **61**, 23-34 (1988).

Crystals, dec 240-250°. uv max (0.1*N* NaOH): 282 nm (% T = 27.0 for 10 mg/l). $[\alpha]_D^{20}$ +14.26° (c = 3.42 as anhydr Ca salt). pKa (3 groups): 3.1, 4.8, and 10.4. Sparingly sol in water. pH of satd aq soln 2.8-3.0 at which pH partial decompn takes place. More stable at neutral or mildly alkaline pH.

Calcium salt pentahydrate. [6035-45-6] Calcium folinate; NSC-3590; Folaren; Foliben; Lederfolat; Lederfolin; Leucovorin; Leucosar; Rescufolin; Rescuvolin; Tonofolin; Wellcovorin. $C_{20}H_{21}CaN_7O_7 \cdot 5H_2O$; mol wt 601.58. Off-white to light beige amorphous, odorless powder, freely sol in water. Practically insol in alc. $[\alpha]_D^{21}$ +14.9° (c = 1 in water).

l-**Form calcium salt.** [80433-71-2] Calcium (6*S*)-folinate; calcium levofolinate; levoleucovorin calcium; Elvorine. $[\alpha]_D^{20}$ −15.1° (c = 1.82).

THERAP CAT: Antidote to folic acid antagonists; antianemic (folate deficiency).

4223. Follicle-Stimulating Hormone. [9002-68-0] FSH; follitropin. Gonadotropic hormone secreted by the anterior pituitary under the regulation of gonadotopin-releasing hormone and inhibin, *q.q.v.* In the female, FSH stimulates estrogen production by the granulosa cells of the ovary and induces maturation of the Graafian follicle. In the male, stimulates the Sertoli cells of the testes and promotes spermatogenesis. Glycoprotein with mol wt ~34 kDa; multiple isoforms exist. Structure is a heterodimer of noncovalently linked α and β subunits; analogous with LH, TSH and chorionic gonadotropin, *q.q.v.* Isoln from pituitary: H. L. Fevold *et al., Endocrinology* **26**, 999 (1940); C. H. Li *et al., Science* **109**, 445 (1949). Prepn of human FSH from pituitaries and from postmenopausal urine: P. Roos, *Acta Endocrinol.* **59**, Suppl. 131, 1-93 (1968). Amino acid sequence of human FSH α-subunit: P. Rathnam, B. B. Saxena, *J. Biol. Chem.* **250**, 6735 (1975); of human β-subunit: B. B. Saxena, P. Rathnam, *ibid.* **251**, 993 (1976). Production in Chinese hamster ovary cells by recombinant DNA technology: J. L. Keene *et al., J. Biol. Chem.* **264**, 4769 (1989). Characterization of isoforms: P. G. Stanton *et al., Mol. Cell. Endocrinol.* **125**, 133 (1996). Review of structure, biosynthesis and receptor binding: J. G. Pierce, T. F. Parsons, *Annu. Rev. Biochem.* **50**, 465-495 (1981). Review of role in spermatogenesis: R. I. McLachlan *et al., J. Endocrinol.* **148**, 1-9 (1996); in ovarian function and clinical use: B. C. Fauser, A. M. Van Heusden, *Endocr. Rev.* **18**, 71-106 (1997).

Solid. Isoelectric point 4.5. Soluble in water, physiological saline soln, 50% alc. uv max: 277 nm (pH 7.0 phosphate buffer); 291 nm (0.1*N* NaOH-8*M* urea).

Follitropin Alfa. Gonal-F. Recombinant human FSH, glycoform α. Clinical pharmacokinetics: J.-Y. le Cotonnec *et al., Fertil. Steril.* **61**, 669, 679 (1994). Clinical trial: T. Strowitzki *et al., Hum. Reprod.* **10**, 3097 (1995).

Follitropin Beta. Org-32489; Follistim; Puregon. Recombinant human FSH, glycoform β. Clinical pharmacokinetics: B. Mannaerts *et al., Fertil. Steril.* **59**, 108 (1993). Clinical trial: B. Hedon *et al., Hum. Reprod.* **10**, 3102 (1995).

Menotropins. Menotrophin; human menopausal gonadotropins; Humegon; Menogon; Pergonal; Repronex. Extract of human postmenopausal urine containing both FSH and LH.

Urofollitropin. [97048-13-0] Urofollitrophin; Fertinorm; Metrodin; Orgafol. Purified extract of human postmenopausal urine containing FSH.

THERAP CAT: Gonad-stimulating principle.

THERAP CAT (VET): Gonad-stimulating principle.

4224. Folpet. [133-07-3] 2-[(Trichloromethyl)thio]-1*H*-isoindole-1,3(2*H*)-dione; *N*-(trichloromethylthio)phthalimide; *N*-(trichloromethylmercapto)phthalimide; Phaltan. $C_9H_4Cl_3NO_2S$; mol wt 296.56. C 36.45%, H 1.36%, Cl 35.86%, N 4.72%, O 10.79%, S 10.81%. *Cf:* Captan. Prepn: Kittleson, US 2553770 (1951 to Standard Oil). Toxicity: T. B. Gaines, R. E. Linder, *Fundam. Appl. Toxicol.* **7**, 299 (1986).

'Crystals from benzene, mp 177°. LD_{50} orally in adult male, female rats: >5000 mg/kg (Gaines, Linder).

Caution: May irritate mucosal surfaces. *See Clinical Toxicology of Commercial Products*, R. E. Gosselin *et al.*, Eds. (Williams & Wilkins, Baltimore, 5th ed., 1984) Section II, p 317.

USE: Agricultural fungicide.

4225. Fomecins. Antibacterial substances produced by several strains of the basidiomycete *Fomes juniperinus* Schrenk. Isoln of fomecin A (major) and fomecin B (minor) from cultures grown in corn steep liquor: M. Anchel *et al., Proc. Natl. Acad. Sci. USA* **38**, 655 (1952). Structures: T. C. McMorris, M. Anchel, *Can. J. Chem.* **42**, 1595 (1964). Synthesis of B: S. M. Al-Mousawi *et al., Bull. Soc. Chim. Belg.* **88**, 883 (1979); of A and B: K. Hayashi *et al., Chem. Pharm. Bull.* **28**, 1971 (1980).

Fomecin A R = CH₂OH
Fomecin B R = CHO

Fomecin A. 2,3,4-Trihydroxy-6-(hydroxymethyl)benzaldehyde. $C_8H_8O_5$; mol wt 184.15. Cream-colored to orange crystals from ethanol-water, ethanol-benzene, acetone-benzene, or ethyl acetate. Dec above 160° without melting. Optically inactive in ethanol. uv max (ethanol): 241, 304 nm (ε 10800, 15300). Weakly acidic. Sparingly sol in water (1 mg/ml); slightly more sol in ethanol, acetone, ethyl acetate. Less sol in chloroform, benzene. Aq solns at neutral or acid pH are stable. The activity is lost around pH 8.

Fomecin B. 3,4,5-Trihydroxy-1,2-benzenedicarboxaldehyde. $C_8H_6O_5$; mol wt 182.13. Yellow needles from ethyl acetate. Darkens on heating; mp ~230°. uv max (ethanol): 263, 336 nm (ε 26400, 9200).

4226. Fomepizole. [7554-65-6] 4-Methyl-1*H*-pyrazole; 4-MP; Antizol. $C_4H_6N_2$; mol wt 82.10. C 58.52%, H 7.37%, N 34.12%. Alcohol dehydrogenase inhibitor. Prepn: H. Pechmann, E. Burkard, *Ber.* **33**, 3590 (1900); D. S. Noyce *et al., J. Org. Chem.* **20**, 1681 (1955); T. Momose *et al., Heterocycles* **30**, 789 (1990). Inhibition of human liver alcohol dehydrogenase: T.-K. Li, H. Theorell, *Acta Chem. Scand.* **23**, 892 (1969). Toxicity study: G. Magnusson *et al., Experientia* **28**, 1198 (1972). GC determn in plasma and urine: R. Achari, M. Mayersohn, *J. Pharm. Sci.* **73**, 690 (1984). Clinical pharmacology: D. Jacobsen *et al., Alcohol. Clin. Exp. Res.* **12**, 516 (1988). Pharmacokinetics: *eidem, Eur. J. Clin. Pharmacol.* **37**, 599 (1989). Clinical trial in ethylene glycol poisoning: J. Brent *et al., N. Engl. J. Med.* **340**, 832 (1999); in methanol poisoning: *idem et al., ibid.* **344**, 424 (2001). *Review:* J. Likforman *et al., J. Toxicol. Clin. Exp.* **7**, 373-382 (1987). Review of use in methanol poisoning: M. B. Mycyk, J. B. Leikin, *Am. J. Therapeut.* **10**, 68-70 (2003).

mp 15.5-18.5°. bp₁₈ₘₘ 98.5-99.5°; bp₇₃₀ 204-205°. n_D^{22} 1.4913. uv max in 95% ethanol: 220 nm (log ε 3.47); in 6*N* HCl: 226 nm (log ε 3.65). Sol in water, alcohol. LD_{50} (7 days) in mice, rats (mmol/kg): 3.8, 3.8 i.v.; 7.8, 6.5 orally (Magnusson).

THERAP CAT: Antidote to methanol and ethylene glycol poisoning.

THERAP CAT (VET): Antidote to ethylene glycol poisoning in dogs.

4227. Fomesafen. [72178-02-0] 5-[2-Chloro-4-(trifluoromethyl)phenoxy]-*N*-(methylsulfonyl)-2-nitrobenzamide; Flex; Reflex. $C_{15}H_{10}ClF_3N_2O_6S$; mol wt 438.76. C 41.06%, H 2.30%, Cl 8.08%, F 12.99%, N 6.38%, O 21.88%, S 7.31%. Post-emergence diphenyl ether herbicide used for early control of broad-leaf weeds in soybean and other legume crops. Prepn: D. Cartwright, D. J. Collins, **EP 3416**; *eidem,* US 4285723 (1979, 1981 both to Imperial Chemical Industries). Properties and field trial in soybeans: S. R. Colby, J. W. Barnes, *Proc. 10th Int. Congr. Plant Prot.* **1**, 295 (1983); in green beans: C. M. Knott, *Brighton Crop Prot. Conf. - Weeds* **1993**, 1053. Mode of selectivity and metabolism in plant crops and weeds: J. D. H. L. Evans *et al., Proc. Br. Crop Prot. Conf. - Weeds* **1987**, 345. Metabolism and hepatoxicity in rodents: J. Krijt *et al., Hum. Exp. Toxicol.* **18**, 338 (1999). Environmental fate in soils: J. B. Weber, *Pestic. Sci.* **39**, 31 (1993); J. Guo *et al., Water Air Soil Pollut.* **148**, 77 (2003). Ecotoxicological effects in aquatic systems: T. Caquet *et al., Environ. Toxicol. Chem.* **24**, 1116 (2005).

White crystalline solid, mp 220-221°. pKa 2.9. Soly in distilled water: ~50 mg/l. LD$_{50}$ orally in male, female rats (mg/kg): 1250-2000, 1600; LC$_{50}$ (48, 96 hr.) in rainbow trout and bluegill (mg/l): 830, 680, 6740, 6030 (Colby).

Sodium salt. [108731-70-0] Flexstar. C$_{15}$H$_{10}$ClF$_3$N$_3$NaO$_6$S; mol wt 461.75. Percutaneous absorption: J. Hilton *et al., Pharm. Res.* **11**, 1396 (1994). Soly at 25° (mg/ml): propylene glycol 631; octanol 12; ethyl decanoate 10. LD$_{50}$ orally (mg/kg) in male, female rats, mice: 1860, 1500, 750, 770; in female guinea pigs: 490-980; in male rabbit: 490 (Colby).

USE: Herbicide.

4228. Fominoben. [18053-31-1] *N*-[3-Chloro-2-[[methyl-[2-(4-morpholinyl)-2-oxoethyl]amino]methyl]phenyl]benzamide; 3'-chloro-α-[methyl[(morpholinocarbonyl)methyl]amino]-*o*-benzotoluidide; 3'-chloro-β-[*N*-methyl-*N*-[(morpholinocarbonyl)methyl]aminomethyl]benzanilide. C$_{21}$H$_{24}$ClN$_3$O$_3$; mol wt 401.89. C 62.76%, H 6.02%, Cl 8.82%, N 10.46%, O 11.94%. Prepn: **FR 1482547**; **FR Addn. 92488** (1967, 1968 both to Thomae), *C.A.* **68**, 95494e (1968); **72**, 21938p (1970); Kruger *et al.,* **US 3661903** (1972 to Boehringer, Ing.); *eidem, Arzneim.-Forsch.* **23**, 290 (1973). Series of articles on pharmacology and clinical findings: *ibid.* 296-375. Metabolism: Zimmer, *ibid.* 1798. Toxicity data: S. Püschmann, R. Engelhorn, *ibid.* 296.

Base, mp 122.5-123°.
Hydrochloride. [24600-36-0] PB-89; Finaten; Nopleptan; Oleptan; Terion; Tussirama. C$_{21}$H$_{24}$ClN$_3$O$_3$.HCl; mol wt 438.35. Crystals, mp 206-208° (dec). Soly in water: 0.1 mg/100 ml; in 0.05*N* aq tartaric acid: 5 g/100 ml. LD$_{50}$ in mice, rats (mg/kg): 630, 1201 i.p.; 2200, 1250 orally (Püschmann, Engelhorn).

THERAP CAT: Antitussive; respiratory stimulant.

4229. Fomivirsen. [144245-52-3] d(*P*-Thio)(G-C-G-T-T-T-G-C-T-C-T-T-C-T-T-C-T-T-G-C-G)deoxyribonucleic acid. C$_{204}$-H$_{263}$N$_{63}$O$_{114}$P$_{20}$S$_{20}$; mol wt 6682.40. C 36.67%, H 3.97%, N 13.21%, O 27.29%, P 9.27%, S 9.60%. Synthetic phosphorothioate antisense oligonucleotide designed to inhibit gene expression in human cytomegalovirus (CMV). Consists of 21 nucleotides in a sequence complementary to the specific portion of CMV messenger RNA which encodes regulatory proteins. Prepn: K. P. Anderson, K. G. Draper, **WO 9203456**; *idem et al.,* **US 5442049** (1992, 1995 both to Isis). Large scale synthesis: M. Andrade *et al., Bioorg. Med. Chem. Lett.* **4**, 2017 (1994). Determn in pharmaceutical formulations by capillary gel electrophoresis: G. S. Srivatsa *et al., J. Chromatogr. A* **680**, 469 (1994). Antiviral activity vs human CMV: R. F. Azad *et al., Antimicrob. Agents Chemother.* **37**, 1945 (1993). Mechanism of action study: K. P. Anderson *et al., ibid.* **40**, 2004 (1996). Pharmacokinetics: J. M. Leeds *et al., Drug Metab. Dispos.* **25**, 921 (1997). Retinal toxicity study: M. Flores-Aguilar *et al., J. Infect. Dis.* **175**, 1308 (1997). Review of pharmacology and therapeutic potential: J. Temsamani *et al., Expert Opin. Invest. Drugs* **6**, 1157-1167 (1997). Series of articles on clinical experience for CMV retinitis in AIDS patients: *Am. J. Ophthalmol.* **133**, 467-498 (2002).

Sodium salt. [160369-77-5] ISIS-2922; Vitravene. C$_{204}$H$_{243}$-N$_{63}$Na$_{20}$O$_{114}$P$_{20}$S$_{20}$; mol wt 7122.04.
THERAP CAT: Antiviral.

4230. Fomocaine. [17692-39-6] 4-[3-[4-(Phenoxymethyl)-phenyl]propyl]morpholine; 4-[3-(α-phenoxy-*p*-tolyl)propyl]morpholine; P-652; Erbocain. C$_{20}$H$_{25}$NO$_2$; mol wt 311.42. C 77.14%, H 8.09%, N 4.50%, O 10.28%. Prepn: **GB 786128** (1957 to Promonta), *C.A.* **52**, 9225h (1958); H. Oelschläger, *Arzneim.-Forsch.* **9**, 313 (1959). Improved synthesis: *eidem, ibid.* **27**, 1625 (1977). Pharmacology: O. Nieschulz *et al., ibid.* **8**, 539 (1958). Metabolism: H. Blume, H. Oelschläger, *ibid.* **28**, 956 (1978). Bioavailability and local anesthetic effect: H. Oelschläger, D. Rothley, *ibid.* **29**, 693 (1979).

Colorless crystals from petr ether, mp 52-53°. bp$_{1.1}$ 238-240°. uv max (ethanol): 220, 269 nm (ε 15820, 1373). LD$_{50}$ i.v. in mice: 175 mg/kg (Nieschulz).
THERAP CAT: Anesthetic (local).

4231. Fonazine. [7456-24-8] 10-[2-(Dimethylamino)propyl]-*N*,*N*-dimethyl-10*H*-phenothiazine-2-sulfonamide; 10-(2-dimethylaminopropyl)-3-dimethylsulfamidophenothiazine; 3-dimethylsulfamido-10-(2-dimethylaminopropyl)phenothiazine; dimethiothiazine; dimethiotazine; dimetiotazine; RP-8599. C$_{19}$H$_{25}$N$_3$O$_2$-S$_2$; mol wt 391.55. C 58.28%, H 6.44%, N 10.73%, O 8.17%, S 16.38%. Serotonin inhibitor. Prepn: **GB 814512** (1959 to Rhône-Poulenc). Pharmacokinetics and distribution in dog and rat: O. R. W. Lewellen, R. Templeton, *Adv. Biochem. Psychopharmacol.* **9**, 213 (1974). Clinical evaluation in spasticity: W. B. Matthews *et al., Acta Neurol. Scand.* **48**, 635 (1972). HPLC determn in plasma: J. Holt *et al., Br. J. Clin. Pharmacol.* **13**, 282 (1982).

Hydrochloride. C$_{19}$H$_{25}$N$_3$O$_2$S$_2$.HCl. Crystals, dec 214°.
Methanesulfonate. [7455-39-2] Dimethothiazine mesylate; fonazine mesylate; Banistyl; Bonpac; Calsekin; Migristène; Neomestine; Promaquid; Yoristen. C$_{19}$H$_{25}$N$_3$O$_2$S$_2$.CH$_3$SO$_3$H; mol wt 487.66.
THERAP CAT: Antimigraine.

4232. Fondaparinux Sodium. [114870-03-0] Methyl *O*-2-deoxy-6-*O*-sulfo-2-(sulfoamino)-α-D-glucopyranosyl-(1 → 4)-*O*-β-D-glucopyranuronosyl-(1 → 4)-*O*-2-deoxy-3,6-di-*O*-sulfo-2-(sulfoamino)-α-D-glucopyranosyl-(1 → 4)-*O*-2-*O*-sulfo-α-L-idopyranuronosyl(1 → 4)-2-deoxy-2-(sulfoamino)-α-D-glucopyranoside 6-(hydrogen sulfate) decasodium salt; fondaparin sodium; SR-90107A; Org-31540; IC-851589; Arixtra. C$_{31}$H$_{43}$N$_3$Na$_{10}$O$_{49}$S$_8$; mol wt 1728.08. C 21.55%, H 2.51%, N 2.43%, Na 13.30%, O 45.37%, S 14.84%. Synthetic pentasaccharide corresponding to the antithrombin binding site of heparin, *q.v.* Prepn: M. Petitou *et al.,* **EP 84999**; *eidem,* **US 4818816** (1983, 1989 both to Choay); M. Petitou *et al., Carbohyd. Res.* **167**, 67 (1987). Review of pharmacology: J. M. Herbert *et al., Cardiovasc. Drug Rev.* **15**, 1-26 (1997). Clinical pharmacokinetics: B. Boneu *et al., Thromb. Haemostasis* **74**, 1468 (1995). Clinical trial for prevention of post-operative deep-vein thrombosis: A. G. G. Turpie *et al., N. Engl. J. Med.* **344**, 619 (2001). Clinical comparison with enoxaparin, *q.v.* in treatment of established deep-vein thrombosis: H. R. Büller *et al., Ann. Intern. Med.* **140**, 867 (2004). Review of clinical safety and efficacy: A. G. G. Turpie, *Expert Opin. Drug Saf.* **4**, 707-721 (2005).

White powder after lyophilisation. $[\alpha]_D^{23}$ +48° (c = 0.61 in water). THERAP CAT: Antithrombotic.

4233. Fonofos. [944-22-9] Ethylphosphonodithioic acid *O*-ethyl *S*-phenyl ester; *O*-ethyl *S*-phenyl ethylphosphonothiolothionate; N-2790; Dyfonate. $C_{10}H_{15}OPS_2$; mol wt 246.33. C 48.76%, H 6.14%, O 6.50%, P 12.57%, S 26.03%. Organophosphorus insecticide; cholinesterase inhibitor. Prepn: Szabo *et al.*, **US 2988474** (1961 to Stauffer); H. M. Pitt, R. A. Simone, **DE 2002629**; *eidem*, **US 3642960** (1970, 1972 both to Stauffer). Toxicity and biochemistry of racemate and isomers: P. W. Lee *et al.*, *Pestic. Biochem. Physiol.* **8**, 146 (1978). Acute toxicity data: R. Ben-Dyke *et al.*, *World Rev. Pest Control* **9**, 119 (1970).

Light yellow liquid, bp$_{0.1}$ 130°. d$_{25}^{25}$ 1.16. n_D^{30} 1.5883. Practically insol in water. Miscible with organic solvents. LD$_{50}$ in mice (mg/kg): 14.0 orally, 4.8 i.p. (Lee). LD$_{50}$ in rats (mg/kg): 3-17 orally, 147 dermally (Ben-Dyke).
Caution: Potential symptoms of overexposure are nausea, vomiting, abdominal cramps, diarrhea, salivation; headache, giddiness, vertigo, weakness; rhinorrhea, chest tightness; blurred vision, miosis; cardiac irregularities; muscle fasciculations; dyspnea. See *NIOSH Pocket Guide to Chemical Hazards* (DHHS/NIOSH 97-140, 1997) p 146.
USE: Soil insecticide.

4234. Foramsulfuron. [173159-57-4] 2-[[[[(4,6-Dimethoxy-2-pyrimidinyl)amino]carbonyl]amino]sulfonyl]-4-(formylamino)-*N*,*N*-dimethylbenzamide; AE-F130360; Option. $C_{17}H_{20}N_6O_7S$; mol wt 452.44. C 45.13%, H 4.46%, N 18.57%, O 24.75%, S 7.09%. Sulfonylurea herbicide for use in corn; acetolactate synthase inhibitor. Prepn: G. Schnabel *et al.*, **DE 4415049**; *eidem*, **US 5922646** (1995, 1999 both to Hoechst Schering AgrEvo). Review of properties and activity: B. Collins *et al.*, *BCPC Conf. - Weeds* **2001**, 35-42.

Light beige solid, mp 199.5°. Vapor pressure (20°): 4.2 × 10^{-11} Pa. Log P (octanol/water): 4.01 (pH 5); 0.166 (pH 7); 0.0106 (pH 8). Soly in water at 20° (g/l): 0.04 (pH 5); 3.3 (pH 7); 94.6 (pH 8). LD$_{50}$ in rats (mg/kg): >5000 orally; >2000 dermally (Collins).
USE: Herbicide.

4235. Formaldehyde. [50-00-0] Methanal; oxomethane; oxymethylene; methylene oxide; formic aldehyde; methyl aldehyde. CH_2O; mol wt 30.03. C 40.00%, H 6.71%, O 53.28%. HCHO. Formed by incomplete combustion of many organic substances. Present in coal and wood smoke, esp in smoke as produced for smoking ham and fish. Found in the atm, esp over large cities. Prepd commercially by catalytic vapor phase oxidation of methanol using air as the oxidizing agent and heated silver, copper, alumina, or coke as catalysts. Process using molybdenum iron oxide catalyst: Allyn *et al.*, **US 2812309** (1957) and **US 2849492** (1958 to Reichhold Chem.). Prepn of stable formaldehyde by heating low molecular polyoxymethylenes with P_2O_5: **DE 1070611** (1959 to BASF). Mfg processes: *Faith, Keyes & Clark's Industrial Chemicals*, F. A. Lowenheim, M. K. Moran, Eds. (Wiley-Interscience, New York, 4th ed., 1975) pp 422-429. Prepn of semicarbazone: M.

Pomerantz *et al.*, *J. Org. Chem.* **47**, 2217 (1982). Toxicity data: H. F. Smyth *et al.*, *J. Ind. Hyg. Toxicol.* **23**, 259 (1941). Carcinogenicity study: J. A. Swenberg *et al.*, *Cancer Res.* **40**, 3398 (1980). Assessment, regulation and evaluation of carcinogenicity: F. Perera, C. Petito, *Science* **216**, 1285 (1982). *Review:* H. R. Gerberich *et al.*, in *Kirk-Othmer Encyclopedia of Chemical Technology* vol. 11 (John Wiley & Sons, New York, 4th ed., 1994) pp 929-951. Review of toxicology: H. d'A. Heck *et al.*, *Crit. Rev. Toxicol.* **20**, 397-426 (1990); of oral toxicity: P. Restani, C. L. Galli, *ibid.* **21**, 315-328 (1991).

Flammable colorless gas at ordinary temp. Pungent suffocating odor. d 1.067 (air = 1.000). d$_4^{-20}$ 0.815. mp −92°. bp$_{760}$ −19.5°; bp$_{400}$ −33.0°; bp$_{200}$ −46.0°; bp$_{100}$ −57.3°; bp$_{60}$ −65.0°; bp$_{40}$ −70.6°; bp$_{20}$ −79.6°; bp$_{10}$ −88.0°. Ignition temp about 300° (572°F). Very sol in water, up to 55%; sol in alcohol, ether. Very reactive, combines readily with many substances, and polymerizes easily. *See also* Paraformaldehyde.

Formaldehyde solution. Formalin; Formol; Morbicid; Veracur. A soln of about 37% by wt of formaldehyde gas in water, usually with 10-15% methanol added to prevent polymerization. This soln is the full strength and also known as Formalin 100% or Formalin 40 which signifies that it contains 40 grams of formaldehyde within 100 ml of the soln. Colorless liq; pungent odor. On standing, esp in the cold, may become cloudy and on exposure to very low temp a ppt of trioxymethylene is formed. When evaporated, some formaldehyde escapes, but most of it is changed to trioxymethylene. It is a powerful reducing agent especially in presence of alkali. In the air it slowly oxidizes to formic acid. d$_{25}^{25}$ 1.081-1.085. One gallon weighs 9.1 lbs. bp$_{760}$ 96°. n$_D^{20}$ 1.3746. Flash pt 60°C (140°F). pH 2.8-4.0. Misc with water, alcohol, acetone. *Keep well closed in a moderately warm place.* LD$_{50}$ orally in rats: 0.80 g/kg (Smyth).

Formaldehyde semicarbazone. $C_2H_5N_3O$; mol wt 87.08. Crystals from ethanol, mp 120-121°. uv max (CH$_3$CN): 227 nm (log ε 3.73).
Caution: Potential symptoms of overexposure to formaldehyde are irritation of eyes, nose, throat and respiratory system; lacrimation; coughing; bronchial spasm. See *NIOSH Pocket Guide to Chemical Hazards* (DHHS/NIOSH 97-140, 1997) p 148. May act as a primary irritant on skin causing erythmatous or eczematous dermatitis. Sensitization can result. *See Patty's Industrial Hygiene and Toxicology vol. 2A*, G. D. Clayton, F. E. Clayton, Eds. (Wiley-Interscience, New York, 3rd ed., 1981) pp 2637-2646. Ingestion may cause immediate intense pain in mouth, pharynx and stomach; nausea, vomiting, hematemesis, abdominal pain, diarrhea; pale, clammy skin and other signs of shock; difficult urination, hematuria, anuria; vertigo, convulsions, stupor, coma; death due to respiratory failure. See *Clinical Toxicology of Commercial Products*, R. E. Gosselin *et al.*, Eds. (Williams & Wilkins, New York, 5th ed., 1984) Section III, pp 196-197. Formaldehyde gas is reasonably anticipated to be a human carcinogen: *Report on Carcinogens, Eleventh Edition* (PB2005-104914, 2004) p III-125.
USE: In the prodn of amino, phenolic, and polyacetal resins, wood products, plastics, fertilizers and foam insulation. As a textile finish, preservative, stabilizer, disinfectant and antibacterial food additive.
THERAP CAT: Solution as disinfectant.
THERAP CAT (VET): Solution as antiseptic; fumigant; has been used in tympany, diarrhea, mastitis, pneumonia, internal bleeding.

4236. Formaldehyde Sodium Bisulfite. [870-72-4] Hydroxymethanesulfonic acid monosodium salt; sodium formaldehydebisulfite; methylolsulfonic acid sodium salt. CH_3NaO_4S; mol wt 134.09. C 8.96%, H 2.26%, Na 17.15%, O 47.73%, S 23.91%. HOCH$_2$SO$_3$Na. Prepn: Skrabal, Skrabal, *Monatsh. Chem.* **69**, 17 (1936); Chhabria *et al.*, **DE 1173059** (1964 to Schill & Seilacher). Structure: Lauer, Langkammerer, *J. Am. Chem. Soc.* **57**, 2360 (1935); Caughlan, Tartar, *ibid.* **63**, 1266 (1941).
Monohydrate. Needles from water. pK (25°): 6.92.
USE: Fixing agent for keratin-containing fibers. Flotation of lead-zinc ores. Protecting color pictures exposed to high humidities against fading and staining.

4237. Formamide. [75-12-7] Methanamide; carbamaldehyde. CH_3NO; mol wt 45.04. C 26.67%, H 6.71%, N 31.10%, O 35.52%. HCONH$_2$. Prepd on a large scale from carbon monoxide and ammonia at high press. and temp: Meyer, Orthner, *Ber.*

54, 1705 (1921); **55**, 857 (1922); Meyer, **DE 390798** (1924); **DE 392409** (1924); **DE 414257** (1925 to BASF); Wietzel, Herbst, **US 1843434** (1932 to I. G. Farben). Toxicity study: Pham-Huu-Chank *et al., Toxicol. Appl. Pharmacol.* **26**, 596 (1973). *Review:* C. L. Eberling in *Kirk-Othmer Encyclopedia of Chemical Technology* vol. 11 (Wiley-Interscience, New York, 3rd ed., 1980) pp 258-263.

Slightly viscous, odorless, colorless liq. Industrial grades may have faint odor of ammonia. mp 2.55°. bp$_{760}$ 210.5° (partial decomp into CO and NH$_3$ at atm pressure beginning at 180°); bp$_{400}$ 193.5°; bp$_{200}$ 175.5°; bp$_{60}$ 147.0°; bp$_{20}$ 122.5°; bp$_{10}$ 109.5°; bp$_{1.0}$ 70.5°. d$_4^{15}$ 1.13756; d$_4^{20}$ 1.13340; d$_4^{30}$ 1.12483. Dielectric constant ε = 84. Viscosity $\eta \times 10^5$ at 15° = 4320, at 30° = 2926. Surface tension γ at 20° = 58.35. n$_D^{15}$ 1.44911; n$_D^{20}$ 1.44754; n$_D^{110}$ 1.4170; n$_D^{130}$ 1.4095. Flash pt, open cup: 310°F (154°C). pH of 0.5 molar aq soln 7.1. Misc with water, methanol, ethanol, acetone, acetic acid, dioxane, ethylene glycol, U.S.P. glycerol, phenol. Very slightly sol in ether, benzene. Dissolves casein, glucose, zein, tannins, starch, lignin, polyvinyl alcohol, cellulose acetate, nylon, the chlorides of copper, lead, zinc, tin, cobalt, iron, aluminum, nickel, the acetates of the alkali metals, some inorganic sulfates and nitrates. LD$_{50}$ in mice, rats (g/kg): 4.6, 5.7 i.p. (Pham-Huu-Chanh).

Caution: Potential symptoms of overexposure are irritation of eyes, skin, mucous membranes; drowsiness, fatigue; nausea, acidosis; skin eruptions. *See NIOSH Pocket Guide to Chemical Hazards* (DHHS/NIOSH 97-140, 1997) p 148.

USE: As ionizing solvent, manuf formic esters, hydrocyanic acid by catalytic dehydration, as softener for paper, animal glues, water-sol gums.

4238. Formanilide. [103-70-8] *N*-Phenylformamide; formylaniline. C$_7$H$_7$NO; mol wt 121.14. C 69.40%, H 5.82%, N 11.56%, O 13.21%. C$_6$H$_5$NHCHO. Review on methods of prepn: de Jonge *et al., Rec. Trav. Chim.* **75**, 5 (1956).

Crystals from ether + petr ether, mp 46.6-47.5°. bp 271°; bp$_{120}$ 216°; bp$_{14}$ 166°. uv max (96% ethanol): 242-243 nm (ε 13700); in water: 239-240 nm (ε 11200); in cyclohexane: 240 nm (ε 12600). Soly in water at 20°: 25.4 g/l; at 25°: 28.6 g/l.

4239. Formebolone. [2454-11-7] 11α,17β-Dihydroxy-17-methyl-3-oxoandrosta-1,4-diene-2-carboxaldehyde; 2-formyl-17α-methylandrosta-1,4-diene-11α,17β-diol-3-one; 2-formyl-11α-hydroxy-Δ^1-methyltestosterone; formyldienolone; Esiclene. C$_{21}$H$_{28}$-O$_4$; mol wt 344.44. C 73.23%, H 8.19%, O 18.58%. Prepn: Canonica *et al., Gazz. Chim. Ital.* **95**, 138 (1968); Gomarasca, **GB 1168931; FR 1584960** (1969, 1970 both to Lab. Prod. Biol. Braglia), *C.A.* **72**, 90742g (1970); **73**, 131212a (1970). Pharmacology: *idem, Minerva Med.* **62**, 842 (1971); Vaccari, Livini, *ibid.* 846; De Marchi *et al., Arzneim.-Forsch.* **23**, 1583 (1973). GC/MS determn of metabolites in urine: R. Massé *et al., Anal. Chim. Acta* **247**, 211 (1991). Toxicological studies: Travella, *Gazz. Int. Med. Chir.* **76**, 400 (1971), *C.A.* **75**, 30792a (1971).

Crystals from ethyl acetate, mp 209-212°. [α]$_D^{25}$ −105° (CHCl$_3$). Water soluble. Approx LD$_{50}$ in rats, mice (mg/kg): 104, 187 i.p.; 270, 293 s.c.; orally in rats: >1000 (Travella).

11-β-Epimer. mp 95-103° from ethyl ether-petr ether.

Note: This is a controlled substance (anabolic steroid): **21 CFR,** 1308.13, as defined in 1300.01.

THERAP CAT: Anabolic.

4240. Formestane. [566-48-3] 4-Hydroxyandrost-4-ene-3,17-dione; 4-OHA; CGP-32349; Lentaron. C$_{19}$H$_{26}$O$_3$; mol wt 302.41. C 75.46%, H 8.67%, O 15.87%. Selective aromatase inhibitor. Prepn: R. D. Burnett, D. N. Kirk, *J. Chem. Soc. Perkin Trans. 1* **1973**, 1830; J. Mann, B. Pietrzak, *ibid.* **1983**, 2681; P. G. Ciattini *et al., Synth. Commun.* **22**, 1949 (1992). Aromatase inhib-

ition and effect on estrogen-dependent processes *in vivo:* A. M. H. Brodie *et al., Endocrinology* **100**, 1684 (1977). Radioimmunoassay in plasma: J. Khubieh *et al., J. Steroid Biochem.* **35**, 377 (1990). GC determn in plasma and urine: P. H. Degen, W. Schneider, *J. Chromatogr.* **565**, 67 (1991). Pharmacokinetics and endocrine effects in breast cancer patients: M. Dowsett *et al., Eur. J. Cancer* **28**, 415 (1992). Clinical evaluation in breast cancer: R. C. Coombes, *J. Steroid Biochem. Mol. Biol.* **43**, 145 (1992).

Needles from aq methanol, mp 199-202° (Burnett, Kirk); also reported as crystals from ethyl acetate, mp 203.5-206° (Brodie). uv max (99.5% ethanol): 278 nm (ε 11030). [α]$_D^{20}$ +181° (c = 7.7 in chloroform).

THERAP CAT: Antineoplastic (hormonal).

4241. Formic Acid. [64-18-6] Ameisensäure (German). CH$_2$O$_2$; mol wt 46.03. C 26.09%, H 4.38%, O 69.52%. HCOOH. Found in the bites and stings of various insects including bees and ants; metabolite of methanol. Observed by S. Fisher in 1670 in the products resulting from the distillation of ants. Production: P. G. Jessop *et al., Nature* **368**, 231 (1994). Acute and chronic toxicity: G. Malorny, *Z. Ernaehrungswiss.* **9**, 332 (1969). Review of metabolism and toxicology: J. Liesivuori, H. Savolainen, *Pharmacol. Toxicol.* **69**, 157-163 (1991). Clinical trial in treatment of warts: R. M. Bhat *et al., Int. J. Dermatol.* **40**, 415 (2001). *Reviews:* A. Aguilo, T. Horlenko, *Hydrocarbon Process. Int. Ed.* **59**, 120-130 (1980); D. J. Drury in *Kirk-Othmer Encyclopedia of Chemical Technology* vol. 11 (Wiley-Interscience, New York, 4th ed., 1994) pp 951-958.

Colorless liq; pungent odor. bp$_{760}$ 100.8°. mp 8.4°. d^{20} 1.220. pKa (20°) 3.75. n$_D^{20}$ 1.3714. Flash point, open cup: 59°C. Surface tension at 20°: 37.67 dyn/cm. Viscosity at 20°: 1.784 cP. Dielectric constant at 20°: 57.9. Vapor pressure at 20°: 33.55 mm Hg. Heat of fusion: 3031 cal/mole; of vaporization at 100°: 104 cal/g. Azeotropic mixture with water: 77.5 wt% formic acid, bp$_{760}$ 107.3°. Strong reducing agent. Misc with water, ether, acetone, ethyl acetate, methanol, ethanol. Partially sol in benzene, toluene, xylenes. LD$_{50}$ in mice (mg/kg): 1100 orally; 145 i.v. (Malorny).

Spirit of Formic Acid. Spirit of ants. Composed of 40 ml of 25% formic acid and 225 ml water in sufficient alcohol to make one liter; corresponds to ~1% formic acid and ~70% abs alcohol by vol. Colorless liquid. Miscible with water, alcohol.

Caution: Potential symptoms of overexposure are eye, skin, throat irritation; skin burns, dermatitis; lacrimation; rhinorrhea; coughing and dyspnea; nausea. *See NIOSH Pocket Guide to Chemical Hazards* (DHHS/NIOSH 97-140, 1997) p 148.

USE: Preservative in foods and silage; acidulant in dyeing of natural and synthetic fibers, leather tanning; coagulating latex in rubber production; chemical synthesis.

THERAP CAT: Caustic.

4242. Formicin. [625-51-4] *N*-(Hydroxymethyl)acetamide; formaldehyde acetamide; methylal acetamide. C$_3$H$_7$NO$_2$; mol wt 89.09. C 40.44%, H 7.92%, N 15.72%, O 35.92%. CH$_3$CONH-CH$_2$OH. Obtained by warming acetamide with formaldehyde and a small amount of potash: Fuchs, *Pharm. Ztg.* **1905**, 803; **DE 164610** (1905 to Kalle).

Colorless, very hygroscopic mass. Marketed only as a slightly yellowish, syrupy liq. d 1.14-1.18. Very sol in water, alcohol; sol in chloroform, glycerol. Insol in ether.

USE: Antiseptic, disinfectant esp for surgical instruments.

4243. Formocortal. [2825-60-7] (11β,16α)-21-(Acetyloxy)-3-(2-chloroethoxy)-9-fluoro-11-hydroxy-16,17-[(1-methylethylidene)bis(oxy)]-20-oxopregna-3,5-diene-6-carboxaldehyde; 3-(2-chloroethoxy)-9-fluoro-11β,16α,17,21-tetrahydroxy-20-oxopregna-

3,5-diene-6-carboxaldehyde, cyclic 16,17-acetal with acetone, 21-acetate; 3-(2-chloroethoxy)-6-formyl-9α-fluoropregna-3,5-diene-11β,16α,17,21-tetrol-20-one 21-acetate 16α,17α-acetonide; 3-(2-chloroethoxy)-9α-fluoro-6-formyl-11β,21-dihydroxy-16α,17α-isopropylidenedioxypregna-3,5-dien-20-one; fluoroformylon; FI-6341; Cortocin-F; Cutisterol; Deflamene; Fluderma. $C_{29}H_{38}ClFO_8$; mol wt 569.06. C 61.21%, H 6.73%, Cl 6.23%, F 3.34%, O 22.49%. Prepn: Camerino et al., **FR 1396602** C.A. **63**, 5713c (1965); **NL 6508458**; **US 3314945** (1965, 1966, 1967 all to Farmitalia); Baldratti et al., Experientia **22**, 468 (1966). Pharmacology: Suchowsky, Baldratti, Proc. 2nd Int. Congr. Horm. Steroids **1966**, L. Martini, F. Fraschini, M. Motta, Eds. (Excerpta Medica Found., Amsterdam, 1967) pp 536-540; Tajima, Otsu, Jpn. J. Pharmacol. **62**, 115 (1966), C.A. **67**, 72329v (1967); Baldratti et al., Arzneim.-Forsch. **21**, 1533 (1971). Toxicity studies: Bertazzoli et al., J. Eur. Toxicol. **4**, 88 (1971).

White crystalline powder from ether-petroleum ether, mp 180-182°. $[\alpha]_D^{20}$ +26° (chloroform). uv max (ethanol): 216, 324 nm (ε 12,100, 17,100). LD_{50} in mice: >2000 mg/kg orally; 490 mg/kg s.c.; 537 mg/kg i.p. (Bertazzoli).

THERAP CAT: Glucocorticoid.

4244. Formononetin. [485-72-3] 7-Hydroxy-3-(4-methoxyphenyl)-4H-1-benzopyran-4-one; 7-hydroxy-4′-methoxyisoflavone; biochanin B; formononetol; neochanin. $C_{16}H_{12}O_4$; mol wt 268.26. C 71.64%, H 4.51%, O 23.86%. Isoln from soy-bean meal (Soja hispida): Walz, Ann. **489**, 118 (1931); from clover species Trifolium subterraneum L. and T. pratense L., Leguminosae in which it is the major estrogenic factor: Bradbury, White, J. Chem. Soc. **1951**, 3447; Bate-Smith, Swain, Chem. Ind. (London) **1953**, 1127. Identity with biochanin B: Bose, J. Sci. Ind. Res. **15B**, 325 (1956). Structure: Baker et al., J. Chem. Soc. **1933**, 274. Synthesis: Wessely et al., Ber. **66**, 685 (1933); Kagal et al., Tetrahedron Lett. **1962**, 593. Biological half-life in Cicer arietinum L., Papilionatae: N. Amrhein, E. Diederich, Naturwissenschaften **67**, 40 (1980). HPLC analysis: R. E. Carlson, J. Chromatogr. **198**, 193 (1980). 13C-NMR study: H. C. Jha et al., Can. J. Chem. **58**, 1211 (1980). Mutagenicity study: R. M. Bartholomew et al., Mutat. Res. **78**, 317 (1980).

Needles from alcohol, mp 258°. uv max (ethanol): 250, 300 nm (ε 27440, 11240).

7-Glucoside. Ononin; 4′-methyldaidzin. $C_{22}H_{22}O_9$. From Ononis spinosa L., Leguminosae: Hlasiwetz, J. Prakt. Chem. **65**, 415 (1855). Synthesis: Farkas, Varady, Ber. **92**, 819 (1959). Needles from water, $C_{22}H_{22}O_9.H_2O$, mp 210-214°. When anhydr, dec 245°. $[\alpha]_D^{25}$ −24.2° (pyridine). Sol in alcohol; slightly sol in water, ether.

4245. Formoterol. [73573-87-2] rel-N-[2-Hydroxy-5-[(1R)-1-hydroxy-2-[[(1R)-2-(4-methoxyphenyl)-1-methylethyl]-amino]ethyl]phenyl]formamide; 3-formylamino-4-hydroxy-α-[N-[1-methyl-2-(p-methoxyphenyl)ethyl]aminomethyl]benzyl alcohol; (±)-2′-hydroxy-5′-[(RS)-1-hydroxy-2-[[(RS)-p-methoxy-α-methyl-

phenethyl]amino]ethyl]formanilide. $C_{19}H_{24}N_2O_4$; mol wt 344.40. C 66.26%, H 7.02%, N 8.13%, O 18.58%. Selective β_2-adrenergic receptor agonist. Mixture of R,R (−) and S,S (+) enantiomers. Prepn: M. Murakami et al., **DE 2305092**; eidem, **US 3994974** (1973, 1976 both to Yamanouchi); K. Murase et al., Chem. Pharm. Bull. **25**, 1368 (1977). Absolute configuration and activity of isomers: eidem, ibid. **26**, 1123 (1978). Toxicity studies: T. Yoshida et al., Pharmacometrics **26**, 811 (1983). HPLC determn in plasma: J. Campestrini et al., J. Chromatogr. B **704**, 221 (1997). Review of pharmacology: G. P. Anderson, Life Sci. **52**, 2145-2160 (1993); and clinical efficacy: R. A. Bartow, R. N. Brogden, Drugs **55**, 303-322 (1998).

R,R-Form

Fumarate dihydrate. [43229-80-7] BD-40A; Atock; Foradil; Oxeze. $(C_{19}H_{24}N_2O_4)_2.C_4H_4O_4.2H_2O$; mol wt 840.91. Crystals from 95% isopropyl alcohol, mp 138-140°. pKa_1 7.9; pKa_2 9.2. Log P (octanol/water): 0.4 (pH 7.4). Freely sol in glacial acetic acid; sol in methanol; sparingly sol in ethanol, isopropanol; slightly sol in water. Practically insol in acetone, ethyl acetate, diethyl ether. LD_{50} in male, female, rats, mice (mg/kg): 3130, 5580, 6700, 8310 orally; 100, 72, 71 i.v.; 1000, 1100, 640, 670 s.c.; 170, 210, 240, 210 i.p. (Yoshida).

R,R-Form. [67346-49-0] Arformoterol.

R,R-Form L-tartrate. [200815-49-2] Arformoterol tartrate. $C_{19}H_{24}N_2O_4.C_4H_6O_6$; mol wt 494.49. Prepn: Y. Gao et al., **WO 9821175**; eidem, **US 6040344** (1998, 2000 both to Sepracor). Pharmacology: D. A. Handley et al., Pulm. Pharmacol. Ther. **15**, 135 (2002). Off-white powder, mp 184°.

THERAP CAT: Antiasthmatic.

4246. Formothion. [2540-82-1] Phosphorodithioic acid S-[2-(formylmethylamino)-2-oxoethyl] O,O-dimethyl ester; phosphorodithioic acid O,O-dimethyl ester S-ester with N-formyl-2-mercapto-N-methylacetamide; S-(N-formyl-N-methylcarbamoylmethyl) O,O-dimethyl phosphorodithioate; J-38; OMS-968; Aflix; Anthio. $C_6H_{12}NO_4PS_2$; mol wt 257.27. C 28.01%, H 4.70%, N 5.44%, O 24.88%, P 12.04%, S 24.93%. Prepn: Lutz, Schuler, **GB 900557** (1962 to Sandoz). Toxicity: K. Liesche, Dtsch. Apoth. **108**, 604 (1968), C.A. **69**, 26287y (1968).

Yellowish liq, mp ~25°. Practically insol in water. Miscible with alcohols, ether, chloroform, benzene. LD_{50} in rats, rabbits (mg/kg): 350, 410 orally (Liesche).

Caution: Cholinesterase inhibitor. See Parathion.

USE: Acaricide, systemic insecticide.

4247. Formyl Fluoride. [1493-02-3] CHFO; mol wt 48.02. C 25.01%, H 2.10%, F 39.56%, O 33.32%. HCOF. Prepn by the interaction of anhydr formic acid, potassium fluoride and benzoyl chloride (16% yield): Nyesmejanov, Kahn, Ber. **67**, 203 (1946); from benzoyl fluoride and formic acid (36% yield): Masentshev, J. Gen. Chem. USSR **16**, 203 (1946); from benzoyl chloride, formic acid, and KHF_2 (35% yield): Olah et al., Ber. **89**, 862 (1956); Olah, Kuhn, J. Am. Chem. Soc. **82**, 2381 (1960); from acetic formic anhydride, $CH_3COOOCH$, and anhydr HF (67% yield): Olah, Kuhn, ibid. 2380.

Gas at ordinary temps and pressure: bp_{760} −29°. mp −142°. Trouton constant 20.8. Heat of vaporization at −24°: 5.175 kcal.

Caution: Strong irritant.

USE: Acylating agent in organic synthesis.

4248. N²-Formylsulfisomidine. [795-13-1] N-(2,6-Dimethyl-4-pyrimidinyl)-4-(formylamino)benzenesulfonamide; 4'-[(2,6-dimethyl-4-pyrimidinyl)sulfamoyl]formanilide; N-[4-[[(2,6-dimethyl-4-pyrimidinyl)amino]sulfonyl]phenyl]formamide; formylsulfamethine; FAK III; Wometin. $C_{13}H_{14}N_4O_3S$; mol wt 306.34. C 50.97%, H 4.61%, N 18.29%, O 15.67%, S 10.47%. Prepd by formylation of sulfisomidine: Brand, Rieckhoff, **DE 1122511**; **DE 1126857** (both 1962 to VEB Farbenfabrik Wolfen).

Crystals, mp 248.5-250.5°.

THERAP CAT: Antibacterial.

4249. Fortimicins. Aminoglycoside antibiotic complex produced by *Micromonospora olivoasterospora*. The main components, fortimicins A and B, both exhibit broad-spectrum antibacterial activity. Isoln of A: T. Nara *et al.*, **JP Kokai 75 29789** (to Kyowa); *eidem*, **US 3976768** (1976 to Abbott). Isoln of B: *eidem*, **DE 2418349** (1974 to Kyowa); *eidem*, **US 3931400** (1976 to Abbott). Isoln and biological properties of A and B: *eidem, J. Antibiot.* **30**, 533 (1977); physical and chromatographic properties: R. Okachi *et al., ibid.* 541. Structures of A and B: R. S. Egan *et al., ibid.* 552. *In vitro* activity: R. Girolami, J. S. Stamm, *ibid.* 564. Isoln and properties of minor components, fortimicins C, D, KE: M. Sugimoto *et al., ibid.* **32**, 868 (1979). Synthesis of B: T. Suami, Y. Honda, *Chem. Lett.* **1980**, 641; Y. Honda, T. Suami, *Bull. Chem. Soc. Jpn.* **55**, 1156 (1982).

Fortimicin A. [55779-06-1] 4-Amino-1-[(aminoacetyl)methylamino]-1,4-dideoxy-3-O-(2,6-diamino-2,3,4,6,7-pentadeoxy-β-L-*lyxo*-heptopyranosyl)-6-O-methyl-L-*chiro*-inositol; astromicin; Abbott 44747. $C_{17}H_{35}N_5O_6$; mol wt 405.49. White amorphous powder, mp >200° (dec). $[\alpha]_D^{25}$ +87.5° (c = 0.1 in water). Sol in water and lower alcohols. Insol in organic solvents. LD_{50} (of the sulfate salt) in mice (mg/kg): 380 i.v.; 400 s.c. (Nara, 1977).

Fortimicin B. [54783-95-8] 4-Amino-1,4-dideoxy-3-O-(2,6-diamino-2,3,4,6,7-pentadeoxy-β-L-*lyxo*-heptopyranosyl)-6-O-methyl-1-(methylamino)-L-*chiro*-inositol. $C_{15}H_{32}N_4O_5$; mol wt 348.44. White amorphous powder, mp 101-103°. $[\alpha]_D^{25}$ +22.2° (c = 0.1 in water). Sol in water and lower alcohols. Insol in organic solvents.

THERAP CAT: Antibacterial.

4250. Fosamprenavir. [226700-79-4] [(1S,2R)-3-[[(4-Aminophenyl)sulfonyl](2-methylpropyl)amino]-1-(phenylmethyl)-2-(phosphonooxy)propyl]carbamic acid C-[(3S)-tetrahydro-3-furanyl] ester; (3S)-tetrahydro-3-furyl [(αS)-α-[(1R)-1-hydroxy-2-(N¹-isobutylsulfanilamido)ethyl]phenethyl]carbamate dihydrogen phosphate (ester); VX-175. $C_{25}H_{36}N_3O_9PS$; mol wt 585.61. C 51.27%, H 6.20%, N 7.18%, O 24.59%, P 5.29%, S 5.48%. HIV protease inhibitor; water soluble prodrug of amprenavir, *q.v.* Prepn: R. D. Tung *et al.*, **WO 9933815**; *eidem*, **US 6559137** (1999, 2003 both to Vertex). Prepn of crystalline calcium salt: I. G. Armitage *et al.*, **WO 0004033** (2000 to Glaxo); *eidem*, **US 6514953** (2003 to SKB). Clinical pharmacokinetics: C. Falcoz *et al., J. Clin. Phar-*

macol. **42**, 887 (2002). Review of pharmacology and clinical experience in HIV: T. M. Chapman *et al., Drugs* **64**, 2101-2124 (2004); C. Arvieux, O. Tribut, *ibid.* **65**, 633-659 (2005).

Calcium salt. [226700-81-8] GW-433908G; Lexiva; Telzir. $C_{25}H_{34}CaN_3O_9PS$; mol wt 623.67. White microcrystalline needles, mp 282-284°. Soly in water (25°): 0.31 mg/ml.

THERAP CAT: Antiviral.

4251. Foscarnet Sodium. [63585-09-1] Dihydroxyphosphinecarboxylic acid oxide trisodium salt; trisodium phosphonoformate; trisodium carboxyphosphate; A-29622; Foscavir. CNa_3O_5P; mol wt 191.95. C 6.26%, Na 35.93%, O 41.68%, P 16.14%. Inhibits viral DNA polymerase and reverse transcriptase. Prepn: P. Nylén, *Ber.* **57B**, 1023 (1924). Crystal structure: R. R. Naqvi *et al., J. Chem. Soc. A* **1971**, 2751; S. C. Abrahams, *Acta Crystallogr.* **B28**, 2886 (1972). Use as antiviral agent: B. F. H. Eriksson *et al.*, **DE 2728685**; *eidem*, **US 4215113** (1978, 1980 both to Astra). Activity against herpes simplex virus: E. Helgstrand *et al., Science* **201**, 819 (1978); J. M. Reno *et al., Antimicrob. Agents Chemother.* **13**, 188 (1978); S. Alenius *et al., Arch. Virol.* **60**, 197 (1979). Mechanism of inhibition of Epstein-Barr virus replication: A. K. Datta, R. E. Hood, *Virology* **114**, 52 (1981). Preclinical evaluation: B. Oeberg *et al., Int. Congr. Ser. - Excerpta Med.* **571**, 175 (1982). Inhibitory effect on HIV-1 (HTLV-III/LAV) virus replication *in vitro*: P. S. Sarin *et al., Biochem. Pharmacol.* **34**, 4075 (1985).

Hexahydrate, mp >250°. LD_{50} i.p. in mice: 2000-4000 μmol/kg (Eriksson).

THERAP CAT: Antiviral.

4252. Fosetyl Al. [39148-24-8] Phosphonic acid monoethyl ester aluminum salt; aluminum tris(ethyl phosphite); aluminum tris(O-ethylphosphonate); efosite Al; phosethyl Al; LS-74-783; Aliette. $C_6H_{18}AlO_9P_3$; mol wt 354.10. C 20.35%, H 5.12%, Al 7.62%, O 40.66%, P 26.24%. Systemic fungicide translocated both upwards and downwards in plants. Prepn: V. V. Orlovskii *et al., J. Gen. Chem. USSR* **42**, 1924 (1972). Alternate prepn, fungicidal properties: J. Ducret *et al.*, **DE 2456627**; *eidem*, **US 4139616** (1975, 1979 both to Rhone-Poulenc); J. Abblard *et al.*, **US 4143059** (1979 to Philagro). Biological properties and field trials against vine mildew and other *Phycomycetes* pathogens: A. Bertrand *et al., Phytiatr.-Phytopharm.* **26**, 3 (1977). Evaluation of carcinogenicity: J. A. Quest *et al., Regul. Toxicol. Pharmacol.* **14**, 3 (1991). Review of properties and fungicidal action on tropical, temperate crops: D. J. Williams *et al., Proc. Br. Crop Prot. Conf. - Pests Dis.* **1977**, 565.

White odorless crystals, mp >300°. Soly in water at 20°: 120 g/l. Practically insol in acetonitrile, propylene glycol (<80 mg/l).

LD$_{50}$ in rats, mice, Japanese quail, rabbits (mg/kg): 5800, 3700, 4997, 2680 orally; LD$_{50}$ i.p. in rats: 550 mg/kg (Williams).

USE: Agricultural fungicide.

4253. Fosfestrol. [522-40-7] 4,4'-[(1E)-1,2-Diethyl-1,2-ethenediyl]bisphenol bis(dihydrogen phosphate); α,α'-diethyl-4,4'-stilbenediol diphosphoric acid ester; diethylstilbestrol diphosphate; diethylstilbestryl diphosphate; diethyldihydroxystilbene diphosphate; stilbestrol diphosphate; Stilphostrol. C$_{18}$H$_{22}$O$_8$P$_2$; mol wt 428.31. C 50.48%, H 5.18%, O 29.88%, P 14.46%. Synthetic, nonsteroidal estrogen. Prepd by treating stilbestrol with phosphorus oxychloride in pyridine: Miescher, Heer, US 2234311 (1941); Arnold, US 2802854 (1957 to Asta-Werke). Prepn of stable solns at pH 10: Fonner, Collins, US 2828244 (1958 to Miles Labs.). Prepn of sodium salts: Dawson, US 2971975 (1961 to Miles Labs.). Clinical pharmacokinetics: H. Oelschläger et al., Arzneim.-Forsch. **36**, 1284 (1986). Review of clinical trials in prostate cancer: J-P. Droz et al, Cancer **71**, 1123-1130 (1993).

Voluminous white cryst powder from dil HCl. Dec 204-206°. Sparingly sol in water.

Disodium salt. [5965-09-3] C$_{18}$H$_{20}$Na$_2$O$_8$P$_2$. Crystals. Softens at 190°, uniform melt at 230°. Sol in water. pH of aq soln 6.5. pH also reported as 4.85 to 5.00.

Tetrasodium salt. [4719-75-9] Honvan; Honvol; ST-52; Stilbostatin. C$_{18}$H$_{18}$Na$_4$O$_8$P$_2$; mol wt 516.24.

THERAP CAT: Antineoplastic (hormonal).

4254. Fosfomycin. [23155-02-4] (2R-cis)-(3-Methyloxiranyl)phosphonic acid; (−)-(1R,2S)-(1,2-epoxypropyl)phosphonic acid; fosfonomycin; phosphonomycin; MK-955. C$_3$H$_7$O$_4$P; mol wt 138.06. C 26.10%, H 5.11%, O 46.35%, P 22.44%. Antibiotic produced by Streptomyces strains: D. Hendlin et al., Science **166**, 122 (1969); B. G. Christensen et al., ibid. 123; also produced by Pseudomonas syringae: J. Shogi et al., J. Antibiot. **39**, 1011 (1986). Isoln: D. Hendlin et al., BE 718507; eidem, US 3914231 (1969, 1975 both to Merck & Co.). Synthesis and resolution: B. G. Christensen et al., BE 723072; BE 723073 (both 1969 to Merck & Co.). Alternate synthesis: Girotra, Wendler, Tetrahedron Lett. **1969**, 4647; Glamkowski et al., J. Org. Chem. **35**, 3510 (1970). Series of articles on characterization, activity and clinical testing: Antimicrob. Agents Chemother. **1969**, 284-351; H. B. Woodruff et al., Chemotherapy **23**, Suppl. 1, 1-22 (1977). Mechanism of action: Kahan et al., Ann. N.Y. Acad. Sci. **235**, 354 (1974). Pharmacokinetics in humans: M. Goto et al., Antimicrob. Agents Chemother. **20**, 393 (1981). Pharmacology of cofosfolactamines, fixed dose combinations of fosfomycin with β-lactam antibiotics: P. Periti, Drugs Exp. Clin. Res. **6**, 305 (1980); and clinical trial: T. Barreca et al., ibid. **10**, 55 (1984). Electrophoretic determn in biological fluids: D. Levêque et al., J. Chromatogr. B **655**, 320 (1994). Clinical trial in cystic fibrosis: A. Mirakhur et al., J. Cyst. Fibr. **2**, 19 (2003).

Crystals, mp ~94°. Soluble in water.

Benzylammonium salt. C$_{10}$H$_{16}$NO$_4$P. mp 170-174°. [α]$_{405}$ −9.1° (c = 5).

Calcium salt monohydrate. [26016-98-8] (anhydrous) Afos; Biocin; Biofos; Endociclina; Faremicin; Fonofos; Fosfobiotic; Fosfocin; Fosfocina; Fosfogram; Fosforal; Fosfotricina; Fosmicin; Foximin; Francital; Gram-Micina; Ipamicina; Lancetina; Lofoxin; Neofocin; Palmofen; Priomicina; Selemicina; Ultramicina; Valemicina. C$_3$H$_5$CaO$_4$P.H$_2$O; mol wt 194.14.

Tromethamine. [78964-85-9] (2R-cis)-(3-Methyloxiranyl)phosphonic acid compd with 2-amino-2-(hydroxymethyl)-1,3-propanediol (1:1); fosfomycin trometamol; Monuril; Monurol. C$_7$H$_{18}$NO$_7$P; mol wt 259.19. Clinical trial in urinary tract infection: G. Bonfiglio et al., Chemotherapy (Basel) **51**, 162 (2005).

THERAP CAT: Antibacterial.

4255. Fosfosal. [6064-83-1] 2-(Phosphonooxy)benzoic acid; salicylic acid dihydrogen phosphate; o-carboxyphenyl phosphate; salicyl phosphate; UR-1521; Disdolen. C$_7$H$_7$O$_6$P; mol wt 218.10. C 38.55%, H 3.24%, O 44.01%, P 14.20%. Salicylic acid deriv. Prepn: A. C. Marin Moga, E. Francia Barra, DE 2641526 (1978 to Uriach), C.A. **88**, 136317h (1978). Pharmacology and comparison with aspirin: J. Garcia Rafanell et al., Arzneim.-Forsch. **30**, 1091 (1980). Toxicity studies: M. S. Sanchez et al., ibid. 1098. Pharmacokinetics: V. Rimbau et al., Arch. Farmacol. Toxicol. **7**, 61 (1981). Double-blind trials in musculoskeletal/articular pain: C. Diaz et al., Clin. Ther. **4**, 121 (1981); L. Madera Cat, J. Garcia Rafanell, Med. Clin. **76**, 18 (1981).

White solid, mp 168-170°. Sol in water, ethanol, acetone. Insol in non-polar organic solvents. Hydrolyzes in aq soln. LD$_{50}$ in male, female mice, male, female rats at pH 1.0, aq soln (mg/kg): 94, 105, 153, 257 i.v.; 352, 253, 338, 360 i.p.; 1455, 1539, 1104, 1213 orally; at pH 3.5 (mg/kg): 117, 118, 207, 215 i.v.; 1592, 1483, 1085, 1128 i.p.; 1702, 2007, 1685, 2225 orally (Sanchez).

THERAP CAT: Analgesic.

4256. Fosinopril. [98048-97-6] (4S)-4-Cyclohexyl-1-[[(R)-[(1S)-2-methyl-1-(1-oxopropoxy)propoxy](4-phenylbutyl)phosphinyl]acetyl]-L-proline; (4S)-4-cyclohexyl-1-[[[(RS)-1-hydroxy-2-methylpropoxy](4-phenylbutyl)phosphinyl]acetyl]-L-proline propionate (ester); fosenopril. C$_{30}$H$_{46}$NO$_7$P; mol wt 563.66. C 63.93%, H 8.23%, N 2.48%, O 19.87%, P 5.50%. Phosphinic acid containing angiotensin converting enzyme (ACE) inhibitor. Prepn: E. W. Petrillo, Jr., US 4337201 (1982 to Squibb); of active diacid form: J. Krapcho et al., J. Med. Chem. **31**, 1148 (1988). Metabolism and pharmacokinetics: S. M. Singhvi et al., Br. J. Clin. Pharmacol. **25**, 9 (1988). GC determn of diacid: M. Jemal et al., J. Chromatogr. **345**, 299 (1985). Clinical trial in hypertension: P. A. Sullivan et al., Am. J. Hypertens. **1**, 280S (1988). Brief description: E. W. Petrillo, Jr., et al., Clin. Exp. Theory Prac. **A9**, 235 (1987). Series of articles on pharmacology, pharmacokinetics, and clinical experience: Drug Invest. **3**, Suppl. 4, 1-53 (1991).

Sodium salt. [88889-14-9] SQ-28555; Dynacil; Elidiur; Fosinorm; Fositen; Fozitec; Monopril; Staril; Tensozide. C$_{30}$H$_{45}$NNaO$_7$P; mol wt 585.64.

Diacid. [95399-71-6] SQ-27519. C$_{23}$H$_{34}$NO$_5$P; mol wt 435.49. mp 149-153°. [α]$_D$ −24° (c = 1 in methanol).

THERAP CAT: Antihypertensive.

4257. Fosmidomycin. [66508-53-0] [3-(Formylhydroxyamino)propyl]phosphonic acid. C$_4$H$_{10}$NO$_5$P; mol wt 183.10. C 26.24%, H 5.50%, N 7.65%, O 43.69%, P 16.92%. Inhibitor of microbial nonmevalonate isoprenoid biosynthesis. Prepn: T. Kamiya et al., US 4206156 (1980 to Fujisawa); K. Hemmi et al., Chem. Pharm. Bull. **29**, 646 (1981); eidem, ibid. **30**, 111 (1982). Synthesis: E. Ohler, S. Kanzler, Synthesis **1995**, 539 (1995). CE

Consult the Name Index before using this section.

determn in serum and urine: S. Bronner *et al., J. Chromatogr. B* **806**, 255 (2004). Mode of action: T. Kuzuyama *et al., Tetrahedron Lett.* **39**, 7913 (1998); H. Jomaa *et al., Science* **285**, 1573 (1999). Pharmacokinetics: T. Murakawa *et al., Antimicrob. Agents Chemother.* **21**, 224 (1982); H.-P. Kuemmerle *et al., Int. J. Clin. Pharmacol. Ther. Toxicol.* **23**, 515, 521 (1985). Clinical evaluation in malaria: M. A. Missinou *et al., Lancet* **360**, 1941 (2002); in combination with clindamycin: S. Borrmann *et al., J. Infect. Dis.* **189**, 901 (2004); *idem et al., ibid.* **190**, 1534 (2004). Interaction with other antimalarial drugs and synergy with clindamycin: J. Wiesner *et al., Antimicrob. Agents Chemother.* **46**, 2889 (2002). *Review: idem et al., Parasitol. Res.* **90**, S71-S76 (2003).

Colorless crystals from methanol, mp 158-160° (dec) (Ohler); also reported as crystals from water-ethanol, mp 160-166° (dec) (Hemmi). LD_{50} in mice and rats (mg/kg): >11000 orally; ~8000 s.c. (Wiesner, 2003).

Monosodium salt. [66508-37-0] FR-31564. $C_4H_{10}NNaO_5P$; mol wt 206.09. C 23.31%, H 4.89%, N 6.80%, Na 11.16%, O 38.82%, P 15.03%. Crystals from methanol-ethanol, mp 189-191° (dec).

THERAP CAT: Antimalarial.

4258. Fosphenytoin. [93390-81-9] 5,5-Diphenyl-3-[(phosphonooxy)methyl]-2,4-imidazolidinedione; 3-(hydroxymethyl)-5,5-diphenylhydantoin phosphate ester; (3-phosphoryloxymethyl)phenytoin; prophenytoin. $C_{16}H_{15}N_2O_6P$; mol wt 362.27. C 53.05%, H 4.17%, O 26.50%, P 8.55%. Prodrug of phenytoin, *q.v.* Prepn: V. J. Stella, K. B. Sloan, **US 4260769** (1981 to INTERx). Series of articles on chemical properties and pharmacokinetics: S. A. Varia *et al., J. Pharm. Sci.* **73**, 1068-1090 (1984). Pharmacology: R. D. Smith *et al., Epilepsia* **30**, Suppl. 2, S15 (1989). Clinical bioavailablilty and pharmacokinetics: B. D. Jamerson *et al., ibid.* **31**, 592 (1990). Series of articles on use in epilepsy: *Neurology* **46**, Suppl. 1, S1-S28 (1996). Clinical trial in epilepsy and neurosurgery: B. J. Wilder *et al., Arch. Neurol.* **53**, 764 (1996).

White crystals from acetone, mp 173-176.5°.

Disodium salt. [92134-98-0] Fosphenytoin sodium; ACC-9653; Cerebyx; Pro-Epanutin. $C_{16}H_{13}N_2Na_2O_6P$; mol wt 406.24. White crystals as the dihydrate from water-ethanol-acetone, mp 220° (softens). pH of a saturated aqueous soln: ~9. Soly at 25° (mg/ml): 142 in water. LD_{50} in mice, rats (mg/kg): 234, 363 i.v. (Smith).

THERAP CAT: Anticonvulsant.

4259. Fospropofol. [258516-89-1] [2,6-Bis(1-methylethyl)phenoxy]methanol dihydrogen phosphate; phosphono-*O*-methyl-2,6-diisopropylphenol. $C_{13}H_{21}O_5P$; mol wt 288.28. C 54.16%, H 7.34%, O 27.75%, P 10.74%. Prodrug of propofol, *q.v.* Prepn: V. J. Stella *et al.,* **WO 0008033**; *eidem,* **US 6204257** (2000, 2001 to Univ. Kansas). Clinical pharmacokinetics and pharmacodynamics: J. Fechner *et al., Anesthesiology* **99**, 303 (2003). Clinical evaluation to induce and maintain sedation: *eidem, Anesth. Analg.* **100**, 701 (2005). Clinical comparison with propofol: E. Gibiansky *et al., Anesthesiology* **103**, 718 (2005); M. M. R. Struys *et al., ibid.* 730. *Review:* M. D. Krasowski, *Curr. Opin. Invest. Drugs* **6**, 90-98 (2005).

Colorless oil, unstable on standing at room temp.

Disodium salt. [258516-87-9] Fospropofol disodium; GPI-15715; Aquavan. $C_{13}H_{19}Na_2O_5P$; mol wt 332.24. White powder. Sol in water.

THERAP CAT: Anesthetic (intravenous).

4260. Fosthiazate. [98886-44-3] (2-Oxo-3-thiazolidinyl)-phosphonothioic acid *O*-ethyl *S*-(1-methylpropyl) ester; *S-sec*-butyl-*O*-ethyl(2-oxo-3-thiazolidinyl)phosphonothioate; IKI-1145; ASC-66824; Nemathorin. $C_9H_{18}NO_3PS_2$; mol wt 283.35. C 38.15%, H 6.40%, N 4.94%, O 16.94%, P 10.93%, S 22.63%. Non-fumigant insecticide and nematicide. Prepn: T. Haga *et al.,* **EP 146748**; *eidem,* **US 4590182** (1985, 1986 both to Ishihara Sangyo Kaisha); and pesticidal activity: T. Koyanagi *et al., J. Pestic. Sci.* **22**, 187 (1997). Activity of isomers: *idem et al., ACS Symp. Ser.* **443**, 387 (1991). Field trial in potatoes: J. Kimpinski *et al., J. Nematol.* **29**, Suppl. 4, 685 (1997). Mode of action: S. R. Woods *et al., Ann. Appl. Biol.* **135**, 409 (1999). Review of physical properties, mode of action, and biological characteristics: T. Toki, O. Imai, *Agrochem. Jpn.* **65**, 13 (1994).

Pale yellow oil. $bp_{0.5}$ 198°. $n_D^{19.6}$ 1.5334. Soly in water at 20°: 9.85 g/l. Vapor pressure at 25°: 4.2×10^{-6} mmHg. LD_{50} in male, female mice, male, female rats (mg/kg): 104, 91, 73, 57 orally; in male, female rats (mg/kg): 2396, 861 dermally. LC_{50} in male, female rats (mg/l): 0.832, 0.558 by inhalation (Toki).

USE: Nematicide.

4261. Fotemustine. [92118-27-9] [1-[[[(2-Chloroethyl)-nitrosoamino]carbonyl]amino]ethyl]phosphonic acid diethyl ester; (±)-diethyl [1-[3-(2-chloroethyl)-3-nitrosoureido]ethyl]phosphonate; 1-[*N*-(2-chloroethyl)-*N*-nitrosoureido]ethylphosphonic acid diethyl ester; S-10036; Muphoran. $C_9H_{19}ClN_3O_5P$; mol wt 315.69. C 34.24%, H 6.07%, Cl 11.23%, N 13.31%, O 25.34%, P 9.81%. Amino acid-linked nitrosourea alkylating agent. Prepn: G. Lavielle, C. Cudennec, **FR 2536075**; *eidem,* **US 4567169** (1984, 1986 both to ADIR). Clinical evaluation in advanced cancers: D. Khayat *et al., Cancer Res.* **47**, 6782 (1987); in disseminated malignant melanoma: D. Khayat *et al., J. Natl. Cancer Inst.* **80**, 1407 (1988).

mp 85°.

THERAP CAT: Antineoplastic.

4262. Francium. [7440-73-5] Eka-cesium. Fr; at. no. 87; valence 1. Group IA (1). No stable nuclides. Naturally occurring isotope: 223, *Actinum K,* (longest lived isotope, $T_{1/2}$ 21.8 min, β^- emitter; rel. at. mass 223.0197) formed by α-decay of actinium ^{227}Ac in ^{235}U series. Known artificial isotopes: 201-222, 224-232. Found in uranium minerals. Terrestial abundance ~2×10^{18} ppm. Also obtainable by proton bombardment of thorium. First obtained in 1939 from an actinium prepn by Perey, *J. Phys. Radium* **10**, 439

(1939); *J. Chim. Phys.* **43**, 155, 262 (1946); Hyde, Ghiorso, *Phys. Rev.* **90**, 267 (1953); Hyde, *J. Am. Chem. Soc.* **74**, 4181 (1952). Isoln by paper chromatography: Perey, Adloff, *Compt. Rend.* **236**, 1163 (1953). *Reviews:* Hyde, *J. Chem. Educ.* **36**, 15-21 (1959); Whaley, "Sodium, Potassium, Rubidium, Cesium and Francium" in *Comprehensive Inorganic Chemistry* vol. **1**, J. C. Bailar Jr., *et al.,* Eds. (Pergamon Press, Oxford, 1973) pp 369-529; *Chemistry of the Elements* N. N. Greenwood, A. Earnshaw, Eds. (Pergamon Press, New York, 1984) pp 75-116.

Most electropositive element. Chemical behavior similar to that of other alkali metals.

4263. Frangula. Buckthorn bark; alder buckthorn; black dogwood; berry alder; arrow wood; Persian berries. Dried bark of *Rhamnus frangula* L., *Rhamnaceae. Habit.* Europe, Russian Asia, Mediterranean coast of Africa. *Constit.* Frangulin, emodin, chrysophanic acid.

4264. Frangulin. [60529-33-1] Franguloside; avornin; Cascarin. In berries, bark, and rootbark of *Rhamnus* spp., especially in alder buckthorn *(Rhamnus frangula* L.), *Rhamnus carthartica* L., and *Rhamnus purshiana* DC. *(Cascara sagrada), Rhamnaceae.* Prepn from bark of alder buckthorn: Bridel, Charaux, *Bull. Soc. Chim. Biol.* **15**, 642 (1933); M. Kubiak, *Herba Pol.* **23**, 217 (1977), *C.A.* **88**, 166260b (1978). Consists of the two glucosides, frangulins A and B, which were originally thought to be isomeric. Structure and synthesis of frangulin A: Hörhammer, Wagner, *Z. Naturforsch.* **27B**, 959 (1972). Structure of frangulin B: Wagner, Demuth, *Tetrahedron Lett.* **1972**, 5013.

Frangulin A   R =

Frangulin B   R =

Frangulin A. [521-62-0] 1,3,8-Trihydroxy-6-methylanthraquinone-*l*-rhamnoside; emodin-*l*-rhamnoside; rhamnoxanthin. $C_{21}H_{20}O_9$; mol wt 416.38. Crystals, mp 228°. Absorption max: 225, 264, 282, 300, 430 nm (log ε 4.52, 4.28, 4.15, 3.97, 4.05).

Frangulin B. [14101-04-3] 6-*O*-(D-Apiofuranosyl)-1,6,8-trihydroxy-3-methylanthraquinone. $C_{20}H_{18}O_9$; mol wt 402.35. mp 196°.

THERAP CAT: Cathartic.

4265. Fraxetin. [574-84-5] 7,8-Dihydroxy-6-methoxy-2*H*-1-benzopyran-2-one; 7,8-dihydroxy-6-methoxycoumarin. $C_{10}H_8O_5$; mol wt 208.17. C 57.70%, H 3.87%, O 38.43%. The aglucon of fraxin. Obtained by heating fraxin with dil H_2SO_4. Structure: Wessely, Demmer, *Ber.* **61**, 1279 (1928). Synthesis: Aghoramurthy, Seshadri, *J. Chem. Soc.* **1954**, 3065.

Plates from alc, mp 228°. Turns yellow at 150° and brown at mp. Sol in 10 liters cold water, in 300 ml boiling water; somewhat more sol in alcohol; hardly sol in ether.

Dimethyl ether. 6,7,8-Trimethoxycoumarin. $C_{12}H_{12}O_5$. Orthorhombic bipyramidal crystals, mp 104°. bp$_{0.2}$ 90-100°.

4266. Fraxin. [524-30-1] 8-(β-D-Glucopyranosyloxy)-7-hydroxy-6-methoxy-2*H*-1-benzopyran-2-one; 7,8-dihydroxy-6-methoxycoumarin-8-β-D-glucoside; 8-(glucosyloxy)-6-methoxyumbelliferone; fraxetin-8-glucoside; fraxoside; paviin. $C_{16}H_{18}O_{10}$; mol wt 370.31. C 51.89%, H 4.90%, O 43.21%. From bark of the common European ash *(Fraxinus excelsior* L.): Salm-Horstmar, *Pogg. Ann.* **100**, 607 (1857); from *F. oxyphylla* Mar., *Oleaceae:* Paris, Stambouli, *Compt. Rend.* **253**, 313 (1961). Identity with paviin: Stokes, *J. Chem. Soc.* **12**, 126 (1859). From the horse chestnut tree *(Aesculus hippocastanum* L., *Hippocastanaceae):* Reppel, *Planta Med.* **4**, 199 (1956); from *Diervilla* spp., *Caprifoliaceae:* Charaux, *J. Pharm. Chim.* [7] **4**, 248 (1911). Structure: Wessely, Demmer, *Ber.* **62**, 120 (1929).

Yellow hydrated needles from water or dil alc. Slightly bitter, astringent taste. The water of crystn (about 3 mols) is removed at 130° and 0.2 mm Hg. The anhydr substance, mp 205° (rapid heating). Sparingly sol in cold water; freely sol in hot water, hot alcohol. Practically insol in ether. Alkaline solns are sulfur-yellow and on dilution show characteristic blue-green fluorescence.

4267. Fredericamycin A. [80455-68-1] (2*S*)-6',7'-Dihydro-4,9,9'-trihydroxy-6-methoxy-3'-[(1*E*,3*E*)-1,3-pentadienyl]spiro[2*H*-benz[*f*]indene-2,8'-[8*H*]cyclopent[*g*]isoquinoline]-1,1',3,5,8(2'*H*)-pentone; FCRC-A48; NSC-305263. $C_{30}H_{21}NO_9$; mol wt 539.49. C 66.79%, H 3.92%, N 2.60%, O 26.69%. Antitumor antibiotic produced by *Streptomyces griseus* (FCRC-48); represents new structural class of antibiotics containing a spiro[4,4]nonane ring system. Isoln together with two biologically inactive components, fredericamycins B and C: R. C. Pandey *et al., J. Antibiot.* **34**, 1389 (1981). Antimicrobial and cytotoxic activity *in vitro* and antitumor activity *in vivo:* D. J. Warnick-Pickle *et al., ibid.* 1402. Prepn and biological activity of water soluble salts: R. Misra, *ibid.* **51**, 976 (1988). Structure determn by x-ray crystallography: R. Misra *et al., J. Am. Chem. Soc.* **104**, 4478 (1982). Spectroscopic and mass spectral characterization: *eidem, J. Antibiot.* **40**, 786 (1987). Synthetic studies: A. V. R. Rao *et al., Chem. Commun.* **1984**, 1119; K. A. Parker *et al., Tetrahedron Lett.* **26**, 2181 (1985). Synthesis of (±)-form: T. R. Kelly *et al., J. Am. Chem. Soc.* **108**, 7100 (1986). Biosynthetic study: K. M. Byrne *et al., Biochemistry* **24**, 478 (1985). Mechanism of action study: B. D. Hilton *et al., ibid.* **25**, 5533 (1986).

Thin, platelet-like crystals from acetonitrile + water, mp >350° (dec). pKa (DMF) 6.80; 8.88. Sol in acetic acid, DMSO, DMF, pyridine; partially sol in acidic methanol, acidic chloroform, acidic ethyl acetate. Insol in water, petr ether, ether. Acts as an indicator: Red in acidic soln, green to blue in basic soln.

Potassium salt. Solubility (mg/ml): water (1.0); DMSO (8/1.5); 1:1 DMSO-H_2O (3.0); also readily sol in DMF, dimethylacetamide, pyridine. Sparingly sol in ethyl acetate, acetonitrile, methanol, chloroform. Insol in hexanes, benzene, acetone, ether.

4268. Fremy's Salt. [14293-70-0] Nitrosodisulfonic acid dipotassium salt; potassium nitrosodisulfonate; potassium peroxylaminedisulfonate. $K_2NO_7S_2$; mol wt 268.33. K 29.14%, N 5.22%, O 41.74%, S 23.90%. $K_2[NO(SO_3)_2]$. Radical oxidizing agent. Prepn: E. Fremy, *Ann. Chim. Phys.* **15**, 408 (1845). Structural studies: W. Moser, R. A. Howie, *J. Chem. Soc. A* **1968**, 3039; R. A. Howie *et al., ibid.* 3043. Mechanism of oxidation: B. Giethlen, J. M. Schaus, *Tetrahedron Lett.* **38**, 8483 (1997). Synthetic applications: H. J. Teuber, G. Jellinek, *Naturwissenschaften* **38**, 259 (1951); H. Schlude, *Tetrahedron* **29**, 4007 (1973); P. M. Deya *et al., ibid.* **43**, 3523 (1987); G. A. Kraus, N. Selvakumar, *Tetrahedron Lett.* **40**, 2039 (1999). EPR studies: B. L. Bales, *Chem. Phys. Lett.* **10**, 361 (1971); M. T. Jones *et al., J. Phys. Chem.* **83**, 1327 (1979); B. L. Bales *et al., J. Magn. Reson.* **118**, 227 (1996). Photochemistry study: H. Kunkely *et al., J. Photochem. Photobiol. A* **112**, 9 (1998). Review of oxidation chemistry: H. Zimmer *et al., Chem. Rev.* **71**, 229-246 (1971).

Occurs in two distinct crystalline forms: as monoclinic yellow-orange needles, and as triclinic orange-brown rhombs. Absorption max (water): 248, 545 nm (ε 1690, 21).

USE: Reagent for the oxidation of anilines and phenols to quinones. EPR standard.

4269. Frenolicin. [10023-07-1] [1*R*-(1α,3β,4aβ,10aβ)]-3,-4,5,10-Tetrahydro-9-hydroxy-5,10-dioxo-1-propyl-4a,10a-epoxy-1*H*-naphtho[2,3-*c*]pyran-3-acetic acid. $C_{18}H_{18}O_7$; mol wt 346.33. C 62.42%, H 5.24%, O 32.34%. Antibiotic produced by *Streptomyces fradiae:* Van Meter *et al., Antimicrob. Agents Annu.* **1960**, 77. Structure: Ellestad *et al., J. Am. Chem. Soc.* **88**, 4109 (1966); **90**, 1325 (1968). Total synthesis: A. Ichihara *et al., Tetrahedron Lett.* **21**, 4469 (1980).

Pale yellow needles from benzene, mp 160-161°. $[\alpha]_D^{25}$ $-37.7°$ (c = 1.5 in methanol). uv max (methanol): 234, 362 nm (ε 18300, 5200). Sol in methanol, ethanol, ethyl acetate, acetone, glacial acetic acid, carbon tetrachloride; slightly sol in benzene. Practically insol in water, cyclohexane, petr ether.

4270. Frequentin. [29119-03-7] 6-(1,3-Heptadienyl)-3,4-dihydroxy-2-oxocyclohexanecarboxaldehyde. $C_{14}H_{20}O_4$; mol wt 252.31. C 66.64%, H 7.99%, O 25.36%. Mold metabolite with antineoplastic and antibiotic activity; isolated from *Penicillium frequentans* Westling and *P. palitans* Westling: Curtis *et al., Nature* **167**, 557 (1951); Birkinshaw, *Biochem. J.* **51**, 271 (1952). Structure: Sigg, *Helv. Chim. Acta* **46**, 1061 (1963). Effect on Ehrlich ascites carcinoma cells: J. Fuska *et al., Int. Congr. Chemother., Proc., 7th, Prague, 1971* vol. 2 (Univ. Park Press, Baltimore, 1972) pp 97-98. Synthetic study: C. G. Unson, *Diss. Abstr. B* **39**, 1296 (1978).

Needles from boiling water, mp 134.5°. When dissolved, exists as the 1-hydroxymethylene tautomer. $[\alpha]_D^{22}$ +65° (c = 0.95 in $CHCl_3$); $[\alpha]_D^{22}$ +61° (c = 0.96 in methanol). uv max (dioxane): 290, 232 nm (log ε 3.74, 4.52). Sol in acetone, dioxane; less sol in chloroform, ethanol, benzene; slightly sol in carbon tetrachloride, water.

4271. Friedelin. [559-74-0] *D:A*-Friedooleanan-3-one; friedelan-3-one. $C_{30}H_{50}O$; mol wt 426.72. C 84.44%, H 11.81%, O 3.75%. Major triterpene constituent of cork, obtained by extraction of ground cork with alc. Isoln: Istrati, Ostrogovich, *Compt. Rend.* **128**, 1581 (1899). Isolated also from *Ceratopetalum apetalum* D. Don, *Cunoniaceae:* Jefferies, *J. Chem. Soc.* **1954**, 473. Structure,

sterochemistry: Brownlie *et al., Chem. Ind. (London)* **1955**, 1156; Kane, Stevenson, *Tetrahedron* **15**, 223 (1961); Stevenson, *J. Org. Chem.* **28**, 188 (1963). Total synthesis of (±)-form: R. E. Ireland, D. M. Walba, *Tetrahedron Lett.* **1976**, 1071.

Needles from ethyl acetate or alcohol, mp 263-263.5°. $[\alpha]_D$ $-27.8°$ (chloroform). One gram dissolves in 8.6 ml chloroform, 264 ml 99% alcohol.

4272. Frovatriptan. [158747-02-5] (3*R*)-2,3,4,9-Tetrahydro-3-(methylamino)-1*H*-carbazole-6-carboxamide; 3-methylamino-6-carboxamido-1,2,3,4-tetrahydrocarbazole; SB-209509. C_{14}-$H_{17}N_3O$; mol wt 243.30. C 69.11%, H 7.04%, N 17.27%, O 6.58%. Serotonin 5-HT$_{1B/1D}$ receptor agonist. Prepn: F. D. King *et al.,* **WO 9300086**; *eidem,* **US 5464864** (1993, 1995 both to SmithKline Beecham). Pharmacology: A. A. Parsons *et al., J. Cardiovasc. Pharmacol.* **30**, 136 (1997). Series of articles on pharmacology, safety and clinical studies: *Headache* **42**, Suppl. 2, S45-S99 (2002). Review of clinical experience in cluster headaches: H. C. Siow *et al., Cephalalgia* **24**, 1045-1048 (2004); in acute migraine: N. Poolsup *et al., J. Clin. Pharm. Ther.* **30**, 521-532 (2005).

Succinate monohydrate. [158930-17-7]; [158930-09-7] (anhydrous). SB-209509AX; VML-251; Frova; Frovelan; Migard; Miguard. $C_{14}H_{17}N_3O.C_4H_6O_4.H_2O$; mol wt 379.41. White to off-white powder. Sol in water.

THERAP CAT: Antimigraine.

4273. Fructose. [57-48-7] D-Fructose; β-D-fructose; levulose; fruit sugar; Fructosteril; Laevoral; Levugen; Laevosan. C_6-$H_{12}O_6$; mol wt 180.16. C 40.00%, H 6.71%, O 53.28%. Occurs in a large number of fruits, honey, and as the sole sugar in bull and human semen: Auerbach, Bodlander, *Angew. Chem.* **36**, 602 (1923); Mann, *Nature* **157**, 79 (1946); Pryde, *ibid.* 660. Prepd by adding abs alcohol to the syrup obtained from the acid hydrolysis of inulin: Bates *et al., Natl. Bur. Std. Circ.* **C440**, 399 (1942). Prepn from dextrose: Cantor, Hobbs, **US 2354664** (1944 to Corn Prod. Refining). From sucrose by enzymatic conversion: Koepsell *et al.,* **US 2729587** (1956 to U.S.A.). Crystal and molecular structure: J. A. Kanters *et al., Acta Crystallogr.* **B33**, 665 (1977). *Review:* Barry, Honeyman, *Adv. Carbohyd. Chem.* **7**, 53-98 (1952); M. Chen, R. L. Whistler, *ibid.* **34**, 285-343 (1977). Occurs in both the furanose and pyranose forms. An aq soln at 20° contains about 20% of the furanose form.

Orthorhombic, bisphenoidal prisms from alc, dec 103-105°. Sweetest of the sugars. Shows mutarotation. $[\alpha]_D^{20}$ $-132°$ to $-92°$ (c = 2). Rapid and anomalous mutarotation involves pyranose-furanose interconversion. The final value is obtained instantly in the presence of hydroxyl ions. pKa (18°): 12.06. Freely sol in water. One gram dissolves in 15 ml alc, in 14 ml methanol. Slightly sol in cold, freely in hot acetone; sol in pyridine, ethylamine, methylamine.

Ferric Form. [12286-76-9] CB-302; Ferritose. Prepn: Stitt *et al., Proc. Soc. Exp. Biol. Med.* **110,** 70 (1962); Saltman, Charley, US 3074927 and US 3275514 (1966).

USE: To prevent sandiness in ice cream.

THERAP CAT: Fluid and nutrient replenisher, and ferric form as hematinic.

THERAP CAT (VET): For bovine ketosis.

4274. DL-Fructose. [6035-50-3] α-Acrose; methose. C_6-$H_{12}O_6$; mol wt 180.16. C 40.00%, H 6.71%, O 53.28%. Component of formose (polymerization product of formaldehyde): Vogel, *Helv. Chim. Acta* **11,** 370 (1928).

Needles from methanol. d_4^{16} 1.665. mp 129-130° (slow heating). Reduces Fehling's soln.

Phenylosazone. $C_{18}H_{22}N_4O_4$. mp 216-217°.

4275. Fructose-1,6-diphosphate. [488-69-7] D-Fructose 1,6-bis(dihydrogen phosphate); 1,6-D-fructosediphosphoric acid; hexose diphosphate; Harden-Young ester. $C_6H_{14}O_{12}P_2$; mol wt 340.12. C 21.19%, H 4.15%, O 56.45%, P 18.21%. Formed from fructose-6-phosphate in the presence of ATP, Mg^{2+} and the enzyme phosphohexokinase. Prepn from glucose, mannose, fructose, sucrose by the action of yeasts: A. Harden, *Alcoholic Fermentation* (Longmans, Green & Co., New York, 4th ed., 1932); v. Lebedev, *Biochem. Z.* **36,** 254 (1911); *cf* **DE 292817; DE 293864; DE 301590.** Fructose-1,6-diphosphate is reversibly split in the presence of aldolase forming 1-phosphodihydroxyacetone and 3-phosphoglyceraldehyde: Meyerhof *et al., Biochem. Z.* **286,** 301 (1936). Metabolism regulation study: M. E. Kirtley, M. McKay, *Mol. Cell. Biochem.* **18,** 141 (1977).

Sodium salt monohydrate. Esafosfina.
THERAP CAT: Roborant; tonic.

4276. Fructose-6-phosphate. [643-13-0] D-Fructose 6-(dihydrogen phosphate); D-fructose-6-phosphoric acid; fructose monophosphate; hexose phosphate; hexose monophosphate; Neuberg ester. $C_6H_{13}O_9P$; mol wt 260.14. C 27.70%, H 5.04%, O 55.35%, P 11.91%. Present in animal tissues as an equilibrium mixture with glucose-6-phosphate. The glucose-6-phosphate may be reversibly transformed into fructose-6-phosphate by the enzyme phosphohexose isomerase. Prepn by hydrolysis of 1,6-fructose diphosphate with dil acid: Neuberg, *Biochem. Z.* **88,** 432 (1917); **DE 334250** (Bayer); *Chem. Zentralbl.* **1921,** II, 961; *Frdl.* **13,** 948. Role in metabolic regulation and heat generation: E. A. Newsholme, *Biochem. Soc. Trans.* **4,** 978 (1976).

Very sol in water. $[\alpha]_D^{21}$ +2.5° (c = 3), Meyerhof, Lohmann, *Biochem. Z.* **185,** 117 (1927). $[\alpha]_D$ +1.2° (c = 0.9), Lohmann, *ibid.* **262,** 145 (1933). The magnesium and zinc salts also are sol in water. The equilibrium mixture of 75-80% glucose-6-phosphate and 20-25% fructose-6-phosphate is called *lactacidogen* or *Embden ester*.

4277. Fucosamine. [24724-90-1] 2-Amino-2,6-dideoxygalactose. $C_6H_{13}NO_4$; mol wt 163.17. C 44.17%, H 8.03%, N 8.58%, O 39.22%. Isoln of D-form from lipopolysaccharide of *Chromobacterium violaceum:* Crumpton, Davies, *Biochem. J.* **70,** 729 (1958); from *Bacillus licheniformis:* Sharon *et al., ibid.* **93,** 210

(1964). Isoln of L-form from type V *Pneumococcus* capsular polysaccharide: Barker *et al., Nature* **189,** 303 (1961). Synthesis of L-form: Kuhn *et al., Ann.* **628,** 186 (1959); J. Lehmann *et al., Ber.* **112,** 1470 (1979); of D-form: Zehavi, Sharon, *J. Org. Chem.* **29,** 3654 (1964).

α-D-Fucosamine

D-Form hydrochloride. $C_6H_{13}NO_4$·HCl. Crystals from aq acetone, dec 170-175°. $[\alpha]_D^{20}$ +91° (water). Absorption max: 400 nm.

N-Acetyl-D-fucosamine. $C_8H_{15}NO_5$. Crystals from ethanol, dec 196-197°. $[\alpha]_D^{22}$ +92° (c = 2 in water).

L-Form hydrochloride. $C_6H_{13}NO_4$·HCl. Rods from methanol + isopropanol, mp 192-193°. $[\alpha]_D^{27}$ −92° (c = 0.89 in water).

N-Acetyl-L-fucosamine. $C_8H_{15}NO_5$. Crystals from ethanol, mp 197-198°. $[\alpha]_D^{26}$ −82° (c = 1.46 in water).

4278. D-Fucose. [3615-37-0] 6-Deoxy-D-galactose; D-galactomethylose; rhodeose. $C_6H_{12}O_5$; mol wt 164.16. C 43.90%, H 7.37%, O 48.73%. Obtained from glucosides found in various species of *Convolvulaceae, e.g.,* convolvulin, jalapin, β-turpethein. Isoln: Votocek, *Z. Zuckerind. Böhmen* **24,** 249; *Chem. Zentralbl.* **1901,** I, 1042; **1902,** II, 1361; **1905,** II, 1528. Isoln from jalap resin: Votocek, Bulir, *ibid.* **1906,** I, 1818. Prepn by acid hydrolysis of chartreusin: Sternbach *et al., J. Am. Chem. Soc.* **80,** 1639 (1958).

α-Form, needles from alc. Sweet taste. mp 144°. Shows mutarotation, $[\alpha]_D^{19}$ +127.0° (7 min) → +89.4° (31 min) → +77.2° (71 min) → +76.0° (final value 146 min, c = 10). Soluble in water; moderately sol in alcohol.

Pentaacetate. $C_{16}H_{22}O_{10}$. mp 115.5°.
Oxime. $C_6H_{13}NO_5$. mp 188.5°.
Phenylhydrazone. $C_{12}H_{18}N_2O_4$. mp 172°.
Phenylosazone. $C_{18}H_{22}N_4O_3$. mp 176.5°.

4279. L-Fucose. [2438-80-4] 6-Deoxy-L-galactose; L-galactomethylose. $C_6H_{12}O_5$; mol wt 164.16. C 43.90%, H 7.37%, O 48.73%. Occurs in seaweed: *Ascophyllum nodosum* (L.) Ledol. *(Fucus nodosus* L.), *Fucus vesiculosus* L., *F. serratus* L., *F. virsoides* (Don) J. Ag., *Fucaceae,* and in gum tragacanth. Isoln from seaweed: Clark, *J. Biol. Chem.* **54,** 65 (1922); Hockett *et al., J. Am. Chem. Soc.* **61,** 1658 (1939). Manuf from fucoidan: Schweiger, US 3240775 (1966 to Kelco). Synthesis from D-galactose: Dejterjuszynski, Flowers, *Carbohydr. Res.* **28,** 144 (1973); from D-glucose: T. Chiba, S. Tejima, *Chem. Pharm. Bull.* **27,** 2838 (1979); from D-mannose: J. Defaye *et al., Carbohydr. Res.* **94,** 131 (1981). Review of chemistry and biochemistry: H. M. Flowers, *Adv. Carbohydr. Chem. Biochem.* **39,** 279-345 (1981).

α-Form. Minute needles from abs alcohol, mp 140°. Shows mutarotation. $[\alpha]_D^{20}$ −124.1° (10 min) → −108.0° (20 min) → −91.5° (36 min) → −78.6° (70 min) → −75.6° (final value, 24 hrs, c = 9). Soluble in water and alcohol.

4280. Fucosterol. [17605-67-3] (3β,24E)-Stigmasta-5,24(28)-dien-3-ol; 24-ethylidenecholest-5-en-3β-ol. $C_{29}H_{48}O$; mol wt 412.69. C 84.40%, H 11.72%, O 3.88%. Isoln from *Fucus* *vesiculosus* L., *Fucaceae:* Heilbron *et al., J. Chem. Soc.* **1934,** 1572; from marine brown algae *(Phaeophyceae):* Tsuda, *Chem. Pharm. Bull.* **6,** 724 (1958). Structure: MacPhillamy, *J. Am. Chem. Soc.* **64,** 1732 (1942). Stereochemistry: C. Brooks *et al., Steroids* **20,** 487 (1972). Synthesis: Hayazu, *Pharm. Bull.* **5,** 452 (1957).

Crystals from methanol, mp 124°. $[\alpha]_D^{20}$ −38.4° (chloroform). Soluble in most organic solvents.

Acetate. $C_{31}H_{50}O_2$. Crystals, mp 120-121°. $[\alpha]_D^{20}$ −45° (chloroform).

4281. Fucoxanthin. [3351-86-8] $(3S,3'S,5R,5'R,6S,6'R)$-3'-(Acetyloxy)-6',7'-didehydro-5,6-epoxy-5,5',6,6',7,8-hexahydro-3,5'-dihydroxy-8-oxo-β,β-carotene; 6',7'-didehydro-5,6-epoxy-4',5,5',6,7,8-hexahydro-3,3',5'-trihydroxy-8-oxo-α-carotene 3'-acetate; *all-trans*-fucoxanthin. $C_{42}H_{58}O_6$; mol wt 658.91. C 76.56%, H 8.87%, O 14.57%. Carotenoid pigment found in fresh brown algae: *Fucus virsoides* (Don) J. Ag., *Fucaceae*. Also found in *Zygnema pectinatum* (Vauch.) Ag., *Zygnemaceae* and in *Polysiphonia nigrescens* (Dillw.) Grev., *Rhodomelaceae*. Isoln: Karrer *et al., Helv. Chim. Acta* **14,** 628 (1931); Willstätter, Page, *Ann.* **404,** 237 (1914). Structure: Bonnet *et al., Chem. Commun.* **1966,** 515; *J. Chem. Soc. C* **1969,** 429. Abs config: DeVille *et al., Chem. Commun.* **1969,** 1311; K. Bernhard *et al., Tetrahedron Lett.* **1976,** 115.

Needles from ether + petr ether, mp 160°. $[\alpha]_D^{18}$ +72.5 ±9° (chloroform). Abs max (chloroform): 492, 457 nm. Abs max (ethanol): 450 nm ($E_{1cm}^{1\%}$ 1140), Antia, *Can. J. Chem.* **43,** 302 (1965). Freely sol in ethanol; less sol in carbon disulfide; sparingly sol in ether. Practically insol in petr ether. 1.66 g dissolves in 100 g boiling methanol.

4282. Fucus. Bladder-wrack; sea-wrack; bladder fucus; kelpware; black-tang; cut-weed; sea-oak. Dried thallus of *Fucus vesiculosus* L., *F. serratus* L., or *F. siliquosus*, L. *Fucaceae*. *Habit*. Atlantic and Pacific Oceans. *Constit*. Algin, about 0.01% iodine and some bromine mannite.

4283. Fuller's Earth. Floridin. A nonplastic variety of kaolin containing an aluminum magnesium silicate. The name is derived from an ancient process of cleaning or fulling wool, to remove the oil and dirt particles, with a water slurry of earth or clay. At the present time, the term fuller's earth is applied to any clay that has adequate decolorizing and purifying capacity to be used commercially in oil refining without chemical treatment. It is sometimes considered to be synonymous with montmorillonite, *q.v.*, **kaolinite** ($Al_2O_3.2SiO_2.2H_2O$) and **Halloysite** ($Al_2O_3.2SiO_2.4H_2O$). A long list of minerals likely to be found in fuller's earth is given by Porter, *U.S. Geol. Surv. Bull.* **315,** 268 (1907), *C.A.* **1,** 1684 (1907), and the opinion is expressed that fuller's earth results from the decompn of hornblendes and augites rather than from feldspars. Fuller's earth has for its base a series of amorphous, hydrous alu-

minum silicates that have a rather persistent colloidal (used in its widest sense) structure. It is to this colloidal structure, which is not lost at 130° and possibly higher, that the bleaching power is due. The bleaching efficiency of fuller's earth is usually increased by treatment with dilute acids.

USE: Decolorizer for oils and other liquids; filtering medium; filler for rubber; in agricultural formulations; also instead of absorbent charcoal.

4284. Fulvestrant. [129453-61-8] $(7\alpha,17\beta)$-7-[9-[(4,4,5,5,-5-Pentafluoropentyl)sulfinyl]nonyl]estra-1,3,5(10)-triene-3,17-diol; ICI-182780; Faslodex. $C_{32}H_{47}F_5O_3S$; mol wt 606.77. C 63.34%, H 7.81%, F 15.66%, O 7.91%, S 5.28%. Novel steroidal estrogen antagonist reported to lack any partial agonist activity. Prepn: J. Bowler, B. S. Tait, **EP 138504**; *eidem,* **US 4659516** (1985, 1987 both to ICI). Pharmacology: A. E. Wakeling *et al., Cancer Res.* **51,** 3867 (1991). Clinical pharmacokinetics: A. Howell *et al., Br. J. Cancer* **74,** 300 (1996). Clinical evaluation in breast cancer vs tamoxifen: J. F. Robertson *et al., Cancer Res.* **61,** 6739 (2001). Clinical trial in advanced breast cancer: J. N. Ingle *et al., J. Clin. Oncol.* **24,** 1052 (2006). Review of mechanism of action and clinical evaluation: *idem, Br. J. Cancer* **85,** Suppl. 2, 11-14 (2001); A. Howell, *Crit. Rev. Oncol. Hematol.* **57,** 265-273 (2006); of tolerability profile: I. Vergote, P. Abram, *Ann. Oncol.* **17,** 200-204 (2006).

THERAP CAT: Antineoplastic (hormonal).

4285. Fulvoplumierin. [20867-01-0] (7E)-7-(2E)-Butenylidene-1,7-dihydro-1-oxocyclopenta[c]pyran-4-carboxylic acid methyl ester; 3-(2-butenylidene)-2-carboxy-α-(hydroxymethylene)-1,4-cyclopentadiene-1-acetic acid δ-lactone methyl ester; methyl 7-crotonylidenecyclopenta[c]pyran-1-(7H)-one-4-carboxylate. $C_{14}H_{12}O_4$; mol wt 244.24. C 68.85%, H 4.95%, O 26.20%. Occurs together with plumieride and plumericin. Isoln from *Plumeria acutifolia* Poir., *Apocynaceae*, also from roots of *P. rubra* var *alba:* Grumbach *et al., Experientia* **8,** 224 (1952). Structure: Schmid, Bencze, *Helv. Chim. Acta* **36,** 206, 1468 (1953). Stereochemistry: Albers-Schönberg *et al., ibid.* **45,** 1406 (1962). Synthesis: Büchi, Carlson, *J. Am. Chem. Soc.* **90,** 5336 (1968); **91,** 6470 (1969).

Orange needles from chloroform + petr ether, ethyl acetate, or alcohol, dec 151-152°. Sublimes in high vacuum. uv max (ethanol): 272, 365 nm (ε 7,000; 33,700). Sol in chloroform, hot ethyl acetate, benzene, alcohol; less sol in pyridine, acetone. Practically insol in water, petr ether.

4286. Fumagillin. [23110-15-8] (2E,4E,6E,8E)-2,4,6,8-Decatetraenedioic acid mono[(3R,4S,5S,6R)-5-methoxy-4-[(2R,3R)-2-methyl-3-(3-methyl-2-butenyl)oxiranyl]-1-oxaspiro[2.5]oct-6-yl] ester; 2,4,6,8-decatetraenedioic acid mono[4-(1,2-epoxy-1,5-dimethyl-4-hexenyl)-5-methoxy-1-oxaspiro[2.5]oct-6-yl] ester. $C_{26}H_{34}O_7$; mol wt 458.54. C 68.10%, H 7.47%, O 24.42%. Antibiotic substance produced by *Aspergillus fumigatus:* T. E. Eble, F. R. Hanson, *Antibiot. Chemother.* **1,** 55 (1951); F. R. Hanson, T. E. Eble, **US 2652356** (1953 to Upjohn). Purification: D. S. Tarbell *et al., J. Am. Chem. Soc.* **77,** 5613 (1955). Structure: *eidem, ibid.* **82,** 1005 (1960); **83,** 3096 (1961). Stereochemistry: N. J. McCorkindale, J. G. Sime, *Proc. Chem. Soc. London* **1961,**

331; J. R. Turner, D. S. Tarbell, *Proc. Natl. Acad. Sci. USA* **48**, 733 (1962). Biosynthesis: A. J. Birch, S. F. Hussain, *J. Chem. Soc. C* **1969**, 1473. Total synthesis of (±)-form: E. J. Corey, B. B. Snider, *J. Am. Chem. Soc.* **94**, 2549 (1972). Anti-amebic activity: M. C. McCowen *et al., Science* **113**, 202 (1951). Acute toxicity: J. A. DiPaolo *et al., Antibiot. Annu.* **1958-1959**, 541. HPLC determn in trout muscle: J. Guyonnet *et al., J. Chromatogr. B* **666**, 354 (1995). Field trial in honey bees: T. C. Webster, *J. Econ. Entomol.* **87**, 601 (1994); in rainbow trout: R. le Gouvello *et al., Aquaculture* **171**, 27 (1999). Clinical evaluation in intestinal microsporidiosis in immunocompromised patients: J.-M. Molina *et al., N. Engl. J. Med.* **346**, 1963 (2002).

Yellow needles from methanol, mp 194-195°. $[\alpha]_D^{25}$ −26.6° (c = 1 in 95% ethanol). Absorptivity: 156.0 at 335 nm and 146.5 at 351 nm (soln of 100 mg in 10 ml chloroform diluted with alcohol to 0.0004% fumagillin and 0.04% chloroform). Practically insol in water, dil acids, satd hydrocarbons. Sol in most other organic solvents, in aq solns of bicarbonates and alkali hydroxides. Best stored in dark, evacuated ampuls at low temps. Stability data: T. E. Eble, E. R. Garrett, *J. Am. Pharm. Assoc.* **43**, 536 (1954); E. R. Garrett, *ibid.* 539. LD$_{50}$ in mice (mg/kg): ~800 s.c. (DiPaolo).

Dicyclohexylamine salt. [41567-78-6] Bicyclohexylammonium fumagillin; Fumidil B.

THERAP CAT: Antiprotozoal.

THERAP CAT (VET): Antiprotozoal. Control of *Nosema apis* in honey bees.

4287. Fumaric Acid. [110-17-8] (2*E*)-2-Butenedioic acid; *trans*-1,2-ethylenedicarboxylic acid; allomaleic acid; boletic acid. C$_4$H$_4$O$_4$; mol wt 116.07. C 41.39%, H 3.47%, O 55.14%. Occurs in many plants, *e.g.*, in *Fumaria officinalis* L., *Fumariaceae*, in *Boletus scaber* Bull., *Boletaceae*, and in *Fomes igniarius* (Fries) Kickx., *Polyporaceae*. Essential to vegetable and animal tissue respiration. Prepd industrially from glucose by the action of fungi such as *Rhizopus nigricans:* Foster, Waksman, *J. Am. Chem. Soc.* **61**, 127 (1939). Laboratory prepn by the oxidation of furfural with sodium chlorate in the presence of vanadium pentoxide: Milas, *Org. Synth.* **coll. vol. II**, 302 (1943). Molecular structure: J. L. Derissen, *J. Mol. Struct.* **38**, 177 (1977). *Review:* W. D. Robinson, R. A. Mount in *Kirk-Othmer Encyclopedia of Chemical Technology* **vol. 14** (Wiley-Interscience, New York, 3rd ed., 1981) pp 770-793.

Monoclinic, prismatic needles or leaflets from water. d 1.625. Sublimes at 200°. Sublimes at 165° at 1.7 mm pressure. Partial carbonization and formation of maleic anhydride occur at 230° (open vessel). mp 287° (closed capillary, rapid heating). pK$_1$ (25°): 3.03; pK$_2$: 4.54. Absorption spectrum: Macbeth, Stewart, *J. Chem. Soc.* **111**, 830 (1917). Soly in 100 g water at 25°: 0.63 g; at 40°: 1.07 g; at 60°: 2.4 g; at 100°: 9.8 g; in 100 g 95% alcohol at 30°: 5.76 g; in 100 g acetone at 30°: 1.72 g; in 100 g ether at 25°: 0.72 g. Almost insol in olive oil, chloroform, carbon tetrachloride, benzene, xylene, molten camphor, liq ammonia.

Monomethyl ester. C$_5$H$_6$O$_4$. Prisms from alc, mp 144.5°.

Dimethyl ester. C$_6$H$_8$O$_4$. Crystals, mp 102°. bp 192°.

USE: Substitute for tartaric acid in beverages and baking powders; as a replacement or partial replacement for citric acid in fruit drinks. As an antioxidant. Manuf polyhydric alcohols, synthetic resins. As mordant in dyeing.

4288. Fumigatin. [484-89-9] 3-Hydroxy-2-methoxy-5-methyl-2,5-cyclohexadiene-1,4-dione; 3-hydroxy-2-methoxy-5-

methyl-*p*-benzoquinone; 6-hydroxy-5-methoxy-*p*-toluquinone; 3-hydroxy-4-methoxy-2,5-toluquinone. C$_8$H$_8$O$_4$; mol wt 168.15. C 57.14%, H 4.80%, O 38.06%. Fungal toxin with antibiotic properties isolated from metabolism soln of *Aspergillus fumigatus* Fres: Anslow, Raistrick, *Biochem. J.* **32**, 687 (1938); Waksman, Geiger, *J. Bacteriol.* **47**, 391 (1944). Synthesis: Baker, Raistrick, *J. Chem. Soc.* **1941**, 670; Posternak, Ruelius, *Helv. Chim. Acta* **26**, 2045 (1943); Seshadri, Venkatasubramanian, *J. Chem. Soc.* **1959**, 1660. Biosynthesis: Pettersson, *Acta Chem. Scand.* **17**, 1323 (1963); Simonart, Verachtert, *Bull. Soc. Chim. Biol.* **49**, 543 (1967). Formation and polarographic assay: J. Lafond-Grellety *et al., Ann. Microbiol.* **129B**, 3 (1978). *Review:* Wilson, "Miscellaneous Aspergillus Toxins," in *Microbial Toxins* **vol. VI**, A. Ciegler *et al.,* Eds. (Academic Press, New York, 1971) p 281.

Maroon-colored needles or hexagonal plates from petr ether, mp 116°. Sublimes *in vacuo.* Volatile with steam. Sparingly sol in water, petr ether; freely sol in acetone, ether, chloroform, benzene, ethyl acetate, alcohol.

4289. Fumonisin B$_1$. [116355-83-0] 1,2,3-propanetricarboxylic acid 1,1′-[1-(12-amino-4,9,11-trihydroxy-2-methyl-tridecyl)-2-(1-methylpentyl)-1,2-ethanediyl] ester; macrofusine; FB$_1$. C$_{34}$H$_{59}$NO$_{15}$; mol wt 721.83. C 56.57%, H 8.24%, N 1.94%, O 33.25%. Most prevalent of a family of mycotoxins produced by *Fusarium moniliforme*, a common mold associated with corn; also isolated from other *Fusarium* species. Isolation: W. C. A. Gelderblom *et al., Appl. Environ. Microbiol.* **54**, 1806 (1988). Structure elucidation of family: S. C. Bezuidenhout *et al., Chem. Commun.* **1988**, 743. Causative agent of pulmonary edema in pig: L. R. Harrison *et al., J. Vet. Diagn. Invest.* **2**, 217 (1990). Association of B$_1$, B$_2$ with human esophageal cancer: J. P. Rheeder *et al., Phytopathology* **82**, 353 (1992). Metabolism: G. S. Shephard *et al., Toxicon* **30**, 768 (1992). Toxicity and carcinogenicity in rat: W. C. A. Gelderblom *et al., Carcinogenesis* **12**, 1247 (1991). Toxicology in pig: W. H. Haschek *et al., Mycopathologia* **117**, 83 (1992). LC determn in corn of B series fumonisins: M. E. Stack, R. M. Eppley, *J. Assoc. Off. Anal. Chem.* **75**, 834 (1992); P. A. Murphy *et al., J. Agric. Food Chem.* **41**, 263 (1993). Review of animal toxicoses: P. F. Ross *et al., Mycopathologia* **117**, 109-114 (1992). Review: W. P. Norred, *J. Toxicol. Environ. Health* **38**, 309-328 (1993).

4290. Fungichromin. [6834-98-6] Antibiotic A 246; cogomycin; lagosin; pentamycin; Cantricin. C$_{35}$H$_{58}$O$_{12}$; mol wt 670.83. C 62.66%, H 8.71%, O 28.62%. Antifungal polyene macrolide antibiotic, related structurally to filipin, *q.v.* Isoln from *Streptomyces cellulosae:* A. A. Tytell *et al., Antibiot. Annu.* **1954-1955**, 716. Isoln (as pentamycin) from *S. penticus:* S. Umezawa, Y. Tanaka, *J. Antibiot.* **11A**, 26 (1958). Isoln (as lagosin) from *S. roseoluteus:* C. J. Bessel *et al.,* US 3013947 (1961 to Glaxo). Isoln from *S. griseus* (FCRC-21): R. C. Pandey *et al., Biomed. Mass Spectrom.* **7**, 93 (1980). Structures: A. C. Cope, H. E. Johnson, *J. Am. Chem. Soc.* **80**, 1504 (1958); A. C. Cope *et al., ibid.* **84**, 2170 (1962); M. L. Dhar *et al., J. Chem. Soc.* **1964**, 842; M. P. Berry, M. C. Whiting, *ibid.* 862; V. Pozgay *et al., J. Antibiot.* **29**, 472 (1976). Identity of fungichromin with lagosin and cogomycin and comparison of reported physico-chemical constants: R. C. Pandey *et al., J. Antibiot.* **35**, 988 (1982). Biosynthesis and NMR assignment: H. Noguchi *et al., J. Am. Chem. Soc.* **110**, 2938 (1988).

Light yellow cryst. mp 157-162° (dec). $[\alpha]_D^{20}$ −227.7° (c = 0.53 in DMF). uv max (methanol): 357, 338, 322 nm ($E_{1cm}^{1\%}$ 1231, 1250, 786). LD_{50} in mice (mg/kg): 1624 orally; 33.3 i.p. (Umezawa, Tanaka).

THERAP CAT: Antifungal (topical).

4291. Fungisterol. [53260-54-1] ($3\beta,5\alpha,22E$)-Ergosta-6,8,22-trien-3-ol. $C_{28}H_{44}O$; mol wt 396.65. C 84.78%, H 11.18%, O 4.03%. Formed from ergosterol by fungi. Isoln from *Penicillium chrysogenum:* A. Saito, *J. Ferment. Technol.* **29**, 457 (1951), *C.A.* **47**, 12507f (1953). Structure: *idem, ibid.* **31**, 141 (1953), *C.A.* **48**, 5276d (1954); *idem, ibid.* **32**, 138, 140 (1954), *C.A.* **49**, 9009i (1955).

Crystals from alcohol + ether + ethyl acetate, mp 147.5°. $[\alpha]_D^{15}$ −21.9° (chloroform).

Acetate. $C_{30}H_{46}O_2$. Crystals, mp 158.5°. $[\alpha]_D^{15}$ −15.7° (chloroform).

4292. Funtumine. [474-45-3] ($3\alpha,5\alpha$)-3-Aminopregnan-20-one; 3α-amino-20-oxo-5α-pregnane. $C_{21}H_{35}NO$; mol wt 317.51. C 79.44%, H 11.11%, N 4.41%, O 5.04%. Steroidal alkaloid isolated from *Funtumia latifolia* Stapf., *Apocynaceae:* Janot *et al., C.R. Hebd. Seances Acad. Sci.* **246**, 3076 (1958); from leaves of *Holorrhena febrifuga* Stapf., *Apocynaceae:* H. Dodoun *et al., Phytochemistry* **12**, 923 (1973). Structure: Janot *et al., Bull. Soc. Chim. Fr.* **1960**, 1640, 1669. Prepn: H. Kapnang *et al., Tetrahedron Lett.* **1977**, 3469. *Review:* R. Goutarel, *Bull. Soc. Chim. Fr.* **1960**, 769. Effect on liver carcinogenesis in rats: A. Lacassagne *et al., C.R. Seances Acad. Sci. Ser. D* **274**, 2830 (1972).

Prisms from ethyl acetate, mp 126°. $[\alpha]_D$ +95° (c = 1.7 in chloroform). pK 9.18. Sol in the usual organic solvents. LD_{50} i.v. in mice: 30 mg/kg (Lacassagne).

4293. Fura-2. [96314-98-6] 2-[6-[Bis(carboxymethyl)amino]-5-[2-[2-[bis(carboxymethyl)amino]-5-methylphenoxy]ethoxy]-2-benzofuranyl]-5-oxazolecarboxylic acid. $C_{29}H_{27}N_3O_{14}$; mol wt 641.54. C 54.29%, H 4.24%, N 6.55%, O 34.91%. Fluorescent calcium imaging agent; structurally related to BAPTA, *q.v.* Ca^{2+} binding causes a spectral shift to shorter wavelengths; ratio of the fluorescence at each wavelength is related to changes in Ca^{2+} binding and is independent of dye concentration. Also used as penta-acetoxymethyl ester, *Fura-2/AM*, to enhance crossing of mem-

branes. Prepn: G. Grynkiewicz *et al., J. Biol. Chem.* **260**, 3440 (1985). Binding kinetics to Ca^{2+}: A. P. Jackson *et al., FEBS Lett.* **216**, 35 (1987). Determn of K_d: D. L. Groden *et al., Cell Calcium* **12**, 279 (1991). Spectra of intracellular forms: C. S. Owen, *ibid.* 385. Photophysics: V. Van den Bergh *et al., Biophys. J.* **68**, 1110 (1995). HPLC determn: M. Castle, E. Neuteboom, *J. Chromatogr. A* **696**, 93 (1995). Determn in tissue: N. N. P. Tran *et al., Cell Calcium* **18**, 420 (1995). Practical aspects of use in intracellular Ca^{2+} measurement: K. R. Sipido, G. Callewaert, *Cardiovasc. Res.* **29**, 717 (1995).

uv max absorption (100 m*M* KCl): 362 nm free dye; 335 nm Ca^{2+} complex. emission max: 512 nm free dye; 505 nm Ca^{2+} complex.

USE: Fluorescent probe for measurement of calcium in biological systems.

4294. Furaltadone. [139-91-3] 5-(4-Morpholinylmethyl)-3-[[(5-nitro-2-furanyl)methylene]amino]-2-oxazolidinone; 5-morpholinomethyl-3-(5-nitrofurfurylideneamino)-2-oxazolidinone; 3-(5-nitro-2-furfurylideneamino)-5-(4-morpholinomethyl)-2-oxazolidone; furmethonol; nitrofurmethone; NF-260; Altafur; Altabactina; Furazolin; Ibifur; Medifuran; Nitraldone; Otifuril; Sepsinol; Ultrafur; Unifur; Valsyn. $C_{13}H_{16}N_4O_6$; mol wt 324.29. C 48.15%, H 4.97%, N 17.28%, O 29.60%. Prepn: Gever, **US 2802002** (1957 to Norwich). LC-MS/MS determn of residues in meat: P. Mottier *et al., J. Chromatogr. A* **1067**, 85 (2005).

Yellow crystals from 95% ethanol, dec 206°. Sparingly sol in water: about 75 mg/100 ml at 25°.

THERAP CAT: Antibacterial.

THERAP CAT (VET): Antibacterial.

4295. Furametpyr. [123572-88-3] 5-Chloro-*N*-(1,3-dihydro-1,1,3-trimethyl-4-isobenzofuranyl)-1,3-dimethyl-1*H*-pyrazole-4-carboxamide; *N*-(1,1,3-trimethyl-2-oxa-4-indanyl)-5-chloro-1,3-dimethylpyrazole-4-carboxamide; S-658; Limber. $C_{17}H_{20}ClN_3O_2$; mol wt 333.81. C 61.17%, H 6.04%, Cl 10.62%, N 12.59%, O 9.59%. Fungicide developed to control rice sheath blight. Prepn: T. Mori *et al.,* **EP 315502**; *idem,* **US 4877441** (1989, 1989 both to Sumitomo). *In vitro* and *in vivo* metabolism studies: H. Nagahori *et al., J. Agric. Food Chem.* **48**, 5754 (2000); *idem, ibid.* 5760. Brief description: Y. Oguri, *Agrochem. Jpn.* **1997**, no. 70, 15-16.

Colorless or light brownish crystals, mp 150.2°. Soly in water (25°): 225 mg/l. Sol in most organic solvents. Vapor pressure (25°): 4.7×10^{-6} Pa. LD_{50} in male, female rats, male, female mice (mg/kg): 640, 590, 660, 730 orally. LD_{50} in rats (mg/kg): >2000 dermally (Oguri).

USE: Fungicide.

4296. Furan. [110-00-9] Furfuran; oxole; tetrole; divinyl-ene oxide. C_4H_4O; mol wt 68.07. C 70.58%, H 5.92%, O 23.50%. Occurs in oils obtained by the distillation of rosin contg pine wood. Prepd by decarboxylation of 2-furancarboxylic acid: Wilson, *Org. Synth.* **coll. vol. I** (2nd ed., 1941), p 274. Has been prepd directly from furfural over hot soda-lime or by dropping furfural on a fused mixt of sodium and potassium hydroxides: Hurd *et al., J. Am. Chem. Soc.* **54**, 2532 (1932). Toxicity data: Henderson, *J. Pharmacol. Exp. Ther.* **57**, 394 (1936). Thermodynamic properties: G. B. Guthrie, Jr. *et al., J. Am. Chem. Soc.* **74**, 4662 (1952).

Liquid. $d_4^{19.4}$ 0.9371. bp_{760} 31.36°; bp_{758} 32°. n_D^{20} 1.4216. Flash pt, closed cup: $-32°F$ ($-35°C$). Absorption spectrum: Purvis, *J. Chem. Soc.* **97**, 1648, 1655 (1910). Insol in water. Freely sol in alcohol and ether. Stable to alkalies; resinifies on evaporation or when in contact with mineral acids. LC (in air) in rats: 30400 ppm (Henderson).

Caution: The vapors are anesthetic. Can be absorbed through skin. *See: Toxicity of Industrial Metals,* E. Browning (Appleton-Century-Crofts, New York, 2nd ed., 1969) p 698. This substance is reasonably anticipated to be a human carcinogen: *Report on Carcinogens, Eleventh Edition* (PB2005-104914, 2004) p III-127.

USE: In organic syntheses.

4297. 2-Furanacrylic Acid. [539-47-9] 3-(2-Furanyl)-2-propenoic acid; β-2-furylacrylic acid; furacrylic acid; 2-furalacetic acid; furfurylidene acetic acid. $C_7H_6O_3$; mol wt 138.12. C 60.87%, H 4.38%, O 34.75%. Prepd by the condensation of furfural with malonic acid in the presence of pyridine. Laboratory procedure: S. Rajagopalan, P. V. A. Raman, *Org. Synth.* **25**, 51 (1945). Large scale procedure: Johnson, *ibid.* **20**, 55 (1940). Acid dissociation determn: C. C. Price, E. A. Dudley, *J. Am. Chem. Soc.* **78**, 68 (1956).

Colorless needles from water, mp 141°. Sublimes in high vacuum at 112°. bp_{760} 286°; also reported as bp_{760} 226°; bp_8 117°. pKa in ethanol (25°): 6.49. Volatile in steam. One gram dissolves in 500 ml water at 15°. 100 ml of a satd benzene soln contains 1.14 g at 19°. Sol in alcohol, ether, glacial acetic acid.
Labile Form. mp 104°. Can be converted to the stable form by exposure to sunlight in benzene soln contg some iodine.

4298. 2-Furanacrylonitrile. [7187-01-1] 3-(2-Furanyl)-2-propenenitrile; 3-(2-furyl)acrylonitrile. C_7H_5NO; mol wt 119.12. C 70.58%, H 4.23%, N 11.76%, O 13.43%. Prepd from furfural and cyanoacetic acid in the presence of ammonium acetate and pyridine: Patterson, *Org. Synth.* **40**, 46 (1960).

Liquid. bp_{760} 95-97°. n_D^{25} 1.5824. Miscible with toluene, dimethylformamide.

4299. Furazabol. [1239-29-8] (5α,17β)-17-Methylandro-stano[2,3-c][1,2,5]oxadiazol-17-ol; 17β-hydroxy-17α-methyl-5α-androstano[2,3-c]furazan; androfurazanol; furazalon; DH-245; Mio-tolon. $C_{20}H_{30}N_2O_2$; mol wt 330.46. C 72.69%, H 9.15%, N 8.48%, O 9.68%. Anabolic steroid with hypocholesterolemic properties. Prepn: G. Ohta *et al., BE 645743; eidem, US 3245988* (1964, 1966 both to Daiichi Seiyaku); Shimizu *et al., Chem. Pharm.*

Bull. **13**, 895 (1965); Ohta *et al., ibid.* 1445. Pharmacological studies: Kasahara *et al., ibid.* **13**, 1460 (1965); **16**, 1456, 1460 (1968). Toxicity: *eidem, ibid.* **14**, 285 (1966). Metabolic studies: Takegoshi *et al., ibid.* **20**, 1243 (1972). GC-MS determn in urine: T. Kim *et al., J. Chromatogr. B* **687**, 79 (1996).

Needles from methanol, mp 152-153°. $[α]_D$ +39.4° (c = 1.42 in $CHCl_3$). uv max (ethanol): 217 nm (ε 4300). LD_{50} in mice (g/kg): 2.330 orally; >4 s.c.; 0.494 i.p. (Kasahara, 1966).
Note: This is a controlled substance (anabolic steroid): **21 CFR**, 1308.13, as defined in 1300.01.

4300. Furazolidone. [67-45-8] 3-[[(5-Nitro-2-furanyl)-methylene]amino]-2-oxazolidinone; 3-(5-nitrofurfurylideneamino)-2-oxazolidinone; *N*-(5-nitro-2-furfurylidene)-3-amino-2-oxazoli-done; NF-180; Furovag; Furoxane; Furoxone; Giarlam; Giardil; Medaron; Neftin; Nicolen; Nifulidone; Ortazol; Roptazol; Tiko-furan; Topazone. $C_8H_7N_3O_5$; mol wt 225.16. C 42.67%, H 3.13%, N 18.66%, O 35.53%. Prepn: **GB 735136**; G. Gever, **US 2742462**; G. D. Drake *et al., US 2759931*; G. Gever, C. J. O'Keefe, **US 2927110** (1955, 1956, 1956, 1960 all to Norwich); G. Gever *et al., J. Am. Chem. Soc.* **77**, 2277 (1955). LC-MS/MS determn of residues in meat: P. Mottier *et al., J. Chromatogr. A* **1067**, 85 (2005). Antimicrobial spectrum and toxicity: J. A. Yurchenco *et al., Antibiot. Chemother.* **3**, 1035 (1953); G. S. Rogers *et al., ibid.* **6**, 231 (1956). Pharmacology and toxicology: B. H. Ali, *Vet. Res. Commun.* **6**, 1 (1983).

Yellow crystals from DMF, mp 256-257°. Darkens under strong light. Soly in water (pH 6): approx 40 mg/l. Dec by alkali.
THERAP CAT: Anti-infective (topical); topical antiprotozoal (Trichomonas).
THERAP CAT (VET): Antimicrobial.

4301. Furazolium Chloride. [5118-17-2] 6,7-Dihydro-3-(5-nitro-2-furanyl)-5*H*-imidazo[2,1-*b*]thiazol-4-ium chloride; NF-963; Dermafur. $C_9H_8ClN_3O_3S$; mol wt 273.70. C 39.49%, H 2.95%, Cl 12.95%, N 15.35%, O 17.54%, S 11.72%. Prepn: **NL 6400380**; H. R. Snyder, Jr., **US 3169970** (1964, 1965, both to Norwich Pharmacal); H. R. Snyder, Jr., L. E. Benjamin, *J. Med. Chem.* **9**, 402 (1966).

Crystals from methanol, dec >250°.
Free base. $C_9H_7N_3O_3S$. Crystals from benzene + hexane, dec 171-172°.
THERAP CAT: Antibacterial.

4302. Furcellaran. [9000-21-9] Furcellaria gum; Danish agar; Burtonite 44. A gum obtained from a seaweed of the *Rho-dophyceae,* the red alga *Furcellaria fastigiata,* fam. *Furcellaria-ceae,* order *Gigartinales.* The weed is found primarily in Northern European waters, especially in the Kattegat (between Sweden and Denmark). The gum is the potassium salt of the sulfuric acid ester of a high molecular weight polysaccharide. Consists mainly of D-galactose, 3,6-anhydro-D-galactose, and the half-ester sulfates of these sugars; one sulfate group occurs for each three or four monomeric units, which are arranged in an alternating sequence of $(1 \rightarrow 3)$ and $(1 \rightarrow 4)$-linked units. *Review:* Bjerre-Petersen *et al.* in *Industrial Gums*, R. L. Whistler, Ed. (Academic Press, New York, 2nd ed., 1973) pp 123-136.

The processed gum is a white, odorless powder. Sol in hot or warm water. Easily dispersed in cold water to a homogeneous suspension without lumps; the furcellaran particles hydrate, swell and become almost invisible but do not dissolve unless heated. Forms agar-like gels at low concns. The strength of the gel can be increased by adding salts, esp potassium salts. Highly viscous. Solns in neutral medium are not adversely affected by prolonged exposure to high heat. However, exposure to heat in acidic media results in rapid hydrolysis and loss of gelling power.

USE: Natural colloid, gelling agent, viscosity control agent used primarily in food products but also in pharmaceuticals. Also in products for diabetics, proprietaries for reducing excess body wt, toothpastes. As carrier for food preservatives, bactericides. In bacteriological culture media.

4303. Furethidine. [2385-81-1] 4-Phenyl-1-[2-[(tetrahydro-2-furanyl)methoxy]ethyl]-4-piperidinecarboxylic acid ethyl ester; 4-phenyl-1-[2-(tetrahydrofurfuryloxy)ethyl]isonipecotic acid ethyl ester; ethyl 1-(tetrahydrofurfuryloxyethyl)-4-phenylpiperidine-4-carboxylate; 1-(2′-tetrahydrofurfuryloxyethyl)norpethidine. $C_{21}H_{31}NO_4$; mol wt 361.48. C 69.78%, H 8.64%, N 3.87%, O 17.70%. Prepn: Frearson, Stern, **GB 797448** (1958 to J. F. Macfarlan & Co.); Frearson *et al., J. Chem. Soc.* **1960**, 2103.

bp$_{0.5}$ 210°; bp$_{0.3}$ 175-183°. mp ~28°. n_D^{20} 1.5219. pKa 7.48.
Methiodide. $C_{22}H_{34}INO_4$. Crystals from ethyl acetate, mp 174°.
Note: This is a controlled substance (opiate): **21 CFR, 1308.11.**

4304. Furfural. [98-01-1] 2-Furancarboxaldehyde; 2-furaldehyde; pyromucic aldehyde; artificial oil of ants; "furfurol". C_5-H_4O_2; mol wt 96.08. C 62.50%, H 4.20%, O 33.30%. Occurs in some essential oils. Prepd industrially from pentosans which are contained in cereal straws and brans. Laboratory prepn from corncobs: R. Adams, V. Voorhees, *Org. Synth.* **coll. vol. I**, 280 (2nd ed., 1941). May also be prepd from pyridine. Toxicity study: P. M. Jenner *et al., Food Cosmet. Toxicol.* **2**, 327 (1964).

Colorless oily liq. Peculiar odor, somewhat resembling the odor of benzaldehyde. Turns yellow to brown on exposure to air and light and resinifies (the polymerization is greatly accelerated by hot alkali). d_4^{25} 1.1563. bp$_{760}$ 161.8°; bp$_{100}$ 103°; bp$_{20}$ 67.8°; bp$_{1.0}$ 18.5° mp −36.5°. Volatile in steam. n_D^{20} 1.5261. Absorption spectrum: Purvis, *J. Chem. Soc.* **97**, 1655 (1910). Sol in 11 parts water; very sol in alcohol, ether. Flash pt, closed cup, 140°F (60°C); open cup, 155°F (68°C). Lower explosive limit: 2.1% by vol in air. Autoignition temp 797°F (392°C). *Keep in airtight container and protect from light.* LD$_{50}$ orally in rats: 127 mg/kg (Jenner).
Caution: Potential symptoms of overexposure are irritation of eyes, skin and upper respiratory system; headache; dermatitis. *See NIOSH Pocket Guide to Chemical Hazards* (DHHS/NIOSH 97-140, 1997) p 150.
USE: In the manufacture of furfural-phenol plastics such as Durite; in solvent refining of petroleum oils; in the prepn of pyro-

mucic acid. As a solvent for nitrated cotton, cellulose acetate, and gums; in the manuf of varnishes; for accelerating vulcanization; as insecticide, fungicide, germicide; as reagent in analytical chemistry. In the synthesis of furan derivatives.

4305. Furfuryl Alcohol. [98-00-0] 2-Furanmethanol; 2-furylcarbinol; 2-furancarbinol; α-furylcarbinol; furfuralcohol; 2-hydroxymethylfuran. $C_5H_6O_2$; mol wt 98.10. C 61.22%, H 6.16%, O 32.62%. Prepd from furfural which is obtained by the processing of corncobs. Has been obtained by yeast reduction of furfural. The oil obtained by steam distillation of roasted coffee bean meal consists of 50% furfuryl alcohol after all organic acids have been removed. Laboratory prepn from furfural by the Cannizzaro reaction: Wilson, *Org. Synth.* **coll. vol. I** (2nd ed., 1941) p 276; *cf.* **US 2041184** (to Quaker Oats), *C.A.* **30**, 4515 (1936). Prepd industrially by the catalytic reduction of furfural using nickel and Cu-CrO catalysts: Peters, **US 1906873** (1933 to Quaker Oats); Wojcik, *Ind. Eng. Chem.* **40**, 210 (1948). Acute toxicity study: K. H. Jacobson *et al., Am. Ind. Hyg. Assoc. J.* **19**, 91 (1958). Toxicology and carcinogenesis: *NTP Technical Report 482* (NIH PB99-3972, 1999) 248 p.

Liquid. Faint burning odor. Bitter taste. *Poisonous!* d_4^{23} 1.1282. bp$_{760}$ 170°; bp$_{400}$ 151.8°; bp$_{200}$ 133.1°; bp$_{100}$ 115.9°; bp$_{60}$ 104.0°; bp$_{40}$ 95.7°; bp$_{20}$ 81.0°; bp$_{10}$ 68.0°; bp$_5$ 56.0°; bp$_{1.0}$ 31.8°. n_D^{23} 1.48515. Miscible with water, but unstable in water. Sol in alcohol, benzene, chloroform. Very sol in ether. Easily resinified by acids. Spontaneous ignition temp +490° (915°F). Flash pt 75°C (167°F). LC$_{50}$ (4 hr) in rats: 233 ppm (Jacobson).
Caution: Potential symptoms of overexposure are irritation of eyes and mucous membranes; dizziness; nausea, diarrhea; diuresis; respiration, body temperature depression; vomiting; dermatitis. *See NIOSH Pocket Guide to Chemical Hazards* (DHHS/NIOSH 97-140, 1997) p 150.
USE: Solvent; manuf wetting agents, resins.

4306. α-Furildioxime. [522-27-0] Di-2-furanylethanedione dioxime. $C_{10}H_8N_2O_4$; mol wt 220.18. C 54.55%, H 3.66%, N 12.72%, O 29.07%.

Monohydrate. Needle-like crystals, mp 166-168°. Very sol in alcohol, ether, slightly sol in benzene, petr ether.
USE: As a reagent, in alcohol soln, for nickel with which it gives an orange-red compd.

4307. 2-Furoic Acid. [88-14-2] 2-Furancarboxylic acid; α-furoic acid; pyromucic acid; Brenzschleimsäure (German). C_5H_4-O_3; mol wt 112.08. C 53.58%, H 3.60%, O 42.82%. Prepd from furfural by a Cannizzaro reaction: Wilson, *Org. Synth.* **coll. vol. I** (2nd ed., 1941) p 276; *cf.* **US 2041184** (to Quaker Oats), *C.A.* **30**, 4515 (1936); Wojcik, *Ind. Eng. Chem.* **40**, 210 (1948); Harrisson, Moyle, *Org. Synth.* **coll. vol. IV**, 493 (1963). Formed in man and several animal species as a metabolite of furfural and related compds.

Elongated monoclinic prisms from water or by sublimation at 130-140° and 50-60 mm pressure. mp 133-134°. bp$_{760}$ 230-232°; bp$_{20}$ 141-144°. pK (25°) 3.12. Absorption spectrum: Hartley, Dobbie, *J. Chem. Soc.* **73**, 600 (1898). One gram dissolves in 26 ml water at 15°; in 4 ml boiling water. More sol in alcohol; freely sol in ether.
Ethyl ester. Ethyl furoate; ethyl pyromucate. $C_7H_8O_3$. Colorless crystals. d_4^{20} 1.117. mp 34-36°. bp$_{706}$ 195°. Insol in water; sol in alcohol.

Methyl ester. Methyl furoate; methyl pyromucate. $C_6H_6O_3$. Liquid. Agreeable odor. bp 181.3°; d_4^{21} 1.1786; n_D^{21} 1.4871. Slightly sol in water; sol in alcohol.

4308. Furonazide. [3460-67-1] 4-Pyridinecarboxylic acid [1-(2-furanyl)ethylidene]hydrazide; isonicotinic acid α-methyl-furfurylidenehydrazide; 2-furyl methyl ketone isonicotinoyl-hydrazone; α-methylfurfurylidenehydrazide of isonicotinic acid; INF; Furilazone; Clitizina; Menazone. $C_{12}H_{11}N_3O_2$; mol wt 229.23. C 62.88%, H 4.84%, N 18.33%, O 13.96%. Prepn: Miyatake *et al.*, *J. Pharm. Soc. Jpn.* **75**, 1066 (1955).

Crystals, mp 199-201.5°.
THERAP CAT: Antibacterial (tuberculostatic).

4309. Furosemide. [54-31-9] 5-(Aminosulfonyl)-4-chloro-2-[(2-furanylmethyl)amino]benzoic acid; 4-chloro-N-furfuryl-5-sulfamoylanthranilic acid; 4-chloro-N-(2-furylmethyl)-5-sulfamoyl-anthranilic acid; frusemide; fursemide; LB-502; Aisemide; Beronald; Desdemin; Discoid; Diural; Dryptal; Durafurid; Errolon; Eutensin; Frusetic; Frusid; Fulsix; Fuluvamide; Furesis; Furo-Puren; Furosedon; Hydro-rapid; Impugan; Katlex; Lasilix; Lasix; Lowpston; Macasirool; Mirfat; Nicorol; Odemase; Oedemex; Profemin; Rosemide; Rusyde; Trofurit; Urex. $C_{12}H_{11}ClN_2O_5S$; mol wt 330.74. C 43.58%, H 3.35%, Cl 10.72%, N 8.47%, O 24.19%, S 9.69%. Prepn: K. Stürm *et al.*, **DE 1122541**; *eidem*, **US 3058882** (both 1962 to Hoechst). Molecular and crystal structure: J. Lamotte *et al.*, *Acta Crystallogr.* **B34**, 1657 (1978). Review of pharmacokinetics: L. Z. Benet, *J. Pharmacokinet. Biopharm.* **7**, 1-27 (1979); R. E. Cutler, A. D. Blair, *Clin. Pharmacokinet.* **4**, 279-296 (1979). Pharmacodynamics and pharmacokinetics of a slow-release formulation in man: A. Ebihara *et al.*, *Arzneim.-Forsch.* **33**, 163 (1983). Toxicity: E. I. Goldenthal, *Toxicol. Appl. Pharmacol.* **18**, 185 (1971). Comprehensive description: A. M. Al-Obaid *et al.*, *Anal. Profiles Drug Subs.* **18**, 153-193 (1989).

Crystals from aq ethanol, mp 206°. uv max (95% ethanol): 288, 276, 336 nm ($E_{1cm}^{1\%}$ 945, 588, 144); (0.1N NaOH): 226, 273, 336 nm ($E_{1cm}^{1\%}$ 1147, 557, 133). Slightly sol in water, chloroform, ether. Sol in acetone, methanol, DMF, aq solns above pH 8.0. Less sol in ethanol. *Pharmaceut. Incompat:* Calcium gluconate, ascorbic acid, tetracyclines, urea, epinephrine. LD_{50} orally in female, male rats: 2600, 2820 mg/kg (Goldenthal).
THERAP CAT: Diuretic; antihypertensive.
THERAP CAT (VET): Diuretic.

4310. Furoyl Chloride. [1300-32-9] Furancarbonyl chloride. $C_5H_3ClO_2$; mol wt 130.53. C 46.01%, H 2.32%, Cl 27.16%, O 24.51%. C_4H_3OCOCl.
Colorless liquid; mp −2°. bp 170°. Dec by water or alcohol. Sol in ether.
Caution: Vapors irritate the eyes.

4311. Fursultiamine. [804-30-8] N-[(4-Amino-2-methyl-5-pyrimidinyl)methyl]-N-[4-hydroxy-1-methyl-2-[[(tetrahydro-2-furanyl)methyl]dithio]-1-butenyl]formamide; thiamine tetrahydrofurfuryl disulfide; Alinamin F; Diteftin; Judolor; TTFD. $C_{17}H_{26}N_4O_3S_2$; mol wt 398.54. C 51.23%, H 6.58%, N 14.06%, O 12.04%, S 16.09%. Prepn: S. Yurugi, T. Fushimi, **US 3016380** (1962 to Takeda). Metabolism: S. Kikuchi *et al.*, *Eur. J. Pharmacol.* **9**, 367 (1970); C. Mitoma, *Drug Metab. Dispos.* **1**, 698 (1973). Series

of papers on function of tetrahydrofurfuryl mercaptan moiety: *J. Biochem.* **74**, 717 (1973). Crystal structure: W. Shin, Y. C. Kim, *Bull. Korean Chem. Soc.* **7**, 331 (1986).

E - form

Colorless prisms from ethyl acetate, mp 132° (dec). d 1.29. Sparingly sol in water; sol in organic solvents, dil mineral acids. LD_{50} in rats (mg/kg): 2200 orally; 540 i.p. (Yurugi, Fushimi).
THERAP CAT: Vitamin (enzyme cofactor).

4312. Furtrethonium. [7618-86-2] N,N,N-Trimethyl-2-furanmethanaminium; furfuryltrimethylammonium; trimethyl-furfurylammonium; furtrimethonium; Furmethide. $[C_8H_{14}NO]^+$. Prepn of salts: Nabenhauer, **US 2185220** (1938 to SK & F); Weilmuenster, Jordan, *J. Am. Chem. Soc.* **67**, 415 (1945); Khromov-Borisov *et al.*, *J. Gen. Chem. USSR* **24**, 2021 (1954).

Iodide. [541-64-0] Furamon; Furanol. $C_8H_{14}INO$; mol wt 267.11. Crystals from ethanol + ethyl acetate, mp 116-117° (Weilmuenster, Jordan); also reported as mp 118-120° (Khromov-Borisov). Soluble in water, alcohol. Practically insol in benzene. pH of 1% aq soln, 5.3-6.0.
Benzenesulfonate. Benzamon. $C_{14}H_{19}NO_4S$; mol wt 297.37. Crystals from ethanol + butyl acetate, mp 134-135° (Kromov-Borisov). Soluble in water, alcohol.
p-**Toluenesulfonate.** Fisostina. $C_{15}H_{21}NO_4S$; mol wt 311.40.
THERAP CAT: Cholinergic. Iodide as parasympathomimetic.

4313. Fusafungine. [1393-87-9] S-314; Biofusal; Fusaloyos; Fusarine; Locabiotal. Antibiotic used as an aerosol for local application. Isoln from *Fusarium* species: Couchoud, **FR 1164181** (1958), *C.A.* **54**, 20074b (1960); Servier, **BE 612474** (1962), *C.A.* **57**, 11320b (1962); *idem*, **GB 1018626** (1966 to Biofarma), *C.A.* **64**, 16585b (1966). Bacteriological activity: D. Haler, *J. Int. Med. Res.* **5**, 61 (1977); *idem*, *Vie Med.* **61**, 507 (1980).
Solid, mp 125-129°. Stable up to 180°. Practically insol in water. Sol in glycols and fats.
THERAP CAT: Antibacterial.

4314. Fusaric Acid. [536-69-6] 5-Butyl-2-pyridinecarboxylic acid; 5-butylpicolinic acid. $C_{10}H_{13}NO_2$; mol wt 179.22. C 67.02%, H 7.31%, N 7.82%, O 17.85%. Antibiotic (wilting agent) first isolated from the fungus *Fusarium heterosporium,* Nees: Yabuta *et al.*, *J. Agric. Chem. Soc. Jpn.* **10**, 1059 (1934). Isoln from other *Fusarium* species and from *Gibberella fujikuroi* and synthesis: Plattner *et al.*, *Helv. Chim. Acta* **37**, 1379 (1954). Prepn: Hardegger, Nikles, *ibid.* **39**, 505 (1956); **40**, 2428 (1957); Schreiber, Adam, *Ber.* **93**, 1848 (1960); Umezawa, Nagatsu, **DE 2005255** (1970 to Microbiochem. Res. Found.); R. Tschesche, W. Führer, *Ber.* **111**, 3502 (1978). Dopamine β-hydroxylase inhibitor and hypotensive activity: Suda *et al.*, *Chem. Pharm. Bull.* **17**, 2377 (1969); Nagatsu *et al.*, *Biochem. Pharmacol.* **19**, 35 (1970). Toxicity study: Ishii *et al.*, *Arzneim.-Forsch.* **25**, 55 (1975).

Colorless crystals, mp 96-98°. LD_{50} orally in mice: 230 mg/kg (Ishii).
Copper salt. Bluish-violet crystals from water, mp 258-259°.

4315. Fusarubin. [1702-77-8] 3,4-Dihydro-3,6,9-trihydroxy-7-methoxy-3-methyl-1H-naphtho[2,3-c]pyran-5,10-dione; 5,8-dihydroxy-2-(hydroxymethyl)-6-methoxy-3-(2-oxopropyl)-1,4-

naphthalenedione; 3-acetonyl-5,8-dihydroxy-2-(hydroxymethyl)-6-methoxy-1,4-naphthoquinone; oxyjavanicin. $C_{15}H_{14}O_7$; mol wt 306.27. C 58.82%, H 4.61%, O 36.57%. Isoln from *Fusarium solani*: Ruelius, Gauhe, *Ann.* **569**, 38 (1950). Structure: Hardeger *et al., Helv. Chim. Acta* **47**, 2027 (1964). Efficient total synthesis: Y. Tanoue *et al., Bull. Chem. Soc. Jpn.* **60**, 2927 (1987).

Red prisms from benzene, dec 218°. Absorption max (ether): 535, 499 nm. Sol in glacial acetic acid, tetrahydrofuran, acetone, dioxane, pyridine; slightly sol in cold chloroform, cold alcohol, ether. Practically insol in carbon disulfide, cyclohexane, cold benzene. Dissolves in dil NaOH with a violet color. Practically insol in bicarbonate soln.

4316. Fusel Oil. [8013-75-0] Fusel alcohols. Mixture of higher alcohols formed as a by-product of carbohydrate fermentation in the production of ethyl alcohol. Flavor constituent of beer, wines and distilled spirits. Varies widely in composition, depending on the fermentation raw material used, but contains chiefly isopentyl alcohol and 2-methyl-1-butanol as well as isobutyl alcohol (20%), *n*-propyl alcohol (3-5%), and small amounts of other alcohols, esters and aldehydes. Composition of grape brandy fusel oil: A. D. Webb *et al., Anal. Chem.* **24**, 1944 (1952). HPLC determn of constituents: M. E. Neale, *J. Chromatogr.* **447**, 443 (1988). *Review:* A. G. Patil *et al., Int. Sugar J.* **104**, 51-58 (2002).

Refined fusel oil is a colorless to pale yellow liquid with wine or whiskey-like odor. bp 128-130°. n_D^{20} 1.405-1.410. d_{25}^{25} 0.807-0.813. Rotation: −0.5° to −2.0°. Sol in propylene glycol, vegetable oils, in 3 parts 70% ethanol. Insol in water.

USE: Flavoring agent, solvent, source of amyl alcohols.

4317. Fusidic Acid. [6990-06-3] (3α,4α,8α,9β,11α,13α,-14β,16β,17Z)-16-(Acetyloxy)-3,11-dihydroxy-29-nordammara-17(20),24-dien-21-oic acid; 3α,11α,16β-trihydroxy-29-nor-8α,9β,-13α,14β-dammara-17(20),24-dien-21-oic acid 16-acetate; 3α,11α,-16β-trihydroxy-4α,8,14-trimethyl-18-nor-5α,8α,9β,13α,14β-cholesta-17(20),24-dien-21-oic acid 16-acetate; 3,11,16-trihydroxy-4,8,-10,14-tetramethyl-17-(1′-carboxyisohept-4′-enylidene)cyclopentanoperhydrophenanthrene 16-acetate; ramycin; Fucithalmic. C_{31}-$H_{48}O_6$; mol wt 516.71. C 72.06%, H 9.36%, O 18.58%. Antibiotic isolated from the fermentation broth of *Fusidium coccineum*; structurally similar to cephalosporin P₁, *q.v.* Inhibits bacterial protein synthesis by interference with elongation factor G. Isoln and structure: W. O. Godtfredsen *et al., Nature* **193**, 987 (1962); *Lancet* **I**, 928 (1962); W. O. Godtfredsen, S. Vangedal, *Tetrahedron* **18**, 1029 (1962). Identity with ramycin: H. Vanderhaeghe *et al., Nature* **205**, 710 (1965). Structure: D. Arigoni *et al., Experientia* **19**, 521 (1963). Stereochemistry: W. O. Godtfredsen *et al., Tetrahedron* **21**, 3505 (1965). Synthetic studies: W. G. Dauben *et al., J. Am. Chem. Soc.* **94**, 8593 (1972); R. E. Ireland, U. Hengartner, *ibid.* 3652; M. Tanabe *et al., Tetrahedron Lett.* **1977**, 1481. Total synthesis: W. G. Dauben *et al., J. Am. Chem. Soc.* **104**, 303 (1982). Review of structure-activity relationships: W. von Daehne *et al., Adv. Appl. Microbiol.* **25**, 95-146 (1979). Series of articles on

pharmacology and clinical experience: *Int. J. Antimicrob. Ag.* **12**, Suppl. 2, S1-S93 (1999). Review of use in *Staphylococcus aureus* infections: D. Dobie, J. Gray, *Arch. Dis. Child.* **89**, 74-77 (2004).

Crystals from ether or benzene, mp 192-193°. $[\alpha]_D^{20}$ −9° (chloroform). uv max: 204 nm (ε 9900). pK: 5.35 in water. Sol in alc, acetone, chloroform, pyridine, dioxane; sparingly sol in water, ether, hexane. LD₅₀ in mice (g/kg): 1.2 s.c.; 1.5 orally (Godtfredsen).

Sodium salt. [751-94-0] Sodium fusidate; ZN-6; Fucidin; Fucidine. $C_{31}H_{47}NaO_6$; mol wt 538.69. Crystals, sol in water. LD₅₀ in mice (g/kg): 0.2 i.v. (Godtfredsen, *Nature* 1962).

THERAP CAT: Antibacterial.

THERAP CAT (VET): Antibacterial.

4318. Fustin. [20725-03-5] (2R,3R)-*rel*-2-(3,4-Dihydroxyphenyl)-2,3-dihydro-3,7-dihydroxy-4*H*-1-benzopyran-4-one; 3,3′,-4′,7-tetrahydroxyflavanone; dihydrofisetin. $C_{15}H_{12}O_6$; mol wt 288.25. C 62.50%, H 4.20%, O 33.30%. From wood of *Rhus cotinus* L. (Venice sumac) and *R. succedanea* L., *Anacardiaceae*: Schmid, *Ber.* **19**, 1734 (1886); from *Gleditsia triacanthos* L., *Leguminosae*: Chadenson *et al., Compt. Rend.* **249**, 1362 (1955). Structure: Oyamada, *Ann.* **538**, 44 (1939). Stereochemistry: Weinges, *Ann.* **627**, 229 (1959); Roux, Paulus, *Biochem. J.* **77**, 315 (1960); Gaffield, *Tetrahedron* **26**, 4093 (1970).

(±)-**Form.** Crystals, mp 226-228°. $[\alpha]_D^{21}$ −2.4°.

(±)-**Form tetraacetate.** $C_{23}H_{20}O_{10}$. Crystals from methanol, mp 147-148°.

(−)-**Form.** Crystals, mp 216-218°. $[\alpha]_D^{25}$ −26° (c = 2 in 1:1 acetone, water).

(−)-**Form tetraacetate.** Crystals, mp 117-118°. $[\alpha]_D^{23}$ −25.2° (c = 0.8 in tetrachloroethane).

(+)-**Form.** Needles from water, mp 228-229°. $[\alpha]_D^{23}$ +28.3° (c = 0.9 in 1:1 acetone, water).

(+)-**Form tetraacetate.** Crystals from ethanol, mp 116-119°. $[\alpha]_D^{25}$ +24.4° (c = 1.3 in tetrachloroethane).

G

4319. Gabapentin. [60142-96-3] 1-(Aminomethyl)cyclo-hexaneacetic acid; CI-945; Gö-3450; GOE-3450; Neurontin. $C_9H_{17}NO_2$; mol wt 171.24. C 63.13%, H 10.01%, N 8.18%, O 18.69%. Calcium channel ligand structurally related to γ-amino-butyric acid (GABA), *q.v.*, designed to cross the blood brain barrier. Prepn: G. Satzinger *et al.*, **DE 2460891** (1976 to Gödecke); *eidem*, **US 4024175** (1977 to Warner-Lambert). Pharmacokinetics and metabolism: K.-O. Vollmer *et al.*, *Arzneim.-Forsch.* **36**, 830 (1986). Clinical pharmacology: B. Saletu *et al.*, *Int. J. Clin. Pharmacol. Ther. Toxicol.* **24**, 362 (1986). GC determn in biological fluids: W. D. Hooper *et al.*, *J. Chromatogr.* **529**, 167 (1990). Clinical trial in treatment of pain in diabetic neuropathy: M. Back-onja *et al.*, *J. Am. Med. Assoc.* **280**, 1831 (1998); in treatment of postherpetic neuralgia: M. Rowbotham *et al., ibid.* 1837. Review of pharmacology and clinical trials in epilepsy: B. Schmidt in *Antiepileptic Drugs*, R. H. Levy *et al.*, Eds. (Raven Press, New York, 3rd ed., 1989) pp 925-935; K. L. Goa, E. M. Sorkin, *Drugs* **46**, 409-427 (1993); of pharmacology and use in pain management: M. A. Rose, P. C. A. Kam, *Anaesthesia* **57**, 451-462 (2002); of interactions with voltage-gated calcium channels: K. G. Sutton, T. P. Snutch, *Drug Dev. Res.* **54**, 167-172 (2002).

Crystals from ethanol/ether, mp 162-166° (Satzinger); also reported as mp 165-167° (Schmidt). pKa_1 (25°) 3.68; pKa_2 10.70. Isoelectric point 7.14. Partition coefficient (octanol/buffer): 0.075 (pH 7.4). Solubility in water at pH 7.4 exceeds 10%.

THERAP CAT: Anticonvulsant; analgesic.

4320. Gabexate. [39492-01-8] 4-[[6-[(Aminoiminometh-yl)amino]-1-oxohexyl]oxy]benzoic acid ethyl ester; *p*-hydroxyben-zoic acid ethyl ester 6-guanidinohexanoate; *p*-carbethoxyphenyl ε-guanidinocaproate. $C_{16}H_{23}N_3O_4$; mol wt 321.37. C 59.80%, H 7.21%, N 13.08%, O 19.91%. Non-peptide proteolytic enzyme inhibitor which also inhibits the hydrolytic effects of thrombin, plasmin, and kallikrein, trypsin but not chymotrypsin; *cf.* aprotinin. Prepn as the *p*-toluenesulfonate salt: S. Fujii, T. Watanabe, **DE 2050484**; *eidem*, **US 3751447** (1971, 1973 both to Ono). Enzyme inhibition: M. Muramatu, S. Fujii, *Biochim. Biophys. Acta* **268**, 221 (1972); S. Tamura *et al., ibid.* **484**, 417 (1977). Pharmacology: T. Okegada *et al.*, *Nippon Yakurigaku Zasshi* **71**, 71 (1975), *C.A.* **84**, 218m (1976). Metabolism: M. Sugiyama *et al.*, *Oyo Yakuri* **9**, 733 (1975), *C.A.* **83**, 188145s (1975). Metabolism of inhibitory effect on platelet aggregation: G. Kosaki *et al.*, *Thromb. Res.* **20**, 587 (1980). Beneficial action in traumatic shock: A. M. Lefer *et al.*, *IRCS Med. Sci. Libr. Compend.* **8**, 278 (1980); in exptl acute pan-creatitis: J. R. Wisner *et al.*, *Pancreas* **2**, 181 (1987). Comparative clinical study in acute pancreatitis: N. Tanaka *et al.*, *Adv. Exp. Med. Biol.* **120**, 367 (1979). Teratology and toxicity study: T. Fujita *et al.*, *Oyo Yakuri* **9**, 743 (1975), *C.A.* **83**, 188322x (1975).

Methanesulfonate. [56974-61-9] Gabexate mesylate; FOY; Megacert. $C_{16}H_{23}N_3O_4.CH_3SO_3H$; mol wt 417.48. White crystals. Sol in water, ethanol, chloroform. Slightly sol in acetone. Practically insol in ether. pH of soln (1:100): 4.0-5.0. LD_{50} in mice (mg/kg): 8000 orally; 4700 s.c.; 25 i.v. (Fujita).

THERAP CAT: Enzyme inhibitor (proteinase).

4321. Gaboxadol. [64603-91-4] 4,5,6,7-Tetrahydro-isoxazolo[5,4-*c*]pyridin-3(2*H*)-one; 4,5,6,7-tetrahydroisoxazolo[5,-4-*c*]pyridin-3-ol; THIP; Lu-02-030; MK-0928. $C_6H_8N_2O_2$; mol wt 140.14. C 51.42%, H 5.75%, N 19.99%, O 22.83%. Selective extrasynaptic GABA agonist (SEGA); structural analog of musci-mol, *q.v.* Prepn: P. Krogsgaard-Larsen, *Acta Chem. Scand. B* **31**, 584 (1977); *idem*, **EP 167**; *idem*, **US 4278676** (1979, 1981 both to H. Lundbeck & Co.). GABA agonist effects: *idem et al., Nature* **268**, 53 (1977). ^{3}H-THIP binding study: E. Falch, P. Krogsgaard-Larsen, *J. Neurochem.* **38**, 1123 (1982). HPLC determn: S. M. Madsen, *J. Chromatogr.* **238**, 509 (1982). Pharmacokinetics: *idem et al., Acta Pharmacol. Toxicol.* **53**, 353 (1983). Pharmacodynam-ics and potential therapeutic uses: A. V. Christensen *et al., Pharm. Weekbl. Sci. Ed.* **4**, 145 (1982). Clinical effects on nocturnal sleep and hormone secretion: M. Lancel *et al., Am. J. Physiol. Endocri-nol. Metab.* **281**, E130 (2001); on night sleep and cognitive perform-ance: S. Mathias *et al., Neuropsychopharmacology* **30**, 833 (2005). Review of clinical development: R. Huckle, *Curr. Opin. Invest. Drugs* **5**, 766-773 (2004).

Colorless cryst, mp 242-244° (dec). uv max (methanol): 212 nm (log ε 3.64). pKa (water, 25°): 4.44 ±0.03; 8.48 ±0.04.

Hydrobromide. [65202-63-3] $C_6H_8N_2O_2.HBr$. Faintly red-dish cryst from methanol-ether, mp 162-163° (dec). LD_{50} in mice (mg/kg): 80 i.v., 145 i.p.; >320 orally (U.S. patent).

Hydrochloride. [85118-33-8] $C_6H_8N_2O_2.HCl$; mol wt 176.60.

USE: As a molecular probe to study GABA receptors.

THERAP CAT: Sedative, hypnotic.

4322. Gadobenate Dimeglumine. [127000-20-8] 1-Deoxy-1-(methylamino)-D-glucitol [4-(carboxy-κO)-5,8,11-tris[(carboxy-κO)methyl]-1-phenyl-2-oxa-5,8,11-triazatridecan-13-oato(5−)-$\kappa N^5,\kappa N^8,\kappa N^{11},\kappa O^{13}$]gadolinate(2−) (2:1); gadolinium benzyloxy-propionictetraacetate dimeglumine; Gd-BOPTA/Dimeg; B-19036/7; MultiHance. $C_{36}H_{62}GdN_5O_{21}$; mol wt 1058.15. C 40.86%, H 5.91%, Gd 14.86%, N 6.62%, O 31.75%. Intravascular paramagnetic MRI contrast agent. Prepn: E. Felder *et al.*, **EP 230893**; *eidem*, **US 4916246** (1987, 1990 both to Bracco); F. Ungerri *et al.*, *Inorg. Chem.* **34**, 633 (1995). HPLC determn in biological samples: T. Arbughi *et al.*, *J. Chromatogr. B* **713**, 415 (1998). Physicochemical properties: C. de Haen *et al.*, *J. Comput. Assist. Tomogr.* **23**, Suppl. 1, S161 (1999). Pharmacology: P. Tirone *et al., ibid.* S195. Pharmacokinetics: V. Lorusso *et al., ibid.* S181. Toxicology: A. Morisetti *et al., ibid.* S207. Clinical study in MRI of liver lesions: J. Petersein *et al. Radiology* **215**, 727 (2000). Review of clinical studies: B. Hamm *et al., J. Comput. Assist. Tomogr.* **23**, Suppl. 1, S53-S60 (1999).

Hygroscopic powder. mp 124°. Freely sol in water, sol in methanol. Practically insol in *n*-butanol, *n*-octanol, chloroform. Abs max 257.8 nm (ε 203). $[\alpha]_{365}^{20}$ −26.9° (c = 1.45 in water). Prepd as 0.5*M* soln, osmolality (37°) 1.97 mol/kg. d^{20} 1.22. Viscosity (mPa.s): 9.2 (20°), 5.3 (37°). LD_{50} i.v. in mice (mmol/kg): 5.7 (at 1 mL/min), 7.9 (at 0.2 mL/min); LD_{50} i.v. in rats (mmol/kg): 6.6 (at 6 mL/min), 9.2 (at 1 mL/min) (Morisetti).

THERAP CAT: Diagnostic aid (MRI contrast agent).

4323. Gadobutrol. [138071-82-6] [10-[2,3-Dihydroxy-1-(hydroxymethyl)propyl]-1,4,7,10-tetraazacyclododecane-1,4,7-tri-acetato(3−)-$N^1,N^4,N^7,N^{10},O^1,O^4,O^7$]gadolinium; Gd-DO3A-butrol; Gadovist. $C_{18}H_{31}GdN_4O_9$; mol wt 604.71. C 35.75%, H 5.17%, Gd 26.00%, N 9.27%, O 23.81%. Neutral, macrocyclic gadolinium chelate. Prepn: J. Platzek *et al.*, **EP 448191** (1991 to Schering AG). Physicochemical properties and *in vivo* imaging studies: H. Vogler *et al.*, *Eur. J. Radiol.* **21**, 1 (1995). Clinical pharmacokinetics: T. Staks *et al.*, *Invest. Radiol.* **29**, 709 (1994). Clinical evaluation of diagnostic use for cerebral metastases: T. J. Vogl *et al.*, *Radiologe* **35**, 508 (1995); for glioblastomas: M. Hartmann *et al.*, *Fortschr. Röntgenstr.* **164**, 119 (1996).

Hydrophilic. Osmolality (osmol/kg): 0.57 (0.5 mol/l); 1.39 (1 mol/l). Viscosity (cP): 1.43 (0.5 mol/l); 3.7 (1 mol/l). Partition coefficient (butanol/water): 0.006. LD_{50} i.v. in mice: 23 mmol/kg (Vogler).

THERAP CAT: Diagnostic aid (MRI contrast agent).

4324. Gadodiamide. [131410-48-5] [5,8-Bis(carboxymethyl)-11-[2-(methylamino)-2-oxoethyl]-3-oxo-2,5,8,11-tetraazatridecan-13-oato(3−)]gadolinium; gadolinium diethylenetriamine pentaacetic acid bismethylamide; Gd-DTPA-BMA; S-041. C_{16}-$H_{26}GdN_5O_8$; mol wt 573.66. C 33.50%, H 4.57%, Gd 27.41%, N 12.21%, O 22.31%. Nonionic, low-osmolar paramagnetic gadolinium chelate complex. Prepn: S. C. Quay, **WO 8602841** (1986 to New Salutar); *idem*, **US 4687659** (1987 to Salutar). Pharmacokinetics, hemodynamics and toxicology: E. S. Harpur *et al.*, *Invest. Radiol.* **28**, Suppl. 1, S28 (1993). Clinical pharmacokinetics: M. VanWagoner, D. Worah, *ibid.* S44. Clinical study of CNS imaging: G. Sze *et al.*, *ibid.* **28**, Suppl. 1, S49 (1993); J. Valk *et al.*, *Neuroradiology* **35**, 173 (1993); of myocardial imaging: M.-C. Dulce *et al.*, *Am. J. Roentgenol.* **160**, 963 (1993). Review of physicochemical properties: C. A. Chang, *Invest. Radiol.* **28**, Suppl. 1, S21-S27 (1993).

Osmolality (37°, 0.1*M*): 111 μmol/kg water. LD_{50} i.v. in mice: 14 mmol/kg (Chang).

Gadodiamide injection. [131410-51-0] Omniscan. $C_{16}H_{28}$-$GdN_5O_9.C_{16}H_{26}CaN_5NaO_8$; mol wt 1071.15. Osmolality (37°, 0.5*M*): 789 mOsm/kg water. Viscosity (cP): 2.0 (20°), 1.4 (37°). d^{20} 1.13. Log P (butanol/water): −2.1. LD_{50} i.v. in mice: 34 mmol/kg (Harpur).

THERAP CAT: Diagnostic aid (MRI contrast agent).

4325. Gadofosveset. [201688-00-8] (*SA*-8-11252634)-[[4-[Bis[(carboxy-κO)methyl]amino-κN]-6,9-bis[(carboxy-κO)methyl]-1-[(4,4-diphenylcyclohexyl)oxy]-1-hydroxy-2-oxa-6,9-diaza-1-phosphaundecan-11-oic acid-$\kappa N^6,\kappa N^9,\kappa O^{11}$]-1-oxidato(6−)]gadolinate(3−) trihydrogen; MS-325. $C_{33}H_{41}GdN_3O_{14}P$; mol wt 891.91. C 44.44%, H 4.63%, Gd 17.63%, N 4.71%, O 25.11%, P 3.47%. Intravascular contrast agent exhibiting strong but reversible binding to human serum albumin, *q.v.*, in plasma. Prepn: T. J. McMurray *et al.*, **WO 9623526** (1996 to Metasyn). Pharmacology and image enhancing characteristics: R. B. Lauffer *et al.*, *Radiology* **207**, 529 (1998). Pharmacokinetics: D. J. Parmelee *et al.*, *Invest. Radiol.* **32**, 741 (1997). Physicochemical properties: R. N. Muller *et al.*, *Eur. J. Inorg. Chem.* **1999**, 1949. Clinical evaluation in cornary artery angiography: D. A. Bluemke *et al.*, *Radiology* **219**, 114 (2001); in peripheral vascular angiography: P. Perreault *et al.*, *ibid.* **229**, 811 (2003).

Trisodium salt. [193901-90-5] Vasovist. $C_{33}H_{38}GdN_3Na_3$-$O_{14}P$; mol wt 957.86.

THERAP CAT: Diagnostic aid (MRI contrast agent).

4326. Gadolinium. [7440-54-2] Gd; at. wt 157.25; at. no. 64; valence 3. A lanthanide; belongs to yttrium group of rare earth metals. Naturally occurring isotopes (mass numbers): 152 (0.20%), radioactive, $T_{1/2}$ 1.08×10^{14} years, α-emitter; 154 (2.18%); 155 (14.80%); 156 (20.47%); 157 (15.65%); 158 (24.84%); 160 (21.86%); known artificial radioactive isotopes: 137, 139, 142-151, 153, 159, 161, 162. Abundance in earth's crust: 6.1-6.36 ppm. Sources: samarskite, gadolinite (ytterbite), xenotime, and other rare earth minerals. Discovered by J. C. G. de Marignac in 1880. Prepn of metal: Trombe, *Compt. Rend.* **200**, 459 (1935); *idem, Bull. Soc. Chim. Fr.* **2**, 660 (1935); Klemm, Bommer, *Z. Anorg. Chem.* **231**, 138 (1937). Sepn from other rare earths: F. H. Spedding *et al.*, *J. Am. Chem. Soc.* **69**, 2812 (1947); **76**, 2557 (1954). Spectrum: Albertson, *Phys. Rev.* **47**, 370 (1935); Spedding *et al.*, *J. Chem. Phys.* **5**, 33 (1937). Toxicity study: Haley, *J. Pharm. Sci.* **54**, 663 (1965). Reviews of prepn, properties and compds: *The Rare Earths*, F. H. Spedding, A. H. Daane (Krieger, Huntington, N.Y., 1971, reprint of 1961 ed.) 641 pp; Hulet, Bode, "Separation Chemistry of the Lanthanides and Transplutonium Actinides" in *MTP Int. Rev. Sci.: Inorg. Chem., Ser. One* vol. 7, K. W. Bagnall, Ed. (University Park Press, Baltimore, l971) pp 1-45; T. Moeller, "The Lanthanides" in *Comprehensive Inorganic Chemistry* vol. 4, J. C. Bailar, Jr. *et al.*, Eds. (Pergamon Press, Oxford, 1973) pp 1-101; F. H. Spedding in *Kirk-Othmer Encyclopedia of Chemical Technology* vol. 19 (John Wiley & Sons, New York, 3rd ed., 1982) pp 833-854; *Chemistry of the Elements*, N. N. Greenwood, A. Earnshaw, Eds. (Pergamon Press, New York, 1984) pp 1423-1449. Brief review of properties: G. T. Seaborg, *Radiochim. Acta* **61**, 115-122 (1993).

Colorless or faintly yellowish metal; tarnishes in moist air. Crystalline forms: hexagonal close-packed α-form, d 7.886, transforms to β-form at 1262°; body-centered cubic β-form exists at >1262°. mp 1312°. bp 3273°. Heat of fusion: 10.05 kJ/mol. Heat of sublimation (25°): 397.5 kJ/mol. $E°$(aq) Gd^{3+}/Gd −2.4 V (calc). Experimental reduction potentials (referred to a normal calomel electrode): −1.810, −1.955 V: Noddack, Brukl, *Angew. Chem.* **50**, 362 (1937).

Oxide. Gadolinia. Gd_2O_3. Colorless, hygroscopic powder; prepd by igniting the hydroxide, nitrate, carbonate or oxalate, d^{15} 7.407, absorbs CO_2 from the air.

Hydroxide. $Gd(OH)_3$. Gelatinous precipitate, prepd by the action of alkali or ammonium hydroxide on a soln of a gadolinium salt. Absorbs CO_2 from the air.

Chloride. $GdCl_3$. White monoclinic crystals, prepd by heating the oxide with excess of ammonium chloride above 200°. d^0 4.52. mp ~609°. Sol in water; forms double salts with platinic and auric chlorides. A hexahydrate, $GdCl_3.6H_2O$, deliquesc crystals, d 2.424, is obtained from the aq soln. LD_{50} in mice (mg/kg): 550 i.p.; >2000 orally (Haley).

Sulfate. $Gd_2(SO_4)_3$. Octahydrate, colorless monoclinic crystals. Soly in water decreases with rise in temp. On heating at 400° yields the anhydr sulfate, d 4.139; begins to dec at 500°.

Nitrate. $Gd(NO_3)_3$. Hexahydrate, deliquesc triclinic crystals. d 2.332. mp 91°. Sol in water, in alcohol. A pentahydrate, prismatic crystals, mp 92°, d 2.406, very insol, has been prepd. LD_{50} (hexahydrate) in rats (mg/kg): 230 i.p.; >5000 orally (Haley).

USE: Oxide in control rods of some nuclear power reactors.

4327. Gadopentetic Acid. [80529-93-7] [*N,N*-Bis[2-[bis(carboxymethyl)amino]ethyl]glycinato(5−)]gadolinate(2−) dihydrogen; *N,N*-bis[2-[bis(carboxymethyl)amino]ethyl]glycine gadolinium complex; gadolinium diethylenetriaminepentaacetic acid; Gd-DTPA. $C_{14}H_{20}GdN_3O_{10}$; mol wt 547.57. C 30.71%, H 3.68%, Gd 28.72%, N 7.67%, O 29.22%. Evaluation as water-soluble paramagnetic relaxation reagent (PARR) for NMR spectrometry: J. J. Dechter, G. C. Levy, *J. Magn. Reson.* **39**, 207 (1980); and prepn: T. J. Wenzel *et al.*, *Anal. Chem.* **54**, 615 (1982). Use as diagnostic medium for NMR imaging: H. Gries *et al.*, **DE 3129906**; *eidem*, **US 4647447** (1983, 1987 both to Schering AG). Physicochemical properties: H. Gries, H. Miklautz, *Physiol. Chem. Phys. Med. NMR* **16**, 105 (1984); E. Roux, L. De Broe, *J. Belge Radiol.* **71**, 31 (1988). Evaluation as NMR contrast-enhancing agent in animals: R. C. Brasch *et al.*, *Am. J. Roentgenol.* **142**, 625 (1984). Pharmacokinetics and toxicity: H. J. Weinmann *et al.*, *ibid.* 619; in humans: H. J. Weinmann *et al.*, *Physiol. Chem. Phys. Med. NMR* **16**, 167 (1984). HPLC determn: M. M. Vora *et al.*, *J. Chromatogr.* **369**, 187 (1986). Exptl use in imaging reperfused myocardium in dogs: S. Schaefer *et al.*, *J. Am. Coll. Cardiol.* **12**, 1064 (1988). Clinical studies of diagnostic use in brain imaging: R. Felix *et al.*, *Radiology* **156**, 681 (1985); J. P. Stack *et al.*, *Neuroradiology* **30**, 145 (1988). Safety and tolerance in humans: H. A. Goldstein *et al.*, *Radiology* **174**, 17 (1990). Reviews of diagnostic use in intracranial lesions: J. R. Hesselink, G. A. Press, *Radiol. Clin. North Am.* **26**, 873-887 (1988); in spinal disease: G. Sze, *ibid.* 1009-1024.

Dimeglumine salt. [86050-77-3] SHL-451A; ZK-93035; Magnevist. $C_{28}H_{54}GdN_5O_{20}$; mol wt 938.00. Freely sol in water. LD_{50} i.v. in rats: 10 mmol/kg (Weinmann).

THERAP CAT: Diagnostic aid (MRI contrast agent).

4328. Gadoteridol. [120066-54-8] [10-(2-Hydroxypropyl)-1,4,7,10-tetraazacyclododecane-1,4,7-triacetato(3−)-$N^1,N^4,N^7,N^{10},O^1,O^4,O^7,O^{10}$]gadolinium; 10-(2-hydroxypropyl)-1,-4,7,10-tetraazacyclododecane-1,4,7-triacetic acid gadolinium complex; gadolinium(III) 1,4,7-tris(carboxymethyl)-10-(2′-hydroxypropyl)-1,4,7,10-tetraazacyclododecane; Gd(HP-DO3A); SQ-32692. $C_{17}H_{29}GdN_4O_7$; mol wt 558.68. C 36.55%, H 5.23%, Gd 28.15%, N 10.03%, O 20.05%. Nonionic, low-osmolar paramagnetic gadolinium (III) chelate. Prepn: M. F. Tweedle *et al.*, **EP 292689**; *eidem*, **US 4885363** (1988, 1989 both to Squibb); D. D. Dischino *et al.*, *Inorg. Chem.* **30**, 1265 (1991). Biodistribution: P. Wedeking *et al.*, *Magn. Reson. Imaging* **10**, 641 (1992). RIA determn in biological fluids: M. D. Ogan *et al.*, *J. Pharm. Sci.* **82**, 475 (1993). Toxicological studies: R. A. Soltys, *Invest. Radiol.* **27**, Suppl. 1, S7 (1992). Symposium on physicochemical properties, pharmacokinetics and clinical use in neurological disease: *ibid.* 1-63. Comprehensive description: K. Kumar *et al.*, *Anal. Profiles Drug Subs. Excip.* **24**, 209-241 (1996).

White solid obtained as an aggregate clump of fine needle-like microcrystals from methanol/acetone, mp >225°. Hydrophilic. At pH 7, log P (octanol/water): −3.68; (butanol/water): −1.98. Soly (mg/ml): water 737, methanol 119, isopropanol 41, dimethylformamide 10.1, acetonitrile 6.1, methylene chloride 5.2, ethyl acetate 0.5, acetone 0.4, hexane 0.2, toluene 0.3. uv max (water): 274 nm (a_m 2.5).

Gadoteridol injection. ProHance. Osmolality (37°): 630 mOsM/kg water. Viscosity (cP): 2.0 (20°), 1.3 (37°). d^{25} 1.140. LD_{50} in mice, rats (mmol/kg): 11-14, >10 i.v. (Soltys).

THERAP CAT: Diagnostic aid (MRI contrast agent).

4329. Gadoversetamide. [131069-91-5] [8,11-Bis(carboxymethyl)-14-[2-[(2-methoxyethyl)amino]-2-oxoethyl]-6-oxo-2-oxa-5,8,11,14-tetraazahexadecan-16-oato(3−)]gadolinium; [*N,N''*-bis[*N*-(2-methoxyethyl)-carbamoylmethyl]diethylenetriamine-*N,N',N''*-triaceto]gadolinium (III); gadolinium diethylenetriamine pentaacetic acid bis(methoxyethylamide); Gd-DTPA-BMEA; MP-1177; OptiMARK. $C_{20}H_{34}GdN_5O_{10}$; mol wt 661.76. C 36.30%, H 5.18%, Gd 23.76%, N 10.58%, O 24.18%. Nonionic paramagnetic contrast agent. Prepn: R. W. Weber, M. P. Periasamy, **WO 9001024**; R. W. Weber, **US 5130120** (1990, 1992 both to Mallinckrodt); M. Periasamy *et al.*, *Invest. Radiol.* **26**, S217 (1991). Paramagentic profile: K. Adzamli *et al.*, *ibid.* **34**, 410 (1999). Clinical pharmacokinetics: S. K. Swan *et al.*, *J. Magn. Reson. Imaging* **9**, 317 (1999). Clinical study in liver imaging: D. L. Rubin *et al.*, *ibid.* 240; in CNS imaging: R. I. Grossman *et al.*, *Invest. Radiol.* **35**, 412 (2000).

Prepd as 0.5 mmol/ml soln, osmolality (37°) 1110 mOsmol/kg water. Viscosity (cP): 3.1 (20°), 2.0 (37°). d^{25} 1.160. Log P (butanol/water): −1.93. LD_{50} i.v. in mice: 30.3 mmol/kg (Periasamy).

THERAP CAT: Diagnostic aid (MRI contrast agent).

4330. Gadoxetic Acid. [135326-11-3] (*SA*-8-11252634)-[*N*-[(2*S*)-2-[bis[(carboxy-κ*O*)methyl]amino-κ*N*]propyl]-*N*-[2-[bis[(carboxy-κ*O*)methyl]amino-κ*N*]ethyl]-glycinato(5−)-κ*N*,κ*O*]gadolinate(2−) dihydrogen; 3,6,9-triaza-3,6,9-tris(carboxymethyl)-4-(4-ethoxybenzyl)-undecanedioic acid gadolinium complex; gadolinium ethoxybenzyldiethylenetriaminepentaacetic acid; Gd-EOB-DTPA. $C_{23}H_{30}GdN_3O_{11}$; mol wt 681.75. C 40.52%, H 4.44%, Gd 23.07%, N 6.16%, O 25.81%. Paramagnetic hepatobiliary contrast agent. Prepn: H. Schmitt-Willich *et al.*, **EP 405704**; *eidem*, **US 5695739** (1991, 1997 both to Schering AG). Pharmacology: H.-J. Weinmann *et al.*, *Magn. Reson. Med.* **22**, 233 (1991); and toxicology: A. Mühler *et al.*, *Invest. Radiol.* **28**, 26 (1993). Physicochemical characterization: L. Vander Elst *et al.*, *Acta Radiol.* **38**, Suppl. 412, 135 (1997). Clinical pharmacokinetics: G. Shuhmann-Giampieri *et al.*, *J. Clin. Pharmacol.* **37**, 587 (1997). Clinical evaluation of hepatic imaging: W. Stern *et al.*, *Acta Radiol.* **41**, 255 (2000). Review of preclinical studies: Y. Ni, G. Marchal, *Top. Magn. Reson. Imaging* **9**, 183-195 (1998).

Sodium salt. [135326-22-6] Gadoxetate; SHL-569B; Eovist. $C_{23}H_{28}GdN_3Na_2O_{11}$; mol wt 725.71. Prepd as 0.5 mol/l soln, osmolality 1.53 osmol/kg. Viscosity (37°) 2.32 mPa·s. Amphiphilic. LD_{50} i.v. in mice: 7.5 mmol/kg (Weinmann).

THERAP CAT: Diagnostic aid (MRI contrast agent).

4331. Galactaric Acid. [526-99-8] Mucic acid; galactosaccharic acid; tetrahydroxyadipic acid; saccharolactic acid; Schleimsäure (German). $C_6H_{10}O_8$; mol wt 210.14. C 34.29%, H 4.80%, O 60.91%. Prepd by oxidation of lactose and of galactose: Kent, Tollens, *Ann.* **227**, 221 (1885); Maurer, Drefahl, *Ber.* **75B**, 1489 (1942). Manuf from wood sawdust: Acree, **GB 160777** (1921). *Review:* B. A. Lewis *et al.,* "Galactaric Acid and Its Derivatives" in Whistler, Wolfrom, *Methods in Carbohydrate Chemistry* vol. **II** (Academic Press, New York, 1963) pp 38-46.

Cryst powder, dec ~255° when rapidly heated, also reported as 225°. Soluble in 300 parts cold water, 60 parts boiling water, alkalies; practically insol in alcohol, ether.

Ammonium salt. $(NH_4)_2C_6H_8O_8$. Acicular crystals. Soluble in water.

USE: Has been proposed to replace potassium bitartrate in baking powder and for manuf of granular effervescing salts.

4332. Galactitol. [608-66-2] Dulcitol; dulcite; dulcose; euonymit; melampyrite; melampyrum; melampyrin. $C_6H_{14}O_6$; mol wt 182.17. C 39.56%, H 7.75%, O 52.70%. Found in dulcite or Madagascar manna (*Melampyrum nemorosum* L.) and in other species of *Melampyrum, Scrophulariaceae,* and *Evonymus atropurpureus* Jacq., *Celastraceae.* Isoln: Hünefeld, *Ann.* **24**, 241 (1837); Bouchardat, *Ann. Chim. Phys.* **27**, 68 (1872); Fischer, Hertz, *Ber.* **25**, 1261 (1892); Rogerson, *J. Chem. Soc.* **101**, 1040 (1912). Prepn by catalytic isomerization of D-glucitol: Wright, Hartmann, *J. Org. Chem.* **26**, 1588 (1961). Synthesis: Lespieau, *Bull. Soc. Chim. Fr.* [5] **1**, 1374 (1934); Delepine, Horeau, *ibid.* **4**, 1524 (1937); Wiemann, Gordon, *ibid.* **1958**, 433. Structure: R. L. Lohmar "The Polyols" in W. Pigman, *The Carbohydrates* (Academic Press, New York, 1957) p 247.

Crystals from methanol + water, mp 188-189°. Slightly sweet taste. d^{20} 1.47. bp_1 275-280°. One gram dissolves in 30 ml water, in 2 ml boiling water. Slightly sol in alc. Ka at 18° = 3.5×10^{-14}.

Hexa-O-acetylgalactitol. $C_{18}H_{26}O_{12}$. Crystals from ethanol, mp 168-169°.

Hexanitrate. Nitrodulcitol. mp 94-95°. Has explosive properties: Taylor, Rinkenbach, *J. Franklin Inst.* **204**, 374 (1927).

4333. Galactoflavin. [5735-19-3] 1-Deoxy-1-(3,4-dihydro-7,8-dimethyl-2,4-dioxobenzo[g]pteridin-10(2H)-yl)-D-galactitol; 7,8-dimethyl-10-(D-*galacto*-2,3,4,5,6-pentahydroxyhexyl)-benzo[g]pteridine-2,4(3H,10H)-dione; 7,8-dimethyl-10-(D-*galacto*-2,3,4,5,6-pentahydroxyhexyl)isoalloxazine; 7,8-dimethyl-10-(d-1'-dulcityl)isoalloxazine; 6,7-dimethyl-9-(d-1'-dulcityl)isoalloxazine; 6,7-dimethyl-9-(1-deoxy-D-galactitol-1-yl)isoalloxazine. $C_{18}H_{22}$-N_4O_7; mol wt 406.39. C 53.20%, H 5.46%, N 13.79%, O 27.56%. Prepd from 1-deoxy-1-(3,4-dimethyl-6-phenylazo)anilino-D-galactitol and barbituric acid: Berezovskii, Eremenko, *Zh. Obshch. Khim.* **32**, 4056 (1962), *C.A.* **59**, 736b (1963). Structure: Emerson *et al., J. Biol. Chem.* **160**, 165 (1945). Pharmacology: Lane, Brindley, *Proc. Soc. Exp. Biol. Med.* **116**, 57 (1964). Produces congenital malformations in animals: Nelson *et al., J. Nutr.* **58**, 125 (1956); Miller *et al., J. Biol. Chem.* **237**, 968 (1962); Mackler, *Pediatrics* **43**, 915 (1969).

Yellow crystals, dec 260°. Absorption max: 223, 267, 370, 445 nm (ε 2730, 28100, 9100, 10800). Compd has yellow-green fluorescence in water.

USE: Riboflavine antagonist.

4334. D-Galactosamine. [7535-00-4] 2-Amino-2-deoxy-D-galactose; chondrosamine; GalN. $C_6H_{13}NO_5$; mol wt 179.17. C 40.22%, H 7.31%, N 7.82%, O 44.65%. Amino sugar isolated from chondroitin sulfate, *q.v.:* P. A. Levene, F. B. La Forge, *J. Biol. Chem.* **18**, 123 (1914). Sepn of α- and β-anomers: P. A. Levene, *ibid.* **57**, 337 (1923). Synthesis: S. P. James *et al., Nature* **156**, 308 (1945) *eidem, J. Chem. Soc.* **1946**, 625; R. Kuhn, W. Kirschenlohr, *Ann.* **600**, 126 (1956); P. A. Gent *et al., J. Chem. Soc. Perkin Trans. 1* **1972**, 277. Chemistry: D. Horton in *The Amino Sugars* Vol. 1A, R. W. Jeanloz, Ed. (Academic Press, New York, 1969) pp 133-145. Inducer of exptl hepatitis: D. Keppler *et al., Exp. Mol. Pathol.* **9**, 279 (1968); K. Decker, D. Keppler in *Progress in Liver Diseases* Vol. IV, H. Popper, F. Schaffner, Eds. (Grune & Stratton, New York, 1972) p 183. Powerful inhibitor of hepatic RNA synthesis: D. Keppler *et al., J. Biol. Chem.* **249**, 211 (1974); T. Anukarahanonta *et al., Eur. J. Cancer* **16**, 1171 (1980).

α-form

Hydrochloride. $C_6H_{14}ClNO_5$. Crystals, mp 180° (dec). Shows mutarotation. α-Form: $[\alpha]_D^{23}$ +124° → +93° (water). β-Form: $[\alpha]_D^{23}$ +47° → +93° (water).

4335. D-Galactose. [59-23-4] Cerebrose; brain sugar. C_6-$H_{12}O_6$; mol wt 180.16. C 40.00%, H 6.71%, O 53.28%. Constituent of many oligo- and polysaccharides occurring in pectins, gums, and mucilages. Prepn: Kent, Tollens, *Ann.* **227**, 224 (1885); E. P. Clark, *J. Biol. Chem.* **47**, 2 (1921). Mutarotation and purification of β-form: C. S. Hudson, E. Yanosky, *J. Am. Chem. Soc.* **39**, 1021 (1917). Structural configuration: J. Pryde, *J. Chem. Soc.* **123**, 1809 (1923); W. Charlton *et al., ibid.* **1926**, 94; W. N. Haworth *et al., ibid.* **1927**, 2428; E. L. Jackson, C. S. Hudson, *J. Am. Chem. Soc.* **59**, 994 (1937); R. M. Hann *et al., ibid.* **66**, 1912 (1944). Isoln in the processing of the red algae, *Porphyra umbilicalis:* S. Peat *et al., J. Chem. Soc.* **1961**, 1590. *Review:* W. Pigman, *The Carbohydrates* (Academic Press, New York, 1957) pp 88-90. Review of diagnostic use: W. J. Schirmer *et al., J. Surg. Res.* **41**, 543 (1986).

α-form

α-Form. Prisms from water or ethanol, mp 167°. $[\alpha]_D$ +150.7° → +80.2° (water). Soluble in about 0.5 parts water; freely sol in hot water; final soly in water at 25° = 68%; sol in pyridine; slightly sol in alcohol.

β-Form. Crystals, mp 167°. $[\alpha]_D$ +52.8° → +80.2° (water). Sol in 1.7 parts water at 17°.

Monohydrate. Prisms from water, mp 118-120°.

Microparticulate Form. [90881-70-2] SH U 454; Echovist. Suspension of galactose microparticle granules in a galactose solution. Prepn: J. S. Rasor, E. G. Tickner, **EP 131540** (1985 to Schering). Series of articles on *in vivo* use in echocardiography: *Arzneim.-Forsch.* **36**, 1030-1040 (1986). Review of formulations and clinical diagnostic use: R. Schürmann, R. Schlief, *Radiol. Med.* **87**, Suppl. 1, 15-23 (1994).

Transpulmonary Microparticulate Form. [144046-30-0] SH U 508A; Levovist. Suspension of galactose microparticle granules containing 0.1% physiologic palmitic acid in a sterile water solution.

THERAP CAT: Diagnostic aid (hepatic function). Microparticulate forms as diagnostic aid (ultrasound contrast agent).

4336. α-Galactosidase A. Ceramide trihexosidase. Lysosomal enzyme that hydrolyzes terminal α-D-galactose residues in oligosaccharides and galactolipids. Genetic deficiency of the enzyme results in the glycosphingolipid storage disorder known as Fabry's disease. Homodimeric glycoprotein, mol wt ~101 kDa. Targeted to lysosomes via the mannose-6-phosphate receptor. Identification and role in disease: R. O. Brady *et al., N. Engl. J. Med.* **276**, 1163 (1967). Identification as an α-galactosidase: J. A. Kint, *Science* **167**, 1268 (1970). Use in enzyme replacement therapy: R. J. Desnick *et al., Proc. Natl. Acad. Sci. USA* **76**, 5326 (1979). *Review:* R. J. Desnick *et al.* in *The Metabolic and Molecular Bases of Inherited Disease,* C. R. Scriver *et al.,* Eds. (McGraw-Hill, New York, 7th Ed., 1995) pp 2741-2784.

Agalsidase alfa. [104138-64-9] α-Galactosidase (human clone λAG18 isoenzyme A subunit protein moiety reduced); Replagal. Human α-galactosidase A produced by recombinant DNA technology in cultured human cells. *See:* R. F. Selden *et al.,* **WO 9811206** (1998 to Transkaryotic Therapies). Clinical pharmacology and pharmacokinetics: R. Schiffmann *et al., Proc. Natl. Acad. Sci. USA* **97**, 365 (2000).

Agalsidase beta. Fabrazyme. Human α-galactosidase A produced by recombinant DNA technology in Chinese hamster ovary cells. *See:* R. J. Desnick *et al.,* **US 5356804** (1994 to Mt. Sinai School of Med.). Clinical trial in Fabry's disease: C. M. Eng *et al., N. Engl. J. Med.* **345**, 9 (2001).

THERAP CAT: Enzyme replacement therapy for Fabry's disease.

4337. D-Galacturonic Acid. [685-73-4] $C_6H_{10}O_7$; mol wt 194.14. C 37.12%, H 5.19%, O 57.69%. Obtained by hydrolysis of pectin where it is present as polygalacturonic acid: Ehrlich, *Chem. Ztg.* **41**, 197 (1917); Ehrlich, Guttmann, *Biochem. Z.* **259**, 100 (1933); *Ber.* **66**, 220 (1933); Niemann, Link, *J. Biol. Chem.* **95**, 203 (1932); **104**, 743 (1934); Morell, Link, *ibid.* **100**, 385 (1933); Anderson, King, *J. Chem. Soc.* **1961**, 5333. Isoln from mustard seeds: Goering, **US 2987448** (1961 to Oil Seed Prod.).

α-Form. Monohydrate, needles, mp 159°. $[\alpha]_D^{20}$ +98.0° → +50.9° (water). Soluble in water; slightly sol in hot alcohol. Practically insol in ether.

β-Form. mp 166°. $[\alpha]_D$ +27° → +55.6° (water).

Phenylhydrazone. mp 141°.

4338. Galanga. Galangal; colic root; East India root; Chinese ginger. Dried rhizome of *Alpinia officinarum* Hance, *Zingiberaceae. Habit.* China. *Constit.* Volatile oil, resin, kaempferid, galangin, dioxyflavanol, galangol.

4339. Galangin. [548-83-4] 3,5,7-Trihydroxy-2-phenyl-4H-1-benzopyran-4-one; 3,5,7-trihydroxyflavone; norizalpinin.

$C_{15}H_{10}O_5$; mol wt 270.24. C 66.67%, H 3.73%, O 29.60%. Isoln from galanga root, *Alpininia officinarum,* Hance and characterization: E. Jahns, *Ber.* **14**, 2807 (1881). Prepn: T. Heap, R. Robinson, *J. Chem. Soc.* **129**, 2336 (1926); J. J. Chavan, R. Robinson, *ibid.* **1933**, 368. Mutagenicity studies: J. T. MacGregor, L. Jurd, *Mutat. Res.* **54**, 297 (1978); J. P. Brown, P. S. Dietrich, *ibid.* **66**, 223 (1979).

Yellowish needles from ethanol, mp 214-215°. Moderately sol in ethanol, ether; insol in water. Very sol in chloroform, benzene.

4340. Galantamine. [357-70-0] (4aS,6R,8aS)-4a,5,9,10,-11,12-Hexahydro-3-methoxy-11-methyl-6H-benzofuro[3a,3,2-ef][2]benzazepin-6-ol; galanthamine; lycoremine. $C_{17}H_{21}NO_3$; mol wt 287.35. C 71.06%, H 7.37%, N 4.87%, O 16.70%. Selective acetylcholinesterase inhibitor. Isoln from Caucasian snowdrops, *Galanthus woronowii* Vel., *Amaryllidaceae:* N. F. Proskurnina, A. P. Yakovleva, *J. Gen. Chem. USSR* **22**, 1899 (1952); from *Narcissus* spp: Boit *et al., Ber.* **90**, 725, 2197 (1957). Structure work: S. Kobayashi *et al., Chem. Ind. (London)* **1956**, 177. Synthesis and stereochemistry: D. H. R. Barton, G. W. Kirby, *Proc. Chem. Soc. London* **1960**, 392; *eidem, J. Chem. Soc.* **1962**, 806. Asymmetric synthesis of isomers from L-tyrosine: K. Shimizu *et al., Heterocycles* **8**, 277 (1977). Biosynthesis studies: D. H. R. Barton *et al., J. Chem. Soc.* **1963**, 4545; W. Döbke, *Heterocycles* **6**, 551 (1977). Toxicology study: S. L. Friess *et al., Toxicol. Appl. Pharmacol.* **3**, 347 (1961). Clinical pharmacokinetics: U. Bickel *et al., Clin. Pharmacol. Ther.* **50**, 420 (1991). Review of pharmacology: A. L. Harvey, *Pharmacol. Ther.* **68**, 113-128 (1995); of clinical experience in Alzheimer's disease: R. Bullock, *Exp. Rev. Neurother.* **4**, 153-163 (2004); of synthesis and pharmacology: J. Marco-Contelles *et al., Chem. Rev.* **106**, 116-133 (2006).

Crystals from benzene, mp 126-127°. $[\alpha]_D^{20}$ −118.8° (c = 1.378 in ethanol). Monoacidic base. Fairly sol in hot water; freely sol in alcohol, acetone, chloroform. Less sol in benzene, ether.

Hydrochloride. $C_{17}H_{21}NO_3 \cdot HCl$. Crystals from water, dec 256-257°. Sparingly sol in cold, more sol in hot water. Very sparingly sol in alcohol, acetone.

Hydrobromide. [1953-04-4] Nivalin; Razadyne; Reminyl. $C_{17}H_{21}NO_3 \cdot HBr$; mol wt 368.27. Crystals from water, dec 246-247°. $[\alpha]_D^{20}$ −93.1° (c = 0.1015 in 15 ml H_2O). Sparingly sol in water. LD_{50} i.v. in mice (mg/kg): 5.2 ± 0.2 (Friess).

THERAP CAT: Cholinesterase inhibitor.

4341. Galegine. [543-83-9] (3-Methyl-2-butenyl)guanidine; N-3,3-dimethylallylguanidine; isoamyleneguanidine. $C_6H_{13}N_3$; mol wt 127.19. C 56.66%, H 10.30%, N 33.04%. Isoprenoid guanidine deriv from seeds of *Galega officinalis* L., *Leguminosae:* Tanret, *Compt. Rend.* **158**, 1182, 1426 (1914); **159**, 108 (1914); Markovic, Dittertová, *Chem. Zvesti* **9**, 576 (1955), *C.A.* **50**, 8137d (1956). Structure: Barger, White, *Biochem. J.* **17**, 827 (1923). Synthesis: Späth, Spitzy, *Ber.* **58**, 2273 (1925); Babor, Jezo, *Chem. Zvesti* **8**, 513 (1954), *C.A.* **49**, 7495f (1955). Metabolic effects: G. Weitzel *et al., Z. Physiol. Chem.* **353**, 535 (1972). Effects on mitochondria: B. Lotina *et al., Arch. Biochem. Biophys.* **159**, 520 (1973). Biosynthetic study: J. Steiniger, G. Reuter, *Bio-*

chem. Physiol. Pflanz. **166,** 275 (1974). Review: Braun, J. Chem. Educ. **8,** 2175 (1931).

Hygroscopic, bitter crystals. mp 60-65°. Freely sol in water or alcohol, slightly in ether. Keep well closed.

4342. Gallacetophenone. [528-21-2] 1-(2,3,4-Trihydroxy-phenyl)ethanone; 2′,3′,4′-trihydroxyacetophenone; Alizarine yellow C; C.I. 57000. $C_8H_8O_4$; mol wt 168.15. C 57.14%, H 4.80%, O 38.06%. Prepn: Hart, Woodruff, J. Am. Chem. Soc. **58,** 1957 (1936); Campbell, Coppinger, US 2686123 (1954 to U.S. Secy. Agr.); Knowles, US 2763691 (1956 to Kodak); Price, Israelstam J. Org. Chem. **29,** 2800 (1964).

White to brownish-gray, cryst powder, mp 173°. uv max (methanol): 237, 296 nm (ε 8560, 12,500). Sol in 600 parts cold water, more in hot water; sol in alcohol, ether, soln of sodium acetate.

USE: Antiseptic.

4343. Gallamine Triethiodide. [65-29-2] 2,2′,2″-[1,2,3-Benzenetriyltris(oxy)]tris[N,N,N-triethylethanaminium] triiodide; [ν-phenenyltris(oxyethylene)]tris[triethylammonium triiodide]; 1,2,3-tris(2-triethylammonium ethoxy)benzene triiodide; 1,2,3-tris(2-diethylaminoethoxy)benzene tris(ethyl iodide); tri(β-diethyl-aminoethoxy)-1,2,3-benzene triiodoethylate; pyrogallol 1,2,3-(di-ethylaminoethyl ether) tris(ethyl iodide); benzcurine iodide; RP-3697; F-2559; Relaxan; Flaxedil. $C_{30}H_{60}I_3N_3O_3$; mol wt 891.53. C 40.42%, H 6.78%, I 42.70%, N 4.71%, O 5.38%. Curarizing properties: D. Bovet et al., Compt. Rend. **225,** 74 (1947); F. Depierre, ibid. 956. Prepn: E. Fourneau, US 2544076 (1951 to Rhone-Poulenc). Comparative clinical pharmacokinetics: W. Buzello, S. Agoston, Anaesthesist **27,** 313 (1978). Mode of action: D. Colquhoun, R. E. Sheridan, Br. J. Pharmacol. **66,** 78 (1979); eidem, Proc. R. Soc. London Ser. B **211,** 181 (1981). Effects in mammalian and amphibian nerve fibers: K. J. Smith, C. L. Schauf, Science **212,** 1170 (1981).

White cryst from acetone/water, mp 152-153° (indefinite). Freely sol in water, alc, dil acetone; sparingly sol in anhydr acetone, ether, benzene, chloroform.

THERAP CAT: Neuromuscular blocking agent.

THERAP CAT (VET): Neuromuscular blocking agent.

4344. Gallein. [2103-64-2] 3′,4′,5′,6′-Tetrahydroxyspiro-[isobenzofuran-1(3H),9′-[9H]xanthen]-3-one; 3′,4′,5′,6′-tetrahy-droxyfluoran; 3′,4′,5′,6′-tetrahydroxyspiro[phthalan-1,9′-xanthen]-3-one; pyrogallolphthalein; C.I. 45445; mordant violet 25. $C_{20}H_{12}-O_7$; mol wt 364.31. C 65.94%, H 3.32%, O 30.74%. Obtained by heating 1 part phthalic anhydride with 2 parts of pyrogallol or gallic acid: Baeyer, Ber. **4,** 457 (1871); Buchka, Ann. **209,** 261 (1881). Use as a biological stain: R. D. Lillie et al., Stain Technol. **49,** 339 (1974); R. Welsh, ibid. **52,** 261 (1977). See also H. J. Conn's

Biological Stains, R. D. Lillie, Ed. (Williams & Wilkins, Baltimore, 9th ed., 1977) p 351.

Brownish-red powder or crystals with 1½ H_2O, or red crystals with greenish-yellow color when anhydr. Loses the water of crystn at about 180° and blackens above this temp. Does not melt even at 300°. pH 3.8 brownish-yellow; pH 6.6 rose-red. Almost insol in water, benzene, chloroform. Slightly sol in ether; sol in alc, acetone, alkalies.

Disodium salt. Alizarin violet. $C_{20}H_{10}Na_2O_7$. pH 10.6 rose; pH 13.0 violet.

USE: Clinical reagent (phosphates in urine). Monophosphates give a yellow, dibasic a red, tribasic a violet color. Used in soln of 0.5 g in 100 ml 50% alc; 2-3 drops for 100 ml liq. As sensitive indicator for acids, alkali hydroxides, NH_3, but not for carbonates. Biological stain.

4345. Gallic Acid. [149-91-7] 3,4,5-Trihydroxybenzoic acid. $C_7H_6O_5$; mol wt 170.12. C 49.42%, H 3.55%, O 47.02%. Obtained by alkaline or acid hydrolysis of the tannins from nutgalls; also by enzymatic hydrolysis using spent broths from Penicillium glaucum or Aspergillus niger which contain tannase: A. G. Perkin, O. Gunnell, J. Chem. Soc. **69,** 1303 (1896); Hsias, Huang Hai **No. 7,** 51 (1946), C.A. **42,** 3901i (1948); Cochrane, Econ. Bot. **2,** 145 (1948); Toth, Henster, Acta Chim. Acad. Sci. Hung. **2,** 209 (1952). Prepn from tannin containing materials: Krueger et al., US 2723992 (1955 to Mallinckrodt). Synthesis from aliphatic materials: Shipchandler et al., J. Chem. Soc. Perkin Trans. 1 **1975,** 1400. Biosynthesis: Haslam et al., J. Chem. Soc. **1961,** 1854. Study of polymorphic forms: E. Lindpainter, Mikrochemie **27,** 21 (1939). Toxicity studies: J. W. Dollahite et al., Am. J. Vet. Res. **23,** 1264 (1962).

Needles from abs methanol or chloroform, formerly reported as dec 235-240° (Perkin, Gunnell). Sublimes at 210° giving a stable form with mp 258-265° (dec) and an unstable form mp 225-230° (Lindpainter). One gram dissolves in 87 ml water, 3 ml boiling water, 6 ml alcohol, 100 ml ether, 10 ml glycerol, 5 ml acetone. Practically insol in benzene, chloroform, petr ether. Protect from light. LD_{50} in rabbits (g/kg): 5.0 orally (Dollahite).

Methyl ester. [99-24-1] Methyl gallate; gallicin. $C_8H_8O_5$. Monoclinic prisms from methanol, often hydrated or solvated. When dry, mp 202°. Sol in hot water, alcohol, methanol, ether.

Propyl ester see Propyl Gallate.

USE: Manuf gallic acid esters, pyrogallol, inks; as photographic developer; in tanning; in dyeing; in testing for free mineral acids, dihydroxyacetone and alkaloids. Esters as antioxidants.

THERAP CAT: Formerly as astringent, styptic.

THERAP CAT (VET): Has been used as intestinal astringent.

4346. Gallium. [7440-55-3] Ga; at. wt 69.723; at. no. 31; valences 3, 2, 1. Group IIIA (13). Natural isotopes: 69 (60.2%); 71 (39.8%); artificial radioactive isotopes: 63-68; 70; 72-76. Best source is the mineral germanite, a copper sulfide ore; occurs in very small quantities in zinc blendes, in aluminum clays, found in ores of iron, chromium, manganese; constitutes 5×10^{-4}% of the crust of the earth. Discovered by L. Boisbaudran, Compt. Rend. **81,** 493, 1100 (1875); **82,** 163, 1036 (1876); isolated pure by L. Boisbaudran and E. Jungfleisch, *Bull. Soc. Chim.* [2] **31**, 50 (1879). Isoln from rhenium-rich copper schist: Feit, *Angew. Chem.* **46**, 216 (1933). From bauxite: *Chem. Eng. News* **34**, 4300 (1956). Purification by zone melting: *Chem. Ztg.* **80**, 787 (1956). Alternate methods of purification: Gebauhr, **US 2928731**; Merkel, **US 2927853** (both 1960 to Siemens-Schuckert). Spectra: L. Boisbaudran *et al.*, cited in *Mellor's* **vol. 5**, 378 (1929). *Reviews:* Wagner, Gitzen, *J. Chem. Educ.* **29**, 162 (1952); Greenwood, *Inorg. Chem. Radiochem.* **5**, 91-134 (1963); Wade, Banister, *Comprehensive Inorganic Chemistry* **vol. 1**, J. C. Bailar, Jr. *et al.*, Eds. (Pergamon Press, Oxford, 1973) pp 997-1000, 1069-1117; P. de la Bretèque in *Kirk-Othmer Encyclopedia of Chemical Technology* **vol. 11** (Wiley-Interscience, New York, 3rd ed., 1980) pp 604-620. Review of antineoplastic properties and clinical applications of gallium salts: P. Collery *et al.*, *Crit. Rev. Oncol. Hematol.* **42**, 283-296 (2002).

Grayish metal; possesses a greenish-blue reflection; tin- or silver-like when molten; has a crystalline orthorhombic texture. mp 29.78°. bp approx 2400°: Cochran, Foster, *J. Electrochem. Soc.* **109**, 144 (1962). Shows a tendency to remain in supercooled state. Contracts on melting: $d^{29.65}$ (solid) 5.9037; $d^{29.8}$ (liq) 6.0947: Richards, Boyer, *J. Am. Chem. Soc.* **43**, 274 (1921). Heat capacity: 0.09 cal/g/°C (0-24°, solid). Latent heat of fusion 19.16 cal/g. Stable in dry air; tarnishes in moist air or oxygen. Reacts with alkalies with evolution of hydrogen; attacked by cold concd hydrochloric acid; rendered passive by hot nitric acid; readily attacked by halogens.

Suboxide. [12024-20-3] Ga_2O. Brown powder; obtained by heating the sesquioxide and the metal at 700°; stable in dry air; dec above 800°; converted to the trivalent state by nitric acid or bromine.

Hydroxide. [12023-99-3] $Ga(OH)_3$. A gelatinous precipitate; obtained by the action of ammonia or alkali hydroxide on a soln of a gallic salt.

Caution: Administration to humans has caused metallic taste, skin rashes, bone marrow depression: H. E. Stokinger in *Patty's Industrial Hygiene and Toxicology* **vol. 2A**, G. D. Clayton, F. E. Clayton, Eds. (Wiley-Interscience, New York, 3rd ed., 1981) pp 1630-1637.

4347. Gallium Arsenide. [1303-00-0] AsGa; mol wt 144.64. As 51.80%, Ga 48.20%. GaAs. Prepd by passing a mixture of hydrogen and arsenic vapor over gallium(III) oxide at 600°: Goldschmidt, *Skr. Akad. Oslo* **1926**, no. 8, pp 34, 100; *Ber.* **60**, 1289 (1927). Simplified procedure: Juza, Schulz, *Z. Anorg. Allg. Chem.* **275**, 65 (1954); Minden, *Sylvania Technol.* **11**, no. 1, p 19 (Jan. 1958). Vapor phase crystal growth: McAleer *et al.*, *J. Electrochem. Soc.* **108**, 1168 (1961). Use in high-speed microcircuits: A. L. Robinson, *Science* **219**, 275 (1983). Review of toxicology and human exposure: *Toxicological Profile for Arsenic* (PB2000-108021, 2000) 468 pp.

Cubic crystals. mp 1238°. Dark gray with metallic sheen. Hardness 4.5. d_4^{25} 5.31. Thermal expansion coefficient: 5.9×10^{-6}. Thermal conductivity 0.52 watt units. Specific heat 0.086 cal/g/°C. Molten gallium arsenide attacks quartz, therefore graphite boats or quartz boats, which are carbon coated by pyrolytic decompn of methane, should be used in zone refining. GaAs single crystals have been grown by the Czochralski technique and by the floating zone method. Extensive twinning occurs. Intrinsic electron concn 10^7. Energy gap at room temp 1.38 electron volts. Electron mobility 8800 cm²/volt sec. Hole mobility 450 cm²/volt sec. Effective mass for electrons 0.06 m_0. Lattice constant 5.654Å. Dielectric constant 11.1. Intrinsic resistivity at 300 K = 3.7×10^8 ohm-cm. Electron lattice mobility at 300 K = 10,000 cm²/volt-sec. Intrinsic charge density at 300 K = $1.4 \times 10^6/cm^3$. Electron diffusion constant at 300 K = 310 cm²/sec. Hole diffusion constant = 11.5 cm²/sec.

USE: In semiconductor applications (transistors, solar cells, lasers).

4348. Gallium Chloride. [13450-90-3] Gallium trichloride; trichlorogallium. Cl_3Ga; mol wt 176.08. Cl 60.40%, Ga 39.60%. $GaCl_3$. Occurs as a bridged dimer, Ga_2Cl_6. Prepn: W. C. Johnson, C. A. Haskew, *Inorg. Synth.* **1**, 26 (1939); R. A. Kovar, *ibid.* **17**, 167 (1977). Vapor phase studies: A. W. Laubengayer, F. B. Schirmer, *J. Am. Chem. Soc.* **62**, 1578 (1940). Crystal structure: S. C. Wallwork, I. J. Worrall, *J. Chem. Soc.* **1965**, 1816. Use in synthesis of organogallium compounds: R. A. Kovar *et al.*, *Inorg.*

Chem. **14**, 2809 (1975). Review of applications in organic synthesis: R. M. Kellogg, *Chemtracts Org. Chem.* **16**, 79-92 (2003); R. Amemiya, M. Yamaguchi, *Eur. J. Org. Chem.* **2005**, 5145-5150.

Hygroscopic solid, mp 78-79°. bp$_{760}$ 200.0°. d 2.47. Very sol in water; sol in hydrocarbons, ether-type solvents. *Reacts with air.*

USE: Lewis acid catalyst in organic synthesis; reagent for generating organogallium compounds, metallic gallium, and gallium semiconductors.

4349. Gallium Citrate. [27905-02-8]; [30403-03-3] (unspecified stoichiometry). 2-Hydroxy-1,2,3-propanetricarboxylic acid gallium salt (1:1). $C_6H_5GaO_7$; mol wt 258.82. C 27.84%, H 1.95%, Ga 26.94%, O 43.27%. $Ga(C_6H_5O_7)$. Organogallium complex administered to provide an aqueous source of gallium that accumulates in specific biological tissues. Prepd from gallium hydroxide and citric acid: P. Neogi, S. K. Nandi, *J. Indian Chem. Soc.* **13**, 399 (1936); H. C. Dudley, *J. Am. Chem. Soc.* **72**, 3822 (1950). Review of early clinical use as radiolabeled form: J. I. Hirsch *et al.*, *Drug Intel. Clin. Pharm.* **7**, 519-523 (1973). Mechanism studies of tumor localization: S. R. Vallabhajosula *et al.*, *Int. J. Nucl. Med. Biol.* **8**, 363 (1981); and metabolism: H. Kriegel, *Nuklearmedizin* **2**, 53 (1984). Clinical management of lymphoma with SPECT/CT system: B. Palumbo *et al.*, *Eur. J. Nucl. Med. Mol. Imaging* **32**, 1011 (2005). Toxicity studies: H. C. Dudley *et al.*, *J. Pharmacol. Exp. Ther.* **98**, 409 (1950); H. D. Brunner, *et al.*, *Radiology* **61**, 550 (1953). Review of diagnostic use as imaging agent in oncology: H. A. Macapinlac *et al.*, *Nucl. Med. Biol.* **21**, 731-738 (1994); in infection: C. J. Palestro, *Semin. Nucl. Med.* **24**, 128-141 (1994); in lymphoma: E. Even-Sapir, O. Israel, *Eur. J. Nucl. Med. Mol. Imaging* **30**, Suppl. 1, S65-S81 (2003).

Crystalline powder. Soly at 20° (g/100ml): water 92.4, 95% ethanol 0.12, abs ethanol 0.07. Insol in ether, benzene, acetone. LD_{50} i.v. in rats: >220 mg Ga/kg (Brunner).

^{67}Ga-Labeled form. [41183-64-6

THERAP CAT: ^{67}Ga-labeled form as diagnostic aid (radioactive imaging agent).

4350. Gallium Nitrate. [13494-90-1] Nitric acid gallium salt; gallium trinitrate; NSC-15200; Ganite. GaN_3O_9; mol wt 255.74. Ga 27.26%, N 16.43%, O 56.31%. $Ga(NO_3)_3$. Formed by the reaction of elemental gallium with nitric acid; alters the mineral, matrix, and cellular properties of bone. Prepn: A. Dupré, *C.R. Hebd. Seances Acad. Sci.* **86**, 720 (1878); of octahydrate: E. Einecke, *Angew. Chem.* **55**, 40 (1942); of nonahydrate: R. Reinmann, A. Tanner, *Z. Naturforsch.* **20b**, 71 (1965). Toxicity and antitumor activity: M. M. Hart *et al.*, *J. Natl. Cancer Inst.* **47**, 1121 (1971). Clinical pharmacokinetics: D. P. Kelsen *et al.*, *Cancer* **46**, 2009 (1980). Clinical trial in Paget's disease: R. S. Bockman *et al.*, *J. Clin. Endocrinol. Metab.* **80**, 595 (1995). Review of properties and clinical development: B. J. Foster *et al.*, *Cancer Treat. Rep.* **70**, 1311-1319 (1986); of clinical studies in treatment of bone metastases: R. P. Warrell, Jr., *Cancer* **80**, 1680-1685 (1997); of therapeutic uses: G. Apseloff, *Am. J. Ther.* **6**, 327-339 (1999). Series of articles on pharmacology and mechanism of action: *Semin. Oncol.* **18**, Suppl. 5, 1-31 (1991); on clinical experience in multiple myeloma, lymphoma, bladder cancer and cancer-related hypercalcemia: *ibid.* **30**, Suppl. 5, 1-41 (2003).

White crystalline powder. Sol in warm and cold aqueous solvents, absolute alcohol, ether.

Nonahydrate. [135886-70-3] White, slightly hygroscopic, crystalline powder. Sol in water. LD_{50} in male mice, female rats (mg/kg): 80.0, 67.5 i.p. (Hart).

Octahydrate. mp ~65°.

THERAP CAT: Antineoplastic; antipagetic; bone resorption inhibitor.

4351. Gallium Nitride. [25617-97-4] Gallium mononitride. GaN; mol wt 83.73. Ga 83.27%, N 16.73%. Semiconductor material. Prepn: W. C. Johnson *et al.*, *J. Phys. Chem.* **36**, 2651 (1932); and wurtzite structure determn: R. Juza, H. Hahn, *Z. Anorg. Allg. Chem.* **239**, 282 (1938). Prepn of single crystalline GaN by vapor deposition: H. P. Maruska, J. J. Tietjen, *Appl. Phys. Lett.* **15**, 327 (1969). Luminescence studies: H. G. Grimmeiss, H. Koelmans, *Z. Naturforsch.* **14a**, 264 (1959). P-type doping: H. Amano *et al.*, *Jpn. J. Appl. Phys.* **28**, L2112 (1989). Fabrication of blue light emitting diodes (LEDs): S. Nakamura *et al.*, *ibid.* **30**, L1998

(1991). Potential use of GaN LEDs in phototherapy for jaundice: D. S. Seidman *et al.*, *J. Pediatr.* **136**, 771 (2000). Review of properties and crystal growth techniques: S. Strite, H. Morkoç, *J. Vac. Sci. Technol. B* **10**, 1237-1266 (1992); and applications: S. Keller, S. P. Denbaars, *Curr. Opin. Solid State Mater. Sci.* **3**, 45-50 (1997); S. J. Pearton *et al.*, *Materials Today* **5**, 24-31 (June, 2002); of thin film growth techniques and optical properties: R. F. Davis *et al.*, *Proc. IEEE* **90**, 993-1004 (2002).

Equilibrium crystal structure is hexagonal wurtzite; lattice constants at 300 K: a = 3.189 Å; c = 5.185 Å. Less thermodynamically stable cubic zinc blende structures can be grown on cubic substrates; lattice constant a = 4.503 Å. mp 2500° (2800 K). Thermal conductivity: 1.3 W/cm K. Bandgap at 300 K: 3.39 eV. n (1 eV) = 2.33. n (3.38 eV) = 2.67. Exceedingly chemically and thermally stable. Insol in H_2O, acids, and bases at room temp. Dissolves slowly in hot alkalis.

USE: Blue and UV light emitter with applications in semiconductor devices including: LEDs, laser diodes, lighting, displays, and data storage.

4352. Gallium Oxide. [12024-21-4] Gallia; gallium(III) oxide; gallium sesquioxide. Ga_2O_3; mol wt 187.44. Ga 74.40%, O 25.61%. Wide band gap material; exhibits both conduction and luminescence properties. Prepn: L. de Boisbaudran, *Compt. Rend.* **86**, 941 (1878). Synthesis of nanostructures: S. Sharma, M. K. Sunkara, *J. Am. Chem. Soc.* **124**, 12288 (2002); and photoluminescence properties of nanowires: X. C. Wu *et al.*, *Chem. Phys. Lett.* **328**, 5 (2000). Polymorphism study: R. Roy *et al.*, *J. Am. Chem. Soc.* **74**, 719 (1952). Crystal structure of β-form: S. Geller, *J. Chem. Phys.* **33**, 676 (1960). Electrical properties: M. R. Lorenz *et al.*, *J. Phys. Chem. Solids* **28**, 403 (1967). Toxicity study: R. K. Wolff *et al.*, *J. Appl. Toxicol.* **8**, 191 (1988). Use as a dehydration catalyst: B. H. Davis *et al.*, *J. Org. Chem.* **44**, 2142 (1979).

Multiple crystal forms exist; β-Ga_2O_3 is the only stable form. mp 1725±15°. d 5.94. Band gap, E_g = 4.9 eV.

USE: In semiconductors; gas sensing; catalysis. Nanostructures as blue and UV light emitters in optoelectronic device applications.

4353. Gallium Phosphide. [12063-98-8] GaP; mol wt 100.70. Ga 69.24%, P 30.76%. Prepn and description: Folberth, Oswald, *Z. Naturforsch.* **9a**, 1050 (1954); Wolff *et al.*, *Phys. Rev.* **94**, 753 (1954); Antell, Effer, *J. Electrochem. Soc.* **106**, 509 (1959); **107**, 252 (1960); Frosch, Derick, *ibid.* **108**, 251 (1961); Addamiano, *J. Am. Chem. Soc.* **82**, 1537 (1960); Gershenzon, Mikulyak, *ibid.* **108**, 548 (1961); Pizzarello, *ibid.* **109**, 226 (1962). Seguin, Gans, **US 2862787** (1958); Chang, **US 2921905** (1960 to Westinghouse).

Translucent, amber-colored crystals of the zinc blende type. Greenish-yellow, opaque cryst mass, when unreacted gallium is present. mp 1465°. Dielectric constant 8.4. Energy gap 2.25 ev. Hole mobility 70. Electron mobility 1200. Current density at 4 volts = 25 amps/cm² at 25° (in rectifier circuitry).

USE: In semiconductor electronics.

4354. Gallium Trifluoride. [7783-51-9] F_3Ga; mol wt 126.72. F 44.98%, Ga 55.02%. GaF_3. Prepd by thermal decompn of ammonium hexafluogallate $(NH_4)_3(GaF_6)$: Hannebohn, Klemm, *Z. Anorg. Allg. Chem.* **229**, 342 (1936); Kwasnik in *Handbook of Preparative Inorganic Chemistry* vol. 1, G. Brauer, Ed. (Academic Press, New York, 2nd ed., 1963) pp 227-228; from Ga and HF: Brewer *et al.*, *J. Inorg. Nucl. Chem.* **9**, 56 (1959); Muetterties, Castle, *ibid.* **18**, 148 (1961).

White powder. d 4.47 (after heating to 630° in a current of F_2). mp >1000°. bp ~950°. Can be sublimed in N_2 current at about 800° without decomp. Soly in water (25°) 0.0024 g/100 ml. Soly in hot dil HCl 0.0028 g/100 ml.

Trihydrate. White substance, mp >140°. More sol in water than anhydr form.

4355. Gallocyanine. [1562-85-2] 1-Carboxy-7-(dimethylamino)-3,4-dihydroxyphenoxazin-5-ium chloride; C.I. Mordant Blue 10; C.I. 51030. $C_{15}H_{13}ClN_2O_5$; mol wt 336.73. C 53.50%, H 3.89%, Cl 10.53%, N 8.32%, O 23.76%. Made by introducing nitrosodimethylaniline hydrochloride into a suspension of gallic acid in boiling methanol: Koechlin, **DE 19580** (1881), *Frdl.* **1**, 269; Nietzki, Otto, *Ber.* **21**, 1740 (1888); *Colour Index* vol. 4 (3rd ed., 1971) p 4460.

Green crystals. Practically insol in cold water. Slightly sol in hot water; sol in alcohol, glacial acetic acid, in alkali carbonates with reddish color, in concd HCl with a blue color which becomes red upon diluting with water.

USE: As a dye; in alkali carbonate soln as a reagent for lead with which it forms a deep violet color.

4356. Gallopamil. [16662-47-8] α-[3-[[2-(3,4-Dimethoxyphenyl)ethyl]methylamino]propyl]-3,4,5-trimethoxy-α-(1-methylethyl)benzeneacetonitrile; 5-[(3,4-dimethoxyphenethyl)methylamino]-2-isopropyl-2-(3,4,5-trimethoxyphenyl)valeronitrile; α-isopropyl-α-[(N-methyl-N-homoveratryl)-γ-aminopropyl]-3,4,5-trimethoxyphenylacetonitrile; methoxyverapamil; D-600. $C_{28}H_{40}N_2$-O_5; mol wt 484.63. C 69.39%, H 8.32%, N 5.78%, O 16.51%. Calcium channel blocking agent; methoxy analog of verapamil, *q.v.* Prepn: F. Dengel, **BE 615861**; *idem*, **US 3261859** (1962, 1966 to Knoll). Stereoselective synthesis of enantiomers: L. J. Theodore, W. L. Nelson, *J. Org. Chem.* **52**, 1309 (1987). Pharmacology: H. Haas, E. Busch, *Arzneim.-Forsch.* **17**, 257 (1967); *eidem, ibid.* **18**, 401 (1968); A. Fleckenstein, *ibid.* **20**, 1317 (1970). Clinical trial in stable angina pectoris: N. S. Khurmi *et al.*, *Am. J. Cardiol.* **53**, 684 (1984). Symposium on pharmacology and clinical efficacy: *J. Cardiovasc. Pharmacol.* **20**, Suppl. 7, S1-S95 (1992). Review of pharmacokinetics and therapeutic potential in ischemic heart disease: R. N. Brogden, P. Benfield, *Drugs* **47**, 93-115 (1994).

Pale yellow viscous oil. n_D^{25} 1.5402.

Hydrochloride. [16662-46-7] Algocor; Procorum. $C_{28}H_{40}$-N_2O_5·HCl; mol wt 521.09. mp 145-148°.

d-Form hydrochloride. [38176-09-9] White crystalline solid from propanol/cyclohexane, mp 160.5-161.5°. $[\alpha]_D^{25}$ +11.7° (c = 5.02 in ethanol).

l-Form hydrochloride. [36222-39-6] White crystalline solid from propanol/cyclohexane, mp 160.5-161.5°. $[\alpha]_D^{23}$ −11.7° (c = 5.04 in ethanol).

THERAP CAT: Antianginal.

4357. Galvinoxyl. [2370-18-5] 4-[[3,5-Bis(1,1-dimethylethyl)-4-oxo-2,5-cyclohexadien-1-ylidene]methyl]-2,6-bis(1,1-dimethylethyl)phenoxy; Coppinger's radical; 2,6-di-*tert*-butyl-α-(3,5-di-*tert*-butyl-4-oxo-2,5-cyclohexadien-1-ylidene)-*p*-tolyloxy radical; 2,6,3′,5′-tetra-*tert*-butyl-4′-phenoxy-4-methylene-2,5-cyclohexadiene-1-one radical. $C_{29}H_{41}O_2$; mol wt 421.63. C 82.61%, H 9.80%, O 7.59%. Stable phenoxyl radical. Prepn: G. M. Coppinger, *J. Am. Chem. Soc.* **79**, 501 (1957); M. S. Kharasch, B. S. Joshi, *J. Org. Chem.* **22**, 1435 (1957). Radical scavenging study: P. D. Bartlett, T. Funahashi, *J. Am. Chem. Soc.* **84**, 2596 (1962). Electrical properties: D. D. Eley *et al.*, *Trans. Faraday Soc.* **62**, 3192 (1966). Structure determn: D. E. Williams, *Mol. Physics* **16**, 145 (1969). Resonance Raman study: G. N. R. Tripathi, *Chem. Phys. Lett.* **81**, 375 (1981). Theoretical study of magnetic interactions: F. Dietz *et al.*, *J. Phys. Chem. B* **102**, 3912 (1998). Ab initio studies of ferromagnetic properties: S. J. Luo, K. L. Yao, *J. Magn. Magnet. Mater.* **257**, 11 (2003). Use in detection of phospholipid phase transitions: M. A. Singer *et al.*, *Anal. Biochem.* **94**, 322 (1979). Use in measurement of hydrogen-donating activity and antioxidant activity in phenols: H. Shi *et al.*, *Methods Enzymol.* **335**, 157 (2001).

Deep blue needles from absolute ethanol, mp 157.5° (Kharasch, Joshi). Also reported as dark blue needles from dry ethanol, mp 153° (Eley). Absorption max (iso-octane): 280, 289, 400, 423 nm ($\varepsilon \times 10^3$ 9.39, 9.4, 24.3, 180.0). Absorption max (benzene): 407 nm, 431 nm (ε 30000, 154000). Absorption max (ethanol): 428 nm. Sol in petr ether, benzene, cyclohexane.

USE: Free radical scavenger.

4358. Gamabufotalin. [465-11-2] ($3\beta,5\beta,11\alpha$)-3,11,14-Trihydroxybufa-20,22-dienolide; gamabufogenin; gamabufagin. C_{24}-$H_{34}O_5$; mol wt 402.52. C 71.61%, H 8.51%, O 19.87%. One of the genins found in the venom of a Japanese toad (gama; *Bufo vulgaris formosus*). Isoln and structure: Kotake, *Ann.* **465**, 11 (1928); Wieland, Vocke, *Ann.* **481**, 215 (1930); Chen *et al.*, *J. Pharmacol. Exp. Ther.* **49**, 26 (1933); Kondo, Ohno, *J. Pharm. Soc. Jpn.* **59**, 186 (1939); Jensen, *J. Am. Chem. Soc.* **59**, 767 (1937); Kuno Meyer, *Helv. Chim. Acta* **32**, 1599 (1949). Also found in Ch'an-Su, A Chinese drug prepared from Chinese toads (*Bufo asiaticus = Bufo gargarizans* Cantor): Ruckstuhl, Meyer, *Helv. Chim. Acta* **40**, 1270 (1957).

Bitter, solvated prisms from alcohol + ether, mp 254°; when dry dec 262-263°. $[\alpha]_D^{18}$ +1.26° (c = 0.793 in methanol). Produces numbness of the tongue. uv max about 300 nm. Very sparingly sol in chloroform, acetone, water. Somewhat more sol in methanol.

4359. Gambir. Catechu; pale catechu; gambir catechu; terra japonica. Dried aqueous extract of leaves and twigs of *Uncaria gambier* (Hunter) Roxb. (*Ourouparia gambier* (Hunter) Baill.), *Rubiaceae*. *Habit.* Southern Asia. *Constit.* 7-30% catechol, 20-50% catechutannic acid; quercetin, catechu-red, gambir-fluorescein, fixed oil, wax. Contains not less than 70% water-sol substance and not less than 60% is sol in alcohol. *Incompat:* Iron compds, gelatin, limewater, mercuric chloride, zinc sulfate, alkalies.

USE: Tanning, dyeing fabrics brown or black.

THERAP CAT: Astringent.

THERAP CAT (VET): Astringent (intestinal).

4360. Gamboge. [9000-25-3] Cambogia. Gum-resin from *Garcinia hanburyi* Hook. f., *Guttiferae*. *Habit.* East Indies. *Constit.* 70-80% resin, cambogic acid, 15-25% gum.

THERAP CAT: Cathartic.

THERAP CAT (VET): Drastic purgative.

4361. Gambogic Acid. [2752-65-0] (2Z)-2-Methyl-4-[(1R,-3aS,5S,11R,14aS)-3a,4,5,7-tetrahydro-8-hydroxy-3,3,11-trimethyl-13-(3-methyl-2-butenyl)-11-(4-methyl-3-pentenyl)-7,15-dioxo-1,5-methano-1H,3H,11H-furo[3,4-g]pyrano[3,2-b]xanthen-1-yl]-2-butenoic acid. $C_{38}H_{44}O_8$; mol wt 628.75. C 72.59%, H 7.05%, O 20.36%. Principal acidic component of gamboge from the latex of *Garcinia hanburyi* Hook. f., *Guttiferae*: Amorosa, Lipparini, *Ann. Chim. (Rome)* **45**, 977 (1955). Structure: Ollis *et al.*, *Tetrahedron* **21**, 1453 (1965); Ahmed *et al.*, *J. Chem. Soc. C* **1966**, 772.

Golden, friable mass. $[\alpha]_D^{20}$ −685° (methanol). uv max (ethanol): 217, 280, 291, 362 nm (ε 26000, 16700, 17000, 14900).

Methyl ester monomethyl ether. $C_{40}H_{48}O_8$. Yellow prisms from methanol, mp 130-131°. $[\alpha]_D^{22}$ −560° (c = 0.7 in chloroform). uv max (ethanol): 224, 299 nm (ε 36000, 13600).

Pyridine salt. $C_{43}H_{49}NO_8$. Orange needles from ether + petr ether, mp 147-149°. $[\alpha]_D$ −550° (chloroform). uv max (ethanol): 291.5, 359.5 nm (ε 22300, 18100).

4362. Ganaxolone. [38398-32-2] ($3\alpha,5\alpha$)-3-Hydroxy-3-methylpregnan-20-one; CCD-1042. $C_{22}H_{36}O_2$; mol wt 332.52. C 79.46%, H 10.91%, O 9.62%. Synthetic analog of the neuroactive steroids known as epalons that allosterically modulate the γ-aminobutyric acid type A (GABA$_A$) receptor. Prepn: M. C. Cook *et al.*, **DE 2162555**; *eidem*, **US 3953429** (1972, 1976 both to Glaxo); D. J. Hogenkamp *et al.*, *J. Med. Chem.* **40**, 61 (1997). Binding study and anticonvulsant activity: R. B. Carter *et al.*, *J. Pharmacol. Exp. Ther.* **280**, 1284 (1997). Clinical pharmacology: E. P. Monaghan *et al.*, *Epilepsia* **38**, 1026 (1997). Determn in serum by HPLC-MS-MS: K. Ramu *et al.*, *J. Chromatogr. B* **751**, 49 (2001).

White crystals from methanol, mp 190-192°. $[\alpha]_D$ +103°. Insol in aqueous media.

THERAP CAT: Anticonvulsant; antimigraine.

4363. Ganciclovir. [82410-32-0] 2-Amino-1,9-dihydro-9-[[2-hydroxy-1-(hydroxymethyl)ethoxy]methyl]-6H-purin-6-one; 9-[(1,3-dihydroxy-2-propoxy)methyl]guanine; 2'-nor-2'-deoxyguanosine; DHPG; 2'NDG; BIOLF-62; BW-B759U; BW-759; BW-759U; RS-21592. $C_9H_{13}N_5O_4$; mol wt 255.23. C 42.35%, H 5.13%, N 27.44%, O 25.07%. Nucleoside analog structurally related to acyclovir, *q.v.* Prepn: J. P. Verheyden, J. C. Martin, **US 4355032** (1982 to Syntex); K. K. Ogilvie *et al.*, *Can. J. Chem.* **60**, 3005 (1982); W. T. Ashton *et al.*, *Biochem. Biophys. Res. Commun.* **108**, 1716 (1982); J. C. Martin *et al.*, *J. Med. Chem.* **26**, 759 (1983). Antiviral spectrum *in vitro*: K. O. Smith *et al.*, *Antimicrob. Agents Chemother.* **22**, 55 (1982). Mode of action study: Y.-C. Cheng *et al.*, *Proc. Natl. Acad. Sci. USA* **80**, 2767 (1983). Clinical treatment of cytomegalovirus infection in immunodeficient patients: S. H. Koretz *et al.*, *N. Engl. J. Med.* **314**, 801 (1986). Symposium on pharmacology and clinical efficacy vs cytomegalovirus: *Rev. Infect. Dis.* **10**, Suppl. 3, S457-S572 (1988). *Review:* C. S. Crumpacker, *N. Engl. J. Med.* **335**, 721-729 (1996).

Consult the Name Index before using this section.

Crystals from methanol, mp 250° (dec) (Verheyden, Martin); also reported as crystalline monohydrate from water, mp 248-249° (dec) (Ashton); crystals from water, mp >300° (Martin). uv max (methanol): 254 nm (ε 12880). Soly in water (25°): 4.3 mg/ml at pH 7. LD$_{50}$ i.p. in mice: 1-2 g/kg (Martin).

Sodium salt. [107910-75-8] Cymevan; Cymevene; Cytovene; Denosine; Vitrasert. $C_9H_{12}N_5NaO_4$; mol wt 277.21.

THERAP CAT: Antiviral.

4364. Gangliosides. Animal glycosphingolipids occurring in highest concentration in the central nervous system but widely distributed in other tissues. Primarily located in the outer surface of mammalian cell plasma membranes, they are also found in the synaptic membrane of the central nervous system. More than 60 gangliosides have been characterized. Each consists of a fatty acid (often stearic acid) and an oligosaccharide moiety, both attached to sphingosine. Sialic acid, *q.v.,* is the identifying sugar. The sialic acid residues of gangliosides and those of glycoprotein are the main cause of cell surface negative charge. Gangliosides are also thought to be involved in many different cell functions, e.g. metabolism, growth, malignant transformation. Ganglioside nomenclature: L. Svennerholm, "Ganglioside Metabolism" in *Comprehensive Biochemistry* vol. 18, M. Florkin, E. H. Stotz, Eds. (Elsevier, Amsterdam, 1970) pp 201-204. Isoln from normal brain and from the brain of patients with Tay-Sachs disease: Klenk, *Z. Physiol. Chem.* **268,** 50 (1941); **273,** 76 (1942); Trams, Lauter, *Biochim. Biophys. Acta* **60,** 350 (1962); Svennerholm, *Acta Chem. Scand.* **17,** 239 (1963). Occurrence of different gangliosides: Kuhn, Egge, *Angew. Chem.* **72,** 805 (1960). Chromatographic studies: Kuhn *et al., ibid.* **73,** 580 (1961); Klenk, Gielen, *Z. Physiol. Chem.* **326,** 144 (1961). Structure of ganglioside G$_I$ (or G$_{M1}$): Kuhn, Wiegandt, *Ber.* **96,** 866 (1963). Structure of gangliosides G$_I$ and G$_{II}$ (or G$_{D1a}$): Kuhn, Egge, *ibid.* **96,** 3338 (1963). Structure of gangliosides G$_{II}$, G$_{III}$ (or G$_{D1b}$) and G$_{IV}$ (or G$_{T1b}$): Kuhn, Wiegandt, *Z. Naturforsch.* **18b,** 541 (1963). Molecular diversity, biological implications of brain and thymus gangliosides: Y. Nogai, M. Iwamori, *Mol. Cell. Biochem.* **29,** 81 (1980). Biosynthesis in tissues: S. Basu *et al., Adv. Exp. Med. Biol.* **125,** 213 (1980). Action as biotransducers of membrane-mediated information: R. O. Brady, P. H. Fishman, *Adv. Enzymol.* **50,** 303 (1979). Reviews: Wiegandt, *Angew. Chem. Int. Ed.* **7,** 87-96 (1968). Collection of articles on structure and function: *Adv. Exp. Med. Biol.* **125,** 1-555 (1980); on structure analysis, function and properties, regeneration and recovery in the nervous system, clinical trials in amyotropic lateral sclerosis and diabetic neuropathy: *ibid.* **174,** 1-649 (1984). Book: *Gangliosides in Neurological and Neuromuscular Function, Development, and Repair* M. M. Rapport, A. Gorio, Eds. (Raven Press, New York, 1981) 267 pp.

Ganglioside G$_{M1}$

Gangliosides are colorless crystallizable substances which melt with decompn. Insol in non-polar solvents. Soly in polar solvents increases with the size of the sugar residue and the sialic acid content. Forms micelles in aq soln, having mol wt of about 200,000-250,000. Forms molecular solns in DMF or tetrahydrofuran, having mol wt of 1000-3000.

Ganglioside G$_{M1}$. [37758-47-7] Siagoside; Sygen. $C_{73}H_{131}$-N_3O_{31}; mol wt 1546.82.

Combination of gangliosides G$_{M1}$, G$_{D1a}$, G$_{D1b}$, and G$_{T1b}$. Cronassial; Gangliovet.

THERAP CAT: In treatment of peripheral neuropathies.

THERAP CAT (VET): In treatment of peripheral neuropathies.

4365. Ganirelix. [124904-93-4] *N*-Acetyl-3-(2-naphthalenyl)-D-alanyl-4-chloro-D-phenylalanyl-3-(3-pyridinyl)-D-alanyl-L-

seryl-L-tyrosyl-N^6-[bis(ethylamino)methylene]-D-lysyl-L-leucyl-N^6-[bis(ethylamino)methylene]-L-lysyl-L-prolyl-D-alaninamide; [*N*-Ac-D-Nal(2)^1-D-*p*Cl-Phe^2-D-Pal(3)^3-D-hArg(Et$_2$)^6-hArg(Et$_2$)^8-D-Ala^{10}]GnRH. $C_{80}H_{113}ClN_{18}O_{13}$; mol wt 1570.32. C 61.19%, H 7.25%, Cl 2.26%, N 16.06%, O 13.25%. Decapeptide LH-RH antagonist. Prepn and structure-activity studies: J. J. Nestor, Jr. *et al.* in *Peptides 1988: Proc. 20th Eur. Peptide Symp.,* G. Jung, E. Bayer, Eds. (Walter de Gruyter, Berlin, 1989) pp 592-594; *eidem, J. Med. Chem.* **35,** 3942 (1992). Improved synthesis: H. B. Arzeno *et al., Int. J. Pept. Protein Res.* **41,** 342 (1993). Degradation in aq soln: R. G. Strickley *et al., Pharm. Res.* **7,** 530 (1990). Clinical pharmacology and pharmacokinetics: J. Rabinovici *et al., J. Clin. Endocrinol. Metab.* **75,** 1220 (1992). Clinical trial in assisted fertilization: P. Devroey *et al., Hum. Reprod.* **13,** 3023 (1998).

Acetate. [129311-55-3] Org-37462; RS-26306; Antagon; Orgalutran. $C_{80}H_{113}ClN_{18}O_{13} \cdot 2C_2H_4O_2$; mol wt 1690.42. pKa: 4.2 (3-pyridinylalanine); 9.8 (tyrosine). Sol in water.

THERAP CAT: In treatment of infertility.

4366. Gardenins. A group of flavones isolated from the resinous exudate of leaf buds of *Gardenia lucida* Roxb. *Rubiaceae,* a small spiny tree occurring throughout India. Isoln of the main flavonoid pigment, gardenin A (originally thought to be single component and referred to in early literature as "gardenin"): J. Stenhouse, C. G. Groves, *J. Chem. Soc.* **1877,** 552; *Ann.* **200,** 311 (1880); K. J. Balakrishna, T. R. Seshadri, *Proc. Indian Acad. Sci.* **27A,** 91 (1948). Isoln and structure of gardenins B, C, D, E: A. V. R. Rao *et al., Indian J. Chem.* **8,** 398 (1970). Isoln of B from *Citrus jambhiri* lush. *Rutaceae* and synthesis: B. P. Chaliha *et al., Tetrahedron* **21,** 1441 (1965). Structure of A: P. K. Bose, *J. Indian Chem. Soc.* **22,** 233 (1945). Revised structure: A. V. R. Rao, K. Venkataraman, *Indian J. Chem.* **6,** 677 (1968). Synthesis of A: M. Krishnamurti *et al., ibid.* **8,** 575 (1970); M. Kamalam, A. V. R. Rao, *ibid.* 573; of C: A. J. Kalra *et al., ibid.* **11,** 96 (1973); of E: *eidem, ibid.* 1092. Antineoplastic activity and cytotoxicity: J. Edwards *et al., J. Nat. Prod.* **42,** 85 (1979). ^{13}C-NMR study: M. Iinuma *et al., Chem. Pharm. Bull.* **28,** 708 (1980).

Gardenin A	R = R' = OCH$_3$
Gardenin B	R = R' = H
Gardenin C	R = OH, R' = OCH$_3$
Gardenin D	R = OH, R' = H
Gardenin E	R = R' = OH

Gardenin A. [21187-73-5] 5-Hydroxy-6,7,8-trimethoxy-2-(3,4,5-trimethoxyphenyl)-4*H*-1-benzopyran-4-one. $C_{21}H_{22}O_9$; mol wt 418.39. Golden yellow needles from ethanol, mp 162-163°. Sol in alcohol, chloroform. All the gardenins give a green color with alcoholic ferric chloride.

Gardenin B. [2798-20-1] 5-*O*-Desmethyltangeretin. $C_{19}H_{18}$-O_7; mol wt 358.34. Fine yellow needles from benzene/petr ether, mp 176-177°. uv max (ethanol): 292, 330 nm (log e 4.40, 4.35); (1% AlCl$_3$): 310, 350 nm (log ε 4.48, 4.49).

Gardenin C. [29550-05-8] $C_{20}H_{20}O_9$; mol wt 404.37. Yellow flakes from ethyl acetate-petr ether, mp 179-180°. uv max (methanol) 304, 323 nm (log ε 4.18, 4.20).

Gardenin D. [29202-00-4] $C_{19}H_{18}O_8$; mol wt 374.34. Cryst, mp 190-192°. uv max (ethanol): 256, 280, 343 nm.

Gardenin E. [29550-07-0] $C_{19}H_{18}O_9$; mol wt 390.34. Golden yellow needles from ethyl acetate/petr ether, mp 234-235°. uv max (methanol): 280, 325 nm (log ε 4.37, 4.36).

4367. Gardinol Type Detergents. A mixture of the sodium salts of sulfated fatty alcohols made by reducing the mixed fatty acids of coconut oil or of cottonseed oil, and of fish oils. Sometimes natural waxes such as spermaceti, wool fat, and beeswax are sulfated directly. The mixture of the sulfated alcohols which goes by the commercial name "lauryl alcohol" consists of about 15% mixed C_8 and C_{10} (octyl and decyl) alcohols, 40% C_{12} (lauryl or dodecyl) alcohol, 30% C_{14} (myristyl or tetradecyl) alcohol, and 15% mixed C_{16} and C_{18} (cetyl, stearyl, and oleyl) alcohols. Some of the tradenames designating this type of detergent are: *Gardinol*; *Duponol*; *Modinal*; *Aurinol*; *Maprofix*; *Tergavon*; *Sadopan*; *Cyclopon*; *Cyclanon*; *Sapidan*; *Lissapol*; *Teepol*. See also Sodium Lauryl Sulfate.

Caution: May cause local sensitivity reactions.

USE: Detergents, wetting, emulsifying, dispersing agents for cosmetics, as dry cleaning aids, in fungicidal sprays, in metal cleaning, leather processing, in textile manuf.

4368. Gardol®. [137-16-6] *N*-Methyl-*N*-(1-oxododecyl)-glycine sodium salt; *N*-lauroylsarcosine sodium salt; sodium *N*-lauroyl sarcosinate; Medialan LL-99. $C_{15}H_{28}NNaO_3$; mol wt 293.38. C 61.41%, H 9.62%, N 4.77%, Na 7.84%, O 16.36%. Prepn: Jungermann *et al., J. Am. Chem. Soc.* **78**, 172 (1956).

Aq soln, *Medialan LL-33*.

USE: Detergent, foaming agent, antienzyme for dentifrices: King, US 2689170 (1954 to Colgate-Palmolive).

4369. Garenoxacin. [194804-75-6] 1-Cyclopropyl-8-(difluoromethoxy)-7-[(1*R*)-2,3-dihydro-1-methyl-1*H*-isoindol-5-yl]-1,4-dihydro-4-oxo-3-quinolinecarboxylic acid; T-3811. $C_{23}H_{20}F_2$-N_2O_4; mol wt 426.41. C 64.78%, H 4.73%, F 8.91%, N 6.57%, O 15.01%. Des-F(6)-quinolone antibacterial; topoisomerase II inhibitor. Prepn: Y. Todo *et al.*, **WO 9729102**; *eidem*, **US 6025370** (1997, 2000 both to Toyama); and antibacterial activity: K. Hayashi *et al., Arzneim.-Forsch.* **52**, 903 (2002). HPLC determn in serum: D. Xuan *et al., J. Chromatogr. B* **765**, 37 (2001). Mechanism of action study: D. Ince *et al., Antimicrob. Agents Chemother.* **46**, 3370 (2002). Comparative antimicrobial spectra: M. Takahata *et al., ibid.* **43**, 1077 (1999); M. Bassetti *et al., ibid.* **46**, 234 (2002). Clinical pharmacokinetics: D. A. Gajjar *et al., ibid.* **47**, 2256 (2003); and pharmacodynamics: S. Van Wart *et al., ibid.* **48**, 4766 (2004). Toxicology study: A. Nagai *et al., J. Toxicol. Sci.* **27**, 219 (2002). Review of pharmacology and therapeutic potential: R. Frechette, *Curr. Opin. Invest. Drugs* **2**, 1706-1711 (2001).

Pale yellow plates from ethanol as 0.25 hydrate, mp 226-227°. $[\alpha]_D^{27}$ −9.0° (c = 0.10 in *N,N*-dimethylformamide). Also reported as hydrate, mp 234-235°.

Methanesulfonate. [223652-82-2]; [223652-90-2] (monohydrate). Garenoxacin mesylate; BMS-284756; T-3811ME. $C_{23}H_{20}$-$F_2N_2O_4 \cdot CH_4O_3S$; mol wt 522.52.

THERAP CAT: Antibacterial.

4370. Garlic. Allium. Strongly scented perennial herb, *Allium sativum* L., *Liliaceae*, used extensively in foods and in traditional medicine to treat respiratory infections. *Habit.* Central Asia, Southern Europe, U.S., cultivated worldwide. *Constit.* Enzymes, volatile oil (0.1-0.36%), carbohydrates (26-30%), protein and amino acids, lipids, minerals,vitamins, saponins. Upon bruising of the bulb, the enzyme allinase converts alliin to allicin, *q.q.v.*, the source of the garlic odor. Description and uses: A. Y. Leung, *Encyclopedia of Common Natural Ingredients* (John Wiley & Sons, New York, 1980) pp 176-178. Review of chemistry: E. Block, *Sci. Am.* **252**, 114-119 (March, 1985). Series of articles on cardiovascular

effects: *Br. J. Clin. Pract.* **44**, Suppl. 69, 1-39 (1990). Review of antioxidant properties and therapeutic potential in aging: K. Rahman, *Ageing Res. Rev.* **2**, 39-56 (2003).

Volatile oil. [8000-78-0] Obtained by steam distillation of the crushed bulb. *Constit.* Ajoene, alliin, allicin, diallyl disulfide, diallyl trisulfide, methyl allyl trisulfide, allyl sulfide, terpenes including citral, geraniol, linalool, *α*- and *β*-phellandrene. Brief review: E. Guenther, *The Essential Oils* vol. 6 (Van Nostrand, New York, 1952) pp 67-69. Comprehensive description: N. A. Shaath *et al., Dev. Food Sci.* **37B**, 2025 (1995). Clear yellow to red-orange liquid; strong garlic odor. d_{25}^{25} 1.050-1.095. n_D^{20} 1.550-1.580. Sol in most fixed oils, mineral oil, incompletely sol in alcohol. Insol in glycerin, propylene glycol. *Keep well closed, cool and protected from light.*

USE: As a spice and seasoning in foods.

THERAP CAT: In treatment of hypertension and hyperlipidemia.

4371. Garner's Aldehyde. [127589-93-9] 4-Formyl-2,2-dimethyl-3-oxazolidinecarboxylic acid 1,1-dimethylethyl ester; 1,1-dimethylethyl 4-formyl-2,2-dimethyloxazolidine-3-carboxylate. $C_{11}H_{19}NO_4$; mol wt 229.27. C 57.63%, H 8.35%, N 6.11%, O 27.91%. Both enantiomers are configurationally stable building blocks for use in asymmetric synthesis. Prepn of *R*-form: P. Garner, *Tetrahedron Lett.* **25**, 5855 (1984); of *S*-form: P. Garner, J. M. Park, *J. Org. Chem.* **52**, 2361 (1987). Improved prepn of *S*-form: A. McKillop *et al., Synthesis* **1994**, 31. Review of chemistry: X. Liang *et al., J. Chem. Soc. Perkin Trans. 1* **2001**, 2136-2157.

(S)-Garner Aldehyde

R-Form. [95715-87-0] (*R*)-Garner aldehyde. $[\alpha]_D^{27}$ +103° (c = 1.0 in CHCl$_3$).

S-Form. [102308-32-7] (*S*)-Garner aldehyde. Colorless liquid, bp$_{1.0-1.4}$ 83-88°; bp$_{0.3}$ 72-75°. $[\alpha]_D$ −91.7° (c = 1.34 in CHCl$_3$).

USE: Chiral, non-racemic synthon for asymmetric synthesis of amino sugars and other nitrogen-containing targets.

4372. Gasoline. Petrol (British); Benzin (German). A mixture of C_4 to C_{12} hydrocarbons. Natural gasoline, obtained by fractional distillation of petroleum, contains mostly saturated hydrocarbons; commercial grades of motor gasoline contain paraffins, olefins, naphthenes, and aromatics, all in substantial concns. Motor gasolines are made chiefly by cracking processes, in which heavier petr fractions are converted into more volatile fractions by thermal or catalytic decompn; have also been made commercially by catalytic high-pressure hydrogenation of soft coal and by catalytic synthesis of hydrocarbons from carbon monoxide and hydrogen. Some gasolines sold in the U.S. contain a minor proportion of tetraethyllead added to motor gasoline to increase the octane numbers and thereby prevent "knock" in engines in which the gasoline is used as fuel. Knock is the audible manifestation of an excessive rate of pressure rise when the gasoline vapor is ignited under compression in an engine. The relative knocking tendencies of gasolines are measured in terms of "Octane Number," which is defined as the percentage of iso-octane, having "100 Octane No.," to be blended with *n*-heptane, having "0 Octane No." by definition, in order to obtain the same degree of knock as is obtained with the gasoline being rated, under standard conditions in a standardized test engine. Additives such as ethanol, methanol, benzene, toluene, MTBE and MMT, *q.q.v.*, are replacing tetraethyllead, and only a small percentage of leaded gasoline is sold in the U.S. *Review:* J. C. Lane in *Kirk-Othmer Encyclopedia of Chemical Technology* vol. 11 (Wiley-Interscience, New York, 3rd ed., 1984) pp 652-695. Review of toxicity: N. K. Weaver, *Ann. N.Y. Acad. Sci.* **534**, 441-451 (1988); of carcinogenicity: M. A. Mehlman, *Toxicol. Ind. Health* **7**, 143-152 (1990); of toxicology and human exposure: *Toxicological*

Profile for Gasoline (PB95-264206, 1995) 224 pp. Symposium on toxicology, exposure and health effects: *Environ. Health Perspect.* **101,** Suppl. 6, 1-212 (1993).

Gasoline is a highly flammable, mobile liq with characteristic odor; evaporates quickly. Flash pt 40-70°C. bp 32-210°C. Explosive limits, vol % in air: lower 1.3, upper 6.0. Insol in water. Freely sol in abs alcohol, ether, chloroform, benzene. Dissolves fats, oils, natural resins. LD_{50} orally in rats: 18.85 ml/kg (Weaver).

Caution: Potential symptoms due to mild overexposure by ingestion may include inebriation, vomiting, vertigo, drowsiness, confusion and fever; severe overexposure by ingestion may result in mild excitation, loss of consciousness, convulsions, cyanosis, congestion, capillary hemorrhaging of the lungs and internal organs, and death due to circulatory failure. Aspiration may cause severe inflammatory reaction and chemical pneumonitis. Direct contact may cause irritation of skin, eye, mucous membranes. Prolonged skin exposure may result in a chemical burn; repeated exposure may cause defatting of the skin. Potential symptoms due to acute overexposure by inhalation of vapor may include irritation and burning in the respiratory system, dizziness, anesthesia, bronchopneumonia, asphyxiation; inhalation of vapor at high levels may induce CNS depression, coma, convulsions, myocardial irritability. Potential symptoms due to chronic overexposure by inhalation may include vomiting, diarrhea, insomnia, headache, dizziness, anemia, impairment of renal function, muscle and neurological symptoms. *See Patty's Industrial Hygiene and Toxicology* vol. **2B,** G. D. Clayton, F. E. Clayton, Eds. (Wiley-Interscience, New York, 4th ed., 1994) p 1395-1406; Weaver *loc. cit.* Potential occupational carcinogen. *See NIOSH Pocket Guide to Chemical Hazards* (DHHS/NIOSH 97-140, 1997) p 150.

USE: As fuel in internal combusion engines of the spark-ignited, reciprocating type; diluent; finishing agent; industrial solvent.

4373. Gastrins. Gastrointestinal hormones isolated from the mucosal lining of the gastric antrum of various mammalian species. Highly potent gastric secretion stimulants, first discovered by J. S. Edkins: *Proc. Roy. Soc. London* **76B,** 376 (1905). Several gastrins have been identified; they are referred to as "little gastrin", "big gastrin" and "minigastrin". "Little gastrin" or G-17 exists in two forms, 18-34-gastrin I or G-17-I and 18-34-gastrin II or G-17-II, which are heptadecapeptides that are identical in amino acid sequence, with the latter having sulfated tyrosine residues. There are relatively small species differences in amino acid sequences of G-17, although there are differences in the ratio of the non-sulfated to the sulfated forms. This ratio is about 3:4 in hog compared to about 2:1 in man. "Big gastrin" or 1-34-gastrin, also found in two forms, consists of the heptadecapeptides of "little gastrins" extended from their *N*-termini by additional heptadecapeptides with amino acid compositions different from G-17. For each species, the G-17-I and G-17-II portions of the G-34 gastrin are identical. Pairs of shorter gastrins, or "minigastrins" (22-34-gastrin) are C-terminal tetradecapeptides. Structure of porcine "little gastrins": Gregory *et al., Nature* **204,** 391 (1964); human: Bentley *et al., ibid.* **209,** 583 (1966). Synthesis of porcine "little gastrins": Anderson *et al., ibid.* **204,** 933 (1964); human: Beecham *et al., ibid.* **209,** 585 (1966); human and canine: Agarwal, Kenner, *J. Chem. Soc. C* **1969,** 2213; ovine: Agarwal *et al., ibid.* 954; feline: *eidem, Experientia* **25,** 346 (1969). General synthetic method: E. Brown *et al., Chem. Commun.* **1980,** 1093. Isoln of "big gastrins" from Zollinger-Ellison tumor tissue: R. A. Gregory, H. J. Tracy, *Lancet* **2,** 797 (1972). Isoln of "minigastrins" from Zollinger-Ellison tumor tissue: *eidem, Gut* **15,** 683 (1974). Amino acid sequences of porcine and human "big gastrins": *eidem,* in *Gastrointestinal Hormones,* J. C. Thompson, Ed. (Univ. Texas Press, Austin, 1975) pp 13-14. Revised sequence of porcine: G. J. Dockray *et al., Bioorg. Chem.* **8,** 465 (1979); of human: A. M. Choudhury *et al., Z. Physiol. Chem.* **361,** 1719 (1980). Synthesis of human: G. Wendlberger *et al., Monatsh. Chem.* **112,** 1297 (1981). Structure and synthesis of "minigastrins": R. A. Gregory *et al., Z. Physiol. Chem.* **360,** 73 (1979). Review of chemical studies: Kenner, Sheppard, *Proc. Roy. Soc. London* **170B,** 89 (1968). Review of physiological advances: Gregory, *ibid.* 81. General reviews: Sanders, Schimmel, *Am. J. Med.* **49,** 380 (1970); McGuigan, *Vitam. Horm.* **32,** 47-88 (1974); V. Mutt, *ibid.* **39,** 231-426 (1982).

5-oxo-Pro-Gly-Pro-Trp-Leu-Glu-Glu-Glu-Glu-Glu-Ala-Tyr-Gly-Trp-Met-Asp-PheNH₂

18-34-Gastrin I (human)

4374. Gastrodia. Chi-jian; red arrow. Parasitic herbaceous plant, *Gastrodia elata* Blume, *Orchidaceae*; used in Asian traditional medicine as an analgesic and anticonvulsant. Medicinal portion is the dried tuber, known as **tianma**. Growth is dependent on 2 fungi, *Armillaria mellea* for nutrients and *Mycena osmundicola* for seed germination. *Habit.* Woodlands of Japan, Korea and the central provinces of China. *Constit.* Gastrodin, vanillin, β-sitosterol, *q.q.v.,* vanillyl alcohol, 4-hydroxybenzyl alcohol, 4-hydroxybenzyl aldehyde, parishin, gastrodioside. Isoln of constituents: H. Taguchi *et al., Chem. Pharm. Bull.* **29,** 55 (1981). HPLC determn of active constituents in tuber extracts: C. L. Liu *et al., Chromatographia* **55,** 317 (2002). Effects on learning and memory in rats: C.-R. Wu *et al., Planta Med.* **62,** 317 (1996); on amyloid β peptide-induced cell death: H.-J. Kim *et al., J. Ethnopharmacol.* **84,** 95 (2003). Review of constituents and pharmacology: W. Tang, *Chinese Drugs of Plant Origin* (Springer-Verlag, Berlin, 1992) pp 545-548. Review of life cycle and cultivation: J. Xu, S. Guo, *Chin. Med. J.* **113,** 686-692 (2000).

4375. Gastrodin. [62499-27-8] 4-(Hydroxymethyl)phenyl-β-D-glucopyranoside; 4-(β-D-glucopyranosyloxy)benzyl alcohol. $C_{13}H_{18}O_7$; mol wt 286.28. C 54.54%, H 6.34%, O 39.12%. Pharmacologically active constituent of the traditional medicinal plant, gastrodia, *q.v.* Prepn: B. Helferich *et al., Ann.* **508,** 192 (1934); A. E. Pavlov *et al., Russ. J. Gen. Chem.* **71,** 1811 (2001). Isoln from *Gastrodia elata* tuber: H. Taguchi *et al., Chem. Pharm. Bull.* **29,** 55 (1981); H.-B. Li, F. Chen, *J. Chromatogr. A* **1052,** 229 (2004). CE determn in medicinal formulations: Y. Zhao *et al., ibid.* **849,** 277 (1999). Pharmacokinetics in rats: R. Wang *et al., J. Liq. Chromatogr. Relat. Technol.* **25,** 857 (2002). Pharmacology in gerbils: S.-J. An *et al., J. Neurosci. Res.* **71,** 534 (2003).

mp 169-170°. $[\alpha]_D^{20}$ −17.5° (c = 1 in pyridine). pKa 9.10. uv max (aq soln): 249 nm (log ε 4.140).

Hemihydrate. Colorless needles from methanol + ethyl acetate, mp 156-157°. $[\alpha]_D^{33}$ −62.1° (in ethanol). uv max (ethanol): 223, 273, 278 (log ε 3.91, 2.88, sh 2.78).

4376. Gatifloxacin. [112811-59-3] 1-Cyclopropyl-6-fluoro-1,4-dihydro-8-methoxy-7-(3-methyl-1-piperazinyl)-4-oxo-3-quinolinecarboxylic acid; Tequin; Zymar. $C_{19}H_{22}FN_3O_4$; mol wt 375.39. C 60.79%, H 5.91%, F 5.06%, N 11.19%, O 17.05%. Fluorinated quinolone antibacterial. Prepn: K. Masuzawa *et al.,* **EP 230295;** *eidem,* **US 4980470** (1987, 1990 both to Kyorin); J. P. Sanchez *et al., J. Med. Chem.* **38,** 4478 (1995); of the sesquihydrate: T. Matsumoto *et al.,* **US 5880283** (1999 to Kyorin). *In vitro* antibacterial activity: A. Bauernfeind, *J. Antimicrob. Chemother.* **40,** 639 (1997); H. Fukuda *et al., Antimicrob. Agents Chemother.* **42,** 1917 (1998). Clinical pharmacokinetics: M. Nakashima *et al., ibid.* **39,** 2635 (1995). Clinical study in urinary tract infection: H. Nito, *10th Mediterranean Congr. Chemother.* **1996,** 327; in respiratory tract infection: S. Sethi, *Expert Opin. Pharmacother.* **4,** 1847 (2003).

Pale yellow prisms from methanol as hemihydrate, mp 162°.

Sesquihydrate. [180200-66-2] AM-1155. $C_{19}H_{22}FN_3$-$O_4.1\frac{1}{2}H_2O$; mol wt 384.40.

THERAP CAT: Antibacterial.

4377. GDNF. Glial cell line-derived neurotrophic factor. Survival factor for dopaminergic neurons and spinal motoneurons. Prototype of a family of neurotrophic factors known as GDNF family ligands (GFL) which also includes *neurturin, persephin,* and *artemin.* Glycosylated, disulfide-linked homodimer; mol wt 40-45 kDa; structurally related to the TGF-β superfamily. Widely expressed in peripheral tissues and brain during embryonic and early postnatal development. Isoln from rat glial cells and prepn of recombinant human form: L. H. Lin *et al., Science* **260,** 1130 (1993). Review of pharmacology and therapeutic potential: P. A. Lapchak, *Rev. Neurosci.* **7,** 165-176 (1996); of neuroprotective and neurorestorative properties: D. M. Gash *et al., Ann. Neurol.* **44,** Suppl. 1, S121-S125 (1998). Analgesic effect in neuropathic pain models: T. J. Boucher *et al., Science* **290,** 124 (2000). *Reviews:* M. C. Bohn *et al., Int. J. Dev. Neurosci.* **18,** 679-684 (2000); M. S. Airaksinen, M. Saarma, *Nat. Rev. Neurosci.*. **3,** 383-394 (2002).

Liatermin. [188630-14-0] Methionyl neurotrophic factor (human glial-derived), dimer. Production in *E. coli* by recombinant DNA technology: L. H. Lin *et al., US 6093802* (2000 to Amgen). Clinical evaluation in Parkinson's disease: S. S. Gill *et al., Nat. Med.* **9,** 589 (2003).

4378. Gefarnate. [51-77-4] (4*E*,8*E*)-5,9,13-Trimethyl-4,8,12-tetradecatrienoic acid (2*E*)-3,7-dimethyl-2,6-octadienyl ester; geranyl farnesylacetate; DA-688; Alsanate; Arsanyl; Dixnalate; Gefanil; Gefarnil; Gefarnyl; Gefulcer; Osteol; Salanil; Zackal. C_{27}-$H_{44}O_2$; mol wt 400.64. C 80.94%, H 11.07%, O 7.99%. Prepn: Cardani *et al., J. Med. Chem.* **6,** 457 (1963); **BE 617994** (1962 to Ist. de Angeli). Metabolism: G. Coppi *et al., Arzneim.-Forsch.* **19,** 1519 (1969). Clinical evaluation in duodenal ulcer: C. R. Newman, D. A. Montgomery, *Br. J. Clin. Pract.* **27,** 85 (1973).

Slightly yellowish liq with weak terpenic smell. $bp_{0.05}$ 165-168°. n_D^{20} 1.4900. uv max: 204 nm ($E_{1cm}^{1\%}$ 486). Sol in alc, ether, dimethylformamide, acetone, fatty oils. Practically insol in water, formamide, ethylene glycol, propylene glycol, glycerine.

THERAP CAT: Antiulcerative.

4379. Gefitinib. [184475-35-2] *N*-(3-Chloro-4-fluorophenyl)-7-methoxy-6-[3-(4-morpholinyl)propoxy]-4-quinazolinamine; 4-(3'-chloro-4'-fluoroanilino)-7-methoxy-6-(3-morpholinopropoxy)quinazoline; ZD-1839; Iressa. $C_{22}H_{24}ClFN_4O_3$; mol wt 446.90. C 59.13%, H 5.41%, Cl 7.93%, F 4.25%, N 12.54%, O 10.74%. Selective epidermal growth factor (EGFR)-tyrosine kinase inhibitor which blocks signal transduction pathways implicated in the proliferation and survival of cancer cells. Prepn: K. H. Gibson, **WO 9633980**; *idem,* **US 5770599** (1996, 1998 both to Zeneca). LC/MS/MS determn in biological samples: M. Zhao *et al., J. Chromatogr. B* **819,** 73 (2005). Clinical pharmacokinetics and tolerability: H. Swaisland *et al., Clin. Pharmacokinet.* **40,** 297 (2001). *In vitro* and *in vivo* inhibition of EGFR-expressing cancer lines: N. G. Anderson *et al., Int. J. Cancer* **94,** 774 (2001). Proposed mechanism of action: A. Hirata *et al., Cancer Res.* **62,** 2554 (2002). Clinical study in non-small cell lung cancer: M. G. Kris *et al., J. Am. Med. Assoc.* **290,** 2149 (2003). *Review:* C. L. Arteaga, D. H. Johnson, *Curr. Opin. Oncol.* **13,** 491-498 (2001). Review of clinical evaluations: D. Raben *et al., Semin. Oncol.* **29,** Suppl. 4, 37-46 (2002); of use in non-small cell lung cancer: K. Tamura, M. Fukuoka, *Expert Opin. Pharmacother.* **6,** 985-993 (2005).

Crystals from toluene, mp 119-120°.

THERAP CAT: Antineoplastic.

4380. Geissoschizoline. [18397-07-4] Curan-17-ol; pereirine. $C_{19}H_{26}N_2O$; mol wt 298.42. C 76.47%, H 8.78%, N 9.39%, O 5.36%. From bark of *Geissospermum vellosii* Allem., *Apocynaceae:* Hesse, *Ann.* **202,** 141 (1880); Bertho, Moog, *ibid.* **509,** 241 (1934). Identity with pereirine: Bertho, Koll, *Naturwissenschaften* **48,** 49 (1961). Structure: Janot *et al., Compt. Rend.* **250,** 4383 (1960); Bertho, Koll *Ber.* **94,** 2737 (1961). Synthesis: Hymon, Schmid, *Helv. Chim. Acta* **49,** 2067 (1966); of *dl*-form: Dadson, Harley-Mason, *Chem. Commun.* **1969,** 665; Harley-Mason, Taylor, *ibid.* **1970,** 812.

Coarse crystals from abs methanol, mp 142.5-143°. $[\alpha]_D^{21}$ +32° (ethanol). uv max in (ethanol): 245, 300 nm (log ε 3.93, 3.47). Sol in alcohol, chloroform, ether. Practically insol in water.

Methyl chloride. $C_{19}H_{26}N_2O.CH_3Cl$. Rods from abs methanol, mp 297°.

Methiodide. $C_{19}H_{26}N_2O.CH_3I$. Rods from abs methanol, mp 254°.

4381. Geissospermine. [427-01-0] (16*R*,19*E*)-19,20-Didehydro-16-[(10β,13β,21β)-23-deoxy-21,22-dihydro-11-oxa-12,14-secostrychnidin-10-yl]corynan-17-oic acid methyl ester; 19,20-didehydro-16-(15-ethyl-3a,5,5a,7,8,13a-hexahydro-4*H*-4,6-ethano-1*H*,3*H*-[1,3]oxazino[3,4,5-*lm*]pyrrolo[2,3-*d*]carbazol-1-yl)-corynan-17-oic acid methyl ester; β,17-epoxy-α-(3-ethylidene-1,2,3,4,-6,7,12,12b-octahydroindole[2,3-a]quinolizin-2-yl)-curan-1-propanoic acid methyl ester. $C_{40}H_{48}N_4O_3$; mol wt 632.83. C 75.92%, H 7.65%, N 8.85%, O 7.58%. From bark of *Geissospermum vellosii* Allem., *Apocynaceae:* Hesse, *Ann.* **202,** 141 (1880). Structure: Puisieux, LeHir, *Compt. Rend.* **252,** 902 (1961); Janot, *Tetrahedron* **14,** 113 (1961). Crystal structure: A. Chiaroni, C. Riche, *Acta Crystallogr.* **35B,** 1820 (1979). Pharmacology: M. M. Aurousseau, *Ann. Pharm. Fr.* **19,** 175 (1961). On hydrolysis with HCl splits into geissoschizine and geissoschizoline, *q.v.*

Anhydr form, crystals from abs acetone, mp 213-214° (dec). $[\alpha]_D^{20}$ −101° (ethanol). uv max (methanol): 251, 285, 293 nm (log ε 4.10, 3.91, 3.90). Slightly sol in water, ether; sol in alcohol.

Dihydrate. mp 207° (sinters at 145°).

4382. Gelatin. [9000-70-8] Gelfilm; Gelfoam. A heterogeneous mixture of water-soluble proteins of high average mol wt. Derived from the denaturation and hydrolysis of collagen, *q.v.* Amino acid composition is variable: glycine or alanine account for one third to half of the amino acid residues; approx 25% is proline or hydroxyproline; close to 25% is basic or acidic; contains no tryptophan. Amino acid composition studies: R. E. Neuman, *Arch. Biochem.* **24**, 289 (1949); J. E. Eastoe, *Biochem. J.* **61**, 589 (1955). Surgical use in hemostasis: R. U. Light, H. R. Prentice, *J. Neurosurg.* **2**, 435 (1945). Review of the chemistry and structure of collagen with emphasis on its transformation to gelatin: A. Veis, *The Macromolecular Chemistry of Gelatin* (Academic Press, New York, 1964) 433 pp. Review of therapeutic use as an embolic agent in neurologic disease: A. Berenstein, E. Russell, *Radiology* **141**, 105-112 (1981); of prepn, properties, and use in food and pharmaceutical industries: K. B. Djagny *et al., Crit. Rev. Food Sci. Nutr.* **41**, 481-492 (2001).

Colorless or slightly yellow, transparent, brittle, practically odorless, tasteless sheets, flakes, or coarse powder. Amphoteric. Swells up and absorbs 5-10 times its weight of water to form a gel in solutions below 35-40°. Sol in hot water, glycerol, acetic acid. Insol in organic solvents.

USE: As stabilizer, thickener and texturizer in food; manuf rubber substitutes, adhesives, cements, lithographic and printing inks, plastic compds, artificial silk, photographic plates and films, matches, light filters for mercury lamps; clarifying agent; in hectographic masters; sizing paper and textiles; for inhibiting crystn in bacteriology, for preparing cultures. Pharmaceutic aid (suspending agent; encapsulating agent; tablet binder; tablet and coating agent).

THERAP CAT: Hemostatic.

THERAP CAT (VET): Plasma expander; hemostasis (sponge).

4383. Gellan Gum. [71010-52-1] Native gellan gum; high acyl gellan gum; polysaccharide S-60; PS-60. Extracellular polysaccharide obtained by aerobic fermentation of *Pseudomonas elodea*. Anionic hydrocolloid composed of acetylated linear tetrasaccharide repeat unit β-D-glucose, β-D-glucuronic acid and α-L-rhamnose in a 2:1:1 molar ratio. Prepn of native form: K. S. Kang, G. T. Veeder, US 4326053; of deacetylated form: K. S. Kang *et al.,* US 4326052 (both 1982 to Merck & Co.); R. Moorhouse *et al., ACS Symp. Ser.* **150**, 111 (1981). Structural studies: M. A. O'Neill *et al., Carbohydr. Res.* **124**, 123 (1983); P.-E. Jansson *et al., ibid.* 135. Gelation properties: H. Grasdalen, O. Smidsrod, *Carbohydr. Polym.* **7**, 371 (1987). Texture profile analysis: G. R. Sanderson *et al.* in *Gums and Stabilizers for the Food Industry* **vol. 4**, G. O. Phillips *et al.*, Eds. (IRL Press, Oxford, 1988) pp 219-229. Determn in food gels: J. K. Baird, W. W. Smith, *Food Hydrocolloids* **3**, 407 (1989); in food products: H. D. Graham, *ibid.* 435 (1990). Use as agar substitute in culture media: D. Shungu *et al., Appl. Environ. Microbiol.* **46**, 840 (1983). Physicochemical properties: M. Milas *et al., Biopolymers* **30**, 451 (1990). Rheological study: P. B. Deasy, K. J. Quigley, *Int. J. Pharm.* **73**, 117 (1991). Comparative review of gelling agents: G. R. Sanderson *et al., Cereal Foods World* **34**, 991-998 (1989). *Reviews:* G. R. Sanderson in *Food Gels*, P. Harris, Ed. (Elsevier Appl. Sci., London, 1990) pp 201-232; W. Gibson in *Thickening and Gelling Agents in Food*, A. Imeson, Ed. (Blackie Academic & Professional, London, 1992) pp 227-249.

Low Acyl form

Readily sol in water. Forms thermoreversible gels.

Low acyl purified gellan gum. Deacylated gellan gum; deacylated PS-60; Gelrite; Kelcogel. Unsubstituted tetrasaccharide. White to tan powder, mol wt ~0.5 × 10^6. Partially sol in cold water; aqueous dispersions dissolve >70°. Forms thermoreversible

gels. Incompat with strong oxidizers. Bulk density ~50 lb/cu ft. LD_{50} orally in rats: >5000 mg/kg (Sanderson, 1990).

USE: In foods, pharmaceuticals, and personal care products as gelling, texturizing, stabilizing, film forming and suspending agent. For microbiological media and plant tissue culture.

4384. Gelsemine. [509-15-9] $C_{20}H_{22}N_2O_2$; mol wt 322.40. C 74.51%, H 6.88%, N 8.69%, O 9.93%. CNS stimulant from roots and rhizome of *Gelsemium sempervirens* (L.) Ait., *Loganiaceae*. Isoln: Gerrard, *Pharm. J.* **13**, 641 (1883); Moore, *J. Chem. Soc.* **97**, 2223 (1910); **99**, 1231 (1911); Sayre, Watson, *J. Am. Pharm. Assoc.* **8**, 708 (1919); Chou, *Chin. J. Physiol.* **5**, 131 (1931), *C.A.* **25**, 4085[6] (1931); Schwarz, Marion, *Can. J. Chem.* **31**, 958 (1953). Structure: Conroy, Chakrabarti, *Tetrahedron Lett.* **1959** (4), 6; Lovell *et al., ibid.* 1; Roe, Gates, *Tetrahedron* **11**, 148 (1960). NMR spectroscopic study: Y. Schun, G. A. Cordell, *J. Nat. Prod.* **48**, 969 (1985). Partial syntheses: W. E. Earley *et al., Tetrahedron Lett.* **29**, 3781, 3785 (1988).

Crystals from acetone, mp 178°. *Poisonous!* $[\alpha]_D^{20}$ +13° (c = 1.2 in chloroform). pKa 7.75 in 80% methylcellosolve. uv max (methanol): 210, 252, 280 nm (log ε 4.50, 3.87, 3.15). Slightly sol in water; sol in alcohol, benzene, chloroform, ether, acetone, dilute acids.

Hydrochloride. $C_{20}H_{23}ClN_2O_2$. Prisms from methanol + ether, mp 326°. $[\alpha]_D$ +5° (c = 1.072 in water). Sol in water, slightly sol in alcohol.

4385. Gelsemium. Yellow jasmine; yellow jessamine; wild woodbine. CNS stimulant from dried rhizome and roots of *Gelsemium sempervirens* (L.) Ait., *Loganiaceae. Habit.* Southern U.S. *Constit.* Gelsemine, gelsemoidine, scopoletin, gelsemic acid, volatile oil, resin.

Poisonous!

4386. Gemcitabine. [95058-81-4] 2′-Deoxy-2′,2′-difluorocytidine; 1-(2-oxo-4-amino-1,2-dihydropyrimidin-1-yl)-2-deoxy-2,2-difluororibose; dFdC; dFdCyd; Gemzar. $C_9H_{11}F_2$-N_3O_4; mol wt 263.20. C 41.07%, H 4.21%, F 14.44%, N 15.97%, O 24.32%. Prepn: L. W. Hertel, **GB 2136425**; *idem*, **US 4808614** (1984, 1989 both to Lilly); L. W. Hertel *et al., J. Org. Chem.* **53**, 2406 (1988); T. S. Chou *et al., Synthesis* **1992**, 565. Antitumor activity: L. W. Hertel *et al., Cancer Res.* **50**, 4417 (1990). Mode of action study: V. W. T. Ruiz *et al., Biochem. Pharmacol.* **46**, 762 (1993). Clinical pharmacokinetics and toxicity: J. L. Abbruzzese *et al., J. Clin. Oncol.* **9**, 491 (1991). Review of clinical studies: B. Lund *et al., Cancer Treat. Rev.* **19**, 45-55 (1993).

Crystals from water, pH 8.5. $[\alpha]_{365}$ +425.36°; $[\alpha]_D$ +71.51° (c = 0.96 in methanol). uv max (ethanol): 234, 268 (ε 7810, 8560). LD_{10} i.v. in rats: 200 mg/m² (Abbruzzese).

Hydrochloride. [122111-03-9] $C_9H_{11}F_2N_3O_4$·HCl. Crystals from water-acetone, mp 287-292° (dec). $[\alpha]_D$ +48°; $[\alpha]_{365}$ +257.9° (c = 1.0 in deuterated water). uv max (water): 232, 268 nm (ε 7960, 9360).

THERAP CAT: Antineoplastic.

4387. Gemeprost. [64318-79-2] (2E,11α,13E,15R)-11,15-Dihydroxy-16,16-dimethyl-9-oxoprosta-2,13-dien-1-oic acid methyl ester; 16,16-dimethyl-*trans*-Δ²-PGE₁ methyl ester; ONO-802; Cergem; Cervagem(e); Preglandin. $C_{23}H_{38}O_5$; mol wt 394.54. C 70.02%, H 9.71%, O 20.28%. Analog of prostaglandin E₁, *q.v.* Prepn: M. Hayashi *et al.*, **DE 2700021**; *eidem*, **US 4052512** (both 1977 to Ono); H. Suga *et al.*, *Prostaglandins* **15**, 907 (1978). Effects on uterine contractility and steroid hormone plasma levels: K. Oshima *et al.*, *J. Reprod. Fertil.* **55**, 353 (1979). Effects on reproductive function: K. Matsumoto *et al.*, *Nippon Yakurigaku Zasshi* **79**, 15 (1982), *C.A.* **96**, 98392 (1982). Use in termination of first trimester pregnancy: O. Reiertsen *et al.*, *Prostaglandins Leukotrienes Med.* **8**, 31 (1982).

THERAP CAT: Abortifacient; oxytocic.

4388. Gemfibrozil. [25812-30-0] 5-(2,5-Dimethylphenoxy)-2,2-dimethylpentanoic acid; 2,2-dimethyl-5-(2,5-xylyloxy)valeric acid; CI-719; Decrelip; Genlip; Gevilon; Lipozid; Lipur; Lopid. $C_{15}H_{22}O_3$; mol wt 250.33. C 71.97%, H 8.86%, O 19.17%. Serum lipid regulating agent. Prepn: P. L. Creger, **DE 1925423**; *eidem*, **US 3674836** (1969, 1972, both to Parke, Davis). Production: O. P. Goel, **US 4126637** (1978 to Warner-Lambert). Pharmacology: A. H. Kissebach *et al.*, *Atherosclerosis* **24**, 199 (1976); M. T. Kahonen *et al.*, *ibid.* **32**, 47 (1979). Series of articles on metabolism, clinical pharmacology, kinetics and toxicology: *Proc. R. Soc. Med.* **69**, Suppl 2, 1-120 (1976). Toxicity data: S. M. Kurtz *et al.*, *ibid.* 15. Clinical trial in hyperlipidemia: J. E. Lewis *et al.*, *Pract. Cardiol.* **9**, 99 (1983). Clinical reduction of cardiovascular risk in patients with low HDL levels: H. B. Rubins *et al.*, *N. Engl. J. Med.* **341**, 410 (1999).

Crystals from hexane, mp 61-63°. bp₀.₀₂ 158-159°. LD₅₀ in mice, rats (mg/kg): 3162, 4786 orally (Kurtz).

THERAP CAT: Antilipemic.

4389. Gemifloxacin. [175463-14-6] 7-[3-(Aminomethyl)-4-(methoxyimino)-1-pyrrolidinyl]-1-cyclopropyl-6-fluoro-1,4-dihydro-4-oxo-1,8-naphthyridine-3-carboxylic acid; SB-265805; LB-20304. $C_{18}H_{20}FN_5O_4$; mol wt 389.38. C 55.52%, H 5.18%, F 4.88%, N 17.99%, O 16.44%. Third generation fluorinated quinolone antibacterial. Prepn: J. H. Kwak *et al.*, **EP 688772**; C. Y. Hong *et al.*, **US 5633262** (1995, 1997 both to LG Chemical); C. Y. Hong *et al.*, *J. Med. Chem.* **40**, 3584 (1997). Antibacterial spectrum *in vitro*: R. Wise, J. M. Andrews, *J. Antimicrob. Chemother.* **44**, 679 (1999). HPLC-tandem MS determn in human plasma: E. Doyle *et al.*, *J. Chromatogr. B* **746**, 191 (2000). Clinical pharmacokinetics: A. Allen *et al.*, *Antimicrob. Agents Chemother.* **44**, 1604 (2000). Review of antibacterial activity, pharmacology, and clinical trials: J. M. Blondeau, B. Missaghi, *Expert Opin. Pharmacother.* **5**, 1117-1152 (2004).

Off-white, amorphous solid from chloroform-ethanol, mp 235-237°.

THERAP CAT: Antibacterial.

4390. Gemtuzumab Ozogamicin. [220578-59-6] CDP-771; CMA-676; Mylotarg. Immunoconjugate of N-acetyl-γ-calicheamicin with the humanized mouse monoclonal IgG4 κ antibody, hP67.6, directed against the human CD33 antigen located on the surface of normal and leukemic myeloid cells, but not on normal hematopoietic stem cells. Designed to deliver antibody-targeted chemotherapy for treatment of acute myelocytic leukemia (AML). Prepn of conjugate: P. R. Hamann *et al.*, **EP 689845**; *eidem*, **US 5773001** (1996, 1998 both to Am. Cyanamid). *In vitro* antineoplastic activity: K. Naito *et al.*, *Leukemia* **14**, 1436 (2000). Clinical evaluation in AML: E. L. Sievers *et al.*, *Blood* **93**, 3678 (1999). Reviews of development and therapeutic potential: I. D. Bernstein, *Leukemia* **14**, 474-475 (2000); I. Niculescu-Duvaz, *Curr. Opin. Mol. Ther.* **2**, 691-696 (2000); of clinical experience: F. J. Giles, *Expert Rev. Anticancer Ther.* **2**, 630-640 (2002).

Sensitive to light; protect from direct and indirect sunlight and unshielded fluorescent light.

THERAP CAT: Antineoplastic

4391. Genistein. [446-72-0] 5,7-Dihydroxy-3-(4-hydroxyphenyl)-4H-1-benzopyran-4-one; 4',5,7-trihydroxyisoflavone; prunetol; genisteol. $C_{15}H_{10}O_5$; mol wt 270.24. C 66.67%, H 3.73%, O 29.60%. Phytoestrogen found in soy products; the aglucon of genistin and of sophoricoside. Specific protein kinase inhibitor. Prepn from the glucoside by hydrolysis with emulsin: Charaux, Rabaté, *J. Pharm. Chim.* [9] **1**, 404 (1941); by hydrolysis with HCl in methanol: Walter, *J. Am. Chem. Soc.* **63**, 3273 (1941). Isoln from *prunus* spp., *Rosaceae:* Hasegawa *ibid.* **79**, 1738 (1957); from *Podocarpus spicata* R.Br., *Podocarpaceae:* Briggs, Cebalo, *Tetrahedron* **6**, 145 (1959). Structure: Baker, Robinson, *J. Chem. Soc.* **1925**, 1981; **1926**, 2713; Walz, *Ann.* **489**, 118 (1931). Synthesis: Baker, Robinson, *J. Chem. Soc.* **1928**, 3115; Narasimhachari *et al.*, *J. Sci. Ind. Res.* **12**, 287 (1953); Yoder *et al.*, *Proc. Iowa Acad. Sci.* **61**, 271 (1954); Zemplén *et al.*, *Acta Chim. Acad. Sci. Hung.* **19**, 277 (1959). HPLC determn in biological fluids: J. G. Supko, L. R. Phillips, *J. Chromatogr. B* **666**, 157 (1995); A. A. Franke *et al*, *Proc. Soc. Exp. Biol. Med.* **208**, 18 (1995). Review of synthesis and isotopic labeling: K. Wähälä *et al.*, *ibid.* 27-32. Series of articles on chemopreventive properties and mechanism of action: *ibid.* 103-115, 120-130; *J. Nutr.* **125**, Suppl. 3, 777S-797S (1995).

Rectangular or six-sided rods from 60% alcohol. Dendritic needles from ether. mp 297-298° (slight decompn). Sol in the usual organic solvents, in dil alkalies with yellow color. Practically insol in water. uv max: 262.5 nm (ε 138).

Sophoricoside. [152-95-4] Genistein-4'-glucoside. $C_{21}H_{20}O_{10}$. From the green pods of *Sophora japonica* L., *Leguminosae:* Charaux, Rabate, *Bull. Soc. Chim. Biol.* **20**, 454 (1938). Structure: Zemplén *et al.*, *Ber.* **76**, 267 (1943). Synthesis: Bognár, Szabo, *Acta Chim. Acad. Sci. Hung.* **4**, 383 (1954); *Chem. Ind. (London)* **1954**, 518. Crystals from alcohol, mp 298°. $[\alpha]_D^{20} -47°$ (pyridine). $[\alpha]_D^{20} -32°$ (10% aq pyridine). uv max (abs ethanol): 262 nm. Sparingly sol in water, alc, acetic acid; more sol in hot alc, hot acetic acid; sol in pyridine, dil alkalies. Practically insol in ethyl acetate, acetone.

Genistin. [529-59-9] Genistein-7-O-β-D-glucoside. $C_{21}H_{20}O_{10}$. For isoln and structure *see* Walter, Hasegawa, Walz, *loc. cit.* Synthesis: Zemplén, Farkas, *Ber.* **76B**, 1110 (1943). Pale yellow plates from 80% ethanol, mp 256°. $[\alpha]_D^{21} -28°$ (c = 0.6 in 0.02N NaOH); $[\alpha]_D^{26} -21.4°$ (pyridine). uv max (85% ethanol): 262.5 nm (a 90.5). Practically insol in cold water. Slightly sol in hot water, hot ethanol, hot methanol; sol in hot 80% ethanol, hot 80% methanol, hot acetone, pyridine.

Olmelin. 5,7-Dihydroxy-4'-methoxyisoflavone; biochanin A; 4'-methyl ether. $C_{16}H_{12}O_5$. Isoln from red clover: Pope *et al.*,

Chem. Ind. (London) **1953**, 1092; Wong, *J. Sci. Food Agric.* **13**, 304 (1962); from *Andira inermis* (Swartz) H.B.K., *Leguminosae:* Crocker *et al., J. Chem. Soc.* **1962**, 4906. Identity with olmelin: Gakhokidze, *J. Appl. Chem. USSR* **23**, 789 (1950), *C.A.* **46**, 9098i (1952). Structure: Bose, Siddiqui, *J. Sci. Ind. Res.* **9B**, no. 1, 25 (1950). Synthesis: Baker *et al., Nature* **169**, 706 (1952). Yellow needles from methanol, mp 212-216°.

USE: Chemical probe to explore signal transduction pathways.

4392. Gentamicin. [1403-66-3] Gentamycin. Antibiotic complex produced by fermentation of *Micromonospora purpurea* or *M. echinospora* and variants thereof: M. J. Weinstein *et al., Antimicrob. Agents Chemother.* **1963**, 1. Isoln, purification and characterization: J. P. Rosselet *et al., ibid.* 14. Industrial pats.: G. M. Luedemann, M. J. Weinstein; Charney, **US 3091572**; **US 3136704** (1963, 1964, both to Schering). Consists of three closely related components, gentamicins C_1, C_2, C_{1a}, and also gentamicin A which differs from the other members of the complex but is similar to kanamycin C, *q.v.* Separation of gentamicin C components: H. Maehr, C. P. Schaffner, *J. Chromatogr.* **30**, 572 (1967); Wagman *et al., ibid.* **34**, 210 (1968). Structures contain 2-deoxy-streptamine, *q.v.*, linked to two saccharide units, these being *garosamine* and a *purpurosamine* in the C series gentamicins. Structure studies: D. J. Cooper *et al., J. Chem. Soc. C* **1971**, 960, 2876, 3126. Structure of gentamicin A: H. Maehr, C. P. Schaffner, *J. Am. Chem. Soc.* **89**, 6787 (1967); **92** 1697 (1969). Sepn and structures of gentamicins A_1 to A_4: Nagabhushan *et al., J. Org. Chem.* **40**, 2830, 2835 (1975). Synthetic studies: W. Meyer zu Reckendorf, Bischof, *Ber.* **105**, 2546 (1972); M. Chmielewski *et al., Carbohydr. Res.* **70**, 275 (1979). Review of activity, toxicity and clinical pharmacology: J. Black *et al., Antimicrob. Agents Chemother.* **1963**, 138-147. Comprehensive description: B. E. Rosenkrantz *et al., Anal. Profiles Drug Subs.* **9**, 295-340 (1980). Determn in serum by immunoassay: H. A. Holt *et al., J. Antimicrob. Chemother.* **34**, 747 (1994). Review of clinical use: S. B. Shrimpton *et al., ibid.* **31**, 599-606 (1993). Clinical effect on chloride transport in cystic fibrosis: M. Wilschanski *et al., Am. J. Respir. Crit. Care Med.* **161**, 860 (2000).

Gentamicin C_1 $R_1 = R_2 = CH_3$
Gentamicin C_2 $R_1 = CH_3$, $R_2 = H$
Gentamicin C_{1a} $R_1 = R_2 = H$

White amorphous powder, mp 102-108°. $[\alpha]_D^{25}$ +146°. Freely sol in water; sol in pyridine, DMF, in acidic media with salt formation; moderately sol in methanol, ethanol, acetone. Practically insol in benzene, halogenated hydrocarbons.

Gentamicin C_1. [25876-10-2] $C_{21}H_{43}N_5O_7$; mol wt 477.60. mp 94-100°. $[\alpha]_D^{25}$ +158°.

Gentamicin C_2. [25876-11-3] $C_{20}H_{41}N_5O_7$; mol wt 463.57. mp 107-124°. $[\alpha]_D^{25}$ +160°.

Gentamicin C_{1a}. [26098-04-4] *O*-3-Deoxy-4-*C*-methyl-3-(methylamino)-β-L-arabinopyranosyl-(1 → 6)-*O*-[2,6-diamino-2,3,-4,6-tetradeoxy-α-D-*erythro*-hexopyranosyl-(1 → 4)]-2-deoxy-D-streptamine; gentamicin D. $C_{19}H_{39}N_5O_7$; mol wt 449.54.

Gentamicin A. [13291-74-2] *O*-2-Amino-2-deoxy-α-D-gluco-pyranosyl-(1 → 4)-*O*-[3-deoxy-3-(methylamino)-α-D-xylopyrano-syl-(1 → 6)]-2-deoxy-D-streptamine. $C_{18}H_{36}N_4O_{10}$; mol wt 468.50.

Hydrochloride. mp 194-209°. $[\alpha]_D^{25}$ +113°. Freely sol in water, methanol; slightly in ether. Practically insol in other organic solvents.

C complex sulfate. [1405-41-0] Alcomicin; Cidomycin; Dura-gentam; Garamycin; Garasol; Genoptic; Gentacin; Gent-Ak; Gen-talline; Gentalyn; Gentibioptal; Genticin; Gentocin; Gentogram; Gent-Ophtal; Lugacin; Ophtagram; Pangram; Refobacin; Septopal; Sulmycin. White, hygroscopic powder, mp 218-237°. $[\alpha]_D^{25}$ +102°. Sol in ethylene glycol, formamide. LD_{50} in mice (mg base/kg): 430 i.p.; 485 s.c.; 75 i.v.; >9050 orally (Black).

THERAP CAT: Antibacterial.

THERAP CAT (VET): Antibacterial.

4393. Gentian. Yellow gentian; pale gentian; bitter root. Dried rhizome and roots of *Gentiana lutea* L., *Gentianaceae. Habit.* Central and Southern Europe. *Constit.* Gentiin, gentiamarin, gen-tisin, gentisic acid, gentiopicrin, gentianose (a sugar), pectin.

THERAP CAT: Bitter tonic.

THERAP CAT (VET): Bitter tonic.

4394. Gentianine. [439-89-4] 5-Ethenyl-3,4-dihydro-1*H*-pyrano[3,4-*c*]pyridin-1-one; 4-(2-hydroxyethyl)-5-vinylnicotinic acid δ-lactone; erythricine. $C_{10}H_9NO_2$; mol wt 175.18. C 68.56%, H 5.18%, N 8.00%, O 18.27%. From *Gentiana kirilowi*, *Gentianaceae:* Proskurnina, *J. Gen. Chem. USSR* **14**, 1148 (1944), *C.A.* **40**, 7213 (1946); from *Anthocleista procera* Afz. and *Fagraea fragrans* Roxb., *Loganiaceae:* Lavie, Taylor-Smith, *Chem. Ind. (London)* **1963**, 781; Wan, Chow, *J. Pharm. Pharmacol.* **16**, 484 (1964). Isoln from *Slevogtia orientalis* Gris., *Gentianaceae*, structure and synthesis: Govindachari *et al., J. Chem. Soc.* **1957**, 551, 2725.

Needles from ether or petr ether, mp 82-83°. uv max: 220 nm (log ε 4.38). Sol in alkali.

Hydrochloride. $C_{10}H_9NO_2$.HCl. Needles from alcohol + ether, dec 169-170°.

Dihydrogentianine. $C_{10}H_{11}NO_2$. Crystals from ether + petr ether, mp 74-76°. uv max: 270 nm (log ε 3.4).

4395. Gentian Violet. [548-62-9] *N*-[4-[Bis[4-(dimethyl-amino)phenyl]methylene]-2,5-cyclohexadien-1-ylidene]-*N*-methyl-methanaminium chloride; C.I. Basic Violet 3; hexamethylpararos-aniline chloride; hexamethyl-*p*-rosaniline chloride; aniline violet; crystal violet; methylrosanilinium chloride; C.I. 42555; Axuris; Badil; Gentiaverm; Pyoktanin. $C_{25}H_{30}ClN_3$; mol wt 407.98. C 73.60%, H 7.41%, Cl 8.69%, N 10.30%. Prepn and properties: *Colour Index* **vol. 4** (3rd ed., 1971) p 4391. Toxicity studies: H. C. Hodge *et al., Toxicol. Appl. Pharmacol.* **22**, 1 (1972). Review of metabolism and mode of action: R. Docampo, S. N. Moreno, *Drug Metab. Rev.* **22**, 161-178 (1990); of use as a biological stain: *Conn's Biological Stains*, R. W. Horobin, J. A. Kiernan, Eds. (BIOS Scien-tific Publishers Ltd, Oxford, UK, 10th ed., 2002) 193-195.

Dark green powder or greenish, glistening pieces with metallic luster. Soly (%): water 0.2-1.7; ethanol 3-14; acetone 0.4; chloro-form 5.1. Insol in xylene. Absorption max (water): 590 nm.

Changes from yellow at pH 0.0 to blue-violet at pH 2.0. LD₅₀ orally in mice, rats: 1.2, 1.0 g/kg (Hodge).

Note: Commercial product, which is usually admixed with **pentamethylpararosaniline chloride** and **tetramethylpararosaniline chloride**, contains not less than 96% gentian violet.

USE: As dye for wood, silk, paper; in inks; as biological stain.

THERAP CAT: Anti-infective (topical). Has been used as anthelmintic (Nematodes). Blood additive to prevent transmission of Chagas' disease by blood transfusion.

THERAP CAT (VET): Antimicrobial (topical); mycostatic agent in poultry feed.

4396. Gentiobiose. [554-91-6] 6-*O*-β-D-Glucopyranosyl-D-glucose; 6-(β-D-glucosido)-D-glucose; amygdalose. $C_{12}H_{22}O_{11}$; mol wt 342.30. C 42.11%, H 6.48%, O 51.41%. From gentianose by partial hydrolysis with 0.2% H_2SO_4 or with invertin. From D-glucose by enzymatic synthesis with emulsin: Helferich, Lette, *Org. Synth.* **22**, 53 (1942). Prepn and structure: Haworth, Wylam, *J. Chem. Soc.* **123**, 3120 (1923); Hudson, *J. Am. Chem. Soc.* **51**, 1708 (1930). Structure: Hassid, Ballou in W. Pigman, *The Carbohydrates* (Academic Press, New York, 1957) p 492. Synthesis: Helferich, Klein, *Ann.* **450**, 219 (1926); Reynolds, Evans, *J. Am. Chem. Soc.* **60**, 2559 (1938). Hydrolysis with almond emulsin gives 2 mols D-glucose.

α-Form. Lentil-shaped crystals with 2CH₃OH from methanol. Bitter taste. Very hygroscopic. mp 86°. Shows mutarotation. $[\alpha]_D^{22}$ +16° (3 min) → +8.3° (3½ hrs c = 4). Sol in water, hot methanol, hot 90% alcohol.

β-Form. Anhydr crystals from alc, mp 190-195°. Shows mutarotation. $[\alpha]_D^{22}$ −5.9° (6 min) → +9.6° (6 hrs, c = 3). Sol in water, hot methanol, hot 90% alcohol.

4397. Gentiopicrin. [20831-76-9] (5*R-trans*)-5-Ethenyl-6-(β-D-glucopyranosyloxy)-5,6-dihydro-1*H*,3*H*-pyrano[3,4-*c*]pyran-1-one; gentiopicroside. $C_{16}H_{20}O_9$; mol wt 356.32. C 53.93%, H 5.66%, O 40.41%. The principal bitter glucoside of common gentians, which was isolated in 1862 from *Gentiana lutea*, L., *Gentianaceae:* Canonica *et al., Tetrahedron* **16**, 192 (1961). Isoln from roots of *G. lutea:* Korte, *Ber.* **87**, 512 (1954); Korte *et al., ibid.* **91**, 759 (1958). Structure: Canonica *et al., Tetrahedron Lett.* **1960**(24), 7; *Tetrahedron* **16**, 192 (1961). Revised structure: Inouye *et al., Tetrahedron Lett.* **1968**, 4429. Absolute configuration: Manitto, Pagnoni, *Gazz. Chim. Ital.* **94**, 229 (1964).

Crystals from anhydr ethyl acetate or abs alcohol, mp 191°. $[\alpha]_D^{20}$ −199° (ethanol). uv max (c = 0.0285 g/l methanol): 270 nm (log ε 3.96).

Hemihydrate. Crystals from 50% ethanol, mp 121°.

Tetraacetate. $C_{24}H_{28}O_{13}$. Crystals from methanol. mp 138.5-139.5°. uv max (c = 0.0214 g/l methanol): 272 nm (log ε 3.84).

THERAP CAT: Antimalarial.

4398. Gentisic Acid. [490-79-9] 2,5-Dihydroxybenzoic acid; 5-hydroxysalicylic acid. $C_7H_6O_4$; mol wt 154.12. C 54.55%, H 3.92%, O 41.52%. Occurs in gentian: Redgrove,

Pharm. J. **122**, 324 (1929). Found in urine of dogs after ingestion of salicylates: Neuberg, *Berl. Klin. Wochenschr.* **48**, 799 (1911). Prepd from hydroquinone: Senhofer, Sarlay, *Monatsh. Chem.* **2**, 448 (1881); Juch, *ibid.* **26**, 839 (1905); Brunner, *Ann.* **351**, 321 (1907); Zeltner, Landau, **DE 258887**; *Frdl.* **11**, 210; Dyson, *Manual of Organic Chemistry* **vol. I** (London, 1950) p 614; by oxidation of salicylic acid with potassium persulfate: **DE 81297** (to Schering AG); *Frdl.* **4**, 127; from *p*-hydroxyphenol: Meyer, **US 2588336** (1952 to Monsanto); from 5-bromo-2-hydroxybenzoic acid: Lowenthal, Pepper, *J. Am. Chem. Soc.* **72**, 3292 (1950); by Kolbe synthesis: Clemens, **US 2816137** (1957 to Eastman Kodak). Metabolic product of *Penicillium patulum:* Tanenbaum, Bassett, *Biochim. Biophys. Acta* **28**, 21 (1958); of *Polyporus tumulosus* Cooke: Crowden, Ralph, *Aust. J. Chem.* **14**, 475 (1961). Biosynthesis: Gatenback, Linnroth, *Acta Chem. Scand.* **16**, 2298 (1962).

Needles, monoclinic prisms from water, mp 199-200°. Crystals are dimorphic and undergo phase inversion upon heating. The stable phase begins to sublime at 200° and melts at 205°. pK (25°): 2.93. Sol in water (about 1 part in 200 parts H_2O at 5°, much more sol in hot water), alcohol, ether. Practically insol in carbon disulfide, chloroform, benzene.

Sodium salt. [4955-90-2] Sodium gentisate; Gentinatre; Gentisod; Legential; Gentisine U.C.B. $C_7H_5NaO_4$; mol wt 176.10. Crystals with 5½H₂O from water. Rapidly loses 3H₂O on exposure to air, but holds ½H₂O tenaciously even at 100°. Sol in water.

THERAP CAT: Analgesic; anti-inflammatory.

4399. Gentisin. [437-50-3] 1,7-Dihydroxy-3-methoxy-9*H*-xanthen-9-one; 4,7-dihydroxy-2-methoxyxanthone; gentianic acid; gentianin; gentiin. $C_{14}H_{10}O_5$; mol wt 258.23. C 65.12%, H 3.90%, O 30.98%. From root of *Gentiana lutea* L., *Gentianaceae:* Henry, Caventou, *J. Pharm. Chim.* **1821**, 178; Canonica, Pelizzoni, *Gazz. Chim. Ital.* **85**, 1007 (1955). Structure: Korte, *Ber.* **87**, 1357 (1954). Synthesis: Anand, Venkataraman, *Proc. Indian Acad. Sci.* **25A**, 438 (1947); Rao, Seshadri, *ibid.* **37A**, 710 (1953).

Yellow needles from alc, mp 266-267°. Absorption max (methanol): 260, 275, 315, 410 nm (log ε 4.35, 4.30, 4.10, 3.70). Very slightly sol in water or organic solvents.

Diacetate. $C_{18}H_{14}O_7$. Crystals from alc, mp 196-197°. uv max (methanol): 240, 270, 300 nm (log ε 4.58, 4.05, 4.10).

4400. Geosmin. [19700-21-1] [4*S*-(4α,4aα,8aβ)]-Octahydro-4,8a-dimethyl-4a(2*H*)-naphthalenol; octahydro-4α,8aβ-dimethyl-4aα(2*H*)-naphthol; 1,10-*trans*-dimethyl-*trans*-(9)-decalol. $C_{12}H_{22}O$; mol wt 182.30. C 79.06%, H 12.16%, O 8.78%. Major volatile component of beet essence, also determined to be the potent earthy odor contaminant of fish, beans, water: A. C. Thaysen, *Ann. Appl. Biol.* **23**, 99 (1936); J. Silvey, A. W. Roach, *J. Am. Water Works Assoc.* **56**, 60 (1964); A. A. Rosen *et al., Water Treat. Exam.* **19** (Pt. 2), 106 (1970); R. G. Buttery *et al., J. Agric. Food Chem.* **24**, 419, 1246 (1976). Isoln from *Actinomycetes*, algae: N. N. Gerber, H. A. Lechevalier, *Appl. Microbiol.* **13**, 935 (1965); A. A. Rosen *et al., ibid.* **16**, 178 (1968); R. S. Safferman *et al., Environ. Sci. Technol.* **1**, 429 (1967). Isoln from beets: K. E. Murray, P. A. Bannister, *Chem. Ind. (London)* **1975**, 973; L. D. Tyler *et al., J. Agric. Food Chem.* **26**, 1466 (1978). Structure: N. N. Gerber, *Biotechnol. Bioeng.* **9**, 321 (1967); *eidem, Tetrahedron Lett.* **1968**, 2971. Biological degradation: L. V. Narayan, W. J. Nunez, *J. Am. Water Works Assoc.* **66** (Pt. 1), 532 (1974).

Colorless neutral oil, bp 270°. $[\alpha]_D^{25}$ −16.5°. Threshold odor conc: 0.1 ppb. Decomp in acid to odorless compds.

4401. Gepefrine. [18840-47-6] 3-[(2S)-2-Aminopropyl]-phenol; α-methyl-*m*-tyramine. $C_9H_{13}NO$; mol wt 151.21. C 71.49%, H 8.67%, N 9.26%, O 10.58%. Sympathomimetic isomer of hydroxyamphetamine, *q.v.* Prepn: W. S. Saari *et al., J. Med. Chem.* **11**, 1115 (1968); G. Petrik *et al.,* **DE 2712860** (1978 to Helopharm), *C.A.* **88**, 136296a (1978). Molecular configuration and biological actions: M. L. Torchiana *et al., Arch. Int. Pharmacodyn. Ther.* **174**, 118 (1968). *In vitro* study of tritium-labeled gepefrine: R. L. Dorris, *Eur. J. Pharmacol.* **35**, 225 (1976). Biochemical-pharmacological study: R. R. Ruffolo *et al., Biochem. Pharmacol.* **25**, 399 (1976).

Crystals from ethanol/hexane, mp 155-158°. $[\alpha]_D^{25}$ +31.8° (c = 2 in methanol). Sublimes at 100° (0.3 mm).

Tartrate. [60763-48-6] Pressionorm; Wintonin. C_9H_{13}-$NO.C_4H_6O_6$; mol wt 301.29.

THERAP CAT: Antihypotensive.

4402. Gephyrotoxin. [55893-12-4] (1R,3aR,5aR,6R,9aS)-Dodecahydro-6-(2Z)-2-penten-4-ynyl-pyrrolo[1,2-*a*]-quinoline-1-ethanol; HTX D; histrionicotoxin D. $C_{19}H_{29}NO$; mol wt 287.44. C 79.39%, H 10.17%, N 4.87%, O 5.57%. Parent member of a class of tricyclic perhydrobenzoindolizine neurotoxin alkaloids isolated from the skin secretions of the Colombian poison-dart frogs *Dendrobates histrionicus* and *Dendrobates occultator,* family *Dendrobatidae.* The name gephyrotoxin was coined from the Greek word "gephyra" meaning "bridge", and refers to the bridge presumably formed by addition of the nitrogen function to one side of a 2,6-disubstituted piperidine precursor to form the bicyclic indolizine. Isolation of naturally occurring *l*-form: T. Tokuyama *et al., Helv. Chim. Acta* **57**, 2597 (1974). Structure and absolute configuration: J. W. Daly *et al., ibid.* **60**, 1128 (1977). Revised configuration: R. Fujimoto, Y. Kishi, *Tetrahedron Lett.* **1981**, 4197. Total synthesis of (±)-form: R. Fujimoto *et al., J. Am. Chem. Soc.* **102**, 7154 (1980); D. J. Hart, *J. Org. Chem.* **46**, 3576 (1981); D. J. Hart, K. Kanai, *J. Am. Chem. Soc.* **105**, 1255 (1983); L. E. Overman *et al., ibid.* 5373. Complete proton and ^{13}C NMR assignment: M. W. Edwards, A. Bax, *ibid.* **108**, 918 (1986). Effect on neuromuscular transmission: C. Souccar *et al., Mol. Pharmacol.* **25**, 384, 395 (1984). Receptor binding study: R. S. Aronstam *et al., Neurochem. Res.* **11**, 1227 (1986). Review including discussion of gephyrotoxin congeners: J. W. Daly, *Fortschr. Chem. Org. Naturst.* **41**, 283-300 (*see also* refs pp 326-340) (1982).

mp 231-232° (dec). uv max (ethanol): 225 nm (ε 8400). $[\alpha]_D^{25}$ −51.5° (c = 1 in ethanol).

4403. Geraniol. [106-24-1] *(E)*-3,7-Dimethyl-2,6-octadien-1-ol; *trans*-3,7-dimethyl-2,6-octadien-8-ol; lemonol. $C_{10}H_{18}O$;

mol wt 154.25. C 77.87%, H 11.76%, O 10.37%. An olefinic terpene alcohol constituting the chief part of oil of rose and oil of palmarosa; also found in many other essential oils such as citronella, lemon grass, etc. Isomeric with linalool. Isoln: Jacobsen, *Ann.* **157**, 234 (1871). Structure: Verley, *Bull. Soc. Chim. Fr.* **25**, 68 (1919); J. L. Simonsen, *The Terpenes* vol. **I** (University Press, Cambridge, 2nd ed., 1947) pp 40-52. Stereochemistry: Burrell *et al., Proc. Chem. Soc. London* **1959**, 263; Bates *et al., J. Org. Chem.* **28**, 1086 (1963). Synthesis: Burrell *et al., J. Chem. Soc. C* **1966**, 2144; K. Takabe *et al., Chem. Lett.* **1977**, 1025; K. K. Mathew *et al., Indian J. Chem.* **B20**, 340 (1981).

Oily liq. Sweet rose odor. bp_{757} 229-230°; bp_{12} 114-115°. d_4^{20} 0.8894. n_D^{20} 1.4766. uv max: 190-195 nm (ε 18000). Practically insol in water. Miscible with alcohol, ether.

Acetate. $C_{12}H_{20}O_2$. Sweet, fragrant liq. bp ~242° with decompn. d_{15}^{15} 0.9174. n_D^{15} 1.4628. Almost insol in water. Very sol in alcohol; miscible with ether.

Butyrate. $C_{14}H_{24}O_2$. Liq. Characteristic fragrant odor. bp_{18} 152°. d_4^{17} 0.901. Almost insol in water. Sol in alc, ether.

Formate. $C_{11}H_{18}O_2$. Liq. Odor of roses and of green rose leaves. bp_{15} 113-114°. d_4^{20} 0.927. Almost insol in alc, ether.

USE: In perfumery. As insect attractant. Butyrate for compounding artificial attar of rose. Formate as constituent of artificial neroli oil and of artificial orange blossom oil.

4404. Geranium. Cranesbill; storksbill; alum root. Dried rhizome of *Geranium maculatum* L., *Geraniaceae. Habit.* Canada and Eastern U.S., south to Georgia. *Constit.* 10-28% tannin, gallic, acid, resin, sugar, pectin.

THERAP CAT: Astringent.

THERAP CAT (VET): Astringent (intestinal).

4405. Geranylhydroquinone. [10457-66-6] 2-[(2E)-3,7-Dimethyl-2,6-octadienyl]-1,4-benzenediol; *trans*-(3,7-dimethyl-2,6-octadienyl)hydroquinone; *trans*-1,4-dihydroxy-2-(3,7-dimethyl-2,6-octadienyl)benzene; geranyl-1,4-benzenediol; geroquinol; Béradia. $C_{16}H_{22}O_2$; mol wt 246.34. C 78.01%, H 9.00%, O 12.99%. Prepn and use: Baranger, **FR M2694** (1964), *C.A.* **61**, 15940e (1964). Radioprotective activity: G. Rudali, *C.R. Seances Soc. Biol. Ses Fil.* **160**, 1365 (1966). Effects on cancers in mice: G. Rudali, L. Menetrier, *Therapie* **22**, 895 (1967). Discovery as a potent contact allergen from trichomes of *Phacelia crenulata* var. *funerea* J. Voss, *Hydrophyllaceae:* G. Reynolds, E. Rodriguez, *Phytochemistry* **18**, 1567 (1979).

Colorless needles from *n*-hexane/ethyl acetate, mp 61-62°, H. Inouye *et al., Ber.* **101**, 4057 (1968).

USE: Exptly as a radioprotective agent.

4406. Germane. [7782-65-2] Germanium hydride. GeH_4; mol wt 76.67. Ge 94.74%, H 5.26%. Prepd by the action of lithium aluminum hydride on a germanium halide in ether soln: Finholt *et al., J. Am. Chem. Soc.* **69**, 2692 (1947); by reduction of GeO_2 by sodium hydoborate: Griffiths, *Inorg. Chem.* **2**, 375 (1963).

Colorless gas. mp −165°, bp −90°, d_4^{-142} 1.523. Slightly sol in hot hydrochloric acid, dec in nitric acid.

Caution: Potential symptoms of overexposure are malaise, headache, giddiness, fainting; dyspnea; nausea, vomiting; kidney injury; hemolytic effects. *See NIOSH Pocket Guide to Chemical Hazards* (DHHS/NIOSH 97-140, 1997) p 150.

4407. Germanium. [7440-56-4] Ge; at. wt 72.61; at. no. 32; valences 4, 2. Group IVA (14). Five naturally occurring isotopes:

70 (20.55%); 72 (27.37%); 73 (7.67%); 74 (36.74%); 76 (7.67%); artificial, radioactive isotopes: 65-69; 71; 75; 77; 78. Extent of occurrence in the earth's crust about 0.0007%. Predicted and called ekasilicon by Mendeléeff. Discovered in 1886 by Clemens Winkler: *J. Prakt. Chem.* **34**, 177 (1886). Obtained industrially from the flue dusts of smelters processing zinc-bearing ores: Jaffee *et al.*, *Trans. Electrochem. Soc.* **89**, 277 (1946). Purification by zone refining: Pfann, *J. Met.* **4**, 747 (1952). Physical properties: Hassion *et al.*, *J. Phys. Chem.* **59**, 1076 (1955). Inhalation toxicity studies: J. H. E. Arts *et al.*, *Food Chem. Toxicol.* **28**, 571 (1990). Review and description of modern isolation techniques: Pirest in L. P. Hunter, *Handbook of Semiconductor Electronics* (McGraw-Hill, New York, 1956), section 6. Comprehensive monograph: V. I. Davydov, *Germanium* (Gordon & Breach, New York, 1966) 417 pp. *Reviews:* Rochow in *Comprehensive Inorganic Chemistry* vol. **2**, J. C. Bailar, Jr. *et al.*, Eds. (Pergamon Press, Oxford, 1973) pp 1-41; J. H. Adams in *Kirk-Othmer Encyclopedia of Chemical Technology* vol. **11** (Wiley-Interscience, New York, 3rd ed., 1980) pp 791-802.

Grayish-white, lustrous, brittle metalloid. Diamond-cubic structure when cryst. Poor conductor of electricity. d_4^{25} 5.323. Reported melting points range from 925-975°; best value 937.2° (Hassion). Vol smaller by a few % when molten. bp 2700°. Thermal expansion coefficient (at ~25°): 6.1×10^{-6}/°C. Thermal conductivity (at 25°): 0.14 cal/sec cm/°C. Specific heat (0-100°): 0.074 cal/g/°C. Lattice constant at 25°: 5.657×10^{-8} cm. Atoms/cc = 4.42×10^{22}. Volume compressibility: 1.3×10^{-12} cm²/dyn. Dielectric constant: 16. Covalent bond ionization energy at 0 K = 1.2 ev. Band gap: 0.67 ev. Impurity atom ionization energy: ~0.01 ev. Intrinsic resistivity at 300 K = 47 ohm-cm. Electron mobility at 300 K = 3900 cm²/v sec. Hole mobility at 300 K = 1900 cm/v sec. Magnetic (mass) susceptibility ($\chi \times 10^6$) = -0.12. Intrinsic charge density at 300 K = 2.4×10^{13}. Electron diffusion constant at 300 K = 100. Hole diffusion constant at 300 K = 49. Insol in water, hydrochloric acid, dil alkali hydroxides. Attacked by aqua regia, concd nitric or sulfuric acids, fused alkalies, alkali peroxides, nitrates, or carbonates. Relatively stable, unaffected by air, becomes oxidized above 600°; is slowly oxidized by hydrogen peroxide at room temp, fairly rapidly at 90°; is attacked by hydrogen above 1000°. When finely divided, burns in chlorine or bromine.

USE: In electronics: Manuf rectifying devices (germanium diodes), transistors, in red-fluorescing phosphors; in dental alloys; in the production of glass capable of transmitting infrared radiation. Review of uses: Aldington, Cumming, *Endeavour* **14**, 200-204 (1955); *New Uses for Germanium*, F. I. Metz, Ed. (Midwest Research Institute, 1974) 120 pp.

THERAP CAT (VET): Astringent (intestinal).

4408. Germanium Dichloride. [10060-11-4] Cl_2Ge; mol wt 143.55. Cl 49.39%, Ge 50.60%. $GeCl_2$. Obtained as residue upon low temp distillation of $GeHCl_3$ (prepd by the reaction of hydrogen chloride with germanium monosulfide): Moulton, Miller, *J. Am. Chem. Soc.* **78**, 2702 (1956).

Unstable substance, dec into polymeric subchlorides even at low temps. Sol in ether, benzene.

4409. Germanium Dioxide. [1310-53-8] Germanium oxide (GeO_2); germanium(IV) oxide. GeO_2; mol wt 104.64. Ge 69.42%, O 30.58%.

White powder. Sol in about 250 parts cold water, 100 parts boiling water; sol in acids or in solns of the fixed alkalies. LD_{50} i.p. in rats: 750 mg/kg, Rosenfeld, Wallace, *Arch. Ind. Hyg. Occup. Med.* **8**, 466 (1953).

4410. Germanium Tetrachloride. [10038-98-9] Tetrachlorogermane; germanium(IV) chloride. Cl_4Ge; mol wt 214.45. Cl 66.13%, Ge 33.87%. $GeCl_4$. Prepd from Ge and Cl_2 or GeO_2 and HCl: Bauer, Burschkies, *Ber.* **66**, 277 (1933); Foster *et al.*, *Inorg. Synth.* **2**, 109 (1946).

Mobile liq. Fumes in air. Peculiar, acidic odor, but can be distinguished from that of concd HCl. Appreciably volatile at room temp. d_{20}^{20} 1.879. bp_{760} 83.1°. mp $-49.5°$. Hydrolyzed by water with a crackling noise. Is stable, but not very sol in 6N HCl. If more concd HCl is used, the soly of $GeCl_4$ is reduced. Sol in benzene, ether, other organic solvents.

Caution: Fumes irritating to eyes, mucous membranes of respiratory tract.

4411. Germanium Tetrafluoride. [7783-58-6] F_4Ge; mol wt 148.63. F 51.13%, Ge 48.87%. GeF_4. Prepd by heating $BaGeF_6$ to around 700°: Dennis, Laubengayer, *Z. Phys. Chem.* **130**, 520 (1927); Dennis, *Z. Anorg. Allg. Chem.* **174**, 119 (1928); Biltz, *ibid.* **207**, 65 (1932); Hoffman, Gutowsky, *Inorg. Synth.* **4**, 147 (1953).

Colorless gas. Odor of garlic. Thermally stable up to about 1000°. d^0 (liq) 2.162; d (solid; $-195°$) 3.148. mp $-15°$ (under 3032 mm pressure). Sublimes at $-36.5°$. On contact with water, hydrolyzes to GeO_2 and H_2GeF_6. Does not attack glass when absolutely dry. Corrodes mercury, grease.

Trihydrate. Obtained by slow evaporation of a soln of germanium dioxide in 20% HF. This is said to be water-soluble.

Caution: Highly irritating to eyes, skin, lungs, mucous membranes.

4412. Germine. [508-65-6] $(3\beta,4\alpha,7\alpha,15\alpha,16\beta)$-4,9-Epoxycevane-3,4,7,14,15,16,20-heptol. $C_{27}H_{43}NO_8$; mol wt 509.63. C 63.63%, H 8.50%, N 2.75%, O 25.12%. Alkamine present in many polyester alkaloids which occur in *Veratrum* and *Zygadenus* species. Isoln: Poethke, *Pharm. Monatsh.* **18**, 77 (1937); *idem, Arch. Pharm.* **275**, 571 (1937); Seiferle *et al.*, *J. Econ. Entomol.* **35**, 35 (1942); Klohs *et al.*, *J. Am. Chem. Soc.* **75**, 4925 (1953); Kupchan, Deliwala, *ibid.* **76**, 5545 (1954); Myers *et al.*, *ibid.* **77**, 3348 (1955); **78**, 1621 (1956). Structure and configuration: Kupchan, Narayanan, *ibid.* **81**, 1913 (1959). Comparative toxicity: O. Krayer *et al.*, *J. Pharmacol. Exp. Ther.* **82**, 167 (1944).

Crystals from methanol, mp 221.5-223°. $[\alpha]_D^{25}$ +4.5° (95% ethanol); $[\alpha]_D^{16}$ +23.1° (c = 1.13 in 10% acetic acid). Sol in chloroform, methanol, ethanol, acetone, water; slightly sol in ether. LD_{50} i.v. in mice: 139.0 mg/kg (Krayer).

3-Acetate. $C_{29}H_{45}NO_9$. Needles from ether, mp 219-221°. $[\alpha]_D^{23}$ +10° (c = 1.05 in pyridine).

16-Acetate. $C_{29}H_{45}NO_9$. Crystals from chloroform, mp 225-227°. $[\alpha]_D^{23}$ $-19°$ (c = 0.93 in pyridine).

3,4,7,15,16-Pentaacetate. $C_{37}H_{53}NO_{13}$. Prisms from acetone + petr ether, dec 285-287°. $[\alpha]_D^{23}$ $-65°$ (c = 0.65 in pyridine).

4413. Gestodene. [60282-87-3] (17α)-13-Ethyl-17-hydroxy-18,19-dinorpregna-4,15-dien-20-yn-3-one; 17α-ethynyl-17β-hydroxy-18-methyl-4,15-estradien-3-one; 17α-ethynyl-13-ethyl-17β-hydroxy-4,15-gonadien-3-one; SH B 331. $C_{21}H_{26}O_2$; mol wt 310.43. C 81.25%, H 8.44%, O 10.31%. Orally active gestogen with progesterone-like profile of activity. Prepn: **BE 847090**; H. Hofmeister *et al.*, **US 4081537** (1977, 1978 both to Schering AG). Pharmacokinetics: B. Duesterberg *et al.*, *Contraception* **24**, 673 (1981); B. Duesterberg, *Steroids* **43**, 43 (1984). Comparative study of anti-aldosterone activity: W. Losert *et al.*, *Arzneim.-Forsch.* **35**, 459 (1985). Clinical trial as oral contraceptive: G. Hoppe, *Adv. Contracep.* **3**, 159 (1987).

Crystals from acetone-hexane, mp 197.9°.

Mixture with ethinyl estradiol. [109852-02-0] Femodene; Femovan; Ginoden; Gynera; Harmonet; Meliane; Milvane; Minulet; Phaeva; Tri-Minulet.

THERAP CAT: Progestogen. In combination with estrogen as oral contraceptive.

4414. Gestonorone Caproate. [1253-28-7] 17-[(1-Oxohexyl)oxy]-19-norpregn-4-ene-3,20-dione; 17-hydroxy-19-norpregn-4-ene-3,20-dione hexanoate; 17α-hydroxy-19-norprogesterone caproate; 17β-acetyl-17-hydroxyestr-4-ene-3-one hexanoate; gestronol caproate; SH-582; Depostat. $C_{26}H_{38}O_4$; mol wt 414.58. C 75.32%, H 9.24%, O 15.44%. Prepn: Popper *et al., Arzneim.-Forsch.* **19**, 352 (1969); Popper *et al.,* **DE 1074582** (1960 to Schering). Pharmacological studies: Junkmann, *Anglo-Ger. Med. Rev.* **1**, 385 (1962). Metabolism: Breuer, Lisboa, *Acta Endocrinol.* **51**, 114 (1966).

Crystals, mp 123-124°. $[\alpha]_D$ +13° (chloroform). uv max: 239 nm (ε 17540).

THERAP CAT: Progestogen; in treatment of prostatic hypertrophy.

4415. Gestrinone. [16320-04-0] (17α)-13-Ethyl-17-hydroxy-18,19-dinorpregna-4,9,11-trien-20-yn-3-one; 13β-ethyl-17α-ethynyl-17β-hydroxy-4,9,11-gonatrien-3-one; 13β-ethyl-17α-ethynyl-Δ⁴,⁹,¹¹-gonatriene-17β-ol-3-one; ethylnorgestrienone; A-46745; R-2323; RU-2323; Dimetriose; Dimetrose; Nemestran; Tridomose. $C_{21}H_{24}O_2$; mol wt 308.41. C 81.78%, H 7.84%, O 10.38%. Steroidal antiestrogen, antiprogestogen, analog of norgestrienone, *q.v.* Prepn: G. Nomine *et al.,* **US 3257278**; **NL 6607609** *C.A.* **67**, 44029d (1967); D. Bertin, A. Pierdet, **US 3478067** (1966, 1966, 1969 all to Roussel-UCLAF). Radioimmunoassay in human plasma: J. Frick *et al., Urol. Res.* **5**, 55 (1977). HPLC-MS-MS determn in plasma: Q. Wang *et al., J. Chromatogr. B* **746**, 151 (2000). Clinical evaluation of contraceptive efficacy: G. Azadian-Boulanger *et al., Am. J. Obstet. Gynecol.* **125**, 1049 (1976); of use in fibrocystic breast disease: E. M. Coutinho, G. Azadian-Boulanger, *Int. J. Gynaecol. Obstet.* **22**, 363 (1984); in endometriosis: E. J. Thomas, I. D. Cooke, *Br. Med. J.* **294**, 272 (1987); E. M. Coutinho, G. Azadian-Boulanger, *Fertil. Steril.* **49**, 418 (1988).

Crystals from ethyl acetate and benzene-cyclohexane (1:1), mp 154°. $[\alpha]_D^{20}$ +84.6° (c = 0.41 in methanol).

THERAP CAT: Antigonadotropin.

4416. Ghatti Gum. [9000-28-6] Gum Ghatti; Indian gum. The gummy exudate from stems of *Anogeissus latifolia* Wall., *Combretaceae*, abundant in India and Ceylon, *cf.* C. L. Mantell, *The Water-Soluble Gums* (New York, 1947). Name derived from the word *ghats,* meaning passes, and given to the gum because of its ancient mountain transportation routes. Structure is a complex water-soluble polysaccharide occurring as a calcium-magnesium salt; composed of L-arabinose, D-galactose, D-mannose, D-xylose, D-glucuronic acid, in a molar ratio of 10:6:2:1:2, and traces of 6-deoxyhexose: Aspinall *et al., J. Chem. Soc.* **1955**, 1160. Early investigation of chemistry and mol wt: Shaw *et al., Proc. S. D. Acad. Sci.* **15**, 46 (1935); **16**, 34 (1936); **17**, 27 (1937); **19**, 130 (1939); **21**, 78 (1941). *Review:* Meer *et al.,* in *Industrial Gums,* R.

L. Whistler, Ed. (Academic Press, New York, 2nd ed., 1973) pp 265-271.

Ghatti gum sold in the U.S. usually has been autoclaved in order to make all of the gum water-sol. The *U.S. Dispensatory* (24th ed.) states that gum Ghatti suitable as clinical laboratory reagent is entirely sol in 5 parts of cold water. Forms a very viscous mucilage, more viscous but less adhesive than acacia. Insol in 90% alcohol. $[\alpha]_D^{25}$ +42° (dil H_2SO_4). Gum ghatti solns may be colored slightly due to traces of pigment remaining in the gum. Does not form a true gel.

USE: As substitute for acacia. As emulsifying agent in pharmaceuticals, oils, waxes.

4417. Ghi. Ghee; samli; clarified butter. Prepd from cream or butter by melting and heating to 122° for about 25 mins. The water evaporates, and lactose, salt, and albuminous substances sink to the bottom. This treatment kills existing microorganisms by heat and deprives incoming microorganisms of moisture and necessary nutrients.

Properly clarified butter is of finely grained consistency, yellow color, mp 30° and retains most of the vitamin A content of the original butter. Keeps much longer than ordinary butter and contains less than 0.7% water. Used in India instead of butter.

4418. Ghrelin. [304853-26-7] Orexigenic hormone secreted primarily by the stomach and duodenum; implicated in meal-time hunger and long-term regulation of body weight. Identified as the endogenous ligand for the growth hormone secretagogue receptor (GHSR). Released in response to fasting, resulting in appetite stimulation by the hypothalamus and growth hormone secretion by the pituitary. Contains 28 amino acid residues of which one is acylated by n-octanoic acid. Octanoylation is essential for bioactivity, possibly to facilitate passage across the blood-brain barrier. Isoln from rat stomach and cloning and synthesis of human ghrelin: M. Kojima *et al., Nature* **402**, 656 (1999). Effect on growth hormone release in humans: E. Arvat *et al., J. Endocrinol. Invest.* **23**, 493 (2000). Structure-activity study: M. A. Bednarek *et al., J. Med. Chem.* **43**, 4370 (2000). Identification of stomach as primary source and effect of feeding state on plasma levels: H. Ariyasu *et al., J. Clin. Endocrinol. Metab.* **86**, 4753 (2001). Clinical role in meal initiation: D. E. Cummings *et al., Diabetes* **50**, 1714 (2001); in regulation of body weight: *idem et al., N. Engl. J. Med.* **346**, 1623 (2002). *Reviews:* A. Inui, *Nat. Rev. Neurosci.* **2**, 1-10 (Aug. 2001); G. Wang *et al., Regul. Pept.* **105**, 75-81 (2002); M. Kojima, K. Kangawa, *Physiol. Rev.* **85**, 495-522 (2005).

Human ghrelin. [258279-04-8] Glycyl-L-seryl-*O*-(1-oxooctyl)-L-seryl-L-phenylalanyl-L-leucyl-L-seryl-L-prolyl-L-α-glutamyl-L-histidyl-L-glutaminyl-L-arginyl-L-valyl-L-glutaminyl-L-glutaminyl-L-arginyl-L-lysyl-L-α-glutamyl-L-seryl-L-lysyl-L-lysyl-L-prolyl-L-prolyl-L-alanyl-L-lysyl-L-leucyl-L-glutaminyl-L-prolyl-L-arginine; ghrelin (human clone CTB-187P1 gene GHRELIN). Recombinant form is identical to the naturally occuring human peptide.

4419. Gibberellic Acid. [77-06-5] (1α,2β,4aα,4bβ,10β)-2,-4a,7-Trihydroxy-1-methyl-8-methylenegibb-3-ene-1,10-dicarboxylic acid 1,4a-lactone; gibberellin X; gibberellin A₃; Activol; Gibrel. $C_{19}H_{22}O_6$; mol wt 346.37. C 65.88%, H 6.40%, O 27.71%. Plant hormone; most outstanding of the plant-growth promoting metabolites of *Gibberella fujikuroi*. Isoln: P. J. Curtis, B. E. Cross, *Chem. Ind. (London)* **1954**, 1066; B. E. Cross, *J. Chem. Soc.* **1954**, 4670; P. W. Brian *et al.,* **US 2842051**; C. T. Calam, P. J. Curtis, **US 2950288**; A. J. Birch *et al.,* **US 2977285** (1958, 1960, 1961, all to ICI). Stereochemistry and structure: G. Stork, H. Newman, *J. Am. Chem. Soc.* **81**, 5518 (1959); B. E. Cross *et al., Proc. Chem. Soc. London* **1959**, 302; F. McCapra *et al., ibid.* **1962**, 185; D. C. Aldridge *et al., J. Chem. Soc.* **1963**, 143; P. M. Bourn *et al., ibid.* **1963**, 154. Partial synthesis: E. J. Corey *et al., J. Am. Chem. Soc.* **93**, 7316 (1971). Stereospecific total synthesis: *eidem, ibid.* **100**, 8034 (1978). Promotes growth of seedlings: M. J. Bukovac, S. H. Wittwer, *Q. Bull. Mich. Agric. Exp. Stn.* **39**, 307 (1956); J. M. Merritt, *J. Agric. Food Chem.* **6**, 184 (1958). *Reviews:* B. E. Cross *et al.* in *Adv. Chem. Ser.* **28**, entitled "Gibberellins," J. M. Merritt, Ed. (ACS, Washington DC, 1961) p 13; series of articles in *Plant Growth Subst., Proc. 7th Int. Conf.,* D. J. Carr, Ed. (Springer-Verlag, Berlin, 1972).

Yellow needles from alcohol, mp 65-67°.

USE: In determination of phenols.

Crystals from ethyl acetate, mp 233-235° (effervescence). $[\alpha]_D^{19}$ +86° (c = 2.12). pK 4.0. Slightly sol in water, ether. Freely sol in methanol, ethanol, acetone. Moderately sol in ethyl acetate. Sol in aq solns of sodium bicarbonate and sodium acetate.

Methyl ester. $C_{20}H_{24}O_6$. Needles from benzene + methanol, mp 209-210°. $[\alpha]_D^{20}$ +75° (c = 0.5).

USE: Plant growth regulator.

4420. Gibberellins. GAs. A class of plant growth hormones first isolated in 1938 from cultures of *Gibberella fujikuroi* (Sawada) Wollenweber *(Fusarium moniliforme* Sheldon) the fungus causing Bakanae disease in rice: Yabuta, Sumiki, *J. Agric. Chem. Soc. Jpn.* **14,** 1526 (1938). Isolated also from higher plants; for source references see review by Lang, *Annu. Rev. Plant Physiol.* **21,** 537 (1970). More than 60 gibberellins are known of which gibberellin A_3, *q.v.*, is the most important. GA_3 and mixtures of GA_4 and GA_7 are available commercially. All gibberellins are diterpenoid acids based on the *gibberellane* skeleton containing the *gibbane* nucleus. Major structural differences lie in the substituents at positions 4a, 7, 8 (gibbane numbering) and the presence or absence of a γ-lactone ring. Total synthesis of racemic gibberellins A_2, A_4, A_9, A_{10}: Mori *et al., Tetrahedron* **25,** 1293 (1969); of gibberellin A_4: A. L. Cossey *et al., Tetrahedron Lett.* **1980,** 4383; of gibberellin A_{15}: Nagata *et al., J. Am. Chem. Soc.* **93,** 5740 (1971); of gibberellins A_{15} and A_{37}: E. Fujita *et al., J. Chem. Soc. Perkin Trans. 1* **1977,** 611. Stereochemistry: Meguro, Fuzimura, *Tetrahedron Lett.* **1968,** 6305. Biosynthesis: Cross *et al., J. Chem. Soc. C* **1968,** 1054; Shechter, West, *J. Biol. Chem.* **244,** 3200 (1969). Nomenclature: MacMillan, Takahasni, *Nature* **217,** 170 (1968). Early reviews: Brian *et al., Fortschr. Chem. Org. Naturst.* **18,** 350 (1960); Paleg, *Annu. Rev. Plant Physiol.* **16,** 291 (1965). Recent reviews: Cleland in *The Physiology of Plant Growth and Development,* M. B. Wilkins, Ed. (McGraw-Hill, New York, 1969) pp 49-81; L. Rappaport, "Applications of Gibberellins in Agriculture", in *Plant Growth Subst., Proc. 10th Int. Conf.,* F. K. Skoog, Ed. (Springer-Verlag, Berlin, 1980) pp 377-391; I. D. Railton, *Cell Biol. Int. Rep.* **6,** 319-337 (1982). Comprehensive synthetic review: E. Fujita, M. Node, *Heterocycles* **7,** 709 (1977).

Gibbane

Gibberellane

USE: Plant growth hormone. For specific agricultural uses *see* review by Turner, *Outlook Agric.* **7,** 14 (1972).

4421. Gibbs Reagent. [101-38-2] 2,6-Dichloro-4-(chloro-imino)-2,5-cyclohexadien-1-one; 2,6-dichloro-*p*-benzoquinone-4-chloroimine; *N*,2,6-trichloro-*p*-quinoneimine; 2,6-dichloroquinone chloroimide; *N*,2,6-trichloroquinoneimine; *N*,2,6-trichlorobenzoquinone imine. $C_6H_2Cl_3NO$; mol wt 210.45. C 34.24%, H 0.96%, Cl 50.54%, N 6.66%, O 7.60%. Reagent used to determine the presence of phenols. The reaction with phenols unsubstituted in the *para* position is called the Gibbs Reaction: H. D. Gibbs, *Chem. Rev.* **3,** 291 (1927). Prepn of the reagent: *idem, J. Biol. Chem.* **72,** 649 (1927); G. I. Mikhailov, *Trans. Inst. Pure Chem. Reagents* **16,** 83 (1939). Analysis of the Gibbs color reaction: J. C. Dacre, *Anal. Chem.* **43,** 589 (1971).

4422. Gilsonite. [12002-43-6] Uintahite; uintaite. Naturally occurring, solid hydrocarbon classified as an asphaltite. Coal-like mineral found almost exclusively in the Uinta valley, near Fort Duchesne, Utah: E. S. Dana, *A System of Mineralogy* (John Wiley, New York, 6th ed., 1901) p 1020. Review: K. R. Neel in *Kirk-Othmer Encyclopedia of Chemical Technology* **vol. 11** (John Wiley & Sons, New York, 3rd ed., 1980) pp 803-806. Review of uses and mining methods: D. Jackson, *Eng. Min. J.* **182,** 88-91 (July, 1981); of health effects from occupational exposure: D. G. Keimig *et al., Am. J. Ind. Med.* **11,** 287-296 (1987); G. J. Kullman *et al., Am. Ind. Hyg. Assoc. J.* **50,** 413-418 (1989).

Black, lustrous masses; streak and powder a rich brown. Softening point: 160°. d_{15}^{15} 1.04. Specific heat (J/kg): 2180 (149°); 2550 (260°). Viscosity (cP): 500 (260°); 140 (316°). Nonconductor of electricity. Sol in heavy lubricating petroleum, warm oil of turpentine, and alc.

USE: In automotive body sealers, photogravure inks, anticorrosive paints, oil drilling fluids, and in nuclear-grade graphite.

4423. Ginger. Perennial plant, *Zingiber officinale* Roscoe, *Zingiberaceae,* with tuberous rhizomes that are widely used in traditional medicine and foods. *Habit.* Tropical Asia; cultivated in Jamaica, Africa, Australia, most tropical countries. *Constit.* Volatile oil (1-3%); oleoresin (4-7.5%) containing the pungent gingerols and shogaols; starch (40-60%); proteins (10%); and fats (10%). Chemistry of oil and oleoresin: D. W. Connell *et al., Flavour Ind.* **1,** 677 (1970). Comprehensive review: V. S. Govindarajan, *Crit. Rev. Food Sci. Nutr.* **17,** 1-96; 189-258 (1982). Review of cultivation, processing and uses: B. M. Lawrence, *Perfum. Flavor.* **9,** 1-40 (1984); of history and use: E. Langner *et al., Adv. Ther.* **15,** 25-44 (1998). Review of medicinal uses: J. Gruenwald *et al., PDR for Herbal Medicines* (Medical Economics, Montvale, 3rd Ed., 2004) pp 362-367; of clinical trials in nausea and vomiting of pregnancy: F. Borrelli *et al., Obstet. Gynecol.* **105,** 849 (2005).

Volatile oil. [8007-08-7] Oil of ginger. Obtained by steam distillation of the dried ground rhizome. *Constit:* Chiefly, zingiberene (30-70%), β-sesquiphellandrene (15-20%), β-bisabolene (10-15%), α-farnesene, *ar*-curcumene, *d*-camphene, phellandrene, borneol, cineol, citral. Yellowish, viscid liquid. d_{25}^{25} 0.870-0.882. Angular rotation: −28 to −47°. n_D^{20} 1.488-1.494. Sol in most fixed oils, mineral oil, in alcohol with turbidity. Insol in glycerin, propylene glycol.

USE: Flavor in foods and beverages.

THERAP CAT: Antiemetic; carminative.

THERAP CAT (VET): Carminative.

4424. [6]-Gingerol. [23513-14-6] (5*S*)-5-Hydroxy-1-(4-hydroxy-3-methoxyphenyl)-3-decanone. $C_{17}H_{26}O_4$; mol wt 294.39. C 69.36%, H 8.90%, O 21.74%. The major phenol and most important of the pungent principles of ginger oil, isolated from rhizome of *Zingiber officinale* Roscoe, *Zingiberaceae:* Thresh, *Pharm. J.* [3] **10,** 171 (1879); **12,** 721 (1881); **14,** 798 (1883); **15,** 208 (1884); Garnett, Grier, *ibid.* [4] **25,** 118 (1907); Nelson, *J. Am. Chem. Soc.* **39,** 1466 (1917). Structure studies: Lapworth *et al., J. Chem. Soc.* **111,** 777 (1917). Review of early literature: Redgrove, *Pharm. J.* **125,** 54 (1930); Jacobs, *Am. Perfum.* **48,** no. 7, 60, 62 (1946). Demonstration of the presence of an homologous series of phenolic ketones in the pungent constituents of ginger, [6]-gingerol being the major member: D. W. Connell, M. D. Sutherland, *Aust. J. Chem.* **22,** 1033 (1969). Synthesis of (±)-form: Hirao *et al., Chem. Pharm. Bull.* **20,** 2287 (1972); K. Banno, T. Mukaiyama, *Bull. Chem. Soc. Jpn.* **49,** 1453 (1976); P. Denniff, D. A. Whiting, *Chem. Commun.* **1976,** 712; P. Denniff *et al., J. Chem. Soc. Perkin Trans. 1* **1981,** 82. Stereoselective synthesis of *S*(+)-form: D.

Enders *et al., Ber.* **112**, 3703 (1979). Biosynthesis of (±)-form: P. Denniff, D. A. Whiting, *Chem. Commun.* **1976**, 711; I. Macleod, D. A. Whiting, *ibid.* **1979**, 1152; P. Denniff *et al., J. Chem. Soc. Perkin Trans. 1* **1980**, 2637. Physical properties and cardiotonic effects of gingerols: N. Shoji *et al., J. Pharm. Sci.* **71**, 1174 (1982). Mutagenicity studies: H. Nakamura, T. Yamamoto, *Mutat. Res.* **103**, 119 (1982); *eidem, ibid.* **122**, 87 (1983).

Normally obtained as pungent, yellow oil. n_D^{25} 1.5224. uv max (ethanol) 282 nm (ε 2560) (Connell, Sutherland). Crystalline form, mp 30-32°. $[\alpha]_D$ +27.8° (c = 1 in CHCl$_3$). uv max (ethanol): 284 nm (ε 2700). Sol in 50% alcohol, ether, chloroform, benzene; moderately sol in hot petr ether.

4425. Ginkgo. Maidenhair tree; kew tree. *Ginkgo biloba* Linn; the only living member of the *Ginkgoaceae*. Valued as a street and park tree, the ripe fruit gives off a foul odor. The seeds and leaves have been used in traditional medicine for asthma and vascular disease. *Habit.* China, Japan, cultivated in Eastern U.S. and Canada. A wide variety of compounds have been identified in the fruit, leaves and bark including: ginkgolides, bilobalide, *q.q.v.*, biflavones, flavonol glycosides. Fruit pulp contains toxic principles: ginkgolic acid, ginkgol, bilobol. Analysis of constituents of leaves: S. Furukawa, *Sci. Papers Inst. Phys. Chem. Res. Jpn.* **19**, 27 (1932); **21**, 273 (1933), *C.A.* **27**, 303, 5745 (1933). Isoln and characterization of biflavonyl constituents of ginkgo leaves: W. Baker *et al., J. Chem. Soc.* **1963**, 1477; of phenolic constituents: K. Weinges *et al., Arzneim.-Forsch.* **18**, 539 (1968). Isoln of gink-golides from root bark: M. Maruyama *et al., Tetrahedron Lett.* **1967**, 299-326. HPLC determn of biflavones in leaf extracts: F. Briançon-Scheid *et al., Planta Med.* **49**, 204 (1983); of terpenes: P. G. Pietta *et al., Chromatographia* **29**, 251 (1990). HPLC fingerprint analysis of leaf extracts: Y.-B. Ji *et al., J. Chromatogr. A* **1066**, 97 (2005). *Reviews:* W. Tang, G. Eisenbrand, *Chinese Drugs of Plant Origin* (Springer-Verlag, Berlin, 1992) pp 555-565; P. Houghton, *Pharm. J.* **253**, 122-123 (1994).

EGb 761. Extractum *Ginkgo biloba* 761; Rökan; Tanakan; Te-bonin. A defined extract obtained from the leaves: P. Kloss, H. Jaggy, **DE 2117429** (1972 to Willmar Schwabe), *C.A.* **78**, 47787 (1973). Clinical evaluation in arterial insufficiency: U. Bauer, *Arzneim.-Forsch.* **34**, 716 (1984). Clinical trial in dementia: P. L. Le Bars *et al., J. Am. Med. Assoc.* **278**, 1327 (1997). *Book:* F. V. DeFeudis, *Ginkgo biloba Extract (EGb 761): Pharmacological Activities and Clinical Applications* (Elsevier, Amsterdam, 1991) 187 pp.

THERAP CAT: Nootropic. In treatment of vascular insufficiency.

4426. Ginkgolides. Family of bioactive terpenes isolated from the root bark and leaves of *Ginkgo biloba* L., *Ginkgoaceae*. Specific platelet activating factor (PAF) antagonists. Isoln from leaves: S. Furukawa, *Sci. Papers Inst. Phys. Chem. Res. Jpn.* **19**, 27 (1932), *C.A.* **27**, 303 (1933). Isoln from root bark and characterization: M. Maruyama *et al., Tetrahedron Lett.* **1967**, 299; K. Nakanishi, *Pure Appl. Chem.* **14**, 89 (1967); from leaves: N. Sakabe *et al., Chem. Commun.* **1967**, 259; K. Okabe *et al., J. Chem. Soc. C* **1967**, 2201. Crystal structure of B: L. Dupont *et al., Acta Crystallogr.* **C42**, 1759 (1986); of A and C: M. Sbit *et al., ibid.* **C43**, 2377 (1987). Total synthesis of (±)-B: E. J. Corey *et al., J. Am. Chem. Soc.* **110**, 649 (1988); of (±)-A: E. J. Corey, A. K. Ghosh, *Tetrahedron Lett.* **29**, 3205 (1988). Enantioselective route to B: E. J. Corey, A. V. Gavai, *ibid.*, 3201. Review of syntheses: E. J. Corey, *Chem. Soc. Rev.* **17**, 111-133 (1988). ¹H- and ¹³C-NMR: C. Roumestand *et al., Tetrahedron* **45**, 1975 (1989). Effect on PAF receptor binding: R. Korth *et al., Eur. J. Pharmacol.* **152**, 101 (1988). *Review:* P. Braquet *et al., Med. Res. Rev.* **11**, 295-355 (1991). Review of physical properties: T. A. van Beek, *Bioorg. Med. Chem.* **13**, 5001-5012 (2005).

Ginkgolide B

Ginkgolides are sol in acetone, ethanol, methanol, ethyl acetate, THF, dioxane, acetic acid, trifluoroacetic acid, acetonitrile, pyridine, DMSO; sparingly sol in ether, water. Insol in hexane, benzene, chloroform, carbon tetrachloride.

Ginkgolide A. [15291-75-5] BN-52020. $C_{20}H_{24}O_9$; mol wt 408.40. Bitter crystals from ethanol, mp ~300° (dec). $[\alpha]_D^{24}$ −53.4° (c = 1 in ethanol). uv max (ethanol): 219 nm (log ε 2.72).

Ginkgolide B. [15291-77-7] (1β)-1-Hydroxyginkgolide A; BN-52021. $C_{20}H_{24}O_{10}$; mol wt 424.40. Review of pharmacology and PAF-antagonism: P. Braquet, R. H. Bourgain, *Adv. Exp. Med. Biol.* **215**, 215-235 (1987). Clinical trial in asthma: K.-H. Hsieh, *Chest* **99**, 877 (1991); in severe sepsis: J. F. Dhainaut *et al., Crit. Care Med.* **22**, 1720 (1994). Bitter crystals from ethanol, mp ~300° (dec). $[\alpha]_D^{24}$ −52.6° (c = 1 in ethanol). uv max (ethanol): 219 nm (log ε 2.37). Log P (water/n-octanol): 1.72. pKa$_1$ 7.14; pKa$_2$ 8.60; pKa$_3$ 11.89.

Ginkgolide C. [15291-76-6] (1α,7β)-1,7-Dihydroxyginkgolide A; BN-52022. $C_{20}H_{24}O_{11}$; mol wt 440.40. Bitter crystals from ethanol, mp ~300° (dec). $[\alpha]_D^{24}$ −14.7° (c = 1 in ethanol). uv max (ethanol): 220 nm (log ε 2.30).

USE: Reference compd for PAF receptors in biological systems.

4427. Ginseng. Panax. Root of *Panax ginseng* C.A. Mey., *Araliaceae*, a perennial herb indigenous to Eastern Asia, *P. quinquefolium* L., found in Eastern U.S. and Canada, and *P. pseudoginseng* Wall, found in India, China and Japan. The biologically active constituents are considered to be a series of saponin glycosides known as **ginsenosides, panaxosides** or **panaquilins**. Review of constituents: J. P. Hov, *Comp. Med. East West* **5**, 123-145 (1977). Isoln and identification of ginseng saponin glycosides: S. Shibata *et al., Tetrahedron Lett.* **1962** 419; G. B. Elyakov *et al., ibid.* **1964**, 3591; R. Kasai *et al., Chem. Pharm. Bull.* **31**, 2120 (1983). Chem-ico-pharmacological study: T. Kaku, *Arzneim.-Forsch.* **25**, 539 (1975). Effect on brain biogenic amines: V. Petkov, *ibid.* **28**, 388 (1978). TLC analysis of saponin content of commercial ginseng products: L. E. Liberti, A. D. Marderosian, *J. Pharm. Sci.* **67**, 1487 (1978). Use in oriental medicine as tonic: K. Chimin Wong, Wu Lien-teh, *History of Chinese Medicine* (Shanghai, 2nd ed., 1936) 906 pp. Comprehensive review of morphology, cultivation and uses: Baranov, *Econ. Bot.* **20**, 403-406 (1966). Review of chemical constituents: J. P. Hou, *Comp. Med. East West* **5**, 123-145 (1977). Brief reviews: W. E. Court, *Pharm. J.* **214**, 180-181 (1975); B. J. Spalding, *Chem. Week* **139**, 19-21 (1986).

Sweet, slightly aromatic taste.

THERAP CAT: Tonic.

4428. Giractide. [24870-04-0] 1-Glycine-18-L-argininamide-$\alpha^{(1-18)}$-corticotropin. $C_{100}H_{156}N_{34}O_{22}S$; mol wt 2218.59. C 54.14%, H 7.09%, N 21.47%, O 15.87%, S 1.45%. Polypeptide corresp to the first 18 amino acid residues in corticotropin, in which the 1-serine is replaced by glycine. Prepn: H. Otsuka *et al., Bull. Chem. Soc. Jpn.* **43**, 196 (1970); of the hexaacetate: *eidem*, **JP 70 19061** (1970 to Shionogi), *C.A.* **73**, 110138r (1970). Adrenocorti-cotropic potency in man: *J. Clin. Endocrinol. Metab.* **33**, 355 (1971). Fluorometric study: T. Muraki *et al., Experientia* **32**, 1605 (1976). Absorption: M. Hirata *et al., Chem. Pharm. Bull.* **26**, 1061 (1978). Chromatographic studies: S. Terabe *et al., J. Chromatogr.* **172**, 163 (1979); M. Schoeneshoefer, A. Fenner, *ibid.* **224**, 472 (1981).

Gly–Tyr–Ser–Met–Glu–His–Phe–Arg–Trp–Gly–Lys–Pro–Val–Gly–Lys–Lys–Arg–ArgNH₂

$[\alpha]_D^{23.5}$ −51.4 ±1.9° (c = 0.472 in 0.1N acetic acid). uv max (0.1N NaOH): 281, 288 nm (ε 6750, 6490).

Hexaacetate salt. [29365-11-5] S-50022; Acthormon. $C_{100}H_{156}N_{34}O_{22}S.6C_2H_4O_2$; mol wt 2578.90.

THERAP CAT: Adrenocorticotropic hormone.

4429. Girard Reagents. Quaternary ammonium acetylhydrazine chlorides which form water-soluble hydrazones with carbonyl compounds. The hydrazones formed can subsequently be hydrolyzed in order to regenerate the original carbonyl compounds. Prepn: A. Girard, G. Sandulesco, *GB* **6640** (1934); *eidem, Helv. Chim. Acta* **19**, 1095 (1936); A. Girard, *Org. Synth.* **coll. vol. II**, 85 (1943). *Review:* Wheeler, *Chem. Rev.* **62**, 205 (1962). Use of Girard reagents in separation of carbonyl compounds: Schubert, Wehrberger, *Endokrinologie* **48**, 70 (1965); R. E. J. Mitchel, H. C. Birnboim, *Anal. Biochem.* **81**, 47 (1977); W. Holstein, D. Severin, *Erdoel Kohle, Erdgas, Petrochem.* **32**, 487 (1979); *C.A.* **92**, 44207b (1980).

$$\left[(H_3C)_3\overset{+}{N}-CH_2-\overset{O}{\underset{\|}{C}}-\overset{H}{\underset{}{N}}-NH_2 \right] Cl^-$$

Girard reagent T

$$\left[\underset{}{\text{(pyridinium)}}\overset{+}{N}-CH_2-\overset{O}{\underset{\|}{C}}-\overset{H}{\underset{}{N}}-NH_2 \right] Cl^-$$

Girard reagent P

Girard reagent T. 2-Hydrazino-*N,N,N*-trimethyl-2-oxoethanaminium chloride; (carboxymethyl)trimethylammonium chloride hydrazide; betaine hydrazide hydrochloride. $C_5H_{14}ClN_3O$; mol wt 167.64. Highly hygroscopic needles. May be stored in well-stoppered containers. Material that has developed an odor should be recrystallized from abs ethanol. mp 192° (slight decomp). Very freely sol in water; sol in about 150 parts of absolute ethanol; more sol in methanol. Also very sol in acetic acid, glycerol, ethylene glycol. Practically insol in organic solvents devoid of hydroxyl groups.

Girard reagent P. 1-(2-Hydrazino-2-oxoethyl)pyridinium chloride. $C_7H_{10}ClN_3O$; mol wt 187.63. Non-hygroscopic crystals from methanol, dec 200°. Less soluble in polar solvents than Girard reagent T.

USE: In the isoln of 17-ketosteroids and other carbonyl compounds.

4430. Gitalin. [1405-76-1] Gitaligin. An extract of *Digitalis purpurea* L., *Scrophulariaceae*, once believed to be a single amorphous compd, is a stable, relatively constant mixture of digitoxin, gitoxin, *q.q.v.,* and *gitaloxin* (**16-formylgitoxin, Cristaloxine**) with smaller amounts of several other glycosides and genins, together with minute amounts of other substances. Review of prepn and composition: Mitchell, *Am. J. Pharm.* **136**, 71 (1964).

Amorphous powder. Readily sol in alcohol, slightly (but slowly) sol in water. A satd aq soln has pH of about 7.0 and an intensely bitter taste. *Ref: N.N.D.* **1960**, 301.

THERAP CAT: Cardiotonic.
THERAP CAT (VET): Cardiotonic.

4431. Gitogenin. [511-96-6] (2α,3β,5α,25R)-Spirostan-2,3-diol; digin. $C_{27}H_{44}O_4$; mol wt 432.64. C 74.96%, H 10.25%, O 14.79%. Obtained from gitonin by heating with dil HCl. Structure: Tschesche, *Ber.* **68**, 1090 (1935); Jacobs, Simpson, *J. Biol. Chem.* **110**, 429 (1935); Marker, Rohrmann, *J. Am. Chem. Soc.* **61**, 2724 (1939); **62**, 647 (1940); Noller, Lieberman, *ibid.* **63**, 2131 (1941); Klass *et al, ibid.* **77**, 3829 (1955). Pharmacological study: H. K. Iwamoto *et al., J. Pharmacol. Exp. Ther.* **91**, 130 (1947).

Leaflets from benzene, dec 271.5-275°. $[\alpha]_D^{20}$ −75° (c = 1.02 in $CHCl_3$). Sol in chloroform, hot alc; sparingly sol in cold ethyl acetate, in ether; practically insol in water. Not precipitated by digitonin.

Diacetate. $C_{31}H_{48}O_6$. Long needles from ether + methanol, mp 251-254°. $[\alpha]_D^{20}$ −96° (c = 1.92 in $CHCl_3$).

4432. F-Gitonin. [28591-01-7] Gitogenin β-lycotetraoside. $C_{50}H_{82}O_{23}$; mol wt 1051.17. C 57.13%, H 7.86%, O 35.01%. Leaf saponin from *Digitalis purpurea* L., *Scrophulariaceae:* Kawasaki, Nishioka, *Chem. Pharm. Bull.* **12**, 1311 (1964). Structure: Kawasaki *et al., Tetrahedron* **21**, 299 (1965). A gitogenin tetraglycoside of which the sugar composition is 2 moles D-glucose, 1 mole D-galactose, and 1 mole D-xylose; differs from **gitonin** (the gitogenin tetraglycoside in *D. purpurea* seeds), in which the sugar composition is 2 galactose, 1 glucose, and 1 xylose: Tschesche, Wulff, *Ber.* **94**, 2019 (1961).

Dihydrate. Needles from butanol + water, dec 252-255°. $[\alpha]_D^{25}$ −58.5° (c = 0.53 in pyridine).

4433. Gitoxigenin. [545-26-6] (3β,5β,16β)-3,14,16-Trihydroxycard-20(22)-enolide; $\Delta^{20,22}$-3,14,16,21-tetrahydroxynorcholenic acid lactone. $C_{23}H_{34}O_5$; mol wt 390.51. C 70.74%, H 8.78%, O 20.49%. The aglycon of gitoxin. By refluxing gitoxin in a mixture of water + alcohol + HCl: Smith, *J. Chem. Soc.* **1931**, 23. Structure: Jacobs, Elderfield, *J. Biol. Chem.* **100**, 671 (1933); Elderfield, *Chem. Rev.* **17**, 217 (1935); Henderson, Chen, *J. Med. Pharm. Chem.* **5**, 988 (1962). Configuration: Moore, *Helv. Chim. Acta* **37**, 659 (1954); Repke, Klesczewski, *Arch. Exp. Pathol. Pharmakol.* **239**, 131 (1960). *Cf.* ref under Digoxigenin.

Sesquihydrate. Plates from dil alc. After drying at 100° *in vacuo* mp 234°. $[\alpha]_{545}^{20}$ +38.5° (c = 0.68 in methanol). Absorption max (96% H_2SO_4): 310, 485, 520 nm. Slightly sol in alcohol, acetone, ethyl acetate. Treatment with alcoholic HCl yields digitaligenin with loss of $2H_2O$.

3,16-Diacetylgitoxigenin. mp 249-250°.
3,16-Dibenzoylgitoxigenin. mp 262°.

4434. Gitoxin. [4562-36-1] (3β,5β,16β)-3-[(*O*-2,6-Dideoxy-β-D-*ribo*-hexopyranosyl-(1 → 4)-*O*-2,6-dideoxy-β-D-*ribo*-hexopyranosyl-(1 → 4)-2,6-dideoxy-β-D-*ribo*-hexopyranosyl)oxy]-14,16-dihydroxycard-20(22)-enolide; anhydrogitalin; bigitalin; pseudodigitoxin. $C_{41}H_{64}O_{14}$; mol wt 780.94. C 63.06%, H 8.26%, O 28.68%. Secondary glycoside mainly from *Digitalis purpurea* L., also from *D. lanata* Ehrh., *Scrophulariaceae*. Byproduct of digitoxin manuf. Isoln: Kraft, *Arch. Pharm.* **250**, 118 (1912); Cloetta, *Arch. Exp. Pathol. Pharmakol.* **112**, 261 (1926); Smith, *J. Chem. Soc.* **1931**, 23. Purification: McChesney *et al., J. Am. Pharm. Assoc.* **37**, 364 (1948). Acid hydrolysis yields 1 mol gitoxigenin + 3 mols digitoxose, *q.q.v.:* Windaus, Schwarte, *Ber.* **58**, 1515 (1925). *See also* Satoh, Aoyama, *Chem. Pharm. Bull.* **18**,

94 (1970). Pharmacokinetics in humans: M. Lesne, *Int. J. Clin. Pharmacol. Biopharm.* **16,** 456 (1978). Prepn of pentaacetate: **BE 668116**; **NL 6506250** (1965, 1966 both to VEB Arzneimittelwerk Dresden), *C.A.* **65,** 23366 (1966); **67,** 91092d (1967). Toxicity study: Foerster *et al., Arch. Int. Pharmacodyn.* **155,** 165 (1965). *Review:* R. Megges *et al., Pharmazie* **32,** 665-667 (1977).

Stout prisms from chloroform + methanol, dec 285° (rapid heating). $[\alpha]_{546}^{20}$ +3.5° (c = 1.02 in pyridine). Absorption max (98% H_2SO_4): 315, 415, 495, 530 nm ($E_{1cm}^{1\%}$ 275, 185, 430, 505). Almost insol in chloroform, ethyl acetate and acetone. Dissolves in a mixture of chloroform and alcohol or in pyridine or in dil alcohol. Less sol in hot 80% alcohol than digoxin.

α- and β-Acetylgitoxin. $C_{43}H_{66}O_{15}$. Obtained by enzymatic hydrolysis of digilanide B. β-Form: Long, thin, hair-like prisms from dil methanol, dec 220-225°. $[\alpha]_D^{20}$ +15.7° (c = 1.28 in pyridine). Sol in 80-100 parts methanol; sparingly sol in water and ether.

Pentaacetate. [7242-04-8] Pengitoxin; penta-*O*-acetylgitoxin; Carnacid-Cor; Cordoval; Pentagit. $C_{51}H_{74}O_{19}$; mol wt 991.12. Mass spectral studies: Blessington, Morton, *Org. Mass Spectrom.* **3,** 95 (1970). Rhomboid crystals, mp 151-155°. $[\alpha]_D^{20}$ +14.0 ±1.5° (c = 1.6 in pyridine). LD_{50} in mice (mg/kg): 6.4 i.p.; in rats (mg/kg): 21.0 i.v. (Foerster).

THERAP CAT: Cardiotonic.

4435. Glatiramer. [28704-27-0] L-Glutamic acid polymer with L-alanine, L-lysine and L-tyrosine; copolymer 1; COP 1 (polyamide); COP 1. Random basic synthetic copolymer of L-alanine, L-lysine, L-glutamic acid and L-tyrosine in a molar ratio of 6:1.9:4.7:1. Mol wt of 14,000 to 23,000 Da. Immunologically cross reactive with myelin basic protein. Prepn: D. Teitelbaum *et al., Eur. J. Immunol.* **1,** 242 (1971). Suppression of exptl. allergic encephalomyelitis (EAE): *eidem, ibid.* **3,** 273 (1973). Inhibition of T-cell response to myelin basic protein: D. Teitelbaum *et al., Proc. Natl. Acad. Sci. USA* **89,** 137 (1992); of binding to major histocompatibility complex: M. Fridkis-Hareli *et al., ibid.* **91,** 4872 (1994). Clinical trials in multiple sclerosis: M. B. Bornstein *et al., Neurology* **41,** 533 (1991); K. P. Johnson *et al., ibid.* **45,** 1268 (1995). Review of pharmacology and early clinical evaluation: L. A. Rolak, *Clin. Neuropharmacol.* **10,** 389 (1987); suppression of EAE: R. Arnon, *Israel J. Med. Sci.* **25,** 686-689 (1989).

Acetate. [147245-92-9] Copaxone.

THERAP CAT: Immunomodulator; in treatment of multiple sclerosis.

4436. Glaucine. [475-81-0] (6aS)-5,6,6a,7-Tetrahydro-1,2,-9,10-tetramethoxy-6-methyl-4*H*-dibenzo[*de,g*]quinoline; 1,2,9,10-tetramethoxyaporphine; boldine dimethyl ether; Bromcholitin; Glauvent. $C_{21}H_{25}NO_4$; mol wt 355.43. C 70.96%, H 7.09%, N 3.94%, O 18.01%. *d*-Form prevalent in nature. Found in *Glaucium flavum* Crantz (*G. luteum* Scop.), *Papaveraceae* and in *Dicentra* and *Corydalis* species, *Fumariaceae*. Isoln: Fischer, *Arch. Pharm.* **239,** 426 (1901). Structure and prepn: Gadamer, *ibid.* **249,** 680 (1911); Späth, Tharrer, *Ber.* **66,** 904 (1933). Configuration: Faltis, Adler, *Arch. Pharm.* **284,** 281 (1951). Synthesis of *dl*-form: Chan, Maitland, *J. Chem. Soc. C* **1966,** 753; Jackson, Martin, *ibid.* 2061; Cava *et al., J. Org. Chem.* **35,** 175 (1970). Pharmacology and toxicity of *dl*-glaucine phosphate: Y. Kasé *et al., Arzneim.-Forsch.* **33,** 936 (1983). Sites of antitussive action: *eidem, ibid.* 947.

d-Glaucine

Orthorhombic plates, prisms from ethyl acetate or ether, mp 120°. $[\alpha]_D^{20}$ +115° (c = 3 in alc). Sol in acetone, alcohol, chloroform, ethyl acetate. Moderately sol in ether, petr ether. Practically insol in water and benzene.

Hydrochloride trihydrate. $C_{21}H_{25}NO_4.HCl.3H_2O$. Needles. mp 232° (anhydrous). Sol in water, alcohol, chloroform.

Hydrobromide. $C_{21}H_{25}NO_4.HBr$. Crystals, mp 235°. Less sol than the hydrochloride.

***dl*-Form phosphate.** DL-832. $(C_{21}H_{25}NO_4)_2.3H_3PO_4$; mol wt 1004.84. Crystalline powder. LD_{50} in mice (mg/kg): 98 i.v.; 401 orally (Kasé).

4437. Gliadin. [9007-90-3] A simple protein, one of the prolamins, derived from the gluten of wheat, rye, etc. May contain up to 43% glutamine (*C.A.* **50,** 15792a (1956)). Studies on the physical nature of gliadin: Holme, Briggs, *Cereal Chem.* **36,** 321 (1959). Use of deamidized gliadin in food products: McDonald, **US 3030211** (1962 to USDA).

Practically insol in water, abs alcohol, and other neutral solvents. Sol in 70-80% alcohol, dil acid, dil alkali.

4438. Glibornuride. [26944-48-9] [1*S*-(*endo,endo*)]-*N*-[[(3-Hydroxy-4,7,7-trimethylbicyclo[2.2.1]hept-2-yl)amino]carbonyl]-4-methylbenzenesulfonamide; (1*R*,2*R*,3*S*,4*S*)-1-(2-hydroxy-3-bornyl)-3-(*p*-tolylsulfonyl)urea; D-3-*endo-p*-tosylureidoborneol; 1-(*p*-tolylsulfonyl)-3-(2-*endo*-hydroxy-3-*endo*-D-bornyl)urea; Ro-6-4563; Gluborid; Glutril. $C_{18}H_{26}N_2O_4S$; mol wt 366.48. C 58.99%, H 7.15%, N 7.64%, O 17.46%, S 8.75%. Prepn: H. Bretschneider *et al., Monatsh. Chem.* **100,** 2133 (1969). *See also: eidem,* **ZA 6706161**; *eidem,* **US 3770761**; *eidem,* **ZA 6902395**; *eidem,* **US 3654357** (1968, 1973, 1969, 1972, all to Hoffmann-La Roche). Comprehensive review of pharmacology: *Arzneim.-Forsch.* **22,** 2153-2222 (1972).

Crystals, mp 192-195° (ethanol-water); also reported as 195-198°. $[\alpha]_D$ +63.8° (ethanol).

THERAP CAT: Antidiabetic.

4439. Gliclazide. [21187-98-4] *N*-[[(Hexahydrocyclopenta[*c*]pyrrol-2(1*H*)-yl)amino]carbonyl]-4-methylbenzenesulfonamide; 1-(hexahydrocyclopenta[*c*]pyrrol-2(1*H*)-yl)-3-(*p*-tolylsulfonyl)urea; *N*-(4-methylbenzenesulfonyl)-*N*'-(3-azabicyclo[3.3.0]oct-3-yl)urea; 1-(3-azabicyclo[3.3.0]oct-3-yl)-3-(*p*-tolylsulfonyl)urea; S-1702; Diamicron; Glimicron; Nordialex. $C_{15}H_{21}N_3O_3S$; mol wt 323.41. C 55.71%, H 6.54%, N 12.99%, O 14.84%, S 9.91%. Prepn: Beregi *et al.,* **FR 1510714** and **US 3501495** (1968 and 1970, both to Sci. Union & Co.-Soc. Franc. Rech. Med.). Series of articles on pharmacology: *Arzneim.-Forsch.* **22,** 1686-1695 (1972). Toxicity data: J. Duhault *et al., ibid.* 1682. Review of pharmacology, efficacy: B. Holmes *et al., Drugs* **27,** 301 (1984).

Crystals from anhydrous ethanol, mp 180-182°. LD$_{50}$ orally in mice: >3 g/kg (Duhault).

THERAP CAT: Antidiabetic.

4440. Glimepiride. [93479-97-1] 3-Ethyl-2,5-dihydro-4-methyl-*N*-[2-[4-[[[[(*trans*-4-methylcyclohexyl)amino]carbonyl]-amino]sulfonyl]phenyl]ethyl]-2-oxo-1*H*-pyrrole-1-carboxamide; *N*-[4-[2-(3-ethyl-4-methyl-2-oxo-3-pyrroline-1-carboxamido)-ethyl]-benzenesulfonyl]-*N'*-4-methylcyclohexylurea; 1-[4-[2-(3-ethyl-4-methyl-2-oxo-3-pyrroline-1-carboxamido)ethyl]phenylsulfonyl]-3-(4-methylcyclohexyl)urea; HOE-490; Amaryl. C$_{24}$H$_{34}$N$_4$O$_5$S; mol wt 490.62. C 58.75%, H 6.99%, N 11.42%, O 16.31%, S 6.54%. Sulfonylurea. Prepn: R. Weyer *et al.*, **DE 2951135**; *eidem*, **US 4379785** (1981, 1983 both to Hoechst). Synthesis: R. Weyer, V. Hitzel, *Arzneim.-Forsch.* **38**, 1079 (1988). Pharmacology: K. Geisen, *ibid.*, 1120. Effects on insulin and glucagon secretion: V. Leclercq-Meyer *et al.*, *Biochem. Pharmacol.* **42**, 1634 (1991). HPLC determn in biological fluids: K. H. Lehr, P. Damm, *J. Chromatogr.* **526**, 497 (1990). Clinical pharmacokinetics: K. Ratheiser *et al.*, *Arzneim.-Forsch.* **43**, 856 (1993). Toxicity study: U. Schollmeier *et al.*, *ibid.* 1038. Series of articles on pharmacology and clinical efficacy: *Diabetes Res. Clin. Pract.* **28** Suppl., S115-S149 (1995).

mp 207°.

THERAP CAT: Antidiabetic.

4441. Gliotoxin. [67-99-2] (3*R*,5a*S*,6*S*,10a*R*)-2,3,5a,6-Tetrahydro-6-hydroxy-3-(hydroxymethyl)-2-methyl-10*H*-3,10a-epidithiopyrazino[1,2-*a*]indole-1,4-dione. C$_{13}$H$_{14}$N$_2$O$_4$S$_2$; mol wt 326.39. C 47.84%, H 4.32%, N 8.58%, O 19.61%, S 19.65%. Antibiotic substance produced by various spp of *Trichoderma*, *Gladiocladium fimbriatum*, *Aspergillus fumigatus*, and *Penicillium* spp: Weindling, Emerson, *Phytopathology* **26**, 1068 (1936); **27**, 1175 (1937); Johnson *et al.*, *J. Am. Chem. Soc.* **65**, 2005 (1943); Menzel *et al.*, *J. Biol. Chem.* **152**, 419 (1944). Structure: Bell *et al.*, *J. Am. Chem. Soc.* **80**, 1001 (1958); Beecham *et al.*, *Tetrahedron Lett.* **1966**, 3131. Crystallographic data: McCrone, *Anal. Chem.* **26**, 1662 (1954). Biosynthesis: Suhadolnik, Chenoweth, *J. Am. Chem. Soc.* **80**, 4391 (1958); Winstead, Suhadolnik, *ibid.* **82**, 1644 (1960); J. D. M. Herscheid *et al.*, *J. Org. Chem.* **45**, 1885 (1980). Synthetic studies: Poisel, Schmidt, *Ber.* **104**, 1714 (1971); *ibid.* **105**, 625 (1972); Oehler *et al.*, *ibid.* 625. Total synthesis of *dl*-form: T. Fukuyama, Y. Kishi, *J. Am. Chem. Soc.* **98**, 6723 (1976); T. Fukuyama *et al.*, *Tetrahedron* **37**, 2045 (1981).

Monoclinic needles from methanol or benzene, dec 221°. [α]$_D^{25}$ −290° (c = 0.08 in ethanol). uv max: 270 nm (ε 4500). Soly in mg/ml at 7°: acetic acid 12; acetone 9.0; acetonitrile 10.2; benzene 5.5; carbon tetrachloride 0.8; chloroform 20; dioxane 73 (decompn); dimethylformamide 17; ethyl acetate 8.5; ethanol 4.7; methanol 1.4; pyridine 77; water (30°): 0.07. Sensitive to oxidation and heat; inactivated by heating for 10 min at 100°.

Monoacetate. C$_{15}$H$_{16}$N$_2$O$_5$S$_2$. Isolated from cultures of *Penicillium terlikowski* Zaleski: Johnson *et al.*, *J. Am. Chem. Soc.* **75**, 2110 (1953). Orthorhombic crystals from benzene, mp 162-163°.

4442. Glipizide. [29094-61-9] *N*-[2-[4-[[[(Cyclohexylamino)carbonyl]amino]sulfonyl]phenyl]ethyl]-5-methylpyrazinecarboxamide; 1-cyclohexyl-3-[[*p*-[2-(5-methylpyrazinecarboxamido)-ethyl]phenyl]sulfonyl]urea; glydiazinamide; K-4024; Glibenese;

Glucotrol; Mindiab; Minidiab; Ozidia. C$_{21}$H$_{27}$N$_5$O$_4$S; mol wt 445.54. C 56.61%, H 6.11%, N 15.72%, O 14.36%, S 7.20%. Second generation sulfonylurea with hypoglycemic activity. Prepn: V. Ambrogi, W. Logemann, **DE 2012138**; *eidem*, **US 3669966** (1970, 1972 both to Carlo Erba); Ambrogi *et al.*, *Arzneim.-Forsch.* **21**, 200 (1971). Pharmacology: *eidem, ibid.* 208; Marigo *et al.*, *ibid.* 215. Metabolism: Goldaniga *et al.*, *ibid.* **23**, 242 (1973); Fuccella *et al.*, *J. Clin. Pharmacol.* **13**, 68 (1973). Toxicity: Ambrogi *et al.*, *Arzneim.-Forsch.* **21**, 208 (1971). Review of pharmacology and therapeutic efficacy: R. N. Brogden *et al.*, *Drugs* **18**, 329-353 (1979); H. E. Lebovitz, *Pharmacotherapy* **5**, 63-77 (1985).

Crystals from ethanol, mp 208-209°. Also reported as mp 200-203°. LD$_{50}$ in mice, rats (g/kg): >3, 1.2 i.p. (Ambrogi).

THERAP CAT: Antidiabetic.

4443. Gliquidone. [33342-05-1] *N*-[(Cyclohexylamino)carbonyl]-4-[2-(3,4-dihydro-7-methoxy-4,4-dimethyl-1,3-dioxo-2(1*H*)-isoquinolinyl)ethyl]benzenesulfonamide; 1-cyclohexyl-3-[[*p*-[2-(3,4-dihydro-7-methoxy-4,4-dimethyl-1,3-dioxo-2(1*H*)-isoquinolyl)ethyl]phenyl]sulfonyl]urea; 1,2,3,4-tetrahydro-2-[*p*-(*N'*-cyclohexylureido-*N*-sulfonyl)phenethyl]-4,4-dimethyl-7-methoxyisoquinoline-1,3-dione; AR-DF 26; Glurenorm. C$_{27}$H$_{33}$N$_3$O$_6$-S; mol wt 527.63. C 61.46%, H 6.30%, N 7.96%, O 18.19%, S 6.08%. Prepn: E. Kutter *et al.*, **DE 2000339** (1971 to Thomae); *eidem*, **US 3708486** (1973 to Boehringer, Ing.); *eidem*, **DE 2011126** (1971 to Thomae), *C.A.* **76**, 14359e (1972). Pharmacokinetics and metabolism: Kopitar, *Arzneim.-Forsch.* **25**, 1455 (1975); Kopitar *et al.*, *ibid.* 1933.

Crystals from boiling methanol, mp 180-182°.

Sodium salt. Sinters at 160°. LD$_{50}$ in mice: >2 g/kg orally; 234 mg/kg i.v. (Kutter, 1973).

THERAP CAT: Antidiabetic.

4444. Glisoxepid. [25046-79-1] *N*-[2-[4-[[[[(Hexahydro-1*H*-azepin-1-yl)amino]carbonyl]amino]sulfonyl]phenyl]ethyl]-5-methyl-3-isoxazolecarboxamide; 1-(hexahydro-1*H*-azepin-1-yl)-3-[[*p*-[2-(5-methyl-3-isoxazolecarboxamido)ethyl]phenyl]sulfonyl]-urea; 4-[4-[β-(5-methylisoxazole-3-carboxamido)ethyl]phenylsulfonyl]-1,1-hexamethylenesemicarbazide; BS-4231; RP-22410; Pro-Diaban. C$_{20}$H$_{27}$N$_5$O$_5$S; mol wt 449.52. C 53.44%, H 6.05%, N 15.58%, O 17.80%, S 7.13%. Prepn: H. Plümpe, W. Puls, **ZA 6806886**; *eidem*, **US 3668215** (1969, 1972 both to Bayer). Pharmacology: Loubatieres *et al.*, *C.R. Seances Acad. Sci. Ser. D* **271**, 1446 (1970); *J. Pharmacol.* **3**, 171, 229 (1972). Toxicity study: Tettenborn, *Arzneim.-Forsch.* **24**, 409 (1974). Series of articles: *ibid.* 363-452.

Colorless crystals from ethanol, mp 189°. LD_{50} in mice, rats, cats, dogs (g/kg): >10.0, >10.0, >4.0, >2.0 orally; in mice, rats (mg/kg): 283, 196 i.v. (Tettenborn).

THERAP CAT: Antidiabetic.

4445. Globin. The colorless, basic protein of hemoglobin. Formed from tissue protein in the body, the globin part of catabolized hemoglobin is re-used (unlike heme, the prosthetic group of hemoglobin). Prepn from ox hemoglobin: Anson, Mirsky, *J. Gen. Physiol.* **13**, 469 (1930). Globin from normal adult human hemoglobin consists of four polypeptide chains: two α-chains and two β-chains. The α-chain contains 141, the β-chain 146 amino acids. Thus globin contains 574 amino acids and has an approx mol wt of 62,000. Abnormal globins may contain γ- and δ-chains. Structure: Braunitzer *et al.*, *Z. Physiol. Chem.* **325**, 283 (1961); **331**, 1 (1963); Konigsberg *et al.*, *J. Biol. Chem.* **237**, 1549, 2547 (1962); **238**, 2016, 2028 (1963). Review of prepn and properties: Rossi Fanelli *et al.*, *Adv. Protein Chem.* **19**, 124 (1964). *Review:* Braunitzer *et al.*, *ibid.* 1.

Denatures rapidly above 17°. At pH values near neutrality, combines with ferroprotoporphyrin to yield hemoglobin, or with ferriprotoporphyrin to yield methemoglobin.

4446. Glucagon. [9007-92-5] Glukagon; hyperglycemic-glycogenolytic factor; HG-factor; HGF. Polypeptide hormone produced in the alpha cells of the islets of Langerhans in the pancreas; stimulates hepatic glucose output. Identification as hyperglycemic factor in pancreatic extracts: J. R. Murlin *et al.*, *J. Biol. Chem.* **56**, 253 (1923); C. P. Kimball, J. R. Murlin, *ibid.* **58**, 337 (1923). Purification and properties: M. Bürger, W. Brandt, *Z. Ges. Exp. Med.* **96**, 375 (1935); A. Staub *et al.*, *Science* **117**, 628 (1953); *eidem, J. Biol. Chem.* **214**, 619 (1955). Amino acid sequence of porcine: W. W. Bromer *et al.*, *J. Am. Chem. Soc.* **79**, 2807 (1957); of bovine: *idem et al.*, *J. Biol. Chem.* **246**, 2822 (1971); of human: J. Thomsen *et al.*, *FEBS Lett.* **21**, 315 (1972). *Review:* O. K. Behrens, W. W. Bromer, *Vitam. Horm.* **16**, 263-301 (1958). *Books:* P. J. Lefèbvre, R. H. Unger, *Glucagon* (Pergamon Press, New York, 1972) 535 pp; *Glucagon* **Pts. I and II**, P. Lefèbvre, Ed. (Springer, New York, 1983) 700 pp. Review of cardiovascular effects and use as antidote to beta-blocker overdose: C. M. White, *J. Clin. Pharmacol.* **39**, 442-447 (1999); of role in glucose homeostasis: G. Jiang, B. B. Zhang, *Am. J. Physiol. Endocrinol. Metab.* **284**, E671-E678 (2003). Review of use to decrease gastrointestinal motility during endoscopy: T. Hashimoto *et al.*, *Aliment. Pharmacol. Ther.* **16**, 111 (2002).

His-Ser-Gln-Gly-Thr-Phe-Thr-Ser-Asp-Tyr-Ser-Lys-Tyr-Leu-Asp-Ser-Arg

Thr-Asn-Met-Leu-Trp-Gln-Val-Phe-Asp-Gln-Ala-Arg

Rhombic dodecahedra. Stable. Practically insol in water. Sol in acidic, basic media, *i.e.* below pH 3 and above pH 9.5.

THERAP CAT: Antihypoglycemic. Diagnostic aid (adjunct for endoscopy).

4447. Glucagon-Like Peptides. Bioactive peptides (GLP-1 and GLP-2) encoded within the preproglucagon gene; formed by tissue-specific, post-translational processing of proglucagon by intestinal L-cells. GLP-1 is a potent glucose-dependent stimulator of insulin secretion (incretin) and is released into the circulation in response to a meal. GLP-1 is also found in the brain and may have a role in regulating food and water intake. GLP-2 has growth-promoting effects on intestinal epithelium. Identification in hamster preproglucagon: G. I. Bell *et al.*, *Nature* **302**, 716 (1983); in human: *idem et al.*, *ibid.* **304**, 368 (1983). *Reviews:* D. J. Drucker, *Diabetes* **47**, 159-169 (1998); T. J. Kieffer, J. F. Habener, *Endocr. Rev.* **20**, 876-913 (1999).

GLP-1. [89750-14-1] Glucagon-like peptide I; glucagon-related peptide I. Originally identified as a 37 amino acid peptide, GLP-1 (1-37), that is truncated to the bioactive forms, GLP-1 (7-37) and GLP-1 (7-36) amide. Stimulates insulin secretion, suppresses glucagon secretion and delays gastric emptying. Identification of active structure: S. Mojsov *et al.*, *J. Clin. Invest.* **79**, 616 (1987). Role in appetite control: I. Gunn *et al.*, *J. Endocrinol.* **155**, 197-200 (1997). Review of physiology and therapeutic potential in diabetes:

M. A. Nauck, *Acta Diabetol.* **35**, 117-129 (1998); J. J. Holst, *Curr. Med. Chem.* **6**, 1005-1017 (1999).

GLP-2. [89750-15-2] Glucagon-like peptide II; glucagon-related peptide II. Sequence contains 33 amino acid residues. Identification of bioactivity: D. J. Drucker *et al.*, *Proc. Natl. Acad. Sci. USA* **93**, 7911 (1996). Review of biological properties and therapeutic potential: *idem et al.*, *J. Parenter. Enteral Nutr.* **23**, Suppl., S98-S100 (1999).

4448. Glucametacin. [52443-21-7] 2-[[[1-(4-Chlorobenzoyl)-5-methoxy-2-methyl-1*H*-indol-3-yl]acetyl]amino]-2-deoxy-D-glucose; 2-[2-[1-(*p*-chlorobenzoyl)-5-methoxy-2-methylindol-3-yl]acetamido]-2-deoxy-D-glucose; glucametacine; glucamethacin; indomethacin glucosamide. $C_{25}H_{27}ClN_2O_8$; mol wt 518.94. C 57.86%, H 5.24%, Cl 6.83%, N 5.40%, O 24.66%. Deriv of indomethacin, *q.v.* Prepn: A. Demetrio *et al.*, *DE 2223051* (1973 to SIR Lab. Chem. Biol. SpA), *C.A.* **80**, 83529e (1974). Pharmacological study: E. Paroli *et al.*, *Arzneim.-Forsch.* **28**, 819 (1978). Clinical studies: P. Petera *et al.*, *Int. J. Clin. Pharmacol. Biopharm.* **15**, 581 (1977); L. Capelli *et al.*, *Curr. Med. Res. Opin.* **7**, 227 (1981).

Monohydrate. Euminex; Teorema; Teoremac. $C_{25}H_{27}ClN_2O_8 \cdot H_2O$; mol wt 536.96.

THERAP CAT: Anti-inflammatory.

4449. Glucamine. [488-43-7] 1-Amino-1-deoxy-D-glucitol; 1-amino-1-deoxysorbitol; glycamine; D-glucamine. $C_6H_{15}NO_5$; mol wt 181.19. C 39.77%, H 8.34%, N 7.73%, O 44.15%. Prepn from D-glucose: Holly *et al.*, *J. Am. Chem. Soc.* **72**, 5416 (1950); from *N*-benzylglycamine: Kagan *et al.*, *ibid.* **79**, 3541 (1957); by catalytic reduction of glucose in the presence of hydrazine: Lemieux, *US 2830983* (1958 to Natl. Res. Council, Ottawa). Commercial prepn: Flint, Salzberg, *US 2016962* (1935 to du Pont); Groggins, Stirton, *Ind. Eng. Chem.* **29**, 1358 (1937).

Crystals from methanol, mp 127°. Sharp, slightly sweet taste. $[\alpha]_D^{15}$ −7.95° (c = 10 in water). Very sol in water; slightly sol in alcohol. Practically insol in ether.

4450. D-Glucaric Acid. [87-73-0] Saccharic acid; D-glucosaccharic acid; D-tetrahydroxyadipic acid. $C_6H_{10}O_8$; mol wt 210.14. C 34.29%, H 4.80%, O 60.91%. Best prepd by nitric acid oxidation of starch; yields as high as 65% are obtained in contrast to much lower yields from glucose or sucrose: Kiliani, *Ber.* **58**, 2344 (1925); Schmidt *et al.*, *ibid.* **70**, 2402 (1937). Prepn from D-glucose: Mehltretter *et al.*, *US 2472168* (1949 to U.S. Secy. Agr.); Truchan, *US 2809989* (1957 to Cowles Chem.); Phillips *et al.*, *J. Chem. Soc.* **1958**, 3522; *BE 615023* (1962 to Ciba).

Needles from 95% ethanol, mp 125-126°. Shows mutarotation. $[\alpha]_D^{19}$ +6.86° → +20.60° (H$_2$O). Ka$_1$ = 1.0 × 10^{-5} at 25°. Soluble in water, ethanol. Sparingly sol in ether.

1,4-Lactone. Saccharolactone. Strong inhibitor of β-glucuronidase: Levvy, *Biochem. J.* **52**, 464 (1952); Boyland, Williams, *ibid.* **64**, 578 (1956). Monohydrate, crystals, mp 90°.

4451. D-Glucoascorbic Acid. [528-88-1] D-*arabino*-Hept-2-enonic acid γ-lactone; 3-keto-D-glucoheptonofuranolactone. C$_7$-H$_{10}$O$_7$; mol wt 206.15. C 40.78%, H 4.89%, O 54.33%. A physiologically inactive homolog of ascorbic acid. Prepn: Ault *et al., J. Chem. Soc.* **1933**, 741; Baird *et al., ibid.* **1934**, 62; Reichstein *et al., Helv. Chim. Acta* **17**, 510 (1934); Stacey, Turton, *J. Chem. Soc.* **1946**, 661; Stedehouder, *Rec. Trav. Chim.* **71**, 831 (1952). Review on analogs of ascorbic acid: Smith, *Adv. Carbohyd. Chem.* **2**, 79 (1946).

Monohydrate. Clusters of rod-like crystals with pointed ends from acetone + methanol + petr ether, mp 101-105° (Reichstein); mp 138° (Baird). Becomes anhydr at 70° under high vacuum, mp 191° (Ault). $[\alpha]_D^{20}$ −14° (c = 1 as hydrate); $[\alpha]_D^{20}$ −22° (c = 1 as hydrate in methanol); $[\alpha]_D^{14.5}$ −37.8° (c = 2.41 in 0.01N HCl); $[\alpha]_D^{20}$ −80° (c = 0.75 neutralized with NaOH). pK$_1$ 4.26; pK$_2$ 11.58. Soluble in water; moderately sol in alcohol.

4452. Glucofrangulin. [52731-38-1] Erbalax-N; Irgalax. C$_{27}$H$_{30}$O$_{14}$; mol wt 578.52. C 56.05%, H 5.23%, O 38.72%. Anthraquinone glycoside from bark of *Rhamnus frangula* L., Rhamnaceae (alder buckthorn): Casparis, Maeder, *Bull. Soc. Chim. Biol.* **9**, 324 (1927); Cucu, Jarpo, *Pharmazie* **14**, 316 (1959); Knap *et al.,* CS 110024 (1964), *C.A.* **61**, 4159e (1964). Consists of two isomers, glucofrangulin A and glucofrangulin B, which differ by the linkage to the sugar moiety at the 3 position of the aglycone. Structure: Schindler, *Helv. Chim. Acta* **29**, 411 (1946); Hörhammer *et al., Naturwissenschaften* **51**, 310 (1964); Longo *et al., Arch. Pharm.* **297**, 248 (1964); Wagner, Hörhammer, *Naturwissenschaften* **53**, 585 (1966). Proof of structure of glucofrangulin A and partial synthesis: *eidem, Z. Naturforsch.* **24B**, 1408 (1969).

Glucofrangulin A

Glucofrangulin A. [21133-53-9] 3-[(6-Deoxy-α-L-manno-pyranosyl)oxy]-1-(β-D-glucopyranosyloxy)-8-hydroxy-6-methyl-9,10-anthracenedione.

Glucofrangulin A octaacetate. C$_{43}$H$_{46}$O$_{22}$. Needles from methanol, mp 228-230°. $[\alpha]_D^{20}$ −124° (c = 1.16 in acetone). uv max: 212, 264, 360 nm (log ε 4.57, 4.56, 4.26).

THERAP CAT: Cathartic.

4453. α-Glucogallin. [53318-36-8] α-D-Glucopyranose 1-(3,4,5-trihydroxybenzoate); α-D-glucopyranose-1-gallate; 1-galloyl-α-D-glucose. C$_{13}$H$_{16}$O$_{10}$; mol wt 332.26. C 46.99%, H 4.85%, O 48.15%. Synthesis: Schmidt, Herok, *Ann.* **587**, 63 (1954); Schmidt, Schmadel, *ibid.* **649**, 149 (1961).

Crystals, dec 179-181°. $[\alpha]_D^{20}$ +83° (c = 3 in methanol).

Dihydrate. Prisms from water, mp 171-173°. $[\alpha]_D^{25}$ +79.1° (water). Freely sol in water, methanol, ethanol, dioxane, acetic acid. Sparingly soluble in ethyl acetate, ether and acetone.

4454. β-Glucogallin. [13405-60-2] β-D-Glucopyranose 1-(3,4,5-trihydroxybenzoate); β-D-glucopyranose-1-gallate; glucogallic acid; 1-galloyl-β-D-glucose. C$_{13}$H$_{16}$O$_{10}$; mol wt 332.26. C 46.99%, H 4.85%, O 48.15%. Glucoside or glucotannoid from chinese rhubarb, *Rheum officinale*, Baill., *Polygonaceae:* Gilson, *Compt. Rend.* **136**, 385 (1903). Structure and synthesis: Fischer, Bergmann, *Ber.* **51**, 1760 (1918); Schmidt, Schmadel, *Ann.* **649**, 149 (1961).

Bitter microscopic prisms from water, methanol or 80% ethanol, mp 207°. $[\alpha]_D^{25}$ −24.5° (c = 1.75 in water). Freely sol in hot water. Sparingly sol in cold water, methanol, ethanol, acetone, ethyl acetate. Practically insol in ether, benzene, chloroform, petr ether.

4455. Glucoheptonic Acid. [87-74-1] D-*glycero*-D-*gulo*-Heptonic acid; α-glucoheptonic acid; glucosemonocarboxylic acid; glucomonocarbonic acid. C$_7$H$_{14}$O$_8$; mol wt 226.18. C 37.17%, H 6.24%, O 56.59%. Obtained by treating glucose with HCN yielding a cyanohydrin which is saponified to glucoheptonic acid: Kiliani, *Ber.* **19**, 769 (1886); Fischer, *Ann.* **270**, 71 (1892); Armestar, *C.A.* **45**, 2865 (1951). Process starting with calcium cyanide and glucose: Clevenot, US 2735866 (1956 to Lab. Clevenot). Diagnostic use of ^{99m}Tc complexes in renal scintigraphy: R. E. Boyd *et al., Br. J. Radiol.* **46**, 604 (1973); in brain scanning: J. Léveillé *et al., J. Nucl. Med.* **18**, 957 (1977); T. W. Ryerson *et al., Radiology* **127**, 429 (1978). Subacute toxicity study: L. Belbeck *et al., Can. J. Comp. Med.* **45**, 299 (1981).

Lactonizes upon evapn. The lactone forms large sweetish crystals, mp 145-148°. $[\alpha]_D^{20}$ −56.0° (shows mutarotation). Sol in water.

Sodium salt. [13007-85-7] Gluceptate sodium; sodium glucoheptonate. C$_7$H$_{13}$NaO$_8$. Prepn from corn syrup: Behnke, US

3022343 (1962 to Pfanstiehl Labs). Crystals (α-form), dec 161°. $[\alpha]_D^{20}$ +6.06° (c = 10 in H_2O). Freely sol in water.

Calcium salt. Gluceptate calcium; calcium glucoheptonate; calcium glucosemonocarbonate; calcium glucomonocarbonate; Calciforte; Calheptose. $C_{14}H_{26}CaO_{16}$; mol wt 490.42. Prepn from Na salt: Holstein, **US 3033900** (1962 to Pfanstiehl Labs.). Hygroscopic crystals, somewhat acrid taste, dec 200°. Sol in water.

Magnesium salt. Magnesium glucoheptonate; magnesium glucosemonocarbonate; magnesium glucomonocarbonate; Navolin. $C_{14}H_{26}MgO_{16}$; mol wt 474.65. Prepn: Cipelli, **US 3063896** (1962 to Merck & Co.). Water-sol crystals, pleasant taste.

Complex with ^{99m}Tc. Technetium ^{99m}Tc gluceptate; technetium ^{99m}Tc gluheptonate; Glucoscan; TechneScan gluceptate.

USE: Pharmaceutic aid.

THERAP CAT: ^{99m}Tc complex as diagnostic aid (radioactive imaging agent).

4456. Gluconic Acid. [526-95-4] D-Gluconic acid; dextronic acid; maltonic acid; glyconic acid; glycogenic acid; pentahydroxycaproic acid. $C_6H_{12}O_7$; mol wt 196.16. C 36.74%, H 6.17%, O 57.09%. Prepd by oxidation of glucose: H. Hlasiwetz, J. Habermann, *Ann.* **155**, 120 (1870); J. Habermann, *ibid.* **162**, 297 (1872). Fermentative prepn using *Aspergillus niger:* K. Bernhauer, L. Schulof, **US 1849053** (1932 to Pfizer); A. J. Moyer *et al., Ind. Eng. Chem.* **32**, 1379 (1940). Review of prepns and uses: F. J. Prescott *et al., ibid.* **45**, 338 (1953); M. Roehr *et al.* in *Biotechnology*, **Vol. 6**, H. Rehm, G. Reed, Eds. (VCH, Weinheim, 2nd ed, 1996) pp 347-362. *See also* Gluconolactone.

Crystals, mp 131°. Mild acid taste. $[\alpha]_D^{20}$ −6.7° (c = 1). pK (25°) 3.60. Freely sol in water, slightly sol in alcohol. Insol in ether and most other organic solvents. In aq solns the acid is partially transformed into an equilibrium mixt with gamma and delta gluconolactones.

Magnesium salt. [3632-91-5] Magnesium gluconate; Almora; Ultra-Mg. $C_{12}H_{22}MgO_{14}$; mol wt 414.60. Clinical pharmacokinetics and use as magnesium supplement: J. White *et al., Clin. Ther.* **14**, 678 (1992). Also occurs as the dihydrate. Sol in water, slightly sol in alcohol. Insol in ether.

Potassium salt. [299-27-4] Potassium gluconate; Gluconsan K; Kalimozan; Kaon; Potasoral; Potassuril; Tumil-K. $C_6H_{11}KO_7$; mol wt 234.25. Yellowish-white crystals. Stable in air. Mild, slightly saline taste. Dec 180°. Freely sol in water. Practically insol in abs alcohol, ether, benzene, chloroform. Aq solns are alkaline to litmus and have a pH of 7.5-8.5.

Sodium salt. [527-07-1] Sodium gluconate. $C_6H_{11}NaO_7$; mol wt 218.14. Crystals. The technical grade may have a pleasant odor. Soly in water at 25°: 59 g/100 ml. Sparingly sol in alcohol. Insol in ether. Aq solns are stable to short boiling periods.

Zinc complex. [4468-02-4] $(T\text{-}4)$-Bis-(D-gluconato-κO^1,-κO^2)zinc; zinc gluconate; Rubozinc. $C_{12}H_{22}O_{14}Zn$; mol wt 455.70. Review of clinical use in treatment of colds: M. L. Garland, K. O. Hagmeyer, *Ann. Pharmacother.* **32**, 63-69 (1998). Clinical trial in inflammatory acne: J. Meynadier, *Eur. J. Dermatol.* **10**, 269 (2000).

USE: Chelating agent. In high alkalinity bottle washes and other cleansers; in finish removers; in the tanning and textile industry.

THERAP CAT: Magnesium salt as magnesium replenisher; potassium salt as potassium supplement; zinc complex as zinc supplement.

THERAP CAT (VET): Potassium salt as potassium supplement.

4457. Gluconolactone. [90-80-2] D-Gluconic acid δ-lactone; glucono delta lactone; delta gluconolactone; Fujiglucon. $C_6H_{10}O_6$; mol wt 178.14. C 40.45%, H 5.66%, O 53.89%. Prepn by

oxidation of glucose with bromine water: Isbell, Pigman, *J. Res. Natl. Bur. Stand.* **10**, 337 (1933); by oxidation of glucose in *Acetobacter suboxydans:* King, Cheldelin, *Biochem. J.* **68**, 31P (1958). Structure: J. Staněk *et al., The Monosaccharides* (Academic Press, New York, 1963) p 271.

Crystals, dec 153°. Sweet taste (different from gluconic acid). $[\alpha]_D^{20}$ +61.7° (c = 1). Soly in water 59 g/100 ml; in alc about 1 g/100 g. Insol in ether. Hydrolyzed to gluconic acid by water. A freshly prepd 1% aq soln has a pH of 3.6 changing to pH 2.5 within 2 hrs.

USE: Component of many cleaning cmpds because of the sequestering ability of the gluconate radical which remains active in alk solns; in the dairy industry to prevent milkstone; in breweries to prevent beerstone; as latent acid catalyst for acid colloid resins, particularly in textile printing; as a coagulant for tofu.

4458. Glucosamine. [3416-24-8] 2-Amino-2-deoxy-D-glucose; chitosamine. $C_6H_{13}NO_5$; mol wt 179.17. C 40.22%, H 7.31%, N 7.82%, O 44.65%. Found in chitin, in mucoproteins, and in mucopolysaccharides. Isoln from chitin: Ledderhose, *Z. Physiol. Chem.* **2**, 213 (1878); Hackman, *Aust. J. Biol. Sci.* **7**, 168 (1954). Synthesis: Fischer, Leuchs, *Ber.* **35**, 3787 (1902); **36**, 24 (1903). Separation of α- and β-forms: Westphal, Holzmann, *ibid.* **75B**, 1274 (1942). Structure: Haworth *et al., J. Chem. Soc.* **1939**, 271; Cutler, Peat, *ibid.* 782; Cox, Jeffrey, *Nature* **143**, 894 (1939). Pharmacokinetics in dog and man: I. Setnikar *et al., Arzneim.-Forsch.* **36**, 729 (1986). Clinical trials in arthrosis: Y. Vajarudal, *Clin. Ther.* **3**, 336 (1981); M. J. Tapadinhas *et al., Pharmatherapeutica* **3**, 157 (1982). *Review:* Foster, Stacey, "The Chemistry of the 2-Amino Sugars" in C. S. Hudson *et al., Advan. Carbohyd. Chem.* **vol. 7** (Academic Press, New York, 1952) pp 247-288. Review of pharmacology, toxicology and clinical efficacy: J. W. Anderson *et al., Food Chem. Toxicol.* **43**, 187-201 (2005).

α-**Form.** [28905-11-5] Crystals, mp 88°. $[\alpha]_D^{20}$ +100° changing to +47.5° after 30 min (water).

β-**Form.** [28905-10-4] Needles from methanol, dec 110°. $[\alpha]_D^{20}$ +28° changing to +47.5° after 30 min (water). Very sol in water, sol in about 38 parts boiling methanol; sparingly sol in cold methanol or ethanol. Practically insol in ether, chloroform.

N-**Acetylglucosamine.** [7512-17-6] $C_8H_{15}NO_6$. Needles from methanol + ether, mp 205°. $[\alpha]_D^{18}$ +64° changing to +40.9° (in water).

Sulfate salt. [29031-19-4] Dona. $C_6H_{13}NO_5.xH_2SO_4$.

USE: Pharmaceutic aid.

THERAP CAT: Antiarthritic.

4459. Glucose. [50-99-7] D-Glucose; dextrose; blood sugar; grape sugar; corn sugar; Dextropur; Dextrosol; Glucolin. $C_6H_{12}O_6$; mol wt 180.16. C 40.00%, H 6.71%, O 53.28%. A main source of energy for living organisms. Occurs naturally and in the free state in fruits and other parts of plants. Combined in glucosides, in di- and oligosaccharides, in the polysaccharides cellulose and starch, and in glycogen. Normal human blood contains 0.08-0.1%. Manuf on a large scale from starch: Dean, Gottfried, *Adv. Carbohydr. Chem.* **5**, 127 (1950). Below 50°, α-D-glucose hydrate is the stable cryst form, above 50° the anhydr form is obtained and at still higher temps β-D-glucose is formed: W. Pigman, *The Carbohydrates* (Academic Press, New York, 1957) p 92. Structure: Kjaer, Lindberg, *Acta Chem. Scand.* **13**, 1713 (1959). Conformation: E.

Percival, *Structural Carbohydrate Chemistry* (J. Garnet Miller, London, 1962) pp 51-57. Comprehensive monograph: H. Bartelheimer *et al.*, *D-Glucose und verwandte Verbindungen in Medizin und Biologie* (Enke, Stuttgart, 1966) 1126 pp.

α-Form monohydrate. Crystals from water, mp 83°. $[\alpha]_D$ +102.0° → +47.9° (water). 0.74 times as sweet as sucrose. One gram dissolves in about 1 ml water and in about 60 ml alcohol.

α-Form anhydr. Crystals from hot ethanol or water, mp 146°. $[\alpha]_D$ +112.2° → +52.7° (c = 10 in water). The final value is obtained instantly in the presence of hydroxyl ions. Formula for varying concns: $[\alpha]_D^{20}$ +52.5° + 0.0188p (p = g/100 ml). pH of 0.5 molar aq soln 5.9. $d_{17.5}^{17.5}$ of water solns w/v: 5% = 1.019; 10% = 1.038; 20% = 1.076; 30% = 1.113; 40% = 1.149. n_D^{20} 10% soln 1.3479. One gram dissolves in 1.1 ml water at 25°; in 0.8 ml at 30°; in 0.41 ml at 50°; in 0.28 ml at 70°; in 0.18 ml at 90°; in 120 ml methanol at 20°. Very sparingly sol in abs alcohol, ether, acetone; sol in hot glacial acetic acid, pyridine, aniline.

β-Form. Crystals from hot water + ethanol, from dil acetic acid, or from pyridine, mp 148-155°. $[\alpha]_D$ +18.7° → +52.7° (c = 10 in water).

THERAP CAT: Antihypoglycemic; fluid and nutrient replenisher.

THERAP CAT (VET): Antihypoglycemic; fluid and nutrient replenisher.

4460. Glucose Oxidase. [9001-37-0] β-D-Glucopyranose aerodehydrogenase; P-FAD; corylophyline; microcide; mikrotsid; notatin. An enzyme obtained from mycelia of fungi, such as *Aspergilli* and *Penicillia*; a typical aerobic dehydrogenase which catalyzes the oxidation of glucose to gluconic acid (molecular oxygen is reduced to hydrogen peroxide). It is a flavoprotein, the prosthetic group being flavine-adenine dinucleotide (FAD). Commercial prepns frequently contain appreciable amounts of another enzyme, catalase, which is desirable for certain uses since it removes hydrogen peroxide aerobically generated by glucose oxidase. Names of some commercial prepns are: *DeeO*, *Fermcozyme*, *OxyBan*, *Ovazyme*. Isoln from *Penicillia* cultures: Coulthard *et al.*, *Biochem. J.* **39**, 24 (1945). Commercial production from *Aspergilli* and *Penicillia*: Goldsmith *et al.*, **US 2926122** (1960); from *Aspergillus niger*: Faucett *et al.*, **US 3102081** (1963 to Miles Labs.). Removal of proteolytic enzymes from glucose oxidase (contg catalase) obtained from *Aspergilli* or *Penicillia* cultures: Ohlmeyer, **US 2940904** (1960 to Ben L. Sarett). Separation from catalase: Pazur *et al.*, *Biochim. Biophys. Acta* **65**, 369 (1962). Properties: Muller, *Enzymologia* **10**, 40 (1941); Keilin, Hartree, *Biochem. J.* **42**, 221 (1948), **50**, 331 (1952). *Reviews:* L. A. Underkofler "Glucose Oxidase: Production, Properties, Present and Potential Applications" in *Soc. Chem. Ind. (London) Monograph* **no. 11**, 72-86 (1961); R. Bentley, "Glucose Oxidase" in *The Enzymes* vol. 7, P. D. Boyer *et al.*, Eds. (Academic Press, New York, 1963) pp 567-586. Review of use as analytical reagent: J. Raba, H. A. Mottola, *Crit. Rev. Anal. Chem.* **25**, 1-42 (1995).

Amorphous powder or crystals. Abs max between 270-280, 375-380, and 450-460 nm (aq soln). Freely sol in water giving yellowish-green solns. Most active at pH 5.5-6.0 and 30-35°. Stable between pH 4.5 and 7.0. Stable to pepsin and trypsin. A glucose oxidase unit is defined as that quantity of enzyme which will cause the uptake of 10 mm³ oxygen per min in a Warburg manometer at 30° in the presence of excess air and excess catalase with a substrate contg 3.3% glucose monohydrate and 0.1*M* phosphate buffer, pH 5.9 with 0.4% sodium dehydroacetate: Scott, *J. Agric. Food Chem.* **1**, 727 (1953).

USE: Analytical reagent for the selective determn of glucose. Food additive for the removal of glucose during the prepn of dried egg products. Antioxidant in food and food wrappers. Stabilizer for ascorbic acid and vitamin B_{12}.

4461. α-Glucose-1-phosphate. [59-56-3] α-D-Glucopyranose 1-dihydrogenphosphate; α-glucose-1-phosphoric acid; α-D-glucopyranose-1-phosphate; Cori ester. $C_6H_{13}O_9P$; mol wt 260.14. C 27.70%, H 5.04%, O 55.35%, P 11.91%. Found widely in both plants and animals. In plants it is the immediate precursor of starch, and in animals of glycogen, being also the first product in the breakdown and utilization of these substances. Isoln from muscle and synthesis using trisilver phosphate: Cori *et al.*, *J. Biol. Chem.* **121**, 465 (1937); Krahl, Cori, *Biochem. Prep.* **1**, 33 (1949). Prepn from α-acetobromglucose + silver diphenyl phosphate: Posternak, *J. Am. Chem. Soc.* **72**, 4824 (1950); by phosphorolysis of starch using phosphorylase and orthophosphate: McCready, Hassid, *Biochem. Prep.* **4**, 63 (1955). Structure: Wolfrom, Pletcher, *J. Am. Chem. Soc.* **63**, 1050 (1941). Configuration: Wolfrom *et al.*, *ibid.* **64**, 23 (1942); Harmon, *Diss. Abstr.* **24**, 4400 (1964); Beevers, Maconochie, *Acta Crystallogr.* **18**, 232 (1965).

Free acid. $[\alpha]_D^{25}$ +120°. pK$_1$ = 1.11; pK$_2$ = 6.13. Stronger acid than H_3PO_4. Extremely sol in water.

Barium salt trihydrate. [6056-70-8] Nonhygroscopic, stable powder. $[\alpha]_D^{25}$ +75° (c = 1.26). Easily sol in water.

Calcium salt. [119119-85-6] Actigam.

Dipotassium salt dihydrate. [5996-14-5] Crystals from ethanol. $[\alpha]_D^{20}$ +78° (c = 4); $[\alpha]_{549}^{20}$ +90° (c = 4). Freely sol in water.

THERAP CAT: Calcium salt as roborant.

4462. Glucose-6-phosphate. [56-73-5] D-Glucose 6-(dihydrogen phosphate); glucose-6-phosphoric acid; Robison ester. $C_6H_{13}O_9P$; mol wt 260.14. C 27.70%, H 5.04%, O 55.35%, P 11.91%. A normal constituent of resting muscle, probably always existing in equilibrium with fructose-6-phosphate. For the enzymatic conversion from the 1-phosphate *see* α-Glucose-1-phosphate. Isoln from a crude mixture of hexose phosphates, obtained by yeast fermentation: Robison, King, *Biochem. J.* **25**, 323 (1931). Prepn by the action of phosphoglucomutase on α-glucose-1-phosphate: Colowick, Sutherland, *J. Biol. Chem.* **144**, 423 (1942); from acetone glucose: Levene, Raymond, *ibid.* **92**, 757 (1931); by phosphorylation of 1,2,3,4-tetraacetylglucose followed by deacetylation: Fischer, Lardy, *ibid.* **164**, 513 (1946); *Biochem. Prep.* **2**, 39 (1952). Prepn from starch: de Chatelperron *et al.*, **FR 1379068** (1964), *C.A.* **62**, 9394b (1965).

Barium salt. $C_6H_{11}O_5PO_4Ba$. Nonhygroscopic, stable powder. $[\alpha]_D^{24}$ +17.9°. Easily sol in water.

Dipotassium salt. $C_6H_{11}O_5PO_4K_2$. Precipitate from methanol. $[\alpha]_D^{24}$ +21.2° (c = 1.3). Freely sol in water.

4463. Glucosulfone Sodium. [554-18-7] 1,1′-[Sulfonylbis(4,1-phenyleneimino)]bis[1-deoxy-1-sulfo-D-glucitol] disodium salt; *p,p*′-sulfonyldianiline *N,N*′-diglucoside disodium disulfonate; *p,p*′-sulfonyldianiline-*N,N*′-di-D-glucose sodium bisulfite compd; *p,p*′-diaminodiphenylsulfone-*N,N*′-di(dextrose sodium sulfonate); disodium *p,p*′-diaminodiphenylsulfone-*N,N*′-diglucose sulfonate; 501-P; Protomin; Promin; Promanide. $C_{24}H_{34}N_2Na_2O_{18}S_3$; mol wt 780.70. C 36.92%, H 4.39%, N 3.59%, Na 5.89%, O 36.89%, S 12.32%. Prepd by refluxing a mixture of 4,4′-diaminodiphenylsulfone, glucose, sodium bisulfite, and 80% ethanol: **CH 234108** (1944 to B. Siegfried), *C.A.* **43**, 4297a (1949); B. C. Jain *et al.*, *Sci. Cult.* **11**, 568 (1946). Structure activity study: W. Logemann, G. P. Miori, *Arzneim.-Forsch.* **5**, 213 (1955). Clinical evaluation in ocular leprosy: A. Bouzas, *Arch. Ophthalmol.* **31**, 629 (1971).

White, amorphous powder. Soluble in water; slightly sol in ethanol. Insol in ether, benzene, methanol, ethyl acetate, pyridine. Aq solns may be sterilized by autoclaving. LD_{50} in rats (g/kg): 3-4 orally, 3-3.5 i.v. (Logemann, Miori).

THERAP CAT: Antibacterial (leprostatic).

4464. Glucovanillin. [494-08-6] 4-(β-D-Glucopyranosyloxy)-3-methoxybenzaldehyde; vanillin-D-glucoside; avenein; vanilloside. $C_{14}H_{18}O_8$; mol wt 314.29. C 53.50%, H 5.77%, O 40.73%. From green fruit of vanilla: Goris, *Compt. Rend.* **179**, 70 (1924). From coniferin by oxidation with CrO_3: Tremann, *Ber.* **18**, 1595 (1885). Structure and synthesis: Fischer, Raske, *Ber.* **42**, 1475 (1909); Thorpe, Williams, *J. Chem. Soc.* **1937**, 494.

Needles from methanol, mp 189-190°. Bitter taste. $[\alpha]_D^{20}$ −89.9° (water). Soluble in hot water, alcohol. Almost insol in ether.

Tetraacetate. $C_{22}H_{26}O_{12}$. Crystals from dil alcohol, mp 142-143°. $[\alpha]_D$ −48.3° (chloroform).

USE: Pharmaceutic aid (flavor).

4465. D-Glucuronic Acid. [6556-12-3] $C_6H_{10}O_7$; mol wt 194.14. C 37.12%, H 5.19%, O 57.69%. Widely distributed in the plant and animal kingdoms. Usually occurs in "paired" form, *i.e.* as a glycosidic combination with phenols, alcohols, etc. Such glucuronides form in the liver to detoxify poisonous hydroxyl-containing substances. The glucuronides present in normal urine are those of phenol, cresol, and indoxyl. After the ingestion of poisons such as morphine, chloral hydrate, camphor, or turpentine, glucuronides formed with the poison or its hydroxylated derivatives appear in the urine. Review and bibliography: Stacey, *Adv. Carbohyd. Chem.* **2**, 161 (1946); Jones, Smith, *ibid.* **4**, 243 (1949). Structure: Pryde, Williams, *Nature* **128**, 187 (1931); Levene, Meyer, *J. Biol. Chem.* **92**, 257 (1931); Levene, Kreider, *ibid.* **120**, 597 (1937). Review of syntheses: Mehltretter, *Adv. Carbohyd. Chem.* **8**, 231 (1953). Prepn by irradiation of D-glucose in dil aq soln: Phillips *et al.*, *J. Chem. Soc.* **1958**, 3522; by γ-irradiation of aq sucrose soln: Phillips, Moody, *ibid.* **1960**, 762. Electrophoretic sepn of D-glucuronic acid and its C-5 epimer, **L-iduronic acid**: I. Miyamoto, S. Nagase, *Anal. Biochem.* **115**, 308 (1981). Monographs: N. E. Artz, E. M. Osman, *Biochemistry of Glucuronic Acid* (Academic Press, New York, 1950); G. J. Dutton, Ed., *Glucuronic Acid, Free and Combined* (Academic Press, New York, 1966) 629 pp.

β-Form. Needles from alcohol or ethyl acetate. mp 165°. Shows mutarotation: $[\alpha]_D^{24}$ +11.7° → +36.3° (2 hrs, c = 6). Soluble in water, alcohol. Reduces Fehling's soln.

4466. β-Glucuronidase. [9001-45-0] Glusulase. Glucuronide-splitting enzyme found in liver, spleen, and certain tissues of the endocrine and reproductive systems. Rats seem to have a higher concn than other mammals. Also found in fish liver, snails, mollusks, and some insects. Isoln from rat livers, kidneys, and spleens: Fishman, Talalay, *Science* **105**, 131 (1947). *Review and bibliography:* Fishman, *Adv. Enzymol.* **16**, 361-409 (1955).

White powder. Soluble in water.

USE: In the determination of urinary steroids and of steroid conjugates in blood.

4467. D-Glucuronolactone. [32449-92-6] D-Glucuronic acid γ-lactone; D-glucofuranurono-6,3-lactone; glucurolactone; glucurone; Dicurone; Glucoxy; Guronsan. $C_6H_8O_6$; mol wt 176.12. C 40.92%, H 4.58%, O 54.51%. Found in many plant gums in polymeric combination with other carbohydrates. Important structural constituent of practically all fibrous and connective tissues in the animal organism, *cf.* D-glucuronic acid. Prepd synthetically from many polysaccharides or suitable glucosides where the hydroxyl at carbon 6 may be oxidized while the other sensitive groups are protected. Prepn: Stacey, *J. Chem. Soc.* **1939**, 1529; Hardegger, Spitz, *Helv. Chim. Acta* **33**, 337 (1950); Marsh, *Proc. Biochem. Soc.* [*Biochem. J.*], **50**, XI (1951); Mehltretter *et al.*, *J. Am. Chem. Soc.* **73**, 2424 (1951); Phillips, Moody, *J. Chem. Soc.* **1960**, 762. Structure: J. Stanek *et al.*, *The Monosaccharides* (Academic Press, New York, 1963) p 259. For isoln procedures see the ref under glucuronic acid.

Crystals from ethanol, mp 176-178°. (Commercial grades, mp 172°.) d_4^{30} 1.76. $[\alpha]_D^{25}$ +19.8° (c = 5.19). Soluble in water (26.9 g/100 ml of soln); slightly sol in methanol (2.8 g/100 ml). Very slightly sol in abs ethanol (0.7 g/100 ml), in glacial acetic acid (0.3 g/100 ml). The free acid is more sol than the lactone. At room temp an aq soln of glucuronolactone reaches an equilibrium of about 20% lactone and 80% acid within 2 months. At 100° an equilibrium of 60% lactone and 40% free acid is reached within 2 hrs. Initial pH of 10% aq soln 3.5, after 1 week the pH is about 2.5.

THERAP CAT: Detoxicant.

4468. Glufosfamide. [132682-98-5] 1-[*N,N*ʹ-Bis(2-chloroethyl)phosphorodiamidate]-β-D-glucopyranose; β-D-glucopyranosyl *N,N*ʹ-di(2-chloroethyl) phosphoric acid diamide; β-D-glucosyl-isophosphoramide mustard; D-19575. $C_{10}H_{21}Cl_2N_2O_7P$; mol wt 383.16. C 31.35%, H 5.52%, Cl 18.51%, N 7.31%, O 29.23%, P 8.08%. Glucose coupled to isophosphoramide mustard, the active metabolite of the alkylating agent ifosfamide, *q.v.* Enters cells through upregulated glucose transport proteins. Prepn: M. Wiessler, M. Dickes, DE **3835772**; *eidem*, US **5622936** (1990, 1997 both to Deutsches Krebsforschungszentrum Stiftung). Pharmacology and toxicity studies: J. Pohl *et al.*, *Cancer Chemother. Pharmacol.* **35**, 364 (1995). Mechanism of action study: H. Seker *et al.*, *Br. J. Cancer* **82**, 629 (2000). Clinical evaluation in pancreatic cancer: E. Briasoulis *et al.*, *Eur. J. Cancer* **39**, 2334 (2003); in non-small cell lung cancer: G. Giaccone *et al.*, *ibid.* **40**, 667 (2004). Review of pharmacology and clinical development: I. Niculescu-Duvaz, *Curr. Opin. Invest. Drugs* **3**, 1527-1532 (2002).

LD_{50} in rats, mice (mg/kg): 1575, 1575 i.v.; 1470, 1470 orally (Pohl).

THERAP CAT: Antineoplastic.

4469. Glutamic Acid. [56-86-0] L-Glutamic acid; Glu; E; glutaminic acid; (S)-2-aminopentanedioic acid; α-aminoglutaric acid; 1-aminopropane-1,3-dicarboxylic acid; Glutacid; Glutaminol. $C_5H_9NO_4$; mol wt 147.13. C 40.82%, H 6.17%, N 9.52%, O 43.50%. Non-essential amino acid for human development; referred to as an excitatory amino acid (EAA) due to its role in neurotransmission. Isoln from wheat gluten: H. Ritthausen, *J. Prakt. Chem.* **99**, 454 (1866). Early chemistry and biochemistry: *Amino Acids and Proteins*, D. M. Greenberg, Ed. (Charles C. Thomas, Springfield, IL, 1951) 950 pp., *passim*; J. P. Greenstein, M. Winitz, *Chemistry of the Amino Acids* vols 1-3 (John Wiley and Sons, Inc., New York, 1961) pp. 1929-1954, *passim*; C. W. Huffman, W. G. Skelly, *Chem. Rev.* **63**, 625-644 (1963). Interconversion from L-proline: S. Yoshifuji *et al., Tetrahedron Lett.* **21**, 2963 (1980). Determn in serum: C. D. Stalikas *et al., Eur. J. Clin. Chem.* **32**, 767 (1994); of naturally occurring levels in food: D. H. Daniels *et al., Food Addit. Contam.* **12**, 21 (1995). Identification as excitatory neurotransmitter: D. R. Curtis *et al., J. Physiol.* **150**, 656 (1960). Review of biosynthesis: A. Hamberger *et al., Adv. Biochem. Psychopharmacol.* **27**, 115-126 (1981); of metabolism and associated disorders: S. B. Prusiner, *Annu. Rev. Med.* **32**, 521-542 (1981). Review of receptor binding: P. A. Briley *et al., Mol. Cell. Biochem.* **39**, 347 (1981). Review as neurotransmitter: B. Engelsen, *Acta Neurol. Scand.* **74**, 337-355 (1986); E. Marmo, *Med. Res. Rev.* **8**, 441-458 (1988). Review of role in learning and memory: W. J. McEntee, T. H. Crook, *Psychopharmacology* **111**, 391-401 (1993); in Parkinson's disease: M. S. Starr, *Synapse* **19**, 264-293 (1995). *Books:* R. Powell, *Monosodium Glutamate and Glutamic Acid* (Noyes Dev. Corp., Park Ridge, N.J., 1968) 256 pp.; *Glutamic Acid: Advances in Biochemistry and Physiology* L. J. Filer, Jr. *et al.*, Eds. (Raven, New York, 1979).

Orthorhombic, bisphenoidal crystals from aq alc. d_4^{20} vac 1.538. Melts 160° with conversion to L-pyrrolidonecarboxylic acid. Sublimes at 200°. $[\alpha]_D^{22.4}$ +31.4° (6N HCl). pK$_1$ 2.19; pK$_2$ 4.25; pK$_3$ 9.67. Soly in water (g/l): 8.64 (25°); 21.86 (50°); 55.32 (75°); 140.00 (100°). Insol in methanol, ethanol, ether, acetone, cold glacial acetic acid and common neutral solvents.

Hydrochloride. [138-15-8] Acidulin; Hypochylin. C_5H_9-NO_4·HCl; mol wt 183.59. Orthorhombic bisphenoidal plates, dec 214°.

Sodium salt *see* Monosodium Glutamate.

Magnesium salt hydrobromide monohydrate. Magnesium glutamate hydrobromide; magnesium bromoglutamate; Psicosoma; Psychoverlan. $C_{10}H_{17}BrMgN_2O_8$·H_2O; mol wt 415.47.

DL-Form. [617-65-2] Orthorhombic crystals from water, 225-227° (dec). d_4^{20} 1.4601. Soly in water (g/l): 20.54 (25°); 49.34 (50°); 118.6 (75°); 284.9 (100°). Sparingly sol in alcohol, ether, petr ether.

D-Form. [6893-26-1] Shiny leaflets from water. $[\alpha]_D^{20}$ −30.5° (c = 1.00 in 6N HCl).

THERAP CAT: Nutritional supplement. Hydrochloride as gastric acidifier. Magnesium salt hydrobromide has been used as anxiolytic.

4470. L-Glutamic Acid 5-Ethyl Ester. [1119-33-1] L-Glutamic acid γ-ethyl ester; γ-ethyl L-glutamate; Glutestere. C_7H_{13}-NO_4; mol wt 175.18. C 47.99%, H 7.48%, N 8.00%, O 36.53%. HOOCCH(NH$_2$)CH$_2$CH$_2$COOC$_2$H$_5$. Prepn from glutamic acid, ethanol, and hydrogen chloride: Hegedus, *Helv. Chim. Acta* **31**, 737 (1948); Pravda, *Collect. Czech. Chem. Commun.* **24**, 2083 (1959); CS 88344 (1959), *C.A.* **54**, 8660h (1960).

Hydrochloride. $C_7H_{13}NO_4$·HCl. Crystals from ethanol + ether, mp 134-136°.

4471. Glutamine. [56-85-9] L-Glutamine; Gln; Q; 2-aminoglutaramic acid; (S)-2,5-diamino-5-oxopentanoic acid; glutamic acid 5-amide; Cebrogen; Glumin; Levoglutamina; Stimulina. C_5-$H_{10}N_2O_3$; mol wt 146.14. C 41.09%, H 6.90%, N 19.17%, O 32.84%. Non-essential amino acid for human development; most

abundant free amino acid in plasma and tissue. Isoln from sugarbeet juice: E. Schulze, E. Bosshard, *Ber.* **16**, 312 (1883). Due to ease of conversion to glutamic acid, *q.v.*, it was not isolated from protein until 1932: M. Damodaran *et al., Biochem. J.* **26**, 1704 (1932). Early chemistry and biochemistry: R. M. Archibald, *Chem. Rev.* **37**, 161-208 (1945); *Amino Acids and Proteins*, D. M. Greenberg, Ed. (Charles C. Thomas, Springfield, IL, 1951) 950 pp., *passim*; J. P. Greenstein, M. Winitz, *Chemistry of the Amino Acids* vol 1-3 (John Wiley and Sons, Inc., New York, 1961) pp. 1929-1954, *passim*. HPLC determn in biotech samples: B. Polanuer *et al., J. Chromatogr.* **594**, 173 (1992). Review of nutritive needs: R. J. Smith, D. W. Wilmore, *J. Parenter. Enteral Nutr.* **14**, (Suppl.) 94S-99S (1990); and metabolism: W. W. Souba, *J. Nutr. Biochem.* **4**, 2-9 (1993); L. M. Castell *et al., Amino Acids* **7**, 231-243 (1994). Review of metabolism and physiologic implications: R. J. Smith, *J. Parenter. Enteral Nutr.* **14**, (Suppl.) 40S-44S (1990); B. Moskovitz *et al., Pharmacol. Res.* **30**, 61-71 (1994).

Fine opaque needles from water or dil ethanol, dec 185-186°. $[\alpha]_D^{23}$ +6.1° (c = 3.6). pK$_1$ 2.17; pK$_2$ 9.13. One gram dissolves in 20.8 ml water at 30°, in 38.5 ml at 18°, in 56.7 ml at 0°. Practically insol in methanol (3.5 mg/100 ml at 25°), ethanol (0.46 mg/100 ml at 23°), ether, benzene, acetone, ethyl acetate, chloroform.

DL-Form. [585-21-7] Synthesis: F. E. King, D. A. A. Kidd, *J. Chem. Soc.* **1949**, 3315; G. B. Kline, S. H. Cox, *J. Org. Chem.* **26**, 1854 (1961). Prisms from dil acetone, mp 185-186° (King); mp 173-174.5° (Kline). One gram dissolves in 38.5 ml water at 18°.

4472. Glutaraldehyde. [111-30-8] Pentanedial; glutaral; glutaric dialdehyde; 1,3-diformylpropane; Cidex; Glutarol; Novaruca; Sonacide; Ucarcide; Verucasep; Verutal. $C_5H_8O_2$; mol wt 100.12. C 59.98%, H 8.05%, O 31.96%. Prepn: C. Harries, L. Tank, *Ber.* **41**, 1701 (1908); A. C. Cope *et al., Org. Synth.* **coll. vol. IV**, 816 (1963). Toxicity data: H. F. Smyth *et al., Am. Ind. Hyg. Assoc. J.* **23**, 95 (1962). Clinical evaluation in treatment of viral warts: R. Hirose *et al., J. Dermatol.* **21**, 248 (1994). Review of role in electron microscopy: M. A. Hayat, *Micron Microsc. Acta* **17**, 115-135 (1986); of toxicology: R. O. Beauchamp, Jr. *et al., Crit. Rev. Toxicol.* **22**, 143-174 (1992); of microbiocidal activity and use as chemosterilizing agent: A. D. Russell, *Infect. Control Hosp. Epidemiol.* **15**, 724-733 (1994).

Oil, fp −14°. bp$_{760}$ 187-189° (dec); bp$_{50}$ 106-108°; bp$_{10}$ 71-72°. n_D^{25} 1.43300. Vapor pressure (20°): 0.0152 torr (50% aq soln); 0.0012 torr (2% aq soln). Sol in ethanol, benzene, ether, water; volatile in steam. Polymerizes in water to a glassy form which regenerates the dialdehyde on vacuum distillation. LD$_{50}$ of 25% soln orally in rats: 2.38 ml/kg; by skin penetration in rabbits: 2.56 ml/kg (Smyth).

Dioxime. $C_5H_{10}N_2O_2$. Crystals from water or pyridine, mp 178°. Sublimes. Treatment with hot mineral acids gives pyridine.

Caution: Potential symptoms of overexposure are irritation of eyes, skin, respiratory system; dermatitis, sensitization of skin; cough, asthma; nausea, vomiting. *See: NIOSH Pocket Guide to Chemical Hazards* (DHHS/NIOSH 97-140, 1997) p 152.

USE: Disinfectant; in sterilization of endoscopic instruments; as a tanning agent for leather; fixative for electron microscopy.

THERAP CAT: Keratolytic.

4473. Glutaric Acid. [110-94-1] Pentanedioic acid; 1,3-propanedicarboxylic acid. $C_5H_8O_4$; mol wt 132.11. C 45.46%, H 6.10%, O 48.44%. COOH(CH$_2$)$_3$COOH. Occurs in green sugar beets; is found in water extracts of crude wool. Manuf from cyclopentanone by oxidative ring fission with hot 50% nitric acid in the presence of vanadium pentoxide. Lab prepn by acid hydrolysis of trimethylene cyanide: Marvel, Tuley, *Org. Synth.* **5**, 69 (1925), or of methylenedimalonic ester: Otterbacher, *ibid.* **10**, 58 (1930). Several new methods: Paris *et al.*, *Org. Synth.* **coll. vol. IV**, 496 (1963); English, Dayan, *ibid.* 499.

Large monoclinic prisms, mp 97.5-98°. d_4^{15} 1.429. bp$_{760}$ 302-304° (very slight decompn); bp$_{20}$ 200°; bp$_{10}$ 195-198°, pK$_1$ (25°): 4.34; pK$_2$: 5.22. n_D^{106} 1.41878. Absorption spectrum: *Compt. Rend.* **189**, 915 (1929). Soly in water (g/l): at 0°: 429; at 20°: 639; at 50°: 957; at 65°: 1118. Freely sol in abs alcohol, ether; sol in benzene, chloroform; slightly in petr ether.

Dimethyl ester. $C_7H_{12}O_4$. Liquid, faint agreeable odor. d_4^{15} 1.0934. bp$_{752}$ 213.5-214°; bp$_{13}$ 93.5-94.5°. n_D^{20} 1.4246. Very sol in alcohol and ether.

4474. Glutaronitrile. [544-13-8] Pentanedinitrile; glutaric acid dinitrile; trimethylene dicyanide; trimethylene cyanide. $C_5H_6N_2$; mol wt 94.11. C 63.81%, H 6.43%, N 29.77%. $CN(CH_2)_3$-CN. Prepd by the action of potassium cyanide on trimethylene bromide: Marvel, McColm, *Org. Synth.* **5**, 103 (1925).

Viscous liquid. Bitter-sweet taste. d^{23} 0.9888. mp −29°. bp$_{760}$ 286°; bp$_{100}$ 206°; bp$_{60}$ 190°; bp$_{40}$ 176°; bp$_{20}$ 157°; bp$_{10}$ 140°; bp$_5$ 124°; bp$_{1.0}$ 91.3°. n_D^{23} 1.4365. Soluble in water, alcohol, chloroform. Insol in ether, carbon disulfide.

4475. Glutathione. [70-18-8] *N*-(*N*-L-γ-Glutamyl-L-cysteinyl)glycine; L-glutathione; glutathione-SH; GSH; Agifutol S; Copren; Deltathione; Glutamed; Glutasan; Glutathin; Glutathiol; Glutathion; Glutinal; Isethion; Neuthion; Tathiclon; Tathion; Tationil; Triptide. $C_{10}H_{17}N_3O_6S$; mol wt 307.32. C 39.08%, H 5.58%, N 13.67%, O 31.24%, S 10.43%. The major low mol wt thiol compound of the living plant or animal cell. Isoln from yeast: Hopkins, *J. Biol. Chem.* **84**, 269 (1929). Synthesis: du Vigneaud, Miller, *Biochem. Prep.* **2**, 87 (1952); Goldschmidt *et al.*, *Ber.* **97**, 2434 (1964); Y. Ozawa *et al.*, *Bull. Chem. Soc. Jpn.* **53**, 2592 (1980). Review of early syntheses: Jeschkeit *et al.*, *Pharmazie* **18**, 658 (1963). Review of metabolism: A. Meister, M. E. Anderson, *Annu. Rev. Biochem.* **52**, 711-760 (1983); of metabolic role in antineoplastic chemotherapy: B. A. Arrick, C. F. Nathan, *Cancer Res.* **44**, 4224-4232 (1984). *Monographs:* S. Colowick *et al.*, *Glutathione* (Academic Press, New York, 1954); *Glutathione*, E. M. Crook, Ed., Biochem. Soc. Symposium No. 17, London, 1958 (Cambridge University Press, 1959); *Glutathione*, L. Flohe *et al.*, Eds. (Academic Press, New York, 1974); *Glutathione: Metabolism & Function* I. M. Arias, W. B. Jackoby, Eds. (Raven, New York, 1976).

Crystals from 50% ethanol, mp 195°. [α]$_D^{25}$ −18.9° (c = 4.653). [α]$_D^{27}$ −21° (c = 2.74). pK$_1'$ 2.12; pK$_2'$ 3.53; pK$_3'$ 8.66; pK$_4'$ 9.12. Freely sol in water, dil alcohol, liq ammonia, dimethylformamide.

Disulfide. [27025-41-8] L-γ-Glutamyl-cysteinyl-glycine disulfide; *N,N'*-[dithiobis[1-[(carboxymethyl)carbamoyl]ethylene]]diglutamine; GSSG; oxidized glutathione. $C_{20}H_{32}N_6O_{12}S_2$; mol wt 612.63. Crystals, mp 123°. [α]$_D$ −108° (c = 2 in water).

4476. Gluten. Protein substance of wheat which is intermixed with the starchy endosperm of the grain. Causes the carbon dioxide produced during dough fermentation to be retained by the dough in a manner which provides the porous and spongy structure of bread. Prepn from wheat: Rist, *Sugar J.* **11**, no. 9, 26 (1949), *C.A.* **43**, 9505c (1949); Christensen, **US 2583684** (1952 to Gateway Chemurgic). Amino acid composition: Pence *et al.*, *Cereal Chem.* **27**, 335 (1950). *Reviews:* M. J. Blish "Wheat Gluten" in M. L. Anson, J. T. Edsall, *Advan. Protein Chem.* **vol. II** (Academic Press, New York, 1945) pp 337-359; Meredith, *Cereal Sci. Today* **9**, 33, 54 (1964).

Yellowish-gray powder. Practically insol in water. Partly sol in alcohol, dil acids; sol in alkalies.

USE: As adhesive and as substitute for flour.

4477. Glutethimide. [77-21-4] 3-Ethyl-3-phenyl-2,6-piperidinedione; 2-ethyl-2-phenylglutarimide; α-ethyl-α-phenylglutarimide; 3-ethyl-3-phenyl-2,6-dioxopiperidine; 3-ethyl-3-phen-

yl-2,6-diketopiperidine; Elrodorm; Doriden. $C_{13}H_{15}NO_2$; mol wt 217.26. C 71.87%, H 6.96%, N 6.45%, O 14.73%. Synthesis: Tagmann *et al.*, *Helv. Chim. Acta* **35**, 1541 (1952); Salmon-Legagneur, Neveu, *Compt. Rend.* **234**, 1060 (1952); *Bull. Soc. Chim. Fr.* **1953**, 70; Hoffmann, Tagmann, **US 2673205** (1954 to Ciba). Resolution: Kukalja *et al.*, *Croat. Chem. Acta* **33**, 41 (1961), *C.A.* **55**, 27193g (1961). Abs config of antipodes: Finch *et al.*, *Experientia* **31**, 1002 (1975). Comprehensive description: H. Y. Aboul-Enein, *Anal. Profiles Drug Subs.* **5**, 139-187 (1976).

dl-Form. Crystals from ether or from ethyl acetate + petr ether, mp 84°. uv max (methanol): 251, 257, 263 nm. Freely sol in ethyl acetate, acetone, ether, chloroform; sol in ethanol, methanol. Practically insol in water.

d-Form. Crystals, mp 102.5-103°. [α]$_D^{20}$ +176° (methanol).

l-Form. Crystals, mp 102-103°. [α]$_D^{20}$ −181° (methanol).

Note: This is a controlled substance (depressant): **21 CFR**, 1308.12.

THERAP CAT: Sedative; hypnotic.

4478. Glyburide. [10238-21-8] 5-Chloro-*N*-[2-[4-[[[(cyclohexylamino)carbonyl]amino]sulfonyl]phenyl]ethyl]-2-methoxybenzamide; 1-[[p-[2-(5-chloro-*o*-anisamido)ethyl]phenyl]sulfonyl]-3-cyclohexylurea; *N*-[4-(β-(2-methoxy-5-chlorobenzamido)ethyl)benzosulfonyl]-*N'*-cyclohexylurea; N^1-[4-[β-(2-methoxy-5-chlorobenzoylamino)ethyl]benzenesulfonyl]-N^2-cyclohexylurea; glybenzcyclamide; glibenclamide; HB-419; U-26452; Azuglucon; Bastiverit; Diabasan; Diabeta; Daonil; Duraglucon; Euglucon; Gilemal; Glimidstada; Glycolande; Libanil; Maninil; Micronase; Praeciglucon. $C_{23}H_{28}ClN_3O_5S$; mol wt 494.00. C 55.92%, H 5.71%, Cl 7.18%, N 8.51%, O 16.19%, S 6.49%. Second generation sulfonylurea with hypoglycemic activity. Prepn: Aumuller *et al.*, *Arzneim.-Forsch.* **16**, 1640 (1966); **NL 6603398** (1966 to Boehringer, Mann.), *C.A.* **66**, 65289h (1967); **NL 6610580**; H. Weber *et al.*, **US 3454635** (1967, 1969 both to Hoechst). Pharmacology: Loubatières, Mariani, *C.R. Seances Acad. Sci. Ser. D* **265**, 643 (1967). Toxicity: Mizukami *et al.*, *Arzneim.-Forsch.* **19**, 1413 (1969). Series of articles on synthesis, pharmacology, toxicology and clinical studies: *ibid.* 1323-1494. Effect on release of insulin, glucagon and somatostatin: S. Efendic *et al.*, *Proc. Natl. Acad. Sci. USA* **76**, 5901 (1979). Symposium on pharmacology, mechanism of action and clinical trials: *Ann. Clin. Res.* **15**, Suppl. 37, 1-35 (1983). Comprehensive description: P. G. Takla, *Anal. Profiles Drug Subs.* **10**, 337-355 (1981). Review of pharmacology and clinical efficacy: J. M. Feldman, *Pharmacotherapy* **5**, 43-62 (1985).

Crystals from methanol, mp 169-170° (Weber); also reported as mp 172-174° (Aumüller). pKa 5.3. Sparingly sol in water, sol in the usual organic solvents. LD$_{50}$ in rats and mice (g/kg): >20 orally; >12.5 i.p.; >20 s.c. (Mizukami).

THERAP CAT: Antidiabetic.

4479. Glybuthiazol(e). [535-65-9] 4-Amino-*N*-[5-(1,1-dimethylethyl)-1,3,4-thiadiazol-2-yl]benzenesulfonamide; N^1-(5-*tert*-butyl-1,3,4-thiadiazol-2-yl)sulfanilamide; sulfatertiobutylthiadiazole; 2-(*p*-aminobenzenesulfamido)-5-tertiobutyl-1,3,4-thiadiazole; glybuthiazol; RP-2259; Glipasol. $C_{12}H_{16}N_4O_2S_2$; mol wt

312.41. C 46.13%, H 5.16%, N 17.93%, O 10.24%, S 20.53%. Prepn: **GB 828963** (1960 to Rhône-Poulenc).

Needles from ethanol, mp 221-223°. Sol in ethanol (1.0 g/65 ml); in acetone (1.0 g/15 ml); in DMF (1.0 g/3 ml). Insol in water, ether, benzene. Forms a water-sol Na salt.

THERAP CAT: Antidiabetic.

4480. Glybuzole. [1492-02-0] *N*-[5-(1,1-Dimethylethyl)-1,3,4-thiadiazol-2-yl]benzenesulfonamide; *N*-(5-*tert*-butyl-1,3,4-thiadiazol-2-yl)benzenesulfonamide; 2-benzenesulfonamido-5-*tert*-butyl-1,3,4-thiadiazole; desaglybuzole; TH-1395; RP-7891; AN-1324; Gludiase. $C_{12}H_{15}N_3O_2S_2$; mol wt 297.40. C 48.46%, H 5.08%, N 14.13%, O 10.76%, S 21.56%. Prepn: Macrae, Drain, **GB 822947** (1959 to Smith & Nephew), *C.A.* **54**, 4622h (1960); **FR M3389** (1965 to Rhône-Poulenc), *C.A.* **64**, 3553a (1966). Pharmacodynamics: Bargeton *et al.*, *Arch. Int. Pharmacodyn.* **153**, 379 (1965).

Needles, mp 163°.
THERAP CAT: Antidiabetic.

4481. Glyceraldehyde. [56-82-6] 2,3-Dihydroxypropanal; DL-glyceraldehyde; glyceric aldehyde; α,β-dihydroxypropionaldehyde. $C_3H_6O_3$; mol wt 90.08. C 40.00%, H 6.71%, O 53.28%. Obtained with its isomer dihydroxyacetone from glycerol by mild oxidation: Witzemann, *J. Am. Chem. Soc.* **36**, 2227 (1914). *See also Org. Synth.* **coll. vol. II**, 305 (1943). The equilibrium mixture of glyceraldehyde and dihydroxyacetone is called *glycerose*. The two isomers are convertible into another through a common enediol resulting from the migration of hydrogen atoms (Lobry de Bruyn-van Eckenstein rearrangement). The equilibrium mixture plays an important role in the fermentation of sugars and in the biogenesis of constituents of the animal organism, *cf.* L.F. Fieser, M. Fieser, *Advanced Organic Chemistry* (Reinhold, New York, 1961) pp 78, 284, 405. Glyceraldehyde is the simplest aldose; the D- and L-forms are the configurational reference standard for carbohydrates. The two forms have been obtained through the action of nitrous acid on the corresponding form of 3-amino-2-hydroxypropanal: Wohl, Momber, *Ber.* **47**, 3346 (1914); Pictet, Barbier, *Helv. Chim. Acta* **4**, 924 (1921); *cf.* Baer, Fischer, *Science* **88**, 108 (1938). Prepn of L-glyceraldehyde from L-sorbose and of D-glyceraldehyde from D-fructose: Perlin, *Methods Carbohydr. Chem.* **1**, 61 (1962).

L-form   D-form

Tasteless crystals from alcohol + ether, d_{18}^{18} 1.455. mp 145°. Distills at 140-150° (bath temp) and 0.8 mm pressure. 100 ml water dissolve 3 g at 18°. Insol in benzene, petr ether, pentane. Osazone, mp 132°.

L-Form. [497-09-6] (*S*)-(−)-2,3-Dihydroxypropanol. $[\alpha]_D^{25}$ −8.7° (c = 2 in H_2O). Its dimethylacetal, bp$_{17-20}$ 126-129°. $[\alpha]_D^{26}$ −20.9° (p = 9.22).

D-Form. [453-17-8] $[\alpha]_D^{25}$ +8.7° (c = 2 in H_2O). Its dimethyl-acetal, bp$_{17}$ 127-129°, bp$_{10}$ 123-126°. $[\alpha]_D^{15}$ +21.2° (c = 18).

4482. Glyceraldehyde 3-Phosphate. [142-10-9] 2-Hydroxy-3-(phosphonooxy)propanal; 3-phosphoglyceraldehyde. C_3-

H_7O_6P; mol wt 170.06. C 21.19%, H 4.15%, O 56.45%, P 18.21%. An intermediate product of carbohydrate metabolism. Prepn of DL-form by enzymatic route: Meyerhof, Junowicz-Kocholaty, *J. Biol. Chem.* **149**, 71 (1943); by reductive cleavage of glyceraldehyde 1-benzyl ether 3-phosphoric acid: Fischer, Baer, *Ber.* **65**, 337, 1040 (1932); by hydrolysis of dimeric glyceraldehyde 1,3-diphosphoric acid: Baer, Fischer, *J. Biol. Chem.* **150**, 213 (1943); by hydrolysis of dimeric glyceraldehyde 1-bromide 3-phosphoric acid: *ibid.* 223. *See also* Baer in *Biochem. Prep.* **1**, 50 (1949). Prepn of D-form by enzymatic route: Meyerhof, Junowicz-Kocholaty, *loc. cit.*; by synthetic route: Ballou, Fischer, *J. Am. Chem. Soc.* **77**, 3329 (1955).

DL-Form calcium salt dihydrate. $C_3H_5CaO_6P.2H_2O$. Crystals, sol in water. Aq solns are not stable, particularly when alkaline. The dioxane addition compd of DL-glyceraldehyde 1-bromide 3-phosphoric acid described by Baer is relatively stable and may be stored in the refrigerator. An aq soln of the Na or K salt of glyceraldehyde-3-phosphoric acid (contg dioxane and bromide ion) is readily obtained by dissolving the dioxane compd in cold water and carefully neutralizing to pH 7.

D-Form calcium salt dihydrate. Amorphous powder. $[\alpha]_D^{25}$ +14.5° (c = 1.2 in 0.1N HCl calcd as the free acid). Prepn of calcium-free aq soln: Ballou, Fischer, *loc. cit.*

4483. Glyceric Acid. [473-81-4] 2,3-Dihydroxypropanoic acid; α,β-dihydroxypropionic acid. $C_3H_6O_4$; mol wt 106.08. C 33.97%, H 5.70%, O 60.33%. $CH_2OHCH(OH)COOH$. Prepn from α,β-dibromopropionic acid by treatment with silver oxide: Karrer, Klarer, *Helv. Chim. Acta* **7**, 931 (1924); from isoserine and nitrous acid: Fischer, Jacobs, *Ber.* **40**, 1069 (1907); from glycerol and nitrous acid: Mulder, *Ber.* **9**, 1902 (1876); Beilstein, *Ann.* **120**, 229 (1861). Dextrorotatory glyceric acid is obtained by the action of *Penicillia* or *Aspergilli* on the DL-form: McKenzie, Harden, *J. Chem. Soc.* **83**, 431 (1903). Levorotatory glyceric acid has been obtained by the oxidation of D(+)-glyceric aldehyde: Wohl, Schellenberg, *Ber.* **55**, 1408 (1922).

DL-Form. Syrup, dec on distn. pK (25°): 3.55. Miscible with water, alcohol, acetone. Nearly insol in ether.

L(+)-Form. Syrup. Its esters and salts are levorotatory and its salts are much more sol in water than those of the DL-form.

L-Form calcium salt. $Ca(C_3H_5O_4)_2.2H_2O$. Monoclinic spheroidal crystals, mp 137°. One gram dissolves in 10 ml water. $[\alpha]_D^{20}$ −14.6° (c = 5).

D(−)-Form. Syrup. Its salts are dextrorotatory.

D-Form calcium salt. $Ca(C_3H_5O_4)_2.2H_2O$. Prisms, mp 138°. $[\alpha]_D^{20}$ +14.5° (c = 5).

4484. Glycerol. [56-81-5] 1,2,3-Propanetriol; glycerin; glycerine; trihydroxypropane; incorporation factor; IFP; Bulbold; Cristal; Glyceol; Ophthalgan. $C_3H_8O_3$; mol wt 92.09. C 39.13%, H 8.76%, O 52.12%. $CH_2OHCHOHCH_2OH$. Obtained from oils and fats as byproduct in the manuf of soaps and fatty acids. During World War I supplementary quantities were produced by the "Protol" fermentation process from sugar, a process based upon the fixation of acetaldehyde by sodium sulfite. Just prior to World War II the synthesis of glycerol from propylene was announced. Production from sugars by fermentation: Onishi, **US 3012945** (1961 to Noda). Identity with incorporation factor: Kuehl *et al.*, *J. Am. Chem. Soc.* **82**, 2079 (1960). In nucleic acid the incorporation factor may exist as a bound form of glycerol. Acute toxicity: W. Bartsch *et al.*, *Arzneim.-Forsch.* **26**, 1581 (1976). Reviews and bibliographies: J. W. Lawrie, *Glycerol and the Glycols* (New York, 1928); G. Leffingwell, M. Lesser, *Glycerin* (Brooklyn, 1945); C. S. Miner, N. N. Dalton, *Glycerol* (New York, 1953); C. Lüttgen, *Glyzerin und glyzerinähnliche Stoffe* (Heidelberg, 2nd ed., 1955); J. C. Kern in *Kirk-Othmer Encyclopedia of Chemical Technology* **vol. 11** (Wiley-Interscience, New York, 3rd ed., 1980) pp 921-932.

Syrupy liquid. Sweet warm taste. About 0.6 times as sweet as cane sugar. Hygroscopic; also absorbs H_2S, HCN, SO_2. *Contact with strong oxidizing agents such as chromium trioxide, potassium chlorate, or potassium permanganate may produce an explosion.* Neutral to litmus. Solidifies after prolonged cooling at 0° forming shiny orthorhombic crystals, mp 17.8°. bp_{760} 290.0° (dec); bp_{263} 263.0°; bp_{200} 240.0°; bp_{100} 220.1°; bp_{60} 208.0°; bp_{20} 182.2°; bp_{10} 167.2°; bp_5 153.8°; $bp_{1.0}$ 125.5°. n_D^{15} 1.4758; n_D^{20} 1.4746; n_D^{25} 1.4730. d_1^{15} 1.26557; d_{20}^{20} 1.26362; d_{25}^{25} 1.26201. Flash point, open cup: 350°F (176°C). Specific gravities of 95% aq soln w/w (U.S.P. grade): d_{15}^{15} 1.25270; d_{20}^{20} 1.25075; d_{25}^{25} 1.24910; 90% aq soln w/w: d_{15}^{15} 1.23950; d_{20}^{20} 1.23755; d_{25}^{25} 1.23585; 80% d_{15}^{15} 1.213; 70% d_{15}^{15} 1.185; 60% d_{15}^{15} 1.157; 50% d_{15}^{15} 1.129; 20% d_{15}^{15} 1.049; 5% d_{15}^{15} 1.0122. Viscosity (cP at 20°): 5% soln 1.143; 10% 1.311; 25% 2.095; 50% 6.050; 60% 10.96; 70% 22.94; 83% 111. Freezing points of aq solns w/w: 10% −1.6°; 30% −9.5°; 50% −23.0°; 66.7% −46.5°; 80% −20.3°; 90% −1.6°. Miscible with water, alcohol. One part dissolves in 11 parts ethyl acetate, in about 500 parts ethyl ether. Insol in benzene, chloroform, carbon tetrachloride, carbon disulfide, petr ether, oils. LD_{50} in rats (ml/kg): >20 orally; 4.4 i.v. (Bartsch).

Caution: Potential symptoms of overexposure to mist are irritation of eyes, skin, respiratory system; headache, nausea, vomiting; kidney injury. *See NIOSH Pocket Guide to Chemical Hazards* (DHHS/NIOSH 97-140, 1997) p 152.

USE: As solvent, humectant, plasticizer, emollient, sweetener, in the manuf of nitroglycerol (dynamite), cosmetics, liq soaps, liqueurs, confectioneries, blacking, printing and copying inks, lubricants, elastic glues, lead oxide cements; to keep fabrics pliable; to preserve printing on cotton; for printing rollers, hectographs; to keep frost from windshields; as antifreeze in automobiles, gas meters and hydraulic jacks, in shock absorber fluids. In fermentation nutrients in the production of antibiotics. Pharmaceutic aid (humectant; solvent, vehicle). Leffingwell and Lesser (*op. cit.*) give 1583 different uses.

THERAP CAT: Diagnostic aid (ophthalmic).

THERAP CAT (VET): Emollient, demulcent. As a source of glucose in bovine ketosis.

4485. Glycerol Formal. Methylidinoglycerol; Glicerinformal; Sericosol N. $C_4H_8O_3$; mol wt 104.10. C 46.15%, H 7.75%, O 46.11%. Mixture of isomeric α,α'- and α,β-forms prepd from glycerin and formaldehyde: M. Schultz, B. Tollens, *Ann.* **289**, 20 (1895). Prepn and separation of isomers: H. Hibbert, N. M. Carter, *J. Am. Chem. Soc.* **50**, 3120 (1928); J. D. van Roon, *Rec. Trav. Chim.* **48**, 173 (1929). Prepn and pharmacology: P. Gimeno, **ES 475962** (1979 to Calipe), *C.A.* **93**, 26445u (1980). Toxicological evaluation for use as pharmaceutical solvent: D. M. Sanderson, *J. Pharm. Pharmacol.* **11**, 150, 446 (1959). Teratogenicity studies: V. Aliverti *et al., Arch. Sci. Biol.* **61**, 89 (1977); E. Giavini, M. Prati, *Acta Anat.* **106**, 203 (1980).

α,α'-form   α,β-form

Liquid, bp_{760} 191-195°, bp_{20} 95-97°. d_4^{20} 1.215; n_D^{20} 1.451. Sol in water, alc, chloroform. pH of 10% soln: 4-6.5. LD_{50} in rats (ml/kg): 8.6 orally, 3.5 i.v. (Gimeno).

α,α'-Form. 1,3-Dioxan-5-ol; α,α'-methylene glycerin; α,α'-formaldehyde glycerol; 5-*m*-dioxanol. bp 193.8°. d_4^{25} 1.2200. n_D^{25} 1.4527.

α,β-Form. 1,3-Dioxolane-4-methanol; α,β-methylene glycerin; α,β-formaldehyde glycerol; 4-(hydroxymethyl)-1,3-dioxolane. bp 192.5°. d_4^{25} 1.2008. n_D^{25} 1.4469.

USE: Pharmaceutic aid (solvent).

4486. Glycerophosphoric Acid. [57-03-4] (DL-α-form); [17181-54-3] (β-form). Phosphoric acid glycerol esters. $C_3H_9O_6$-P; mol wt 172.07. C 20.94%, H 5.27%, O 55.79%, P 18.00%. Three isomers exist: **β-glycerophosphoric acid**, the D(+)- and L(−)-forms of **α-glycerophosphoric acid**. The L-α-acid is the natu-

rally occurring form; the β-acid, present in hydrolyzates of lecithins from natural sources, arises from migration of the phosphoryl group from the α-carbon atom. See review: Dawson, *Annu. Rep. Prog. Chem.* **55**, 365 (1958). Prepn by phosphorylation of glycerol results in a mixture of the α- and β-acids: Cherbuliez, Weniger, *Helv. Chim. Acta* **29**, 2006 (1946). Prepn and configuration of L-α-acid: Baer, Fischer, *J. Biol. Chem.* **128**, 491 (1939). Prepn of D-α-acid: *eidem, ibid.* **135**, 321 (1940). Separation of α-acid from β- and polyglycerophosphoric acids: Carrara, *IT 460219* (1950), *C.A.* **46**, 5077a (1952).

α–L-form

Absolute acid (commercial mixture of α- and β-acids); clear syrupy liq, mp −25°. d_4^{14} 1.59. Tends to dec during concn; hence, usually marketed as a 25-50% soln. Soluble in water, alcohol.

α-Acid L-form. [5746-57-6] (2S)-1-(Dihydrogen phosphate)-1,2,3-propanetriol. Syrup. Readily sol in water, methanol, ethanol. Practically insol in ether. $[α]_D$ −1.45° (barium salt, c = 10.3 in 2N HCl).

Note: **Phosphatidic acids** are fatty acid diesters of glycerophosphoric acid.

USE: Absolute acid used to manuf certain glycerophosphates or to impart taste to solns of glycerophosphates which are generally used medicinally. *See also:* Calcium Glycerophosphate.

4487. Glyceryl p-Aminobenzoate. [136-44-7] 1,2,3-Propanetriol 1-(4-aminobenzoate); *p*-aminobenzoic acid monoglyceryl ester; monoglycerol *p*-aminobenzoate; Escalol 106. $C_{10}H_{13}NO_4$; mol wt 211.21. C 56.87%, H 6.20%, N 6.63%, O 30.30%. Prepd by controlled esterification of *p*-aminobenzoic acid with glycerol.

Semisolid, waxy mass or syrup. Faint aromatic odor. Liquefies and congeals very slowly. Soluble in methanol, ethanol, isopropanol, glycerol, propylene glycol. Insol in water, oils, fats.

USE: In cosmetic sunscreen prepns (up to 1%).

4488. Glyceryl Iodide. [554-10-9] 3-Iodo-1,2-propanediol; γ-iodopropyleneglycol; 3-iodo-1,2-dihydroxypropane. $C_3H_7IO_2$; mol wt 201.99. C 17.84%, H 3.49%, I 62.83%, O 15.84%. ICH_2-$CH(OH)CH_2OH$. Prepd from 2,3-epoxy-1-propanol: Kratzl *et al., Monatsh. Chem.* **93**, 49 (1962).

Crystals, mp 48-49°. Freely sol in water, alcohol.

4489. Glyceryl Monostearate. [31566-31-1] Octadecanoic acid monoester with 1,2,3-propanetriol; Monostearin. The commercial product is a mixture of variable proportions of glyceryl monostearate and glyceryl monopalmitate.

White, wax-like solid or wax-like beads, or flakes, mp 56-58°. Saponification value 164-170. Iodine value not more than 6. Soluble in hot organic solvents such as alcohol, benzene, ether, acetone, mineral or fixed oils. Insol in water, but may be dispersed in hot water with the aid of a small amount of soap or other suitable surface active agent.

USE: In pharmaceutical dispensing, see Green, *J. Am. Pharm. Assoc. Pract. Pharm. Ed.* **7**, 299 (1946).

4490. Glycidol. [556-52-5] Oxiranemethanol; 2,3-epoxy-1-propanol; 3-hydroxypropylene oxide. $C_3H_6O_2$; mol wt 74.08. C 48.64%, H 8.16%, O 43.19%. Prepd by the action of perbenzoic acid on allyl alc: Prileshajew, *Ber.* **42**, 4813 (1909); from glycerol-1-monochlorohydrin by the action of KOH in alc, or by the action of sodium in ether: Rider, Hill, *J. Am. Chem. Soc.* **52**, 1521 (1930). L-form prepd from L-1-(*p*-toluenesulfonyl)glycerol: Sowden, Fischer, *ibid.* **64**, 1291 (1942). Acute toxicity data: E. D. Thompson, R. A. Hiles, *Food Cosmet. Toxicol.* **19**, 347 (1981); E. D. Thompson, D. P. Gibson, *Food Chem. Toxicol.* **22**, 665 (1984).

DL-Form. Slightly viscous liq. d_4^{25} 1.1143. bp_{760} 167° (decompn); $bp_{2.5}$ 66°; $bp_{0.9}$ 25°. Miscible with water. LD_{50} in female rats (g/kg): 0.42 orally, 0.20 i.p. (Thompson, Hiles). LD_{50} in male, female rats (g/kg): 0.35, 0.21 i.p.; 0.76, 0.64 orally (Thompson, Gibson).

L-Form. $[\alpha]_D^{20}$ +15° (neat).

Caution: Potential symptoms of overexposure are irritation of eyes, nose, throat and skin; narcosis. *See NIOSH Pocket Guide to Chemical Hazards* (DHHS/NIOSH 97-140, 1997) p 152. *See also Patty's Industrial Hygiene and Toxicology* vol. **2A**, G. D. Clayton, F. E. Clayton, Eds. (John Wiley & Sons, New York, 4th ed., 1994) 422-425. This substance is reasonably anticipated to be a human carcinogen: *Report on Carcinogens, Eleventh Edition* (PB2005-104914, 2004) p III-130.

USE: Stabilizer in manuf of vinyl polymers; intermediate in synthesis of glycerol, glycidyl ethers, and amines; additive for oil and synthetic hydraulic fluids; epoxy resin diluent.

4491. Glycine. [56-40-6] Gly; G; aminoacetic acid; aminoethanoic acid; glycocoll; Gyn-Hydralin. $C_2H_5NO_2$; mol wt 75.07. C 32.00%, H 6.71%, N 18.66%, O 42.63%. Non-essential amino acid for human development. Only amino acid with no asymmetric carbon. Major inhibitory neurotransmitter. Isoln from gelatin: H. Braconnot, *Ann. Chim. Phys.* **13**, 113 (1820). Early chemistry and biochemistry: *Amino Acids and Proteins,* D. M. Greenberg, Ed. (Charles C. Thomas, Springfield, IL, 1951) 950 pp., *passim*; J. P. Greenstein, M. Winitz, *Chemistry of the Amino Acids* vols **1-3**, (John Wiley and Sons, Inc., New York, 1961) pp. 1955-1970, *passim.* Exists in three polymorphic forms, α-, β-, and γ-: Y. Iitaka, *Nature* **183**, 390 (1959). Review of metabolism and radioprotection: S. Capalna, *Rev. Roum. Physiol.* **9**, 17-34 (1972); of metabolism in humans: A. A. Jackson, M. H. Golden, *Clin. Sci.* **58**, 517-522 (1980); in anerobes: J. R. Andreesen, *Antonie van Leeuwenhoek* **66**, 223-227 (1994). Review of role in neurotransmission: S. M. Paul in *Psychopharmacology: The Fourth Generation of Progress,* F. E. Bloom, D. J. Kupfer, Eds. (Raven Press, New York, 1995) pp 87-94. *Book: Glycine Neurotransmission,* O. P. Ottersen, J. Storm-Mathisen, Eds. (John Wiley & Sons, Chichester, U.K., 1990) pp 489.

Sweet, monoclinic prisms from alc, starts to dec at 233°, completely sintered at 290°. d 1.1607. pK_1 2.34; pK_2 9.60. pH of 0.2 molar soln in H_2O = 4.0. Adsorption on various chromatographic agents: Grettie, Williams, *J. Am. Chem. Soc.* **50**, 671 (1928). Soly in 100 ml water at 25°: 25.0 g; at 50°: 39.1 g; at 75°: 54.4 g; at 100°: 67.2 g. 100 g of abs alc dissolve about 0.06 g. Sol in 164 parts pyridine. Almost insol in ether.

Hydrochloride. $C_2H_5NO_2 \cdot HCl$. Hygroscopic prisms from HCl, mp 182°.

4492. Glycine Sulfate. [513-29-1] Triglycine sulfate. $C_6H_{17}N_3O_{10}S$; mol wt 323.28. C 22.29%, H 5.30%, N 13.00%, O 49.49%, S 9.92%. $(NH_2CH_2COOH)_3 \cdot H_2SO_4$. Prepn: Horsford, *Ann.* **60**, 1 (1846); *see also* Matthias, Miller, Remeika, *Phys. Rev.* **104**, 849 (1956). Crystal growing during prepn: Konstantinova *et al., Kristallografiya* **4**, 69-73 and 125-129 (1959).

Orthorhombic crystals. Very freely sol in water. Has ferroelectric properties: Curie point 47°. Spontaneous polarization at room temp: 2.2×10^{-6} coul/cm². Coercive field 220 v/cm.

USE: In electronics research.

4493. Glycinin. [9007-93-6] Chief protein constituent of soybeans: Osborne, Campbell, *J. Am. Chem. Soc.* **20**, 419 (1898); Smith, Circle, *Ind. Eng. Chem.* **31**, 1282 (1939). *Review:* H. Neurath, K. Bailey, Eds., *The Proteins* vol. **I**, Part A (Academic

Press, New York, 1953) pp 208-209, 223; *eidem, ibid.* vol. **II**, part A, (1954) pp 503, 506.

Soluble in water in the pH range 1-4, as well as above 7.

4494. Glycocholic Acid. [475-31-0] N-[(3α,5β,7α,12α)-3,7,12-trihydroxy-24-oxocholan-24-yl]glycine; N-cholylglycine. $C_{26}H_{43}NO_6$; mol wt 465.62. C 67.07%, H 9.31%, N 3.01%, O 20.62%. The product of conjugation of cholic acid with glycine; chief ingredient of the bile of herbivorous animals. In the weakly alkaline bile fluid glycocholic acid exists as the sodium salt. Prepn from bile: Hammarsten in *Abderhalden's Handbuch der Biol. Arbeitsmethoden,* Abt. **I**, Teil 6, p 211 (1925). Prepn from cholic acid: Cortese, *J. Am. Chem. Soc.* **59**, 2532 (1937). Synthesis: Cortese, Bauman, *ibid.* **57**, 1393 (1935); Bergstrom, Norman, *Acta Chem. Scand.* **7**, 1126 (1953). Separation: Antonides, **GB 928635** (1963 to Armour). Metabolism: Norman, *Scand. J. Gastroenterol.* **5**, 231 (1970).

Sesquihydrate. Crystals from 5% alc, mp about 130°. $[\alpha]_D^{23}$ +30.8° (c = 7.5 in 95% ethanol). Anhydr form, mp 165-168°. pK 4.4. Soly in water at 15°: 0.33 g/l; in boiling water: 8.3 g/l. Is hydrolyzed to cholic acid and glycine by acids and alkalies. Forms addition compds with nitrobenzene, aniline, benzyl alcohol, benzaldehyde, triolein.

Sodium salt. $C_{26}H_{42}NNaO_6$. Crystals from 95% alcohol + ether, mp 230-240°. $[\alpha]_D^{24}$ +32° (water). Soly at 15° in water >274 g/l; in alcohol >340 g/l.

4495. Glycocyamine. [352-97-6] N-(Aminoiminomethyl)-glycine; N-amidinoglycine; guanidineacetic acid; guanidoacetic acid. $C_3H_7N_3O_2$; mol wt 117.11. C 30.77%, H 6.02%, N 35.88%, O 27.32%. Prepd from S-ethylthiourea hydrobromide, sodium hydroxide, and glycine: Brand, Brand, *Org. Synth.* **coll. vol. III**, 440 (1955). Crystal and molecular structure: Guha, *Acta Crystallogr.* **B29**, 2163 (1973); J. Berthou *et al., ibid.* **B32**, 1529 (1976).

Crystals, dec 280-284°. Appreciably sol in water.

THERAP CAT: In combination with betaine as cardiotonic.

4496. Glycogen. [9005-79-2] Animal starch; liver starch. $(C_6H_{10}O_5)_n$; mol wt from about 2.7×10^5 to 3.5×10^6. Reserve carbohydrate of the animal organism. High molecular wt polymer having branched-chain structure composed of D-glucopyranose residues. Distributed through the cell protoplasm. Found esp in the liver and in rested muscle. Occurs also in insects and lower plants including fungi and yeasts. Isoln by alkaline destruction of the other cell constituents: Claude Bernard, *Lecons sur le diabete* (Paris, 1877) p 553; by destruction with trichloroacetic acid: Bell, Young, *Biochem. J.* **28**, 882 (1934); by centrifugation: Meyer, Jeanloz, *Adv. Enzymol.* **3**, 112 (1943); by hydraulic pressure: Stockhausen, Silbereisen, *Biochem. Z.* **287**, 276 (1936). For biological synthesis and lysis from the Cori ester (glucose-1-phosphate) *see* the review and bibliography by Meyer, *Adv. Enzymol.* **3**, 109 (1943); *see also* Nord, *Chem. Rev.* **26**, 423 (1940); Kalckar, *ibid.* **28**, 71 (1941). Isoln from the causal agent of cotton root rot, *Phymatotrichum omnivorum* (Shear) Duggar: Ergle, *J. Am. Chem. Soc.* **69**, 2061 (1947). Studies on linkages: Bahl, Smith, *J. Org. Chem.* **31**, 2915 (1966).

White powder. $[\alpha]_D^{25}$ +196 to +197°. Sol in water with opalescence. Insol in alc. Does not reduce Fehling's soln. With iodine, brown to violet colors are produced.

4497. Glycol Dilaurate. [624-04-8] Dodecanoic acid 1,2-ethanediyl ester; ethylene dilaurate. $C_{26}H_{50}O_4$; mol wt 426.67. C 73.19%, H 11.81%, O 15.00%. $C_{11}H_{23}COOCH_2CH_2OOCC_{11}H_{23}$.
Colorless, amorphous mass, mp 50-52°. bp_{20} 188°. Insol in alcohol, ether.
USE: In lacquers and varnishes as a plasticizer.

4498. Glycolic Acid. [79-14-1] Hydroxyacetic acid; hydroxyethanoic acid. $C_2H_4O_3$; mol wt 76.05. C 31.59%, H 5.30%, O 63.11%. $HOCH_2COOH$. Constituent of sugar cane juice. Made by the action of NaOH on monochloroacetic acid; also by electrolytic reduction of oxalic acid. *Review*: Sales brochure on hydroxyacetic acid from E. I. du Pont.
Odorless, somewhat hygroscopic crystals, mp 80°. pK (25°) 3.83. Sol in water, methanol, alcohol, acetone, acetic acid, ether. pH of aq solns: 2.5 (0.5%); 2.33 (1.0%); 2.16 (2.0%); 1.91 (5.0%); 1.73 (10.0%). LD_{50} orally in rats: 1.95 g/kg, H. F. Smyth *et al.*, *J. Ind. Hyg. Toxicol.* **23**, 259 (1941).
Caution: Mild irritant to skin, mucous membranes.
USE: In the processing of textiles, leather, and metals; in pH control, and wherever a cheap organic acid is needed, e.g. in the manuf of adhesives, in copper brightening, decontamination cleaning, dyeing, electroplating, in pickling, cleaning and chemical milling of metals.

4499. Glycol Salicylate. [87-28-5] 2-Hydroxybenzoic acid 2-hydroxyethyl ester; monoglycol salicylate; ethylene glycol monosalicylate; 2-hydroxyethyl salicylate; glysal; GL-7; Lumbinon; Phardol; Phlogont. $C_9H_{10}O_4$; mol wt 182.17. C 59.34%, H 5.53%, O 35.13%. $C_6H_4(OH)COOCH_2CH_2OH$.
Almost colorless, odorless liq. bp_{12} 169-172°. Soluble in about 110 parts water, 8 parts olive oil; very sol in alcohol, benzene, chloroform, ether.
THERAP CAT: Counterirritant, anti-inflammatory (topical).

4500. Glyconiazide. [3691-74-5] D-Glucuronic acid γ-lactone 1-[(4-pyridinylcarboxyl)hydrazone]; D-glucuronolactone isonicotinoylhydrazone; isonicotinoylhydrazone of D-glucuronic acid lactone; isonicotinic acid hydrazide hydrazone with glucuronic acid lactone; Galatone; Gatalone; Glucazide; Gluconiazide; Gluronazide; Guidazide; Hydronsan; INH-G; Mycobactyl. $C_{12}H_{13}N_3O_6$; mol wt 295.25. C 48.82%, H 4.44%, N 14.23%, O 32.51%. Prepd by heating isonicotinic acid hydrazide with D-glucuronolactone in methanol: Sah, *J. Am. Chem. Soc.* **75**, 2512 (1953); Sah, US 2940899 (1960 to U. of Calif.).

Plates and rods from methanol, needles from abs ethanol. Dec 150-160°. Freely sol in water. Practically insol in cold alc; 1.2 g dissolve in 100 ml methanol at 66°.
THERAP CAT: Antibacterial (tuberculostatic).

4501. Glycopyrrolate. [596-51-0] 3-[(Cyclopentylhydroxyphenylacetyl)oxy]-1,1-dimethylpyrrolidinium bromide; 3-hydroxy-1,1-dimethylpyrrolidinium bromide α-cyclopentylmandelate; α-cyclopentylmandelic acid ester with 3-hydroxy-1,1-dimethylpyrrolidinium bromide; 1-methyl-3-pyrrolidyl α-cyclopentylmandelate methobromide; 1-methyl-3-pyrrolidyl α-phenyl-α-cyclopentylglycolate methobromide; 3-(2-phenyl-2-cyclopentylglycoloyloxy)-1,1-dimethylpyrrolidinium bromide; glycopyrronium bromide; AHR-504; Nodapton; Robanul; Robinul; Tarodyl; Tarodyn. $C_{19}H_{28}BrNO_3$; mol wt 398.33. C 57.29%, H 7.09%, Br 20.06%, N 3.52%, O 12.05%. Synthetic, quaternary ammonium anticholinergic. Prepn: Franko, Lunsford, *J. Med. Pharm. Chem.* **2**, 523 (1960); Lunsford, US 2956062 (1960 to A. H. Robins). Pharmacodynamics: E. Kaltiala *et al.*, *J. Pharm. Pharmacol.* **26**, 352 (1974).

Toxicology: B. V. Franko *et al.*, *Toxicol. Appl. Pharmacol.* **17**, 361 (1970). Clinical comparison with atropine in anaesthetic practice: F. Kongsrud, S. Sponheim, *Acta Anaesthesiol. Scand.* **26**, 620 (1982); A. I. Webb, R. M. McMurphy, *Am. J. Vet. Res.* **48**, 1733 (1987); B. V. G. Malling *et al.*, *Br. J. Anaesth.* **60**, 426 (1988). Brief review of pharmacology and clinical use: R. K. Mirakhur, J. W. Dundee, *Anaesthesia* **38**, 1195-1204 (1983).

White crystals from butanone, mp 193.2-194.5°. Sol in water. LD_{50} (72 hr.) in female mice, female rats (mg/kg): 107, 196 i.p.; in male rats (mg/kg): 1150 orally (Franko).
THERAP CAT: Antispasmodic; preanesthetic medicant.
THERAP CAT (VET): Preanesthetic medicant.

4502. Glycosine. [6873-15-0] 1-Methyl-2-(phenylmethyl)-4(1H)-quinazolinone; 2-benzyl-1-methylquinazol-4-one; arborine. $C_{16}H_{14}N_2O$; mol wt 250.30. C 76.78%, H 5.64%, N 11.19%, O 6.39%. Found in the toothbrush plant, *Glycosmis pentaphylla* (Retz.) Corr., and *G. arborea* Corr., *Rutaceae*. Isoln from dried, powdered leaves: Chatterjee, Majumdar, *J. Am. Chem. Soc.* **76**, 2459 (1954). Identity of arborine and glycosine, structure: Chakravarti *et al.*, *Tetrahedron* **16**, 224 (1961). Synthesis: Pakrashi *et al.*, *Indian J. Chem.* **6**, 472 (1968); Ziegler *et al.*, *Monatsh. Chem.* **100**, 948 (1969); T. Kametani *et al.*, *Heterocycles* **9**, 1585 (1978).

Rhombohedral prisms from chloroform + ethyl acetate, mp 155-156°. uv max (ethanol): 231, 268, 277, 306 nm. Freely sol in chloroform, ethyl acetate, benzene, ethanol. Sparingly sol in ether.
Hydrochloride. $C_{16}H_{14}N_2O.HCl$. Leaflets from 90% ethanol, dec 209-210°.

4503. N-Glycylglycine. [556-50-3] $C_4H_8N_2O_3$; mol wt 132.12. C 36.36%, H 6.10%, N 21.20%, O 36.33%. $NH_2CH_2CONHCH_2COOH$. The simplest of all peptides. Prepn from 2,5-diketopiperazine: Schott *et al.*, *J. Org. Chem.* **12**, 490 (1947); Greenstein, Winitz, *Chemistry of the Amino Acids* vol. 2, (New York, 1961) p 803. From tritylglycylglycine: Zervas *et al.*, *J. Am. Chem. Soc.* **78**, 1359 (1956). From phthalylglycylglycine: Sheehan, Frank, *ibid.* **71**, 1856 (1949). From the dicyclohexylamine salt of trifluoroacetylglycylglycine: Weygand, Reiher, *Ber.* **88**, 26 (1955).
Crystals from dil alc. Crystal shape described as small tetrahedral leaves with a lustrous ball in center. Dec 262-264°. pK_1' 3.12; pK_2' 8.17. Heat of combustion: 472.4 kcal/mole. Soluble in hot water; slightly sol in ethanol. Practically insol in ether.
Hydrochloride monohydrate. $C_4H_8N_2O_3.HCl.H_2O$. Crystals from water + ethanol.
Ethyl ester hydrochloride. Crystals from abs ethanol, dec 182°.
USE: In the synthesis of more complicated peptides.

4504. Glycyrrhiza. Licorice; liquorice; sweet root. Dried rhizome and roots of *Glycyrrhiza glabra* L., var. *typica* Regel & Herder (Spanish licorice), or of *G. glabra* L., var. *glandulifera* (Waldst. & Kit.) Regel & Herder (Russian licorice), or of other varieties of *G. glabra* yielding a yellow and sweet wood, *Leguminosae*. *Habit*. Southern Europe to Central Asia. *Constit*. 6-14% glycyrrhizin (the glucoside of glycyrrhetic acid), asparagine, sugars, resin. Used chiefly in the form of glycyrrhiza syrup. *Incompat*. Acids, metallic salts.
USE: Extract and syrup as pharmaceutic aids (flavor and flavored vehicles).

4505. Glycyrrhizic Acid. [1405-86-3] (3β,20β)-20-Car-
boxy-11-oxo-30-norolean-12-en-3-yl 2-*O*-β-D-glucopyranurono-
syl-α-D-glucopyranosiduronic acid; glycyrrhizin; glycyrrhizinic
acid; glycyrrhetinic acid glycoside. $C_{42}H_{62}O_{16}$; mol wt 822.93.
C 61.30%, H 7.59%, O 31.11%. Triterpene saponin used in traditional Chinese medicinal preparations for its anti-inflammatory,
antiulcerous and antiallergic effects. Extraction from *Glycyrrhiza
glabra* L., *Leguminosae:* Karrer, Chao, *Helv. Chim. Acta* **4**, 100
(1921); Ruzicka, Louenberger, *ibid.* **19**, 1402 (1936). From commercial glycyrrhizinum ammoniacale: Tschirch, Cederberg, *Arch.
Pharm.* **245**, 97 (1907); Voss *et al., Ber.* **70**, 122 (1937). Revised
method of isoln: Conn, Conn, *J. Lab. Clin. Med.* **47**, 20 (1956).
Structure: Lythgoe, Trippett, *J. Chem. Soc.* **1950**, 1983. Revised
structure: Marsh, Levvy, *Biochem. J.* **63**, 9 (1956). See also: I.
Kitagawa *et al., Chem. Pharm. Bull.* **36**, 3710 (1988); T. Hatano *et
al., ibid.* **39**, 1238 (1991). Synthesis of derivatives: Brieskorn, Sax,
Arch. Pharm. **303**, 905 (1970). LC-MS/MS determn in plasma: Z.
J. Lin *et al., J. Chromatogr. B* **814**, 201 (2005). *Review:* Nieman,
Chem. Weekbl. **48**, 213 (1952).

Crystals from glacial acetic acid. Intensely sweet taste. $[\alpha]_D^{17}$
+46.2° (c = 1.5 in alc). Freely sol in hot water, alcohol; practically
insol in ether.

Ammonium glycyrrhizinate pentahydrate. $C_{42}H_{65}NO_{16}.5H_2-$
O. Needles from 75% aqueous ethanol, decomp 212-217°. $[\alpha]_D^{20}$
+46.9° (c = 1.5 in 40% ethanol). uv max: 248 nm (ε 11400). Sol
in ammonia water, glacial acetic acid.

Dipotassium salt. Rizinsan K2 A2. $C_{42}H_{60}K_2O_{16}$; mol wt
899.11.

4506. Glyhexamide. [451-71-8] *N*-[(Cyclohexylamino)car-
bonyl]-2,3-dihydro-1*H*-indene-5-sulfonamide; 1-cyclohexyl-3-(5-
indanylsulfonyl)urea; 1-cyclohexyl-3-(5-hydrindenylsulfonyl)urea;
SQ-15860; Subose. $C_{16}H_{22}N_2O_3S$; mol wt 322.42. C 59.60%,
H 6.88%, N 8.69%, O 14.89%, S 9.95%. Prepd from hydrindene-5-
sulfonamide and cyclohexyl isocyanate: Hoehn, Breuer, **US
3097242** (1963 to Olin Mathieson). Clinical pharmacology: Grinnell *et al., Am. J. Med. Sci.* **253**, 312 (1967).

Crystals from 70% acetone, mp 153-155°.
THERAP CAT: Antidiabetic.

4507. Glymidine. [339-44-6] *N*-[5-(2-Methoxyethoxy)-2-
pyrimidinyl]benzenesulfonamide; 2-benzenesulfonamido-5-(β-
methoxyethoxy)pyrimidine; glycodiazine. $C_{13}H_{15}N_3O_4S$; mol wt
309.34. C 50.47%, H 4.89%, N 13.58%, O 20.69%, S 10.37%.
Prepn: **BE 609270**; H. Priewe *et al., US 3275635** (1962, 1966 both
to Schering, AG); Gutsche *et al., Arzneim.-Forsch.* **14**, 373 (1964).
Series of articles on pharmacology: *ibid.* 377-412. Activity:
Losert *et al., ibid.* **23**, 1251 (1973). Metabolism: Soyfer *et al.,
Chim. Ther.* **5**, 441 (1970). Toxicity data: Kramer *et al., Arzneim.-
Forsch.* **14**, 377 (1964).

Crystals, mp 152-154°. Soly in ethanol: 0.91%; in toluene:
0.67%.

Sodium salt. [3459-20-9] SH-717; Glyconormal; Gondafon;
Lycanol; Redul. $C_{13}H_{14}N_3NaO_4S$; mol wt 331.32. Crystals, mp
221-226°. Sparingly sol in alc. Soly in water at 37°: 70.5%.
LD_{50} in mice, rats (g/kg): 1.48, 2.00 i.v.; 5.30, 2.85 orally
(Kramer).

THERAP CAT: Antidiabetic.

4508. Glyodin. [556-22-9] 2-Heptadecyl-4,5-dihydro-1*H*-
imidazole monoacetate; 2-heptadecylglyoxalidine acetate; Crag
Fruit Fungicide 341. $C_{22}H_{44}N_2O_2$; mol wt 368.60. C 71.69%,
H 12.03%, N 7.60%, O 8.68%. Prepn from stearic acid and ethylenediamine: Kiff, **US 2540171** (1951 to Union Carbide and Carbon).

Light orange crystals, mp 62-68°. d^{20} 1.035. Insol in water,
acetone, toluene. Sol in isopropanol.

Base. Soft greasy wax, mp 94°.
USE: Agricultual fungicide.

4509. Glyoxal. [107-22-2] Ethanedial; biformyl; diformyl;
oxalaldehyde. $C_2H_2O_2$; mol wt 58.04. C 41.39%, H 3.47%, O
55.13%. OHCCHO. Prepd by the oxidation of acetaldehyde by
nitric or selenious acid: Lubawin, *Ber.* **8**, 768 (1875); Wyss, *Ber.* **10**,
1366 (1877); Kölln, *Ann.* **416**, 230 (1918); Riley *et al., J. Chem. Soc.*
1932, 1881; Ronzio, Waugh, *Org. Synth.* **coll. vol. III**, 438 (1955);
by hydrolysis of dichlorodioxane: Butler, Cretcher, *J. Am. Chem.
Soc.* **54**, 2988 (1932). Review of commercial development: J. F.
Bohmfalk *et al., Ind. Eng. Chem.* **43**, 786 (1951). Toxicity study:
H. F. Smyth *et al., J. Ind. Hyg. Toxicol.* **23**, 259 (1941). *Review:* A.
B. Boese *et al.* in *Glycols,* G. O. Curme, F. Johnston, Eds. (Reinhold,
New York, 1952) pp 125-128.

Yellow prisms or irregular pieces turning white on cooling. d^{20}
1.14. Opaque at 10°, mp 15°. bp_{776} 51°. The vapors are green and
burn with a purple flame. *Explosive:* Mixtures with air may explode! $n_D^{20.5}$ 1.3826. Sol in anhydr solvents. pH of a 40% aq soln:
2.1-2.7; d_4^{20} 1.27. Polymerizes quickly on standing, on contact with
water (violent reaction), or when dissolved in solvents contg water.
The anhydr polymer changes to the monomer on heating. Solns of
the monomer are obtained on heating the polymer with anethole,
phenetole, safrole, methyl nonyl ketone, or benzaldehyde. LD_{50} in
rats, guinea pigs (mg/kg): 2020, 760 orally (Smyth).

Dihydrate. $(OHCCHO)_3.2H_2O$. Crystalline powder, nonhygroscopic. More sol in hot water than in cold water. Commercially
available in anhydr form as crystalline dihydrate, or as a 40% aq soln
which may contain polymerization inhibitors.

Caution: Moderately irritating to skin, mucous membranes.
USE: In textiles, organic synthesis, glues, biocides.

4510. Glyoxal-Sodium Bisulfite. [517-21-5] 1,2-Dihy-
droxy-1,2-ethanedisulfonic acid disodium salt; glyoxal compd
with sodium bisulfite. $C_2H_4Na_2O_8S_2$; mol wt 266.16. C 9.03%,
H 1.51%, Na 17.28%, O 48.09%, S 24.09%. Prepn: Ronzio,
Waugh, *Org. Synth.* **coll. vol. III**, 438 (1955).

Monohydrate. Hard crystals. Faint SO_2 odor. Freely sol in
water. Practically insol in alcohol.

4511. Glyoxylic Acid. [298-12-4] Oxoacetic acid; formylformic acid; glyoxalic acid; oxoethanoic acid. $C_2H_2O_3$; mol wt
74.04. C 32.44%, H 2.72%, O 64.83%. OHCCOOH. Occurs in
unripe fruit and in young green leaves; has also been found in very
young sugar beets. Prepd by heating dibromoacetic acid with some
water: Grimaux, *Bull. Soc. Chim.* [2] **26**, 483; Cramer, *Ber.* **25**, 714
(1892); by electrolytic reduction of oxalic acid: Meyer, *Ber.* **37**,
3592 (1904); by the action of *Aspergillus niger* on calcium acetate,

malonic or citric acid: Challenger *et al., J. Chem. Soc.* **1927,** 205, 207. Prepn of glyoxylic acid soln for analytical use: *Beilstein* vol. **III,** 594.

Hemihydrate. Crystals from water, mp 70-75°. Also obtained in anhydr form as monoclinic crystals from water, mp 98°. Obnoxious odor. Strong, corrosive acid. K = 4.6 × 10⁻⁴. Deliquesces rapidly and forms a syrup on short exposure to air. Sparingly sol in alc, ether, benzene. Freely sol in water; aq solns tend to acquire a yellowish tint. Attacks most base metals except certain stainless steel alloys.

Monohydrate. Crystals, mp ~50°. Highly hygroscopic.
Caution: Irritant, corrosive.

4512. Glyphosate. [1071-83-6] *N*-(Phosphonomethyl)glycine; MON-0573. C₃H₈NO₅P; mol wt 169.07. C 21.31%, H 4.77%, N 8.28%, O 47.32%, P 18.32%. Broad-spectrum post-emergence, translocated herbicide. Prepn: J. E. Franz, **DE 2152826;** *idem,* **US 3799758** and **US 3853530** (1972, 1974, 1974 all to Monsanto). Metabolism and degradation in soil and water: M. L. Rueppel *et al., J. Agric. Food Chem.* **25,** 517 (1977). Toxicity study: E. A. Bababunmi *et al., Toxicol. Appl. Pharmacol.* **45,** 319 (1978).

White solid, mp 230° (dec). Soly in water at 25°: 12 g/l. Insol in most organic solvents. LD₅₀ in rats, mice (mg/kg): 4873, 1568 orally (Bababunmi).

Mono(isopropylamine) salt. [38641-94-0] MON-2139; Accord; Durango; Glyphomax; Glypro; Rodeo; Roundup. C₃H₈NO₅-P.C₃H₉N; mol wt 228.18. Very sol in water.

Trimethylsulfonium salt. [81591-81-3] Sulfosate; glyphosate-trimesium; Avans-330; SC-0224; ICIA-0224; Touchdown. C₃H₇-NO₅P.C₃H₉S; mol wt 245.23. Description of biological and physical properties: B. Trousland, *Phytoma* **429,** 47 (1991); A. D. Baylis *et al., J. Biosci.* **8,** 173 (1997). bp₇₆₀ 110°. d 1.27. Soly in water (20°): 1050 g/l. LD₅₀ in rats, mice (mg/kg): 748, 1383 orally; in rabbits (mg/kg): >2000 dermally. LC₅₀ in rainbow trout (48 hrs): 4800 mg/l (Trousland).
USE: Herbicide.

4513. Goitrin. [500-12-9] (5*S*)-5-Ethenyl-2-oxazolidine-thione; 5-vinyl-2-thiooxazolidone; (−)-5-vinyl-2-oxazolidine-thione. C₅H₇NOS; mol wt 129.18. C 46.49%, H 5.46%, N 10.84%, O 12.39%, S 24.82%. An antithyroid compd isolated from seeds of different species of *Brassica, Cruciferae:* Astwood *et al., J. Biol. Chem.* **181,** 121 (1949); Greer, *J. Am. Chem. Soc.* **78,** 1260 (1956). Stereochemistry: Kjaer *et al., Acta Chem. Scand.* **13,** 144 (1959). Activity: Langer *et al., Endokrinologie* **57,** 225 (1971).

Large prisms from ether, mp 50°. [α]ᴅ³¹ −70.5° (c = 2 in methanol). Behaves as a weak acid; pKa 10.5. Stable in alkali, but not in acid.

4514. Gold. [7440-57-5] Au; at. wt 196.966569; at. no. 79; valences 1, 3. Group IB (11). Occurrence in the earth's crust: 0.005 ppm. One natural isotope: 197; artificial isotopes (mass numbers): 177-179, 181, 183, 185-196, 198-203. Probably the first pure metal known to man. Occurs in nature in its native form and in minute quantities in almost all rocks and in seawater. Gold ores include *calaverite,* (AuTe₂), *sylvanite,* [(Ag,Au)Te₂], *petzite,* [(Ag,Au)₂Te]. Methods of mining, extracting and refining: Hull, Stent in *Modern Chemical Processes* Vol. 5 (Reinhold, New York, 1958) pp 60-71. Lab prepn of gold powder from gold pieces: Block, *Inorg. Synth.* **4,** 15 (1953). Chemistry of gold drugs in the treatment of rheumatoid arthritis: D. H. Brown, W. E. Smith, *Chem. Soc. Rev.* **9,** 217 (1980). Use as catalyst in oxidation of organic compds by NO₂: R. E. Sievers, S. A. Nyarady, *J. Am. Chem. Soc.*

107, 3726 (1985). Least reactive metal at interfaces with gas or liquid: B. Hammer, J. K. Norskov, *Nature* **376,** 238 (1995). Reviews: *Gmelins, Gold* (8th ed.) **62,** parts 2, 3 (1954); Johnson, Davis, "Gold" in *Comprehensive Inorganic Chemistry* vol. **3,** J. C. Bailar Jr. *et al.,* Eds. (Pergamon Press, Oxford, 1973) pp 129-186; J. G. Cohn, E. W. Stern in *Kirk-Othmer Encyclopedia of Chemical Technology* vol. **11** (Wiley-Interscience, New York, 3rd ed., 1980) pp 972-995.

Yellow, soft metal; face-centered cubic structure; when prepared by volatilization or precipitation methods, deep violet, purple, or ruby powder, mp 1064.76°; bp 2700°. d 19.3. Hardness (Mohs') 2.5-3.0; (Brinell's) 18.5. Extremely inactive; not attacked by acids, air or oxygen. Superficially attacked by aq halogens at room temp. Reacts with aqua regia, with mixtures contg chlorides, bromides, or iodides if they can generate nascent halogens, with many oxidizing mixtures especially those contg halogens. Also with alkali cyanides, solns of thiocyanates and double cyanides.

USE: In manuf jewelry; in gold plating other metals; as a standard of currency; most frequently alloyed with silver and copper. For use in medicine, *see* Gold, Radioactive, Colloidal.

4515. Gold Monochloride. [10294-29-8] Aurous chloride. AuCl; mol wt 232.42. Au 84.75%, Cl 15.25%. Prepd by thermal decompn of gold trichloride: Biltz, Wein, *Z. Anorg. Allg. Chem.* **148,** 192 (1925); Capella, Schwab, *C.R. Hebd. Seances Acad. Sci.* **260,** 4337 (1965).

Yellowish powder. d 7.57. Dec at about 289° into gold and Cl₂. Practically insol in water, but slowly dec by it, more rapidly on heating, with formation of gold trichloride and separation of metallic gold; sol in alkali cyanides. With solns of alkali bromides, metallic gold and potassium auribromide are formed.

4516. Gold Monocyanide. [506-65-0] Aurous cyanide; gold cyanide. CAuN; mol wt 222.98. C 5.39%, Au 88.33%, N 6.28%. AuCN. May be prepd by decompn of Na[Au(CN)₂] with HCl: Wogrinz, *Metalloberflaeche* **8,** B162 (1954).

Yellow, odorless powder; iridescent in sunlight; slowly dec in presence of moisture. When warmed with HCl, HCN is evolved. When ignited, dec into metal Au and CN. d₄²⁰ 7.14. Hexagonal when cryst. Practically insol in water, alcohol, ether, dil acids; sol in ammonia, soln of NaCN; dissolved by aqua regia. On warming with concd H₂SO₄ half of the gold separates as metal.
Caution: May liberate HCN.

4517. Gold, Radioactive, Colloidal. [10043-49-9] Radioactive colloidal gold; colloidal gold ¹⁹⁸Au; radio-gold (¹⁹⁸Au) colloid; gold colloid ¹⁹⁸Au; Aurcoloid-198; Aurcoscan-198; Aureotope. Colloidal dispersion of radioactive gold (¹⁹⁸Au) for parenteral administration.

Particle diameter range, 3-7 mμ. Has half-life of 2.7 days and emits beta and gamma radiation. Stable to heat except autoclaving under pressure. Compatible with saline solns, radiopaque media and other agents; flocculated by polyvalent metal ion.
THERAP CAT: Antineoplastic.

4518. Gold Sodium Thiomalate. [12244-57-4] Mercapto-butanedioic acid monogold(1+) sodium salt; sodium aurothiomalate; Myochrysine; Shiosol; Tauredon. Disease modifying antirheumatic drug (DMARD). Mixture of the mono- (C₄H₄AuNaO₄S) and di-sodium (C₄H₃AuNa₂O₄S) salts of gold thiomalic acid. Prepn as the monohydrate of the disodium salt: M. Delépine, **US 1994213** (1935 to Rhone Poulenc). Detection in blood by atomic absorption spectroscopy: A. I. A. Rodgers *et al., Anal. Proc.* **19,** 87 (1982). Clinical pharmacokinetics: K. L. N. Blocka *et al., Clin. Pharma-cokinet.* **11,** 133 (1986). Discussion of mechanisms of action: H. A. Capell, *Agents Actions Suppl.* **24,** 158 (1988). Clinical trial in rheumatoid arthritis: R. Munro *et al., Ann. Rheum. Dis.* **57,** 88 (1998).

White to yellowish-white powder, metallic taste. Very sol in water. Practically insol in alcohol, ether. Aq solns are colorless to pale yellow. pH of a 5% aq soln: 5.8-6.5.
THERAP CAT: Antirheumatic.

4519. Gold Sodium Thiosulfate. [15283-45-1] Trisodium (*T*-4)-bis[monothiosulfato(2−)-*κO,κS*]-aurate(3−); hyposulfite of gold and sodium; sodium aurothiosulfate; Aurocidin; Aurolin; Crisalbine; Fosfocrisolo; Sanocrysin. $AuNa_3O_6S_4$; mol wt 490.19. Au 40.18%, Na 14.07%, O 19.58%, S 26.17%. $Na_3Au(S_2O_3)_2$. Prepn of dihydrate: Fordos, Gélis, *Ann. Chim. Phys.* **13**, 394 (1845); H. Brown, *J. Am. Chem. Soc.* **49**, 958 (1927); *Roger's Inorganic Pharmaceutical Chemistry,* T. O. Soine, C. O. Wilson, Eds. (Lea & Febiger, Philadelphia, 8th ed., 1967) pp 343-345. Crystal structure of dihydrate: H. Ruben *et al., Inorg. Chem.* **13**, 1836 (1974). Efficacy of antidotes: M. A. Basinger *et al., J. Rheumatol.* **12**, 274 (1985). Clinical study of contact allergy patch test reactions: K. E. McKenna *et al., Contact Dermatitis* **32**, 143 (1995). Clinical evaluation in rheumatoid arthritis: M. L. Ciompi *et al., Reumatismo* **54**, 251 (2002).

Dihydrate. [33614-49-2] White, glistening, needle-like or prismatic crystals. d 3.14. Darkens slowly on exposure to light. One gram dissolves in 2 ml water. Insol in alc and most other organic solvents. A 1:20 aq soln is neutral or slightly alkaline to litmus. LD_{50} i.p. in mice: 110 mg/kg (Basinger).

Caution: Potential symptoms of overexposure via therapeutic i.m. administration are dermatitis, nausea, vomiting, diarrhea, nephritis, blood disorders, peripheral neuritis, hepatitis, encephalitis. *See Clinical Toxicology of Commercial Products,* R. E. Gosselin *et al.,* Eds. (Williams & Wilkins, Baltimore, 5th ed., 1984) p II-144.

THERAP CAT: Antirheumatic; diagnostic aid (contact allergen).

4520. Gold Stannate. [1345-24-0] Aurous stannate; C.I. Pigment Red 109; C.I. 77482; gold-tin precipitate; gold-tin purple; purple of Cassius. Contains gold, tin and oxygen; composition of commercial products varies and in some cases may be a complex mixture of gold and stannic acid. Prepn: *Colour Index* vol. 4 (3rd ed., 1971) p 4669.

Brown powder. Practically insol in water. Sol in ammonia.

USE: Manuf ruby glass, colored enamels, and painting porcelain.

4521. Gold Trichloride. [13453-07-1] Auric chloride. $AuCl_3$; mol wt 303.33. Au 64.93%, Cl 35.06%. Conveniently prepd in the laboratory from metallic gold and iodine monochloride: Gutmann, *Z. Anorg. Allg. Chem.* **264**, 169 (1951).

Dihydrate. Dark orange-red crystals, deliquesc in moist air. d_4^{20} 3.9. Sublimes at 180° (760 mm). bp 229°. Decomp 254°. Soluble in water, alcohol, ether. *Keep well closed and protected from light.*

4522. Gold Trichloride, Acid. [16903-35-8] (*SP*-4-1)-Hydrogen tetrachloroaurate(1−); hydrochloroauric acid; aurochlorohydric acid; chloroauric acid. $AuCl_4H$; mol wt 339.79. Au 57.97%, Cl 41.74%, H 0.30%. $HAuCl_4$. Prepd according to the equation $2Au + 3Cl_2 + 2HCl \rightarrow 2HAuCl_4$: Thomsen, *Ber.* **16**, 1585 (1883); Biltz, Wein, *Z. Anorg. Allg. Chem.* **148**, 192 (1925).

Tetrahydrate. Golden-yellow to reddish-yellow, very hygroscopic and deliquesc monoclinic crystals; readily affected by sunlight. (Also available as brown crystals or cryst masses, contg 50-51% gold, and having the same properties as the yellow crystals.) Has caustic action on the skin (blisters) and then on exposure to light leaves violet-brown spots. Dec on strong heating to Cl_2, HCl, and metallic gold. d about 3.9. Very sol in water, alcohol; sol in ether. *Keep tightly closed and protected from light.*

USE: Photography, gold-plating, gilding glass and porcelain; manuf ruby glass; as a reagent for alkaloids.

4523. Gold Trihydroxide. [1303-52-2] Auric hydroxide. AuH_3O_3; mol wt 247.99. Au 79.43%, H 1.22%, O 19.35%. $Au(OH)_3$. Usually contains about $3H_2O$ and hence about 65% gold. May be prepd in lab according to the equation $2KAuCl_4 + 3Na_2CO_3 + 3H_2O \rightarrow 2Au(OH)_3 + 6NaCl + 2KCl + 3CO_2$: Lydén, *Z. Anorg. Allg. Chem.* **240**, 157 (1939).

Brown powder; dec by sunlight to metallic gold; also slowly dec with age or at 100°, and completely at 250°. Practically insol in water. Sol in solns of NaCN, in HCl or concd HNO_3. With NH_3 yields gold fulminate which *explodes easily in dry form. Protect from light.*

USE: In gold-plating solns; for decorating porcelains.

4524. Gold Trioxide. [1303-58-8] Auric oxide; gold sesquioxide; gold oxide. Au_2O_3; mol wt 441.93. Au 89.14%, O 10.86%.

Prepd from the hydroxide: Roseveare, Buehner, *J. Am. Chem. Soc.* **49**, 1221 (1927).

Brown powder; begins to evolve oxygen at 110°; at 250° it is entirely dec to metallic gold; also slowly dec by sunlight. Practically insol in water. Sol in HCl, concd HNO_3 and in NaCN soln. *Keep protected from light.*

4525. Gold Trisulfide. [1303-61-3] Auric sulfide. Au_2S_3; mol wt 490.13. Au 80.37%, S 19.63%. Prepd by treating dry lithium aurichloride $Li(AuCl_4)$ with hydrogen sulfide at −10°. The reaction product consists of HCl, lithium chloride, and auric sulfide. The lithium chloride can be removed by extraction with alcohol. *Ref:* Antony, Lucchesi, *Gazz. Chim. Ital.* **19**, 552 (1889). Prepd from $AuCl_3$ or $HAuCl_4$ and H_2S in abs ether at low temp: Guthier, Dürrwachter, *Z. Anorg. Allg. Chem.* **121**, 266 (1922).

Black powder. Heating to 200° dec it into its elements.

USE: In photography.

4526. Goserelin. [65807-02-5] 6-[*O*-(1,1-Dimethylethyl)-D-serine]-10-deglycinamideluteinizing hormone-releasing factor (pig) 2-(aminocarbonyl)hydrazide; D-Ser(Bu^t)^{6}Azgly^{10}-gonadorelin; D-Ser(Bu^t)^{6}Azgly^{10}-luliberin; ICI-118630. $C_{59}H_{84}N_{18}O_{14}$; mol wt 1269.41. C 55.82%, H 6.67%, N 19.86%, O 17.65%. Synthetic peptide agonist analog of LH-RH, *q.v.* Prepn: A. S. Dutta *et al.,* **DE 2720245**; *eidem,* **US 4100274** (1977, 1978 both to I.C.I.); *eidem, J. Med. Chem.* **21**, 1018 (1978). Radioimmunoassay in serum: R. N. Clayton *et al., Clin. Endocrinol.* **22**, 453 (1985). Endocrine effects in women: C. P. West, D. T. Baird, *ibid.* **26**, 213 (1987). Review of pharmacokinetics and therapeutic efficacy in sex hormone related disorders: P. Chrisp, K. L. Goa, *Drugs* **41**, 254-288 (1991). Clinical trial in treatment of uterine fibroids: J. Gerris *et al., Horm. Res.* **45**, 279 (1996); in prostate cancer: M. Bolla *et al., N. Engl. J. Med.* **337**, 295 (1997).

5-oxoPro–His–Trp–Ser–Tyr–D-Ser(*t*-Bu)–Leu–Arg–Pro–NHNHCONH$_2$

Acetate. Zoladex. $C_{59}H_{84}N_{18}O_{14} \cdot xC_2H_4O_2$, where x = 1 to 2.4. Off-white powder. Freely sol in acetic acid; sol in water, 0.1M HCl, 0.1M NaCl, DMF, DMSO. Insol in acetone, chloroform, ether.

THERAP CAT: Antineoplastic (hormonal).

4527. Gossyplure. [50933-33-0] 7,11-Hexadecadien-1-ol acetate. $C_{18}H_{32}O_2$; mol wt 280.45. C 77.09%, H 11.50%, O 11.41%. Sex pheromone of pink bollworm, *Pectinophora gossypiella* (Saunders): Hummel *et al., Science* **181**, 873 (1973). Isoln and prepn of 1:1 mixture of (*Z,Z*) and (*Z,E*) isomers: B. A. Bierl *et al., J. Econ. Entomol.* **67**, 211 (1974). Improved prepn: R. J. Anderson, C. A. Hendrick, **US 3919329** (1975 to Zoecon); *eidem, J. Am. Chem. Soc.* **97**, 4327 (1975). Stereoselective synthesis of isomers: K. Mori *et al., Agric. Biol. Chem.* **38**, 1551 (1974); *eidem, Tetrahedron* **31**, 1846 (1975); H. Su, P. G. Mahany, *J. Econ. Entomol.* **67**, 319 (1974); H. J. Bestmann *et al., Tetrahedron Lett.* **1976**, 353; J. M. Muchowski, M. C. Venuti, *J. Org. Chem.* **46**, 459 (1981). Activity of isomers: H. M. Flint *et al., Environ. Entomol.* **6**, 274 (1977). Degradn: R. D. Henson, *ibid.* 821.

(Z,Z) - form

Yellow liquid. Sol in most org solvents. Extremely flammable.
(*Z,Z*)-Form. [52207-99-5] bp 130-132°. n_D^{21} 1.4592.
(*Z,E*)-Form. [53042-79-8] bp 132-134°. n_D^{21} 1.4591.
USE: Insect attractant.

4528. Gossypol. [303-45-7] 1,1′,6,6′,7,7′-Hexahydroxy-3,3′-dimethyl-5,5′-bis(1-methylethyl)[2,2′-binaphthalene]-8,8′-dicarboxaldehyde; 2,2′-bis[1,6,7-trihydroxy-3-methyl-5-isopropyl-8-aldehydonaphthalene]; 2,2′-bis[8-formyl-1,6,7-trihydroxy-5-isopropyl-3-methylnaphthalene]. $C_{30}H_{30}O_8$; mol wt 518.55. C 69.49%, H 5.83%, O 24.68%. Yellow pigment found in cottonseed; functions as a natural insecticide in plants. Name derived from the botanical name of the cotton plant, *Gossypium* L., *Malvaceae.* Isoln: J. Longmore, *J. Soc. Chem. Ind.* **5**, 200 (1886); L. Marchlewski, *J. Prakt. Chem.* **60**, 84 (1899); K. N. Campbell *et al.*, *J. Am. Chem. Soc.* **59**, 1723 (1937). Structural studies: R. Adams *et al.*, *ibid.* **60**, 2193 (1938). Synthesis: Edwards, *J. Am. Oil Chem. Soc.* **47**, 441 (1970). NMR studies: J. W. Jaroszewski *et al.*, *NMR Spectrosc. Drug Res.* **26**, 75 (1988). Vibrational CD structural studies: T. B. Freedman *et al.*, *Chirality* **15**, 196 (2003). Prepn of enantiomers: M. K. Dowd, *ibid.* 486. HPLC determn: G. B. Marcelle *et al.*, *J. Pharm. Sci.* **73**, 396 (1984). Metabolism studies: M. B. Abou-Donia *et al.*, *Lipids* **5**, 938 (1970). Mechanism of action study: C.-Y. G. Lee *et al.*, *Mol. Cell. Biochem.* **47**, 65 (1982). Structure-activity study in tumor cell lines: M. D. Shelley *et al.*, *Anti-Cancer Drugs* **11**, 209 (2000). Clinical evaluation in malignant glioma: P. Bushunow *et al.*, *J. Neuro-Oncol.* **43**, 79 (1999); in male contraception: E. M. Coutinho *et al.*, *Contraception* **61**, 61 (2000). Review of chemistry: R. Adams *et al.*, *Chem. Rev.* **60**, 555-574 (1960); of toxicity in livestock: S. E. Morgan, *Vet. Clinics North Am.: Food Anim. Pract.* **5**, 251-262 (1989); of clinical pharmacology and use as a male contraceptive agent: D. Wu, *Drugs* **38**, 333-341 (1989); E. M. Coutinho, *Contraception* **65**, 259-263 (2002).

Exists in 3 tautomeric forms. Yellow crystals from ether, mp 184°; from chloroform, mp 199°; from ligroin, mp 214°. *Light sensitive.* Very sol in methanol, ethanol, cold dioxane, diethylene glycol, ether, ethyl acetate, acetone, carbon tetrachloride, pyridine, chloroform, DMF, lipids. Freely sol (with slow decompn) in dil aq solns of ammonia and sodium carbonate. Slightly sol in glycerol, cyclohexane. Insol in water. Absorption max: 385 nm (ε 18000).

***R*-Form.** [90141-22-3] (−)-gossypol. Bright yellow crystals from acetone, mp 181-184° (dec). $[\alpha]_D^D$ −386 to −390° (c = 0.5 g/100 g soln in CHCl$_3$) (Dowd).

***S*-Form.** [20300-26-9] (+)-gossypol. Isoln from *Thespesia populnea*: T. J. King, L. B. de Silva, *Tetrahedron Lett.* **9**, 261 (1968); S. C. Datta *et al.*, *Indian J. Chem.* **10**, 263 (1972). Synthesis: A. I. Meyers, J. J. Willemsen, *Tetrahedron* **54**, 10493 (1998). Bright yellow crystals from acetone, mp 181-184° (dec). $[\alpha]_D^{28}$ +386 to +390° (c = 0.5 g/100 g soln in CHCl$_3$) (Dowd). uv max (ethanol): 237.5, 277. 378 nm (log ε 4.8, 4.4, 4.2) (Datta).

Gossypol Acetic Acid. [12542-36-8] Bright yellow plates, mp 187° (Adams *et al.*).

Caution: Potentially toxic to animals overfed cottonseed products; symptoms of overexposure may include cardiac failure, shortness of breath, pulmonary edema, and reproductive effects (Morgan).

4529. Gougerotin. [2096-42-6] 1-(4-Amino-2-oxo-1(2*H*)-pyrimidinyl)-1,4-dideoxy-4-[[*N*-(*N*-methylglycyl)-D-seryl]amino]-β-D-glucopyranuronamide; 1-(4-amino-2-oxo-1(2*H*)-pyrimidinyl)-1,4-dideoxy-4-[D-2-[2-(methylamino)acetamido]hydracrylamido]-glucopyranuronamide; 1-[4-deoxy-4-(sarcosyl-D-seryl)amino-β-D-glucopyranuronamide]cytosine; aspiculamycin; asteromycin. C$_{16}$H$_{25}$N$_7$O$_8$; mol wt 443.41. C 43.34%, H 5.68%, N 22.11%, O 28.87%. Antibiotic substance with antibacterial and antineoplastic activity. Isoln from *Streptomyces gougerotii*: Kanzaki *et al.*, *J. Antibiot.* **15A**, 93 (1962). Identity with asteromycin: Ikeuchi *et al.*, *ibid.* **25**, 548 (1972). Structure: Iwasaki, *Yakugaku Zasshi* **82**, 1358 (1962). Revised structure: Fox *et al.*, *Tetrahedron Lett.* **1968**, 6029; Watanabe *et al.*, *Chem. Pharm. Bull.* **17**, 416 (1969). Total synthesis: *eidem*, *J. Am. Chem. Soc.* **94**, 3272 (1972); Lichtenthaler *et al.*, *Tetrahedron Lett.* **1975**, 3527. Identity with aspiculamycin: Lichtenthaler *et al.*, *ibid.* 665. Mechanism of action study: J. C. Lacal *et al.*, *J. Antibiot.* **33**, 441 (1980). *Reviews:* Clark in *Antibiotics* vol. 1, D. Gottlieb, P. D. Shaw, Eds. (Springer-

Verlag, New York, 1967) pp 278-282; Yukioka, *ibid.* vol. 3, J. W. Corcoran, F. E. Hahn, Eds. (1975) pp 448-458.

Needles, mp 211-217° (dec). $[\alpha]_D^{27}$ +53° (c = 0.8). uv max (water): 267, 235 nm (ε 9400, 9300); in 0.1*N* HCl: 275 nm (ε 13600); in 0.1*N* NaOH: 267 nm (ε 9800). LD$_{50}$ in mice (mg/kg): 57 i.v. (Kanzaki).

4530. G-Proteins. GTP binding proteins. Distinct class of membrane associated *guanine nucleotide binding proteins* characterized by their function as couplers between a wide variety of receptors and their effector molecules in transmembrane signalling pathways. An example is the retinal G-protein, *transducin*, which links the photon receptor, rhodopsin, *q.v.*, to cGMP phosphodiesterase. G-Proteins are heterotrimeric, with apparent mol wt of 100 kDa and composed of α, β, γ subunits. The α subunit contains the guanine nucleotide binding site, possesses GTPase activity, and is specific for each G-protein. β and γ subunits form a noncovalent, membrane attached complex. *Reviews:* A. M. Spiegel, *Mol. Cell. Endocrinol.* **49**, 1-16 (1987); idem, *Annu. Rep. Med. Chem.* **23**, 235-242 (1988); P. J. Casey, A. G. Gilman, *J. Biol. Chem.* **263**, 2577-2580 (1988); H. R. Bourne, *Nature* **337**, 504-505 (1989); L. Birnbaumer, *Annu. Rev. Pharmacol. Toxicol.* **30**, 675-705 (1990); M. E. Linder, A. G. Gilman, *Sci. Am.* **267**, 56-65 (July, 1992). Review of role in disease: A. C. Dolphin, *Trends Neurosci.* **10**, 53-57 (1987).

4531. Gramicidin S. [113-73-5] Gramicidin S (Soviet); gramicidin C (Soviet). C$_{60}$H$_{92}$N$_{12}$O$_{10}$; mol wt 1141.45. C 63.13%, H 8.12%, N 14.73%, O 14.02%. Cyclic decapeptide antibiotic produced by a strain of *Bacillus brevis*. Isoln: Gause *et al.*, *Compt. Rend. Acad. Sci. USSR* **43**, 217 (1944), *C.A.* **39**, 1195 (1945); Gause, Brazhnikova, *Lancet* **247**, 715 (1944). More closely related to tyrocidines in biological and chemical properties than to true gramicidins, *q.q.v.* Structure: Synge, *Biochem. J.* **39**, 363 (1945); Consden *et al.*, *ibid.* **40**, xliii (1946); **41**, 596 (1947); Battersby, Craig, *J. Am. Chem. Soc.* **73**, 1887 (1951); Erlanger, Goode, *Nature* **174**, 840 (1954). Synthesis and absorption spectrum: Schwyzer, Sieber, *Helv. Chim. Acta* **40**, 624 (1957); Waki, Izuniya, *Bull. Chem. Soc. Jpn.* **40**, 1687 (1967). Solid phase synthesis: Losse, Neubert, *Tetrahedron Lett.* **1970**, 1267; M. Ohno *et al.*, *J. Am. Chem. Soc.* **93**, 5251 (1971). Improved synthesis via a linear pentapeptide: Y. Minematsu *et al.*, *Tetrahedron Lett.* **1980**, 2179; via a linear decapeptide: T. Mukaiyama *et al.*, *Chem. Lett.* **1981**, 1367. Industrial procedure: GB 836725 (1960 to Ciba). *Review:* Y. A. Ovchinnikov, V. T. Ivanov, "The Cyclic Peptides: Structure, Conformation, and Function" in *The Proteins* vol. V, H. Neurath, R. L. Hill, Eds. (Academic Press, New York, 3rd ed., 1982) pp 547-555.

Hydrochloride. C$_{60}$H$_{92}$N$_{12}$O$_{10}$.2HCl. Prisms from ethanol + aq HCl, dec 277-278°. $[\alpha]_D^{24}$ −289° (c = 0.43 in 70% ethanol). Freely sol in alcohol; slightly sol in acetone. Practically insol in water, acids, alkalies. LD$_{50}$ i.p. in rats: 17 mg/kg (Gause, Brazhnikova).

THERAP CAT: Topical antibacterial.

4532. Gramicidin(s). Gramicidin D (Dubos); linear gramicidins; Gramoderm. Polypeptide antibiotic complex first isolated from the mixture tyrothricin along with tyrocidine, *q.q.v.* from cultures of *Bacillus brevis:* Dubos, Hotchkiss, *J. Exp. Med.* **73,** 629 (1941); *eidem, J. Biol. Chem.* **141,** 155 (1941). Commercial extraction: Baron, **US 2534541** (1950 to Penick). Commercial preparation is a mixture of the four components, gramicidin A, B, C, and D, comprising about 87.5, 7.1, 5.1, 0.3 percent resp: Gross, Witkop, *Biochemistry* **4,** 2495 (1965). Each of the components A, B, and C consist of 2 chains, one with valine in position 1, comprising 80-95% of the component, and the other with isoleucine in position 1. Structure, characterization, and synthesis of the two isoforms of gramicidin A, *N*-formylvaline and isoleucine: Sarges, Witkop, *J. Am. Chem. Soc.* **86,** 1862 (1964); **87,** 2011, 2020 (1965); Bauer *et al., Biochemistry* **11,** 3266 (1972). Structure of gramicidin B: Sarges, Witkop, *J. Am. Chem. Soc.* **87,** 2027 (1965); of gramicidin C: *eidem, Biochemistry* **4,** 2491 (1965). Synthesis of valine-gramicidin B and C: K. Noda, E. Gross in *Chemistry and Biology of Peptides, Proc. 3rd Am. Peptide Symp.,* J. Meienhofer Ed. (Ann Arbor Science Publishers, Michigan, 1972) pp 241-250. *Review:* Hunter, Schwartz, "Gramicidins" in *Antibiotics* I, S. Gottlieb, P. Shaw, Eds. (Springer-Verlag, New York, 1967) pp 642-648. Comprehensive description: G. A. Brewer, *Anal. Profiles Drug Subs.* **8,** 179-218 (1979).

HC–Val–Gly–Ala–D-Leu–Ala–D-Val–Val–D-Val–Trp–D-Leu–Trp–D-Leu–Trp–D-Leu–Trp–NHCH₂CH₂OH
|
O

Valine-Gramicidin A

Spear-shaped or lenticular platelets, mp 229-230°. Almost insol in water (0.6 mg/100 ml). Soluble in the lower alcohols, acetic acid, pyridine. Moderately sol in dry acetone and dioxane. Practically insol in ether, hydrocarbons. Tends to form colloidal suspensions in water.

THERAP CAT: Antibacterial.

THERAP CAT (VET): Antimicrobial.

4533. Gramine. [87-52-5] *N,N*-Dimethyl-1*H*-indole-3-methanamine; 3-(dimethylaminomethyl)indole; Donaxine. $C_{11}H_{14}N_2$; mol wt 174.24. C 75.83%, H 8.10%, N 16.08%. In chlorophyll-deficient mutants of barley: Euler *et al., Z. Physiol. Chem.* **217,** 23 (1933). In the Asiatic reed *Arundo donax* L., *Gramineae:* Orechoff, Norkina, *Ber.* **68,** 436 (1935). From *Acer saccharinum* L. (the Silver Maple) and *A. rubrum* L., *Aceraceae:* Pachter *et al., J. Org. Chem.* **24,** 1285 (1959); Pachter, *J. Am. Pharm. Assoc. Sci. Ed.* **48,** 670 (1959). Synthesis: Kühn, Stein, *Ber.* **70,** 567 (1937). Biosynthesis from tryptophan in barley: Bowden, Marion, *Can. J. Chem.* **29,** 1037 (1951); O'Donovan, Leete, *J. Am. Chem. Soc.* **85,** 461 (1963); Gower, Leete, *ibid.* 3683; *see also* Gross *et al., Tetrahedron Lett.* **1971,** 4047.

Shiny, flat needles or plates from acetone, mp 138-139°. Absorption spectrum: Kanakoa *et al., Chem. Pharm. Bull.* **8,** 294 (1960). Sol in alcohol, ether, chloroform; slightly sol in cold acetone. Practically insol in petr ether, water.

Hydrochloride. $C_{11}H_{14}N_2 \cdot HCl$. Crystals from ethanol + ether, dec 191°. Sol in water.

Methiodide. $C_{11}H_{14}N_2 \cdot CH_3I$. Crystals from methanol + benzene, mp 168-169°. Sol in water: Geissman, Armen, *J. Am. Chem. Soc.* **74,** 3916 (1952).

4534. Granaticin. [19879-06-2] (3a*S*,5*S*,8*S*,9*R*,11*R*,13b*S*,-15*R*)-3,3a,5,8,11,13b-Hexahydro-7,8,12,15-tetrahydroxy-5,9-dimethyl-8,11-ethanofuro[2,3-*e*]naphtho[2,3-*c*:6,7-*c'*]dipyran-2,6,-13(9*H*)-trione; antibiotic WR 141; litmomycin. $C_{22}H_{20}O_{10}$; mol wt 444.39. C 59.46%, H 4.54%, O 36.00%. Antibiotic substance produced by *Streptomyces olivaceus* from soil of Portuguese West Africa. Isoln and antibacterial activity: R. Corbaz *et al., Helv. Chim. Acta* **40,** 1262 (1957). Determn by microbiological diffusion assay: A. Ricicova, M. Podojil, *Folia Microbiol.* **10,** 299 (1965). Isoln of granaticin B, the α-L-rhodinoside of granaticin: S. Barcza *et al., Helv. Chim. Acta* **49,** 1736 (1966); **FR 1525993**; W. Keller, H. Zaehner, **US 3836642** (1968, 1974 both to Ciba-Geigy). Structure

of granaticin and granaticin B: W. Keller-Schierlein *et al., Helv. Chim. Acta* **51,** 1257 (1968); M. Brufani, M. Dobler, *ibid.* 1269; *Naturally Occurring Quinones,* R. H. Thomson, Ed. (Academic Press, New York, 2nd ed., 1971) pp 298-302. Identity of granaticin with antibiotic litmomycin: C.-J. Chang *et al., J. Antibiot.* **28,** 156 (1975). Biosynthesis: C. E. Snipes *et al., J. Nat. Prod.* **42,** 627 (1979); *eidem, J. Am. Chem. Soc.* **101,** 701 (1979). Total synthesis of (±)-form: K. Nomura *et al., ibid.* **109,** 3402 (1987); of the natural (−)-form: K. Okazaki *et al., Chem. Commun.* **1989,** 354. Cytotoxic action on carcinoma cells: E. Sturdik, L. Drobnica, *Neoplasma* **30,** 3 (1983). Inhibition of RNA synthesis: A. Ogilvie *et al., Biochem. J.* **152,** 517 (1975); P. Heinstein, *J. Pharm. Sci.* **71,** 197 (1982).

Deep red, garnet-like crystals from acetone, dec 204-206°. Also reported as mp 211-213° (dec). Acts as an indicator: red in acids, blue in alkalies. Absorption max (abs ethanol): 223, 286, 532, 576 nm (log ε 4.58, 3.76, 3.87, 3.75).

Tetraacetylgranaticin. [1401-59-8] $C_{30}H_{28}O_{14}$. Yellow crystals from alc, mp 242-243°. $[\alpha]_D^{20} -100°$ (c = 0.818 in chloroform).

Granaticin B. [19879-03-9] $C_{28}H_{30}O_{12}$; mol wt 558.53. Red crystalline solid from methanolic-HCl, mp 117-119°. $[\alpha]_D^{22} +17.2°$ (c = 0.83 in pyridine). Absorption max (methanol): 223, 285, 527, 566 nm (log ε 4.42, 3.68, 3.76, 3.57).

4535. Grandisol. [26532-22-9] (1*R-cis*)-1-Methyl-2-(1-methylethenyl)cyclobutaneethanol; *cis*-(+)-2-isopropenyl-1-methylcyclobutaneethanol; (+)-(1*R*,2*S*)-1-(2'-hydroxyethyl)-1-methyl-2-isopropenylcyclobutane. $C_{10}H_{18}O$; mol wt 154.25. C 77.87%, H 11.76%, O 10.37%. Major component of *grandlure,* the sex pheromone of the boll weevil (*Anthonomus grandis,* Boheman). Isoln and synthesis: J. H. Tumlinson *et al., Science* **166,** 1010 (1969); *eidem, J. Org. Chem.* **36,** 2616 (1971). Synthesis of optically active grandisol: P. D. Hobbs, P. D. Magnus, *Chem. Commun.* **1974,** 856; *eidem, J. Am. Chem. Soc.* **98,** 4594 (1976); K. Mori, *Tetrahedron* **34,** 915 (1978); of enantiomerically pure grandisol: J. B. Jones *et al., Can. J. Chem.* **60,** 2007 (1982). Synthesis of racemate: B. M. Trost *et al., J. Am. Chem. Soc.* **99,** 3088 (1977). Short stereoselective synthesis of (±)-grandisol: I. Aljancic-Solaja *et al., Helv. Chim. Acta* **70,** 1302 (1987). Review of syntheses: J. A. Katzenellenbogen, *Science* **194,** 139-148 (1976); J. M. Brand *et al., Fortschr. Chem. Org. Naturst.* **37,** 18-29 (1979), *see also* refs pp 157-190; K. Mori, "The Synthesis of Insect Pheromones" in *The Total Synthesis of Natural Products* vol. 4, J. ApSimon, Ed. (Wiley-Interscience, New York, 1981) pp 80-85.

Liquid, $bp_{1.0}$ 50-60°. $[\alpha]_D^{21.5} +18.5°$ (c = 1 in hexane). n_D^{20} 1.4748.

4536. Granisetron. [109889-09-0] 1-Methyl-*N*-[(3-*endo*)-9-methyl-9-azabicyclo[3.3.1]non-3-yl]-1*H*-indazole-3-carboxamide. $C_{18}H_{24}N_4O$; mol wt 312.41. C 69.20%, H 7.74%, N 17.93%, O 5.12%. Specific serotonin (5HT₃) receptor antagonist. Prepn: F. D. King, **EP 200444**; *idem,* **US 4886808** (1986, 1989 both to Beecham). 5HT₃ receptor binding study: G. J. Kilpatrick *et al., Nature* **330,** 746 (1987). Series of articles on pharmacology and clinical trials to prevent chemotherapy-induced emesis: *Semin. Oncol.* **22,** Suppl. 10, 1-30 (1995).

Hydrochloride. [107007-99-8] BRL-43694A; Kytril. C_{18}-$H_{24}N_4O.HCl$; mol wt 348.87. White to off-white solid, mp 290-292°. Readily sol in water at 20°.

THERAP CAT: Antiemetic.

4537. Granulocyte Colony-Stimulating Factor. [143011-72-7] CSF-β; G-CSF; GM-DF; MGI-2; pluripoietin. Hematopoietic growth factor that stimulates the development of committed progenitor cells to neutrophils and enhances the functional activities of the mature end-cell. Glycoprotein of mol wt 18-22 kDa; produced in response to specific stimulation by a variety of cells including monocytes, fibroblasts and endothelial cells. Murine and human molecules exhibit cross species reactivity. Originally identified as a differentiation factor for murine leukemic cells. Characterization in mouse serum: J. Lotem et al., Int. J. Cancer **25**, 763 (1980); A. W. Burgess, D. Metcalf, ibid. **26**, 647 (1980). Purification of murine G-CSF: N. A. Nicola et al., J. Biol. Chem. **258**, 9017 (1983); of human G-CSF: K. Welte et al., Proc. Natl. Acad. Sci. USA **82**, 1526 (1985); N. Nicola et al., Nature **314**, 625 (1985); H. Nomura et al., EMBO J. **5**, 871 (1986). Production of human G-CSF by recombinant DNA technology: L. M. Souza et al., Science **232**, 61 (1986); S. Nagata et al., Nature **319**, 415 (1986). Review of clinical potential and comparison with GM-CSF: W. P. Steward, Lancet **342**, 153-157 (1993). Reviews: G. D. Demetri, J. D. Griffin, Blood **78**, 2791-2808 (1991); L. S. Tkatch, D. J. Tweardy, Lymphokine Cytokine Res. **12**, 477-488 (1993). Review of role in infectious diseases: D. C. Dale et al., J. Infect. Dis. **172**, 1061-1075 (1995).

Filgrastim. [121181-53-1] N-L-Methionylcolony-stimulating factor (human clone 1034); recombinant methionyl human G-CSF; r-metHuG-CSF; KRN-8601; Neupogen. 175 amino acid peptide produced in E. coli by recombinant DNA technology; mol wt 18.8 kDa. Differs from endogenous human G-CSF by the addition of an N-terminal methionine and the absence of glycosylation. Prepn: L. M. Souza, EP 237545 (1987 to Kirin-Amgen); idem, US 5580755 (1996 to Amgen). Clinical trial in severe chronic neutropenia: D. C. Dale et al., Blood **81**, 2496 (1993). Book: Filgrastim in Clinical Practice, G. Morstyn, T. M. Dexter, Eds. (Marcel Dekker, New York, 1994) 351 pp.

Pegfilgrastim. [208265-92-3] 3-Hydroxypropyl-N-methionyl-colony-stimulating factor (human) 1-ether with α-methyl-ω-hydroxypoly(oxy-1,2-ethanediyl); Neulasta. Pegylated form of filgrastim; modified by the addition of a 20 kDa linear molecule of polyethylene glycol. Pharmacology: G. Molineux et al., Exp. Hematol. **27**, 1724 (1999). Series of articles on chemistry, pharmacokinetics and clinical efficacy: Pharmacotherapy **23**, 1S-19S (2003). Review of prepn and development: G. Molineux, Curr. Pharm. Des. **10**, 1235-1244 (2004); of clinical experience in chemotherapy-induced neutropenia: A.-R. Waladkhani, Eur. J. Cancer Care **13**, 371-379 (2004).

Lenograstim. [135968-09-1] Granocyte; Neutrogin. Glycoprotein with 174 amino acids and 4% sugar chains produced in Chinese hamster ovary cells by recombinant DNA technology; mol wt ~20 kDa. Closely resembles endogenous human G-CSF. Prepn: M. Ono et al., WO 8604605; eidem, EP 215126 (1986, 1987 both to Chugai). Clinical trial in bone-marrow transplantation: C. Gisselbrecht et al., Lancet **343**, 696 (1994). Review of pharmacology and clinical experience: C. J. Dunn, K. L. Goa, Drugs **59**, 681-717 (2000).

Nartograstim. [134088-74-7] 1-(N-L-Methionyl-L-alanine)-3-L-threonine-4-L-tyrosine-5-L-arginine-17-L-serinecolony-stimulating factor (human clone 1034); marograstim; KW-2228; Neu-up. G-CSF mutein of 175 amino acids produced in E. coli by recombinant DNA technology; mol wt 18.9 kDa. Prepn: Y. Yokoo et al., JP 2234692 (1990 to Kyowa), C.A. **114**, 183900 (1991). In vitro activity: T. Suzuki et al., Acta Haematol. **87**, 181 (1992). ELISA determn in plasma: T. Kuwabara et al., J. Pharmacobio-Dyn. **25**, 121 (1992).

THERAP CAT: Hematopoietic; antineutropenic.

4538. Granulocyte-Macrophage Colony-Stimulating Factor. [83869-56-1] Colony-stimulating factor-2; CSF-2; CSFα; GM-CSF; NIF-T. Hematopoietic growth factor that stimulates the development of neutrophils and macrophages and promotes the proliferation and development of early erythroid, megakaryocytic and eosinophilic progenitor cells. Produced by endothelial cells, monocytes, fibroblasts and T lymphocytes. Inhibits neutrophil migration and enhances the functional activities of the mature end-cells. Purification of murine GM-CSF: A. W. Burgess et al., J. Biol. Chem. **252**, 1998 (1977); of human GM-CSF: N. A. Nicola et al., Blood **54**, 614 (1979); and identity with neutrophil migration inhibition factor (NIF-T): J. C. Gasson et al., Science **226**, 1339 (1984). Partial amino acid sequence of murine: L. G. Sparrow et al., Proc. Natl. Acad. Sci. USA **82**, 292 (1985). Cloning and expression of murine GM-CSF: N. M. Gough et al., Nature **309**, 763 (1984); of human: G. G. Wong et al., Science **228**, 810 (1985); F. Lee et al., Proc. Natl. Acad. Sci. USA **82**, 4360 (1985); M. A. Cantrell et al., ibid. 6250. Pharmacokinetics: W. P. Petros, Pharmacotherapy **12**, Suppl 2-2, 32S (1992). Clinical comparison with G-CSF: S. Blackwell, J. Crawford, ibid. 20S. Review: J. C. Gasson, Blood **77**, 1131-1145 (1991). Review of clinical and biological effects: S. G. Louie, B. Jung, Am. J. Hosp. Pharm. **50**, Suppl 3, S10-S18 (1993).

Molgramostim. [99283-10-0] Colony-stimulating factor 2 (human clone pHG25 protein moiety reduced); Sch-39300; Leucomax. Nonglycosylated peptide of 127 amino acids produced in E. coli by recombinant DNA technology. Mol wt 14.5 kDa. Pharmacokinetics in AIDS and ARC: R. G. Hewitt et al., Antimicrob. Agents Chemother. **37**, 512 (1993).

Regramostim. [127757-91-9] Colony-stimulating factor 2 (human clone pCSF-1 protein moiety reduced) glycoform GMC 89-107. Glycoprotein of 127 amino acids produced in Chinese hamster ovary cells by recombinant DNA technology. Mol wt 21-34 kDa.

Sargramostim. [123774-72-1] 23-L-Leucinecolony-stimulating factor 2 (human clone pHG25 protein moiety); BI 61.012; Leukine; Prokine. Variably glycosylated glycoprotein of 127 amino acids produced in yeast by recombinant DNA technology. Mol wt 15.5-19.5 kDa. Differs from endogenous human GM-CSF by the substitution of a leucine moiety at position 23 of the amino acid sequence. Clinical evaluation in myelodysplasia: W. J. Gradishar et al., Blood **80**, 2463 (1992); in Crohn's disease: J. R. Korzenik et al., N. Engl. J. Med. **352**, 2193 (2005).

THERAP CAT: Hematopoietic; antineutropenic.

4539. Graphite. [7782-42-5] Plumbago; black lead; mineral carbon. Obtained by mining, especially in Canada and Ceylon. Monograph: A. R. Ubbelohde, F. A. Lewis, Graphite and Its Crystal Compounds (Oxford, 1960). Review: Holliday et al. in Comprehensive Inorganic Chemistry vol. 1, J. C. Bailar, Jr. et al., Eds. (Pergamon Press, Oxford, 1973) pp 1250-1294.

Crystallized carbon with traces of Fe, SiO_2, etc. Usually soft, black scales, crystals rare. d 2.09-2.23. Mohs' hardness = 1.0. Commercial varieties usually withstand temps up to 2820°. Sol in molten iron.

Caution: Potential symptoms of overexposure are coughing, dyspnea, black sputum, decreased pulmonary function and lung fibrosis. See NIOSH Pocket Guide to Chemical Hazards (DHHS/-NIOSH 97-140, 1997) p 154.

USE: For "lead" pencils, refractory crucibles, stove polish; as pigment, lubricant, graphite cement; for matches and explosives; commutator brushes, anodes, arc-lamp carbons, electroplating; polishing compds, rust and needle-paper; coating for cathode ray tubes; moderator in nuclear piles.

4540. Graphite Fluoride. [11113-63-6] Fluorine compd with graphite. Non-wettable layered solid, CF_x, (0.5<x<1.3), obtained by direct fluorination of graphite at high temp. Two covalent forms have been produced by controlling the quality of the graphite and the reaction temp: $(CF)_n$ at (300°-600°) and $(C_2F)_n$ at (350°-400°). Composition and color are a function of the fluorination temp; the F/C ratio increases with increasing temp, and color changes from black to gray to white. Prepn: O. Ruff, O. Bretschneider, Z. Anorg. Allg. Chem. **217**, 1 (1934); and thermal/electrical characteristics: C.-C. Hung et al., SAMPE Q. **19**, 12 (1988). Evaluation as solid lubricant of $(CF_x)_n$: R. L. Fusaro, H. E. Sliney, ASLE Trans. **13**, 56 (1970); of $(C_2F)_n$: H. Miyake et al., Proc. JSLE Int. Tribiol. Conf. **2**, 395 (1985). Lubrication mechanism and wear life: R. L. Fusaro, *Wear* **53**, 303 (1979). Brief review of physical properties: Central Glass Co. in *Proc. BMRA Symp.*, Brussels 1983, A. Kozawa, M. Nagayama, Eds. (Battery Mat. Res. Assoc., 1984) 135-141; of prepn, properties and uses: T. Nakajima, N. Watanabe, *Chemtech* **1990**, 426-430. Book: N. Watanabe *et al.*, *Graphite Fluorides* (Elsevier Press, Amsterdam, 1988), 262 pp.

(**CF**)ₙ. Poly(carbon monofluoride); Cefbon-CF. Gray-white (commercial). d 2.58 g/cm³; packed bulk density 0.7 g/cm³. Insol in all solvents. Fluorine content: 61-64 wt%.

(**C₂F**)ₙ. Poly(dicarbon monofluoride); Cefbon-C₂F. Dark gray-black (commercial). d 2.79 g/cm³; packed bulk density 0.8 g/cm³. Insol in all solvents. Fluorine content: 49-53 wt%.

USE: Solid lubricant; as cathode material in lithium-fluoride batteries; in controlling wettability of surfaces.

4541. Graphitic Acid. [1399-57-1] Graphite oxide; graphitic oxide. This material, obtained by oxidation of graphite, was first prepd by Brodie in 1859; Hummers, Offeman, *J. Am. Chem. Soc.* **80**, 1339 (1958). Its composition is not well defined but usually given as C₄O(OH): Aragon de la Cruz, Cowley, *Nature* **196**, 468 (1962), *Acta Crystallogr.* **16**, 531 (1963). Prepn and manufacture: Hummers, **US 2798878** (1957 to National Lead); Hummers, Offeman, *loc. cit.*; Ruskin, **US 2933381** and **US 2944881** (both 1960 to Union Carbide). Crystal structure: Aragon de la Cruz, Cowley, *loc. cit.*

Very light to dark brown, or yellowish-brown solid.

USE: In rocket propellant mixtures.

4542. Gravitol(e). [6006-09-3] 2-(2-Allyl-6-methoxyphenoxy)triethylamine; 2-methoxy-6-allylphenol diethylaminoethyl ether; Clavitol; Uterol. C₁₆H₂₅NO₂; mol wt 263.38. C 72.96%, H 9.57%, N 5.32%, O 12.15%. Prepn: Slotta, *Grundriss der modernen Arzneistoff-Synthese* (Stuttgart, 1931) p 118; H. Hahl, **DE 433182** (1926 to I.G. Farbenind.), *Frdl.* **15**, 1500; *Chem. Zentralbl.* **1926**, II, 2223; H. Pal'gi, *Zh. Obshch. Khim. Eng. Ed.* **28**, 2275 (1958). Pharmacology: E. Käer, G. Barkan, *Arch. Exp. Pathol. Pharmakol.* **170**, 111 (1933).

Oily liq. bp₁₀ 160-161°; bp₂.₃ 141-144°. nᴅ²⁴·⁵ 1.5075. Slightly sol in water.

Hydrochloride. C₁₆H₂₆ClNO₂. Crystals, freely sol in water.

4543. Grayanotoxins. Toxic diterpenoids present in leaves of the various species of *Rhododendron*, *Kalmia*, and *Leucothoe*, *Ericaceae*; also found in honey from rhododendron flowers. Eighteen grayanotoxins have been isolated, the first three being the most important. Isoln of grayanotoxins I, II, III: Kakisawa *et al.*, *Tetrahedron* **21**, 3091 (1965); of IV and V: Okuno *et al.*, *ibid.* **26**, 4765 (1970); of V, VI, and VII: Hikino *et al.*, *Chem. Pharm. Bull.* **18**, 2357 (1970); of VIII, IX, X, and XI: Hikino *et al.*, *ibid.* **19**, 1289 (1971); of XII and XIII: Hikino *et al.*, *ibid.* **20**, 422 (1972). Approaches to synthesis of the grayanotoxin skeleton: T. Shiozaki *et al.*, *Tetrahedron Lett.* **1972**, 657; T. Kametani *et al.*, *Chem. Pharm. Bull.* **27**, 152 (1979); *eidem*, *Tetrahedron Lett.* **22**, 2379 (1981); *eidem*, *Tetrahedron* **37**, 3813 (1981). Toxicity study: H. Hikino *et al.*, *Toxicol. Appl. Pharmacol.* **35**, 303 (1976).

	R₁	R₂	R₃
Grayanotoxin I	OH	CH₃	COCH₃
Grayanotoxin III	OH	CH₃	H
Grayanotoxin II	R₁R₂ = =CH₂		R₃ = H

Grayanotoxin I. [4720-09-6] (3β,6β,14R)-Grayanotoxane-3,-5,6,10,14,16-hexol 14-acetate; G-I; acetylandromedol; andromedotoxin; rhodotoxin; asebotoxin. C₂₂H₃₆O₇; mol wt 412.52. From *Leucothoe grayana* Max., *Ericaceae:* Miyajimi, Takei, *J. Agric. Chem. Soc. Jpn.* **10**, 1093 (1934); from *Rhododendron maximum* L., *Ericaceae:* Wood *et al.*, *J. Am. Chem. Soc.* **76**, 5689 (1954). Identity with acetylandromedol, andromedotoxin, rhodotoxin: Tallent *et al.*, *ibid.* **79**, 4548 (1957). Stereochemistry: Iwasa, Nakamura, *Tetrahedron Lett.* **1969**, 3973; Narayanan *et al.*, *ibid.* **1970**, 3943; Hikino *et al.*, *Chem. Pharm. Bull.* **18**, 1071 (1970). Approach to synthesis: Okuno, Matsumoto, *Tetrahedron Lett.* **1969**, 4077. Has hypotensive action: Moran *et al.*, *J. Pharmacol. Exp. Ther.* **110**, 415 (1954). Crystals from ethyl acetate, mp 258-260 to 267-270°, depending on rate of heating. [α]ᴅ²⁵ −8.8° (c = 2.3 in ethanol). Sol in hot water, alcohol, acetic acid, hot chloroform; very slightly sol in benzene, ether, petr ether. LD₅₀ i.p. in mice: 1.31 mg/kg (Hikino, 1976).

Grayanotoxin II. [4678-44-8] (3β,6β,14R)-Grayanotox-10(20)-ene-3,5,6,14,16-pentol; G-II; deacetylanhydroandromedotoxin. C₂₀H₃₂O₅; mol wt 352.47. From *L. grayana* Max., *Ericaceae:* Miyajimi, Takei, *loc. cit.* Identity with deacetylanhydromedotoxin: Meguri, *Yakugaku Zasshi* **79**, 1060 (1959); *C.A.* **54**, 5599g (1960). Stereochemistry: Iwasa, Nakamura, *loc. cit.*; Kumazawa, Iriye, *Tetrahedron Lett.* **1970**, 927; Yasue *et al.*, *Chem. Pharm. Bull.* **18**, 2586 (1970). Synthesis: S. Gasa *et al.*, *Tetrahedron Lett.* **1976**, 553. Columnar crystals, mp 199-200°. [α]ᴅ²⁸ −41.88°. LD₅₀ i.p. in mice: 26.1 mg/kg (Hikino, 1976).

Grayanotoxin III. [4678-45-9] (3β,6β,14R)-Grayanoxane-3,5,6,10,14,16-hexol; G-III; deacetylandromedotoxin. C₂₀H₃₄O₆; mol wt 370.48. From *L. grayana* Max., *Ericaceae:* Miyajimi, Takei, *J. Agric. Chem. Soc. Jpn.* **12**, 947 (1936), *C.A.* **30**, 6747⁹ (1936). Stereochemistry: Hikino *et al.*, *Chem. Pharm. Bull.* **18**, 1071 (1970). LD₅₀ i.p. in mice: 0.84 mg/kg (Hikino, 1976).

4544. Green Fluorescent Protein. GFP. Class of autofluorescent proteins found in bioluminescent coelenterates where they function as energy transfer acceptors, emitting a green fluorescent light (λ_max = 509 nm). Acidic globular proteins consisting of 238 amino acids, monomeric mol wt ~30,000. Developed commercially as a biochemical tool to visualize cellular structure and monitor dynamic cellular events via fluorescence resonance energy transfer (FRET) assays. Purifn, characterization and energry transfer studies from *Aequorea victoria:* H. Morise *et al.*, *Biochemistry* **13**, 2656 (1974); from *Renilla reniformis:* W. W. Ward, M. J. Cormier, *J. Biol. Chem.* **254**, 781 (1979). Properties of naturally occurring proteins: M. Chalfie, *Photochem. Photobiol.* **62**, 651 (1995). Structural studies of chromophore fragment: G. N. Phillips, Jr., *Curr. Opin. Struct. Biol.* **7**, 821 (1997); B. R. Branchini *et al.*, *J. Am. Chem. Soc.* **120**, 1 (1998). Fluorescence and spectral properties of variants genetically engineered for enhanced fluorescence: G. H. Patterson *et al.*, *Biophys. J.* **73**, 2782 (1997); R. H. Stauber *et al.*, *BioTechniques* **24**, 462 (1998); for Ca²⁺ visualization: T. Nagai *et al.*, *Proc. Natl. Acad. Sci. USA* **98**, 3197 (2001). Review of expression and detection: S. R. Kain, P. Kitts, *Methods Mol. Biol.* **63**, 305-324 (1997). Review of research applications: T. Misteli, D. L. Spector, *Nat. Biotechnol.* **15**, 961-964 (1997); as reporter gene: S. R. Kain *et al.*, *BioTechniques* **19**, 650-655 (1995); as fluorescent protein tag: H.-H. Gerdes, C. Kaether, *FEBS Lett.* **389**, 44-47 (1996). Bibliography: L. J. Kricka, P. E. Stanley, *J. Biolumin. Chemilumin.* **12**, 113-134 (1997).

USE: Research tool in cell biology.

4545. Grepafloxacin. [119914-60-2] 1-Cyclopropyl-6-fluoro-1,4-dihydro-5-methyl-7-(3-methyl-1-piperazinyl)-4-oxo-3-quinolinecarboxylic acid. C₁₉H₂₂FN₃O₃; mol wt 359.39. C 63.50%, H 6.17%, F 5.29%, N 11.69%, O 13.36%. Fluorinated quinolone antibacterial. Prepn: J. M. Domagala *et al.*, **WO 8906649**; *eidem*, **US 4920120** (1989, 1990 both to Warner-Lambert); S. E. Hagen *et al.*, *J. Med. Chem.* **34**, 1155 (1991). Comparative *in vitro* activity: F. Marco *et al.*, *J. Antimicrob. Chemother.* **33**, 647 (1994); R. C. Arduino *et al.*, *ibid.* **34**, 403. HPLC determn in human bronchoalveolar lavage samples: J. M. Woodcock *et al.*, *FEMS Microbiol. Lett.* **119**, 315 (1994). Clinical pharmacokinetics: J. Child *et al.*, *Antimicrob. Agents Chemother.* **39**, 513 (1995). Tissue concentration in lung: P. J. Cook *et al.*, *J. Antimicrob.*

Chemother. **35,** 317 (1995). Review of pharmacology and clinical trials: A. J. Wagstaff, J. A. Balfour, *Drugs* **53,** 817-824 (1997).

Dihydrate. mp 190-192°.

Hydrochloride. [161967-81-3] OPC-17116; Raxar. $C_{19}H_{22}$-$FN_3O_3 \cdot HCl$; mol wt 395.86.

THERAP CAT: Antibacterial.

4546. Grindelia. Gum-plant (of California). Dried leaves and flowering tops of *Grindelia camporum* Greene or of *G. humilis* H. & A. (*G. cuneifolia* Auth.), *Compositae. Habit.* North America (California). *Constit.* Volatile oil, over 20% resin, grindelol, saponin, tannin, robustic acid.

THERAP CAT: Expectorant.

4547. Grindelic Acid. [1438-57-9] (1′*R*,4′a*S*,5*S*,8′a*S*)-4,-4′a,5,5′,6′,7′,8′,8′a-Octahydro-2′,5,5′,5′,8′a-pentamethylspiro[furan-2(3*H*),1′(4′*H*)-naphthalene]-5-acetic acid; 9,13-epoxylabd-7-en-15-oic acid. $C_{20}H_{32}O_3$; mol wt 320.47. C 74.96%, H 10.06%, O 14.98%. Major grindelane diterpenoid isolated from the resin of *Grindelia robusta* Nutt., *Compositae.* Isoln and structure: L. Panizzi *et al., Gazz. Chim. Ital.* **92,** 522 (1962). Stereochemical studies: L. Mangoni, M. Belardini, *ibid.* **92,** 1379 (1962); **93,** 455, 465 (1963). Synthesis: M. Adinolfi *et al., ibid.* **106,** 625 (1976). Absolute configuration: M. Adinolfi *et al., Phytochemistry* **27,** 1878 (1988); L. A. Paquette, H.-L. Wang, *J. Org. Chem.* **61,** 5352 (1996).

Crystals from acetic acid, mp 100-101°. $[\alpha]_D$ −102.2°.

Methyl ester. $C_{21}H_{34}O_3$. Crystals from methanol, mp 70-70.5°. $[\alpha]_D$ −134.1° (c = 1.46 in methanol).

4548. Grisein. [1391-82-8] Antibiotic substance produced by strains of *Streptomyces griseus.* Isoln: Reynolds *et al., Proc. Soc. Exp. Biol. Med.* **64,** 50 (1947); Reynolds, Waksman, *J. Bacteriol.* **55,** 739 (1948). Improved method of isoln: F. A. Kuehl, L. Chaiet, US 2505053 (1950 to Merck & Co.); F. A. Kuehl *et al., J. Am. Chem. Soc.* **73,** 1770 (1951). Analysis of composition: C_{40}-$H_{61}FeN_{10}O_{20}S$. Degradation of grisein by acid hydrolysis yielded 3-methyluracil and at least two amino acids. One of the acids appears to be glutamic acid: F. A. Kuehl *et al., loc. cit.* Probably is a mixture of components; similar or identical to albomycin, *q.v.*: Stapley, Ormond, *Science* **125,** 587 (1957); Turková *et al., Collect. Czech. Chem. Commun.* **31,** 2444 (1966). Toxicity study: V. I. Aksenov, *Veterinariya (Moscow)* **12,** 93 (1974), *C.A.* **83,** 54127d (1975). Biosynthesis: V. V. Kuklin *et al., Antibiotiki* **25,** 403 (1980), *C.A.* **93,** 146173a (1980).

Amorphous red powder. Sol in water; slightly sol in 95% alcohol. Practically insol in abs alcohol, ether, acetone, chloroform, benzene. The activity remains unchanged when an aq soln is heated to 100° for 10 min. LD_{50} in mice (mg/kg): 600 orally; 34 s.c. (Aksenov).

4549. Griseofulvin. [126-07-8] (1′*S*,6′*R*)-7-Chloro-2′,4,6-trimethoxy-6′-methylspiro[benzofuran-2(3*H*),1′-[2]cyclohexene]-3,4′-dione; 7-chloro-4,6-dimethoxycoumaran-3-one-2-spiro-1′-(2′-methoxy-6′-methylcyclohex-2′-en-4′-one); amudane; Curling factor; Fulcin; Fulvicin; Grifulvin; Grisactin; Griséfuline; Grisovin; Gris-PEG; Grysio; Lamoryl; Likuden; Polygris; Poncyl-FP; Spiro-

fulvin; Sporostatin. $C_{17}H_{17}ClO_6$; mol wt 352.77. C 57.88%, H 4.86%, Cl 10.05%, O 27.21%. Antibiotic substance produced by *Penicillium griseofulvum* Dierckx and by *P. janczewskii* Zal. [same as *P. nigricans* (Banier)Thom]. Isoln: Oxford *et al., Biochem. J.* **33,** 240 (1939); Brian *et al., Trans. Br. Mycol. Soc.* **29,** 173 (1946); Hockenhull, Dorey *et al.,* US 3069328, US 3069329 (both 1962 to Glaxo). Structure: Grove *et al., Chem. Ind. (London)* **1951,** 219; *J. Chem. Soc.* **1952,** 3977. Stereochemistry: MacMillan, *ibid.* **1959,** 1823; Brown, Sim, *ibid.* **1963,** 1050. Total synthesis: Brossi *et al., Helv. Chim. Acta* **43,** 1444, 2071 (1960); Taub *et al., Tetrahedron* **19,** 1 (1963); Stork, Tomasz, *J. Am. Chem. Soc.* **86,** 471 (1964); S. Danishefsky, F. J. Walker, *ibid.* **101,** 7018 (1979). Conformation: Levine, Hicks, *Tetrahedron Lett.* **1971,** 311. Crystal structure: G. Malmros *et al., Cryst. Struct. Commun.* **6,** 463 (1977). Review and evaluation of studies of carcinogenic action in laboratory animals: *IARC Monographs* **10,** 153-161 (1976). *Review:* Grove, *Q. Rev. Chem. Soc.* **17,** 1 (1963); Huber in *Antibiotics* vol. 3, J. W. Corcoran, F. E. Hahn, Eds. (Springer-Verlag, New York, 1975) pp 606-613. Comprehensive description: E. R. Townley, *Anal. Profiles Drug Subs.* **8,** 219-249 (1979).

Stout octahedra or rhombs from benzene, mp 220°. $[\alpha]_D^{17}$ +370° (satd $CHCl_3$ soln). uv max: 286, 325 nm. Soly in DMF at 25°: 12 to 14 g/100 ml. Slightly sol in ethanol, methanol, acetone, benzene, $CHCl_3$, ethyl acetate, acetic acid. Practically insol in water, pet ether.

THERAP CAT: Antifungal.

THERAP CAT (VET): Antifungal.

4550. Grubbs' Catalyst. [172222-30-9] (*SP*-5-31)-Dichloro(phenylmethylene)bis(tricyclohexylphosphine)ruthenium; benzylidenebis(tricyclohexylphosphine)ruthenium dichloride. C_{43}-$H_{72}Cl_2P_2Ru$; mol wt 822.96. C 62.76%, H 8.82%, Cl 8.62%, P 7.53%, Ru 12.28%. Transition metal catalyst. Prepn: P. Schwab *et al., Angew. Chem. Int. Ed.* **34,** 2039 (1995); and of related catalysts: *eidem, J. Am. Chem. Soc.* **118,** 100 (1996). Ring-closing metathesis intoduction of carbon-carbon crosslinks in peptides: S. J. Miller *et al., ibid.* 9606. Mechanism of ring-opening metathesis: J. A. Tallarico *et al., ibid.* **119,** 7157 (1997). Yne-ene cross metathesis: M. Schuster, S. Blechert, *Tetrahedron Lett.* **39,** 2295 (1998). Review of use and prepn: A. Fürstner, *Angew. Chem. Int. Ed.* **39,** 3012-3043 (2000).

Purple air-stable microcrystalline solid.

USE: Catalysis of olefin metathesis including ring-closing of dienes, cross metathesis and ring-opening metathesis polymerizations (ROMP).

4551. Grundmann's Ketone. [66251-18-1] (1*R*,3a*R*,7a*R*)-1-[(1*R*)-1,5-Dimethylhexyl]octahydro-7a-methyl-4*H*-inden-4-one; (1*R*,3a*R*,7a*R*)-7a-methyl-1-((*R*)-6-methylheptan-2-yl)-octahydro-inden-4-one; Windaus-Grundmann ketone. $C_{18}H_{32}O$; mol wt 264.45. C 81.75%, H 12.20%, O 6.05%. Prepd by ozonolysis of vitamin D_3, *q.v.* Preparative method: A. Windaus, W. Grundmann, *Ann.* **524,** 295 (1936). Prepn: H. H. Inhoffen *et al., Ber.* **90,** 664 (1957). Synthetic applications: H. Nemoto *et al., J. Org. Chem.* **51,** 5311 (1986); P. Bovicelli *et al., ibid.* **57,** 5052 (1992); M. C. Clasby, D. Craig, *Synth. Commun.* **24,** 481 (1994); R. R. Sicinski, H. F. DeLuca, *Bioorg. Med. Chem. Lett.* **5,** 159 (1995); W. H. Okamura *et al., J. Org. Chem.* **67,** 1637 (2002).

Colorless oil, bp$_{0.001}$ 115-120°. [α]$_D^{20}$ +8.9°.

USE: Intermediate in the synthesis of vitamin D active compounds.

4552. Guaiac. [9000-29-7] Gum guaiac; resin guaiac; guaiacum. Resin from *lignum vitae*, the wood of *Guajacum officinale* L. or *G. sanctum* L., *Zygophyllaceae. Constit.* About 70% α- and β-guaiaconic acids, about 11% guaiacic acid, related compds and guaiaretic acid, 15% vanillin, guaiac yellow, guaiac saponin (guaiacin). Use as clinical reagent for occult blood: R. H. Wilkinson, W. A. F. Penfold, *Lancet* **2**, 847 (1969). Acute toxicity: P. M. Jenner *et al., Food Cosmet. Toxicol.* **2**, 327 (1964).

Brown or greenish-brown, irregular lumps. mp 85-90°. Insol in water. Freely sol in alcohol, chloroform, ether, creosote, soln of chloral hydrate, alkalies; slightly sol in benzene, carbon disulfide. LD$_{50}$ orally in rats: >5000 mg/kg (Jenner).

USE: Clinical reagent (blood or hemoglobin).

4553. Guaiacol. [90-05-1] 2-Methoxyphenol; methylcatechol; *o*-hydroxyanisole; 1-hydroxy-2-methoxybenzene; Anastil. C$_7$H$_8$O$_2$; mol wt 124.14. C 67.73%, H 6.50%, O 25.78%. Isolated from guaiac resin: Sobrero, *Ann.* **48**, 19 (1843); from hardwood tar: McGinness *et al., Tappi* **43**, 1027 (1960). Prepd by mercuric oxide oxidation of lignin: Lewis, Pearl, US 2433227 (1947 to Sulphite Prod.); by oxidation of anisole with trifluoroperoxyacetic acid: McClure, Williams, *J. Org. Chem.* **27**, 627 (1962); from acetovanillone + ZnCl$_2$: Read, US 3057927 (1962 to Ontario Res. Found.); from the diazonium salt of *o*-anisidine: Herbst, DE 1148236 (1963 to Hoechst). Toxicity data: Taylor *et al., Toxicol. Appl. Pharmacol.* **6**, 378 (1964).

White or slightly yellow cryst mass or colorless to yellowish, very refractive liquid; characteristic odor. Darkens on exposure to air and light. d (crystals) 1.129; d (liq) ~1.112. Solidif 28°, but may remain liq for a long time even at a much lower temp. bp 204-206°; bp$_4$ 53-55°. One gram dissolves in 60-70 ml water, 1 ml glycerol; miscible with alcohol, chloroform, ether, oils, glacial acetic acid. Slightly sol in petr ether; sol in NaOH soln; with moderately concd KOH it forms a sparingly sol compd. *Protect from light.* LD$_{50}$ orally in rats: 725 mg/kg (Taylor).

Phenylacetate. [4112-89-4] Gujaphenyl; Gunyl. C$_{15}$H$_{14}$O$_3$; mol wt 242.27.

THERAP CAT: Expectorant.

THERAP CAT (VET): Expectorant.

4554. Guaiazulene. [489-84-9] 1,4-Dimethyl-7-(1-methylethyl)azulene; 7-isopropyl-1,4-dimethylazulene; *S*-guaiazulene; AZ 8; AZ 8 Beris; Eucazulen; Kessazulen; Vaumigan. C$_{15}$H$_{18}$; mol wt 198.30. C 90.85%, H 9.15%. Isoln from chamomile oil: Sorm *et al., Collect. Czech. Chem. Commun.* **16**, 626 (1951); from guaiac wood oil: Joos, CH 314487 (1956), *C.A.* **52**, 443b (1958). Total synthesis: Plattner *et al., Helv. Chim. Acta* **32**, 2452 (1949); Sorm *et al., Collect. Czech. Chem. Commun.* **16**, 168 (1951); Jacob *et al., Tetrahedron* **20**, 2821 (1964); J. Mukherjee *et al., J. Am. Chem. Soc.* **101**, 251 (1979). Pharmacokinetics of guaiazulene soluble in animals: H. Mukai *et al., J. Pharmacobio-Dyn.* **8**, 329, 337 (1985). Effect on gastric and duodenal ulcers in rats: S. Okabe *et al., Nippon Yakurigaku Zasshi* **88**, 467 (1986), *C.A.* **106**, 43769 (1987).

Blue oil. bp$_{10}$ 165-170°.

3-Sulfonate sodium salt. [6223-35-4] 5-Isopropyl-3,8-dimethyl-1-azulenesulfonic acid sodium salt; sodium gualenate; guaiazulene soluble; Azulon. C$_{15}$H$_{17}$NaO$_3$S; mol wt 300.35.

Trinitrobenzene deriv. [4968-29-0] C$_{15}$H$_{18}$·C$_6$H$_3$N$_3$O$_6$. Violet to black needles from ethanol, mp 151°.

THERAP CAT: Anti-inflammatory; antiulcerative.

4555. Guaifenesin. [93-14-1] 3-(2-Methoxyphenoxy)-1,2-propanediol; glycerol mono(2-methoxyphenyl) ether; glycerol α-(2-methoxyphenyl) ether; guaiacyl glyceryl ether; glyceryl guaiacyl ether; glycerol guaiacolate; α-glyceryl guaiacol ether; *o*-methoxyphenyl glyceryl ether; guaiphenesin; guaiacuran; MY-301; XL-90; Colrex; Mucinex; Myoscain; Relaxil G; Resyl; Robitussin. C$_{10}$H$_{14}$O$_4$; mol wt 198.22. C 60.59%, H 7.12%, O 32.29%. Centrally acting muscle relaxant with expectorant properties. Prepn: Marle, *J. Chem. Soc.* **101**, 305 (1912); Yale *et al., J. Am. Chem. Soc.* **72**, 3710 (1950); Roviralta, Astoul, ES 212920 (1954), *C.A.* **49**, 8332b (1955). Prepn from 2-methoxyphenol and glycidol: W. Merk *et al.,* DE 3106995; *eidem,* US 4390732 (1982, 1983 to Degussa AG). GLC determn in blood: W. R. Maynard, R. B. Bruce, *J. Pharm. Sci.* **59**, 1346 (1970). Clinical use in chronic respiratory disease: D. G. Workman *et al., Curr. Ther. Res.* **7**, 665 (1965). Clinical efficacy as antitussive: J. J. Kuhn *et al., Chest* **82**, 713 (1982). Pharmacokinetics and cardiopulmonary effects in horses: J. A. E. Hubbell *et al., Am. J. Vet. Res.* **41**, 1751 (1980). Use in equine anesthesia: J. L. Grandy, W. N. McDonell, *J. Am. Vet. Med. Assoc.* **176**, 619 (1980); G. J. Brouwer, *Equine Vet. J.* **17**, 133 (1985).

Minute rhombic prisms from ether, mp 78.5-79°. bp$_{19}$ 215°. Slightly bitter aromatic taste. One gram dissolves in 20 ml water at 25°. Much more sol in hot water; freely sol in ethanol; sol in chloroform, glycerol, propylene glycol, DMF; moderately sol in benzene. Practically insol in petr ether.

THERAP CAT: Expectorant

THERAP CAT (VET): Expectorant; muscle relaxant.

4556. Guaiol. [489-86-1] [3S-(3α,5α,8α)]-1,2,3,4,5,6,7,8-Octahydro-α,α,3,8-tetramethyl-5-azulenemethanol; 3,8-dimethyl-5-(α-hydroxyisopropyl)-Δ^9-octahydroazulene; champaca camphor; champacol; guaiac alcohol; Guajol. C$_{15}$H$_{26}$O; mol wt 222.37. C 81.02%, H 11.79%, O 7.19%. A sesquiterpene alc from guaiac wood: *Michelia champaca* L., *Magnoliaceae:* also from oil of wood of *Bulnesia sarmienti* Lorentz, *Zygophyllaceae.* Isoln: Plattner, Lemay, *Helv. Chim. Acta* **23**, 897 (1940). Structure: Plattner, Magyar, *ibid.* **25**, 581 (1942). Stereochemistry: Takeda, Minato, *Tetrahedron Lett.* **1960** (22), 33; Minato, *Chem. Pharm. Bull.* **9**, 625 (1961); *idem, Tetrahedron* **18**, 365 (1962). Total synthesis of *dl*-form: Buchanan, Young, *Chem. Commun.* **1971**, 643; *eidem, J. Chem. Soc. Perkin Trans. 1* **1973**, 2404; Marshall *et al., Tetrahedron Lett.* **1971**, 885; Marshall, Greene, *J. Org. Chem.* **37**, 982 (1972); Andersen, Uh, *Tetrahedron Lett.* **1973**, 2079.

Trigonal pyramidal crystals from alc, mp 91°. d_{20}^{100} 0.9074. bp_{760} 288° (slight decompn); bp_{17} 165°; bp_{10} 148°. $[\alpha]_D^{20}$ −30° (c = 4 in alc). n_D^{100} 1.4716. Sol in alc, ether. Insol in water.

Methyl ether. $C_{16}H_{28}O$. Liq, d_4^{25} 0.9332. bp_9 142°. $[\alpha]_D^{20}$ −31.8°. $n_D^{18.5}$ 1.4896.

Note: The name "guaiol" is also applied to 1,2-dimethylacrolein, isolated from guaiacum resin.

4557. Guamecycline. [16545-11-2] [4S-(4α,4aα,5aα,6β,-12aα)]-N-[[4-[[(Aminoiminomethyl)amino]iminomethyl]-1-piperazinyl]methyl]-4-(dimethylamino)-1,4,4a,5,5a,6,11,12a-octahydro-3,6,10,12,12a-pentahydroxy-6-methyl-1,11-dioxo-2-naphthacenecarboxamide; tetrabiguanide; "xanthomycin"; xantomicina. $C_{29}H_{38}N_8O_8$; mol wt 626.66. C 55.58%, H 6.11%, N 17.88%, O 20.42%. Prepn: **GB 1042207** (1966 to Societa Prodotti Antibiotici), *C.A.* **65**, 16922g (1966). Clinical studies: O. Restivo, G. Sindoni, *Gazz. Med. Ital.* **127**, 17 (1968).

Dihydrochloride. [13040-98-7] Terratrex; Xantociclina. $C_{29}H_{38}N_8O_8 \cdot 2HCl$; mol wt 699.58.

THERAP CAT: Antibacterial.

4558. Guanabenz. [5051-62-7] 2-[(2,6-Dichlorophenyl)-methylene]hydrazinecarboximidamide; [(2,6-dichlorobenzylidene)-amino]guanidine; N-(2,6-dichlorobenzylidene)-N′-amidino-hydrazine; NSC-68982. $C_8H_8Cl_2N_4$; mol wt 231.08. C 41.58%, H 3.49%, Cl 30.68%, N 24.25%. α₂-Adrenergic agonist. Prepn: J. Yates, E. Haddock, **GB 1019120** (1966 to Shell), *C.A.* **64**, 11132h (1966). Use as antihypertensive: W. J. Houlihan *et al.,* **DE 1804634** (1969 to Sandoz), *C.A.* **71**, 89976j (1969). Pharmacology: T. Baum *et al., J. Pharmacol. Exp. Ther.* **171**, 276 (1970); E. Lampa *et al., Experientia* **36**, 228 (1980). Disposition of ¹⁴C-guanabenz in humans: R. H. Meacham *et al., Clin. Pharmacol. Ther.* **27**, 44 (1980). Mechanism of action: G. F. DiBona, *J. Cardiovasc. Pharmacol.* **6**, Suppl. 3, S543 (1984). Radioimmunoassay determn in plasma: H. Tatsumi, *Arzneim.-Forsch.* **34**, 1704 (1984). Clinical studies: A. Reppelli *et al., Boll. Soc. Ital. Cardiol.* **23**, 177 (1978); C. V. Ram *et al., J. Clin. Pharmacol.* **19**, 148 (1979). Clinical studies in opiate withdrawal: F. S. Tennant, R. A. Rawson, *NIDA Res. Monogr. Ser.* **49**, 338 (1984); J. T. Murphy, *Drug Intell. Clin. Pharm.* **19**, 32 (1985). Review of pharmacodynamic properties and therapeutic efficacy: B. Holmes *et al., Drugs* **26**, 212-229 (1983). Comprehensive description: C. M. Shearer, *Anal. Profiles Drug Subs.* **15**, 319-336 (1986).

White solid from acetonitrile, mp 227-229° (dec).

Monoacetate. [23256-50-0] Wy-8678; Rexitene; Tenelid; Wytensin. $C_{10}H_{12}Cl_2N_4O_2$; mol wt 291.13. Solid, mp 192.5° (dec). Soly at 25° (mg/ml): water 11; alcohol 50; propylene glycol 100; chloroform 0.6; ethyl acetate 1.

THERAP CAT: Antihypertensive.

4559. Guanadrel. [40580-59-4] (1,4-Dioxaspiro[4.5]dec-2-ylmethyl)guanidine. $C_{10}H_{19}N_3O_2$; mol wt 213.28. C 56.31%, H 8.98%, N 19.70%, O 15.00%. Orally active postganglionic sympathetic inhibitor. Prepn: W. R. Hardie, J. E. Aaron, **ZA 6706328**; *eidem,* **US 3547951** (1968, 1970 both to Cutter). Antihypertensive activity: L. Hansson *et al., Clin. Pharmacol. Ther.* **14**, 204 (1973). *In vitro* adrenergic neuron blocking activity: L. Roller, *Aust. J. Pharm. Sci.* **5**, 35 (1976). Pharmacologic study: E. M. Johnson, F. E. Hunter, *Biochem. Pharmacol.* **28**, 1525 (1979). Effect on patients with thyrotoxicosis: S. Rubenfeld *et al., Arch. Intern. Med.*

138, 1106 (1978). Review of pharmacology and efficacy in hypertension: F. A. Finnerty Jr., R. N. Brogden, *Drugs* **30**, 22-31 (1985).

Sulfate. [22195-34-2] CL-1388R; U-28288D; Hylorel. $(C_{10}H_{19}N_3O_2)_2 \cdot H_2SO_4$; mol wt 524.63. Cryst from methanol/ethanol, mp 213.5-215°.

THERAP CAT: Antihypertensive.

4560. Guanethidine. [55-65-2] [2-(Hexahydro-1(2H)-azocinyl)ethyl]guanidine; [2-(octahydro-1-azocinyl)ethyl]guanidine; 1-(2-guanidinoethyl)octahydroazocine; 2-(1′-azacyclooctyl)ethyl-guanidine; N-(2-perhydroazocin-1-ylethyl)guanidine; 2-(1-N,N-heptamethylenimino)ethylguanidine; oktadin; oktatenzin. $C_{10}H_{22}N_4$; mol wt 198.31. C 60.57%, H 11.18%, N 28.25%. Prepn: R. A. Maxwell *et al., Experientia* **15**, 267 (1959); R. P. Mull, **US 2928829** (1960 to Ciba). Pharmacology: H. J. Sah *et al., Arzneim.-Forsch.* **16**, 53 (1966). Clinical trial in hypertension: E. A. Ramirez *et al., Circulation* **55**, 519 (1977); in glaucoma: R. A. Hitchings, D. Glover, *Br. J. Ophthalmol.* **66**, 247 (1982).

Sulfate. [60-02-6] Su-5864. $(C_{10}H_{22}N_4)_2 \cdot H_2SO_4$; mol wt 494.70. Crystals from dil ethanol, mp 276-281° (dec).

Monosulfate. [645-43-2] Sanotensin; Ismelin. $C_{10}H_{22}N_4 \cdot H_2SO_4$; mol wt 296.39. Colorless, crystalline, almost odorless powder. Sol in 1.5 parts water at 20°. Very slightly sol in alcohol. Practically insol in ether, chloroform.

THERAP CAT: Antihypertensive; antiglaucoma.

4561. Guanfacine. [29110-47-2] N-(Aminoiminomethyl)-2,6-dichlorobenzeneacetamide; N-amidino-2-(2,6-dichlorophenyl)-acetamide; [(2,6-dichlorophenyl)acetyl]guanidine. $C_9H_9Cl_2N_3O$; mol wt 246.09. C 43.93%, H 3.69%, Cl 28.81%, N 17.08%, O 6.50%. Centrally acting α₂-adrenoceptor agonist. Prepn: J. B. Bream, C. W. Picard, **FR 1584670**; *eidem,* **US 3632645** (1969, 1972, both to Wander). Pharmacology: D. M. Coward *et al., Arzneim.-Forsch.* **27**, 2326 (1977); H. F. Oates *et al., Arch. Int. Pharmacodyn. Ther.* **231**, 148 (1979); *eidem, Clin. Exp. Pharmacol. Physiol.* **6**, 61 (1979). Determn in biological fluids: M. Guerrat *et al., J. Pharm. Sci.* **68**, 219 (1979). Kinetics: Y. A. Weiss *et al., Clin. Pharmacol. Ther.* **25**, 283 (1979). Clinical studies: U. C. Dubach *et al., Arzneim.-Forsch.* **27**, 674 (1977); P. MacCarthy *et al., Clin. Exp. Pharmacol. Physiol.* **5**, 187 (1978). Symposium on pharmacology, pharmacokinetics, clinical efficacy and comparison with clonidine: *Am. J. Cardiol.* **57**, 1E-61E (1986). *Review:* Br. J. Clin. Pharmacol. **10**, Suppl. 1, 1S-208S (1980).

White grains from methanol/ether, mp 225-227°.

Hydrochloride. [29110-48-3] BS-100-141; LON-798; Estulic; Tenex. $C_9H_9Cl_2N_3O \cdot HCl$; mol wt 282.55. White needles, mp 213-216°. LD_{50} in mice: 165 mg/kg orally (Coward).

THERAP CAT: Antihypertensive.

4562. Guanidine. [113-00-8] Aminomethanamidine; carbamamidine; carbamidine; aminoformamidine; iminourea. CH_5N_3; mol wt 59.07. C 20.33%, H 8.53%, N 71.14%. $(NH_2)_2C=NH$. Strong organic base existing primarily as guanidinium ion at physiological pH. Found in turnip juice, mushrooms, corn germ, rice hulls, mussels, earthworms. Prepn of nitrate from dicyanodiamide + ammonium nitrate: Smith *et al., Ind. Eng. Chem.* **23**, 1124

(1931); Davis, *Org. Synth.* **coll. vol. I** (2nd ed., 1941) p 302; from SO_2, CO_2, + NH_3: Boivin, **US 2762843** (1956); from urea: Mackay, **US 2590257** (1952 to Am. Cyanamid); Craig, Minor, **US 3009949** (1961 to Deere); Shaver, **US 3108999** (1963 to Monsanto); from ammonium thiocyanate or thiourea + ammonia: Watt, Makosky, *Ind. Eng. Chem.* **46**, 2599 (1954). Pharmacology as muscle stimulant: A. I. Podlesnaya, *Bull. Exp. Biol. Med.* **61**, 291 (1966). Clinical evaluation with pyridostigmine in Lambert-Eaton myasthenic syndrome: S. J. Oh *et al.*, *Muscle Nerve* **20**, 1146 (1997). Review of mode of action: D. R. Tershak *et al.*, "Guanidine" in *Handbook of Experimental Pharmacology* Vol. 61, G. V. R. Born *et al.*, Eds. entitled "Chemotherapy of Viral Infections" P. E. Came, L. A. Caliguiri, Eds. (Springer-Verlag, New York, 1982) pp 343-375. Review of structure activity studies: F. Davidoff, *N. Engl. J. Med.* **289**, 141-146 (1973). General reviews: M. Schenck, *Pharmazie* **3**, 5 (1948); G. Schaefer, "Guanidines and Biguanidines" in *International Encyclopedia of Pharmacology and Therapeutics* **107**, M. Erecinska, Ed. (Pergamon, Oxford 1981) pp 165-185.

Deliquescent, cryst mass, mp ~50°. pKa ~12.5. Absorbs CO_2 from air. Very sol in water, alcohol. On heating to 160° it is converted to melamine and NH_3. *Keep well closed.* LD_{50} i.p. in mice: 350 mg/kg (Podlesnaya).

Hydrochloride. [50-01-1] CH_5N_3.HCl. Cryst powder. Freely sol in water, alcohol. Aq soln is neutral.

Nitrate. [506-93-4] CH_5N_3.HNO_3. Cryst powder, mp 214°. Soluble in 10 parts water; in alcohol. Aq soln is neutral.

THERAP CAT: Cholinergic.

4563. Guanidinium Aluminum Sulfate Hexahydrate. [10199-21-0] Sulfuric acid aluminum salt compd with guanidine (2:1:1) hexahydrate; GASH. $CH_{18}AlN_3O_{14}S_2$; mol wt 387.28. C 3.10%, H 4.68%, Al 6.97%, N 10.85%, O 57.84%, S 16.56%. Prepd from an aq soln of an equimolecular mixture of guanidine sulfate and aluminum sulfate: Ferraboschi, *Proc. Cambridge Philos. Soc.* **14**, 473 (1908); Holden *et al.*, *Phys. Rev.* **101**, 962 (1956); Wieder, *Proc. IRE* **45**, 1094 (1957). Crystal structure: Schein *et al.*, *J. Chem. Phys.* **47**, 5183 (1967). Crystal growth: T. A. Zarembovskaya, *Zh. Fiz. Khim.* **45**, 2504 (1971). Optical properties: P. M. Nikolic *et al.*, *Fizika (Zagreb)* **12**, Suppl. 1, 165 (1980).

Large hexagonal plates belonging to the trigonal system with perfect basal cleavage. Has ferroelectric properties.

4564. Guanine. [73-40-5] 2-Amino-1,7-dihydro-6*H*-purin-6-one; 2-aminohypoxanthine. $C_5H_5N_5O$; mol wt 151.13. C 39.74%, H 3.33%, N 46.34%, O 10.59%. Constituent of nucleic acids; widespread in animal and plant kingdom. First isolated from guano. Syntheses: Fisher, *Ber.* **30**, 2226 (1897); Traube, *ibid.* **33**, 1371 (1900); **DE 134984** (1903); **DE 158591** (1903); **DE 162336** (1904). Prepn of ^{15}N-isotopic guanine following Traube's synthesis: Plentl, Schoenheimer, *J. Biol. Chem.* **153**, 203 (1944). Several desmotropic forms. Crystal structure of hydrochloride monohydrate: Broomhead, *Acta Crystallogr.* **4**, 92 (1951). Reviews: Shapiro, *Prog. Nucleic Acid Res. Mol. Biol.* **8**, 73-112 (1968); Ts'o, "Bases, Nucleosides and Nucleotides" in *Basic Principles in Nucleic Acid Chemistry* vol. 1, P. O. P. Ts'o, Ed. (Academic Press, New York, 1974) pp 453-584.

Usually amorphous. Small rhombic crystals by slow evaporation of aq soln contg large excess of NH_3. Dec above 360° with partial sublimation. uv max (pH 6.2): 246, 275 nm ($\varepsilon \times 10^{-3}$ 10.7, 8.1). Freely sol in ammonia water, aq KOH solns, dil acids; sparingly sol

in alcohol, ether. Almost insol in water. pKb 3.22; pKa 9.92, detd at 40°. Many compds with acids, bases and metals have been prepared.

Hydrochloride monohydrate. $C_5H_5N_5O$.HCl.H_2O. Cryst powder. Loses H_2O at 100°, HCl at 200°. Practically insol in water, alcohol, ether; sol in acidulated water.

4565. Guano. Bird manure. The dried excrements of sea birds (cormorants) and bats from coastal islands of Peru, Chile, West Indies, and Africa. Usually mixed with feathers and bones. Contains about 9% nitrogen, 6% phosphorus, 2% potassium, and 15-20% moisture. Used as fertilizer.

4566. Guanosine. [118-00-3] 2-Amino-9-β-D-ribofuranosyl-9*H*-purine-6(1*H*)-one; guanine riboside; vernine. $C_{10}H_{13}N_5$-O_5; mol wt 283.24. C 42.40%, H 4.63%, N 24.73%, O 28.24%. Constituent of nucleic acids. Prepn from yeast nucleic acid: P. A. Levene, L. W. Bass, *Nucleic Acids* (New York, 1931) p 163. Prepn from polynucleotides: P. A. Levene, E. Jorpes, *J. Biol. Chem.* **86**, 389 (1930). Prepn from plants: H. Stendel, E. Peiser in G. Klein, *Handbuch der Pflanzenanalyse* **IV** (Vienna, 1933) p 448. Structure: Levene, Tipson, *J. Biol. Chem.* **97**, 491 (1932); Gulland *et al.*, *J. Chem. Soc.* **1934**, 1639; Tsuboi *et al.*, *Biochim. Biophys. Acta* **55**, 1 (1962). Synthesis: Davoll, *J. Chem. Soc.* **1958**, 1593. Tautomerism in aq soln: Miles *et al.*, *Science* **142**, 1458 (1963). Crystal structure and conformation: Bugg *et al.*, *Biochem. Biophys. Res. Commun.* **3**, 436 (1968). *Review: Basic Principles in Nucleic Acid Chemistry* vol. 1, P. O. P. Ts'o, Ed. (Academic Press, New York, 1974) *passim.*

Dihydrate. Needles from water. Anhydr at 110°. Dec 240° in sealed tube (rapid heating). $[\alpha]_D^{20}$ −61° (in water); $[\alpha]_D^{24}$ −72° (c = 0.96 in 0.1*N* NaOH). uv max (pH 5.5): 188.3, 252.5 nm ($\varepsilon \times 10^{-3}$ 26.8, 13.7), Voet *et al.*, *Biopolymers* **1**, 193 (1963). One gram dissolves in 1320 ml water at 18°, in 33 ml boiling water. Soluble in dil mineral acids, in hot acetic acid, and in dil bases. Insol in alcohol, ether, chloroform, benzene.

4567. Guanoxabenz. [24047-25-4] 2-[(2,6-Dichlorophenyl)methylene]-*N*-hydroxyhydrazinecarboximidamide; 1-[(2,6-dichlorobenzylidene)amino]-3-hydroxyguanidine; Compd 43-663. $C_8H_8Cl_2N_4O$; mol wt 247.08. C 38.89%, H 3.26%, Cl 28.70%, N 22.68%, O 6.48%. Prepn: W. J. Houlihan, R. E. Manning, **DE 1902449**; *eidem*, **US 3591636** (1969, 1971 both to Sandoz). Pharmacological study: J. C. Doxey, A. S. Hersom, *Br. J. Pharmacol.* **70**, 171 (1980).

Hydrochloride. [23256-40-8] Benzerial. $C_8H_8Cl_2N_4O$.HCl; mol wt 283.54. Crystals from ethanol/ether, mp 173-175°.

THERAP CAT: Antihypertensive.

4568. Guanoxan. [2165-19-7] [(2,3-Dihydro-1,4-benzodioxin-2-yl)methyl]guanidine; (1,4-benzodioxan-2-ylmethyl)guanidine; 2-guanidinomethyl-1,4-benzodioxan. $C_{10}H_{13}N_3O_2$; mol wt 207.23. C 57.96%, H 6.32%, N 20.28%, O 15.44%. Prepn: **BE 632701**; J. Augstein, S. M. Green, **US 3247221** (1963, 1966, both to Pfizer); Monro, *Chem. Ind. (London)* **1964**, 1806; Gardner, **GB 996708** (1965 to SKF), *C.A.* **63**, 14877d (1965); Yu, Shen, *C.A.* **66**, 94969k (1967). Prepn and properties of (+) and (−)-forms:

Stenlake *et al., J. Pharm. Pharmacol.* **20** (Suppl), 82 (1968). Pharmacology: Augstein *et al., J. Med. Chem.* **8**, 446 (1965); Cession-Fossion, *Arch. Int. Pharmacodyn. Ther.* **164**, 419 (1966); Vidal-Beretewide *et al., Arzneim.-Forsch.* **19**, 947 (1969). Metabolic studies: Jack *et al., J. Pharm. Pharmacol.* **23**, 2225 (1971); *Xenobiotica* **2**, 35 (1972).

Crystals, mp 164-165°.

Sulfate. [5714-04-5] Envacar. $(C_{10}H_{13}N_3O_2)_2.H_2SO_4$; mol wt 512.54.

THERAP CAT: Antihypertensive.

4569. 3′-Guanylic Acid. [117-68-0] Guanosine 3′-monophosphate; guanine riboside-3-phosphoric acid; guanylic acid b. $C_{10}H_{14}N_5O_8P$; mol wt 363.22. C 33.07%, H 3.89%, N 19.28%, O 35.24% P 8.53%. From yeast or pancreas. Prepn: P. A. Levene, L. W. Bass, *Nucleic Acids* (New York, 1931) pp 224-227. Structure: Levene, Jorpes, *J. Biol. Chem.* **81**, 579 (1929); Levene, Harris, *ibid.* **95**, 755 (1932); **98**, 9 (1932). Early work probably done on a mixture of 2′- and 3′-guanylic acids; see physical data below. Separation of two isomers: Cohn, *J. Am. Chem. Soc.* **72**, 1471 (1950); Khym, Cohn, *ibid.* **76**, 1818 (1954); *eidem, Biol. Prepn.* **5**, 40 (1957). Absorption spectrum: Voet *et al., Biopolymers* **1**, 193 (1963). *Reviews: see* Guanine.

Dihydrate. Long prisms from water. The water of crystn is given up at 118° and is taken up again at room temp. When anhydrous, dec 180° (closed tube). $[\alpha]_D^{25}$ −8° (c = 2); −65° (c = 2 in 5% NaOH). Acid to litmus. Soluble in cold water, freely sol in hot water. Boiling with dil mineral acids yields guanine, H_3PO_4, and D-ribose.

Neutral sodium salt. $Na_2C_{10}H_{12}N_5O_8P$. Flakes from water, contains 21.1% H_2O. Sol in cold, freely sol in hot water.

Brucine salt heptahydrate. $C_{10}H_{14}N_5O_8P.(C_{23}H_{26}N_2O_4)_2.$7H$_2$O. Rectangular leaflets from alc. When anhyd, dec 233-240°. $[\alpha]_D^{20}$ −26° (35% alc). One gram dissolves in 100 ml water.

4570. 5′-Guanylic Acid. [85-32-5] Guanosine 5′-monophosphate; GMP; guanosine 5′-phosphate; guanine riboside-5-phosphoric acid. $C_{10}H_{14}N_5O_8P$; mol wt 363.22. C 33.07%, H 3.89%, N 19.28%, O 35.24%, P 8.53%. Nucleotide widely distributed in nature; found in hydrolyzates of RNA. Isolated together with inosinic acid from sardines or yeast extract: Kuninaka *et al., New Food Ind.* **3**, no. 1, 21 (1961). Also by direct biosynthesis using microorganisms or enzymes: Abrams, Bentley, *Arch. Biochem. Biophys.* **79**, 91 (1959); Magasanik, Karibian, *J. Biol. Chem.* **235**, 2672 (1960); Okumura *et al.,* US 3249511 (1966). Chemical synthesis: Michelson, Todd, *J. Chem. Soc.* **1949**, 2483; Chambers *et al., J. Am. Chem. Soc.* **79**, 3747 (1957); Gilham, Tener, *Chem. Ind. (London)* **1959**, 542; Tener, *J. Am. Chem. Soc.* **83**, 159 (1961); Koransky *et al., Z. Naturforsch.* **17B**, 291 (1962). Prepn of Na salt: Ishibashi, Ito, US 3190877 (1965 to Takeda). Monograph on synthesis of nucleotides: G. R. Pettit, *Synthetic Nucleotides* vol. 1 (Van Nostrand Reinhold, New York, 1972) 252 pp. *Reviews: See* Guanidine.

Microcrystals, dec 190-200°. Sparingly sol in cold water.

Barium salt octahydrate. $C_{10}H_{12}N_5O_8PBa.8H_2O$. White powder. uv max (pH 2): 256 nm (ε 12400); (pH 12): 260 nm (ε 12100).

Disodium salt monohydrate. $C_{10}H_{12}N_5O_8PNa_2.H_2O$. Hygroscopic crystals, decomp at about 250°. Characteristic meaty taste. a_M (molar absorbancy): 13.7×10^3 at 252.5 nm (pH 7). Soly in water at 25° about 25 g/100 ml. Practically insol in alcohol, acetone, ether.

USE: The disodium salt as flavor intensifier, like sodium inosinate and sodium glutamate. Said to be more effective than either.

4571. Guaran. [9000-30-0] Principal polysaccharide from endosperm of guar seeds, *Cyamopsis tetragonaloba* (L.) Taub., *Leguminosae:* Heyne, Whistler, *J. Am. Chem. Soc.* **70**, 2249 (1948). Structure: Whistler, Durso, *ibid.* **74**, 5140 (1952). Configuration: Koleske, Kurath, *J. Polym. Sci. A* **2**, 4123 (1964). *Review:* Deuel *et al., Chimia* **8**, 64 (1954).

$[\alpha]_D^{25}$ +53° (1N NaOH). Sol in cold water.

Triacetate. Fibrous material, mp 226-227°. Can be formed into strong films which can be elongated 550%. Becomes birefringent and does not develop crystallinity.

USE: In textile and paper industry.

4572. Guar Gum. [9000-30-0] Guar flour; gum cyamopsis; cyamopsis gum; Burtonite V-7-E; Decorpa; Guarina; Glucotard; Guarem. Mol wt about 220,000. The ground endosperms of *Cyamopsis tetragonolobus* (L.) Taub., *Leguminosae* which is cultivated in India as livestock feed. The water soluble fraction (85%) of guar flour is called guaran which consists of linear chains of (1 → 4)-β-D-mannopyranosyl units with α-D-galactopyranosyl units attached by (1 → 6) linkages. Ratio of D-galactose to D-mannose is 1:2. Effect on lipid metabolism: D. J. A. Jenkins *et al., Br. Med. J.* **2**, 1555 (1979); on glucose and lipid levels in diabetic and healthy volunteers: U. Smith, G. Holm, *Atherosclerosis* (Shannon, Ire.) **45**, 1 (1982); on renal tumors in diabetic rats: B. C. Chin *et al., Biomed. Res.* **5**, 273 (1984). As source of fiber in patients with non-insulin dependent diabetes: M. E. McIvor *et al., Am. J. Clin. Nutr.* **41**, 891 (1985). Toxicology studies: S. L. Graham *et al., Food Cosmet. Toxicol.* **19**, 287 (1981). Comprehensive monograph: F. Smith, R. Montgomery, *The Chemistry of Plant Gums and Mucilages* (Reinhold, New York, 1959) 627 pp. *Review:* Goldstein *et al.* in *Industrial Gums*, R. L. Whistler, Ed. (Academic Press, New York, 2nd ed., 1973) p 303-321. Comprehensive description: K. Yu *et al., Anal. Profiles Drug Subs. Excip.* **24**, 243-276 (1996).

White to yellowish white, nearly odorless, free flowing powder. Dispersible in hot or cold water, forming a colloidal solution.

Slightly sol in water but not in organic solvents. Water solns are tasteless, odorless, nontoxic, of a pale, translucent gray color, and neutral. Stable to heat. Has five to eight times the thickening power of starch. Water solns may be converted to a gel by small amounts of borax. Aq dispersions are neutral. *Cf.* "A Comparative Study of Commercially Available Guar Gums" by I. A. Schlakman, A. J. Bartilucci, *Drug Stand.* **25**, 149-154 (1957). LD_{50} in male, female rats (g/kg): 7.35, 6.77 orally (Graham).

USE: In paper sizing; as a protective colloid, stabilizer, thickening and film forming agent for cheese, salad dressings, ice cream, soups; as a binding and disintegrating agent in tablet formulations; in pharmaceutical jelly formulations; in suspensions, emulsions, lotions, creams, toothpastes; in the mining industry as a flocculant, as a filtering agent; in water treatment as a coagulant aid.

THERAP CAT: Adjunct to diet, insulin or oral hypoglycemics in control of diabetes.

4573. Guggulsterone. [95975-55-6] Pregna-4,17(20)-diene-3,16-dione. $C_{21}H_{28}O_2$; mol wt 312.45. C 80.72%, H 9.03%, O 10.24%. Bioactive component in guggulu, *q.v.*, the gum resin of the Ayurvedic medicinal plant, *Commiphora mukul, Burseraceae*, used in treatment of lipid disorders. Both the *E*- and *Z*- isomers are naturally occurring and bioactive. Synthesis and stereochemistry: W. R. Benn, R. M. Dodson, *J. Org. Chem.* **29**, 1142 (1964). Isoln from guggulu: V. D. Patil *et al., Tetrahedron* **28**, 2341 (1972). HPLC determn of isomers in serum: N. Verma *et al., J. Chromatogr. B* **708**, 243 (1998). LC determn of isomers in commercial guggulu formulations: M. Nagarajan *et al., J. AOAC Int.* **84**, 24 (2001). Inhibition of the bile acid receptor FXR and cholesterol lowering activity: N. L. Urizar *et al., Science* **296**, 1703 (2002). Brief review of proposed mechanism of action: C. J. Sinal, F. J. Gonzalez, *Trends Endocrinol. Metab.* **13**, 275-276 (2002).

Z-form

E-Form. [39025-24-6] Prisms from aq methanol, mp 170-171.5°. $[\alpha]_D^{26}$ −30° (c = 1 in chloroform). uv max (methanol): 241 nm (ε 27600).

Z-Form. [39025-23-5] Crystals from aq methanol, mp 188-190°. $[\alpha]_D^{26}$ −61° (c = 1 in chloroform). uv max (methanol): 241 nm (ε 25000).

4574. Guggulu. Guggul; gum guggulu; gum guggul. Oleoresin exudate of the guggul tree, *Commiphora mukul* (Hook, ex Stocks), also known as *C. wightii* (Arnott), *Burseraceae*. Used in Aruyvedic medicine for treatment of lipid disorders, obesity and arthritis. *Constit.* Ethyl acetate-soluble fraction containing guggulsterone, *q.v.*, guggulsterols, diterpenoids, ferulic acid esters of guggultetrols, lignins; essential oil consisting primarily of myrcene, camphorene, insoluble carbohydrate gum. Identification of steroidal constituents: V. D. Patil *et al., Tetrahedron* **28**, 2341 (1972). Review of chemical constituents and bioactivity: S. Dev in *Studies in Natural Products Chemistry* Vol. 5, A. Rahman, Ed. (Elsevier, New York, 1989) pp 695-719. Clinical evaluation in hyperlipidemia: S. K. Verma, A. Bordia, *Indian J. Med. Res.* **87**, 356 (1988). Review of medicinal uses: G. V. Satyavati, *ibid.* 327-335 (1988); of pharmacognosy: A. K. Tajuddin *et al., Curr. Res. Med. Aromat. Plants* **16**, 75-86 (1994); of clinical studies in hyperlipidemia: C. Ulbricht *et al., Comp. Ther. Med.* **13**, 279-290 (2005).

Ethyl acetate extract. Gugulipid; Guglip. Standardized to contain 4.0% guggulsterones. Clinical evaluation in hypercholesterolemia: R. B. Singh *et al., Cardiovasc. Drugs Ther.* **8**, 659 (1994); P. O. Szapary *et al., J. Am. Med. Assoc.* **290**, 765 (2003). LD_{50} in mice (mg/kg): 1600 i.p. and orally (Dev).

THERAP CAT: Antilipemic.

4575. Guinea Green B. [4680-78-8] *N*-Ethyl-*N*-[4-[[4-[ethyl[(3-sulfophenyl)methyl]amino]phenyl]phenylmethylene]-2,5-cyclohexadien-1-ylidene]-3-sulfobenzenemethanaminium inner salt, sodium salt; C.I. Acid Green 3; C.I. Food Green 1; FD & C Green 1; C.I. 42085. $C_{37}H_{35}N_2NaO_6S_2$; mol wt 690.80. C 64.33%, H 5.11%, N 4.06%, Na 3.33%, O 13.90%, S 9.28%. Prepn: Jones *et al., J. Assoc. Off. Agric. Chem.* **38**, 977 (1955). Toxicity studies: F. C. Lu, A. Lavalle, *Can. Pharm. J.* **97**, 30 (1964); W. H. Hansen *et al., Food Cosmet. Toxicol.* **4**, 389 (1966). *See also: Colour Index* vol. 4 (3rd ed., 1971) p 4385.

A dull, dark green powder, or a bright, crystalline solid. Sol in water to a green soln which becomes brownish-yellow on addn of HCl and blackish-green with NaOH. An excess of NaOH decolorizes the soln. Sparingly sol in alcohol; it dissolves in concd H_2SO_4 to a yellow soln which, when diluted with water, turns first yellowish-red, then green. LD_{50} orally in rats: >2 g/kg (Lu, Lavalle).

USE: Limited use as a dye for silk and wool fabrics; as biological stain.

4576. D-Gulonic Acid. [20246-33-7] $C_6H_{12}O_7$; mol wt 196.16. C 36.74%, H 6.17%, O 57.09%. Prepd as the sodium salt by reduction of sodium glucuronate with sodium amalgam in alkaline medium: Fischer, Piloty, *Ber.* **24**, 525 (1891); from D-gulonic acid γ-lactone: Rehorst, Naumann, *ibid.* **77**, 24 (1944).

$[\alpha]_D^{20}$ −6° (10 min) → −38.6° (15 days). The free acid forms the lactone spontaneously. pK (25°): 3.68.

Sodium salt. $C_6H_{11}NaO_7$. Crystals. $[\alpha]_D^{20}$ +11.5°. Sol in water.

Calcium salt. $Ca(C_6H_{11}O_7)_2$. $[\alpha]_D^{21}$ −14.45° (c = 1.73). Precipitated from aq soln by alc.

4577. L-Gulonic Acid. [526-97-6] Xylosecarboxylic acid. $C_6H_{12}O_7$; mol wt 196.16. C 36.74%, H 6.17%, O 57.09%. Prepd from L-xylose and HCN followed by hydrolysis of the nitrile: Fischer, Stahel, *Ber.* **24**, 529 (1891). Prepn from D-glucuronic acid: DE 618907 (1935 to Hoffmann-La Roche); from L-gulonolactone: Ishidate *et al., Chem. Pharm. Bull.* **13**, 173 (1965).

Crystallizes as the lactone on evapn of an aq soln.
Sodium salt. $[\alpha]_D^{20}$ +12.7° (c = 9). Freely sol in water.

4578. D-Gulose. [4205-23-6] $C_6H_{12}O_6$; mol wt 180.16. C 40.00%, H 6.71%, O 53.28%. Prepd by sodium amalgam reduction of an acid soln of D-gulonic acid: Fischer, Stahel, *Ber.* **24**, 532 (1891); van Ekenstein, Blanksma, *Rec. Trav. Chim.* **27**, 3 (1908). Alternate synthesis: Meyer zu Reckendorf, *Angew. Chem. Int. Ed.* **6**, 177 (1967); *idem, Methods Carbohydr. Chem.* **6**, 129 (1972); R. Köster *et al., Angew. Chem. Int. Ed.* **19**, 547 (1980).

Syrup. Sweet taste. $[\alpha]_D^{20}$ $-20.4°$. Sol in water, slightly sol in alcohol. Not fermentable by yeast.

4579. L-Gulose. [6027-89-0] $C_6H_{12}O_6$; mol wt 180.16. C 40.00%, H 6.71%, O 53.28%. Prepd by sodium amalgam reduction of an acid soln of the γ-lactone of L-gulonic acid: Fischer, Piloty, *Ber.* **24,** 526 (1891). *See also* van Ekenstein, Blanksma, *Rec. Trav. Chim.* **27,** 3 (1908); Levene, LaForge, *J. Biol. Chem.* **20,** 430 (1915); Talen, *Rec. Trav. Chim.* **44,** 891 (1925); Isbell, *J. Am. Chem. Soc.* **55,** 2167 (1933). Synthesis from D-mannose: Evans, Parrish, *Carbohydr. Res.* **28,** 359 (1973); from D-glucose: D. K. Minster, S. M. Hecht, *J. Org. Chem.* **43,** 3987 (1978).

Syrup. $[\alpha]_D^{20}$ $+61.6°$. $[\alpha]_D$ $+21.3°$ (c = 4.58) (Evans, Parrish). Freely sol in water; slightly sol in alcohol. Not fermentable by yeast.

4580. Gum Benzoin. [9000-05-9] Resin benzoin; resin benjamin; gum benjamin. Balsamic resin from *Styrax benzoin* Dryand., known as Sumatra benzoin, or from *S. tonkinensis* (Pierre) Craib, *Styracaceae,* or other species of *Styrax* known as Siam benzoin. *Habit.* Thailand, Cambodia, S. Vietnam, Sumatra, Java, and Sunda Islands. *Constit.* Ethereal oil, free and combined benzoic and cinnamic acids up to 39%, vanillin, coniferyl benzoate, resin (a mixture of benzoresinol and benzoresinotannol) esterified with benzoic acid, styrol, styracin. Not less than 90% of Siam and not less than 75% of Sumatra benzoic is sol in alc (U.S.P.). *Ref:* Reinitzer, *Arch. Pharm.* **264,** 131 (1926); Brans, *Pharm. Weekbl.* **73,** 374 (1936); Freudenberg, Bittner, *Ber.* **83,** 600 (1950).

USE: Preserving ointments; preparing natural benzoic acid; for fumigating pastilles; in perfumery and cosmetics.

THERAP CAT: Topical protectant.

THERAP CAT (VET): Tincture is used topically as an antiseptic and to promote healing; as an inhalant for bronchitis, and orally as an expectorant.

4581. Gum Tragacanth. [9000-65-1] Tragacanth. Mol wt about 840,000. The dried gummy exudation from *Astragalus gummifer* Labill. (white gavan) or other Asiatic species of *Astragalus, Leguminosae,* found largely in Iran, also in Asia Minor and in Syria. When mixed with water gives a soluble fraction, as a hydrosol, called *tragacanthin* which is a complex mixture of polysaccharides containing D-galacturonic acid, other sugars, and traces of starch and cellulose. The insoluble fraction swells to a gel and consists of 60-70% bassorin. Structural studies: Norman, *Biochem. J.* **25,** 200 (1931); James, Smith, *J. Chem. Soc.* **1945,** 739, 749; Aspinall, Baillie, *ibid.* **1963,** 1702, 1714. *Reviews:* D. C. Beach in *Adv. Chem. Ser.* **11,** entitled "Natural Plant Hydrocolloids," (ACS, Washington DC, 1954) pp 38-44; Meer *et al.* in *Industrial Gums,* R. L. Whistler, Ed. (Academic Press, New York, 2nd ed., 1973) pp 289-299. *Book:* F. Smith, R. Montgomery, *The Chemistry of Plant Gums and Mucilages* (Reinhold, New York, 1959) 627 pp.

Odorless. Insipid, mucilaginous taste. Acid reaction. One gram requires 0.9 ml 0.1N NaOH for neutralization to phenolphthalein: Gabel, *J. Am. Pharm. Assoc.* **23,** 341 (1934). Viscosity of tragacanth mucilages is reduced by adding acid, alkali, and NaCl particularly if the mucilage is heated: Mantell, *The Water-Soluble Gums* (New York, 1947). Maximum initial viscosity of solns at pH 8; maximum stable viscosity near pH 5. Forms a deep yellow stringy precipitate when a soln is boiled with a few drops of 10% aqueous ferric chloride soln. A stringy precipitate formed also on heating a soln with Schweitzer reagent. Tragacanth is entirely insol in alcohol.

USE: In pharmaceutical compounding and dispensing, *e.g.,* to suspend heavy insol powders, as an excipient for tablets and to impart consistence to troches; also in making emulsions and emulsifying agents; as stabilizer, thickener, texturizer in food; in adhesives (mucilages, pastes); in textile sizing, textile printing and general printing inks, and in dyeing with insol color lakes.

4582. Gusperimus. [104317-84-2] 7-[(Aminoiminomethyl)amino]-*N*-[2-[[4-[(3-aminopropyl)amino]butyl]amino]-1-hydroxy-2-oxoethyl]heptanamide; ($\pm$)-*N*-[[[4-[(3-aminopropyl)-amino]butyl]carbamoyl]hydroxymethyl]-7-guanidinoheptanamide; 1-amino-19-guanidino-11-hydroxy-4,9,12-triazanonadecane-10,13-dione; deoxyspergualin; ($\pm$)-15-deoxyspergualin. $C_{17}H_{37}N_7O_3$; mol wt 387.52. C 52.69%, H 9.62%, N 25.30%, O 12.39%. Synthetic derivative of the antitumor antibiotic **spergualin.** Prepn: **BE 894651;** H. Umezawa *et al.,* **US 4518532** (1983, 1985 both to Microbiochem. Res. Found.); Y. Umeda *et al., J. Antibiot.* **38,** 886 (1985). Prepn of the active ($-$)-isomer: H. Iwasawa *et al., ibid.* **35,** 1665 (1982); H. Umezawa *et al.,* **EP 94632;** *eidem,* **US 4525299** (1983, 1985 both to Microbiochem. Res. Found.). Synthesis and bioactivity of isomers: Y. Umeda *et al., J. Antibiot.* **40,** 1316 (1987). Mechanism of action study: W. E. G. Müller *et al., ibid.* 1028. HPLC determn in plasma: R. Nakanuma *et al., J. Chromatogr.* **527,** 208 (1990). Pharmacokinetics: J. F. Muindi *et al., Cancer Res.* **51,** 3096 (1991). Preliminary evaluation in renal transplant rejection: H. Amemiya *et al., Transplant. Proc.* **25,** 730 (1993). Series of articles on synthesis and immunomodulating activity: *Ann. N.Y. Acad. Sci.* **685,** 123-206 (1993).

Trihydrochloride. [85468-01-5] BMS-181173; NKT-01; NSC-356894; Spanidin. $C_{17}H_{37}N_7O_3 \cdot 3HCl$; mol wt 496.90. White powder, prepd as the sesquihydrate. Sol in water. pH of 50 mg/ml saline soln: ~4.9. LD_{50} in mice (mg/kg): 25-50 i.p. (Umezawa).

($-$)-Form trihydrochloride. [84937-45-1] Prepd as the dihydrate. Colorless syrup, no def mp. $[\alpha]_D^{25}$ $-7.3°$ (c = 1 in H_2O). LD_{50} in mice (mg/kg): 35-40 i.v. or i.p. (Iwasawa).

THERAP CAT: Immunosuppressant.

4583. Gutta-Percha. [9000-32-2] The purified, coagulated, milky exudate of various trees of the genus *Palaquium, Sapotaceae. Habit.* Malayan Archipelago. Extensive review: Williams, *Econ. Bot.* **18,** 5-26 (1964). Defined as a *trans* isomer of rubber. Rubber has a repeat period of 8.2 Å, whereas α-gutta-percha has 8.7 Å and β-gutta-percha has 4.8 Å. The short period of β-gutta-percha identifies it almost uniquely as an all-*trans* polyisoprene.

Becomes pliable at 25-30°, plastic at 60°. mp 100° (partial dec). On exposure to air and sunlight, it absorbs oxygen and becomes brittle. Insol in water; partially sol in hot alcohol; 90% or more dissolves in chloroform, carbon disulfide, petr ether, oil of turpentine. *Keep under water and protected from light.*

USE: Insulator in electrotechnics, as dental cement; in orthopedics for fracture splints; manuf surgical instruments; covering golf balls.

4584. Guvacine. [498-96-4] 1,2,5,6-Tetrahydro-3-pyridinecarboxylic acid; 1,2,5,6-tetrahydronicotinic acid. $C_6H_9NO_2$; mol wt 127.14. C 56.68%, H 7.14%, N 11.02%, O 25.17%. From betel nuts, the seeds of *Areca catechu* L., *Palmae.* Extraction: Jahns, *Ber.* **24,** 2615 (1891). Synthesis: Freudenberg, *ibid.* **51,** 976, 1669 (1918); Hess, Leibbrandt, *ibid.* **51,** 806; **52,** 206 (1919).

Prisms from water, dec 295°. Neutral to litmus. Sol in water. Almost insol in abs alc, ether, chloroform, benzene.

Hydrochloride. $C_6H_{10}ClNO_2$. Needles from water, dec 318°. Sol in water.

Hydrobromide. $C_6H_{10}BrNO_2$. Needles from abs alcohol, dec 280°. Almost insol in acetone.

USE: Has been proposed as growth factor for *Staphylococcus aureus* and *Proteus vulgaris* instead of nicotinic acid.

4585. Gymnemic Acid. [1399-64-0] Gymnemin. Antisaccharin principle occurring in the leaves of *Gymnema sylvestre* R. Br. and allied *Asclepiadaceae:* Hooper, *Chem. News* **59**, 159 (1889); Mhaskar, Caius, *Indian J. Med. Res.* No. **16**, 1 (1930); Warren, Pfaffman, *J. Appl. Physiol.* **14**, 40 (1959); Stöcklin *et al., Helv. Chim. Acta* **50**, 474 (1967). A complex mixture of at least nine closely related acidic glycosides, the major active component being gymnemic acid A_1: Stöcklin, *J. Agric. Food Chem.* **17**, 704 (1969); Dateo, Long, *ibid.* **21**, 899 (1973). Separation of major components: Sinsheimer *et al., J. Pharm. Sci.* **59**, 622, 629 (1970). Completely obtunds taste for several hours for sweet but not for bitter, sour, or salty substances: G. Hellekant *et al., Acta Physiol. Scand.* **124**, 399 (1985).

The acid is a yellow to brown amorphous, bitter powder. Almost insol in water; sol in alcohol. The potassium salt is a reddish-brown cryst mass, sol in water or alcohol.

Consult the Name Index before using this section.

H

4586. Hachimycin. [1394-02-1] Trichomycin; Trichonat. Heptaene macrolide antibiotic substance produced by *Streptomyces hachijoensis* from soil of the Pacific Island Hachijo Jima: S. Hosoya *et al., J. Antibiot.* **5,** 564 (1952); T. Yamaguchi, *ibid.* **7A,** 10 (1954). Purification and prepn of insol derivs: S. Hosoya *et al., ibid.* **8A,** 5 (1955). At one time, trichomycin was believed to be identical to candicidin and hamycin, *q.q.v.:* H. Burrows, D. Calam, *J. Chromatogr.* **53,** 566 (1970). Subsequent HPLC studies have shown the three polyene antibiotics to be different entities: P. Helboe *et al., ibid.* **189,** 249 (1980). Active against *Trichomonas vaginalis, Treponema pallidum, Trichophyton, Candida,* and yeast, weak activity against *Aspergillus* and *Penicillium:* T. Yamaguchi, *J. Antibiot.* **7A,** 10 (1954). Toxicity: S. Hosoya *et al., J. Antibiot.* **6A,** 98 (1953). *Review:* S. A. Waksman, H. A. Lechevalier, *The Actinomycetes* vol. **III** (Williams & Wilkins, Baltimore, 1962) pp 397-399.

Yellow crystals. Acid reaction. Forms a water-sol sodium salt. Can be pptd as a water-insol salt by acridine derivs such as acriflavine, by sulfa drugs such as homosulfanilamide, by basic antibiotics such as streptomycin base, by enzymes such as papain and lysozyme, by dyes such as methylene blue, and by metallic salts such as $CaCl_2$. LD_{50} i.p. in mice: 0.05 mg/10-12 g mouse (Hosoya).

THERAP CAT: Antifungal. Antiprotozoal (Trichomonas).

4587. Hadacidin. [689-13-4] *N*-Formyl-*N*-hydroxyglycine; *N*-formyl-*N*-hydroxyaminoacetic acid; *N*-hydroxyformamidoacetic acid. $C_3H_5NO_4$; mol wt 119.08. C 30.26%, H 4.23%, N 11.76%, O 53.74%. Antitumor antibiotic originally isolated from cultures of *Penicillium frequentans* Westling. Synthesis: Kaczka *et al., Biochemistry* **1,** 340 (1962); Kinnel, Schoenewaldt, **US 3154578** (1964 to Merck & Co.). Biosynthesis: Stevens, Emery, *Biochemistry* **5,** 74 (1966). *Review:* Shigeura, "Hadacidin" in *Antibiotics* **I,** D. Gottlieb, P. Shaw, Eds. (Springer-Verlag, New York, 1967) pp 451-456.

Unstable crystals, mp 119-120°. Turns brown and liquefies on standing. The decompn products are formic acid and *N*-hydroxyglycine. Dibasic acid, potentiometric titration shows pH peak at 3.5 and 9.1. Soluble in water, methanol, ethanol, acetone, ether.

Monosodium salt. $C_3H_4NNaO_4$. Crystals. Easily forms a hydrate, very freely sol in water.

4588. Hafnium. [7440-58-6] Hf; at. wt 178.49; at. no. 72; valences 4; also 2, 3. Group IVB (4). Six naturally occurring isotopes: 180 (35.22%); 178 (27.1%); 177 (18.56%); 179 (13.75%); 176 (5.21%); 174 (0.163%; α-emitter, $T_{1/2}$ 2 × 10^{15} years); artificial isotopes: 157; 158; 168-173; 175; 181-183. Abundance in earth's crust: 5 ppm. Found in all zirconium-contg minerals. Discovered in 1923 by Coster and Hevesy: *Nature* **111,** 79 (1923). Extraction from the mineral cyrtolite: Larsen *et al., Inorg. Synth.* **3,** 67 (1950). Prepd by thermal decompn of its iodide; by reduction of the tetrachloride or of the hydrofluohafniate with metallic sodium; by reduction of the oxide with a mixture of calcium and sodium: van Arkel, de Boer, *Z. Anorg. Chem.* **148,** 345 (1925); de Boer, Fast, *ibid.* **187,** 193 (1930); **US 2741628.** Spectra: Coster *et al.,* cited by Mellor, *A Comprehensive Treatise on Inorganic and Theoretical Chemistry* **7,** 170 (1930). A dibromide and tribromide have been prepd: Schumb, Morehouse, *J. Am. Chem. Soc.* **69,** 2696 (1947). Reviews of hafnium and its compds: Larsen, "Zirconium and Hafnium Chemistry" in *Adv. Inorg. Chem. Radiochem.* **13,** 1-133 (1970); Bradley, Thornton, "Zirconium and Hafnium" in *Comprehensive Inorganic Chemistry* vol. **3,** J. C. Bailar, Jr. *et al.,* Eds. (Pergamon Press, Oxford, 1973) pp 419-490; R. H. Nielson in *Kirk-Othmer Encyclopedia of Chemical Technology* vol. **12** (Wiley-Interscience, New York, 3rd ed., 1980) pp 67-80.

Highly lustrous, ductile metal of hexagonal cryst structure. mp 2227°; d 13.3. Resembles zirconium and thorium.

Dioxide. HfO_2. Obtained by igniting the hydroxide, the oxalate, or the sulfate. d^{20} 9.68. mp 2774°.

Tetrachloride. $HfCl_4$. White cryst mass, obtained by heating the oxide in the presence of chlorine and a reducing agent. Hydrolyzed to hafnyl chloride, $HfOCl_2$, by water. Volatilizes appreciably at 250°.

Sulfate. $Hf(SO_4)_2$. Prepd by the action of fuming sulfuric acid on the tetrachloride, dec above 500°.

Caution: Potential symptoms of overexposure to hafnium in exptl animals are irritation of eyes, skin, mucous membranes; liver damage. *See NIOSH Pocket Guide to Chemical Hazards* (DHHS/-NIOSH 97-140, 1997) p 156.

4589. Halazepam. [23092-17-3] 7-Chloro-1,3-dihydro-5-phenyl-1-(2,2,2-trifluoroethyl)-2*H*-1,4-benzodiazepin-2-one; Sch-12041; Paxipam. $C_{17}H_{12}ClF_3N_2O$; mol wt 352.74. C 57.88%, H 3.43%, Cl 10.05%, F 16.16%, N 7.94%, O 4.54%. Polyfluoroalkyl analog of diazepam, *q.v.* Prepn: J. G. Topliss, **US 3429874** (1969 to Schering); M. Steinman *et al., J. Med. Chem.* **16,** 1354 (1973). Pharmacology: J. B. Petel *et al., Psychopharmacology* **61,** 25 (1979). Use in schizophrenia: K. Y. Ota *et al., Curr. Ther. Res.* **15,** 327 (1973); in anxiety: K. Rickels *et al., Int. Pharmacopsychiatry* **13,** 118 (1978).

Crystals from acetone-hexane, mp 164-166°. LD_{50} in mice: >4000 mg/kg orally (Steinman).

Note: This is a controlled substance (depressant): **21 CFR,** 1308.14.

THERAP CAT: Anxiolytic.

4590. Halazone. [80-13-7] 4-[(Dichloroamino)sulfonyl]-benzoic acid; *p*-(dichlorosulfamoyl)benzoic acid; *p*-sulfondichloramidobenzoic acid; *p*-carboxybenzenesulfondichloroamide; Pantocid. $C_7H_5Cl_2NO_4S$; mol wt 270.09. C 31.13%, H 1.87%, Cl 26.25%, N 5.19%, O 23.69%, S 11.87%. Prepd by chlorination of *p*-sulfamylbenzoic acid in alkaline medium; product is a mixture of mono- and dichloroamides with the dichloro compd predominating: Proschko, **DE 492249**; *Chem. Zentralbl.* **101,** I, 2630 (1930); **US 1697139** *C.A.* **23,** 1138 (1929); Claas, **DE 318899**; *Chem. Zentralbl.* **91,** IV, 14 (1920). Water disinfection study: R. Kfir *et al., Water Sci. Technol.* **21,** 207 (1989). Review of use as antiseptic in water disinfection: J. T. O'Connor, S. K. Kapoor, *J. Am. Water Works Assoc.* **62,** 80-84 (1970).

Crystals or white powder, dec about 195°. Odor of chlorine. Slightly sol in water, chloroform (differing from chloramine-T which is very sol in chloroform). Sol in glacial acetic acid and in solns of alkali hydroxides and of alkali carbonates with the formation of a salt.

USE: Water disinfectant.

4591. Halcinonide. [3093-35-4] (11β,16α)-21-Chloro-9-fluoro-11-hydroxy-16,17-[(1-methylethylidene)bis(oxy)]pregn-4-ene-3,20-dione; 21-chloro-9-fluoro-11β,16α,17-trihydroxypregn-4-ene-3,20-dione cyclic 16,17-acetal with acetone; 21-chloro-9α-fluoro-11β-hydroxy-16α,17α-isopropylidenedioxy-4-pregnene-3,20-dione; 9α-fluoro-21-chloro-11β,16α,17α-trihydroxypregn-4-ene-3,20-dione 16,17-acetonide; SQ-18566; Halciderm; Halcimat; Halog.

$C_{24}H_{32}ClFO_5$; mol wt 454.96. C 63.36%, H 7.09%, Cl 7.79%, F 4.18%, O 17.58%. Prepn: Bernstein *et al., J. Org. Chem.* **27**, 690 (1962); L. T. Difazio, M. A. Augustine, **DE 2355710**; *eidem,* **US 3892857** (1972, 1975 both to Squibb). Pharmacological evaluation: Bagatell, Augustine, *Curr. Ther. Res.* **16**, 748 (1974); R. C. Millonig, E. Yiakas, in *Pharmacological and Biochemical Properties of Drug Substances* vol. 1, M. E. Goldberg, Ed. (Am. Pharmaceut. Assoc., Washington, DC, 1977) pp 215-231. Comprehensive description: J. Kirshbaum, *Anal. Profiles Drug Subs.* **8**, 251-281 (1979).

Crystals from acetone-petr ether, mp 264-265° (dec). uv max (methanol): 238 nm (ε 16400). $[\alpha]_D^{25}$ +155° (CHCl$_3$). Sol in acetone, chloroform, DMSO. Slightly sol in benzene, ethanol, ethyl ether, methanol. Insol in water, 0.1M HCl, 0.1M NaOH, hexanes. LD$_{50}$ i.p. in mice: 150 mg/kg (Millonig, Yiakas).

THERAP CAT: Anti-inflammatory (topical).

4592. Halibut Liver Oil. From the liver of the halibut, *Hippoglossus hippoglossus* L. It usually contains not less than 60,000 U.S.P. vitamin A units and not less than 500 U.S.P. vitamin D units per gram.

Pale yellow liq; slight fishy odor and taste. d 0.922-0.925. n_D^{40} 1.470-1.478. Sapon no. 170-180. Iodine no. 120-136. Unsaponifiable matter 8-13%.

THERAP CAT: Source of vitamins A and D.

THERAP CAT (VET): Source of vitamins A and D.

4593. Halobetasol Propionate. [66852-54-8] (6α,11β,16β)-21-Chloro-6,9-difluoro-11-hydroxy-16-methyl-17-(1-oxopropoxy)pregna-1,4-diene-3,20-dione; 21-chloro-6α,9-difluoro-11β,17-dihydroxy-16β-methylpregna-1,4-diene-3,20-dione 17-propionate; ulobetasol propionate; BMY-30056; CGP-14458; Ultravate. $C_{25}H_{31}ClF_2O_5$; mol wt 484.96. C 61.92%, H 6.44%, Cl 7.31%, F 7.84%, O 16.50%. Trihalogenated corticosteroid structurally related to clobetasol, *q.v.* Prepn: J. Kalvoda, G. Anner, **DE 2743069**; *eidem,* **US 4619921** (1978, 1986 both to Ciba-Geigy). Clinical pharmacology in psoriatic patients: W. A. Watson *et al., Pharmacotherapy* **10**, 107 (1990). Clinical trial in localized vitiligo: L. Xunquan *et al., Int. J. Dermatol.* **29**, 295 (1990).

Crystals from methylene chloride/ether, mp 220-221°.
THERAP CAT: Anti-inflammatory.

4594. Halofantrine. [69756-53-2] 1,3-Dichloro-α-[2-(dibutylamino)ethyl]-6-(trifluoromethyl)-9-phenanthrenemethanol; 1-(1,3-dichloro-6-trifluoromethyl-9-phenanthryl)-3-di(*n*-butyl)aminopropanol; γ-(dibutylamino)-1,3-dichloro-6-(trifluoromethyl)-9-phenanthrenepropanol. $C_{26}H_{30}Cl_2F_3NO$; mol wt 500.42. C 62.40%, H 6.04%, Cl 14.17%, F 11.39%, N 2.80%, O 3.20%. Prepn of the hydrochloride: W. T. Colwell *et al., J. Med. Chem.* **15**, 771 (1972); of the β-glycerophosphate salt: J. F. Rossignol, **EP 138374**; *idem,* **US 4507288** (both 1985 to Smithkline Beckman). Antimalarial activity *in vivo:* L. H. Schmidt *et al., Antimicrob. Agents Chemother.* **14**, 292 (1978). HPLC determn in human blood: J. W. Hines *et al., J. Pharm. Sci.* **74**, 433 (1985). Antimalarial activity in clinically-induced infection in humans: J. Rinehart *et al., Am. J. Trop. Med. Hyg.* **25**, 769 (1976); T. M. Cosgriff *et al., ibid.* **31**,

1075 (1982); in naturally acquired disease: J. P. Coulaud *et al., Trans. R. Soc. Trop. Med. Hyg.* **80**, 615 (1986). Review of pharmacology and therapeutic potential: H. M. Bryson, K. L. Goa, *Drugs* **43**, 236-258 (1992).

Hydrochloride. [36167-63-2] SKF-102886; WR-171669; Halfan. $C_{26}H_{30}Cl_2F_3NO.HCl$; mol wt 536.88. Two crystalline forms have been reported: mp 93-96°, mp 203-204°.

β-Glycerophosphate. $C_{29}H_{39}Cl_2F_3NO_7P$. White crystals, mp 60-65°.

THERAP CAT: Antimalarial.

4595. Halofenozide. [112226-61-6] 4-Chlorobenzoic acid 2-benzoyl-2-(1,1-dimethylethyl)hydrazide; RH-0345; Mach 2. $C_{18}H_{19}ClN_2O_2$; mol wt 330.81. C 65.35%, H 5.79%, Cl 10.72%, N 8.47%, O 9.67%. Ecdysone agonist causing premature molting; insect growth regulator. Prepn: R. W. Addor *et al.,* **EP 228564** (1987 to Am Cyanamid). Susceptibility study in insects: R. S. Cowles, M. G. Villani, *J. Econ. Entomol.* **89**, 1556 (1996). LC determn of residues in grass: S. S. Skorczynski, *J. AOAC Int.* **80**, 418 (1997). Review of biological activity and efficacy: T. S. Dhadialla *et al., Annu. Rev. Entomol.* **43**, 545-569 (1998).

mp 198.0-199.0°.
USE: Insecticide.

4596. Halofuginone. [55837-20-2] *rel*-7-Bromo-6-chloro-3-[3-[(2R,3S)-3-hydroxy-2-piperidinyl]-2-oxopropyl]-4(3H)-quinazolinone; ($\pm$)-*trans*-7-bromo-6-chloro-3-[3-(3-hydroxy-2-piperidyl)acetonyl]-4(3H)-quinazolinone; 7-bromo-6-chlorofebrifugine; HAL. $C_{16}H_{17}BrClN_3O_3$; mol wt 414.68. C 46.34%, H 4.13%, Br 19.27%, Cl 8.55%, N 10.13%, O 11.57%. Halogenated deriv of febrifugine, *q.v.* Prepn: E. Waletzky *et al.,* **US 3320124** (1967 to Am. Cyanamid). *In vivo* and *in vitro* activity: J. G. Ryley *et al., Parasitology* **70**, 203 (1975). Toxicity to fresh water organisms: *Bull. Environ. Contam. Toxicol.* **15**, 720 (1976). HPLC determn in chicken feed: A. Anderson *et al., J. Chromatogr.* **168**, 471 (1979); in chicken serum: R. C. Beier *et al., J. Liq. Chromatogr.* **17**, 2961 (1994). Evaluation as coccidiostat: P. E. Waibel *et al., Poult. Sci.* **66**, 1629 (1987). Inhibition of collagen synthesis and effect on skin tearing: I. Granot *et al., ibid.* **70**, 1559 (1991).

Hydrobromide. [64924-67-0] RU-19110; Stenorol. $C_{16}H_{17}$-$BrClN_3O_3.HBr$; mol wt 495.59. Crystals, mp 247° (dec).
THERAP CAT (VET): Antiprotozoal (coccidiostat).

4597. Halometasone. [50629-82-8] (6α,11β,16α)-2-Chloro-6,9-difluoro-11,17,21-trihydroxy-16-methylpregna-1,4-diene-3,20-dione; 2-chloroflumethasone; C-48401-Ba. $C_{22}H_{27}ClF_2O_5$; mol wt 444.90. C 59.39%, H 6.12%, Cl 7.97%, F 8.54%, O 17.98%. Synthetic corticosteroid. Prepn: G. G. Anner *et al.,* **NL 540244**; *eidem,* **US 3652554**; *eidem,* **CH 551399**, *C.A.* **81**, 120864d (1974) (1968, 1972, 1974 all to Ciba-Geigy). Series of clinical trials in eczema, psoriasis, dermatomycoses, bacterial infections: *J. Int. Med. Res.* **11**, Suppl. 1 (1983).

mp 220-222° (dec).
Monohydrate. Sicorten. $C_{22}H_{27}ClF_2O_5 \cdot H_2O$; mol wt 462.91.
THERAP CAT: Anti-inflammatory (topical); antipruritic.

4598. Haloperidol. [52-86-8] 4-[4-(4-Chlorophenyl)-4-hydroxy-1-piperidinyl]-1-(4-fluorophenyl)-1-butanone; 4-[4-(p-chlorophenyl)-4-hydroxypiperidino]-4'-fluorobutyrophenone; 4'-fluoro-4-(4-hydroxy-4-p-chlorophenylpiperidino)butyrophenone; 1-(3-p-fluorobenzoylpropyl)-4-p-chlorophenyl-4-hydroxypiperidine; R-1625; Aloperidin; Bioperidolo; Brotopon; Dozic; Einalon S; Eukystol; Haldol; Halosten; Keselan; Linton; Peluces; Serenace; Serenase; Sigaperidol. $C_{21}H_{23}ClFNO_2$; mol wt 375.86. C 67.11%, H 6.17%, Cl 9.43%, F 5.05%, N 3.73%, O 8.51%. Prepn: P. A. J. Janssen et al., J. Med. Pharm. Chem. **1**, 281 (1959); P. A. J. Janssen, **BE 577977** (1959), C.A. **54**, 4630c (1960); idem, **GB 895309**; idem, **US 3438991** (1962, 1969 both to Janssen). Toxicity: E. I. Goldenthal, Toxicol. Appl. Pharmacol. **18**, 185 (1971); A. J. Collins, M. Horlington, Br. J. Pharmacol. **37**, 140 (1969). Metabolism in man: A. Forsman et al., Curr. Ther. Res. **21**, 606 (1977). Comprehensive description: C. A. Janicki, C. Y. Ko, Anal. Profiles Drug Subs. **9**, 341-369 (1980). Review of pharmacology and therapeutic efficacy of decanoate in psychosis: R. Beresford, A. Ward, Drugs **33**, 31-49 (1987).

Crystals, mp 148.0-149.4°. uv max (9:1 0.1M HCl:methanol): 247, 221 nm (ε 13300, 15000). pKa 8.3. Soly in water: 1.4 mg/100 ml. Freely sol in chloroform, methanol, acetone, benzene, dil acids. LD_{50} orally in rats: 165 mg/kg (Goldenthal); i.p. in mice: 60 mg/kg (Collins, Horlington).
Hydrochloride. [1511-16-6] $C_{21}H_{23}ClFNO_2 \cdot HCl$. Crystals, mp 226-227.5°. Soly in water: 300 mg/100 ml.
Decanoate. [74050-97-8] KD-136; Haldol Decanoate; Halomonth; Neoperidole. $C_{31}H_{41}ClFNO_3$; mol wt 530.11.
THERAP CAT: Antidyskinetic (in Gilles de la Tourette's disease); antipsychotic.

4599. Halopredone Acetate. [57781-14-3] (6β,11β)-17,21-Bis(acetyloxy)-2-bromo-6,9-difluoro-11-hydroxypregna-1,4-diene-3,20-dione; 2-bromo-6β,9-difluoro-11β,17,21-trihydroxypregna-1,4-diene-3,20-dione 17,21-diacetate; Haloart. $C_{25}H_{29}BrF_2O_7$; mol wt 559.39. C 53.68%, H 5.23%, Br 14.28%, F 6.79%, O 20.02%. Prepn: M. Riva, L. Toscano, **DE 2508136**; M. Riva et al., **US 4226862** (1975, 1980 both to Pierrel); L. Toscano et al., J. Med. Chem. **20**, 213 (1977). Physico-chemical and analytical studies: eidem, Arzneim.-Forsch. **27**, 1636 (1977). Pharmacology: A. Bianchetti et al., ibid. 2096. Clinical study: B. Palmerio, P. Magnani, ibid. 2404. Toxicological study: L. Casilli et al., ibid. 2102.

Crystals from benzene, mp 290-292° (dec). $[\alpha]_D^{24}$ −36° (c = 1 in chloroform). uv max (methanol): 246 nm (ε 12500).
THERAP CAT: Anti-inflammatory (topical).

4600. Haloprogin. [777-11-7] 1,2,4-Trichloro-5-[(3-iodo-2-propynyl)oxy]benzene; 3-iodo-2-propynyl 2,4,5-trichlorophenyl ether; 2,4,5-trichlorophenyl γ-iodopropargyl ether; M-1028; Halotex; Mycanden. $C_9H_4Cl_3IO$; mol wt 361.39. C 29.91%, H 1.12%, Cl 29.43%, I 35.12%, O 4.43%. Prepn: S. Seki et al., Agric. Biol. Chem. **27**, 150 (1963), C.A. **58**, 14635g (1963); eidem, **JP 64 19791**; eidem, **US 3322813** (1964, 1967 both to Meiji Seika). Pharmacology: S. Seki et al., Antimicrob. Agents Chemother. **1963**, 569; E. F. Harrison et al., Appl. Microbiol. **19**, 746 (1970).

White or pale yellow crystals, mp 113-114°; dec 190°. uv max (anhydr ethanol): 288.5, 298.5 nm. Easily soluble in methanol, ethanol; very slightly sol in water. LD_{50} in mice: >3 g/kg orally and s.c.; 510 mg/kg i.p. (Seki, 1963).
THERAP CAT: Antifungal.

4601. Halostachine. [495-42-1] (αR)-α-[(Methylamino)methyl]benzenemethanol; (−)-α-(methylaminomethyl)benzyl alcohol; 1-hydroxy-1-phenyl-2-methylaminoethane; (−)-phenyl(methylaminomethyl)carbinol; 2-methylamino-1-phenylethanol. C_9H_{13}-NO; mol wt 151.21. C 71.49%, H 8.67%, N 9.26%, O 10.58%. Isoln from Halostachis caspica (Halostachis caspia): Menshikov, Rubinshtein, J. Gen. Chem. USSR **13**, 801 (1943), C.A. **39**, 1172 (1945). Synthesis: Menshikov, Borodina, J. Gen. Chem. USSR **17**, 1569 (1947), C.A. **42**, 2245 (1948). Configuration: Lukes et al., Collect. Czech. Chem. Commun. **26**, 466 (1961). As a possible cause of ryegrass staggers: Aasen et al., Aust. J. Agric. Res. **20**, 71 (1969). TLC determn in rye and fescue grasses: L. P. Bush, J. A. D. Jeffreys, J. Chromatogr. **111**, 165 (1975). Vasoactive potential: C. B. Davis et al., Vet. Hum. Toxicol. **25**, 6 (1983). One pot synthesis: P. Zandbergen et al., Tetrahedron **48**, 3977 (1992).

Crystals, mp 43-45°. $[\alpha]_D^{20}$ −47.03°. Soluble in water, alc, ether.
Hydrochloride. Crystals from alcohol, mp 113-114°. $[\alpha]_D^{20}$ −52.46°. Freely sol in water.

4602. Halosulfuron-methyl. [100784-20-1] 3-Chloro-5-[[[[(4,6-dimethoxy-2-pyrimidinyl)amino]carbonyl]amino]sulfonyl]-1-methyl-1H-pyrazole-4-carboxylic acid methyl ester; methyl 3-chloro-5-(4,6-dimethoxypyrimidin-2-ylcarbamoylsulfamoyl)-1-methylpyrazole-4-carboxylate; MON-12000; MON-12037; NC-319; Manage; Permit. $C_{13}H_{15}ClN_6O_7S$; mol wt 434.81. C 35.91%, H 3.48%, Cl 8.15%, N 19.33%, O 25.76%, S 7.37%. Sulfonylurea herbicide. Prepn: S. Yamamoto et al., **JP Kokai 85 208977**; eidem, **US 4668277** (1985, 1987 both to Nissan); S. Yamamoto et al., ACS Symp. Ser. **504**, 34 (1992). Physical properties and field trials in corn: K. Suzuki et al., Brighton Crop Prot. Conf. - Weeds **1991**, 31. Field trials in landscape plants: R. T. Hurt, W. K. Vencill, J. Environ. Hort. **12**, 135 (1994).

White powder, mp 172-173°. Vapor pressure (25°): 2.8 × 10^{-12} mm Hg. Soly in water (25°): 36 mg/l. LD_{50} orally in rats: 8865 mg/kg; dermally in rabbits: >2000 mg/kg; LC$_{50}$ (4 hr) in rats: >4.3 mg/l (Suzuki).

USE: Herbicide.

4603. Halothane. [151-67-7] 2-Bromo-2-chloro-1,1,1-trifluoroethane; bromochlorotrifluoroethane; 1,1,1-trifluoro-2,2-chlorobromoethane; Fluothane; Rhodialothan. C$_2$HBrClF$_3$; mol wt 197.38. C 12.17%, H 0.51%, Br 40.48%, Cl 17.96%, F 28.88%. CF$_3$CHClBr. Prepn from a mixt of F$_3$CCH$_2$Cl and F$_3$CCBr$_2$Cl: Suckling, Raventos, **US 2921098** (1960 to I.C.I.); by rearrangement of F$_2$BrCCHFCl: Scherer, Kühn, **US 2959624** (1960 to Hoechst); from BrClCHCBrCl$_2$: Chapman, McGinty, **GB 805764** (1958 to I.C.I.); from Br$_2$ClCCF$_3$: McGinty, **US 3082263** (1963 to I.C.I.); Madai, Muller, *J. Prakt. Chem.* **19,** 83 (1963). Enantiomeric resolution: J. Meinwald *et al., Science* **251,** 560 (1991). Comprehensive description: R. D. Daley, *Anal. Profiles Drug Subs.* **1,** 119-147 (1972).

Non-flammable, highly volatile liquid. Characteristic, sweetish, not unpleasant odor. d$_4^{20}$ 1.871. bp 50.2°; bp$_{243}$ 20°. n$_D^0$ 1.3697. Sensitive to light, may be stabilized with 0.01% thymol. Soly in water 0.345%. Miscible with petr ether, other fat solvents.

Caution: Potential symptoms of overexposure are irritation of eyes, skin, respiratory system; confusion, drowsiness, dizziness, nausea, analgesia, anesthesia; cardiac arrhythmia; liver and kidney damage; decreased audio visual performance. *See NIOSH Pocket Guide to Chemical Hazards* (DHHS/NIOSH 97-140, 1997) p 156.

THERAP CAT: Anesthetic (inhalation).

THERAP CAT (VET): Anesthetic (inhalation).

4604. Haloxazolam. [59128-97-1] 10-Bromo-11b-(2-fluorophenyl)-2,3,7,11b-tetrahydrooxazolo[3,2-*d*][1,4]benzodiazepin-6(5*H*)-one; CS-430; Somelin. C$_{17}$H$_{14}$BrFN$_2$O$_2$; mol wt 377.21. C 54.13%, H 3.74%, Br 21.18%, F 5.04%, N 7.43%, O 8.48%. Sleep-inducing agent, related structurally to oxazolam and cloxazolam, *q.q.v.* Prepn of analogous compounds: T. Miyadera *et al., J. Med. Chem.* **14,** 520 (1971). Structure-activity study: M. Yoshimoto *et al., Chem. Pharm. Bull.* **25,** 1378 (1977). Pharmacological studies: T. Kamioka *et al., Arzneim.-Forsch.* **28,** 838 (1978). Metabolism in animals: R. Hayashi *et al., Oyo Yakuri* **17,** 617 (1979), *C.A.* **91,** 204161s (1979).

Colorless cryst, mp 185°. Sparingly sol in water. LD$_{50}$ in mice: 1850 mg/kg orally (Kamioka).

Note: This is a controlled substance (depressant): **21 CFR,** 1308.14.

THERAP CAT: Sedative, hypnotic.

4605. Haloxon. [321-55-1] Phosphoric acid bis(2-chloroethyl) 3-chloro-4-methyl-2-oxo-2*H*-1-benzopyran-7-yl ester; 7-[[bis(2-chloroethoxy)phosphinyl]oxy]-3-chloro-4-methyl-2*H*-1-benzopyran-2-one; 3-chloro-7-hydroxy-4-methylcoumarin bis(2-chloroethyl) phosphate; *O,O*-bis(β-chloroethyl) *O*-(3-chloro-4-methyl-7-coumarinyl) phosphate; 3-chloro-7-hydroxy-4-methyl-2*H*-1-benzopyran-2-one bis(chloroethyl) phosphate; 3-chloro-4-methylumbelliferone di(2-chloroethyl) phosphate; galoxone; Galloxon; Loxon; Luxon. C$_{14}$H$_{14}$Cl$_3$O$_6$P; mol wt 415.59. C 40.46%, H 3.40%, Cl 25.59%, O 23.10%, P 7.45%. Prepn: **BE 610896** (1962 to Cooper, McDougall & Robertson), *C.A.* **57,** 13729g (1962). Toxicity data: Brown *et al., Nature* **194,** 379 (1962).

Crystals from ethanol, mp 91°. LD$_{50}$ orally in rats: 900 mg/kg (Brown).

THERAP CAT (VET): Anthelmintic.

4606. Hamamelis. Witch hazel; winter bloom; snapping hazel; striped alder; spotted alder; tobacco wood. Dried leaves of *Hamamelis virginiana* L., *Hamamelidaceae,* collected in autumn. History of hamamelis extract and distillate: Lloyd, Lloyd, *J. Am. Pharm. Assoc.* **24,** 220 (1935). *Habit.* North America (New England to Minnesota, southward to Louisiana). *Constit.* Hamamelitannin, gallic acid, volatile oil, bitter principle.

THERAP CAT: Astringent.

THERAP CAT (VET): Has been used as astringent, hemostatic, sedative.

4607. Hamamelitannin. [469-32-9] 2-*C*-[[(3,4,5-Trihydroxybenzoyl)oxy]methyl]-D-ribofuranose 5-(3,4,5-trihydroxybenzoate); 2-*C*-(hydroxymethyl)-D-ribofuranose 2′,5-digallate. C$_{20}$H$_{20}$O$_{14}$; mol wt 484.36. C 49.59%, H 4.16%, O 46.24%. From bark of *Hamamelis virginiana* L., *Hamamelidaceae:* Grüttner, *Arch. Pharm.* **236,** 278 (1898); from bark of *Castanea dentata* (Marsh.) Borkh., *Fagaceae:* Mayer, Kunz, *Naturwissenschaften* **46,** 206 (1959). Structure: Mayer *et al., Ann.* **688,** 232 (1965). Synthesis: Ezekiel *et al., Carbohyd. Res.* **11,** 233 (1969).

Prisms from water, mp 145-147°. [α]$_D^{19}$ +32.6° (c = 1.5).

Hexamethyl ether. C$_{26}$H$_{32}$O$_{14}$. Needles from dioxane + water, mp 73-76°. [α]$_{578}^{25}$ +10.0° (c = 2.0 in dioxane). Sol in acetone, dioxane, methanol. Practically insol in water.

4608. Hamamelose. [4573-78-8] 2-*C*-(Hydroxymethyl)-D-ribose. C$_6$H$_{12}$O$_6$; mol wt 180.16. C 40.00%, H 6.71%, O 53.28%. From tannin of witch hazel *(Hamamelis virginiana* L., *Hamamelidaceae):* Fischer, Freudenberg, *Ber.* **45,** 2709 (1912); Freudenberg, Peters, *ibid.* **53,** 953 (1920); Anderson, *U.S.A.E.C.* **UCRL-8870,** 114 (1959). Structure: Schmidt, *Ann.* **476,** 250 (1929). Configuration: Schmidt, Heintz, *ibid.* **515,** 77 (1934). Synthesis: Novák, Sorm, *Collect. Czech. Chem. Commun.* **30,** 3303 (1965); Paulsen *et al., Ber.* **105,** 1978 (1972). Synthesis of L-hamamelose: Burton *et al., Proc. Chem. Soc. London* **1962,** 181. Synthesis and ^{1}H, ^{13}C NMR study of aqueous equilibrium: W. A. Szarek *et al., Can. J. Chem.* **61,** 461 (1983).

D-Form. Crystals from abs ethanol, mp 111°. [α]$_D^{21}$ −7.4° (equilib in water).

L-Form. Crystals from ethanol + ethyl acetate, mp 110-111°. [α]$_D^{22}$ +1.3° (3 min) → +7.3° (equilib after 17 min).

4609. Hamycin. [1403-71-0] Primamycin. Polyene antibiotic complex produced by *Streptomyces pimprina:* M. J. Thirumalachar *et al., Hind. Antibiot. Bull.* **3,** 136 (1961), *C.A.* **55,** 27515i (1961); M. J. Thirumalachar, **US 3261751** (1966 to Hindustan Antibiot.). Formerly believed to be identical to trichomycin and candicidin, *q.q.v.:* H. Burrows, D. Calam, *J. Chromatogr.* **53,** 566 (1970). Subsequent HPLC studies have shown the three polyene antibiotics to be different entities: P. Helboe *et al., ibid.* **189,** 249 (1980). Structural study showing hamycin to be a mixture of components A, B, C, D: R. C. Pandey, K. L. Rinehart, *16th Interscience Conference on Antimicrob. Ag. Chemother.,* Chicago, 1976, *Abstracts of Papers,* no. 41. Absorption, excretion, tissue concentration: M. G.

Phatak *et al.*, *Indian J. Exp. Biol.* **12**, 284 (1974), *C.A.* **82**, 118703j (1975). Toxicity studies: Williams *et al.*, *Antimicrob. Agents Chemother.* **1964**, 737; antifungal activity: A. C. Parekh, C. V. Dave, *Life Sci.* **19**, 1737 (1976). HPLC study: W. Mechlinski, C. P. Schaffner, *J. Antibiot.* **33**, 591 (1980). Review of clinical use in mycoses: M. J. Thirumalachar, *J. Sci. Ind. Res.* **31**, 542-544 (1972), *C.A.* **79**, 13308 (1973).

Yellow amorphous powder, no definite mp, decomp 160°. $[\alpha]_D^{25}+216°$. uv max (80% methanol): 383 nm ($E_{1cm}^{1\%}$ 916). An amphoteric compd. Almost insol in water, benzene, chloroform, dry lower aliphatic alcohols, ether. Sol in basic solvents such as pyridine, collidine, and in aq lower alcohols. In concd H_2SO_4 gives stable blue color; no coloration with ferric chloride or with HCl. LD_{50} i.v. in mice (using sodium carboxymethyl cellulose as a vehicle): 6.16 mg/kg (Williams). Also reported as LD_{50} i.v. in Swiss mice (using a colloidal suspension): 1.20 mg/kg (Parekh, Dave).

Hamycin A. mp >300° (dec), $[\alpha]_D^{24}$ +181.1° (c = 0.6 in DMF). uv max: 380 nm ($E_{1cm}^{1\%}$ 989).

THERAP CAT: Antifungal.

4610. Hanatoxins. [253687-10-4] HaTx. Peptide toxins isolated from the venom of the Chilean tarantula, *Phrixotrichus spatulata*, originally named *Grammostola spatulata*; modifies voltage-dependent K^+ channels by shifting channel opening to more depolarized voltages. 35 amino acids long with 3 disulfide linkages, mol wt ~4.1 kDa. Isoln and characterization: K. J. Swartz, R. MacKinnon, *Neuron* **15**, 941 (1995). Mechanism of action and identification of receptor binding sites: *eidem, ibid.* **18**, 665, 675 (1997). Use as probe for determn of channel structure: Y. Li-Smerin, K. J. Swartz, *Proc. Natl. Acad. Sci. USA* **95**, 8585 (1998); V. Ruta *et al.*, *Nature* **422**, 180 (2003). Reagent for measurement of channel current in myocytes: H. M. Himmel *et al.*, *Am. J. Physiol.* **277**, H107 (1999).

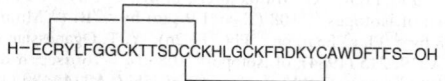

Hanatoxin 1. [281212-01-9] (native)]; [170780-00-4] (reduced). $HaTx_1$. NMR determn of 3d-structure: H. Takahashi *et al.*, *J. Mol. Biol.* **297**, 771 (2000).
Hanatoxin 2. [170780-01-5] (reduced) $HaTx_2$.
USE: Inhibition of voltage-gated K^+ channels.

4611. Haplophytine. [16625-20-0] [15(3a*S*,7*R*)]-3,4-Didehydro-19-hydroxy-16,17-dimethoxy-1-methyl-15-(2,3,5,6-tetrahydro-11-hydroxy-4-methyl-1,13-dioxo-1*H*-3a,7-methanopyrrolo[1,-2-*a*][1,3]benzodiazocin-7(4*H*)-yl)aspidospermidin-21-oic acid γ-lactone. $C_{37}H_{40}N_4O_7$; mol wt 652.74. C 68.08%, H 6.18%, N 8.58%, O 17.16%. Insecticidal alkaloid from the Mexican plant *Haplophyton cimicidum* A. DC., *Apocynaceae*: Rogers *et al., J. Am. Chem. Soc.* **74**, 1987 (1952); **76**, 2819 (1954). Partial structure: Snyder *et al., ibid.* **80**, 3708 (1958). Structure: Rae *et al., ibid.* **89**, 3061 (1967). Crystal structure and absolute config.: Zacharias, *Acta Crystallogr.* **26B**, 1455 (1970). Synthetic approaches: P. Yates, D. A. Schwartz, *Can. J. Chem.* **61**, 509 (1983). *Review:* Yates *et al., J. Am. Chem. Soc.* **95**, 7842 (1973).

Crystals from ethanol + chloroform, mp 290-293° (rapid heating, starting at 250°). Also reported as mp 300-302° (Yates *et al., loc. cit.*). $[\alpha]_D^{25}$ +109.0° (chloroform). uv max (ethanol): 220, 265, 305 nm (ε 48500, 14300, 4500). Very sol in chloroform, benzene,

dioxane, ethyl acetate. Moderately sol in acetone, methanol, somewhat less in ethanol. Practically insol in water, ether, petr ether. Readily sol in dil acids or alkalies.
Dihydrochloride. $C_{27}H_{31}N_3O_5.2HCl$. Dec 208-218° (darkens at 200°).
O-Methylhaplophytine. $C_{28}H_{33}N_3O_5$. Crystals from ether + ethanol, dec 288-291°. $[\alpha]_D^{24}$ +12° (c = 4.37 in chloroform).

4612. Haptoglobins. α_2-Globulins which combine with hemoglobin to form a weak peroxidase and which constitute about one-quarter of the α_2-globulin fraction of human plasma: Jayle, Conas, *Bull. Soc. Chim. Biol.* **34**, 65 (1952). Prepn: Herman-Boussier *et al., ibid.* **48**, 817, 837 (1960). For each individual there are three genetic types of haptoglobins, each reacting identically with antibodies to each of the others. Structure of this serum glycoprotein is a tetramer composed of α- and β-polypeptide chains, the α-chain varying in the three phenotypes, the β-chains being identical. Amino acid sequence of α-chains: Black, Dixon, *Nature* **218**, 736 (1968); Malchy, Dixon, *Can. J. Biochem.* **51**, 321 (1973). *C*- and *N*-terminal sequences of the β-chain: Barnett *et al., Biochemistry* **11**, 1189 (1972); A. Kurosky *et al., Comp. Biochem. Physiol.* **55B**, 453 (1976); *eidem, Biochemistry* **15**, 5326 (1976). Lowered levels of haptoglobins found in individuals with acute hepatitis and pernicious anemia. *Review:* Laurell, Grönvall, *Adv. Clin. Chem.* **5**, 135-172 (1962). Monograph: Kirk, *The Haptoglobin Groups in Man* (S. Karger, New York, 1968) 77 pp. Review on genetics, biochemistry and physiology of human haptoglobins: J. Javid, *Curr. Top. Hematol.* **1**, 151-192 (1978).

4613. Harmaline. [304-21-2] 4,9-Dihydro-7-methoxy-1-methyl-3*H*-pyrido[3,4-*b*]indole; 1-methyl-7-methoxy-3,4-dihydro-β-carboline; 3,4-dihydroharmine; harmidine; harmalol methyl ether; *O*-methylharmalol. $C_{13}H_{14}N_2O$; mol wt 214.26. C 72.87%, H 6.59%, N 13.07%, O 7.47%. CNS stimulant from seeds of *Peganum harmala* L., *Zygophyllaceae:* Goebel, *Ann.* **38**, 363 (1841); from *Banisteria caapi* Spruce, *Malpighiaceae:* Hochstein, Paradies, *J. Am. Chem. Soc.* **79**, 5735 (1957). Structure: Manske *et al., J. Chem. Soc.* **1927**, 1. Synthesis: Späth, Lederer, *Ber.* **63**, 120, 2102 (1930); Spenser, *Can. J. Chem.* **37**, 1851 (1959). Identity with harmidine: Robinson, *Chem. Ind. (London)* **1965**, 605. Pharmacology: Fuentes, Longo, *Neuropharmacology* **10**, 15 (1971). Metabolism: Ho *et al., Biochem. Pharmacol.* **20**, 1313 (1971). Review of structure and synthesis work: Hofmann, *Sven. Farm. Tidskr.* **75**, 933 (1971), *C.A.* **76**, 149609g (1972).

Orthorhombic bipyramidal prisms, tablets from methanol, rhombic octahedra from ethanol, mp 229-231°. pK 4.2. uv max (methanol): 218, 260, 376 nm (log ε 4.27, 3.90, 4.02). Slightly sol in water, alcohol, ether; quite sol in hot alcohol, dil acids.
Hydrochloride dihydrate. Slender, yellow needles, moderately sol in water, alcohol.
N-Acetylharmaline. Needles, mp 204-205°.

4614. Harmalol. [525-57-5] 4,9-Dihydro-1-methyl-3*H*-pyrido[3,4-*b*]indol-7-ol; 3,4-dihydro-1-methyl-9*H*-pyrido[3,4-*b*]indol-7-ol. $C_{12}H_{12}N_2O$; mol wt 200.24. C 71.98%, H 6.04%, N 13.99%, O 7.99%. From seeds of *Peganum harmala* L., *Zygophyllaceae:* Göbel, *Ann.* **38**, 363 (1841); Fischer, *Ber.* **18**, 400 (1885); by demethylation of harmaline: Coulthard *et al., Biochem. J.* **27**, 727 (1933). HPLC determn in *Peganum harmala* L. seeds: M. Kartal *et al., J. Pharm. Biomed. Anal.* **31**, 263 (2003). *In vitro* neuroprotective effects: D. H. Kim *et al., Eur. J. Neurosci.* **13**, 1861 (2001).

Trihydrate. [6027-99-2] Red needles from water. Dec 212° (anhydr). Readily sol in hot water, acetone, chloroform, alkali hydroxides, but not carbonates. Aq solns are yellow with green fluorescence.

Lactate. [6028-08-6] $C_{12}H_{12}N_2O.C_3H_6O_3$. mp 174-176°; monohydrate as bright yellow leaflets, mp 116-120°. Sol in water and alcohol.

O-Ethylharmalol. [6010-17-9] $C_{14}H_{16}N_2O$. Brown needles from alc, mp 237-239°.

O-n-Propylharmalol. [6028-01-9] $C_{15}H_{18}N_2O$. Brown needles from alc, mp 195-197°.

O-n-Butylharmalol. [6197-42-8] $C_{16}H_{20}N_2O$. Colorless needles from alc, mp 173°.

O-Methylharmalol *see* Harmaline.

4615. Harman. [486-84-0] 1-Methyl-9*H*-pyrido[3,4-*b*]indole; 3-methyl-4-carboline; 2-methyl-β-carboline; aribine; loturine; passiflorin. $C_{12}H_{10}N_2$; mol wt 182.22. C 79.10%, H 5.53%, N 15.37%. From bark of *Sickingia rubra* (Mart.) K. Schum. (*Arariba rubra* Mart.), *Rubiaceae; Symplocus racemosa* Roxb., *Symplocaceae;* and *Passiflora incarnata* L., *Passifloraceae:* Rieth, Wohler, *Ann.* **120**, 247 (1861); Späth, *Monatsh. Chem.* **40**, 351; **41**, 401 (1920); Neu, *Arzneim.-Forsch.* **4**, 601 (1954). Structure: Neu, *ibid.* **6**, 94 (1956). Synthesis: Harvey, Robson, *J. Chem. Soc.* **1938**, 97; Snyder *et al., J. Am. Chem. Soc.* **70**, 222 (1948); Clemo, Holt, *J. Chem. Soc.* **1953**, 1313; Kametani *et al., ibid. (C)* **1968**, 1006. Isoln from cigarette smoke: Poindexter, Carpenter, *Chem. Ind. (London)* **1962**, 176. Toxicity study: E. B. Sigg *et al., Arch. Int. Pharmacodyn.* **149**, 164 (1964).

Bitter orthorhombic crystals from heptane + cyclohexane, mp 237-238°. Exhibits bright blue fluorescence in uv light. pKa: 7.37, 14.6. uv max (methanol): 234, 287, 347 nm (log ε 4.57, 4.21, 3.66). Absorption and fluorescence spectra: O. S. Wolfbeis *et al., Monatsh. Chem.* **113**, 509 (1982). Practically insol in water. Sol in dil acids. LD$_{50}$ i.p. in mice: 50 mg/kg (Sigg).

Hydrochloride. $C_{12}H_{10}N_2.HCl$. Rosettes of needles from ethanol + 20% HCl in water, sublimes at 120-130°.

4616. Harmine. [442-51-3] 7-Methoxy-1-methyl-9*H*-pyrido[3,4-*b*]indole; banisterine; yageine; telepathine; leucoharmine. $C_{13}H_{12}N_2O$; mol wt 212.25. C 73.56%, H 5.70%, N 13.20%, O 7.54%. CNS stimulant isolated from seeds of *Peganum harmala* L., *Zygophyllaceae:* Göbel, *Ann.* **38**, 363 (1841); Reinhard *et al., Phytochemistry* **7**, 503 (1968); from *Banisteria caapi* Spruce, *Malpighiaceae:* Hochstein, Paradies, *J. Am. Chem. Soc.* **79**, 5735 (1957); from *Banisteriopsis inebrians* Morton, *Malpighiaceae:* O'Connell, Lynn, *J. Am. Pharm. Assoc.* **42**, 753 (1953). Structure: Manske *et al., J. Chem. Soc.* **1927**, 1, 240. Synthesis: Späth, Lederer, *Ber.* **63B**, 120 (1930); Akaboro, Saito, *ibid.* 2245; Hahn *et al., Ber.* **67B**, 2031 (1934), *Ann.* **520**, 107, 123 (1935), *Ber.* **71B**, 2163, 2175 (1938); Harvey, Robson, *J. Chem. Soc.* **1938**, 97. Metabolism: Slotkin, DiStefano, *J. Pharmacol. Exp. Ther.* **174**, 456 (1970). Toxicity study: K. K. Chen *et al., J. Pharmacol. Exp. Ther.* **79**, 127 (1943).

Slender, orthorhombic prisms from methanol, mp 261° (dec). Sublimes. pKa 7.70. uv max (methanol): 241, 301, 336 nm (log ε 4.61, 4.21, 3.69). Absorption and fluorescence spectra: O. S. Wolfbeis, E. Fürlinger, *Z. Phys. Chem.* **129**, 171 (1982). Slightly sol in water, alcohol, chloroform, ether.

Hydrochloride dihydrate. Crystals, mp 262° (dec), mp 321° when anhydrous. Sol in 40 parts water, freely sol in hot water. Aq solns have blue fluorescence. LD$_{50}$ i.v. in mice: 38 mg/kg (Chen).

4617. Harpin. [151438-54-9] Messenger. Protein product of the *hrp*N gene of *Erwinia amylovora,* a phytopathogenic bacterium that causes fire blight disease. Composed of 403 amino acid residues; mol wt ~44 kDa. Member of a class of glycine-rich, acidic, heat stable proteins that elicit the hypersensitive response as part of the plant's defense mechanism vs pathogenic bacteria. Induces systemic acquired resistance to fire blight and many other plant pathogens, enhances plant growth, and promotes insect repellency. Isoln: Z.-M. Wei *et al., Science* **257**, 85 (1992). Prepn: S. V. Beer *et al.,* **WO 9401546**; *eidem,* **US 5849868** (1994, 1998 both to Cornell Research Foundation). Elicitation of hypersensitive response: S. V. Beer *et al.* in *Curr. Plant Sci. Biotechnol. Agric.* **vol. 14,** E. W. Nester, D. P. S. Verma, Eds. (Kluwer, Dordrecht, 1993) pp 281-286. Induction of plant resistance: Z.-M. Wei, S. V. Beer, *Acta Hortic.* **411**, 223 (1996); and mode of action of disease resistance: H. Dong *et al., Plant J.* **20**, 207 (1999). Effects on tobacco leaf cell membranes: S. M. Pike *et al., Physiol. Mol. Plant Pathol.* **53**, 39 (1998). Blue mold resistance study in apples: G. de Capdeville *et al., Plant Dis.* **87**, 39 (2003). Review of *hrp* genes and harpin proteins: J. F. Kim, S. V. Beer in *Fire Blight,* J. Vanneste, Ed. (CABI Publishing, Wallingford, 2000) pp. 141-161; of commercial product: *Biopesticide Regulatory Action Document: Harpin Protein* (U.S. EPA, 2002) 32 pp.

pI 4.3. Mean bulk density: 0.452 g/ml. uv max: 204 nm (pH 7). LD$_{50}$ in rats orally; rabbits dermally (g/kg): >2; >6. LC$_{50}$ in rainbow trout (mg/l): >3270 (U.S. EPA).

USE: Biodegradable plant health regulator effective in vegetables, field crops, small grains, trees, vines, specialty crops, turf and ornamentals.

4618. Hassium. [54037-57-9] Element 108; unniloctium. Hs, Uno; at. no. 108. Group VIII (8). No stable nuclides. Prepn of isotope $^{265}108$ (T$_½$ ~1.8 msec, α-decay, rel. at. mass 265.1306) by ^{208}Pb (^{58}Fe,n): G. Münzenberg *et al., Z. Phys.* **A317**, 235 (1984); of isotopes $^{263}108$ (T$_½$ ~1.9 sec) by ^{209}Bi (^{55}Mn,n) and $^{264}108$ by ^{207}Pb (^{58}Fe,n) or ^{208}Pb(^{58}Fe,2n): Y. T. Oganessian *et al., ibid.* **A319**, 215 (1984); of isotope $^{264}108$ (T$_½$ ~76 μsec, α-decay) by ^{207}Pb(^{58}Fe,n): G. Münzenberg *et al., ibid.* **A324**, 489 (1986). Review of synthesis: *eidem, ibid.* **A328**, 49-59 (1987); G. N. Flerov, G. M. Ter-Akopian, *Prog. Particle Nucl. Phys.* **19**, 197-239 (1987); G. T. Seaborg in *Transuranium Elements: A Half Century,* L. R. Morss, J. Fuger, Eds. (Am. Chem. Soc., Washington DC, 1992) p 40-41.

4619. Hasubanonine. [1805-85-2] 7,8-Didehydro-3,4,7,8-tetramethoxy-17-methylhasuban-6-one. $C_{21}H_{27}NO_5$; mol wt 373.44. C 67.54%, H 7.29%, N 3.75%, O 21.42%. Alkaloid having a modified morphinan skeleton with a five membered heterocyclic ring, hitherto unknown in natural sources. (Alkaloids with this unique skeleton are called *hasubanan* alkaloids; *see* S. Shiotani, T. Kometani, *Tetrahedron Lett.* **1976**, 767 for synthesis of hasubanan skeleton). Isolated from *Stephania japonica* Miers, *Menispermaceae:* Kondo *et al., Annu. Rep. Itsuu Lab.* **2**, 35 (1951); Satomi, *ibid.* **3**, 37 (1953); Kondo, Satomi, *ibid.* **8**, 41 (1957); *C.A.* **47**, 5951f (1953); **48**, 2728c (1954); **51**, 17956i (1957). Structure: Tomita *et al., Tetrahedron Lett.* **1964**, 2937; *eidem, Chem. Pharm. Bull.* **13**, 538 (1965). Total synthesis: Ibuka *et al., Tetrahedron Lett.* **1970**, 4811; *Chem. Pharm. Bull.* **22**, 782 (1974). Biosynthesis: A. R. Battersby *et al., Chem. Commun.* **1974**, 773; *eidem, J. Chem. Soc. Perkin Trans. 1* **1981**, 2010, 2016, 2030. *Review:* Y. Inubushi, T. Ibuka in *The Alkaloids* vol. **XVI**, R. H. F. Manske, Ed. (Academic Press, New York, 1977) pp 393-428.

Prisms from methanol, mp 116°. [α]$_D$ −219° (ethanol).

4620. HCS. [11085-36-2] Lactogen (human placental); lactogenic hormone (placental human); human chorionic somatomammotropin; chorionic growth hormone-prolactin; CGP; human placental lactogen; HPL. Growth hormone from human placenta. Exhibits lactogenic as well as growth-promoting activity: Josimovich, MacLearen, *Endocrinology* **71**, 209 (1962); Kaplan, Grumbach, *J. Clin. Endocrinol. Metab.* **24**, 80 (1964). Structure is a single polypeptide chain containing 190 amino acid residues: Li *et al., Science* **173**, 56 (1971); Sherwood *et al., Nature New Biol.* **233**, 59 (1971). Structural revision to 191 amino acid residues and comparison with human growth hormone and human prolactin: Li *et al., Arch. Biochem. Biophys.* **155**, 95 (1973); Niall *et al., Recent Prog. Horm. Res.* **29**, 387 (1973). Purification: Parcells, Dahlgren, US 3687833 (1972 to Upjohn). Terminology: Li *et al., Experientia* **24**, 1288 (1968). *Review:* M. Chatterjee, H. N. Munro in *Vitamins and Hormones* vol. **35**, P. L. Munson *et al.*, Eds. (Academic Press, New York, 1977) pp 149-208.

4621. Hecameg®. [115457-83-5] Methyl-α-D-glucopyranoside 6-(heptylcarbamate); 6-*O*-(*N*-heptylcarbamoyl)-methyl-α-D-glucopyranoside. $C_{15}H_{29}NO_7$; mol wt 335.39. C 53.72%, H 8.72%, N 4.18%, O 33.39%. Glycolipid surfactant. Prepn: D. Plusquellec *et al., Anal. Biochem.* **179**, 145 (1989). Kinetics of surfactant exchange; effect on micelle aggregation: M. Frindi *et al., J. Phys. Chem.* **96**, 8137 (1992). Crystal structure: S. B. Engelsen *et al., Carbohydr. Res.* **264**, 161 (1994). Assessment as detergent in biochemical applications: M. B. Ruiz *et al., Biochim. Biophys. Acta* **1193**, 301 (1994). Use in protein purification: M. C. Sanders *et al., J. Biol. Chem.* **271**, 2651 (1996); P. Bron *et al., J. Mol. Biol.* **287**, 117 (1999).

Orthorhombic white needles, mp 108-110°. d 1.229 g/cm³. $[\alpha]_D^{22}$ +89 ±2° (c = 9.42 x 10^{-3} in water). Neutral, non-ionic.
USE: Detergent, primarily for protein purification.

4622. Hecogenin. [467-55-0] (3β,5α,25R)-3-Hydroxyspirostan-12-one. $C_{27}H_{42}O_4$; mol wt 430.62. C 75.31%, H 9.83%, O 14.86%. A steroidal sapogenin which has been isolated from plants, particularly from numerous *Agave* species. Isoln: Marker *et al., J. Am. Chem. Soc.* **69**, 2167 (1947); Rubin, US 3303186 (1967). Synthesis and configuration: Mazur *et al., J. Am. Chem. Soc.* **82**, 5889 (1960). Separation of an optically inactive product from sapogenin mixtures: Cardenas, US 3013010 (1961 to Searle). *Review:* L. F. Fieser, M. Fieser, *Steroids* (Reinhold, New York, 1959) pp 667-671 sqq.

Crystals from acetone, mp 264-266°. $[\alpha]_D$ +8° (CHCl₃) (Mazur *et al.*); mp 245°, 253°, 268° (Marker *et al.*); mp 240-245°, 245-250°. $[\alpha]_D$ ±0° (CHCl₃) (Cardenas).
Pseudohecogenin. [11005-20-2] (3β,5α,25R)-3,26-Dihydroxyfurost-20(22)-en-12-one. $C_{27}H_{42}O_4$; mol wt 430.62. Prepn from hecogenin: Cameron *et al., J. Chem. Soc.* **1955**, 2807; Wall, Serota, US 2870143 (1959 to USDA). Plates from aq acetone, mp 190-

191°. $[\alpha]_D^{20}$ +103° (c = 1.5 in chloroform), +96° (c = 1 in dioxane). uv max (ethanol): 213 nm (ε 6400).
USE: In prepn of steroidal hormones.

4623. Hectorite. [12173-47-6] Strese & Hofmann's hectorite. Swelling and gelling clay of the montmorillonite group. Approx formula: $Na_{0.67}(Mg,Li)_6Si_8O_{20}(OH,F)_4$. Some analyses show neither Li nor F, whether by oversight or by variation in the mineral is uncertain: M. H. Hey, *Mineral Species and Varieties* (Brit. Museum, London, 2nd ed., 1962) p 205.
Caution: Dust can be irritating to respiratory tract.
USE: In the chill-proofing of beer: Shaler *et al.*, US 3100707 (1963 to American Tansul).

4624. Hederagenin. [465-99-6] (3β,4α)-3,23-Dihydroxyolean-12-en-28-oic acid; caulosapogenin; melanthigenin. $C_{30}H_{48}O_4$; mol wt 472.70. C 76.23%, H 10.24%, O 13.54%. Occurs as glycoside in many saponins, see α-Hederin. Isoln and structure: van der Haar, *Arch. Pharm.* **250**, 424 (1912); Ruzicka *et al., Helv. Chim. Acta* **28**, 380 (1945); Haynes *et al., J. Chem. Soc.* **1963**, 744. Identity with melanthigenin: Mustafa, Soliman, *ibid.* **1943**, 70. Identity with caulosapogenin: McShefferty, Stenlake, *ibid.* **1956**, 2314. Molecular and crystal structure: R. Roques *et al., Acta Crystallogr.* **B34**, 1634 (1978). *See also* α- and β-Amyrin and Oleanolic Acid.

Crystals from alc, mp 332-334°. $[\alpha]_D^{20}$ +81° (c = 0.7 in pyridine). Freely sol in pyridine; sol in chloroform-alcohol mixtures; slowly sol in alcohol; practically insol in water; sol in dil alcoholic NaOH, but not in water solns of alkalies.
Diacetate. mp 172-174°. $[\alpha]_D^{20}$ +64° (CHCl₃).
Methyl ester. mp 240°. $[\alpha]_D^{23}$ +76° (c = 0.8 in CHCl₃).

4625. α-Hederin. [27013-91-8] Helixin (the saponin). $C_{41}H_{66}O_{12}$; mol wt 750.96. C 65.57%, H 8.86%, O 25.57%. Isoln from ivy leaves *(Hedera helix* L., *Araliaceae):* van der Haar, *Arch. Pharm.* **250**, 424 (1912); **251**, 632, 650; *idem, Biochem. Z.* **76**, 335 (1916); *idem, Ber.* **54**, 3142 (1921). Isoln and structure: Tschesche *et al., Z. Naturforsch.* **20b**, 708 (1965).

Precipitated from ethanol by addition of ether, mp 256-259°. $[\alpha]_D^{20}$ +14.5° (c = 0.92 in methanol).

4626. Helenalin. [6754-13-8] [3aS-(3aα,4α,4aβ,7aα,8α,-9aα)]-3,3a,4,4a,7a,8,9,9a-Octahydro-4-hydroxy-4a,8-dimethyl-3-methyleneazuleno[6,5-*b*]furan-2,5-dione; 6α,8β-dihydroxy-4-oxo-ambrosa-2,11(13)-dien-12-oic acid 12,8-lactone. $C_{15}H_{18}O_4$; mol wt 262.30. C 68.68%, H 6.92%, O 24.40%. Pseudoguaianolide sesquiterpenoid lactone from *Helenium autumnale* L., *H. amarum* (Raf.) H. Roch, *H. microcephalum* DC., *Compositae.* Isoln: Clark, *J. Am. Chem. Soc.* **58**, 1982 (1936); and characterization: Adams,

Herz, *ibid.* **71**, 2546 (1949). Structure: Büchi, Rosenthal, *ibid.* **78**, 3860 (1956); Barton, de Mayo, *Q. Rev. Chem. Soc.* **11**, 189 (1957); Herz, *J. Org. Chem.* **27**, 4043 (1962). Abs config studies: Herz, Kagan, *ibid.* **32**, 216 (1967). Synthesis of racemic form: Y. Ohfune *et al., J. Am. Chem. Soc.* **100**, 5946 (1978); M. R. Roberts, R. H. Schlessinger, *ibid.* **101**, 7626 (1979); C. H. Heathcock *et al., ibid.* **104**, 1907 (1982). Toxicity study: D. A. Witzel *et al., Am. J. Vet. Res.* **37**, 859 (1976).

Bitter, sternutative crystals from benzene, mp 167-168°. $[\alpha]_D^{25}$ −102.8° (c = 3.64 in 95% ethanol). uv max: 223 nm (ε 11900). Slightly sol in water; sol in alcohol, chloroform, hot benzene. LD_{50} in mice, rats (mg/kg): 150, 125 orally (Witzel).

Acetylhelenalin. $C_{17}H_{20}O_5$. Crystals from aq methanol, mp 184°. uv max: 221, 316 nm (ε 12600, 61).

4627. Helenynolic Acid. [7309-58-2] (9*S*,10*E*)-9-Hydroxy-10-octadecen-12-ynoic acid. $C_{18}H_{30}O_3$; mol wt 294.43. C 73.43%, H 10.27%, O 16.30%. From seed oil of *Helichrysum bracteatum* Andr., *Compositae:* R. G. Powell *et al., J. Am. Oil Chem. Soc.* **42**, 165 (1965). Structure: *eidem, J. Org. Chem.* **30**, 610 (1965). Absolute configuration: J. C. Craig *et al., ibid.* 4342. Partial synthesis of racemic helenynolic acid: H. R. S. Conacher, Gunstone, *Lipids* **5**, 137 (1970). Synthesis of (±)-form: T. B. Patrick, G. F. Melm, *J. Org. Chem.* **44**, 645 (1979).

Methyl ester. $C_{19}H_{32}O_3$. uv max (isooctane): 228, 238 nm (ε 17400, 14300). $[\alpha]_{600}^{26}$ −7° (c = 3.6 in ethanol).

4628. Helicin. [618-65-5] 2-(β-D-Glucopyranosyloxy)-benzaldehyde; salicylaldehyde β-D-glucoside. $C_{13}H_{16}O_7$; mol wt 284.26. C 54.93%, H 5.67%, O 39.40%. Prepn by the oxidation of salicin with dil nitric acid: Schiff, *Ann.* **154**, 19 (1870); from salicylaldehyde + *O*-tetraacetyl-α-glucosidyl bromide: Robertson, Waters, *J. Chem. Soc.* **1930**, 2729. ORD and stereochemical studies: Tsuzuki *et al., Bull. Chem. Soc. Jpn.* **44**, 526 (1971).

Needles with 0.75 mol H_2O from H_2O; mp 175-176° when dried at 100°. $[\alpha]_D^{20}$ −60° (c = 1.4). One gram dissolves in 55 ml water; freely sol in hot water, alcohol. Forms compds with urea, thiourea, certain amino acids.

Tetraacetate. $C_{21}H_{24}O_{11}$. Needles from alc, mp 142°. $[\alpha]_D^{20}$ −37° (acetone).

Note: The same formula is ascribed to **spirein**, found in *Spiraea camtschatica* Pall. and in *S. ulmaria* L., *Rosaceae.* Emulsin hydrolyzes helicin and spirein, yielding D-glucose and salicylaldehyde.

4629. Heliosupine. [32728-78-2] 2-Methyl-2-butenoic acid 7-[[2,3-dihydroxy-2-(1-hydroxyethyl)-3-methyl-1-oxobutoxy]-methyl]-2,3,5,7a-tetrahydro-1*H*-pyrrolizin-1-yl ester; cynoglossophine. $C_{20}H_{31}NO_7$; mol wt 397.46. C 60.44%, H 7.86%, N 3.52%, O 28.18%. Hepatotoxic pyrrolizidine alkaloid isolated from *Heliotropium supinum* L., *Boraginaceae:* Denisova *et al., Dokl. Akad. Nauk SSSR* **93**, 59 (1953); from *Cynoglossum officinale* L., *Boraginaceae:* Man'ko, Borisyuk, *Ukr. Khim. Zh.* **23**, 362 (1957), *C.A.* **52**, 2188a (1958); Man'ko, Marchenko, *Khim. Prir.*

Soedin. **7**, 537 (1971), *C.A.* **75**, 126598t (1971). Identity with cynoglossophine: Man'ko, *Ukr. Khim. Zh.* **25**, 627 (1959), *C.A.* **54**, 12494d (1960). Structure: Crowley, Culvenor, *Aust. J. Chem.* **12**, 694 (1959). Biosynthesis studies: Crout, *J. Chem. Soc. C* **1967**, 1233. *Reviews: see* Lasiocarpine.

Colorless gum. $[\alpha]_D^{20}$ −4.3° (c = 5.1 in ethanol).
Methyl ether *see* Lasiocarpine.

4630. Helium. [7440-59-7] He; at. wt 4.002602; at. no. 2. Group VIIIA (18), also known as Group 0. A noble gas characterized by an electronic structure in which the outer *p* subshell is entirely filled. Natural isotopic mixture (mass numbers): 4 (99.999862%), 3 (1.38 × 10^{-4}%). Known artificial radioactive isotopes: 5-8. Longest-lived isotope: ^{6}He ($T_{1/2}$ 806.7 msec, β-emitter). Abundance in igneous rock of earth's crust: 3 × 10^{-3} ppm by wt; concentration in air: 5.24 ppm by vol. Identified in the spectrum of the sun's chromosphere by Lockyer and Frankland in 1868. Obtained by Hillebrand in 1890 by heating uranium minerals and identified by Ramsay in 1895. Found in natural gas from which it is extracted on a commercial scale. Produced in the decay of radioactive elements: 1 kg of uranium in its conversion into 865 g of lead forms 756 l of helium; also produced in nature by the bombardment of beryllium, lithium, and other light elements with cosmic rays, x-rays and high-speed protons and deuterons. Monograph: G. A. Cook, *Argon, Helium and the Rare Gases* (Interscience, New York, 1961). *Reviews:* Cockett, Smith, "The Monatomic Gases" in *Comprehensive Inorganic Chemistry* **vol. 1**, J. C. Bailar, Jr. *et al.,* Eds. (Pergamon Press, Oxford, 1973) pp 139-211; E. Cook, *Science* **206**, 1141-1146 (1979); S.-C. Hwang, W. R. Weltmer, Jr. in *Kirk-Othmer Encyclopedia of Chemical Technology* **vol. 13** (John Wiley & Sons, 4th ed., 1995) pp 1-38; *Chemistry of the Elements* N. N. Greenwood, A. Earnshaw, Eds. (Pergamon Press, New York, 1984) pp 1042-1059. Review of use in inductively coupled plasma-mass spectrometry: S. F. Durrant, *Fresenius J. Anal. Chem.* **347**, 389-392 (1993).

Colorless, odorless, tasteless, nonflammable, monatomic, inert gas; will form compds with highly electronegative elements such as O, F, Cl. Cannot be frozen by lowering the temp at ordinary press.; no triple point. Very slightly sol in water (ml/100 ml): 0.97 at 0°; 1.08 at 50°. Trouton's const 4.64.

^{4}**He.** Critical temp 5.2014 K, critical press 227.5 kPa, critical d 69.64 kg/m^3. Gas: d^0 (101.3 kPa) 0.17850 kg/m^3, d (normal bp) 16.89 kg/m^3. Liquid: normal bp −268.926°, d (normal bp) 125.0 kg/m^3, heat of vaporization (normal bp) 81.70 J/mol. Two liq forms exist: He I above ~2.2 K; He II below ~2.2 K. He II is a superconducting liq; has very low viscosity; superfluid.

^{3}**He.** Critical temp 3.324 K, critical press 116.4 kPa, critical d 41.3 kg/m^3. Gas: d^0 (101.3 kPa) 0.1347 kg/m^3, d (normal bp) 23.64 kg/m^3. Liquid: normal bp −269.959°, d (normal bp) 58.9 kg/m^3, heat of vaporization (normal bp) 25.48 J/mol.

Caution: Can act as a simple asphyxiant by displacing air. *See: Matheson Gas Data Book* (Matheson Co., Inc., 4th ed., East Rutherford, NJ, 1966) pp 249-253.

USE: Liquid helium (the most volatile liq known) as cryogen for the production of low temps, in MRI machines. Gas in manuf of semiconducting devices; in detection devices for leaks in vacuum systems; in Ne-He lasers; in gas mixtures as the working fluid in plasma devices; in mixtures with Ne and Ar in Geiger counters. *Q-Gas,* a mixture of 98.7% He and 1.3% butane, has been used as a filling for gas-flow Geiger counters. Gas as a shield in gas tungsten-arc welding, in metal processing; substitute for N_2 in synthetic breathing gas for deep sea divers and workers in high pressure conditions; coolant in high temp nuclear reactors; carrier gas in gas-liquid and gas-solid chromatography; inert diluent; to create inert atmosphere; to fill balloons and airships, lifting power is 0.93 if hydrogen is taken as 1.00.

4631. Helonias. False unicorn; blazing star; starwort. Rhizome and roots of *Chamaelirium luteum* (L.) A. Gray, *Liliaceae*. *Habit.* Ontario and Eastern U.S.

4632. Helveticoside. [630-64-8] $(3\beta,5\beta)$-[(2,6-Dideoxy-β-D-*ribo*-hexopyranosyl)oxy]-5,14-dihydroxy-19-oxocard-20(22)-enolide; erisimin; erysimin; alleoside A. $C_{29}H_{42}O_9$; mol wt 534.64. C 65.15%, H 7.92%, O 26.93%. A β-glycoside consisting of one mole strophanthidin and one mole D-digitoxose. Isoln from *Erysimum helveticum* (Jacq.) DC. and *Erysimum crepidifolium* Reichenb., *Cruciferae*, and structure: Nagata *et al.*, *Helv. Chim. Acta* **40**, 41 (1957); *eidem, Festschr. Arthur Stoll* **1957**, 715; Gmelin, **DE 1221764** (1966). From *Erysimum* spp.: Kowalewski, *Helv. Chim. Acta* **43**, 1314 (1960). Toxicity study: Graebner, Giesel, *Arzneim.-Forsch.* **22**, 1854 (1972).

Dihydrate. Needles from dil methanol, mp 153-157°. $[\alpha]_D^{25}$ +30.7° (c = 1.5 in methanol); $[\alpha]_D^{24}$ +26.0° (c = 1.1 in chloroform). uv max (ethanol): 217, 304 nm (log ε 4.27, 1.55). *Violent poison!* LD_{100} i.v. in cats: 0.104 mg/kg (Graebner, Giesel).

3',4'-Diacetate. $C_{33}H_{46}O_{11}$. Prisms from methanol + ether, mp 237-244°. $[\alpha]_D^{25}$ +41.3° (chloroform).

4633. Helvolic Acid. [29400-42-8] $(4\alpha,6\beta,8\alpha,9\beta,13\alpha,14\beta,$-$16\beta,17Z)$-6,16-Bis(acetyloxy)-3,7-dioxo-29-nordammara-1,17(20),24-trien-21-oic acid; (Z)-6β,16β-dihydroxy-3,7-dioxo-29-nor-8α,9β,13α,14β-dammara-1,17(20),24-trien-21-oic acid diacetate; fumigacin. $C_{33}H_{44}O_8$; mol wt 568.70. C 69.69%, H 7.80%, O 22.51%. Antibiotic substance of the fusidane class. Produced by *Aspergillus fumigatus*: Waksman *et al.*, *J. Bacteriol.* **45**, 233 (1943); by *A. fumigatus* mut. *helvola*: Chain *et al.*, *Br. J. Exp. Pathol.* **24**, 108 (1943). Structural studies: Okuda *et al.*, *Chem. Pharm. Bull.* **12**, 121 (1964); Oxley, *Chem. Commun.* **1966**, 729; Okuda *et al.*, *Tetrahedron Lett.* **1967**, 2295. Revised structure and stereochemistry: Iwaki *et al.*, *Chem. Commun.* **1970**, 1119. Chemical and biological data: Reshetova, *Antibiotiki* **14**, 554 (1969). Review of literature until 1960: Wilson, "Miscellaneous *Aspergillus* Toxins" in *Microbial Toxins* **vol. VI**, A. Ciegler *et al.*, Eds. (Academic Press, New York, 1971) p 265.

Needles from methanol, mp 215°. $[\alpha]_D^{25}$ $-121°$ (chloroform). uv max (ethanol): 231 nm (log ε 4.24). Very slightly sol in water; slightly sol in petr ether, methanol, ethanol. More sol in hot methanol, ethanol; sol in chloroform, acetone, ethyl acetate, benzene, pyridine, glacial acetic acid, dioxane, ether.

Methyl ester. Methyl helvolate. $C_{34}H_{46}O_8$. Crystals from methanol, mp 257°. $[\alpha]_D^{25}$ $-140°$ (chloroform).

4634. Hematein. [475-25-2] 6a,7-Dihydro-3,4,6a,10-tetrahydroxybenz[*b*]indeno[1,2-*d*]pyran-9(6*H*)-one; hydroxybrasilein; hydroxybrazilein. $C_{16}H_{12}O_6$; mol wt 300.26. C 64.00%, H 4.03%, O 31.97%. Not to be confused with hematin. From hematoxylin or logwood extract and NH_3 by treatment with air: Engels *et al.*, *J. Chem. Soc.* **93**, 1115 (1908); Rolland, *Teintex* **3**, 261, 322, 460 (1938); Justin-Mueller, *Melliand Textilber.* **30**, 26, 63 (1949), *C.A.* **46**, 8375h (1952).

Reddish-brown crystals with yellowish-green metallic luster. mp >200°; also stated as 250° with decompn. Sol in about 1700 parts water; slightly sol in alcohol, ether; insol in benzene, chloroform; freely sol in ammonia with brownish-violet color and in dil NaOH with bright red color. Forms salts with heavy metals.

USE: As an indicator like hematoxylin; for staining animal tissue, particularly cell nuclei.

4635. Hematin. [15489-90-4] $(SP$-5-13)-[7,12-Diethenyl-3,8,13,17-tetramethyl-21H,23H-porphine-2,18-dipropanoato(4$-$)-$N^{21},N^{22},N^{23},N^{24}$]hydroxyferrate(2$-$) dihydrogen; [dihydrogen 3,-7,12,17-tetramethyl-8,13-divinyl-2,18-porphinedipropionato(2$-$)]-hydroxyiron; hydroxy[dihydrogen protoporphyrin IX-ato(2$-$)]iron; ferriheme hydroxide; ferriporphyrin hydroxide; ferriprotoporphyrin basic; hydroxyhemin; phenodin. $C_{34}H_{33}FeN_4O_5$; mol wt 633.49. C 64.46%, H 5.25%, Fe 8.82%, N 8.84%, O 12.63%. Found in the body in pathological conditions, *e.g.*, after phosgene poisoning, in pernicious anemia. Prepn: Fischer-Orth, *Die Chemie des Pyrrols* **II**, 1, 386 (Leipzig, 1937). Brief review including structure: J. E. Falk, *Porphyrins and Metalloporphyrins* (Elsevier, New York, 1964) pp 17, 23, 46. Toxicology: D. L. Lips *et al.*, *Toxicol. Lett.* **2**, 329 (1978). Use in treatment of hepatic porphyria: C. J. Watson *et al.*, *Ann. Intern. Med.* **79**, 80 (1973); G. J. Dhar *et al.*, *ibid.* **83**, 20 (1975); J. M. Lamon *et al.*, *Medicine* **58**, 252 (1979).

Solvated crystals from pyridine, dry at 40° *in vacuo*. Freely sol in dil solns of alkali hydroxides, slightly sol in hot pyridine. Unstable. Absorption max (10% aq NaOH): 580 nm (E_{mM} 10.5). LD_{50} i.v. in rats: 4.32 mg/100 g (Lips).

4636. Hematoporphyrin. [14459-29-1] 7,12-Bis(1-hydroxyethyl)-3,8,13,17-tetramethyl-21H,23H-porphine-2,18-dipropanoic acid; 7,12-bis(1-hydroxyethyl)-3,8,13,17-tetramethyl-2,18-porphinedipropionic acid; 1,3,5,8-tetramethyl-2,4-bis(α-hydroxyethyl)porphine-6,7-dipropionic acid; hematoporphyrin IX; Photodyn. $C_{34}H_{38}N_4O_6$; mol wt 598.69. C 68.21%, H 6.40%, N 9.36%, O 16.03%. Prepd from hemin by the action of hydrobromic acid in glacial acetic acid: Fischer-Orth, *Die Chemie des Pyrrols* **II**, 1, 421 (Leipzig, 1937). Review and prepn: J. E. Falk, *Porphyrins and Metalloporphyrins* (Elsevier, New York, 1964) pp 175-177.

Deep red crystals. Absorption max (0.1N KOH): 615.5, 565, 534.4, 499.5 nm. Insol in water. Sol in alc. Sparingly sol in ether, chloroform.

Hydrochloride monohydrate. [6033-08-5] Sensibion. C_{34}-$H_{38}N_4O_6$·HCl·H_2O; mol wt 653.16. Prepn of a stable product: Woods, Steigman, **US 2858320** (1958 to Baxter Labs.). Dark red crystals.

THERAP CAT: Antidepressant.

4637. Hematoxylin. [517-28-2] *cis*-(+)-7,11b-Dihydro-benz[*b*]indeno[1,2-*d*]pyran-3,4,6a,9,10(6*H*)-pentol; hematoxiline;

hydroxybrazilin; hydroxybrasilin. $C_{16}H_{14}O_6$; mol wt 302.28. C 63.57%, H 4.67%, O 31.76%. From the heart-wood of logwood *(Haematoxylon campechianum* Linn., *Leguminosae):* Chevreul, *Ann. Chim. Phys.* **82**, 54, 126 (1810). Structure: Perkin, Robinson, *J. Chem. Soc.* **93**, 489 (1908). Synthesis: Dann, Hofmann, *Angew. Chem.* **75**, 1125 (1963); Morsingh, Robinson, *Tetrahedron* **26**, 281 (1970); Kirkiacharian, Billet, *Bull. Soc. Chim. Fr.* **1972**, 3292. Stereochemistry: Craig *et al., J. Org. Chem.* **30**, 1573 (1965). Spectroscopic and physico-chemical properties: C. Bettinger, H. W. Zimmerman, *Histochemistry* **95**, 279 (1991). Prepn for staining: R. B. Bosma *et al., J. Histotechnol.* **16**, 371 (1993). Use in determn of ruthenium: A.-A. Y. El-Sayed, *Fresenius J. Anal. Chem.* **349**, 830 (1994). *Review:* Robinson, *Bull. Soc. Chim. Fr.* **1958**, 125. Review of theory and application as histological stain: B. B. Hrapchak, *Am. J. Med Technol.* **42**, 371-379 (1976).

Trihydrate. White to yellowish crystals; redden on exposure to light, mp 100-120°; also stated as 140°. Slightly sol in cold water, ether; sol in hot water, hot alc, also in alkali hydroxides, borax, glycerol. Its solns darken on standing.

USE: Chiefly as a stain in microscopy; also in manufacture of ink.

4638. Hematoxylon. Logwood. Heart-wood of *Haematoxylon campechianum* L., *Leguminosae*. *Habit.* Central America; grown in the West Indies. *Constit.* About 10% hematoxylin; tannin, resin.

USE: Largely as dye.

4639. Heme. [14875-96-8] $(SP-4-2)$-[7,12-Diethenyl-3,8,-13,17-tetramethyl-21H,23H-porphine-2,18-dipropanoato(4−)-$N^{21},N^{22},N^{23},N^{24}$]ferrate(2−) dihydrogen; [dihydrogen 3,7,12,17-tetramethyl-8,13-divinyl-2,18-porphinedipropionato(2−)]iron; 1,-3,5,8-tetramethyl-2,4-divinylporphine-6,7-dipropionic acid ferrous complex; ferroheme; hem; protoheme; protoheme IX; reduced hematin; ferroprotoporphyrin. $C_{34}H_{32}FeN_4O_4$; mol wt 616.49. C 66.24%, H 5.23%, Fe 9.06%, N 9.09%, O 10.38%. Heme occurs free in tissues in the presence of certain pathological conditions, and in normal tissues; it occurs as the prosthetic group of a number of hemoproteins. It has been identified as the prosthetic group of hemoglobins, erythrocruorins (the hemoglobin analog of many invertebrates), myoglobins, some peroxidases, catalases, and cytochromes b. It is the color-furnishing portion of hemoglobin. Obtained when a soln of hematin in alkali is reduced in absence of nitrogenous substances: Bertin-Sans, de Moitessier, *Compt. Rend.* **114**, 923 (1892); Dhéré *et al., ibid.* **165**, 515 (1917). Synthesis: Fischer-Orth, *Die Chemie des Pyrrols* **II**, 1, 384 (Leipzig, 1937). Biosynthesis: Shemin, *Naturwissenschaften* **57**, 185 (1970). *Review:* J. E. Falk, *Porphyrins and Metalloporphyrins* (Elsevier, NewYork, 1964) pp 8, 94, 183. Comprehensive monograph: Chance *et al., Hemes and Hemoproteins* (Academic Press, New York, 1966) 624 pp; *Handbook of Experimental Pharmacology* **vol. 44**, entitled "Heme and Hemoproteins", F. DeMatteis, W. N. Aldridge, Eds. (Springer-Verlag, New York, 1978) 449 pp.

Fine brown needles with a dark violet sheen. Absorption max in phosphate buffer at pH 7: ~550, 575 nm (E_{mM}^{572} 5.5). Sparingly sol in glacial acetic acid; freely sol in the presence of oxygen. Very unstable.

4640. Hementin. [87041-58-5] Anticoagulant enzyme from the salivary glands of the South American giant leech *Haementeria ghiliarii*. Extraction: R. T. Sawyer *et al.,* US 4390630 (1983 to Univ. California, Berkeley). Anticoagulant, fibrinolytic properties: A. Z. Budzynski *et al., Proc. Soc. Exp. Biol. Med.* **168**, 266 (1981). Purification and identification as single polypeptide chain with mol wt approx 120000: S. M. Malinconico *et al., J. Lab. Clin. Med.* **103**, 44 (1984). Proteolytic degradation of fibrinogen by hementin: *eidem, ibid.* **104**, 842 (1984). Protease inhibition: E. H. Murer *et al., Thromb. Haemostasis* **51**, 24 (1984).

4641. Hemerythrin. A non-heme, oxygen-carrying protein found in members of four invertebrate phyla: sipunculids, polychaetes, priapulids and brachiopods. Oxygenated form is called *oxyhemerythrin.* Isoln from the sipunculid, *Golfingia goldii* (or *Phascolosoma goldii):* Klotz *et al., Arch. Biochem. Biophys.* **68**, 284 (1957). Consists of eight subunits, each containing two ferrous ions which form a complex with one molecule of oxygen: Klotz, Keresztes-Nagy, *Biochemistry* **2**, 445, 923 (1963). Each subunit is built up from 113 amino acids. Amino acid sequence: Klippenstein *et al., ibid.* **7**, 3868 (1968); Klippenstein, *ibid.* **11**, 372 (1972). Structure of trimeric hemerythrin: J. L. Smith *et al., Nature* **303**, 86 (1983). *Reviews:* Okamura, Klotz, "Hemerythrin" in *Inorganic Biochemistry* **vol. 1**, G. L. Eichhorn, Ed. (Elsevier, New York, 1973) pp 320-343; Klotz *et al., Science* **192**, 335-344 (1976); J. S. Loehr, T. M. Loehr in *Advances in Inorganic Biochemistry* **vol. 1**, G. L. Eichhorn, L. G. Marzilli, Eds. (Elsevier, New York, 1979) pp 235-252.

Hemerythrin is colorless. Oxyhemerythrin forms violet-pink crystals. Spectral data: Garbett *et al., Arch. Biochem. Biophys.* **135**, 419 (1969).

4642. Hemicelluloses. Large group of polysaccharides found, in association with lignin, in the primary and secondary cell walls of all plants and of some seaweeds. Whether lignin and hemicellulose are chemically bonded or lignin mechanically entraps hemicellulose molecules is still unknown. There are variations in the hemicellulosic composition of plants and even between the organs of the same plant. Hemicellulosic composition of plants changes with growth and maturation and is influenced also by environmental factors during growth. Principal sugar residues present in hemicellulose are: D-xylose, D-glucose, D-galactose, D-mannose, L-arabinose, D-glucuronic acid, D-galacturonic acid, 4-O-methyl-D-glucuronic acid, L-rhamnose and L-fucose. The most ubiquitous and abundant hemicelluloses are the *xylans* which are composed of linear and/or branched chains of β-$(1 \rightarrow 4)$ linked D-xylopyranosyl units. Hemicelluloses from woods: T. E. Timell, *Adv. Carbohyd. Chem.* **19**, 247 (1964); *idem, ibid.* **20**, 409 (1965). Hemicelluloses from grasses and cereals: K. C. B. Wilke, *ibid.* **36**, 215 (1979).

4643. Hemicholinium. [16478-59-4] 2,2′-[1,1′-Biphenyl]-4,4′-diylbis[2-hydroxy-4,4-dimethylmorpholinium]; 2,2′-(4,4′-biphenylylene)bis[2-hydroxy-4,4-dimethylmorpholinium]. [C_{24}-$H_{34}N_2O_4$]$^{2+}$. Specific, competitive inhibitor of the sodium-dependent high-affinity choline uptake system (HACU) localized on cholinergic presynaptic nerve terminals, resulting in the inhibition of acetylcholine synthesis. Prepn of seco tautomer: J. P. Long, F. W. Schueler, *J. Am. Pharm. Assoc.* **43**, 79 (1954). *In vitro* pharmacology and revised hemiacetal structure: F. W. Schueler, *J. Pharmacol. Exp. Ther.* **115**, 127 (1955). Structure-activity studies: R. P. DiAugustine, V. B. Haarstad, *Biochem. Pharmacol.* **19**, 559 (1970); J. G. Cannon *et al., Pharm. Res.* **5**, 359 (1988). Pharmacology: J. J. Freeman *et al., J. Pharmacol. Exp. Ther.* **210**, 91 (1979); J. J. Hagan *et al., Psychopharmacology* **98**, 347 (1989). Receptor binding studies in human brain: J. Pascual *et al., J. Neurochem.* **54**, 792 (1990); in rat brain: *eidem, Pharmacol. Res.* **24**, 345 (1991). Potential uses of tritium labeled compound: T. W. Vickroy *et al.* in *Synth. Appl. Isotop. Labeled Compd. 1985*, R. R. Muccino, Ed. (Elsevier, Amsterdam, 1986) pp 145-150; H. K. Happe, L. C. Murrin, *J. Neurochem.* **60**, 1191 (1993).

Consult the Name Index before using this section.

Dibromide. [312-45-8] Hemicholinium-3; HC-3. $C_{24}H_{34}Br_2$-N_2O_4. mp 180°. Moderately soluble in water, soluble in ethanol. Occurs as the monohydrate, white solid from ethanol/ether, mp 226-228° (dec). LD_{50} i.p. in female mice: 0.048-0.082 mg/kg (DiAugustine, Haarstad).

USE: Research tool as cholinergic probe, to deplete acetylcholine stores.

4644. Hemin. [16009-13-5] (*SP*-5-13)-Chloro[7,12-diethenyl-3,8,13,17-tetramethyl-21*H*,23*H*-porphine-2,18-dipropanoato(4−)-$N^{21},N^{22},N^{23},N^{24}$]ferrate(2−) dihydrogen; chloro[dihydrogen 3,7,12,17-tetramethyl-8,13-divinyl-2,18-porphinedipropionato(2−)]iron; chlorohemin; 1,3,5,8-tetramethyl-2,4-divinylporphine-6,7-dipropionic acid ferrichloride; Teichmann's crystals; ferriheme chloride; ferriprotoporphyrin chloride; ferriporphyrin chloride. $C_{34}H_{32}ClFeN_4O_4$; mol wt 651.94. C 62.64%, H 4.95%, Cl 5.44%, Fe 8.57%, N 8.59%, O 9.82%. Prepd from hemoglobin soln by heating with acetic acid and sodium chloride. Practical procedure for its prepn from ox blood: Schalfejeff, *J. Russ. Phys. Chem. Soc.* **1885**, 30; *Ber.* **18**, 232 (1885); Gattermann-Wieland, *Praxis des Organischen Chemikers* 23rd ed., p 407; Fischer-Orth, *Die Chemie des Pyrrols* **II**, 1, 377 (Leipzig, 1937); H. Fischer, *Org. Synth.* coll. vol. **III**, 442 (1955); Labbe, Nishida, *Biochim. Biophys. Acta* **26**, 437 (1957). Biosynthesis: Karlzeile, *Angew. Chem.* **66**, 729 (1954). *Review:* Stoll, *Experientia* **4**, 6 (1948); H. H. Inhoffen, *Naturwissenschaften* **55**, 457 (1968); W. S. Caughey in *Inorganic Biochemistry* **vol. 2**, G. L. Eichhorn, Ed. (Elsevier, New York, 1973) pp 797-831.

Long, thin blades from glacial acetic acid or from chloroform-pyridine-acetic acid, appearing brown in transmitted light and steel-blue in reflected light. Sinters at 240° but is not melted at 300°. Absorption spectrum: Fischer-Orth, *loc. cit.* Freely sol in dil ammonia water, also in solns of sodium hydroxide with hematin formation, *i.e.*, the chlorine is displaced by an OH group. Practically insol in carbonate solns, dil acid solns. Sol in strong organic bases such as trimethylamine, *p*-toluidine, dimethylaniline. Sol in concd H_2SO_4 with loss of Fe. Sparingly sol in 70-80% alc. Practically insol but stable in water.

Dimethyl ester. $C_{36}H_{36}ClFeN_4O_4$. Needles from benzene, not melted at 300°. Freely sol in acetic acid, benzene, chloroform, acetone.

Diethyl ester. $C_{38}H_{40}ClFeN_4O_4$. Crystals, freely sol in chloroform.

4645. Hemipyocyanine. [528-71-2] 1-Phenazinol; α-hydroxyphenazine; 1-hydroxy-5,10-diazoanthracene; pyoxanthose. $C_{12}H_8N_2O$; mol wt 196.20. C 73.46%, H 4.11%, N 14.28%, O 8.15%. Found in old cultures of *Pseudomonas pyocyanea*. Isoln: Fordos, *Compt. Rend.* **56**, 1128 (1863). Prepd from pyocyanine by the action of 2% NaOH: Wrede, Strack, *Z. Physiol. Chem.* **140**, 12 (1924); by the reaction of pyrogallol monomethyl ether and *o*-phenylenediamine followed by demethylation of the formed α-methoxyphenazine: Surrey, *Org. Synth.* coll. vol. III, 753 (1955). Alternate syntheses: Hegedüs, *Helv. Chim. Acta* **33**, 766 (1950); Vivian, *Nature* **178**, 753 (1956).

Yellow needles from benzene, mp 159-160°. Sublimes easily *in vacuo*. Slightly sol in hot water; freely sol in the usual organic solvents except petr ether. Sol in aq alkaline solns with purplish-red color which turns yellow on neutralization. Forms red salts with mineral acids.

4646. Hemisulfur Mustard. [693-30-1] 2-(2-Chloroethylthio)ethanol; 2-chloro-2'-hydroxydiethyl sulfide; 2-chloroethyl 2-hydroxyethyl sulfide; β-chloroethyl β-hydroxyethyl thioether; mustard chlorohydrin; semi-mustard gas; semisulfur mustard. C_4H_9-ClOS; mol wt 140.63. C 34.16%, H 6.45%, Cl 25.21%, O 11.38%, S 22.80%. $ClCH_2CH_2SCH_2CH_2OH$. Prepn: Ogston *et al., Trans. Faraday Soc.* **44**, 45 (1948); Grant, Kinsey, *J. Am. Chem. Soc.* **68**, 2075 (1946); Fuson, Ziegler, *J. Org. Chem.* **11**, 510 (1946); Rueggeberg *et al., ibid.* **13**, 110 (1948); Tsou *et al., ibid.* **26**, 4987 (1961).

Oily, somewhat hygroscopic liquid. $bp_{0.6}$ 100° (Fuson); $bp_{0.5-0.75}$ 87°; bp_6 44.5° (Rueggeberg). n_D^{20} 1.5188; $n_D^{24.5}$ 1.5205. Sol in water; miscible with bis(2-chloroethyl) sulfide, thiodiglycol. Unstable, forming sulfonium salts at room temp or in solns with ethanol or chloroform.

4647. Hemocyanins. A non-heme, oxygen carrying copper protein found in arthropods and mollusca of which *keyhole-limpet hemocyanin* (*KLH*) is an example. Dissolved in the hemolymph; not found in blood cells. Mol wt ranges from 4.5×10^5 to 1.3×10^7. One molecule of oxygen is bound by two copper atoms. The oxygenated form, *oxyhemocyanin* is blue, while *deoxyhemocyanin* is colorless. The copper can be removed reversibly to form *apo-hemocyanin*. Structure of snail, *Helix pomatia*, hemocyanin: J. E. Mellema, A. Klug, *Nature* **239**, 146 (1972). The role of copper in hemocyanin: R. Lontie, L. Vanquickenborne, *Met. Ions Biol. Syst.* **3**, 183 (1974). *Reviews:* K. E. van Holde, E. F. J. van Bruggen in *Subunits in Biological Systems* **vol. 5**, pt. A, S. N. Timasheff, G. D. Fasman, Eds. (Dekker, New York, 1971) pp 1-53; R. Lontie, R. Witters in *Inorganic Biochemistry* **vol. I**, G. L. Eichhorn, Ed. (Elsevier, New York, 1973) pp 344-358; E. F. J. van Bruggen, *Trends Biochem. Sci.* **5**, 185-8 (1980). Review of respiratory function: J. Bonaventura, C. Bonaventura, *Am. Zool.* **20**, 7-17 (1980); C. P. Magnum, *ibid.* 19-38.

USE: KLH as an experimental antigen in animals.

4648. Hemoglobin. Hb; ferrohemoglobin. The major component of red blood cells which transports oxygen from the lungs to body tissues and facilitates the return transport of carbon dioxide. Mammalian hemoglobins have mol wts of about 64,500. Composed of four peptide chains called globins, each of which is bound to a heme, *q.q.v.* Normal human hemoglobin is composed of a pair of two identical chains. Iron is coordinated to four pyrrole nitrogens of protoporphyrin IX, and to an imidazole nitrogen of a histidine residue from the globin side of the porphyrin. The sixth coordination position is available for binding with oxygen and other small molecules. Called *oxyhemoglobin*, HbO_2, in the oxygenated form and *carboxyhemoglobin*, HbCO, when oxygen is displaced by carbon monoxide. Binds reversibly with oxygen while the heme iron remains in the ferrous state. Autoxidation is prevented by the cover of hydrophobic groups of the globin. When the iron in hemoglobin is oxidized from the ferrous to the ferric state the compd is called methemoglobin, *q.v.* and is accompanied by a loss of oxygen-binding capacity. Hemoglobin is usually prepd by separating the red blood corpuscles from the lighter plasma by centrifuging; the plasma is siphoned off, and on adding ether to the blood corpuscle paste, the cells burst. After another centrifugation to remove the ruptured cell envelopes, a clear red soln of the protein is obtained [Fieser, Fieser, *Org. Chem.* (New York, 3rd ed., 1956) p 455]. Prepn of cryst HbO_2 from washed horse or dog erythrocytes: Heidelberger, *J. Biol. Chem.* **53**, 31 (1922); *see also* Ferry, Green, *ibid.* **81**, 175 (1929); from human blood: Drabkin, *ibid.* **164**, 703 (1946). Structure studies: Muirhead, Perutz, *Nature* **199**, 633 (1963); Perutz *et al., ibid.* **219**, 131 (1968); Perutz, *Proc. Roy. Soc. London*

173B, 113 (1969). Respiratory properties of hemoglobin and its function as a carrier of oxygen and carbon dioxide: Peters, Van Slyke, *Quantitative Clinical Chemistry* **vol. I** (Baltimore, 1932). Mechanism of action: Arnone in *Annu. Rev. Med.* **25,** 123-130 (1974). *Reviews:* Lemberg, Legge, *Hematin Compounds and Bile Pigments* (New York, 1949); F. W. Sunderman, *Hemoglobin: its Precursors and Metabolites* (Lippincott, Philadelphia, 1964); H. Lehmann, R. G. Huntsman, *Man's Hemoglobins* (*ibid.* 1966); Huisman, Schroeder, *New Aspects of the Structure, Function, and Synthesis of Hemoglobins* (Butterworth, London, 1971); M. F. Perutz, *Annu. Rev. Biochem.* **48,** 327-386 (1979); G. Fermi, M. F. Perutz, *Haemoglobin & Myoglobin* (Oxford Univ. Press, New York, 1982) 104 pp; R. E. Dickerson, I. Geis, *Hemoglobin: Structure, Function, Evolution, and Pathology* (Benjamin-Cummings, Menlo Park, Calif., 1983) 176 pp.

Crystal form, solubility, affinity for oxygen, absorption spectra differ quantitatively in hemoglobins of different species, due to the variation in amino acid sequence of the protein moiety since the same heme group is present in all vertebrate and many invertebrate hemoglobins. Human HbO_2 = tetragonal crystals; horse HbO_2 = orthorhombic crystals from citrated blood, monoclinic crystals from oxalated blood. Absorption spectra, *see* Lemberg, Legge, *loc. cit.,* 228. Oxyhemoglobin is an article of commerce where it is called hemoglobin. Brownish-red powder or scales. Soluble in about 7 parts water, slowly sol in glycerol.

4649. Hemozoin. [39404-00-7] β-Hematin; malaria pigment; haemozoin; HZ. Polymerized heme produced as a detoxification response by malaria parasites and by blood-sucking insects. It is the end product of hemoglobin digestion in intraerythrocytic malaria parasites. Constituents include hematin and protein but the exact composition remains unclear. Identification: T. Carbone, *Giorn. Regia. Acad. Med. Torino* **39,** 901 (1891). Biochemical characterization: P. Goldie *et al., Am. J. Trop. Med. Hyg.* **43,** 584 (1990). Identification in tissue: A D. Sullivan, S. R. Meshnick, *Parasitol. Today* **12,** 161 (1996); of formation in insects: M. F. Oliveira *et al., Nature* **400,** 517 (1999). Depression of cellular immunity: F. Turrini *et al., ibid.* **9,** 297 (1993). Effect of antimalarials on depolymerization: A. V. Pandey, B. L. Tekwani, *FEBS Lett.* **402,** 236 (1997). *Review:* P. Arese, E. Schwarzer, *Ann. Trop. Med. Parasitol.* **91,** 501 (1997).

Insoluble, black-brown, crystalline pigment.

4650. Hendrickson's Reagent. [72450-51-2] μ-Oxohexaphenyldiphosphorus(2+) salt with trifluoromethanesulfonic acid (1:2); triphenylphosphonium anhydride trifluoromethanesulfonate; POP. $C_{36}H_{30}OP_2 \cdot 2CF_3O_3S$; mol wt 838.71. C 54.42%, H 3.61%, O 13.35%, P 7.39%, F 13.59%, S 7.65%. Alternative to Mitsunobu reagents for the esterification of primary alcohols. Synthesis method: J. B. Hendrickson, S. M. Schwartzman, *Tetrahedron Lett.* **16,** 277 (1975). Prepn: A. Aaberb *et al., ibid.* **20,** 2263 (1979). Synthetic applications as a dehydration agent: J. B. Hendrickson, Md. S. Hussoin, *J. Org. Chem.* **52,** 4137 (1987); *eidem et al., Synlett* **1996,** 661; and X-ray crystal structure determn: S.-L. You *et al., Angew. Chem. Int. Ed.* **42,** 83 (2003). Mechanism of dehydration reactions vs the Mitsunobu reaction: K. E. Elson *et al., Org. Biomol. Chem.* **1,** 2958 (2003).

White crystalline solid, mp 74-75°. Sol in pyridine, THF. *Water and air sensitive.*

USE: Dehydration reagent in organic synthesis.

4651. Henna. Dried powdered leaves of *Lawsonia alba* Lam., *L. inermis* L., and *L. spinosa* L., *Lythraceae.* Obtained from North Africa or India. Contains about 1% of lawsone, *q.v.* Ref: Cox, *Analyst* **63,** 397 (1938); Talaat, *Br. Med. J.* **II,** 944 (1960).

USE: For dyeing hair and nails auburn to red, in the Orient together with "reng," the dried, powdered leaves of the indigo plant, in order to produce darker and even bluish-black shades. For relatively permanent dyeing the pH must be about 5.5; this is achieved by the addition of citric, boric, or adipic acid. Ingredient of many commercial hair rinses.

4652. Heparamine. [53260-52-9] *N*-Desulfoheparin. The —$NHSO_3H$ groups in heparin are replaced by —NH_2 groups. Prepn of sodium salt by methanolysis of sodium heparinate and saponification: Velluz *et al., Compt. Rend.* **247,** 1521 (1958); from sodium heparinate heated with HCl, neutralized with $NaHCO_3$ and dialyzed against running water: Foster *et al., J. Chem. Soc.* **1961,** 1204; from sodium heparinate demineralized with Dowex 50 resin: GB **863235** (1961 to UCLAF).

Sodium salt. Solid, sol in water. $[\alpha]_D^{20}$ +67 ± 2°.

N-**Acyl derivatives.** Heparides. Similar to heparin in clearing alimentary lipemia but are practically devoid of its anticoagulant activity.

4653. Heparin. [9005-49-6] Heparinic acid; Arteven; Leparan. Glycosaminoglycan with anticoagulant activity. Heterogenous mixture of variably sulfated polysaccharide chains composed of repeating units of D-glucosamine and either L-iduronic or D-glucuronic acids. Mol wt ranges from 6000-30000 Da. Biosynthesized and stored in mast cells of various animal tissues, particularly liver, lung or gut. Commercial heparin is isolated from beef lung or pork intestinal mucosa. Isoln from mammalian tissue: Howell, *Am. J. Physiol.* **63,** 434 (1922-23); **71,** 553 (1924-25); Korn, *J. Biol. Chem.* **234,** 1325 (1959); L. B. Jaques, *Can. J. Biochem. Physiol.* **37,** 1183 (1959); J. A. Bush *et al., US **2884358*** (1959 to So. Calif. Gland). Purification: G. Nominé *et al., US **2989438*** (1961 to UCLAF); Toccaceli, US **3016331** (1962 to Ormonoterapia Richter); L. Roden *et al., Methods Enzymol.* **26,** 73 (1972). Structural studies: M. L. Wolfrom, *J. Am. Chem. Soc.* **72,** 5796 (1950); Velluz *et al., Compt. Rend.* **247,** 1521 (1958); M. L. Wolfrom *et al., J. Org. Chem.* **29,** 540 (1964). Configuration of glycosidic linkages: M. L. Wolfrom *et al., ibid.* **31,** 1173 (1966); A. S. Perlin *et al., Can. J. Chem.* **48,** 2260 (1970); T. Helting, U. Lindahl, *J. Biol. Chem.* **246,** 5442 (1971). Identification of L-iduronic acid residues: A. S. Perlin *et al., Carbohydr. Res.* **7,** 369 (1968). Antithrombotic activity results from the binding and activation of *antithrombin III*, a plasma protein which inhibits several enzymes in the coagulation cascade: R. D. Rosenberg, *Fed. Proc.* **36,** 10 (1977). Anticoagulant activity is related to the mol wt of the polysaccharide fragments; low molecular weight components exhibit decreased hemorrhagic effects while retaining antithrombin binding ability: L.-O. Andersson *et al., Thromb. Res.* **15,** 531 (1979); T. W. Barrowcliffe *et al., Br. J. Haematol.* **41,** 573 (1979); J. Hirsch *et al., Semin. Thromb. Hemostasis* **11,** 13 (1985). Characterization of the antithrombin binding site: U. Lindahl *et al., Proc. Natl. Acad. Sci. USA* **76,** 3198 (1979); J. Choay *et al., Thromb. Res.* **18,** 573 (1980). Synthesis of the pentasaccharide corresponding to the binding site sequence: *eidem, Biochem. Biophys. Res. Commun.* **116,** 492 (1983). Symposium on structure, activity and clinical applications: *Fed. Proc.* **36,** 9-116 (1977). Review of mechanism of action: I. Björk, U. Lindahl, *Mol. Cell. Biochem.* **48,** 161-182 (1982); of structure-activity relationships and prepn of low mol wt fractions: B. Casu, *Adv. Carbohydr. Chem. Biochem.* **43,** 51-134 (1985); of biosynthesis: U. Lindahl *et al., Trends Biochem. Sci.* **11,** 221-225 (1986). Comprehensive description: F. Nachtmann *et al., Anal. Profiles Drug Subs.* **12,** 215-276 (1983). Overview of clinical results in pulmonary embolism and venous thrombosis: R. Collins *et al., N. Engl. J. Med.* **318,** 1162-1170 (1988); J. Hirsh, *ibid.* **324,** 1565-1574 (1991); of clinical studies with low mol wt heparinoids: H. ten Cate *et al., Am. J. Hematol.* **27,** 146-153 (1988).

Antithrombin binding site of Heparin

Heparin has a rotation of $[\alpha]_D^{20}$ +55°.

Calcium salt. [37270-89-6] Calciparine; Ecasolv.

Magnesium salt. [54479-70-8] Magnesium heparinate; Cutheparine. Sol in water. Insol in organic solvents.

Potassium salt. [9005-48-5] Clarin (formerly).

Sodium salt. [9041-08-1] Heparin sodium; Hepsal; Lipo-Hepin; Liquémin; Longheparin; Monoparin; Panheprin; Pularin; Liquaemin Sodium; Minihep; Thromboliquine; Thrombophob; Unihep. White to grayish-brown amorphous powder. Odorless, hygroscopic. $[\alpha]_D^{25}$ +47° (c = 1.5 in water). One gram dissolves in 20 ml water. Sol in saline soln. Practically insol in alcohol, acetone, benzene, chloroform, ether. pH of 1% aq soln = 6.0 to 7.5. Absorption spectrum: Burson *et al.*, *J. Am. Chem. Soc.* **78**, 5874 (1956). Ampuled solns may be stored at room temp for at least 12 months. Commercially available ampuled, sterile solns contain 0.5% phenol or chlorobutanol as preservative.

THERAP CAT: Anticoagulant.

THERAP CAT (VET): Anticoagulant.

4654. HEPES. [7365-45-9] 4-(2-Hydroxyethyl)-1-piperazineethanesulfonic acid; *N*-(2-hydroxyethyl)piperazine-*N'*-2-ethanesulfonic acid. $C_8H_{18}N_2O_4S$; mol wt 238.30. C 40.32%, H 7.61%, H 11.76%, O 26.86%, S 13.46%. One of several zwitterionic *N*-substituted aminosulfonic acids known as *Good Buffers*, active in the pH range of 6-8.5. Prepn: N. E. Good *et al.*, *Biochemistry* **5**, 467 (1966). Buffering characteristics: W. J. Ferguson *et al.*, *Anal. Biochem.* **104**, 300 (1980). Temperature effects on pKa and pH: R. N. Roy *et al.*, *Cryo-Lett.* **6**, 285 (1985). Interaction with hydroxyl radicals: M. Hicks, J. M. Gebicki, *FEBS Lett.* **199**, 92 (1986). Interference with Lowry protein determination: H. M. Himmel, W. Heller, *J. Clin. Chem. Clin. Biochem.* **25**, 909 (1987). Use as biological buffer: H. Eagle, *Science* **174**, 500 (1971); K. V. Rao, *Indian J. Exp. Biol.* **15**, 552 (1977); E. D. Lalague *et al.*, *J. Microsc.* **127**, 307 (1982); G. I. McFadden, M. Melkonian, *Phycologia* **25**, 551 (1986).

Crystals from alcohol + water, mp 234°. $pKa_1 \simeq 3$, pKa_2 (20°) 7.55. $\Delta pKa/°C$ −0.014. Saturated aqueous soln is 2.25M at 0°.

USE: Biological buffer.

4655. Heptabarbital. [509-86-4] 5-(1-Cyclohepten-1-yl)-5-ethyl-2,4,6(1*H*,3*H*,5*H*)-pyrimidinetrione; 5-(1-cyclohepten-1-yl)-5-ethylbarbituric acid; 5-ethyl-5-cycloheptenylbarbituric acid; heptabarb; Heptadorm; Medomin. $C_{13}H_{18}N_2O_3$; mol wt 250.29. C 62.38%, H 7.25%, N 11.19%, O 19.18%. Prepn: FR 870714 (1942 to Geigy); Taub, US 2501551 (1950).

Crystals, mp 174°. Slightly bitter taste. uv max (0.2*N* NaOH): 218.5, 254 nm. Very sparingly sol in water, more sol in alcohol. At 25° 100 ml of soln contains: 4.0 g in alcohol; 5.7 g in acetone; 1.4 g. in chloroform. Soluble in alkaline solns. Forms water-soluble sodium, magnesium, and calcium salts.

Note: This is a controlled substance (depressant): **21 CFR**, 1308.13.

THERAP CAT: Sedative, hypnotic.

4656. Heptachlor. [76-44-8] 1*H*-1,4,5,6,7,8,8-Heptachloro-3a,4,7,7a-tetrahydro-4,7-methanoindene; E-3314; Velsicol 104; Drinox; Heptamul. $C_{10}H_5Cl_7$; mol wt 373.32. C 32.17%, H 1.35%, Cl 66.48%. Insecticide for soil and seed treatment. Prepn: Bluestone *et al.*, US 2576666 (1951 to Julius Hyman); McKenna *et al.*, US 2661377-8 (1953 to Shell); Kleiman, Tapas, US 2904599 (1959 to Velsicol). Toxicity data: T. B. Gaines, *Toxicol. Appl. Pharmacol.* **14**, 515 (1969). Review of toxicology and human exposure: *Toxicological Profile for Heptachlor/Heptachlor Epoxide* (PB93-182467, 1993) 162 pp.

Crystals, mp 95-96°. Camphor-like odor. Vapor pressure at 25° = 3 × 10⁻⁴ mm Hg. Soly in g/100 ml solvent at 27°: acetone 75, benzene 106, carbon tetrachloride 112, cyclohexanone 119, alcohol 4.5, xylene 102. LD_{50} in male, female rats (mg/kg): 100, 162 orally (Gaines).

Caution: Poisoning may occur by ingestion, inhalation, skin contamination. May cause blood dyscrasias and liver necrosis. *See: Clinical Toxicology of Commercial Products*, R. E. Gosselin *et al.*, Eds. (Williams & Wilkins, Baltimore, 5th ed., 1984) Section II, pp 285-286.

USE: Formerly as insecticide for control of cotton boll weevil.

4657. Heptaminol. [372-66-7] 6-Amino-2-methyl-2-heptanol; 2-methyl-6-amino-2-heptanol; 6-methyl-2-amino-6-heptanol. $C_8H_{19}NO$; mol wt 145.24. C 66.16%, H 13.19%, N 9.64%, O 11.02%. Prepn: H. T. F. Givens, R. M. Herbst, US 2457656 (1948 to Bilhuber); of hydrochloride: J. Doeuvre, J. Poizat, *Compt. Rend.* **224**, 286 (1947). Pharmacokinetics and metabolism: F. Chanoine *et al.*, *Arzneim.-Forsch.* **31**, 1430 (1981). HPLC determn in biological fluids: R. R. Brodie *et al.*, *J. Chromatogr.* **274**, 179 (1983). Clinical trial in hypotension: D. Milon *et al.*, *Fundam. Clin. Pharmacol.* **4**, 695 (1990). Review of mode of action: B. Pourrias *Ann. Pharm. Fr.* **49**, 127-138 (1991).

Colorless liquid, bp₉₂ 92-93°.

Hydrochloride. [543-15-7] RP-2831; Cortensor; Eoden; Hepta-myl; Heptylon. $C_8H_{19}NO.HCl$; mol wt 181.70. Crystals, mp 150°. Freely sol in water. Sol in alcohol. Practically insol in acetone, benzene, ether. pH of 2% aq soln: 4.5-5.5.

5'-Adenylate. [57249-13-5] Ampecyclal.

THERAP CAT: Antihypotensive.

4658. Heptanal. [111-71-7] Heptaldehyde; Aldehyde C-7; heptylaldehyde; oenanthal; enanthal; oenanthol; oenanthaldehyde; enanthaldehyde. $C_7H_{14}O$; mol wt 114.19. C 73.63%, H 12.36%, O 14.01%. $CH_3(CH_2)_5CHO$. Obtained by distilling castor oil under reduced pressure: Rogers, *J. Am. Pharm. Assoc. Sci. Ed.* **12**, 503 (1923); Dominguez *et al.*, *J. Chem. Educ.* **29**, 446 (1952). Catalytic dehydration of ricinoleic acid methyl ester yields heptanal as a cleavage product in almost quantitative yield: Panjutin, *Chem. Zentralbl.* **1928**, II, 747.

Liquid. Penetrating fruity odor. d_4^0 0.83423; d_4^{15} 0.82162; d_4^{30} 0.80902. mp −43.3°. bp_{760} 152.8°; bp_{30} 59.6°; bp_{10} 42.5°. n_D^{20} 1.42571. Viscosity at 15°: 0.977 cP; at 30°: 0. 791 cP. Surface tension (γ) at 30° = 25.68. Surface tension against water at 30°: 14.41. Heat of combustion (liq) −1062.4 kcal/mol. Slightly sol in water. Misc with alc, ether. Sol in 3 vols of 60% alc.

USE: Manufacture of 1-heptanol; ethyl oenanthate.

4659. *n*-Heptane. [142-82-5] C_7H_{16}; mol wt 100.20. C 83.91%, H 16.09%. $CH_3(CH_2)_5CH_3$. A hydrocarbon from petroleum. Toxicity data: Lazarew, *Arch. Exp. Pathol. Pharmakol.* **143**, 223 (1929).

Volatile, flammable liquid. d^{20} 0.684. bp 98.4°. mp −90.7°. Flash pt, open cup: 30°F (−1°C); closed cup: 25°F (−4°C). n_D^{25} 1.3855. Insol in water. Sol in alcohol, chloroform, ether. LC (2 hr in air) in mice: 75 mg/l (Lazarew).

Caution: Potential symptoms of overexposure are lightheadedness, giddiness, stupor, vertigo, incoordination; loss of appetite, nausea; unconsciousness. Direct contact may cause dermatitis; aspiration of liquid may cause chemical pneumonia. *See NIOSH Pocket Guide to Chemical Hazards* (DHHS/NIOSH 97-140, 1997) p 156.

USE: As standard in testing knock of gasoline engines.

4660. Heptanoic Acid. [111-14-8] Enanthic acid; oenanthic acid; oenanthylic acid; n-heptoic acid; n-heptylic acid. $C_7H_{14}O_2$; mol wt 130.18. C 64.58%, H 10.84%, O 24.58%. $CH_3(CH_2)_5$-COOH. Found in the various fusel oils in appreciable amounts. Has been observed in rancid oils. Prepd by the oxidation of heptaldehyde with potassium permanganate in dil sulfuric acid: Ruhoff, *Org. Synth.* **coll. vol. II**, 315 (1943). Toxicity study: L. Orö, A. Wretlind, *Acta Pharmacol. Toxicol.* **18**, 141 (1961).

Oily liquid. Disagreeable, rancid odor. Faint, tallow-like odor when spectroscopically pure. d_4^0 0.9345; d_4^{15} 0.9222; d_4^{20} 0.9181; d_4^{30} 0.9099. mp −7.5°. bp_{760} 223.01°, also reported as 221.9°; bp_{256} 187.5°; bp_{64} 150.8°. Specific heat 0.54 cal/g. Heat of combustion −986.1 cal/g (20°). n_D^{20} 1.42162. Viscosity 3.40 cP at 30°; 0.82 cP at 120°. Interfacial tension against water: 7.0 dynes/cm. pka (25°): 4.4. Soly in water (15°): 0.2419 g/100 ml H_2O. Sol in ethanol, ether, DMF, DMSO. LD_{50} i.v. in mice: 1200±56 mg/kg (Orö, Wretlind).

Methyl ester. $C_8H_{16}O_2$. Liquid. d_4^{20} 0.8815; mp −55.8°; bp 173.8°. n_D^{20} 1.41152.

Ethyl ester *see* Ethyl Oenanthate.

4661. 1-Heptanol. [111-70-6] n-Heptyl alcohol; enanthic alcohol; 1-hydroxyheptane. $C_7H_{16}O$; mol wt 116.20. C 72.35%, H 13.88%, O 13.77%. $CH_3(CH_2)_5CH_2OH$. Prepd from heptaldehyde by reduction with iron filings in dil acetic acid: Clarke, Dreger, *Org. Synth.* **6**, 52 (1926); *cf.* Noller, Bannerot, *ibid.* **14**, 91 (1934); **coll. vol. I** (2nd ed., 1941) p 304. Other methods include the reaction between pentane and ethylene oxide in the presence of anhyd aluminum bromide: I. G. Farbenind., **FR 716604** *C.A.* **26**, 2198 (1932); and the action of amyl magnesium bromide on ethylene oxide: Vaughn *et al.*, *J. Am. Chem. Soc.* **55**, 4207 (1933).

Liquid. d_4^{25} 0.8187. mp −34.6°. bp_{760} 176.15°; bp_{400} 155.6°; bp_{200} 136.6°; bp_{100} 119.5°; bp_{40} 9.98°; bp_{20} 85.8°; bp_{10} 74.7°; bp_5 64.3°; $bp_{1.0}$ 42.4°. n_D^{25} 1.4224. Water solns are colloidal: Traube, Klein, *Kolloid-Z.* **29**, 236 (1921), *Chem. Zentralbl.* **1922, I,** 233. One liter of water dissolves 1.0 g at 18°; 2.85 g at 100°; 5.15 g at 130°. Miscible with alcohol, ether.

4662. 2-Heptanol. [543-49-7] Amylmethylcarbinol; 2-hydroxyheptane. $C_7H_{16}O$; mol wt 116.20. C 72.35%, H 13.88%, O 13.77%. $CH_3CH(OH)(CH_2)_4CH_3$. Occurs in oil of cloves: Masson, *Compt. Rend.* **149**, 630 (1907). Prepd by the action of amylmagnesium bromide on acetaldehyde: Henry, de Wael, *Rec. Trav. Chim.* **28**, 446 (1909); by the reduction of methyl amyl ketone with sodium in alcoholic soln: Thoms, Mannich, *Ber.* **36**, 2544 (1903); Pickard, Kenyon, *J. Chem. Soc.* **99**, 58 (1911); **105**, 849 (1914); Whitmore, Otterbacher, *Org. Synth.* **10**, 60 (1930); by the action of *Penicillium palitans* on coconut oil: Stokoe, *Biochem. J.* **22**, 82, 84 (1928). Toxicity data: Smyth *et al.*, *Arch. Ind. Hyg. Occup. Med.* **10**, 61 (1954).

dl-**Form.** Liquid. d^0 0.8344; d^{20} 0.8193. bp_{760} 158-160°, n_D 1.42131. Almost insol in water: 3.5 g/l. Sol in alc, ether, benzene. LD_{50} orally in rats: 2.58 g/kg (Smyth).

d-**Form.** Liquid. d_4^{20} 0.8190; d_4^{35} 0.8050; d_4^{51} 0.7920; d_4^{64} 0.7815; d_4^{110} 0.7417. bp_{20} 73.5°. $[\alpha]_D^{20}$ +11.45° (1.039 g in 20 ml abs ethanol); $[\alpha]_4^{20}$ +13.71° (0.992 in 20 ml benzene).

l-**Form.** Liquid. d_4^{20} 0.8184. bp_{23} 74.5°. $[\alpha]_D^{17}$ −10.48°.

4663. 2-Heptanone. [110-43-0] Methyl amyl ketone. $C_7H_{14}O$; mol wt 114.19. C 73.63%, H 12.36%, O 14.01%. CH_3-$(CH_2)_4COCH_3$. Found in oil of cloves and in cinnamon-bark oil. Responsible for the "peppery" odor in cheeses of the Roquefort type: Hammer, Bryant, *Iowa State Coll. J. Sci.* **11**, 281 (1937). Prepd by the ketone decompn of ethyl butylacetoacetate: Drake, Riemenschneider, *J. Am. Chem. Soc.* **52**, 5005 (1930); Dehn, Jackson, *ibid.* **55**, 4285 (1933); Johnson, Hager, *Org. Synth.* **coll. vol. I** (2nd ed., 1941) p 351; by hydration of 1-heptyne and 2-heptyne: Thomas *et al.*, *J. Am. Chem. Soc.* **60**, 719 (1938). Toxicity study: Smyth *et al.*, *Am. Ind. Hyg. Assoc. J.* **23**, 95 (1962).

Liquid. Penetrating fruity odor. d_4^0 0.8324; d_4^{15} 0.8197; d_4^{30} 0.8068. bp_{760} 151.5°; bp_{21} 111°. n_D^{15} 1.41156; n_D^{25} 1.40729. Very slightly sol in water. Sol in alc, ether. LD_{50} orally in rats: 1.67 g/kg (Smyth).

Caution: Potential symptoms of overexposure are irritation of eyes, skin and mucous membranes; headache; narcosis, coma; dermatitis. *See NIOSH Pocket Guide to Chemical Hazards* (DHHS/NIOSH 97-140, 1997) p 200.

USE: In perfumery as constituent of artificial carnation oils; as industrial solvent.

4664. Heptenophos. [23560-59-0] Phosphoric acid 7-chlorobicyclo[3.2.0]hepta-2,6-dien-6-yl dimethyl ester; 7-chlorobicyclo[3.2.0]hepta-2,6-dien-6-yl dimethylphosphate; HOE-2982; Ragadan; Hostaquick. $C_9H_{12}ClO_4P$; mol wt 250.62. C 43.13%, H 4.83%, Cl 14.15%, O 25.54%, P 12.36%. Systemic and contact insecticide of short persistence. Prepn: B. Böhner, K. Rüfenacht, **ZA 6706947**; *eidem*, **US 3600474** (1968, 1971 both to Geigy). Activity: R. T. Hewson, *Proc. 8th Br. Insectic. Fungic. Conf.* **2**, 697 (1975); W. Bonin, *ibid.* 705.

Pale amber liquid, $bp_{0.001}$ 94-95°. d_4^{20} 1.294. Vapor pressure at 20°: 7.5×10^{-4} mm Hg. Sol in xylene, acetone, methanol. LD_{50} orally in rats: 96-117 mg/kg (Hewson).

USE: Insecticide.

THERAP CAT (VET): Ectoparasiticide.

4665. Heptoxime. [530-97-2] 1,2-Cycloheptanedione dioxime. $C_7H_{12}N_2O_2$; mol wt 156.18. C 53.83%, H 7.74%, N 17.94%, O 20.49%. Prepn from cycloheptanone: Vander *et al.*, *J. Org. Chem.* **14**, 836 (1949); Belcher *et al.*, *J. Chem. Soc.* **1958**, 2743. *Review:* Banks, Nicholas, *USAEC* **ISC-737** (1956).

Crystals from benzene, mp 182°. pK_1: 10.65 ± 0.2; pK_2: 12.21 ±0.2.

Monohydrate. Crystals from water, mp 179-180°.

USE: As reagent in quantitative determination of nickel.

4666. D-manno-Heptulose. [3615-44-9] D-*manno*-Ketoheptose. $C_7H_{14}O_7$; mol wt 210.18. C 40.00%, H 6.71%, O 53.29%. Isoln from the wet pulp of the fruit of the avocado tree, *Persea gratissima* Gaertn. f. (*P. americana* Mill.), *Lauraceae:* LaForge, *J. Biol. Chem.* **28**, 511 (1917); Montgomery, Hudson, *J. Am. Chem. Soc.* **61**, 1654 (1939); Richtmyer in *Methods in Carbohydrate Chemistry* R. L. Whistler *et al.*, Eds. **vol. 1**, 173 (1962).

Large, transparent prisms from methanol, mp 151-152°. $[\alpha]_D^{20}$ +29° (c = 2 in H_2O). Sol in water. Usually accompanied by perseitol. Although perseitol is much more insol in water and methanol than D-*manno*-heptulose, clean separation of the two substances is not always easy and may require patient fractional crystn.

4667. Hercynine. [534-30-5] (αS)-α-Carboxy-N,N,N-trimethyl-1H-imidazole-4-ethanaminium inner salt; L-(1-carboxy-2-imidazol-4-ylethyl)trimethyl ammonium hydroxide inner salt; histidine-betaine; histidine trimethylbetaine. $C_9H_{15}N_3O_2$; mol wt 197.23. C 54.81%, H 7.67%, N 21.31%, O 16.22%. Present in many fungi, especially in *Amanita muscaria* Fr. and *Agaricus campestris* L., *Agaricaceae*. Isoln: Kutscher, *Zentralbl. Physiol.* **24**, 775 (1910); **26**, 569 (1912); Barger, Ewins, *J. Chem. Soc.* **99**, 2340 (1911); Küng, *Z. Physiol. Chem.* **91**, 249 (1914). Occurrence in the *Limulus polyphemus* L. (king crab), and prepn: Ackermann, List, *ibid.* **313**, 30 (1958). Synthesis: Reinhold *et al.*, *J. Med. Chem.* **11**, 258 (1968). Biosynthesis by fungi and *Actinomycetales:* Genghof, *J. Bacteriol.* **103**, 475 (1969).

Consult the Name Index before using this section.

White crystals from methanol and ether, mp 237-238° (dec). $[\alpha]_D^{22}$ +44.5° (5N HCl). Sol in water, alc.

4668. Herqueinone. [26871-30-7] (7a*S*,9*R*)-8,9-Dihydro-4,6,7a-trihydroxy-5-methoxy-1,8,8,9-tetramethyl-3*H*-phenaleno[1,-2-*b*]furan-3,7(7a*H*)-dione. $C_{20}H_{20}O_7$; mol wt 372.37. C 64.51%, H 5.41%, O 30.08%. Red fungal pigment isolated from *Penicillium herquei*: Stodola *et al., Nature* **167**, 773 (1951); Galarraga *et al., Biochem. J.* **61**, 456 (1955); Harman *et al., J. Org. Chem.* **20**, 1260 (1955). Structure: Cason *et al., Tetrahedron* **18**, 839 (1962); Paul, Sim, *Proc. Chem. Soc. London* **1962**, 352; Cason *et al., J. Org. Chem.* **35**, 179 (1970); J. S. Brooks, G. A. Morrison, *Tetrahedron Lett.* **1970**, 963; *eidem, J. Chem. Soc. Perkin Trans. 1* **1972**, 421; **1974**, 2114. Crystal structure and abs config: A. Quick *et al., Chem. Commun.* **1980**, 1051. ^{13}C-NMR study: T. Suga *et al., Chem. Lett.* **1981** 1063.

Red needles from alc, dec 226°. Sublimes in high vacuum at 175-190°. Absorption max (ethanol): 220, 250, 314, 416 nm (log ε 4.29, 4.09, 4.47, 3.66). Sol in acetone, DMF, 2N NaOH, concd HCl, cold concd H_2SO_4; fairly sol in methanol, ethanol, ether, ethyl acetate, chloroform; slightly sol in benzene, carbon disulfide. Practically insol in petr ether, carbon tetrachloride, water, aq Na_2CO_3.

4669. Herrmann-Beller Catalyst. [172418-32-5] Bis[μ-(acetato-κO:$\kappa O'$)]bis[[2-[bis(2-methylphenyl)phosphino-κP]phenyl]methyl-κC]dipalladium stereoisomer; *trans*-di(μ-acetato)bis[*o*-(di-*o*-tolylphosphino)benzyl]dipalladium(II); Herrmann's palladacycle. $C_{46}H_{46}O_4P_2Pd_2$; mol wt 937.64. C 58.92%, H 4.94%, O 6.83%, P 6.61%, Pd 22.70%. Highly efficient palladacycle catalyst; exists in a monomer/dimer equilibrium in soln. Prepn: M. Beller *et al.,* **DE 4421753** (1995 to Hoechst); *eidem,* **US 5831107** (1998 to Aventis); and catalytic applications: W. A. Herrmann *et al., Angew. Chem. Int. Ed.* **34**, 1844 (1995); *eidem, Chem. Eur. J.* **3**, 1357 (1997); W. A. Herrmann *et al., J. Chem. Educ.* **77**, 92 (2000). EXAFS characterization: S. G. Fiddy *et al., Chem. Commun.* **2003**, 2682. Catalysis mechanism in the Heck reaction: V. P. W. Böhm, W. A. Herrmann, *Chem. Eur. J.* **7**, 4191 (2001). Review of catalytic applications: A. Speicher *et al., J. Prakt. Chem.* **341**, 605-608 (1999).

Yellow crystals from toluene/hexane or CH_2Cl_2/hexane, mp 229-231° (dec). Air stable; thermally stable; becomes catalytically active at ~80°.

USE: Homogeneous catalyst in carbon-carbon bond forming reactions such as the Heck and Suzuki reactions.

4670. Hesperetin. [520-33-2] (2*S*)-2,3-Dihydro-5,7-dihydroxy-2-(3-hydroxy-4-methoxyphenyl)-4*H*-1-benzopyran-4-one; 3′,5,7-trihydroxy-4′-methoxyflavanone; cyanidanon 4′-methyl ether 1626. $C_{16}H_{14}O_6$; mol wt 302.28. C 63.57%, H 4.67%, O 31.76%. The aglucon of hesperidin. Prepd by hydrolysis of hesperidin or by synthesis: Shinoda, Kawagoye, *C.A.* **23**, 2957 (1929); Seka, Prosche, *Monatsh. Chem.* **69**, 284 (1936). Sepn of isomers: Arthur *et al., J. Chem. Soc.* **1956**, 632. Structure and configuration: Arakawa, Nakazaki, *Ann.* **636**, 111 (1960). *See also* Bioflavonoids.

(±)-Form, prisms from alc, mp 226-228°. Freely sol in alc, moderately in ether. Slightly sol in water, chloroform, benzene; sol in dil alkalies. Precipitated by carbonates.

4671. Hesperidin. [520-26-3] (2*S*)-7-[[6-*O*-(6-Deoxy-α-L-mannopyranosyl)-β-D-glucopyranosyl]oxy]-2,3-dihydro-5-hydroxy-2-(3-hydroxy-4-methoxyphenyl)-4*H*-1-benzopyran-4-one; hesperetin 7-rhamnoglucoside; cirantin; hesperetin-7-rutinoside. $C_{28}H_{34}O_{15}$; mol wt 610.56. C 55.08%, H 5.61%, O 39.31%. Predominant flavonoid in lemons and sweet oranges (*Citrus sinensis*). Extraction procedures: Higby, *J. Am. Pharm. Assoc. Sci. Ed.* **30**, 629 (1941); **US 2421061** (1947); Baier, **US 2442110** (1948 to Calif. Fruit Growers Exchange). Structure: King, Robertson, *J. Chem. Soc.* **1931**, 1704; Arthur *et al., ibid.* **1956**, 632; Horowitz, Gentili, *Tetrahedron* **19**, 773 (1963). Synthesis: Zemplen, Bognar, *Ber.* **75**, 1043 (1943); **76**, 773 (1943). Identity with cirantin: Manwaring *et al., Phytochemistry* **7**, 1881 (1968). *See also* Bioflavonoids, Rutinose.

Fine, dendritic needles by precipitation at pH 6-7, mp 258-262° (softens at 250°). $[\alpha]_D^{20}$ −76° (c = 2 in pyridine). One gram dissolves in 50 l water. Sol in formamide, DMF at 60°. Slightly sol in methanol, hot glacial acetic acid. Almost insol in acetone, benzene, chloroform. Freely sol in dil alkalies, pyridine.

4672. Hetacillin. [3511-16-8] (2*S*,5*R*,6*R*)-6-[(4*R*)-2,2-Dimethyl-5-oxo-4-phenyl-1-imidazolidinyl]-3,3-dimethyl-7-oxo-4-thia-1-azabicyclo[3.2.0]heptane-2-carboxylic acid; 6-(2,2-dimethyl-5-oxo-4-phenyl-1-imidazolidinyl)penicillanic acid; phenazacillin; BRL-804; Versapen. $C_{19}H_{23}N_3O_4S$; mol wt 389.47. C 58.59%, H 5.95%, N 10.79%, O 16.43%, S 8.23%. Semi-synthetic antibiotic related to penicillin. Prepn and structure: Hardcastle *et al., J. Org. Chem.* **31**, 897 (1966); Johnson, Panetta, **US 3198804** (1965 to Bristol-Myers). Pharmacology: Kirby, Kind, *Ann. N.Y. Acad. Sci.* **145**, 291 (1967); Ueda *et al., J. Antibiot.* **20B**, 206 (1967), *C.A.* **69**, 95016w (1968). Stability studies: Saccani, Pansera, *Boll. Chim. Farm.* **107**, 640 (1968). Epimerization at C-6 to *epihetacillin*: Johnson *et al., Tetrahedron Lett.* **1968**, 1903.

Rectangular plates from water + methyl isobutyl ketone, dec 182.8-183.9°; also reported as mp 189.2-191.0°. $[\alpha]_D^{25}$ +366° (pyridine). Practically insol in most organic solvents and water; sol in dil aq NaOH soln (pH 7-8), DMF, DMSO, pyridine, methanol (with dec).

Potassium salt. [5321-32-4] Hetacin-K; Natacillin; Versatrex. $C_{19}H_{22}KN_3O_4S$; mol wt 427.56.

Methyl ester. $C_{20}H_{25}N_3O_4S$. Crystals from carbon tetrachloride, mp 101.5-102°. Sol in most organic solvents.

Epihetacillin. Crystals, mp 164-165°. $[\alpha]_D^{23}$ +232° (pyridine).

THERAP CAT: Antibacterial.

THERAP CAT (VET): Antibacterial.

4673. Hetastarch. [9004-62-0] Starch 2-hydroxyethyl ether; hydroxyethyl starch; HES; 6-H.E.S.; Hespan; Hespander; Hestar; Plasmasteril. A starch derivative of undetermined exact composition. Comprised of more than 90% amylopectin and etherified to the extent that an average of 7 to 8 of the OH groups present in every ten D-glucopyranose units of the polymer have been converted to OCH_2CH_2OH groups. Preparation by treating starch with pyridine and ethylene chlorohydrin: Mima, Yokoyama, **JP 70 6556** (1970 to Green Cross), *C.A.* **73**, 36822r (1970). Structure evaluation studies: Banks *et al., Br. J. Pharmacol.* **47**, 172 (1973). Physicochemical and biological properties: Tamada *et al., Chem. Pharm. Bull.* **19**, 286 (1971); Banks *et al., Staerke* **24**, 181 (1972). Pharmacology: Irikura *et al., Oyo Yakuri* **6**, 985 sqq (1972). Metabolism: Bogan *et al., Toxicol. Appl. Pharmacol.* **15**, 206 (1969); Ryan *et al., Xenobiotica* **2**, 141 (1972). Toxicity studies: Irikura *et al., Oyo Yakuri* **6**, 1023 (1972). Introduction as a plasma expander: Wiedersheim, *Arch. Int. Pharmacodyn.* **111**, 353 (1957). Review of production and uses: Hjermstad, *Starch Chem. Technol.* **2**, 423-432 (1967).

R or R' = H or CH₂CH₂OH

White powder. Very sol in water. Insol in alcohol.

Amylopectin derivative. The sequence is frequently interrupted by a unit in which R' is the residue of an additional O-hydroxyethylated α-D-glucopyranosyl moiety that constitutes the first unit in a branch or sub-branch of the polymer.

USE: Cryoprotective agent for erythrocytes.

THERAP CAT: Plasma volume expander.

THERAP CAT (VET): Plasma volume expander.

4674. 5-HETE. [70608-72-9] (5S,6E,8Z,11Z,14Z)-5-Hydroxy-6,8,11,14-eicosatetraenoic acid; (S)-5-hydroxy-6-*trans*-8,11,14-*cis*-eicosatetraenoic acid. $C_{20}H_{32}O_3$; mol wt 320.47. C 74.96%, H 10.06%, O 14.98%. Important intermediate in a series of biosynthetic processes leading from arachidonic acid, *q.v.*, to a number of biologically active compounds. First discovered during the transformation of arachidonic acid by rabbit peritoneal polymorphonuclear leukocytes: P. Borgeat *et al., J. Biol. Chem.* **251**, 7816 (1976). Revised description: *eidem, ibid.* **252**, 8772 (1977). It has also been found during metabolism of arachidonic acid by human peripheral blood polymorphonuclear leukocytes: P. Borgeat, B. Samuelsson, *Proc. Natl. Acad. Sci. USA* **76**, 2148 (1979); and has been shown to be strongly chemotactic for human eosinophils and neutrophils: E. J. Goetzl *et al., Immunology* **39**, 491 (1980); E. J. Goetzl, *N. Engl. J. Med.* **303**, 822 (1980). 5-HETE is formed via **5-HPETE (5-hydroperoxy-6,8,11,14-eicosatetraenoic acid)**, a precursor of the leukotrienes, *q.v.* Chemical and enzymic syntheses of 5-HETE and 5-HPETE: E. J. Corey *et al., J. Am. Chem. Soc.* **102**, 1435 (1980). Synthesis via phenylselenylation of arachidonic acid: J. E. Baldwin *et al., Tetrahedron* **37**, Suppl. 1, 263 (1981). Large-scale synthesis of 5-HETE: E. J. Corey, S. Hashimoto, *Tetrahedron Lett.* **22**, 299 (1981). Biosynthetic study: R. C. Mebane, *Diss. Abstr. B* **42**, 2839 (1982). Selected synthesis of octadeuterated (±)-5-HETE: W. C. Hubbard *et al., Prostaglandins* **23**, 61 (1982). Stereospecific syntheses of 5-

(S)- and 5-*(R)*-HETE and transformation to (±)-5-HPETE: R. Zamboni, J. Rokach, *Tetrahedron Lett.* **24**, 999 (1983). Review of syntheses: J. G. Atkinson, J. Rokach, in *Handbook of Prostaglandins and Related Lipids: The Eicosanoids,* A. L. Willis *et al.,* Eds. (CRC Press, Boca Raton, in press).

Methyl ester. $C_{21}H_{34}O_3$. Colorless oil. $[\alpha]_D^{23}$ +14.0°; $[\alpha]_{436}^{23}$ +35.7° (c = 2.02 in benzene).

4675. Hexaaminecobalt Trichloride. [10534-89-1] Luteocobaltic chloride; hexammino-cobalt chloride. $Cl_3CoH_{18}N_6$; mol wt 267.48. Cl 39.76%, Co 22.03%, H 6.78%, N 31.42%. $[Co(NH_3)_6]Cl_3$. Prepd from $CoCl_2$, NH_4Cl, NH_3 and O_2: Bjerrum, McReynolds, *Inorg. Synth.* **2**, 217 (1946).

Wine-red or brownish-orange-red, monoclinic crystals. Sol in water; on long boiling with water, NH_3 is evolved and $Co(OH)_3$ pptd.

USE: As reagent for pyrophosphoric acid, for the estimation of phosphate.

4676. Hexaborane(10). [23777-80-2] Hexaboron decahydride; borohexane. B_6H_{10}; mol wt 74.95. B 86.55%, H 13.45%. Prepd by the reaction of magnesium boride with hydrochloric or phosphoric acid: Stock, Kuss, *Ber.* **56B**, 789 (1923).

Liquid. mp $-62.3°$; bp 108°; vapor pressure (0°): 7.5 mm: Burg, Kratzer, *Inorg. Chem.* **1**, 725 (1962). d^0 0.69. Slowly dec at room temp. Hydrolyzes in water after long heating.

4677. Hexachlorobenzene. [118-74-1] Perchlorobenzene; Anticarie; Bunt-cure; Bunt-no-more; Julin's carbon chloride. C_6Cl_6; mol wt 284.78. C 25.31%, Cl 74.70%. Prepn: Becke, Sperber, **US 2792434** (1957 to BASF). Teratogenicity study: K. D. Courtney *et al., Toxicol. Appl. Pharmacol.* **35**, 239 (1976). Carcinogenicity studies: J. R. P. Cabral *et al., Nature* **269**, 510 (1977); D. L. Arnold *et al., Food Chem. Toxicol.* **23**, 779 (1985) (corr. *ibid.* **26**, 169 (1988)). uv spectrum: H. Conrad-Billroth, *Z. Phys. Chem.* **19**, 76 (1932); O. Schnepp, R. Kopelman, *J. Chem. Phys.* **30**, 868 (1959). Toxicology: G. Vettorazzi, *Residue Rev.* **56**, 107 (1975); R. Ockner, R. Schmid, *Nature* **189**, 499 (1961). Review of toxicology and human exposure: *Toxicological Profile for Hexachlorobenzene* (PB2003-100139, 2002) 403 pp.

Needles. d^{23} 2.044. mp 231°. bp 323-326°. Vapor pressure at 20°: 1.09×10^{-5} mm Hg. Sublimable. Insol in water. Sparingly sol in cold alcohol; sol in benzene, chloroform, ether. Flash point 242°C.

Note: Not to be confused with benzene hexachloride, *see* Lindane.

Caution: Potential symptoms of chronic oral overexposure are dermal lesions, hypertrichosis, anorexia, weight loss, focal alopecia, corneal opacity, atrophic hands, hepatomegaly, porphyria, skeletal muscle wasting. *See Clinical Toxicology of Commercial Products,* R. E. Gosselin *et al.,* Eds. (Williams & Wilkins, 5th ed., 1984) Section II, pp 170-171; *Patty's Industrial Hygiene and Toxicology* vol. **2B**, G. D. Clayton, F. E. Clayton, Eds. (John Wiley & Sons, New York, 4th ed., 1994) pp 1477-1492. This substance is reasonably anticipated to be a human carcinogen: *Report on Carcinogens, Eleventh Edition* (PB2005-104914, 2004) p III-138.

USE: In organic syntheses. Formerly as agricultural fungicide.

4678. Hexachlorobutadiene. [87-68-3] 1,1,2,3,4,4-Hexachloro-1,3-butadiene; perchlorobutadiene. C_4Cl_6; mol wt 260.76. C 18.42%, Cl 81.58%. $Cl_2C=CCl-CCl=CCl_2$. Prepn: F.

Krafft, *Ber.* **10**, 801 (1877); E. T. McBee, R. E. Hatton, *Ind. Eng. Chem.* **41**, 809 (1949); J. Jelinek, M. Hudlicky, *Collect. Czech. Chem. Commun.* **22**, 651 (1957). GC determn in blood: P. E. Kastl, E. A. Hermann, *J. Chromatogr.* **280**, 390 (1983). Toxicity study: D. Gradiski *et al.*, *Eur. J. Toxicol. Environ. Hyg.* **8**, 180 (1975). Review of toxicology and human exposure: *Toxicological Profile for Hexachlorobutadiene* (PB95-100160, 1994) 135 pp. Review: G. Choudhary, *Environ. Carcinog. Ecotoxicol. Rev.* **C13**, 179-203 (1995).

Colorless liquid with faint turpentine-like odor. mp −21°; bp$_{760}$ 215°. d$_4^{20}$ 1.6820; n$_D^{20}$ 1.5542. Viscosity (cP): 2.446 at 37.8°; 1.131 at 98.9°. Soly in water (20°): 0.0005%. Sol in ethanol, ether. LD$_{50}$ in male, female mice, rats (mg/kg): 105, 76, 216, 175 i.p.; 80, 65, 250, 270 orally (Gradiski).

Caution: Potential symptoms of overexposure in exptl animals are irritation of eyes, skin, respiratory system; kidney damage. Potential occupational carcinogen. *See: NIOSH Pocket Guide to Chemical Hazards* (DHHS/NIOSH 97-140, 1997) p. 158; *Patty's Industrial Hygiene and Toxicology* vol. **2E**, G. D. Clayton, F. E. Clayton, Eds. (John Wiley & Sons, New York, 4th ed., 1994) p 4240-4247.

USE: Intermediate in the manuf of rubber compds, chlorofluorocarbons, and lubricants. Hydraulic fluid, fluid for gyroscopes, heat transfer fluid, solvent, laboratory reagent. Soil fumigant for vineyards.

4679. Hexachloroethane. [67-72-1] Carbon hexachloride; perchloroethane. C$_2$Cl$_6$; mol wt 236.74. C 10.15%, Cl 89.85%. CCl$_3$CCl$_3$. Prepn: *Beilstein* **1**, 87 (1918) and suppls. Toxicity data: Barsoum, Saad, *Q. J. Pharm. Pharmacol.* **7**, 205 (1934). Review of toxicology and human exposure: *Toxicological Profile for Hexachloroethane* (PB98-101041, 1997) 190 pp.

Crystals; camphorous odor. d 2.09. Readily sublimes without melting. bp 186.8° (triple point). Heat of sublimation 12.2 kcal/mol. Sol in alcohol, benzene, chloroform, ether, oils. Insol in water. MLD i.v. in dogs: 325 mg/kg (Barsoum, Saad).

Caution: Potential symptoms of overexposure are irritation of eyes, skin, mucous membranes. *See NIOSH Pocket Guide to Chemical Hazards* (DHHS/NIOSH 97-140, 1997) p 158. *See also Patty's Industrial Hygiene and Toxicology* vol. **2E**, G. D. Clayton, F. E. Clayton, Eds. (John Wiley & Sons, New York, 4th ed., 1994) p 4144-4151. This substance is reasonably anticipated to be a human carcinogen: *Report on Carcinogens, Eleventh Edition* (PB2005-104914, 2004) p III-140.

USE: In metallurgy for refining aluminum alloys, removing impurities from molten metals, recovering metal from ores or smelting products. Degassing agent for magnesium; to inhibit explosiveness of methane and combustion of ammonium perchlorate. Smoke generator in grenades; in pyrotechnics. Ignition suppressant, in fire extinguishing fluids, polymer additive, flame-proofing agent, vulcanizing agent. In prodn of synthetic diamonds.

THERAP CAT (VET): Anthelmintic (flukicide).

4680. Hexachlorophene. [70-30-4] 2,2′-Methylenebis[3,4,-6-trichlorophenol]; 2,2′-dihydroxy-3,3′,5,5′,6,6′-hexachlorodiphenylmethane; bis(3,5,6-trichloro-2-hydroxyphenyl)methane; AT-7; G-11; Bilevon; Dermadex; Exofene; Hexosan; pHisohex; Surgi-Cen; Surofene. C$_{13}$H$_6$Cl$_6$O$_2$; mol wt 406.90. C 38.37%, H 1.49%, Cl 52.28%, O 7.86%. Prepd by the condensation of 2 mols of 2,4,5-trichlorophenol with 1 mol formaldehyde in the presence of concd sulfuric acid: Gump, **US 2250480** (1941 to Burton T. Bush). Improved procedures: **US 2435593** (1948) and **US 2812365** (1957 to Givaudan). Acute toxicity: T. B. Gaines, R. E. Linder, *Fundam. Appl. Toxicol.* **7**, 299 (1986).

Crystals from benzene, mp 164-165°. Practically insol in water. Sol in alcohol, acetone, ether, chloroform, propylene glycol; polyethylene glycols; olive oil; cottonseed oil; dil aq solns of the alka-

lies. Forms salts with alkalies and alkaline earths. Phenol coefficient ~125 (monopotassium salt). Incompatible with Tweens from bacteriological point of view. LD$_{50}$ in adult male, female rats (mg/kg): 66, 57 orally (Gaines, Linder).

Monophosphate. Hepadist.

Caution: Excessive dosage to animals results in symptoms of neurotoxicity. Reversible vacuolar changes mainly affecting the myelin of the brain and spinal cord have been reported. Because of potential neurotoxicity in humans, the FDA has regulated use. *See* Lockhart, *Pediatrics* **50**, 229 (1972).

USE: Chiefly in the manuf of germicidal soaps.

THERAP CAT: Antiseptic; disinfectant.

THERAP CAT (VET): Anthelmintic (flukicide).

4681. Hexaconazole. [79983-71-4] α-Butyl-α-(2,4-dichlorophenyl)-1H-1,2,4-triazole-1-ethanol; (RS)-2-(2,4-dichlorophenyl)-1-(1H-1,2,4-triazol-1-yl)hexan-2-ol; PP-523; ICIA-0523; Anvil; Planete. C$_{14}$H$_{17}$Cl$_2$N$_3$O; mol wt 314.21. C 53.52%, H 5.45%, Cl 22.57%, N 13.37%, O 5.09%. Ergosterol biosynthesis inhibitor. Prepn: H. K. Spencer, **BE 886128** (1981 to Sandoz); and resolution of isomers: P. A. Worthington, *Pestic. Sci.* **31**, 457 (1991). Properties and fungicidal activity in vines and food crops: M. C. Shephard *et al.*, *Proc. Br. Crop Prot. Conf. - Pests Dis.* **1986**, 19. Review of analytical methods: K. J. Harradine *et al.* in *Comprehensive Analytical Profiles of Important Pesticides*, J. Sherma, T. Cairns, Eds. (CRC Press, Boca Raton, 1993) pp 43-57.

White crystalline solid, mp 111°. d^{25} 1.29. Log P (octanol/water): −3.9 at 20°. Vapor pressure (20°): 2 × 10^{-8} kPa. Soly at 20° (g/l): water 0.017; methanol 246; acetone 164; toluene 59; hexane 0.8. LD$_{50}$ orally in mallard ducks, male rats, female rats: >4000, 2189, 6071 mg/kg; dermally in rats: >2000 mg/kg. LC$_{50}$ (96 hour) in rainbow trout: >6.7 mg/l (Shephard).

USE: Agricultural fungicide.

4682. Hexadimethrine Bromide. [28728-55-4] N,N,N′,N′-Tetramethyl-1,6-hexanediamine polymer with 1,3-dibromopropane; polymer of N,N,N′,N′-tetramethylhexamethylenediamine and trimethylene bromide; poly(N,N,N′,N′-tetramethyl-N-trimethylene-hexamethylenediammonium dibromide); Polybrene. (C$_{13}$H$_{30}$Br$_2$-N$_2$)$_x$. Toxicity study: Kimura *et al.*, *Toxicol. Appl. Pharmacol.* **1**, 185 (1959).

White, hygroscopic, amorphous polymer. Soluble in water up to 10%. pH of 1% saline soln 5-9. Stable in soln and when autoclaved. Polymers with mol wt of 5000-10,000 have LD$_{50}$ i.v. in mice: 25-40 mg/kg (Kimura).

THERAP CAT: Heparin antagonist.

4683. Hexaflumuron. [86479-06-3] N-[[[3,5-Dichloro-4-(1,1,2,2-tetrafluoroethoxy)phenyl]amino]carbonyl]-2,6-difluorobenzamide; 1-[3,5-dichloro-4-(1,1,2,2-tetrafluoroethoxy)phenyl]-(2,6-difluorobenzoyl)urea; DE-473; XRD-473; Consult; Recruit; Recruit II. C$_{16}$H$_8$Cl$_2$F$_6$N$_2$O$_3$; mol wt 461.14. C 41.67%, H 1.75%, Cl 15.38%, F 24.72%, N 6.07%, O 10.41%. Insect growth regulator; inhibits chitin synthesis. Prepn: R. H. Rigterink, R. J. Sbragia, **EP 71279**; *eidem*, **US 4468405** (1983, 1984 both to Dow). Physical properties and activity: R. J. Sbragia *et al.*, *Proc. 10th Int. Congr. Plant Prot.* **1**, 417 (1983). Chromatographic determn in soil: A. Khoshab, R. Teasdale, *J. Chromatogr. A* **660**, 195 (1994). Environmental distribution: D. Yon *et al.*, *Brighton Crop Prot. Conf. -*

Pests Dis. **1992**, 907. Field trials in food crops: K. N. Komblas, R. C. Hunter, *Proc. Br. Crop Prot. Conf. - Pests Dis.* **1986**, 907; vs subterranean termites: N.-Y. Su, *J. Econ. Entomol.* **87**, 389 (1994).

White solid, mp 197-199°. Soly in water (23°): 0.7 mg/l. vapor pressure (298 K): 5.87×10^{-9}.

USE: Insecticide.

4684.   Hexafluorenium Bromide. [317-52-2] *N,N'*-Di-9*H*-fluoren-9-yl-*N,N,N',N'*-tetramethyl-1,6-hexanediaminium dibromide; hexamethylenebis[9-fluorenyldimethylammonium bromide]; hexamethylenebis(dimethyl-9-fluorenylammonium bromide); Mylaxen. $C_{36}H_{42}Br_2N_2$; mol wt 662.54. C 65.26%, H 6.39%, Br 24.12%, N 4.23%. Neuromuscular blocking agent with pseudocholinesterase inhibitory activity. Prepn: Cavallito *et al., J. Am. Chem. Soc.* **76**, 1862 (1954); Cavallito, Gray, US 2783237 (1957 to Irwin, Neisler). Clinical trial for prolongation of succinylcholine muscular block: L. F. Walts *et al., Anesthesiology* **33**, 503 (1970). Review: R. M. Britton, M. Figueroa, *Anesth. Analg.* **52**, 100-105 (1973).

Crystals from *n*-propanol, mp 188-189°.

THERAP CAT: Succinylcholine synergist.

4685.   Hexafluoroacetone. [684-16-2] 1,1,1,3,3,3-Hexafluoro-2-propanone. C_3F_6O; mol wt 166.02. C 21.70%, F 68.66%, O 9.64%. CF_3COCF_3. Synthon in organic and inorganic reactions with an exceptionally electron deficient carbonyl group. Prepn: N. Fukuhara, L. A. Bigelow, *J. Am. Chem. Soc.* **63**, 788 (1941). Comprehensive review: C. G. Krespan, W. J. Middleton in *Fluorine Chem. Rev.* vol. 1, P. Tarrant, Ed. (Marcel Dekker, New York, 1967) pp 145-196. Review of reactivity: H. W. Roesky, *J. Fluorine Chem.* **30**, 123-139 (1985); of use in inorganic chemistry: M. Witt *et al., Adv. Inorg. Chem. Radiochem.* **30**, 223-312 (1986); in polymer chemistry: P. E. Cassidy *et al., J. Macromol. Sci. Rev. Macromol. Chem. Phys.* **C29**, 365-429 (1989); in peptide chemistry: K. Burger *et al., Amino Acids* **8**, 195-199 (1995); of toxicology: G. L. Kennedy, Jr., *Crit. Rev. Toxicol.* **21**, 149-170 (1990).

bp$_{760}$ -27.4°. mp -122°. d$^{23.3}$ 1.323; d$^{44.4}$ 1.149. uv max: 302 nm (ε 16.9). Critical pressure: 411 psia. Critical temp: 84.1°. Heat capacity (Btu/lb/°F) of liquid at 0°: 0.192; of vapor: 0.23. Reacts with water to form hydrates. LD$_{50}$ (mg/kg) in rats: 190 orally (trihydrate), 670 dermally (sesquihydrate); in mice: 250 i.p., 180 i.v.; in rabbits: 113 dermally (trihydrate) (Kennedy).

USE: Protecting and activating reagent in peptide chemistry; in synthesis of high performance fluoropolymers, pharmaceutical and agricultural chemicals; in ^{19}F NMR. Solvent for polyamides, polyesters, polyacetals, polyols.

4686.   Hexafluorobenzene. [392-56-3] Perfluorobenzene. C_6F_6; mol wt 186.05. C 38.73%, F 61.27%. Prepn: E. T. McBee *et al., Ind. Eng. Chem.* **39**, 378 (1947); J. A. Godsell *et al., Nature* **178**, 199 (1956). Toxicology: C. F. B. Nhachi, *Toxicology* **39**, 317 (1986). Mechanistic study of metabolite formation: I. M. C. M. Rietjens, J. Vervoort, *Chem. Res. Toxicol.* **5**, 10 (1992).

mp -13 to -11°. bp$_{743}$ 81.0-82.0° (McBee); also reported as bp 80° (Godsell). n$_D^{20}$ 1.3760; n$_D^{18}$ 1.3746. d$_4^{25}$ 1.612.

USE: Solvent; intermediate in chemical synthesis.

4687.   Hexalure. [23192-42-9] (*Z*)-7-Hexadecen-1-ol acetate; *cis*-7-hexadecenyl acetate; *cis*-1-acetoxy-7-hexadecene; hexalene. $C_{18}H_{34}O_2$; mol wt 282.46. C 76.54%, H 12.13%, O 11.33%. Synthetic sex pheromone for pink bollworm moths, *Pectinophora gossypiella* (Saunders). Discovery and prepn: N. Green *et al., Experientia* **25**, 682 (1969); N. Green, J. C. Keller, DE **1960155**; *eidem,* US **3586712** (1970, 1971 both to U.S. Sec. Agric.). Field trials: J. C. Keller *et al., J. Econ. Entomol.* **62**, 1520 (1969). Acute toxicity study: M. Beroza *et al., Toxicol. Appl. Pharmacol.* **31**, 421 (1975). *See also* Gossyplure, Propylure.

Clear oily liquid, bp$_{0.001}$ 100-104°. n$_D^{25}$ 1.4484. Insol in water. Sol in hexane, ether, acetone, benzene. LD$_{50}$ in rats (mg/kg): >34600 orally; in rabbits (mg/kg): >2025 dermally (Beroza).

USE: Insect attractant.

4688.   Hexamethonium. [60-26-4] *N,N,N,N',N',N'*-Hexamethyl-1,6-hexanediaminium; hexamethylenebis(trimethylammonium); α,ω-bis(trimethylammonium)hexane; hexathonide; hexamethone. $[C_{12}H_{30}N_2]^{2+}$. $[(CH_3)_3N(CH_2)_6N(CH_3)_3]^{2+}$. Prepn: H. J. Barber, US **2641610** (1953 to May & Baker); H. J. Barber, K. Gaimster, *J. Pharm. Pharmacol.* **3**, 663 (1951). Ganglion blocking agent: R. Wien, D. F. J. Mason, *Br. J. Pharmacol.* **6**, 611 (1951).

Bromide. [55-97-0] C-6; Bistrium bromide; Esametina; Gangliostat; Hexameton bromide; Hexanium bromide; Simpatoblock; Vegolysin; Vegolysin. $C_{12}H_{30}Br_2N_2$; mol wt 362.19. Hygroscopic crystals, mp 274-276°. Sol in water, alc. Insol in acetone, chloroform, ether. pH of 1% soln: 6.2-7.0.

Chloride. Bistrium chloride; Chloor-hexaviet; Hestrium chloride; Hexameton chloride; Hexone chloride; Hiohex chloride; Methium chloride; Meton. $C_{12}H_{30}Cl_2N_2$; mol wt 273.29. Hygroscopic crystals, dec 289-292°. Sol in water, alc. Practically insol in chloroform, ether. pH of 10% soln: 5.5-6.5.

Iodide. Hexathide. $C_{12}H_{30}I_2N_2$; mol wt 456.19. Hygroscopic cryst powder. Sol in water. Practically insol in alc.

Tartrate. Vegolysen-T. $C_{20}H_{40}N_2O_{12}$; mol wt 500.54. Hygroscopic powder, dec 186°. Sol in water. Practically insol in alc. pH of 10% soln: 3.8.

THERAP CAT: Antihypertensive.

4689.   Hexamethyldisilazane. [999-97-3] 1,1,1-Trimethyl-*N*-(trimethylsilyl)silanamine; HMDS. $C_6H_{19}NSi_2$; mol wt 161.39. C 44.65%, H 11.87%, N 8.68%, Si 34.80%. $(CH_3)_3SiNHSi$-$(CH_3)_3$. Silylating agent. Prepn: R. O. Sauer, *J. Am. Chem. Soc.* **66**, 1707 (1944). Surface tension and density as a function of temperature: R. S. Myers, H. L. Clever, *J. Chem. Eng. Data* **14**, 161 (1969). Mass spec. study: J. Tamás, P. Miklos, *Org. Mass Spectrom.* **10**, 859 (1975). Raman, IR and NMR spectra: K. Hamada, H. Morishita, *Spectrosc. Lett.* **16**, 717 (1983). Molecular structure and conformation: T. Fjeldberg, *J. Mol. Struct.* **112**, 159 (1984). Use in deactivation of chromatography columns: T. Welsch *et al., J. Chromatogr.* **241**, 41 (1982); R. C. Kong *et al., Chromatographia* **18**, 362 (1984). Use as adhesion promoter for photoresists: J. N. Helbert, H. G. Hughes in *Proc. Symp. Adhesion Aspects Polymeric Coatings,* K. L. Mittal, Ed. (Plenum Press, New York, 1983) pp 499-508; D. Freeman, W. Kern, *J. Vac. Sci. Technol. A* **7**, 1446 (1989). Physical properties, toxicity and technical data: Petrarch Systems Inc. Product Information Sheets. Brief review of chemistry and applications: R. J. De Pasquale, *Am. Lab.* **5**(6), 35-39 (1973).

Colorless liquid with an ammonia-like odor. bp 126.0°. d$_4^{20}$ 0.7742. n$_D^{20}$ 1.4080. Flash pt, closed cup: 81°F (27°C). pKa 7.55. Vapor pressure at 50°C: 79 mm. Viscosity: 0.90 cSt. Ignition pt: 380°. Dielectric constant (1000 Hz): 2.27. Insol in water, reacts slowly. LD$_{LO}$ i.p. in mice: 650 mg/kg (Petrarch Systems Inc. Product Information Sheets).

Caution: Causes severe burns to eyes and irritation of the skin (Petrarch Systems Inc. Product Information Sheets).

USE: Deactivation of chromatographic support materials. In electronic industry as an adhesion promoter for photoresists on silicon.

4690. Hexamethylene Glycol. [629-11-8] 1,6-Hexanediol; 1,6-dihydroxyhexane. $C_6H_{14}O_2$; mol wt 118.17. C 60.98%, H 11.94%, O 27.08%. $HOCH_2(CH_2)_4CH_2OH$. Prepd by reduction of ethyl adipate with copper chromite: Lazier *et al., Org. Synth.* **coll. vol. II,** 325 (1943); from 2,5-tetrahydrofurandimethanol: Utne *et al.,* US 3070633 (1962 to Merck & Co.). Toxicity study: C. P. Carpenter *et al., Toxicol. Appl. Pharmacol.* **28,** 313 (1974).

Crystals, mp 42.8°. bp_{760} 208°; bp_{10} 134°. n_D^{25} 1.4579. Dipole moment: 2.48 (dioxane). Sol in water, alcohol; sparingly sol in hot ether. LD_{50} orally in rats: 3.73 g/kg (Carpenter).

Bis(3,5-dinitrobenzoate). $C_{20}H_{18}N_4O_{12}$. Crystals from dioxane + ethanol, mp 169-171°.

USE: Intermediate in the production of nylon; to make hexamethylenediamine, polyesters, polyurethans; in gasoline refining; as plasticizer.

4691. Hexamethylolmelamine. [531-18-0] (1,3,5-Triazine-2,4,6-triyltrinitrilo)hexakismethanol; (*s*-triazine-2,4,6-triyltrinitrilo)hexamethanol; hexakis(hydroxymethyl)melamine; Resloom M 75. $C_9H_{18}N_6O_6$; mol wt 306.28. C 35.29%, H 5.92%, N 27.44%, O 31.34%. Prepn: Gams *et al., Helv. Chim. Acta* **24,** 302E (1941); Widmer, Fisch, US 2387547 (1945 to Ciba).

Amorphous to cryst, white mass, mp 135-139°. Sol in water. Easily forms insol polymerization products. For the prepn of aq solns double distilled water and hard glass vessels are recommended. A 1.4-2% aq soln is thus possible.

USE: In fireproofing and creaseproofing of cottons, rayons.

4692. Hexamidine. [3811-75-4] 4,4'-[1,6-Hexanediylbis(oxy)]bisbenzenecarboximidamide; 4,4'-(hexamethylenedioxy)dibenzamidine; 4,4'-diamidino-α,ω-diphenoxyhexane. $C_{20}H_{26}N_4O_2$; mol wt 354.45. C 67.77%, H 7.39%, N 15.81%, O 9.03%. Prepn: A. J. Ewins *et al.,* GB 507565 (1939 to May & Baker); and trypanocidal activity: J. N. Ashley *et al., J. Chem. Soc.* **1942,** 103. Activity in fibrinolytic systems: J. D. Geratz, *Thromb. Diath. Haemorrh.* **29,** 154 (1973). Antibacterial activity: G. Michel *et al., J. Int. Med. Res.* **14,** 205 (1986). Antifungal activity: M. C. Reynaud, C. Chauve, *Bull. Soc. Fr. Mycol. Med.* **15,** 269 (1986). HPLC determn in pharmaceutics: P. Taylor *et al., J. Pharm. Sci.* **72,** 1477 (1983); in cosmetics: B. Wyhowski de Bukanski, M. O. Masse, *Int. J. Cosmet. Sci.* **6,** 283 (1984). Clinical use as a topical antiseptic: M. J. Fénelon, *Bordeaux Med.* **3,** 867 (1970). Use in treatment of acne: P. Taylor, A. A. Levy, EP 93186 (1983 to Richardson-Vicks). Amebicidal effects: D. Perrine *et al., Antimicrob. Agents Chemother.* **39,** 339 (1995).

Isethionate. [659-40-5] RF-2535; Desomedine; Hexomedin. $C_{24}H_{38}N_4O_{10}S_2$; mol wt 606.71. Prisms from HCl, mp 246-247° (dec).

USE: Preservative in cosmetics.

THERAP CAT: Antiseptic (topical).

4693. Hexaminolevulinate. [140898-97-1] 5-Amino-4-oxopentanoic acid hexyl ester; 5-aminolevulinic acid hexyl ester; hexyl 5-aminolevulinate. $C_{11}H_{21}NO_3$; mol wt 215.29. C 61.37%, H 9.83%, N 6.51%, O 22.29%. Prodrug of δ-aminolevulinic acid, *q.v.*; induces production of intracellular protoporphyrin IX. Prepn:

H. Takeya, JP Kokai 92 9360 (1992 to Cosmo Sogo Kenkyusho); and use as photosensitizer: K. E. Gierskcky *et al.,* WO 9628412 (1996 to Norwegian Radium Res. Found.); *eidem,* US 6034267 (2000 to PhotoCure). Synthesis and pharmacology: C. J. Whitaker *et al., Anti-Cancer Drug Des.* **15,** 161 (2000). Clinical evaluation for photodetection of bladder cancer: N. Lange *et al., Br. J. Cancer* **80,** 185 (1999).

Hydrochloride. [140898-91-5] P-1206; Hexvix. $C_{11}H_{21}$-NO_3.HCl; mol wt 251.75. Crystals from methanol/ethyl acetate, mp 94°.

THERAP CAT: Diagnostic aid (fluorescence imaging agent).

4694. *n*-Hexane. [110-54-3] C_6H_{14}; mol wt 86.18. C 83.62%, H 16.37%. $CH_3(CH_2)_4CH_3$. Chief constituent of petr ether, ligroin, and commercial hexane. Review of toxicity and metabolism: D. Couri, M. Milk, *Annu. Rev. Pharmacol. Toxicol.* **22,** 145-166 (1982). Book: *Technology and Solvents for Extracting Oilseeds and Nonpetroleum Oil,* P. J. Wan, P. J. Wakelyn, Eds. (AOCS Press, Champaign, 1987) 350 pp.

Colorless, very volatile liquid; faint, peculiar odor. d_4^{20} 0.6591. bp 69°. mp −100 to −95°. n_D^{20} 1.375. Flash point: −18.0°C. Vapor pressure (mmHg): 186.1 at 30°, 400.6 at 50°. Partition coefficient (1-octanol/water) at 25°: >4100. Spec heat at 22.0°: 0.536 cal/g/°C. Viscosity at 15°: 0.337 cP. Heat of vaporization: 79.4 cal/g. Surface tension at 20°: 18.41 dyne/cm. Insol in water. Miscible with alcohol, chloroform, ether. LC_{50} (4 hr) in mice by inhalation: 48000 ppm; LD_{50} orally in rats: 32.0 g/kg (Couri, Milks).

Caution: Potential symptoms of overexposure are lightheadedness; giddiness; nausea, headache; peripheral neuropathy; numbness of extremities, muscle weakness; irritation of eyes and nose; dermatitis; aspiration of liquid may cause chemical pneumonia. See *NIOSH Pocket Guide to Chemical Hazards* (DHHS/NIOSH 97-140, 1997) p 162.

USE: Determining refractive index of minerals; filling for thermometers instead of mercury, usually with a blue or red dye; extraction solvent for oilseed processing.

4695. 1,6-Hexanediamine. [124-09-4] Hexamethylenediamine; 1,6-diaminohexane. $C_6H_{16}N_2$; mol wt 116.20. C 62.02%, H 13.88%, N 24.11%. $NH_2(CH_2)_6NH_2$. Prepd by reducing adiponitrile with sodium and alcohol: Slotta, Tschesche, *Ber.* **62,** 1404 (1929). Manuf: *Faith, Keyes & Clark's Industrial Chemicals,* F. A. Lowenheim, M. K. Moran, Eds. (Wiley-Interscience, New York, 4th ed., 1975) pp 442-444.

Platelets, leaflets. Sublimes as long needles. Odor of piperidine. Absorbs water and carbon dioxide from air. mp 42°. bp 205°; bp_{20} 100°. Freely sol in water; slightly sol in alcohol, benzene.

Dihydrochloride. $C_6H_{16}N_2$.2HCl. Needles from water or alcohol, mp 248°. Freely sol in water.

USE: Intermediate in the manuf of nylon.

4696. Hexanitrohexaazaisowurtzitane. [135285-90-4] Octahydro-1,3,4,7,8,10-hexanitro-5,2,6-(iminomethenimino)-1*H*-imidazo[4,5-*b*]pyrazine; CL-20; HNIW; 2,4,6,8,10,12-hexanitro-2,-4,6,8,10,12-hexaazatetracyclo[5.5.0.0^{5,9}.0^{3,11}]dodecane. C_6H_6-$N_{12}O_{12}$; mol wt 438.19. C 16.45%, H 1.38%, N 38.36%, O 43.81%. Symmetric polyazacyclic nitramine explosive. Polymorphs α, β, γ, ε, ζ have been identified and confirmed by x-ray diffraction or IR techniques. A sixth polymorph δ has been identified, but not confirmed. First synthesized by A. T. Nielsen in 1987; modified by R. Wardle and J. C. Hinshaw. Gas phase dissociation: R. J. Doyle, Jr., *Org. Mass Spectrom.* **26,** 723 (1991). EPR spectra: M. D. Pace, *J. Phys. Chem.* **95,** 5858 (1991). Identification of δ polymorph by high-pressure phase transition and verification of ζ by ir: T. P. Russell *et al., ibid.* **96,** 5509 (1992). Pressure-temperature phase diagrams: *eidem, ibid.* **97,** 1993 (1993). Thermal decomposition: J. C. Oxley *et al., ibid.* **98,** 7004 (1994). High-pressure/thermal shock matrix isolation deflagration and detonation study: J. K. Rice, T. P. Russell, *Chem. Phys.*

Lett. **234**, 195 (1995). Review: S. Borman, *Chem. Eng. News* **72**, 18-22 (Jan. 17, 1994).

Explosive! Crystalline.

USE: Rocket propellants. Munitions. Construction or demolition explosive.

4697. 1-Hexanol. [111-27-3] *n*-Hexyl alcohol; amylcarbinol; pentylcarbinol; 1-hydroxyhexane. $C_6H_{14}O$; mol wt 102.17. C 70.53%, H 13.81%, O 15.66%. $CH_3(CH_2)_4CH_2OH$. Occurs as the acetate in seeds and fruits of *Heracleum sphondylium* L. and *H. giganteum* Fisch., *Umbelliferae*. Lab prepn by the action of butylmagnesium bromide on ethylene oxide: Dreger, *Org. Synth.* **coll. vol. I**, 306 (2nd ed., 1941). Reduction of 1,3-hexadienal with iron wire in the presence of nickel acetate: Zeisel, Neuwirth, *Ann.* **433**, 127 (1923); *cf.* Baumgarten, Glatzel, *Ber.* **59**, 2659 (1926); Kuhn, Hoffer, *Ber.* **63**, 2165 (1930). Industrial prepn by reducing ethyl caproate with sodium in abs alcohol: Bouveault, Blanc, **DE 164294** (1903). Toxicity study: H. F. Smyth *et al., Arch. Ind. Hyg. Occup. Med.* **4**, 119 (1951).

Liquid. d_4^{25} 0.8153; d_4^{35} 0.8082. mp −51.6°. bp_{760} 157°; bp_{400} 138°; bp_{200} 119.6°; bp_{100} 102.8°; bp_{60} 92°; bp_{40} 83.7°; bp_{20} 70.3°; bp_{10} 58.2°; bp_5 47.2°; $bp_{1.0}$ 24.4°. n_D^{25} 1.4162. Absorption spectrum: Massol, Faucon, *Bull. Soc. Chim.* [4] **11**, 932. Flash pt, closed cup: 145°F (63°C). Slightly sol in water; miscible with alcohol, ether. LD_{50} orally in rats: 4.59 g/kg (Smyth).

USE: Manuf antiseptics, hypnotics.

4698. Hexapropymate. [358-52-1] 1-(2-Propynyl)cyclohexanol carbamate; carbamic acid 1-(2-propynyl)cyclohexyl ester; 1-(2-propynyl)cyclohexyl carbamate; 1-carbamoyloxy-1-(2-propynyl)cyclohexane; hexopropynate; L-2103; Merinax. $C_{10}H_{15}NO_2$; mol wt 181.23. C 66.27%, H 8.34%, N 7.73%, O 17.66%. Prepn: Lauger *et al., Helv. Chim. Acta* **42**, 2379 (1959); Prost, **US 2931828** (1960 to Soc. Belge des Labs. Labaz).

Crystals from petr ether or dioxane, mp 99°. Slight characteristic odor. Sol in ethanol, glycerol, propylene glycol.

THERAP CAT: Sedative, hypnotic.

4699. Hexazinone. [51235-04-2] 3-Cyclohexyl-6-(dimethylamino)-1-methyl-1,3,5-triazine-2,4(1*H*,3*H*)-dione; DPX-3674; Velpar. $C_{12}H_{20}N_4O_2$; mol wt 252.31. C 57.12%, H 7.99%, N 22.21%, O 12.68%. Broad spectrum, pre- and post-emergence herbicide effective against woody and herbaceous weeds. Prepn: **NL 7307218**; J. J. Fuchs, J. B. Wommack, **US 3850924**; K. Lin, **US 3983116** (1973, 1974, 1976 all to Du Pont). Herbicidal activity: J. A. Allison, T. D. Joyce, *Proc. Brit. Weed Control Conf.,* **1974**, 279; J. D. Riggleman, *Proc. South. Weed Sci. Soc.* **31**, 141 (1978). Field trials: S. J. B. Hay, R. G. Jones, *Proc. Symp. Methods Weed Control* **1977**, 139; D. E. Yarborough *et al., Weed Sci.* **34**, 723 (1986). HPLC determn in soil and water: D. C. Bouchard, T. L. Lavy, *J. Chromatogr.* **270**, 396 (1983). Residues in ground water: D. G. Neary, *South. J. Appl. For.* **7**, 217 (1983). Retention and degradation in soil: K. I. N. Jensen, E. R. Kimball, *Bull. Environ. Contam. Toxicol.* **38**, 232 (1987).

White crystalline solid. mp 97-100.5°. Very soluble in water, 330 g/l at 25°. LD_{50} orally in rats: 1690 mg/kg (Neary).

USE: Herbicide.

4700. 3-Hexen-1-ol. [544-12-7] Leaf alcohol; Blätteralkohol. $C_6H_{12}O$; mol wt 100.16. C 71.95%, H 12.08%, O 15.97%. $CH_3CH_2CH=CHCH_2CH_2OH$. Occurs in leaves of odoriferous plants (including shrubs and trees). Isoln from Japanese oil of peppermint: Walbaum *J. Prakt. Chem.* [2] **96**, 245 (1917); Walbaum, Rosenthal, *Ber. Schimmel* 1929 Jubiläums-Ausg., p 205; from raspberry juice: Bohnsack, *Ber.* **75**, 72 (1942). The natural product has the *cis* configuration: Crombie, Harper, *J. Chem. Soc.* **1950**, 873; Harper, Smith, *ibid.* **1955**, 1512.

Liquid. Strong odor resembling that of isoamyl alc, approaching the odor of green leaves when highly dil. d_{15}^{22} 0.846. bp 156-157°; bp_9 55-56°. n_D^{20} 1.4389.

4701. Hexestrol. [84-16-2] 4,4′-(1,2-Diethyl-1,2-ethanediyl)bisphenol; 4,4′-(1,2-diethylethylene)diphenol; *meso*-3,4-bis(*p*-hydroxyphenyl)-*n*-hexane; 4,4′-dihydroxy-γ,δ-diphenylhexane; 4,4′-dihydroxy-α,β-diethyldiphenylethane; dihydrodiethylstilbestrol; hexoestrol; Synthovo; Cycloestrol; Hexanoestrol; Hormoestrol; Syntrogène; Syntrogèn. $C_{18}H_{22}O_2$; mol wt 270.37. C 79.96%, H 8.20%, O 11.84%. From anethole HBr: Campbell *et al., Proc. Roy. Soc.* **B128**, 253 (1940); Bernstein, Wallis, *J. Am. Chem. Soc.* **62**, 2871 (1940); **US 2357985** (1944); Buu-Hoi, Hoán, *J. Org. Chem.* **14**, 1023 (1949). By the reduction of Grignard compds with cobaltous chloride: Kharasch *et al., J. Am. Chem. Soc.* **65**, 491 (1943). Proof of meso configuration: Wessely, Welleba, *Ber.* **74**, 777 (1941). Comprehensive description: H. Y. Aboul-Enein *et al., Anal. Profiles Drug Subs.* **11**, 347-374 (1982).

Needles from benzene, thin plates from dil alc, mp 185-188°. Freely sol in ether; sol in acetone, alcohol, methanol; slightly sol in benzene, chloroform. Sol in vegetable oils upon slight warming, also in dil solns of alkali hydroxides. Practically insol in water and in dil mineral acids.

Diacetate. Retalon-Lingual. Crystals, mp 137-139°.

Dipropionate. Retalon Oleosum. Crystals from petr ether, mp 127-128°.

Diphosphate. [14188-82-0] Hexestrol 4,4′-diphosphoric ester; Cytostatin. $C_{18}H_{24}O_8P_2$; mol wt 430.33. Prepn: **GB 593480** (1947 to Roche); Atherton *et al.,* **US 2490573** (1949 to Hoffmann-La Roche).

THERAP CAT: Estrogen; antineoplastic (hormonal).

THERAP CAT (VET): Estrogen.

4702. Hexestrol Bis(β-diethylaminoethyl ether). [2691-45-4] 2,2′-[(1,2-Diethyl-1,2-ethanediyl)bis(4,1-phenyleneoxy)]bis[*N*,*N*-diethylethanamine]; 2,2′′′-[(1,2-diethylethylene)bis(*p*-phenyleneoxy)]bis(triethylamine); 4,4′-bis(β-diethylaminoethoxy)-α,β-diethyldiphenylethane; 3,4-bis[*p*-(β-diethylaminoethoxy)phenyl]hexane; α,α′-diethyl-4,4′-bis(β-diethylaminoethoxy)bibenzyl. $C_{30}H_{48}$-N_2O_2; mol wt 468.71. C 76.88%, H 10.32%, N 5.98%, O 6.83%. Prepn: Lowe *et al., J. Chem. Soc.* **1951**, 3286.

Dihydrochloride. [69-14-7] Coralgil; Coralgina. $C_{30}H_{48}N_2$-O_2.2HCl; mol wt 541.64. Needles from alc + ethyl acetate, mp 226-227°. Freely sol in water, methanol, chloroform, hot alc.

THERAP CAT: Vasodilator (coronary).

4703. Hexetidine. [141-94-6] 1,3-Bis(2-ethylhexyl)hexahydro-5-methyl-5-pyrimidinamine; 5-amino-1,3-bis(2-ethylhexyl)-

hexahydro-5-methylpyrimidine; 1,3-bis(β-ethylhexyl)-5-methyl-5-aminohexahydropyrimidine; 5-amino-1,3-di(β-ethylhexyl)hexahydro-5-methylpyrimidine; Glypesin; Hexigel; Hexocil; Hexoral; Hextril; Oraldene; Oraseptic; Sterisil; Steri/Sol. $C_{21}H_{45}N_3$; mol wt 339.60. C 74.27%, H 13.36%, N 12.37%. Prepn: Senkus, *J. Am. Chem. Soc.* **68**, 1611 (1946); US 2415047; Bell, Necker, US 3054797 (1947, 1962 both to Comm. Solvents Corp.). Comprehensive description: G. Satzinger *et al., Anal. Profiles Drug Subs.* **7**, 277-295 (1978).

Liquid. d_{20}^{20} 0.8889. $bp_{0.4}$ 160°. n_D^{20} 1.4668. Sol in petr ether, methanol, benzene, acetone, ethanol, *n*-hexane, chloroform. Practically insol in water. pKa 8.3. Has good thermal stability.

THERAP CAT: Antiseptic.

THERAP CAT (VET): Antiseptic.

4704. Hexobarbital. [56-29-1] 5-(1-Cyclohexen-1-yl)-1,5-dimethyl-2,4,6($1H,3H,5H$)-pyrimidinetrione; 5-(1-cyclohexen-1-yl)-1,5-dimethylbarbituric acid; 5-cyclohexenyl-3,5-dimethylbarbituric acid; methylhexabital; methexenyl; enhexymal; hexobarbitone; Citodon; Citopan; Cyclonal; Dorico; Evipal; Evipan; Hexanastab Oral; Noctivane; Sombucaps; Sombulex; Somnalert. $C_{12}H_{16}N_2O_3$; mol wt 236.27. C 61.00%, H 6.83%, N 11.86%, O 20.31%. Prepd by condensation of monomethylurea with methyl cyclohexenylmethylcyanoacetate in abs alcohol in the presence of sodium: US 1947944; *cf.* DE 595175; FR 753178. Comparative clinical trial in anesthesia: D. W. Barron *et al., Br. J. Anaesth.* **38**, 802 (1966). GC determn in human plasma: D. D. Breimer, J. M. Van Rossum, *J. Chromatogr.* **88**, 235 (1974). Pharmacokinetics: N. P. E. Vermeulen *et al., Br. J. Clin. Pharmacol.* **15**, 459 (1983); M. Van der Graaff *et al., Biopharm. Drug Dispos.* **7**, 265 (1986).

Prismatic crystals, practically tasteless, mp 145-147°. Practically insol in water. One gram dissolves in about 3 liters of water. Sol in methanol, hot ethanol, ether, chloroform, acetone, benzene, aq solns of alkali hydroxides, but not carbonates.

Sodium salt. [50-09-9] Hexobarbital soluble; Cyclonal Sodium; Dorico Soluble; Evipal Sodium; Evipan Sodium; Hexanastab; Hexenal; Methexenyl Sodium; Noctivane Sodium; Narcosan Soluble; Privenal. $C_{12}H_{15}N_2NaO_3$; mol wt 258.25. White, bitter, very hygroscopic powder. Very sol in water, freely sol in alcohol, methanol, acetone. Practically insol in chloroform, ether, benzene. A soln in water absorbs carbon dioxide from the air, causing precipitation of the insol free acid. Aq and alcoholic solns are alkaline to litmus and phenolphthalein. The pH of a 10% w/v soln of hexobarbital soluble is about 11.5.

Note: This is a controlled substance (depressant): 21 CFR, 1308.13.

THERAP CAT: Sedative, hypnotic. Anesthetic (intravenous).

THERAP CAT (VET): Sedative, hypnotic.

4705. Hexobendine. [54-03-5] 3,4,5-Trimethoxybenzoic acid 1,2-ethanediylbis[(methylimino)-3,1-propanediyl] ester; 3,4,5-trimethoxybenzoic acid diester with 3,3'-[ethylenebis(methylimino)]di-1-propanol; *N,N'*-dimethyl-*N,N'*-bis[3-(3',4',5'-trimethoxybenzoxy)propyl]ethylenediamine; hexabendin. $C_{30}H_{44}N_2O_{10}$; mol wt 592.68. C 60.80%, H 7.48%, N 4.73%, O 27.00%. Prepn: O. Kraupp, K. Schlögl, AT 231432; *eidem*, US 3267103 (1964, 1966 both to OSSW). Pharmacology: Rudolph *et al., Arzneim.-Forsch.* **20**, 637 (1970); Kolassa, Pfleger, *Biochem. Pharmacol.* **20**, 490 (1971); H. Rameis *et al., Arzneim.-Forsch.* **30**, 671 (1980).

mp 75-77°.

Dihydrochloride. [50-62-4] ST-7090; Reoxyl; Ustimon; Andiamine. $C_{30}H_{44}N_2O_{10} \cdot 2HCl$; mol wt 665.60. Crystals, mp 170-174°. uv max: 267 nm. Freely sol in water, less sol in alc. Practically insol in ether.

THERAP CAT: Vasodilator (coronary).

4706. Hexocyclium Methyl Sulfate. [115-63-9] 4-(2-Cyclohexyl-2-hydroxy-2-phenylethyl)-1,1-dimethylpiperazinium methyl sulfate (salt); *N*-(β-cyclohexyl-β-hydroxy-β-phenylethyl)-*N*^{l}-methylpiperazine methosulfate; *N*-(β-cyclohexyl-β-hydroxy-β-phenylethyl)-*N*^{l}-methylpiperazine dimethylsulfate; 4-(β-cyclohexyl-β-hydroxy-β-phenethyl)-1,1-dimethylpiperazinium methyl sulfate; Tral; Tralin. $C_{21}H_{36}N_2O_5S$; mol wt 428.59. C 58.85%, H 8.47%, N 6.54%, O 18.67%, S 7.48%. Anticholinergic. Description: Helgren *et al., J. Am. Pharm. Assoc. Sci. Ed.* **46**, 639 (1957). Prepn: Weston, US 2907765 (1959 to Abbott).

Crystals, mp 200-210°. uv max ($0.1N$ H_2SO_4): 252, 257, 263 nm. Soly in water about 50% w/v. Slightly sol in chloroform. Insol in ether.

THERAP CAT: Antispasmodic.

4707. Hexoprenaline. [3215-70-1] 4,4'-[1,6-Hexanediyl-bis[imino(1-hydroxy-2,1-ethanediyl)]]bis-1,2-benzenediol; α,α'-[hexamethylenebis(iminomethylene)]bis[3,4-dihydroxybenzyl alcohol]; *N,N'*-bis[2-(3,4-dihydroxyphenyl)-2-hydroxyethyl]hexamethylenediamine; BYK 1512. $C_{22}H_{32}N_2O_6$; mol wt 420.50. C 62.84%, H 7.67%, N 6.66%, O 22.83%. β_2-Adrenergic agonist. Prepn: O. Schmid *et al.*, AT 241436; *eidem*, US 3329709 (1965, 1967, both to OSSW); Schmid *et al.*, DE 1215729 (1966 to Lentia GmbH). Pharmacology: Thiede *et al., Arzneim.-Forsch.* **21**, 416 (1971). Clinical studies: Schindl, *ibid.* **20**, 1755 (1970); several authors in *Wien. Klin. Wochenschr.* **83**, 75, 80, 101, 114, 117, 130 (1971). Clinical evaluation for interruption of labor: J. Lipshitz *et al., J. Reprod. Med.* **31**, 1023 (1986).

Crystals, mp 162-165° (hemihydrate).

Dihydrochloride. [4323-43-7] ST-1512; Ipradol. $C_{22}H_{32}N_2O_6 \cdot 2HCl$; mol wt 493.42. Crystals from methanol-ether, mp 197.5-198°.

Sulfate. [32266-10-7] Bronalin; Delaprem; Etoscol; Gynipral; Ipradol; Leanol. $C_{22}H_{32}N_2O_6 \cdot H_2SO_4$; mol wt 518.58. Crystals from water-alcohol, mp 222-228°.

THERAP CAT: Bronchodilator; tocolytic.

4708. Hexylcaine Hydrochloride. [532-76-3] 1-(Cyclohexylamino)-2-propanol benzoate (ester) hydrochloride; D-109; Cyclaine. $C_{16}H_{24}ClNO_2$; mol wt 297.82. C 64.53%, H 8.12%, Cl 11.90%, N 4.70%, O 10.74%. Prepn: Cope, Hancock, *J. Am. Chem. Soc.* **66**, 1453 (1944); Cope, US 2486374 (1949 to Sharp & Dohme). Pharmacokinetics: R. M. Rodgers *et al., Res. Commun. Chem. Pathol. Pharmacol.* **29**, 99 (1980).

• HCl

Crystals from abs alc, mp 177-178.5°. Soluble in water to the extent of about 12% w/w. A 1% soln is stable to boiling and autoclaving for sterilization purposes.

THERAP CAT: Anesthetic (local).

THERAP CAT (VET): Anesthetic (local).

4709. 2-Hexyldecanoic Acid. [25354-97-6] $C_{16}H_{32}O_2$; mol wt 256.42. C 74.94%, H 12.58%, O 12.48%. Prepn: Lederer *et al., Bull. Soc. Chim. Fr.* **1952,** 413.

Viscous oil, bp$_{0.02}$ 140-150°. n_D^{24} 1.4432.

Sodium salt. [536-37-8] Devaricin. White powder. Sol in water.

THERAP CAT: Sclerosing agent.

4710. Hexylene Glycol. [107-41-5] 2-Methyl-2,4-pentanediol; α,α,α'-trimethyltrimethyleneglycol; pinakon. $C_6H_{14}O_2$; mol wt 118.17. C 60.98%, H 11.94%, O 27.08%. Prepn: Franke, *Monatsh. Chem.* **22,** 1067 (1901); Leopold, **DE 486767** (1925 to I. G. Farben), *Frdl.* **16,** 679; Adkins, Cramer, *J. Am. Chem. Soc.* **52,** 4349 (1930); Arundale, Mikeska, **US 2367324** (1945 to Standard Oil). Toxicity study: Smyth, Carpenter, *J. Ind. Hyg. Toxicol.* **30,** 63 (1948).

Liquid. Mild sweetish odor. d$_{15}^{15}$ 0.924. bp$_{760}$ 198°; bp$_{10}$ 97°. Flash pt (open cup): 93°C (200°F). n_D^{20} 1.4276. Dipole moment: 2.8. Viscosity at 20° = 34 cP. Sol in water, alcohol, ether, lower aliphatic hydrocarbons. LD$_{50}$ orally in rats: 4.70 g/kg (Smyth, Carpenter).

Diacetate. $C_{10}H_{18}O_4$. Liquid. bp$_{12}$ 95°.

Caution: Potential symptoms of overexposure are irritation of eyes, skin, respiratory system; headache, dizziness, nausea, incoordination, CNS depression; dermatitis, skin sensitization. *See NIOSH Pocket Guide to Chemical Hazards* (DHHS/NIOSH 97-140, 1997) p 164.

USE: Cosmetics, hydraulic brake fluids (as coupling agent to castor oil).

4711. Hexyl Methyl Ketone. [111-13-7] 2-Octanone; methyl hexyl ketone. $C_8H_{16}O$; mol wt 128.21. C 74.94%, H 12.58%, O 12.48%. $CH_3(CH_2)_5COCH_3$.

Liquid; apple odor; camphor taste. d$_4^{20}$ 0.820. mp −16°. bp 172-173°. n_D^{20} 1.41512. Insol in water. Miscible with alc, ether.

4712. 4-Hexylresorcinol. [136-77-6] 4-Hexyl-1,3-benzenediol; 4-hexyl-1,3-dihydroxybenzene; ST-37; Ascaryl; Caprokol; Crystoids; Gelovermin; Sucrets; Worm-Agen. $C_{12}H_{18}O_2$; mol wt 194.27. C 74.19%, H 9.34%, O 16.47%. Prepd by reduction of hexanoylresorcinol with zinc amalgam + dil HCl: Dohme *et al., J. Am. Chem. Soc.* **48,** 1688 (1926); Twiss, *ibid.* 2206; **DE 488419** and **DE 489117** (both 1929 to Sharp & Dohme). Toxicity: Lamson *et al., J. Pharmacol. Exp. Ther.* **53,** 198 (1935).

Pale yellow, heavy liq becoming solid on standing at room temp. Needles from benzene or petr ether, mp 67.5-69°; bp$_{6-7}$ 178-180°; bp$_{13-14}$ 198-200°; bp$_{760}$ 333-335°. Pungent odor; sharp astringent taste. Sol in ether, chloroform, acetone, alcohol, vegetable oils; slightly sol in petr ether; sol in about 2000 parts water. LD$_{50}$ orally in rats: 550 mg/kg (Lamson).

Caution: Concd solns can cause irritation of skin, mucous membranes: *Clinical Toxicology of Commercial Products*, R. E. Gosselin *et al.,* Eds. (Williams & Wilkins, Baltimore, 5th ed., 1984) Section II, p 190.

THERAP CAT: Anthelmintic (Nematodes). Antiseptic (topical).

THERAP CAT (VET): Anthelmintic.

4713. Hexythiazox. [78587-05-0] (4*R*,5*R*)-*rel*-5-(4-Chlorophenyl)-*N*-cyclohexyl-4-methyl-2-oxo-3-thiazolidinecarboxamide; *trans*-4-methyl-5-(4-chlorophenyl)-3-cyclohexylcarbamoyl-2-thiazolidone; HTZ; NA-73; DPX-Y5893-9; Nissorun; Acariflor; Cesar; Savey; Zeldox. $C_{17}H_{21}ClN_2O_2S$; mol wt 352.88. C 57.86%, H 6.00%, Cl 10.05%, N 7.94%, O 9.07%, S 9.09%. Prepn: I. Iwataki *et al.,* **DE 3037105**; *eidem,* **US 4442116** (1981, 1984 to Nippon Soda). Miticidal activity: M. A. Hoy, Y.- L. Ouyang, *J. Econ. Entomol.* **79,** 1377 (1986); C. Welty *et al., ibid.* **81,** 586 (1988). Residue determn in crops: M. Tokieda *et al., J. Pestic. Sci.* **12,** 711 (1987), *C.A.* **108,** 162770b (1988). Brief description of physical properties, toxicity and efficacy: Nippon Soda Co., Ltd., *Jpn. Pestic. Inf.* **44,** 21 (1984).

White odorless crystals, mp 105.5°. Vapor pressure at 20°: 2.54 × 10^{-8} mm Hg. Soly at 20° (g/100 ml): acetone 16, chloroform 137.9, methanol 2.06, *n*-hexane 0.39, xylene 36.2, acetonitrile 2.86; water 0.5 ppm. LD$_{50}$ in male, female mice, male, female rats (mg/kg): all >5000 orally; all >5000 dermally (Nippon Soda Co.).

USE: Acaricide.

4714. HFC-134a. [811-97-2] 1,1,1,2-Tetrafluoroethane; 1,-2,2,2-tetrafluoroethane; refrigerant 134a; R134a; HFA-134a. C_2-H_2F_4; mol wt 102.03. C 23.54%, H 1.98%, F 74.48%. F_3CCH_2F. Environmentally acceptable alternative to chlorofluorocarbons used as a refrigerant, solvent and propellant. Overview of commercial development: L. E. Manzer, *Catal. Today* **13,** 13-22 (1992). General description: D. Mayer *et al., Jt. Assess. Commod. Chem.* **1995,** 1-36. Dielectric data: Y. Tanaka *et al., Fluid Phase Equilib.* **80,** 107 (1992); pressure-volume data: M.-S. Zhu *et al., ibid.* 149. Density measurements of HFC-134a and its mixtures: P. S. Fialho *et al., High Temp. - High Pressures* **27/28,** 569 (1996). Chemistry of atmospheric degradation: J. Sehested, T. J. Wallington, *Environ. Sci. Technol.* **27,** 146 (1993). Catalytic synthesis and kinetics: F. H. Ribeiro *et al., Catal. Lett.* **45,** 149 (1997). Review of catalytic synthesis: L. E. Manzer, V. N. M. Rao, *Adv. Catal.* **39,** 329-350 (1993). Review of toxicology: D. J. Alexander, S. E. Libretto, *Hum. Exp. Toxicol.* **14,** 715-720 (1995). Review of viscosity measurements: C. M. B. Oliveira, W. A. Wakeham, *High Temp. - High Pressures* **27/28,** 91-98 (1996). Review of use as refrigerant: E. Preisegger, R. Henrici, *Int. J. Refrig.* **15,** 326-331 (1992); as blowing agent: R. E. Morgan *et al., UTECH Asia '97, Int. Polyurethanes Conf. Exhib. Asia-Pac.* (Crain Communications, London, UK, 1997) pp 1-8.

Non-flammable, colorless gas with a faint ethereal odor. bp$_{1atm}$ −26.15°. mp −101°. Critical temp: 101.05°. Critical pressure: 40.64 atm. Critical density: 0.508 g/cm^3. d$_{25}$ 1.202. log P (octanol/water): 1.06. Heat of vaporization (0°): 47.52 cal/g. Viscosity (25°): 0.204 cP. Surface tension (25°): 8.466 dynes/cm. LC$_{50}$ (15 min) in rats: 3400000 mg/m^3 (>800000 ppm); LC$_{50}$ (4 hr) in rats: 2215000 mg/m^3 (>500000 ppm) (Mayer).

USE: Refrigerant, propellant for pharmaceuticals; blowing agent for foams.

Consult the Name Index before using this section.

4715. HHCB. [1222-05-5] 1,3,4,5,6,7,8-Hexahydro-4,6,6,-7,8,8-hexamethylcyclopenta[g]-2-benzopyran; 6-oxa-1,1,2,3,3,8-hexamethyl-2,3,5,6,7,8-hexahydro-1*H*-benz[*f*]-indene; Galaxolide. $C_{18}H_{26}O$; mol wt 258.40. C 83.67%, H 10.14%, O 6.19%. Isochroman musk odorant; scent is primarily due to the (−)-(4*S*,7*R*) and (−)-(4*S*,7*S*) isomers. Prepn: L. G. Heeringa, M. G. J. Beets, **GB 991146**; *eidem*, **US 3360530** (1965, 1967 both to International Flavors & Fragrances). Prepn and olfactory characterization of enantiomers: G. Fráter *et al.*, *Helv. Chim. Acta* **82**, 1656 (1999). Synthesis of olfactorally active stereoisomers: A. Ciappa *et al.*, *Tetrahedron: Asymmetry* **13**, 2193 (2002). HPLC determn: W. Schüssler, L. Nitschke, *Fresenius J. Anal. Chem.* **361**, 220 (1998). Subchronic toxicity study: A. M. Api, R. A. Ford, *Toxicol. Lett.* **111**, 143 (1999).

(4*S*,7*R*)-Form

Colorless crystals from methanol, mp 57-58°. bp$_{0.8}$ 129°. Strong musk odor. n_D^{20} 1.5342. d_4^{20} 1.0054. Crystal density: 1.087 g/cm³.

(−)-(4*S*,7*R*)-Form. [252332-95-9] Colorless crystals from methanol, mp 78-78.5°. $[\alpha]_D^{24}$ −23.5°; $[\alpha]_{546}^{24}$ −27.3° (c = 5.0 in ethanol). Powerful typical musk odor.

(−)-(4*S*,7*S*)-Form. [172339-62-7] Colorless crystals from hexane, mp 57-58°. $[\alpha]_D^{23}$ −25.1°; $[\alpha]_{546}^{23}$ −29.2° (c = 5.0 in ethanol). Musky odor with dry aspects; slightly less powerful than (−)-(4*S*,7*R*)-form.

(+)-(4*R*,7*S*)-Form. [172339-63-8] Colorless crystals from methanol, mp 77-78°. $[\alpha]_D^{24}$ +24.1°; $[\alpha]_{546}^{24}$ +28.0° (c = 5.2 in ethanol). Weak, musky, uncharacteristic odor.

(+)-(4*R*,7*R*)-Form. [252332-96-0] Colorless crystals from hexane, mp 52-53°. $[\alpha]_D^{23}$ +25.2°; $[\alpha]_{546}^{23}$ +29.3° (c = 5.0 in ethanol). Very weak, mainly fruity odor.

USE: Fragrance ingredient in perfumes, soaps, cosmetics, and detergents.

4716. Hippuric Acid. [495-69-2] *N*-Benzoylglycine; benzoylaminoacetic acid; benzamidoacetic acid. $C_9H_9NO_3$; mol wt 179.17. C 60.33%, H 5.06%, N 7.82%, O 26.79%. C_6H_5-CONHCH$_2$COOH. Present in the urine of herbivorous animals; also in smaller amounts in human urine. Prepd from benzoyl chloride and glycine in NaOH soln: Ingersoll, Babcock, *Org. Synth.* **coll. vol. II**, 328 (1943).

Crystals. mp 187-188°. One gram dissolves in about 250 ml cold water, 1000 ml chloroform, 400 ml ether, 60 ml amyl alcohol; slightly sol in cold, freely in hot alcohol or hot water; also sol in aq soln of sodium phosphate. Practically insol in benzene, carbon disulfide, petr ether.

Ammonium salt. $NH_4C_9H_8NO_3$. Crystals. Freely sol in water; sol in alcohol.

Potassium salt monohydrate. $KC_9H_{10}NO_4.H_2O$. Cryst powder. Very sol in water; sol in alcohol.

4717. Hirsutic Acid C. [3650-17-7] (1a*R*,2*R*,3a*R*,3b*R*,5*S*,-6a*R*,7a*S*)-Decahydro-2-hydroxy-3a,5-dimethyl-3-methylenecyclopenta[4,5]pentaleno[1,6a-*b*]oxirene-5-carboxylic acid; 6β,6aβ-epoxy-2,3,3aα,3b,4,5,6,6a,7,7aα-decahydro-5β-hydroxy-2β,3bβ-dimethyl-4-methylene-1*H*-cyclopenta[*a*]pentalene-2-carboxylic acid. $C_{15}H_{20}O_4$; mol wt 264.32. C 68.16%, H 7.63%, O 24.21%. Antibiotic metabolite isolated from the fungus *Stereum hirsutum*: Heatley *et al.*, *Br. J. Exp. Pathol.* **28**, 35 (1947). Structure and stereochemistry: Comer *et al.*, *Chem. Commun.* **1965**, 310; Comer, Trotter, *J. Chem. Soc. B* **1966**, 11; Comer *et al.*, *Tetrahedron* **23**, 4761 (1967). Synthesis of (±)-form: Hashimoto *et al.*, *Tetrahedron Lett.* **1974**, 3745; M. Yamazaki *et al.*, *Chem. Lett.* **1981**, 1245. Stereosynthesis: B. M. Trost *et al.*, *J. Am. Chem. Soc.* **101**, 1284 (1979); of (+)-form: M. Shibasaki *et al.*, *Tetrahedron Lett.* **23**, 5311 (1982).

Prisms from ethanol, mp 179-182°. $[\alpha]_D^{23}$ +116° (c = 1.05).

Methyl ester. $C_{16}H_{22}O_4$. Colorless prisms, mp 161-162°. $[\alpha]_D^{20}$ +119° (c = 2.25).

4718. Hirudin. [8001-27-2] Exhirud; Hirudex. Anticoagulant protein extracted from the salivary glands of the medicinal leech, *Hirudo medicinalis* Linn. Hirudin is a single chain polypeptide containing 65 amino acids; mol wt approximately 7000 daltons. Several isoforms have been identified. A specific inhibitor of thrombin, *q.v.*, hirudin does not require the presence of other coagulation factors. Isoln: J. B. Haycraft, *Arch. Exp. Pathol. Pharmakol.* **18**, 209 (1884). Initial characterization: F. Markwardt, *Naturwissenschaften* **42**, 537 (1955). Improved isoln: P. Walsmann, F. Markwardt, *Thromb. Res.* **40**, 563 (1985). Amino acid sequence: T. E. Petersen *et al.* in *Protides of the Biological Fluids* vol. 23, H. Peeters, Ed. (Pergamon Press, London, 1976) pp 145-149. Antithrombin activity: F. Markwardt, *Methods Enzymol.* **19**, 924 (1970). Pharmacokinetics in humans: F. Markwardt *et al.*, *Thromb. Haemostasis* **52**, 160 (1984). Chromogenic assay in plasma: U. Griessbach *et al.*, *Thromb. Res.* **37**, 347 (1985). Series of articles on development, pharmacology, and therapeutic potential of natural and recombinant hirudins: *Semin. Thromb. Hemostasis* **15**, 261-333 (1989). Review of pharmacology and therapeutic potential: P. H. Johnson, *Annu. Rev. Med.* **45**, 165-177 (1994); of therapeutic use in myocardial infarction: U. Zeymer, K.-L. Neuhaus, *Drug Saf.* **12**, 234-239 (1995).

Gray or white flakes or powder. pI 3.9. Sol in water, physiol saline soln, in pyridine. Practically insol in alcohol, ether, acetone, benzene. Deteriorates on storage in sealed ampuls, on exposure to heat and when in soln with dil acids.

Desirudin. [120993-53-5] 63-Desulfohirudin (*Hirudo medicinalis* isoform HV1); ds-hirudin; CGP-39393; Revasc. Identical in amino acid sequence to natural hirudin variant 1 (HV1) except that it lacks a sulfate group on Tyr at residue 63. Production by recombinant DNA technology: M. Liersch *et al.*, **EP 168342** (1986 to Ciba-Geigy); *eidem*, **US 5422249** (1995 to Ciba-Geigy; UCP GenPharma); E. Fortkamp *et al.*, *DNA* **5**, 511 (1986); J. Dodt *et al.*, *FEBS Lett.* **202**, 373 (1986). Physicochemical properties: A. Electricwala *et al.*, *Thromb. Haemostasis* **63**, 499 (1990). Clinical pharmacology: M. Verstraete *et al.*, *J. Am. Coll. Cardiol.* **22**, 1080 (1993). Clinical trial in coronary angioplasty: A. A. van den Bos *et al.*, *Circulation* **88**, 2058 (1993); in acute coronary syndromes: E. J. Topol *et al.*, *N. Engl. J. Med.* **335**, 775 (1996).

Lepirudin. [138068-37-8] 1-L-Leucine-2-L-threonine-63-desulfohirudin (*Hirudo medicinalis* isoform HV1); HBW-023; Refludan. Peptide of 65 amino acids produced by recombinant DNA technology. Prepn: P. Crause *et al.*, **EP 324712**; *eidem*, **US 5180668** (1989, 1993 both to Hoechst AG). Clinical pharmacology: H. J. Roethig *et al.*, *Int. Congr. Ser. - Excerpta Med.* **944**, 227 (1991). Clinical trial as adjunctive therapy with TPA: U. Zeymer *et al.*, *Am. J. Cardiol.* **76**, 997 (1995); in heparin-induced thrombocytopenia: F. Schiele *et al.*, *Am. J. Hematol.* **50**, 20 (1995).

THERAP CAT: Antithrombotic.

4719. Histamine. [51-45-6] 1*H*-Imidazole-4-ethanamine; 2-(4-imidazolyl)ethylamine; 4-imidazoleethylamine; 5-imidazoleethylamine; β-aminoethylimidazole; β-aminoethylglyoxaline. $C_5H_9N_3$; mol wt 111.15. C 54.03%, H 8.16%, N 37.80%. Biogenic amine widely distributed in nature; decarboxylation product of histidine, *q.v.* Present in most mammalian tissues; primarily stored in mast cells and basophils. Exhibits multiple biological effects through at least 3 specific receptors. Induces bronchoconstriction and vasodilation; stimulates gastric acid secretion; and acts as a neurotransmitter. Synthesis: A. Windaus, W. Vogt, *Ber.* **40**, 3691 (1907); F. L. Pyman, *J. Chem. Soc.* **101**, 530 (1912). Identification as vasodilator: H. H. Dale, P. P. Laidlaw, *J. Physiol.* **41**, 318 (1910). Toxicity data: K. Nagai *et al.*, *Arzneim.-Forsch.* **17**, 1575 (1967). Diagnostic use in pheochromocytoma: T. Nakai, R. Yamada, *J. Clin. Endocrinol. Metab.* **57**, 19 (1983); in airway responsiveness:

A. James, G. Ryan, *Respirology* **2**, 97 (1997). Clinical efficacy in combination with interleukin-2, *q.v.*, in treatment of acute myelogenous leukemia: K. Hellstrand *et al.*, *Leuk. Lymphoma* **27**, 429 (1997). Mechanism of antineoplastic activity: *eidem, Acta Oncol.* **37**, 347 (1998). Review of assay methods for determn in plasma: E. Oosting *et al.*, *Clin. Exp. Allergy* **20**, 349-357 (1990). Review of role in allergic disease: M. V. White, *J. Allergy Clin. Immunol.* **86**, 599-605 (1990); in gastric acid secretion: K. J. Obrink, *Scand. J. Gastroenterol.* **26**, Suppl. 180, 4-8 (1991); in homeostatic energy metabolism: T. Sakata *et al.*, *Nutrition* **13**, 403-411 (1997). Review of pharmacology and classification of receptors: S. J. Hill *et al.*, *Pharmacol. Rev.* **49**, 253-278 (1997).

Deliquescent needles from chloroform, mp 83-84°. bp$_{18}$ 209-210°. Freely sol in water, alcohol, hot chloroform. Practically insol in ether. LD$_{50}$ i.p. in mice: 2020 mg/kg (Nagai).

Dihydrochloride. [56-92-8] Maxamine. $C_5H_9N_3$.2HCl; mol wt 184.07. Prisms from ethanol, mp 244-246°. Freely sol in water, methanol; sol in ethanol.

Phosphate. [51-74-1] $C_5H_9N_3$.2H$_3$PO$_4$. Clear, colorless prisms from water, mp 132-133°. Readily sol in hot water.

THERAP CAT: Antineoplastic (immunomodulator); diagnostic aid (gastric secretion, pheochromocytoma, bronchial hyperreactivity).

4720. Histidine. [71-00-1] L-Histidine; His; H; *(S)*-α-amino-1*H*-imidazole-4-propanoic acid; α-amino-4(or 5)-imidazolepropionic acid; glyoxaline-5-alanine. $C_6H_9N_3O_2$; mol wt 155.15. C 46.45%, H 5.85%, N 27.08%, O 20.62%. Essential amino acid for human development; precursor to histamine and a component of carnosine, *q.v.* Independently isolated in 1896 by both A. Kossel and S. G. Hedin, *Zeit. Physiol.* **22**, 176, 191 (1896). Early chemistry and biochemistry: *Amino Acids and Proteins*, D. M. Greenberg, Ed. (Charles C. Thomas, Springfield, IL, 1951) 950 pp., *passim*; J. P. Greenstein, M. Winitz, *Chemistry of the Amino Acids* **vols 1-3** (John Wiley and Sons, Inc., New York, 1961) pp. 1971-1995, *passim*. NMR spectra: D. H. Sachs *et al.*, *J. Biol. Chem.* **246**, 6576 (1971). HPLC determn in dipeptides: E. Kasziba *et al.*, *J. Chromatogr.* **432**, 315 (1988). Often found at the active site of proteins: W. T. Morgan *et al.*, *J. Biol. Chem.* **268**, 6256 (1993); J.-W. P. Boots *et al.*, *Biochim. Biophys. Acta* **1248**, 27 (1995). Role in proton translocation – a model: J. E. Morgan *et al.*, *J. Bioenerg. Biomembr.* **26**, 599 (1994). Review of metabolism: F. B. Stifel, R. H. Herman, *Am. J. Clin. Nutr.* **24**, 207-217 (1971). Review of role in nutrition: *eidem, ibid.* **25**, 182-185 (1972); L. P. Mercer *et al.*, *Nutrition* **6**, 273-277 (1990).

Sweet needles or plates, dec 287° (softens at 277°). $[\alpha]_D^{20}$ −10.9° (c = 0.77 in 0.5*N* NaOH); $[\alpha]_D^{25}$ −38.95° (c = 0.75 to 3.77); $[\alpha]_D^{25}$ +13.34° (c = 1.00-4.05 in 6.1*N* HCl). pK$_1$ 1.82; pK$_2$ 6.00; pK$_3$ 9.17. Soly in water at 25°: 41.9 g/l. Insol in common neutral solvents except water.

Monohydrochloride. Ecristidine; Laristine; Larostidin; Plexamine. $C_6H_9N_3O_2$.HCl; mol wt 191.62. Rhombic crystals, dec 251-252° (also forms a monohydrate, mp 80°, anhydrous, mp at 140°). $[\alpha]_D^{26}$ +8.0° (c = 2 in 3 mols HCl). Fairly sol in water. Insol in alcohol, ether.

DL-Form. Quadrilateral plates or tetragonal prisms, dec 285°. Sol in water.

4721. Histones. Small chromosomal proteins (mol wt 12,000-20,000) possessing an open, unfolded structure, attached to DNA of cell nuclei by ionic linkages. First isolated from bird erythrocytes: Kossel, *Z. Physiol. Chem.* **8**, 511 (1884). Prepd also from cell nuclei of calf thymus, spleen, and liver, liver and spleen of leukemic rats, bovine spermatozoa: Hnilica, *Biochem. J.*

82, 123 (1962); Berry, Mayer, *Exp. Cell Res.* **20**, 116 (1960). Classification is based on relative amounts of lysine and arginine: Histone I is very rich in lysine and has several subtypes; histone II, moderately rich in lysine with two subtypes; histone III, moderately rich in arginine, contains cysteine; histone IV, very rich in arginine and in glycine. Histones of the same type obtained from various plant and animal sources are very similar in amino acid sequence. Amino acid composition of animal histones: Hnilica *et al.*, *Biochim. Biophys. Acta* **124**, 109 (1966); of plant histones and similarity of plant and animal histones: Fambrough, Bonner, *Biochemistry* **5**, 2563 (1966). Complete amino acid sequence of calf thymus histone IV: DeLange *et al.*, *J. Biol. Chem.* **244**, 319 (1969); Ogawa *et al.*, *ibid.* 4387; of histone III: DeLange *et al.*, *Proc. Natl. Acad. Sci. USA* **69**, 882 (1972); *eidem, J. Biol. Chem.* **248**, 3261 (1973); Hooper *et al., ibid.* 3275; of the two subtypes of histone II: Iwai *et al., Nature* **226**, 1056 (1970); Yeoman *et al.*, *J. Biol. Chem.* **247**, 6018 (1972). Toxicity study: Starbuck *et al.*, *Arch. Int. Pharmacodyn. Ther.* **165**, 374 (1967). Review of structural studies: DeLange, *Acc. Chem. Res.* **5**, 368 (1972). Review of histone in the chromosome structure: Bradbury *et al.*, *Ann. N.Y. Acad. Sci.* **222**, 266 (1973). Review of biological functions: Binner, Garrard, *Life Sci.* **14**, 209 (1974). General review: Butler *et al.*, *Prog. Biophys. Mol. Biol.* **18**, 211 (1968); R. J. DeLange, E. L. Smith in *Proteins* **vol. 4**, H. Neurath, R. L. Hill, Eds. (Academic, New York, 3rd ed., 1979) pp 134-243.

Histones are susceptible to enzymatic cleavage; sol in an Hg$_2$-SO$_4$/H$_2$SO$_4$ medium. Infrared spectra: de Lozé, *Compt. Rend.* **246**, 417 (1958). LD$_{50}$ i.v. in rats of lysine-rich, slightly lysine-rich, and arginine-rich histones: 90, 60-70, 60 mg/kg (Starbuck).

4722. Histrelin. [76712-82-8] 6-[1-(Phenylmethyl)-D-histidine]-9-(*N*-ethyl-L-prolinamide)-10-deglycinamide luteinizing hormone-releasing factor (pig); 5-oxo-L-prolyl-L-histidyl-L-tryptophyl-L-seryl-L-tyrosyl-N^7-benzyl-D-histidyl-L-leucyl-L-arginyl-*N*-ethyl-L-prolinamide; L-pyroglutamyl-L-histidyl-L-tryptophyl-L-seryl-L-tyrosyl-D-N^{im}-benzyl-histidyl-L-leucyl-L-arginyl-L-proline ethylamide; [(im-Bzl)-D-His^6,Pro^9-NEt]-gonadotropin-releasing hormone; ORF-17070; RWJ-17070. $C_{66}H_{86}N_{18}O_{12}$; mol wt 1323.50. C 59.89%, H 6.55%, N 19.05%, O 14.51%. Synthetic nonapeptide agonist analog of LH-RH, *q.v.* Prepn: J. E. F. Rivier, W. W. Vale, Jr., **EP 21620**; *eidem*, **US 4244946** (both 1981 to Salk Inst.). *See also:* J. E. Rivier, W. W. Vale, *Life Sci.* **23**, 869 (1978). Pharmacology: Y.-Q. Cao *et al.*, *Int. J. Androl.* **5**, 158 (1982); J. W. Gunnet *et al.*, *J. Endocrinol.* **131**, 211 (1991). HPLC purification: J. Rivier *et al.*, *J. Chromatogr.* **288**, 303 (1984). Amino acid sequence: C. J. Shaw, M. L. Cotter, *Chromatographia* **21**, 197 (1986). Clinical evaluations in polycystic ovarian disease: K. Steingold *et al.*, *J. Clin. Endocrinol. Metab.* **65**, 773 (1987); in endometriosis: *idem et al.*, *Obstet. Gynecol.* **69**, 403 (1987); in porphyria: K. E. Anderson *et al.*, *Arch. Int. Med.* **150**, 1469 (1990); in PMS: J. F. Mortola *et al.*, *J. Clin. Endocrinol. Metab.* **72**, 252A (1991). Review of pharmacology and therapeutic use in central precocious puberty: L. B. Barradell, D. McTavish, *Drugs* **45**, 570-588 (1993).

5-oxoPro–His–Trp–Ser–Tyr–...–Leu–Arg–ProNHCH$_2$CH$_3$

$[\alpha]_D^{20}$ −33.9° (c = 1 in acetic acid).

Acetate. Supprelin. $C_{66}H_{86}N_{18}O_{12}$.xC$_2$H$_4$O$_2$.yH$_2$O

THERAP CAT: Treatment of central precocious puberty.

4723. Histrionicotoxin. [34272-51-0] (2*S*,6*R*,7*S*,8*S*)-7-(1*Z*)-1-Buten-3-ynyl-2-(2*Z*)-2-penten-4-ynyl-1-azaspiro[5.5]undecan-8-ol; HTX; (−)-HTX 1; (−)-histrionicotoxin. $C_{19}H_{25}NO$; mol wt 283.41. C 80.52%, H 8.89%, N 4.94%, O 5.65%. One of a family of piperidine alkaloids isolated from the skin of the poison arrow frog *Dendrobates histrionicus*. Noncompetitive inhibitor of nicotinic acetylcholine receptors characterized by an unusual spirocyclic *cis*-enyne structure. Virtually nontoxic, the family was originally misnamed because of the source. Isoln: J. W. Daly *et al.*, *Proc. Natl. Acad. Sci. USA* **68**, 1870 (1971). Isoforms: *idem et al.*,

Helv. Chim. Acta **60,** 1128 (1977). Acetylcholine antagonism: M. Glavinovic *et al., Can. J. Physiol. Pharmacol.* **52,** 1220 (1974); as allosteric inhibitor: S. M. Sine, P. Taylor, *J. Biol. Chem.* **257,** 8106 (1982). Total synthesis: S. C. Carey *et al., Tetrahedron Lett.* **26,** 5887 (1985); stereospecific synthesis: G. M. Williams *et al., J. Am. Chem. Soc.* **121,** 4900 (1999). *Review:* J. W. Daly, *J. Nat. Prod.* **61,** 162-172 (1997).

Viscous oil; on storage at $-15°C$ crystals slowly form, mp 75-76°. uv max: 224 nm (ε 15500). $[\alpha]_D^{20}$ $-112°$ (c = 0.34 in ethanol).

USE: Biochemical probe for neuromuscular transmission.

4724. HLö-7. [120103-35-7] 1-[[[4-(Aminocarbonyl)pyridinio]methoxy]methyl]-2,4-bis[(hydroxyimino)methyl]pyridinium diiodide; HLoe-7. $C_{15}H_{17}I_2N_5O_4$; mol wt 585.14. C 30.79%, H 2.93%, I 43.38%, N 11.97%, O 10.94%. Bisquaternary Hagedorn oxime; acetylcholinesterase reactivator. *In vitro* reactivation of tabun and soman acetylcholinesterase inhibition: L. P. A. de Jong *et al., Biochem. Pharmacol.* **38,** 633 (1989). Stability and decomposition: P. Eyer *et al., Arch. Toxicol.* **63,** 59 (1989). Synthesis, pharmacology and toxicity: *eidem, ibid.* **66,** 603 (1992). Pharmacokinetics: U. Spöhrer *et al., ibid.* **68,** 480 (1994). Efficacy in nerve agent poisoning: B. P. C. Melchers *et al., Pharmacol. Biochem. Behav.* **49,** 781 (1994). MS determn: P. A. D'Agostino *et al., Rapid Commun. Mass Spectrom.* **10,** 805 (1996). Comparative reactivation studies in human acetylcholinesterase inhibition: F. Worek *et al., Biochem. Pharmacol.* **68,** 2237 (2004).

Crystals from hot water, mp 160° (dec). Soly in water: 20 mg/ml. Aq solns are unstable and liberate iodine even when protected from light. uv max (pH 2): 298, 252, 224 nm (log ε 4.20, 4.20, 4.15); (pH 11) 368 nm (log ε 4.35). pKa_1 7.04, pKa_2 8.52. LD_{50} i.m. in female mice: 744 μmol/kg (Eyer, 1992).

Dimethanesulfonate. [145613-73-6] $C_{15}H_{17}N_5O_4.2CH_3O_3S$; mol wt 521.52. Crystals from warm methanol, 173-174 (dec). pH (1% aq soln) ~4. Soly in water: 0.68 g/ml. LD_{50} i.m. in female mice: 799 μmol/kg (Eyer, 1992).

THERAP CAT: Antidote (organophosphate poisoning).

4725. HMPA. [680-31-9] Hexamethylphosphoric triamide; hexamethylphosphoramide; hexametapol; hempa; HMPT; ENT-50882. $C_6H_{18}N_3OP$; mol wt 179.20. C 40.21%, H 10.12%, N 23.45%, O 8.93%, P 17.28%. $[(CH_3)_2N]_3PO$. Prepn: Saul, Godfrey, US 2752392 (1956 to Monsanto); Godfrey, US 2852550 (1958 to Monsanto); Miller, Lomonte, US 3084190 (1963 to Dow); Vetter, Noeth, *Ber.* **96,** 1308 (1963). Solvation effects: J. E. Dubois, A. Bienvenue, *Tetrahedron Lett.* **1966,** 1809. Toxicity studies: T. B. Gaines, *Toxicol. Appl. Pharmacol.* **14,** 515 (1969). Carcinogenicity studies: J. A. Zapp, *Science* **190,** 422 (1975); *IARC Monographs* **15,** 211 (1977). *Review:* H. Normant, *Angew. Chem. Int. Ed.* **6,** 1047 (1967).

Colorless liquid, completely miscible with water. mp 7.20°. bp_{760} 235°. bp_{11} 105-107°, bp_6 97-99°; $bp_{2.5}$ 78°. n_D^{21} 1.4572. d_{20} 1.03. Dipole moment at 25°: 5.37D. LD_{50} in male, female rats (mg/kg): 2650, 3360 orally (Gaines).

Caution: Potential symptoms of overexposure are irritation of eyes, skin, respiratory system; dyspnea; abdominal pain. *See NIOSH Pocket Guide to Chemical Hazards* (DHHS/NIOSH 97-140, 1997) p 162. This substance is reasonably anticipated to be

a human carcinogen: *Report on Carcinogens, Eleventh Edition* (PB2005-104914, 2004) p III-141.

USE: Aprotic solvent in organic synthesis. Solvent for polymers, gases; polymerization catalyst; thermal stabilizer in polystyrene; protective additive for polyvinyl and polyolefin resins against uv light degradation. De-icing additive for jet fuels. Chemosterilant for a number of insect pests; chemical mutagen.

4726. HNE. [18286-49-2] (*E*-form); [29343-52-0] (undefined). (2*E*)-4-Hydroxy-2-nonenal; 4-HNE. $C_9H_{16}O_2$; mol wt 156.22. C 69.19%, H 10.32%, O 20.48%. Toxic aldehyde formed during lipid peroxidation in response to oxidative stress. Reacts primarily with the amino acids His or Lys to form an adduct which may alter protein function. Increased levels of the HNE-adduct are seen in Alzheimer's disease and after ozone exposure. Identification of cytotoxic activity of lipid oxidative products: E. Schauenstein, H. Esterbauer, *Monatsh. Chem.* **94,** 164 (1963). Prepn: H. Esterbauer, W. Weger, *ibid.* **98,** 1994 (1967). Synthesis: H. W. Gardner *et al., Lipids* **27,** 686 (1992). Quantitative analysis by uv, GC/MS, HPLC: M. Kinter in *Free Radicals* N. A. Punchard, F. J. Kelly, Eds. (IRL Press, Oxford, UK, 1996) pp 133-145. Cytotoxicity: A. Benedetti *et al., Biochim. Biophys. Acta* **620,** 281 (1980). Structural definition of adduct sites: D. V. Nadkarni, L. M. Sayre, *Chem. Res. Toxicol.* **8,** 284 (1995); by MS: M. S. Bolgar, S. J. Gaskell, *Anal. Chem.* **68,** 2325 (1996). Ozone-induced formation: A. Kirichenko *et al., Toxicol. Appl. Pharmacol.* **141,** 416 (1996). Role in Alzheimer's disease: R. J. Mark *et al., J. Neurochem.* **68,** 255 (1997); L. M. Sayre *et al., ibid.* 2092.

$bp_{0.4 \text{ torr}}$ 84-87°. n_D 1.471. d_4^{20} 0.944. uv max (water): 447 nm; (ethanol) 452.5 nm; (hexane) 465 nm (ε 13750, 13100, 14400). Soly at 20° (g/l): water 6.6. Partition coefficient K_{20} (H_2O/$CHCl_3$): 0.04.

4727. Holmium. [7440-60-0] Ho; at. wt 164.93032; at. no. 67; valence 3. A rare earth metal of the yttrium group; member of the lanthanide series. Naturally occurring isotope (mass number): 165; known artificial radioactive isotopes: 146-164; 166-170. Estimated abundance in earth's crust 1.15-1.4 ppm; occurs in rare earth minerals. Discovered by Soret in 1878 and independently by Cleve in 1879: Cleve, *Compt. Rend.* **89,** 478, 708 (1879). Purification of salts: Holmberg, *Z. Anorg. Chem.* **71,** 226 (1911). Separation from erbium: Driggs, Hopkins, *J. Am. Chem. Soc.* **47,** 363 (1925); from other rare earths: Spedding *et al., ibid.* **69,** 2812 (1947); **76,** 2557 (1954). Absorption spectrum: Severin, *Z. Phys.* **125,** 455 (1949). Analysis by means of emission spectra: Smith, Wiggins, *Analyst* **74,** 95 (1949). Toxicity study: Haley *et al., Toxicol. Appl. Pharmacol.* **8,** 37 (1966). Reviews of prepn, properties and compds: *The Rare Earths,* F. H. Spedding, A. H. Daane, Eds. (Krieger, Huntington, N.Y., 1971, reprint of 1961 ed.) 641 pp; Hulet, Bode, "Separation Chemistry of the Lanthanides and Transplutonium Actinides" in *MTP Int. Rev. Sci.: Inorg. Chem., Ser. One* vol. 7, K. W. Bagnall, Ed. (University Park Press, Baltimore, 1972) pp 1-45; Moeller, "The Lanthanides" in *Comprehensive Inorganic Chemistry* vol. 4, J. C. Bailar, Jr. *et al.,* Eds. (Pergamon Press, Oxford, 1973) pp 1-101; F. H. Spedding in *Kirk-Othmer Encyclopedia of Chemical Technology* vol. 19, (John Wiley & Sons, New York, 3rd ed., 1982) pp 833-854; *Chemistry of the Elements,* N. N. Greenwood, A. Earnshaw, Eds. (Pergamon Press, New York, 1984) pp 1423-1449. Brief review of properties: G. T. Seaborg, *Radiochim. Acta* **61,** 115-122 (1993).

Metal; hexagonal close-packed crystals. d 8.7947. mp 1474°. bp 2700°. Heat of fusion: 16.874 kJ/mol. Heat of sublimation (25°): 300.8 kJ/mol. Forms yellow-green salts.

Oxide. Holmia. Ho_2O_3. Yellow solid. Obtained by igniting the hydroxide, nitrate, sulfate, oxalate. Dissolves in acids with formation of a yellow salt.

Chloride. $HoCl_3$. Bright yellow, crystalline solid, mp 718°. Formed by heating the hydrated salt in a current of hydrogen chloride at 350°. LD_{50} in mice: 560 mg/kg i.p.; 7.2 g/kg orally (Haley).

Bromide. $HoBr_3$. mp 914°.

Iodide. HoI₃. Obtained by passing hydrogen iodide over the anhydr chloride at 600°: Jantsch *et al., Z. Anorg. Chem.* **207**, 353 (1932). Light-yellow solid. mp 1010 ±10°.

4728. Holomycin. [488-04-0] *N*-(4,5-Dihydro-5-oxo-1,2-dithiolo[4,3-*b*]pyrrol-6-yl)acetamide; *N*-(4,5-dihydro-5-oxo-1,2-dithiolo[4,3-*b*]pyrrol-6-yl)-*N*-methylformamide; 6-acetamido-1,2-dithiolo[4,3-*b*]pyrrol-5(4*H*)-one; *N*-demethylthiolutin. $C_7H_6N_2$-O_2S_2; mol wt 214.26. C 39.24%, H 2.82%, N 13.07%, O 14.93%, S 29.93%. Antibiotic substance produced by a strain of *Streptomyces griseus* (Krainski) Waksman et Henrici. Isoln and structure: Ettlinger *et al., Helv. Chim. Acta* **42**, 563 (1959). Crystal structure: Jensen, *J. Antibiot.* **22**, 231 (1969). Activity: Von Daehne *et al., ibid.* 233. Manuf process: Gaumann *et al.,* **US 3014922** (1961 to Ciba). Total synthesis: Schmidt, Geiger, *Ann.* **664**, 168 (1963); Büchi, Lukas, *J. Am. Chem. Soc.* **86**, 5654 (1964); Hagio, Yoneda, *Bull. Chem. Soc. Jpn.* **47**, 1484 (1974); J. E. Ellis *et al., J. Org. Chem.* **42**, 2891 (1977).

Orange-yellow flakes from methanol + ethyl acetate, dec 268-270. uv max: 245, 302, 290 nm (log ε 3.78, 3.51, 4.05). LD₅₀ i.v. in mice: 5-10 mg/kg (Von Daehne).

4729. Homarine. [445-30-7] 2-Carboxy-1-methylpyridinium inner salt; 1-methyl-2-pyridinium carboxylate; picolinic acid *N*-methylbetaine; *N*-methylpicolinic acid. $C_7H_7NO_2$; mol wt 137.14. C 61.31%, H 5.14%, N 10.21%, O 23.33%. Quaternary ammonium base occurring in tissues of marine animals such as sea urchin, *Arabacia pustulosa*, jellyfish, *Velella spirans*, lugworm, *Arenicola marina*. Isoln: Hoppe-Seyler, *Z. Physiol. Chem.* **222**, 105 (1933). Prepn: Kosower, Patton, *J. Org. Chem.* **26**, 1318 (1961); Quast, Schmitt, *Ann.* **732**, 64 (1970). Review of distribution and function in animals: Brodzicki, *Kosmos (Warsaw)* **16A**, 431-438 (1967), *C.A.* **68**, 18617v (1968).

Crystals from methanol. Does not have a melting point, slowly carbonizes when heated. Absorption spectrum: Gasteiger *et al., Ann. N.Y. Acad. Sci.* **90**, 624 (1962).

Hydrochloride. $C_7H_7NO_2$.HCl. Fine needles, dec 170-175°. Freely sol in water, less sol in methanol and ethanol.

4730. Homatropine. [87-00-3] *endo*-(±)-α-Hydroxybenzeneacetic acid 8-methyl-8-azabicyclo[3.2.1]oct-3-yl ester; 1α*H*,-5α*H*-tropan-3α-ol mandelate; mandelyltropeine; tropine mandelate. $C_{16}H_{21}NO_3$; mol wt 275.34. C 69.79%, H 7.69%, N 5.09%, O 17.43%. Ophthalmic anticholinergic. Prepd from mandelic acid and tropine: Ladenburg, *Ann.* **217**, 82 (1883); Chemnitius, *J. Prakt. Chem.* **117**, 142 (1927). Prepn of D(−)- and L(+)-forms: Werner, Miltenberger, *Ann.* **631**, 163 (1960). Comprehensive description: F. J. Muhtadi *et al., Anal. Profiles Drug Subs.* **16**, 245-290 (1987). Toxicity: R. L. Cahen, K. Tvede, *J. Pharmacol. Exp. Ther.* **105**, 166 (1952).

DL-Form. Prisms from ether, mp 99-100°. *Poisonous!* Hygroscopic, but only slightly sol in water; sol in alcohol, benzene, chloroform, ether, acetone, dil acids.

DL-Hydrobromide. [51-56-9] Homatrisol; Bufopto Homatrocel. $C_{16}H_{21}NO_3$.HBr; mol wt 356.25. Orthorhombic, bipyramidal prisms from water, mp ~212° (partial decompn). *Poisonous!* One gram dissolves in 6 ml water, 40 ml alcohol (12 ml at 60°), 420 ml chloroform. Insol in ether. pH (1% aq soln): 5.4.

DL-Hydrochloride. $C_{16}H_{21}NO_3$.HCl. Prisms from water, mp 217-220° (dec). *Poisonous!* Freely sol in water, alcohol. pH (1% aq soln): 5.4.

DL-Methylbromide. [80-49-9] Arkitropin; Homapin; Malcotran; Mesopin; Novatrin; Novatropine; Sethyl. $C_{16}H_{21}NO_3$.CH₃-Br; mol wt 370.28. Minute needles from alc + ether, mp 191-192° (slight dec). *Poisonous!* Freely sol in water, dil alc; slightly sol in abs alc. Insol in ether. pH (1% aq soln) 5.9; pH (10% aq soln) 4.5. LD₅₀ in mice (mg/kg): 1400 orally, 60 i.p. (Cahen, Tvede).

THERAP CAT: Mydriatic.

4731. Homidium. [3546-21-2] 3,8-Diamino-5-ethyl-6-phenylphenanthridinium; 2,7-diamino-9-phenyl-10-ethylphenanthridinium; 2,7-diamino-10-ethyl-9-phenylphenanthridinium; ethidium; RD-1572; Novidium; Babidium. $[C_{21}H_{20}N_3]^+$. Prepn: T. I. Watkins, *J. Chem. Soc.* **1952**, 3059; Short *et al.,* **US 2662082** (1953 to Boots Pure Drug). uv spectrum: B. Hudson, R. Jacobs, *Biopolymers* **14**, 1309 (1975). Inhibition of DNA synthesis: B. A. Newton, *J. Gen. Microbiol.* **17**, 718 (1957); of DNA polymerase: W. H. Elliott, *Biochem. J.* **86**, 562 (1963). Intercalation of double-stranded DNA: M. J. Waring, *J. Mol. Biol.* **13**, 269 (1965); J.-B. LePecq, C. Paoletti, *ibid.* **27**, 87 (1967). Mutagenicity studies: J. T. MacGregor, I. J. Johnson, *Mutat. Res.* **48**, 103 (1977); G. S. Probst *et al., Environ. Mutagen.* **3**, 11 (1981). Review of interactions with nucleic acids: J.-B. LePecq in *Methods of Biochemical Analysis* **vol. 20**, D. Glick, Ed. (Wiley-Interscience, New York, 1971) pp 41-86; M. Waring in *Antibiotics* **vol. 3**, J. W. Corcoran, F. E. Hahn, Eds. (Springer-Verlag, New York, 1975) pp 141-165.

Bromide. [1239-45-8] Dromilac. $C_{21}H_{20}BrN_3$; mol wt 394.31. Bitter tasting dark red crystals from alc, mp 238-240°. uv max in water: 210, 285, 316, 343 nm (ε 200-500, 5000-10000, 50000, 40000). Sol in 20 parts water and 750 parts chloroform at 20°.

Chloride. $C_{21}H_{20}ClN_3$. Dark red cryst powder. Crystallizes with 1 mol of ethanol. Sol in 5 parts of water at room temp.

USE: In sepn and determn of nucleic acids.

THERAP CAT (VET): Antiprotozoal (Trypanosoma).

4732. Homochelidonine. [476-33-5] 4b,5,6,11b,12,13-Hexahydro-1,2-dimethoxy-12-methyl[1,3]benzodioxolo[5,6-*c*]phenanthridin-5-ol; α-homochelidonine. $C_{21}H_{23}NO_5$; mol wt 369.41. C 68.28%, H 6.28%, N 3.79%, O 21.66%. From root of *Chelidonium majus* L., *Papaveraceae*: Schmidt, Selle, *Arch. Pharm.* **228**, 441 (1890). Structure: Späth, Kuffner, *Ber.* **64**, 1123 (1931); H. W. Bersch, *Arch. Pharm.* **291**, 491 (1958). Total synthesis: I. Ninomiya *et al., Heterocycles* **7**, 137 (1977).

Orthorhombic prisms from ethyl acetate, mp 182°. $[\alpha]_D$ +118° (alc). Very sol in chloroform. Sol in alcohol, acetic acid, ethyl acetate, dil mineral acids; sparingly sol in ether.

4733. Homochlorcyclizine. [848-53-3] 1-[(4-Chlorophenyl)phenylmethyl]hexahydro-4-methyl-1*H*-1,4-diazepine; *N*-(*p*-chlorobenzhydryl)-*N'*-methylhomopiperazine; 1-(4-chlorodiphenylmethyl)-4-methyl-2,3,4,5,6,7-hexahydro-1,4-diazepine; 1-(*p*-chloro-α-phenylbenzyl)-4-methylhomopiperazine; SA-97. $C_{19}H_{23}$-ClN_2; mol wt 314.85. C 72.48%, H 7.36%, Cl 11.26%, N 8.90%. Prepn: Weston, Sommers, **US 2655498** (1953 to Abbott); *eidem, J. Am. Chem. Soc.* **76,** 5805 (1954). HPLC determn of enantiomers in urine: M. Nishikata *et al., J. Chromatogr.* **612,** 239 (1993).

$bp_{0.8}$ 177°. n_D^{25} 1.5804.

Dihydrochloride. [1982-36-1] Curosajin; Homoclomin. C_{19}-$H_{23}ClN_2$.2HCl; mol wt 387.77. Crystals from ethanol, mp 227-228°.

THERAP CAT: Antihistaminic.

4734. Homocysteine. [6027-13-0] 2-Amino-4-mercaptobutyric acid. $C_4H_9NO_2S$; mol wt 135.18. C 35.54%, H 6.71%, N 10.36%, O 23.67%, S 23.72%. $HSCH_2CH_2CH(NH_2)COOH$. A sulfur containing amino acid, produced by the demethylation of methionine and an intermediate in the biosynthesis of cysteine from methionine. Originally obtained from the liver of mammals. Has also been obtained from cystathionine: Binkley, *Methods Enzymol.* **2,** 314 (1955). D-Homocysteine may be prepd from *S*-benzyl-D-homocysteine, while L-homocysteine is best obtained from L-homocystine: du Vigneaud, Brown, *Biochem. Prep.* **5,** 93 (1957); *see also* Patterson, du Vigneaud, *J. Biol. Chem.* **111,** 393 (1935); Riegel, du Vigneaud, *ibid.* **112,** 149 (1935). Origin and biochemical conversions in review by Shapiro, Schlenk, *Adv. Enzymol.* **22,** 264-268 (1960). Use of L-form sodium salt as flavor enhancer similar to monosodium glutamate: Kaneko *et al.,* **US 3259505** (1966 to Ajinomoto Kabushiki Kaisha).

DL-Form. Platelets from dil ethanol, mp 232-233°. pK_1 2.22; pK_2 8.87; pK_3 10.86.

Thiolactone hydrochloride. C_4H_8ClNOS. Crystals from abs ethanol. L-form: $[\alpha]_D^{26}$ +21.5° (c = 1); D-form: $[\alpha]_D^{26}$ −21.5° (c = 1).

4735. Homocystine. [462-10-2] 4,4'-Dithiobis[2-aminobutanoic acid]; 4,4'-dithiobis[2-aminobutyric acid]. $C_8H_{16}N_2O_4$-S_2; mol wt 268.35. C 35.81%, H 6.01%, N 10.44%, O 23.85%, S 23.90%. Synthesis by the "malonate" method: Patterson, du Vigneaud, *J. Biol. Chem.* **111,** 393 (1935); Shiroishi *et al., Rep. Food Res. Inst. (Tokyo)* **5,** 75 (1951); du Vigneaud, Brown, *Biochem. Prep.* **5,** 93 (1957); from 3,6-bis(β-chloroethyl)-2,5-dioxopiperazine: Snyder, Cannon, *J. Am. Chem. Soc.* **66,** 511 (1944).

DL-Form. Platelets from water, dec 263-265°. pK_1 1.59; pK_2 2.54; pK_3 8.52; pK_4 9.44.

L-Form. Crystals, dec 281-284°. $[\alpha]_D^{21}$ −16° (H_2O); $[\alpha]_D^{26}$ +79° (1.0*N* HCl).

D-Form. Crystals, dec 281-284°. $[\alpha]_D^{21}$ +16° (H_2O); $[\alpha]_D^{26}$ −79° (1.0*N* HCl).

4736. Homoeriodictyol. [446-71-9] 2,3-Dihydro-5,7-dihydroxy-2-(4-hydroxy-3-methoxyphenyl)-4*H*-1-benzopyran-4-one;

4',5,7-trihydroxy-3'-methoxyflavanone; eriodictyonone; cyanidanon-3-methyl ether 1625. $C_{16}H_{14}O_6$; mol wt 302.28. C 63.57%, H 4.67%, O 31.76%. From *Eriodictyon californicum* (H. & A.) Torr., and *E. angustifolium* Nutt., *Hydrophyllaceae:* Geissman, *J. Am. Chem. Soc.* **62,** 3258 (1940); Hadley, Gisvold, *J. Am. Pharm. Assoc.* **33,** 275 (1944). Purification: Seka, Prosche, *Monatsh. Chem.* **69,** 284 (1936). Structure: Shinoda, Sato, *J. Pharm. Soc. Jpn.* **49,** 64 (1929), *C.A.* **23,** 4210 (1929). Synthesis: Farooq *et al., Naturwissenschaften* **46,** 76 (1959).

Crystals from 70% acetic acid. Needles by sublimation in high vacuum (0.003-0.005 mm Hg) at 190-195°. Plates from dil alc, dec 225° (after drying *in vacuo* at 110°). $[\alpha]_D^{20}$ −28° (alc). uv max (alc): 290, 328 nm (log ε 2.26, 2.33). Moderately sol in alcohol, acetic acid. Nearly insol in water, ethyl acetate; practically insol in benzene, chloroform.

Triacetate. mp 115-116°.

4737. Homogentisic Acid. [451-13-8] 2,5-Dihydroxybenzeneacetic acid; 2,5-dihydroxyphenylacetic acid; 2,5-dihydroxy-α-toluic acid. $C_8H_8O_4$; mol wt 168.15. C 57.14%, H 4.80%, O 38.06%. An important intermediate in metabolism of tyrosine and phenylalanine, *q.q.v.*. Occurs in plants and in the urine of alkaptonurics: Garrod, *Inborn Errors of Metabolism* (Oxford Medical Publications, London, 1923, and later). Isoln from alkaptonuric urine: Mörner, *Z. Physiol. Chem.* **117,** 85 (1921). Synthesis from 2,5-dihydroxymandelic acid or from 2,5-dihydroxyphenylglyoxylic acid by boiling with fuming HI: Neubauer, Flatow, *ibid.* **52,** 395 (1907). Alternate syntheses: L. DeForrest Abbott, J. D. Smith, *J. Biol. Chem.* **179,** 365 (1949); S. B. Bostock, A. H. Renfrew, *Synthesis* **1978,** 66; J. L. Bloomer, K. M. Damodaran, *ibid.* **1980,** 111. Biosynthesis from tyrosine: Davies *et al., J. Chem. Soc.* **1964,** 3126. Metabolic studies: W. E. Knox, M. LeMay-Knox, *Biochem. J.* **49,** 686 (1951); B. N. LaDu, V. G. Zannoni, *J. Biol. Chem.* **217,** 777 (1955).

Monohydrate. Prisms from water. Anhydrous leaflets from hot alcohol + chloroform, mp 152°. Freely sol in water, alcohol, ether; insol in chloroform, benzene. Easily dehydrated to the lactone. Aq solns are stable.

Dimethyl ether. $C_{10}H_{12}O_4$. mp 124.5°.

Methyl ester dimethyl ether. $C_{11}H_{14}O_4$. mp 45°.

4738. Homosalate. [118-56-9] 2-Hydroxybenzoic acid 3,3,5-trimethylcyclohexyl ester; salicylic acid 3,3,5-trimethylcyclohexyl ester; 3,3,5-trimethylcyclohexyl salicylate; homomenthyl salicylate; Eusolex HMS; Neo Heliopan HMS; Parsol HMS. C_{16}-$H_{22}O_3$; mol wt 262.34. C 73.25%, H 8.45%, O 18.30%. UV-B absorber in cosmetics and sunscreens. Prepn: Stockelbach, **US 2369084** (1945 to Fries Bros.).

bp_4 161-165°. n^{20} 1.516 to 1.518. d_{25}^{25} 1.045. Sol in oil.

THERAP CAT: Ultraviolet screen.

4739. Homoserine. [672-15-1] 2-Amino-4-hydroxybutanoic acid; 2-amino-4-hydroxybutyric acid; α-amino-γ-hydroxy-*n*-butyric acid. $C_4H_9NO_3$; mol wt 119.12. C 40.33%, H 7.62%, N 11.76%, O 40.29%. Principal free amino acid occurring in pea plants: A. I. Virtanen, *Acta Chem. Scand.* **7**, 1423 (1953); J.A. Bakhuis, *Nature* **180**, 713 (1957). Prepn: Fischer, Blumenthal, *Ber.* **40**, 106 (1907); Armstrong *J. Am. Chem. Soc.* **70**, 1756 (1948); Birnbaum, Greenstein, *Arch. Biochem. Biophys.* **42**, 212 (1953); M. Frankel, Y. Knobler, *J. Am. Chem. Soc.* **80**, 3147 (1958). Review of homoserine production by fermentation: T. Nara in *Microbial Prod. Amino Acids*, K. Yamada, Ed. (Wiley, New York, 1972) pp 417-434.

L-form

L-Homoserine. Flat prisms from 90% alc. Dec 203°. $[M]_D$ +21.8° (5*N* HCl), $[M]_D$ +14.3° (glacial acetic acid). $[\alpha]_D^{26}$ −8.8° (c = 5 in H_2O); $[\alpha]_D^{26}$ +18.3° (c = 2 in 2*N* HCl). On standing for 8 hrs at 26° the $[\alpha]_D$ of the HCl soln decreases to nearly zero as the corresponding levorotatory-γ-butyrolactone is formed.

L-Homoserine γ-lactone monohydrochloride. Prepd by refluxing L-homoserine with 2*N* HCl for 2 hrs, crystals, $[\alpha]_D^{26}$ −27.0° (c = 5).

D-Homoserine. Crystals, dec 203°. $[\alpha]_D^{26}$ +8.8° (c = 5).

DL-Homoserine. Crystals from dil ethanol, dec 186-187°.

4740. Homovanillic Acid. [306-08-1] 4-Hydroxy-3-methoxybenzeneacetic acid; (4-hydroxy-3-methoxyphenyl)acetic acid; 4-hydroxy-3-methoxy-α-toluic acid. $C_9H_{10}O_4$; mol wt 182.17. C 59.34%, H 5.53%, O 35.13%. Metabolite found in human urine. Prepn: F. Tiemann, N. Nagai, *Ber.* **10**, 201 (1877); F. Mauthner, *Ann.* **370**, 368 (1909); H. E. Fisher, H. Hibbert, *J. Am. Chem. Soc.* **69**, 1208 (1947). End product of dopamine, *q.v.*: K. Shaw *et al.*, *J. Biol. Chem.* **226**, 255 (1957); M. Goodall, H. Alton, *Biochem. Pharmacol.* **25**, 2635 (1968).

White crystals, mp 143°. Sol in water, benzene. Slightly sol in alcohol, ether. Insol in cyclohexane.

4741. HON. [4439-84-3] 5-hydroxy-4-oxonorvaline; 2-amino-5-hydroxylevulinic acid; δ-hydroxy-γ-oxo-L-norvaline; 2-amino-5-hydroxy-4-oxopentanoic acid. $C_5H_9NO_4$; mol wt 147.13. C 40.82%, H 6.17%, N 9.52%, O 43.50%. $HOCH_2CO$-$CH_2CH(NH_2)COOH$. Antitubercular antibiotic substance isolated from *Streptomyces akiyoshiensis nova* sp.: Tatsuoka *et al.*, *J. Antibiot.* **14A**, 39 (1961). Synthesis and structure: Miyake, *Chem. Pharm. Bull.* **8**, 1071, 1074, 1079 (1960).

Needles from water + acetone, no definite mp. $[\alpha]_D^{20}$ −6° (water); $[\alpha]_D^{17}$ −8.2° (c = 3.4 in water). pKa 2.91. uv max (water): 271 nm (ε 24). Stable in pure, dry state. Less stable in basic than in acidic solns. Colors red when heated in caustic soln, losing antibiotic activity. The DL-form is half as active as L-HON. LD_{50} in mice (mg/kg): 5200 i.v.; 8000 s.c.; 7600 orally (Tatsuoka).

4742. Honokiol. [35354-74-6] 3′,5-Di-2-propenyl-[1,1′-biphenyl]-2,4′-diol; 3′,5-diallyl-2,4′-biphenyldiol; 5,3′-diallyl-2,4′-dihydroxydiphenyl. $C_{18}H_{18}O_2$; mol wt 266.33. C 81.17%, H 6.81%, O 12.01%. Bioactive principle isolated from the bark of *Magnolia obovata*, Thunb., *Magnoliaceae* and other *Magnolia* species used in Japanese and Chinese traditional medicine. Name derived from "Honoki", the Japanese name of *M. obovata*. Isomeric with magnolol, *q.v.* Identification in methanolic extracts of *M. obovata* bark: M. Fujita *et al.*, *Chem. Pharm. Bull.* **20**, 212 (1972). Isoln from seeds of *M. grandiflora* L.: F. S. El-Feraly, W.-S. Li, *Lloydia* **41**, 442 (1978). Synthesis: T. Takeya *et al.*, *Chem. Pharm. Bull.* **34**, 2066 (1986). CNS depressant effects *in vivo*: K. Watanabe *et al.*,

Planta Med. **49**, 103 (1983). HPLC determn in *M. officinalis* extracts: T.-H. Tsai, C.-F. Chen, *J. Chromatogr.* **598**, 143 (1992).

Colorless needles, mp 86-86.5° (El-Feraly, Li); also reported as mp 87.5° (Fujita). Sol in usual organic solvents and caustic alkali. uv max (ethanol): 294 nm (ε 8200).

4743. Hoodia. Genus of succulent plants in the family *Apocynaceae*, primarily *Hoodia gordonii* (Masson) Sweet ex Decne. or *H. pilifera* (L.f.) Plowes (syn. *Trichocaulon piliferum*); used traditionally by the Bushman of the Kalahari desert as an appetite suppressant, thirst quencher and as a cure for digestive disturbances. *Habit.* Angola, Botswana, Namibia, and South Africa. Brief review: B.-E. van Wyk, M. Wink, *Medicinal Plants of the World* (Timber Press, Portland, 2004) p 171. Description of the genus: D. Court, *Succulent Flora of Southern Africa* (Balkema Press, Rotterdam, 2000) pp 169-172.

P57AS3

P57AS3. [384329-61-7] (3β,12β,14β)-3-[(*O*-6-Deoxy-3-*O*-methyl-β-D-glucopyranosyl-(1 → 4)-*O*-2,6-dideoxy-3-*O*-methyl-β-D-*ribo*-hexopyranosyl-(1 → 4)-2,6-dideoxy-3-*O*-methyl-β-D-*ribo*-hexopyranosyl)oxy]-14-hydroxy-12-[[(2*E*)-2-methyl-1-oxo-2-butenyl]oxy]pregn-5-en-20-one; P57. $C_{47}H_{74}O_{15}$; mol wt 879.08. Steroid glycoside thought to be the anorectic principle. Isoln and activity: F. R. Van Heerden *et al.*, **WO 9846243**; *eidem*, **US 6376657** (1998, 2002 both to CSIR). Mechanism of action study: D. B. Mac Lean, L.-G. Luo, *Brain Res.* **1020**, 1 (2004). mp 147-152°. $[\alpha]_D^{20}$ +12.67° (c = 3 in chloroform).

USE: Appetite suppressant.

4744. Hopantenic Acid. [18679-90-8] 4-[[(2*R*)-2,4-Dihydroxy-3,3-dimethyl-1-oxobutyl]amino]butanoic acid; D-(+)-4-(2,4-dihydroxy-3,3-dimethylbutyramido)butyric acid; D-homopantothenic acid. $C_{10}H_{19}NO_5$; mol wt 233.26. C 51.49%, H 8.21%, N 6.00%, O 34.30%. Homolog of pantothenic acid, *q.v.* Prepn: R. Fuerst, L. L. Li, *Biochim. Biophys. Acta* **86**, 26 (1964); C. M. DeSha, R. Fuerst, *ibid.* 33. Prepn of the calcium salt: Y. Nishizawa *et al.*, **JP 66 732** (1966 to Tanabe), *C.A.* **64**, 12555c (1965). Series of articles on analysis, physicochemical properties, electrophysiology, pharmacology, toxicity studies, teratology: *Bitamin* **33**, 603-632 (1966), *C.A.* **65**, 5949a-g (1966). Colorimetric determn, properties: T. Kodama *et al.*, *J. Vitaminol.* **13**, 298 (1967), *C.A.* **68**, 62755n (1968). Peri- and postnatal studies in rats: Y. Asano *et al.*, *Oyo Yakuri* **19**, 1011 (1980), *C.A.* **94**, 58160 (1981). Mechanism of action: V. M. Arakumov, M. A. Kovler, *Farmakol. Toksikol.* **44**, 30 (1981), *C.A.* **94**, 114577 (1981). Determn in plasma: Y. Umeno *et al.*, *J. Chromatogr.* **226**, 333 (1981). Toxicology studies: Y. Nishizawa *et al.*, *J. Vitaminol.* **15**, 26 (1969). Pharmacology and acute toxicity study: Y. Nishizawa, *Med. J. Osaka Univ.* **35**, 41 (1984).

Sol in water; stable at pH 5-6. $[\alpha]_D^{20}$ +23.8°. pKa 4.52 at 25°. LD_{50} in male, female mice, male, female rats (mg/kg): 850, 954,

1575, 1458 i.p.; 2063, 2495, 5940, 7348 s.c.; 6297, 7935, 16810, 13350 orally (Nishizawa).

Calcium salt hemihydrate. Calcium homopantothenate; hopantenate calcium; pantogam; Hopate. $C_{20}H_{36}CaNO_5 \cdot \frac{1}{2}H_2O$; mol wt 419.59. White powder, mp 155-165°. $[\alpha]_D^{20}$ +24.19° (c = 2 in water). Bitter taste. Sol in water, slightly sol in methanol. Practically insol in organic solvents. Stable at pH 5-6.

THERAP CAT: Cerebral activator.

4745. Hops. Carefully dried strobiles of *Humulus lupulus* L., *Moraceae,* bearing their glandular trichomes. *Habit.* Europe, Asia, North America, cultivated widely. *Constit.* Volatile oil (0.3-1%), bitter acids incl. lupulone, humulone; flavonoids incl. xanthohumol; ferulic, caffeic and chlorogenic acids; tannins, resins. Review of chemistry and constituents: R. Stevens, *Chem. Rev.* **67**, 19-71 (1967); of botany, chemistry and use in beer brewing: M. Moir, *J. Am. Soc. Brew. Chem.* **58**, 131-146 (2000); of medicinal uses: J. Barnes *et al., Herbal Medicines* (Pharmaceutical Press, London, 2nd Ed., 2002) pp 290-292.

Volatile oil. [8007-04-3] Oil of hops. *Constit.* Complex mixture of more than 100 terpenoid components, primarily humulene, β-caryophyllene, farnescene. Light yellow to green-yellow liquid. Darkens and becomes viscous with aging. d_{25}^{25} 0.825-0.926. n_D^{20} 1.470-1.494. Acid value not more than 11.0. Saponification value between 14 and 69. Sol in most fixed oils. Practically insol in glycerin, propylene glycol. *Keep well closed, cool and protected from light.*

USE: In beer brewing; oil in hair rinses and bath prepns.

THERAP CAT: Sedative.

4746. Hordenine. [539-15-1] 4-[2-(Dimethylamino)ethyl]-phenol; *N,N*-dimethyltyramine; *p*-hydroxy-*N,N*-dimethylphenethylamine; anhaline; eremursine; peyocactine. $C_{10}H_{15}NO$; mol wt 165.23. C 72.69%, H 9.15%, N 8.48%, O 9.68%. Isoln from barley germs: Leger, *Compt. Rend.* **142**, 108 (1906); **143**, 234, 916 (1906); **144**, 488 (1907); Erspamer, Falconieri, *Naturwissenschaften* **39**, 431 (1952). Structure: Leger, *Bull. Soc. Chim. Fr.* [3] **35**, 868 (1906); [4] **1**, 148 (1907); Gaebel, *Arch. Pharm.* **244**, 441 (1906). Synthesis from phenethyl alcohol: Barger, *J. Chem. Soc.* **95**, 2193 (1909); from tyrosine: Raoul, *Compt. Rend.* **204**, 74 (1937); from *p*-(β-hydroxyethyl)anisole: Cheng *et al., J. Am. Chem. Soc.* **73**, 4081 (1951).

Orthorhombic prisms from alcohol or from benzene + petr ether, needles from water, mp 117-118°. bp$_{11}$ 173°. Sublimes 140-150°. Very sol in alcohol, chloroform, ether. 7 grams dissolve in 1000 ml water. Sparingly sol in benzene, toluene, xylene. Practically insol in petr ether.

Hydrochloride. [6027-23-2] $C_{10}H_{15}NO \cdot HCl$. Needles from alcohol, mp 177°. Very sol in water.

4747. Horehound. Hoarhound. *Marrubium vulgare* (Tourn.) L., *Labiatae. Habit.* Europe, Asia, naturalized in the U.S. *Constit.* Bitter principle marrubiin, volatile oil.

THERAP CAT: Expectorant.

4748. Horse Chestnut. Deciduous, flowering tree, *Aesculus hippocastanum* L., *Hippocastanaceae,* bearing spiny, globular fruit capsules that contain up to 3 reddish brown, inedible seeds. Medicinal portions are the dried leaves and an extract prepared from the seeds. *Habit.* Balkan peninsula; widely cultivated in Northern hemisphere as a shade tree. *Constit.* Mixture of triterpene saponins known as escin, *q.v.* (3-5%); coumarins such as esculetin, fraxin, scopolin; flavonoids incl. astragalin, isoquercetin, rutin, leucocyanidin; tannins, starch, fatty acids; also contains the toxic glycoside, esculin. Comprehensive description: N. Tiffany *et al., J. Herb. Pharmacother.* **2**, 71-85 (2002). Review of constituents and uses: J. Barnes *et al., Herbal Medicines* (Pharmaceutical Press, London, 2nd Ed., 2002) pp 296-299; A. Y. Leung, S. Foster, *Encyclopedia of Common Natural Ingredients,* (Wiley-Interscience, Hoboken, 2nd Ed., 2003) pp 304-306; J. Gruenwald *et al., PDR for Herbal Medicines* (Medical Economics, Montvale, 3rd Ed., 2004) pp 445-448.

Dried extract. [8053-39-2] Horse chestnut seed extract; Aescorin; Aescusan; Essaven; Venalot; Venoplant; Venopyronum; Venostasin. Principle constituent is escin which is used to calculate potency. Clinical pharmacokinetics and bioavailability of formulations: D. Bässler *et al., Adv. Ther.* **20**, 295 (2003). Review of clinical trials in chronic venous insufficiency: U. Siebert *et al., Int. Angiol.* **21**, 305-315 (2002).

Caution: Potential symptoms of toxicity following ingestion of leaves, bark, flowers or raw seeds are vomiting, diarrhea, headache, stupor, coma, paralysis (Tiffany).

USE: In shampoos, skin care products, body and hand creams, lotions.

THERAP CAT: Seed extract in treatment of chronic venous insufficiency.

4749. Horse-radish. Raphanus rusticanus; Kren; Maliner Kren. The root of *Radicula armoracia* (L.) Robinson [*Cochlearia armoracia* L.; *Armoracia lopathifolia* Gilib.; *Roripa armoracia* Hitch.; *Nasturtium armoracia* Fries], *Cruciferae. Habit.* Europe, naturalized in North America. Contains ascorbic acid and sinigrin which yields allyl isothiocyanate on hydrolysis with peroxidase or myrosinase, an enzyme from black mustard: Stoll, Seebeck, *Helv. Chim. Acta* **31**, 1432 (1948).

Active ingredient of **Rasapen**, a urinary antiseptic.

USE: Condiment.

4750. HPA-23. [89899-81-0] Hexaoctacontaoxononoantimonateheneicosatungstate(19−) heptadecaammonium disodium; ammonium 5-tungsto-2-antimonate; 5-tungsto-2-antimonate; 21-tungsto-9-antimonate. $H_{68}Na_2N_{17}O_{86}Sb_9W_{21}$; mol wt 6685.06. H 1.03%, Na 0.69%, N 3.56%, O 20.58%, Sb 16.39%, W 57.75%. $(NH_4)_{17}Na(NaSb_9W_{21}O_{86})$. One of the condensed mineral heteropolyanions, also called polyoxotungstates. Synthesis: M. Michelon, G. Hervé, *C.R. Seances Acad. Sci. Ser. C* **274**, 209 (1972); M. Michelon *et al., J. Inorg. Nucl. Chem.* **42**, 1583 (1980). Crystal structure: J. Fischer *et al., J. Am. Chem. Soc.* **98**, 3050 (1976). Laser Raman studies of intracellular localization: C. Cibert, C. Jasmin, *Biochem. Biophys. Res. Commun.* **108**, 1424 (1982). Antiviral activity in mice: C. Jasmin *et al., J. Natl. Cancer Inst.* **53**, 469 (1974); G. H. Werner *et al., J. Gen. Virol.* **31**, 59 (1976). In vitro inhibition of rabies virus: H. Tsiang *et al., J. Gen. Virol.* **40**, 665 (1978). Effects in scrapie model systems: R. H. Kimberlin, C. A. Walker, *Lancet* **2**, 591 (1979); eidem, *Arch. Virol.* **78**, 9 (1983). Structure-activity study: M. Hervé *et al., Biochem. Biophys. Res. Commun.* **116**, 222 (1983). Clinical evaluation in AIDS: W. Rozenbaum *et al., Lancet* **1**, 450 (1985); B. L. Moskovitz, *Antimicrob. Agents Chemother.* **32**, 1300 (1988).

Crystals from water. Solution has pH near 6.7, and is stable around neutrality. LD$_{50}$ i.p. in mice: 750 mg/kg (Werner).

Note: Formerly known as **ammonium antimony tungsten oxide**.

4751. HQNO. [341-88-8] 2-Heptyl-4-quinolinol 1-oxide; 2-heptyl-4-hydroxyquinoline *N*-oxide. $C_{16}H_{21}NO_2$; mol wt 259.34. C 74.10%, H 8.16%, N 5.40%, O 12.34%. Inhibitor of electron transport through the cytochrome bc_1 segment of the respiratory chain. Isoln of the naturally occurring antagonist to dihydrostreptomycin from *Pseudomonas pyocyanea*: Hays *et al., J. Biol. Chem.* **159**, 725 (1948); J. Lightbown, *J. Gen. Microbiol.* **11**, iv (1954). Properties: J. W. Cornforth, A. T. James, *Biochem. J.* **58**, xlviii (1954). Synthesis: *eidem, ibid.* **63**, 124 (1956); D. E. Ames *et al., J. Chem. Soc.* **1956**, 3079. Inhibition of electron transport: J. W. Lightbown, F. L. Jackson, *Biochem. J.* **63**, 130 (1956); M. Avron, *ibid.* **78**, 735 (1961); N. J. Jacobs, J. M. Wolin, *Biochim. Biophys. Acta* **69**, 29 (1963). Effect on proton permeability of the mitochondrial membrane: K. Krab, M. Wikström, *Biochem. J.* **186**, 637 (1980). Sites of inhibition: G. Izzo *et al., FEBS Lett.* **93**, 320 (1978); M. Droppa *et al., Z. Naturforsch.* **36C**, 109 (1981).

Crystals from methylethyl ketone, mp 156-157°.

4752. Humic Acids. Allomelanins found in soils, coals, and peat, resulting from the decompn of organic matter, particularly dead plants. Consists of a mixture of complex macromolecules having polymeric phenolic structures with the ability to chelate with metals, esp iron. *Review:* R. A. Nicolaus, *Melanins* (Hermann, Paris, 1968) pp 147-153; W. Flaig *et al.* in *Soil Components* **vol. 1,** J. E. Gieseking, Ed. (Springer, New York, 1975) pp 1-211.

Chocolate-brown, dust-like powder. Slightly sol in water, usually with much swelling; sol in alkali hydroxides and carbonates; also sol in hot concd HNO_3 with dark-red color.

USE: In mud baths, drilling muds, pigments for printing inks, fertilizers, growth hormones for plants, transporters of trace minerals in soil: Steelnick, *J. Chem. Educ.* **40,** 379 (1963).

4753. Humulene. [6753-98-6] (1*E,4E,8E*)-2,6,6,9-Tetramethyl-1,4,8-cycloundecatriene; α-humulene; α-caryophyllene. $C_{15}H_{24}$; mol wt 204.35. C 88.16%, H 11.84%. Sesquiterpenoid isomer of caryophyllene, *q.v.* occurring in many essential oils, especially oil of hops *(Humulus lupulus* L. *Moraceae)* and leaves of *Lindera strychnifolia* (F.) Will *Lauraceae.* Occurs in nature as a mixture with β-humulene. Isolation of mixture: A. C. Chapman, *J. Chem. Soc.* **67,** 54, 780 (1895). Identity with α-caryophyllene: F. Sorm *et al., Collect. Czech. Chem. Commun.* **14,** 693, 699, 716 (1949). Structure: F. Sorm *et al., ibid.* **19,** 570 (1954). Stereochemistry: A. T. McPhail, G. A. Sim, *J. Chem. Soc. B* **1966,** 112. Synthesis: E. J. Corey, E. Hanamaka, *J. Am. Chem. Soc.* **89,** 2758 (1967). Stereoselective synthesis: Y. Kitagawa *et al., ibid.* **99,** 3864 (1977); E. J. Corey *et al., Tetrahedron Lett.* **34,** 3675 (1993). Chromatographic conversion to β-humulene: V. Benesova *et al., Collect. Czech. Chem. Commun.* **26,** 1832 (1961). *Reviews:* F. Sorm in *Fortschr. Chem. Org. Naturst.* **19,** 1-32 (1961); *Rodd's Chemistry of Carbon Compounds* **vol. IIC,** S. Coffey, Ed., (Elsevier, New York, 2nd ed., 1969) pp 282-283.

Liquid. bp$_5$ 106-107°. n_D^{30} 1.5004, N. P. Damodaran, S. Dev, *Tetrahedron* **24,** 4113 (1968). Also reported as bp$_{10}$ 123°. n_D^{25} 1.5015. d$_4^{25}$ 0.8865, R. P. Hildebrand *et al., Chem. Ind. (London)* **1959,** 489. NMR spectrum: S. Dev *et al., J. Am. Chem. Soc.* **90,** 1246 (1968).

Silver nitrate complex. $C_{15}H_{24}.2AgNO_3$. Crystals from aq ethanol, mp 175°.

β-Humulene. [116-04-1] (*E,E*)-1,4,4-Trimethyl-8-methylene-1,5-cycloundecadiene. Liquid. n_D^{20} 1.5014. d$_4^{20}$ 0.8905.

4754. Humulon. [26472-41-3] (6*R*)-3,5,6-Trihydroxy-4,6-bis(3-methyl-2-butenyl)-2-(3-methyl-1-oxobutyl)-2,4-cyclohexadien-1-one; α-bitter acid; α-lupulic acid; humulone. $C_{21}H_{30}O_5$; mol wt 362.46. C 69.59%, H 8.34%, O 22.07%. Antibiotic constituent of hops *(Humulus lupulus* L., *Moraceae). See also* Lupulon. Isoln from commercial hops: Bungener, *Bull. Soc. Chim.* [2] **45,** 487 (1886); Barth, Lintner, *Ber.* **31,** 2022 (1898); Wollmer, *Ber.* **49,** 780 (1916); Lewis *et al., J. Clin. Invest.* **28,** 916 (1949). Structure: Riedl, *Ber.* **85,** 692 (1952); Carson, *J. Am. Chem. Soc.* **73,** 4652 (1951). Absolute configuration and structure of preferred isomer: DeKeukeleire, Verzele, *Tetrahedron* **26,** 385 (1970).

Crystals from ether, mp 65-66.5°. Bitter taste, esp in alcoholic soln. More stable to air than lupulon. Monobasic acid. $[α]_D^{20}$

−212° (1.0 g in 15.5 g 96% alc). uv max (ethanol): 237, 282 nm (ε 13,760; 8330). Soluble in the usual organic solvents. Slightly sol in boiling water from which it separates as a milky precipitate on cooling. Forms a sodium salt which is readily sol in water. Suffers no loss of bacteriostatic potency against *Staphylococcus aureus* upon autoclaving 40 ppm in phosphate buffer at pH 6.5 or 8.5. The presence of ascorbic acid in low concns extends the duration of bacteriostatic action.

4755. Huperzine A. [102518-79-6] [5*R*-(5α,9β,11*E*)]-5-Amino-11-ethylidene-5,6,9,10-tetrahydro-7-methyl-5,9-methanocycloocta[*b*]pyridin-2(1*H*)-one; selagine; HUP. $C_{15}H_{18}N_2O$; mol wt 242.32. C 74.35%, H 7.49%, N 11.56%, O 6.60%. Reversible alkaloid inhibitor of AChE which crosses the blood-brain barrier. Occurs as the (−)-form in the vegetative part of clubmosses; teas brewed from these mosses have traditionally been used in China to alleviate memory problems. Isolated as selagine from *Lycopodium selago* L., *Lycopodiaceae:* J. Muszynski, *Q. J. Pharm. Pharmacol.* **21,** 34 (1948); from *Huperzia serrata* as huperzine: Chin. Co-op Res. Group, *J. Tradit. Chin. Med.* **2,** 45 (1982). Original structure: Z. Valenta *et al., Tetrahedron Lett.* **1960,** 26; revised structure as huperzine A: J.-S. Liu *et al., Can. J. Chem.* **64,** 837 1986. Identity with selagine: W. A. Ayer *et al., ibid.* **67,** 1538 (1989). Synthesis of (±)-form: A. P. Kozikowski *et al., J. Org. Chem.* **56,** 4636 (1991); G. Campiani *et al., ibid.* **58,** 7660 (1993). NMR spectra: B. N. Zhou *et al., Phytochemistry* **34,** 1425 (1993). HPLC determn in serum: J. Ye *et al., J. Chromatogr. B* **817,** 187 (2005). Anticholinesterase activity: Y.-E. Wang *et al., Acta Pharmacol. Sin.* **7,** 110 (1986); binding profile of enantiomers: M. McKinney *et al., Eur. J. Pharmacol.* **203,** 303 (1991); binding specificity: Y. Ashani *et al., Mol. Pharmacol.* **45,** 555 (1994). Clinical evaluation in senile dementia: R.-W. Zhang *et al., Acta Pharmacol. Sin.* **12,** 259 (1991). Brief review of chemistry and clinical use: D. Bai, *Pure Appl. Chem.* **65,** 1103-1112 (1993).

Monoclinic crystals from acetone, mp 214-215°. $[α]_D$ −147° (c = 0.36 in CH_3OH) (Ayer). Also reported as mp 230°. $[α]_D^{24.5}$ −150.4° (c = 0.498 in MeOH) (Liu). uv max (EtOH): 231, 313 nm (log ε 4.01, 3.89).

THERAP CAT: In treatment of memory disorders.

4756. Hyalobiuronic Acid. [499-15-0] 2-Amino-2-deoxy-3-*O*-β-D-glucopyranuronosyl-D-glucose; 3-*O*-(β-D-glucopyranosyl-uronic acid)-2-amino-2-deoxy-D-glucose. $C_{12}H_{21}NO_{11}$; mol wt 355.30. C 40.57%, H 5.96%, N 3.94%, O 49.53%. Disaccharide unit of hyaluronic acid. Isoln from hyaluronic acid: Rapport *et al., Nature* **168,** 996 (1951). Structure: Weissman, Meyer, *J. Am. Chem. Soc.* **76,** 1753 (1954). Synthesis: Takanashi *et al., ibid.* **84,** 3029 (1962).

Rectangular prisms from water, darken at 190° with no characteristic melting or dec point. pK$_1'$ = 2.6, pK$_2'$ = 7.1. Shows mutarotation: $[α]_D^{20}$ +34° → +30° (c = 1.08 in 0.1*N* HCl). Sparingly sol in hot water, dilute HCl, dil $NaHCO_3$. Practically insol in water, glacial acetic acid, ethanol, methanol and pyridine.

N-Acetylhyalobiuronic acid. $C_{14}H_{23}NO_{12}$. Amorphous. pK' = 3.3. $[α]_D^{24}$ −32° (c = 2.0 in water).

4757. Hyaluronic Acid. [9004-61-9] Unbranched high molecular weight polysaccharide made up of alternating glucuronic acid and *N*-acetyl glucosamine units. Present in the connective tissue of all vertebrates as the hyaluronate; in man high concentrations are found in skin, cartilage, in the umbilical cord, in vitreous body and in synovial fluid. Isoln and characterization: K. Meyer, J. W. Palmer, *J. Biol. Chem.* **107**, 629 (1934); *eidem, ibid.* **114**, 689 (1936). Structure: K. Meyer, *Fed. Proc.* **17**, 1075 (1958). Crystal structure: I. C. M. Dea *et al., Science* **179**, 560 (1973); E. D. T. Atkins, J. K. Sheehan, *ibid.* 562. *Reviews:* Tauber, *Chemistry and Technology of Enzymes* (New York, 1946); Meyer, Rapport in *Adv. Enzymol.* **13**, 199 (1952); R. L. Whistler, E. J. Olson in *Adv. Carbohydr. Chem.* **12**, 299 (1957). Review of role in various developmental processes: B. P. Toole, *Cell Biology of Extracellular Matrix*, E. D. Hay, Ed. (Plenum Press, New York, 1981) pp 259-288.

Sodium salt. [9067-32-7] ARTZ; Connettivina; Equron; Healon; Healonid; Hyacid; Hyalgan; Hyalovet; Hyonate; Ial; Opegan; Provisc; Synacid. $[\alpha]_D^{25}$ −74° (c = 0.25 in water): Rapport *et al., J. Am. Chem. Soc.* **73**, 2416 (1951).

USE: Surgical aid (ophthalmological).

THERAP CAT (VET): Adjunct in treatment of noninfectious synovitis. Osteoarthritis in dogs and horses.

4758. Hyaluronidases. [9001-54-1] Spreading factor; diffusing factor; invasin; Alidase; Apertase; Diffusin; Enzodase; Harodase; Hyalase; Hyalozima; Hyalidase; Hyasmonta; Hyason; Hyazyme; Jalovis; Kinaden; Kinetin; Luronase; Permease; Rondase; Ronidase; Thiomucase; Unidasa; Wydase. Enzymes which have in common the cleavage of glycosidic bonds of hyaluronic acid, *q.v.*, and, to a variable degree, of some other acid mucopolysaccharides of connective tissue. The skin is probably the largest store of hyaluronidase in the body; the enzyme although generally present in an inactive form, may be supposed to regulate the velocity of water and metabolite exchange by decreasing the viscosity of the intercellular matrix. Also has a physiological role in fertilization: The sperm is rich in the enzyme and can thus advance better in the cervical canal and reach the ovum. Found in the type II pneumococci, in group A and C hemolytic streptococci, *Staphylococcus aureus* and *Clostridium welchii:* Linker *et al., J. Biol. Chem.* **219**, 13 (1956); in heads of leeches: Linker *et al., Nature* **180**, 810 (1957); in snake venoms: Favilli, *ibid.* **145**, 866 (1940); in testes: Hahn, *Biochem. Z.* **315**, 83 (1943); Högberg, *Acta Chem. Scand.* **8**, 1098 (1954). Biochemical properties: D. Platt, *Arzneim.-Forsch.* **20**, 1836 (1970). *Review:* Meyer, Rapport in *Adv. Enzymol.* **13**, 199-236 (1952); Meyer *et al., The Enzymes* **vol. 4**, P. D. Boyer *et al.*, Eds. (Academic Press, New York, 2nd ed., 1960) pp 447-460; Meyer, *ibid.* **vol. 5** (3rd ed., 1971) pp 307-320. Reviews of clinical trials in myocardial infarction: G. S. May *et al., Prog. Cardiovasc. Dis.* **25**, 335-359 (1983); A. B. Saunders, *Emerg. Med. Clin. North Am.* **6**, 361-372 (1988). Hyaluronidase manufacturers define their product in terms of turbidity-reducing (TR) units or in viscosity units. Prepd solns for injection usually contain 150 turbidity-reducing units or 500 viscosity units dissolved in 1 ml of isotonic NaCl soln.

USE: Pharmaceutic aid (diffusing agent in s.c. injections).

THERAP CAT: Spreading agent.

THERAP CAT (VET): To promote diffusion, absorption, resorption.

4759. Hycanthone. [3105-97-3] 1-[[2-(Diethylamino)ethyl]amino]-4-(hydroxymethyl)-9*H*-thioxanthen-9-one. $C_{20}H_{24}N_2O_2S$; mol wt 356.48. C 67.38%, H 6.79%, N 7.86%, O 8.98%, S 8.99%. Metabolite of lucanthone, *q.v.*: Rosi *et al., Nature* **208**, 1005 (1965). Prepn by oxidative fermentation of lucanthone and schistosomicidal activity: Rosi *et al., J. Med. Chem.* **10**, 867 (1967); *NL* 6410359, and Rosi, Peruzzotti, *US* 3294803; *US* 3312598 (1965, 1966, 1967 all to Sterling Drug). Alternate synthesis: Laidlaw *et al., J. Org. Chem.* **38**, 1743 (1973).

Crystals, mp 100.6-102.8°. Absorption max (ethanol): 233, 258, 329, 438 nm (ε 19400, 37000, 9700, 6600). Extremely sensitive to acid.

Hydrochloride. mp 173-176° (dec).

Mesylate. [23255-93-8] Etrenol.

THERAP CAT: Anthelmintic (Schistosoma).

4760. Hydantoin. [461-72-3] 2,4-Imidazolidinedione; 2,4-(3*H*,5*H*)-imidazoledione; glycolylurea. $C_3H_4N_2O_2$; mol wt 100.08. C 36.00%, H 4.03%, N 27.99%, O 31.97%. Prepn: Baeyer, *Ann.* **130**, 129 (1864). Manuf: Gresham, Schweitzer, *US* 2402134 (1946 to du Pont); White, Wysong, *US* 2663713 (1953 to Dow). *Review:* J. H. Bateman in *Kirk-Othmer Encyclopedia of Chemical Technology* **vol. 12** (Wiley-Interscience, New York, 3rd ed., 1980) pp 692-711.

Needles from methanol, mp 220°. Slightly sol in water or ether; sol in alcohol, in solns of fixed alkali hydroxides.

4761. Hydnocarpic Acid. [459-67-6] (1*R*)-2-Cyclopentene-1-undecanoic acid; 11-(2-cyclopenten-1-yl)undecanoic acid. $C_{16}H_{28}O_2$; mol wt 252.39. C 76.14%, H 11.18%, O 12.68%. Component of chaulmoogra oil; naturally occurring in *d*-form. Isoln from seeds of *Hydnocarpus wightiana* Blume or *H. anthelmintica* Pierre, *Flacourtiaceae*, or from the seeds of *Taraktogenos kurzii* King, *Bixaceae:* F. B. Power, M. Barrowcliff, *J. Chem. Soc.* **87**, 884 (1905); *ibid.* **91**, 557 (1907). Structure: R. L. Shriner, R. Adams, *J. Am. Chem. Soc.* **47**, 2727 (1925). Synthesis of *dl*-hydnocarpic acid: D. G. M. Diaper, J. C. Smith, *Biochem. J.* **42**, 581 (1948). Toxicity data: Anderson, *Int. J. Lepr.* **2**, 39 (1934). Antimicrobial spectrum: P. L. Jacobsen, L. Levy, *Proc. West. Pharmacol. Soc.* **15**, 44 (1972). Mechanism of action: *eidem, Antimicrob. Agents Chemother.* **3**, 373 (1973). Chromatographic determn in seed oils: W. W. Christie *et al., Lipids* **24**, 116 (1989).

Colorless, glistening leaflets from petr ether + ethyl acetate, mp 59-60°. $[\alpha]_D$ +68.3° (chloroform). Sparingly sol in usual organic solvents; sol in chloroform.

***dl*-Form.** Pearly plates from alcohol, ethyl actate or petr ether + ethyl acetate, mp 59-59.5°.

Sodium salt. Sodium hydnocarpate; hydnocarpate sodium; sodium gynocardate. Yellowish powder. Sol in water, alc. The aq soln is alkaline. MLD in rats (mg/kg): 100-125 i.v. (Anderson).

THERAP CAT: Antibacterial (leprostatic).

4762. Hydracrylic Acid. [503-66-2] 3-Hydroxypropanoic acid; β-hydroxypropionic acid; ethylene lactic acid. $C_3H_6O_3$; mol wt 90.08. C 40.00%, H 6.71%, O 53.28%. CH_2OHCH_2COOH. Prepd by alkaline hydrolysis of the nitrile: R. R. Read, *Org. Synth.* **coll. vol. I**, 321 (2nd ed., 1941).

Viscous liq. Strong acid, pK (25°): 4.51. On distn or boiling with 50% H_2SO_4 dec into water and acrylic acid. Very sol in water, sol in alcohol, miscible with ether.

Sodium salt. $NaC_3H_5O_3$. Deliquescent crystals, mp 143°.

Calcium salt dihydrate. $Ca(C_3H_5O_3)_2.2H_2O$. Prisms, mp 140-145°; freely sol in cold water.

4763. Hydralazine. [86-54-4] 1(2H)-Phthalazinone hydrazone; 1-hydrazinophthalazine; Ciba 5968; Präparat 5968; C-5968. $C_8H_8N_4$; mol wt 160.18. C 59.99%, H 5.03%, N 34.98%. Prepd by the action of hydrazine hydrate on 1-chloro- or 1-phenoxyphthalazine: Hartmann, Druey, **US 2484029** (1949 to Ciba); Druey, Ringier, *Helv. Chim. Acta* **34**, 204 (1951). Metabolism: Z. H. Israile, P. G. Dayton, *Drug Metab. Rev.* **6**, 283 (1977); K. Schmid *et al., Arzneim.-Forsch.* **31**, 1143 (1981). Pharmacology: J. L. Cangiano *et al., J. Lab. Clin. Med.* **92**, 516 (1978). Clinical paper: R. F. Albrecht *et al., Int. Anesthesiol. Clin.* **16**, 299 (1978). Acute toxicity: L. Dorigotti *et al., Pharmacol. Res. Commun.* **8**, 295 (1976). Comprehensive description: C. E. Orzech *et al., Anal. Profiles Drug Subs.* **8**, 283-314 (1979).

Yellow needles from methanol, mp 172-173° (rapid heating). One gram dissolves in 3 ml 2N acetic acid, in 12 ml warm methanol. Forms a red compd (phthalazinylhydrazone) with acetone at 60° in presence of 2N acetic acid. LD_{50} in mice, rats (mg/kg): 122, 90 orally; 101, 40 i.p. (Dorigotti).

Hydrochloride. [304-20-1] Alphapress; Apresoline. C_8H_8-N_4.HCl; mol wt 196.64. Yellow crystals, dec 273°. Soly in water (g/100 ml) at 15°: 3.01; at 25°: 4.42; in 95% ethanol: 0.2 g/100 ml. Very slightly sol in ether. pH of a 2% aq soln 3.5 to 4.5. uv max (0.001% aq soln): 211, 240, 260, 304, 315 nm. Aq solns containing 20 mg/ml may be preserved with 0.5% chlorobutanol.

THERAP CAT: Antihypertensive.

4764. Hydrallostane. [516-41-6] (5α,11β)-11,17,21-Trihydroxypregnane-3,20-dione; 11β,17α,21-trihydroxyallopregnane-3,20-dione; allodihydrohydrocortisone; allopregnane-11β,17α,21-triol-3,20-dione; 4,5α-dihydrocortisol; allodihydro F. $C_{21}H_{32}O_5$; mol wt 364.48. C 69.20%, H 8.85%, O 21.95%. Isoln from beef and hog adrenals: Neher, Wettstein, *Helv. Chim. Acta* **39**, 2062 (1956). Prepn: Pataki *et al., J. Biol. Chem.* **195**, 753 (1952); Fukushima, Daum, *J. Org. Chem.* **26**, 520 (1961); Gould, Oliveto, **US 2783254; US 2897216** (1957; 1959 to Schering); Gould, Herzog, **US 2783226** (1957 to Schering); **GB 742888** (1956 to Syntex).

Crystals, mp 234-240°. $[\alpha]_D^{25}$ +83° (acetone). Practically insol in water. Sol in methanol, acetone, chloroform.

21-Acetate. $C_{23}H_{34}O_6$. Crystals from hexane + ethyl acetate, mp 211-213°. $[\alpha]_D^{20}$ +69° (chloroform).

21-*tert*-Butylacetate. $C_{27}H_{42}O_6$. Crystals from ethanol, mp 256-264° (also crystallizes as a hydrate). Sol in chloroform, oils, fats.

4765. Hydramethylnon. [67485-29-4] Tetrahydro-5,5-dimethyl-2(1H)-pyrimidinone[3-[4-(trifluoromethyl)phenyl]-1-[2-[4-(trifluoromethyl)phenyl]ethenyl]-2-propenylidene]hydrazone; 1,5-bis(α,α,α-trifluoro-*p*-tolyl)-1,4-pentadiene-3-one (1,4,5,6-tetrahydro-5,5-dimethyl-2-pyrimidinyl)hydrazone; AC-217300; Amdro; Combat; Maxforce. $C_{25}H_{24}F_6N_4$; mol wt 494.48. C 60.72%, H 4.89%, F 23.05%, N 11.33%. Slow-activating stomach poison insecticide. Prepn: J. B. Lovell, **US 4087525** (1975 to Am. Cyanamid). Activity: *idem, Proc. Br. Crop Prot. Conf. - Pests Dis.* **1979**, 575. Field trials for control of red imported fire ant: D. P.

Harlan *et al., Southwest. Entomol.* **6**, 150 (1981); W. A. Banks *et al., ibid.* 158; for control of cockroaches: J. F. Milio *et al., J. Econ. Entomol.* **79**, 1280 (1986).

Crystals from isopropanol, mp 189-191°. Insol in water. Sol in alc, acetone.

USE: Insecticide.

4766. Hydrangea. Seven barks. Dried rhizome and roots of *Hydrangea arborescens* L., *Saxifragaceae. Habit.* Eastern U.S. *Constit.* The glucoside hydrangin, saponin, resins, fixed and volatile oils, starch.

4767. Hydrastine. [118-08-1] (3S)-6,7-Dimethoxy-3-[(5R)-5,6,7,8-tetrahydro-6-methyl-1,3-dioxolo[4,5-g]isoquinolin-5-yl]-1(3H)-isobenzofuranone; *l*-β-hydrastine. $C_{21}H_{21}NO_6$; mol wt 383.39. C 65.79%, H 5.52%, N 3.65%, O 25.04%. Isoln of naturally occurring *l*-β-form from *Hydrastis canadensis* L., *Ranunculaceae* together with berberine and canadine. Synthesis of diastereoisomeric mixtures of hydrastines: Hope *et al., J. Chem. Soc.* **1931**, 236; Marshall *et al., ibid.* **1934**, 1315; M. Hanaoka *et al., Chem. Pharm. Bull.* **27**, 1947 (1979); J. R. Falck, S. Manna, *Tetrahedron Lett.* **22**, 619 (1981). Resolution to the *l*-β-form: Haworth, Pinder, *J. Chem. Soc.* **1950**, 1776; Haworth *et al., Nature* **165**, 529 (1950). Structure: Knabe, *Arch. Pharm.* **293**, 121 (1960). Abs config: Ohta *et al., Tetrahedron Lett.* **1963**, 859; Blaha *et al., Collect. Czech. Chem. Commun.* **29**, 2328 (1964); Snatzke *et al., Tetrahedron* **25**, 5059 (1969). Biosynthesis: Gear, Spenser, *Can. J. Chem.* **41**, 783 (1963).

Orthorhombic prisms from alc, mp 132°. $[\alpha]_D^{20}$ −50° (c = 0.3 in abs alc). uv max (ethanol): 202, 218, 238, 298, 316 nm (log ε 4.79, 4.53, 4.15, 3.86, 3.63). pK 7.8. Freely sol in acetone and benzene; insol in water. The salts hydrolyze easily and do not crystallize well.

Hydrochloride. [5936-28-7] $C_{21}H_{21}NO_6$.HCl. Prepn: R. Paech, M. V. Tracy, *Modern Methods of Plant Analysis* **vol. IV** (Springer-Verlag, Berlin, 1955) p 383. Powder, mp 116°. $[\alpha]_D^{17}$ +127° (c = 4 in dil HCl). Very sol in water, alcohol; slightly sol in $CHCl_3$; very slightly sol in ether. pH (0.5% aq soln): 4.2. Hygroscopic. *Keep well closed.*

THERAP CAT: Hydrochloride formerly as uterine hemostatic, antiseptic.

4768. Hydrastinine. [6592-85-1] 5,6,7,8-Tetrahydro-6-methyl-1,3-dioxolo[4,5-g]isoquinolin-5-ol; 1-hydroxy-6,7-methylenedioxy-2-methyl-1,2,3,4-tetrahydroisoquinoline. $C_{11}H_{13}NO_3$; mol wt 207.23. C 63.75%, H 6.32%, N 6.76%, O 23.16%. By oxidation of hydrastine: Freund, Will, *Ber.* **20**, 88 (1887). From berberine: Freund, **DE 241136** (1910), *C.A.* **6**, 2145 (1912). From cotarnine: Pyman, Remfry, *J. Chem. Soc.* **101**, 1595 (1912); Topchiev, *J. Appl. Chem. USSR* **6**, 529 (1933). From formylhomopiperonylamine: Decker *et al., Ann.* **395**, 299, 321, 328 (1913); Rosenmund, *Ber. Dtsch. Pharm. Ges.* **29**, 200 (1919). From safrole: Kindler, Peschke, *Arch. Pharm.* **270**, 353 (1932). Structure study: Schneider, Müller, *Ann.* **615**, 34 (1958).

Needles from petr ether, mp 117°. Freely sol in alcohol, chloroform, ether, dil acids; practically insol in cold, moderately sol in hot water. Solns with water or alcohol are yellow and fluorescent, those with nonpolar organic solvents are colorless. pK 2.62. Absorption spectra: Dobbie, Tinkler, *J. Chem. Soc.* **85**, 1005 (1904).

THERAP CAT: The hydrochloride as cardiotonic; uterine hemostatic.

4769. Hydrastis. Golden seal; orange root; yellow root; yellow puccoon; Indian turmeric. Dried rhizome and roots of *Hydrastis canadensis* L., *Ranunculaceae*, contg not less than 2.5% ether-soluble alkaloids. *Habit.* North America. *Constit.* 2-4% hydrastine, 2-3% berberine; canadine, volatile oil, resin.

4770. Hydrazine. [302-01-2] Hydrazine anhydrous. H_4N_2; mol wt 32.05. H 12.58%, N 87.41%. H_2NNH_2. Prepn from hydrazine hydrate: Sisler *et al., J. Am. Chem. Soc.* **76**, 3914 (1954); Schenk in *Handbook of Preparative Inorganic Chemistry* vol. 1, G. Brauer, Ed. (Academic Press, New York, 1963) pp 469-472. Toxicity data: Witkin, *Arch. Ind. Health* **13**, 34 (1956). Toxicology study: Back, Thomas, *Annu. Rev. Pharmacol.* **10**, 395 (1970). Review of carcinogenic risk: *IARC Monographs* **4**, 127-136 (1974); of toxicology: R. von Burg, T. Stout, *J. Appl. Toxicol.* **11**, 447-450 (1991); and human exposure: *Toxicological Profile for Hydrazines* (PB98-101025, 1997) 224 pp. Books: L. F. Audrieth, B. A. Ogg, *The Chemistry of Hydrazine* (Wiley, New York, 1951); C. C. Clark, *Hydrazine* (Mathieson Chem., Baltimore, 1953). *Reviews:* Troyan, *Ind. Eng. Chem.* **45**, 2608-2612 (1953); Zimmer, *Chem. Ztg.* **79**, 599-605 (1955); Hudson *et al.,* "Hydrazine" in *Mellor's* vol. VIII, suppl. II, *Nitrogen* (Part 2), 69-114 (1967); Jones in *Comprehensive Inorganic Chemistry* vol. 2, J. C. Bailar, Jr. *et al.,* Eds. (Pergamon Press, Oxford, 1973) p 250-265; H. W. Schiessl in *Kirk-Othmer Encyclopedia of Chemical Technology* vol. 13 (John Wiley & Sons, New York, 4th ed., 1995) pp 560-606.

Colorless oily liq, fuming in air. Penetrating odor resembling that of ammonia. Burns with violet flame. Explodes during distn if traces of air are present, also affected by uv and metal ion catalysts. Can be stored for years if sealed in glass and kept in a cool, dark place. Flash and fire pt 126°F (52°C). Contracts on freezing. d_4^{-5} 1.146; d_4^0 1.0253; d_4^2 1.024; d_4^{15} 1.011; d_4^{25} 1.0036; d_4^{35} 0.9955. One gallon of commercial product weighs 8.38 lbs. mp 2.0°. bp_{760} 113.5°; bp_{71} 56°; $bp_{5\ atm}$ 170°; $bp_{10\ atm}$ 200°; $bp_{20\ atm}$ 236°. $n_D^{22.3}$ 1.46979; n_D^{25} 1.46444. Dipole moment 1.83-1.90. Dielectric constant (25°): 51.7. Latent heat of fusion (mp): 3.025 kcal/mole; latent heat of vaporization (bp): 9760 kcal/mole (calc). Crit temp 380°; crit pressure 14 atm. Diacidic base. pK_1 (25°): ~6.05. Forms salts with inorganic acids. Highly polar solvent. Powerful reducing agent. Dissolves many inorganic substances. Misc with water, methyl, ethyl, propyl, isobutyl alcohols. Forms an azeotropic mixture with water, bp_{760} 120.3°, which contains 55 mole-% (68.5 weight-%) N_2H_4. LD_{50} in mice (mg/kg): 57 i.v.; 59 orally (Witkin).

Dihydrochloride. [5341-61-7] $H_4N_2\cdot 2HCl$. White crystalline powder, mp 198°. d 1.42. Freely sol in water, slightly in alcohol.

Caution: Potential symptoms of overexposure to hydrazine are irritation of eyes, skin, nose and throat; temporary blindness; dizziness, nausea; dermatitis; burns skin and eyes. *See NIOSH Pocket Guide to Chemical Hazards* (DHHS/NIOSH 97-140, 1997) p 166. *See also Patty's Industrial Hygiene and Toxicology* vol. **2E**, G. D. Clayton, F. E. Clayton, Eds. (John Wiley & Sons, Inc., New York, 4th ed., 1994) pp 3435-3441. Hydrazine is reasonably anticipated to be a human carcinogen: *Report on Carcinogens, Eleventh Edition* (PB2005-104914, 2004) p III-145.

USE: Chemical intermediate in manuf of agricultural chemicals, spandex fibers and antioxidants. Reducing agent; organic hydrazine derivs; rocket fuel. Dihydrochloride as chlorine scavenger for HCl gas streams.

4771. Hydrazine Hydrate. [7803-57-8] H_6N_2O; mol wt 50.06. H 12.08%, N 55.96%, O 31.96%. $H_2NNH_2\cdot H_2O$. Prepd

from hydrazine sulfate by the action of NaOH, followed by distn under nitrogen.

Fuming refractive liquid, faint characteristic odor. *Violent poison!* d^{21} 1.03. mp −51.7° or below −65° (two eutectics). bp_{740} 118-119°; bp_{26} 47°. n_D^{20} 1.42842. Strong base, very corrosive, attacks glass, rubber, cork, but not stainless V_2A steel or Allegheny stainless 304 and 347. Molybdenum steels such as Allegheny stainless 316 should not be used. Very powerful reducing agent. Miscible with water and alcohol. Insol in chloroform and ether.

Mixture with methanol. C-Stuff.

Caution: Causes delayed eye irritation.

USE: Reducing agent, solvent for inorganic materials. Manuf "Helman" catalyst, consisting of 80% hydrazine hydrate, 19.5% ethanol, 0.5 to 0.05% copper, used to dec hydrogen peroxide in V-2 type rockets. Mixture with methanol as propellant for rocket engines.

4772. Hydrazine Sulfate. [10034-93-2] Hydrazinium sulfate; hydrazonium sulfate. $H_6N_2O_4S$; mol wt 130.12. H 4.65%, N 21.53%, O 49.18%, S 24.64%. $H_2NNH_2\cdot H_2SO_4$. Prepd by Raschig synthesis: $2NH_3\cdot aq + [Ca(OCl)_2/Na_2CO_3/colloid]$ and treatment with H_2SO_4. Starch, glue, or gelatin are used as colloids, and sodium hypochlorite may be used instead of bleaching powder: Adams, Brown, *Org. Synth.* **2**, 37 (1922); Audrieth, Nickles, *Inorg. Synth.* **1**, 90 (1939). Industrial prepn by the action of sodium hypochlorite on urea in the presence of NaOH: *BIOS Final Report* **369**; Moncrieff, *Manuf. Chem.* **18**, 177 (1947). Revised lab procedures: Pfeiffer, Simons, *Ber.* **80**, 127 (1947); Adams, Brown, *Org. Synth.* **coll. vol. I**, 2nd ed. (1941), p 309. Crystal structure: Nitta *et al., Acta Crystallogr.* **4**, 289 (1951); Jönsson, Hamilton, *ibid.* **26B**, 536 (1970). Review of activity and clinical studies in cancer cachexia: J. Gold, *Nutr. Cancer* **9**, 59-66 (1987).

Orthorhombic crystals. Glass-like plates or prisms. d 1.378: Curtis, Jay, *J. Prakt. Chem.* **39**, 39 (1889); d^7 2.016. mp 254°. Sol in about 33 parts water; freely sol in hot water. Insol in alcohol. pH of 0.2 molar aq soln 1.3.

Caution: This substance is reasonably anticipated to be a human carcinogen: *Report on Carcinogens, Eleventh Edition* (PB2005-104914, 2004) p III-145.

USE: In the gravimetric estimation of nickel, cobalt and cadmium; in the refining of rare metals; as antioxidant in soldering flux for light metals; as reducing agent in the analysis of minerals and slags; in separating polonium from tellurium; in tests for blood; for destroying fungi and molds; in the prepn of hydrazine hydrate.

4773. 4-Hydrazinobenzenesulfonic Acid. [98-71-5] *p*-Sulfophenylhydrazine; phenylhydrazine-*p*-sulfonic acid. $C_6H_8N_2O_3$-S; mol wt 188.20. C 38.29%, H 4.28%, N 14.88%, O 25.50%, S 17.04%. Prepn by sulfonation of phenylhydrazine: L. Claisen, P. Roosen, *Ann.* **278**, 296 (1894); by the reduction of *p*-diazobenzenesulfonic acid: Th. Zincke, A. Kuchenbecker, *Ann.* **330**, 1 (1903); L. V. Lazeeva *et al.,* SU 1057493 (1983 to Tambov Pigment), *C.A.* **100**, 138755q (1984). Used in resoln of 2-pyrazoline cmpds: M. Mukai *et al., Can. J. Chem.* **57**, 360 (1979); in isoln of volatile ketones: W. Treibs, H. Röhnert, *Ber.* **84**, 433 (1951); in analysis of trace amounts of selenium: T. Kawashima *et al., Anal. Chim. Acta* **49**, 443 (1970); *eidem, ibid.* **89**, 65 (1977).

Needles from water, mp 286°. Slightly sol in water, alcohol.

4774. Hydrazoic Acid. [7782-79-8] Hydrogen azide; hydronitric acid; triazoic acid; stickstoffwasserstoffsäure (German). HN_3; mol wt 43.03. H 2.34%, N 97.65%. Produced by the action of sulfuric acid on sodium azide: L. F. Audrieth, C. F. Gibbs, *Inorg. Synth.* **7** (1939); using stearic acid: Günther, Meyer, *Z. Elektrochem.* **41**, 541 (1935). Prepn of water and ether solns of hydrazoic acid: W. S. Frost *et al., J. Am. Chem. Soc.* **55**, 3516 (1933); L. F. Audrieth, C. F. Gibbs, *loc. cit.;* P. W. Schenk in *Handbook of Preparative Inorganic Chemistry* vol. 1, G. Brauer, Ed. (Academic Press, New York, 2nd ed., 1963) pp 472-474. GC determn: J. M. Zehner, R.A. Simonaitis, *J. Chromatogr. Sci.* **14**, 493 (1976). Toxicity study: Graham *et al., J. Ind. Hyg. Toxicol.* **30**, 98 (1948).

Review of toxicology: C. F. Reinhardt, M. R. Brittelli, in *Patty's Industrial Hygiene and Toxicology* Vol. 2A, G. D. Clayton, F. E. Clayton, Eds. (Wiley-Interscience, New York, 1981) pp 2779-2784. *Reviews:* Mason in *Mellor's* vol. **VIII**, suppl. II, *Nitrogen* (part II), 1-15 (1967); Jones in *Comprehensive Inorganic Chemistry* vol. 2, J. C. Bailar Jr. *et al.,* Eds. (Pergamon Press, Oxford, 1973) pp 276-293.

Mobile liquid. Intolerable pungent odor. *Extremely explosive!* mp −80°. bp 37°. pKa 4.72. LD$_{50}$ in mice (mg/kg): 21.5 i.p. (Graham).

Caution: Acute exposure: eye irritation, cough, headache, fall in blood pressure, weakness, collapse. *Chronic exposure:* hypotension, weakness, palpitation, ataxia (Graham).

USE: Industrially in prepn of heavy metal azides for shell detonators.

4775. Hydrindantin. [5103-42-4] 2,2′-Dihydroxy-[2,2′-bi-1*H*-indene]-1,1′,3,3′-(2*H*,2′*H*)-tetrone; 2,2′-dihydroxy-[2,2′-biindan]-1,1′,3,3′-tetrone; reduced ninhydrin. C$_{18}$H$_{10}$O$_6$; mol wt 322.27. C 67.08%, H 3.13%, O 29.79%. Formed by the action of potassium cyanide on ninhydrin: Bruice, Richards, *J. Org. Chem.* **23,** 145 (1958). Convenient prepn by reduction of ninhydrin with ascorbic acid: Moore, Stein, *J. Biol. Chem.* **211,** 907 (1954).

Dihydrate. Prisms from acetone, anhyd at 100°, turns reddish-brown at 200°, dec 249-254°. Very sparingly sol in hot water; sol in Methyl Cellosolve. Sol with decompn in aq Na$_2$CO$_3$ solns (deep red color), and in NaOH solns (deep blue color). Can be precipitated from carbonate solns by the addn of acid. Deep purple color with ammonia and blue color with amino acids.

USE: Reagent for the photometric determination of amino acids and similar compds.

4776. Hydriodic Acid. [10034-85-2] HI; mol wt 127.91. A soln of hydrogen iodide in water. Marketed in various concns, *e.g.,* 57% HI, d 1.7; 47%, d 1.5; 10%, d 1.1. Prepd by absorption of hydrogen iodide gas in water or by the action of iodine on hydrogen sulfide according to the eq H$_2$S + I$_2$ → 2HI + S: Heisig, Frykholm, *Inorg. Synth.* **1,** 157 (1939). *See also* Hydrogen Iodide.

Colorless when freshly made, but rapidly turns yellowish or brown on exposure to light and air. This discoloration can be prevented by the addition of about 1.5% hypophosphorous acid (H$_3$-PO$_2$). Concd solns that have been stored for some time are usually opaque from oxidation, they may be regenerated with hypophosphorous acid: Foster, Nahas, Jr., *Inorg. Synth.* **2,** 210 (1946). *Keep protected from light and air, preferably not above 30°.* Miscible with water or alcohol. Dissolves iodine. The azeotrope (constant-boiling acid) bp$_{760}$ 127°, d 1.70, contains 56.9% HI. Strong, corrosive acid, attacks natural rubber. 0.1 molar soln, pH 1.0.

Caution: Strong irritant.

USE: Reducing agent, manuf of inorganic iodides, pharmaceuticals, disinfectants. The 57% acid is also used for analytical purposes, such as methoxyl determinations.

THERAP CAT: Expectorant.

4777. Hydrobenzoin. [492-70-6] 1,2-Diphenyl-1,2-ethanediol; diphenylethyleneglycol. C$_{14}$H$_{14}$O$_2$; mol wt 214.26. C 78.48%, H 6.59%, O 14.93%. Prepn of *d-, l-, dl-* and *meso-*forms: Forst, Zincke, *Ann.* **182,** 262, 275 (1876); Irvine, Weir, *J. Chem. Soc.* **91,** 1390 (1907); Buck, Jenkins, *J. Am. Chem. Soc.* **51,** 2163 (1929); L. F. Fieser, *Organic Experiments* (D. C. Heath, Boston, 1964) pp 210, 214, 216-217, 229-231. Improved method for prepn of *dl-*form from the *meso* isomer: Collet, *Synthesis* **1973,** 664.

*dl-*Form. Crystals from ether + petr ether, mp 120°. Resolved into *d-* and *l-*forms by slow, repeated crystallizations from ether.

*d-*Form. [α]$_D^{20}$ +97.6° (chloroform).

*l-*Form. [α]$_D^{20}$ −97.0° (chloroform).

*meso-*Form. Monoclinic leaflets from alcohol or water, mp 139°. Soly in water: 0.25% at 20°, 1.25% at 100°. Freely sol in hot alcohol, chloroform. Infrared absorption (chloroform): 2.82, 2.96μ. Dipole moment 2.67.

4778. Hydrobromic Acid. [10035-10-6] HBr; mol wt 80.91. A soln of hydrogen bromide gas in water. Marketed in various concns, e.g., 50% HBr, d 1.517; 40% HBr, d 1.38; 34%, d 1.31; 10%, d 1.08. Lab prepn according to the eq H$_2$SO$_4$ + KBr → KHSO$_4$ + HBr: Heisig, Amdur, *Inorg. Synth.* **1,** 155 (1939). *See also* Hydrogen Bromide.

Colorless or faintly yellow; slowly darkens on exposure to air and light. Miscible with water, alcohol. *Keep protected from light.* When dil hydrobromic acid is distilled, a weaker acid comes over first and when a very concd acid is boiled, HBr gas chiefly distills over first; in both cases a "constant boiling" acid contg about 47.5% HBr remains which distills unchanged at 126°. The bp and compn of the azeotrope varies with pressure: at 100 mm, bp 74.12°, compn 49.80% HBr; at 400 mm, bp 107.00°, compn 48.47%; at 700 mm, bp 122°, compn 47.74%; at 800 mm, bp 125.79°, compn 47.56%: Bonner *et al., J. Am. Chem. Soc.* **55,** 1406 (1933). Aq solns are strongly acid. The satd aq soln contains 68.85% HBr at 0° and 66% at 25°.

Caution: Strong irritant.

USE: The concd acid is used principally in analytical chemistry and organic prepns.

THERAP CAT: Sedative.

THERAP CAT (VET): Has been used as a sedative.

4779. Hydrocarbostyril. [553-03-7] 3,4-Dihydro-2(1*H*)-quinolinone; 3,4-dihydrocarbostyril; 3,4-dihydro-2-quinolinol; *o*-aminohydrocinnamic acid lactam; 2-oxo-1,2,3,4-tetrahydroquinoline; dihydro-α-quinolone. C$_9$H$_9$NO; mol wt 147.17. C 73.45%, H 6.16%, N 9.52%, O 10.87%. Prepd by the catalytic reduction of *o*-nitrocinnamic acid: Blout, Silverman, *J. Am. Chem. Soc.* **66,** 1442 (1944).

Prisms from methanol + water, mp 165-166.5°. Freely sol in alcohol, ether, dimethylformamide. Practically insol in water. Sol in hot aq NaOH solns.

4780. Hydrochloric Acid. [7647-01-0] Muriatic acid. HCl; mol wt 36.46. A soln of hydrogen chloride gas (HCl) in water. Prepn and reviews: *see* Hydrogen Chloride.

Fumes in air. May be colored yellow by traces of iron, chlorine, and organic matter. Reagent grade concd hydrochloric acid contains close to 38.0% HCl. 83 ml of concd HCl poured into sufficient water to make 1 liter yields approx 1.0*N* HCl. The pH of 1.0*N* HCl is 0.10; of 0.1*N* = 1.10; of 0.01*N* = 2.02; of 0.001*N* = 3.02; of 0.0001*N* = 4.01. n_D^{18} (1.0*N* soln) 1.34168. d$_4^{15}$ 1.05 (10.17% w/w soln); 1.10 (20%); 1.15 (29.57%); 1.20 (39.11%). Freezing pt: −17.14° (10.81% soln); −62.25° (20.69%); −46.2° (31.24%); −25.4° (39.17%), Gmelins, Chlorine (8th ed.) **6,** 136-137 (1927). Constant boiling azeotrope with water bp$_{760}$ 108.58° contg 20.22% HCl, d$_4^{15}$ 1.096. Boiling weaker or stronger aq solns results in loss of either component until the constant boiling acid is obtained.

Caution: Corrosive burns may result from the inhalation of acid fumes and from skin contact with or the ingestion of strong acid. Symptoms after ingestion or skin contact include immediate pain and ulceration of all membranes and tissues which come in contact with the acid. Ingestion may be associated with nausea, vomiting and intense thirst; corrosion of the stomach may lead within a few hours or a few days to gastric perforation and peritonitis. Late esophageal, gastric and pyloric strictures and stenoses should be anticipated. Contact of conc acid with the eye can cause extensive necrosis of the conjunctiva and corneal epithelium, resulting in perforation or opaque scarring. Chemical pneumonitis can be expected after respiratory exposure to acid vapors or after tracheo-bronchial aspiration of ingested acid. Death may occur due to complications such as circulatory shock, asphyxia due to glottic or laryngeal edema, perforation of the stomach with peritonitis, gastic hemorrhage, infection or anition due to stricture formation. *See: Clinical Toxicology of Commercial Products*, R. E. Gosselin *et al.*, Eds. (Williams & Wilkins, Baltimore, 5th ed., 1984) Section III, pp 8-11.

USE: In the production of chlorides; refining ore in the production of tin and tantalum; for the neutralization of basic systems; as laboratory reagent; hydrolyzing of starch and proteins in the prepn of various food products; pickling and cleaning of metal products; as catalyst and solvent in organic syntheses. Also used for oil- and gas-well treatment and in removing scale from boilers and heat-exchange equipment. Pharmaceutic aid (acidifier).

THERAP CAT (VET): Has been used as gastric acidifier.

4781. Hydrochlorothiazide. [58-93-5] 6-Chloro-3,4-dihydro-2*H*-1,2,4-benzothiadiazine-7-sulfonamide 1,1-dioxide; 6-chloro-3,4-dihydro-7-sulfamoyl-2*H*-1,2,4-benzothiadiazine 1,1-dioxide; 6-chloro-7-sulfamyl-3,4-dihydro-1,2,4-benzothiadiazine 1,1-dioxide; 3,4-dihydrochlorothiazide; chlorsulfonamidodihydrobenzothiadiazine dioxide; chlorosulthiadil; Aquarius; Bremil; Cidrex; Dichlorosal; Dichlotride; Diclotride; Direma; Diu-melusin; Disalunil; Esidrex; Esidrix; Fluvin; Hidroronol; Hydril; Hydro-Aquil; Hydro-Diuril; Hydrosaluric; Hydrothide; Hydrozide; Hypothiazide; Ivaugan; Maschitt; Nefrix; Neo-Codema; Neoflumen; Oretic; Panurin; Thiaretic; Thiuretic; Urodiazin. $C_7H_8ClN_3O_4S_2$; mol wt 297.74. C 28.24%, H 2.71%, Cl 11.91%, N 14.11%, O 21.49%, S 21.54%. Prepn: de Stevens *et al.*, *Experientia* **14**, 463 (1958); Werner *et al.*, *J. Am. Chem. Soc.* **82**, 1161 (1960); Jones, Novello, **US 3025292** (1962 to Merck & Co.); de Stevens, Werner, **US 3163645** (1964 to Ciba); Klosa, **DE 1163332** (1964); J. S. Irons, T. M. Cook, **US 3164588** (1965 to Merck & Co.). Purification: Downing, **US 3043840** (1962 to Merck & Co.). Toxicity data: J. J. Piala *et al.*, *J. Pharmacol. Exp. Ther.* **134**, 273 (1961). Comprehensive description: H. P. Deppeler, *Anal. Profiles Drug Subs.* **10**, 405-441 (1981).

Crystals, mp 273-275°. uv max (methanol + trace HCl): 317, 271, 226 nm ($A_{1cm}^{1\%}$ 130, 654, 1280). pKa 7.9, 9.2. Sol in dil ammonia, or sodium hydroxide; also sol in methanol, ethanol, acetone. Practically insol in water. LD_{50} in mice (mg/kg): 590 i.v.; >8000 orally (Piala).

THERAP CAT: Diuretic.

THERAP CAT (VET): Diuretic.

4782. Hydrocinchonidine. [485-64-3] (8α,9R)-10,11-Dihydrocinchonan-9-ol; (−)-dihydrocinchonidine; cinchamidine. $C_{19}H_{24}N_2O$; mol wt 296.41. C 76.99%, H 8.16%, N 9.45%, O 5.40%. Found in cinchona barks: Forst, Böhringer, *Ber.* **14**, 1270 (1881); Hesse, *ibid.* 1683; *idem*, *Ann.* **214**, 1 (1882); Skita, Nord, *Ber.* **45**, 3312 (1912); Heidelberger, Jacobs, *J. Am. Chem. Soc.* **41**, 817 (1919). Configuration: Ochiai *et al.*, *J. Pharm. Soc. Jpn.* **67**, 211 (1947). Stereospecific synthesis from secologanin: R. T. Brown, D. Curless, *Tetrahedron Lett.* **27**, 6005 (1986). Total synthesis: M. Ihara *et al.*, *J. Chem. Soc. Perkin Trans. 1* **1988**, 1277. Stereoisomer of hydrocinchonine, *q.v.*

Needles or leaflets, mp 230°. $[\alpha]_D^{15}$ −98° (alcohol). Practically insol in water. Sol in alcohol, chloroform; slightly sol in ether.

4783. Hydrocinchonine. [485-65-4] (9S)-10,11-Dihydrocinchonan-9-ol; cinchotine; cinconifine; (+)-dihydrocinchonine; pseudocinchonine. $C_{19}H_{24}N_2O$; mol wt 296.41. C 76.99%, H 8.16%, N 9.45%, O 5.40%. From cinchona barks: Caventou, Willm, *Compt. Rend.* **69**, 284 (1869). Prepn from cinchonine: Hesse, *Ann.* **300**, 46 (1898); Pum, *Monatsh. Chem.* **16**, 68 (1895); Arlt, *ibid.* **20**, 426, 439 (1899); Heidelberger, Jacobs, *J. Am. Chem. Soc.* **41**, 817 (1919). Structure: Rabe, *Ber.* **55**, 522 (1922). Conversion of hydroquinidine to hydrocinchonine: King, *J. Chem. Soc.* **1946**, 523. HPLC determn: C.-T. A. Chung, E. J. Staba, *J. Chromatogr.* **295**, 276 (1984). Stereospecific synthesis from secologanin: R. T. Brown, D. Curless, *Tetrahedron Lett.* **27**, 6005 (1986). Total synthesis: M. Ihara *et al.*, *J. Chem. Soc. Perkin Trans. 1* **1988**, 1277.

Prisms, mp 268-269°. $[\alpha]_D^{14}$ +204° (c = 0.6 in alc). Almost insol in water, ether. Sol in alcohol.

Hydrochloride. $C_{19}H_{24}N_2O \cdot HCl$. Crystals, mp 220-221°. $[\alpha]_D^{23}$ +155° (c = 0.8 in water).

4784. Hydrocinnamic Acid. [501-52-0] Benzenepropanoic acid; 3-phenylpropionic acid; β-phenylpropionic acid; benzylacetic acid. $C_9H_{10}O_2$; mol wt 150.17. C 71.98%, H 6.71%, O 21.31%. $C_6H_5CH_2CH_2COOH$. Prepn by reduction of cinnamic acid: Ingersoll, *Org. Synth.* **9**, 42 (1929); from propiophenone: Schwenk, Papa, *J. Org. Chem.* **11**, 798 (1946); by Mauer oxidation of 1-phenyl-3-propanol: Langenbeck, Richter, *Ber.* **89**, 202 (1956); by chromate oxidation of propylbenzene: Reitsema, Allphin, *J. Org. Chem.* **27**, 27 (1962).

White, cryst powder, mp 47-48°. bp 280°; bp_{75} 194-197°; bp_{18} 145-147°; bp_6 125-129°. Sol in 170 parts cold, more sol in hot water, in alcohol, benzene, chloroform, ether, glacial acetic acid, petr ether, carbon disulfide.

4785. Hydrocodone. [125-29-1] 4,5-Epoxy-3-methoxy-17-methylmorphinan-6-one; dihydrocodeinone; Bekadid; Dicodid. $C_{18}H_{21}NO_3$; mol wt 299.36. C 72.22%, H 7.07%, N 4.68%, O 16.03%. Prepn by hydrogenation of codeinone: Mannich, Löwenheim, *Arch. Pharm.* **258**, 295 (1920); by oxidation of dihydrocodeine, **DE 415097** (1925 to E. Merck), *Frdl.* **15**, 1518 (1925-1927); by catalytic rearrangement of codeine: **DE 623821**. Industrial prepn from dihydrocodeine: K. Pfister, M. Tishler, **US 2715626** (1955 to Merck & Co.). Pharmacology and toxicity data: N. B. Eddy, J. G. Reid, *J. Pharmacol. Exp. Ther.* **52**, 468 (1934). Brief description: A. Stein, *Pharmazie* **10**, 180 (1955). *Review:* Small, Lutz, "Chemistry of the Opium Alkaloids" in *U.S. Public Health Reports* **Suppl. No. 103** (Washington, 1932).

Prisms from alcohol, mp 198°. Sol in alcohol, dil acids. Insol in water. uv max: 280 nm (ε 1310). LD_{50} s.c. in mice: 85.7 mg/kg (Eddy, Reid).

Hydrochloride monohydrate. $C_{18}H_{21}NO_3.HCl.H_2O$. Crystals, mp 185-186° dec. $[\alpha]_D^{27}$ −130° (c = 2.877). Very sol in water.

Bitartrate hemipentahydrate. [34195-34-1] Calmodid; Codinovo; Duodin; Kolikodal; Orthoxycol; Mercodinone; Synkonin; Norgan; Hydrokon. $C_{18}H_{21}NO_3.C_4H_6O_6.2\tfrac{1}{2}H_2O$; mol wt 494.49. Needles, mp 118-128°. One gram dissolves in 16 ml water, in 150 g 95% ethanol. Almost insol in ether, chloroform. pH of a 2% aq soln about 3.6.

Hydriodide. $C_{18}H_{21}NO_3.HI$. mp 219-220°.
Methiodide. $C_{18}H_{21}NO_3.CH_3I$. mp 250-255°.

Note: This is a controlled substance (opiate): **21 CFR**, 1308.12.

THERAP CAT: Analgesic (narcotic); antitussive.

4786. Hydrocortamate. [76-47-1] *N,N*-Diethylglycine (11β)-11,17-dihydroxy-3,20-dioxopregn-4-en-21-yl ester; cortisol 21-ester with *N,N*-diethylglycine; cortisol 21-(*N,N*-diethyl)glycinate; hydrocortisone 21-diethylaminoacetate; Ulcort. $C_{27}H_{41}NO_6$; mol wt 475.62. C 68.18%, H 8.69%, N 2.94%, O 20.18%. Prepn: Pinson, Laubach, **DE 1016708** (1957 to Pfizer), *C.A.* **54**, 22737a (1960); Richter, Schenck, **DE 1037451** (1958 to Schering AG), *C.A.* **54**, 22730h (1960).

Crystals from ethyl acetate, mp 162-163°.

Hydrochloride. [125-03-1] Ethamicort; Magnacort. $C_{27}H_{41}NO_6.HCl$; mol wt 512.08. Crystals from ethyl acetate, dec 222°.

THERAP CAT: Glucocorticoid.

4787. Hydrocortisone. [50-23-7] (11β)-11,17,21-Trihydroxypregn-4-ene-3,20-dione; cortisol; 4-pregnene-11β,17α,21-triol-3,20-dione; 17-hydroxycorticosterone; anti-inflammatory hormone; Kendall's compound F; Reichstein's substance M; Aeroseb-HC; Ala-Cort; Anflam; Cetacort; Cort-Dome; Cortef; Cortenema; Cortril; Dermacort; Dermocortal; Dermolate; Dioderm; Efcortelan; Evacort; Ficortril; Hydracort; Hydro-Adreson; Hydrocort; Hydrocortisyl; Hydrocortone; Hytone; Lacticare-HC; Medicort; Mildison; Nutracort; Penecort; Proctocort; Scheroson F; Synacort; Texacort; Timocort; Zenoxone. $C_{21}H_{30}O_5$; mol wt 362.46. C 69.59%, H 8.34%, O 22.07%. Principal glucocorticoid hormone produced by the adrenal cortex. Biosynthesis stimulated by ACTH, *q.v.* Circulates in plasma primarily bound to *corticosteroid-binding globulin*, also known as *transcortin*, and to albumin. Isoln from adrenal glands: Reichstein, *Helv. Chim. Acta* **20**, 953 (1937); Mason *et al., J. Biol. Chem.* **124**, 459 (1938); from urine: Mason, Sprague, *ibid.* **175**, 451 (1948); from blood: Reich *et al., ibid.* **187**, 411 (1950). Configuration: von Euw, Reichstein, *Helv. Chim. Acta* **25**, 988 (1942); **30**, 205 (1947). Synthesis: N. L. Wendler *et al., J. Am. Chem. Soc.* **72**, 5793 (1950). Biosynthesis by isolated adrenal glands: O. Hechter *et al., Arch. Biochem. Biophys.* **25**, 457 (1950); A. Zaffaroni *et al., J. Am. Chem. Soc.* **73**, 1390 (1951). Prepn by microbial transformation: H. C. Murray, D. H. Peterson, **US 2602769** (1952 to Upjohn); D. R. Colingsworth *et al., J. Biol. Chem.* **203**, 807 (1953). Total biosynthesis in yeast: F. M. Szczebara *et al., Nat. Biotechnol.* **21**, 143 (2003). Comprehensive description: K. Florey, *Anal. Profiles Drug Subs.* **12**, 277-324 (1983). Review of clinical use in dermatoses: A. M. Kligman, K. H. Kaidbey, *Cutis* **22**, 232-244 (1978). Review of clinical assays in serum and urine: A. Moore *et al., Ann. Clin. Biochem.* **22**, 435-454 (1985). Physiological role in immunity: W. M. Jefferies, *Med. Hypotheses* **34**, 198-208 (1991); in fetal maturation: G. C. Liggins, *Reprod. Fertil. Dev.* **6**, 141-150 (1994).

Bitter-tasting crystalline, striated blocks from abs ethanol or isopropanol, mp 217-220° with some decompn. $[\alpha]_D^{22}$ +167° (abs ethanol). uv max: 242 nm ($E_{1cm}^{1\%}$ 445). Soly (mg/ml) at 25°: water 0.28; ethanol 15.0; methanol 6.2; acetone 9.3; chloroform 1.6; propylene glycol 12.7; ether about 0.35. Sol in concd sulfuric acid with intense green fluorescence.

21-Acetate. [50-03-3] Colifoam; Colofoam; Cortaid; Cordes; Cortifoam; Hc45; Hydrocal; Hydrocortistab; Lanacort; Lenirit; Sigmacort; Sintotrat; Velopural. $C_{23}H_{32}O_6$; mol wt 404.50. Monoclinic, sphenoidal, tabular crystals from dil acetone. Tasteless. d_4^{20} 1.289; dec 223°. $[\alpha]_D^{25}$ +166° (c = 0.4 in dioxane); $[\alpha]_D^{25}$ +150.7° (c = 0.5 in acetone). uv max (methanol): 242 nm ($E_{1cm}^{1\%}$ 390). Somewhat hygroscopic. Soly in water: 1 mg/100 ml; in ethanol: 0.45 g/100 ml; in methanol: 3.9 mg/ml; in acetone: 1.1 mg/g; in ether: 0.15 mg/ml. One gram dissolves in about 200 ml chloroform. Very sol in DMF; sol in dioxane.

17-Butyrate. [13609-67-1] Alfason; Laticort; Locoid; Plancol. $C_{25}H_{36}O_6$; mol wt 432.55.

21-Phosphate disodium salt. [6000-74-4] Hydrocortisone sodium phosphate; Cleiton; Efcortesol. $C_{21}H_{29}Na_2O_8P$; mol wt 486.40. White powder. uv max (methanol): 242 nm ($A_{1cm}^{1\%}$ 298-341). $[\alpha]_D^{25}$ +120° (H_2O). Soly in water (25°): >500 mg/ml. pH of a 1% aq soln: 7.5-8.5.

21-Sodium succinate. [125-04-2] Hydrocortisone hemisuccinate sodium salt; A-hydroCort; Buccalsone; Corlan; Efcortelan Soluble; Saxizon; Solu-Cortef; Solu-Glyc. $C_{25}H_{33}NaO_8$; mol wt 484.51. Amorphous, hygroscopic, white powder, mp 169.0-171.2°. Soly in water: ~500 mg/ml. Similarly sol in methanol, ethanol; sparingly sol in chloroform.

17-Valerate. [57524-89-7] Hydrocortisone valerate; Westcort. $C_{26}H_{38}O_6$; mol wt 446.58.

THERAP CAT: Glucocorticoid.
THERAP CAT (VET): Glucocorticoid.

4788. Hydrocotarnine. [550-10-7] 5,6,7,8-Tetrahydro-4-methoxy-6-methyl-1,3-dioxolo[4,5-g]isoquinoline; 8-methoxy-5,6-methylenedioxy-2-methyl-1,2,3,4-tetrahydroisoquinoline. $C_{12}H_{15}NO_3$; mol wt 221.25. C 65.14%, H 6.83%, N 6.33%, O 21.69%. Found in mother liquors from morphine extraction. It is not certain whether it is formed from narcotine during the extraction or whether it exists in the poppy plant. May also be prepd by reduction of cotarnine: Topchiev, *J. Appl. Chem. USSR* **6**, 529 (1933), *C.A.* **28**, 2718 (1934); Schneider, Müller, *Ann.* **615**, 34 (1958); Knabe, *Arch. Pharm.* **292**, 652 (1959). Reduction of hydrocotarnine with sodium in alcohol leads to replacement of the methoxyl group by hydrogen, with formation of hydrohydrastinine. Review and bibliography: Small, Lutz, "Chemistry of the Opium Alkaloids," Suppl. No. 103, *Public Health Reports,* Washington (1932).

Hemihydrate. Plates from petr ether, mp 56°. Loses water of crystn at 60°. May be distilled with little decompn at 100°: Hesse, *Ber.* **4**, 693 (1871). Absorption spectrum: Hantzsch, *Ber.* **44**, 1816 (1911); Steiner, *Compt. Rend.* **176**, 244, 1379 (1923); Csokán, *Z. Anal. Chem.* **124**, 344 (1942). Almost insol in water, alkaline solns; sol in alcohol, acetone, chloroform, benzene, ether.

Hydrochloride monohydrate. Prisms; sol in water.
Hydrobromide. Crystals, mp 237°; sparingly sol in water.
Hydriodide. Needles from methanol, mp 196°; sol in hot water.
Methiodide. Needles from water, plates from alc, mp 206°.
Methobromide. Needles from chloroform, dec 221°.

4789. Hydroflumethiazide. [135-09-1] 3,4-Dihydro-6-(tri-fluoromethyl)-2*H*-1,2,4-benzothiadiazine-7-sulfonamide 1,1-diox-ide; 6-trifluoromethyl-3,4-dihydro-7-sulfamoyl-2*H*-1,2,4-benzo-thiadiazine 1,1-dioxide; 3,4-dihydro-7-sulfamyl-6-trifluoromethyl-1,2,4-benzothiadiazine 1,1-dioxide; trifluoromethylhydrothiazide; dihydroflumethiazide; methforylthiazidine; metflorylthiazidine; Diucardin; Elodrine; Finuret; Hydol; Hydrenox; Leodrine; NaClex; Rodiuran; Rontyl; Saluron; Sisuril; Vergonil. $C_8H_8F_3N_3O_4S_2$; mol wt 331.29. C 29.00%, H 2.43%, F 17.20%, N 12.68%, O 19.32%, S 19.36%. Synthesis: Holdrege et al., *J. Am. Chem. Soc.* **81**, 4807 (1959); Close et al., *ibid.* **82**, 1132 (1960); Yale et al., *ibid.* 2042; Novello et al., *J. Org. Chem.* **25**, 970 (1960). Numerous patents, e.g., Lund et al., US 3254076 (1966 to Lövens Kemiske Fabrik). Pharmacology: J. J. Piala et al., *J. Pharmacol. Exp. Ther.* **134**, 273 (1961). Comprehensive description: C. E. Orzech et al., *Anal. Profiles Drug Subs.* **7**, 297-317 (1978).

Crystals, mp 272-273°. uv max (methanol): 272.5 nm (log ε 4.286). Soly in mg/ml at 25°: acetone >100; methanol 58; aceto-nitrile 43; water 0.3; ether 0.2; benzene <0.1. pK_1 8.9; pK_2 10.7. Forms water-sol salts with bases. LD_{50} in mice (mg/kg): >8000 orally, 750 i.v., 6280 i.p. (Piala).

THERAP CAT: Antihypertensive; diuretic.

4790. Hydrofluoric Acid. [7664-39-3] Fluohydric acid. HF; mol wt 20.01. Soln of hydrogen fluoride gas in water. Ob-tained by distilling calcium fluoride with H_2SO_4. Vapor pressure data: Brosheer et al., *Ind. Eng. Chem.* **39**, 423 (1947). Compn of liq and vapor: Munter et al., *ibid.* 427. Review of toxicology and human exposure: *Toxicological Profile for Fluorides, Hydrogen Fluoride, and Fluorine* (PB2004-100002, 2003) 404 pp. *See also* Hydrogen Fluoride.

Colorless or almost colorless, fuming liquid. *Poisonous! Han-dle with care.* Miscible with water. Weak acid: pKa 3.19. The 38.2% (w/w HF) soln is a binary azeotrope; bp 112.2°. Attacks glass or stoneware, dissolving the silica. *Keep in plastic, lead, wax, or paraffin paper bottles.* Has been marketed in concns of about 47% and 53%. d 1.15-1.18.

Caution: Potential symptoms of overexposure are pulmonary edema, skin and eye burns, rhinitis, bronchitis, bone changes. Direct contact may cause irritation of eyes, skin, nose and throat. *See NIOSH Pocket Guide to Chemical Hazards* (DHHS/NIOSH 97-140, 2003) p 168. *See also Patty's Industrial Hygiene and Toxicol-ogy* vol. 2B, G. D. Clayton, F. E. Clayton, Eds. (Wiley-Interscience, New York, 3rd ed., 1981) pp 2945-2948.

USE: Cleaning cast iron, copper, brass; removing efflorescence from brick and stone, or sand particles from metallic castings; working over too heavily weighted silks; frosting, etching glass and enamel; polishing crystal glass; decomposing cellulose; enam-eling and galvanizing iron; increasing porosity of ceramics. Its salts are used as insecticides and to arrest undesirable fermentation in brewing. Also used in analytical work to determine SiO_2, etc.

4791. Hydrofuramide. [494-47-3] 1-(2-Furanyl)-*N,N'*-bis(2-furanylmethylene)methanediamine; *N,N'*-difurfurylidene-2-furanmethanediamine; furfuramide. $C_{15}H_{12}N_2O_3$; mol wt 268.27. C 67.16%, H 4.51%, N 10.44%, O 17.89%. Prepn: Hartley, Dobbie, *J. Chem. Soc.* **73**, 598 (1898); Taniyama, *J. Chem. Soc. Jpn. Ind. Chem. Sect.* **51**, 33 (1948); Kapur et al., *J. Sci. Ind. Res.* **19B**, 509 (1960); Kamal et al., *Tetrahedron* **19**, 869 (1963). Structure: Soundararajan, Anantakrishnan, *Proc. Indian Acad. Sci.* **38A**, 176 (1953).

Brownish crystals from abs alcohol, mp 117°. bp ~250° with decompn. uv max: 259, 215 nm (log ε 4.18, 4.16). Practically insol in water; freely sol in alc, ether; readily dec by acids.

USE: Vulcanization accelerator.

4792. Hydrogen. [1333-74-0] Protium. H; at. wt 1.00794; at. no. 1; valence 1. Group IA (1). Elemental state: H_2. Exists in two forms, distinguished by the nuclear spins of the atoms: *ortho* has parallel spins, *para* has antiparallel spins. Normal hydrogen is a 3:1 equilibrium ratio of *ortho* to *para* at rm temp. Naturally occur-ring isotopes: 1 (protium 99.985%); 2 (deuterium 0.015%); 3 (tritium, traces only). The most abundant element in the known universe. Occurrence in the earth's atmosphere 0.00005% H_2. First recognized as an element by Cavendish in 1766; named by Lavoisier. Obtained by passing H_2O vapors over heated iron; by electrolysis of water or by action of HCl or H_2SO_4 on Fe or Zn; by hydrolysis of metal hydrides. Produced industrially by steam re-forming, partial oxidation, coal gasification and water electrolysis. *Reviews: Nouveau Traité de Chimie Minérale* vol. 1, P. Pascal, Ed. (Masson, Paris, 1956) pp 565-675; Mackay in *Comprehensive In-organic Chemistry* vol. 1, J. C. Bailar, Jr. et al., Eds. (Pergamon Press, Oxford, 1973) pp 1-76; *Chemistry of the Elements* N. N. Greenwood, A. Earnshaw, Eds. (Pergamon Press, New York, 1984) pp 38-74; T. A. Czuppon et al. in *Kirk-Othmer Encyclopedia of Chemical Technology* vol. **13** (Wiley-Interscience, New York, 4th ed., 1995) pp 838-894. *See also* Deuterium and Tritium.

Colorless, odorless, tasteless gas; flammable or explosive when mixed with air, oxygen, chlorine, etc. mp -259.2° (13.96 K) at 54 mm (triple point). bp -252.77° (20.39 K). d_{gas} 0.069 (air = 1); d_{liq} 0.0700 (at bp); d_{sol} 0.0763 (13 K). A liter of the gas at 0° weighs 0.08987 g. Crit. temp -239.9°; crit press. 12.8 atm. Sol in about 50 vols of water at 0°. Ionization potential of H atom 13.59 eV.

Caution: Can act as an asphyxiant by displacing air. *See: Matheson Gas Data Book* (Matheson, 6th ed., Lyndhurst, NJ, 1980) pp 366-371.

USE: In oxy-hydrogen blowpipe (welding) and limelight; autog-enous welding of steel and other metals; manuf ammonia, synthetic methanol, HCl, NH_3; hydrogenation of oils, fats, naphthalene, phe-nol; in balloons and airships; in metallurgy to reduce oxides to metals; in petroleum refining; in thermonuclear reactions (ionizes to form protons, deuterons (D) or tritons (T)). Liq hydrogen used in bubble chambers to study subatomic particles; as a coolant.

4793. Hydrogen Bromide. [10035-10-6] Anhydrous hydro-bromic acid. BrH; mol wt 80.91. Br 98.76%, H 1.25%. HBr. Prepd commercially by direct combination of the elements at 375° preferably over a catalyst such as platinized silica gel or platinized asbestos: Richards, Hönigschmid, *J. Am. Chem. Soc.* **32**, 1581 (1910); Smyth, Hitchcock, *ibid.* **55**, 1830 (1933); Schneider, John-son, *Inorg. Synth.* **1**, 152 (1939). Lab procedure from tetrahydro-naphthalene and bromine: Müller, *Monatsh. Chem.* **49**, 29 (1928); Duncan, *Inorg. Synth.* **1**, 151 (1939); Schmeisser in *Handbook of Preparative Inorganic Chemistry* vol. **1**, G. Brauer, Ed. (Academic Press, New York, 2nd ed., 1963) pp 282-286. Detailed description of laboratory methods of prepn: Houben-Weyl, *Methoden der or-ganischen Chemie* vol 5/4 (Thieme, Stuttgart, 4th ed., 1960) p 16-20. Review of prepn and properties of HBr and other hydrogen halides: Woolf in *Mellor's* vol. II, Suppl I (originally published as Suppl II, part 1) 724-741 (1956); John in *Bromine and its Com-pounds*, Z. E. Jolles, Ed. (Ernest Benn, London, 1966) pp 81-105; Downs, Adams in *Comprehensive Inorganic Chemistry* vol. **2**, J. C. Bailar, Jr. et al., Eds. (Pergamon Press, Oxford, 1973) pp 1280-1329.

Colorless, corrosive, nonflammable gas. Acrid odor. Fumes in moist air forming clouds which have a sour taste. d 2.71 (air = 1.00). mp -86.9°. bp$_{760}$ -66.8°; bp$_{11.0 atm}$ -4.8°; bp$_{17.1 atm}$ 12°; bp$_{30.0 atm}$ 36°; bp$_{59.2 atm}$ 70°. Crit temp 89.8°; crit press. 84.5 atm. Sp heat (cal/g/°C): solid (-91°) 0.152; liq 0.176; gas (27°) 0.085. Heat of fusion at mp: 7.44 cal/g. Heat of vaporization at bp: 51.3 cal/g. Freely sol in water: One vol H_2O dissolves 600 vols HBr gas at 0°. Also sol in alc. Soly in organic solvents: Fernandes, *J. Chem. Eng. Data* **17**, 377 (1972); Gerrard, *Chem. Ind. (London)* **1969**, 295; Ahmed et al., *J. Appl. Chem.* **20**, 109 (1970). Aq solns are strongly acid. The satd aq soln contains 68.85% HBr at 0° and 66% at 25°. The boiling point of a constant-boiling mixture is 122.5° at 740 mm and 126° at 760 mm. The composition of the constant-boiling mixture is 47.38% HBr at 752 mm. For complete tables *see* Bonner *et al., J. Am. Chem. Soc.* **55,** 1406 (1943). *See also* Hydrobromic Acid. Anhydr HBr is marketed in steel cylinders in the form of a gas over liquid. LC$_{50}$ in mice, rats: 814, 2858 ppm by inhalation, K. C. Back *et al., Reclassification of Materials Listed as Transportation Health Hazards* (TSA-20-72-3, PB 214-270, 1972).

Caution: Potential symptoms of overexposure are irritation of eyes, skin, nose and throat; direct contact with solutions may cause skin and eye burns; direct contact with liquid may cause frostbite. *See NIOSH Pocket Guide to Chemical Hazards* (DHHS/NIOSH 97-140, 1997) p 166.

USE: Mfg organic and inorganic bromides, hydrobromic acid, as reducing agent and as catalyst in controlled oxidations, in the alkylation of aromatic compds, in the isomerization of conjugated diolefins.

4794. Hydrogen Chloride. [7647-01-0] Anhydrous hydrochloric acid. ClH; mol wt 36.46. Cl 97.24%, H 2.76%. HCl. *See also* Hydrochloric Acid. Produced industrially by the interaction of NaCl and H$_2$SO$_4$; from NaCl, SO$_2$, air and water vapor; by controlled combination of the elements; or as a by-product of the synthesis of chlorinated hydrocarbons: A. C. Cumming, *Hydrochloric Acid and Salt Cake* (Gurney and Jackson, London, 1923); N. A. Laury, *Hydrochloric Acid and Sodium Sulfate* (Chem. Catalog Co., New York, 1927); Maude, *Chem. Eng. Prog.* **44,** 179 (1948); *Faith, Keyes & Clark's Industrial Chemicals,* F. A. Lowenheim, M. K. Moran, Eds. (Wiley-Interscience, New York, 4th ed., 1975) pp 454-461. Prepn of pure HCl for research purposes: Hönigschmid *et al., Z. Anorg. Allg. Chem.* **163,** 315 (1927); Kemp, *J. Chem. Educ.* **37,** 142 (1960); Schmeisser in *Handbook of Preparative Inorganic Chemistry* **vol. 1,** G. Brauer, Ed. (Academic Press, New York, 2nd ed., 1963) pp 280-282. Toxicity: K. I. Darmer *et al., Am. Ind. Hyg. Assoc. J.* **35,** 623 (1974). Reviews of prepn and properties: Addison, Lewis in *Mellor's* **vol. II,** suppl. I (originally published as suppl. II, part I) 402-475 (1956); Downs, Adams in *Comprehensive Inorganic Chemistry* **vol. 2,** J. C. Bailar, Jr. *et al.,* Eds. (Pergamon Press, Oxford, 1973) pp 1280-1329; D. S. Rosenberg in *Kirk-Othmer Encyclopedia of Chemical Technology* **vol. 12** (Wiley-Interscience, New York, 3rd ed., 1980) pp 983-1015.

Colorless, corrosive, nonflammable gas. Characteristic pungent odor. Fumes in air. d 1.268 (air = 1.000). d 1.639 g/l. mp −114.22°. bp$_{760}$ −85.05°; bp$_{100}$ −114.61°; bp$_{10}$ −137.77°; bp$_{1.0}$ −154.37°. Critical temp 51.4°; critical pressure 81.6 atm; critical density 0.42 g/ml. n_D^{20} (liquid under pressure) 1.256. Heat capacity at constant volume (15°): 0.1939 cal/g/°C. Heat capacity at constant pressure (15°): 0.1375 cal/g/°C. Heat of vaporization at −85°: 3860 cal/mole; heat of soln (infinite dilution) −17.88 kcal/mole; heat of formation of gas at 25°: −22.063 kcal/mole. Dielectric constant (gas at 0°) 1.0046; dipole moment 1.07. Soln in water (g/100 g H$_2$O): 82.3 (0°); 67.3 (30°); 63.3 (40°); 59.6 (50°); 56.1 (60°). Forms a const boiling mixture: 20.22 g/100 g soln; *see* Hydrochloric Acid. Soly in methanol (g/100 g soln): 54.6 (−10°); 51.3 (0°); 47.0 (20°); 43.0 (30°); in ethanol: 45.4 (0°); 42.7 (10°); 41.0 (20°); 38.1 (30°); in ether: 37.52 (−10°); 35.6 (0°); 24.9 (20°); 19.47 (30°). LC$_{50}$ (30 min) in mice, rats: 2142, 5666 ppm (Darmer).

Caution: Potential symptoms of overexposure are irritation of nose, throat and larynx; coughing, choking; dermatitis; direct contact with solutions may cause eye and skin burns; direct contact with liquid may cause frostbite. *See NIOSH Pocket Guide to Chemical Hazards* (DHHS/NIOSH 97-140, 1997) p 166. *See also Patty's Industrial Hygiene and Toxicology* **vol. 2B,** G. D. Clayton, F. E. Clayton, Eds. (Wiley-Interscience, New York, 3rd ed., 1981) pp 2959-2961.

USE: In the manuf of pharmaceutical hydrochlorides, vinyl chloride from acetylene, alkyl chlorides from olefins, and arsenious chloride from arsenious oxide. In the chlorination of rubber, as a gaseous flux for babbitting operations. In organic reactions involving isomerization, polymerization, and alkylation. For making chlorine where economical.

4795. Hydrogen Cyanide. [74-90-8] Hydrocyanic acid; prussic acid. CHN; mol wt 27.03. C 44.43%, H 3.73%, N 51.82%. HCN. Prepd on a large scale by the catalytic oxidation of ammonia-methane mixtures (Andrussow Process): *see* Andrussow, *Angew. Chem.* **48,** 593 (1935); Maffezzoni, *Chim. Ind. (Milan)*

34, 460 (1952); *Faith, Keyes & Clark's Industrial Chemicals,* F. A. Lowenheim, M. K. Moran, Ed. (Wiley-Interscience, New York, 4th ed., 1975) pp 482-486. Prepd in the lab by acidifying NaCN or K$_4$[Fe(CN)$_6$]: Glemser in *Handbook of Preparative Inorganic Chemistry* **vol. 1,** G. Brauer, Ed. (Academic Press, New York, 2nd ed., 1963) pp 658-660. Review of toxicology and human exposure: *Toxicological Profile for Cyanide* (PB98-101207, 1997) 291 pp.

Colorless gas or liquid; characteristic odor. Burns in air with a blue flame. *Flammable. Intensely poisonous even when mixed with air. Must be handled by specially trained experts.* mp −13.4°. bp 25.6°. d(gas) 0.941 (air = 1); d(liq) 0.687. Very weakly acid (does not redden litmus). Miscible with water, alc; slightly sol in ether. LC$_{50}$ in rats, mice, dogs: 544 ppm (5 min), 169 ppm (30 min), 300 ppm (3 min) by inhalation, K. C. Back *et al., Reclassification of Materials Listed as Transportation Health Hazards* (TSA-20-72-3; PB214-270, 1972).

Caution: Potential symptoms of acute overexposure are asphyxia; lassitude, headache, confusion; nausea, vomiting; increased rate and depth of respiration, or slow and gasping respiration. *See NIOSH Pocket Guide to Chemical Hazards* (PB2003-100121, 2003) p 168; *Patty's Industrial Hygiene and Toxicology* **vol. 2D,** G. D. Clayton, F. E. Clayton, Eds. (Wiley-Interscience, New York, 4th ed., 1994) pp 3119-3127.

USE: Compressed gas as rodenticide, and insect fumigant.

4796. Hydrogen Fluoride. [7664-39-3] Hydrofluoric acid gas; fluohydric acid gas; anhydr hydrofluoric acid. FH; mol wt 20.01. F 94.94%, H 5.04%. HF. Obtained by the action of sulfuric acid on fluorspar (calcium fluoride): *Faith, Keyes & Clark's Industrial Chemicals,* F. A. Lowenheim, M. K. Moran, Eds. (Wiley-Interscience, New York, 4th ed., 1975) pp 462-467; prepn of pure HF: Simons, *Inorg. Synth.* **1,** 134 (1939); Shamir, Netzer, *J. Sci. Instrum.* (Ser. 2) **1,** 770 (1968). Exists as hydrogen-bonded polymers: Simons, Hildebrand, *J. Am. Chem. Soc.* **46,** 2183 (1924); Jarry, Davis, *J. Phys. Chem.* **57,** 600 (1953); Atoji, Lipscomb, *Acta Crystallogr.* **7,** 173 (1954). pKa determn: N. E. Vanderborgh, *Talanta* **15,** 1009 (1968). Cryoscopic determn: R. J. Gillespie, D. A. Humphreys, *J. Chem. Soc. A* **1970,** 2311. Toxicity study: M. J. Rosenholtz *et al., Am. Ind. Hyg. Assoc. J.* **24,** 253 (1963). Review of prepn, properties and chemistry: Simons in *Fluorine Chemistry* **vol. 1,** J. H. Simons, Ed. (Academic Press, New York, 1950); Hyman, Katz, "Liquid Hydrogen Fluoride" in *Non-aqueous Solvent Systems,* T. C. Waddington, Ed. (Academic Press, New York, 1965) pp 47-81; O'Donnell in *Comprehensive Inorganic Chemistry* **vol. 2,** J. C. Bailar, Jr. *et al.,* Eds. (Pergamon Press, Oxford, 1973) pp 1038-1054; J. F. Gall in *Kirk-Othmer Encyclopedia of Chemical Technology* **vol. 10** (Wiley-Interscience, New York, 3rd ed., 1980) pp 733-753; of toxicology and human exposure: *Toxicological Profile for Fluorides, Hydrogen Fluoride, and Fluorine* (PB2004-100002, 2003) 404 pp.

Colorless gas. Fumes in air. *Highly irritating, corrosive and poisonous!* d^{34} 1.27 (air = 1); d$_4^0$ 1.002. mp −83.57°. bp 19.51°; bp$_{400}$ 2.5°; bp$_{200}$ −13.2°; bp$_{100}$ −28.2°; bp$_{40}$ −45.0°; bp$_{20}$ −56.0°; bp$_5$ −74.7°. Very sol in water and alcohol. Slightly sol in ether. Sol in many organic solvents; soly (wt % at 5°): benzene 2.54; toluene 1.80; *m*-xylene 1.28; tetralin 0.27. Many compds are sol in HF. Anhydr HF is one of the most acidic substances known; Hammett acidity function (H$_0$) −10.98. Weak acid in aqueous soln. pKa 3.189. Forms a constant boiling mixture with water, *see* hydrofluoric acid. Dissolves silica, silicic acid, glass. *Store in steel cylinders.* LC$_{50}$ (15 min.) in rats, guinea pigs: 2689, 4327 ppm (Rosenholtz).

Caution: Potential symptoms of overexposure are irritation of eyes, skin, nose and throat; pulmonary edema; skin and eye burns; rhinitis; bronchitis; bone changes. *See NIOSH Pocket Guide to Chemical Hazards* (DHHS/NIOSH 97-140, 1997) p 168. *See also Patty's Industrial Hygiene and Toxicology* **vol. 2B,** G. D. Clayton, F. E. Clayton, Eds. (Wiley-Interscience, New York, 3rd ed., 1981) pp 2945-2948.

USE: Catalyst, especially in the petroleum industry (paraffin alkylation); in fluorination processes, especially in the aluminum industry; in the manuf of fluorides; for separating uranium isotopes; in making fluorine contg plastics; in dye chemistry.

4797. Hydrogen Iodide. [10034-85-2] Anhydrous hydriodic acid. HI; mol wt 127.91. H 0.79%, I 99.21%. Prepd by catalytic union of the elements: Caley, Burford, *Inorg. Synth.* **1**, 159 (1939); Powell, Campbell, *J. Am. Chem. Soc.* **69**, 1227 (1947). May also be prepd by treating concd hydriodic acid solns with P_2O_5: Schmeisser in *Handbook of Preparative Inorganic Chemistry* **vol. 1**, G. Brauer, Ed. (Academic Press, New York, 2nd ed., 1963) pp 286-289. Lab prepn: Hoffman, *Inorg. Synth.* **7**, 180 (1963). Purification: A. Klemenc, *Die Behandlung und Reindarstellung von Gasen* (Vienna, 2nd ed., 1948) p 239; Irving, Wilson, *Chem. Ind. (London)* **1964**, 653. Reviews of prepn and properties of HI and other hydrogen halides: Hills in *Mellor's* **vol. II**, suppl. 1 (originally published as suppl. II, part 1) 857-869 (1956); Downs, Adams, in *Comprehensive Inorganic Chemistry* **vol. 2**, J. C. Bailar, Jr. *et al.*, Eds. (Pergamon Press, Oxford, 1973) pp 1280-1329.

Colorless, acrid, non-flammable gas. Fumes in moist air. Decomposed by light. mp $-50.8°$. bp_{760} $-35.1°$; $bp_{2 \text{ atm}}$ $-18.9°$; $bp_{5 \text{ atm}}$ $7.3°$; $bp_{10 \text{ atm}}$ $32.0°$; $bp_{60 \text{ atm}}$ $127.5°$. d^0 5.66; d^{25} 5.23 g/l. Crit temp $151.0°$, crit press. 82.0 atm. Sp heat $(25°)$ 0.0545 cal/g/°C. Extremely sol in water. Soly (g/100 g H_2O): 234 $(10°)$; 900 $(0°)$. Soly in organic solvents: Gerrard, *Chem. Ind. (London)* **1969**, 295; Ahmed *et al.*, *J. Appl. Chem.* **20**, 109 (1970). Forms an azeotrope with water, *see* Hydriodic Acid. Reacts with the lower aliphatic alcohols forming the corresponding iodo compds. Forms a colorless liquid at atm pressure when cooled with dry ice and ether or similar cooling mixture. Attacks natural rubber.

Caution: Strong irritant.

USE: Manuf of hydriodic acid, organic iodo compds, to remove iodine from iodo compds.

4798. Hydrogen Peroxide. [7722-84-1] Hydrogen dioxide; hydroperoxide; Albone; Hioxyl; Lensan A; Mirasept; Oxysept; Pegasyl. H_2O_2; mol wt 34.01. H 5.93%, O 94.09%. First reported by Thenard in 1818; prepd by treating barium peroxide with acid. Manuf of aqueous solns: *Faith, Keyes & Clark's Industrial Chemicals*, F. A. Lowenheim, M. K. Moran, Eds. (Wiley-Interscience, New York, 4th ed., 1975) pp 487-495; R. Powell, *Hydrogen Peroxide Manufacture* (Noyes Dev. Corp., Park Ridge, N.J., 1968) 221 pp. Production of anhydr hydrogen peroxide by continuous fractional crystn: Crewson, Ryan, US 2724640 (1955 to Becco). Production and green reactions in liquid CO_2, *q.v.*: D. Hâncu *et al., Acc. Chem. Res.* **35**, 757 (2003). Use in green oxidation reactions: R. Noyori *et al., Chem. Commun.* **2003**, 1977. *Reviews:* ACS Monograph Series **no. 128**, entitled "Hydrogen Peroxide," W. C. Schumb, Ed. (Reinhold, New York, 1955) 759 pp; Ebsworth *et al.,* in *Comprehensive Inorganic Chemistry* **vol. 2**, J. C. Bailar, Jr. *et al.*, Eds. (Pergamon Press, Oxford, 1973) pp 771-778; J. R. Kirchner in *Kirk-Othmer Encyclopedia of Chemical Technology* **vol. 13** (Wiley-Interscience, New York, 3rd ed., 1981) pp 12-38.

Colorless, rather unstable liquid; bitter taste. Distillable in high vacuum. May dec violently if traces of impurities are present. d^0 1.463. mp $-0.43°$. bp $152°$. Misc with water; sol in ether. Insol in petr ether. Decomposed by many organic solvents. Marketed as a soln in water in concns of 3-90% by wt. Solns of hydrogen peroxide gradually deteriorate and are usually stabilized by the addition of acetanilide or similar organic materials. Agitation or contact with rough surfaces, metals or many other substances accelerates decomposition. Rapidly dec by alkalies, finely divided metals; the presence of mineral acid renders it more stable. *Strong oxidizing agent! Keep protected from light and in a cool place.*

3% Solution. Oxydol. Contains 2.5-3.5% by wt of H_2O_2 = 8-12 vols oxygen. Colorless, slightly acid liq. d ~1.00.

30% Solution. Contains 30% by wt of H_2O_2 = 100 vols of oxygen. Clear, colorless liquid. d ~1.11. Miscible with water. Now replacing the 3% soln for industrial uses; diluted to the required strength immediately before use. It also is used for making the 3% soln.

Caution: Potential symptoms of overexposure are irritation of eyes, nose and throat; corneal ulceration; erythema, vesicles on skin; bleaching of hair. *See NIOSH Pocket Guide to Chemical Hazards* (DHHS/NIOSH 97-140, 1997) p 168.

USE: Environmentally friendly oxidant. Bleaching agent in foods, textiles, and personal care products; oxidant in wastewater treatment. A 90% soln is used in rocket propulsion.

THERAP CAT: Antiseptic; disinfectant.

THERAP CAT (VET): Topical antiseptic and cleansing agent (as a dilute soln).

4799. Hydrogen Selenide. [7783-07-5] Selenium hydride. H_2Se; mol wt 80.98. H 2.49%, Se 97.51%. Prepd by heating selenium and hydrogen in a sealed tube at $440°$: Hautefeuille, *Bull. Soc. Chim.* [2] **7**, 198 (1867); by passing a mixture of hydrogen and selenium vapor over pumice stone at $440°$: Corenwinder, *Ann. Chim. Phys.* [3] **34**, 77 (1852); by warming potassium or ferrous selenide with hydrochloric acid: Berzelius, *Acad. Handl. Stockholm* **39**, 13 (1818); by the action of water on aluminum selenide: Fonzes-Diacon, *Traité de Chimie Minérale, Paris* **1**, 469 (1904); Waitkins, Shutt, *Inorg. Synth.* **2**, 183 (1946). Review of chemistry and toxicity: *Medical and Biologic Effects of Environmental Pollutants: Selenium* (Nat. Acad. Sci., Washington D.C., 1976) 203 p.

Gas. Disagreeable odor. Highly toxic and reactive gas that decomposes rapidly in presence of oxygen to form elemental Se and H_2O. d_4^{-42} 2.12. bp $-41.3°$. Liquefies at $0°$ under a pressure of 6.6 atm; at $18°$, 8.6 atm; at $52°$, 21.5 atm; at $100°$, 47.1 atm; at the crit temp $137°$, 91.0 atm. mp $-65.73°$. v.p. at $-30°$, 1.75 atm; v.p. at $0.2°$, 4.5 atm; v.p. at $30.8°$, 12 atm. K_1 at $25° = 1.30 \times 10^{-4}$; K_2 at $25° = 1 \times 10^{-11}$. Soly in water (ml/100 ml): 377 $(4°)$; 270 $(22.5°)$. Sol in carbonyl chloride and carbon disulfide. Unites directly with most metals to form metal selenides.

Caution: Potential symptoms of overexposure are irritation of eyes, nose and throat; nausea, vomiting and diarrhea; metallic taste, garlic breath; dizziness, lassitude and fatigue; direct contact with liquid may cause frostbite. *See NIOSH Pocket Guide to Chemical Hazards* (DHHS/NIOSH 97-140, 1997) p 168.

4800. Hydrogen Sulfide. [7783-06-4] Sulfureted hydrogen; "hydrosulfuric acid". H_2S; mol wt 34.08. H 5.92%, S 94.09%. Evolved from numerous environmental natural sources such as bacterial decomposition of vegetable and animal proteinaceous material. Occurs naturally as a component of crude petroleum, natural gas, volcanic gas and sulfur springs. Also a pollutant released into the environment as a by-product of a variety of industrial operations. Lab prepn: Bickford, Wilkinson, *Inorg. Synth.* **1**, 111 (1939). Purification: Ward *et al., ibid.* **3**, 14 (1950). Toxicity studies: E. H. Vernot *et al., Toxicol. Appl. Pharmacol.* **42**, 417 (1977); M. F. Tansy *et al., J. Toxicol. Environ. Health* **8**, 71-88 (1981). Review of toxicity and properties: R. O. Beauchamp, Jr., *et al., Crit. Rev. Toxicol.* **13**, 25-97 (1984); of toxicology: R. J. Reiffenstein *et al., Annu. Rev. Pharmacol. Toxicol.* **32**, 109-134 (1992); and human exposure: *Toxicological Profile for Hydrogen Sulfide* (PB99-166696, 1999) 217 pp.

Gas with characteristic odor of rotten eggs, perceptible in air at concns of 0.02-0.13 ppm, sweetish taste. *Flammable, poisonous.* Burns in air with pale blue flame. Ignition temp $260°$. Explosive limits when mixed with air: lower limit 4.3% by vol, upper limit 46% by vol. mp $-85.49°$; bp $-60.33°$: Giauque, Blue, *J. Am. Chem. Soc.* **58**, 831 (1936). Heavier than air; 1.5392 g/l $(0°$; 760 mm). d^{gas} 1.19 (air = 1.00). Vapor pressure 18.75×10^5 Pa. One gram H_2S dissolves in 187 ml water at $10°$, in 242 ml water at $20°$, 314 ml water at $30°$; in 94.3 ml abs alcohol at $20°$; in 48.5 ml ether at $20°$. Sol in glycerol, gasoline, kerosene, carbon disulfide, crude oil. Water solns of H_2S are not stable, absorbed oxygen causes the formation of elemental sulfur, and the solns become turbid rapidly. In a 50:50 v/v mixture of glycerol and water the precipitation of sulfur is retarded considerably. pH of freshly prepd satd water soln 4.5. pKa_1 7.04; pKa_2 11.96. LC_{50} in mice, rats (ppm): 634, 712 (1 hr inhalation) (Vernot). LC_{50} in rats (ppm): 444 (4 hr inhalation) (Tansy).

Caution: Highly toxic irritant and chemical asphyxiant; overexposure can be fatal. Insidious poison, since sense of smell may be fatigued and fail to give warning of high concns. Direct contact with gas may cause irritation of eyes and respiratory tract resulting in keratoconjunctivitis, photophobia, lacrimation, corneal opacity; rhinitis, laryngitis, cough, bronchopneumonia. Direct contact with solution may cause skin irritation, erythema. Potential symptoms of overexposure by inhalation include salivation, GI disturbances; giddiness, headache, vertigo, confusion, unconsciousness; tachypnea, tachycardia, sweating, fatigue. Exposure to very high vapor concentrations may result in systemic intoxication leading to paralysis of respiratory center of brain, apnea and sudden collapse. *See Clinical Toxicology of Commercial Products*, R. E. Gosselin *et al.*, Eds. (Williams & Wilkins, Baltimore, 5th ed., 1984) Section III, pp 198-202; *NIOSH Pocket Guide to Chemical Hazards* (DHHS/-NIOSH 97-140, 1997) p 170.

USE: To produce elemental sulfur and sulfuric acid; in manuf of heavy water and other chemicals; in metallurgy; as analytical reagent.

4801. Hydrogen Telluride. [7783-09-7] H_2Te; mol wt 129.62. H 1.56%, Te 98.44%. Prepd by the action of H_2O or HCl on aluminum telluride; by electrolysis of a 50% soln of sulfuric or phosphoric acid with a Te cathode: Dennis, Anderson, *J. Am. Chem. Soc.* **36**, 882 (1914); Fehér in *Handbook of Preparative Inorganic Chemistry* vol. 1, G. Brauer, Ed. (Academic Press, New York, 2nd ed., 1963) pp 438-441.

Colorless gas. Offensive, garlic-like odor. *Highly poisonous!* mp −49°. bp −2°. d_{liq}^{-12} 2.68. Wt of one liter of the gas: 6.234 g. Liquid H_2Te is dec immediately by light. The dry gas is stable to light, but dec in the presence of dust, traces of moisture, rubber, cork, etc. Sol in water with fairly quick decompn. A satd aq soln is about 0.1N.

Caution: Imparts offensive odor to breath. Symptoms similar to hydrogen selenide, *q.v.*

4802. Hydrohydrastinine. [494-55-3] 5,6,7,8-Tetrahydro-6-methyl-1,3,dioxolo[4,5-g]isoquinoline. $C_{11}H_{13}NO_2$; mol wt 191.23. C 69.09%, H 6.85%, N 7.32%, O 16.73%. Prepn from cotarnine, *q.v.*: Topchiev, *J. Appl. Chem. USSR* **6**, 529 (1933), *C.A.* **28**, 2718 (1934); Clayson, *J. Chem. Soc.* **1949**, 2016; Schneider, Müller, *Ann.* **615**, 34 (1958); Knabe, *Arch. Pharm.* **292**, 652 (1959). *See also:* Hydrastinine, Hydrocotarnine.

Crystals from petr ether, mp 66°. bp_{752} 303°. Sol in alc, ether, acetone, benzene, CS_2, ethyl acetate. Absorption spectrum: Dobbie, Tinkler, *J. Chem. Soc.* **85**, 1007 (1904).

Hydrochloride. [5985-04-6] $C_{11}H_{13}NO_2$.HCl. Crystals from water or alcohol, dec 278°. Sol in water.
Hydrobromide. [5985-05-7] $C_{11}H_{13}NO_2$.HBr. Needles from water, dec 272°.
Hydriodide. $C_{11}H_{13}NO_2$.HI. Crystals from water, dec 242°. Sol in water or alc.
Platinichloride. [5985-06-8] $(C_{11}H_{13}NO_2)_2$.H_2PtCl_6. Yellow tablets, dec 222°. Sparingly sol in alc.

4803. Hydromorphone. [466-99-9] 4,5-Epoxy-3-hydroxy-17-methylmorphinan-6-one; dihydromorphinone; Dimorphone; Novolaudon. $C_{17}H_{19}NO_3$; mol wt 285.34. C 71.56%, H 6.71%, N 4.91%, O 16.82%. Prepn by electrolytic reduction of morphine: Takagi, Ueda, *J. Pharm. Soc. Jpn.* **56**, 44 (1936); Nakamura, *ibid.* **62**, 347 (1942); by oxidation of dihydromorphine: Rapoport *et al.*, *J. Org. Chem.* **15**, 1103 (1950); Homeyer, De la Mater, **US 2628962** and **US 2654756** (both 1953 to Mallinckrodt); Rapoport, **US 2649454** (1953 to Univ. of California). Crystal structure: Steinmetz, *Z. Kristallogr.* **67**, 434 (1928). Toxicity data: M. E. Buchwald, G. S. Eadie, *J. Pharmacol. Exp. Ther.* **71**, 197 (1941). *Review:* King *et al.*, *U.S. Public Health Reports* Suppl. no. 113, 38 pp (1935).

Crystals from ethanol, mp 266-267°. $[\alpha]_D^{25}$ −194° (c = 0.98 in dioxane).
Hydrochloride. [71-68-1] Dilaudid; Laudicon; Hymorphan; Palladone. $C_{17}H_{19}NO_3$.HCl; mol wt 321.80. Crystals, dec 305-315° (evacuated tube). $[\alpha]_D^{25}$ −133°. Sol in 3 parts water; sparingly sol in alc. LD_{50} in mice (mg/kg): 61-96 i.v. (Buchwald, Eadie).
Note: This is a controlled substance (opiate): **21 CFR**, 1308.12.
THERAP CAT: Analgesic (narcotic).

4804. Hydroorotic Acid. [155-54-4] Hexahydro-2,6-dioxo-4-pyrimidinecarboxylic acid; 4,5-dihydroorotic acid. $C_5H_6N_2O_4$; mol wt 158.11. C 37.98%, H 3.82%, N 17.72%, O 40.48%. Prepn from carbethoxyasparagine: Miller *et al.*, *J. Am. Chem. Soc.* **75**, 6086 (1953); **US 2773872** (1956 to Merck & Co.).

L-Form. Crystals, dec 266°. $[\alpha]_D^{25.3}$ +33.23° (c = 1.992 in 1% $NaHCO_3$).
D-Form. Crystals from water, dec 266°. $[\alpha]_D^{25.3}$ −31.54° (c = 2.01 in 1% $NaHCO_3$).
DL-Form. Crystals, dec 259°. Forms a water-sol salt.
USE: The L- and DL-dihydroorotic acids are precursors to the biological pyrimidines, such as thymine, uracil, cytosine and hydroxymethylcytosine. When employed in large amounts D-dihydroorotic acid is an antimetabolite of L-dihydroorotic acid in pyrimidine utilization. It has also been found to inhibit the orotic acid utilization of those organisms which have a requirement for it in order to grow. In general it may be said to inhibit bacterial growth.

4805. Hydroprene. [41096-46-2] (2E,4E)-3,7,11-Trimethyl-2,4-dodecadienoic acid ethyl ester; ethyl (2E,4E)-3,7,11-trimethyldodeca-2,4-dienoate; OMS-1696; SHA-486300; ZR-512; Gencor; Gentrol. $C_{17}H_{30}O_2$; mol wt 266.42. C 76.64%, H 11.35%, O 12.01%. Juvenile hormone mimic. Prepn: C. A. Henrick, **US 4021461** (1977 to Zoecon); *idem et al.*, *J. Agric. Food Chem.* **21**, 354 (1973); and insecticidal activity of enantiomers: *idem et al.*, *ibid.* **26**, 542 (1978). Effect on sweet potato weevil: G. M. Ram, A. C. Sekhar, *Indian J. Comp. Anim. Physiol.* **2**, 87 (1991); cockroach: B. L. Reid, G. W. Bennett, *J. Econ. Entomol.* **87**, 1537 (1994). Effect of (S)-enantiomer on cockroach: J. P. Edwards, J. E. Short, *ibid.* **86**, 436 (1993). Review and use in food industries: M. Martinez, *Cereal Foods World* **38**, 818-820 (1993).

$bp_{0.03}$ 95°. uv max (hexane): 262 nm (ε 28300). LD_{50} orally in rats: >34000 mg/kg (Edwards).
(S)-form. [65733-18-8] $bp_{0.05}$ 80°. $[\alpha]_D^{25}$ +2.9° (c = 0.020 in methanol).
USE: Insect growth regulator; insecticide.

4806. Hydroquinidine. [1435-55-8] (9S)-10,11-Dihydro-6'-methoxycinchonan-9-ol; dihydroquinidine; hydroconchinine. $C_{20}H_{26}N_2O_2$; mol wt 326.43. C 73.59%, H 8.03%, N 8.58%, O 9.80%. An alkaloid of cinchona, stereoisomeric with hydroquinine. Usually prepd by hydrogenation of quinidine: Heidelberger, Jacobs, *J. Am. Chem. Soc.* **41**, 826 (1919). Conversion to dihydrocinchonine by removal of the methoxy group: King, *J. Chem. Soc.* **1946**, 523. Manuf pat.: Gutzwiller, Uskokovic, **DE 1933599** (1970 to Hoffmann-La Roche), *C.A.* **72**, 90696v (1970). Pharmacology: Cosnier *et al.*, *Therapie* **26**, 97 (1971).

Plates from ether, needles from alcohol, mp 169°. $[\alpha]_D^{20}$ +231° (c = 2.02 in alc); +299° (c = 0.82 in 0.1N H_2SO_4). Readily sol in hot alcohol; slightly sol in water and ether.

Hydrochloride. [1476-98-8] Serecor. $C_{20}H_{26}N_2O_2 \cdot HCl$; mol wt 362.89. Rhombic plates, mp 273-274°. $[\alpha]_D^{26} +184°$ (c = 1.3). Freely sol in methanol, chloroform; less readily in water or abs alcohol; difficultly sol in dry acetone.

THERAP CAT: Antiarrhythmic.

4807. Hydroquinine. [522-66-7] $(8\alpha,9R)$-10,11-Dihydro-6'-methoxycinchonan-9-ol; dihydroquinine. $C_{20}H_{26}N_2O_2$; mol wt 326.43. C 73.59%, H 8.03%, N 8.58%, O 9.80%. An alkaloid of cinchona, found in quinine sulfate mother liquors. Stereoisomeric with hydroquinidine, *q.v.* Usually prepd by careful hydrogenation of quinine: Heidelberger, Jacobs, *J. Am. Chem. Soc.* **41,** 819 (1919). Total synthesis: Rabe *et al., Ber.* **64B,** 2487 (1931). Synthesis of isomers: Rubtsov, *J. Gen. Chem. USSR* **9,** 1493 (1939), *C.A.* **34,** 2850 (1940); *ibid.* **13,** 593, 702 (1943), *C.A.* **39,** 705 (1945). LC determn in quinine beverages: L. P. Valenti, *J. Assoc. Off. Anal. Chem.* **68,** 782 (1985).

Needles from ether or benzene, mp 172°. $[\alpha]_D^{18} -142°$ (alc); $[\alpha]_D^{20} -236°$ (c = 0.82 in 0.1N H_2SO_4). $pK_1 = 5.33$. Freely sol in acetone, alcohol, chloroform, ether, petr ether; fairly sol in ammonia water. Almost insol in water (290 mg/l).

Hydrochloride hemihydrate. $C_{20}H_{27}ClN_2O_2 \cdot \frac{1}{2}H_2O$. Prisms from water, mp 208° (Heidelberger). $[\alpha]_D^{21} -124°$ (c = 1.1). pH of 0.005 molar soln 5.85. Freely sol in water, alcohol, methanol, acetone. Almost insol in ether. Crystallizes also with 2 mols H_2O. Infrared spectrum: J. Suszko, Z. Dega-Szafran, *Bull. Acad. Pol. Sci. Ser. Sci. Chim.* **12,** 607 (1964), *C.A.* **62,** 7819b (1965).

THERAP CAT: Depigmentor.

4808. Hydroquinone. [123-31-9] 1,4-Benzenediol; *p*-dihydroxybenzene; hydroquinol; quinol; Aida; Black and White Bleaching Cream; Eldoquin; Eldopaque; Tecquinol. $C_6H_6O_2$; mol wt 110.11. C 65.45%, H 5.49%, O 29.06%. Prepd by the oxidation of aniline: L. Gattermann, T. Wieland, *Die Praxis des Organischen Chemikers* (de Gruyter, Berlin, 40th ed., 1961) p 266; by reduction of quinone: Kitchen, **US 1322580** (1920); Seyewetz, Miodon, *Bull. Soc. Chim. Fr.* **33,** 449 (1923); by Elbs persulfate oxidation of phenol: Baker, Brown, *J. Chem. Soc.* **1948,** 2303; Forrest, Petrow, *ibid.* **1950,** 2340; from acetylene + CO: Howk, Sauer, **US 3055949** (1962 to du Pont). Toxicity data: Woodard *et al., Fed. Proc.* **8,** 348 (1949). Toxicology and carcinogenicity study: F. W. Kari *et al., Food Chem. Toxicol.* **30,** 737 (1992). *Review:* J. Varagnat in *Kirk-Othmer Encyclopedia of Chemical Technology* **vol. 13** (Wiley-Interscience, New York, 3rd ed., 1981) pp 39-69.

Crystals, mp 170-171°. d_{15} 1.332. bp 285-287°. Sol in 14 parts water; freely sol in alcohol, ether, slightly in benzene. Its soln becomes brown in the air due to oxidation; the oxidation is very rapid in presence of alkali. *Keep well closed and protected from light. Handle with caution. Avoid contact with skin and eyes.* LD_{50} orally in rats: 320 mg/kg (Woodard).

Caution: Harmful effects may occur following overexposure to dust and vapors by inhalation or by contact with skin or eyes. Contact with skin may cause dermatitis. Contact with eyes may cause eye irritation, keratitis, discoloration of conjunctiva and corneal changes. Ingestion may cause tinnitus, nausea, dizziness, sense of suffocation, increased respiration rate, vomiting, pallor,

muscle twitching, headache, dyspnea, cyanosis, delirium, and collapse. Urine is usually green or brownish green in color and continues to darken on standing. *See Patty's Industrial Hygiene and Toxicology* **vol. 2B,** G. D. Clayton, F. E. Clayton, Eds. (Wiley-Interscience, New York, 4th ed., 1994) pp 1590-1592. *See also NIOSH Pocket Guide to Chemical Hazards* (DHHS/NIOSH 97-140, 1997) p 170.

USE: As photographic reducer and developer; as reagent in the determination of small quantities of phosphate; as antioxidant.

THERAP CAT: Depigmentor.

4809. Hydroxocobalamin. [13422-51-0] Cobinamide hydroxide dihydrogen phosphate (ester) inner salt 3'-ester with 5,6-dimethyl-1-α-D-ribofuranosyl-1H-benzimidazole; α-(5,6-dimethyl-benzimidazolyl)hydroxocobamide; vitamin B_{12a}; hydroxocobemine; OHB_{12}; Cobalin-H; Dodécavit; Duradoce; Neo-Cytamen; Redisol H. $C_{62}H_{89}CoN_{13}O_{15}P$; mol wt 1346.36. C 55.31%, H 6.66%, Co 4.38%, N 13.52%, O 17.83%, P 2.30%. Physiological analog of vitamin B_{12} where the CN group is replaced with OH. Exists in aq soln as an equilibrium mixture of the hydroxy isomer and the ionic aqua isomer (aquacobalamin). Precursor of the coenzymes methylcobalamin and cobamamide, *q.q.v.* Prepn: E. A. Kaczka *et al., J. Am. Chem. Soc.* **71,** 1514 (1949); *eidem, ibid.* **73,** 335 (1951); *eidem,* **US 2738301** (1956 to Merck & Co.). Acids replace the hydroxo group with the anion of the acid: *eidem, Science* **112,** 354 (1950). Prepn from cyanocobalamin: R. Bieganowski, G. Klar, *Chem. Ztg.* **106,** 235 (1982). Clinical evaluation as antidote to cyanide: J. C. Forsyth *et al., Clin. Toxicol.* **31,** 277 (1993). *Review:* "Vitamin B_{12}" in *Vitamins,* W. Friedrich, Ed. (de Gruyter, Berlin, 1988) pp 837-928.

Dark red, orthorhombic needles or platelets from water + acetone. Darkens at 200°, but not melted at 300°. Absorption max (H_2O): 279, 325, 359, 516, 537 nm (ε 19000, 11400, 20600, 8900, 9500). Moderately sol in water and in the lower aliphatic alcohols. Practically insol in acetone, ether, petr ether, halogenated hydrocarbons, benzene.

Aquacobalamin. [13422-52-1] Cobinamide hydroxide monohydrate dihydrogen phosphate (ester) inner salt 3'-ester with 5,6-dimethyl-1-α-D-ribofuranosyl-1H-benzimidazole; aquacobalamin; vitamin B_{12b}; vitamin B_{12d}. $C_{62}H_{90}CoN_{13}O_{15}P \cdot OH$; mol wt 1364.37. Absorption max (H_2O): 274, 317, 351, 499, 527 nm (ε 20600, 6100, 26500, 8100, 8500).

Acetatocobalamin. [22465-48-1] Cobinamide acetate (salt) dihydrogen phosphate (ester) inner salt 3'-ester with 5,6-dimethyl-1-α-D-ribofuranosyl-1H-benzimidazole; Depogamma; Docelan; Novidroxin. $C_{64}H_{91}CoN_{13}O_{16}P$; mol wt 1388.39. Prepn of stable solns: Marcus *et al.,* **FR 1336671** (1963 to Merck & Co.), *C.A.* **60,** 380a (1964).

Nitrocobalamin. [20623-13-6] Cobinamide nitrite (salt) dihydrogen phosphate (ester) inner salt 3'-ester with 5,6-dimethyl-1-α-D-ribofuranosyl-1*H*-benzimidazole; nitritocobalamin; vitamin B$_{12c}$. C$_{62}$H$_{88}$CoN$_{14}$O$_{16}$P; mol wt 1375.35. Prepn: E. A. Kaczka *et al., J. Am. Chem. Soc.* **73**, 3569 (1951). Red crystalline solid. Absorption max in water: 352, 527.5 nm (E$_{1cm}^{1\%}$ 153.2, 59.5); in 0.01*N* NaOH: 357, 535 nm (E$_{1cm}^{1\%}$ 139, 62.5).

Sulfitocobalamin. [15671-27-9] Cobinamide sulfite (1:1) (salt) dihydrogen phosphate (ester) inner salt 3′-ester with 5,6-dimethyl-1-α-D-ribofuranosyl-1*H*-benzimidazole; cobalaminsulfonic acid. C$_{62}$H$_{89}$CoN$_{13}$O$_{17}$PS; mol wt 1410.42. Prepn: Fricke, **US 2721162** (1955 to Abbott). Absorption max: 275, 365, 418, 516 nm (E$_{1cm}^{1\%}$ 328, 130, 49, 61).

THERAP CAT: Vitamin (hematopoietic).

THERAP CAT (VET): Vitamin (hematopoietic).

4810. Hydroxyamphetamine. [1518-86-1] 4-(2-Amino-propyl)phenol; *dl-p*-hydroxy-α-methylphenethylamine; *dl*-1-*p*-hydroxyphenyl-2-propylamine; *p*-hydroxyphenylisopropylamine; α-methyltyramine; Paredrine; Paredrinex; Pulsoton. C$_9$H$_{13}$NO; mol wt 151.21. C 71.49%, H 8.67%, N 9.26%, O 10.58%. Prepn from oxime of *p*-methoxyphenyl acetone: Mannich, Jacobsohn, *Ber.* **43**, 189 (1910), **DE 243546**. From *p*-nitrobenzyl chloride and a salt of nitroethane: Hoover, Hass, *J. Org. Chem.* **12**, 501 (1947).

Crystals (rosettes) from benzene, mp 125-126°. Sol in water, alcohol, chloroform, ethyl acetate.

Iodide. C$_9$H$_{14}$INO. Stout prisms, mp 155°. Freely sol in water, alcohol, acetone.

Hydrochloride. C$_9$H$_{14}$ClNO. Crystals from HCl, mp 171-172°. Sol in water, alcohol. Practically insol in ether.

Hydrobromide. [306-21-8] C$_9$H$_{14}$BrNO. Crystals. Freely sol in water, alcohol, acetone. Prepd as Paredrine Hydrobromide Aqueous—a 1% aq soln made isotonic with sodium chloride and preserved with sodium ethylmercuri thiosalicylate. Also prepd as Paredrine Hydrobromide Ophthalmic 1%, with boric acid—a 1% aq soln made tear-isotonic with 2% boric acid and preserved with sodium ethylmercuri thiosalicylate.

THERAP CAT: Adrenergic (ophthalmic); mydriatic.

4811. *p*-Hydroxybenzaldehyde. [123-08-0] 4-Formylphenol. C$_7$H$_6$O$_2$; mol wt 122.12. C 68.85%, H 4.95%, O 26.20%. Widely distributed in plants in very small amounts. Obtained as a byproduct from the Reimer-Tiemann reaction for salicylaldehyde from phenol: L. F. Fieser, M. Fieser, *Organic Chemistry* (Reinhold, New York, 3rd ed., 1956) p 681; *cf.* Reimer, Tiemann, *Ber.* **9**, 824 (1876); Herzfeld, Tiemann, *Ber.* **10**, 64 (1877).

Needles from water. Slight, agreeable, aromatic odor, mp 116°. Sublimes at atmospheric pressure without decomposition. Reacts like a weak monobasic acid: Ka at 25° = 2.2×10^{-8}. Dipole moment: 4.19. Sparingly sol in cold water: 1.38 g/100 ml H$_2$O at 30.5°; more sol in hot water. Freely sol in alc, ether. Slightly sol in benzene: 3.68 g/100 ml C$_6$H$_6$ at 65°.

4812. *p*-Hydroxybenzoic Acid. [99-96-7] C$_7$H$_6$O$_3$; mol wt 138.12. C 60.87%, H 4.38%, O 34.75%. Prepn from *p*-bromophenol: Gilinan, Arntzen, *J. Am. Chem. Soc.* **69**, 1537 (1947); from *p*-hydroxybenzaldehyde: Pearl, *J. Org. Chem.* **12**, 85 (1947); from phenol + potassium ethyl carbonate: Jones, *Chem. Ind. (London)* **1958**, 228; from potassium phenolate + CO$_2$: **GB 942418** (1963 to Inventa). A metabolic product of *Penicillium patulum*: Tanenbaum, Bassett, *Biochim. Biophys. Acta* **28**, 21 (1958).

Crystals, mp 213-214°. d 1.46. Soluble in about 125 parts water, freely in alcohol, slightly in chloroform; sol in ether, acetone. Practically insol in carbon disulfide. Ferric chloride does not color its aq soln.

USE: In org. syntheses; intermediate for dyes, fungicides.

4813. α-Hydroxybenzylphosphinic Acid. [52705-43-8] C$_7$H$_9$O$_3$P; mol wt 172.12. C 48.85%, H 5.27%, O 27.89%, P 18.00%. Prepd from benzaldehyde (3 moles) and H$_3$PO$_2$ (1 mole): Ville, *Ann. Chim. (Paris)* [6] **23**, 305 (1891); *Beilstein* **7**, 232; Viout, *J. Rech. Cent. Nat. Rech. Sci.* no. **28**, 15-31 (1954), *C.A.* **50**, 7078d (1956).

Leaflets from butanol, mp 110°. Freely sol in water, alcohol; also sol in benzene. Practically insol in anhydr ether.

Sodium salt. Phos; Phoselit; Phosilite. Very freely sol in water. The pH is on the acid side, but aq solns are suitable for injection.

THERAP CAT: Sodium salt as nutrient.

4814. 4′-Hydroxybutyranilide. [101-91-7] *N*-(4-Hydroxyphenyl)butanamide; *p*-hydroxybutyranilide; *N*-butyroyl-*p*-aminophenol; Suconox-4. C$_{10}$H$_{13}$NO$_2$; mol wt 179.22. C 67.02%, H 7.31%, N 7.82%, O 17.85%. Prepn: Kuhn *et al., Z. Physiol. Chem.* **247**, 197 (1937); Fierz-David, Kuster, *Helv. Chim. Acta* **22**, 82 (1939); Rohmann, Friedrich, *Arch. Pharm.* **278**, 456 (1940).

Needles from water, mp 139-140°. Slightly sol in cold water, more sol in hot water, sol in alcohol.

USE: As antioxidant: Young, Cottle, **US 2654722** (1953 to Standard Oil).

4815. γ-Hydroxybutyrate. [591-81-1] 4-Hydroxybutanoic acid; γ-hydroxybutyric acid; 4-hydroxybutyrate; gamma-hydroxybutyrate; GHB. C$_4$H$_8$O$_3$; mol wt 104.10. C 46.15%, H 7.75%, O 46.11%. HOCH$_2$CH$_2$CH$_2$COOH. Endogenous constituent of mammalian brain; thought to function as a neurotransmitter or neuromodulator. Biosynthesized from γ-aminobutyric acid, *q.v.*; freely crosses the blood-brain barrier. Prepn of salts: A. Saytzeff, *Ann.* **171**, 258 (1874); C. S. Marvel, E. R. Birkhimer, *J. Am. Chem. Soc.* **51**, 260 (1929). Acute toxicity: B. Bruguerolle *et al., Therapie* **32**, 375 (1977). GC-MS determn in biological fluids: S. D. Ferrara *et al., J. Pharm. Biomed. Anal.* **11**, 483 (1993). Clinical pharmacokinetics: *idem et al., Br. J. Clin. Pharmacol.* **34**, 231 (1992). Clinical studies in narcolepsy: L. Scrima *et al., Sleep* **13**, 479 (1990); in opiate withdrawal: L. Gallimberti *et al., Neuropsychopharmacology* **9**, 77 (1993). Review of efficacy in alcoholism: G. Biggio *et al., Adv. Biochem. Psychopharmacol.* **47**, 281-288 (1992). Review of potential role as neurotransmittor: G. Tunnicliff, *Gen. Pharmacol.* **23**, 1027-1034 (1992); of neuropharmacology and abuse potential: R. Bernasconi *et al., Trends Pharmacol. Sci.* **20**, 135-141 (1999); of clinical experience in narcolepsy: M. J. Thorpy, *Expert Opin. Pharmacother.* **6**, 329-335 (2005).

Sodium salt. [502-85-2] γ-OH; sodium oxybate; sodium γ-oxybutyrate; Wy-3478; NSC-84223; Somsanit; Gamma-OH; Xyrem. C$_4$H$_8$NaO$_3$; mol wt 127.09. Crystals from alcohol. Highly sol in aq solns. LD$_{50}$ in male, female rats (mg/kg): 2,000, 1,650 i.p. (Bruguerolle).

Note: This is a controlled substance (depressant): **21 CFR**, 1308.11.

THERAP CAT: Anesthetic (intravenous). In treatment of narcolepsy; in treatment of alcoholism.

4816. β-Hydroxybutyric Acid. [300-85-6] 3-Hydroxybutanoic acid. C$_4$H$_8$O$_3$; mol wt 104.10. C 46.15%, H 7.75%, O 46.11%. CH$_3$CHOHCH$_2$COOH.

d-Form. Prepd by the action of *Aspergillus griseus* on the *dl*-form: McKenzie, Harden, *J. Chem. Soc.* **83**, 430 (1903). Crystals. $[\alpha]_D^{10}$ +24.3° (c = 2.226). Sol in water, alcohol, ether.

l-Form. Found in the urine of diabetics (as much as 30 g per day). Isoln: Fischer, Scheibler, *Ber.* **42**, 1221 (1909); Shaffer, Marriott, *J. Biol. Chem.* **16**, 268 (1913). Hygroscopic, monoclinic crystals, mp 45.5-48°. $[\alpha]_D^{25}$ −24.5° (c = 5). K at 22° = 3.86×10^{-5}. Freely sol in water, alcohol, ether. Sparingly sol in benzene. On distn it dec into crotonic acid and water.

dl-Form. Prepd from acetoacetic ester by the action of sodium amalgam: Wislicenus, *Ann.* **149**, 207 (1869); Marian, *Biochem. Z.* **150**, 283 (1924); by the oxidation of aldol: Wurtz, *Compt. Rend.* **76**, 1167 (1873); from crotonic acid by heating with dil acid: Wacker, *DE 441003*; *Frdl.* **15**, 135; by heating crotonitrile with KOH soln: Bruylants, *Bull. Soc. Chim. Belg.* **31**, 182 (1922). Hygroscopic syrup. Volatile with steam. Sol in water, alcohol, ether. On distn it dec into crotonic acid and water.

4817. 3-Hydroxycamphor. [10373-81-6] 3-Hydroxy-1,7,7-trimethylbicyclo[2.2.1]heptan-2-one; oxycamphor; Oxaphor. $C_{10}H_{16}O_2$; mol wt 168.23. C 71.39%, H 9.59%, O 19.02%. Prepn: Lucius, Brüning, *DE 91718* (1897); Manasse, *Ber.* **30**, 659 (1897); Lapworth, Chapman, *J. Chem. Soc.* **79**, 377 (1901).

Needles from benzene + petr ether, mp 205-206°. Sol in 50 parts water, more in hot water; very sol in alcohol, chloroform, ether.
THERAP CAT: Antipruritic (topical).

4818. Hydroxychloroquine. [118-42-3] 2-[[4-[(7-Chloro-4-quinolinyl)amino]pentyl]ethylamino]ethanol; 7-chloro-4-[4-[eth-yl(2-hydroxyethyl)amino]-1-methylbutylamino]quinoline; 7-chloro-4-[4-[(N-ethyl-N-β-hydroxyethylamino)-1-methylbutylamino]-quinoline; 7-chloro-4-[5-(N-ethyl-N-2-hydroxyethylamino)-2-pen-tyl]aminoquinoline; oxychloroquine; oxichlorochine. $C_{18}H_{26}ClN_3O$; mol wt 335.87. C 64.37%, H 7.80%, Cl 10.56%, N 12.51%, O 4.76%. Prepd by reacting a mixture of 4,7-dichloro-quinoline, phenol and N '-ethyl-N '-β-hydroxyethyl-1,4-pentadia-mine at 125-130°: Surrey, Hammer, *J. Am. Chem. Soc.* **72**, 1814 (1950); Surrey, *US 2546658* (1951 to Sterling Drug). Use in combination with cyclophosphamide and azathioprine, *q.q.v.* in the treatment of rheumatoid arthritis: D. J. McCarty, G. F. Carrera, *J. Am. Med. Assoc.* **248**, 1718 (1982). Reassessment in the treatment of rheumatoid arthritis: *Am. J. Med.* **75**, no. 1A, 1-56 (1983). Series of articles on clinical use: *ibid.* **85**, Suppl. 4A, 1-71 (1988).

Crystals from ethylene dichloride and Skellysolve B; mp 89-91°.
Diphosphate. $C_{18}H_{26}ClN_3O.2H_3PO_4$. Recrystallized from ethanol, mp 168-170° (dec).
Sulfate. [747-36-4] Ercoquin; Plaquenil Sulfate; Quensyl. $C_{18}H_{26}ClN_3O.H_2SO_4$; mol wt 433.95. White crystalline powder; odorless but has a bitter taste. pH of aq solns about 4.5. Exists in two forms, the usual form mp ~240°, the other mp ~198°. Freely sol in water. Practically insol in alcohol, chloroform, ether.
THERAP CAT: Antimalarial; antirheumatic; lupus erythematosus suppressant.

4819. 1α-Hydroxycholecalciferol. [41294-56-8] (1α,3β,-5Z,7E)-9,10-Secocholesta-5,7,10(19)-triene-1,3-diol; 1α-hydroxy-vitamin D₃; 1α-OH-CC; alfacalcidol; Alfarol; Alpha D₃; EinsAlpha; Etalpha; One-Alpha; Vetalpha. $C_{27}H_{44}O_2$; mol wt 400.64. C

80.94%, H 11.07%, O 7.99%. Synthetic analog of calcitriol, *q.v.*, the hormonal form of vitamin D₃, which shows identical potency with respect to stimulation of intestinal calcium absorption and bone mineral mobilization. This common activity is thought to be due either to the presence in both of a 1α hydroxy group or more likely, to the conversion of the 1α-OH-CC *in vivo* to 1α,25-dihydroxycho-lecalciferol: Haussler *et al., Proc. Natl. Acad. Sci. USA* **70**, 2248 (1973). Synthesis from cholesterol: Holick *et al., Science* **180**, 190 (1973); Barton *et al., J. Am. Chem. Soc.* **95**, 2748 (1973); Fürst *et al., Helv. Chim. Acta* **56**, 1708 (1973); M. Morisaki *et al., Chem. Pharm. Bull.* **23**, 3272 (1975); T. Sato *et al., ibid.* **26**, 2933 (1979). Total synthesis: R. G. Harrison *et al., Tetrahedron Lett.* **1973**, 3649; *eidem, J. Chem. Soc. Perkin Trans. 1* **1974**, 2654; P. J. Kocienski, B. Lythgoe, *ibid.* **1980**, 1400. Synthesis of the 1β-epimer from the 1α-form and biological properties: H. E. Paaren *et al., Chem. Commun.* **1977**, 890.

mp 134-136° (Harrison); also reported as mp 138-139.5° (Fürst). $[\alpha]_D^{25}$ +28° (ether). uv max (ether): 264 nm (ε 18000) (Harrison); also reported as ε 20200 (Barton).
1β-Epimer. 1β-Hydroxycholecalciferol; 1β-hydroxyvitamin D₃.
THERAP CAT: Vitamin D source.
THERAP CAT (VET): Vitamin D source.

4820. 24-Hydroxycholesterol. [474-73-7] (3β,24S)-Cho-lest-5-ene-3,24-diol. $C_{27}H_{46}O_2$; mol wt 402.65. C 80.54%, H 11.52%, O 7.95%. Two stereoisomers exist: **cholest-5-ene-3β,24β-diol** and **cholest-5-ene-3β,24α-diol**. Isoln of the naturally occurring 24β-epimer, from horse brain: Ercoli *et al., Boll. Soc. Ital. Biol. Sper.* **29**, 494 (1953), *C.A.* **49**, 4744i (1955); from beef spinal cord: Fieser *et al., J. Org. Chem.* **22**, 1380 (1957). Prepn and separation of isomers: Ercoli, Ruggieri, *Gazz. Chim. Ital.* **83**, 720 (1953); *eidem, J. Am. Chem. Soc.* **75**, 3284 (1953). Configurations at C-24: Klyne, Stokes, *J. Chem. Soc.* **1954**, 1979.

24β-Epimer. Cerebrostenediol; cerebrosterol. Needles from acetone, mp 175-176°. $[\alpha]_D^{20}$ −48.2° (c = 1.06 in CHCl₃).
24β-Epimer dibenzoate. $C_{41}H_{54}O_4$. Crystals from ether + acetone, mp 182-183°. α_D −19° (c = 1.20 in CHCl₃).
24α-Epimer. Crystals, mp 182-183°. $[\alpha]_D^{20}$ −26.8° (c = 0.672 in CHCl₃).
24α-Epimer dibenzoate. Crystals, mp 141-142°. $[\alpha]_D^{26}$ −11.8° (c = 1 in CHCl₃).

4821. 25-Hydroxycholesterol. [2140-46-7] (3β)-Cholest-5-ene-3,25-diol; Δ⁵-cholestene-3β,25-diol. $C_{27}H_{46}O_2$; mol wt 402.65. C 80.54%, H 11.52%, O 7.95%. An important intermediate in the synthesis of 25-hydroxycholecalciferol, *q.v.* Synthesis: A. Ryer *et al., J. Am. Chem. Soc.* **72**, 4247 (1950); W. G. Dauben, H. L. Bradlow, *ibid.* 4248. Isoln from autoxidation products of cholesterol, *q.v.*: L. F. Fieser *et al., J. Org. Chem.* **22**, 1380 (1957). Prepn from pregnenolone, *q.v.*: T. A. Narwid, M. R. Uskokovic, US **3856780** (1974). Alternate syntheses: M. Morisaki *et al., Chem. Pharm. Bull.* **21**, 457 (1973); A. Rotman, Y. Mazur, *Chem. Commun.* **1974**, 15; J. J. Partridge *et al., Helv. Chim. Acta* **57**, 764 (1974); T. A. Narwid *et al., ibid.* 771; W. G. Salmond *et al., Tetrahedron Lett.* **1977**, 987, 1237, 1695; K. Ochi *et al., Chem. Pharm. Bull.* **27**, 252 (1979); M. Riediker, J. Schwartz, *Tetrahedron Lett.* **22**, 4655 (1981).

Colorless needles from methanol, mp 178-180°. $[\alpha]_D^{25}$ −39.0° (c = 1.05 in chloroform).

20(S)-isomer. Crystals from chloroform, mp 189.5-190.5°. $[\alpha]_D^{25}$ −41.50°(c = 0.9278 in chloroform).

4822. Hydroxycodeinone. [508-54-3] 5α-7,8-Didehydro-4,5α-epoxy-14-hydroxy-3-methoxy-17-methylmorphinan-6-one; 14-hydroxycodeinone. $C_{18}H_{19}NO_4$; mol wt 313.35. C 68.99%, H 6.11%, N 4.47%, O 20.42%. Preparation from thebaine: Freund, Speyer, *J. Prakt. Chem.* **94**, 135 (1916). From codeine: Merck, **DE 411530**; *Frdl.* **15**, 1516; K. W. Bentley, *The Chemistry of the Morphine Alkaloids* (Oxford, 1954). Improved synthesis: F. M. Hauser *et al., J. Med. Chem.* **17**, 1117 (1974). Isoln from *Papaver bracteatum* Lindl.: H. G. Theuns *et al., Phytochemistry* **16**, 753 (1977).

Plates from 96% alcohol + few drops chloroform, dec 275°. Freely sol in $CHCl_3$, methyl Cellosolve, petr ether, ethyl acetate; slightly sol in alcohol. Practically insol in water, ether; also insol in aq alkaline solns.

Hydrochloride monohydrate. $C_{18}H_{19}NO_4 \cdot HCl \cdot H_2O$. Rods from water, dec 285-286°. $[\alpha]_D^{20}$ −150° (c = 2.5).

Note: This is a controlled substance (opiate): **21 CFR**, 1308.12.

4823. Hydroxydione Sodium. [53-10-1] 21-(3-Carboxy-1-oxopropoxy)-5β-pregnane-3,20-dione sodium salt; 21-hydroxypregnane-3,20-dione sodium hemisuccinate; hydroxydione succinate; Presuren; Viadril. $C_{25}H_{35}NaO_6$; mol wt 454.53. C 66.06%, H 7.76%, Na 5.06%, O 21.12%. Prepd by palladium reduction of deoxycorticosterone followed by treatment with succinic anhydride and formation of the sodium salt: Laubach, US **2708651** (1955 to Pfizer); Laubach *et al., Science* **122**, 78 (1955).

Lyophilized, fluffy white powder. Dec 193-203°. uv max: 280 nm (ε 93.2). Sol in water, in mildly alkaline buffer solns, acetone, chloroform. pH of 2% aq soln 8.5-9.8.

Free acid. mp 195-197°. $[\alpha]_D^{20}$ +95° in chloroform.

THERAP CAT: Anesthetic (intravenous).

4824. *p*-Hydroxyephedrine. [365-26-4] 4-Hydroxy-α-[1-(methylamino)ethyl]benzenemethanol; *p*-hydroxy-α-[1-(methylamino)ethyl]benzyl alcohol; 1-(4-hydroxyphenyl)-2-methylaminopropanol; α-(1-methylaminoethyl)-*p*-hydroxybenzyl alcohol; oxyephedrin; Carnigen; Edornat; Methylsympatol; Suprifen. $C_{10}H_{15}$-NO_2; mol wt 181.23. C 66.27%, H 8.34%, N 7.73%, O 17.66%. Prepn: Stolz, US **1878021** (1932 to Winthrop). Prepn of hydrochlorides of *d*- and *l*-forms: Takamatsu, Minaki, *J. Pharm. Soc. Jpn.* **76**, 1230 (1956), *C.A.* **51**, 4305e (1957).

Cryst powder, mp 152-154°. Sparingly sol in water, alcohol, ether; readily sol in NaOH soln and dil acids.

Hydrochloride. $C_{10}H_{15}NO_2 \cdot HCl$. Crystals, mp 209-211°. Sol in 3 parts water, 5 parts glycerol, 10 parts 90% alcohol. Sparingly sol in abs alcohol, acetone.

***d*-Form hydrochloride.** Crystals, dec 223-224°. $[\alpha]_D^{22}$ +33.8°.

***l*-Form hydrochloride.** Crystals, dec 222-223°. $[\alpha]_D^{22}$ −35.5°.

THERAP CAT: Adrenergic.

4825. Hydroxyglutamic Acid. [533-62-0] β-Hydroxyglutamic acid; α-amino-β-hydroxyglutaric acid. $C_5H_9NO_5$; mol wt 163.13. C 36.81%, H 5.56%, N 8.59%, O 49.04%. An amino acid classified as nonessential with respect to its growth effect in rats. Not among the naturally occurring hydrolytic products of proteins, *see* Schmidt, *Chemistry of the Amino Acids and Proteins* (Springfield, Ill., 2nd ed., 1944) p 1090. Synthesis from ethyl α-isonitrosoacetone dicarboxylate: Harington, Randall, *Biochem. J.* **25**, 1917 (1931); Levene, Schormüller, *J. Biol. Chem.* **106**, 595 (1934).

L-Form. Prisms from water. Dec 135° (if completely anhydrous; hydrated crystals soften at 100-105°). $[\alpha]_D^{20}$ +1.2° (c = 2); $[\alpha]_D^{20}$ +17.6° (c = 2 in 6N HCl). pK$_1$' 2.09; pK$_2$' 4.18; pK$_3$' 9.20. Freely sol in water, acetic acid. Insol in alc, ether.

DL-Form. Orthorhombic prisms, needles from water. Dec 198°. Very sol in hot water.

4826. 8-Hydroxy-7-iodo-5-quinolinesulfonic Acid. [547-91-1] 7-Iodo-8-hydroxyquinoline-5-sulfonic acid; *m*-iodo-*o*-hydroxyquinolineanasulfonic acid; Ferron; Loretin. $C_9H_6INO_4S$; mol wt 351.12. C 30.79%, H 1.72%, I 36.14%, N 3.99%, O 18.23%, S 9.13%. Obtained from the potassium salt of 8-hydroxy-5-quinolinesulfonic acid by the action of KI, bleaching powder, and HCl: Claus, *Arch. Pharm.* **231**, 704 (1893); **DE 72942** (1893); by the action of KI and Ca(OCl)$_2$ on 8-hydroxy-5-quinolinesulfonic acid: Botton, *C.A.* **52**, 18407e (1958).

Sulfur yellow, almost odorless and tasteless, crystalline powder. mp 260-270° (dec). One gram dissolves in 500 ml cold, 170 ml boiling water; slightly sol in alcohol. Practically insol in ether or oils.

Compd with chloroquine (2:1). [7270-12-4] Chloquinate; chlochinate; cloquinate; Resotren. Prepn: Koenig, Andersag, US **2650224** (1953 to Schenley Industries).

Mixture of 80% of 8-hydroxy-7-iodo-5-quinolinesulfonic acid and 20% sodium bicarbonate. Chiniofon; quiniofon; Quinoxyl; Sefona; Yatren; Yochinol.

USE: As colorimetric reagent for ferric ion.
THERAP CAT: Antiamebic; antiseptic.

4827. 4-Hydroxyisophthalic Acid. [636-46-4] 4-Hydroxy-1,3-benzenedicarboxylic acid. $C_8H_6O_5$; mol wt 182.13. C 52.76%, H 3.32%, O 43.92%. Prepd by high pressure carbonation of potassium phenate (Kolbe-Schmitt reaction): Baine *et al., J. Org. Chem.* **19**, 510 (1954) or by boiling salicylic acid with carbon tetrachloride in alkaline medium in the presence of Cu powder: **DE 258887** (1913 to Zeltner & Landau); *Chem. Zentralbl.* **1913**, I, 1641; *Frdl.* **11**, 210. Major constituent of the brown dust residue from sublimation of salicylic acid: Hunt *et al., Chem. Ind. (London)* **1955**, 417.

Branched needles from water, platelets from dil alc. Dec 314-315°. One gram dissolves in 3 liters of water at 24°, in 160 ml at 100°. Freely sol in alcohol, ether.
Dimethyl ester. Crystals, mp 97.5°.
Diethyl ester. Crystals, mp 54-55°.
Note: 4-Hydroxyisophthalic acid has been proposed as an improvement over aspirin: Chesher *et al., Nature* **175**, 206 (1955).

4828. Hydroxylamine. [7803-49-8] H_3NO; mol wt 33.03. H 9.15%, N 42.41%, O 48.44%. NH_2OH. Prepn as the hydrochloride: W. L. Semon, *Org. Synth.* **coll. vol. I**, 318 (1932). Prepn: Hurd, *Inorg. Synth.* **1**, 87 (1939); Benson *et al., J. Am. Chem. Soc.* **78**, 4202 (1956). Crystal structure: Meyers, Lipscomb, *Acta Crystallogr.* **5**, 583 (1955). Toxicity data: Riemann, *Acta Pharmacol. Toxicol.* **6**, 285 (1950); R. P. Smith, W. R. Layne, *J. Pharmacol. Exp. Ther.* **165**, 30 (1969). Mutagenic action: Phillips, Brown in *Prog. Nucleic Acid Res. Mol. Biol.* **7**, 349-368 (1967). *Reviews:* Mason, "Hydroxylamine" in *Mellor's* **vol. VIII**, supplement 2, *Nitrogen* (part 2), 115-157 (1967); Jones in *Comprehensive Inorganic Chemistry* **vol. 2**, J. C. Bailar, Jr. *et al.*, Eds. (Pergamon Press, Oxford, 1973) pp 265-276.

Unstable, large white flakes or needles, mp 33°, bp_{22} 58°. d_4^0 1.2255; d_4^{40} 1.204. pK (20°) 7.97. Very sol in water, liq ammonia and methanol. The soly in the higher alcohols decreases with increasing mol wt. Sparingly sol in ether, benzene, carbon disulfide, chloroform. Very hygroscopic. Dec by hot water. Undergoes rapid decompn at room temps esp in the presence of atm moisture and CO_2. Detonates in test tube heated with flame. LD_{50} i.p. in mice: 1.83 mmol/kg (Smith, Layne).
Hydrochloride. [5470-11-1] Oxammonium hydrochloride. $H_3NO.HCl$. Monoclinic columnar crystals; slowly dec when moist. d_{17} 1.67. mp about 151°. One gram dissolves in about 1 ml water (83 g in 100 ml water at 17°); 19 ml alcohol; 8 ml methanol. Sol in glycerol, propylene glycol. Insol in cold ether. pH of 0.2 molar aq soln 3.2. Keep well closed. LD_{50} orally in mice: 408 mg/kg (Riemann).
Sulfate. [10039-54-0] Oxammonium sulfate. $(H_3NO)_2.H_2SO_4$. Crystals, mp about 170°. Freely sol in water.
Caution: Skin irritant. May cause methemoglobinemia, sulfhemoglobinemia, cyanosis, convulsions, hypotension and coma. See *Clinical Toxicology of Commercial Products*, R. E. Gosselin *et al.*, Eds. (Williams & Wilkins, Baltimore, 5th ed., 1984) Section II, p 117.

USE: As reducing agent in photography; in synthetic and analytical chemistry; to purify aldehydes and ketones. As antioxidant for fatty acids and soaps. As dehairing agent for hides.

4829. Hydroxylupanine. [15358-48-2] [2S-(2α,7β,7aβ,-14β,14aα)]-Dodecahydro-2-hydroxy-7,14-methano-2H,11H-dipyrido[1,2-a:1',2'-e][1,5]diazocin-11-one; octalupine; oxylupanine; 13-hydroxylupanine. $C_{15}H_{24}N_2O_2$; mol wt 264.36. C 68.15%, H 9.15%, N 10.60%, O 12.10%. From seed of *Lupinus perennis* L., *L. angustifolius* L. and *L. polyphyllus* Lindl., *Leguminosae:* Rink, Schäfer, *Arch. Pharm.* **287**, 290 (1954); Winterfeld, Pies, *ibid.* **290**, 537 (1957); Bohlmann, Winterfeldt, *Ber.* **93**, 1956 (1960). Structure: Galinovsky *et al., Monatsh. Chem.* **81**, 77 (1950). Biosynthesis: Schuette *et al., Arch. Pharm.* **296**, 438 (1963).

Crystals from dry acetone, mp 169-170°. $[α]_D^{20}$ +45.6° (c = 1.49 in ethanol); $[α]_D^{20}$ +65.1° (c = 1.09 in water). Sol in water, alc, chloroform; slightly sol in benzene, ether.
Methiodide. $C_{15}H_{24}N_2O_2.CH_3I$. Needles from methanol + ether, mp 254-255°.

4830. Hydroxymercurichlorophenols. Prepared from *o*-chlorophenol and mercuric oxide or mercuric salts: F. C. Whitmore, *Organic Compounds of Mercury* (Chemical Catalog Co., New York, 1921) p 269; **DE 234851** (1910 to Bayer), *Frdl.* **10**, 1272.

2-Chloro-4-(hydroxymercuriphenol). [538-04-5] (3-Chloro-4-hydroxyphenyl)hydroxymercury; Semesan. $C_6H_5ClHgO_2$; mol wt 345.15. (n = 1).
USE: Fungicide.

4831. 1-(Hydroxymethyl)-5,5-dimethylhydantoin. [116-25-6] 1-(Hydroxymethyl)-5,5-dimethyl-2,4-imidazolidinedione; monomethyloldimethylhydantoin; MDMH; methylol dimethylhydantoin. $C_6H_{10}N_2O_3$; mol wt 158.16. C 45.56%, H 6.37%, N 17.71%, O 30.35%. Prepd by treating 5,5-dimethylhydantoin with formaldehyde: Mackey, **US 2762708** (1956 to GAF).

Crystals, mp 100°. Freely sol in water, methanol, ethanol, acetone; slightly sol in ethyl acetate. Practically insol in ether, trichloroethylene, carbon tetrachloride.
USE: As preservative in cosmetic prepns. The compound liberates formaldehyde steadily at a very slow rate in the presence of water at pH 6. The available formaldehyde is about 19% (w/w), and 0.1-10% is usuallly mixed with the cosmetic product. When heated in the dry state MDMH forms a water-soluble *dimethylhydantoin formaldehyde resin*, compatible with gelatin, polyvinyl acetate, ethyl cellulose. The resin is used in hair lacquers.

4832. 5-(Hydroxymethyl)-2-furaldehyde. [67-47-0] 5-(Hydroxymethyl)-2-furancarboxaldehyde; 5-(hydroxymethyl)-2-furancarbonal; 5-(hydroxymethyl)-2-furfural; HMF; 5-hydroxymethyl-2-formylfuran. $C_6H_6O_3$; mol wt 126.11. C 57.14%, H 4.80%, O 38.06%. Prepn from the fructose portion of the sugar molecule in 57% yield: Haworth, Jones, *J. Chem. Soc.* **1944**, 667; Haworth, Wiggins, **GB 591858** (1947); **GB 600871** (1948). Improved process: Garber, Jones, **US 2929823** (1960 to Merck & Co.). Purification: Jones, Lange, **US 2994645** (1961 to Merck & Co.). Outline of process using cornstarch, glucose and sucrose as raw materials: Medwick, *Chem. Eng. News* 75 (Sept. 11, 1961). Prepn from molasses: Jones, Lange, **US 3066150** (1962 to Merck & Co.); Hales *et al.*, **US 3071599** (1963 to Atlas Chem.).

Needles from ether + petr ether, mp 31.5°. Avoid contact with eyes. Produces harmless yellow stains on skin. Odor of chamomile flowers. Very slightly volatile with steam (as compared with furfural). d_4^{25} 1.2062. $bp_{0.02}$ 110°. n_D^{18} 1.5627. uv max: 283 nm. Heat of combustion: 665 kcal/mol. Freely sol in water, methanol,

ethanol, acetone, ethyl acetate, dimethylformamide. Sol in ether, benzene, chloroform. Less sol in carbon tetrachloride. Sparingly sol in petr ether. *Keep protected from light and air.*

USE: In the synthesis of dialdehydes, glycols, ethers, amino-alcohols, acetals. Aq acid catalyzes ring opening.

4833. *N*-(Hydroxymethyl)nicotinamide. [3569-99-1] *N*-(Hydroxymethyl)-3-pyridinecarboxamide; 3-pyridinecarboxylic acid hydroxymethylamide; pyridine-3-carboxylic acid *N*-methyl-olamide; Bilamid(e); Felosan; Nikoform; Choligen. $C_7H_8N_2O_2$; mol wt 152.15. C 55.26%, H 5.30%, N 18.41%, O 21.03%. Prepn: Graf, *J. Prakt. Chem.* **138**, 292 (1933); Chechelska, Urbanski, *Rocz. Chem.* **27**, 396 (1953), *C.A.* **49**, 1033f (1955).

Crystals, mp 141-142°. Freely sol in hot alcohol and water; sparingly sol in cold alcohol and water.

Hydrochloride. $C_7H_8N_2O_2 \cdot HCl$. Crystals, mp >120° (dec).

THERAP CAT: Cholagogue.

4834. 1-Hydroxy-2-naphthoic Acid. [86-48-6] 1-Naphthol-2-carboxylic acid. $C_{11}H_8O_3$; mol wt 188.18. C 70.21%, H 4.29%, O 25.51%. Obtained by the action of CO_2 on the sodium salt of α-naphthol under pressure at 120-140°.

White to reddish crystals. mp 191-192°. Almost insol in cold water; freely sol in alcohol, benzene, ether, alkalies.

4835. 3-Hydroxy-2-naphthoic Acid. [92-70-6] 3-Hydroxy-2-naphthalenecarboxylic acid; 3-naphthol-2-carboxylic acid. $C_{11}H_8O_3$; mol wt 188.18. C 70.21%, H 4.29%, O 25.51%. Obtained by the action of CO_2 on the sodium salt of β-naphthol under pressure at 280-290°: Schmitt, Burkard, *Ber.* **20**, 2702 (1887); DE 50341; *Frdl.* **2**, 133; DE 436034; *Chem. Zentralbl.* **1926, I**, 1717; *Frdl.* **15**, 295; DE 436524; *Chem. Zentralbl.* **1927, I**, 182; *Frdl.* **15**, 298; Schwenk, *Chem. Ztg.* **53**, 335 (1929).

Very pale yellow crystals, mp 222-223°. Practically insol in cold water. Slightly sol in hot water. Sol in benzene, chloroform. Freely sol in alc, ether. Sol in alkaline solns.

Magnesium salt. Regacholyl.

USE: The water-sol sodium salt has been used to solubilize riboflavin: Arnold *et al., Poult. Sci.* **31**, 350 (1952).

4836. Hydroxypethidine. [468-56-4] 4-(3-Hydroxyphen-yl)-1-methyl-4-piperidinecarboxylic acid ethyl ester; 4-(*m*-hydroxyphenyl)-1-methylisonipecotic acid ethyl ester; ethyl 4-(*m*-hydroxyphenyl)-1-methylisonipecotate; demidone; oxipethidine; oxypeti-din; Hoechst 10446; Win-771; Bemidone; Biphenal. $C_{15}H_{21}NO_3$; mol wt 263.33. C 68.42%, H 8.04%, N 5.32%, O 18.23%. Prepn: Morrison, Rinderknecht, *J. Chem. Soc.* **1950**, 1467; Eisleb, DE 752755 (1952 to I. G. Farben), *C.A.* **52**, 7361e (1958).

Crystals from ethanol, mp 110°.

Hydrochloride. $C_{15}H_{21}NO_3 \cdot HCl$. Crystals, mp 173-174°. Soluble in water; slightly sol in alc.

Note: This is a controlled substance (opiate): **21 CFR**, 1308.11.

THERAP CAT: Analgesic (narcotic).

4837. *N*-(4-Hydroxyphenyl)glycine. [122-87-2] *p*-Hydroxyphenylaminoacetic acid; *p*-hydroxyanilinoacetic acid; photoglycine; Glycin; Iconyl; Monazol. $C_8H_9NO_3$; mol wt 167.16. C 57.48%, H 5.43%, N 8.38%, O 28.71%. Prepd from *p*-aminophenol and chloracetic acid: Vater, *J. Prakt. Chem.* **29**, 291 (1884); Meldola *et al., J. Chem. Soc.* **111**, 552 (1917); Galatis, *Helv. Chim. Acta* **4**, 576 (1921).

Shiny leaflets from water, browns at 200°, begins to melt at 220°, completely melted at 245-247° (decompn). Sparingly sol in water, alcohol, acetone, ether, chloroform, ethyl acetate, benzene, glacial acetic acid. Sol in alkalies and mineral acids. Freely sol in warm 20% hydrochloric acid.

USE: Photographic developer. In determination of iron; detection and determination of phosphorus and silicon. Acid indicator in bacteriology.

4838. *N*-Hydroxyphthalimide. [524-38-9] 2-Hydroxy-1*H*-isoindole-1,3(2*H*)-dione; NHPI. $C_8H_5NO_3$; mol wt 163.13. C 58.90%, H 3.09%, N 8.59%, O 29.42%. Mediates oxidative catalytic transformations of organic compounds with molecular oxygen. Prepn: L. Cohn, *Ann.* **205**, 295 (1880); H. Gross, I. Keitel, *J. Prakt. Chem.* **311**, 692 (1969). Crystal structure: F.-M. Miao *et al., Acta Crystallogr.* **C51**, 712 (1995). Transition metal free oxidation reactions: C. Einhorn *et al., Chem. Commun.* **1997**, 447; epoxidation of alkenes: T. Iwahama *et al., Heterocycles* **52**, 693 (2000). Transition metal cocatalysis in alkane oxidation: Y. Ishii *et al., J. Org. Chem.* **61**, 4520 (1996); in hydroxylation of fatty acids: M. A. Oakley *et al., J. Mol. Catal. A* **150**, 105 (1999). Description of catalytic mechanisms: Y. Ishii, S. Sakaguchi, *Catal. Surv. Jpn.* **3**, 27 (1999).

Yellowish needles from water, mp 227-229°. Also reported as colorless monoclinic crystals from water. d 1.59 mg m⁻³.

USE: Catalyst for oxidation reactions.

4839. 17α-Hydroxyprogesterone. [68-96-2] 17-Hydroxypregn-4-ene-3,20-dione; 4-pregnen-17α-ol-3,20-dione. $C_{21}H_{30}O_3$; mol wt 330.46. C 76.33%, H 9.15%, O 14.52%. Isoln from adrenal glands: Pfiffner, North, *J. Biol. Chem.* **132**, 459 (1940); **139**, 855 (1941); von Euw, Reichstein, *Helv. Chim. Acta* **24**, 879 (1941). Prepn: Julian *et al.*, US 2648662 (1953 to Glidden); Ringold *et al.*, US 2802839; Stork *et al.*, US 2805203 (both 1957 to Syntex); Chemerda *et al.*, US 2777843; Cutler, Chemerda, US 2786856; US 2786857; Dulaney, McAleer, US 2813060 (all 1957 to Merck & Co.); Cutler *et al., J. Org. Chem.* **24**, 1629 (1959); Pederson, US 3000883 (1961 to Upjohn).

Rhombic or hexagonal leaflets from acetone or alcohol, mp 222-223° (rapid heating). With slow heating the substance undergoes molecular rearrangement accompanied by partial resolidification and becomes completely molten only at 276°. $[\alpha]_D^{17}$ +105.6° (c = 1.0417 in chloroform).

Acetate. 17α-Acetoxyprogesterone. $C_{23}H_{32}O_4$. Crystals from chloroform + methanol, mp 239-240°. uv max: 240 nm (log ε 4.33).

Caproate. [630-56-8] 17α-Hydroxyprogesterone hexanoate; Lentogest; Proge; Proluton Depot. $C_{27}H_{40}O_4$; mol wt 428.60. Prepn: Kaspar *et al.*, **US 2753360** (1956 to Schering AG). Comprehensive description: K. Florey, *Anal. Profiles Drug Subs.* **4** 209-224 (1975). Dense needles from isopropyl ether or methanol, mp 119-121°. $[\alpha]_D^{20}$ +61° (c = 1 in chloroform). Soly (mg/ml): sesame oil 25-29; levulinic acid butyl ester 350-400.

THERAP CAT: Progestogen.

THERAP CAT (VET): Estrus regulator.

4840. Hydroxyproline. [51-35-4] (4R)-4-Hydroxy-L-proline; Hyp; L$_s$-hydroxyproline; (−)-(2S,4R)-4-hydroxyproline; *trans*-4-hydroxyproline; 4(R)-hydroxy-2(S)-pyrrolidinecarboxylic acid. $C_5H_9NO_3$; mol wt 131.13. C 45.80%, H 6.92%, N 10.68%, O 36.60%. Amino acid analog of proline, *q.v.*; non-essential for human development. Shows *cis-trans* isomerism. Constituent of collagen, *q.v.* Isoln from gelatin: E. Fischer, *Ber.* **35**, 2660 (1902). Synthesis: H. Leuchs, *Ber.* **38**, 1937 (1905); and structure determn: H. Leuchs, J. F. Brewster, *Ber.* **46**, 986 (1913). Stereochemistry: Hudson, Neuberger, *J. Org. Chem.* **15**, 24 (1950). Early chemistry and biochemistry: *Amino Acids and Proteins*, D. M. Greenberg, Ed. (Charles C. Thomas, Springfield, IL, 1951) 950 pp., *passim*; J. P. Greenstein, M. Winitz, *Chemistry of the Amino Acids* vols 1-3 (John Wiley and Sons, Inc., New York, 1961) pp. 2018-2042, *passim*. Flow sheets of four different syntheses: *Chem. Eng. News* **40**, 40 (Nov. 12, 1962). One pot synthesis: S. G. Ramaswamy, E. Adams, *J. Org. Chem.* **42**, 3440 (1977). Proof of occurence in plants: D. Ashford, A. Neuberger, *Trends Biochem. Sci.* **5**, 245 (1980). Effects of *cis-trans* isomerism on protein structure: N. Panasik, Jr. *et al.*, *Int. J. Pept. Protein Res.* **44**, 262 (1994). *Review*: R. Kuttan, A. N. Radhakrishnan, *Adv. Enzymol.* **37**, 273-348 (1973). Review of metabolism: E. Adams, L. Frank, *Annu. Rev. Biochem.* **49**, 1005-1061 (1980).

Rhombs or needles from water, mp 274°. $[\alpha]_D$ −76.5° (c = 2.5 in water). pK$_1$' 1.82; pK$_2$' 9.65. Soly in water at 0°: 288.6 g/l; at 25°: 361.1 g/l; at 50°: 451.8 g/l; at 65°: 516.7 g/l. Very slightly sol in alcohol. Insol in ether.

cis-**Form.** [618-27-9] Allohydroxyproline; (2S,4S)-4-hydroxy-proline. mp 238-241°. $[\alpha]_D^{18}$ −58.1° (c = 5.2 in water).

4841. Hydroxypropyl Cellulose. [9004-64-2] Cellulose 2-hydroxypropyl ether; oxypropylated cellulose; Klucel; Lacrisert. Nonionic water soluble ether of cellulose, *q.v.* that produces solns having a wide range of viscosity (200-2500 cp). Prepn: **NL 6401036**; E. D. Klug, **US 3278520**, **US 3278521** (1964, 1966, 1966 all to Hercules). Use in the treatment of dry eye syndrome: T. P. Werblin *et al.*, *Ophthalmology* **88**, 78 (1981); P. Huguet *et al.*, *Bull. Soc. Ophthalmol. Fr.* **81**, 1173 (1981). Review of chemistry, physical properties and uses: E. D. Klug in *Encyclopedia of Polymer Science and Technology* vol. 15 (Interscience, New York, 1971) pp 307-314; A. J. Desmarais, *Industrial Gums*, R. L. Whistler, Ed. (Academic Press, New York, 2nd ed., 1973) pp 649-672.

Off-white powder, softens at 130°. Sol in many polar organic solvents. Ppts from water at 40-45°. Thermoplastic.

USE: As emulsifier, stabilizer, whipping aid, protective colloid, film former or thickener in foods; as binder in ceramics and glazes; in hair and cosmetic prepns; in vacuum-formed containers and blow-molded bottles; as suspending agent in PVC polymerization. Pharmaceutic aid (tablet coating agent).

THERAP CAT: Topical protectant.

4842. Hydroxypropyl Methylcellulose. [9004-65-3] Cellulose 2-hydroxypropyl methyl ether; hypromellose; HPMC; Artelac; Benecel MP; GenTeal; Gonak; Goniosol; Methocel (E, F, J, K); Ocucoat. Derivative of methylcellulose, *q.v.*, that also contains 3-12% hydroxypropyl substitution. Prepn: A. B. Savage, **US 2949452** (1960 to Dow). Review of chemistry, physical properties and use: *idem, Encyclopedia of Polymer Science and Technology* vol. 3 (Interscience, New York, 1965); pp 496-511; G. K. Greminger, A. B. Savage, *Industrial Gums*, R. L. Whistler, Ed. (Academic Press, New York, 1973) pp 619-647. Clinical efficacy as ocular lubricant in Sjogren's syndrome: I. Toda *et al.*, *Cornea* **15**, 120 (1996); in contact lens solutions: P. A. Simmons *et al.*, *CLAO J.* **27**, 192 (2001). Review of production and uses in foods: P. de Mariscal, D. A. Bell in *Handbook of Fat Replacers*, S. Roller, S. A. Jones, Eds. (CRC Press, Boca Raton FL, 1996) pp 145-159. Review of drug release from HPMC-based pharmaceutical systems: J. Siepmann, N. A. Peppas, *Adv. Drug Delivery Rev.* **48**, 139-157 (2001).

Powder. Dissolves slowly in cold water. Insol in hot water. Sol in most polar organics. Solns have a wide range of viscosity (400-60,000 mPa.s).

USE: As emulsifier, film former, protective colloid, stabilizer, suspending agent, or thickener in foods. Pharmaceutic aid (suspending agent; tablet excipient; demulcent; viscosity increasing agent); hydrophilic carrier in drug delivery systems. In adhesives, asphalt emulsions, caulking compounds, tile mortars, plastic mixes, cements, paints.

THERAP CAT: Ocular lubricant.

4843. 8-Hydroxyquinoline. [148-24-3] 8-Quinolinol; oxyquinoline; hydroxybenzopyridine; oxybenzopyridine; phenopyridine; oxychinolin; oxine. C_9H_7NO; mol wt 145.16. C 74.47%, H 4.86%, N 9.65%, O 11.02%. Prepn: Z. H. Skraup, *Monatsh. Chem.* **1**, 316 (1880); **3**, 536 (1882); R. H. F. Manske *et al.*, *Can. J. Res.* **27F**, 359 (1949). Toxicity study: Bernstein *et al.*, *Toxicol. Appl. Pharmacol.* **5**, 599 (1963). *Review*: J. P. Phillips, *Chem. Rev.* **56**, 271-297 (1956). Book: R. G. W. Hollingshead, *Oxine and Its Derivatives* **I-IV** (Butterworth, London, 1954/56).

White crystals or crystalline powder. mp 76°. bp ~267°. Almost insol in water, ether. Freely sol in alc, acetone, chloroform, benzene, aq mineral acids. LD$_{50}$ i.p. in mice: 48 mg/kg (Bernstein).

Sulfate. [134-31-6] Chinosol. $(C_9H_7NO)_2.H_2SO_4$; mol wt 388.39. Pale yellow, cryst powder; slight saffron odor; burning taste. mp 175-178°. Freely sol in water; sol in about 100 parts glycerol, slightly in alcohol. Insol in ether.

Aluminum sulfate. [153-77-5] Nyxolan; Aloxyn. $C_{27}H_{24}AlN_3O_{15}S_3$; mol wt 753.67.

USE: As fungistat; chelating agent in determn of trace metal ions. Aluminum sulfate as antiperspirant, deodorant.

THERAP CAT: Antiseptic. Aluminum sulfate as anthelmintic (Nematodes).

THERAP CAT (VET): THERAP VET (VET): Antiseptic.

4844. 8-Hydroxy-5-quinolinesulfonic Acid. [84-88-8] $C_9H_7NO_4S$; mol wt 225.22. C 48.00%, H 3.13%, N 6.22%, O 28.42%, S 14.24%. Prepn: K. Matsumura, *J. Am. Chem. Soc.* **49**, 810 (1927); N. K. Chawla, M. M. Jones, *Inorg. Chem.* **3**, 1549 (1964).

Pale yellow, needle-like crystals or cryst powder; odorless. mp 322-324°. Freely sol in water, slightly in organic solvents.

USE: In determn of trace metal ions.

4845. Hydroxystilbamidine. [495-99-8] 4-[2-[4-(Amino-iminomethyl)phenyl]ethenyl]-3-hydroxybenzenecarboximidamide; 2-hydroxy-4,4′-stilbenedicarboxamidine; 2-hydroxy-4,4′-diamidi-nostilbene; 2-hydroxy-4,4′-diguanylstilbene; 2-hydroxystilbamide. $C_{16}H_{16}N_4O$; mol wt 280.32. C 68.55%, H 5.75%, N 19.99%, O 5.71%. Prepn: J. N. Ashley, J. O. Harris, *J. Chem. Soc.* **1946**, 567; A. J. Ewins *et al.*, **GB 574486**; A. J. Ewins, **US 2510047** (1946, 1950 both to May & Baker). Organ and tissue distribution in animals: I. Snapper *et al.*, *Cancer* **4**, 1246 (1951). Pharmacology and antiprotozoal activity: I. Snapper *et al.*, *Trans. N.Y. Acad. Sci.* **14**, 269 (1952). Probe for studying nucleic acid conformation: B. Festy, *C.R. Seances Acad. Sci. Ser. D* **266**, 1433 (1968); B. Festy, M. Daune, *Biochemistry* **12**, 4827 (1973); B. Festy *et al.*, *Biochim. Biophys. Acta* **407**, 24 (1975). Crystal structure: C. Courseille *et al.*, *C.R. Seances Acad. Sci. Ser. C* **274**, 1921 (1972). Use as a fluorochrome for selective staining of nuclei: L. B. Murgatroyd, *Histochemistry* **74**, 107 (1982). *Review:* B. Festy in *Antibiotics* vol. 5, pt. 2, F. E. Hahn, Ed. (Springer-Verlag, New York, 1979) pp 223-235.

Yellow microcrystals from nitrobenzene, mp 235°. LD_{50} in mice (mg/g); 0.027 i.v.; 0.14 s.c. (Ewins, 1950).

Isethionate. [533-22-2] $C_{20}H_{28}N_4O_9S_2$. Yellow crystals, discolored by light, mp 286° (dec). Freely sol in water. Soly in alcohol ~1.0 g/100 ml. Practically insol in ether. pH of a 1% aq soln 3.3 to 5.3. Solns show strong yellow fluorescence under uv light. Solns should be freshly prepared. Although the hydroxy compd is more stable in soln, such solns should not be stored and must not be used if cloudy.

THERAP CAT: Antiprotozoal (Leishmania).

4846. Hydroxytetracaine. [490-98-2] 4-Butylamino-2-hydroxybenzoic acid 2-dimethylaminoethyl ester; *p*-butylaminosalicylic acid 2-dimethylaminoethyl ester; 2-dimethylaminoethyl *p*-butylaminosalicylate; hydroxamethocaine; Rhenocain; Salicain. $C_{15}H_{24}N_2O_3$; mol wt 280.36. C 64.26%, H 8.63%, N 9.99%, O 17.12%. Prepn: **GB 736960** (1955); **GB 760003** (1956 to Rheinpreussen AG); Grimme, Schmitz, *Ber.* **84**, 734 (1951).

Hydrochloride. $C_{15}H_{24}N_2O_3$·HCl. Crystals from water, mp 157°. Soly in water at 20°: about 4%.

Hemihydrate. Prisms from ligroin, mp 48°.

THERAP CAT: Anesthetic (local).

4847. 5-Hydroxytryptophan. [56-69-9] 5-HTP. $C_{11}H_{12}N_2O_3$; mol wt 220.22. C 59.99%, H 5.49%, N 12.72%, O 21.80%. Precursor of serotonin. Synthesis from 5-benzyloxy-indole: Ek, Witkop, *J. Am. Chem. Soc.* **76**, 5579 (1954); Shaw, Morris, *Biochem. Prep.* **9**, 92 (1962); from 5-benzyloxytryptophan: Frangatos, Chubb, *Can. J. Chem.* **37**, 1374 (1959); Frangatos, **CA 619472** (1961 to Frank W. Horner); Ash, **GB 845034** (1960 to May & Baker); from tryptophan: Renson *et al.*, *Biochem. Biophys. Res. Commun.* **6**, 20 (1961). Prepn of L- and D-forms: A. J. Morris, M. D. Armstrong, *J. Org. Chem.* **22**, 306 (1957). Crystal and molecular structure of DL-form: Wakahara *et al.*, *Tetrahedron Lett.* **1970**, 3003. Use of L-5HTP in treatment of myoclonus: M. H. Van Woert, D. Rosenbaum, *Adv. Neurol.* **26**, 107 (1979). Clinical trial in migraine: F. Titus *et al.*, *Eur. Neurol.* **25**, 327 (1986). *Review:* M. H. Van Woert, *Orphan Drugs*, F. E. Karch, Ed. (Marcel Dekker, New York, 1982) pp 13-31. Review of antidepressant efficacy: W. F. Byerley *et al.*, *J. Clin. Psychopharmacol.* **7**, 127-137 (1987); of

metabolism and clinical experience: T. C. Birdsall, *Altern. Med. Rev.* **3**, 271-280 (1998).

DL-Form. Minute rods or needles from ethanol, dec 298-300°. uv max (H_2O at pH 6.0): 278 nm. Soly in water at 5°: 1.0 g/100 ml; at 100°: 5.5 g/100 ml. Soly in 50% boiling alc: 2.5 g/100 ml. Aq solns are stable at low pH.

L-Form. [4350-09-8] Oxitriptan; L-5HTP; Cincofarm; Levothym; Lévotonine; Oxyfan; Telesol; Tript-Oh. Crystals, $[\alpha]_D^{20}$ −32.5° (H_2O); $[\alpha]_D^{20}$ +16.0° (4N HCl).

D-Form. [4350-07-6] Crystals, $[\alpha]_D^{20}$ +32.2° (H_2O).

THERAP CAT: Antidepressant; in treatment of myoclonus.

4848. Hydroxyurea. [127-07-1] Hydroxycarbamide; Droxia; Hydrea; Litalir. $CH_4N_2O_2$; mol wt 76.05. C 15.79%, H 5.30%, N 36.84%, O 42.08%. $H_2NCONHOH$. Ribonuleotide reductase inhibitor; blocks DNA synthesis and repair. Induces fetal hemoglobin production in patients with sickle cell anemia. Prepn: W. F. C. Dressler, R. Stein, *Ann.* **150**, 242 (1869). Alternate route: P. J. Graham, **US 2705727** (1955 to Du Pont). Symposium on mechanism of action and clinical experience in cancer: *Semin. Oncol.* **19**, Suppl. 9, 1-116 (1992). Clinical trials in sickle cell crises in adults: S. Charache *et al.*, *N. Engl. J. Med.* **332**, 1317 (1995); in children: T. R. Kinney *et al.*, *Blood* **94**, 1550 (1999). Review of clinical pharmacokinetics: P. R. Gwilt, W. G. Tracewell, *Clin. Pharmacokinet.* **34**, 347-358 (1998); of pharmacology and potential therapeutic indications: P. Navarra, P. Preziosi, *Crit. Rev. Oncol. Hematol.* **29**, 249-255 (1999). Clinical trial in essential thrombocythemia: C. N. Harrison *et al.*, *N. Engl. J. Med.* **353**, 33 (2005).

Needles from alc, mp 133-136°. Freely sol in water, hot alcohol.

THERAP CAT: Antineoplastic; in treatment of sickle cell anemia.

4849. Hydroxyzine. [68-88-2] 2-[2-[4-[(4-Chlorophenyl)-phenylmethyl]-1-piperazinyl]ethoxy]ethanol; 1-(*p*-chloro-α-phenylbenzyl)-4-(2-hydroxyethoxyethyl)piperazine; 1-(*p*-chlorodiphenylmethyl)-4-[2-(2-hydroxyethoxy)ethyl]piperazine; *N*-(4-chlorobenzhydryl)-*N*′-(hydroxyethyloxyethyl)piperazine; 1-(*p*-chlorobenzhydryl)-4-[2-(2-hydroxyethoxy)ethyl]diethylenediamine; UCB-4492; Tran-Q; Tranquizine. $C_{21}H_{27}ClN_2O_2$; mol wt 374.90. C 67.28%, H 7.26%, Cl 9.46%, N 7.47%, O 8.54%. H_1 receptor antagonist. Outline of commercial prepn: *Chem. Week* **79** (5), 70 (Aug. 4, 1956); Morren, **US 2899436** (1959 to UCB). Pharmacology and metabolism: Cannizaro, *Boll. Chim. Farm.* **104**, 39 (1965); Close *et al.*, *Ind. Chim. Belge* **33**, 94 (1968); *eidem, Proc. Eur. Soc. Study Drug Toxic.* **9**, 144 (1968); S. F. Pong, C. L. Huang, *J. Pharm. Sci.* **63**, 1527 (1974). Pharmacokinetics and antihistaminic activity: F. E. R. Simons *et al.*, *J. Allergy Clin. Immunol.* **73**, 69 (1984); S. Ting *et al.*, *ibid.* **75**, 63 (1985). Clinical trials of efficacy in allergic rhinitis: L. Wong *et al.*, *ibid.* **67**, 223 (1981); in urticaria, R. P. Harvey *et al.*, *ibid.* **68**, 262 (1981); as anti-emetic: R. McKenzie *et al.*, *Anesth. Analg.* **60**, 783 (1981); as pre-surgical sedative: G. Wallace, L. J. Mindlin, *ibid.* **63**, 571 (1984). Toxicity data: E. I. Goldenthal, *Toxicol. Appl. Pharmacol.* **18**, 185 (1971). Comprehensive description: J. Tsau, N. DeAngelis, *Anal. Profiles Drug Subs.* **7**, 319-341 (1978).

Dihydrochloride. [2192-20-3] Alamon; Atarax; Aterax; Durrax; Orgatrax; Quiess; Vistaril Parenteral. $C_{21}H_{27}ClN_2O_2$·2HCl;

mol wt 447.83. Crystals, mp 193°. Bitter taste. Soly in mg/ml: water <700; chloroform 60; acetone 2; ether <0.1. Solns are unstable to intense uv light. LD_{50} in rats (mg/kg): 126 i.p.; 950 orally (Goldenthal).

Pamoate. [10246-75-0] Equipose; Masmoran; Paxistil; Vistaril Pamoate. $C_{21}H_{27}ClN_2O_2 \cdot C_{23}H_{16}O_6$; mol wt 763.27. Crystals. Practically insol in water.

THERAP CAT: Anxiolytic. Antihistaminic.

THERAP CAT (VET): Has been used as a tranquilizer.

4850. Hygrine. [496-49-1] 1-[(2*R*)-1-Methyl-2-pyrrolidinyl]-2-propanone; (+)-*N*-methyl-2-acetonylpyrrolidine. $C_8H_{15}NO$; mol wt 141.21. C 68.04%, H 10.71%, N 9.92%, O 11.33%. Occurs in leaves of *Erythroxylon coca* Lam., *Erythroxylaceae* of diverse origin: Liebermann, *Ber.* **22**, 677 (1889). Synthesis: Galinovsky *et al.*, *Monatsh. Chem.* **82**, 551 (1951); Lukes *et al.*, *Collect. Czech. Chem. Commun.* **24**, 2433 (1959); Leonard, Cook, *J. Am. Chem. Soc.* **81**, 5627 (1959). Enzymatic synthesis: Tuppy, Faltaous, *Monatsh. Chem.* **91**, 167 (1960). Stereochemistry: Galinovsky *et al.*, *ibid.* **84**, 798 (1953). Absolute configuration: Lukes *et al.*, *Collect. Czech. Chem. Commun.* **25**, 483 (1960).

Liquid. bp_{11} 76.5°; bp_{14} 81°. n_D^{20} 1.4555. Sol in alcohol, chloroform, dil acids; slightly sol in water.

Oxime. $C_8H_{16}N_2O$. Crystals from ether, mp 123-124°.

4851. Hygromycin. [6379-56-2] (*E*)-5-Deoxy-5-[[3-[4-[(6-deoxy-β-D-*arabino*-hexofuranos-5-ulos-1-yl)oxy]-3-hydroxyphenyl]-2-methyl-1-oxo-2-propenyl]amino]-1,2-*O*-methylene-D-*neo*-inositol; homomycin; hygromycin A; 1703-18B; ST-4331. $C_{23}H_{29}NO_{12}$; mol wt 511.48. C 54.01%, H 5.71%, N 2.74%, O 37.54%. Antibiotic substance produced by *Streptomyces hygroscopicus* (Jensen) Waksman & Henrici, from forest soil near Indianapolis, Ind: R. L. Mann *et al.*, *Antibiot. Chemother.* **3**, 1279 (1953). Produced also by *Streptomyces noboritoensis* from soil collected in Kanawaga Prefecture. Identity of homomycin and hygromycin: K. Isono *et al.*, *J. Antibiot.* **10A**, 21 (1957). Structure: *eidem, ibid.* 160; R. L. Mann, D. O. Woolf, *J. Am. Chem. Soc.* **79**, 120 (1957). Abs config: K. Kakinuma, Y. Sakagami, *Agric. Biol. Chem.* **42**, 279 (1978). Synthesis of the sugar component: M. Nakajima, S. Takahashi, *ibid.* **31**, 1082 (1967). Total synthesis: N. Chida *et al.*, *Chem. Commun.* **1989**, 436. Peptide synthesis inhibitor: M. Guerrero, J. Modolell, *Eur. J. Biochem.* **107**, 409 (1980).

Amorphous white powder. mp 105-109°, dec above 160°. Also reported as mp 110-112° (dec) (Chida). Weakly acidic. pKa 8.9. $[\alpha]_D^{25}$ −126° (c = 1 in water). Freely sol in water, alc. Practically insol in the less polar solvents. uv max (dil HCl): 272, 214 nm ($E_{1cm}^{1\%}$ 306, 416).

4852. Hygromycin B. [31282-04-9] *O*-6-Amino-6-deoxy-L-*glycero*-D-*galacto*-heptopyranosylidene-(1 → 2-3)-*O*-β-D-talopyranosyl-(1 → 5)-2-deoxy-*N*³-methyl-D-streptamine; Hygromix. $C_{20}H_{37}N_3O_{13}$; mol wt 527.52. C 45.54%, H 7.07%, N 7.97%, O 39.43%. Antibiotic substance produced by *Streptomyces hygroscopicus* (Jensen) Waksman & Henrici, from soil samples from Nebraska and Indiana: Mann, Bromer, *J. Am. Chem. Soc.* **80**, 2714 (1958). Prodn: McGuire, Mann, US 3018220 (1962 to Lilly). Structure: Neuss *et al.*, *Helv. Chim. Acta* **53**, 2314 (1970). Studies on mode of action: A. Gonzalez *et al.*, *Biochim. Biophys. Acta* **521**, 459 (1978).

Amorphous powder, dec 160-180°. Weakly basic. pKa 7.1, 8.8. $[\alpha]_D^{20}$ +20.2° (c = 1 in water). Freely sol in water, methanol and ethanol. Practically insol in less polar solvents. Absorption spectrum: Mann, Bromer, *loc. cit.*

THERAP CAT (VET): Anthelmintic (swine and chicken).

4853. Hygrophylline. [3573-82-8] (1α,14α)-1,2-Dihydro-12,14-dihydroxysenecionan-11,16-dione. $C_{18}H_{27}NO_6$; mol wt 353.41. C 61.17%, H 7.70%, N 3.96%, O 27.16%. Pyrrolizidine alkaloid isolated from *Senecio hygrophyllus* Dyer and Sm., *Compositae*: Richardson, Warren, *J. Chem. Soc.* **1943**, 452. Structure and stereochemistry: Schlosser, Warren, *ibid.* **1965**, 5707. NMR spectrum: S. E. Drewes *et al.*, *J. Chem. Soc. Perkin Trans. 1* **1981**, 287. X-ray crystallography: M. F. Mackay *et al.*, *Acta Crystallogr.* **C41**, 395 (1985).

Prisms from acetone, mp 173-174°. $[\alpha]_D^{20}$ −67.3° (c = 2.9 in ethanol).

4854. Hymecromone. [90-33-5] 7-Hydroxy-4-methyl-2*H*-1-benzopyran-2-one; 7-hydroxy-4-methylcoumarin; 7-hydroxy-4-methyl-2-oxo-3-chromene; 4-methylumbelliferone; β-methylumbelliferone; imecromone; 4-MU; Bilcolic; Biliton H; Cantabilin; Cantabiline; Cholonerton; Cholspasmin; Cumarote C; Himecol; Medilla; Mendiaxon. $C_{10}H_8O_3$; mol wt 176.17. C 68.18%, H 4.58%, O 27.25%. Prepd from resorcinol and ethyl acetoacetate: Pechmann, Duisberg, *Ber.* **16**, 2119 (1883); Russell, Frye, *Org. Synth.* **21**, 23 (1941); Woods, Sapp, *J. Org. Chem.* **27**, 3703 (1962). Use in determn of nitric acid: F. J. Welcher, *Organic Analytical Reagents* vol. 1 (Van Nostrand, New York, 1947) pp 214-215.

Crystals from alc, mp 194-195° (Woods, Sapp), formerly reported as 185-186° (Pechmann, Duisberg). uv max (methanol): 221, 251, 322.5 nm. Blue fluorescence in alcohol + water. Sol in methanol, glacial acetic acid; slightly sol in ether, chloroform. Practically insol in cold water.

USE: Analytical reagent.

THERAP CAT: Choleretic; antispasmodic.

4855. Hymecromone *O,O*-Diethyl Phosphorothioate. [299-45-6] 7-Hydroxy-4-methylcoumarin *O*-ester with *O,O*-diethyl phosphorothioate; *O,O*-diethyl *O*-(4-methyl-7-coumarinyl) phosphorothioate; *O,O*-diethyl *O*-(4-methyl-7-coumarinyl) thiophosphate; *O,O*-diethyl *O*-(4-methylumbelliferone) phosphorothioate; 4-methylumbelliferone *O,O*-diethyl phosphorothioate; E-838; Potasan. $C_{14}H_{17}O_5PS$; mol wt 328.32. C 51.22%, H 5.22%, O 24.37%, P 9.43%, S 9.77%. Cholinesterase inhibitor. Dechlorination product of coumaphos, *q.v.* Prepn: Schrader, Kükenthal, US 2583744 (1952 to Bayer). Pharmacology and toxicology: J. P. Frawley *et al.*, *J. Pharmacol. Exp. Ther.* **105**, 156 (1952). Water partition and molecular interactions: A. Lopes *et al.*, *Environ. Sci. Technol.* **29**, 562 (1995). *Review:* G. Schrader, *Die En-*

twicklung neuer insektizider Phosphorsäure-Ester (Verlag Chemie, 1963) p 187.

Long needles from petr ether. Weak aromatic odor. mp 39.5-41.3°. bp$_{1.0}$ 210° (dec). d$_4^{38}$ 1.260 (liq); n$_D^{37}$ 1.5685 (liq). Log P (1-octanol/water): 14. Very sparingly sol in water. Slightly sol in petr ether. Sol in most other organic solvents. Aq solns of emulsions adjusted to pH 7 to 8 show a blue fluorescence. LD$_{50}$ in mice, guinea pigs, male, female rats (mg/kg): 98.5 ±5.0, 25.0 ±2.3, 42.0 ±3.1, 19.0 ±2.5 orally (Frawley).

USE: Systemic insecticide, especially effective against the Colorado beetle.

4856. Hymexazol. [10004-44-1] 5-Methyl-3(2*H*)-isoxazolone; 3-hydroxy-5-methylisoxazole; F-319; RTY-319; Tachigaren. C$_4$H$_5$NO$_2$; mol wt 99.09. C 48.48%, H 5.09%, N 14.14%, O 32.29%. Prepn: NL 6511925; I. Iwai *et al.*, US 3544584 (1966, 1970 both to Sankyo); I. Iwai, N. Nakamura, *Chem. Pharm. Bull.* **14**, 1277 (1966). Metabolism in plants: S. Kamimura *et al.*, *Phytopathology* **64**, 1273 (1974). Properties and analytical methods: T. Nakamura *et al.*, *Anal. Methods Pestic. Plant Growth Regul.* **10**, 215 (1978). GC determn in plants and soils: *idem et al.*, *Annu. Rep. Sankyo Res. Lab.* **28**, 130 (1976). Plant growth promoting activity: Y. Ota, *Jpn. Agric. Res. Q.* **9**, 1 (1975). Mode of fungicidal action: T. Nakanishi, H. D. Sisler, *J. Pestic. Sci.* **8**, 173 (1983). Field studies: P. A. Payne, G. E. Williams, *Crop Prot.* **9**, 371 (1990). Series of articles on chemistry, biological activity and metabolism: *Annu. Rep. Sankyo Res. Lab.* **25**, 1-51 (1973). Brief review: R. Ishitsuka, *Jpn. Pestic. Inf.* **18**, 27-30 (1974).

White needles from *n*-hexane, mp 84-85°. Also reported as mp 86-87° (Nakamura, 1983). Vapor pressure (25°) 1.01 × 10^{-3} Torr. Soly at 25° (g/100 ml): ~8.5 in water. Very sol in methanol, ethanol, isopropanol, acetone, methyl isobutyl ketone, tetrahydrofuran, dioxane, DMF, ethylene glycol, chloroform. Fairly sol in diethyl ether, benzene, xylene, trichloroethylene. Slightly sol in *n*-hexane, carbon disulfide. LD$_{50}$ in male, female mice, rats (mg/kg): 2148, 1968, 4678, 3909 orally; 1297, 1167, 1924, 1884 s.c.; 445, 514, >1000, >1000 i.v.; in rats, rabbits (mg/kg): >10000, >2000 dermally (Nakamura, 1978).

USE: Agricultural fungicide and plant growth regulator.

4857. Hyodeoxycholic Acid. [83-49-8] (3α,5β,6α)-3,6-Dihydroxycholan-24-oic acid; 3α,6α-dihydroxy-5β-cholanic acid; α-hyodeoxycholic acid; hyodesoxycholic acid. C$_{24}$H$_{40}$O$_4$; mol wt 392.57. C 73.43%, H 10.27%, O 16.30%. Isoln from pig bile: Wieland, Gumlich, *Z. Physiol. Chem.* **215**, 18 (1933); Trickey, US 2547726 (1951 to U.S. Rubber); Fogle, US 2745849 (1956 to Armour); Buckley, Ziegler, US 2758120 (1956 to Canada Packers); Liebig, US 3006927 (1961 to Riedel-de Haen). Configuration: Moffett, Hoehn, *J. Am. Chem. Soc.* **69**, 1995 (1947).

Crystals from ethyl acetate, mp 196-197°. [α]$_D^{20}$ +8° (alc). Moderately sol in ethanol, glacial acetic acid. Less sol in ether, acetone, ethyl acetate, benzene.

4858. Hyoscyamine. [101-31-5] [3(*S*)-*endo*]-α-(Hydroxymethyl)benzeneacetic acid 8-methyl-8-azabicyclo[3.2.1]oct-3-yl ester; 1α*H*,5α*H*-tropan-3α-ol(−)-tropate (ester); 3α-tropanyl *S*-(−)-tropate; *l*-tropic acid ester with tropine; *l*-tropine tropate; duboisine; *l*-hyoscyamine; Cystospaz; Levsin. C$_{17}$H$_{23}$NO$_3$; mol wt 289.37. C 70.56%, H 8.01%, N 4.84%, O 16.59%. Anticholinergic. From *Hyoscyamus niger* L., *Atropa belladonna* L., *Datura stramonium* L., and other *Solanaceae*: Ladenburg, *Ann.* **206**, 274 (1881). Identity with duboisine and daturine: Beckurts, *Apoth. Ztg.* **27**, 683 (1912). Obtained by resolution of atropine: Werner, Miltenberger, *Ann.* **631**, 163 (1960). Prepd from (−)-acetyltropoyl chloride and atropine hydrochloride: Fodor *et al.*, *Acta Chim. Acad. Sci. Hung.* **28**(4), 409 (1961), *C.A.* **61**, 1903g (1964). Configuration: Fodor, Csepreghy, *Tetrahedron Letters* no. 7, 16 (1959). Comprehensive description: F. J. Muhtadi, *Anal. Profiles Drug Subs. Excip.* **23**, 153-228 (1994).

Silky, tetragonal needles from evaporating alc. *Keep well closed and protect from light and heat;* easily racemized. mp 108.5°. [α]$_D^{20}$ −21.0° (alc). pKa (21°) 9.7. One gram dissolves in 281 ml water (pH 9.5), 69 ml ether, 150 ml benzene, 1 ml chloroform. Freely sol in alcohol, dil acids. uv max (methanol): 247, 252, 258, 264 nm (A$_{1cm}^{1\%}$ 5.18, 5.70, 6.12, 5.10). Absorption spectra: Dobbie, Fox, *J. Chem. Soc.* **103**, 1194, 1195 (1913).

Hydrobromide. [306-03-6] C$_{17}$H$_{23}$NO$_3$.HBr. Deliquescent crystals, mp 152°. pH 5.4 (1 in 100). Levorotatory. Very sol in water. One gram dissolves in 3 ml alcohol, 1.2 ml chloroform, 2260 ml ether.

Hydrochloride. C$_{17}$H$_{23}$NO$_3$.HCl. Crystals. *Poisonous!* mp 149-151°. Freely sol in water, alcohol.

Methyl bromide. *N*-Methylhyoscyaminium bromide. C$_{17}$H$_{23}$-NO$_3$.CH$_3$Br. Crystals, mp 210-212°. Freely sol in water, dil alc; slightly sol in abs alc.

Sulfate dihydrate. [6835-16-1] Egacene; Egazil Duretter; Peptard. (C$_{17}$H$_{23}$NO$_3$)$_2$.H$_2$SO$_4$.2H$_2$O; mol wt 712.85. Needles from alcohol, mp 206° when dry. [α]$_D^{15}$ −29° (c = 2). pH 5.3 (1 in 100). One gram dissolves in 0.5 ml water, about 5.0 ml alcohol. Very slightly sol in chloroform, ether.

THERAP CAT: Antispasmodic.

4859. Hyoscyamus. Henbane; hog's bean; insane root; poison tobacco; black henbane. Dried leaves, with or without the tops, of *Hyoscyamus niger* L., *Solanaceae,* yielding 0.040% hyoscyamus alkaloids (chiefly hyoscyamine and scopolamine). The leaves and seeds have been used as smooth muscle relaxants. The alkaloid content of the seeds is less than that of the leaves. Egyptian henbane *(Hyoscyamus muticus* L., *Solanaceae)* contains about 0.5% alkaloids. *Habit.* Europe, Africa, Asia, naturalized in U.S.; cultivated in England. *Constit.* Leaves: scopolamine, hyoscyamine, hyoscipicrin, choline.

4860. Hypalon®. [9008-08-6] Elastomer made by substituting chlorine and sulfonyl chloride groups into polyethylene. Prepd from polyethylene of average mol wt of about 20,000; contains approx one chlorine atom for each seven carbon atoms and one sulfonyl chloride group for every ninety carbon atoms. Three types of Hypalon are available: 20, 30, and 40 with sp gr of 1.12, 1.28, and 1.18, respectively. Prepn: Reed, Horn, US 2046090 (1933). *Reviews: Ullmanns Encyklopädie der technischen Chemie* vol. 9, 342 (1957); Keeley, "Hypalon Synthetic Rubber" in *Introduction to Rubber Technology,* Morton, Ed. (Reinhold, New York, 1959) p 349.

4861. Hypaphorine. [487-58-1] (αS)-α-Carboxy-N,N,N-tri-methyl-1H-indole-3-ethanaminium inner salt; 1-trimethylammonio-3-(3-indolyl)propionate. $C_{14}H_{18}N_2O_2$; mol wt 246.30. C 68.27%, H 7.37%, N 11.37%, O 12.99%. The trimethylbetaine of trypto-phan. Poisonous alkaloid from seeds of *Erythrina americana* Mill., *E. sandwicensis* Degener, *E. crista-galli* L., and *Abrus precatorius* Linn., *Leguminosae*: Folkers, Koniuszy, *J. Am. Chem. Soc.* **61**, 1232 (1939); **62**, 1677 (1940); Deulofeu *et al., J. Chem. Soc.* **1939**, 1841; Tung, Lao, *C.A.* **55**, 17770i (1961). Structure and synthesis: von Romburgh, Barger, *J. Chem. Soc.* **99**, 2068 (1911).

Crystals from dil alc, dec 237°; after purification through the nitrate, dec 255°. $[\alpha]_D^{27}$ +113° (c = 0.52). Sol in 12 parts water, slightly in alc. Almost insol in other usual solvents.

Hydrochloride. $C_{14}H_{18}N_2O_2$.HCl. Crystals from water, dec 231-232°, $[\alpha]_D^{32}$ +90° (c = 0.5). Moderately sol in water.

Nitrate. $C_{14}H_{18}N_2O_2$.HNO$_3$. Dec 224°, $[\alpha]_D^{20}$ +95°. Sol in 170 parts water.

4862. Hyperforin. [11079-53-1] (1R,5S,6R,7S)-4-Hy-droxy-6-methyl-1,3,7-tris(3-methyl-2-butenyl)-5-(2-methyl-1-oxo-propyl)-6-(4-methyl-3-pentenyl)bicyclo[3.3.1]non-3-ene-2,9-dione. $C_{35}H_{52}O_4$; mol wt 536.78. C 78.31%, H 9.76%, O 11.92%. Principal acylphloroglucinol component in St. John's wort. Inhibits synaptosomal uptake of serotonin, norephinephrine and dopamine; thought to be responsible for the antidepressant activity of medicinal preparations of hypericum, *q.v.* Isoln and antibacterial activity: A. I. Gurevich *et al., Antibiotiki* **16**, 510 (1971), *C.A.* **75**, 95625 (1971). Improved isoln procedure: C. A. J. Erdelmeier, *Pharmacopsychiatry* **31**, Suppl 1, 2 (1998). Structure: N. S. Bystrov *et al., Tetrahedron Lett.* **1975**, 2791. Abs config: I. Brondz *et al., Acta Chem. Scand.* **A37**, 263 (1983). HPLC determn in plasma: J. D. Chi, M. Franklin, *J. Chromatogr. B* **735**, 285 (1999). Series of articles on psychopharmacology and neurotransmitter reuptake inhibition: *Pharmacopsychiatry* **31**, Suppl 1, 7-29 (1998).

mp 79-80°. $[\alpha]_D^{18}$ +41° (in ethanol). pKa 4.8 (50% aq ethanol). uv max (methanol): 275.5 nm (log ε 3.95). Unstable when exposed to air and light.

4863. Hypericin. [548-04-9] 1,3,4,6,8,13-Hexahydroxy-10,11-dimethylphenanthro[1,10,9,8-*opqra*]perylene-7,14-dione; 4,-5,5′,4′,5′,7′-hexahydroxy-2,2′-dimethylnaphthodianthrone; hypericum red. $C_{30}H_{16}O_8$; mol wt 504.44. C 71.43%, H 3.20%, O 25.37%. Characteristic principal of hypericum, *q.v.* (St. John's wort). Isoln from *Hypericum perforatum* L., *Hypericaceae*: Brockmann *et al., Ann.* **553**, 1 (1942). Synthesis from bromo-emodin trimethylether: Brockmann, Muxfeld, *Naturwissenschaften* **40**, 411 (1953). Structure: Brockmann *et al., ibid.* **37**, 540 (1950); Brockmann, Sanne, *ibid.* **40**, 509 (1953). Total synthesis: Brockmann, Kluge, **US 2707704** (1955 to Schenley); Brockmann *et al., Ber.* **90**, 2302 (1957); Brockmann, Eggers, *ibid.* **91**, 547 (1958). Clinical pharmacokinetics and evaluation of phototoxic potential: J. Brockmöller *et al., Pharmacopsychiatry* **30**, Suppl 2, 94 (1997). HPLC determn in plasma: J. D. Chi, M. Franklin, *J. Chromatogr. B* **724**, 195 (1999).

Solvated blue-black needles from pyridine + methanolic HCl, dec 320°. Freely sol in pyridine and other organic bases yielding cherry-red solns with red fluorescence. Almost insol in most other organic solvents. Sol in alkaline aq solns; below pH 11.5 solns are red, above pH 11.5 they are green with red fluorescence. Absorption and fluorescence spectra: Scheibe, Schöntag, *Ber.* **75**, 2019 (1942); Brockmann, Neef, *loc. cit.*

THERAP CAT: Antidepressant.

4864. Hypericum. St. John's wort; hyperici herba. Herbaceous, perennial plant, *Hypericum perforatum* L. (*Hypericaceae*), widely used in traditional medicine. *Habit.* Europe, Asia, North Africa; naturalized in the U.S. *Constit.* Hyperforin, hypericin, *q.q.v.*, pseudohypericin; flavonoids such as hyperin, rutin, quercetin; biapigenins; essential oil; tannins; procyanidins. Medicinal formulations are prepared from the dried flowering tops. Description of botany, constituents and medicinal uses: E. Bombardelli, P. Morazzoni, *Fitoterapia* **66**, 43-68 (1995). HPLC analysis and effect of cultivation on components: B. Büter *et al., Planta Med.* **64**, 431 (1998). HPLC determn of constituents in dietary supplements: W. Li, J. F. Fitzloff, *J. Chromatogr. B* **765**, 99 (2001). Pharmacology of extracts: S. Perovic, W. E. G. Müller, *Arzneim.-Forsch.* **45**, 1145 (1995); J. T. Neary, Y. Bu, *Brain Res.* **816**, 358 (1999). Clinical trial in comparison with imipramine for depression: M. Philipp *et al., Br. Med. J.* **319**, 1534 (1999). Reviews of clinical experience: E. Ernst *et al., Eur. J. Clin. Pharmacol.* **54**, 589-594 (1998); B. Gaster, J. Holroyd, *Arch. Int. Med.* **160**, 152-156 (2000).

THERAP CAT: Antidepressant.

4865. Hypochlorous Acid. [7790-92-3] ClHO; mol wt 52.46. Cl 67.58%, H 1.92%, O 30.50%. HClO. Known in aq soln only. Formed by the action of water on chlorine: Cady, *Inorg. Synth.* **5**, 160 (1957). A 25% soln of hypochlorous acid is obtained when chlorine hydrate and mercuric oxide are distilled at low pressure: Goldschmidt, *Ber.* **52**, 753 (1919). *Review:* J. A. Wojtowicz, "Chlorine Monoxide, Hypochlorous Acid, and Hypochlorites", in *Kirk-Othmer Encyclopedia of Chemical Technology* vol. 5 (Wiley-Interscience, New York, 3rd ed., 1979) pp 580-611.

Aq soln (25%), greenish yellow liquid. May be stored for a few days if kept at $-20°$. Dec slowly to Cl_2, O_2 and $HClO_4$. Very weak acid. pK (25°) 7.49. Strong oxidizing agent. When a 25% soln is evapd in a vacuum, chlorine monoxide, Cl_2O, is given off. Cl_2O in soln with HClO may be removed by shaking with carbon tetrachloride, but will form again. *Protect from light.*

Note: An aqueous soln of the potassium salt is known as **Javelle water** or **Eau de Javelle** (also used for sodium hypochlorite, *q.v.*).

USE: Disinfectant.

4866. Hypoglycine A. [156-56-9] ($\alpha S,1R$)-α-Amino-2-methylenecyclopropanepropanoic acid; 2-methylenecyclopropane-alanine; 2-amino-4,5-methylenehex-5-enoic acid; α-amino-β-(2-methylenecyclopropyl)propionic acid; hypoglycin; hypoglycin A. $C_7H_{11}NO_2$; mol wt 141.17. C 59.56%, H 7.85%, N 9.92%, O 22.67%. Hypoglycemic principle from the akee plant, *Blighia sapida* Kon., *Sapindaceae*: Hassall *et al., Nature* **173**, 356 (1954); Hassall, Reyle, *Biochem. J.* **60**, 334 (1955). Structure: de Ropp *et al., J. Am. Chem. Soc.* **80**, 1004 (1958); Renner *et al., Helv. Chim. Acta* **41**, 589 (1958); Ellington *et al., J. Chem. Soc.* **1959**, 80. Synthesis: Carbon *et al., J. Am. Chem. Soc.* **80**, 1002 (1958); Black, Landor, *Tetrahedron Lett.* **1963**, 1065.

Yellow plates from methanol + water, mp 280-284°. $[\alpha]_D^{32}$ +9.2°.
Methyl ester hydrochloride. $C_8H_{13}NO_2.HCl$. Needles from methanol + ether, mp 151-152°. $[\alpha]_D^{22}$ +36° (c = 2.0).

Hypoglycine B. [502-37-4] *N*-L-γ-Glutamyl-3-(2-methylene-cyclopropyl)alanine; γ-L-glutamylhypoglycine. $C_{12}H_{18}N_2O_5$. Structure: Jöhl, Stoll, *Helv. Chim. Acta* **42**, 156 (1959); Hassall, John, *J. Chem. Soc.* **1960**, 4112. Synthesis: Jöhl, Stoll, *Helv. Chim. Acta* **42**, 716 (1959). Yellow needles from acetone + water, mp 194-195°, 200-206°. $[\alpha]_D^{32}$ +9.6° (c = 1.12). Neutralization equivalent 175.

4867.　Hypophosphoric Acid. [7803-60-3] $H_4O_6P_2$; mol wt 161.98. H 2.49%, O 59.26%, P 38.24%. Prepn from its salts: Salzer, *Ann.* **187**, 322 (1877); **211**, 1 (1882). *Review:* Ohashi, "Lower Oxo Acids of Phosphorus and Their Salts" in *Topics in Phosphorus Chemistry* **Vol. 1**, M. Grayson, E. J. Griffith, Eds. (Interscience, New York, 1964) pp 113-187.

Orthorhombic plates, mp 70° (easily forms a dihydrate, mp 55°), usually available only in aq soln. The aq acid is colorless and odorless; dec on concn at atm pressure. Readily forms crystallizable normal and acid sodium salts.

USE: Acid sodium salts in baking powders.

4868.　Hypophosphorous Acid. [6303-21-5] H_3O_2P; mol wt 66.00. H 4.58%, O 48.48%, P 46.93%. Conveniently prepd by treating NaH_2PO_2 with an ion-exchange resin: Klement, *Z. Anorg. Allg. Chem.* **260**, 267 (1949). *Review:* Ohashi, "Lower Oxo Acids of Phosphorus and Their Salts" in *Topics in Phosphorus Chemistry* **Vol. 1**, M. Grayson, E. J. Griffith, Eds. (Interscience, New York, 1964) pp 113-187.

The water-free acid forms deliquesc crystals; supercools to a colorless, odorless, oily liquid. d 1.493. mp 26.5°. Dec by heat into H_3PO_4 and spontaneously flammable PH_3. Miscible with water, alcohol, ether. Oxidized by hot H_2SO_4; SO_2 and S formed. It is a powerful reducing agent. Marketed in aq solns of various concns, *e.g.*, 50%, d 1.274; 30-32%, d 1.13; 10%, d 1.04. pK₁ 1.1.

4869.　Hypoxanthine. [68-94-0] 1,7-Dihydro-6*H*-purin-6-one; purin-6(1*H*)-one; sarcine; sarkin. $C_5H_4N_4O$; mol wt 136.11. C 44.12%, H 2.96%, N 41.16%, O 11.75%. Desmotropic forms: purin-6-ol; 1*H*-purin-6-ol; 3*H*-purin-6-ol; 9*H*-purin-6-ol; purin-6(3*H*)-one; 9*H*-purin-6(1*H*)-one. Formed in the animal body during the breakdown of nucleic acids; formation from adenosine continues after death. Also widely distributed in the vegetable kingdom. Numerous syntheses, *e.g.*, from 2,6,8-trichloropurine:

Fischer, *Ber.* **30**, 2226 (1897); by oxidation of adenine: Krüger, *Z. Physiol. Chem.* **18**, 445 (1894). By reduction of uric acid: Sundwik, *ibid.* **76**, 486 (1912); by condensing ethyl cyanoacetate and thiourea in the presence of Na-ethoxide: Traube, *Ann.* **331**, 64 (1904); from mercapto-4-hydroxy-6-aminopyrimidine: Taylor, Cheng. *J. Org. Chem.* **25**, 148 (1960). *Reviews:* Levene, Bass, *ACS Monograph Series* **no. 56**, entitled "Nucleic Acids" (New York, 1931); Chargaff, Davidson, *Nucleic Acids* **vols. I & II** (Academic Press, New York, 1955).

Small octahedra, needles from water, dec 150° without melting. Sol in 1400 parts water, 70 parts boiling water; sol in dil acids, alkalies. Combines with one equivalent of acid or with two equivalents of base. pK_b (25°): 8.7. Absorption spectrum: Dhere, *Compt. Rend.* **141**, 720.

4870.　Hypusine. [34994-11-1] N^6-[(2*R*)-4-Amino-2-hydroxybutyl]-L-lysine; (2*S*,9*R*)-2,11-diamino-9-hydroxy-7-azaundecanoic acid; N^6-(4-amino-2-hydroxybutyl)-2,6-diaminohexanoic acid. $C_{10}H_{23}N_3O_3$; mol wt 233.31. C 51.48%, H 9.94%, N 18.01%, O 20.57%. Naturally occurring L-amino acid formed by the post-translational modification of lysine. Name coined to indicate the condensation product of hydroxyputrescine with lysine. Isoln: T. Shiba *et al.*, *Biochim. Biophys. Acta* **244**, 523 (1971); from archaebacteria: H. Schümann, F. Klink, *Syst. Appl. Microbiol.* **11**, 103 (1989). In eukaryotes occurs only at a single position in one protein, eukaryotic protein synthesis initiation factor 5A, (eIF-5A, formerly eIF-4D): M. H. Park *et al.*, *Proc. Natl. Acad. Sci. USA* **78**, 2869 (1981); H. L. Cooper *et al.*, *ibid.* **80**, 1854 (1983). Biosynthesis: M. H. Park *et al.*, *J. Biol. Chem.* **257**, 7217 (1982); M. H. Park *et al.*, *ibid.* **259**, 12123 (1984). Synthesis and stereochemistry: T. Shiba *et al.*, *Bull. Chem. Soc. Jpn.* **55**, 899 (1982). Total synthesis: C. M. Tice, B. Ganem, *J. Org. Chem.* **48**, 5045, 5048 (1983); R. J. Bergeron *et al.*, *ibid.* **58**, 6804 (1993). Biological significance in eukaryotes: J. W. B. Hershey *et al.*, *Biochim. Biophys. Acta* **1050**, 160 (1990). HPLC determn in eukaryotic samples: S. Beninati *et al.*, *Anal. Biochem.* **184**, 16 (1990). Chromatographic determn in archaebacteria: D. Bartig, F. Klink, *J. Chromatogr.* **606**, 43 (1992). Review of biological significance: M. H. Park *et al.*, *Trends Biochem. Sci.* **18**, 475-479 (1993).

Dihydrochloride. [82310-93-8] $C_{10}H_{23}N_3O_3.2HCl$. White crystals, mp 239-241° (dec). $[\alpha]_D^{23}$ +8.3° (c = 0.96 in 6*M* HCl).

I

4871. IACFT. [180468-34-2] (1*R*,2*S*,3*S*,5*S*)-3-(4-Fluorophenyl)-8-[(2*E*)-3-(iodo-2-propenyl)]-8-azabicyclo[3.2.1]octane-2-carboxylic acid methyl ester; 2β-carboxymethoxy-3β-(4-fluorophenyl)-*N*-(1-iodoprop-1-en-3-yl)nortropane; Altropane. C₁₈H₂₁- — $C_{18}H_{21}FINO_2$; mol wt 429.27. C 50.36%, H 4.93%, F 4.43%, I 29.56%, N 3.26%, O 7.45%. Cocaine analog with dopamine transport inhibitor activity. Radiolabeled form designed for SPECT brain imaging. Prepn: D. R. Elmaleh *et al.*,**WO 9511901**; *eidem*, **US 5493026** (1995, 1996 both to Gen. Hosp. Corp., Harvard College, Organix and Northeastern Univ.); and receptor binding studies: *eidem*, *J. Nucl. Med.* **37**, 1197 (1996). Series of articles on pharmacology and binding studies: B. K. Madras *et al.*, *Synapse* **29**, 93-127 (1998). Clinical evaluation in Parkinson's disease: A. J. Fischman *et al.*, *ibid.* 128. CE determn in plasma: K. Hettiarachchi *et al.*, *J. Chromatogr. A* **895**, 87 (2000).

White solid, mp 115-116°.
¹²³I-Labeled form. [208517-65-1]
¹²⁵I-Labeled form. [180268-78-4]
THERAP CAT: ¹²³I-labeled form as diagnostic aid (radioactive imaging agent).

4872. Ibafloxacin. [91618-36-9] 9-Fluoro-6,7-dihydro-5,8-dimethyl-1-oxo-1*H*,5*H*-benzo[*ij*]quinolizine-2-carboxylic acid; R-835; S-25930. C₁₅H₁₄FNO₃; mol wt 275.27. C 65.45%, H 5.13%, F 6.90%, N 5.09%, O 17.44%. Tricyclic fluorinated quinolone-type antibacterial; related to flumequine, *q.v.* Prepn: R. M. Stern, **EP 109284**; *idem*, **US 4472405** (both 1984 to Riker Labs.). Antimicrobial spectrum: L. J. V. Piddock *et al.*, *Eur. J. Clin. Microbiol.* **5**, 303 (1986); K. V. I. Rolston *et al.*, *Eur. J. Clin. Microbiol. Infect. Dis.* **7**, 681 (1988). Synthesis, absolute configuration and antibacterial activity of enantiomers: J. F. Gerster *et al.*, *J. Med. Chem.* **30**, 839 (1987).

Off-white solid, mp 269-272°.
S-Form. Colorless crystals from DMF, mp 274-276°. [α]D −107.4° (c = 0.1109 g/10mL in dichloroethane).
R-Form. Colorless crystals from DMF, mp 274-276°. [α]D +106.8° (c = 0.1165 g/10mL in dichloroethane).
THERAP CAT (VET): Antibacterial.

4873. Ibandronic Acid. [114084-78-5] [1-Hydroxy-3-(methylpentylamino)propylidene]bisphosphonic acid. C₉H₂₃NO₇P₂; mol wt 319.23. C 33.86%, H 7.26%, N 4.39%, O 35.08%, P 19.41%. Bisphosphonate antiresorptive agent. Prepn: R. Gall, E. Bosies, **DE 3623397**; *idem*, **US 4927814** (1988, 1990 both to Boehringer Mann.). Inhibition of bone resorption: R. C. Mühlbauer *et al.*, *J. Bone Miner. Res.* **6**, 1003 (1991). Mechanism of action study: C. Vitté *et al.*, *Endocrinology* **137**, 2324 (1996). Clinical trial in cancer-associated hypercalcemia: M. Pecherstorfer *et al.*, *J. Clin. Oncol.* **14**, 268 (1996); in osteoporosis: P. Ravn *et al.*, *Bone* **19**, 527 (1996). Review of pharmacology and clinical efficacy: M. Dooley *et al.*, *Drugs* **57**, 101-108 (1999); of clinical experience in osteoporosis: R. D. Chapurlat, P. D. Delmas, *Expert Opin. Pharmacother.* **4**, 391-396 (2003); of development and therapeutic potential: L. Gennari, *IDrugs* **8**, 155-169 (2005).

Dec 84°.
Sodium salt. [138926-19-9] (monohydrate)]; [138844-81-2] (anhydrous). Ibandronate sodium; BM-21.0955; Bondronat; Boniva; Bonviva. C₉H₂₂NNaO₇P₂; mol wt 341.21. Occurs as the monohydrate.
THERAP CAT: Bone resorption inhibitor.

4874. Iberiotoxin. [129203-60-7] IbTX. Peptide inhibitor of K⁺ channels isolated from the venom of the scorpion, *Buthus tamulus*. Single polypeptide chain of 37 amino acids with 3 disulfide bridges; mol wt 4.23 kDa. Isoln, purification and characterization: A. Galvez *et al.*, *J. Biol. Chem.* **265**, 11083 (1990). 3D structure determn by NMR: B. A. Johnson, E. E. Sugg, *Biochemistry* **31**, 8151 (1992). Mode of action: S. Candia *et al.*, *Biophys. J.* **63**, 583 (1992). Synthesis of labeled mutant: A. Koschak *et al.*, *Biochemistry* **36**, 1943 (1997). Use as probe: W. A. A. Kunze *et al.*, *Pflügers Arch.* **428**, 300 (1994); G. Fauaz *et al.*, *Vascul. Pharmacol.* **40**, 127 (2003); Y. Tanaka *et al.*, *Arch. Pharmacol.* **367**, 35 (2003).

```
pyroE-F-T-D-V-D-C-S-V-S-K-E-C-W-  S-V-C-K-D-L-F-G-V-D-R-G-K-C-M- G-K-K-C-R-C-Y-Q
```

USE: Selective probe for high-conductance calcium-activated potassium channels.

4875. Ibogaine. [83-74-9] 12-Methoxyibogamine. C₂₀-H₂₆N₂O; mol wt 310.43. C 77.38%, H 8.44%, N 9.02%, O 5.15%. Indole alkaloid of the *iboga* group. Isoln from root (1.27%), rootbark (2 to 6%), stems (1.95%) and leaves (0.35%) of the shrub *Tabernanthe iboga* Baill., *Apocynaceae*, found in Africa: Dybowski, Landrin, *Compt. Rend.* **133**, 748 (1901); Haller, Heckel, *ibid.* 850, 1236; from other *Apocynaceae*: H. Achenbach, B. Raffelsberger, *Z. Naturforsch.* **35B**, 219, 885 (1980); N. Ghorbel *et al.*, *J. Nat. Prod.* **44**, 717 (1981); T. Mulamba *et al.*, *ibid.* 184; B. Richard *et al.*, *ibid.* **46**, 283 (1983). Purification: Schlittler *et al.*, *Helv. Chim. Acta* **36**, 1341 (1953). Revised extraction procedure: Dickel *et al.*, *J. Am. Chem. Soc.* **80**, 123 (1958). Review of early isolation work: Lebeau, Janot, *Traité de Pharmacie Chimique* **vol. 4** (Masson et Cie., Paris, 1956) pp 2982-2988. Structure: Bartlett *et al.*, *J. Am. Chem. Soc.* **80**, 126 (1958). Mass spectrum: Biemann, Friedmann-Spiteller, *ibid.* **83**, 4805 (1961). Synthesis: Büchi *et al.*, *ibid.* **88**, 3099 (1966); Rosenmund *et al.*, *Ber.* **108**, 1871 (1975). Derivs: Taylor, **US 2877229** (1959 to Ciba). Absolute configuration: K. Blàha *et al.*, *Tetrahedron Lett.* **1972**, 2763. Interatomic distances similar to those of serotonin: J. M. Kelley, R. H. Adamson, *Pharmacology* **10**, 28 (1973). NMR spectrum: E. Wenkert *et al.*, *Helv. Chim. Acta* **59**, 2437 (1976). Determn in biological fluids: E. Bertol *et al.*, *J. Chromatogr.* **117**, 239 (1976). Iboga extracts said to be used by African natives while stalking game, to enable them to remain motionless for as long as 2 days while retaining mental alertness. Neuropharmacological studies: Schneider, Sigg, *Ann. N.Y. Acad. Sci.* **66**, 765 (1957); S. Gershon, W. J. Lang, *Arch. Int. Pharmacodyn. Ther.* **135**, 31 (1962). Cardiovascular effects: J. A. Schneider, R. K. Rinehart, *ibid.* **110**, 92 (1957). Serotonergic properties: R. S. Sloviter *et al.*, *J. Pharmacol. Exp. Ther.* **214**, 231 (1980). Experimental use in treatment of heroin addiction: H. S. Lotsof, **US 4499096** (1985). *Reviews*: W. I. Taylor, "The Iboga and Voacanga Alkaloids" in *The Alkaloids, Chemistry and Physiology* **Vol. 8**, R. H. F. Manske, Ed. (Academic Press, New York, 1965) p 203-235, *idem*, *ibid.* **Vol. 11** (1968), pp 79-98.

Prismatic needles from abs ethanol, mp 152-153°. Sublimes$_{0.01}$ 150°. $[\alpha]_D^{20}$ −53° (in 95% ethanol). pKa 8.1 in 80% methylcellosolve. uv max (methanol): 226, 298 nm (log ε 4.39, 3.93). Sol in ethanol, ether, chloroform, acetone, benzene. Practically insol in water.

Hydrochloride. $C_{20}H_{26}N_2O\cdot HCl$. Crystals. Dec 299-300°. $[\alpha]_D^{25}$ −63° (ethanol); $[\alpha]_D^{25}$ −49° (H_2O). Soluble in water, methanol, ethanol. Slightly sol in acetone, chloroform. Practically insol in ether.

Note: This is a controlled substance (hallucinogen): **21 CFR, 1308.11.**

4876. Ibopamine. [66195-31-1] 2-Methylpropanoic acid 4-[2-(methylamino)ethyl]-1,2-phenylene ester; 4-[2-(methylamino)-ethyl]-*o*-phenylene diisobutyrate; *N*-methyldopamine diisobutyric ester; 3,4-di-*o*-isobutyryl epinine. $C_{17}H_{25}NO_4$; mol wt 307.38. C 66.43%, H 8.20%, N 4.56%, O 20.82%. Inotropic agent with dopaminergic and adrenergic agonist activities; converted to active metabolite, deoxyepinephrine, *q.v.* Prepn: C. Casagrande, G. Ferrari, **DE 2734678**; *eidem,* **US 4218470** (1978, 1980 both to Simes). Pharmacology: G. F. Melloni *et al., Curr. Ther. Res.* **25,** 406 (1979); *eidem, ibid.* **26,** 466 (1979). Series of articles on synthesis, pharmacology, clinical efficacy: *Arzneim.-Forsch.* **36,** 285-408 (1986). Review of pharmacodynamics, pharmacokinetics and therapeutic efficacy: J. M. Henwood, P. A. Todd, *Drugs* **36,** 11-31 (1988). Series of articles on clinical use in congestive heart failure: *Cardiology* **77,** Suppl. 5, 1-95 (1990). Clinical efficacy and safety in heart failure: J. R. Hampton *et al., Lancet* **349,** 971 (1997). Clinical evaluation in diagnosis of glaucoma: G. Marchini *et al., J. Ocul. Pharmacol. Ther.* **17,** 215 (2001); in treatment of ocular hypertony: L. C. Ugahary *et al., Am. J. Ophthalmol.* **141,** 571 (2006).

Hydrochloride. [75011-65-3] SB-7505; Inopamil; Scandine; Trazyl. $C_{17}H_{25}NO_4\cdot HCl$; mol wt 343.85. Crystals from ethyl acetate, mp 132°.

THERAP CAT: Cardiotonic. Diagnostic aid (glaucoma).

4877. Ibotenic Acid. [2552-55-8] α-Amino-2,3-dihydro-3-oxo-5-isoxazoleacetic acid; α-amino-3-hydroxy-5-isoxazoleacetic acid; amino-(3-hydroxy-5-isoxazolyl)acetic acid. $C_5H_6N_2O_4$; mol wt 158.11. C 37.98%, H 3.82%, N 17.72%, O 40.48%. Fly-killing and narcosis-potentiating amino acid structurally similar to kainic acid, *q.v.*, extracted from poisonous mushroom species. Isoln from *Amanita pantherina* (DC.) Fr., and *A. muscaria* (L.) Fr., *Agaricaceae:* Takemoto *et al., J. Pharm. Soc. Jpn.* **84,** 1233 (1964); Eugster *et al., Tetrahedron Lett.* **1965,** 1813. Structure: Takemoto *et al., J. Pharm. Soc. Jpn.* **84,** 1186, 1232 (1964). Syntheses: Gagneux *et al., Tetrahedron Lett.* **1965,** 2081; Sirakawa *et al., Chem. Pharm. Bull.* **14,** 89 (1966); Kishida *et al., ibid.* **14,** 92 (1966); **15,** 1025 (1967). Improved synthesis: Nakamura, *ibid.* **19,** 46 (1971). Industrial pats: **BE 665249** *C.A.* **65,** 2266e (1966); Gagneux *et al.,* **US 3459862** (1965, 1969 both to Geigy); Kishida *et al.,* **JP 68 15975**; **JP 69 25780** (1968, 1969 both to Sankyo); *C.A.* **70,** 77944p (1969); **72,** 13054g (1970). Pharmacology: Theobald *et al., Arzneim.-Forsch.* **18,** 311 (1968); Johnston *et al., Biochem. Pharmacol.* **17,** 2488 (1968). Exhibits potent neuroexcitatory activity: *eidem, Nature* **248,** 804 (1974). Chemistry review: Eugster, *Fortschr. Chem. Org. Naturst.* **27,** 261-321 (1969); Catalfomo, Eugster, *Bull. Narc.* **22,** 33-41 (1970). Excitatory and possible sedative actions on spinal neurons: D. R. Curtis *et al., J. Physiol.* **291,** 19 (1979); in cerebral cortex: E. Puil, *Can. J. Physiol. Pharmacol.* **59,** 1025 (1981). Use as experimental neurotoxic agent: A. Contestabile *et al., Experientia* **40,** 524 (1984).

Crystals from water or methanol, mp 151-152° (anhydrous); mp 144-146° (monohydrate). LD$_{50}$ in mice, rats (mg/kg): 15, 42 i.v.; 38, 129 orally (Theobald).

USE: Neurobiological tool.

4878. Ibritumomab Tiuxetan. [206181-63-7] Anti-(human CD20 antigen) immunoglobulin G1 (mouse monoclonal IDEC-Y2B8 γ$_1$-chain) disulfide with mouse monoclonal IDEC-Y2B8 κ-chain, dimer *N*-[2-[bis(carboxymethyl)amino]-3-(4-isothiocyanato-phenyl)propyl]-*N*-[2-[bis(carboxymethyl)amino]propyl]glycine conjugate. Murine monoclonal antibody targeted against CD-20 antigen on mature B lymphocytes, conjugated to linker-chelator tiuxetan. Radiolabeled form designed for antibody-targeted treatment of non-Hodgkin's lymphoma (NHL). Prepn of monoclonal antibody: M. E. Reff *et al., Blood* **83,** 435 (1994). Prepn of radiolabeled conjugate: D. R. Anderson *et al.,* **WO 9411026**; *eidem,* **US 5736137** (1994, 1998 both to IDEC); P. C. Chinn *et al., Int. J. Oncol.* **15,** 1017 (1999). Clinical pharmacology: S. J. Knox *et al., Clin. Cancer Res.* **2,** 457 (1996). Clinical evaluation in NHL: T. E. Witzig *et al., J. Clin. Oncol.* **17,** 3793 (1999). Review of development and therapeutic potential: G. A. Wiseman *et al., Clin. Cancer Res.* **5** Suppl., 3281s-3286s (1999); of clinical experience: A. J. Grillo-López, *Expert Rev. Anticancer Ther.* **2,** 485-493 (2002).

^{90}Y-Labeled form. Y2B8-MX-DTPA; IDEC-Y2B8; Zevalin.

THERAP CAT: ^{90}Y-Labeled form as antineoplastic.

4879. Ibudilast. [50847-11-5] 2-Methyl-1-[2-(1-methyl-ethyl)pyrazolo[1,5-*a*]pyridin-3-yl]-1-propanone; 3-isobutyryl-2-isopropylpyrazolo[1,5-*a*]pyridine; KC-404; Ketas. $C_{14}H_{18}N_2O$; mol wt 230.31. C 73.01%, H 7.88%, N 12.16%, O 6.95%. Leukotriene D$_4$ antagonist. Prepn: T. Irikura *et al.,* **DE 2315801**; *eidem,* **US 3850941** (1973, 1974 both to Kyorin). Pharmacology and antiallergic activity: K. Nishino *et al., Jpn. J. Pharmacol.* **33,** 267 (1983); H. Nagai *et al., ibid.* 1215. *In vitro* cerebral vasodilating activity: M. Ohashi *et al., Arch. Int. Pharmacodyn.* **280,** 216 (1986); *in vivo* activity: W. M. Armstead *et al., J. Pharmacol. Exp. Ther.* **244,** 138 (1988). Bronchodilating activity in animals: S. Mue *et al., Arch. Int. Pharmacodyn.* **283,** 153 (1986). Antiplatelet activity in animals: M. Ohashi *et al., ibid.* 321; M. Ohashi *et al., Gen. Pharmacol.* **17,** 385 (1986).

Crystals from hexane, mp 53.5-54°. Slightly sol in water, freely sol in organic solvents. LD$_{50}$ i.v. in mice: 260 mg/kg (Irikura, 1973).

THERAP CAT: Antiallergic; antiasthmatic; vasodilator (cerebral).

4880. Ibufenac. [1553-60-2] 4-(2-Methylpropyl)benzene-acetic acid; (*p*-isobutylphenyl)acetic acid; *p*-isobutyl-α-toluic acid; Dytransin; Ibunac. $C_{12}H_{16}O_2$; mol wt 192.25. C 74.97%, H 8.39%, O 16.64%. Prepn: J. S. Nicholson, S. S. Adams, **GB 971700**; *eidem,* **US 3385887** (1964, 1968 both to Boots Pure Drug). Pharmacology: S. S. Adams *et al., J. Pharm. Pharmacol.* **20,** 305 (1968). Toxicity data: S. S. Adams *et al., Nature* **200,** 271 (1962).

Crystals, mp 85-87°. Very slightly sol in water. Freely sol in many organic solvents. LD$_{50}$ orally in mice: 1.8 g/kg (Adams).

THERAP CAT: Analgesic, anti-inflammatory.

4881. Ibuprofen. [15687-27-1] α-Methyl-4-(2-methylpropyl)benzeneacetic acid; *p*-isobutylhydratropic acid; (±)-2-(4-isobutylphenyl)propionic acid; RD-13621; Advil; Brufen; Brufort; Dolgit; Dolocyl; Epobron; Fenbid; Gynofug; Ibumetin; Ibutop; Ipren; Motrin; Napacetin; Novogent; Nuprin; Nurofen; Opturem; Proflex; Solufen; Tabalon; Urem. $C_{13}H_{18}O_2$; mol wt 206.28. C 75.69%, H 8.80%, O 15.51%. Nonsteroidal anti-inflammatory drug (NSAID); activity resides primarily in the (*S*)-isomer. Prepn: J. S. Nicholson, S. S. Adams, **GB 971700**; *eidem*, **US 3385886** (1964, 1968 both to Boots Pure Drug); T. Shiori, N. Kawai, *J. Org. Chem.* **43**, 2936 (1978); J. T. Pinhey, B. A. Rowe, *Tetrahedron Lett.* **21**, 965 (1980). Methods for resolution of enantiomers: R. Bhushan, J. Martens, *Biomed. Chromatogr.* **12**, 309 (1998). HPLC determn in plasma: R. Canaparo *et al.*, *ibid.* **14**, 219 (2000). Pharmacology: S. S. Adams *et al.*, *Arch. Int. Pharmacodyn. Ther.* **178**, 115 (1969). Acute toxicity: G. Orzalesi *et al.*, *Arzneim.-Forsch.* **27**, 1006 (1977). Clinical trial for closure of patent ductus arteriosus: B. Van Overmeire *et al.*, *N. Engl. J. Med.* **343**, 674 (2000). Review of pharmacology and clinical experience: M. Busson *et al.*, *J. Int. Med. Res.* **14**, 53-62 (1986); of clinical pharmacokinetics and metabolism: N. M. Davies, *Clin. Pharmacokinet.* **34**, 101-154 (1998).

Colorless, crystalline stable solid, mp 75-77°. Relatively insol in water. Readily sol in most organic solvents. LD_{50} in male mice, rats (mg/kg): 495, 626 i.p.; 1255, 1050 orally (Orzalesi).

Lysine salt. Arfen; Imbun. $C_{13}H_{18}O_2 \cdot C_6H_{14}N_2O_2$; mol wt 352.47.

S-Form L-lysine salt monohydrate. [141505-32-0] Dexibuprofen lysine; MK-223. $C_{13}H_{18}O_2 \cdot C_6H_{14}N_2O_2 \cdot H_2O$; mol wt 370.48.

THERAP CAT: Anti-inflammatory; analgesic; antipyretic.

THERAP CAT (VET): Anti-inflammatory.

4882. Ibuproxam. [53648-05-8] *N*-Hydroxy-α-methyl-4-(2-methylpropyl)benzeneacetamide; *dl*-2-(4-isobutylphenyl)propionohydroxamic acid; G-277; Ibudros. $C_{13}H_{19}NO_2$; mol wt 221.30. C 70.56%, H 8.65%, N 6.33%, O 14.46%. Hydroxylamine deriv of ibuprofen, *q.v.*, to which it is converted *in vivo*. Prepn: G. Orzalesi, R. Selleri, **DE 2400531**; *eidem*, **US 4082707** (1974, 1978 both to Manetti & Roberts). Metabolism in rats: G. Orzalesi *et al.*, *Arzneim.-Forsch.* **27**, 1012 (1977); in humans: *eidem*, *ibid.* **30**, 1607 (1980). Pharmacological study: *eidem*, *ibid.* **27**, 1006 (1977). Thermal decomposition: S. Chimichi *et al.*, *J. Pharm. Sci.* **69**, 521 (1980). Physico-chemical properties: M. Mannelli *et al.*, *Boll. Chim. Farm.* **119**, 203 (1980).

Crystals from acetone/petr ether, mp 119-121°. Sol in methanol, ethanol, acetone, ethyl ether. Practically insol in water and petr ether. LD_{50} in mice, rats (g/kg): >2, >3 orally (Orzalesi, Selleri, 1978).

THERAP CAT: Anti-inflammatory.

4883. Ibutilide. [122647-31-8] *N*-[4-[4-(Ethylheptylamino)-1-hydroxybutyl]phenyl]methanesulfonamide. $C_{20}H_{36}N_2O_3S$; mol wt 384.58. C 62.46%, H 9.44%, N 7.28%, O 12.48%, S 8.34%. Methanesulfonanilide antiarrhythmic agent; prolongs myocardial action potential duration, predominantly by activation of slow inward sodium current. Prepn: J. B. Hester, **EP 164865**; *idem*, **US 5155268** (1985, 1992 both to Upjohn); *idem et al.*, *J. Med. Chem.* **34**, 308 (1991). HPLC determn of enantiomers: C. L. Hsu, R. R. Walters, *J. Chromatogr. B* **667**, 115 (1995); determn of racemate in plasma: L. Tian *et al.*, *J. Chromatogr. B* **816**, 81 (2005). Review of electrophysiology and pharmacology: G. V. Naccarelli *et al.*, *Am. J. Cardiol.* **78**, Suppl. 8A, 12-16 (1996); of pharmacology

and clinical potential: R. H. Foster *et al.*, *Drugs* **54**, 312-330 (1997). Clinical trial in atrial flutter or fibrillation: B. S. Stambler *et al.*, *Circulation* **94**, 1613 (1996); J. T. VanderLugt *et al.*, *ibid.* **100**, 369 (1999); in elderly patients: R. M. Gowda *et al.*, *Am. J. Ther.* **11**, 95 (2004).

Fumarate. [122647-32-9] U-70226E; Corvert. $(C_{20}H_{36}N_2O_3S)_2 \cdot C_4H_4O_4$; mol wt 885.23. Crystals from acetone, mp 117-119°. uv max (95% ethanol): 228, 267 nm (ε 16670, 894) Soly (mg/ml): aqueous >100 (pH ≤ 7).

THERAP CAT: Antiarrhythmic (class III).

4884. Iceland Moss. *Cetraria islandica* (L.) Ach., *Parmeliaceae*, a lichen growing in all northern countries. Exported from Iceland, Norway, and Sweden. The gum from the powdered plant appears to be a hemicellulose contg uronic acid, galactose, mannose, and glucose; *cf.* Mantell, *The Water-Soluble Gums*, New York, 1947.

About 60% of dried Iceland moss dissolves when boiled with water contg a little sodium bicarbonate. The soln forms a jelly when cold.

USE: Manuf sea biscuits which are somewhat more resistant to weevil infestation than when wheat flour alone is used. In foods for convalescents. Manuf sizing agents for rayon; hair-setting lotions, other cosmetics.

4885. Ichthammol. [8029-68-3] Ammonium bituminosulfonate; ammonium ichthosulfonate; ammonium sulfobituminate; ammonium sulfoichthyolate; bitumol; bituminol; ichthammonium; ammonium bithiolicum; ichthosulfol; Ichthyol; Hirathiol; Ichden; Ichtammon; Ichthadone; Ichthymall; Ichthysalle; Ichthalum; Ichthium; Ichtopur; Ichthosan; Ichthynat; Ichthyopon; Lithol; Petrosulpho; Perichthol; Piscarol; Pisciol; Saurol; Subitol; Sulfogenol; Thilaven; Thiolin; Thiozin; Trasulphane; Tumenol; Leukochthol; Ichthosauran; Amsubit; Bitulan. Obtained by sulfation and ammoniation of a distillate from mineral deposits (bituminous schists) originally found near Seefeld, Tyrol. Contains satd and unsatd hydrocarbons, nitrogenous bases, acids, and several thiophene derivs. Analysis shows at least 2.5% NH_3 and at least 10% S. Also contains traces of some 20 minerals and *"zoomelanoidic" acids*. Method of prepn: Schröter, **DE 35216** (1885); Helmers, **DE 76128** (1892). Similar deposits occur in Asia east of Lake Baikal where the oil is known as *stone oil, barakshin, Asil*; sold in India for remedial purposes as *saladjidi*: Gerbrein, *Photo-Journal* (Montreal, 1969, July 2-9) p 19. *Review:* Wernicke, *Chem. Ztg.* **60**, 85-87 (1936).

Pale yellow or (usually) brownish-black, thick, viscous liquid. Bituminous odor. Miscible with water, glycerol, propylene glycol, fats, oils, carbowaxes, lanolin. Partially sol in alcohol, ether.

An injectable form is marketed as *Adnexol*.

THERAP CAT: Anti-infective (topical).

THERAP CAT (VET): Demulcent, emollient, antiseptic.

4886. Idarubicin. [58957-92-6] (7*S*,9*S*)-9-Acetyl-7-[(3-amino-2,3,6-trideoxy-α-L-*lyxo*-hexopyranosyl)oxy]-7,8,9,10-tetrahydro-6,9,11-trihydroxy-5,12-naphthacenedione; (1*S*,3*S*)-3-acetyl-1,2,3,4,6,11-hexahydro-3,5,12-trihydroxy-6,11-dioxo-1-naphthacenyl-3-amino-2,3,6-trideoxy-α-L-*lyxo*-hexopyranoside; 4-demethoxydaunomycin; 4-demethoxydaunorubicin; DMDR; IMI-30; NSC-256439. $C_{26}H_{27}NO_9$; mol wt 497.49. C 62.77%, H 5.47%, N 2.82%, O 28.94%. Orally active anthracycline; analog of daunorubicin, *q.v.* Prepn: B. Patelli *et al.* **DE 2525633**; *eidem*, **US 4046878** (1976, 1977 both to Soc. Farmac. Ital.); and antitumor activity: F. Arcamone *et al.*, *Cancer Treat. Rep.* **60**, 829 (1976). Total synthesis for larger scale preparation: M. J. Broadhurst *et al.*, *Chem. Commun.* **1982**, 158. Synthesis of optically pure isomers: Y. Kimura *et al.*, *Bull. Chem. Soc. Jpn.* **59**, 423 (1986). Metabolism and biodistribution in rats: G. Zini *et al.*, *Cancer Chemother. Pharmacol.* **16**, 107 (1986). HPLC determn in plasma: S. S. N. De Graaf *et al.*, *J. Chromatogr.* **491**, 501 (1989). Clinical pharmacokinetics: H. C. Gillies *et al.*, *Br. J. Clin. Pharmacol.* **23**, 303

(1987). Clinical evaluation of cardiac toxicity: F. Villani *et al.*, *Eur. J. Cancer Clin. Oncol.* **25**, 13 (1989). Reviews of pharmacology and antitumor efficacy: A. M. Casazza, *Cancer Treat. Rep.* **63**, 835-844 (1979); F. Ganzina *et al.*, *Invest. New Drugs* **4**, 85-105 (1986). Symposium on clinical experience in acute leukemias: *Semin. Oncol.* **17**, Suppl. 2, 1-36 (1989).

Hydrochloride. [57852-57-0] Idamycin; Zavedos. $C_{26}H_{27}$-$NO_9 \cdot HCl$; mol wt 533.95. Orange crystalline powder, mp 183-185° (Arcamone); also reported as mp 172-174° (Broadhurst). $[\alpha]_D^{20}$ +205° (c = 0.1 in methanol) (Arcamone); also reported as $[\alpha]_D^{20}$ +188° (c = 0.10 in methanol) (Kimura).

THERAP CAT: Antineoplastic.

4887. Idazoxan. [79944-58-4] 2-(2,3-Dihydro-1,4-benzodioxin-2-yl)-4,5-dihydro-1*H*-imidazole; 2-[2-(1,4-benzodioxanyl)]-2-imidazoline. $C_{11}H_{12}N_2O_2$; mol wt 204.23. C 64.69%, H 5.92%, N 13.72%, O 15.67%. α_2-Adrenergic blocker. Prepn: J. Krapcho, W. A. Lott, US 2979511 (1961 to Olin Mathieson); and confirmation of structure: C. B. Chapleo, P. L. Myers, *Tetrahedron Lett.* **22**, 4839 (1981). Structure-activity study: C. B. Chapleo *et al.*, *J. Med. Chem.* **26**, 823 (1983). Pharmacology: M. Dabiré, *J. Pharmacol.* **17**, 113 (1986). Clinical evaluation in progressive supranuclear palsy: D. G. Cole, J. H. Growdon, *J. Neural Transm. Suppl.* **42**, 283 (1994); as adjunct to fluphenazine in schizophrenia: R. E. Litman *et al.*, *Br. J. Psychiatry* **168**, 571 (1996).

Hydrochloride. [79944-56-2] RX-781094. $C_{11}H_{12}N_2O_2 \cdot$HCl; mol wt 240.69. White, crystalline solid from isopropanol, mp 207-208°.

THERAP CAT: Antiparkinsonian.

4888. Idebenone. [58186-27-9] 2-(10-Hydroxydecyl)-5,6-dimethoxy-3-methyl-2,5-cyclohexadiene-1,4-dione; 6-(10-hydroxydecyl)-2,3-dimethoxy-5-methyl-1,4-benzoquinone; 2,3-dimethoxy-5-methyl-6-(10'-hydroxydecyl)-1,4-benzoquinone; 6-(10-hydroxydecyl)ubiquinone; CV-2619; Avan; Daruma; Lucebanol; Mnesis. $C_{19}H_{30}O_5$; mol wt 338.44. C 67.43%, H 8.93%, O 23.64%. Ubiquinone derivative with protective effects against cerebral ischemia. Prepn: H. Morimoto *et al.*, **DE 2519730**; *eidem*, **US 4271083** (1975, 1981 both to Takeda); K. Okamoto *et al.*, *Chem. Pharm. Bull.* **30**, 2797 (1982); C.-A. Yu, L. Yu, *Biochemistry* **21**, 4096 (1982). Effect on ischemia-induced amnesia in rats: N. Yamazaki *et al.*, *Jpn. J. Pharmacol.* **36**, 349 (1984). Metabolism in animals: T. Kobayashi *et al.*, *J. Pharmacobio-Dyn.* **8**, 448 (1985). Disposition: H. Torii *et al.*, *ibid.* 457. Pharmacokinetics and tolerance in humans: M. F. Barkworth *et al.*, *Arzneim.-Forsch.* **35**, 1704 (1985). Series of articles on pharmacology and clinical studies: *Arch. Gerontol. Geriatr.* **8**, 193-366 (1989). Review of chemistry, toxicology and pharmacology: I. Zs-Nagy, *Arch. Gerontol. Geriatr.* **11**, 177-186 (1990).

Orange needles from ligroin, mp 46-50° (Morimoto); also reported as crystals from hexane + ethyl acetate, mp 52-53° (Okamoto). Sol in organic solvents. Practically insol in water.

THERAP CAT: Nootropic.

4889. Idose. [2152-76-3] $C_6H_{12}O_6$; mol wt 180.16. C 40.00%, H 6.71%, O 53.28%. Prepn of D-idose by reduction of D-idonolactone: Fischer, Fay, *Ber.* **28**, 1975 (1895); from D-galactose: Sorking, Reichstein, *Helv. Chim. Acta* **28**, 1 (1945); from tri-*O*-acetyl-1,6-anhydro-β-D-idopyranose: *eidem, ibid.* 662. Prepn of L-idose by reduction of L-idonolactone: Fischer, Fay, *loc. cit.*; by hydrolysis of 1,2-*O*-isopropylidene-L-idofuranose: Meyer, Reichstein, *Helv. Chim. Acta* **29**, 152 (1946); von Vargha, *Ber.* **87**, 1351 (1954). Improved synthesis: M. Blanc-Muesser, J. Defaye, *Synthesis* **1977**, 568. Structure: S. F. Dyke, *The Carbohydrates* (Interscience, New York, 1960) p 45. Conformation: Reeves, *J. Am. Chem. Soc.* **72**, 1499 (1950). *Review:* R. L. Whistler, M. L. Wolfrom, *Methods in Carbohydrate Chemistry* (Academic Press, New York, 1962) pp 140-145.

β-D-Idose

D-Form. Syrup. $[\alpha]_D^{13}$ +15.8° (c = 2.3).
Phenylosazone. $C_{18}H_{22}N_4O_4$. Yellow needles from alc, mp 168-169°.
L-Form. Syrup. $[\alpha]_D^{20}$ −17.4° (c = 3.6).
1,2-*O*-Isopropylidene-L-idofuranose. Plates from ethyl acetate, mp 113-114°. $[\alpha]_D^{26}$ −20° (c = 2.7 in methanol).

4890. Idoxifene. [116057-75-1] 1-[2-[4-[(1*E*)-1-(4-Iodophenyl)-2-phenyl-1-butenyl]phenoxy]ethyl]pyrrolidine; 1-[2-[*p*-[(*E*)-β-ethyl-α-(*p*-iodophenyl)styryl]phenoxy]ethyl]pyrrolidine; CB-7432. $C_{28}H_{30}INO$; mol wt 523.45. C 64.25%, H 5.78%, I 24.24%, N 2.68%, O 3.06%. Nonsteroidal estrogen antagonist; structurally analogous to tamoxifen, *q.v.* Prepn: R. McCague, **EP 260066**; *idem*, **US 4839155** (1988, 1989 both to Nat. Res. Dev. Corp.); and structural activity: R. McCague *et al., J. Med. Chem.* **32**, 2527 (1989). Stereochemistry: C. M. Nunn, E. J. Parker, *Acta Crystallogr.* **C50**, 2043 (1994). Modulating effects on multidrug resistance: J. Kirk *et al., Biochem. Pharmacol.* **48**, 277 (1994); S. Y. Sharp *et al., Br. J. Cancer* **70**, 409 (1994). Clinical evaluation in breast cancer: R. C. Coombes *et al., Cancer Res.* **55**, 1070 (1995).

Crystals from light petroleum (pet. ether), mp 108-109° (McCague *et al.*); also reported as colorless monoclinic prisms from methanol (Nunn).

THERAP CAT: Antineoplastic.

4891. Idoxuridine. [54-42-2] 2'-Deoxy-5-iodouridine; 1-(2-deoxy-β-D-ribofuranosyl)-5-iodouracil; 5-iodo-2'-deoxyuridine; IdU; IdUR; IUdR; IdUrd; Dendrid; Emanil; Herpes-Gel; Herplex; Idexur; Idoxene; Idulea; Iduridin; Kerecid; Ophthalmadine; Stoxil; Virudox. $C_9H_{11}IN_2O_5$; mol wt 354.10. C 30.53%, H 3.13%, I 35.84%, N 7.91%, O 22.59%. Cytotoxic nucleoside with antiviral and antineoplastic activity. Prepn: Prusoff, *Biochim. Biophys. Acta* **32**, 295 (1959); Cheong *et al., J. Biol. Chem.* **235**, 1441

(1960); Chang, Welch, *J. Med. Chem.* **6**, 428 (1963); Amiard, Torelli, **FR 1336866** (1963 to Roussel-UCLAF), *C.A.* **60**, 3082g (1964); **GB 1024156**; Prystas, Sorm, *Collect. Czech. Chem. Commun.* **29**, 121 (1964). Crystal and molecular structure: Camerman, Trotter, *Acta Crystallogr.* **18**, 203 (1965). *Review:* W. H. Prusoff *et al.* in *Antibiotics* vol. 5 (pt. 2), F. E. Hahn, Ed. (Springer-Verlag, New York, 1979) pp 236-261.

Crystals from water, triclinic, dec 160° (Prusoff; Chang, Welch), 190-195° (Cheong *et al.*), 240° (Amiard, Torelli), over 175° (Prystas, Sorm). uv max (water): 288 nm (log ε 3.87). $[\alpha]_D^{25}$ +7.4° (c = 0.108 in water); $[\alpha]_D^{20}$ +29° (*N* soda). Physical properties: Ravin, Gulesich, *J. Am. Pharm. Assoc.* [NS] **4**, 122 (1964). pKa 8.25. pH of 0.1% aq soln, about 6. Soly at 25° in mg/ml: 2.0 in water; 2.0 in 0.2*N* HCl; 74.0 in 0.2*N* NaOH; 4.4 in methanol; 2.6 in alc; 0.014 in ether; 0.003 in chloroform; 1.6 in acetone; 1.8 in ethyl acetate; 5.7 in dioxane. LD_{50} i.p. in mice: 2.5 g/kg (Prusoff, 1979).

α-Anomer. 1-(2-Deoxy-α-D-*erythro*-pentofuranosyl)-5-iodouracil; 1-(2-deoxy-α-D-ribofuranosyl)-5-iodouracil; α-2'-deoxy-5-iodouridine. Crystals from water, dec 170°. $[\alpha]_D^{25}$ +21.8° (c = 0.170). uv max (water): 288 nm (log ε 3.88).

THERAP CAT: Antiviral.

4892. Idraparinux Sodium. [149920-56-9]; [162610-17-5] (Idraparinux). Methyl *O*-2,3,4-tri-*O*-methyl-6-*O*-sulfo-α-D-glucopyranosyl-(1 → 4)-*O*-2,3-di-*O*-methyl-β-D-glucopyranuronosyl-(1 → 4)-*O*-2,3,6-tri-*O*-sulfo-α-D-glucopyranosyl-(1 → 4)-*O*-2,3-di-*O*-methyl-α-L-idopyranuronosyl-(1 → 4)-α-D-glucopyranoside 2,3,6-tris(hydrogen sulfate) nonasodium salt; Org-34006; SANORG-34006; SR-34006. $C_{38}H_{55}Na_9O_{49}S_7$; mol wt 1727.18. C 26.42%, H 3.21%, Na 11.98%, O 45.39%, S 13.00%. Synthetic pentasaccharide that inhibits factor Xa; analog of fondaparinux sodium, *q.v.* Prepn: M. Petitou, C. A. van Boeckel, **EP 0529715**; *eidem*, **US 5378829** (1993, 1995 both to Akzo; Sanofi); P. Westerduin *et al.*, *Bioorg. Med. Chem.* **2**, 1267 (1994). Biochemical and pharmacological properties: J. M. Herbert *et al.*, *Blood* **91**, 4197 (1998). Comparative pharmacokinetics in rats: J. P. Hérault *et al.*, *Thromb. Haemostasis* **87**, 985 (2002). Clinical pharmacology and reversal by factor VIIa: N. R. Bijsterveld *et al.*, *Br. J. Haematol.* **124**, 653 (2004). Review of clinical development: Q. Ma, J. Fareed, *IDrugs* **7**, 1028-1034 (2004).

$[\alpha]_D^{20}$ +55° (c = 1 in water).
THERAP CAT: Antithrombotic.

4893. Idrocilamide. [6961-46-2] *N*-(2-Hydroxyethyl)-3-phenyl-2-propenamide; *N*-(2-hydroxyethyl)cinnamamide; LCB-29; Brolitène; Srilane. $C_{11}H_{13}NO_2$; mol wt 191.23. C 69.09%, H 6.85%, N 7.32%, O 16.73%. Prepn: M. Bayssat *et al.*, **DE 2015447**; *eidem*, **US 3659014** (1970, 1972 to LIPHA); *Chim. Ther.* **8**, 202 (1973). Pharmacology: Grand *et al.*, *Eur. J. Med. Chem.* **9**, 205 (1974). Metabolism: Belleville *et al.*, *Therapie* **29**, 829 (1974).

White crystals from ethyl acetate or acetone, mp 100-102°. Soluble in alcohol; slightly sol in water. LD_{50} orally in mice, rats: >2950, >3000 mg/kg (Grand).

THERAP CAT: Muscle relaxant (skeletal).

4894. α-L-Iduronidase. [9073-56-7] α-L-Iduronide iduronohydrolase; IDUA; Hurler corrective factor. Lysosomal enzyme that hydrolyzes nonreducing terminal α-L-iduronide glycosidic bonds in heparan sulfate and dermatan sulfate. Genetic deficiency of the enzyme results in the lysosomal storage disorder mucopolysaccharidosis-I (MPS-I) also known as Hurler and Scheie syndromes. Identification in human fibroblasts and liver: R. Matalon *et al.*, *Biochem. Biophys. Res. Commun.* **42**, 340 (1971); in human urine: R. W. Barton, E. F. Neufeld, *J. Biol. Chem.* **246**, 7773 (1971). Localization in lysosomes: B. Weissmann, R. Santiago, *Biochem. Biophys. Res. Commun.* **46**, 1430 (1972). Identification as enzymatic defect in Hurler's syndrome: R. Matalon, A. Dorfman, *ibid.* **47**, 959 (1972); G. Bach *et al.*, *Proc. Natl. Acad. Sci. USA* **69**, 2048 (1972). Purification and characterization of multiple forms: P. R. Clements *et al.*, *Biochem. J.* **259**, 199 (1989). Cloning and expression in Chinese hamster ovary cells: H. S. Scott *et al.*, *Proc. Natl. Acad. Sci. USA* **88**, 9695 (1991).

Laronidase. [250378-38-2] Alronidase; Aldurazyme. Human α-L-iduronidase produced by recombinant DNA technology in Chinese hamster ovary cells. Prepn and pharmacology: E. D. Kakkis *et al.*, *Protein Expression Purif.* **5**, 225 (1994). *See also:* E. D. Kakkis, B. Tanamachi, **WO 9958691** (1999 to Harbor-UCLA). Clinical evaluation in MPS-I: *idem et al.*, *N. Engl. J. Med.* **344**, 182 (2001).

THERAP CAT: Enzyme replacement therapy in mucopolysaccharidosis-I.

4895. Ifenprodil. [23210-56-2] α-(4-Hydroxyphenyl)-β-methyl-4-(phenylmethyl)-1-piperidineethanol; 4-benzyl-α-(*p*-hydroxyphenyl)-β-methyl-1-piperidineethanol; 2-(4-benzylpiperidino)-1-(4-hydroxyphenyl)-1-propanol; 1-methyl-2-hydroxy-2-(4-hydroxyphenyl)ethyl-1-(4-benzylpiperidine); RC-61-91. $C_{21}H_{27}$-NO_2; mol wt 325.44. C 77.50%, H 8.36%, N 4.30%, O 9.83%. Prepn and pharmacology: M. Carron *et al.*, **FR M5733**; **US 3509164** (1968, 1970 to Robert et Carrière); C. Carron *et al.*, *Arzneim.-Forsch.* **21**, 1992 (1971).

mp 114°.
Neutral tartrate. Cerocral; Dilvax; Vadilex. $(C_{21}H_{27}NO_2)_2$.-$C_4H_6O_6$; mol wt 800.98. Crystals from methanol, mp 178-180°. Sol in alc, water. Very slightly sol in acetone, chloroform. Practically insol in ether. LD_{50} in male Swiss mice (mg/kg): 17 i.v.; 120 i.p.; 275 orally (Carron, 1970).

THERAP CAT: Vasodilator (cerebral and peripheral).

4896. Ifosfamide. [3778-73-2] *N*,3-Bis(2-chloroethyl)-tetrahydro-2*H*-1,3,2-oxazaphosphorin-2-amine 2-oxide; 3-(2-chloroethyl)-2-[(2-chloroethyl)amino]tetrahydro-2*H*-1,3,2-oxazaphosphorin-2-oxide; iphosphamid(e); isoendoxan; isophosphamide; A-4942; Asta Z-4942; MJF-9325; NSC-109724; Z-4942; Holoxan; Ifex; Ifomide; Mitoxana. $C_7H_{15}Cl_2N_2O_2P$; mol wt 261.09. C 32.20%, H 5.79%, Cl 27.16%, N 10.73%, O 12.26%, P 11.86%. Cytostatic agent, related structurally to cyclophosphamide, *q.v.* Prepn: **FR 1530962** (1968 to Asta), *C.A.* **71**, 49998m (1969); H. Arnold *et al.*, **US 3732340** (1973 to Asta). Chemical properties: H. Arnold, *Proc. 5th Int. Congr. Chemother. Vienna* (Verhandlungen, Vienna, 1967) **2**, pp 751-754. Pharmacology: N. Brock, *ibid.* pp 155-161. Molecular structure and conformation: H. A. Brassfield *et al.*, *J. Am. Chem. Soc.* **97**, 4143 (1975). Mass spectrometry: M.

Przybylski *et al., Biomed. Mass Spectrom.* **4**, 209 (1977). Mechanism of action: S. Tomita *et al., Chemotherapy (Tokyo)* **25**, 3014 (1977). Metabolism: A. Takamizawa *et al., Chem. Pharm. Bull.* **25**, 2900 (1977); *eidem, J. Med. Chem.* **17**, 1237 (1974). Toxicity studies: R. Marcy *et al., IRCS Med. Sci. Libr. Compend.* **5**, 427, 478 (1977). Mutagenicity studies: D. Wald, *J. Mutat. Res.* **56**, 319 (1978); G. R. Mohn, J. Ellenberger, *ibid.* **32**, 331 (1976). Clinical studies: P. J. Creaven *et al., Cancer Treat. Rep.* **60**, 445, 451 (1976); J. Schnitker *et al., Arzneim.-Forsch.* **26**, 1793 (1976). Symposium on clinical efficacy and comparison with cyclophosphamide: *Cancer Chemother. Pharmacol.* **18**, Suppl. 2, S1-S58 (1986). Reviews of pharmacology, toxic effects and clinical activity: M. Zalupski, L. H. Baker, *J. Natl. Cancer Inst.* **80**, 556-566 (1988); S. E. Schoenike, W. J. Dana, *Clin. Pharm.* **9**, 179-191 (1990).

Crystals from anhyd ether, mp 39-41°. LD_{50} in rats (mg/kg): 160 i.p. (Arnold, 1973); also reported as 150 i.p. (Brock).

THERAP CAT: Antineoplastic.

4897. Ignatia. Ignatius bean; St. Ignatius' bean. Dried, ripe seed of *Strychnos ignatii* Berg., *Loganiaceae. Habit.* Philippine Islands, naturalized in Vietnam, Cambodia. *Constit.* 2-3% strychnine, about 1% brucine, igasuric acid, loganin.

THERAP CAT: Bitter tonic.

4898. Ilimaquinone. [71678-03-0] 3-[[(1*R*,2*S*,4a*S*,8a*S*)-Decahydro-1,2,4a-trimethyl-5-methylene-1-naphthalenyl]methyl]-2-hydroxy-5-methoxy-2,5-cyclohexadiene-1,4-dione; IQ. $C_{22}H_{30}$-O_4; mol wt 358.47. C 73.71%, H 8.44%, O 17.85%. Sesquiterpenoid quinone isolated from the marine sponge, *Hippiospongia metachromia*; naturally occurring as (−)-form. Inhibits cellular secretions by selective breakdown of the Golgi apparatus. Isoln and structure determn: R. T. Luibrand *et al., Tetrahedron* **35**, 609 (1979). Revised stereochemistry: R. J. Capon, J. K. MacLeod, *J. Org. Chem.* **52**, 5059 (1987). Total stereosynthesis: S. D. Bruner *et al., ibid.* **60**, 1114 (1995); increased yield: S. Poigny *et al., ibid.* **63**, 5890 (1998). Photoaffinity study on cellular targets: H. S. Radeke, M. N. L. Snapper, *Bioorg. Med. Chem.* **6**, 1227 (1998). Mechanism of action studies: P. A. Takizawa *et al., Cell* **73**, 1079 (1993); H. S. Radeke *et al., Chem. Biol.* **6**, 639 (1999). Use as inhibitor of protein secretion: P. A. Feldman *et al., J. Membr. Biol.* **155**, 275 (1997).

Orange needles from hexane, mp 113-114°. $[\alpha]_D^{23}$ −23.2° (c = 1.12 in $CHCl_3$).

USE: Biological probe for intracellular communications and vesicle-mediated transport.

4899. Illudins. Anti-tumor antibiotic substances produced by the poisonous basidiomycetes *Clitocybe illudens* (now called *Omphalotus illudens*): Anchel *et al., Proc. Natl. Acad. Sci. USA* **36**, 300 (1950); **38**, 927 (1952); and *Lampteromyces japonicus*: Nakanishi *et al., Nature* **197**, 292 (1963); Endo *et al., Chem. Commun.* **1970**, 309. Structure: McMorris, Anchel, *J. Am. Chem. Soc.* **87**, 1594 (1965); Matsumoto *et al., Tetrahedron* **21**, 2671 (1965); Tada *et al., Chem. Pharm. Bull.* **12**, 853 (1964). Stereochemistry: Nakanishi *et al., ibid.* 856; *Tetrahedron* **21**, 1231 (1965); Matsumoto *et al., Bull. Chem. Soc. Jpn.* **37**, 1716 (1964). Abs config of illudin S: Harada, Nakanishi, *Chem. Commun.* **1970**, 310. Total synthesis

of illudin M: Matsumoto *et al., J. Am. Chem. Soc.* **90**, 3280 (1968); *Tetrahedron Lett.* **1970**, 1171; of illudin S: *eidem, ibid.* **1971**, 2049. *In vitro* antitumor activity in human cancer cells: M. J. Kelner *et al., J. Natl. Cancer Inst.* **82**, 1562 (1990).

Illudin M   R = H
Illudin S   R = OH

Illudin M. [1146-04-9] (3′*S-trans*)-2′,3′-Dihydro-3,6-dihydroxy-2′,2′,4′,6′-tetramethylspiro[cyclopropane-1,5′-[5*H*]inden]-7′(6′*H*)-one. $C_{15}H_{20}O_3$; mol wt 248.32. Rods, mp 120-122.5° (Matsumoto); from ethanol-water, mp 128-130° (McMorris). uv max (ethanol): 228, 318 nm (ε 13900, 3600).

Monoacetate. $C_{17}H_{22}O_4$. mp 75-76° from petr ether.

Illudin S.[1149-99-1][2′*S*-(2′α,3′β,6′α)]-2′,3′-Dihydro-3′,6′-dihydroxy-2′-(hydroxymethyl)-2′,4′,6′-trimethylspiro[cyclopropane-1,5′-[5*H*]inden]-7′(6′*H*)-one; lampterol; lunamycin (obsolete). $C_{15}H_{20}O_4$; mol wt 264.32. Needles from acetone, mp 124-126°. uv max (ethanol): 233, 319 nm (ε 13200, 3600). Sol in polar organic solvents.

Diacetate. $C_{19}H_{24}O_5$. Crystals from petr ether, mp 99-100°. uv max (ethanol): 227, 313 nm (ε 12900, 3400).

4900. Iloperidone. [133454-47-4] 1-[4-[3-[4-(6-Fluoro-1,2-benzisoxazol-3-yl)-1-piperidinyl]propoxy]-3-methoxyphenyl]-ethanone; HP-873; ILO-522; Zomaril. $C_{24}H_{27}FN_2O_4$; mol wt 426.48. C 67.59%, H 6.38%, F 4.45%, N 6.57%, O 15.01%. Combined dopamine (D_2) and serotonin (5HT$_2$) receptor antagonist. Prepn: J. T. Strupczewski *et al.,* **EP 402644**; *eidem,* **US 5364866** (1990, 1994 both to Hoechst-Roussel); *eidem, J. Med. Chem.* **38**, 1119 (1995). Pharmacology: M. R. Szewczak *et al., J. Pharmacol. Exp. Ther.* **274**, 1404 (1995). Clinical pharmacokinetics: S. M. Sainati *et al., J. Clin. Pharmacol.* **35**, 713 (1995). HPLC determn in plasma: A. E. Mutlib, J. T. Strupczewski, *J. Chromatogr. B* **669**, 237 (1995). Receptor binding study: S. Kongsamut *et al., Eur. J. Pharmacol.* **317**, 417 (1996). Review of pharmacology and therapeutic potential in schizophrenia: J. M. K. Hesselink, *Curr. Opin. Cent. Peripher. Nerv. Syst. Invest. Drugs* **2**, 71-78 (2000); K. K. Jain, *Expert Opin. Invest. Drugs* **9**, 2935-2943 (2000).

Crystals from ethanol, mp 118-120°.

THERAP CAT: Antipsychotic.

4901. Iloprost. [78919-13-8] 5-[Hexahydro-5-hydroxy-4-(3-hydroxy-4-methyl-1-octen-6-ynyl)-2(1*H*)-pentalenylidene]pentanoic acid; 5-(*E*)-(1*S*,5*S*,6*R*,7*R*)-7-hydroxy-6-[(*E*)-(3*S*,4*RS*)-3-hydroxy-4-methyl-1-octenyl]bicyclo[3.3.0]octan-3-ylidenepentanoic acid; (*E*)-(3a*S*,4*R*,5*R*,6a*S*)-hexahydro-5-hydroxy-4-[(*E*)-(3*S*,4*RS*)-3-hydroxy-4-methyl-1-octen-6-ynyl]-$\Delta^{2(1H),\delta}$-pentalenevaleric acid; ciloprost; ZK-36374. $C_{22}H_{32}O_4$; mol wt 360.49. C 73.30%, H 8.95%, O 17.75%. Prostacyclin analog; 1:1 mixture of 16α- and 16β-methyl diastereomers. Prepn: W. Skuballa *et al.,* **DE 2845770**; *eidem,* **US 4692464** (1980, 1987 both to Schering AG); W. Skuballa, H. Vorbrüggen, *Adv. Prostaglandin Thromboxane Leukotriene Res.* **11**, 299 (1983). Antithrombotic and cardiovascular pharmacology: K. Schrör *et al., Arch. Pharmacol.* **316**, 252 (1981).

Review of clinical pharmacology and pharmacokinetics: S. M. Grant, K. L. Goa, *Drugs* **43**, 889-924 (1992). Clinical study in limb ischemia: J. Dormandy, *Therapie* **46**, 319 (1991); in Raynaud phenomenon: F. M. Wigley *et al.*, *Ann. Intern. Med.* **120**, 199 (1994); in pulmonary hypertension: H. Olschewski *et al.*, *N. Engl. J. Med.* **347**, 322 (2002).

Colorless oil.

Tromethamine. Endoprost; Ilomedin; Ventavis. $C_{22}H_{32}O_4 \cdot C_4H_{11}NO_3$; mol wt 481.62.

THERAP CAT: Vasodilator (peripheral). In treatment of pulmonary hypertension.

4902. Imatinib. [152459-95-5] 4-[(4-Methyl-1-piperazinyl)methyl]-*N*-[4-methyl-3-[[4-(3-pyridinyl)-2-pyrimidinyl]amino]phenyl]benzamide; *N*-[5-[4-(4-methylpiperazinomethyl)benzoylamido]-2-methylphenyl]-4-(3-pyridyl)-2-pyrimidineamine. $C_{29}H_{31}N_7O$; mol wt 493.60. C 70.57%, H 6.33%, N 19.86%, O 3.24%. Tyrosine kinase inhibitor; highly specific for BCR-ABL, the enzyme associated with chronic myelogenous leukemia (CML) and certain forms of acute lymphoblastic leukemia (ALL). Also shown to inhibit the transmembrane receptor KIT and platelet-derived growth factor (PDGF) receptors. Prepn: J. Zimmermann, **EP 564409**; *idem*, **US 5521184** (1993, 1996 both to Ciba-Geigy); *idem et al.*, *Bioorg. Med. Chem. Lett.* **7**, 187 (1997). Structural mechanism of ABL specificity: T. Schindler *et al.*, *Science* **289**, 1938 (2000). Activity vs KIT and PDGF receptor kinases: E. Buchdunger *et al.*, *J. Pharmacol. Exp. Ther.* **295**, 139 (2000). Clinical trial in CML: H. Kantarjian *et al.*, *N. Engl. J. Med.* **346**, 645 (2002); in gastrointestinal stromal tumors related to KIT: G. D. Demetri *et al.*, *ibid.* **347**, 472 (2002). Review of clinical experience: D. G. Savage, K. H. Antman, *ibid.* **346**, 683-693 (2002); and pharmacology: V. K. Pindolia *et al.*, *Pharmacotherapy* **22**, 1249-1265 (2002); and development of therapeutic target: B. J. Druker, *Adv. Cancer Res.* **91**, 1-30 (2004).

mp 211-213°. pKa_1 8.07; pKa_2 3.73; pKa_3 2.56; pKa_4 1.52.

Methanesulfonate. [220127-57-1] STI-571; CGP-57148B; Gleevec; Glivec. $C_{29}H_{31}N_7O \cdot CH_3SO_3H$; mol wt 589.71. Prepn of crystalline form: J. Zimmermann *et al.*, **WO 9903854** (1999 to Novartis). Occurs in 2 crystalline modifications. α-form, begins to melt at 226°; β-form, mp 217°. Lipophilic at pH 7.4. Soly in water: >100 g/l (pH 4.2); 49 mg/l (pH 7.4).

THERAP CAT: Antineoplastic.

4903. Imazamethabenz. [81405-85-8] 2-[4,5-Dihydro-4-methyl-4-(1-methylethyl)-5-oxo-1*H*-imidazol-2-yl]-4(and 5)-methylbenzoic acid methyl ester; imazamethabenz methyl; imazamethabenz; AC-222293; AC-293; CL-222293; Assert; Dagger. $C_{16}H_{20}N_2O_3$; mol wt 288.34. C 66.65%, H 6.99%, N 9.72%, O 16.65%. Selective, post-emergence imidazolinone herbicide; mixture of ***methyl 2-(4-isopropyl-4-methyl-5-oxo-2-imidazolin-2-yl)-p-toluate*** and ***methyl 6-(4-isopropyl-4-methyl-5-oxo-2-imidazolin-2-yl)-m-toluate*** (approx 3:2). Prepn of isomeric mixture: M. Los, **US 4188487** (1980 to American Cyanamid). Activity, physical properties and toxicity: D. L. Shaner *et al.*, *Proc. Br. Crop Prot. Conf. - Weeds* **1982**, 25; K. Hedlund, L. Andersson, *Weeds Weed Control* **28**, 1 (1987). Activity of component isomers: D. L. Shaner *et al.*,

Proc. Br. Crop Prot. Conf. - Weeds **1982**, 333. Mechanism of action: J. B. Pillmoor, J. C. Caseley, *Pestic. Biochem. Physiol.* **27**, 340 (1987). Persistence and mobility in soil: R. Allen, J. C. Caseley, *Proc. Br. Crop Prot. Conf. - Weeds* **1987**, 569. Field studies: K. Kirkland, N. E. Shafer, *ibid.* **1982**, 33; A. A. Hudson, S. C. E. Townsend, *ibid.* **1985**, 923; in food crops: S. D. Miller, H. P. Alley, *Weed Technol.* **1**, 29 (1987).

m - form   *p* - form

Off-white fine powder with a tendency to form easily friable aggregates; slight musty odor. Softening begins at 108-117°, melting starts at 113-122° and is completed at 144-153°. Soly (g/100 ml) at 25°: acetone 18.2, DMSO 23.8, distilled water 0.13 (*p*-isomer), 0.22 (*m*-isomer), *n*-heptane 0.04, isopropyl alcohol 14.4, methanol 24.4, methylene chloride 30.0, toluene 3.9. Soly (g/100 g) at 25°: xylene <5, DMF 30. Partition coefficient (*n*-octanol/water): 35 (*p*-isomer), 66 (*m*-isomer). LD_{50} in rats, rabbits (mg/kg): >5000, 4500 orally, >2000, >2000 dermally (Hedlund, Anderson).

USE: Herbicide.

4904. Imazamox. [114311-32-9] 2-[4,5-Dihydro-4-methyl-4-(1-methylethyl)-5-oxo-1*H*-imidazol-2-yl]-5-(methoxymethyl)-3-pyridinedicarboxylic acid; 2-(4-isopropyl)-4-methyl-5-oxo-2-imidazolin-2-yl-5-(methoxymethyl)nicotinic acid; AC-299263; CL-299263; Raptor. $C_{15}H_{19}N_3O_4$; mol wt 305.33. C 59.01%, H 6.27%, N 13.76%, O 20.96%. Acetohydroxyacid synthase (AHAS) inhibitor. Prepn: R. F. Doehner, Jr., **EP 254951**; *idem et al.*, **US 5334576** (1988, 1994 both to Am. Cyanamid). Chemical and physical properties: G. R. Glover, *Proc. South. Weed Sci. Soc.* **48**, 269 (1995). Metabolism study: B. Tecle *et al.*, *Brighton Crop Prot. Conf. - Weeds* **1997**, 605. CE determn in beans: K. Ohba *et al.*, *J. Pestic. Sci.* **22**, 277 (1997). Field trials: K. A. Nelson, K. A. Renner, *Weed Technol.* **12**, 137 (1998); R. E. Blackshaw, *ibid.* **64**. Soil persistence: T. Cobucci *et al.*, *Weed Sci.* **46**, 258 (1998). *Review:* T. M. Brady *et al.*, *ACS Symp. Ser.* **686**, 30-37 (1998).

mp 166.0-166.7°. Soly (g/100 ml): hexane 0.0006; methanol 6.68; acetonitrile 1.85; toluene 0.21; acetone 2.93; dichloromethane 14.3; ethyl acetate 1.02. Soly in water: 4160 ppm. Volatility: $<1.0 \times 10^{-7}$ torr. Partition coefficient (octanol/water): 0.004 (pH 7). pK_1 2.3; pK_2 3.3. LD_{50} (technical grade) orally in rats: >5000 mg/kg; dermally in rabbits: >4000 mg/kg; LC_{50} by inhalation in rats: >6.3 mg/l (Glover).

USE: Herbicide.

4905. Imazapyr. [81334-34-1] 2-[4,5-Dihydro-4-methyl-4-(1-methylethyl)-5-oxo-1*H*-imidazol-2-yl]-3-pyridinecarboxylic acid; 2-(4-isopropyl-4-methyl-5-oxo-2-imidazolin-2-yl)nicotinic acid. $C_{13}H_{15}N_3O_3$; mol wt 261.28. C 59.76%, H 5.79%, N 16.08%, O 18.37%. Inhibitor of acetolactate synthase, a key enzyme in branched chain amino acid biosynthesis. Prepn: M. Los, **EP 41623**; *idem*, **US 4798619** (1981, 1989 both to Am. Cyanamid). Description: R. Paxman *et al.*, *Proc. 38th N. Z. Weed Pest Control Conf.*, 73 (1985). Mode of action: D. Shaner *et al.*, *Proc. Br. Crop Prot. Conf. - Weeds* **1985**, 147. Determn in soil: O. Nováková, *Chromatographia* **39**, 62 (1994). Persistence in soil: S. Vizantinopoulos, P. Lolos, *Bull. Environ. Contam. Toxicol.* **52**, 404 (1994). Field trials in sod: K. A. Griffin *et al.*, *Crop Sci.* **34**, 202 (1994).

Crystals from acetone + hexane, mp 170-172.5°. pK_1 1.9; pK_2 3.6. Soly in water (pH 7): ~1.0 g/l. LD_{50} orally in rats: >5000 mg/kg; dermally in rabbits: >2000 mg/kg (Paxman).

Isopropylamine salt. [81510-83-0] AC-252925; CL-252925; Arsenal; Chopper. $C_{13}H_{15}N_3O_3 \cdot C_3H_9N$; mol wt 320.39. mp 160-180° (dec).

USE: Herbicide.

4906. Imazaquin. [81335-37-7] 2-[4,5-Dihydro-4-methyl-4-(1-methylethyl)-5-oxo-1H-imidazol-2-yl]-3-quinolinecarboxylic acid; 2-(5-isopropyl-5-methyl-4-oxo-2-imidazolin-2-yl)-3-quino-linecarboxylic acid; AC-252214. $C_{17}H_{17}N_3O_3$; mol wt 311.34. C 65.58%, H 5.50%, N 13.50%, O 15.42%. Pre- and post-emergence imidazolinone herbicide especially for use in soybean crops. Prepn: M. Los, **EP 41623** (1981 to Am. Cyanamid), *C.A.* **96,** 199687q (1982). Alternate prepn: D. R. Maulding, R. F. Doehner, Jr., **US 4459408** (1984 to Am. Cyanamid). Inhibition of branched-chain amino acid biosynthesis: D. L. Shaner *et al., Plant Physiol.* **76,** 545 (1984). Metabolism by plants: D. L. Shaner, P. A. Robson, *Weed Sci.* **33,** 469 (1985). Persistence in soil: G. Basham *et al., ibid.* **35,** 576 (1987). Herbicidal activity: M. W. Beale *et al., Proc. Annu. Meet. Northeast. Weed Sci. Soc.* **38,** 36 (1984); W. F. Congleton *et al., Weed Technol.* **1,** 186 (1987).

Crystals from hexane + ethyl acetate, mp 219-222° (dec). Slightly sol in some organic solvents. Soly in water at 25°: 60-120 ppm. LD_{50} orally in rats: 5000 mg/kg; LC_{50} (96 hr) in rainbow trout: 100 mg/l (Congleton).

Ammonium salt. Scepter. $C_{17}H_{20}N_4O_3$; mol wt 328.37. Sol in water.

USE: Herbicide.

4907. Imazethapyr. [81335-77-5] 2-[4,5-Dihydro-4-methyl-4-(1-methylethyl)-5-oxo-1H-imidazol-2-yl]-5-ethyl-3-pyridine-carboxylic acid; (±)-5-ethyl-2-(4-isopropyl-4-methyl-5-oxo-1H-imidazolin-2-yl)nicotinic acid; AC-263499; CL-263499. $C_{15}H_{19}$-N_3O_3; mol wt 289.33. C 62.27%, H 6.62%, N 14.52%, O 16.59%. Selective imidazolinone herbicide. Inhibitor of acetolactate synthase, a key enzyme in the biosynthesis of branched chain amino acids. Prepn: M. Los, **EP 41623**; *idem,* **US 4798619** (1981, 1989 both to Am. Cyanamid). Comprehensive description: T. R. Peoples *et al., Proc. Br. Crop Prot. Conf. - Weeds* **1985,** 99-106. Determn in soil: O. Nováková, *Chromatographia* **39** 62 (1994). Metabolism in corn: N. M. Mallipudi *et al., J. Agric. Food Chem.* **42,** 1213 (1994).

White to off-white crystalline solid, mp 172-175°. pK_1 2.1; pK_2 3.9. Soly in water (25°): 1415 ppm. LD_{50} orally in rats and mice: >5000 mg/kg; dermally in rabbits: >2000 mg/kg (Peoples).

Ammonium salt. [101917-66-2] Pivot; Pursuit. $C_{15}H_{22}N_4O_3$; mol wt 306.36.

USE: Herbicide.

4908. Imazosulfuron. [122548-33-8] 2-Chloro-N-[[(4,6-di-methoxy-2-pyrimidinyl)amino]carbonyl]imidazo[1,2-a]pyridine-3-sulfonamide; 1-(2-chloroimidazo[1,2-a]pyridin-3-ylsulfonyl)-3-(4,6-dimethoxypyrimidin-2-yl)urea; TH-913; Brazzos; Takeoff. $C_{14}H_{13}ClN_6O_5S$; mol wt 412.81. C 40.73%, H 3.17%, Cl 8.59%, N 20.36%, O 19.38%, S 7.77%. Acetolactate-synthase (ALS) inhibitor; sulfonylurea herbicide for weed control in rice crops. Prepn: Y. Ishida *et al.,* **EP 238070;** *eidem,* **US 5017212** (1987, 1991 both to Takeda); *eidem, J. Pestic. Sci.* **18,** 175 (1993). Mechanism of action study: Y. Tanaka, H. Yoshikawa, *J. Weed Sci. Technol.* **43,** 291 (1998). Soil degradation studies: K. Mikata *et al., J. Pestic. Sci.* **26,** 376 (2001). LC determn in water and soil: M. Ventriglia *et al., J. Chromatogr. A* **857,** 327 (1999); in rice: Y. Akiyama *et al., J. Food Hyg. Soc. Jpn.* **43,** 99 (2002). Review of development: H. Nagase, *Agrochem. Jpn.* **64,** 15-16 (1994); and biological activity: Y. Ishida *et al., J. Pestic. Sci.* **21,** 247-258 (1996).

Crystalline solid, mp 183-184° (dec). d^{25} 1.574. pK_a 4.0. Log P (octanol/water): 0.05. Vapor pressure (25°): 3.4×10^{-10} mmHg. Soly at 25° (mg/l): water 308 (pH 7.0), 67 (pH 6.1), 5 (pH 5.1), acetonitrile 2500, ethyl acetate 2200, acetone 7600, dichloromethane 12800, xylene 400.

USE: Herbicide.

4909. Imibenconazole. [86598-92-7] N-(2,4-Dichlorophen-yl)-1H-1,2,4-triazole-1-ethanimidothioic acid (4-chlorophenyl)-methyl ester; 1,2,4-triazol-1-yl-isothioacetic acid 2',4'-dichloro-anilide S-p-chlorobenzyl ether; 4-chlorobenzyl-N-(2,4-dichloro-phenyl)-2-(1H-1,2,4-triazol-1-yl)thioacetimidate; HF-6305; HF-8505; Manage. $C_{17}H_{13}Cl_3N_4S$; mol wt 411.74. C 49.59%, H 3.18%, Cl 25.83%, N 13.61%, S 7.79%. Broad spectrum triazole fungicide. Prepn: H. Ohyama *et al.,* **FR 2514766;** *eidem,* **US 4512989** (1983, 1985 both to Hokko Chem. Ind.). HPLC determn of metabolite in fruits and vegetables: A. Kaihara *et al., J. Health Sci.* **46,** 336 (2000). Review of physical properties, biological activity and field trials: H. Ohyama *et al., Brighton Crop Prot. Conf. - Pests Dis.* **1988,** 519-526; and mode of action: Y. Ogawa, *Agrochem. Jpn.* **1995,** no. 67, 20-21.

White crystalline solid, mp 89.5-90°. Vapor pressure (25°): 85 nPa. Soly in water (25°): 1.7 mg/l. Soly at 25° (g/l): acetone 1063; benzene 580; xylene 250; methanol 120. LD_{50} in male, female rats, male, female mice (mg/kg): 2800, 3000, >5000, >5000 orally; in male, female rats (mg/kg): >2000, >2000 dermally; in honey bees (μg/bee): >125 orally. LC_{50} (48 hr) in carp: 1.02 ppm. LC_{50} (6 hr) in water fleas: >102 ppm (Ogawa).

USE: Fungicide.

4910. Imidacloprid. [105827-78-9] 1-[(6-Chloro-3-pyri-dinyl)methyl]-4,5-dihydro-N-nitro-1H-imidazol-2-amine; 1-[(6-chloro-3-pyridinyl)methyl]-N-nitro-2-imidazolidinimine; 1-(6-chloro-3-pyridylmethyl)-*N*-nitroimidazolidin-2-ylideneamine; 1-(2-chloro-5-pyridylmethyl)-2-(nitroimino)imidazolidine; BAY NTN 33893; Admire; Advantage; Confidor; Gaucho; Marathon; Merit; Premier; Provado; Trimax. $C_9H_{10}ClN_5O_2$; mol wt 255.66. C 42.28%, H 3.94%, Cl 13.87%, N 27.39%, O 12.52%. Chloronicotinyl insecticide; targets the nicotinic acetylcholine receptor. Prepn: K. Shiokawa *et al.*, **EP 192060**; *eidem*, **US 4742060** (1986, 1988 both to Nihon Tokushu Noyaku Seizo KK). Properties and bioactivity: A. Elbert *et al.*, *Brighton Crop Prot. Conf. - Pests Dis.* **1990**, 21. Field trials: H. E. Schmeer *et al.*, *ibid.* 29. LC-MS determn in fruits and vegetables: D. Zywitz *et al.*, *Deutsche Lebens.-Rundschau* **99**, 188 (2003). Review of mode of action and agricultural uses: W. Leicht, *Pestic. Outlook* **4**, 17-21 (1993); of chemistry, toxicology, and veterinary use vs flea infestation: N. Mencke, P. Jeschke, *Curr. Top. Med. Chem.* **2**, 701-715 (2002).

Crystals, mp 143.8°; second crystalline modification, mp 136.4°. Vapor pressure (20°): 2.0×10^{-9} mbar. Soly in water (20°): 0.51 g/l. Log P (octanol/water): 0.57. LD_{50} in rats (mg/kg): ~450 orally; >5000 dermally (Elbert).

USE: Insecticide.

THERAP CAT (VET): Ectoparasiticide.

4911. Imidapril. [89371-37-9] (4*S*)-3-[(2*S*)-2-[[(1*S*)-1-(Ethoxycarbonyl)-3-phenylpropyl]amino]-1-oxopropyl]-1-methyl-2-oxo-4-imidazolidinecarboxylicacid;(4*S*)-3-[(2*S*)-2-[*N*-[(1*S*)-1-(ethoxycarbonyl)-3-phenylpropyl]amino]propionyl]-1-methyl-2-oxoimidazolidine-4-carboxylic acid. $C_{20}H_{27}N_3O_6$; mol wt 405.44. C 59.25%, H 6.71%, N 10.36%, O 23.68%. Angiotensin converting enzyme (ACE) inhibitor. Prepn: N. Yoneda *et al.*, **EP 95163**; *eidem*, **US 4508727** (1983, 1985 both to Tanabe Seiyaku); K. Hayashi *et al.*, *J. Med. Chem.* **32**, 289 (1989). Series of articles on pharmacology, pharmacokinetics and metabolism in animals: *Arzneim.-Forsch.* **42**, 446-512 (1992). HPLC determn in plasma and urine: K. Tagawa *et al.*, *J. Chromatogr.* **617**, 95 (1993). Clinical pharmacology: P. Démolis *et al.*, *Fundam. Clin. Pharmacol.* **8**, 80 (1994). Clinical trial in hypertension: M. J. Vandenburg *et al.*, *Br. J. Clin. Pharmacol.* **37**, 265 (1994).

Colorless crystals from ethyl acetate + *n*-hexane, mp 139-140°. $[\alpha]_D^{20} -71.7°$ (c = 0.5 in ethanol).
Monohydrochloride. [89396-94-1] TA-6366; Novaloc; Tanatril. $C_{20}H_{27}N_3O_6 \cdot HCl$; mol wt 441.91. Colorless crystals, mp 214-216° (dec). $[\alpha]_D^{20} -64.1°$ (c = 0.5 in ethanol).
Diacid. [89371-44-8] Imidaprilat. $C_{18}H_{23}N_3O_6$. Crystals, mp 239-241° (dec). $[\alpha]_D^{19} -88.4°$ (c = 1 in 5% $NaHCO_3$).
THERAP CAT: Antihypertensive.

4912. Imidazole. [288-32-4] Glyoxaline; 1,3-diazole; iminazole; miazole; pyrro[*b*]monazole; 1,3-diaza-2,4-cyclopentadiene. $C_3H_4N_2$; mol wt 68.08. C 52.93%, H 5.92%, N 41.15%. Prepd by the action of ammonia on glyoxal: Debus, *Ann.* **107**, 204 (1858); from glyoxal, ammonia, and formaldehyde: Radziszewski, *Ber.* **15**, 1493 (1882); Behrend, Schmitz, *Ann.* **277**, 338 (1893); vapor phase synthesis from formamide and ethylenediamine in presence of a dehydrogenation catalyst: Green, **US 3255200** (1966 to Air Products and Chemicals). Crystal structure: B. M. Craven *et al.*, *Acta Crystallogr.* **33B**, 2585 (1977). Acute toxicity: Nishie *et al.*, *Toxicol. Appl. Pharmacol.* **14**, 301 (1969). *Review:* Pyman, *J. Soc. Dyers Colour.* **36**, 107 (1920). *Monograph:* K. Hofmann, *Imidazole and Its Derivatives* (Interscience, New York, 1953). Review of imidazole chemistry: Grimmett, *Adv. Heterocycl. Chem.* **12**, 103-183 (1970).

Stout prisms from benzene. mp 90-91°. bp_{760} 257°; bp_{20} 165-168°; bp_{12} 138.2°. Weak base. pK (25°): 6.92. Absorption spectrum: Rosanov, *J. Russ. Phys. Chem. Soc.* **48**, 1241 (1916); *Chem. Zentralbl.* **1923**, III, 1080. Freely sol in water, alcohol, ether, chloroform, pyridine; slightly sol in benzene; very sparingly sol in petr ether. LD_{50} in mice (mg/kg): 610 i.p.; 1880 orally (Nishie).

4913. Imidazole Salicylate. [36364-49-5] 2-Hydroxybenzoic acid compd with 1*H*-imidazole (1:1); mono(2-hydroxybenzoate)-1*H*-imidazole; salizolo; ITF-182; Flogozen; Selezen. $C_{10}H_{10}N_2O_3$; mol wt 206.20. C 58.25%, H 4.89%, N 13.59%, O 23.28%. Prepn from equimolar amounts of salicylic acid with imidazole: M. Brissemoret, *Bull. Soc. Chim. Fr.* [3] **35**, 316 (1906). Use as anti-inflammatory agent: **BE 889704**; G. Sportoletti, **US 4329340** (1981, 1982 both to Italfarmaco). Pharmacology: P. G. Pagella *et al.*, *Arzneim.-Forsch.* **33**, 716 (1983). Penetration of inflamed sites: *eidem, ibid.* **34**, 208 (1984). Pharmacokinetics: H. P. Kuemmerle *et al.*, *Int. J. Clin. Pharmacol. Ther. Toxicol.* **22**, 521 (1984). Series of clinical studies: *Boll. Chim. Farm.* **122**, 37S-63S (1983). *Review:* R. Fantozzi, *Drugs Exp. Clin. Res.* **10**, 853-856 (1984).

Crystals from methanol-ether, mp 123-124°. uv max: 300 nm ($E_{1cm}^{1\%}$ 182.5). Soly in water >100 mg/cc. LD_{50} in male, female rats, mice (mg/kg): 763, 724, 595, 685 s.c.; 422, 434, 462, 435 i.v.; 1211, 1430, 1034, 1091 orally (Pagella).

THERAP CAT: Anti-inflammatory; antipyretic; analgesic.

4914. 2-Imidazolidinone. [120-93-4] 2-Imidazolidone; ethylene urea. $C_3H_6N_2O$; mol wt 86.09. C 41.85%, H 7.02%, N 32.54%, O 18.58%. Prepd from ethylenediamine and carbon dioxide under the influence of heat and pressure: Mulvaney, Evans, *Ind. Eng. Chem.* **40**, 393 (1948); from ethylenediamine and urea: Schweitzer, *J. Org. Chem.* **15**, 471 (1950). Systematic survey and bibliography: Klaus Hofmann, *Imidazole*, Part I (Interscience, New York, 1953).

Needles from chloroform, mp 131°. Very sol in water and in hot alc; difficultly sol in ether.

USE: Manuf high polymers, finishing agents for textiles and leather. In the formulation of plasticizers, lacquers, and adhesives. Insecticide: Simkover, **US 3242044** (1966 to Shell).

4915. Imidocarb. [27885-92-3] *N,N*′-Bis[3-(4,5-dihydro-1*H*-imidazol-2-yl)phenyl]urea; 3,3′-di-2-imidazolin-2-ylcarbanilide. $C_{19}H_{20}N_6O$; mol wt 348.40. C 65.50%, H 5.79%, N 24.12%, O 4.59%. Prepn: **GB 1007334**; R. Fischer, R. Hirt, **US 3338917** (1965, 1967 both to Wander). Babesicidal effect in mice and rats: G. Schmidt *et al.*, *Res. Vet. Sci.* **10**, 530 (1969); E. Beveridge, *ibid.* 534. Effect on exptl anaplasmosis in calves: T. O. Roby, *ibid.* **13**, 519 (1972). Comparison of the dipropionate and tetracycline, *q.v.*, in canine ehrlichiosis: J. E. Price, T. T. Dolan, *Vet. Rec.* **107**, 275 (1980). Efficacy in *Babesia felis* infection: F. T. Potgieter, *J. S. Afr. Vet. Assoc.* **52**, 289 (1981). Effect on *B. ovis* infection in sheep: S. A. Michael, A. H. El Refaii, *Trop. Anim. Health Prod.* **14**, 1 (1982), *C.A.* **96**, 192991 (1982).

Dihydrochloride. [5318-76-3] Imizocarb; 4A65. $C_{19}H_{20}N_6 \cdot 0.2HCl$; mol wt 421.32. Solid, mp 350° (dec). LD$_{50}$ in mice, rats (mg/kg): 107, 150 s.c. (Beveridge).

Dipropionate. Imizol; Imizad Equine Injection. $C_{25}H_{32}N_6O_7$; mol wt 528.56.

THERAP CAT (VET): Antiprotozoal (Babesia).

4916. Imidurea. [39236-46-9] *N,N''*-Methylenebis[*N '*-[3-(hydroxymethyl)-2,5-dioxo-4-imidazolidinyl]urea]; methanebis[*N,-N '*-(5-ureido-2,4-diketotetrahydroimidazole)-*N,N*-dimethylol]; imidazolidinyl urea; Abiol; Biopure 100; Germall 115; Sepicide CI; Tri-Stat IU; Unicide U-13. $C_{11}H_{16}N_8O_8$; mol wt 388.29. C 34.03%, H 4.15%, N 28.86%, O 32.96%. Condensation product of formaldehyde and allantoin, *q.q.v.* Member of a family of heterocyclic substituted urea compounds with formaldehyde releasing activity. Prepn: P. A. Berke, **US 3248285** (1966 to Sutton). Description, toxicity and antimicrobial activity: P. A. Berke, W. E. Rosen, *Am. Perfum. Cosmet.* **85**, 55 (1970). Kinetics of formaldehyde release: M. Johansen, H. Bundgaard, *Arch. Pharm. Chemi Sci. Ed.* **9**, 117 (1981). Determn in cosmetic products: G. M. Michalakis, E. F. Barry, *J. Soc. Cosmet. Chem.* **45**, 193 (1994). Review of use and safety assessment: *J. Environ. Pathol. Toxicol.* **4**, 133-146 (1980); of properties and preservative activity: W. E. Rosen, P. A. Berke, *Cosmet. Sci. Technol. Ser.* **1**, 191-205 (1984).

Exists as a monohydrate. White, free-flowing fine powder, dec at temps >160°. Odorless, tasteless. Non-uv absorbing. Polar, hydrophilic. Soly (g/100 g solvent): water 200; ethylene glycol 150; propylene glycol 120; glycerin 100; methanol 0.05; ethanol <0.05; sesame oil <0.05.

USE: Antimicrobial preservative in cosmetics and topical pharmaceutical preparations.

4917. Iminodiacetic Acid. [142-73-4] *N*-(Carboxymethyl)-glycine; iminodiethanoic acid; diglycine; IDA. $C_4H_7NO_4$; mol wt 133.10. C 36.10%, H 5.30%, N 10.52%, O 48.08%. HOOCCH$_2$-NHCH$_2$COOH. Obtained from nitrilotriacetic acid, N(CH$_2$-COOH)$_3$, by HCl-hydrolysis in a bomb tube: Schwarzenbach *et al., Helv. Chim. Acta* **28**, 1133 (1945); by oxygenation in presence of palladium/carbon catalyst: Tetenbaum, Stone, *Chem. Commun.* **1970**, 1699. Iminodiacetic acid and nitrilotriacetic acid are formed upon boiling chloroacetic acid with concd aq ammonia: Heintz, *Ann.* **149**, 88 (1869). *See also* Martell, Bersworth, *J. Org. Chem.* **15**, 46 (1950).

Orthorhombic crystals, dec 247.5° (commercial grade, mp 220-250°). pKa$_1$ 2.98; pKa$_2$ 9.89. Forms salts with acids and bases. Soly in water at 5°: 2.43 g/100 ml. Practically insol in acetone, methanol, ether, benzene, carbon tetrachloride, heptane.

Hydrochloride. $C_4H_7NO_4 \cdot HCl$. Crystals, dec 238-239°. Concd aq solns yield the free acid when adjusted to pH 2 with NaOH.

Sodium salt monohydrate. $C_4H_6NNaO_4 \cdot H_2O$. Freely sol in water. Forms complexes with Mg, Ca, Ba.

USE: Has been suggested as intermediate in the manuf of surface active agents, complex salts, chelating agents.

4918. Iminodisuccinic Acid. [7408-20-0]; [70543-06-5] (stereo unspecified). *N*-[(1S)-1,2-Dicarboxyethyl]-L-aspartic acid; 2,2'-iminodisuccinic acid. $C_8H_{11}NO_8$; mol wt 249.17. C 38.56%, H 4.45%, N 5.62%, O 51.37%. Synthesis of ester from fumaric acid, ammonia and water: G. Stadnikoff, *Ber.* **44**, 44 (1911). Industrial processes: **GB 1306331** (1971 to Pfizer); T. Groth *et*

al., **US 6107518** (2000 to Bayer). Synthesis and complex forming properties: E. D. Malakhaev *et al., J. Gen. Chem. USSR* **48**, 2361 (1978). Thermochemical study: V. P. Vasil'ev *et al., Russ. J. Phys. Chem.* **63**, 1566 (1989). Formation constants with metal cations: C. K. Gangoda, D. R. Williams, *Chem. Speciation Bioavailab.* **9**, 101 (1997).

White solid, mp 206-208°. pK$_1$ 2.96 ±0.05; pK$_2$ 3.84 ±0.02; pK$_3$ 4.83 ±0.05; pK$_4$ 10.12 ±0.04 (25°). Heat of combustion: 2974.3 ±0.6 kJ/mol. Sol in water; insol in alcohol, ether, acetone, benzene.

Tetrasodium salt. [144538-83-0] Baypure CX 100. Review of commercial product: *NICNAS New chemical assessment: Aspartic acid, N-(1,2-dicarboxyethyl)-tetrasodium salt,* (Sydney, Nat. Ind. Chem. Notif. Assess. Scheme, 2002) 22 pp. White solid, mp >300°. Bulk density (kg/m^3): ~740. Vapor pressure at 20°: 1.5×10^{-16} kPa. Sol at 20° (g/l): water 564 (pH 13.1). LD$_{50}$ in rats (mg/kg): >2000 orally; >2000 dermally (NICNAS).

USE: Biodegradable metal chelator in detergents, cleaners and personal care products; in photographic applications; in trace nutrient agricultural fertilizers. In mfr of textiles and newspaper. Scale deposit remover, water softener, bleaching agent stabilizer.

4919. Imipenem. [74431-23-5]; [64221-86-9] (anhydrous). (5*R*,6*S*)-6-[(1*R*)-1-Hydroxyethyl]-3-[[2-[(iminomethyl)amino]ethyl]thio]-7-oxo-1-azabicyclo[3.2.0]hept-2-ene-2-carboxylic acid monohydrate; *N*-formimidoylthienamycin monohydrate; imipemide; MK-787. $C_{12}H_{17}N_3O_4S \cdot H_2O$; mol wt 317.36. C 45.41%, H 6.03%, N 13.24%, O 25.21%, S 10.10%. Extremely broad-spectrum semi-synthetic antibiotic; first stable derivative of thienamycin, *q.v.* Prepn: W. J. Leanza *et al., J. Med. Chem.* **22**, 1435 (1979); T. W. Miller, **EP 6639** (1980 to Merck & Co.), *C.A.* **93**, 155845y (1980); B. G. Christensen *et al.*, **US 4194047** (1980 to Merck & Co.). Totally synthetic prepn without formation of thienamycin: I. Shinkai *et al., Tetrahedron Lett.* **23**, 4903 (1982). HPLC determn in serum: C. M. Myers, J. L. Blumer, *Antimicrob. Agents Chemother.* **26**, 78 (1984). Series of articles on *in vitro* activity, pharmacokinetics, clinical efficacy of combination with cilastatin sodium, *q.v.*, a renal dehydropeptidase I inhibitor: *J. Antimicrob. Chemother.* **12**, Suppl. D, 1-155 (1983); *Rev. Infect. Dis.* **7**, Suppl. 3, S389-S536 (1985); *Am. J. Med.* **78**, Suppl. 6A, 1-167 (1985); *Infection* **14**, Suppl. 2, S111-S180 (1986). Comprehensive description: E. R. Oberholtzer, *Anal. Profiles Drug Subs.* **17**, 73-114 (1988).

Crystals from water-ethanol. $[\alpha]_D^{25}$ +86.8° (c = 0.05 in 0.1*M* phosphate, pH 7). pKa$_1$ ~3.2, pKa$_2$ ~9.9. uv max (water): 299 nm (ε 9670, 98% NH$_2$OH ext). Soly (mg/ml): water 10, methanol 5, ethanol 0.2, acetone <0.1, dimethylformamide <0.1, dimethylsulfoxide 0.3.

Combination with cilastatin sodium. [85960-17-4] Imipem; Primaxin; Tenacid; Tienam; Zienam.

THERAP CAT: Antibacterial.

4920. Imipramine. [50-49-7] 10,11-Dihydro-*N,N*-dimethyl-5*H*-dibenz[*b,f*]azepine-5-propanamine; 5-(3-dimethylaminopropyl)-10,11-dihydro-5*H*-dibenz[*b,f*]azepine; *N*-(γ-dimethylaminopropyl)iminodibenzyl; imizin; G-22355. $C_{19}H_{24}N_2$; mol wt 280.41. C 81.38%, H 8.63%, N 9.99%. Tricyclic antidepressant. Prepn: Haefliger, Schindler, **US 2554736** (1951 to Geigy); *eidem, Helv. Chim. Acta* **37**, 472 (1954). Reviews of pharmacology: Crismon, *Psychopharmacol. Bull.* **4**, 151 pp (Oct. 1967); Glassman,

Perel, *Arch. Gen. Psychiatry* **28**, 649 (1973). Toxicity data: A. Tobe *et al.*, *Arzneim.-Forsch.* **31**, 1278 (1981). Comprehensive description: D. N. Kender, R. E. Schiesswohl, *Anal. Profiles Drug Subs.* **14**, 37-75 (1985). Comparative clinical trials in depression: R. S. Lipman *et al.*, *Arch. Gen. Psychiatry* **43**, 68 (1986); in anxiety: R.J. Kahn *et al.*, *ibid.* 79. Clinical trial for panic disorder: D. H. Barlow *et al.*, *J. Am. Med. Assoc.* **283**, 2529 (2000).

Free base, bp$_{0.1}$ 160°.

Hydrochloride. [113-52-0] Chrytemin; Deprinol; Feinalmin; Imidol; Imilanyle; Imiprin; Janimine; Melipramine; Presamine; Pryleugan; Tofranil. C$_{19}$H$_{24}$N$_2$.HCl; mol wt 316.87. Crystals from acetone, mp 174-175°. Acquires a yellow to reddish discoloration under the influence of light. Freely sol in water, less sol in alcohol, sparingly sol in acetone. LD$_{50}$ in mice, rats (mg/kg): 400, 490 orally; 110, 90 i.p. (Tobe).

Pamoate. [10075-24-8] Tofranil-PM. (C$_{19}$H$_{24}$N$_2$)$_2$.C$_{23}$H$_{16}$-O$_6$; mol wt 949.18.

THERAP CAT: Antidepressant.

4921. Imipramine *N*-Oxide. [6829-98-7] 10,11-Dihydro-*N*,*N*-dimethyl-5*H*-dibenz[*b,f*]azepine-5-propanamine *N*-oxide; 5-[3-(dimethylamino)propyl]-10,11-dihydro-5*H*-dibenz[*b,f*]azepine *N*-oxide; *N*-(γ-dimethylaminopropyl)iminodibenzyl *N*-oxide; IPNO. C$_{19}$H$_{24}$N$_2$O; mol wt 296.41. C 76.99%, H 8.16%, N 9.45%, O 5.40%. Identification as a metabolite of imipramine, *q.v.*: V. Fishman, H. Goldenberg, *Proc. Soc. Exp. Biol. Med.* **110**, 187 (1962). Prepn: **FR M2508**; H. Dyrsting, J. B. Pedersen, **US 3574852** (1964, 1971, both to Dumex). Pharmacology: W. Theobald *et al.*, *Med. Pharmacol. Exp.* **15**, 187 (1966). Metabolism: M. H. Bickel, M. Baggiolini, *Biochem. Pharmacol.* **15**, 1155 (1966); R. Minder *et al.*, *Arch. Pharmakol.* **268**, 334 (1971). GLC determn in biological samples: H. J. Weder, M. H. Bickel, *J. Chromatogr.* **37**, 181 (1968); HPLC determn: E. Koyama *et al.*, *Ther. Drug Monit.* **15**, 224 (1993). Clinical trial: W. Rapp *et al.*, *Acta Psychiatr. Scand.* **49**, 77 (1973). Clinical pharmacokinetics: A. Nagy, T. Hansen, *Acta Pharmacol. Toxicol.* **42**, 58 (1978).

White needle-shaped crystals, mp 120-123° (dec). Sol in methanol, ether, acetone and benzene. Strongly hygroscopic.

Monohydrate. mp 75-79°.

Hydrochloride. [20438-98-6] Imiprex. C$_{19}$H$_{24}$N$_2$O.HCl; mol wt 332.87. Colorless crystalline powder, mp 167-174° (dec). Very bitter taste. An aq. soln is moderately acidic. Sol in 75 parts water, in 12 parts 95% ethanol, 4.5 parts chloroform. Nearly insol in ether. LD$_{50}$ in rats, mice (mg/kg): 90, 150 i.p. (Dyrsting, Pedersen).

THERAP CAT: Antidepressant.

4922. Imiquimod. [99011-02-6] 1-(2-Methylpropyl)-1*H*-imidazo[4,5-*c*]quinolin-4-amine; 4-amino-1-isobutyl-1*H*-imidazo[4,5-*c*]quinoline; R-837; S-26308; Aldara. C$_{14}$H$_{16}$N$_4$; mol wt 240.30. C 69.97%, H 6.71%, N 23.32%. Immune response modifier; stimulates production of interferon-α, *q.v.* Prepn: J. F. Gerster, **EP 145340**; *idem*, **US 4689338** (1985, 1987 both to Riker). Mechanism of action study: K. Megyeri *et al.*, *Mol. Cell. Biol.* **15**, 2207 (1995). Clinical pharmacology: P. L. Witt *et al.*, *Cancer Res.* **53**, 5176 (1993). Clinical trial for genital warts: L. Edwards *et al.*,

Arch. Dermatol. **134**, 25 (1998). Series of articles on pharmacology and clinical experience in cutaneous viral infections: *J. Am. Acad. Dermatol.* **43**, S1-S30 (2000).

Crystals from DMF, mp 292-294°.

THERAP CAT: Antiviral; immunomodulator.

4923. Imolamine. [318-23-0] 4-[2-(Diethylamino)ethyl]-5-imino-3-phenyl-Δ^2-1,2,4-oxadiazoline; 3-phenyl-4-diethylamino-ethyl-5-imino-1,2,4-oxadiazoline. C$_{14}$H$_{20}$N$_4$O; mol wt 260.33. C 64.59%, H 7.74%, N 21.52%, O 6.15%. Prepn: Aron-Samuel, Sterne, **FR M2023** (1963), *C.A.* **60**, 2952f (1964). Pharmacology: Molino, Belluardo, *Gazz. Int. Med. Chir.* **71**, 2100 (1966), *C.A.* **66**, 74830e (1967).

bp$_{0.2}$ 165°.

Hydrochloride. [15823-89-9] LA-1211; Irrigor. C$_{14}$H$_{20}$N$_4$-O.HCl; mol wt 296.80. Crystals, mp 154-155°.

THERAP CAT: Antianginal.

4924. IMPA. [1832-54-8] Methylphosphonic acid mono(1-methylethyl) ester; *i*PMPA; *O*-isopropyl methyl phosphonic acid; neutralized sarin. C$_4$H$_{11}$O$_3$P; mol wt 138.10. C 34.79%, H 8.03%, O 34.76%, P 22.43%. Degradation product of the nerve gas, sarin, *q.v.* Identification as hydrolysis product: F. C. G. Hoskin, *Can. J. Biochem. Physiol.* **34**, 75 (1956). Prepn as silver salt: *idem, Can. J. Chem.* **35**, 581 (1957); of ester: J. I. G. Cadogan *et al.*, *J. Chem. Soc.* **1971**, 1988. Biodisposition in mice: P. J. Little *et al.*, *Toxicol. Appl. Pharmacol.* **83**, 412 (1986). Biological monitoring in human urine after sarin exposure: M. Minami *et al.*, *J. Toxicol. Sci.* **23**, Suppl. II, 250 (1998). Biodegradation: Y. Zhang *et al.*, *Biotechnol. Bioeng.* **64**, 221 (1999). Determn in ground water by GC with flame photometric detection: G. A. Sega *et al.*, *J. Chromatogr. A* **790**, 143 (1997); LC-MS rapid determn: R. W. Read, R. M. Black, *ibid.* **862**, 169 (1999).

bp$_{0.02}$ 88°. n$_D^{25}$ 1.4210.

USE: Marker for the detection of sarin.

4925. Imperatorin. [482-44-0] 9-[(3-Methyl-2-butenyl)-oxy]-7*H*-furo[3,2-*g*][1]benzopyran-7-one; 6-hydroxy-7-(3-methyl-2-butenyloxy)-5-benzofuranacrylic acid δ-lactone; 8-isoamyl-enoxypsoralen; marmelosin; ammidin; pentosalen. C$_{16}$H$_{14}$O$_4$; mol wt 270.28. C 71.10%, H 5.22%, O 23.68%. From roots of *Imperatoria osthruthium* L., *Umbelliferae*: Späth, Holzen, *Ber.* **66**, 1137 (1933); from seeds of *Angelica archangelica* L.: Späth, Vierhapper, *ibid.* **71**, 1667 (1938); from fruit of *Pastinaca sativa* L., *Umbelliferae*: Soine *et al.*, *J. Am. Pharm. Assoc.* **45**, 426 (1956). Identity with marmelosin: Späth *et al.*, *Ber.* **70**, 1021 (1937). Identity with ammidin: Fahmy, Abu-Shady, *Q. J. Pharm. Pharmacol.* **21**, 499 (1948). Partial synthesis: Späth, Holzen, *Ber.* **68**, 1123 (1935). Synthesis: Späth, Vierhapper, *ibid.* **70**, 248 (1937).

Prisms from ether, long fine needles from hot water, mp 102°. Practically insol in cold water. Very sparingly sol in boiling water; freely sol in chloroform; sol in benzene, alcohol, ether, petr ether, alkali hydroxides. uv max: 302, 265, 250 nm (log ε 3.95, 4.00, 4.24).

4926. Imperialine. [18059-10-4] 3,20-Dihydroxycevan-6-one; raddeamine; sipeimine. $C_{27}H_{43}NO_3$; mol wt 429.64. C 75.48%, H 10.09%, N 3.26%, O 11.17%. Isolation from bulb of *Fritillaria imperialis* L., *Liliaceae:* Fragner, *Ber.* **21**, 3284 (1888); Boit, *ibid.* **87**, 472 (1954); from *Petilium eduardi:* Shakirov *et al., C.A.* **60**, 13280h (1964). Identity with sipeimine and raddeamine: Chu *et al., C.A.* **53**, 7503e (1959); Nurridinov, Yunusov, *C.A.* **57**, 15165h (1962). Structure: Nuriddinov *et al., Khim. Prir. Soedin.* **3**, 316 (1967); *C.A.* **68**, 69168g (1968). Prepn of the β-D-glucopyranoside: Shakirov *et al., C.A.* **63**, 1858e (1965). Isolation and structure of the β-D-glucopyranoside: *eidem, C.A.* **63**, 3007f (1965). Absolute configuration: S. Itô *et al., Tetrahedron Lett.* **1976**, 3161.

Prisms from methanol, mp 267°. [α]$_D^{22}$ −38.5° (c = 1.5 in chloroform).

β-D-Glucopyranoside. Edpetiline. $C_{33}H_{53}NO_8$. Crystals from methanol, mp 272-276°. [α]$_D$ −57.89° (c = 0.449 in methanol).

4927. Improsulfan. [13425-98-4] 3,3′-Iminobis-1-propanol dimethanesulfonate (ester); *N,N*-bis(3-methylsulfonyloxypropyl)-amine; bis(3-mesyloxypropyl)amine. $C_8H_{19}NO_6S_2$; mol wt 289.37. C 33.21%, H 6.62%, N 4.84%, O 33.17%, S 22.16%. Alkylating agent related to busulfan, *q.v.* Prepn and antitumor activity of the hydrochloride: M. M. El-Merzabani, Y. Sakurai, *Gann* **56**, 589 (1965), *C.A.* **64**, 8793b (1965); Y. Sakurai, *JP 67 26616* (1967), *C.A.* **69**, 51596f (1968). Prepn of the tosylate: M. Nakanishi *et al., DE 2059377* (1971 to Yoshitomi), *C.A.* **75**, 63127r (1972). Absorption, distribution, excretion, metabolism: Y. Kato *et al., Yakugaku Zasshi* **94**, 1107 (1974), *C.A.* **82**, 38441a (1975). Pharmacology: N. Brock, J. Kuhlmann, *Arzneim.-Forsch.* **24**, 1139 (1974); H. Imamura *et al., Oyo Yakuri* **9**, 861 (1975), *C.A.* **84**, 12492j (1976). Antitumor effect: T. Okumoto *et al., Chem. Pharm. Bull.* **25**, 3003 (1977); T. Iwaguchi, H. Kitagawa, *Gann* **69**, 123 (1968), *C.A.* **89**, 157282 (1978). Clinical study: S. J. Altman *et al., Cancer* **35**, 1145 (1975). Toxicity study: N. Rakieten *et al., U.S. NTIS Report* **PB-196468** (1970) 17 pp, *C.A.* **75**, 47359n (1971). Mutagenicity study: W. F. Benedict *et al., Cancer Res.* **37**, 2209 (1977).

Hydrochloride. [3458-22-8] Yoshi 864; NSC-102627. $C_8H_{19}NO_6S_2$·HCl; mol wt 325.83. Crystals, mp 94-95°. LD$_{50}$ i.v. in rats: 75 mg/kg (Brock, Kuhlmann).

Tosylate. [32784-82-0] 864T; NSC-140117; Protecton. $C_8H_{19}NO_6S_2$·$C_7H_8O_3S$; mol wt 461.57. White crystals, mp 113-118°. Faint, characteristic odor and bitter taste. Sol in water, methanol, acetonitrile. Slightly sol in chloroform.

THERAP CAT: Antineoplastic.

4928. Inaperisone. [99323-21-4] 1-(4-Ethylphenyl)-2-methyl-3-(1-pyrrolidinyl)-1-propanone; (±)-4′-ethyl-2-methyl-3-(1-pyrrolidinyl)propiophenone. $C_{16}H_{23}NO$; mol wt 245.36. C 78.32%, H 9.45%, N 5.71%, O 6.52%. Prepn: *JP Kokai 84 33276*; Y. Itho *et al., US 4638009* (1984, 1987 both to Hokuriku). Pharmacology: K. Morikawa *et al., Arzneim.-Forsch.* **37**, 331 (1987); *idem et al., Eur. J. Pharmacol.* **213**, 409 (1992). Pharmacokinetics in rats: O. Nagata *et al., Drug Metab. Dispos.* **18**, 902 (1990). GC/MS determn in human serum: *idem et al., J. Chromatogr.* **496**, 456 (1989). Series of articles on toxicology: *Yakuri to Chiryo* **20**, 1027-1115 (1992). Comparative clinical evaluation: K. Hiraga *et al., Rinsho Yakuri* **23**, 635 (1992), *C.A.* **118**, 247431y (1993).

Hydrochloride. [118230-97-0] HSR-770; HY-770; Riran. $C_{16}H_{23}NO$·HCl; mol wt 281.82. Colorless needles from methyl ethyl ketone (isolated as ¼ hydrate), mp 152-153°. Also reported as a white to yellowish white crystalline powder. Bitter taste. Very sol in water and methanol. LD$_{50}$ orally in mice: 425 mg/kg (Itho).

THERAP CAT: Muscle relaxant (skeletal).

4929. Incadronic Acid. [124351-85-5] [(Cycloheptylamino)methylene]bisphosphonic acid. $C_8H_{19}NO_6P_2$; mol wt 287.19. C 33.46%, H 6.67%, N 4.88%, O 33.43%, P 21.57%. Bisphosphonate antiresorptive agent. Prepn: Y. Isomura *et al., EP 325482*; *eidem, US 4970335* (1989, 1990 both to Yamanouchi); M. Takeuchi *et al., Chem. Pharm. Bull.* **41**, 688 (1993). HPLC determn in plasma, urine and bone: T. Usui *et al., J. Chromatogr.* **584**, 213 (1992). Effect on bone mineral density in dogs: H. Motoie *et al., J. Bone Miner. Res.* **10**, 910 (1995). Toxicology: A. Okazaki *et al., J. Toxicol. Sci.* **20**, Suppl. 1, 15 (1995). Clinical pharmacokinetics: T. Usui *et al., Int. J. Clin. Pharmacol. Ther.* **35**, 239 (1997). Clinical evaluation in hypercalcemia of malignancy: S. Fukumoto *et al., J. Clin. Endocrinol. Metab.* **79**, 165 (1994).

Crystals from methanol-water, mp 232-233°.

Disodium salt. [138330-18-4] Cimadronate sodium; incadronate sodium; YM-175; Bisphonal. $C_8H_{17}NNa_2O_6P_2$; mol wt 331.15. Occurs as the monohydrate. White, odorless crystalline powder. Easily sol in water. LD$_{50}$ in male, female rats (mg/kg): 23, 21 i.v. (Okazaki).

THERAP CAT: Bone resorption inhibitor.

4930. Indalpine. [63758-79-2] 3-[2-(4-Piperidinyl)ethyl]-1*H*-indole; 4-[2-(3-indolyl)ethyl]piperidine; LM-5008; Upstene. $C_{15}H_{20}N_2$; mol wt 228.33. C 78.90%, H 8.83%, N 12.27%. Selective serotonin uptake inhibitor. Prepn: A. A. Champseix *et al., DE 2618152*; *eidem, US 4064255* (both 1977 to Mar-Pha Soc. Etud. Exploit. Marques). HPLC determn: C. Jozefczak *et al., J. Chromatogr.* **230**, 87 (1982). Spectrofluorimetric determn and clinical pharmacology: A. Iliopoulou *et al., Pharmatherapeutica* **2**, 613 (1981). Pharmacology: G. LeFur *et al., Life Sci.* **23**, 1959 (1978); C. Gueremy *et al., J. Med. Chem.* **23**, 1306 (1980); R. Ashkenazi *et al., Br. J. Pharmacol.* **79**, 765, 915 (1983). Clinical study: A. Wauters, *Acta Psychiatr. Belg.* **83**, 69 (1983).

Monohydrochloride. $C_{15}H_{20}N_2 \cdot HCl$. mp 167°.

THERAP CAT: Antidepressant.

4931. Indan. [496-11-7] 2,3-Dihydro-1H-indene; hydrindene. C_9H_{10}; mol wt 118.18. C 91.47%, H 8.53%. Occurs in coal tar: Krämer, Spilker, *Ber.* **29**, 552 (1896). Prepn: *eidem, ibid.* **33**, 2257 (1900); Grosse *et al., Ind. Eng. Chem.* **38**, 1041 (1946); Carpenter, Easter, *J. Org. Chem.* **19**, 87 (1954); Juday, *ibid.* **22**, 532 (1957); Hunter, Aldridge, **US 3082267** (1963 to Esso); Bestmann *et al., Ann.* **718**, 33 (1968).

Liquid. d_4^{20} 0.9639; d_4^{50} 0.9378. mp −51.4°. bp_{762} 176.5°; bp_{12} 61-64°. n_D^{20} 1.5383. uv max (isooctane): 272, 265, 258 nm (log ε 3.18, 3.08, 2.90). Insol in water. Sol in organic solvents.

1-Methylindan. $C_{10}H_{12}$. Liq, d_4^{20} 0.9402. bp_{760} 186-190°; bp_{10} 60°. n_D^{20} 1.5222.

4932. Indanazoline. [40507-78-6] *N*-(2,3-Dihydro-1H-inden-4-yl)-4,5-dihydro-1H-imidazol-2-amine; *N*-(2-imidazolin-2-yl)-*N*-(4-indanyl)amine. $C_{12}H_{15}N_3$; mol wt 201.27. C 71.61%, H 7.51%, N 20.88%. Prepn: H. J. May, A. Berg, **DE 2136325**; *eidem*, **US 3882229** (1973, 1975 both to Nordmark); H. J. May, *Arzneim.-Forsch.* **30**, 1733 (1980). Toxicity data: W. Worstmann *et al., ibid.* 1760. Series of articles on galenical development, pharmacology, pharmacokinetics and toxicity: *ibid.* 1738-1787.

Crystals from petr ether, mp 109-113°.

Hydrochloride. [40507-80-0] E-VA-16; Farial. $C_{12}H_{15}N_3 \cdot$ HCl; mol wt 237.73. Crystals from isopropanol, mp 182-184°. LD_{50} in male, female mice (mg/kg): 179, 233 orally; 22.3, 26.9 i.v.; in male, female rats: 481, 542 orally; 16.3, 17.6 i.v. (Worstmann).

THERAP CAT: Decongestant (nasal).

4933. Indanofan. [133220-30-1] 2-[[2-(3-Chlorophenyl)oxiranyl]methyl]-2-ethyl-1H-indene-1,3(2H)-dione; MK-243; MX-70906; NH-502; Trebiace. $C_{20}H_{17}ClO_3$; mol wt 340.80. C 70.49%, H 5.03%, Cl 10.40%, O 14.08%. Herbicide developed for use in paddy rice and turf. Prepn: T. Jikihara *et al.*, **EP 398258**; *eidem*, **US 5076830** (1990, 1991 both to Mitsubishi); K. Tanaka *et al.*, *Synthesis* **1999**, 249. Review of physical and biological properties: K. Yagi, K. Inoue, *Agrochem. Jpn.* **76**, 12-14 (2000).

Colorless crystals from methanol-water, mp 60.4-61.3°; also reported as off-white crystals. Soly in water at 25°: 17.1 mg/l. Vapor pressure at 25°: 2.8×10^{-6} Pa. LD_{50} male, female (mg/kg): 631, 460 orally; >2000, >2000 dermally. LC_{50} in rats (mg/l): 1.57 by inhalation (Yagi).

USE: Herbicide.

4934. Indanthrene. [81-77-6] 6,15-Dihydro-5,9,14,18-anthrazinetetrone; *N,N'*-dihydro-1,2,1',2'-anthraquinonazine. C_{28}-$H_{14}N_2O_4$; mol wt 442.42. C 76.01%, H 3.19%, N 6.33%, O 14.47%. Vat dye discovered by René Bohn (1901). Prepn: Fierz-David, Blangey, *Grundlegende Operationen der Farbenchemie* (Vienna, 5th ed., 1943) pp 304-305; Thielert, Bauman, **US 2693469** (1954 to Bayer); Sutter, Fioroni, **US 2831860** (1958 to Ciba); Kastner, **US 3138612** (1964 to Allied Chem.). Structure: Weinstein, Merrit, *J. Am. Chem. Soc.* **81**, 3759 (1959).

Blue powder, dec 470-500°. uv max on cellophane film: 278 nm. Practically insol in organic solvents. Sol in concd H_2SO_4, in dil alkali solns. *Indanthrene Blue R*, the usual commercial grade, is extremely stable to light and heat, but sensitive to chlorine. A purer grade, which is not as sensitive to chlorine, is sold as *Indanthrene Brilliant Blue FF*.

USE: Mainly to dye cotton.

4935. Indapamide. [26807-65-8] 3-(Aminosulfonyl)-4-chloro-*N*-(2,3-dihydro-2-methyl-1H-indol-1-yl)benzamide; 4-chloro-*N*-(2-methyl-1-indolinyl)-3-sulfamoylbenzamide; *N*-(3-sulfamyl-4-chlorobenzamido)-2-methylindoline; S-1520; SE-1520; Bajaten; Fludex; Indaflex; Indamol; Lozol; Noranat; Tandix; Veroxil. $C_{16}H_{16}ClN_3O_3S$; mol wt 365.83. C 52.53%, H 4.41%, Cl 9.69%, N 11.49%, O 13.12%, S 8.77%. Prepn: Beregi *et al.*, **FR 2003311**; *eidem*, **US 3565911** (1969, 1971, both to Sci. Union et Cie, Soc. Franc. Recherche Med.). LC/MS determn in plasma: F. Albu *et al., J. Chromatogr. B* **816**, 35 (2005). Pharmacology: Leary *et al., Curr. Ther. Res.* **15**, 571 (1973); D. B. Campbell, R. A. Moore, *Postgrad. Med. J. Suppl.* **57**, 7 (1981). Acute toxicity data: J. Kyncl *et al., Arzneim.-Forsch.* **25**, 1491 (1975). Symposium on pharmacology and clinical efficacy: *Am. J. Med.* **84**, Suppl. 1B, 1-111 (1988); *Am. J. Cardiol.* **65**, Suppl. H, 1H-80H (1990). Comprehensive description: T. J. DiFeo, J. E. Shuster, *Anal. Profiles Drug Subs. Excip.* **23**, 229-268 (1994).

Crystals from isopropanol/water, mp 160-162°. uv max (methanol): 242, 278, 286 nm ($A_{1cm}^{1\%}$ 630, 98, 100). Sol in methanol, acetic acid, ethyl acetate. Very slightly sol in chloroform. pKa (25°) 8.8 ± 0.2. LD_{50} in rats, mice, guinea pigs (mg/kg): 393-421, 410-564, 347-416 i.p.; 394-440, 577-635, 272-358 i.v.; >3000 all species orally (Kyncl).

Hemihydrate. Damide; Ipamix; Natrilix; Pressural. $C_{16}H_{16}$-$ClN_3O_3S \cdot \frac{1}{2}H_2O$; mol wt 374.84.

THERAP CAT: Antihypertensive; diuretic.

4936. 1H-Indazole. [271-44-3] Isoindazole; benzopyrazole. $C_7H_6N_2$; mol wt 118.14. C 71.17%, H 5.12%, N 23.71%. Prepn: Stephenson, *Org. Synth.* **coll. vol. III**, 475 (1955); Ainsworth, *Org. Synth.* **39**, 27 (1959); Huisgen, Bast, *ibid.* **42**, 69 (1962).

Needles from hot water, mp 146.5°. bp_{743} 267-270°. Sol in hot water, alcohol, ether.

4937. Indecainide. [74517-78-5] 9-[3-[(1-Methylethyl)-amino]propyl]-9*H*-fluorene-9-carboxamide; 9-carbamoyl-9-(3-isopropylaminopropyl)fluorene; 9-[3-(isopropylamino)propyl]-9-(aminocarboyl)fluorene; ricainide. $C_{20}H_{24}N_2O$; mol wt 308.42. C 77.89%, H 7.84%, N 9.08%, O 5.19%. Prepn: W. B. Lacefield, R. L. Simon, **US 4197313** and **US 4452745** (1980, 1984 both to Lilly). Pharmacokinetics in animals: T. L. Lindstrom, G. W. Whitaker, *Drug Metab. Dispos.* **12**, 683 (1984). Metabolism: *eidem, ibid.* 691. LC determn in biological fluids: K. Z. Farid *et al., J. Chromatogr.* **337**, 329 (1985). Toxicological studies: G. E. Sandusky, Jr., D. B. Meyers, *Fundam. Appl. Toxicol.* **5**, 175 (1985). Clinical evaluation in cardiac arrhythmias: P. F. Nestico *et al., Am. J. Cardiol.* **59**, 1332 (1987); P. J. Podrid *et al., ibid.* **61**, 764 (1988).

Crystals from Skelly B, mp 94-95°.

Hydrochloride. [73681-12-6] LY-135837; Decabid. $C_{20}H_{24}$-N_2O.HCl; mol wt 344.88. Crystals from chloroform, mp 216.5-217°; also reported as crystals from fresh ethanol and diethyl ether, mp 203-204°. LD_{50} orally in male, female mice, rats: 100, 96, 103, 82 mg/kg (Sandusky, Meyers).

THERAP CAT: Antiarrhythmic (cardiac depressant).

4938. Indeloxazine Hydrochloride. [65043-22-3] 2-[(1*H*-Inden-7-yloxy)methyl]morpholine hydrochloride; (±)-2-[(7-indenyloxy)methyl]morpholine hydrochloride; YM-08054-1; Elen; Noin. $C_{14}H_{18}ClNO_2$; mol wt 267.75. C 62.80%, H 6.78%, Cl 13.24%, N 5.23%, O 11.95%. Serotonin uptake inhibitor. Prepn: M. Masuo *et al.*, **DE 2601703**; *eidem*, **US 4109088** (1976, 1978 both to Yamanouchi). Synthesis and resolution of isomers: T. Kojima *et al., Chem. Pharm. Bull.* **33**, 3766 (1985). Pharmacology and toxicity: S. Tachikawa *et al., Arch. Int. Pharmacodyn.* **238**, 81 (1979). Inhibition of synaptosomal uptake of serotonin and noradrenaline: M. Harada, H. Maeno, *Biochem. Pharmacol.* **28**, 2645 (1979). GLC determn in human plasma: A. G. Hayes, T. Chang, *J. Chromatogr.* **272**, 176 (1983).

Polymorphic; pale yellow needles from methanol, mp 169-170°; colorless, acicular crystals from acetone, mp 155-156°. LD_{50} in mice (mg/kg): 47 i.v. (Tachikawa).

(+)-Form. Crystals from ethanol, mp 112-113°. $[\alpha]_D^{21}$ +4.9° (c = 5 in methanol).

(−)-Form. Crystals from isopropanol, mp 142-142.5°. $[\alpha]_D^{20}$ −4.9° (c = 5 in methanol).

THERAP CAT: Antidepressant; nootropic.

4939. Indene. [95-13-6] Indonaphthene. C_9H_8; mol wt 116.16. C 93.06%, H 6.94%. Found in the tars from coal, lignite, and crude petr. Isoln from coal tar: Weissgerber, *Ber.* **42**, 569 (1909); *Brennst.-Chem.* **5**, 208 (1924); Weissgerber, Seidler, *Ber.* **60**, 2088 (1927). Prepn from acetylene over activated charcoal at 625°: Zelinsky, *Ber.* **57**, 264 (1924). Manuf from tetrahydronaphthalene by passing over SiO_2-Al_2O_3 catalyst at 670°: **GB 578083** (1946). Prepn from *o*-BrCH_2C_6H_4CH_2CH_2Br and triphenylphosphine: Bestmann *et al., Ann.* **718**, 33 (1968).

Liquid. d_4^4 1.0081; d_4^{20} 0.9968; d_4^{50} 0.9692. mp −1.8°. bp_{760} 181.6°; bp_{400} 157.8°; bp_{200} 135.6°; bp_{100} 114.7°; bp_{60} 100.8°; bp_{40} 90.7°; bp_{20} 73.9°; bp_{10} 58.5°; bp_5 44.3°; $bp_{1.0}$ 16.4°. $n_D^{18.5}$ 1.5773.

Absorption spectrum: Morton, de Gouveia, *J. Chem. Soc.* **1934**, 911. Insol in water. Miscible with most organic solvents. Polymerizes and oxidizes on standing. Concd H_2SO_4 forms metaindene, $(C_9H_8)_{16-22}$.

Caution: Potential symptoms of overexposure in exptl animals are irritation of eyes, skin, mucous membranes; dermatitis, skin sensitization; liver, kidney and spleen injury; aspiration of liquid may cause chemical pneumonia. *See NIOSH Pocket Guide to Chemical Hazards* (DHHS/NIOSH 97-140, 1997) p 170.

4940. Indenolol. [60607-68-3] 1-[1*H*-Inden-4(or 7)-yloxy]-3-[(1-methylethyl)amino]-2-propanol; (±)-1-[inden-4(or 7)-yloxy]-3-(isopropylamino)-2-propanol; YB-2; Sch-28316Z. $C_{15}H_{21}NO_2$; mol wt 247.33. C 72.84%, H 8.56%, N 5.66%, O 12.94%. Nonselective β-adrenergic blocker. Prepn: M. Murakami *et al.*, **DE 1955229**; *eidem*, **US 4045482** (1970, 1977 both to Yamanouchi); K. Murase *et al., Yakugaku Zasshi* **92**, 1358 (1972), *C.A.* **78**, 71723 (1973). Indenolol is a tautomeric mixture of the 7- and 4-indenyloxy isomers in a 2:1 ratio, respectively. Unambiguous synthesis of the two isomers: *eidem, Chem. Pharm. Bull.* **24**, 552 (1976). β-Blocking and cardiovascular properties: T. Takenaka, S. Tachikawa, *Arzneim.-Forsch.* **22**, 1864 (1972). General pharmacology: M. Takeda *et al., Oyo Yakuri* **7**, 469 (1973), *C.A.* **80**, 44015 (1974). Comparative pharmacological study with other β-blockers: W. Bartsch *et al., Arzneim.-Forsch.* **27**, 1022 (1977). Dose-response studies: F. E. Okupa *et al., Clin. Pharmacol. Ther.* **29**, 434 (1981). Pharmacokinetics: R. Sega *et al., J. Clin. Pharmacol.* **25**, 337 (1985). Clinical evaluation in hypertension: B. Trimarco *et al., ibid.* 328; L. Poggesi *et al., Clin. Pharmacol. Ther.* **41**, 344 (1987).

Crystals from *n*-hexane/ether, mp 88-89°.

Hydrochloride. [81789-85-7] Pulsan; Securpres. $C_{15}H_{21}$-NO_2.HCl; mol wt 283.79. Crystals from ethanol/ether, mp 147-148°. LD_{50} in mice: 26 mg/kg i.v. (Bartsch).

THERAP CAT: Antihypertensive, antiarrhythmic, antianginal.

4941. Indican (Metabolic Indican). [487-94-5] 1*H*-Indol-3-ol hydrogen sulfate ester; indol-3-yl sulfate; 3-indoxylsulfuric acid. $C_8H_7NO_4S$; mol wt 213.21. C 45.07%, H 3.31%, N 6.57%, O 30.02%, S 15.04%. Unstable as the free acid. Occurs in urine of mammals, also in blood plasma. Prepn of potassium salt from potassium indoxyl and potassium bisulfate: Baeyer, *Ber.* **14**, 1745 (1881); from chlorosulfonic acid and *N*-acetylindoxyl in pyridine: Schwenk, Jolles, *Biochem. Z.* **69**, 467 (1915); by persulfate oxidation of indole: Boyland *et al., Biochem. J.* **62**, 546 (1956).

Potassium salt. Indol-3-yl potassium sulfate; urinary indican; potassium indoxyl sulfate. $C_8H_6KNO_4S$. Light brown plates from aq alc, dec 179-180° with sublimation. Very sol in water. Practically insol in cold alcohol.

4942. Indican (Plant Indican). [487-60-5] 1*H*-Indol-3-yl-β-D-glucopyranoside; 3-(β-glucosido)indole; indoxyl-β-D-glucoside. $C_{14}H_{17}NO_6$; mol wt 295.29. C 56.94%, H 5.80%, N 4.74%, O 32.51%. Isolated from *Indigofera* spp., *Leguminosae* and from *Polygonum tinctorium* Ait., *Polygonaceae*. Extraction procedure for the glucoside: Hoogewerff, Meulen, *Rec. Trav. Chim.* **19**, 166 (1900); Perkin, Bloxam, *J. Chem. Soc.* **91**, 1715 (1907); Perkin, Thomas, *ibid.* **95**, 793 (1909). About 3% indican is found in 4-day old air-dried leaves of *Indigofera tinctoria*. Synthesis: Robertson, *J. Chem. Soc.* **1927**, 1937; Robertson, Waters, *ibid.* **1933**, 30; Freudenberg *et al., Ber.* **85**, 641 (1952).

O—β-D-glucose

Trihydrate. Orthorhombic spear-shaped needles, mp 57-58°. $[\alpha]_{546}^{19}$ −66°. After heating *in vacuo* (oil pump) over H_2SO_4 for 48 hrs the hemihydrate is obtained, mp 101°. Robertson obtained the anhydrous compound by heating in the steam oven for 3 hrs, at 110° for 1 hr, and at 160° for 5 minutes. Perkin and Bloxam obtained anhydr indican by treating the trihydrate with boiling alcohol and boiling benzene. Anhydr indican decomposes at 178-180°. $[\alpha]_D^{15}$ −66° (c = 2); $[\alpha]_{546}^{19}$ −78° (c = 0.6). Sol in water, methanol, alcohol, acetone; slightly sol in ether, benzene, chloroform, ethyl acetate, carbon disulfide. Anhydr indican is sparingly sol in anhydr alcohol.

4943. Indigo. [482-89-3] 2-(1,3-Dihydro-3-oxo-2*H*-indol-2-ylidene)-1,2-dihydro-3*H*-indol-3-one; [$\Delta^{2,2'}$-biindoline]-3,3'-dione; $\Delta^{2,2'}$-bipseudoindoxyl; indigotin; indigo blue; D & C Blue No. 6; C.I. Pigment Blue 66; C.I. Vat Blue 1; C.I. 73000. $C_{16}H_{10}$-N_2O_2; mol wt 262.26. C 73.28%, H 3.84%, N 10.68%, O 12.20%. Probably the oldest known coloring matter. Originally obtained from various species of *Indigofera, Leguminosae*, indigenous to Bengal, Java, Guatemala, in which it occurs as a glucoside. First synthesis: Baeyer, *Ber.* **11**, 1296 (1878); **12**, 456 (1879). First commercial process: Heumann, *Ber.* **23**, 3043, 3431 (1890). Newer prepns: Harley-Mason, *J. Chem. Soc.* **1950**, 2907; Ziegler, Kappe, *Monatsh. Chem.* **96**, 889 (1965); J. Gosteli, *Helv. Chim. Acta* **60**, 1980 (1977). Indigo occurs in *cis* and *trans* forms, in solid state it is in the *trans* form: Posner, *Ber.* **56**, 31 (1923); **57**, 1313 (1924); **59**, 1799 (1926). Reviews on indigo and indigoid dyes: Lubs, *The Chemistry of Synthetic Dyes*, ACS Monograph Series no. **127** (Reinhold, New York, 1955) pp 551-576; Schweizer, *Künstliche Organische Farbstoffe und ihre Zwischenprodukte* (Springer Verlag, 1964) pp 320-334; *Colour Index* **vol. 4** (3rd ed., 1971) p 4595.

Dark-blue powder with coppery luster. Sublimes at about 300°; dec 390°. Practically insol in water, alcohol, ether, and dil acids. Dissolves in nonpolar solvents with red and in polar solvents with blue color. With fuming H_2SO_4 it forms a sol sulfonic acid.

USE: As textile dye. In sutures.

4944. Indigo Carmine. [860-22-0] 2-(1,3-Dihydro-3-oxo-5-sulfo-2*H*-indol-2-ylidene)-2,3-dihydro-3-oxo-1*H*-indole-5-sulfonic acid disodium salt; 3,3'-dioxo-[$\Delta^{2,2'}$-biindoline]-5,5'-disulfonic acid disodium salt; disodium 5,5'-indigotin disulfonate; sodium indigotin disulfonate; soluble indigo blue; indigotine; Acid Blue 74; C.I. Acid Blue 74; C.I. Food Blue 1; FD & C Blue No. 2; C.I. 73015. $C_{16}H_8N_2Na_2O_8S_2$; mol wt 466.35. C 41.21%, H 1.73%, N 6.01%, Na 9.86%, O 27.45%, S 13.75%. Synthesis and structure determination: Vorlander, Schubart, *Ber.* **34**, 1860 (1901). Prepn and properties: Matthews, *Color Trade J.* **6**, 96 (1920). *See also Colour Index* **vol. 4** (3rd ed., 1971) p 4597.

Dark-blue powder with coppery luster. Sensitive to light. Its solns have a blue or bluish-purple color. One gram dissolves in about 100 ml water at 25°. Slightly sol in alcohol. Practically insol in most other organic solvents. It is also marketed as a paste with water, the dye contents varying according to specification or requirements of the user. It almost always contains sodium chloride or sulfate used for "salting" it out. Indigo carmine is very sensitive to oxidizing agents. The color is readily discharged by nitric acid, chlorates, etc. The color of the aq soln fades on standing.

USE: Colorant for nylon, surgical sutures, foods and ingested drugs. As a reagent for functional kidney tests, for detection of nitrates, chlorates and in testing milk.

4945. Indinavir. [150378-17-9] 2,3,5-Trideoxy-*N*-[(1*S*,2*R*)-2,3-dihydro-2-hydroxy-1*H*-inden-1-yl]-5-[(2*S*)-2-[[(1,1-dimethylethyl)amino]carbonyl]-4-(3-pyridinylmethyl)-1-piperazinyl]-2-(phenylmethyl)-D-*erythro*-pentonamide; (α*R*,γ*S*,2*S*)-α-benzyl-2-(*tert*-butylcarbamoyl)-γ-hydroxy-*N*-[(1*S*,2*R*)-2-hydroxy-1-indanyl]-4-(3-pyridylmethyl)-1-piperazinevaleramide; *N*-(2(*R*)-hydroxy-1(*S*)-indanyl)-2(*R*)-(phenylmethyl)-4(*S*)-hydroxy-5-[1-[4-(3-pyridylmethyl)-2(*S*)-(*N-tert*-butylcarbamoyl)piperazinyl]]pentanamide. $C_{36}H_{47}N_5O_4$; mol wt 613.79. C 70.45%, H 7.72%, N 11.41%, O 10.43%. Member of the novel hydroxyaminopentane amide class of HIV-1 protease inhibitors. Prepn: J. P. Vacca *et al.*, **EP 541168**; *eidem*, **US 5413999** (1993, 1995 both to Merck & Co.); B. D. Dorsey *et al.*, *J. Med. Chem.* **37**, 3443 (1994). Diastereoselective synthesis: D. Askin *et al.*, *Tetrahedron Lett.* **35**, 673 (1994); P. E. Maligres *et al.*, *ibid.* **36**, 2195 (1995). Crystal structure of HIV-II protease complex: Z. Chen *et al.*, *J. Biol. Chem.* **269**, 26344 (1994). Antiviral activity and pharmacokinetics: J. P. Vacca *et al.*, *Proc. Natl. Acad. Sci. USA* **91**, 4096 (1994). HPLC determn in plasma and urine: E. Woolf *et al.*, *J. Chromatogr. A* **692**, 45 (1995). Metabolism in humans: S. K. Balani *et al.*, *Drug Metab. Dispos.* **23**, 266 (1995).

Occurs as monohydrate, crystals from wet ethyl or isopropyl acetate, loss of water below 100° followed by recrystallization of anhydrous form with mp 153-154°; second anhydrous form, mp 167.5-168°. Soly in water (mg/ml): 0.015 (unbuffered), >1.5 (pH 4.0). $[\alpha]_D^{22}$ +24.1° (c = 0.0133 in chloroform).

Sulfate. [157810-81-6] MK-639; Crixivan. $C_{36}H_{47}N_5O_4.H_2$-SO_4; mol wt 711.87. Occurs as the monoethanolate, crystals from absolute ethanol, softens at 135°, mp 150-153° (dec). Converts to hydrate upon loss of ethanol and exposure to moist air.

THERAP CAT: Antiviral.

4946. Indiplon. [325715-02-4] *N*-Methyl-*N*-[3-[3-(2-thienylcarbonyl)pyrazolo[1,5-*a*]pyrimidin-7-yl]phenyl]acetamide; CL-285489; NBI-34060. $C_{20}H_{16}N_4O_2S$; mol wt 376.43. C 63.81%, H 4.28%, N 14.88%, O 8.50%, S 8.52%. Short-acting nonbenzodiazepine sedative; high-affinity α_1-selective allosteric potentiator of $GABA_A$ receptor function. Prepn: J. P. Dusza *et al.*, **US 4521422** (1985 to Am. Cyanamid). *See also: idem et al.*, **US 6399621** (2002 to Am. Cyanamid). Receptor binding studies: S. K. Sullivan *et al.*, *J. Pharmacol. Exp. Ther.* **311**, 537 (2004). *In vivo* pharmacology: A. C. Foster *et al.*, *ibid.* 547. Review of clinical development: D. N. Neubauer, *Expert Opin. Invest. Drugs* **14**, 1269-1276 (2005).

Yellow solid.

Note: This is a controlled substance (depressant): **21 CFR,** 1308.14.

THERAP CAT: Sedative, hypnotic.

4947.   Indium. [7440-74-6] In; at. wt 114.818; at. no. 49; valence 3, 2, 1. Group IIIA(13). Natural isotopes: 115 (95.77%); 113 (4.23%); ^{115}In is a β^- emitter, $T_{\frac{1}{2}}$ 6 × 10^{14} years. Artificial radioactive isotopes: 107-112; 114; 116-124. Occurrence in the earth's crust: 1 × 10^{-5}%. Discovered in sphalerite ore by Reich and Richter in 1863. Generally found in zinc blendes. Monograph: M. T. Ludwick, *Indium* (Indium Corp. of America, Utica, N.Y., 1950). *Review:* Wade, Banister in *Comprehensive Inorganic Chemistry* vol. 1, J. C. Bailar, Jr. *et al.,* Eds. (Pergamon Press, Oxford, 1973) pp 997-1000, 1065-1117; E. F. Milner, C. E. T. White in *Kirk-Othmer Encyclopedia of Chemical Technology* vol. 13 (Wiley-Interscience, New York, 3rd ed., 1981) pp 207-212.

Soft, white metal with bluish tinge. Emits a "tin cry" on bending. Ductile, malleable, softer than lead, leaves a mark on paper. Quite stable in air. Crystallizes and is diamagnetic. d^{20} 7.3. mp 155°. bp 2000°. Sp heat: 0.0568 cal/g/°C. Hardness (Mohs') = 1.2. Unaffected by water; attacked by mineral acids. Very resistant to alkalies.

Caution: Indium salts are relatively nontoxic when administered orally; highly toxic when administered subcutaneously or intravenously. Experimental animal poisoning has produced injury to blood, heart, liver, kidneys: E. Browning, *Toxicity of Industrial Metals* (Appleton-Century-Crofts, New York, 2nd ed., 1969) pp 164-168.

USE: In bearing alloys; as a thin film on moving surfaces made from other metals. In dental alloys. In semiconductor research. In nuclear reactor control rods (in the form of an Ag-In-Cd alloy).

4948.   Indium Antimonide. [1312-41-0] InSb; mol wt 236.58. In 48.53%, Sb 51.47%. Prepd by melting together stoichiometric amounts of indium and antimony in evacuated ampuls or in zone-refining apparatus: Kleppa, *J. Am. Chem. Soc.* **77,** 897 (1955); Harmon, *J. Electrochem. Soc.* **103,** 128 (1956). *Reviews:* Welker, Weiss in *Solid State Physics* vol. 3 (Academic Press, New York, 1956); Minden, *Sylvania Technol.* **11,** no. 1, 13-25 (Jan. 1958); Hulme, Mullin, *Solid State Electron.* **5** (Pergamon Press, 1962) 211-247.

Crystals (zinc blende structure). mp 535°. d at mp 5.74 (solid); 6.48 (liq). Dielectric constant = 15.9. Energy gap at 25° = 0.18 ev. Hole mobility 1250 cm^2/volt-sec. Electron mobility approx 80,000 cm^2/volt-sec.

USE: In semiconductor electronics. Grown p-n junctions have been made by doping a melt with an acceptor impurity such as zinc or cadmium, and dipping in an n-type crystal. Rate-grown junctions have also been made. Broad-area surface junctions have been produced by out-diffusing antimony in vacuum from the surface of an n-type crystal, producing a p-n junction just inside the surface. Also has photoconductive, photoelectromagnetic, and magnetoresistive properties. Useful as an infrared detector and filter, and in Hall effect devices.

4949.   Indium Arsenide. [1303-11-3] AsIn; mol wt 189.74. As 39.49%, In 60.51%. InAs. Prepd by fusion of the elements in an evacuated, sealed tube: Gans *et al., Compt. Rend.* **237,** 310 (1953); Talley, Enright, *Phys. Rev.* **94,** 1931 (1954); Harmon *et al., ibid.* **104,** 1562 (1956); Minden, *Sylvania Technol.* **11,** no. 1, 17 (Jan. 1958).

Metallic appearance. Small single crystals have been grown by a modification of the Czochralski technique: Gremmelmaier, *Z. Naturforsch.* **11A,** 463 (1956). mp 943°. Hardly attacked by mineral acids. Energy gap: 0.35 ev. Electron mobility: approx 33,000 cm^2/volt-sec. Hole mobility: 460 cm^2/volt-sec. Dielectric constant 11.7.

USE: In semiconductor electronics.

4950.   Indium Gallium Aluminum Phosphide. [108424-49-3]; [108730-13-8]. InGaAlP. Crystal lattice matched to GaAs substrates for production of visible (670-690 nm) light lasers. Conforms to the general formula In$_{0.5}$(Ga$_{(1-x)}$Al$_x$)$_{0.5}$P. Prepn by molecular beam epitaxy: H. Asahi *et al., J. Appl. Phys.* **53,** 4928 (1982); M. J. Hafich *et al., J. Vac. Sci. Technol. B* **10,** 969 (1992).

Refractive indices: H. Tanaka *et al., J. Appl. Phys.* **59,** 985 (1986). Photoluminescence studies: S. Naritsuka *et al., J. Electron. Mater.* **20,** 687 (1991). Schottky barrier energy: A. Nanda *et al., Appl. Phys. Lett.* **61,** 81 (1992). Thermal analysis: G. Hatakoshi *et al., Trans. Inst. Electron. Inf. Commun. Eng.* **E71,** 315 (1988); K. Itaya *et al., IEEE J. Quantum Electron.* **29,** 2068 (1993). Use in lasers: G. Hatakoshi *et al., Jpn. J. Appl. Phys.* **31,** 501 (1992); J. Rennie *et al., IEEE J. Quantum Electron.* **29,** 1857 (1993).

USE: Laser diode arrays for high-density optical systems and information processing systems such as barcode readers.

4951.   Indium Nitride. [25617-98-5] Indium mononitride. InN; mol wt 128.82. In 89.13%, N 10.87%. Semiconductor material. Prepn and structure determn: R. Juza, H. Hahn, *Z. Anorg. Allg. Chem.* **239,** 282 (1938). Low-temperature organometallic chemical vapor deposition: R. A. Fischer *et al., Chem. Mater.* **8,** 1356 (1996). Prepn and characterization of nanocrystalline forms: J. Xiao *et al., Inorg. Chem.* **42,** 107 (2003). Physical properties of films: G. V. Samsonov, A. F. Andreeva, *Sci. Sintering* **12,** 155 (1980). Thermal properties: S. Krukowski *et al., J. Phys. Chem. Solids* **59,** 289 (1998). Optical and electronic properties: V. V. Sobolev, M. A. Zlobina, *Semiconductors* **33,** 385 (1999).

Usually crystallizes as a hexagonal wurtzite lattice. T_{dec} 427-550°. mp ~1900°. Bandgap = 1.89 eV. n (4.80 eV) = 2.78. d 6.78±0.05.

USE: In manuf of optoelectronic devices such as light-emitting diodes, laser diodes, and solar cells.

4952.   Indium Oxide. [1312-43-2] Indium sesquioxide. In$_2$O$_3$; mol wt 277.63. In 82.71%, O 17.29%.

White to pale-yellow powder. d 7.18. Volatilizes at 850°. Insol in water. Sol in hot mineral acids.

USE: In glass manufacture.

4953.   Indium Phosphide. [22398-80-7] InP; mol wt 145.79. In 78.76%, P 21.25%. Prepd from white phosphorus and indium iodide at 400°: Thiel, Koelsch, *Z. Anorg. Chem.* **66,** 319 (1910); from phosphorus vapor and heated indium metal: Jandelli, *Gazz. Chim. Ital.* **71,** 58 (1941). Synthesis in zone melting furnace at 1010° from a non-stoichiometric melt: Minden, *Sylvania Technol.* **11,** no. 1, 18 (Jan. 1958).

Brittle mass with metallic appearance, not easily attacked by mineral acids. mp 1070°. Dielectric constant: 10.8. Energy gap: 1.3 ev at 25°. Electron mobility: approx 4600 cm^2/volt-sec. Hole mobility: approx 150 cm^2/volt-sec. Solid solns of InP can cover the energy gap continuously from 0.3 to 1.3 ev. Rectification has been observed in InP although it is more characteristic of a Schottky type barrier than the minority carrier injection phenomenon observed in germanium.

USE: In electronics for research on semiconductors.

4954.   Indium Selenide. [1312-42-1] InSe; mol wt 193.78. In 59.25%, Se 40.75%. Prepd from the elements: Klemm *et al., Z. Anorg. Allg. Chem.* **219,** 45 (1934); Schubert *et al., Naturwissenschaften* **41,** 448 (1954).

Black crystals, rhombohedric structure, mp 660°.

USE: In semiconductor research.

4955.   Indium Sulfate. [13464-82-9] In$_2$O$_{12}$S$_3$; mol wt 517.82. In 44.35%, O 37.08%, S 18.58%. In$_2$(SO$_4$)$_3$.

White, hygroscopic powder. d 3.44. Sol in water. *Keep well closed.* MLD in rabbits: 1.8 g/kg orally; 0.67 mg/kg i.v., McCord *et al., J. Ind. Hyg. Toxicol.* **24,** 243 (1942).

4956.   Indium Telluride. [1312-45-4] In$_2$Te$_3$; mol wt 612.44. In 37.50%, Te 62.50%. Prepn of black brittle crystals by double furnace technique: Inuzuka, Sugaike, *Proc. Jpn. Acad.* **30,** 383 (1954), *C.A.* **49,** 2922e (1955).

Pycnometric d 5.78; x-ray d 5.798. mp 667°: Klemm, Ulrich, *Z. Anorg. Allg. Chem.* **219,** 45 (1934), *C.A.* **29,** 1730 (1935). Activation energies: 0.94 ev at 300-600 K, 2.4 ev at 600-900 K.

USE: In semiconductor research.

4957.   Indium Tribromide. [13465-09-3] Indium bromide (InBr$_3$). Br$_3$In; mol wt 354.53. Br 67.61%, In 32.39%. InBr$_3$. Water-stable, green Lewis acid catalyst. Prepn: G. P. Baxter, C. M. Alter, *J. Am. Chem. Soc.* **55,** 1943 (1933). Hydrolysis constants: T. Moeller, *ibid.* **64,** 953 (1942). Raman spectroscopy of aqueous solns: M. A. Marques *et al., J. Chem. Soc. Faraday Trans.* **86**, 3883 (1990). Chemical bonding analysis of binary indium bromides: R. Dronskowski, *Inorg. Chem.* **33**, 6201 (1994). Catalytic applications in organic synthesis: J. S. Yadav, B. V. S. Reddy, *Synthesis* **2002**, 511; *eidem et al., Synlett* **2003**, 396; C. Peppe *et al., ibid.* **2004**, 1723; L. Yin *et al., ibid.* 1727; Z.-H. Zhang *et al., Adv. Synth. Catal.* **348**, 184 (2006). Review of synthetic applications: Z.-H. Zhang, *Synlett* **2005**, 711-712.

White crystalline solid.

USE: Regio-, chemo-, and stereoselective Lewis acid catalyst in organic synthesis.

4958. Indium Trichloride. [10025-82-8] Indium chloride. Cl_3In; mol wt 221.18. Cl 48.09%, In 51.91%. $InCl_3$.

Yellowish, deliquesc crystals. d 4.0. mp 586°; sublimes at 500°. Freely sol in water. *Keep tightly closed.* MLD s.c. in rats: 10.2 mg/kg; MLD i.v. in rabbits: 0.64 mg/kg, McCord *et al., J. Ind. Hyg. Toxicol.* **24**, 243 (1942).

USE: In electroplating using a soln of the salt with dextrose and NaCN. This soln is stable, though it turns dark on standing and deposits a mud which, however, contains no indium.

4959. Indium Trifluoride. [7783-52-0] Indium fluoride; indic fluoride. F_3In; mol wt 171.81. F 33.17%, In 66.83%. InF_3. Prepd by heating In_2O_3 or $(NH_4)_3InF_6$ in a current of fluorine: Hannebohn, Klemm, *Z. Anorg. Allg. Chem.* **229**, 342 (1936); Ensslin, Dreyer, *ibid.* **249**, 119 (1942); Kwasnik in *Handbook of Preparative Inorganic Chemistry* **vol. 1**, G. Brauer, Ed. (Academic Press, New York, 2nd ed., 1963) pp 228-229; from In and HF: Brewer *et al., J. Inorg. Nucl. Chem.* **9**, 56 (1959); Muetterties, Castle, *ibid.* **18**, 148 (1961).

Colorless substance, d 4.39. mp 1170°. bp >1200°. Soly in water (25°) 0.040 g/100 ml. Freely sol in dil acids. Stable in hot and cold water.

Trihydrate. Crystals. Soly in water (22°) 8.49 g/100 ml, indicating a complex.

4960. Indo-1. [96314-96-4] 2-[4-[Bis(carboxymethyl)amino]-3-[2-[2-[bis(carboxymethyl)amino]-5-methylphenoxy]ethoxy]phenyl]-1*H*-indole-6-carboxylic acid; 1-[2-amino-5-(6-carboxyindol-2-yl)phenoxy]-2-(2′-amino-5-methylphenoxy)ethane-*N,N,N′,N′*-tetraacetic acid. $C_{32}H_{31}N_3O_{12}$; mol wt 649.60. C 59.17%, H 4.81%, N 6.47% O 29.56%. Fluorescent calcium imaging agent; structurally related to BAPTA, *q.v.* Ca^{2+} binding causes a spectral shift to shorter wavelengths; ratio of the fluorescence at each wavelength is related to changes in Ca^{2+} binding and independent of dye concentration. Synthesis and characterization: G. Grynkiewicz *et al., J. Biol. Chem.* **260**, 3440 (1985). Acid-base and calcium binding properties: F. Bancel *et al., J. Photochem. Photobiol. A* **53**, 397 (1990); spectral properties: H. Szmacinski *et al., Biophys. J.* **70**, 547 (1996). Practical aspects of use in intracellular measurements: K. R. Sipido, G. Callewaert, *Cardiovasc. Res.* **29**, 717 (1995). Detection of other metal cations: G. A. Peeters *et al., Am. J. Physiol.* **256**, C351 (1989); J. R. Jefferson *et al., Anal. Biochem.* **187**, 328 (1990). Review of use in plant cells: D. S. Bush, R. L. Jones, *Plant Physiol.* **93**, 841-845 (1990).

uv max absorption (100mM KCl): 349 nm free dye; 331 nm Ca^{2+} complex; emission maxima: 485 nm free dye; 410 nm Ca^{2+} complex. pKa_1: 6.2; pKa_2: 4.35.

USE: Fluorescent probe primarily for measuring calcium in biological systems.

4961. Indobufen. [63610-08-2] 4-(1,3-Dihydro-1-oxo-2*H*-isoindol-2-yl)-α-ethylbenzeneacetic acid; (±)-2-[*p*-(1-oxo-2-isoindolinyl)phenyl]butyric acid; 1-oxo-2-[*p*-[(α-ethyl)carboxymethyl]phenyl]isoindoline; 2-[4-(1-carboxypropyl)phenyl]-1-isoindolinone; K-3920; Ibustrin. $C_{18}H_{17}NO_3$; mol wt 295.33. C 73.20%, H 5.80%, N 4.74%, O 16.25%. Platelet aggregation inhibitor. Prepn: R. W. J. Carney, G. de Stevens, **DE 2034240** (1971 to Ciba), *C.A.* **74**, 12547p (1971); P. N. Giraldi *et al.*, **DE 2154525**; *eidem*, **US 4118504** (1972, 1978 both to Carlo Erba); G. Nannini *et al., Arzneim.-Forsch.* **23**, 1090 (1973). Pharmacology: M. Bergameaschi *et al., Pharmacol. Res. Commun.* **16**, 979 (1984). HPLC determn in plasma: E. Wahlin-Boll *et al., Eur. J. Clin. Pharmacol.* **20**, 375 (1981). Review of clinical pharmacokinetics and efficacy in vascular disease: L. R. Wiseman *et al., Drugs* **44**, 445-464 (1992); in atherothrombosis: N. Bhana, K. J. McClellan, *Drugs Aging* **18**, 369-388 (2001).

Crystals from ethanol, mp 182-184°.

THERAP CAT: Antithrombotic.

4962. Indocyanine Green. [3599-32-4] 2-[7-[1,3-Dihydro-1,1-dimethyl-3-(4-sulfobutyl)-2*H*-benz[*e*]indol-2-ylidene]-1,3,5-heptatrienyl]-1,1-dimethyl-3-(4-sulfobutyl)-1*H*-benz[*e*]indolium inner salt, sodium salt; anhydro-3,3,3′,3′-tetramethyl-1,1′-bis(4-sulfobutyl)-4,5,4′,5′-dibenzoindotricarbocyanine hydroxide inner salt sodium salt; Fox green; Cardio-Green. $C_{43}H_{47}N_2NaO_6S_2$; mol wt 774.96. C 66.64%, H 6.11%, N 3.61%, Na 2.97%, O 12.39%, S 8.28%. Prepn: Heseltine, Brooker, **US 2895955** (1959 to Kodak).

A tricarbocyanine type of dye with infrared absorbing properties; peak absorption at about 800 nm. Has little or no absorption in the visible. Commercial product contains moisture and about 5% sodium iodide as contaminant.

USE: In infrared photography; in prepn of Wratten filters.

THERAP CAT: Diagnostic aid (blood volume determination, cardiac output, hepatic function).

4963. Indole. [120-72-9] 2,3-Benzopyrrole. C_8H_7N; mol wt 117.15. C 82.02%, H 6.02%, N 11.96%. Obtained from the 240-260° fraction from coal tar: Weissgerber, *Ber.* **43**, 3520 (1910); from feces: Bergeim, *J. Biol. Chem.* **32**, 17 (1917). Prepn from *o*-formotoluide: Tyson, *Org. Synth.* **coll. vol. III**, 479 (1955); by dehydrocyclizing ortho alkyl anilines: Erner *et al.*, **US 2953575** (1960 to Houdry Process); from *N*-(2-tolyl)-*N*′-methyl-*N*′-phenylformamidine: Lorenz *et al., J. Org. Chem.* **30**, 2531 (1965). Toxicity data: Smyth *et al., Am. Ind. Hyg. Assoc. J.* **23**, 95 (1962). Comprehensive review: Van Order, Lindwall, *Chem. Rev.* **30**, 69 (1942); D. W. Bannister in *Kirk-Othmer Encyclopedia of Chemical Technology* **vol. 13** (Wiley-Interscience, New York, 3rd ed., 1981) pp 213-222.

Leaflets, mp 52°. bp$_{762}$ 253°; bp$_{28}$ 128-133°. Intense fecal odor. Volatile with steam. Soluble in hot water, hot alcohol, ether, benzene. LD$_{50}$ orally in rats: 1 g/kg (Smyth).

USE: In highly dil solns the odor is pleasant, hence indole has been used in perfumery.

4964. Indoleacetic Acid. [87-51-4] 1H-Indole-3-acetic acid; heteroauxin; IAA. C$_{10}$H$_9$NO$_2$; mol wt 175.18. C 68.56%, H 5.18%, N 8.00%, O 18.27%. Plant hormone; recognized as the principal auxin of higher plants. Prepd by the reaction of indole with potassium glycolate at 250°: Johnson, Crosby, *J. Org. Chem.* **28**, 1246 (1963). From indole and chloroacetic acid: Shagalov *et al.*, **US 3320281** (1967). *Reviews:* Leopold in *The Hormones* vol. IV, G. Pincus *et al.*, Eds. (Academic Press, New York, 1964) pp 1-66; Thimann in *The Physiology of Plant Growth and Development*, M. B. Wilkins, Ed. (McGraw-Hill, New York, 1969) pp 1-45.

Leaflets or cryst powder from water, mp 168-170°. pK 4.75. Sparingly sol in water or chloroform; freely sol in alc; sol in acetone, ether.

USE: Plant growth regulator.

4965. Indolebutyric Acid. [133-32-4] 1H-Indole-3-butanoic acid; indole-3-butyric acid; 4-(3-indolyl)butyric acid; Seradix. C$_{12}$H$_{13}$NO$_2$; mol wt 203.24. C 70.92%, H 6.45%, N 6.89%, O 15.74%. Prepn: Jackson, Manske, *J. Am. Chem. Soc.* **52**, 5029 (1930); by heating indole, γ-butyrolactone, and sodium hydroxide, followed by acidification of the product: Fritz, **US 3051723** (1962 to Union Carbide); by decarboxylation of 2-carboxyindole-3-butyric acid: Bowman, Islip, *Chem. Ind. (London)* **1971**, 154. Toxicity studies: Anderson *et al.*, *Proc. Soc. Exp. Biol. Med.* **34**, 138 (1936); Pesonen, *Acta Endocrinol.* **5**, 409 (1950). Hypoglycemic effect in rats: Mirsky *et al.*, *Endocrinology* **59**, 715 (1956).

White or slightly yellow crystals. Slight characteristic odor. mp 123-125°. Practically insol in water, chloroform. Sol in alc, ether, acetone. LD$_{50}$ i.p. in mice: 100 mg/kg (Anderson).

USE: To stimulate root formation of plant clippings.

4966. Indolmycin. [21200-24-8] (5S)-5-[(1R)-1-(1H-Indol-3-yl)ethyl]-2-(methylamino)-4(5H)-oxazolone; (1R,5S)-5-(1-indol-3-ylethyl)-2-(methylamino)-2-oxazolin-4-one; 2-methylamino-5α-(β-indolyl)ethyl-2-oxazolin-4-one; PA-155A. C$_{14}$H$_{15}$N$_3$O$_2$; mol wt 257.29. C 65.35%, H 5.88%, N 16.33%, O 12.44%. Antibiotic substance produced by *Streptomyces albus*: Rao, *Antibiot. Chemother.* **10**, 312 (1960); Marsh *et al., ibid.* 316; **GB 862685** (1961 to Pfizer). Structure: M. Schach von Wittenau, H. Els, *J. Am. Chem. Soc.* **83**, 4678 (1961). Total synthesis: *eidem, ibid.* **85**, 3425 (1963); Preobrazhenskaya *et al., Tetrahedron* **24**, 6131 (1968); T. Takeda, T. Mukaiyama, *Chem. Lett.* **1980**, 163. Abs config: T. H. Chan, R. K. Hill, *J. Org. Chem.* **35**, 3519 (1970). Biosynthetic studies: Hornemann *et al., Chem. Commun.* **1969**, 245; *eidem, J. Am. Chem. Soc.* **93**, 3028 (1971).

Long rectangular prisms from methanol or ethyl acetate, mp 209-210°. [α]$_D^{25}$ −214° (c = 2 in methanol). uv max: 218 nm (E$_{1cm}^{1\%}$ 1960). Weakly basic, stable to heat. Slightly sol in water, benzene, ether; moderately in lower alcohols, acetone.

4967. 3-Indolylacetone. [1201-26-9] Indol-3-yl-2-propanone. C$_{11}$H$_{11}$NO; mol wt 173.21. C 76.28%, H 6.40%, N 8.09%, O 9.24%. Prepn: Brown *et al., J. Chem. Soc.* **1952**, 3172; Williamson, *ibid.* **1962**, 2834; Morris *et al.*, **GB 974895** (1964 to Parke, Davis).

Brownish rhombs from benzene or needles from aq methanol. mp 115-117.5°. uv max (ethanol): 221, 280, 289 nm (ε 35100, 6400, 5300).

4968. Indomethacin. [53-86-1] 1-(4-Chlorobenzoyl)-5-methoxy-2-methyl-1H-indole-3-acetic acid; 1-(p-chlorobenzoyl)-5-methoxy-2-methyl-3-indolylacetic acid; indometacin; Bonidon; Catlep; Chrono-Indocid; Confortid; Dolcidium; Elmetacin; Idomethine; Inacid; Indacin; Indocid; Indocin; Indomed; Indomee; Indomod; Indoptic; Indoptol; Indoxen; Inflazon; Inteban; Mikametan; Rheumacin LA; Serastar; Vonum. C$_{19}$H$_{16}$ClNO$_4$; mol wt 357.79. C 63.78%, H 4.51%, Cl 9.91%, N 3.91%, O 17.89%. Nonsteroidal anti-inflammatory agent (NSAID); inhibits prostaglandin synthesis. Prepn: T. Y. Shen *et al., J. Am. Chem. Soc.* **85**, 488 (1963); T. Y. Shen, **US 3161654** (1964 to Merck & Co.). Alternate process: **BE 679678** (1966 to Sumitomo). Anti-inflammatory and antipyretic activity: C. A. Winter *et al., J. Pharmacol. Exp. Ther.* **141**, 369 (1963). Metabolic studies: D. W. Yesair *et al., Biochem. Pharmacol.* **19**, 1579 (1970). Toxicity: C. D. Klaassen, *Toxicol. Appl. Pharmacol.* **38**, 127 (1976). Review of discovery, pharmacology and mechanism of action: T. Y. Shen, C. A. Winter in *Advances in Drug Research* vol. **12**, A. B. Simmons, Ed. (Academic Press, New York, 1977) pp 89-245; of clinical trials in osteoarthritis: W. M. O'Brien, *Clin. Pharmacol. Ther.* **9**, 94-107 (1968); of role in ductus closure: S. M. Douidar *et al., Dev. Pharmacol. Ther.* **11**, 196-212 (1988).

Crystals exhibiting polymorphism, mp for one form ~155°, for the other ~162°. uv max (ethanol): 230, 260, 319 nm (ε 20800, 16200, 6290). pKa 4.5. Sol in ethanol, ether, acetone, castor oil. Practically insol in water. Stable in neutral or slightly acidic media; dec by strong alkali. LD$_{50}$ i.p. in rats: 13 mg/kg (Klaassen).

Sodium salt trihydrate. [74252-25-8] Indocin I.V.; Indocid PDA. C$_{19}$H$_{15}$ClNNaO$_4$.3H$_2$O. Pale yellow crystalline powder. pH of 1% soln: 8.4. Very sol in methanol; sol in water, ethanol. Very slightly sol in chloroform, acetone.

Meglumine salt. Liometacen.

THERAP CAT: Anti-inflammatory; analgesic. For closure of patent ductus arteriosus in preterm infants.

4969. Indoramin. [26844-12-2] N-[1-[2-(1H-Indol-3-yl)ethyl]-4-piperidinyl]benzamide; 3-[2-(4-benzamidopiperidino)ethyl]indole; Wy-21901. C$_{22}$H$_{25}$N$_3$O; mol wt 347.45. C 76.05%, H 7.25%, N 12.09%, O 4.60%. α$_1$-Adrenergic blocking agent with antihypertensive and bronchodilating activity. Prepn: J. L. Archibald, J. L. Jackson, **ZA 6803204**; *eidem,* **US 3527761** (1969, 1970 both to Wyeth); J. L. Archibald *et al., J. Med. Chem.* **14**, 1054 (1971). Pharmacological study: R. B. Royds *et al., Clin. Pharmacol. Ther.* **13**, 380 (1972). Pharmacokinetics: G. H. Draffan *et al., Br. J. Clin. Pharmacol.* **3**, 489 (1976). Antihypertensive activity: G. S. Stokes *et al., Clin. Pharmacol. Ther.* **25**, 783 (1979). Cardiovascular effects in man: A. J. Coleman *et al., J. Int. Med. Res.* **7**, 511 (1979). Effects on respiration in guinea pigs: C. Hamer, D. M. Temple, *Agents Actions* **10**, 399 (1980). Determn of therapeutic concentrations: A. J. Swaisland, *Analyst* **106**, 717 (1981). Symposium on pharmacology and clinical studies: *Br. J. Clin. Pharmacol.* **12**, Suppl. 1, 1S-140S (1981). Review of pharmacology, therapeutic efficacy: B. Holmes, E. M. Sorkin, *Drugs* **31**, 467-499 (1986).

Crystals from ethanol, mp 208-210°.

Hydrochloride. [38821-52-2] Baratol; Doralese; Vidora; Wydora; Wypresin. $C_{22}H_{25}N_3O.HCl$; mol wt 383.91. Crystals, mp 230-232°. Recryst from isopropanol gives different cryst modification, mp 258-260°.

THERAP CAT: Antihypertensive.

4970. Indospicine. [16377-00-7] (2*S*)-2,7-Diamino-7-iminoheptanoic acid; L-6-amidinonorleucine; L-2-amino-6-amidinohexanoic acid; L-α-amino-ε-amidinocaproic acid. $C_7H_{15}N_3O_2$; mol wt 173.21. C 48.54%, H 8.73%, N 24.26%, O 18.47%. H_2-NC=NH(CH$_2$)$_4$CH(NH$_2$)COOH. Teratogenic and hepatotoxic factor found in extracts of *Indigofera spicata* Forsk (*Indogofera endecaphylla* Jacq.), *Leguminosae*. Isoln: Hegarty, Pound, *Nature* **217**, 354 (1968). Isoln, structure and biological studies: *eidem, Aust. J. Biol. Sci.* **23**, 831 (1970). Total synthesis: Culvenor *et al., Aust. J. Chem.* **24**, 371 (1971). *Review:* Hegarty: *Australas. J. Dermatol.* **14**, 35-38 (1973).

Monohydrochloride monohydrate. $C_7H_{15}N_3O_2.HCl.H_2O$. Needle-like crystals from aq ethanol, mp 131-134°. $[\alpha]_D^{22}$ +18° (c = 1.1 in 5*N* HCl).

4971. Indoxacarb. [173584-44-6] (4a*S*)-7-Chloro-2,5-dihydro-2-[[(methoxycarbonyl)[4-(trifluoromethoxy)phenyl]amino]-carbonyl]indeno[1,2-*e*][1,3,4]oxadiazine-4a(3*H*)-carboxylic acid methyl ester; DPX-KN128; Steward. $C_{22}H_{17}ClF_3N_3O_7$; mol wt 527.83. C 50.06%, H 3.25%, Cl 6.72%, F 10.80%, N 7.96%, O 21.22%. Oxadiazine pro-insecide; bioactivated in lepidoptera to the decarbomethoxylated metabolite that inhibits neuronal sodium channels. Prepn: G. D. Annis *et al.,* **WO 9211249** (1992 to DuPont); *eidem,* **US 5462938** (1995). Physical properties and field trials: H. H. Harder *et al., Brighton Crop Prot. Conf. - Pests Dis.* **1996**, 449. Efficacy of *DPX-MP062*, a 3:1 mixture of active (*S*)- to inactive (*R*)-isomer: U. Pluschkell *et al., Pestic. Sci.* **54**, 85 (1998). Metabolism and mode of action: K. D. Wing *et al., Arch. Insect Biochem. Physiol.* **37**, 91 (1998).

(*RS*)-Form. [144171-61-9] DPX-JW062. mp 140-141°. Partition coefficient (octanol/water): ~40000. Vapor pressure (20-25°): <10^{-5} Pa. Soly (mg/l): water <0.5; 1-octanol 480; methanol 390; acetonitrile 76000; acetone 140000. LD_{50} orally in rat: >5000 mg/kg; dermally in rabbit: >2000 mg/kg; LC_{50} in rat by inhalation: >2 mg/l; LC_{50} (96 hr) in bluegill sunfish, rainbow trout: >1.0, >0.5 mg/l (Harder).

USE: Insecticide.

4972. Infliximab. [170277-31-3] Anti-(human tumor necrosis factor) immunoglobulin G (human-mouse monoclonal cA2 heavy chain) disulfide with human-mouse monoclonal cA2 light chain, dimer; chimeric A2 antibody; cA2; Remicade. Chimeric monoclonal antibody that binds and neutralizes soluble and transmembrane tumor necrosis factor α (TNFα). Consists of constant

regions of human (Hu)IgG1κ coupled to Fv region of a high-affinity neutralizing murine anti-HuTNFα antibody (A2). Prepn: J. Le *et al.,* **WO 9216553** (1992 to New York Univ.; Centocor); D. M. Knight *et al., Mol. Immunol.* **30**, 1443 (1993). Pharmacology: S. A. Siegel *et al., Cytokine* **7**, 15 (1995). Mechanism of action: B. J. Scallon *et al., ibid.* 251. Clinical study in rheumatoid arthritis: R. Maini *et al., Lancet* **354**, 1932 (1999); in psoriasis: U. Chaudhari *et al., ibid.* **357**, 1842 (2001); in Crohn's disease: B. E. Sands *et al., N. Engl. J. Med.* **350**, 876 (2004). Review of use in early rheumatoid arthritis: R. C. Geletka, E. W. St. Clair, *Expert Opin. Biol. Ther.* **5**, 405-417 (2005); of use in Crohn's disease: M. Bewtra, G. R. Lichtenstein, *ibid.,* 589-599 (2005).

THERAP CAT: Anti-inflammatory.

4973. Infusorial Earth. Siliceous earth; diatomaceous earth; fossil flour; kieselguhr; Celite; Super-Cel. Siliceous frustules and fragments of various species of diatoms. *See also* Silicon Dioxide.

White to light gray to pale buff powder. Insol in water, acids, or dil alkalies. Capable of taking up and holding about four times its wt of water.

USE: Clarifying agent. Largely used as an absorbent for liquids and for dispensing fluid extracts in powder form; also in cataplasms and as constituent of and excipient for pill masses. Clarifying oils, varnishes; filtering liquids; manuf heat insulators, fire brick, and fire- and acid-proof packing materials; filler for paper, paints; adsorbent dynamite; in metal polishes, dentifrices, nail polishes; in chromatography.

4974. Inhibins. Gonadal polypeptide hormones produced by Sertoli cells in males and granulosa cells in females, which selectively inhibits the secretion of FSH, *q.v.* Dimer, mol wt 32,000 Da, isolated in two isoforms, inhibin A and inhibin B, which have the same α subunit linked to similar but distinct β subunits. Dimers of the β subunits have been isolated which stimulate the secretion of FSH, *see* activins. Name "inhibin" coined upon identification as a water-soluble, testicular factor with pituitary inhibitory activity: D. R. McCullagh, *Science* **76**, 19 (1932). Specific inhibition of FSH: H. F. Klinefelter *et al., J. Clin. Endocrinol.* **2**, 615 (1942); B. P. Setchell, F. Jacks, *J. Endocrinol.* **62**, 675 (1974). Identification in ovarian follicular fluid: F. H. de Jong, R. M. Sharpe, *Nature* **263**, 71 (1976); N. B. Schwartz, C. P. Channing, *Proc. Natl. Acad. Sci. USA* **74**, 5721 (1977). Localization of production to Sertoli cells: A. Steinberger, E. Steinberger, *Endocrinology* **99**, 918 (1976); to granulosa cells: G. F. Erickson, A. J. W. Hsueh, *ibid.* **103**, 1960 (1978). Immunohistochemical confirmation of production sites: P. Cuevas *et al., Biochem. Biophys. Res. Commun.* **142**, 23 (1987). Identification of inhibin-like proteins from human seminal plasma: N. G. Seidah *et al., FEBS Lett.* **175**, 349 (1984); C. H. Li *et al., Proc. Natl. Acad. Sci. USA* **82**, 4041 (1985). Isolation of inhibins and higher mol wt precursors: K. Miyamoto *et al., Biochem. Biophys. Res. Commun.* **129**, 396 (1985). Purification and characterization of inhibins A and B: J. Rivier *et al., ibid.* **133**, 120 (1985); N. Ling *et al., Proc. Natl. Acad. Sci. USA* **82**, 7217 (1985). Each subunit is synthesized as a larger precursor molecule, then processed to the mature form. Complete amino acid sequence of mature form α, β_A and β_B subunits: A. J. Mason *et al., Nature* **318**, 659 (1985); A. J. Mason *et al., Biochem. Biophys. Res. Commun.* **135**, 957 (1986). Demonstration of negative feedback mechanism between secretion of FSH and inhibin: S.-Y. Ying *et al., Proc. Natl. Acad. Sci. USA* **84**, 4631 (1987). Proposed nomenclature: H. G. Burger, *J. Endocrinol.* **117**, 159 (1988). Approach to nonradiometric assays: R. Schwall *et al., Prog. Clin. Biol. Res.* **285**, 205 (1988). Review of early bioassays: B. Hudson *et al., J. Reprod. Fertil. Suppl.* **26**, 17-29 (1979). Reviews of purification and physiology: C. P. Channing *et al., Proc. Soc. Exp. Biol. Med.* **178**, 339-361 (1985); F. H. de Jong, D. M. Robertson, *Mol. Cell. Endocrinol.* **42**, 95-103 (1985). Review of possible use as contraceptive: A. R. Sheth, S. B. Moodbidri, *Adv. Contracept.* **2**, 131-139 (1986); P. Franchimont, *Male Contraception: Advances and Future Prospects,* G. I. Zatuchni *et al.,* Eds. (Harper & Row, Philadelphia, 1986) pp 408-418. *Reviews:* F. H. de Jong, *Oxford Rev. Reprod. Biol.* **9**, 1-53 (1987); N. Ling *et al., Vitam. Horm.* (New York) **44**, 1-46 (1988).

4975. Inosine. [58-63-9] Hypoxanthine riboside; 9-β-D-ribofuranosylhypoxanthine; hypoxanthosine; Inosie; Oxiamine; Ribonosine; Trophicardyl. $C_{10}H_{12}N_4O_5$; mol wt 268.23. C 44.78%,

H 4.51%, N 20.89%, O 29.82%. In meat and meat extracts, in sugar beets. Prepd from adenosine by incubation with purified adenosine deaminase from intestine: Kalckar, *J. Biol. Chem.* **167**, 445 (1947); also by the action of sodium nitrite and acetic acid on adenosine: Levene, Jacobs, *Ber.* **43**, 3161 (1910); by the use of barium nitrite and H_2SO_4: Reiff *et al.,* **US 3049536** (1962 to Zellstoff-Fabrik Waldhof). Fermentation method: Motozaki *et al.,* **US 3111459** (1963 to Ajinomoto). Structure: Bredereck, *Ber.* **66**, 198 (1933); *Z. Physiol. Chem.* **223**, 61 (1934); Gulland, Holiday, *J. Chem. Soc.* **1936**, 765.

Dihydrate. Long rectangular plates from water, mp 90°. Anhydrous needles from 80% alc, dec 218° (rapid heating). $[\alpha]_D^{18}$ −49.2° (c = 0.9 in H_2O). $[\alpha]_{white}^{20}$ −73° (0.5 g + 2 ml *N* NaOH + 3 ml H_2O). 100 ml of the satd water soln at 20° contain 1.6 g inosine. Absorption spectrum: Kalckar, *loc. cit.* uv max (pH 6.0): 248.5 nm (ε 12200). Boiling with 0.1*N* H_2SO_4 yields hypoxanthin and D-ribose.

THERAP CAT: Activates cellular functions.

4976. Inosine Pranobex. [36703-88-5] Inosine mono[4-(acetylamino)benzoate] (salt) compd with 1-(dimethylamino)-2-propanol (1:3); inosine:dimethylaminoisopropanol acetamidobenzoate (1:3); inosiplex; methisoprinol; NP-113; NPT-10381; Aviral; Delimmun; Imunoviral; Isoprinosin; Isoprinosina; Isoprinosine; Isoviral; Modimmunal; Pranosina; Pranosine; Viruxan. $C_{52}H_{78}$-$N_{10}O_{17}$; mol wt 1115.23. C 56.00%, H 7.05%, N 12.56%, O 24.39%. Immunostimulant complex formed from the *p*-acetamidobenzoate salt of dimethylaminoisopropanol and inosine in a 3:1 molar ratio. Prepn: P. Gordon, **DE 1965431**; *idem,* **US 3646007** (1971, 1972 both to Newport Pharm.). Antiviral activity: E. R. Brown, P. Gordon, *Can. J. Microbiol.* **18**, 1463 (1972); R. L. Muldoon *et al., Antimicrob. Agents Chemother.* **2**, 224 (1972). Stimulatory effect on T-cell function: L. Binderup, *Int. J. Immunopharmacol.* **7**, 93 (1985). Pharmacology and therapeutic potential: D. M. Campoli-Richards *et al., Drugs* **32**, 383 (1986). Clinical immunopharmacology: A. J. Glasky, J. F. Gordon, *Cancer Detect. Prev. Suppl.* **1**, 597 (1987). Clinical trial in subacute sclerosing panencephalitis (SSPE): C. E. Jones *et al., Lancet* **1**, 1034 (1982); G. Gascon *et al., Brain Dev.* **15**, 346 (1993). Clinical trial in pre-AIDS patients: C. Pedersen *et al., N. Engl. J. Med.* **322**, 1757 (1990). Review of efficacy in HIV infection: C. De Simone *et al., Int. J. Immunopharmacol.* **13**, Suppl. 1, 19-27 (1991).

Neutral water-soluble solid. LD_{50} in mice and rats (mg/kg): >4000 orally and i.p. (Gordon).

THERAP CAT: Immunomodulator; antiviral.

4977. Inosinic Acid. [131-99-7] 5′-Inosinic acid; 5-inosinic acid; muscle inosinic acid; t-inosinic acid; hypoxanthine riboside-5-phosphoric acid; IMP. $C_{10}H_{13}N_4O_8P$; mol wt 348.21. C 34.49%, H 3.76%, N 16.09%, O 36.76%, P 8.90%. Prepn from meat extract: Levene, Bass, *Nucleic Acids* (New York, 1931) p 229; from dried sardines: Yoshida, Kageyama, **JP 56 732** (1956 to Ajinomoto), *C.A.* **51**, 3870b (1957). Structure: Levene, Bass, *op. cit.,* pp 187-192; Bredereck, *Ber.* **66**, 198 (1933); Levene, Tipson, *J. Biol. Chem.* **111**, 313 (1935). Also prepd from muscle by enzymatic deamina-

tion of muscle adenylic acid: Ostern, *Biochem. Z.* **254**, 65 (1932); by hydrolysis of inosine triphosphate: Kleinzeller, *Biochem. J.* **36**, 729 (1942). Studies on the enzymatic synthesis: Greenberg, *J. Biol. Chem.* **190**, 611 (1951); Korn *et al., ibid.* **217**, 875 (1955). Microbial fermentation method using mutant strains of *Micrococcus glutamicus:* Kinoshita *et al.,* **US 3232844** (1966 to Kyowa).

Syrup, solidifies to a glass when dried over H_2SO_4. Agreeable sour taste. pK_1 = 2.4; pK_2 = 6.4. Absorption spectrum: Kalckar, *J. Biol. Chem.* **167**, 445 (1947). Freely sol in water, in formic acid; very sparingly sol in alcohol, ether. On boiling with acid hydrolyzes to 1 mol H_3PO_4, 1 mol hypoxanthine, 1 mol D-ribose.

Disodium salt dihydrate. $C_{10}H_{11}N_4Na_2O_8P.2H_2O$. Barely sol in alcohol, ether, acetone; soly in water at 20° about 13 g/100 ml. Kawasaki, *New Food Ind.* **3**, no. 1, 17 (1961).

Barium salt. $C_{10}H_{11}BaN_4O_8P$. Hemipentadecahydrate, lustrous leaflets. Becomes anhyd at 100° *in vacuo.* $[\alpha]_D^{20}$ −18.5° (0.3 g of anhydr Ba salt in 10 ml of 2.5% HCl).

USE: Its salts as flavor intensifiers, like sodium glutamate. Examples of mixtures of sodium inosinate and sodium glutamate or other salts: Toi *et al.,* **US 3109741** (1963 to Ajinomoto).

4978. Inositol. [87-89-8] *myo*-Inositol; *meso*-inositol; *i*-inositol; hexahydroxycyclohexane; cyclohexanehexol; cyclohexitol; meat sugar; inosite; mesoinosite; phaseomannite; dambose; nucite; bios I; rat antispectacled eye factor; mouse antialopecia factor. C_6-$H_{12}O_6$; mol wt 180.16. C 40.00%, H 6.71%, O 53.28%. Widely distributed in plants and animals. Growth factor for animals and microorganisms. Isoln from heart muscle: Scherer, *Ann.* **73**, 322 (1850); from liver: Woolley, *J. Biol. Chem.* **139**, 29 (1941). Synthesis: Wieland, Wishart, *Ber.* **47**, 2082 (1914); Anderson, Wallis, *J. Am. Chem. Soc.* **70**, 2931 (1948). Obtained commercially from corn steep liquor, since inositol is present as phytic acid in corn: Bartow, Walker, *Ind. Eng. Chem.* **30**, 300 (1938); **US 2112553** (1938); Hoglan, Bartow, *J. Am. Chem. Soc.* **62**, 2397 (1940); Elkin, Meadows, **US 2414365** (1947); **GB 601273** (1948 to Corn Prod. Refining). Nine possible stereoisomers: Seven are optically inactive or *meso.* Two optically active forms, the racemic form, and several *cis,trans*-isomers occur naturally. The prevalent natural form is *cis*-1,2,3,5-*trans*-4,6-cyclohexanehexol which is described here. *Reviews:* R. Beckmann, *m-Inosit* (Editio Cantor, Aulendorf, 1953); several authors in *The Vitamins* vol. 2, W. H. Sebrell, Jr., R. S. Harris, Eds. (Academic Press, New York, 1954) pp 321-386; *ibid.* **vol. 3** (2nd ed., 1971) pp 340-415.

Anhydr, non-hygroscopic crystals from water or acetic acid above 80°. Sweet taste. d 1.752. mp 225-227°. Optically inactive. Soly in water at 25°: 14 g/100 ml soln; at 60°: 28 g/100 ml soln. Slightly sol in alc. Practically insol in ether and other common organic solvents. Aq solns are neutral to litmus.

Dihydrate. Efflorescent crystals from water below 50°. d 1.524. mp 218°. Becomes anhyd at 100°.

Monophosphate. [573-35-3] $C_6H_{13}O_9P$. Prepn: Posternak, Posternak, *Helv. Chim. Acta* **12**, 1165 (1929); McCormick, Carter, *Biochem. Prep.* **2**, 65 (1952). Crystals from water + alcohol, dec 195-197°. Titrates as a dibasic acid. Freely soluble in water (1 g dissolves in 3 ml H_2O). Practically insol in abs ethanol, ether. Remarkably resistant to hydrolysis by boiling with strong alkali. May be hydrolyzed by boiling with 6*N* HCl for 14 hrs.

THERAP CAT: Vitamin B complex; lipotropic.

4979. Inositol Niacinate. [6556-11-2] *myo*-Inositol hexa-3-pyridinecarboxylate; hexanicotinoyl inositol; hexanicotinyl *cis*-1,-2,3,5-*trans*-4,6-cyclohexane; inositol hexanicotinate; *meso*-inositol hexanicotinate; Dilcit; Dilexpal; Mesotal; Esantene; Hämovannid; Hexanicit; Hexopal; Linodil; Mesonex; Palohex. $C_{42}H_{30}N_6O_{12}$; mol wt 810.72. C 62.22%, H 3.73%, N 10.37%, O 23.68%. Prepn: Badgett, Woodward, *J. Am. Chem. Soc.* **69**, 2907 (1947).

Crystals, mp 254.3-254.9°. Practically insol in water. Sol in dil acids.

THERAP CAT: Vasodilator (peripheral).

4980. Insulin. [9004-10-8]; [11061-68-0] (human). Polypeptide hormone produced by pancreatic beta cells that regulates carbohydrate homeostasis. Converted by proteolysis from the single chain proinsulin, *q.v.*, to the active dimer composed of 51 amino acid residues; mol wt ~6000. Regulates carbohydrate and lipid metabolism, and influences protein synthesis. Insulin was the first protein for which the chemical structure and mol wt were determined. Also the first commercial health care product produced by recombinant DNA technology. Because of its solubility at physiological pH, insulin is rapidly absorbed after subcutaneous injection. Various complexes with protamine and/or zinc have been prepd to improve drug delivery. In addition to biological source (human, porcine or bovine), insulin formulations for therapeutic use are classified according to onset and duration of action. Isoln: F. G. Banting, C. H. Best, *J. Lab. Clin. Med.* **7**, 251 (1921-22). Crystallization: Abel, *Proc. Natl. Acad. Sci. USA* **12**, 132 (1926). Purification and properties: J. Lens, *Biochim. Biophys. Acta* **2**, 76 (1948). Complete amino acid sequence of bovine insulin: F. Sanger, H. Tuppy, *Biochem. J.* **49**, 463, 481 (1951); F. Sanger, E. O. P. Thompson, *ibid.* **53**, 353, 366 (1953). Identification of 2 chain structure: A. P. Ryle *et al.*, *ibid.* **60**, 541 (1955). Review of structure determination: F. Sanger, *Science* **129**, 1340 (1959). Structure of human insulin: D. Nichol, L. F. Smith, *Nature* **187**, 483 (1960). Crystal structure: D. C. Hodgkin, *Verh. Schweiz. Naturforsch. Ges.* **150**, 93 (1970). Synthesis of human insulin: P. G. Katsoyannis *et al.*, *J. Am. Chem. Soc.* **88**, 164, 166 (1966); by the enzymatic modification of porcine insulin: M. A. Ruttenberg, *Science* **177**, 623 (1972). Review of synthetic insulins: P. G. Katsoyannis, *Recent Prog. Horm. Res.* **23**, 505-563 (1967). Synthesis of human insulin gene: H. M. Hsiung *et al.*, *Nucleic Acids Res.* **6**, 1371 (1979); **7**, 2199 (1979); **8**, 5753 (1980); S. A. Narang *et al.*, *Nucleic Acids Symp. Ser.* **7**, 377 (1980). Review of the development and production of human insulin by recombinant DNA technology: I. S. Johnson, *Science* **219**, 632-637 (1983). Molecular basis of insulin action: M. P. Czech, *Annu. Rev. Biochem.* **46**, 359 (1977). History: M. Bliss, *The Discovery of Insulin* (Univ. Chicago Press, Chicago, 1982) 304 pp. Review of biosynthesis: D. F. Steiner *et al.*, *Recent Prog. Horm. Res.* **25**, 207-282 (1969). Review of the structure and function of the insulin receptor: J. Lee, P. F. Pilch, *Am. J. Physiol.* **266**, C319-C334 (1994). Symposium on the physiological regulation of insulin secretion and the pathogenesis of diabetes: *Diabetologia* **37**, Suppl. 2, S1-S187 (1994). Review of bioactivity, pharmacokinetics and therapeutic efficacy of human insulin: R. N. Brogden, R. C. Heel, *Drugs* **34**, 350-371 (1987). Review of insulin formulations and therapy: J. A. Galloway, R. E. Chance, *Horm. Metab. Res.* **26**, 591-598 (1994); of analogs and

alternative delivery methods: J. E. Gerich, *Am. J. Med.* **113**, 308-316 (2002).

HUMAN INSULIN

Crystals, hexagonal system, usually obtained as flat rhombohedra and contg 0.4% Zn. Readily sol in dil acids and alkalies. Isoelectric point 5.30 to 5.35.

Bovine insulin. [11070-73-8] Hypurin.

Porcine insulin. [12584-58-6] Iletin II; Velosulin. Differs from human insulin by a single amino acid substitution.

Recombinant human insulin. Biosynthetic human insulin; insulin (prb); Huminsulin; Humulin; Humulina. Human insulin prepd by recombinant DNA technology. Clinical evaluation of inhaled intrapulmonary delivery in type 1 diabetes: J. S. Skyler *et al.*, *Lancet* **357**, 331 (2001); in type 2 diabetes: W. T. Cefalu *et al.*, *Ann. Intern. Med.* **134**, 203 (2001).

Semi-synthetic human insulin. Insulin (emp); Biohulin; Novolin; Orgasuline. Human insulin prepd by enzymatic modification of porcine insulin.

Zinc insulin. [8049-62-5] Crystalline prepn of insulin containing 0.45-0.9% zinc. Formulated as suspensions in physiological saline; size of the particles determines the duration of action. Formulations are designated as prompt (or semilente), lente and extended (or ultralente).

Protamine zinc insulin. [9004-17-5] PZI insulin. Suspensions of insulin modified by the addition of zinc chloride and protamine sulfate. White or almost white suspension, pH 7.1-7.4. Onset of action occurs in 4-6 hrs after s.c. injection; duration of action is 36 hrs.

Isophane insulin. NPH insulin; neutral protein Hagedorn insulin. Crystallized prepn of protamine, zinc and insulin. Prepn: H. C. Hagedorn *et al.*, *J. Am. Med. Assoc.* **106**, 177 (1936). *Review:* P. Felig, *ibid.* **251**, 393-396 (1984). White suspensions of rod-shaped crystals ~30 nm in length, pH 7.1-7.4. Onset of action is 3-4 hrs following s.c. injection; duration of action is 18-28 hrs.

Insulin ^{131}I. Radio-iodinated insulin. Prepn: Burrows *et al.*, *J. Clin. Invest.* **36**, 393 (1957); Grodsky *et al.*, *Arch. Biochem. Biophys.* **81**, 264 (1959).

USE: Insulin ^{131}I used in the study of insulin binding factors from insulin resistant sera.

THERAP CAT: Antidiabetic.

4981. Insulinase. [9013-83-6] An enzyme that hydrolyzes insulin and is prepd from hog pancreas: Brink, Lewis, *US 2957809* (1960 to Merck & Co.). May be obtained from commercial pancreatin or trypsin. Even the purified crystals contain large amounts of elastase. *Review:* Thomas, *Postgrad. Med. J. Suppl.* **49**, 940 (1973).

4982. Insulin Aspart. [116094-23-6] 28^B-L-Aspartic acid-insulin (human); AspB28-insulin (human); B28-asp-insulin; INA-X14; Novorapid. Rapid-acting insulin analog produced by recombinant DNA technology. Identical to human insulin except for one amino acid substitution. Prepn: J. Brange *et al.*, *Nature* **333**, 679 (1988). Pharmacology and safety: V. Dall, *Arzneim.-Forsch.* **49**, 463 (1999). Clinical pharmacokinetics and dynamics: S. R. Mudaliar *et al.*, *Diabetes Care* **22**, 1501 (1999). Clinical trial for postprandial glycemic control in type 1 diabetics: P. Raskin *et al.*, *ibid.* **23**, 583 (2000). Review of pharmacology and clinical experience: K. L. Simpson, C. M. Spencer, *Drugs* **57**, 759-765 (1999).

THERAP CAT: Antidiabetic.

4983. Insulin Detemir. [169148-63-4] 29^B-[N^6-(1-Oxo-tetradecyl)-L-lysine](1^A-21^A),(1^B-29^B)-insulin (human); 29^B-(N^6-myristoyl-L-lysine)-30^B-de-L-threonineinsulin (human); Lys^{B29}-tetradecanoyl, des(B30)-insulin; NN-304; Levemir. $C_{267}H_{402}N_{64}$-$O_{76}S_6$; mol wt 5916.82. C 54.20%, H 6.85%, N 15.15%, O 20.55%, S 3.25%. Soluble long-acting basal insulin analog. Prepn: S. Havelund *et al.*, *WO 9507931* (1995 to Novo Nordisk); and albumin binding affinity: P. Kurtzhals *et al.*, *Biochem. J.* **312**, 725 (1995). Clinical pharmacokinetics: T. Danne *et al.*, *Diabetes Care* **26**, 3087 (2003). Pharmacodynamic profile: J. Plank *et al.*, *ibid.* **28**, 1107 (2005). Clinical comparison with NPH insulin in type 1 diabetes: P. Home *et al.*, *ibid.* **27**, 1081 (2004). Review of pharmacology and clinical experience: P. Home, P. Kurtzhals, *Expert Opin. Pharmacother.* **7**, 325-343 (2006).

THERAP CAT: Antidiabetic.

4984. Insulin Glargine. [160337-95-1] 21^A-Glycine-30^Ba-L-arginine-30^Bb-L-arginine-insulin (human); [Gly(A21),Arg(B31),-Arg(B32)]insulin (human); HOE-901; Lantus. Long-acting analog of human insulin produced by recombinant DNA technology. Prepn: M. Dörschug, *DE 3837825*; *idem*, *US 5656722* (1990, 1997 both to Hoechst). Characterization of receptor interaction: L. Berti *et al.*, *Horm. Metab. Res.* **30**, 123 (1998). Clinical pharmacodynamics: L. Heinemann *et al.*, *Diabetes Care* **23**, 644 (2000); pharmacokinetics: D. R. Owens *et al.*, *ibid.* 813. Clinical trial in type 1 diabetics: R. E. Ratner *et al.*, *ibid.* 639. Review of clinical experience: P. S. Gillies *et al.*, *Drugs* **59**, 253-260 (2000).

pI 6.7. Sol in acid pH. Insol at physiological pH.

THERAP CAT: Antidiabetic.

4985. Insulin Glulisine. [207748-29-6] 3^B-L-Lysine-29^B-L-glutamic acid-insulin (human); [Lys(B3),Glu(B29)]-insulin (human); HMR-1964; Apidra. $C_{258}H_{384}N_{64}O_{78}S_6$; mol wt 5822.58. C 53.22%, H 6.65%, N 15.40%, O 21.43%, S 3.30%. Rapid-acting insulin analog produced in *E. coli* by recombinant DNA technology. Identical to human insulin except for 2 amino acid substitutions. Prepn: J. Ertl *et al.*, *EP 885961* (1998 to Hoechst Marion Roussel); *idem*, *US 6221633* (2001 to Aventis). Evaluation of mitogenic potential: I. Rakatzi *et al.*, *Diabetes* **52**, 2227 (2003); of β-cell protective effect: *idem et al.*, *Biochem. Biophys. Res. Commun.* **310**, 852 (2003). Clinical trial in type 2 diabetes: G. Dailey *et al.*, *Diabetes Care* **27**, 2363 (2004). *Review*: S. K. Garg *et al.*, *Expert Opin. Pharmacother.* **6**, 643-651 (2005).

THERAP CAT: Antidiabetic.

4986. Insulin-like Growth Factors. IGFs. Family of conserved peptide hormones structurally homologous with insulin. Two major circulating forms mediate the growth promoting effects of somatotropin, *q.v.* IGF-I regulates both prenatal and postnatal growth; IGF-II is a key factor in fetal development. IGFs are produced primarily in the liver under the regulation of growth hormone; also produced locally by most tissues. Transported in the serum by *IGF binding proteins* (or *IGFBP*) that prolong the half-life and regulate the metabolic effects of IGFs. Discovered and termed *sulphation factors* because of their ability to stimulate the incorporation of sulfate by cartilage: W. D. Salmon, W. H. Daughaday, *J. Lab. Clin. Med.* **49**, 825 (1957). These peptides have also been referred to as *NSILA-S*, or non-suppressible insulin-like activity substance. The designation *somatomedin* was proposed to connote the intermediary relationship to somatotropin: W. H. Daughaday *et al.*, *Nature* **235**, 107 (1972). Discussion of nomenclature: *idem et al.*, *J. Clin. Endocrinol. Metab.* **65**, 1075 (1987). Isoln, chemical characterization, biological properties of IGF-I and IGF-II: E. Rinderknecht, R. E. Humbel, *Proc. Natl. Acad. Sci. USA* **73**, 2365, 4379 (1976). Amino acid sequence of IGF-I: *eidem*, *J. Biol. Chem.* **253**, 2769 (1978); of IGF-II: *eidem*, *FEBS Lett.* **89**, 283 (1978). Total synthesis of human IGF-I: C. H. Li *et al.*, *Proc. Natl. Acad. Sci. USA* **80**, 2216 (1983); of human IGF-II: *eidem*, *Biochem. Biophys. Res. Commun.* **127**, 420 (1985). Review of molecular biology: W. H. Daughaday, P. Rotwein, *Endocr. Rev.* **10**, 68-91 (1989); of mechanism of action: A. Spagnoli, R. C. Rosenfeld, *Endocrinol. Metab. Clin. North Am.* **25**, 615-631 (1996). Review of IGF binding proteins: D. R. Clemmons, *Cyto-*

kine Growth Factor Rev. **8**, 45-62 (1997). *Reviews:* C. E. H. Stewart, P. Rotwein, *Physiol. Rev.* **76**, 1005-1026 (1996); D. Le Roith, *N. Engl. J. Med.* **336**, 633-640 (1997).

Insulin-like Growth Factor I. [67763-96-6] IGF-I; somatomedin 1; somatomedin C; SM-C. Single chain, basic protein containing 70 amino acid residues. Review of physiology and potential therapeutic uses: E. R. Froesch *et al.*, *Diabetes Metab. Rev.* **12**, 195-215 (1996).

Insulin-like Growth Factor II. [67763-97-7] IGF-II; multiplication-stimulating activity III-2; MSA III-2. Single chain, slightly acidic protein containing 66 or 67 amino acid residues depending on the species.

Mecasermin. [68562-41-4] Human insulin-like growth factor I. $C_{331}H_{512}N_{94}O_{101}S_7$; mol wt 7648.63. *Myotrophin* and *Somason* are recombinant forms. Clinical trial in amyotrophic lateral sclerosis: D. J. Lange *et al.*, *Neurology* **47**, Suppl. 2, S93 (1996).

THERAP CAT: In treatment of growth hormone insensitivity syndrome and insulin resistance.

4987. Insulin Lispro. [133107-64-9] 28^B-L-Lysine-29^B-L-prolineinsulin (human); [Lys(B28),Pro(B29)]-insulin (human); LY-275585; Humalog. Rapid-acting insulin analog produced in *E. coli* by recombinant DNA technology. Identical to human insulin except for the transposition of proline and lysine at positions 28 and 29 on the B chain. Prepn: R. E. Chance *et al.*, *EP 383472*; *eidem*, *US 5514646* (1990, 1996 both to Lilly). Study of immunogenicity: C. M. Zwickl *et al.*, *Arzneim.-Forsch.* **45**, 524 (1995). General pharmacology: D. R. Helton *et al.*, *ibid.* **46**, 91 (1996). Clinical comparison with regular human insulin: J. H. Anderson, Jr. *et al.*, *Diabetes* **46**, 265 (1997). Review of development and pharmacokinetics: F. Holleman, J. B. L. Hoekstra, *N. Engl. J. Med.* **337**, 176-183 (1997); of clinical trials: V. A. Koivisto, *Ann. Med.* **30**, 260-266 (1998). Series of articles on pharmacology and clinical experience: *Acta Clin. Belg.* **54**, 233-254 (1999).

THERAP CAT: Antidiabetic.

4988. Integrins. Family of transmembrane glycoproteins involved in cellular adhesion and signal transduction. Name derived from their ability to "integrate" activities of the extracellular matrix (ECM) and the cytoskeleton. Integrins exhibit widespread evolutionary distribution: identified in mammals and other vertebrates, insects, and yeast; homologues have been identified in plants. At least 20 have been identified in mammals; composed of αβ heterodimers selected from among 16 α and 8 β subunits. The α subunits vary in size from 120-200 kDa with ~1000 amino acid residues and usually consist of a heavy and light chain joined by a disulfide bond; β subunits generally range from 90-120 kDa with ~800 amino acids. Three major subfamilies have been characterized. Most integrins bind to the Arg-Gly-Asp (RGD) amino acid sequence found on components of the ECM, such as fibronectin, *q.v.* Others bind to cell membrane proteins, such as the intercellular cell adhesion molecules (ICAMs), or to soluble ligands, such as fibrinogen, *q.v.* Several recognize more than one ligand. Integrins anchor cells to the ECM or to adjacent cells, regulate cell spreading and motility, and transduce extracellular stimuli into a variety of intracellular signals. Implicated in a variety of physiological processes including embryological development, wound healing, immune functions, thrombosis, and metastasis. Identification of membrane glycoproteins involved in cell adhesion: D. E. Wylie *et al.*, *J. Cell Biol.* **80**, 385 (1979). Identification of the transmembrane link between the ECM and the cytoskeleton: J. W. Tamkun *et al.*, *Cell* **46**, 271 (1986). Description of integrin family: R. O. Hynes, *ibid.* **48**, 549 (1987); C. A. Buck, A. F. Horwitz, *Annu. Rev. Cell Biol.* **3**, 179-205 (1987). Role of RGD sequence in cell adhesion: E. Ruoslahti, M. D. Pierschbacher, *Science* **238**, 491 (1987). Review of integrin structure and ligand binding: A. Sonnenberg, *Curr. Top. Microbiol. Immunol.* **184**, 7-35 (1993); D. S. Tuckwell, M. J. Humphries, *Crit. Rev. Oncol. Hematol.* **15**, 149-171 (1993). Review of pharmacology: D. Cox *et al.*, *Med. Res. Rev.* **14**, 195-228 (1994). Review of role in signal transduction: A. Richardson, J. T. Parsons, *BioEssays* **17**, 229-236 (1995); E. A. Clark, J. S. Brugge, *Science* **268**, 233-239 (1995).

β₁-Integrins. VLA antigens; VLA integrins; very late activation antigens. Widely distributed on various cell types. Share a common $β_1$ chain complexed with various α chains. Bind to ECM components such as fibronectin, collagen, laminin. Ca^{2+}/Mg^{2+}-dependent. Review: L. G. M. Baldini, L. M. Cro, *Leuk. Lymphoma* **12,** 197-203 (1994).

β₂-Integrins. Leukocyte integrins; Leu-Cam proteins; leukocyte adhesion molecules. Contain the β_2 chain; found on leukocytes. Bind to ICAMs, complement 3, and fibrinogen. Play an important role in regulating the immune system.

β₃-Integrins. Cytoadhesins. Contain the β_3 subunit; found on platelets, megakaryocytes and some melanoma cells. Ligands include fibrinogen, fibronectin, von Willebrand factor, vitronectin, and thrombospondin. Includes $\alpha_{IIb}\beta_3$, also known as *platelet glycoprotein IIb/IIIa (GPIIb-IIIa)*, a fibrinogen receptor involved in platelet aggregation. Review: M. H. Ginsberg *et al., Thromb. Haemostasis* **70,** 87-93 (1993).

4989. Interferon. IFN. A family of species-specific vertebrate proteins that confer non-specific resistance to a broad range of viral infections, affect cell proliferation and modulate immune responses. Discovered by A. Isaacs and J. Lindenmann, *Proc. Roy. Soc.* **B147,** 258 (1957) while studying viral interference. Originally produced by the interaction of inactivated influenza virus with chick chorioallantoic membranes; subsequently found to be inducible by viable virus in a variety of cells: D. C. Burke, A. Isaacs, *Br. J. Exp. Pathol.* **39,** 452 (1958); in human leukocytes: I. Gresser, *Proc. Soc. Exp. Biol. Med.* **108,** 799 (1961). Host cell specificity and physical properties: D. A. J. Tyrrell, *Nature* **184,** 452 (1959); T. C. Merigan, *Science* **145,** 811 (1964). Production of acid-labile interferon by mitogen-stimulated human leukocytes: E. F. Wheelock, *ibid.* **149,** 310 (1966). Three major interferons, alpha, beta and gamma, *q.q.v.,* have been identified based on antigenic and physicochemical properties, the nature of the inducer, and the cellular source from which they are derived, *cf. Nature* **286,** 110 (1980). Known collectively as type I interferon, IFNs-α and -β are structurally related, are stable at pH 2, and compete for the same cell surface receptor. IFN-γ, also known as type II interferon, is structurally unrelated to type I IFNs, is acid labile, and has a different receptor. Receptor binding study: A. A. Branca, C. Baglioni, *Nature* **294,** 768 (1981). *Reviews:* S. Baron, F. Dianzoni, Eds., *Tex. Rep. Biol. Med.* **35,** 1-573 (1977); *Ann. N.Y. Acad. Sci.* **350,** entitled "Regulatory Function of Interferons", J. Vilcek *et al.,* Eds. (1980) 643 pp; S. Baron *et al.,* Eds., *Tex. Rep. Biol. Med.* **41,** 1-715 (1982). Review of immunobiology and clinical significance: E. R. Stiem *et al., Ann. Intern. Med.* **96,** 80-93 (1982); of pharmacology and toxicology: G. J. Mannering, L. B. Deloria, *Annu. Rev. Pharmacol. Toxicol.* **26,** 455-515 (1986); of IFN-gene family: C. Weissmann, H. Weber, *Prog. Nucleic Acid Res. Mol. Biol.* **33,** 251-300 (1986). Symposium on antiviral activity of natural and recombinant IFNs: *Antiviral Res.* **5,** Suppl. 1, 131-257 (1985). Review of structure, function and nomenclature: K. C. Zoon, *Interferon* **9,** 1-12 (1987). Books: *Interferons and Interferon Inducers*, N. Finter, Ed. (North Holland Publ. Co., Amsterdam, 1973) 598 pp; W. E. Stewart, *The Interferon System* (Springer, New York, 1979) 421 pp; *Interferons*, T. C. Merigan, R. M. Friedman, Eds. (Academic Press, New York, 1982) 481 pp; *Interferon*, K. Munk, H. Kirchner, Eds. (S. Karger, New York, 1982) 233 pp; H. Strander, *Interferon Treatment of Human Neoplasia* (Academic Press, New York, 1986) 265 pp.

4990. Interferon-α. Alfa-interferon; alpha-interferon; IFN-α; LeIF; leukocyte interferon; lymphoblastoid interferon. Cytokine with antiviral, antiproliferative, and immunomodulatory activity. Produced by leukocytes stimulated by virus, bacteria, or protozoa as part of the immune response; artificially induced by double-stranded RNA. Inhibits protein synthesis and viral replication; enhances cytotoxic activity. Multiple subtypes have been identified which contain ~166 amino acids and are variably glycosylated; mol wt 16-27.5 kDa. Identification of interferon produced by human leukocytes exposed to virus: I. Gresser, *Proc. Soc. Exp. Biol. Med.* **108,** 799 (1961). Purification and characterization: M. Rubinstein *et al., Proc. Natl. Acad. Sci. USA* **76,** 640 (1979). Prepn by recombinant DNA technology: S. Nagata *et al., Nature* **284,** 316 (1980); D. V. Goeddel *et al., ibid.* **287,** 411 (1980). Comparison of structures and activities of HuIFN-α subtypes: M. Streuli *et al., Science* **209,** 1343 (1980); D. V. Goeddel *et al., Nature* **290,** 20 (1981). *Review:* A. Meager in *Cytokines,* A. R. Mire-Sluis, R. Thorpe, Eds. (Academic Press, San Diego, 1998) pp 361-389. Review of pharmacology and clinical efficacy in malignant and viral disease: R. T. Dorr, *Drugs* **45,** 177-211 (1993); in chronic

viral hepatitis: M. H. Woo, T. G. Burnakis, *Ann. Pharmacother.* **31,** 330-337 (1997); of use in metastatic renal cell carcinoma: A. Ravaud, M.-S. Dilhuydy, *Expert Opin. Biol. Ther.* **5,** 749-762 (2005).

Interferon alfa-2a. [77907-69-8] Interferon-αA (human leukocyte protein moiety); IFN-αA; Ro-22-8181; Canferon; Laroféron; Roferon-A. Recombinant HuIFN-α produced in *E. coli.* Contains 165 amino acids; mol wt ~19 kDa. Symposium on clinical antineoplastic activity: *Semin. Oncol.* **12,** Suppl. 5, 1-34 (1985). Review of clinical efficacy in hepatitis C: C. M. Perry, M. I. Wilde, *BioDrugs* **10,** 65-89 (1998).

Interferon alfa-2b. [98530-12-2] Interferon α2 (human leukocyte clone pM21 protein moiety reduced); interferon α2 (human leukocyte clone Hif-SN206 protein moiety reduced); IFN-α2; Sch-30500; YM-14090; Introna; Intron A; Viraferon. Recombinant HuIFN-α produced in *E. coli.* Mol wt ~19 kDa. Symposium on clinical antineoplastic activity: *Invest. New Drugs* **5,** Suppl, S1-S77 (1987). Clinical trial in hepatitis C: S. Schenker *et al., J. Interferon Cytokine Res.* **17,** 665 (1997).

Interferon alfa-2c. [142192-09-4] Interferon α2 (human clone pAD19B-IFN protein moiety reduced); Berofor. Clinical trial in chronic myelogenous leukemia: J. Thaler *et al., Leuk. Res.* **21,** 75 (1997); in lung cancer: C. Prior *et al., Eur. Respir. J.* **10,** 392 (1997).

Interferon alfacon-1. [118390-30-0] N-L-Methionyl-22-L-arginine-76-L-alanine-78-L-aspartic acid-79-L-glutamic acid-86-L-tyrosine-90-L-tyrosine-156-L-threonine-157-L-asparagine-158-L-leucine-interferon α1 (human lymphoblast reduced); consesus interferon; CIFN; Infergen. Synthetic, recombinant interferon derived by assigning the most commonly observed amino acid in each position of several alpha IFN subtypes to create a consensus sequence. Contains 166 amino acids; mol wt 19.5 kDa. Molecular characterization and bioactivity: L. M. Blatt *et al., J. Interferon Cytokine Res.* **16,** 489 (1996). Clinical trial in hepatitis C: M. J. Tong *et al., Hepatology* **26,** 747 (1997).

Interferon alfa-n1. NSC-339140; Sumiferon; Wellferon. Mixture of natural human α-interferons derived from lymphoblastoid cells exposed to Sendai virus. Review of clinical trials in hepatitis C: G. C. Farrell, *Hepatology* **26,** Suppl. 1, 96S-100S (1997); of pharmacology and clinical efficacy: C. M. Perry, A. J. Wagstaff, *BioDrugs* **9,** 125-154 (1998).

Interferon alfa-n3. Alferon. Mixture of natural, human α-interferons produced by human leukocytes exposed to Sendai virus. mol wt 16-27 kDa. Clinical trial in hepatitis C: D. M. Simon *et al., Hepatology* **25,** 445 (1997).

THERAP CAT: Antiviral; antineoplastic.

4991. Interferon-β. Beta-interferon; fibroblast interferon; FIF; IFN-β; IFN-β_1. Cytokine with antiviral, antiproliferative and immunomodulatory activity produced by fibroblasts in response to stimulation by live or inactivated virus or by certain synthetic polynucleotides. One of the type I interferons. Glycoprotein containing 166 amino acids; mol wt ~20 kDa. Production by human fibroblast cell cultures: E. A. Havell, J. Vilcek, *Antimicrob. Agents Chemother.* **2,** 476 (1972). Purification and initial characterization: E. Knight, Jr., *Proc. Natl. Acad. Sci. USA* **73,** 520 (1976). Amino acid analysis, partial sequence: *idem et al., Science* **207,** 525 (1980); S. Stein *et al., Proc. Natl. Acad. Sci. USA* **77,** 5716 (1980). Production by recombinant DNA technology: T. Taniguchi *et al., Proc. Natl. Acad. Sci. USA* **77,** 5230 (1980); R. Derynck *et al., Nature* **285,** 542 (1980); D. V. Goeddel *et al., Nucleic Acids Res.* **8,** 4057 (1980). Review of therapeutic activity in viral disease and in multiple sclerosis (MS): J. J. Alam, *Curr. Opin. Biotechnol.* **6,** 688-691 (1995).

Interferon Beta (human). Feron; Fiblaferon; Frone; Naferon. Natural interferon produced by cell cultured human fibroblasts. Clinical evaluation in MS: L. Jacobs *et al., Arch. Neurol.* **44,** 589 (1987); in herpes simplex infections: M. Glezerman *et al., Lancet* **1,** 150 (1988). Review of industrial prepn: M. Morandi, A. Valeri, *Adv. Biochem. Eng. Biotechnol.* **37,** 57-72 (1988).

Interferon Beta-1a. [145258-61-3] Avonex; Rebif. Recombinant human IFN-β produced in Chinese Hamster ovary cells. Glycoprotein consisting of 166 amino acid residues; contains ~11% carbohydrate by weight. Clinical trial in MS: L. D. Jacobs *et al., Ann. Neurol.* **39,** 285 (1996).

Interferon Beta-1b. [145155-23-3] IFN-beta$_{ser}$; Betaferon; Betaseron. Nonglycosylated polypeptide produced in *E. coli.* Consists of 165 amino acid residues; mol wt ~18.5 kDa. Synthetic mutein having a serine substituted for the cysteine residue at position 17 of the native molecule. Prepn: D. F. Mark *et al., Proc. Natl. Acad. Sci. USA* **81,** 5662 (1984). Review of clinical use in MS: D. E. Goodkin, *Lancet* **344,** 1057-1060 (1994). Clinical pharmacokinetics: O. A. Khan *et al., Neurology* **46,** 1639 (1996).

THERAP CAT: Antiviral; immunomodulator.

4992. Interferon-γ. [82115-62-6] Gamma-interferon; IFN-γ; immune IFN; ImIFN. Immunomodulatory cytokine produced by T-cells and natural killer (NK) cells as part of the immune response. Stimulates cellular immunity: activates macrophages, promotes antigen presentation, and enhances NK-cell activity. Regulates production of immunoglobulin G2a by B cells. Natural human IFN-γ is a glycoprotein containing 143 amino acids; mol wt 16-25 kDa. Forms non-covalent homodimers under physiological conditions. A type II interferon, IFN-γ is structurally unrelated to interferons-α and -β, *q.q.v.,* is acid-labile and has a different cell surface receptor. Discovery of interferon produced by non-infected human leukocytes stimulated by mitogen: E. F. Wheelock, *Science* **149,** 310 (1965). Production by antigen-stimulated leukocytes: J. A. Green *et al., ibid.* **164,** 1415 (1969). Large-scale production by cell culture: M. P. Langford *et al., Infect. Immun.* **26,** 36 (1979). Purification and characterization: Y. K. Yip *et al., Proc. Natl. Acad. Sci. USA* **79,** 1820 (1982). Prepn of recombinant human IFN-γ: P. W. Gray *et al., Nature* **295,** 503 (1982). Amino acid sequence: E. Rinderknecht *et al., J. Biol. Chem.* **259,** 6790 (1984). Review of biological activities: E. M. Bonnem, R. K. Oldham, *J. Biol. Response Modif.* **6,** 275-301 (1987); U. Boehm *et al., Annu. Rev. Immunol.* **15,** 749-795 (1997). Review of clinical experience in antimicrobial defense: H. W. Murray, *Intensive Care Med.* **22,** Suppl. 4, S456-S461 (1996). *Review:* E. De Maeyer, J. De Maeyer-Guignard, in *Cytokines* (Academic Press, San Diego, 1998) pp 391-400.

Interferon Gamma-1a. [98059-18-8] N^2-[N-(N-L-Cysteinyl-L-tyrosyl)-L-cysteinyl]-interferon γ (human lymphocyte protein moiety reduced); Cys-Tyr-Cys-interferon γ; S-6810; Immuneron; Polyferon. Nonglycosylated HuIFN-γ produced in *E. coli* by recombinant DNA technology. Consists of 146 amino acid residues; mol wt ~17 kDa. Clinical trial in rheumatoid arthritis: E. M. Lemmel *et al., Rheumatol. Int.* **8,** 87 (1988).

Interferon Gamma-1b. [98059-61-1] N^2-L-Methionyl-1-139-interferon γ (human lymphocyte protein moiety reduced); interferon gamma-2a; Actimmune; Immukin. Nonglycosylated HuIFN-γ produced in *E. coli* by recombinant DNA technology. Consists of 140 amino acid residues; mol wt ~16.5 kDa. Review of pharmacology and therapeutic potential in chronic granulomatous disease: P. A. Todd, K. L. Goa, *Drugs* **43,** 111-122 (1992).

THERAP CAT: Immunomodulator.

4993. Interleukin-1. IL-1; lymphocyte activating factor; LAF; B-cell activating factor; BAF; T-cell replacing factor; TRF; endogenous pyrogen; leukocytic endogenous mediator; mononuclear cell factor. Immunoenhancing, pyrogenic, polypeptide factor produced in blood and in a variety of tissues by mononuclear phagocytes responding to antigens or inflammatory agents. Responsible for a wide variety of bioactivities. Elicits a non-antigen specific amplification of cellular and humoral immune responses. Induces production of interleukin-2 (IL-2), collagenase and prostaglandins, *q.q.v.* Initial identification of factor inducing T-cell proliferation: I. Gery *et al., J. Exp. Med.* **136,** 128, 143 (1972); of factor enhancing antibody production: D. D. Wood, S. L. Gaul, *J. Immunol.* **113,** 925 (1974). Isoln and preliminary chemical characterization: I. Gery, R. E. Handschumacher, *Cell. Immunol.* **11,** 162 (1974); D. D. Wood, *J. Immunol.* **123,** 2395 (1979). Definition and nomenclature: L. A. Aarden *et al., ibid.* 2928. Identity with endogenous pyrogen: L. J. Rosenwasser, C. A. Dinarello, *Cell. Immunol.* **63,** 134 (1981). Purification of murine IL-1: S. B. Mizel, D. Mizel, *J. Immunol.* **126,** 834 (1981); of human IL-1: J. A. Schmidt, *J. Exp. Med.* **160,** 772 (1984). Exists in several biochemically distinct forms exhibiting charge heterogeneity and differing in amino acid sequence. Produced as ~30,000 mol wt precursor which is subsequently converted to low mol wt form. Cloning and expression of cDNA for murine precursor IL-1: P. T. Lomedico *et al., Nature* **312,** 458 (1984); for human precursor IL-1: P. E. Auron *et al., Proc. Natl. Acad. Sci. USA* **81,** 7907 (1984); for 2

distinct forms of human IL-1 (IL-1α and IL-1β): C. J. March *et al., Nature* **315,** 641 (1985). Amino acid sequence of dominant species corresponding to IL-1β: P. Cameron *et al., J. Exp. Med.* **162,** 790 (1985). Crystallization of recombinant human IL-1β: D. B. Carter *et al., Proteins: Struct. Funct. Genet.* **3,** 121 (1988). Characterization of membrane-associated IL-1: E. A. Kurt-Jones *et al., Proc. Natl. Acad. Sci. USA* **82,** 1204 (1985). Induction of IL-2 production by IL-1: K. A. Smith *et al., J. Exp. Med.* **151,** 1551 (1980); S. Gillis, S. B. Mizel, *Proc. Natl. Acad. Sci. USA* **78,** 1122 (1981). Effect on B-cells in antibody production: D. D. Wood, *J. Immunol.* **123,** 2400 (1979); P. Lipsky, *Contemp. Top. Mol. Immunol.* **10,** 195 (1985). Effect in inflammatory response: S. B. Mizel *et al., Proc. Natl. Acad. Sci. USA* **78,** 2474 (1981). Role in the pathogenesis of the acute-phase response: C. A. Dinarello, *N. Engl. J. Med.* **311,** 1413 (1984). Comparison of bioactivity of 4 forms of human IL-1: D. D. Wood *et al., J. Immunol.* **134,** 895 (1985). Review of interrelationship with lymphokines: N. M. Kouttab *et al., Clin. Chem.* **30,** 1539-1545 (1984). *Reviews:* J. J. Oppenheim *et al., Fed. Proc.* **41,** 257-262 (1982); S. B. Mizel, *Immunol. Rev.* **63,** 51-72 (1982); K. Bendtzen, *Allergy* **38,** 219-226 (1983); C. A. Dinarello, *Rev. Infect. Dis.* **6,** 51-95 (1984).

Isoelectric point (human): 6.8-7.3 (dominant species); 5.3-5.8 (minor species). Isoelectric point (murine): 4.5-5.5. Sensitive to trypsin, chymotrypsin, sodium dodecyl sulfate. Insensitive to 2-mercaptoethanol, neuraminidase, sodium periodate, iodacetamide. Stable at pH 3-10; stable at 56° for 60 min; unstable after 2 min at 100°.

4994. Interleukin-2. [85898-30-2] T-Cell growth factor; TCGF; thymocyte stimulating factor; costimulator; lymphocyte mitogenic factor; IL-2. Pleiotropic cytokine produced by T-lymphocytes following activation by antigens or mitogens in the presence of IL-1, *q.v.* Native, human IL-2 is a glycoprotein containing 133 amino acid residues; mol wt ~15 kDa. Potent immunomodulator with important role in activating and maintaining the immune response. Induces growth and proliferation of CD4+ and CD8+ T cells; enhances natural killer cell activity; stimulates antigen secretion; potentiates the release of γ-interferon and other cytokines. Also serves to down-regulate the immune system to prevent autoimmunity. Identification of soluble mitogenic factor produced by T-cells in response to antigen: R. S. Geha, E. Merler, *Cell. Immunol.* **10,** 86 (1974). Identification of T-cell growth promoting factor produced by mitogen stimulated lymphocytes: D. A. Morgan *et al., Science* **193,** 1007 (1976). Definition and nomenclature: L. A. Aarden *et al., J. Immunol.* **123,** 2928 (1979). Induction of IL-2 production by IL-1: K. A. Smith *et al., J. Exp. Med.* **151,** 1551 (1980). Review of early studies: J. Watson, D. Mochizuki, *Immunol. Rev.* **51,** 257 (1980). Purification and partial amino acid sequence: R. J. Robb *et al., Proc. Natl. Acad. Sci. USA* **80,** 5990 (1983). Expression of cloned cDNA for human IL-2 and predicted amino acid sequence: T. Taniguchi *et al., Nature* **302,** 305 (1983). Isolation of human IL-2 gene: S. Mita *et al., Biochem. Biophys. Res. Commun.* **117,** 114 (1983). Purification and cloning of the T-cell surface receptor for IL-2: W. J. Leonard *et al., Nature* **311,** 626 (1984). Review of recombinant IL-2 muteins: L. T. Vlasveld, E. M. Rankin, *Cancer Treat. Rev.* **20,** 275-311 (1994). Review of pharmacology and therapeutic use in cancer: R. Whittington, D. Faulds, *Drugs* **46,** 446-514 (1993); of function, production and clinical applications: S. L. Gaffen, K. D. Liu, *Cytokine* **28,** 109-123 (2004).

Isoelectric point: 6.5-6.8 (human); 3.9-5.0 (mouse). Sensitive to trypsin, chymotrypsin, sodium dodecyl sulfate. Stable in 2-mercaptoethanol, urea (2-4 mol/liter), neuraminidase. Stable at pH 3-10; at 56°C for 60 min. Unstable after 30 min. at 70°C.

Aldesleukin. [110942-02-4] 125-L-Serine-2-133-interleukin 2 (human reduced); Proleukin. Nonglycosylated interleukin-2 mutein produced by expressing the human IL-2 gene from Jurkat leukemia cells in *E. coli.* Production and bioactivity: S. A. Rosenberg *et al., Science* **223,** 1412 (1984). Clinical trial in metastatic melanoma: M. B. Atkins *et al., J. Clin. Oncol.* **17,** 2105 (1999). Review of clinical trials in HIV-infection: A. K. Pau, J. A. Tavel, *Curr. Opin. Pharmacol.* **2,** 433-439 (2002); in renal cell carcinoma: M. Schmidinger *et al., Expert Rev. Anticancer Ther.* **4,** 957-980 (2004).

Teceleukin. [136279-32-8] N-L-Methionylinterleukin 2 (human); BG-8301; Ro-23-6019; Imunace. Human interleukin-2 produced by recombinant DNA technology. Clinical evaluation of combination with interferon-α in renal cell carcinoma: H. Miyake *et al., Int. J. Oncol.* **10**, 338 (2005).

THERAP CAT: Antineoplastic; immunomodulator.

4995. Interleukin-3. Multipotent colony stimulating factor; IL-3; multi-CSF. Hematopoietic growth factor that promotes the survival, differentiation and proliferation of multipotent hematopoietic stem cells and of committed progenitor cells of the megakaryocyte, granulocyte-macrophage, erythroid, eosinophil, basophil and mast cell lineages. Enhances thrombopoiesis, phagocytosis, antibody-mediated cellular cytotoxicity and eosinophil metabolism. Species-specific, variably glycosylated peptide; human: 14-28 kDa, 133 amino acids; murine: 22-32 kDa, 140 amino acids. Produced primarily by activated T-lymphocytes; also by natural killer cells and mast cells. Undetectable in normal serum, postulated to be involved in the immune response. Purification from murine myelomonocytic leukemia cells (WEHI-3): J. N. Ihre *et al., J. Immunol.* **129**, 2431 (1982). Cloning of murine IL-3: M. C. Fung *et al., Nature* **307**, 233 (1984); T. Yokota *et al., Proc. Natl. Acad. Sci. USA* **81**, 1070 (1984); of human: Y.-C. Yang *et al., Cell* **47**, 3 (1986). Review of molecular and cellular biology: C. F. Morris *et al., Immunol. Ser.* **49**, 177-214 (1990); of structure and function: A. Lindemann, R. Mertelsmann, *Cancer Invest.* **11**, 609-623 (1993). Review of clinical pharmacology: A. Ganser, *ibid.* 212-218.

Muplestim. [148641-02-5] SDZ-ILE-964; Hemokine. Human IL-3 produced in *E. coli* by recombinant DNA technology. Clinical pharmacokinetics: B. Biesma *et al., Cancer Res.* **53**, 5915 (1993). Clinical evaluation in chemotherapy induced neutropenia: S. Kudoh *et al., Cancer Chemother. Pharmacol.* **38**, Suppl., S89 (1996).

Fusion protein with GM-CSF. [137463-76-4] PIXY321; GM-CSF/IL-3 fusion protein. Hybrid molecule consisting of the active domains of human GM-CSF and IL-3 coupled by a flexible amino acid sequence. Construction and expression in yeast: B. M. Curtis *et al., Proc. Natl. Acad. Sci. USA* **88**, 5809 (1991). Evaluation in cancer patients: S. Vadhan-Raj *et al., J. Clin. Oncol.* **12**, 715 (1994). Review: *idem, Stem Cells* **12**, 253-261 (1994).

THERAP CAT: Hematopoietic; antineutropenic.

4996. Interleukin-4. B-cell growth factor; BCGF-1; B-cell stimulatory factor-1; BSF-1; IL-4. Pleiotropic cytokine produced primarily by activated T-cells; also produced by mast cells and basophils. Directs the immune response toward humoral immunity and mediates the allergic response. Enhances the development of T_{H2} helper cells; regulates the B-cell immunoglobulin class switch to IgE and IgG$_4$. Also promotes mast cell development and eosinophil adherence. Exhibits anti-inflammatory effects on macrophages and monocytes. Mature human IL-4 is a glycoprotein containing 129 amino acids; mol wt ~20 kDa. Identification as a growth factor for B-cells: M. Howard *et al., J. Exp. Med.* **155**, 914 (1982). Initial characterization: J. J. Farrar *et al., J. Immunol.* **131**, 1838 (1983). Review of molecular characterization and function of IL-4 and its receptor: W. E. Paul, *Blood* **77**, 1859-1870 (1991); R. K. Puri, *Cancer Treat. Res.* **80**, 143-185 (1995). Inhibitory role in hematopoiesis and therapeutic potential in hematologic malignancies: K. Akashi, *Leuk. Lymphoma* **9**, 205 (1993). Mechanism of antitumor activity: R. I. Tepper, *J. Allergy Clin. Immunol.* **94**, 1225 (1994). Clinical evaluation with IL-2 in malignancy: T. Olencki *et al., J. Immunother.* **19**, 69 (1996). Review of role in asthma: M. Wills-Karp *et al., Adv. Exp. Med. Biol.* **409**, 343-347 (1996); in allergy: J. J. Ryan, *J. Allergy Clin. Immunol.* **99**, 1-5 (1997).

4997. Interleukin-5. Eosinophil differentiation factor; T cell replacing factor; B-cell growth factor II; IL-5; EDF; TRF; BCGFII. Essential cytokine for the maturation, growth, activation and survival of eosinophils; also acts on basophils. Produced primarily by activated T cells; other sources include natural killer cells, bone marrow endothelial cells and eosinophils. Exists as a variably glycosylated homodimer; mol wt 45-60 kDa. The mature, human monomer consists of 115 amino acid residues. Originally characterized as a T cell replacing factor: K. Takatsu *et al., J. Immunol.* **125**, 2646 (1980). Identity with BCGFII: N. Harada *et al., ibid.* **134**, 3944 (1985); with EDF: C. J. Sanderson *et al., Proc. Natl. Acad. Sci. USA* **83**, 437 (1986). Review of discovery and characterization of IL-5 and its receptor: K. Takatsu *et al., Adv. Immunol.* **57**, 145-190 (1994). Review of bioactivity and relevance to allergic disease: R. W. Egan *et al., Allergy* **51**, 71-81 (1996); of potential as

therapeutic target: F. Cuss, *ibid.* **53**, 89-92 (1998). *Reviews:* S. Karlen *et al., Int. Rev. Immunol.* **16**, 227-247 (1998); G. J. Roboz, S. Rafii, *Curr. Opin. Hematol.* **6**, 164-168 (1999).

4998. Interleukin-6. B-cell stimulatory factor-2; BSF-2; hepatocyte stimulating factor; hybridoma growth factor; interferon-β_2; IFN-β_2; IL-6. Pleiotropic cytokine produced by T-cells, monocytes, fibroblasts, endothelial cells, and keratinocytes. Glycoprotein occurring in at least 5 isoforms; mol wt 23-30 kDa. Human IL-6 contains 184 amino acid residues. Critical factor in host defense, regulating immune and inflammatory responses. Stimulates B-cell differentiation and antibody production; induces production of hepatic acute-phase protein synthesis; regulates bone metabolism; and synergizes with IL-3, *q.v.*, in megakaryocyte development and platelet production. Identification of factor produced by fibroblasts under conditions for IFN-β production: P. B. Sehgal, A. D. Sagar, *Nature* **288**, 95 (1980). Identification of multiple identities and proposed designation as IL-6: J. Van Damme *et al., Eur. J. Biochem.* **168**, 543 (1987); P. Poupart *et al., EMBO J.* **6**, 1219 (1987). Use as predictor of mortality in coronary artery disease: E. Lindmark *et al., J. Am. Med. Assoc.* **286**, 2107 (2001). Review of discovery and biological significance: M. C. J. Wolvekamp, R. L. Marquet, *Immunol. Lett.* **24**, 1-10 (1990). Role in aging processes: W. B. Ershler, *J. Am. Geriatr. Soc.* **41**, 176-181 (1993). Clinical potential in chemotherapy-induced thrombocytopenia: G. J. Veldhuis *et al., Leuk. Lymphoma* **20**, 373-379 (1996). Comprehensive review: M. Lotz, *Cancer Treat. Res.* **80**, 209-233 (1995). Review of role in lymphoproliferative disorders: J. F. Seymour, R. Kurzrock, *ibid.* **84**, 167-206 (1996).

4999. Interleukin-10. Cytokine synthesis inhibitory factor; CSIF; IL-10. Immunomodulatory cytokine produced by a wide variety of mammalian cell types including macrophages, monocytes, T cells, B cells and keratinocytes. Inhibits the synthesis of proinflammatory cytokines such as interleukin-1 and tumor necrosis factor α. Upregulates humoral immune responses and attenuates cell-mediated immune reactions. Protein composed of 160 amino acid residues; mol wt 18.5 kDa. Exists as a homodimer; the native human form has little or no glycosylation. A viral analog has been identified that is produced by Epstein Barr virus (EBV). Discovery: D. F. Fiorentino *et al., J. Exp. Med.* **170**, 2081 (1989). Cloning and expression of murine form and homology with product of EBV gene BCRFI: K. W. Moore *et al., Science* **248**, 1230 (1990). Review of discovery, properties and biological function: T. R. Mosmann, *Adv. Immunol.* **56**, 1-26 (1994). Review of potential clinical applications in inflammatory disease: I. Lalani *et al., Ann. Allergy Asthma Immunol.* **79**, 469-483 (1997); in infectious diseases: S. M. Opal *et al., Clin. Infect. Dis.* **27**, 1497-1507 (1998); in inflammatory bowel disease: M. W. Leach *et al., Toxicol. Pathol.* **27**, 123-133 (1999). *Review:* K. Asadullah *et al., Pharmacol. Rev.* **55**, 241-269 (2003).

Ilodecakin. [149824-15-7] Interleukin-10 (human clone pH15C); rhIL-10; Sch-52000; Tenovil. Human form produced in *E. coli* by recombinant DNA technology. Production: T. R. Mosmann *et al., EP 405980; eidem, US 5231012* (1991, 1993 both to Schering). Clinical pharmacokinetics: E. Radwanski *et al., Pharm. Res.* **15**, 1895 (1998). Clinical effect on circulating leukocyte populations: R. D. Huhn *et al., Immunopharmacology* **41**, 109 (1999).

5000. Interleukin-11. IL-11; adipogenesis inhibitory factor; AGIF. Multifunctional cytokine produced by stromal cells such as fibroblasts, epithelial cells, and osteoblasts. Expressed in a wide variety of tissues, including CNS, thymus, lung, bone, and connective tissue. Nonglycosylated protein containing 178 amino acid residues; mol wt 19 kDa. Important regulator of hematopoiesis; stimulates growth of myeloid, erythroid, and megakaryocyte progenitor cells. Regulates bone metabolism; inhibits production of proinflammatory mediators; and protects against gastromucosal injury. Identification: S. R. Paul *et al., Proc. Natl. Acad. Sci. USA* **87**, 7512 (1990). Identity with AGIF: I. Kawashima *et al., FEBS Lett.* **283**, 199 (1991). Review of biological activity and clinical studies: X. Du, D. A. Williams, *Blood* **89**, 3897-3908 (1997); A. J. Dorner *et al., BioDrugs* **8**, 418-429 (1997). *Review:* P. F. Schendel, K. J. Turner in *Cytokines*, A. R. Mire-Sluis, R. Thorpe, Eds. (Academic Press, San Diego, 1998) pp 169-182.

Highly basic protein, pI 11.7. Rich in leucine (23%) and proline (12%). Has no disulfide bonds as it does not contain cysteine. Heat stable; melting temp 90°. Highly sol at physiologic pH.

Oprelvekin. [145941-26-0] 2-178-Interleukin 11 (human clone pXM/IL-11); Neumega. Human IL-11 produced in *E. coli* by recombinant DNA technology. Differs from naturally occurring protein only in the absence of the amino-terminal proline residue. Clinical pharmacokinetics: K. Aoyama *et al., Br. J. Clin. Pharmacol.* **43**, 571 (1997). Clinical trial in chemotherapy-induced thrombocytopenia: I. Tepler *et al., Blood* **87**, 3607 (1996); C. Isaacs *et al., J. Clin. Oncol.* **15**, 3368 (1997). *Review:* J. A. Kaye, *Curr. Opin. Hematol.* **3**, 209-215 (1996).

THERAP CAT: Hematopoietic.

5001. Interleukin-1 Receptor Antagonist. IL-1ra; interleukin-1 inhibitor protein; IRAP. Endogenous inhibitor of interleukin-1, *q.v.*; modulates the normal, acute inflammatory response to infection and injury. First known naturally occurring protein that functions as a specific receptor antagonist of a cytokine. Variably glycosylated, 152 amino acid protein; mol wt 17-25 kDa. Secreted (glycosylated) and intracellular (nonglycosylated) forms have been identified. Structurally homologous with IL-1 and produced by the same cells. Isoln of an IL-1 inhibitor produced by human monocytes: W. P. Arend *et al., J. Immunol.* **134**, 3868 (1985). Isoln from human urine: P. Seckinger *et al., ibid.* **139**, 1541 (1987). Purification: C. H. Hannum *et al., Nature* **343**, 336 (1990). Cloning and expression of human IL-1ra: S. P. Eisenberg *et al., ibid.* 341. Study of biological function: E. Hirsch *et al., Proc. Natl. Acad. Sci. USA* **93**, 11008 (1996). Therapeutic potential in IL-1-mediated disease: R. C. Thompson *et al., Int. J. Immunopharmacol.* **14**, 475 (1992); C. A. Dinarello, *Nutrition* **11**, 492 (1995). *Reviews:* W. P. Arend, *Adv. Immunol.* **54**, 167-227 (1993); A. C. Lennard, *Crit. Rev. Immunol.* **15**, 77-105 (1995). Prognostic value in percutaneous coronary intervention: G. Patti *et al., Am. J. Cardiol.* **89**, 372 (2002).

Anakinra. [143090-92-0] N^2-L-Methionyl-interleukin 1 receptor antagonist (human isoform x reduced); Kineret. Nonglycosylated, recombinant human IL-1ra expressed in *E. coli*; mol wt 17 kDa. Prepn: C. H. Hannum *et al., EP 343684; eidem, US 5075222* (1989, 1991 both to Synergen). Biological properties: W. P. Arend *et al., J. Clin. Invest.* **85**, 1694 (1990). Clinical trial in sepsis syndrome: C. J. Fisher, Jr. *et al., Crit. Care Med.* **22**, 12 (1994); in rheumatoid arthritis: R. M. Fleischmann *et al., Arthritis Rheum.* **48**, 927 (2003). Series of articles on safety and clinical experience in rheumatoid arthritis: *Rheumatology* **42**, Suppl. 2, ii22-ii40 (2003).

THERAP CAT: Anti-inflammatory.

5002. Interleukin-4 Receptor. IL-4R. Endogenous receptor for interleukin-4, *q.v.*, expressed on the surface of B and T lymphocytes, mast cells and macrophages, that mediates the bioactivities of the cytokine. mol wt ~140 kDa. Also secreted as a soluble, truncated form (*sIL-4R*) which lacks the transmembrane and intracellular domains and is capable of binding and sequestering circulating IL-4. Identification of membrane bound receptors: J. Ohara, W. E. Paul, *Nature* **325**, 537 (1987). Characterization of murine: L. S. Park *et al., Proc. Natl. Acad. Sci. USA* **84**, 1669 (1987); of human: *idem et al., J. Exp. Med.* **166**, 476 (1987). Cloning of murine and identification of soluble form: B. Mosley *et al., Cell* **59**, 335 (1989). Detection of sIL-4R in biological fluids: R. Fernandez-Botran, E. S. Vitetta, *Proc. Natl. Acad. Sci. USA* **87**, 4204 (1990). Immunoregulatory effects of recombinant sIL-4R: C. R. Maliszewski *et al., Proc. Soc. Exp. Biol. Med.* **206**, 233 (1994). Review of signaling mechanisms of membrane receptor: A. D. Keegan *et al., Immunol. Today* **15**, 423-432 (1994). Review of bioactivity and therapeutic potential of sIL-4R: K. Enssle *et al., Behring Inst. Mitt.* **96**, 103-117 (1995).

Altrakincept. [239076-74-5] Recombinant human soluble interleukin-4 receptor; Nuvance. Soluble form of the human IL-4 receptor produced by recombinant DNA technology in Chinese hamster ovary cells. Glycoprotein; mol wt 54 kDa. Prepn: D. J. Cosman *et al., EP 367566;* B. Mosley *et al., US 5599905* (1990, 1997 both to Immunex). Clinical evaluation in atopic asthma: L. C. Borish *et al., Am. J. Respir. Crit. Care Med.* **160**, 1816 (1999). *Review:* R. Lange, *Curr. Opin. Cardiovasc. Pulm. Renal Invest. Drugs* **1**, 526-531 (1999).

THERAP CAT: Soluble form as antiasthmatic.

5003. Inula. Elecampane; scabwort; elfwort; horseheal. Dried rhizome and roots of *Inula helenium* L., *Compositae. Habit.* Central Asia, Europe; naturalized in U.S. *Constit.* Inulin, volatile oil, alantol, helenin, alantic acid, acrid resin.

5004. Inulin. [9005-80-5] Dahlin; alantin; alant starch. Mol wt approx 5000. Polysaccharide of *Compositae* which partially or completely replaces starch as a reserve food. Isoln from dahlia tubers: McDonald, "Polyfructosans and Difructose Anhydrides" in *Advan. Carbohyd. Chem.* **vol. 2**, 254 (1946); from Jerusalem artichoke tubers: Bacon, Edelman, *Biochem. J.* **48**, 114 (1951). Structure: E. G. V. Percival, *Structural Carbohydrate Chemistry* (J. Garnet Miller, London, 2nd ed., 1962) p 274.

R = CH₂OH
n = approx 35

Spherical crystals from water. Hygroscopic in moist air. $[\alpha]_D^{20}$ −40° (c = 2) for the anhydr. Sol in hot water; slightly sol in cold water and organic solvents. Yields D-fructose and D-glucose upon acid hydrolysis.

Acetate. Fine powder from methanol. $[\alpha]_D^{20}$ −34° (c = 1.5 in chloroform); $[\alpha]_D^{20}$ −43° (c = 1.8 in acetic acid).

Trimethylinulin. Powder from hot water + acetone, mp 140°. $[\alpha]_D^{20}$ −55° (c = 1.03 in chloroform); $[\alpha]_D^{20}$ −54° (c = 1.09 in benzene).

THERAP CAT: Diagnostic aid (renal function).

5005. Invertase. [9001-57-4] Invertin; saccharase; sucrase. Enzymes, obtained primarily from yeast as well as other sources, which catalyze the hydrolysis of sucrose into fructose and glucose. Since sucrose is both a β-fructofuranoside and an α-glucoside, it is split by two different types of enzymes, *β-fructofuranosidases* or *β-h-fructosidases* and certain *α-glucosidases* or *α-n-glucosidoinvertases*, which attack the sucrose molecule from the fructose and glucose end, respectively. β-Fructofuranosidase, generally obtained from yeast, is characterized by its ability to hydrolyze raffinose, while α-glucosidase is inactive toward raffinose. *Reviews:* K. Myrbäck, "Invertases" in *The Enzymes* **vol. 4**, P. D. Boyer *et al.,* Eds. (Academic Press, New York, 1960) pp 379-396; Lampen, "Yeast and Neurospora Invertases", *ibid.* **vol. 5** (3rd ed., 1971) pp 291-305; Cochrane, *Soc. Chem. Ind. Monogr.* no. **11**, 25-31 (1959) (Pub. 1961); Meister, *Wallerstein Lab. Commun.* **28**, 7 (1965).

USE: For preparation of invert sugar from sucrose; as analytical reagent for sucrose.

5006. Invert Sugar. [8013-17-0] Nulomoline; Calorose; Invesol; Insubeta; Travert. A mixture of about 50% glucose (dextrose) and 50% fructose (levulose) obtained by hydrolysis of sucrose. Hydrolysis of the sucrose may be carried out with acids or enzymes. Invert sugar is slightly levorotatory, reduces Fehling's soln and can be fermented. Honey is mostly invert sugar. Due to the levulose, it is somewhat sweeter than sucrose. The commercial product is obtained by inversion of a 96% cane sugar soln. The inversion is carried out at pH 3 to 4 by means of invertase and dil HCl. The acid is usually neutralized with sodium carbonate to pH 6.5. At this point, the dextrose crystallizes and the entire mass is beaten into a creamy, plastic product.

USE: In food products, in confectionery. As a humectant, like glycerol, to hold moisture and to prevent drying out. In brewing.

THERAP CAT: Nutrient (parenteral).

Consult the Name Index before using this section.

5007. Iobenguane. [80663-95-2] [(3-Iodophenyl)methyl]-guanidine; *m*-iodobenzylguanidine; MIBG. $C_8H_{10}IN_3$; mol wt 275.09. C 34.93%, H 3.66%, I 46.13%, N 15.28%. Norepinephrine analog with specific affinity for tissues of sympathetic nervous system and related tumors; prepd as ^{123}I and ^{131}I labeled forms. Prepn and imaging studies: D. M. Wieland *et al., J. Nucl. Med.* **21,** 349 (1980); *eidem,* **US 4584187** (1986). Improved synthesis: P. A. P. M. van Doremalen, A. G. M. Janssen, *J. Radioanal. Nucl. Chem. Lett.* **96,** 97 (1985). Metabolism in man: T. J. Mangner *et al., J. Nucl. Med.* **27,** 37 (1986). HPLC determn in serum and urine: D. Schwabe *et al., J. Chromatogr.* **487,** 177 (1989). Radiopharmacokinetics: S. Ertl *et al., Nucl. Med. Commun.* **8,** 643 (1987). Clinical evaluation of myocardial imaging: D. Fagret *et al., Eur. J. Nucl. Med.* **15,** 624 (1989). Diagnostic use in pheochromocytoma: B. Shapiro *et al., J. Nucl. Med.* **26,** 576 (1985); therapeutic use: M. Krempf *et al., J. Clin. Endocrinol. Metab.* **72,** 455 (1991). Symposia on therapeutic and diagnostic use in neuroblastoma: *Advances in Neuroblastoma Research* **2,** A. E. Evans *et al.,* Eds. (Alan R. Liss, Inc., New York, 1988) p 643-726; *Med. Pediatr. Oncol.* **15,** 157-228 (1987). Review of pharmacology: J. C. Sisson, D. M. Weiland, *Am. J. Physiol. Imaging* **1,** 96-103 (1986); of biodistribution and clinical studies: A. R. Wafelman *et al., Eur. J. Nucl. Med.* **21,** 545-559 (1994); of therapeutic use in neural crest tumors: L. Troncone, V. Rufini, *Anticancer Res.* **17,** 1823-1832 (1997).

Sulfate. $(C_8H_{10}IN_3)_2.H_2SO_4$. Colorless crystals from water + ethanol, mp 166-167°.

THERAP CAT: Radiolabeled forms as antineoplastic; diagnostic aid (radioactive imaging agent).

5008. Iobitridol. [136949-58-1] *N,N*′-Bis(2,3-dihydroxypropyl)-5-[[3-hydroxy-2-(hydroxymethyl)-1-oxopropyl]amino]-2,4,6-triiodo-*N,N*′-dimethyl-1,3-benzenedicarboxamide; 5-[3-hydroxy-2-(hydroxymethyl)-propionamido]-*N,N*′-dimethyl-*N,N*′-bis-(2,3-dihydroxypropyl)-2,4,6-triiodoisophthalamide; Xenetix. $C_{20}H_{28}I_3N_3O_9$; mol wt 835.16. C 28.76%, H 3.38%, I 45.59%, N 5.03%, O 17.24%. Nonionic, monomeric, low-osmolality x-ray contrast medium for urography and angiography. Prepn: M. Schaefer *et al.,* **EP 437144**; *eidem,* **US 5043152** (both 1991 to Guerbet). Biodistribution studies: P. Bourrinet *et al., Invest. Radiol.* **29,** 1057 (1994). HPLC determn in biological fluids: *idem et al., J. Chromatogr. B* **670,** 369 (1995). Toxicology: A.-M. Donadieu *et al., Acta Radiol.* **37,** Suppl. 400, 17 (1996). Series of articles on pharmacology, pharmacokinetics and clinical studies: *ibid.* 1-92.

Hydrophilic. Log P (octanol/water): −2.63 at 37°. LD_{50} in male, female mice (g I/kg): 16.8, 16.6 i.v. (Donadieu).

THERAP CAT: Diagnostic aid (radiopaque medium).

5009. Iocarmic Acid. [10397-75-8] 3,3′-[(1,6-Dioxo-1,6-hexanediyl)diimino]bis[2,4,6-triiodo-5-[(methylamino)carbonyl]-benzoic acid]; 5,5′-(adipoyldiimino)bis[2,4,6-triiodo-*N*-methyliso-phthalamic acid]; Myelotrast. $C_{24}H_{20}I_6N_4O_8$; mol wt 1253.86. C 22.99%, H 1.61%, I 60.73%, N 4.47%, O 10.21%. Prepn: **GB 1033695**; **US 3290366** (both 1966 to Mallinckrodt); G. B. Hoey *et al., J. Med. Chem.* **9,** 964 (1966). Clinical studies: Kunze, Schiefer, *Dtsch. Med. Wochenschr.* **97,** 245 (1972). Diagnostic use in myelography: P. Ahlgren, *Acta Radiol. Diagn.* **13,** 753 (1972); in hysterosalpingography: H. E. Schutte, *Diagn. Imaging* **51,** 277

(1982). Spinal toxicity in rats: I. O. Skalpe, A. Torvik, *Invest. Radiol.* **10,** 154 (1975).

Crystals from dimethylformamide, mp 302° (dec).

Di-*N*-methylglucamine salt. [54605-45-7] Dimeglumine iocarmate; LM-280; Dimeray; Dimer-X; Dirax. $C_{38}H_{54}I_6N_6O_{18}$; mol wt 1644.29. Soly in water (25°): 65 g/100 ml.

THERAP CAT: Diagnostic aid (radiopaque medium).

5010. Iocetamic Acid. [16034-77-8] 3-[Acetyl-(3-amino-2,4,6-triiodophenyl)amino]-2-methylpropanoic acid; *N*-acetyl-*N*-(3-amino-2,4,6-triiodophenyl)-2-methyl-β-alanine; *N*-acetyl-*N*-(2,4,6-triiodo-3-aminophenyl)-β-aminoisobutyric acid; DRC-1201; MP-620; Cholebrine; Cholimil. $C_{12}H_{13}I_3N_2O_3$; mol wt 613.96. C 23.48%, H 2.13%, I 62.01%, N 4.56%, O 7.82%. Prepn: **NL 6515305**; **NL 6607275** (both 1967 to Dagra), *C.A.* **67,** 108422m (1967); **69,** 10263b (1968); Korver, *Rec. Trav. Chim.* **87,** 308 (1968). Pharmacology and toxicology: J. M. Janbroers *et al., Toxicol. Appl. Pharmacol.* **14,** 232, 246 (1969). Metabolic studies: Neleman, *Pharm. Weekbl.* **102,** 1039 (1967). Clinical studies: Hekster, *Radiol. Clin. Biol.* **37,** 338 (1968). Use in cholecystography: B. Goldberg, *Radiol. Clin.* **46,** 42 (1977).

White to light cream-colored powder, mp 224-225° (**NL 6515305**). Also reported as mp range 191-212° (Korver). Practically insol in water. Very slightly sol in ether, ethanol, benzene; slightly sol in acetone, chloroform (Janbroers). LD_{50} in rats (g/kg): 7.1 orally; 0.70 i.v. (Janbroers). Consists of 2 isomers having mps 232° and 200-201° and pKa's of 4.25 and 4.0 respectively. The lower melting compd is approx two times as soluble.

THERAP CAT: Diagnostic aid (radiopaque medium).

5011. Iodamide. [440-58-4] 3-(Acetylamino)-5-[(acetylamino)methyl]-2,4,6-triiodobenzoic acid; α,5-diacetamido-2,4,6-triiodo-*m*-toluic acid; 3-acetamido-5-(acetamidomethyl)-2,4,6-triiodobenzoic acid; ametriodinic acid; SH-926. $C_{12}H_{11}I_3N_2O_4$; mol wt 627.94. C 22.95%, H 1.77%, I 60.63%, N 4.46%, O 10.19%. Prepn: Felder, Pitre, **FR 1382277** and **US 3360436** (1964 and 1967 to Eprova); Felder *et al., Helv. Chim. Acta* **48,** 259 (1965). Pharmacology and toxicology: F. Bonati *et al., Arzneim.-Forsch.* **15,** 222 (1965); Z. B. Zsebök, L. Szlavy, *ibid.* **17,** 1380 (1967); *eidem, Int. Z. Klin. Pharmakol. Ther. Toxikol.* **3,** 157 (1970). Clinical trials: Grothuesmann, *Arzneim.-Forsch.* **15,** 233 (1965). Comprehensive description: D. Pitré, *Anal. Profiles Drug Subs.* **15,** 337-365 (1986).

Crystals from acetic acid, mp 255-257°. Soly in water: 0.3 g/100 ml (22°).

N-Methyl-D-glucamine salt. [18656-21-8] Iodamide meglumine; Isteropac E.R.; Jodomiron; Opacist E.R.; Renovue-65; Renovue-DIP; Uromiro. $C_{19}H_{28}I_3N_3O_9$; mol wt 823.15. Sparingly sol in methanol, slightly sol in water, ethanol. Practically insol in ether, chloroform. LD_{50} in mice, rats, rabbits (g/kg): 9.0, 11.4, 13.2 i.v.; in rats, guinea pigs (g/kg): 17.9, 15.0 i.p. (Bonati).

THERAP CAT: Diagnostic aid (radiopaque medium).

5012. Iodic Acid. [7782-68-5] HIO_3; mol wt 175.91. H 0.57%, I 72.14%, O 27.29%. Prepd by the oxidation of iodine with nitric acid, perchloric acid, or hydrogen peroxide: Baxter, Tilley, *Z. Anorg. Allg. Chem.* **61**, 295 (1909); Lamb *et al., J. Am. Chem. Soc.* **42**, 1643 (1920); Bray, Caulkins, *ibid.* **53**, 44 (1931). Electrolytic method: Willard, Ralston, *Trans. Am. Electrochem. Soc.* **62**, 239 (1932).

Orthorhombic crystals. Darkens upon exposure to light. d_4^0 4.629. mp 110° (dec). Decompn to $HIO_3.I_2O_5$ starts at 70° and decompn to I_2O_5 is complete at 220°. Not hygroscopic, yet very freely sol in water: 269 g/100 ml H_2O at 20°; 295 g/100 ml H_2O at 40°. Density of aq solns (w/w) at 18°: 1% = 1.0071; 10% = 1.0900; 20% = 1.1969; 40% = 1.4640; 75% = 2.4710. Strong electrolyte, especially when dil. Sol in nitric acid, dil alcohol. Insol in abs alc, ether, chloroform. *Keep well closed and protected from light.*

THERAP CAT: Astringent, disinfectant.

5013. Iodinated Glycerol. [5634-39-9] Iodopropylidene glycerol. $C_6H_{11}IO_3$; mol wt 258.05. C 27.93%, H 4.30%, I 49.18%, O 18.60%. Isomeric mixture of 67-75% of **2-(1-iodo-ethyl)-1,3-dioxolane-4-methanol** or **2,3-(2-iodopropylidenedioxy)-propanol** and 33-25% of **2-(2-iodoethyl)-1,3-dioxolane-4-methanol** or **2,3-(3-iodopropylidenedioxy)propanol**. Prepn: Manchey *et al.*, US 2872378 (1959 to The Denver Chem. Manuf.).

Pale yellow liquid. Pungent, bitter aftertaste. d 1.797. n_D 1.547. Sol in ether, chloroform, isobutyl alc, methyl acetate, ethyl acetate, methyl formate, tetrahydrofuran.

THERAP CAT: Has been used as expectorant.

5014. Iodine. [7553-56-2] I; at. wt 126.90447; at. no. 53; valences −1, 1, 3, 5, 7. A halogen; Group VIIA (17). Does not occur as elemental state, I_2, in nature. Abundance in igneous rocks: 3×10^{-5}% by wt; in seawater: 5×10^{-8}% by wt. Naturally occurring stable isotope (mass number): 127 (100%); known artificial radioactive isotopes: 108 to 141; commonly used radioactive tracer elements: 123 ($T_{1/2}$ 13.27 hrs, EC decay), 125 ($T_{1/2}$ 59.408 days, EC decay), 129 ($T_{1/2}$ 1.57×10^7 years, β^- decay), 131 ($T_{1/2}$ 8.02070 days, β^- decay). Discovered in 1811 by Courtois. Classed among the rarer elements. Trace element essential to animal and plant life. Extracted commercially from natural subterranean brines, and Chilean nitrate-bearing earth (caliche); formerly from seaweed. *Reviews: MTP Int. Rev. Sci.: Inorg. Chem., Ser. One* Vol. **3**, V. Gutmann, Ed. (Butterworths, London, 1972); A. J. Downs, C. J. Adams, "Chlorine, Bromine, Iodine and Astatine" in *Comprehensive Inorganic Chemistry* vol. **2**, J. C. Bailar, Jr. *et al.*, Eds. (Pergamon Press, Oxford, 1973) p 1107-1573; *Chemistry of the Elements* N. N. Greenwood, A. Earnshaw, Eds. (Pergamin Press, New York, 1984) pp 920-1041; A. Lauterbach, G. Ober in *Kirk-Othmer Encyclopedia of Chemical Technology* vol. **14** (Wiley-Interscience, New York, 4th ed., 1995) pp 709-737. Review of geochemistry: R. Fuge, C. C. Johnson, *Environ. Geochem. Health* **8**, 31-54 (1986); of human toxicity: *Iodine Toxicity* (PB89-183016, 1989) 107 pp; of metabolism and nutritional deficiency: J. T. Dunn in *Contemporary Endocrinology: Diseases of the Thyroid*, L. E. Braverman, Ed. (Humana Press Inc., Totowa, NJ, 1997) pp 349-360; of toxicology and human exposure: *Toxicological Profile for Iodine* (PB2004-104399, 2004) 580 pp.

Bluish-black scales or plates; diatomic; metallic luster; characteristic odor; sharp acrid taste. Readily sublimes at rm temp, forming violet corrosive vapor. mp 113.60°. bp 185.24°. d (solid, 25°) 4.93, d (liq 120°) 3.960. Vapor pressure (solid): 0.030 mm (0°); 0.305 mm (25°); 2.154 mm (50°); 26.78 mm (90°). Heat capacity at constant pressure (25°) 13.011 cal/mole/°C: Shirley, Giauque, *J.*

Am. Chem. Soc. **81**, 4778 (1959). Total soly in water (25°) 0.0013 moles/l with negligible formation of HOI (6.4×10^{-6} moles/l); freely sol in aq solns of HI or iodides. Soly in organic solvents (g I_2/100 g soln, 25°): benzene 14.09; CS_2 16.47; ethanol 21.43; ethyl ether 25.20; cyclohexane 2.719; heptane 1.702; CCl_4 (35°) 2.603: Hildebrand, Jenks, *J. Am. Chem. Soc.* **42**, 2180 (1920); Hildebrand *et al., ibid.* **72**, 1017 (1950); sol in chloroform, glacial acetic acid, glycerol oils. Solutions of iodine in aq solns of inorganic iodides are brown or deep brown, depending on the concn of the iodine. Solvents contg nitrogen atoms, such as pyridine, amines, or quinoline form brown solns. Aliphatic hydrocarbons, chloroform, carbon tetrachloride, carbon disulfide, phosphorus trichloride and fluorinated amines give violet solns. Aromatic hydrocarbons give pink or reddish-brown solns. Alcohols and ethers give deep brown solns. Soly in water is increased by alkali bromides, but decreased by sulfates and nitrates. Less reactive than bromine; E° (aq) $\frac{1}{2}I_2/I^-$ 0.535 V dissociation energy (25°): 36.115 kcal. Iodine stains may be removed with sodium thiosulfate soln or ammoniated alc.

Tamed Iodine see Iodophors.

Caution: Potential symptoms of overexposure are irritation of eyes, skin, and nose; lacrimation; headache; tight chest; skin burns, rash; cutaneous hypersensitivity. *See NIOSH Pocket Guide to Chemical Hazards* (DHHS/NIOSH 97-140, 1997) p 172. Ingestion of large quantities causes abdominal pain, vomiting and diarrhea due to the highly corrosive action of iodine on the GI tract. *See Clinical Toxicology of Commercial Products*, R. E. Gosselin *et al.*, Eds. (Williams & Wilkins, Baltimore, 5th ed., 1984) Sect. III, pp 213-214.

USE: Manuf of organic and inorganic chemicals, pharmaceuticals, radiopaque contrast agents, animal feed supplements, disinfectants, stabilizers, inks, colorants, photographic chemicals. Catalyst in the alkylation and condensation of aromatic amines; in sulfations and sulfonations; for prodn of synthetic rubber. Microbicide for drinking water and swimming pools. Artificial radioisotopes as tracers in biological, biochemical and chemical research; in medical imaging. Reagent in analytical chemistry.

THERAP CAT: Antihyperthyroid; anti-infective (topical).

THERAP CAT (VET): Internally for goiter, hypothyroidism, in iodine deficiency. Topically as antiseptic, disinfectant, counterirritant and to promote absorption.

5015. Iodine Heptafluoride. [16921-96-3] F_7I; mol wt 259.89. F 51.17%, I 48.83%. IF_7. Prepd by passing fluorine through liq IF_5 at 90°, then heating the vapors to 270°: Ruff, Keim, *Z. Anorg. Allg. Chem.* **193**, 176 (1930); Kwasnik in *Handbook of Preparative Inorganic Chemistry* vol. **1**, G. Brauer, Ed. (Academic Press, New York, 2nd ed., 1963) pp 160-161. May also be prepd from fluorine and dried PdI_2 or KI to minimize formation of the impurity, IOF_5: Bartlett, Levchuk, *Proc. Chem. Soc. London* **1963**, 342; Selig *et al., J. Phys. Chem.* **71**, 2739 (1967). *Reviews:* Kemmitt, Sharp, *Adv. Fluorine Chem.* **4**, 246-247 (1965); Stein, "Physical and Chemical Properties of Halogen Fluorides" in *Halogen Chemistry* Vol. **1**, V. Gutmann, Ed. (Academic Press, New York, 1967) pp 133-224; Meinert, *Z. Chem.* **7**, 41-57 (1967).

Colorless gas. Crystals when solid. Moldy, acrid odor. *Attacks glass and quartz.* d (liq; 6°) 2.8. mp 6.45°. Sublimes at 4.77°. Easily forms a supercooled liquid which boils at +4.5°. Trouton constant 26.4. Water dissolves the gas without violence, some decompn. Readily absorbed by NaOH soln.

Caution: Highly irritating to skin, mucous membranes. *See also* Fluorine.

USE: Fluorinating agent.

5016. Iodine Monobromide. [7789-33-5] BrI; mol wt 206.81. Br 38.64%, I 61.36%. IBr. Prepd from the elements, excess Br is removed by heating to 50° in a current of CO_2: Bornemann, *Ann.* **189**, 202 (1877); Terwogt, *Z. Anorg. Allg. Chem.* **47**, 203 (1905); *Gmelins, Iodine* (8th ed.) **8**, p 631 (1933); Schmeisser in *Handbook of Preparative Inorganic Chemistry* vol. **1**, G. Brauer, Ed. (Academic Press, New York, 2nd ed., 1963) p 291-292. Crystal structure: Swink, Carpenter, *Acta Crystallogr.* **24B**, 429 (1968).

Brownish-black crystals or very hard solid. d 4.416. mp 40°. bp 116° (decompn). Sol in water, alcohol, ether, carbon disulfide, glacial acetic acid. May be stored in brown glass-stoppered bottles. *Keep in a cool place.*

Caution: Vapors are corrosive to the eyes and mucous membranes.

5017. Iodine Monochloride. [7790-99-0] Wijs' chloride. ClI; mol wt 162.36. Cl 21.84%, I 78.16%. ICl. Prepd from the elements: Cornog, Karges, *Inorg. Synth.* **1**, 165 (1939); Buckles, Bader, *ibid.* **9**, 130 (1967).

Black crystals or reddish-brown liquid. The crystals occur in two modifications: α-form (stable), black needles (ruby red by transmitted light), mp 27.2°; β-form (labile), black platelets (brownish red by transmitted light), mp 13.9°. bp 97° (decompn). d_4^4 3.10. Sol in water, alc, ether, CS_2, acetic acid. May be stored in brown glass-stoppered bottles. Not hygroscopic, but forms I_2O_5 in the presence of air.

Caution: Attacks the skin, forming dark, painful patches (effective countermeasure: immediate washing with 20% HCl).

USE: In Wijs' soln (iodine monochloride in glacial acetic acid), used to determine iodine values of fats and oils.

THERAP CAT: Anti-infective (topical).

5018. Iodine Pentafluoride. [7783-66-6] F_5I; mol wt 221.90. F 42.81%, I 57.19%. IF_5. Prepd by passing fluorine over iodine with cooling: Gore, *Philos. Mag.* [4] **41**, 309 (1871); Moissan, *Compt. Rend.* **135**, 563 (1902); *Bull. Soc. Chim. Fr.* [3] **29**, 6 (1903); Ruff, Keim, *Z. Anorg. Allg. Chem.* **201**, 245 (1931); Ruff, Braida, *ibid.* **220**, 43 (1934); Kwasnik in *Handbook of Preparative Inorganic Chemistry* **vol. 1**, G. Brauer, Ed. (Academic Press, New York, 2nd ed., 1963) pp 159-160. *Reviews:* Kemmitt, Sharp, *Adv. Fluorine Chem.* **4**, 247-248 (1965); Stein, "Physical and Chemical Properties of Halogen Fluorides" in *Halogen Chemistry* **Vol. 1**, V. Gutmann, Ed. (Academic Press, New York, 1967) pp 133-224; Meinert, *Z. Chem.* **7**, 41-57 (1967).

Liquid. mp 9.43°. bp 100.5°. d^{25} 3.19. Thermodynamic data: Osborne *et al., J. Chem. Phys.* **54**, 3790 (1971). *Fumes in air!* Attacks glass, especially when hot. Violent reaction with water. Organic compds carbonize on contact, sometimes with conflagration. Instant reaction with S, P, Si, Bi, W, As, usually with incandescence.

USE: Mild fluorinating agent.

5019. Iodine Pentoxide. [12029-98-0] Iodic anhydride. I_2O_5; mol wt 333.81. I 76.03%, O 23.96%. Prepd by thermal dehydration of iodic acid at 195°: Lamb *et al., J. Am. Chem. Soc.* **42**, 1644 (1920). Crystal structure: Selte, Kjekshus, *Acta Chem. Scand.* **24**, 1912 (1970).

Needle shaped, hygroscopic crystals (an impure product may have a pink cast). d^{25} 5.08. Decompn into I_2 and O_2 begins at 275° and proceeds rapidly at 350°. Very sol in water (187.4 g/100 ml at 13°) forming HIO_3. Insol in abs alc, ether, chloroform, carbon disulfide. Dissolves in nitric acid from which it crystallizes as I_2O_5 if the HNO_3 concn is >50%. Strong oxidizing agent, may detonate when triturated with oxidizable matter. *Keep well closed and protected from light.*

USE: Oxidizes carbon monoxide to carbon dioxide with the formn of iodine (Ditte's reaction, which proceeds rapidly at 65° or above, but slowly at room temp). This reaction is used in gas analysis and for removing carbon monoxide from the air (in respirators preferably in presence of some H_2SO_4).

5020. Iodine Trichloride. [865-44-1] Cl_3I; mol wt 233.26. Cl 45.60%, I 54.40%. ICl_3. Prepd by adding finely powdered iodine to an excess of liq chlorine, which is then boiled away: Thomas, Depuis, *Compt. Rend.* **143**, 282 (1906); Booth, Morris, *Inorg. Synth.* **1**, 167 (1939). Alternate process: Birk, *Angew. Chem.* **41**, 751 (1928); *Z. Anorg. Allg. Chem.* **172**, 399 (1928); Wilke-Dörfurt, Wolff, *ibid.* **185**, 333 (1930).

Long yellow or brownish needles or fluffy powder. Pungent, irritating odor. *Corrosive to human skin. Must be stored in well closed amber glass bottles, preferably in refrigerator.* d^{-4} 3.203. mp ~33°. Volatile at room temp. mp 101° at 16 atm (pressure of its satd vapor). A pressure of 1 atm is reached at 64°. Complete decompn into ICl and Cl_2 at 77°. Generally used as a 20 to 35% soln in concd HCl.

Caution: Concd solns are strongly irritating.

USE: Chlorinating and oxidizing agent.

THERAP CAT: Anti-infective (topical).

5021. Iodinin. [68-81-5] 1,6-Phenazinediol 5,10-dioxide; 1,5-dihydroxyphenazine *N,N'*-dioxide. $C_{12}H_8N_2O_4$; mol wt 244.20. C 59.02%, H 3.30%, N 11.47%, O 26.21%. Antibiotic pigment from *Chromobacterium iodinum:* Clemo, McIlwain, *J. Chem. Soc.* **1938**, 479; Hegedüs in *Emil Barell Jubilee Volume* (1946), p 388; from *Waksmania aerata* and *Pseudomonas iodinum:* Gerber, Lechevalier, *Biochemistry* **3**, 598 (1964). Structure: Clemo, Daglish, *J. Chem. Soc.* **1950**, 1481. Synthesis: Matsumura, Takeda, *Nippon Kagaku Zasshi* **81**, 515 (1960), *C.A.* **56**, 470a (1962). Biosynthetic studies on incorporation of shikimic acid, *q.v.,* into iodinin: U. Hollstein *et al., Tetrahedron Lett.* **1978**, 2987; R. B. Herbert *et al., J. Chem. Soc. Perkin Trans. 1* **1979**, 2411; T. Etherington *et al., ibid.* 2416.

Purple crystals with coppery sheen from chloroform, dec 236°. pK 12.5. Stable in acid, unstable in alkali. Sol in benzene, toluene, xylene, carbon disulfide, chloroform, ethyl acetate. Slightly sol in hot alc. Practically insol in cold alc, ether, acetic acid, petr ether, amyl alcohol. Insol in water. Sol in concd sulfuric acid and in glacial acetic acid with red color. Sol in NaOH solns giving brilliantly blue solns which deposit green crystals of the unstable sodium deriv.

5022. Iodipamide. [606-17-7] 3,3'-[(1,6-Dioxo-1,6-hexanediyl)diimino]bis[2,4,6-triiodobenzoic acid]; 3,3'-(adipoyldiimino)bis[2,4,6-triiodobenzoic acid]; *N,N'*-adipylbis(3-amino-2,4,6-triiodobenzoic acid); adipic acid di(3-carboxy-2,4,6-triiodoanilide); adipiodone; Cholografin; Cholospect. $C_{20}H_{14}I_6N_2O_6$; mol wt 1139.76. C 21.08%, H 1.24%, I 66.81%, N 2.46%, O 8.42%. Prepn: Priewe, Rutkowski, *US 2776241* (1957 to Schering AG); Kotler-Brajtburg *et al., Rocz. Chem.* **36**, 763 (1962), *C.A.* **58**, 5568a (1963). Purification: Cassebaum, Drux, **DD 33738** (1964), *C.A.* **63**, 11441b (1965). Pharmacology: E. Fischer, F. Varga, *Acta Physiol. Acad. Sci. Hung.* **38**, 135 (1970). Metabolic studies: Kiyono *et al., Radioisotopes* **20**, 78 (1971). Pharmacology and toxicity study: F. J. Rosenberg *et al., Invest. Radiol.* **15**, S142 (1980). Comprehensive description: H. H. Lerner, *Anal. Profiles Drug Subs.* **3**, 333-363 (1974).

Crystals, dec 306-308°. $n_D^{21.5}$ 1.3294 (c = 0.445 in methanol). Soly at 20°: methanol 0.8%; ethanol 0.3%; acetone 0.2%; ether 0.1%. Practically insol in water, benzene. LD_{50} in mice, rats (mg/kg): 2380 ±290, 4430 ±310 i.v. (Rosenberg).

Disodium salt. [2618-26-0] $C_{20}H_{12}I_6N_2Na_2O_6$. Prepd by dissolving the free acid in a dil aq soln of NaOH and buffering to pH 6.5- 7.7. Used as 20% soln.

Bis[*N*-methylglucamine] salt. [3521-84-4] Iodipamide meglumine; Biligrafin; Endocistobil; Endografin; Intrabilix; Transbilix. $C_{34}H_{48}I_6N_4O_{16}$; mol wt 1530.19. More sol in water than the disodium salt. Used as 40% soln.

THERAP CAT: Diagnostic aid (radiopaque medium—cholecystographic).

THERAP CAT (VET): Diagnostic aid (radiopaque medium).

5023. Iodixanol. [92339-11-2] 5,5'-[(2-Hydroxy-1,3-propanediyl)bis(acetylimino)]bis[*N,N'*-bis(2,3-dihydroxypropyl)-

2,4,6-triiodo-1,3-benzenedicarboxamide]; 5,5'-[(2-hydroxytrimethylene)bis(acetylimino)]bis[N,N'-bis(2,3-dihydroxypropyl)-2,4,6-triiodoisophthalamide]; 1,3-bis(acetylamino)-N,N'-bis[3,5-bis(2,3-dihydroxypropylaminocarbonyl)-2,4,6-triiodophenyl]-2-hydroxypropane; 2-5410-3A; Visipaque. $C_{35}H_{44}I_6N_6O_{15}$; mol wt 1550.18. C 27.12%, H 2.86%, I 49.12%, N 5.42%, O 15.48%. Nonionic, dimeric x-ray contrast medium. Prepn: P. E. Hansen et al., **EP 108638** (1984 to Nyegaard), C.A. **101**, 151599g (1984). HPLC determn in plasma: H. Nomura et al., J. Chromatogr. **572**, 333 (1991). Clinical pharmacokinetics: M. G. Svaland et al., Invest. Radiol. **27**, 130 (1992). Clinical studies in cerebral arteriography: Y. Palmers et al., Eur. J. Radiol. **17**, 203 (1993); in cardiac angiography: J. A. Hill et al., Am. J. Cardiol. **74**, 57 (1994); in urography: R. M. Conroy et al., Clin. Radiol. **49**, 337 (1994). Use as density gradient medium: T. Ford et al., Anal. Biochem. **220**, 360 (1994); J. Graham et al., ibid. 367.

mp 240-250°. Soluble in water. Viscosity (37°) 11.1 mPa; osmolality 290 mOsm/kg H_2O; pH 7.2-7.6 (c = 320 mgI/ml). 50% aqueous soln (w/v): viscosity 8.3 mPa; n 1.4128 ±0.0003; d 1.266 ±0.003; osmolality 200 ±5 mOsm. LD_{50} i.v. in mice: 21 gI/kg (Palmers).

THERAP CAT: Diagnostic aid (radiopaque medium).

5024. Iodized Oil. [8001-40-9] Lipiodol. An iodine addition product of vegetable oils, contg 38-42% organically combined iodine.

Thick, viscous, oily liq; alliaceous odor; oleaginous taste; dec on exposure to air and light, becoming brown. *Keep in small, nearly full containers, protected from light.*

THERAP CAT: Diagnostic aid (radiopaque medium).

THERAP CAT (VET): X-ray contrast medium.

5025. Iodoacetic Acid. [64-69-7] $C_2H_3IO_2$; mol wt 185.95. C 12.92%, H 1.63%, I 68.25%, O 17.21%. CH_2ICOOH. Prepd by treating chloroacetic acid in acetone soln with NaI.

Colorless or white crystals. mp 82-83°. Sol in water, alc; very slightly sol in ether.

5026. Iodoalphionic Acid. [577-91-3] 4-Hydroxy-3,5-diiodo-α-phenylbenzenepropanoic acid; β-(4-hydroxy-3,5-diiodophenyl)-α-phenylpropionic acid; 3,5-diiodo-α-phenylphloretic acid; Coletrast; Priodax; Pheniodol; Dikol; Iodobil; Jodobil; Biliognost; Tenicid; Biliselectan. $C_{15}H_{12}I_2O_3$; mol wt 494.06. C 36.47%, H 2.45%, I 51.37%, O 9.72%. Prepd by iodinating β-(4-hydroxyphenyl)-α-phenylpropionic acid with iodine in an aq soln of alkali iodide in the presence of NH_3 or with iodine in acetic anhydride as the iodinating agent, cf. **GB 559024** (1944), C.A. **40**, 1883 (1946). Prepn of optically active forms: Tullar, Hoppe, US **2552696** (1951 to Sterling Drug). Toxicity data: J. O. Hoppe, S. Archer, Am. J. Roentgenol. Radium Ther. **69**, 630 (1953).

dl-Form. Faintly yellowish powder. dec 157-162°. Crystals from acetic acid, mp 163.5-163.8°. Insol in water. Sol in alcohol, ether, alkali carbonate and in alkali hydroxide solns; slightly sol in benzene and chloroform. Forms a water-sol disodium salt. LD_{50} in mice (g/kg): 3.8 orally (Hoppe, Archer).

l-Form. Hydrated crystals, mp 80-85°, $[\alpha]_D^{25}$ −59° (c = 1.5 in 95% alcohol).

l-Form disodium salt. mp >230°, $[\alpha]_D^{26}$ −56.6° (c = 1.5 in water).

d-Form. Hydrated crystals, mp 80-85°, $[\alpha]_D^{25}$ +59° (c = 1.5 in 95% alcohol).

d-Form disodium salt. mp >230°, $[\alpha]_D^{26}$ +56.6° (c = 1.5 in water).

THERAP CAT: Diagnostic aid (radiopaque medium —cholecystographic).

5027. p-Iodoaniline. [540-37-4] C_6H_6NI; mol wt 219.02. C 32.90%, H 2.76%, N 6.40%, I 57.94%.

White crystals. mp 67-68°. Slightly sol in water, freely in alcohol, chloroform, ether.

5028. o-Iodoanisole. [529-28-2] C_7H_7IO; mol wt 234.03. C 35.92%, H 3.01%, I 54.23%, O 6.84%. Prepd by diazotizing o-anisidine and decomposing the diazonium salt with KI.

Yellow liquid; darkens on exposure to air. d^{20} 1.80. bp_{730} 238-240°. Insol in water; miscible with alcohol, chloroform, ether. *Protect from light.*

5029. Iodobenzene. [591-50-4] C_6H_5I; mol wt 204.01. C 35.32%, H 2.47%, I 62.21%. Obtained by diazotizing aniline and then treating with aq soln of KI, or by the action of HNO_3 on a mixture of C_6H_6 and iodine.

Colorless liquid; rapidly becomes yellow; characteristic odor. d_4^{15} 1.8384. bp 188-189°. mp −30°. n_D^{18} 1.621. Insol in water; miscible with alcohol, chloroform, ether. *Protect from light.*

5030. o-Iodobenzoic Acid. [88-67-5] $C_7H_5IO_2$; mol wt 248.02. C 33.90%, H 2.03%, I 51.17%, O 12.90%. C_6H_4ICOOH. Prepd by diazotizing o-aminobenzoic acid and treating the resulting diazonium compound with aq KI.

White needles. d 2.25. mp 162°. Sparingly sol in water; sol in alcohol, ether.

5031. Iodochlorhydroxyquin. [130-26-7] 5-Chloro-7-iodo-8-quinolinol; 5-chloro-8-hydroxy-7-iodoquinoline; chloroiodoquin; iodochlorohydroxyquinoline; iodochloroxyquinoline; clioquinol; Amebil; Alchloquin; Amoenol; Bactol; Barquinol; Budoform; Chinoform; Cliquinol; Eczecidin; Enteroquinol; Entero-Septol; Enterozol; Entrokin; Hi-Enterol; Iodoenterol; Nioform; Quinambicide; Rometin; Vioform. C_9H_5ClINO; mol wt 305.50. C 35.38%, H 1.65%, Cl 11.60%, I 41.54%, N 4.58%, O 5.24%. Prepn: **DE 117767** (1899 to Ciba); **US 641491** (1900); A. Das, S. L. Mukherji, J. Org. Chem. **22**, 1111 (1957). Toxicity study: Davis et al., Am. J. Trop. Med. **24**, 29 (1944). Comprehensive description: G. Padmanabhan et al., Anal. Profiles Drug Subs. **18**, 57-90 (1989).

Brownish-yellow, bulky powder. Practically odorless. Dec ~178-179°. uv max (water/conc. HCl): 266 nm ($A_{1cm}^{1\%}$ 990); (0.1N methanolic NaOH): 269 nm ($A_{1cm}^{1\%}$ 1120); (ethanol): 255 nm ($A_{1cm}^{1\%}$ 1570). One part dissolves in 43 parts of boiling alc, 128 parts chloroform, 17 parts of boiling ethyl acetate, 170 parts of cold acetic acid, 13 parts of boiling acetic acid. Almost insol in water, cold alc, ether. Soly at room temp (mg/ml): water <0.01, methanol 1.9, ethanol 1.3, ether 5.4, chloroform 14.9, 0.1N NaOH 17.3, 0.1N

Consult the Name Index before using this section.

HCl 0.02, acetonitrile between 1.7-2.5, tetrahydrofuran between 20-100, ethyl acetate between 6.7-10, carbon disulfide between 10-20, dimethyl sulfoxide between 20-100, dimethyl acetamide between 20-100. Darkens upon exposure to light. LD_{50} orally in cats: 400 mg/kg (Davis).

Caution: Has been linked with the occurrence of subacute myelooptic neuropathy (S.M.O.N. syndrome) in Japan, T. Tsubaki *et al.,* *Lancet* **1,** 696 (1971); *see also ibid.* **1,** 534 (1977); J. Tateishi in *Drug-Induced Sufferings* T. Soda, Ed. (Excerpta Medica, New York, 1980) pp 464-472.

THERAP CAT: Anti-infective (topical); antiamebic.

THERAP CAT (VET): Has been used as an intestinal anti-infective.

5032. Iodofenphos. [18181-70-9] Phosphorothioic acid *O*-(2,5-dichloro-4-iodophenyl) *O,O*-dimethyl ester; *O*-(2,5-dichloro-4-iodophenyl) *O,O*-dimethyl phosphorothioate; C-9491; Nuvanol N. $C_8H_8Cl_2IO_3PS$; mol wt 413.00. C 23.27%, H 1.95%, Cl 17.17%, I 30.73%, O 11.62%, P 7.50%, S 7.76%. Organophosphorous insecticide with stomach and contact activity. Prepn: E. Beriger *et al.,* **ZA 6506107**; *eidem,* **US 3468984** (1965, 1969 both to Ciba). Metabolism and anti-cholinesterase activity: F. R. Johannsen, C. O. Knowles, *J. Econ. Entomol.* **63,** 693 (1970). GLC determn in cattle urine and tissues: M. C. Ivey, D. D. Oehler, *J. Agric. Food Chem.* **24,** 1049 (1976). Crystal and molecular structure: R. G. Baughman, P.-J. Yu, *ibid.* **30,** 293 (1982). Use to control flies and ticks in cattle: R. O. Drummond *et al., J. Econ. Entomol.* **65,** 1354 (1972). *Review:* B. C. Haddow, T. G. Marks, *Proc. 5th Br. Insectic. Fungic. Conf.* **2,** 531 (1970).

Pale yellow oil, solidifies to crystals, mp 72-73° (Beriger). Also reported as white crystals, mp 75° (Haddow). Sol in acetone, xylene. Slightly sol in alcohol. Soly in water: <2 ppm. LD_{50} in rats, female mice (mg/kg): 2100, >10000, orally (Haddow, Marks).

USE: Insecticide.

THERAP CAT (VET): Ectoparasiticide.

5033. Iodoform. [75-47-8] Triiodomethane. CHI_3; mol wt 393.73. C 3.05%, H 0.26%, I 96.69%. Prepn from acetone, sodium hypochlorite, potassium iodide, and sodium hydroxide: Glass, *Q. J. Pharm. Pharmacol.* **8,** 351 (1935); from chloroform + methyl iodide: Soroos, Hinkamp, *J. Am. Chem. Soc.* **67,** 1642 (1945); by electrolysis: Glasstone, *Ind. Chem.* **7,** 315 (1931). Description of the iodoform reaction: Seelye, Turney, *J. Chem. Educ.* **36,** 572 (1959). Toxicity study: Kutob, Plaa, *Toxicol. Appl. Pharmacol.* **4,** 354 (1962).

Yellow powder or crystals; mp ~120°; dec at high temp with evolution of iodine. Unctuous touch; characteristic, disagreeable odor. Volatile with steam. d 4.1. Very slightly sol in water. One gram dissolves in 60 ml cold alcohol, 16 ml boiling alcohol, 10 ml chloroform, 7.5 ml ether, 80 ml glycerol, 3 ml carbon disulfide, 34 ml olive oil; freely sol in benzene, acetone, slightly sol in petr ether. LD_{50} s.c. in mice: 1.6 mmoles/kg (Kutob, Plaa).

Caution: Potential symptoms of overexposure are irritation of eyes and skin; lightheadedness, dizziness, nausea, incoordination, CNS depression; dyspnea; liver, kidney and heart damage; visual disturbances. *See NIOSH Pocket Guide to Chemical Hazards* (DHHS/NIOSH 97-140, 1997) p 172.

THERAP CAT: Anti-infective (topical).

THERAP CAT (VET): Antiseptic, disinfectant for superficial lesions and in the female reproductive tract.

5034. *o*-Iodohippurate Sodium. [133-17-5] *N*-(2-Iodobenzoyl)glycine monosodium salt; sodium *o*-iodohippurate; Hippodin; Jodairol. $C_9H_7INNaO_3$; mol wt 327.05. C 33.05%, H 2.16%, I 38.80%, N 4.28%, Na 7.03%, O 14.68%. "Contains not less than 38.5% nor more than 39% iodine, when calcd to the dried substance." Prepd by the condensation of *o*-iodobenzoic acid with

glycine, and treatment with NaOH soln: A. P. Sachs, **US 2135474** (1938 to Zonite Prods.). Diagnostic use in post-transplant renography: H. Huland, K. Bischoff, *J. Urol.* **129,** 925 (1983); J.-I. D. Jorgensen, J. Ladefoged, *Dan. Med. Bull.* **34,** 50 (1987).

Dihydrate. Crystals. Freely sol in water; sol in alcohol and in dil solns of alkalies. An aq soln is neutral or faintly alkaline to litmus.

^{131}**I-Labeled form.** [881-17-4] Hippuran I 131; Hipputope.

^{123}**I-Labeled form.** [56254-07-0] Nephroflow.

THERAP CAT: Diagnostic aid (radiopaque medium); labeled form as diagnostic aid (radioactive imaging agent).

5035. *o*-Iodophenol. [533-58-4] C_6H_5IO; mol wt 220.01. C 32.75%, H 2.29%, I 57.68%, O 7.27%. Prepd by the action of iodine on *o*-chloromercuriphenol in chloroform: Whitmore, Hanson, *Org. Synth.* **4,** 37 (1925).

Plates from ligroin, mp 43°. d^{80} 1.8757. bp_{160} 186-187°. Sol in alcohol, ether, chloroform, carbon disulfide, benzene; fairly sol in hot water.

5036. *p*-Iodophenol. [540-38-5] C_6H_5IO; mol wt 220.01. C 32.75%, H 2.29%, I 57.68%, O 7.27%. Obtained by action of iodine in alkaline KI upon phenol; or by diazotization of *p*-aminophenol and subsequent replacement of the diazonium group by iodine.

White or reddish crystals; characteristic odor. mp 93-94°. Slightly sol in water, freely in alc, ether. *Protect from light.*

Note: The designation "phenol iodide", or more properly "iodized phenol", is applied to a soln of 1 part iodine in 4 parts phenol.

5037. Iodophors. Tamed Iodine. The term iodophor may be applied to any product in which surface active agents (such as nonoxynol, *q.v.*) or polymers (such as polyvinylpyrrolidone, *cf.* povidone-iodine) act as carriers and solubilizing agents for iodine. Other examples: *Biopal CVL-10; Dermevan; Idonyx; Iobac; Ioprep; Iosan; Kleenodyne; Rhudane; Showersan; Wescodyne; Westamine X.* An iodophor usually enhances the bactericidal activity of iodine, reduces vapor pressure and odor. Staining is almost nonexistent and wide dilution with water is possible. Examples of prepn: Shelanski, Winicov, **US 2710277** (1955 to West Labs); Scheib *et al.,* **US 2977315** (1961 to Lazarus Labs). Germicidal activity: C. A. Lawrence *et al., J. Am. Pharm. Assoc.* **46,** 500 (1957). Reviews of manufacture, properties and use: D. R. Batey, *Aust. J. Dairy Technol.* **31,** 5-7 (1976); A. Leitmanova *et al., Pharmazie* **42,** 809-813 (1987).

USE: Germicide.

THERAP CAT: Antiseptic; disinfectant.

THERAP CAT (VET): Antiseptic; disinfectant.

5038. Iodophthalein Sodium. [2217-44-9] Soluble iodophthalein; tetraiodophenolphthalein sodium; T.I.P.P.S.; tetraiodophthalein sodium; tetiothalein sodium; Iodeikon; Cholepulvis; Keraphen; Shadocol; Bilitrast; Iodognost; Stipolac; Tetraiode; Foriod; Iodtetragnost; Antinosin; Cholumbrin; Iodorayoral; Opacin; Photobiline; Piliophen; Videophel; Radiotetrane; Nosophene sodium; Iodophene sodium. $C_{20}H_8I_4Na_2O_4$; mol wt 865.87. C 27.74%, H 0.93%, I 58.63%, Na 5.31%, O 7.39%. Isomeric with phentetiothalein sodium, *q.v.* Prepd by the action of iodine (in KI soln) on phenolphthalein in aq alk soln: Classen, Löb, *Ber.* **28,** 1603 (1895); **DE 85930** (1894); **DE 88390** (1895). Also obtained by treating an alk soln of phenolphthalein with iodine monochloride: Kalle, **DE**

143596 (1900). Prepn of free acid: Orndorff, Mahood, *J. Am. Chem. Soc.* **40**, 937 (1918). Toxicity data: J. O. Hoppe *et al., J. Med. Chem.* **13**, 997 (1970). Metabolism in rabbits: D. Pitre, L. Fumagalli, *Farmaco Ed. Sci.* **32**, 76 (1977).

Trihydrate. Pale-blue to violet crystals. Saline and astringent taste. Somewhat hygroscopic. Gradually decomp on exposure to air due to absorption of CO_2 and becomes incompletely sol. One g dissolves in about 7 ml water, forming a clear, deep-blue dichroic soln. Slightly sol in alc. *Keep well closed.* LD_{50} in mice (mg/kg): 360 i.v., 3800 orally (Hoppe).

Free acid. [386-17-4] Iodophthalein; tetraiodophthalein; Iodophene; Nosophen. $C_{20}H_{10}I_4O_4$; mol wt 821.91. Light-yellow, odorless, tasteless powder; dec at about 200°. Practically insol in water. Slightly sol in alcohol; sol in alkalies, chloroform, ether.

THERAP CAT: Diagnostic aid (radiopaque medium—cholecystographic).

5039. Iodopsin. [1415-94-7] One of 3 visual pigments found in retinal cone cells. Absorption maximum approx 560 nm. Biological activity is similar to that of rhodopsin, *q.v.* Composed of the chromophore, 11-*cis* retinal, *q.v.*, bound to photopsin, the specific protein component of cone pigments. (*See* Opsins). Isoln from chicken retinas: G. Wald, *Nature* **140**, 545 (1937). Prepn from 11-*cis* retinal and opsin: G. Wald *et al., J. Gen. Physiol.* **38**, 623 (1955). Methods for purification, prepn, and assay: R. Hubbard *et al., Methods Enzymol.* **18**, 615-653 (1971). Exposure to light initiates the conversion of iodopsin through a series of distinct intermediates to yield opsin and *trans*-retinal. Photochemistry: R. Hubbard, A. Kropf, *Nature* **183**, 448 (1959); T. Yoshizawa, G. Wald, *ibid.* **214**, 566 (1967). Studies on the iodopsin binding site: H. Matsumoto *et al., Biochim. Biophys. Acta* **404**, 300 (1975). Three distinct pigments are responsible for color vision: W. B. Marks *et al., Science* **143**, 1181 (1964); P. K. Brown, G. Wald, *ibid.* **144**, 45 (1964). The variation in the absorption maximum of the 3 pigments is regulated by differences in the apoprotein portion of the molecule: R. Hubbard, L. Sperling, *Exp. Eye Res.* **17**, 581 (1973); B. Honig *et al., J. Am. Chem. Soc.* **101**, 7084 (1979). *Reviews:* G. Wald, *Science* **162**, 230-239 (1968); H. Matsumoto, T. Yoshizawa, *Methods Enzymol.* **81**, 154-160 (1982). General review of the visual process: P. S. Zurer, *Chem. Eng. News* **61**, 24-35 (Nov. 28, 1983).

5040. Iodopyracet. [300-37-8] 3,5-Diiodo-4-oxo-1(4*H*)-pyridineacetic acid compound with 2,2′-iminobis[ethanol] (1:1); bis(hydroxyethyl)ammonium 3,5-diiodo-4-pyridone-*N*-acetate; diethanolamine 3,5-diiodo-4-pyridone-*N*-acetate; 3,5-diiodo-4-pyridone-*N*-acetic acid diethanolamine salt; diodone; RP-3203; Diatrast; Diodrast; Iopyracil; Nosylan; Neo-Methiodal; Neo-Skiodan; Neo-Tenebryl; Nosydrast; Oparenol; Per-Abrodil; Per-Radiographol; Pyelosil; Pylumbrin; Savac; Umbradil; Uriodone; Vasiodone; Xumbradil. $C_{11}H_{16}I_2N_2O_5$; mol wt 510.06. C 25.90%, H 3.16%, I 49.76%, N 5.49%, O 15.68%. Prepn: **FR 728634** (1931 to I. G. Farbenhind AG); J. Reitmann, **US 1993039** (1935 to Winthrop). Pharmacology, toxicology and radiographic studies: R. St. A. Heathcote, R. A. Gardner, *Br. J. Radiol.* **6**, 304 (1933). HPLC determn in biological fluids: P. Hekman, C. A. M. Van Ginneken, *J. Chromatogr.* **182**, 492 (1980).

Odorless powder, dec 155-157°. Soly: about 36% in water; about 12% in methanol, much less sol in ice-cold methanol. Practically insol in acetone, ether, chloroform. pH of aq solns: 5 to 8, depending on concn. 3,5-Diiodo-4-pyridone-*N*-acetic acid separated by pptn with dil HCl and dried at 100°, mp 245-249°, and contains not less than 61.5% and not more than 63.5% iodine: *N.F. XI.*

Iodopyracet Injection. 35% (w/v) soln of the diethanolamine salt of 3,5-diiodo-4-pyridone-*N*-acetic acid. Contains about 22% I (w/v). d_4^{25} 1.185. Neutral to litmus.

Iodopyracet Concentrated Solution. Diodrast Concentrated Solution. 70% soln (w/v) of the diethanolamine salt of 3,5-diiodo-4-pyridone-*N*-acetic acid. Contains about 44% I (w/v). Neutral to litmus.

Iodopyracet Compound Solution. Diodrast Compound Solution. Soln contg approx 40.5% (w/v) of the diethanolamine salt and approx 9.5% (w/v) of the diethylamine salt of 3,5-diiodo-4-pyridone-*N*-acetic acid. Contains about 25% I. Neutral to litmus. d_4^{25} 1.270.

THERAP CAT: Diagnostic aid (radiopaque medium—urographic).

THERAP CAT (VET): Diagnostic aid (radiopaque medium).

5041. Iodopyrrole. [87-58-1] 2,3,4,5-Tetraiodo-1*H*-pyrrole; Iodol. C_4HI_4N; mol wt 570.68. C 8.42%, I 88.95%, N 2.45%. Prepd by iodination of pyrrole: Potts, *J. Chem. Soc.* **1953**, 3711; Treibs, Kolm, *Ann.* **614**, 176 (1958). Isoln from shale-oil naphtha: Janssen *et al., J. Am. Chem. Soc.* **73**, 4040 (1951).

Needles from ethanol, dec 162-164°, also reported as dec 150-160° and 140-150°. One gram dissolves in 4900 ml water, 9 ml alcohol. 1.5 ml ether, 105 ml chloroform, 155 ml glycerol; sol in fixed oils.

THERAP CAT: Antiseptic (local).

THERAP CAT (VET): Antiseptic, disinfectant for superficial lesions and in the female reproductive tract.

5042. Iodoquinol. [83-73-8] 5,7-Diiodo-8-quinolinol; diiodohydroxyquin; diiodo-oxyquinoline; 5,7-diiodo-8-hydroxyquinoline; SS-578; Diodoquin; Disoquin; Floraquin; Dyodin; Dinoleine; Searlequin; Diodoxylin; Rafamebin; Ioquin; Direxiode; Stanquinate; Yodoxin; Zoaquin; Enterosept; Embequin. $C_9H_5I_2NO$; mol wt 396.95. C 27.23%, H 1.27%, I 63.94%, N 3.53%, O 4.03%. Prepd by the action of iodine monochloride on 8-hydroxyquinoline: Papesch, Burtner, *J. Am. Chem. Soc.* **58**, 1314 (1936); by the action of KIO_3 on 8-hydroxyquinoline: Zeifman, *C.A.* **34**, 3745. Electrolytic prepn: Brown, Berkowitz, *Trans. Electrochem. Soc.* **75**, 385 (1939). *See also* Claus, **DE 78880**; Passek, **DE 411050**; Matsumura, *C.A.* **21**, 1461 (1927); Pirrone, Cherubino, *C.A.* **28**, 3073 (1934).

Crystals from xylene. The medicinal grade is a yellowish-brown powder. mp 200-215° (extensive decompn). Almost insol in water. Sparingly sol in alcohol, ether, and acetone; sol in hot pyridine and in hot dioxane.

THERAP CAT: Antiamebic.

5043. *N*-Iodosaccharin. [86340-94-5] 2-Iodo-1,2-benziso-thiazol-3(2*H*)-one 1,1-dioxide; NISac. $C_7H_4INO_3S$; mol wt 309.08. C 27.20%, H 1.30%, I 41.06%, N 4.53%, O 15.53%, S 10.37%. Iodination reagent. Prepn: M. Papadopoulou, A. Varvoglis, *J. Chem. Res. Synop.* **1983**, 66. Synthesis and use for iodination of aromatics and alkenes: D. Dolenc, *Synlett* **2000**, 544. As an activator of thioglycosides: M. Aloui, A. J. Fairbanks, *ibid.* **2001**, 797; *eidem, Chem. Commun.* **2001**, 1406. Iodination of enol acetates and diones: D. Dolenc, *Synth. Commun.* **33**, 2917 (2003); of isatins: S. P. L. de Souza *et al., Heterocycl. Commun.* **9**, 31 (2003).

Crystallizes in small pale yellow crystals as the monohydrate, mp 206-208°. Reprecipitation from THF, then drying produces a white powder which can be stored indefinitely in a dark freezer. pKa: 1.30. Sol in common organic solvents (better in more polar ones such as acetone, acetonitrile). Insol in water.

USE: Iodination reagent; activator of thioglycosides.

5044. Iodosobenzene. [536-80-1] Iodosylbenzene; PhIO. C_6H_5IO; mol wt 220.01. C 32.75%, H 2.29%, I 57.68%, O 7.27%. Versatile oxidizing agent. Prepn: C. Willgerodt, *Ber.* **26**, 357 (1893). Synthesis: H. Saltzman, J. G. Sharefkin, *Org. Synth.* **5**, 658 (1973). Mechanistic study: R. M. Moriarty *et al., J. Am. Chem. Soc.* **103**, 686 (1981). Use as oxidant: S. Mukerjee *et al., ibid.* **119**, 8097 (1997); G. Mielniczak, A. Lopusinski, *Synlett* **2001**, 505; as mediator: P. Dauban *et al., J. Am. Chem. Soc.* **123**, 7707 (2001); C.-C. Guo *et al., Appl. Catal. A* **230**, 53 (2002). Brief review: A. Minatti, *Synlett* **2003**, 140-141.

Yellowish amorphous powder. *Explosive* if heated to 210° due to disproportion into phenyliodide and iodylbenzene.

USE: Oxygen transfer reagent for stiochiometric or catalytic cross-functionalization of alkenes, alcohols, sulfides, and organometallo compds.

5045. N-Iodosuccinimide. [516-12-1] Succiniodimide; NIS. $C_4H_4INO_2$; mol wt 224.98. C 21.35%, H 1.79%, I 56.41%, N 6.23%, O 14.22%. Prepd by iodination of silver succinimide: Djerassi, Lenk, *J. Am. Chem. Soc.* **75**, 3493 (1953). Structural studies: K. Padmanabhan *et al., Acta Crystallogr.* **C46**, 88 (1990). Use as synthetic reagent for cysteine peptides: H. Shih, *J. Org. Chem.* **58**, 3003 (1993); in oxidation and halogenation reactions: A. Speicher, T. Eicher, *J. Prakt. Chem.* **340**, 278 (1998).

Needles from dioxane + carbon tetrachloride. mp 200-201°. Sol in acetone, methanol; moderately sol in dioxane. Practically insol in CCl_4, ether. Dec in water. *Protect from light.*

Caution: Avoid contact with skin and mucous membranes.

USE: Iodination of ketones and aldehydes.

5046. Iodosulfuron-methyl-sodium. [144550-36-7] 4-Iodo-2-[[[[(4-methoxy-6-methyl-1,3,5-triazin-2-yl)amino]carbonyl]amino]sulfonyl]benzoic acid methyl ester monosodium salt; methyl 4-iodo-2-[3-(4-methoxy-6-methyl-1,3,5-triazin-2-yl)ureido-sulfonyl]benzoate sodium salt; AE-F115008. $C_{14}H_{13}IN_5NaO_6S$; mol wt 529.24. C 31.77%, H 2.48%, I 23.98%, N 13.23%, Na 4.34%, O 18.14%, S 6.06%. Sulfonylurea herbicide for post-emergence use in cereals; acetolactate synthase inhibitor. Prepn: O. Ort *et al., WO 9213845; eidem, US 5688745* (1992, 1997 both to Hoechst). Comprehensive description and use with the safener, mefenpyr-diethyl: E. Hacker *et al., Brighton Crop Prot. Conf. - Weeds* **1999**, 15-22. Field trials in wheat: H. L. Crooks *et al., Weed Technol.* **18**, 93 (2004).

Almost colorless to light beige crystalline powder, mp 152°. Vapor pressure (25°): 6.7×10^{-9} Pa. Soly in water at 20° (g/l): 0.16 (pH 5); 25 (pH 7); 65 (pH 9). Log P (octanol/water): 1.07 (pH 5); -0.70 (pH 7); -1.22 (pH 9). LD_{50} in rats (mg/kg): 2678 orally; >2000 dermally (Hacker).

Combination with mefenpyr-diethyl. Husar; Hussar.

USE: Herbicide.

5047. 3-Iodotyrosine. [70-78-0] Monoiodotyrosine. $C_9H_{10}INO_3$; mol wt 307.09. C 35.20%, H 3.28%, I 41.32%, N 4.56%, O 15.63%. Prepn of L-form: Hillman, Hillman-Elies, *Z. Physiol. Chem.* **305**, 177 (1956); Pitt-Rivers, *Chem. Ind. (London)* **1956**, 21. Prepn of L- and DL-form: Harington, Rivers, *Biochem. J.* **38**, 320 (1944).

L-Form. Crystals from water, dec 204-206°. $[\alpha]_D^{20}$ -4.4° (c = 5 in 1N HCl). Dissolves in 15 parts boiling water.

DL-Form monohydrate. Crystals from water, dec 200-201°.

5048. o-Iodoxybenzoic Acid. [64297-64-9]; [61717-82-6] (cyclic tautomer). 2-Iodylbenzoic acid; 1-hydroxy-1,2-benzio-doxol-3(1H)-one 1-oxide; IBX; 2-iodoxybenzoic acid. $C_7H_5IO_4$; mol wt 280.02. C 30.02%, H 1.80%, I 45.32%, O 22.85%. Hypervalent 10-I-4 iodine reagent; cyclic tautomer is the predominant molecular structure. Prepn: C. Hartmann, V. Meyer, *Ber.* **26**, 1727 (1893); F. R. Greenbaum, *Am. J. Pharm.* **108**, 17 (1936); and conversion to stable 12-I-5 periodinanes: D. B. Dess, J. C. Martin, *J. Am. Chem. Soc.* **113**, 7277 (1991). Improved prepn: M. Frigerio *et al., J. Org. Chem.* **64**, 4537 (1999). Prepn of a stabilized, nonexplosive formulation: D. Depernet, B. Francois, *US 6462227* (2002 to Simafex). IR analysis: R. Bell, K. J. Morgan, *J. Chem. Soc.* **1960**, 1209. Crystal structure: J. Z. Gougoutas, *Acta Crystallogr.* **10**, 489 (1981). ^{13}C NMR analysis: A. R. Katritzky *et al., Magn. Reson. Chem.* **27**, 1007 (1989). Oxidizing properties and reaction conditions: M. Frigerio *et al., J. Org. Chem.* **60**, 7272 (1995). Kinetics and mechanism of oxidation reactions: S. De Munari *et al., ibid.* **61**, 9272 (1996). Characterization of crystallographic forms: P. J. Stevenson *et al., J. Chem. Soc. Perkin Trans. 2* **1997**, 589. Brief review of chemistry: T. Wirth, *Angew. Chem. Int. Ed.* **40**, 2812-2814 (2001).

White crystalline solid, mp 233° (dec). Virtually insol in common organic solvents; insol in water. Soly in DMSO: 1.5 M. Sol in aq pyridine, aq sodium hydroxide (dec).

Caution: Explosive under impact or heating >200°: J. B. Plumb, D. J. Harper, *Chem. Eng. News* **68**, 3 (July 16, 1990).

USE: Mild, chemoselective, environmentally friendly oxidizing agent. In prepn of Dess-Martin periodinane, *q.v.*

5049. Iofetamine ^{123}**I.** [75917-92-9] 4-(Iodo-^{123}I)-α-methyl-N-(1-methylethyl)benzeneethanamine; (±)-p-iodo-^{123}I-N-iso-propyl-α-methylphenethylamine; [^{123}I](±)-N-isopropyl-p-iodoamphetamine. $C_{12}H_{18}{}^{123}IN$. Lipid soluble radioactive brain imaging agent. Prepn: R. M. Baldwin *et al.*, **EP 11858** (1980 to Hoffmann-La Roche); *eidem*, **US 4360511** (1982 to Medi-Physics). Detailed synthesis: L. Carlsen, K. Andresen, *Eur. J. Nucl. Med.* **7**, 280 (1982). Modified synthesis for improved yields: A. Najafi, *J. Labelled Compd. Radiopharm.* **24**, 1167 (1987). Preparative HPLC purification: J. Mertens *et al.*, *Nucl. Med. Commun.* **5**, 705 (1984). Brain uptake and localization: H. S. Winchell *et al.*, *J. Nucl. Med.* **21**, 940 (1980); H. S. Winchell *et al.*, *ibid.* 947. Distribution kinetics in animals: P. Som *et al.*, *Int. J. Nucl. Med. Biol.* **12**, 185 (1985); in humans: B. L. Holman *et al.*, *J. Nucl. Med.* **25**, 25 (1984). Diagnostic use for cerebral function in Alzheimer's disease: K. A. Johnson *et al.*, *Arch. Neurol.* **45**, 392 (1988). Reviews of radiopharmaceutical production and diagnostic use with single photon emission computed tomography (SPECT) imaging: M. B. Cohen *et al.*, *Appl. Radiat. Isot.* **37**, 749-763 (1986); of diagnostic applications in stroke: C. H. Park *et al.*, *RadioGraphics* **8**, 305-326 (1988); of metabolism and kinetics: R. M. Baldwin, J.-L. Wu, *J. Nucl. Med.* **29**, 122-124 (1988).

bp$_{0.05}$ 91-92°. Also reported as bp$_{0.6}$ 98-99° (Najafi).
Hydrochloride. [85068-76-4] IMP; ^{123}I labeled IMP; ^{123}I-M123; Perfusamine; Spectamine. $C_{12}H_{18}{}^{123}IN.HCl$. Crystals from ether, mp 156-158°.
THERAP CAT: Diagnostic aid (radioactive imaging agent).

5050. Ioflupane ^{123}I. [155798-07-5] [1*R*-(*exo,exo*)]-8-(3-Fluoropropyl)-3-[4-(iodo^{123}I)phenyl]-8-azabicyclo[3.2.1]octane-2-carboxylic acid methyl ester; *N*-(3-fluoropropyl)-2β-carbomethoxy-3β-(4-^{123}I-iodophenyl)nortropane; methyl 8-(3-fluoropropyl)-3β-(*p*-iodo-^{123}I-phenyl)-1α*H*,5α*H*-nortropane-2β-carboxylate; ^{123}I-FP-CIT; DaTSCAN. $C_{18}H_{23}FINO_2$; mol wt 431.28. C 50.13%, H 5.38%, F 4.41%, I 29.43%, N 3.25%, O 7.42%. Analog of cocaine, *q.v.*, that binds specifically to the dopamine transporters (DAT) in the membrane of the presynaptic dopaminergic neuron; designed as SPECT imaging agent to determine nigrostriatal neuronal integrity. Prepn: J. L. Neumeyer *et al.*, **US 5310912** (1994 to Research Biochemicals); *idem et al.*, *J. Med. Chem.* **37**, 1558 (1994). HPLC determn in biological fluids: K. A. Bergstroem *et al.*, *Hum. Psychopharmacol.* **11**, 483 (1996). Binding study: J. L. Neumeyer *et al.*, *J. Med. Chem.* **39**, 543 (1996). Clinical biodistribution: J. Booij *et al.*, *Eur. J. Nucl. Med.* **25**, 24 (1998). Clinical imaging for tremor differentiation: H. T. S. Benamer *et al.*, *Mov. Disord.* **15**, 503 (2000); for dementia differentiation: D. C. Costa *et al.*, *ibid.* **18**, Suppl. 7, S34 (2003). Functional imaging for dopaminergic deficit: H. T. S. Benamer *et al.*, *ibid.* **18**, 977 (2003). Clinical use in diagnosis of parkinsonism: A. M. Catafau *et al.*, *ibid.* **19**, 1175 (2004). Review of role in dopaminergic imaging: P. M. Kemp, *Nucl. Med. Commun.* **26**, 87-96 (2005).

mp 82-83°. $[\alpha]_D^{24}$ −12.8°.
THERAP CAT: Diagnostic aid (radioactive imaging agent).

5051. Ioglycamic Acid. [2618-25-9] 3,3'-[Oxybis[(1-oxo-2,1-ethanediyl)imino]]bis[2,4,6-triiodobenzoic acid]; 3,3'-[oxybis(methylenecarbonylimino)]bis[2,4,6-triiodobenzoic acid]; 3,3'-(diglycoloyldiimino)bis(2,4,6-triiodobenzoic acid); diglycolic acid bis(2,4,6-triiodo-3-carboxanilide); *N,N*-(oxydiacetyl)bis[3-amino-2,4,6-triiodobenzoic acid]. $C_{18}H_{10}I_6N_2O_7$; mol wt 1127.71. C 19.17%, H 0.89%, I 67.52%, N 2.48%, O 9.93%. Prepn: Priewe *et al.*, *Ber.* **87**, 651 (1954); Priewe, Rutkowski, **US 2776241**; **US 2853424** (1957, 1958 both to Schering AG).

Occurs in three cryst modifications: Neudert, Röpke, *Helv. Chim. Acta* **41**, 855 (1958). mp with baking at 222°, sintering at 227°, splitting of iodine at 245°, dec 281°.
Meglumine salt. [14317-18-1] Dimeglumine ioglycamide; Biligram. $C_{18}H_{10}I_6N_2O_7 \cdot 2(C_7H_{17}NO_5)$; mol wt 1518.14. Water soluble.
THERAP CAT: Diagnostic aid (radiopaque medium—cholecystographic).

5052. Iohexol. [66108-95-0] 5-[Acetyl(2,3-dihydroxypropyl)amino]-*N,N'*-bis(2,3-dihydroxypropyl)-2,4,6-triiodo-1,3-benzenedicarboxamide; *N,N'*-bis(2,3-dihydroxypropyl)-5-[*N*-(2,3-dihydroxypropyl)acetamido]-2,4,6-triiodoisophthalamide; Win-39424; Compd 545; Omnipaque. $C_{19}H_{26}I_3N_3O_9$; mol wt 821.14. C 27.79%, H 3.19%, I 46.36%, N 5.12%, O 17.54%. Nonionic radio-contrast medium. Prepn: V. Nordal, H. Holtermann, **DE 2726196**; *eidem*, **US 4250113** (1977, 1981 both to Nyegaard). HPLC-UV determn in plasma: R. S. Soman *et al.*, *J. Chromatogr. B* **816**, 339 (2005). Pharmacology and toxicology: *Acta Radiol. Suppl.* **362**, 1-134 (1980). Acute toxicity: S. Salvesen, *ibid.* **73**. Fibrillatory potential in dogs: G. L. Wolf *et al.*, *Invest. Radiol.* **16**, 320 (1981). Comparative clinical studies in coronary angiography: G. B. J. Mancini *et al.*, *Am. J. Cardiol.* **51**, 1218 (1983); I. D. Sullivan *et al.*, *Br. Heart J.* **51**, 643 (1984); M. A. Bettmann *et al.*, *Radiology* **153**, 583 (1984). *Review*: T. Almén, *Acta Radiol. Suppl.* **366**, 9-19 (1983).

Crystals from butanol, mp 174-180°. Sol in water. Stable in aqueous solutions. Viscosity (cP): 6.2 at 37°; 12.6 at 20° (c = 200 mg Iodine/ml). LD$_{50}$ in male, female rats, mice (g Iodine/kg): 15.0, 12.3, 24.3, 25.1 i.v. (Salvesen).
THERAP CAT: Diagnostic aid (radiopaque medium).

5053. Iomeglamic Acid. [25827-76-3] 5-[(3-Amino-2,4,6-triiodophenyl)methylamino]-5-oxopentanoic acid; 3'-amino-2',4',6'-triiodo-*N*-methylglutaranilic acid; *N*-methyl-*N*-(3-amino-2,4,6-triiodophenyl)glutaramic acid; *N*-methyl-*N*-(2,4,6-triiodo-3-aminophenyl)glutaramidic acid; RG-270; Falignost. $C_{12}H_{13}I_3N_2O_3$; mol wt 613.96. C 23.48%, H 2.13%, I 62.01%, N 4.56%, O 7.82%. Prepn: Cassebaum, Dierbach, **DD 67209** (1969), *C.A.* **72**, 66654j (1970). Biotransformation: Pfeifer *et al.*, *Pharmazie* **27**, 403 (1972). Pharmacology: H. Bekker *et al.*, *ibid.* 411. Clinical evaluation: Barke, *Zentralbl. Pharm. Pharmakother. Laboratoriumsdiagn.* **110**, 1117 (1971).

Yellow to brown crystals from acetic acid, mp 169°. Freely sol in DMF; slightly sol in ethanol, chloroform. Practically insol in water. LD$_{50}$ i.v. in mice: 500 mg/kg (Bekker).

THERAP CAT: Diagnostic aid (radiopaque medium—cholecystographic).

5054. Iomeprol. [78649-41-9] *N,N*'-Bis(2,3-dihydroxypropyl)-5-[(hydroxyacetyl)methylamino]-2,4,6-triiodo-1,3-benzenedicarboxamide; *N,N*'-bis(2,3-dihydroxypropyl)-2,4,6-triiodo-5-(*N*-methylglycolamido)isophthalamide; B-16880; Imeron; Iomeron. $C_{17}H_{22}I_3N_3O_8$; mol wt 777.09. C 26.28%, H 2.85%, I 48.99%, N 5.41%, O 16.47%. Nonionic x-ray contrast media. Prepn: E. Felder, D. Pitrè, **EP 026281**; *eidem*, **US 4352788** (1981, 1982 both to Bracco). HPLC determn in plasma and urine: V. Lorusso *et al., J. Chromatogr.* **525**, 401 (1990). Series of articles on properties, pharmacology, pharmacokinetics and clinical experience in angiography and urography: *Eur. J. Radiol.* **18**, Suppl. 1, S1-S124 (1994). Toxicology study: A. Morisetti *et al., ibid.* S21.

Crystalline powder, mp 285-291° (dec). Extremely sol in water, very sol in methanol, poorly sol in ethanol. Practically insol in chloroform. Aqueous soln of 150 mg I/ml: d_4^{20} 1.166, d_4^{37} 1.161; osmolality (37°) 0.27 osmol/kg H_2O; viscosity at 20° (mPa.s) 1.9, at 37° 1.3; n_D^{20} 1.3828. Aqueous soln of 300 mg I/ml: d_4^{20} 1.334, d_4^{37} 1.329; osmolality (37°) 0.52 osmol/kg H_2O; viscosity at 20° (mPa.s) 8.4, at 37° 4.8; n_D^{20} 1.4327. Aqueous soln of 400 mg I/ml: d_4^{20} 1.446, d_4^{37} 1.441; osmolality (37°) 0.72 osmol/kg H_2O; viscosity at 20° (mPa.s) 28.9, at 37° 13.9; n_D^{20} 1.4660. LD_{50} (400 mgI/ml soln) i.v. in mice, rats (gI/kg): 19.9, 14.5; LD_{50} (370 mgI/ml soln) i.v. in dogs (gI/kg): >12.5 (Morisetti).

THERAP CAT: Diagnostic aid (radiopaque medium).

5055. Ionic Liquids. Liquids composed entirely of ions; molten salts with melting points below 100°. Commonly consist of organic cations and inorganic anions. The cations most frequently used to generate ionic liquids are alkyl derivatives of imidazolium, pyridinium, ammonium and phosphonium. Early development: S. Sugden, H. Wilkins, *J. Chem. Soc.* **1929**, 1291. Environmental risk assessment: B. Jastorff *et al., Green Chem.* **5**, 136 (2003). Comprehensive description: R. D. Rogers, K. R. Seddon, Eds., *ACS Symp. Ser.* **818**, 1-474 (2002). Review of prepn, properties and uses in synthesis and catalysis: T. Welton, *Chem. Rev.* **99**, 2071-2083 (1999); P. Wasserscheid, W. Keim, *Angew. Chem. Int. Ed.* **39**, 3772-3789 (2000); of applications in organic synthesis: H. Zhao, S. V. Malhotra, *Aldrichim. Acta***35**, 75-83 (2002); of use as reaction media for catalytic reactions: R. Sheldon, *Chem. Commun.* **2001**, 2399-2407; for biocatalytic transformations: F. van Rantwijk *et al., Trends Biotechnol.* **21**, 131-138 (2003); of commercial uses: J. H. Davis, Jr., P. A. Fox, *Chem. Commun.* **2003**, 1209-1212.

Many are colorless, some are pale yellow to orange in color. No measurable vapor pressure. Thermally stable; many have liquid ranges of more than 300°. Dissolve a wide range of organic and inorganic compounds; soly of gases is generally good. Immisc with many organic solvents, forming biphasic systems.

USE: Highly polar, noncoordinating solvents with a broad range of green chemistry applications in organic synthesis and catalysis.

5056. Ionone. Irisone. $C_{13}H_{20}O$; mol wt 192.30. C 81.20%, H 10.48%, O 8.32%. Mixture in which the major constituents are *α*-ionone, *(E)-4-(2,6,6-trimethyl-2-cyclohexen-1-yl)-3-buten-2-one*, and *β*-ionone, *(E)-4-(2,6,6-trimethyl-1-cyclohexen-1-yl)-3-buten-2-one.* The latter is a key intermediate in the synthesis of vitamin A. Isoln from the volatile oil of *Boronia megastigma* Nees., *Rutaceae:* Naves, Parry, *Helv. Chim. Acta* **30**, 419 (1946). Prepn by condensing citral with acetone: Tiemann, Schmidt, *Ber.* **33**, 3703 (1900); Hibbert, Cannon, *J. Am. Chem. Soc.* **46**, 119 (1924); Krishna, Joshi, *J. Org. Chem.* **22**, 224 (1957). Prepn from isobutylene and vinyl methyl ketone: Pasedach, Seefelder, **DE 1000374** (1957 to BASF), *C.A.* **54**, 1595g (1960). Prepn

by cyclization of pseudoionone with H_2SO_4: Kimel *et al., J. Org. Chem.* **22**, 1611 (1957); Kaiser, Kimel, **US 2877271** (1959 to Hoffmann-La Roche). *Review:* Naves, *J. Soc. Cosmet. Chem.* **22**, 439 (1971).

α-Form   β-Form

Liquid. Odor reminiscent of cedar wood; in very dilute alcoholic soln it resembles the odor of violets. d_{25}^{25} 0.933-0.937. n_D^{20} 1.503-1.508. bp_{12} 126-128°. uv max: α-ionone 228.5 nm (ε 14300); β-ionone 293.5 nm (ε 8700). Miscible with abs alc. Soluble in 2 to 3 parts of 70% alcohol, ether, chloroform, benzene. Very slightly sol in water.

Caution: May cause allergic reactions, Shultheiss, *Dermatol. Wochenschr.* **135**, 629 (1967).

USE: In perfumery.

5057. Iopamidol. [60166-93-0] *N,N*'-Bis[2-hydroxy-1-(hydroxymethyl)ethyl]-5-[[(2S)-2-hydroxy-1-oxopropyl]amino]-2,4,6-triiodo-1,3-benzenedicarboxamide; *(S)-N,N*'-bis[2-hydroxy-1-(hydroxymethyl)ethyl]-2,4,6-triiodo-5-lactamidoisophthalamide; 5-(α-hydroxypropionylamino)-2,4,6-triiodoisophthalic acid di(1,3-dihydroxyisopropylamide); iomidol; B-15000; SQ-13396; Iopamiro; Iopamiron; Isovue; Jopamiro; Niopam; Solutrast. $C_{17}H_{22}I_3N_3O_8$; mol wt 777.09. C 26.28%, H 2.85%, I 48.99%, N 5.41%, O 16.47%. Nonionic radiocontrast medium. Prepn: E. Felder, D. Pitre, **DE 2547789**; *eidem*, **US 4001323** (1976, 1977 both to Savac). Physicochemical properties, preclinical studies: E. Felder *et al., Farmaco Ed. Sci.* **32**, 835 (1977). Determn of optical purity: *eidem, Farmaco Ed. Prat.* **32**, 3 (1982). *In vitro* effects: B. Schulze, H. K. Beyer, *Arzneim.-Forsch.* **31**, 1067 (1981). Development, initial testing: M. Sovak *et al., Radiology* **142**, 115 (1982). Clinical studies in angiography: A. J. Molyneux, P. W. Sheldon, *Br. J. Radiol.* **55**, 117 (1982); G. H. Whitehouse, S. L. Snowdon, *Clin. Radiol.* **33**, 231 (1982); in myelography: B. Drayer *et al., Am. J. Neuroradiol.* **3**, 59 (1982). Comprehensive description: E. Felder *et al., Anal. Profiles Drug Subs.* **17**, 115-154 (1988).

White, odorless cryst powder. Dec at about 300° without melting. $[\alpha]_D^{20}$ −2.01° (c = 10 in water). pKa (25°) 10.70. Very sol in water, methanol. Practically insol in chloroform. Miscible with boiling ethanol. LD_{50} in mice, rats, rabbits, dogs (g/kg): 44.5, 28.2, 19.6, 34.7 i.v. (Felder). Also reported as: LD_{50} in mice (mg iodine/kg body wt): 21,800 i.v.; 20,000 i.p.; 1500 intracerebral (Felder, Pitre).

THERAP CAT: Diagnostic aid (radiocontrast medium).

5058. Iopanoic Acid. [96-83-3] 3-Amino-α-ethyl-2,4,6-triiodobenzenepropanoic acid; 3-amino-α-ethyl-2,4,6-triiodohydrocinnamic acid; iodopanoic acid; 3-(3-amino-2,4,6-triiodophenyl)-2-ethylpropanoic acid; 3-(3-amino-2,4,6-triiodophenyl)-2-ethylpropionic acid; Cistobil; Colepax; Telepaque; Teletrast. $C_{11}H_{12}I_3$-NO_2; mol wt 570.93. C 23.14%, H 2.12%, I 66.68%, N 2.45%, O 5.60%. Oral radiocontrast medium. Prepn: S. Archer, **US 2705726** (1955 to Sterling Drug). Optical resolution: Pitré, Boveri, *J. Med. Chem.* **11**, 406 (1968). Toxicity data: P. Tirone, G. Rosati, *Farmaco Ed. Prat.* **31**, 397 (1976). Review of pharmacology and clinical efficacy in oral cholecystography: R. N. Berk *et* *al., N. Engl. J. Med.* **290,** 204 (1974). Comprehensive description: D. Pitre, *Anal. Profiles Drug Subs.* **14,** 181-206 (1985).

dl-**Form.** Cream-colored solid, mp 155.2-157°. pKa 4.8. Insol in water. Sol in dil alkali, in 95% alc, in other organic solvents. LD$_{50}$ in mice, rats (mg/kg): 285, 320 i.v.; 1540, 2870 orally (Tirone).

l-**Form.** [17879-97-9] Crystals, mp 162-163°. $[\alpha]_D^{20}$ −5.2 ± 0.1° (c = 2 in ethanol).

d-**Form.** [17879-96-8] Crystals, mp 162°. $[\alpha]_D^{20}$ +5.1 ± 0.1° (c = 2 in ethanol).

Sodium salt. [2497-78-1] Bilijodon-Natrium.

THERAP CAT: Diagnostic aid (radiopaque medium —cholecystographic).

5059. Iopentol. [89797-00-2] 5-[Acetyl(2-hydroxy-3-methoxypropyl)amino]-*N,N*′-bis(2,3-dihydroxypropyl)-2,4,6-triiodo-1,3-benzenedicarboxamide; *N,N*′-bis(2,3-dihydroxypropyl)-5-[*N*-(2-hydroxy-3-methoxypropyl)acetamido]-2,4,6-triiodoisophthalamide; Imagopaque. C$_{20}$H$_{28}$I$_3$N$_3$O$_9$; mol wt 835.16. C 28.76%, H 3.38%, I 45.59%, N 5.03%, O 17.24%. Nonionic, water soluble vascular contrast medium. Prepn: K. Wille, **EP 105752** (1984 to Nyegaard A/S), *C.A.* **101,** 72456e (1984). Synthesis and preparative LC purification: W. Skjold, A. Berg, *J. Chromatogr.* **366,** 299 (1986). Effects on blood-brain barrier in animals: A. A. Michelet, *Acta Radiol.* **28,** 329 (1987). Series of articles on clinical experience: *Eur. Radiol.* **7,** Suppl. 4, S104-S161 (1997).

Osmolality (300 mg I/ml): 0.64 mol/kg H$_2$O. Viscosity at 20° (300 mg I/ml): 13.2 mPa. Partition coefficient (1-octanol/water): 0.007.

THERAP CAT: Diagnostic aid (radiopaque medium).

5060. Iophendylate. [99-79-6] 4-Iodo-ι-methylbenzenedecanoic acid ethyl ester; ethyl 10-(*p*-iodophenyl)undecylate; ethyl 10-(*p*-iodophenyl)hendecanoate. C$_{19}$H$_{29}$IO$_2$; mol wt 416.34. C 54.81%, H 7.02%, I 30.48%, O 7.69%. Chief component of *Ethiodan, Mulsopaque, Myodil, Neurotrast, Pantopaque*; may also contain other isomers including 11-(*p*-iodophenyl)undecylate. Prepn: W. H. Strain *et al., J. Am. Chem. Soc.* **64,** 1436 (1942); *eidem,* **US 2348231** (1944 to Noned Corp. and Kodak); W. Baker *et al., J. Soc. Chem. Ind.* **63,** 223 (1944). Pharmacology and toxicity: T. B. Steinhausen *et al., Radiology* **43,** 230 (1944). Clinical evaluation of diagnostic use in myelography: G. H. Ramsey *et al., ibid.* **236.** Clinical comparison with metrizamide, *q.v.,* in diagnostic radiology: S. A. Keiffer *et al., ibid.* **129,** 695 (1978). Evaluation of use in MR imaging of the spine: I. F. Braun *et al., Am. J. Neuroradiol.* **7,** 997 (1986); A. K. Anand *et al., Comput. Radiol.* **11,** 165 (1987).

Viscous liquid. Darkens slowly in air. d$_{20}^{20}$ 1.240-1.263. n_D^{25} 1.5230-1.5280. Saponif equiv 395-420. Very slightly sol in water. Freely sol in alcohol, benzene, chloroform, ether. LD$_{50}$ in mice, rats (g/kg): 4.6, 19 i.p. (Steinhausen).

THERAP CAT: Diagnostic aid (radiopaque medium).

THERAP CAT (VET): Diagnostic aid (radiopaque medium).

5061. Iophenoxic Acid. [96-84-4] α-Ethyl-3-hydroxy-2,4,6-triiodobenzenepropanoic acid; α-ethyl-3-hydroxy-2,4,6-triiodohydrocinnamic acid; α-(2,4,6-triiodo-3-hydroxybenzyl)butyric acid; α-ethyl-β-(3-hydroxy-2,4,6-triiodophenyl)propionic acid; α-ethyl-β-(2,4,6-triiodo-3-hydroxyphenyl)propionic acid; triiodoethionic acid; Teridax. C$_{11}$H$_{11}$I$_3$O$_3$; mol wt 571.92. C 23.10%, H 1.94%, I 66.57%, O 8.39%. Prepn: Papa *et al., J. Am. Chem. Soc.* **75,** 1107 (1953); **GB 726987** (1955 to Sterling Drug). Toxicity data: J. O. Hoppe *et al., J. Med. Chem.* **13,** 997 (1970).

Crystals from benzene + petr ether, mp 143-144°. LD$_{50}$ i.v. in mice: 374 mg/kg (Hoppe).

THERAP CAT: Diagnostic aid (radiopaque medium —cholecystographic).

5062. Iopromide. [73334-07-3] *N,N*′-Bis(2,3-dihydroxypropyl)-2,4,6-triiodo-5-[(methoxyacetyl)amino]-*N*-methyl-1,3-benzenedicarboxamide; *N,N*′-bis(2,3-dihydroxypropyl)-2,4,6-triiodo-5-(2-methoxyacetamido)-*N*-methylisophthalamide; 5-methoxyacetylamino-2,4,6-triiodoisophthalic acid [(2,3-dihydroxy-*N*-methylpropyl)-(2,3-dihydroxypropyl)]diamide; Ultravist. C$_{18}$H$_{24}$I$_3$N$_3$O$_8$; mol wt 791.11. C 27.33%, H 3.06%, I 48.12%, N 5.31%, O 16.18%. Nonionic, injectable radio-contrast medium. Prepn: U. Speck *et al.,* **DE 2909439**; *eidem,* **US 4364921** (1980, 1982 both to Schering AG). Physicochemical properties and pharmacological profile: W. Muetzel, U. Speck, *Am. J. Neuroradiol.* **4,** 350 (1983); P. Dawson *et al., Acta Radiol. Diagn.* **25,** 253 (1984). Clinical experience: K.-J. Wolf *et al., ibid.* **24,** 55 (1983).

Colorless solid. Stable in aqueous solutions. Viscosity (cP): 4.8 at 37°; 10.2 at 20° (c = 300 mg iodine/ml). LD$_{50}$ in mice, rats (g iodine/kg body weight): 16.5, 11.4 i.v. (Muetzel).

THERAP CAT: Diagnostic aid (radiopaque medium).

5063. Iopronic Acid. [41473-08-9] 2-[[2-[3-(Acetylamino)-2,4,6-triiodophenoxy]ethoxy]methyl]butanoic acid; (±)-2-[[2-(3-acetamido-2,4,6-triiodophenoxy)ethoxy]methyl]butyric acid; 3-[2-(3-acetylamino-2,4,6-triiodophenoxy)ethoxy]-2-ethylpropionic acid; B-11420; SQ-21983; Bilimiro; Bilimiron; Oravue; Videobil. C$_{15}$H$_{18}$I$_3$NO$_5$; mol wt 673.02. C 26.77%, H 2.70%, I 56.57%, N 2.08%, O 11.89%. Oral cholecystographic agent. Prepn: E. Felder, D. Pitre, **DE 2128902**; *eidem,* **US 3842124** (1972, 1974 both to Bracco); E. Felder *et al., Farmaco Ed. Sci.* **31,** 349 (1976). Pharmacology, toxicology: P. Tirone, G. Rosati, *Farmaco Ed. Prat.* **31,** 397, 437 (1976). Series of articles on metabolism: *ibid.* 516-546; 755. Intestinal absorption: J. R. Amberg *et al., Invest. Radiol.* **15,** S136 (1980). Effect on bile flow and composition: J. L. Barnhart *et al., ibid.* S124. Toxicity: P. Tirone, G. Rosati, *Farmaco Ed. Prat.* **31,** 397 (1976).

Crystals from 50% ethanol, mp 130°. LD$_{50}$ in mice, rats, dogs (mg/kg): 1950, 5650, >3000 orally; 1090, 1000, 835 i.v. (Tirone).

THERAP CAT: Diagnostic aid (radiopaque medium—cholecystographic).

5064. Iothalamic Acid. [2276-90-6] 3-(Acetylamino)-2,4,6-triiodo-5-[(methylamino)carbonyl]benzoic acid; 5-acetamido-2,4,6-triiodo-N-methylisophthalamic acid. $C_{11}H_9I_3N_2O_4$; mol wt 613.91. C 21.52%, H 1.48%, I 62.01%, N 4.56%, O 10.42%. Synthesis: Hoey et al., J. Med. Chem. **6**, 24 (1963).

Crystals, dec about 285°.

N-Methylglucamine salt. [13087-53-1] Meglumine iothalamate; Conray; Contrix "28"; Cysto-Conray. $C_{18}H_{26}I_3N_3O_9$; mol wt 809.13.

Sodium salt. [1225-20-3] Sodium iothalamate; Angio-Conray; Angio-Contrix "48"; Conray-400; Medio-Contrix "38". $C_{11}H_8$-$I_3N_2NaO_4$; mol wt 635.90.

^{131}I-Labeled sodium salt. [15845-98-4] Glofil-131.

THERAP CAT: Diagnostic aid (radiopaque medium).

5065. Iotrolan. [79770-24-4] 5,5'-[(1,3-Dioxo-1,3-propanediyl)bis(methylimino)]bis[N,N'-bis[2,3-dihydroxy-1-(hydroxymethyl)propyl]-2,4,6-triiodo-1,3-benzenedicarboxamide]; 5,5'-[malonylbis(methylimino)]bis[N,N'-bis[2,3-dihydroxy-1-(hydroxymethyl)propyl]-2,4,6-triiodoisophthalamide]; iotrol; DL-3117; SH-437; ZK-39482; Isovist. $C_{37}H_{48}I_6N_6O_{18}$; mol wt 1626.23. C 27.33%, H 2.98%, I 46.82%, N 5.17%, O 17.71%. Nonionic, isotonic contrast medium. Prepn: M. Sovak, R. Ranganathan, **EP 33426**; idem, **US 4341756** (1981, 1982 both to Univ. Cal., Berkeley). Neurotoxicity study: M. Sovak et al., Radiology **142**, 115 (1982). Neuropharmacology: M. Sovak et al., Am. J. Neuroradiol. **4**, 319 (1983); and cerebral distribution: J.-C. Castel et al., Neuroradiology **29**, 206 (1987). Arthrographic evaluation in animals: J. Guerra et al., Invest. Radiol. **19**, 228 (1983). Cardiovascular effects in animals: P. Lanzer et al., ibid. **20**, 746 (1985). Clinical study of patient tolerance and diagnostic adequacy for intrathecal use: B. Hammer, E. Deisenhammer, Neuroradiology **27**, 337 (1985); B. Hoffmann et al., ibid. **29**, 380 (1987); M. D. Malnor et al., Radiology **158**, 845 (1986).

Colorless glassy solid. Soly at 20° (mg/ml): water >400. LD$_{50}$ in mice, rats (g/kg): >26, 12.7 i.v. (Sovak, 1982).

THERAP CAT: Diagnostic aid (radiopaque medium).

5066. Ioversol. [87771-40-2] N,N'-Bis(2,3-dihydroxypropyl)-5-[(hydroxyacetyl)(2-hydroxyethyl)amino]-2,4,6-triiodo-1,3-benzenedicarboxamide; N,N'-bis(2,3-dihydroxypropyl)-5-[N-(2-hy-

droxyethyl)glycolamido]-2,4,6-triiodoisophthalamide; MP-328; Optiray. $C_{18}H_{24}I_3N_3O_9$; mol wt 807.11. C 26.79%, H 3.00%, I 47.17%, N 5.21%, O 17.84%. Nonionic, low osmolality, radiographic contrast agent. Prepn: Y. Lin, **EP 83964**; idem, **US 4396598** (both 1983 to Mallinckrodt). Clinical pharmacokinetics: R. A. Wilkins et al., Invest. Radiol. **24**, 781 (1989). Comparative clinical study in intravenous urography: A. J. Kaufman et al., Urol. Radiol. **12**, 56 (1990). Toxicity studies: W. H. Ralston et al., Invest. Radiol. **24**, Suppl. 1, S2 (1989). Symposium on pharmacology, toxicology and diagnostic use in contrast enhanced computed tomographic scanning and angiography: ibid. S1-S76.

mp 186-198°. Soly in water >125% wt/vol. Partition coefficient (octanol/water): 0.0004 (c = 0.01 mgI/ml). Osmolality: 702 mOsm/kg H_2O (c = 320 mgI/ml). Viscosity (cP): 11.6 (20°); 9.9 (25°); 5.8 (37°) (c = 320 mgI/kg). d^{37} 1.371 (c = 320 mgI/ml). LD$_{50}$ in mice, rats, rabbits, dogs (gI/kg): 17, 15, >25, >12 i.v.; in male, female rats (mgI/kg): 1000, >1200 intracisternally (Ralston).

THERAP CAT: Diagnostic aid (radiopaque medium).

5067. Ioxaglic Acid. [59017-64-0] 3-[[[[3-(Acetylmethylamino)-2,4,6-triiodo-5-[(methylamino)carbonyl]benzoyl]amino]acetyl]amino]-5-[[(2-hydroxyethyl)amino]carbonyl]-2,4,6-triiodobenzoic acid; N-(2-hydroxyethyl)-2,4,6-triiodo-5-[2-[2,4,6-triiodo-3-(N-methylacetamido)-5-(methylcarbamoyl)benzamido]acetamido]isophthalamic acid; P-286. $C_{24}H_{21}I_6N_5O_8$; mol wt 1268.88. C 22.72%, H 1.67%, I 60.01%, N 5.52%, O 10.09%. Ionic contrast medium of low osmolality. Prepn: G. Tilly et al., **DE 2523567**; idem, **US 4014986** (1975, 1977 both to Guerbet). Effect on peripheral arterial blood flow in dogs: R. M. Steiner et al., Clin. Radiol. **31**, 621 (1980). Effect on thyroid function: R. G. Grainger, G. W. Pennington, Br. J. Radiol. **54**, 768 (1981). Clinical study in femoral angiography: S. Suzuki et al., Acta Radiol. **23**, 87 (1982); in cardiac radiology: R. L. Feldman, Am. J. Cardiol. **61**, 1334 (1988). Toxicity study: M. Sovak, Invest. Radiol. **16**, 438 (1981). Mutation study: W. Hadnagy et al., Mutat. Res. **104**, 249 (1982).

Mixture of meglumine and sodium salts. [76820-74-1] MP-302; Hexabrix.

THERAP CAT: Diagnostic aid (radiopaque medium).

5068. Ioxilan. [107793-72-6] 5-[Acetyl(2,3-dihydroxypropyl)amino]-N-(2,3-dihydroxypropyl)-N'-(2-hydroxyethyl)-2,4,6-triiodo-1,3-benzenedicarboxamide; N-(2,3-dihydroxypropyl)-5-[N-(2,3-dihydroxypropyl)acetamido]-N'-(2-hydroxyethyl)-2,4,6-triiodoisophthalamide; ioxitol; Oxilan. $C_{18}H_{24}I_3N_3O_8$; mol wt 791.14. C 27.33%, H 3.06%, I 48.12%, N 5.31%, O 16.18%. Nonionic iodinated contrast medium. Prepd not claimed: M. Sovak, R. Ranganathan, **WO 8700757**; idem, **US 5035877** (1987, 1991 both to Cook Imaging). HPLC analysis of isomers: S. J. Foster, M. Sovak, Invest. Radiol. **23**, Suppl. 1, S106 (1988). Pharmacology: R. W. Katzberg et al., ibid. **25**, 46 (1990). Clinical evaluation: M. R. Callantine et al., ibid. Suppl. 1, S107; C. L. McIntosh, R. Reed, ibid. **29**, Suppl. 2, S40 (1994). Brief review of physical properties: M. Sovak, ibid. **23**, Suppl. 1, S79-S83 (1988).

Sol in water. Osmolality (mOsm/kg H_2O): 690 (c = 350 mgI/ml); 570 (c = 300 mgI/ml). Viscosity (37°): 4.6-4.7 cP (c = 300 mgI/ml).

THERAP CAT: Diagnostic aid (radiopaque medium).

5069. IPBC. [55406-53-6] Butylcarbamic acid 3-iodo-2-propynyl ester; 3-iodo-2-propynyl butylcarbamate; Glycacil; Polyphase P-100. $C_8H_{12}INO_2$; mol wt 281.09. C 34.18%, H 4.30%, I 45.15%, N 4.98%, O 11.38%. Prepn: BE 817530; W. Singer, US 3923870 (both 1975 to Troy Chemical). Aquatic toxicities: A. P. Farrell et al., Arch. Environ. Contam. Toxicol. **35**, 472 (1998); fate and behavior: L. Juergensen et al., Environ. Toxicol. **15**, 201 (2000). HPLC-MS determn in cosmetic formulations: M. Frauen et al., J. Pharm. Biomed. Anal. **25**, 965 (2001). GC-MS determn of degradation products: K. G. Karaisz, N. H. Snow, J. Microcol. Separat. **13**, 1 (2001). Review of use in wood protection: J. Hansen, Mod. Paint Coat. **74**, 50-56, 90 (1984); of microbial activities and commerical uses: R. Gruening, Cosmet. Toiletries **112**, 59-65 (1997).

White crystalline powder with a specific odor. mp 66°. Specific gravity: 1.575 g mL^{-1}. Vapor pressure (Pa): <0.002 (20°); 0.007 (30°). pH 7.01. Good soly in ionic and non-ionic surfactants, emulsifying agents and polar solvents. LD_{50} orally in rats: 1580 mg/kg; dermally in rabbit: >2000 mg/kg. LC_{50} (96 hr) in bluegill sunfish, rainbow trout, bobwhite quail: 1.12, 0.31, >7683 ppm. LC_{50} (8 day) in mallard duck: >7182 ppm (Hansen).

USE: Fungicide; mildewcide; preservative in cosmetics, paints and coatings, metal working fluids; wood protection.

5070. Ipecac. Ipecacuanha. Dried rhizome and roots of Cephaelis ipecacuanha (Brot.) A. Rich., Rubiaceae, known as Rio or Brazilian Ipecac; or of Cephaelis acuminata Karsten, known as Cartagena, Nicaragua or Panama Ipecac. Habit. Brazil to Bolivia; cultivated in India and Malaysia. Constit. Emetine, cephaeline, emetamine, psychotrine, methyl psychotrine, protoemetine and resin. Cartagena ipecac contains ~2.2-2.5% total alkaloids, with twice as much cephaeline as emetine. Determn of major alkaloids in ipecacuanha root: A. G. Davidson, S. M. Hassan, J. Pharm. Biomed. Anal. **2**, 441 (1984); in pharmaceutical preparations by HPLC: D. A. Elvidge et al., J. Chromatogr. **463**, 107 (1989). Review of distribution and chemistry of ipecac alkaloids: M.-M. Janot in The Alkaloids vol. 3, R. H. F. Manske, H. L. Holmes, Eds. (Academic Press, New York, 1953) pp 363-394; A. Brossi, S. Teitel, ibid. vol. 13, 189-212 (1971). Review of use in acute poisoning: W. D. King, Clin. Toxicol. **17**, 353-358 (1980).

THERAP CAT: Emetic; expectorant.

THERAP CAT (VET): Emetic; expectorant.

5071. Ipodate. [5587-89-3] 3-[[(Dimethylamino)methylene]amino]-2,4,6-triiodobenzenepropanoic acid; 3-[(dimethylaminomethylene)amino]-2,4,6-triiodohydrocinnamic acid; 2,4,6-triiodo-3-[(dimethylaminomethylene)amino]hydrocinnamic acid; β-(3-dimethylaminomethyleneamino-2,4,6-triiodophenyl)propionic acid. $C_{12}H_{13}I_3N_2O_2$; mol wt 597.96. C 24.10%, H 2.19%, I 63.67%, N 4.68%, O 5.35%. Prepn: Priewe, Poljak, Ber. **93**, 2347 (1960). Toxicity data: J. O. Hoppe et al., J. Med. Chem. **13**, 997 (1970).

Crystals, mp 168-169° (dec 225°). Practically insol in water. Very sol in methanol, ethanol, chloroform, acetone, dil sulfuric acid. Estimated pK 5-5.5.

Sodium salt. [1221-56-3] Sodium ipodate; Biloptin; Oragrafin Sodium. $C_{12}H_{12}I_3N_2NaO_2$; mol wt 619.94. Bitter leaflets from water + acetone, mp 303-304° (decompn with evolution of iodine). Very freely sol in water; freely sol in methanol, ethanol. Practically insol in acetone, ether. Soly in DMF and DMSO about 33 g/100 ml; in dimethylacetamide about 66 g/100 ml. LD_{50} in mice (mg/kg): 290 i.v.; 2570 orally (Hoppe).

Calcium salt. [1151-11-7] Calcium ipodate; Solu-Biloptin; Oragrafin Calcium. $C_{24}H_{24}CaI_6N_4O_4$; mol wt 1233.98. Crystals, mp 298-302°. Soly in water at 20°: 0.1%. Sol in chloroform, dimethylformamide, hot propylene glycol.

Ethyl ester. SH-617L. $C_{14}H_{17}I_3N_2O_2$; mol wt 626.01.

THERAP CAT: Diagnostic aid (radiopaque medium —cholecystographic).

5072. Ipomea. Mexican scammony (root); Orizaba jalap root. Dried root of Ipomoea orizabensis Ledenois, Convolvulaceae. Active constituent is the resin. Yields not less than 15% total ipomea resins. Different from Ipomoea violacea var. Pearly Gates Hort., Convolvulaceae and Ipomoea rubrocoerulea var. praecox, **morning-glory**, ololiuqui, which contain ergot alkaloids. Occurrence of lysergic acid derivatives and ergolines in Ipomea: A. Hofmann, H. Tscherter, Experientia **16**, 414 (1960); D. Stauffacher et al., Helv. Chim. Acta **48**, 1379 (1965).

THERAP CAT: Cathartic.

5073. Ipratropium Bromide. [22254-24-6] (3-endo,8-syn)-3-(3-Hydroxy-1-oxo-2-phenylpropoxy)-8-methyl-8-(1-methylethyl)-8-azoniabicyclo[3.2.1]octane bromide; 3α-hydroxy-8-isopropyl-1αH,5αH-tropanium bromide (±)-tropate; 8-isopropylnoratropine methobromide; N-isopropylnoratropinium bromomethylate; Sch-1000; Atem; Atrovent; Bitrop; Itrop; Narilet; Respontin; Rinatec. $C_{20}H_{30}BrNO_3$; mol wt 412.36. C 58.25%, H 7.33%, Br 19.38%, N 3.40%, O 11.64%. Anticholinergic. Prepn: K. Zeile et al., ZA 6707766; eidem, US 3505337 (1968, 1970, both to Boehringer, Ing.); W. Schulz et al., Arzneim.-Forsch. **26**, 960 (1976). Chemistry and pharmacokinetics: W. Deckers, Postgrad. Med. J. **51**, Suppl. 7, 76 (1975). Pharmacology and toxicology: A. Engelhardt, H. Klupp, ibid. 82. Series of articles on pharmacology, toxicology, pharmacokinetics and clinical studies: Arzneim.-Forsch. **26**, 974-985, 989-1020 (1976). Toxicity data: L. Sarafana et al., ibid. 985. Review: R. Bauer et al., in Pharmacological and Biochemical Properties of Drug Substances vol. 2, M. E. Goldberg, Ed. (Am. Pharm. Assoc., Washington, DC, 1979) pp 489-515. Symposium on pharmacology, toxicology and clinical efficacy: Am. J. Med. **81**(5A), 1-102 (1986). Review of clinical toxicology: J. D. Truwit, Crit. Care Clin. **7**, 639-657 (1991).

White crystals from n-propanol, mp 230-232°. Freely sol in water and lower alcohols. Insol in ether, chloroform and fluorohydrocarbons. Fairly stable in neutral and acid solns; rapidly hydrolyzed in alkaline soln. LD_{50} in male, female mice (mg/kg): 1001,

Consult the Name Index before using this section.

1083 orally; 12.29, 14.97 i.v.; 300, 340 s.c. LD$_{50}$ in male, female rats (mg/kg): 1663, 1779 orally; 15.89, 15.70 i.v. (Sarafana).

THERAP CAT: Bronchodilator; antiarrhythmic.

5074. Ipriflavone. [35212-22-7] 7-(1-Methylethoxy)-3-phenyl-4H-1-benzopyran-4-one; 7-isopropoxy-3-phenyl-4H-1-benzopyran-4-one; 7-isopropoxy-3-phenylchromone; 7-isopropoxyisoflavone; FL-113; TC-80; Iprosten; Osten; Osteofix; Yambolap. C$_{18}$H$_{16}$O$_3$; mol wt 280.32. C 77.12%, H 5.75%, O 17.12%. Isoflavone derivative with anti-anginal and anti-osteopenic activity. Prepn: L. Feuer et al., DE 2125245 (1971 to Chinoin), C.A. 76, 72407e (1972). Use as anabolic in animals: eidem, US 3833730; in humans; eidem, US 3949085 (1974, 1976 both to Chinoin). Cardiovascular properties in stable angina: V. Grubich et al., Lancet 1, 211 (1979). Cardiological effects in animals: L. Feuer et al., Arzneim.-Forsch. 31, 953 (1981). Metabolism and disposition in rats: K. Yoshida et al., Radioisotopes 34, 612, 618 (1985). Effect in rats on estrogen-stimulated calcitonin secretion: I. Yamazaki, Life Sci. 38, 757 (1986); I. Yamazaki, M. Kinoshita, ibid. 1535; on glucocorticoid-induced osteoporosis: I. Yamazaki et al., ibid. 951.

Crystals from acetone, mp 115-117°.
THERAP CAT: Calcium regulator.

5075. Iprindole. [5560-72-5] 6,7,8,9,10,11-Hexahydro-N,N-dimethyl-5H-cyclooct[b]indole-5-propanamine; 5-[3-(dimethylamino)propyl]-6,7,8,9,10,11-hexahydro-5H-cyclooct[b]indole; 1-(3-dimethylaminopropyl)-2,3-hexamethyleneindole; pramindole (obsolete); Tertran. C$_{19}$H$_{28}$N$_2$; mol wt 284.44. C 80.23%, H 9.92%, N 9.85%. Prepn: L. M. Rice, M. E. Freed, BE 623933; eidem, US 3282942 (1963, 1966, both to Am. Home Prods.); Rice et al., J. Med. Chem. 7, 313 (1964). Pharmacology: Gluckman, Baum, Psychopharmacologia 15, 169 (1969); Baum et al., Eur. J. Pharmacol. 13, 287 (1971). Mechanism of action: Miller et al., Experientia 26, 863 (1970); Lemberger et al., Biochem. Pharmacol. 19, 3021 (1970). Freeman, Sulser, J. Pharmacol. Exp. Ther. 183, 307 (1972).

Hydrochloride. [20432-64-8] Wy-3263; Prondol; Galatur. C$_{19}$H$_{28}$N$_2$·HCl; mol wt 320.90. Crystals from methanol + acetone, mp 146-147°.
THERAP CAT: Antidepressant.

5076. Iproclozide. [3544-35-2] 4-(Chlorophenoxy)acetic acid 2-(1-methylethyl)hydrazide. C$_{11}$H$_{15}$ClN$_2$O$_2$; mol wt 242.70. C 54.44%, H 6.23%, Cl 14.61%, N 11.54%, O 13.18%. Monoamine oxidase inhibitor. Prepn: Libermann, Denis, Bull. Soc. Chim. Fr. 1961, 1952. GC determn in urine: R. M. DeSagher et al., Anal. Chem. 47, 1144 (1976).

Crystals, mp 93-94°.
THERAP CAT: Antidepressant.

5077. Iprodione. [36734-19-7] 3-(3,5-Dichlorophenyl)-N-(1-methylethyl)-2,4-dioxo-1-imidazolidinecarboxamide; glycophene; promidione; RP-26019; ROP-500F; NRC-910; LFA-2043; FA-2071; Rovral; CHIPCO-26019. C$_{13}$H$_{13}$Cl$_2$N$_3$O$_3$; mol wt 330.17. C 47.29%, H 3.97%, Cl 21.48%, N 12.73%, O 14.54%. Prepn: M. Sauli, DE 2149923; idem, US 3755350 (1972, 1973 to Rhône-Poulenc). Biological properties: L. Lacroix et al., Phytiatr.-Phytopharm. 23, 165 (1974). Structural rearrangement: B. K. Cooke et al., Pestic. Sci. 10, 393 (1979). Thermal degradn: J. Gomez et al., J. Agric. Food Chem. 30, 180 (1982). HPLC determn in surface water: C. E. Goewie, E. A. Hogendoorn, Sci. Total Environ. 47, 349 (1985). GC-MS determn in chicory and leek: F. Rouberty, J. Fournier, Chromatographia 41, 693 (1995). Field study: T. B. Brenneman et al., Plant Dis. 71, 546 (1987). Degradation in soil: A. Walker, Pestic. Sci. 21, 219 (1987). Review: L. Lacroix et al., Anal. Methods Pestic. Plant Growth Regul. 11, 247-261 (1980).

Colorless, odorless, nonhygroscopic crystals, mp ~136°. Vapor press. at 20°: <10^{-6} mm Hg. Soly in water at 20°: 13 mg/l. Soly at 20° (g/l): ethanol 25; methanol 25; acetone 300; dichloromethane 500; DMF 500. LD$_{50}$ in mice, rats (g/kg): 4, 3.5 orally (Lacroix, 1980).
USE: Fungicide.

5078. Iproniazid. [54-92-2] 4-Pyridinecarboxylic acid 2-(1-methylethyl)hydrazide; isonicotinic acid 2-isopropylhydrazide; 1-isonicotinoyl-2-isopropylhydrazine; 1-isonicotinyl-2-isopropylhydrazine. C$_9$H$_{13}$N$_3$O; mol wt 179.22. C 60.31%, H 7.31%, N 23.45%, O 8.93%. Monoamine oxidase inhibitor. Prepd by treating isoniazid with isopropyl bromide in abs alcohol in the presence of sodium: McMillan et al., J. Am. Pharm. Assoc. Sci. Ed. 42, 457 (1953). Alternate synthesis: Fox, Gibas, J. Org. Chem. 18, 994 (1953). Comprehensive description: F. Belal, H. Abdel-Aliem, Anal. Profiles Drug Subs. 20, 337-368 (1991).

Needles from benzene + ligroin, mp 112.5-113.5°. Freely sol in water, alcohol; pH of aq solns about 6.7.
Dihydrochloride. C$_9$H$_{13}$N$_3$O·2HCl. Rhomboid crystals from isopropanol, dec at 227-228°. Freely sol in water; aq solns are very acidic.
Phosphate. [305-33-9] Marsilid. C$_9$H$_{13}$N$_3$O·H$_3$PO$_4$; mol wt 277.21. White to slightly yellowish powder, melting range 175-184°. pH of a 5% soln: 2.7-3.6. uv spectrum: J. Kracmar, J. Kracmarova, Pharmazie 34, 27 (1979). uv max (methanol): 265 nm (A$_{1cm}^{1\%}$ 166); (water): 264 nm (A$_{1cm}^{1\%}$ 176); (0.1N HCl): 267 nm (A$_{1cm}^{1\%}$ 179); (0.1N KOH): 244, 272, 308 nm (A$_{1cm}^{1\%}$ 113, 121, 135). Soly at 25° (mg/ml): water ~188; methanol ~21; ethanol (96%) ~9; chloroform ~0.6; diethyl ether <0.1; hexane <0.1.
THERAP CAT: Antidepressant.

5079. Ipronidazole. [14885-29-1] 1-Methyl-2-(1-methylethyl)-5-nitro-1H-imidazole; 2-isopropyl-1-methyl-5-nitroimidazole; Ro-7-1554; Ipropran. C$_7$H$_{11}$N$_3$O$_2$; mol wt 169.18. C 49.70%, H 6.55%, N 24.84%, O 18.91%. Prepn: GB 1119636; M. Hoffer, M. Mitrovic, US 3634446 (1968, 1972 both to Hoffmann-La Roche); K. Butler, ZA 6607466 (1968 to Pfizer), C.A. 71, 3384e (1969). Structure-activity relationship: K. Butler et al., J.

Med. Chem. **10**, 891 (1967). Activity studies as an antihistomonal agent: M. Mitrovic *et al., Antimicrob. Agents Chemother.* **1968**, 445; M. Mitrovic, E. G. Schildknecht, *Poult. Sci.* **49**, 86 (1970); as a growth promotant: W. L. Marusich *et al., ibid.* 98. Toxicity studies: *eidem, ibid.* 92.

White plates, mp 60°. LD$_{50}$ orally in poults: 640 ± 25 mg/kg (Marusich, p 92).

Hydrochloride. mp 177-182°. Water-soluble.

THERAP CAT (VET): Antiprotozoal (Histomonas).

5080. Iprovalicarb. [140923-17-7] [(1S)-2-Methyl-1-[[[1-(4-methylphenyl)ethyl]amino]carbonyl]propyl]carbamic acid 1-methylethyl ester; isopropyl-2-methyl-1-[(1-p-tolyethyl)carbamoyl]-(S)-propylcarbamate; N-(isopropyloxycarbonyl)-L-valine-4-methylphenylethylamide; SZX-722; Melody. C$_{18}$H$_{28}$N$_2$O$_3$; mol wt 320.43. C 67.47%, H 8.81%, N 8.74%, O 14.98%. Fungicide for use in food crops; commercial product is a mixture of two diastereomers (SS, SR). Prepn: T. Seitz *et al.*, **DE 4026966**; *eidem*, **US 5453531** (1992, 1995 both to Bayer). Comprehensive description: K. Stenzel *et al., Brighton Crop Prot. Conf. - Pests Dis.* **2**, 367 (1998). Series of articles on prepn, structure, field studies, ecological profile and metabolism: *Pflanzenschutz-Nachr. Bayer* **52**, 5-114 (1999). LC-MS determn: R. Brennecke *ibid.* **53**, 5 (2000). ELISA method for residue detection: J. K. Lee *et al., J. Agric. Food Chem.* **52**, 6680 (2004).

(S,R)-form

White powder, mp 163-165° (mixture), 183° (SR), 199° (SS). d^{20} 1.11. Log P (octanol/water): 3.2. Vapor pressure: 7.7 × 10^{-10} hPa (20°), 2.1 × 10^{-9} hPa (25°). LD$_{50}$ in rats (mg/kg): >5000 orally; >5000 dermally; in bobwhite quail (mg/kg): >2000 orally. LC$_{50}$ in rats (mg/m^3): >4977 by inhalation (Stenzel).

USE: Fungicide.

5081. Ipsapirone. [95847-70-4] 2-[4-[4-(2-Pyrimidinyl)-1-piperazinyl]butyl]-1,2-benzisothiazolin-3(2H)-one 1,1-dioxide; isapirone. C$_{19}$H$_{23}$N$_5$O$_3$S; mol wt 401.48. C 56.84%, H 5.77%, N 17.44%, O 11.96%, S 7.99%. Nonbenzodiazepine anxiolytic; 5-hydroxytryptamine (5-HT$_1$) receptor agonist. Prepn: W. Dompert *et al.*, **DE 3321969**; P.-R. Seidel *et al.*, **US 4818756** (1984, 1989 both to Troponwerke). Pharmacology and serotonin (5-HT$_1$) receptor binding study: J. Traber *et al., Brain Res. Bull.* **12**, 741 (1984). 5-HT$_1$ specific binding activity: W. U. Dompert *et al., Arch. Pharmacol.* **328**, 467 (1985); T. Glaser, J. Traber, *ibid.* **329**, 211 (1985). Behavioral effects in mice: R. J. DeSouza *et al., Br. J. Pharmacol.* **89**, 377 (1986). Neurophysiological effects in comparison with buspirone. M. J. Rowan, R. Anwyl, *Eur. J. Pharmacol.* **132**, 93 (1987). HPLC determn in biological samples: G. Bianchi, S. Caccia, *J. Chromatogr.* **431**, 477 (1988).

Crystals from isopropanol, mp 137-138°.

Hydrochloride. [92589-98-5] Bay q 7821; TVX Q 7821. C$_{19}$H$_{23}$N$_5$O$_3$S.HCl; mol wt 437.94. Crystals from isopropanol, mp 221-222°.

THERAP CAT: Anxiolytic.

5082. IPTG. [367-93-1] 1-Methylethyl 1-thio-β-D-galactopyranoside; isopropyl β-D-thiogalactopyranoside. C$_9$H$_{18}$O$_5$S; mol wt 238.30. C 45.36%, H 7.61%, O 33.57%, S 13.46%. Artificial, slow-hydrolyzing inducer of the lactose (lac) operon. Prepn: B. Helferich, D. Türk, *Ber.* **89**, 2215 (1956); U. Carlsson *et al., Protein Eng.* **4**, 1019 (1991). Induction of β-galactosidase: V. Paces *et al., Collect. Czech. Chem. Commun.* **38**, 2983 (1973). Binding to β-D-galactosidase: C. K. De Bruyne, M. Yde, *Carbohydr. Res.* **56**, 153 (1977). Concentration effects on lac operon induction in *E. coli*: S. Cho *et al., Biochem. Biophys. Res. Commun.* **128**, 1268 (1985). Effect of lactose permease on induction by IPTG: L. H. Hansen *et al., Curr. Microbiol.* **36**, 341 (1998).

mp 109.5-110.5°. [α]$_D^{22}$ −31.4° (c = 5 in water). Also reported as crystals from dioxane, mp 118-119°. [α]$_D$ −26.4° (c = 1 in water) (Carlsson). Log P (octanol/water): −1.26.

USE: Induces protein synthesis in *E. coli* when transcription is controlled by the lac-promoter. In conjunction with X-gal, *q.v.*, in detection of lac gene activity during cloning experiments.

5083. Irbesartan. [138402-11-6] 2-Butyl-3-[[2′-(1H-tetrazol-5-yl)[1,1′-biphenyl]-4-yl]methyl]-1,3-diazaspiro[4.4]non-1-en-4-one; 2-butyl-3-[p-(o-1H-tetrazol-5-ylphenyl)benzyl]-1,3-diazaspiro[4.4]non-1-en-4-one; 2-n-butyl-4-spirocyclopentane-1-[(2′-(tetrazol-5-yl)biphenyl-4-yl)methyl]-2-imidazolin-5-one; BMS-186295; SR-47436; Aprovel; Avapro. C$_{25}$H$_{28}$N$_6$O; mol wt 428.53. C 70.07%, H 6.59%, N 19.61%, O 3.73%. Angiotensin II type 1 (AII$_1$)-receptor antagonist. Prepn: C. Bernhart *et al.*, **WO 9114679**; *eidem*, **US 5270317** (1991, 1993 both to Sanofi); *eidem et al., J. Med. Chem.* **36**, 3371 (1993). HPLC determn in plasma and urine: S.-Y. Chang *et al., J. Chromatogr. B* **702**, 149 (1997). Metabolism: T. J. Chando *et al., Drug Metab. Dispos.* **26**, 408 (1998). Review of pharmacology and clinical efficacy: J. C. Gillis, A. Markham, *Drugs* **54**, 885-902 (1997). Renoprotective effect in diabetic nephropathy: E. J. Lewis *et al., N. Engl. J. Med.* **345**, 851 (2001); H.-H. Parving *et al., ibid.* 870.

Crystals from 96% ethanol, mp 180-181°.

THERAP CAT: Antihypertensive.

5084. Irgarol®. [28159-98-0] N-Cyclopropyl-N′-(1,1-dimethylethyl)-6-(methylthio)-1,3,5-triazine-2,4-diamine; 2-(tert-butylamino)-4-(cyclopropylamino)-6-(methylthio)-s-triazine. C$_{11}$H$_{19}$N$_5$S; mol wt 253.37. C 52.14%, H 7.56%, N 27.64%, S 12.66%. Photosystem-II (PSII) herbicide, inhibits photosynthetic electron transport in chloroplasts. Prepn: D. Berrer, C. Vogel, **DE 1914014** (1969 to Agripat); *eidem*, **US 3629256** (1971 to Geigy). Photodegradation and persistence in water: H. Okamura *et al., J. Environ. Sci. Health* **B34**, 225 (1999). Review of analytical methods: N. Voulvoulis *et al., Chemosphere* **38**, 3503-3516 (1999).

Ecological risk assessment: L. W. Hall, Jr. *et al.*, *Crit. Rev. Toxicol.* **29**, 367-437 (1999).

Crystals from water, mp 128-133°. Soly (ppm): 9.0 in water; 5.9 in 0.3 mol/l salinity; 1.8 in 0.6 mol/l salinity. Vapor pressure 6.6×10^{-7} mm Hg. Log P (*n*-octanol/water): 3.95; also reported as 2.8 (Hall). LC_{50} (96 hr in salt water) in mysid shrimp, inland silverside, sheepshead minnow (ng/l): 400000, 1580000, 3500000; LC_{50} (96 hr in fresh water) in rainbow trout, bluegill sunfish (ng/l): 790000, 2600000 (Hall).

USE: Booster algicide in antifouling paint.

5085. Iridium. [7439-88-5] Ir; at. wt 192.217; at. no. 77; valences 1, 3, 4; also 2, 5, 6. Group VIII (9). Two naturally occurring isotopes: 191 (38.5%); 193 (61.5%); artificial, radioactive isotopes: 182-190; 191; 192; 194-198. Occurrence in earth's crust about 0.001 ppm. Discovered in 1804 by Tennant. Occurs in nature in the metallic state, usually as a natural alloy with osmium (osmiridium); found in small quantities alloyed with native platinum (platinum mineral) or with native gold. Recovery and purification from osmiridium: Deville, Debray, *Ann. Chim. Phys.* **61**, 84 (1861); from the platinum mineral: Wichers, *J. Res. Natl. Bur. Stand.* **10**, 819 (1933). Reviews of prepn, properties and chemistry of iridium and other platinum metals: Gilchrist, *Chem. Rev.* **32**, 277-372 (1943); W. P. Griffith, *The Chemistry of the Rarer Platinum Metals* (John Wiley, New York, 1967) pp 1-41, 227-312; Livingstone in *Comprehensive Inorganic Chemistry* vol. 3, J. C. Bailar Jr. *et al.*, Eds. (Pergamon Press, Oxford, 1973) pp 1163-1189, 1254-1274.

Silver-white, very hard metal; face-centered cubic lattice. mp 2450°; bp ~4500°. d_4^{20} 22.65; highest sp gr of all elements. Specific heat 0.0307 cal/g/°C. Mohs' hardness 6.5. Pure iridium is not attacked by any acids including aqua regia; only slightly by fused (non-oxidizing) alkalies. It is superficially oxidized on heating in the air. Is attacked by fluorine and chlorine at a red heat; attacked by potassium sulfate or by a mixture of potassium hydroxide and nitrate on fusion; attacked by lead, zinc or tin. The powdered metal is oxidized by air or oxygen at a red heat to the dioxide, IrO_2, but on further heating the dioxide dissociates into its constituents.

USE: In manufacturing crucibles; in hardening platinum; in making nibs for fountain-pen points.

5086. Iridium Hexafluoride. [7783-75-7] F_6Ir; mol wt 306.21. F 37.23%, Ir 62.77%. IrF_6. Prepd by direct fluorination of iridium: Ruff, Fischer, *Z. Anorg. Allg. Chem.* **179**, 161 (1929); Robinson, Westland, *J. Chem. Soc.* **1956**, 4481. Crystal structure: Siegel, Northrop, *Inorg. Chem.* **5**, 2187 (1966).

Golden yellow, cubic crystals. d (calc) 4.82. Very hygroscopic. mp 44.4°. bp 53°. Volatilizes on slow heating. Reduced to IrF_4 by halogens. Decomposes in aqueous soln. Does not react with dry glass below 150°. May be stored in evacuated quartz ampuls.

5087. Iridium Sesquioxide. [1312-46-5] Ir_2O_3; mol wt 432.43. Ir 88.90%, O 11.10%.

Blue-black powder. Decomposes at about 1000° into metal and oxygen. Insol in water; slowly dissolved by boiling HCl. Oxidized to IrO_2 by HNO_3.

5088. Iridium Trichloride. [10025-83-9] Cl_3Ir; mol wt 298.58. Cl 35.62%, Ir 64.38%. $IrCl_3$. Prepn: Dillamore, Edwards, *J. Inorg. Nucl. Chem.* **31**, 2427 (1969). Several known modifications. Crystal structure: Brodersen *et al.*, *Naturwissenschaften* **52**, 205 (1966); Babel, Deigner, *Z. Anorg. Allg. Chem.* **339**, 57 (1965).

α-Form. Brown, monoclinic crystals. β-Form; red, orthorhombic crystals. Olive-green modification also prepd: Dillamore, Edwards, *loc. cit.* Decomposes at 763°. Insol in water, acids, alkalies.

USE: Catalyst for chlorination and polymerization reactions.

5089. Iridomyrmecin. [485-43-8] [4S-(4α,4aβ,7β,7aβ)]-Hexahydro-4,7-dimethylcyclopenta[c]pyran-3(1H)-one; 2-(hydroxymethyl)-α,3-dimethylcyclopentaneacetic acid δ-lactone; iridomyrmexin. $C_{10}H_{16}O_2$; mol wt 168.23. C 71.39%, H 9.59%, O 19.02%. Iridolactone isolated from the Argentine ant *Iridomyrmex humilis* Mayr., *Dolichoderinae*. Exhibits antibacterial and insect antifeedant activity. Isoln: Pavan, *Ric. Sci.* **19**, 1011 (1949); *Chim. Ind. (Milan)* **37**, 625 (1955); Fusco *et al.*, *ibid.* **251**, 958; Cavill *et al.*, *Aust. J. Chem.* **9**, 288 (1956); **10**, 352 (1957). Synthesis: Korte *et al.*, *Tetrahedron* **6**, 201 (1959); Sisido *et al.*, *J. Org. Chem.* **29**, 3361 (1964); R. S. Matthews, J. K. Whitesell, *ibid.* **40**, 3312 (1975); Y. Yamada *et al.*, *Chem. Lett.* **1978**, 1405; P. Callant *et al.*, *Tetrahedron* **37**, 2085 (1981). Stereochemistry: Korte *et al.*, *Ber.* **94**, 1952 (1961); McConnell *et al.*, *Tetrahedron Lett.* **1962**, 445; Büchi, Manning, *Tetrahedron* **18**, 1049 (1962). Activity as bactericide and insecticide: M. Pavan, *Z. Hyg. Infektionskrankh.* **134**, 136 (1952), *C.A.* **46**, 9796f (1952).

Prisms from petr ether. Aromatic odor, resembling catnip. Salty taste. mp 60-61°. Sublimes$_{0.01}$ 50-55°. bp$_{1.5}$ 104-108°. $[α]_D^{20}$ +210° (c = 4 in ethanol); $[α]_D^{17}$ +205° (c = 0.223 in carbon tetrachloride). n_D^{65} 1.4607. Sparingly sol in water: 0.2 g/100 ml H_2O (25°). Sol in fats and fat solvents. Freely sol in ether.

5090. Irigenin. [548-76-5] 5,7-Dihydroxy-3-(3-hydroxy-4,5-dimethoxyphenyl)-6-methoxy-4H-1-benzopyran-4-one; 3′,5,7-trihydroxy-4′,5′,6-trimethoxyisoflavone. $C_{18}H_{16}O_8$; mol wt 360.31. C 60.00%, H 4.48%, O 35.52%. From rhizome of *Iris florentina* L., *Iridaceae*: de Laire, Tiemann, *Ber.* **26**, 2010 (1893). Structure: Baker, *J. Chem. Soc.* **1928**, 1022. Synthesis: Baker *et al.*, *Tetrahedron Lett.* no. **5**, 6 (1960); Farkas, Várady, *Ber.* **93**, 2685 (1960); Baker *et al.*, *J. Chem. Soc. C* **1970**, 1219.

Yellow plates or needles from dil alc, mp 185°. uv max (abs ethanol): 267 nm. Sol in warm alcohol, benzene, chloroform; practically insol in water, ether, petr ether.

Triacetate. $C_{24}H_{22}O_{11}$. Prisms from dil acetic acid, mp 127-128°.

7-Glucoside. Iridin; 7-(glucosyloxy)-3′,5-dihydroxy-4′,5′,6-trimethoxyisoflavone. $C_{24}H_{26}O_{13}$. Monohydrate, needles from dil alc, mp 208°. When anhydrous, mp 217°. One gram of anhydrous iridin dissolves in 500 ml water, 43 ml acetone. Sol in hot alcohol; practically insol in ether, ethyl acetate, benzene, chloroform.

Note: There also is an oleoresin called *iridin* (Extractum Iridis) from *Iris versicolor* (blue flag) by extraction with 60% alc. Another substance named *iridine* is a protamine from the sperm of rainbow trout: Felix, Mager, *Z. Physiol. Chem.* **249**, 124 (1937).

5091. Irinotecan. [97682-44-5] [1,4′-Bipiperidine]-1′-carboxylic acid (4S)-4,11-diethyl-3,4,12,14-tetrahydro-4-hydroxy-3,14-dioxo-1H-pyrano[3′,4′:6,7]indolizino[1,2-b]quinolin-9-yl ester; 7-ethyl-10-[4-(1-piperidino)-1-piperidino]carbonyloxycamptothecin; (+)-7-ethyl-10-hydroxycamptothecine 10-[1,4′-bipiperidine]-1′-carboxylate; (+)-(4S)-4,11-diethyl-4-hydroxy-9-[(4-piperidinopiperidino)carbonyloxy]-1H-pyrano[3′,4′:6,7]indolizino[1,2-b]quinoline-3,14-(4H,12H)-dione. $C_{33}H_{38}N_4O_6$; mol wt 586.68. C 67.56%, H 6.53%, N 9.55%, O 16.36%. DNA topoisomerase I inhibitor. Semisynthetic derivative of camptothecin, *q.v.*; de-esterified *in vivo* to the active metabolite, *7-ethyl-10-hydroxy-*

camptothecin (*SN-38*). Prepn: **JP Kokai 85 19790**; T. Miyasaka *et al., US 4604463* (1985, 1986 both to Yakult Honsha); S. Sawada *et al., Chem. Pharm. Bull.* **39**, 1446 (1991). Antitumor activity and toxicity data: T. Kunimoto *et al., Cancer Res.* **47**, 5944 (1987). Mechanism of action study: Y. Kawato *et al., ibid.* **51**, 4187 (1991). Clinical trial in colorectal cancer: J. Y. Douillard *et al., Lancet* **355**, 1041 (2000). Review of pharmacology and clinical experience: N. Masuda *et al., Crit. Rev. Oncol. Hematol.* **24**, 3-26 (1996); S. O'Reilly, E. K. Rowinsky, *ibid.* 47-70; of clinical toxicity: K. Seiter, *Expert Opin. Drug Safety* **4**, 45-53 (2005).

Pale yellow powder, mp 222-223°.

Hydrochloride trihydrate. [136572-09-3]; [100286-90-6] (hydrochloride). CPT-11; DQ-2805; Campto; Camptosar. $C_{33}H_{38}N_4$-$O_6.HCl.3H_2O$; mol wt 677.18. Slightly pale yellow needles or crystalline powder from water, mp 256.5°. $[\alpha]_D^{20}$ +67.7° (c = 1 in water). uv max (ethanol): 221, 254, 359, 372 nm (ε 53800, 36600, 26200, 25300). Slightly sol in water and organic solvents. pH of 2% aqueous soln = 4. LD_{50} in mice (mg/kg): 177.5 i.p.; 765.3 orally (Kunimoto).

THERAP CAT: Antineoplastic.

5092. Irofulven. [158440-71-2] (6'*R*)-6'-Hydroxy-3'-(hydroxymethyl)-2',4',6'-trimethylspiro[cyclopropane-1,5'-[5*H*]inden]-7'(6'*H*)-one; (hydroxymethyl)acylfulvene; HMAF; MGI-114; NSC-683863. $C_{15}H_{18}O_3$; mol wt 246.30. C 73.15%, H 7.37%, O 19.49%. Semi-synthetic antitumor agent derived from illudin S, *q.v.* Inhibits DNA synthesis and induces apoptosis in tumor cells. Prepn: M. J. Kelner *et al., US 5523490* (1996 to Univ. California); T. C. McMorris *et al., J. Nat. Prod.* **59**, 896 (1996). Enantioselective synthesis: *idem et al., J. Org. Chem.* **69**, 619 (2004). Effect on DNA integrity and apoptosis: J. M. Woynarowski *et al., Biochem. Pharmacol.* **54**, 1181 (1997). Clinical pharmacokinetics and toxicology: J. Alexandre *et al., Clin. Cancer Res.* **10**, 3377 (2004). Clinical evaluation in hormone-refractory prostate cancer: N. Senzer *et al., Am. J. Clin. Oncol.* **28**, 36 (2005). Review: M. Baekelandt, *Curr. Opin. Invest. Drugs* **3**, 1517-1526 (2002).

Crystals from ether, mp 127-129°. $[\alpha]_D^{25}$ −639° (c = 0.096 in ethanol). Crystal density: 1.262 g/cm³. uv max (ethanol): 235, 330 nm (ε 15100, 9200) with tailing to 480 nm.

THERAP CAT: Antineoplastic.

5093. Iron. [7439-89-6] Fe; at. no. 26; at. wt 55.845; valences 2, 3; seldom 1, 4, 6. Group VIII (8). Four naturally occurring isotopes: 54 (5.82%); 56 (91.66%); 57 (2.19%); 58 (0.33%); artificial, radioactive isotopes: 52; 53; 55; 59-61. Second most abundant metal in earth's crust after aluminum: about 5%. The earth's core is believed to consist mainly of iron. Important ores include hematite (Fe_2O_3), magnetite (Fe_3O_4), limonite [FeO(OH).nH_2O] and *siderite* ($FeCO_3$). Essential dietary nutrient. Study of iron and its compds by Mössbauer spectroscopy: Danon, "^{57}Fe: Metal, Alloys and Inorganic Compounds" in *Chemical Applications of Mössbauer Spectroscopy*, V. I. Goldanskii, R. H. Herber, Eds. (Aca-

demic Press, New York, 1968) p 159-313. Ions involved in oxygen transport, electron transport, nitrogen fixation and a number of other biological processes: Nielands, "Evolution of Biological Iron Binding Centers" in *Struct. Bonding* **11**, 145-170 (1972). Review of biology, pharmacology and toxicity of iron compounds: several authors, *Clin. Toxicol.* **4**, 525-642 (1971); of metabolism and homeostasis: G. Papanikolaou, K. Pantopoulos, *Toxicol. Appl. Pharmacol.* **202**, 199-211 (2005). Comprehensive reviews: Feldmann, Schenck in *Ullmanns Encyklopädie der technischen Chemie* vol. 6 (München-Berlin, 1955) pp 261-407; Nicholls in *Comprehensive Inorganic Chemistry* vol. 3, J. C. Bailar, Jr. *et al.,* Eds. (Pergamon Press, Oxford, 1973) pp 979-1051; W. A. Knepper in *Kirk-Othmer Encyclopedia of Chemical Technology* vol. 13 (Wiley-Interscience, New York, 3rd ed., 1981) pp 735-753. Review of use in cereal flour fortification: R. Hurrell *et al., Nutr. Rev.* **60**, 391-406 (2002).

Silvery-white or gray, soft, ductile, malleable, somewhat magnetic metal. Holds magnetism only after hardening (as alloy steel, *e.g.,* Alnico). Supplied as ingots, powder, wire, sheets, etc. Takes a bright polish; can be rolled, hammered, bent, particularly when red hot. Stable in dry air but readily oxidizes in moist air, forming "rust" (chiefly oxide, hydrated). In powder form it is black to gray. Commercial iron usually contains some C, P, Si, S and Mn. d pure 7.86; cast 7.76; wrought 7.25-7.78; steel 7.6-7.78. mp pure 1535°; cast 1000-1300°; wrought 1500°; steel 1300°. bp 3000°. Electrical resistivity (20°): 9.71 microhm-cm. Readily attacked by dil mineral acids and attacked or dissolved by organic acids; not appreciably attacked by cold concd H_2SO_4 or HNO_3, but is attacked by the hot acids.

USE: Alloyed with C, Mn, Cr, Ni, and other elements to form steels. Nutritional supplement in wheat flours, corn meal, grits and other cereal products. ^{55}Fe and ^{59}Fe used in tracer studies; the former in biological studies.

5094. Iron Dextran. [9004-66-4] Dextran iron complex; DexFerrum; Imferon; INFeD. Complex of ferric hydroxide with dextran, *q.q.v.* Prepn: E. London, G. D. Twigg, *US 2820740* (1958 to Benger); *US RE 24642* (1959); J. R. Herb, *US 2885393* (1959 to Laros). Use in treatment of iron-deficiency anemia: I. M. Baird, D. A. Podmore, *Lancet* **264**, 942 (1954). Acute toxicity: R. P. Beliles, *Toxicol. Appl. Pharmacol.* **23**, 537 (1972). Comparison of different formulations: R. Lawrence, *PDA J. Pharm. Sci. Technol.* **52**, 190 (1998). Mössbauer spectroscopy and x-ray diffraction study: B. Knight *et al., J. Inorg. Biochem.* **73**, 227 (1999). Use as an iron supplement for anemic piglets: A. K. Egeli, T. Framstad, *Res. Vet. Sci.* **66**, 179 (1999). Clinical evaluation in iron deficiency: J. C. Barton *et al., Am. J. Med.* **109**, 27 (2000). Review of carcinogenicity studies: *IARC Monographs* **2**, 161-178 (1973); of clinical experience: D. L. Burns *et al., Nutrition* **11**, 163-168 (1995); of toxicity profile: D. L. Burns, J. J. Pomposelli, *Kidney Int.* **55**, S119-S124 (1999).

Commercial product is a dark brown, slightly viscous soln. Very sol in water, DMSO. Dec in 95% ethanol and acetone. LD_{50} i.v. in mice: 2240 mg Fe/kg (Beliles).

Caution: This substance is reasonably anticipated to be a human carcinogen: *Report on Carcinogens, Eleventh Edition* (PB2005-104914, 2004) p III-155.

THERAP CAT: Hematinic.

THERAP CAT (VET): Nutritional factor (parenteral). Used in iron deficiency anemia, chiefly in pigs.

5095. Irone. [1335-94-0] 6-Methylionone. The fragrant principle of violets, best isolated from the rhizomes of iris or from orris oil: F. Tiemann, P. Kruger, *Ber.* **26**, 2675 (1893); Ruzicka *et al., Helv. Chim. Acta* **16**, 1143 (1933); Naves, Mazuyer, *Les Parfums Naturels* (Paris, 1939). Irone, as isolated, is an isomeric mixture of α-, β-, and γ-irones, *q.q.v.,* with each having the same molecular formula, $C_{14}H_{22}O$. Synthesis of isomeric mixture: Eschinazi, *US 3019265* (1962 to Givaudan).

Light yellow, slightly viscous liquid. Very stable, does not discolor. In dil alcoholic soln the characteristic odor of violets is best appreciated.

USE: In perfumery for orris and violet compositions.

5096. α-Irone. [79-69-6] 4-(2,5,6,6-Tetramethyl-2-cyclo-hexen-1-yl)-3-butene-2-one. $C_{14}H_{22}O$; mol wt 206.32. C 81.50%, H 10.75%, O 7.75%. Main perfume ingredient of violets.

Both the d-(1,5)-cis- and d-(1,5)-trans-forms occur in nature. Isoln from irone mixture and synthesis: Naves, *Helv. Chim. Acta* **31**, 893, 1103 (1948); Ruzicka et al., ibid. **31**, 257 (1948). Synthesis: Barton, Mousseron-Canet, *J. Chem. Soc.* **1960**, 271. Industrial preparation: Kaiser, Kimel, *US 2877271* (1959 to Hoffmann-La Roche); Eschenmoser et al., *US 3413351; US 3470241* (1968, 1969 to Firmenich & Cie). Nomenclature in early papers: Naves, *Helv. Chim. Acta* **32**, 969 (1949). Stereochemistry: Tribolet, Schinz, ibid. **37**, 2184 (1954); Naves, Ardizio, *Bull. Soc. Chim. Fr.* **1955**, 1479; V. Rautenstrauch, G. Ohloff, *Helv. Chim. Acta* **54**, 1776 (1971); V. Rautenstrauch et al., ibid. **67**, 325 (1984). Stereoselective synthesis of cis- and trans-α-irones: S. Torii et al., *J. Org. Chem.* **45**, 16 (1980); of (±)-cis-α-irone: C. Nussbaumer, G. Fráter, ibid. **52**, 2096 (1987).

(+)-cis-α-Irone   (+)-trans-α-Irone

All forms are viscous liquids with characteristic odors.
dl-cis-α-Irone. d_4^{20} 0.9360; n_D^{20} 1.50098. uv max (ethanol): 227 nm (ε 15400), Naves, Bachmann, *Helv. Chim. Acta* **32**, 394 (1949).
d-cis-α-Irone. [35124-13-1] $[\alpha]_D^{20}$ +109° (CH_2Cl_2).
dl-trans-α-Irone. d_4^{20} 0.9347; n_D^{20} 1.50119. uv max (ethanol): 229 (ε 15450).
d-trans-α-Irone. [90242-81-2] $[\alpha]_D^{20}$ +420° (CH_2Cl_2).

5097. β-Irone. [79-70-9] 4-(2,5,6,6-Tetramethyl-1-cyclohexen-1-yl)-3-buten-2-one. $C_{14}H_{22}O$; mol wt 206.32. C 81.50%, H 10.75%, O 7.75%. Frequent byproduct in synthesis of α-irone. Stereoselective synthesis of (±)-form: S. Torii et al., *J. Org. Chem.* **45**, 16 (1980). For general refs see α-irone.

(+)-β-Irone

Oil with odor similar to that of β-ionone. $bp_{0.1}$ 85-90°; $bp_{0.7}$ 99-104°; bp_{11} 125°. $[\alpha]_D^{20}$ +59° (CH_2Cl_2). d_4^{21} 0.9434; n_D^{21} 1.5178; n_D^{25} 1.5162. uv max: 295 nm (log ε 4.05).

5098. γ-Irone. [79-68-5] 4-(2,2,3-Trimethyl-6-methylenecyclohexyl)-3-buten-2-one. $C_{14}H_{22}O$; mol wt 206.32. C 81.50%, H 10.75%, O 7.75%. Principal fragrant constituent of natural iris oil. Isoln from irone mixture: Ruzicka et al., *Helv. Chim. Acta* **30**, 1807 (1947); Ruzicka et al., ibid. **31**, 257 (1948). Synthesis of dl-γ-irone: Favre, Schinz, ibid. **41**, 1368 (1958). Synthesis of (±)-cis- and trans-γ-irone: F. Leyendecker, M.-T. Comte, *Tetrahedron* **43**, 85 (1987); T. Kawanobe et al., *Agric. Biol. Chem.* **51**, 791 (1987). Stereoselective synthesis of (±)-cis-γ-irone: C. Nussbaumer, G. Fráter, *Helv. Chim. Acta* **71**, 619 (1988). Stereochemistry: See α-irone.

(+)-cis-γ-Irone

Oil. $bp_{0.06}$ 85-88°. bp_2 114-116°. d_4^{15} 0.939; n_D^{15} 1.505. $[\alpha]_D^{20}$ +2° (methylene chloride). uv max: 230 nm (log ε 4.2).
USE: In perfumery.

5099. Iron Pentacarbonyl. [13463-40-6] Iron carbonyl; pentacarbonyliron. C_5FeO_5; mol wt 195.90. C 30.66%, Fe 28.51%, O 40.84%. $Fe(CO)_5$. Prepn from CO and Fe ore: Wallis, Townshend, *US 2378053* (1945 to International Nickel); from CO and Fe or $FeSO_4.7H_2O$: Reppe et al., *Ann.* **582**, 116 (1953); from CO and Fe amalgams: Ettmayer, Jangg, *Monatsh. Chem.* **92**, 834 (1961); from CO and steel turnings: Shipman, *GB 897204* (1962 to ICI). Convenient lab prepn of small quantities of $Fe(CO)_5$ from $Fe(CO)_4I_2$: Hieber, Lagally, *Z. Anorg. Allg. Chem.* **245**, 295 (1940). Thermodynamic data: Cotton et al., *J. Am. Chem. Soc.* **81**, 800 (1959); Leadbetter, Spice, *Can. J. Chem.* **37**, 1923 (1959). Toxicity: Sunderman et al., *Arch. Ind. Health* **19**, 11 (1959); Gage, *Br. J. Ind. Med.* **27**, 1 (1970). Reviews: Cable, Sheline, *Chem. Rev.* **56**, 1 (1956); Wender et al., *The Chemistry and Catalytic Properties of Cobalt and Iron Carbonyls* (U.S. Govt. Printing Office, Washington, 1962) 83 pp; H. Alper, "Organic Syntheses with Iron Pentacarbonyl" in *Organic Syntheses via Metal Carbonyls* vol. 2, I. Wender, P. Pino, Eds. (John Wiley, New York, 1977) pp 545-593. Review of *iron tetracarbonyl*, the photochemically produced intermediate: M. Poliakoff, *Chem. Soc. Rev.* **7**, 527-540 (1978).
Colorless to yellow, oily liquid. *Pyrophoric in air;* burns to Fe_2O_3. Dec by light to $Fe_2(CO)_9$ and CO. mp -20°. bp 103°. d_4^{20} 1.46-1.52; n_D^{22} 1.453. Critical temp 285-288°; critical pressure 29.6 atm. Flash pt -15°C. Heat capacity at constant pressure (14°) 56.9 cal/mole/°C. Latent heat of fusion 3161 cal/mol; latent heat of vaporization 9.6 kcal/mole. Heat of combustion -386.9 kcal/mole; heat of formation [$Fe(CO)_5$(liq)] -182.6 kcal/mole. Practically insol in water, liquid ammonia. Readily sol in most organic solvents including ether, benzene, petr ether, acetone, ethyl acetate, carbon tetrachloride, carbon disulfide; slightly sol in alcohol. *Protect from light and air.* LD_{50} in mice, rats (mg/l): 2.19, 0.91 inhalation for 30 min. (Sunderman).
Caution: Potential symptoms of overexposure are irritation of eyes, mucous membranes, respiratory system; headache, dizziness, nausea, vomiting; fever, cyanosis, cough, dyspnea; liver, kidney, lung injury; degenerative CNS changes. See *NIOSH Pocket Guide to Chemical Hazards* (DHHS/NIOSH 97-140, 1997) p 174.
USE: To make finely divided iron, so-called carbonyl iron, which is used in the manuf of powdered iron cores for high frequency coils used in the radio and television industry; as antiknock agent in motor fuels; as catalyst and reagent in organic reactions.

5100. Iron Sorbitex. [1338-16-5] Glucitol iron complex, compd with citric acid; iron sorbitol; iron sorbitol citrate; Jectofer. Sterile soln (pH 7.2-7.9) of a complex of iron, sorbitol, and citric acid, stabilized with dextrin in a dil soln of sorbitol. Contains 50 ±2 mg/ml of elemental iron. Average mol wt <5000. Prepn: Lindvall, Andersson, *Br. J. Pharmacol. Chemother.* **17**, 358 (1961).
The prepn is hypertonic, stable in serum and rapidly absorbed from muscle, does not produce hemolysis, affects coagulation only at very high concns.
THERAP CAT: Hematinic.

5101. Iron Sucrose. [8047-67-4] Iron saccharate; iron(III) hydroxide sucrose complex; saccharated ferric oxide; Ferrivenin; Venofer. Composed of a polynuclear ferric hydroxide inner sphere surrounded by sucrose molecules; mol wt 34 to 60 kDa. Prepn: C. Mannich, C. A. Rojahn, *Ber. Dtsch. Pharm. Ges.* **32**, 158 (1922); and use in i.v. treatment of anemia: H. G. B. Slack, J. F. Wilkinson, *Lancet* **256**, 11, 163 (1949). Histological properties: P. Geisser et al., *Arzneim.-Forsch.* **42**, 1439 (1992). Pharmacokinetics: B. G. Danielson et al., ibid. **46**, 615 (1996). Clinical evaluation in dialysis-associated anemia: C. Charytan et al., *Am. J. Kidney Dis.* **37**, 300 (2001). Review of clinical experience: J. Yee, A. Besarab, ibid. **40**, 1111-1121 (2002).
Brown powder. Sol in water (pH 10.5 to 11.1; 1430 mOsm/l). LD_{50} in mice (mg Fe/kg): >2500 orally; >200 i.v. (Geisser).
THERAP CAT: Hematinic.

5102. Irsogladine. [57381-26-7] 6-(2,5-Dichlorophenyl)-1,3,5-triazine-2,4-diamine; 2,4-diamino-6-(2,5-dichlorophenyl)-s-triazine; dicloguamine. $C_9H_7Cl_2N_5$; mol wt 256.09. C 42.21%, H 2.76%, Cl 27.69%, N 27.35%. Gastric cytoprotectant with benzoguanamine skeleton. Prepn: H. Murai et al., *DE 2506814*; eidem, *US 3966728* (1975, 1976 both to Nippon Shinyaku). Series of articles on pharmacology: F. Ueda et al., *Arzneim.-Forsch.* **34**,

474-491 (1984). Tissue distribution studies: T. Ando *et al., ibid.* **36**, 1221 (1984). Metabolism: M. Sugiyama *et al., ibid.* 1229. Phase I study: M. Nakashima *et al., ibid.* **34**, 492 (1984). Mechanism of antiulcer action study: F. Ueda *et al., Oyo Yakuri* **33**, 157 (1987), *C.A.* **107**, 17604a (1987).

Colorless crystals from dioxane, mp 268-269°.

Maleate. [84504-69-8] MN-1695; Gaslon. $C_9H_7Cl_2N_5.C_4H_4O_4$; mol wt 372.16. Crystals from dioxane, mp 205° (dec). LD_{50} in male, female mice, rats (mg/kg): 6035, 5697, 3898, 2917 orally; 2841, 3216, 1600, 1524 s.c.; 775, 1006, 558, 545 i.p. (Ueda, 1984 p 474).

THERAP CAT: Antiulcerative.

5103. Isanic Acid. [506-25-2] 17-Octadecene-9,11-diynoic acid; bolecic acid; erythrogenic acid. $C_{18}H_{26}O_2$; mol wt 274.40. C 78.79%, H 9.55%, O 11.66%. $CH_2=CH(CH_2)_4C\equiv C-C\equiv C(CH_2)_7COOH$. Found in vegetable oils obtained from tropical and equatorial regions. Isoln from boleko oil: De Vries, *Oleagineux* **12**, 427 (1957); US 2789993 (1957 to UCB). Structure: Steger, Van Loon, *Rec. Trav. Chim.* **59**, 1156 (1940); Gunstone, Sealy, *J. Chem. Soc.* **1963**, 5772; Morris, *ibid.* 5779. Synthesis: Black, Weedon, *ibid.* **1953**, 1785.

Crysts from petr ether, mp 39.5°. d_4^{45} 0.9309; d_4^{60} 0.91966; d_4^{78} 0.9095; n_D^{50} 1.49148; n_D^{78} 1.4860. Turns pink on exposure to air and light. Tendency to polymerize and explode, especially when heated above 250°. Sol in acetone, ethanol, isopropanol. Moderately sol in petr ether.

5104. Isatin. [91-56-5] Indole-2,3-dione; 2,3-indolinedione; 2,3-diketoindoline. $C_8H_5NO_2$; mol wt 147.13. C 65.31%, H 3.43%, N 9.52%, O 21.75%. May be obtained by oxidation of indigo or of oxygenated indoles such as indoxyl, oxindole, or dioxindole: Erdmann, *J. Prakt. Chem.* [1] **24**, 1 (1841); Laurent, *ibid.* **25**, 430 (1842); DE 229815 in *Frdl.* **10**, 353 (1910); JP 152932 (1942 to ICI); *C.A.* **44**, 1544d (1950). Synthesis: Sandmeyer, *Helv. Chim. Acta* **2**, 234 (1919); GB 128122 in *C.A.* **13**, 2375 (1919); Marvel, Hiers, *Org. Synth.* **coll. vol. I** (2nd ed., 1941) p 327; Wibaut, Gerling, *Rec. Trav. Chim.* **50**, 41 (1931); Neunhoeffer, Lehmann, *Ber.* **94**, 2960 (1961); Ziegler *et al., Monatsh. Chem.* **94**, 453 (1963). May be isolated from the urine of rabbits that are fed *o*-nitrophenylglyoxylic acid: Bohm, *Z. Physiol. Chem.* **265**, 210 (1940). Pharmacology: Singh, *Indian Vet. J.* **48**, 672 (1971). *Reviews:* Heller, *Ueber Isatin, Isatyd, Dioxindol und Indophenin* (F. Enke, Stuttgart, 1931); Sumpter, *Chem. Rev.* **34**, 393 (1944). Discussion of chemistry of isatin: Morton, *Chemistry of Heterocyclic Compounds* (New York, 1946) pp 126-132.

Orange-colored monoclinic prisms. mp 203.5° (partial sublimation). Absorption spectrum: Hartley, Dobbie, *J. Chem. Soc.* **75**, 647, 656. Freely sol in boiling alcohol; sol in ether and in boiling water with reddish-brown color; sol in alkali hydroxide solns with a violet color becoming yellow on standing. The alc soln imparts a persistent, disagreeable odor to the human skin. Extremely weak base, forms a crystalline perchlorate, $C_8H_5NO_2.HClO_4.2H_2O$.

USE: Manuf vat dyes. In analytical chemistry as a reagent for cuprous ions, mercaptans, thiophene, and indican.

5105. Iseganan. [257277-05-7] Cyclic (5 → 14),(7 → 12)-L-arginylglycylglycyl-L-leucyl-L-cysteinyl-L-tyrosyl-L-cysteinyl-L-

arginylglycyl-L-arginyl-L-phenylalanyl-L-cysteinyl-L-valyl-L-cysteinyl-L-valylglycyl-L-argininamide; IB-367. $C_{78}H_{126}N_{30}O_{18}S_4$; mol wt 1900.29. C 49.30%, H 6.68%, N 22.11%, O 15.16%, S 6.75%. Cationic antibacterial cyclic peptide composed of 17 amino acid residues with 2 disulfide linkages; synthetic protegrin analog based on the sequence of Protegrin-1 as isolated from porcine neutrophils. Prepn: C. Chang *et al.*, WO 9718826; *eidem*, US 5994306 (1997, 1999 both to IntraBiotics). CE characterization and purification: J. Chen *et al., J. Chromatogr. A* **853**, 197 (1999). Structure activity study: *eidem et al., Biopolymers* **55**, 88 (2000). *In vitro* and *in vivo* antibacterial activity: D. A. Mosca *et al., Antimicrob. Agents Chemother.* **44**, 1803 (2000). Clinical study in oral mucositis: F. J. Giles *et al., Leuk. Lymphoma* **44**, 1165 (2003). Review of pharmacology and clinical experience: *idem et al., Expert Opin. Invest. Drugs* **11**, 1161-1170 (2002).

Arg–Gly–Gly–Leu–Cys–Tyr–Cys–Arg–Gly–Arg–Phe–Cys–Val–Cys–Val–Gly–ArgNH$_2$

Hydrochloride. [256475-21-5]; [244015-05-2] (hydrate). IB-367-03

THERAP CAT: Antibacterial.

5106. Isepamicin. [58152-03-7] *O*-6-Amino-6-deoxy-α-D-glucopyranosyl-(1 → 4)-*O*-[3-deoxy-4-*C*-methyl-3-(methylamino)-β-L-arabinopyranosyl-(1 → 6)]-N^1-[(2S)-3-amino-2-hydroxy-1-oxopropyl]-2-deoxy-D-streptamine; 1-*N*-[(S)-3-amino-2-hydroxypropionyl]gentamicin B; HAPA-B; Sch-21420. $C_{22}H_{43}N_5O_{12}$; mol wt 569.60. C 46.39%, H 7.61%, N 12.30%, O 33.71%. Aminoglycoside antibiotic; semisynthetic derivative of gentamicin B. Prepn: M. J. Weinstein *et al.*, BE 818431; J. J. Wright, P. J. L. Daniels, BE 824657 (both 1975 to Sherico); J. J. Wright *et al.*, US 4002742 (1977 to Schering Corp.); T. L. Nagabhushan *et al., J. Antibiot.* **31**, 681 (1978). Antibacterial spectrum *in vitro* and *in vivo*: G. H. Miller *et al., ibid.* 688. Comparison with amikacin of nephrotoxic potential: L. I. Rankin *et al., Antimicrob. Agents Chemother.* **16**, 491 (1979). Series of articles on antibacterial activity, toxicology and clinical efficacy: *Chemotherapy (Tokyo)* **35**, Suppl 5, 1-610 (1985); on toxicology: *Jpn. J. Antibiot.* **39**, 3164-3328 (1986), *C.A.* **107**, 32666r-32673r (1987). Acute toxicity: T. Morino *et al., ibid.* 3164, *C.A.* **107**, 32667s (1987).

Sulfate. [67814-76-0] Exacin; Isepacin; Isépalline. $[\alpha]_D^{26}$ +110.9° (c = 1 in water as the disulfate hydrate). LD_{50} in male, female mice, rats (mg/kg): 234, 236, 489, 476 i.v.; 3312, 3320, 3451, 3392 s.c.; >5000 orally both species (Morino).

THERAP CAT: Antibacterial.

5107. Isethionic Acid. [107-36-8] 2-Hydroxyethanesulfonic acid; hydroxyethylsulfonic acid. $C_2H_6O_4S$; mol wt 126.13. C 19.04%, H 4.79%, O 50.74%, S 25.42%. $HOCH_2CH_2SO_3H$. Obtained by heating ethylene, chlorosulfonic acid, and water: Klason, *J. Prakt. Chem.* [2] **19**, 234 (1879); from ether and SO_3: Hubner, *Ann.* **223**, 198 (1884); from ethylenesulfite + $NaHCO_3$: Smith, US 2899461 (1959 to Dow).

Colorless, syrupy, strongly acid liquid. Kept over H_2SO_4, it solidifies to a very hygroscopic, cryst mass. Miscible with water, alc. Forms readily cryst salts with organic bases.

Caution: Irritating to skin, mucous membranes.

5108. Ishikawa Reagent. [309-88-6] *N,N*-Diethyl-1,1,2,3,-3,3-hexafluoro-1-propanamine; PPDA. $C_7H_{11}F_6N$; mol wt 223.16. C 37.67%, H 4.97%, F 51.08%, N 6.28%. Reagent for the fluorination of alcohols and esters; prepd from perfluoropropene and diethylamine. Prepn: I. L. Knunyants *et al., Bull. Acad. Sci. USSR Div. Chem. Sci.* **1953**, 255; D. C. England *et al., J. Am. Chem. Soc.* **82**, 5116 (1960); A. Y. Yakubovich *et al., Dokl. Akad. Nauk SSSR (Engl. Transl.)* **161**, 399 (1965); and use as a fluorinating agent: A. Takaoka *et al., Bull. Chem. Soc. Jpn.* **52**, 3377 (1979). Synthetic applications: S. Watanabe *et al., J. Fluorine Chem.* **31**, 135, 247 (1986); **36**, 361 (1987); **38**, 243 (1988); **39**, 17 (1988); **47**, 187 (1990); K. Ogu *et al., Tetrahedron Lett.* **39**, 305 (1998); G. Koch *et al., Synlett* **2004**, 693.

bp$_{50}$ 54° (England). Also reported as bp$_{20}$ 38-39° (Yakubovich). n_D^{24} 1.2160. d_4^{24} 1.2127.

USE: Fluorinating agent.

5109. Isinglass. Ichthyocolla; fish glue. The inner membrane of the swimming bladder of *Acipenser huso* and other species of sturgeon and of hake. *Constit.* Chiefly glutin.

Thin, white or yellowish, semi-transparent, pearly iridescent, horny sheets. Sol in hot water, hot dil alcohol. In cold water, softens and becomes adhesive.

USE: As nutrient and food instead of gelatin; as adhesive, in "court plaster"; for clarifying (fining) wine and beer; as protective colloid in manuf various chemicals; in glass and porcelain cements; for lustering and stiffening silks and other fabrics; with pyroxylin for waterproofing fabrics.

5110. Isoaminile. [77-51-0] α-[2-(Dimethylamino)propyl]-α-(1-methylethyl)benzeneacetonitrile; 4-(dimethylamino)-2-isopropyl-2-phenylvaleronitrile; 3-cyano-5-dimethylamino-3-phenyl-2-methylhexane; α-(β-dimethylaminopropyl)-α-isopropylphenylacetonitrile; Aprecon; Dimyril; Nullatuss. $C_{16}H_{24}N_2$; mol wt 244.38. C 78.64%, H 9.90%, N 11.46%. Prepn: **GB 822695**; Stühmer, Funke, **US 2934557** (1959, 1960, both to Kali-Chemie).

Liquid, bp$_3$ 138-146°.
Citrate. [28416-66-2] Perocan. $C_{16}H_{24}N_2 \cdot C_6H_8O_7$; mol wt 436.50. Crystals from alcohol + ether, mp 63-64°.
Cyclamate. [10075-36-2] Mucalan; Peracon. $C_{22}H_{37}N_3O_3S$; mol wt 423.61. Prepn: Dickinson, **US 3074996** (1963 to Abbott).
Tartrate. $C_{16}H_{24}N_2 \cdot C_4H_6O_6$. Crystals, mp 64°.
THERAP CAT: Antitussive.

5111. Isoamyl Acetate. [123-92-2] Amylacetic ester. $C_7H_{14}O_2$; mol wt 130.18. C 64.58%, H 10.84%, O 24.58%. CH_3-$COOCH_2CH_2CH(CH_3)_2$. The technical product is also known as *pear oil* or *banana oil.*

Colorless, neutral liq; pear-like odor and taste. d_4^{15} 0.876. Pure isoamyl acetate bp 142°. n_D^{21} 1.400; the ordinary grade of commerce boils between 120-145°. Flash pt, closed cup: 92°F (33°C); open cup: 100°F (38°C). Sol in 400 parts water; miscible with alcohol, ether, ethyl acetate, amyl alcohol. Soly of water in isoamyl acetate (25°) 1.6% by volume.

Caution: Potential symptoms of overexposure are irritation of eyes, skin, nose and throat; dermatitis. *See NIOSH Pocket Guide to Chemical Hazards* (DHHS/NIOSH 97-140, 1997) p 174.

USE: In alcohol solution as a pear flavor in mineral waters and syrups; as solvent for old oil colors, for tannins, nitrocellulose, lacquers, celluloid, and camphor; swelling bath sponges; covering

unpleasant odors, perfuming shoe polish; manuf artificial silk, leather or pearls, photographic films, celluloid cements, waterproof varnishes, bronzing liquids, and metallic paints; dyeing and finishing textiles. A special grade of the amyl acetate has been used for burning in the Hefner lamp serving as a photometric standard.

5112. Isoamylamine. [107-85-7] 3-Methyl-1-butanamine; isopentylamine; isobutylcarbylamine; 3-methylbutylamine. $C_5H_{13}N$; mol wt 87.16. C 68.90%, H 15.03%, N 16.07%. $(CH_3)_2$-$CHCH_2CH_2NH_2$. Prepn from acetamide + isoamylbromide: Erickson, *Ber.* **59B**, 2665 (1926); from α-methylhydroxylamine + isoamylmagnesium chloride: Sheverdina, Kocheshkov, *J. Gen. Chem. USSR* **8**, 1825 (1938). Isoln from *Clostridium sordelli:* Prevot, Thouvenot, *Ann. Inst. Pasteur* **103**, 925 (1962).

Colorless liq; strong ammonia odor. d^{18} 0.751. bp 95°. n_D^{18} 1.4096. Miscible with water, alcohol, chloroform, ether.
Hydrochloride. $C_5H_{13}N \cdot HCl$. Crystals from acetone, mp 215°. One gram dissolves in 0.5 ml water, 20 ml chloroform; sol in alcohol.
Caution: Irritating to skin, mucous membranes.

5113. Isoamyl Benzoate. [94-46-2] $C_{12}H_{16}O_2$; mol wt 192.25. C 74.97%, H 8.39%, O 16.64%. $C_6H_5COOCH_2CH_2CH$-$(CH_3)_2$.

Colorless liquid, d_4^{15} 0.993. bp 260-262°. Insol in water; miscible with alcohol.

USE: In perfumery and cosmetics.

5114. Isoamyl Bromide. [107-82-4] 1-Bromo-3-methylbutane. $C_5H_{11}Br$; mol wt 151.04. C 39.76%, H 7.34%, Br 52.90%. $(CH_3)_2CHCH_2CH_2Br$. Prepd from isoamyl alcohol, bromine and phosphorus or by refluxing isoamyl alcohol with HBr in presence of H_2SO_4: Kamm, Marvel, *Org. Synth.* **vol. 1**, p 4 (1921).

Colorless liquid. d_4^{15} 1.210. bp 120-121°. mp −112°. n_D^{15} 1.4433. Slightly sol in water (0.02 g/100 ml at 16.5°); miscible with alcohol, ether.

USE: In organic synthesis.

5115. Isoamyl Butyrate. [106-27-4] $C_9H_{18}O_2$; mol wt 158.24. C 68.31%, H 11.47%, O 20.22%. $CH_3(CH_2)_2COOCH_2$-$CH_2CH(CH_3)_2$.

Colorless liq; aromatic pear-like odor. d_{15}^{19} 0.866. bp 179°. Slightly sol in water; miscible with alcohol, ether.

USE: Manuf artficial rum and fruit essences.

5116. Isoamyl Chloride. [107-84-6] 1-Chloro-3-methylbutane. $C_5H_{11}Cl$; mol wt 106.59. C 56.34%, H 10.40%, Cl 33.26%. $(CH_3)_2CHCH_2CH_2Cl$. Prepd by refluxing isoamyl alcohol and HCl in presence of $ZnCl_2$; also by direct chlorination of isopentane.

Liquid. d^0 0.893. bp ~100°. n_D^{20} 1.4103. Slightly sol in water; miscible with alcohol, ether.

5117. Isoamyl Cyanide. [542-54-1] 4-Methylpentanenitrile; isocapronitrile. $C_6H_{11}N$; mol wt 97.16. C 74.17%, H 11.41%, N 14.42%. $(CH_3)_2CHCH_2CH_2CN$. Prepd from KCN and isoamyl chloride in boiling alcohol.

Liquid, very disagreeable odor. d_4^{20} 0.806. bp 155-156°. mp −51°. n_D^{20} 1.406. Insol in water; miscible with alc, ether.

5118. Isoamyl Ether. [544-01-4] 1,1'-Oxybis[3-methylbutane]; isoamyl oxide; diisoamyl ether. $C_{10}H_{22}O$; mol wt 158.28. C 75.88%, H 14.01%, O 10.11%. $[(CH_3)_2CHCH_2CH_2]_2O$.

Colorless liquid; pleasant, fruity odor. d_4^{12} 0.783. bp 172°. n_D^{20} 1.408. Insol in water; miscible with alc, chloroform, ether.

USE: Solvent in Grignard reaction; also as solvent of odorous principles; manuf lacquers; regenerating rubber.

5119. Isoamyl Formate. [110-45-2] $C_6H_{12}O_2$; mol wt 116.16. C 62.04%, H 10.41%, O 27.55%. $HCOOCH_2CH_2CH$-$(CH_3)_2$.

Colorless liquid; fruity odor. d^{20} 0.877. bp 123-124°. n_D^{20} 1.391. Sol in 300 parts water; miscible with alc, ether. LD_{50} orally in rats: 9840 mg/kg, P. M. Jenner *et al., Food Cosmet. Toxicol.* **2**, 327 (1964).

USE: Artificial fruit syrups.

5120. Isoamyl Iodide. [541-28-6] 1-Iodo-3-methylbutane. $C_5H_{11}I$; mol wt 198.05. C 30.32%, H 5.60%, I 64.08%.

$(CH_3)_2CHCH_2CH_2I$. Obtained from isoamyl alcohol, iodine, and phosphorus, or by distillation of the alcohol with HI.

Liquid; quickly becomes brown on exposure to air and light. d_{15}^{18} 1.515. bp 147°. Slightly sol in water; miscible with alc, ether. *Keep well closed and protected from light.*

5121. Isoamyl Isovalerate. [659-70-1] Isoamyl valerianate; amyl valerate; amyl isovalerate; apple oil. $C_{10}H_{20}O_2$; mol wt 172.26. C 69.72%, H 11.70%, O 18.58%. $(CH_3)_2CHCH_2$-$COOCH_2CH_2CH(CH_3)_2$.

Colorless liquid; apple-like odor. d_4^{19} 0.858. bp 191-194°. n_D^{19} 1.413. Very slightly sol in water; miscible with alc, ether.

USE: As apple essence for flavoring liqueurs and candy.

5122. Isoamyl Nitrate. [543-87-3] 3-Methyl-1-butanol nitrate. $C_5H_{11}NO_3$; mol wt 133.15. C 45.10%, H 8.33%, N 10.52%, O 36.05%. $(CH_3)_2CHCH_2CH_2NO_3$.

Colorless liquid. d_4^{22} 0.996. bp 147-148°. n_D^{22} 1.4122. Slightly sol in water; miscible with alcohol, ether.

Caution: Do not confuse with isoamyl nitrite, *q.v.*

5123. Isoamyl Nitrite. [110-46-3] Isopentyl nitrite. C_5-$H_{11}NO_2$; mol wt 117.15. C 51.26%, H 9.46%, N 11.96%, O 27.31%. $(CH_3)_2CHCH_2CH_2ONO$. Prepd by nitrosation of isopentyl alcohol: Bevillard, Choucroun, *Bull. Soc. Chim. Fr.* **1957**, 337.

Yellowish, transparent, flammable liquid; penetrating fragrant, somewhat fruity odor. Unstable and dec on exposure to air and light. The pure nitrite has d_{25}^{25} 0.875. bp 97-99°, but volatilizes readily at much lower temps. n_D^{21} 1.3871. Very slightly sol in water; miscible with alc, chloroform, ether. *Forms an explosive mixture with air or oxygen. Keep in tightly closed containers protected from light and in cool place.* Incompat. Alcohol, antipyrine, caustic alkalies, alkaline carbonates, potassium iodide, bromides, ferrous salts.

5124. Isoamyl Phthalate. [605-50-5] 1,2-Benzenedicarboxylic acid bis(3-methylbutyl) ester; diisoamyl phthalate; amyl phthalate. $C_{18}H_{26}O_4$; mol wt 306.40. C 70.56%, H 8.55%, O 20.89%.

Colorless, practically odorless liquid. d 1.028. bp$_{40}$ 225°. Insol in water; sol in organic solvents.

USE: Plasticizer for nitrocellulose and resin lacquers; preventing foam in manuf of glue; in rubber cements.

5125. Isoamyl Salicylate. [87-20-7] $C_{12}H_{16}O_3$; mol wt 208.25. C 69.21%, H 7.74%, O 23.05%. $C_6H_4(OH)COOC_5H_{11}$.

Colorless liquid; pleasant odor. d_{15}^{19} 1.048. bp 274-278°. n_D^{20} 1.506. Almost insol in water; miscible with alcohol, chloroform, ether.

USE: In perfumery and soaps.

5126. Isoascorbic Acid. [89-65-6] D-*erythro*-Hex-2-enonic acid γ-lactone; D-araboascorbic acid; erythorbic acid; isovitamin C; saccharosonic acid; glucosaccharonic acid; D-*erythro*-3-ketohexonic acid lactone; D-*erythro*-3-oxohexonic acid lactone; erycorbin; Mercate "5"; Neo-Cebicure. $C_6H_8O_6$; mol wt 176.12. C 40.92%, H 4.58%, O 54.51%. Epimer of L-ascorbic acid. Has one-twentieth of the vitamin C activity of L-ascorbic acid. Prepd by treating methyl 2-keto-D-gluconate with sodium methoxide: Maurer, Schiedt, *Ber.* **66**, 1054 (1933); **67**, 1239 (1934); Ohle *et al., ibid.* **67**, 324 (1934); Baird *et al., J. Chem. Soc.* **1934**, 63; Reichstein *et al., Helv. Chim. Acta* **17**, 516 (1934). Synthesis from sucrose: Heimann, Reiff, *Pharm. Zentralhalle* **93**, 97 (1954). Production by *Penicillium* spp: Takahashi *et al., Nature* **188**, 411 (1960); **US 3052609** (1962 to Sankyo); *Bull. Agric. Chem. Soc. Jpn.* **24**, 533 (1960), *C.A.* **55**, 1788 (1961). Conformation: Matsui *et al., Agric. Biol. Chem.* **27**, 185 (1963).

Shiny granular crystals from water or dioxane. Dec 174°. $[\alpha]_D^{16.5}$ $-17°$ (c = 1.8 in 0.01*N* HCl); $[\alpha]_D^{20}$ $-16.6°$ (H_2O). Soluble in water, alc, pyridine. Moderately sol in acetone. Slightly sol in glycerol.

Sodium salt. Sodium erythorbate; Mercate "20"; Neo-Cebitate. Crystals, sol in water. pH of aq solns of the sodium salt between 5 and 6. A 10% soln, made from commercial grade, may have a pH of 7.2 to 7.9. The free acid is more sol in water (40 g/100 ml H_2O) than the sodium salt (16 g/100 ml H_2O).

USE: Antioxidant and antimicrobial agent for foods: Kadin, Osadca, *J. Agric. Food Chem.* **7**, 358 (1959).

5127. Isobenzan. [297-78-9] 1,3,4,5,6,7,8,8-Octachloro-1,-3,3a,4,7,7a-hexahydro-4,7-methanoisobenzofuran; 1,3,4,5,6,7,10,-10-octachloro-4,7-endomethylene-4,7,8,9-tetrahydrophthalan; SD-4402; R-6700; Omtan; Telodrin. $C_9H_4Cl_8O$; mol wt 411.75. C 26.25%, H 0.98%, Cl 68.88%, O 3.89%. Prepn: **GB 772212** (1957 to Ruhrchemie); Korte, Stiasni, *Ann.* **656**, 140 (1962); Feichtinger, Linden, *Chem. Ind. (London)* **1965**, 1938. Toxicity study: Tauberger, *Arch. Exp. Pathol. Pharmakol.* **232**, 227 (1957).

Crystals from heptane, mp 120-122°. Sol in acetone, benzene, toluene, ether, xylene, heavy aromatic naphtha. LD_{50} i.v. in rats: 1.8 mg/kg (Tauberger).

USE: Insecticide.

5128. Isoborneol. [124-76-5] *exo*-1,7,7-Trimethylbicyclo-[2.2.1]heptan-2-ol; *exo*-2-bornanol; *exo*-2-camphanol. $C_{10}H_{18}O$; mol wt 154.25. C 77.87%, H 11.76%, O 10.37%. Prepn of *dl*-form: Pickard, Littlebury, *J. Chem. Soc.* **91**, 1973 (1907); Truett, Moulton, *J. Am. Chem. Soc.* **73**, 5913 (1951); Ziegler, **GB 803178** (1958). Prepn of the *l*-form by reduction of *d*-camphor with lithium aluminum hydride: Trevoy, Brown, *J. Am. Chem. Soc.* **71**, 1675 (1949). Separation of isoborneol from its *endo*-isomer, borneol, via the *p*-nitrobenzoate deriv: Truett, Moulton, *loc. cit.* Resolution of the *dl*-form: Pickard, Littlebury, *loc. cit.*; Kenyon, Priston, *ibid.* **127**, 1472 (1925). Configuration (isoborneol = *exo*-form; borneol = *endo*-form): Toivonen *et al., Acta Chem. Scand.* **3**, 991 (1949). *Review:* J. L. Simonsen, *The Terpenes* vol. II (University Press, Cambridge, 2nd ed., 1949) pp 365-367; A. R. Pinder, *The Chemistry of the Terpenes* (Chapman & Hall, London, 1960) pp 22-24, 101, 103, 105-107, 111.

l-Isoborneol

dl-**Form.** Crystals from petr ether. Sublimes on heating, mp 212° (in a sealed tube). Practically insol in water. Readily sol in alcohol, ether, chloroform.

d-**Form.** Crystals from petr ether, mp 214°. Approx $[\alpha]_D$ +34.3° in alc soln: Picard, Littlebury, *loc. cit.*

l-**Form.** Crystals from petr ether, mp 214°. Approx $[\alpha]_D$ $-34.3°$ in alc soln.

5129. Isobornyl Thiocyanoacetate. [115-31-1] Thiocyanatoacetic acid *exo*-1,7,7-trimethylbicyclo[2.2.1]hept-2-yl ester; terpinyl thiocyanoacetate; Thanite. $C_{13}H_{19}NO_2S$; mol wt 253.36. C 61.63%, H 7.56%, N 5.53%, O 12.63%, S 12.66%. *See also* Borneol. May be prepared by treating isoborneol with chloroacetyl chloride and KCNS: J. N. Borglin, **US 2217611** (1940 to Hercules).

Technical grade, yellow oily liquid with terpene-like odor. Contains 82% or more of isobornyl thiocyanoacetate with other terpenes. $bp_{0.06}$ 95°. Flash pt 82°C (180°F). d_4^{25} 1.1465. Acid no. 1.19. n_D^{25} 1.512. Very sol in alcohol, benzene, chloroform, ether. Practically insol in water.

USE: Insecticide, especially in cattle sprays.

5130. Isobutyl Acetate. [110-19-0] $C_6H_{12}O_2$; mol wt 116.16. C 62.04%, H 10.41%, O 27.55%. CH_3COOCH_2CH-$(CH_3)_2$. Prepn from isobutyl alcohol + acetic acid: **BE 505023** (1951 to Soc. Belge de l'Azote et des Prod. Chim. du Marly); from methyl isobutyl ketone: White, Emmons, *Tetrahedron* **17**, 31 (1962). Isoln from wood-rotting fungus, *Endoconidiophora coerulescens* Münch.: Birkinshaw, Morgan, *Biochem. J.* **47**, 55 (1950).

Colorless liquid. d_4^{20} 0.871. bp 118°. mp −99°. Flash pt, closed cup: 64°F (18°C). n_D^{19} 1.3907. Sol in 180 parts water, freely in alc.

Caution: Potential symptoms of overexposure are headache; drowsiness; irritation of eyes, upper respiratory system and skin; anesthesia. *See NIOSH Pocket Guide to Chemical Hazards* (DHHS/NIOSH 97-140, 1997) p 176.

USE: Flavoring, solvent.

5131. Isobutyl Alcohol. [78-83-1] 2-Methyl-1-propanol; isopropylcarbinol; 1-hydroxymethylpropane; fermentation butyl alcohol. $C_4H_{10}O$; mol wt 74.12. C 64.82%, H 13.60%, O 21.59%. $(CH_3)_2CHCH_2OH$. Present in fusel oil; also produced by fermentation of carbohydrates: Baraud, Genevois, *Compt. Rend.* **247**, 2479 (1958); Sukhodol, Chatskii, *Spirt. Promst.* **28**, 35 (1962), *C.A.* **57**, 5124e (1962). Prepn: Wender *et al.*, *J. Am. Chem. Soc.* **71**, 4160 (1949); Schreyer, **US 2564130** (1951 to du Pont); Pistor, **US 2753366**; Harrer, Rühl, **DE 1011865**; Himmler, Schiller, **US 2787628** (1956, 1957, 1957 all to BASF). Toxicity study: Smyth *et al.*, *Arch. Ind. Hyg. Occup. Med.* **10**, 61 (1954).

Colorless, refractive liq; flammable; odor like that of amyl alcohol, but weaker. d^{15} 0.806. bp 108°. mp −108°. Flash pt, closed cup: 82°F (28°C). n_D^{15} 1.3976. Sol in about 20 parts water; misc with alcohol, ether. LD_{50} orally in rats: 2.46 g/kg (Smyth).

Caution: Potential symptoms of overexposure are irritation of eyes and throat; headache, drowsiness; skin cracking. *See NIOSH Pocket Guide to Chemical Hazards* (DHHS/NIOSH 97-140, 1997) p 176.

USE: Manuf esters for fruit flavoring essences; solvent in paint, varnish removers.

5132. Isobutylamine. [78-81-9] 2-Methyl-1-propanamine; 2-methylpropylamine; 1-amino-2-methylpropane. $C_4H_{11}N$; mol wt 73.14. C 65.69%, H 15.16%, N 19.15%. $(CH_3)_2CHCH_2NH_2$. Prepn from isobutyl alcohol + NH_3: **GB 847799** (1960 to Cellulose-Polymères et Dérivés "Cepede"); Shirley, Speranza, **US 3128311** (1964 to Jefferson Chem.). Isoln from fungi: von Kamienski, *Planta* **50**, 331 (1958). Acute toxicity: K. L. Cheever *et al.*, *Toxicol. Appl. Pharmacol.* **62**, 150 (1982).

Liquid. d_4^{25} 0.724. mp −85°. bp 68-69°. n_D^{17} 1.3988. Miscible with water, alcohol, ether. LD_{50} (14 day) in male, female rats (mg/kg): 224.4, 231.8 orally (Cheever).

Caution: Skin contact can result in erythema, blistering. Inhalation causes headache, dryness of nose and throat.

5133. Isobutyl *p*-Aminobenzoate. [94-14-4] 4-Aminobenzoic acid 2-methylpropyl ester; Cycloform; Isobutyl Keloform; Isocaine. $C_{11}H_{15}NO_2$; mol wt 193.24. C 68.37%, H 7.82%, N 7.25%, O 16.56%. Prepn: Adams *et al.*, *J. Am. Chem. Soc.* **48**, 1758 (1926).

Crystals from benzene, mp 65°. Slightly sol in water; sol in alcohol, benzene, ether, acetone, olive oil.

USE: Sunscreen.

THERAP CAT: Anesthetic (topical).

5134. Isobutylbenzene. [538-93-2] (2-Methylpropyl)benzene; 2-methyl-1-phenylpropane. $C_{10}H_{14}$; mol wt 134.22. C 89.49%, H 10.51%. $C_6H_5CH_2CH(CH_3)_2$. Prepd from bromobenzene, isobutyl iodide, and sodium preferably in the presence of benzene: Wreden, Znatovicz, *Ber.* **9**, 1606 (1876); Schramm, *Monatsh. Chem.* **9**, 616 (1888); by passing vapors of dimethylbenzyl carbinol and hydrogen over activated charcoal: Zelinsky, Gawerdowskaya, *Ber.* **61**, 1052 (1928).

Liquid. d_4^{20} 0.8673. bp_{760} 170.5°; bp_{400} 145.2°; bp_{200} 120.7°; bp_{100} 99.0°; bp_{60} 84.1°; bp_{40} 73.2°; bp_{20} 54.7°; bp_{10} 37.3°; bp_5 21.1°; $bp_{1.0}$ −9.8°. n_D^{20} 1.4928. Critical temp 377.1°; crit pressure 23,636 mm Hg.

5135. Isobutyl Bromide. [78-77-3] 1-Bromo-2-methylpropane. C_4H_9Br; mol wt 137.02. C 35.06%, H 6.62%, Br 58.32%. $(CH_3)_2CHCH_2Br$. Obtained from isobutyl alc and PBr_3: Noller, Dinsmore, *Org. Synth.* **coll. vol. II**, 358 (1943).

Colorless liquid. d^{15} 1.272. bp 91.5°. mp −119°. n_D^{15} 1.4391. Slightly sol in water (0.6 g/l); miscible with alcohol, ether.

5136. Isobutyl *n*-Butyrate. [539-90-2] $C_8H_{16}O_2$; mol wt 144.21. C 66.63%, H 11.18%, O 22.19%. $CH_3CH_2CH_2COOCH_2$-$CH(CH_3)_2$.

Liquid. d 0.866. bp 157°. n_D^{20} 1.4035. Slightly sol in water; miscible with alcohol, ether.

5137. Isobutyl Carbamate. [543-28-2] $C_5H_{11}NO_2$; mol wt 117.15. C 51.26%, H 9.46%, N 11.96%, O 27.31%. H_2NCOO-$CH_2CH(CH_3)_2$. Prepd from isobutyl chloroformate and NH_3 in benzene soln.

Crystals, d 0.956. mp 67°; also stated at 61°. bp 206-207°. Insol in water. Sol in alcohol, ether.

5138. Isobutyl Chloride. [513-36-0] 1-Chloro-2-methylpropane. C_4H_9Cl; mol wt 92.57. C 51.90%, H 9.80%, Cl 38.30%. $(CH_3)_2CHCH_2Cl$. Formed by the action of HCl or PCl_5 on isobutyl alcohol.

Liquid. d^{15} 0.883. bp 68-69°. mp −131°. n_D^{15} 1.40096. Insoluble in water. Miscible with alcohol, ether.

5139. Isobutyl Chlorocarbonate. [543-27-1] Carbonochloridic acid 2-methylpropyl ester; isobutyl chloroformate. C_5H_9-ClO_2; mol wt 136.58. C 43.97%, H 6.64%, Cl 25.96%, O 23.43%. $ClCO_2CH_2CH(CH_3)_2$. Prepd from isobutyl alcohol and phosgene.

Clear liquid; vapors irritate eyes and mucous membranes. d 1.040. bp 130°. Gradually dec by water and alcohol. Miscible with benzene, chloroform, ether.

5140. Isobutyl Cyanoacrylate. [1069-55-2] 2-Cyano-2-propenoic acid 2-methylpropyl ester; 2-cyanoacrylic acid isobutyl ester; bucrilate; bucrylate; IBC; IBCA. $C_8H_{11}NO_2$; mol wt 153.18. C 62.73%, H 7.24%, N 9.14%, O 20.89%. Monomer rapidly polymerizes upon contact with fluid or tissue. Preparative method: A. E. Ardis, **US 2467926** (1949 to B. F. Goodrich). Development of polymer nanoparticles as a magnetic drug carrier: A. Ibrahim *et al.*, *J. Pharm. Pharmacol.* **35**, 59 (1983). Clinical experience in treatment of varicocele-associated infertility by transcatheter embolization: F. H. Comhaire, M. Kunnen, *Fertil. Steril.* **43**, 781 (1985); in treatment of arteriovenous malformations: H. V. Vinters *et al.*, *N. Engl. J. Med.* **314**, 477 (1986). Review of 2-cyanoacrylic ester polymers: J. T. O'Connor in *Kirk-Othmer Encyclopedia of Chemical Technology* vol. 1 (Wiley-Interscience, New York, 4th ed., 1991) pp 344-352; of use in treatment of bleeding gastric varices: R. Kind *et al.*, *Endoscopy* **32**, 512-519 (2000).

Liquid, bp 71-73°. d 0.99. n_D^{20} 1.4352. Viscosity: 2.0 cP. Flash pt: 199°F (93°C). Heat of polymerization: 66.9 kJ/mol.

Polymer. [26809-38-1] Poly(isobutyl 2-cyanoacrylate); PIBCA. LD$_{50}$ i.v. in mice (mg/kg): 242 (Ibrahim).

USE: Adhesive; polymer nanoparticles as pharmaceutic aid for controlled release drug delivery.

THERAP CAT: Tissue adhesive.

5141. Isobutylene. [115-11-7] 2-Methylpropene; isobutene. C$_4$H$_8$; mol wt 56.11. C 85.62%, H 14.37%. CH$_2$=C(CH$_3$)$_2$. Obtained from refinery streams by absorption on 65% H$_2$SO$_4$ at about 15°: Packie, Rupp, **US 2424186, US 2509885**; Draeger, **US 2456260**; Steele, Epps Jr., **US 2497191** (1947, 1950, 1948, 1950, all to Standard Oil); Peters, Gothman; Edwards, Wesselhoft, **US 2962537; US 3129265** (1960, 1964, both to Esso). Separation from a mixed C$_4$ stream using 50% H$_2$SO$_4$: **GB 824573, GB 858645** and **FR 1337232** (1959, 1961 and 1963 to Compagnie Francaise de Raffinage); Valet *et al., Hydrocarbon Process. Petr. Refin.* **41,** No. 5, 119 (1962); Martel, *Chem. Eng.* **72,** No. 7, 66 (1965). Prepn: Verdol, **US 3170000** (1965 to Sinclair). *Review:* Kennedy, Kirshenbaum, "Isobutylene" in *Vinyl and Diene Monomers* (part 2), E. C. Leonard, Ed. (Wiley-Interscience, New York, 1971) pp 691-756.

Gas. bp$_{760}$ −6.900°; bp$_{100}$ −49.309°; bp$_{30}$ −67.90°; bp$_{10}$ −81.95°; bp$_1$ −105.06°. d$_4^{20}$ 0.5942; d$_4^{25}$ 0.5879; d$_4^{30}$ 0.5815. Practically insol in water. Very sol in alc, ether, sulfuric acid.

Caution: Simple asphyxiant.

USE: Primarily used to produce diisobutylene, trimers, butyl rubber, and other polymers; also to produce antioxidants for foods, packaging, food supplements, and for plastics: Hatch, *Pet. Refin.* **39,** No. 6, 207 (1960).

5142. Isobutyl Ether. [628-55-7] 1,1′-Oxybis[2-methylpropane]; diisobutyl ether. C$_8$H$_{18}$O; mol wt 130.23. C 73.78%, H 13.93%, O 12.29%. (CH$_3$)$_2$CHCH$_2$OCH$_2$CH(CH$_3$)$_2$. Colorless liquid, characteristic odor. d^{15} 0.761. bp 122-124°. Insol in water. Miscible with alcohol, ether.

5143. Isobutyl Formate. [542-55-2] Tetryl formate. C$_5$-H$_{10}$O$_2$; mol wt 102.13. C 58.80%, H 9.87%, O 31.33%. HCOOCH$_2$CH(CH$_3$)$_2$. Liquid. d$_4^{20}$ 0.885. bp 98°. mp −95°. n$_D^{20}$ 1.3858. Sol in 100 parts water; miscible with alc, ether.

5144. Isobutyl Iodide. [513-38-2] 1-Iodo-2-methylpropane. C$_4$H$_9$I; mol wt 184.02. C 26.11%, H 4.93%, I 68.96%. (CH$_3$)$_2$CHCH$_2$I. Obtained by distilling isobutyl alcohol and HI, or from isobutyl alcohol, iodine and phosphorus.
Liquid; becomes brown on exposure. d^{20} 1.605. bp 120°. mp −93°. n$_D^{20}$ 1.4960. Insol in water. Miscible with alcohol, ether. *Keep well closed and protected from light.*

5145. Isobutyl Isobutyrate. [97-85-8] 2-Methylpropanoic acid 2-methylpropyl ester. C$_8$H$_{16}$O$_2$; mol wt 144.21. C 66.63%, H 11.18%, O 22.19%. (CH$_3$)$_2$CHCOOCH$_2$CH(CH$_3$)$_2$. Liquid. d$_4^0$ 0.875. bp 147°. mp −81°. n$_D^{20}$ 1.3999. Insol in water. Miscible with alcohol.

5146. Isobutyl Isovalerate. [589-59-3] Isobutyl valerate. C$_9$H$_{18}$O$_2$; mol wt 158.24. C 68.31%, H 11.47%, O 20.22%. (CH$_3$)$_2$CHCH$_2$COOCH$_2$CH(CH$_3$)$_2$. Liquid; ethereal odor. d^{20} 0.853. bp 170-172°. n$_D^{20}$ 1.4064. Insol in water. Miscible with alcohol, ether.

USE: Flavoring and manuf fruit essences.

5147. Isobutyl Mercaptan. [513-44-0] 2-Methyl-1-propanethiol. C$_4$H$_{10}$S; mol wt 90.19. C 53.27%, H 11.18%, S 35.55%. (CH$_3$)$_2$CHCH$_2$SH. May be prepd from isobutyl bromide and KHS in alcohol, *see ref under* other butyl mercaptans.
Mobile liq. Heavy skunk odor. mp −79°. bp 88°. Flammable. d$_4^{20}$ 0.8357. n$_D^{20}$ 1.43859. Slightly sol in water; very sol in alcohol, ether, liquid hydrogen sulfide.

5148. Isobutyl Nitrate. [543-29-3] C$_4$H$_9$NO$_3$; mol wt 119.12. C 40.33%, H 7.62%, N 11.76%, O 40.29%. (CH$_3$)$_2$CH-CH$_2$ONO$_2$. Liquid. d$_4^{20}$ 1.015. bp 123-125°. n$_D^{20}$ 1.4028. Insol in water. Miscible with alcohol, ether.

5149. Isobutyl Nitrite. [542-56-3] C$_4$H$_9$NO$_2$; mol wt 103.12. C 46.59%, H 8.80%, N 13.58%, O 31.03%. (CH$_3$)$_2$-CHCH$_2$NO$_2$. Prepd from isobutyl alcohol, NaNO$_2$, and dil H$_2$SO$_4$. Colorless liq. d$_4^{22}$ 0.870. bp 67°. n$_D^{22}$ 1.3715. Slightly sol and gradually dec by water. Miscible with alcohol.

5150. Isobutyl Propionate. [540-42-1] C$_7$H$_{14}$O$_2$; mol wt 130.18. C 64.58%, H 10.84%, O 24.58%. CH$_3$CH$_2$COOCH$_2$-CH(CH$_3$)$_2$. Liquid; agreeable, ethereal odor. d$_4^0$ 0.888. bp 137°. mp −71°. n$_D^{20}$ 1.3975. Insol in water. Miscible with alc.

USE: Manuf fruit essences.

5151. Isobutyl Stearate. [646-13-9] C$_{22}$H$_{44}$O$_2$; mol wt 340.58. C 77.58%, H 13.02%, O 9.40%. CH$_3$(CH$_2$)$_{16}$COOCH$_2$-CH(CH$_3$)$_2$. Paraffin-like, crystal substance at low temp, mp about 20°.

USE: Waterproof coatings, polishes, face creams, rouges, ointments, soaps, rubber manuf, dye solns, inks, lubricants.

5152. Isobutyl Sulfide. [592-65-4] 1,1′-Thiobis[2-methylpropane]; diisobutyl sulfide. C$_8$H$_{18}$S; mol wt 146.29. C 65.68%, H 12.40%, S 21.92%. [(CH$_3$)$_2$CHCH$_2$]$_2$S. Obtained by heating isobutyl chloride or potassium isobutyl sulfate with K$_2$S.
Liquid. d$_4^{10}$ 0.836. bp 171-173°. Insol in water. Miscible with alcohol, ether.

5153. Isobutyl Urethane. [539-89-9] (2-Methylpropyl)carbamic acid ethyl ester. C$_7$H$_{15}$NO$_2$; mol wt 145.20. C 57.90%, H 10.41%, N 9.65%, O 22.04%. (CH$_3$)$_2$CHCH$_2$NHCOOC$_2$H$_5$. Obtained by shaking isobutylamine with ethyl chloroformate and aq KOH in the cold.
Liquid; apple-like odor. d$_4^{20}$ 0.943. Solidif below −65°. bp$_{17}$ 96°. n$_D^{20}$ 1.4288. Insol in water. Sol in alcohol.

5154. Isobutyraldehyde. [78-84-2] 2-Methylpropanal; isobutylaldehyde; isobutyric aldehyde. C$_4$H$_8$O; mol wt 72.11. C 66.62%, H 11.18%, O 22.19%. (CH$_3$)$_2$CHCHO. Manuf by the oxo process from propylene, carbon monoxide, and hydrogen at 130-160° and 1500-3000 psi in the presence of a cobalt catalyst: Roelen, **US 2327066** (1943); also prepared by air oxidation of isobutyl alcohol: Fossek, *Monatsh. Chem.* **2,** 614 (1881); Lipp, *Ann.* **205,** 2 (1880). Toxicity study: Smyth *et al., Arch. Ind. Hyg. Occup. Med.* **10,** 61 (1954). *Review:* P. D. Sherman in *Kirk-Othmer Encyclopedia of Chemical Technology* vol. 4 (Wiley-Interscience, New York, 3rd ed., 1978) pp 376-386.
Flammable liq. Pungent odor. d$_4^{20}$ 0.7938. mp −65.9°. bp$_{760}$ 64°. n$_D^{20}$ 1.3730. Heat of combustion 599.9 kcal. Flash pt (open cup) <20°F. Soly in water at 20°: 11 g/100 ml H$_2$O. Miscible with ethanol, ether, carbon disulfide, acetone, benzene, toluene, chloroform. Forms an azeotrope with water contg 94% isobutyraldehyde. The azeotrope bp$_{760}$ 59°. Weight per gallon of isobutyraldehyde: 6.55 lbs. Oxidizes slowly on exposure to air, forming isobutyric acid. LD$_{50}$ orally in rats: 3.7 g/kg (Smyth).

USE: In the synthesis of pantothenic acid, valine, leucine, cellulose esters, perfumes, flavors, plasticizers, resins, gasoline additives.

5155. Isobutyric Acid. [79-31-2] 2-Methylpropanoic acid; isopropylformic acid. C$_4$H$_8$O$_2$; mol wt 88.11. C 54.53%, H 9.15%, O 36.32%. (CH$_3$)$_2$CHCOOH. Prepn from 1-nitroisobutane: Lippincott, Hass, *Ind. Eng. Chem.* **31,** 118 (1939); from methallyl chloride: Towle, Hall, **US 2667508** (1954 to Standard Oil Co. of Indiana); from propylene: Alderson, **US 3020314** (1962 to du Pont); from 2-methylpropane + CO with HF catalyst: Friedman, Cotton, *J. Org. Chem.* **27,** 481 (1962).
Liquid; pungent odor like that of butyric acid, but not as unpleasant. bp$_{760}$ 152-155°. mp −47°. d$_4^{20}$ 0.950. n$_D^{20}$ 1.3930. Flash pt, open cup: 170°F (77°C). Sol in 6 parts of water; misc with alcohol, chloroform, ether.

Caution: Mild irritant.

5156. Isobutyronitrile. [78-82-0] 2-Methylpropanenitrile; isopropyl cyanide; 2-cyanopropane. C$_4$H$_7$N; mol wt 69.11. C 69.52%, H 10.21%, N 20.27%. (CH$_3$)$_2$CHCN. Prepn: E. A. Letts, *Ber.* **5,** 669 (1872); A. E. Arbusow, *ibid.* **43,** 2296 (1910); R. E. Kent *et al., Org. Synth.* **coll. vol. III,** 493 (1955); A. Ahmad, *Synthesis* **1976,** 418. Acute toxicity and human industrial experience: H. Zeller *et al., Zentralbl. Arbeitsmed. Arbeitsschutz* **19,** 225

(1969), *C.A.* **71,** 128340 (1969). Acute toxicity and metabolism: H. Tanii, K. Hashimoto, *Arch. Toxicol.* **55,** 47 (1984).

Colorless liquid. bp_{740} 99-102°. bp 101-103° (Kent); also reported as bp 103-103.5° (Arbusow), bp 104° (Ahmad), bp 107-108° (Letts). $d_0^{16.25}$ 0.7731. n_D^{25} 1.3713. Log P (*n*-octanol/water): 0.46. LD_{50} (mg/kg): 25 i.p. in mice; 200 orally in rats (Zeller). LD_{50} orally in male mice: 0.3652 mmol/kg (Tanii).

Caution: Potential symptoms of overexposure are irritation of eyes, skin, nose, throat; headache, dizziness, weakness, giddiness, confusion, convulsions; dyspnea; abdominal pain, nausea, vomiting. *See NIOSH Pocket Guide to Chemical Hazards* (DHHS/NIOSH 97-140, 1997) p 178.

USE: Solvent.

5157. Isocarboxazid. [59-63-2] 5-Methyl-3-isoxazole-carboxylic acid 2-benzylhydrazide; 3-(*N*-benzylhydrazinocarbonyl)-5-methylisoxazole; 1-benzyl-2-(5-methyl-3-isoxazolylcarbonyl)hydrazine; Ro-5-0831; Marplan. $C_{12}H_{13}N_3O_2$; mol wt 231.25. C 62.33%, H 5.67%, N 18.17%, O 13.84%. Monoamine oxidase inhibitor. Prepn: Gardner, Wenis, **US 2908688** (1959 to Hoffmann-La Roche); *J. Med. Pharm. Chem.* **2,** 133 (1960). Comprehensive description: B. C. Rudy, B. Z. Senkowski, *Anal. Profiles Drug Subs.* **2,** 295-314 (1973).

Crystals from methanol, practically tasteless. mp 105-106°. Very sparingly sol in hot water (0.05%), somewhat more (1 to 2%) in 95% alc, in glycerol, in propylene glycol.

THERAP CAT: Antidepressant.

5158. Isochondrodendrine. [477-62-3] $O^7,O^{7'}$-Didemethylcycleanine; isobebeerine. $C_{36}H_{38}N_2O_6$; mol wt 594.70. C 72.71%, H 6.44%, N 4.71%, O 16.14%. From *Chondodendron tomentosum* Ruiz and Pav., *Menispermaceae:* Faltis, *Monatsh. Chem.* **33,** 873 (1912); Faltis, Neumann, *ibid.* **42,** 311 (1921); Dutcher, *J. Am. Chem. Soc.* **68,** 419 (1946); from the drug *Radix pareirae bravae:* King, *J. Chem. Soc.* **1940,** 737. Structure: Faltis, Dietreich, *Ber.* **67,** 231 (1934); Jeffreys, *J. Chem. Soc.* **1956,** 4451.

Needles from methanol, dec 288°. $[\alpha]_D^{20}$ −29° (c = 1.3 in chloroform). Sol in alcohol, benzene, chloroform.

5159. Isocinchomeronic Acid. [100-26-5] 2,5-Pyridinedicarboxylic acid. $C_7H_5NO_4$; mol wt 167.12. C 50.31%, H 3.02%, N 8.38%, O 38.29%. Prepd by treating 5-ethyl-2-picoline (aldehyde-collidine) with suitable oxidizing agents such as HNO_3, $KMnO_4$, or H_2SeO_3: Meyer, Staffen, *Monatsh. Chem.* **34,** 517 (1913); Jordan, *Ind. Eng. Chem.* **44,** 332 (1952); Kato, *Bull. Chem. Soc. Jpn.* **34,** 636 (1961); by oxidation of 5-acetyl-2-methylpyridine: Binns, Swan, *J. Chem. Soc.* **1962,** 2831; from the lutidine fraction of coal tar lutidine: Lukes *et al., Collect. Czech. Chem. Commun.* **26,** 3044 (1961).

Triclinic leaflets or prisms from dilute HCl, mp 254°. Sublimes as nicotinic acid when heated above mp. Practically insol in cold water, alcohol, ether, benzene. Slightly sol in boiling water, boiling alcohol. Appreciably sol in hot, dil aq solns of mineral acids.

Monohydrate. Crystals from water or alcohol, dec 238°.

Dihydrazide. Crystals, mp 268-269°.

USE: Intermediate in the manuf of nicotinic acid.

5160. Isoconazole. [27523-40-6] 1-[2-(2,4-Dichlorophenyl)-2-[(2,6-dichlorophenyl)methoxy]ethyl]-1*H*-imidazole; 1-[2,4-dichloro-β-[(2,6-dichlorobenzyl)oxy]phenethyl]imidazole. $C_{18}H_{14}Cl_4N_2O$; mol wt 416.13. C 51.95%, H 3.39%, Cl 34.08%, N 6.73%, O 3.84%. Prepn: E. F. Godefroi *et al., J. Med. Chem.* **12,** 784 (1969); *eidem,* **DE 1940388**; *eidem,* **US 3717655** and **US 3839574** (1970, 1973, 1974 all to Janssen). *In vitro* activity: H. J. Kessler, *Arzneim.-Forsch.* **29,** 1344 (1979). Animal study: H. J. Kessler *et al., ibid.* 1352. Antimicrobial activity in humans: H. Wendt, H. J. Kessler, *ibid.* 846. Bioavailability: U. Täuber, M. Rzadkiewicz, *Mykosen* **22,** 201 (1979).

Nitrate. [24168-96-5] R-15454; Fazol; Gyno-Travogen; Travogen; Travogyn. $C_{18}H_{14}Cl_4N_2O.HNO_3$; mol wt 479.14. Solid, mp 182-183°.

THERAP CAT: Antibacterial; antifungal.

5161. Isocorybulbine. [22672-74-8] (13*S-trans*)-5,8,13,-13a-Tetrahydro-3,9,10-trimethoxy-13-methyl-6*H*-dibenzo[*a,g*]-quinolizin-2-ol; 3,9,10-trimethoxy-13α-methyl-13aβ-berbin-2-ol; 2-hydroxy-13-methyl-3,9,10-trimethoxyberbine. $C_{21}H_{25}NO_4$; mol wt 355.43. C 70.96%, H 7.09%, N 3.94%, O 18.01%. From tubers of *Corydalis cava* (L.) Schweigg. & Korte (*C. tuberosa* DC., *Fumariaceae):* Gadamer, *Arch. Pharm.* **240,** 19 (1902). Structure: Späth, Dobrowsky, *Ber.* **58,** 1274 (1925). Synthesis: Späth, Holter, *ibid.* **59,** 2800 (1926). Abs configuration: P. W. Jeffs, *Experientia* **21,** 690 (1965); K. Iwasa *et al., J. Org. Chem.* **46,** 4744 (1981).

Leaflets, mp 179-180°; also given as 187-188°. $[\alpha]_D^{15}$ +301° in chloroform. Sol in alcohol, dil acids.

Methiodide. $C_{21}H_{25}NO_4.CH_3I$. Crystals, mp 218-221°.

5162. Isocorydine. [475-67-2] (6a*S*)-5,6,6a,7-Tetrahydro-1,2,10-trimethoxy-6-methyl-4*H*-dibenzo[*de,g*]quinolin-11-ol; 1,2,10-trimethoxy-6aα-aporphin-11-ol; 11-hydroxy-1,2,10-trimethoxyaporphine; artabotrine; luteanine. $C_{20}H_{23}NO_4$; mol wt 341.40. C 70.36%, H 6.79%, N 4.10%, O 18.75%. From tubers of *Corydalis cava* (L.) Schweigg. & Korte (*C. tuberosa* DC., *Fumariaceae); Artabotrys suaveolens* Blume, *Anonaceae; Papaver oreophilum* Rupr.; *Phoebe clemensii* Allen (*Lauraceae)* and others. Isoln: Gadamer, *Arch. Pharm.* **249,** 669 (1911); Johns, Lamberton, *Aust. J. Chem.* **20,** 1277 (1967); Pfeifer, Mann, *Pharmazie* **23,** 82 (1968). Structure: Späth, Berger, *Ber.* **64,** 2038 (1931); Gulland *et al., J. Chem. Soc.* **1931,** 2885; Barger, Sargent, *ibid.* **1939,** 991. Identity with artabotrine: Schlittler, Huber, *Helv. Chim. Acta* **35,** 111 (1952); with luteanine: Manske, *Can. J. Res.* **21B,** 13 (1943). Total synthesis: Kametani *et al., Tetrahedron* **27,** 5367 (1971). Pharmacology: Berezhinskaya *et al., Farmakol. Toksikol. (Moscow)* **31,** 44 (1968), *C.A.* **68,** 94521z (1968).

Plates from ethanol or acetone, mp 185°. $[\alpha]_D^{20}$ +195° (chloroform). Sol in ether, chloroform, alcohol, acetone, alkali hydroxide. Practically insol in water, alkali carbonates.

5163.   Isocorypalmine. [53447-14-6] 5,8,13,13a-Tetrahydro-3,9,10-trimethoxy-6H-dibenzo[a,g]quinolizin-2-ol; 3,9,10-trimethoxy-13aα-berbin-2-ol; d-tetrahydrocolumbamine. $C_{20}H_{23}$-NO_4; mol wt 341.40. C 70.36%, H 6.79%, N 4.10%, O 18.75%. From tubers of Corydalis cava (L.) Schweigg. & Korte (C. tuberosa DC.) and C. nobilis Pers., Fumariaceae: Gadamer et al., Arch. Pharm. **265**, 675 (1927); Manske, Can. J. Res. **18B**, 288 (1940). Structure: Späth, Burger, Ber. **59**, 1486 (1926). Synthesis of dl-form: Govindachari et al., ibid. **92**, 1654 (1959). Configuration: Corrodi, Hardegger, Helv. Chim. Acta **39**, 889 (1956).

Crystals, mp 239-241°. $[\alpha]_D^{20}$ +30.3° (c = 0.4 in chloroform). Sol in alcohol, ether.

dl-**Form.** Crystals from methanol, mp 216°.

5164.   Isocrotonic Acid. [503-64-0] (2Z)-2-Butenoic acid; cis-2-butenoic acid; cis-crotonic acid. $C_4H_6O_2$; mol wt 86.09. C 55.81%, H 7.02%, O 37.17%. $CH_3CH=CHCOOH$. Prepd by reacting acetaldehyde with malonic acid in the presence of pyridine: v. Auwers et al., Ann. **432**, 46 (1923); from ethyl acetoacetate: Hatch, Nesbitt, J. Am. Chem. Soc. **72**, 727 (1950); from but-2-ynoic acid: Allan et al., J. Chem. Soc. **1955**, 1862; from CH_3-$CH=CHMgBr + CO_2$: Normant, Maitte, Bull. Soc. Chim. Fr. **1956**, 1439. Structure: v. Auwers, Wissebach, Ber. **56**, 715 (1923); Plisov, Bogatskii, Zh. Obshch. Khim. **27**, 360 (1957), C.A. **51**, 15401c (1957). Review: W. Blau et al., in Ullmann's Encyclopedia of Industrial Chemistry vol. **A8** (VCH, Weinheim, 5th ed., 1987) pp 83-89.

Liquid. bp_5 55-56°; bp_{10} 62-64°; bp_{760} 168-169°. mp 15°; crystallized from pentane. d_4^{20} 1.0267. n_D^{14} 1.4483. n_D^{20} 1.4450. uv max (95% ethanol): 205.5 nm (ε 13500).

Methyl ester. $C_5H_8O_2$. Liquid. bp 118°. n_D^{20} 1.4175. uv max (95% ethanol): 205.5 nm (ε 14000).

Benzyl ester. $C_{11}H_{12}O_2$. Liquid. bp_{10} 121-122°. n_D^{20} 1.5110.

Caution: Can cause severe irritation of skin, mucous membranes.

5165.   Isocyanic Acid. [75-13-8] Carbimide. CHNO; mol wt 43.02. C 27.92%, H 2.34%, N 32.56%, O 37.19%. $HN=C=O$. Prepn: J. Liebig, F. Wöhler, Ann. **39**, 29 (1846); Steyermark, J. Org. Chem. **28**, 586 (1963); R. Vorhoeve, L. E. Trimble, Science **202**, 525 (1978). Crystal structure: Von Dohlen, Carpenter, Acta Crystallogr. **8**, 646 (1955). Review of prepn and properties: D. J. Belson, A. N. Strachan, Chem. Soc. Rev. **11**, 41-56 (1982). See also Cyanic Acid.

Store in dil solns of carbon tetrachloride or ether at −30° to slow polymerization. The free acid in the vapor phase or in ether soln gives no indication of being a mixture, and all the evidence supports the iso structure, HNCO, whereas in aq soln cyanic acid HOCN is present: N. V. Sidgwick, The Chemical Elements and Their Compounds vol. **I** (Oxford, 1950) p 673.

Caution: Strongly acidic, will blister skin.

5166.   Isodurene. [527-53-7] 1,2,3,5-Tetramethylbenzene. $C_{10}H_{14}$; mol wt 134.22. C 89.49%, H 10.51%. Occurs in coal tar. Prepd by the action of dimethyl sulfate on 2,4,6-trimethylphenylmagnesium bromide: Smith, Org. Synth. **11**, 66 (1931).

Liquid. d_4^0 0.8961; d_4^{20} 0.8906. mp −24°. bp_{760} 197.9°; bp_{400} 173.7°; bp_{200} 149.9°; bp_{100} 128.3°; bp_{60} 115.4°; bp_{40} 105.8°; bp_{20} 91.0°; bp_{10} 77.8°; bp_5 65.8°; $bp_{1.0}$ 40.6°. n_D^{20} 1.5134; n_{He}^{20} 1.51126. Insol in water. Sol in alcohol; very sol in ether.

5167.   Isoestradiol. [517-04-4] (8α,17β)-Estra-1,3,5(10)-triene-3,17-diol; $\Delta^{1,3,5}$-8α-epiestratriene-3,17β-diol; 8α-estradiol; 8-epiestradiol; 8-isoestradiol-17β. $C_{18}H_{24}O_2$; mol wt 272.38. C 79.37%, H 8.88%, O 11.75%. Prepn by high pressure hydrogenation of dihydroequilin: Serini, Logemann, Ber. **71**, 186 (1938); by hydrogenation of equilenin with Raney nickel at 2800 psi and 85°: Dauben, Ahramjian, J. Am. Chem. Soc. **78**, 633 (1956). Prepn of dl-form from dl-equilenin and stereochemistry: Johnson et al., ibid. **80**, 661 (1958).

d-**Form.** Crystals from dil methanol + chloroform, mp 181°. $[\alpha]_D^{20}$ +18° (16 mg in 2 ml dioxane).

3-Benzoate. $C_{25}H_{28}O_3$. Crystals from ethyl acetate, mp 190°. $[\alpha]_D^{20}$ +9.5° (17 mg in 2 ml dioxane).

dl-**Form.** Needles from dil methanol, mp 213.5-214°.

5168.   8-Isoestrone. [517-06-6] (8α)-3-Hydroxyestra-1,3,5(10)-trien-17-one; $\Delta^{1,3,5}$-8-epiestratrien-3-ol-17-one; 8α-estrone; 8-epiestrone. $C_{18}H_{22}O_2$; mol wt 270.37. C 79.96%, H 8.20%, O 11.84%. Prepn: Serini, Logemann, Ber. **71**, 186 (1938); Johnson et al., J. Am. Chem. Soc. **80**, 661 (1958); Ananchenko, Torgov, Tetrahedron Lett. **1963**, 1553.

dl-**Form.** Prisms from methanol, mp 254-255°.

dl-**Methyl ether.** $C_{19}H_{24}O_2$. Blades from methanol, mp 153-155°.

dl-**Benzoate.** $C_{25}H_{26}O_3$. Prisms from methanol, mp 197-198°.

5169.   Iso E Super®. [54464-57-2] (unspecified); [59056-94-9] (trans-form). 1-(1,2,3,4,5,6,7,8-Octahydro-2,3,8,8-tetramethyl-2-naphthalenyl)ethanone. $C_{16}H_{26}O$; mol wt 234.38. C 81.99%, H 11.18%, O 6.83%. Synthetic woody odorant. Prepn: J. B. Hall, J. M. Sanders, **DE 2408689**; eidem, **US 3911018** (1974, 1975 both to Int. Flavor Fragrance). Patch testing for contact allergies: P. J. Frosch et al., Contact Dermatitis **33**, 333 (1995). Adherence and duration to fabric: S. Widder, Dragoco Rep. **1999**, 69. Isoln of major odor producing "impurity": C. Nussbaumer et al., Helv. Chim. Acta **82**, 1016 (1999). Brief description: M. Gras, Perfum. Flavor. **17**, 2-12 (1992). Review of synthesis and use: G. Fráter et al., Tetrahedron **54**, 7633-7703 (1998).

Rich, warm-woody odor with a shade of amber. $bp_{2.8\ mm}$ 134-135°.

USE: Scent in perfumes, laundry products and cosmetics.

5170. Isoetharine. [530-08-5] 4-[1-Hydroxy-2-[(1-methylethyl)amino]butyl]-1,2-benzenediol; 3,4-dihydroxy-α-[1-(isopropylamino)propyl]benzyl alcohol; α-(1-isopropylaminopropyl)-protocatechuyl alcohol; *N*-isopropylethylnorepinephrine; 1-(3,4-dihydroxyphenyl)-2-isopropylamino-1-butanol; etyprenaline; isoetarine; Win-3046; Dilabron; Neoisuprel. $C_{13}H_{21}NO_3$; mol wt 239.31. C 65.25%, H 8.84%, N 5.85%, O 20.06%. Prepn: Bockmühl *et al.,* **DE 638650** (1936 to I. G. Farben.), *C.A.* **31,** 3209[4] (1937). Pharmacology: Lands *et al., J. Pharmacol. Exp. Ther.* **99,** 45 (1950); *eidem, J. Am. Pharm. Assoc.* **47,** 744 (1958).

Hydrochloride. [2576-92-3] Numotac. $C_{13}H_{21}NO_3 \cdot HCl$; mol wt 275.77. Crystals from methanol + ether. mp 212-213° (dec).

THERAP CAT: Bronchodilator.

5171. Isoeugenol. [97-54-1] 2-Methoxy-4-(1-propenyl)-phenol; 4-hydroxy-3-methoxy-1-propenylbenzene; 4-propenylguaiacol; $C_{10}H_{12}O_2$; mol wt 164.20. C 73.15%, H 7.37%, O 19.49%. Occurs in ylang-ylang and other essential oils. Prepd from eugenol: West, *J. Soc. Chem. Ind.* **59,** 275 (1940); Pal'gi, *Zh. Obshch. Khim.* **28,** 2239 (1958). Stereochemistry: von Auwers, *Ber.* **68,** 1346 (1935); Puxeddu, Rattu, *Gazz. Chim. Ital.* **67,** 647 (1937). Toxicity study: P. M. Jenner *et al., Food Cosmet. Toxicol.* **2,** 327 (1964).

trans-form

Oily liquid; easily becomes somewhat yellow. d_4^{25} 1.080. bp 266°; bp_8 128-130°. mp −10°. n_D^{19} 1.5739. Slightly sol in water; misc with alcohol, ether. LD_{50} orally in rats: 1560 mg/kg (Jenner).

***trans*-Form.** [5932-68-3] Crystals, mp 33°, bp_{12} 140°. d_4^{20} 1.087. n_D^{20} 1.5778.

***cis*-Form.** [5912-86-7] Liquid, bp_{11} 133°. d_4^{20} 1.088. n_{He}^{20} 1.5724.

USE: Manuf vanillin.

5172. Isofenphos. [25311-71-1] 2-[[Ethoxy[(1-methylethyl)amino]phosphinothioyl]oxy]benzoic acid 1-methylethyl ester; salicylic acid isopropyl ester *O*-ester with *O*-ethyl isopropylphosphoramidothioate; 1-methylethyl 2-[[ethoxy[(1-methylethyl)amino]phosphinothioyl]oxy]benzoate; *O*-ethyl *O*-2-isopropoxycarbonylphenyl isopropylphosphoramidothioate; isophenphos; Amaze; Bay 92114; SRA-12869; Lighter; Oftanol. $C_{15}H_{24}NO_4PS$; mol wt 345.39. C 52.16%, H 7.00%, N 4.06%, O 18.53%, P 8.97%, S 9.28%. Selective soil insecticide. Prepn: G. Schrader *et al.,* **FR 1600932;** *eidem,* **US 3621082** (1970, 1971 both to Bayer). Physical and biological properties: B. Homeyer, *Meded. Fac. Landbouwwet. Rijksuniv. Gent* **39,** 789 (1974). Determn of residues: M. J. Brown,

I. H. Williams, *Pestic. Sci.* **7,** 545 (1976). MS determn: T. Cairns *et al., Anal. Chem.* **56,** 2547 (1984). Persistence in soil: A. Felsot, *J. Environ. Sci. Health* **B19,** 13 (1984).

Oil, $bp_{0.01}$ 120°. d_4^{20} 1.339. Vapor pressure at 20°: 3×10^{-6} Torr; at 40°: 3.8×10^{-5} Torr. Soly in water at 20°: 23.8 ppm. Sol in dichloromethane, cyclohexanone, acetone, alc, ether, benzene. LD_{50} orally in rats, mice (mg/kg): 30-40, 90-130 (Homeyer).

USE: Insecticide.

5173. Isoflavone. [574-12-9] 3-Phenyl-4*H*-1-benzopyran-4-one; 3-phenylchromone. $C_{15}H_{10}O_2$; mol wt 222.24. C 81.07%, H 4.54%, O 14.40%. Prepn from *o*-hydroxyphenyl benzyl ketone, sodium dust and ethyl formate: Joshi, Venkataraman, *J. Chem. Soc.* **1934,** 513. Structure: Warburton, *Q. Rev. Chem. Soc.* **8,** 67 (1954).

Leaflets and needles from petr ether, mp 148°. uv max: 245, 307 nm (log ε 4.41, 3.82).

5174. Isoflupredone. [338-95-4] (11β)-9-Fluoro-11,17,21-trihydroxypregna-1,4-diene-3,20-dione; 1-dehydro-9α-fluorohydrocortisone; 9-fluoroprednisolone. $C_{21}H_{27}FO_5$; mol wt 378.43. C 66.65%, H 7.19%, F 5.02%, O 21.14%. Prepn: J. Fried *et al., J. Am. Chem. Soc.* **77,** 4181 (1955). Microbiological prepn: A. Nobile *et al., J. Am. Chem. Soc.* **77,** 4184 (1955); E. Vischer *et al., Helv. Chim. Acta* **38,** 1502 (1955); T. H. Stoudt *et al., Arch. Biochem. Biophys.* **59,** 304 (1955). Prepn of the 21-acetate: R. F. Hirschmann *et al., ibid.* 3166; J. A. Hogg *et al., ibid.* 4438; Ch. Meystre *et al., Helv. Chim. Acta* **39,** 734 (1956); A. Wellstein *et al.,* **DE 1020329** (1957 to Ciba), *C.A.* **54,** 25562h (1960); **GB 843214** (1960 to Schering), *C.A.* **55,** 5597b (1961). Absorption spectra: L. L. Smith, W. H. Muller, *J. Org. Chem.* **23,** 960 (1958). Mass spectrometry: P. Toft *et al., Can. J. Pharm. Sci.* **7,** 53 (1972). Urinary excretion in horses: D. I. Chapman *et al., Vet. Rec.* **100,** 447 (1977).

Crystals from acetone, mp 263-266° (dec). $[\alpha]_D^{23}$ +108° (c = 0.611 in ethanol). uv max (ethanol): 240 nm (ε 15800) (Vischer), also reported as mp 274-275° (dec), $[\alpha]_D^{23}$ +94° (alcohol)(Fried).

21-Acetate. [338-98-7] U-6013; Predef. $C_{23}H_{29}FO_6$; mol wt 420.47. Crystals from acetone/isopropyl ether or methanol, mp 244-246° (dec). $[\alpha]_D^{23}$ +108° (c = 0.735 in dioxane). uv max (ethanol): 240 (ε 16250).

THERAP CAT (VET): Anti-inflammatory.

5175. Isoflurane. [26675-46-7] 2-Chloro-2-(difluoromethoxy)-1,1,1-trifluoroethane; 1-chloro-2,2,2-trifluoroethyl difluoromethyl ether; compd 469; Aerrane; Forane; Forene. $C_3H_2ClF_5O$; mol wt 184.49. C 19.53%, H 1.09%, Cl 19.22%, F 51.49%, O 8.67%. $CF_3CHClOCHF_2$. Prepn: Croix, Terrell, **DE 1814962** (1969); Terrell, **US 3535388; US 3535425** (both 1970 to Air Reduction); Terrell *et al., J. Med. Chem.* **14,** 517 (1971). Series of articles on pharmacology: *Anesthesiology* **35,** 8-53 (1971); Byles *et al., Can. Anaesth. Soc. J.* **18,** 376-407 (1971). Enantiomeric resolution: J. Meinwald *et al., Science* **251,** 560 (1991).

Clear, colorless liquid having a slight odor. bp 48.5°. Vapor pressure at 25°: 330 mm. sp gr 1.45. n_D^{20} 1.3002. Nonflammable; soda lime stable. Easily miscible with organic liquids including fats and oils.

USE: Solvent and dispersant for fluorinated materials.

THERAP CAT: Anesthetic (inhalation).

THERAP CAT (VET): Anesthetic (inhalation).

5176. Isoflurophate. [55-91-4] Phosphorofluoridic acid bis(1-methylethyl) ester; phosphorofluoridic acid diisopropyl ester; isopropyl fluophosphate; diisopropyl fluorophosphonate; diisopropyl fluorophosphate; diisopropylphosphorofluoridate; fluostigmine; isofluorphate; DFP; Diflupyl; Dyflos; Floropryl; Fluropryl. C_6H_{14}-FO_3P; mol wt 184.15. C 39.13%, H 7.66%, F 10.32%, O 26.06%, P 16.82%. Prepd by the action of PCl_3 on isopropanol, chlorinating the resulting intermediate, and converting the diisopropyl chlorophosphate by means of sodium fluoride: Hardy, Kosolapoff, **US 2409039** (1946); *see also* Edgewood Arsenal, *Chemical Warfare Service TDMR 832* (April, 1944); **GB 601210** (1948); Lange, von Krueger, *Ber.* **65,** 1598 (1932); Saunders, Stacey, *J. Chem. Soc.* **1948,** 695; B. C. Saunders, *Some Aspects of the Chemistry and Toxic Action of Organic Compounds Containing Phosphorus and Fluorine* (Cambridge, 1957) p 46. Toxicity data: R. G. Horton *et al., J. Pharmacol. Exp. Ther.* **87,** 414 (1946).

Liquid. Forms HF in presence of moisture. d 1.055. mp −82°. bp₅ 46°; bp₉ 62°; bp₇₆₀ 183° (by extrapolation). Vapor pressure at 20°: 0.579 mm. n_D^{25} 1.3830. Soly in water at 25°: 1.54% w/w (dec; pH about 2.5). Sol in vegetable oils. Not very sol in mineral oils. The anhyd compd or oil solns are stable in glass containers at room temp. LD_{50} in mice (mg/kg): 3.71 s.c.; 36.8 orally (Horton).

Caution: Highly toxic; cholinesterase inactivator. Do not inhale vapors. Avoid contact with skin.

THERAP CAT: Cholinergic (ophthalmic).

THERAP CAT (VET): Has been used as a miotic.

5177. L-Isoglutamine. [636-65-7] (4*S*)-4,5-Diamino-5-oxopentanoic acid; 4-amino-L-glutaramic acid; glutamic acid α-amide. $C_5H_{10}N_2O_3$; mol wt 146.14. C 41.09%, H 6.90%, N 19.17%, O 32.84%. Prepn by the action of NH_3 on *N*-carbobenzyloxy-L-glutamic acid anhydride: Kozo Narita, *J. Chem. Soc. Jpn. Pure Chem. Sect.* **74,** 832 (1953); from 1-tosylpyroglutamide by reduction with Na in NH_3: Swan, du Vigneaud, *J. Am. Chem. Soc.* **76,** 3110 (1954); from the γ-methyl ester of *N*-tritylglutamic acid: Amiard, Heymes, **US 2927118** (1960 to UCLAF).

Crystals from acetone, dec 181°. $[\alpha]_D^{21}$ +20.5° (c = 6.1 in H_2O). pK_1' 3.81; pK_2' 7.88. Sol in water. Sparingly sol in organic solvents.

5178. Isolan. [119-38-0] Dimethylcarbamic acid 3-methyl-1-(1-methylethyl)-1*H*-pyrazol-5-yl ester; 1-isopropyl-3-methyl-5-pyrazolyl dimethylcarbamate; G-23611. $C_{10}H_{17}N_3O_2$; mol wt 211.26. C 56.85%, H 8.11%, N 19.89%, O 15.15%. Carbamate insecticide: Gerguson, Alexander, *J. Agric. Food Chem.* **1,** 288 (1953); Muller, Spindler, *Experientia* **10,** 91 (1954). Prepd by treating the K salt of the enol form of 1-isopropyl-3-methyl-5-pyrazolone with dimethylcarbamoyl chloride: **CH 279553** and **CH 282655; GB 681376** (all 1952 to Geigy); Kost, Sagitullin, *Zh. Obshch. Khim.* **33,** 867 (1963), *C.A.* **59,** 8724 (1963). Toxicity studies: T. B. Gaines *et al., Nature* **209,** 88 (1966); T. B. Gaines, *Toxicol. Appl. Pharmacol.* **14,** 515 (1969).

Liquid, bp₀.₇ 103°, bp₂.₅ 117.5-118°. d 1.07. Vapor pressure at 20° = 0.001 mm Hg. Unlike most insecticides, Isolan is more toxic to rats dermally than orally (Gaines, 1966). LD_{50} in male, female rats (mg/kg): 23, 13 orally (Gaines, 1969).

USE: Insecticide.

5179. Isoleucine. [73-32-5] L-Isoleucine; Ile; I; 2-amino-3-methylvaleric acid; α-amino-β-methylvaleric acid; (2*S*,3*S*)-2-amino-3-methylpentanoic acid. $C_6H_{13}NO_2$; mol wt 131.17. C 54.94%, H 9.99%, N 10.68%, O 24.39%. An essential amino acid for human development. Isoln from beet-sugar mother liquors: F. Ehrlich, *Ber.* **37,** 1809 (1904). Structure and identification of isomers: *idem, Ber.* **40,** 2538 (1907); J. P. Greenstein *et al., J. Biol. Chem.* **204,** 307 (1953). Early chemistry and biochemistry: *Amino Acids and Proteins,* D. M. Greenberg, Ed. (Charles C. Thomas, Springfield, IL, 1951) 950 pp., *passim;* J. P. Greenstein, M. Winitz, *Chemistry of the Amino Acids* **vol 1-3** (John Wiley and Sons, Inc., New York, 1961) pp. 2043-2074, *passim.* TLC determ in serum from patients with maple sugar urine disease (MSDU): R. J. Allen *et al., Clin. Chem.* **18,** 413 (1972). Metabolism of Ile and isomers in MSDU: U. Wendel *et al., Pediatr. Res.* **25,** 11 (1989); and clinical consequences: T. Mogos *et al., Rev. Roum. Med. Interne* **32,** 57 (1994). Review of biosynthesis: M. Iaccarino *et al., Curr. Top. Cell. Regul.* **14,** 29-73 (1978).

Waxy, shiny, rhombic leaflets from alc. Bitter taste. Sublimes 168-170°. Dec 284°. $[\alpha]_D^{20}$ +40.61° (c = 4.6 in 6.1*N* HCl); +11.09° (c = 3.3 in 0.33*N* NaOH). $[M]_D$ +53.5° (5*N* HCl); +64.2° (glacial acetic acid). pK_1 2.36; pK_2 9.68. Soly in water (g/l): 37.9 at 0°; 41.2 at 25°; 48.2 at 50°; 60.8 at 75°; 82.6 at 100°. Sparingly sol in hot alc (0.13% w/w at 80°), hot acetic acid. Insol in ether.

DL-Form. (±)-*erythro*-2-Amino-3-methylpentanoic acid. Glistening rhombic or monoclinic plates from dil alc. Dec 292°. pK_1 2.32; pK_2 9.76. Soly in water (g/l): 18.3 at 0°; 22.3 at 25°; 30.3 at 50°; 46.1 at 75°; 78.0 at 100°.

L-allo-Form. α-Ile; L(+)-alloisoleucine; (+)-*threo*-2-amino-3-methylpentanoic acid . Waxy leaflets. Sweet taste. Dec 280°. $[\alpha]_D^{20}$ +14.0° (c = 2); +38.1° (c = 2 in 6*N* HCl). $[M]_D$ +53.1° (5*N* HCl); +55.7° (glacial acetic acid). pK_1 2.27; pK_2 9.62. One part dissolves in 34.2 parts water at 20°; 0.82 part dissolves in 100 parts 80% alcohol at 20°; 1.97 parts dissolve in 100 parts 80% alcohol; 0.19 part dissolves in 100 parts abs alcohol at 90°.

5180. Isolysergic Acid. [478-95-5] (8α)-9,10-Didehydro-6-methylergoline-8-carboxylic acid. $C_{16}H_{16}N_2O_2$; mol wt 268.31. C 71.62%, H 6.01%, N 10.44%, O 11.93%. Parent compd of the ergotinine group of alkaloids from ergot. Prepn: Smith, Timmis, *J. Chem. Soc.* **1936,** 1440; Craig *et al., J. Biol. Chem.* **125,** 289 (1938). Differs from lysergic acid by the α-configuration at C-8. Stereochemical studies: Stenlake, *J. Chem. Soc.* **1955,** 1626; Leemann, Fabbri, *Helv. Chim. Acta* **42,** 2696 (1959).

Dihydrate from water, mp 218° (dec). $[\alpha]_D^{20}$ +281° (pyridine). pKa 3.44, pKb 8.61. More sol in water and pyridine than lysergic acid.

Methyl ester. Rods from benzene, mp 170-174°. $[\alpha]_D^{20}$ +179° (c = 0.5 in chloroform).

5181. Isomaltol. [3420-59-5] 1-(3-Hydroxy-2-furanyl)-ethanone; 3-hydroxy-2-furyl methyl ketone. $C_6H_6O_3$; mol wt 126.11. C 57.14%, H 4.80%, O 38.06%. Trace constituent of bread. Obtained by the action of enzymes on starch: Backe, *Compt. Rend.* **151,** 78 (1910). Synthesis from α-lactose and a secondary amine: Hodge, Nelson, **US 3054805** (1962 to USDA). Structure: Hodge, Nelson, *Cereal Chem.* **38,** 207 (1961); Fischer, Hodge, *J. Org. Chem.* **29,** 776 (1964).

Crystals from water or ether, mp 98-103°. uv max (abs methanol): 280 nm ($E_{1cm}^{1\%}$ 1270). Sol in alcohols, acetone, chloroform, benzene, ethyl acetate, hot water. Practically insol in cold water and petr ether.

Benzoate. $C_{13}H_{10}O_4$. Crystals from benzene-toluene, mp 100-101°.

p-Nitrophenylhydrazone. $C_{12}H_{11}N_3O_4$. Deep red crystals from nitrobenzene, mp 100-101°.

5182. Isomaltulose. [13718-94-0]; [58024-13-8] (monohydrate). 6-O-α-D-Glucopyranosyl-D-fructose; 6-O-α-D-glucopyranosyl-D-fructofuranose; Palatinose. $C_{12}H_{22}O_{11}$; mol wt 342.30. C 42.11%, H 6.48%, O 51.41%. Reducing disaccharide occurring naturally in honey and sugar cane juice; commercially available in crystalline (42% of the sweetness of sucrose) and molasses (70% of the sweetness of sucrose) forms. Prepn: D. Weidenhagen, S. Lorenz, **DE 1049800** (1959 to Süddeutsche Zucker-Aktiengesellschaft); *eidem, Z. Zuckerind.* **7,** 533 (1957); E. S. Sharpe *et al., J. Org. Chem.* **25,** 1062 (1960). Clinical effects on glucose levels in diabetic patients: K. Kawai *et al., Horm. Metab. Res.* **21,** 338 (1989). Review of cariological studies: D. Birkhed *et al., Dtsch. Zahnaerztl. Z.* **42,** S124-S127 (1987). Review of development and properties: W. E. Irwin, P. J. Sträter in *Alternative Sweeteners,* L. O'Brien Nabors, R. C. Gelardi, Eds. (Marcel Dekker, Inc., New York, 1991) pp 299-307; and production and clinical activity: I. Takazoe in *Progress in Sweeteners,* T. H. Grenby, Ed. (Elsevier, Barking, UK, 1989) pp 143-167. Review of toxicology and metabolism: B. A. R. Lina *et al., Food Chem. Toxicol.* **40,** 1375-1381 (2002).

Crystals as monohydrate, mp 123-124°. $[\alpha]_D^{20}$ +97.2° (Weidenhagen, 1957); also reported as $[\alpha]_D^{20}$ +103° (c = 1.9 in water) (Sharpe). Nonhygroscopic, acid stable, low glycemic index.

USE: Non-cariogenic sweetener; sugar substitute in foods and beverages.

5183. Isometamidium Chloride. [34301-55-8] 3-Amino-8-[3-[3-(aminoiminomethyl)phenyl]-1-triazenyl]-5-ethyl-6-phenyl-phenanthridinium chloride; 8-[3-(m-amidinophenyl)-2-triazeno]-3-amino-5-ethyl-6-phenylphenanthridinium chloride; 7-m-amidino-phenyldiazoamino-2-amino-10-ethyl-9-phenylphenanthridinium chloride; M & B 4180 A; Samorin. $C_{28}H_{26}ClN_7$; mol wt 496.01.

C 67.80%, H 5.28%, Cl 7.15%, N 19.77%. Prepn: Wragg *et al., Nature* **182,** 1005 (1958). Structure: Berg, *ibid.* **188,** 1106 (1960).

Red crystals from aq methanol, dec 244-245°.
THERAP CAT (VET): Antitrypanosomal agent.

5184. Isomethadone. [466-40-0] 6-(Dimethylamino)-5-methyl-4,4-diphenyl-3-hexanone; 6-dimethylamino-4,4-diphenyl-5-methyl-3-hexanone; 1-dimethylamino-2-methyl-3,3-diphenyl-4-hexanone; isoamidone; Isoadanone. $C_{21}H_{27}NO$; mol wt 309.45. C 81.51%, H 8.79%, N 4.53%, O 5.17%. Prepn of dl-form: Easton *et al., J. Am. Chem. Soc.* **70,** 76 (1948); Walton *et al., J. Chem. Soc.* **1949,** 648; Larsen, Tullar, **US 2773901** (1956 to Sterling Drug). Prepn of d- and l-forms and resolution of dl-form: Larsen *et al., J. Am. Chem. Soc.* **70,** 4194 (1948); Howe, Sletzinger, *ibid.* **71,** 2935 (1949); Larsen, Tullar, *loc. cit.* Configuration of l-form, the isomer with greater analgesic activity: Beckett *et al., Chem. Ind. (London)* **1960,** 1418. Pharmacology: Eddy *et al., J. Pharmacol. Exp. Ther.* **98,** 121 (1950); Winter, Flataker, *ibid.* 305.

dl-Form. [116836-09-0] Slightly yellow, very viscous liq, bp_{12} 215°.

dl-Form hydrobromide. $C_{21}H_{27}NO.HBr$. Crystals from water, mp 149-150°.

d-Form. [26594-41-2] Oil, $[\alpha]_D^{25}$ +20.8°.

d-Form hydrochloride. [63814-06-2] $C_{21}H_{27}NO.HCl$. mp 231-232°. $[\alpha]_D^{25}$ +70°.

d-Form hydrochloride monohydrate. $C_{21}H_{27}NO.HCl.H_2O$. mp 176-177°. $[\alpha]_D^{25}$ +66°.

l-Form. [561-10-4] Liden. Oily liq, $bp_{0.6}$ 162-165°. $[\alpha]_D^{25}$ −20° (c = 1.5 in 95% ethanol).

l-Form hydrobromide. Crystals, mp 217-218°. $[\alpha]_D^{25}$ −59° (c = 1.5).

l-Form hydrochloride. [7487-81-2] mp 231-233°. $[\alpha]_D^{25}$ −70° (c = 1.5 in water), −90° (methanol). Sol in water, alcohol. pH of 1% aq soln: 5 to 6.5. Solutions and tablets are stable. LD_{50} s.c. in mice: 21 mg/kg (Winter, Flataker).

l-Form hydrochloride monohydrate. mp 173-174°.
Note: This is a controlled substance (opiate): **21 CFR,** 1308.12.
THERAP CAT: Analgesic (narcotic).

5185. Isometheptene. [503-01-5] N,6-Dimethyl-5-hepten-2-amine; N,1,5-trimethyl-4-hexenylamine; 6-methylamino-2-methylheptene; 2-methyl-6-methylamino-2-heptene; methylisooctenyl-amine; methyloctenylamine; Octin; Octon; Octanil. $C_9H_{19}N$; mol wt 141.25. C 76.53%, H 13.56%, N 9.92%. $(CH_3)_2C=CHCH_2$-$CH_2CH(NHCH_3)CH_3$. Prepn: Klavehn, Wolf, **US 2230753; US 2230754** (both 1941 to E. Bilhuber). Toxicity data: Walton *et al., J. Pharmacol. Exp. Ther.* **92,** 214 (1948).

Colorless, oily liq; characteristic amine odor. Strong base. Volatile with steam. d 0.795. bp 176-178°; bp_7 58-59°. n_D^{15} 1.4472. Practically insol in water. Freely sol in alc, ether, acetone, chloroform.

Hydrochloride. [6168-86-1] $C_9H_{19}N.HCl$. Crystals, very hygroscopic, mp 68-69°. Sol in water, alc. LD_{50} in mice (mg/kg): 17.5 i.v.; 171 s.c. (Walton).

Bitartrate (acid tartrate). $C_{13}H_{25}NO_6$. Crystals, mp 78-80° (preliminary sintering). Freely sol in water, alcohol.

Mucate. $C_{24}H_{48}N_2O_8$. Bitter crystals, mp 152° (rapid heating). Freely sol in water. Soly in alc about 5 g/100 ml. Almost insol in ether, chloroform. LD_{50} orally in dogs: 148 mg/kg (Walton).

THERAP CAT: Adrenergic.

THERAP CAT (VET): Sympathomimetic. Antispasmodic for gut and urinary tract.

5186. Isoniazid. [54-85-3] 4-Pyridinecarboxylic acid hydrazide; isonicotinic acid hydrazide; isonicotinoylhydrazine; isonicotinylhydrazine; INH; rimitsid; tubazid; RP-5015; FSR-3; Isonex; Isotamine; Isozid; Neoteben; Nicizina; Nicozid; Nydrazid; Rimifon; tebesium; Tibinide; Valifol. $C_6H_7N_3O$; mol wt 137.14. C 52.55%, H 5.14%, N 30.64%, O 11.67%. Prepn: Meyer, Mally, *Monatsh. Chem.* **33**, 400 (1912); Lock, *Pharm. Ind.* **14**, 366 (1952); Urbanski *et al., Rocz. Chem.* **27**, 161 (1953); Gasson, **US 2830994** (1958 to Distillers). Compositions for combating tuberculosis: H. H. Fox, **US 2596069** (1952 to Hoffmann-La Roche). Pharmacokinetics: W. W. Weber, D. W. Hein, *Clin. Pharmacokinet.* **4**, 401 (1979). Mechanism of action study: K. Johnsson *et al., J. Am. Chem. Soc.* **117**, 5009 (1995). Toxicity data: E. H. Jenney, C. C. Pfeiffer, *J. Pharmacol. Exp. Ther.* **122**, 110 (1958). Evaluation of carcinogenic risk: *IARC Monographs* **4**, 159 (1974). Comprehensive description: G. A. Brewer, *Anal. Profiles Drug Subs.* **6**, 183-258 (1977). Clinical trial in HIV-positive patients: J. W. Pape *et al., Lancet* **342**, 268 (1993). Review of use in prevention and treatment of TB: American Thoracic Society, *Am. Rev. Respir. Dis.* **134**, 355-363 (1986); T. J. Jordan *et al., ibid.* **144**, 1357-1360 (1991).

Crystals from alc, mp 171.4°. uv max (water): 266 nm ($E_{1cm}^{1\%}$ 378); (0.01*N* HCl): 265 nm ($E_{1cm}^{1\%}$ ~420). Soly in water at 25°: about 14%; at 40°: about 26%; in alc at 25°: about 2%, in boiling alc: about 10%; in chloroform: about 0.1%. Practically insol in ether, benzene. pH of a 1% aq soln 5.5 to 6.5. Aqueous solns may be sterilized at 120° for 30 min. LD_{50} in mice (mg/kg): 151 i.p., 149 i.v. (Jenney, Pfeiffer).

4-Aminosalicylate. [2066-89-9] Pasiniazide; GEWO-399. $C_{13}H_{14}N_4O_4$; mol wt 290.27. An equimolecular salt produced by dissolving the components in hot dil alc, followed by cooling and evapn: Charonnat, Boime, *Compt. Rend.* **236**, 2140 (1953). Prepn: **CH 303085** (1955 to Hoffmann-La Roche). Yellow crystals from methanol or ethanol, mp 142-144°. Sparingly sol in water. uv max 272, 303 nm ($E_{1cm}^{1\%}$ 550, 445).

Methanesulfonate. [13447-95-5] 4-Pyridinecarboxylic acid 2-(sulfomethyl)hydrazide; methaniazide. $C_7H_9N_3O_4S$; mol wt 231.23. Prepn: Logemann, **US 2759944** (1956 to Carlo Erba). Crystals, dec 187-189°.

Methanesulfonate sodium. [3804-89-5] Sodium isonicotinylhydrazide methanesulfonate. $C_7H_8N_3NaO_4S$; mol wt 253.21. Yellow crystals from water, dec 164-167°.

THERAP CAT: Antibacterial (tuberculostatic).

THERAP CAT (VET): Antibacterial (tuberculostatic); anti-actinomycotic agent.

5187. Isonicotinic Acid. [55-22-1] 4-Pyridinecarboxylic acid; γ-pyridinecarboxylic acid; γ-picolinic acid. $C_6H_5NO_2$; mol wt 123.11. C 58.54%, H 4.09%, N 11.38%, O 25.99%. Prepd by permanganate oxidation of γ-picoline: Gilman, Broadbent, *J. Am. Chem. Soc.* **70**, 2757 (1948); Fields, **US 2946801** (1960 to Standard Oil); from 4-ethylpyridine: Wibaut, Arens, *Rec. Trav. Chim.* **60**, 137 (1941); from citric acid to citrazinic acid to 2,6-dichloroisonicotinic acid: Behrmann, Hofmann, *Ber.* **17**, 2681 (1884); Wibaut, *Rec. Trav. Chim.* **63**, 141 (1944). Prepn of ethyl ester: Burrus, Powell, *J. Am. Chem. Soc.* **67**, 1469 (1945).

Platelets, mp 319°. Sublimes at 260° and 15 mm pressure. pK (25°) 4.96. pH of satd aq soln 3.6. Sparingly sol in cold water (0.52 g/100 ml at 20°), more sol in hot water. Practically insol in benzene, ether, boiling alcohol.

Methyl ester. $C_7H_7NO_2$. Liq, slight odor, similar to mint or oil of wintergreen. mp 8.5°. bp_{21} 104°; bp_{760} 209° (slight decompn).

Ethyl ester. Liq, ester-like odor. Needles, when cooled by salt-ice mixture, mp 23°. d_4^{15} 1.0091 (liq). bp_5 78.5°; bp_{15} 110°; bp_{760} 220°. Sol in alcohol, ether, chloroform, benzene. Practically insol in water.

5188. Isonicotinic Acid Diethylamide. [530-40-5] *N,N*-Diethylisonicotinamide; pyridine-4-carboxylic acid diethylamide. $C_{10}H_{14}N_2O$; mol wt 178.23. C 67.39%, H 7.92%, N 15.72%, O 8.98%. Prepd by the action of phosphorus oxychloride upon a mixture of isonicotinic acid and diethylamine: Carrara, **US 2858317** (1958 to Lepetit).

Slightly viscous liq. $bp_{1.0}$ 119-120°. n_D^{20} 1.525. Miscible with water, ether, chloroform, acetone, alcohol.

5189. Isonipecotic Acid. [498-94-2] 4-Piperidinecarboxylic acid; hexahydroisonicotinic acid. $C_6H_{11}NO_2$; mol wt 129.16. C 55.79%, H 8.58%, N 10.84%, O 24.77%. Prepd by reduction of isonicotinic acid in glacial acetic acid in the presence of platinum oxide: Wibaut, *Rec. Trav. Chim.* **63**, 141 (1944); by reduction of isonicotinic acid in H_2O and concd HCl with PtO_2: Sperber *et al.,* **US 2739968** (1956 to Schering); Freifelder, **US 3159639** (1964 to Abbott).

Needles. Darkens at about 300°; mp 336°.

Hydrochloride. $C_6H_{11}NO_2$.HCl. mp 300° (Wibaut); mp 293° with decompn (Sperber). Sol in ethanol and methanol; freely sol in water.

5190. Isonitrosoacetone. [306-44-5] 2-Oxopropanal 1-oxime; pyruvaldoxime; propanone 1-oxime. $C_3H_5NO_2$; mol wt 87.08. C 41.38%, H 5.79%, N 16.08%, O 36.75%. Prepd from acetone by treatment with sodium nitrite in acetic acid at 0°: Küster, *Z. Physiol. Chem.* **155**, 174 (1926); by the action of methyl nitrite on acetone in ether in the presence of HCl: Slater, *J. Chem. Soc.* **117**, 589 (1920).

Leaflets from ether + petr ether or from carbon tetrachloride, mp 69°. Sublimes easily forming shiny needles. Volatile with steam. Freely sol in water, ether. Moderately sol in warm chloroform, benzene, carbon tetrachloride. Practically insol in petr ether. Sol in alkalies forming yellow solns. Faintly acid to litmus. pK (25°) 8.39.

5191. Isonitrosoacetophenone. [532-54-7] α-Oxobenzeneacetaldehyde aldoxime; benzoylformaldoxime. $C_8H_7NO_2$; mol wt 149.15. C 64.42%, H 4.73%, N 9.39%, O 21.45%.

Plates or prisms, mp 126-128°. Slightly sol in cold water; more sol in hot water; sol in alkalies and alkali carbonates.

USE: As a reagent for the detection of ferrous ions with which it gives a blue color sol in chloroform.

5192. Isonixin. [57021-61-1] N-(2,6-Dimethylphenyl)-1,2-dihydro-2-oxo-3-pyridinecarboxamide; 2-pyridone-3-carboxylic acid 2,6-xylidide; 2-hydroxy-2',6'-nicotinoxylidide; Nixyn. $C_{14}H_{14}N_2O_2$; mol wt 242.27. C 69.41%, H 5.82%, N 11.56%, O 13.21%. Non-steroidal anti-inflammatory agent. Prepn: J.-A. Canicio Chimeno, **BE 820578**; idem, **US 4031105** (1975, 1977 both to Hermes). Prepn, pharmacology and toxicity: R. Cadena et al., Arzneim.-Forsch. **27**, 1457 (1977). Toxicological study: M. T. Mitjavila et al., ibid. 1460. Absorption, excretion studies: G. Carrera et al., ibid. **29**, 1401 (1979). Tolerance in humans: T. M. Serra et al., Therapie **35**, 173 (1980). HPLC determn in plasma: F. González Lopez et al., Farmaco Ed. Prat. **38**, 273 (1983).

White crystalline powder from ethanol, mp 266-267°. Sol in chloroform and strong alkali. Practically insol in acids and water. LD_{50} in male, female mice, male, female rats (mg/kg): 7000, 8000, >6000, >6000 orally; all >2000 i.p. (Cadena).

THERAP CAT: Analgesic, anti-inflammatory.

5193. Isooctane. [540-84-1] 2,2,4-Trimethylpentane; isobutyltrimethylmethane. C_8H_{18}; mol wt 114.23. C 84.12%, H 15.88%. $(CH_3)_3CCH_2CH(CH_3)_2$. Produced by the refining of petroleum.

Highly flammable, mobile liquid. Odor of gasoline. Antiknock octane no. 100. mp −107.45°. bp 99.3°. d_4^{20} 0.69194. n_D^{20} 1.39157. Dipole moment: 0. Flash pt, closed cup: 10°F (−12°C). Practically insol in water; somewhat sol in abs alcohols; sol in benzene, toluene, xylene, chloroform, ether, carbon disulfide, carbon tetrachloride, DMF and oils, except castor oil.

Note: The name isooctane has also been applied to 2-methylheptane.

USE: In determining octane numbers of fuels; in spectrophotometric analysis; as solvent and thinner.

5194. Isooctyl Alcohol. [26952-21-6] $C_8H_{18}O$; mol wt 130.23. C 73.78%, H 13.93%, O 12.29%. A mixture of closely related isomeric branched-chain primary alcohols: RCH_2OH where R represents a branched heptyl radical. The branching consists mostly of methyl groups located in the 3-, 4-, or 5-positions.

Caution: Potential symptoms of overexposure are irritation of eyes, skin, nose, throat; eye and skin burns. See NIOSH Pocket Guide to Chemical Hazards (DHHS/NIOSH 97-140, 1997) p 178.

5195. Isopentyl Alcohol. [123-51-3] 3-Methyl-1-butanol; isoamyl alcohol; isobutyl carbinol; primary isoamyl alcohol; fermentation amyl alcohol. $C_5H_{12}O$; mol wt 88.15. C 68.13%, H 13.72%, O 18.15%. $(CH_3)_2CHCH_2CH_2OH$. A major component of commercial amyl alcohol, fusel oil, q.v., and **potato-spirit oil**. Prepn from butadiene, CO, H_2O, plus catalyst: Alderson, **US 3020314** (1962 to du Pont); from methylbutenes: Brown, Zweifel, J. Am. Chem. Soc. **82**, 1504 (1960). Early review of metabolism and toxicity: H. W. Haggard et al., J. Ind. Hyg. Toxicol. **27**, 1 (1945). Review of manuf by fractionation of fusel oil and via chlorination of pentanes, and properties: W. L. Faith et al., Eds., Industrial Chemicals (John Wiley, New York, 2nd ed., 1957) pp 107-114. Acute toxicity data: Smyth et al., Am. Ind. Hyg. Assoc. J. **30**, 470 (1969).

Liquid; characteristic, disagreeable odor; pungent, repulsive taste. bp_{760} 130.5°. mp −117.2°. d_4^{15} 0.813. n_D^{20} 1.4075. Flash pt, closed cup: 114°F (45°C); open cup: 132°F (55°C). Slightly sol in water (2 g/100 ml at 14°); misc with alcohol, ether, benzene, chloroform, petr ether, glacial acetic acid, oils. LD_{50} orally in rats: 7.07 ml/kg (Smyth).

Caution: Potential symptoms of overexposure are irritation of eyes, skin, nose and throat; headache, dizziness; coughing, dyspnea, nausea, vomiting and diarrhea; skin cracking. See NIOSH Pocket Guide to Chemical Hazards (DHHS/NIOSH 97-140, 1997) p 174. See also Patty's Industrial Hygiene and Toxicology vol. 2C, G. D. Clayton, F. E. Clayton, Eds. (Wiley-Interscience, New York, 3rd ed., 1982) pp 4588-4599.

USE: Solvent for fats, resins, alkaloids, etc.; manuf isoamyl (amyl) compds, isovaleric acid, mercury fulminate, pyroxylin, artificial silk, lacquers, smokeless powders; in microscopy; for dehydrating celloidin solns; for determining fat in milk.

5196. Isophorone. [78-59-1] 3,5,5-Trimethyl-2-cyclohexen-1-one; α-isophorone; 1,5,5-trimethyl-3-oxocyclohexene; 1,3,3-trimethylcyclohexen-5-one; isoforon; isoacetophorone. $C_9H_{14}O$; mol wt 138.21. C 78.21%, H 10.21%, O 11.58%. Prepn: E. Knoevenagel, Ann. **297**, 113 (1897). Synthesis: H. Ueda et al., Agric. Biol. Chem. **30**, 1004 (1966); D. S. Torok, W. J. Scott, Tetrahedron Lett. **34**, 3067 (1993). Colorimetric field test for determn in air: P. Andrew, R. Wood, Analyst **95**, 691 (1970). Solid-phase microextraction/GC determn in aq. samples: J.-Y. Horng, S.-D. Huang, J. Chromatogr. A **678**, 313 (1994). Brief description: P. D. Sherman, Jr., A. J. Papa in Kirk-Othmer Encyclopedia of Chemical Technology vol. **13** (Wiley-Interscience, New York, 3rd ed., 1981) pp 918-922. Review of prepn and purification: G. S. Salvapati, M. Janardanarao, J. Sci. Ind. Res. **42**, 261-267 (1983). Review of toxicology and human exposure: Toxicological Profile for Isophorone (PB90-180225, 1989) pp 101.

Clear liquid with peppermint-like odor. bp 215.3°. Freezing pt −8.1°. Flash pt (open cup): 184°F (84°C). Autoignition pt: 864°F (462°C). d_{20}^{20} 0.9229. d_4^{20} 0.9613. n_4^{20} 1.4778. uv max (MeOH): 235.5 nm (ε 14300). Vapor pressure at 20°: 0.3 mm Hg. Soly in water (mg/l): 12000 (20°); 14500 (25°). Sol in ether, acetone alcohol. LD_{50} in male, female rats and male mice (mg/kg): 2700 ±200, 2100 ±200, 2200 ±200 orally (PB90-180225).

Caution: Potential symptoms of overexposure are irritation of eyes, nose, throat; headache, nausea, dizziness, fatigue, malaise, narcosis; dermatitis. See NIOSH Pocket Guide to Chemical Hazards (DHHS/NIOSH 97-140, 1997) p 178.

USE: Solvent in some printing inks, paints, lacquers and adhesives.

5197. Isophthalic Acid. [121-91-5] 1,3-Benzenedicarboxylic acid; m-phthalic acid. $C_8H_6O_4$; mol wt 166.13. C 57.84%, H 3.64%, O 38.52%. Obtained by the oxidation of m-xylene: Smith, J. Am. Chem. Soc. **43**, 1920 (1921); Weisemann, Fragen, Proc. 5th World Petrol. Congr. **4**, 197 (1960); Brill, Ind. Eng. Chem. **52**, 837 (1960); Bhattacharyya, Ganguly, J. Indian Chem. Soc. **38**, 463 (1961); Saffer, Barker, **US 3089906** (1963 to Mid-Century Corp.); Hay, **GB 951192** (1964 to General Electric).

Cryst powder, mp 345-348°; sublimes without decompn. Sol in 8000 parts cold water, 460 boiling water; freely sol in alcohol, glacial acetic acid; practically insol in benzene, petr ether.

5198. Isophytol. [505-32-8] 3,7,11,15-Tetramethyl-1-hexadecen-3-ol; 2,6,10,14-tetramethylhexadec-15-en-14-ol; 2,6,10-trimethyl-14-vinylpentadecan-14-ol. $C_{20}H_{40}O$; mol wt 296.53. C 81.01%, H 13.60%, O 5.40%. Decompn product of chlorophyll. Synthesis from linalool or citral: Fischer, Löwenberg, *Ann.* **475**, 183 (1929); Karrer *et al., Helv. Chim. Acta* **26**, 1741 (1943); Sarycheva *et al., Zh. Obshch. Khim.* **28**, 647 (1958); Maurit *et al., ibid.* **32**, 2483 (1962); from acetylene: Nazarov *et al., ibid.* **28**, 1444 (1958); Blaha, Weichet, *CS* **88887** (1959), *C.A.* **54**, 2167c (1960); from pseudoionone and propargyl alcohol: Sato *et al., J. Org. Chem.* **28**, 45 (1963).

Oily liquid. d_4^{20} 0.8519. n_D^{20} 1.4571. $bp_{0.01}$ 107-110°; $bp_{0.06}$ 125-128°. Practically insol in water; sol in the usual organic solvents.

USE: Prepn of vitamins E and K_1.

5199. Isopilosine. [491-88-3] (3S,4R)-Dihydro-3-[(R)-hydroxyphenylmethyl]-4-[(1-methyl-1H-imidazol-5-yl)methyl]-2(3H)-furanone; carpiline; carpidine. $C_{16}H_{18}N_2O_3$; mol wt 286.33. C 67.12%, H 6.34%, N 9.78%, O 16.76%. This compound was originally called pilosine (the *cis*-isomer of isopilosine): H. W. Voigtländer, W. Rosenberg, *Arch. Pharm.* **292**, 579 (1959). Isoln from leaves of *Pilocarpus microphyllus* Stapf, *Rutaceae:* F. L. Pyman, *J. Chem. Soc.* **101**, 2260 (1912). Synthesis and abs config: Link, Bernauer, *Helv. Chim. Acta* **55**, 1053 (1972). Crystal structure: W. E. Oberhaensli, *Cryst. Struct. Commun.* **1**, 203 (1972).

Needles from alcohol, mp 182-182.5°. $[\alpha]_D^{20}$ +37.6° (alcohol).
Pilosine. [13640-28-3] Needles from alcohol, mp 179°. $[\alpha]_D^{20}$ +83.9° (alcohol). uv max (alcohol): 210 nm (log ε 4.10).

5200. Isopimaric Acid. [5835-26-7] [1R-(1α,4aβ,4bα,7α,-10aα)]-7-Ethenyl-1,2,3,4,4a,4b,5,6,7,8,10,10a-dodecahydro-1,4a,7-trimethyl-1-phenanthrenecarboxylic acid; 13β-methyl-13-vinylpodocarp-7-ene-15-oic acid; miropinic acid. $C_{20}H_{30}O_2$; mol wt 302.45. C 79.42%, H 10.00%, O 10.58%. Isoln from *Dacrydium biforme* Pilg., *Podocarpaceae:* Hosking, Brandt, *Ber.* **68**, 1311 (1935); from the bled resin of *Podocarpus ferrugineus, Podocarpaceae:* Brandt, Neubauer, *J. Chem. Soc.* **1940**, 683; from *Pimus palustris* Mill., *Pinaceae:* Harris, Sanderson, *J. Am. Chem. Soc.* **70**, 2079, 2081 (1948). Identity of isopimaric and miropinic acids: Brossi, Jeger, *Helv. Chim. Acta* **33**, 722 (1950). Structure: Antkowiak *et al., J. Org. Chem.* **27**, 1930 (1962). Stereochemistry: Ireland, Newbould, *ibid.* 1931; Antkowiak *et al., Can. J. Chem.* **43**, 1257 (1965); Bose *et al., Indian J. Chem.* **5**, 228 (1967).

Needles from methanol or ethanol, mp 160°. $[\alpha]_D^{16}$ −3.6° (10.4% soln in 1:1 alcohol:chloroform). Freely sol in chloroform, benzene; moderately sol in ether, alcohol; slightly sol in light petroleum. Absorption spectrum: Brossi, Jeger, *loc. cit.*

5201. Isoprene. [78-79-5] 2-Methyl-1,3-butadiene. C_5H_8; mol wt 68.12. C 88.16%, H 11.84%. Isoln from the products of the pyrolysis of natural rubber: Williams, *Trans. R. Soc. London* **150**, 241 (1860); Boonstra, van Amerongen, *Ind. Eng. Chem.* **41**, 161

(1949). Structure: Euler, *Ber.* **30**, 1989 (1897). Prepn from turpentine: Tilden, *J. Chem. Soc.* **45**, 410 (1884); Bibb, *US* **2386537** (1945 to Newport Ind.); from terpenes: Davis *et al., Ind. Eng. Chem.* **38**, 53 (1946); Bourbon, *US* **2547684** (1951 to Manufacture de Caoutchouc Michelin); by condensation of isobutylene and formaldehyde in acetic acid: Blomquist, Verdol, *J. Am. Chem. Soc.* **77**, 78 (1955); Chaffe *et al.,* **FR 1294716** (1962 to Inst. Francais du Petrole); by dehydrogenation of isoamylenes from cracked gasolines: **GB 875346** (Apr. 21, 1960 to Shell Int. Res. Maatschappij); Voge *et al., US* **3110746** (1963 to Shell); by dimerization of propylene followed by pyrolysis of the resulting 2-methyl-2-pentene: Gorin, Oblad, *US* **2404056** (1946 to Socony-Vacuum Oil); **GB 913852** (1962 to Goodyear); by dehydrogenation of isopentane: Dempsey, *US* **2914588** (1959 to Sun Oil); Owen, *US* **2982795** (1961 to Phillips Petroleum); Stevenson, *US* **3088986** (1963 to Air Products & Chem.); by reacting isoamylenes with methanol and pyrolizing and dehydrogenating the resulting tertiary ethers: Verdol, Walker, *US* **2972645** (1961 to Sinclair Refining). Toxicity: Gostinskii, *C.A.* **62**, 15338a (1965). Reviews of isoprene and its polymers: Bean *et al.,* "Isoprene Polymers" in *Encyclopedia of Polymer Science and Technology* vol. 7 (Interscience, New York, 1967) pp 782-855; Bailey, "Isoprene" in *Vinyl and Diene Monomers* (part 2), E. C. Leonard, Ed. (Wiley-Interscience, New York, 1971) pp 997-1148; W. M. Saltman in *Kirk-Othmer Encyclopedia of Chemical Technology* vol. 13 (Wiley-Interscience, New York, 3rd ed., 1981) pp 818-837; of carcinogenic risk: *IARC Monographs* **60**, 215-232 (1994).

Colorless, volatile liquid. Unstable, oxidizable, flammable. bp_{760} 34.067°. mp −145.95°. d_4^{20} 0.681; d_{20}^{20} 0.6805. n_D^{20} 1.42160. Practically insol in water. Miscible with alcohol or ether. LD_{50} for mice: 144 mg isoprene vapors/l air (Gostinskii).
Caution: Respiratory irritation is a potential symptom of overexposure. May act as a CNS depressant and asphyxiant at high concns. *See Patty's Industrial Hygiene and Toxicology* **vol. 2B,** G. D. Clayton, F. E. Clayton, Eds. (John Wiley & Sons, New York, 4th ed., 1994) p 1252-1253. This substance is reasonably anticipated to be a human carcinogen: *Report on Carcinogens, Eleventh Edition* (PB2005-104914, 2004) p III-156.

USE: Manuf "synthetic" natural rubber, butyl rubber. Copolymer in the production of synthetic elastomers.

5202. Isopropamide Iodide. [71-81-8] γ-(Aminocarbonyl)-N-methyl-N,N-bis(1-methylethyl)-γ-phenylbenzenepropanaminium iodide; (3-carbamoyl-3,3-diphenylpropyl)diisopropylmethylammonium iodide; 2,2-diphenyl-4-diisopropylaminobutyramide methiodide; R-79; Darbid; Priamide; Tyrimide. $C_{23}H_{33}IN_2O$; mol wt 480.43. C 57.50%, H 6.92%, I 26.41%, N 5.83%, O 3.33%. Anticholinergic. Prepn: P. Janssen *et al., Arch. Int. Pharmacodyn.* **103**, 82 (1955); M. E. Speeter, *US* **2823233** (1958 to Bristol). Crystal and molecular structure: N. Datta *et al., J. Chem. Soc. Perkin Trans. 2* **1977**, 781. Comprehensive description: R. S. Santoro *et al., Anal. Profiles Drug Subs.* **2**, 315-338 (1973); A. Post, R. S. Santoro, *ibid.* **12**, 721-732 (1983).

Crystals or amorphous powder, mp 198-201° (dec) (Janssen); also reported as mp 189.0-191.5° (Santoro). Sensitive to light. Freely sol in boiling water, in methanol, ethanol, chloroform. Practically insol in ether.
Free base. $C_{22}H_{30}N_2O$. mp 84-86°.
Note: Ingredient of **Stelabid** (also contg trifluoperazine, *q.v.*).
THERAP CAT: Antispasmodic.
THERAP CAT (VET): Antiemetic; antidiarrheal.

5203. Isopropenyl Acetate. [108-22-5] 1-Propen-2-ol acetate; 1-propen-2-yl acetate. $C_5H_8O_2$; mol wt 100.12. C 59.98%, H 8.05%, O 31.96%. Prepn from ketene + acetone: Hull, Agett; Hagemeyer, **US 2481669**; **US 2476860** (both 1949 to Eastman Kodak); Young, **US 2461016**; **US 2511423** (1949, 1950 both to Carbide & Carbon Chem.); Mawer, **US 2684980** (1954 to I.C.I.); Buttner, Enk, **US 2867653** (1959 to Wacker-Chemie). Use as reagent for acylation of potential enols: Hagemeyer, Hull, *Ind. Eng. Chem.* **41**, 2920 (1949); Hull, Agett, **US 2482066** (1949 to Eastman Kodak); Jeffery, Satchell, *J. Chem. Soc.* **1962**, 1876, 1906. Toxicity study: Smyth *et al., J. Ind. Hyg. Toxicol.* **31**, 60 (1949).

Liquid. bp 97°; bp_{200} 58-60°. n_D^{20} 1.4001. LD_{50} orally in rats: 3.0 g/kg (Smyth).

Caution: Mild irritant. Narcotic in high concns.

USE: Reagent for acylation of potential enols.

5204. 4-(5-Isopropenyl-2-methyl-1-cyclopenten-1-yl)-2-butanone. [87-45-6] 4-[2-Methyl-5-(1-methylethenyl)-1-cyclopenten-1-yl]-2-butanone; 4-(2-methyl-5-isopropenyl-1-cyclopenten-1-yl)-2-butanone; Pentione. $C_{13}H_{20}O$; mol wt 192.30. C 81.20%, H 10.48%, O 8.32%. Prepn: Kimel, Sax, **US 2799706** (1957 to Hoffmann-La Roche).

Pale yellow liquid. Citrus-like odor with woody background. d_{25}^{25} 0.9218. $bp_{0.5}$ 72-75°. n_D^{25} 1.4800. Freely sol in diethyl phthalate. At least 10% soly in 70% ethanol, in mineral oil and in corn oil.

USE: In perfumery, i.e., in milled soaps, in modified eau de Cologne, in neroli and orange-blossom compositions. Blends well with ionones.

5205. Isopropyl Acetate. [108-21-4] $C_5H_{10}O_2$; mol wt 102.13. C 58.80%, H 9.87%, O 31.33%. $CH_3COOCH(CH_3)_2$. Toxicity study: Smyth *et al., Arch. Ind. Hyg. Occup. Med.* **10**, 61 (1954).

Colorless liquid. d_4^{20} 0.870. bp 89°. Flash pt, open cup: 40°F (4°C); closed cup: 36°F (2°C). Sol in 23 parts water at 27°; miscible with alc, ether. LD_{50} orally in rats: 6.75 g/kg (Smyth).

Caution: Potential symptoms of overexposure are irritation of eyes, nose and skin; dermatitis. *See NIOSH Pocket Guide to Chemical Hazards* (DHHS/NIOSH 97-140, 1997) p 180.

USE: Solvent for cellulose derivatives, plastics, oils and fats; in perfumery.

5206. Isopropyl Acetoacetate. [542-08-5] 3-Oxobutanoic acid 1-methylethyl ester. $C_7H_{12}O_3$; mol wt 144.17. C 58.32%, H 8.39%, O 33.29%. $CH_3COCH_2COOC_3H_7$.

Liquid. d_4^{25} 0.957. bp ~205° with decompn. Slightly sol in water, freely in alcohol, ether.

5207. Isopropylacetone. [108-10-1] 4-Methyl-2-pentanone; methyl isobutyl ketone; hexone. $C_6H_{12}O$; mol wt 100.16. C 71.95%, H 12.08%, O 15.97%. $CH_3COCH_2CH(CH_3)_2$. Manuf: *Faith, Keyes & Clark's Industrial Chemicals,* F. A. Lowenheim, M. K. Moran, Eds. (Wiley-Interscience, New York, 4th ed., 1975) pp 543-546. Toxicity data: Smyth *et al., Arch. Ind. Hyg. Occup. Med.* **4**, 119 (1951).

Colorless liquid; faint, ketonic and camphor odor. d_4^{20} 0.801. bp 117-118°. n_D^{20} 1.396. Flash pt, closed cup: 73°F (23°C). mp −84.7°. Moderately sol in water (1.91%); misc with alcohol, benzene, ether. LD_{50} orally in rats: 2.08 g/kg (Smyth).

Caution: Potential symptoms of overexposure are irritation of eyes, skin and mucous membranes; headache; narcosis, coma; der-

matitis. *See NIOSH Pocket Guide to Chemical Hazards* (DHHS/NIOSH 97-140, 1997) p 164.

USE: Solvent for gums, resins, nitrocellulose, etc.

5208. Isopropyl Alcohol. [67-63-0] 2-Propanol; isopropanol; secondary propyl alcohol; dimethyl carbinol; petrohol. C_3H_8O; mol wt 60.10. C 59.95%, H 13.42%, O 26.62%. CH_3-$CHOHCH_3$. Manuf from propylene: *Faith, Keyes & Clark's Industrial Chemicals,* F. A. Lowenheim, M. K. Moran, Eds. (Wiley-Interscience, New York, 4th ed., 1975) pp 496-501. Monograph: L. F. Hatch, *Isopropyl Alcohol* (McGraw-Hill, New York, 1961) 184 pp. Toxicity: Smyth, Carpenter, *J. Ind. Hyg. Toxicol.* **30**, 63 (1948).

Flammable liq. Slight odor resembling that of a mixture of ethanol and acetone. Slightly bitter taste (*not potable!*). mp −88.5°; fp −89.5°. bp_{760} 82.5°; bp_{400} 67.8°; bp_{200} 53.0°; bp_{100} 39.5°; bp_{60} 30.5°; bp_{40} 23.8°; bp_{20} 12.7°; bp_{10} 2.4°; bp_5 −7.0°; $bp_{1.0}$ −26.1°. d_4^{20} 0.78505; d_4^{25} 0.78084; d_4^{83} 0.728. Flash pt, closed cup: 11.7°C (53°F). Autoignition temp 455.6°C (852°F). Lower explosive limit in air: 2.5% (v/v). n_D^8 1.3852; n_D^{15} 1.3802; n_D^{20} 1.37723; n_D^{25} 1.3749. Absorption spectrum: Brode, *J. Phys. Chem.* **30**, 61 (1926). Miscible with water, alcohol, ether, chloroform. Insol in salt solns. May be recovered from aq mixtures by salting out with sodium chloride, sodium sulfate, sodium hydroxide, etc. Forms an azeotrope with water (bp_{760} 80.37°, d_4^0 0.83361) isopropanol 87.7% (w/w). Freezing points of mixtures with water (v/v, per cent by volume): Isopropanol 15% = −3.3°; 25% = −6.7°; 30% = −8.3°; 35% = −11.1°; 40% = −13°; 45% = −17.8°; 50% = −23°; 60% = −32°. LD_{50} orally in rats: 5.8 g/kg (Smyth, Carpenter).

Caution: Potential symptoms of overexposure are irritation of eyes, nose and throat; drowsiness, dizziness and headache; dry cracking skin. *See NIOSH Pocket Guide to Chemical Hazards* (DHHS/NIOSH 97-140, 1997) p 180.

USE: In antifreeze compositions; as solvent for gums, shellac, essential oils; in the extraction of alkaloids; in quick-drying oils; in quick-drying inks; in denaturing ethyl alcohol; in body rubs; hand lotions, after-shave lotions and similar cosmetics. Solvent for creosote, resins, gums; in manuf of acetone, glycerol, isopropyl acetate. Pharmaceutic aid (solvent).

THERAP CAT: Antiseptic.

THERAP CAT (VET): Antiseptic, rubefacient.

5209. Isopropylamine. [75-31-0] 2-Propanamine; 2-aminopropane. C_3H_9N; mol wt 59.11. C 60.96%, H 15.35%, N 23.70%. $(CH_3)_2CHNH_2$. Prepn from acetone + NH_3: Skita, Keil, *Ber.* **61**, 1682 (1928); Norton *et al., J. Org. Chem.* **19**, 1054 (1954); from acetone oxime: Winans, Adkins, *J. Am. Chem. Soc.* **55**, 2056 (1933). Toxicity study: H. F. Smyth *et al., Arch. Ind. Hyg. Occup. Med.* **4**, 119 (1951).

Colorless, flammable liquid; ammonia odor; strong base. d_4^{15} 0.694. mp −101°. bp 33-34°. n_D^{15} 1.3770. Flash pt, open cup: −15°F (−26°C). Miscible with water, alcohol, ether. LD_{50} orally in rats: 820 mg/kg (Smyth).

Caution: Potential symptoms of overexposure are irritation of eyes, nose, throat and skin; pulmonary edema; visual disturbance; skin and eye burns; dermatitis. *See NIOSH Pocket Guide to Chemical Hazards* (DHHS/NIOSH 97-140, 1997) p 180.

5210. Isopropyl Bromide. [75-26-3] 2-Bromopropane. C_3H_7Br; mol wt 122.99. C 29.30%, H 5.74%, Br 64.97%. CH_3-$CHBrCH_3$. Obtained by heating isopropyl alcohol with HBr.

Colorless liquid. d_4^{20} 1.31. mp −89°. bp 59-60°. n_D^{20} 1.4251. Slightly sol in water; miscible with alcohol, benzene, chloroform, ether.

5211. Isopropyl Chloride. [75-29-6] 2-Chloropropane. C_3H_7Cl; mol wt 78.54. C 45.88%, H 8.98%, Cl 45.14%. CH_3-$CHClCH_3$. Prepd by refluxing isopropyl alcohol with concd HCl and $ZnCl_2$.

Liquid. d^{15} 0.868. mp −117°. bp 35-36°. Flash pt, closed cup: −26°F (−32°C). Slightly sol in water; miscible with alcohol, ether.

5212. Isopropyl Ether. [108-20-3] 2,2′-Oxybispropane; 2-isopropoxypropane; diisopropyl ether; DIPE. $C_6H_{14}O$; mol wt 102.17. C 70.53%, H 13.81%, O 15.66%. $(CH_3)_2CHOCH$-$(CH_3)_2$. Prepn: E. Erlenmeyer, *Ann.* **126**, 305 (1863). Physical properties and solubility: H. R. Fife, E. W. Reid, *Ind. Eng. Chem.* **22**, 513 (1930). Manuf process: M. N. Harandi, H. Owen, US 5208387 (1993 to Mobil). GC determn in gasolines: N. G. Johansen, *J. High Resolut. Chromatogr. Chromatogr. Commun.* **7**, 487 (1984). Acute toxicity: E. T. Kimura *et al.*, *Toxicol. Appl. Pharmacol.* **19**, 699 (1971). Comparison with MTBE, ETBE and TAME, *q.q.v.*, as gasoline oxygenate: M. J. McNally *et al.*, *Oil Gas J.* **90**, 39 (May 25, 1992).

Liquid. bp$_{760}$ 68.27°. fp -85.89°. d$_4^{20}$ 0.72813. n$_D^{20}$ 1.36888. Surface tension in air (23°): 32 dynes/cm. Viscosity (25°): 0.379 cP. Vapor pressure (20°): 158 mm Hg. Specific heat (22-27°): 0.526 cal/g. Flash pt, closed cup: -6.7°F. Latent heat of vaporization (67.5°): 68.2 cal/g. Soly of commercial grade in water (19°): 1.71 wt%. Misc with most organic solvents. Ethanolamines, glycols, glycerol and their monoesters have limited soly; diesters are sol. Readily forms peroxides when exposed to oxygen unless stabilized with inhibitors such as hydroquinone or BHT. LD$_{50}$ in 14 day old, young adult, adult rats (ml/kg): 6.4, 16.5, 16.0 orally (Kimura).

Caution: Potential symptoms of overexposure are irritation of eyes, skin and nose; respiratory discomfort; dermatitis. *See NIOSH Pocket Guide to Chemical Hazards* (DHHS/NIOSH 97-140, 1997) p 182.

USE: As solvent; fuel additive.

5213. Isopropylidene Glycerol. [100-79-8] 2,2-Dimethyl-1,3-dioxolane-4-methanol; 2,2-dimethyl-4-hydroxymethyl-1,3-dioxolane; glycerol dimethylketal; acetone glycerol; Solketal. C$_6$H$_{12}$O$_3$; mol wt 132.16. C 54.53%, H 9.15%, O 36.32%. Prepn: Fisher, *Ber.* **28**, 1167 (1895); Fisher, Pfähler, *Ber.* **53**, 1607 (1920); Hibbert, Morazain, *Can. J. Res.* **2**, 38 (1930); Smith, Lindberg, *Ber.* **64**, 510 (1931); M. M. Maglio, C. A. Burger, *J. Am. Chem. Soc.* **68**, 529 (1946); M. Renoll, M. S. Newman, *Org. Synth.* **coll. vol. III**, 502 (1955); Mikschik, AT 180926 (1955 to Chemomedica Chemikalien), *C.A.* **49**, 15951 (1955); Williams, GB 802022 (1958 to Peter Spence & Sons); GB 819835 (1959 to Bayer); Perez *et al.*, ES 499129 (1982 to Calipe), *C.A.* **97**, 55794v (1982). Synthesis of D(+)-form: E. Baer, H. Fischer, *J. Biol. Chem.* **128**, 463 (1939); of L(−)-form: *eidem*, *J. Am. Chem. Soc.* **61**, 761 (1939). Conversion of D(+)- to L(−)-form: *eidem*, *ibid.* **67**, 944 (1945).

Practically odorless liq of medium mobility. d$_4^{20}$ 1.064. bp$_{10}$ 82°. n$_D^{20}$ 1.4383. Viscosity (20°): 11 cP. Practically nonflammable at ordinary storage temps: Flash pt 90°C (194°F). Evaporation no. about 600 (ether = 1). Miscible with water, alcohols, acetals, esters, ethers, aromatic hydrocarbons, chlorinated hydrocarbons, gasolines, petr ether, turpentine, oils. LD$_{50}$ in rats (g/kg): 7 orally; 3 i.p. (Perez).

D(+)-Form. [α]$_D$ +13.6°; [α]$_D$ +10.8° (c = 15.19 in benzene).
L(−)-Form. [α]$_D$ −13.6°; [α]$_D$ −10.8° (c = 15.19 in benzene).

USE: Versatile solvent and plasticizer. Pharmaceutic aid (solubilizing and suspending agent).

5214. Isopropyl Iodide. [75-30-9] 2-Iodopropane. C$_3$H$_7$I; mol wt 169.99. C 21.20%, H 4.15%, I 74.65%. CH$_3$CHICH$_3$. Prepared by distilling isopropyl alcohol with HI; or from glycerol, iodine, water, and phosphorus.

Colorless liquid but readily discolors in air and light. d$_4^{20}$ 1.703. mp -90°. bp 89-90°. n$_D^{20}$ 1.5026. Sol in 720 parts water; miscible with alcohol, benzene, chloroform, ether.

5215. Isopropyl Myristate. [110-27-0] Tetradecanoic acid 1-methylethyl ester. C$_{17}$H$_{34}$O$_2$; mol wt 270.45. C 75.50%, H 12.67%, O 11.83%. CH$_3$(CH$_2$)$_{12}$COOCH(CH$_3$)$_2$. The commercial product usually appears as a mixture of myristate with small amounts of esters of palmitic and other satd fatty acids. Physical properties: Bonhorst *et al.*, *Ind. Eng. Chem.* **40**, 2379 (1948).

Liquid of low viscosity, practically odorless. mp ~3°. bp$_2$ 140.2°; bp$_{20}$ 192.6°; dec 208°. d^{20} 0.8532; d^{99} 0.7942. n$_D^{20}$ 1.432-1.434. Withstands oxidation and does not readily become rancid. Sol in castor oil, cottonseed oil, acetone, chloroform, ethyl acetate, ethanol, toluene, and mineral oil. Practically insol in water,

glycerol, propylene glycol. Dissolves many waxes, cholesterol, lanolin.

USE: In cosmetic and topical medicinal prepns where good absorption through the skin is desired. A jellied isopropyl myristate was marketed as *Estergel*.

5216. Isopropyl Nitrite. [541-42-4] Nitrous acid 1-methylethyl ester; 2-propanol nitrite; nitrous acid isopropyl ester. C$_3$H$_7$NO$_2$; mol wt 89.09. C 40.44%, H 7.92%, N 15.72%, O 35.92%. (CH$_3$)$_2$CHONO. Prepd by treating isopropyl alcohol with nitrosyl chloride: Kornblum *et al.*, *J. Am. Chem. Soc.* **77**, 5531 (1955); by adding concd sulfuric acid and isopropyl alcohol to sodium nitrite: Levin, Hartung, *Org. Synth.* **24**, 26 (1944).

Pale yellow oil. d$_4^0$ 0.856; d$_4^{25}$ 0.844. bp$_{752}$ 39-39.5°; bp$_{745}$ 39-40°. n$_D^{20}$ 1.3520.

Caution: Can cause vasodilation with fall in blood pressure, tachycardia, headache. Large doses can cause methemoglobinuria with cyanosis. Severe poisoning results in shock which can end fatally.

USE: Jet propellant.

5217. Isoproterenol. [7683-59-2] 4-[1-Hydroxy-2-[(1-methylethyl)amino]ethyl]-1,2-benzenediol; 3,4-dihydroxy-α-[(isopropylamino)methyl]benzyl alcohol; α-(isopropylaminomethyl)-protocatechuyl alcohol; isoprenaline; isopropylarterenol; 1-(3,4-dihydroxyphenyl)-2-isopropylaminoethanol; isopropylaminomethyl-(3,4-dihydroxyphenyl)carbinol; N-isopropyl-β-dihydroxyphenyl-β-hydroxyethylamine; dihydroxyphenylethanolisopropylamine; N-isopropylnoradrenaline; epinephrine isopropyl homolog; A-21; Aludrine; Aleudrin; Isuprel; Norisodrine; Asiprenol; Asmalar; Neo-Epinine; Novodrin; Isupren; Neodrenal; Isopropydrin; Assiprenol; Respifral; Bellasthman; Saventrine; Proternol; Isorenin; Vapo-N-Iso; Isonorin. C$_{11}$H$_{17}$NO$_3$; mol wt 211.26. C 62.54%, H 8.11%, N 6.63%, O 22.72%. β-Adrenergic agonist. Catecholamine derivative prepd by the reaction of 3,4-dihydroxy-α-haloacetophenone with an excess of isopropylamine: Scheuing, Thomä, DE 723278 (1942 to Boehringer, Ing.); US 2308232 (1943); from guaiacol and chloral hydrate: Beke *et al.*, *Pharm. Zentralhalle* **92**, 237 (1953). Resolution: Kerschbaum, Benedikt, *Monatsh. Chem.* **83**, 1090 (1952); Beccari *et al.*, *Science* **118**, 249 (1953); Delmar *et al.*, US 2715141 (1955 to Delmar Chem.). Configuration: Pratesi *et al.*, *Farmaco Ed. Sci.* **15**, 3 (1960). Toxicity: E. I. Goldenthal, *Toxicol. Appl. Pharmacol.* **18**, 185 (1971). Effect on gastric acid secretion: M. J. Daly, *Scand. J. Gastroenterol.* **89**, 3 (1984). Use in treatment of primary pulmonary hypertension: D. A. Pietro *et al.*, *N. Engl. J. Med.* **310**, 1032 (1984). Review of pharmacology and comparison with other β-adrenoceptor agonists: V. T. Popa, *J. Asthma* **21**, 183-207 (1984). Comprehensive description: M. Tariq, A. A. Al-Badr, *Anal. Profiles Drug Subs.* **14**, 391-422 (1985).

dl-Form. Crystals from alc, mp 155.5°. pKa 8.64. LD$_{50}$ in male, female rats (mg/kg): 3675, 4282 orally (Goldenthal).

dl-Form hydrochloride. Aerolone; Aerotrol; Euspiran; Isomenyl; Isovon; Mistarel; Suscardia. C$_{11}$H$_{17}$NO$_3$.HCl; mol wt 247.72. Crystals from alc, mp 170-171°. Soly: one gram dissolves in 3 ml water, in 50 ml ethanol (95%). Less sol in abs ethanol. Practically insol in chloroform, ether, benzene. pH of 1% aq soln about 5. Aq solns turn brownish-pink upon prolonged exposure to air or upon addition of alkali. LD$_{50}$ orally in rats: 2221 ±93 mg/kg (Goldenthal).

dl-Form sulfate dihydrate. [6700-39-6] Aludrin; Isomist; Propal. (C$_{11}$H$_{17}$NO$_3$)$_2$.H$_2$SO$_4$.2H$_2$O; mol wt 556.62. Crystals from acetone + methanol, mp 128° (some decomp). One gram dissolves in about 4 ml water. Slightly sol in alc. Practically insol in chloroform, ether, benzene. pH of a 1% aq soln about 5.

l-Form. Crystals, mp 164-165°. [α]$_D^{19}$ -45.0° (c = 2 in 2N HCl).

l-Form hydrochloride. Crystals, dec 162-164°. [α]$_D^{20}$ -50°.

l-Form d-bitartrate dihydrate. Isolevin. Crystals, mp 80-83° (sinters at 78°). [α]$_D^{19}$ -14.9° (c = 2.31).

THERAP CAT: Bronchodilator.

THERAP CAT (VET): Sympathomimetic. Chiefly as bronchodilator.

5218. Isoproturon. [34123-59-6] N,N-Dimethyl-N'-[4-(1-methylethyl)phenyl]urea; 3-p-cumenyl-1,1-dimethylurea; N-(4-isopropylphenyl)-N',N'-dimethylurea; I.P.U.; HOE-16410; CGA-18731; Arelon; Protugan. $C_{12}H_{18}N_2O$; mol wt 206.28. C 69.87%, H 8.80%, N 13.58%, O 7.76%. Pre- and post-emergence herbicide for control of annual grasses and broad-leaved weeds. Prepn and herbicidal properties: C. W. Todd, US 2655447 (1953 to du Pont); BE 770928 (1971 to Pepro); A. Thizy et al., US 4295877 (1981 to Philagro). Physical properties, herbicidal activity: eidem, C.R. Seances Acad. Sci. Ser. D 274, 2053 (1972); J. Rognon et al., Meded. Fac. Landbouwwet. Rijksuniv. Gent 37, 663 (1972), C.A. 79, 1260c (1973). Microbial degradation of labelled isoproturon: J.-C. Fournier et al., Chemosphere 4, 207 (1975). Efficacy in winter cereals: R. T. Hewson, Proc. 12th Br. Weed Control Conf. 75 (1974); P. Gonzales et al., Weed Res. 23, 39 (1983). HPLC determn in soil: G. Kulshrestha, R. Khazanchi, J. Chromatogr. 318, 144 (1985).

White crystals from benzene, mp 158°. Soly in water at 22°: 70 mg/l. LD_{50} in mice, rats (mg/kg): 3350, 3600 orally (Thizy, 1972).
USE: Herbicide.

5219. Isopyrocalciferol. [474-70-4] (3β,9β,22E)-9-Ergosta-5,7,22-trien-3-ol; 9β-ergosterol. $C_{28}H_{44}O$; mol wt 396.65. C 84.78%, H 11.18%, O 4.03%. Differs sterically from pyrocalciferol at C-10, from ergosterol at C-9. See ref under Pyrocalciferol. Stereochemistry: Castells et al., J. Chem. Soc. 1959, 1159. Selenium dehydrogenation gives Diel's hydrocarbon (3'-methyl-1,2-cylopentenophenanthrene).

Prisms from ether-methanol. mp 112-115°. uv max: 262, 280 nm. $[\alpha]_D^{20}$ +332°, $[\alpha]_{546}^{20}$ +415° (c = 1.5 in chloroform). Precipitated by digitonin.
Acetate. $C_{30}H_{46}O_2$. mp 113-115°. $[\alpha]_D^{20}$ +333°, $[\alpha]_{546}^{20}$ +423° (c = 2 in chloroform).

5220. Isoquassin. [21293-20-9] Picrasmin. $C_{22}H_{28}O_6$; mol wt 388.45. C 68.02%, H 7.27%, O 24.71%. Bitter principle from Jamaica quassia, Picrasma excelsa (Sw.) Planch., Simaroubaceae. Isoln: Clark, J. Am. Chem. Soc. 60, 1146 (1938). Identity of isoquassin and picrasmin: Adams, Whaley, ibid. 72, 375 (1950). Isomer of quassin, q.v.: Valenta et al., Tetrahedron 18, 1433 (1962).

Crystals from methanol, mp 222-225°. $[\alpha]_D^{20}$ +45.4° (chloroform). uv max: 258 nm (ε 12500).

5221. Isoquercitrin. [21637-25-2] 2-(3,4-Dihydroxyphenyl)-3-(β-D-glucofuranosyloxy)-5,7-dihydroxy-4H-1-benzopyran-4-one; 3,3',4',5,7-pentahydroxyflavone-3-glucoside; quercetin-3-glucoside; isotrifoliin; trifoliin. $C_{21}H_{20}O_{12}$; mol wt 464.38. C 54.31%, H 4.34%, O 41.34%. From flowers of Gossypium herbaceum L., Malvaceae: Perkin, J. Chem. Soc. 95, 2181 (1909); from flowers of Aesculus hippocastanum L., Hippocastanaceae: Hörhammer, Wagner, Arch. Pharm. 290, 224 (1957); from Tropaeolum majus L., Tropaeolaceae: Delaveau, Compt. Rend. 252, 1510 (1961); from Arnica montana L., Compositae: Friedrick, Naturwissenschaften 49, 541 (1962). Structure: Attree, Perkin, J. Chem. Soc. 1927, 234. Identity with trifoliin and isotrifoliin: Hattori et al., J. Chem. Soc. Jpn. 58, 844 (1937), C.A. 32, 219c (1938). Synthesis: Ice, Wender, J. Am. Chem. Soc. 74, 4606 (1952); eidem, US 2727890 (1955 to the USAEC).

Yellow needles from water, mp 225-227°. uv max: 257, 369 nm. Practically insol in cold but sparingly sol in boiling water. Sol in alkaline solns with a deep yellow tint.

5222. Isoquinoline. [119-65-3] 2-Benzazine; benzo[c]pyridine. C_9H_7N; mol wt 129.16. C 83.69%, H 5.46%, N 10.84%. Occurs in coal tar: Hoogewerff, van Dorp, Rec. Trav. Chim. 4, 125, 285 (1885); Weissgerber, Ber. 47, 3175 (1914); Harris, Pope, J. Chem. Soc. 121, 1029 (1922). Modern isoln processes: H. J. V. Winkler, Der Steinkohlenteer und seine Aufarbeitung (Essen, 1951). Isoln by a freeze-out method: Kjellman, US 2483420 (1946 to Koppers). Purification: Freiser, Glowacki, J. Am. Chem. Soc. 71, 514 (1949). Synthesis: D. L. Boger et al., Tetrahedron 37, 3977 (1981). Toxicity data: Smyth et al., Arch. Ind. Hyg. Occup. Med. 4, 119 (1951). Comprehensive survey of isoquinoline alkaloids: Gensler, Heterocyclic Compounds vol. 4, R. C. Elderfield, Ed. (Wiley, New York, 1952) pp 344-490; T. Kametani, Total Synthesis of Natural Products vol. 3, J. ApSimon, Ed. (Wiley, New York, 1977) pp 1-272.

Liquid. Pungent odor resembling that of a mixture of anise oil and benzaldehyde. Hygroscopic platelets when solid. d_4^{30} 1.09101; d_4^{80} 1.05143. mp 26.48°. n_D^{30} 1.62078. Viscosity (cP): 3.2528 (30°); 1.0230 (100°); 0.4223 (200°). bp_{743} 242.2°; bp_{760} 243.25°. Dipole moment: 2.49. More basic than quinoline, pKa (25°): 8.60. Almost insol in water. Miscible with many organic solvents. Sol in dil acids. LD_{50} orally in rats: 360 mg/kg (Smyth).
Sulfate. $C_9H_7N.H_2SO_4$. Crystals, mp 209-209.5°. Sol in water.
USE: Synthesis of dyes, insecticides, antimalarials, rubber accelerators.

5223. Isosafrole. [120-58-1] 5-(1-Propenyl)-1,3-benzodioxole; 1,2-(methylenedioxy)-4-propenylbenzene. $C_{10}H_{10}O_2$; mol wt 162.19. C 74.05%, H 6.21%, O 19.73%. Purification and separation from safrole: Balbiano, Ber. 42, 1505 (1911); Hoering, Baum, ibid. 3082. Prepn: Bert, Compt. Rend. 213, 873 (1941); Naves, Ardizio, Bull. Soc. Chim. Fr. 1957, 1053; Fengeas, ibid. 1964, 1892; Cabiddu et al., Ann. Chim. (Rome) 52, 1261 (1962). Review and evaluation of studies of carcinogenic action in laboratory animals: IARC Monographs 10, 231-241 (1976).

trans-Form. Liquid, odor of anise. bp_{760} 253°; bp_{100} 179.5°; bp_{20} 135.6°; $bp_{3.4}$ 85-86°. mp 8.2°. d_4^{20} 1.1206. n_D^{20} 1.5782. uv max (96% alc): 305, 267, 259.5 nm (ε 5340; 11600; 12160). Miscible with alc, ether, benzene. Sol in 8 parts of 90% alcohol.

cis-Form. Liq. $bp_{3.5}$ 77-79°. mp −21.5°. d_4^{20} 1.1182. n_D^{20} 1.5691. uv max (96% alc): 296.5, 259 nm (ε 4450; 10000).

USE: Manuf heliotropin; to modify oriental perfumes; to strengthen soap perfumes; in small quantities together with methyl salicylate in root beer and sarsaparilla flavors.

5224. Isosorbide. [652-67-5] 1,4:3,6-Dianhydro-D-glucitol; 1,4:3,6-dianhydrosorbitol; AT-101; NSC-40725; Hydronol; Ismotic; Isobide. $C_6H_{10}O_4$; mol wt 146.14. C 49.31%, H 6.90%, O 43.79%. Prepd by acid dehydration of D-glucitol: Haworth, Wiggins, **GB 600870** (1948). Purification: Hartmann, **US 3160641** (1964 to Atlas Chemical Industries). Review of prepn, structure, properties: Wiggins, *Adv. Carbohydr. Chem.* **5**, 191-228 (1950). Stereochemistry: Cope, Shen, *J. Am. Chem. Soc.* **78**, 3177 (1956). Conformation studies: Hopton, Thomas, *Can. J. Chem.* **47**, 2395 (1969). Pharmacodynamics in man: Nodine *et al.*, *Clin. Pharmacol. Ther.* **14**, 196 (1973).

Crystals, mp 61-64°. $[\alpha]_D$ +44°.
THERAP CAT: Diuretic.

5225. Isosorbide Dinitrate. [87-33-2] 1,4:3,6-Dianhydro-D-glucitol dinitrate; dinitrosorbide; 1,4:3,6-dianhydrosorbitol 2,5-dinitrate; Carvasin; Cedocard; Coroviss; Dignonitrat; Dilatrate; Diniket; Frandol; Imtack; Isocard; Isoket; IsoMack; Isorbid; Isordil; Isostenase; Isotrate; Langoran; Maycor; Myorexon; Nitorol; Nitrol; Nitrosorbon; Rifloc; Risordan; Sorbangil; Sorbichew; Sorbidilat; Sorbid SA; Sorbitrate; Vascardin; Vasorbate. $C_6H_8N_2O_8$; mol wt 236.14. C 30.52%, H 3.41%, N 11.86%, O 54.20%. Coronary vasodilator. Prepn from sorbitol: Goldberg, *Acta Physiol. Scand.* **15**, 173 (1948), *C.A.* **42**, 5564 (1948); Kochergin, Titkova, *C.A.* **54**, 8647h (1960). Absorption and disposition in man: H. Laufen *et al.*, *Arzneim.-Forsch.* **33**, 980 (1983). Comprehensive description: L. A. Silvieri, N. J. DeAngelis, *Anal. Profiles Drug Subs.* **4**, 225-244 (1975).

Hard colorless crystals, mp 70°. $[\alpha]_D^{20}$ +135° (alc). Sparingly sol in water (1.089 mg/ml, also given as 1.0 g dissolves in 900 ml H_2O). Freely sol in organic solvents, such as acetone, alc, ether.

Isosorbide-5-mononitrate. [16051-77-7] Corangin; Elan; Elantan; Imdur; Ismo; Isomonat; Monicor; Monit; Mono-Cedocard; Monoclair; Monoket; Mono Mack; Monosorb; Olicard; Pentacard. $C_6H_9NO_6$; mol wt 191.14. Metabolite of isosorbide dinitrate.
THERAP CAT: Antianginal.

5226. Isothebaine. [568-21-8] (6aS)-5,6,6a,7-Tetrahydro-2,11-dimethoxy-6-methyl-4H-dibenzo[de,g]quinolin-1-ol; 2,11-dimethoxy-6aα-aporphin-1-ol; 1-hydroxy-2,11-dimethoxyaporphine. $C_{19}H_{21}NO_3$; mol wt 311.37. C 73.29%, H 6.80%, N 4.50%, O 15.42%. Occurs as d-form in the root and whole plant of *Papaver orientale* L., *Papaveraceae*, collected in late autumn. Isoln: Gadamer, *Arch. Pharm.* **249**, 39 (1911). Structure: Bentley, Blues, *J.*

Chem. Soc. **1956**, 1732; Bentley, Dyke, *J. Org. Chem.* **22**, 429 (1957). Synthesis of dl-form: Battersby, Brown, *Proc. Chem. Soc. London* **1964**, 85; H. Hara *et al.*, *Chem. Pharm. Bull.* **29**, 1083 (1981). Synthesis of natural and racemic forms: Battersby *et al.*, *J. Chem. Soc.* **1965**, 4550. Biosynthesis: *eidem, Chem. Commun.* **1965**, 230.

Light-sensitive, rhombic crystals. mp 203-204°. $[\alpha]_D^{18}$ +285° in alc. Sol in alcohol, chloroform, slightly in ether.

5227. Isothipendyl. [482-15-5] N,N,α-Trimethyl-10H-pyrido[3,2-b][1,4]benzothiazine-10-ethanamine; 10-(2-dimethylamino-2-methylethyl)-10H-pyrido[3,2-b][1,4]benzothiazine; 10-(2-dimethylaminopropyl)-1-azaphenothiazine; N-dimethylaminoisopropylthiophenylpyridylamine; D-201. $C_{16}H_{19}N_3S$; mol wt 285.41. C 67.33%, H 6.71%, N 14.72%, S 11.23%. Prepn: H. L. Yale, F. Sowinski, *J. Am. Chem. Soc.* **80**, 1651 (1958). Pharmacology: A. von Schlichtegroll, *Arzneim.-Forsch.* **8**, 489 (1958). Clinical evaluation: N. W. Klehr *et al.*, *Therapiewoche* **34**, 6050 (1984); E. Milsmann, P. Rohdewald, *Dermatologica* **170**, 230 (1985). Spectroscopic determn: M. H. Abdel-Hay *et al.*, *J. Pharm. Belg.* **45**, 259 (1990). HPLC determn: A. Turcant *et al.*, *Clin. Chem.* **37**, 1210 (1991).

$bp_{0.4mm}$ 171-174°. LD_{50} in mice (mg/kg): 65 ±2 i.p.; 222 ±18 orally (Schlichtegroll).
Hydrochloride. [1225-60-1] Andantol; Andanton; Nilergex. $C_{16}H_{19}N_3S$.HCl; mol wt 321.87. Sol in water.
THERAP CAT: Antihistaminic.

5228. Isotretinoin. [4759-48-2] 13-cis-Retinoic acid; 2-cis-vitamin A acid; neovitamin A acid; Ro-4-3780; Accutane; Isotrex; Oratane; Roaccutane. $C_{20}H_{28}O_2$; mol wt 300.44. C 79.95%, H 9.39%, O 10.65%. Naturally occurring metabolite of vitamin A, q.v.; inhibits sebum production. Prepn: C. D. Robeson *et al.*, *J. Am. Chem. Soc.* **77**, 4111 (1955). Stereoselective process: R. Lucci, **EP 111325**; idem, **US 4556518** (1984, 1985 both to Hoffmann-La Roche). Toxicology and teratogenicity study: J. J. Kamm, *J. Am. Acad. Dermatol.* **6**, 652 (1982). Identification as endogenous metabolite of all-trans-retinoic acid: M. E. Cullum, M. H. Zile, *J. Biol. Chem.* **260**, 10590 (1985). HPLC determn in serum: G. Tang, R. M. Russell, *J. Lipid Res.* **31**, 175 (1990). Review of pharmacology and clinical efficacy in acne: A. R. Shalita *et al.*, *Cutis* **42**, Suppl. 6A, 1-19 (1988). Symposium on clinical experience: *Dermatology* **195**, Suppl. 1, 1-37 (1997).

Reddish-orange plates from isopropyl alcohol, mp 174-175°. uv max: 354 nm (ε 39800). LD_{50} (20 day) in mice, rats (mg/kg): 904, 901 i.p.; 3389, >4000 orally (Kamm).
THERAP CAT: Antiacne.

Consult the Name Index before using this section.

5229. Isovaleraldehyde. [590-86-3] 3-Methylbutanal; iso-valeral; isovaleric aldehyde. $C_5H_{10}O$; mol wt 86.13. C 69.72%, H 11.70%, O 18.58%. $(CH_3)_2CHCH_2CHO$. Occurs in orange, lemon, peppermint, eucalyptus and other oils. Made by oxidation of isoamyl alcohol with $Na_2Cr_2O_7$ and H_2SO_4.

Colorless liquid; pungent apple-like odor. d_{20}^{20} 0.785. mp −51°. bp 92-93°. n_D^{20} 1.3902. Sparingly sol in water; miscible with alcohol, ether.

USE: In artificial flavors and perfumes.

5230. Isovaleramide. [541-46-8] $C_5H_{11}NO$; mol wt 101.15. C 59.37%, H 10.96%, N 13.85%, O 15.82%. $(CH_3)_2CH-CH_2CONH_2$.

Crystals. d 0.965. mp 135-137°. bp 232°. Sol in water, alcohol.

5231. Isovaleric Acid. [503-74-2] 3-Methylbutanoic acid; isovalerianic acid; isopropylacetic acid; delphinic acid. $C_5H_{10}O_2$; mol wt 102.13. C 58.80%, H 9.87%, O 31.33%. $(CH_3)_2CHCH_2-COOH$. Occurs in hop oil, tobacco and several other plants: Schmeltz et al., J. Assoc. Off. Agric. Chem. **46**, 779 (1963). Prepn: Caldwell, US 2484486 (1949 to Kodak); Gustak, Sajko, Ark. Kemi **24**, 11 (1952), C.A. **49**, 163e (1955); L'vov et al., Zh. Prikl. Khim. **35**, 700 (1962). "Valeric" acid of commerce is isovaleric acid. Toxicity data: L. Orö, A. Wretlind, Acta Pharmacol. Toxicol. **18**, 141 (1961).

Liquid. Acid taste; disagreeable, rancid-cheese odor. d_4^{20} 0.931. mp −37°. bp 175-177°. n_D^{20} 1.4043. Sol in 24 parts water; sol in alcohol, chloroform, ether. Keep tightly closed. LD_{50} i.v. in mice: 1120±30 mg/kg (Orö, Wretlind).

USE: In flavors, perfumes, manuf sedatives.

5232. Isovaleryl Chloride. [108-12-3] C_5H_9ClO; mol wt 120.58. C 49.80%, H 7.52%, Cl 29.40%, O 13.27%. $(CH_3)_2-CHCH_2COCl$.

Liquid. d_4^{20} 0.985. bp 114-116°. n_D^{20} 1.4156. Dec by water, alcohol.

5233. 2-Isovalerylindane-1,3-dione. [83-28-3] 2-(3-Meth-yl-1-oxobutyl)-1H-indene-1,3(2H)-dione; PMP; Valone. $C_{14}H_{14}-O_3$; mol wt 230.26. C 73.03%, H 6.13%, O 20.85%. Prepn: Shapiro et al., J. Org. Chem. **25**, 1860 (1960).

Yellow solid from methanol, mp 68-69°. Practically insol in water, sol in most organic solvents.

USE: Insecticide, rodenticide.

5234. Isovaline. [595-39-1] DL-2-Amino-2-methylbutyric acid; α-amino-α-methylbutyric acid. $C_5H_{11}NO_2$; mol wt 117.15. C 51.26%, H 9.46%, N 11.96%, O 27.31%. Prepn: Kurono, Biochem. Z. **134**, 427 (1922); Levene, Steiger, J. Biol. Chem. **76**, 299 (1928); Bucherer, Steiner, J. Prakt. Chem. **141**, 5 (1934); Upham, Dermer, J. Org. Chem. **22**, 799 (1957). Optical enantiomorphs: Ehrlich, Wendel, Biochem. Z. **8**, 438 (1908); Fischer, von Gravenitz, Ann. **406**, 5 (1914); Baker et al., J. Am. Chem. Soc. **74**, 4701 (1952); Greenstein et al., J. Biol. Chem. **204**, 307 (1953).

Monoclinic prisms, mp 307-308° (closed tube). Sublimes at around 300°. Soly in cold water about 39 g/100 ml; in alc about 6.6 g/100 g alc at 75°. Slightly sol in ether.

L-Form. [595-40-4] Crystals. $[\alpha]_D^{25}$ +11.13° (c = 5 in H_2O). $[M]_D$ +9.7° (5N HCl); $[M]_D$ +26.3° (glacial acetic acid).

D-Form. [3059-97-0] Long needles from water + acetone. $[\alpha]_D^{25}$ −11.28° (c = 5 in H_2O).

5235. Isoxaben. [82558-50-7] N-[3-(1-Ethyl-1-methylpro-pyl)-5-isoxazolyl]-2,6-dimethoxybenzamide; benzamizole; EL-107; NA-8318; Flexidor; Gallery. $C_{18}H_{24}N_2O_4$; mol wt 332.39. C 65.04%, H 7.28%, N 8.43%, O 19.25%. Selective, pre-emergent herbicide for broadleaf weeds and annual grasses. Prepn: K. W. Burow, GB 2084140; see also: idem, US 4636243 (1982, 1987 both to Lilly). Physical properties and herbicidal activity: F. Huggenberger et al., Proc. Br. Crop Prot. Conf. - Weeds **1982**, 47. Mobility and degradation in soil: F. Huggenberger, P. J. Ryan, ibid. **1985**, 947. Effect on cellular growth and metabolism: A. Lefebvre et al., Weed Res. **27**, 125 (1987). Field trials: F. Huggenberger, F. Gueguen, Crop Prot. **6**, 75 (1987); F. O. Colbert, D. H. Ford, Proc. West. Soc. Weed Sci. **40**, 155 (1987).

White crystalline solid, mp 176-179°. Soly at 25° (mg/ml): methanol 50-100; ethyl acetate 50-100; acetonitrile 30-50; toluene 4-5; hexane 0.07-0.08; water 0.001-0.002. Vapor pressure at 30°: <3.9 × 10^{-7} mm Hg. LD_{50} in mice, rats (mg/kg): >10000 orally both species; LC_{50} in rats by inhalation: >1.99 mg/l (Huggenberger, 1982).

USE: Herbicide.

5236. Isoxaflutole. [141112-29-0] (5-Cyclopropyl-4-isox-azolyl)[2-(methylsulfonyl)-4-(trifluoromethyl)phenyl]methanone; 5-cyclopropyl-1,2-oxazol-4-yl α,α,α-trifluoro-2-mesyl-p-tolyl ketone; 5-cyclopropylisoxazol-4-yl 2-mesyl-4-trifluoromethylphenyl ketone; 5-cyclopropyl-4-(2-methanesulfonyl-4-trifluoromethyl-benzoyl)isoxazole; 264-EUP-99; RPA-201772; Balance; Merlin. $C_{15}H_{12}F_3NO_4S$; mol wt 359.32. C 50.14%, H 3.37%, F 15.86%, N 3.90%, O 17.81%, S 8.92%. Pre-emergent herbicide designed for use in maize. Disrupts pigment biosynthesis via an inhibition of 4-hydroxyphenylpyruvate dioxygenase. Prepn: P. A. Cain et al., EP 527036 (1993 to Rhone-Poulenc). Properties and biological activity: B. M. Luscombe et al., Brighton Crop Prot. Conf. - Weeds **1995**, 35. Weed control in maize: B. M. Luscombe, K. E. Pallett, Pestic. Outlook **7**, 29 (1996). Mechanism of action: K. E. Pallett et al., Pestic. Sci. **50**, 83 (1997). Soil persistence: J. Rouchaud et al., Bull. Environ. Contam. Toxicol. **60**, 577 (1998).

Off-white or pale yellow solid, mp 138-138.5° (Cain); also reported as mp 140° (Luscombe). Vapor pressure at 25°: 1×10^{-6} Pa. Soly in water: 6.2 mg/l. LD_{50} in rats, quails, mallard ducks (mg/kg): >5000, >2150, >2150 orally; in rabbits (mg/kg): >2000 dermally (Luscombe).

USE: Herbicide.

5237. Isoxepac. [55453-87-7] 6,11-Dihydro-11-oxodi-benz[b,e]oxepin-2-acetic acid; oxepinac; HP-549; P-720549; Artil. $C_{16}H_{12}O_4$; mol wt 268.26. C 71.64%, H 4.51%, O 23.86%. Non-steroidal anti-inflammatory with analgesic and antipyretic activity. Prepn: K. Ueno et al., JP Kokai 74 124086 (1974 to Daiichi), C.A. **82**, 170735d (1975); G. C. Helsley et al., DE 2442060; eidem, US 4585788 (1975, 1986 both to Hoechst); K. Ueno et al., J. Med. Chem. **19**, 941 (1976); D. E. Aultz et al., ibid. **20**, 66 (1977). Pharmacology: H. B. Lassman et al., Arch. Int. Pharmacodyn. Ther. **227**, 142 (1977). Disposition and metabolism in animals and humans: H. P. A. Illing, J. M. Fromson, Drug Metab. Dispos. **6**, 510 (1978). HPLC determn in plasma: J. A. Slack, J. Chromatogr. **221**, 431 (1980); H. K. L. Hundt, L. W. Brown, ibid. **225**, 482 (1981). Clinical studies: S. Sasaki, Arzneim.-Forsch. **28**, 462

(1978); L. B. Svendsen *et al., Scand. J. Rheumatol.* **10**, 186 (1981); J. Scott, E. C. Huskisson, *Rheumatol. Rehabil.* **21**, 48 (1982).

Crystals from ethyl acetate, mp 131-132.5°. LD$_{50}$ orally in rats: 199 mg/kg (Ueno).

THERAP CAT: Anti-inflammatory.

5238. Isoxsuprine. [395-28-8] 4-Hydroxy-α-[1-[(1-methyl-2-phenoxyethyl)amino]ethyl]benzenemethanol; *p*-hydroxy-α-[1-[(1-methyl-2-phenoxyethyl)amino]ethyl]benzyl alcohol; *p*-hydroxy-*N*-(1-methyl-2-phenoxyethyl)norephedrine; 1-(*p*-hydroxyphenyl)-2-(1-methyl-2-phenoxyethylamino)-1-propanol; 2-(3-phenoxy-2-propylamino)-1-(*p*-hydroxyphenyl)-1-propanol. C$_{18}$H$_{23}$-NO$_3$; mol wt 301.38. C 71.73%, H 7.69%, N 4.65%, O 15.93%. Prepn: Moed, van Dijk, *Rec. Trav. Chim.* **75**, 1215 (1956); **GB 832286** and **GB 832287** (both 1960 to N. V. Philip Gloeilampenfabrieken); Moed, **US 3056836** (1962 to N. Am. Philips). Configuration: Dirkx, *Rec. Trav. Chim.* **83**, 535 (1964). Toxicity data: Goldenthal, *Toxicol. Appl. Pharmacol.* **18**, 185 (1971). Clinical evaluation in Raynaud's phenomenon: H. Wesseling *et al., Eur. J. Clin. Pharmacol.* **20**, 329 (1981); in intermittent claudication: S. H. Skotnicki *et al., Angiology* **35**, 685 (1984). Veterinary trial in navicular disease: A. S. Turner, C. M. Tucker, *Equine Vet. J.* **21**, 338 (1989).

Crystals, mp 102.5-103.5°.

Hydrochloride. [579-56-6] Dilavase; Duvadilan; Duviculine; Navilox; Suprilent; Vadosilan; Vasodilan; Vasotran. C$_{18}$H$_{23}$NO$_3$.-HCl; mol wt 337.84. Bitter crystals from water, mp 203-204°. Soly in water at 25° about 2.0% w/v; also sol in ethanol. LD$_{50}$ in rats (mg/kg): 1750 orally; 164 i.p. (Goldenthal).

THERAP CAT: Vasodilator (peripheral).

THERAP CAT (VET): In treatment of navicular disease.

5239. Ispronicline. [252870-53-4] (2*S*,4*E*)-*N*-Methyl-5-[5-(1-methylethoxy)-3-pyridinyl]-4-penten-2-amine; RJR-1734; TC-1734. C$_{14}$H$_{22}$N$_2$O; mol wt 234.34. C 71.75%, H 9.46%, N 11.95%, O 6.83%. Specific $\alpha_4\beta_2$ nicotinic receptor agonist. Prepn: W. S. Caldwell *et al., WO 9965876* (1999 to R. J. Reynolds); *eidem,* **US 6958399** (2005 to Targacept). Effect on cortical acetylcholine release in rats: M. C. Obinu *et al., Prog. Neuro-Psychopharmacol. Biol. Psychiatry* **26**, 913 (2002). Review of pharmacology: G. J. Gatto *et al., CNS Drug Rev.* **10**, 147-166 (2004); and clinical experience: H. Geerts, *Curr. Opin. Invest. Drugs* **7**, 60-69 (2006).

Colorless oil, bp$_{0.5}$ 90-100°.

Hemigalactarate. [252870-54-5] C$_{28}$H$_{44}$N$_4$O$_2$.C$_6$H$_{10}$O$_8$; mol wt 678.81. White crystalline powder, mp 140-143°.

THERAP CAT: Nootropic.

5240. Isradipine. [75695-93-1] 4-(4-Benzofurazanyl)-1,4-dihydro-2,6-dimethyl-3,5-pyridinedicarboxylic acid methyl 1-methylethyl ester; isopropyl 4-(2,1,3-benzoxadiazol-4-yl)-1,4-dihydro-5-methoxycarbonyl-2,6-dimethyl-3-pyridinecarboxylate; 4-(2,1,3-benzoxadiazol-4-yl)-2,6-dimethyl-1,4-dihydro-3-isopropyloxycarbonylpyridine-5-carboxylic acid methyl ester; isrodipine; PN-200-110; Clivoten; DynaCirc; Esradin; Lomir; Prescal. C$_{19}$-

H$_{21}$N$_3$O$_5$; mol wt 371.39. C 61.45%, H 5.70%, N 11.31%, O 21.54%. Dihydropyridine calcium channel blocker. Prepn: P. Neumann, **DE 2949491**; *idem,* **US 4466972** (1980, 1984 both to Sandoz). Prepn of enantiomers: A. Vogel, **DE 3320616** (1983 to Sandoz), *C.A.* **101**, 7162s (1984). Comparative study of *in vitro* effects on human and canine cerebral arteries: E. Müller-Schweinitzer, P. Neumann, *J. Cereb. Blood Flow Metab.* **3**, 354 (1983). Effect on α-adrenoceptor mediated vasoconstriction in rats: K. Jie *et al., Arch. Int. Pharmacodyn.* **278**, 72 (1985). Pharmacokinetics: F. L. S. Tee, J. M. Jaffe, *Eur. J. Clin. Pharmacol.* **32**, 361 (1987). Clinical evaluation in angina and coronary artery disease: C. E. Handler, E. Sowton, *ibid.* **27**, 415 (1984); in hypertension: E. B. Nelson *et al., Clin. Pharmacol. Ther.* **40**, 694 (1986). Comparison of hemodynamic effects of enantiomers: R. P. Hof *et al., J. Cardiovasc. Pharmacol.* **8**, 221 (1986). Series of articles on pharmacology and clinical use: *Am. J. Med.* **86**, 1-146 (1989).

mp 168-170°.

S(+)-**Form.** PN-205-033. Crystals from ether + hexane, mp 142°. $[\alpha]_D^{20}$ +6.7° (c = 1.5 in ethanol).

R(−)-**Form.** PN-205-034. Crystals from ether + hexane, mp 140°. $[\alpha]_D^{20}$ −6.7° (c = 1.67 in ethanol).

THERAP CAT: Antihypertensive; antianginal.

5241. Israpafant. [117279-73-9] 4-(2-Chlorophenyl)-6,9-dimethyl-2-[2-[4-(2-methylpropyl)phenyl]ethyl]-6*H*-thieno[3,2-*f*][1,2,4]triazolo[4,3-*a*][1,4]diazepine; ($\pm$)-4-(*o*-chlorophenyl)-2-(*p*-isobutylphenethyl)-6,9-dimethyl-6*H*-thieno[3,2-*f*]-*s*-triazolo[4,-3-*a*][1,4]diazepine; Y-24180; Pafnol. C$_{28}$H$_{29}$ClN$_4$S; mol wt 489.07. C 68.76%, H 5.98%, Cl 7.25%, N 11.46%, S 6.56%. Platelet activating factor (PAF) antagonist. Prepn: T. Tahara *et al., EP 268242; eidem,* **US 4820703** (1988, 1989 both to Yoshitomi). Pharmacology: M. Terasawa *et al., Prostaglandins* **40**, 553 (1990). Receptor binding study: S. Takehara *et al., ibid.* 571. Clinical evaluation in asthma: S. Hozawa *et al., Am. J. Respir. Crit. Care Med.* **152**, 1198 (1995).

Colorless crystals from isopropyl ether, mp 129.5-131.5°. Sol in propylene glycol.

THERAP CAT: Antiasthmatic.

5242. Itaconic Acid. [97-65-4] Methylenesuccinic acid; propylenedicarboxylic acid. C$_5$H$_6$O$_4$; mol wt 130.10. C 46.16%, H 4.65%, O 49.19%. Obtained from distillation of citric acid and subsequent treatment of the anhydride with water. Produced on a large scale by submerged aerobic fermentation using *Aspergillus terreus* and low cost carbohydrates from beet or cane: Kane *et al., US 2385283* (1945 to Pfizer). Synthesis from propargyl chloride, carbon monoxide, nickel carbonyl and water: Chiusoli, **US 3025320** (1962 to Montecatini).

Hygroscopic crystals; characteristic odor. d 1.63. mp 162-164° with decompn. Also reported as mp 172° [Kinoshita, *Acta Phytochim.* **5,** 273 (1931)]. One gram dissolves in 12 ml water, 5 ml alcohol; very slightly sol in benzene, chloroform, ether, carbon disulfide, petr ether. *Keep well closed.*

5243. Itasetron. [123258-84-4] 2,3-Dihydro-*N*-[(3-*endo*)-8-methyl-8-azabicyclo[3.2.1]oct-3-yl]-2-oxo-1*H*-benzimidazole-1-carboxamide; 2-oxo-*N*-1α*H*,5α*H*-tropan-3α-yl-1-benzimidazoline-1-carboxamide. $C_{16}H_{20}N_4O_2$; mol wt 300.36. C 63.98%, H 6.71%, N 18.65%, O 10.65%. Serotonin (5-HT$_3$) receptor antagonist. Prepn: M. Turconi *et al.,* **EP 309423** (1989 to Istituto De Angeli); *eidem,* **US 5223511** (1993 to Boehringer, Ing.); M. Turconi *et al., J. Med. Chem.* **33,** 2101 (1990). Pharmacology: *idem et al., Eur. J. Pharmacol.* **203,** 203 (1991). Mode of action: M. B. Passani *et al., Br. J. Pharmacol.* **112,** 695 (1994). Clinical efficacy and tolerability: H. Goldschmidt *et al., Anti-Cancer Drugs* **8,** 436 (1997). Review of therapeutic potential: M. B. Passani, R. Corradetti, *CNS Drug Reviews* **2,** 195-213 (1996).

Crystals from acetonitrile, mp 205-207°. LD$_{50}$ in mice, rats (mg/kg): 56, 62 i.v. (Passani).
Hydrochloride. [127618-28-4] DAU 6215. $C_{16}H_{20}N_4O_2$·HCl; mol wt 336.82. Colorless crystals, mp 270°.
THERAP CAT: Antiemetic.

5244. Itopride. [122898-67-3] *N*-[[4-[2-(Dimethylamino)-ethoxy]phenyl]methyl]-3,4-dimethoxy benzamide; *N*-[*p*-[2-(di-methylamino)ethoxy]benzyl]veratramide. $C_{20}H_{26}N_2O_4$; mol wt 358.43. C 67.02%, H 7.31%, N 7.82%, O 17.85%. Dopamine D$_2$-receptor antagonist with anticholinesterase activity. Prepn: Y. Itoh *et al.,* **EP 306827**; *eidem,* **US 4983633** (1989, 1991 both to Hokuriku Pharm.); J. Sakaguchi *et al., Chem. Pharm. Bull.* **40,** 202 (1992). Pharmacology: Y. Iwanaga *et al., Jpn. J. Pharmacol.* **56,** 261 (1991). Toxicity studies: M. H. Barker *et al., Yakuri to Chiryo* **21,** 1685, 1669 (1993). Metabolism study: T. Mushiroda *et al., Drug Metab. Dispos.* **28,** 1231 (2000). HPLC determn in serum and clinical pharmacokinetics: S. S. Singh *et al., J. Chromatogr. B* **818,** 213 (2005). Clinical study in postoperative ileus: R. Gürlich *et al., Chir. Gastroenterol. Interdiszip.* **20,** 61 (2004); in dyspepsia: D. N. Amarapurkar, P. Rane, *J. Indian Med. Assoc.* **102,** 735 (2004).

Crystals from ethanol + isopropyl ether, mp 111-112°.
Hydrochloride. [122892-31-5] HSR-803; HC-803; Itax; Ganaton. $C_{20}H_{26}N_2O_4$·HCl; mol wt 394.89. Crystals from ethanol, mp 194-195°. Also reported as prisms from ethanol, mp 190.5-191.5° (Sakaguchi). Readily sol in water.
THERAP CAT: Gastroprokinetic.

5245. Itraconazole. [84625-61-6] 4-[4-[4-[4-[[2-(2,4-Di-chlorophenyl)-2-(1*H*-1,2,4-triazol-1-ylmethyl)-1,3-dioxolan-4-yl]methoxy]phenyl]-1-piperazinyl]phenyl]-2,4-dihydro-2-(1-methyl-propyl)-3*H*-1,2,4-triazol-3-one; (±)-1-*sec*-butyl-4-[*p*-[4-[*p*-[[(2*R**,4*S**)-2-(2,4-dichlorophenyl)-2-(1*H*-1,2,4-triazol-1-ylmeth-yl)-1,3-dioxolan-4-yl]methoxy]phenyl]-1-piperazinyl]phenyl]-Δ^2-1,2,4-triazolin-5-one; oriconazole; R-51211; Itrizole; Sporanox; Tri-

asporin. $C_{35}H_{38}Cl_2N_8O_4$; mol wt 705.63. C 59.57%, H 5.43%, Cl 10.05%, N 15.88%, O 9.07%. Orally active antimycotic structurally related to ketoconazole, *q.v.* Prepn: J. Heeres, L. J. J. Backx, **EP 6711**; *eidem,* **US 4267179** (1980, 1981 both to Janssen); J. Heeres *et al., J. Med. Chem.* **27,** 894 (1984). *In vitro* activity: A. Espinel-Ingroff *et al., Antimicrob. Agents Chemother.* **26,** 5 (1984). HPLC determn in biological samples: R. Woestenborghs *et al., J. Chromatogr.* **413,** 332 (1987). Symposium on pharmacology and clinical efficacy: *Rev. Infect. Dis.* **9,** Suppl 1, S1-S152 (1987). Toxicity data: H. Van Cauteren *et al., ibid.* S43. Review of clinical pharmacokinetics: J. Heykants *et al., Mycoses* **32,** Suppl 1, 67-87 (1989); of clinical efficacy in dermatophytosis: P. De Doncker, G. Cauwenbergh, *Br. J. Clin. Pract.* **Suppl. 71,** 118-122 (1990). *Review:* A. M. Sugar, *Curr. Clin. Top. Infect. Dis.* **13,** 74-98 (1993).

Crystals from toluene, mp 166.2°. pKa 3.7. Lipophilic; partition coefficient (*n*-octanol/aq buffer of pH 8.1): 5.66. Practically insol in water and dil acidic solns. LD$_{50}$ (14 day) in mice, rats, dogs (mg/kg): >320, >320, >200 orally (Van Cauteren).
THERAP CAT: Antifungal.

5246. Itramin Tosylate. [13445-63-1] 2-Aminoethanol nitrate mono(4-methylbenzenesulfonate); 2-aminoethanol nitrate mono-*p*-toluenesulfonate; 2-nitratoethylaminotoluene-*p*-sulfonate; Cardisan; Tostram; Nilatil. $C_9H_{14}N_2O_6S$; mol wt 278.28. C 38.84%, H 5.07%, N 10.07%, O 34.50%, S 11.52%. Prepn: **SE 168308** (1959 to Aktiebolaget Pharmacia), *C.A.* **54,** 24405d (1960).

Crystals from ethanol, mp 132-133°.
THERAP CAT: Vasodilator.

5247. Ivabradine. [155974-00-8] 3-[3-[[[(7*S*)-3,4-Dimeth-oxybicyclo[4.2.0]octa-1,3,5-trien-7-yl]methyl]methylamino]pro-pyl]-1,3,4,5-tetrahydro-7,8-dimethoxy-2*H*-3-benzazepin-2-one; 7,8-dimethoxy-3-[3-[[(1*S*)-(4,5-dimethoxybenzocyclobutan-1-yl)-methyl]methylamino]propyl]-1,3,4,5-tetrahydro-2*H*-benzazepin-2-one; S-16257. $C_{27}H_{36}N_2O_5$; mol wt 468.59. C 69.21%, H 7.74%, N 5.98%, O 17.07%. Selective bradycardic agent with direct effect on the pacemaker I_f current of the sinoatrial node. Prepn: J.-L. Peglion *et al.,* **EP 534859**; *eidem,* **US 5296482** (1993, 1994 both to ADIR). *In vitro* electrophysiological effects: C. Thollon *et al,. Br. J. Pharmacol.* **112,** 37 (1994). LC-MS determn in plasma: M. François-Bouchard *et al., J. Chromatogr. B* **745,** 261 (2000). Clinical pharmacokinetics: I. Ragueneau *et al., Clin. Pharmacol. Ther.* **64,** 192 (1998). Clinical trial in stable angina: J. S. Borer *et al., Circulation* **107,** 817 (2003). Series of articles on pharmacology and clinical experience: *Eur. Heart J. Suppl.* **5,** Suppl. G, G26-G56 (2003). Review of mechanism of action: D. DiFrancesco, J. A. Camm, *Drugs* **64,** 1757-1765 (2004).

Hydrochloride. [148849-67-6] S-16257-2; Procoralan; Corlentor. $C_{27}H_{36}N_2O_5$·HCl; mol wt 505.05. Crystals from acetonitrile, mp 135-140°. $[\alpha]_{589}^{21}$ +7.8°; $[\alpha]_{365}^{21}$ +27.8° (c = 1% in DMSO).
(±)-Form. [149470-60-0] $C_{27}H_{36}N_2O_5$. Crystals from ethyl acetate, mp 101-103°.
THERAP CAT: Antianginal.

5248. Ivermectin. [70288-86-7] 22,23-Dihydroabamectin; 22,23-dihydroavermectin B_1; 22,23-dihydro C-076B_1; MK-933; Eqvalan; Heartgard 30; Ivomec; Mectizan; Noromectin; Stromectol. Semi-synthetic deriv of abamectin, *q.v.*, consists of a mixture of not less than 80% component B_{1a} and not more than 20% component B_{1b}. Prepn: **JP Kokai 79 61198**; J. C. Chabala, M. H. Fisher, **US 4199569** (1979, 1980 both to Merck & Co.); J. C. Chabala *et al., J. Med. Chem.* **23,** 1134 (1980). Irreversible effects on adult parasites in onchocerciasis: A. P. Plaisier *et al., J. Infect. Dis.* **172,** 204 (1995). Metabolism in animals: S.-H. L. Chiu *et al., Drug Metab. Dispos.* **14,** 590 (1986). Pharmacokinetics in horses and sheep: S. E. Marriner *et al., J. Vet. Pharmacol. Ther.* **10,** 175 (1987). HPLC determn in cattle and sheep tissues: P. C. Tway *et al., J. Agric. Food Chem.* **29,** 1059 (1981); in human plasma and milk: R. Chiou *et al., J. Chromatogr.* **416,** 196 (1987). Review of early chemistry and biology: W. C. Campbell *et al., Science* **221,** 823-828 (1983). Review of clinical use and pharmacology: W. C. Campbell, G. W. Benz, *J. Vet. Pharmacol. Ther.* **7,** 1-16 (1984); T. B. Barragry, *Can. Vet. J.* **28,** 512-517 (1987); of pharmacology: J. L. Bennett *et al., Parasitol. Today* **4,** 226-228 (1988). Book: *Ivermectin and Abamectin,* W. C. Campbell, Ed. (Springer-Verlag, New York, 1989) 363 pp. Review in filariasis: D. Richard-Lenoble *et al., Fundam. Clin. Pharmacol.* **17,** 199-203 (2003). *See also:* Avermectins.

Component B_{1a} R = CH$_2$CH$_3$
Component B_{1b} R = CH$_3$

Clear, moist, off-white to slightly yellow powder. $[\alpha]_D$ +71.5 ± 3° (c = 0.755 in chloroform). uv max (methanol): 238, 245 nm (ε 27100, 30100). Soly in water: ~4 μg/ml. Virtually insol in satd hydrocarbons such as cyclohexane. Highly sol in methyl ethyl ketone, propylene glycol, polyethylene glycol. LD$_{50}$ in dogs, rhesus monkeys (mg/kg): about 80, more than 24 orally. (MSDS Merck & Co. Inc., 2003).

Component B_{1a}. [71827-03-7] 5-*O*-Demethyl-22,23-dihydroavermectin A_{1a}; 22,23-dihydroavermectin B_{1a}; 22,23-dihydro C-076B_{1a}. $C_{48}H_{74}O_{14}$; mol wt 875.09. Crystals from ethanol/water, mp 155-157°.

Component B_{1b}. [70209-81-3] 5-*O*-Demethyl-25-*de*(1-methylpropyl)-22,23-dihydro-25-(1-methylethyl)avermectin A_{1a}; 22,23-dihydroavermectin B_{1b}. $C_{47}H_{72}O_{14}$; mol wt 861.07.

THERAP CAT: Anthelmintic (Onchocerca).

THERAP CAT (VET): Anthelmintic, insecticide, acaricide.

5249. Ixabepilone. [219989-84-1] (1*S*,3*S*,7*S*,10*R*,11*S*,12*S*,16*R*)-7,11-Dihydroxy-8,8,10,12,16-pentamethyl-3-[(1*E*)-1-methyl-2-(2-methyl-4-thiazolyl)ethenyl]-17-oxa-4-azabicyclo[14.1.0]heptadecane-5,9-dione; azaepothilone B; BMS-247550; NSC-710428. $C_{27}H_{42}N_2O_5S$; mol wt 506.70. C 64.00%, H 8.35%, N 5.53%, O 15.79%, S 6.33%. Microtubule stabilizing semisynthetic lactam analog of epothilone B, *q.v.* Prepn: G. D. Vite *et al.,* **WO 9902514**; *eidem,* **US 6605599** (1999, 2003 both to Bristol-Myers Squibb); R. M. Borzilleri *et al., J. Am. Chem. Soc.* **122,** 8890 (2000). Antineoplastic activity *in vitro* and *in vivo*: F. Y. F. Lee *et al., Clin. Cancer Res.* **7,** 1429 (2001). Clinical evaluation with estramustine in prostate cancer: J. E. Rosenberg *et al., Cancer* **106,** 58 (2006). Clinical pharmacokinetics and evaluation in solid tumors: S. Mani *et al., Clin. Cancer Res.* **10,** 1289 (2004). Clinical evaluation in breast cancer: J. A. Low *et al., J. Clin. Oncol.* **23,** 2726 (2005); in prostate cancer: M. Hussain *et al., ibid.* 8724. Review of pharmacology and clinical development: N. Lin *et al., Curr. Opin. Invest. Drugs* **4,** 746-756 (2003).

Colorless oil or white lyopholizate; $[\alpha]_D^{22}$ −40.7° (c = 1.0 in chloroform).

THERAP CAT: Antineoplastic.

5250. Ixbut. A native name for *Euphorbia lancifolia* Schlecht, *Euphorbiaceae.* Used as a galactagogue: Serrano, *Time,* August 1st, **1949,** p 38; F. Rosengarten, Jr., *Bot. Mus. Leafl. Harv. Univ.* **26** (9-10), 277-309 (Nov.-Dec. 1978).

5251. Ixodin. Hirudin-like anticoagulant from *Ixodes ricinus* L., *Acari* and other blood-sucking ticks: Sabbatani, *Arch. Ital. Biol.* **31,** 37 (1899). Thrombokinase inhibitor. Extraction procedure: F. Markwardt, *Blutgerinnungshemmende Wirkstoffe aus blutsaugenden Tieren* (Jena, 1963) pp 88-92.

White powder. Soluble in 80% ethanol, 90% methanol and 75% acetone. Practically insol in ether. Stable at pH 1.0-12.0. Adsorbed on Amberlite IRC 50 (H-form). Acts like a high-molecular weight polypeptide. Attacked by papain.

J

5252. Jacobsen's Catalyst. [149656-63-3] (*SP*-5-13)-Chloro[[*rel*-2,2'-[(1*R*,2*R*)-1,2-cyclohexanediylbis[(nitrilo-κ*N*)methylidyne]]bis[4,6-bis(1,1'-dimethylethyl)phenolato-κ*O*]](2−)]manganese. C$_{36}$H$_{52}$ClMnN$_2$O$_2$; mol wt 635.20. C 68.07%, H 8.25%, Cl 5.58%, Mn 8.65%, N 4.41%, O 5.04%. Manganese-salen Schiff base complex used as a catalyst in asymmetric syntheses. Prepn: E. N. Jacobsen *et al., J. Am. Chem. Soc.* **113**, 7063 (1991); large-scale: J. F. Larrow *et al., J. Org. Chem.* **59**, 1939 (1994). Synthesis and enantioselectivity of dimer: K. B. M. Janssen *et al., Tetrahedron: Asymmetry* **8**, 3481 (1997). HPLC determn of enantiomeric purity in commercial samples: J. Zukowski, *Chirality* **10**, 362 (1998). Mechanism of asymmetric epoxidation of indenes: D. L. Hughes *et al., J. Org. Chem.* **62**, 2222 (1997). Use in epoxidation of isoflavones: W. Adam *et al., Tetrahedron: Asymmetry* **9**, 1121 (1998).

(R,R)-form

(*R,R*)-form. [138124-32-0] (*R,R*)-[*N,N'*-Bis(3,5-di-*tert*-butylsalicylidene)-1,2-cyclohexanediamine]manganese (III) chloride. mp 324-326°. [α]$_D^{23}$ +580° (c = 0.01 in ethanol).
USE: Chiral catalyst for epoxidation of olefins.

5253. Jalap. Dried tuberous root of *Exogonium purga* (Hayne) Lindl. (*E. jalapa* Baill., *Ipomoea purga* Hayne), *Convolvulaceae. Habit.* Mexico; culivated in India. *Constit.* 7-12% resin, gum, sugar.
THERAP CAT: Cathartic.

5254. Jambul. Jamboo; Java plum; jumbul. Bark, fruit and seeds of *Syzygium jambolanum* (Lam.) DC. (*Eugenia jambolana* Lam.), *Myrtaceae. Habit.* East Indies. *Constit.* Bark: resin, tannin. Fruit: volatile and fixed oils, resin, tannin. Seeds: resin, fat, gallic acid, albumin.
THERAP CAT: Antidiarrheal.

5255. Janus Green B. [2869-83-2] 3-(Diethylamino)-7-[[4-(dimethylamino)phenyl]azo]-5-phenylphenazinium chloride; C.I. 11050. C$_{30}$H$_{31}$ClN$_6$; mol wt 511.06. C 70.50%, H 6.11%, Cl 6.94%, N 16.44%. Prepd by diazotizing 3-amino-7-(diethylamino)-5-phenylphenazinium chloride (*N,N*-diethylphenosafranine) and coupling resulting diazo compd with *N,N*-dimethylaniline: *Colour Index* vol. 4 (3rd ed., 1971) p 4015.

USE: As dye for cotton, wool; as biological stain; in electrodeposition of copper, Brown, Fellows, **US 2882209** (1959 to Udylite Res. Corp.).

5256. Japan Wax. [8001-39-6] Vegetable wax; sumach wax; Japan tallow. A fat expressed from mesocarp of the fruit of *Rhus succedanea* L., *Anacardiaceae. Habit.* Japan and China. *Constit.* 10-15% palmitin; stearin, olein; 1% japanic acid and homologs. Brief review: C. S. Letcher in *Kirk-Othmer Encyclopedia of Chemical Technology* **vol. 24** (Wiley-Interscience, New York, 3rd ed., 1984) p 470.

Pale yellow, flat cakes, disks or squares with a greasy feel; somewhat tallow-like, rancid odor and taste. d 0.97-0.98. mp 53.5-55°. Acid number 22-23. Saponification number 217-237. Iodine number 10-15. Insol in water or cold alcohol; sol in benzene, carbon disulfide, petr ether, ether, hot alc, alkalies.
USE: As a substitute for beeswax in wax varnishes or candles, ingredients in plasters, ointments; floor waxes, furniture polish. As a plasticizer in dental impression compounds.

5257. Japonilure. [64726-91-6] [*R*-(*Z*)]-5-(1-Decenyl)-dihydro-2(3*H*)-furanone; [(4*R*,5*Z*)]-tetradecen-4-olide; (*R,Z*)-5-(dec-1-enyl)oxacyclopentan-2-one; IN-60. C$_{14}$H$_{24}$O$_2$; mol wt 224.34. C 74.95%, H 10.78%, O 14.26%. Sex pheromone produced by the female Japanese beetle, *Popillia japonica* Newman (Coleoptera: Scarabaeidae); biological activity is inhibited by its antipode. Isoln and synthesis: J. H. Tumlinson *et al., Science* **197**, 789 (1977). Description of attractant activity: J. H. Tumlinson in *Adv. Pest. Sci., 4th Int. Congr. Pest. Chem.* **2**, H. Geissbühler, Ed (Pergamon Press, Oxford, England, 1979) 315-322. Use in beetle traps: T. L. Ladd, Jr., M. G. Klein, *J. Econ. Entomol.* **79**, 84 (1986); A. Martins *et al., Ecol. Bull.* **39**, 101 (1988). Stereospecific synthesis: S. Chattopadhyay *et al., Synth. Commun.* **20**, 1299 (1990); T. Ebata *et al., Biosci. Biotech. Biochem.* **56**, 818 (1992). Isolation from *Anomala spp.* as component of pheromone system and field evaluation: W. S. Leal *et al., J. Chem. Ecol.* **20**, 1643 (1994); W. S. Leal *et al., ibid.* 1667.

bp$_{0.1mm}$ 130-134°. [α]$_D^{21}$ −69.0° (c = 1.42 in CHCl$_3$). [α]$_D^{25}$ −70.2° (c = 0.5 in CHCl$_3$).

5258. Jasmolins. Active insecticidal constituents of pyrethrum flowers. Isoln and structure: Godin *et al., J. Econ. Entomol.* **58**, 548 (1965); Godin *et al., J. Chem. Soc. C* **1966**, 322. Stereochemistry: Begley *et al., Chem. Commun.* **1972**, 1276. Review of toxicology and human exposure: *Toxicological Profile for Pyrethrins and Pyrethroids* (PB2004-100004, 2003) 332 pp.

Jasmolin I   R = CH$_3$
Jasmolin II   R = COOCH$_3$

Jasmolin I. [4466-14-2] (1*R*,3*R*)-2,2-Dimethyl-3-(2-methyl-1-propenyl)cyclopropanecarboxylic acid (1*S*)-2-methyl-4-oxo-3-(2*Z*)-2-pentenyl-2-cyclopenten-1-yl ester; 4',5'-dihydropyrethrin I. C$_{21}$H$_{30}$O$_3$; mol wt 330.46. Liquid. uv max (Spectrosol hexane): 219 nm (ε 21500).
Jasmolin II. [1172-63-0] (1*R*,3*R*)-3-[(1*E*)-3-Methoxy-2-methyl-3-oxo-1-propenyl]-2,2-dimethylcyclopropanecarboxylic acid (1*S*)-2-methyl-4-oxo-3-(2*Z*)-2-pentenyl-2-cyclopenten-1-yl ester; 4',5'-dihydropyrethrin II. C$_{22}$H$_{30}$O$_5$; mol wt 374.47. Liquid. uv max (Spectrosol hexane): 229 nm (ε 22900).

5259. Jasmone. [488-10-8] 3-Methyl-2-(2-pentenyl)-2-cyclopenten-1-one. C$_{11}$H$_{16}$O; mol wt 164.24. C 80.44%, H 9.82%, O 9.74%. Found in the volatile portion of oil from jasmine flowers. Natural jasmone is the *cis*-ketone. Isoln and structure: Ruzicka, Pfeiffer, *Helv. Chim. Acta* **16**, 1208 (1933). Stereochemistry: Crombie, Harper, *J. Chem. Soc.* **1952**, 869. Synthesis of *cis*-jasmone: H. Hunsdiecker, *Ber.* **75**, 447 (1942); Stork, Borch, *J. Am. Chem. Soc.* **86**, 936 (1964); Büchi, Wuest, *J. Org. Chem.* **31**, 977 (1966); Sakan *et al., Chem. Lett.* **1973**, 713; P. Bakuzis, M. L. F. Bakuzis, *J. Org. Chem.* **42**, 2362 (1977). Synthesis of dihydrojasmone and *cis*-jasmone: C. S. Subramaniam *et al., J. Chem. Soc. Perkin Trans. 1* **1979**, 2346; T. Kato *et al., Chem. Pharm. Bull.* **28**, 349 (1980). Synthesis of *trans*-jasmone: Sisido *et al., J. Org. Chem.* **29**, 2290 (1964). Comprehensive synthetic reviews: R. A.

Ellison, *Synthesis* **1973**, 397; T. L. Ho, *Synth. Commun.* **4**, 265 (1974).

cis - Form

cis-Form. Oil, odor of jasmine, bp$_{27}$ 146°. n_D^{20} 1.4978. uv max: 235 nm (ε 12,000).

trans-Form. Oil, odor of jasmine, bp$_{23}$ 142°. n_D^{20} 1.4974. uv max: 234 nm (ε 12,300).

USE: In perfumery.

5260.　Jasmonic Acid. [6894-38-8] (1*R*,2*R*)-3-Oxo-2-(2*Z*)-2-penten-ylcyclopentaneacetic acid; (1*S*,2*S*)-3-oxo-2-(2'-*cis*-pentenyl)cyclopentan-1-acetate; JA. $C_{12}H_{18}O_3$; mol wt 210.27. C 68.54%, H 8.63%, O 22.83%. Naturally occurring plant growth inhibitor. Orginally isolated from jasmin flowers as the methyl ester, the major aroma component: E. Demole *et al., Helv. Chim. Acta* **45**, 675 (1962). Isoln of the free acid from *Lasiodiplodia theobromae*: D. C. Aldridge *et al., J. Chem. Soc.* **1971**, 1623; by fermentation: D. Broadbent *et al.*, **GB 1286266** (1972 to ICI). Occurrence in plants: A. Meyer *et al., J. Plant Growth Regul.* **3**, 1 (1984). NMR characterization: A. Husain *et al., J. Nat. Prod.* **56**, 2008 (1993). Quantification by GC/MS: M. J. Mueller, W. Brodschelm, *Anal. Biochem.* **218**, 425 (1994). Resoln of racemate: R. Kramell *et al., Phytochem. Anal.* **7**, 209 (1996). Review of role in plant development: Y. Koda, *Int. Rev. Cytol.* **135**, 155-199 (1992); of biochemisty and physiology: G. Sembdner, B. Parthier, *Annu. Rev. Plant Physiol. Plant Mol. Biol.* **44**, 569-589 (1993); of signaling in plants: P. Staswick, *Curr. Top. Plant Physiol.* **11**, 14-23 (1993).

Colorless oil. n_D^{23} 1.486. [α]$_D^{25}$ −73° (c = 1 in CH$_3$OH).

Methyl ester. [1211-29-6] (−)-Methyl *cis*-2-pent-2'-enyl-3-oxocyclopentylacetate; JA-ME; MeJA; methyl jasmonate. $C_{13}H_{20}O_3$. Colorless liquid with a sharp persistent odor. $n_D^{21.8}$ 1.4730. [α]$_D$ −76.5° (c = 3.4 in CH$_3$OH). d$_4^{22.6}$ 1.021.

USE: Methyl ester in perfumes.

5261.　Jatrorrhizine. [3621-38-3] 5,6-Dihydro-3-hydroxy-2,9,10-trimethoxydibenzo[*a,g*]quinolizinium; 7,8,13,13a-tetradehydro-3-hydroxy-2,9,10-trimethoxyberbinium; jateorrhizine; neprotin; [C$_{20}$H$_{20}$NO$_4$]$^+$. From root of *Jateorhiza palmata* (DC.) Miers (*J. columba* Miers), *Menispermaceae:* Feist, *Arch. Pharm.* **245**, 586 (1907); from *Berberis asiatica* Roxb. ex DC. and *B. thunbergii* DC., *Berberidaceae:* Chatterjee *et al., J. Indian Chem. Soc.* **31**, 83 (1954); Tomita, Kikuchi, *J. Pharm. Soc. Jpn.* **76**, 597 (1956); from *Coptis teeta* Wall., *Ranunculaceae:* Chatterjee *et al., J. Indian Chem. Soc.* **29**, 97 (1952); from *Mahonia acanthifolia* Wall., *M. borealis* Takeda and *M. simonsii* Takeda, *Berberidaceae:* Chatterjee, Guha, *J. Am. Pharm. Assoc.* **39**, 577 (1950); Chatterjee *et al., ibid.* **40**, 36 (1951). Structure: Späth, Duschinsky, *Ber.* **58**, 1939 (1925).

Iodide. C$_{20}$H$_{20}$INO$_4$. Reddish-yellow needles, mp 208-210°. Sol in water and alcohol.

5262.　Javanicin. [476-45-9] 5,8-Dihydroxy-6-methoxy-2-methyl-3-(2-oxopropyl)-1,4-naphthalenedione; 3-acetonyl-5,8-dihydroxy-6-methoxy-2-methyl-1,4-naphthoquinone. $C_{15}H_{14}O_6$; mol wt 290.27. C 62.07%, H 4.86%, O 33.07%. Antibiotic substance produced by *Fusarium javanicum:* Arnstein, Cook, *J. Chem. Soc.* **1947**, 1021. Prepd by reduction of fusarubin: Ruelius, Gauhe, *Ann.* **569**, 38 (1950). Structure: Birch, Donovan, *Chem. Ind. (London)* **1954**, 1047; Whalley, *ibid.* **1958**, 131; Hardegger *et al., Helv. Chim. Acta* **47**, 2027 (1964).

Red crystals with a coppery luster from ethanol, decomp 207.5-208°. Absorption max (alc): 303, 305 nm (log ε 3.97, 3.90); in chloroform: 307, 510 nm (log ε 3.99, 3.86).

Diacetyljavanicin. C$_{19}$H$_{18}$O$_8$. Needles from dil acetone, dec 207-208°. Absorption max (alc): 221, 290, 426 nm (log ε 4.57, 4.17, 3.79).

5263.　Jerusalem Artichoke. Topinambur. The subterranean stem tuber of *Helianthus tuberosus* L., *Compositae*, a kind of sunflower native to North America. Used as food by American Indians. Contains up to 20% (wet basis) of polysaccharides usable as sweetening agents: Rubin, **US 2782123** (1957).

5264.　Jervine. [469-59-0] (3β,23β)-17,23-Epoxy-3-hydroxyveratraman-11-one. C$_{27}$H$_{39}$NO$_3$; mol wt 425.60. C 76.20%, H 9.24%, N 3.29%, O 11.28%. Steroidal alkaloid found in *Veratrum grandiflorum* (Maxim.) Loes F., *V. album* L., *V. viride* Sol., *Liliaceae:* Saito, *Bull. Chem. Soc. Jpn.* **9**, 15 (1934), *C.A.* **28**, 2463 (1934); Poethke, *Arch. Pharm.* **275**, 357, 571 (1937); **276**, 170 (1938); **282**, 56 (1944); Seiferle *et al., J. Econ. Entomol.* **35**, 35 (1942); Jacobs, Craig, *J. Biol. Chem.* **160**, 555 (1945). Structure: Fried *et al., J. Am. Chem. Soc.* **73**, 2970 (1951). *Reviews:* Wintersteiner in Graff, *Essays in Biochemistry* (Wiley, New York, 1956) pp 308-321; idem, *Festschrift Arthur Stoll* (Basel, 1957) pp 166-176; L. F. Fieser, M. Fieser, *Steroids* (Reinhold, New York, 1959) pp 870-877. Stereochemistry: Sicher, Tichy, *Tetrahedron Lett.* no. 12, 6 (1959); Augustine, *Chem. Ind. (London)* **1961**, 1448; Mitsuhashi, Shimizu, *Tetrahedron* **19**, 1027 (1963); Bailey *et al., Tetrahedron Lett.* **1963**, 555; Masamune *et al., ibid.* **1965**, 489. Revised stereochemistry: Scott *et al., ibid.* **1967**, 2381; Kupchan, Suffness, *J. Am. Chem. Soc.* **90**, 2730 (1968); Sprague *et al., Tetrahedron* **27**, 4857 (1971). Total synthesis: Kutney *et al., Can. J. Chem.* **53**, 1796 (1975). Comparative toxicity: O. Krayer *et al., J. Pharmacol. Exp. Ther.* **82**, 167 (1944); K. Tanaka, *ibid.* **113**, 89 (1955).

Needles from methanol + water, mp 243.5-244.5° (Saito). [α]$_D^{20}$ −150° (ethanol) (Saito); [α]$_D^{20}$ −167.6° (chloroform) (Poethke). uv max: 250, 360 nm (ε 15000, 60). LD$_{50}$ i.v. in mice: 9.3 mg/kg (Krayer). LD$_{50}$ s.c. in male mice: 29 mg/kg (Tanaka).

Diacetyljervine. C$_{31}$H$_{43}$NO$_5$. mp 173-175°. [α]$_D$ −112°. uv max (ethanol): 250, 360 nm (ε 16400, 80).

Hydrochloride. mp 300-302°.

5265.　Jesaconitine. [16298-90-1] (1α,3α,6α,14α,15α,16β)-20-Ethyl-1,6,16-trimethoxy-4-(methoxymethyl)aconitane-3,8,13,-

14,15-pentol 8-acetate 14-(4-methoxybenzoate). $C_{35}H_{49}NO_{12}$; mol wt 675.76. C 62.21%, H 7.31%, N 2.07%, O 28.41%. From *Aconitum fischeri* Reich. and *A. sachalinense* F. Schmidt, *Ranunculaceae:* Makoshi, *Arch. Pharm.* **247**, 243 (1909); Majima, Morio, *Ber.* **57**, 1472 (1924). Structure: Ochiai *et al., J. Pharm. Soc. Jpn.* **75**, 545 (1955); Keith, Pelletier, *Chem. Commun.* **1967**, 993 (corr. *ibid.* **1968**, 1739); *eidem, J. Org. Chem.* **33**, 2497 (1968).

Amorphous powder, dec 128-131°. Sol in ether, dil acids. **Perchlorate.** $C_{35}H_{49}NO_{12} \cdot HClO_4$. Prisms from alcohol, dec 230-232°. $[\alpha]_D$ −16.7° (methanol).

5266. Jojoba Oil. Oil of jojoba. A liquid wax ester mixture extracted from ground or crushed seeds from *Simmondsia chinensis* and *S. californica* Nutt. *Buxaceae*, desert shrubs native to Arizona, California, and northern Mexico: Greene, Foster, *Bot. Gaz.* **94**, 826 (1933); Green *et al., J. Chem. Soc.* **1936**, 1750; McKinney, Jamieson, *Oil Soap (Chicago)* **13**, 289 (1936). Similar to sperm whale oil, it is composed essentially of C_{20} and C_{22} straight chain monoethylene acids and alcohols in the form of esters: Molaison *et al., J. Am. Oil Chem. Soc.* **36**, 379 (1959); Miwa, *ibid.* **48**, 259 (1971). Solvent effects in extraction: Knoepfler *et al., ibid.* **36**, 644 (1959). Comparison of sulfurized jojoba and sperm whale oils as high pressure lubricants: T. K. Miwa *et al., ibid.* **56**, 765 (1979). Potential chemical utilization studies: Fore *et al., ibid.* **37**, 387 (1960); J. D. Johnson, C. W. Hinman, *Science* **208**, 460 (1980). Possible uses: J. H. Brown, *Manuf. Chem.* **50**(6), 47 (1979). *Reviews:* Knoepfler, Vix, *J. Agric. Food Chem.* **6**, 118 (1958); *Products from Jojoba: A Promising New Crop for Arid Lands*, Committee on Jojoba Utilization, Natl. Res. Council, 1975; *Jojoba: New Crop for Arid Lands, New Raw Material for Industry* Natl. Res. Council, 1985.

Liquid wax. fp 10.6 to 7°; mp 6.8 to 7°, bp_{757} (under N_2) 398°. Fire point 338°. Pour point 10°. d^{25} 0.8642. n^{25} 1.4648. Iodine no. 81.7. Saponification value 92.2. Acid value 0.32. Avg mol wt of wax esters: 606. Highly stable, and resistant to bacterial degradation; can be stored for years without becoming rancid.

USE: Potentially as lubricant, fuel, chemical feedstock, substitute for sperm whale oil. For other potential uses *see* Fore *et al., loc. cit.,* Knoepfler, Vix, *loc. cit*, Johnson, Hinman, *loc. cit.*

5267. Josamycin. [16846-24-5] Leucomycin V 3-acetate 4^B-(3-methylbutanoate); leucomycin A_3; EN-141; Iosalide; Jomybel; Josamina. $C_{42}H_{69}NO_{15}$; mol wt 827.99. C 60.92%, H 8.40%, N 1.69%, O 28.98%. Macrolide antibiotic produced by *Streptomyces narbonensis* var. *josamyceticus* nov. var. Isoln and characterization: T. Osono *et al., J. Antibiot.* **20A**, 174 (1967). Manuf process: H. Umezawa, T. Osono, *JP 66 21759* (1966 to Microbiochemical Res. Found.), *C.A.* **66**, 54258w (1967). Prepn: Y. Oka *et al., JP Kokai 76 41497* (1976 to Yamanouchi), *C.A.* **85**, 121788b (1976). Identification with leucomycin A_3: S. Omura *et al., J. Antibiot.* **23**, 511 (1970). Structure: *eidem, ibid.* **27**, 366 (1974). Absolute configuration: A. Ducruix *et al., Chem. Commun.* **1976**, 947. Stereospecific total synthesis: K. Tatsuta *et al., Tetrahedron Lett.* **1980**, 2837. Retrosynthetic studies: K. C. Nicolaou *et al., J. Am. Chem. Soc.* **103**, 1222 (1981). A 17-membered aglycone was proposed at one time, *see* T. Osono, H. Umezawa in *Drug Action and Drug Resistance in Bacteria* **1**, S. Mitsuhashi, Ed. (University Park Press, Baltimore, 1971) pp 41-120; T. Osono *et al., J. Antibiot.* **27**, 366 (1974). Pharmacology: K. Kuriaki *et al., Jpn. J. Antibiot.* **22**, 232 (1969). *Review:* T. Osono, H. Umezawa, *loc. cit.*

Colorless needles from benzene, mp 130-133° (after drying under reduced pressure at 100° for 5 hrs). $[\alpha]_D^{25}$ −70° (c = 1 in ethanol). uv max (0.001N HCl): 232 nm ($E_{1cm}^{1\%}$ 325). pKa 7.1 (40% aq methanol). Very sol in methanol, ethanol, acetone, chloroform, ethyl acetate, dioxane, acidic water. Sol in butanol, ether, CCl_4, benzene, toluene. Practically insol in water, petr ether, ligroin, *n*-hexane.

Propionate. [51016-68-3] Josacine; Josamy; Josaxin; Wilprafen. $C_{45}H_{73}NO_{16}$; mol wt 884.06.

THERAP CAT: Antibacterial.

THERAP CAT (VET): Antibacterial.

5268. Juglans. Butternut; white walnut; lemon walnut; oil nut. Dried inner root bark of *Juglans cinerea* L., *Juglandaceae,* collected in the autumn. *Habit.* North America. *Constit.* Resinoid juglandin, juglone, juglandic acid, fixed and volatile oils, tannin.

5269. Juglone. [481-39-0] 5-Hydroxy-1,4-naphthalenedione; 5-hydroxy-1,4-naphthoquinone; 8-hydroxy-1,4-naphthoquinone; C.I. 75500; C.I. Natural Brown 7; nucin; regianin. $C_{10}H_6O_3$; mol wt 174.15. C 68.97%, H 3.47%, O 27.56%. Coloring matter occurring in various *Juglandaceae* spp: Brissemoret, Combes, *Compt. Rend.* **141**, 838 (1905). Isoln from walnut shells: Combes, *Bull. Soc. Chim.* **1**(4), 800 (1907). Isoln and description of sedative properties in fish, mammals: B. A. Westfall *et al., Science* **134**, 1617 (1961). Isoln from pecans and identification as inhibitory agent of mycelial growth of *Fusicladium effusum:* P. A. Hedin *et al., J. Agric. Food Chem.* **28**, 340 (1980). Synthesis: Bernthsen, Semper, *Ber.* **20**, 938 (1887); Willstätter, Wheeler, *Ber.* **47**, 2798 (1914); Teuber, Götz, *Ber.* **87**, 1236 (1954); C. Grundmann, *Synthesis* **1977**, 644. Tumor-promoting activity study: B. L. Van Duuren *et al., J. Med. Chem.* **21**, 26 (1978). Use as pH indicator: S. S. Sawhney, B. M. L. Bhatia, *J. Indian Chem. Soc.* **57**, 438 (1980).

Yellow needles from benzene + petr ether, mp 155°. Sublimes. Absorption max (methanol): 420 nm (log ε 3.56). Volatile with steam. Slightly sol in hot water; freely sol in chloroform, benzene; sol in alcohol, ether; sol in aq solns of alkalies giving a purplish-red soln.

5270. Juniper. Dioecious, evergreen shrub, *Juniperus communis* L., *Cupressaceae*, bearing tangy, bitter, blue berries. Medicinal portions inlude the ripe berries, berry cones and essential oil. *Habit.* Europe, northern Africa, northern Asia, North America. *Constit.* Volatile oil (1-2%), diterpenes, catechin tannins, flavonoids, inverted sugar (20-30%), oligomeric proanthocyanidins. Analysis by GLC of the oil of six western North American species: F. C. Vasec, R. W. Scora, *Am. J. Bot.* **54**, 781 (1967). Botanical description and medicinal uses: J. Gruenwald *et al., PDR for Herbal Medicines* (Medical Economics, Montvale, 2nd Ed., 2000) pp 440-441. Review of pharmacology: J. Barnes *et al., Herbal Medicines* (Pharmaceutical Press, London, 2nd Ed., 2002) pp 317-319.

Volatile oil. [8002-68-4] Juniperberry oil; oil of juniper. Obtained by steam distillation of the dried ripe fruit (berries). *Constit.* Primarily monoterpenes incl. α-pinene, β-myrcene, sabinine, camphene, terpineol. Colorless, faintly green or yellow liquid with characteristic odor and aromatic, bitter taste. Odor and taste as of the berries. d_{25}^{25} 0.854-0.879. $[\alpha]_D^{25}$ 0 to $-15°$. n_D^{20} 1.474-1.484. Sol in most fixed oils, mineral oil. Insol in glycerin, propylene glycol. *Keep cool in well-closed and well-filled bottles, protected from light.*

USE: Volatile oil as flavor component of gin; in perfumery.
THERAP CAT: Diuretic; carminative.

5271. Juniper Tar. Oil of cade; empyreumatic oil of juniper; oil of juniper tar; Haarlem oil; Harlem oil; Tilly drops; Holland balsam; silver drops; silver balsam; Kaparlem; Caparlem. Volatile oil from wood of *Juniperus oxycedrus* L., *Cupressaceae. Constit.* Chiefly cadinene. Toxicity data: P. M. Jenner *et al., Food Cosmet. Toxicol.* **2**, 327 (1964). *Review:* D. L. J. Opdyke, *ibid.* **13**, 733-734 (1975).

Dark brown, more or less viscid liq; smoky odor; acrid, slightly aromatic taste. d_{25}^{25} 0.950-1.055. n_D^{20} 1.510-1.530. Very slightly sol in water; sol in 3 vols ether, in chloroform, amyl alcohol, glacial acetic acid, oil turpentine; partly sol in alcohol or petr ether. LD_{50} orally in rats: 8014 mg/kg (Jenner).

USE: As a gin-like flavor; in perfumery.
THERAP CAT: Anti-eczematic (topical).

5272. Justicidins. Lignans from various species of *Justicia, Acanthaceae.* Isoln and structures for justicidins A, B, C, D, E and F have been elucidated. Isoln of A and B: Munakata *et al., Tetrahedron Lett.* **1965**, 4167; Ohta *et al., Agric. Biol. Chem.* **33**, 610 (1969); Okigawa *et al., Tetrahedron* **26**, 4301 (1970). Structure of A: Govindachari *et al., Tetrahedron Lett.* **1967**, 3517; Horii *et al., Chem. Pharm. Bull.* **19**, 535 (1971). Synthesis of B: Munakata *et al., Tetrahedron Lett.* **1967**, 2831; Munakata, Katsura, **GB 1178341** (1970), *C.A.* **72**, 100365c; T. Momose *et al., Chem. Pharm. Bull.* **26**, 3195 (1978). Isoln and structures of C and D: Ohta, Munakata, *Tetrahedron Lett.* **1970**, 923. Synthesis of C: Horii *et al., Chem. Pharm. Bull.* **17**, 1878 (1969). Structure of E: Wada, Munakata, *Tetrahedron Lett.* **1970**, 2017. Synthesis of E: Holmes, Stevenson, *J. Org. Chem.* **36**, 3450 (1971). Synthesis of D, E, and F: Z. I. Horii *et al., Chem. Pharm. Bull.* **25**, 1803 (1977).

Justicidin A   R = OCH₃
Justicidin B   R = H

Justicidin A. [25001-57-4] 9-(1,3-Benzodioxol-5-yl)-4,6,7-trimethoxynaphtho[2,3-*c*]furan-1(3*H*)-one; diphyllin methyl ether. $C_{22}H_{18}O_7$; mol wt 394.37. Crystals, mp 263°. uv max (CHCl₃): 265, 295, 315, 335 nm (log ε 4.35, 4.13, 4.13, 3.33).

Justicidin B. [17951-19-8] 9-(1,3-Benzodioxol-5-yl)-6,7-dimethoxynaphtho[2,3-*c*]furan-1(3*H*)-one; dehydrocollinusin. $C_{21}H_{16}O_6$; mol wt 364.35. Crystals, mp 240°. uv max (CHCl₃): 260, 295, 310, 350 nm (log ε 4.52, 4.13, 4.13, 3.41).

USE: Piscicidal agent.

5273. Juvenile Hormones. JH. Family of hormones, secreted by the corpora allata, controlling the larval metamorphosis of insects; so named since they induce the retention of insects' juvenile characteristics and prevent maturation. Isoln from the abdomen of the male wild silk moth, *Hyalophora cecropia* L.: C. M. Williams, *Nature* **178**, 212 (1956); H. Röller, J. S. Bjerke, *Life Sci.* **4**, 1617 (1965). Structure elucidation of JH I: H. Röller *et al., Angew. Chem. Int. Ed.* **6**, 179 (1967). Racemic synthesis of JH I: K. H. Dahm *et al., J. Am. Chem. Soc.* **89**, 5292 (1967). Toxicity of racemic JH I: J. B. Siddall, M. Slade, *Nature New Biol.* **229**, 158 (1971). Abs config of JH I: K. Nakanishi *et al., Chem. Commun.* **1971**, 1235; A. S. Meyer *et al., Proc. Natl. Acad. Sci. USA* **68**, 2312 (1971). Stereoselective syntheses of JH I: E. J. Corey *et al., ibid.* **90**, 5618 (1968); W. S. Johnson *et al., ibid.* 6225. Enantioselective syntheses of JH I: P. Loew, W. S. Johnson, *ibid.* **93**, 3765 (1971); D. J. Faulkner, M. R. Petersen, *ibid.* 3766. Isoln, structure, and abs config of JH II and III: K. J. Judy *et al., Proc. Natl. Acad. Sci. USA* **70**, 1509 (1973). Isoln and structure of *JH 0*: B. J. Bergot *et al., Science* **210**, 336 (1980); and *iso-JH 0* (MeJH I): *idem et al.* in *Juvenile Hormone Biochemistry*, G. E. Pratt, G. T. Brooks, Eds. (Elsevier-North Holland Biomedical Press, Amsterdam, 1981) pp 33-45. Biosynthesis, isoln, and structure elucidation of *JH III bisepoxide* (JHB₃): D. S. Richard *et al., Proc. Natl. Acad. Sci. USA* **86**, 1421 (1989). Abs config of JHB₃: A. J. Herlt *et al., Chem. Commun.* **1993**, 1497. Enantioselective synthesis of JH III: K. Mori, H. Mori, *Tetrahedron* **43**, 4097 (1987); of JH I and II: K. Mori, M. Fujiwhara, *ibid.* **44**, 343 (1988); of JHB₃: R. W. Rickards, R. D. Thomas, *Tetrahedron Lett.* **34**, 8369 (1993). Study of regulatory role: M. Cusson *et al., Arch. Insect Biochem. Physiol.* **25**, 329 (1994). Book: *The Juvenile Hormones*, L. I. Gilbert, Ed. (Plenum Press, New York, 1976) 572 pp. Review of biosynthesis: D. A. Schooley, F. C. Baker in *Comprehensive Insect Physiology, Biochemistry and Pharmacology* vol. 8, G. A. Kerkut, L. I. Gilbert, Eds. (Pergamon Press, New York, 1985) pp 363-389. Review of techniques for identification and quantification: F. C. Baker in *Morphogenetic Hormones of Arthropods* Part 1, A. P. Gupta, Ed. (Rutgers Univ. Press, New Brunswick, 1990) pp 389-453. Review of discovery and identification of JHB₃: C.-M. Yin, *Zool. Stud.* **33**, 237-245 (1994). Review of molecular mechanisms of action: G. Jones, *Annu. Rev. Entomol.* **40**, 147-169 (1995).

	R	R'
JH I	CH₂CH₃	CH₂CH₃
JH II	CH₂CH₃	CH₃
JH III	CH₃	CH₃

Juvenile hormone I. [13804-51-8] [2*R*-[2α(2*E*,6*E*),3α]]-7-Ethyl-9-(3-ethyl-3-methyloxiranyl)-3-methyl-2,6-nonadienoic acid methyl ester; methyl (2*E*,6*E*,10*R*,11*S*)-10,11-epoxy-7-ethyl-3,11-dimethyl-2,6-tridecadienoate; C-18 JH. $C_{18}H_{30}O_3$; mol wt 294.43. n_D^{24} 1.4732. $[\alpha]_D^{23}$ +14.9° (c = 0.935 in chloroform). $[\alpha]_D^{22.5}$ +14.5° (c = 0.78 in methanol).

Juvenile hormone II. [34218-61-6] [2*R*-[2α(2*E*,6*E*),3α]]-9-(3-Ethyl-3-methyloxiranyl)-3,7-dimethyl-2,6-nonadienoic acid methyl ester; methyl (2*E*,6*E*,10*R*,11*S*)-10,11-epoxy-3,7,11-trimethyl-2,6-tridecadienoate; C-17 JH. $C_{17}H_{28}O_3$; mol wt 280.40. $n_D^{23.5}$ 1.4774. $[\alpha]_D^{24.5}$ +17.6° (c = 0.590 in methanol).

Juvenile hormone III. [22963-93-5] [*R*-(*E,E*)]-9-(3,3-Dimethyloxiranyl)-3,7-dimethyl-2,6-nonadienoic acid methyl ester; methyl (2*E*,6*E*,10*R*)-10,11-epoxy-3,7,11-trimethyl-2,6-dodecadienoate; C-16 JH. $C_{16}H_{26}O_3$; mol wt 266.38. Colorless oil. n_D^{24} 1.4736. $[\alpha]_D^{24}$ +6.71° (c = 0.57 in methanol).

K

5274. Kaempferol. [520-18-3] 3,5,7-Trihydroxy-2-(4-hydroxyphenyl)-4*H*-1-benzopyran-4-one; 3,4′,5,7-tetrahydroxyflavone; nimbecetin; pelargidenolon 1497; populnetin; rhamnolutein; robigenin; swartziol; trifolitin. $C_{15}H_{10}O_6$; mol wt 286.24. C 62.94%, H 3.52%, O 33.54%. Plant flavonoid isolated from *Delphinium consolida* L., *Ranunculaceae:* A. G. Perkin, E. J. Wilkinson, *J. Chem. Soc.* **81**, 585 (1902); from grapefruit *(Citrus paradisi* Macf., *Rutaceae):* Dunlap, Wender, *Anal. Biochem.* **4**, 110 (1962); from stems and seeds of *Cuscuta reflexa* Roxb., *Convolvulaceae:* K. W. Gopinath *et al., J. Sci. Ind. Res.* **21B**, 601 (1962), *C.A.* **58**, 7134e (1963). Identity with swartziol: M. R.-R. Paris, L. Bézanger-Beauquesne, *Compt. Rend.* **242**, 1761 (1956). Structure: S. von Kostanecki, A. Rozycki, *Ber.* **34**, 3721 (1901). Total synthesis: Y.-H. Lu *et al., Yao Hsueh Hsueh Pao* **15**, 477 (1980), *C.A.* **94**, 174808a (1981). Convenient synthesis: M. Ichikawa *et al., Org. Prep. Proced. Int.* **14**, 183 (1982). Mutagenicity studies: J. T. MacGregor, L. Jurd, *Mutat. Res.* **54**, 297 (1978); A. A. Hardigree, J. L. Epler, *ibid.* **58**, 231 (1978). HPLC determination in soybean: J. D. Gaynor *et al., Chromatographia* **25**, 1049 (1988).

Yellow needles, mp 276-278°; also reported as light yellow powder from ethanol-water, mp 278-280° (dec) (Ichikawa). uv max: 265, 365 nm. Slightly sol in water; sol in hot alcohol, ether or alkalies.

3,7-Dirhamnoside. Kaemferitrin; lespedin. $C_{27}H_{30}O_{14}$. Isoln from the leaves of *Indigo arrecta* Benth., *Leguminosae:* Perkin, *J. Chem. Soc.* **91**, 435 (1907); from leaves of *Trichosanthus cucumeroides* Maxim., *Cucurbitaceae:* Nakaoki, Morita, *J. Pharm. Soc. Jpn.* **77**, 108 (1957). Identity with lespedin: Hatlori, *Nature* **168**, 788 (1952). Crystals from dil alc, mp 201-203°. Slightly sol in boiling water and cold alcohol.

3-Glucoside. Astragalin. $C_{21}H_{20}O_{11}$. From *Podophyllum peltatum* L. and *P. emodi* Wall., *Berberidaceae.* Isoln and structure: von Wartburg, Kuhn, *Experientia* **21**, 67 (1965). Crystals from methanol, mp 175-178°. $[\alpha]_D^{20} -16.9°$ (c = 0.45 in methanol).

5275. Kahalalide F. [149204-42-2] PM-92102. $C_{75}H_{124}$-$N_{14}O_{16}$; mol wt 1477.87. C 60.95%, H 8.46%, N 13.27%, O 17.32%. One of a family of cyclic depsipeptides isolated from the Hawaiian marine mollusk, *Elysia rufescens.* First reported diet-derived chemical defense peptide; production of which depends on consumption of the green alga, *Bryopsis* sp. Isoln: P. J. Schauer *et al.,* **EP 610078** (1994 to Pharma Mar); M. T. Hamann, P. J. Scheuer, *J. Am. Chem. Soc.* **115**, 5825 (1993); of the family: M. T. Hamann *et al., J. Org. Chem.* **61**, 6594 (1996). Synthesis: A. López-Macià *et al., J. Am. Chem. Soc.* **123**, 11398 (2001). Stereochemistry: G. Goetz *et al., Tetrahedron* **55**, 7739 (1999). Updated stereochemistry: I. Bonnard *et al., J. Nat. Prod.* **66**, 1466 (2003). Identification as defensive peptide: M. A. Becerro *et al., J. Chem. Ecol.* **27**, 2287 (2001). LC/MS/MS determ in plasma: E. Stokvis *et al., J. Mass Spectrom.* **37**, 992 (2002). Toxicology: A. P. Brown *et al., Cancer Chemother. Pharmacol.* **50**, 333 (2002). *In vitro* cytotoxic activity: Y. Suárez *et al., Mol. Cancer Ther.* **2**, 863 (2003). Mechanism of cytotoxicity: J. M. Sewell *et al., Eur. J. Cancer* **41**, 1637 (2005). Clinical pharmacology in prostate cancer: J. M. Rademaker-Lakhai *et al., Clin. Cancer Res.* **11**, 1854 (2005). Review of development and therapeutic potential: M. T. Hamann, *Curr. Opin. Mol. Ther.* **6**, 657-665 (2004).

White amorphous powder. $[\alpha]_D -8°$ (c = 4.32 in CH_3OH). LD_{50} in male, female rats (μg/kg): 375, 600 i.v. (Brown).

THERAP CAT: Antineoplastic.

5276. Kainic Acid. [487-79-6] [2*S*-(2α,3β,4β)]-2-Carboxy-4-(1-methylethenyl)-3-pyrrolidineacetic acid; 2-carboxy-3-carboxymethyl-4-isopropenylpyrrolidine; digenic acid; α-kainic acid; L$_S$-*xylo*-kainic acid; Digenin; Helminal. $C_{10}H_{15}NO_4$; mol wt 213.23. C 56.33%, H 7.09%, N 6.57%, O 30.01%. Anthelmintic principle from the dried red alga *Digenea simplex* (Wulf.) Ag., *Rhodomelaceae:* Murakami *et al., J. Pharm. Soc. Jpn.* **73**, 1026 (1953); **JP 54 4947** (1954), *C.A.* **49**, 13604i (1955); Katsuya *et al.,* **JP 64 1942** (1964 to New-Japan Pharmaceutical Co). Structure: Watase, Nitta, *Bull. Chem. Soc. Jpn.* **30**, 889 (1957); Watase *et al., ibid.* **31**, 714 (1958). Eight theoretical stereoisomers, Nitta *et al., Nature* **181**, 761 (1958). Synthesis: Ueno, **US 2902492**; Tatsuoka *et al.,* **US 2954384** (1959, 1960 both to Takeda); W. Oppolzer, H. Andres, *Helv. Chim. Acta* **62**, 2282 (1979). Excitotoxic amino acid used to identify a specific subset of EAA receptors. Consequently the receptors are known as kainate receptors. Neurotoxic activity: J. V. Nadler, *Life Sci.* **24**, 289 (1979). Mechanism of neurotoxicity: E. G. McGeer *et al., Adv. Neurol.* **23**, 577 (1979); J. T. Coyle *et al., ibid.* 593; J. W. Ferkany *et al., Nature* **298**, 757 (1982); J. Garthwaite, G. Garthwaite, *ibid.* **305**, 138 (1983). Induces epileptogenic lesions: J. V. Nadler, *Neurosci. Res. Program Bull.* **19**, 369 (1981). Autoradiographic characterization of binding sites: J. T. Greenamyre *et al., J. Pharmacol. Exp. Ther.* **233**, 254 (1985). *Book: Kainic Acid as a Tool in Neurobiology,* E. G. McGeer *et al.,* Eds. (Raven Press, New York, 1978). *Review:* J. T. Coyle, *Ciba Found. Symp.* **126**, 186-203 (1987).

Needles, dec 251°. $[\alpha]_D^{24} -14.8°$ (c = 1.01). Intense absorption at 6.05 and 11.2 μ. Sol in water. Insol in ethanol. Stable in boiling aq solns.

USE: Neurobiological tool.

THERAP CAT: Anthelmintic (Nematodes).

5277. Kalkitoxin. [247184-89-0] (2*R*)-*N*-[(3*S*,5*S*,6*R*)-7-[(4*R*)-4-Ethenyl-4,5-dihydro-2-thiazolyl]-3,5,6-trimethylheptyl]-*N*,2-dimethylbutanamide. $C_{21}H_{38}N_2OS$; mol wt 366.60. C 68.80%, H 10.45%, N 7.64%, O 4.36%, S 8.75%. Neurotoxic lipopeptide isolated from the Caribbean marine algae, *Lyngbya majuscula.* Isoln, structure determn and synthesis: M. Wu *et al., J. Am. Chem. Soc.* **122**, 12041 (2000). NMDA-receptor based neurotoxicity: F. W. Berman *et al., Toxicon* **37**, 1645 (1999). Total synthesis: T. Asano *et al., Tennen Yuki Kagobutsu Toronkai Koen Yoshishu* **2000**, 691. Brief review: J. Fricker, *Drug Devel. Today* **6**, 223-224 (2001).

$[\alpha]_D^{25}$ +16° (c = 0.07 in CHCl$_3$). uv max (methanol): 250 nm (ε 2600). LC$_{50}$ in common goldfish, brine shrimp: 700, 150 nM (Wu).

5278. Kallidin. [342-10-9] N^2-L-Lysylbradykinin; kallidin-10; kallidin II. C$_{56}$H$_{85}$N$_{17}$O$_{12}$; mol wt 1188.38. C 56.60%, H 7.21%, N 20.04%, O 16.16%. A hypotensive and smooth muscle-stimulating principle formed by the proteolysis of kininogen by glandular and other kallikreins, q.v. The decapeptide structure is a homologue of bradykinin, q.v.: Werle et al., Z. Physiol. Chem. **326**, 174 (1961). Synthesis: Nicolaides et al., Biochem. Biophys. Res. Commun. **6**, 210 (1961); Pless et al., Helv. Chim. Acta **45**, 394 (1962).

Lys–Arg–Pro–Pro–Gly–Phe–Ser–Pro–Phe–Arg

Amorphous precipitate. $[\alpha]_D^{21}$ −57° (c = 1 in N acetic acid). R$_f$ value in a butanol/acetic acid/water system (70:10:20) 0.15.

THERAP CAT: Vasodilator.

5279. Kallikrein. [9001-01-8] Kallidinogenase; Callicrein; Padreatin; Padukrein; Glumorin; Depot-Glumorin; Circuletin; Kalirechin; Onokrein P; Padutin; Prokrein; Promotin. Hypotensive enzyme which releases kinins from plasma proteins. Major sources in the body are blood plasma, glandular tissues, and urine, occurring abundantly in the pancreas, parotid and submaxillary glands, in intestinal wall, in feces, in duodenal juice, and to a lesser degree in kidney. Isoln from mammalian pancreas or urine: Abelous, Bardier, C.R. Seances Soc. Biol. Ses Fil. **64**, 848 (1908); Webster et al., Proc. Soc. Exp. Biol. Med. **93**, 181 (1956). Separation into two components, kallikreins A and B: E. Habermann, Z. Physiol. Chem. **328**, 15 (1962); F. Fiedler, E. Werle, ibid. **348**, 1087 (1967); C. Kutzbach, G. Schmidt-Kastner, ibid. **353**, 1099 (1972). Prepn of high purity material: Werle, Trautschold, **DE 1102973** (1960 to Bayer). Review on pig pancreatic kallikrein: F. Fiedler, Methods Enzymol. **45B**, 289-303 (1976); on human kallikrein and prekallikrein: R. W. Colman, A. Bagdasarian, ibid. 303-322. Plasma kallikrein differs from glandular or urinary kallikrein. The latter two liberate kallidin, q.v.; the former releases bradykinin, q.v., both from the common precursor, kininogen. Pharmacology: Franz, Marquardt, Arzneim.-Forsch. **10**, 779 (1960). Reviews: Schachter, Physiol. Rev. **49**, 509 (1969); Suzuki et al., Adv. Exp. Med. Biol. **8**, 15 (1970).

THERAP CAT: Vasodilator.

5280. Kamala. Kamila; kameela; spoonwood. Glands and hairs covering the fruits of Mallotus philippinensis (Lam.) Muell. Arg., (also known as Rottlera tinctoria Roxb.) Euphorbiaceae. Habit. Philippine Islands, India, China, Australia. Constit. Rottlerin, isoallorottlerin, flavanoids, resins, wax. Detemn of constituents: Khorana, Motiwala, Indian J. Pharm. **11**, 37 (1949); M. Lounasmaa et al., Planta Med. **28**, 16 (1975); C. J. Widén, H. S. Puri, ibid. **40**, 284 (1980); V. K. Ahluwalia et al., Indian J. Chem. **27B**, 238 (1988). Anthelmintic effects: S. S. Gupta et al., Indian J. Physiol. Pharmacol. **28**, 63 (1984).

THERAP CAT: Anthelmintic (Cestodes).

THERAP CAT (VET): Has been used as anthelmintic.

5281. Kanamycin. [8063-07-8] Antibiotic complex produced by Streptomyces kanamyceticus Okami & Umezawa from Japanese soil: Umezawa et al., J. Antibiot. **10A**, 181 (1957); **US 2931798** (1960). Comprised of three components, kanamycin A, the major component (usually designated as kanamycin) and kanamycins B and C, two minor congeners. Isoln and purification of kanamycins A and B and their salts: Johnson et al., and Johnson, Hardcastle, **US 2936307** and **US 2967177** (1960, 1961 both to Bristol-Myers). Separation process: Rothrock, Putter, **US 3032547** (1962 to Merck & Co.). Prepn of kanamycin C: Murase et al., J. Antibiot. **14A**, 156 (1961). Studies on kanamycin B: Wakazawa et al., ibid. 180, 187. Structure of kanamycin A: Ogawa et al., ibid. **11A**, 169 (1958); Cron et al., J. Am. Chem. Soc. **80**, 4741 (1958). Structure of kanamycin B: Ito et al., J. Antibiot. **17A**, 189 (1964). Structure of kanamycin C: Murase, ibid. **14A**, 367 (1961). Abs config of kanamycin A: Hichens, Rinehart, J. Am. Chem. Soc. **85**, 1547 (1963); Umezawa et al., Bull. Chem. Soc. Jpn. **39**, 1244 (1966). Crystal structure of kanamycin A: Koyama et al., Tetrahedron Lett. **1968**, 1875. Mono-

graph: Ann. N.Y. Acad. Sci. **76**, 17-408 (1958). Synthesis of kanamycin A: Umezawa et al., J. Antibiot. **21**, 367 (1968); Nakajima et al., Tetrahedron Lett. **1968**, 623; Umezawa et al., Bull. Chem. Soc. Jpn. **42**, 533 (1969). Synthesis of kanamycin B: eidem, J. Antibiot. **21**, 424 (1968); Bull. Chem. Soc. Jpn. **42**, 537 (1969). Chemical conversion of kanamycin B to kanamycin C: S. Toda et al., J. Antibiot. **30**, 1002 (1977). Synthesis of kanamycin C: Umezawa et al., Bull. Chem. Soc. Jpn. **41**, 533 (1968); J. Antibiot. **21**, 162 (1968). Effects on protein synthesis: Suzuki et al., ibid. **23**, 99 (1970). Toxicity data (kanamycin A sulfate): Zel'tser et al., Antibiotiki **19**, 552 (1974). Comprehensive description: P. J. Claes et al., Anal. Profiles Drug Subs. **6**, 259-296 (1977).

	R	R'
Kanamycin A	NH$_2$	OH
Kanamycin B	NH$_2$	NH$_2$
Kanamycin C	OH	NH$_2$

Kanamycin A. [59-01-8] O-3-Amino-3-deoxy-α-D-glucopyranosyl-(1 → 6)-O-[6-amino-6-deoxy-α-D-glucopyranosyl-(1 → 4)]-2-deoxy-D-streptamine. C$_{18}$H$_{36}$N$_4$O$_{11}$; mol wt 484.50. Crystals from methanol + ethanol. $[\alpha]_D^{24}$ +146° (0.1N H$_2$SO$_4$). LD$_{50}$ i.v. in mice: 583 mg/kg (Wakazawa).

Kanamycin A sulfate. [25389-94-0] Cantrex; Cristalomicina; Enterokanacin; Kamycine; Kamynex; Kanacedin; Kanamytrex; Kanasig; Kanatrol; Kanicin; Kannasyn; Kantrex; Klebcil; Otokalixin; Resistomycin; Kanescin; Kanaqua. (U.S.P. requires that kanamycin sulfate contains not less than 75% kanamycin A on an anhydr basis). Irregular prisms, dec over a wide range above 250°C. Freely sol in water. Practically insol in the common alcohols and nonpolar solvents. LD$_{50}$ in mice: 20.7 g/kg orally; 1450 mg/kg i.p. (Zel'tser).

Kanamycin B. [4696-76-8] Bekanamycin; aminodeoxykanamycin; NK-1006. C$_{18}$H$_{37}$N$_5$O$_{10}$; mol wt 483.51. Crystals, mp 178-182° (dec). $[\alpha]_D^{18}$ +130° (c = 0.5 in water). $[\alpha]_D^{21}$ +114° (c = 0.98 in water). Sol in water, formamide; slightly sol in chloroform, isopropyl alcohol. Practically insol in the common alcohols and nonpolar solvents. LD$_{50}$ i.v. in mice: 136 mg/kg (Wakazawa).

Kanamycin B sulfate. [29701-07-3] Coltericin; Kanendomycin; Kanendos. Pharmacokinetics: F. Di Nola et al., Minerva Med. **70**, 1803 (1979).

Kanamycin C. [2280-32-2] C$_{18}$H$_{36}$N$_4$O$_{11}$; mol wt 484.50. Crystals from methanol + ethanol, dec above 270°. $[\alpha]_D^{20}$ +126° (H$_2$O). Sol in water; slightly sol in formamide. Practically insol in the common alcohols and nonpolar solvents.

THERAP CAT: Antibacterial.

THERAP CAT (VET): Antibacterial.

5282. Kaolin. Bolus alba; China clay; porcelain clay; white bole; argilla. Essentially a hydrated aluminum silicate, approximately H$_2$Al$_2$Si$_2$O$_8$.H$_2$O. Prepared for pharmaceutical and medicinal purposes by levigating with water to remove sand, etc.

White or yellowish-white, earthy mass or white powder; unctuous when moist. Insol in water, cold acids or in alkali hydroxides.

Caution: Potential symptoms of overexposure are chronic pulmonary fibrosis, stomach granuloma. See NIOSH Pocket Guide to Chemical Hazards (DHHS/NIOSH 97-140, 1997) p 182.

USE: Manuf porcelain, pottery, bricks, Portland cement; ultramarine, color lakes, refractory mortar; plaster material, filler for paper; electric and heat insulators; clarifying liquids; drying and emollient agent.

THERAP CAT: Adsorbent.

THERAP CAT (VET): Topical and G.I. adsorbent. Poultice.

5283. Karanjin. [521-88-0] 3-Methoxy-2-phenyl-4*H*-furo[2,3-*h*]-1-benzopyran-4-one. $C_{18}H_{12}O_4$; mol wt 292.29. C 73.97%, H 4.14%, O 21.90%. From *Pongamia glabra* Vent., *Leguminosae:* Beal, Katti, *J. Am. Pharm. Assoc.* **14**, 1086 (1925); Rao, Rao, *J. Indian Chem. Soc.* **17**, 526 (1940); Bhat *et al., J. Am. Oil Chem. Soc.* **33**, 197 (1956). Structure: Limaye, *Rasayanam* **1**, 1 (1936), *C.A.* **31**, 2206⁹ (1937); Manjunath *et al., Ber.* **72B**, 39 (1939). Synthesis: Seshadri, Venkateswarlu, *Proc. Indian Acad. Sci.* **13A**, 404 (1941); **17A**, 16 (1943); Kawase *et al., Bull. Chem. Soc. Jpn.* **28**, 273 (1955); Rao, Seshadri, *Proc. Indian Acad. Sci.* **33A**, 168 (1951); Aneja *et al., Tetrahedron* **2**, 203 (1958); Raizada *et al., J. Sci. Ind. Res.* **19B**, 76 (1960).

Needles from methanol, mp 157-158°. Sol in methanol, ethanol, chloroform, benzene, ether, concd H_2SO_4, HNO_3, HOAc, HCl; practically insol in petr ether, dil mineral acids.

5284. Karaya Gum. [9000-36-6] Gum karaya; kadaya; katilo; kullo; kuteera; sterculia; Indian tragacanth; mucara. The dried exudate of the tree *Sterculia urens* Roxb., *Sterculiaceae,* found in India, especially in the Gujerat region and in the central provinces: Toothaker, *The Soluble Gums* (Philadelphia, 1921); Mantell, *The Water-Soluble Gums* (New York, 1947). Constituents and structure: Hirst, Dunstan, *J. Chem. Soc.* **1953**, 2332. Structure is a partially acetylated polysaccharide containing about 8% acetyl groups and about 37% uronic acid residues. *Reviews:* F. Smith, R. Montgomery, *The Chemistry of Plant Gums and Mucilages* (Reinhold, New York, 1959); Goldstein, Alter, in *Industrial Gums,* R. L. Whistler, Ed. (Academic Press, New York, 2nd ed., 1973) pp 273-287.

Finely ground white powder, faint odor of acetic acid. Acid to litmus. Absorbs water rapidly to form viscous mucilages at low concs. Viscosity decreases on addn of acid or alkali. Color of the soln lightens in acidic media and darkens in alkaline soln due to the presence of tannins. Gum karaya loses viscosity forming ability when stored in the dry state, the loss being greater for a powdered material than for the crude gum. Cold storage inhibits this degradation.

Note: Karaya gum occurring in broken irregular pieces having a somewhat crystalline appearance has been referred to commercially as 'crystal' gum.

USE: As denture adhesive; as binder in paper manuf; as stabilizer, thickener, texturizer, emulsifier in foods; as thickening agent for dyes in textile industry. A substitute for gum tragacanth.

THERAP CAT: Cathartic.

5285. Karsil. [2533-89-3] *N*-(3,4-Dichlorophenyl)-2-methylpentanamide; 3′,4′-dichloro-2-methylvaleranilide; Niagara 4562. $C_{12}H_{15}Cl_2NO$; mol wt 260.16. C 55.40%, H 5.81%, Cl 27.25%, N 5.38%, O 6.15%. Prepd from 3,4-dichloroaniline and 2-methylvaleryl chloride: Dorschner *et al.,* **GB 869169** (1961 to FMC).

Crystals, mp 106-107°.
USE: Herbicide.

5286. Kava. Kava-kava; ava-ava; kawa. Dried rhizome and roots of *Piper methysticum* Forst., *Piperaceae.* *Habit.* Polynesia. Most important constituents are: kawain, dihydrokawain, methysticin, dihydromethysticin, and yangonin: Borsche, Lewinsohn, *Ber.* **66**, 1792 (1933) and references to preceding papers therein. Chemical and pharmacological investigation of the kava constituents: Klohs *et al., J. Med. Pharm. Chem.* **1**, 95 (1959); Meyer, Kretzschmar, *Klin. Wochenschr.* **44**, 902 (1966). Review of chem-

istry, pharmacology and historical sketch: *U.S. Public Health Service Publ. No. 1645,* D. H. Efron, Ed., pp 103-181 (1967).

Note: Kava is also the popular name for the intoxicating drink prepared from the plant's roots.

5287. Kawain. [500-64-1] (6*R*)-5,6-Dihydro-4-methoxy-6-[(1*E*)-2-phenylethenyl]-2*H*-pyran-2-one; 5-hydroxy-3-methoxy-7-phenyl-2,6-heptadienoic acid δ-lactone; 4-methoxy-6-(β-phenyl-vinyl)-5,6-dihydro-α-pyrone; 4-methoxy-6-styryl-5,6-dihydro-α-pyrone; kavain; gonosan. $C_{14}H_{14}O_3$; mol wt 230.26. C 73.03%, H 6.13%, O 20.85%. From the rhizome and roots of *Piper methysticum* Forst., *Piperaceae* (kava): Borsche, Peitzsch, *Ber.* **63**, 2414 (1930); Hänsel, Beiersdorff, *Naturwissenschaften* **45**, 573 (1958); *eidem, Arzneim.-Forsch.* **9**, 581 (1959). Synthesis: Fowler, Henbest, *J. Chem. Soc.* **1950**, 3642; Kostermans, *Nature* **166**, 788 (1950); *idem, Rec. Trav. Chim.* **70**, 79 (1951); Z. H. Israili, E. E. Smissman, *J. Org. Chem.* **41**, 4070 (1976). Abs config: Snatzke, Hänsel, *Tetrahedron Lett.* **1968**, 1797. Crystal and molecular structure: A. Yoshino, W. Nowacki, *Z. Kristallogr. Kristallgeom. Kristallphys. Kristallchem.* **136**, 66 (1972), *C.A.* **78**, 63591z (1973).

Rods from methanol + ether, mp 105-106°. bp₀.₁ 195-197°. $[\alpha]_D^{20}$ +105° (abs alc). uv max (methanol): 210, 245, 282 nm (log ε 4.38, 4.44, 2.81). Practically insol in water. Sol in acetone, ether, methanol; slightly sol in hexane.

(±)-**Form.** [3155-48-4] Needles from methanol, mp 146-147°.
Dihydrokawain. [587-63-3] Marindinin. $C_{14}H_{16}O_3$; mol wt 232.28. Crystals from ether, mp 58-60°. $[\alpha]_D^{24}$ +31° (methanol). uv max (methanol): 236 nm (log ε 4.14). Sol in alc, chloroform; moderately sol in ether. Practically insol in petr ether, water.

5288. Kebuzone. [853-34-9] 4-(3-Oxobutyl)-1,2-diphenyl-3,5-pyrazolidinedione; 1,2-diphenyl-4-(γ-ketobutyl)-3,5-pyrazolidinedione; 1,2-diphenyl-4-(3′-oxobutyl)-3,5-dioxopyrazolidine; ketophenylbutazone; KPB; Chebutan; Chepirol; Chetazolidin; Chetil; Copirene; Ketason; Ketazone; Pecnon; Phloguron; Recheton. $C_{19}H_{18}N_2O_3$; mol wt 322.36. C 70.79%, H 5.63%, N 8.69%, O 14.89%. Prepn: Deuss *et al.,* **US 2910481** (1959 to Geigy). Review of pharmacology: Horakova *et al., Pharmacotherapeutica* **1950-1959**, 335-350 (1963), *C.A.* **60**, 6072g (1964). Metabolism: Nemecek *et al., Arzneim.-Forsch.* **16**, 1339 (1966); Queisnerova, Nemecek, *Cesk. Farm.* **20**, 55 (1971), *C.A.* **75**, 47077u (1971).

Crystals, mp 115.5-116.5° or 127.5-128.5° depending on cryst form.
THERAP CAT: Antirheumatic.

5289. Kefir Fungi. Kefir grains; kefir seeds. A conglomeration of various fungi, including *Dispora caucasica, Schizomyces* and a species of *Saccharomyces.*

Grayish-yellow lumps, irregular in size; firm, toughly gelatinous consistency, becoming cartilaginous and brittle when dry.

USE: Preparing a nutritious beverage of fermented milk known as kefir.

5290. Kenaf. Both the annual herbaceous plant and the resulting fiber are known as Kenaf. Believed to have orginated in Western Sudan around 4000 BC, the fiber, primarily produced from

Hibiscus cannibinus L., was traditionally used for ropes, canvas, sacks and carpets. Structural characterization of fibers: S. M. A. Shah *et al., Pakistan J. Sci. Ind. Res.* **23**, 213 (1980); of bark and lignins: A. M. L. Seca *et al., J. Agric. Food Chem.* **46**, 3100 (1998). Genetic diversity: Z. Cheng *et al., Hereditas* **136**, 231 (2002). Evaluation in laminated products: G. N. Ramaswamy *et al., Indust. Crops Products* **17**, 1 (2003). Brief review: C. L. Webber, III, R. E. Bledsoe, "Kenaf: Production, Harvesting, Processing, and Products" in *New Crops*, J. Janick, J. E. Simon, Eds. (John Wiley and Sons, New York, 1993) pp 416-421. *Review:* H. P. Stout, "Jute and Kenaf" in *Handbook of Fiber Science and Technology* **4,** M. Lewin, E. M. Pearce, Eds. (Marcel Dekker, New York, 1985) pp 701-726; R. K. Maiti, N. Samajpati, *Indian Agric.* **44**, 105-146 (2000).

USE: Traditionally in fiber production; more recently in pulping and papermaking, potting and filtration media, animal feed and as a jute substitute.

5291. Keratin. A protein obtained from hair, wool, horn, nails, claws, beaks, scales, membranes of egg shells and nerve tissue. There are two types of keratins—hard keratin of hair, horn, nails, etc., and soft keratin (pseudokeratin) of the epidermis, and whalebone: Rudall, *Adv. Protein Chem.* **7**, 253-290 (1952). The keratins contain all of the common amino acids and differ from other fibrous structural proteins chiefly by their high cystine content. Sequence studies revealed no preferable grouping or periodicity. Amino acid compn of a few keratins: Tristram in H. Neurath, K. Bailey, *The Proteins* vol. 1A (Academic Press, New York, 1953) p 220. Stability of the protein is due to frequent primary valence cross-links (disulfide bonds) and secondary valence cross-links (hydrogen bonds) between neighboring polypeptide chains. Prepn of different forms for different purposes: Grassmann, **DE 673203** and **DE 682257** (both 1939). Molecular structure of α-keratin: Fraser *et al., Nature* **203**, 1231 (1964); of β-keratin: M. L. Huggins, *Macromolecules* **13**, 465 (1980). *Reviews:* Ward, Lundgren, *Adv. Protein Chem.* **9**, 243-297 (1954); Crewther *et al., ibid.* **20**, 191 (1965); Bradbury, *ibid.* **27**, 111 (1973).

Characteristic properties ascribed to keratins: *(a)* insolubility in water, including aq solns of salts, hydrotropic substances, and dil acids and bases at temps not much above room temp; *(b)* resistance to proteolytic enzymes; *(c)* resistance to hydrolysis; *(d)* solvolysis by mixtures of substances which break the —S—S— bonds and the hydrogen bonds.

USE: Coating "enteric" pills which are unaffected in the stomach, but dissolved by the alkaline intestinal secretions. Detailed coating instructions: Dale, *Pharm. J.* **129**, 494 (1932). Other uses are in formulations of foam type extinguishers and in the production of protein hydrolyzates.

5292. Keratinase. [9025-41-6] M-Zyme. A proteolytic enzyme, commercially produced by a strain of *Streptomyces fradiae:* Nickerson, Noval, **US 2988487** (1961 to Rutgers Res. and Educ. Found.). Can convert about 50% of the dry wt of wool into a water-sol form, permitting hair separation from hides. The amount of enzyme needed to dehair hides is not enough to cause much digestion of the hair itself, which is recovered and used in felt making. The enzyme attacks at the base of the hair shaft, which is particularly sensitive to the action of keratinase.

Soluble in water. Non-dialyzable. Optimum efficiency at pH 8.5-9.5. Becomes inactive by heating to 100° for 5 min. The ability to digest keratin appears to be dependent on the presence of at least trace amounts of metal ions which form chelates.

USE: In the dehairing of hides and skins: Robison, Nickerson, **US 2988488** (1961 to Mearl). In depilatory compositions for human use: Mattin, Greenstein, **US 2988485** (1961 to Mearl).

5293. Kermesic Acid. [18499-92-8] 9,10-Dihydro-3,5,6,8-tetrahydroxy-1-methyl-9,10-dioxo-2-anthracenecarboxylic acid; C.I. Natural Red 3; C.I. 75460. $C_{16}H_{10}O_8$; mol wt 330.25. C 58.19%, H 3.05%, O 38.76%. Principle constituent of kermes, one of the oldest known insect dyes. Isoln and characterization: O. Dimroth, *Ber.* **43**, 1387 (1910); O. Dimroth, W. Scheurer, *Ann.* **399**, 43 (1913). Structure: O. Dimroth, R. Fick, *Ann.* **411**, 315 (1916). Revised structure: D. D. Gadgil *et al., Tetrahedron Lett.* **1968**, 2223. Synthesis: D. W. Cameron *et al., Chem. Commun.* **1978**, 688; *idem, Aust. J. Chem.* **34**, 2401 (1981).

Dark red rosettes from acetic acid, mp >320° (dec). Absorption max: 276, 312, 498 nm (log ε 4.52, 4.12, 3.96). Slightly sol in cold water; sol in hot water (yellowish-red soln). Violet-red in conc H_2SO_4, turning blue on addn of boric acid. Violet in aq NaOH.

USE: As brilliant scarlet dye.

5294. Kerosene. [8008-20-6] Kerosine. A mixture of petroleum hydrocarbons, chiefly of the methane series having from 10 to 16 carbon atoms per molecule. It constitutes the fifth fraction in the distillation of petroleum (after the petr ethers and before the oils). A typical analysis of the kerosene fraction from Midcontinent crude includes *n*-dodecane, three alkyl derivatives of benzene, naphthalene, 1- and 2-methyl-5,6,7,8-tetrahydronaphthalene. Toxicity study: W. B. Deichmann *et al., Ann. Intern. Med.* **21**, 803 (1944). Toxicological studies and recommended treatment of kerosene poisoning: H. W. Gerarde, *Toxicol. Appl. Pharmacol.* **1**, 462 (1959).

Pale yellow or water-white, mobile, oily liquid. Characteristic, not altogether disagreeable odor. d ~0.80. bp 175-325°. Flash pt 150-185°F. (65-85°C). Insol in water. Misc with other petroleum solvents. A water-white, deodorized form of kerosene is marketed under the trade name *Deobase*. Kerosene is deodorized and decolorized by washing with (fuming) sulfuric acid, followed by sodium plumbite soln and sulfur (Doctor sweetening). LD_{50} orally in rabbits: 28 ml/kg (Deichmann).

Caution: Potential symptoms of overexposure are irritation of eyes, skin, nose, throat; burning sensation in chest; headache, nausea, weakness, restlessness, incoordination, confusion, drowsiness; vomiting, diarrhea; dermatitis; aspiration of liquid may cause chemical pneumonia. *See NIOSH Pocket Guide to Chemical Hazards* (DHHS/NIOSH 97-140, 1997) p 184.

USE: In kerosene lamps, flares, and stoves; as degreaser and cleaner; Deobase formerly used as a solvent in cosmetics and in fly spray.

5295. Ketamine. [6740-88-1] 2-(2-Chlorophenyl)-2-(methylamino)cyclohexanone. $C_{13}H_{16}ClNO$; mol wt 237.73. C 65.68%, H 6.78%, Cl 14.91%, N 5.89%, O 6.73%. Prepn: C. L. Stevens, **BE 634208**; *idem,* **US 3254124** (1963, 1966 both to Parke, Davis). Isoln of optical isomers: T. W. Hudyma *et al.,* **DE 2062620** (1971 to Bristol-Myers), *C.A.* **75**, 118119x (1971). Clinical pharmacology of racemate and enantiomers: P. F. White *et al., Anesthesiology* **52**, 231 (1980). Toxicity: E. J. Goldenthal, *Toxicol. Appl. Pharmacol.* **18**, 185 (1971). Enantioselective HPLC determn in plasma: G. Geisslinger *et al., J. Chromatogr.* **568**, 165 (1991). Comprehensive description: W. C. Sass, S. A. Fusari, *Anal. Profiles Drug Subs.* **6**, 297-322 (1977). Review of pharmacology and use in veterinary medicine: M. Wright, *J. Am. Vet. Med. Assoc.* **180**, 1462-1471 (1982). Review of pharmacology and clinical experience: D. L. Reich, G. Silvay, *Can. J. Anaesth.* **36**, 186-197 (1989); in pediatric procedures: S. M. Green, N. E. Johnson, *Ann. Emerg. Med.* **19**, 1033-1046 (1990).

Crystals from pentane-ether, mp 92-93°. uv max (0.01*N* NaOH in 95% methanol): 301, 276, 268, 261 nm ($A_{1cm}^{1\%}$ 5.0, 7.0, 9.8, 10.5). pKa 7.5. pH of 10% aq soln 3.5.

Hydrochloride. [1867-66-9] CI-581; Ketalar; Ketanest; Ketaset; Ketavet; Vetalar. $C_{13}H_{16}ClNO.HCl$; mol wt 274.19. White crystals, mp 262-263°. Soly in water: 20 g/100 ml. LD_{50} in adult mice, rats (mg/kg): 224 ±4, 229 ±5 i.p. (Goldenthal).

Note: This is a controlled substance (depressant): **21 CFR**, 1308.13.

THERAP CAT: Anesthetic (intravenous).

THERAP CAT (VET): Anesthetic (intravenous).

5296. Ketanserin. [74050-98-9] 3-[2-[4-(4-Fluoro-benzoyl)-1-piperidinyl]ethyl]-2,4[1H,3H]-quinazolinedione; R-41468; Ketensin; Serefrex; Taseron. $C_{22}H_{22}FN_3O_3$; mol wt 395.43. C 66.82%, H 5.61%, F 4.80%, N 10.63%, O 12.14%. Specific serotonin (5HT$_2$)-receptor antagonist. Prepn: J. Vandenbeck *et al.*, *EP 13612*; *eidem*, *US 4335127* (1980, 1982 both to Janssen). X-ray structure: O. M. Peeters *et al.*, *Cryst. Struct. Commun.* **11**, 375 (1982). Receptor binding profile: J. E. Leysen *et al.*, *Life Sci.* **28**, 1015 (1981). Pharmacology: J. M. Van Neuten *et al.*, *J. Pharmacol. Exp. Ther.* **218**, 217 (1981). HPLC determn in plasma: A. T. Kacprowicz *et al.*, *J. Chromatogr.* **272**, 417 (1983). Clinical efficacy in intermittent claudication: J. De Cree *et al.*, *Lancet* **2**, 775 (1984); in Raynaud's phenomenon: J. R. Seibold, A. H. M. Jageneau, *Arthritis Rheum.* **27**, 139 (1984); in hypertension: A. Amery *et al.*, *J. Cardiovasc. Pharmacol.* **6**, 182 (1984). Series of articles on pharmacology and clinical studies: *ibid.* **7**, Suppl. 7, S1-S182 (1985); on pharmacokinetics and metabolism: *Arzneim.-Forsch.* **38**, 775-800 (1988). Review of pharmacology and clinical efficacy in hypertension and vascular disease: R. N. Brogden, E. M. Sorkin, *Drugs* **40**, 903-949 (1990).

Crystals from 4-methyl-2-pentanone, mp 227-235°. Soly (g/100 ml): 0.001 in water; 0.038 in ethanol; 2.34 in DMF. pKa 7.5.

Tartrate. [83846-83-7] R-49945; Ket; Perketan; Serepress; Sufrexal. $C_{22}H_{22}FN_3O_3 \cdot C_4H_6O_6$; mol wt 545.51.

THERAP CAT: Antihypertensive.

5297. Ketazolam. [27025-33-4] 11-Chloro-8,12b-dihydro-2,8-dimethyl-12b-phenyl-4H-[1,3]oxazino[3,2-d][1,4]benzodiazepine-4,7(6H)-dione; U-28774; Anseren; Unakalm. $C_{20}H_{17}$-ClN$_2$O$_3$; mol wt 368.81. C 65.13%, H 4.65%, Cl 9.61%, N 7.60%, O 13.01%. Prepn: J. Szmuszkovicz, *DE 1947226*; *idem*, *US 3573282* (1970, 1971 both to Upjohn). Synthesis and structure: J. Szmuszkovicz *et al.*, *Tetrahedron Lett.* **1971**, 3665. Analysis by HPLC: D. J. Weber, *J. Pharm. Sci.* **61**, 1797 (1972). Pharmacology: V. H. Sethy, *Arch. Exp. Pathol. Pharmakol.* **301**, 157 (1978). Clinical studies: L. F. Fabre, *J. Int. Med. Res.* **4**, 50 (1976); L. A. Gottschalk, J. B. Cohn, *Psychopharmacol. Bull.* **14**, 39 (1978).

Colorless prisms from chloroform/ether, mp 182-183.5° (sinters at 170°). uv max (ethanol): 202, 241 nm (ε 40600; 18400).

Note: This is a controlled substance (depressant): 21 CFR, 1308.14.

THERAP CAT: Anxiolytic.

5298. Ketene. [463-51-4] Ethenone; carbomethene. C_2H_2-O; mol wt 42.04. C 57.14%, H 4.80%, O 38.06%. $CH_2\!=\!C\!=\!O$. Prepd by the thermal decompn of acetone, diketene or acetic anhydride: Hurd, *Org. Synth.* **coll. vol. I**, 330 (2nd ed., 1941); S. Andreades, H. D. Carlson, *ibid.* **coll. vol. V**, 679 (1973). Structure of ketene dimer as 3-buteno-β-lactone: Blomquist, Baldwin, *J. Am. Chem. Soc.* **70**, 29 (1948); Hurd, Blanchard, *ibid.* **72**, 1461 (1950); Katz, Lipscomb, *J. Org. Chem.* **17**, 515 (1953). Toxicology: J. F.

Treon *et al.*, *J. Ind. Hyg. Toxicol.* **31**, 209 (1949). *Review* on the prepn of stable ketenes: R. S. Ward in *The Chemistry of Ketenes, Allenes and Related Compounds* **Part 1,**, S. Patai, Ed. (Wiley, New York, 1980) pp 223-277; on synthetic uses of ketenes: W. T. Brady, *ibid.* pp 279-308.

Gas. Penetrating odor. mp $-150°$. bp $-56°$. Electron diffraction pictures: Beach, Stevenson, *J. Chem. Phys.* **6**, 75 (1938). Fairly sol in acetone. All operations with ketene should be carried out in an efficient hood (Andreades, Carlson).

Caution: Potential symptoms of overexposure are irritation of skin, eyes, nose, throat and respiratory system; pulmonary edema. *See NIOSH Pocket Guide to Chemical Hazards* (DHHS/NIOSH 97-140, 1997) p 184.

USE: For the conversion of higher acids into their anhydrides; for acetylation in the manuf of cellulose acetate and aspirin.

5299. Kethoxal. [27762-78-3] 3-Ethoxy-1,1-dihydroxy-2-butanone; β-ethoxy-α-ketobutyraldehyde; 3-ethoxy-2-oxobutyraldehyde hydrate; U-2032. $C_6H_{12}O_4$; mol wt 148.16. C 48.64%, H 8.16%, O 43.19%. Also depicted as $CH_3CH(OC_2H_5)COCHO$ monohydrate. Prepn: Rappen, *J. Prakt. Chem.* **157**, 177 (1941); Tiffany *et al.*, *J. Am. Chem. Soc.* **79**, 1682 (1957). Antiviral activity: H. E. Rennis, *Ann. N.Y. Acad. Sci.* **173/1**, 527 (1970).

Yellow oil. bp$_{11}$ 54-58°. bp$_{760}$ 145°. Initial $n_D^{23.7}$ 1.4348. Miscible with alc; sol in benzene with yellow color; one part dissolves in ten parts of water.

Bis(thiosemicarbazone). [2507-91-7] 2,2'-[1-(1-Ethoxyethyl)-1,2-ethanediylidene]bishydrazinecarbothioamide; gloxazone; BW-356-C-61; NSC-82116; Contrapar. $C_8H_{16}N_6OS_2$; mol wt 276.38.

THERAP CAT: Antiviral.

THERAP CAT (VET): Bis(thiosemicarbazone) as anaplasmodastat.

5300. Ketipic Acid. [533-76-6] 3,4-Dioxohexanedioic acid; 2,3-diketoadipic acid; oxalodiacetic acid. $C_6H_6O_6$; mol wt 174.11. C 41.39%, H 3.47%, O 55.14%. Prepn: Fittig *et al.*, *Ann.* **249**, 182 (1888); Stachel, *Arch. Pharm.* **295**, 735 (1932); **296**, 479 (1963). Structure studies; occurs in the solid form as the γ-lactol: Stachel, *Ann.* **689**, 118 (1965).

Dec at 150° forming diacetyl. Sparingly sol in ether. Sol in glacial acetic acid, concd hydrochloric acid. Practically insol in water, alc, chloroform, CS_2, benzene, petr ether.

Diethyl ester. $C_{10}H_{14}O_6$. Prisms from alcohol, mp 83°. bp$_{30}$ 230°. Soluble in ether, chloroform.

5301. Ketobemidone. [469-79-4] 1-[4-(3-Hydroxyphenyl)-1-methyl-4-piperidyl]-1-propanone; 4-(*m*-hydroxyphenyl)-1-methyl-4-piperidyl ethyl ketone. $C_{15}H_{21}NO_2$; mol wt 247.33. C 72.84%, H 8.56%, N 5.66%, O 12.94%. Prepn: Suter, *Abstracts of First National Medicinal Chemistry Symposium of the A.C.S.* (Ann Arbor, 1948) p 20; **GB 591992** and **GB 609763** (1947 and 1948 to Ciba); Eisleb, **US 2167351**; **US 2242575** and **US 2248018** (1939 and 1941 to Winthrop); **DE 752755** (1952 to I. G. Farben). Metabolism in man: U. Bondesson *et al.*, *Drug Metab. Dispos.* **9**, 376 (1981).

Crystals, mp 156-157°.

Hydrochloride. [5965-49-1] Hoechst 10720; Win-1539; Cliradon; Cymidon; Ketogan; Ketogin. $C_{15}H_{21}NO_2 \cdot HCl$; mol wt 283.79. Crystals, mp 201-202°. Sol in water; slightly sol in alcohol. Aq solns may be sterilized by boiling for short periods.

Note: This is a controlled substance (opiate): **21 CFR,** 1308.11.

THERAP CAT: Analgesic (narcotic).

5302. Ketoconazole. [65277-42-1] *cis*-1-Acetyl-4-[4-[[2-(2,4-dichlorophenyl)-2-(1*H*-imidazol-1-ylmethyl)-1,3-dioxolan-4-yl]methoxy]phenyl]piperazine; R-41400; Fungarest; Fungoral; Ketoderm; Ketoisdin; Nizoral; Orifungal M; Panfungol. $C_{26}H_{28}Cl_2N_4O_4$; mol wt 531.43. C 58.76%, H 5.31%, Cl 13.34%, N 10.54%, O 12.04%. Orally active, broad-spectrum antimycotic. Prepn: J. Heeres *et al.*, **DE 2804096**, *eidem*, **US 4144346** and **US 4223036** (1978, 1979, 1980, all to Janssen); *eidem, J. Med. Chem.* **22,** 1003 (1979). Pharmacokinetics: E. W. Gascoigne *et al., Clin. Res. Rev.* **1,** 177 (1981); C. Brass *et al., Antimicrob. Agents Chemother.* **21,** 151 (1982). HPLC determn in human serum: V. L. Pascucci *et al., J. Pharm. Sci.* **72,** 1467 (1983). Series of articles on animal and human studies: *Rev. Infect. Dis.* **2,** 519-692 (1980). Effect on hepatic enzymes *in vitro* and *in vivo:* K. N. Buchi *et al., Biochem. Pharmacol.* **35,** 2845 (1986); J. K. Ritter, M. R. Franklin, *Toxicol. Lett.* **36,** 51 (1987). Case reports of hepatic toxicity: J. K. Heiberg, E. Svejgaard, *Br. Med. J.* **283,** 825 (1981); R. Rollman, L. Loof, *Br. J. Dermatol.* **108,** 376 (1983). Controlled clinical trials: E. A. Petersen *et al., Ann. Intern. Med.* **93,** 791 (1980); W. T. Hughes *et al., J. Infect. Dis.* **147,** 1060 (1983); H. W. Jolly *et al., Cutis* **31,** 208 (1983). Clinical evaluation as inhibitor of steroid synthesis: N. Sonino, *N. Engl. J. Med.* **317,** 812 (1987). Review of pharmacology and therapeutic efficacy: C. A. Sohn, *Clin. Pharm.* **1,** 217 (1982); R. C. Heel *et al., Drugs* **23,** 1-36 (1982). Series of articles on clinical efficacy and therapeutic experience: *Drugs Exp. Clin. Res.* **12,** 397-427 (1986).

Crystals from 4-methyl-2-pentanone, mp 146°. LD_{50} in mice, rats, guinea pigs, dogs (mg/kg): 44, 86, 28, 49 i.v.; 702, 227, 202, 780 orally (Heel).

THERAP CAT: Antifungal.

5303. α-Ketoglutaric Acid. [328-50-7] 2-Oxopentanedioic acid; 2-oxoglutaric acid; 2-oxo-1,5-pentanedioic acid. $C_5H_6O_5$; mol wt 146.10. C 41.10%, H 4.14%, O 54.75%. HOOCCH$_2$CH$_2$-COCOOH. Plays an important role in amino acid metabolism (transamination) *see* Severo Ochoa, "Enzymic Mechanisms in the Citric Acid Cycle" in *Adv. Enzymol.* **15,** 183-270 (1954). Prepn: Friedman, Kosower, *Org. Synth.* **coll. vol. III,** 510 (1955); Bottorff, Moore, *ibid.* **coll. vol. V,** 687 (1973). Microbial synthesis using a strain of *Pseudomonas:* Lockwood *et al.*, **US 2443919** (1948); Berger, Witt, **US 2841616** (1958).

Crystals from acetone-benzene, mp 113.5°. Freely sol in water, alcohol. Very sparingly sol in ether.

Diethyl ester. $C_9H_{14}O_5$. Liq, bp$_{23}$ 160°, bp$_{13}$ 144°.

Compound with L(+)-ornithine. L(+)-Ornithine α-ketoglutarate; Ornicetil. $C_{10}H_{18}N_2O_7$; mol wt 278.26.

USE: Can be converted to L-glutamic acid by *Aeromonas* spp. *see* Good, **US 2933434** (1960 to International Minerals & Chem. Corp.).

5304. 2-Keto-L-gulonic Acid. [526-98-7] L-*xylo*-2-Hexulosonic acid; 2-oxo-L-gulonic acid. $C_6H_{10}O_7$; mol wt 194.14. C 37.12%, H 5.19%, O 57.69%. Important intermediate in vitamin C manufacture. Prepn from sorbitol: Reichstein, Grüssner, *Helv. Chim. Acta* **17,** 311 (1934); Reichstein, **US 2301811** (1942); from L-sorbose: Haworth *et al.*, **GB 443901** (1936); by microbial conversion: Huang, **US 3043749** (1962 to Pfizer); Motizuki *et al.*, **US 3234105** (1966 to Takeda); Z. Y. Yuan *et al., Ann. N.Y. Acad. Sci.* **672,** 628 (1992). Biosynthesis and metabolism in bacteria: S.

Makover *et al., Biotechnol. Bioeng.* **17,** 1485 (1975). NMR structure determn: T. C. Crawford *et al., J. Am. Chem. Soc.* **102,** 2220 (1980). HPLC separation in fermentation broth: R. A. Lazarus, J. L. Seymour, *Anal. Biochem.* **157,** 360 (1986). Review of early syntheses: T. C. Crawford, S. A. Crawford, *Adv. Carbohydr. Chem. Biochem.* **37,** 79-159 (1980).

Crystals from water (may be washed with acetone). mp 171° (slight dec). $[\alpha]_D^{18}$ −48° (c = 1). Moderately sol in water. Strong acid. Reduces boiling Fehling's soln rapidly.

Methyl ester. Crystals, mp 155-157°. $[\alpha]_D^{18}$ −25° (c = 1 in methanol).

Ethyl ester. Crystals, $[\alpha]_D^{20}$ −14.5° (c = 0.63 in abs alc).

5305. Ketoprofen. [22071-15-4] 3-Benzoyl-α-methylbenzeneacetic acid; *m*-benzoylhydratropic acid; 2-(3-benzoylphenyl)propionic acid; RP-19583; Alreumat; Alrheumun; Capisten; Epatec; Fastum; Iso-K; Ketofen; Ketopron; Menamin; Meprofen; Orudis; Oruvail; Profenid; Toprec; Toprek. $C_{16}H_{14}O_3$; mol wt 254.28. C 75.57%, H 5.55%, O 18.88%. Prepn: D. Farge *et al.*, **ZA 6800524**; *eidem*, **US 3641127** (1968, 1972 both to Rhône-Poulenc); G. A. Pinna *et al., Farmaco Ed. Sci.* **35,** 684 (1980). Resolution of isomers: S. Rendic *et al., Chimia* **29,** 170 (1975). Enantioselective synthesis and absolute configuration of (+)-form: G. Comisso *et al., Gazz. Chim. Ital.* **110,** 123 (1980). Pharmacology of enantiomers: P. J. Hayball *et al., Chirality* **4,** 484 (1992). HPLC determn in plasma: R. Lovlin *et al., J. Chromatogr. B* **679,** 196 (1996). Toxicity data: K. Ueno *et al., J. Med. Chem.* **19,** 941 (1976). Comprehensive description: G. G. Liversidge, *Anal. Profiles Drug Subs.* **10,** 443-471 (1981). Review of pharmacokinetics: F. Jamali, D. R. Brocks, *Clin. Pharmacokinet.* **19,** 197-217 (1990); of clinical experience: E. M. Veys, *Scand. J. Rheumatol.* **Suppl. 90,** 3-44 (1991).

Crystals from 6:20 benzene-petr ether, mp 94°. uv max (methanol): 255 nm (log ε 4.33). Sol in ether, alc, acetone, chloroform, DMF, ethyl acetate. Slightly sol in water. LD_{50} orally in rats: 101 mg/kg (Ueno).

Lysine salt. [57469-78-0] Artrosilene. $C_{16}H_{14}O_3 \cdot C_6H_{14}N_2O_2$; mol wt 400.47.

(S)-(+)-Form tromethamine salt. [156604-79-4] Dexketoprofen trometamol; Enantyum; Keral. $C_{16}H_{14}O_3 \cdot C_4H_{11}NO_3$; mol wt 375.42. Prepn: G. Carganico *et al.*, **WO 9411332** (1994 to Menarini). Clinical trial: C. Gay *et al., Clin. Drug Invest.* **11,** 320 (1996). White crystalline solid from ethanol-ethyl acetate, mp 104.8-105.1°. $[\alpha]_D^{20}$ −5.2° (c = 1.47 in methanol).

THERAP CAT: Anti-inflammatory; analgesic.

THERAP CAT (VET): Anti-inflammatory; analgesic.

5306. Ketorolac. [74103-06-3] 5-Benzoyl-2,3-dihydro-1*H*-pyrrolizine-1-carboxylic acid; 5-benzoyl-1,2-dihydro-3*H*-pyrrolo-[1,2-a]pyrrole-1-carboxylic acid; RS-37619. $C_{15}H_{13}NO_3$; mol wt 255.27. C 70.58%, H 5.13%, N 5.49%, O 18.80%. Prostaglandin biosynthesis inhibitor. Prepn and separation of isomers: **BE 856681**; J. M. Muchowski, A. F. Kluge, **US 4089969** (both 1978 to Syntex). Alternate processes: J. M. Muchowski, R. Greenhouse, **US 4347186** (1982 to Syntex); F. Franco *et al., J. Org. Chem.* **47,** 1682 (1982); J. B. Doherty, **US 4496741** (1985 to Merck & Co.). Absolute configuration: A. Guzman *et al., J. Med. Chem.* **29,** 589 (1986). Structure-activity relationships: J. M. Muchowski *et al.*, *ibid.* **28,** 1037 (1985). Pharmacology and analgesic, anti-inflammatory profile of ketorolac and its tromethamine salt: W. H. Rooks *et al., Agents Actions* **12,** 684 (1982); *eidem, Drugs Exp. Clin. Res.* **11,** 479 (1985). Clinical comparison with acetaminophen in postoperative pain: H. J. McQuay *et al., Clin. Pharmacol. Ther.* **39,** 89 (1986).

Crystals from ethyl acetate + ether, mp 160-161°. uv max in methanol: 245, 312 nm (ε 7080, 17400). pKa 3.49 ±0.02. LD$_{50}$ orally in mice: ~200 mg/kg (Rooks).

(±)-Form tromethamine salt. [74103-07-4] Acular; Dolac; Lixidol; Tarasyn; Toradol; Toratex. C$_{19}$H$_{24}$N$_2$O$_6$; mol wt 376.40.

(+)-Form. Crystals from hexane + ethyl acetate, mp 174° (Guzman); also reported as mp 154-156° (Muchowski, Kluge). [α]$_D$ +173° (c = 1 in methanol).

(−)-Form. Crystals from hexane + ethyl acetate, mp 169-170° (Guzman); also reported as mp 153-155° (Muchowski, Kluge). [α]$_D$ −176° (c = 1 in methanol).

THERAP CAT: Analgesic; anti-inflammatory.

5307. Ketotifen. [34580-13-7] 4,9-Dihydro-4-(1-methyl-4-piperidinylidene)-10*H*-benzo[4,5]cyclohepta[1,2-*b*]thiophen-10-one. C$_{19}$H$_{19}$NOS; mol wt 309.43. C 73.75%, H 6.19%, N 4.53%, O 5.17%, S 10.36%. Prepn: J. P. Bourquin *et al.,* **DE 2111071**; *eidem,* **US 3682930** (1971, 1972 both to Sandoz); E. Waldvogel *et al., Helv. Chim. Acta* **59,** 866 (1976). Pharmacology: U. Martin, D. Roemer, *Arzneim.-Forsch.* **28,** 770 (1978). Clinical studies: B. Wüthrich, P. Radielovic, *Dtsch. Med. Wochenschr.* **103,** 1865 (1978); H. Gmür, M. Scherrer, *Schweiz. Med. Wochenschr.* **109,** 881 (1979). *Review:* U. Martin *et al.,* in *Pharmacological and Biochemical Properties of Drug Substances* vol. 3, M. E. Goldberg, Ed. (Am. Pharm. Assoc., Washington, DC, 1981) pp 424-460. Review of clinical experience in asthma and allergy: S. M. Grant *et al., Drugs* **40,** 412-448 (1990).

Crystals from ethyl acetate, mp 152-153°.

Fumarate. [34580-14-8] HC-20511; Totifen; Zaditen; Zaditor; Zasten. C$_{19}$H$_{19}$NOS.C$_4$H$_4$O$_4$; mol wt 425.50. Crystals, mp 192° (dec).

THERAP CAT: Antiasthmatic; antiallergic.

5308. Khat. Chat; quat. Leaves of *Catha edulis* Forsk., Celastraceae. *Habit.* East Africa, Arabia. *Constit.* Cathinone, norpseudoephedrine, *q.q.v.,* (−)-norephedrine, cathidine, cathedulin. Widely used in E. Africa and Yemen as an amphetamine-like stimulant. Isoln and characterization of constituents: O. Wolfes, *Arch. Pharm.* **268,** 81 (1930); H. Friebel, R. Brilla, *Naturwissenschaften* **50,** 354 (1963); M. Cais *et al., Tetrahedron* **31,** 2727 (1975); R. L. Baxter *et al., Chem. Commun.* **1976,** 463. Isoln of cathinone, the major psychoactive alkaloid: X. Schorno, E. Steinegger, *Experientia* **35,** 572 (1979). Review of botany, cultivation and use: A. Getahun, A. D. Krikorian, *Econ. Bot.* **27,** 353-377 (1973); of chemistry: *eidem, ibid.* 378-389; of pharmacology and abuse potential: P. Nencini, A. M. Ahmed, *Drug Alcohol Depend.* **23,** 19-29 (1989); P. Kalix, *Pharm. World Sci.* **18,** 69-73 (1996).

5309. Khellin. [82-02-0] 4,9-Dimethoxy-7-methyl-5*H*-furo[3,2-*g*][1]benzopyran-5-one; 5,8-dimethoxy-2-methyl-4′,5′-

furo-6,7-chromone; 5,8-dimethoxy-2-methyl-6,7-furanochromone; 4,9-dimethoxy-7-methyl-5-oxofuro[3,2-*g*]-1,2-chromene; 4,9-dimethoxy-7-methyl-5-oxo-1,8-dioxabenz[*f*]indene; visammin; Ammivin; Lynamine; Vasokellina. C$_{14}$H$_{12}$O$_5$; mol wt 260.24. C 64.61%, H 4.65%, O 30.74%. Found in seeds of *Ammi visnaga* Lam., *Umbelliferae;* one of the active principles of the Egyptian traditional medicine known as "khella." *See also:* visnadine, visnagin. Isoln and structure: Späth, Gruber, *Ber.* **71,** 106 (1938). Synthesis: Baxter *et al., J. Chem. Soc.* **1949,** S 30; Gardner *et al., J. Org. Chem.* **15,** 841 (1950); Schönberg, Sina, *J. Am. Chem. Soc.* **72,** 1611, 3396 (1950); M. W. Reed, H. W. Moore, *J. Org. Chem.* **53,** 4166 (1988). Crystal structure: J. P. Beale, *Cryst. Struct. Commun.* **2,** 125 (1973). Toxicity data: E. Busch *et al., Arzneim.-Forsch.* **11,** 915 (1961). GC determn in serum: A. S. Carlin *et al., J. Chromatogr.* **614,** 324 (1993). Clinical evaluation in vitiligo: B. Ortel *et al., J. Am. Acad. Dermatol.* **18,** 693 (1988). Comprehensive description: M. A. Hassan, M. U. Zubair, *Anal. Profiles Drug Subs.* **9,** 371-396 (1980).

Crystals from methanol. Bitter taste. mp 154-155°. bp$_{0.05}$ 180-200°. uv max (alc): 250, 338 nm (E$_{1cm}^{1\%}$ 1600, 200). Soly in g/100 ml at 25°: water 0.025; acetone 3.0; methanol 2.6; isopropanol 1.25; ether 0.5. Much more sol in hot water and hot methanol. LD$_{50}$ in mice, rats (mg/kg): 30.6, 34.4 i.v.; 50.8, 68.8 orally (Busch).

THERAP CAT: Vasodilator (coronary). Photosensitizer in treatment of vitiligo.

5310. Kiku Oil. Obtained by distillation from leaves and flowers of *Chrysanthemum indicum* L., *Compositae.* Produced in Japan: Perrier, *Bull. Soc. Chim. Fr.* [3] **23,** 216 (1900). *Constit. l*-Camphene, camphor carvone, xanthophyll, coumarin, angelic acid esters. Used as a folk remedy in Japan in a manner comparable with the use of chamomile and mint in Europe, but also against intestinal worms.

Colorless or greenish oil. Odor reminiscent of oil of Eucalyptus. d$_4^{15}$ 0.932. n$_D^{18}$ 1.4931. Acid to moist litmus paper. Ten grams dissolves in 100 grams abs alc at 95°. Almost insol in alc at 70°.

5311. Kinetin. [525-79-1] *N*-(2-Furanylmethyl)-1*H*-purin-6-amine; *N*^{6}-furfuryladenine; 6-furfurylaminopurine. C$_{10}$H$_9$N$_5$O; mol wt 215.21. C 55.81%, H 4.22%, N 32.54%, O 7.43%. A cell division factor found in various plant parts and in yeast. Isoln from autoclaved water slurries of deoxyribonucleic acid: Miller *et al., J. Am. Chem. Soc.* **77,** 1392 (1955). Structure and synthesis from furfurylamine and 6-methylmercaptopurine: Miller *et al., ibid.* 2662; **78,** 1375 (1956); **US 2903455** (1959 to Wisc. Alumni Res. Found.). Physiologically active at very great dilutions, but only in presence of auxin, *see* Indoleacetic Acid. Crystal structure: M. Soriano-Garcia, R. Parthasarathy, *Acta Crystallogr.* **33B,** 2674 (1977). *Review:* Miller, *Annu. Rev. Plant Physiol.* **12,** 395 (1961).

Platelets from abs ethanol, mp 266-267° (sealed tube). Sublimes at 220°. pKa$_1$ 2.7; pKa$_2$ 9.9. uv max (ethanol): 268 nm (ε 18,650). Slightly soluble in cold water, methanol, ethanol. Freely soluble in dil aq HCl or NaOH. Can be extracted from neutral aq solns by shaking with ether.

Note: Kinetin is also a brand of hyaluronidase, *q.v.*

USE: Plant growth regulator. To augment growth of microbial cultures: **BE 632589** (1963 to Hoechst).

5312. Kininogens. [12244-26-7] Precursor molecules of the vasoactive kinins. Also serve as endogenous cysteine proteinase inhibitors known as type 3 cystatins and are essential cofactors for the contact activation of blood clotting. Single chain glycoproteins synthesized by hepatocytes and secreted into plasma. Three forms have been identified in mammals: H-kininogen (HK) having a molecular mass of 88-115 kDa, L-kininogen (LK) with molecular mass of 50-68 kDa, and T-kininogen, mol wt 68 kDa, which has been found only in rats. Structures consist of an amino-terminal heavy chain portion linked to a carboxy terminal light chain by the kinin segment which is released by kallikrein, *q.v.* The heavy chain contains 3 tandemly repeated domains that are structurally homologous to the type-2 cystatins, *q.v.* The HK light chain contains 2 additional domains that are responsible for the procoagulant activity. Purification from bovine serum: E. Habermann *et al., Z. Phys. Chem.* **332**, 121 (1963); *eidem, Biochem. Z.* **337**, 440 (1963). Isoln of 2 forms from human plasma: F. M. Habal *et al., Biochem. Pharmacol.* **23**, 2291 (1974). Review of purification methods and structure: H. Kato *et al., Methods Enzymol.* **80**, Part C, 172-199 (1981). Identity with α-cysteine proteinase inhibitors: W. Müller-Esterl *et al., FEBS Lett.* **182**, 310 (1985). Review of structure and function: R. A. DeLa Cadena, R. W. Colman, *Trends Pharmacol. Sci.* **12**, 272-275 (1991); of biological role: K. D. Bhoola *et al., Pharmacol. Rev.* **44**, 1-80 (1992); C. Blais, Jr. *et al., Peptides* **21**, 1903-1940 (2000).

H-Kininogen. [308068-04-3] α_1-CPI; α_1-cysteine proteinase inhibitor; high molecular weight kininogen. Preferred substrate for plasma kallikrein to release bradykinin, *q.v.* α-globulin; isoelectric point 4.3. Plasma conc in humans: 90 μg/ml.

L-Kininogen. α_2-CPI; α_2-cysteine proteinase inhibitor; low molecular weight kininogen. Preferred substrate for tissue kallikrein to release kallidin, *q.v.* β-globulin; isoelectric point 4.7. Plasma conc in humans: 170 μg/ml.

5313. Kino. [8052-27-5] Resin kino; gum kino. Dried juice from trunk of *Pterocarpus marsupium* Roxb., *Leguminosae. Habit.* Western Africa, East India, Ceylon. *Constit.* 70-80% kinotannic acid; kino-red, pyrocatechol, kinoin, gum. Contains not less than 45% alcohol-soluble and not less than 80% water-soluble material.

THERAP CAT: Astringent.

THERAP CAT (VET): Has been used as astringent.

5314. Kistrin. [127829-86-1] Kistrin (*Agkistrodon rhodostoma* reduced). Member of a homologous family of low molecular weight, cysteine-rich proteins known as **disintegrins**. Isolated from various viper venoms; characterized by an Arg-Gly-Asp (RGD) binding site and by inhibition of platelet aggregation by antagonism of glycoprotein IIb-IIIa integrin receptors. A single chain polypeptide, mol wt ~7318, consists of 68 amino acids with six intramolecular disulfide bonds; no regular secondary structure. Isolated from the venom of the Malayan pit viper *Agkistrodon rhodostoma.* Purification, chemical and biological characterization: M. S. Dennis *et al., Proc. Natl. Acad. Sci. USA* **87**, 2471 (1989); R. A. Lazarus, M. S. Dennis, **WO 9015072** (1990 to Genentech). Preliminary structural study: M. Adler *et al., Science* **253**, 445 (1991). NMR structural study: M. Adler, G. Wagner, *Biochemistry* **31**, 1031 (1992). Enhancement of coronary arterial thrombolysis in dogs: T. Yasuda *et al., Circulation* **83**, 1038 (1991). Binding interaction with glycoprotein IIb-IIIa: M. S. Dennis *et al., Proteins* **15**, 312 (1993). Brief review: R. J. Gould *et al., Proc. Soc. Exp. Biol. Med.* **195**, 168-171 (1990).

5315. Kitol. [4626-00-0] [1α,2α,5α(1*E*,3*E*),6β(1*E*,3*E*,5*E*)]-3,6-Dimethyl-5-[2-methyl-4-(2,6,6-trimethyl-1-cyclohexen-1-yl)-1,3-butadienyl]-6-[4-methyl-6-(2,6,6-trimethyl-1-cyclohexen-1-yl)-1,3,5-hexatrienyl]-3-cyclohexene-1,2-dimethanol. $C_{40}H_{60}O_2$; mol wt 572.90. C 83.86%, H 10.56%, O 5.59%. One of the provitamins A. Obtained from mammalian liver oil: Embree, Shantz, *J. Am. Chem. Soc.* **65**, 910 (1943); Clough *et al., Science* **105**, 436 (1947); Barua, Morton, *Biochem. J.* **45**, 309 (1949); Chatan, Fridenson, *Compt. Rend.* **234**, 1094 (1952). Purification: Tawara, Fukazawa, *C.A.* **47**, 12483e (1953). Conversion to vitamin A: Libermann, Grundland, *Compt. Rend.* **224**, 1033 (1947). Structure: Burger *et al., Chem. Commun.* **1965**, 588; Giannotti *et al., ibid.* **1966**, 28; Giannotti *et al., Bull. Soc. Chim. Fr.* **1966**, 3299; Burger, Garbers, *J. Chem. Soc. Perkin Trans. 1* **1973**, 590.

Crystals from methanol, mp 88-90° (Embree); 98-100° (Chatan); 72° (Tawara). $[\alpha]_D$ −2.6° (c = 1.1 in chloroform). Labile in light, air, petr ether. Kitol has no vitamin A activity. uv max: 290 nm ($E_{1cm}^{1\%}$ 586).

Diphenylazobenzoate. Exists in two forms, probably geometric isomers, one mp 125-126°, the other 153-155°.

5316. Kodel®. Polyester staple and filament fiber. Prepn from dimethyl terephthalate and 1,4-cyclohexanedimethanol: Kibler *et al., US 2901466* (1959 to Eastman-Kodak). Review and structure: R. W. Moncrieff, *Man-Made Fibres* (John Wiley, New York, 4th ed., 1963) pp 389-393.

Solid, mp 290-295°. Burns slowly. Sp gr 1.22. Fiber has good resistance to acids and alkalies. Treatment of fabric with trichloroethylene and methylene chloride causes it to shrink; boiling water and perchloroethylene induce slight shrinkage. Fabric has good crease resistance.

5317. Kojic Acid. [501-30-4] 5-Hydroxy-2-(hydroxymethyl)-4*H*-pyran-4-one; 5-hydroxy-2-(hydroxymethyl)-4-pyrone; 2-hydroxymethyl-5-hydroxy-γ-pyrone. $C_6H_6O_4$; mol wt 142.11. C 50.71%, H 4.26%, O 45.03%. Antibiotic substance produced in an aerobic process by a variety of microorganisms from a wide range of carbon sources. Isoln from *Aspergillus oryzae:* Saito, *Bot. Mag. Tokyo* **21**, 249 (1907). Structure: Yabuta, *J. Chem. Soc.* **125**, 575 (1924); Heyns, Vogelsang, *Ber.* **87**, 13 (1954). Synthesis: Stacey, Turton, *J. Chem. Soc.* **1946**, 661; Lichtenthaler, Heidel, *Angew. Chem. Int. Ed.* **8**, 978 (1968). Industrial prepn: *GB 826244* (1959 to Pfizer), *C.A.* **54**, 11372e (1960). Mutagenicity study: C. I. Wei *et al., Toxicol. Lett.* **59**, 213 (1991). *Review:* Beélik, *Adv. Carbohydr. Chem.* **11**, 145-183 (1956); Wilson, "Miscellaneous *Aspergillus* Toxins" in *Microbial Toxins* vol. **VI**, A. Ciegler *et al.,* Eds. (Academic Press, New York, 1971) pp 235-250.

Prismatic needles from acetone, ethanol + ether or methanol+ ethyl acetate, mp 153-154°. pKa 7.90, 8.03. Freely sol in water, ethanol, acetone; sparingly sol in ether, ethyl acetate, chloroform, pyridine. Absorption spectrum: Stacey, Turton.

USE: Converted to maltol and ethyl maltol, flavor-enhancing additives. Food additive to inhibit tyrosinase.

5318. Kola. Cola; Soudan coffee; Bissy nuts; gooroo nuts; guru nuts. Dried cotyledons of *Cola nitida* Schott and Endl. or of other species of *Cola, Sterculiaceae. Habit.* West Africa; naturalized in West Indies, India, Ceylon. *Constit.* About 1.5% caffeine; theobromine, kola-red, kolatin; glucoside kolanin; kolazyme; kolatannin, glucose, gum.

THERAP CAT: Analeptic.

5319. Konjac. Konnyaku. Flowering perennial plant with tuberous roots, *Amorphophallus konjac* K. Koch, *Araceae* or closely related species such as *A. bulbifer* B., *A. oncophyllys* Prain ex Hook. f., or *A. variabilis* Blume. *Habit.* Southeast Asia. The tubers are ground to produce a flour used in traditional Asian cooking. *Constit.* Konjac mannan (8-10%), starch, lipid, minerals. Review of plant cultivation, production of flour and properties of konjac mannan: S. Takigami in *Handbook of Hydrocolloids*, G. O. Phillips, P. A. Williams, Eds. (CRC Press, Boca Raton, 2000) pp 413-424.

Konjac mannan. [37220-17-0] Konjac glucomannan. Nonionic, slightly branched polysaccharide. Consists of β-1,4 linked D-glucose and D-mannose in a ratio of approx 1 to 1.6, some branching at C3 of mannose, and an acetyl group attached to one per 19 sugar residues. Average mol wt 200-2000 kDa. Review of properties and applications: R. J. Tye, *Food Technol.* **45**, 82-92 (1991); K. Nishinari in *Novel Macromolecules in Food Systems*, G. Doxastakis, V. Kiosseoglou, Eds. (Elsevier Science, Amsterdam, 2000) pp 309-330. Light tan powder. Dispersible in hot or cold water; forms highly viscous solutions. Viscosity (cP): 31,600 (1% in water); 341,000 (2% in water). A heat-stable gel is formed in the presence of mild alkali.

USE: Source of dietary fiber; as thickening and gelling agent in foods.

5320. Kopsine. [559-48-8] 3-Hydroxy-22-oxokopsan-1-carboxylic acid methyl ester. $C_{22}H_{24}N_2O_4$; mol wt 380.44. C 69.46%, H 6.36%, N 7.36%, O 16.82%. From *Kopsia fructicosa* A.D., *Apocynaceae*: Bhattacharya *et al.*, *J. Am. Chem. Soc.* **71**, 3370 (1949). Structure: Spiteller, *Monatsh. Chem.* **93**, 1220 (1962); Govindachari *et al.*, *Helv. Chim. Acta* **45**, 1146 (1962); **46**, 572 (1963); Guggisberg *et al.*, *ibid.* **52**, 76 (1969).

Crystals from alc, dec 217-218°. $[\alpha]_D^{27}$ −14.3 ± 1° (c = 2 in chloroform). uv max (ethanol): 240, 278, 285-286 nm (log ε 4.08, 3.37, 3.35). Sol in chloroform; sparingly sol in methanol, ethanol, ethyl acetate, benzene, ether. Practically insol in petr ether, water.

Methiodide. $C_{23}H_{27}IN_2O_4$. Crystals from methanol, dec 194-196°.

Oxalate. $C_{24}H_{26}N_2O_8$. Prisms from alcohol + acetone, dec 154°. Sol in water.

5321. Koser's Reagent. [27126-76-7] Hydroxy(4-methylbenzenesulfonato-κO)phenyliodine; [hydroxy(tosyloxy)iodo]benzene; HTIB; phenyliodoso hydroxide tosylate; phenylhydroxytosyloxyiodine. $C_{13}H_{13}IO_4S$; mol wt 392.21. C 39.81%, H 3.34%, I 32.36%, O 16.32%, S 8.18%. Unsymmetrical aryl λ^3-iodane. Prepn: O. Y. Neiland, B. Y. Karele, *J. Org. Chem. USSR* **6**, 889 (1970). Solid state structure determn by single-crystal x-ray analysis: G. F. Koser *et al.*, *J. Org. Chem.* **41**, 3609 (1976). Review of use in organic synthesis: R. M. Moriarty *et al.*, *Synlett* **1990**, 365-383; of chemistry: G. F. Koser, *Aldrichim. Acta* **34**, 89-102 (2001).

Stable, nonhygroscopic crystalline solid. Colorless fine needles from dichloroethane, mp 140-142° (Neiland), also reported as color-

less prisms from diethyl ether + methanol, mp 136-138.5° (Koser *et al.*). Sparingly sol in acetonitrile and dichloromethane at room temp. Readily dissolves in acetonitrile near the reflux temp. to give a yellow soln. Sol in dimethylformamide, alcohols and water with the formation of a yellow color. Sol in chloroform and acetic acid to give a colorless soln. Soly in water at 22°: ca. 1 g/42 mL.

USE: Versatile synthetic reagent in phenyliodination and/or tosylation of a range of organic substrates; in oxidative transformations including oxidative rearrangements.

5322. Kosins. Phloroglucinols from flowers of *Hagenia abyssinica* J. J. Gmel. (*Brayera anthelmintica* Kunth.), *Rosaceae*. Isoln and early characterization: M. Leichsenring, *Arch. Pharm.* **232**, 50 (1894); A. Lobeck, *ibid.* **239**, 672 (1901); B. A. Hems, A. R. Todd, *J. Chem. Soc.* **1937**, 562. Structure of α-kosin: W. Riedl, *Ber.* **89**, 2600 (1956). Orginally identified as α- and β-kosins; ultimately shown to be a mixture of compds differing only in their acyl side chains. Structural elucidation of kosins and protokosin: M. Lounasmaa *et al.*, *Acta Chem. Scand.* **B28**, 1200 (1974). Mass spectrometry: *idem*, P. Varenne, *Planta Med.* **34**, 153 (1978). Identificaton and proportions in male and female flowers: T. Z. Woldemariam *et al.*, *Anal. Proc.* **27**, 178 (1990). Antitumor activity: *idem, et al.*, *J. Pharm. Biomed. Anal.* **10**, 555 (1992).

α-Kosin

α-Kosin. 5,5'-Methylenebis[4,6-dihydroxy-2-methoxy-3-methylisobutyrophenone]. $C_{25}H_{32}O_8$. Yellow needles from ethanol, mp 160-160.5°. uv max: 227, 290 nm (ε 30800, 24400). Soluble in alcohol, benzene, chloroform, ether, glacial acetic acid, alkalies.

Protokosin. [1392-97-8] Structurally related phloroglucinol. Exists in several tautomeric forms and is a mixt of isobutyryl, isovaleryl, and 2-methylbutyryl side chain homologues. Colorless needles from acetone, mp 181-183°. $[\alpha]_D^{25}$ +13.9° (c = 0.610 in chloroform). uv max (cyclohexane): 224, 285 nm (ε 28200, 36400). Practically insol in water. Slightly sol in alcohol, light petroleum; freely sol in ether, acetone, ethyl acetate, chloroform.

THERAP CAT: Has been used as anthelmintic (Cestodes).

5323. Krebiozen. [9008-19-9] A white powder "chemically separated from horses' serum after stimulation of their cell network by the injection of *Actinomyces bovis*." Claimed to be a lipopolysaccharide. Developed by Stevan Durovic. Used experimentally in the treatment of cancer: Szujewski, *J. Am. Med. Assoc.* **148**, 929 (1952). Quackery Congress Symposium: James F. Holland, "The Krebiozen Story", *J. Am. Med. Assoc.* **200**, 213-218 (1967). *See also:* W. F. Janssen, *Anal. Chem.* **50**, 197A (1978); G. A. Curt, "Unsound Methods of Cancer Treatment" in *Cancer: Principles and Practice of Oncology*, V. T. DeVita, Jr. *et al.*, Eds. (J. B. Lippincott, Philadelphia, 4th ed., 1993) pp 2734-2747.

5324. Kresoxim-methyl. [143390-89-0] (αE)-α-(Methoxyimino)-2-[(2-methylphenoxy)methyl]benzeneacetic acid methyl ester; methyl-(E)-methoxyimino[α-(o-tolyloxy)-o-tolyl]acetate; BAS-490 F; BAS-490-02F; Candit; Sovran; Stroby. $C_{18}H_{19}NO_4$; mol wt 313.35. C 68.99%, H 6.11%, N 4.47%, O 20.42%. Synthetic strobilurin fungicide which inhibits mitochondrial respiration by blocking electron transfer at bc_I complex. Prepn: B. Wenderoth *et al.*, DE 3623921; *idem*, US 4829085 (1988, 1989 both to BASF). Description of chemical properties and biological activities: E. Ammermann *et al.*, *Brighton Crop Prot. Conf. - Pests Dis.* **1992**, 403. Fungicidal effects on spore germination: R. E. Gold, G. M. Leinhos, *Pestic. Sci.* **43**, 250 (1995). Field trials against scab and powdery mildew on fruit: P. Creemers *et al.*, *Meded. Fac. Landbouwwet. Univ. Gent* **61**, 431 (1996); A. Brunelli *et al.*, *Brighton Crop Prot. Conf. - Pests Dis.* **1996**, 137. *Review:* R. E. Gold *et al.*, *Mod. Fungic. Antifungal Compd.*, 11th Int. Symp. **1996**, 79-92.

Colorless, odorless crystals, mp 97.2-101.7°. Vapor pressure at 20°: 2.3×10^{-8} mbar. Soly at 20° (mg/l): 2 water. log P at 25° (n-octanol/water, pH 7): 3.4. LD_{50} in rats (mg/kg): >5000 orally; >2000 dermally (Ammerman).

USE: Agricultural fungicide.

5325. Krypton. [7439-90-9] Kr; at. wt 83.798; at. no. 36. Group VIIIA (18), also known as Group 0. A noble gas characterized by an electronic structure in which the outer p subshell is entirely filled. Naturally occurring stable isotopes (mass numbers): 78 (0.35%); 80 (2.25%); 82 (11.6%); 83 (11.5%); 84 (57.0%); 86 (17.3%); known artificial radioactive isotopes: 71-77; 79; 81; 85; 87-95; 97. Isoln from the final residues obtained after evaporation of liq air: Ramsay, Travers, *Proc. Roy. Soc.* **63 [A]**, 405 (1898). Concentration in air: 1.14 ppm by vol. Obtained commercially from the atmosphere by distillation-liquefaction process. Prepn: Lepape, *Compt. Rend.* **187**, 231 (1928); Claude, *ibid.* 581. Monograph: *Argon, Helium and the Rare Gases* vols. **1, 2**, G. A. Cook, Ed. (Interscience, New York, 1963) 818 pp. Diagnostic use of ^{81m}Kr in lung ventilation imaging: A. Zwijnenburg *et al., Clin. Phys. Physiol. Meas.* **9**, 147 (1988). Reviews: A. H. Cockett, K. C. Smith, "The Monatomic Gases" in *Comprehensive Inorganic Chemistry* vol. **1**, J. C. Bailar, Jr. *et al.,* Eds. (Pergamon Press, Oxford, 1973) pp 139-211; N. Bartlett, F. O. Sladky, "The Chemistry of Krypton, Xenon and Radon" *ibid.* pp 213-249; S.-C. Hwang, W. R. Weltmer, Jr. in *Kirk-Othmer Encyclopedia of Chemical Technology* vol. **13** (John Wiley & Sons, 4th ed., 1995) pp 1-38; G. J. Schröbilgen, J. M. Whalen, *ibid.* pp 38-53; *Chemistry of the Elements,* N. N. Greenwood, A. Earnshaw, Eds. (Pergamon Press, New York, 1984) pp 1042-1059.

Colorless, odorless, inert, monatomic gas; will form compds with highly electronegative elements such as O, F, Cl. Condenses to a colorless liquid. Triple pt temp 115.95 K, press 73.15 kPa. Critical temp 209.4 K, critical press 5502 kPa, critical d 908 kg/m³. Gas: d^0 (101.3 kPa) 3.7493 kg/m³, d (normal bp) 8.6 kg/m³. Liquid: normal bp $-153.35°$, d (normal bp) 2415 kg/m³, d (triple pt) 2451 kg/m³, heat of vaporization (normal bp) 9.050 kJ/mol. Solid: d (triple pt) 2826 kg/m³, heat of vaporization (triple pt) 10.77 kJ/mol, heat of fusion (triple pt) 1.64 kJ/mol; solid form exists as face-centered cubic crystals at normal pressure. Excitation potentials: 9.91; 10.03; 10.56; 10.64 ev; ionization potentials: 14.00; 14.66 ev: Brocklehurst, *Q. Rev. Chem. Soc.* **22**, 147 (1968). Soly of gas in water (20°): 59.4 cm³/kg water. Slightly soluble in water with formation of a hydrate; ideal formula Kr.5.75H$_2$O. A hexadeuterate has been prepd. Soluble in liquid oxygen. Emission spectra: T. Jacksier, R. M. Barnes, *Appl. Spectrosc.* **48**, 65 (1994).

Krypton difluoride. [13773-81-4] F_2Kr; mol wt 121.79. Prepn: Turner, Pimentel, *Science* **140**, 974 (1963). Colorless solid; decomposes rapidly at room temperature. d (calc) 3.24. Vapor pressure (mm Hg): 10 ±1 at $-15.5°$; 29 ±2 at 0°; 73 ±3 at 15°.

Caution: Can act as a simple asphyxiant by displacing air. *See: Matheson Gas Data Book* (Matheson Co., Inc., 4th ed., East Rutherford, NJ, 1966) pp 313-314.

USE: As gas filler in special purpose electric bulbs. To initiate and sustain the arc in metal-vapor discharge tubes, such as mercury and sodium vapor lamps. To determine surface areas of fine solids by adsorption techniques.

THERAP CAT: ^{81m}Kr as diagnostic aid (radioactive imaging agent).

5326. Kyanmethin. [461-98-3] 2,6-Dimethyl-4-pyrimidinamine; 4-amino-2,6-dimethylpyrimidine; 6-amino-2,4-dimethylpyrimidine; $C_6H_9N_3$; mol wt 123.16. C 58.51%, H 7.37%, N 34.12%. Prepn from acetonitrile and potassium methoxide: Ronzio, Cook, *Org. Synth.* **coll. vol. III**, 71 (1955).

Needles from alcohol or scales from benzene, mp 182-183°. One gram dissolves in 0.64 ml water at 18° or in 5.25 parts alcohol at 18°.

5327. Kynurenic Acid. [492-27-3] 4-Hydroxy-2-quinolinecarboxylic acid; 4-hydroxyquinaldic acid. $C_{10}H_7NO_3$; mol wt 189.17. C 63.49%, H 3.73%, N 7.40%, O 25.37%. Found in the urine of some animals as a metabolic product of tryptophan; its excretion is stepped up in avitaminoses B_1, B_2 and B_6. Isoln and syntheses: Späth, *Monatsh. Chem.* **42**, 89 (1921); Besthorn, *Ber.* **54**, 1330 (1921). Alternate syntheses: Benassi, *Gazz. Chim. Ital.* **91**, 1097 (1961); Wald, Joullie, *J. Org. Chem.* **31**, 3369 (1966); Jordanides, *Ann.* **729**, 244 (1969).

Yellow needles, mp 282-283°. Soly in water: about 0.9% at 100°. Sol in hot alc. Insol in ether.

Methyl ester. $C_{11}H_9NO_3$. Yellow crystals, mp 224°. *Cf.* xanthurenic acid.

USE: In nutrition studies, specifically in vitamin B deficiency diseases.

5328. Kynurenine. [343-65-7] α,2-Diamino-γ-oxobenzenebutanoic acid; 3-anthraniloylalanine. $C_{10}H_{12}N_2O_3$; mol wt 208.21. C 57.69%, H 5.81%, N 13.45%, O 23.05%. An amino acid produced in the body from tryptophan. Isoln from urine of rabbits that had been fed tryptophan: Matsuoka, Yoshimatsu, *Z. Physiol. Chem.* **143**, 206 (1925); Butenandt *et al., ibid.* **279**, 27 (1943); Heidelberger *et al., J. Biol. Chem.* **179**, 143 (1949). Structure and synthesis: Butenandt *et al., loc. cit.* Laboratory prepn by oxidation of L-tryptophan with a *Pseudomonas* sp.: Hayaishi, Meister, *Biochem. Prep.* **3**, 108 (1953). From acetyltryptophan: Warnell, Berg, *J. Am. Chem. Soc.* **76**, 1708 (1954); Auerbach, Knox, *Methods Enzymol.* **3**, 620 (1957).

L-Kynurenine hydrate. $3C_{10}H_{12}N_2O_3.H_2O$. Leaflets from water, dec 180-190°. $[\alpha]_D^{20} -29°$ (c = 0.4). Slightly sol in water (more sol than the DL-form). Forms a molecular compound with sucrose, $C_{22}H_{34}N_2O_{14}.H_2O$, rosettes; dec 145-153°, $[\alpha]_D +14.5°$ (c = 0.7). Soluble in water.

L-Kynurenine sulfate monohydrate. $C_{10}H_{12}N_2O_3.H_2SO_4.H_2O$. Needles from water + alcohol. Darkens at 165°, dec 195°. $[\alpha]_D^{20} +7.3°$ (c = 1). uv max (pH 7.0): 230, 257, 360 nm (ϵ 18,900, 7500, 4500). Soluble in water, slightly in alcohol. Kynurenine sulfate requires 3 molecules alkali for neutralization in alcoholic soln.

L-Kynurenine diacetate. $C_{14}H_{16}N_2O_5$. Obtained by acetylating L-kynurenine with ketene. Needles, mp 198°.

Anhydro-L-kynurenine monoacetate. $C_{12}H_{12}N_2O_3$. Obtained by acetylating L-kynurenine with acetic anhydride in pyridine. Needles from alc, darkens at 215°, dec 237°.

DL-Kynurenine sulfate. $C_{10}H_{12}N_2O_3.H_2SO_4$. Crystals from water + alcohol. Darkens at 166°, dec 194°. Soluble in water. Slightly sol in alcohol.

USE: In biochemical investigations.

Consult the Name Index before using this section.

L

5329. Labetalol. [36894-69-6] 2-Hydroxy-5-[1-hydroxy-2-[(1-methyl-3-phenylpropyl)amino]ethyl]benzamide; 5-[1-hydroxy-2-[(1-methyl-3-phenylpropyl)amino]ethyl]salicylamide; ibidomide. $C_{19}H_{24}N_2O_3$; mol wt 328.41. C 69.49%, H 7.37%, N 8.53%, O 14.62%. Specific competitive antagonist at both α- and β-adrenergic receptor sites. Prepn: L. H. Lunts, D. T. Collin, **DE 2032642**; *eidem*, **US 4012444** (1971, 1977 both to Allen & Hanburys). Synthesis of labetalol and enantiomers: J. E. Clifton *et al., J. Med. Chem.* **25**, 670 (1982); and comparison of cardiovascular properties: E. H. Gold *et al., ibid.* 1363. Abs config of dilevalol: P. Murray-Rust *et al., Acta Crystallogr.* **C40**, 825 (1984). Adrenoceptor blocking properties: E. J. Sybertz *et al., J. Pharmacol. Exp. Ther.* **218**, 435 (1981). HPLC determn in serum or plasma: T. F. Woodman, B. Johnson, *Ther. Drug Monit.* **3**, 371 (1981). Metabolism in animals and man: R. Hopkins *et al., Biochem. Soc. Trans.* **4**, 726 (1976). Toxicity: K. Shimpo *et al., Hokkaido Igaku Zasshi* **53**, 15 (1978), *C.A.* **90**, 66465v (1974). Review of pharmacology: R. Donnelly, G. J. A. Macphee, *Clin. Pharmacokinet.* **21**, 95-109 (1991); of therapeutic applications in hypertension and ischemic heart disease: K. L. Goa *et al., Drugs* **37**, 583-627 (1989).

Hydrochloride. [32780-64-6] AH-5158A; Sch-15719W; Amipress; Ipolab; Labelol; Labrocol; Normodyne; Presdate; Pressalolo; Trandate. $C_{19}H_{24}N_2O_3$·HCl; mol wt 364.87. White crystalline solid from ethanol-ethyl acetate, mp 187-189°. Sol in water, ethanol. Insol in ether, chloroform. LD_{50} in male, female mice, male, female rats (mg/kg): 114, 120, 113, 107 i.p.; 47, 54, 60, 53 i.v.; 1450, 1800, 4550, 4000 orally (Shimpo).

(R,R)-Form hydrochloride. [75659-08-4]; [75659-07-3] (free base). Dilevalol hydrochloride; Sch-19927. Polymorphic crystals from ethanol, mp 133-134° (dec); mp 192-193.5° (dec). $[\alpha]_D^{26}$ −30.6° (c = 1.0 in ethanol).

THERAP CAT: Antihypertensive.

5330. Laccaic Acid. C.I. Natural Red 25; lac dye; C.I. 75450. Pigment found in the lac resin produced by the insect *Coccus laccae (Laccifer lacca* Kerr) on certain trees in India. Isoln: R. E. Schmidt, *Ber.* **20**, 1285 (1887). Chemistry: O. Dimroth, S. Goldschmidt, *Ann.* **399**, 62 (1913). Originally thought to be one compound, laccaic acid has been separated into four components: A (major), B, C and D. Isoln of A: R. Burwood *et al., J. Chem. Soc. C* **1965**, 6067. Structure of A: *eidem, Tetrahedron Lett.* **1966**, 3059; *eidem, J. Chem. Soc. C* **1967**, 842; E. D. Pandhare *et al., Indian J. Chem.* **7**, 977 (1969). Isoln and structure of B: *eidem, Tetrahedron Lett.* **1967**, 2437; N. S. Bhide *et al., Indian J. Chem.* **7**, 987 (1969); of C: A. V. R. Rao *et al., ibid.* 188; of D: A. R. Mehandale *et al., Tetrahedron Lett.* **1968**, 2231. Synthesis of D: D. W. Cameron *et al., Chem. Commun.* **1978**, 688; *eidem, Aust. J. Chem.* **34**, 2401 (1981).

Laccaic Acid A   R = CH₂CH₂NHCOCH₃
Laccaic Acid B   R = CH₂CH₂OH
Laccaic Acid C   R = CH₂CH(NH₂)COOH
Laccaic Acid D

Laccaic acid A. Laccaic acid A_1. $C_{26}H_{19}NO_{12}$; mol wt 537.43. Red platelets from methanol, chars at 230°. Absorption max (conc H_2SO_4): 302, 361, 518, 558 nm (log ε 4.33, 4.11, 4.32, 4.37).

Laccaic acid B. $C_{24}H_{16}O_{12}$; mol wt 496.38. Red needles from methanol.

Laccaic acid C. $C_{25}H_{17}NO_{13}$; mol wt 539.40. Dark red needles from methanol, dec >360°.

Laccaic acid D. Xanthokermesic acid. $C_{16}H_{10}O_7$; mol wt 314.25. Yellow needles from water, dec >300°.

USE: As crimson dye.

5331. Lacidipine. [103890-78-4] (*E*)-4-[2-[3-(1,1-Dimethylethoxy)-3-oxo-1-propenyl]phenyl]-1,4-dihydro-2,6-dimethyl-3,5-pyridinedicarboxylic acid diethyl ester; diethyl (*E*)-4-[2-[2-(*tert*-butoxycarbonyl)vinyl]phenyl]-2,6-dimethyl-1,4-dihydropyridine-3,5-dicarboxylate; 4-[*o*-[(*E*)-2-carboxyvinyl]phenyl]-1,4-dihydro-2,6-dimethyl-3,5-pyridinedicarboxylic acid 4-*tert*-butyl diethyl ester; GR-43659X; GX-1048; Caldine; Lacimen; Lacipil; Lacirex; Midotens; Motens. $C_{26}H_{33}NO_6$; mol wt 455.54. C 68.55%, H 7.30%, N 3.07%, O 21.07%. Dihydropyridine calcium channel blocker. Prepn: C. Semeraro *et al.*, **DE 3529997**; *eidem*, **US 4801599** (1986, 1989 both to Glaxo). Clinical pharmacology: M. Safar *et al., Clin. Pharmacol. Ther.* **46**, 94 (1989). HPTLC determn in urine: V. R. Kharat *et al., J. Pharm. Biomed. Anal.* **28**, 789 (2002). Clinical trial in atherosclerosis: A. Zanchetti *et al., Circulation* **106**, 2422 (2002). Review of use in hypertension: P. L. McCormack, A. J. Wagstaff, *Drugs* **63**, 2327-2356 (2003).

Crystalline solid from ethyl acetate, mp 174-175°.

THERAP CAT: Antihypertensive.

5332. Lacmoid. Resorcin blue; Iris Blue B; Fluorescent Blue; C.I. 51400. Prepn: Traub, Hock, *Ber.* **17**, 2615 (1884); Musso *et al., Angew. Chem.* **73**, 434 (1961). Discussion of structure controversy: *H. J. Conn's Biological Stains*, R. D. Lillie, Ed. (Williams & Wilkins, Baltimore, 8th ed., 1969) pp 283-284. *See also: Colour Index* **vol. 4** (3rd ed., 1971) p 4468.

Dark-violet, lustrous scales or granules. Freely sol in methanol, ethanol, amyl alcohol, glacial acetic acid, acetone, phenol. Sparingly sol in water, ether. Practically insol in chloroform, benzene, petr ether.

USE: As acid-base indicator in 0.2% soln in alcohol. pH: 4.4 red; 6.4 blue. Satisfactory for titrating mineral acids, strong bases, many alkaloids; determining alkalinity and temporary hardness in water analysis. Biological stain; dye for wool, silk. Not adapted for carbonates, weak inorganic and organic acids, weak bases. Lacmoid is more sensitive than litmus, particularly in form of test paper.

5333. Lacosamide. [175481-36-4] (2*R*)-2-(Acetylamino)-3-methoxy-*N*-(phenylmethyl)propanamide; (*R*)-*N*-benzyl-2-acetamido-3-methoxypropionamide; erlosamide; harkoseride; ADD-234037; SPM-927. $C_{13}H_{18}N_2O_3$; mol wt 250.29. C 62.38%, H 7.25%, N 11.19%, O 19.18%. Functionalized amino acid with demonstrated anticonvulsant and analgesic activity. Prepn: D. Choi *et al., J. Med. Chem.* **39**, 1907 (1996); H. Kohn, **WO 9733861**; *idem*, **US 5773475** (1997, 1998 both to Research Corp. Technol.). Improved prepn and anticonvulsant activity: S. V. Andurkar *et al., Tetrahedron: Asymmetry* **9**, 3841 (1998). Mode of action study: G. Lees *et al., Neuropharmacology* **50**, 98 (2006). Evaluation in animal models of seizure: G. E. Duncan, H. Kohn, *Epilepsy Res.* **67**, 81 (2005); of inflammatory pain: T. Stöhr *et al., Eur. J. Pain* **10**, 241 (2006). Clinical evaluation in neuropathic pain: G. McCleane *et al., Neurosci. Lett.* **352**, 117 (2003). Review of clinical development: C. A. Hovinga, *IDrugs* **6**, 479-485 (2003).

White solid, mp 143-144°. $[\alpha]_D^{23}$ +16.0° (c = 1 in CH_3OH).

THERAP CAT: Analgesic; anticonvulsant.

5334. Lactate Dehydrogenase. [9001-60-9] Lactic dehydrogenase; serum lactic dehydrogenase. Enzyme found in almost all animal tissues, in microorganisms, and in plants. Isoln from heart muscle, rat skeletal muscle, and Jensen sarcoma: Straub, *Biochem. J.* **34**, 483 (1940); Kubowitz, Ott, *Biochem. Z.* **314**, 94 (1943); Meister, *Biochem. Prep.* **2**, 18 (1952). Catalyzes the equilibrium reaction of pyruvic acid to lactic acid. Plays an important role in the equilibrium of carbohydrate catabolism and anabolism. Used as fuel for aerobic tissues such as the heart. Structure is a tetramer of mol wt about 140,000. Consists of units of mol wt about 35,000. Two types of subunits are distinguishable: M (muscle) type and H (heart) type. Lactate dehydrogenases of heart and muscle are mainly H_4 and M_4; all other possible hybrids have been found in various tissues. Elevations of lactate dehydrogenase activity have been found in myocardial infarction, hepatocellular necrosis, metastatic carcinoma, diabetic ketosis, sickle cell anemia, malignant lymphoma, infectious mononucleosis, and cerebral infarction: Standjord *et al.*, *J. Am. Med. Assoc.* **182**, 1099 (1962). Comprehensive reviews: Everse, Kaplan, *Adv. Enzymol. Relat. Areas Mol. Biol.* **37**, 61 (1973); Holbrook *et al.*, in *The Enzymes* vol. XI (part A), P. D. Boyer, Ed. (Academic Press, New York, 3rd ed., 1975) pp 191-292.

USE: In the determination of pyruvate (used in conjunction with reduced coenzyme). In the diagnosis of myocardial infarction and leukemia.

5335. D-Lactic Acid. [10326-41-7] (2R)-2-Hydroxypropanoic acid; D(−)-lactic acid; levorotatory lactic acid; *l*-lactic acid; D-Milchsäure (German). $C_3H_6O_3$; mol wt 90.08. C 40.00%, H 6.71%, O 53.28%. Obtained by resolution of DL-lactic acid: Purdie, Walker, *J. Chem. Soc.* **61**, 754 (1892); Borsook *et al.*, *J. Biol. Chem.* **102**, 449 (1933). Convenient laboratory prepn from glucose using *Lactobacillus leichmannii*: Brin, *Biochem. Prep.* **3**, 61 (1953).

Crystals from ether + isopropyl ether, mp 52.8°. $[\alpha]_{546}^{21.5}$ −2.6° (c = 8). pK = 3.83. Sol in water, alcohol, acetone, ether, glycerol. Practically insol in chloroform. Forms salts with many metals. Most of these salts are dextrorotatory.

Zinc D(+)-lactate. $Zn(C_3H_5O_3)_2.2H_2O$. Crystals, $[\alpha]_D^{14}$ +8.18° (c = 2.5).

5336. DL-Lactic Acid. [598-82-3] 2-Hydroxypropanoic acid; racemic lactic acid; ordinary lactic acid; α-hydroxypropionic acid; Milchsäure (German); Lactovagan; Tonsillosan (Lösung). $C_3H_6O_3$; mol wt 90.08. C 40.00%, H 6.71%, O 53.28%. Occurs in sour milk as a result of lactic acid bacteria; also found in molasses due to partial conversion of sugars, in apples and other fruits, tomato juice, beer, wines, opium, ergot, foxglove, and several higher plants, especially during germination. Lactic acid is prepd technically by "lactic acid fermentation" of carbohydrates such as glucose, sucrose, lactose with *Bacillus acidi lacti* or related organisms such as *Lactobacillus delbrueckii, L. bulgaricus* etc. The fermentation is carried out at relatively high temps. Produced commercially by fermentation of whey, cornstarch, potatoes, molasses. Review on the production of lactic acid by fermentation: S. C. Prescott, C. G. Dunn, *Industrial Microbiology* (McGraw-Hill, New York, 3rd ed., 1959) pp 304-331. Chem prepns from acetaldehyde and CO in dil H_2SO_4 at 130-200° and 900 atm: Loder, **US 2265945** (1938 to du Pont); by hydrolysis of hexoses with NaOH: Lock, **US 2382889** (1943). Prepn of crystalline lactic acid: Borsook *et al.*, *J. Biol. Chem.* **102**, 449 (1933). Toxicity data: Smyth *et al.*, *J. Ind. Hyg. Toxicol.* **23**, 259 (1941). Comprehensive description: F. J. Al-Shammary *et al.*, *Anal. Profiles Drug Subs. Excip.* **22**, 263-316 (1993).

Crystals, mp 16.8°. bp_{14-15} 122°; $bp_{0.5-1}$ 82-85°. pKa at 25° 3.86. n_D^{20} 1.4262. Heat of combustion at constant pressure 3615 cal/kg. Volatile with superheated steam. Sol in water, alc, furfurol; less sol in ether. Practically insol in chloroform, petr ether, carbon disulfide. Caustic in concd solns. LD_{50} orally in rats: 3.73 g/kg (Smyth).

Barium salt. [54983-89-0] Barium lactate. $C_6H_{10}BaO_6$. Powder. *Poisonous!* Sol in water, dil alcohol.

Copper salt dihydrate. [5893-61-1] Cupric lactate. C_6H_{10}-$CuO_6.2H_2O$. Green to blue crystals. Readily sol in water. Practically insol in alcohol.

USE: In dyeing baths, as mordant in printing woolen goods, solvent for water-insoluble dyes (alcohol-soluble induline, nigrosine, spirit-blue); reducing chromates in mordanting wool; manuf cheese, confectionery; acidulant in beverages; for acidulating worts in brewing, for removing *Clostridium butyricum* in manuf of yeast; dehairing, plumping, and decalcifying hides; solvent for cellulose formate; flux for soft solder; manuf lactates which are used in food products, in medicine, and as solvents; plasticizer, catalyst in the casting of phenolaldehyde resins.

THERAP CAT: Acidulant.

THERAP CAT (VET): Has been used as a caustic, and in dilute solutions to irrigate tissues; as an intestinal antiseptic and antiferment.

5337. L-Lactic Acid. [79-33-4] (2S)-2-Hydroxypropanoic acid; L(+)-lactic acid; dextrorotatory lactic acid; *d*-lactic acid; sarcolactic acid; paralactic acid; Fleishmilchsäure; L-Milchsäure. C_3-H_6O_3; mol wt 90.08. C 40.00%, H 6.71%, O 53.28%. Occurs in small quantities in the blood and muscle fluid of man and animals. The lactic acid concn increases in muscle and blood after vigorous activity. L(+)-Lactic acid is also present in liver, kidney, thymus gland, human amniotic fluid, and other organs and body fluids. Obtained by resolution of DL-lactic acid: Purdie, Walker, *J. Chem. Soc.* **61**, 754 (1892); Borsook *et al.*, *J. Biol. Chem.* **102**, 449 (1933). Convenient laboratory prepn from glucose by fermentation by *Lactobacillus delbrueckii*: Brin, *Biochem. Prep.* **3**, 61 (1953). Prepn from hexoses using *B. dextrolacticus*: Andersen, Greaves, *Ind. Eng. Chem.* **34**, 1522 (1942). Monograph: M. Brin, R. H. Dunlop, "Chemistry and Metabolism of L- and D-Lactic Acids" in *Ann. N.Y. Acad. Sci.* **119**, 851-1165 (1965).

Crystals from acetic acid or chloroform, mp 53°. $[\alpha]_{546.1}^{21-22}$ +2.6° (c = 2.5). pK at 25°, 3.79. Forms salts with many metals. The salts are more sol in water than the salts of the racemic acid. Most of the salts are levorotatory.

Zinc L(−)-lactate dihydrate. $Zn(C_3H_5O_3)_2.2H_2O$. Prisms. $[\alpha]_D^{25}$ −8.2° (c = 2.5 in water).

5338. Lactic Acid Homopolymer. [26023-30-3]; [26161-42-2] (L-form); [26917-25-9] (D-form). Poly[oxy(1-methyl-2-oxo-1,2-ethanediyl)]; poly(lactic acid); PLA; EcoPLA; Lacea; Lactron; Lacty. Biodegradable thermoplastic polymer which can be derived from entirely renewable resources; degrades *in vivo* to lactic acid. Prepn: W. H. Carothers *et al.*, *J. Am. Chem. Soc.* **54**, 761 (1932); J. Kleine, H.-H. Kleine, *Makromol. Chem.* **30**, 23 (1959). Synthesis of L-form by lactide ring-opening polymerization: H. R. Kricheldorf, S.-R. Lee, *Polymer* **36**, 2995 (1995); by lactic acid melt/solid polycondensation: R. Miyoshi *et al.*, *Int. Polym. Process.* **11**, 320 (1996); S.-I. Moon *et al.*, *High Perform. Polym.* **13**, S189 (2001). Kinetics and mechanism of ring-opening polymerization: W. Dittrich, R. C. Schulz, *Angew. Makromol. Chem.* **15**, 109 (1971). Comparison of properties from different synthetic methods: M. Ajioka *et al.*, *J. Environ. Polym. Degrad.* **3**, 225 (1995). Compar-

Consult the Name Index before using this section.

ison of melt-spun and solution-spun L-form fibers: B. Eling *et al.,* *Polymer* **23,** 1587 (1982). Thermal properties: K. Jamshidi *et al.,* *ibid.* **29,** 2229 (1988). ^{13}C solid state NMR study of crystallinity and morphology: K. A. M. Thakur *et al., Macromolecules* **29,** 8844 (1996). ^{1}H NMR determn of lactide composition: *idem et al.,* *Anal. Chem.* **69,** 4303 (1997). Study to assess potential use in surgical implants: R. K. Kulkarni *et al., Arch. Surg.* **93,** 839 (1966). Brief reviews: M. Matsui, *Chem. Fibers Int.* **46,** 318-319 (1996); M. Dartee *et al., ibid.* **50,** 546, 548, 551 (2000). Review of properties and uses: M. Vert *et al., J. Macromol. Sci.-Pure Appl. Chem.* **A32,** 787-796 (1995); of material design systems: M. Spinu *et al., ibid.* **A33,** 1497-1530 (1996); of biocompatibility and clinical orthopaedic applications: K. A. Athanasiou *et al., Biomaterials* **17,** 93-102 (1996); of mfr, properties and commercial applications: J. Lunt, *Polym. Degrad. Stab.* **59,** 145-152 (1998); of use in drug delivery with polyglycolide: R. A. Jain, *ibid.* **21,** 2475-2490 (2000).

$$* \overset{\displaystyle CH_3 \quad O}{{-}O{-}CH{-}C{-}} *$$

Glassy material. mp 175°. Glass transition temperature: 55-60°. d 1.25 g/cm[3]. *n* 1.45. Contact angle: 0.254.

USE: In packaging (primarily food), biomedical, film and fiber applications.

5339. Lactic Acid Lactate. [617-57-2] 2-Hydroxypropanoic acid 1-carboxyethyl ester; 2-(lactoyloxy)propanoic acid; 2-(2-hydroxypropanoyloxy)propanoic acid. $C_6H_{10}O_5$; mol wt 162.14. C 44.45%, H 6.22%, O 49.34%. Prepd by heating lactic acid at 120° for 10 hours: Dietzel, Krug, *Ber.* **58,** 1307 (1925).

HOOC–CH(CH_3)–O–CO–CH(OH)–CH_3

Pale yellow, clear, odorless oil. Sol in water and in the usual organic solvents.

Methyl ester. $C_7H_{12}O_5$. Prepn: Claborn, **US 2371281** (1945 to the people of the U.S.). bp$_{7.8}$ 107°; n_D^{20} 1.4313.

USE: The methyl ester as a solvent or plasticizer.

5340. Lactitol. [585-86-4] 4-O-β-D-Galactopyranosyl-D-glucitol; β-galactoside sorbitol; lactit; lactit M; lactite; lactobiosit; lactosit; lactositol. $C_{12}H_{24}O_{11}$; mol wt 344.31. C 41.86%, H 7.03%, O 51.11%. Polyol sweetener; relative sweetness compared to sucrose is 36%. Prepd by hydrogenation of lactose, *q.v.*: M. J. B. Senderens, *Compt. Rend.* **170,** 47 (1920); M. L. Wolfrom *et al., J. Am. Chem. Soc.* **60,** 571 (1938). Pharmacology: D. H. Patil *et al., Br. J. Nutr.* **57,** 195 (1987). Crystal structure: J. A. Kanters *et al., Acta Crystallogr.* **C46,** 2408 (1990); J. Kivikoski *et al., Carbohydr. Res.* **223,** 45 (1992). Toxicology: E. J. Sinkeldam *et al., J. Am. Coll. Toxicol.* **11,** 165 (1992). Clinical trial in chronic hepatic encephalopathy: O. Riggio *et al., Hepatogastroenterology* **37,** 524 (1990); as a laxative: L. Goovaerts, G. P. Ravelli, *Acta Ther.* **19,** 61 (1993). Review of properties and applications: J. A. van Velthuijsen, *J. Agric. Food Chem.* **27,** 680-686 (1979); of chemistry and use in foods: C. H. den Uyl, *Dev. Sweeteners* **3,** 65-81 (1987).

Crystals from absolute ethanol, mp 146°. $[\alpha]_D^{23}$ +14° (c = 4 in water). Sol in water, dimethyl sulfoxide, *N,N*-dimethylformamide; slightly sol in ethanol, ether. Strongly hygroscopic.

Monohydrate. [81025-04-9] Importal; Portolac. White, sweet, odorless, crystalline solid. Non-hygroscopic. mp 94-97° (van Velthuijsen), water of crystallization evaporates 145°-185°;

also reported as mp 120° (den Uyl). $[\alpha]_D^{22}$ +12.3°. Soly at 25° (g/100 g solvent): water 206; ethanol 0.75; ether 0.4; DMSO 233; DMF 39; at 50°: water 512; ethanol 0.88; at 75°: water 917.

Dihydrate. [81025-03-8] Lacty. White, sweet, odorless, crystalline powder. Data for food grade, mp 75°. $[\alpha]_D^{25}$ +13.5-15.0°. pH of 10% solution 4.5 - 8.5. 140 g will dissolve in 100 ml water at 25°.

USE: Sweetener in food.

THERAP CAT: Laxative. In treatment of hepatic encephalopathy.

5341. Lactobacillic Acid. [19625-10-6] 2-Hexylcyclopropanedecanoic acid; 11,12-methyleneoctadecanoic acid; phytomonic acid. $C_{19}H_{36}O_2$; mol wt 296.49. C 76.97%, H 12.24%, O 10.79%. A lipid constituent of various microorganisms. Isoln from *Lactobacillus arabinosus*: K. Hofmann, R. A. Lucas, *J. Am. Chem. Soc.* **72,** 4328 (1950); from *Agrobacterium tumefaciens* and identity of phytomonic acid with lactobacillic acid: K. Hofmann, F. Tausig, *J. Biol. Chem.* **213,** 425 (1955). Structure: K. Hofmann *et al., J. Am. Chem. Soc.* **80,** 5717 (1958). Abs config: J. F. Tocanne, *Tetrahedron* **28,** 363 (1972).

H_3C–(chain)–cyclopropane–$(CH_2)_8$COOH

Crystals from acetone, mp 27.8-28.8°. Soluble in acetone, petr ether.

Methyl ester. $C_{20}H_{38}O_2$. Liq, bp$_3$ 187-187.5°. Soluble in many fat solvents.

Amide. Lactobacillamide. $C_{19}H_{37}NO$. Crystals, mp 79.4-81.5°. Soluble in dimethylformamide.

5342. Lactobionic Acid. [96-82-2] 4-O-β-D-Galactopyranosyl-D-gluconic acid; 4-(β-D-galactosido)-D-gluconic acid. $C_{12}H_{22}O_{12}$; mol wt 358.30. C 40.23%, H 6.19%, O 53.58%. Obtained by oxidation of lactose: Fischer, Meyer, *Ber.* **22,** 362 (1889); Ruff, Ollendorff, *ibid.* **33,** 1806 (1900); Isbell, *J. Res. Natl. Bur. Stand.* **11,** 713 (1933); Margariello, **US 2746916** (1956 to Nat. Dairy Res. Labs.); Eddy, *Nature* **181,** 904 (1958); Nishizuka *et al., J. Biol. Chem.* **235,** PC13 (1960). Manuf from lactose: Y. Sato *et al.,* **DE 2038230** (1971 to Hayashibara Co.), *C.A.* **74,** 142296c (1971). Crystal structure of calcium salt: W. J. Cook, C. E. Bugg, *Acta Crystallogr.* **B29,** 215 (1973). NMR studies: T. Taga *et al., Bull. Chem. Soc. Jpn.* **51,** 2278 (1978). For therapeutic use *see* Erythromycin Lactobionate.

COOH
H–C–OH
HO–C–H
H–C–OH
H–C–OH
CH_2OH (with galactopyranosyl ring)

Syrup. Freely sol in water, slightly sol in methanol, ethanol, glacial acetic acid. Dehydration by distillation with dioxane yields *lactobionic δ-lactone*, $C_{12}H_{20}O_{11}$, non-deliquescent crystals, dec 195-196°. Shows mutarotation. $[\alpha]_D^{20}$ +53.0° initial (c = 8.8) → $[\alpha]_D^{20}$ +22.6° final (240 minutes).

Calcium salt. Calcium lactobionate. $C_{24}H_{42}CaO_{24}$. Pentahydrate, hairlike needles in brushlike groups. When anhydr, slender needles from small amts of anhydr ethanol. $[\alpha]_D^{20}$ +23.7° (c = 6.28). n_D^{20} 1.4583 (concd syrup just before crystallization). Freely sol in water.

5343. Lactose. [63-42-3] 4-O-β-D-Galactopyranosyl-D-glucose; 4-(β-D-galactosido)-D-glucose; milk sugar. $C_{12}H_{22}O_{11}$; mol wt 342.30. C 42.11%, H 6.48%, O 51.41%. Present in milk of mammals: human 6.7%; cow's 4.5%. Milk at body temp contains lactose as an equilibrium mixture of 2 parts of α-lactose and 3 parts of β-lactose. By-product of the cheese industry, produced from whey: Davis, *Can. Dairy and Ice Cream J.* **19,** 52 (1940); *Milk Trade Gaz.* **12,** 4 (1941); F. Ullmann, *Encyklopädie der Technischen*

Chemie, **VII**, 579 (2nd ed., 1931). Structure and configuration: Zemplén, *Ber.* **59**, 2402 (1926); Levene, Sobotka, *J. Biol. Chem.* **71**, 471 (1926); Levene, Wintersteiner, *ibid.* **75**, 315 (1927); Haworth, Long, *J. Chem. Soc.* **1927**, 544; Hudson, *J. Am. Chem. Soc.* **52**, 1712 (1930); Hassid, Ballou in *The Carbohydrates*, W. Pigman, Ed. (Academic Press, New York, 1957) p 495. Synthesis: Haskins *et al., J. Am. Chem. Soc.* **64**, 1852 (1942). *Reviews:* Whittier, *Chem. Rev.* **2**, 85-125 (1926); *J. Dairy Sci.* **27**, 505-537 (1944); Weisberg, *ibid.* **37**, 1106-1115 (1954); L. A. W. Thelwall, *Dev. Food Carbohydr.* **2**, 275-326 (1980). Comprehensive description: H. G. Brittain *et al., Anal. Profiles Drug Subs.* **20**, 369-398 (1991).

On hydrolysis with 2% H_2SO_4 or with emulsin lactose yields 1 mol D-glucose and 1 mol D-galactose. Reduces Fehling's soln.

α-Lactose monohydrate. Is the usual milk sugar and the lactose of pharmacy. Monoclinic sphenoidal crystals from water. Faintly sweet taste. Stable in air, but readily absorbs odors. d^{20} 1.53. Becomes anhydrous at 120°. mp 201-202° (rapid heating). Shows mutarotation. $[\alpha]_D^{20}$ +92.6° → +83.5° (10 min.) → +69° (50 min) → +52.3° (22 hrs, c = 4.5). The final value is obtained instantly in the presence of a trace of NH_3. U.S.P. requires +54.4° to +55.9° (c = 10). One gram dissolves in 5 ml water, in 2.6 ml boiling water; very slightly sol in alcohol. Insol in chloroform, ether. Ka at 16.5° = 6.0×10^{-13}. d_4^{20} of aq solns calcd for the monohydrate: 5.2% = 1.018; 10.2% = 1.038; 20.0% = 1.078; 30.2% = 1.123; 50.9% = 1.226; 60.8% = 1.281; 69.1% = 1.330.

β-Lactose. $C_{12}H_{22}O_{11}$. Obtained by crystallizing concd solns of α-lactose above 93.5°. Somewhat sweeter than the α-form. $[\alpha]_D^{25}$ +34° (3 min) → +39° (6 min) → +46° (1 hr) → +52.3° (22 hrs). One gram dissolves in 2.2 ml water at 15°, in 1.1 ml boiling water. After a few days crystals of the less sol α-monohydrate appear from satd solns.

USE: Both forms of lactose are employed, with the α-form predominating: as a nutrient in preparing modified milk and food for infants and convalescents (Whittier). In baking mixtures. Pharmaceutic aid (tablet and capsule excipient and diluent). To produce lactic acid fermentation in ensilage and food products. As chromatographic adsorbent in analytical chemistry. In culture media. For many additional uses *see* Weisberg.

THERAP CAT (VET): Added to cow's milk for feeding orphan foals.

5344. Lactucarium. Lettuce opium. Dried milky juice or latex of several species of lettuce, primarily *Lactuca virosa* L., Asteraceae (wild lettuce); garden lettuce, *L. sativa* L., and related species, *L. serriola* and *L. sagittata* have also been used. Thought to possess sleep-inducing and pyschotropic properties. *Constit.* Lactucin, lactucopicrin, lactucerol, lactucic acid. Brief description: V. E. Tyler in *The Honest Herbal* (Pharmaceutical Products Press, New York, 3rd ed.) pp 193-195.

Similar to opium in odor, taste and appearance.

5345. Lactucin. [1891-29-8] [3a*R*-(3aα,4β,9aα,9bβ)]-3,3a,-4,5,9a,9b-Hexahydro-4-hydroxy-9-(hydroxymethyl)-6-methyl-3-methyleneazuleno[4,5-*b*]furan-2,7-dione. $C_{15}H_{16}O_5$; mol wt 276.28. C 65.21%, H 5.84%, O 28.96%. From various *Lactuca* spp and *Cichorium intybus* L., *Compositae*. Isoln: Schenck, Graf, *Arch. Pharm.* **274**, 537 (1936); **275**, 36 (1937); Schenck *et al., ibid.* **294**, 17 (1961). Purification: Späth *et al., Monatsh. Chem.* **82**, 114 (1951). Structure: Dolejs *et al., Collect. Czech. Chem. Commun.* **23**, 2195 (1958); Barton, Narayanan, *J. Chem. Soc.* **1958**, 963; Michl, Högenauer, *Monatsh. Chem.* **89**, 317 (1958). Revised stereochemistry: Bachelor, Itô, *Can. J. Chem.* **51**, 3626 (1973).

Crystals from methanol, sinters at 218°, mp 228-233°. $[\alpha]_D$ +49° (c = 0.90 in methanol), +77.9° (c = 3.44 in pyridine). uv max: 257 nm (ε 14,000). Soluble in water, ethanol, methanol, ethyl acetate, dioxane anisol.

p-Hydroxyphenylacetate hydrate. Intybin; lactucopicrin. $C_{23}H_{22}O_7$. Identity with intybin: Schmitt, *Bot. Arch.* **40**, 516 (1940), *C.A.* **36**, 5616 (1942). Structure: Michl, Högenauer, *Monatsh. Chem.* **91**, 500 (1960). Crystals from water, dec 148-151°. $[\alpha]_D^{17.5}$ +67.3° (pyridine).

5346. Lactulose. [4618-18-2] 4-*O*-β-D-Galactopyranosyl-D-fructose; 4-D-galactopyranosyl-4-D-fructofuranose; 4-*O*-β-D-galactosyl-D-fructose; 4-β-D-galactosido-D-fructose; Cephulac; Cholac; Constilac; Duphalac; Generlac; Lactuflor; Laevilac; Normase. $C_{12}H_{22}O_{11}$; mol wt 342.30. C 42.11%, H 6.48%, O 51.41%. Prebiotic, synthetic disaccharide composed of galactose and fructose. Prepn: E. M. Montgomery, C. S. Hudson, *J. Am. Chem. Soc.* **52**, 2101 (1930); Oosten, *Rec. Trav. Chim.* **86**, 673 (1967); K. B. Hicks, F. W. Parrish, *Carbohydr. Res.* **82**, 393 (1980). Clinical evaluation of effects on fecal bifidobacteria and selected metabolic indices: Y. Bouhnik *et al., Eur. J. Clin. Nutr.* **58**, 462 (2004).

Hexagonal clustered plates from methanol, mp 168-171°. Sweeter than lactose, but not as sweet as sucrose. Shows mutarotation; constant value after 24 hrs: $[\alpha]_D^{22}$ −51.5°. Soly in water (w/w) at 30°: 76.4%; at 60°: 81%; at 90°: >86%. Acid hydrolysis yields galactose and fructose.

THERAP CAT: Laxative.

5347. Lafutidine. [118288-08-7] 2-[(2-Furanylmethyl)-sulfinyl]-*N*-[(2*Z*)4-[[4-(1-piperidinylmethyl)-2-pyridinyl]oxy]-2-butenyl]-acetamide; 2-(furfurylsulfinyl)-*N*-[(*Z*)-4-[[4-(piperidinomethyl)-2-pyridyl]oxy]-2-butenyl]acetamide; FRG-8813; Protecadin; Stogar. $C_{22}H_{29}N_3O_4S$; mol wt 431.55. C 61.23%, H 6.77%, N 9.74%, O 14.83%, S 7.43%. Second generation histamine H_2-receptor antagonist. Prepn of racemate: N. Hirakawa *et al., EP 282077; eidem, US 4912101* (1988, 1990 both to Fujirebio); and pharmacology: *eidem, Chem. Pharm. Bull.* **46**, 616 (1998). Pharmacology: S. Onodera *et al., Jpn. J. Pharmacol.* **68**, 161 (1995). Mode of action study: M. Umeda *et al., J. Gastroenterol. Hepatol.* **14**, 859 (1999). Gastroprotective effects in rats: H. Ajioka *et al., Pharmacology* **61**, 83 (2000). Clinical pharmacokinetics: S. Haruki *et al., Yakuri to Chiryo* **23**, 3049 (1995). Toxicology study: A. Broadmeadow *et al., Oyo Yakuri* **50**, 167 (1995).

Prepd as the (±) mixture, crystals from benzene-hexane, mp 92.7-94.9°. Slightly bitter taste. Freely sol in DMF, glacial acetic acid; sol in methanol; sparingly sol in dehydrated ethanol; very slightly sol in ether. Practically insol in water.

THERAP CAT: Antiulcerative.

5348. Laidlomycin. [56283-74-0] 16-Deethyl-3-*O*-demethyl-16-methyl-3-*O*-(1-oxopropyl)monensin. $C_{37}H_{62}O_{12}$; mol wt 698.88. C 63.59%, H 8.94%, O 27.47%. Polyether ionophore antibiotic; structurally related to monensin, *q.v.* Isoln from *Streptomyces spp.* and antimicrobial activity: F. Kitame *et al., J. Antibiot.* **27**, 884 (1974). Structure determn: F. Kitame, N. Ishida, *ibid.* **29**, 759 (1976). Prepn of esters: A. F. Kluge, R. D. Clark, **EP 24189** (1981 to Syntex). ^{13}C-NMR study and enhancement of biological activities: R. D. Clark *et al., J. Antibiot.* **35**, 1527 (1982). Mechanism of action study: U. Gräfe *et al., J. Basic Microbiol.* **29**, 391 (1989). HPLC determn in fermentation broth: M. Beran *et al., Chromatographia* **31**, 603 (1991). Effect on cattle growth: M. T. Van Koevering *et al., 1991 Animal Science Research*

Report (Agricultural Experiment Station, Oklahoma State University, Stillwater, OK, 1991) 241; M. L. Galyean *et al., J. Anim. Sci.* **70**, 2950 (1992).

Colorless prisms from chloroform-ethyl acetate. mp 151-153°. $[\alpha]_D^{22}$ +51.3° (c=0.2 in $CHCl_3$). Sol in $CHCl_3$, acetone, alcohols. Insol in water, *n*-hexane. LD_{50} in mice (mg/kg): 5 i.p.; 1 i.v.; 2.5 s.c. (Kitame).

Propionate potassium. [84799-02-0] RS-11988; Cattlyst. $C_{40}H_{65}KO_{13}$; mol wt 793.03. mp 190-192°.

THERAP CAT (VET): Growth promotant.

5349. Lamifiban. [144412-49-7] (*S*)-[[1-[2-[[4-(Aminoiminomethyl)benzoyl]amino]-3-(4-hydroxyphenyl)-1-oxopropyl]-4-piperidinyl]oxy]acetic acid; [[1-[*N*-(*p*-amidinobenzoyl)-L-tyrosyl]-4-piperidinyl]oxy]acetic acid; Ro-44-9883. $C_{24}H_{28}N_4O_6$; mol wt 468.50. C 61.53%, H 6.02%, N 11.96%, O 20.49%. Specific nonpeptide platelet fibrinogen receptor (GPIIb/IIIa) antagonist. Prepn: L. Alig *et al.*, EP 505868; *eidem*, US 5378712 (1992, 1995 both to Hoffmann-La Roche); L. Alig *et al., J. Med. Chem.* **35**, 4393 (1992). Pharmacology: J.-P. Carteaux *et al., Thromb. Haemostasis* **70**, 817 (1993); Y. Takiguchi *et al., ibid.* **73**, 683 (1995).

Crystals (zwitterionic form) from water, mp above 200° (dec). $[\alpha]_D^{20}$ +29.8° (c = 0.86 in 1*N* HCl).

Trifluoroacetate salt. [144412-50-0] $C_{24}H_{28}N_4O_6 \cdot C_2HF_3O_2$. mp 125-130° (dec). LD_{50} i.v. in mice: 250 mg/kg (Alig, 1995).

THERAP CAT: Antithrombotic.

5350. Laminaran. [9008-22-4] Laminarin. A polysaccharide found in brown seaweed and occurring principally in the *Laminaria* spp. Linear polymer composed of β-(1 → 3)-linked glucose residues; may contain small amounts of β-(1 → 6) linkages as interresidue linkages or as branch points and 2-3% D-mannitol as end groups. Two forms of laminaran are recognized; they are referred to as soluble and insoluble laminaran: Percival, Ross, *J. Chem. Soc.* **1951**, 720. Structure: Peat *et al., ibid.* **1958**, 724, 729; **1960**, 175; Goldstein *et al., Chem. Ind. (London)* **1959**, 124; Annan *et al., ibid.* **1962**, 984; Annan *et al., J. Chem. Soc.* **1965**, 885; Maeda, Nisizawa, *Carbohyd. Res.* **7**, 97 (1968). Structure of soluble laminaran from *Eisenia bicyclis*: T. Usui *et al., Agric. Biol. Chem.* **43**, 603 (1979). NMR studies of laminaran: D. Gagnaire, *Org. Magn. Reson.* **11**, 344 (1978); H. Friebolin *et al., ibid.* **12**, 216 (1979). *Review*: W. A. P. Black, E. T. Dewar in *Industrial Gums*, R. L. Whistler, Ed. (Academic Press, New York, 2nd ed., 1973) pp 137-145.

Water-insoluble laminaran. Isolated from *L. cloustoni* Edmondst., *Laminariaceae,* is pptd spontaneously from the aq acid extract of the plant. Has lower degree of branching than the sol form. Typical analysis of the dry material: 92.5% polyglucose, 0.4% non-volatile matter; $[\alpha]_D^{16}$ −13.4° (c = 0.9). Amorphous triacetate, $(C_{12}H_{16}O_8)_n$, $[\alpha]_D^{16}$ −63.5° (c = 0.4 in chloroform).

Soluble form. Isolated from *L. digitata,* is separated from the acidified extract only after addition of a precipitant such as ethanol. Typical analysis (on dry basis): 91.2% polyglucose, 1.0% nonvolatile matter; $[\alpha]_D^{18}$ −11.9° (c = 2.1).

Sulfate. Laminaran hydrogen sulfate. Laminaran can be sulfated to varying degrees. Highly sulfated products have anticoagulant properties comparable to heparin, while laminarans with few sulfate groups are antilipemic only: Besterman, Evans, *Br. Med. J.* **I**, 310 (1957).

5351. Laminin. Abundant structural component of the basal lamina; critical to the stability of the extracellular matrix and to the adhesion of cells to the basement membrane. Family of heterotrimeric glycoproteins composed of a heavy chain, designated α (also known as A) and 2 light chains, designated β (B1) and γ (B2), which are linked by disulfide bonds to form an asymmetrical cross-shaped structure. Eight genetically distinct laminin subunits have been identified: α1, α2, α3, β1, β2, β3, γ1, and γ2. Seven different assembly forms (laminins-1 to -7) are known and appear to be tissue specific and developmentally regulated. Exhibits diverse biological activities. Influences adhesion, growth, morphology and differentiation of a variety of cells via specific receptors including several of the integrin type. Isoln from murine Engelbreth-Holm-Swarm (EHS) tumor: R. Timpl *et al., J. Biol. Chem.* **254**, 9933 (1979). Review of biological activities: H. K. Kleinman *et al., J. Cell. Biochem.* **27**, 317-325 (1985); of role in neural development: V. Nurcombe, *Pharmacol. Ther.* **56**, 247 (1992). Tissue distribution: E. Engvall *et al., Cell Regul.* **1**, 731 (1990). Review of laminin binding proteins and receptors: R. P. Mecham, *Annu. Rev. Cell Biol.* **7**, 71-91 (1991); and role in metastasis: V. Castronovo, *Invasion Metastasis* **13**, 1-30 (1993). Structure and function of laminin isoforms: E. Engvall, *Kidney Int.* **43**, 2-6 (1993); K. Tryggvason, *Curr. Opin. Cell Biol.* **5**, 877-882 (1993). Nomenclature: R. E. Burgeson *et al., Matrix Biol.* **14**, 209 (1994). Review of structure: R. Timpl, J. C. Brown, *ibid.* 275-281.

Laminin-1. EHS-laminin. Prototype laminin produced by murine EHS tumor. Contains α1 (also known as A or Ae), β1 (B1, B1e) and γ1 (B2, B2e) subunits.

Laminin-2. Merosin; laminin M. Variant found in striated muscle, placental trophoblast and Schwann cell basement membranes. Contains α2 (also known as M or Am), β1 and γ1 subunits. Identification: I. Leivo, E. Engvall, *Proc. Natl. Acad. Sci. USA* **85**, 1544 (1988); K. Ehrig *et al., ibid.* **87**, 3264 (1990).

Laminin-3. S-laminin; synaptic laminin. Contains α1, β2 (also known as s or B1s), and γ1 chains. Identification in neuromuscular junction: D. D. Hunter *et al., Nature* **338**, 229 (1989).

Laminin-5. Kallinin; nicein. Contains α3, β3, and γ2 subunits. Isoln from human keratinocytes: P. Rousselle *et al., J. Cell Biol.* **114**, 567 (1991). Review of role in progression of cancer: J. Lohi, *Int. J. Cancer* **94**, 763-767 (2001).

5352. Lamivudine. [134678-17-4] (2*R-cis*)-4-Amino-1-[2-(hydroxymethyl)-1,3-oxathiolan-5-yl]-2(1*H*)-pyrimidinone; (−)-2′-deoxy-3′-thiacytidine; (−)-1-[(2*R*,5*S*)-2-(hydroxymethyl)-1,3-oxathiolan-5-yl]cystosine; 3′-thia-2′,3′-dideoxycytidine; 3TC; (−)-BCH-189; GR-109714X; Epivir; Zeffix. $C_8H_{11}N_3O_3S$; mol wt 229.26. C 41.91%, H 4.84%, N 18.33%, O 20.94%, S 13.99%. Reverse transcriptase inhibitor. Prepn: J. A. V. Coates *et al.*, WO 9117159 *C.A.* **117**, 111989 (1991). Synthesis of enantiomers: J. W. Beach *et al., J. Org. Chem.* **57**, 2217 (1992); of (−)-enantiomer: D. C. Humber *et al., Tetrahedron Lett.* **33**, 4625 (1992). HPLC determn in urine: D. M. Morris, K. Selinger, *J. Pharm. Biomed. Anal.* **12**, 255 (1994). Clinical trial in hepatitis B: F. Nevens *et al., Gastroenterology* **113**, 1258 (1997). Review of pharmacology and clinical efficacy in HIV infection: C. M. Perry, D. Faulds, *Drugs* **53**, 657-680 (1997).

Crystals from boiling ethanol. mp 160-162°. $[\alpha]_D^{21}$ −135° (c = 0.38 in methanol). Soly in water (20°): ~70 mg/ml.

THERAP CAT: Antiviral.

5353. Lamotrigine. [84057-84-1] 6-(2,3-Dichlorophenyl)-1,2,4-triazine-3,5-diamine; 3,5-diamino-6-(2,3-dichlorophenyl)-1,2,4-triazine; LTG; BW-430C; Lamictal. $C_9H_7Cl_2N_5$; mol wt 256.09. C 42.21%, H 2.76%, Cl 27.69%, N 27.35%. Prepn: M. G. Baxter et al., **EP 21121** (1981 to Wellcome Foundation); D. A. Sawyer et al., **US 4602017** (1986). HPLC determn in plasma: C.-L. Cheng et al., J. Chromatogr. B **817**, 199 (2005). Anticonvulsant activity: A. A. Miller et al., Epilepsia **27**, 483 (1986). Mechanism of action studies: M. J. Leach et al., ibid. 490; X. Xie, R. M. Hagan, Neuropsychobiology **38**, 119 (1998). Series of articles on clinical pharmacology, antiepileptic efficacy and safety: Epilepsia **32**, Suppl. 2, S1-S21 (1991). Clinical trial in bipolar depression: J. R. Calabrese et al., J. Clin. Psychiatry **60**, 79 (1999). Review of clinical experience in epilepsy: H. Choi, M. J. Morrell, Expert Opin. Pharmacother. **4**, 243-251 (2003); in bipolar disorder: Z. Bhagwagar, G. M. Goodwin, Expert Opin. Pharmacother. **6**, 1401-1408 (2005).

White to pale cream-colored powder. Crystals from isopropanol, mp 216-218° (uncorr). pKa 5.7. Soly at 25° (mg/ml): water 0.17; 0.1M HCl 4.1. LD_{50} in mice, rats (mg/kg): 250, >640 orally (Sawyer).

THERAP CAT: Anticonvulsant. In treatment of bipolar depression.

5354. Lanatosides. Family of four glycosides, A, B, C, D, isolated from various species of Digitalis including D. lanata Ehrh., Scrophulariaceae: Stoll, Kreis, Helv. Chim. Acta **16**, 1049 (1933); Ligeti, Pharmazie **12**, 433 (1957); **14**, 162 (1959); Angliker et al., Ann. **607**, 131 (1957); D. Lutea L., Scrophulariaceae: Cole, Gisvold, J. Am. Pharm. Assoc. Sci. Ed. **47**, 654 (1958). Structure: Tschesche et al., Ber. **92**, 2258 (1959); Uskert, Ann. **638**, 199 (1960); Kuhn et al., Helv. Chim. Acta **45**, 881 (1962). Absorption spectrum: Bell, J. Am. Pharm. Assoc. Sci. Ed. **49**, 277 (1960). Cardioactivity of lanatoside C: K.-O. Haustein, Pharmacology **11**, 117 (1974). Mitogenicity: L. L. G. Hammarström, C. I. E. Smith, J. Immunol. **120**, 694 (1978). HPLC determn: V. Y. Davydov et al., J. Chromatogr. **248**, 49 (1982); of lanatoside C: F. Orosz et al., Anal. Biochem. **156**, 171 (1986).

Lanatoside A	R = digitoxigenin
Lanatoside B	R = gitoxigenin
Lanatoside C	R = digoxigenin
Lanatoside D	R = diginatigenin

Lanatoside A. [17575-20-1] (3β,5β)-3-[(O-β-D-Glucopyranosyl-(1 → 4)-O-3-O-acetyl-2,6-dideoxy-β-D-ribo-hexopyranosyl-(1 → 4)-O-2,6-dideoxy-β-D-ribo-hexopyranosyl-(1 → 4)-2,6-dideoxy-β-D-ribo-hexopyranosyl)oxy]-14-hydroxycard-20(22)-enolide; digilanide A; Adigal. $C_{49}H_{76}O_{19}$; mol wt 969.12. Long, flat prisms from methanol, dec 245-248°. $[\alpha]_D^{20}$ +31.6° (0.48 g in 25 ml 95% alc); $[\alpha]_D^{20}$ +23.2° (0.95 g in 25 ml dioxane). Soluble in 20

parts methanol, 40 parts alcohol, 225 parts chloroform, 16,000 parts water.

Lanatoside B. [17575-21-2] (3β,5β,16β)-3-[(O-β-D-Glucopyranosyl-(1→4)-O-3-O-acetyl-2,6-dideoxy-β-D-ribo-hexopyranosyl-(1 → 4)-O-2,6-dideoxy-β-D-ribo-hexopyranosyl-(1 →4)-2,6-dideoxy-β-D-ribo-hexopyranosyl)oxy]-14,16-dihydroxycard-20(22)-enolide; digilanide B. $C_{49}H_{76}O_{20}$; mol wt 985.12. Long, flat prisms from alcohol, dec 245-248° after drying in high vacuum at 150°. $[\alpha]_D^{20}$ +36.7° (0.47 g in 25 ml 95% alc); $[\alpha]_D^{20}$ +31.8° (0.25 g in 14.1 ml dioxane). Soluble in 20 parts methanol, 40 parts alcohol, 550 parts chloroform. Nearly insol in water.

Lanatoside C. [17575-22-3] (3β,5β,12β)-3-[(O-β-D-Glucopyranosyl-(1→4)-O-3-O-acetyl-2,6-dideoxy-β-D-ribo-hexopyranosyl-(1 → 4)-O-2,6-dideoxy-β-D-ribo-hexopyranosyl-(1 →4)-2,6-dideoxy-β-D-ribo-hexopyranosyl)oxy]-12,14-dihydroxycard-20(22)-enolide; digilanide C; Allocor; Cedilanid; Ceglunat; Celadigal; Cetosanol; Lanimerck. $C_{49}H_{76}O_{20}$; mol wt 985.12. Long, flat prisms from alcohol, dec 248-250°, after drying in vacuum at 150°. $[\alpha]_D^{20}$ +33.4 to +33.7° (200 mg dry weight in 10 ml alcohol). One gram dissolves in 20,000 ml methanol, in 2000 ml chloroform. Freely sol in pyridine, dioxane. Practically insol in ether, petr ether.

Lanatoside D. [11030-31-2] (3β,5β,12β,16β)-3-[(O-β-D-Glucopyranosyl-(1 → 4)-O-3-O-acetyl-2,6-dideoxy-β-D-ribo-hexopyranosyl-(1 → 4)-O-2,6-dideoxy-β-D-ribo-hexopyranosyl-(1 → 4)-2,6-dideoxy-β-D-ribo-hexopyranosyl)oxy]-12,14,16-trihydroxycard-20(22)-enolide; digilanide D. $C_{49}H_{76}O_{21}$; mol wt 1001.12. Needles from methanol and water, dec 242-250°. $[\alpha]_D^{20}$ +40.5° (c = 5.95 in methanol). uv max: 220 nm (log ε 4.16).

THERAP CAT: Cardiotonic.

5355. Landiolol. [133242-30-5] 4-[(2S)-2-Hydroxy-3-[[2-[(4-morpholinylcarbonyl)amino]ethyl]amino]propoxy]benzenepropanoic acid [(4S)-2,2-dimethyl-1,3-dioxolan-4-yl]methyl ester; (−)-2,2-dimethyl-1,3-dioxolan-4S-ylmethyl 3-[4-[3-[2-(morpholinocarbonylamino)ethylamino]-2S-hydroxypropoxy]phenyl]propionate. $C_{25}H_{39}N_3O_8$; mol wt 509.59. C 58.92%, H 7.71%, N 8.25%, O 25.12%. Cardioselective β-adrenergic blocker. Prepn: S. Iguchi et al., **EP 397031**; **US 5013734** (1990, 1991 both to Ono Pharm.); idem et al., Chem. Pharm. Bull. **40**, 462 (1992). Electrophysiology: A. Sugiyama et al., J. Cardiovasc. Pharmacol. **34**, 70 (1999). Clinical pharmacology: A. Kitamura et al., Eur. J. Clin. Pharmacol. **51**, 467 (1997). Clinical pharmacokinetics in patients with cardiac tachyarrhythmias: H. Atarashi et al., Clin. Pharmacol. Ther. **68**, 143 (2000).

Hydrochloride. [144481-98-1] ONO-1101; Onoact. $C_{25}H_{39}$-N_3O_8·HCl; mol wt 546.05. mp 125.4°. LD_{50} in mice (mg/kg): 290 i.v. (Iguchi).

THERAP CAT: Antiarrhythmic.

5356. Lankamycin. [30042-37-6] Kujimycin B. $C_{42}H_{72}$-O_{16}; mol wt 833.01. C 60.56%, H 8.71%, O 30.73%. Macrolide antibiotic produced by Streptomyces violaceoniger from soil of Ceylon. Isolation: Gaumann et al., Helv. Chim. Acta **43**, 601 (1960). Yields on hydrolysis an aglucone, monoacetyllankolid, $C_{26}H_{48}O_{10}$, and two sugar-like substances, lankavose (D-chalcose, q.v.) and acetylarcanose: Keller-Schierlein, Roncari, ibid. **45**, 138 (1962). Structure: eidem, ibid. **47**, 78 (1964); Egan, Martin, J. Am. Chem. Soc. **92**, 4129 (1970). Stereochemistry: Muntwyler, Keller-Schierlein, Helv. Chim. Acta **55**, 460 (1972). Identity with kujimycin B: Omura et al., J. Antibiot. **22**, 629 (1969).

Consult the Name Index before using this section.

Crystals from ether + petr ether. Double mp, 147-150° and 181-182°. $[\alpha]_D^{20}$ −94° (c = 1.23 in alc.). uv max: 289 nm (log ε 1.50).

5357. Lanoconazole. [101530-10-3] (E)-(±)-α-[4-(2-Chlorophenyl)-1,3-dithiolan-2-ylidene]-1H-imidazole-1-acetonitrile; latoconazole; TJN-318; NND-318; Astat. $C_{14}H_{10}ClN_3S_2$; mol wt 319.83. C 52.57%, H 3.15%, Cl 11.08%, N 13.14%, S 20.05%. Prepn: A. Soe et al., **JP Kokai 85 218387**; idem et al., **US 4636519** (1985, 1987 both to Nihon Nohyaku). In vivo antifungal activity: H. Oka et al., Arzneim.-Forsch. **42**, 345 (1992); Y. Niwano et al., Antimicrob. Agents Chemother. **38**, 2204 (1994). Toxicity study: P. L. Munt et al., Oyo Yakuri **43**, 195 (1992).

Light yellow crystals, mp 141.5°. LD_{50} in male, female mice, rats (mg/kg): 3224, 2715, 993, 652 orally; 2158, 1743, 1655, 2596 i.p.; >5000 both species s.c. LD_{50} dermally in rats: >5000 mg/kg (Munt).

THERAP CAT: Antifungal.

5358. Lanolin. [8006-54-0] Wool fat; anydrous lanolin; Emery 1600. Refined form of wool wax, the unctuous secretion of the sebaceous glands of sheep which is deposited onto the wool fibers. Known since antiquity for its emollient properties. Chemically a wax consisting of a complex mixture of esters and polyesters of lanolin alcohols, q.v., and higher fatty acids, including α- and ω-hydroxy acids. Lanolin can be separated by solvent fractionation into lanolin oil and lanolin wax. Analytical methods: C. W. Spilker, T. B. Richey, Cosmet. Perfum. **88**, 43 (Sept. 1973). Discussion of lanolin allergy: R. Wolf, Dermatology **192**, 198 (1996). Review of prepn, derivatives and uses: G. Barnett, Cosmet. Toiletries **101**, 23-44 (Mar. 1986); J. Thewlis, Agro-Food-Ind. Hi-Tech **8**, no. 3, 14-20 (1997).

Translucent, pale yellow, soft tenacious solid; slight odor or practically odorless. mp 38-42°. Sp gr at 25° 0.935. Iodine no. 27. Hydroxyl no. 32. Practically insol in water. Sparingly sol in cold, more in hot alcohol; freely sol in chloroform, ether.

Hydrous lanolin. Ointment base prepared by the addition of about 25-30% water. Yellowish-white unctuous mass; slight odor. Practically insol in water. Sol in chloroform or ether with the separation of the water.

Acetylated lanolin. [61788-48-5] Acylan; Fancol ACEL; Modulan; Ritacetyl. Prepn: L. I. Conrad, K. Motiuk, J. Soc. Cosmet. Chem. **6**, 344 (1955). Almost odorless, pale yellow, soft, unctuous solid. mp 36°. Sp gr at 25° 0.935. Iodine no. 27. Hydroxyl no. 2. Sol in mineral oils, in some vegetable oils. Readily dispersed in oil-in-water emulsions.

Lanolin oil. Liquid lanolin; dewaxed lanolin; Lanogene; Lantrol 1673; Ritalan. Amber viscous liquid. Odorless, tasteless. Sol in mineral oil. Rich in lower molecular weight, branched aliphatic acids and alcohols.

Lanolin wax. Lanfrax. Light yellow waxy solid. Insol in water; emulsifies in ~3 parts water.

USE: Pharmaceutic aid (ointment base). Emulsifier, emollient, conditioner and lubricant in cosmetics and toiletries.

5359. Lanolin Alcohols. [8027-33-6] Wool alcohols; Amerchol 400; Ceralan; Emery 1780; Eucerin; Fancol LA; Hartolan; Ritawax. Complex combination of organic alcohols obtained by the saponification of lanolin. Composed of monohydric and dihydric aliphatic alcohols and sterols, primarily cholesterol and lanosterol, q.q.v. Prepn: L. I. Conrad, K. Motiuk, J. Soc. Cosmet. Chem. **6**, 344 (1955). Composition: M. L. Schlossman, J. P. McCarthy, Contact Dermatitis **5**, 65 (1979). Clinical evaluation of moisturizing capacity: J. Sindhvananda et al., J. Soc. Cosmet. Chem. **44**, 279 (1993).

Golden-brown solid, plastic when warm, but brittle when cold; faint characteristic odor. mp >56°. Practically insol in water. Very slightly sol in alcohol; sol in ether, chloroform and light petroleum.

Acetylated Lanolin Alcohols. [61788-49-6] Acetulan; Fancol ALA. Pale yellow, practically odorless liquid. Sp gr at 25°: 0.867. Neutral to litmus. Acid no. 0.35. Hydroxyl no. 2.0. Saponification no. 190.0. Hydrophobic, practically insol in water with no emulsification. Miscible with mineral oil, castor oil, vegetable oils, isopropanol, 95% ethanol, isopropyl myristate, isopropyl palmitate, butyl stearate.

USE: Emulsifier, stabilizer, emollient and lubricant in cosmetics, toiletries and pharmaceuticals.

5360. Lanosterol. [79-63-0] (3β)-Lanosta-8,24-dien-3-ol; kryptosterol. $C_{30}H_{50}O$; mol wt 426.72. C 84.44%, H 11.81%, O 3.75%. The core steroid from which all others are derived by biological modification. From wool fat of sheep: Windaus, Tschesche, Z. Physiol. Chem. **190**, 51 (1930). Identity with kryptosterol: Ruzicka et al., Helv. Chim. Acta **28**, 759 (1945). Structure: Voser et al., ibid. **35**, 2414 (1952); Barnes et al., J. Chem. Soc. **1953**, 571. Stereochemistry: eidem, ibid. **1953**, 576. Prepn from isocholesterol: Bloch, Urech, Biochem. Prep. **6**, 32 (1958). Prepn by cyclization of squalene: Cornforth et al., Ciba Found. Symp. Terpenes Sterols **1958**, 119; van Tamelen et al., J. Am. Chem. Soc. **88**, 4752 (1966). Mechanism of the squalene to lanosterol conversion: eidem, ibid. **104**, 6479, 6480 (1982).

Crystals, mp 138-140°. $[\alpha]_D^{20}$ +62.0° (chloroform). .
Lanosteryl acetate. Crystals, mp 131.5-133°, $[\alpha]_D^{20}$ +62.5° (c = 1.12 in chloroform).

5361. Lanreotide. [108736-35-2] 3-(2-Naphthalenyl)-D-alanyl-L-cysteinyl-L-tyrosyl-D-tryptophyl-L-lysyl-L-valyl-L-cysteinyl-L-threoninamide cyclic (2 → 7)-disulfide; angiopeptin; DC 13-116; BIM-23014. $C_{54}H_{69}N_{11}O_{10}S_2$; mol wt 1096.32. C 59.16%, H 6.34%, N 14.05%, O 14.59%, S 5.85%. Octapeptide somatostatin analog. Prepn: D. H. Coy et al., **EP 215171**; eidem, **US 4853371** (1987, 1989 both to Tulane Educational Fund). Clinical pharmacokinetics and hormonal effects: J. M. Kuhn et al., Br. J. Clin. Pharmacol. **38**, 213 (1994). Clinical evaluation in acromegaly: P. Caron et al., Eur. J. Endocrinol. **132**, 320 (1995).

Acetate. [127984-74-1] BIM-23014C; Somatuline LP. C_{54}-$H_{69}N_{11}O_{10}S_2.xC_2H_4O_2$

THERAP CAT: Antineoplastic.

5362. Lansoprazole. [103577-45-3] 2-[[[3-Methyl-4-(2,2,2-trifluoro-ethoxy)-2-pyridinyl]methyl]sulfinyl]-1*H*-benzimidazole; 2-(2-benzimidazolylsulfinylmethyl)-3-methyl-4-(2,2,2-trifluoroethoxy)pyridine; A-65006; AG-1749; Agopton; Lansox; Lanzor; Limpidex; Ogast; Prevacid; Takepron; Zoton. $C_{16}H_{14}F_3N_3$-O_2S; mol wt 369.36. C 52.03%, H 3.82%, F 15.43%, N 11.38%, O 8.66%, S 8.68%. Gastric proton-pump inhibitor. Prepn: A. Nohara, Y. Maki, *EP 174726*; *eidem, US 4628098* (both 1986 to Takeda). HPLC determn in plasma: T. Uno *et al., J. Chromatogr. B 816,* 309 (2005). Pharmacology: H. Satoh *et al., J. Pharmacol. Exp. Ther.* **248,** 806 (1989). Mechanism of action study: H. Nagaya *et al., ibid.* **252,** 1289 (1990). Clinical pharmacology and effect on human gastric acid secretion: P. Müller *et al., Aliment. Pharmacol. Ther.* **3,** 193 (1989). Review of pharmacology and clinical experience: H. D. Langtry, M. I. Wilde, *Drugs* **54,** 473-500 (1997). Comparative clinical trial with esomeprazole in erosive esophagitis: C. W. Howden *et al., Clin. Drug Invest.* **22,** 99 (2002).

mp 178-182° (dec).

THERAP CAT: Antiulcerative.

5363. Lanthanum. [7439-91-0] La; at. wt 138.90547; at. no. 57; valence 3. Group IIIB (3). A rare earth metal; member of the lanthanide series. Naturally occurring isotopes (mass numbers): 139 (99.91%); 138 (0.09%), radioactive, $T_{1/2}$ 1.06×10^{11} years; known artificial radioactive isotopes: 123-137; 140-149. Estimated abundance in earth's crust: 18-35 ppm. Found in association with cerium and other light lanthanons. Sources of commercial importance are the rare earth minerals monazite and bastnaesite; also found in cerite. Discovery and isoln: Mosander, *Pogg. Ann.* **47,** 207 (1839). Sepn: James, *J. Am. Chem. Soc.* **34,** 757 (1912). Prepn of metal: Mazzi, *Atti X Congr. Int. Chim.* **3,** 604 (1938); Spedding *et al., Ind. Eng. Chem.* **44,** 553 (1952). Toxicity study: Cochran *et al., Arch. Ind. Hyg. Occup. Med.* **1,** 637 (1950). Reviews of prepn, properties and compds: *The Rare Earths* F. H. Spedding, A. H. Daane, Eds. (Krieger, Huntington, N.Y., 1971, reprint of 1961 ed.) 641 pp; Hulet, Bode, "Separation Chemistry of the Lanthanides and Transplutonium Actinides" in *MTP Int. Rev. Sci.: Inorg. Chem., Ser. One* Vol. 7, K. W. Bagnall, Ed. (University Park Press, Baltimore, 1972) pp 1-45; Vickery, "Scandium, Yttrium, Lanthanum" in *Comprehensive Inorganic Chemistry* vol. 3, J. C. Bailar Jr. *et al.,* Eds. (Pergamon Press, Oxford, 1973) pp 329-353; Moeller, "The Lanthanides" *ibid.* vol. 4, 1-101; F. H. Spedding in *Kirk-Othmer Encyclopedia of Chemical Technology* vol. 19 (John Wiley & Sons, New York, 3rd ed., 1982) pp 833-854; *Chemistry of the Elements* N. N. Greenwood, A. Earnshaw, Eds. (Pergamon Press, New York, 1984) pp 1102-1110, 1423-1449. Brief review of properties: G. T. Seaborg, *Radiochim. Acta* **61,** 115-122 (1993).

White, malleable metal; tarnishes in air. Three crystalline forms: hexagonal α-form, d 6.162, transforms to β-form at 310°; face-centered cubic β-form, d 6.19, transforms to γ-form at 864°; body-centered cubic γ-form, d 5.97, exists at >864°. mp 920°. bp 3464°. Heat of fusion: 6.201 kJ/mol. Heat of sublimation (25°): 431.0 kJ/mol. E°(aq) La^{3+}/La -2.52 V (calc). Very active; dec water slowly in the cold, more readily on heating. Readily attacked by mineral acids; not attacked by cold concd H_2SO_4. Burns in air at about 450° producing a mixture of oxide and nitride; forms the hydride on heating in hydrogen. Forms alloys with several metals.

Oxide. Lanthana; lanthanum sesquioxide; lanthanum trioxide. La_2O_3. Almost white, amorphous powder. d 6.51. mp >2000°. Insol in water. Sol in dil mineral acids with formation of salts. Absorbs CO_2 from the air.

Hydroxide. La(OH)$_3$. White, amorphous precip, prepd by adding excess of caustic alkali to a lanthanum salt soln. Strongly basic; displaces ammonia from ammonium salts, absorbs CO_2 from air. On dehydration yields $La_2O_3.H_2O$.

Chloride. LaCl$_3$. Heptahydrate, triclinic crystals. Sol in water or alc. On heating in HCl the anhyd salt (mp 852°) is formed. LD$_{50}$ in rats: 4.2 g/kg orally; 350 mg/kg i.p. (Cochran).

Carbonate octahydrate. Artificial lanthanite. $C_3La_2O_9$. White, crystalline powder. Practically insol in water. Freely sol in dil mineral acids.

Sulfate. La$_2$(SO$_4$)$_3$. Nonahydrate, hexagonal prisms. Prepd by treating a lanthanum salt with a slight excess of sulfuric acid. Dec at white heat. Is the least sol of the rare earth sulfates; soly in water decreases with increase in temp. Insol in alc. Forms double salts with alkali or ammonium hydroxide. Anhyd salt prepd by heating hydrate. LD$_{50}$ in rats: >5000 g/kg orally; 275 mg/kg i.p. (Cochran).

Nitrate. La(NO$_3$)$_3$. Hexahydrate, white deliquesc crystals, mp $\sim$40°, at higher temp forms a basic salt. bp 126°. Very sol in water, alc. Forms double salts with bivalent ion nitrates and ammonium nitrates. *Keep well closed.* LD$_{50}$ in rats: 4.5 g/kg orally; 450 mg/kg i.p. (Cochran).

USE: Oxide in glass to improve optical properties. La^{3+} used in experimental biology as a specific antagonist of calcium: Weiss, *Annu. Rev. Pharmacol.* **14,** 343 (1974).

5364. Lanthanum Carbonate. [587-26-8] Carbonic acid lanthanum(3+) salt (3:2); lanthanum sesquicarbonate; Fosrenol; Foznol. $C_3La_2O_9$; mol wt 457.84. C 7.87%, La 60.68%, O 31.45%. La$_2$(CO$_3$)$_3$. Binds dietary phosphate to reduce hyperphosphatemia in patients with chronic renal failure. Occurs in various hydrated forms. Prepn of hydrated forms: M. L. Salutsky, L. L. Quill, *J. Am. Chem. Soc.* **72,** 3306 (1950); and use of hydrated pharmaceutical compositions: B. A. Murrer, N. A. Powell, *US 5968976* (1999 to AnorMed Inc.). Crystal structure of octahydrate: D. B. Shinn, H. A. Eick, *Inorg. Chem.* **7,** 1340 (1968). Soly equilibrium of octahydrate: D. Ferri, F. Salvatore, *Acta Chem. Scand.* **37,** 531 (1983). Clinical trial in hyperphosphatemia: M. S. Joy, W. F. Finn, *Am. J. Kidney Dis.* **42,** 96 (2003). Review of clinical development: T. S. Harrison, L. J. Scott, *Drugs* **64,** 985-996 (2004); and clinical efficacy: F. Albaaj, A. J. Hutchison, *Expert Opin. Pharmacother.* **6,** 319-328 (2005).

THERAP CAT: In treatment of hyperphosphatemia.

5365. Lanthionine. [922-55-4] *S*-[(2*R*)-2-Amino-2-carboxyethyl]-L-cysteine; 3,3'-thiodi-L-alanine; L-lanthionine; [*R*-(*R***,*R***)]-bis(2-amino-2-carboxyethyl)sulfide. $C_6H_{12}N_2O_4S$; mol wt 208.24. C 34.61%, H 5.81%, N 13.45%, O 30.73%, S 15.40%. A rare amino acid found in proteins; sulfide analog of cystine. First isolated as artifacts of wool hydrolysates. Isoln: M. J. Horn *et al., J. Biol. Chem.* **138,** 141 (1941); from chick embryo: N. H. Sloane, K. G. Untch, *Biochemistry* **5,** 2658 (1966); from silkworm and Japanese oak moth: D. R. Rao *et al., ibid.* **6,** 1208. Synthesis: V. du Vigneaud, G. B. Brown, *J. Biol. Chem.* **138,** 151 (1941). Structure studies: I. W. Stapleton, O. A. Weber, *Int. J. Pept. Protein Res.* **3,** 243 (1971). Crystal structure: G. R. Desiraju, D. R. Rao, *Acta Crystallogr.* **C46,** 627 (1990).

Elongated hexagonal plates. mp 295-296° (dec). $[\alpha]_D^{25}$ +9.4° (c = 1.4 in 2.4N NaOH); $[\alpha]_D^{22}$ +8.6° (c = 5 in 2.4N NaOH); $[\alpha]_D^{22}$ +6.0° (c = 1 in 1N NaOH).

meso-**Form.** Six-sided plates having a triangular appearance from dil NH$_3$. Softens at 270°, dec 304°. Stable to alkalies. Sol in dil acids and alkalies. Sparingly sol in water. Insol in alcohol, ether, chloroform, acetone.

DL-**Form.** Elongated hexagonal plates. Chars at 240°, dec 286-292°.

D-**Form.** Elongated hexagonal plates. Darkens at 245°, dec 293-295°. $[\alpha]_D^{21}$ $-8.0°$ (c = 5 in 2.4N NaOH).

5366. Lapachol. [84-79-7] 2-Hydroxy-3-(3-methyl-2-butenyl)-1,4-naphthalenedione; lapachic acid; taiguic acid; tecomin; greenhartin; NSC-11905. $C_{15}H_{14}O_3$; mol wt 242.27. C 74.36%, H 5.82%, O 19.81%. Yellow crystalline material derived from the

Consult the Name Index before using this section.

heartwood of Asian and South American bignoniaceous plants, esp Surinam greenheart, Taigu wood, Lapacho heartwood and Bethabarra wood: Arnoudon, *Compt. Rend.* **41**, 1152 (1857); Stein, *J. Prakt. Chem.* **99**, 1 (1866); Paterno, *Gazz. Chim. Ital.* **9**, 506 (1879); Greene, Hooker, *Am. Chem. J.* **11**, 267 (1889). Structure: Paterno, *Gazz. Chim. Ital.* **12**, 337 (1882); Hooker *J. Chem. Soc.* **61**, 611 (1892); **69**, 1355 (1896); *J. Am. Chem. Soc.* **58**, 1168 (1936). Synthesis: Fieser, *ibid.* **49**, 857 (1927); Hooker, *ibid.* **58**, 1181 (1936); G. R. Pettit, L. E. Houghton, *J. Chem. Soc. C* **1971**, 509. Although it is related structurally to vitamin K, *q.v.*, it does not possess antihemorrhagic activity: H. J. Almquist, A. A. Klose, *J. Am. Chem. Soc.* **61**, 1923 (1939); L. F. Fieser *et al.*, *J. Biol. Chem.* **137**, 659 (1941). It is reported to be an inhibitor of respiratory processes: E. G. Ball *et al.*, *ibid.* **168**, 257 (1947). Lapachol has also exhibited antitumor activity vs Walker 256 carcinoma: K. V. Rao *et al.*, *Proc. Am. Assoc. Cancer Res.* **8**, 55 (1967). Mass spectrometry: T. A. Elwood *et al.*, *Org. Mass Spectrom.* **3**, 841 (1970). Chromatographic detection: M. H. Simatupang *et al.*, *J. Chromatogr.* **52**, 180 (1970). Pharmacology: S. M. Sieber *et al.*, *Cancer Treat. Rep.* **60**, 1127 (1976). Toxicity study: R. K. Morrison *et al.*, *Toxicol. Appl. Pharmacol.* **17**, 1 (1970). Review of antitumor activity: K. V. Rao, *Cancer Chemother. Rep. Part 2* **4** (4), 11-17 (1974).

Yellow prisms from alcohol or ether, mp 140°. uv max: 251.5, 278, 331 nm (log ε 4.38, 4.28, 3.43). Soluble in alcohol, chloroform, benzene, acetic acid, slightly sol in ether, hot water. Sol in aq NaOH solns forming a bright red sodium salt. LD_{50} in male, female BALB/c mice (g/kg): 0.487; 0.792 orally (Morrison).

5367. Lapatinib. [231277-92-2] *N*-[3-Chloro-4-[(3-fluorophenyl)methoxy]phenyl]-6-[5[[[2-(methylsulfonyl)ethyl]amino]-methyl]-2-furanyl]-4-quinazolinamine; GW-572016; Tykerb. C_{29}-$H_{26}ClFN_4O_4S$; mol wt 581.06. C 59.94%, H 4.51%, Cl 6.10%, F 3.27%, N 9.64%, O 11.01%, S 5.52%. Reversible dual inhibitor of ErbB1 and ErbB2 tyrosine kinases. Prepn: M. C. Carter *et al.*, *WO 9935146* (1999 to Glaxo); *eidem*, *US 6727256* (2004 to SmithKline Beecham). Mechanism of action study: W. Xia *et al.*, *Oncogene* **21**, 6255 (2002); and crystal structure in complex with epidermal growth factor receptor (EGFR, ErbB1): E. R. Wood *et al.*, *Cancer Res.* **64**, 6652 (2004). *In vitro* antitumor activity in combination with anti-ErbB2 antibodies: W. Xia *et al.*, *Oncogene* **24**, 6213 (2005). Biologic effects on tumor growth: N. L. Spector *et al.*, *J. Clin. Oncol.* **23**, 2502 (2005). Pharmacokinetics and clinical activity in metastatic carcinomas: H. A. Burris III *et al.*, *ibid.* **5305**. Review of clinical development: T. E. Kim, J. R. Murren, *IDrugs* **6**, 886-893 (2003); H. A. Burris III, *Oncologist* **9**, Suppl. 3, 10-15 (2004).

Ditoluenesulfonate monohydrate. [388082-78-8]; [388082-77-7] (anhydrous). Lapatinib ditosylate; GW-572016F. $C_{29}H_{26}$-$ClFN_4O_4S.2C_7H_8O_3S.H_2O$; mol wt 943.48. Yellow solid.
    THERAP CAT: Antineoplastic.

5368. Lappa. Burdock; clotbur; bardana. Dried first-year root of *Arctium lappa* L., or of *Arctium minus* Bernh., *Compositae*. *Habit.* Europe, Northern Asia; naturalized in N. America. *Constit.* Volatile oil, bitter principle, inulin, tannin.
    THERAP CAT: Dermatologic.

5369. Lappaconitine. [32854-75-4] (1α,14α,16β)-20-Ethyl-1,14,16-trimethoxyaconitane-4,8,9-triol 4-[2-(acetylamino)-benzoate]. $C_{32}H_{44}N_2O_8$; mol wt 584.70. C 65.73%, H 7.58%, N 4.79%, O 21.89%. From tubers and herb of *Aconitum septentrionale* Kölle, *A. orientale* Mill., *A. excelsum* Reichb., *A. ranunculaefolium, Ranunculaceae*: Schulze, Ulfert, *Arch. Pharm.* **260**, 230 (1922); Kuzovkov, Massagetov; Platonova *et al.*, *Zh. Obshch. Khim.* **25**, 178 (1955); **28**, 258 (1958), *C.A.* **50**, 1852e (1956), *C.A.* **52**, 12883i (1958), resp.; Mollov *et al.*, *Compt. Rend. Acad. Bulgare Sci.* **17**, 251 (1964), *C.A.* **61**, 12324g (1964). Structure: Khaimova *et al.*, *Tetrahedron Lett.* **1964**, 2711. Revised structure: V. A. Tel'nov *et al.*, *Khim. Prir. Soedin.* **6**, 583 (1970), *C.A.* **74**, 42527k (1971). Analgesic activity studies in mice and rats: N. Ono, J. Satoh, *Arzneim.-Forsch.* **38**, 892 (1988). Toxicology: F. Dybing *et al.*, *Acta Pharmacol. Toxicol.* **7**, 337 (1951).

Bitter crystals, mp 217-218°. $[\alpha]_D^{18}$ +27° (chloroform). Sol in benzene; slightly sol in alcohol, ether. Practically insol in water. LD_{50} in mice (mg/kg): 6.9 i.v.; 9.1 i.p.; approx 20 orally (Dybing).

5370. Lapyrium Chloride. [6272-74-8] 1-[2-Oxo-2-[[2-[(1-oxododecyl)oxy]ethyl]amino]ethyl]pyridinium chloride; 1-[(2-dodecanoyloxyethylcarbamoyl)methyl]pyridinium chloride; 1-[[(2-hydroxyethyl)carbamoyl]methyl]pyridinium chloride laurate (ester); *N*-(lauroylcolaminoformylmethyl)pyridinium chloride; *N*-(acylcolaminoformylmethyl)pyridinium chloride; emulsept (obsolete); E-607; DG-6; Emcol E-607. $C_{21}H_{35}ClN_2O_3$; mol wt 398.97. C 63.22%, H 8.84%, Cl 8.89%, N 7.02%, O 12.03%. Cationic surfactant. Prepn: A. K. Epstein, B. R. Harris, *US 2290173* (1942). Bactericidal potency: A. K. Epstein *et al.*, *Proc. Soc. Exp. Biol. Med.* **53**, 238 (1943). Toxicity study: A. E. Vivino, T. Koppanyi, *J. Am. Pharm. Assoc. Sci. Ed.* **35**, 169 (1946). Chemoenzymatic synthesis: E. M. Rustoy, A. Baldessari, *Eur. J. Org. Chem.* **2005**, 4628.

Powder, mp 141-144°.
    Stearoyl analog. [14492-68-3] Quaternium-7; steapyrium chloride; Emcol E-607S. $C_{27}H_{47}ClN_2O_3$; mol wt 483.13.
    USE: Surfactant ingredient in personal care products; in wastewater treatment; in corrosion inhibition formulations. Pharmaceutic aid (surfactant).
    THERAP CAT: Antiseptic, disinfectant.

5371. Lard. Adeps; axungia porci. Purified internal fat from abdomen of the hog.
    Soft, white unctuous mass; slight characteristic odor, bland taste. d 0.917. mp 36-42°. Insoluble in water. Very slightly sol in alcohol, freely in benzene, chloroform, ether, carbon disulfide, petr ether. Sapon. no. 195-203. Iodine no. 46-70. *Keep cool and in tight containers.*
    Benzoinated lard. Prepd by heating lard with 1% benzoin powder at temps not above 60°. Less likely to become rancid than pure lard.
    Lard oil. The oil expressed from lard at a low temp. *Constit.* Olein, stearin. Colorless or pale yellow liq. d 0.905-0.915. Solidif

$-2°$ to $+4°$. n_D^{20} 1.470-1.472. Sapon no. 195-197. Iodine no. 56-74. Acid no. 1.5-2.5. Insol in water or cold alc. Freely sol in benzene.

USE: As vehicle for medicinal agents and in manufacture of ointments. Oil as lubricant, manuf soap, oiling wool, illuminant.

5372. Larkspur. Delphinium; knight's spur; lark's-heel; lark's-claw; staggerweed. Dried ripe seeds of *Delphinium ajacis* L., *Ranunculaceae*. *Habit.* Central Europe, cultivated in U.S. *Constit.* Calcatripine, volatile oil, gum, resin, fixed oil, gallic and aconitic acids. Identification and toxicity of alkaloids: G. D. Manners *et al., J. Range Manage.* **45,** 63 (1992).

Caution: Toxic. Poisoning from percutaneous absorption may occur.

THERAP CAT: Pediculicide.

5373. Lasalocid A. [25999-31-9] 6-[(3R,4S,5S,7R)-7-[(2S,-3S,5S)-5-Ethyl-5-[(2R,5R,6S)-5-ethyltetrahydro-5-hydroxy-6-methyl-2H-pyran-2-yl]tetrahydro-3-methyl-2-furanyl]-4-hydroxy-3,5-dimethyl-6-oxononyl]-2-hydroxy-3-methylbenzoic acid; 3-methyl-6-[7-ethyl-4-hydroxy-3,5-dimethyl-6-oxo-7-[5-ethyl-3-methyl-5-(5-ethyl-5-hydroxy-6-methyl-2-tetrahydropyranyl)-2-tetrahydro-furyl]heptyl]salicylic acid; antibiotic X-537A; ionophore X-4537A; Ro-2-2985; X-537A; Bovatec. $C_{34}H_{54}O_8$; mol wt 590.79. C 69.12%, H 9.21%, O 21.67%. Ionophorous (transport-inducing) antibiotic isolated from an unidentified *Streptomyces* from soil samples of Hyde Park, Mass.: Berger *et al., J. Am. Chem. Soc.* **73,** 5295 (1951). Prepn and activity of title compd and derivs: A. Stempel, J. Westley, **DE 2040998**; *eidem,* **US 3715372** (1971, 1973 to Hoffmann-La Roche); Westley *et al., J. Med. Chem.* **16,** 397 (1973). Structure: *eidem, Chem. Commun.* **1970,** 71. Crystal and molecular structure studies: Johnson *et al., ibid.* 72; *J. Am. Chem. Soc.* **92,** 4428 (1970). Total synthesis: T. Nakata *et al., ibid.* **100,** 2933 (1978); R. E. Ireland *et al., ibid.* **102,** 1155 (1980). Complete assignment of ^{13}C-NMR spectra of lasalocid A and its sodium salt: H. Seto *et al., J. Antibiot.* **31,** 289 (1978). Effect in coccidiosis: G. M. J. Horton, P. H. G. Stockdale, *Am. J. Vet. Res.* **42,** 433 (1981). Biosynthesis: Westley *et al., Chem. Commun.* **1970,** 1467; C. R. Hutchinson *et al., J. Am. Chem. Soc.* **103,** 5953, 5956 (1981). Mode of action studies: Lin, Kun, *Biochem. Biophys. Res. Commun.* **50,** 820 (1973). Isoln and structure of four homologs, lasalocids B, C, D, E from *Streptomyces lasaliensis*: J. W. Westley *et al., J. Antibiot.* **27,** 744 (1974).

Crystals, mp 110-114°; also reported as mp 100-109° (unsharp). $[\alpha]_D^{25}$ $-7.55°$ (methanol). uv max (50% aq isopropanol): 248, 318 nm (ε 6750, 4200). Sol in organic solvents. Insol in water. LD_{50} in mice (mg/kg): 40 i.p. (Berger); also reported as LD_{50} in mice (mg/kg): 146 orally, 64 i.p., J. W. Westley, "Antibiotics (Polyether)" in *Kirk-Othmer Encyclopedia of Chemical Technology* **Vol. 3** (Interscience, New York, 3rd ed., 1978) p 61.

Sodium salt. Avatec. $C_{34}H_{53}NaO_8$; mol wt 612.77. Crystals from benzene-ligroin, mp (open capillary) 191-192° (dec), also reported as mp 168-171°. $[\alpha]_D^{25}$ $-30°$ (c = 1 in methanol). uv max (50% aq isopropanol): 308 nm (ε 4100).

THERAP CAT (VET): Coccidiostat (for poultry).

5374. Laserpitin. [7067-12-1] [1R-[1α,3aα,4β(Z),6β,-8β(Z),8aβ]]-2-Methyl-2-butenoic acid decahydro-1,6-dihydroxy-3a,6-dimethyl-1-(1-methylethyl)-5-oxo-4,8-azulenediyl ester. $C_{25}H_{38}O_7$; mol wt 450.57. C 66.64%, H 8.50%, O 24.86%. From root of *Laserpitium latifolium* L., *Umbelliferae*: Külz, *Arch. Pharm.* **221,** 161 (1883); Morgenstern, *Monatsh. Chem.* **33,** 709 (1912). Structure: M. Holub *et al., Tetrahedron Lett.* **1965,** 1441, 2855. Absolute configuration: M. Holub *et al., Collect. Czech. Chem. Commun.* **35,** 3597 (1970).

Crystals, mp 118°. Practically insol in water. Sol in alcohol, chloroform, ether, petr ether, fatty oils.

USE: Used as seasoning and flavoring agent in antiquity (Greece and Rome).

5375. Lasiocarpine. [303-34-4] (2Z)-2-Methyl-2-butenoic acid (1S,7aR)-7-[[(2R)-2,3-dihydroxy-2-[(1S)-1-methoxyethyl]-3-methyl-1-oxobutoxy]methyl]-2,3,5,7a-tetrahydro-1H-pyrrolizin-1-yl ester. $C_{21}H_{33}NO_7$; mol wt 411.49. C 61.30%, H 8.08%, N 3.40%, O 27.22%. Hepatotoxic pyrrolizidine alkaloid isolated from *Heliotropium lasiocarpum* Fish. et C. Mey. *Boraginaceae:* G. Menschikoff, *Ber.* **65,** 974 (1932), *C.A.* **26,** 4818[3] (1932), G. Menschikoff, J. Schdanowitsch, *Ber.* **69,** 1110 (1936), *C.A.* **30,** 5227[9] (1936). Structure: L. J. Drummond, *Nature* **167,** 41 (1951); R. Adams, B. L. VanDuvren, *J. Am. Chem. Soc.* **76,** 6379 (1954). Review and evaluation of studies of carcinogenicity and toxicity in laboratory animals: *IARC Monographs* **10,** 281-290, 333-342 (1976). Comprehensive reviews: L. Bull *et al., The Pyrrolizidine Alkaloids* (North-Holland, Amsterdam, 1965) 293 pp; F. L. Warren in *The Alkaloids* vol. 12, R. H. F. Manske, Ed. (Academic Press, New York, 1970) pp 245-331; D. J. Robins, *Fortschr. Chem. Org. Naturst.* **41,** 115-203 (1982).

Colorless leaflets from petr ether. mp 94-95.5°. $[\alpha]_D$ $-4°$ (10% alc). Sol on ether, alc, benzene; difficultly sol in water.

5376. Latanoprost. [130209-82-4] (5Z)-7-[(1R,2R,3R,5S)-3,5-Dihydroxy-2-[(3R)-3-hydroxy-5-phenylpentyl]cyclopentyl]-5-heptenoic acid 1-methylethyl ester; isopropyl (Z)-7-[(1R,2R,3R,5S)-3,5-dihydroxy-2-[(3R)-3-hydroxy-5-phenylpentyl]cyclopentyl]-5-heptenoate; 13,14-dihydro-17-phenyl-18,19,20-trinor-PGF$_{2\alpha}$-isopropyl ester; PhXA-41; Xalatan. $C_{26}H_{40}O_5$; mol wt 432.59. C 72.19%, H 9.32%, O 18.49%. Prostaglandin analog; prodrug of active acid metabolite. Prepd (not claimed): J. Ivanics *et al.,* **WO 9300329** (1993 to Kabi Pharmacia; Chinoin). Prepn: B. Resul *et al., J. Med. Chem.* **36,** 243, 2242 (corr.) (1993). Clinical pharmacology: C. B. Toris *et al., Ophthalmology* **100,** 1297 (1993). Clinical evaluation in glaucoma: P. Rácz *et al., Arch. Ophthalmol.* **111,** 657 (1993); as single therapy and in combination with timolol, q.v.: A. H. Rulo *et al., Br. J. Ophthalmol.* **78,** 899 (1994). Review of preclinical pharmacology: J. Stjernschantz *et al., Adv. Prostaglandin Thromboxane Leukotriene Res.* **23,** 513-518 (1995).

Colorless oil. $[\alpha]_D^{20}$ +31.57° (c = 0.91 in acetonitrile). Very sol in acetonitrile; freely sol in acetone, ethanol, ethyl acetate, isopropanol, methanol, octanol. Practically insol in water.

THERAP CAT: Antiglaucoma.

5377. α-Latrotoxin. [65988-34-3] Neurotoxic protein isolated from the venom of black widow spiders, *Latrodectus sp.* Mol wt of monomer ~130 KDa. Active tetrameric form induces a massive release of neurotransmitters from neurosecretory cells; its mode of action involves receptor-mediated calcium dependent binding and calcium independent binding as well as pore formation. Identification of toxin as a peptide: S. Bettini, N. Toschi-Frontali, *Proc. 11th Int. Congr. Entomol.* **1960**, 115-121. Purification: N. Frontali *et al., J. Cell Biol.* **68**, 462 (1976). 3D-structure: E. V. Orlova *et al., Nat. Struct. Biol.* **7**, 48 (2000). Possible mechanism of transmitter release: M. Khvotchev, T. C. Südhof, *EMBO J.* **19**, 3250 (2000). Brief review: A. Malgaroli, J. Meldolesi, "α-Latrotoxin (black widow spider)" in *Guide to Protein Toxins and Their Use in Cell Biology*, R. Rappuoli, C. Montecucco, Eds. (Oxford University Press, Oxford, 1997) pp 233-235. *Review:* A. Grasso *et al., Cell Mol. Mech. Toxin Action* **2**, 333-355 (1998); of mechanisms of action: A. W. Henkel, S. Sankaranarayanan, *Cell Tissue Res.* **296**, 229-233 (1999).

USE: Neurobiological tool for studying exocytosis, toxin-binding sites and pre-synaptic organization.

5378. Latrunculins. Highly potent toxins which disrupt microfilament organization by binding the actin monomer. Isolated from the Red Sea sponge *Latrunculia magnifica* Keller; also found in the Pacific nudibranch *Chromodoris elisabethina* and the Fijian sponge *Spongia mycofijiensis.* Isoln and biological activities: I. Néeman *et al., Mar. Biol.* **30**, 293 (1975). First family of natural products possessing the 2-thiazolidinone moiety; latrunculins A-D are 14- or 16- membered macrolides, infrastructures previously unknown in marine isolates. Structure elucidation of A and B: A. Groweiss *et al., J. Org. Chem.* **48**, 3512 (1983); of A through D: Y. Kashman *et al., Tetrahedron* **41**, 1905 (1985). Chemistry of A and B: D. Blasberger *et al., Ann.* **1989**, 1171. Total synthesis of B: R. Zibuck *et al., J. Am. Chem. Soc.* **108**, 2451 (1986); of A: J. D. White, M. Kawasaki, *J. Am. Chem. Soc.* **112**, 4991 (1990); of A, B, C and M: A. B. Smith, III *et al., ibid.* **114**, 2995 (1992). Comparative study with cytochalasin D, *q.v.*, on the effects actin organization and cell processes: I. Spector *et al., Cell Motil. Cytoskel.* **13**, 127 (1989). Inhibition of the actin monomer: W. M. Morton *et al., Nat. Cell. Biol.* **2**, 376 (2000). Review of use as research tool: K. Ayscough, *Methods Enzymol.* **298**, 18-25 (1998).

Latrunculin A   Latrunculin B

Latrunculin A. [76343-93-6] (4R)-4-[(1R,4Z,8E,10Z,12S,-15R,17R)-17-Hydroxy-5,12-dimethyl-3-oxo-2,16-dioxabicyclo[13.3.1]nonadeca-4,8,10-trien-17-yl]-2-thiazolidinone; LAT-A. $C_{22}H_{31}NO_5S$; mol wt 421.55. Foam. $[\alpha]_D^{24}$ +152° (c = 1.2 in chloroform). uv max (methanol): 218 nm (ε 23500).

Latrunculin B. [76343-94-7] (4R)-4-[(1R,4Z,8Z,10S,13R,-15R)-15-Hydroxy-5,10-dimethyl-3-oxo-2,14-dioxabicyclo[11.3.1]-heptadeca-4,8-dien-15-yl]-2-thiazolidinone; LAT-B. $C_{20}H_{29}NO_5$-S; mol wt 395.51. Major toxin. Localization within the Red Sea sponge: O. Gillor *et al., Mar. Biotechnol.* **2.** 213 (2000). Crystals. $[\alpha]_D^{24}$ +112° (c = 0.48 in chloroform). uv max (methanol): 212 nm (ε 17200).

USE: In elucidation of molecular mechanisms of motile processes.

5379. Laudanidine. [301-21-3] 2-Methoxy-5-[[(1R)-1,2,3,-4-tetrahydro-6,7-dimethoxy-2-methyl-1-isoquinolinyl]methyl]-phenol; *l*-laudanine; tritopine. $C_{20}H_{25}NO_4$; mol wt 343.42. C 69.95%, H 7.34%, N 4.08%, O 18.64%. The *l*-form of laudanine, *q.v.* Traces in opium: Hesse, *Ann.* **282**, 208 (1894); Kauder, *Arch. Pharm.* **228**, 419 (1890). Structure and synthesis: Späth, Bernhauer, *Ber.* **58**, 200 (1925); Späth, Seka, *ibid.* 1272; Späth, Burger, *Monatsh. Chem.* **47**, 733 (1926); Frydman *et al., Tetrahedron* **4**, 342 (1958). Configuration: Corrodi, Hardegger, *Helv. Chim. Acta* **39**, 889 (1956).

Prisms from alcohol, mp 185°. $[\alpha]_D^{15}$ −88° (p = 5 in chloroform). $[\alpha]_D$ −94.7 ± 1.3°. The hydrochloride is more sol than laudanine hydrochloride and makes possible a separation of the two alkaloids.

5380. Laudanine. [85-64-3] 2-Methoxy-5-[(1,2,3,4-tetra-hydro-6,7-dimethoxy-2-methyl-1-isoquinolinyl)methyl]phenol; *dl*-laudanidine. $C_{20}H_{25}NO_4$; mol wt 343.42. C 69.95%, H 7.34%, N 4.08%, O 18.64%. In the alkaline mother liquors from morphine extraction, in amounts corresp to about 0.005% of the opium employed: L. F. Small, R. E. Lutz, *Chemistry of the Opium Alkaloids*, Supplement No. 103, Public Health Reports, Washington (1932) p 34. Structure: Späth, *Monatsh. Chem.* **41**, 297 (1920). Synthesis: Späth, Lang, *ibid.* **42**, 273 (1921); Frydman *et al., Tetrahedron* **4**, 342 (1958).

Orthorhombic prisms from alcohol or chloroform, mp 167°. d_4^{20} 1.26. uv max: 284 nm (log ε 3.78). Sol in benzene, chloroform, hot alcohol; sparingly sol in ether. Practically insol in water.

5381. Laudanosine. [2688-77-9] (1S)-1-[(3,4-Dimethoxy-phenyl)methyl]-1,2,3,4-tetrahydro-6,7-dimethoxy-2-methylisoquinoline; 1,2,3,4-tetrahydro-6,7-dimethoxy-2-methyl-1-veratryl-isoquinoline; N-methyltetrahydropapaverine. $C_{21}H_{27}NO_4$; mol wt 357.44. C 70.56%, H 7.61%, N 3.92%, O 17.90%. Occurs in opium (0.0008%). It is the last alkaloid to be separated from morphine extraction mother liquors; occurs as (+)-form. Synthesis: Pictet, Finkelstein, *Ber.* **42**, 1979 (1909); Frydman *et al., Tetrahedron* **4**, 342 (1958); Elliott, *J. Heterocycl. Chem.* **9**, 853 (1972). Asymmetric synthesis: M. Konda *et al., Chem. Pharm. Bull.* **23**, 1025 (1975); of (R)-(−)-laudanosine: M. Konda *et al., ibid.* **25**, 69 (1977); R. E. Gawley, G. A. Smith, *Tetrahedron Lett.* **29**, 301 (1988). Configuration: Leithe, *Ber.* **64**, 2827 (1931); Faltis, Adler, *Arch. Pharm.* **284**, 281 (1951); Corrodi, Hardegger, *Helv. Chim. Acta* **39**, 889 (1956).

Crystals from light petr (30-60°), mp 89°. $[\alpha]_D^{16}$ +106° (c = 1.6 in 97% alc); $[\alpha]_D^{16}$ +130° (chloroform); $[\alpha]_D^{22}$ +52.2 ±1.3° (chloroform). $[\alpha]_D^{20}$ +82.5° (ethanol). Absorption spectrum: Dobbie, Lauder, *J. Chem. Soc.* **83**, 626 (1903). Practically insol in water. Freely sol in alcohol, chloroform, ether, hot petr ether.

(−)-Form. Colorless needles from ethanol, mp 83-85°. $[\alpha]_D^{20}$ −84.8° (c = 0.466 in ethanol).

(±)-Form. Crystals from dil alc, mp 114-115.5°.

5382. Laurel. Bay laurel; Roman laurel; Turkish laurel; sweet bay. Evergreen shrub, *Laurus nobilis* L., *Lauraceae*, bearing pale yellow flowers, shiny black berries and glossy aromatic foliage. Known since ancient times as a medicinal plant and spice; often used as a symbol of victory or achievement. *Habit.* Mediterrean region. *Constit.* Leaves: volatile oil (1-3%), costunolide, laurenobiolide, catechins, proanthocyanidins, alkaloids, plant acids. Fruit: fatty oil (25-55%), sesquiterpine lactones, volatile oil (1-4%). Comprehensive description: S. Kumar *et al.* in *Handbook of Herbs and Spices*, K. V. Peter, Ed., (CRC Press, Boca Raton, 2001) pp 52-61. Composition of essential oil: M. Ozcan, J.-C. Chalchat, *J. Med. Food*, **8**, 408 (2005). Reviews of composition and uses: A. Y. Leung, S. Foster, *Encyclopedia of Common Natural Ingredients*, (Wiley-Interscience, Hoboken, 2nd Ed., 2003) pp 69-72; J. Gruenwald *et al., PDR for Herbal Medicines* (Medical Economics, Montvale, 3rd Ed., 2004) p 500.

Laurel berry oil. [8002-41-3] Fixed oil from fresh fruit. *Constit.* Chiefly lauric, palmitic, oleic acids, volatile oil, sesquiterpene lactones. Greenish, fatty solid. d ~0.88. mp ~40°. n_D^{25} 1.4783. Sapon no. 198-199. Iodine no. 68-80. Insol in water. Sparingly sol in alcohol; sol in benzene, ether, carbon disulfide.

Laurel leaf oil. Oil of sweet bay; bay leaf oil; volatile oil of laurel. Obtained by steam distillation from leaves of *Laurus nobilis* L., *Lauraceae. Constit.* Eucalyptol (30-60%), α- and β-pinene, α-terpineol, sabinene, linalool. Light yellow to yellow liquid with aromatic spicy odor. d_{25}^{25} 0.905-0.929. n_D^{20} 1.465-1.470. Rotation: −10° to −19°. Acid no. not >3.0. Sapon no. 15-45; 36-85 after acetylation. Sol in most fixed oils, in 1 vol 80% alcohol, with cloudiness in mineral oil, propylene glycol. Insol in glycerin. *Keep well closed, cool and protected from light.*

Note: Should not be confused with West Indian bay, *Pimenta racemosa*, or California laurel, *Umbellularia californica*.

USE: Culinary herb (bay leaf), component of bouquet garni; flavoring agent. Fragrance component in soaps, creams, lotions, detergents, perfumes.

THERAP CAT: Rubefacient; in treatment of rheumatism and gout; carminative.

5383. Laureline. [81-38-9] (7a*R*)-6,7,7a,8-Tetrahydro-11-methoxy-7-methyl-5*H*-benzo[*g*]-1,3-benzodioxolo[6,5,4-*de*]quinoline; 10-methoxy-1,2-(methylenedioxy)aporphine. $C_{19}H_{19}NO_3$; mol wt 309.36. C 73.77%, H 6.19%, N 4.53%, O 15.52%. From bark of *Laurelia novae-zelandiae* A. Cunn., *Lauraceae*: Aston, *J. Chem. Soc.* **97**, 1381 (1910). Synthesis: Schlittler, *Helv. Chim. Acta* **15**, 394 (1932); Faltis *et al., Ber.* **77B**, 686 (1945); Gibson *et al., J. Chem. Soc. C* **1970**, 2234; Govindachari *et al., Indian J. Chem.* **8**, 475 (1970).

Cubes from petr ether. $[\alpha]_D^{20}$ −99.2° (c = 0.736 in 50% alc). Absorption spectrum: Girardet, *J. Chem. Soc.* **1931**, 2636. Feebly basic. Readily oxidizes in air. Sol in alcohol, ether. Practically insol in water.

Hydrochloride. $C_{19}H_{19}NO_3$.HCl. Crystals, mp 280°. $[\alpha]_D^{20}$ −57°. Sparingly sol in water.

(S)-Form. [65981-49-9] Cubes from petr ether, mp 114-115°. $[\alpha]_D^{20}$ +97.9° (c = 1.12 in abs alc); $[\alpha]_D^{20}$ +100° (c = 0.560 in CS₂).

(±)-Form. [3749-97-1] Rough needles from petr ether, mp 115-116°.

Nitrate. $C_{19}H_{19}NO_3$.HNO₃. Crystals, mp 238-240°. Sparingly sol in water.

Hydriodide. $C_{19}H_{19}NO_3$.HI. Crystals. Practically insol in water.

Oxalate. $(C_{19}H_{19}NO_3)_2$.(COOH)₂. Moderately sol in water.

5384. Lauric Acid. [143-07-7] Dodecanoic acid; laurostearic acid; dodecoic acid. $C_{12}H_{24}O_2$; mol wt 200.32. C 71.95%, H 12.08%, O 15.97%. $CH_3(CH_2)_{10}COOH$. Isoln from coconut oil: Dale, Meara, *J. Sci. Food Agric.* **6**, 162 (1955); Naudet *et al., Bull. Soc. Chim. Fr.* **1959**, 718; from arecanut fat: Pathak, Mathur, *J. Sci. Food Agric.* **5**, 461 (1954); from *Holoptelea integrifolia* seed oil: Badami, *ibid.* **13**, 297 (1962). Synthesis: Ballard *et al., US 2572238* (1951 to Shell); Langenbeck, Richter, *Ber.* **89**, 202 (1956); Sprowls, *US 2782214* (1957 to Baker Castor Oil); Zapesochnoya *et al., Zh. Obshch. Khim.* **33**, 2552 (1963). Toxicity study: L. Orö, A. Wretlind, *Acta Pharmacol. Toxicol.* **18**, 141 (1961).

White, crystalline powder; slight odor of bay oil, mp 44°; also reported as 48°. d_5^4 0.869. bp_{100} 225°; bp_{20} 160-165°. n_D^{82} 1.4183. Insol in water. 1 g dissolves in 1 ml alcohol, 2.5 ml propyl alcohol; freely sol in benzene, ether. LD_{50} i.v. in mice: 131 ±5.7 mg/kg (Orö, Wretlind).

5385. Laurocapram. [59227-89-3] 1-Dodecylhexahydro-2*H*-azepin-2-one; 1-dodecylazacycloheptan-2-one; *N*-dodecyl-ε-caprolactam; N-0252; Azone. $C_{18}H_{35}NO$; mol wt 281.48. C 76.81%, H 12.53%, N 4.98%, O 5.68%. Caprolactam derivative used to enhance percutaneous absorption of physiologically active agents. Also exhibits intrinsic anti-inflammatory activity. Prepn: A. P. Swain *et al., J. Org. Chem.* **18**, 1087 (1953). Improved synthesis: V. J. Rajadhyaksha *et al., EP 95096; eidem, US 4422970* (both 1983 to Nelson). Use as skin penetrant: V. J. Rajadhyaksha, *US 3989816; US 4405616* (1976, 1983 to Nelson). Anti-inflammatory activity: E. L. Nelson, *US 4310525* (1982 to Nelson). Pharmacology: R. B. Stoughton, *Arch. Dermatol.* **118**, 474 (1982). Comprehensive description: *idem, Drug Dev. Ind. Pharm.* **9**, 725 (1983). Topical antiviral activity *in vivo*: M. F. Leonard *et al., Chemotherapy (Basel)* **33**, 151 (1987).

Clear, colorless liquid, mp −7°. $bp_{50\mu}$ 160°. d 0.91; n 1.4701. Insol in water. Freely sol in most organic solvents. LD_{50} rats, mice (g/kg): 8 i.v., i.p. (Stoughton).

USE: Pharmaceutic aid (excipient).

5386. Lauroguadine. [135-43-3] *N,N'''*-[4-(Dodecyloxy)-1,3-phenylene]bisguanidine; 1,1'-[4-(dodecyloxy)-*m*-phenylene]diguanidine; 2,4-diguanidinophenyl lauryl ether; 2,4-diguanidino-1-dodecyloxybenzene; 2,4-diguanidino-1-lauryloxybenzene; 2,4-diguanidinophenyl dodecyl ether; dodecyl 2,4-diguanidinophenyl ether. $C_{20}H_{36}N_6O$; mol wt 376.54. C 63.80%, H 9.64%, N 22.32%, O 4.25%. Prepn of the dihydrochloride: Pasini, *Farmaco Ed. Sci.* **8**, 646 (1953); *idem, Rend. Sci. Farmitalia* **1**, 405 (1954); **GB 730394** (1955 to Farmitalia).

Dihydrochloride monohydrate. P-7; Farmidril. $C_{20}H_{36}N_6O$·2HCl.H₂O; mol wt 467.48. Crystals from water + ethanol. Sinters from 135-210°, dec 250°. Soly (g/100 ml): 0.2 in cold water; ~10 in boiling water; 84.2 in methanol (25°). Practically insol in acetone, benzene. Aq solns are neutral to litmus.

THERAP CAT: Antiprotozoal (Trichomonas).

5387. Laurolinium Acetate. [146-37-2] 4-Amino-1-dodecyl-2-methylquinolinium acetate; 4-amino-1-dodecylquinaldinium acetate; 1-dodecyl-4-aminoquinaldinium acetate; Laurodin. $C_{24}H_{38}N_2O_2$; mol wt 386.57. C 74.57%, H 9.91%, N 7.25%, O 8.28%. Prepn: D. Caldwell *et al., J. Pharm. Pharmacol.* **13**, 554 (1961); D. Caldwell, L. R. Rowe, *US 2997476* (1961 to Allen & Hanburys). Toxicity data: W. A. Cox, P. F. D'Arcy, *J. Pharm. Pharmacol.* **15**, 129 (1963).

Crystals from acetone, mp 170-171°. Freely sol in water. About 1 g dissolves in 2 ml of water at 20°. LD_{50} in mice (mg/kg): 131 ±36.2 orally; 30.2 ±5.6 s.c.; 6.0 ±04 i.v.; 2.3 ±0.2 i.p. (Cox, D'Arcy).

THERAP CAT: Antiseptic.

5388. Laurotetanine. [128-76-7] (6aS)-5,6,6a,7-Tetrahydro-1,2,10-trimethoxy-4H-dibenzo[de,g]quinolin-9-ol; 1,2,10-trimethoxy-6aα-noraporphin-9-ol; Litsoeine. $C_{19}H_{21}NO_4$; mol wt 327.37. C 69.71%, H 6.47%, N 4.28%, O 19.55%. From the bark of *Litsea citrata* Blume (*Tetranthera citrata* (Blume) Nees), *Lauraceae* and allied plants. Isoln: Greshoff, *Ber.* **23**, 3537 (1890); Filippo, *Arch. Pharm.* **236**, 601 (1898). Structure: Barger *et al.*, *Ber.* **66**, 450 (1933). Synthesis: Kikkawa, *C.A.* **53**, 17163i (1959).

Monohydrate. Needles, mp 125°. $[\alpha]_D^{25}$ +98.5°. Practically insol in water. Freely sol in alcohol, chloroform, ethyl acetate, slightly in ether.

5389. Lauryl Bromide. [143-15-7] 1-Bromododecane; dodecyl bromide. $C_{12}H_{25}Br$; mol wt 249.23. C 57.83%, H 10.11%, Br 32.06%. $CH_3(CH_2)_{10}CH_2Br$. Prepd by the action of hydrobromic acid on primary *n*-lauryl alcohol in the presence of sulfuric acid: Kamm, Marvel, *Org. Synth.* **1**, 7 (1921).

Liquid. bp_{45} 175-180°. Insol in water. Sol in alc, ether.

5390. Lavender. Garden lavender; true lavender. Aromatic, woody perennial, *Lavandula angustifolia* Mill. (syn. *L. officinalis* Chaix.), *Labiatae*. Parts used are the fresh or dried flowering tops and the essential oil. Also used for oil production are *spike lavender* (*L. latifolia*, syn. *L. spica*) and *lavandin* referring to hybrid varieties including *L. abrialis* and *L. hybridia*. Habit. Mediterranean region; cultivated widely. Constit. Volatile oil (1-3%), tannins, coumarin, umbelliferone, herniarin, flavonoids. Comprehensive description: M. T. Lis-Balchin in *Handbook of Herbs and Spices*, Vol. 2, K. V. Peter, Ed., (CRC Press, Boca Raton, 2004) pp 179-195. Characterization of essential oil: R. Shellie *et al.*, *J. Chromatogr. A* **970**, 225 (2002); A. R. Fakhari *et al.*, *ibid.* **1098**, 14 (2005). Review of clinical studies of psychological effects: M. Kirk-Smith, *Int. J. Aromather.* **13**, 82-89 (2003); of medicinal uses: J. Gruenwald *et al.*, *PDR for Herbal Medicines* (Medical Economics, Montvale, 3rd Ed., 2004) pp 285-288.

Lavender oil. [8000-28-0] Oil of lavender. Volatile oil obtained by steam distillation of fresh flowering tops of *L. angustifolia*. Constit. Complex mixture of components, chiefly linalool (20-50%), linalyl acetate (30-40%), terpinen-4-ol, lavandulyl acetate, lavandulol. Colorless or yellow liquid. d_{25}^{25} 0.875-0.888. n_D^{20} 1.459-1.470. Rotation: −3° to −10°. Slightly sol in water; sol in 4 vols 70% alcohol. Insol in propylene glycol. *Keep well closed, cool and protected from light.*

Lavandin oil. [8022-15-9] Abrial lavandin oil. Volatile oil obtained from flowering tops of *L. abrialis* or other hybrid varieties. Constit. Linalool, linalyl acetate, eucalyptol, camphor. Pale yellow to yellow liquid with a slight, camphoraceous odor. d_{25}^{25} 0.885-0.893. n_D^{20} 1.460-1.464. Rotation: −2° to −5°. Sol in most fixed oils, propylene glycol, with opalescence in mineral oil, in 2 vols 70% alcohol. Relatively insol in glycerin.

Spike lavender oil. [8016-78-2] Oil of spike. Volatile oil from dried flowers of *L. latifolia*. Constit. 40-60% eucalyptol and camphor, linalool, linalyl acetate (1%). Pale yellow to yellow liquid; camphoraceous lavender odor. d_{25}^{25} 0.893-0.909. Rotation: −5° to +5°. n_D^{20} 1.463-1.468. Sol in most fixed oils, propylene glycol, in 3 vols 70% alcohol; slightly sol in glycerin, mineral oil. *Keep well closed, cool and protected from light.*

USE: Fragrance component in cosmetics, soaps, lotions, perfumes. Flavor in beverages, desserts, aromatic vinegars. Oil in aromatherapy for a soothing, calming effect.

THERAP CAT: Carminative, astringent, antiseptic.

5391. Lawesson's Reagent. [19172-47-5] 2,4-Bis(4-methoxyphenyl)-1,3,2,4-dithiadiphosphetane 2,4-disulfide; anisyldithiophosphinic anhydride. $C_{14}H_{14}O_2P_2S_4$; mol wt 404.47. C 41.57%, H 3.49%, O 7.91%, P 15.32%, S 31.71%. Thionating agent for conversion of carbonyls to thiocarbonyls. Prepn: H. Z. Lecher *et al.*, *J. Am. Chem. Soc.* **78**, 5018 (1956); and delineation of use: B. S. Pedersen *et al.*, *Bull. Soc. Chim. Belg.* **87**, 223 (1978); S. Scheibye *et al.*, *ibid.*, 229. Mechanistic study: T. B. Rauchfuss, G. A. Zank, *Tetrahedron Lett.* **27**, 3445 (1986). Use in thionations: A. Z.-Q. Khan, J. Sandström, *J. Chem. Soc. Perkin Trans. 1* **1988**, 2085; S. Araki *et al.*, *Bull. Chem. Soc. Jpn.* **61**, 2977 (1988); as reducing agent for sulfoxides: H. Bartsch, T. Erker, *Tetrahedron Lett.* **33**, 199 (1992). Review of thionation reactions: M. P. Cava, M. I. Levinson, *Tetrahedron* **41**, 5061-5087 (1985); of applications in organic and organometallic syntheses: M. Jesberger *et al.*, *Synthesis* **2003**, 1929-1958.

mp 229°, should be stored under anhydrous conditions.

USE: Thiation reagent.

5392. Lawrencium. [22537-19-5] Lr; formerly Lw; at. no. 103; valence 3. Man-made radioactive element. No stable nuclides; known isotopes (mass numbers): 253-262. Longest-lived known isotope: 262 (T½ 216 minutes, rel. at. mass 262.110). Prepn of first isotope ^{257}Lr (T½ 0.65 sec, α-emitter): A. Ghiorso *et al.*, *Phys. Rev. Lett.* **6**, 473 (1961). Prepn of isotope originally assigned mass number 257, later changed to 258 (T½ 4.3 seconds, α-emitter) by bombardment of Cf with boron ions: Eskola *et al.*, *Phys. Rev. C* **4**, 632 (1971). Prepn of isotopes including ^{256}Lr (T½ 28 seconds) by irradiating ^{243}Am with ^{18}O ions: Donets *et al.*, *At. Energ.* **19**, 109 (1965), *C.A.* **64**, 1542c (1966). *Reviews:* C. Keller, *The Chemistry of the Transuranium Elements* (Verlag Chemie, Weinheim, English Ed., 1971) pp 609-612; Silva, "Trans-Curium Elements" in *MTP Int. Rev. Sci.: Inorg. Chem., Ser. One* vol. 8, A. G. Maddock, Ed. (University Park Press, Baltimore, 1972) pp 71-105; Ghiorso, *Handb. Exp. Pharmakol.* **36**, 691-715 (1973); Taylor, *ibid.* 717-738; R. J. Silva in *The Chemistry of the Actinide Elements* vol. 2, J. J. Katz *et al.*, Eds. (Chapman and Hall, New York, 1986) pp 1099-1103; *The Elements Beyond Uranium*, G. T. Seaborg, W. D. Loveland, Eds. (John Wiley & Sons, Inc., New York, 1990) p 49-51.

Caution: Radiation hazard; handling requires special equipment and shielding facilities (Katz *et al., loc. cit.* vol. 2, p. 1128).

5393. Lawsone. [83-72-7] 2-Hydroxy-1,4-naphthalenedione; 2-hydroxy-1,4-naphthoquinone. $C_{10}H_6O_3$; mol wt 174.15. C 68.97%, H 3.47%, O 27.56%. From leaves of *Lawsonia inermis* L. and *L. alba* Lam., *Lythraceae*: Latif, *Indian J. Agric. Sci.* **29**, No. 2-3, 147 (1959), *C.A.* **55**, 14828g (1961). Synthesis: Fieser, *J. Am. Chem. Soc.* **70**, 3165 (1948); Jain, Seshadri, *Proc. Indian Acad. Sci.* **35A**, 233 (1952); Eistert, Müller, *Ber.* **92**, 2071 (1959).

Yellow prisms from acetic acid, dec 195-196°.

THERAP CAT: Ultraviolet screen.

5394. Lazabemide. [103878-84-8] N-(2-Aminoethyl)-5-chloro-2-pyridinecarboxamide; N-(2-aminoethyl)-5-chloropicolinamide. $C_8H_{10}ClN_3O$; mol wt 199.64. C 48.13%, H 5.05%, Cl 17.76%, N 21.05%, O 8.01%. Member of a novel class of potent, reversible, and extremely selective monoamine oxidase type B (MAO-B) inhibitors. Prepn: R. Imhof, E. Kyburz, **GB 2163746**; *eidem*, **US 4764522** (1986, 1988 both to Hoffmann-LaRoche). HPLC determn in plasma: R. Wyss, W. Philipp, *J. Chromatogr.* **507**, 187 (1990). Neurochemical profile: W. E. Haefely *et al.*, *Adv. Neurol.* **53**, 505 (1990). Enzyme binding studies: J. Saura *et al.*, *J. Neurosci.* **12**, 1977 (1992). Clinical trial: Parkinson Study Group, *Ann. Neurol.* **33**, 350 (1993).

Monohydrochloride. [103878-83-7] Ro-19-6327. C_8H_{10}-$ClN_3O.HCl$; mol wt 236.10. Crystals from methanol/ether, mp 193-195°. Partition coefficient (*n*-octanol/water) ~0.1. pKa 8.9. LD_{50} orally in mice: 1000-2000 mg/kg (Imhof, Kyburz, 1986).

THERAP CAT: Antiparkinsonian.

5395. Lazurite. [1302-83-6] Lapis lazuli; lasurite. Composition: $(Na,Ca)_4(AlSiO_4)_3(SO_4,S,Cl)$, E. S. Dana, *A System of Mineralogy* (John Wiley, New York, 6th ed., 1901) pp 432-433; C. S. Hurlbut, Jr., *Dana's Manual of Mineralogy* (John Wiley, New York, 17th ed., 1959) p 503.

Blue, blue-violet or greenish-blue, translucent, cubic or dodecahedral crystals. d 2.4. Dec by HCl with pptn of SiO_2 and evolution of H_2S.

USE: In manuf of vases, ornamental furniture, mosaics; in paints, jewelry.

5396. Lead. [7439-92-1] Pb; at. wt 207.2; at. no. 82; valence 2, 4. Group IVA (14). Four naturally occurring isotopes: 204 (1.40%); 206 (25.2%); 207 (21.7%); 208 (51.7%); artificial, radioactive isotopes: 195-203; 205; 209-214. One of the metals known to the ancient world. Extent of occurrence in earth's crust about 15 g/ton, also expressed as 0.002% (depth of crust: 16 km). Occurs chiefly as sulfide in *galena*, other minerals include *anglesite* ($PbSO_4$), *cerussite* ($PbCO_3$), *mimetite* [$PbCl_2.3Pb_3(AsO_4)_2$] and *pyromorphite* [$PbCl_2.3Pb_3(PO_4)_2$]. Recovery from ore and purification: Heuser, *Metall.* **9**, 675 (1955), *C.A.* **49**, 14609 (1955); Ziegfeld, *Eng. Min. J.* **153**, 82 (1952), *C.A.* **46**, 2975 (1952). Prepn of high purity lead: Piontelli, Fagnani, *Chim. Ind. (Milan)* **34**, 629 (1952), *C.A.* **47**, 12062 (1953); Giesen, *Technik* **2**, 393 (1947), *C.A.* **42**, 852 (1948); Hughes *J. Electrochem. Soc.* **101**, 267 (1954); Baralis, Marone, *Met. Ital.* **59**, 494 (1967), *C.A.* **67**, 119613a (1967). Review of uses, corrosion metallurgy: Mullarkey, *Ind. Eng. Chem.* **49**, 1607 (1957). Reviews of lead, its alloys and compds: W. Hofmann, *Lead and Lead Alloys, Properties and Technology* (Springer, New York, Eng. Ed., 1970) 551 pp; Abel in *Comprehensive Inorganic Chemistry* **vol. 2**, J. C. Bailar, Jr. *et al.*, Eds. (Pergamon Press, Oxford, 1973) pp 105-146; H. E. Howe in *Kirk-Othmer Encyclopedia of Chemical Technology* **vol. 14** (Wiley-Interscience, New York, 3rd ed., 1981) pp 98-139. Review of carcinogenic risk: *IARC Monographs* **23**, 325-415 (1980); of toxicology and human exposure: *Toxicological Profile for Lead* (PB99-166704, 1999) 640 pp.

Bluish-white, silvery, gray metal. Highly lustrous when freshly cut, tarnishes upon exposure to air. Very soft and malleable, easily melted, cast, rolled, and extruded. Cubic crystal structure. mp 327.4°; bp 1740°. d_4^{20} 11.34; d (at mp) 10.65: Schneider *et al.*, *Naturwissenschaften* **41**, 326 (1954). Heat of vaporization (1740°) 206 cal/g. Heat capacity (20°): 0.031 cal/g/°C. Resistivity (μ-ohm-cm) at 20°: 20.65; at 100°: 27.02; at 320°: 54.76; at 330°: 96.74. Vapor pressure at 1000°: 1.77 mm Hg. $E°$ (aq) Pb/Pb^{2+} +0.126 v. Coefficient of linear expansion (0-100°) 29×10^{-6}, (20-300°) 31.3×10^{-6}, ($-183°$ to $+14°$) 27×10^{-6}; thermal conductiv-

ity varies from 0.083 at 50° to 0.077 at 225°: Francl, Kingery, *J. Am. Ceram. Soc.* **37**, 80 (1954). Viscosity of molten lead (cP): 3.2 (327.4°); 2.32 (400°); 1.54 (600°); 1.23 (800°). Heat capacity and heat of fusion study: Douglas, Dever, *J. Am. Chem. Soc.* **76**, 4824 (1954); hardness 1 on Mohs' scale; Brinell hardness (high purity Pb) 4.0: McLellan, *Am. Mineral.* **30**, 635 (1945). Reacts with hot concd nitric acid, with boiling concd hydrochloric or sulfuric acid. Attacked by pure water, weak organic acids in the presence of oxygen. Resistant to tap water, hydrofluoric acid, brine, solvents.

Caution: Potential symptoms of overexposure are lassitude, insomnia; facial pallor; anorexia, weight loss, malnutrition; constipation, abdominal pain, colic; anemia; gingival lead line; tremor; paralysis of wrists or ankles; kidney disease; hypotension. Symptoms in children include encephalopathy, behavioral and learning deficits; in adults, peripheral motor neuropathy. *See NIOSH Pocket Guide to Chemical Hazards* (PB2003-100121, 2003) p 184; *Patty's Industrial Hygiene and Toxicology* **vol 2C**, G. D. Clayton, F. E. Clayton, Eds. (Wiley-Interscience, New York, 4th ed., 1994) pp 2065-2087.

USE: Construction material for tank linings, piping, and other equipment handling corrosive gases and liqs used in the manuf of sulfuric acid, petr refining, halogenation, sulfonation, extraction, condensation; for x-ray and atomic radiation protection; manuf of tetraethyllead, pigments for paints, and other organic and inorganic lead compds; bearing metal and alloys; storage batteries; in ceramics, plastics, and electronic devices; in building construction; in solder and other lead alloys; in the metallurgy of steel and other metals.

5397. Lead Acetate. [301-04-2] Neutral lead acetate; normal lead acetate; sugar of lead; salt of Saturn. $C_4H_6O_4Pb$; mol wt 325.29. C 14.77%, H 1.86%, O 19.67%, Pb 63.70%. Pb(CH_3-COO$)_2$. Toxicity data: W. R. Bradley, W. G. Fredrick, *Ind. Med.* **10**, *Ind. Hyg. Sect.* **2**, 15 (1941). Review of safety assessment in hair coloring: A. J. Cohen, F. J. C. Roe, *Food Chem. Toxicol.* **29**, 485-507 (1991); of toxicology and human exposure: *Toxicological Profile for Lead* (PB99-166704, 1999) 640 pp.

Occurs as trihydrate, colorless crystals or white granules or powder; slight acetic odor; slowly effloresces. *Poisonous!* Takes up CO_2 from air and becomes incompletely sol. d 2.55. mp 75° when rapidly heated; at a little above 100° it begins to lose acetic acid; dec completely above 200°. One gram dissolves in 1.6 ml water, 0.5 ml boiling water, 30 ml alcohol; freely sol in glycerol. Aq solns of lead acetate dissolve lead monoxide. pH of 5% aq soln at 25° = 5.5-6.5. *Keep well closed.* LD_{50} i.p. in rats: 15 mg Pb/100g (Bradley, Fredrick).

Caution: This substance is reasonably anticipated to be a human carcinogen: *Report on Carcinogens, Eleventh Edition* (PB2005-104914, 2004) p III-158.

USE: Mordant in cotton dyes; lead coating for metals; drier in paints, varnishes and pigment inks; colorant in hair dyes. Weighting silks; manuf lead salts, chrome-yellow; as analytical reagent for detection of sulfide, determination of CrO_3, MoO_3.

THERAP CAT: Astringent.

THERAP CAT (VET): Astringent and sedative (usually in lotions) for bruises and superficial inflammation. Has been used internally in diarrheas.

5398. Lead Antimonate(V). [13510-89-9] Naples yellow. Approx $Pb_3(SbO_4)_2$.

Orange-yellow powder. Insol in water, dil acids.

USE: As pigment in oil painting, staining glass, crockery and porcelain.

5399. Lead Arsenate. [7784-40-9] Approx $PbHAsO_4$. Occurs in nature as the mineral *schultenite*. Toxicity studies: Voigt *et al.*, *J. Am. Pharm. Assoc.* **37**, 122 (1948); T. B. Gaines, *Toxicol. Appl. Pharmacol.* **14**, 515 (1969).

White, heavy powder. *Poisonous!* d 5.79. At ~280° loses H_2O and is converted into pyroarsenate. Insol in water. Sol in HNO_3, caustic alkalies. LD_{50} in rats, rabbits (mg/kg): 825, 125 orally (Voigt). LD_{50} in female rats (mg/kg): 1050 orally, >2400 dermally (Gaines).

USE: As constituent of various insecticides for larvae of gypsy moth, boll weevil, etc.

THERAP CAT (VET): Has been used as a teniacide; insecticide.

5400. Lead Arsenite. [10031-13-7] Approx Pb(AsO$_2$)$_2$.
White powder. *Poisonous!* d 5.85. Insol in water; sol in dil HNO$_3$.
USE: As insecticide like the arsenate.

5401. Lead Azide. [13424-46-9] N$_6$Pb; mol wt 291.24. N 28.86%, Pb 71.14%. Pb(N$_3$)$_2$. Prepd from sodium azide and lead nitrate: Schenk in *Handbook of Preparative Inorganic Chemistry* vol. 1, G. Brauer, Ed. (Academic Press, New York, 2nd ed., 1963) p 763. Review: B. T. Fedoroff *et al., Encyclopedia of Explosives and Related Items* vol. 1 (Picatinny Arsenal, Dover, N.J., 1960) pp A545-A587. Review of toxicology and human exposure: *Toxicological Profile for Lead* (PB99-166704, 1999) 640 pp.
Needles or white powder. Explodes at 350° or on percussion. Heat of formation (25°): +110.5 kcal/mol. Soly in water: 0.023% at 18°; 0.09% at 70°. Freely sol in acetic acid. Insol in NH$_4$OH.
USE: As primer in explosives. In the form of dextrinated lead azide.

5402. Lead Borate. [10214-39-8] Approx Pb(BO$_2$)$_2$.H$_2$O.
White powder. *Poisonous!* Insoluble in water; soluble in dil HNO$_3$.
USE: Drier for varnishes and paints; with other metals (e.g., Ag) in galvanoplasty for production of conducting coatings on glass, pottery, porcelain, and chinaware.

5403. Lead Bromide. [10031-22-8] Br$_2$Pb; mol wt 367.01. Br 43.54%, Pb 56.46%. PbBr$_2$. Review of toxicology and human exposure: *Toxicological Profile for Lead* (PB99-166704, 1999) 640 pp.
White, cryst powder. *Poisonous!* d 6.66. mp 373°. On solidifying forms a horn-like mass. Sol in about 200 parts cold water, 20 parts boiling water; insol in alcohol.

5404. Lead Chloride. [7758-95-4] Cl$_2$Pb; mol wt 278.11. Cl 25.50%, Pb 74.50%. PbCl$_2$. Occurs in nature as the mineral *cotunnite*. Toxicity data: Tartler, *Arch. Hyg.* **125,** 273 (1941). Review of toxicology and human exposure: *Toxicological Profile for Lead* (PB99-166704, 1999) 640 pp.
White, cryst powder. *Poisonous!* d 5.85. mp 501°. bp 950°. Sol in 93 parts cold water, 30 parts boiling water; readily sol in soln of NH$_4$Cl, NH$_4$NO$_3$, alkali hydroxides; slowly in glycerol. MLD in guinea pigs (mg/kg): 1500-2000 orally (Tartler).
USE: Manuf Pattison's white lead, Verona Yellow, Turner's Patent Yellow, lead oxychloride; as solder and flux.

5405. Lead Chromate(VI). [7758-97-6] Chrome yellow; Cologne yellow; King's yellow; Leipzig yellow; Paris yellow; C.I. Pigment Yellow 34; C.I. 77600. CrO$_4$Pb; mol wt 323.19. Cr 16.09%, O 19.80%, Pb 64.11%. PbCrO$_4$. Occurs in nature as the minerals *crocoite, phoenicochroite*. Ref: *Colour Index* vol. 4 (3rd ed., 1971) p 4677. Evaluation of carcinogenic risk: *IARC Monographs* **23,** 205-324 (1980); *ibid.* **49,** 49-256 (1990). Review of environmental exposure and bioavailability: D. Waldron, *Am. Ink Maker* **72,** 50-60 (1994); of toxicology and human exposure: *Toxicological Profile for Lead* (PB99-166704, 1999) 640 pp.
Yellow or orange-yellow powder. d 6.3. mp 844°. It is one of the most insol salts (0.2 mg/l H$_2$O). Insol in acetic acid. Sol in solns of fixed alkali hydroxides, in dil HNO$_3$.
Caution: Chromium hexavalent compounds are listed as known human carcinogens: *Report on Carcinogens, Eleventh Edition* (PB2005-104914, 2004) p III-63.
USE: Pigment for paints and inks; in oil and water colors; printing fabrics, decorating china and porcelain; in chemical analysis of organic substances; in traffic paints.

5406. Lead Chromate(VI) Oxide. [18454-12-1] Chromic acid lead(2+) salt (1:2); basic lead chromate; red lead chromate; chrome red; chromium lead oxide; Persian red; Austrian cinnabar. CrPb$_2$O$_5$; mol wt 546.39. Cr 9.52%, Pb 75.84%, O 14.64%. PBCrO$_4$.PbO. *See: Colour Index* vol. 4, (3rd ed., 1971) p 4677.
Red powder. Insol in water.
USE: As pigment.

5407. Lead Dioxide. [1309-60-0] Lead oxide (PbO$_2$); lead (IV) oxide; lead oxide brown; lead peroxide; lead superoxide. O$_2$Pb; mol wt 239.20. O 13.38%, Pb 86.62%. Occurs in nature as the mineral *plattnerite*. Lab prepn from lead acetate and calcium

hypochlorite: Newell, Maxson, *Inorg. Synth.* **1,** 45 (1939); by hydrolysis of lead acetate: Kuhn, Hammer, *Ber.* **83,** 413 (1950). Review of toxicology: B. Venugopal, T. D. Luckey, *Environ. Qual. Safety* Suppl. 1, 4-73 (1975).
Dark-brown powder; evolves oxygen when heated, first forming Pb$_3$O$_4$, at high temp PbO. d 9.38. Insol in water. Sol in HCl with evolution of Cl; in dil HNO$_3$ in presence of H$_2$O$_2$, oxalic acid, or other reducers; sol in alkali iodide solns with liberation of iodine; soluble in hot caustic alkali solns. LD$_{50}$ i.p. in guinea pigs: 220 mg/kg (Venugopal, Luckey).
USE: Electrodes in batteries; oxidizing agent in manuf dyes; as discharge in dyeing with indigo; manuf rubber substitutes; with amorphous phosphorus as ignition surface for matches; pyrotechny; manuf pigments; in anal. chemistry.

5408. Lead Fluoride. [7783-46-2] Lead difluoride; plumbous fluoride. F$_2$Pb; mol wt 245.20. F 15.50%, Pb 84.50%. PbF$_2$. Prepd by treating lead carbonate or hydroxide with hydrogen fluoride and evaporating the soln; by mixing solns of potassium fluoride and lead acetate; by precipitation from the soln of a lead salt by HF; by the action of fluorine on lead: Ruff, *Die Chemie des Fluors* (Springer, Berlin, 1920) p 33; Emeléus in *Fluorine Chemistry* vol. 1, J. H. Simons, Ed. (Academic Press, New York, 1950) p 51; Kwasnik in *Handbook of Preparative Inorganic Chemistry* vol. 1, G. Brauer, Ed. (Academic Press, New York, 1963) pp 218-219. *Review:* Kemmitt, Sharp, *Adv. Fluorine Chem.* **4,** 188 (1965).
White to colorless crystals. *Poisonous!* Dimorphous: orthorhombic, converted to cubic above 316°. d (orthorhombic) 8.445; d (cubic) 7.750. mp 824°. bp 1293°. Soly in water (g/100 ml): 0.057 (0°); 0.065 (20°). The soly increases in the presence of HNO$_3$ or nitrates.

5409. Lead Formate. [811-54-1] C$_2$H$_2$O$_4$Pb; mol wt 297.23. C 8.08%, H 0.68%, O 21.53%, Pb 69.71%. Pb(CHO$_2$)$_2$.
White, lustrous prisms or needles. *Poisonous!* d 4.63. Dec at 190°. Sol in 65 parts cold water, 6 parts boiling water; insol in alcohol.

5410. Lead Hexafluorosilicate. [25808-74-6] Lead fluosilicate; lead silicofluoride. F$_6$PbSi; mol wt 349.28. F 32.64%, Pb 59.32%, Si 8.04%. PbSiF$_6$.
Dihydrate. Colorless crystals. Sol in water. *Poisonous!*
USE: In refining lead by electrolytic methods.

5411. Lead Iodide. [10101-63-0] I$_2$Pb; mol wt 461.01. I 55.05%, Pb 44.94%. PbI$_2$. Review of toxicology and human exposure: *Toxicological Profile for Lead* (PB99-166704, 1999) 640 pp.
Bright yellow, heavy odorless powder. *Poisonous!* d 6.16. mp 402°. One gram dissolves in 1350 ml cold, 230 ml boiling water; sol in concd solns of alkali iodides; freely sol in soln of sodium thiosulfate; sol in 200 parts cold 90 parts hot aniline; insol in alcohol or cold HCl. *Protect from light.*
USE: Bronzing, gold pencils, mosaic gold, printing, photography.

5412. Lead Molybdate(VI). [10190-55-3] MoO$_4$Pb; mol wt 367.14. Mo 26.13%, O 17.43%, Pb 56.44%. PbMoO$_4$. Occurs as the mineral *wulfenite*.
Yellow powder. Insol in water; sol in HNO$_3$ or NaOH when freshly pptd.
USE: In pigments.

5413. Lead Monoxide. [1317-36-8] Lead oxide (PbO); lead (II) oxide; lead oxide yellow; plumbous oxide; litharge; massicot; lead protoxide. OPb; mol wt 223.20. O 7.17%, Pb 92.83%. PbO. Prepn of high purity PbO: Kwestroo, Huizing, *J. Inorg. Nucl. Chem.* **27,** 1591 (1965); Kwestroo *et al., ibid.* **29,** 39 (1967). Mfg processes: *Faith, Keyes & Clark's Industrial Chemicals*, F. A. Lowenheim, M. K. Moran, Eds. (Wiley-Interscience, New York, 4th ed., 1975) pp 509-513. Toxicity study: W. R. Bradley, W. G. Fredrick, *Ind. Med.* **10,** *Ind. Hyg. Sect.* **2,** 15 (1941). Review of toxicology and human exposure: *Toxicological Profile for Lead* (PB99-166704, 1999) 640 pp.
Exists in two forms: red to reddish-yellow, tetragonal crystals, stable at ordinary temp; yellow, orthorhombic crystals, stable above 489°: Petersen, *J. Am. Chem. Soc.* **63,** 2617 (1941). *Poisonous!* At 300-450° in the air, it converts slowly into Pb$_3$O$_4$, but at higher

temp reverts to PbO. d 9.53. mp 888°. Insol in water, alcohol. Sol in acetic acid, dil HNO_3, in warm solns of fixed alkali hydroxides. LD_{50} i.p. in rats: 40 mg Pb/100g (Bradley, Fredrick).

USE: In ointments, plasters; preparing soln of lead subacetate. Glazing pottery; glass flux for painting on porcelain and glass; lead glass; varnishes; with glycerol as metal cement; producing iridescent colors on brass and bronze; coloring sulfur-containing substances, *e.g.*, hair, nails, wool, horn; manuf artificial tortoise shell and horn; pigment for rubber; manuf boiled linseed oil; in assay of gold and silver ores.

5414. Lead Nitrate. [10099-74-8] N_2O_6Pb; mol wt 331.21. N 8.46%, O 28.98%, Pb 62.56%. $Pb(NO_3)_2$. Review of toxicology and human exposure: *Toxicological Profile for Lead* (PB99-166704, 1999) 640 pp.

White or colorless translucent crystals. *Poisonous!* d 4.53. One g dissolves in 2 ml cold, 0.75 ml boiling water, in 2500 ml abs alcohol, 75 ml abs methanol; insol in concd HNO_3. The aq soln is slightly acid. pH of 20% aq soln at 25° = 3.0-4.0.

USE: Manuf matches and special explosives; as mordant in dyeing and printing on textiles; mordant for staining horn, mother-of-pearl; oxidizer in dye industry; sensitizer in photography; process engraving.

THERAP CAT (VET): Has been used as a caustic in equine canker.

5415. Lead Oxalate. [814-93-7] C_2O_4Pb; mol wt 295.22. C 8.14%, O 21.68%, Pb 70.18%.

White, heavy powder. Dec at 300°. d 5.28. *Poisonous!* Insol in water; sol in dil HNO_3, fixed alkali hydroxides; sparingly sol in acetic acid.

5416. Lead Phosphate. [7446-27-7] $O_8P_2Pb_3$; mol wt 811.54. O 15.77%, P 7.63%, Pb 76.60%. $Pb_3(PO_4)_2$. Review of toxicology and human exposure: *Toxicological Profile for Lead* (PB99-166704, 1999) 640 pp.

White powder. d 6.9. mp 1014°. *Poisonous!* Insol in water, alcohol. Sol in HNO_3, fixed alkali hydroxides.

Caution: This substance is reasonably anticipated to be a human carcinogen: *Report on Carcinogens, Eleventh Edition* (PB2005-104914, 2004) p III-158.

USE: Stabilizer for styrene and casein plastics; in special glasses.

5417. Lead Sesquioxide. [1314-27-8] Lead trioxide; plumbous plumbate. O_3Pb_2; mol wt 462.40. O 10.38%, Pb 89.62%. Pb_2O_3.

Reddish-yellow powder; converted at 370° in air to Pb_3O_4, dec at ~530° to PbO. Insol in water; dec by concd HCl or H_2SO_4 with the liberation of Cl or oxygen, respectively.

5418. Lead Stearate. [1072-35-1] Octadecanoic acid lead (2+) salt; lead distearate; stearic acid lead salt. $C_{36}H_{70}O_4Pb$; mol wt 774.14. C 55.85%, H 9.11%, O 8.27%, Pb 26.77%. $Pb(C_{18}H_{35}O_2)_2$.

White powder, mp ~125°. *Poisonous!* Insol in water; sol in hot alcohol.

USE: In extreme pressure lubricants; as drier in varnishes.

5419. Lead Subacetate. [1335-32-6] Lead monosubacetate; monobasic lead acetate. $C_4H_{10}O_8Pb_3$; mol wt 807.72. C 5.95%, H 1.25%, O 15.85%, Pb 76.96%. $Pb(C_2H_3O_2)_2 \cdot 2Pb(OH)_2$.

White, heavy powder. *Poisonous!* Sol in 16 parts cold, 4 parts boiling water with alkaline reaction. On exposure to air absorbs CO_2 and becomes incompletely sol. *Keep well closed.*

USE: In sugar analysis to remove coloring matters, etc., from solns before polarizing; for clarifying and decolorizing other solns of organic substances.

5420. Lead Sulfate. [7446-14-2] O_4PbS; mol wt 303.26. O 21.10%, Pb 68.32%, S 10.57%. $PbSO_4$. Occurs as the minerals: *anglesite, lanarkite*. Review of toxicology and human exposure: *Toxicological Profile for Lead* (PB99-166704, 1999) 640 pp.

White, heavy, cryst powder. *Poisonous!* d 6.2. mp 1170°. Sol in about 2225 parts water; more soluble in dil HCl or HNO_3, less in dil H_2SO_4; sol in NaOH, ammonium acetate or tartrate soln; sol in concd hydriodic acid. Insol in alcohol.

USE: As pigment instead of white lead; manuf of galvanic and lead-acid batteries; manuf minium, in lithography; preparing rapidly drying oil varnishes; weighting fabrics.

5421. Lead Sulfide. [1314-87-0] PbS; mol wt 239.27. Pb 86.60%, S 13.40%. Occurs as the mineral *galena*. Toxicity study: W. R. Bradley, W. G. Fredrick, *Ind. Med.* **10**, *Ind. Hyg. Sect.* **2**, 15 (1941). Review of toxicology and human exposure: *Toxicological Profile for Lead* (PB99-166704, 1999) 640 pp.

Black powder. Insol in water. Sol in HNO_3, hot, dil HCl. LD_{50} i.p. in rats: 160 mg Pb/100 g (Bradley, Fredrick).

USE: Glazing earthenware.

5422. Lead Telluride. [1314-91-6] PbTe; mol wt 334.80. Pb 61.89%, Te 38.11%. Found in nature as the mineral *altaite*. Prepd from lead nitrate, sodium carbonate and powdered tellurium: Montignie, *Bull. Soc. Chim. Fr.* **1947**, 750. Prepn of single crystals by heating stoichiometric quantities of the elements in a graphite cup or fused quartz tube: Brady, *J. Electrochem. Soc.* **101**, 466 (1954).

Silver-gray cubic crystals. d_4^{20} 8.16. mp 905°. Most of the crystal is *p*-type, the *n*-type material being present in the surface layer. Energy gap 0.27 ev. Electron mobility 2240 cm^2/volt-sec. Hole mobility 860 cm^2/volt-sec. Resistivity 0.005 ohm-cm (*p*-type), 0.00090 ohm-cm (*n*-type). Not attacked by hydrochloric, hydrofluoric, perchloric and acetic acids or their mixtures; not attacked by solns of 30% potassium hydroxide or of alkali metal sulfides. Dil nitric acid turns the surface black, while concd nitric acid produces lighter gray surface and turns the black surface to gray. Hot concd sulfuric acid produces a reddish-violet surface.

USE: In photoconductor cells; in semiconductor research.

5423. Lead Tetraacetate. [546-67-8] $C_8H_{12}O_8Pb$; mol wt 443.38. C 21.67%, H 2.73%, O 28.87%, Pb 46.73%. $Pb(CH_3COO)_4$. Prepd from Pb_3O_4 and glacial acetic acid preferably in the presence of some acetic anhydride: Dimroth, Schweizer, *Ber.* **56**, 1375 (1923); Bailar, *Inorg. Synth.* **1**, 47 (1939); Baudler in *Handbook of Preparative Inorganic Chemistry* vol. 1, G. Brauer, Ed. (Academic Press, New York, 2nd ed., 1963) p 767. Prepn by electrolysis: Fioshin, Gus'kov, *Dokl. Akad. Nauk SSSR* **112**, 303 (1957), *C.A.* **51**, 16146 (1957); Sataev *et al., Khim. Prom. (Moscow)* **46**, 892 (1970), *C.A.* **74**, 49005x (1971). Reviews of prepn and use as oxidizing agent: Criegee "Oxidations with Lead Tetraacetate" in *Oxidation in Organic Chemistry,* Part A, K. B. Wiberg, Ed. (Academic Press, New York, 1965) pp 277-366; Zyka, *Pure Appl. Chem.* **13**, 569-581 (1966).

Colorless monoclinic prisms from glacial acetic acid. Turns pink easily. Unstable in air. Hydrolyzed by water with the formation of brown lead dioxide and acetic acid. *Avoid contact with skin.* d_4^{17} 2.228. mp 175-180°. Sol in hot glacial acetic acid, benzene, chloroform, tetrachloroethane, nitrobenzene. Dissolves in concd halogen acids with the formation of haloplumbic acids, H_2PbX_6. The dry material can be stored in sealed, evacuated ampuls.

USE: Selective oxidizing agent in organic syntheses: Criegee, *Angew. Chem.* **53**, 321 (1940); *Newer Methods of Preparative Organic Chemistry* (Interscience, N. Y., 1948) pp 1-17.

5424. Lead Tetrafluoride. [7783-59-7] Plumbic fluoride. F_4Pb; mol wt 283.19. F 26.83%, Pb 73.17%. PbF_4. Prepd by passing fluorine diluted with CO_2 or N_2 over PbF_2 at 300°: v. Wartenberg, *Z. Anorg. Allg. Chem.* **244**, 339 (1940). *Review:* Kemmitt, Sharp, *Adv. Fluorine Chem.* **4**, 187 (1965).

White, tetragonal crystals, d 6.7. mp ~600°. Readily hydrolyzes and turns brown (forms PbO₂) in the presence of moisture.

USE: Has been proposed as a fluorinating agent for hydrocarbons.

5425. Lead Tetroxide. [1314-41-6] Lead oxide red; red lead; minium; lead orthoplumbate; mineral orange; mineral red; Paris red; Saturn red; C.I. Pigment Red 105; C.I. 77578. O_4Pb_3; mol wt 685.60. O 9.33%, Pb 90.67%. Pb_3O_4. The article of commerce contains about 90% Pb_3O_4; the remainder being chiefly lead monoxide. Prepn: M. Baudler in *Handbook of Preparative Inorganic Chemistry* vol. 1, G. Brauer, Ed. (Academic Press, New York, 1963) pp 755-757. Structure: S. T. Gross, *J. Am. Chem. Soc.* **65**, 1107 (1943). *Review: Mellor's* vol. 7 (1930) pp 672-680. Book: *Biologic Effects of Atmospheric Pollutants: Lead* (Nat. Acad. Sci., Washington, D.C., 1972) 330 p.

Bright-red, heavy powder. *Poisonous!* Dec at ~500° with evolution of oxygen. d 9.1. Insol in water or alcohol. Sol in excess glacial acetic acid, in hot HCl with evolution of Cl, in dil HNO_3 in presence of H_2O_2. LD_{50} i.p. in rats: 45 mg Pb/100 g (*Lead*, 1972).

USE: Plasters and ointments; manuf colorless glass; glaze for faience; flux for porcelain painting, protective paint for iron and steel; oil-color for ship paints, varnishes; coloring rubber; cement for glass, gas and steam pipes; storage batteries; pencils for writing on glass; manuf lead peroxide; matches.

5426. Lead Thiocyanate. [592-87-0] Lead sulfocyanate. $C_2N_2PbS_2$; mol wt 323.36. C 7.43%, N 8.66%, Pb 64.08%, S 19.83%. $Pb(SCN)_2$. Prepn: Gardner, Weinberger, *Inorg. Synth.* **1**, 85 (1939).

White, odorless powder. d 3.82. *Poisonous!* Sol in ~200 parts cold, 50 parts boiling water; also sol in alkali hydroxide and thiocyanate solns.

USE: Reverse dyeing with aniline black; manufacture of safety matches and cartridges.

5427. Lead Vanadate(V). [10099-79-3] Lead metavanadate. O_6PbV_2; mol wt 405.08. O 23.70%, Pb 51.15%, V 25.15%. $Pb(VO_3)_2$.

Yellow powder. Insol in water. Dec by HNO_3.

USE: Manuf other vanadium compds; as pigment.

5428. Lecithins. [8002-43-5] Phosphatidylcholine; Lecithol; Vitellin; Kelecin; Granulestin. Phosphatides found in all living organisms (plants and animals). Significant constituent of nervous tissue and brain substance. A mixture of the diglycerides of stearic, palmitic, and oleic acids, linked to the choline ester of phosphoric acid. Commercial grades contain 2.2% P. Isoln from eggs: Sinclair, *Can. J. Res.* **26B**, 777 (1948). Product of commerce is predominantly soybean lecithin obtained as a by-product in the manuf of soybean oil: Stanley in K. S. Markley, *Soybeans* **vol. II** (Interscience, New York, 1951) pp 593-647. Soybean lecithin contains palmitic acid 11.7%, stearic 4.0%, palmitoleic 8.6%, oleic 9.8%, linoleic 55.0%, linolenic 4.0%, C_{20} to C_{22} acids (includes arachidonic) 5.5%. Synthesis of a mixed acid α-lecithin: de Haas, van Deenen, *Tetrahedron Lett.* **1960** (no. 9), 1. Synthetic L-α-(distearoyl)lecithin is identical with hydrogenated egg yolk lecithin and L-α-(dipalmitoyl)lecithin is identical with colfosceril palmitate, *q.v.*, a natural phosphatide of brain, lung, and spleen. Commercial grades of natural lecithin are reported to contain a potent vasodepressor substance: McQuarrie, Andersen, *US 2931818* (1960 to Cutter Labs.). Comprehensive monograph: G. B. Ansell, J. N. Hawthorne, *Phospholipids* (Elsevier, New York, 1964) 439 pp; A. Wendel, "Lecithin" in *Kirk-Othmer Encyclopedia of Chemical Technology* **vol. 15** (Wiley-Interscience, New York, 4th ed., 1995) pp 192-210.

R = fatty acids

Waxy mass when the acid value is about 20. Pourable, thick fluid when the acid value is around 30. Color is nearly white when freshly made, but rapidly becomes yellow to brown in air. d_4^{24} 1.0305. Iodine value 95; saponification value 196. Insoluble but swells up in water and in NaCl soln forming a colloidal suspension. Soluble in about 12 parts cold, abs alcohol; sol in chloroform, ether, petr ether, in mineral oils and fatty acids; sparingly sol in benzene. Insol in acetone; practically insol in cold vegetable and animal oils.

USE: Edible and digestible surfactant and emulsifier of natural origin. Used in margarine, chocolate and in the food industry in general. In pharmaceuticals and cosmetics. Many other industrial uses, e.g. treating leather and textiles.

THERAP CAT: Lipotropic.

5429. Lectins. Agglutinins; affinitins; phytoagglutinins; phasins; protectins. A group of proteins, widely distributed in nature, that have the ability to agglutinate erythrocytes and many other types of cells. Although their existence has been known since 1899, when Stillmark isolated a hemagglutinin from castor beans, the term "lectin" (from the Latin *legere*, to choose) was first introduced by W. C. Boyd and E. Slapleigh in *Science* **119**, 419 (1954). It is now used to designate "a sugar-binding protein or glycoprotein of non-immune origin which agglutinates cells and/or precipitates glycoconjugates", I. J. Goldstein *et al.*, *Nature* **285**, 66 (1980). Lectins are found primarily in seeds of plants, but also occur in roots, leaves and bark. In addition, they are present in invertebrates such as clams, snails, and horseshoe crabs, and in several vertebrate species. The term *phytohemagglutinin* is used to refer to plant lectins. Important members of the lectin family include concanavalin A, abrin, ricin, *q.q.v.*, as well as *soybean agglutinin* or *SBA* and *wheat germ agglutinin* or *WGA*. Lectins vary considerably in chemical and physical properties; only a limited number have been purified. Mol wts of 17,000 to 400,000 have been reported and most lectins have been found to contain Mn^{2+} and Ca^{2+}. Nearly all lectins can be inhibited by free oligo- or monosaccharides of appropriate specificity. Although their physiological functions in plants or in other organisms are unknown, lectins exhibit a variety of unusual biological properties. Some are specific in their reactions with human blood groups; some induce mitosis in lymphocytes. WGA from wheat germ lipase has been shown to agglutinate mouse tumor cells more readily than cells from normal tissue: J. C. Aub *et al.*, *Proc. Natl. Acad. Sci. USA* **50**, 613 (1963); M. M. Burger, A. R. Goldberg, *ibid.* **57**, 359 (1967). Soybean agglutinin and concanavalin A have been shown to agglutinate cell lines transformed by viral or chemical carcinogens: M. Inbar, L. Sachs, *Nature* **223**, 710 (1969); *eidem, Proc. Natl. Acad. Sci. USA* **63**, 1418 (1969); B. A. Sela *et al.*, *J. Membr. Biol.* **3**, 267 (1970). Some plant lectins mimic the direct effects of insulin on nuclear envelope phosphorylation: F. Purrello *et al.*, *Science* **221**, 462 (1983). Soybean agglutinin has also been used in bone marrow transplants in patients with severe combined immunodeficiency: Y. Reisner *et al.*, *Blood* **61**, 341 (1983). Reviews: N. Sharon, H. Lis, *Science* **177**, 949-955 (1972); *eidem, Annu. Rev. Biochem.* **42**, 541-574 (1973); L. Sequeira, *Annu. Rev. Phytopathol.* **16**, 453-481 (1978). Book: *Lectins: Biology, Biochemistry, Clinical Biochemistry* vol. 1, T. C. Bog-Hansen, Ed. (de Gruyter, New York, 1981) 414 pp.

USE: As tools for studying cell surface properties; in cancer research.

5430. Ledol. [577-27-5] [1aR-(1aα,4α,4aβ,7α,7aβ,7bα)]-Decahydro-1,1,4,7-tetramethyl-1H-cycloprop[e]azulen-4-ol; "Ledum camphor". $C_{15}H_{26}O$; mol wt 222.37. C 81.02%, H 11.79%, O 7.19%. Occurs in the essential oil from leaves of *Ledum palustre* L.: Grassmann, *Repert. Pharm.* **38**, 53 (1931); Hjelt, *Ber.* **28**, 3087 (1895); from *L. groenlandicum* Veder; *L. columbianum* Piper, *Ericaceae:* Cain, Lynn, *J. Am. Pharm. Assoc.* **23**, 666 (1934); Penfold, *J. Proc. R. Soc. N.S.W.* **59**, 206 (1925). Structure: G. Büchi *et al., Tetrahedron Lett.* **1959** (no. 6), 14. Stereochemistry: L. Dolejs, F. Sorm, *Tetrahedron Lett.* **1959** (no. 17), 1; revised stereochemistry: G. Büchi *et al., J. Am. Chem. Soc.* **91**, 6473 (1969).

Needles from alc, mp 104-105°. Sublimes easily, even below the mp. bp$_{760}$ 292°. n_D^{110} 1.4667. $[\alpha]_D^{20}$ +28° (c = 10 in chloroform). Practically insol in water. Sol in alc (about 10% w/v). Soluble in other organic solvents.

Chromate. $C_{30}H_{50}O_4Cr$. Ruby-red prisms, mp 92°. $[\alpha]_{671}^{20}$ +30° (c = 2 in chloroform).

5431. Lefetamine. [7262-75-1] (αR)-N,N-Dimethyl-α-phenylbenzeneethanamine; (−)-N,N-dimethyl-1,2-diphenylethylamine; (−)-N,N-dimethyl-α-phenylphenethylamine. $C_{16}H_{19}$-N; mol wt 225.33. C 85.28%, H 8.50%, N 6.22%. Centrally acting analgesic with stereochemical resemblance to morphine, *q.v.* Prepn and activity: K. Ogiu *et al.*, *J. Pharm. Soc. Jpn.* **80**, 283 (1960); *eidem,* **JP 61 23087** (1961 to Res. Found. Practical Life). Absolute configuration: M. Nakazaki, *Chem. Ind. (London)* **1962**, 1577.

NMR data indicates 22% eclipsed conformation which appears to enhance stereoselectivity for morphine receptors: T. Sasaki *et al., J. Med. Chem.* **9**, 847 (1966). Pharmacology: H. Nakamura, M. Shimizu, *Arch. Int. Pharmacodyn. Ther.* **221**, 105 (1976). Clinical study: J. P. Famaey, T. L. Peeters, *Brux. Med.* **56**, 21 (1976). Analgesic activity: M. Nozaki *et al., Life Sci.* **33**, Suppl. 1, 431 (1983). Opiate agonist activity: M. Graziella de Montis *et al., Pharmacol. Res. Commun.* **17**, 471 (1985).

bp$_6$ 142-147°. $[\alpha]_D^{20}$ −124.2° (ethanol).

Hydrochloride. [14148-99-3] Santenol; SPA. C$_{16}$H$_{19}$N.HCl; mol wt 261.79. mp 218-219°. $[\alpha]_D^{20}$ −91.7° (water).

Note: This is a controlled substance (stimulant): **21 CFR**, 1308.14.

THERAP CAT: Analgesic.

5432. Leflunomide. [75706-12-6] 5-Methyl-*N*-[4-(trifluoromethyl)phenyl]-4-isoxazolecarboxamide; α,α,α-trifluoro-5-methyl-4-isoxazolecarboxy-*p*-toluidide; 5-methylisoxazole-4-carboxylic acid trifluoromethylanilide; HWA-486; Arava. C$_{12}$H$_9$F$_3$N$_2$O$_2$; mol wt 270.21. C 53.34%, H 3.36%, F 21.09%, N 10.37%, O 11.84%. Disease modifying antirheumatic drug (DMARD) with immunosuppressant activity. Converted *in vivo* to its active open ring metabolite, teriflunomide, *q.v.* Inhibits *de novo* pyrimidine biosynthesis in immune cells. Prepn: F. J. Kaemmerer, R. Schleyerbach, **DE 2854439**; *eidem*, **US 4284786** (1980, 1981 both to Hoechst); and pharmacology: P. Fossa *et al., Farmaco* **46**, 789 (1991). HPLC determn of active metabolite in plasma: V. C. Dias *et al., Ther. Drug Monit.* **17**, 84 (1995). Review of mechanisms of action: R. I. Fox, *J. Rheumatol.* **25**, Suppl. 53, 20-26 (1998); of clinical pharmacology: B. Rozman, *ibid.* 27-32. Clinical trial in rheumatoid arthritis: V. Strand *et al., Arch. Intern. Med.* **159**, 2542 (1999). *Reviews:* C. Miceli-Richard, M. Dougados, *Expert Opin. Pharmacother.* **4**, 987-997 (2003); J. P. Kaltwasser, F. Behrens, *ibid.* **6**, 787-801 (2005).

Crystals from toluene, mp 166.5°. pKa 10.8. Soly in water (25°): 25 - 27 mg/l. Sol in methanol, ethanol, acetone.

THERAP CAT: Antirheumatic.

5433. Leghemoglobin. Legoglobin. Hemoglobin-like red pigment present in the root nodules of leguminous plants. Isolation from soya beans: Keilin, Wang, *Nature* **155**, 227 (1945); Appleby, *Biochim. Biophys. Acta* **60**, 226 (1962). Mol wt is approx one-fourth that of hemoglobin: Ehrenberg, Ellfolk, *Acta Chem. Scand.* **17**, S343 (1963). Resolved into four components on DEAE-cellulose column: Ellfolk, *ibid.* **14**, 609 (1960). Suggested to act as an oxido-reduction catalyst in the symbiotic nitrogen fixation: *idem, ibid.* **15**, 975 (1961). Primary structure of soybean leghemoglobin: Ellfolk, Sievers, *ibid.* **25**, 3532 (1971).

5434. Lemon Peel. Outer rind of fresh ripe fruit of *Citrus limonum* (L.) Risso (*C. medica* var. *limon* L.), Rutaceae. Habit. Northern India; cultivated in California, West Indies, Italy, Spain. *Constit.* Volatile oil, hesperidin, bitter extractive.

USE: As a flavor in medicines; also in beverages, confectionery, and cooking.

5435. Lenacil. [2164-08-1] 3-Cyclohexyl-6,7-dihydro-1*H*-cyclopentapyrimidine-2,4-(3*H*,5*H*)-dione; 3-cyclohexyl-5,6-tri-

methyleneuracil; 3-cyclohexyl-1,5,6,7-tetrahydro-2*H*-cyclopentapyrimidine-2,4(3*H*)-dione; Du Pont 634; Venzar. C$_{13}$H$_{18}$N$_2$O$_2$; mol wt 234.29. C 66.64%, H 7.74%, N 11.96%, O 13.66%. Prepn: S. Senda, H. Fujimura, **JP 62 4892** (1962), *C.A.* **59**, 642g (1963); and herbicidal activity: E. J. Soboczenski, **US 3235360** (1966 to duPont Nemours). Synthesis: S. Senda *et al., Chem. Pharm. Bull.* **21**, 1894 (1973). Mode of action: C. E. Hoffmann, *Pestic. Chem., Proc. 2nd Int. Congr. Pestic.* **5**, A. S. Tahori, Ed., (Gordon and Breach Science Publishers, New York, 1972) pp 65-85. Field evaluation: J. G. Hilton, W. E. Bray, *Proc. 12th Brit. Weed Contr. Conf.* 485 (1974). GC determn in soils: D. J. Caverly, R. C. Denney, *Analyst* **102**, 576 (1977). Soil persistence: M. Tena *et al., Weed Res.* **23**, 245 (1982). Field tolerance: D. V. Clay, *Tests Agrochem. Cultiv.* **11**, 80 (1990).

Crystals from methanol or dioxane, mp >290° (Senda, Fujimura). Also reported as light grey crystals from DMF, mp 310-313° (Soboczenski). Technical product properties: odorless, white to tan crystalline solid. d^{20} 1.32 kg/l. Vapor pressure (25°): 0.2 μPa. Soly in water 6 mg/l; in xylene: 2 g/l. LD$_{50}$ (80% wettable powder) orally in rats: >11,000 mg/kg. LC$_{50}$ 96 hr in bluegill sunfish; rainbow trout: 100-1000; 135 mg/l. LC$_{50}$ 8 day in bobwhite quail, Peking duck (mg/kg): 2300, >5620. (DuPont technical data sheet).

USE: Herbicide.

5436. Lenalidomide. [191732-72-6] 3-(4-Amino-1,3-dihydro-1-oxo-2*H*-isoindol-2-yl)-2,6-piperidinedione; 1-oxo-2-(2,6-dioxopiperidin-3-yl)-4-aminoisoindoline; CC-5013; Revimid; Revlimid. C$_{13}$H$_{13}$N$_3$O$_3$; mol wt 259.26. C 60.22%, H 5.05%, N 16.21%, O 18.51%. Immunomodulatory drug; analog of thalidomide, *q.v.* Prepn: G. W. Muller *et al., US 5635517* (1997 to Celgene); and *in vitro* TNF-α inhibition: *eidem, Bioorg. Med. Chem. Lett.* **9**, 1625 (1999). LC-MS determn in plasma: T. M. Tohnya *et al., J. Chromatogr. B* **811**, 135 (2004). Clinical evaluation in multiple myeloma: P. G. Richardson *et al., Blood* **100**, 3063 (2002); in myelodysplastic syndromes: A. List *et al., N. Engl. J. Med.* **352**, 549 (2005). Review of development, pharmacology and therapeutic potential: J. B. Bartlett *et al., Nature Rev.* **4**, 314-322 (2004); C. S. Mitsiades, N. Mitsiades, *Curr. Opin. Invest. Drugs* **5**, 635-647 (2004).

THERAP CAT: Immunomodulator.

5437. Lenampicillin. [86273-18-9] (2*S*,5*R*,6*R*)-6-[[(2*R*)-Aminophenylacetyl]amino]-3,3-dimethyl-7-oxo-4-thia-1-azabicyclo[3.2.0]heptane-2-carboxylic acid (5-methyl-2-oxo-1,3-dioxol-4-yl)methyl ester; ampicillin (5-methyl-2-oxo-1,3-dioxolen-4-yl)methyl ester; 6-[D(−)-α-aminophenylacetamido]penicillanic acid (5-methyl-2-oxo-1,3-dioxol-4-yl)methyl ester. C$_{21}$H$_{23}$N$_3$O$_7$S; mol wt 461.49. C 54.65%, H 5.02%, N 9.11%, O 24.27%, S 6.95%. Orally active ampicillin prodrug. Prepn: F. Sakamoto *et al., EP 39086*; *eidem*, **US 4342693** (1981, 1982 both to Kanebo); F. Sakamoto *et al., Chem. Pharm. Bull.* **32**, 2241 (1984); S. Ikeda *et al., ibid.* 4316. Metabolism in man, dogs, rats: N. Awata *et al., Jpn. J. Antibiot.* **38**, 1776, 1785, *C.A.* **104**, 161479u, 122550r (1985). Human pharmacokinetics: A. Saito, M. Nakashima, *Antimicrob. Agents Chemother.* **29**, 948 (1986). Series of articles on antibacterial activity, mutagenicity, pharmacology, clinical trials: *Chemotherapy (Tokyo)* **32**, Suppl. 8, pp 1-772 (1984). Acute toxicity data: F. Ogino *et al., ibid.* 31.

Hydrochloride. [80734-02-7] KB-1585; KBT-1585; Takacillin; Varacillin. $C_{21}H_{23}N_3O_7S.HCl$; mol wt 497.95. Crystals from isopropanol-ethyl acetate, mp 145° (dec). LD_{50} in male, female rats, male, female mice (mg/kg): approx 10000, approx 10000, 8294, 8492 orally; 4362, 4471, 3576, 4284 s.c.; 876, 838, 711, 775 i.v.; in dogs (mg/kg): >300 orally (Ogino).

THERAP CAT: Antibacterial.

5438. Lenthionine. [292-46-6] 1,2,3,5,6-Pentathiepane. $C_2H_4S_5$; mol wt 188.38. C 12.75%, H 2.14%, S 85.11%. Odorous principle from the edible mushroom *Shiitake Lentinus edodes* (Berk.) Sing. Isoln and synthesis: Morita, Kobayashi, *Tetrahedron Lett.* **1966**, 573. Simple, efficient synthesis: I. Still, G. W. Kutney, *ibid.* **22**, 1939 (1981).

Crystals from methylene chloride, mp 60-61°.

5439. Lentinan. [37339-90-5] LC-33; $(C_6H_{10}O_5)_n$; mol wt 400,000-800,000. Neutral polysaccharide isolated from the edible mushroom, *Lentinus edodes* (Berk.) Sing. Primary structure is a β-1,3-D-glucan having 2 β-1,6-glucopyranoside branchings for every 5 β-1,3 linear linkages. Isoln and antitumor activity: G. Chihara *et al., Nature* **222**, 637 (1969); *eidem, Cancer Res.* **30**, 2776 (1970). Immunostimulant activity: Y. Y. Maeda, G. Chihara, *Nature* **229**, 634 (1971). Prepn of stable aqueous solution: M. Fujii *et al., NL 7601114*; *eidem, US 4207312* (1976, 1980 both to Ajinomoto; Morishita). Structural study: T. Sasaki *et al., Carbohydr. Res.* **47**, 99 (1976). Preclinical evaluation and toxicity studies: G. Chihara, *Adv. Exp. Med. Biol.* **166**, 189 (1983). Mechanism of action studies: H. Miyakoshi, T. Aoki, *Int. J. Immunopharmacol.* **6**, 365, 373 (1984). Clinical trial in gastric and colorectal cancer: T. Taguchi *et al., Adv. Exp. Med. Biol.* **166**, 181 (1983); K. Okuyama *et al., Cancer* **55**, 2498 (1985). *Review:* G. Chihara, *Int. J. Tissue Res.* **4**, 207-225 (1982).

White powder, dec 250°. Sol in aqueous alkali, formic acid. Slightly sol in hot water, DMSO. Insol in cold water, alcohol, ether, chloroform, pyridine, hexamethylphosphoramide. Stable against sulfuric and hydrochloric acids. $[\alpha]_D^{20}$ +13.5-14.5° (in 2% NaOH); +19.5-21.5° (in 10% NaOH).

THERAP CAT: Antineoplastic; immunomodulator.

5440. Leonurine. [24697-74-3] 4-Hydroxy-3,5-dimethoxybenzoic acid 4-[(aminoiminomethyl)amino]butyl ester; 4-hydroxy-3,5-dimethoxybenzoic acid δ-guanidinobutyl ester; syringic acid δ-guanidinobutyl ester; [4-(4-hydroxy-3,5-dimethoxybenzoyloxy)butyl]guanidine; 4-guanidino-1-butanol syringate. $C_{14}H_{21}N_3O_5$; mol wt 311.33. C 54.01%, H 6.80%, N 13.50%, O 25.70%. Isoln from leaves of *Leonurus sibiricus* L., *Labiatae:* Kubota, Nakajima, *C.A.* **25**, 771 (1931). Structure: Goto *et al., Tetrahedron Lett.* **1962**, 545. Revised structure: Kishi *et al., ibid.* **1968**, 637. Structure

and synthesis: Sugiura *et al., Tetrahedron* **25**, 5155 (1969). Alternate synthesis: K. F. Cheng *et al., Experientia* **35**, 571 (1979). Biological effect: H. W. Yeung *et al., Planta Med.* **31**, 51 (1977).

Hydrochloride monohydrate. $C_{14}H_{21}N_3O_5.HCl.H_2O$. mp 193-194°. pKa 7.9 in water.

5441. Lepidine. [491-35-0] 4-Methylquinoline; cincholepidine. $C_{10}H_9N$; mol wt 143.19. C 83.88%, H 6.34%, N 9.78%. Prepn from 2-chlorolepidine: Neumann *et al., Org. Synth.* **26**, 45 (1946); from aniline hydrochloride: Campbell, *US 2451611* (1948 to du Pont); Bach, Rast, *J. Prakt. Chem.* **17**, 63 (1962); from ethylacetanilide: Ardashev, Minkin, *Zh. Obshch. Khim.* **28**, 1578 (1958).

Colorless, oily liq; quinoline odor; turns reddish-brown in light. bp 261-263°; bp_{14-15} 126-127°; bp_{6-7} 115-120°; $bp_{1.5-2}$ 90-95°. d_4^{20} 1.0826. n_D^{20} 1.6190. mp 0°. Slightly sol in water; miscible with alc, benzene, ether. *Protect from light.*

5442. Leptandra. Culver's root; black root. Dried rhizome and roots of *Veronicastrum virginicum* (L.) Farw. (*Leptandra virginica* (L.) Nutt.), *Scrophulariaceae. Habit.* North America. *Constit.* A sterol; esters of cinnamic, methoxycinnamic and fatty acids; resin saponin, tannin, sugars.

THERAP CAT: Cathartic.

5443. Leptin. OB protein. Peptide hormone produced by adipose tissue that is thought to act on receptors in the brain to regulate body weight and fat deposition. Name derived from the Greek word "leptos" meaning "thin." Protein product of the *obese* (*ob*) gene, mutation of which causes marked obesity and diabetes in mice. Secreted by adipocytes; mol wt 16 kDa. Identification of weight-regulating substance in blood of normal mice: D. L. Coleman, *Diabetologia* **9**, 294 (1973). Cloning of mouse and human *ob* genes: Y. Zhang *et al., Nature* **372**, 425 (1994). Biological activity as regulator of body weight in mice: M. A. Pelleymounter *et al., Science* **269**, 540 (1995); J. L. Halaas *et al., ibid.* 543. Identification of brain as target tissue: L. A. Campfield *et al., ibid.* 546. Increased *ob* gene expression in obese humans: R. V. Considine *et al., J. Clin. Invest.* **95**, 2986 (1995). Review of discovery and role in energy homeostasis: M. Rosenbaum, R. L. Leibel, *Trends Endocrinol. Metab.* **9**, 117-124 (1998).

5444. Leptomycin B. [87081-35-4] (2E,5S,6R,7S,9R,10E,-12E,15R,16Z,18E)-19-[(2S,3S)-3,6-Dihydro-3-methyl-6-oxo-2H-pyran-2-yl]-17-ethyl-6-hydroxy-3,5,7,9,11,15-hexamethyl-8-oxo-2,10,12,16,18-nonadecapentaenoic acid; elactocin; CL-1957A; NSC-364372; PD-114720. $C_{33}H_{48}O_6$; mol wt 540.73. C 73.30%, H 8.95%, O 17.75%. Antibiotic compound with antifungal and antitumor activity. Inhibits the CRM1/exportin1 pathway of nuclear transport in eukaryotic cells, facilitating its use in the study of nuclear export. Isoln from *Streptomyces* sp. ATS1287: T. Hamamoto *et al., J. Antibiot.* **36**, 639 (1983); from actinomycete ATCC 39366: G. C. Hokanson *et al., EP 139458*; *eidem, US 4771070* (1985, 1988 both to Warner Lambert). Antitumor activity: B. J. Roberts *et al., Cancer Chemother. Pharmacol.* **16**, 95 (1986); and antimicrobial activity: J. B. Tunac *et al., J. Antibiot.* **38**, 460 (1985). Synthesis and abs config: M. Kobayashi *et al., Tetrahedron Lett.* **39**, 8291 (1998). HPLC determn in fermentation extracts: M. Stadler *et al., J. Chromatogr. A* **818**, 187 (1998). Review of use as inhibitor of nuclear export: M. Yoshida *et al., Actinomycetologica* **12**, 120-128 (1998).

Isolated as yellow sticky oil (Hamamoto). Sol in methanol, ethanol, ethyl acetate and ethyl ether. Insol in *n*-hexane, water. $[\alpha]_D$ −24.5° (c = 0.70 in MeOH). uv max (ethanol): 225 nm (ε 20000); shoulder 240 nm (ε 15000). Purified as a pale yellow solid foam, mp 41-44°, with prior softening (Hokanson). $[\alpha]_D^{23}$ −157 ° (c = 0.7% in chloroform).

USE: Biological tool for studying nuclear localization and protein trafficking in eukaryotic cells.

5445. Leptophos. [21609-90-5] Phenylphosphonothioic acid *O*-(4-bromo-2,5-dichlorophenyl) *O*-methyl ester; *O*-(4-bromo-2,5-dichlorophenyl) *O*-methyl phenylphosphonothioate; *O*-methyl *O*-2,5-dichloro-4-bromophenyl phenylthiophosphonate; VCS-506; Abar; Phosvel. $C_{13}H_{10}BrCl_2O_2PS$; mol wt 412.07. C 37.89%, H 2.45%, Br 19.39%, Cl 17.21%, O 7.77%, P 7.52%, S 7.78%. Prepn and use as an insecticide: Richter, Hanna; US 3459836, US 3551563, US 3577482 (1969, 1970, 1971, all to Velsicol). Metabolism in mice and on cotton plants: Holmstead *et al., Arch. Environ. Contam. Toxicol.* **1**, 133 (1973). Toxicological studies in mammals: Kamel *et al., J. Eur. Toxicol.* **6**, 70 (1973); Abou-Donia *et al., Experientia* **30**, 63 (1974); T. B. Gaines, R. E. Linder, *Fundam. Appl. Toxicol.* **7**, 299 (1986).

Tan waxy solid. mp range 55-67°. Sp gr at 25° = 1.53. Solubility at 25° (gm/100 ml): benzene, 133; xylene, 73; acetone, 62; cyclohexane,14; heptane, 7; isopropanol, 2.4; water, 0.03 ppm. Stable to acids; hydrolyzed slowly under strongly alkaline conditions. LD_{50} in adult male, female rats (mg/kg): 19, 20 orally (Gaines, Linder).

USE: Insecticide.

5446. Lercanidipine. [100427-26-7] 1,4-Dihydro-2,6-dimethyl-4-(3-nitrophenyl)-3,5-pyridinedicarboxylic acid 2-[(3,3-diphenylpropyl)methylamino]-1,1-dimethylethyl methyl ester; methyl 1,1,*N*-trimethyl-*N*-(3,3-diphenylpropyl)-2-aminoethyl 1,4-dihydro-2,6-dimethyl-4-(3-nitrophenyl)pyridine-3,5-dicarboxylate; methyl 1,1-dimethyl-2-[*N*-(3,3-diphenylpropyl)-*N*-methylamino]ethyl 2,6-dimethyl-4-(3-nitrophenyl)-1,4-dihydropyridine-3,5-dicarboxylate; masnidipine. $C_{36}H_{41}N_3O_6$; mol wt 611.73. C 70.68%, H 6.76%, N 6.87%, O 15.69%. Dihydropyridine calcium channel blocker. Prepn: D. Nardi *et al.*, **EP 153016**; *eidem*, **US 4705797** (1985, 1987 both to Recordati). Pharmacology: G. Bianchi *et al., Pharmacol. Res.* **21**, 193 (1989). Clinical evaluation in hypertension: E. Rimoldi *et al., Acta Ther.* **20**, 23 (1994).

Hydrochloride. [132866-11-6] Rec-15-2375; R-75; Lerdip; Zanidip. $C_{36}H_{41}N_3O_6 \cdot HCl$; mol wt 648.19. Prepd as the hemi-

hydrate, mp 119-123°. LD_{50} in mice (mg/kg): 83 i.p.; 657 orally (Nardi).

THERAP CAT: Antihypertensive.

5447. Lesopitron. [132449-46-8] 2-[4-[4-(4-Chloro-1*H*-pyrazol-1-yl)butyl]-1-piperazinyl]pyrimidine. $C_{15}H_{21}ClN_6$; mol wt 320.82. C 56.16%, H 6.60%, Cl 11.05%, N 26.20%. Selective serotonin $5HT_{1A}$-receptor agonist. Prepn: A. Colombo Pinol *et al.*, **EP 382637**; *eidem*, **US 5128343** (1990, 1992 both to Esteve). Receptor binding studies and pharmacology: B. Costall *et al., J. Pharmacol. Exp. Ther.* **262**, 90 (1992); M. Ballarin *et al., Br. J. Pharmacol.* **113**, 425 (1994). Gastroprotective effects: A. J. Farré *et al., J. Pharmacol. Exp. Ther.* **272**, 832 (1995).

Dihydrochloride. [132449-89-9] E-4424. $C_{15}H_{21}ClN_6 \cdot 2HCl$; mol wt 393.74. Crystals, mp 194-197.5°.

THERAP CAT: Anxiolytic.

5448. Leteprinim. [138117-50-7] 4-[[3-(1,6-Dihydro-6-oxo-9*H*-purin-9-yl)-1-oxopropyl]amino]benzoic acid. $C_{15}H_{13}N_5O_4$; mol wt 327.29. C 55.05%, H 4.00%, N 21.40%, O 19.55%. Synthetic purine derivative with neuroprotective effects. Prepn: A. J. Glasky, **WO 9114434** (1991); *idem*, **US 5091432** (1992). Effect on working memory in mice: *idem et al., Pharmacol. Biochem. Behav.* **47**, 325 (1994). Mode of action study: P. J. Middlemiss *et al., Neurosci. Lett.* **199**, 131 (1995). Mechanism of brain efflux: R. Yan, E. M. Taylor, *Drug Metab. Dispos.* **30**, 513 (2002). Reviews of pharmacology: M. P. Rathbone *et al., Drug Dev. Res.* **45**, 356-372 (1998); *idem et al., Expert Opin. Invest. Drugs* **8**, 1255-1262 (1999).

White solid, mp 319-321°.

Potassium salt. [192564-13-9] AIT-082; Neotrofin. $C_{15}H_{13}KN_5O_4$; mol wt 366.39.

THERAP CAT: Nootropic.

5449. Letosteine. [53943-88-7] 2-[2-[(2-Ethoxy-2-oxoethyl)thio]ethyl]-4-thiazolidinecarboxylic acid; 2-[2-[(carboxymethyl)thio]ethyl]-4-thiazolidinecarboxylic acid 2-ethyl ester; Viscotiol. $C_{10}H_{17}NO_4S_2$; mol wt 279.38. C 42.99%, H 6.13%, N 5.01%, O 22.91%, S 22.95%. Cyclic cysteine derivative. Prepn: M. X. Chodkiewicz, **DE 2410307**; *eidem*, **US 4032534** (1974, 1979 to Ferlux-Chemie). Effect on viscoelasticity of mucus: E. Puchelle *et al., Eur. J. Respir. Dis.* **61** (Suppl 110), 195 (1980). In treatment of bronchitis: V. Macquet *et al., Lille Med.* **24**, 735 (1979); P. Freour, J. Vergeret, *Bordeaux Med.* **12**, 1553 (1979); P. Freour, ibid. **13**, 1431 (1980); P. Meroni *et al., Clin. Ter.* **105**, 109 (1983). Comparison with sulfur-containing compounds in bronchitis: D. Rodde, *C.R. Ther. Pharmacol. Clin.* **1**(5), 31 (1983).

Crystals from ethanol, mp 142°.

THERAP CAT: Mucolytic.

5450. Letrozole. [112809-51-5] 4,4'-(1*H*-1,2,4-Triazol-1-ylmethylene)bisbenzonitrile; 1-[bis(4-cyanophenyl)methyl]-1,2,4-

triazole; 4-[1-(4-cyanophenyl)-1-(1,2,4-triazol-1-yl)methyl]-benzonitrile; CGS-20267; Femara. $C_{17}H_{11}N_5$; mol wt 285.30. C 71.57%, H 3.89%, N 24.55%. Nonsteroidal aromatase inhibitor; structurally related to fadrozole, q.v. Prepn: R. M. Bowman et al., **EP 236940**; eidem, **US 4978672** (1987, 1990 both to Ciba-Geigy). Pharmacology: A. S. Bhatnagar et al., J. Steroid Biochem. Mol. Biol. **37**, 1021 (1990). Clinical suppression of estrogen biosynthesis: L. M. Demers et al., ibid. **44**, 687 (1993). EIA and HPLC determn in biological fluids: C. U. Pfister et al., J. Pharm. Sci. **83**, 520 (1994). Clinical evaluation in breast cancer: A. Lipton et al., Cancer **75**, 2132 (1995). Review of clinical efficacy: P. E. Goss, R. E. Smith, Expert Rev. Anticancer Ther. **2**, 249-260 (2002).

mp 181-183°.
THERAP CAT: Antineoplastic.

5451. Leucine. [61-90-5] L-Leucine; Leu; L; 2-amino-4-methylvaleric acid; α-aminoisocaproic acid; (S)-2-amino-4-methylpentanoic acid. $C_6H_{13}NO_2$; mol wt 131.17. C 54.94%, H 9.99%, N 10.68%, O 24.39%. An essential amino acid for human development. Discovery of leucine is attributed to Proust in 1819 who reported its separation from fermented milk curds. Early chemistry and biochemistry: Amino Acids and Proteins, D. M. Greenberg, Ed. (Charles C. Thomas, Springfield, IL, 1951) 950 pp., passim; J. P. Greenstein, M. Winitz, Chemistry of the Amino Acids **vols 1-3** (John Wiley and Sons, Inc., New York, 1961) pp. 2075-2096, passim. Chromatographic determn of specific activity in biological fluids: E. P. Donahue et al., J. Chromatogr. **571**, 29 (1991); separation of isotopes: P. Q. Baumann et al., ibid. **573**, 11 (1992). Metabolism in humans: K. J. Motil et al., Metabolism **30**, 783 (1981); in children receiving parenteral nutrition: O. Goulet et al., Am. J. Physiol. **265**, E540 (1993). Kinetics modelling in humans: C. Cobelli et al., ibid. **261**, E539 (1991).

White glistening hexagonal plates from aq alc. d_{18} 1.293. Sublimes at 145-148°. Dec 293-295° (rapid heating, sealed tube). $[M]_D$ +21.0° (5N HCl); $[M]_D$ +29.5° (glacial acetic acid); $[\alpha]_D^{25}$ −10.8° (c = 2.2); $[\alpha]_D^{25}$ +15.1° in 6N HCl (38 mols HCl per mol leucine); $[\alpha]_D^{20}$ +7.6° in 3N NaOH (30 mols NaOH per mol leucine). R_f value 0.79. Soly in water (g/l): 22.7 (0°); 24.26 (25°); 28.87 (50°); 38.23 (75°); 56.38 (100°); in 99% alcohol: 0.72; in acetic acid: 10.9. Insol in ether.

DL-Form. Leaflets fom water. Sweet taste. Dec 332° (also reported as 290°). Sublimes. pK_1 2.36; pK_2 9.60. Soly in water (g/l): 7.97 (0°); 9.91 (25°); 14.06 (50°); 22.76 (75°); 42.06 (100°); in 90% alcohol: 1.3. Insol in ether.

Hydrochloride. $C_6H_{13}NO_2 \cdot HCl$. Crystals. Freely sol in water.

USE: Nutrient.

5452. Leucocyanidin. [480-17-1] 2-(3,4-Dihydroxyphenyl)-3,4-dihydro-2H-1-benzopyran-3,4,5,7-tetrol; 3,3′,4,4′,5,7-flavanhexol; 3,3′,4,4′,5,7-hexahydroxyflavane; leucocyanidol; Flavan; Hamaméliode P; Résivit. $C_{15}H_{14}O_7$; mol wt 306.27. C 58.82%, H 4.61%, O 36.57%. From petals of Asiatic cotton flowers (Gossypium spp): Stephens, Arch. Biochem. Biophys. **18**, 449 (1948); from Butea frondosa Koen. ex Roxb., Leguminosae: Ganguly, Seshadri, Tetrahedron **6**, 21 (1959). Prepn from quercetin: Bauer et al., Chem. Ind. (London) **1954**, 433; from taxifolin: Freudenberg, Weinges, Ann. **613**, 61 (1958). Metabolism: Claveau, Masquelier, Can. J. Pharm. Sci. **1**, 74 (1966). See also Bioflavonoids.

Monohydrate. Crystals from ethyl acetate + petr ether, mp above 355°. uv max (ethanol): 285 nm. Soluble in water, alcohol, acetone. Practically insol in ether, chloroform, petr ether.

THERAP CAT: Capillary protectant.

5453. Leucomycins. [1392-21-8] Kitasamycin; C-637; Ayermicina; Sineptina; Stereomycin; Syneptine. Macrolide antibiotic complex similar to carbomycin, q.v. and erythromycin, q.v., produced by Streptomyces kitasatoensis Hata: T. Hata et al., J. Antibiot. **6A**, 87 (1953); Sano, ibid. **7A**, 93 (1954). Early work performed on a mixture of at least six components, A_1, A_2, B_1-B_4, of which A_1 was the most biologically active: J. Abe et al., J. Chem. Soc. Jpn. Pure Chem. Sect. **81**, 969 (1960); T. Watanabe et al., Bull. Chem. Soc. Jpn. **33**, 1100, 1104 (1960). Leucomycin isolated from an improved strain of S. kitasatoensis is a mixture of at least eight biologically active components, A_1 and new substances A_3-A_9: Hata et al., **US 3535309** (1970 to Kitasato Institute and Toyo Jozo). Leucomycins A_1, A_3-A_9, U and V are substituted variations of the structure represented below. Structure of A_1: T. Watanabe et al., Angew. Chem. **76**, 792 (1964); T. Hata et al., Chem. Pharm. Bull. **15**, 358 (1967); of A_3: S. Omura et al., Tetrahedron Lett. **1967**, 609, 1267; of A_4 through A_9: eidem, J. Antibiot. **20A**, 234 (1967); **21**, 272 (1968). Conformation: eidem, Tetrahedron **28**, 2839 (1972). Revised configuration at C-9: L. A. Freiberg et al., J. Org. Chem. **39**, 2474 (1974). Liquid chromatography of A_1, A_{3-9}, U, V: S. Omura et al., J. Antibiot. **26**, 795 (1973). Antibacterial and antimycoplasmal activity: Iwata, Akiba, ibid. **15A**, 258 (1962); Omura et al., ibid. **21**, 532 (1968); **25**, 105 (1972). In vitro and preliminary clinical studies: B. C. Stratford, S. Dixson, Med. J. Aust. **1**, 1029 (1974). Antimicrobial transformation of A_5 to V: K. Singh, S. Rakhit, ibid. **32**, 78 (1979). Biosynthesis: C. Kitao et al., ibid. **32**, 1055 (1979); S. Omura et al., ibid. **36**, 611 (1983). Reviews: Desvignes, Ann. Pharm. Fr. **21**, 569 (1963); Toju, Omura, "Chemical and Biological Studies on Leucomycins (Kitasamycins)" in Drug Action and Drug Resistance in Bacteria **vol. I**, S. Mitsuhashi, Ed. (University Park Press, Baltimore, 1971) pp 267-291; Keller-Schierlein in Fortschr. Chem. Org. Naturst. **30**, 313-460 (1973); S. Omura, A. Nakagawa, J. Antibiot. **28**, 401-433 (1975).

Leucomycin A₁

Leucomycin A_1, A_2, B_1-B_4 complex. (Sano, loc. cit.). Powder from acetone; stable at room temp; dec 125°. $[\alpha]_D^{20}$ −67.1° (ethanol). uv max (ethanol): 232, 285 nm ($E_{1cm}^{1\%}$ 228, 8.6). Freely sol in most organic solvents. Insol in petr ether. Slightly sol in water.

Leucomycin A_3-A_9 complex. White powder; mp 128-145°. uv max (methanol): 231 nm ($E_{1cm}^{1\%}$ 353). $[\alpha]_D^{25}$ −53° (c = 1 in chloroform). Sol in methanol, ethanol, ethyl acetate, butyl acetate, acetone, benzene, and chloroform; difficultly sol in water. Insol in petr ether. LD_{50} in mice (mg/kg): >650 i.v., >1000 orally (**US 3535309**).

Leucomycin A_1. $C_{40}H_{67}NO_{14}$; mol wt 785.96. $[\alpha]_D^{25}$ −66.0° ($CHCl_3$). uv max (methanol): 232 nm ($E_{1cm}^{1\%}$ 400). pKa′ (50% ethanol): 6.69.

Triacetylleucomycin A_1. $C_{46}H_{73}NO_{17}$. Crystals, mp 125-126°. $[\alpha]_D^{25}$ −82.5° (c = 1.3 in $CHCl_3$).

Leucomycin A_3 see Josamycin.

THERAP CAT: Antibacterial.

5454. Leucopterin. [492-11-5] 2-Amino-5,8-dihydro-4,6,-7(1*H*)-pteridinetrione; 2-amino-4,6,7-pteridinetriol; 2-amino-4,6,7-trihydroxypteridine; 2-amino-4,6,7-trihydroxypyrimido[4,5-*b*]pyrazine. $C_6H_5N_5O_3$; mol wt 195.14. C 36.93%, H 2.58%, N 35.89%, O 24.60%. A colorless substance found in the wings of butterflies (especially of white-winged butterflies). May be obtained from xanthopterin by dehydrogenation: Wieland, Purrmann, *Ann.* **544**, 172 (1940). Synthesis by fusing 2,4,5-triamino-6-hydroxypyrimidine with an excess of oxalic acid: Purrmann, *ibid.* 188. *See also* ref *under* Xanthopterin and review on pterins by Purrmann, *Fortschr. Chem. Org. Naturst.* **4**, 64 (1945).

Fine colorless crystals forming yellow Na and Ag salts, and a sparingly sol NH_4 salt. Soluble in alkaline solns with blue fluorescence.

5455. Leukotrienes. LTs. A family of endogenous metabolites of arachidonic acid via the lipoxygenase pathway, chemically related to the prostaglandins and thromboxanes, *q.q.v.* The name leukotrienes was applied because of their origin in leukocytes and their conjugated triene structures. [For a description of the nomenclature of individual leukotrienes *see* B. Samuelsson, S. Hammarström, *Prostaglandins* **19**, 645 (1980)]. Members of the group are potent bronchoconstrictors that play an important pathophysiological role in immediate hypersensitivity reactions; they have been proposed as mediators of the inflammatory process and some are potent chemotactic agents. Initial studies of novel arachidonate metabolites in rabbit polymorphonuclear leukocytes: P. Borgeat *et al., J. Biol. Chem.* **251**, 7816 (1976); **252**, 8772 (1977). Subsequent studies and structure of a dihydroxyeicosatetraenoic acid (leukotriene B, LTB₄): P. Borgeat, B. Samuelsson, *ibid.* **254**, 2643 (1979). LTB₄ is formed from an unstable intermediate oxido-eicosatetraenoic acid, leukotriene A or LTA₄: *eidem, Proc. Natl. Acad. Sci. USA* **76**, 3213 (1979). Stereochemistry and enzymatic conversion of LTA₄ to LTB₄: O. Radmark *et al., Biochem. Biophys. Res. Commun.* **92**, 954 (1980). Synthesis of the four optical isomers of LTA₄: J. Rokach *et al., Tetrahedron Lett.* **22**, 2759, 2763 (1981). Total synthesis of LTB₄: E. J. Corey *et al., J. Am. Chem. Soc.* **102**, 7984 (1980); Y. Guindon *et al., Tetrahedron Lett.* **23**, 739 (1982). Formation of the 20-hydroxy and 20-carboxy metabolites of LTB₄: G. Hansson *et al., FEBS Lett.* **130**, 107 (1981); total synthesis: R. Zamboni, J. Rokach, *Tetrahedron Lett.* **23**, 4751 (1982). Earlier studies had described a "slow-reacting substance of anaphylaxis" (*SRS-A* or *SRS*) released from guinea pig and cat lung by cobra venom and in guinea pig lung after anaphylactic shock, *cf.* W. S. Feldberg, C. H. Kellaway, *J. Physiol.* **94**, 187 (1938); C. H. Kellaway, E. R. Trethewie, *Q. J. Exp. Physiol.* **30**, 121 (1940). The relationship between SRS and members of the leukotriene family was established following publication of the uv spectrum of purified SRS-A, which showed the presence of the conjugated triene, *cf.* H. R. Morris *et al., FEBS Lett.* **87**, 203 (1978). Purification and structure of LTC₄, an SRS from mouse mastocytoma cells: R. C. Murphy *et al., Proc. Natl. Acad. Sci. USA* **76**, 4275 (1979); S. Hammarström *et al., Biochem. Biophys. Res. Commun.* **91**, 1266 (1979). Total synthesis of LTC₄: E. J. Corey *et al., J. Am. Chem. Soc.* **102**, 1436, 3663 (1980); J. Rokach *et al., Tetrahedron Lett.* **21**, 1485 (1980). Identity of synthetic LTC₄ with SRS from mouse mastocytoma cells: S. Hammarström *et al., Biochem. Biophys. Res. Commun.* **92**, 946 (1980). Structure of the SRS from rat basophil leukemia cells (RBL-1) and identification as a leukotriene (LTD₄): H. R. Morris *et al., Prostaglandins* **19**, 185 (1980).It was subsequently proposed that LTC₄ was an intermediate in the biosynthesis of LTD₄. Identity of SRS-A released in sensitized guinea pig lung perfusates and LTD₄: *eidem, Nature* **285**, 104 (1980). Assignment of stereochemistry: *eidem, Prostaglandins* **20**, 601 (1980). Detection of LTA₄ as an intermediate in the biosynthesis of LTC₄ and LTD₄: S. Hammarström, B. Samuelsson, *FEBS Lett.* **122**, 83

(1980). The sulfone of LTC₄, which has also been proposed as a natural product, *cf.* H. Ohnishi *et al., Prostaglandins* **20**, 655 (1980), has been found to be as potent as LTC₄: T. Jones *et al., ibid.* **24**, 279 (1982). Synthesis: Y. Girard *et al., Tetrahedron Lett.* **23**, 1023 (1982). Discovery of LTF₄: M. E. Anderson *et al., Proc. Natl. Acad. Sci. USA* **79**, 1088 (1982). Synthesis: F. Ellis *et al., Tetrahedron Lett.* **23**, 3735 (1982). It is now known that SRS-A is made up of varying amounts of cysteine-containing members of the leukotrienes, *i.e.* leukotrienes C₄, D₄, and E₄. These three LTs are generally found to be 100 to 1000 times more potent, on a molar basis, than histamine or prostaglandins in their effects on pulmonary airways. Review of chemistry and structure elucidation: D. A. Clark, A. Marfat, *Annu. Rep. Med. Chem.* **17**, 291-300 (1982). Comprehensive review of synthesis of leukotrienes and other lipoxygenase-derived products: J. G. Atkinson, J. Rokach, in *Handbook of Eicosanoids: Prostaglandins and Related Lipids* IB, A. L. Willis, Ed. (CRC Press, Boca Raton, 1987) pp 175-263. General reviews: P. Sirois, P. Borgeat, *Int. J. Immunopharmacol.* **2**, 281-293 (1980); P. Borgeat, P. Sirois, *J. Med. Chem.* **24**, 121-126 (1981); B. Samuelsson, *Int. Arch. Allergy Appl. Immunol.* **66**, Suppl. 1, 98-106 (1981); L. S. Wolfe, *J. Neurochem.* **38**, 1-14 (1982); J. L. Marx, *Science* **215**, 1380-1384 (1982); B. Samuelsson, S. Hammarström, *Vitam. Horm.* **39**, 1-30 (1982). Books: *SRS-A and Leukotrienes*, P. J. Piper, Ed. (Research Studies Press, London, 1981) 279 pp; *Advances in Prostaglandin, Thromboxane, and Leukotriene Research* vol. 9, B. Samuelsson, R. Paoletti, Eds. (Raven Press, New York, 1982) 341 pp.

Leukotriene A₄. [72059-45-1] (2*S*,3*S*)-3-(1*E*,3*E*,5*Z*,8*Z*)-1,3,5,-8-Tetradecatetraenyloxiranebutanoic acid; leukotriene A; LTA₄. $C_{20}H_{30}O_3$; mol wt 318.45. Unstable. Characterized as its methyl ester: mp 28-32°. $[\alpha]_D^{25} -27°$ (hexane). uv max (methanol): 270, 278, 290 nm (ε 43900, 56700, 43100), *cf.* J. Rokach *et al., Tetrahedron Lett.* **22**, 2759 (1981); I. Ernest *et al., ibid.* **23**, 167 (1982).

Leukotriene B₄. [71160-24-2] (5*S*,6*Z*,8*E*,10*E*,12*R*,14*Z*)-5,12-Dihydroxy-6,8,10,14-eicosatetraenoic acid; leukotriene B; LTB₄.

$C_{20}H_{32}O_4$; mol wt 336.47. uv max (methanol): 260, 270.5, 281 nm (ε 38000, 50000, 39000).

Leukotriene C₄. [72025-60-6] L-γ-Glutamyl-S-[(1R,2E,4E,-6Z,9Z)-1-[(1S)-4-carboxy-1-hydroxybutyl]-2,4,6,9-pentadecate-traenyl]-L-cysteinylglycine; leukotriene C; leukotriene C_1; LTC₄. $C_{30}H_{47}N_3O_9S$; mol wt 625.77. uv max (methanol): 270, 280, 290 nm (ε 32000, 40000, 31000). Can be stored for several days without appreciable decomposition in frozen ($-20°$) pH 6.8 phosphate buffer under argon or as the tripotassium salt frozen in water. Biological activity destroyed after incubation with soybean lipoxygenase and uv max shifts to 308 nm.

Leukotriene D₄. [73836-78-9] S-[(1R,2E,4E,6Z,9Z)-1-[(1S)-4-Carboxy-1-hydroxybutyl]-2,4,6,9-pentadecatetraenyl]-L-cysteinyl-glycine; leukotriene D; LTD₄. $C_{25}H_{40}N_2O_6S$; mol wt 496.66. uv max (methanol): 270, 280, 290 nm (ε 31000, 40000, 31000). Storage, destruction of biological activity, uv shift are the same as for LTC₄.

Leukotriene E₄. [75715-89-8] (5S,6R,7E,9E,11Z,14Z)-6-[[(2R)-2-Amino-2-carboxyethyl]thio]-5-hydroxy-7,9,11,14-eicosa-tetraenoic acid; leukotriene E; LTE₄. $C_{23}H_{37}NO_5S$; mol wt 439.61. uv max (ethanol) of methyl ester: 269, 280, 291 nm (ε 28200, 35200, 28900).

5456. Leupeptins. Class of modified tripeptide protease inhibitors produced by various species of *Actinomycetes*. Two major components, *leupeptin Ac-LL* and *leupeptin Pr-LL*, consisting of L-leucyl-L-leucyl-DL-argininal modified at the amino terminal by acetyl- or propionyl-, respectively, have been isolated. Various minor analogs, in which valine or isoleucine replaces either or both leucines, have also been found. Isolation from *Actinomycetes*: T. Aoyagi *et al.*, *J. Antibiot.* **22**, 283 (1969); S.-I. Kondo *et al.*, *Chem. Pharm. Bull.* **17**, 1896 (1969). Structure and synthesis of leupeptins Ac-LL and Pr-LL: K. Kawamura *et al.*, *ibid.* 1902; K. Maeda *et al.*, *J. Antibiot.* **24**, 402 (1971). Improved purification of leupeptin Ac-LL: M. C. Y. Ning, R. J. Beynon, *Int. J. Biochem.* **18**, 813 (1986). Inhibition of proteases: T. Aoyagi *et al.*, *J. Antibiot.* **22**, 558 (1969); and synthesis of analogs: G. Borin *et al.*, *Z. Physiol. Chem.* **362**, 1435 (1981). Effects on protein degradation in normal and diseased muscle: P. Libby, A. L. Goldberg, *Science* **199**, 534 (1978); I. Nonaka *et al.*, *Acta Neuropathol.* **58**, 279 (1982); R. P. Hummel, III *et al.*, *J. Surg. Res.* **45**, 140 (1988). HPLC determn of leupeptin Ac-LL in serum and muscle: M. Kai *et al.*, *J. Chromatogr.* **345**, 259 (1985).

Note: In some sources leupeptin refers only to leupeptin Ac-LL.

USE: Enzyme inhibitor in biological preparations.

5457. Leuprolide. [53714-56-0] 6-D-Leucine-9-(*N*-ethyl-L-prolinamide)-10-deglycinamideluteinizing hormone-releasing factor (pig); leuprorelin; [D-Leu⁶]-des-Gly¹⁰-LH-RH-ethylamide. $C_{59}H_{84}N_{16}O_{12}$; mol wt 1209.40. C 58.59%, H 7.00%, N 18.53%, O 15.88%. Synthetic nonapeptide agonist analog of LH-RH, *q.v.* Prepn: M. Fujino *et al.*, *DE 2446005* (1975 to Takeda), *C.A.* **83**, 10895y (1975); R. L. Gendrich *et al.*, *US 4005063* (1977 to Abbott). Synthesis: J. A. Vilchez-Martinez *et al.*, *Biochem. Biophys. Res. Commun.* **59**, 1226 (1974); M. Fujino *et al.*, *ibid.* **60**, 406 (1974). Comparison of biological activity with natural LH-RH: D. H. Coy *et al.*, *ibid.* **67**, 576 (1975). Pharmacokinetics: L. T. Sennello *et al.*, *J. Pharm. Sci.* **75**, 158 (1986). Clinical efficacy in prostatic carcinoma: M. B. Garnick *et al.*, *N. Engl. J. Med.* **311**, 1281 (1984); in benign prostatic hypertrophy: L. M. Eri, K. J. Tveter, *J. Urol.* **150**, 359 (1993). Clinical trial in endometriosis: J. M. Wheeler *et al.*, *Am. J. Obstet. Gynecol.* **167**, 1367 (1992).

5-oxoPro–His–Trp–Ser–Tyr–D-Leu–Leu–Arg–ProNHC₂H₅

Fluffy solid. $[\alpha]_D^{25}$ $-31.7°$ (c = 1 in 1% acetic acid).

Monoacetate (salt). [74381-53-6] Leuprolide acetate; Abbott 43818; A-43818; TAP-144; Carcinil; Eligard; Enantone; Leuplin; Lucrin; Lupron; Prostap; Viadur. $C_{59}H_{84}N_{16}O_{12}.C_2H_4O_2$; mol wt 1269.44.

THERAP CAT: Antineoplastic (hormonal); LH-RH agonist.

5458. Levallorphan. [152-02-3] 17-(2-Propenyl)morphinan-3-ol; *l*,*N*-allyl-3-hydroxymorphinan; *l*-3-hydroxy-*N*-allyl-morphinan. $C_{19}H_{25}NO$; mol wt 283.41. C 80.52%, H 8.89%, N 4.94%, O 5.65%. Prepn from 3-hydroxy-*N*-methylmorphinan:

Schnider, Grüssner, *Helv. Chim. Acta* **34**, 2211 (1951). Alternate route: Hellerbach *et al.*, *ibid.* **39**, 429 (1956). Comprehensive description: B. C. Rudy, B. Z. Senkowski, *Anal. Profiles Drug Subs.* **2**, 339-361 (1973).

Crystals from dilute ethanol, mp 180-182°. $[\alpha]_D^{20}$ $-88.9°$ (c = 3 in methanol).

Tartrate. [71-82-9] Lorfan. $C_{19}H_{25}NO.C_4H_6O_6$; mol wt 433.49. Crystals from ethanol, mp 176-177°. $[\alpha]_D^{20}$ $-39°$. Soluble in water.

THERAP CAT: Narcotic antagonist.

THERAP CAT (VET): Narcotic antagonist.

5459. Levamisole. [14769-73-4] (6S)-2,3,5,6-Tetrahydro-6-phenylimidazo[2,1-b]thiazole; ($-$)-6-phenyl-2,3,5,6-tetrahydro-imidazo[2,1-b]thiazole; Levovermax; Totalon. $C_{11}H_{12}N_2S$; mol wt 204.29. C 64.67%, H 5.92%, N 13.71%, S 15.70%. Biological response modifier with anthelmintic activity. Prepn of racemate: A. H. M. Raeymaekers *et al.*, *US 3274209* (1966 to Janssen); *eidem*, *J. Med. Chem.* **9**, 545 (1966). Pharmacology: D. Thienpoint *et al.*, *Nature* **209**, 1084 (1966). Prepn and abs config of isomers: A. H. M. Raeymaekers *et al.*, *Tetrahedron Lett.* **1967**, 1467. *See also:* M. W. Bullock *et al.*, *J. Med. Chem.* **11**, 169 (1968); *US 3565907* (1971 to Am. Cyanamid); Dewar *et al.*, *US 3579530* (1971 to ICI). Stereospecific inhibition of succinic dehydrogenase: H. Van den Bossche, P. A. J. Janssen, *Biochem. Pharmacol.* **18**, 35 (1969). Exptl effect on IL-1 production: E. S. Kimball, *Ann. N.Y. Acad. Sci.* **685**, 259 (1993). Review of pharmacology: H. Schneiden, *Int. J. Immunopharmacol.* **3**, 9 (1981); of clinical use in parasitic infections: M. J. Miller, *Drugs* **20**, 122-130 (1980). Determn in animal tissues by ELISA: J. J. Silverlight, R. Jackman: *Analyst* **119**, 2705 (1994); by LC-MS: A. Cannavan *et al.*, *ibid.* **120**, 331 (1995). Clinical trial with fluorouracil in colon cancer: C. G. Moertel *et al.*, *Ann. Intern. Med.* **122**, 321 (1995). Review of immunopharmacology and clinical trials in cancer treatment: H. C. Stevenson *et al.*, *J. Clin. Oncol.* **9**, 2052-2066 (1991); M. De Brabander *et al.*, *Anticancer Res.* **12**, 177-188 (1992); W. K. Amery, J. P. Bruynseels, *Int. J. Immunopharmacol.* **14**, 481-486 (1992).

mp 60-61.5°. $[\alpha]_D^{25}$ $-85.1°$ (c = 10 in chloroform).

Hydrochloride. [16595-80-5] R-12564; Ascaridil; Decaris; Ergamisol; Levacide; Levadin; Levasole; Meglum; Nemicide; Nilverm; Ripercol; Solaskil; Spartakon; Tramisol. $C_{11}H_{12}N_2S.HCl$; mol wt 240.75. mp 227-229°. $[\alpha]_D^{20}$ $-124 \pm 2°$ (c = 0.9, water). Sol in water. Stable in aq acid media.

DL-Form. [5036-02-2] Tetramisole; tetramizole. Crystals, mp 87-89°.

DL-Form hydrochloride. [5086-74-8] Bayer 9051; McN-JR-8299; R-8299. Crystals, mp 264-265°. Sol in water (21 g/100 ml at 20°), methanol, propylene glycol; sparingly sol in ethanol. Slightly sol in chloroform, hexane, acetone. LD₅₀ in mice, rats (mg/kg): 22, 24 i.v.; 84, 130 s.c.; 210, 480 orally (Thienpoint).

D-(+)-Form. Dexamisole. mp 60-61.5°. $[\alpha]_D^{25}$ $+85.1°$ (c = 10 in chloroform).

D-(+)-Form hydrochloride. R-12563. mp 227-227.5°. $[\alpha]_D^{20}$ $+125°$ (c = 0.7 in water).

THERAP CAT: Anthelmintic (nematodes); immunomodulator.

THERAP CAT (VET): Anthelmintic (Nematodes).

5460. Levcromakalim. [94535-50-9] (3S-*trans*)-3,4-Dihydro-3-hydroxy-2,2-dimethyl-4-(2-oxo-1-pyrrolidinyl)-2H-1-benzo-pyran-6-carbonitrile; (3S,4R)-3-hydroxy-2,2-dimethyl-4-(2-oxo-1-

pyrrolidinyl)-6-chromancarbonitrile; (−)-6-cyano-3,4-dihydro-2,2-dimethyl-*trans*-4-(2-oxo-1-pyrrolidinyl)-2*H*-benzo[*b*]pyran-3-ol; lemakalim; (−)-cromakalim; BRL-38227. $C_{16}H_{18}N_2O_3$; mol wt 286.33. C 67.12%, H 6.34%, N 9.78%, O 16.76%. Potassium channel opener. Prepn of racemate: J. M. Evans *et al.*, **EP 76075**; *eidem*, **US 4446113** (1983, 1984 both to Beecham); of isomers: E. Faruk, **EP 120428** (1984 to Beecham); V. A. Ashwood *et al.*, *J. Med. Chem.* **29**, 2194 (1986). Mechanism of action and hemodynamic effects: R. P. Hof *et al.*, *Circ. Res.* **62**, 679 (1988). Pharmacology: J. C. Clapham *et al.*, *Arzneim.-Forsch.* **41**, 385 (1991). Clinical evaluation in hypertension: S. Suzuki *et al.*, *ibid.* **45**, 859 (1995).

Crystals from ethyl acetate, mp 242-244°. $[\alpha]_D^{26}$ −52.2° (c = 1 in chloroform).

(+)-**Form**. Crystals from ethyl acetate, mp 243-245°. $[\alpha]_D^{26}$ +53.5° (c = 1 in chloroform).

(±)-**Form**. [94470-67-4] Cromakalim; BRL-34915. Crystals from ethyl acetate, mp 230-231°.

THERAP CAT: Antihypertensive.

5461. Levetiracetam. [102767-28-2] (*αS*)-α-Ethyl-2-oxo-1-pyrrolidineacetamide; 2(*S*)-(2-oxopyrrolidin-1-yl)butyramide; UCB-L059; SIB-S1; Keppra. $C_8H_{14}N_2O_2$; mol wt 170.21. C 56.45%, H 8.29%, N 16.46%, O 18.80%. (*S*)-Enantiomer of the ethyl analog of piracetam, *q.v.* Prepn: J. Gobert *et al.*, **EP 162036**; *eidem*, **US 4943639** (1985, 1990 both to UCB). HPLC-UV determn in plasma: J. Martens-Lohnhoffer, S. M. Bode-Böger, *J. Chromatogr. B* **819**, 197 (2005). Clinical evaluation in refractory partial seizures: S. D. Shorvon *et al.*, *Epilepsia* **41**, 1179 (2000); E. Ben-Menachem, U. Falter, *ibid.* 1276. Review of pharmacokinetics: P. N. Patsalos, *Pharmacol. Ther.* **85**, 77-85 (2000); of clinical efficacy: E. Ben-Menachem, *Expert Opin. Pharmacother.* **4**, 2079-2088 (2003); of safety and tolerability: D. E. Briggs, J. A. French, *Expert Opin. Drug Saf.* **3**, 415-424 (2004).

Crystals from ethyl acetate, mp 117°. $[\alpha]_D^{25}$ −90.0° (c = 1 in acetone). Soly (g/100 ml): water 104.0; chloroform 65.3; methanol 53.6; ethanol 16.5; acetonitrile 5.7. Practically insol in *n*-hexane. LD_{50} in male mice, male rats (mg/kg): 1081, 1038 i.v. (Gobert, 1990).

THERAP CAT: Anticonvulsant.

5462. Levobunolol. [47141-42-4] 5-[(2*S*)-3-[(1,1-Dimethylethyl)amino]-2-hydroxypropoxy]-3,4-dihydro-1(2*H*)-naphthalenone; (−)-5-[3-(*tert*-butylamino)-2-hydroxypropoxy]-3,4-dihydro-1(2*H*)-naphthalenone; *l*-bunolol; W-6421A. $C_{17}H_{25}NO_3$; mol wt 291.39. C 70.07%, H 8.65%, N 4.81%, O 16.47%. Nonselective β-adrenoceptor antagonist. Prepn of racemate: C. F. Schwender *et al.*, *J. Med. Chem.* **13**, 684 (1970); J. Shavel, Jr., S. Farber, **DE 1948144**; *eidem*, **US 3641172** (1970, 1972 both to Warner-Lambert). Resolution of enantiomers: J. Shavel, Jr., C. F. Schwender, **DE 2046043**; *eidem*, **US 3649691** (1971, 1972 both to Warner-Lambert); R. D. Dennis *et al.*, **US 4463176** (1984 to Bristol Myers, Mead Johnson). Cardiovascular pharmacology, anti-arrhythmic activity of racemate and isomers: R. D. Robson, H. R. Kaplan, *J. Pharmacol. Exp. Ther.* **175**, 157, 168 (1970). Adrenoceptor blocking activity: H. R. Kaplan *et al.*, *Eur. J. Pharmacol.* **16**, 237 (1971). Metabolism in humans: F. J. DiCarlo *et al.*, *Clin. Pharmacol. Ther.* **22**, 858 (1977); F.-J. Leinweber *et al.*, *Pharmacology* **16**, 70 (1978). Corneal permeability: R. D. Schoenwald, H.-S. Huang, *J. Pharm.*

Sci. **72**, 1266, 1272 (1983). HPLC determn in biological fluids: H. Hengy, E. U. Kolle, *J. Chromatogr.* **338**, 444 (1985); D. D. S. Tang-Liu *et al.*, *J. Liq. Chromatogr.* **9**, 2237 (1986). Clinical evaluation in hypertension: E. Arce-Gomez *et al.*, *Curr. Ther. Res.* **19**, 386 (1976); comparison with timolol, *q.v.*, in glaucoma and ocular hypertension: A. Cinotti *et al.*, *Am. J. Ophthalmol.* **99**, 11 (1985); D. Long *et al.*, *ibid.* 18. *Review:* H. R. Kaplan, "Levobunolol" in *Pharmacology of Antihypertensive Drugs*, A. Scriabine, Ed. (Raven Press, New York, 1980) pp 317-323. Brief review of long-term treatment of glaucoma: G. D. Novack, *Gen. Pharmacol.* **17**, 373-377 (1986).

LD_{50} in male, female rats, mice (mg/kg): 700, 800, 1530, 1220 orally; 25, 28, 78, 84 i.v.; LD_{50} in male, female hamsters, dogs (mg/kg): 435, 500, 100, 100 orally (Kaplan, 1980).

Hydrochloride. [27912-14-7] W-7000A; Betagan; Vistagan. $C_{17}H_{25}NO_3 \cdot HCl$; mol wt 327.85. Crystals from methanol-ether, mp 209-211°. $[\alpha]_{589}^{24}$ −19.6±0.7° (c = 2.90 in methanol). uv max (NaOH): 221, 253, 310 nm (ε 24700, 9000, 2400).

THERAP CAT: Antiglaucoma.

5463. Levocabastine. [79516-68-0] [3*S*-[1(*cis*),3α,4β]]-1-[4-Cyano-4-(4-fluorophenyl)cyclohexyl]-3-methyl-4-phenyl-4-piperidinecarboxylic acid; (−)-*trans*-1-[*cis*-4-cyano-4-(*p*-fluorophenyl)cyclohexyl]-3-methyl-4-phenylisonipecotic acid; (−)-cabastine. $C_{26}H_{29}FN_2O_2$; mol wt 420.52. C 74.26%, H 6.95%, F 4.52%, N 6.66%, O 7.61%. Histamine H_1-receptor antagonist. Prepn: R. Stokbroekx *et al.*, **EP 34415**; *eidem*, **US 4369184** (1981, 1983 both to Janssen); and pharmacology: R. A. Stokbroekx *et al.*, *Drug Dev. Res.* **8**, 87 (1986). Pharmacology: K. Tasaka *et al.*, *Arzneim.-Forsch.* **40**, 1295 (1990). Clinical pharmacology: N. Rombaut *et al.*, *Ann. Allergy* **67**, 75 (1991). Clinical trial in children with allergic conjunctivitis: M. Rimas *et al.*, *Allergy* **45**, 18 (1990); in allergic rhinitis: M. Schata *et al.*, *J. Allergy Clin. Immunol.* **87**, 873 (1991). Review of pharmacology and therapeutic use: K. L. Dechant, K. L. Goa, *Drugs* **41**, 202-224 (1991).

Hydrochloride. [79547-78-7] R-50547; Levophta; Livostin. $C_{26}H_{29}FN_2O_2 \cdot HCl$; mol wt 456.98.

THERAP CAT: Antihistaminic.

5464. Levodopa. [59-92-7] 3-Hydroxy-L-tyrosine; (−)-3-(3,4-dihydroxyphenyl)-L-alanine; L-dopa; β-(3,4-dihydroxyphenyl)-L-alanine; (−)-2-amino-3-(3,4-dihydroxyphenyl)propanoic acid; Bendopa; Deadopa; Dopaflex; Dopal; Dopaidan; Dopalina; Dopar; Doparkine; Doparl; Dopasol; Dopaston; Dopastral; Cidandopa; Doprin; Eldopal; Eldopar; Eldopatec; Eurodopa; Laradopa; Maipedopa; Larodopa; Ledopa; Parda; Lepova; Veldopa (formerly Weldopa). $C_9H_{11}NO_4$; mol wt 197.19. C 54.82%, H 5.62%, N 7.10%, O 32.45%. Naturally occurring form of dopa, *q.v.*, the biological precursor of the catecholamines. Prepn from *l*-3-nitrotyrosin: Wasser, Lewandowski, *Helv. Chim. Acta* **4**, 657 (1921); from 3-(3,4-methylenedioxyphenyl)-L-alanine: Yamada *et al.*, *Chem. Pharm. Bull.* **10**, 693 (1962); from L-tyrosine: Vorbrüggen, Krolikiewicz, *Ber.* **105**, 1168 (1972); Bretschneider *et al.*, *Helv. Chim. Acta* **56**, 2857 (1973); from *Vicia faba* beans: Wysong, **US 3253023** (1966 to Dow Chem.); by fermentation of L-tyrosine: Sih *et al.*, *J. Am. Chem. Soc.* **91**, 6204 (1969); Florent, Renaut, **DE 2102793** (1971 to Rhône-Poulenc), *C.A.* **75**, 108505f (1971). Sepn from racemate: Vogler, Baumgartner, *Helv. Chim. Acta* **35**, 1776

(1952); **NL 6514950**; **US 3405159** (1966, 1968 both to Merck & Co.). Molecular conformation: Becker *et al., Biochem. Biophys. Res. Commun.* **41**, 444 (1970). Metabolism studies: Shaw *et al., J. Biol. Chem.* **226**, 255 (1957); Calne *et al., Br. J. Pharmacol.* **37**, 57 (1969). Hemodynamic effects in congestive heart failure: S. I. Rajfer *et al., N. Engl. J. Med.* **310**, 1357 (1984). Series of articles on clinical efficacy in Parkinson's disease: *Adv. Neurol.* **45**, 457-510 (1986). Reviews on L-dopa and parkinsonism: Barbeau, *Can. Med. Assoc. J.* **101**, 791 (1969); Pletscher *et al., Schweiz. Med. Wochenschr.* **100**, 797 (1970); Calne, Sandler, *Nature* **226**, 21 (1970); *L-Dopa and Parkinsonism*, A. Barbeau, Ed. (F. A. Davis, Philadelphia, 1970). Review of acute toxicity data: W. G. Clark *et al., Toxicol. Appl. Pharmacol.* **28**, 1-7 (1974). Comprehensive description: R. Gomez *et al., Anal. Profiles Drug Subs.* **5**, 189-223 (1976).

Colorless to white, odorless and tasteless crystals or crystalline powder. Needles from water, mp 276-278° (dec) (Yamada); also reported as mp 284-286° (Wysong). $[\alpha]_D^{13}$ −13.1° (c = 5.12 in 1*N* HCl). uv max (0.001*N* HCl): 220.5, 280 nm (log ε 3.79, 3.42). Readily sol in dil HCl and formic acid. Soly in water: 66 mg/40 ml. Practically insol in ethanol, benzene, chloroform and ethyl acetate. In the presence of moisture, L-dopa is rapidly oxidized by atmospheric oxygen and darkens. LD$_{50}$ in mice (mg/kg): 3650 ±327 orally, 1140 ±66 i.p., 450 ±42 i.v., >400 s.c.; in male, female rats (mg/kg): >3000, >3000 orally; 624, 663 i.p.; >1500, >1500 s.c. (Clark).

THERAP CAT: Antiparkinsonian.

5465. Levoglucosenone. [37112-31-5] (1*S*,5*R*)-6,8-Dioxabicyclo[3.2.1]oct-2-en-4-one; 1,6-anhydro-3,4-dideoxy-β-D-*glycero*-hex-3-enopyranos-2-ulose; 1,6-anhydro-3,4-dideoxy-Δ³-β-D-pyranosen-2-one. C$_6$H$_6$O$_3$; mol wt 126.11. C 57.14%, H 4.80%, O 38.06%. (−)-Form is a pyrolysis product of cellulose and cellulose-containing materials including pulp and paper waste products. Prepn from cellulosic materials: Y. Halpern *et al., J. Org. Chem.* **38**, 204 (1973); and decompn reactions: F. Shafizadeh, P. P. S. Chin, *Carbohydr. Res.* **46**, 149 (1976). Prepn from Kraft paper: *eidem, ibid.* **58**, 79 (1977). Synthesis of (−)-form: M. Shibagaki *et al., Chem. Lett.* **1990**, 307; of (+) and (−) enantiomers: T. Taniguchi *et al., Synlett* **1996**, 971. MS analysis: Y. Halpern, J. P. Hoppesch, *J. Org. Chem.* **50**, 1556 (1985). Electrochemistry: C. Z. Smith *et al., J. Chem. Res. Synop.* **1987**, 88. Stereoselective reactivity: F. Shafizadeh *et al., Carbohydr. Res.* **71**, 169 (1979). Cycloaddition reactions: *idem et al., ibid.* **114**, 71 (1983); A. J. Blake *et al., Tetrahedron* **48**, 8053 (1992). Michael addition reactions: M. G. Essig, *Carbohydr. Res.* **156**, 225 (1986); A. V. Samet *et al.*, **61**, 8786 (1996). Applications in chiral carbohydrate synthesis: Y. Gelas-Mialhe *et al., Heterocycles* **24**, 931 (1986); Z. J. Witczak, *Pure Appl. Chem.* **66**, 2189 (1994); R. Blattner, D. M. Page, *J. Carbohydr. Chem.* **13**, 27 (1994).

Faintly greenish-yellow liquid. n_D^{25} 1.5084. uv max (*n*-hexane): 211, 275 nm (log E$_{1cm}^{1\%}$ 2.82, 1.5). uv max (95% ethanol): 218, 275 nm (log E$_{1cm}^{1\%}$ 2.78, 1.5). $[\alpha]_D^{25}$ −460° (c = 1.0 in CHCl$_3$) (Halpern, 1973); also reported as $[\alpha]_D^{31}$ −514.8° (c = 0.3 in CHCl$_3$) (Taniguchi).

USE: Chiral building block in organic synthesis.

5466. Levomethadyl Acetate. [1477-40-3] (α*S*)-β-[(2*S*)-2-(Dimethylamino)propyl]-α-ethyl-β-phenylbenzeneethanol acetate (ester); (−)-6-(dimethylamino)-4,4-diphenyl-3-heptanol acetate

(ester); α-*l*-acetylmethadol; *levo*-α-acetylmethadol; LAAM. C$_{23}$H$_{31}$NO$_2$; mol wt 353.50. C 78.15%, H 8.84%, N 3.96%, O 9.05%. Longest-acting enantiomer of methadyl acetate, *q.v.* Duration of action due to active metabolites. Prepn: A. Pohland *et al., J. Am. Chem. Soc.* **71**, 460 (1949). Synthesis of metabolites: F. I. Carroll *et al., J. Org. Chem.* **41**, 3521 (1976). Metabolism in rats: G. L. Henderson *et al., Drug Metab. Dispos.* **5**, 321 (1977); M. Man *et al., ibid.* **8**, 55 (1980); in man: B. S. Finkle *et al., J. Anal. Toxicol.* **6**, 100 (1982). Determn of LAAM and metabolites by HPLC: C.-H. Kiang *et al., J. Chromatogr.* **222**, 81 (1981); by GLC: K. Verebey *et al., ibid.* **343**, 339 (1985). Analgesic activity in mice: N. B. Eddy *et al., J. Org. Chem.* **17**, 321 (1952); in man: A. S. Keats, H. K. Beecher, *J. Pharmacol. Exp. Ther.* **105**, 210 (1952). Pharmacology in monkeys: S. J. Mule, A. L. Misra, *Ann. N.Y. Acad. Sci.* **311**, 199 (1978). Comparison with methadone in the treatment of heroin addiction: T. J. Crowley *et al., Psychopharmacology* **86**, 458 (1985). Review of use in treatment of narcotic addiction: J. D. Blaine *et al., Ann. N.Y. Acad. Sci.* **362**, 101-115 (1981).

Hydrochloride. [43033-72-3] ORLAAM. C$_{23}$H$_{31}$NO$_2$.HCl; mol wt 389.96. Crystals from ethanol-ether, mp 215°. $[\alpha]_D^{25}$ −60° (c = 0.2). Sol in water. LD$_{50}$ in mice (mg/kg): 110.0 s.c., 172.8 orally (Eddy).

Note: This is a controlled substance (opiate): **21 CFR**, 1308.12.

THERAP CAT: In treatment of narcotic addiction.

5467. Levophacetoperane. [24558-01-8] α-Phenyl-2-piperidinemethanol acetate; *threo*-1-acetoxy-1-phenyl-1-(2-piperidyl)methane; acetic acid α-phenyl-2-piperidylmethyl ester; 1-phenyl-1-(2'-piperidyl)-1-acetoxymethane; phacetoperane; RP-8228. C$_{14}$H$_{19}$NO$_2$; mol wt 233.31. C 72.07%, H 8.21%, N 6.00%, O 13.72%. Prepn: Jacob, Joseph, **US 2928835** (1960 to Rhône-Poulenc).

Hydrochloride. [23257-56-9] Lidepran. C$_{14}$H$_{19}$NO$_2$.HCl; mol wt 269.77. Crystals from acetone + ether, mp 229-230°. Levorotatory.

THERAP CAT: Antidepressant; anorexic.

5468. Levopimaric Acid. [79-54-9] [1*R*-(1α,4aβ,4bα,-10aα)]-1,2,3,4,4a,4b,5,9,10,10a-Decahydro-1,4a-dimethyl-7-(1-methylethyl)-1-phenanthrenecarboxylic acid; 13-isopropylpodocarpa-8(14),12-dien-15-oic acid; Δ⁶,⁸⁽¹⁴⁾-abietadienoic acid; *l*-pimaric acid; β-pimaric acid; *l*-sapietic acid. C$_{20}$H$_{30}$O$_2$; mol wt 302.45. C 79.42%, H 10.00%, O 10.58%. Isolation from American pine oleoresin: Palkin, Harris, *J. Am. Chem. Soc.* **55**, 3677 (1933); from French galipot, from *Pinus maritima*: Ruzicka, Bacon, *Helv. Chim. Acta* **20**, 1542 (1937); from *Pinus palustris*: Harris, Sanderson, *J. Am. Chem. Soc.* **70**, 334, 3671 (1948). Structure: Ruzicka, Kaufmann, *Helv. Chim. Acta* **23**, 1346 (1940): *cf.* Arbuzov, *Chem. Zentralbl.* **1942**, II, 893. Stereochemistry: Schuller, Lawrence, *J. Am. Chem. Soc.* **83**, 2563 (1961); Burgstahler *et al., ibid.* **83**, 4660 (1961); Weiss *et al., Chem. Ind. (London)* **1962**, 1286; Dauben, Coates, *J. Org. Chem.* **28**, 1698 (1963). Conformation: Burgstahler *et al., Chem. Commun.* **1971**, 121; Weiss *et al., ibid.* **1972**, 17.

Orthorhombic crystals, mp 150°; $[\alpha]_D^{20}$ −280.4° (c = 0.7 in alcohol); $[\alpha]_D^{14}$ −266.6° (c = 0.4 in chloroform). Absorption max 273 nm: Kraft, *Ann.* **520**, 133 (1935). Practically insol in water, sol in most organic solvents. Forms a crystalline ammonium salt.

Methyl ester. $C_{21}H_{32}O_2$. Crystals from methanol, mp 64°. $[\alpha]_D^{20}$ −268° (c = 1 in ether).

Molecular compd with quinone. $C_{26}H_{34}O_4$. Yellow prisms from methanol, mp 214°. $[\alpha]_D^{20}$ −148° (c = 0.7 in chloroform).

5469. Levopropoxyphene. [2338-37-6] (αR)-α-[(1*S*)-2-(Dimethylamino)-1-methylethyl]-α-phenylbenzeneethanol propanoate (ester); α-*l*-4-dimethylamino-3-methyl-1,2-diphenyl-2-butanol propionate; α-*l*-4-dimethylamino-1,2-diphenyl-3-methyl-2-butanol propionate; *l*-propoxyphene. $C_{22}H_{29}NO_2$; mol wt 339.47. C 77.84%, H 8.61%, N 4.13%, O 9.43%. Prepn: Pohland, Sullivan, *J. Am. Chem. Soc.* **77**, 3400 (1955). Stereoselective synthesis: Pohland *et al.*, *J. Org. Chem.* **28**, 2483 (1963). Toxicity data: E. I. Goldenthal, *Toxicol. Appl. Pharmacol.* **18**, 185 (1971). *See also* Propoxyphene.

Crystals from petr ether, mp 75-76°. $[\alpha]_D^{25}$ −68.2° (c = 0.6 in chloroform).

Hydrochloride. [1596-70-9] $C_{22}H_{29}NO_2$·HCl. Crystals from methanol + ethyl acetate, mp 163-164°. $[\alpha]_D^{25}$ −60.1° (c = 0.7).

2-Naphthalenesulfonate. [5714-90-9] Levopropoxyphene napsylate; Novrad; Letusin; Contratuss. $C_{22}H_{29}NO_2$·$C_{10}H_8SO_3$; mol wt 547.70. LD$_{50}$ orally in female rats: 1455 ±77 mg/kg (Goldenthal).

THERAP CAT: Antitussive.

5470. Levorphanol. [77-07-6] 17-Methylmorphinan-3-ol; (−)-3-hydroxy-*N*-methylmorphinan; levorphan; lemoran; Ro-1-5431. $C_{17}H_{23}NO$; mol wt 257.37. C 79.33%, H 9.01%, N 5.44%, O 6.22%. Orally active synthetic morphine analog. Prepn of racemate from 2-methyl-1-benzyl-1,2,3,4,5,6,7,8-octahydro-isoquinoline: Grewe, *Naturwissenschaften* **33**, 333 (1946); *Angew. Chem.* **A59**, 198 (1947); Grewe, Mondon, *Ber.* **81**, 279 (1948); **CH 280674** (1952 to Hoffmann-La Roche), *C.A.* **47**, 7554 (1953). Prepn of isomers: Schnider, Grüssner, *Helv. Chim. Acta* **34**, 2211 (1951); Vogler, **US 2744112** (1956 to Hoffmann-La Roche). Absolute configuration: Corrodi *et al.*, *Helv. Chim. Acta* **42**, 212 (1959). Analgesic activity and toxicity data: L. O. Randall, G. Lehmann, *J. Pharmacol. Exp. Ther.* **99**, 163 (1950). HPLC determn in plasma: R. Lucek, R. Dixon, *J. Chromatogr.* **341**, 239 (1985). Clinical pharmacokinetics: R. Dixon *et al.*, *Res. Commun. Chem. Pathol. Pharmacol.* **41**, 3 (1983).

Crystals, mp 198-199°. $[\alpha]_D^{20}$ −56° (c = 3 in absolute alcohol).

Tartrate dihydrate. [5985-38-6] Ro-1-5431/7; Dromoran; Levo-Dromoran. $C_{17}H_{23}NO$·$C_4H_6O_6$·$2H_2O$; mol wt 443.49. Crystals, mp 113-115° (when anhydrous, mp 206-208°). $[\alpha]_D^{20}$ −14° (c = 3 in water). pH of a 0.2% aq soln 3.4 to 4.0. One gram dissolves in 45 ml water, in 110 g alcohol, in 50 g ether.

***dl*-Form.** [297-90-5] Racemorphan; methorphinan. Crystals from anisole and dil alcohol, mp 251-253°.

***dl*-Form hydrobromide.** [5985-35-3] Nu-2206. $C_{17}H_{23}$-NO·HBr; mol wt 338.28. Crystals, mp 193-195°. Sol in water; sparingly sol in alcohol. Practically insol in ether. LD$_{50}$ i.v. in mice: 41 mg/kg (Randall, Lehmann).

***d*-Form.** [125-73-5] Dextrorphan; Ro-1-6794. HPLC-MS/MS determn in urine: M. L. Constanzer *et al.*, *J. Chromatogr. B* **816**, 297 (2005). Crystals, mp 198-199°. $[\alpha]_D^{20}$ +56.3° (c = 3 in abs alcohol).

***d*-Form tartrate monohydrate.** $C_{17}H_{23}NO$·$C_4H_6O_6$·H_2O. Crystals, mp 183-185°. $[\alpha]_D^{20}$ +34.6° (c = 3 in water). Sol in water.

Note: Levorphanol and racemorphan are controlled substances (opiates): **21 CFR**, 1308.12.

THERAP CAT: Analgesic (narcotic).

5471. Levosimendan. [141505-33-1] [[4-[(4*R*)-1,4,5,6-Tetrahydro-4-methyl-6-oxo-3-pyridazinyl]phenyl]hydrazono]propanedinitrile; (−)-[*p*[(*R*)-1,4,5,6-tetrahydro-4-methyl-6-oxo-3-pyridazinyl]phenyl]hydrazone mesoxalonitrile; (*R*)-simendan; OR-1259; Simdax. $C_{14}H_{12}N_6O$; mol wt 280.28. C 59.99%, H 4.32%, N 29.98%, O 5.71%. Bioactive enantiomer of racemate, simendan. Positive inotropic agent with vasodilating activity. Binds to and sensitizes the myocardial contractile protein, troponin C, to calcium, thereby stabilizing the troponin conformation needed to trigger muscle contraction. Prepn: R. J. Backstrom *et al.*, **GB 2251615**; P. Nore *et al.*, **US 5569657** (1992, 1996 both to Orion). Pharmacology: A. F. E. Rump *et al.*, *Pharmacol. Toxicol.* **74**, 244 (1994). Binding studies: P. Pollesello *et al.*, *J. Biol. Chem.* **269**, 28584 (1994). HPLC determn in plasma: M. Karlsson *et al.*, *Biomed. Chromatogr.* **11**, 54 (1997). Clinical pharmacokinetics: E.-P. Sandell *et al.*, *J. Cardiovasc. Pharmacol.* **26**, Suppl. 1, S57 (1995). Review of mechanism of action: H. Haikala, I.-B. Lindén, *ibid.*, S10-S19 (1995); of pharmacology, toxicology and clinical evaluation: P. S. Pagel *et al.*, *Cardiovasc. Drug Rev.* **14**, 286-316 (1996). Comparison with dobutamine, *q.v.*, in heart failure: F. Follath *et al.*, *Lancet* **360**, 196 (2002).

Yellow crystalline powder, mp 210-214°. $[\alpha]_D^{25}$ −566° (tetrahydrofuran/methanol). Soluble in water. pKa 6.3. LD$_{50}$ in male, female mice, male rats (mg/kg): 156, 152, 103 orally; 32, 50, 57 i.v. (Pagel).

THERAP CAT: Cardiotonic.

5472. Levulinic Acid. [123-76-2] 4-Oxopentanoic acid; laevulinic acid; β-acetylpropionic acid. $C_5H_8O_3$; mol wt 116.12. C 51.72%, H 6.94%, O 41.33%. $CH_3COCH_2CH_2COOH$. Laboratory procedure from starch or cane sugar by boiling with HCl: McKenzie, *Org. Synth.* **coll. vol. I**, 335 (1941). Produced commercially from low grade cellulose. By-product of furfural manuf. Extensive review: Leonard, *Ind. Eng. Chem.* **48**, 1331 (1956).

Plates or leaflets (commercial product is yellow), mp 33-35°. bp 245-246°. d 1.1447. n_D^{16} 1.442. Freely sol in water, alcohol, ether; essentially insol in aliphatic hydrocarbons. *Protect from light.*

Phenylhydrazone. Antithermin. $C_{11}H_{14}N_2O_2$; mol wt 206.24. Leaflets, mp 108°. Slightly sol in cold water, more sol in hot water; freely sol in alcohol, chloroform, ether, dil acids.

USE: In organic syntheses; in the manuf of nylon, synthetic rubbers, plastics, and medicinals.

5473. Lexipafant. [139133-26-9] *N*-Methyl-*N*-[[4-[(2-methyl-1*H*-imidazo[4,5-*c*]pyridin-1-yl)methyl]phenyl]sulfonyl]-L-leucine ethyl ester; *N*-methyl-*N*-[[α-(2-methyl-1*H*-imidazo[4,5-*c*]-

Consult the Name Index before using this section.

pyridin-1-yl)-*p*-tolyl]sulfonyl]-L-leucine ethyl ester; BB-882; Zacutex. $C_{23}H_{30}N_4O_4S$; mol wt 458.57. C 60.24%, H 6.59%, N 12.22%, O 13.96%, S 6.99%. Platelet activating factor (PAF) antagonist. Prepn: M. Whittaker, A. Miller, **WO 9203422**; *eidem*, **US 5200412** (1992, 1993 both to British Bio-Technology). Structure-activity report: M. Whittaker *et al., J. Lipid Mediators Cell Signalling* **10**, 151 (1994). Pharmacology: F. M. Abu-Zidan *et al., Pharmacol. Toxicol.* **78**, 23 (1996). Clinical evaluation in acute pancreatitis: A. N. Kingsnorth *et al., Br. J. Surg.* **82**, 1414 (1995).

White crystalline solid from ethyl acetate, mp 105°. $[\alpha]_D^{20} -6.7°$ (c = 2.0 in $CDCl_3$).

THERAP CAT: Anti-inflammatory.

5474. LH-RH. [9034-40-6] Luteinizing hormone-releasing factor; LH-RF; luteinizing hormone-releasing hormone; LRF; LRH; gonadorelin; gonadotropin-releasing factor; gonadoliberin; luliberin; LH-RH/FSH-RH; Fertagyl; Fertiral; Kryptocur; Relefact LH-RH. $C_{55}H_{75}N_{17}O_{13}$; mol wt 1182.29. C 55.87%, H 6.39%, N 20.14%, O 17.59%. Neurohumoral hormone produced in the hypothalamus which stimulates the secretion of the pituitary hormones, LH (luteinizing hormone) and FSH (follicle-stimulating hormone) *q.q.v.*, which in turn produce changes resulting in the induction of ovulation. Isoln from porcine hypothalamic extracts: A. V. Schally *et al., Biochem. Biophys. Res. Commun.* **43**, 393 (1971). Structure: Matsuo *et al., ibid.* 1334; Baba *et al., ibid.* **44**, 459 (1971); Burgus *et al., C.R. Seances Acad. Sci. Ser. D* **273**, 1611 (1971). Solid phase synthesis: Monahan *et al., ibid.* 508; Monahan, Rivier, *Biochem. Biophys. Res. Commun.* **48**, 1100 (1972); Coy *et al., Methods Enzymol.* **37**, 416 (1975); D. H. Rich, S. K. Gurwara, *Tetrahedron Lett.* **1975**, 301. Industrial prepn: Geiger *et al.*, **DE 2213737** (1973 to Hoechst). Confirmation of biological activity: A. V. Schally *et al., Science* **173**, 1036 (1971). Pharmacokinetics: T. W. Redding, *J. Clin. Endocrinol. Metab.* **37**, 626 (1973). Reviews of physiology and implications in fertility control: A. V. Schally *et al., Fertil. Steril.* **22**, 703 (1971); R. Guillemin, *Contraception* **6**, 1 (1972). Review of LH-RH and other hypothalamic hormones: A. V. Schally *et al., Science* **179**, 341 (1973); A. V. Schally, *ibid.* **202**, 18-28 (1978); of LH-RH and somatostatin, *q.v.*: S. M. McCann, *Annu. Rev. Pharmacol. Toxicol.* **22**, 491-515 (1982). General reviews: J. Sandow, *Clin. Endocrinol.* **18**, 571-592 (1983); S. M. McCann, *J. Endocrinol. Invest.* **6**, 243-251 (1983).

5-oxoPro–His–Trp–Ser–Tyr–Gly–Leu–Arg–Pro–GlyNH₂

$[\alpha]_D^{25} -50°$ (1% acetic acid). Chymotrypsin, papain, subtilisin, thermolysin destroy the pituitary hormone releasing action of LH-RH.

Acetate (salt) hydrate. Gonadorelin acetate; Cystorelin; Hypocrine; Lutrelef; Lutrepulse. $C_{55}H_{75}N_{17}O_{13}.xC_2H_4O_2.yH_2O$, as the diacetate tetrahydrate or a mixture of monoacetate and diacetate hydrates.

Hydrochloride. [51952-41-1] AY-24031; HRF; Factrel.

THERAP CAT: Gonad-stimulating principle.

THERAP CAT (VET): Gonad-stimulating principle.

5475. Liarozole. [115575-11-6] 5-[(3-Chlorophenyl)-1*H*-imidazol-1-ylmethyl]-1*H*-benzimidazole; (±)-5-(*m*-chloro-α-imidazol-1-ylbenzyl)benzimidazole. $C_{17}H_{13}ClN_4$; mol wt 308.76. C 66.13%, H 4.24%, Cl 11.48%, N 18.15%. Inhibits cytochrome P450-dependent enzymes involved in steroid biosynthesis and ret-

inoic acid catabolism. Prepn: A. H. M. Raeymaekers *et al.*, **EP 260744**; *eidem*, **US 4859684** (1988, 1989 both to Janssen). *In vivo* antitumor activity: R. Van Ginckel *et al., Prostate* **16**, 313 (1990). Pharmacology and effect on steroid synthesis: J. Bruynseels *et al., ibid.*, 345; and effect on retinoic acid: R. De Coster *et al., J. Steroid Biochem. Mol. Biol.* **43**, 197 (1992). Clinical evaluation in prostate cancer: C. Mahler *et al., Cancer* **71**, 1068 (1993); in psoriasis: P. Dockx *et al., Br. J. Dermatol.* **133**, 426 (1995); in combination therapy for malignant brain tumors: M. E. Westarp *et al., Onkologie* **16**, 22 (1993).

mp 108.2°.

Fumarate. [145858-52-2] R-85246; Liazal. $2C_{17}H_{13}ClN_4.-3C_4H_4O_4$; mol wt 965.75.

Hydrochloride. [145858-50-0] R-75251. $C_{17}H_{13}ClN_4.HCl$; mol wt 345.23.

THERAP CAT: Antineoplastic.

5476. Liatris. Deer's tongue; vanilla plant. Leaves of *Trilisa odoratissima* (Walt.) Cass. (*Liatris odoratissima* (Walt.) Willd.), *Compositae. Habit.* U.S., Virginia to Florida and Louisiana. *Constit.* Volatile oil, coumarin.

USE: In perfumery and for perfuming smoking, chewing and snuff tobacco.

5477. Licheniformins. Antibiotic substances produced by *Bacillus licheniformis.* Isoln: Callow *et al., Br. J. Exp. Pathol.* **28**, 418 (1947). Separation of licheniformins A, B, and C: Callow, Work, *Biochem. J.* **51**, 558 (1952). Mol wt as measured by sedimentation: licheniformin A, 4400; licheniformin B, 3800; and licheniformin C, 4800: Ogston, *ibid.* **51**, 569 (1952).

All three constituents in the form of hydrochlorides are white, amorphous, slightly hygroscopic powders, melting with decompn at indefinite temperatures.

5478. Lichenin. [1402-10-4] Moss starch. $C_6H_{10}O_5$; mol wt 162.14. C 44.45%, H 6.22%, O 49.34%. Polyglucan from *Cetraria islandica* (L.) Ach., *Parmeliaceae* (Iceland Moss). Isoln: Peat *et al., J. Chem. Soc.* **1957**, 3916. Linear polysaccharide structure composed of regular sequences of two $(1 \rightarrow 4)$- and one $(1 \rightarrow 3)$-β-D-glucopyranosyl residues: Perlin, Suzuki, *Can. J. Chem.* **40**, 50 (1962); Fleming, Manners, *Biochem. J.* **100**, 4, 24 (1966). Exhibits antineoplastic activity: Shibata, **JP 71 17147** (1971), *C.A.* **75**, 67474z (1971); Tadahiro *et al., Chem. Pharm. Bull.* **20**, 2445 (1972). NMR spectrum: D. Gagnaire, M. Vincedon, *Bull. Soc. Chim. Fr.* **1977**, 479.

White powder. Sol in boiling water, in HCl. $[\alpha]_D +18.4°$.

5479. Licochalcones. Oxygenated chalcones isolated from licorice root, a traditional medicine prepared from various species of *Glycyrrhiza* (Leguminosae). Exhibit antiparasitic and antitumor activity and appear to interfere with mitochondrial respiration. Four have been identified, A-D, as well as a closely related compound, *echinatin*. Isoln of A and B from *G. glabra* L. and structure: T. Saitoh, S. Shibata, *Tetrahedron Lett.* **50**, 4461 (1975); of C and D from *G. inflata*: K. Kajiyama *et al., Phytochemistry* **31**, 3229 (1992). Mechanism of action study: H. Haraguchi *et al., ibid.* **48**, 125 (1998); L Zhai *et al., J. Antimicrob. Chemother.* **43**, 793 (1999).

Licochalcone A

Licochalcone A. [58749-22-7] (2E)-3-[5-(1,1-Dimethyl-2-propenyl)-4-hydroxy-2-methoxyphenyl]-1-(4-hydroxyphenyl)-2-propen-1-one. $C_{21}H_{22}O_4$; mol wt 338.40. Synthesis: A. Islam, M. A. Hossain, *Indian J. Chem.* **32B**, 713 (1993). HPLC determn in biological fluids: L. Nadelmann *et al., J. Chromatogr. B* **695**, 389 (1997). Antileishmanial activity: M. Chen *et al., Antimicrob. Agents Chemother.* **38**, 1339 (1994). Antimalarial activity: *eidem, ibid.* 1470. Effect on human cancer cell lines: E. J. Park *et al., Planta Med.* **64**, 464 (1998). Yellow needles from methanol-water, mp 100°. uv max in methanol: 264, 308, 378 nm (log ε 3.96, 3.97, 4.31).

Licochalcone B. [58749-23-8] (2E)-3-(3,4-Dihydroxy-2-methoxyphenyl)-1-(4-hydroxyphenyl)-2-propen-1-one. $C_{16}H_{14}O_5$; mol wt 286.28. Yellow needles from methanol-water, mp 197°. uv max in methanol: 262, 366 nm (log ε 3.71, 4.27).

Licochalcone C. [144506-14-9] (2E)-3-[4-Hydroxy-2-methoxy-3-(3-methyl-2-butenyl)phenyl]-1-(4-hydroxyphenyl)-2-propen-1-one. $C_{21}H_{22}O_4$; mol wt 338.40. Amorphous. uv max in methanol: 250, 308sh, 358 nm (log ε 3.88, 3.95, 4.24).

Licochalcone D. [144506-15-0] (2E)-3-(3,4-Dihydroxy-2-methoxyphenyl)-1-[4-hydroxy-3-(3-methyl-2-butenyl)phenyl]-2-propen-1-one. $C_{21}H_{22}O_5$; mol wt 354.40. Pale yellow needles from methanol-water, mp 113°. uv max in methanol: 254, 359 nm (log ε 3.86, 4.30).

5480. Licofelone. [156897-06-2] 6-(4-Chlorophenyl)-2,3-dihydro-2,2-dimethyl-7-phenyl-1*H*-pyrrolizine-5-acetic acid; ML-3000. $C_{23}H_{22}ClNO_2$; mol wt 379.88. C 72.72%, H 5.84%, Cl 9.33%, N 3.69%, O 8.42%. Dual inhibitor of cyclooxygenase and 5-lipoxygenase. Prepn: G. Dannhardt *et al.,* **EP 397175**; *eidem,* **US 5260451** (1990, 1993 both to Merckle); S. A. Laufer *et al., J. Med. Chem.* **37**, 1894 (1994); J. Cossy, D. Belotti, *Tetrahedron* **55**, 5145 (1999). Mechanism of action: S. Tries *et al., Inflamm. Res.* **51**, 135 (2002). Experience in experimental dog osteoarthritis: D. Lajeunesse *et al., Ann. Rheum. Dis.* **63**, 78 (2004). Gastrointestinal safety profile in dogs: M. Moreau *et al., J. Vet. Pharmacol. Ther.* **28**, 81 (2005). Review of clinical development: S. Laufer, *Inflammopharmacology* **9**, 101-112 (2001); J. M. Alvaro-Gracia, *Rheumatology* **43**, Suppl. 1, i21-i25 (2004).

Slightly yellowish solid, mp 162-163°.
THERAP CAT: Anti-inflammatory.
THERAP CAT (VET): Anti-inflammatory.

5481. Lidamidine. [66871-56-5] *N*-(2,6-Dimethylphenyl)-*N*′-[imino(methylamino)methyl]urea; 1-(2,6-dimethylphenyl)-3-methylamidinourea. $C_{11}H_{16}N_4O$; mol wt 220.27. C 59.98%, H 7.32%, N 25.44%, O 7.26%. Amidinourea with antisecretory, antimotility properties. Prepn as hydrochloride: **BE 844832** (1977 to Rorer), *C.A.* **88**, 22432m (1977). *See also:* J. Diamond, G. H. Douglas, **US 4147804** (1979 to Rorer). Prepn, structure activity relationship: G. H. Douglas *et al., Arzneim.-Forsch.* **28**, 1435 (1978). Physical-chemical properties: J. J. Zalipsky *et al., ibid.* 1441. Effect on α_2-adrenergic receptors and electrolyte absorption: T. Durbin *et al., Gastroenterology* **82**, 1352 (1982). Series of articles on pharmacology, metabolism, pharmacokinetics: *Arzneim.-Forsch.* **28**, 1448-1480 (1978). Toxicity: B. J. Chou *et al., ibid.* 1471. Clinical comparison with loperamide, *q.v.,* in acute diarrhea: G. Gasbarrini *et al., ibid.* **36**, 1843 (1986). Brief review: G. Friedman, *Am. J. Gastroenterol.* **80**, 143 (1985).

Hydrochloride. [65009-35-0] WHR-1142A; Lidarral; Smodin. $C_{11}H_{16}N_4O\cdot HCl$; mol wt 256.73. White powder, mp 194-197°. uv max (H_2O): 262, 271 nm (ε 626, 524). Soly at 25° (mg/ml): water 153.55, methanol 297.94, ethanol 88.55, chloroform 4.62, hexane 0.01. LD_{50} in male mice, male, female rats (mg/kg): 260, 267, 160 orally; in mice (mg/kg): 56 i.v. (Chou).

THERAP CAT: Antiperistaltic; antidiarrheal.

5482. Lidocaine. [137-58-6] 2-(Diethylamino)-*N*-(2,6-dimethylphenyl)acetamide; 2-diethylamino-2′,6′-acetoxylidide; ω-diethylamino-2,6-dimethylacetanilide; lignocaine; Cuivasil; Lidoderm; LidoPosterine; Vagisil. $C_{14}H_{22}N_2O$; mol wt 234.34. C 71.75%, H 9.46%, N 11.95%, O 6.83%. Long-acting, membrane stabilizing agent against ventricular arrhythmia. Originally developed as a local anesthetic. Prepn: N. M. Löfgren, B. J. Lundqvist, **US 2441498** (1948 to Astra); A. D. H. Self, A. P. T. Easson, **GB 706409** (1954 to May & Baker); I. P. S. Hardie, E. S. Stern, **GB 758224** (1956 to J. F. Macfarlane & Co.); Zhuravlev, Nikolaev, *Zh. Obshch. Khim.* **30**, 1155 (1960). Toxicity studies: E. R. Smith, B. R. Duce, *J. Pharmacol. Exp. Ther.* **179**, 580 (1971); G. H. Kronberg *et al., J. Med. Chem.* **16**, 739 (1973). Review of pharmacokinetics: N. L. Benowitz, W. Meister, *Clin. Pharmacokinet.* **3**, 177 (1978). Review of action as local anesthetic: Löfgren, *Studies on Local Anesthetics: Xylocaine, A New Synthetic Drug* (Hoeggstroms, Stockholm, 1948); Cooper, *Pharm. J.* **171**, 68 (1953). Reviews of anti-arrhythmic agents: J. L. Anderson *et al., Drugs* **15**, 271 (1978); L. H. Opie, *Lancet* **1**, 861 (1980); E. Carmeliet, *Ann. N.Y. Acad. Sci.* **427**, 1 (1984). Comprehensive description: K. Groningsson *et al., Anal. Profiles Drug Subs.* **14**, 207-243 (1985); M. F. Powell, *ibid.* **15**, 761-779 (1986). Review of use in treatment of postherpetic neuralgia: P. S. Davies, B. S. Galer, *Drugs* **64**, 937-947 (2004).

Needles from benzene or alcohol, mp 68-69°. bp_4 180-182°; bp_2 159-160°. Insol in water. Sol in alcohol, ether, benzene, chloroform, oils. Partition coefficient (octanol/water, pH 7.4): 43.

Hydrochloride. [73-78-9]; [6108-05-0] (monohydrate). Basicaina; Batixim; Dynexan; Heweneural; Licain; Lidesthesin; Lidofast; Lidoject; Lidrian; Odontalg; Sedagul; Xylocaine; Xylocard; Xylocitin; Xyloneural. $C_{14}H_{22}N_2O\cdot HCl$; mol wt 270.80. Crystals, mp 127-129°; monohydrate, mp 77-78°. Very sol in water, alcohol; sol in chloroform. Insol in ether. pH of 0.5% aq soln: 4.0-5.5. LD_{50} in mice (mg/kg): 292 orally (Smith, Duce); 105 i.p.; 19.5 i.v. (Kronberg).

THERAP CAT: Anesthetic (local); antiarrhythmic (class IB).
THERAP CAT (VET): Anesthetic (local).

5483. Lidofenin. [59160-29-1] *N*-(Carboxymethyl)-*N*-[2-[(2,6-dimethylphenyl)amino]-2-oxoethyl]glycine; *N*-(2,6-dimethylphenyl)-2-oxoethylglycine; *N*-(2,6-dimethylacetanilide)iminodiacetic acid; *N*-(2,6-dimethylphenylcarbamoylmethyl)iminodiacetic acid; [[(2,6-xylylcarbamoyl)methyl]imino]diacetic acid; HIDA. $C_{14}H_{18}N_2O_5$; mol wt 294.30. C 57.14%, H 6.16%, N 9.52%, O 27.18%. Iminodiacetic acid analog. Prepn of compd and ^{99m}Tc-complex: M. D. Loberg *et al.,* **BE 840556**; *eidem,* **US 4017596** (1976, 1977 both to Research Corp.); and imaging studies: M. D. Loberg *et al., J. Nucl. Med.* **17**, 633 (1976). Structural studies: M. D. Loberg, A. T. Fields, *Int. J. Appl. Radiat. Isot.* **29**, 167 (1978). Chromatographic determn of radiochemical purity: A. M. Zimmer *et al., Eur. J. Nucl. Med.* **7**, 88 (1982). Biodistribution and clinical kinetics: J. Ryan *et al., J. Nucl. Med.* **18**, 995 (1977). Clinical studies of diagnostic use as hepatobiliary imaging agent: H. S. Weissmann *et al., Am. J. Roentgenol.* **132**, 523 (1979); R. W. Nicholson *et al., Br. J. Radiol.* **53**, 878 (1980).

Crystals from water, mp 201-203°. LD$_{50}$ i.v. in male mice: 168 mg/kg (Ryan).

^{99m}Tc-complex. ^{99m}Tc-HIDA; TechneScan HIDA.

THERAP CAT: ^{99m}Tc-complex as diagnostic aid (radioactive imaging agent).

5484. Lidoflazine. [3416-26-0] 4-[4,4-Bis(4-fluorophenyl)-butyl]-*N*-(2,6-dimethylphenyl)-1-piperazineacetamide; 4-[4,4-bis(*p*-fluorophenyl)butyl]-1-piperazineaceto-2′,6′-xylidide; 1-[4,4-di(4-fluorophenyl)butyl]-4-[(2,6-dimethylanilinocarbonyl)methyl]-piperazine; McN-JR-7094; R-7904; Angex; Clinium; Klinium; Ordiflazine; Corflazine. C$_{30}$H$_{35}$F$_2$N$_3$O; mol wt 491.62. C 73.29%, H 7.18%, F 7.73%, N 8.55%, O 3.25%. Calcium blocking agent. Prepn: **NL 6507312**; H. K. F. Hermans, W. K. Schaper, **US 3267104** (1965, 1966, both to Janssen). Crystal structure: G. Germain *et al., Acta Crystallogr.* **33B**, 1971 (1977). Tissue specificity of calcium-blocking properties: J. M. Van Neuten, D. Wellens, *Arch. Int. Pharmacodyn. Ther.* **242**, 329 (1979). Cardioprotective effects: W. Daenen, W. Flameng, *Angiology* **32**, 543 (1981). Effects in angina: F. L. Gobel *et al., Circulation* **65**, 1 Pt. 2, 127 (1982); W. Shapiro *et al., ibid.* 143.

Crystals, mp 159-161°. Almost insol in water (<0.01%), very sol in chloroform (>50%), but much less sol in other common organic solvents: W. K. Schaper *et al., J. Pharmacol. Exp. Ther.* **152**, 265 (1966).

THERAP CAT: Vasodilator (coronary).

5485. Light Green SF Yellowish. [5141-20-8] *N*-Ethyl-*N*-[4-[[4-[ethyl](3-sulfophenyl)methyl]amino]phenyl](4-sulfophenyl)-methylene]-2,5-cyclohexadien-1-ylidene]-3-sulfobenzenemethan-aminium inner salt, disodium salt; C.I. Acid Green 5; ethyl[4-[*p*-[ethyl(*m*-sulfobenzyl)amino]-α-(*p*-sulfophenyl)benzylidene]-2,5-cyclohexadien-1-ylidene](*m*-sulfobenzyl)ammonium hydroxide inner salt disodium salt; C.I. 42095; FD & C Green No. 2; Lissamine Green SF. C$_{37}$H$_{34}$N$_2$Na$_2$O$_9$S$_3$; mol wt 792.85. C 56.05%, H 4.32%, N 3.53%, Na 5.80%, O 18.16%, S 12.13%. Prepn and refs: *Colour Index* **vol. 4** (3rd ed., 1971) p 4385. Biological use: *H. J. Conn's Biological Stains*, R. D. Lillie, Ed. (Williams & Wilkins, Baltimore, 9th ed., 1977) pp 257-258, 582. Toxicity data: F. C. Lu, A. Lavalle, *Can. Pharm. J.* **97**, 30 (1964). Chronic toxicity study: W. H. Hansen *et al., Food Cosmet. Toxicol.* **4**, 389 (1966).

A reddish-brown powder. Sol in water to a green soln which turns yellowish-brown with HCl and then gradually fades. Addition of NaOH almost completely decolorizes the soln yielding a dull violet ppt. LD$_{50}$ orally in rats: >2 g/kg (Lu, Lavalle).

USE: As dye, biological stain.

5486. Lignans. Plant products of low molecular weight formed primarily by the oxidative coupling of *p*-hydroxyphenyl-propene units in which the two units may be linked by an oxygen

bridge. The monomeric precursor units are cinnamic acid, cinnamyl alcohol, propenylbenzene and allylbenzene. The term lignan or *Haworth lignan* is applied to compounds derived by coupling acid and/or alcohol while the compounds derived by coupling propenyl and/or allyl derivatives are called *neolignans*: O. R. Gottlieb, *Fortschr. Chem. Org. Naturst.* **35**, 1-72 (1978). Lignans occur widely and have been obtained from roots, heartwood, foliage, fruit and resinous exudates of plants. Lignans are optically active compounds. They represent the dimer stage intermediate between monomeric propylphenol units and lignin. Naturally occurring trimers and tetramers have not been reported. Occurrence of lignans, enterolactone, *q.v.*, and enterodiol, in man and animal species: S. R. Stitch *et al., Nature* **287**, 238 (1980); K. D. R. Setchell, *ibid.* 740. Synthesis of first lignans found in man and animals: G. Cooley *et al., Tetrahedron Lett.* **22**, 349 (1981).

5487. Lignin. [9005-53-2] The most abundant natural aromatic organic polymer found in all vascular plants. Lignin together with cellulose and hemicellulose, *q.q.v.*, are the major cell wall components of the fibers of all wood and grass species. Lignin is composed of coniferyl, *p*-coumaryl and sinapyl alcohols in varying ratios in different plant species. Monographs: F. E. Brauns, D. A. Brauns, *The Chemistry of Lignin,* Supplement Volume covering the literature 1949-1958 (Academic Press, New York, 1960) 804 pp; I. A. Pearl, *The Chemistry of Lignin* (Marcel Dekker, New York, 1967) 360 pp. Structural aspects and applications: H. Veeramani, G. A. Wani, *Chem. Ind. Dev.* **11**, 13-25 (1977). Chemistry and structure: C. A. Reddy, L. Forney, *Dev. Ind. Microbiol.* **19**, 27-34 (1978). *Reviews:* Nord, Shubert, *Sci. Am.* **199**, no. 4, 104-113 (Oct. 1958); I. A. Pearl, "Lignin as a Raw Material for the Production of Pure Chemicals," *J. Chem. Educ.* **35**, 502 (1958); D. W. Goheen, C. H. Hoyt in *Kirk-Othmer Encyclopedia of Chemical Technology* **vol. 14**, (Wiley-Interscience, New York, 3rd ed., 1981) pp 294-312.

USE: Source of vanillin, syringic aldehyde, dimethyl sulfoxide. Extender for phenolic plastics, to strengthen rubber (esp for shoe soles), as oil mud additive, to stabilize asphalt emulsions, to precipitate proteins.

5488. Lignoceric Acid. [557-59-5] Tetracosanoic acid. C$_{24}$H$_{48}$O$_2$; mol wt 368.64. C 78.19%, H 13.12%, O 8.68%. C$_{23}$-H$_{47}$COOH. Obtained from beechwood tar or by the distillation of rotten oak wood: Sullivan, *Ind. Eng. Chem.* **8**, 1027 (1916). Most natural fats contain small amounts (0.2-1%). The seed fat of the Indian tree *Adenanthera pavonina* is said to contain 25%. Synthesis: Fieser, Szmuszkovicz, *J. Am. Chem. Soc.* **70**, 3352 (1948).

Crystals, mp 84.15°. n_D^{100} 1.4287. Soly in 91.53% ethanol: 0.182 g/100 ml. Neutralization value 152.2.

Methyl ester. C$_{25}$H$_{50}$O$_2$. Platelets, mp 58-59.8°.

5489. Ligroin. [8032-32-4] V.M.&P. naphtha; varnish makers' and painters' naphtha; refined solvent naphtha; solvent naphtha; Benzoline; Canadol. Term that has been applied to petroleum fractions of the same nature as described for petroleum benzin, *q.v.*, but of higher density, higher boiling range and higher flash pt. Defined by ASTM prior to 1950 as synonymous with petroleum benzin and petroleum ether: *ASTM Standard Specifications* D 288-49, 865-867 (1949).

Refined solvent, mobile, flammable liquid. d$_{15.6}^{15.6}$ 0.850 to 0.870. Distillation range at 760 mm: percentage recovered at 130° = not more than 5; percentage recovered at 145° = not less than 90. End point (dry point) = not above 155°. Technical benzin (high boiling petr ether) usually has a d$_{15.6}^{15.6}$ 0.730-0.750 and bp$_{760}$ 90-120°.

Caution: Potential symptoms of overexposure are irritation of eyes, upper respiratory system; dermatitis, CNS depression; aspiration of liquid may cause chemical pneumonia. *See NIOSH Pocket Guide to Chemical Hazards* (DHHS/NIOSH 97-140, 1997) p 332.

5490. Limaprost. [74397-12-9] (2*E*,11α,13*E*,15*S*,17*S*)-11,15-Dihydroxy-17,20-dimethyl-9-oxoprosta-2,13-dien-1-oic acid; 17*S*,20-dimethyl-*trans*-2,3-didehydro-PGE$_1$; 9-oxo-11α,15α-dihydroxy-17*S*,20-dimethylprosta-*trans*-2,*trans*-13-dienoic acid; 17*S*-methyl-ω-homo-*trans*-Δ^2-PGE$_1$; ONO-1206; OP-1206; Opalmon; Prorenal. C$_{22}$H$_{36}$O$_5$; mol wt 380.52. C 69.44%, H 9.54%, O 21.02%. Derivative of prostaglandin E$_1$, *q.v.* Prepn: M. Hayashi *et al.*, **DE 3002677** (1980 to Ono); *eidem*, **US 4294849** (1981 to Warner-Lambert). Cardiovascular pharmacology in animals: T.

Tsuboi *et al., Arch. Int. Pharmacodyn.* **247,** 89 (1980). Effect on smooth muscle *in vitro:* P. G. Adaikan, S. M. M. Karim, *Prostaglandins Med.* **6,** 449 (1981). Coronary vasodilating effects in primates: S. R. Kottegoda *et al., Prostaglandins Leukotrienes Med.* **8,** 343 (1982). Clinical hemodynamics in chronic lung disease: T. Ishizaki *et al., Chest* **85,** 382 (1984).

White crystals, mp 97-100°.

THERAP CAT: Antianginal.

5491. Limestone. Natural calcium carbonate; agricultural limestone; Agstone; lithographic stone; Solnhofen stone. A term originally applied only to minerals consisting largely of $CaCO_3$, such as Portland stone, dolomite, marble, and chalk, now used indiscriminately to designate technical and agricultural grades of calcium carbonate. *Review:* R. S. Boynton in *Kirk-Othmer Encyclopedia of Chemical Technology* **vol. 14** (Wiley-Interscience, New York, 3rd ed., 1981) pp 343-382.

Caution: Potential symptoms of overexposure are irritation of eyes, skin, mucous membranes; cough, sneezing, rhinorrhea; lacrimation. *See NIOSH Pocket Guide to Chemical Hazards* (DHHS/NIOSH 97-140, 1997) p 186.

5492. Limettin. [487-06-9] 5,7-Dimethoxy-2*H*-1-benzopyran-2-one; 5,7-dimethoxycoumarin; citropten. $C_{11}H_{10}O_4$; mol wt 206.19. C 64.08%, H 4.89%, O 31.04%. From rind of fruit of *Citrus lima* Lunan (*C. limetta* Auth.), *Rutaceae* (lime): Tilden, Beck, *J. Chem. Soc.* **57,** 323 (1890); from W. Indian lime oil: Caldwell, Jones, *ibid.* **1945,** 570; from citrus oils: Stanley, Vannier, **US 2889337** (1959 to U.S.D.A.). Synthesis: Schmidt, *Arch. Pharm.* **242,** 288 (1904); Heyes, Robertson, *J. Chem. Soc.* **1936,** 1831.

Needles from methanol, mp 147-148°. uv max (alcohol): 222, 247, 250.5, 324 nm (log ε 4.03, 3.84, 3.84, 4.18). Almost insol in boiling water, ether, petr ether. Freely sol in alcohol, chloroform, acetone.

5493. Limonene. [138-86-3] 1-Methyl-4-(1-methylethenyl)cyclohexene; *p*-mentha-1,8-diene; cinene; cajeputene; kautschin. $C_{10}H_{16}$; mol wt 136.23. C 88.16%, H 11.84%. Occurs in various ethereal oils, particularly in oils of lemon, orange, caraway, dill and bergamot. Isoln of *d*-limonene from mandarin peel oil (*Citrus reticulata* Blanco, *Rutaceae):* Kugler, Kováts, *Helv. Chim. Acta* **46,** 1480 (1963). *Review:* J. L. Simonsen, *The Terpenes* **vol. I** (University Press, Cambridge, 2nd ed., 1947) pp 143-165.

dl-**Form.** Inactive limonene; dipentene. Liquid. Pleasant lemon-like odor. bp_{763} 175.5-176.5°. $d_4^{20.85}$ 0.8402. n_D 1.4744. Practically insol in water. Miscible with alcohol. With dry HCl or HBr it forms monohalides, with aq HCl or HBr, the dihalide.

d-**Form.** Liquid. bp_{763} 175.5-176°. d_4^{21} 0.8402. n_D^{21} 1.4743. $[α]_D^{19.5}$ +123.8°.

l-**Form.** Liquid. bp_{763} 175.5-176.5°. $d_4^{20.5}$ 0.8407. n_D^{21} 1.474. $[α]_D^{19.5}$ −101.3°.

Caution: Skin irritant, sensitizer.

USE: Solvent, manuf resins; wetting and dispersing agent.

5494. Limonin. [1180-71-8] Limonoic acid di-δ-lactone; 8-(3-furyl)decahydro-2,2,4a,8a-tetramethyl-11*H*,13*H*-oxireno[*d*]-pyrano[4′,3′:3,3a]isobenzofuro[5,4-*f*][2]benzopyran-4,6,13(2*H*,-5a*H*)-trione; limonoic acid 3,19:16,17-dilactone. $C_{26}H_{30}O_8$; mol wt 470.51. C 66.37%, H 6.43%, O 27.20%. Tetracyclic triterpenoid; bitter principle of citrus fruits. Isoln: Bernays, *Ann.* **40,** 317 (1841). Improved isoln and purification: P. G. Pifferi *et al., Ital. J. Food Sci.* **5,** 269 (1993). Structure: A. Melera *et al., Helv. Chim. Acta* **40,** 1420 (1957). Stereochemistry: D. Arigoni *et al., Experientia* **16,** 41 (1960); S. Arnott *et al., ibid.* **49.** Partial synthesis: C. Lüthy *et al., Helv. Chim. Acta* **57,** 1060 (1974). HPLC determn in citrus juice: W. W. Widmer, *J. Agric. Food Chem.* **39,** 1472 (1991). Review of chemistry: V. P. Maier *et al., ACS Symp. Ser.* **143,** 63-82 (1980); and removal of juice bitterness: R. F. H. Dekker, *Aust. J. Biotechnol.* **2,** 65 (1988).

Bitter crystals from methylene chloride + isopropanol or acetic acid, mp 298°. $[α]_D$ −128° (c = 1.21 in acetone). uv max: 207, 285 nm (ε 7000, 38). Slightly sol in water, ether; sol in alcohol, glacialaceticacid.

5495. Linalool. [78-70-6] 3,7-Dimethyl-1,6-octadien-3-ol; 2,6-dimethyl-2,7-octadien-6-ol; linalol. $C_{10}H_{18}O$; mol wt 154.25. C 77.87%, H 11.76%, O 10.37%. $(CH_3)_2C=CHCH_2CH_2-C(CH_3)(OH)CH=CH_2$. Chief constituent of linaloe oil; also occurs in oils of Ceylon cinnamon, sassafras, orange flower, bergamot, *Artemisia balchanorum*, ylang ylang, etc.: Tiemann, *Ber.* **31,** 808 (1898); Walbaum, Stephan, *ibid.* **33,** 2305 (1900); Hesse, Zeitschel, *J. Prakt. Chem.* **66,** 493 (1902); Rafanova *et al.,* **SU 103725** (1956), *C.A.* **51,** 3656c (1957); Naves, *Helv. Chim. Acta* **42,** 1692 (1959). Presence in essential oils: *idem, Compt. Rend.* **251,** 900 (1960). Absolute configuration: Prelog, Watanabe, *Ann.* **603,** 1 (1957). Synthesis of *dl*-linalool: Ruzicka, Fornasir, *Helv. Chim. Acta* **2,** 182 (1919); Surmatis, **US 2848502** (1958 to Hoffmann-La Roche); Nair, Pandit, *Tetrahedron Lett.* **1966,** 5097. *Review:* J. L. Simonsen, *The Terpenes* **vol. I** (University Press, Cambridge, 2nd ed., 1947), pp 57-68.

l-**Form.** Licareol. Colorless liq. bp_{760} 198°; bp_{25} 98-98.3°; bp_{14} 86-87°. d^{20} 0.8622. n_D^{22} 1.4604. $[α]_D^{20}$ −20.1°. Practically insol in water. Miscible with alcohol, ether.

d-**Form.** Coriandrol. bp_{760} 198-200°; bp_{26} 114-114.5°; bp_{15.5} 93-94°; bp_{12} 86°. d_4^{20} 0.8733. n_D^{20} 1.4673. $[α]_D^{20}$ +19.3°. Soluble in 10 vol 50% alc, 4 vol 60% alc.

dl-**Form.** bp_{720} 194-197°; bp_{14} 89-91°. d^{15} 0.865.

USE: In perfumery instead of bergamot or French lavender oil since it has an odor similar to these oils.

5496. Linalyl Acetate. [115-95-7] 3,7-Dimethyl-1,6-octadien-3-yl acetate; Bergamol. $C_{12}H_{20}O_2$; mol wt 196.29. C 73.43%, H 10.27%, O 16.30%. $CH_3COOC_{10}H_{17}$. Most valuable constituent of bergamot and lavender oils, also found in many other volatile oils.

Liquid; bergamot odor. d_4^{20} 0.895. bp 220°. n_D^{20} 1.4460. Insol in water. Miscible with alcohol, ether.

USE: In perfumery.

5497. Linamarin. [554-35-8] 2-(β-D-Glucopyranosyloxy)-2-methylpropanenitrile; phaseolunatin. $C_{10}H_{17}NO_6$; mol wt 247.25. C 48.58%, H 6.93%, N 5.66%, O 38.83%. From the seed skins or embryos of flax: Jorissen, Hairs, *Bull. Acad. Roy. Sci. Belg.* [3] **21**, 529 (1891); André *et al., Compt. Rend.* **231**, 590 (1950); Lüdtke, *Biochem. Z.* **323**, 428 (1953). Synthesis: Fischer, Anger, *Ber.* **52**, 854 (1919). Biosynthesis in white clover: Butler, Butler, *Nature* **187**, 780 (1960).

Bitter needles, mp 142-143°. $[\alpha]_D^{18}$ −29°. Freely sol in water, cold alcohol, hot acetone; slightly in hot ethyl acetate, ether, benzene, chloroform. Practically insol in petr ether. Evolves HCN with linseed meal but not with emulsin.

Tetraacetate. $C_{18}H_{25}NO_{10}$. Needles from alcohol, mp 140-141°. $[\alpha]_D^{14}$ −10.8° (acetone). Sol in acetone, ethyl acetate, chloroform, glacial acetic acid, benzene, warm methanol and ethanol. Practically insol in petr ether.

5498. Linarin. [480-36-4] 7-[[6-*O*-(6-Deoxy-α-L-mannopyranosyl)-β-D-glucopyranosyl]oxy]-5-hydroxy-2-(4-methoxyphenyl)-4*H*-1-benzopyran-4-one; acacetin-β-rutinoside; linarigenin-glucoside; 5,7-dihydroxy-4′-methoxyflavone-D-glucosido-L-rhamnoside; buddleoflavonoloside. $C_{28}H_{32}O_{14}$; mol wt 592.55. C 56.75%, H 5.44%, O 37.80%. From the flowers of *Linaria vulgaris* Mill., *Scrophulariaceae:* Merz, Wu, *Arch. Pharm.* **274**, 126 (1936); from *Cirsium oleraceum* Scop., *Compositae:* Wagner *et al., ibid.* **293**, 1053 (1960). Structure: Baker *et al., J. Chem. Soc.* **1951**, 691. Synthesis: Zemplén, Bognàr, *Ber.* **74**, 1818 (1941).

Monohydrate. Needles from methanol, mp 268-270°. $[\alpha]_D^{26}$ −100° (0.07 g in 10 ml glacial acetic acid); $[\alpha]_D^{24}$ −87° (0.05 g in pyridine). Practically insol in water and the usual organic solvents. Sol in nitrobenzene, phenol, aniline, pyridine, concd acids and alkalies. The water of crystn cannot be removed at 100° *in vacuo* over P_2O_5 (Merz); may be removed at 138° in high vacuum (Zemplén). Hydrolysis gives 5,7-dihydroxy-4′-methoxyflavone, D-glucose, and L-rhamnose.

5499. Linatine. [10139-06-7] 1-[(4-Amino-4-carboxy-1-oxobutyl)amino]-D-proline; *N*-(D-2-carboxy-1-pyrrolidinyl)-L-glutamine; 1-[*N*-(γ-L-glutamyl)amino]-D-proline. $C_{10}H_{17}N_3O_5$; mol wt 259.26. C 46.33%, H 6.61%, N 16.21%, O 30.86%. A vitamin B_6 antagonist. The first reported naturally occurring hydrazino acid having antibacterial properties. Isoln from flaxseed *(Linum usitatissimum),* characterization, and synthesis: Klosterman *et al., Biochemistry* **6**, 170 (1967); Lamoureux, *Diss. Abstr. B* **28**, 4908 (1968). Bacterial inhibition: Parsons *et al., Antimicrob. Agents Chemother.* **1967**, 415.

Amorphous powder. $[\alpha]_D^{25}$ +46.4° (c = 2.8 in water). Attempts to obtain well-defined crystals have failed; melts with dec over a wide temperature range. Very sol in water. Practically insol in anhydr organic solvents.

L-Isomer. Amorphous solid. $[\alpha]_D^{24}$ −34.6° (c = 2 in water).

5500. Lincomycin. [154-21-2] (2*S-trans*)-Methyl 6,8-dideoxy-6-[[(1-methyl-4-propyl-2-pyrrolidinyl)carbonyl]amino]-1-thio-D-*erythro*-α-D-*galacto*-octopyranoside; lincolnensin; U-10149; NSC-70731. $C_{18}H_{34}N_2O_6S$; mol wt 406.54. C 53.18%, H 8.43%, N 6.89%, O 23.61%, S 7.89%. Antibiotic produced by *Streptomyces lincolnensis* var. *lincolnensis.* Isoln: D. J. Mason *et al., Antimicrob. Agents Chemother.* **1962**, 555; R. R. Herr, M. E. Bergy, *ibid.* 560; M. E. Bergy *et al.,* US 3086912 (1963 to Upjohn). Structure: Hoeksema *et al., J. Am. Chem. Soc.* **86**, 4223 (1964). Synthesis: Magerlein, *Tetrahedron Lett.* **1970**, 33. Stereoselective synthesis: S. Knapp, P. J. Kukkola, *J. Org. Chem.* **55**, 1632 (1990). Mechanism of action: F. N. Chang in *Antibiotics* vol. 5(pt. 1), F. E. Hahn, Ed. (Springer-Verlag, New York, 1979) pp 127-134. Clinical study: F. Puleo *et al., Gazz. Med. Ital.* **138**, 401 (1979). Toxicity data: Gray *et al., Toxicol. Appl. Pharmacol.* **6**, 476 (1964). Comprehensive description: H. Y. Muti, F. H. Al-Hajjar, *Anal. Profiles Drug Subs. Excip.* **23**, 269-319 (1994).

Free base, pKa′ 7.6. More stable in salt form. Sol in methanol, lower alcohols, ethyl acetate, acetone, chloroform. Slightly sol in water (Bergy).

Hydrochloride hemihydrate. Lincocin. $C_{18}H_{34}N_2O_6$·S.HCl.½H_2O; mol wt 452.01. Crystals from acetone, mp 135-140°. Also reported as mp 146-148°. $[\alpha]_D^{25}$ +137° (water). No uv absorption. pKa′ 7.60. Freely sol in water, methanol, ethanol; sparingly sol in most organic solvents other than hydrocarbons. LD_{50} in mice, rats (g/kg): 1 i.p.; 4 orally (Gray).

Hydrochloride monohydrate. [7179-49-9] Albiotic; Lincomix. White or almost white crystalline powder. odorless or with a slight mercaptan-like odor and a bitter taste. mp 156-158°. $[\alpha]_D^{25}$ +143° (water). pH of a 1% aq. soln: 4.8.

THERAP CAT: Antibacterial.

THERAP CAT (VET): Antibacterial.

5501. Lindane. [58-89-9] (1α,2α,3β,4α,5α,6β)-1,2,3,4,5,6-Hexachlorocyclohexane; γ-HCH; γ-benzene hexachloride; gamma benzene hexachloride; gamma hexachlor; γ-BHC; ENT-7796; Aphtiria; Gamma-Col; Gammexane; Jacutin; Kwell; Lintox; Lorexane; Quellada; Scabecid. $C_6H_6Cl_6$; mol wt 290.83. C 24.78%, H 2.08%, Cl 73.14%. Active isomer among the eight well-described stereoisomers of hexachlorocyclohexane. Prepn: T. Hardie, US 2218148 (1940 to ICI); R. E. Slade, *Chem. Ind. (London)* **1945**, 314; F. A. Gunther, *ibid.* **1946**, 399. Metabolism: R. Engst *et al., Residue Rev.* **68**, 59 (1977); **72**, 71 (1979). Acute toxicity: T. B. Gaines, *Toxicol. Appl. Pharmacol.* **14**, 515 (1969). Review of isomers: I. Hornstein, *Science* **121**, 206 (1955); S. H. Safe in *Kirk-Othmer Encyclopedia of Chemical Technology* vol. 6 (John Wiley & Sons, New York, 4th ed., 1993) pp 135-139. Reviews of carcinogenic risk: M. D. Reuber, *Environ. Res.* **19**, 460-481 (1979); S. D. Vesselinovitch, F. W. Carlborg, *Toxicol. Pathol.* **11**, 12 (1983); of toxicology and human exposure: *Toxicological Profile for Alpha, Beta, Gamma, and Delta-Hexachlorocyclohexane* (PB2006-100003, 2005) 377 pp.

Crystals, mp 112.5°. Slight musty odor. Vapor pressure at 20°: 9.4×10^{-6} mm Hg. n_D^{20} 1.644. Soly in g/100 g at 20°: acetone 43.5, benzene 28.9, $CHCl_3$ 24.0, ether 20.8, ethanol 6.4. Insol in water. LD_{50} in male, female rats (mg/kg): 88, 91 orally (Gaines).

Caution: Poisoning may occur by ingestion, inhalation, or percutaneous absorption. Potential symptoms of overexposure are irritation of eyes, skin, nose, throat; dizziness, headache, nausea, vomiting, diarrhea, tremors, weakness, convulsions, dyspnea, cyanosis; aplastic anemia; muscle spasms. *See NIOSH Pocket Guide to Chemical Hazards* (DHHS/NIOSH 97-140, 1997) p 186; *Clinical Toxicology of Commercial Products*, R. E. Gosselin *et al.*, Eds. (Williams & Wilkins, Baltimore, 5th ed., 1984) Section III, pp 239-241. Lindane and other hexachlorocyclohexane isomers are reasonably anticipated to be human carcinogens: *Report on Carcinogens, Eleventh Edition* (PB2005-104914, 2004) p III-162.

USE: Insecticide.

THERAP CAT: Pediculicide; scabicide.

THERAP CAT (VET): Ectoparasiticide.

5502. Lindlar Catalyst. [53092-86-7] $Pd\text{-}Pb\text{-}CaCO_3$. Prepn: Lindlar, *Helv. Chim. Acta* **35,** 446 (1952); Lindlar, Dubuis cited by Fieser, Fieser, *Reagents for Organic Synthesis* (New York, 1967) p 566.

USE: In selective hydrogenation of triple bonds to *cis*-double bonds.

5503. Lineatin. [65035-34-9] [1*R*-(1α,2β,5α,7β)]-3,3,7-Trimethyl-4,9-dioxatricyclo[3.3.1.0^{2,7}]nonane; 3,3,7-trimethyl-2,9-dioxatricyclo[3.3.1.0^{4,7}]nonane; 4,6,6-lineatin. $C_{10}H_{16}O_2$; mol wt 168.23. C 71.39%, H 9.59%, O 19.02%. Isoln of the unique tricyclic aggregation pheromone from ambrosia beetles, *Trypodendron lineatum* (Olivier): J. G. MacConnell *et al.*, *J. Chem. Ecol.* **3,** 549 (1977). Synthesis of (±)-form: K. Mori, M. Sasaki, *Tetrahedron Lett.* **1979,** 1329; K. N. Slessor *et al.*, *J. Org. Chem.* **45,** 2290 (1980); K. Mori *et al.*, *Tetrahedron Lett.* **23,** 1921 (1982); L. Skattebol, Y. Stenstrom, *ibid.* **24,** 3021 (1983); B. D. Johnston *et al.*, *J. Org. Chem.* **50,** 114 (1985). Synthesis of racemate and optical isomers: K. Mori, M. Sasaki, *Tetrahedron* **36,** 2197 (1980). Short stereoselective synthesis: I. Aljancic-Solaja *et al.*, *Helv. Chim. Acta* **70,** 1302 (1987). Comparative activity of the isomers: J. H. Borden *et al.*, *Can. Entomol.* **112,** 107 (1980).

Oil, bp$_{10}$ 70°. $[\alpha]_D^{24}$ +66.3° (c = 3.1 in CHCl$_3$).

USE: Insect sex attractant.

5504. Linezolid. [165800-03-3] *N*-[[(5*S*)-3-[3-Fluoro-4-(4-morpholinyl)phenyl]-2-oxo-5-oxazolidinyl]methyl]acetamide; PNU-100766; U-100766; Zyvox; Zyvoxid. $C_{16}H_{20}FN_3O_4$; mol wt 337.35. C 56.96%, H 5.98%, F 5.63%, N 12.46%, O 18.97%. Prototype of the oxazolidinone antimicrobials; inhibits bacterial mRNA translation. Prepn: M. R. Barbachyn *et al.*, **WO 9507271** (1995 to Upjohn); *eidem*, **US 5688792** (1997 to Pharmacia & Upjohn); S. J. Brickner *et al.*, *J. Med. Chem.* **39,** 673 (1996). Antibacterial spectrum: C. W. Ford *et al.*, *Antimicrob. Agents Chemother.* **40,** 1508 (1996). Mechanism of action study: D. L. Shinabarger *et al.*, *ibid.* **41,** 2132 (1997). HPLC determn in plasma: C. Buerger *et al.*, *J. Chromatogr. B* **796,** 155 (2003). Clinical comparison with vancomycin, *q.v.*, for MRSA infections: D. L. Stevens *et al.*, *Clin. Infect. Dis.* **34,** 1481 (2002). Review of pharmacology: L. D. Dresser, M. J. Rybak, *Pharmacotherapy* **18,** 456-462 (1998); and clinical experience: R. Norrby, *Expert Opin. Pharmacother.* **2,** 293-302 (2001).

White crystals from ethyl acetate and hexanes, mp 181.5-182.5°. $[\alpha]_D^{20}$ −9° (c = 0.919 in chloroform).

THERAP CAT: Antibacterial.

5505. Linoleic Acid. [60-33-3] (*Z,Z*)-9,12-Octadecadienoic acid; 9,12-linoleic acid; linolic acid. $C_{18}H_{32}O_2$; mol wt 280.45. C 77.09%, H 11.50%, O 11.41%. An essential fatty acid. Major constituent of many vegetable oils, *e.g.*, cottonseed, soybean, peanut, corn, sunflower seed, safflower, poppy seed, linseed, and perilla oils, where it occurs as a glyceride. Characteristic ingredient of semi-drying oils. Isoln: Swern, Parker, *J. Am. Oil Chem. Soc.* **30,** 5 (1953); Parker *et al.*, *Biochem. Prep.* **4,** 86 (1955); McCutcheon, *Org. Synth.* **coll. vol. III,** 526 (1955). Summary of work on structure: T. P. Hilditch, *The Chemical Constitution of Natural Fats* (Chapman & Hall, London, 2nd ed. 1956). Synthesis: Raphael, Sondheimer, *J. Chem. Soc.* **1950,** 2102; Gensler, Thomas, *J. Am. Chem. Soc.* **73,** 4601 (1951); Walborsky *et al.*, *ibid.* 2590; Nigam, Weedon, *J. Chem. Soc.* **1956,** 4052; Osbond, Wickens, *Chem. Ind. (London)* **1959,** 1288. Review of physiological role in mammals: H. S. Hansen, *Trends Biochem. Sci.* **11,** 263 (1986).

Colorless oil. Easily oxidized by air, cannot be distilled without decompn. Storage in ester form is recommended. d_4^{18} 0.9038; d_4^{22} 0.9007. mp −12°. bp$_{1.4}$ 202°; bp$_{16}$ 230°. $n_D^{11.5}$ 1.4715; n_D^{20} 1.4699; $n_D^{21.5}$ 1.4683; n_D^{50} 1.4588. Iodine value: 181.1. Thiocyanogen value 96.7. Freely sol in ether. Sol in abs alc. One ml dissolves in 10 ml petr ether. Miscible with dimethylformamide, fat solvents, oils.

Aluminum salt. [645-17-0] $Al(C_{18}H_{31}O_2)_3$. Yellow lumps or powder; linseed oil odor. Practically insol in water. Sol in oils, fixed alkali hydroxides.

Methyl ester *see* Methyl Linoleate.

Ethyl ester *see* Ethyl Linoleate.

Cyclohexylamide. [3207-50-9] Linolexamide; *N*-cyclohexyllinoleamide; Clinolamide; $C_{24}H_{43}NO$; mol wt 361.60.

USE: Manuf paints, coatings, emulsifiers, vitamins. Aluminum salt used to manuf lacquers.

THERAP CAT: Nutrient (essential fatty acid).

THERAP CAT (VET): Dietary supplement.

5506. Linolenic Acid. [463-40-1] (*Z,Z,Z*)-9,12,15-Octadecatrienoic acid; α-linolenic acid. $C_{18}H_{30}O_2$; mol wt 278.43. C 77.65%, H 10.86%, O 11.49%. An essential fatty acid. Occurs as the glyceride in most drying oils. Synthesis: Nigam, Weedon, *J. Chem. Soc.* **1956,** 4049; Osbond, Wickens, *Chem. Ind. (London)* **1959,** 1288. Biosynthetic studies: C. G. Kannangara *et al.*, *Biochem. Biophys. Res. Commun.* **52,** 648 (1973); B. S. Jacobson *et al.*, *ibid.* 1190; C. J. Bedord *et al.*, *Arch. Biochem. Biophys.* **185,** 15 (1978). Effects on lipid metabolism in rat tissue: M. L. Garg *et al.*, *Lipids* **23,** 847 (1988). Review of dietary linolenic acid in mammals: J. Tinoco *et al.*, *ibid.* **14,** 166-171 (1979); in man: N. Zöllner, *Prog. Lipid Res.* **25,** 177-180 (1986).

Colorless liquid. d_4^{18} 0.914. bp$_1$ 230-232°. Insol in water. Sol in organic solvents.

THERAP CAT: Nutrient (essential fatty acid).

5507. γ-Linolenic Acid. [506-26-3] (6*Z*,9*Z*,12*Z*)-6,9,12-Octadecatrienoic acid; *cis*-6,*cis*-9,*cis*-12-octadecatrienoic acid; gamolenic acid; GLA; Viacutan. $C_{18}H_{30}O_2$; mol wt 278.43. C 77.65%, H 10.86%, O 11.49%. Polyunsaturated fatty acid produced in the body as the Δ^6-desaturase metabolite of linoleic acid, *q.v.* Converted to dihomo-γ-linolenic acid, a biosynthetic precursor of monoenoic prostaglandins such as PGE$_1$. Present to varying extents in the fatty acid fraction of evening primrose oil (7-10%), in borage oil (18-26%), in black currant oil (15-20%) and in oils from different fungal sources (6-24%). Isoln from evening primrose oil, *q.v.*: A. Heiduschka, K. Luft, *Arch. Pharm.* **257,** 33 (1919). Proposed structure: Eibner *et al.*, *Chem. Umschau.* **34,** 312 (1927). Confirmation of structure: J. P. Riley, *J. Chem. Soc.* **1949,** 2728. Discussion of occurrence, esp. in fungi: R. Shaw, *Biochim. Biophys. Acta* **98,** 230 (1965). Synthesis: J. M. Osbond *et al.*, *J. Chem. Soc.* **1961,** 2779; J. M. Osbond, *ibid.* 5270. Metabolism studies: J.

F. Mead, D. R. Howton, *J. Biol. Chem.* **229**, 575 (1957); K. J. Stone *et al., Lipids* **14**, 174 (1979). Effect of source on essential fatty acid and prostanoid metabolite formation: D. K. Jenkins *et al., Med. Sci. Res.* **16**, 525 (1988).

Hexabromide deriv. $C_{18}H_{30}Br_6O_2$. Crystals from ethyl methyl ketone, mp 201-202°.

USE: Nutrient.

THERAP CAT: In treatment of atopic eczema.

THERAP CAT (VET): Dermatological.

5508. Linseed. Flaxseed; linum. Dried ripe seeds of *Linum usitatissimum* L., Linaceae. *Constit.* 30-40% oil, about 6% mucilage, about 25% proteins and linamarin. Brief review of medicinal uses: M. Wichtl, N. G. Bisset, *Herbal Drugs and Phytopharmaceuticals*, English Ed. (CRC Press, Boca Raton, 1994) pp 298-300

Linseed oil. A drying oil obtained by expression of linseed. *Constit.* Glycerides of linolenic, linoleic, oleic, stearic, palmitic and myristic acids. *Ref:* T. P. Hilditch, *The Chemical Constitution of Natural Fats* (London, 3rd ed., 1956) p 175 sqq; E. W. Eckey, *Vegetable Fats and Oils* (New York, 1954) pp 535-547. Yellowish liquid, peculiar odor, bland taste. Exposed to air it gradually thickens, becomes darker, and acquires a more pronounced odor and taste. d 0.925-0.935. n_D^{40} 1.4725-1.4750. Does not congeal above −20°. Sapon no.: 187-195. Iodine no. not below 170. Unsaponifiable matter not over 1.5%. Slightly sol in alcohol, miscible with chloroform, ether, petr ether, carbon disulfide, oil turpentine.

USE: Emollient. Oil in varnishes, paints, putty, oilcloths, linoleum, printing inks, artificial rubber, tracing cloth, tanning and enameling leather; applied to paper and fabrics to render them waterproof and tough.

THERAP CAT: Laxative; externally as poultice.

THERAP CAT (VET): Laxative.

5509. Linuron. [330-55-2] N'-(3,4-Dichlorophenyl)-N-methoxy-N-methylurea; methoxydiuron; Du Pont Herbicide 326; HOE-2810; Afalon; Linurex; Lorox. $C_9H_{10}Cl_2N_2O_2$; mol wt 249.09. C 43.40%, H 4.05%, Cl 28.47%, N 11.25%, O 12.85%. Selective pre- and post-emergence herbicide. Preparation: Sherer, Heller, US 2960534 (1960 to Hoechst). Degradn in soil: G. F. Kempson-Jones, R. J. Hance, *Pestic. Sci.* **10**, 449 (1979). Toxicity study: G. W. Bailey, J. L. White, *Residue Rev.* **10**, 97 (1965).

mp 93-94°. Vapor pressure at 24°: 1.5×10^{-5} mm Hg. Soly in water: 75 ppm. Partially sol in acetone, alcohol, benzene, toluene, xylene. LD_{50} orally in rats: 1500 mg/kg (Bailey, White).

USE: Herbicide.

5510. Liothyronine. [6893-02-3] O-(4-Hydroxy-3-iodophenyl)-3,5-diiodo-L-tyrosine; L-3-[4-(4-hydroxy-3-iodophenoxy)-3,5-diiodophenyl]alanine; 4-(3-iodo-4-hydroxyphenoxy)-3,5-diiodophenylalanine; 3,5,3'-triiodothyronine; T_3. $C_{15}H_{12}I_3NO_4$; mol wt 650.97. C 27.68%, H 1.86%, I 58.48%, N 2.15%, O 9.83%. One of the hormones produced by the thyroid gland that is involved in the maintenance of metabolic homeostasis. Also produced in peripheral tissues as the active metabolite of thyroxine, *q.v.* Identification in serum: J. Gross, R. Pitt-Rivers, *Lancet* **I**, 439 (1952). Prepn from diiodothyronine: J. Roche *et al., Biochim. Biophys. Acta* **11**, 215 (1953). Isoln from thyroid gland and synthesis: J. Gross, R. Pitt-Rivers, *Biochem. J.* **53**, 645 (1953). Bioactivity: *eidem, ibid.* 652. Elevated levels of T_3 have been noted in victims of sudden infant death syndrome: G. Kocsard-Varo, *Med. J. Aust.* **2**, 789 (1973); M. A. Chacon, J. T. Tildon, *J. Pediatr.* **99**, 758 (1981). Direct determn in serum by RIA: I. J. Chopra *et al., Thyroid* **6**, 255 (1996). Clinical trial in combination with thyroxine: R. Bunevicius *et al., N. Engl. J. Med.* **340**, 424 (1999). Review of pharmacology and clinical uses: E. Sypniewski, *Ann. Thorac. Surg.* **56**, S2-S8 (1993); of clinical trials in depression: R. Aronson *et al., Arch. Gen. Psychiatry* **53**, 842-848 (1996); of use in heart trans-

plantation: V. Jeevanandam, *Thyroid* **7**, 139-145 (1997). Review of T_3-receptors and molecular mechanism of action: M. A. Lazar, *Endocr. Rev.* **14**, 184-193 (1993); G. A. Brent, *N. Engl. J. Med.* **331**, 847-853 (1994). Review of biological effects: H. C. Freake, J. H. Oppenheimer, *Annu. Rev. Nutr.* **15**, 263-291 (1995).

Crystals, dec 236-237°. $[\alpha]_D^{29.5}$ +21.5° (c = 4.75 in a mixture of 1 part N HCl + 2 parts ethanol). Insol in water, alc, propylene glycol. Sol in dil alkalies with the formation of a brownish, water-soluble, sodium salt.

Sodium salt. [55-06-1] Liothyronine sodium; sodium L-triiodothyronine; Cytobin; Cytomel; Cynomel; Tertroxin. $C_{15}H_{11}I_3$-NNaO$_4$; mol wt 672.96.

Hydrochloride. [6138-47-2] Thybon. $C_{15}H_{12}I_3NO_4 \cdot HCl$; mol wt 687.43. Long birefringent needles, dec 202-203°. $[\alpha]_D^{29.5}$ +21.5° (c = 4.75 in a mixture of 1 vol N HCl and 2 vols ethanol).

THERAP CAT: Thyroid hormone.

THERAP CAT (VET): Thyroid hormone.

5511. Lipase. [9001-62-1] Triacylglycerol lipase. An enzyme (or more exactly a group of enzymes) belonging to the esterases. Hydrolyzes fat (present in ester form, such as glycerides) yielding fatty acids and glycerol. Catalyzes digestion. Widely distributed in the plant world, also in molds, bacteria, milk and milk products, and in animal tissues, especially in the pancreas. Isoln from castor beans: H. Gibian in *Ullmanns Encyklopädie der technischen Chemie*, 3rd ed., **vol. 7**, 406-407 (1956). Purification of pancreatic lipase: Marchis-Mouren *et al., Arch. Biochem. Biophys.* **83**, 309 (1959). Review of milk lipases: Chandan, Shahani, *J. Dairy Sci.* **47**, 471 (1964). Comprehensive reviews: Wills, *Adv. Lipid Res.* **3**, 197-240 (1965); Desnuelle in *The Enzymes* vol. 7, P. D. Boyer, Ed. (Academic Press, New York, 3rd ed., 1972) pp 575-616.

The optimum temp for enzyme action is between 35° and 37° at pH 5-6. Lipase contains sulfhydryl groups and is inactivated by substances that inhibit such compds. It is activated by substances that keep SH groups in the reduced state, such as glutathione, cysteine, and ascorbic acid. The addition of acid activates lipase preparations. Castor-oil lipase is activated by sulfuric, oxalic, formic, acetic and butyric acids. Acetic, salicylic and hydrochloric acids increase the action of lipase derived from various organs of the pig. Caprylic and caproic acids increase the action of lipase derived from certain mold fungi. Almost all organic solvents decrease lipase activity, petr ether being an exception.

USE: To split fats without damaging sensitive constituents, such as vitamins or unsaturated fatty acids. In food processing for flavor improvement; in detergents for the improvement of cleaning action. For review of industrial applications of microbial lipases, *see* Seitz, *J. Am. Oil Chem. Soc.* **51**, 12 (1974).

THERAP CAT: Digestive enzyme.

5512. Lipoprotein Lipase. [9004-02-8] Diacylglycerol lipase; clearing factor. A specific lipase which preferentially hydrolyzes triglycerides in the presence of a lipoprotein complex, forming glycerol and unesterified fatty acids: Korn, *Methods Enzymol.* **5**, 542 (1962). The normal substrate is turbid lipemic or chylomicron-containing plasma. This substance is clarified by the enzyme, hence the term clearing factor. First detected in the plasma of animals injected intravenously with heparin: Hahn, *Science* **98**, 19 (1943); Robinson, French, *Pharmacol. Rev.* **12**, 241 (1960). Prepn from post heparin human plasma: Baskys, *Diss. Abstr.* **20**, 1146 (1959). It has since been prepd from several tissues of normal, untreated animals. Prepn from chicken adipose tissue: Korn, Quigley, *J. Biol. Chem.* **226**, 833 (1957); from human heart: Schnatz *et al., Am. J. Physiol.* **205**, 401 (1963). Role in the metabolism of triglycerides by adipose tissues: Rodbell, Scow in K. Rodahl, *Fat as a Tissue* (McGraw-Hill, New York, 1964) pp 110-126. *Reviews:* Jensen, *Prog. Chem. Fats Other Lipids* **11**, 347 (1971); Desnuelle in *The Enzymes* **vol. 7**, P. D. Boyer, Ed. (Academic Press, New York, 3rd ed., 1972) pp 606-609.

Lipotropic Hormone

5513. Lipotropic Hormone. [9035-55-6] Lipotropin; pituitary lipotropic hormone; lipid-mobilizing hormone; adipokinetic hormone; lipolytic hormone; lipotrophin; LPH. Hypophyseal hormone which stimulates the release of fatty acids from adipose tissue. **β-LPH** is a single chain polypeptide containing 89-93 amino acid residues and has been proposed as the biosynthetic precursor for β-MSH and β-endorphin, *q.q.v., see* M. Chretien *et al., Can. J. Biochem.* **57,** 1111 (1979). **γ-LPH** consists of 58 amino acids and is identical to the sequence of the first 58 residues of β-LPH. Both contain sequences common to ACTH and β-melanotropin, *q.q.v.* Sequences differ slightly among mammalian species. Isoln and proposed structure of ovine β-LPH: C. H. Li, *Nature* **201,** 924 (1964); Y. Birk, C. H. Li, *J. Biol. Chem.* **239,** 1048 (1964); C. H. Li *et al., Nature* **208,** 1093 (1965); C. H. Li, *Arch. Biol. Med. Exp.* **5,** 55 (1968); revised structure: Chretien *et al., Int. J. Pept. Protein Res.* **4,** 263 (1972). Isoln and characterization of porcine β-LPH: Gilardeau, Chretien, *Can. J. Biochem.* **48,** 1017 (1970). Amino acid sequence of porcine γ-LPH: Graf *et al., Acta Biochim. Biophys.* **5,** 305 (1970). Isoln, characterization of bovine β-LPH: P. Lohmar, C. H. Li, *Biochem. Biophys. Res. Commun.* **77,** 1088 (1977); of rat β-LPH: M. Rubinstein *et al., Proc. Natl. Acad. Sci. USA* **74,** 3052 (1977); of whale β-LPH: H. Kawauchi *et al., Int. J. Pept. Protein Res.* **15,** 171 (1980); of turkey γ-LPH: W. C. Chang *et al., ibid.* 261. Initial isoln, partial structure of human β-LPH: G. Cseh *et al., FEBS Lett.* **2,** 42 (1968); *eidem, ibid.* **21,** 344(1972). Isoln, characterization, amino acid sequence of human β-LPH: C. H. Li, D. Chung, *Int. J. Pept. Protein Res.* **17,** 131 (1981). *Review:* D. T. Krieger *et al., Recent Prog. Horm. Res.* **36,** 277-344 (1980).

5514. Liraglutide. [204656-20-2] N^{26}-(Hexadecanoyl-γ-glutamyl)-(34-arginine)GLP-1-(7-37)-peptide; Lys^{26}($N^{ε}$-(γ-glutamyl-($N^{α}$-hexadecanoyl))), Arg^{34}-GLP-1(7-37); NN-2211. $C_{172}H_{265}$-$N_{43}O_{51}$; mol wt 3751.20. C 55.07%, H 7.12%, N 16.06%, O 21.75%. Acylated derivative of glucagon-like peptide 1, *q.v.* Prepn: L. B. Knudsen *et al., WO 9808871; idem et al., US 6268343* (1998, 2001 both to Novo Nordisk); *eidem, J. Med. Chem.* **43,** 1664 (2000). Clinical effect on glucose and insulin homeostasis: H. Agerso, P. Vicini, *Eur. J. Pharm. Sci.* **19,** 141 (2003). Clinical pharmacokinetics: B. Elbrond *et al., Diabetes Care* **25,** 1398 (2002). Clinical trial in type 2 diabetes: S. Madsbad *et al., ibid.* **27,** 1335 (2004); M. N. Feinglos *et al., Diabetic Med.* **22,** 1016 (2005).

Glu-Gly-Thr-Phe-Thr-Ser-Asp-Val-Ser-Ser-Tyr-Leu-Glu-Gly-Gln-Ala-Ala-Lys-Glu
|
Ala   Phe
|
His   Gly-Arg-Gly-Arg-Val-Leu-Trp-Ala-Ile

THERAP CAT: Antidiabetic.

5515. Liranaftate. [88678-31-3] (6-Methoxy-2-pyridinyl)-methylcarbamothioic acid *O*-(5,6,7,8-tetrahydro-2-naphthalenyl) ester; *O*-5,6,7,8-tetrahydro-2-naphthyl *N*-(6-methoxy-2-pyridyl)-*N*-methylthiocarbamate; piritetrate; M-732; Zefnart. $C_{18}H_{20}N_2O_2S$; mol wt 328.43. C 65.83%, H 6.14%, N 8.53%, O 9.74%, S 9.76%. Squalene epoxidase inhibitor. Prepn: **BE 897021;** T. Takematsu *et al., US 4554012* (1983, 1985 both to Toyo Soda Manufacturing Co., Ltd.). Mode of action study: T. Morita *et al., J. Med. Vet. Mycol.* **27,** 17 (1989). Antifungal spectrum: K. Iwata *et al., Antimicrob. Agents Chemother.* **33,** 2118 (1989). Physicochemical properties and stability: H. Awano *et al., Iyakuhin Kenkyu* **23,** 558 (1992).

White crystalline powder, mp 98.5-99.5°. Soly (ml/g): acetone 10; chloroform 2; dehydrated ethanol 152; dichloromethane 2; ether 21; hexane 233; methanol 175; water >10000. Soly (mg/l): 0.10 (distilled water); 0.07 (buffer pH 1); 0.08 (buffer pH 4); 0.07 (buffer pH 7); 0.08 (buffer pH 11). Sol in benzene, dimethyl sulfoxide, *N,N*-dimethylformamide.

THERAP CAT: Antifungal.

5516. Lisinopril. [83915-83-7] (*S*)-1-[N^2-(1-Carboxy-3-phenylpropyl)-L-lysyl]-L-proline dihydrate; MK-521; Acerbon; Alapril; Carace; Coric; Novatec; Prinil; Prinivil; Vivatec; Zestril. $C_{21}H_{31}N_3O_5$.2H$_2$O; mol wt 441.52. C 57.13%, H 7.99%, N 9.52%, O 25.37%. Orally active angiotensin-converting enzyme (ACE) inhibitor. Prepn: A. A. Patchett *et al., EP 12401;* E. E. Harris *et al., US 4374829* (1980, 1983 both to Merck & Co.); M. T. Wu *et al., J. Pharm. Sci.* **74,** 352 (1985). Comprehensive description: D. P. Ip *et al., Anal. Profiles Drug Subs. Excip.* **21,** 233-276 (1992). HPLC determn in urine: Y. C. Wong, B. G. Charles, *J. Chromatogr. B* **673,** 306 (1995). Series of articles in hypertension and congestive heart failure: *Am. J. Med.* **85,** Suppl. 3B, 1-59 (1988). Review of clinical efficacy in myocardial infarction: K. L. Goa *et al., Drugs* **52,** 564-588 (1996). Clinical trial in diabetic retinopathy: N. Chaturvedi *et al., Lancet* **351,** 28 (1998).

• 2 H$_2$O

White to off-white crystalline, odorless powder. pKa$_1$ (25°) 2.5; pKa$_2$ 4.0; pKa$_3$ 6.7; pKa$_4$ 10.1. Approx uv max (0.1*N* NaOH): 246, 254, 258, 261, 267 nm (A$_{1cm}^{1\%}$ 4.0, 4.5, 5.1, 5.1, 3.7); (0.1*N* HCl): 246, 253, 258, 264, 267 nm (A$_{1cm}^{1\%}$ 3.2, 3.9, 4.5, 3.0, 2.8). [α]$_{405}^{25}$ −120° (c = 1 in 0.25*M* pH 6.4 zinc acetate); [α]$_{436}^{25}$ −96° (c = 1 in 0.25*M* pH 6.4 zinc acetate). Partition coefficient at room temp (*n*-octanol/0.1*M* pH 7 phosphate buffer): 10.2 ±0.5. Soly (mg/ml): water 97; methanol 14; ethanol <0.1; acetone <0.1; acetonitrile <0.1; chloroform <0.1; DMF <0.1.

Mixture with hydrochlorothiazide. Prinzide; Zestoretic.
THERAP CAT: Antihypertensive.

5517. Lisofylline. [100324-81-0] 3,7-Dihydro-1-[(5*R*)-5-hydroxyhexyl]-3,7-dimethyl-1*H*-purine-2,6-dione; 1-[(*R*)-5-hydroxyhexyl]theobromine; 1-(5*R*-hydroxyhexyl)-3,7-dimethylxanthine; CT-1501R; ProTec. $C_{13}H_{20}N_4O_3$; mol wt 280.32. C 55.70%, H 7.19%, N 19.99%, O 17.12%. Methylxanthine that inhibits production of phosphatidic acid during the inflammatory response. Identification as metabolite of pentoxifylline: H.-J. Hinze *et al., Arzneim.-Forsch.* **22,** 1144 (1972). Enantioselective process: W. Aretz *et al., DE 3942872; eidem, US 5310666* (1991, 1994 both to Hoechst). Asymmetric synthesis: J. P. Klein *et al., WO 9531450* (1995 to Cell Therapeutics). Study of mechanism of action in septic shock: G. C. Rice *et al., Proc. Natl. Acad. Sci. USA* **91,** 3857 (1994). Enhancement of hematopoietic recovery following 5-fluorouracil treatment in mice: E. Clarke *et al., Cancer Res.* **56,** 105 (1996).

mp 110°. [α]$_D^{20}$ −5.6° (c = 6.7 in ethanol).
THERAP CAT: Immunomodulator.

5518. Lisuride. [18016-80-3] *N'*-[(8α)-9,10-didehydro-6-methylergolin-8-yl]-*N,N*-diethylurea; 9-(3,3-diethylureido)-4,6,6a,-7,8,9-hexahydro-7-methylindolo[4,3-*f,g*]quinoline; 1,1-diethyl-3-

Consult the Name Index before using this section.

(D-6-methylisoergolen-8-yl)urea; N-(D-6-methyl-8-isoergolenyl)-N,N-diethylurea; methylergol carbamide; lysuride. $C_{20}H_{26}N_4O$; mol wt 338.45. C 70.97%, H 7.74%, N 16.55%, O 4.73%. Dopamine D_2-receptor agonist. Prepn: V. Zikan, M. Semonsky, *Collect. Czech. Chem. Commun.* **25**, 1922 (1960); *eidem, Pharmazie* **23**, 147 (1968). Pharmacology and toxicity: Z. Votava, I. Lamplova, *Physiol. Bohemoslov.* **12**, 37 (1963), *C.A.* **59**, 9221d (1963).

Crystals from benzene, mp 186°. $[\alpha]_D^{20}$ +313° (c = 0.60 in pyridine).

Maleate. [19875-60-6] Apodel; Cuvalit; Dopergin; Eunal; Lysenyl; Revanil. $C_{20}H_{26}N_4O.C_4H_4O_4$; mol wt 454.52. Prisms from ethanol, mp 200° (dec). $[\alpha]_D^{20}$ +288° (c = 0.5 in methanol). uv max (methanol): 313 nm. LD_{50} i.v. in mice: 14.4 mg/kg (Votava, Lamplova).

THERAP CAT: Antimigraine; prolactin inhibitor; antiparkinsonian.

5519. Lita®. Protein-based fat mimetic consisting of water-dispersible microparticles of zein, *q.v.*, a hydrophobic prolamine derived from corn. Prepn: L. E. Stark, A. T. Gross, US 5021248 (1991 to Enzytech); *eidem*, US 5145702 (1992 to Opta Food Ingred.). Brief description: R. Iyengar, A. Gross in *Biotechnology and Food Ingredients*, I. Goldberg, R. Williams, Eds. (Van Nostrand Reinhold, New York, 1991) pp 287-313; M. S. Miller in *Protein Functionality in Food Systems*, N. S. Hettiarachchy, G. R. Zeigler, Eds. (Marcel Dekker, New York, 1994) pp 435-465.

Hydrophobic, smooth spheroidal particles. Size distribution: 0.3-3.0 μm. Insol in water. Sol in ethanol. Colloidal suspensions stable to 95°.

USE: Fat substitute for food products.

5520. Lithium. [7439-93-2] Li; at. wt 6.941; at. no. 3; valence 1. Group IA (1). Alkali metal. Occurrence in earth's crust: 20 ppm. Naturally occurring isotopes: 7 (92.5%); 6 (7.5%); artificial radioactive isotopes: 5, 8-11; all are unstable ($T_{1/2}$ < 1 sec). Discovered as salt in 1817 by Arfvedson: *Ann. Chim. Phys.* [2] **10**, 82 (1819); metal prepared independently by Davy and Brandé in 1818. Occurs in a number of minerals: *spodumene* ($LiAlS_2O_6$), *lepidolite* [$K(Li,Al)_3(Si,Al)_4O_{10}(F,OH)_2$], *petalite* ($LiAlSi_4O_{10}$), *amblygonite* ($AlPO_4$,LiF), and *triphylite* ($LiFePO_4$). Also recovered from natural brines. Prepn of the metal by electrochemical processes: Guntz, *Compt. Rend.* **117**, 732 (1893); Ruff, Johannsen, *Z. Elektrochem.* **12**, 186 (1906); by reduction of the oxide with magnesium or aluminum: Warren, *Chem. News* **74**, 6 (1896); Hanson, US 2028390 (1936). Reviews of biology, pharmacology and toxicity of lithium ion: Schou, "Lithium in Psychiatry: A Review" in *Psychopharmacology, A Review of Progress 1957-1967*, D. H. Efron, Ed. (Public Health Service Publication No. 1836, 1968) pp 701-718; Doig *et al., J. Chem. Educ.* **50**, 343-345 (1973); Samuel, Gottesfeld, *Endeavour* **32**, 122-128 (1973); Saran, Gaind, *Clin. Toxicol.* **6**, 257-269 (1973); Schou, *Annu. Rev. Pharmacol. Toxicol.* **16**, 231-243 (1976). *Reviews:* Hart, Beumel, "Lithium and its Compounds" in *Comprehensive Inorganic Chemistry* **vol. 1**, J. C. Bailar, Jr. *et al.*, Eds. (Pergamon Press, Oxford, 1973) pp 331-367; C. W. Kamienski *et al.* in *Kirk-Othmer Encyclopedia of Chemical Technology* **vol. 15** (Wiley-Interscience, New York, 4th ed., 1995) pp 434-463; *Chemistry of the Elements* N. N. Greenwood, A. Earnshaw, Eds. (Pergamon Press, New York, 1984) pp 75-116; *Patty's Industrial Hygiene and Toxicology* **vol. 2C**, G. D. Clayton, F. E. Clayton, Eds. (John Wiley & Sons, Inc., New York, 4th ed., 1994) pp 2087-2097. *Review of pharmacology:* N. J. Birch, J. D. Phillips, *Adv. Inorg. Chem.* **36**, 49-75 (1991); and clinical use: L. H. Price, G. R. Heninger, *N. Engl. J. Med.* **331**, 591-598 (1994).

Silvery-white metal; body-centered cubic structure; becomes yellowish on exposure to moist air. mp 180.54°. bp 1347°. Also reported as bp 1336 ± 5°: Hartman, Schneider, *Z. Anorg. Chem.* **180**, 275 (1929). d^{20} 0.534. Hardest of the alkali metals; Mohs' hardness 0.6. Heat capacity at constant pressure (25°): 5.892 cal/mole deg. *See:* Douglass *et al., J. Am. Chem. Soc.* **77**, 2144 (1955). E° (aqueous) Li/Li⁺ 3.045 V. Reacts with H_2O forming the hydroxide and H_2. Reacts violently with inorganic acids; reacts slowly with cold H_2SO_4. Sol in liq ammonia forming a blue soln. Does not react with oxygen at room temp; forms Li_2O when heated to 100° or higher. Emits characteristic crimson color (670.8 nm) in flame. *Flammable. Keep under mineral oil or other liquid free from oxygen or water.* Li metal ignites in air near its mp; presents fire and explosion risk when exposed to water, N, acids or oxidizing reagents.

Caution: Potential symptoms of mild overexposure to the Li ion by ingestion of lithium salts are impaired concentration, lethargy, irritability, muscle weakness; moderate overexposure may cause disorientation, confusion, drowsiness; severe overexposure may cause impaired consciousness with progression to coma, convulsions, and impaired renal function (Price, Heninger). Direct contact with metal may be corrosive and cause skin and eye burns. *See: Fire Protection Guide to Hazardous Materials* (National Fire Protection Assoc., Quincy, MA, 12th ed., 1997) Section 49, p 82. *See also: Clinical Toxicology of Commercial Products*, R. E. Gosselin *et al.*, Eds. (Williams & Wilkins, Baltimore, 5th ed., 1984) Section III, pp 241-245.

USE: In prodn of organometallic alkyl and aryl lithium compounds; in prodn of high-strength, low-density aluminum alloys for the aircraft industry; extremely tough, low-density alloys with aluminum and magnesium used for armour plate and aerospace components. In polymerization catalysts for the polyolefin plastics industry; manuf of high-strength glass and glass-ceramics. As anode in electrochemical cells and batteries; as chemical intermediate in organic syntheses. Lithium stearate as thickener and gelling agent to transform oils into lubricating greases.

5521. Lithium Acetate. [546-89-4] Quilonum. $C_2H_3LiO_2$; mol wt 65.99. C 36.40%, H 4.58%, Li 10.52%, O 48.49%. Prepn: *Gmelins, Lithium* (8th Ed.) **20**, pp 230-232 (1927). Prepn and solubilities: N. V. Sidgwick, J. A. H. R. Gentle, *J. Chem. Soc.* **121**, 1837 (1922). Crystal structure of anhydrous: C. Saunderson, R. B. Ferguson, *Acta Crystallogr.* **14**, 321 (1961). Pharmacokinetics in psychiatric patients: J.-L. Evrard *et al., Acta Psychiatr. Scand.* **58**, 67 (1978).

mp 286° (slight dec). Changes to dihydrate at 56.5°.

Dihydrate. [6108-17-4] Quilonorm. Rhombic crystals. Begins to melt at 49° (Gmelin). Congruent mp 57.8° (Sidgwick). Freely sol in water or alcohol. Its aq soln is practically neutral.

THERAP CAT: Antimanic.

5522. Lithium Amide. [7782-89-0] Lithamide. H_2LiN; mol wt 22.96. H 8.78%, Li 30.23%, N 61.00%. $LiNH_2$. Prepd from Li + NH_3: Titherley, *J. Chem. Soc.* **65**, 517 (1894); Ruff, Geisel *Ber.* **39**, 840 (1906); **44**, 505 (1911); Campbell *et al., Proc. Indiana Acad. Sci.* **50**, 123 (1940); Schenk in *Handbook of Preparative Inorganic Chemistry* **vol. 1**, G. Brauer, Ed. (Academic Press, New York, 2nd ed., 1963) p 463. *See also Inorg. Synth.* **2**, 135. Crystal structure: Juza, Opp, *Z. Anorg. Allg. Chem.* **266**, 313 (1951).

Tetragonal crystal structure, d 1.18. mp 380-400°. Sublimes in NH_3 current. When heated *in vacuo* to 450°, NH_3 is given off and Li_2NH forms, which dec ~750-800°. Heat of formation: 42 kcal/mole at 18° and 760 mm Hg. Stable in air-tight containers at room temp. Dec by water to form $LiOH + NH_3$, slowly when in lumps, faster as the particle size decreases. Insol in anhyd ether, benzene, toluene.

USE: In Claisen condensations, alkylation of nitriles and ketones, synthesis of ethynyl compds, acetylenic carbinols.

5523. Lithium Benzoate. [553-54-8] $C_7H_5LiO_2$; mol wt 128.05. C 65.66%, H 3.94%, Li 5.42%, O 24.99%.

White, cryst powder. One gram dissolves in 3 ml water, 13 ml alcohol, 10 ml boiling alcohol. Soly in water is increased by sodium benzoate. The aq soln is slightly alkaline to litmus; pH ~8.

USE: Has been used as a lubricant for compressing tablets.

5524. Lithium Borate. [12007-60-2] Boron lithium oxide ($B_4Li_2O_7$); lithium biborate; lithium tetraborate. $B_4Li_2O_7$; mol wt 169.12. B 25.57%, Li 8.21%, O 66.22%. $Li_2B_4O_7$.

Pentahydrate. [1303-94-2] White, cryst powder. Slightly sol in water. Practically insol in alcohol.

USE: In enamels.

5525. Lithium Borohydride. [16949-15-8] Lithium tetrahydroborate. BH_4Li; mol wt 21.78. B 49.64%, H 18.51%, Li 31.87%. $LiBH_4$. Prepd by the action of diborane on ethyllithium; by the action of aluminum borohydride on ethyllithium: Schlesinger, Brown, *J. Am. Chem. Soc.* **62,** 3429-35 (1940). Review of lithium and other metal tetrahydroborates: James, Wallbridge, *Prog. Inorg. Chem.* **11,** 99-231 (1970).

Orthorhombic crystals, mp 268°; dec 380°. d 0.66. Stable under ordinary conditions, but dec in moist air. Reacts with hydrogen chloride to form hydrogen, diborane, and lithium chloride; forms lithium boromethoxide and hydrogen with methyl alcohol. Sol in water at pH >7. Aq solns dec slowly if the pH is >7, and rather vigorously when acidified. Sol in ether, tetrahydrofuran, aliphatic amines.

USE: Strong reducing agent. Used in the reduction of compds contg ketonic, aldehydic, or ester carbonyls and a nitrile group, where reduction of the carbonyl, but not of the nitrile group, is wanted. In the determination of free carboxyl groups in peptides and proteins; after esterification and acetylation, only the ester groups, and none of the peptide bonds are reduced.

5526. Lithium Bromide. [7550-35-8] BrLi; mol wt 86.85. Br 92.00%, Li 7.99%. LiBr. Usually contains water and 85-90% LiBr.

White, very deliquesc, slightly bitter, granular powder. mp 547° when anhydr. Sol in 0.6 part water, 0.4 part boiling water; freely sol in alcohol, glycol; sol in ether, amyl alcohol. The aq soln is neutral or only slightly alkaline to litmus. *Keep well closed.*

Caution: Large doses may cause CNS depression. Chronic absorption may cause skin eruptions and CNS disturbances due to bromide. May also cause disturbed blood electrolyte balance.

USE: As humectant, in air-conditioning systems.

THERAP CAT: Sedative, hypnotic.

5527. Lithium Carbonate. [554-13-2] Camcolit; Carbolith; Eskalith; Hypnorex; Limas; Liskonum; Lithane; Lithicarb; Lithobid; Plenur; Priadel; Quilonum-retard; Téralithe. CLi_2O_3; mol wt 73.89. C 16.25%, Li 18.79%, O 64.96%. Li_2CO_3. Purification: Caley, Elving, *Inorg. Synth.* **1,** 1 (1939). Initial report of effect in mental illness: J. F. J. Cade, *Med. J. Aust.* **2,** 349 (1949). Early review of biology and pharmacology of lithium: M. Schou, *Pharmacol. Rev.* **9,** 17-58 (1957); of toxicity: *idem, Acta Pharmacol. Toxicol.* **15,** 70-84 (1958). Thermal behavior: A. Reisman, *J. Am. Chem. Soc.* **80,** 3558 (1958). Acute toxicity data: H. F. Smyth *et al., Am. Ind. Hyg. Assoc. J.* **30,** 470 (1969). Toxicological studies in mammals: Gralla, McIlhenny, *Toxicol. Appl. Pharmacol.* **21,** 428 (1972). Pharmacokinetics: J. S. Ku *et al., Int. J. Clin. Pharmacol. Ther. Toxicol.* **25,** 648 (1987). Clinical studies: J. Rybakowski *et al., Int. Pharmacopsychiatry* **15,** 86 (1980); B. F. Kjellman *et al., Acta Psychiatr. Scand.* **62,** 32 (1980). Review of development of use: G. Chouinard, *Union Med. Can.* **109,** 221-224, 226, 304 (1980). Comprehensive description: H. C. Stober, *Anal. Profiles Drug Subs.* **15,** 367-391 (1986).

White, light, alkaline powder. d 2.11. mp 720 ±1°. One gram dissolves in 78 ml cold, 140 ml boiling water; dissolved by dil acids. Practically insol in alcohol. LD$_{50}$ orally in rats: 0.71 g/kg (Smyth).

USE: In the production of glazes on ceramic and electrical porcelain.

THERAP CAT: Antimanic.

5528. Lithium Chloride. [7447-41-8] ClLi; mol wt 42.39. Cl 83.64%, Li 16.37%. LiCl. Prepn: Pray, *Inorg. Synth.* **5,** 153 (1957). Review of prepn and properties: Oliver in *Mellor's* vol. II, supplement II, *The Alkali Metals* (part 1) 179-215 (1961). Pharmacology: M. Wielosz, *Pol. J. Pharmacol. Pharm.* **26,** 399 (1974).

Deliquesc, cubic crystals, granules or cryst powder; sharp saline taste. mp 613° when anhydr; bp 1360°; d 2.07. One gram dissolves in 1.3 ml cold, 0.8 ml boiling water; sol in alcohol, acetone, amyl

alcohol, pyridine. The aq soln is neutral or slightly alkaline. *Keep well closed.* LD$_{50}$ in mice (mg/kg): 990 i.p.; in rats (mg/kg): 600 i.p., 4.8 i.v. (Wielosz).

Caution: Prolonged absorption may cause disturbed electrolyte balance, impaired renal function, CNS disturbances.

USE: Manuf mineral waters; in pyrotechnics; soldering aluminum; in refrigerating machines.

THERAP CAT: Antidepressant.

5529. Lithium Chromate(VI). [14307-35-8] $CrLi_2O_4$; mol wt 129.88. Cr 40.03%, Li 10.69%, O 49.27%. Li_2CrO_4.

The anhydr salt is appreciably sol in methanol and ethanol. Eutectic with water below −60°. *Keep well closed.*

Dihydrate. Yellow, deliquesc, cryst powder. Becomes anhydr at 74.6°. Very sol in water.

USE: Corrosion inhibitor for water-cooled atomic reactors. Soln as low temp heat transfer medium.

5530. Lithium Citrate. [919-16-4] 2-Hydroxy-1,2,3-propanetricarboxylic acid trilithium salt; citric acid trilithium salt; Litarex; Lithonate S. $C_6H_5Li_3O_7$; mol wt 209.92. C 34.33%, H 2.40%, Li 9.92%, O 53.35%.

Tetrahydrate. White granules or cryst powder; feebly alkaline taste; deliquesces on exposure to moist air; loses all of its water at 105°. Sol in 1.5 parts water, slightly in alc. pH ~8. *Keep well closed.*

USE: Formerly in soft drinks.

THERAP CAT: Antidepressant.

5531. Lithium Fluoride. [7789-24-4] FLi; mol wt 25.94. F 73.24%, Li 26.76%. LiF. Prepd from LiOH and HF or by dissolving Li_2CO_3 in excess HF, evaporating to dryness, and heating to red heat: v. Wartenberg, Schultz, *Z. Elektrochem.* **27,** 568 (1921); Kwasnik in *Handbook of Preparative Inorganic Chemistry* vol. 1, G. Brauer, Ed. (Academic Press, New York, 2nd ed., 1963) p 235. Review of toxicology of fluoride compounds: G. L. Waldbott, *Acta Med. Scand. Suppl.* **400,** 1-44 (1963).

Cubic crystals (NaCl lattice) or white fluffy powder. d^{20} 2.640. mp 848°; bp 1681°. Volatilizes at 1100-1200°. Soly in water (25°): 0.13 g/100 ml. Soluble in acids. With hydrofluoric acid it forms lithium bifluoride, LiHF$_2$. With lithium hydroxide it forms a double salt LiF.LiOH, mp 462°. LD in guinea pigs (mg/kg): 200 orally, 2000 s.c. (Waldbott).

USE: As flux for soldering and welding aluminum, in the manuf of vitreous enamels and glazes. Lithium fluoride prisms are used in infrared spectrophotometers.

5532. Lithium Formate. [556-63-8] $CHLiO_2$; mol wt 51.96. C 23.12%, H 1.94%, Li 13.36%, O 61.58%. HCOOLi.

Monohydrate. Colorless or white crystals. d 1.46. Sol in 3 parts water. The aq soln is practically neutral.

5533. Lithium Hydride. [7580-67-8] HLi; mol wt 7.95. H 12.68%, Li 87.31%. LiH. Prepd by the direct combination of hydrogen and lithium: Gibb, *Trans. Electrochem. Soc.* **93,** 198-211 (1948). Review of prepn and properties: Truter in *Mellor's* vol. II, supplement II, *The Alkali Metals* (part 1) 131-145 (1961).

Cubic crystals, darkens rapidly on exposure to light, the commercial product is usually gray. mp 680°. d 0.76-0.77. No solvent known. Rapidly dec in water to form lithium hydroxide and hydrogen. Reacts with the lower alcohols, carboxylic acids, chlorine, and ammonia at 400° to liberate hydrogen.

Caution: Potential symptoms of overexposure are irritation and burns of eyes and skin; burns of mouth and esophagus (if ingested); nausea; muscle twitches; mental confusion; blurred vision. See *NIOSH Pocket Guide to Chemical Hazards* (DHHS/NIOSH 97-140, 1997) p 186.

USE: Reducing agent; condensing agent with ketones and acid esters; desiccant; in hydrogen generators; 1 g in water liberates ~2.8 liters of hydrogen at STP.

5534. Lithium Hydroxide. [1310-65-2] Lithium hydrate. HLiO; mol wt 23.95. H 4.21%, Li 28.98%, O 66.80%. LiOH. Prepn: Barnes, *J. Chem. Soc.* **1931,** 2605; Cohen, *Inorg. Synth.* **5,** 3 (1957); Bravo, *ibid.* **7,** 1 (1963). Review of prepn, properties and uses: Oliver in *Mellor's* vol. II, supplement II, *The Alkali Metals* (part 1) 159-171 (1961).

Granular, free-flowing powder; acrid, strongly alkaline. Readily absorbs CO_2 and water from air. d 2.54. mp 471°. Sol in water, slightly sol in alcohol. *Keep tightly closed.*

Monohydrate. Small monoclinic crystals. d_4^{20} 1.51. Heat of formation −188.9 kcal/mol at 25°. Heat of soln −0.87 kcal/mol at 25°. Soly in water (w/w) at 0°: 10.7%; at 20°: 10.9%; at 100°: 14.8%. Slightly sol in alcohol. pH of a 1.0N soln about 14.

Caution: Strongly alkaline and hence caustic. Very irritating to skin. Systemic toxicity similar to other lithium compds. *See Lithium.*

USE: In photographic developers; in alkaline storage batteries; in prepn of other lithium salts where use of carbonate is not practical; as catalyst in the production of alkyd resins, in esterifications; in the production of lithium soaps, sulfonates, greases.

5535. Lithium Iodide. [10377-51-2] ILi; mol wt 133.85. I 94.81%, Li 5.19%. LiI.

Trihydrate. White, deliquesc granules or fused masses; becomes yellow on exposure to air, due to liberation of iodine. mp 73°; mp 446° when anhydr. Sol in about 0.5 part water or alcohol, freely in amyl alcohol or acetone. The aq soln is neutral or slightly alkaline. *Keep tightly closed and protected from light.*

USE: In photography.

5536. Lithium Nitrate. [7790-69-4] LiNO$_3$; mol wt 68.95. Li 10.07%, N 20.31%, O 69.61%.

Colorless, deliquesc granules. d 2.38. mp ~255°. Sol in ~2 parts water; sol in alcohol. The aq soln is neutral. *Keep well closed.*

5537. Lithium Oxalate. [553-91-3] $C_2Li_2O_4$; mol wt 101.90. C 23.57%, Li 13.62%, O 62.80%. $Li_2C_2O_4$.

White crystals. d 2.12. Sol in 15 parts water.

5538. Lithium Oxide. [12057-24-8] Li_2O; mol wt 29.88. Li 46.46%, O 53.55%. Prepd from lithium peroxide: Cohen, *Inorg. Synth.* **5,** 5 (1957); from lithium hydroxide: Bravo, *ibid.* **7,** 3 (1963). Review of prepn and properties: Oliver in *Mellor's* vol. II, supplement II, *The Alkali Metals* (part 1) 146-158 (1961).

Finely divided powder or crusty material. d_4^{25} 2.013. mp 1570°: van Arkel *et al., Can. J. Chem.* **31,** 1009 (1953); 1427° (1700°K): Brewer, Margrave, *J. Phys. Chem.* **59,** 421 (1955). Readily absorbs carbon dioxide and water from the atm. At elevated temp attacks glass, silica, many metals.

5539. Lithium Perchlorate. [7791-03-9] ClLiO$_4$; mol wt 106.39. Cl 33.32%, Li 6.52%, O 60.15%. LiClO$_4$.

Small crystals. d_4^{25} 2.43. mp 236°. Decompn starts at ~400° and becomes rapid at 430° yielding lithium chloride and oxygen. Heat of formation: −99.94 kcal/mol at 25°. Soly in water (w/w) at 0°: 29.9%; at 25°: 37.5%; at 100°: 71.5%. Appreciably sol in alcohol, acetone, ether, ethyl acetate.

Caution: May be irritating on contact with skin, mucous membranes.

USE: Oxidizing agent.

5540. Lithium Silicate. [10102-24-6] Lithium metasilicate. Li_2O_3Si; mol wt 89.97. Li 15.43%, O 53.35%, Si 31.22%. Li_2SiO_3. Prepd by fusing Li_2CO_3 with SiO_2: Schwarz, Sturm, *Ber.* **47,** 1737 (1914).

Orthorhombic needles. d_4^{25} 2.52. mp 1201°. Heat of formation (solid): −434.9 kcal/mol. Heat of formation (liq) −374.6 kcal/mol. Latent heat of fusion (1177°) = 7.24 kcal/mol, also reported as −80.2 cal/g. Insol in cold water, dec by boiling water, dilute hydrochloric acid.

USE: To calibrate thermoelements.

5541. Lithium Sulfate. [10377-48-7] Lithiophor; Lithium-Duriles. Li_2O_4S; mol wt 109.94. Li 12.63%, O 58.21%, S 29.17%. Li_2SO_4.

Monohydrate, colorless crystals; loses the water at 130°. d 2.06. Sol in 2.6 parts water. Almost insol in alcohol. The aq soln is neutral.

THERAP CAT: Antidepressant.

5542. Lithium Tetracyanoplatinate(II). [14402-73-4] Platinous lithium cyanide; lithium platinocyanide. $C_4Li_2N_4Pt$;

mol wt 313.04. C 15.35%, Li 4.43%, N 17.90%, Pt 62.32%. $Li_2-Pt(CN)_4$.

Pentahydrate. Greenish-yellow crystals. Slightly sol in water.

USE: In x-ray photography.

5543. Lithium Tetrafluoroborate. [14283-07-9] Lithium fluoroboride; lithium fluoborate. BF$_4$Li; mol wt 93.75. B 11.53%, F 81.06%, Li 7.40%. LiBF$_4$. Mild Lewis acid. Prepn: P. Baumgarten, W. Bruns, *Ber.* **72,** 1753 (1939); I. Shapiro, H. G. Weiss, *J. Am. Chem. Soc.* **75,** 1753 (1953). NMR structural study: E. C. Reynhardt, J. A. J. Lourens, *J. Chem. Phys.* **80,** 6240 (1984); ^{19}F NMR study of soln behavior: V. N. Plakhotnik *et al., J. Fluorine Chem.* **98,** 133 (1999). Catalytic use in Diels-Alder reactions: D. A. Smith, K. N. Houk, *Tetrahedron Lett.* **32,** 1549 (1991); J. S. Yadav *et al., Synthesis* **2001,** 1065. Review of applications in organic synthesis: B. S. Babu, K. K. Balasubramanian, *Acros Org. Acta* **7,** 1-3 (2000).

White, crystalline, hygroscopic solid. Sol in water, methanol, acetonitrile. Soly in ether at 25°: 1.3 g/100 ml.

USE: Catalyst in organic synthesis; electrolyte for lithium ion batteries.

5544. Lithium Triethylborohydride. [22560-16-3] (*T*-4)-Lithium triethylhydroborate(1−); Super-Hydride. $C_6H_{16}BLi$; mol wt 105.94. C 68.02%, H 15.22%, B 10.20%, Li 6.55%. LiBH(C$_2$H$_5$)$_3$. Commercial product is available in THF solution. Prepn: H. C. Brown *et al., J. Am. Chem. Soc.* **75,** 192 (1953); P. Binger *et al., Ann.* **717,** 21 (1968); H. C. Brown *et al., Inorg. Chem.* **16,** 2229 (1977). Mechanism of reduction of organic halides: E. C. Ashby *et al., J. Org. Chem.* **49,** 4505 (1984). Use as a reducing agent in organic and inorganic synthesis: H. C. Brown *et al., J. Org. Chem.* **45,** 1 (1980); S. Krishnamurthy, H. C. Brown, *ibid.* **48,** 3085 (1983); H. C. Brown, S.-C. Kim, *ibid.* **49,** 1064 (1984); B. E. Blough, F. I. Carroll, *Tetrahedron Lett.* **34,** 7239 (1993); C. K. Yee *et al., Langmuir* **15,** 3486 (1999); H. Tanaka, K. Ogasawara, *Tetrahedron Lett.* **43,** 4417 (2002).

Colorless crystals, mp 66-67° (Binger). Also reported as white needles from benzene, mp 78-83° (dec) (Brown, 1977). Moderately sol in benzene, toluene, *n*-hexane. *Unstable in air. Reacts violently with water.*

USE: Powerful and selective reducing agent.

5545. Lithocholic Acid. [434-13-9] (3α,5β)-3-Hydroxycholan-24-oic acid; 3α-hydroxycholanic acid; 17β-(1-methyl-3-carboxypropyl)etiocholan-3α-ol. $C_{24}H_{40}O_3$; mol wt 376.57. C 76.55%, H 10.71%, O 12.75%. Found in ox bile, human bile, rabbit bile, and in ox and pig gallstones. Isoln: Fischer, *Z. Physiol. Chem.* **73,** 234 (1911). Characterization: Wieland, Weyland, *ibid.* **110,** 123 (1920). Prepn from cholic or from desoxycholic acid: Hoehn, Mason, *J. Am. Chem. Soc.* **62,** 569 (1940); Sarel, Yanuka, *J. Org. Chem.* **24,** 2018 (1959). Crystal and molecular structure by x-ray diffraction: S. K. Arora *et al., Acta Crystallogr.* **32B,** 415 (1976).

Hexagonal leaflets from alcohol, prisms from acetic acid, mp 184-186°. $[\alpha]_D^{20}$ +33.7° (c = 1.5 in abs ethanol); $[\alpha]_D^{19}$ +23.3° (Wieland); $[\alpha]_D^{20}$ +32.1° (Fischer). Freely sol in hot alc. More sol in ether than cholic or desoxycholic acid. Sol in about 10 times its weight of ethyl acetate. Slightly sol in glacial acetic acid (about 0.2 g in 3 ml). More sol in benzene than desoxycholic acid. Insol in petr ether, gasoline, ligroin, water.

Methyl ester. $C_{25}H_{42}O_3$. Crystallizes with ½ mol methanol, mp 125-127°.

Ethyl ester. $C_{26}H_{44}O_3$. Crystals, mp 92-93°.

Benzyl ester. $C_{31}H_{46}O_3$. Crystals, mp 145-148°.

Acetyllithocholic acid. $C_{26}H_{42}O_4$. Crystals, mp 169°.

Lithopone

Acetyllithocholic acid methyl ester. $C_{27}H_{44}O_4$. Flat needles from pentane, mp 123-130°.

Acetyllithocholic acid ethyl ester. $C_{28}H_{46}O_4$. Crystals, mp 90-91°.

5546. Lithopone. [1345-05-7] C.I. Pigment White 5; Griffith's zinc white. A white pigment consisting of a mixture of zinc sulfide, barium sulfate and some zinc oxide. Several grades of lithopone are commercially available. The zinc sulfide content varies from 26 to 60%. The commercial importance of lithopone has decreased since the introduction of titanium pigments.

USE: In water and oil paints to provide thixotropy, improve gloss and flow.

5547. Litmus. Lacmus; tournesol; turnsole; lacca musica; lacca coerulea. Mol wt about 3300. Blue coloring matter from various species of lichens, particularly *Variolaria, Lecanora,* and *Roccella. Habit.* Scandinavia, shores of Mediterranean, Azores, California, East India, Madagascar. *Constit.* Chiefly azolitmin and erythrolitmin combined with alkalies: lecanoric acid, orcein, erythrolein. Manuf almost exclusively in Holland. Structure studies: Beecken *et al., Angew. Chem.* **73**, 665 (1961). Contains in small amounts α,β,γ-amino and hydroxyorcein.

Blue powder, lumps or cubes. Partly soluble in water or alcohol.

USE: As acid-base indicator; pH: 4.5 red, 8.3 blue. For preparing litmus papers; in microscopy to color culture media for diagnostic purposes. Has been used for coloring beverages.

5548. Livetins. Major water-soluble proteins found in egg yolk: Shepard, Hottle, *J. Biol. Chem.* **179**, 349 (1949). Prepn and mol wts of α- and β-livetin: Martin *et al., Can. J. Biochem. Physiol.* **35**, 241 (1957). Prepn and mol wt of γ-livetin: Martin, Cook, *ibid.* **36**, 153 (1958). Separation of four fractions, α_1-, α_2-, β-, and γ-livetins, and preparation of β- and γ-livetins: Oberdorfer, *Z. Physiol. Chem.* **331**, 280 (1963). Protein constituents of the livetin fraction of egg yolk were identified as follows: α-livetin identified as serum albumin; β-livetin as an α_2-glycoprotein with a sedimentation coeff of 2.95; and γ-livetin as serum γ-globulin: Williams, *Biochem. J.* **83**, 346 (1962). Heterogeneity of livetin proteins in egg yolk: S. F. Hui, R. H. Common, *Can. J. Biochem.* **44**, 1357 (1966); W. M. McIndoe, J. Culbert, *Int. J. Biochem.* **10**, 659 (1979).

5549. Lobaplatin. [135558-11-1] (*SP*-4-3)-[*rel*-(1*R*,2*R*)-1,2-Cyclobutanedimethanamine-$\kappa N,\kappa N'$][(2*S*)-2-(hydroxy-κO)propanoato(2−)-κO]platinum; *cis*-[*trans*-1,2-cyclobutanebis(methylamine)][(*S*)-lactato-O^1,O^2]platinum; D-19466. $C_9H_{18}N_2O_3Pt$; mol wt 397.33. C 27.21%, H 4.57%, N 7.05%, O 12.08%, Pt 49.10%. Water-soluble platinum compound; mixture of two *trans* diastereoisomers. Prepn: W. Schumacher *et al., EP 324154; eidem,* US 5023335 (1989, 1991 both to ASTA Pharma); and pharmacology: R. Voegeli *et al., J. Cancer Res. Clin. Oncol.* **116**, 439 (1990). HPLC determn of diastereoisomers in plasma: J. Welink *et al., J. Chromatogr. B* **675**, 107 (1996). Clinical evaluation: M. Degardin *et al., Invest. New Drugs* **13**, 253 (1995); and pharmacokinetics: J. A. Gietema *et al., Br. J. Cancer* **71**, 1302 (1995). Evaluation in canine osteosarcoma: J. Kirpensteijn *et al., Anticancer Res.* **22**, 2765 (2002). Review of clinical development: M. J. McKeage, *Expert Opin. Invest. Drugs* **10**, 119-128 (2001).

Crystals from diethyl ether, mp 220° (dec). Sol in water. LD$_{50}$ i.p. in mice: 46 mg/kg (Voegeli).

THERAP CAT: Antineoplastic.

THERAP CAT (VET): Antineoplastic.

5550. Lobelia. Indian tobacco; wild tobacco; emetic herb; asthma weed; bladder pod; vomit wort. Dried leaves and tops of *Lobelia inflata* L., *Lobeliaceae.* (The seeds are also used.) *Habit.* Canada, U.S. *Constit.* Leaves and tops: chiefly lobeline, also lobelidine, lobelanine, lobelanidine, and other alkaloids. Seeds: lobeline, fixed oil.

THERAP CAT: Expectorant.

THERAP CAT (VET): Has been used as an expectorant.

5551. Lobeline. [90-69-7] 2-[(2*R*,6*S*)-6-[(2*S*)-2-Hydroxy-2-phenylethyl]-1-methyl-2-piperidinyl]-1-phenylethanone; 2-[6-(β-hydroxyphenethyl)-1-methyl-2-piperidyl]acetophenone; α-lobeline; inflatine. $C_{22}H_{27}NO_2$; mol wt 337.46. C 78.30%, H 8.06%, N 4.15%, O 9.48%. High affinity nicotinic ligand. From herb and seeds of *Lobelia inflata* L., *Lobeliaceae* (Indian tobacco): H. Wieland, *Ber.* **54**, 1784 (1921). Structure: H. Wieland, O. Dragendorff, *Ann.* **473**, 83 (1929). Synthesis: H. Wieland, I. Drishaus, *ibid.* 102; G. Schering, L. Winterhalder, *ibid.* 126. Absolute configuration: Schöpf, Müller, *Ann.* **687**, 241 (1965). Pharmacology: M. I. Damaj *et al., J. Pharmacol. Exp. Ther.* **282**, 410 (1997). Receptor binding study: D. Flammia *et al., J. Med. Chem.* **42**, 3726 (1999). Comprehensive description: F. J. Muhtadi, *Anal. Profiles Drug Subs.* **19**, 261-313 (1990). Review of mechanism of action and therapeutic potential in psychostimulant abuse: L. P. Dwoskin, P. A. Crooks, *Biochem. Pharmacol.* **63**, 89-98 (2002).

Needles from alc, ether, benzene, mp 130-131°. $[\alpha]_D^{15}$ −43° (alc). Very slightly sol in water or in petr ether; sol in hot alcohol, or in chloroform, benzene, ether.

Hydrochloride. [134-63-4] $C_{22}H_{27}NO_2.HCl$; mol wt 373.92. Rosettes of slender needles from alcohol, mp 178-180°. $[\alpha]_D^{20}$ −43° (c = 2). uv max (methanol) 245, 280 nm (log ε 4.08, 3.05). One gram dissolves in 40 ml water, 12 ml alcohol; very sol in chloroform; very slightly sol in ether. Water solns are slightly acid to litmus. A 1% soln in water has a pH of 4.0-6.0.

Sulfate. [134-64-5] $(C_{22}H_{27}NO_2)_2.H_2SO_4$; mol wt 772.99. Hygroscopic. Crystals from alc. $[\alpha]_D^{20}$ −25° (c = 2). Soluble in about 30 parts water, slightly in alcohol.

(±)-Form. [134-65-6] Lobelidine. Prisms, mp 110°.

THERAP CAT: CNS stimulant.

THERAP CAT (VET): Has been used as a respiratory stimulant, ruminatoric.

5552. Lobenzarit. [63329-53-3] 2-[(2-Carboxyphenyl)amino]-4-chlorobenzoic acid; *N*-(2-carboxyphenyl)-4-chloroanthranilic acid; 4-chloro-2,2'-iminodibenzoic acid; CCA. $C_{14}H_{10}ClNO_4$; mol wt 291.69. C 57.65%, H 3.46%, Cl 12.15%, N 4.80%, O 21.94%. Disease modifying antirheumatic drug (DMARD) with immunomodulating activity. Prepn: M. Tanemura *et al., DE 2526092; eidem,* US 4092426 (1976, 1978 both to Chugai). HPLC determn in plasma: F. J. Schwende, S. W. Turner, *Pharm. Res.* **8**, 523 (1991). Immunosuppression of B cell activity: S. Hirohata *et al., Arthritis Rheum.* **35**, 168 (1992). Clinical trial in rheumatoid arthritis: Y. Shiokawa *et al., J. Rheumatol.* **11**, 615 (1984); in systemic lupus erythematosus: S. Hirohata *et al., Clin. Exp. Rheumatol.* **12**, 261 (1994). Review of pharmacology: R. González, D. Remirez, *Invest. Allergol. Clin. Immunol.* **7**, 77-82 (1997).

Crystals, mp >306°. LD$_{50}$ in male, female rats (mg/kg): 2100, 2600 orally (Tanemura).

Disodium salt. [64808-48-6] Carfenil. $C_{14}H_8ClNNa_2O_4$; mol wt 335.65. Solid, mp 388° (dec).

THERAP CAT: Antirheumatic.

5553. Lochnericine. [72058-36-7] (5α,6α,7α,12β,19α)-2,3-Didehydro-6,7-epoxyaspidospermidine-3-carboxylic acid methyl ester. $C_{21}H_{24}N_2O_3$; mol wt 352.43. C 71.57%, H 6.86%, N

7.95%, O 13.62%. Indole alkaloid. From *Vinca rosea* Linn. (*Catharanthus roseus* G. Don.), *Apocynaceae:* Gorman *et al., J. Am. Pharm. Assoc.* **48,** 256 (1959); Svoboda *et al., ibid.* **48,** 659 (1959); Moza, Trojánek, *Collect. Czech. Chem. Commun.* **28,** 1419 (1963). Structure: Moza *et al., Tetrahedron Lett.* **1964,** 2561.

Crystals from methanol, dec 190-193°. $[\alpha]_D^{27}$ $-432°$ (chloroform). pKa in 66% DMF: 4.2. uv max (ethanol): 227, 299, 328 nm (log ε 4.10, 4.15, 4.32).

5554. Locust Bean Gum. Carob flour; Johannisbrotmehl; Arobon. The ground kernel endosperms of tree pods of *Ceratonia siliqua* L., *Leguminosae* (St. John's bread). Consists of proteins such as albumins, globulins, prolamins, gluteline; carbohydrates such as reducing sugars, sucrose, dextrins, pentosans; ash; fat; crude fiber; moisture. *Refs:* Plaut *et al., Bull. Res. Counc. Isr.* **3,** No. 11, 129 (1953), *C.A.* **48,** 5397 (1954); Griffiths, *Manuf. Chem.* **20,** 321 (1949); Coit, *Econ. Bot.* **5,** 82 (1951). Use as coffee, chocolate, cocoa substitute, extender: W. A. Meer, *Manuf. Confect.* **59,** 41 (1979). Caffeine, theobromine content: W. J. Craig, T. T. Nguyen, *J. Food Sci.* **49,** 302 (1984). *Review:* F. Rol in *Industrial Gums,* R. L. Whistler, Ed. (Academic Press, New York, 2nd ed., 1973) pp 323-337.

Yellow-green color, is odorless and tasteless, but acquires a leguminous taste when boiled in water.

USE: Stabilizer, thickener, and binder in foods and cosmetics. Coffee, chocolate, cocoa substitute. Sizing and finishing agent in textiles. As fiber bonding in paper manuf. Drilling mud additive.

THERAP CAT: Adsorbent-demulcent.

5555. Lodoxamide. [53882-12-5] 2,2′-[(2-Chloro-5-cyano-1,3-phenylene)diimino]bis(2-oxoacetic acid); *N,N′*-(2-chloro-5-cyano-*m*-phenylene)dioxamic acid. $C_{11}H_6ClN_3O_6$; mol wt 311.63. C 42.40%, H 1.94%, Cl 11.38%, N 13.48%, O 30.80%. Mast cell stabilizer. Prepn: C. M. Hall, J. B. Wright, **DE 2362409**; *idem,* **US 3993679** (1974, 1976 both to Upjohn); J. B. Wright *et al., J. Med. Chem.* **21,** 930 (1978). HPLC determn in human plasma: I. L. Honigberg *et al., J. Chromatogr.* **276,** 213 (1983). Mechanism of action study: M. K. Church, J. Hiroi, *Br. J. Pharmacol.* **90,** 421 (1987). Clinical evaluation in asthma: R. L. Case *et al., J. Am. Med. Assoc.* **247,** 661 (1982); in allergic eye disease: G. T. Fahy *et al., Eur. J. Ophthalmol.* **2,** 144 (1992).

mp 212° (dec). uv max (0.1*N* NaOH) 239.5 (ε 23800).

Diethyl ester. [53882-13-6] Diethyl *N,N′*-(2-chloro-5-cyano-*m*-phenylene)dioxamate; lodoxamide ethyl; U-42718. $C_{15}H_{14}$-ClN_3O_6; mol wt 367.74. Crystals from ethanol, mp 177-179°.

Tromethamine salt. [63610-09-3] Lodoxamide tromethamine; lodoxamide trometamol; U-42585E; Alomide. $C_{11}H_6ClN_3O_6$·$2C_4H_{11}NO_3$; mol wt 553.90.

THERAP CAT: Antiallergic; topically in allergic conjunctivitis.

5556. Lofentanil. [61380-40-3] *cis*-(−)-3-Methyl-4-[(1-oxopropyl)phenylamino]-1-(2-phenylethyl)-4-piperidinecarboxylic acid methyl ester; (−)-*cis*-3-methyl-1-phenethyl-4-(*N*-phenylpropionamido)isonipecotic acid methyl ester. $C_{25}H_{32}N_2O_3$; mol wt 408.53. C 73.50%, H 7.90%, N 6.86%, O 11.75%. Prepn: P. A. J. Janssen, G. H. P. Van Daele, **DE 2610228**; *idem,* **US 3998834** (both 1976 to Janssen). Receptor affinity and pharmacological

potency: K. D. Stahl *et al., Eur. J. Pharmacol.* **46,** 199 (1977). Structural study: C. De Ranter *et al., Arch. Int. Physiol. Biochim.* **87,** 1031 (1979). Antinociceptive effects in cats: A. S. Tung, T. L. Yaksh, *Pain* **12,** 343 (1982). Opiate receptor binding studies of ³H-lofentanil: W. Gommeren, J. E. Leysen, *Arch. Int. Pharmacodyn. Ther.* **258,** 171 (1982); B. Ilien *et al., ibid.* 313; P. M. Laduron, P. Janssen, *Life Sci.* **31,** 457 (1982).

Oxalate. [61380-41-4] R-34995. $C_{27}H_{34}N_2O_7$; mol wt 498.57. Solid, mp 177°.

THERAP CAT: Analgesic (narcotic).

5557. Lofepramine. [23047-25-8] 1-(4-Chlorophenyl)-2-[[3-(10,11-dihydro-5*H*-dibenz[*b,f*]azepin-5-yl)propyl]methyl-amino]ethanone; 4′-chloro-2-[[3-(10,11-dihydro-5*H*-dibenz[*b,f*]azepin-5-yl)propyl]methylamino]acetophenone; *N*-methyl-*N*-(4-chlorobenzoylmethyl)-3-(10,11-dihydro-5*H*-dibenzo[*b,f*]azepin-5-yl)propylamine; lopramine. $C_{26}H_{27}ClN_2O$; mol wt 435.00. C 74.54%, H 6.50%, Cl 8.46%, N 6.69%, O 3.82%. Psychotropic drug related to imipramine, *q.v.* Prepn: E. Eriksoo *et al.,* **GB 1177525**; *idem,* **US 3637660** (1970, 1972 both to AB Leo). Chemistry and pharmacology: E. Eriksoo, O. Rohte, *Arzneim.-Forsch.* **20,** 1561 (1970). Absorption and metabolism: J. R. Tulic *et al., Acta Pharmacol. Toxicol.* **32,** 304 (1973). Distribution and excretion: G. Plym Forshell, *Xenobiotica* **5,** 73 (1975). Pharmacokinetics: G. Plym Forshell *et al., Eur. J. Clin. Pharmacol.* **9,** 291 (1976). Clinical study: S. Wright, L. Herrmann, *Arzneim.-Forsch.* **26,** 1167 (1976).

Crystals from methanol or acetone, mp 104-106°. Easily oxidized by air and other oxidizing agents to desipramine and *p*-chlorobenzoic acid.

Hydrochloride. [26786-32-3] Leo 640; Amplit; Gamanil; Gamonil; Timelit; Tymelyt. $C_{26}H_{27}ClN_2O$·HCl; mol wt 455.42. Crystals from butanone, mp 152-154°. Sol in methanol, ethanol, chloroform. Practically insol in water. LD_{50} in mice, rats (mg/kg): >2500, >1000 orally; 920, >1000 i.p.; >1000, >1000 s.c. (Eriksoo, Rohte).

THERAP CAT: Antidepressant.

5558. Lofexidine. [31036-80-3] 2-[1-(2,6-Dichlorophenoxy)ethyl]-4,5-dihydro-1*H*-imidazole; 2-[1-(2,6-dichlorophenoxy)ethyl]-2-imidazoline. $C_{11}H_{12}Cl_2N_2O$; mol wt 259.13. C 50.99%, H 4.67%, Cl 27.36%, N 10.81%, O 6.17%. α_2-Adrenoceptor agonist related structurally to clonidine, *q.v.* Prepn of the HCl salt: H. Baganz, H. J. May, **ZA 6800850**; *idem,* **US 3966757** (1968, 1976 both to Nordmark); of the free base: *idem,* **DE 1935479** (1971 to Nordmark), *C.A.* **74,** 87979 (1971). Pharmacological studies: J. Velly, *J. Pharmacol.* **8,** 351 (1977); B. Jarrot *et al., Biochem. Pharmacol.* **28,** 141 (1979). NMR data and cardiovascular effects: P. B. M. Timmermans, P. A. Van Zwieten, *Eur. J. Med. Chem.* **15,** 323 (1980). Hypotensive and sedative properties: P. Birch *et al., Br. J. Pharmacol.* **68,** 107 (1980). Effects in hypertension: N. D. Vlachakis *et al., Fed. Proc.* **39,** 4844 (1980). Series of articles on pharmacology, toxicology, clinical studies: *Arzneim.-Forsch.* **32**, 915-993 (1982). Toxicity studies: T. H. Tsai *et al., ibid.* 955. Review of clinical trials in treatment of opiate withdrawal: J. Strang *et al., Am. J. Addict.* **8**, 337-348 (1999).

Crystals, mp 126-128°.

Hydrochloride. [21498-08-8] MDL-14042A; Ba-168; BritLofex; Lofetensin. $C_{11}H_{12}Cl_2N_2O\cdot HCl$; mol wt 295.59. Crystals from ethanol/ether or 2-propanol, mp 221-223° (**U.S.** patent); also reported as mp 230-232° (**Ger.** patent). Very sol in water, ethanol. Slightly sol in 2-propanol. Practically insol in ether. LD_{50} in mice, rats, dogs (mg/kg): between 74-147 orally (all species); between 8-18 i.v. (all species) (Tsai).

THERAP CAT: In treatment of opioid withdrawal symptoms; antihypertensive.

5559. Loflucarban. [790-69-2] *N*-(3,5-Dichlorophenyl)-*N*′-(4-fluorophenyl)thiourea; 3,5-dichloro-4′-fluorothiocarbanilide; Fluonilid. $C_{13}H_9Cl_2FN_2S$; mol wt 315.19. C 49.54%, H 2.88%, Cl 22.50%, F 6.03%, N 8.89%, S 10.17%. Prepd from *p*-fluorophenyl isothiocyanate and 3,5-dichloroaniline or from 3,5-dichlorophenyl isothiocyanate and *p*-fluoroaniline: **BE 613154** (1962 to Madan), *C.A.* **58**, 474f (1963).

Crystals from ethanol, mp 148°. Soluble in ethyl oleate, isopropyl myristate.

THERAP CAT: Antifungal.

5560. Loganin. [18524-94-2] 1-(β-D-Glucopyranosyloxy)-1,4a,5,6,7,7a-hexahydro-6-hydroxy-7-methylcyclopenta[*c*]pyran-4-carboxylic acid methyl ester; 7-hydroxy-7-desoxyverbenalin. $C_{17}H_{26}O_{10}$; mol wt 390.38. C 52.30%, H 6.71%, O 40.98%. Key intermediate in the biosynthesis of indole alkaloids. First isolated from the seeds but chiefly from the pulp of the fruit of *Strychnos nux-vomica* L., *Loganiaceae:* Dunstan, Short, *Pharm. J.* **14**, 1025 (1883); Merz, Krebs, *Arch. Pharm.* **275**, 217 (1937); Merz, Lehmann, *ibid.* **290**, 543 (1957). Structure: Sheth *et al., Tetrahedron Lett.* **1961**, 394; Büchi, Manning, *Tetrahedron* **18**, 1049 (1962). Crystal structure: Lentz, Rossmann, *Chem. Commun.* **1969**, 1269; P. G. Jones *et al., Acta Crystallogr.* **B36**, 481 (1980). Abs config: Inouye *et al., Tetrahedron* **26**, 3905 (1970). Total synthesis: Büchi *et al., J. Am. Chem. Soc.* **92**, 2165 (1970); Partridge *et al., ibid.* **95**, 532 (1973); Büchi *et al., ibid.* 540; B.-W. Au-Yeung, I. Fleming, *Chem. Commun.* **1977**, 81; I. Fleming, B.-W. Au-Yeung, *Tetrahedron* **37**, Suppl. 9, 13 (1981); K. Hiroi *et al., Chem. Lett.* **1981**, 559. Biosynthetic studies: Battersby, "Biosynthesis II: Terpenoid Indole Alkaloids", in *The Alkaloids* vol. **1,** The Chemical Society (Burlington House, London, 1971) pp 31-47.

Crystals, mp 222-223°. $[\alpha]_D^{20}$ −82.1° (water). Freely sol in water; less sol in 96% alcohol; sparingly in abs alcohol. Practically insol in ether, petr ether, ligroin, ethyl acetate, acetone, chloroform.

5561. Loline. [25161-91-5] [2*R*-(2α,3α,3aβ,4α,6aβ)]-Hexahydro-*N*-methyl-2,4-methano-4*H*-furo[3,2-*b*]pyrrol-3-amine;festucine; methyl-*N*-depropionyldecorticasine. $C_8H_{14}N_2O$; mol wt 154.21. C 62.31%, H 9.15%, N 18.17%, O 10.38%. One of a group of pyrrolizidine alkaloids whose common feature is a unique oxygen bridge. Isoln from seeds of *Lolium cuneatum* Nevski, *Gramineae:* S. Y. Yunusov, S. T. Akramov, *J. Gen. Chem. USSR* **25**, 1765 (1955); from tall fescue hay, *Festuca arundinaceae* Schreb., *Gramineae:* Yates, Tookey, *Aust. J. Chem.* **18**, 53 (1965). Identity with festucine: Aasen, Culvenor, *ibid.* **22**, 2021 (1969). Identity with methyl-*N*-depropionyldecorticasine: Ribas *et al., An. Quim.* **64**, 516 (1968), *C.A.* **69**, 109764c (1968). Abs config: R. B. Bates, S. R. Morehead, *Tetrahedron Lett.* **1972**, 1629. Synthesis of bisquaternary salts: N. P. Abdullaev *et al., Khim. Prir. Soedin.* **3**, 371 (1977), *C.A.* **88**, 23216 (1978). Synthetic and structural studies: S. R. Wilson *et al., J. Org. Chem.* **46**, 3887 (1981).

Dihydrochloride. $C_8H_{14}N_2O\cdot 2HCl$. Needles from abs ethanol, dec 237-242°. $[\alpha]_D^{25}$ +4.6° (c = 4.37 in water). pKa 8.25 and 2.5-3.0.

5562. Lomefloxacin. [98079-51-7] 1-Ethyl-6,8-difluoro-1,4-dihydro-7-(3-methyl-1-piperazinyl)-4-oxo-3-quinolinecarboxylic acid. $C_{17}H_{19}F_2N_3O_3$; mol wt 351.35. C 58.11%, H 5.45%, F 10.81%, N 11.96%, O 13.66%. Fluorinated quinolone antibacterial. DNA gyrase antagonist. Prepn: Y. Itoh *et al.,* **DE 3433924**; *eidem,* **US 4528287** (both 1985 to Hokuriku Pharm.). *In vitro* and *in vivo* activity: T. Hirose *et al., Antimicrob. Agents Chemother.* **31**, 854 (1987). Comparative antibacterial spectrum *in vitro:* R. Wise *et al., ibid.* **32**, 617 (1988). HPLC determn in urine and bile and preliminary pharmacokinetics in rats: A. Saito *et al., ibid.* 156. Photochemistry study: E. Fasani *et al., Eur. J. Org. Chem.* **2004**, 5075. Supplement on antibacterial spectrum, pharmacokinetics and clinical efficacy: *Chemotherapy (Tokyo)* **36**, Suppl. 2, 1-1418 (1988). Comprehensive description: Y. D. Sanzgiri *et al., Anal. Profiles Drug Subs. Excip.* **23**, 321-369 (1994).

Colorless needles from ethanol, mp 239-240.5°. Soly at 25° (mg/ml): 1.03 at ionic strength 0.15 *M* NaCl. uv max (0.15 *M* acetate buffer, pH 5): 226, 288, 320 nm ($a_M \times 10^{-3}$ 15.5, 36.7, 13.5); uv max (0.05 *M* phosphate buffer, pH 7): 282, 326 nm ($a_M \times 10^{-3}$ 31.5, 13.3); uv max (0.15 *M* borate buffer, $\mu = 0.15$ *M* with NaCl, pH 9): 282, 328 nm ($a_M \times 10^{-3}$ 29.3, 13.2). LD_{50} in mice (mg/kg): 245.6 i.v.; >4000 orally (Itoh).

Monohydrochloride. [98079-52-8] NY-198; SC-47111; Bareon; Chimono; Lomebact; Maxaquin; Okacin; Okacyn. $C_{17}H_{19}F_2N_3O_3\cdot HCl$; mol wt 387.81. Colorless needles from water, mp 290-300° (dec).

THERAP CAT: Antibacterial.

5563. Lomerizine. [101477-55-8] 1-[Bis(4-fluorophenyl)methyl]-4-[(2,3,4-trimethoxyphenyl)methyl]piperazine; 1-[bis(*p*-fluorophenyl)methyl]-4-(2,3,4-trimethoxybenzyl)piperazine; 1-(2,3,4-trimethoxybenzyl)-4-[bis(4-fluorophenyl)methyl]piperazine. $C_{27}H_{30}F_2N_2O_3$; mol wt 468.54. C 69.21%, H 6.45%, F 8.11%, N 5.98%, O 10.24%. Diphenylpiperazine calcium channel blocker; selective cerebral vasodilator. Prepn: H. Ohtaka *et al.,* **EP 159566**; *eidem,* **US 4663325** (1985, 1987 both to Kanebo); *eidem et al., Chem. Pharm. Bull.* **35**, 3270 (1987). Structure-activity study: H. Ohtaka, G. Tsukamoto, *ibid.* 4117. HPLC determn in plasma and brain tissue: H. Waki, S. Ando, *J. Chromatogr.* **494**, 408 (1989). Pharmacology: T. Kanazawa *et al., J. Cardiovasc. Pharmacol.* **16**, 430 (1990). Protective effect in cerebral ischemia: H. Hara *et al., Arch. Int. Pharmacodyn.* **304**, 206 (1990); V. Danielisova, M. Chavko, *Neurochem. Res.* **19**, 1503 (1994).

Dihydrochloride. [101477-54-7] KB-2796; Terranas. C_{27}-$H_{30}F_2N_2O_3 \cdot 2HCl$; mol wt 541.46. Colorless crystals from acetonitrile, mp 214-218° (dec). Also reported as mp 204-207° (dec). LD_{50} orally in mice: 300 mg/kg (Ohtaka).

THERAP CAT: Antimigraine.

5564. Lomustine. [13010-47-4] *N*-(2-Chloroethyl)-*N'*-cyclohexyl-1-nitrosourea; 1-(2-chloroethyl)-3-cyclohexyl-1-nitrosourea; NSC-79037; RB-1509; Belustine; CCNU; Cecenu; CeeNU; CiNU. $C_9H_{16}ClN_3O_2$; mol wt 233.70. C 46.25%, H 6.90%, Cl 15.17%, N 17.98%, O 13.69%. Chloroethylnitrosourea derivative with antitumor activity. Similar to carmustine, chlorozotocin, nimustine, ranimustine, *q.q.v.* Synthesis: T. P. Johnston *et al., J. Med. Chem.* **9**, 892 (1966). Clinical review: S. K. Carter, J. W. Newman, *Cancer Chemother. Rep. Part 3* **1**, 136 (1968). Physiological disposition: V. T. Oliverio *et al., Cancer Res.* **30**, 1330 (1970). Toxicology and pharmacology: G. R. Thompson, R. E. Larson, *Toxicol. Appl. Pharmacol.* **21**, 405 (1972); V. T. Oliverio, *Cancer Chemother. Rep. Part 3* **4**, 13 (1973). Comprehensive description: F. J. Al-Shammary, *Anal. Profiles Drug Subs.* **19**, 315-340 (1990).

Yellow powder, mp 90°. Freely sol in chloroform; sol in ethanol, acetone. Soly in water, 0.1*N* NaOH, 0.1*N* HCl or 10% ethanol: <0.05 mg/ml; in absolute ethanol: 70 mg/ml. The bulk drug should be stored in a deep freeze and protected from moisture. LD_{50} in male mice (mg/kg): 51 orally; 56 i.p.; 61 s.c. (Thompson, Larson).

Caution: This substance is reasonably anticipated to be a human carcinogen: *Report on Carcinogens, Eleventh Edition* (PB2005-104914, 2004) p III-52.

THERAP CAT: Antineoplastic.

5565. Lonafarnib. [193275-84-2] 4-[2-[4-[(11*R*)-3,10-Dibromo-8-chloro-6,11-dihydro-5*H*-benzo[5,6]cyclohepta[1,2-*b*]pyridin-11-yl]-1-piperidinyl]-2-oxoethyl]-1-piperidinecarboxamide; Sch-66336; Sarasar. $C_{27}H_{31}Br_2ClN_4O_2$; mol wt 638.82. C 50.76%, H 4.89%, Br 25.02%, Cl 5.55%, N 8.77%, O 5.01%. Tricyclic farnesyl protein transferase inhibitor. Prepn: R. J. Doll *et al.,* **WO 9723478**; *eidem,* **US 5874442** (1997, 1999 both to Schering-Plough); F. G. Njoroge *et al., J. Med. Chem.* **41**, 4890 (1998). Improved prepn: S.-C. Kuo *et al., J. Org. Chem.* **68**, 4984 (2003). Crystal structure of complex with farnesyl protein transferase: C. L. Strickland *et al., J. Med. Chem.* **42**, 2125 (1999). LC/MS/MS determn in plasma: N. M. G. Appels *et al., Rapid Commun. Mass Spectrom.* **19**, 2187 (2005). Antitumor activity in human xenograft and transgenic mouse cancer models: M. Liu *et al., Cancer Res.* **58**, 4947 (1998). Clinical evaluation in cancer: A. A. Adjei *et al., ibid.* **60**, 1871 (2000). Inhibition of P-glycoprotein mediated drug efflux: E. Wang *et al., ibid.* **61**, 7525 (2001). Clinical evaluation with paclitaxel in non-small cell lung cancer: E. S. Kim *et al., Cancer* **104**, 561 (2005).

White solid. Crystals from acetone, mp 214.5-215.9° (monohydrate); anhydrous form mp 222-223°. $[\alpha]_D^{25} = +49.1°$ (c = 0.21 in methanol).

THERAP CAT: Antineoplastic.

5566. Lonazolac. [53808-88-1] 3-(4-Chlorophenyl)-1-phenyl-1*H*-pyrazole-4-acetic acid. $C_{17}H_{13}ClN_2O_2$; mol wt 312.75. C 65.29%, H 4.19%, Cl 11.34%, N 8.96%, O 10.23%. Prepn: R. A. Newberry, **GB 1373212** (1974 to Wyeth), *C.A.* **82**, 72987t (1975); G. Rainer, **US 4146721** (1979 to Byk Gulden); G. Rainer *et al., Arzneim.-Forsch.* **31**, 649 (1981). Pharmacology: R. Riedel, *ibid.* 655. Clinical studies: G. Lonauer *et al., Z. Rheumatol.* **40**, 161 (1981); W. Siegmeth, P. Placheta, *Wien. Klin. Wochenschr.* **94**, 145 (1982).

Crystals from ethanol/water, mp 150-151°. uv max (methanol): 281 nm (ε 24800); (0.1*N* NaOH): 281 nm (ε 23700). pKa 4.3. LD_{50} in male mice, rats (mg/kg): 195, 165 i.v. (Riedel).

Calcium salt. [75821-71-5] Argun L; Irritren. $C_{34}H_{24}CaCl_2$-N_4O_4; mol wt 663.56. Solid, melts between 270-290° (dec). uv max (0.1*N* NaOH): 280 nm (ε 46400). LD_{50} in male, female mice, male, female rats (mg/kg): 670, 845, 730, 1000 orally (Riedel).

THERAP CAT: Anti-inflammatory.

5567. Longifolene. [475-20-7] [1*S*-(1α,3aβ,4α,8aβ)]-Decahydro-4,8,8-trimethyl-9-methylene-1,4-methanoazulene; junipene; kuromatsuene. $C_{15}H_{24}$; mol wt 204.35. C 88.16%, H 11.84%. Tricyclic sesquiterpene present to the extent of 5-10% in Indian turpentine oil which is produced commercially from the Himalayan pine, *Pinus longifolia* Roxb., *Pinaceae:* J. L. Simonsen, *J. Chem. Soc.* **117**, 570 (1920). Structure: R. H. Moffett, D. Rogers, *Chem. Ind. (London)* **1953**, 916; P. Naffa, G. Ourisson, *ibid.* 917. Abs config: G. Ourisson, *Bull. Soc. Chim. Fr.* **1955**, 895. Identity of longifolene with junipene and kuromatsuene: S. Akiyoshi *et al., Tetrahedron* **9**, 237 (1960). Total synthesis of naturally occurring (+)-form: E. J. Corey *et al., J. Am. Chem. Soc.* **86**, 478 (1964); of the (±)-form: *eidem, ibid.* **83**, 1251 (1961); J. E. McMurray, S. J. Isser, *ibid.* **94**, 7132 (1972); R. A. Volkmann *et al., ibid.* **97**, 4777 (1975). Review of chemistry of longifolene and its derivs: S. Dev, *Acc. Chem. Res.* **14**, 82-88 (1981); *idem, Fortschr. Chem. Org. Naturst.* **40**, 50-104 (1981).

Viscous oil, bp$_{706}$ 254-256°, bp$_{15}$ 126-127°. $[\alpha]_D^{18}$ +42.73°. d$_4^{18}$ 0.9319; n$_D^{20}$ 1.5040. Insol in water; sol in benzene.

Borane deriv. Dilongifolylborane. $C_{30}H_{51}B$. Heavy, snow-white, shiny plates, mp 160-161° (sealed, evacuated capillary). Strongly dimeric. Sparingly sol in common organic solvents. Prepn and use in hydroboration: P. K. Jadhav, H. C. Brown, *J. Org. Chem.* **46**, 2988 (1981).

USE: Borane deriv as a chiral hydroborating agent.

5568. Lonidamine. [50264-69-2] 1-[(2,4-Dichlorophenyl)-methyl]-1*H*-indazole-3-carboxylic acid; 1-(2,4-dichlorobenzyl)-1*H*-indazole-3-carboxylic acid; diclondazolic acid; DICA; AF-1890; Doridamina. $C_{15}H_{10}Cl_2N_2O_2$; mol wt 321.16. C 56.10%, H 3.14%, Cl 22.08%, N 8.72%, O 9.96%. Antitumor agent with antispermatogenic activity; inhibits cellular respiration in neoplastic cells. Prepn: G. Palazzo, B. Silvestrini, DE 2310031; *eidem*, US 3895026 (1973, 1975 both to Angelini Francesco); G. Corsi, G. Palazzo, *J. Med. Chem.* **19**, 778 (1976). Antispermatogenic activity: T. J. Lobl, *Arch. Androl.* **2**, 353 (1979). *In vitro* and *in vivo* antitumor activity: B. Silvestrini *et al.*, *Br. J. Cancer* **47**, 221 (1983). Mechanism of action in neoplastic cells: A. Floridi *et al.*, *Exp. Mol. Pathol.* **42**, 293 (1985). Pharmacology: V. Cioli *et al.*, *Arzneim.-Forsch.* **34**, 455 (1984). HPLC determn in plasma and urine: R. Leclaire *et al.*, *J. Chromatogr.* **277**, 427 (1983). Toxicological study: R. Heywood *et al.*, *Chemotherapy (Basel)* **27**, Suppl. 2, 91 (1981). Series of articles on mechanism of action, pharmacokinetics and clinical applications in spermatogenesis and tumors: *ibid.* 5-120; on pharmacology and clinical evaluation in cancers: *Oncology* **41**, Suppl. 1, 1-121 (1984). Symposium on clinical evaluations in cancers: *Semin. Oncol.* **18**, Suppl 4, 1-72 (1991).

COOH structure image

Crystals from ethanol, mp 207°. Sol in methanol, acetic acid. LD_{50} in mice, rats (mg/kg): 900, 1700 orally; 435, 525 i.p. (Heywood).

THERAP CAT: Antineoplastic.

5569. Lonomycins. Polyether antibiotics active against gram-positive bacteria, esp. coccidia. The major component is lonomycin A (initially named lonomycin). Lonomycin B and C are minor congeners. Isoln from *Streptomyces ribosidificus* strain TM-481 as sodium salt: M. Shibata *et al.*, **JP Kokai 75 49495** (1975 to Taisho Pharm.), *C.A.* **83**, 191339p (1975); S. Omura *et al.*, *J. Antibiot.* **29**, 15 (1976). Identity of A with antibiotic DE-3936; fermentation, isolation, physicochemical properties and biological activity: M. Ohshima *et al.*, *ibid.* 354. Structure of A: N. Otake, M. Koenuma, *Tetrahedron Lett.* **1975**, 4147; C. Riche, C. Pascard-Billy, *Chem. Commun.* **1975**, 951; of B, C: H. Seto *et al.*, *J. Antibiot.* **31**, 929 (1978); T. Mizutani *et al.*, *ibid.* **33**, 1224 (1980). ^{13}C-NMR spectrum of A: H. Seto *et al.*, *ibid.* 979. Ionophorous activity of A: M. Mitani, N. Otake, *ibid.* **31**, 750 (1978). Cardiovascular effects of A: K. Kaneko *et al.*, *Res. Commun. Chem. Pathol. Pharmacol.* **67**, 17 (1990); K. Tsuchida *et al.*, *Arch. Int. Pharmacodyn.* **314**, 25 (1991). Total synthesis of A: D. A. Evans *et al.*, *J. Am. Chem. Soc.* **117**, 3448 (1995).

Lonomycin A structure image

Lonomycin A

Sodium salts are sol in lower alcohols, acetone, ethyl acetate, benzene, chloroform, ether. Slightly sol in *n*-hexane, petr ether. Insol in water.

Lonomycin A. [58785-63-0] Antibiotic DE-3936; emericid. $C_{44}H_{76}O_{14}$. Colorless prisms from benzene-petr ether, mp 109-114°. $[\alpha]_D^{20}$ +66.6° (c = 1 in $CHCl_3$); $[\alpha]_D^{23}$ +57.5° (c = 0.40 in CH_2Cl_2). pKa' (66% acetone) 5.9. Sol in most organic solvents. Insol in water.

Lonomycin A sodium salt. [58845-80-0] $C_{44}H_{75}NaO_{14}$. Colorless prisms from benzene-petr ether, mp 173-176° (dec) (Ohshima); also reported as mp 188-189° (Omura). $[\alpha]_D^{25}$ +49.8° (c = 1 in CH_3OH), $[\alpha]_D^{25}$ +67.0° (c = 1 in $CHCl_3$) (Ohshima); also reported as $[\alpha]_D^{25}$ +47° (c = 1 in CH_3OH) (Omura). LD_{50} in mice (mg/kg): 45.8 orally; 13.0 i.p.; 37.5 s.c. (Ohshima).

Lonomycin B sodium salt. $C_{44}H_{75}NaO_{14}$. White prisms from *n*-hexane-benzene, mp 181-182°. $[\alpha]_D$ +48.2° (c = 0.5 in CH_3OH).

Lonomycin C sodium salt. $C_{43}H_{73}NaO_{14}$. White prisms from *n*-hexane-benzene, mp 186-187°. $[\alpha]_D$ +49.2° (c = 0.5 in CH_3OH).

5570. Looplure. [14959-86-5] (*Z*)-7-Dodecen-1-ol acetate; *cis*-7-dodecenyl acetate; *cis*-1-acetoxy-7-dodecene; ENT-33266. $C_{14}H_{26}O_2$; mol wt 226.36. C 74.28%, H 11.58%, O 14.14%. Sex pheromone of the female cabbage looper moth, *Trichoplusia ni* (Hübner). Isoln, identification and synthesis: R. S. Berger, *Ann. Entomol. Soc. Am.* **59**, 767 (1966). Synthesis and activity of isomers: N. Green *et al.*, *J. Med. Chem.* **10**, 533 (1967); H. H. Toba *et al.*, *J. Econ. Entomol.* **63**, 1048 (1970). Alternate syntheses: W. Seidel *et al.*, *Ber.* **110**, 3544 (1977); H. J. Bestmann *et al.*, *Ber.* **112**, 1923 (1979); M. Horiike, C. Hirano, *Agric. Biol. Chem.* **44**, 2229 (1980); D. Basavaiah *et al.*, *J. Org. Chem.* **47**, 1792 (1982). Acute toxicity study: M. Beroza *et al.*, *Toxicol. Appl. Pharmacol.* **31**, 421 (1975).

Looplure structure image

Oil, $bp_{0.05}$ 98-100°. n_D^{25} 1.4420. LD_{50} in rats (mg/kg): >13430 orally; in rabbits (mg/kg): >2025 dermally; LC_{50} (24 hr) in rainbow trout, bluegill sunfish (ppm): >100, >100 (Beroza).

USE: Insect attractant.

5571. Loperamide. [53179-11-6] 4-(4-Chlorophenyl)-4-hydroxy-*N,N*-dimethyl-α,α-diphenyl-1-piperidinebutanamide; 4-(*p*-chlorophenyl)-4-hydroxy-*N,N*-dimethyl-α,α-diphenyl-1-piperidinebutyramide. $C_{29}H_{33}ClN_2O_2$; mol wt 477.04. C 73.01%, H 6.97%, Cl 7.43%, N 5.87%, O 6.71%. Prepn: Janssen *et al.*, **FR 2100711**; *eidem*, US 3714159 (1972, 1973 to Janssen); Stokbroekx *et al.*, *J. Med. Chem.* **16**, 782 (1973). LC-MS/MS determn in plasma: B. Streel *et al.*, *J. Chromatogr. B* **814**, 263 (2005). Series of articles on pharmacology, toxicology, metabolism, and clinical studies: *Arzneim.-Forsch.* **24**, 1640-1665 (1974). Toxicity studies: C. J. E. Niemegeers *et al.*, *ibid.* 1633, 1636. Review: D. A. Shriver *et al.*, in *Pharmacological and Biochemical Properties of Drug Substances* vol. 3, M. E. Goldberg, Ed. (Am. Pharm. Assoc., Washington, DC, 1981) pp 461-476. Comprehensive description: J. Van Rompay, J. E. Carter, *Anal. Profiles Drug Subs.* **19**, 341-365 (1990).

Loperamide structure image

Hydrochloride. [34552-83-5] PJ-185; R-18553; Arret; Blox; Brek; Dissenten; Fortasec; Imodium; Imosec; Imossel; Lopemid; Lopemin; Loperyl; Suprasec; Tebloc. $C_{29}H_{33}ClN_2O_2·HCl$; mol wt 513.50. Crystals from isopropanol, mp 222-223°. uv max (0.1*N* HCl/2-propanol, 10/90 v/v): 253, 259, 265, 273 nm (ε 532, 648, 581, 233). Soly (g/100ml): water (pH 1.7) 0.14; citrate-phosphate (pH 6.1) 0.008; citrate-phosphate (pH 7.9) <0.001; methanol 28.6; ethanol 5.37; 2-propanol 1.11; dichloromethane 35.1; acetone 0.20; ethyl acetate 0.035; diethyl ether <0.001; hexane <0.001; toluene 0.001; *N,N*-dimethylformamide 10.3; tetrahydrofuran 0.32; 4-methyl-2-pentanone 0.020; propylene glycol 5.64; polyethylene glycol 400 1.40; dimethylsulfoxide 20.5; 2-butanone 0.18. pKa 8.66. Practically insol in H_2O at physiological pH (0.002%). Stable, can be stored for several years under normal conditions; not hygroscopic; not affected by light. LD_{50} in mice (mg/kg): 75 s.c.; 28 i.p.; 105 orally; in rats (mg/kg): 185 orally (Niemegeers).

THERAP CAT: Antidiarrheal.

5572. Lophotoxin. [78697-56-0] (1R,2S,4S,10R,12R,14R,-15R)-2-(Acetyloxy)-12-methyl-4-(1-methylethyl)-17-oxo-11,16,-18,19-tetraoxapentacyclo[12.2.2.1^{6,9}.0^{1,15}.0^{10,12}]nonadeca-6,8-diene-7-carboxaldehyde; LTX. $C_{22}H_{24}O_8$; mol wt 416.42. C 63.45%, H 5.81%, O 30.74%. A novel neuromuscular toxin isolated from several spp of Pacific gorgonians (sea fans and whips) of the genus *Lophogorgia*. Although it belongs to the cembrene class of diterpenoids, the ability of LTX to cause irreversible postsynaptic blockade at the neuromuscular junction resembles the mode of action of the protein snake venom α-bungarotoxin (cf. bungarotoxins). Isoln and structure: W. Fenical et al., Science **212**, 1512 (1981). Molecular mode of action: J. R. Smythies, Med. Hypotheses **7**, 1457 (1981), C.A. **96**, 137527 (1982). Toxicity study: P. Culver, R. S. Jacobs, Toxicon **19**, 825 (1981). Description of the cytotoxic, ichthyotoxic, and antibacterial activity of alcoholic extracts of gorgonians: R. S. Jacobs et al., Fed. Proc. **40**, 26 (1981); V. J. Paul, W. Fenical, J. Org. Chem. **45**, 3401 (1981).

White needles, mp 164-166°. [α]$_D^{27}$ +14.2° (c = 1.7 in chloroform). LD$_{50}$ in mice (mg/kg): 8.9 s.c. (Culver, Jacobs).

5573. Lopinavir. [192725-17-0] (αS)-N-[(1S,3S,4S)-4-[[(2,6-Dimethylphenoxy)acetyl]amino]-3-hydroxy-5-phenyl-1-(phenylmethyl)pentyl]tetrahydro-α-(1-methylethyl)-2-oxo-1(2H)-pyrimidineacetamide; (αS)-tetrahydro-N-[(αS)-α-[(2S,3S)-2-hydroxy-4-phenyl-3-[2-(2,6-xylyloxy)acetamido]butyl]phenethyl]-α-isopropyl-2-oxo-1(2H)-pyrimidineacetamide; (2S,3S,5S)-2-(2,6-dimethylphenoxyacetyl)amino-3-hydroxy-5-[2S-(1-tetrahydropyrimid-2-onyl)-3-methylbutanoyl]amino-1,6-diphenylhexane; ABT-378; A-157378. $C_{37}H_{48}N_4O_5$; mol wt 628.80. C 70.67%, H 7.69%, N 8.91%, O 12.72%. HIV protease inhibitor; analog of ritonavir, q.v. Prepn: H. L. Sham et al., **WO 9721685**; idem et al., **US 5914332** (1997, 1999 both to Abbott); E. J. Stoner et al., Org. Process Res. Dev. **3**, 145 (1999). Protease inhibition and pharmacokinetics: H. L. Sham et al., Antimicrob. Agents Chemother. **42**, 3218 (1998). In vitro metabolism study: G. N. Kumar et al., Drug Metab. Dispos. **27**, 86 (1999). Pharmacokinetic enhancement by ritonavir: G. N. Kumar et al., ibid. 902. Clinical trial with ritonavir in HIV infection: S. Walmsley et al., N. Engl. J. Med. **346**, 2039 (2002).

Colorless solid from ethyl acetate, mp 124-127°.
Mixture with ritonavir. Kaletra.
THERAP CAT: Antiviral.

5574. Loprazolam. [61197-73-7] (Z)-6-(2-Chlorophenyl)-2,4-dihydro-2-[(4-methyl-1-piperazinyl)methylene]-8-nitro-1H-imidazo[1,2-a][1,4]benzodiazepin-1-one. $C_{23}H_{21}ClN_6O_3$; mol wt 464.90. C 59.42%, H 4.55%, Cl 7.63%, N 18.08%, O 10.32%. Annelated 1,4-benzodiazepine deriv. Prepn: J. B. Taylor, D. R.

Harrison, **DE 2605652**; eidem, **US 4044142** (1976, 1977 both to Roussel-UCLAF). CNS activity: J. R. Agar et al., J. Med. Chem. **20**, 1035 (1977). Pharmacological profile: T. G. Johns et al., Arch. Int. Pharmacodyn. Ther. **240**, 53 (1979). Effects on sleep in normal volunteers: I. Hindmarch, C. A. Clyde, Drugs Exp. Clin. Res. **2**, 61 (1980). Review of pharmacology and efficacy in insomnia: B. G. Clark et al., Drugs **31**, 500-516 (1986).

Crystals from chloroform/ether, mp 214-215°. LD$_{50}$ in mice: >1000 mg/kg orally (Agar).
Methanesulfonate. [70111-54-5] Loprazolam mesylate; HR-158; RU-31158; Dormonoct; Havlane; Somnovit; Sonin. $C_{23}H_{21}$-ClN$_6$O$_3$.CH$_3$SO$_3$H; mol wt 561.01. Crystals from methylene chloride, mp 205-210°.
Note: This is a controlled substance (depressant): **21 CFR**, 1308.14.
THERAP CAT: Sedative, hypnotic.

5575. Loprinone. [106730-54-5] 1,2-Dihydro-5-imidazo-[1,2-a]pyridin-6-yl-6-methyl-2-oxo-3-pyridinecarbonitrile; 1,2-dihydro-5-imidazo[1,2-a]pyridin-6-yl-6-methyl-2-oxonicotinonitrile; olprinone. $C_{14}H_{10}N_4O$; mol wt 250.26. C 67.19%, H 4.03%, N 22.39%, O 6.39%. Inotropic agent which inhibits cAMP phosphodiesterase. Prepn: M. Yamanaka et al., **JP Kokai 86 218589**; eidem, **US 4751227** (1986, 1988 both to Eisai). Synthesis: M. Yamanaka et al., J. Labelled Compd. Radiopharm. **31**, 125 (1992). Pharmacology: M. Tajimi et al., Arch. Pharmacol. **344**, 602 (1991). Pharmacokinetics in dogs: Y. Uemura et al., J. Pharm. Pharmacol. **45**, 1077 (1993). Review of pharmacology, toxicology and clinical evaluation: M. Endoh, Cardiovasc. Drug Rev. **11**, 432-450 (1993).

Crystals from DMF, mp >300°.
Hydrochloride monohydrate. E-1020. $C_{14}H_{10}N_4O.HCl.H_2$-O; mol wt 304.73. White to yellowish-white odorless crystalline powder, mp >300°. Sol in water (pH 3-5) up to 3 mg/ml. LD$_{50}$ in male, female rats, mice (mg/kg): 7,804, >10,000, >10,000, >10,000 orally; 176, 240, 242, 269 i.v.; 2,133, 2,890, 3,898, 4,479 s.c. (Endoh).
THERAP CAT: Cardiotonic.

5576. Loracarbef. [121961-22-6] (6R,7S)-7-[[(2R)-Aminophenylacetyl]amino]-3-chloro-8-oxo-1-azabicyclo[4.2.0]oct-2-ene-2-carboxylic acid monohydrate; (6R,7S)-3-chloro-7-[(R)-phenylglycinamido]-8-oxo-1-azabicyclo[4.2.0]oct-2-ene-2-carboxylic acid monohydrate; carbacefaclor; KT-3777; LY-163892 monohydrate; Lorabid. $C_{16}H_{16}ClN_3O_4.H_2O$; mol wt 367.78. C 52.25%, H 4.93%, Cl 9.64%, N 11.43%, O 21.75%. Carbacephem analog of cefaclor, q.v. Prepn: T. Hirata et al., **EP 14476**; eidem, **US 4708956** (1980, 1987 both to Kyowa Hakko); I. Matsukuma et al., Chem. Pharm. Bull. **37**, 1239 (1989). Prepn of the crystalline monohydrate: C. E. Pasini, **EP 311366** (1989 to Lilly). Enantioselective synthesis: C. C. Bodurow et al., Tetrahedron Lett. **30**, 2321 (1989). Antibacterial spectrum: K. Sato et al., J. Antibiot.

42, 1844 (1989). β-Lactamase stability: R. N. Jones, A. L. Barry, *Eur. J. Clin. Microbiol.* **6,** 570 (1987). Pharmacology in animals: T. Shetler *et al., Arzneim.-Forsch.* **43,** 60 (1993). Pharmacokinetics in children: J. D. Nelson *et al., Antimicrob. Agents Chemother.* **32,** 1738 (1988).

mp 205-215° (dec) (Matsukuma). $[\alpha]_D^{21}$ +34.0° (c = 0.35 in water).

THERAP CAT: Antibacterial.

5577. Lorajmine. [47562-08-3] (17*R*,21α)-Ajmalan-17,21-diol 17-(chloroacetate); 17-monochloroacetylajmaline; 17-chloroacetylajmaline; MCAA. $C_{22}H_{27}ClN_2O_3$; mol wt 402.91. C 65.58%, H 6.75%, Cl 8.80%, N 6.95%, O 11.91%. Semi-synthetic ajmaline derivative. Prepn from ajmaline: **BE 622395** (1962 to Inverni Della Beffa), *C.A.* **59,** 8816d (1963); A. Bonati, A. Bocchia, *Farmaco Ed. Sci.* **18,** 84 (1963). Improved prepn: A. Bonati, **DE 2023949;** *eidem,* **US 3741972** (1970, 1973 both to Inverni Della Beffa). *In vitro* and *in vivo* anti-arrhythmic activity: C. Capra, *Farmaco Ed. Sci.* **19,** 865 (1964); cardiac action: Y. Katano *et al., Arzneim.-Forsch.* **23,** 483 (1973); cardiovascular effects and toxicity: C. Capra *et al., Farmaco Ed. Prat.* **35,** 49 (1980). Determination in plasma by TLC fluorescence: L. J. Dombrowski *et al., J. Pharm. Sci.* **64,** 643 (1975). GC-MS determination in blood: St. D. Clemans *et al., Arzneim.-Forsch.* **27,** 1128 (1977). Comparison with other ajmaline esters: M. Salmona *et al., J. Pharm. Sci.* **64,** 1561 (1975); P. Jaillon *et al., Arch. Int. Pharmacodyn.* **224,** 310 (1976). Clinical studies: M. Cafiero *et al., Minerva Cardioangiol.* **32,** 59 (1984). Book: G. G. Gensini, Ed., *Concepts on the Mechanism and Treatment of Arrhythmias* (Futura Publishing Co., Mount Kisco, N.Y., 1974) 281 pp.

Crystals, mp 232-238°. $[\alpha]_D^{20}$ +27.5° (c = 1 in chloroform).
Hydrochloride. [40819-93-0] Win-11831; Nevergor; Ritmos Elle. $C_{22}H_{27}ClN_2O_3 \cdot HCl$; mol wt 439.38. Crystals from methyl ethyl ketone, mp 243-246°. $[\alpha]_D^{20}$ +29° (c = 1 in ethanol). LD_{50} in mice, rats (mg/kg): 176, 139 i.p.; 370, 480 orally (Capra).

THERAP CAT: Antiarrhythmic (cardiac depressant).

5578. Loratadine. [79794-75-5] 4-(8-Chloro-5,6-dihydro-11*H*-benzo[5,6]cyclohepta[1,2-*b*]pyridin-11-ylidene)-1-piperidinecarboxylic acid ethyl ester; 11-[*N*-(ethoxycarbonyl)-4-piperidylidene]-8-chloro-6,11-dihydro-5*H*-benzo[5,6]cyclohepta[1,2-*b*]pyridine; Sch-29851; Alavert; Claritin; Clarityn; Clarytin; Lisino. $C_{22}H_{23}ClN_2O_2$; mol wt 382.88. C 69.01%, H 6.05%, Cl 9.26%, N 7.32%, O 8.36%. Nonsedating-type histamine H_1-receptor antagonist. Prepn: F. J. Villani, **US 4282233** (1981 to Schering); F. J. Villani *et al., Arzneim.-Forsch.* **36,** 1311 (1986). Pharmacology: A. Barnett *et al., Agents Actions* **14,** 590 (1984). Evaluation of CNS effects in humans: C. M. Bradley, A. N. Nicholson, *Eur. J. Clin. Pharmacol.* **32,** 419 (1987). Clinical pharmacokinetics: E. Radwanski *et al., J. Clin. Pharmacol.* **27,** 530 (1987). Clinical trial in allergic rhinitis: R. J. Dockhorn *et al., Ann. Allergy* **58,** 407 (1987); in comparison with terfenadine, *q.v.:* F. Horak *et al., Arzneim.-*

Forsch. **38,** 124 (1988); G. Bruttmann *et al., J. Allergy Clin. Immunol.* **83,** 411 (1989). HPLC determn in plasma: O. Q. P. Yin *et al., J. Chromatogr. B* **796,** 165 (2003). Review of pharmacology and therapeutic efficacy: M. Haria *et al., Drugs* **48,** 617-637 (1994).

Crystals from acetonitrile, mp 134-136°.
THERAP CAT: Antihistaminic.

5579. Lorazepam. [846-49-1] 7-Chloro-5-(2-chlorophenyl)-1,3-dihydro-3-hydroxy-2*H*-1,4-benzodiazepin-2-one; Wy-4036; Ativan; Emotival; Lorax; Lorsilan; Pro Dorm; Psicopax; Punktyl; Quait; Sedatival; Sedazin; Somagerol; Tavor; Temesta; Wypax. $C_{15}H_{10}Cl_2N_2O_2$; mol wt 321.16. C 56.10%, H 3.14%, Cl 22.08%, N 8.72%, O 9.96%. Prepn: S. C. Bell, **BE 621819;** *idem,* **US 3296249** (1963, 1967 both to Am. Home Prod.); and structure-activity study: *idem et al., J. Med. Chem.* **11,** 457 (1968). Determn by HPLC: I. Jane, A. McKinnon, *J. Chromatogr.* **323,** 191 (1985). Series of articles on pharmacology, metabolism, clinical studies: *Arzneim.-Forsch.* **21,** 1047-1102 (1971). Toxicity study: G. Owen *et al., ibid.* 1065. Comprehensive description: J. G. Rutgers, C. M. Shearer, *Anal. Profiles Drug Subs.* **9,** 397-426 (1980). Review of clinical pharmacology and therapeutic use: B. Ameer, D. J. Greenblatt, *Drugs* **21,** 161-200 (1981). Clinical trial to prevent recurrent alcohol-related seizures: G. D'Onofrio *et al., N. Engl. J. Med.* **340,** 915 (1999).

Crystals, mp 166-168°. uv max (methanol): 229 nm, (1*N* NaOH): 233 nm, (1*N* HCl): 237 nm. Soly (mg/ml): water 0.08, chloroform 3, alcohol 14, propylene glycol 16, ethyl acetate 30. pK_1 1.3; pK_2 11.5. LD_{50} in mice, rats (mg/kg): 3178, >5000 orally (Owen).

Note: This is a controlled substance (depressant): **21 CFR,** 1308.14.

THERAP CAT: Anxiolytic; anticonvulsant.

5580. Lorcainide. [59729-31-6] *N*-(4-Chlorophenyl)-*N*-[1-(1-methylethyl)-4-piperidinyl]benzeneacetamide; 4'-chloro-*N*-(1-isopropyl-4-piperidyl)-2-phenylacetanilide. $C_{22}H_{27}ClN_2O$; mol wt 370.92. C 71.24%, H 7.34%, Cl 9.56%, N 7.55%, O 4.31%. Prepn: S. Sanczuk, H. K. F. Hermans, **DE 2642856** (1977 to Janssen), *C.A.* **87,** 53094 (1977); *eidem,* **US 4126689** (1978 to Janssen). Determn of lorcainide and its metabolites by GLC: R. Woestenborghs *et al., J. Chromatogr.* **164,** 169 (1979). Disposition and anti-arrhythmic effects: U. Klotz *et al., Int. J. Clin. Pharmacol. Biopharm.* **17,** 152 (1979). Pharmacokinetics and tissue distribution: U. Klotz, E. Golbs, *Arzneim.-Forsch.* **30,** 619 (1980). Clinical study: P. Somani, S. di Giorgi, *Chest* **78,** 658 (1980). Toxicology: G. J. Barton, R. Marsboom, "A Brief Summary of Animal Toxicology Studies on Lorcainide", in *Prognosis and Pharmacotherapy of Life-Threatening Arrhythmias,* Jähnchen *et al.,* Eds. (Royal Soc. Med. London, 1981) pp 23-25. Review of pharmacology and efficacy: C. E. Eriksson, R. N. Brogden, *Drugs* **27,** 279-300 (1984). Symposium: *Am. J. Cardiol.* **54,** 1B-54B (1984).

LD$_{50}$ in male mice, male and female rats (mg/kg): 18.8, 19.3, 18.6 i.v.; 483, 395, 435 orally (Barton, Marsboom).

Hydrochloride. [58934-46-6] R-15889; Ro-13-1042; Lopantrol; Lorivox; Remivox. C$_{22}$H$_{27}$ClN$_2$O.HCl; mol wt 407.38. Crystals from 2-propanone and 2-propanol, mp 263°.

THERAP CAT: Antiarrhythmic (class IC).

5581. Lormetazepam. [848-75-9] 7-Chloro-5-(2-chlorophenyl)-1,3-dihydro-3-hydroxy-1-methyl-2H-1,4-benzodiazepin-2-one; N-methyllorazepam; Wy-4082; Ergocalm; Loramet; Noctamid. C$_{16}$H$_{12}$Cl$_2$N$_2$O$_2$; mol wt 335.18. C 57.33%, H 3.61%, Cl 21.15%, N 8.36%, O 9.55%. Analog of lorazepam, *q.v.* Prepn: S. C. Bell, **BE 621819** *C.A.* **60**, 2993b (1964); *idem,* **US 3296249** (1963, 1967 both to Am. Home Products); *idem, J. Med. Chem.* **11**, 457 (1968); A. Nudelman *et al., J. Pharm. Sci.* **63**, 1886 (1974). Pharmacokinetics and biotransformation in humans: M. Hümpel *et al., Eur. J. Drug Metab. Pharmacokinet.* **4**, 237 (1979). Hypnotic effect: A. Doenicke *et al., Anaesthesist* **28**, 578 (1979). Comparative study: H. Ott *et al., ibid.* 29. Absorption, distribution, excretion of ^{14}C-lormetazepam: R. Girkin *et al., Xenobiotica* **10**, 401 (1980). Radioimmunologic study: M. Hümpel *et al., Clin. Pharmacol. Ther.* **28**, 673 (1980).

Crystals from ethanol/THF, mp 205-207°.

Note: This is a controlled substance (depressant): **21 CFR,** 1308.14.

THERAP CAT: Sedative, hypnotic.

5582. Lornoxicam. [70374-39-9] 6-Chloro-4-hydroxy-2-methyl-N-2-pyridinyl-2H-thieno[2,3-e]-1,2-thiazine-3-carboxamide 1,1-dioxide; 6-chloro-4-hydroxy-2-methyl-3-(2-pyridylcarbamoyl)-2H-thieno[2,3-e]-1,2-thiazine-1,1-dioxide; chlortenoxicam; Ro-13-9297; TS-110; Xefo. C$_{13}$H$_{10}$ClN$_3$O$_4$S$_2$; mol wt 371.82. C 41.99%, H 2.71%, Cl 9.53%, N 11.30%, O 17.21%, S 17.25%. Cyclooxygenase inhibitor; structurally similar to tenoxicam, *q.v.* Prepn: R. Pfister *et al.,* **DE 2838851**; *eidem,* **US 4180662** (both 1979 to Hoffmann-La Roche). Clinical pharmacokinetics: S. I. Ankier *et al., Postgrad. Med. J.* **64**, 752 (1988). Symposium on pharmacology and clinical experience: *ibid.* **66**, Suppl. 4, S1-S50 (1990). Overview of pharmacology and safety assessment: T. P. Pruss *et al., ibid.* S18.

Orange to yellow crystals, mp 225-230° (dec). pKa$_2$ 4.7. uv max: 371 nm. Partition coefficient (*n*-octanol/pH 7.4 buffer): 1.8.

LD$_{50}$ orally in mice, rats, rabbits, dogs, monkeys: >10 mg/kg (Pruss).

THERAP CAT: Anti-inflammatory; analgesic.

5583. Losartan. [114798-26-4] 2-Butyl-4-chloro-1-[[2′-(1H-tetrazol-5-yl)[1,1′-biphenyl]-4-yl]methyl]-1H-imidazole-5-methanol; 2-*n*-butyl-4-chloro-5-hydroxymethyl-1-[[2′-(1*H*-tetrazol-5-yl)biphenyl-4-yl]methyl]imidazole; 2-butyl-4-chloro-1-[*p*-(*o*-1*H*-tetrazol-5-ylphenyl)benzyl]imidazole-5-methanol. C$_{22}$H$_{23}$ClN$_6$O; mol wt 422.91. C 62.48%, H 5.48%, Cl 8.38%, N 19.87%, O 3.78%. Non-peptide angiotensin II receptor antagonist. Prepn: D. J. Carini, J. J. V. Duncia, **EP 253310**; D. J. Carini *et al,* **US 5138069** (1988, 1992 both to Du Pont); D. J. Carini *et al., J. Med. Chem.* **34**, 2525 (1991). Angiotensin receptor binding study: A. T. Chiu *et al., J. Pharmacol. Exp. Ther.* **252**, 711 (1990); receptor subtype specificity: A. T. Chiu *et al., Biochem. Biophys. Res. Commun.* **172**, 1195 (1990). Pharmacology of active metabolite, **EXP-3174**: P. C. Wong *et al., J. Pharmacol. Exp. Ther.* **255**, 211 (1990). Symposium on pharmacology: *Am. J. Hypertens.* **4**, 271S-353S (1991). Review of clinical experience in hypertension: M. McIntyre *et al., Pharmacol. Ther.* **74**, 181-194 (1997). Clinical effect on mortality in heart failure: B. Pitt *et al., Lancet* **355**, 1582 (2000). Renoprotective effect in diabetic nephropathy: B. M. Brenner *et al., N. Engl. J. Med.* **345**, 861 (2001).

Light yellow solid, mp 183.5-184.5°. pKa: 5-6.

Monopotassium salt. [124750-99-8] Du Pont 753; DUP-753; MK-954; Cozaar; Lortaan; Lorzaar; Losaprex; Neo-Lotan. C$_{22}$-H$_{22}$ClKN$_6$O; mol wt 461.00.

Monopotassium salt mixture with hydrochlorothiazide. Fortzaar; Hyzaar.

THERAP CAT: Antihypertensive.

5584. Loteprednol Etabonate. [82034-46-6] (11β,17α)-17-[(Ethoxycarbonyl)oxy]-11-hydroxy-3-oxoandrosta-1,4-diene-17-carboxylic acid chloromethyl ester; chloromethyl 17α-ethoxycarbonyloxy-11β-hydroxyandrosta-1,4-diene-3-one-17β-carboxylate; 17α-ethoxycarbonyloxy-Δ'-cortienic acid chloromethyl ester; CDDD-5604; HGP-1; P-5604; Alrex; Lotemax. C$_{24}$H$_{31}$ClO$_7$; mol wt 466.95. C 61.73%, H 6.69%, Cl 7.59%, O 23.98%. Ophthalmic corticosteroid. Prepn: N. S. Bodor, **BE 889563** (1981 to Otsuka); *idem,* **US 4996335** (1991). Physicochemical properties: M. Alberth *et al., J. Biopharm. Sci.* **2**, 115 (1991). HPLC determn in plasma and urine: G. Hochhaus *et al., J. Pharm. Sci.* **81**, 1210 (1992). NMR structural studies: S. Rachwal *et al., Steroids* **61**, 524 (1996); *idem et al., ibid.* **63**, 193 (1998). Metabolism and transdermal permeability: N. Bodor *et al., Pharm. Res.* **9**, 1275 (1992). Evaluation of effect on intraocular pressure: J. D. Bartlett *et al., J. Ocul. Pharmacol.* **9**, 157 (1993). Clinical trial in keratoconjunctivitis sicca: S. C. Pflugfelder *et al., Am. J. Ophthalmol.* **138**, 444 (2004). Review of ophthalmic clinical studies: J. F. Howes, *Pharmazie* **55**, 178-183 (2000).

Crystals from THF + hexane, mp 220.5-223.5°. Soly at 25° (mg/ml): 0.0005 in water; 0.037 in 50% propylene glycol + water. Lipophilicity (log K): 3.04.

THERAP CAT: Anti-inflammatory (topical).

5585. Lotrifen. [66535-86-2] 2-(4-Chlorophenyl)-(1,2,-4)triazolo[5,1-*a*]isoquinoline; 2-(*p*-chlorophenyl)-*s*-triazolo[5,1-*a*]isoquinoline; L-12717; DL-717-IT; Canocenta; Privaprol. C$_{16}$-H$_{10}$ClN$_3$; mol wt 279.72. C 68.70%, H 3.60%, Cl 12.67%, N 15.02%. Non-hormonal antifertility agent. Prepn: **BE 815498**; A. Omodei-Salé *et al.*, **US 4075341** (1974, 1978 both to Lepetit). Pharmacokinetics: G. GalliZani *et al.*, *J. Pharmacobio-Dyn.* **5**, 55 (1981). Pregnancy-terminating effect in dogs: G. Galliani, A. Omodei-Salé, *J. Small Anim. Pract.* **23**, 295 (1982). Effect on subsequent fertility: G. Galliani *et al.*, *IRCS Med. Sci.* **12**, 433, 435 (1984). *Review:* A. Assandri *et al.*, *Rev. Drug Metab. Drug Interact.* **4**, 237 (1982).

Crystals mp 238-240°.

THERAP CAT (VET): Abortifacient.

5586. Lovastatin. [75330-75-5] (2*S*)-2-Methylbutanoic acid (1*S*,3*R*,7*S*,8*S*,8a*R*)-1,2,3,7,8,8a-hexahydro-3,7-dimethyl-8-[2-[(2*R*,4*R*)-tetrahydro-4-hydroxy-6-oxo-2*H*-pyran-2-yl]ethyl]-1-naphthalenyl ester; (1*S*,3*R*,7*S*,8*S*,8a*R*)-1,2,3,7,8,8a-hexahydro-3,7-dimethyl-8-[2-[(2*R*,4*R*)-tetrahydro-4-hydroxy-6-oxo-2*H*-pyran-2-yl]ethyl]-1-naphthalenyl (*S*)-2-methylbutyrate; 1,2,6,7,8,8a-hexahydro-β,δ-dihydroxy-2,6-dimethyl-8-(2-methyl-1-oxobutoxy)-1-naphthaleneheptanoic acid δ-lactone; 2β,6α-dimethyl-8α-(2-methyl-1-oxobutoxy)mevinic acid lactone; mevinolin; 6α-methylcompactin; monacolin K; MK-803; Lovalip; Mevacor; Mevinacor; Mevlor; Sivlor. C$_{24}$H$_{36}$O$_5$; mol wt 404.54. C 71.26%, H 8.97%, O 19.77%. Fungal metabolite; potent inhibitor of HMG-CoA reductase, the rate controlling enzyme in cholesterol biosynthesis. Isoln from *Monascus ruber:* A. Endo, *J. Antibiot.* **32**, 852 (1979); from *Aspergillus terreus:* R. L. Monaghan *et al.*, **US 4231938** (1980 to Merck & Co.). Structure and biochemical properties: A. W. Alberts *et al.*, *Proc. Natl. Acad. Sci. USA* **77**, 3957 (1980). Total synthesis: M. Hirama, M. Iwashita, *Tetrahedron Lett.* **24**, 1811 (1983). Review of syntheses: T. Rosen, C. H. Heathcock, *Tetrahedron* **42**, 4909-4951 (1986). Biosynthesis: M. D. Greenspan, J. B. Yudkovitz, *J. Bacteriol.* **162**, 704 (1985); R. N. Moore *et al.*, *J. Am. Chem. Soc.* **107**, 3694 (1985). HPLC determn in plasma and bile: R. J. Stubbs *et al.*, *J. Chromatogr.* **383**, 438 (1986). Clinical pharmacology: S. M. Grundy, G. L. Vega, *J. Lipid Res.* **26**, 1464 (1985). Clinical comparison with gemfibrozil, *q.v.:* M. J. Tikkanen *et al.*, *Am. J. Cardiol.* **62**, 35J (1988). Review of clinical experience: J. A. Tobert, *Am. J. Cardiol.* **62**, 28J-34J (1988). Comprehensive description: G. S. Brenner *et al.*, *Anal. Profiles Drug Subs. Excip.* **21**, 277-305 (1992). Prevention of acute coronary events in men and women with average cholesterol levels: J. R. Downs *et al.*, *J. Am. Med. Assoc.* **279**, 1615 (1998).

White crystals, mp (under N$_2$): 174.5°. [α]$_D^{25}$ +323° (c = 0.5 g in 100 ml acetonitrile). uv max: 231, 238, 247 nm (A$^{1\%}$ 532, 621,

418). Soly at room temp (mg/ml): acetone 47, acetonitrile 28, *n*-butanol 7, *i*-butanol 14, chloroform 350, *N*,*N*-dimethylformamide 90, ethanol 16, methanol 28, *n*-octanol 2, *n*-propanol 11, *i*-propanol 20, water 0.4 × 10^{-3}. LD$_{50}$ orally in mice: >1000 mg/kg (Endo).

THERAP CAT: Antilipemic.

5587. Loxapine. [1977-10-2] 2-Chloro-11-(4-methyl-1-piperazinyl)dibenz[*b*,*f*][1,4]oxazepine; oxilapine; CL-62362; S-805; SUM-3170. C$_{18}$H$_{18}$ClN$_3$O; mol wt 327.81. C 65.95%, H 5.53%, Cl 10.82%, N 12.82%, O 4.88%. Prepn: **NL 6406089**; Schmutz *et al.*, **US 3546226** (1964, 1970 both to Wander); *eidem Helv. Chim. Acta* **50**, 245 (1967); Coppola, **US 3412193** (1968 to Am. Cyanamid). Crystal structure: D. B. Cosulich, F. M. Lovell, *Acta Crystallogr.* **33B**, 1147 (1977). Pharmacology: Schmutz *et al.*, *Chim. Ther.* **2**, 424 (1967); Latimer, *J. Pharmacol. Exp. Ther.* **166**, 151 (1969). Toxicity data: Stille *et al.*, *Arzneim.-Forsch.* **15**, 841 (1965). Toxicity studies: Mineshita *et al.*, *Oyo Yakuri* **4**, 293 (1970), *C.A.* **76**, 81145v (1972). Review of pharmacology and therapeutic efficacy: R. C. Heel *et al.*, *Drugs* **15**, 198-217 (1978).

Pale yellowish crystals from petr ether, mp 109-110°. LD$_{50}$ orally in mice: 65 mg/kg (Stille).

Succinate. [27833-64-3] CL-71563; Loxapac; Loxitane. C$_{18}$-H$_{18}$ClN$_3$O.C$_4$H$_6$O$_4$; mol wt 445.90.

THERAP CAT: Anxiolytic.

5588. Loxiglumide. [107097-80-3] 4-[(3,4-Dichlorobenzoyl)amino]-5-[(3-methoxypropyl)pentylamino]-5-oxopentanoic acid; (±)-4-(3,4-dichlorobenzamido)-*N*-(3-methoxypropyl)-*N*-pentylglutaramic acid; CR-1505. C$_{21}$H$_{30}$Cl$_2$N$_2$O$_5$; mol wt 461.38. C 54.67%, H 6.55%, Cl 15.37%, N 6.07%, O 17.34%. Cholecystokinin type-1 (CCK-1) antagonist. Prepn: F. Makovec *et al.*, **WO 8703869**; *eidem*, **US 4769389** (1987, 1988 both to Rotta). Pharmacology and receptor binding: I. Setnikar *et al.*, *Arzneim.-Forsch.* **37**, 703 (1987). Pharmacokinetics: *idem et al.*, *ibid.* **38**, 716 (1988). Effect on bilio-pancreatic secretion: W. E. Schmidt *et al.*, *Digestion* **46**, Suppl. 2, 232 (1990). Clinical evaluation in irritable bowel syndrome: P. A. Cann *et al.*, *Ann. N.Y. Acad. Sci.* **713**, 449 (1994); in nonulcer dyspepsia: A. S. B. Chua *et al. ibid.* 451; in pancreatitis: K. Shiratori *et al.*, *Pancreas* **25**, e1 (2002).

(*R*)-Form

Crystals from acetone, mp 113-115°. pKa ~5. Soly in water: 0.01%.

(*R*)-**Form.** [119817-90-2] Dexloxiglumide; CR-2017. HPLC determn in plasma: R. Brodie *et al.*, *J. Chromatogr. B* **784**, 91 (2003). *In vitro* biopharmaceutical properties: S. Tolle-Sander *et al.*, *J. Pharm. Sci.* **92**, 1968 (2003). Clinical pharmacokinetics: C. Webber *et al.*, *Xenobiotica* **33**, 625 (2003). Clinical evaluation in irritable bowel syndrome: F. Cremonini *et al.*, *Am. J. Gastroenterol.* **100**, 652 (2005). Soly (μg/ml): 33 (pH 3.4), 533 (pH 7.5). pKa 4.48.

THERAP CAT: Gastroprokinetic.

5589. Loxoprofen. [68767-14-6] α-Methyl-4-[(2-oxocyclopentyl)methyl]benzeneacetic acid; (±)-*p*-[(2-oxocyclopentyl)methyl]hydratropic acid. C$_{15}$H$_{18}$O$_3$; mol wt 246.30. C 73.15%, H 7.37%, O 19.49%. Non-steroidal anti-inflammatory pro-drug; the active metabolite is the *trans*-cyclohydroxypentane. Prepn of race-mate: A. Terada *et al.*, **DE 2814556**; *eidem*, **US 4161538** (1978, 1979 both to Sankyo); of enantiomers: A. Terada, E. Misaka, **EP 55588**; *eidem*, **US 4400534** (1982, 1983 both to Sankyo). Use as topical anti-inflammatory: A. Terada *et al.*, **BE 889149** (1981 to Sankyo), *C.A.* **96**, 199326w (1982). Metabolism: Y. Tanaka *et al.*, *Chem. Pharm. Bull.* **31**, 3656 (1983); *eidem, ibid.* **32**, 1040 (1984). Structure of metabolites: S. Naruto *et al., ibid.* 258. Optical inversion of (2*R*)- to (2*S*)-isomer after oral administration to rats: H. Nagashima *et al., ibid.* 251. Inhibition of *in vivo* and *in vitro* prostaglandin synthesis: K. Matsuda *et al., Biochem. Pharmacol.* **33**, 2473 (1984).

Colorless oil. bp$_{0.3}$ 190-195°. mp 108.5-111°.

Sodium salt. [80382-23-6] CS-600; Loxonin. C$_{15}$H$_{17}$NaO$_3$; mol wt 268.28.

THERAP CAT: Anti-inflammatory; analgesic.

5590. Lubeluzole. [144665-07-6] (α*S*)-4-(2-Benzothiazol-ylmethylamino)-α-[(3,4-difluorophenoxy)methyl]-1-piperidine-ethanol; R-87926; Prosynap. C$_{22}$H$_{25}$F$_2$N$_3$O$_2$S; mol wt 433.51. C 60.95%, H 5.81%, F 8.76%, N 9.69%, O 7.38%, S 7.40%. Modulates the glutamate-activated nitric oxide synthase (NOS) pathway. Prepn: R. A. Stokbroekx, G. A. J. Grauwels, **EP 501552**; **US 5434168** (1992, 1995 both to Janssen). Mechanism of action study: M. De Ryck *et al., J. Pharmacol. Exp. Ther.* **279**, 748 (1996); A. S. Lesage *et al., ibid.* 759. Clinical pharmacokinetics: J. De Keyser *et al., Clin. Ther.* **19**, 1340 (1997). Clinical trial in acute ischemic stroke: J. Grotta *et al., Stroke* **28**, 2338 (1997).

Crystals from 2,2'-oxybispropane, mp 65.8°. [α]$_D^{20}$ +4.38° (c = 1 in methanol).

THERAP CAT: Neuroprotective.

5591. Lucanthone Hydrochloride. [548-57-2] 1-[[2-(Di-ethylamino)ethyl]amino]-4-methyl-9*H*-thioxanthen-9-one hydro-chloride; 1-(2-diethylaminoethylamino)-4-methylthiaxanthone hy-drochloride; MS-752; RP-3735; Miracil D; Nilodin; Miracol; Tix-antone. C$_{20}$H$_{25}$ClN$_2$OS; mol wt 376.94. C 63.73%, H 6.69%, Cl 9.41%, N 7.43%, O 4.24%, S 8.51%. Prepd by the reaction of 1-chloro-4-methylthiaxanthone with *asym*-diethylethylenediamine: Mauss, *Naturwissenschaften* **33**, 253 (1946); *idem, Ber.* **81**, 19 (1948); Sharp, *J. Chem. Soc.* **1951**, 2961; Archer, Suter, *J. Am. Chem. Soc.* **74**, 4296 (1952). Review of mode of action: Weinstein, Hirschberg, *Prog. Mol. Subcell. Biol.* **2**, 232 (1971). *Review:* Hirschberg in *Antibiotics* vol. **3**, J. W. Corcoran, F. E. Hahn, Eds. (Springer-Verlag, New York, 1975) pp 274-303.

Yellow crystals from alcohol, mp 195-196°. Freely sol in water. Aq soln (orange) is neutral. Slightly sol in alcohol.

Free base. mp 64-65°. Sol in the usual organic solvents.

THERAP CAT: Anthelmintic (Schistosoma).

5592. Lucensomycin. [13058-67-8] Antibiotic FI 1163; FI-1163; Etruscomicina; Etruscomycin. C$_{36}$H$_{53}$NO$_{13}$; mol wt 707.80. C 61.09%, H 7.55%, N 1.98%, O 29.39%. Polyene antifungal antibiotic isolated from cultures of *Streptomyces lucensis:* Arca-mone *et al., G. Microbiol.* **4**, 119 (1957); Arcamone, Perego, *Ann. Chim. (Rome)* **49**, 345 (1959); Marini, Pennella, *Proc. Symp. Anti-biotics Prague* (May 1959) p 148; Arcamone *et al.*, **US 3170837** (1965 to Farmitalia). Structure: Guadiano *et al., Tetrahedron Lett.* **1966**, 3559, 3567; *Gazz. Chim. Ital.* **96**, 1470 (1966); *Chim. Ind. (Milan)* **48**, 1327 (1966). Revised structure: R. C. Pandey, K. L. Rinehart, *J. Antibiot.* **29**, 1035 (1976).

Crystalline powder. [α]$_D^{20}$ +296° (pyridine), +50° (methanolic 0.1*N* HCl). uv max: 218, 278, 290, 303, 318 nm (E$_{1cm}^{1\%}$ 300, 370, 780, 1170, 1098). Practically insol in water, anhydr alcohol, non-polar solvents. Sol in pyridine, dimethylformamide. Unstable beyond pH 6-8, and to heat, light, or air.

THERAP CAT: Antifungal.

5593. Luciferin. A generic term referring to a substrate which, upon oxidation by the enzyme luciferase, produces biolumi-nescence. Luciferins isolated from different species may vary greatly in structure, although in many cases identical structures have been found in widely diverse animals. The most widely studied luciferins are those isolated from the sea pansey, *Renilla reniformis,* the ostracod, *Cypridina hilgendorfii,* the limpet, *Latia neritoides,* and the firefly, *Photinus pyralis (see* separate entry, Fire-fly Luciferin). Structure of *Renilla reniformis* luciferin: K. Hori *et al., Proc. Natl. Acad. Sci. USA* **74**, 4285 (1977). *Review:* M. J. Cormier *et al., Fortschr. Chem. Org. Naturst.* **30**, 1-60 (1973).

5594. Lucifer Yellow(s). Water soluble fluorescent dyes. Description of properties and potential uses: W. W. Stewart, *Cell* **14**, 741 (1978). Prepn: *idem, J. Am. Chem. Soc.* **103**, 7615 (1981). Use in flux kinetics: C. L. Bowman, H. Tedeschi, *Biochim. Bio-phys. Acta* **731**, 261 (1983); in intercellular communications: M. H. El-Fouly *et al., Exp. Cell Res.* **168**, 422 (1987); as covalent marker: K. M. Lowe, R. E. McCarty, *Biochemistry* **37**, 2507 (1998).

Lucifer Yellow CH   R = HN—C(=O)—NH—NH$_2$

Lucifer Yellow VS   R =

Lucifer Yellow CH. [67769-47-5] 6-Amino-2-[(hydrazino-carbonyl)amino]-2,3-dihydro-1,3-dioxo-1*H*-benz[*de*]isoquinoline-5,8-disulfonic acid dilithium salt; lucifer yellow carbohydrazide; 4-amino-*N*-[(hydrazinocarbonyl)amino]-2,3-naphthalimide-3,6-disulfonate. $C_{13}H_9Li_2N_5O_9S_2$; mol wt 457.25. Fluffy orange hygroscopic powder. uv max (water, excitation max): 280, 428 nm (ε 24200, 11900); emission max: 540 nm. Quantum yield: 0.21.

Lucifer Yellow VS. [71231-14-6] 6-Amino-2-[3-(ethenyl-sulfonyl)phenyl]-2,3-dihydro-1,3-dioxo-1*H*-benz[*de*]isoquinoline-5,8-disulfonic acid dilithium salt; lucifer yellow vinylsulfone. $C_{20}H_{12}Li_2N_2O_{10}S_3$; mol wt 550.39. Crystals. uv max (water, excitation max): 280, 428 nm (ε 24600, 12200); emission max: 540 nm. Quantum yield: 0.24.

USE: Fluoroprobe for biological tracing.

5595. Lufenuron. [103055-07-8] *N*-[[[2,5-Dichloro-4-(1,-1,2,3,3,3-hexafluoropropoxy)phenyl]amino]carbonyl]-2,6-difluoro-benzamide; 1-[2,5-dichloro-4-(1,1,2,3,3,3-hexafluoropropoxy)-phenyl]-3-(2,6-difluorobenzoyl)urea; fluphenacur; CGA-184699; Program. $C_{17}H_8Cl_2F_8N_2O_3$; mol wt 511.15. C 39.95%, H 1.58%, Cl 13.87%, F 29.73%, N 5.48%, O 9.39%. Chitin synthesis inhibitor. Prepn: J. Drabek, M. Böger, **EP 179022**; *eidem*, **US 4798837** (1986, 1989 both to Ciba-Geigy). Effect on fleas following oral administration in cats: W. F. Hink *et al.*, *J. Med. Entomol.* **28**, 424 (1991). HPLC determn: M. Zakson *et al.*, *Pestic. Sci.* **35**, 117 (1992). Review of properties and field trials in crops: F. Buholzer *et al.*, *Meded. Fac. Landbouwwet. Univ. Gent* **57**, 781-790 (1992).

Colorless, odorless, crystalline solid, mp 174.1°. Vapor pressure (25°): <4 × 10^{-6} Pa. Soly (20°): water <0.1 ppm; acetone 40%; cyclohexanone 35%; xylene 5%; methanol 4.5%. Log P (*n*-octanol/water): 5.12. LD$_{50}$ in rats (mg/kg): >2000 orally; LC$_{50}$ in rats (mg/m³): >2350 (Buholzer).

THERAP CAT (VET): Ectoparasiticide.

5596. Lumazine. [487-21-8] 2,4(1*H*,3*H*)-Pteridinedione. $C_6H_4N_4O_2$; mol wt 164.12. C 43.91%, H 2.46%, N 34.14%, O 19.50%. Prepn from 4,5-diamino-2,6-dihydoxypyrimidine and glyoxal sodium bisulfate in the presence of ammonia: Weijlard *et al.*, *J. Am. Chem. Soc.* **67**, 804 (1945); **US 2479442** (1950 to Merck & Co.); from 5,6-diaminouracil hydrosulfite + ethylene glycol disulfonic acid disodium salt + HCl: Dallacker, Steiner, *Ann.* **660**, 98 (1962).

Yellow to orange needles from water, mp 348-349°. Soly in water at 25° = 0.125%. Sol in acetic acid. Aq solns have a bluish-green fluorescence when neutral, a green fluorescence when alkaline, and a blue fluorescence when acid.

5597. Lumefantrine. [82186-77-4] (9*Z*)-2,7-Dichloro-9-[(4-chlorophenyl)methylene]-α-[(dibutylamino)methyl]-9*H*-fluo-rene-4-methanol; 2-dibutylamino-1-[2,7-dichloro-9-(4-chloroben-zylidene)-9,11-fluoren-4-yl]ethanol; *dl*-benflumelol; benflumetol; BFL; CGP-56695. $C_{30}H_{32}Cl_3NO$; mol wt 528.94. C 68.12%, H 6.10%, Cl 20.11%, N 2.65%, O 3.02%. Racemic aryl alcohol originally synthesized in the 1970's by the Academy of Military Medical Sciences in Beijing, China. Inhibits hemozoin formation. Prepn: R. Deng *et al.*, **CN 1042535** (1990 to Acad. Military Med. Sci., Microbiol. & Epidemic Dis. Instit.); *C.A.* **114**, 6046 (1991).

LC determn in plasma: A. Annerberg *et al.*, *J. Chromatogr. B* **822**, 330 (2005). In vitro activity against *Plasmodium falciparum:* B. Pradines *et al.*, *Antimicrob. Agents Chemother.* **43**, 418 (1999).

Odorless, yellow powder. Poorly sol in water, oil, and most organic solvents. Sol in unsaturated fatty acids.

Co-artemether. [141204-94-6] CPG-56697; Coartem; Riamet. Fixed 6:1 mixture with artemether, *q.v.* Clinical pharmacokinetics and bioavailability: F. Ezzet *et al.*, *Br. J. Clin. Pharmacol.* **46**, 553 (1998). Clinical trial in children against *P. falciparum* malaria: C. Hatz *et al.*, *Trop. Med. Int. Health* **3**, 498 (1998); in adults: S. Looareesuwan *et al.*, *Am. J. Trop. Med. Hyg.* **60**, 238 (1999). Review of comparative clinical trials in malaria: A. A. Omari *et al.*, *Trop. Med. Int. Health* **9**, 192-199 (2004).

THERAP CAT: Antimalarial.

5598. Lumichrome. [1086-80-2] 7,8-Dimethylbenzo[*g*]-pteridine-2,4-(1*H*,3*H*)-dione; 7,8-dimethylalloxazine; 6,7-dimethyl-alloxazine. $C_{12}H_{10}N_4O_2$; mol wt 242.23. C 59.50%, H 4.16%, N 23.13%, O 13.21%. Irradiation product of riboflavine. Isoln: Karrer *et al.*, *Helv. Chim. Acta* **17**, 1010 (1934). Prepn: Tishler, Wellman, **US 2417143** (1947 to Merck & Co.); Cresswell, Wood, *J. Chem. Soc.* **1960**, 4768; Bardos *et al.*, **US 3057865** (1962 to Armour Pharm. Co.); Seng, Ley, *Angew. Chem.* **84**, 1061 (1972).

Pale yellow crystals from pyridine or pyridine + alcohol, mp >300°. Sparingly sol in methanol and 90% hot ethanol, water and chloroform. The aqueous, alcoholic and chloroformic solns fluoresce blue. Absorption spectrum: Karrer *et al.*, *loc. cit.*

5599. Lumiflavine. [1088-56-8] 7,8,10-Trimethylbenzo[*g*]-pteridine-2,4(3*H*,10*H*)-dione; 7,8,10-trimethylisoalloxazine. $C_{13}H_{12}N_4O_2$; mol wt 256.26. C 60.93%, H 4.72%, N 21.86%, O 12.49%. Irradiation product of riboflavine. Isoln: Warburg, Christian, *Biochem. Z.* **266**, 377 (1933). Structure: Kuhn, Rudy, *Ber.* **67**, 1298 (1934). Prepn: Tishler, Wellman, **US 2417143** (1947 to Merck & Co.); Birch, Moye, *J. Chem. Soc.* **1958**, 2622; Yoneda *et al.*, *Chem. Pharm. Bull.* **20**, 1832 (1972).

Orange crystals from 12% acetic acid, mp 320°. Purified by sublimation in vacuum, mp 330°. Freely sol in chloroform; very sparingly sol in water and most organic solvents. Aq and chloroformic solns fluoresce green. uv max: 269, 355, 445 nm (ε 38,800, 11,700, 11,800) in 0.1*N* NaOH and 264, 373, 440 nm (ε 34,700, 11,400, 10,400) in 0.1*N* HCl.

5600. Luminol. [521-31-3] 5-Amino-2,3-dihydro-1,4-phthalazinedione; *o*-aminophthalylhydrazide; 3-aminophthalic hydrazide; *o*-aminophthaloyl hydrazide. $C_8H_7N_3O_2$; mol wt 177.16. C 54.24%, H 3.98%, N 23.72%, O 18.06%. Prepn from 3-nitrophthalic acid: Huntress *et al., J. Am. Chem. Soc.* **56**, 241 (1934); Redemann, Redemann, *Org. Synth.* **29**, 78, 8 (1949); L. Fieser, *Organic Experiments* (Boston, 1964) pp 240-242. Chemiluminescent: Weber, *Ber.* **75**, 565 (1942); Weber *et al., ibid.* **76**, 366 (1943).

Crystals, mp 319-320°. Oxidation of luminol is accompanied by a striking emission of light.

Note: Not to be confused with Luminal.

USE: Detection of copper, iron, peroxides, cyanides.

5601. Lumiracoxib. [220991-20-8] 2-[(2-Chloro-6-fluorophenyl)amino]-5-methylbenzeneacetic acid; 5-methyl-2-(2′-chloro-6′-fluoroanilino)phenylacetic acid; COX-189; Prexige. $C_{15}H_{13}$-ClFNO$_2$; mol wt 293.72. C 61.34%, H 4.46%, Cl 12.07%, F 6.47%, N 4.77%, O 10.89%. Selective cyclooxygenase-2 (COX-2) inhibitor. Prepn: R. A. Fujimoto *et al.,* **WO 9911605**; *eidem,* **US 6310099** (1999, 2001 both to Novartis). Clinical evaluation of gastroduodenal tolerability: C. Rordorf *et al., Aliment. Pharmacol. Ther.* **18**, 533 (2003). Clinical experience in dysmenorrhea: M. Bitner *et al., Int. J. Clin. Pract.* **58**, 340 (2004); in rheumatoid arthritis: P. Geusens *et al. ibid.* 1033; in tension headache: E. Packman *et al., Headache* **45**, 1163 (2005). Review of clinical pharmacology: C. M. Rordorf *et al., Clin. Pharmacokinet.* **44**, 1247-1266 (2005); of clinical experience in osteoarthritis: F. Berenbaum *et al., J. Int. Med. Res.* **33**, 21-41 (2005); in osteoarthritis, rheumatoid arthritis, and dental pain: T. J. Schnitzer *et al., Curr. Med. Res. Opin.* **21**, 151-161 (2005).

mp 158-159°.

THERAP CAT: Anti-inflammatory.

5602. Lumisterol. [474-69-1] (3β,9β,10α,22E)-Ergosta-5,7,22-trien-3-ol. $C_{28}H_{44}O$; mol wt 396.65. C 84.78%, H 11.18%, O 4.03%. Differs from ergosterol by spatial arrangement involving the methyl group at C-10. Prepd by ultraviolet irradiation of a benzene-alcohol soln of ergosterol: Askew *et al., Proc. Roy. Soc. (London)* **B109**, 488 (1932). Stereochemistry: Castells *et al., J. Chem. Soc.* **1959**, 1159. Dehydrogenation with selenium gives Diel's hydrocarbon, 3′-methyl-1,2-cyclopentenophenanthrene.

Needles from acetone-methanol, mp 118°. $[\alpha]_D^{19}$ +191.5°, $[\alpha]_{546}^{19}$ +235.4° (c = 2 in acetone). uv max: 265, 280 nm: Windaus *et al., Ann.* **493**, 259 (1932); Heilbron *et al., J. Chem. Soc.* **1937**, 411.

Practically insol in water. Sol in organic solvents. Forms a monomolecular compd with calciferol, mp 122°.

Acetate. $C_{30}H_{46}O_2$. mp 100°. $[\alpha]_D^{19}$ +130.5°, $[\alpha]_{546}^{19}$ +163° (c = 1.8 in acetone).

5603. Lunacridine. [83-58-9] 3-[(2R)-2-Hydroxy-3-methylbutyl]-4,8-dimethoxy-1-methyl-2(1*H*)-quinolinone. $C_{17}H_{23}$-NO$_4$; mol wt 305.37. C 66.86%, H 7.59%, N 4.59%, O 20.96%. From bark of *Lunasia costulata* Miq., and *L. quercifolia* K. Schum. et Lauterb., *Rutaceae.* (+)-Form is naturally occurring. Isoln: Boorsma, *Bull. Inst. Bot. Buitenzorg* **21**, 8 (1904). Structure: Goodwin, Horning, *J. Am. Chem. Soc.* **81**, 1908 (1959). Synthesis: Clarke, Grundon, *J. Chem. Soc.* **1964**, 438. Synthesis and stereochemistry: R. M. Bowman *et al., J. Chem. Soc. Perkin Trans. 1* **1973**, 1051. Short synthesis of racemate: M. Ramesh, P. Shanmugam, *Indian J. Chem.* **24B**, 767 (1985).

Crystals from methanol/water, mp 86-87°. $[\alpha]_D^{25}$ +28.1°; $[\alpha]_{436}^{25}$ +76.5° (c = 0.935 in ethanol). uv spectra: Goodwin, Horning, *loc. cit.* Very slightly sol in water; freely sol in alcohol, benzene, chloroform, ether, ethyl acetate, carbon disulfide, petr ether.

Hydroperchlorate. $C_{17}H_{24}ClNO_8$. Shiny flakes from methanol/ether, mp 146-148°; remelts at 193-195°. $[\alpha]_D^{25}$ +22.3°; $[\alpha]_{436}^{25}$ +60.7° (c = 0.750 in ethanol).

(±)-**Form.** [52306-35-1] Prisms from petr ether, mp 72-74°. uv max (methanol): 239, 258, 285, 292, 333 nm (ε 24000, 26300, 8300, 7800, 3100).

5604. Lunacrine. [82-40-6] (2R)-3,9-Dihydro-8-methoxy-9-methyl-2-(1-methylethyl)furo[2,3-*b*]quinolin-4(2*H*)-one. C_{16}-H$_{19}$NO$_3$; mol wt 273.33. C 70.31%, H 7.01%, N 5.12%, O 17.56%. From bark of *Lunasia costulata* Miq., and *L. amara* Blanco, *Rutaceae.* Isoln: Boorsma, *Bull. Inst. Bot. Buitenzorg* **6**, 15 (1900). Structure: Goodwin, Horning, *J. Am. Chem. Soc.* **81**, 1908 (1959). Synthesis: Clarke, Grundon, *J. Chem. Soc.* **1964**, 438. Stereochemistry: Bowman *et al., J. Chem. Soc. Perkin Trans. 1* **1973**, 1051.

Fine needles from ethyl acetate, mp 117-119°. $[\alpha]_D^{25}$ −50.4°; $[\alpha]_{436}^{25}$ −116° (c = 0.806 in ethanol). Practically insol in water. Freely sol in alcohol, benzene, chloroform, ether, carbon disulfide, ethyl acetate; slightly sol in petr ether.

dl-**Form.** [95723-59-4] Prisms from ethyl acetate + pentane, mp 146-148°. $[\alpha]_D^{25}$ +2.3°; $[\alpha]_{436}^{25}$ +4.2° (c = 0.864 in ethanol).

5605. Lunasine. [6901-22-0] (2R)-2,3-Dihydro-4,8-dimethoxy-9-methyl-2-(1-methylethyl)furo[2,3-*b*]quinolinium. $[C_{17}H_{22}NO_3]^+$. From bark of *Lunasia costulata* Miq., and *L. quercifolia* K. Schum. et Lauterb., *Rutaceae.* Isoln: Boorsma, *Bull. Inst. Bot. Buitenzorg* **6**, 14 (1900). Structure: Price, *Aust. J. Chem.* **12**, 458 (1959). Stereochemistry: Bowman *et al., J. Chem. Soc. Perkin Trans. 1* **1973**, 1051.

(−)-**Form perchlorate.** [121543-68-8] $C_{17}H_{22}NO_3 \cdot ClO_4$. Microcrystalline powder from methanol + ether, mp 195-196°. $[\alpha]_D^{20}$ −29.3° (c = 0.46 in methanol).

5606. Lunularic Acid. [23255-59-6] 2-Hydroxy-6-[2-(4-hydroxyphenyl)ethyl]benzoic acid; 6-(p-hydroxyphenethyl)-salicylic acid. $C_{15}H_{14}O_4$; mol wt 258.27. C 69.76%, H 5.46%, O 24.78%. Dihydrostilbene growth inhibitor isolated from liverworts and algae. Isoln from *Lunularia cruciata* (L.) Dum., *Lunulariaceae*, and characterization: I. F. M. Valio *et al.*, *Nature* **223**, 1178 (1969); I. F. M. Valio, W. W. Schwab, *J. Exp. Bot.* **21**, 138 (1970); from more than 70 species of liverwort: J. Gorham, *Phytochemistry* **16**, 249 (1977); from cultures of *Marchantia polymorphia*: S. Abe, Y. Ohta, *ibid.* **22**, 1917 (1983). Synthesis: Y. Arai *et al.*, *Tetrahedron Lett.* **1972**, 1615; S. Haneck, K. Schreiber, **DD 126866** (1977 to Akad. Wissenschaft. D.D.R.), *C.A.* **88**, 152249t (1978). Effect on liverwort growth: J. Gorham, *Phytochemistry* **17**, 99 (1978). Metabolism by *L. cruciata*: R. J. Pryce, *ibid.* **11**, 1355 (1972).

Pale yellow crystals from methanol/water, mp 192°. uv max in neutral ethanol: 280, 287, 308 nm (ε 3300, 3600, 4200); in weakly alkaline ethanol: 300 nm (ε 6600).

USE: Growth inhibitor for lower plants.

5607. Lupanine. (7α,7aα,14α,14aβ)-Dodecahydro-7,14-methano-2H,11H-dipyrido[1,2-a:1',2'-e][1,5]diazocin-11-one; dodecahydro-7,14-methano-4H,6H-dipyrido[1,2-a:1',2'-e][1,5]-diazocin-4-one. $C_{15}H_{24}N_2O$; mol wt 248.36. C 72.54%, H 9.74%, N 11.28%, O 6.44%. Racemic lupanine is found in white lupins, d-lupanine is found in blue lupins, l-lupanine has been prepd from the natural racemic form. Structure: Davis, *Arch. Pharm.* **235**, 199, 218, 229 (1897); Clemo, Leitch, *J. Chem. Soc.* **1928**, 1811; Clemo *et al.*, *ibid.* **1931**, 429; **1933**, 644; Ing, *ibid.* **1933**, 504; Karrer *et al.*, *Helv. Chim. Acta* **11**, 1062 (1928), **13**, 1292 (1930); Winterfeld, Holschneider, *Ber.* **64**, 137, 2415 (1931), **66**, 1751 (1933); *Ann.* **499**, 109 (1932); Winterfeld, Kneuer, *Ber.* **64**, 150 (1931); Winterfeld, Hoffman, *Arch. Pharm.* **275**, 5, 65 (1937). Abs config of l-form: Okuda *et al.*, *Chem. Ind. (London)* **1961**, 1116. Crystal structure of dl-form: H. Doucerain *et al.*, *Acta Crystallogr.* **B32**, 3213 (1976). Biosynthetic study of d-form: W. M. Golebewski, I. D. Spenser, *J. Am. Chem. Soc.* **106**, 7925 (1984). *See also* sparteine, q.v.

d- form

dl-Form. [4356-43-8] Orthorhombic prisms from acetone, mp 98-99°. bp$_{1.0}$ 185-195°. Sol in water, alcohol, ether, chloroform. Insol in petr ether. *See:* Soldaini, *Arch. Pharm.* **231**, 321 (1893); Couch, *J. Am. Chem. Soc.* **56**, 1423 (1934).

Dihydrochloride. $C_{15}H_{24}N_2O \cdot 2HCl$. Deliquescent prisms, mp 185° (dec).

Hydrochloride dihydrate. $C_{15}H_{24}N_2O \cdot HCl \cdot 2H_2O$. Crystals, mp 177-178°. mp 250-252° (dry).

d-Form. [550-90-3] 2-Oxosparteine. Syrup crystallizing difficultly in hygroscopic needles, mp 40-44°. bp$_3$ 190-193°. n_D^{24} 1.5444. $[\alpha]_D^{25}$ +84° (c = 4.8 in alc). Freely sol in water, alcohol, chloroform, ether. Sol in petr ether.

Hydrochloride dihydrate. $C_{15}H_{24}N_2O \cdot HCl \cdot 2H_2O$. Rhombic crystals from water, mp 127° (dry).

l-Form. [486-88-4] Hydrorhombinine. Viscous oil, bp$_{1.0}$ 186-188°. $[\alpha]_D$ about −61° in acetone.

α-Isolupanine. [486-87-3] cis-cis-Isomer of lupanine: Marion, Leonard, *Can. J. Chem.* **29**, 355 (1951). Isoln of d-form from *Lupinus sericeus* Pursh., *L. perennis* L. and *L. augustifolius, Leguminosae*: Marion *et al.*, *ibid.* **31**, 181 (1953); Rink, Schäfer, *Arch. Pharm.* **287**, 290 (1954). Needles from petr ether, mp 75-76°. $[\alpha]_D^{26}$ +39° (c = 0.77). $[\alpha]_D^{26}$ +65.9° (c = 3.4 in abs ethanol).

5608. Lupeol. [545-47-1] (3β)-Lup-20(29)-en-3-ol; monogynol B; β-viscol; fagarasterol. $C_{30}H_{50}O$; mol wt 426.72. C 84.44%, H 11.81%, O 3.75%. Abundant plant triterpene. Occurs in the skin of lupin seeds, in chicle, in the latex of fig trees and of rubber plants. Was detected in cocoons of *Bombyx mori*. Isoln: Cohen, *Rec. Trav. Chim.* **28**, 368 (1909); Ruzicka *et al.*, *Helv. Chim. Acta* **20**, 1567 (1937). Identity with β-viscol: Meyer, Jeger, *ibid.* **31**, 1868 (1948). Identity with monogynol B: Chatterji *et al.*, *J. Sci. Ind. Res.* **18B**, 262 (1959). Structure: Ruzicka *et al.*, *Helv. Chim. Acta* **28**, 942 (1945); Ames *et al.*, *J. Chem. Soc.* **1951**, 450. Structure of hydrochloride: Halsall *et al.*, *ibid.* **1952**, 2862. Configuration: Barton, Holmes, *ibid.* **1952**, 78; Djerassi *et al.*, *J. Am. Chem. Soc.* **77**, 5330 (1955). NMR studies: Buckley *et al.*, *Chem. Ind. (London)* **1971**, 298. Total synthesis: Stork *et al.*, *J. Am. Chem. Soc.* **93**, 4945 (1971).

Needles from alcohol or acetone, mp 215°. $[\alpha]_D^{20}$ +27.2° (c = 4.8 in chloroform). Freely sol in ether, benzene, petr ether, warm alcohol. Practically insol in water, dil acid and alkalies.

Acetate. $C_{32}H_{52}O_2$. Needles from acetone, mp 218°. $[\alpha]_D^{20}$ +47.3° (c = 2 in chloroform).

Benzoate. $C_{37}H_{54}O_2$. Prisms from acetone, mp 273-274°. $[\alpha]_D^{20}$ +61° (0.78 g in 25 ml chloroform).

Hydrochloride. $C_{30}H_{50}O \cdot HCl$. Needles from ethanol, mp 211-212°. $[\alpha]$ −31° (c = 1.1 in chloroform).

5609. Lupinine. [486-70-4] [1R-trans]-Octahydro-2H-quinolizine-1-methanol; l-lupinine; (−)-lupinine. $C_{10}H_{19}NO$; mol wt 169.26. C 70.96%, H 11.31%, N 8.28%, O 9.45%. Naturally occurring l-form isolated from seeds and herb of *Lupinus luteus* L. and other *L.* species, *Leguminosae* also found in *Anabasis aphylla* L., *Chenopodiaceae*. Extraction procedure: J. F. Couch, *J. Am. Chem. Soc.* **56**, 2434 (1934). Structure and synthesis: R. W. Willstätter, E. Fourneau, *Ber.* **35**, 1910 (1902); P. Karrer *et al.*, *Helv. Chim. Acta* **11**, 1062 (1928); K. Winterfeld, F. W. Holschneider, *Ber.* **64B**, 137, 692 (1931); K. Winterfeld, *ibid.* 692. Synthesis of racemic lupinine: F. W. Holschneider, K. Winterfeld, *Arch. Pharm.* **277**, 192 (1939); G. C. Gerrans *et al.*, *Tetrahedron Lett.* **1975**, 4171; T. Iwashita *et al.*, *J. Org. Chem.* **47**, 230 (1982). Synthesis of racemic lupinine and **epi-lupinine**: G. R. Clemo *et al.*, *J. Chem. Soc.* **1937**, 965; H. Takahata *et al.*, *Chem. Pharm. Bull.* **34**, 4523 (1986); of l-**epi-lupinine**: M. L. Bremmer, S. M. Weinreb, *Tetrahedron Lett.* **24**, 261 (1983). Absolute configuration of (−)-form: R. C. Cookson, *Chem. Ind. (London)* **1953**, 339. Crystal structure: A. Koziol *et al.*, *Acta Crystallogr.* **B34**, 3491 (1978). Biosynthesis: Soucek, Schutte, *Angew. Chem.* **74**, 901 (1962); W. M. Golebiewski, I. D. Spenser, *J. Am. Chem. Soc.* **106**, 1441 (1984).

Stout, orthorhombic prisms from acetone, mp 68.5-69.2°. bp$_4$ 160-164°; bp$_{755}$ 269-270°. $[\alpha]_D^{26}$ −25.9° (c = 3 in water); $[\alpha]_D^{28}$ −21° (c = 9.5 in alcohol). Sol in water, alcohol, chloroform, ether. It is a strong base.

l-Form hydrochloride. $C_{10}H_{20}ClNO$. Orthorhombic prisms, mp 208-213°. $[\alpha]_D$ −14°.

dl-Form. Crystals from acetone, mp 58.5-59.5°.

5610. Luprostiol. [73523-00-9] (5Z)-7-[(1S,2R,3R,5S)-2-[[(2S)-3-(3-Chlorophenoxy)-2-hydroxypropyl]thio]-3,5-dihydroxy-cyclopentyl]-5-heptenoic acid; 9α,11α,15-trihydroxy-16-*m*-chloro-phenoxy-13-thia-17,18,19,20-tetranor-5-prostenoic acid; prostianol; EMD-34946; Prosolvin; Reprodin. $C_{21}H_{29}ClO_6S$; mol wt 444.97. C 56.68%, H 6.57%, Cl 7.97%, O 21.57%, S 7.21%. Analog of prostaglandin $F_{2\alpha}$, *q.v.* Prepn: J. Kraemer *et al.*, **DE 2513371** (1976 to E. Merck), *C.A.* **86**, 55069k (1977); *eidem*, **US 4309441** (1982 to E. Merck). Luteolytic study in cattle: H. De Vries, H. Feenstra, *J. Vet. Pharmacol. Ther.* **2**, 223 (1979). Estrus cycle regulation: D. Schams, H. Karg, *Theriogenology* **17**, 499 (1982), *C.A.* **97**, 50430p (1982).

THERAP CAT (VET): Luteolytic.

5611. Lupulin. Glandular trichomes separated from strobiles of *Humulus lupulus* L., *Moraceae* (hops). *Habit.* Europe, Asia, North America; widely cultivated. *Constit.* Lupamaric acid, humulol, about 3% volatile oil; resin, choline, wax (myricin), tannin, asparagin. Not less than 60% of lupulin is sol in ether.

THERAP CAT: Aromatic bitter, sedative.

THERAP CAT (VET): Formerly in nymphomania.

5612. Lupulon. [468-28-0] 3,5-Dihydroxy-2,6,6-tris(3-methyl-2-butenyl)-4-(3-methyl-1-oxobutyl)-2,4-cyclohexadien-1-one; β-bitter acid; β-lupulic acid. $C_{26}H_{38}O_4$; mol wt 414.58. C 75.32%, H 9.24%, O 15.44%. Antimicrobial constituent of hops. Isoln from commercial hops: Bungener, *Bull. Soc. Chim. Fr.* [2] **45**, 487 (1886); Barth, Lintner, *Ber.* **31**, 2022 (1898); Wöllmer, *Ber.* **49**, 780 (1916); Lewis, *et al.*, *J. Clin. Invest.* **28**, 916 (1949). Structure: Wöllmer, *Ber.* **58**, 672 (1925); Wieland, *ibid.* **102**, 2012 (1949); Govaert, Verzele, *Bull. Soc. Chim. Belg.* **58**, 432 (1949); Riedl, *Ber.* **85**, 692 (1952). Toxicity study: R. Hänsel, H. H. Wagener, *Arzneim.-Forsch.* **17**, 79 (1967).

Prisms from 90% methanol, mp 92-94°. Bitter taste esp in alc soln. Turns yellow and amorphous within a few days with development of an odor. Perfectly stable *in vacuo* even at 60°. Slightly acid reaction. Monobasic acid. Optically inactive. Soluble in methanol, ethanol, petr ether, hexane, isooctane. Slightly sol in neutral or acidic aq solns. Forms a sodium salt which is readily sol in water. The addition of 0.1% ascorbic acid exerts a marked protective action on the bacteriostatic activity of lupulon steamed or autoclaved at a concentration of 4 ppm in phosphate buffers at pH 6.5 and 8.5. LD$_{50}$ in mice, rats (mg/kg): 525, 100 orally (Hänsel, Wagener).

5613. Luteinizing Hormone. [9002-67-9] LH; ICSH; interstitial cell stimulating hormone. Gonadotropic hormone secreted by the anterior pituitary under the regulation of LH-RH, *q.v.* Together with follicle-stimulating hormone, *q.v.*, is critical to the growth and maturity of ovarian follicles. Stimulates androgen production by ovarian theca cells that is converted to estrogen by granulosa cells. Induces ovulation and the development of the corpus luteum. In males, stimulates production of testosterone by Leydig cells of the testes. Structure is a heterodimer of non-covalently linked α and β subunits; analogous with FSH, TSH and chorionic gonadotropin, *q.q.v.* Isoln from sheep pituitaries: C. H. Li *et al.*, *Endocrinology* **27**, 803 (1940); *eidem*, *Science* **92**, 355 (1940); *eidem*, *J. Am. Chem. Soc.* **64**, 367 (1942). Isoln from pig pituitaries: T. Shedlovsky *et al.*, *Science* **138** (1940); B. F. Chow *et al.*, *Endocrinology* **30**, 650 (1942). Complete amino acid sequence of ovine LH subunits: H. Papkoff *et al.*, *J. Am. Chem. Soc.* **93**, 1531 (1971); W.-K. Liu *et al.*, *J. Biol. Chem.* **247**, 4351, 4365 (1972); of human LH subunits: H. T. Keutmann *et al.*, *Endocr. Res. Commun.* **5**, 57 (1978); *eidem*, *Biochem. Biophys. Res. Commun.* **90**, 842 (1979). Reviews of structural studies: D. N. Ward *et al.*, *Recent Prog. Horm. Res.* **29**, 533-561 (1973); H. Papkoff *et al.*, *ibid.* 563-590. Review of physiological roles: M. Filicori, *Fertil. Steril.* **71**, 405-414 (1999); C. V. Rao, *ibid.* **76**, 1097-1100 (2001); of clinical experience in ovulation induction: M. Filicori, G. E. Cognigni, *J. Clin. Endocrinol. Metab.* **86**, 1437-1441 (2001); Z. Shoham, *Fertil. Steril.* **77**, 1170-1177 (2002).

White powder. Isoelectric point 4.6 (sheep), 7.45 (pig). Soluble in water. Chymotrypsin, trypsin and pepsin destroy the gonadotropic action of LH. Picrolonic, flavianic, picric, and trichloroacetic acids precipitate LH with retention of its physiological activity.

Lutropin alfa. [152923-57-4] Luteinizing hormone (human α-subunit reduced) complex with luteinizing hormone (human β-subunit reduced) glycoform α; Luveris. Recombinant human LH produced in genetically engineered Chinese hamster ovary cells. Review of prepn: S. Chappel, *Int. Congr. Symp. Sem. Ser.* **12**, 147-152 (1997). Series of articles on pharmacokinetics and bioavailability: *Fertil. Steril.* **69**, 189-209 (1998). Clinical trial in assisted reproductive procedures: E. Loumaye *et al.*, *J. Clin. Endocrinol. Metab.* **86**, 2607 (2001).

THERAP CAT: Gonad-stimulating principle.

5614. Luteolin. [491-70-3] 2-(3,4-Dihydroxyphenyl)-5,7-dihydroxy-4*H*-1-benzopyran-4-one; 3′,4′,5,7-tetrahydroxyflavone; digitoflavone; cyanidenon 1470. $C_{15}H_{10}O_6$; mol wt 286.24. C 62.94%, H 3.52%, O 33.54%. Found in many plants in glycosidic combination, *e.g.*, as the arabinoside: Perkin, *J. Chem. Soc.* **69**, 800 (1896); Fleischer, *Ber.* **32**, 1186 (1899); Perkin, Horsfall, *J. Chem. Soc.* **77**, 1315 (1900); Hayashi, Inoue, *Acta Phytochim.* **15**, 53 (1949); *C.A.* **43**, 8450 (1949). Identity with digitoflavone: Kiliani, Mayer, *Ber.* **34**, 3577 (1901). Synthesis: Hutchins, Wheeler, *J. Chem. Soc.* **1939**, 91. *See also* Bioflavonoids.

Monohydrate. Yellow needles from alc, dec 328-330°. Sublimes in high vacuum. Sparingly sol in water. Sol in alkalies forming yellow solns.

5-Glucoside. Galuteolin. $C_{21}H_{20}O_{11}$. From seeds of *Galega officinalis* L., *Leguminosae*: Barger, White, *Biochem. J.* **17**, 836 (1923). Structure: Nakamura, Hukuti, *J. Pharm. Soc. Jpn.* **60**, 449 (1940); *C.A.* **34**, 7910^3 (1940); Nordström, Swain, *J. Chem. Soc.* **1953**, 2764. Yellow needles from hot dil alc, dec 280°. Practically insol in water. Slightly sol in abs alcohol; sol in hot dil alcohol.

7-Glucoside. Cynaroside. $C_{21}H_{20}O_{11}$. From *Achillea millefolium* L., *Compositae*: Hörhammer *et al.*, *Acta Chim. Acad. Sci. Hung.* **40**, 463 (1964). Yellow needles from alc, mp 254-256°. uv max (CH$_3$OH): 350, 255 nm (log ε 4.30, 4.27).

5615. Lutetium. [7439-94-3] Lutecium. Lu; at. wt 174.967; at. no. 71; valence 3. A lanthanide; belongs to the yttrium group of rare earth metals. Naturally occurring isotopes (mass numbers): 175 (97.41%), 176 (2.59%), radioactive, $T_{1/2}$ 3.59 × 10^{10} years, β^- emitter. Known artificial radioactive isotopes: 151; 153-174; 177-181. Abundance in earth's crust: 0.75-0.8 ppm. Occurs in xenotime, gadolinite and other rare earth minerals. Discovered independently: Urbain, *Compt. Rend.* **145,** 759 (1907); **146,** 406 (1908); **152,** 141 (1911); and called *cassiopeium*: von Welsbach, *Sitzungsber. Akad. Wiss. Wien* **1907,** 468; *idem, Monatsh. Chem.* **29,** 181 (1908); **30,** 695 (1909). Isoln in form of salt: Prandtl, *Z. Anorg. Chem.* **238,** 321 (1938); Marsh, *J. Chem. Soc.* **1952,** 4804. Sepn by ion exchange: Spedding *et al., J. Am. Chem. Soc.* **76,** 2557 (1954). Toxicity study: Haley, *J. Pharm. Sci.* **54,** 663 (1965). Reviews of prepn, properties and compds: *The Rare Earths,* F. H. Spedding, A. H. Daane, Eds. (Krieger, Huntington, N.Y., 1971, reprint of 1961 ed.) 641 pp; Hulet, Bode, "Separation Chemistry of the Lanthanides and Transplutonium Actinides" in *MTP Int. Rev. Sci.: Inorg. Chem., Ser. One* vol. 7, K. W. Bagnall, Ed. (University Park Press, Baltimore, 1972) pp 1-45; Moeller, "The Lanthanides" in *Comprehensive Inorganic Chemistry* vol. 4, J. C. Bailar, Jr. *et al.,* Eds. (Pergamon Press, Oxford, 1973) pp 1-101; F. H. Spedding in *Kirk-Othmer Encyclopedia of Chemical Technology* vol. **19** (John Wiley & Sons, New York, 3rd ed., 1982) pp 833-854; *Chemistry of the Elements,* N. N. Greenwood, A. Earnshaw, Eds. (Pergamon Press, New York, 1984) pp 1423-1449. Brief review of properties: G. T. Seaborg, *Radiochim. Acta* **61,** 115-122 (1993).

Silvery-white metal. Hexagonal close-packed crystals. d 9.8404. mp 1663°. bp 3402°. Heat of fusion: 18.65 kJ/mol. Heat of sublimation (25°): 427.6 kJ/mol.

Oxide. Lu_2O_3. Cubic crystals.

Chloride. $LuCl_3$. Colorless crystals. Sublimes above 750°. mp 892 ±2°; sol in water. LD_{50} in mice: 315 mg/kg i.p.; 7.1 g/kg orally (Haley).

Sulfate. $Lu_2(SO_4)_3$. Octahydrate, soly in water (g/100 g): 42.27 (20°); 16.93 (40°).

5616. 2,6-Lutidine. [108-48-5] 2,6-Dimethylpyridine; α,α'-lutidin. C_7H_9N; mol wt 107.15. C 78.46%, H 8.47%, N 13.07%. Isolated from the basic fraction of coal tar: Heap *et al., J. Am. Chem. Soc.* **43,** 1936 (1921); from a bone oil fraction: Ladenburg, Roth, *Ber.* **18,** 51 (1885). Synthesis from ethyl acetoacetate, formaldehyde, and ammonia: Singer, McElvain, *Org. Synth.* **coll. vol. II,** 214 (1943).

Oily liquid. Odor of pyridine + peppermint. d_4^{20} 0.9252. mp −5.8°. bp_{760} 144°; bp_{87} 79°. n_D^{20} 1.49797. Solubility in water at 45.3° = 27.2% (w/w); at 48.1° = 18.1%; at 57.5° = 12.1%; at 74.5° = 9.5%. Also sol in alcohol, ether. Miscible with dimethylformamide and tetrahydrofuran.

5617. Lyapolate Sodium. [25053-27-4] Ethenesulfonic acid homopolymer sodium salt; sodium lyapolate; sodium apolate; sodium polyethylene sulfonate; polyethylene sodium sulfonate; PES; Peson. $[CH_2CH(SO_3Na)]_n$.

THERAP CAT: Anticoagulant.

5618. Lycoctonine. [26000-17-9] $(1\alpha,6\beta,14\alpha,16\beta)$-20-Ethyl-4-(hydroxymethyl)-1,6,14,16-tetramethoxyaconitane-7,8-diol; royline. $C_{25}H_{41}NO_7$; mol wt 467.60. C 64.21%, H 8.84%, N 3.00%, O 23.95%. Isomeric with delsoline. Originally isolated from *Aconitum lycoctonum* L., *Ranunculaceae*: Hubschmann, *Schweiz. Wochschr. Pharm.* **3,** 269 (1865). Widely distributed in *Aconitum* and *Delphinium* spp., *Ranunculaceae.* Structure: Edwards *et al., Can. J. Chem.* **34,** 1315 (1956); Anet *et al., ibid.* **35,** 400 (1957). Identity with royline: Edwards, Rodger, *ibid.* **37,** 1187 (1959). Stereochemistry: Przybylska, Marion, *ibid.* **1843.** Revised configuration: S. W. Pelletier *et al., J. Am. Chem. Soc.* **103,** 6536 (1981).

Crystals. Bitter taste. mp 143°. $[\alpha]_D^{20}$ +53° (ethanol). Slightly sol in water, ether, benzene; freely sol in alcohol, chloroform.

Ajacine. [509-17-1] *N*-Acetylanthranilic acid ester. $C_{34}H_{48}$-N_2O_9; mol wt 628.75. Needles from 70% alcohol, mp 154°. $[\alpha]_D$ +49.5° (c = 2 in abs alcohol); $[\alpha]_D^{16}$ +53° (c = 0.66 in chloroform). uv max: 223, 252, 310 nm (ε 28400, 16600, 5400). Slightly sol in water; sol in ether, alcohol with blue fluorescence.

Lycaconitine. [25867-19-0] *N*-Succinylanthranilic acid ester. $C_{36}H_{48}N_2O_{10}$. Isoln: Schulze, Bierling, *Arch. Pharm.* **251,** 8 (1913). White, amorphous powder, mp 111-114°. $[\alpha]_D$ +42°; also reported as +31.5°. Insol in water. Sol in alcohol, chloroform, ether.

5619. Lycodine. [20316-18-1] [4a*R*-(4aα,5α,10bα,12*R**)]-2,3,4,4a,5,6-Hexahydro-12-methyl-1*H*-5,10b-propano-1,7-phenanthroline. $C_{16}H_{22}N_2$; mol wt 242.36. C 79.29%, H 9.15%, N 11.56%. Isoln from *Lycopodium annotinum* L., *Lycopodiaceae*: F. A. L. Anet, C. R. Eves, *Can. J. Chem.* **36,** 902 (1958). Structure: W. A. Ayer, G. G. Iverach, *ibid.* **38,** 1823 (1960); F. A. L. Anet, M. V. Rao, *Tetrahedron Lett.* **1960,** 9. Synthesis of (±)-form: E. Kleinman, C. H. Heathcock, *ibid.* **1979,** 4125; C. H. Heathcock *et al., J. Am. Chem. Soc.* **104,** 1054 (1982).

Cryst powder, mp 118-119°. $[\alpha]_D$ −10° (c = 1.01 in ethanol). pKa's 3.97, 8.08.

5620. Lycopene. [502-65-8] ψ,ψ-Carotene; (*all-trans*)-lycopene. $C_{40}H_{56}$; mol wt 536.87. C 89.49%, H 10.51%. Carotenoid antioxidant occurring in ripe fruit, especially in tomatoes. One kg of fresh ripe tomatoes yields 0.02 g lycopene. Isoln procedure: R. Willstätter, H. H. Escher, *Z. Physiol. Chem.* **64,** 47 (1910). Chromatographic sepn from other carotenoids: A. Winterstein, *ibid.* **215,** 51 (1933); A. Winterstein, G. Stein, *ibid.* **220,** 247 (1933). HPLC determn in plasma: M. V. Vertzoni *et al., J. Chromatogr. B* **819,** 149 (2005). Structure: Willstätter, Escher, *loc. cit.;* Karrer and collaborators: *Helv. Chim. Acta* **11,** 751, 1201 (1928); **12,** 285 (1929); **13,** 1084 (1930); **14,** 435 (1931); Kuhn, Grundmann, *Ber.* **65,** 898, 1880 (1932). Synthesis: P. Karrer *et al., Helv. Chim. Acta* **33,** 1349 (1950); O. Isler *et al., ibid.* **39,** 463 (1956). Commercial prepn: Kabbe *et al., DE 1168890* (1964 to Bayer). Oral toxicity study: W. Mellert *et al., Food Chem. Toxicol.* **40,** 1581 (2002). Review of antioxidant activity and role in human health: A. V. Rao, S. Agarwal, *Nutr. Res.* **19,** 305-323 (1999).

Long, deep red needles from carbon disulfide + ethanol, from methylene chloride + methanol, mp 172-173°. Absorption max,

Consult the Name Index before using this section.

trans-form (petroleum ether): 446, 472, 505 nm ($E_{1cm}^{1\%}$ 2250, 3450, 3150). One gram dissolves in 50 ml carbon disulfide, in 3 l boiling ether, in 12 l boiling petr ether, in 14 l hexane at 0°. Sol in chloroform, benzene. Almost insol in methanol, ethanol, water.

15,15'-*cis*-Form. [59092-07-8] mp ~105° then solidifies again. Absorption max (petroleum ether): 361, 444, 470, 502 nm ($E_{1cm}^{1\%}$ 1110, 1280, 1660, 1280).

5621. Lycophyll. [19891-75-9] ψ,ψ-Carotene-16,16'-diol; (*all-trans*)-lycopene-16,16'-diol. $C_{40}H_{56}O_2$; mol wt 568.87. C 84.45%, H 9.92%, O 5.62%. Carotenoid pigment, isoln from *Solanum dulcamara* L. and *Lycopersicum esculentum* Mill., *Solanaceae* and structure: Zechmeister, Cholnoky, *Ber.* **69**, 422 (1936). Revised structure: Cholnoky, Szabolcs, *Tetrahedron Lett.* **1968**, 1931. Stereochemistry: Kelly *et al.*, *Acta Chem. Scand.* **25**, 1607 (1971). Synthesis: Kjosen, Liaaen-jensen, *ibid.* 1500.

Purple leaflets from benzene + methanol, needles from benzene + petr ether, mp 179°. Absorption max (benzene): 521, 487, 456 nm. Freely sol in carbon disulfide, less in benzene, ethanol, very slightly sol in petr ether.

Dipalmitate. Purple needles from benzene + methanol, mp 76°.

5622. Lycopodine. [466-61-5] (15*R*)-15-Methyllycopodan-5-one. $C_{16}H_{25}NO$; mol wt 247.38. C 77.68%, H 10.19%, N 5.66%, O 6.47%. From herb of *Lycopodium complanatum* L., *Lycopodiaceae*: Bödeker, *Ann.* **208**, 363 (1881). Structure: Harrison *et al.*, *Can. J. Chem.* **39**, 2086 (1961). Stereochemistry: Anet, *Tetrahedron Lett.* **1960**, no. 20, 13. Synthesis of (±)-form: G. Stork *et al.*, *J. Am. Chem. Soc.* **90**, 1647 (1968); W. A. Ayer *et al.*, *ibid.* 1648; C. H. Heathcock *et al.*, *ibid.* **100**, 8036 (1978); **104**, 1054 (1982); D. Schumann *et al.*, *Ann.* **1982**, 1700. Review of synthetic studies: Stork, *Pure Appl. Chem.* **17**, 383 (1968).

Bitter prisms, mp 114-115°; mp (racemate) 130-131°. $[\alpha]_D$ −24° (alc). Sol in water, alc, benzene, chloroform, ether.

5623. Lycopodium. Club-moss spores; Lycopodium seed (spores); vegetable sulfur. Spores of *Lycopodium clavatum* L., *Lycopodiaceae*. The spores of *Lycopodium annotinum* L., and of *L. anceps* Wall., *Lycopodiaceae* can also be used. The spores contain a substance called *selagnine*. *Habit.* North America, Europe, Asia; cultivated in Russia.

The spores are a fine yellowish powder which is highly flammable. Odorless and tasteless. Unctuous to the touch and easily sticking to the fingers. Lycopodium powder is very mobile and when poured on a flat surface should form an even layer, without visible lumps or dimples. When observed in chloral hydrate soln it is seen that the powder consists of unicellular lycopod spores, about 30 μ in diameter, in the shape of triangular pyramids with a convex base and rounded angles; a three-radical suture runs from the top of the pyramid along its facets. After warming and crushing the spores between glass slides, they burst along the suture and yield drops of oil, assuming a red color with alkalies. Adulteration usually consists of the admixture of flour (detected microscopically with iodine soln which stains the starch grains of the flour violet). Other admixtures may be pine pollen and sawdust. When mounted with chloral hydrate, pine pollen is larger than lycopodium, it is oval and has two lateral flying sacs, filled with air, and appearing black at the beginning of the observation. Sawdust is easily detected by the phloroglucinol test.

USE: As covering for pills or suppositories; in explosives, pyrotechnics, flashlight powders; as "dry parting compound" in foundry work for ornamental and nameplate castings. Review: Appel, *Sci. Mon.* **78**, 268 (1954).

THERAP CAT: Adsorbent.

5624. Lycopus. Bugleweed; sweet bugle; water bugle. Whole plant of *Lycopus virginicus* L., *Labiatae*. *Habit.* N. America. *Constit.* Volatile oil, resin, tannin, glucoside.

5625. Lycoramine. [21133-52-8] 1,2-Dihydrogalanthamine; 3,4-dihydrogalanthamine. $C_{17}H_{23}NO_3$; mol wt 289.37. C 70.56%, H 8.01%, N 4.84%, O 16.59%. One of the minor alkaloids of *Lycoris radiata* Herb., *Amaryllidaceae*: Kondo, Ishiwata, *Ber.* **70B**, 2427 (1937). From *Narcissus* spp.: Boit *et al.*, *ibid.* **90**, 725 2197 (1957). Tentative structure: Kobayashi, Uyeo, *Chem. Ind. (London)* **1956**, 177. Structure elucidation: William, Rogers, *Proc. Chem. Soc. London* **1964**, 357. Synthesis of the naturally occurring (−)-form: Barton, Kirby, *J. Chem. Soc.* **1962**, 806; of the (±)-form: N. Hazama *et al.*, *J. Chem. Soc. C* **1968**, 2947; Y. Misaka *et al.*, *ibid.* 2954; A. G. Schultz *et al.*, *J. Am. Chem. Soc.* **99**, 8065 (1977); S. F. Martin, P. J. Garrison, *J. Org. Chem.* **46**, 3567 (1981); **47**, 1513 (1982).

Plates from acetone, mp 121°. $[\alpha]_D^{27}$ −98° (alcohol). Freely sol in water; sol in alc, acetone. Its salts hydrolyze easily.

5626. Lycorine. [476-28-8] (1α,2β)-3,12-Didehydro-9,10-[methylenebis(oxy)]galanthan-1,2-diol; 3,3a-didehydrolycoran-1α,2β-diol; 2,4,5,7,12b,12c-hexahydro-1*H*-[1,3]dioxolo[4,5-*j*]pyrrolo[3,2,1-*de*]phenanthridine-1,2-diol; amarylline; belamarine; narcissine; galanthidine. $C_{16}H_{17}NO_4$; mol wt 287.31. C 66.89%, H 5.96%, N 4.88%, O 22.27%. Alkaloid isolated from the bulbs of *Lycoris radiata* L., *Narcissus pseudonarcissus* L., *N. tazetta* L., from *Buphane disticha* Herb., in *Crinum* spp., *Amaryllis belladonna* L., *Clivia miniata* Regel and other *Amaryllidaceae*. Extraction procedure: Cook, Loudon in Manske-Holmes, *Alkaloids* vol. II (Academic Press, 1952) p 336. Identity of lycorine and galanthidine: Proskurnina, *Dokl. Akad. Nauk SSSR* **90**, 565 (1953), *C.A.* **49**, 12500c (1955). Structure: Takeda *et al.*, *J. Am. Chem. Soc.* **80**, 2562 (1958). Stereochemistry: Nakagawa, Uyeo, *J. Chem. Soc.* **1959**, 3736; K. Kotera *et al.*, *Tetrahedron Lett.* **1966**, 2009. Crystal structure: R. Roques, *Acta Crystallogr.* **30B**, 296 (1974). Attempted synthesis: Dyke *et al.*, *Tetrahedron* **29**, 213 (1973). Synthesis: Y. Tsuda *et al.*, *Chem. Commun.* **1975**, 933; *eidem*, *J. Chem. Soc. Perkin Trans. 1* **1979**, 1358; T. Sano *et al.*, *Heterocycles* **14**, 1097 (1980); S. F. Martin, C. Tu, *J. Org. Chem.* **46**, 3763 (1981). Biosynthesis: Archer *et al.*, *Proc. Chem. Soc. London* **1963**, 168; Fugati, Mazza, *Chem. Commun.* **1972**, 936. Review: W. C. Wildman in *The Alkaloids* vol. XI, R. H. F. Manske, Ed. (Academic Press, New York, 1968) pp 307-400.

Stout prisms from alcohol, mp 275-280° (dec). $[\alpha]_D^{16}$ −129° (c = 0.16 in 98% alc). Alkaline reaction to litmus; salts hydrolyze easily. Sparingly sol in alcohol, chloroform, petr ether. Sol in dilute acids. Practically insol in water, alkalies.

Hydrochloride. $C_{16}H_{17}NO_4 \cdot HCl$. Long needles from water, mp 217° (dec with slight preliminary sintering). $[\alpha]_D^{20}$ +43°.

Hydrochloride monohydrate. Elongated prisms from water, mp 206°. Soluble in 20 parts water.

Methiodide. $C_{16}H_{17}NO_4 \cdot CH_3I$. Two forms exist which may be stereoisomeric about the nitrogen atom. α- Form: polyhedra from alc, dec 247°. $[\alpha]_D^{20}$ −46° (c = 1.52). Freely sol in water; sparingly sol in hot alcohol. β-Form: prisms contg $1H_2O$ from water, dec 198°, after recryst from alcohol, dec 281°. $[\alpha]_D^{20}$ +123° (c = 2.44). Freely sol in water and hot alcohol.

5627. Lycoxanthin. [19891-74-8] ψ,ψ-Carotene-16-ol; (all-trans)-lycopen-16-ol. $C_{40}H_{56}O$; mol wt 552.87. C 86.90%, H 10.21%, O 2.89%. Carotenoid isolated from *Solanum dulcamara* L., *Lycopersicum esculentum* Mill., *Solanaceae; Tamus communis* L., *Dioscoreaceae.* Isoln by chromatography and structure: Zechmeister, Cholnoky, *Ber.* **69**, 422 (1936). Structure: Karrer *et al., Helv. Chim. Acta* **13**, 268, 1084 (1930); **14**, 614, 843 (1931); Winterstein, *Angew. Chem.* **72**, 902 (1960). Revised structure: Cholnoky, Szabolcs, *Tetrahedron Lett.* **1968**, 1931. Stereochemistry: Kelly *et al., Acta Chem. Scand.* **25**, 1607 (1971). Total synthesis: Kjosen, Liaaen-jensen, *ibid.* 1500.

Purple needles from carbon disulfide. Reddish-brown round or acicular cryst aggregates from benzene + petr ether, mp 168°. Absorption max (acetone): 448, 474 ($E_{1cm}^{1\%}$ 3080), 505 nm. Sol in carbon disulfide and benzene. Moderately sol in petr ether. Sparingly sol in alc.

Monoacetate. Deep purple needles from benzene+ methanol, mp 137°. Freely sol in carbon disulfide; sparingly sol in alcohol, petr ether.

5628. Lymecycline. [992-21-2] N^6-[[[[(4S,4aS,5aS,6S,-12aS)-4-(Dimethylamino)-1,4,4a,5,5a,6,11,12a-octahydro-3,6,10,-12,12a-pentahydroxy-6-methyl-1,11-dioxo-2-naphthacenyl]carbonyl]amino]methyl]-L-lysine; tetracyclinemethylene lysine; N-lysinomethyltetracycline; Tetralisal; Tetralysal. $C_{29}H_{38}N_4O_{10}$; mol wt 602.63. C 57.80%, H 6.36%, N 9.30%, O 26.55%. Semi-synthetic antibiotic related to tetracycline, *q.v.* Prepn: R. K. Blackwood, K. J. Brunings, US 3042716 (1962 to Pfizer); F. Lauria, W. Logemann, DE 1134071 (1962 to Carlo Erba), *C.A.* **58**, 492 (1963); E. Tubaro, E. Raffaldoni, *Boll. Chim. Farm.* **100**, 9 (1961). Clinical pharmacokinetics: A. Schreiner, A. Digranes, *Chemotherapy (Basel)* **31**, 261 (1985). Comparison with doxycycline of phototoxic potential: M. Bjellerup, B. Ljunggren, *Br. J. Dermatol.* **130**, 356 (1994). Clinical trial in acne: L. Bossuyt *et al., Eur. J. Dermatol.* **13**, 130 (2003); of combination with adapalene: W. J. Cunliffe *et al., J. Am. Acad. Dermatol.* **49**, S218 (2003).

Sodium salt. $C_{29}H_{37}N_4NaO_{10}$; mol wt 624.61. uv max (CH_3-OH): 376 nm.

THERAP CAT: Antibacterial.

5629. Lynestrenol. [52-76-6] (17α)-19-Norpregn-4-en-20-yn-17-ol; 17α-ethinyl-17β-hydroxyestr-4-ene; 17α-ethynylestr-4-en-17β-ol; 3-desoxynorlutin; ethinylestrenol; Exluton(a); Exlutena; Orgametril; Orgametil; $C_{20}H_{28}O$; mol wt 284.44. C 84.45%, H

9.92%, O 5.62%. Prepn: de Winter *et al., Chem. Ind. (London)* **1959**, 905. Metabolism: Kamyab *et al., Biochem. J.* **103**, 14P (1967); *J. Endocrinol.* **42**, 337 (1968). Pharmacokinetics and metabolism: H. Kuhl *et al., Contraception* **26**, 303 (1982). Clinical trial of use in normophasic oral contraceptives: N. Dombrowicz *et al., ibid.* **22**, 537 (1980). Review of carcinogenicity studies: *IARC Monographs* **21**, 407-415 (1979).

Solid, mp 158-160°. $[\alpha]_D$ −13° (chloroform).

Mixture with ethinyl estradiol. [8064-76-4] Fysionorm; Minilyn; Ovanon; Ovoresta; Yermonil.

Mixture with mestranol. [8015-14-3] Lyndiol.

THERAP CAT: Progestogen. In combination with estrogen as oral contraceptive.

5630. Lypressin. [50-57-7] 8-L-Lysinevasopressin; Schweine-Vasopressin; Phe³-Lys⁸-oxytocin; Diapid; Postacton; Syntopressin. $C_{46}H_{65}N_{13}O_{12}S_2$; mol wt 1056.22. C 52.31%, H 6.20%, N 17.24%, O 18.18%, S 6.07%. Purification after isolation from hog pituitary glands: Ward, du Vigneaud, *J. Biol. Chem.* **222**, 951 (1956). Structure: du Vigneaud *et al., J. Am. Chem. Soc.* **75**, 4880 (1953); Bartlett *et al., ibid.* **78**, 2905 (1956). Synthesis: du Vigneaud *et al., loc. cit.;* Bartlett *et al., loc. cit.;* Bodanszky *et al., ibid.* **82**, 3195 (1960); Boissonnas, Huguenin, *Helv. Chim. Acta* **43**, 182 (1960); Zaoral, *Collect. Czech. Chem. Commun.* **30**, 1853 (1965); Meienhofer, Sano, *J. Am. Chem. Soc.* **90**, 2996 (1968); Meienhofer, Trzeciak, *Proc. Natl. Acad. Sci. USA* **68**, 1006 (1971). Configuration: Schally, Barret, *J. Am. Chem. Soc.* **87**, 2497 (1965). *Review:* E. Schröder, K. Lübke, *The Peptides* vol. II (Academic Press, New York, 1966) pp 336-350.

Cys–Tyr–Phe–Gln–Asn–Cys–Pro–Lys–GlyNH₂

THERAP CAT: Antidiuretic; vasopressor.

5631. Lysalbinic Acid. [9006-58-0] A colloidal substance prepd by the action of caustic alkalies on albumin, usually egg albumin, although it also may be obtained from serum albumin or from casein (caseolysalbinic acid): Paal, *Ber.* **35**, 2195 (1902); DE 129031 (1902); DE 132322 (1902). Composition: C 52.9%, H 7.0%, N 14.9%, S 1.2%.

Usually isolated as the Na salt, a brittle yellowish mass, readily sol in water, forming a colloidal soln which foams. It is precipitated by alc, and it may be purified by dialysis.

Colloidal gold. Prepd by adding a soln of gold chloride to a soln of lysalbinic acid. The intensely red hydrosol is precipitated with alcohol and dried. The precipitate forms hard, bronze-colored granules which may be stored for a long time, yielding a red, colloidal gold soln upon addn of water. Analysis of dried granules shows about 30% Au. See Paal, *Ber.* **35**, 2236-2244 (1902); DE 170433; DE 180730 (1906, 1907 to Kalle).

USE: As a protective colloid for metal sols, especially gold, silver, and mercury sols.

5632. Lysergamide. [478-94-4] 9,10-Didehydro-6-methyl-ergoline-8β-carboxamide; lysergic acid amide; ergine. $C_{16}H_{17}N_3$-O; mol wt 267.33. C 71.89%, H 6.41%, N 15.72%, O 5.98%. Isoln from *Rivea corymbosa* (L.) and from *Ipomoea tricolor* Cav., *Convolvulaceae:* Hofmann, Tscherter, *Experientia* **16**, 414 (1964). Prepn from lysergic acid hydrazide: Ainsworth, US 2756235 (1956 to Lilly); from lysergic acid and phosgene-dimethylformamide complex: Patelli, Bernardi, US 3141887 (1964 to Farmitalia). Microbiological production: Rutschmann, Kobel, US 3219545 (1965 to Sandoz).

Consult the Name Index before using this section.

Prisms from methanol, dec 242°. $[\alpha]_{5461}^{20}$ +15° (c = 0.5 in pyridine).

Methanesulfonate. $C_{16}H_{17}N_3O.CH_3SO_3H$. Prisms from methanol + acetone, dec 232°.

Note: This is a controlled substance (depressant): **21 CFR, 1308.13.**

5633. Lysergic Acid. [82-58-6] 9,10-Didehydro-6-methyl-ergoline-8-carboxylic acid. $C_{16}H_{16}N_2O_2$; mol wt 268.31. C 71.62%, H 6.01%, N 10.44%, O 11.93%. Lysergic acid and isolysergic acid are the main cleavage products formed on alkaline hydrolysis of the alkaloids which are characteristic of ergot. Jacobs, Craig *et al., J. Biol. Chem.* **104,** 547 (1934); **125,** 289 (1938); **130,** 399 (1939); **145,** 487 (1942); *J. Org. Chem.* **10,** 76 (1945). High-yield production by *Claviceps paspali:* Arcamone *et al., Proc. R. Soc. London Ser. B* **155,** 26 (1961). Total synthesis: Kornfeld *et al., J. Am. Chem. Soc.* **76,** 5256 (1954); **78,** 3087 (1956); M. Julia *et al., Tetrahedron Lett.* **1969,** 1569; V. W. Armstrong *et al., ibid.* **1976,** 4311; W. Oppolzer *et al., Helv. Chim. Acta* **64,** 478 (1981); R. Ramage *et al., Tetrahedron* **37,** Suppl. 9, 157 (1981); J. Rebek, D. F. Tai, *Tetrahedron Lett.* **24,** 859 (1983). Stereochemistry: Stoll *et al., Helv. Chim. Acta* **37,** 2039 (1954); Stenlake, *J. Chem. Soc.* **1955,** 1626; Leeman, Fabbri, *Helv. Chim. Acta* **42,** 2696 (1959). Absolute configuration: Stadler, Hofmann, *ibid.* **45,** 2005 (1962).

Hexagonal scales, plates with one or two moles H_2O from water, mp 240° (dec). $[\alpha]_D^{20}$ +40° (c = 0.5 in pyridine). Behaves as an acid and base, pKa 3.44, pKb 7.68. Moderately sol in pyridine. Sparingly sol in water and in neutral organic solvents; sol in NaOH, NH_4OH, Na_2CO_3, and HCl solns. Slightly sol in dil H_2SO_4.

Methyl ester. Thin leaflets from benzene, mp 168°.

Note: This is a controlled substance (depressant): **21 CFR, 1308.13.**

5634. Lysergide. [50-37-3] 9,10-Didehydro-*N,N*-diethyl-6-methylergoline-8β-carboxamide; *N,N*-diethyl-D-lysergamide; D-lysergic acid diethylamide; LSD; LSD-25; lysergsäure diethylamid. $C_{20}H_{25}N_3O$; mol wt 323.43. C 74.27%, H 7.79%, N 12.99%, O 4.95%. Microbial formation by *Claviceps paspali* over the hydroxyethylamide: Arcamone *et al., Proc. Roy. Soc. (London)* **155B,** 26 (1961). Partial synthesis: Stoll, Hofmann, *Helv. Chim. Acta* **26,** 944 (1943); **38,** 421 (1955). Industrial prepn: Pioch, **US 2736728**; Garbrecht, **US 2774763** (both 1956 to Lilly); Patelli, Bernardi, **US 3141887** (1964 to Farmitalia). Isotope-labeled LSD: Stoll *et al., Helv. Chim. Acta* **37,** 820 (1954). LC-MS determn in biological fluids: J. Canezin *et al., J. Chromatogr. B* **765,** 15 (2001). Toxicity data: E. Rothlin, *Ann. N.Y. Acad. Sci.* **66,** 668 (1957). *Review:* Hoffer, *Clin. Pharmacol. Ther.* **6,** 183 (1965). Book: *The Use of LSD in Psychotherapy and Alcoholism,* H. A. Abramson, Ed. (Bobbs-Merrill, Indianapolis, 1967) 697 pp.

Pointed prisms from benzene, mp 80-85°. $[\alpha]_D^{20}$ +17° (c = 0.5 in pyridine). uv max (ethanol): 311 nm ($E_{1cm}^{1\%}$ 257). LD_{50} in mice, rats, rabbits (mg/kg): 46, 16.5, 0.3 i.v. (Rothlin).

D-Tartrate. $C_{46}H_{64}N_6O_{10}$. Solvated, elongated prisms from methanol, mp 198-200°. $[\alpha]_D^{20}$ +30°. Soluble in water.

Note: This is a controlled substance (hallucinogen): **21 CFR, 1308.11.**

USE: In biochemical research as antagonist to serotonin. Has been used experimentally as adjunct in study and treatment of mental disorders.

5635. Lysidine. [534-26-9] 4,5-Dihydro-2-methyl-1*H*-imidazole; 2-methyl-2-imidazoline; methylglyoxalidine. $C_4H_8N_2$; mol wt 84.12. C 57.11%, H 9.59%, N 33.30%. Prepn: Chitwood, Reid, *J. Am. Chem. Soc.* **57,** 2424 (1935); King, McMillan, *ibid.* **68,** 1774 (1946); Kyrides, **US 2392326** and **US 2404299** (both 1946 to Monsanto); Ahrens, **US 2813862** (1957 to Organon).

Needles from benzene, mp 105°. bp 198-200°. Soluble in water, alc, chloroform; less sol in benzene, carbon tetrachloride, petr ether; practically insol in ether. *Keep well closed. Incompat:* Acids, metallic salts, alkaloids.

5636. Lysine. [56-87-1] L-Lysine; Lys; K; (*S*)-2,6-diamino-hexanoic acid; α,ε-diaminocaproic acid. $C_6H_{14}N_2O_2$; mol wt 146.19. C 49.29%, H 9.65%, N 19.16%, O 21.89%. An essential amino acid for human development; probably the most limited in the food chain. Identified in a hydrolysate of casein by Drechsel in 1889. Named "lysatine" from the Greek for "loosing", as it produced urea on treatment with barium hydroxide; changed to "lysine" in 1891. Verification of structure: E. Fischer, F. Weigert, *Ber.* **35,** 3772 (1902). Early chemistry and biochemistry: *Amino Acids and Proteins,* D. M. Greenberg, Ed. (Charles C. Thomas, Springfield, IL, 1951) 950 pp, *passim;* J. P. Greenstein, M. Winitz, *Chemistry of the Amino Acids* vols. **1-3** (John Wiley & Sons, Inc., New York, 1961) pp 2097-2124, *passim.* Review of supplementation of cereals: C. Feldberg, C. P. Hetzel, *Food Technol.* **12,** 496 (1958); of wheat proteins: S. B. Vaghefi *et al., Am. J. Clin. Nutr.* **27,** 1231-1246 (1974). Review of metabolism in mammals: F. C. Fellows, M. H. R. Lewis, *Biochem. J.* **136,** 329-334 (1973); of metabolic errors: N. A. J. Carson, *Clin. Endocrinol. Metab.* **3,** 71-86 (1974). Brief review of production by fermentation: *Nutr. Rev.* **43,** 88-90 (1985). Review of synthesis: G. Galili, *Plant Cell* **7,** 899-906 (1995).

Needles from water, hexagonal plates from dil alcohol. Darkens at 210°; dec 224.5°. $[\alpha]_D^{20}$ +14.6° (c = 6.5); $[\alpha]_D^{23}$ +25.9° (c = 2 in 6.0*N* HCl). pK_1 2.18; pK_2 8.95; pK_3 10.53. Very freely sol in water. Insol in common neutral solvents.

Dihydrochloride. $C_6H_{14}N_2O_2.2HCl$. Crystals from ethanol + ether, mp 193°. $[\alpha]_D^{20}$ +15.3° (c = 2).

Monohydrochloride. [657-27-2] Darvyl; Enisyl. $C_6H_{14}N_2$-O_2.HCl; mol wt 182.65. Crystals from dil ethanol. mp 263-264° when anhydrous. $[\alpha]_D^{25}$ +14.6° (c = 2 in 0.6N HCl).

Monoorotate. Lysortine. $C_{11}H_{18}N_4O_6$; mol wt 302.28. Prepn: GB 922361 (1962 to A.E.C. Soc. Chim. Org. Biol.). Crystals, dec 315°.

USE: Enrichment of cereals and feeds.

5637. Lysine Acetylsalicylate. [62952-06-1] DL-Lysine mono[2-(acetyloxy)benzoate]; lysine monosalicylate acetate; aspirin lysine salt; LAS; Aspidol; Aspisol; Delgesic; Flectadol; Lysal; Quinvet; Venopirin; Vetalgina. $C_{15}H_{22}N_2O_6$; mol wt 326.34. C 55.21%, H 6.79%, N 8.58%, O 29.42%. Water soluble, injectable aspirin derivative. Prepn: **FR 1295304** (1962 to Equilibre Biologique), *C.A.* **58,** 1536f (1963). Prepn of D,L isomers and racemate: **FR 2115060** (1972 to Metabio), *C.A.* **78,** 75877k (1972). Comparison with aspirin: S. Rampon *et al., Rhumatologie* **24,** 141 (1972). Pharmacokinetics: H. von Ross *et al., Klin. Wochenschr.* **56,** 1119 (1978); F. Gentit, *Gaz. Med. Fr.* **86,** 4539 (1979). Veterinary use as analgesic: P. Richez *et al., J. Vet. Pharmacol. Ther.* **2,** 231 (1979); *eidem, ibid.* **3,** 121 (1980). Analgesic activity in post-operative pain: K. Korttila *et al., Br. J. Anaesth.* **52,** 613 (1980); in articular pain: C. Diaz *et al., Clin. Ther.* **4,** 121 (1981). Use in treatment of premature labor: F. Wolff *et al., Arch. Gynecol.* **233,** 15 (1982). Comparison with aspirin in production of gastromucosal damage: J.-F. Bretagne *et al., Gastroenterol. Clin. Biol.* **8,** 28 (1984).

Crystals from ethanol, mp 154-156°. Sol in water; slightly sol in ethanol. Insol in methanol, acetone, ether.

THERAP CAT: Analgesic; antipyretic; anti-inflammatory.

THERAP CAT (VET): Analgesic; antipyretic; anti-inflammatory.

5638. L-Lysine L-Glutamate. [5408-52-6] L-Glutamic acid L-lysine salt. $C_{11}H_{23}N_3O_6$; mol wt 293.32. C 45.04%, H 7.90%, N 14.33%, O 32.73%. $H_2N(CH_2)_4CH(NH_2)COOH.HOOC$-$(CH_2)_2CH(NH_2)COOH$. Prepd from DL-lysine and L-glutamic acid as an intermediate in the resolution of DL-lysine: Emmick, Rogers, **US 2556907; US 2657230** (1951, 1953 both to du Pont).

Monohydrate. Crystals, $[\alpha]^{22}$ +3.73° (12% in water).

USE: As a flavor and nutritive additive to food: **GB 882163** (1961 to Stamicarbon N.V.).

5639. Lysostaphin. [9011-93-2] Antibiotic protein complex produced by *Staphylococcus staphyloliticus* with highly specific lytic activity against other *Staphylococcus* species. Contains three enzymes: a hexosaminidase, an amidase, and the major component, an endopeptidase which cleaves the polyglycine cross-linkages in the staphylococcal cell wall. Isoln and antibacterial spectrum: Schindler, Schuhardt, *Proc. Natl. Acad. Sci. USA* **51,** 414 (1964). Prepn by fermentation: *eidem,* **US 3278378** (1966); Zygmunt, Browder, **US 3398056** (1968 to Mead Johnson). The endopeptidase is a single polypeptide chain of mol wt 25,000: H. R. Trayer, C. E. Buckley, *J. Biol. Chem.* **245,** 4842 (1970). Identification of active principle: H. P. Browder *et al., Biochem. Biophys. Res. Commun.* **19,** 383 (1965). Characterization of three enzyme components: T. Wadstrom, O. Vesterberg, *Acta Pathol. Microbiol. Scand.* **79,** 248 (1971); O.-J. Iversen, A. Grov, *Eur. J. Biochem.* **38,** 293 (1973). Clinical studies to eradicate *Staph. aureus* from nasal carriers: R. L. Harris *et al., Antimicrob. Agents Chemother.* **1967,** 110; K. E. Quickel *et al., Appl. Microbiol.* **1971,** 446. Use as identification method for *Staphylococcus* sp.: K. H. Schleifer, W. E. Kloos, *J. Clin. Microbiol.* **1,** 337 (1975); P. J. Severance *et al., ibid.* **11,** 724 (1980); disk modification: B. Poutrel, J.-P. Caffin, *ibid.* **13,** 1023 (1982). *Review:* Zygmunt, Tavormina, *Progress in Drug Research* **Vol. 16,** E. Jucker, Ed. (Birkhauser Verlag, Basel, 1972) pp 309-333.

Isoelectric pt: pH 10.4-11.4. uv max: 278 nm. Sedimentation coeff 2.35 S. Destroyed by pepsin or trypsin. Inhibited by Hg^{2+}, Cu^{2+}, Zn^{2+}. LD_{50} (7-day) in mice, rats (mg/kg): 820, 530 i.v. (Zygmunt).

5640. Lysozyme. [9001-63-2] Muramidase; *N*-acetylmuramide glycanohydrolase; *N*-acetylmuramyl hydrolase; globulin G_1. Mol wt about 14,400 ± 100. Mucolytic enzyme with antibiotic properties, first discovered by A. Fleming: *Proc. Roy. Soc. London* **93B,** 306 (1922). Found in tears, nasal mucus, milk, saliva, blood serum, in a great number of tissues and secretions of different animals, vertebrates and invertebrates, in egg white, in some molds, and in the latex of different plants. Isoln from egg white: Alderton *et al., J. Biol. Chem.* **157,** 43 (1945); Alderton, Fevold, *ibid.* **164,** 1 (1946); *Biochem. Prep.* **1,** 67 (1949); Sophianopoulos *et al., J. Biol. Chem.* **237,** 1107 (1962); from *Ficus* latex: Meyer *et al., ibid.* **163,** 733 (1946). Structure consists of a single polypeptide chain of 129 amino acid subunits of 20 different kinds cross-linked by four disulfide bridges. Chromatographic studies: Goncalves *et al., Arch. Biochem. Biophys.* **60,** 171 (1956); King, Craig, *J. Am. Chem. Soc.* **80,** 3366 (1958). Complete amino acid sequence of egg white lysozyme: Jolles *et al., Biochim. Biophys. Acta* **78,** 668 (1963); Canfield, *J. Biol. Chem.* **238,** 2698 (1963). Synthetic studies of egg white lysozyme: L. E. Barston *et al.* in *Chemistry and Biology of Peptides, Proc. Am. Peptide Symp.,* J. Meienhofer, Ed. (Ann Arbor Science Publishers, Inc., Michigan, 1972) pp 231-233; J. J. Sharp *et al., J. Am. Chem. Soc.* **95,** 6097 (1973). Three dimensional structure: Blake *et al., Nature* **206,** 757 (1965); North, *Sci. J.* **2**(11), 55 (1966); Phillips, *Sci. Am.* **215,** 78 (Nov. 1966); Blake *et al., Proc. Roy. Soc. London* **167B,** 365 (1967). Primary chemical structure and tentative complete sequence of human milk lysozyme: Jolles, Jolles, *Helv. Chim. Acta* **52,** 2671 (1969). Complete primary structure of human milk lysozyme and comparison with lysozymes of various origins: *eidem, ibid.* **54,** 2668 (1971). Dissolves bacterial cell wall mucopolysaccharides by hydrolyzing the β-(1 → 4) linkages between *N*-acetyl-D-muramic acid and 2-acetylamino-2-deoxy-D-glucose residues. Also acts on chitin. *Reviews:* Salton, *Bacteriol. Rev.* **21,** 82 (1957); Acker, Hartsell, *Sci. Am.* **202,** 132 (June 1960); Jolles, "Lysozyme" in P. D. Boyer, H. Lardy, K. Myrback, *The Enzymes* **vol. 4,** (Academic Press, New York, 2nd ed., 1960) pp 431-445; *idem, Angew. Chem.* **76,** 20 (1964); Raftery, Dahlquist, *Fortschr. Chem. Org. Naturst.* **27,** 340 (1969); Hamaguchi, Hayashi, "Lysozyme" in *Proteins, Structure and Function* **vol. 1,** M. Funatsu *et al.,* Eds. (Kodansha, Tokyo, Wiley, New York, 1972) pp 85-222. Book: *Lysozyme,* E. F. Osserman *et al.,* Eds. (Academic Press, New York, 1974).

Crystals. Isoelectric pt: pH 10.5-11.0. Fairly stable in acid soln. Not affected by heat up to 55°: Cotterill, Winter, *Poult. Sci.* **33,** 1185 (1954).

Hydrochloride. [9066-59-5] Acdeam; Antalzyme; Immunozima; Lanzyme; Leftose; Likinozym; Lisozima; Murazyme; Neutase; Neuzyme; Toyolysom-DS.

THERAP CAT: Mucolytic enzyme. Antiviral.

5641. D-Lyxose. [1114-34-7] α-D-Lyxose. $C_5H_{10}O_5$; mol wt 150.13. C 40.00%, H 6.71%, O 53.29%. Prepd by the oxidation of calcium D-galactonate: Clark, *J. Biol. Chem.* **31,** 605 (1917); Fletcher *et al., J. Am. Chem. Soc.* **72,** 4546 (1950); by γ-irradiation of lactose: Adachi, *J. Dairy Sci.* **45,** 1427 (1962). Structure of β-D-lyxose: Hordvik, *Acta Chem. Scand.* **15,** 1781 (1961).

α-D-Lyxose

Hygroscopic monoclinic prisms from ethanol + ether, mp 106-107°. Sweet taste. d^{20} 1.545. Shows mutarotation: $[\alpha]_D^{20}$ +5.5° → −14.0° (c = 0.82 in water). Freely sol in water. One part dissolves in 38 parts abs alc at 17°; 100 ml of 90% alc satd at 20° contain 7.9 g.

Consult the Name Index before using this section.

M

5642. Mabuterol. [56341-08-3] 4-Amino-3-chloro-α-[[(1,1-dimethylethyl)amino]methyl]-5-(trifluoromethyl)benzene-methanol; 4-amino-α-[(*tert*-butylamino)methyl]-3-chloro-5-(trifluoromethyl)benzyl alcohol; 1-(4′-amino-3′-chloro-5′-trifluoromethyl-phenyl)-2-*tert*-butylaminoethanol; ambuterol. $C_{13}H_{18}ClF_3N_2O$; mol wt 310.74. C 50.25%, H 5.84%, Cl 11.41%, F 18.34%, N 9.02%, O 5.15%. Orally active β_2-adrenergic agonist related to clenbuterol, *q.v.* Prepn and resolution of isomers: **BE 808743** (1974 to Thomae); G. Engelhardt *et al.,* **US 4119710** (1978 to Boehringer Ing.); *eidem, Arzneim.-Forsch.* **34,** 1612 (1984). Series of articles on pharmacology, pharmacokinetics, toxicology and clinical studies: *ibid.* 1625-1700. Toxicity data: K. Amemiya *et al., ibid.,* 1680. Teratological study: A. M. Hoberman *et al., J. Am. Coll. Toxicol.* **4,** 91 (1985). Determn in human urine and plasma by enzyme immunoassay: I. Yamamoto *et al., J. Immunoassay* **6,** 261 (1985).

dl-Form hydrochloride. [95656-48-7] KF-868; PB-868Cl; Broncholin. $C_{13}H_{18}ClF_3N_2O.HCl$; mol wt 347.20. Crystals from ethyl acetate + ether, mp 205-206°. Fairly sol in water.LD$_{50}$ in male, female mice, male, female rats (mg/kg): 41.5, 51.1, 26.4, 28.1 i.v.; 60.3, 60.0, 76.3, 78.3 i.p.; 113.0, 125.7, 117.2, 123.1 s.c.; 220.8, 199.9, 319.3, 305.6 orally (Amemiya).
d-Form hydrochloride. [95656-54-5] mp >194° (slow dec). $[\alpha]_{364}^{20}$ +154.9° (c = 1 in methanol).
l-Form hydrochloride. [95656-55-6] mp >194° (slow dec). $[\alpha]_{364}^{20}$ −154.8° (c = 1 in methanol).
THERAP CAT: Bronchodilator; antiasthmatic.

5643. Macassar Oil. Kusum oil; Kon oil; Paka oil. From the nut kernels of *Schleichera trijuga* Willd., *Sapindaceae* (Ceylon oak). *Habit.* India, Burma, Ceylon, Java. *Constit.* Glycerides of oleic acid 60%, arachidic 20-25%, palmitic 5-8% stearic 2-6%; free acetic acid 1-2%. Unsaponifiable matter 1.5-3% (this may include cyanide-containing glycosides which are removed by careful refining). *Reviews:* Sen-Gupta, *J. Soc. Chem. Ind. London* **39,** 88T (1920); Dhingra *et al., ibid.* **48,** 281T (1929).

Yellowish-white oil. Pleasant odor. Melting range: 21-31° (initial to complete transparency). d_{15}^{99} 0.860. n_D^{21} 1.46757; n_D^{27} 1.46655; $n_D^{31.5}$ 1.4646; n_D^{45} 1.4636. Acid value 10-70; saponification value 220-230; iodine value 48-58; Reichert-Meissl value 16. Miscible with ether, chloroform, other vegetable oils, petrolatum, lanolin.
USE: In hair oil formulations.

5644. Maclurin. [519-34-6] (3,4-Dihydroxyphenyl)(2,4,6-trihydroxyphenyl)methanone; 2,3′,4,4′,6-pentahydroxybenzophenone; morintannic acid; moritannic acid; laguncurin; kino-yellow; C.I. Natural Yellow 11; C.I. 75240. $C_{13}H_{10}O_6$; mol wt 262.21. C 59.55%, H 3.84%, O 36.61%. From wood of *Chlorophora tinctoria* (L.) Gaud. (*Morus tinctoria* L., *Maclura tinctoria* (L.) D. Don), *Moraceae* (old fustic): Haley, Bassin, *J. Am. Pharm. Assoc.* **40,** 111 (1951); Laidlow, Smith, *Chem. Ind. (London)* **1959,** 1604; from *Morus alba* Linn., *Moraceae:* Spada *et al., Gazz. Chim. Ital.* **86,** 46 (1956). Identity with laguncurin and kino-yellow: Nierenstein, *Q. J. Pharm. Pharmacol.* **16,** 11 (1943). *See also Colour Index* **vol. 4** (3rd ed., 1971) p 4627.

Yellow needles from ethanol, mp 222-222.5°. Sol in 190 parts water; freely sol in alcohol or ether.
USE: Dyeing fabrics.

5645. Macromerine. [2970-95-8] α-[(Dimethylamino)-methyl]-3,4-dimethoxybenzenemethanol; α-[(dimethylamino)methyl]veratryl alcohol; 3,4-dimethoxy-α-[(dimethylamino)methyl]benzyl alcohol; dimethylaminomethyl 3,4-dimethoxyphenyl carbinol. $C_{12}H_{19}NO_3$; mol wt 225.28. C 63.98%, H 8.50%, N 6.22%, O 21.31%. Prepn of *dl*-form: La Manna *et al., Farmaco Ed. Sci.* **15,** 9 (1960); Chapman *et al., Proc. R. Soc. London Ser. B* **163,** (990), 116 (1965); Hodgkins *et al., Tetrahedron Lett.* **1967,** 1321; of *d*- and *l*-form: La Manna *et al., loc. cit.* Isoln of *l*-form from cactus, *Coryphantha macromeris* (Engelm.) Lem., Britton and Rose, *Cactaceae:* Hodgkins *et al., loc. cit.*

dl-Form. Crystals, mp 46-47°.
l-Form. Crystals, mp 66-67.5°. $[\alpha]_D^{25}$ −147.01° (c = 0.0390 g/ml chloroform), −42.61° (c = 0.0200 g/ml abs alcohol).
d-Form. Crystals, mp 60-62°.
dl-Form hydrochloride. $C_{12}H_{19}NO_3.HCl$. Crystals from ethanol, mp 163-164°.
l-Form hydrochloride. Crystals, mp 178-179°. $[\alpha]_D^{18}$ −41.3° (c = 2.04 in 50% ethanol).
d-Form hydrochloride. Crystals from ethanol, mp 178- 179°. $[\alpha]_D^{18}$ +51.5° (c = 2.2 in 50% ethanol).
Note: Both the *dl*- and *l*-forms are physiologically active, and caused hallucinogenic reactions when tested in animals (Hodgkins *et al., loc. cit.*).

5646. Macrophage Colony-Stimulating Factor. [81627-83-0] Colony-stimulating factor 1; M-CSF; CSF-1. Species specific hematopoietic growth factor which stimulates the development of committed progenitor cells to monocytes/macrophages. Also potentiates phagocytic activity and monocyte-mediated tumor cell cytotoxicity. Heavily glycosylated homodimer; produced in response to specific activating agents by a variety of cell types including monocytes, fibroblasts and endothelial cells. In humans, several molecular species have been identified which are produced via alternative splicing mechanisms from a single-copy gene. The primary transcripts include a 90 kDa glycoprotein, which is the principle form detected in serum and urine, and a fully bioactive, membrane-associated 40-50 kDa dimer. Murine M-CSF is similar to the human long form. Isoln from human urine: E. R. Stanley *et al., Fed. Proc.* **34,** 2272 (1975); from cultured human pancreatic carcinoma cells: M. Wu *et al., J. Biol. Chem.* **254,** 6226 (1979). Purification of murine M-CSF: E. R. Stanley, P. M. Heard, *ibid.* **252,** 4305 (1977). Characterization of human M-CSF: S. K. Das *et al., Blood* **58,** 630 (1981); K. Motoyoshi *et al., ibid.* **60,** 1378 (1982). Cloning of short form (human clone pcCSF-17): E. S. Kawasaki *et al., Science* **230,** 291 (1985); of long form (human clone p3ACSF-69): G. G. Wong *et al., ibid.* **235,** 1504 (1987). Review of molecular biology: E. S. Kawasaki, M. B. Ladner, *Immunol. Ser.* **49,** 155-176 (1990); of bioactivity and clinical studies: D. H. Munn, N.-K. V. Cheung, *Semin. Oncol.* **19,** 395-407 (1992).

Mirimostim. [121547-04-4] 1-214-Colony-stimulating factor 1 (human clone p3ACSF-69 protein moiety reduced) homodimer; Costilate; Leukoprol.

4-221-Colony-stimulating factor 1 (human clone p3ACSF-69 protein moiety reduced). [117276-75-2] Nonglycosylated, 218 amino acid polypeptide produced in *E. coli* by recombinant DNA technology. Prepn and renaturation into bioactive homodimer: R. Halenbeck *et al., BioTechnology* **7,** 710 (1989). Clinical evaluation in invasive fungal infections: J. Nemunaitis *et al., Blood* **82,** 1422 (1993). Immunomodulatory effects and pharmacokinetics: R. M. Bukowski *et al., J. Clin. Oncol.* **12,** 97 (1994).
THERAP CAT: Immunomodulator.

5647. Maddrell's Salt. [10361-03-2] Polymeric sodium metaphosphate. Upon heating NaH_2PO_4 or $NaNH_4HPO_4$ to 250°

and then slowly to 350°, first $Na_2H_2P_2O_7$ and then the insol Maddrell's salt is obtained, which is stable to about 500°; at 505° it changes to sodium trimetaphosphate, and above 607° to sodium hexametaphosphate. According to Maddrell, *Ann.* **61**, 63 (1847) the salt may be prepd by heating two parts $NaNO_3$ with one part H_3PO_4. An improved procedure is described by v. Knorre, *Z. Anorg. Chem.* **24**, 397 (1900). Structure: Jost, *Acta Crystallogr.* **16**, 428 (1963). *Reviews: see* Sodium Metaphosphate.

White powder. Practically insol in water and in aq solns of pyrophosphates and hexametaphosphates. Sol in mineral acids. Does not form complexes with Fe(II), Fe(III), U(IV) salts.

USE: In dentifrices, polishing agents, abrasive detergents.

5648. Maduramicin. [84878-61-5] (2R,3S,4S,5R,6S)-6-[(1R)-1-[(2S,5R,7S,8R,9S)-2-[(2S,2'R,3'S,5R,5'R)-3'-[(2,6-Dideoxy-3,4-di-O-methyl-β-L-*arabino*-hexopyranosyl)oxy]octahydro-2-methyl-5'-[(2S,3S,5R,6S)-tetrahydro-6-hydroxy-3,5,6-trimethyl-2H-pyran-2-yl][2,2'-bifuran]-5-yl]-9-hydroxy-2,8-dimethyl-1,6-dioxaspiro[4.5]dec-7-yl]ethyl]tetrahydro-2-hydroxy-4,5-dimethoxy-3-methyl-2H-pyran-2-acetic acid, monoammonium salt; antibiotic X-14868A ammonium salt; CL-273703; Cygro; $C_{47}H_{83}NO_{17}$; mol wt 934.16. C 60.43%, H 8.96%, N 1.50%, O 29.12%. Polyether antibiotic chemically related to the Ionomycins, *q.v.* Isoln as sodium salt from *Nocardia* sp X-14868 and biological activity: C.-M. Liu *et al., US 4278663* (1981 to Hoffmann-La Roche); as free acid hydrate from *Actinomadura yumaense* sp nov.: D. P. Labeda *et al., US 4407946* (1983 to Am. Cyanamid). Fermentation and properties: C.-M. Liu *et al., J. Antibiot.* **36**, 343 (1983). ^{13}C-NMR spectrum: S. Rajan, *ibid.* **37**, 1495 (1984). Biosynthetic studies: H.-R. Tsou *et al., ibid.* 1651; H.-R. Tsou *et al., ibid.* **40**, 94 (1987). Antimalarial activity: L. Oronsky, *US 4496549* (1985 to Am. Cyanamid). Nematocidal activity: I. B. Wood, *US 4510134* (1985 to Am. Cyanamid).

Sodium salt. $C_{47}H_{79}NaO_{17}$. Crystals from ethyl acetate + *n*-hexane, mp 193-195°. $[α]_D$ +40.6° (chloroform). $[α]_D$ +23.8° (methanol).

Note: Not to be confused with *maduramycin* isolated from *Actinomadura rubra,* by: W. F. Fleck *et al., 16th Interscience Conference on Antimicrob. Ag. Chemother.,* Chicago, 1976, *Abstracts of Papers,* no. 51.

THERAP CAT (VET): Coccidiostat.

5649. Mafenide. [138-39-6] 4-(Aminomethyl)benzenesulfonamide; α-amino-*p*-toluenesulfonamide; *p*-(aminomethyl)benzenesulfonamide; 4-homosulfanilamide; maphenide; Marfanil; Mesudrin; Mesudin; Sulfamylon; Homosulfamine; Ambamide; Neofamid; Septicid; Emilene; Homonal; Paramenyl. $C_7H_{10}N_2O_2S$; mol wt 186.23. C 45.15%, H 5.41%, N 15.04%, O 17.18%, S 17.22%. Prepn: Miller *et al., J. Am. Chem. Soc.* **62**, 2099 (1940); Klarer, *US 2288531* (1942 to Winthrop); Bergeim, Braker, *J. Am. Chem. Soc.* **66**, 1459 (1944); Kusami *et al., J. Pharm. Soc. Jpn.* **64**, no. 9a, 51 (1944); Komokina *et al., J. Appl. Chem. (USSR)* **21**, 681 (1948); Angyal, Jenkin, *Aust. J. Sci. Res.* **3A**, 461 (1950). Toxicity study: T. W. Skulan, J. O. Hoppe, *Life Sci.* **5**, 2279 (1966). Comprehensive description: A. K. Dash, S. Saha, *Anal. Profiles Drug Subs. Excip.* **24**, 277-305 (1996).

Crystals from alc, mp 151-152°. Sol in dil alkali, acid.

Hydrochloride. [138-37-4] $C_7H_{10}N_2O_2S.HCl$. Crystals from 95% alc, mp 256°. Neutral in soln. LD_{50} in rats, mice (mg/kg): 1170, 900 i.v. (Skulan, Hoppe).

Acetate. [13009-99-9] Mafatate; Mefamide. $C_7H_{10}N_2O_2$-$S.C_2H_4O_2$; mol wt 246.28. mp 151-152°. Freely sol in water, methanol. LD_{50} in rats, mice (mg/kg): 2040, 1580 i.v. (Skulan, Hoppe).

Propionate. [12001-72-8] Sulfomyl. $C_7H_{10}N_2O_2S.C_3H_6O_2$; mol wt 260.31. Crystals, mp 158°. Readily sol in water.

THERAP CAT: Antibacterial.

5650. Magainins. A class of potent antimicrobial peptides isolated from the granular gland of clawed toad *Xenopus laevis.* Name coined by Zasloff from the Hebrew word for "shield". Consists of magainins I and II, both containing 23 amino acid residues and differing only at the 10 (I: Gly, II: Lys) and 22 (I: Lys, II: Asn) positions. Isolation and characterization: M. Zasloff, *Proc. Natl. Acad. Sci. USA* **84**, 5449 (1987). Identification of post-secretory degradation product: T. W. Schwartz *et al., Nature* **329**, 494 (1987). Brief overview: J. Alper, *Chem. Week* 66 (November 4, 1987); M. Cannon, *Nature* **328**, 478 (1987).

Gly–Ile–Gly–Lys–Phe–Leu–His–Ser–Ala–Gly–Lys–Phe
|
Ser–Lys–Met–Ile–Glu–Gly–Val–Phe–Ala–Lys–Gly

Magainin I

5651. Magaldrate. [74978-16-8] Aluminum magnesium hydroxide sulfate ($Al_5Mg_{10}(OH)_{31}(SO_4)_2$) hydrate; magnesium aluminate hydrate; monalium hydrate; AY-5710; Dynese; Riopan; Ripon. Formerly treated as $[Mg(OH)]_4[(HO)_4Al(OH)(HO)Al-(OH)_4].2H_2O$. Prepd by mixing together and allowing to react at 0° to 50° an alkali aluminate soln (contg 3-5 mols of Na_2O or K_2O per mol Al_2O_3) with a magnesium salt soln in such proportions that 1 g of Al combines with 0.9 to 3.0 g of Mg, and washing the pptd product: Hallmann, *US 2923660* (1960 to Byk-Gulden Lomberg). Characterization: C. L. Peterson *et al., Pharm. Res.* **10**, 998 (1993).

White, odorless, crystalline powder which contains the equivs of not <28.0% and not >39.0% MgO and not <17.0% and not >25.0% Al_2O_3.

THERAP CAT: Antacid.

5652. Magenta I. [632-99-5] 4-[(4-Aminophenyl)(4-imino-2,5-cyclohexadien-1-ylidene)methyl]-2-methylbenzenamine monohydrochloride; C.I. Basic Violet 14; $α^4$-(*p*-aminophenyl)-$α^4$-(4-imino-2,5-cyclohexadien-1-ylidene)-2,4-xylidine hydrochloride; 2-methyl-4,4'-[(4-imino-2,5-cyclohexadien-1-ylidene)methylene]dianiline hydrochloride; fuchsine; magenta; rosaniline hydrochloride; C.I. 42510. $C_{20}H_{20}ClN_3$; mol wt 337.85. C 71.10%, H 5.97%, Cl 10.49%, N 12.44%. Prepn: Fischer, Fischer, *Ann.* **194**, 276, 290 (1878); *Ber.* **13**, 2204 (1880); J. T. Scalan, *J. Am. Chem. Soc.* **57**, 887 (1935). Evaluation of carcinogenicity studies: *IARC Monographs* **4**, 57 (1974). *See also: Colour Index vol. 4* (3rd ed., 1971) p 4389.

Metallic green, lustrous crystals, dec above 200°. Absorption max (ethanol): 543 nm (ε 93000). 2.65 parts dissolve in 1000 parts water. Practically insol in ether. Sol in alcohol with a carmine red color.

USE: As a dye or in manuf of other dyes.

THERAP CAT: Antifungal.

5653. Magnesium. [7439-95-4] Mg; at. wt 24.3050; at. no. 12; valence 2. Group IIA (2). Alkaline earth metal. One of the most common elements in the earth's crust: 27,640 ppm. Naturally occurring isotopes: 24 (78.99%); 25 (10.00%); 26 (11.01%). Known radioactive isotopes: 20-23, 27-34. Found naturally only in the form of its compounds in *magnesite, carnallite, dolomite* [CaMg(CO$_3$)$_2$], *epsomite, kieserite,* and many other minerals; found in sea-water, underground natural brines and salt deposits. Essential nutrient for most plant and animal life. Commercial production by electrolytic reduction of magnesium chloride or thermal reduction of magnesium oxide. First obtained in metallic form by Davy in 1808 by electrolyte reduction of magnesium oxide with mercury cathode. Prepn: Deville *et al.* in *Gmelins, Magnesium* (8th ed.) **27A,** 121 (1937). Review of magnesium and its compounds: Goodenough, Stenger, "Magnesium, Calcium, Strontium, Barium and Radium" in *Comprehensive Inorganic Chemistry* vol. 1, J. C. Bailar, Jr. *et al.,* Eds. (Pergamon Press, Oxford, 1973) pp 591-664; *Chemistry of the Elements* N. N. Greenwood, A. Earnshaw, Eds. (Pergamon Press, New York, 1984) pp 117-154; C. B. Wilson *et al.* in *Kirk-Othmer Encyclopedia of Chemical Technology* vol. 15 (Wiley-Interscience, New York, 4th ed., 1995) pp 622-674.

Silvery-white metal; hexagonal close-packed structure. Slowly oxidizes in moist air. Available as bars, ribbons, wire, castings, sheets and powder. mp 651°. bp 1100°. d^{20} 1.738. Specific heat (20°) 0.245 cal/g. Heat of fusion 88 cal/g. Electrical resistivity 4.46 μohm-cm. E° (aq) Mg^{2+}/Mg −2.37 V. Reacts very slowly with water at ordinary temp, less slowly at 100°. Reacts readily with dil acids with liberation of hydrogen; reacts with aq solns of ammonium salts, forming a double salt. Reduces carbon monoxide, carbon dioxide, sulfur dioxide, nitric oxide, and nitrous oxide at a red heat. Fine powder, thin sheets, chips and turnings are easily ignited and burn with intense heat and brilliant white flame. Combines directly with nitrogen, sulfur, the halogens, phosphorus, and arsenic. Reacts vigorously with anhydrous methyl alcohol.

Caution: Direct contact may cause irritation of skin, eyes, respiratory system. *See: Fire Protection Guide to Hazardous Materials* (National Fire Protection Assoc., Quincy, MA, 12th ed., 1997) Section 49, p 83.

USE: In alloys to produce light weight structural metals. In aluminum alloys to improve mechanical properties; in Grignard reagents; in dry cell batteries; in pyrotechnics. For hot metal desulfurization, esp. molten iron; prodn of ductile iron; metal reduction to produce elemental boron, titanium, zirconium; corrosion protection of steel structures; sacrificial anodes for corrosion protection.

5654. Magnesium Acetate. [142-72-3] Cromosan. C$_4$H$_6$-MgO$_4$; mol wt 142.39. C 33.74%, H 4.25%, Mg 17.07%, O 44.95%. Mg(C$_2$H$_3$O$_2$)$_2$.

Tetrahydrate. [16674-78-5] Colorless or white, deliquesc crystals. d 1.45. mp about 80°. Very sol in water or alcohol. The aq soln is neutral or slightly acid. *Keep well closed.*

5655. Magnesium Acetylsalicylate. [132-49-0] 2-(Acetyloxy)benzoic acid magnesium salt; magnesium aspirin; Apyron; Fyracyl; Magisal; Magnespirin; Novacetyl. C$_{18}$H$_{14}$MgO$_8$; mol wt 382.60. C 56.51%, H 3.69%, Mg 6.35%, O 33.45%. (CH$_3$COOC$_6$-H$_4$COO)$_2$Mg.

White, nonhygroscopic, almost tasteless and odorless powder. Freely soluble in water; less sol in alcohol.

THERAP CAT: Has been used as analgesic, antipyretic.

5656. Magnesium Amide. [7803-54-5] Magnesium diamide. H$_4$MgN$_2$; mol wt 56.35. H 7.15%, Mg 43.13%, N 49.71%. Mg(NH$_2$)$_2$. Prepd by the action of ammonia on an ether soln of magnesium diethyl or on magnesium activated with iodine (at 400°): Terentiew, *Z. Anorg. Chem.* **162,** 351 (1927); Schlenk, Jr., *Ber.* **64,** 738 (1931). Prepd from metal and liquid ammonia at high pressure: Juza, Jacobs, *Angew. Chem. Int. Ed.* **5,** 247 (1966); *eidem, Z. Anorg. Allg. Chem.* **370,** 245 (1969).

White powder or crystals. d$_4^{25}$ 1.39. Catches fire in air. Dec on heating. Reacts violently with water, evolving ammonia.

USE: Polymerization catalyst.

5657. Magnesium Benzoate. [553-70-8] C$_{14}$H$_{10}$MgO$_4$; mol wt 266.53. C 63.09%, H 3.78%, Mg 9.12%, O 24.01%. Mg(C$_7$H$_5$O$_2$)$_2$.

Trihydrate. White, odorless powder. mp about 200°. Sol in 20 parts water, freely in hot water, alcohol. The aq soln is neutral or slightly acid.

5658. Magnesium Borate. [13703-82-7] "Antifungin". B$_2$MgO$_4$; mol wt 109.92. B 19.67%, Mg 22.11%, O 58.22%. Mg(BO$_2$)$_2$. Various magnesium borate minerals occur in nature. These include: *ascharite, camsellite, inderite, kotoite, kurnakovite, paternoite, pinnoite, szaibelyite.*

Octahydrate. White powder. Slightly sol in water.

USE: Antiseptic; fungicide.

5659. Magnesium Bromide. [7789-48-2] Br$_2$Mg; mol wt 184.11. Br 86.80%, Mg 13.20%. MgBr$_2$.

Hexahydrate. Colorless, very deliquesc crystals or white granules; bitter taste. mp about 165° with decompn. Sol in 0.3 part water; sol in alcohol. The aq soln is neutral. *Keep well closed.*

USE: In organic syntheses.

THERAP CAT: Sedative, anticonvulsant.

5660. Magnesium Carbonate Hydroxide. [39409-82-0] Carbonic acid, magnesium salt (1:1), mixt. with magnesium hydroxide, hydrate; Marinco C. Usually a basic carbonate, approx (MgCO$_3$)$_4$.Mg(OH)$_2$.5H$_2$O; approx mol wt 485; contains 40-42% MgO. Prepn of various hydrates: Pond, Heneghan, US 3169826 (1965 to Merck & Co.). Magnesium carbonate minerals include *magnesite* and *lansfordite.*

White, odorless, bulky powder or light friable masses; at about 700° is converted into MgO. Sol in about 3300 parts CO$_2$-free water; more sol in water contg CO$_2$; sol in dil acids with effervescence. Insol in alcohol. Imparts slight alkaline reaction to water.

Hydrotalcite. [12304-65-3] Altacite; Hi-Ti; Nacid; Talcid. an aluminum magnesium hydroxide carbonate hydrate of the general formula Al$_2$O$_3$.6MgO.CO$_2$.12H$_2$O. Prepn: Kumuru *et al., US 3539306* (1970 to Kyowa).

Caution: Potential symptoms of overexposure to magnesite are irritation of eyes, skin, respiratory system; cough. *See NIOSH Pocket Guide to Chemical Hazards* (DHHS/NIOSH 97-140, 1997) p 188.

USE: Fireproofing, heat insulating; preparing effervescent magnesium citrate; clarifying liqs by filtration; in tooth and face powders, in polishing compds; manuf mineral waters, pigments, paper; filler for rubber.

THERAP CAT: Magnesium carbonate hydroxide as antacid, cathartic; hydrotalcite as antacid.

THERAP CAT (VET): Laxative.

5661. Magnesium Chlorate. [10326-21-3] Cl$_2$MgO$_6$; mol wt 191.21. Cl 37.08%, Mg 12.71%, O 50.20%. Mg(ClO$_3$)$_2$.

Hexahydrate. White, very deliquesc crystals or cryst powder; bitter taste; d 1.80. mp ~35°. Sol in 0.9 part water; slightly sol in alcohol. *Keep well closed.* LD$_{50}$ orally in rats: 5.25 g/kg, Ulrich, *J. Pharmacol. Exp. Ther.* **35,** 1 (1929).

5662. Magnesium Chloride. [7786-30-3] Magnogene. Cl$_2$Mg; mol wt 95.21. Cl 74.47%, Mg 25.53%. MgCl$_2$. Prepd from magnesium ammonium chloride hexahydrate in the presence of HCl: Bryce-Smith, *Inorg. Synth.* **6,** 9 (1960). Toxicity study: H. F. Smyth *et al., Am. Ind. Hyg. Assoc. J.* **30,** 470 (1969).

Soft, highly deliquescent leaflets. mp 712° (rapid heating). d 2.41, also reported as d 2.325. Slow heating releases chlorine at 300°. Can be distilled in a stream of hydrogen. Attacks fused silica when melted. Sol in water, with the evolution of much heat, giving a clear soln. Easily forms alcoholates and etherates.

Hexahydrate. Deliquescent crystals. d 1.56. At 100° loses 2H$_2$O (17.7%); at 110° begins to lose some HCl. By strong ignition is converted into oxychloride. mp, when rapidly heated, ~118° with decompn. One gram dissolves in 0.6 ml water, 0.3 ml boiling water, 2 ml alcohol. Its aq soln is neutral. *Keep well closed.* LD$_{50}$ orally in rats: 8.1 g/kg (Smyth).

USE: Fireproofing wood; in disinfectants; various magnesia cements; fire extinguishers; dressing cotton fabrics; in floor-sweeping compds; carbonizing wool; manuf parchment paper or artificial leather; as addition to casein glue; as a reagent in analytical chemistry.

THERAP CAT: Cathartic.

THERAP CAT (VET): Has been used in bovine hypomagnesemia.

5663. Magnesium Citrate. [7779-25-1] 2-Hydroxy-1,2,3-propanetricarboxylic acid magnesium salt; Citramag. Mg$_x$(C$_6$H$_5$-O$_7$)$_y$. Prepn of stable, soluble form: J. L. Davenport, C. F. De

Costa, US 2260004 (1941 to Pfizer). Clinical evaluation of cathartic efficacy in pediatric toxic ingestions: Y.-J. Sue et al., Ann. Emerg. Med. **24**, 709 (1994); of colonoscopic prepn with magnesium citrate + bisacodyl vs castor oil, q.q.v.: C.-C. Chen et al., J. Gastroenterol. Hepatol. **14**, 1219 (1999).

Magnesium citrate dibasic. [144-23-0] Magnesium hydrogen citrate. $C_6H_6MgO_7$; mol wt 214.41.

Magnesium citrate tribasic. [3344-18-1]; [153531-96-5] (nonahydrate)]; [6150-79-4] (tetradecahydrate). Trimagnesium dicitrate. $C_{12}H_{10}Mg_3O_{14}$; mol wt 451.11. Soly of hydrated forms: A. Apelblat, J. Chem. Thermodyn. **25**, 1443 (1993). Thermal decomposition of tetradecahydrate: S. A. A. Mansour, Thermochim. Acta **233**, 231 (1994). Soly in water at 298 K (m): nonahydrate 0.0482; tetradecahydrate 0.0446.

THERAP CAT: Cathartic.

5664. Magnesium Diboride. [12007-25-9] B_2Mg; mol wt 45.93. B 47.08%, Mg 52.92%. MgB_2. Prepn and crystal structure: V. Russell et al., Acta Crystallogr. **6**, 870 (1953); M. E. Jones, R. E. Marsh, J. Am. Chem. Soc. **76**, 1434 (1954). Use as reagent in metathesis reactions: E. G. Gillan, R. B. Kaner, Chem. Mater. **8**, 333 (1996). Superconductive properties: J. Nagamatsu et al., Nature **410**, 63 (2001). Brief review: R. J. Cava, ibid. 23-24.

Sol in dilute hydrochloric acid. Becomes superconductive at 39 K.

USE: Chemical reagent.

5665. Magnesium Fluoride. [7783-40-6] Sellaite. F_2Mg; mol wt 62.30. F 60.99%, Mg 39.01%. MgF_2. Prepd from $MgCO_3$ + HF: Klemm et al., Z. Anorg. Allg. Chem. **176**, 13 (1928). Review of toxicology of fluoride compounds: G. L. Waldbott, Acta Med. Scand. Suppl. **400**, 1-44 (1963).

Colorless substance (rutile-type lattice). Slight violet fluorescence. d 3.148. Mohs' hardness: 6. mp 1248°. bp 2260°. Very sparingly sol in water 87 mg/l (18°). Slightly sol in dil acids, especially nitric acid. May be stored in glass bottles. LD in guinea pigs (mg/kg): 1000 orally, 3000 s.c. (Waldbott).

USE: In the ceramics and glass industry.

5666. Magnesium Formate. [557-39-1] $C_2H_2MgO_4$; mol wt 114.34. C 21.01%, H 1.76%, Mg 21.26%, O 55.97%. $Mg(HCOO)_2$.

Dihydrate. Crystals or granules. Sol in water; insol in alcohol. Its aq soln is practically neutral.

5667. Magnesium Germanide. [1310-52-7] $GeMg_2$; mol wt 121.25. Ge 59.91%, Mg 40.09%. Mg_2Ge. Prepd by fusion of the components: Winkler, Helv. Phys. Acta **28**, 633 (1955).

Crystals, mp 1115°.

USE: In semiconductor research.

5668. Magnesium Hexafluorosilicate. [16949-65-8] Magnesium silicofluoride; magnesium fluosilicate. F_6MgSi; mol wt 166.38. F 68.51%, Mg 14.61%, Si 16.88%. $MgSiF_6$. Review of toxicology of fluorine compounds: G. L. Waldbott, Acta Med. Scand. Suppl. **400**, 1-44 (1963).

LD in guinea pigs (mg/kg): 200 orally, 400 s.c. (Waldbott).

Hexahydrate. [18972-56-0] $F_6MgSi.6H_2O$. White, efflorescent, odorless crystals. d 1.788. At ~120° loses SiF_4. Soluble in water. Insol in alcohol. pH of 1% aq soln: 3.1.

USE: For mothproofing of textile fabrics.

5669. Magnesium Hydride. [60616-74-2] H_2Mg; mol wt 26.32. H 7.66%, Mg 92.34%. Prepd by thermal decompn of diethylmagnesium at 200° in high vacuum: Wiberg, Bauer, Ber. **85**, 593 (1952); from the elements: Ellinger et al., J. Am. Chem. Soc. **77**, 2647 (1955).

White, nonvolatile mass or tetragonal crystals. d 1.45. Dec at 280° in high vacuum. Strong reducing agent. Ignites spontaneously on contact with air, forming MgO and H_2O. On contact with water a violent evolution of hydrogen takes place. On contact with methanol, magnesium alcoholate and hydrogen are formed. Forms double hydrides with boron hydride and aluminum hydride.

5670. Magnesium Hydroxide. [1309-42-8] Magnesium hydrate; Carmilax; Emgesan; Marinco H. H_2MgO_2; mol wt 58.32. H 3.46%, Mg 41.68%, O 54.87%. $Mg(OH)_2$. Occurs in nature as the mineral **brucite**. Prepn from magnesium chloride or

sulfate and NaOH: Perlard, Waldron, US 3127241 (1964 to Dow). Industrial method for producing magnesium hydroxide having variable particle sizes: Chisholm, US 3232708 (1966 to FMC).

Amorphous powder. Practically insol in water (1:80,000). Sol in dil acids. Imparts slight alkaline reaction to water. pH of aq slurry: 9.5-10.5. Absorbs CO_2 in the presence of water. *Keep well closed.*

THERAP CAT: Antacid; cathartic.

THERAP CAT (VET): Laxative.

5671. Magnesium Iodide. [10377-58-9] I_2Mg; mol wt 278.11. I 91.26%, Mg 8.74%. MgI_2.

Octahydrate. White, deliquesc powder; readily discolors in air and light. Very sol in water; sol in alcohol. The aq soln is neutral or slightly alkaline. *Keep well closed and protected from light.*

5672. Magnesium Lactate. [18917-93-6] 2-Hydroxypropanoic acid magnesium salt. $C_6H_{10}MgO_6$; mol wt 202.45. C 35.60%, H 4.98%, Mg 12.01%, O 47.42%. $(CH_3CHOHCOO)_2Mg$.

Trihydrate. White cryst, very bitter powder. One gram dissolves in 25 ml cold water, 3.5 ml boiling water; slightly sol in alcohol. The aq soln is slightly acid.

THERAP CAT: Cathartic.

5673. Magnesium Monoperoxyphthalate. [78948-87-5] (T-4)-Bis[2-carboxybenzenecarboperoxoato(2−)-$κO,κOO$]magnesate(2−) dihydrogen; magnesium bis(monoperoxyphthalate); H48; MMPP. $C_{16}H_{10}MgO_{10}$; mol wt 386.55. C 49.71%, H 2.61%, Mg 6.29%, O 41.39%. Versatile, mild peroxygen product; stable alternative to **m-chloroperoxybenzoic acid** (**MCPBA**) in oxidation reactions. Prepn: G. J. Hignett, EP 27693; idem, US 4385008 (1981, 1983 both to Interox). Thermal decompn studies: B. M. Kariuki, W. Jones, Mol. Cryst. Liq. Cryst. **186**, 45 (1990); eidem, ibid. **248**, 21 (1994). Decontamination studies with warfare agents and insecticides: C. Lion et al., Phosphorus Sulfur Silicon Relat. Elem. **56**, 213 (1991). Antimicrobial properties: M. G. C. Baldry, J. Appl. Bacteriol. **57**, 499 (1984). Clinical evaluation as an anti-plaque mouthrinse and dentifrice: C. Scully et al., J. Clin. Periodontol. **26**, 234 (1999). Review of synthetic applications in oxidation reactions: P. Brougham et al., Synthesis **1987**, 1015-1017; H. Heaney, Aldrichim. Acta **26**, 35-45 (1993).

Hexahydrate. [131391-55-4] $C_{16}H_{10}MgO_{10}.6H_2O$; mol wt 494.64. White granular solid, mp 96°. Soly in water (15°): 160 g/l. Sol in low mol wt alcohols; very low soly in common organic solvents.

USE: Oxidizing agent in organic synthesis. Bleaching agent. Decontaminant reagent for nerve gases and insecticides.

5674. Magnesium Nitrate. [10377-60-3] MgN_2O_6; mol wt 148.31. Mg 16.39%, N 18.89%, O 64.73%. $Mg(NO_3)_2$. Hydrated form occurs in nature as the mineral **nitromagnesite**.

Hexahydrate, colorless, clear, deliquesc crystals. d 1.464. mp ~95°. Sol in 0.8 part water; freely sol in alcohol. The aq soln is neutral. *Keep well closed.*

USE: In pyrotechnics; in the concentration of nitric acid.

5675. Magnesium Oleate. [1555-53-9] 9-Octadecenoic acid magnesium salt. $C_{36}H_{66}MgO_4$; mol wt 587.21. C 73.63%, H 11.33%, Mg 4.14%, O 10.90%. $Mg(C_{18}H_{33}O_2)_2$. Commercial form usually contains some stearate and palmitate.

Yellowish powder or mass. Insol in water; partly sol in alcohol, ether, petr ether.

USE: As an addition to naphtha to prevent spontaneous ignition in cleaning establishments.

5676. Magnesium Oxalate. [547-66-0] Ethanedioic acid magnesium salt. C_2MgO_4; mol wt 112.32. C 21.39%, Mg 21.64%, O 56.98%. MgC_2O_4.

Dihydrate. White powder. Sol in about 1500 parts water, in dil mineral acid; insol in alcohol.

5677. Magnesium Oxide. [1309-48-4] Magnesia; calcined magnesia; magnesia usta; Magcal; Maglite. MgO; mol wt 40.30. Mg 60.31%, O 39.70%. Occurs in nature as the mineral *periclase*. Commercial prepn from magnesite ores: Adams, US 3320029 (1967 to Northwest Magnesite).

White, very fine, odorless powder. Available in a very bulky form termed "Light" or in a dense form termed "Heavy." Takes up CO_2 and H_2O from the air, the light form more readily than the heavy. mp 2800°. Highly reflective in visible and near uv region. Combines with water to form magnesium hydroxide. Very slightly sol in pure water, soly increased by CO_2; sol in dil acids; insol in alcohol. Imparts a slight alkaline reaction to water. pH of satd aq soln 10.3. *Keep well closed.*

Caution: Potential symptoms of overexposure to fumes are irritation of eyes and nose; metal fume fever (coughing, chest pain and flu-like fever). *See NIOSH Pocket Guide to Chemical Hazards* (DHHS/NIOSH 97-140, 1997) p 188.

USE: Manuf refractory crucibles, fire bricks, magnesia cements and boiler scale compounds, "powdered" oils, casein glue. Reflector in optical instruments; white color standard. Insulator at low temp.

THERAP CAT: Antacid.

THERAP CAT (VET): Antacid, laxative, in hypomagnesemia.

5678. Magnesium Perchlorate. [10034-81-8] Anhydrone; Dehydrite. Cl_2MgO_8; mol wt 223.21. Cl 31.77%, Mg 10.89%, O 57.34%. $Mg(ClO_4)_2$.

White, very hygroscopic, granular or flaky powder; dec above 250°. Dissolves in water with evolution of a considerable amount of heat. Crystallizes from water with $6H_2O$. *Keep tightly closed.*

Caution: Can cause irritation of skin, mucous membranes.

USE: As a drying agent for gases. The article of commerce may contain an amount of water equivalent to a dihydrate, but even the trihydrate is said to be effective for drying gases.

5679. Magnesium Permanganate. [10377-62-5] $MgMn_2O_8$; mol wt 262.18. Mg 9.27%, Mn 41.91%, O 48.82%. $Mg(MnO_4)_2$. As polymerization catalyst: Pengilly *et al.*, US 3576790 (1971 to Goodyear). In purification of benzene: Ingwalson *et al.*, US 3478092 (1969 to Velsicol).

Bluish-black, deliquesc crystals. Freely sol in water. *Keep well closed.*

USE: Catalyst.

5680. Magnesium Peroxide. [14452-57-4] Magnesium dioxide; Magnesium Perhydrol; Magnesium Superoxol. MgO_2; mol wt 56.30. Mg 43.17%, O 56.84%. The article of commerce contains 15-25% MgO_2, the balance being magnesium hydroxide. For medicinal use the 25% article is preferred.

White, tasteless, odorless powder. Insol in water and gradually dec by it with liberation of oxygen; sol in dil acids, forming hydrogen peroxide; when strongly heated loses all the peroxide oxygen. *Keep well closed.*

THERAP CAT: Antacid, anti-infective.

5681. Magnesium Phosphate, Dibasic. [7757-86-0] Magnesium hydrogen phosphate; secondary magnesium phosphate. $HMgO_4P$; mol wt 120.28. H 0.84%, Mg 20.21%, O 53.21%, P 25.75%. $MgHPO_4$. Trihydrate occurs in nature as the minerals *newberyite, phosphor-roesslerite.*

Trihydrate. White, cryst powder. d 2.13. Slightly sol in water; sol in dil acids.

THERAP CAT: Cathartic.

5682. Magnesium Phosphate, Monobasic. [13092-66-5] Magnesium biphosphate; acid magnesium phosphate; primary magnesium phosphate. $H_4MgO_8P_2$; mol wt 218.28. H 1.85%, Mg 11.13%, O 58.64%, P 28.38%. $Mg(H_2PO_4)_2$.

Trihydrate. White powder. Soluble in water.

USE: In fireproofing wood.

5683. Magnesium Phosphate, Tribasic. [7757-87-1] "Neutral" magnesium phosphate; tertiary magnesium phosphate; trimagnesium phosphate. $Mg_3O_8P_2$; mol wt 262.86. Mg 27.74%,

O 48.69%, P 23.57%. $Mg_3(PO_4)_2$. Octahydrate occurs in nature as the mineral *bobierrite*.

Pentahydrate. White, cryst powder. Loses last mol of water at ~400°. Insol in water; sol in dil mineral acids.

THERAP CAT: Antacid.

5684. Magnesium Pyrophosphate. [13446-24-7] $Mg_2O_7P_2$; mol wt 222.55. Mg 21.84%, O 50.32%, P 27.84%. $Mg_2P_2O_7$.

Trihydrate. White powder; loses its water at 100°. d 2.56. Insol in water. Sol in dil mineral acids.

5685. Magnesium Salicylate. [18917-89-0] 2-Hydroxybenzoic acid magnesium salt; Analate; Lorisal; Magan; Mobidin; Tri-act. $C_{14}H_{10}MgO_6$; mol wt 298.53. C 56.33%, H 3.38%, Mg 8.14%, O 32.16%. $Mg[C_6H_4(OH)COO]_2$.

Tetrahydrate. White, odorless, efflorescent, cryst powder. Sol in 13 parts water; sol in alc. The aq soln is slightly acid.

THERAP CAT: Anti-infective (intestinal).

5686. Magnesium Selenide. [1313-04-8] MgSe; mol wt 103.27. Mg 23.54%, Se 76.46%. Prepd by the action of hydrogen selenide on anhydr magnesium chloride at a red heat and by the action of selenium vapor carried in a current of nitrogen on powdered magnesium: Fonzes-Diacon, *Contribution a l' Etude des Séléniures Métalliques* (Montpellier, 1901); by dropping selenium into molten magnesium: Liddell, *Chem. Metall. Eng.* **25**, 102, 263, 453 (1921).

Light brown powder. d 4.21. Unstable in air. Dec in water.

5687. Magnesium Silicates. Several varieties of magnesium silicate are known. *See also* asbestos, talc.

Magnesium metasilicate. [13776-74-4] $MgSiO_3$; mol wt 100.39. Occurs in nature as the minerals *clinoenstatite, enstatite, protoenstatite.* White monoclinic crystals, dec at 1557°. d_4^{25} 3.192. Practically insol in water; very slightly sol in HF.

Magnesium orthosilicate. [10034-94-3] Mg_2SiO_4; mol wt 140.69. Occurs in nature as the mineral *forsterite.* White orthorhombic crystals. mp 1910°; d 3.21. Practically insol in water.

Magnesium trisilicate. [14987-04-3] Magnesium mesotrisilicate; Magnosil; Petimin; Trisomin. $Mg_2Si_3O_8$; mol wt 260.86. Occurs in nature as the minerals *meerschaum, parasepiolite, sepiolite.* Prepd from sodium silicate and magnesium sulfate: Glass, *Q. J. Pharm. Pharmacol.* **9**, 445 (1936); Uyeda, US 3272594 (1966 to Merck & Co.). Odorless, tasteless, slightly hygroscopic powder. Usually contains some water of hydration. Practically insol in water.

Magnesium trisilicate pentahydrate. Sellagen.

Serpentine (mineral). $Mg_3O_7Si_2$; mol wt 241.08. Occurs in nature as the dihydrate, $(OH)_4MgSi_2O_5$; exists in two forms: *antigorite*, a platy variety, and *chrysotile*, a fibrous variety. The latter is the most common form of asbestos.

USE: An activated magnesium silicate, *Florisil*, a hard, porous, granular substance, is used in vitamin analysis, chromatography, antibiotic processing: Simons, US 2393625 (1946 to Floridin).

THERAP CAT: Trisilicate as antacid.

THERAP CAT (VET): Trisilicate as antacid; gastric sedative.

5688. Magnesium Silicide. [22831-39-6] Mg_2Si; mol wt 76.70. Mg 63.38%, Si 36.62%. Prepd by heating finely powdered Mg and Si in a proportion of 20 to 6: Gire, *Compt. Rend.* **196**, 1404 (1933), *C.A.* **27**, 3678 (1933); Winkler, *Helv. Phys. Acta* **28**, 633 (1955), *C.A.* **50**, 6908c (1956). Prepn and conversion to silanes: Emeleus, Maddock, *J. Chem. Soc.* **1946**, 1131.

Slate-blue, cubic crystals. d_4^{20} ~2.0. mp 1085°. Dec at 550° *in vacuo* yielding Mg_3Si_2. Heat of formation: 18.5 cal/mol. Dec by water, HCl.

USE: In semiconductor research. Has been used to build Mg-Si rectifiers.

5689. Magnesium Stannide. [1313-08-2] Mg_2Sn; mol wt 167.32. Mg 29.05%, Sn 70.95%. Prepn by fusion of a stoichiometric mixture of the elements: Winkler, *Helv. Phys. Acta* **28**, 633 (1955); Korenblit, Kolesnikov, *Zh. Tekh. Fiz.* **26**, 941 (1956), *C.A.* **50**, 11475b (1956). Magnetic susceptibility and electrical conductivity measurements: Boltaks, *Dokl. Akad. Nauk SSSR* **64**, 487, 653, (1949), *C.A.* **43**, 4528f, 4533f (1949). Electrical conductivity, magnetoresistance: Frederikse *et al., Phys. Rev.* **103**, 67 (1956).

Bluish-white, metallic substance. Calcium fluoride crystal structure. mp 778°. Resistivity (25°): 42,000 microhm-cm; thermoelectric power 90 microvolts per degree for 15-100°. Energy of activation: 22,100 cal/mole. Soluble in water, dilute HCl.

USE: In semiconductor research.

5690. Magnesium Stearate. [557-04-0] Octadecanoic acid magnesium salt. $C_{36}H_{70}MgO_4$; mol wt 591.24. C 73.13%, H 11.93%, Mg 4.11%, O 10.82%. $Mg(C_{18}H_{35}O_2)_2$. The commercial preparation also contains palmitate.

White powder. Insoluble in water; dec by dil acids.

USE: In baby dusting powders; as tablet lubricant.

5691. Magnesium Sulfate. [7487-88-9] MgO_4S; mol wt 120.37. Mg 20.19%, O 53.17%, S 26.64%. $MgSO_4$. Monohydrate occurs in nature as the mineral *kieserite*. *Review: Gmelins, Magnesium* (8th ed) **27**, 210-211, 223-226 (1939). Review of clinical experience: R. Swain, B. Kaplan-Machlis, *South. Med. J.* **92**, 1040-1047 (1999); of toxicology: J. W. Van Hook, *Crit. Care Clin.* **7**, 215-223 (1991); R. B. Birrer *et al., J. Emerg. Med.* **22**, 185-188 (2002). Clinical trial in prevention of eclamptic convulsions: L. Duley *et al., Lancet* **359**, 1877 (2002).

Trihydrate. [15320-30-6] Prepn: Bennett, US 3297413 (1967 to Dow). Odorless crystals.

Heptahydrate. [10034-99-8] Bitter salts; epsom salts; Mg 5-Sulfat. Occurs in nature as the mineral *epsomite*. Efflorescent crystals or powder; bitter, saline, cooling taste. d 1.67. Soly in water (g/100 ml): at 20° = 71; at 40° = 91. Slightly sol in alcohol. Its aq soln is neutral. pH 6-7. On exposure to dry air at ordinary temp it loses ~$1H_2O$; at 70-80° loses $4H_2O$; at 100° loses $5H_2O$; at 120° loses $6H_2O$, rapidly reabsorbing water when exposed to moist air; loses the last mol of water at ~250°.

Dried magnesium sulfate. Prepd by heating the heptahydrate until ~25% of its weight is lost. Used in *Morison's paste. Keep well closed.*

Caution: Parenteral use or use in presence of renal insufficiency may lead to magnesium intoxication. *See:* M. J. Ellenhorn *et al., Ellenhorn's Medical Toxicology: Diagnosis and Treatment of Human Poisoning* (Williams & Wilkins, Baltimore, 2nd ed., 1997) pp 1013-1014. Potential symptoms of overexposure are pseudocoma, hyporeflexia, muscle weakness, ataxia, confusion, nausea, vomiting, flushing, bradycardia, hypotension, widened QRS, AV block and respiratory arrest (Swain, Kaplan-Machlis).

USE: Weighting cotton and silk; increasing the bleaching action of chlorinated lime; manuf mother-of-pearl and frosted papers; fireproofing fabrics; dyeing and printing calicos; in fertilizers; explosives, matches; mineral water; tanning leather.

THERAP CAT: Anticonvulsant; cathartic; magnesium replenisher.

THERAP CAT (VET): Anticonvulsant; cathartic; magnesium replenisher.

5692. Magnesium Sulfite. [7757-88-2] MgO_3S; mol wt 104.37. Mg 23.29%, O 45.99%, S 30.72%. $MgSO_3$. Occurs as tri- and hexahydrates.

Hexahydrate. Colorless crystals or white, cryst powder; gradually oxidizes to sulfate on exposure to air; loses all its water at 200°; dec at higher temp. Sol in ~150 parts water, slightly more in boiling water.

USE: A soln of magnesium sulfite in sulfurous acid (magnesium bisulfite) is used in the manuf of paper pulp.

5693. Magnesium Thiocyanate. [306-61-6] Magnesium sulfocyanate. $C_2MgN_2S_2$; mol wt 140.47. C 17.10%, Mg 17.30%, N 19.94%, S 45.65%. $Mg(SCN)_2$.

Tetrahydrate. Colorless or white deliquesc crystals. Freely sol in water or alcohol. *Keep well closed.*

5694. Magnesium Thiosulfate. [10124-53-5] Magnesium hyposulfite; Magnosulf; Antichoc Hipmag. MgO_3S_2; mol wt 136.43. Mg 17.81%, O 35.18%, S 47.01%. MgS_2O_3.

Hexahydrate. Colorless or white crystals; loses $3H_2O$ at 170°. d 1.82. Sol in 2 parts water; insol in alcohol. Its aq soln is neutral.

5695. Magneson. [74-39-5] 4-[(4-Nitrophenyl)azo]-1,3-benzenediol; 4-(*p*-nitrophenylazo)resorcinol; 2,4-dihydroxy-4'-nitroazobenzene. $C_{12}H_9N_3O_4$; mol wt 259.22. C 55.60%, H 3.50%, N 16.21%, O 24.69%. *Ref:* Suitzu, Okuma, *J. Soc.*

Chem. Ind. Jpn. **29**, 132 (1926); Ruigh, *J. Am. Chem. Soc.* **51**, 1456 (1929); Engel, *ibid.* **52**, 1812 (1930).

Brownish-red powder. Practically insol in water; sol in dil aq NaOH.

USE: For the detection of magnesium with which it yields a bright blue color in alkaline soln. Also used to determine molybdenum with which it forms a red-violet complex: Nikitina, Andrianova, *C.A.* **75**, 136789v (1971).

5696. Magnoflorine. [2141-09-5] (6a*S*)-5,6,6a,7-Tetrahydro-1,11-dihydroxy-2,10-dimethoxy-6,6-dimethyl-4*H*-dibenzo[*de,-g*]quinolinium; thalictrine. $[C_{20}H_{24}NO_4]^+$. From *Magnolia grandiflora* L., *Magnoliaceae.* Isoln and structure: Nakano, *Chem. Pharm. Bull.* **2**, 329 (1954). From *Cocculus trilobus* D.C., *Menispermaceae:* Nakano, *ibid.* **4**, 69 (1956); from *Thalictrum thunbergii* D.C., *Ranunculaceae:* Fujita, Tomimatsu, *ibid.* **6**, 107 (1958); from *Aristolochia clematitis* L., *Aristolochiaceae:* Pailer, Pruckmayr, *Monatsh. Chem.* **90**, 145 (1959). Identity with thalictrine: Gopinath *et al., J. Sci. Ind. Res.* **18B** 444 (1959). Synthesis: Tomita, Kikkawa, *J. Pharm. Soc. Jpn.* **77**, 195 (1957).

Iodide. $C_{20}H_{24}INO_4$. Crystals from methanol + acetone, dec 248-249°. $[\alpha]_D^{15}$ +220.1° (methanol). uv max: 270, 310 nm (log ε 3.75, 3.59).

5697. Magnolol. [528-43-8] 5,5'-Di-2-propenyl-[1,1'-biphenyl]-2,2'-diol; 5,5'-diallyl-2,2'-biphenyldiol; 2,2'-bichavicol; dehydrodichavicol; 2,2'-dihydroxy-5,5'-diallylbiphenyl. $C_{18}H_{18}O_2$; mol wt 266.33. C 81.17%, H 6.81%, O 12.01%. Bioactive constituent of *Magnoliae Cortex*, the bark of *Magnolia officinalis*, Rehd. et Wils., *Magnoliaceae*, known in Chinese traditional medicine as *houpo*, or of *M. obovata*, Thunb., called *wakoboku* in Japanese. Isoln: Y. Sugii, *Yakugaku Zasshi* **50**, 183 (1930), *C.A.* **24**, 3505 (1930). Synthesis: H. Erdtman, J. Runeberg, *Acta Chem. Scand.* **11**, 1060 (1957); J. Runeberg, *ibid.* **12**, 188 (1958). Isoln from seeds of *M. grandiflora* L.: F. S. El-Feraly, W.-S. Li, *Lloydia* **41**, 442 (1978). CNS depressant effects: K. Watanabe *et al., Jpn. J. Pharmacol.* **25**, 605 (1975); *eidem, Planta Med.* **49**, 103 (1983). Anti-inflammatory and analgesic effects: J.-P. Wang *et al., Arch. Pharmacol.* **346**, 707 (1992). HPLC determn: T.-H. Tsai, C.-F. Chen, *J. Chromatogr.* **598**, 143 (1992).

mp 101.5-102°. uv max: 293 nm (log ε 3.90). Sol in ethanol.

5698. Maitotoxin. [59392-53-9] MTX. $C_{164}H_{256}Na_2O_{68}$-S_2; mol wt 3425.86. C 57.50%, H 7.53%, Na 1.34%, O 31.76%, S 1.87%. Polycyclic ether toxin involved in ciguatera fish poisoning of humans. From the Tahitian for the surgeon fish (maito) from which it was orginally isolated; later found to be a product of the dinoflagellate, *Gamberdiscus toxicus*. One of the most toxic and the largest (mol wt 3422 Da) natural products known to date besides the biopolymers. Isoln from surgeon fish: T. Yasumoto *et al., Bull. Jpn. Soc. Sci. Fish.* **42**, 359 (1976); from dinoflagellate: *idem et al.,*

"A New Toxic Dinoflagellate Found in Association with Ciguatera" in *Toxic Dinoflagellate Blooms*, D. L. Taylor, H. Seliger, Eds. (Elsevier/North Holland, Inc., NY, 1979) pp 65-70. Toxicity and channel activation: M. Takahashi *et al.*, *J. Biol. Chem.* **257**, 7287 (1982). Structure: M. Murata *et al.*, *J. Am. Chem. Soc.* **115**, 2060 (1993); and stereochemistry: L. R. Cook *et al.*, *ibid.* **119**, 7928 (1997). Use as activator of calcium influx: J. W. Daly *et al.*, *Biochem. Pharmacol.* **50**, 1187 (1995); H. M. Brereton *et al.*, *Biochim. Biophys. Acta* **1540**, 107 (2001); as receptor differentiator: P. M. Lundy *et al.*, *Eur. J. Pharmacol.* **487**, 17 (2004). Effect of cations on MTX response: V. Morales-Tlalpan, L. Vaca, *Toxicon* **40**, 493 (2002). Determn by capillary zone electrophoresis: N. Bouaïcha *et al.*, *ibid.* **35**, 955 (1997). Review of use as tool for calcium flux: F. Gusovsky, J. W. Daly, *Biochem. Pharmacol.* **39**, 1633-1639 (1990); of mechanism of action and pharmacology: M. Estacion, *Food. Sci. Technol.* **103**, 473-503 (2000).

Sol in water, methanol, ethanol, 1-butanol saturated with water. Insol in diethyl ether, acetone and chloroform.

USE: Calcium channel activator; research tool for ion flux.

5699. Malachite Green. [569-64-2]; [510-13-4] (carbinol base). *N*-[4-[[4-(Dimethylamino)phenyl]phenylmethylene]-2,5-cyclohexadien-1-ylidene]-*N*-methylmethanaminium chloride; bis-[*p*-(dimethylamino)phenyl]phenylmethylium chloride; C.I. Basic Green 4; C.I. 42000; aniline green; benzal green; benzaldehyde green; china green; diamond green B; diamond green Bx; diamond green P extra; fast green; light green N; new victoria green extra O; new victoria green extra I; new victoria green extra II; solid green O; victoria green W; victoria green B. $C_{23}H_{25}ClN_2$; mol wt 364.91. C 75.70%, H 6.91%, Cl 9.72%, N 7.68%. Triphenylmethane dye with fungicidal and limited antiseptic activity. Prepn: *Colour Index* **Vol. 4** (3rd ed., 1971) p 4380. Conformational changes in excited state: S. Saikan, J. Sei, *J. Chem. Phys.* **79**, 4154 (1983). Use in electron microscopy: R. G. Pourcho *et al.*, *Stain Technol.* **53**, 29 (1978); as stain in determn of prostaglandin E and F compounds: E. J. Singh *et al.*, *J. Chromatogr.* **105**, 195 (1975); in determn of inorganic phosphate: W. Hohenwallner, E. Wimmer, *Clin. Chim. Acta* **45**, 169 (1973); S. G. Carter, D. W. Karl, *J. Biochem. Biophys. Methods* **7**, 7 (1982). Antiseptic activity: J. E. Madden *et al.*, *Surg. Forum* **22**, 63 (1971). Toxicology: N. Brock, A. Erhardt, *Arzneim.-Forsch.* **1**, 5 (1951); T. D. Bills, L. L. Marking, *Invest. Fish Control* **75**, 6 (1977); S. Clemmensen *et al.*, *Arch. Toxicol.* **56**, 43 (1984). Reviews of use as fungicide in fish culture: N. C. Nelson, *U.S. NTIS Report* (PB-235450, 1974) 79 pp, *C.A.* **82**, 150006p (1975), (PB-235451, 1974) 33 pp, *C.A.* **83**, 1547j (1975); and as biological stain: *Conn's Biological Stains*, R. W. Horobin, J. A. Kiernan, Eds. (BIOS Scientific Publishers Ltd, Oxford, UK, 10th ed., 2002) 189-190. Review of toxicological effects: S. Srivastava *et al.*, *Aquat. Toxicol.* **66**, 310-329 (2004).

Green crystals with metallic luster. Very sol in water; sol in alcohol, methanol, amyl alcohol. Water solns are blue-green, absorption max 616.9 nm; yellow below pH 2. pK 6.90. LD_{50} in mice (mg/kg): 80 orally; 4.2 i.p. (Brock, Erhardt). LC_{50} (6 hr, 12°C) in bluegill sunfish, channel catfish, rainbow trout, coho salmon (mg/l): 2.19 (pH 7.5), 0.960 (pH 7.5), 6.8 (pH 8.0), 3.0 (pH 7.5) (Bills, Marking).

Oxalate salt. [2437-29-8] $C_{46}H_{50}N_4 \cdot 2HC_2O_4 \cdot C_2H_2O_4$; mol wt 927.00. Sol to 4% in water, 5% in ethanol. Insol in xylene.

Leucomalachite green. [129-73-7] Bis(*p*-dimethylaminophenyl)phenylmethane. $C_{23}H_{26}N_2$; mol wt 330.47. Colorless, reduced form of malachite green. Practically insol in water. Slightly sol in ethanol.

Note: The term malachite green applies to the oxalate as well as the chloride.

USE: For directly dyeing silk, wool, jute and leather; dyeing cotton after mordanting. Biological stain. Clinical reagent (inorganic phosphate assay). As spot test reagent for detecting sulfurous acid and cerium. As acid-base indicator: pH 0.0 yellow, 2.0 green; 11.6 green, 14 colorless.

THERAP CAT (VET): Fungicide and parasiticide in fish.

5700. Malathion. [121-75-5] [(Dimethoxyphosphinothioyl)thio]butanedioic acid diethyl ester; diethyl mercaptosuccinate S-ester with O,O-dimethyl phosphorothioate; S-(1,2-dicarbethoxyethyl) O,O-dimethyldithiophosphate; insecticide no. 4049; carbofos; malathon (obsolete); mercaptothion; phosphothion; ENT-17034; Cython; Derbac-M; Malamar 50; Malaspray; Organoderm; Prioderm; Suleo-M. $C_{10}H_{19}O_6PS_2$; mol wt 330.36. C 36.36%, H 5.80%, O 29.06%, P 9.38%, S 19.41%. Cholinesterase inhibitor. Prepn: Johnson *et al.*, *J. Econ. Entomol.* **45**, 279 (1952); Cassaday, US **2578652** (1951 to Am. Cyanamid). Purification: Usui, US **2962521** (1960 to Sumitomo). Treatment of *Pediculus humanus* (head lice) infestation: D. Taplin *et al.*, *J. Am. Med. Assoc.* **247**, 3103 (1982). Toxicity data: T. B. Gaines, *Toxicol. Appl. Pharmacol.* **14**, 515 (1969). Review of distribution, transport and fate in the environment: M. S. Mulla *et al.*, *Residue Rev.* **81**, 1-159 (1981); of carcinogenic risk: *IARC Monographs* **30**, 103-129 (1983); of toxicology and human exposure: *Toxicological Profile for Malathion* (PB2004-100003, 2003) 327 pp.

Deep brown to yellow liq, mp 2.9°. bp$_{0.7}$ 156-157°. Characteristic odor. d_4^{25} 1.23. n_D^{25} 1.4985. Vapor pressure at 30°: 4×10^{-5} mm Hg. Slightly sol in water (145 ppm). Misc with many organic solvents including alcohols, esters, ketones, ethers, aromatic and alkylated aromatic hydrocarbons and vegetable oils. Limited soly in certain paraffin hydrocarbons. Petroleum ether is sol to about 35% in malathion. Hydrolyzed at pH >7.0 or <5.0. Stable in an aq soln buffered to pH 5.26. LD_{50} in female, male rats (mg/kg): 1000, 1375 orally (Gaines).

Caution: Potential symptoms of overexposure are miosis, aching eyes, blurred vision and lacrimation; eye and skin irritation; salivation; anorexia, nausea, vomiting, abdominal cramps, diarrhea, giddiness, confusion and ataxia; rhinorrhea, headache; tightening of chest, wheezing and laryngeal spasms. *See NIOSH Pocket Guide to Chemical Hazards* (DHHS/NIOSH 97-140, 1997) p 188.

USE: Insecticide.
THERAP CAT: Pediculicide.
THERAP CAT (VET): Ectoparasiticide.

5701. Maleamic Acid. [557-24-4] (Z)-4-Amino-4-oxo-2-butenoic acid; maleic acid monoamide. $C_4H_5NO_3$; mol wt 115.09. C 41.74%, H 4.38%, N 12.17%, O 41.70%. Prepd by passing ammonia into a mixture of maleic anhydride and an inert solvent such as xylene, dioxane, etc.: Robinson, Humburger, **US 2459964** (1949 to Beck, Koller).

Crystals from alcohol, mp 172-173°. Also reported as mp 178-180° (dec). Very sol in water, hot alcohol. Practically insol in ether, chloroform, benzene.

5702. Maleanilic Acid. [555-59-9] (Z)-4-Oxo-4-(phenyl-amino)-2-butenoic acid; N-phenylmaleamic acid. $C_{10}H_9NO_3$; mol wt 191.18. C 62.82%, H 4.74%, N 7.33%, O 25.11%. Use of esters as fungicides: Ligett et al., **US 2885319** (1959 to Pittsburgh Coke & Chem.).

Monoclinic yellow crystals, dec 192°. Apparent density 1.418 g/ml at 30°. Soly in g/100 ml soln at 27°: acetonitrile 0.2; acetone 0.3; benzene <0.1; butyl Cellosolve 1.1; carbon tetrachloride <0.1; chloroform <0.1; dimethylformamide 12.9; dioxane 0.9; ethanol 0.2; ether <0.1; methanol 0.3; toluene <0.1; water <0.1. Shows hydrolysis in aq soln. Dissociates to maleic anhydride and aniline when heated above 100° *in vacuo*.
USE: Esters as fungicides.

5703. Maleic Acid. [110-16-7] (Z)-Butenedioic acid; toxilic acid; cis-1,2-ethylenedicarboxylic acid. $C_4H_4O_4$; mol wt 116.07. C 41.39%, H 3.47%, O 55.14%. Prepd by the catalytic oxidation of benzene over vanadium pentoxide: Bhattacharyya, Venkataraman, J. Appl. Chem. **8**, 728 (1958); Saffer, Olenberg, **FR 1321416** (1963 to Scientific Design), C.A. **59**, 11265d (1963). Crystal structure: Shahat, Acta Crystallogr. **5**, 763 (1952). Review: W. D. Robinson, R. A. Mount in Kirk-Othmer Encyclopedia of Chemical Technology vol. 14 (Wiley-Interscience, New York, 3rd ed., 1981) pp 770-793.

White crystals from water, mp 138-139°; from alcohol and benzene, mp 130-131°. Faint, acidulous odor; characteristic repulsive, astringent taste. d 1.59. Is converted in part into the much higher-melting fumaric acid (mp 287°) when heated to a temp slightly above the melting point. Freely sol in water or alcohol. Sol in acetone, glacial acetic acid. Slightly sol in ether. Practically insol in benzene.
Caution: Strong irritant.
USE: Manuf artificial resins; to retard rancidity of fats and oils in 1:10,000 (these are said to keep 3 times longer than those without the acid); dyeing and finishing wool, cotton, and silk; preparing the maleate salts of antihistamines and similar drugs.

5704. Maleic Anhydride. [108-31-6] 2,5-Furandione; cis-butenedioic anhydride; toxilic anhydride. $C_4H_2O_3$; mol wt 98.06. C 48.99%, H 2.06%, O 48.95%. May be prepd by sublimation of maleic acid and P_2O_5 under reduced pressure: Kempf, J. Prakt. Chem. [2] **78**, 239 (1908). Commercial production by catalytic vapor-phase oxidation of benzene or other suitable hydrocarbons: Weiss, Downs, Ind. Eng. Chem. **12**, 228 (1920); **US 1318633** (1920

to Barrett Co.). Many other syntheses. Review of commercial methods of manufacture: Ashcroft, Clifford, Chem. Prod. **24**, 11 (1961), C.A. **55**, 9724d (1961); Faith, Keyes & Clark's Industrial Chemicals, F. A. Lowenheim, M. K. Moran, Eds. (Wiley-Interscience, New York, 4th ed., 1975) pp 514-518. Review: W. D. Robinson, R. A. Mount in Kirk-Othmer Encyclopedia of Chemical Technology vol. 14 (Wiley-Interscience, New York, 3rd ed., 1981) pp 770-793. Book: B. C. Trivedi, B. M. Culbertson, Maleic Anhydride (Plenum, New York, 1982) 872 pp.

Orthorhombic needles from chloroform; also readily by sublimation. Commercial grades are furnished in fused form, as briquettes. d 1.48. mp 52.8°. bp_{760} 202.0°; bp_{400} 179.5°; bp_{200} 155.9°; bp_{100} 135.8°; bp_{60} 122.0°; bp_{40} 111.8°; bp_{20} 95.0°; bp_{10} 78.7°; bp_5 63.4°. Specific heat: 0.285 (solid); 0.396 (liq). Sol in water, forming maleic acid. Soly at 25° (g/100 g): acetone 227; ethyl acetate 112; chloroform 52.5; benzene 50; toluene 23.4; o-xylene 19.4; carbon tetrachloride 0.60; ligroin 0.25. Sol in dioxane. Sol in alc with ester formation.
Caution: Potential symptoms of overexposure are conjunctivitis; photophobia, double vision; nasal and upper respiratory irritation; bronchial asthma; dermatitis. See NIOSH Pocket Guide to Chemical Hazards (DHHS/NIOSH 97-140, 1997) p 188.
USE: In Diels-Alder syntheses (as a dienophile), manuf alkyd-type of resins, dye intermediates, pharmaceuticals, agricultural chemicals (maleic hydrazide, malathion), in copolymerization reactions.

5705. Maleic Hydrazide. [123-33-1] 1,2-Dihydro-3,6-pyridazinedione; maleic acid hydrazide; MH; Fazor; Malazide; Regulox. $C_4H_4N_2O_2$; mol wt 112.09. C 42.86%, H 3.60%, N 24.99%, O 28.55%. Prepd by treating maleic anhydride with hydrazine hydrate in alcohol: Arndt et al., C.A. **43**, 579 (1949); see also Curtius, Foerstinger, J. Prakt. Chem. [2] **51**, 391 (1895). From maleic acid and a hydrazine salt of a strong inorganic acid: Harris, Schoene, **US 2575954** (1951 to U.S. Rubber). Alternate prepn from hydrazine sulfate and maleic anhydride in aqueous NaOH: Amatsu, Karasawa, C.A. **51**, 18014c (1957); from hydrazine hydrate and maleic anhydride in glacial acetic acid: Feuer et al., J. Am. Chem. Soc. **80**, 3790 (1958). Has the ability to inhibit growth of plants without killing them: Schoene, Hoffmann, Science **109**, 588 (1949). Toxicity data: R. Ben-Dyke et al., World Rev. Pest Control **9**, 119 (1970). Review: Massey, Manuf. Chem. **26**, 197-200 (1955). Review and chromatographic studies: Fishbein, Chromatography of Environmental Hazards (Elsevier, New York, 1972) pp 161-166. Review of toxicology: R. Ponnampalam et al., Regul. Toxicol. Pharmacol. **3**, 38-47 (1983).

Crystals from water, dec 260°. Also reported as mp >300° (Feuery). Slightly sol in hot alcohol, more sol in hot water. LD_{50} orally in rats: 3800-6800 mg/kg; dermally in rabbits: >4000 mg/kg (Ben-Dyke).
USE: Experimentally in horticulture and agriculture. To control suckering of tobacco. In the synthesis of pyridazine.

5706. Maleuric Acid. [105-61-3] (Z)-4-[(Aminocarbonyl)-amino]-4-oxo-2-butenoic acid; N-carbamoylmaleamic acid; maleyl-urea. $C_5H_6N_2O_4$; mol wt 158.11. C 37.98%, H 3.82%, N 17.72%, O 40.48%. Prepd from maleic anhydride and urea: Dunlap, Phelps, Am. Chem. J. **19**, 492 (1897); Batt et al., J. Am. Chem. Soc. **76**, 3663 (1954).

Crystals from hot water, dec 158.5°. uv max: 235 nm (ε 8720). Sol in hot acetic acid. Practically insol in cold water, cold acetic acid, acetone, ligroin, chloroform, alc, ether.

Methyl ester. Crystals, mp 113-114°. Sol in hot water, methanol, ethanol, acetone, dioxane.

Butyl ester. Crystals, mp 95-98°. Sol in ethanol, acetone, benzene, chloroform.

5707. Malic Acid. [6915-15-7] Hydroxybutanedioic acid; hydroxysuccinic acid. $C_4H_6O_5$; mol wt 134.09. C 35.83%, H 4.51%, O 59.66%. The naturally occurring isomer is the L-form which has been found in apples and many other fruits and plants. Prepn of D- and DL-forms, and resolution of racemic mixture: McKenzie et al., J. Chem. Soc. **123**, 2875 (1923). Solubilities: Descamps, Bull. Soc. Chim. Belg. **49**, 91 (1940). Microbial production of L-form: Kitahara; Abe et al., US 2972566; US 3063910 (1961, 1962, both to Kyowa). Configuration: J. A. Mills, W. Klyne in Progress in Stereochemistry vol. 1, W. Klyne, Ed. (Academic Press, New York, 1954) pp 182-183; E. L. Eliel, Stereochemistry of Carbon Compounds (McGraw-Hill, New York, 1962) pp 97-98; Cymerman-Craig, Roy, Tetrahedron **21**, 1847 (1965). Review of uses: Manuf. Chem. Aerosol News **35**, 56 (December, 1964). Review: S. E. Berger, "Hydroxy Dicarboxylic Acids" in Kirk-Othmer Encyclopedia of Chemical Technology vol 13 (Wiley-Interscience, New York, 3rd ed., 1981) pp 103-110.

L-Malic Acid

DL-Form. [617-48-1] Crystals, mp 131-132°. Soly in g/100 g solvent at 20°: methanol 82.70, diethyl ether 0.84, ethanol 45.53, acetone 17.75, dioxane 22.70, water 55.8. Practically insol in benzene.

D-(+)-Form. [636-61-3] Crystals, mp 101°.

L-(−)-Form. [97-67-6] Apple acid. Crystals from acetone, or acetone + CHCl₃, mp 100°. Dec ~140°. $[\alpha]_D$ −2.3° (c = 8.5). Soly in g/100 g solvent at 20°: methanol 197.22, diethyl ether 2.70, ethanol 86.60, acetone 60.66, dioxane 74.35, water 36.35. Practically insol in benzene.

USE: Intermediate in chemical synthesis. Chelating and buffering agent. Flavoring agent, flavor enhancer and acidulant in foods.

5708. Mallow. Common mallow; high mallow; cheeseflower. Leaves of Malva sylvestris L., and M. rotundifolia L., Malvaceae. Habit. Europe, Asia, naturalized in U.S. Constit. Pectin, tannin, coloring matter.

5709. Malondialdehyde. [542-78-9] Propanedial; malonaldehyde. $C_3H_4O_2$; mol wt 72.06. C 50.00%, H 5.60%, O 44.41%. Endogenous product of lipid peroxidation and prostaglandin biosynthesis in mammals; also formed by oxidation of polyunsaturated fatty acids in foods. Reacts with functional groups of a variety of cellular compounds including DNA and amino acids, forming genotoxic adducts and crosslinks. Associated with detrimental protein modifications and decreased nutritional value in foods. Prepn: L. Claisen, Ber. **36**, 3664 (1903); R. Hüttel, ibid. **74**, 1825 (1941). Chemistry and reactions with amino acids: V. Nair et al., J. Am. Chem. Soc. **103**, 3030 (1981). NMR spectroscopy: S. H. Bertz, G. Dabbagh, J. Org. Chem. **55**, 5161 (1990). Determn methods using thiobarbituric acid: H. H. Draper et al., Free Radical Biol. Med. **15**, 353 (1993). HPLC determn in foods: P. Bergamo et al., J. Agric. Food Chem. **46**, 2171 (1998); in biological samples: R. Mateos et al., J. Chromatogr. B **827**, 76 (2005). Acute toxicity study: D. L. Crawford et al., Toxicol. Appl. Pharmacol. **7**, 826 (1965). Clinical use as biomarker in neurodegenerative disease: M. Dib et al., J. Neurol. **249**, 367 (2002); in coronary artery disease: H. H. Jung et al., Am. J. Nephrol. **24**, 537 (2004). Review of metabolism: H. H. Draper, M. Hadley, Xenobiotica **20**, 901-907 (1990); of biochemistry: H. Esterbauer et al., Free Radical Biol. Med. **11**, 81-128 (1991). Review of carcinogenic risk: IARC Monographs **71**, Part 3, 1037-1047 (1999); of toxicity of DNA adducts: L. J. Marnett, IARC Sci. Publ. **150**, 17-27 (1999); and pathological significance: D. Del Rio et al., Nutr. Metab. Cardiovasc. Dis. **15**, 316-328 (2005).

Needles, mp 72-74°. pKa (enolate) 4.46. Stable in neutral conditions but not in acidic. LD_{50} orally in rats: 632 mg/kg (Crawford).

Sodium salt. [24382-04-5] $C_3H_4NaO_2$; mol wt 95.05. White needles from ethanol/ether, mp 246° (dec). uv max (0.01M HCl): 245 nm (ε 12800).

Direct contact may cause irritation of eyes, skin and respiratory system; potential symptom of overexposure is CNS depression. Potential occupational carcinogen. See NIOSH Pocket Guide to Chemical Hazards (2003-100121, 2003) p 190.

USE: Biomarker for oxidative stress. Index of oxidative rancidity in foods.

5710. Malonic Acid. [141-82-2] Propanedioic acid; methanedicarboxylic acid. $C_3H_4O_4$; mol wt 104.06. C 34.63%, H 3.87%, O 61.50%. HOOCCH₂COOH. Prepd from malic acid: Dessaignes, Ann. **107**, 251 (1858). Made by the interaction of monochloroacetic acid and NaCN followed by hydrolysis of the resulting cyanoacetic acid: Weiner, Org. Synth. coll. vol. II, 376 (1943). Prepn from diethyl malonate: Britton, Monroe, US 2373011 (1945 to Dow); from ligneous wastes: Grangaard, US 2928868 (1960 to Kimberly-Clark); from sodium acetate: Normant, Angelo, Bull. Soc. Chim. Fr. **1962**, 810. Review: D. W. Hughes in Kirk-Othmer Encyclopedia of Chemical Technology vol. 14 (Wiley-Interscience, New York, 3rd ed., 1981) pp 794-810.

Small crystals, mp ~135° with decompn; sublimes in vacuo. d 1.63. One gram dissolves in 0.65 ml water, about 2 ml alcohol, 1.1 ml methanol, 3 ml propyl alcohol, 13 ml ether, 7 ml pyridine.

Diethyl Ester see Ethyl Malonate.

Caution: Strong irritant.

USE: In manuf of barbiturates.

5711. Malononitrile. [109-77-3] Propanedinitrile; methylene cyanide; dicyanomethane; cyanoacetonitrile. $C_3H_2N_2$; mol wt 66.06. C 54.54%, H 3.05%, N 42.41%. CH₂(CN)₂. Prepn: Henri, Compt. Rend. **102**, 1394 (1886); B. B. Corson et al., Org. Synth. coll. vol. 2, 379 (1943); A. R. Surrey, J. Am. Chem. Soc. **65**, 2471 (1943); idem, US 2389217 (1945 to Winthrop); idem, Org. Synth. coll. vol. 3, 535 (1955). Toxicity study: G. R. N. Jones, M. S. Israel, Nature **228**, 1315 (1970). Reviews: F. Freeman, Chem. Rev. **69**, 591-624 (1969); A. J. Fatiadi, Synthesis **1978**, 165-204, 241-282.

Colorless solid, mp 32°. bp_{760} 218-219°, bp_{20} 109°. d_4^{20} 1.1910; n_D^{34} 1.4146. Very sol in alc, ether; sol in water, acetone, benzene. LD_{50} i.p. in mice: 12.9 mg/kg (Jones, Israel).

Caution: Potential symptoms of overexposure are irritation of eyes, skin, nose, throat; headache, dizziness, weakness, giddiness, confusion, convulsions; dyspnea; abdominal pain, nausea, vomiting. See NIOSH Pocket Guide to Chemical Hazards (DHHS/NIOSH 97-140, 1997) p 190.

USE: In organic synthesis.

5712. Malotilate. [59937-28-9] 1,3-Dithiol-2-ylidenepropanedioic acid bis(1-methylethyl) ester; diisopropyl 1,3-dithiol-2-ylidenemalonate; NKK-105; Hepation; Kantec. $C_{12}H_{16}O_4S_2$; mol wt 288.38. C 49.98%, H 5.59%, O 22.19%, S 22.24%. Prepn from diisopropyl malonate: K. Taninaka et al., DE 2545569; eidem, US 4035387 (1976, 1977 both to Nihon Nohyaku); from the corresponding ketene mercaptide: H. Matsui et al., US 4327223 (1982 to Nihon Nohyaku). Effect on CCl₄-induced liver injury in rats: Y. Imaizumi et al., Jpn. J. Pharmacol. **31**, 15 (1981). Enhancement of rat liver protein synthesis: eidem, ibid. **32**, 369 (1982). Pharmacokinetics and pharmacodynamics: M. Buhrer et al., Eur. J. Clin. Pharmacol. **30**, 407 (1986). Clinical evaluation in liver cirrhosis: S. Takase et al., Gastroenterol. Jpn. **23**, 639 (1988).

Pale yellow crystals, mp 60.5°. Sol in benzene, cyclohexane, *n*-hexane, ether.

THERAP CAT: Hepatoprotectant.

5713. Maltol. [118-71-8] 3-Hydroxy-2-methyl-4*H*-pyran-4-one; 3-hydroxy-2-methyl-4-pyrone; 3-hydroxy-2-methyl-γ-pyrone; larixinic acid; palatone; veltol. $C_6H_6O_3$; mol wt 126.11. C 57.14%, H 4.80%, O 38.06%. Found in the bark of young larch trees (*Larix decidua* Mill.), in pine needles (*Abies alba* Mill., *Pinaceae*), in chicory, in wood tars and oils, in roasted malt. Isoln from these sources and structure: Kiliani, Bazlen, *Ber.* **27**, 3115 (1894); Feuerstein, *Ber.* **34**, 1804 (1901); Erdmann, Schaefer, *Ber.* **43**, 2398 (1910); Reichstein, Beitter, *Ber.* **63**, 824 (1930), *cf.* Peratoner, Tamburello, *Chem. Zentralbl.* **76**, II 680 (1905). Also obtained by alkaline hydrolysis of streptomycin salts: Schenck, Spielman, *J. Am. Chem. Soc.* **67**, 2276 (1945). Synthesis: Spielman, Freifelder, *ibid.* **69**, 2908 (1947); Chawla, McGonigal, *J. Org. Chem.* **39**, 3281 (1974). Novel high-yield synthesis: T. M. Brennan *et al.*, *Tetrahedron Lett.* **1978**, 331; P. D. Weeks *et al.*, *J. Org. Chem.* **45**, 1109 (1980). History and comparison with isomaltol: Hodge, Nelson, *Cereal Chem.* **38**, 207 (1961).

Monoclinic prisms from chloroform, orthorhombic bipyramidal crystals + monoclinic prisms from 50% alcohol, mp 161-162°. Fragrant, caramel-like odor. Begins to sublime at 93°. Volatile with steam. uv max (0.1*N* HCl): 274 nm (E_m 8400); (0.1*N* NaOH): 317 nm (E_m 7300). pH of 0.5% aq soln 5.3. One gram dissolves in 85 ml water. Freely sol in hot water, chloroform; sol in alcohol; sparingly sol in benzene, ether, petr ether; sol in aq alkali hydroxides giving yellow solns.

USE: Flavoring agent, to impart "freshly baked" odor and flavor to bread and cakes.

5714. Maltose. [69-79-4] 4-*O*-α-D-Glucopyranosyl-D-glucose; malt sugar; maltobiose; 4-(α-D-glucosido)-D-glucose; Maltos; Martos-10. $C_{12}H_{22}O_{11}$; mol wt 342.30. C 42.11%, H 6.48%, O 51.41%. Monohydrate obtained in about 80% yield by enzymatic (diastase) degradation of starch: Gore, US 1657079 (1928). Structure: Haworth, Peat, *J. Chem. Soc.* **1926**, 3094; Hassid, Ballou in W. Pigman, *The Carbohydrates* (Academic Press, New York, 1957) p 498. Crystal and molecular structure: F. Takusagawa, R. A. Jacobson, *Acta Crystallogr.* **B34**, 213 (1978). *Review:* E. Tarelli, *Dev. Food Carbohydr.* **2**, 187-227 (1980); R. Khan, *Carbohydr. Chem. Biochem.* **39**, 213-278 (1981).

Monohydrate. Crystals from water or dil alc, mp 102-103°. Does not lose its water of crystn by drying at room temp *in vacuo* over H_2SO_4 or P_2O_5. About one-third as sweet as sucrose. *Cf.* Isbell, Pigman, *J. Res. Natl. Bur. Stand.* **18**, 141 (1937). Shows mutarotation. $[\alpha]_D^{20}$ +111.7° → +130.4° (c = 4). pKa (21°): 12.05. Sol in water, slightly sol in alcohol. Practically insol in ether.

USE: Nutrient, sweetener, in culture media, in prepd bee food. Parenteral supplement of sugar for diabetics. Fermentable intermediate in brewing. Stabilizer for polysulfides. In pharmaceutical dispensing.

5715. Malvidin Chloride. [643-84-5] 3,5,7-Trihydroxy-2-(4-hydroxy-3,5-dimethoxyphenyl)-1-benzopyrylium chloride; 3,4',5,7-tetrahydroxy-3',5'-dimethoxyflavylium chloride; enidin; primulidin; syringidin; 3,4',5,7-tetrahydroxy-3',5'-dimethoxy-2-phenylbenzopyrrylium chloride. $C_{17}H_{15}ClO_7$; mol wt 366.75. C 55.67%, H 4.12%, Cl 9.67%, O 30.54%. Found as the diglucoside

(malvin) in wild malve (*Primula viscosa* All., *Primulaceae*) and as the monoglucoside in blue grapes: Willstätter, Mieg, *Ann.* **408**, 122 (1915); Karrer, Widmer, *Helv. Chim. Acta* **10**, 5 (1927). Structure: Anderson, Nabenhauer, *J. Am. Chem. Soc.* **48**, 2997 (1926). Synthesis: Bradley, Robinson, *J. Chem. Soc.* **1928**, 1541.

Prisms or rhombic tablets, appearing red by transmitted light with a green luster when dry or with a steel-blue luster when in contact with solvent. Usually obtained as the mono- or dihydrate. The anhydr salt is very hygroscopic. Not melted at 300°. Sol in abs alc, giving a violet-red soln. Sparingly sol in water. Also sol in amyl alc. In methanol the substance is first sol with purple color, then begins to separate as red crystals which are violet by transmitted light.

3-β-Glucoside tetrahydrate. 3-(Glucosyloxy)-4',5,7-trihydroxy-3',5'-dimethoxyflavylium chloride; enin; cyclamin. $C_{23}H_{25}ClO_{12}$.$4H_2O$. Synthesis: Levy *et al.*, *J. Chem. Soc.* **1931**, 2701. Dark prisms with a green metallic shine, from alcohol + HCl. Sparingly sol in water, alcohol, glycerol. Practically insol in benzene, chloroform, ether.

3,5-Diglucoside. 3,5-Bis(glucosyloxy)-4',7-dihydroxy-3',5'-dimethoxyflavylium chloride; malvin; malvoside. $C_{29}H_{35}ClO_{17}$. Synthesis: Robinson, Todd, *ibid.* **1932**, 2299. Reddish-brown prisms or needles with a green shine from dil HCl, dec 165°.

3-Galactoside hemihendecahydrate. Primulin. $C_{23}H_{25}ClO_{12}$.$5\frac{1}{2}H_2O$. Bronze metallic needles or prisms from methanol + HCl. Bluish-violet by transmitted light. Very sol in methanol, ethanol, cold water, forming deep red solns; slightly sol in acetone. Practically insol in ethyl acetate.

5716. Mancozeb. [8018-01-7] [[1,2-Ethanediylbis(carbamodithioato)](2−)]manganese mixt. with [[1,2-ethanediylbis(carbamodithioato)](2−)]zinc; ethylenebis(dithiocarbamic acid) manganese zinc complex; manzeb; manganese ethylenebis(dithiocarbamate) (polymeric) complex with zinc salt; zinc manganese ethylenebisdithiocarbamate; Dithane M-45; Fore; Manzate; Manzin; Nemispor; Penncozeb; Vondozeb. Polymeric salt of ethylenebisdithiocarbamic acid containing approx 20% manganese and 2.5% zinc; related to maneb and zineb, *q.q.v.* Displays activity against a wide range of foliage fungal diseases. Prepn: NZ 131543; C. B. Lyon *et al.*, US 3379610 (1965, 1968 both to Rohm & Haas). Metabolic fate in plants, animals: W. R. Lyman, "Metabolic fate of Dithane M-45," in *Pestic. Terminal Residues, Invited Pap. Int. Symp.*, A. S. Tahori, Ed. (Butterworth, New York, 1971) pp 243-256. Residue studies: *WHO Pestic. Residues Ser.* **vol. 4**, (WHO, FAO, 1975) 451; W. H. Newsome, *J. Agric. Food Chem.* **27**, 1188 (1979). HPLC determn: K. Gustafsson *et al.*, *ibid.* **29**, 729 (1981). Demonstrates low phytotoxicity: L. H. Cornford, *Proc. 36th N. Z. Weed Pest Control Conf.* 258 (1983). In potato blight: H. W. Platt, *Can. J. Plant Pathol.* **5**, 38 (1984). *In vitro* activity against *Alternaria alternata*: V. A. Bourbos *et al.*, *Br. Crop Prot. Counc. Monogr.* **2**, No. 31, 461 (1985). Aquatic toxicology: C. J. Van Leeuwen *et al.*, *Aquat. Toxicol.* **7**, 145 (1985).

x : y   10:1

Insol in water.

USE: Fungicide.

5717. Mandelic Acid. [90-64-2] α-Hydroxybenzeneacetic acid; *dl*-mandelic acid; racemic mandelic acid; α-hydroxy-α-toluic acid; α-hydroxyphenylacetic acid; phenylhydroxyacetic acid; phenylglycolic acid; amygdalic acid; amygdalinic acid; paramandelic acid; Uromaline. $C_8H_8O_3$; mol wt 152.15. C 63.15%, H 5.30%, O 31.55%. $C_6H_5CH(OH)COOH$. Prepd by the action of warm, dil alkali upon dichloroacetophenone: *Org. Synth.* **23**, 48 (1943); by hydrolysis of mandelonitrile (prepd from benzaldehyde and hydrogen cyanide or from benzaldehyde, sodium bisulfite, and sodium cyanide): *Org. Synth.* **coll. vol. I**, 336 (1941); *ibid.* **coll. vol. III**, 538 (1955); L. F. Fieser, *Organic Experiments* (Boston, 1964) p 109. May be prepd by boiling amygdalin with HCl.

Orthorhombic plates from water, mp 119°. Darkens and dec on prolonged exposure to light. d 1.30. Can be distilled rapidly *in vacuo* at 2 mm without much decompn. Acid to litmus. pK (25°) 3.37. One gram dissolves in 6.3 ml water, 1 ml alc; freely sol in ether, isopropyl alcohol.

Calcium salt. [134-95-2] Calcium mandelate; Camdelate. $C_{16}H_{14}CaO_6$; mol wt 342.36. Contains 88.88% mandelic acid. White powder. One gram dissolves in 80 ml boiling water. Slightly sol in cold water. Insol in alc. The aq soln is slightly acid.

Sodium salt. [114-21-6] Sodium mandelate. $C_8H_7NaO_3$. Cryst powder; slight aromatic odor. Very sol in water; sol in alcohol; the aq soln is neutral or slightly alkaline to litmus.

THERAP CAT: Antiseptic (urinary).

5718. Mandelic Acid Isoamyl Ester. [5421-04-5] α-Hydroxybenzeneacetic acid 3-methylbutyl ester; mandelic acid isopentyl ester; isoamyl mandelate; Atractyl; Spasmol; Vermiparin; Spasmostenyl. $C_{13}H_{18}O_3$; mol wt 222.28. C 70.24%, H 8.16%, O 21.59%. Prepd by esterification of DL-mandelic acid with an excess of isoamyl alcohol in the presence of concd H_2SO_4: Rona *et al., Biochem. Z.* **181**, 50 (1927). Improved procedure and spasmolytic activity: N. Brock *et al., Arzneim.-Forsch.* **2**, 165 (1952).

Oily liquid. bp_{11} 172° (Rona); bp_{12} 155° (Brock). Practically insol in water. Miscible with fat solvents. Easily hydrolyzed by esterases.

Caution: The pure, undiluted liquid is a skin irritant.

THERAP CAT (VET): Has been used as an anthelmintic.

5719. Mandelonitrile. [532-28-5] α-Hydroxybenzeneacetonitrile; mandelic acid nitrile; benzaldehyde cyanohydrin. C_8H_7-NO; mol wt 133.15. C 72.16%, H 5.30%, N 10.52%, O 12.02%. Isoln of *d*-form from peach flower buds: Jones, Enzie, *Science* **134**, 284 (1961). Prepn of *d*-form by hydrolysis of amygdalin: Auld, *J. Chem. Soc.* **95**, 927 (1909); Smith, *Ber.* **64**, 427 (1931). Resolution of *dl*-form: Feist, *Arch. Pharm.* **247**, 226 (1909). Synthesis of *l*-form using cotton fibers: Bredig, Gerstner, *Biochem. Z.* **250**, 414 (1932). Asymmetric synthesis: Krieble, Wieland, *J. Am. Chem. Soc.* **43**, 164 (1921); Prelog, Wilhelm, *Helv. Chim. Acta* **37**, 1634 (1954); Tsuboyama, *Bull. Chem. Soc. Jpn.* **35**, 1004 (1962). It has been suggested that mandelonitrile may be responsible for the alleged anticancer activity of Laetrile, *q.v.: see* Culliton, *Science* **182**, 1000 (1973). Metabolism study: P. D. A. Singh *et al., Biochem. Pharmacol.* **34**, 2207 (1985).

dl-**Form.** Yellow, oily liquid, mp −10°. Decomp at 170°. d 1.115-1.120. Almost insol in water. Freely sol in alcohol, chloroform, ether.

d-**Form.** $[\alpha]_D^{25}$ +43.75° (c = 5.006 in benzene).

USE: Preparing bitter almond water, by mixing 11 g with 500 g alc and 1489 g water; the mixture contains 0.1% HCN.

5720. Mandelonitrile Glucoside. [138-53-4] α-(β-D-Glucopyranosyloxy)benzeneacetonitrile. $C_{14}H_{17}NO_6$; mol wt 295.29. C 56.94%, H 5.80%, N 4.74%, O 32.51%. Prepn of *d*-form by action of yeast on amygdalin: Fischer, *Ber.* **28**, 1508 (1895); Auld, *J. Chem. Soc.* **93**, 1276 (1908). Isoln of *d*-form from *Prunus serotina,* Ehrk, *P. macrophylla* Sieb et Zucc., *Rosaceae:* Power, Moore, *ibid.* **95**, 243 (1909); **97**, 1099 (1910); Kariyone, Matsushima, *J. Pharm. Soc. Jpn.* No. **514**, 1061 (1924); from *Eucalyptus corynocalyx* F.v.M., *Myrtaceae:* Finnemore *et al., J. Proc. R. Soc. N.S.W.* **69**, 209 (1936); from *Pteridium aquilinum* (L.) Kühn, *Polypodiaceae:* Kofod, Eyjolfssen, *Tetrahedron Lett.* **1966**, 1289. Isoln of *dl*-form from *Prunus laurocerasus* L. and *Cotoneaster microphylla* Wall., *Rosaceae:* Winkler, Simon, *Ann.* **31**, 263 (1839); Hérissey, *J. Pharm. Chim.* **24**, 537 (1906). Isoln of *l*-form from *Sambucus nigra* L., *Caprifoliaceae:* Guignart, *Compt. Rend.* **141**, 16 (1905); Bourquelot, Danjot, *ibid.* 598 (1905). Prulaurasin is *dl*-mandelonitrile glucoside and sambunigrin is *l*-mandelonitrile glucoside: Caldwell, Courtauld, *J. Chem. Soc.* **91**, 671 (1907). Biosynthesis of *d*-mandelonitrile glucoside: Mentzer, Favre-Bonvin, *Compt. Rend.* **253**, 1072 (1961). Abs config of isomers: U. Schwarzmaier, *Ber.* **109**, 3250 (1976).

d-**Form.** Prunasin. Needles from chloroform, mp 147-148°. $[\alpha]_D^{14}$ −29.94°. Soluble in water, alcohol, acetone. Converted by alkalies to prulaurasin.

dl-**Form.** Prulaurasin. Slightly bitter needles from ethyl acetate + ether, mp 123-125°. $[\alpha]_D$ −54° (water). Soluble in water, alcohol. Practically insol in ether. On hydrolysis yields *dl*-mandelic acid.

l-**Form.** Sambunigrin. Bitter needles from hot ethyl acetate, mp 151-152°. $[\alpha]_D^{18}$ −75.1°. Soluble in water, alcohol, ethyl acetate. On hydrolysis yields *l*-mandelic acid.

5721. Maneb. [12427-38-2] [[1,2-Ethanediylbis[carbamodithioato]](2−)]manganese; [ethylenebis(dithiocarbamato)]manganese; ethylenebis[dithiocarbamic acid] manganous salt; manganous ethylenebis[dithiocarbamate]; Dithane M-22; Manex; Trimangol. $(C_4H_6MnN_2S_4)_n$. Polymeric salt of ethylenebisdithiocarbamic acid; related to zineb and mancozeb, *q.q.v.* Prepd from aq nabam, *q.v.,* by neutralizing with acetic acid and adding $MnCl_2$ soln: A. L. Flenner, US 2504404 (1950 to Du Pont), *see also* W. F. Hester, US 2317765 (1943 to Rohm & Haas). Fungicidal activity is due to degradation products, principally **ethylenethiuram monosulfide**: R. A. Ludwig *et al., Can. J. Bot.* **32**, 42 (1955). *In vitro* activity against *Alternaria alternata:* V. A. Bourbos *et al., Br. Crop Prot. Counc. Monogr.* **2**, No. 31, 461 (1985). Decomposition of maneb to ethylenebisdithiocarbamate and ethylene thiourea, *q.v.:* W. J. Trotter, J. Pardue, *J. Food Saf.* **4**, 59 (1982). HPLC determn: K. Gustafsson *et al., J. Agric. Food Chem.* **29**, 729 (1981). Toxicological studies in rats: D. W. R. Bleyl, H. Seidler, *Nahrung* **29**, 421 (1985); in aquatic organisms: C. J. Van Leeuwen *et al., Aquat. Toxicol.* **7**, 145 (1985).

Yellow powder. Crystals from alcohol. Moderately sol in water. Sol in chloroform, pyridine.

USE: Agricultural fungicide.

5722. Mangafodipir. [118248-94-5] (free acid); [155319-91-8] (hexahydrogen). (*OC*-6-13)-[[*N*,*N* '-1,2-Ethanediylbis[*N*-[[3-(hydroxy-κ*O*)-2-methyl-5-[(phosphonooxy)methyl]-4-pyridinyl]methyl]glycinato-κ*N*,κ*O*]](8−)]manganate(6−); manganese(II)-*N*,*N* '-dipyridoxylethylenediamine-*N*,*N* '-diacetate-5,5-bis(phosphonate); manganese dipyridoxal diphosphate; MnDPDP; S-095. C$_{22}$H$_{24}$MnN$_4$O$_{14}$P$_2$; mol wt 685.33. C 38.56%, H 3.53%, Mn 8.02%, N 8.18%, O 32.68%, P 9.04%. Paramagnetic manganese (II) chelate designed as a tissue specific imaging agent taken up by normal liver parenchyma. Prepn: S. M. Rocklage, S. C. Quay, **EP 290047**; *eidem*, **US 4933456** (1988, 1990 both to Salutar); *idem et al., Inorg. Chem.* **28**, 477 (1989). Pharmacology, toxicity and image enhancement studies: G. Elizondo *et al., Radiology* **178**, 73 (1991). HPLC determn in plasma: K. G. Toft *et al., J. Pharm. Biomed. Anal.* **15**, 973 (1997). Series of articles on clinical studies, toxicology and physicochemical properties: *Acta Radiol.* **38**, 626-789 (1997). Review of use as contrast agent for liver lesion detection: N. M. Rofsky, J. P. Earls, *MRI Clin. North Am.* **4**, 73-85 (1996).

LD$_{50}$ i.v. in mice: 5.4 mmol/kg (Elizondo).
Trisodium salt. [140678-14-4] Magnafodipir trisodium; Win-59010; Teslascan. C$_{22}$H$_{27}$MnN$_4$Na$_3$O$_{14}$P$_2$; mol wt 757.32. Pale yellow, triclinic hygroscopic crystals. d 1.537. uv max (water): 220, 257, 319 nm (ε 37600, 10300, 13400). Soly (g/ml): 0.4596 water, 0.0230 methanol, 0.0008 ethanol, 0.0006 acetone, 0.0011 chloroform. Log P (1-octanol:water) −5.62; (1-butanol: water) −3.68. Prepd as 0.01 mmol/ml aqueous infusion: bright yellow, clear soln, pH 7.5. Viscosity (mPa.s): 1.0 at 20°, 0.7 at 37°. Osmolality (37°): 290 mosmol/kg. d^{20} 1.01 g/ml.
THERAP CAT: Diagnostic aid (MRI contrast agent).

5723. Manganese. [7439-96-5] Mn; at. wt 54.938045; at. no. 25; valences 2, 4, 7; 1, 3, 5, 6 rare. Group VIIB (7). One stable isotope: 55; artificial radioactive isotopes 49-54; 56-58. Widely-distributed, abundant element; constitutes 0.085% of earth's crust. Occurs in the minerals pyrolusite, hausmannite, manganite, **braunite** (3Mn$_2$O$_3$.MnSiO$_3$), **manganosite** (MnO), and in several others; occurs in minute quantities in water, plants and animals. Essential dietary nutrient. First isolated by Gahn in 1774. Prepn of the metal: John *et al.*, cited by Mellor, *A Comprehensive Treatise on Inorganic and Theoretical Chemistry* **12**, 163 (1932); A. H. Sully, *Manganese* (Academic Press, New York, 1955) 305 pp. Review of physical properties: Meaden, *Met. Rev.* **13**, 97-114 (1968). Review of manganese and its compds: Kemmitt in *Comprehensive Inorganic Chemistry* vol. **3**, J. C. Bailar Jr. *et al.*, Eds. (Pergamon Press, Oxford, 1973) pp 771-876; L. R. Matricardi, J. H. Downing in *Kirk-Othmer Encyclopedia of Chemical Technology* vol. **14**, (Wiley-Interscience, New York, 3rd ed., 1981) pp 824-843. Review of toxicology and human exposure: *Toxicological Profile for Manganese* (PB2000-108025, 2000) 504 pp.
Steel gray, lustrous, hard, brittle metal. Exists in four allotropic forms: α-form, body-centered cubic, stable below 710° (approx), d^{20} 7.47; β-form, cubic, stable in the range 710-1079°, d^{20} 7.26; γ-form or electrolytic Mn, face-centered cubic, stable in the range 1079-1143°C, d^{1100} 6.37; δ-form, body-centered cubic, stable from 1143° to mp, d^{1143} 6.28. γ-Mn when stabilized at room temp is face-centered tetragonal, d^{20} 7.21. mp 1244°. bp 2095°. Sp heat 0.115 cal/g/°C; latent heat of fusion: 3.5 kcal/g-atom. Mohs' hardness 5.0. Superficially oxidized on exposure to air. Burns with an intense white light when heated in air. Dec water slowly in the cold, rapidly on heating; pure electrolytic manganese is not attacked by water at ordinary temp; slightly attacked by steam. Reacts with dil mineral acids with evolution of hydrogen and formation of divalent manganous salts. Reacts with aq solns of sodium or potassium

bicarbonate. When heated in nitrogen above 2000° burns to form a nitride. Converted by fluorine into the di- and trifluoride, by chlorine into the dichloride. In form of powder reduces most metallic oxides on heating. On heating, reacts directly with carbon, phosphorus, antimony or arsenic.
Caution: Potential symptoms of overexposure are parkinsonism; asthenia, insomnia and mental confusion; metal fume fever (dry throat, coughing, tight chest, dyspnea, rales and flu-like fever); lower back pain; vomiting; malaise; fatigue; kidney damage. See *NIOSH Pocket Guide to Chemical Hazards* (DHHS/NIOSH 97-140, 1997) p 190.
USE: In manuf of steel; for rock crushers, railway points and crossings, wagon buffers; as a constituent of several alloys, *e.g.*, ferromanganese, copper manganese, Manganin.

5724. Manganese Acetate. [638-38-0] C$_4$H$_6$MnO$_4$; mol wt 173.03. C 27.77%, H 3.50%, Mn 31.75%, O 36.99%. Mn(CH$_3$-COO)$_2$.
Tetrahydrate. Pale red, transparent monoclinic crystals. d 1.59. Sol in water or alcohol. LD$_{50}$ orally in rats: 3.73 g/kg, Smyth *et al., Am. Ind. Hyg. Assoc. J.* **30**, 470 (1969).
USE: As mordant in dyeing; manuf bister; drier for paints and varnishes (1-1.5:1000).

5725. Manganese Bromide. [13446-03-2] Manganese dibromide. Br$_2$Mn; mol wt 214.75. Br 74.42%, Mn 25.58%. MnBr$_2$.
Tetrahydrate. Rose-red, slightly deliquesc crystals. mp 64° with some decompn. Sol in 0.5 parts water; sol in alcohol. The aq soln is slightly acid. *Keep well closed.*

5726. Manganese Carbonate. [598-62-9] CMnO$_3$; mol wt 114.95. C 10.45%, Mn 47.79%, O 41.76%. MnCO$_3$. (Usually contains some H$_2$O). Occurs in nature as the mineral *rhodochrosite.*
Pink to almost white powder when freshly pptd, but gradually becomes light brown in the air. Rhombohedral, calcite structure. d 3.1. Insol in water or alcohol. Sol in dil acid. *Keep well closed.*
USE: As pigment —"manganese white"; drier for varnishes; in feeds.

5727. Manganese Carbonyl. [10170-69-1] Decacarbonyldimanganese. C$_{10}$Mn$_2$O$_{10}$; mol wt 389.98. C 30.80%, Mn 28.17%, O 41.03%. Mn$_2$(CO)$_{10}$. First prepd by reduction of MnI$_2$ with a Grignard reagent under CO pressure: Hurd *et al., J. Am. Chem. Soc.* **71**, 1899 (1949). Improved prepns: Brimm *et al., ibid.* **76**, 3831 (1954); Closson, *ibid.* **80**, 6167 (1958); Podall *et al., ibid.* **82**, 1325 (1960); Calderazzo, *Inorg. Chem.* **4**, 293 (1965). Crystal structure: Dahl, Rundle, *Acta Crystallogr.* **16**, 419 (1963); molecular structure: Almenningen *et al., Acta Chem. Scand.* **23**, 685 (1969). *Reviews: Organic Syntheses via Metal Carbonyls* vol. **1**, I. Wender, P. Pino, Eds. (Interscience, New York, 1968) *passim*; Anisimov *et al., Usp. Khim.* **37**, 380-408 (1968); *Russ. Chem. Rev.* **37**, 184-197 (1968) (English translation).
Golden yellow, monoclinic crystals. d^{25} 1.75. mp 154-155°. Stable under an atm of CO. In absence of CO, begins to dec at 110°. Sol in organic solvents. Insol in water. Less stable to air, heat and light in soln.
USE: Catalyst; antiknock additive.

5728. Manganese Chloride. [7773-01-5] Manganous chloride; manganese dichloride. Cl$_2$Mn; mol wt 125.84. Cl 56.35%, Mn 43.66%. MnCl$_2$. Acute toxicity studies: D. J. Holbrook, Jr. *et al., Environ. Health Perspect.* **10**, 95 (1975); P. P. Singh, A. Y. Junnarkar, *Indian J. Pharmacol.* **23**, 153 (1991).
LD$_{50}$ in mice, rats (mg/kg): 1330.0, 1470.0 orally; 126.0, 147.0 i.p.; 171.0, 92.6 i.v. (Singh, Junnarkar).
Tetrahydrate. [13446-34-9] Cl$_2$Mn.4H$_2$O. Reddish, slightly deliquesc, monoclinic crystals. d 2.01. mp 58°. Sol in 0.7 part water; sol in alcohol. Insol in ether. pH of 0.2 molar aq soln 5.5. *Keep well closed.* LD$_{50}$ in rats (mmole/kg): 7.5 orally; 0.70 i.p. (Holbrook).
USE: In dyeing (manganese bister); disinfecting; purifying natural gas; linseed oil drier; in electric batteries.

5729. Manganese Difluoride. [7782-64-1] Manganous fluoride; manganese fluoride. F$_2$Mn; mol wt 92.93. F 40.89%,

Mn 59.12%. MnF$_2$. Prepd from manganese carbonate and hydrogen fluoride: Moissan, Venturi, *Compt. Rend.* **130,** 1158 (1900); Kwasnik in *Handbook of Preparative Inorganic Chemistry* Vol. 1, G. Brauer, Ed. (Academic Press, New York, 2nd ed., 1963) pp 262-263. Review of toxicology of fluoride compounds: G. L Waldbott, *Acta Med. Scand. Suppl.* **400,** 1-44 (1963).

Pink, quadratic prisms (tetragonal structure, rutile type) or reddish powder. *Poisonous!* d 3.98. mp 856°. Soly in water (g/100 ml): 0.66 (40°); 0.44 (60°); 0.48 (100°). Insol in alc. Sol in dil hydrofluoric acid, concd hydrochloric or nitric acid. LD in guinea pigs (mg/kg): 200 orally, 700 s.c. (Waldbott).

Tetrahydrate. Obtained by dissolving manganese carbonate in hydrofluoric acid, evaporating, and drying *in vacuo*.

5730. Manganese Dioxide. [1313-13-9] Manganese binoxide; manganese peroxide; manganese superoxide; black manganese oxide. MnO$_2$; mol wt 86.94. Mn 63.19%, O 36.81%. Occurs in nature as the mineral *pyrolusite*, or made artificially (pptd). The native product is heavy, steel-gray when in lumps, black when powdered; the pptd product is a brownish-black, fine powder. Both usually contain some Mn$_3$O$_4$ and some water. When ignited evolves oxygen, leaving Mn$_3$O$_4$. Lab prepn: Moore *et al., J. Am. Chem. Soc.* **72,** 856 (1950); Covington *et al., Trans. Faraday Soc.* **58,** 1975 (1962). Toxicity study: D. J. Holbrook, Jr. *et al., Environ. Health Perspect.* **10,** 95 (1975). Review of use as reagent: J. S. Pizey, *Synthetic Reagents* **vol.** 2 (John Wiley, New York, 1974) pp 143-174.

Tetragonal crystals (rutile structure). Insol in water, nitric or cold sulfuric acid. Slowly dissolves in cold HCl with evolution of Cl$_2$; in presence of hydrogen peroxide or oxalic acid it dissolves in dil H$_2$-SO$_4$ or HNO$_3$. *Strong oxidizer; should not be heated or rubbed with organic matter or other oxidizable substances, e.g., sulfur, sulfides, phosphides, hypophosphites, etc.* LD$_{50}$ orally in rats: >40 mmole/kg (Holbrook).

USE: The mineral is the source of manganese and all its compds; largely used in manuf manganese steel; oxidizer; in alkaline batteries (dry cells); for making amethyst glass, decolorizing glass; painting on porcelain, faience and majolica. The ppt is used in electrotechnics, pigments, browning gun barrels, drier for paints and varnishes, printing and dyeing textiles.

5731. Manganese Hypophosphite. [10043-84-2] H$_4$-MnO$_4$P$_2$; mol wt 184.91. H 2.18%, Mn 29.71%, O 34.61%, P 33.50%. Mn(H$_2$PO$_2$)$_2$.

Monohydrate. Pink, odorless, almost tasteless crystals or powder. When heated evolves spontaneously flammable phosphine. One gram dissolves in 6.5 ml water, 6 ml boiling water. Insol in alcohol.

5732. Manganese Iodide. [7790-33-2] Manganese diiodide. I$_2$Mn; mol wt 308.75. I 82.21%, Mn 17.79%. MnI$_2$.

Tetrahydrate. Rose-red crystals; rapidly becomes brown on exposure to air and light, due to liberation of iodine. Very sol in water with gradual decompn; sol in alcohol. The aq soln is slightly acid. *Keep tightly closed and protected from light.*

5733. Manganese Nitrate. [10377-66-9] MnN$_2$O$_6$; mol wt 178.95. Mn 30.70%, N 15.65%, O 53.64%. Mn(NO$_3$)$_2$. Prepn: Dehnicke, Strähle, *Ber.* **97,** 1502 (1964). *Review: Gmelins, Manganese* (8th ed.) **56,** part C3, 267-281 (1975).

Colorless; hygroscopic. Sol in water, dioxane, tetrahydrofuran, acetonitrile.

Tetrahydrate. Pink, deliquesc cryst masses at temp below 20°. d 2.129. mp 37.1°. Very sol in water, sol in alcohol. The aq soln is slightly acid.

Hexahydrate. Rose-colored, deliquesc, monoclinic needles (colorless after several crystns). d 1.8. mp 25.0°. Freely sol in water, alcohol.

USE: Intermediate in manuf of reagent grade MnO$_2$; in prepn of porcelain colorants.

5734. Manganese Oxalate. [640-67-5] C$_2$MnO$_4$; mol wt 142.96. C 16.80%, Mn 38.43%, O 44.77%. MnC$_2$O$_4$.

Dihydrate. White cryst powder; dec at 150°. Slightly sol in water; sol in acids.

5735. Manganese Oxide. [1317-35-7] Manganomanganic oxide; manganese tetroxide. Mn$_3$O$_4$; mol wt 228.81. Mn 72.03%, O 27.97%. Occurs in nature as the mineral *hausmannite*. Prepn: Moore *et al., J. Am. Chem. Soc.* **72,** 856 (1950).

Brownish-black powder. d 4.7. Insol in water. Sol in HCl with evolution of chlorine.

Caution: Potential symptoms of overexposure are asthenia, insomnia, mental confusion; low back pain, vomiting, malaise, fatigue; kidney damage; pneumonitis. *See NIOSH Pocket Guide to Chemical Hazards* (DHHS/NIOSH 97-140, 1997) p 192.

5736. Manganese Selenide. [1313-22-0] MnSe; mol wt 133.90. Mn 41.03%, Se 58.97%. Prepd by the action of manganese salts on alkali selenides: Berzelius *et al.,* cited by Mellor, *A Comprehensive Treatise on Inorganic and Theoretical Chemistry* **10,** 798 (1930); by the action of a manganese salt on a soln of hydrogen selenide out of contact with air: Moser, Atynsky, *Monatsh. Chem.* **45,** 235 (1925).

Gray-black cubic crystals. d^{15} 5.59. Completely oxidized when heated to redness in oxygen. Insol in cold water. Dec in hot water and dil acids.

5737. Manganese Sesquioxide. [1317-34-6] Mn$_2$O$_3$; mol wt 157.87. Mn 69.60%, O 30.40%. Occurs in nature as the mineral *manganite*, Mn$_2$O$_3$.H$_2$O. Prepn: Moore *et al., J. Am. Chem. Soc.* **72,** 856 (1950).

Black, fine powder. d 4.50. Insol in water. Sol in HCl with evolution of chlorine.

5738. Manganese Silicate. [7759-00-4] Approx MnSiO$_3$. Occurs in nature as the minerals *rhodonite, manganjustite, tephroite*.

Red crystals or yellowish-red powder. The pptd article is a yellowish-red powder. d of the mineral 3.48. Insol in water.

USE: As color for special glass; producing red glazes on pottery.

5739. Manganese Sulfate. [7785-87-7] MnO$_4$S; mol wt 151.00. Mn 36.38%, O 42.38%, S 21.24%. MnSO$_4$. Forms several hydrates. The article of commerce is usually a mixture of the tetra- and pentahydrates.

Monohydrate. Pale red, slightly efflorescent crystals; loses all water at 400-450°. Sol in about 1 part cold, 0.6 part boiling water; insol in alcohol.

USE: In dyeing; for red glazes on porcelain; boiling oils for varnishes; in fertilizers for vines, tobacco; in feeds.

THERAP CAT (VET): Nutritional factor (essential trace element in all animals); prevention of perosis in poultry.

5740. Manganese Sulfide. [18820-29-6] Manganese monosulfide. MnS; mol wt 87.00. Mn 63.15%, S 36.86%. Occurs in nature as the mineral *alabandite* or *manganblende*. Prepn: Mehmed, Haraldsen, *Z. Anorg. Chem.* **235,** 194 (1938).

Pink, green or brown-green powder. Three cryst modifications: α-form, green cubic crystals; β-form, red cubic crystals; γ-form, red hexagonal crystals. Practically insol in water; sol in dil acids. In moist condition it readily oxidizes in air to the sulfate.

5741. Manganese Trifluoride. [7783-53-1] Manganic fluoride. F$_3$Mn; mol wt 111.93. F 50.92%, Mn 49.08%. MnF$_3$. Prepd by fluorination of manganese iodide according to the equation 2MnI$_2$ + 13F$_2$ → 2MnF$_3$ + 4IF$_5$: Moissan, *Compt. Rend.* **130,** 622 (1900); v. Wartenberg, *Z. Anorg. Allg. Chem.* **244,** 346 (1940); Kwasnik in *Handbook of Preparative Inorganic Chemistry* **vol.** 1, G. Brauer, Ed. (Academic Press, New York, 2nd ed., 1963) pp 263-264.

Red mass; monoclinic crystals. d 3.54. Stable to 600°. Hydrolyzed by water. May be stored in glass ampuls.

USE: Fluorinating agent in organic chemistry.

5742. Mangostin. [6147-11-1] 1,3,6-Trihydroxy-7-methoxy-2,8-bis-(3-methyl-2-butenyl)-9H-xanthen-9-one; 1,3,6-trihydroxy-7-methoxy-2,8-di(3-methyl-2-butenyl)xanthone. C$_{24}$H$_{26}$O$_6$; mol wt 410.46. C 70.23%, H 6.38%, O 23.39%. From various parts of the mangosteen tree *(Garcinia mangostana* L., *Guttiferae):* Schmid, *Ann.* **93,** 83 (1855); Dragendorff, *ibid.* **482,** 280 (1930).

Structure: Yates, Stout, *J. Am. Chem. Soc.* **80**, 1691 (1958); Scheinmann, *Chem. Commun.* **1967**, 1015; Stout *et al., ibid.* **1968**, 211.

Yellow crystals from benzene, mp 181.6-182.6°. uv max (ethanol): 243, 259, 318, 351 nm (log ε 4.54, 4.44, 4.38, 3.86). Practically insol in water; sol in alcohol, ether, acetone, chloroform, ethyl acetate.

3,6-Dimethylmangostin. $C_{26}H_{30}O_6$. Pale yellow needles from ethanol, mp 123.3-123.8°. uv max (ethanol): 245, 262, 314, 350 nm (log ε 4.50, 4.53, 4.36, 3.81).

5743. Manidipine. [89226-50-6] 1,4-Dihydro-2,6-dimethyl-4-(3-nitrophenyl)-3,5-pyridinedicarboxylic acid 2-[4-(diphenylmethyl)-1-piperazinyl]ethyl methyl ester; 2-[4-(diphenylmethyl)-1-piperazinyl]ethyl methyl (±)-1,4-dihydro-2,6-dimethyl-4-(*m*-nitrophenyl)-3,5-pyridinecarboxylate; franidipine. $C_{35}H_{38}N_4O_6$; mol wt 610.70. C 68.83%, H 6.27%, N 9.17%, O 15.72%. Dihydropyridine calcium channel blocker. Prepn: K. Meguro, A. Nagaoka, **EP 94159**; *eidem*, **US 4892875** (1983, 1990, both to Takeda); K. Meguro *et al., Chem. Pharm. Bull.* **33**, 3787 (1985). Synthesis and bioactivity of optical isomers: M. Kajino *et al., ibid.* **37**, 2225 (1989). Acute toxicity study: S. Chiba *et al., Yakuri to Chiryo* **17**, Suppl. 4, 961 (1989), *C.A.* **111**, 146499b (1989). Determn of enantiomers in human serum: M. Yamaguchi *et al., J. Chromatogr.* **575**, 123 (1992). Clinical evaluation in hypertension: K. Mizuno *et al., Curr. Ther. Res.* **52**, 248 (1992).

Light yellow crystals from isopropyl ether + hexane, mp 125-128°.

Dihydrochloride. [89226-75-5] CV-4093; Calslot. $C_{35}H_{38}N_4O_6 \cdot 2HCl$; mol wt 683.62. Two crystalline forms. α-form: yellow crystals, mp 157-163°. β-form: light yellow, fine crystals, mp 174-180°. Also prepd as the monohydrate, mp 167-170°. LD_{50} in male, female mice, male, female rats (mg/kg): 387, 340, 222, 199 s.c.; 62.2, 68.0, 66.5, 48.8 i.p.; 190, 171, 247, 156 orally (Chiba).

THERAP CAT: Antihypertensive.

5744. Manna. Dried exudation of *Fraxinus ornus* L., *Oleaceae. Habit.* Mediterranean Basin, Asia Minor, Spain. *Constit.* 40-60% mannitol; 10-16% mannotetrose; 6-16% mannotriose; glucose, mucilage, fraxin.

One gram dissolves in 5 ml water, 150 ml 90% alcohol.

THERAP CAT: Cathartic.

5745. Mannitol. [69-65-8] D-Mannitol; mannite; manna sugar; cordycepic acid; Manicol; Mannidex; Osmitrol; Osmosal; Resectisol. $C_6H_{14}O_6$; mol wt 182.17. C 39.56%, H 7.75%, O 52.70%. Widespread in plants and plant exudates; obtained from manna and seaweeds: *The Carbohydrates*, W. Pigman, Ed. (Academic Press, New York, 1957) pp 249-250. Forms a stable, equimolar compound with H_2O_2: S. Tanatar, *J. Russ. Phys. Chem. Soc.* **40**, 376, *C.A.* **3**, 883 (1909). Prepd by electrolytic reduction of glucose: Creighton, *Can. Chem. Process Ind.* **26**, 690 (1942), *C.A.* **37**, 1088⁵ (1943); Wolfrom *et al., J. Am. Chem. Soc.* **68**, 578 (1946).

Prepn from seaweed: Sorensen, Kristensen, **US 2516350** (1950); by hydrogenation of invert sugar, monosaccharides, and sucrose: Kasehagen, and Kasehagen, Luskin, **US 2642462**, **US 2749371**, and **US 2759024** (1953, 1956, and 1956, all to Atlas Powder). Review of prepn: Pigman, *loc. cit.* Novel synthesis: M. Makkee *et al., Chem. Commun.* **1980**, 930.

Orthorhombic needles from alc, mp 166-168°. Sweetish taste. d^{20} 1.52. $bp_{3.5}$ 290-295°. Is inactive or very slightly levorotatory in distilled water. Forms sodium mannitoborate on addition of borax giving a greater rotation: $[\alpha]_D^{20}$ +23° → +24° after 1 hr in a soln of 10 g mannitol +12.8 g borax + sufficient H_2O to make 100 ml. One gram dissolves in ~5.5 ml water, 83 ml alcohol; more sol in hot water. Insol in ether. Sol in pyridine, aniline, aq solns of alkalies. One gram dissolves in 18 ml glycerol (d 1.24). Soly tables: Creighton, Klauder, *J. Franklin Inst.* **195**, 687 (1923). pKa (18°): 13.50.

USE: Used with boric acid in the manuf of dry electrolytic condensers for radio applications; in making artificial resins and plasticizers; in pharmacy as excipient and diluent for solids and liqs; in analytical chemistry for boron determinations; in the manuf of mannitol hexanitrate. Used in the food industry as anticaking and free-flow agent, flavoring agent, lubricant and release agent, stabilizer and thickener and nutritive sweetener.

THERAP CAT: Diuretic. Diagnostic aid (renal function).

5746. D-Mannitol Hexanitrate. [15825-70-4] Mannitol nitrate; nitromannite; nitromannitol; Medemanol; Dilangil; Moloid; Mannitrin; Manexin. $C_6H_8N_6O_{18}$; mol wt 452.16. C 15.94%, H 1.78%, N 18.59%, O 63.69%. Made by nitration of mannitol: Fleury *et al., Mem. Poudres* **31**, 107 (1949).

Long needles in regular clusters from alc. mp 106-108°. Soluble in alc, in ether; insol in water. Explodes on percussion. Its stability at ordinary temps is such that it may be used commercially, but it is distinctly less stable than nitroglycerol at 75°. Its employ for pharmaceutical prepns is only in admixture with carbohydrate substances in dilutions corresponding to 1 part of mannitol hexanitrate to 9 or more parts of carbohydrate. In such dilutions mannitol hexanitrate is considered nonexplosive.

THERAP CAT: Vasodilator.

5747. D-Mannose. [3458-28-4] Seminose; carubinose. $C_6H_{12}O_6$; mol wt 180.16. C 40.00%, H 6.71%, O 53.28%. Prepn of α-form by treating ivory nut shavings with H_2SO_4: Isbell, *J. Res. Natl. Bur. Stand.* **26**, 47 (1941); Isbell, Frush in *Methods in Carbohydrate Chemistry*, R. L. Whistler, M. L. Wolfrom, Eds. (Academic Press, New York, 1962) pp 145-147. Prepn and stability of α- and β-forms: Reeves, *J. Am. Chem. Soc.* **72**, 1499 (1950); J. Sowden in *The Carbohydrates*, W. Pigman, Ed. (Academic Press, New York, 1957) pp 94-95.

α-Form. Crystals from methanol, mp 133°. $[\alpha]_D$ +29.3° → +14.2° (water).

β-Form. Orthorhombic, bisphenoidal needles from alcohol or acetic acid, dec 132°. Sweet taste with bitter aftertaste. d^{20} 1.54. Shows mutarotation. $[\alpha]_D^{20}$ −17.0° → +14.2° (c = 4). One gram dissolves in 0.4 ml water, 120 ml methanol, 250 ml abs ethanol, 3.5 ml pyridine. pKa (18°): 11.98. Reduces Fehling's soln; is fermented by yeast.

Phenylhydrazone. $C_{12}H_{18}N_2O_5$. Crystals from dil ethanol, mp 199-200°. $[\alpha]_D^{20}$ +26.3° → +33.8° (pyridine).
CaCl₂-addition compd tetrahydrate. $C_6H_{12}O_6.CaCl_2.4H_2O$. mp 101-102°. $[\alpha]_D^{20}$ −31.3° → +6.0° (c = 9).

5748. Maprotiline. [10262-69-8] *N*-Methyl-9,10-ethanoanthracene-9(10*H*)-propanamine; 9-(γ-methylaminopropyl)-9,10-dihydro-9,10-ethanoanthracene; 1-(3-methylaminopropyl)dibenzo[*b,-e*]bicyclo[2.2.2]octadiene. $C_{20}H_{23}N$; mol wt 277.40. C 86.59%, H 8.36%, N 5.05%. Prepn: P. Schmidt *et al.*, **US 3399201** (1968 to Ciba). Synthesis, NMR, mass spectra: M. Wilhelm, P. Schmidt, *Helv. Chim. Acta* **52**, 1385 (1969). Toxicity: R. Hess *et al.*, *Boll. Chim. Farm.* **112**, 782 (1973), *C.A.* **81**, 33479p (1974). Review of pharmacology and therapeutic efficacy: R. M. Pinder *et al.*, *Drugs* **13**, 321 (1977). Comprehensive description: S. K. Suh, J. B. Smith, *Anal. Profiles Drug Subs.* **15**, 393-426 (1986).

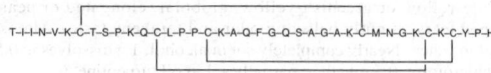

mp 92-94°.
Hydrochloride. [10347-81-6] Ba-34276; Deprilept; Ludiomil; Psymion. $C_{20}H_{23}N.HCl$; mol wt 313.86. Crystals from isopropanol, mp 230-232°. Freely sol in methanol and chloroform, slightly sol in water. Practically insol in isooctane. LD₅₀ in mice, rats (mg/kg): ~750, ~900 orally (Hess).
THERAP CAT: Antidepressant.

5749. Maraviroc. [376348-65-1] 4,4-Difluoro-*N*-[(1*S*)-3-[(3-*exo*)-3-[3-methyl-5-(1-methylethyl)-4*H*-1,2,4-triazol-4-yl]-8-azabicyclo[3.2.1]oct-8-yl]-1-phenylpropyl]-cyclohexanecarboxamide; *N*-[(1*S*)-3-[3-(3-isopropyl-5-methyl-4*H*-1,2,4-triazol-4-yl)-*exo*-8-azabicyclo[3.2.1]oct-8-yl]-1-phenylpropyl]-4,4-difluorocyclohexanecarboxamide; UK-427857. $C_{29}H_{41}F_2N_5O$; mol wt 513.67. C 67.81%, H 8.05%, F 7.40%, N 13.63%, O 3.11%. Potent, noncompetitive CCR5 receptor antagonist; inhibits binding of HIV viral coat protein gp120. Prepn: M. Perros *et al.*, **WO 0190106**; *eidem*, **US 020013337** (2001, 2002 both to Pfizer); D. A. Price *et al.*, *Tetrahedron Lett.* **46**, 5005 (2005). Overview of structure identification and development: A. Wood, D. Armour, *Prog. Med. Chem.* **43**, 239-271 (2005). Pharmacokinetics and metabolism in humans and animals: D. K. Walker *et al.*, *Drug Metab. Dispos.* **33**, 587 (2005).

White solid from toluene/hexane (2:1), mp 197-198°. pKa 7.3.
THERAP CAT: Antiviral.

5750. Marbofloxacin. [115550-35-1] 9-Fluoro-2,3-dihydro-10-methyl-10-(4-methyl-1-piperazinyl)-7-oxo-7*H*-pyrido[3,2,1-*ij*][4,1,2]benzoxadiazine-6-carboxylic acid; Marbocyl; Zeniquin. $C_{17}H_{19}FN_4O_4$; mol wt 362.36. C 56.35%, H 5.29%, F 5.24%, N 15.46%, O 17.66%. Fluorinated quinolone antibacterial. Prepn: M. Aoki *et al.*, **EP 259804**; K. Yokose *et al.*, **US 4801584** (1987, 1989 both to Hoffmann-LaRoche). HPLC determn in plasma: M. A. Garcia *et al.*, *J. Chromatogr. B* **729**, 157 (1999). Evaluation of experimental surgical infection in dogs: P. Gruet *et al.*, *Vet. Rec.* **140**, 199 (1997). Pharmacokinetics and efficacy in cattle: C. Eyett-Burton *et al.*, *Cattle Practice* **5**, 289 (1997). Pharmacokinetics in renally impaired dogs: H. P. Lefebvre *et al.*, *J. Vet. Pharmacol. Ther.* **21**, 453 (1998).

Crystals from methanol, mp 268-269° (dec).
THERAP CAT (VET): Antibacterial.

5751. Margaric Acid. [506-12-7] Heptadecanoic acid. $C_{17}H_{34}O_2$; mol wt 270.45. C 75.50%, H 12.67%, O 11.83%. $CH_3(CH_2)_{15}COOH$. Prepn: Kaufmann, Stamm, *Ber.* **91**, 2121 (1958); Bhattacharyya *et al.*, *Chem. Ind. (London)* **1959**, 1352; Hünig, Ledle, *Ber.* **93**, 913 (1960). Metabolism: Boyer, Scheig, *Lipids* **4**, 615 (1969). Toxicity study: L. Orö, A. Wretlind, *Acta Pharmacol. Toxicol.* **18**, 141 (1961).

Crystals from alcohol, mp 61°. d 0.853. bp₁₀₀ 227°. n_D^{60} 1.4342. Insol in water. Freely sol in ether; slightly sol in alcohol. LD₅₀ i.v. in mice: 360.3 mg/kg (Orö, Wretlind).

5752. Margatoxin. [145808-47-5] MgTX. $C_{178}H_{286}N_{52}O_{50}S_7$; mol wt 4178.95. C 51.16%, H 6.90%, N 17.43%, O 19.14%, S 5.37%. Peptide toxin isolated from the new world scorpion, *Centruroides margaritatus*, consists of 39 amino acids with 3 disulfide bridges. Selectively inhibits voltage-gated potassium channels. Isoln and characterization: M. Garcia-Calvo *et al.*, *J. Biol. Chem.* **268**, 18866 (1993). Synthesis: M. A. Bednarek *et al.*, *Biochem. Biophys. Res. Commun.* **198**, 619 (1994). NMR determn of three dimensional structure: B. A. Johnson *et al.*, *Biochemistry* **33**, 15061 (1994). Use as an affinity label for potassium channels: H.-G. Knaus *et al.*, *ibid.* **34**, 13627 (1995); H. S. Fischer, A. Saria, *Neurosci. Lett.* **263**, 208 (1999).

T-I-I-N-V-K-C-T-S-P-K-Q-C-L-P-P-C-K-A-Q-F-G-Q-S-A-G-A-K-C-M-N-G-K-C-K-C-Y-P-H

USE: Biochemical probe.

5753. Marimastat. [154039-60-8] (2*S*,3*R*)-*N*⁴-[(1*S*)-2,2-Dimethyl-1-[(methylamino)carbonyl]propyl]-*N*¹-2-dihydroxy-3-(2-methylpropyl)butanediamide; *N*²-[3*S*-hydroxy-4-(*N*-hydroxyamino)-2*R*-isobutylsuccinyl]-L-*tert*-leucine-*N*¹-methylamide; BB-2516. $C_{15}H_{29}N_3O_5$; mol wt 331.41. C 54.36%, H 8.82%, N 12.68%, O 24.14%. Synthetic matrix metalloproteinase inhibitor (MMPI). Prepn: J. P. Dickens *et al.*, **WO 9402447**; *eidem*, **US 5700838** (1994, 1997 both to British Biotech) and structure-activity study: D. E. Levy *et al.*, *J. Med. Chem.* **41**, 199 (1998). Improved synthesis: R. J. Davenport, R. J. Watson, *Tetrahedron Lett.* **41**, 7983 (2000). Clinical study in pancreatic cancer: S. R. Bramhall *et al.*, *J. Clin. Oncol.* **19**, 3447 (2001); in gastric cancer: *idem et al.*, *Br. J. Cancer* **86**, 1864 (2002). Review of pharmacology: H. S. Rasmussen, P. P. McCann, *Pharmacol. Ther.* **75**, 69-75 (1997); and clinical development: A. L. Thomas, W. P. Steward, *Expert Opin. Invest. Drugs* **9**, 2913-2922 (2000). Review of structure-activity and mechanism of action: M. Whittaker *et al.*, *Chem. Rev.* **99**, 2735-2776 (1999).

Soly in water: 1.4 mg/ml.
THERAP CAT: Antineoplastic.

5754. Marrubiin. [465-92-9] [2a*S*-(2aα,5aβ,6α,7α,8aα,-8bα)]-6-[2-(3-Furanyl)ethyl]decahydro-6-hydroxy-2a,5a,7-trimethyl-2*H*-naphtho[1,8-*bc*]furan-2-one; 15,16-epoxy-6β,9-dihydroxy-8βH-labda-13(16),14-dien-19-oic acid γ-lactone; 5-[2-(3-furyl)ethyl]decahydro-5,8-dihydroxy-1,4a,6-trimethyl-1-naphthoic acid γ-lactone. $C_{20}H_{28}O_4$; mol wt 332.43. C 72.26%, H 8.49%, O 19.25%. Diterpene lactone principle isolated from white horehound, *Marrubium vulgare* (Tourn.) L., *Labiatae:* Harms, *Arch. Pharm.* **83**, 144 (1842); Ludwig, Kromayer, *ibid.* **158**, 257 (1861); Nicholas, *J. Pharm. Sci.* **53**, 895 (1964). Alternate view that marrubiin is an artefact generated from *premarrubiin* during the isoln: Henderson, McCrindle, *J. Chem. Soc. C* **1969**, 2014. Structure and stereochemistry: Cocker *et al., J. Chem. Soc.* **1953**, 2540; *Chem. Ind. (London)* **1954**, 1561; **1955**, 1484; Fulke, McCrindle, *ibid.* **1965**, 647. Total stereochemistry: Wheeler *et al., Tetrahedron* **23**, 3909 (1967); Appleton *et al., J. Chem. Soc. C* **1967**, 1943. Synthesis: Mangoni *et al., Tetrahedron* **28**, 611 (1972).

Crystals from alc, mp 160°. $[\alpha]_D^{20}$ +35.8° (c = 3.1 in chloroform); $[\alpha]_D^{24}$ +45° (acetone). uv max: 208, 212, 216 nm (log ε 3.75, 3.75, 3.70). One gram dissolves in 60 ml alc. Freely sol in chloroform, acetone, hot alc, pyridine; sparingly sol in ether, benzene. Practically insol in water.

5755. Mastic. Balsam tree; pistachia galls; mastiche; mastix; lentisk; Mastisol. Concrete resinous exudation from *Pistacia lentiscus* L., *Anacardiaceae. Habit.* Mediterranean Islands, especially Chios. *Constit.* Volatile oil (about 2%); masticinic, masticonic acids; masticoresene.

Pale yellow or greenish-yellow, globular, elongated or pear-shaped tears; slightly balsamic odor and terebene taste. Almost insol in water. Nearly completely sol in alcohol; 1 g dissolves in 0.5 ml chloroform, 0.5 ml ether; partially sol in oil turpentine.

USE: In tooth cements, plasters, lacquers, chewing gums, and incense; also for retouching negatives.

5756. Maté. Paraguay tea; yerba maté; St. Bartholomew's tea; Jesuit's tea. Leaves of *Ilex paraguensis* St. Hil., *Aquifoliaceae,* grown in Brazil, Uruguay, Argentina, and Paraguay. *Review:* Cheney, *Econ. Bot.* **1**, 243 (1947). For constituents see: Siesto, *Quad. Nutr.* **18**, 35 (1959), *C.A.* **57**, 13133d (1962); Roberts, *Chem. Ind. (London)* **1956**, 985; Paula, *Rev. Bras. Quim.* (Sao Paulo) **42**, 202 (1956), *C.A.* **51**, 3167i (1957). Among its constituents are caffeine, other purines, tannins or tannoid substances, such as chlorogenic acid and derivatives.

5757. Matico. Dried leaves of *Piper elongatum* Vahl. (*P. angustifolium* R. & P.), *Piperaceae. Habit.* Peru, Bolivia, Brazil, Mexico, Cuba. *Constit.* 1-3.5% volatile oil, maticin (a bitter principle); artanthic acid, tannin, mucilage, resin.

THERAP CAT: Astringent.

5758. Matricarin. [5989-43-5] (3S,3aR,4S,9aS,9bR)-4-(Acetyloxy)-3,3a,4,5,9a,9b-hexahydro-3,6,9-trimethylazuleno[4,5-b]furan-2,7-dione. $C_{17}H_{20}O_5$; mol wt 304.34. C 67.09%, H 6.62%, O 26.29%. Isoln from *Matricaria chamomilla* L. and *Artemisia tilesii* Ledeb, *Compositae:* Z. Cekan *et al., Collect. Czech. Chem. Commun.* **24**, 1554 (1959). Structure: W. Herz, K. Ueda, *J. Am. Chem. Soc.* **83**, 1139 (1961). Molecular conformation: M. Martinez V. *et al., J. Nat. Prod.* **51**, 221 (1988).

Plates from benzene + petr ether and acetone + petr ether, mp 190-191°. $[\alpha]_D^{23}$ +23.5° (c = 0.65 in chloroform). uv max: 255 nm (ε 15,100).

Desacetoxymatricarin. [17946-87-1] $C_{15}H_{18}O_3$. Isoln from *Artemisia* spp.: M. Holub, V. Herout, *Collect. Czech. Chem. Commun.* **27**, 2980 (1962); H. H. A. Linde, M. S. Ragab, *Helv. Chim. Acta* **50**, 1961 (1967). Synthesis and stereochemistry: E. H. White *et al., Tetrahedron* **25**, 2099 (1969). Crystals from ether, mp 205-205.5°, also reported as mp 202-203° (Holub). $[\alpha]_D^{24}$ +52.5° (c = 1 in chloroform).

Desacetylmatricarin monohydrate. $C_{15}H_{18}O_4 \cdot H_2O$. Crystals from benzene + acetone, mp 123-125°, resolidifies and mp 143-146°.

Tetrahydromatricarin. $C_{17}H_{24}O_5$. Needles from benzene + petr ether, mp 175-178°. $[\alpha]_D^{22}$ +32.3° (c = 1.92 in chloroform).

5759. Matrine. [519-02-8] Matridin-15-one; sophocarpidine. $C_{15}H_{24}N_2O$; mol wt 248.36. C 72.54%, H 9.74%, N 11.28%, O 6.44%. Occurs naturally as the (+)-form in the Chinese drug *Kuh Seng* or the Japanese *Shinkyogan,* the dried roots of *Sophora angustifolia* Sieb. & Zucc., *S. flavescens* Ait. and other *Sophora* spp., *Leguminosae.* Isomeric with lupanine, *q.v.* Isoln: Kondo, *Arch. Pharm.* **266**, 1 (1928); Winterfeld, Knener, *Ber.* **64**, 150 (1931); Orechov, Proskurnina, *Ber.* **67**, 77 (1934); Briggs, Ricketts, *J. Chem. Soc.* **1937**, 1795. Identity with sophocarpidine: Orechov *et al., Ber.* **68**, 429 (1935). Alternate method of isoln: F. Bohlmann *et al., Ber.* **91**, 2189 (1958). Structure: Tsuda, Murakami, *Ber.* **69**, 429 (1936). Configuration: Bohlmann *et al., Ber.* **91**, 2176 (1958). Absolute configuration: Okuda *et al., Chem. Pharm. Bull.* **14**, 314 (1966); Cervinka, *Z. Chem.* **7**, 190 (1967). Synthetic studies: Tsuda *et al., J. Org. Chem.* **21**, 1481 (1956); **23**, 1179 (1958). Synthesis of *matridine* (*deoxymatrine*): Mandell, Singh, *J. Am. Chem. Soc.* **83**, 1766 (1961). Total synthesis of (±)-matrine: Mandell *et al., ibid.* **87**, 5234 (1965); J. Chen *et al., Chem. Commun.* **12**, 905 (1986). Synthesis of (+)-matrine: Okuda *et al., Chem. Pharm. Bull.* **14**, 275 (1966). Biosynthesis: Schütte *et al., Arch. Pharm.* **295**, 34 (1962).

Has been obtained in four forms: α-Form: needles or flat prisms, mp 76°. β-Form: orthorhombic prisms, mp 87°, $[\alpha]_D^{20}$ +38° (alc). γ-Form: liquid, bp$_6$ 223°, d_4^{20} 1.088, n_D^{85} 1.5287. δ-Form: prisms, mp 84°. Sol in water, benzene, chloroform, ether, carbon disulfide; slightly sol in petr ether.

5760. Maxacalcitol. [103909-75-7] (1R,3S,5Z)-4-Methylene-5-[(2E)-[(1S,3aS,7aS)-octahydro-1-[(1S)-1-(3-hydroxy-3-methylbutoxy)ethyl]-7a-methyl-4H-inden-4-ylidene]ethylidene]-1,3-cyclohexanediol; (+)-(5Z,7E,20S)-20α-(3-hydroxy-3-methylbutoxy)-9,10-secopregna-5,7,10(19)-trien-1α,3β-diol; 1α,25-dihydroxy-22-oxavitamin D_3; 22-oxa-1α,25-dihydroxyvitamin D_3; 22-oxacalcitriol; 22-oxa-1,25(OH)$_2D_3$; MC-1275; Sch-209579; Oxarol; Prezios. $C_{26}H_{42}O_4$; mol wt 418.61. C 74.60%, H 10.11%, O 15.29%. Noncalcemic analog of vitamin D. Prepn: N. Kubodera *et al.,* **EP 184112**; *eidem,* **US 4891364** (1986, 1990 both to Chugai); E. Murayama *et al., Chem. Pharm. Bull.* **34**, 4410 (1986). Industrial synthesis: H. Shimizu *et al., Org. Process Res. Dev.* **9**, 278 (2005). Pharmacology: A. J. Brown *et al., J. Clin. Invest.* **84**, 728 (1989). Immunomodulatory effects: M. Komine *et al., Arch. Dermatol. Res.* **291**, 500 (1999). Metabolism study: M. Ishigai *et al., J. Steroid Biochem. Mol. Biol.* **66**, 281 (1998). LC-MS determn in serum: *idem et al., J. Chromatogr. B* **706**, 261 (1998). Clinical evaluation in psoriasis: J. Barker *et al., Br. J. Dermatol.* **141**, 274 (1999); in secondary hyperparathyroidism: Y. Tsukamoto *et al., Am. J. Kidney Dis.* **35**, 458 (2000).

Colorless crystals from hexane + ethyl acetate, mp 122°. $[\alpha]_D^{20}$ +49.4° (c = 1.00 in ethanol). uv max (ethanol): 263 nm.

THERAP CAT: Antihyperparathyroid; antipsoriatic.

5761. Maytansine. [35846-53-8] Maitansine; NSC-153858. $C_{34}H_{46}ClN_3O_{10}$; mol wt 692.20. C 59.00%, H 6.70%, Cl 5.12%, N 6.07%, O 23.11%. Anti-leukemic ansa macrolide, member of a class of compounds that includes the rifamycins, streptovaricins etc. First ansa compound isolated from a plant rather than produced by a microorganism. Isoln from *Maytenus ovatus* Loes., *Celastraceae* and structure elucidation: S. M. Kupchan *et al., J. Am. Chem. Soc.* **94,** 1354 (1972); S. M. Kupchan, **DE 2241418** (1974); S. M. Kupchan *et al.*, **US 3896111** (1975 to Research Corp.). Crystal structure and absolute configuration of the (3-bromopropyl) ether: R. F. Bryan *et al., J. Chem. Soc. Perkin Trans. 2* **1973,** 897. Synthetic studies: A. I. Meyers *et al., Tetrahedron Lett.* **1974,** 717; **1975,** 1745, 1749; E. J. Corey, M. G. Bock, *ibid.* **1975,** 2643; E. J. Corey *et al., ibid.* **1978,** 1051; A. I. Meyers, J. P. Hudspeth, *ibid.* **22,** 3925 (1981). Total synthesis of (±)-form: A. I. Meyers *et al., J. Am. Chem. Soc.* **102,** 6597 (1980); of naturally occurring (−)-form: E. J. Corey *et al., ibid.* 6613. Cytotoxic action: M. K. Wolpert-Defilippes, *Biochem. Pharmacol.* **24,** 751 (1975). Clinical studies in carcinoma, melanoma: J. A. Neidhart *et al., Cancer Treat. Rep.* **64,** 675 (1980); D. L. Ahmann *et al., ibid.* 721. Toxicity: G. M. Mugera, J. M. Ward, *ibid.* **61,** 1333 (1977).

mp 171-172°. $[\alpha]_D^{26}$ −145° (c = 0.055 in chloroform). uv max (ethanol): 233, 254, 282, 290 nm (ε 29800, 27200, 5690, 5520). LD$_{50}$ in rats (mg/kg): 0.48 s.c. (Mugera, Ward).

5762. Mazindol. [22232-71-9] 5-(4-Chlorophenyl)-2,5-dihydro-3*H*-imidazo[2,1-*a*]isoindol-5-ol; 5-(4-chlorophenyl)-2,3-dihydro-5-hydroxy-5*H*-imidazo[2,1-*a*]isoindole; SaH-42548; Magrilon; Mazildene; Sanorex; Teronac. $C_{16}H_{13}ClN_2O$; mol wt 284.74. C 67.49%, H 4.60%, Cl 12.45%, N 9.84%, O 5.62%. Prepn: W. J. Houlihan, **DE 1814540** *C.A.* **71,** 81368s (1969); W. J. Houlihan, M. K. Eberle, **DE 1930488**; *eidem*, **US 3597445** (1969, 1970, 1970 all to Sandoz); T. S. Sulkowski, **US 3763178** (1973 to American Home Prod.). Clinical trials as appetite depressant: C. Sirtori *et al., Am. J. Med. Sci.* **261,** 341 (1971); A. J. Hadler, *J. Clin. Pharmacol.* **12,** 453 (1972). Effect on human prolactin and growth hormone responses: D. A. Thompson *et al., Metabolism* **30,** 1015 (1981). Clinical evaluation in Duchenne muscular dystrophy: P. J. Collipp *et al., J. Med. Genet.* **21,** 254 (1984).

White crystalline solid from ethanol, mp 215-217° (Sulkowski); also reported as crystals from acetone-hexane, mp 198-199° (Houlihan, Eberle). uv max (95% ethanol): 223, 268.5, 272 nm (ε 19000, 4400, 4400). Sol in ethanol. Insol in water.

Note: This is a controlled substance (stimulant): **21 CFR,** 1308.14.

THERAP CAT: Anorexic; CNS stimulant.

5763. Mazipredone. [13085-08-0] (11β)-11,17-Dihydroxy-21-(4-methyl-1-piperazinyl)pregna-1,4-diene-3,20-dione; 11β,17α-dihydroxy-3,20-dioxo-21-(4-methyl-1-piperazinyl)pregna-1,4-diene; 11β,17-dihydroxy-21-(4-methyl-1-piperazinyl)-Δ^1-progesterone. $C_{26}H_{38}N_2O_4$; mol wt 442.59. C 70.56%, H 8.65%, N 6.33%, O 14.46%. Prepn: Tuba *et al.*, **HU 150350** (1963 to Gedeon Richter), *C.A.* **60,** 3057h (1964).

Crystals from tetrahydrofuran + ligroin, dec 199°.

Hydrochloride. [60-39-9] Depersolone. $C_{26}H_{38}N_2O_4$.HCl; mol wt 479.05. Crystals, dec 246°. Sol in water.

THERAP CAT: Anti-inflammatory.

5764. MCPA. [94-74-6] (4-Chloro-2-methylphenoxy)acetic acid; (4-chloro-*o*-toloxy)acetic acid; 2-methyl-4-chlorophenoxyacetic acid; MCP; Agritox; Agroxone; Cornox; Methoxone. C_9H_9-ClO_3; mol wt 200.62. C 53.88%, H 4.52%, Cl 17.67%, O 23.92%. Prepn: Synerholm, Zimmerman, *Contrib. Boyce Thompson Inst.* **14,** 91 (1945); Templeman, Sexton, *Proc. Roy. Soc.* **133B,** 300 (1946); Foster, **GB 573479** and **GB 573510** (both 1945 to ICI); Skeeters, **US 2740810** (1956 to Diamond Alkali). Toxicity study: Rowe, Hymas, *Am. J. Vet. Res.* **15,** 622 (1954). Review of carcinogenic risk: *IARC Monographs* **30,** 255-269 (1983); of genotoxicity studies: B. Elliott, *Mutagenesis* **20,** 3-13 (2005).

Plates from benzene, mp 120°. Practically insol in water. LD$_{50}$ orally in rats: 700 mg/kg (Rowe, Hymas).

Sodium salt. [3653-48-3] Chiptox. $C_9H_8ClNaO_3$; mol wt 222.60. Very sol in water.

USE: Herbicide.

5765. MDA. [4764-17-4] α-Methyl-1,3-benzodioxole-5-ethanamine; 3,4-methylenedioxyamphetamine; 3,4-methylenedioxy-α-methyl-β-phenylethylamine; 3,4-methylenedioxyphenylisopropylamine; "Love"; EA-1299. $C_{10}H_{13}NO_2$; mol wt 179.22. C 67.02%, H 7.31%, N 7.82%, O 17.85%. Entactogen; synthetic amphetamine derivative with stimulant and hallucinogenic properties. Metabolite of MDMA, *q.v.* Prepn: C. Mannich, W. Jacobsohn, *Ber.* **43,** 189 (1910); U. Braun *et al., J. Pharm. Sci.* **69,** 192 (1980). Pharmacology: L. E. Markert, D. C. S. Roberts, *Pharmacol. Biochem. Behav.* **39,** 569 (1991); K. M. Hegadoren *et al., Psychopharmacology* **118,** 295 (1995). HPLC determn in whole blood: R. E. Michel *et al., J. Neurosci. Methods* **50,** 61 (1993). GC/MS determn in hair: P. Kintz *et al., J. Chromatogr. B* **670,** 162

(1995). Acute toxicity studies: P. N. Thiessen, D. A. Cook, *Clin. Toxicol.* **6**, 193 (1973); H. F. Hardman *et al.*, *Toxicol. Appl. Pharmacol.* **25**, 299 (1973). Review of toxicity, mechanism of action, and psychoactive effects: R. P. Climko *et al.*, *Int. J. Psychiatry Med.* **16**, 359-372 (1986-1987).

Almost colorless oil. bp_{22} 157°. $bp_{0.2}$ 80-90°.

Hydrochloride. [6292-91-7] $C_{10}H_{13}NO_2$.HCl. Crystals from isopropanol/ether, mp 187-188° (Braun); also reported as mp 180-181° (Mannich, Jacobsohn). Easily sol in water, alcohol. LD_{50} in mice, rats, guinea pigs (mg/kg): 68, 27, 28 i.p. (Hardman).

Note: This is a controlled substance (hallucinogen): **21 CFR,** 1308.11.

5766. MDE. [82801-81-8] *N*-Ethyl-α-methyl-1,3-benzodioxole-5-ethanamine; (±)-*N*-ethyl-3,4-methylenedioxyamphetamine; *N*-ethyl-3,4-methylenedioxyphenylisopropylamine; 3,4-methylenedioxyethamphetamine; MDEA; "Eve". $C_{12}H_{17}NO_2$; mol wt 207.27. C 69.54%, H 8.27%, N 6.76%, O 15.44%. Entactogen; *N*-ethyl derivative of MDA, *q.v.* Prepn: U. Braun *et al.*, *J. Pharm. Sci.* **69**, 192 (1980); F. T. Noggle, Jr. *et al*, *J. Assoc. Off. Anal. Chem.* **70**, 981 (1987). Pharmacology: M. Johnson *et al.*, *Biochem. Pharmacol.* **38**, 4333 (1989); K. M. Hegadoren *et al.*, *Psychopharmacology* **118**, 295 (1995). Determn in human urine using immunoassays and GC/MS: G. W. Kunsman *et al.*, *J. Anal. Toxicol.* **14**, 149 (1990). HPLC determn in tablets: M. Longo *et al.*, *J. Liq. Chromatogr.* **17**, 649 (1994). Impact on public health and abuse potential: G. P. Dowling *et al.*, *J. Am. Med. Assoc.* **257**, 1615 (1987); R. O. Bost, *J. Forensic Sci.* **33**, 576 (1988); B. Tehan *et al.*, *Anaesthesia* **48**, 507 (1993). Psychological effects in humans: L. Hermle *et al.*, *Neuropsychopharmacology* **8**, 171 (1993). Neuroendocrine and cardiovascular effects in humans: E. Gouzoulis *et al.*, *ibid.* 187.

Viscous, colorless oil. $bp_{0.2}$ 85-95°.

Hydrochloride. [74341-78-9] Fine white granular solid from ethanol-ether, mp 197-198° (Noggle). Also reported as white solid from isopropanol-ether, mp 201-202° (Braun). LD_{50} i.p. in mice: 102 mg/kg (Noggle).

Note: This is a controlled substance (hallucinogen): **21 CFR,** 1308.11.

5767. MDMA. [42542-10-9] *N*,α-Dimethyl-1,3-benzodioxole-5-ethanamine; (±)-3,4-methylenedioxymethamphetamine; *N*-methyl-3,4-methylenedioxyphenylisopropylamine; "Ecstasy"; "E"; "XTC"; "Adam". $C_{11}H_{15}NO_2$; mol wt 193.24. C 68.37%, H 7.82%, N 7.25%, O 16.56%. Entactogen; *N*-methyl derivative of MDA, *q.v.* (*S*)-Form possesses more potent CNS activity. Prepn: **DE 274350** (1914 to E. Merck), *C.A.* **8**, 3350 (1914); U. Braun *et al.*, *J. Pharm. Sci.* **69**, 192 (1980). Spectral and chromatographic analyses: K. Bailey *et al.*, *J. Assoc. Off. Anal. Chem.* **58**, 62 (1975). GC/MS determn in urine: B. K. Gan *et al.*, *J. Forensic Sci.* **36**, 1331 (1991). HPLC determn in whole blood: R. E. Michel *et al.*, *J. Neurosci. Methods* **50**, 61 (1993). Acute toxicity study: H. F. Hardman *et al.*, *Toxicol. Appl. Pharmacol.* **25**, 299 (1973). Series of articles on history, pharmacology, and neurotoxicity: *Ann. N.Y. Acad. Sci.* **600**, 601-715 (1990). Review of biochemical actions: M. Rattray, *Essays Biochem.* **26**, 77-87 (1991); of pharmacology, toxicology, and human experience: T. D. Steele *et al.*, *Addiction* **89**, 539-551 (1994); A. R. Green *et al.*, *Psychopharmacology* **119**, 247-260 (1995); H. Kalant, *Can. Med. Assoc. J.* **165**, 917-928 (2001).

Oil, $bp_{0.4}$ 100-110°.

Hydrochloride. [64057-70-1] $C_{11}H_{15}NO_2$.HCl. Crystals from isopropanol/*n*-hexane, mp 147-148° (Bailey). Crystals from isopropanol/ether, mp 152-153° (Braun). uv max (ethanol): 286 nm (ε 3843). LD_{50} in mice, rats, guinea pigs (mg/kg): 97, 49, 98 i.p. (Hardman).

Note: This is a controlled substance (hallucinogen): **21 CFR,** 1308.11.

5768. Mebendazole. [31431-39-7] (5-Benzoyl-1*H*-benzimidazol-2-yl)carbamic acid methyl ester; 5-benzoyl-2-benzimidazolecarbamic acid methyl ester; methyl 5-benzoyl-2-benzimidazolecarbamate; R-17635; Bantenol; Equivurm Plus; Lomper; Mebenvet; Noverme; Ovitelmin; Pantelmin; Telmin; Vermicidin; Vermirax; Vermox. $C_{16}H_{13}N_3O_3$; mol wt 295.29. C 65.08%, H 4.44%, N 14.23%, O 16.25%. Prepn: J. L. H. Van Gelder *et al.*, **DE 2029637**; *eidem*, **US 3657267** (1971, 1972 to Janssen). Activity studies: Walker, Knight, *Vet. Rec.* **90**, 58 (1972). Clinical studies: Brugmans *et al.*, *J. Am. Med. Assoc.* **217**, 313 (1971); Callear, Neave, *Br. Vet. J.* **127**, xli (1971); *eidem*, *ibid.* **129**, 79 (1973). Comprehensive description: A. A. Al-Badr, M. Tariq, *Anal. Profiles Drug Subs.* **16**, 291-326 (1987).

Crystals from acetic acid and methanol, mp 288.5°. Soluble in formic acid. Practically insol in water, ethanol, ether, chloroform. LD_{50} orally: >80 mg/kg in sheep; >40 mg/kg in mice, rats and chickens (Van Gelder).

THERAP CAT: Anthelmintic (Nematodes).

THERAP CAT (VET): Anthelmintic.

5769. Mebeverine. [3625-06-7] 3,4-Dimethoxybenzoic acid 4-[ethyl[2-(4-methoxyphenyl)-1-methylethyl]amino]butyl ester; veratric acid 4-[ethyl(*p*-methoxy-α-methylphenethyl)amino]butyl ester; 3,4-dimethoxybenzoic acid 4-[ethyl(*p*-methoxy-α-methylphenethyl)amino]butyl ester; 4-[ethyl(*p*-methoxy-α-methylphenethyl)amino]butyl 3,4-dimethoxybenzoate; 4-[*N*-[2-(*p*-methoxyphenyl)-1-methylethyl]-*N*-ethylamino]butyl 3,4-dimethoxybenzoate. $C_{25}H_{35}NO_5$; mol wt 429.55. C 69.90%, H 8.21%, N 3.26%, O 18.62%. Smooth muscle relaxant. Prepn: **BE 609490** *C.A.* **59**, 517b (1963) and T. Kralt *et al.*, **DE 1126889**; *eidem*, **US 3265577** (1962, 1962, 1966 to N. V. Philips). Pharmacology: G. Bertaccini *et al.*, *Farmaco Ed. Sci.* **30**, 823 (1975).

Hydrochloride. [2753-45-9] Colofac; Duspatalin; Duspatal. $C_{25}H_{35}NO_5$.HCl; mol wt 466.01. Crystals from ethyl methyl ketone, mp 105-107° (Ger. patent); also reported as mp 129-131° (Belg. patent).

THERAP CAT: Antispasmodic.

5770. Mebhydroline. [524-81-2] 2,3,4,5-Tetrahydro-2-methyl-5-(phenylmethyl)-1*H*-pyrido[4,3-*b*]indole; 5-benzyl-2,3,4,5-tetrahydro-2-methyl-1*H*-pyrido[4,3-*b*]indole; 3-methyl-9-benzyl-1,2,3,4-tetrahydro-γ-carboline; 5-benzyl-1,2,3,4-tetrahydro-2-methyl-γ-carboline; *N*-methyl-9-benzyltetrahydro-γ-carboline; Incidal. $C_{19}H_{20}N_2$; mol wt 276.38. C 82.57%, H 7.29%, N 10.14%. Prepn: Hörlein, *Ber.* **87**, 463 (1954); **GB 721171** (1954 to Bayer); Hörlein, **US 2786059** (1957 to Schenley). Pharmacology of Diazoline: Kharkevich, *Farmakol. Toksikol.* **20**(no. 6), 46 (1957).

Minute crystals, mp 95°. bp_1 207-215°. Practically insol in water. Freely sol in methanol, ethanol, acetone, chloroform. Slightly sol in ether.

1,5-Naphthalenedisulfonate salt. [6153-33-9] Diazoline; Fabahistin; Omeril. $(C_{19}H_{20}N_2)_2 . C_{10}H_8O_6S_2$; mol wt 841.05. White powder, dec 280°. Practically insol in water. Sparingly sol in hot glacial acetic acid. Sol in hot formamide, giving a yellow soln.

THERAP CAT: Antihistaminic.

5771. MeBmt. [59865-23-5] (2S,3R,4R,6E)-3-Hydroxy-4-methyl-2-(methylamino)-6-octenoic acid; (4R)-4-[(E)-2-butenyl]-4,N-dimethyl-L-threonine. $C_{10}H_{19}NO_3$; mol wt 201.26. C 59.68%, H 9.52%, N 6.96%, O 23.85%. Characteristic C_9 amino acid of cyclosporins, q.v. Identification in cyclosporin A: A. Ruegger et al., Helv. Chim. Acta 59, 1075 (1976). Syntheses: R. M. Wenger, ibid. 66, 2308 (1983); D. A. Evans, A. E. Weber, J. Am. Chem. Soc. 108, 6757 (1986); U. Schmidt, W. Siegel, Tetrahedron Lett. 28, 2849 (1987). Appears to be necessary for full biological activity of cyclosporin: R. M. Wenger, Angew. Chem. Int. Ed. 24, 77 (1985); D. H. Rich et al., J. Med. Chem. 29, 978 (1986).

Crystals from ethanol, mp 240-241° (Wenger). $[\alpha]_D^{20}$ +13.5° (c = 0.50 in water, pH 7). Also reported as mp 242-243° (Evans, Weber). $[\alpha]_D$ +17° (c = 0.51 in 0.4N aq HCl).

5772. Mebrofenin. [78266-06-5] N-[2-[(3-Bromo-2,4,6-trimethylphenyl)amino]-2-oxoethyl]-N-(carboxymethyl)glycine; [[[(3-bromomesityl)carbamoyl]methyl]imino]diacetic acid; N-(3-bromo-2,4,6-trimethylacetanilide)iminodiacetic acid; trimethyl-bromo-IDA; Choletec. $C_{15}H_{19}BrN_2O_5$; mol wt 387.23. C 46.53%, H 4.95%, Br 20.63%, N 7.23%, O 20.66%. Prepn: A. D. Nunn, M. D. Loberg, BE 891534; eidem, US 4418208 (1982, 1983 both to Squibb). Physicochemical properties of ^{99m}technetium complex used for hepatobiliary tract imaging: A. D. Nunn et al., J. Nucl. Med. 24, 423 (1983). Pharmacokinetics in rats: A. R. Fritzberg et al., J. Pharm. Sci. 73, 1861 (1984). Evaluation as cholescintigraphic imaging agent in animals: A. van Aswegen et al., Nucl. Med. Biol. 13, 509 (1986); J. Kapuscinski et al., Nucl. Med. 25, 188 (1986); in humans: W. C. Klingensmith et al., Radiology 146, 181 (1983). Toxicity study: M. Jiang et al., Zhonghua Heyixue Zazhi 4, 214 (1984), C.A. 102, 42241j (1985).

Crystals from ethanol, mp 198-200°. LD_{50} in mice, rats (mg/kg): 213.8, 226.4 i.v. (Jiang).

THERAP CAT: ^{99m}Tc complex as diagnostic aid (radioactive imaging agent).

5773. Mebutamate. [64-55-1] 2-Methyl-2-(1-methylpropyl)-1,3-propanediol dicarbamate; 2-sec-butyl-2-methyl-1,3-propanediol dicarbamate; carbamic acid 2-sec-butyl-2-methyl-

trimethylene ester; 2-sec-butyl-2-methyltrimethylenecarbamate; 2-methyl-2-sec-butyl-1,3-propanediol dicarbamate; 2,2-dicarbamoyloxymethyl-3-methylpentane; dicamoylmethane; W-583; Capla; Butatensin; Carbuten; Dormate; Mebutina; Prean; Sigmafon; Vallene; Mega; No-Press; Axiten; Ipotensivo. $C_{10}H_{20}N_2O_4$; mol wt 232.28. C 51.71%, H 8.68%, N 12.06%, O 27.55%. Prepn: Berger, Ludwig, US 2878280 (1959 to Carter Prod.). Mechanism of action: Kletzkin, Arch. Int. Pharmacodyn. Ther. 164, 71 (1966). Metabolism: Edelson, Douglas, ibid. 173, 182 (1968).

Crystals, mp 77-79°. Soly in water: ~0.1%. Sol in most organic solvents. On heating or boiling with acid or alkali, hydrolyzes to the alcohol, ammonia and carbon dioxide.

Note: This is a controlled substance (depressant): **21 CFR**, 1308.14.

THERAP CAT: Antihypertensive.

5774. Mecamylamine. [60-40-2] N,2,3,3-Tetramethylbicyclo[2.2.1]heptan-2-amine; N,2,3,3-tetramethyl-2-norbornanamine; N,2,3,3-tetramethyl-2-norcamphanamine; 3-methylaminoisocamphane; 2-methylaminoisocamphane; 2-methylamino-2,3,3-trimethylnorbornane; N-methyl-2-isocamphanamine; 3β-methylamino-2,2,3-trimethylbicyclo[2.2.1]heptane; mecamine. $C_{11}H_{21}N$; mol wt 167.29. C 78.98%, H 12.65%, N 8.37%. Nicotinic receptor antagonist; orally active ganglionic blocker. Prepn: G. A. Stein et al., J. Am. Chem. Soc. 78, 1514 (1956); K. Pfister, III, G. A. Stein, US 2831027 (1958 to Merck & Co.). Structure activity study: C. A. Stone et al., J. Med. Pharm. Chem. 5, 665 (1962). GC-MS determn in plasma: P. Jacob, III et al., J. Pharm. Biomed. Anal. 23, 653 (2000). Receptor binding study of isomers: R. L. Papke et al., J. Pharmacol. Exp. Ther. 297, 646 (2001). Review of pharmacology and clinical experience: J. M. Young et al., Clin. Ther. 23, 532-565 (2001).

Oily liquid. $bp_{4.0}$ 72°. n_D^{25} 1.4881. Slightly sol in water.

Hydrochloride. [826-39-1] Inversine. $C_{11}H_{21}N.HCl$; mol wt 203.75. Crystals, dec 245.5-246.5°. Bittersweet. Soly (g/100 ml): water 21.2; ethanol 8.2; glycerol 10.4; isopropanol 2.1. pH of 1% aq soln 6.0-7.5.

THERAP CAT: Antihypertensive.

5775. Mechlorethamine. [51-75-2] 2-Chloro-N-(2-chloroethyl)-N-methylethanamine; 2,2'-dichloro-N-methyldiethylamine; N-methyl-2,2'-dichlorodiethylamine; di(chloroethyl)methylamine; methylbis(β-chloroethyl)amine; methyldi(2-chloroethyl)amine; chlormethine; nitrogen mustard; stickstofflost; MBA; HN2. $C_5H_{11}Cl_2N$; mol wt 156.05. C 38.48%, H 7.10%, Cl 45.44%, N 8.98%. A nitrogen mustard prepd by action of thionyl chloride on 2,2'-(methylimino)diethanol in trichloroethylene: Prelog, Stepan, Collect. Czech. Chem. Commun. 7, 93 (1935); Hanby, Rydon, J. Chem. Soc. 1947, 513; Abrams et al., J. Soc. Chem. Ind. London 68, 280 (1949); T. W. Doyle, D. M. Vyas in Kirk-Othmer Encyclopedia of Chemical Technology vol. 5 (John Wiley & Sons, New York, 4th ed., 1993) pp 876-879, 900-901. Toxicity data: W. P. Anslow et al., J. Pharmacol. Exp. Ther. 91, 224 (1947).

Mobile liquid. Faint odor of herring. *Vesicant, necrotizing irritant. Never use without appropriate gas mask.* Volatility at 25° = 3.581 mg/l. d_4^{25} 1.118. mp −60°. bp_{18} 87°; bp_{10} 75°; bp_5 64°; bp_2

59°. Very slightly sol in water. Miscible with DMF, CS_2, CCl_4, many other organic solvents and oils. The undiluted liq dec on standing and forms polymeric quaternary ammonium salts which are insol in the free base.

Hydrochloride. [55-86-7] Caryolysine; Mustargen; Mustine hydrochloride; Nitrogranulogen. $C_5H_{11}Cl_2N.HCl$; mol wt 192.51. Hygroscopic leaflets from acetone or chloroform, mp 109-111°. Very sol in water; sol in alcohol. Initial pH of a 2% aq soln: 3.0-4.0. Dry crystals are stable at temps up to 40°. LD_{50} in rats (mg/kg): 1.1 i.v.; 1.9 s.c. (Anslow).

Caution: Direct contact may cause severe skin and eye irritation; injury to deeper ocular structures, particularly the iris and lens. *See Patty's Industrial Hygiene and Toxicology* vol. **2E**, G. D. Clayton, F. E. Clayton, Eds. (John Wiley & Sons, Inc., New York, 4th ed., 1994) pp 3297-3299. Mechlorethamine hydrochloride is reasonably anticipated to be a human carcinogen: *Report on Carcinogens, Eleventh Edition* (PB2005-104914, 2004) p III-192.

N-**Oxide hydrochloride** *see* Mechlorethamine Oxide Hydrochloride.

USE: Base as a gas warfare agent.

THERAP CAT: Hydrochloride as an antineoplastic.

THERAP CAT (VET): Hydrochloride has been used as an antineoplastic.

5776. **Mechlorethamine Oxide Hydrochloride.** [302-70-5] 2-Chloro-*N*-(2-chloroethyl)-*N*-methylethanamine *N*-oxide hydrochloride; 2,2'-dichloro-*N*-methyldiethylamine *N*-oxide hydrochloride; *N*-methyl-2,2'-dichlorodiethylamine *N*-oxide hydrochloride; methylbis(β-chloroethyl)amine *N*-oxide hydrochloride; methyl-di(2-chloroethyl)amine *N*-oxide hydrochloride; Nitromin; Mitomen; Mustron. $C_5H_{12}Cl_3NO$; mol wt 208.51. C 28.80%, H 5.80%, Cl 51.01%, N 6.72%, O 7.67%. Prepd by treating 2,2'-dichloro-*N*-methyldiethylamine with hydrogen peroxide and acetic anhydride in ether, followed by shaking with 10% hydrochloric acid: Aiko *et al., J. Pharm. Soc. Jpn.* **72**, 1297 (1952, English Text), *C.A.* **47**, 1289 (1953). *Cf.* Stahmann, Bergmann, *J. Org. Chem.* **11**, 586 (1946).

Prisms from acetone, mp 109-110°. Sol in water.

THERAP CAT: Antineoplastic.

5777. **Meclizine.** [569-65-3] 1-[(4-Chlorophenyl)phenylmethyl]-4-[(3-methylphenyl)methyl]piperazine; 1-(*p*-chloro-α-phenylbenzyl)-4-(*m*-methylbenzyl)piperazine; 1-(*p*-chlorobenzhydryl)-4-(*m*-methylbenzyl)piperazine; 1-(*p*-chlorobenzhydryl)-4-(*m*-methylbenzyl)diethylenediamine; meclozine; parachloramine. $C_{25}H_{27}ClN_2$; mol wt 390.95. C 76.80%, H 6.96%, Cl 9.07%, N 7.17%. Synthesis: Morren, **BE 502889** (1951); **GB 705979** (1954), **US 2709169** (1955 to U.C.B.). Outline of reactions: Grivsky, *Ind. Chim. Belge* **17**, 735 (1952). Clinical evaluation in vertigo: B. Cohen, J. M. B. Vianney de Jong, *Arch. Neurol.* **27**, 129 (1972).

bp$_2$ 230°.

Dihydrochloride monohydrate. [31884-77-2] UCB-5062; Ancolan; Antivert; Bonamine; Bonine; Calmonal; Peremesin; Postafen. $C_{25}H_{27}ClN_2.2HCl.H_2O$; mol wt 481.89. Freely sol in chloroform, pyridine; slightly sol in dil acids, alc. Practically insol in water (0.1 gm/100 ml), ether.

THERAP CAT: Antiemetic.

THERAP CAT (VET): Antiemetic.

5778. **Meclocycline.** [2013-58-3] [4*S*-(4α,4aα,5α,5aα,-12aα)]-7-Chloro-4-(dimethylamino)-1,4,4a,5,5a,6,11,12a-octahydro-3,5,10,12,12a-pentahydroxy-6-methylene-1,11-dioxo-2-naph-

thacenecarboxamide; 7-chloro-6-methylene-5-hydroxytetracycline; GS-2989; NSC-78502. $C_{22}H_{21}ClN_2O_8$; mol wt 476.86. C 55.41%, H 4.44%, Cl 7.43%, N 5.87%, O 26.84%. Semi-synthetic antibiotic derived from tetracycline, *q.v.* Prepn: R. K. Blackwood *et al.,* **US 2984686** (1961 to Pfizer); *eidem, J. Am. Chem. Soc.* **83**, 2773 (1961); of the free base and 5-sulfosalicylate salt: *eidem, ibid.* **85**, 3943 (1963). *In vitro* study: L. Lucca, G. Vittadini, *G. Ital. Chemioter.* **26**, 203 (1979). ^{13}C-NMR study: E. Mazzola *et al., J. Pharm. Sci.* **69**, 229 (1980). Toxicity study: F. Bernardi *et al., G. Ital. Chemioter.* **17**, 276 (1970).

uv max (methanol, 0.01*N* HCl): 245, 347 nm (log ε 4.34, 410). LD_{50} in mice (mg/kg): >5000 orally, 425 i.p. (Bernardi).

5-Sulfosalicylate. [73816-42-9] Meclan; Mecloderm; Meclosorb; Meclutin; Traumatociclina. $C_{29}H_{27}ClN_2O_{14}S$; mol wt 695.05. uv max (methanol, 0.01*N* HCl): 239, 268, 346 nm (log ε 4.46, 4.07, 4.11).

THERAP CAT: Antibacterial.

5779. **Meclofenamic Acid.** [644-62-2] 2-[(2,6-Dichloro-3-methylphenyl)amino]benzoic acid; *N*-(2,6-dichloro-*m*-tolyl)-anthranilic acid; meclophenamic acid; CI-583; INF-4668; Arquel. $C_{14}H_{11}Cl_2NO_2$; mol wt 296.15. C 56.78%, H 3.74%, Cl 23.94%, N 4.73%, O 10.80%. Prepn: Scherrer, Short, **DE 1149015** *C.A.* **61**, 1801d (1964) and **US 3313848** (1963, 1967 to Parke, Davis); Juby *et al., J. Med. Chem.* **11**, 111 (1968). Pharmacology and toxicology: Winder *et al., J. Pharmacol. Exp. Ther.* **148**, 422 (1965); Winder, *Ann. Phys. Med.* **1966**, 7; Kaump, *ibid.* 16. Series of articles on structure-activity relationships, mechanism of action, clinical studies: *Arzneim.-Forsch.* **33**, 619-680 (1983). Effect on prostaglandin E receptor binding: M. C. P. Rees *et al., Lancet* **2**, 541 (1988).

White crystals from acetone-water, mp 257-259°; also reported as mp 248-250°. Soly (mg/ml): water 0.03; 0.1*N* NaOH 28. pH of satd aq soln: ~6.9.

Sodium salt monohydrate. Lenidolor; Meclodol; Meclomen; Movens. $C_{14}H_{10}Cl_2NNaO_2.H_2O$; mol wt 336.15. mp 289-291°. Soly in water: 15 mg/ml (slightly turbid). pH 8.7.

THERAP CAT: Anti-inflammatory; antipyretic.

THERAP CAT (VET): Anti-inflammatory.

5780. **Meclofenoxate.** [51-68-3] (4-Chlorophenoxy)acetic acid 2-(dimethylamino)ethyl ester; dimethylaminoethyl *p*-chlorophenoxyacetate; centrophenoxine; meclofenoxane; acephen; ANP-235; Analux; Cetrexin; Proseryl. $C_{12}H_{16}ClNO_3$; mol wt 257.71. C 55.93%, H 6.26%, Cl 13.76%, N 5.44%, O 18.62%. Prepn: Rumpf, Thuillier, **FR M398** (1962 to Centre Nat'l. Recherche Sci.), *C.A.* **57**, 16768e (1962); Thuillier *et al., Compt. Rend.* **249**, 2081 (1959); Thuillier, Rumpf, *Bull. Soc. Chim. Fr.* **1960**, 1786. Pharmacology: Petkov, *C.A.* **65**, 20717g (1966); Liberman, *Farmakol. Toksikol.* **30**, 409 (1967). Auxin activity: Conti, *Boll. Chim. Farm.* **107**, 325 (1968).

Hydrochloride. [3685-84-5] Cellative; Clocete; Lucidril; Methoxynal; Proserout; Brenal; Marucotol; Helfergin. $C_{12}H_{16}$-$ClNO_3.HCl$; mol wt 294.17. Crystals from isopropyl alcohol or acetone, mp 135-139°. Sol in cold water. Sparingly sol in cold isopropyl alcohol, acetone. Practically insol in benzene, ether, chloroform. A 5% soln in water has pH 6. LD_{50} in mice (mg/kg): 330 i.v.; 1750 orally; 845 i.p. (Rumpf, Thuillier).

USE: Plant growth regulator.

THERAP CAT: Cerebral stimulant.

5781. Mecloqualone. [340-57-8] 3-(2-Chlorophenyl)-2-methyl-4(3H)-quinazolinone; 2-methyl-3-(2-chlorophenyl)-4-quinazolone; Nubarene. $C_{15}H_{11}ClN_2O$; mol wt 270.71. C 66.55%, H 4.10%, Cl 13.10%, N 10.35%, O 5.91%. Prepd from acetylanthranilic acid and o-chloroaniline in the presence of $POCl_3$: Jackman et al., J. Pharm. Pharmacol. **12**, 529 (1960); Closa, J. Prakt. Chem. [4] **14**, 84 (1961). Metabolism: Dubnick, Towne, Toxicol. Appl. Pharmacol. **22**, 82 (1972); Daenens, Van Bovan, Arzneim.-Forsch. **24**, 195 (1974).

Crystals mp 126-128°.
Hydrochloride. $C_{15}H_{11}ClN_2O.HCl$. Crystals, mp 239-241°.
Note: This is a controlled substance (depressant): **21 CFR**, 1308.11.

THERAP CAT: Sedative; hypnotic.

5782. Meconic Acid. [497-59-6] 3-Hydroxy-4-oxo-4H-pyran-2,6-dicarboxylic acid; oxychelidonic acid. $C_7H_4O_7$; mol wt 200.10. C 42.02%, H 2.01%, O 55.97%. From opium which contains 4 to 6%. Prepn: Thoms, Pietrulla, Ber. Pharm. Ges. **31**, 4 (1921); Wibaut, Kleinpool, Rec. Trav. Chim. **66**, 24 (1947).

Monohydrate. Prisms from concd aq solns. One gram dissolves in 4 ml hot water, 50 ml methanol, 50 ml ethyl acetate, 100 ml acetone; freely sol in ethanol, benzene.
Trihydrate. Orthorhombic pyramidal prisms from dil aq solns. Becomes anhydr when heated to 100-102° for 20 min. Dec with evolution of CO_2 when heated to 120° or when boiled with water. The slight brown tint often characteristic of meconic acid prepns is due to traces of iron.

5783. Meconin. [569-31-3] 6,7-Dimethoxy-1(3H)-isobenzofuranone; 6,7-dimethoxyphthalide; opianyl; meconinic acid lactone. $C_{10}H_{10}O_4$; mol wt 194.18. C 61.85%, H 5.19%, O 32.96%. Isolated from opium by Dublanc in 1832. Occurs also in the root of Hydrastis canadensis L., Ranunculaceae: Freund, Ber. **22**, 456, 459 (1889). Is formed in oxidation of noscapine with HNO_3. Synthesis from o-veratric acid: Edwards et al., J. Chem. Soc. **1925**, 195; Wilson et al., J. Org. Chem. **16**, 792 (1951). From opianic acid: Brown, Newbold, J. Chem. Soc. **1952**, 4878.

White, optically inactive needles; sharp bitter taste. mp 102-103°. uv max: 213, 308 nm (ε 25000, 3800). Sol in 700 parts cold, 22 parts boiling water; sol in alcohol, benzene, chloroform, ether, glacial acetic acid; slowly sol in alkalies with formation of alkali salt of meconinic acid, $(CH_2OH)(CH_3O)_2C_6H_2COOH$. The acid itself is unstable, rapidly changing to lactone.

5784. Mecoprop. [7085-19-0] 2-(4-Chloro-2-methylphenoxy)propanoic acid; (±)-2-[(4-chloro-o-tolyl)oxy]propionic acid; mechlorprop; MCPP; CMPP; RD-4593; Astix CMPP; Iso-Cornox; Compitox; Compitox Plus; Proponex-Plus. $C_{10}H_{11}ClO_3$; mol wt

214.65. C 55.95%, H 5.17%, Cl 16.52%, O 22.36%. Prepn: M. E. Synerholm, P. W. Zimmerman, Contrib. Boyce Thompson Inst. **14**, 91 (1945). Studies on plant growth regulation: C. H. Fawcett et al., Ann. Appl. Biol. **40**, 231 (1953); and comparison of enantiomers: M. Matell, Kungl. Lantbruks-Hogsk. Ann. **20**, 207 (1953); B. Aberg, ibid. 241. GLC determn: H. G. Higson, D. Butler, Analyst **85**, 657 (1960). Crystal structure: G. Smith et al., Acta Crystallogr. **B36**, 992 (1980). Herbicidal activity: G. B. Lush, Proc. 3rd Br. Weed Control Conf. 625 (1956); E. L. Leafe, ibid. 633; B. Wallgren, Weeds Weed Contr. **24th** Swedish Weed Conf. 30 (1983); of (+)-enantiomer: J. Toll, Weeds Weed Contr. **28th** Swedish Weed Conf. 100 (1987). Degradation in soils: L. Lindholm et al., Acta Agric. Scand. **32**, 429 (1982); A. E. Smith, Bull. Environ. Contam. Toxicol. **34**, 656 (1985). Toxicological studies: M. R. Gurd et al., Food Cosmet. Toxicol. **3**, 883 (1965); H. G. Verschuuren et al., Toxicology **3**, 349 (1975); R. Roll, G. Matthiaschk, Arzneim.-Forsch. **33**, 1479 (1983). EC-GLC determn in tissues and biological fluids: J. De Beer et al., Vet. Hum. Toxicol. **21**, Suppl., 172 (1979). HPLC resolution of enantiomers: B. Blessington et al., J. Chromatogr. **396**, 177 (1987).

Solid, mp 93-94°. LD_{50} in rats (mg/kg): 1210 orally, 402 i.p. (Verschuuren).
(+)-Form. Mecoprop-P; Duplosan KV. Solid, mp 95-96°. $[\alpha]_D^{25}$ +19° (alcohol).
Sodium salt. $C_{10}H_{11}ClNaO_3$. LD_{50} i.p. in rats, mice: 500, 600 mg/kg; orally in mice: 650 mg/kg (Gurd).
Diethylamine salt. Mecopar. $C_{14}H_{22}ClNO_3$; mol wt 287.78. LD_{50} in rats, mice (mg/kg): 1060 ±120, 600 ±35 orally; 350, 400 i.p. (Gurd).
Potassium salt. Mecomec; Hedonal MCPP. $C_{10}H_{11}ClKO_3$; mol wt 253.74.

USE: Herbicide.

5785. Mecysteine Hydrochloride. [18598-63-5] L-Cysteine methyl ester hydrochloride; methyl cysteine hydrochloride; methyl β-mercaptoalanine hydrochloride; methyl α-amino-β-mercaptopropionate hydrochloride; LJ-48; Visclair. $C_4H_{10}ClNO_2S$; mol wt 171.65. C 27.99%, H 5.87%, Cl 20.65%, N 8.16%, O 18.64%, S 18.68%. $HSCH_2CH(NH_2)COOCH_3.HCl$. Prepn: Bergmann, Michalis, Ber. **63**, 987 (1930); Zervas, Theodoropoulos, J. Am. Chem. Soc. **78**, 1359 (1956).

Crystals from methanol, mp 140-141°. $[\alpha]_D^{20}$ −2.9° (methanol).
THERAP CAT: Mucolytic.

5786. Medazepam. [2898-12-6] 7-Chloro-2,3-dihydro-1-methyl-5-phenyl-1H-1,4-benzodiazepine; Ansilan; Diepin; Medazepol; Megasedan; Narsis; Nobrium; Psiquium; Resmit; Rudotel; Tranquilax. $C_{16}H_{15}ClN_2$; mol wt 270.76. C 70.97%, H 5.58%, Cl 13.09%, N 10.35%. Prepn: L. H. Sternbach et al., J. Org. Chem. **28**, 2456 (1963); G. A. Archer et al., **BE 620773** C.A. **59**, 10095b (1963); E. Reeder, L. H. Sternbach, **US 3243427** (1963, 1966 both to Hoffmann-La Roche); S. Inaba et al., Chem. Pharm. Bull. **20**, 1628 (1972); M. Mihalic et al., J. Heterocycl. Chem. **14**, 941 (1977). Pharmacology: L. O. Randall et al., Arch. Int. Pharmacodyn. Ther. **185**, 135 (1970). Crystal structure: G. Gilli et al., Acta Crystallogr. **B34**, 3793 (1978).

Colorless prismatic crystals from ether + petr ether, mp 95-97°. LD_{50} in mice (mg/kg): 360 i.p., 1070 orally (Randall).
Hydrochloride. [2898-11-5] $C_{16}H_{15}ClN_2.HCl$. Orange-red crystalline powder. Freely sol in water, alcohol.

Note: This is a controlled substance (depressant): **21 CFR,** 1308.14.

THERAP CAT: Anxiolytic.

5787. Medetomidine. [86347-14-0] 4-[1-(2,3-Dimethylphenyl)ethyl]-1*H*-imidazole; (±)-4-(α,2,3-trimethylbenzyl)imidazole; 4-[(α-methyl)-2,3-dimethylbenzyl]imidazole. C$_{13}$H$_{16}$N$_2$; mol wt 200.28. C 77.96%, H 8.05%, N 13.99%. α$_2$-Adrenergic agonist. Prepn: A. J. Karjalainen *et al.,* **GB 2101114**; A. J. Karjalainen, K. O. A. Kurkela, **US 4544664** (1983, 1985 both to Farmos). Receptor binding study: R. Virtanen *et al., Eur. J. Pharmacol.* **150,** 9 (1988). Sedative and cardiovascular effects in humans: M. Scheinin *et al., Br. J. Clin. Pharmacol.* **24,** 443 (1987). Veterinary evaluation in cats: D. Stenberg *et al., J. Vet. Pharmacol. Ther.* **10,** 319 (1987). Review of pharmacology and use in dogs and cats: L. K. Cullen, *Br. Vet. J.* **152,** 519-535 (1996).

Hydrochloride. [86347-15-1] MPV-785; Domitor. C$_{13}$H$_{16}$-CN$_2$.HCl; mol wt 248.75. White or almost white crystalline substance. Sol in water.

d-Form see Dexmedetomidine.

THERAP CAT (VET): Sedative; analgesic.

5788. Medicagol. [1983-72-8] 3-Hydroxy-6*H*-[1,3]dioxolo[5,6]benzofuro[3,2-*c*][1]benzopyran-6-one; 7-hydroxy-11,12-(methylenedioxy)coumestan; 7-hydroxy-5',6'-methylenedioxybenzofurano(3',2':3,4)coumarin. C$_{16}$H$_8$O$_6$; mol wt 296.23. C 64.87%, H 2.72%, O 32.41%. Occurs in alfalfa having viral leafspot infections. Synthesis: Livingston *et al., J. Org. Chem.* **30,** 2353 (1965); Jurd, *J. Pharm. Sci.* **54,** 1221 (1965); Fukui *et al., Experientia* **24,** 536 (1968).

mp 326-327°. uv max (ethanol): 245, 270, 297, 310, 348 nm (log ε 4.29, 3.91, 3.85, 4.03, 4.46).

5789. Medicarpin. [32383-76-9] (6a*R*,11a*R*)-6a,11a-Dihydro-9-methoxy-6*H*-benzofuro[3,2-*c*][1]benzopyran-3-ol; (−)-3-hydroxy-9-methoxypterocarpan; demethylhomopterocarpin. C$_{16}$H$_{14}$-O$_4$; mol wt 270.28. C 71.10%, H 5.22%, O 23.68%. Antifungal phytoalexin produced by leguminous species. Isoln from the heartwood of *Swartzia madagascariensis* Desv., *Caesalpinioidae:* S. H. Harper *et al., Chem. Ind. (London)* **1965,** 562; from alfalfa, *Medicago sativa* L., *Leguminosae:* D. G. Smith *et al., Physiol. Plant Pathol.* **1,** 41, (1971); from red clover, *Trifolium pratense* L., *Leguminosae:* V. J. Higgins, D. G. Smith, *Phytopathology* **62,** 235 (1972). ^{13}C-NMR: A. A. Chalmers *et al., Tetrahedron* **33,** 1735 (1977). HPLC: J. Koster *et al., J. Chromatogr.* **270,** 392 (1983). Synthesis of racemic form: W. Cocker *et al., J. Chem. Soc. C* **1965,** 1034. Biosynthetic studies: P. M. Dewick, *Chem. Commun.* **1975,** 656; S. W. Banks *et al., ibid.* **1982,** 157; H. A. M. Al-Ani, P. M. Dewick, *J. Chem. Soc. Perkin Trans. 1* **1984,** 2831. Antifungal properties: L. J. Duczek, V. J. Higgins, *Can. J. Bot.* **54,** 2620 (1976); H. D. Van Etten, *Phytochemistry* **15,** 655 (1976); A. O. Latunde-Dada, J. A. Lucas, *Physiol. Plant Pathol.* **26,** 31 (1985).

Prisms from benzene, mp 127.5-128.5°. [α]$_D^{22}$ −226° (chloroform). uv max: 207, 282, 287, 310 nm (log ε 4.86, 3.97, 4.01, 3.38).

(±)-Form. Prisms from ethyl acetate/light petroleum, mp 194-195°.

5790. Medifoxamine. [32359-34-5] *N,N*-Dimethyl-2,2-diphenoxyethanamine; (dimethylamino)acetaldehyde diphenyl acetal; *N,N*'-dimethyl-2,2-diphenoxyethylamine. C$_{16}$H$_{19}$NO$_2$; mol wt 257.33. C 74.68%, H 7.44%, N 5.44%, O 12.43%. Prepn: **FR M5498** (1967 to Gerda), *C.A.* **72,** 12358x (1970); M. A. Brunet *et al., Bull. Soc. Chim. Fr.* **6,** 2000 (1967). Pharmacology and toxicity: A. Vagne *et al., Therapie* **26,** 553 (1971). Clinical pharmacology: M. A. Randhawa *et al., Hum. Psychopharmacol.* **3,** 195 (1988). Comparative clinical trial with clomipramine, *q.v.,* in depression: H. Scharbach *et al., Psychol. Med.* **18,** 1485 (1986).

Fumarate. [16604-45-8] LG-152; Clédial; Gerdaxyl. C$_{16}$H$_{19}$-NO$_2$.C$_4$H$_4$O$_4$; mol wt 373.40. Crystals from 95% ethanol, mp 128.5°. LD$_{50}$ orally in rats: 750 mg/kg (Vagne).

THERAP CAT: Antidepressant.

5791. Medrogestone. [977-79-7] 6,17-Dimethylpregna-4,6-diene-3,20-dione; 6,17α-dimethyl-6-dehydroprogesterone; AY-62022; Colpro; Colprone; Prothil. C$_{23}$H$_{32}$O$_2$; mol wt 340.50. C 81.13%, H 9.47%, O 9.40%. Prepn: Deghenghi, Gaudry, *J. Am. Chem. Soc.* **83,** 4668 (1961); Deghenghi *et al., Tetrahedron* **19,** 289 (1963); *J. Med. Chem.* **6,** 301 (1963); Deghenghi, **US 3133913, US 3210387**; Morand, Deghenghi, **US 3170936** (1964, 1965, and 1965, all to Am. Home Prod.). HPLC determn in serum: W. T. Robinson, L. Cosyns, *Arzneim.-Forsch.* **29,** 882 (1979). Comparative clinical evaluation in benign prostatic hyperplasia: D. F. Paulson, R. D. Kane, *J. Urol.* **113,** 811 (1975); in endometrial carcinoma: K. C. Podratz *et al., Obstet. Gynecol.* **66,** 106 (1985).

Crystals from ether, mp 144-146°. [α]$_D^{23}$ +79° (c = 1 in chloroform). uv max: 288 nm (ε 25000).

THERAP CAT: Progestogen.

5792. Medronic Acid. [1984-15-2] Methylenebisphosphonic acid; methylenediphosphonic acid; methanebisphosphonic acid; methanediphosphonic acid; MDP. CH$_6$O$_6$P$_2$; mol wt 176.00. C 6.82%, H 3.44%, O 54.54%, P 35.20%. Prepn: G. Schwarzenbach, J. Zurc, *Monatsh. Chem.* **81,** 202 (1950), *C.A.* **44,** 8205f (1950); V. A. Ginsburg, A. Y. Yakubovich, *J. Gen. Chem. USSR* **28,** 710 (1958), *C.A.* **52,** 17091g (1958); J. A. Cade, *J. Chem. Soc.* **1959,** 2266. Physical properties: K. Moedritzer, R. R. Irani, *J. Inorg. Nucl. Chem.* **22,** 297 (1961). Prepn of ^{99m}Tc-complexes: G. Subramanian, J. G. McAfee, **US 4032625** (1977 to Research Corp.); J. Kroesbergen *et al., Int. J. Nucl. Med. Biol.* **12,** 419 (1986). HPLC separation of ^{99m}Tc-complexes: D. J. Hoch, T. C. Pinkerton, *Appl. Radiat. Isot.* **37,** 593 (1986). Biodistribution, toxicity and clinical evaluation for skeletal imaging: G. Subramanian *et al., J. Nucl. Med.* **16,** 744 (1975). Comparative biodistribution studies: G. Subramanian *et al., Radiology* **149,** 823 (1983). Clinical pharmacokinetics: L. Rosenthall *et al., Clin. Nucl. Med.* **2,** 232 (1977). Clinical studies for bone imaging: U. Büll *et al., Br. J. Radiol.* **50,** 629 (1977); for neuroblastoma imaging: I. Garty *et al., Clin. Nucl. Med.* **14,** 515 (1989).

Crystals from acetic acid, mp 199-200°. LD_{50} in mice, rabbits (mg/kg): 45-50 i.v. (Subramanian, 1975).

99mTc-Complex. 99mTc-MDP; Amerscan MDP; Osteolite; TechneScan MDP.

THERAP CAT: 99mTc complex as diagnostic aid (radioactive imaging agent).

5793. Medroxyprogesterone. [520-85-4] (6α)-17-Hydroxy-6-methylpregn-4-ene-3,20-dione; 17α-hydroxy-6α-methylprogesterone; 6α-methyl-17α-hydroxyprogesterone; 6α-methyl-4-pregnen-17α-ol-3,20-dione. $C_{22}H_{32}O_3$; mol wt 344.49. C 76.70%, H 9.36%, O 13.93%. Orally active progestogen; formerly used in combinations as oral contraceptive. Prepn: J. C. Babcock *et al., J. Am. Chem. Soc.* **80**, 2904 (1958); **GB 866381**; G. B. Spero, **US 3377364** (1961, 1968 both to Upjohn); P. Ruggieri, C. Ferrari, **US 3043832** (1962 to Ormonoterapia Richter); B. Camerino *et al.,* **US 3061616** (1962 to Farmitalia). HPLC determn in plasma: J. Read, G. Mould, *J. Chromatogr.* **341**, 437 (1985). Comparative clinical trial with norethisterone as injectable contraceptive: H. K. Toppozada *et al., Contraception* **28**, 1 (1983). Clinical trial in advanced breast cancer: M. Izuo *et al., Cancer* **56**, 2576 (1985). Review of pharmacology and clinical uses: I. S. Fraser, E. Weisberg, *Med. J. Aust.* **1**, Suppl. 1, 3-19 (1981).

Crystals from chloroform, mp 220-223.5°. $[\alpha]_D^{25}$ +75° (in chloroform). uv max (ethanol): 241 nm (ε 16000).

17-Acetate. [71-58-9] 17α-Acetoxy-6α-methylprogesterone; 6α-methyl-17α-acetoxyprogesterone; MAP; Amen; Clinovir; Cycrin; Depo-Clinovir; Depo-Prodasone; Depo-Provera; Farlutal; Gestoral; Hysron; Oragest; Perlutex; Provera; Veramix. $C_{24}H_{34}O_4$; mol wt 386.52. Crystals from methanol, mp 207-209°. $[\alpha]_D$ +61° (in chloroform). uv max (ethanol): 240 nm (ε 15900). Freely sol in chloroform; sol in acetone, dioxane; sparingly sol in ethanol, methanol; slightly sol in ether. Insol in water.

THERAP CAT: Progestogen; contraceptive (injectable); antineoplastic (hormonal).

THERAP CAT (VET): Progestogen; estrus regulator.

5794. Medrysone. [2668-66-8] (6α,11β)-11-Hydroxy-6-methylpregn-4-ene-3,20-dione; 11β-hydroxy-6α-methylprogesterone; 6α-methyl-11β-hydroxyprogesterone; hydroxymesterone; U-8471; HMS. $C_{22}H_{32}O_3$; mol wt 344.49. C 76.70%, H 9.36%, O 13.93%. Prepn and use as an intermediate: Sebek *et al.,* Spero, Thompson, **US 2864837** and **US 2968655** (1958 and 1961, both to Upjohn). In treatment of ocular inflammation: Bedrossian, *Arch. Ophthalmol.* **81**, 184 (1969).

Crystals, mp 155-158°. $[\alpha]_D$ +189° (in chloroform).
THERAP CAT: Glucocorticoid.

5795. Medullipin. [97621-73-3] Medullipin I; antihypertensive neutral renomedullary lipid; ANRL. Antihypertensive lipid prohormone produced by the renomedullary interstitial cells of the renal papilla under the control of the renal artery perfusion pressure. Converted to the active form, *medullipin II*, by the cytochrome P-450 dependent enzyme system of the liver. Medullipin II acts as as vasodilator that suppresses sympathetic activity, causes diuresis-natriuresis, and has a suppressive action on the CNS. Constitutes a feedback control of the renin-angiotensin system. Extraction from renomedullary interstitial cells: E. E. Muirhead *et al., Lab. Invest.* **35**, 162 (1977); from renal venous effluent: E. E. Muirhead *et al., J. Lab. Clin. Med.* **99**, 64 (1982). Biological activity: E. E. Muirhead *et al., Hypertension* **5**, Suppl I, I-112 (1983); G. Karlström *et al., Acta Physiol. Scand.* **137**, 521 (1989). Activation by the liver: E. E. Muirhead *et al., Trans. Assoc. Am. Physicians* **101**, 226 (1988). Effect in spontaneously hypertensive rats: E. E. Muirhead *et al., Hypertension* **17**, 1092 (1991). Review of medullipin system of blood pressure control: E. E. Muirhead, *Am. J. Hypertens.* **4**, 556S-568S (1991).

5796. Meerwein's Reagent. [368-39-8] Triethyloxonium tetrafluoroborate (1−); triethyloxonium fluoborate. $C_6H_{15}BF_4O$; mol wt 189.99. C 37.93%, H 7.96%, B 5.69%, F 40.00%, O 8.42%. Powerful ethylating agent; converts alcohols to ethyl ethers at neutral pH. Prepn: H. Meerwein *et al., J. Prakt. Chem.* **147**, 257 (1937); *idem et al., ibid.* **154**, 83 (1939); H. Meerwein, *Org. Synth.* **46**, 113 (1966). Synthetic applications: N. Kornblum, G. P. Coffey, *J. Org. Chem.* **31**, 3449 (1966); R. Kreher, *Angew. Chem. Int. Ed.* **12**, 1022 (1973); D. G. McMinn, *Synthesis* **1976**, 824; D. Crich, H. Dyker, *Tetrahedron Lett.* **30**, 475 (1989); Y. Yamamoto *et al., Synthesis* **1995**, 571; A. J. Kiessling, C. K. McClure, *Synth. Commun.* **27**, 923 (1997). *Brief review:* S. Pichlmair, *Synlett* **2004**, 195-196.

Colorless solid, mp 91-92° (dec). *Hygroscopic. Store at 0-5° in dichloromethane or diethyl ether.*

USE: Alkylating agent for nucleophilic functional groups in organic synthesis.

5797. Mefenacet. [73250-68-7] 2-(2-Benzothiazolyloxy)-N-methyl-N-phenylacetamide; 2-(1,3-benzothiazol-2-yloxy)-N-methylacetanilide; FOE-1976; NTN-801; Hinochloa; Rancho. $C_{16}H_{14}N_2O_2S$; mol wt 298.36. C 64.41%, H 4.73%, N 9.39%, O 10.72%, S 10.75%. Oxyacetamide herbicide; inhibits cell division and growth in meristematic plant tissue. Prepn: H. Förster *et al.,* **EP 5501**; *eidem,* **US 4509971** (1979, 1985 both to Bayer). Properties and field trials in rice: R. R. Schmidt *et al., Meded. Fac. Landbouwwet. Rijksuniv. Gent* **49**, 1075 (1984). Properties and toxicity studies: *J. Pestic. Sci.* **13**, 633 (1988). Distribution and metabolism: B. Krauskopf *et al., Proc. 4th Symposium on Weed Problems in Mediterranean Climates* **2**, 386 (1989). GC determn in agricultural products: Y. Nakamura *et al., J. Agric. Food Chem.* **42**, 2508 (1994).

Crystals, mp 134.8°. Vapor pressure at 20°: 4.8×10^{-11} mm Hg. Partition coefficient (octanol/water): log P 3.23. Soly at 20° (g/l): 0.004 water; 0.1-1 *n*-hexane; 20-50 toluene; >200 dichloromethane; 5-10 2-propanol. LD_{50} in rats, mice (mg/kg): >5000, >5000 orally; >1000, >1000 s.c.; >5000, >5000 dermally; LC_{50} (4 hr) in rats: 134 mg/m³ (Schmidt).

USE: Herbicide.

5798. Mefenamic Acid. [61-68-7] 2-[(2,3-Dimethylphenyl)amino]benzoic acid; N-(2,3-xylyl)anthranilic acid; CI-473; INF-3355; Lysalgo; Mefenacid; Parkemed; Ponalar; Ponstan; Ponstel;

Ponstyl; Pontal. $C_{15}H_{15}NO_2$; mol wt 241.29. C 74.67%, H 6.27%, N 5.80%, O 13.26%. Prepn: **BE 605302**; R. A. Scherrer, **US 3138636** (1961, 1964 both to Parke-Davis). Pharmacology: C. V. Winder *et al., J. Pharmacol. Exp. Ther.* **138**, 405 (1962); C. V. Winder *et al., Arthritis Rheum.* **12**, 472 (1969); and toxicology: Mokhort, Korkhova, *Farmakol. Toksikol. (Kiev)* **1968**, 85, *C.A.* **71**, 29080c (1969); U. Jahn, R. W. Adrian, *Arzneim.-Forsch.* **19**, 36 (1969). Crystal structure: J. F. McConnell, F. Z. Company, *Cryst. Struct. Commun.* **5**, 861 (1976). Clinical trial in primary dysmenorrhea: P. W. Budoff, *J. Am. Med. Assoc.* **241**, 2713 (1979). HPLC determn in human plasma: I. Niopas, K. Mamzoridi, *J. Chromatogr. B* **656**, 447 (1994).

Crystals, mp 230-231° (effervescence). pKa 4.2. uv max (0.1N NaOH): 285, 340 nm. Soly in H_2O, pH 7.1 (g/100 ml): 0.0041 (25°); 0.008 (37°). Soluble in solns of alkali hydroxides; sparingly sol in ether, chloroform; slightly sol in ethanol. LD_{50} orally in mice, rats: 630, 790 mg/kg (Jahn, Adrian).

Sodium salt. $C_{15}H_{14}NNaO_2$. White powder. Soly in H_2O: >5 g/100 ml. LD_{50} in mice (mg/kg): 600 orally; 150 i.p. (Mokhort, Korkhova).

THERAP CAT: Anti-inflammatory; analgesic.

5799. Mefenorex. [17243-57-1] *N*-(3-Chloropropyl)-α-methylbenzeneethanamine; *N*-(3-chloropropyl)-α-methylphenethylamine; 1-phenyl-2-(3-chloropropylamino)propane. $C_{12}H_{18}ClN$; mol wt 211.73. C 68.07%, H 8.57%, Cl 16.74%, N 6.62%. Prepn: Beschke *et al.*, **DE 1210873** (1966 to Hoffmann-La Roche), *C.A.* **64**, 19486c (1966). Clinical pharmacology: P. Netter *et al., Arzneim.-Forsch.* **28**, 1310 (1978). GC-MS determn in urine: A. Franceschini *et al., J. Chromatogr.* **541**, 109 (1991). Pharmacokinetics and metabolism: S. Rendic *et al., Eur. J. Drug Metab. Pharmacokinet.* **19**, 107 (1994). *Review:* J. Engel *et al., Drug Alcohol Depend.* **17**, 229-234 (1986).

Hydrochloride. [5586-87-8] Ro-4-5282; Incital; Pondinil; Pondinol. $C_{12}H_{18}ClN.HCl$; mol wt 248.19. Solid, mp 128-130°. *Note:* This is a controlled substance (stimulant): **21 CFR, 1308.14.**

THERAP CAT: Anorexic.

5800. Mefenpyr-diethyl. [135590-91-9] 1-(2,4-Dichlorophenyl)-4,5-dihydro-5-methyl-1*H*-pyrazole-3,5-dicarboxylic acid diethyl ester; diethyl 1-(2,4-dichlorophenyl)-5-methyl-2-pyrazoline-3,5-dicarboxylate; AE-F107892; HOE-107892. $C_{16}H_{18}Cl_2N_2O_4$; mol wt 373.23. C 51.49%, H 4.86%, Cl 19.00%, N 7.51%, O 17.15%. Herbicide safener that enhances metabolism of herbicides and exhibits selective control of grass weeds in wheat and barley. Prepn: W. Rösch *et al.*, **WO 9107874**; *idem*, **US 5700758** (1991, 1997 both to Hoechst). Comprehensive description: E. Hacker *et al., Brighton Crop Prot. Conf. - Weeds* **1999**, 15-22. Effects on glutathione *S*-transferase activity on dark-grown barley: R. Scalla, A. Roulet, *Physiol. Plant.* **116**, 336 (2002). Field study of mixture with iodosulfuron-methyl-sodium in barley: S. R. King, E. S. Hagood, Jr., *Weed Technol.* **19**, 372 (2005).

mp 50-52°. Vapor pressure at 25°: 1.4×10^{-5} Pa. Soly in water (20°): 20 mg/ml (pH 6.2). Log P (octanol/water): 3.83 (pH 6.3, 21°). LD_{50} in rats (mg/kg): >5000 orally, >4000 dermally; LC_{50} in carp (mg/l): 2.4 (Hacker).

USE: Herbicide safener.

5801. Mefloquine. [53230-10-7] (α*S*)-*rel*-α-(2*R*)-2-Piperidinyl-2,8-bis(trifluoromethyl)-4-quinolinemethanol; DL-*erythro*-α-2-piperidyl-2,8-bis(trifluoromethyl)-4-quinolinemethanol; Ro-21-5998. $C_{17}H_{16}F_6N_2O$; mol wt 378.31. C 53.97%, H 4.26%, F 30.13%, N 7.40%, O 4.23%. Quinoline methanol antimalarial agent. Prepn (stereo unspec): C. J. Ohnmacht *et al., J. Med. Chem.* **14**, 926 (1971). Prepn, activity, and abs config of isomers: F. I. Carroll, J. T. Blackwell, *J. Med. Chem.* **17**, 210 (1974). Prepn of *erythro*-form: G. Grethe, T. Mitt, **DE 2806909**; H. Bömches, B. Hardegger, **US 4507482** (1978, 1985 both to Hoffmann-La Roche). X-ray crystal structure: A. Skórska *et al., Bioorg. Med. Chem. Lett.* **16**, 850 (2006). Mechanism of action studies: M. W. Davidson *et al., J. Med. Chem.* **20**, 1117 (1977); R. E. Brown *et al., Life Sci.* **25**, 1857 (1979). Photochemistry: G. A. Epling, U. C. Yoon, *Chem. Lett.* **1982** (2), 211. Pharmacokinetics: D. E. Schwartz *et al., Chemotherapy (Basel)* **28**, 70 (1982). HPLC determn in blood and plasma: I. M. Kapetanovic *et al., J. Chromatogr.* **277**, 209 (1983). Comprehensive description: P. Lim, *Anal. Profiles Drug Subs.* **14**, 157-180 (1985). Review of development: *Bull. WHO* **61**, 169-178 (1983); of clinical trials in malaria prophylaxis: A. Croft, P. Garner, *Br. Med. J.* **315**, 1412-1416 (1997).

mp 174-176°. Crystal density: 1.432 g/cm³.

Hydrochloride. [51773-92-3] WR-142490; Lariam. $C_{17}H_{16}F_6N_2O.HCl$; mol wt 414.77. C 49.23%, H 4.13%, F 27.48%, N 6.75%, O 3.86%, Cl 8.55%. Odorless, white powder, mp 259-260° (dec). Sol in ethanol, ethyl acetate; slightly sol in water. uv max (methanol): 222, 283, 304, 318 nm (ε 46700, 6600, 4000, 3100).

THERAP CAT: Antimalarial.

5802. Mefluidide. [53780-34-0] *N*-[2,4-Dimethyl-5-[[(trifluoromethyl)sulfonyl]amino]phenyl]acetamide; 5-acetamido-2,4-dimethyltrifluoromethanesulfonanilide; methafluoridamid; MBR-12325; VEL-3973; Vistar; Embark. $C_{11}H_{13}F_3N_2O_3S$; mol wt 310.29. C 42.58%, H 4.22%, F 18.37%, N 9.03%, O 15.47%, S 10.33%. Prepn: T. L. Fridinger, **DE 2406475**; *idem*, **US 3894073** (1974, 1975 to 3M). Metabolism: G. W. Ivie, *J. Agric. Food Chem.* **28**, 1286 (1980).

Cryst solid, mp 183-185°. Vapor press at 25°: $<10^{-4}$ mm Hg. pKa 4.6. Soly at 25° (g/l): water 0.18; benzene 0.31; dichloromethane 2.1; 1-octanol 17; methanol 310; acetone 350. Aq solns decomp in uv light. Mildly corrosive to metals.

USE: Plant growth regulator; herbicide.

5803. Mefruside. [7195-27-9] 4-Chloro-*N*¹-methyl-*N*¹-[(tetrahydro-2-methyl-2-furanyl)methyl]-1,3-benzenedisulfonamide; 4-chloro-*N*¹-methyl-*N*¹-(tetrahydro-2-methylfurfuryl)-*m*-benzenedisulfonamide; 2-[(4-chloro-*N*¹-methyl-3-sulfamoylbenzenesulfonamido)methyl]-2-methyltetrahydrofuran; *N*-(4-chloro-3-sulfamoylbenzenesulfonyl)-*N*-methyl-2-furfurylamine; B-1500; Baycaron. $C_{13}H_{19}ClN_2O_5S_2$; mol wt 382.88. C 40.78%, H 5.00%, Cl 9.26%, N 7.32%, O 20.89%, S 16.75%. Prepn: H. Horstmann *et al.*, **GB 1031916**; *idem*, **US 3356692** (1966, 1967 to Bayer AG); of *dl*-, *d*-, and *l*-forms, *idem, Arzneim.-Forsch.* **17**, 653 (1967).

dl-Form. Crystals, mp 149-150°.

d-Form. Crystals, mp 146°. $[\alpha]_{578}^{20}$ +5.4° (c = 2.026 in methanol).

l-Form. Crystals, mp 146°. $[\alpha]_{578}^{20}$ −5.5° (c = 2.100 in methanol). More active as a diuretic than the d-form.

THERAP CAT: Diuretic.

5804. Megacins. Antibiotic proteins produced by strains of *Bacillus megaterium,* which are highly specific in their antibacterial activity against strains of homologous species. Isoln of megacin A from *B. megaterium:* Ivanovics, Alföldi, *Nature* **174,** 465 (1954); Holland, *Biochem. J.* **78,** 641 (1961). Destroys the cytoplasmic membrane of sensitive bacteria: Nagy, *Acta Microbiol. Acad. Sci. Hung.* **6,** 337 (1959). Isoln of megacin C from *B. megaterium:* Holland, Roberts, *J. Gen. Microbiol.* **35,** 271 (1964). Has a mode of action quite different from megacin A and is more reminiscent of colicins, *q.v.* Review: Holland in *Antibiotics* vol. 1, D. Gottlieb, P. Shaw, Eds. (Springer-Verlag, New York, 1967) pp 688-695.

5805. Megestrol Acetate. [595-33-5] 17-Hydroxy-6-methylpregna-4,6-diene-3,20-dione acetate; 17α-acetoxy-6-methylpregna-4,6-diene-3,20-dione; 6-dehydro-6-methyl-17α-acetoxyprogesterone; 6-methyl-Δ^{4,6}-pregnadien-17α-ol-3,20-dione acetate; Maygace; Megace; Megestat; Megestil; Nia; Niagestin; Ovaban. $C_{24}H_{32}O_4$; mol wt 384.51. C 74.97%, H 8.39%, O 16.64%. Orally active progestogen; formerly used in combinations as oral contraceptive. Prepn: Ringold *et al., J. Am. Chem. Soc.* **81,** 3712 (1959); Dodson, Sollman, US 2891079 (1959 to Searle); Kirk *et al.,* GB 870286 *C.A.* **56,** 10248i (1962), and US 3356573 (1967 to Brit. Drug Houses); Cross, US 3400137 (1968 to Syntex). Biological effectiveness studies: Chang, Kincl, *Steroids* **12,** 689 (1968). Metabolic studies: Cooper, Kellie, *ibid.* **11,** 133 (1968). Soly and diffusion studies: Sundaram, Kincl, *ibid.* **12,** 517 (1968). Comparative clinical trial with tamoxifen in metastatic breast cancer: J. C. Allergra *et al., Semin. Oncol.* **12,** Suppl. 6, 61 (1985). Evaluation in prevention of hot flashes: C. L. Loprinzi *et al., N. Engl. J. Med.* **331,** 347 (1994). Review of carcinogenicity studies: *IARC Monographs* **21,** 431-439 (1979).

Crystals from methanol, mp 214-216°. Soly at 37°: in water (2 μg/ml); in plasma (24 μg/ml). $[\alpha]_D^{24}$ +5° (chloroform). uv max (ethanol): 287 nm (log ε 4.40).

Mixture with ethinyl estradiol. [8064-66-2] Co-Ervonum; Kombiquens; Noval; Nuvacon; Planovin; Tri-Ervonum; Volidan; Weradys.

Mixture with mestranol. [8064-51-5] Delpregnin.

THERAP CAT: Progestogen. Palliative treatment of breast and endometrial carcinoma.

THERAP CAT (VET): Progestogen. Estrus regulator.

5806. Meglumine Acetrizoate. [22154-43-4] 1-Deoxy-1-(methylamino)-D-glucitol 3-(acetylamino)-2,4,6-triiodobenzoate (salt); 3-acetamido-2,4,6-triiodobenzoic acid methylglucamine salt; 3-acetylamino-2,4,6-triiodobenzoate of methylglucamine; methylglucamine 3-acetylamino-2,4,6-triiodobenzoate; methylglucamine acetrizoate; Fortombrine M; Fortoshade M; Jodozoat Meglumin; Vasurix. $C_{16}H_{23}I_3N_2O_8$; mol wt 752.08. C 25.55%, H 3.08%, I 50.62%, N 3.72%, O 17.02%. $C_9H_6I_3NO_3 \cdot C_7H_{17}NO_5$.

Minute crystals. Freely sol in water. Aq solns have a pH of ~7.0. The iodine content of the dry powder is reported as 50.67%.

THERAP CAT: Diagnostic aid (radiopaque medium).

5807. Meglumine Diatrizoate. [131-49-7] 1-Deoxy-1-(methylamino)-D-glucitol 3,5-bis(acetylamino)-2,4,6-triiodobenzoate salt; 3,5-diacetamido-2,4,6-triiodobenzoic acid methylglucamine salt; urografic acid methylglucamine salt; diatrizoate meglumine; diatrizoate methylglucamine; methylglucamine diatrizoate; meglumine amidotrizoate; Angiografin; Cardiografin; Cystografin; Hypaque Cysto; Hypaque Meglumine; Reno M; Urovist. $C_{18}H_{26}I_3N_3$-O_9; mol wt 809.13. C 26.72%, H 3.24%, I 47.05%, N 5.19%, O 17.80%. $C_{11}H_9I_3N_2O_4 \cdot C_7H_{17}NO_5$. Distribution and metabolism: H. Langecker *et al., Arch. Exp. Pathol. Pharmakol.* **222,** 584 (1954). Clinical evaluation of diagnostic use in contrast enhanced computer tomography: J. S. Morrow, *Curr. Ther. Res.* **27,** 229 (1980).

Rhombic needles, slightly sweet taste. mp 189-193° (dec). Soly in water at 20°: 89 g/100 ml.

Mixture with sodium diatrizoate. [8064-12-8] MD-76; Gastrografin; Renografin; Renovist; Urografin.

THERAP CAT: Diagnostic aid (radiopaque medium).

THERAP CAT (VET): X-ray contrast medium.

5808. Meglutol. [503-49-1] 3-Hydroxy-3-methylpentanedioic acid; 3-hydroxy-3-methylglutaric acid; dicrotalic acid; medroglutaric acid; HMG; HMGA; CB-337; Lipoglutaren; Mevalon. C_6-$H_{10}O_5$; mol wt 162.14. C 44.45%, H 6.22%, O 49.34%. Hypolipidemic agent that decreases the rate of cholesterol synthesis. Prepn via Reformatsky reaction between ethyl acetoacetate and ethyl bromoacetate: R. Adams, B. L. Van Duuren, *J. Am. Chem. Soc.* **75,** 2377 (1953). Synthesis via oxidation of diallylmethylcarbinol with ozone and hydrogen peroxide: H. J. Klosterman, F. Smith, *ibid.* **76,** 1229 (1954); J. L. Rabinowitz, *Biochem. Prep.* **6,** 25 (1958). *Caution:* attempts to increase batch size of the ozonolysis resulted in an explosion, *cf. Chem. Eng. News* **51**(6), 29 (1973). Improved synthesis: A. Yavrouian *et al., Synthesis* **1981,** 791. Hypocholesteremic properties: Z. H. Beg, M. Siddiqi, *Experientia* **23,** 380 (1967); M. Siddiqi, Z. H. Beg, US 3629449 (1971); Z. H. Beg, P. J. Lupien, *Biochim. Biophys. Acta* **260,** 439 (1972); A. N. K. Yusufi, M. Siddiqi, *Atherosclerosis* **20,** 517 (1974); C. D. Padova *et al., Life Sci.* **30,** 1907 (1982). Biosynthetic studies: L. W. White, H. Rudney, *Biochemistry* **9,** 2713 (1970); L. Hagenfeldt, K. Hellstrom, *Life Sci.* **9,** Pt. 2, 991 (1970). Organ distribution: L. L. Savoie, P. J. Lupien, *Can. J. Physiol. Pharmacol.* **53,** 638 (1975). Effectiveness in familial hypercholesteremia: P. J. Lupien *et al., J. Clin. Pharmacol.* **19,** 120 (1979). GC study in patients with organic acidurias: K. Tanaka, D. J. Hine, *J. Chromatogr.* **239,** 301 (1982). Toxicological study: L. L. Savoie, P. J. Lupien, *Arzneim.-Forsch.* **25,** 1284 (1975).

Cryst from ether/petr ether, mp 108-109°. Sol in water. Stable when stored dry. LD$_{50}$ in mice (g/kg): 7.33 orally; 3.23 i.p. (Savoie, Lupien).

THERAP CAT: Antilipemic.

5809. Meitnerium. [54038-01-6] Element 109; unnilennium. Mt, Une; at. no. 109. Group VIII(9). No stable nuclides. Prepn of isotope ^{266}109 (T$_{½}$ ~3.5 msec, α-decay) by ^{209}Bi(^{58}Fe,n): G. Münzenberg *et al., Z. Phys.* **A309,** 89 (1982); *eidem, ibid.* **A315,** 145 (1984). Review of synthesis: G. N. Flerov, G. M. Ter-Akopian, *Prog. Particle Nucl. Phys.* **19,** 197-239 (1987); G. T. Seaborg in *Transuranium Elements: A Half Century,* L. R. Morss, J. Fuger, Eds. (Am. Chem. Soc., Washington DC, 1992) p 41-42.

5810. Melagatran. [159776-70-2] N-[(1R)-2-[(2S)-2-[[[[4-(Aminoiminomethyl)phenyl]methyl]amino]carbonyl]-1-azetidinyl]-1-cyclohexyl-2-oxoethyl]glycine; N-[(R)-[[(2S)-2-[[p-amidinobenzyl]carbamoyl]-1-azetidinyl]carbonyl]cyclohexylmethyl]glycine; H-319/68. $C_{22}H_{31}N_5O_4$; mol wt 429.51. C 61.52%, H 7.27%, N 16.31%, O 14.90%. Synthetic thrombin inhibitor. Prepn: K. T. Antonsson *et al.,* WO 9429336; *eidem,* US 5939392 (1994, 1999 both to Astra AB). Pharmacology: D. Gustafsson *et al., Thromb. Haemostasis* **79,** 110 (1998). Clinical evaluation in patients with deep vein thrombosis: H. Eriksson *et al., ibid.* **81**, 358 (1999).

THERAP CAT: Antithrombotic.

5811. Melamine. [108-78-1] 1,3,5-Triazine-2,4,6-triamine; 2,4,6-triamino-*s*-triazine; cyanurotriamide. $C_3H_6N_6$; mol wt 126.12. C 28.57%, H 4.80%, N 66.64%. Usually prepd by heating dicyandiamide, $H_2NC(=NH)NHC\equiv N$, under pressure: Mackay, US **2737513** (1956 to Am. Cyanamid). Alternate methods starting with urea: Mackey, US **2760961** (1956 to Am. Cyanamid); Pomot *et al.*, US **3111519** (1963 to Office Natl. Ind. de l'Azote). X-ray and neutron crystal structure: J. N. Varghese *et al., Acta Crystallogr.* **33B**, 2102 (1977). Review of mfg processes: *Faith, Keyes & Clark's Industrial Chemicals*, F. A. Lowenheim, M. K. Moran, Eds. (Wiley-Interscience, New York, 4th ed., 1975) pp 519-523.

Monoclinic prisms. mp <250°. Sublimes. d^{250} 1.573. Slightly sol in water; very slightly sol in hot alc; insol in ether.

USE: Forms synthetic resins with formaldehyde.

5812. Melanins. Pigments responsible for the dark color of skin, hair, feathers, fur, insect cuticle, soil; found also in fungi, bacteria, and pathological human urine where it is an indication of melanotic tumors. Structures are highly irregular polymers produced in the form of granules which may be bound to protein material. *Allomelanins* are found in the plant kingdom and are produced from nitrogen-free precursors. *See:* aspergillin, humic acid. *Eumelanins* and *phaeomelanins* are found in the animal kingdom. Eumelanins are black or brown, insoluble, nitrogenous pigments produced by the oxidative polymerization of 5,6-dihydroxyindoles derived enzymatically from tyrosine via dopa. One of the best characterized is sepiomelanin, *q.v.* Phaeomelanins are sulfur-containing, alkali-soluble, yellow to reddish-brown pigments produced by oxidative polymerization of cysteinyldopas via 1,4-benzothiazine intermediates. Biosynthesis from tyrosine: H. S. Raper, *Physiol. Rev.* **8**, 245 (1928); H. S. Mason, *J. Biol. Chem.* **172**, 83 (1948). *In vitro* prepn from dopa: L. E. Arnow, *Science* **87**, 308 (1938). Series of articles on structure and biosynthesis: M. Piattelli, R. A. Nicolaus, *Tetrahedron* **15**, 66 (1961); M. Piattelli *et al., ibid.* **18**, 941 (1962); *eidem, ibid.* **19**, 2061 (1963); R. A. Nicolaus *et al., ibid.* **20**, 1163 (1964). NMR-study: G. A. Duff *et al., Biochemistry* **27**, 7112 (1988). Determn of eumelanin metabolites in human urine: S. Pavel, W. van der Slik, *J. Chromatogr.* **375**, 392 (1986). Review of biosynthesis: J. M. Pawelek, A. M. Körner, *Am. Sci.* **70**, 136-145 (1982); of photochemistry and photobiology: M. R. Chedekel, *Photochem. Photobiol.* **35**, 881-885 (1982); M. R. Chedekel, L. Zeise, *Lipids* **23**, 587-591 (1988). *Reviews:* R. A. Nicolaus, *Melanins* (Hermann, Paris, 1968); G. Prota, *Med. Res. Rev.* **8**, 525-556 (1988).

5813. Melanostatin. [9083-38-9] Melanocyte-stimulating hormone release-inhibiting factor; MIF; MRIH; MSH release-inhibiting hormone; melanotropin inhibiting factor. An inhibiting factor which mediates hypothalamic control of MSH, *q.v.*, a pituitary hormone: A. J. Kastin, A. V. Schally, *Gen. Comp. Endocrinol.* **7**, 452 (1966); A. V. Schally, A. J. Kastin, *Endocrinology* **79**, 768 (1966). Although several substances have MIF activity, the exact nature of MSH release inhibition is not known, *cf.* A. J. Kastin *et al., Yale J. Biol. Med.* **46**, 617 (1973); *eidem, Fed. Proc.* **39**, 2931 (1980). The first factor with melanocyte-release inhibiting activity to be

isolated was the side-chain tripeptide of oxytocin, *q.v.*, now referred to as MIF-I: M. E. Celis *et al., Proc. Natl. Acad. Sci. USA* **68**, 1428 (1971). Isoln of bovine MIF-I and identity with the tripeptide (Pro-Leu-GlyNH_2): R. M. G. Nair *et al., Biochem. Biophys. Res. Commun.* **43**, 1376 (1971). Synthesis: H. Irie *et al., Chem. Lett.* **1980**, 705. Extrapituitary effects of MIF-I are known, particularly potentiation of DOPA-induced behavioral changes: N. P. Plotnikoff *et al., Life Sci.* **10**, 1279 (1971); *eidem, Neuroendocrinology* **14**, 271 (1974). Clinical studies in Parkinson's disease: A. J. Kastin, A. Barbeau, *Can. Med. Assoc. J.* **107**, 1079 (1972); A. Barbeau, *Lancet* **2**, 683 (1975); V. E. Schneider *et al., Arzneim.-Forsch.* **28**, 1296 (1978). *Reviews:* A. V. Schally *et al., Recent Prog. Horm. Res.* **24**, 497-581 (1968); A. J. Kastin *et al., Life Sci.* **25**, 401-414 (1979); *eidem* in *Polypeptide Hormones*, R. F. Beers, E. G. Bassett, Eds. (Raven Press, New York, 1980) pp 223-224; *eidem, Fed. Proc.* **39**, 2931-2936 (1980).

Pro–Leu–Gly–NH_2

MIF-I

MIF-I. [2002-44-0] L-Prolyl-L-leucylglycinamide; melanostatin I (ox); MSH release-inhibiting factor I. $C_{13}H_{24}N_4O_3$; mol wt 284.35.

5814. Melanotan. [75921-69-6] 4-L-Norleucine-7-D-phenylalanine-α-melanotropin (swine); [Nle^4,D-Phe^7]-α-MSH; melanotan-1. $C_{78}H_{111}N_{21}O_{19}$; mol wt 1646.85. C 56.89%, H 6.79%, N 17.86%, O 18.46%. Synthetic analog of human α-melanocyte-stimulating hormone, *see* MSH. Stimulates melanin production which protects skin from UV radiation. Prepn and bioactivity: T. K. Sawyer *et al., Proc. Natl. Acad. Sci. USA* **77**, 5754 (1980); *idem et al., J. Med. Chem.* **25**, 1022 (1982); V. J. Hruby *et al.*, US **4457864** (1984 to University Patents). Review of pharmacology and development: M. E. Hadley *et al., Pharmaceut. Biotechnol.* **11**, 575-595 (1998). Clinical induction of skin tanning: N. Levine *et al., J. Am. Med. Assoc.* **266**, 2730 (1991); R. T. Dorr *et al., Arch. Dermatol.* **140**, 827 (2004).

Ac–Ser–Tyr–Ser–Nle–Glu–His–D-Phe–Arg–Trp–Gly–Lys–Pro–Val–NH_2

THERAP CAT: Prevention of sunburn injury.

5815. Melarsoprol. [494-79-1] 2-[4-[(4,6-Diamino-1,3,5-triazin-2-yl)amino]phenyl]-1,3,2-dithiarsolane-4-methanol; *p*-[(4,6-diamino-*s*-triazin-2-yl)amino]dithiobenzenearsonous acid 3-hydroxypropylene ester; 2-*p*-(4,6-diamino-*s*-triazin-2-ylamino)-phenyl-4-hydroxymethyl-1,3,2-dithiarsoline; 2-(4-melamin-2-yl-phenyl)-4-hydroxymethyl-1,3-dithia-2-arsolane; Mel B; Arsobal. $C_{12}H_{15}AsN_6OS_2$; mol wt 398.34. C 36.18%, H 3.80%, As 18.81%, N 21.10%, O 4.02%, S 16.10%. Prepn: Friedheim, US **2659723** (1953); US **2772303** (1956).

Practically insol in water, cold ethanol, methanol. Sol in propylene glycol.

THERAP CAT: Antiprotozoal (Trypanosoma).

5816. Melatonin. [73-31-4] *N*-[2-(5-Methoxy-1*H*-indol-3-yl)ethyl]acetamide; *N*-acetyl-5-methoxytryptamine; Regulin. $C_{13}H_{16}N_2O_2$; mol wt 232.28. C 67.22%, H 6.94%, N 12.06%, O 13.78%. A hormone of the pineal gland, also produced by extrapineal tissues, that lightens skin color in amphibians by reversing the darkening effect of MSH, *q.v.* Melatonin has been postulated as the mediator of photic-induced antigonadotrophic activity in photoperiodic mammals and has also been shown to be involved in thermoregulation in some ectotherms and in affecting locomotor activity rhythms in sparrows. Isoln from the pineal glands of beef cattle: Lerner *et al., J. Am. Chem. Soc.* **80**, 2587 (1958); Wurtman *et al., Science* **141**, 277 (1963). Structure: Lerner *et al., J. Am. Chem. Soc.* **81**, 6084 (1959). Crystal and molecular structure: A. Wakahara, *Chem. Lett.* **1972**, 1139. Synthesis from 5-methoxyindole as starting material by two different routes: Szmuszkovicz *et al., J. Org. Chem.* **25**, 857 (1960). Biochemical role of melatonin: *Chem. Eng. News* **45**, 40 (May 1, 1967). Pharmacological studies: Barchas *et al., Nature* **214**, 919 (1967). Identification of antigonadal action sites in mouse brain: J. D. Glass, G. R. Lynch, *Science* **214**, 821 (1981). Binding studies in human hypothalamus: S. M. Reppert *et al., Science* **242**, 78 (1988). Efficacy in control of estrus in red deer: G. W. Asher, *Anim. Reprod. Sci.* **22**, 145 (1990). *Reviews:* M. K. Vaughn, *Int. J. Rev. Physiol.* **24**, 41-95 (1981); D. C.Klein *et al., Life Sci.* **28**, 1975-1986 (1981). Book: *Advan. Biosci.* **vol. 29**, N. Birau, W. Schlott, Eds. (Pergamon Press, New York, 1981) 420 pp. Review of etiological role in clinical disease: A. Miles, D. Philbrick, *Crit. Rev. Clin. Lab. Sci.* **25**, 231-253 (1987); in psychiatric disorders: *eidem, Biol. Psychiatry* **23**, 405-425 (1988).

Pale yellow leaflets from benzene, mp 116-118°. uv max: 223, 278 nm (ε 27550, 6300).

THERAP CAT (VET): Control of estrus.

5817. Meldrum's Acid. [2033-24-1] 2,2-Dimethyl-1,3-dioxane-4,6-dione; malonic acid cyclic isopropylidene ester; isopropylidene malonate; 2,2-dimethyl-4,6-diketo-1,3-dioxane. $C_6H_8O_4$; mol wt 144.13. C 50.00%, H 5.59%, O 44.40%. Prepd from malonic acid and acetone in the presence of acetic anhydride: Meldrum, *J. Chem. Soc.* **93**, 598 (1908). Prepn and structure: Davidson, Bernhard, *J. Am. Chem. Soc.* **70**, 3426 (1948); P. Schuster *et al., Monatsh. Chem.* **95**, 53 (1964); G. H. Bihlmayer *et al., ibid.* **98**, 564 (1967). *Review:* H. McNab, *Chem. Soc. Rev.* **7**, 345-358 (1978).

Crystals from acetone + water, dec 94-95°. pKa 5.1.

USE: In organic synthesis as a substitute for acyclic malonic esters and generally as a C_3O_2 synthon.

5818. Melengestrol Acetate. [2919-66-6] 17-(Acetyloxy)-6-methyl-16-methylenepregna-4,6-diene-3,20-dione; 6α-methyl-6-dehydro-16-methylene-17-acetoxyprogesterone; MGA. $C_{25}H_{32}$-O_4; mol wt 396.52. C 75.73%, H 8.13%, O 16.14%. Orally active progestational steroid. Prepn: D. N. Kirk *et al.,* **GB 886619**; *eidem,* **US 3332940** (1962, 1967 both to British Drug Houses). Environmental degradation study: B. Schiffer *et al., Environ. Health Perspect.* **109**, 1145 (2001). Receptor binding study: G. A. Perry *et al., Domest. Anim. Endocrinol.* **28**, 147 (2005). Review of pharmacology in animals: R. G. Zimbelman *et al., J. Am. Vet. Med. Assoc.* **157**, 1528-1536 (1970); of use in control of bovine estrus: D. J. Patterson *et al., J. Anim. Sci.* **67**, 1895-1906 (1989).

Needles from acetone/hexane, mp 224-226°. $[\alpha]_D^{23}$ $-127°$ (c = 0.31 in chloroform). uv max (ethanol): 287.5 nm (log ε 4.35).

LD$_{50}$ (mg/kg): >8000 orally in rats; >2500 i.p. in mice (Zimbelman).

THERAP CAT (VET): Progestogen; growth promotant.

5819. Melezitose. [597-12-6] *O*-α-D-Glucopyranosyl-(1 → 3)-β-D-fructofuranosyl-α-D-glucopyranoside. $C_{18}H_{32}O_{16}$; mol wt 504.44. C 42.86%, H 6.39%, O 50.75%. Trisaccharide built from 2 mols glucose and 1 mol fructose. Acid hydrolysis yields at first glucose and turanose. Occurs in a manna that forms upon the Douglas fir, jack pine *(Pinus virginiana* Mill., *Pinaceae)* and other trees. During periods of drought, bees collect it from the manna in sufficient quantity to change the character of the honey, making it unsuitable for maintaining the bees, but providing a source of melezitose: Hudson, Sherwood, *J. Am. Chem. Soc.* **42**, 116 (1920). Procedure: Bates, *Natl. Bur. Std. Circ.* **C440**, p 472 (1942). Structure: Hehre, Carlson, *Arch. Biochem. Biophys.* **36**, 158 (1952); Hehre, *Adv. Carbohydr. Chem.* **8**, 277 (1953). *Review:* E. B. Rathbone, *Dev. Food Carbohydr.* **2**, 145-185 (1980).

Dihydrate. Crystals from water. The water of crystn is given up at 110°. When anhydr, mp 153-154°. $[\alpha]_D^{20}$ +88° (c = 4). Sol in water, very sparingly sol in alc. Not fermented by baker's yeast; does not reduce Fehling's soln.

5820. Melibiose. [585-99-9] 6-*O*-α-D-Galactopyranosyl-D-glucose; 6-(α-D-galactosido)-D-glucose. $C_{12}H_{22}O_{11}$; mol wt 342.30. C 42.11%, H 6.48%, O 51.41%. Prepd from raffinose by fermentation with top yeast which removes the fructose: Hudson, Harding, *J. Am. Chem. Soc.* **37**, 2734 (1915); Fletcher, Diehl, *ibid.* **74**, 5774 (1952). Structure: Haworth, Leitch, *J. Chem. Soc.* **113**, 188 (1918); Charlton *et al., ibid.* **1926**, 99; Charlton *et al., ibid.* **1927**, 1527; Haworth *et al., ibid.* 3146; Levene, Jorpes, *J. Biol. Chem.* **86**, 403 (1930). Synthesis: Helferich, Bredereck, *Ann.* **465**, 166 (1928).

Dihydrate. Monoclinic crystals from water or dil alcohol. mp 84-85°. Shows mutarotation. $[\alpha]_D^{20}$ +111.7° → +129.5° (c = 4). One gram dissolves in 0.4 ml water, 8.5 ml methanol, 220 ml abs alcohol. Dilute acids hydrolyze melibiose to D-glucose and D-galactose. Also split by emulsin and by bottom yeast. Reduces Fehling's soln. 3.5 g melibiose dihydrate are about as sweet as 1.0 g sucrose.

5821. Melilot. Sweet clover; yellow Melilot; yellow sweet clover. Dried leaves and flowering tops of *Melilotus officinalis* (L.) Lam., *Leguminosae. Habit.* Europe, Asia, natural to some extent in U.S. *Constit.* Coumarin, resin, volatile oil.

An extract is marketed as *Esberiven.*

5822. Melinamide. [14417-88-0] (Z,Z)-*N*-(1-Phenylethyl)-9,12-octadecadienamide; *N*-(α-methylbenzyl)linoleamide; MBLA; AC-223; Artes. $C_{26}H_{41}NO$; mol wt 383.61. C 81.41%, H 10.77%, N 3.65%, O 4.17%. Linoleic acid derivative. Prepn and use in lowering blood cholesterol levels: **FR 1476596**; T. Seki *et al.,* **US 3621043** (1967, 1971 both to Sumitomo). Physical properties and effect on cholesterol levels in rabbits: K. Toki *et al., J.*

Melitracen

Atheroscler. Res. **7**, 708 (1967). Comparative activity of melinamide and its optical isomers: H. Fukushima, K. Nakatani, *ibid.* **9**, 65 (1969); H. Fukushima *et al., ibid.* **10**, 403 (1969). Mechanism of action studies: D. Kritchevsky, S. A. Tepper, *Arzneim.-Forsch.* **21**, 1024 (1971); D. Kritchevsky *et al., Lipids* **12**, 16 (1977); K. Natori *et al., Jpn. J. Pharmacol.* **42**, 517 (1986). Metabolism: A. Hirohashi *et al., Xenobiotica* **6**, 329 (1976).

Oil. mp <4°. bp$_{0.03}$ 200-215°; bp$_{0.07}$ 200-204°. n_D^{23} 1.5050; n_D^{30} 1.4863. Saponification value 0.9. Iodine value 127.0.

THERAP CAT: Antilipemic.

5823. Melitracen. [5118-29-6] 3-(10,10-Dimethyl-9(10*H*)-anthracenylidene)-*N,N*-dimethyl-1-propanamine; *N,N*,10,10-tetramethyl-Δ$^{9(10H),\gamma}$-anthracenepropylamine; 9,10-dihydro-10,10-dimethyl-9-(3-dimethylaminopropylidene)anthracene; 9-[3-(dimethylamino)propylidene]-10,10-dimethyl-9,10-dihydroanthracene; *N,N*-dimethyl-3-(10,10-dimethyl-9(10*H*)-anthrylidene)propylamine. C$_{21}$H$_{25}$N; mol wt 291.43. C 86.55%, H 8.65%, N 4.81%. Prepn of the hydrochloride: Holm, *Acta Chem. Scand.* **17**, 2437 (1963); *idem*, **GB 939856** corresp to **US 3177209** (1963, 1965, both to Kefalas A/S). Crystal structure: J. Lopez de Lerma *et al., Acta Crystallogr.* **B35**, 1739 (1979). Toxicity data: P. V. Petersen *et al., Acta Pharmacol. Toxicol.* **24**, 121 (1966).

Hydrochloride. [10563-70-9] U-24973A; Melixeran; Trausabun; Dixeran. C$_{21}$H$_{25}$N.HCl; mol wt 327.89. Crystals from acetone, mp 245-248°. LD$_{50}$ i.v. in mice: 52 mg/kg (Petersen).

THERAP CAT: Antidepressant.

5824. Melittin. [20449-79-0] Melittin I; mellitin; Forapin. C$_{131}$H$_{229}$N$_{39}$O$_{31}$; mol wt 2846.46. C 55.28%, H 8.11%, N 19.19%, O 17.42%. Strongly basic polypeptide, the principal component of the venom of the honey bee, *Apis mellifica (mellifera)*, comprising 40-50% of the dried venom. A "direct" hemolysin, one of the hemolytic principles present in the venom, the other being "indirect" acting **phospholipase A**. Sepn and isoln: Neumann *et al., Naturwissenschaften* **39**, 286 (1952); Neumann, Haberman, *Arch. Exp. Pathol. Pharmakol.* **222**, 367 (1954); Habermann, Reiz, *Biochem. Z.* **341**, 451 (1965). Melittin is the first polypeptide whose biological effects can be understood on the basis of its primary structure. Elucidation of structure and correlation with activity: E. Habermann, J. Jentsch, *Z. Physiol. Chem.* **348**, 37 (1967). Conformation studies: R. Bazzo *et al., Eur. J. Biochem.* **173**, 139 (1988). About 10% of the melittin is thought to be formylated at the *N*-terminus: Kreil, Kreil-Kiss, *Biochem. Biophys. Res. Commun.* **27**, 275 (1967). Isoln and structure of *N$^\alpha$-formyl melittin*: Lübke *et al., Experientia* **27**, 765 (1971). Synthesis of melittin and related peptides: Lübke, Schröder, *Peptides*, H. C. Beyerman, A. van der Linde, W. M. van den Brink, Eds. (North-Holland Publishing Company, Amsterdam, 1967) pp 271-279; Dorman, Markley, *J. Med. Chem.* **14**, 5 (1970); Schröder *et al., Experientia* **27**, 764 (1971). Solid phase synthesis and purification: M. T. Tosteson *et al., Biochemistry* **26**, 6627 (1987). Review of biochemistry and pharmacology: Habermann, *Science* **177**, 314 (1972).

[1]
Gly–Ile–Gly–Ala–Val–Leu–Lys–Val–Leu–Thr–Thr–Gly–Leu–Pro

[26]
NH$_2$Gln–Gln–Arg–Lys–Arg–Lys–Ile–Trp–Ser–Ile–Leu–Ala

Cream white, water soluble powder. $[\alpha]_D^{21}$ −89.52° (c = 0.409).

THERAP CAT: Antirheumatic.

5825. Mellitic Acid. [517-60-2] Benzenehexacarboxylic acid; mellic acid. C$_{12}$H$_6$O$_{12}$; mol wt 342.17. C 42.12%, H 1.77%, O 56.11%. C$_6$(COOH)$_6$. Preparation from carbonaceous material: M. Kiebler, **US 2461740** (1949 to Carnegie Inst. of Tech.); Germain *et al., Bull. Soc. Chim. Fr.* **1962**, 779; from tetrahalophthalic acid: Brusset, Uny, *ibid.* **1951**, 565; Juettner, **US 3067246** (1962).

Crystals. mp 286-288° in sealed tube with decompn. Freely sol in water or alcohol; sol in boiling concd H$_2$SO$_4$ without decompn.

5826. Meloxicam. [71125-38-7] 4-Hydroxy-2-methyl-*N*-(5-methyl-2-thiazolyl)-2*H*-1,2-benzothiazine-3-carboxamide 1,1-dioxide; Metacam; Mobec; Mobic; Mobicox; Movalis; Movatec; Parocin. C$_{14}$H$_{13}$N$_3$O$_4$S$_2$; mol wt 351.40. C 47.85%, H 3.73%, N 11.96%, O 18.21%, S 18.25%. Preferential cyclooxygenase (COX-2) inhibitor. Prepn: G. Trummlitz *et al.*, **DE 2756113** (1979 to Thomae); *eidem*, **US 4233299** (1980 to Boehringer Ingelheim). Pharmacology in horses: P. Lees *et al., Br. Vet. J.* **147**, 97 (1991). Physicochemical properties: R.-S. Tsai *et al., Helv. Chim. Acta* **76**, 842 (1993). Veterinary trial in dogs: A. J. Henderson *et al., Prakt. Tierarzt* **75**, 179 (1994). Series of articles on pharmacology, mechanism of action and clinical efficacy: *Br. J. Rheumatol.* **35**, Suppl. 1, 1-77 (1996). Clinical trials of GI tolerability in arthritis: C. Hawkey *et al., ibid.* **37**, 937 (1998); J. Dequeker *et al., ibid.* 946. Review of clinical experience: R. Fleischmann *et al., Expert Opin. Pharmacother.* **3**, 1501-1512 (2002).

Crystals from ethylene chloride, mp 254° (dec). pKa: 4.08 in water; 4.24 ± 0.01 in water/ethanol (1:1); 4.63 ± 0.03 in water/-ethanol (1:4). Log P (octanol/water): 3.02. LD$_{50}$ orally in mice: 470 mg/kg (Trummlitz, 1980).

THERAP CAT: Anti-inflammatory.

THERAP CAT (VET): Anti-inflammatory.

5827. Melperone. [3575-80-2] 1-(4-Fluorophenyl)-4-(4-methyl-1-piperidinyl)-1-butanone; 4′-fluoro-4-(4-methylpiperidino)butyrophenone; γ-(4-methylpiperidino)-*p*-fluorobutyrophenone; methylperone; flubuperone. C$_{16}$H$_{22}$FNO; mol wt 263.35. C 72.97%, H 8.42%, F 7.21%, N 5.32%, O 6.08%. Neuroleptic agent related structurally to haloperidol, *q.v.* Prepn: **BE 651144**; S. E. H. Hernestam *et al.*, **US 3816433** (1964, 1974 both to Ferrosan). Distribution of ^{14}C melperone: N. Einer-Jensen, E. Hansson, *Acta Pharmacol. Toxicol.* **23**, 65 (1965). Pharmacological and toxicological studies: J. A. Christensen *et al., ibid.* 109; R. Heywood, A. K. Palmer, *Farmaco Ed. Prat.* **29**, 586 (1974). Dopamine-receptor binding in relation to clinical effect: I. Creese *et al., Science* **192**, 481 (1976). Sedative and sleep-inducing properties: R. Kretzschmer *et al., Arzneim.-Forsch.* **26**, 1073 (1976). Clinical studies in anxiety: W. J. Poeldinger, *Therapiewoche* **30**, 4862 (1980); L. F. Fabre, M. J. Napoliello, *Curr. Ther. Res.* **30**, 427 (1981).

Liquid, bp$_{0.1}$ 120-125°.

Hydrochloride. [1622-79-3] FG-5111; Buronil; Eunerpan. C$_{16}$H$_{22}$FNO.HCl; mol wt 299.81. Crystals, mp 209-211°. LD$_{50}$ in rats, mice (mg/kg): 330, 230 orally; 40, 35 i.v. (Christensen).

THERAP CAT: Antipsychotic.

5828. Melphalan. [148-82-3] 4-[Bis(2-chloroethyl)amino]-L-phenylalanine; *p*-di(2-chloroethyl)amino-L-phenylalanine; L-phenylalanine mustard; alanine nitrogen mustard; L-PAM; melfalan; L-sarcolysine; NSC-8806; CB-3025; Alkeran; Sarcoclorin. C_{13}-$H_{18}Cl_2N_2O_2$; mol wt 305.20. C 51.16%, H 5.94%, Cl 23.23%, N 9.18%, O 10.48%. Syntheses: Bergel, Stock, *J. Chem. Soc.* **1954**, 2409; **1955**, 1223; *eidem*, US 3032584; US 3032585 (both 1962 to NRDC); Larionov, *Lancet* **2**, 169 (1955). Toxicity: W. C. J. Ross, *Biochem. Pharmacol.* **13**, 969 (1964). Neurotoxicity study: M. G. Donelli *et al., J. Pharm. Pharmacol.* **18**, 760 (1966). Mutation study: J. McCann *et al., Proc. Natl. Acad. Sci. USA* **72**, 5135 (1975). Biliary excretion in rats: K. H. Byington *et al., Biochem. Pharmacol.* **29**, 2518 (1980). Review of carcinogenicity studies: *IARC Monographs* **9**, 167-180 (1975). *Review:* R. L. Furner, R. K. Brown, *Cancer Treat. Rep.* **64**, 559-574 (1980).

Needles from methanol (monosolvate), mp 182-183° (dec.) $[\alpha]_D^{25}$ +7.5° (c = 1.33 in 1.0N HCl); $[\alpha]_D^{22}$ −31.5° (c = 0.67 in methanol). Soluble in ethanol, propylene glycol. Practically insol in water. LD_{50} i.p. in rats: 14.7 μmol/kg (Ross).

D-Form. D-Sarcolysine; medphalan; CB-3026; NSC-35051. Needles from methanol (monosolvate), mp 181.5-182° (dec.) $[\alpha]_D^{21}$ −7.5° (c = 1.26 in 1.0N HCl).

DL-Form. Merphalan; sarcolysine. Tiny needles from methanol, mp 180-181°.

Caution: This substance is listed as a known human carcinogen: *Report on Carcinogens, Eleventh Edition* (PB2005-104914, 2004) p III-164.

THERAP CAT: Antineoplastic.

5829. Memantine. [19982-08-2] 3,5-Dimethyltricyclo-$[3.3.1.1^{3,7}]$decan-1-amine; 3,5-dimethyl-1-adamantanamine; 1-amino-3,5-dimethyladamantane; DMAA; D-145. $C_{12}H_{21}N$; mol wt 179.30. C 80.38%, H 11.81%, N 7.81%. NMDA-receptor antagonist; deriv of adamantane, *q.v.* Prepn of the hydrochloride: K. Gerzon *et al., J. Med. Chem.* **6**, 760 (1963); of the free base and hydrochloride: J. Mills, E. Krumkalns, US 3391142 (1968 to Lilly). Series of articles on pharmacology and metabolism: *Arzneim.-Forsch.* **27**, 1471-1489 (1977); on neuropharmacology and clinical efficacy: *ibid.* **32**, 1236-1276 (1982). Pharmacodynamics and pharmacokinetics: W. Wesemann *et al., ibid.* **33**, 1122 (1983). NMDA-receptor binding study: J. Kornhuber *et al., Eur. J. Pharmacol.* **166**, 589 (1989); and neuroprotective properties: *idem et al., J. Neural Transm.* **43**, Suppl., 91 (1994). Clinical studies as antispasmodic: H. Rohde, *Fortschr. Med.* **100**, 2023 (1982); in senile dementia: R. Görtelmeyer, H. Erbler, *Arzneim.-Forsch.* **42**, 904 (1992). Review of clinical experience in neurodegenerative disorders: K. K. Jain, *Expert. Opin. Invest. Drugs* **9**, 1397-1406 (2000).

Oil, n_D^{25} 1.4941.

Hydrochloride. [41100-52-1] Akatinol; Auxura; Ebixa; Namenda. $C_{12}H_{21}N.HCl$; mol wt 215.76. Fine white to off-white powder. Crystals from alcohol/ether, mp 258° (Mills, Krumkalns); also reported as mp 290-295° (Gerzon). Sol in water.

THERAP CAT: Neuroprotective; antispasmodic; antiparkinsonian.

5830. Menadiol. [481-85-6] 2-Methyl-1,4-naphthalenediol; 2-methyl-1,4-naphthohydroquinone; 2-methyl-1,4-naphthoquinol; dihydrovitamin K_3. $C_{11}H_{10}O_2$; mol wt 174.20. C 75.84%, H 5.79%, O 18.37%. Synthetic naphthoquinol derivative having physiological properties of Vitamin K, *q.v.*; starting material for prepn of menaquinones, *q.v.* Prepn: K. Fries, W. Lohmann, *Ber.* **54**, 2912 (1921); D. W. MacCorquodale *et al., J. Biol. Chem.* **131**,

357 (1939); C. D. Snyder, H. Rapoport, *J. Am. Chem. Soc.* **96**, 8046 (1974). Crystal structure: J. Gaultier, C. Hauw, *Acta Crystallogr.* **25B**, 51 (1969). Bioactivity and tissue distribution: M. J. Thierry, J. W. Suttie, *J. Nutr.* **97**, 512 (1969).

White needles from dil alc, mp 168-170° (MacCorquodale); also reported as mp 181° (Gaultier, Hauw). Slightly sol in benzene, chloroform; easily sol in acetone, alcohol.

Diacetate. [573-20-6] 1,4-Diacetoxy-2-methylnaphthalene; acetomenaphthone; vitamin K_4; Kapilin; Prokayvit Oral; Vitavel K. $C_{15}H_{14}O_4$; mol wt 258.27. Prepn: Sah *et al., Ber.* **73**, 762 (1940); *Rec. Trav. Chim.* **59**, 461 (1940). Crystals, mp 112-114°. Practically insol in water. Slightly sol in cold alc; sol in 3.3 parts boiling alc, in acetic acid.

Sodium diphosphate. [131-13-5] 2-Methyl-1,4-naphthalenediol diphosphoric acid ester tetrasodium salt; Kappadione; Synkavit; Synkayvite. $C_{11}H_8Na_4O_8P_2$; mol wt 422.08. Prepn: Fieser, Fry, *J. Am. Chem. Soc.* **62**, 228 (1940). Prepd as the hexahydrate, white to pinkish powder. Salty taste. Very sol in water. Practically insol in methanol, ethanol, ether, acetone.

THERAP CAT: Vitamin (prothrombogenic).

5831. Menadione. [58-27-5] 2-Methyl-1,4-naphthalenedione; 2-methyl-1,4-naphthoquinone; menaphthone; vitamin $K_{2(0)}$; vitamin K_3; Kappaxin; Kayquinone; Thyloquinone. $C_{11}H_8O_2$; mol wt 172.18. C 76.73%, H 4.68%, O 18.58%. Synthetic naphthoquinone derivative having physiologic properties of vitamin K, *q.v.* Prepn: Fieser, *J. Biol. Chem.* **133**, 391 (1940). Toxicity study: Molitor, Robinson, *Proc. Soc. Exp. Biol. Med.* **43**, 725 (1940). Alkylated *in vivo* to the bioactive metabolite, menaquinone-4, *q.v.*: C. Martius, H. O. Esser, *Biochem. Z.* **331**, 1 (1958). Metabolism and tissue distribution: W. V. Taggart, J. T. Matschiner, *Biochemistry* **8**, 1141 (1969). Improved synthesis: W. Adam *et al., Angew. Chem. Int. Ed.* **33**, 2475 (1994).

Bright yellow crystals. Very faint acrid odor. mp 105-107°. Stable in air; dec by sunlight. Insol in water. One gram dissolves in about 60 ml alcohol, in 10 ml benzene, in 50 ml vegetable oils; moderately sol in chloroform, carbon tetrachloride. The alcoholic soln is neutral to litmus. Solutions may be heated to 120° without dec. Destroyed by alkalies and reducing agents. *Keep protected from light.* LD_{50} orally in mice: ~0.5 g/kg (Molitor, Robinson).

Sodium bisulfite. [130-37-0]; [6147-37-1] (trihydrate). 1,2,3,-4-Tetrahydro-2-methyl-1,4-dioxo-2-naphthalenesulfonic acid sodium salt; Hykinone; Klotogen; K-Thrombin. $C_{11}H_9NaO_5S$; mol wt 276.24. Prepn: Moore, *J. Am. Chem. Soc.* **63**, 2049 (1941). Structure: Carmack *et al., ibid.* **72**, 844 (1950). Occurs as the trihydrate. White, hygroscopic crystals. Discolors and may turn purple under the influence of light. One gram dissolves in ~2 ml water. Slightly sol in alcohol. Almost insol in ether, benzene.

Dimethylpyrimidinol bisulfite. [14451-99-1] Hetrazeen. $C_{17}H_{18}N_2O_6S$; mol wt 378.40. Prepn: J. B. Nanninga *et al.,* US 3328169 (1967 to Heterochemical). Efficacy in swine diets: R. W. Seerley *et al., J. Anim. Sci.* **42**, 599 (1976). Cryst powder, mp 215-217°. Soly in water ~1 g/100 ml. Slightly sol in alcohol. Insol in ether, benzene.

THERAP CAT: Vitamin (prothrombogenic).

THERAP CAT (VET): Vitamin (prothrombogenic); antidote to bishydroxycoumarin poisoning, including sweet clover poisoning.

5832. Menadoxime. [573-01-3] [[(3-Methyl-4-oxo-1(4*H*)-naphthalenylidene)amino]oxy]acetic acid ammonium salt; menadione carboxymethoxime ammonium salt; menaphthone carboxymethoxime ammonium salt; carboxymethylmenadione monoxime ammonium salt; Kapilon injectable. $C_{13}H_{14}N_2O_4$; mol wt 262.26. C 59.54%, H 5.38%, N 10.68%, O 24.40%. Prepn: Holland, **GB 621934** (1949 to Glaxo).

Crystals from alc. Sol in water. Aq solns are neutral. May be sterilized by autoclaving and stored in ampuls if protected from light. Shows high antihemorrhagic activity.

Free acid. $C_{13}H_{11}NO_4$. Yellow platelets from alc, mp 162-163°. Forms water-sol salts.

THERAP CAT: Vitamin (prothrombogenic).

5833. Menaquinones. Vitamin K_2; 2-methyl-3-*all-trans*-polyprenyl-1,4-naphthoquinones. Group of prenylated naphthoquinone derivatives having the physiological activity of vitamin K, *q.v.* Nomenclature is based on the number of isoprene residues comprising the side chain. Compds of varying chain length are produced by bacteria, particularly by normal intestinal flora, and may serve as a source of vitamin K for humans. Birds and animals are capable of alkylating menadione, *q.v.*, to produce menaquinone 4. Originally isolated from putrefied fish meal: R. W. McKee *et al.*, *J. Biol. Chem.* **131**, 327 (1939). Identification of menaquinone 6: S. B. Binkley *et al.*, *ibid.* **133**, 721 (1940). Isoln of menaquinone 7 from cultures of *Bacillus brevis:* M. Tishler, W. L. Sampson, *Proc. Soc. Exp. Biol. Med.* **68**, 136 (1948). Structures and syntheses of series of menaquinones: O. Isler *et al.*, *Helv. Chim. Acta* **41**, 786 (1958). Review of isoln, props, synthesis: O. Isler, O. Wiss, *Vitam. Horm.* **17**, 53-90 (1959); H. Mayer, O. Isler, *Methods Enzymol.* **18C**, 469-547 (1971); of biosynthesis: D. R. Threlfall, *Vitam. Horm.* **29**, 153-200 (1971); R. Bentley, R. Meganathan, *Microbiol. Rev.* **46**, 241-280 (1982). Menaquinones with side chains of up to 15 repeating units have been described: T. Sakano *et al.*, *Chem. Pharm. Bull.* **34**, 4322 (1986). HPLC determn in bone: S. J. Hodges *et al.*, *J. Bone Miner. Res.* **8**, 1005 (1993). Metabolism and distribution: H. H. W. Thijssen, M. J. Drittij-Reijnders, *Br. J. Nutr.* **72**, 415 (1994). Absorption and bioavailability in humans: J. M. Conly *et al.*, *Am. J. Gastroenterol.* **89**, 915 (1994).

Menaquinone 4

Menaquinone 4. [863-61-6] *(E,E,E)*-2-Methyl-3-(3,7,11,15-tetramethyl-2,6,10,14-hexadecatetraenyl)-1,4-naphthalenedione; menatetrenone; MK 4; Vitamin $K_{2(20)}$; Kaytwo. $C_{31}H_{40}O_2$; mol wt 444.65. Yellow crystals from alcohol, mp 35°. uv max: 248 nm ($E_{1cm}^{1\%}$ 439).

Menaquinone 6. [84-81-1] *(all-E)*-2-(3,7,11,15,19,23-Hexamethyl-2,6,10,14,18,22-tetracosahexaenyl)-3-methyl-1,4-naphthalenedione; 2-difarnesyl-3-methyl-1,4-naphthoquinone; farnoquinone; MK 6; Vitamin $K_{2(30)}$. $C_{41}H_{56}O_2$; mol wt 580.88. Yellow crystals from acetone + alcohol or petr ether, mp 50°. uv max (petr ether): 243, 248, 261, 270, 325-328 nm ($E_{1cm}^{1\%}$ 304, 320, 290, 292, 53).

Menaquinone 7. [2124-57-4] *(all-E)*-2-(3,7,11,15,19,23,27-Heptamethyl-2,6,10,14,18,22,26-octacosaheptaenyl)-3-methyl-1,4-naphthalenedione; Vitamin $K_{2(35)}$. $C_{46}H_{64}O_2$; mol wt 649.00. Light yellow microcrystalline plates from petr ether, mp 54°. bp$_{0.0002}$ 200° (some dec). uv max (petr ether): 243, 248, 261, 270, 325-328 nm ($E_{1cm}^{1\%}$ 278, 195, 266, 267, 48). Slightly less sol than vitamin K_1 in the same organic solvents.

THERAP CAT: Vitamin (prothrombogenic).

5834. Menbutone. [3562-99-0] 4-Methoxy-γ-oxo-1-naphthalenebutanoic acid; 3-(4-methoxy-1-naphthoyl)propionic acid; β-(1-methoxy-4-naphthoyl)propionic acid; γ-oxo-4-methoxy-1-naphthalenebutyric acid; Ictéryl. $C_{15}H_{14}O_4$; mol wt 258.27. C 69.76%, H 5.46%, O 24.78%. Prepn: Ruzicka, Waldman, *Helv. Chim. Acta* **15**, 907 (1932); Fieser, Hershberg, *J. Am. Chem. Soc.* **58**, 2314 (1936); Burtner, **US 2623065** (1952 to Searle).

Crystals, mp 172-173°.

Magnesium salt. [16643-66-6] Hepalande. $C_{30}H_{26}MgO_8$; mol wt 538.83.

THERAP CAT: Choleretic.

5835. Mendelevium. [7440-11-1] Md; formerly Mv; at. no. 101; valence 3, 2. Man-made radioactive element. No stable nuclides; known isotopes (mass numbers): 247-252, 254-259. Longest-lived known isotope 258 ($T_{1/2}$ 55 days, α-emitter, rel. at. mass 258.0984). Prepn of isotope [256]Md ($T_{1/2}$ 1.27 hrs, rel. at. mass 256.0941; decays by electron capture to [256]Fm) by bombarding [253]Es with helium ions: A. Ghiorso *et al.*, *Phys. Rev.* **98**, 1518 (1955). Prepn of isotope [258]Md by bombardment of [255]Es with [4]He ions: Fields *et al.*, *Nucl. Phys. A* **154**, 407 (1970). *Reviews:* C. Keller, *The Chemistry of the Transuranium Elements* (Verlag Chemie, Weinheim, English Ed., 1971) pp 595-600; Silva, "Trans-Curium Elements" in *MTP Int. Rev. Sci.: Inorg. Chem., Ser. One* vol. 8, A. G. Maddock, Ed. (University Park Press, Baltimore, 1972) pp 71-105; *Comprehensive Inorganic Chemistry* vol. 5, J. C. Bailar, Jr. *et al.*, Eds. (Pergamon Press, Oxford, 1973) *passim; Handb. Exp. Pharmakol.* **36**, 689-738 (1973); R. J. Silva in *The Chemistry of the Actinide Elements* vol. 2, J. J. Katz *et al.*, Eds. (Chapman and Hall, New York, 1986) pp 1092-1095; *The Elements Beyond Uranium*, G. T. Seaborg, W. D. Loveland, Eds. (John Wiley & Sons, Inc., New York, 1990) p 38-46.

Caution: Radiation hazard; handling requires special equipment and shielding facilities (Katz *et al.*, *loc. cit.* vol. 2, p. 1128).

5836. Menhaden Oil. Pogy oil; mossbunker oil. Obtained along the East Coast of North America from the menhaden fish, *Brevoortia tyrannis*, somewhat larger than a herring. The oil contains (in the form of glycerides) about 6% myristic acid, 16% palmitic acid, 30% linoleic acid, 19% C_{20}- and 11% C_{22}-acids (highly unsaturated).

Reddish oil. Characteristic, distasteful fishy odor and taste. d 0.925-0.933. mp 38.5-47.2°. n_D^{20} 1.480. Sapon no. 191-200. Iodine no. 139-180. Acid no. 3.0-11.6. Sol in ether, benzene, petr ether, naphtha, kerosene, CS_2.

USE: Substitute for linseed oil. In leather dressing formulations. Hydrogenated menhaden oil can be used as a substitute for tallow in soap-making.

5837. Menthol. [89-78-1] (1α,2β,5α)-5-Methyl-2-(1-methylethyl)cyclohexanol; 3-*p*-menthanol; *l*-menthol; hexahydrothymol; peppermint camphor. $C_{10}H_{20}O$; mol wt 156.27. C 76.86%, H 12.90%, O 10.24%. Obtained from peppermint oil or other mint oils, or prepd synthetically by hydrogenation of thymol. Chromatographic sepn from mint oils: Chang, **US 2760993** (1956 to Iowa State College). Toxicity data: P. M. Jenner *et al.*, *Food Cosmet. Toxicol.* **2**, 327 (1964).

Crystals or granules; peppermint taste and odor. d 0.890. mp 41-43°. bp 212°. n_D^{25} 1.458. $[\alpha]_D^{18}$ −50° (10% alc soln). Slightly sol in water; very sol in alcohol, chloroform, ether, petr ether; freely sol in glacial acetic acid, liq petrolatum. LD_{50} orally in rats: 3180 mg/kg (Jenner). *Incompat:* Butylchloral hydrate, camphor, phenol, chloral hydrate, Exalgine, betanaphthol, resorcinol or thymol in triturations; potassium permanganate, chromium trioxide, pyrogallol.

USE: In liqueurs, confectionery, perfumery, cigarettes, cough drops, and nasal inhalers.

THERAP CAT: Antipruritic (topical).

THERAP CAT (VET): Has been used as a mild local anesthetic, antiseptic; internally as a carminative and gastric sedative.

5838. *l*-Menthone. [14073-97-3] (2S-*trans*)-5-Methyl-2-(1-methylethyl)cyclohexanone; (1R,4S)-(−)-*p*-menthan-3-one; 1-methyl-4-isopropylcyclohexan-3-one. $C_{10}H_{18}O$; mol wt 154.25. C 77.87%, H 11.76%, O 10.37%. Of the four optically active isomers of methone, the one occurring most frequently in nature. Found in various volatile oils, such as pennyroyal, peppermint, geranium: Simonsen, *The Terpenes* **vol. I** (University Press, Cambridge, 2nd ed., 1947) pp 314-327. Prepd by chromic acid oxidation of *l*-menthol: Hussey, Baker, *J. Org. Chem.* **25**, 1434 (1960); Brown, Garg, *J. Am. Chem. Soc.* **83**, 2952 (1961).

Bitter liq; slight peppermint odor. bp 207°. bp_{41} 116-119°. mp −6°. d_4^{20} 0.895. n_D^{20} 1.4505; n_D^{23} 1.4490. $[\alpha]_D^{20}$ −24.8°; $[\alpha]_D^{27}$ −28.9°. Slightly sol in water; sol in organic solvents.

Apinol. Obtained by dry distln of wood of *Pinus palustris* Mill. (*P. australis* Michx.), *Pinaceae* is chiefly *l*-menthone: *J. Pharm. Chim.* **18**, 139, 177, 208 (1918), *C.A.* **13**, 56⁹ (1919). Amber-colored oil, bp ∼182.2°, d 0.946.

USE: In perfume and flavor compositions.

5839. Menthyl Acetate. [89-48-5] 5-Methyl-2-(1-methylethyl)cyclohexanol acetate. $C_{12}H_{22}O_2$; mol wt 198.30. C 72.68%, H 11.18%, O 16.14%. $CH_3COOC_{10}H_{19}$. Present in peppermint oil.

Colorless liquid, characteristic odor. d_4^{20} 0.919. bp 227°. n_D^{20} 1.4468. $[\alpha]_D^{20}$ −79.42°. Slightly sol in water; miscible with alcohol, ether.

USE: In perfumery; emphasizes floral notes, especially that of rose, used in toilet waters having a lavender odor. Has been suggested for flavoring extracts having caraway or mint flavors.

5840. Menthyl Anthranilate. [134-09-8] 5-Methyl-2-(1-methylethyl)cyclohexanol 2-aminobenzoate; anthranilic acid *p*-menth-3-yl ester; menthyl *o*-aminobenzoate; meradimate; Neo Heliopan MA. $C_{17}H_{25}NO_2$; mol wt 275.39. C 74.14%, H 9.15%, N 5.09%, O 11.62%. UV-A absorber in cosmetics and sunscreens. Prepn: H. G. Rule, W. E. MacGillivray, *J. Chem. Soc.* **1929**, 401; M. S. Carpenter, US 2170185 (1939 to Givaudan-Delawanna). Photophysical properties and use as sunscreen: A. Beeby, A. E. Jones, *Photochem. Photobiol.* **72**, 10 (2000). Photostability study: O. Ozer *et al., Cosmet. Toiletries* **116**, 67 (2001). Review of sunscreen formulations: K. Klein, H. A. Finkelmeier, *ibid.* **105**, 75-77 (1990).

Colorless or pale yellow oil with distinct bluish fluorescence, bp_3 177-179° (Carpenter). Also reported as mp 62.5-63.5°; $bp_{0.33}$ 156° (Rule, MacGillivray). d^{35} 1.037. Sol in oil. Dissolves readily in alcohol, dilute aq acids. uv max (ethanol): 220, 249, 340 nm. Fluorescence emission max (ethanol): 405 nm.

THERAP CAT: Ultraviolet screen.

5841. Menthyl Valerate. [89-47-4] (1α,2β,5α)-3-Methylbutanoic acid 5-methyl-2-(1-methylethyl)cyclohexyl ester; isovaleric acid *p*-menth-3-yl ester; Validol. $C_{15}H_{28}O_2$; mol wt 240.38. C 74.95%, H 11.74%, O 13.31%. Contains about 30% free menthol.

Liquid; menthol and valerian odor; cooling, faintly bitter taste. d 0.906-0.908. Insol in water. Freely sol in alcohol, chloroform, ether, oils; dec by alkalies.

THERAP CAT: Sedative.

5842. Menyanthes. Buck bean; bog bean; marsh trefoil; water shamrock. Dried leaves or roots of *Menyanthes trifoliata* L., *Gentianaceae*. Habit. Europe, Asia, N. America. *Constit.* Menyanthin.

5843. Meobentine. [46464-11-3] N-[(4-Methoxyphenyl)-methyl]-N′,N″-dimethylguanidine; 1-(*p*-methoxybenzyl)-2,3-dimethylguanidine. $C_{11}H_{17}N_3O$; mol wt 207.27. C 63.74%, H 8.27%, N 20.27%, O 7.72%. Antidysrhythmic, antifibrillatory deriv of guanidine, *q.v.* Prepn of the sulfate: R. A. Maxwell, E. Walton, DE 2030693 corresp to US 3949089 (1971, 1976 both to Burroughs Wellcome). Antidysrhythmic effects and tissue concentration: K. B. Touw *et al., Pharmacologist* **19**, 268 (1977); K. B. Touw, *Diss. Abstr. B* **39**, 5340 (1979). Pharmacokinetics by radioimmunoassay: J. W. A. Findlay *et al., Pharmacologist* **21**, 337 (1979). Pharmacological study: W. B. Wastila *et al., J. Pharm. Pharmacol.* **33**, 594 (1981).

Sulfate. [58503-79-0] Rythmatine. $(C_{11}H_{17}N_3O)_2 \cdot H_2SO_4$; mol wt 512.62. Cryst, mp 273-274°.

THERAP CAT: Antiarrhythmic (class III).

5844. Mepact. [83461-56-7] N-(N-Acetylmuramoyl)-L-alanyl-N-[(7R)-4-hydroxy-4-oxido-10-oxo-7-[(1-oxohexadecyl)oxy]-3,5,9-trioxa-4-phosphapentacos-1-yl]-L-alaninamide; N-acetylmuramyl-L-alanyl-D-isoglutaminyl-L-alanine-2-(1′,2′-dipalmitoyl-*sn*-glycero-3′-hydroxyphosphoryloxy)ethylamide; muramyl tripeptide phosphatidylethanolamine; MTP-cephalin; MTP-PE; CGP-19835. $C_{59}H_{109}N_6O_{19}P$; mol wt 1237.50. C 57.26%, H 8.88%, N 6.79%, O 24.56%, P 2.50%. Synthetic, lipophilic analog of muramyl dipeptide, *q.v.* Immunostimulant promoting cancer cell destruction by *in vivo* macrophage activation. Prepn: L. Tarcsay *et al.*, EP 25495; *eidem*, US 4406890 (1981, 1983 both to Ciba-Geigy). Synthesis of labeled form: D. E. Brundish, R. Wade, *J. Labelled Compd. Radiopharm.* **22**, 29 (1985). Liposomal encapsulation: R. Natar *et al., Methods Enzymol.* **132**, 594 (1986). Activation of tumoricidal properties in monocytes: E. S. Kleinerman *et al., Cancer Res.* **43**, 2010 (1983). Potentiation of antitumor immunity: I. J. Fidler *et al., J. Immunol.* **138**, 4509 (1987). Immunoassay in plasma: B. Gay *et al., J. Biolumin. Chemilumin.* **6**, 73 (1991). Comparative pharmacokinetics of free and liposomal forms: B. Gay *et al., J. Pharm. Sci.* **82**, 997 (1993). Mechanism of action study: T. Asano *et al., J. Pharmacol. Exp. Ther.* **268**, 1032 (1994). Clinical study as chemotherapy adjuvant: P. A. Meyers *et al., J. Clin. Oncol.* **23**, 2004 (2005). Review of phamacology and clinical studies as immune adjuvant in osteosarcoma: E. S. Kleinerman, *Hematol. Oncol. Clinics North Am.* **9**, 927-938 (1995); A. Nardin *et al., Curr. Cancer Drug Targets* **6** 123-133 (2006).

Sodium salt. [90825-43-7] CGP-19835A; Junovan. $C_{59}H_{108}N_6NaO_{19}P$; mol wt 1259.48.

THERAP CAT: Antineoplastic (immunomodulator).

5845. Mepanipyrim. [110235-47-7] 4-Methyl-N-phenyl-6-(1-propynyl)-2-pyrimidinamine; 2-anilino-4-methyl-6-(1-propynyl)pyrimidine; N-(4-methyl-6-prop-1-ynylpyrimidin-2-yl)aniline; KIF-3535; KUF-6201; Frupica. $C_{14}H_{13}N_3$; mol wt 223.27. C 75.31%, H 5.87%, N 18.82%. Antifungal for use in food crops; inhibits secretion of host-cell wall degrading enzymes. Prepn: S. Ito *et al., EP 224339; eidem,* **US 4814338** (1987, 1989 both to Kumiai; Ihara); and biological activity: S. Hayashi *et al., J. Pestic. Sci.* **22,** 165 (1997). Fungicidal activity and field trials: S. Maeno *et al., Brighton Crop Prot. Conf. - Pests Dis.* **1990,** 415. Mode of action study: I. Miura *et al., Pestic. Biochem. Physiol.* **48,** 222 (1994). GC-MS determn in grapes, must and wine: P. Cabras *et al., J. AOAC Int.* **81,** 1185 (1998). Metabolism in tomato seedlings: M. Ikeda *et al., J. Pestic. Sci.* **23,** 9 (1998).

White solid with two crystalline modifications. mp 125-126° (Maeno); also reported as 132.8° (Hayashi). Specific gravity 1.2025. Soly in water at 20°: 5.58 mg/l. Sol in most organic solvents. Vapor pressure at 20°: 1.03×10^{-5} torr. Log P (octanol/water): 3.42. LD_{50} in mice, rats, bobwhite, mallard (mg/kg): >5000, >5000, >2250, >2250 orally; in rats (mg/kg): >2000 dermally. LC_{50} in bluegill, rainbow trout (mg/l): 3.8, 3.1 (Maeno).

USE: Agricultural fungicide.

5846. Meparfynol. [77-75-8] 3-Methyl-1-pentyn-3-ol; ethyl ethynyl methyl carbinol; 2-ethynyl-2-butanol; methylparafynol; methylpentynol; Allotropal; Anti-Stress; Apridol; Atemorin; Atempol; Dalgol; Dorison; Dormalest; Dormidin; Dormigen; Dormiphen; Dormison; Dormosan; Formison; Hesofen; Hexofen; Imnudorm; Oblivon; Pentadorm; Perlopal; Seral; Somnesin. $C_6H_{10}O$; mol wt 98.14. C 73.43%, H 10.27%, O 16.30%. Prepd from methyl ethyl ketone and sodium acetylide in liquid ammonia or by a Grignard reaction: **DE 285770** (1913 to Bayer); also **DE 289800** and **DE 291185** *see Frdl.* **12,** 55, 56, 57; Sung Wouseng, *Ann. Chim.* [10] **1,** 343 (1924); Rupe, Vonaesch, *Ann.* **442,** 80 (1925); Carothers, Coffman, *J. Am. Chem. Soc.* **54,** 4071 (1932); Campbell *et al., ibid.* **60,** 2882 (1938); Campbell, Campbell, *Proc. Indiana Acad. Sci.* **50,** 123-127 (1940), *C.A.* **35,** 5471; Smith, **US 2385547** (1945 to Commercial Solvents); A. W. Johnson, *The Chemistry of the Acetylenic Compounds* vol. I (Edward Arnold & Co., London, 1946) p 278; Hurd, McPhee, *J. Am. Chem. Soc.* **69,** 239 (1947); P. Piganiol, *Acetylene Homologs and Derivatives* (Brooklyn, 1950); Papa *et al., Arch. Biochem. Biophys.* **33,** 482 (1951); Thiele, Martinez, *Ciencia (Mexico City)* **15,** 70 (1955). An optically active form has been described by Hickmann, Kenyon, *J. Chem. Soc.* **1955,** 2051. Toxicity data: Margolin *et al., Science* **114,** 384 (1951).

Mobile liquid. Acrid odor, burning taste. d_4^{20} 0.8688. d_{20}^{20} 0.8721; 7.28 lbs/U.S. gal. bp_{760} 121-122°; bp_{37} 50°; $bp_{6.5}$ 20°. mp −30.6°. n_D^{20} 1.4318. Flash pt 101.3°F. Surface tension at 25°: 23.8 dynes/cm; 5% aq soln: 34.1 dynes/cm. Soly in water at 25°: 12.8 g/100 ml. Sol in ether. Miscible with acetone, benzene, carbon tetrachloride, Cellosolve, cyclohexanone, diethylene glycol, ethyl acetate, kerosene, methyl ethyl ketone, mineral spirits, ethanolamine, neatsfoot oil, petr ether, soybean oil, Stoddard solvent. LD_{50} orally in mice, rats, guinea pigs: 600-900 mg/kg (Margolin).

Carbamate. [302-66-9] N-Oblivon; Oblivon C; Trusono. $C_7H_{11}NO_2$; mol wt 141.17. Prepn: McLamore *et al., J. Org. Chem.* **20,** 1379 (1955); from 3-methyl-1-pentyn-3-ol, trichloroacetic acid, KOCN: McCrea *et al., GB 761817* (1956 to British Schering). Acute toxicity: Soehring *et al., Arzneim.-Forsch.* **5,** 161 (1955). Crystals from ether + petr ether. mp 55.8-57° (McLamore); from

cyclohexane, mp 53.5-55° (McCrea). bp_{16} 120-121°; $bp_{0.01}$ 95°. Solubility in water: 1.6 g/100 ml. LD_{50} (4 hr) s.c. in mice: 0.56 g/kg (Soehring).

THERAP CAT: Hypnotic; sedative.

5847. Mepartricin. [11121-32-7] Partricin methyl ester; methylpartricin; SN-654; SPA-S-160; Ipertrofan; Orofungin; Tricandil; Tricangine. Methyl ester of the heptaene macrolide antibiotic complex, partricin, *q.v.* Prepn: T. Bruzzese *et al., Experientia* **28,** 1515 (1972); T. Bruzzese, R. Ferrari, **DE 2154436** (1972 to SPA); *eidem,* **US 3780173** (1973). Alternate prepn: R. C. Pandey, *J. Antibiot.* **30,** 158 (1977); R. C. Tweit *et al., ibid.* **35,** 997 (1982). Structure of mepartricins A and B: J. Golik *et al., ibid.* **33,** 904 (1980). Antimycotic activity: W. Ritzerfield, *Farmaco Ed. Sci.* **27,** 235 (1972); activity vs *Trichomonas vaginalis:* G. Pucci, S. Ripa, *Farmaco Ed. Prat.* **28,** 293 (1973). Hemolytic activity studies: B. Cybulska *et al., Biochem. Pharmacol.* **33,** 41 (1984). Stability data: S. Mizuba, K. Lee, *Dev. Ind. Microbiol.* **16,** 380 (1975). Use of mepartricin and its complexes in treatment of benign prostatic hypertrophy: T. Bruzzese, L. Ferrari, **US 4237117** (1980 to SPA). Clinical studies: M. De Bernardi *et al., Curr. Ther. Res.* **43,** 1159 (1988); T. Lotti *et al., ibid.* **44,** 402 (1988).

Mepartricin A R' = CH_3
Mepartricin B R' = H

Deep yellow crystalline material. uv max (ethanol): 401, 378, 359, 340 nm. Slightly sol in water, aq alkali, ether, petr ether, benzene. Sol in acetone, alcohols, pyridine, DMF, DMSO. LD_{50} in mice: >2 g/kg orally; 200 mg/kg i.p. (Bruzzese, 1972).

Mepartricin A. [62534-68-3] 40-Demethyl-3,7-dideoxo-3,7-dihydroxy-N^{47}-methyl-5-oxocandicidin D methyl ester cyclic 15,19-hemiacetal; gedamycin methyl ester. $C_{60}H_{88}N_2O_{19}$; mol wt 1141.34. Lemon yellow powder from ether, mp 145-149° (dec). uv max (methanol): 400, 377, 357, 339, 287, 240, 234, 204 nm (ε 79326, 92454, 68094, 51685, 14199, 24612, 26505, 16092).

Mepartricin B. [62534-69-4] $C_{59}H_{86}N_2O_{19}$; mol wt 1127.32. Lemon yellow powder from ether, mp 154-158° (dec). uv max (methanol): 402, 379, 359, 340, 285, 233, 204 nm (ε 81101, 94729, 64171, 41558, 16196, 23835, 21696).

Complex with sodium lauryl sulfate. SPA-S-222; Montricin.

THERAP CAT: Antifungal; antiprotozoal (Trichomonas). In treatment of benign prostatic hypertrophy.

5848. Mepenzolate Bromide. [76-90-4] 3-[(Hydroxydiphenylacetyl)oxy]-1,1-dimethylpiperidinium bromide; N-methyl-3-piperidyl benzilate methyl bromide; N-methyl-3-piperidyl diphenylglycolate methobromide; Cantil; Trancolon. $C_{21}H_{26}BrNO_3$; mol wt 420.34. C 60.00%, H 6.23%, Br 19.01%, N 3.33%, O 11.42%. Anticholinergic. Prepn: Biel, **US 2918408** (1959 to Lakeside Labs.). Prepn of base: Biel *et al., J. Am. Chem. Soc.* **77,** 2250 (1955). Crystal structure: J. M. Leger *et al., Acta Crystallogr.* **B35,** 886 (1979). Toxicity data: E. I. Goldenthal, *Toxicol. Appl. Pharmacol.* **18,** 185 (1971).

Consult the Name Index before using this section.

Crystals, mp 228-229° (dec). LD_{50} orally in rats: 742±47 mg/kg (Goldenthal).

Free base. [25990-43-6] $bp_{0.03}$ 175-176°.

Note: N-Methyl-3-piperidyl benzilate is a controlled substance (hallucinogen): **21 CFR,** 1308.11.

THERAP CAT: Antispasmodic.

5849. Meperidine. [57-42-1] 1-Methyl-4-phenyl-4-piperidinecarboxylic acid ethyl ester; 1-methyl-4-phenylisonipecotic acid ethyl ester; N-methyl-4-phenyl-4-carbethoxypiperidine; ethyl 1-methyl-4-phenylpiperidine-4-carboxylate; isonipecaine; pethidine. $C_{15}H_{21}NO_2$; mol wt 247.33. C 72.84%, H 8.56%, N 5.66%, O 12.94%. Prepn: Eisleb, **US 2167351** (1939 to Winthrop); Smissman, Hite, *J. Am. Chem. Soc.* **81,** 1201 (1959). Pharmacokinetics: L. E. Mather, P. J. Meffin, *Clin. Pharmacokinet.* **3,** 352 (1978). Metabolism: S. Y. Yeh *et al., J. Pharm. Sci.* **70,** 867 (1981). GC-MS/MS determn in biological fluids: A. Ishii *et al., J. Chromatogr. B* **792,** 117 (2003). Toxicity data: O. W. Barlow, J. R. Lewis, *J. Pharmacol. Exp. Ther.* **103,** 147 (1951). Comprehensive description: N. P. Fish, N. J. DeAngelis in *Anal. Profiles Drug Subs.* **1,** 175-205 (1972).

Hydrochloride. [50-13-5] Algil; Alodan; Centralgin; Demerol hydrochloride; Dispadol; Dolantin; Dolestine; Dolosal; Mefedina. $C_{15}H_{21}NO_2.HCl$; mol wt 283.79. Minute crystals, mp 186-189°. Slightly bitter taste. Stable to air. Just acid to litmus (1:10 soln). Sol in water, acetone, ethyl acetate; slightly sol in alcohol, isopropanol. Insol in benzene, ether. Aq solns may be sterilized by boiling for short periods without dec. LD_{50} orally in rats: 170 mg/kg (Barlow, Lewis).

Note: This is a controlled substance (opiate): **21 CFR,** 1308.12.

THERAP CAT: Analgesic (narcotic).

THERAP CAT (VET): Analgesic (narcotic); sedative; anesthetic.

5850. Mephenesin. [59-47-2] 3-(2-Methylphenoxy)-1,2-propanediol; 3-(o-tolyloxy)-1,2-propanediol; 1,2-dihydroxy-3-(2-methylphenoxy)propane; α-(o-tolyl)glyceryl ether; glyceryl o-tolyl ether; o-cresyl glycerol ether; cresoxypropanediol; cresoxydiol; α:β-dihydroxy-γ-(2-methylphenoxy)propane; BDH-312; Atensin; Avosyl; Avoxyl; Curythan; Daserol; Decontractyl; Dioloxol; Glyotol; Glykresin; Lissephen; Memphenesin; Mepherol; Mephesin; Mephson; Mervaldin; Myanesin; Myanol; Myodetensine; Myolysin; Myopan; Myoserol; Myoten; Oranixon; Prolax; Relaxar; Relaxil; Renarcol; Rhex; Sansdolor; Sinan; Spasmolyn; Stilalgin; Thoxidil; Tolansin; Tolcil; Tolhart; Tolosate; Toloxyn; Tolserol; Tolulexin; Tolulox; Tolyspaz; Walconesin. $C_{10}H_{14}O_3$; mol wt 182.22. C 65.91%, H 7.74%, O 26.34%. Prepn: P. Morch, *Arch. Pharm. Chemi* **54,** 327 (1947), *C.A.* **42,** 2058 (1948); **GB 589821** (1947 to Carroll and Boake Roberts); of the carbamate: W. A. Lott, E. Pribyl, **US 2609386** (1952 to Squibb). Pharmacology: F. M. Berger, W. Bradley, *Br. J. Pharmacol.* **1,** 265 (1946); and toxicity data: P. E. Dresel, I. H. Slater, *Proc. Soc. Exp. Biol. Med.* **79,** 286 (1952); A. P. Roszkowski, *J. Pharmacol. Exp. Ther.* **129,** 75 (1960).

Crystals. Bitter taste. Produces numbness of the tongue. mp 70-71°. uv max (0.005% aq soln): 270 nm (E 0.395). Freely sol in alcohol, propylene glycol, chloroform. At 20° one part dissolves in 85 parts water, in 11 parts ether. Urea and its derivatives, particularly urethan, increase the water soly. One part dissolves in 60 parts of 5% urethan soln, in 40 parts of 10%, in 4.5 parts of 25%. Aq solns are stable, can be sterilized by heating, and are compatible and freely miscible with solns of sodium chloride, glucose, and derivatives of barbituric and thiobarbituric acids. pH of satd aq soln ~6. LD_{50} in mice, rats, hamsters (mg/kg): 471, 283, 322 i.p.; 990, 945, 821 orally (Roszkowski). LD_{50} in mice (mM/kg): 2.83 i.p.; 10.53 orally (Dresel, Slater).

Carbamate. [533-06-2] Tolseram. $C_{11}H_{15}NO_4$; mol wt 225.24. Crystals from water, mp about 93°. (Also a hemihydrate, mp 80-84°.) uv max (ethanol): 271, 277 nm ($A_{1cm}^{1\%}$ 72.7, 64.1). Has a lower water-solubility and a higher oil-solubility than mephenesin. Soly in water about 0.3%, in chloroform about 2.0%. Freely sol in alcohol. LD_{50} in mice (mM/kg): 2.77 i.p.; 7.67 orally (Dresel, Slater).

THERAP CAT: Muscle relaxant (skeletal).

THERAP CAT (VET): Muscle relaxant.

5851. Mephenoxalone. [70-07-5] 5-[(2-Methoxyphenoxy)-methyl]-2-oxazolidinone; 5-(o-methoxyphenoxymethyl)-2-oxazolidinone; metoxadone; methoxydon(e); methoxadone; AHR-233; OM-518; Dorsiflex; Control-Om; Xerene. $C_{11}H_{13}NO_4$; mol wt 223.23. C 59.18%, H 5.87%, N 6.27%, O 28.67%. Prepn: Lunsford *et al., J. Am. Chem. Soc.* **82,** 1166 (1960); Lunsford, **US 2895960** (1959 to A. H. Robins). Toxicity data: E. I. Goldenthal, *Toxicol. Appl. Pharmacol.* **18,** 185 (1971). Determn in pharmaceutical formulations: N. Erk, *J. Pharm. Biomed. Anal.* **21,** 429 (1999).

Crystals from 95% ethanol, mp 143-145°. Water insol. LD_{50} orally in rats: 3820 ±17 mg/kg (Goldenthal).

THERAP CAT: Muscle relaxant (skeletal).

5852. Mephentermine. [100-92-5] N,α,α-Trimethylbenzeneethanamine; 2-methylamino-2-methyl-1-phenylpropane; N-methyl-ω-phenyl-*tert*-butylamine; N,α,α-trimethylphenethylamine. $C_{11}H_{17}N$; mol wt 163.26. C 80.92%, H 10.50%, N 8.58%. α-Adrenergic agonist. Prepd by hydrogenating 1-chloro-2-methyl-amino-2-methyl-1-phenylpropane hydrochloride in methanol in the presence of palladium barium carbonate: Bruce, Szabo, **US 2597445** (1952 to Wyeth). Alternate process: Abel *et al.,* **US 2590079** (1952 to Wyeth). Pharmacology: D. K. Eckfeld *et al., J. Am. Pharm. Assoc.* **43,** 705 (1954).

Liquid. Fishy amine odor. bp_{7mm} 82-83°. n_D^{20} 1.5110. d_{20}^{20} 0.9231. pKa (30°) 10.35. Alkaline reaction. Freely sol in alc. Sol in ether. Practically insol in water.

Sulfate dihydrate. [6190-60-9] Wyamine; Mephine. ($C_{11}H_{17}$-$N)_2.H_2SO_4.2H_2O$; mol wt 460.63. Crystals, mp 215-217° (dec). One gram dissolves in 20 ml water, about 150 ml ethanol (95%). Practically insol in chloroform. pH of aq soln about 6. LD_{50} (calc as base) intra-abdominally in mice: 89.4 mg/kg (Eckfeld).

THERAP CAT: Antihypotensive.

5853. Mephenytoin. [50-12-4] 5-Ethyl-3-methyl-5-phenyl-2,4-imidazolidinedione; 5-ethyl-3-methyl-5-phenylhydantoin; 3-methyl-5,5-phenylethylhydantoin; "methyl hydantoin"; phenylethylmethylhydantoin; 3-ethylnirvanol; methoin; Insulton; Mesontoin; Mesantoin; Phenantoin; Sedantoinal; Gerot-Epilan; Sacerno. C_{12}-$H_{14}N_2O_2$; mol wt 218.25. C 66.04%, H 6.47%, N 12.84%, O 14.66%. Prepn: **FR 769667; CH 166004** (both 1934 to Sandoz); **CH 179692** (1935 to Sandoz). Pharmacology: I. A. Dzhagatspanyan *et al., Pharm. Chem. J.* **25,** 181 (1991).

Crystals, mp 136-137°. Insol in water. Forms a water-soluble sodium salt which has an alkaline reaction. LD$_{50}$ i.p. in mice: 300 mg/kg (Dzhagatspanyan).

THERAP CAT: Anticonvulsant.

5854. Mephobarbital. [115-38-8] 5-Ethyl-1-methyl-5-phenyl-2,4,6(1H,3H,5H)-pyrimidinetrione; 5-ethyl-1-methyl-5-phenylbarbituric acid; 5-phenyl-5-ethyl-3-methylbarbituric acid; N-methylethylphenylbarbituric acid; methylphenobarbital; Phemiton; Prominal; Mebaral. C$_{13}$H$_{14}$N$_2$O$_3$; mol wt 246.26. C 63.40%, H 5.73%, N 11.38%, O 19.49%. Prepn: Taub, Kropp, **DE 537366** (1929 to I. G. Farben.).

White, tasteless crystals. mp 176°. Slightly sol in cold, freely in hot water or in alcohol.

Note: This is a controlled substance (depressant): **21 CFR, 1308.14.**

THERAP CAT: Anticonvulsant; sedative; hypnotic.

THERAP CAT (VET): Anticonvulsant; sedative; hypnotic.

5855. Mephosfolan. [950-10-7] (4-Methyl-1,3-dithiolan-2-ylidene)phosphoramidic acid diethyl ester; phosphonodithioimidocarbonic acid cyclic propylene P,P-diethyl ester; 2-diethoxyphosphinylimino-4-methyl-1,3-dithiolane; cyclic propylene (diethoxyphosphinyl)dithioimidocarbonate; EI-47470; ENT-25991; Cytrolane. C$_8$H$_{16}$NO$_3$PS$_2$; mol wt 269.32. C 35.68%, H 5.99%, N 5.20%, O 17.82%, P 11.50%, S 23.81%. Insecticidal contact and stomach poison with systemic activity: D. L. Bull *et al., J. Econ. Entomol.* **57**, 112 (1964). Prepn: J. B. Lovell, **US 3197365** (1965 to Am. Cyanamid). Metabolism: J. Zulalian, R. C. Blinn, *J. Agric. Food Chem.* **25**, 1033 (1977). Photodegradation: C. C. Ku *et al., ibid.* **27**, 1046 (1979).

Yellow to amber liquid, bp$_{0.001}$ 120°. n_D^{26} 1.5354. Soly in water at 25°: 57 g/kg. Sol in acetone, ethanol, benzene, 1,2-dichloroethane. Stable at neutral pH; hydrolyzed by acid or alkali.

USE: Insecticide, acaricide.

5856. Mepindolol. [23694-81-7] 1-[(1-Methylethyl)amino]-3-[(2-methyl-1H-indol-4-yl)oxy]-2-propanol; 1-(isopropylamino)-3-[(2-methylindol-4-yl)oxy]-2-propanol. C$_{15}$H$_{22}$N$_2$O$_2$; mol wt 262.35. C 68.67%, H 8.45%, N 10.68%, O 12.20%. β-Adrenergic blocker; the 2-methyl analog of pindolol, *q.v.* Prepn: F. Troxler, **CH 469002** and **CH 472404** (both 1969 to Sandoz); F. Seeman *et al., Helv. Chim. Acta* **54**, 2411 (1971). Pharmacokinetics: R. Gugler *et al., Arzneim.-Forsch.* **25**, 1067 (1975). Pharmacodynamics: J. Bonelli *et al., Eur. J. Clin. Pharmacol.* **15**, 1 (1979). Clinical studies: H. M. Beumer *et al., Int. J. Clin. Pharmacol. Biopharm.* **16**, 249 (1978); M. Sukerman *et al., Curr. Ther. Res.* **25**, 384 (1979).

Crystals from ethyl acetate, mp 100-102° (Seeman). Also reported as 95-97° (Troxler).

Sulfate salt. [56396-94-2] SH-E-222; Betagon; Corindolan; Mepicor. (C$_{15}$H$_{22}$N$_2$O$_2$)$_2$.H$_2$SO$_4$; mol wt 622.77.

THERAP CAT: Antihypertensive; antianginal.

5857. Mepiquat Chloride. [24307-26-4] 1,1-Dimethylpiperidinium chloride; BAS-083; BAS-85559X; Pix. C$_7$H$_{16}$ClN; mol wt 149.66. C 56.18%, H 10.78%, Cl 23.69%, N 9.36%. Prepn: B. Zeeh *et al.,* **DE 2207575**; *eidem,* **US 3905798** (1973, 1975 both to BASF). IC determn: A. Fegert *et al., Fresenius J. Anal. Chem.* **339**, 441 (1991). Toxicity study: BASF Agric. Chem. Div., *J. Pestic. Sci.* **17**, S269 (1992). Field study on cotton: J. S. McConnell *et al., J. Plant Nutr.* **15**, 457 (1992); R. K. Boman, R. L. Westerman, *J. Prod. Agric.* **7**, 70 (1994). Review: P. E. Schott, F. R. Rittig, in *Chemical Manipulation of Crop Growth and Development* J. S. McLaren, Ed. (Butterworth Scientific, London, 1982) pp 415-424.

White crystals, mp 285°. Soly at 20° g/100g: water >50; methyl alcohol 25.0; ethyl alcohol 16.2; chloroform 1.1; acetone <0.1; benzene <0.1; cyclohexane <0.1; diethyl ether <0.1; olive oil <0.1. Log P (n-octanol:water): −2.83. LD$_{50}$ in mice, rats (mg/kg): 780, 464 orally; in rats (mg/kg): >2000 dermally (BASF Agric. Chem. Div.).

USE: Plant growth regulator.

5858. Mepitiostane. [21362-69-6] (2α,3α,5α,17β)-2,3-Epithio-17-[(1-methoxycyclopentyl)oxy]androstane; cyclopentanone 2α,3α-epithio-5α-androstan-17β-yl methyl acetal; 10364-S; Thiodelone; Thioderon. C$_{25}$H$_{40}$O$_2$S; mol wt 404.65. C 74.20%, H 9.96%, O 7.91%, S 7.92%. Orally active deriv of epitiostanol, *q.v.* Prepn: T. Komeno, **ZA 6800565** corresp to **US 3567713** (1968, 1971 both to Shionogi); T. Komeno *et al., Shionogi Kenkyusho Nempo* **19**, 3 (1969), *C.A.* **72**, 28554u (1970). Inhibitory effect on mammary tumors in rats: O. Takatani, S. Kumaoka, *Gann* **68**, 337 (1977), *C.A.* **87**, 112187u (1977). Clinical study in advanced breast cancer: K. Inoue *et al., Cancer Treat. Rep.* **62**, 743 (1978). Toxicity studies: *Oyo Yakuri* **16**, 739-812 (1978), *C.A.* **90**, 146152f, 146153g (1979).

Cryst, mp 98-101°. [α]$_D^{20}$ +22.5 ±0.5° (c = 1 in chloroform).

THERAP CAT: Antineoplastic.

5859. Mepivacaine. [96-88-8] *N*-(2,6-Dimethylphenyl)-1-methyl-2-piperidinecarboxamide; 1-methyl-2′,6′-pipecoloxylidide; *dl-N*-methylpipecolic acid 2,6-dimethylanilide; *dl-N*-methyl-hexahydropicolinic acid 2,6-dimethylanilide. $C_{15}H_{22}N_2O$; mol wt 246.35. C 73.13%, H 9.00%, N 11.37%, O 6.49%. Prepn: Ekenstam *et al., Acta Chem. Scand.* **11**, 1183 (1957); US 2799679 (1957 to A. B. Bofors). Prepn of other salts: Rinderknecht, *Helv. Chim. Acta* **42**, 1324 (1959); GB 826668 (1960 to Crookes Labs.). Resolution of isomers: Tullar, *J. Med. Chem.* **14**, 891 (1971); Friberger, Aberg, *Acta Pharm. Suec.* **8**, 361 (1971). Pharmacology: Helmy *et al., J. Egypt. Med. Assoc.* **50**, 688 (1967). Metabolism: Reynolds, *Br. J. Anaesth.* **43**, 33 (1971). Toxicity data: G. Aberg, *Acta Pharmacol. Toxicol.* **31**, 273 (1972).

Crystals from ether, mp 150-151°.
Hydrochloride. [1722-62-9] Carbocaina; Carbocaine hydrochloride; Chlorocain; Meaverin; Mepicaton; Mepident; Mepivastesin; Optocain; Scandicain. $C_{15}H_{22}N_2O \cdot HCl$; mol wt 282.81. mp 262-264°. Sol in water. LD_{50} in mice, rats (mg/kg): 280, 500 s.c. (Aberg).
(+)-Form. Dexivacaine.
THERAP CAT: Anesthetic (local).
THERAP CAT (VET): Anesthetic (local).

5860. Mepixanox. [17854-59-0] 3-Methoxy-4-(1-piperidinylmethyl)-9*H*-xanthen-9-one; 3-methoxy-4-piperidinylmethyl-9-oxo-10-oxa-9,10-dihydroanthracene; mepixanthone; Pimexone. $C_{20}H_{21}NO_3$; mol wt 323.39. C 74.28%, H 6.55%, N 4.33%, O 14.84%. Prepn: M. Sparaci, ZA 6902150 (1969 to Mondi), *C.A.* **72**, 111,300d (1970). Alternate process: D. Milani, US 3646030 (1972 to Mondi). CNS activity: P. Da Re *et al., J. Med. Chem.* **13**, 527 (1970). Pharmacology: R. Guira *et al., Minerva Pneumolog.* **21**, 317 (1982). Pharmacokinetics in man: G. Grossi *et al., Curr. Ther. Res.* **38**, 141 (1985). HPLC determn in serum: G. Grossi *et al., J. Chromatogr.* **309**, 214 (1984). Clinical comparison with doxapram, *q.v.,* in chronic bronchopulmonary disease: M. Parziale *et al., G. Ital. Mal. Torace* **38**, 323 (1984). Clinical evaluations in chronic obstructive lung disease: D. Olivieri *et al., Arch. Monaldi Tisiol. Mal. Appar. Respir.* **35**, 117 (1980); L. Bertoli *et al., Minerva Pneumolog.* **23**, 323 (1984).

White crystalline powder from ethyl acetate, mp 159-160°. LD_{50} i.p. in mice: 70.73 mg/kg (Sparaci).
Hydrochloride. $C_{20}H_{22}ClNO_3$. White crystalline solid from ethanol, mp >200° (dec).
THERAP CAT: Respiratory stimulant.

5861. Meprednisone. [1247-42-3] (16β)-17,21-Dihydroxy-16-methylpregna-1,4-diene-3,11,20-trione; 16β-methylprednisone; Betapred; Betapar; Betalone; Deltisona B. $C_{22}H_{28}O_5$; mol wt 372.45. C 70.95%, H 7.58%, O 21.48%. Prepn: E. P. Oliveto *et al., J. Am. Chem. Soc.* **80**, 4428 (1958); D. Taub *et al., ibid.* 4435; D. Taub *et al., ibid.* **82**, 4012 (1960); G. G. Nathansohn *et al., Experientia* **17**, 448 (1961); GB 901092 (1962 to Scherico); R. Rausser, E. P. Oliveto, US 3164618 (1965 to Schering).

Crystals, mp 200-205°. $[\alpha]_D$ +200° (dioxane). uv max (methanol): 239 nm ($E_{1cm}^{1\%}$ 416).
21-Acetate. $C_{24}H_{30}O_6$. mp 232-235°. $[\alpha]_D$ +210° (dioxane). uv max (methanol): 238 nm ($E_{1cm}^{1\%}$ 358).
THERAP CAT: Glucocorticoid.

5862. Meprobamate. [57-53-4] 2-Methyl-2-propyl-1,3-propanediol dicarbamate; carbamic acid 2-methyl-2-propyl-trimethylene ester; 2,2-di(carbamoyloxymethyl)pentane; 2-methyl-2-propyltrimethylene carbamate; procalmadiol; procalmidol; Andaxin; Artolon; Atraxin; Cyrpon; Ecuanil; Equanil; Mepavlon; Meprodil; Meprospan; Meprotabs; Miltaun; Miltown; Nervonus; Oasil; Perequil; Pertranquil; Probamyl; Quaname; Quanil; Restenil; Trancot; Tranquilan; Urbilat; Visano. $C_9H_{18}N_2O_4$; mol wt 218.25. C 49.53%, H 8.31%, N 12.84%, O 29.32%. Prepn: Ludwig, Piech, *J. Am. Chem. Soc.* **73**, 5779 (1951); Berger, Ludwig, US 2724720 (1955 to Carter Prod.). Pharmacology: F. M. Berger, *J. Pharmacol. Exp. Ther.* **112**, 413 (1954). Comprehensive description: C. Shearer, P. Rulon, *Anal. Profiles Drug Subs.* **1**, 207-232 (1972); C. Shearer, *ibid.* **11**, 587-591 (1982).

Crystals from hot water, mp 104-106°. Characteristic bitter taste. Soly in water at 20°: 0.34% (w/w), at 37°: 0.79% (w/w). Easily forms supersatd solns with hot water. Freely sol in most organic solvents. Aq solns are neutral. Stable in dilute acid and alkali. LD_{50} i.p. in mice: 800 mg/kg (Berger).
Note: This is a controlled substance (depressant): **21 CFR,** 1308.14.
THERAP CAT: Anxiolytic.

5863. Meptazinol. [54340-58-8] 3-(3-Ethylhexahydro-1-methyl-1*H*-azepin-3-yl)phenol; 1-methyl-3-ethyl-3-(*m*-hydroxy-phenyl)hexahydro-1*H*-azepine. $C_{15}H_{23}NO$; mol wt 233.35. C 77.21%, H 9.93%, N 6.00%, O 6.86%. Mixed opioid agonist-antagonist. Prepn of the hydrobromide: J. F. Cavalla, A. C. White, DE 1941534 corresp to US 3729465 (1970, 1973 both to Wyeth); of the free base: *eidem,* US 4197241 (1980 to Wyeth). Properties: P. G. Goode, A. C. White, *Br. J. Pharmacol.* **43**, 462 (1971). HPLC determn in plasma: T. Frost, *Analyst* **106**, 999 (1981). Pharmacokinetics in man: G. Davies, *Eur. J. Clin. Pharmacol.* **23**, 535 (1982). Human pharmacology and abuse potential: R. E. Johnson, D. R. Jasinski, *Clin. Pharmacol. Ther.* **41**, 426 (1987). Clinical studies: R. K. Price, A. N. Latham, *Curr. Med. Res. Opin.* **8**, 54 (1982); C. E. Parker, A. F. Langrick, *J. Int. Med. Res.* **10**, 408 (1982). Symposium on clinical studies: *Postgrad. Med. J.* **59**, Suppl. 1, 1-94 (1983). Review of pharmacology and clinical efficacy: B. Holmes, A. Ward, *Drugs* **30**, 285-312 (1985).

Cryst from acetonitrile, mp 127.5-133°.

Hydrochloride. [59263-76-2] Wy-22811; Meptid. $C_{15}H_{23}$-NO.HCl; mol wt 269.81.

THERAP CAT: Analgesic (narcotic).

5864. Mequitazine. [29216-28-2] 10-(1-Azabicyclo[2.2.2]-oct-3-ylmethyl)-10H-phenothiazine; 10-(3-quinuclidinylmethyl)-phenothiazine; LM-209; Butix; Metaplexan; Mircol; Primalan; Zesulan. $C_{20}H_{22}N_2S$; mol wt 322.47. C 74.49%, H 6.88%, N 8.69%, S 9.94%. Prepn: G. Gueremy *et al., DE 2009555* corresp to US 3987042 (1970, 1976 to Sogeras). Absorption, distribution, and excretion: A. Uzan *et al., Xenobiotica* **6,** 633 (1976). Biotransformation: *eidem, ibid.* 649. Pharmacologic study: *eidem, J. Pharm. Pharmacol.* **31,** 701 (1979). Clinical studies: J. Blamoutier, *Curr. Med. Res. Opin.* **5,** 366 (1978); P. Laugier, M. Orusco, *ibid.* 371.

Crystals from acetonitrile, mp 130-131°.

THERAP CAT: Antihistaminic.

5865. Meralein Sodium. [4386-35-0] (3',6'-Dihydroxy-2',7'-diiodospiro[3H-2,1-benzoxanthiole-3,9'-[9H]xanthen]-4'-yl)-hydroxymercury S,S-dioxide monosodium salt; o-[6-hydroxy-5-(hy-droxymercuri)-2,7-diiodo-3-oxo-3H-xanthen-9-yl]benzenesulfonic acid sodium salt; 2,7-diiodo-4-hydroxymercuriresorcinsulfonphtha-lein monosodium salt; monohydroxymercuridiiodoresorcinsul-fonphthalein sodium salt; sodium meralein; Merodicein. $C_{19}H_9$-HgI_2NaO_7S; mol wt 858.72. C 26.57%, H 1.06%, Hg 23.36%, I 29.56%, Na 2.68%, O 13.04%, S 3.73%. Prepn: Dunning, Farin-holt, *J. Am. Chem. Soc.* **51,** 804 (1929). Pharmacology and tox-icology: Macht, Cook, *J. Pharmacol. Exp. Ther.* **43,** 571 (1931).

Green scales, turn dark red on pulverizing. Sol in water; aq soln slightly fluorescent.

THERAP CAT: Antiseptic, disinfectant.

5866. Meralluride. [8069-64-5] [3-[[[(3-Carboxylato-1-oxopropyl)amino]carbonyl]amino]-2-methoxypropyl]hydroxymer-curate(1−) sodium, mixture with 3,7-dihydro-1,3-dimethyl-1H-pu-rine-2,6-dione; N-[[2-methoxy-3-[(1,2,3,6-tetrahydro-1,3-dimethyl-2,6-dioxopurin-7-yl)mercuri]propyl]carbamoyl]succinamic acid; Mercuhydrin; Mercuretin. $C_{16}H_{23}HgN_6NaO_8$; mol wt 650.97. C 29.52%, H 3.56%, Hg 30.81%, N 12.91%, Na 3.53%, O 19.66%. Structure: Pearson, Sigal, *J. Org. Chem.* **15,** 1055 (1950). Toxicity data: E. I. Goldenthal, *Toxicol. Appl. Pharmacol.* **18,** 185 (1971).

White to slightly yellow powder, slowly dec on exposure to light. Saturated soln is acid to litmus. Slightly sol in water; sol in hot water, glacial acetic acid, and solns of alkali hydroxides. Almost

insol in alc, chloroform, ether. LD_{50} s.c. in rats: 28±7 mg/kg (Goldenthal).

THERAP CAT: Diuretic.

THERAP CAT (VET): Diuretic.

5867. Merbromin. [129-16-8] (2'7'-Dibromo-3',6'-dihydr-oxy-3-oxospiro[isobenzofuran-1(3H),9'-[9H]xanthen]-4'-yl)hydr-oxymercury disodium salt; [2,7-dibromo-9-(o-carboxyphenyl)-6-hydroxy-3-oxo-3H-xanthen-4-yl]hydroxymercury disodium salt; mercurochrome; dibromohydroxymercurifluorescein disodium salt; no. 220 sol; Chromargyre; Planochrome; Flavurol; D.O.M.F.; Mercurophage; Mercurocol; Gallochrome; Gynochrome; Mercu-rome; Asceptichrome; Mercuranine. $C_{20}H_8Br_2HgNa_2O_6$; mol wt 750.65. C 32.00%, H 1.07%, Br 21.29%, Hg 26.72%, Na 6.13%, O 12.79%. Prepd by treating dibromofluorescein with mercuric ace-tate and sodium hydroxide: White, *J. Am. Chem. Soc.* **42,** 2355 (1920); also prepd by the action of mercuric acetate on dibromo-fluorescein sodium: Rymill, Corran, *Q. J. Pharm. Pharmacol.* **7,** 543 (1934), *see also* US 1535003 (1925).

Trihydrate, iridescent green scales or granules. Freely sol in water, giving a carmine-red soln. Very dil solns (1:2000) possess a yellow-green fluorescence. pH of 0.5% soln: 8.8. One gram dissolves in 50 grams of 94% alcohol, in 8.1 grams methanol: Denoel, *J. Pharm. Belg.* **22,** 423 (1940); **23,** 75 (1941). Practically insol in alcohol, acetone, chloroform, ether. *Incompat.* Acids, most alkaloidal salts and most local anesthetics. Colors the skin carmine-red. The stains may be removed by washing first with permanganate soln and then with oxalic acid soln.

THERAP CAT: Antibacterial.

THERAP CAT (VET): Antiseptic.

5868. 2-Mercaptobenzothiazole. [149-30-4] 2(3H)-Benzo-thiazolethione; 2-benzothiazolethiol; MBT; Captax; Dermacid; Mertax; Thiotax. $C_7H_5NS_2$; mol wt 167.25. C 50.27%, H 3.01%, N 8.37%, S 38.34%. Prepd industrially by reacting aniline, carbon disulfide, and sulfur at elevated press. and temps: Kelly, US 1631871. Purification by treatment with a per-acid salt in alkaline medium: Weyker, Ebel, US 2730528 (1956 to Am. Cyanamid). Improved process: Szlatinay, US 3031073 (1962 to Monsanto).

Pale yellow, monoclinic needles or leaflets. Disagreeable odor. d 1.42. mp 180.2-181.7° (the technical product mp 170-175°). Practically insol in water. Soly at 25° (g/100 ml) in alcohol: 2.0; ether 1.0; acetone 10.0; benzene 1.0; carbon tetrachloride <0.2; naphtha <0.5. Moderately sol in glacial acetic acid. Sol in alkalies and alkali carbonate solns.

Zinc salt. Bantex. Light yellow powder, d_4^{25} 1.70.

Sodium salt. Nuodex 84.

USE: Rubber vulcanization accelerator. Salts used as fungicide.

5869. 2-Mercaptoethanol. [60-24-2] β-Mercaptoethanol; 2-hydroxy-1-ethanethiol; 2-hydroxyethyl mercaptan; monothioeth-yleneglycol; thioglycol. C_2H_6OS; mol wt 78.13. C 30.75%, H 7.74%, O 20.48%, S 41.04%. $SHCH_2CH_2OH$. Prepn: Wood-ward, *J. Chem. Soc.* **1948,** 1892; Peppel, Signaigo; Jones, US 2402665; US 3394192 (1946, 1968 both to du Pont). Properties: Bennett, *J. Chem. Soc.* **121,** 2139 (1922). IR: Thompson, *J. Am. Chem. Soc.* **61,** 1398 (1939). Toxicology: K. White *et al., J. Pharm. Sci.* **62,** 237 (1973).

Liquid with very strong, disagreeable odor. bp$_{742}$ 157-158° (dec). d$_4^{20}$ 1.1143. n$_D^{20}$ 1.4996. The pure liquid is miscible with water, alc, ether and benzene. LD$_{50}$ in mice (mg/kg): 322.0 i.p.; 344.8 orally (White).

Caution: Irritating to eyes, nose and skin.

USE: In organic synthesis; as biochemical research tool.

5870. Mercaptomerin Sodium. [21259-76-7] (*T*-4)-[3-[[(3-Carboxylato-2,2,3-trimethylcyclopentyl)carbonyl]amino]-2-methoxypropyl][mercaptoacetato(2−)-*O,S*]mercurate(2−) disodium; *N*-(γ-carboxymethylmercaptomercuri-β-methoxy)propyl-camphoramic acid disodium salt; Diucardyn sodium; Thiomerin sodium. C$_{16}$H$_{25}$HgNNa$_2$O$_6$S; mol wt 606.01. C 31.71%, H 4.16%, Hg 33.10%, N 2.31%, Na 7.59%, O 15.84%, S 5.29%. Prepn: Lehman, **US 2576349** (1951 to Wyeth); Wendt, Bruce, *J. Org. Chem.* **23**, 1448 (1958); Wendt, **US 2834795** (1958 to Am. Home Prod.).

Hygroscopic white powder. Dec 150-155°. Freely soluble in water. Soluble in alcohol. Practically insoluble in ether, benzene, chloroform.

THERAP CAT: Diuretic.

THERAP CAT (VET): Diuretic.

5871. 6-Mercaptopurine. [50-44-2] 1,7-Dihydro-6*H*-purine-6-thione; purine-6-thiol; 6MP; Leukerin; Mercaleukin; Puri-Nethol; Purinethol. C$_5$H$_4$N$_4$S; mol wt 152.18. C 39.46%, H 2.65%, N 36.82%, S 21.07%. Prepd from hypoxanthine and phosphorus pentasulfide: G. B. Elion *et al.*, *J. Am. Chem. Soc.* **74**, 411 (1952); G. H. Hitchings, G. B. Elion, **US 2697709** (1954 to Burroughs Wellcome). Improved procedure: A. G. Beaman, R. K. Robins, *J. Am. Chem. Soc.* **83**, 4042 (1961). Prepn from 7-aminothiazolo[5,4-*d*]pyrimidine: G. H. Hitchings, G. B. Elion, **US 2721866** (1955 to Burroughs Wellcome). Metabolized in the body to 6-thiouric acid (6-mercapto-2,8-purinediol): G. B. Elion *et al.*, *J. Am. Chem. Soc.* **81**, 3042 (1959). Pharmacology: H. Froberg, M. S. Schencking, *Arch. Toxicol.* **32**, 1 (1974). HPLC determn in body fluids: J. L. Rudy *et al.*, *Ann. Clin. Biochem.* **25**, 504 (1988). Clinical trial with methotrexate in acute lymphoblastic leukemia: S. Koizumi *et al.*, *Cancer* **61**, 1292 (1988). Comprehensive description: S. A. Benezra, P. R. B. Foss, *Anal. Profiles Drug Subs.* **7**, 343-357 (1978). Review in treatment of Crohn's disease and ulcerative colitis: D. H. Present, *Gastroenterol. Clin. North Am.* **18**, 57-71 (1989); in treatment of leukemia: B. A. Kamen, *Semin. Hematol.* **28**, 12-14 (1991).

Monohydrate. Yellow prisms from water. Becomes anhydrous at 140°, dec 313-314°. uv max (0.1*N* NaOH): 230, 312 nm (ε 14000, 19600); (0.1*N* HCl): 222, 327 nm (ε 9240, 21300); (methanol): 216, 329 nm (ε 8940, 19300). pKa$_1$ 7.77, pKa$_2$ 11.17. Insol in water, acetone, ether. Sol in hot ethanol, in alkaline solns with slow decompn. LD$_{50}$ in mice, hamsters (mg/kg): 157, 364 i.p. (Froberg, Schencking).

THERAP CAT: Antineoplastic; immunosuppressant.

THERAP CAT (VET): Antineoplastic.

5872. Mercumallylic Acid. [86-36-2] [3-(3-Carboxy-2-oxo-2*H*-1-benzopyran-8-yl)-2-methoxypropyl]hydroxymercurate(1−) hydrogen; [3-[3-(3-hydroxymercuri)-2-methoxypropyl]-salicylidene]malonic acid δ-lactone; 8-[3-(hydroxymercuri)-2-methoxypropyl]-2-oxo-2*H*-1-benzopyran-3-carboxylic acid; 8-(2-methoxy-3-hydroxymercuripropyl)coumarin-3-carboxylic acid; 8-[3-(hydroxymercuri)-2-methoxypropyl]-3-carboxycoumarin; 8-[3-(hydroxymercuri)-2-methoxypropyl]coumarin-3-carboxylic acid.

C$_{14}$H$_{14}$HgO$_6$; mol wt 478.85. C 35.12%, H 2.95%, Hg 41.89%, O 20.05%. Prepn: A. Schlesinger *et al.*, **US 2667442** (1954 to Endo); L. H. Werner, C. R. Scholz, *J. Am. Chem. Soc.* **76**, 2453 (1954). Toxicology of mercumatalin sodium: H. Blumberg *et al.*, *J. Pharmacol. Exp. Ther.* **105**, 336 (1952).

Powder, bitter taste. mp 155-160° (Schlesinger); mp 197° (Werner, Scholz). One gram dissolves in about 4.2 parts of 1*N* NaOH. Slightly sol in acetic acid. Very slightly sol in water, alcohol, chloroform. Practically insol in ether.

Sodium salt compd with theophylline. [8018-15-3] Mercumatilin sodium; Cumertilin Sodium. C$_{21}$H$_{21}$HgN$_4$NaO$_8$; mol wt 680.99. Dry, light yellow powder. Very sol in water. LD$_{50}$ in rats (mg Hg/kg): 9.8 i.v.; 238 orally (Blumberg).

THERAP CAT: Diuretic.

5873. Mercuric Acetate. [1600-27-7] C$_4$H$_6$HgO$_4$; mol wt 318.68. C 15.08%, H 1.90%, Hg 62.94%, O 20.08%. Hg(CH$_3$COO)$_2$. Prepd from HgO and acetic acid: Wagenknecht, Juza in *Handbook of Preparative Inorganic Chemistry* vol. 2, G. Brauer, Ed. (Academic Press, New York, 2nd ed., 1965) pp 1120-1121.

Crystals or cryst powder; slight acetic odor; sensitive to light. *Poisonous!* d 3.28. mp 178-180° (overheating results in decompn). One g dissolves in 2.5 ml cold, 1 ml boiling water; sol in alcohol. *Keep well closed and protected from light.* Aq solns decomp on standing, yielding a yellow ppt.

USE: Chiefly for mercuration of organic compounds; for the absorption of ethylene.

5874. Mercuric Benzoate. [583-15-3] C$_{14}$H$_{10}$HgO$_4$; mol wt 442.82. C 37.97%, H 2.28%, Hg 45.30%, O 14.45%. Hg(C$_7$H$_5$O$_2$)$_2$.

Monohydrate. Odorless, cryst powder; sensitive to light. *Poisonous!* Sol in 90 parts cold, 40 parts boiling water; freely sol in NaCl soln; slightly sol in alcohol. When boiled with water or alc it hydrolyzes to a basic salt and free benzoic acid. *Protect from light.*

THERAP CAT: Formerly as antisyphilitic.

5875. Mercuric Bromide. [7789-47-1] Br$_2$Hg; mol wt 360.40. Br 44.34%, Hg 55.66%. HgBr$_2$. Usually prepd from the elements: Jander, Brodersen, *Z. Anorg. Chem.* **261**, 261 (1950).

White crystals or cryst powder; sensitive to light. *Poisonous!* d 6.05. mp 237°; sublimes at higher temp. Sol in about 200 parts cold, 25 parts boiling water; freely sol in hot alcohol, in methanol, HCl, HBr, alkali bromide solns; slightly sol in chloroform. *Protect from light.*

5876. Mercuric Chloride. [7487-94-7] Mercury bichloride; corrosive sublimate; mercury perchloride; corrosive mercury chloride. Cl$_2$Hg; mol wt 271.50. Cl 26.12%, Hg 73.88%. HgCl$_2$.

Crystals or white granules or powder. *Violent poison! May be fatal if swallowed.* d 5.4. mp 277°; volatilizes unchanged at about 300°; also slightly volatile at ordinary temp; appreciably so at 100°. One gram dissolves in 13.5 ml water (soly is increased by HCl or alkali chlorides), in 2.1 ml boiling water, 3.8 ml alc, 1.6 ml boiling alc, 200 ml benzene, 22 ml ether, 12 ml glycerol, 40 ml acetic acid; also sol in methanol, acetone, ethyl acetate; slightly sol in carbon disulfide, pyridine. pH about 4.7. Also reported as 3.2 for 0.2 molar aq soln. Coagulates albumin; produces with NaOH a yellow ppt (difference from calomel, which turns black). *Incompat:* Formates, sulfites, hypophosphites, phosphates, sulfides, albumin, gelatin, alkalies, alkaloid salts, ammonia, lime water, antimony and arsenic, bromides, borax, carbonates; reduced iron; copper, iron, lead, silver salts; infusions of cinchona, columbo, oak bark or senna; tannic acid; vegetable astringents.

Caution: Highly toxic. Corrosive to mucous membranes. Ingestion may cause severe nausea, vomiting, hematemesis, abdominal pain, diarrhea, melena, renal damage, prostration. 1 or 2 g is frequently fatal. Poisoning and death also have occurred from intrauterine douches and application of alcoholic soln to large areas of skin. Do not breathe dust. Keep away from feed or food products. Wash hands before eating or smoking. *Antidote:* Dimercaprol (BAL). Review of clinical toxicology of mercury and its compounds: H. B. Gerstner, J. E. Huff, *J. Toxicol. Environ. Health* **2**, 491-526 (1977).

USE: Preserving (kyanizing) wood and anatomical specimens; also embalming; disinfecting; browning and etching steel and iron; intensifier in photography; white reserve in fabric printing; tanning leather; electroplating aluminum; depolarizer for dry batteries; freeing gold from lead; magic photograms; mordant for rabbit and beaver furs; staining wood and vegetable ivory pink; manuf of ink for mercurography; treating seed potatoes; manuf other mercury compds. As an important reagent in anal. chemistry.

THERAP CAT: Topical antiseptic, disinfectant.

THERAP CAT (VET): Caustic, antiseptic, disinfectant.

5877. Mercuric Cyanide. [592-04-1] Cianurina. C_2HgN_2; mol wt 252.62. C 9.51%, Hg 79.40%, N 11.09%. $Hg(CN)_2$. Obtained by evaporating a soln of HgO in aq HCN: Biltz, *Z. Anorg. Allg. Chem.* **170**, 161 (1928).

Colorless, odorless, tetragonal crystals or white powder; darkens on exposure to light. *Violent poison!* d 3.996. Dec at 320°. One gram dissolves in 13 ml water, 3 ml boiling water, 13 ml alcohol, 4 ml methanol; slowly sol in glycerol; slightly sol in ether. *Protect from light.*

THERAP CAT: Topical antiseptic.

THERAP CAT (VET): Has been used as a topical antiseptic.

5878. Mercuric Fluoride. [7783-39-3] Mercury difluoride. F_2Hg; mol wt 238.59. F 15.93%, Hg 84.07%. HgF_2. Prepd from $HgCl_2$ and F_2: Henne, Midgley, *J. Am. Chem. Soc.* **58**, 886 (1936).

White powder or cubic crystals. Very sensitive to moisture. d^{15} 8.95. mp 645°. bp >650°. Turns yellow and hydrolyzes in the prolonged presence of water.

Dihydrate. Obtained when mercuric oxide is dissolved in excess of 50% HF.

USE: In the fluorination of organic compds.

5879. Mercuric Iodide, Red. [7774-29-0] Mercury biniodide. HgI_2; mol wt 454.40. Hg 44.14%, I 55.86%.

Scarlet-red, heavy, odorless, almost tasteless powder; sensitive to light; at 130° becomes yellow, and then red on cooling. *Poisonous!* d 6.28. mp 259°. bp ~350° and sublimes. Soly in water (25°) 0.006 g/100 g. 1 g dissolves in 115 ml alcohol, 20 ml boiling alcohol, about 120 ml ether, about 60 ml acetone, 910 ml chloroform, 75 ml ethyl acetate, 260 ml carbon disulfide, readily in alkali iodides, $HgCl_2$, $Na_2S_2O_3$; sol in 230 ml olive oil, 50 ml castor oil. *Protect from light.*

USE: In anal. chemistry for preparation of Nessler's Reagent (alkaline mercuric potassium iodide solution).

THERAP CAT: Antiseptic (topical).

THERAP CAT (VET): Has been used as a topical antiseptic, counterirritant, vesicant.

5880. Mercuric Nitrate. [10045-94-0] Mercury pernitrate. HgN_2O_6; mol wt 324.60. Hg 61.80%, N 8.63%, O 29.57%. $Hg(NO_3)_2$.

Hydrate. White or slightly yellow, deliquesc, cryst powder; odor of nitric acid. *Poisonous!* d 4.3. Sol in a small amount of water; with much water or on boiling with water, an insol basic salt is formed; sol in dil acids. *Keep well closed and protect from light.*

USE: Manufacture of felt; mercury fulminate; destroying phylloxera.

5881. Mercuric Oleate. [1191-80-6] 9-Octadecenoic acid mercury salt; oleate of mercury. $C_{36}H_{66}HgO_4$; mol wt 763.50. C 56.63%, H 8.71%, Hg 26.27%, O 8.38%. $Hg(C_{17}H_{33}COO)_2$. Commercial product prepd by dissolving yellow mercuric oxide in oleic acid; contains 24-26% HgO and about 10% excess oleic acid.

Yellowish-brown, somewhat transparent, ointment-like mass; odor of oleic acid. *Poisonous!* On keeping, the mercury is partly reduced to mercurous state or metal. Practically insol in water. Slightly sol in alcohol or ether, freely in fixed oils. *Protect from light.*

THERAP CAT: Has been used as ectoparasiticide.

5882. Mercuric Oxide, Red. [21908-53-2] Red precipitate. HgO; mol wt 216.59. Hg 92.61%, O 7.39%. Contains 99-99.5% HgO.

Bright red or orange-red, heavy, odorless, crystalline powder or scales; orthorhombic structure; yellow when finely powdered. *Poisonous!* Dec on exposure to light into mercury and oxygen; at 400° becomes almost black, but red again on cooling; at 500° dec into mercury and oxygen. d 11.14. Practically insol in water; sol in dil HCl or HNO_3 or in solns of alkali cyanides or iodides, slowly in solns of alkali bromides; insol in alcohol. *Protect from light.*

USE: In marine bottom paints, diluting pigments for painting on porcelain, with graphite as depolarizer in dry batteries. In Kjeldahl nitrogen determination; and as reagent for citric acid, thiophene, glucose, aldehyde, urea, acetone. As reagent and catalyst in organic reactions: J. S. Pizey, *Synthetic Reagents* **vol. 1** (John Wiley, New York, 1974) pp 295-319.

THERAP CAT: Antiseptic (topical).

THERAP CAT (VET): Has been used as a topical antiseptic.

5883. Mercuric Oxide, Yellow. [21908-53-2] Yellow precipitate. HgO; mol wt 216.59. Hg 92.61%, O 7.39%. Contains 99-99.5% HgO.

Yellow or orange-yellow, heavy, odorless powder, orthorhombic structure. *Poisonous!* Becomes red on heating and yellow again on cooling; more finely divided and more reactive than red mercuric oxide. Other physical properties and solubilities: *see* Mercuric Oxide, Red. *Protect from light. Incompat:* Reducing agents.

USE: Similar to that of the red oxide; in the mfr of organic mercurials. In anal. chemistry for determining Zn or HCN; detecting acetic acid in formic acid, CO in gas mixtures.

THERAP CAT: Topical antiseptic (ophthalmic).

THERAP CAT (VET): Has been used as a topical antiseptic, fungicide, in chronic skin conditions, conjunctivitis, corneal ulcers.

5884. Mercuric Oxycyanide. [1335-31-5] Mercury cyanide oxide. $C_2Hg_2N_2O$; mol wt 469.21. C 5.12%, Hg 85.50%, N 5.97%, O 3.41%. $HgO.Hg(CN)_2$. For reasons explained below, the article of commerce contains about 33% mercuric oxycyanide and about 67% mercuric cyanide.

White, orthorhombic crystals or cryst powder d 4.44. One gram dissolves in 80 ml cold water, more sol in hot water. *Violent poison! It explodes when touched with a flame or by percussion;* hence for commerce it is made with an excess of mercuric cyanide which eliminates the danger of explosion.

THERAP CAT: Antiseptic (topical).

5885. Mercuric Salicylate. [5970-32-1] [2-(Hydroxy-κO)-benzoato(2−)-κO]mercury; mercury subsalicylate. $C_7H_4HgO_3$; mol wt 336.69. C 24.97%, H 1.20%, Hg 59.58%, O 14.26%. Article of commerce contains 54-58% Hg. Prepn: C. H. Rogers *et al., Inorganic Pharmaceutical Chemistry* (Lea & Febriger, Philadelphia, 4th ed., 1948) pp 409-411.

White or slightly yellowish or pinkish, odorless powder. *Poisonous!* Insol in water or alcohol. Sol in warm solns of alkali halides, fixed alkali hydroxides and carbonates. *Incompat:* Alkali iodides.

THERAP CAT: Topical antiseptic.

5886. Mercuric Sodium p-Phenolsulfonate. [535-55-7] Mercury and sodium phenolsulfonate; mercuriphenoldisulfonate sodium; Hermophényl. $C_{12}H_8HgNa_2O_8S_2$; mol wt 590.89. C 24.39%, H 1.36%, Hg 33.95%, Na 7.78%, O 21.66%, S 10.85%. Prepd by the action of the sodium salt of p-phenolsulfonic acid on yellow mercuric oxide: Lumière, Chevrottier, *Compt. Rend.* **132**, 145 (1901); Lumière, Perrin, *Pharmacie* **1**, 102 (1943). The commercial product is a mixture of the monosulfonate (80%) and the disulfonate.

$$Na^+\ {}^-O_3S - \!\!\!\!\bigcirc\!\!\!\!- O - Hg - O -\!\!\!\!\bigcirc\!\!\!\!- SO_3^-\ Na^+$$

White powder. One gram dissolves in 5 ml water. The aq soln does not coagulate albuminous matter.

Caution: Ingestion or percutaneous absorption may cause mercury poisoning.

USE: As germicide in soaps and lotions. Usual concn in soap about 1:100.

THERAP CAT: Antiseptic (local).

5887. Mercuric Sulfate. [7783-35-9] Mercury bisulfate. HgO_4S; mol wt 296.65. Hg 67.62%, O 21.57%, S 10.81%. $HgSO_4$.

White, odorless granules or cryst powder. *Poisonous!* d 6.47. Dec by water into a yellow insol, basic sulfate and free H_2SO_4; sol in HCl, hot dil H_2SO_4, concd soln of NaCl. *Protect from light.*

USE: Electrolyte for primary batteries; with NaCl for extracting gold and silver from roasted pyrites; as a reagent for wine coloring, barbital, and cystine.

5888. Mercuric Sulfide, Black. [1344-48-5] Ethiops mineral. HgS; mol wt 232.66. Hg 86.22%, S 13.78%. Occurs as a mineral in California. Prepd by passing hydrogen sulfide through a soln of mercuric chloride in hydrochloric acid.

Black or grayish-black, heavy, odorless, tasteless, amorphous powder. Also occurs as black, cubic crystals (β-form). Transition temp (red to black) 386°. Black form can exist indefinitely in metastable state at room temp. Insol in water, alcohol, dil mineral acids.

USE: As pigment for horn, rubber, etc.

5889. Mercuric Sulfide, Red. [1344-48-5] Vermilion; Chinese red; C.I. Pigment Red 106; C.I. 77766. HgS; mol wt 232.66. Hg 86.22%, S 13.78%. Occurs in nature as the mineral *cinnabar*. Prepd from mercuric acetate, ammonium thiocyanate, glacial acetic acid and hydrogen sulfide: Newell *et al., Inorg. Synth.* **1**, 19 (1939). *See also Colour Index* **vol. 4** (3rd ed., 1971) p 4682.

Bright scarlet-red powder, lumps, hexagonal crystals (α-form); blackens on exposure to light, particularly in presence of H_2O or alkali hydroxides. At about 250° becomes brownish, at higher temp black, but red again on cooling. When ignited in air it dec into metal and sulfur, the latter burning to SO_2. Practically insol in water; not attacked by HNO_3 or cold HCl; dec by hot concd H_2SO_4; sol in aqua regia with separation of S, in warm hydriodic acid with evolution of H_2S. *Protect from light.*

USE: For coloring plastics, sealing wax, and with $FeSO_4$ for marking linen; manuf fancy colored papers; as pigment.

THERAP CAT: Antibacterial.

5890. Mercuric Thiocyanate. [592-85-8] Mercuric sulfocyanate; mercuric sulfocyanide. $C_2HgN_2S_2$; mol wt 316.75. C 7.58%, Hg 63.33%, N 8.84%, S 20.25%. $Hg(SCN)_2$. Prepd from $Hg(NO_3)_2$ + KSCN: Peters, *Z. Anorg. Allg. Chem.* **77**, 157 (1912).

Odorless powder. When crystalline, usually in radially arranged needles. *Poisonous!* When heated it swells up to many times its original vol, decomposing finally into mercury, nitrogen, etc., at about 165°. Slightly sol in cold water (0.069 g/100 ml H_2O at 25°), more sol in boiling water with decompn; sol in dil HCl, in solns of alkali cyanides, chlorides. *Protect from light.*

USE: For Pharaoh's serpents (fireworks); intensifier in photography.

5891. Mercurophen. [52486-78-9] Sodium 4-(hydroxymercuri)-2-nitrophenolate; sodium hydroxymercuri-*o*-nitrophenolate; 4-(hydroxymercuri)-2-nitrophenol sodium salt. $C_6H_4HgN\text{-}NaO_4$; mol wt 377.68. C 19.08%, H 1.07%, Hg 53.11%, N 3.71%, Na 6.09%, O 16.94%. Prepn from *o*-nitrophenol and $Hg(OCOCH_3)_2$: Schamberg *et al.*, **US 1390972** (1922). Structure: Malcolm, *J. Bacteriol.* **22**, 403 (1931).

Brick-red, odorless powder. *Poisonous!* Sol in hot water. Solns are deep amber in color.

THERAP CAT: Antiseptic, disinfectant.

THERAP CAT (VET): Antiseptic, disinfectant.

5892. Mercurous Acetate. [631-60-7] $C_4H_6Hg_2O_4$; mol wt 519.27. C 9.25%, H 1.16%, Hg 77.26%, O 12.32%. $Hg_2(CH_3\text{-}COO)_2$. Prepd from $Hg_2(NO_3)_2$ + CH_3COONa: Wagenknecht, Juza, in *Handbook of Preparative Inorganic Chemistry* **vol. 2**, G. Brauer, Ed. (Academic Press, New York, 2nd ed., 1965) p 1120.

Lustrous leaflets or cryst powder. Darkens on exposure to light. Sol in about 100 parts water; sol in dil acetic acid. Practically insol in alcohol, ether. Aq solns dec quickly under the influence of light and heat. *Keep well closed and protected from light.*

THERAP CAT: Antibacterial.

5893. Mercurous Bromide. [10031-18-2] Br_2Hg_2; mol wt 560.99. Br 28.49%, Hg 71.51%. Hg_2Br_2.

White, odorless powder; darkens on exposure to light. d 7.3. Sublimes at approx 390° (dec). Insol in water, alcohol, ether; dec by hot HCl or alkali bromides. *Protect from light.*

5894. Mercurous Chloride. [10112-91-1] Calomel; mild mercury chloride; mercury monochloride; mercury protochloride; mercury subchloride; precipité blanc; Calogreen. Cl_2Hg_2; mol wt 472.09. Cl 15.02%, Hg 84.98%. Hg_2Cl_2.

White, odorless, tasteless, heavy powder; slowly dec by sunlight into mercuric chloride and metallic mercury; sublimes at 400-500° without melting. d 7.15. Practically insol in water (0.00020 g/100 ml H_2O at 25°). HCl or alkali and alkaline earth chlorides increase soly in water. Insol in alcohol, ether. Dec by solns of alkali iodides, bromides or cyanides into the mercuric salt and metallic mecury; solns of alkali chlorides act similarly but slowly. Blackened by ammonia, caustic alkali and alkaline earth solns. *Protect from light.*

USE: Dark green Bengal lights; calomel paper, mixed with gold in painting on porcelain; for calomel electrodes; as fungicide; in agriculture to control root maggots on cabbage and onions.

THERAP CAT: Cathartic, diuretic, antiseptic, antisyphilitic.

THERAP CAT (VET): Has been used as cathartic, and locally as an antiseptic and desiccant.

5895. Mercurous Iodide. [15385-57-6] Yellow mercury iodide; mercury protoiodide. Hg_2I_2; mol wt 654.99. Hg 61.25%, I 38.75%.

Bright-yellow, amorphous, heavy, odorless powder. Darkens or becomes greenish on exposure to light, HgI$_2$ and metallic mercury being formed. d 7.70. mp 290° when rapidly heated with partial decompn into Hg and HgI$_2$. Insol in water, alcohol or ether. Sol in solns of mercurous or mercuric nitrates; cold ammonia, its solns or alkali iodide dec it into mercury and mercuric iodide. *Protect from light.* "Green" mercury iodide is made from metallic mercury and iodine, the green color being due to presence of some uncombined mercury.

5896. Mercurous Nitrate. [10415-75-5] Mercury protonitrate. $Hg_2N_2O_6$; mol wt 525.19. Hg 76.39%, N 5.33%, O 18.28%. $Hg_2(NO_3)_2$. Normally exists as dihydrate. Prepn of anhydr salt: Potts, Allred, *Inorg. Chem.* **5**, 1066 (1966).

Dihydrate. Colorless crystals, usually with slight odor of HNO_3. mp $\sim$70° with decompn. *Poisonous!* d 4.78. Sol in 13 parts water contg 1% HNO_3; with water alone a basic salt is formed. Blackened by ammonia, caustic alkali, and alkaline earth solns. *Keep well closed and protected from light.*

USE: Fire gilding, blackening brass.

5897. Mercurous Sulfate. [7783-36-0] Hg_2O_4S; mol wt 497.24. Hg 80.68%, O 12.87%, S 6.45%. Hg_2SO_4.

White to slightly yellow cryst powder. Becomes gray on exposure to light with production of mercury and mercuric sulfate. d 7.56. Slightly sol in water (0.06 g/100g at 25°); sol in dil HNO_3.

USE: For making electric batteries; with zinc sulfate in the standard Clark cell and with cadmium sulfate in the standard Weston cell.

5898. Mercury. [7439-97-6] Hydrargyrum; liquid silver; quicksilver. Hg; at. wt 200.59; at. no. 80; valences 1, 2. Group IIB(12). Abundance in earth's crust 0.5 ppm. Natural isotopes: 202 (29.80%); 200 (23.13%); 199 (16.84%); 201 (13.22%); 198 (10.02%); 204 (6.85%); 196 (0.146%); known isotopes range in mass number from 189 to 206. Obtained by roasting cinnabar (mercuric sulfide). General reviews: Roberts, *Adv. Inorg. Chem. Radiochem.* **11** (Academic Press, New York, 1968) pp 309-339; Aylett, "Group IIB" in *Comprehensive Inorganic Chemistry* **vol. 3** (Pergamon Press, Oxford, 1973) pp 187-328; H. J. Drake in *Kirk-Othmer Encyclopedia of Chemical Technology* **vol. 15** (Wiley-Interscience, New York, 3rd ed., 1981) pp 143-156. Review of clinical toxicology: H. B. Gerstner, J. E. Huff, *J. Toxicol. Environ. Health* **2**, 491-526 (1977); and human exposure: *Toxicological Profile for Mercury* (PB99-142416, 1999) 676 pp.

Silver-white, heavy, mobile, liquid metal; slightly volatile at ordinary temp; solid mercury is a tin-white, ductile, malleable mass which may be cut with a knife. mp $-38.87°$; bp $356.72°$; d^{25} 13.534. Heat capacity at constant pressure (25°) 6.687 cal/mole deg. Vapor pressure (25°): 2×10^{-3} mm; heat of vaporization (25°): 14.652 kcal/mole: Busey, Giauque, *J. Am. Chem. Soc.* **75**, 806 (1953). Surface tension (25°): 484 dynes/cm; electrical resistivity (20°): 95.76 μohm cm. When pure does not tarnish on exposure to air at ordinary temp, but when heated to near the boiling point slowly oxidizes to HgO. Forms alloys with most metals except iron and combines with sulfur at ordinary temperatures. E^0 (aq) Hg/Hg^{2+} -0.854 V; E^0 (aq) 2 Hg/Hg_2^{2+} -0.789 V. Soly in water (25°): 0.28 μmoles/l; data on soly in organic solvents: Spencer, Voigt, *J. Phys. Chem.* **72**, 464 (1968). Reacts with HNO_3 and hot, concd H_2SO_4; does not react with dil HCl, cold H_2SO_4, or alkalies. Reacts with ammonia solns in air to form Hg_2NOH, *Millon's base*. Mercury salts when heated with Na_2CO_3 yield metallic Hg and are reduced to metal by H_2O_2 in the presence of alkali hydroxide. Cu, Fe, Zn and many other metals ppt metallic Hg from neutral or slightly acid solns of mercury salts. Soluble ionized *mercuric* salts give a yellow ppt of HgO with NaOH and a red ppt of HgI_2 with alkali iodide. *Mercurous* salts give a black ppt with alkali hydroxides and a white ppt of calomel with HCl or sol chlorides. They are slowly dec by sunlight. *Poisonous!*

Caution: Readily absorbed via respiratory tract (elemental mercury vapor, mercury compd dusts), intact skin, and G.I. tract, although occasional incidental swallowing of metallic mercury is without harm. Spilled and heated elemental mercury is particularly hazardous. *Acute:* sol salts have violent corrosive effects on skin and mucous membranes; severe nausea, vomiting, abdominal pain, bloody diarrhea; kidney damage; death usually within 10 days. *Chronic:* inflammation of mouth and gums, excessive salivation, loosening of teeth; kidney damage; muscle tremors, jerky gait, spasms of extremities; personality changes, depression, irritability, nervousness. Phenyl and alkyl mercurials can cause skin burns and be absorbed by the skin. Burning sensation is delayed several hours and thus gives no warning. Alkyls have affinity for brain tissue and may cause permanent damage. Phenyls are no more toxic than inorganic Hg. *Antidote:* Dimercaprol (BAL). *See* E. Browning, *Toxicity of Industrial Metals* (Appleton-Century Crofts, New York, 2nd ed., 1969) pp 226-242.

USE: In barometers, thermometers, hydrometers, pyrometers; in mercury arc lamps producing ultraviolet rays; in switches, fluorescent lamps; in mercury boilers; manuf all mercury salts, mirrors; as catalyst in oxidation of organic compds; extracting gold and silver from ores; making amalgams, electric rectifiers, mercury fulminate; also in dentistry; in determining N by Kjeldahl method, for Millon's reagent; as cathode in electrolysis, electroanalysis, and many other uses. Also in pharmaceuticals, agricultural chemicals, anti-fouling paints.

5899. Merimepodib. [198821-22-6] [[3-[[[[3-Methoxy-4-(5-oxazolyl)phenyl]amino]carbonyl]amino]phenyl]methyl] carbamic acid (3*S*)-tetrahydro-3-furanyl ester; VX-497. $C_{23}H_{24}N_4O_6$; mol wt 452.46. C 61.05%, H 5.35%, N 12.38%, O 21.22%. Inosine 5'-monophosphate dehydrogenase (IMPDH) inhibitor. Prepn (stereochemistry unspecified): D. M. Armistead *et al.*, **WO 9740028**; *eidem*, **US 5807876** (1997, 1998 both to Vertex). *In vitro* antiviral spectrum: W. Markland *et al.*, *Antimicrob. Agents Chemother.* **44**, 859 (2000); immunosuppressive activity: J. Jain *et al.*, *J. Pharm. Sci.* **90**, 625 (2001). Clinical evaluation in hepatitis C: J. G. McHutchison *et al.*, *Antiviral Ther.* **10**, 635 (2005). Review of structure-activity and mechanism of action: M. D. Sintchak, E. Nimmesgern, *Immunopharmacology* **47**, 163-184 (2000); of development and therapeutic potential: G. Tossing, *IDrugs* **6**, 372-376 (2003).

THERAP CAT: Antiviral.

5900. Meropenem. [96036-03-2] (4*R*,5*S*,6*S*)-3-[[(3*S*,5*S*)-5-[(Dimethylamino)carbonyl]-3-pyrrolidinyl]thio]-6-[(1*R*)-1-hydroxyethyl]-4-methyl-7-oxo-1-azabicyclo[3.2.0]hept-2-ene-2-carboxylic acid; (1*R*,5*S*,6*S*)-2-[(3*S*,5*S*)-5-(dimethylaminocarbonyl)-pyrrolidin-3-ylthio]-6-[(*R*)-1-hydroxyethyl]-1-methylcarbapen-2-em-3-carboxylic acid. $C_{17}H_{25}N_3O_5S$; mol wt 383.46. C 53.25%, H 6.57%, N 10.96%, O 20.86%, S 8.36%. Carbapenem antibiotic. Prepn: M. Sunagawa *et al.*, **EP 126587**; M. Sunagawa, **US 4943569** (1984, 1990 both to Sumitomo). Structure-activity study: M. Sunagawa *et al.*, *J. Antibiot.* **43**, 519 (1990). Crystal structure: K. Yanagi *et al.*, *Acta Crystallogr.* **C48**, 1737 (1992). HPLC determn in serum and bronchial secretions: M. Ehrlich *et al.*, *J. Chromatogr.* B **751**, 357 (2001). Pharmacokinetics: R. Wise *et al.*, *Antimicrob. Agents Chemother.* **34**, 1515 (1990). Series of articles on antimicrobial activity, metabolism: *J. Antimicrob. Chemother.* **24**, Suppl. A, 1-320 (1989); and clinical performance: *ibid.* **36**, Suppl. A, 1-223 (1995). Review of clinical experience in intensive care: M. Hurst, H. M. Lamb, *Drugs* **59**, 653-680 (2000).

Trihydrate. [119478-56-7] ICI-194660; SM-7338; Meronem; Meropen; Merrem. White to pale yellow crystalline powder. Sparingly sol in water; very slightly sol in hydrated ethanol. Practically insol in acetone, ether.

THERAP CAT: Antibacterial.

5901. Mersalyl. [492-18-2] [3-[[2-(Carboxylatomethoxy)benzoyl]amino]-2-methoxypropyl]hydroxymercurate(1−) sodium; *o*-[[3-(hydroxymercuri)-2-methoxypropyl]carbamoyl]phenoxyacetic acid sodium salt; sodium *o*-[(3-hydroxymercuri-2-methoxypropyl)carbamoyl]phenoxyacetate; *N*-(γ-hydroxymercuri-β-methoxypropyl)salicylamide-*O*-acetic acid sodium salt; mercuramide; Salyrgan. $C_{13}H_{16}HgNNaO_6$; mol wt 505.85. C 30.87%, H 3.19%, Hg 39.65%, N 2.77%, Na 4.54%, O 18.98%. Prepn: Diels, Beccard, *Ber.* **39**, 4125 (1906); Bockmühl, Schwarz, **DE 423031** (1925 to Hoechst); *Frdl.* **15**, 1609. Use as diuretic: F. Brunn, *Wien. Klin. Wochenschr.* **37**, 901 (1924). Toxicity data: E. B. Robbins, K. K. Chen, *J. Am. Pharm. Assoc.* **40**, 249 (1951). Use of acid as physiological sulfhydryl inhibitor: P. Mavier, J. Hanoune, *Eur. J. Biochem.* **59**, 593 (1975).

Bitter crystals. Somewhat deliquescent. Gradually dec by light. One gram dissolves in about 1 ml water, in about 3 ml ethanol (95%), in 2 ml abs methanol. Practically insol in ether, chloroform. Aq solns are alkaline to litmus. LD_{50} i.v. in mice, rats: 72.6, 17.7 mg/kg (Robbins, Chen).

Mersalyl Acid. [486-67-9] $C_{13}H_{17}HgNO_6$; mol wt 483.87. Odorless, white, slightly hygroscopic powder. Slightly sol in water, dil mineral acids; sol in solutions of alkali hydroxides.

USE: Sulfhydryl specific biochemical probe.

THERAP CAT: Diuretic.

THERAP CAT (VET): Diuretic.

5902. MES. [4432-31-9] 4-Morpholineethanesulfonic acid; 2-(4-morpholino)ethyl sulfonate; 2-(*N*-morpholino)ethanesulfonic acid. $C_6H_{13}NO_4S$; mol wt 195.24. C 36.91%, H 6.71%, N 7.17%, O 32.78%, S 16.42%. One of the zwitterionic *N*-substituted aminosulfonic acids known as *Good Buffers*, active in the pH range 6-8. Prepn as sodium salt: S. Malkiel, J. P. Mason, *J. Org. Chem.* **8**, 199 (1943); as acid: N. E. Good *et al.*, *Biochemistry* **5**, 467 (1966). Thermodynamic parameters: C. D. McGlothlin, J. Jordan, *Anal.*

Lett. **9,** 245 (1976). Acid-base properties: A. Balikungeri, *Chimia* **43,** 13 (1989). Interference with protein determn: P. L. Lleu, G. Rebel, *Anal. Biochem.* **192,** 215 (1991). Use as buffer: S. C. Lee *et al., J. AOAC Int.* **75,** 395 (1992); P. J. Henney *et al., Anim. Genet.* **25,** 363 (1994).

Colorless crystals from alcohol/water, dec >300°. Apparent pKa at 0.1*M* ionic: 0°, 6.38; 20°, 6.15; 37°, 5.98. At 0.1*M* ionic, 25.0° ±0.1°: pKa$_1$ 1.99; pKa$_2$ 6.21. Δ pKa/°C −0.011. Saturation at 0°: 0.65*M.*

USE: Biological buffer.

5903. Mesaconic Acid. [498-24-8] (*E*)-2-Methyl-2-butene-dioic acid; methylfumaric acid; *trans*-1-propene-1,2-dicarboxylic acid. C$_5$H$_6$O$_4$; mol wt 130.10. C 46.16%, H 4.65%, O 49.19%. Prepd by heating citraconic anhydride with nitric acid: Shriner *et al., Org. Synth.* **11,** 74 (1931); from ethyl itaconate: Jones *et al., J. Chem. Soc.* **1954,** 1865; from *N,N*-diethyl-5-diethylamino-2,3-dihydro-3-furamide: Sauer *et al., J. Am. Chem. Soc.* **81,** 693 (1959). Obtained almost instantly by the action of sunlight on citraconic acid in ether + chloroform in the presence of a little bromine: Fittig, Langworthy, *Ber.* **26,** 46 (1893); *Ann.* **304,** 119, 149 (1899); by action of β-radiation on citraconic acid + bromine: Lavigne, Levine, **US 2979445** (1961 to California Res. Corp.).

Orthorhombic needles from alcohol, monoclinic tablets from ethyl acetate, mp 204-205°. d 1.466. Sublimes. bp 250° (decompn). K$_1$ at 25° = 8.5 × 10^{-4}; K$_2$ = 15 × 10^{-6}. 100 g water dissolves 2.7 g at 18° and 117.9 g at the boiling point; 100 g 90% alc dissolves 30.6 g at 17° and 95.7 g at the boiling point. Sol in ether; sparingly sol in chloroform, carbon disulfide and ligroin.

Dimethyl ester. C$_7$H$_{10}$O$_4$. Liq, bp 206°. d$_4^{21}$ vac 1.12011. n$_D^{20}$ 1.45575. Sol in 122 parts water at 15°.

Diethyl ester. C$_9$H$_{14}$O$_4$. Liq, bp 229°. d$_4^{20}$ vac 1.04675. n$_4^{20}$ 1.44936.

5904. Mesalamine. [89-57-6] 5-Amino-2-hydroxybenzoic acid; 5-aminosalicylic acid; 5-amino-2-hydroxybenzene-1-carboxylic acid; *m*-aminosalicylic acid; fisalamine; mesalazine; 5-ASA; Asacol; Asacolitin; Claversal; Lixacol; Mesasal; Pentasa; Rowasa; Salofalk. C$_7$H$_7$NO$_3$; mol wt 153.14. C 54.90%, H 4.61%, N 9.15%, O 31.34%. Prepn by reduction of *m*-nitrobenzoic acid with Zn dust and HCl: H. Weil *et al., Ber.* **55B,** 2664 (1922); by electrolytic reduction: Le Guyader, Peltier, *Compt. Rend.* **253,** 2544 (1961). Use in manufacture of dyes: **GB 751386** (1956 to J. R. Geigy). Identification as active metabolite of sulfasalazine, *q.v.:* A. K. Azad Khan *et al., Lancet* **2,** 892 (1977); P. A. M. Van Hees *et al., Gut* **21,** 632 (1980). HPLC determn in serum: E. Brendel *et al., J. Chromatogr.* **385,** 299 (1987). Bioavailability, plasma level and excretion: S. N. Rasmussen *et al., Gastroenterology* **83,** 1062 (1982). Clinical evaluation in Crohn's disease: *eidem, ibid.* **85,** 1350 (1983). Clinical trials in ulcerative colitis: M. Campieri *et al., Lancet* **2,** 270 (1981); L. S. Friedman *et al., Am. J. Gastroenterol.* **81,** 412 (1986); in comparison with olsalazine, *q.v.:* S. S. Rao *et al., Scand. J. Gastroenterol.* **22,** 332 (1987). Brief review: G. Friedman, *Am. J. Gastroenterol.* **81,** 141-144 (1986). Review of clinical efficacy in colonic diverticulosis: A. Tursi, *Expert Opin. Pharmacother.* **6,** 69-74 (2005).

White to pinkish crystals, dec ~280°. Slightly sol in cold water, alc; more sol in hot water; sol in HCl.

USE: In manuf of light-sensitive paper, azo and sulfur dyes.
THERAP CAT: Anti-inflammatory (gastrointestinal).

5905. Mescaline. [54-04-6] 3,4,5-Trimethoxybenzene-ethanamine; 3,4,5-trimethoxyphenethylamine; mezcaline. C$_{11}$H$_{17}$-NO$_3$; mol wt 211.26. C 62.54%, H 8.11%, N 6.63%, O 22.72%. Psychotomimetic alkaloid isolated from *peyote* (mescal buttons), the flowering heads of *Lophophora williamsii* (Lemaire) Coult., *Cactaceae.* Isoln: A. Heffter, *Ber.* **29,** 221 (1896). Structure and synthesis: E. Späth, *Monatsh. Chem.* **40,** 129 (1919); K. H. Slotta, H. Heller, *Ber.* **63,** 3029 (1930); E. Späth, F. Becke, *Monatsh. Chem.* **66,** 327 (1935); M. U. Tsao, *J. Am. Chem. Soc.* **73,** 5495 (1951); K. Banholzer *et al., Helv. Chim. Acta* **35,** 1577 (1952). Novel synthesis: M. N. Aboul-Enein, A. I. Eid, *Acta Pharm. Suec.* **16,** 267 (1979). MS determn: S. P. Jindal, T. Lutz, *Eur. J. Mass Spectrom. Biochem. Med. Environ. Res.* **2,** 117 (1982). Pharmacokinetics in rabbits: C. Van Peteghem *et al., Eur. J. Drug Metab. Pharmacokinet.* **7,** 1 (1982). Mode of action study: M. E. Trulson *et al., Eur. J. Pharmacol.* **96,** 151 (1983). Use in evaluating serotonin S$_2$ antagonists: C. J. E. Niemegeers *et al., Drug Dev. Res.* **3,** 123 (1983). Evaluation of use with chlorpromazine, *q.v.,* in various psychoses: H. C. B. Denber, S. Merlis: *J. Nerv. Ment. Dis.* **122,** 463 (1955). Toxicity data: L. B. Speck, *J. Pharmacol. Exp. Ther.* **119,** 78 (1957); H. F. Hardman *et al., Toxicol. Appl. Pharmacol.* **25,** 299 (1973). *Reviews:* A. R. Patel, *Progress in Drug Research* **vol. 11,** E. Jucker, Ed. (Birkhäuser Verlag, Basel, 1968) pp 11-47; G. J. Kapadia, M. B. E. Fayez, *J. Pharm. Sci.* **59,** 1699-1727 (1970).

Crystals, mp 35-36°. bp$_{12}$ 180°. Moderately sol in water; sol in alcohol, chloroform, benzene. Practically insol in ether, petr ether. Takes up CO$_2$ from the air and forms a crystalline carbonate. LD$_{50}$ i.p. in rats: 370 mg/kg (Speck).

Hydrochloride. C$_{11}$H$_{17}$NO$_3$.HCl. Needles, mp 181°. Sol in water, alcohol. LD$_{50}$ in mice, rats, guinea pigs (mg/kg): 212, 132, 328 i.p. (Hardman).

Sulfate dihydrate. (C$_{11}$H$_{17}$NO$_3$)$_2$.H$_2$SO$_4$.2H$_2$O. Prisms, mp 183-186°. Sol in hot water, methanol; sparingly sol in cold water, ethanol.

Acid sulfate. C$_{11}$H$_{17}$NO$_3$.H$_2$SO$_4$. Crystals, mp 158°.

N-Benzoylmescaline. Needles from aq alc, mp 121°. Very sol in alcohol, ether.

N-Methylmescaline. Occurs naturally, bp 130-140°.

N-Acetylmescaline. Occurs naturally, mp 94°.

Note: This is a controlled substance (hallucinogen): **21 CFR,** 1308.11.

5906. Mesembrine. [24880-43-1] (3a*S-cis*)-3a-(3,4-Dimethoxyphenyl)octahydro-1-methyl-6*H*-indol-6-one; 3a-(3,4-dimethoxyphenyl)tetrahydro-1-methyl-6(3a*H*)-indolinone. C$_{17}$H$_{23}$-NO$_3$; mol wt 289.37. C 70.56%, H 8.01%, N 4.84%, O 16.59%. Alkaloid used in preparing *Channa,* a drug of Southwest Africa. Occurs naturally as the (−)-form. From *Sceletium expansum* L., *S. tortuosum* L., *Aizoaceae:* Hartwick, Zwicky, *Apoth. Ztg.* **29,** 925 (1914); Rimington *et al., J. Vet. Sci. Animal Ind.* **9,** 187 (1938), *C.A.* **32,** 4279^9 (1938). Structure: Popelak *et al., Naturwissenschaften* **47,** 156 (1960). Configuration: P. W. Jeffs *et al., J. Am. Chem. Soc.* **91,** 3831 (1969). Synthesis of (±) form: Shamma, Rodriguez, *Tetrahedron Lett.* **1965,** 4847; O. Hoshino *et al., Heterocycles* **10,** 61 (1978); of (±)-form and *trans* isomer: Oh-Ishi, Kugita, *Chem. Pharm. Bull.* **18,** 299 (1970). Synthesis of (+)-form: Yamada, Otani, *Tetrahedron Lett.* **1971,** 1133; *eidem, Chem. Pharm. Bull.* **21,** 2130 (1973). Stereoselective synthesis of (±)-form: Wijnberg, Speckamp, *Tetrahedron Lett.* **1975,** 3963; *eidem, Tetrahedron* **34,** 2579 (1978); S. F. Martin *et al., J. Org. Chem.* **44,** 3391 (1979); S. Takano *et al., Chem. Lett.* **1981,** 1385. Enantioselective synthesis of natural mesembrine: *eidem, Tetrahedron Lett.* **24,** 4479 (1981). Biosynthesis: Jeffs *et al., J. Am. Chem. Soc.* **93,** 3752 (1971); *eidem, Chem. Commun.* **1977,** 60. Review of mesembrine alkaloids: A. Popelak, G. Lettenbauer in *The Alkaloids* **vol. IX,** R. H.

F. Manske, Ed. (Academic Press, New York, 1967) pp 467-481; R. V. Stevens in *The Total Synthesis of Natural Products* vol. 3, J. ApSimon, Ed. (Wiley, New York, 1977) pp 443-453.

Pale yellow oil. $bp_{0.3}$ 186-190°. $[\alpha]_D^{20}$ −55.4° (CH_3OH). Freely sol in alcohol, chloroform, acetone; slightly sol in ether. Practically insol in benzene, petr ether, alkalies.

Hydrochloride. $C_{17}H_{23}NO_3 \cdot HCl$. mp 205-206°. $[\alpha]_D^{20}$ −8.4° (CH_3OH).

(+)-Form. (Partially optically active). Pale yellow oil. $[\alpha]_D^{20}$ +16.1° (c = 1.32 in CH_3OH).

(+)-Form hydrochloride. $C_{17}H_{23}NO_3 \cdot HCl$. Crystals from 2-propanol, mp 206.5-207.5°. $[\alpha]_D^{20}$ +7.3° (c = 0.465 in CH_3OH).

(±)-Form. Colorless oil. $bp_{0.07}$ 178°.

(±)-Form hydrochloride. $C_{17}H_{23}NO_3 \cdot HCl$. mp 179-181°.

5907. Mesitylene. [108-67-8] 1,3,5-Trimethylbenzene; *sym*-trimethylbenzene. C_9H_{12}; mol wt 120.19. C 89.94%, H 10.06%. Occurs in coal tar and in petroleum crudes; prepd by dehydrating acetone with H_2SO_4: Adams, Hufferd, *Org. Synth.* **2**, 41 (1922).

Liquid; peculiar odor. d_4^{20} 0.8637. mp −44.8°. n_D^{18} 1.49541. bp_{760} 164.7°; bp_{100} 98.9°; bp_{20} 61°; bp_{10} 47.4°; $bp_{1.0}$ 9.6°. Practically insol in water (100 g H_2O dissolve 0.002 g). Miscible with alcohol, ether, benzene.

Caution: Potential symptoms of overexposure are irritation of eyes, skin, nose, throat, respiratory system; bronchitis; hypochromic anemia, headache, drowsiness, fatigue, dizziness, nausea, incoordination; vomiting, confusion; aspiration of liquid may cause chemical pneumonia. *See NIOSH Pocket Guide to Chemical Hazards* (DHHS/NIOSH 97-140, 1997) p 320.

5908. Mesityl Oxide. [141-79-7] 4-Methyl-3-penten-2-one; isopropylideneacetone. $C_6H_{10}O$; mol wt 98.14. C 73.43%, H 10.27%, O 16.30%. $(CH_3)_2C$=$CHCOCH_3$. Made by distilling diacetone alcohol with a small amount of iodine: Conant, Tuttle, *Org. Synth.* **1**, 53 (1921). Condensation of acetone to mesityl oxide using sulfonated polystyrene-divinylbenzene resin as ion exchange catalyst: Klein, Banchero, *Ind. Eng. Chem.* **48**, 1278 (1956). Believed to be a mixture of two isomers. Toxicity data: N. F. Izmerov *et al.*, *Toxicometric Parameters of Industrial Toxic Chemicals Under Single Exposure* (Centre Internat. Projects, Moscow, 1982) p 81. Brief review of toxicity: *Dangerous Prop. Ind. Mater. Rep.* **9**, 58-65 (1989).

Colorless, oily liq; honey-like odor. d_4^{15} 0.8592. bp_{760} 130°; bp_{100} 72.1°; bp_{20} 26°; $bp_{1.0}$ −8.7°. mp −41.5°; also reported as mp −59°. Can be made to crystallize at low temp in petr ether. n_D^{22} 1.4425. Absorption spectrum: Morton, *J. Chem. Soc.* **1926**, 719. Sol in about 30 parts water; miscible with most organic liqs. Flash pt: 87°F (30.6°C). LD_{50} in mice (mg/kg): 710 ±85 intragastric; LC_{50} in mice (2 hr), rats (4 hr) (mg/m³): 10000 ±270, 9000 ±600 (Ismerov).

Caution: Potential symptoms of overexposure are irritation of eyes, skin and mucous membranes; narcosis, coma. *See NIOSH Pocket Guide to Chemical Hazards* (DHHS/NIOSH 97-140, 1997) p 194.

USE: Solvent for nitrocellulose, many gums and resins, particularly vinyl resins. In lacquers, varnishes and enamels. In making methyl isobutyl ketone.

5909. Mesna. [19767-45-8] 2-Mercaptoethanesulfonic acid sodium salt; sodium mercaptoethanesulfonate; D-7093; UCB-3983; Mesnex; Mistabron; Mistabronco; Mucofluid; Uromitexan. C_2H_5-NaO_3S_2; mol wt 164.18. C 14.63%, H 3.07%, Na 14.00%, O 29.24%, S 39.06%. $[HSCH_2CH_2SO_3]^-Na^+$. Sulfhydryl donor used to reduce the urotoxic effects of antineoplastic alkylating agents; also has mucolytic activity. Prepn: I. M. Lipovich, *J. Appl. Chem. USSR* **18**, 718 (1945); C. H. Schramm *et al.*, *J. Am. Chem. Soc.* **77**, 6231 (1955). Synthesis and properties: V. E. Petrun'kin, *C.A.* **51**, 5693a (1957); *ibid.* **54**, 24379c (1960). Use as mucolytic: NL 6605816; H. Morren, US 3567835 (1966, 1971 both to U.C.B.); as uroprotective agent: N. Brock, DE 2756018; *idem*, US 4220660 (1979, 1980 both to Asta-Werke AG). Pharmacology, toxicity, and uroprotective effects in animals: N. Brock *et al.*, *Eur. J. Cancer Clin. Oncol.* **18**, 1377 (1982). HPLC determn in plasma and urine: C. A. James, H. J. Rogers, *J. Chromatogr.* **382**, 394 (1986). Clinical pharmacokinetics: C. A. James *et al.*, *Br. J. Clin. Pharmacol.* **23**, 561 (1987). Clinical study of mucolytic effects: M. Tekeres *et al.*, *Clin. Ther.* **4**, 56 (1981). Symposium on pharmacology, toxicity and clinical uroprotective efficacy: *Cancer Treat. Rev.* **10**, Suppl. A, 1-192 (1983). *Reviews:* I. C. Shaw, M. I. Graham, *ibid.* **14** 67-86 (1987); S. E. Schoenike, W. J. Dana, *Clin. Pharm.* **9**, 179-191 (1990).

Freely sol in water, sparingly sol in organic solvents. LD_{50} in male, female mice, male, female rats (mg/kg): 1887, 2048, 2098, 1683 i.v.; 2005, 2098, 1529, 1251 i.p.; 6102, >7200, 4440, 4679 orally (Brock).

THERAP CAT: Mucolytic; antineoplastic adjunct (uroprotective).

5910. Mesoridazine. [5588-33-0] 10-[2-(1-Methyl-2-piperidinyl)ethyl]-2-(methylsulfinyl)-10*H*-phenothiazine; thioridazine-2-sulfoxide; TPS-23. $C_{21}H_{26}N_2OS_2$; mol wt 386.57. C 65.25%, H 6.78%, N 7.25%, O 4.14%, S 16.59%. Dopamine receptor blocking agent; analog of thioridazine. Prepn: Renz *et al.*, US 3084161 (1963 to Sandoz). Pharmacology and toxicology: Loew *et al.*, *Boll. Chim. Farm.* **106**, 332-371 (1967). Effects on dopaminergic function in comparison with sulforidazine and thioridazine, *q.q.v.*: D. M. Niedzwiecki *et al.*, *J. Pharmacol. Exp. Ther.* **228**, 636 (1984); C. D. Kilts *et al.*, *ibid.* **231**, 334 (1984). GLC determn in plasma: E. C. Dinovo *et al.*, *J. Pharm. Sci.* **65**, 667 (1976). Clinical evaluation in sleep disorders: K. Adam *et al.*, *Br. J. Clin. Pharmacol.* **3**, 157 (1976); as antipsychotic: R. Axelsson, *Curr. Ther. Res.* **21**, 587 (1977). Toxicity studies: S. Maruyama *et al.*, *Niigata Igakkai Zasshi* **81**, 611 (1967), *C.A.* **68**, 76856h (1968). Brief description: *J. Am. Med. Assoc.* **216**, 313 (1971).

Oily product.

Benzenesulfonate. [32672-69-8] Mesoridazine besylate; NC-123; Lidanar; Lidanil; Serentil. $C_{27}H_{32}N_2O_4S_3$; mol wt 544.75. LD_{50} in mice (mg/kg): 33 i.v.; 611 s.c.; 346 orally (Maruyama).

Tartrate. $C_{25}H_{32}N_2O_7S_2$. Crystals from ethyl acetate, mp 115-120°.

THERAP CAT: Antipsychotic.

5911. Mesosulfuron-methyl. [208465-21-8] 2-[[[[(4,6-Dimethoxy-2-pyrimidinyl)amino]carbonyl]amino]sulfonyl]-4-[[(methylsulfonyl)amino]methyl]benzoic acid methyl ester; methyl 2-[3-(4,6-dimethoxypyrimidin-2-yl)ureidosulfonyl]-4-methanesulfonamidomethylbenzoate; AE-F130060; Osprey; Silverado. C_{17}-$H_{21}N_5O_9S_2$; mol wt 503.51. C 40.55%, H 4.20%, N 13.91%, O

28.60%, S 12.74%. Sulfonylurea herbicide; acetolactate synthase inhibitor. Prepn: K. Lorenz *et al., WO 9510507; eidem* **US 5648315** (1995, 1997 both to Hoechst Schering AgrEvo). Comprehensive description: E. Hacker *et al., BCPC Conf. - Weeds* **2001**, 43-48. Greenhouse trial of combination with iodosulfuron-methyl-sodium in winter wheat: W. A. Bailey *et al., Weed Sci.* **51**, 515 (2003).

Cream-colored solid, mp 195.4°. Vapor pressure (25°): 1.1 × 10^{-11} Pa. Log P (octanol/water): 1.39 (pH 5); −0.48 (pH 7); −2.06 (pH 9). Soly in water at 20° (g/l): 7.24 × 10^{-3} (pH 5); 0.483 (pH 7); 15.39 (pH 9). LD$_{50}$ in rats (mg/kg): >5000 orally; >5000 dermally. LC$_{50}$ in rats: >1.33 mg/l air (Hacker).

USE: Herbicide.

5912. Mesotrione. [104206-82-8] 2-[4-(Methylsulfonyl)-2-nitrobenzoyl]-1,3-cyclohexanedione; ZA-1296; Callisto. $C_{14}H_{13}$-NO_7S; mol wt 339.32. C 49.55%, H 3.86%, N 4.13%, O 33.01%, S 9.45%. Triketone herbicide for use in maize; inhibits *p*-hydroxy-phenylpyruvate dioxygenase (HPPD). Synthetic mimic of *leptospermone*, a natural herbicide produced by the bottlebrush plant, *Callistemon citrinus* Stapf. Prepn: C. G. Carter, **EP 186118** (1986 to Stauffer); *idem,* **US 5006158** (1991 to ICI). Comprehensive description: R. A. Wichert *et al., Brighton Crop Prot. Conf. - Weeds* **1999**, 105-110. HPLC determn in crops, soil, water: P. Alferness, L. Wiebe, *J. Agric. Food Chem.* **50**, 3926 (2002). Adsorption and degradation in soil: J. S. Dyson *et al., J. Environ. Qual.* **31**, 613 (2002). *Review:* G. Mitchell *et al., Pest Manage. Sci.* **57**, 120-128 (2001).

Opaque solid, mp 165°. pKa (20°): 3.12. Vapor pressure (20°): 4.27 × 10^{-8} mm Hg. Soly in water at 20° (g/l): 2.2 (pH 4.8); 15 (pH 6.9); 22 (pH 9). LD$_{50}$ in rats (mg/kg): >5000 orally; >2000 dermally. LC$_{50}$ in rats (mg/l): >5 by inhalation. LC$_{50}$ (96 hr) in bluegill sunfish, rainbow trout (mg/l): >120, >120 (Wichert).

USE: Herbicide.

5913. Mesoxalic Acid. [473-90-5] Oxopropanedioic acid; ketomalonic acid; oxomalonic acid. $C_3H_2O_5$; mol wt 118.04. C 30.53%, H 1.71%, O 67.77%. HOOCCOCOOH. Occurs in *Medicago sativa* L., *Leguminosae;* has been found in beet molasses. Prepd by boiling a soln of alloxan and lead acetate: Deichsel, *J. Prakt. Chem.* [1] **93**, 194 (1864). By electrolysis of *d*-tartaric acid in alkaline soln: *Chem. Zentralbl.* **1922, III,** 871. Laboratory prepn from dibromomalonic acid: Conrad, Reinbach, *Ber.* **35**, 1819 (1902); from malonic ester and N_2O_3: Curtiss, *Am. Chem. J.* **35**, 477 (1906).

Monohydrate. Dihydroxymalonic acid. $C_3H_2O_5.H_2O$. Begins to melt at 113-114° and is clear at 121°. Very sol in water; sol in alc, ether.

Diethyl ester. Ethyl oxomalonate. $C_7H_{10}O_5$. Liquid. bp$_{19}$ 105-107°. d$_4^{15.6}$ 1.1419. n$_D^{15.6}$ 1.419. Prepn: A. W. Dox, *Org. Synth.* **coll. vol. I,** 266 (2nd ed., 1941). Diethyl ester of dihydroxy-malonic acid ($C_7H_{12}O_6$) is obtained from the crude ester mixture by fractional distn. Crystals, mp 57°. Sol in water, alcohol.

5914. Mesquite Gum. [9000-47-9] Sonora; Prosopis gum. Collected from small thorny trees abundant in the arid regions of the Western United States and as far south as Chile: *Prosopis juliflora* (Swartz) DC., *P. dulcis* Kunth., *P. horrida* Kunth., *P. inermis* H.B.K., *P. glandulosa* Torr., *P. pubescens* Benth., *P. spicigera* L., and other species of *Prosopis, Leguminosae.* Mesquite gum resembles acacia (gum arabic) in its physical and chemical characteristics. Review of structure work: F. Smith, R. Montgomery, *The Chemistry of Plant Gums and Mucilages* (Reinhold, New York, 1959) pp 175, 288-291.

USE: Substitute for acacia. Potential source of L-arabinose and D-glucuronic acid, *cf.* C. L. Mantell, *The Water-Soluble Gums* (Reinhold, New York, 1947) pp 72-73.

5915. Mestanolone. [521-11-9] (5α,17β)-17-Hydroxy-17-methylandrostan-3-one; 17β-hydroxy-17α-methyl-3-androstanone; 17α-methylandrostan-17β-ol-3-one; 17α-methylandrostan-3-on-17β-ol; Anabo; Antalone; Duramin; Mechiaron; Prohormo; Protenolon; Tantarone. $C_{20}H_{32}O_2$; mol wt 304.47. C 78.90%, H 10.59%, O 10.51%. Prepd by the oxidation of 17-methyl-3,17-androstanediol: Ruzicka *et al., Helv. Chim. Acta* **18**, 1487 (1935); **CH 208080** (1940 to Ciba).

Crystals from ethyl acetate, mp 192-193°. Insol in water. Sol in acetone, alcohol, ether, ethyl acetate.

Note: This is a controlled substance (anabolic steroid): **21 CFR,** 1308.13, as defined in 1300.01.

THERAP CAT: Anabolic.

5916. Mesterolone. [1424-00-6] (1α,5α,17β)-17-Hydroxy-1-methylandrostan-3-one; 1α-methyl-5α-androstan-17β-ol-3-one; 1α-methyl-5α-dihydrotestosterone; Androviron; Proviron; Mestoranum. $C_{20}H_{32}O_2$; mol wt 304.47. C 78.90%, H 10.59%, O 10.51%. Prepn of acetate: R. Wiechert, **DE 1122944** corresp to **US 3361773** (1962, 1968 to Schering, AG).

Crystals from ethyl acetate, mp 203.5-205.0°. [α]$_D^{20}$ +17.6° (c = 0.875 in CHCl$_3$).

Acetate. 17β-Acetoxy-1α-methyl-5α-androstan-3-one. C_{22}-$H_{34}O_3$. Crystals, mp 169-170°. [α]$_D^{25}$ +16.5° (c = 0.88 in CHCl$_3$).

Note: This is a controlled substance (anabolic steroid): **21 CFR,** 1308.13, as defined in 1300.01.

THERAP CAT: Androgen.

5917. Mestranol. [72-33-3] (17α)-3-Methoxy-19-norpregna-1,3,5(10)-trien-20-yn-17-ol; 17α-ethynyl-3-methoxy-1,3,5(10)-estratrien-17β-ol; 17α-ethynylestradiol 3-methyl ether; Menophase; Norquen; Ovastol. $C_{21}H_{26}O_2$; mol wt 310.43. C 81.25%, H 8.44%, O 10.31%. Orally active estrogenic steroid. Prepn: F. B. Colton, **US 2666769** (1954 to Searle); *J. Am. Chem. Soc.* **79**, 1123 (1957). Comprehensive description: H. A. El-Obeid, A. A. Al-Badr, *Anal. Profiles Drug Subs.* **11**, 375-406 (1982). Clinical pharmacokinetics: J. W. Goldzieher *et al., Contraception* **21**, 17 (1980). Effect on carbohydrate metabolism: W. N. Spellacy *et al., Metabolism* **31**, 106 (1982). Randomized, double-blind clinical trials: S. Koetsawang *et al., Contraception* **25**, 231 (1982); A. Sheth *et al., ibid.* 243. Evaluation of carcinogenic risk: *IARC Monographs* **21**, 257 (1979).

Crystals from methanol or acetone, mp 150-151°. uv max (methanol): 279, 287.5 nm ($E_{1cm}^{1\%}$ 82, 14.4). Sol in ethanol, ether, chloroform, dioxane, acetone. Slightly sol in methanol. Practically insol in water.

Note: Also used in combination with chlormadinone acetate, ethynodiol, lynestrenol, norethindrone or norethynodrel, *q.q.v.* Has been used in combination with megestrol acetate, *q.v.*

Caution: This substance is listed as a known human carcinogen: *Report on Carcinogens, Eleventh Edition* (PB2005-104914, 2004) p III-115.

THERAP CAT: Estrogen; in combination with progestogen as oral contraceptive.

5918. Mesulfen. [135-58-0] 2,7-Dimethylthianthrene; 2,6-dimethylthianthrene; 2,6-dimethyldiphenylene disulfide; mesulphen; Mitigal; Odylen; Sudermo; Peligal; Neosulfine. $C_{14}H_{12}S_2$; mol wt 244.38. C 68.81%, H 4.95%, S 26.24%. Prepn: Cohen, Skirrow, *J. Chem. Soc.* **75**, 890 (1899); Barber, Smiles, *ibid.* **1928**, 1149; Rumpf, *Bull. Soc. Chim. Fr.* **7**, 632 (1940).

Needles from acetic acid, ethyl acetate, or alcohol, mp 123°. bp₃ 184°; bp₁₄ 228-231°. Freely sol in acetone, chloroform, ether, petr ether; moderately sol in abs alcohol, ethyl acetate; practically insol in water.

THERAP CAT: Scabicide, antipruritic.
THERAP CAT (VET): Scabicide, antipruritic.

5919. Metachrome Yellow. [584-42-9] 2-Hydroxy-5-[(3-nitrophenyl)azo]benzoic acid monosodium salt; C.I. Mordant Yellow 1; C.I. 14025; alizarine yellow GG; salicyl yellow; sodium *m*-nitrobenzeneazosalicylate. $C_{13}H_8N_3NaO_5$; mol wt 309.21. C 50.50%, H 2.61%, N 13.59%, Na 7.44%, O 25.87%. Prepd from diazotized *m*-nitroaniline and salicylic acid in alkaline medium: R. Nietzki, *US 424019*; *Colour Index* **vol. 4** (3rd ed., 1971) p 4058.

Yellow powder. Slightly sol in cold water; more sol in hot water.
USE: Biological stain and acid-base indicator. pH: 10.2 colorless, 12.0 yellow.

5920. Metaclazepam. [84031-17-4] 7-Bromo-5-(2-chlorophenyl)-2,3-dihydro-2-(methoxymethyl)-1-methyl-1*H*-1,4-benzodiazepine; brometazepam; metuclazepam; Ka-2547; KC-2547. $C_{18}H_{18}BrClN_2O$; mol wt 393.71. C 54.91%, H 4.61%, Br 20.30%, Cl 9.00%, N 7.12%, O 4.06%. Benzodiazepine deriv with alkoxymethyl group replacing carbonyl in parent compd. Prepn: W. Milkowski *et al.*, **DE 2221558**; *eidem*, **US 4098786** (1973, 1978 both to Kali-Chemie). Effect on psychomotor performance and memory in volunteers: Z. Subhan, I. Hindmarch, *Drugs Exp. Clin. Res.* **9**, 567 (1983). Interaction with ethanol: H. R. Musch, M. Ruhland, *Arzneim.-Forsch.* **32**, 567 (1982); H. J. Mallach *et al.*, *Blutalkohol* **20**, 196 (1983); V. Schmidt *et al.*, *Med. Welt* **35**, 32 (1984). Clinical studies: G. Laakman *et al.*, *Arzneim.-Forsch.* **30**, 1233 (1980).

Hydrochloride. [61802-93-5] Talis. $C_{18}H_{18}BrClN_2O \cdot HCl$; mol wt 430.17. Crystals from ethanol, mp 193-196°. LD_{50} orally in NMRI white mice: 1578 mg/kg (Milkowski).
THERAP CAT: Anxiolytic.

5921. [2.2]Metacyclophane. [2319-97-3] Tricyclo-[9.3.1.1⁴,⁸]hexadeca-1(15),4,6,8(16),11,13-hexaene; di-*m*-xylylene; *m*-dixylylene. $C_{16}H_{16}$; mol wt 208.30. C 92.26%, H 7.74%. Prepd by the action of phenyllithium on *m*-xylene dibromide: Allinger *et al.*, *J. Am. Chem. Soc.* **83**, 1974 (1961); *eidem, J. Org. Chem.* **32**, 2272 (1967).

Orthorhombic prisms from ether, mp 132.5°. bp₇₆₀ 290°; bp₁₂ 170°. Sparingly sol in alc. More sol in ether, benzene.

5922. Metalaxyl. [57837-19-1] N-(2,6-Dimethylphenyl)-N-(methoxyacetyl)-DL-alanine methyl ester; methyl N-(2-methoxyacetyl)-N-(2,6-xylyl)-DL-alaninate; metaxanin; CGA-48988; Ridomil. $C_{15}H_{21}NO_4$; mol wt 279.33. C 64.50%, H 7.58%, N 5.01%, O 22.91%. Phenylamide fungicide for use in food crops, shrubs and turf. Prepn: A. Hubele, **DE 2515091**; *idem*, **US 4151299** (1975, 1979 to Ciba-Geigy). Comprehensive description: P. A. Urech, F. J. Schwinn, *Phytiatr.-Phytopharm.* **27**, 239-247 (1978). Antifungal spectrum: A. Kerkenaar, A. K. Sijpesteijn, *Pestic. Biochem. Physiol.* **15**, 71 (1981). Enzyme-linked immunosorbent assay of residues in foods: W. H. Newsome, *J. Agric. Food Chem.* **33**, 528 (1985).

Whitish crystals, mp 71-72°. Vapor pressure (20°): 2.2×10^{-6} mm Hg. Soly in water (20°): 7.1 g/l. Readily sol in most organic solvents. LD_{50} in rats (mg/kg): 669 orally (Urech).

R-form. [70630-17-0] N-(2,6-Dimethylphenyl)-N-(methoxyacetyl)-D-alanine methyl ester; (R)-[(2,6-dimethylphenyl)methoxyacetylamino]propionic acid methyl ester; metalaxyl-M; mefenoxam; CGA-329351; Apron; Ridomil Gold; Subdue. Enantioselective prepn: H.-U. Blaser, F. Spindler, *Top. Catal.* **4**, 275 (1997). Comprehensive description: C. Nuninger *et al.*, *Brighton Crop Prot. Conf. - Pests Dis.* **1996**, 41-46. Pale yellow to light brown viscous liquid. dec ~270°. Log P (n-octanol/water): 1.71. Soly in water (25°): 26 g/l.
USE: Agricultural fungicide.

5923. Metaldehyde. [9002-91-9] Metacetaldehyde. Polymer of acetaldehyde. $(C_2H_4O)_n$. Prepd by polymerization of acetaldehyde in the presence of HCl, H_2SO_4 at low temp: Kekule, Zincke, *Ann.* **162**, 125 (1872); in the presence of pyridine and HBr: R. S. Wilder, **US 2426961** (1947 to Publicker Ind.). Use as molluscicide: R. M. Coloso *et al.*, *Crop Prot.* **17**, 669 (1998).

Prisms, mp 246° in sealed tube. Sublimes at about 112°, but dec with partial regeneration of aldehyde above 80°. Practically insol in water. Sol in benzene, chloroform; sparingly sol in alcohol, ether.

Caution: Potential symptoms of overexposure by ingestion are severe abdominal pain, nausea, vomiting, diarrhea, convulsions, coma. *See Clinical Toxicology of Commercial Products*, R. E. Gosselin *et al.*, Eds. (Williams & Wilkins, Baltimore, 5th ed., 1984) p II-187.

USE: In compressed form as a fuel instead of alcohol; molluscicide.

5924. Metamitron. [41394-05-2] 4-Amino-3-methyl-6-phenyl-1,2,4-triazin-5(4*H*)-one; BAY DRW 1139; Goltix. $C_{10}H_{10}$-N_4O; mol wt 202.21. C 59.40%, H 4.98%, N 27.71%, O 7.91%. Prepn: K. Dickore *et al.*, **DE 2107757**; *eidem*, **US 3847914** (1972, 1974 both to Bayer); W. Draber *et al.*, *Ann.* **1976**, 2206. Chemistry and mode of action: *idem et al., Proc. 8th Int. Plant Prot. Congress* **1**, 203 (1975). Comprehensive description: H. Lembrich, *Pflanzenschutz-Nachr.* **31**, 197 (1978). Degradation in soil: R. Allen, A. Walker, *Pestic. Sci.* **18**, 95 (1987). HPLC determn in surface water: R. B. Geerdink, *J. Chromatogr.* **543**, 244 (1991).

Crystals from isopropanol/water, mp 169°. uv max (methanol): 312 nm (log ε 4.06). Vapor pressure (20-70°): $<1 \times 10^{-4}$ mbar. Soly (g/100g): water 0.18; isopropanol 0-1; methylene chloride 1-5; toluene 0-1; ligroin (80-110°) 0-1. Stable in acid media; rapidly decomp at pH >10. LD_{50} orally in male, female rats, male, female mice: 3343, 1832, 1450, 1463 mg/kg; dermally in rats: >500 mg/kg. LC_{50} (4 hr) in rats, mice, hamsters (mg/m^3): >331, >206, >206 by inhalation (Lembrich).

USE: Herbicide.

5925. Metampicillin. [6489-97-0] (2*S*,5*R*,6*R*)-3,3-Dimethyl-6-[[(2*R*)-(methyleneamino)phenylacetyl]amino]-7-oxo-4-thia-1-azabicyclo[3.2.0]heptane-2-carboxylic acid; D-6-[α-(methyleneamino)phenylacetamido]penicillanic acid; methampicillin; Bonopen; Fedacilina; Micinovo; Pravacilin; Ruticina; Suvipen; Viderpen. $C_{17}H_{19}N_3O_4S$; mol wt 361.42. C 56.49%, H 5.30%, N 11.63%, O 17.71%, S 8.87%. Semi-synthetic antibiotic related to penicillin. Prepn: **BE 661232**, *C.A.* **65**, 3884e (1966); Gradnik, **GB 1081093**, *C.A.* **68**, 114595g (1968) (1965, 1967 both to E.R.A.S.M.E.). Synthesis: Gradnik *et al., Farmaco Ed. Sci.* **26**, 20 (1971). Antibacterial activity studies: Sutherland *et al., Chemotherapy* **17**, 145 (1972). Pharmacokinetics: Fleischmann *et al., Farmaco Ed. Prat.* **26**, 106 (1971). Clinical studies: Farina, *Minerva Med.* **60**, 1999 (1969); Ginocchi, *ibid.* 2003; Cardinale, Arrotta, *ibid.* 2011.

Sodium salt. [6489-61-8] Ocelina; Magnipen; Venzoquimpe. $C_{17}H_{18}N_3NaO_4S$; mol wt 383.40.

THERAP CAT: Antibacterial.

5926. Metanephrine. [5001-33-2] 4-Hydroxy-3-methoxy-α-(methylaminomethyl)benzenemethanol; α-(methylaminomethyl)-vanillyl alcohol; 3-*O*-methylepinephrine; 3-*O*-methyladrenaline; 1-(4-hydroxy-3-methoxyphenyl)-2-methylaminoethanol. $C_{10}H_{15}$-NO_3; mol wt 197.23. C 60.90%, H 7.67%, N 7.10%, O 24.34%. A naturally occurring derivative of epinephrine, found in the urine and in certain tissues. Various methods of prepn: Külz, Hornung, **DE 682394** (1939); *Chem. Zentralbl.* **1940, I**, 1078, *C.A.* **36**, 3011 (1942); Axelrod *et al., J. Biol. Chem.* **233**, 697 (1958); Heacock, Hutzinger, *Chem. Ind. (London)* **1961**, 595.

dl-**Form hydrochloride.** $C_{10}H_{15}NO_3$·HCl. Prisms from ethanol + ether (also reported as crystals from dil acetone). Dec 175°. uv max (ethanol): 231, 280 nm (ε 7600, 3100).

5927. Metanilic Acid. [121-47-1] 3-Aminobenzenesulfonic acid; *m*-sulfanilic acid; aniline-*m*-sulfonic acid. $C_6H_7NO_3S$; mol wt 173.19. C 41.61%, H 4.07%, N 8.09%, O 27.71%, S 18.51%. Usually obtained by reduction of 3-nitrobenzenesulfonic acid: Fierz-David, Blangey, *Fundamental Processes of Dye Chemistry* (Interscience, New York, 1949) pp 120-123; A. I. Vogel, *Practical Organic Chemistry* (Longmans, London, 3rd ed., 1959) p 589. Large-scale process: *FIAT Final Rept.* **1313** (I), 187-191 (1948). The industrial reduction with iron filings and dil acid gives up to 90% yields, in the lab it seldom exceeds 55%. Better yields with small amounts are claimed for a hydrazine-Raney nickel reduction (about 75%): Gialdi *et al., Farmaco Ed. Sci.* **14**, 765 (1959) or by using WS$_2$ (about 94%): Ehrmann, **FR 1336648** (1963 to BASF), *C.A.* **60**, 2846d (1964).

Anhydrous, orthorhombic needles from water. d 1.69. Very slow crystn yields triclinic prisms of the sesquihydrate. Crystallographic data for both forms: Hall, Maslen, *Acta Crystallogr.* **18**, 301-306 (1965). Photomicrograph of the sesquihydrate: *Helv. Chim. Acta* **12** (1929), facing page 666. Both forms dec on heating without melting. pK (25°) 3.70. Soly of the sesquihydrate in water (16.8°): 2.37% (w/w). The soly of the anhydr form in water is given as 0.79% (w/w) at 0° and as 6.50% (w/w) at 85°. Sparingly sol in methanol, ethanol.

Sodium salt. $H_2NC_6H_4SO_3Na$. Minute crystals from water, dec 302-304°.

USE: The sodium salt in the manuf of azo dyes. In the synthesis of certain sulfa drugs.

5928. Metanil Yellow. [587-98-4] 3-[[4-(Phenylamino)-phenyl]azo]benzenesulfonic acid monosodium salt; C.I. Acid Yellow 36; *m*-[(*p*-anilinophenyl)azo]benzenesulfonic acid sodium salt; sodium salt of metanilylazodiphenylamine; Ext. D & C Yellow No. 1; C.I. 13065; Tropaeolin G. $C_{18}H_{14}N_3NaO_3S$; mol wt 375.38. C 57.59%, H 3.76%, N 11.19%, Na 6.12%, O 12.79%, S 8.54%. Prepn: Welcher, *Organic Analytical Reagents* **vol. 4** (Van Nostrand, 1948) p 516; *Colour Index* **vol. 4** (3rd ed., 1971) p 4045.

Brownish-yellow powder. Sol in water, alc; moderately sol in benzene, ether; slightly sol in acetone.

USE: As indicator in 0.1% soln, of which 2 drops are required for 10 ml liquid. pH: 1.2 red to 2.3 yellow.

5929. Metaphanine. [1805-86-3] (8β,10β)-8,10-Epoxy-8-hydroxy-3,4-dimethoxy-17-methylhasuban-7-one. $C_{19}H_{23}NO_5$; mol wt 345.39. C 66.07%, H 6.71%, N 4.06%, O 23.16%. A member of the hasubanan alkaloids; also possesses an intramolecular hemiketal ring. Isolated from stems of *Stephania japonica* Miers, *Menispermaceae* from which the alkaloids **stephanine** and protostephanine, *q.v.* are also obtained: Kondo, Sanada, *J. Pharm. Soc. Jpn.* **514**, 5 (1924); *Yakugaku Zasshi* **44**, 5, 1034 (1924); **48**, 177, 930 (1927); Kondo, Watanabe, *ibid.* **58**, 268 (1938). Structure and stereochemistry: Tomita *et al., Tetrahedron Lett.* **1964**, 3605; *Chem. Pharm. Bull.* **13**, 695 (1965). Synthesis of *dl*-form: Ibuka *et* *al., Tetrahedron Lett.* **1972,** 1393; *eidem, Chem. Pharm. Bull.* **22,** 907 (1974).

Needles, mp 232°. Also reported as colorless prisms, mp 205-206° for the *dl*-form (Ibuka). pKa 6.03. Sol in water, alcohol.

Dihydrometaphanine. $C_{19}H_{25}NO_5$. Cryst, mp 211°. $[\alpha]_D^{20}$ +72° (in chloroform). pKa 6.76.

5930. Metapramine. [21730-16-5] 10,11-Dihydro-*N*,5-dimethyl-5*H*-dibenz[*b,f*]azepin-10-amine; 10,11-dihydro-5-methyl-10-(methylamino)-5*H*-dibenz[*b,f*]azepine; RP-19560; Timaxel. $C_{16}H_{18}N_2$; mol wt 238.33. C 80.63%, H 7.61%, N 11.75%. Psychotropic agent, related structurally to imipramine, *q.v.* Prepn: J. C. Fouche, C. G. A. Gueremy, **ZA 6800345** corresp to **US 3622565** (1968, 1971 both to Rhone-Poulenc). Determn in plasma by GC: A. R. Viala *et al., Anal. Chem.* **49,** 2354 (1977). HPLC method: J. P. Sommadossi *et al., J. Chromatogr.* **228,** 205 (1982). Pharmacological and clinical effects: P. Dick, *Encephale* **4,** 41 (1978). Clinical studies: L. F. Gayral *et al., ibid.* 365; E. J. Caille, J.-P. Brun, *Psychol. Med.* **13,** 1879 (1981). Biotransformation in animals and man: B. Decouvelaere *et al., Therapie* **37,** 249 (1982).

Hydrochloride. $C_{16}H_{19}ClN_2$. Crystals from isopropanol + ether, mp 238-240°. Injectable formulation. The fumarate is used for tablet formulations.

THERAP CAT: Antidepressant.

5931. Metaproterenol. [586-06-1] 5-[1-Hydroxy-2-[(1-methylethyl)amino]ethyl]-1,3-benzenediol; 3,5-dihydroxy-α-[(iso-propylamino)methyl]benzyl alcohol; 1-(3,5-dihydroxyphenyl)-2-isopropylaminoethanol; 1-(3,5-dihydroxyphenyl)-1-hydroxy-2-iso-propylaminoethane; orciprenaline. $C_{11}H_{17}NO_3$; mol wt 211.26. C 62.54%, H 8.11%, N 6.63%, O 22.72%. Prepn and resolution of *d*- and *l*-forms: **BE 611502**; O. Thoma, K. Zeile, **US 3341594** (1961, 1967 both to Boehringer, Ing.). Pharmacology: H. H. Pelz, *Am. J. Med. Sci.* **253,** 321 (1967). Metabolism: K. Tatsumi *et al., Yakugaku Zasshi* **90,** 639 (1970); *ibid.* **91,** 680 (1971). Toxicity: E. I. Goldenthal, *Toxicol. Appl. Pharmacol.* **18,** 185 (1971). Review of clinical toxicology: J. D. Truwit, *Crit. Care Clin.* **7,** 639-657 (1991).

Crystals, mp 100°.

Sulfate. [5874-97-5] TH-152; Alotec; Alupent; Metaprel; No-vasmasol. $(C_{11}H_{17}NO_3)_2 \cdot H_2SO_4$; mol wt 520.59. Crystals from 90% ethanol, mp 202-203°. LD_{50} in rats (mg/kg): 42 orally (Goldenthal).

d-**Form hydrochloride.** Crystals, mp 212-213°. $[\alpha]_D$ +45.2° (c = 5 in methanol).

l-**Form hydrochloride.** Crystals, mp 212°. $[\alpha]_D$ −45°.

THERAP CAT: Bronchodilator.

5932. Metaraminol. [54-49-9] (α*R*)-α-[(1*S*)-1-Aminoethyl]-3-hydroxybenzenemethanol; (−)-α-(1-aminoethyl)-*m*-hydroxybenzyl alcohol; *m*-hydroxynorephedrine; *m*-hydroxypropadrine; *m*-hydroxyphenylpropanolamine; *m*-hydroxy-α-(1-aminoethyl)benzyl alcohol; 2-amino-1-(*m*-hydroxyphenyl)-1-propanol; 1-(*m*-hydroxyphenyl)-2-amino-1-propanol; α-(*m*-hydroxyphenyl)-β-aminopropanol; metadrine. $C_9H_{13}NO_2$; mol wt 167.21. C 64.65%, H 7.84%, N 8.38%, O 19.14%. Prepn from *m*-hydroxy-isonitrosopropiophenone: **GB 353361** (1930 to I. G. Farben); *l*-form: **GB 396951** (1932 to I. G. Farben); from *l*-*m*-hydroxyphenylacetylcarbinol: **CH 162367** (1931 to I. G. Farben); *see also* **US 1948162** and **US 1951302**; Hartung, **US 1995709** (1935 to Sharp & Dohme). Pharmacology: A. Cession-Fossion, *Arch. Int. Pharmacodyn. Ther.* **172,** 421 (1968). Toxicity data: O. H. Siegmund *et al., J. Pharmacol. Exp. Ther.* **92,** 207 (1948).

Bitartrate. [33402-03-8] Aramine; Araminon. $C_{13}H_{19}NO_8$; mol wt 317.29. Crystals, mp 176-177°. Freely sol in water. pH of 1% aq soln about 3.5.

Hydrochloride. [5967-52-2] $C_9H_{13}NO_2 \cdot HCl$. Hygroscopic crystals, $[\alpha]_D^{20}$ −19.75°. Freely sol in water. LD_{50} i.p. in mice: 440 mg/kg (Siegmund).

Oxalate dihydrate. [5967-53-3] $C_9H_{13}NO_2 \cdot C_2H_2O_4 \cdot 2H_2O$. Crystals, mp 190°. $[\alpha]_D^{20}$ −21.66°. Sol in water.

THERAP CAT: Adrenergic.

5933. Metazocine. [3734-52-9] 1,2,3,4,5,6-Hexahydro-3,6,11-trimethyl-2,6-methano-3-benzazocin-8-ol; 2'-hydroxy-2,5,9-trimethyl-6,7-benzomorphan; methobenzmorphan. $C_{15}H_{21}NO$; mol wt 231.33. C 77.88%, H 9.15%, N 6.05%, O 6.92%. Prepd from 3,4-lutidine methiodide: May, Fry, *J. Org. Chem.* **22,** 1366 (1957); May, Ager, *ibid.* **24,** 1432 (1959).

Plates from dil methanol, mp 232-235°.

Hydrochloride monohydrate. $C_{15}H_{21}NO \cdot HCl \cdot H_2O$. Rods from abs alcohol + ether, mp 194-196°.

Note: This is a controlled substance (opiate): **21 CFR**, 1308.12.

THERAP CAT: Analgesic (narcotic).

5934. Metconazole. [125116-23-6] 5-[(4-Chlorophenyl)-methyl]-2,2-dimethyl-1-(1*H*-1,2,4-triazol-1-ylmethyl)cyclopentanol; (1*RS*,5*RS*;1*RS*,5*SR*)-5-(4-chlorobenzyl)-2,2-dimethyl-1-(1*H*-1,2,4-triazol-1-ylmethyl)cyclopentanol; Caramba. $C_{17}H_{22}ClN_3O$; mol wt 319.83. C 63.84%, H 6.93%, Cl 11.08%, N 13.14%, O 5.00%. Broad spectrum triazole antifungal; mixture of two racemic diastereomers. Prepn: S. Kumazawa *et al.,* **EP 267778**; *eidem,* **US 4938792** (1987, 1990 both to Kureha); and structure activity study: A. Ito *et al., J. Pestic. Sci.* **24,** 262 (1999). Efficacy in wheat and barley: B. T. Grayson *et al., Pestic. Sci.* **45,** 153 (1995); A. J. Sampson *et al., ibid.* 161. Review: *idem et al., Brighton Crop Prot. Conf. - Pests Dis.* **1992,** 419-426.

cis-**Form.** [115850-27-6] WL-136184. Mixture of (1*R*,5*S*) and (1*S*,5*R*) isomers and is more bioactive than the *trans* form. Colorless crystals from hexane-ethyl acetate, mp 113-114°. Soly in water: 15 mg/kg.

trans-Form. [115850-28-7] mp 90-92°.

USE: Agricultural fungicide.

5935. Meteloidine. [526-13-6] [1α,3β(E),5α,6α,7α]-2-Methyl-2-butenoic acid 6,7-dihydroxy-8-methyl-8-azabicyclo-[3.2.1]oct-3-yl ester; (E)-1αH,5αH-tropane-3α,6β,7β-triol 3-(2-methylcrotonate); 3-(3,6,7-tropanetriol) tiglate; 6,7-dihydroxy-tropinetiglic acid ester; 6,7-dihydroxy-3-tiglyloxytropane. $C_{13}H_{21}$-NO_4; mol wt 255.31. C 61.16%, H 8.29%, N 5.49%, O 25.07%. From leaves of *Datura meteloides* DC., *Solanaceae:* Pyman, Reynolds, *J. Chem. Soc.* **93,** 2077 (1908); King, *ibid.* **115,** 487 (1919); from *D. ferox* L.: Evans, Wellendorf, *ibid.* **1959,** 1406. Stereochemistry: Heusner, *Z. Naturforsch.* **9b,** 683 (1954). Synthesis: Zeile, Heusner, *Arch. Pharm.* **292,** 238 (1959).

Flat needles from benzene, mp 141-142°. uv max: 217 nm (ε 12,200). Freely sol in alcohol, chloroform, acetone; sparingly sol in water, ether, benzene.

Hydrobromide dihydrate. $C_{13}H_{22}BrNO_4 \cdot 2H_2O$. Chisel-shaped needles, when anhydr, mp 250°.

5936. Metepa. [57-39-6] 1,1′,1″-Phosphinylidynetris[2-methylaziridine]; tris[2-methyl-1-aziridinyl]phosphine oxide; tris[1-methylethylene]phosphoric triamide; methyl aphoxide; methapoxide; MAPO; $C_9H_{18}N_3OP$; mol wt 215.23. C 50.22%, H 8.43%, N 19.52%, O 7.43%, P 14.39%. Prepd by treatment of 2-methylethyleneimine with $POCl_3$ in alk medium: Parke *et al., US 2606902* (1952 to Am. Cyanamid). Toxicity study: Gaines, *Toxicol. Appl. Pharmacol.* **14,** 515 (1969).

Liquid, bp 90-92° (0.15-0.3 mm). LD_{50} in male, female rats (mg/kg): 136, 213 orally (Gaines).

USE: Chemosterilant; in creaseproofing and flameproofing textiles.

5937. Metergoline. [17692-51-2] [[(8β)-1,6-Dimethyl-ergolin-8-yl]methyl]carbamic acid phenylmethyl ester; D-8β-[(car-bobenzoxyamino)methyl]-1,6-dimethyl-10α-ergoline; D-*N*-carbo-benzoxydihydro-1-methyllysergamine I; D-8β-[(carboxyamino)-methyl]-1,6-dimethylergoline I benzyl ester; D-*N*-carboxydihydro-1-methyllysergamine I benzyl ester; D-[(4,6,6a,7,8,9,10,10a-octahy-dro-4,7-dimethyl-10aα-indolo[4,3-*fg*]quinolin-9β-yl)methyl]-carbamic acid benzyl ester; methergoline; Liserdol; Contralac. C_{25}-$H_{29}N_3O_2$; mol wt 403.52. C 74.41%, H 7.24%, N 10.41%, O 7.93%. Serotonin 5HT-receptor antagonist. Prepn: Bernardi *et al., Gazz. Chim. Ital.* **94,** 936 (1964); Camerino *et al., US 3238211* (1966 to Farmitalia). Pharmacology: C. Beretta *et al., Nature* **207,** 421 (1965). Metabolic studies: Arcamone *et al., Boll. Chim. Farm.* **110,** 704 (1971). Mode of action study: L. Krulich *et al., Endocrinology* **108,** 1115 (1981). Clinical antiprolactin activity: F. Scapin *et al., Eur. J. Clin. Pharmacol.* **22,** 181 (1982); A. Caballero *et al., J. Reprod. Med.* **32,** 115 (1987).

Crystals from benzene + ether, mp 146-149°. $[\alpha]_D^{28}$ −7 ±2°. uv max: 291 nm ($E_{1cm}^{1\%}$ 165). Very sol in pyridine; sol in alc, acetone, chloroform. Practically insol in benzene, ether, water. LD_{50} in mice (mg/kg): 85 i.p., 430 orally; in rats (mg/kg): >800 orally (Beretta).

THERAP CAT: Prolactin inhibitor.

THERAP CAT (VET): Prolactin inhibitor.

5938. Metformin. [657-24-9] *N,N*-Dimethylimidodicar-bonimidic diamide; 1,1-dimethylbiguanide; *N,N*-dimethyldigua-nide; *N′*-dimethylguanylguanidine; DMGG; LA-6023. $C_4H_{11}N_5$; mol wt 129.16. C 37.20%, H 8.58%, N 54.22%. Oral hypoglycemic agent. Prepn: Werner, Bell, *J. Chem. Soc.* **121,** 1790 (1922); Shapiro *et al., J. Am. Chem. Soc.* **81,** 3728 (1959). Use as antidiabetic: J. J. Sterne, **US 3174901** (1965 to Jan Marcel Didier Aron-Samuel). Toxicity: *Rx Bulletin* **3,** 25 (1972). Determn in plasma: S. AbuRuz *et al., J. Chromatogr. B* **798,** 203 (2003). Clinical pharmacokinetics: G. T. Tucker *et al., Br. J. Clin. Pharmacol.* **12,** 235 (1981). Review of pharmacology: L. S. Hermann, *Diabete Metab.* **5,** 233-245 (1979). Metabolic effects and mechanism of action study: M. Stumvoll *et al., N. Engl. J. Med.* **333,** 550 (1995). Review of efficacy in polycystic ovary syndrome: J. M. Lord *et al., Br. Med. J.* **327,** 951-955 (2003); in type 2 diabetes mellitus: S. M. Setter *et al., Clin. Ther.* **25,** 2991-3026 (2003).

Hydrochloride. [1115-70-4] Debeone; Diabex; Glucophage; Metiguanide. $C_4H_{11}N_5 \cdot HCl$; mol wt 165.62. Prisms from water, mp 232° (Werner, Bell); crystals from propanol, mp 218-220° (uncorr) (Shapiro). Sol in water, 95% alcohol. Practically insol in ether, chloroform. LD_{50} in rats (mg/kg): 1000 orally, 300 s.c. (*Rx Bulletin*).

p-Chlorophenoxyacetate (salt). [25672-33-7] Glucinan. C_4-$H_{11}N_5 \cdot C_8H_7ClO_3$; mol wt 315.76.

Embonate. [34461-22-8] Metformin pamoate; Stagid. (C_4-$H_{11}N_5)_2 \cdot C_{23}H_{16}O_6$; mol wt 646.70.

THERAP CAT: Antidiabetic. In treatment of polycystic ovary syndrome.

5939. Methabenzthiazuron. [18691-97-9] *N*-2-Benzothia-zolyl-*N,N′*-dimethylurea; 1-(2-benzothiazolyl)-1,3-dimethylurea; metabenzthiazuron; MBU; Bayer 5633; Bayer 74283; Tribunil. $C_{10}H_{11}N_3OS$; mol wt 221.28. C 54.28%, H 5.01%, N 18.99%, O 7.23%, S 14.49%. Derivative of urea. Prepn and use as pre-emergence herbicide: N. E. Searle, **US 2756135** (1956 to du Pont). Use *et al., GB 1085430* (1967 to Bayer). Herbicidal properties: H. Hack, *Pflanzenschutz-Nachr.* **22,** 331 (1969). Toxicity studies: G. Kimmerle, E. Löser, *ibid.* 351. Use in winter cereals: D. C. Clark *et al., Proc. 12th Brit. Weed Control Conf.* 163 (1974). Mode of action: G. F. Collet, *Weed Res.* **9,** 340 (1969). Long-term effect on soil: P. L. Huge, *Pflanzenschutz-Nachr.* **34,** 97 (1981). Brief review: P. Lours, *Def. Veg.* **24,** 91 (1970).

White crystals from benzene, mp 119-120.5°. Soly in water at 20°: 59 ppm. Sol in organic solvents. Vapor pressure at 20°: $<10^{-6}$ mm Hg. LD_{50} in mice (mg/kg): >1000 orally; in male, female rats (mg/kg): >2500, >2500 orally; 540, 315 i.p. (Kimmerle, Löser).

USE: Selective herbicide.

5940. Methacholine Chloride. [62-51-1] 2-(Acetyloxy)-N,N,N-trimethyl-1-propanaminium chloride; acetyl-β-methylcholine chloride; O-acetyl-β-methylcholine chloride; (2-hydroxypropyl)trimethylammonium chloride acetate; (2-acetoxypropyl)trimethylammonium chloride; trimethyl-β-acetoxypropylammonium chloride; Amechol; Provocholine. $C_8H_{18}ClNO_2$; mol wt 195.69. C 49.10%, H 9.27%, Cl 18.12%, N 7.16%, O 16.35%. Parasympathomimetic bronchoconstrictor. Prepn: R. T. Major, J. K. Cline, **US 2040146** (1936 to Merck & Co.). Mechanism of ganglionic blockade in cats: R. L. Volle, *J. Pharmacol. Exp. Ther.* **158**, 66 (1967). Clinical diagnostic efficacy in bronchial asthma: S. L. Spector, R. S. Farr, *J. Allergy Clin. Immunol.* **56**, 308 (1975); J. G. Easton, I. Hirata, *Ann. Allergy* **50**, 171 (1983).

White, hygroscopic needles from ether, mp 172-173°. Slight odor of dead fish. Freely sol in water, alcohol, chloroform. Insol in ether. Aq solns are neutral to litmus. Should not be handled in very moist atmosphere. Bromide is less hygroscopic.

Antidote: Atropine.

THERAP CAT: Cholinergic. Diagnostic aid (bronchial asthma).

5941. Methacrylic Acid. [79-41-4] 2-Methyl-2-propenoic acid; α-methylacrylic acid. $C_4H_6O_2$; mol wt 86.09. C 55.81%, H 7.02%, O 37.17%. Occurs in oil from Roman chamomile. Prepd by dehydration of α-hydroxyisobutyric acid: Crawford, **US 2143941** (1939 to I.C.I.); by hypochlorite oxidation of methyl α-alkylvinyl ketone: Meitzner, **US 2192142** (1940 to Rohm & Haas); by hydrolysis of acetone cyanohydrin: Crawford, **GB 405699** (1932 to I.C.I.); by oxidation of methacrolein: Bauer, **US 2153406** (1939 to Rohm & Haas). Toxicity study: W. Deichmann, *J. Ind. Hyg. Toxicol.* **23**, 343 (1941). *Review:* J. W. Nemec, L. S. Kirch in *Kirk-Othmer Encyclopedia of Chemical Technology* **vol. 15** (Wiley-Interscience, New York, 3rd ed., 1981) pp 346-376.

Long prisms, mp 16°, forming a corrosive liquid. Acrid, repulsive odor. d_4^{20} 1.0153. bp_{760} 163°; bp_{30} 81°; bp_{12} 63°. n_D^{20} 1.43143. Flash pt, open cup: 170°F (76°C). Sol in warm water; miscible with alc, ether. Polymerizes easily, especially on heating or in the presence of traces of HCl. The polymer forms a ceramic-looking mass, sol in abs alc, from which it is precipitated by ether.

Methyl ester. [80-62-6] Methyl methacrylate. Review of carcinogenic risk: *IARC Monographs* **60**, 445-474 (1994). Polymerizes easily, forming a clear plastic known as *Lucite*, *Plexiglas*, *Perspex*. Sol in methyl ethyl ketone, tetrahydrofuran, esters, aromatic and chlorinated hydrocarbons. LD_{50} orally in rats: 8.4 g/kg (Deichmann).

Caution: Potential symptoms of overexposure to methacrylic acid or methyl methacrylate are irritation of eyes, skin, nose, throat, mucous membranes; dermatitis; eye and skin burns. *See NIOSH Pocket Guide to Chemical Hazards* (DHHS/NIOSH 97-140, 1997) pp 194, 214.

USE: In the manuf of methacrylate resins and plastics.

5942. Methacrylonitrile. [126-98-7] 2-Methyl-2-propenenitrile; isopropenylnitrile; α-methylacrylonitrile; isopropene cya-

nide. C_4H_5N; mol wt 67.09. C 71.61%, H 7.51%, N 20.88%. $CH_2=C(CH_3)C\equiv N$. Prepd by vapor-phase catalytic oxidation of methallylamine: Peters *et al.*, *Ind. Eng. Chem.* **40**, 2046 (1948); **US 2375016** (1945 to Shell); by the dehydration of methacrylamide: Kung, **US 2373190** (1945 to Goodrich); from isopropylene oxide and ammonia: Spillane, Kayser, **US 2557703** (1951 to Allied Chem.). Toxicity study: Smyth *et al.*, *Am. Ind. Hyg. Assoc. J.* **23**, 95 (1962).

Liquid. d_4^{20} 0.8001; d_4^{30} 0.7896. mp $-35.8°$. bp_{760} 90.3°. n_D^{20} 1.4007; n_D^{30} 1.3954. Flash pt, open cup: 55°F (13°C). Viscosity (20°): 0.392 cP. Surface tension at 20°, 24.4 dynes/cm. Soly in water at 20° = 2.57 wt-%, at 50° = 2.69 wt-%. Soly of water in methacrylonitrile at 20° = 1.62 wt-%, at 50° = 2.83 wt-%. Misc with acetone, octane, toluene at 20-25°. LD_{50} orally in rats: 0.25 ml/kg (Smyth).

Caution: Potential symptoms of overexposure are irritation of eyes, skin; lacrimation. *See NIOSH Pocket Guide to Chemical Hazards* (DHHS/NIOSH 97-140, 1997) p 198.

USE: In prepn of homopolymers and copolymers; as an intermediate in the prepn of acids, amides, amines, esters, nitriles.

5943. Methacycline. [914-00-1] [4S-(4α,4aα,5α,5aα,-12aα)]-4-Dimethylamino-1,4,4a,5,5a,6,11,12a-octahydro-3,5,10,-12,12a-pentahydroxy-6-methylene-1,11-dioxo-2-naphthacenecarboxamide; 6-methyleneoxytetracycline; 6-methylene-5-hydroxytetracycline; metacycline. $C_{22}H_{22}N_2O_8$; mol wt 442.42. C 59.73%, H 5.01%, N 6.33%, O 28.93%. Broad spectrum, semisynthetic antibiotic related to tetracycline, *q.v.* Prepn from oxytetracycline, *q.v.:* R. K. Blackwood *et al.*, **US 2984686** (1961 to Pfizer); *eidem, J. Am. Chem. Soc.* **83**, 2773 (1961); **85**, 3943 (1963). Solubility data: J. R. Marsh, P. J. Weiss, *J. Assoc. Off. Anal. Chem.* **50**, 257 (1967). Toxicity data: E. I. Goldenthal, *Toxicol. Appl. Pharmacol.* **18**, 185 (1971). Comparative clinical study with ampicillin, *q.v.*, in chronic bronchitis: S. Chodosh *et al.*, *Chest* **69**, 587 (1976).

Hydrochloride. [3963-95-9] Adriamicina; Ciclobiotic; Germiciclin; Metadomus; Metilenbiotic; Londomycin; Optimycin; Physiomycine; Rindex; Rondomycin. $C_{22}H_{22}N_2O_8\cdot HCl$; mol wt 478.88. Obtained as crystals containing 0.5 mol water and 0.5 mol methanol from methanol + acetone + concd HCl + ether. Yellow, crystalline powder, dec $\sim$205°. Bitter taste. Soluble in water, sparingly sol in alcohol. Practically insol in ether, chloroform. uv max (methanol + 0.01N HCl): 253, 345 nm (log ε 4.37, 4.19). LD_{50} in rats, mice (mg/kg): 252, 288 i.p. (Goldenthal).

THERAP CAT: Antibacterial.

5944. Methadone. [76-99-3] 6-Dimethylamino-4,4-diphenyl-3-heptanone; 1,1-diphenyl-1-(2-dimethylaminopropyl)-2-butanone; 4,4-diphenyl-6-dimethylamino-3-heptanone. $C_{21}H_{27}NO$; mol wt 309.45. C 81.51%, H 8.79%, N 4.53%, O 5.17%. Prepn: Eisleb, *Office of Publication Board, Department of Commerce* **Report no. PB-981**, 96A; Schultz *et al.*, *J. Am. Chem. Soc.* **69**, 2454 (1947); Easton *et al.*, *ibid.* 2941 (1947). Resolution: Larsen *et al.*, *ibid.* **70**, 4194 (1948); Howe, Sletzinger, *ibid.* **71**, 2935 (1949); Brode, Hill, *J. Org. Chem.* **13**, 191 (1948); Howe, Tishler, **US 2644010** (1953 to Merck & Co.); Zaugg, **US 2983757** (1961 to Abbott). Pharmacokinetics in patients with chronic pain: C. E. Inturrisi *et al.*, *Clin. Pharmacol. Ther.* **41**, 392 (1987). Toxicity data: Finnegan *et al.*, *J. Pharmacol. Exp. Ther.* **92**, 269 (1948); Winter, Flataker, *ibid.* **98**, 305 (1950). *Review:* Eddy, *J. Am. Pharm. Assoc. Pract. Pharm. Ed.* **8**, 536 (1947). Comprehensive description: R. H. Bishara, *Anal. Profiles Drug Subs.* **3**, 365-439 (1974). Review of use in opioid dependence: E. C. Senay, *Int. J. Addict.* **20**, 803-821 (1985). Clinical trial of methadone maintenance vs long-term detoxification: K. L. Sees *et al.*, *J. Am. Med. Assoc.* **283**, 1303 (2000).

mp 78°; pptd from solns of pH >6.

Hydrochloride. [1095-90-5] AN-148; Hoechst 10820; Depridol; Dolophine; Fenadone; Heptadon; Heptanon; Ketalgin; Mephenon; Methadose; Physeptone. Platelets from alcohol + ether, mp 235°. Bitter taste. uv max: 292 nm. Soly (g/100 ml): water 12; alcohol 8; isopropanol 2.4. Practically insol in ether, glycerol. The pH of a 1% aq soln: 4.5-5.6. LD$_{50}$ orally in rats: 95 mg/kg (Finnegan).

***l*-Form Hydrochloride.** [5967-73-7] Levomethadone hydrochloride; L-Polamidon. Crystals, mp 241°. $[\alpha]_D^{20}$ −145° (c = 2.5); $[\alpha]_D^{20}$ −169° (c = 2.1 in alc). LD$_{50}$ s.c. in rats: 44 mg/kg (Winter, Flataker).

Note: This is a controlled substance (opiate): **21 CFR**, 1308.12.

THERAP CAT: Analgesic (narcotic); in treatment of opioid dependence.

5945. Methadyl Acetate. [509-74-0] β-[2-(Dimethylamino)propyl]-α-ethyl-β-phenylbenzeneethanol acetate (ester); 6-(dimethylamino)-4,4-diphenyl-3-heptanol acetate (ester); O-acetyl-6-dimethylamino-4,4-diphenyl-3-heptanol; 3-acetoxy-6-dimethylamino-4,4-diphenylheptane; 5-acetoxy-2-dimethylamino-4,4-diphenylheptane; acetylmethadol; acemethadone; amidolacetate; race-acetylmethadol. C$_{23}$H$_{31}$NO$_2$; mol wt 353.50. C 78.15%, H 8.84%, N 3.96%, O 9.05%. Congener of methadone, *q.v.* Prepn of β-*dl*-form: M. Bockmühl, G. Ehrhart, *Ann.* **561**, 52 (1948); of α-*dl*-form: M. E. Speeter *et al., J. Am. Chem. Soc.* **71**, 57 (1949); R. L. Clark, **US 2565592**; **US 2668814** (1951, 1954 to Merck & Co.); M. E. Speeter, **US 2649445** (1953 to Bristol); of α-*d* and α-*l*-forms: A. Pohland *et al., J. Am. Chem. Soc.* **71**, 460 (1949). The α-*dl*-form is more active and less toxic than the β-*dl*-form. The α-*l*-form, levomethadyl acetate, *q.v.* is less active than the α-*d*-form but is longer acting. Metabolism of the α-*dl*-form: R. E. McMahon *et al., J. Pharmacol. Exp. Ther.* **149**, 436 (1965). Analgesic, depressant activity of α-*dl*-form in mice, rats: N. B. Eddy *et al., ibid.* **98**, 121 (1950); of enantiomers: N. B. Eddy *et al., J. Org. Chem.* **17**, 321 (1952). Comparison of methadone with α-*dl*-form in the treatment of heroin addiction: J. H. Jaffe *et al., J. Am. Med. Assoc.* **211**, 1834 (1970).

α-*dl*-Form hydrochloride. C$_{23}$H$_{32}$ClNO$_2$. Crystals from ethyl acetate, mp 213-214°. Sol in water. pH 4-5. LD$_{50}$ in mice (mg/kg): 61.0 s.c., 118.3 orally (Eddy, 1952).

α-*dl*-Form hydrobromide. C$_{23}$H$_{32}$BrNO$_2$. Crystals, mp 193-194.5°. Sol in water.

α-*d*-Form. Alphacetylmethadol.

α-*d*-Form hydrochloride. Crystals from ethanol-ether, mp 215°. $[\alpha]_D^{25}$ +61.2° (c = 0.2). Sol in water. LD$_{50}$ in mice (mg/kg): 72.2 s.c., 130.4 orally (Eddy, 1952).

α-*l*-Form *see* Levomethadyl Acetate.

β-*l*-Form. Betacetylmethadol.

β-*dl*-Form hydrochloride. Crystals, mp 215-217°. Sol in water. LD$_{50}$ in mice (mg/kg): 42.0 s.c., 80.2 orally (Eddy, 1952).

Note: This is a controlled substance (opiate): **21 CFR**, 1308.11.

5946. Methallibure. [926-93-2] N-Methyl-N'-(1-methyl-2-propenyl)-1,2-hydrazinedicarbothioamide; 1-methyl-6-(1-methyl-

allyl)-2,5-dithiobiurea; N-methylthiocarbamoyl-N'-[(1-methylallyl)thiocarbamoyl]hydrazine; metallibure; ICI-33828; Aimax. C$_7$H$_{14}$N$_4$S$_2$; mol wt 218.34. C 38.51%, H 6.46%, N 25.66%, S 29.37%. Prepn: Paget *et al.,* **GB 878177** (1961 to I.C.I.). Inhibition of pituitary gonadotropic function in animals: Paget *et al., Nature* **192**, 1191 (1961). Prevention of fetus nidation when given orally to rats: Harper, *J. Reprod. Fertil.* **7**, 211 (1964).

Crystals, dec 198-200°.

THERAP CAT (VET): Anterior pituitary activator (for swine).

5947. Methamidophos. [10265-92-6] Phosphoramidothioic acid O,S-dimethyl ester; O,S-dimethyl phosphoramidothioate; Bayer 71628; ENT-27396; Ortho 9006; SRA-5172; Monitor; Tamaron. C$_2$H$_8$NO$_2$PS; mol wt 141.13. C 17.02%, H 5.71%, N 9.92%, O 22.67%, P 21.95%, S 22.72%. Prepn: W. Lorenz *et al.,* **BE 666143** (1965 to Bayer), *C.A.* **65**, 16864f (1966); **NL 6602588**; P. S. Magee, **US 3309266** (both 1967 to Chevron). Activity: I. Hammann, *Pflanzenschutz-Nachr.* **23**, 140 (1970). Acute toxicity: T. B. Gaines, R. E. Linder, *Fundam. Appl. Toxicol.* **7**, 299 (1986). Review of properties and metabolism: A. M. A. Khasawinah *et al., Pestic. Biochem. Physiol.* **9**, 211-221 (1978).

Crystals from ether, mp 54°. n_D^{40} 1.5092; d$^{44.5}$ 1.31. Vapor pressure at 30°: 3×10^{-4} mm Hg. Readily sol in water, ethanol. LD$_{50}$ in adult male, female rats (mg/kg): 25, 27 orally (Gaines, Linder).

USE: Insecticide; acaricide.

5948. Methamphetamine. [537-46-2] (αS)-N,α-Dimethylbenzeneethanamine; (S)-(+)-N,α-dimethylphenethylamine; *d*-N-methylamphetamine; *d*-deoxyephedrine; *d*-desoxyephedrine; 1-phenyl-2-methylaminopropane; *d*-phenylisopropylmethylamine; methyl-β-phenylisopropylamine; Norodin. C$_{10}$H$_{15}$N; mol wt 149.23. C 80.48%, H 10.13%, N 9.39%. Central stimulant. Can be prepd by reducing ephedrine or pseudoephedrine: Emde, *Helv. Chim. Acta* **12**, 365 (1929). Prepn by reducing the condensation product of benzyl methyl ketone and methylamine: A. Ogata, *J. Pharm. Soc. Jpn.* **451**, 751 (1919), *C.A.* **14**, 745 (1920). Synthesis from D-phenylalanine: D. B. Repke *et al., J. Pharm. Sci.* **67**, 1167 (1978). Stereochemistry-pharmacology aspects: Patil *et al., J. Pharmacol. Exp. Ther.* **155**, 1, 13 (1967). Toxicity data: A. M. Lands *et al., J. Pharmacol. Exp. Ther.* **89**, 382 (1947). Review of clinical trials in bulimia: H. G. Pope, Jr., J. I. Hudson, *J. Clin. Psychiatry* **47**, 339 (1986). Review of pharmacology and abuse potential: A. K. Cho, *Science* **249**, 631-634 (1990).

Hydrochloride. [51-57-0] "Speed"; "meth"; "ice"; Amphedroxyn; Desfedrin; Desoxyfed; Desoxyn; Destim; Doxephrin; Drinalfa; Gerobit; Hiropon; Isophen; Madrine; Methampex; Methedrine; Methylisomyn; Pervitin; Soxysympamine; Syndrox; Tonedron. C$_{10}$H$_{15}$N.HCl; mol wt 185.69. Crystals, mp 170-175°. Bitter taste. $[\alpha]_D^{25}$ +14 to +20°. Sol in water, alcohol, chloroform. Practically insol in ether. A 1% aq soln is neutral or slightly acid to litmus. LD$_{50}$ i.p. in mice: 70 mg/kg (Lands).

Note: This is a controlled substance (stimulant): **21 CFR**, 1308.12.

THERAP CAT: Anorexic. In attention deficit disorder with hyperactivity.

THERAP CAT (VET): Sympathomimetic, CNS stimulant.

5949. Metham Sodium. [137-42-8] Methylcarbamodithioic acid sodium salt; methyldithiocarbamic acid sodium salt; *N*-methylaminodithioformic acid sodium salt; sodium *N*-methylaminomethanethionothiolate; metam sodium; SMDC; carbathione; trimaton; VPM. $C_2H_4NNaS_2$; mol wt 129.18. C 18.60%, H 3.12%, N 10.84%, Na 17.80%, S 49.64%. $CH_3NHCSSNa$. Prepn: Compin, *Bull. Soc. Chim. Fr.* [4] **27**, 464 (1920). Use as soil fumigant: S. C. Dorman, A. B. Lindquist, US 2766554 (1956 to Stauffer). Conversion to methyl isothiocyanate, *q.v.*, in soil: N. J. Turner, M. E. Corden, *Phytopathology* **53**, 1388 (1963); J. H. Smelt, M. Leistra, *Pestic. Sci.* **5**, 401 (1974). Field study: J. A. Bunt, *Meded. Fac. Landbouwwet. Rijksuniv. Gent* **42**, 1529 (1977); L. P. Moreno *et al.*, *Tests of Agrochemicals and Cultivars* No. 17, (*Ann. Appl. Biol.* **128** Supplement), pp 6-13 (1996). Determn of efficacy: J. Krikun, *Can. J. Plant Pathol.* **8**, 345 (1986).

Dihydrate. N-869; Maposol; Sistan; Vapam. Crystals, anhydr at 130°. Unpleasant odor, similar to that of carbon disulfide. Nonflammable. Soly in water at 20°: 72.2 g/100 ml H_2O. Moderately sol in alc. Sparingly sol in other solvents. Concd aq solns are stable.

Caution: Irritating to skin, mucous membranes: *Clinical Toxicology of Commercial Products*, R.E. Gosselin *et al.*, Eds. (Williams & Wilkins, Baltimore, 5th ed., 1984) Section II, pp 312.

USE: Soil fumigant to control weeds and weed seeds, nematodes, fungi, and soil insects.

5950. Methandriol. [521-10-8] ($3\beta,17\beta$)-17-Methylandrost-5-ene-3,17-diol; methylandrostenediol; MAD; mestenediol; Masdiol; Metocryst; Metildiolo; Androdiol; Metidione; Nabadial; Neosteron; Diolandrone; Stenediol; Neostene; Crestabolic; Diolostene; Metendiol; Metandiol; Methandiol; Methanabol; Methostan; Neutrormone; Neutrosteron; Androteston-M; Megabion (Japanese); Notandron. $C_{20}H_{32}O_2$; mol wt 304.47. C 78.90%, H 10.59%, O 10.51%. Prepd by the action of methylmagnesium iodide on 3β-hydroxy-5-androsten-17-one, also called 5,6-dehydroandrosterone: Ruzicka *et al.*, *Helv. Chim. Acta* **18**, 1487 (1935); Miescher, Klarer, *ibid.* **22**, 962 (1939). Absorption spectrum in H_2SO_4: Bernstein, Lenhard, *J. Org. Chem.* **18**, 1153 (1953). NMR: Hampel, Kraemer, *Tetrahedron* **22**, 1601 (1966).

Crystals from ethyl acetate, mp 205.5-206.5°. $[\alpha]_D^{20}$ −73° (alc). Insol in water. Slightly sol in some organic solvents.

Diacetate. [2061-86-1] $C_{24}H_{36}O_4$. Crystals from hexane, mp 145-146°. $[\alpha]_D^{21}$ −59° (c = 0.984 in alc).

Dipropionate. [3593-85-9] Probolin. $C_{26}H_{40}O_4$; mol wt 416.59.

Note: This is a controlled substance (anabolic steroid): **21 CFR**, 1308.13, as defined in 1300.01.

THERAP CAT: Anabolic.

5951. Methandrostenolone. [72-63-9] (17β)-17-Hydroxy-17-methylandrosta-1,4-dien-3-one; 17α-methyl-17β-hydroxyandrosta-1,4-dien-3-one; 1-dehydro-17α-methyltestosterone; methandienone; Danabol; Nerobol; Nabolin; Stenolon; Dianabol. $C_{20}H_{28}O_2$; mol wt 300.44. C 79.95%, H 9.39%, O 10.65%. Anabolic steroid. Prepn by microbial dehydrogenation of 17α-methyltestosterone: Vischer *et al.*, *Helv. Chim. Acta* **38**, 1502 (1955); by reduction of 17α-methyltestosterone with selenium dioxide: Meystre *et al.*, *ibid.* **39**, 734 (1956); Wettstein *et al.*, US 2900398 (1959 to Ciba).

Crystals from acetone + ether. mp 163-164°. uv max: 245 nm (ϵ 15600).

Note: This is a controlled substance (anabolic steroid): **21 CFR**, 1308.13, as defined in 1300.01.

THERAP CAT: Androgen.

THERAP CAT (VET): Anabolic.

5952. Methane. [74-82-8] Marsh gas; methyl hydride. CH_4; mol wt 16.04. C 74.88%, H 25.14%. Widely distributed in nature. American natural gas is about 85% methane. The earth's atm contains 0.00022% by vol. Major constituent of the atm of the outer planets (Jupiter, Saturn, Uranus, Neptune), exact figures in *Landolt-Börnstein* vol. **III** (Springer, 6th ed., 1952) p 59; G. P. Kuiper, *The Atmospheres of the Earth and the Planets* (University of Chicago Press, 1949). Pure carbon combines directly with pure hydrogen at temperatures above 1100° forming methane. Above 1500° amount of methane formed increases with temperature: Pring, *J. Chem. Soc.* **97**, 498 (1910). Can be prepd from sodium acetate and sodium hydroxide, or from aluminum carbide and water: Matthews, *J. Am. Chem. Soc.* **21**, 647 (1899); Carroll, *J. Phys. Chem.* **22**, 148 (1918). Prepd commercially from natural gas or by fermentation of cellulose and sewage sludge: Cost, US 2583090 (1952 to Elliott Co.); Le Paige, de Dommartin, FR 994032 (1951), *C.A.* **51**, 10836i (1957); Oswald, Golueke, *Mech. Eng.* **86**, 40 (1964).

Colorless, odorless, non-poisonous, flammable gas. Burns with a pale, faintly luminous flame. d_4^0 0.554 (air = 1) or 0.7168 g/liter. mp −182.6°. bp −161.4°. Crit temp −82.25°; crit pressure 45.8 atm. Heat of combustion 978 Btu/cu ft at 25° (a kilogram of CH_4 yields 13,300 kcal). Forms exposive mixtures with air, the loudest explosions occur when one vol of methane is mixed with 10 vols of air (or 2 vols of oxygen). Air contg less than 5.53% methane no longer explodes. Air contg more than 14% methane burns without noise. Autoignition temp 650°. Soly in water at 17°: 3.5 ml/100 ml H_2O. Sol in alc, ether, other organic solvents.

Caution: Simple asphyxiant.

USE: Constituent of illuminating and cooking gas, in the manuf of hydrogen, hydrogen cyanide, ammonia, acetylene, formaldehyde, in organic syntheses.

5953. Methanearsonic Acid. [124-58-3] Methylarsonic acid; methylarsinic acid; monomethylarsinic acid. CH_5AsO_3; mol wt 139.97. C 8.58%, H 3.60%, As 53.53%, O 34.29%. CH_3-$AsO(OH)_2$. Prepd from sodium arsenite and methyl iodide: Quick, Adams, *J. Am. Chem. Soc.* **44**, 809 (1922). The disodium salt is easily prepd by treating sodium arsenite with dimethyl sulfate at 85°: Uhlinger, Cook, *Ind. Eng. Chem.* **11**, 105 (1919). Other routes are by the reaction of methyl chloride with sodium arsonate under pressure: Miller *et al.*, US 2442372 (1948); by the reaction of dimethyl sulfate with a solution of arsenic trioxide in sodium hydroxide: Schwerdle, US 2889347 (1959). Acute toxicity: T. B. Gaines, R. E. Linder, *Fundam. Appl. Toxicol.* **7**, 299 (1986). Review of toxicology and human exposure: *Toxicological Profile for Arsenic* (PB2000-108021, 2000) 468 pp.

Monoclinic, spear-shaped plates from abs alcohol. Pleasant acid taste. mp 161°. Strong dibasic acid. Freely sol in water; sol in alcohol.

Monosodium salt. Monosodium methanearsonate; MSMA; Ansar 6.6; Bueno; Daconate; Weed Hoe. CH_4AsNaO_3; mol wt 161.95. LD_{50} in adult male, female rats (mg/kg): 1105, 1059 orally (Gaines, Linder).

Disodium salt. Disodium monomethanearsonate; DSMA; Ansar 8100; Arrhenal; Arsinyl; Clout; Crab-E-Rad; Dal-E-Rad; Sodar. $CH_3AsNa_2O_3$; mol wt 183.93. Hydrated crystals contg $5H_2O$ or $6H_2O$. One gram dissolves in about one ml water; slightly sol in alcohol. LD_{50} in adult male, female rats (mg/kg): 928, 821 orally (Gaines, Linder).

USE: Herbicide.

5954. Methanesulfonic Acid. [75-75-2] Methylsulfonic acid. CH_4O_3S; mol wt 96.11. C 12.50%, H 4.19%, O 49.94%, S 33.36%. CH_3SO_2OH. Prepd from sulfur trioxide and methane: Snyder, Grosse, US 2493038 (1950 to Houdry Process); by oxidation of dimethyl disulfide: Johnson, Wolff, US 2697722 (1954 to Standard Oil of Indiana); Proell *et al.*, *Ind. Eng. Chem.* **40**, 1129 (1948). Other prepns and chemistry: Suter, *The Organic Chemistry of Sulfur* (Wiley, New York, 1944).

Solid. d_4^{18} 1.4812. mp 20°. bp$_{10}$ 167°; bp$_1$ 122°. Soly at 26-28° in wt %: hexane, 0; methylcyclopentane, 0; benzene, 1.50; toluene, 0.38; o-chlorotoluene, 0.23; ethyl disulfide, 0.47. Thermally stable at moderately elevated temps. Not hydrolyzed by boiling water or hot aq alkali. Corrosive to iron, steel, brass, copper, lead.

Ethyl ester *see* Ethyl Methanesulfonate.
Methyl ester *see* Methyl Methanesulfonate.
Caution: Strong irritant.
USE: As catalyst in polymerization, alkylation and esterification reactions; as a solvent.

5955. Methanesulfonyl Chloride. [124-63-0] Mesyl chloride. CH$_3$ClO$_2$S; mol wt 114.55. C 10.49%, H 2.64%, Cl 30.95%, O 27.93%, S 27.99%. CH$_3$SO$_2$Cl. Reagent used in solution with pyridine to introduce mesyl groups in organic synthesis. Prepn: L. Carius, *Ann.* **114**, 140 (1860); T. B. Johnson, J. M. Sprague, *J. Am. Chem. Soc.* **58**, 1348 (1936); C. R. Noller, P. J. Hearst, *ibid.* **70**, 3955 (1948). Environmentally-friendly synthesis: S. Mukhopadhyay *et al., Chem. Commun.* **2004**, 472. Thermodynamics: J. P. Guthrie *et al., Can. J. Chem.* **76**, 929 (1998). Synthetic applications: J. H. Looker, *J. Org. Chem.* **17**, 510 (1952); W. E. Truce, C. W. Vriesen, *J. Am. Chem. Soc.* **75**, 5032 (1953); Y. Morimoto *et al., Chem. Lett.* **1998**, 829; P. A. Jacobi, E. H. Sessions, Jr., *Synth. Commun.* **33**, 2575 (2003).
Liquid. d_4^{18} 1.4805. bp$_{730}$ 161°; bp$_{21}$ 60°. n_D^{23} 1.451. Practically insol in water; sol in alcohol, ether.
USE: In the synthesis of photographic and agricultural chemicals, pharmaceutical intermediates. As a stabilizer; catalyst; curing and chlorinating agent; precursor to methanesulfonic acid.

5956. Methanethiol. [74-93-1] Methyl mercaptan; mercaptomethane; thiomethyl alcohol; methyl sulfhydrate. CH$_4$S; mol wt 48.11. C 24.97%, H 8.38%, S 66.65%. CH$_3$SH. Occurs in "sour" gas of W. Texas, in coal tar, and in petroleum distillates. Isolated from roots of *Raphanus sativus*. Produced in the intestinal tract by the action of anaerobic bacteria on albumin. Evolved from *Penicillium brevicaule* bread cultures containing disulfides. Prepn from sodium methyl sulfate and KHS: Klason, *Ber.* **20**, 3409 (1887); Arndt, *ibid.* **54**, 2236 (1921); catalytically from methanol and hydrogen sulfide: Kramer, Reid, *J. Am. Chem. Soc.* **43**, 880 (1921); from methyl chloride and sodium hydrosulfide: Scott *et al., Ind. Eng. Chem.* **47**, 876 (1955). Review of occurrence, preparation, properties and reactions: E. E. Reid, *Organic Chemistry of Bivalent Sulfur* **vol. I** (Chemical Publishing Co., New York, 1958) pp 15-261; of toxicology and human exposure: *Toxicological Profile for Methyl Mercaptan* (PB93-110799, 1992) 92 pp.
Flammable gas; odor of rotten cabbage. mp −123°. bp$_{760}$ 5.95°; d_4^{20} 0.8665; d_4^{25} 0.9600. Critical temp 196.8°. Critical pressure 71.4 atm. Heat capacity (solid at 14.97-146.57 K): 0.773-17.47 cal/deg/mole; (liq at 154.16-271.06 K): 21.27-21.13 cal/deg/mole, Russell *et al., J. Am. Chem. Soc.* **64**, 165 (1942). Azeotrope with isobutane (14.9% methanethiol) bp −13.00°. Soly in water at 20°: 23.30 g/l. Forms a cryst hydrate.
Sodium salt heminonahydrate. CH$_3$SNa.4½H$_2$O. Needles. Freely sol in water, methanol. Practically insol in ether.
Copper salt. CH$_3$SCu. Pale yellow crystals. Practically insol in water, ethanol, ether, benzene.
Caution: Potential symptoms of overexposure to methanethiol are irritation of eyes, skin and respiratory system; narcosis; cyanosis; convulsions; direct contact with liquid may cause frostbite. *See NIOSH Pocket Guide to Chemical Hazards* (DHHS/NIOSH 97-140, 1997) p 214.
USE: Intermediate in manuf of jet fuels, pesticides, fungicides, plastics; synthesis of methionine.

5957. Methanol. [67-56-1] Methyl alcohol; carbinol; wood spirit; wood alcohol. CH$_4$O; mol wt 32.04. C 37.49%, H 12.58%, O 49.94%. CH$_3$OH. Originally obtained by the destructive distillation of wood, now usually manuf from hydrogen and carbon monoxide or carbon dioxide, also by oxidation of hydrocarbons. *Review:* Faith, Keyes & Clark's *Industrial Chemicals*, F. A. Lowenheim, M. K. Moran, Eds. (Wiley-Interscience, New York, 4th ed., 1975) pp 524-529; L. E. Wade *et al.*, in *Kirk-Othmer Encyclopedia of Chemical Technology* **vol. 15** (Wiley-Interscience, New York, 3rd

ed., 1981) pp 398-415. Review of metabolism and toxicology: J. Liesivuori, H. Savolainen, *Pharmacol. Toxicol.* **69**, 157-163 (1991).
Flammable, poisonous, mobile liq. Slight alcoholic odor when pure; crude material may have a repulsive, pungent odor. Burns with a non-luminous, bluish flame. d_4^0 0.8100; d_4^{15} 0.7960; d_4^{20} 0.7915; d_4^{25} 0.7866. mp −97.8°. bp$_{760}$ 64.7°; bp$_{400}$ 49.9°; bp$_{200}$ 34.8°; bp$_{100}$ 21.2°; bp$_{60}$ 12.1°; bp$_{40}$ 5.0°; bp$_{20}$ −6.0°; bp$_{10}$ −16.2°; bp$_5$ −25.3°; bp$_{1.0}$ −44.0°; n_D^{15} 1.33066; n_D^{20} 1.3292. Vapor density: 1.11 (air = 1). Flash pt, closed cup: 54°F (12°C). Ignition temp 470°C (878°F). Explosive limits (%-vol in air): 6.0 to 36.5. Crit temp 240.0°; crit pressure 78.5 atm. Specific heat at 20-25° = 0.595 to 0.605. Dipole moment 1.69. Miscible with water, ethanol, ether, benzene, ketones, and most other organic solvents. Forms azeotropes with many compds. *Density, freezing and boiling point data of methanol-water mixtures:* 10% methanol by vol (d_4^{25}, fp, bp): 0.9836, −5°, 92.8°; 20% methanol: 0.9695, −12°, 87.8°; 30% methanol: 0.9572, −21°, 84.0°; 40% methanol: 0.9423, −33°, 80.9°; 50% methanol: 0.9259, −47°, 78.3°; 60% methanol: 0.9082, −57°, 75.9°. Methanol usually is a better solvent than ethanol, dissolves many inorganic salts, *e.g.,* sodium iodide 43%, calcium chloride 22%, ammonium nitrate 14%, copper sulfate 13%, silver nitrate 4%, ammonium chloride 3.2%, sodium chloride 1.4%.
Caution: Potential symptoms of overexposure are irritation of eyes, skin, upper respiratory system; dermatitis; headache, drowsiness, dizziness, vertigo, light headedness, nausea, vomiting, anorexia; weakness, fatigue; abdominal, back and leg pain; visual disturbances, dimness of vision, dilated pupils; optic nerve damage, bilateral blindness. *See NIOSH Pocket Guide to Chemical Hazards* (DHHS/NIOSH 97-140, 1997) p 200; *Clinical Toxicology of Commercial Products*, R. E. Gosselin *et al.*, Eds. (Williams & Wilkins, Baltimore, 5th ed., 1984) Section III, pp 275-279.
USE: Industrial solvent. Raw material for making formaldehyde and methyl esters of organic and inorganic acids. Antifreeze for automotive radiators and air brakes; ingredient of gasoline and diesel oil antifreezes. Octane booster in gasoline. As fuel for picnic stoves and soldering torches. Extractant for animal and vegetable oils. To denature ethanol. Softening agent for pyroxylin plastics. Solvent and solvent adjuvant for polymers. Solvent in the manuf of cholesterol, streptomycin, vitamins, hormones, and other pharmaceuticals.

5958. Methantheline Bromide. [53-46-3] *N,N*-Diethyl-*N*-methyl-2-[(9*H*-xanthen-9-ylcarbonyl)oxy]ethanaminium bromide; diethyl(2-hydroxyethyl)methylammonium bromide xanthene-9-carboxylate; β-diethylaminoethyl 9-xanthenecarboxylate methobromide; MTB-51; SC-2910; Banthine Bromide; Avagal; Uldumont; Vagantin; Metaxan; Methanide; Xanteline; Gastron; Gastrosedan; Methanthine Bromide; Vagamin; Metanyl; Doladene; Asabaine. C$_{21}$H$_{26}$BrNO$_3$; mol wt 420.34. C 60.00%, H 6.23%, Br 19.01%, N 3.33%, O 11.42%. Anticholinergic. Prepn from 9-xanthenecarboxylic acid and 2-diethylaminoethanol: J. W. Cusic, R. A. Robinson, *J. Org. Chem.* **16**, 1921 (1951); *eidem,* US 2659732 (1952 to Searle). Pharmacology: W. E. Hambourger *et al., J. Pharmacol. Exp. Ther.* **99**, 245 (1950).

Crystals from isopropanol, mp 175-176°. Bitter taste. Very slightly hygroscopic. Freely sol in water, alcohol. Practically insol in ether. pH (2% aq soln): 5.0-5.5. Aq solns tend to hydrolyze after a few days. The corresponding chloride is very hygroscopic. uv max (alc): 246, 282 nm (E$_{1cm}^{1\%}$ 135, 69). LD$_{50}$ i.p. in mice: 76 mg/kg (Hambourger).
THERAP CAT: Antispasmodic. In treatment of urinary incontinence.

5959. Methapyrilene. [91-80-5] *N,N*-Dimethyl-*N*′-2-pyridinyl-*N*′-(2-thienylmethyl)-1,2-ethanediamine; 2-[(2-dimethylaminoethyl)-2-thenylamino]pyridine; *N,N*-dimethyl-*N*′-(2-pyridyl)-*N*′-(2-thenyl)ethylenediamine; *N,N*-dimethyl-*N*′-(α-pyridyl)-*N*′-(2-

methylthienyl)ethylenediamine; thenylpyramine; AH-42; Thenylene; Pyrathyn; Thionylan; Histadyl (formerly); Restryl; Rest-On; Sleepwell; Paradormalene; Pyrinistab; Pyrinistol; Lullamin. C_{14}-$H_{19}N_3S$; mol wt 261.39. C 64.33%, H 7.33%, N 16.08%, S 12.27%. Prepd by heating a 2-thenyl halide with an alkali metal salt of N,N-dimethyl-N'-(2-pyridyl)ethylenediamine: Kyrides, **US 2581868** (1952 to Monsanto). Alternate syntheses: Weston, *J. Am. Chem. Soc.* **69**, 980 (1947); Clapp *et al., ibid.* 1549. Toxicity data: H. M. Lee *et al., Proc. Soc. Exp. Biol. Med.* **80**, 458 (1952). Carcinogenicity study: W. Lijinsky *et al., Science* **209**, 817 (1980). Study of mechanism of hepatocarcinogenicity: K. L. Steinmetz *et al., Carcinogenesis* **9**, 959 (1988). Clinical pharmacokinetics: E. P. Calandre *et al., Clin. Pharmacol. Ther.* **29**, 527 (1981). HPLC determn in feed and sleep aid tablets: B. Shaikh, M. R. Hallmark, *J. Assoc. Off. Anal. Chem.* **64**, 889 (1981); in feed, urine and wastewater: H. C. Thompson, Jr., C. L. Holder, *J. Chromatogr.* **283**, 251 (1984).

Liquid. $bp_{0.45}$ 125-135°; bp_3 173-175°. n_D^{25} 1.5842 (also reported as 1.5835). LD_{50} in mice, guinea pigs (mg/kg): 182.2 ±12.8, 374.9 ±34.5 orally; in mice (mg/kg): 19.85 ±0.69 i.v. (Lee).

Hydrochloride. [135-23-9] $C_{14}H_{19}N_3S.HCl$. Bitter crystals, mp 162°. uv max: 238 nm ($E_{1cm}^{1\%}$ 623); min: 272 nm. One gram dissolves in about 0.5 ml water, in 5 ml alcohol, in 3 ml chloroform. Practically insol in ether, benzene.

Fumarate. [33032-12-1] $(C_{14}H_{19}N_3S)_2 \cdot 3C_4H_4O_4$. Prepn: Meyer, **GB 694805** (1953 to Monsanto). Crystals, mp 135-136°.

THERAP CAT: Antihistaminic.

THERAP CAT (VET): Antihistaminic.

5960. Methaqualone. [72-44-6] 2-Methyl-3-(2-methylphenyl)-4(3H)-quinazolinone; 2-methyl-3-o-tolyl-4(3H)-quinazolinone; 3,4-dihydro-2-methyl-4-oxo-3-o-tolylquinazoline; metolquizolone; QZ-2; CI-705; R-148; TR-495; Parest; Quaalude; Somnafac. $C_{16}H_{14}N_2O$; mol wt 250.30. C 76.78%, H 5.64%, N 11.19%, O 6.39%. Quinazoline sedative-hypnotic. Prepn: Kacker, Zaheer, *J. Indian Chem. Soc.* **28**, 344 (1951); Klosa, *J. Prakt. Chem.* **14**, 84 (1961); **20**, 283 (1963). Review of syntheses: E. F. van Zyl, *Forensic Sci. Int.* **122**, 142-149 (2001). GC determn in serum: M. A. Evenson, G. L. Lensmeyer, *Clin. Chem.* **20**, 249 (1974). Metabolism: W. G. Stillwell *et al., Drug Metab. Dispos.* **3**, 287 (1975). Toxicity data: E. I. Goldenthal, *Toxicol. Appl. Pharmacol.* **18**, 185 (1971). Reports of abuse potential: D. S. Inaba *et al., J. Am. Med. Assoc.* **224**, 1505 (1973); E. M. Pascarelli, *ibid.* 1512. Review of pharmacology: S. S. Brown, S. Goenechea, *Clin. Pharmacol. Ther.* **14**, 314-324 (1973). Comprehensive description: D. M. Patel *et al., Anal. Profiles Drug Subs.* **4**, 245-267 (1975). Comparison of abuse potential with benzodiazepines: M. H. Orzack *et al., Int. J. Addict.* **23**, 449-467 (1988).

Crystals, mp 120°; also given as mp 114-116°. uv max (ethanol): 225, 263, 304, 316 nm; (0.01N HCl): about 234, 269 nm. Sol in ethanol, ether, chloroform. Practically insol in water. LD_{50} orally in rats: 255 mg/kg (Goldenthal).

Hydrochloride. [340-56-7] $C_{16}H_{14}N_2O.HCl$; mol wt 286.76. Crystals, mp 255-265°. Sol in ether, ethanol. Practically insol in water.

Note: This is a controlled substance (depressant): **21 CFR,** 1308.11.

5961. Metharbital. [50-11-3] 5,5-Diethyl-1-methyl-2,4,-6(1H,3H,5H)-pyrimidinetrione; 5,5-diethyl-1-methylbarbituric acid; Gemonil. $C_9H_{14}N_2O_3$; mol wt 198.22. C 54.53%, H 7.12%, N 14.13%, O 24.21%. Prepn: Halpern, Jones, *J. Am. Pharm. Assoc.* **38**, 352 (1949); Snyder, Link, *J. Am. Chem. Soc.* **75**, 1881 (1953).

Crystals from benzene + petr ether, mp 155°. Solubility (g/100 ml soln) in water 0.12; in alcohol 4.3; in ether 2.6. pH of satd aq solns: 5.6-5.7. pK 8.45: Fox, Shugar, *Bull. Soc. Chim. Belg.* **61**, 44 (1952).

Note: This is a controlled substance (depressant): **21 CFR,** 1308.13.

THERAP CAT: Anticonvulsant.

5962. Methazolamide. [554-57-4] N-[5-(Aminosulfonyl)-3-methyl-1,3,4-thiadiazol-2(3H)-ylidene]acetamide; N-(4-methyl-2-sulfamoyl-Δ^2-1,3,4-thiadiazolin-5-ylidene)acetamide; 5-acetylamino-4-methyl-Δ^2-1,3,4-thiadiazoline-2-sulfonamide; Neptazane. $C_5H_8N_4O_3S_2$; mol wt 236.27. C 25.42%, H 3.41%, N 23.71%, O 20.31%, S 27.14%. Carbonic anhydrase inhibitor. Prepn: Young *et al., J. Am. Chem. Soc.* **78**, 4649 (1956); **US 2783241** (1957 to Am. Cyanamid); Pala, *Farmaco Ed. Sci.* **13**, 650 (1958).

Crystals from water, mp 213-214°. pKa 7.30. uv max (95% ethanol): 254 nm (log ε 3.66); (0.1N NaOH): 247 nm (log ε 3.61).

THERAP CAT: Diuretic.

5963. Methcathinone. [5650-44-2] 2-(Methylamino)-1-phenyl-1-propanone; α-methylaminopropiophenone; monomethylpropion; ephedrone; Jeff; mulka; cat; cosmos; Jee cocktail. C_{10}-$H_{13}NO$; mol wt 163.22. C 73.59%, H 8.03%, N 8.58%, O 9.80%. Oxidation product of ephedrine possessing amphetamine-like central stimulant properties. Prepn: J. F. Hyde *et al., J. Am. Chem. Soc.* **50**, 2287 (1928); K. Y. Zhingel *et al., J. Forensic Sci.* **36**, 915 (1991). Prepn of enantiomers and chromatographic analysis: J. DeRuiter *et al., J. Chromatogr. Sci.* **32**, 552 (1994). Comparative pharmacology: R. Young, R. A. Glennon, *Pharmacol. Biochem. Behav.* **45**, 229 (1993). Pharmacology of enantiomers: R. A. Glennon *et al., ibid.* **50**, 601 (1995). Absorption and metabolism: S. L. Markantonis *et al., J. Pharm. Pharmacol.* **38**, 515 (1986). GLC/MS determn in urine: *eidem, Chim. Chron.* **14**, 211 (1985). Impact on public health: T. S. Emerson, J. E. Cisek, *Ann. Emerg. Med.* **22**, 1897 (1993).

Hydrochloride. [49656-78-2] $C_{10}H_{13}NO.HCl$. Crystals from alcohol-acetone, mp 176-177°.

l-Form hydrochloride. $C_{10}H_{13}NO.HCl$. Prepn: Y. J. L'Italien, M. C. Rebstock, **US 2802865** (1957 to Parke, Davis). Crystals from ethanol-ether or chloroform-petr ether, mp 182-183°. Pungent taste. $[\alpha]_D^{25}$ −53° (c = 1 in water). Sol in water. LD_{50} in mice, rats (mg/kg): 106, 90 iv; 233, 86 sc; 342, 99 orally (Emerson).

Note: This is a controlled substance (stimulant): **21 CFR,** 1308.11.

5964. Methdilazine. [1982-37-2] 10-[(1-Methyl-3-pyrrolidinyl)methyl]-10*H*-phenothiazine. $C_{18}H_{20}N_2S$; mol wt 296.43. C 72.93%, H 6.80%, N 9.45%, S 10.82%. Prepn: Feldkamp, Wu, **US 2945855** (1960 to Mead Johnson). Toxicity data: E. I. Goldenthal, *Toxicol. Appl. Pharmacol.* **18,** 185 (1971).

Crystals, mp 87-88°.
Hydrochloride. [1229-35-2] Dilosyn; Disyncran; Tacaryl. $C_{18}H_{20}N_2S.HCl$; mol wt 332.89. Crystals from isopropyl alc, mp 187.5-189°. LD_{50} orally in rats: 320 mg/kg (Goldenthal).
THERAP CAT: Antipruritic.

5965. Methemoglobin. Hemiglobin; ferrihemoglobin; met Hb. Oxidation product of the normal blood pigment, hemoglobin, in which the iron is present in the ferric state. Methemoglobin may be formed through the direct action of oxidants, through the coaction of hydrogen donors and atmospheric oxygen, or through the autoxidation of hemoglobin which occurs to a small extent in normal blood. Methemoglobin does not have the capacity to combine with molecular oxygen. *Reviews:* Bodansky, *Pharmacol. Rev.* **3,** 144 (1951); Jaffé in *The Red Blood Cell,* Bishop, Surgenor, Eds. (Academic Press, 1964) pp 397-422.
Cleaved by acids and bases to yield globin and ferriprotoporphyrin.

5966. Methenamine. [100-97-0] 1,3,5,7-Tetraazatricyclo-[3.3.1.1³,⁷]decane; hexamethylenetetramine; HMT; HMTA; hexamine; 1,3,5,7-tetraazaadamantane; hexamethylenamine. C_6H_{12}-N_4; mol wt 140.19. C 51.40%, H 8.63%, N 39.96%. Prepn: A. Butlerow, *Ann.* **115,** 322 (1860); from formaldehyde and ammonia: F. Meissner, E. Schwiedessen, **US 2762799; US 2762800** (both 1956); *Faith, Keyes & Clark's Industrial Chemicals,* F. A. Lowenheim, M. K. Moran, Eds. (Wiley-Interscience, New York, 4th ed., 1975) pp 445-448. Comprehensive reviews: J. F. Walker, *Formaldehyde* (Reinhold, New York, 3rd ed., 1964) pp 511-551; J. M. Dreyfors *et al., Am. Ind. Hyg. Assoc. J.* **50,** 579-585 (1989). Review of therapeutic use: R. Gleckman *et al., Am. J. Hosp. Pharm.* **36,** 1509-1512 (1979); of toxicology: H. J. Trochimowicz *et al.* in *Patty's Industrial Hygiene and Toxicology* vol. 2E, G. D. Clayton, F. E. Clayton, Eds. (John Wiley & Sons, New York, 1994) pp 3324-3327.

Colorless, odorless crystalline solid with sweet, metallic taste. Sublimes at about 263° without melting and with partial decompn; somewhat volatile at lower temp. Flammable. Specific heat: 36.4 cal/°C. d 1.331. Soly at 20° (g/100g): chloroform 13.4; methanol 7.25; abs ethanol 2.89; acetone 0.65; benzene 0.23; xylene 0.14; ether 0.06. Practically insol in petr ether. pH of 0.2 molar aq sol 8.4.
Anhydromethylenecitrate. [6190-43-8] Helmitol. C_6H_{12}-$N_4.C_7H_8O_7$; mol wt 344.32. White, cryst powder. mp 175° with decompn. Sol in 10 parts water; very slightly sol in alcohol, ether.
Hippurate. [5714-73-8] Hiprex; Urex; Urotractan. $C_6H_{12}N_4$.-$C_9H_9NO_3$; mol wt 319.36. Crystals, mp 105-110°. Freely sol in water, alcohol.
Mandelate. [587-23-5] Mandelamine; Uronamin. $C_6H_{12}N_4$.-$C_8H_8O_3$; mol wt 292.33. Crystals or white, crystalline powder. mp 128-130°. Slightly sol in acetone, ether; sol in alcohol, chloroform; very sol in water.
Sulfosalicylate. [20480-93-7] $C_6H_{12}N_4.C_7H_6O_6S$; mol wt 358.37. Occurs as the monohydrate. Odorless, cryst powder, mp ~190° with decompn. Sol in 8 parts water; slightly sol in alcohol.

USE: In adhesives, coatings, and sealing compounds; as crosslinking agent for hardening phenol-formaldehyde resin and vulcanizing rubber; as corrosion inhibitor for steel; as fuel tablets for camping stoves; as stabilizer for lubricating and insulating oils; for the manufacture of explosive compounds (*see* Cyclonite); antimicrobial food additive.
THERAP CAT: Antibacterial (urinary).
THERAP CAT (VET): Antibacterial (urinary).

5967. Methenolone. [153-00-4] (5α,17β)-17-Hydroxy-1-methylandrost-1-en-3-one; 1-methyl-Δ¹-androsten-17β-ol-3-one; méténolone. $C_{20}H_{30}O_2$; mol wt 302.45. C 79.42%, H 10.00%, O 10.58%. Prepn: Wiechert, Kaspar, *Ber.* **93,** 1710 (1960); Popper, **DE 1023764** (1958 to Schering, AG).

Crystals from isopropyl ether, mp 149.5-152°. mp 160-161° (Popper). $[\alpha]_D$ +58.9°.
17-Acetate. [434-05-9] Primobolan Tablets; Primonabol. C_{22}-$H_{32}O_3$; mol wt 344.49. Crystals from isopropyl ether, mp 138-139°. uv max (methanol): 240 nm (ε 13300). Sol in methanol, ether, chloroform.
17-Enanthate. [303-42-4] Methenolone enanthate; 17β-heptanoyloxy-1-methyl-5α-androst-1-en-3-one; Primobolan-Depot; Primonabol Depot. $C_{27}H_{42}O_3$; mol wt 414.62. Used as repository form.
Note: This is a controlled substance (anabolic steroid): **21 CFR,** 1308.13, as defined in 1300.01.
THERAP CAT: Anabolic.

5968. Methestrol. [130-73-4] 4,4′-(1,2-Diethyl-1,2-ethanediyl)bis[2-methylphenol]; 4,4′-(1,2-diethylethylene)di-*o*-cresol; 3,4-bis(3-methyl-4-hydroxyphenyl)hexane; dimethylhexestrol; promethestrol; γ-promethestrol. $C_{20}H_{26}O_2$; mol wt 298.42. C 80.50%, H 8.78%, O 10.72%. Prepd by hydrolysis of the dipropionate: Niederl *et al., J. Am. Chem. Soc.* **70,** 508 (1948). Chromatographic identification and determn: R. W. Roos, *J. Pharm. Sci.* **63,** 594 (1974). Pharmacologic study: P. H. Jellinck, A. M. Newcombe, *Biochem. Pharmacol.* **29,** 3031 (1980). Pharmacotherapeutic study: C. B. Hammond, W. S. Maxson, *Fertil. Steril.* **37,** 5 (1982).

Crystals from dil acetic acid, mp 145°.
Dipropionate. Meprane Dipropionate. $C_{26}H_{34}O_4$; mol wt 410.55. Cryst, mp 115°. Freely sol in ether, ethyl acetate, benzene; slightly sol in alc. Practically insol in water, dil acids.
THERAP CAT: Estrogen.

5969. Methicillin Sodium. [132-92-3] (2S,5R,6R)-6-[(2,6-Dimethoxybenzoyl)amino]-3,3-dimethyl-7-oxo-4-thia-1-azabicyclo[3.2.0]heptane-2-carboxylic acid monosodium salt; 6-(2,6-dimethoxybenzamido)penicillanic acid sodium salt; sodium 2,6-dimethoxyphenylpenicillin; 2,6-dimethoxyphenylpenicillin sodium salt; sodium 6-(2,6-dimethoxybenzamido)penicillinate; 2,6-dimethoxybenzoylpenin sodium salt; dimethoxyphenecillin sodium; sodium methicillin; BRL-1241; X-1497; Azapen; Belfacillin; Celpillina; Celbenin; Cinopenil; Flabelline; Penistaph; Staphcillin. $C_{17}H_{19}$-N_2NaO_6S; mol wt 402.40. C 50.74%, H 4.76%, N 6.96%, Na 5.71%, O 23.86%, S 7.97%. Semi-synthetic antibiotic related to penicillin. Prepn starting with 6-aminopenicillanic acid: Doyle *et* al., *J. Chem. Soc.* **1962**, 1457; Doyle *et al.*, **US 2951839** (1960); Glombitza, *Ann.* **673**, 166 (1964). Physical-chemical properties: Cotta-Ramusino, Intonti, *Farmaco Ed. Prat.* **16**, 227 (1961).

Monohydrate. Crystals from acetone, mp 196-197° (dec). $[\alpha]_D^{20}$ +230° (c = 5); +225° (c = 1). uv max: 281 nm ($E_{1cm}^{1\%}$ 55); min 264 nm. Solubilities (mg/ml) at 20°: water >300; ethanol 40; ether <0.03; acetone 0.35; chloroform 0.06; isooctane <0.03.

THERAP CAT: Antibacterial.

THERAP CAT (VET): Antimicrobial.

5970. Methidathion. [950-37-8] Phosphorodithioic acid *S*-[(5-methoxy-2-oxo-1,3,4-thiadiazol-3(2*H*)-yl)methyl] *O,O*-dimethyl ester; phosphorodithioic acid *O,O*-dimethyl ester *S*-ester with 4-(mercaptomethyl)-2-methoxy-Δ^2-1,3,4-thiadiazolin-5-one; dithiophosphoric acid *O,O'*-dimethyl-*S*-[(5-methoxy-1,3,4-thiadiazol-2(3*H*)-one-3-yl)methyl] ester; *O,O'*-dimethyl-*S*-[(2-methoxy-1,3,4-thiadiazol-5(4*H*)-one-4-yl)methyl] dithiophosphate; GS-13005; Supracid(e); Ultracid(e). $C_6H_{11}N_2O_4PS_3$; mol wt 302.33. C 23.84%, H 3.67%, N 9.27%, O 21.17%, P 10.25%, S 31.82%. Synthesis and degradation products: Rüfenacht, *Helv. Chim. Acta* **51**, 518 (1968); **FR 1335755** (1963 to Geigy), *C.A.* **60**, 1764g (1964). Metabolism in rats: Esser *et al.*, *Helv. Chim. Acta* **51**, 513 (1968). Acute toxicity: T. B. Gaines, R. E. Linder, *Fundam. Appl. Toxicol.* **7**, 299 (1986). Carcinogenicity studies: J. A. Quest *et al.*, *Regul. Toxicol. Pharmacol.* **12**, 117 (1990).

Crystals from methanol, mp 39-40°. Soly in water <1%. Readily sol in benzene, acetone, methanol, xylene and other org solvents. LD_{50} in adult male, female rats (mg/kg): 31, 32 orally (Gaines, Linder).

USE: Insecticide, acaricide.

5971. Methimazole. [60-56-0] 1,3-Dihydro-1-methyl-2*H*-imidazole-2-thione; 1-methylimidazole-2-thiol; 1-methyl-2-mercaptoimidazole; mercazolyl; thiamazole; Basolan; Danantizol; Favistan; Frentirox; Mercazole; Metazolo; Tapazole; Thacapzol; Thycapsol; Strumazol. $C_4H_6N_2S$; mol wt 114.17. C 42.08%, H 5.30%, N 24.54%, S 28.09%. Prepd by treating aminoacetaldehyde diethyl acetal with methyl isothiocyanate: Wohl, Marckwald, *Ber.* **22**, 1354 (1889); from thiocyanic acid and *N*-substituted amino acetals: Jones *et al.*, *J. Am. Chem. Soc.* **71**, 4000 (1949). Metabolism: D. S. Sitar, D. P. Thornhill, *J. Pharmacol. Exp. Ther.* **184**, 432 (1973). Comprehensive description: H. Y. Aboul-Enein, A. A. Al-Badr, *Anal. Profiles Drug Subs.* **8**, 351-370 (1979). Review of pharmacology and clinical experience: D. S. Cooper, *N. Engl. J. Med.* **311**, 1353-1362 (1984).

Leaflets from alc, mp 146-148°. bp 280° (some decompn). uv max (0.1*N* H_2SO_4): 211, 251.5 nm ($E_{1cm}^{1\%}$ 593, 1528). Freely sol in water. Sol in alcohol, chloroform. Sparingly sol in ether, petr ether, benzene.

Methiodide. Jomezol.

USE: In cyanide-free silver electroplating.

THERAP CAT: Antihyperthyroid.

5972. Methiocarb. [2032-65-7] 3,5-Dimethyl-4-(methyl-thio)phenol methylcarbamate; methylcarbamic acid 4-(methyl-thio)-3,5-xylyl ester; 4-(methylthio)-3,5-xylyl methylcarbamate; 4-methylthio-3,5-dimethylphenyl *N*-methylcarbamate; mercaptodimethur; metmercapturon; Bayer 37344; H-321; Draza; Mesurol. $C_{11}H_{15}NO_2S$; mol wt 225.31. C 58.64%, H 6.71%, N 6.22%, O 14.20%, S 14.23%. Prepn: E. Schegk *et al.*, **GB 912895**; *eidem*, **US 3313684** (1962, 1967 both to Bayer); E. E. Gilbert, J. A. Otto, **US 3358012** (1967 to Allied). Molluscicidal activity: H. H. Crowell, *J. Econ. Entomol.* **60**, 1048 (1967). Bird repellent properties: E.W. Schafer, R. B. Brunton, *J. Wildl. Manage.* **35**, 569 (1971). Toxicity study: T. B. Gaines, *Toxicol. Appl. Pharmacol.* **14**, 515 (1969).

White crystalline powder, mp 121.5°. Insol in water. Sol in organic solvents. Unstable in alk media. LD_{50} in male, female rats (mg/kg): 70, 60 orally (Gaines).

USE: Insecticide; molluscicide; bird repellent.

5973. Methiodal Sodium. [126-31-8] Iodomethanesulfonic acid sodium salt; sodium iodomethanesulfonate; Skiodan; Abrodil; Radiographol; Segosin; Diagnorenol. CH_2INaO_3S; mol wt 243.98. C 4.92%, H 0.83%, I 52.01%, Na 9.42%, O 19.67%, S 13.14%. CH_2ISO_3Na. Prepd by the action of sodium sulfite on methylene iodide at 70° in water-alcohol soln: Ossenbeck *et al.*, **US 1842626** (1932 to Winthrop); from iodoform + sodium sulfite: Allardt, **US 1867793** (1932 to Schering-Kahlbaum AG).

Crystals. Slightly saline taste followed by sweetish aftertaste. Freely sol in water (70 g/100 ml); slightly sol in alcohol (2.5 g/100 ml), benzene, ether, acetone.

THERAP CAT: Diagnostic aid (radiopaque medium—urographic).

5974. Methionic Acid. [503-40-2] Methanedisulfonic acid. $CH_4O_6S_2$; mol wt 176.17. C 6.82%, H 2.29%, O 54.49%, S 36.40%. $CH_2(SO_3H)_2$. Prepn from methane + sulfur trioxide: Snyder, Grosse, **US 2493038** (1950 to Houdry Process); by H_2SO_4 oxidation of acetic acid: Schwab, Neuwirth, *Ber.* **90**, 567 (1957); from $MeSO_3H + SO_3$: Crowder, Gilbert, **US 2842589** (1958 to Allied Chem.). Prepn of aluminum salt: Christian, Jenkins, *J. Am. Pharm. Assoc.* **39**, 633 (1950); **US 2504107** (1950 to Purdue Res. Found.).

Crystals, mp 96-100°.

Aluminum salt. $C_3H_6Al_2O_{18}S_6$. Crystals from water + alcohol. Hygroscopic. Soly in water at 27°: 69 w/v. pH of 5% aq soln = 3.5.

USE: Antiperspirant.

THERAP CAT: Aluminum salt as topical astringent.

5975. Methionine. [63-68-3] L-Methionine; Met; M; 2-amino-4-(methylthio)butyric acid; α-amino-γ-methylmercaptobutyric acid; (*S*)-2-amino-4-(methylthio)butanoic acid; γ-methylthio-α-aminobutyric acid; Acimethin. $C_5H_{11}NO_2S$; mol wt 149.21. C 40.25%, H 7.43%, N 9.39%, O 21.45%, S 21.49%. Essential amino acid for human development. Universal translation start signal although usually missing from mature protein. Isoln from casein: J. H. Mueller, *Proc. Soc. Exp. Biol. Med.* **19**, 161 (1922). Early chemistry and biochemistry: *Amino Acids and Proteins*, D. M. Greenberg, Ed. (Charles C. Thomas, Springfield, IL, 1951) 950 pp., *passim*; J. P. Greenstein, M. Winitz, *Chemistry of the Amino Acids* vols. 1-3 (John Wiley and Sons, Inc., New York, 1961) pp. 2125-2155, *passim*. Determn and distribution in non-protein fractions: J. Giovanelli, S. H. Mudd, *J. Biochem. Biophys. Methods* **11**, 1 (1985). GC-MS determn in biological fluids: S. P. Stabler *et al.*, *Anal. Biochem.* **162**, 185 (1987). Evaluation as tracer in cancer imaging in mice: R. Kubota, *J. Nucl. Med.* **36**, 484 (1995). Clinical evaluation in acetaminophen overdose: A. N. Hamlyn *et al.*, *J. Int. Med. Res.* **9**, 226 (1981). Clinical use as radiolabel in hyperparathyroidism: P. Hellman *et al.*, *Surgery* **116**, 974 (1994). Review of metabolism and clinical significance in man: L. D. Fleisher,

G. E. Gaull, *Clin. Endocrinol. Metab.* **3**, 37-55 (1974); and in carcinogenesis: T. L. Gatton-Umphress, *Hosp. Pract.* **28**, 83-90 (1993). Review of toxicity: N. J. Benevenga, *J. Agric. Food Chem.* **22**, 2-9 (1974). Review of biosynthesis: I. G. Old *et al.*, *Prog. Biophys. Mol. Biol.* **56**, 145-185 (1991). Review as translation start signal: T. Meinnel *et al.*, *Biochimie* **75**, 1061-1075 (1993).

Minute hexagonal plates from dil alc, mp 280-282° (dec, sealed capillary). $[\alpha]_D^{25}$ −8.11° (c = 0.8). $[\alpha]_D^{20}$ +23.40° (c = 5.0 in 3*N* HCl). Sol in water, but the crystals are somewhat water-repellent at first. Sol in warm, dil alcohol. Insol in abs alcohol, ether, petr ether, benzene, acetone.

D-Form. [348-67-4] Converted by deamination, followed by transamination with resultant inversion to the L-form. Comparative study with L-form of metabolism in plants: M. Pokorny *et al.*, *Phytochemistry* **9**, 2175 (1970). Evaluation in parenteral nutrition: K J. Printen *et al.*, *Am. J. Clin. Nutr.* **32**, 1200 (1979). *Review:* L. D. Stegink, D-Amino Acids in *Clin. Nutr. Update: Amino Acids* H. L. Greene *et al.*, Eds. (American Medical Association, Chicago, IL, 1977) pp 198-206. $[\alpha]_D^{25}$ +8.12° (c = 0.8). $[\alpha]_D^{25}$ −21.18° (c = 0.8 in 0.2*N* HCl).

DL-Form. [59-51-8] Racemethionine; Banthionine; Dyprin; Lobamine; Metione; Pedameth; Urimeth. Platelets from alc, mp 281° (decomp). d 1.340. pK$_1$ 2.28; pK$_2$ 9.21. pH of 1% aq soln 5.6-6.1. R$_f$ value 0.77. Soly in water (g/l) at 0°: 18.18; at 25°: 33.81; at 50°: 60.70; at 75°: 105.2; at 100°: 176.0. Sol in dil acids, alkalies. Very slightly sol in 95% alcohol. Insol in ether.

THERAP CAT: Hepatoprotectant; antidote (acetaminophen poisoning); urinary acidifier.

THERAP CAT (VET): Nutritional supplement; urinary acidifier.

5976. Methionine Hydroxy Analog. [583-91-5] 2-Hydroxy-4-(methylthio)butanoic acid; 2-hydroxy-4-(methylthio)butyric acid; 2-hydroxy-4-(methylmercapto)butyric acid; Alimet. C$_5$H$_{10}$O$_3$S; mol wt 150.20. C 39.98%, H 6.71%, O 31.96%, S 21.35%. CH$_3$SCH$_2$CH$_2$CH(OH)COOH. Prepn (not claimed) and use as poultry feed additive: E. S. Blake, R. J. Wineman, US 2745745 (1956 to Monsanto). HPLC determn in feeds: A. Baudichau *et al.*, *J. Sci. Food Agric.* **38**, 1 (1987). Use as a feed additive for livestock: A. Papas *et al.*, *J. Nutr.* **104**, 653 (1974); A. K. Clark, A. H. Rakes, *J. Dairy Sci.* **65**, 1493 (1982); D. H. Reifsnyder *et al.*,*J. Nutr.* **114**, 1705 (1984). Efficacy of calcium salt vs free acid: K. P. Boebel, D. H. Baker, *Poult. Sci.* **61**, 1167 (1982).

Calcium salt. MHA. C$_{10}$H$_{18}$CaO$_6$S$_2$; mol wt 338.45.

USE: Dietary supplement in livestock.

5977. Methisazone. [1910-68-5] 2-(1,2-Dihydro-1-methyl-2-oxo-3*H*-indol-3-ylidene)hydrazinecarbothioamide; 1-methyl-indole-2,3-dione 3-thiosemicarbazone; *N*-methylisatin 3-thiosemicarbazone; BW-33-T-57; Marboran; Viruzona. C$_{10}$H$_{10}$N$_4$OS; mol wt 234.28. C 51.27%, H 4.30%, N 23.91%, O 6.83%, S 13.69%. Prepn: Bauer, Sadler, *Br. J. Pharmacol.* **15**, 101 (1960); GB 975357 (1964 to Wellcome Found.).

Crystals from butanol, mp 245°.

THERAP CAT: Antiviral.

5978. Methitural. [467-43-6] Dihydro-5-(1-methylbutyl)-5-[2-(methylthio)ethyl]-2-thioxo-4,6(1*H*,5*H*)-pyrimidinedione; 5-(1-methylbutyl)-5-[2-(methylthio)ethyl]-2-thiobarbituric acid; 5-(2-methylthioethyl)-5-(2-pentyl)-2-thiobarbituric acid. C$_{12}$H$_{20}$N$_2$O$_2$S$_2$; mol wt 288.43. C 49.97%, H 6.99%, N 9.71%, O 11.09%, S

22.23%. Prepn: Zima, Von Werder, US 2802827 (1957 to E. Merck).

Sodium salt. [730-68-7] Methioturiate; AM-109; Sch-3132; Neraval; Thiogenal. C$_{12}$H$_{19}$N$_2$NaO$_2$S$_2$; mol wt 310.41. Very hygroscopic, yellow crystals. Slight odor of mercaptans. Freely sol in water. pH of a 10% aq soln ~9.5. Water solns are unstable as evidenced by a deepening of color and formation of a cloudy precipitate upon autoclaving and exposure to light. The addition of sodium carbonate has a stabilizing effect and prevents precipitation for about 24 hrs: Irwin *et al.*, *J. Pharmacol. Exp. Ther.* **116**, 317 (1956).

Note: This is a controlled substance (depressant): **21 CFR,** 1308.13.

THERAP CAT: Sedative, hypnotic.

5979. Methixene. [4969-02-2] 1-Methyl-3-(9*H*-thioxanthen-9-ylmethyl)piperidine; 9-(*N*-methyl-3-piperidylmethyl)thioxanthene. C$_{20}$H$_{23}$NS; mol wt 309.47. C 77.62%, H 7.49%, N 4.53%, S 10.36%. Anticholinergic. Prepn: Caviezel *et al.*, *Pharm. Acta Helv.* **33**, 447 (1958); J. Schmutz, US 2905590 (1959 to Wander). Metabolism and toxicity study: H. Lehner *et al.*, *Arzneim.-Forsch.* **14**, 89 (1964). Crystal structure: S. S. C. Chu, *Acta Crystallogr.* **B28**, 3625 (1972). Spectrofluorimetric determn: F. Belal *et al.*, *Anal. Chim. Acta* **255**, 103 (1991). Comprehensive description: E. M. Abdel-Moety *et al.*, *Anal. Profiles Drug Subs. Excip.* **22**, 317-358 (1993).

Slightly yellow viscous liquid, bp$_{0.07}$ 171-175°. Insol in water.

Hydrochloride monohydrate. [7081-40-5] Tremoquil; Methixart; Trest; Tremonil; Tremaril; Tremarit; Cholinfall; Methyloxan. C$_{20}$H$_{23}$NS.HCl.H$_2$O; mol wt 363.94. Flakes from ether, mp 215-217°. uv max (dil HCl): 268 nm (ε 10250). Sol in water, alcohol, chloroform. Insol in ether.

THERAP CAT: Antiparkinsonian.

5980. Methocarbamol. [532-03-6] 3-(2-Methoxyphenoxy)-1,2-propanediol 1-carbamate; 3-(*o*-methoxyphenoxy)-2-hydroxypropyl 1-carbamate; 2-hydroxy-3-(*o*-methoxyphenoxy)propyl 1-carbamate; guaiacol glyceryl ether carbamate; AHR-85; Neuraxin; Miolaxene; Lumirelax; Etroflex; Delaxin; Robamol; Traumacut; Tresortil; Relestrid; Robaxin. C$_{11}$H$_{15}$NO$_5$; mol wt 241.24. C 54.77%, H 6.27%, N 5.81%, O 33.16%. Prepn from 3-(*o*-methoxyphenoxy)-2-hydroxypropyl chlorocarbonate: Murphey, US 2770649 (1956 to A. H. Robins). Comprehensive description: S. Alessi-Severini *et al.*, *Anal. Profiles Drug Subs. Excip.* **23**, 371-399 (1994).

Crystals from benzene, mp 92-94°. uv max (water): 222, 274 nm (E$_{1cm}^{1\%}$ 298, 94). log P −0.06. Soly in water at 20°: 2.5 g/100 ml.

Sol in alcohol, propylene glycol. Sparingly sol in chloroform. Practically insol in *n*-hexane.

THERAP CAT: Muscle relaxant (skeletal).

THERAP CAT (VET): Muscle relaxant (skeletal).

5981. Methohexital Sodium. [22151-68-4] 1-Methyl-5-(1-methyl-2-pentynyl)-5-(2-propenyl)-2,4,6(1*H*,3*H*,5*H*)-pyrimidine-trione sodium salt; 5-allyl-1-methyl-5-(1-methyl-2-pentynyl)-barbituric acid sodium salt; α-*dl*-1-methyl-5-(1-methyl-2-pentynyl)-5-allylbarbituric acid sodium salt; α-*dl*-1-methyl-5-allyl-5-(1-methyl-2-pentynyl)barbituric acid sodium salt; methohexitone sodium; Brevital; Brevital Sodium; Brevimytal Sodium; Brietal Sodium. $C_{14}H_{17}N_2NaO_3$; mol wt 284.29. C 59.15%, H 6.03%, N 9.85%, Na 8.09%, O 16.88%. Prepn: Doran, US 2872448 (1959 to Lilly).

Minute crystals. Soluble in water.

Note: This is a controlled substance (depressant): **21 CFR**, 1308.14.

THERAP CAT: Anesthetic (intravenous).

THERAP CAT (VET): Ultra-short acting anesthetic.

5982. Methomyl. [16752-77-5] *N*-[[(Methylamino)carbonyl]oxy]ethanimidothioic acid methyl ester; *N*-[(methylcarbamoyl)oxy]thioacetimidic acid methyl ester; *S*-methyl *N*-[(methylcarbamoyl)oxy]thioacetimidate; methyl *O*-(methylcarbamoyl)thioacetohydroxamate; Insecticide 1179; Lannate; Nudrin. $C_5H_{10}N_2O_2S$; mol wt 162.21. C 37.02%, H 6.21%, N 17.27%, O 19.73%, S 19.77%. Prepn: A. G. Jelinek, ZA 6800093; *idem*, US 3506698 (1968, 1970 both to du Pont). Metabolism studies: J. Harvey *et al.*, *J. Agric. Food Chem.* **21**, 769, 775, 781 (1973). Crystal structure: Sim, Waite, *J. Chem. Soc. B* **1971**, 752. Acetylcholinesterase activity: Pickering, Pickering, *Arch. Toxicol.* **27**, 292 (1971). Toxicity studies: A. M. Kaplan, H. Sherman, *Toxicol. Appl. Pharmacol.* **40**, 1 (1977).

Crystals, mp 78-79°. d_4^{24} 1.2946. Soly at 25° (w/w): water 5.8; methanol 100; ethanol 42; isopropanol 22; acetone 73. LD_{50} orally in male rats: 17 mg/kg (Kaplan, Sherman).

Caution: Potential symptoms of overexposure are eye irritation; blurred vision, miosis; salivation; abdominal cramps, nausea, vomiting; dyspnea; weakness, muscle twitching; liver and kidney damage. *See NIOSH Pocket Guide to Chemical Hazards* (DHHS/NIOSH 97-140, 1997) p 194.

USE: Insecticide.

5983. Methoprene. [40596-69-8] (2*E*,4*E*)-11-Methoxy-3,7,11-trimethyl-2,4-dodecadienoic acid 1-methylethyl ester; isopropyl (2*E*,4*E*,7*RS*)-11-methoxy-3,7,11-trimethyl-2,4-dodecadienoate; ZR-515. $C_{19}H_{34}O_3$; mol wt 310.47. C 73.50%, H 11.04%, O 15.46%. Juvenile hormone mimic. Prepn: BE 778242; *see also* C. A. Henrick, US 3818047 (1972, 1974 both to Zoecon); *idem et al.*, *J. Org. Chem.* **40**, 1 (1975); L. Novák *et al.*, *Ann.* **1982**, 1173. Effect on mustard aphid: P. J. Rup, R. K. Gill, *Insect Sci. Applic.* **14**, 173 (1993). Field trial in a saltwater marsh against mosquitoes: V. L. Kramer *et al.*, *J. Am. Mosq. Control Assoc.* **9**, 127 (1993). Mechanism of action study: E. M. Berger *et al.*, *Dev. Biol.* **151**, 410 (1992). HPLC determn in tobacco: S. S. Yang, *Chromatographia* **33**, 309 (1992). GC determn in aquatic microcosms: D. H. Ross *et al.*, *J. Am. Mosq. Control Assoc.* **10**, 202 (1994). Impact on the fathead minnow: *idem et al.*, *ibid.* 211. Review of properties, metabolism, toxicology, and use: J. B. Siddall, *Environ. Health*

Perspect. **14**, 119-126 (1976). Review of analytical methods: L. L. Dunham, W. W. Miller in *Analytical Methods for Pesticides and Plant Growth Regulators* vol. X, G. Zweig, Ed. (Academic Press, New York, 1978) pp 95-109.

Amber liquid, $bp_{0.06}$ 135-136°. d^{20} 0.9261 g/ml. Vapor pressure at 25°: 2.37×10^{-5} mm Hg. Soly in water at 25°: 1.39 ppm. Sol in org solvents. Temperature stable up to at least 42° for 24 months. Stable in water, org solvents, and in the presence of dil alkali and acid. LD_{50} orally in rats: >34500 mg/kg (Siddall).

(7S)-Form. [65733-16-6] *S*-Methoprene; ZR-2458; Altosid; Precor; Extinguish; Pharorid.

USE: Insecticide; insect growth regulator.

THERAP CAT (VET): Ectoparasiticide.

5984. Methopterin. [2410-93-7] *N*-[4-[[(2-Amino-1,4-dihydro-4-oxo-6-pteridinyl)methyl]methylamino]benzoyl]-L-glutamic acid; *N*-[4-[[(2-amino-4-hydroxy-6-pteridinyl)methyl]methylamino]benzoyl]glutamic acid; 10-methylpteroylglutamic acid; N^{10}-methylfolic acid. $C_{20}H_{21}N_7O_6$; mol wt 455.42. C 52.75%, H 4.65%, N 21.53%, O 21.08%. Prepn: Cosulich, Smith, *J. Am. Chem. Soc.* **70**, 1922 (1948); Cosulich, US 2563707 (1951 to Am. Cyanamid).

Monohydrate. Yellow spherulites. uv max (0.1*N* NaOH): 255, 302, 368 nm (ε × 10^{-3} 26, 27, 9); (0.1*N* HCl): 307 nm (ε × 10^{-3} 25).

5985. Methotrexate. [59-05-2] *N*-[4-[[(2,4-Diamino-6-pteridinyl)methyl]methylamino]benzoyl]-L-glutamic acid; 4-amino-N^{10}-methylpteroylglutamic acid; 4-amino-10-methylfolic acid; methylaminopterin; amethopterin; MTX; CL-14377; Ledertrexate; Maxtrex. $C_{20}H_{22}N_8O_5$; mol wt 454.44. C 52.86%, H 4.88%, N 24.66%, O 17.60%. Folic acid antagonist. Prepn: D. R. Seeger *et al.*, *J. Am. Chem. Soc.* **71**, 1753 (1949); J. M. Smith, D. B. Cosulich, US 2512572 (1950 to American Cyanamid). Metabolism: M. V. Freeman, *J. Pharmacol. Exp. Ther.* **122**, 154 (1958); E. S. Henderson *et al.*, *Cancer Res.* **25**, 1008, 1018 (1965). Toxicity data: H. R. Scherf *et al.*, *Arzneim.-Forsch.* **20**, 1467 (1970). Comprehensive description: A. R. Chamberlin *et al.*, *Anal. Profiles Drug Subs.* **5**, 283-306 (1976). Review of metabolism and pharmacokinetics: W. E. Evans, *Appl. Pharmacokinet.* **1980**, 518-548; of clinical pharmacology and toxicity: J. R. Bertino, *Cancer Chemother.* **3**, 359-375 (1981); J. Jolivet *et al.*, *N. Engl. J. Med.* **309**, 1094-1104 (1983). Symposium on clinical experience in rheumatoid arthritis: *J. Rheumatol.* **12**, Suppl. 12, 1-44 (1985). Review of use in leukemia: O. G. Jonsson, B. A. Kamen, *Cancer Invest.* **9**, 53-60 (1991). Clinical trials in Crohn's disease: B. G. Feagan *et al.*, *N. Engl. J. Med.* **332**, 292 (1995); *idem et al.*, *ibid.* **342**, 1627 (2000). CE determn in blood: C.-Y. Kuo *et al.*, *J. Chromatogr. A* **1014**, 93 (2003). Review of pulmonary toxicity: O. Lateef *et al.*, *Expert Opin. Drug Saf.* **4**, 723-730 (2005).

Monohydrate. [6745-93-3] Yellow crystals from dil HCl, dec 185-204° (bath preheated to 160°). uv max (0.1N HCl): 244, 307 nm; (0.1N NaOH): 257, 302, 370 nm. Soluble in alkaline solns with decompn. LD$_{50}$ i.v. in rats: 14 mg/kg (Scherf).

Disodium salt. [7413-34-5] Folex; Mexate; Rheumatrex. C$_{20}$H$_{20}$N$_8$Na$_2$O$_5$; mol wt 498.40.

THERAP CAT: Antineoplastic; antirheumatic.

5986. Methotrimeprazine. [60-99-1] (βR)-2-Methoxy-N,-N,β-trimethyl-10H-phenothiazine-10-propanamine; (−)-10-(3-dimethylamino-2-methylpropyl)-2-methoxyphenothiazine; levomepromazine; 2-methoxytrimeprazine; levomeprazine; RP-7044; Sinogan-Debil; Tisercin; Neozine; Nirvan; Nozinan; Levoprome. C$_{19}$H$_{24}$N$_2$OS; mol wt 328.47. C 69.47%, H 7.36%, N 8.53%, O 4.87%, S 9.76%. Prepn: Courvoisier et al., C.R. Seances Soc. Biol. Ses Fil. **151**, 1378 (1957); Jacob, Robert, US 2837518 (1958 to Rhône-Poulenc).

Maleate. [7104-38-3] Minozinan; Milezin; Neuractil; Neurocil; Sofmin; Veractil. C$_{19}$H$_{24}$N$_2$OS.C$_4$H$_4$O$_4$; mol wt 444.54. Crystals, darkened by light. Dec about 190°. Sparingly sol in water (0.3% at 20°) and in ethanol (0.4%). pH of a 0.3% aq soln is 4.3. The free base is levorotatory: [α]$_D^{20}$ −17° (c = 5 in chloroform).

THERAP CAT: Analgesic.

5987. Methoxamine. [390-28-3] α-(1-Aminoethyl)-2,5-dimethoxybenzenemethanol; α-(1-aminoethyl)-2,5-dimethoxybenzyl alcohol; 2-amino-1-(2,5-dimethoxyphenyl)-1-propanol; β-hydroxy-β-(2,5-dimethoxyphenyl)isopropylamine; β-(2,5-dimethoxyphenyl)-β-hydroxyisopropylamine; 2,5-dimethoxynorephedrine. C$_{11}$H$_{17}$NO$_3$; mol wt 211.26. C 62.54%, H 8.11%, N 6.63%, O 22.72%. α_1-Adrenergic agonist. Prepn: Baltzly et al., US 2359707 (1944 to Burroughs Wellcome). Metabolism: A. Klutch, M. Bordun, J. Med. Chem. **10**, 860 (1967). Clinical pharmacology: N. T. Smith, C. Whitcher, Anesthesiology **28**, 735 (1967); P. D. Snashall et al., Clin. Sci. Mol. Med. **54**, 283 (1978). HPLC determn in plasma: I. A. Al-Meshal et al., J. Liq. Chromatogr. **12**, 1589 (1989). Therapeutic use: P. M. C. Wright et al., Anesth. Analg. **75**, 56 (1992); L. Cabanes et al., N. Engl. J. Med. **326**, 1661 (1992). Comprehensive description: A. M. Al-Obaid, M. M. El-Domiaty, Anal. Profiles Drug Subs. **20**, 399-431 (1991).

Hydrochloride. [61-16-5] Vasoxine; Vasoxyl; Vasylox. C$_{11}$H$_{17}$NO$_3$.HCl; mol wt 247.72. Crystals, mp 212-216°. pKa (25°C) 9.2. Very sol in water: One gram dissolves in 2.5 ml water, in 12 ml ethanol. Practically insol in ether, benzene, chloroform. pH of a 2% aq soln between 4.5 and 5.5.

THERAP CAT: Antihypotensive.

5988. Methoxsalen. [298-81-7] 9-Methoxy-7H-furo[3,2-g][1]benzopyran-7-one; 6-hydroxy-7-methoxy-5-benzofuranacrylic acid δ-lactone; 9-methoxypsoralen; 8-methoxy-4′,5′:6,7-furocoumarin; 8-methoxy[furano-3′,2′:6,7-coumarin]; ammoidin; xanthotoxin; 8-methoxypsoralen; 8-MOP; Meladinine; 8-MOP; Oxsoralen. C$_{12}$H$_8$O$_4$; mol wt 216.19. C 66.67%, H 3.73%, O 29.60%. Naturally occurring analog of psoralen, q.v., found in spp. of Leguminosae, Umbelliferae, and Rutaceae. Isolation: Priess, Ber. Dtsch. Pharm. Ges. **21**, 227 (1911); Thoms, Ber. **44**, 3325 (1911); **45**, 3705 (1912); Jois et al., J. Indian Chem. Soc. **10**, 41 (1933); Späth et al., Ber. **73**, 1361 (1933); Schonberg, Sina, Nature

160, 468 (1947); **161**, 481 (1948); J. Am. Chem. Soc. **72**, 4826 (1950). Synthesis: Späth, Pailer, Ber. **69**, 767 (1936); Lagercrantz, Acta Chem. Scand. **10**, 647 (1956); Stanley, Vannier, US 2889337 (1959 to USDA); P. Nore, E. Honkanen, J. Heterocycl. Chem. **17**, 985 (1980). Use in treatment of psoriasis and mycosis fungoides: J. A. Parrish et al., Int. J. Dermatol. **19**, 379 (1980). Acute toxicity data: Hakim et al., J. Pharmacol. Exp. Ther. **131**, 394 (1961). Phototoxicity study: A. Kornhauser et al., Science **217**, 733 (1982). Comprehensive description: M. A. Loutfy, M. A. Hassan, Anal. Profiles Drug Subs. **9**, 427-454 (1980). Review of use in photochemotherapy: T. F. Anderson, J. J. Voorhees, Annu. Rev. Pharmacol. Toxicol. **20**, 235-258 (1980); Acta Derm. Venereol. Suppl. **106**, 9-42 (1982).

Silky needles from hot water or benzene + petr ether, long rhombic prisms from alcohol + ether. mp 148°. Odorless. Bitter taste followed by tingling sensation. pH 5.5. uv max: 219, 249, 300 nm (log ε 4.32, 4.35, 4.06). Practically insol in cold water. Sparingly sol in boiling water, liq petrolatum, ether. Sol in boiling alcohol, acetone, acetic acid, vegetable fixed oils, propylene glycol, benzene. Freely sol in chloroform. Sol in aq alkalies with ring cleavage, but is reconstituted upon neutralization. LD$_{50}$ i.p. in rats: 470 ±30 mg/kg (Hakim).

Caution: Methoxsalen with ultraviolet A (long wave light) therapy (PUVA) is listed as a known human carcinogen: *Report on Carcinogens, Eleventh Edition* (PB2005-104914, 2004) p III-165.

THERAP CAT: Pigmentation agent.

5989. Methoxyamine. [67-62-9] O-Methylhydroxylamine; methoxylamine; α-methylhydroxylamine; hydroxylamine methyl ether. CH$_5$NO; mol wt 47.06. C 25.52%, H 10.71%, N 29.76%, O 34.00%. CH$_3$ONH$_2$. Prepd by treating hydroxylamine disulfonic acid with methyl sulfate: Goldfarb, J. Am. Chem. Soc. **67**, 1852 (1945). May also be prepd from hydroxyurethan. Use as reagent for carbonyl compounds: A. H. Blatt, J. Am. Chem. Soc. **61**, 3494 (1939).

Free base. Mobile liquid. Fishy, amine odor. *Highly poisonous!* bp$_{760}$ 49-50°. Miscible with water, alcohol, ether.

Hydrochloride. CH$_5$ON.HCl. Nacreous scales from alcohol+ether, mp 149-151°. Sol in water, alcohol.

Caution: Strong irritant.

USE: Analytical reagent for aldehydes and ketones.

5990. Methoxychlor. [72-43-5] 1,1′-(2,2,2-Trichloroethylidene)bis[4-methoxybenzene]; 1,1,1-trichloro-2,2-bis(p-methoxyphenyl)ethane; 2,2-di-p-anisyl-1,1,1-trichloroethane; DMDT; methoxy-DDT; Marlate. C$_{16}$H$_{15}$Cl$_3$O$_2$; mol wt 345.65. C 55.60%, H 4.37%, Cl 30.77%, O 9.26%. Commercial prepn by the condensation of anisole with chloral in the presence of sulfuric acid: Schneller, Smith, Ind. Eng. Chem. **41**, 1027 (1949). Activity: P. Läuger et al., Helv. Chim. Acta **27**, 892 (1944). Toxicity study: H. C. Hodge et al., J. Pharmacol. Exp. Ther. **99**, 140 (1950). Review of toxicology and human exposure: *Toxicological Profile for Methoxychlor* (PB2003-100140, 2002) 290 pp.

Dimorphic crystals, mp 78-78.2° or 86-88°. Practically insol in water. Soluble in alc. The solubilities are approx those of DDT, q.v. LD$_{50}$ orally in rats: 5.0 g/kg (Hodge).

Caution: Potential symptoms of overexposure in exptl animals are fasciculations; trembling, convulsions; kidney and liver damage. Potential occupational carcinogen. See *NIOSH Pocket Guide to Chemical Hazards* (DHHS/NIOSH 97-140, 1997) p 194. See also *Clinical Toxicology of Commercial Products*, R. E. Gosselin et al.,

Eds. (Williams & Wilkins, Baltimore, 5th ed., 1984) Section II, p 284.

USE: Insecticide.

THERAP CAT (VET): Ectoparasiticide.

5991.   5-Methoxy-*N*,*N*-diisopropyltryptamine. [4021-34-5] 5-Methoxy-*N*,*N*-bis(1-methylethyl)-1*H*-indole-3-ethanamine; 3-[2-(diisopropylamino)ethyl]-5-methoxyindole; 5-MeO-DIPT; "Methoxy Foxy"; "Foxy". $C_{17}H_{26}N_2O$; mol wt 274.40. C 74.41%, H 9.55%, N 10.21%, O 5.83%. Synthetic hallucinogen. Prepn: D. Desaty, D. Keglevic, *Croat. Chem. Acta* **36**, 103 (1964); M. Julia, P. Manoury, *Bull. Soc. Chim. Fr.* **1965**, 1411; and clinical psychopharmacology: A. T. Shulgin, M. F. Carter, *Commun. Psychopharmacol.* **4**, 363 (1980). GC-MS and HPLC-MS determn in blood and urine: S. P. Vorce, J. H. Sklerov, *J. Anal. Toxicol.* **28**, 407 (2004). Determn in forensic samples: C. Huhn *et al.*, *Electrophoresis* **26**, 2391 (2005). Case reports of intoxication: A. A. Muller, *J. Emerg. Nurs.* **30**, 507 (2004); J. M. Wilson *et al.*, *Forensic Sci. Int.* **148**, 31 (2005).

Hydrochloride. [2426-63-3] $C_{17}H_{26}N_2O$.HCl; mol wt 310.86. Crystals from ethanol + ether, mp 180-181°.

Note: This is a controlled substance (hallucinogen): **21 CFR**, 1308.11.

5992.   Methoxyethylbenzeneboronic Acid. [159752-39-3] [2-[(1*R*)-1-Methoxyethyl]phenyl]boronic acid. $C_9H_{13}BO_3$; mol wt 180.01. C 60.05%, H 7.28%, B 6.01%, O 26.66%. Synthesis of (+)-form and use: K. Burgess, A. M. Porte, *Angew. Chem. Int. Ed.* **33**, 1182 (1994). Chemoenzymatic stereosynthesis of both enantiomers and use: S. M. Resnick *et al.*, *J. Org. Chem.* **60**, 3546 (1995).

White solid from *n*-hexane, mp 72-74°. $[\alpha]_D^{25}$ +27 (c = 0.5 in CH_2Cl_2) (Burgess); $[\alpha]_D$ +27.2° (c = 4.6 in CH_2Cl_2) (Resnick).

(−)-*S*-Form. [166191-23-7] $[\alpha]_D$ −28.7° (c = 2.3 in CH_2Cl_2).

USE: NMR shift reagent for enantiomeric assay of diols.

5993.   Methoxyfenozide. [161050-58-4] 3-Methoxy-2-methylbenzoic acid 2-(3,5-dimethylbenzoyl)-2-(1,1-dimethylethyl)-hydrazide; *N'*-*tert*-butyl-*N'*-(3,5-dimethylbenzoyl)-3-methoxy-2-methylbenzohydrazide; *N*-*tert*-butyl-*N'*-(3-methoxy-*o*-toluoyl)-3,5-xylohydrazide; RH-112485; RH-2485; Intrepid; Runner; Prodigy. $C_{22}H_{28}N_2O_3$; mol wt 368.47. C 71.71%, H 7.66%, N 7.60%, O 13.03%. Synthetic nonsteroidal ecdysone agonist. Prepn: Z. Lidert *et al.*, **EP 602794**; *eidem*, **US 5530028** (1994, 1996 both to Rhom & Haas). Comparative insecticidal activity: A. Trisyono, G. M. Chippendale, *J. Econ. Entomol.* **90**, 1486 (1997). Mechanism of action and metabolism: G. Smagghe *et al.*, *Pestic. Sci.* **55**, 386 (1999). Review of physical properties, biological activity and field studies: D. P. Le *et al.*, *Brighton Crop Prot. Conf. - Pests Dis.* **1996**, 481-486; of physical properties and insecticidal activity: G. R. Carlson *et al.*, *Pest Manage. Sci.* **57**, 115-119 (2001).

White powder, mp 204-205°. Vapor pressure (25°): <4.0 × 10^{-8} torr. Soly in water: 3.3 mg/l; in acetone: 9%. Soly (g/l): crop oil <10, cyclohexanone 90, DMSO 110, *N*-methylpyrrolidone 380, xylene <10. Soly in acetone 9%. LD_{50} in rats, mice (mg/kg): >5000, >5000 orally; in rats (mg/kg): >2000 dermally. LC_{50} in rats (mg/l): >4.3 by inhalation. LC_{50} (8 day dietary) in mallard duck, bobwhite quail (mg/kg diet): >5620, >5620. LC_{50} in bluegill sunfish, *Daphnia magna* (mg/l): >4.3 (96 hr); 3.7 (48 hr) (Le).

USE: Insecticide.

5994.   Methoxyflurane. [76-38-0] 2,2-Dichloro-1,1-difluoro-1-methoxyethane; 2,2-dichloro-1,1-difluoroethyl methyl ether; 1,1-difluoro-2,2-dichloroethyl methyl ether; DA-759; Metofane; Penthrane; Pentrane. $C_3H_4Cl_2F_2O$; mol wt 164.97. C 21.84%, H 2.44%, Cl 42.98%, F 23.03%, O 9.70%. $CH_3OCF_2CHCl_2$. Prepn and properties: Miller *et al.*, *J. Am. Chem. Soc.* **70**, 431 (1948); Park *et al.*, *ibid.* **73**, 861 (1951); **GB 754976** (1956 to Standard Tele. & Cable).

Liquid, bp 105°; bp_{100} 51°. mp −35°. n_D^{20} 1.3861; n_D^{25} 1.3839. d_4^{20} 1.4262 (Miller); d_4^{20} 1.4226 (Park).

Caution: Potential symptoms of overexposure are eye irritation; CNS depression, analgesia; anesthesia, seizures, respiratory depression; liver and kidney injury. *See NIOSH Pocket Guide to Chemical Hazards* (DHHS/NIOSH 97-140, 1997) p 196.

THERAP CAT: Anesthetic (inhalation).

THERAP CAT (VET): Anesthetic.

5995.   10-Methoxyharmalan. [3589-73-9] 4,9-Dihydro-6-methoxy-1-methyl-3*H*-pyrido[3,4-*b*]indole; 1-methyl-6-methoxy-3,4-dihydro-2-carboline; 3,4-dihydromethoxyharman. $C_{13}H_{14}N_2$O; mol wt 214.26. C 72.87%, H 6.59%, N 13.07%, O 7.47%. Prepn from 5-methoxytryptamine: Späth, Lederer, *Ber.* **63**, 2102 (1930); Petrova *et al.*, *Zh. Obshch. Khim.* **33**, 1333 (1963), *C.A.* **59**, 10149b (1963). Weak serotonin inhibitor: M. M. Airaksinen *et al.*, *Acta Pharmacol. Toxicol.* **46**, 308 (1980).

Crystals, mp 208-209°. R_f 0.74 in 4:1:5 butanol, acetic acid, water.

5996.   3-Methoxy-4-hydroxyphenylglycol. [534-82-7] 1-(4-Hydroxy-3-methoxyphenyl)-1,2-ethanediol; (4-hydroxy-3-methoxyphenyl)ethylene glycol; vanylglycol; MHPG. $C_9H_{12}O_4$; mol wt 184.19. C 58.69%, H 6.57%, O 34.75%. Major metabolite of norepinephrine, *q.v.* Isoln from rat urine: J. Axelrod *et al.*, *Biochim. Biophys. Acta* **36**, 576 (1959); from cat liver and kidney: M. Goldstein, S. B. Gertner, *Nature* **187**, 147 (1960). Metabolism studies on urinary MHPG levels in patients with affective disorders: K. Greenspan *et al.*, *J. Psychiatr. Res.* **7**, 171 (1970); J. W. Maas *et al.*, *Biochem. Pharmacol.* **1974**, Suppl., pt. 2, 907; J. J. Schildkraut *et al.*, *Biol. Markers Psychiatry Neurol.*, *Proc. Conf.* **1981**, E. Usdin, I. Hanin, Eds. (Pergamon, Oxford, 1982) pp 23-33. Studies on MHPG levels in cerebrospinal fluid (CSF): E. Garelis *et al.*, *Brain Res.* **79**, 1 (1974); P. Frattini *et al.*, *Clin. Chim. Acta* **125**, 97 (1982); in CSF of patients with CNS disorders: T. N. Chase *et al.*, *J. Neurochem.* **21**, 581 (1973); M. G. Ziegler *et al.*, *Am. J. Psychiatry* **134**, 565 (1977). Direct method to estimate rate of prodn of MHPG by human brain *in vivo:* J. W. Maas *et al.*, *Science* **205**, 1025 (1979). Review of origin and distribution in body fluids: E. M. DeMet, A. E. Halaris, *Biochem. Pharmacol.* **28**, 3043-3050 (1979). Use as biochemical marker to identify mental disorders: T. H. Maugh, *Science* **214**, 39 (1981).

USE: As biochemical tool.

5997. 2-Methoxynaphthalene. [93-04-9] Methyl β-naphthyl ether; nerolin "old"; Yara yara. $C_{11}H_{10}O$; mol wt 158.20. C 83.51%, H 6.37%, O 10.11%. Prepn: Hiers, Hager, *Org. Synth.* **coll. vol. I,** 59 (1941).

Leaflets from ether, mp 72°. bp 272°. Practically insol in water. Sparingly sol in alc; sol in ether, carbon disulfide, benzene.

5998. Methoxyphenamine. [93-30-1] 2-Methoxy-*N*,α-dimethylbenzeneethanamine; *o*-methoxy-*N*,α-dimethylphenethylamine; β-(*o*-methoxyphenyl)isopropylmethylamine; α-(2-methoxyphenyl)-β-methylaminopropane. $C_{11}H_{17}NO$; mol wt 179.26. C 73.70%, H 9.56%, N 7.81%, O 8.93%. β-Adrenergic agonist. Prepn: Woodruff *et al., J. Am. Chem. Soc.* **62,** 922 (1940); Heinzelman, *ibid.* **75,** 921 (1953); Morishita, **JP 61 2921** (1961 to Nippon Shinyaku), *C.A.* **55,** 24677f (1961).

Oil, bp$_2$ 97-99°.
Hydrochloride. [5588-10-3] Orthoxine. $C_{11}H_{17}NO.HCl$; mol wt 215.72. Bitter crystals from ether + alcohol, mp 129-131°. Freely sol in water, alcohol, chloroform. Slightly sol in ether, benzene. pH 5.3-5.7 (5% aq soln).
THERAP CAT: Bronchodilator.

5999. *N*-(*p*-Methoxyphenyl)-*p*-phenylenediamine. [101-64-4] *N*-(4-Methoxyphenyl)-1,4-benzenediamine; 4-amino-4'-methoxydiphenylamine; 4-methoxy-4'-aminodiphenylamine; Variamine Blue base. $C_{13}H_{14}N_2O$; mol wt 214.26. C 72.87%, H 6.59%, N 13.07%, O 7.47%. Prepd from the corresp nitroso compd: Willstätter, Kubli, *Ber.* **42,** 4139 (1909).

Needles from ligroin, mp 102°. bp$_{12}$ 238°. Freely sol in alcohol, ether, benzene. Slightly sol in water, petr ether.
Sulfate. $(C_{13}H_{14}N_2O)_2.H_2SO_4$. Crystals, sol in water. Addition of ferric chloride produces intensely blue solns.

6000. 6-Methoxy-α-tetralone. [1078-19-9] 3,4-Dihydro-6-methoxy-1(2*H*)-naphthalenone; 6-methoxy-3,4-dihydro-1(2*H*)-naphthalenone; 1-keto-6-methoxy-1,2,3,4-tetrahydronaphthalene; 5-keto-2-methoxy-5,6,7,8-tetrahydronaphthalene. $C_{11}H_{12}O_2$; mol wt 176.21. C 74.98%, H 6.86%, O 18.16%. Prepn: Papa, *J. Am. Chem. Soc.* **71,** 3246 (1949); Ananchenko *et al., Tetrahedron* **18,** 1355 (1962).

Crystals from methanol or ligroin, mp 80°. bp$_1$ 135-139°, bp$_{11}$ 171°.
USE: In the synthesis of derivatives of estrane and 19-norsteroids (Ananchenko *et al., loc. cit.*).

6001. 1-Methoxy-3-(trimethylsilyloxy)-1,3-butadiene. [54125-02-9] (*E*-form); [59414-23-2] (unspecified stereo). [[(2*E*)-3-Methoxy-1-methylene-2-propenyl]oxy]trimethylsilane; Danishefsky's diene. $C_8H_{16}O_2Si$; mol wt 172.30. C 55.77%, H 9.36%, O 18.57%, Si 16.30%. A silyl enol ether used in Diels-Alder reactions; highly reactive and nucleophilic diene. Prepn and ^{1}H-NMR: S. Danishefsky, T. Kitahana, *J. Am. Chem. Soc.* **96,** 7807 (1974); S. Danishefsky *et al., Org. Synth.* **61,** 147 (1983). In synthesis of

vernolepin, *q.v.: eidem, J. Am. Chem. Soc.* **99,** 6066 (1977); of pentalenolactone: *eidem, ibid.* **100,** 6536 (1978). Regiospecific addition to juglone, *q.v.:* R. K. Boeckman *et al., ibid.* 7098. *Review:* S. Danishefsky, *Acc. Chem. Res.* **14,** 400 (1981).

Oil. bp$_{23}$ 78-81°.
USE: In organic syntheses.

6002. 5-Methoxytryptamine. [608-07-1] 5-Methoxy-1*H*-indole-3-ethanamine; 3-(2-aminoethyl)-5-methoxyindole; meksamin; mexamine. $C_{11}H_{14}N_2O$; mol wt 190.24. C 69.45%, H 7.42%, N 14.73%, O 8.41%. Prepn: Supniewski *et al., C.A.* **55,** 15458 (1961). Proposed as potentiator for hypnotics, sedatives. Claimed to be more active than serotonin: Mashkovsky, Arutyunyan, *Farmakol. Toksikol.* **26** (no. 1), 10 (1963).

Crystals from ethanol, mp 121-122°.
Hydrochloride. $C_{11}H_{14}N_2O.HCl$. Crystals, dec 248°.

6003. Methscopolamine Bromide. [155-41-9] (1α,2β,4β,-5α,7β)-7-[(2*S*)-3-Hydroxy-1-oxo-2-phenylpropoxy]-9,9-dimethyl-3-oxa-9-azoniatricyclo[3.3.1.0^{2,4}]nonane bromide; 6β,7β-epoxy-3α-hydroxy-8-methyl-1α*H*,5α*H*-tropanium bromide tropate (ester); *N*-methylscopolammonium bromide; hyoscine methyl bromide; scopolamine methobromide; scopolamine methyl bromide; epoxymethamine bromide; Holopon; Pamine. $C_{18}H_{24}BrNO_4$; mol wt 398.29. C 54.28%, H 6.07%, Br 20.06%, N 3.52%, O 16.07%. Anticholinergic. Prepd by the action of methyl bromide on scopolamine base: Visscher, **US 2753288** (1956 to Upjohn). Treatment of duodenal ulcer by transdermally administered methscopolamine bromide: R. P. Walt *et al., Br. Med. J.* **284,** 1736 (1982).

Crystals from ethanol, dec 214-217°. Freely sol in water, in dil ethanol. Slightly sol in abs ethanol.
THERAP CAT: Antispasmodic.

6004. Methsuximide. [77-41-8] 1,3-Dimethyl-3-phenyl-2,5-pyrrolidinedione; *N*,2-dimethyl-2-phenylsuccinimide; 1,3-dimethyl-3-phenyl-2,5-dioxopyrrolidine; mesuximide; Celontin; Petinutin. $C_{12}H_{13}NO_2$; mol wt 203.24. C 70.92%, H 6.45%, N 6.89%, O 15.74%. Prepd by the action of methylamine on α-methyl-α-phenylsuccinic acid: Miller, Long, *J. Am. Chem. Soc.* **73,** 4895 (1951); *eidem,* **US 2643257** (1953 to Parke, Davis). Pharmacology: P. G. Marshall, D. K. Vallance, *J. Pharm. Pharmacol.* **6,** 740 (1954).

Crystals from dil alc, mp 52-53°. bp$_{0.1}$ 121-122°. Freely sol in methanol, alc. LD$_{50}$ orally in mice: 0.9 g/kg (Marshall, Vallance).
THERAP CAT: Anticonvulsant.

6005. Methyclothiazide. [135-07-9] 6-Chloro-3-(chloromethyl)-3,4-dihydro-2-methyl-2H-1,2,4-benzothiadiazine-7-sulfonamide 1,1-dioxide; 6-chloro-3-chloromethyl-3,4-dihydro-2-methyl-7-sulfamoyl-1,2,4-benzothiadiazine 1,1-dioxide; 6-chloro-3-chloromethyl-2-methyl-7-sulfamyl-3,4-dihydro-1,2,4-benzothiadiazine 1,1-dioxide; Aquatensen; Duretic; Enduron; Enduronum; Naturon. C$_9$H$_{11}$Cl$_2$N$_3$O$_4$S$_2$; mol wt 360.24. C 30.01%, H 3.08%, Cl 19.68%, N 11.66%, O 17.77%, S 17.80%. Prepn: Close et al., J. Am. Chem. Soc. **82**, 1132 (1960). Description: Ford, Curr. Ther. Res. **2**, 422 (1960). Comprehensive description: J. A. Raihle, Anal. Profiles Drug Subs. **5**, 307-326 (1976).

Crystals from alcohol + water, mp 225°. uv max (methanol): 226, 267, 311 nm (ε 39300, 21250, 3300). pKa 9.4. Very sol in acetone, pyridine; slightly sol in methanol, ethanol. Almost insol in water, chloroform, benzene.
THERAP CAT: Diuretic; antihypertensive.

6006. Methyl Abietate. [127-25-3] Abalyn. C$_{21}$H$_{32}$O$_2$; mol wt 316.48. C 79.70%, H 10.19%, O 10.11%. C$_{19}$H$_{29}$-COOCH$_3$. The article of commerce is a mixture of the methyl esters of the rosin acids.
Colorless to yellow, almost odorless, thick liquid. d$_{20}^{20}$ 1.040. bp 360-365° with decompn. n$_D^{20}$ 1.530. Flash pt 180-218°C. Insol in water. Miscible with usual organic solvents, also with aliphatic hydrocarbons. Dissolves ester gums, rosin, many synthetic resins as well as ethyl cellulose, rubber, etc.
USE: As a solvent for ester gums, rosin, many synthetic resins, ethyl cellulose, rubber, etc.; in the manuf of varnish resins; as ingredient in adhesives.

6007. N-Methylacetanilide. [579-10-2] N-Methyl-N-phenylacetamide; acetomethylanilide; Exalgin. C$_9$H$_{11}$NO; mol wt 149.19. C 72.46%, H 7.43%, N 9.39%, O 10.72%. Made by the action of acetic anhydride on methylaniline.

Orthorhombic rods from alcohol, plates from ether or petr ether. mp 102-104°. bp$_{712}$ 253°. One gram dissolves in 60 ml water, 2 ml boiling water, 2 ml alcohol, 1.5 ml chloroform, 10 ml ether.

6008. Methyl Acetate. [79-20-9] C$_3$H$_6$O$_2$; mol wt 74.08. C 48.64%, H 8.16%, O 43.19%. CH$_3$COOCH$_3$.
Colorless liquid; pleasant odor. mp −98°. bp 56.9°. d$_4^{20}$ 0.9342; d$_4^{25}$ 0.9279. n$_D^{20}$ 1.3614: Mumford, Phillips, J. Chem. Soc. **1950**, 75. Flash pt, closed cup: 14°F (−10°C). Sol in water; miscible with alcohol, ether.
Caution: Potential symptoms of overexposure are irritation of eyes, skin, nose and throat; headache, drowsiness; optic nerve atrophy; chest tightness. See NIOSH Pocket Guide to Chemical Hazards (DHHS/NIOSH 97-140, 1997) p 196.
USE: Solvent for nitrocellulose, acetylcellulose, and many resins and oils; manuf artificial leather.

6009. Methyl Acetoacetate. [105-45-3] 3-Oxobutanoic acid methyl ester. C$_5$H$_8$O$_3$; mol wt 116.12. C 51.72%, H 6.94%, O 41.33%. CH$_3$COCH$_2$COOCH$_3$. Toxicity data: H. F. Smyth, C. P. Carpenter, J. Ind. Hyg. Toxicol. **30**, 63 (1948).
Liquid. d 1.078-1.080. bp 169-171° (slight dec). mp −80°. n$_D^{20}$ 1.418. Flash pt 82°C. Sol in 2 parts water; miscible with alc,

ether; gives a deep red color with FeCl$_3$. LD$_{50}$ orally in rats: 3.0 g/kg (Smyth, Carpenter).

6010. Methyl Acetylsalicylate. [580-02-9] 2-(Acetyloxy)-benzoic acid methyl ester; acetylsalicylic acid methyl ester; methylaspirin; Methylrodin; Methylrhodine. C$_{10}$H$_{10}$O$_4$; mol wt 194.18. C 61.85%, H 5.19%, O 32.96%. Prepd from acetylsalicylic acid and diazomethane: Herzig, Tichatschek, Ber. **39**, 1559 (1906); from methyl salicylate and acetic anhydride: Erdmann, J. Prakt. Chem. [2] **56**, 154 (1897); Thorp, US **1255950** (1918).

Plates from petr ether. mp 51-52°. bp$_9$ 134-136°. Very sparingly sol in water; sol in alc, ether, chloroform, glycerol, propylene glycol, oils.
USE: Fixative for perfumes.

6011. Methyl Acrylate. [96-33-3] 2-Propenoic acid methyl ester; acrylic acid methyl ester. C$_4$H$_6$O$_2$; mol wt 86.09. C 55.81%, H 7.02%, O 37.17%. CH$_2$=CHCOOCH$_3$. Convenient prepn from ethylene chlorohydrin: DE **571123** (1928 to Rohm & Haas). For direct syntheses from acetylene and carbon monoxide see W. Reppe, Chemie & Technik der Acetylen-Druck-Reaktionen (Weinheim, 2nd ed., 1952). Toxicity study: H. F. Smyth, C. P. Carpenter, J. Ind. Hyg. Toxicol. **30**, 63 (1948).
Liquid. Acrid odor. Lacrimator. d$_4^{20}$ 0.9561; d$_{20}^{20}$ 0.9574; d$_4^0$ 0.9702; d$_4^{-5}$ 0.9868; d$_4^{-10}$ 0.9929. Weighs 8.0 lbs/gal. mp −76.5°. bp$_{608}$ 70°; bp$_{428}$ 60°; bp$_{298}$ 50°; bp$_{200}$ 40°; bp$_{88}$ 20°; bp$_{54}$ 10°; bp$_{41.5}$ 5°; bp$_{32}$ 0°; bp$_{24.5}$ −5°; bp$_{18.5}$ −10°. n$_D^{20}$ 1.401. Sp heat at −60° = 0.444 cal/g/°C; heat of vaporization 8.25 kcal/mol; heat of combustion 502.88 kcal/mol. Soly in water at 20° = 6 g/100 ml, at 40° = 5 g/100 ml. Soly of water in methyl acrylate at 20° = 1.8 ml/100 g. Sol in alc, ether. Azeotropes: 9.5% water = bp 73°; 49.0% methanol = bp 61°. Easily polymerizes on standing. The polymerization process can be speeded up by heat, light, and peroxides. If pure, the monomer can be stored below +10° without incurring polymerization. LD$_{50}$ orally in rats: 0.3 g/kg (Smyth, Carpenter).
Polymer. Transparent, elastic substance. Practically no odor. Little adhesive power. Resists the usual solvents.
Caution: Potential symptoms of overexposure to the monomer are irritation of eyes, upper respiratory system and skin. See NIOSH Pocket Guide to Chemical Hazards (DHHS/NIOSH 97-140, 1997) p 198. See also Clinical Toxicology of Commercial Products, R. E. Gosselin et al., Eds. (Williams & Wilkins, Baltimore, 5th ed., 1984) Section II, p 409.
USE: The monomer in manuf leather finish resins, textile and paper coatings, and plastic films. Produces the hardest resin of the acrylate ester series.

6012. Methylal. [109-87-5] Dimethoxymethane; formal; formaldehyde dimethyl acetal. C$_3$H$_8$O$_2$; mol wt 76.09. C 47.35%, H 10.60%, O 42.05%. CH$_2$(OCH$_3$)$_2$. Prepn by catalytic vapor-phase oxidation of methanol in the presence of small amts of HCl; from methanol and formaldehyde: Frevel, Hedelund, US **2663742**; US **2691684** (1953, 1954, both to Dow); from paraformaldehyde + methanol in the presence of CaCl$_2$ + HCl: R. Rambaud, D. Besserre, Bull. Soc. Chim. Fr. **1955**, 45.
Colorless, clear, volatile, flammable liq; chloroform odor; pungent taste. bp$_{760}$ 41.6°; bp$_{754}$ 41.5°. mp −105°. d$_4^{14}$ 0.8669; d$_4^{20}$ 0.8593. n$_D^{18}$ 1.3589. Flash pt, closed cup: 0°F (−18°C). Sol in 3 parts water; miscible with alcohol, ether, oils.
Caution: Potential symptoms of overexposure are irritation of eyes, skin and upper respiratory system; anesthesia. See NIOSH Pocket Guide to Chemical Hazards (DHHS/NIOSH 97-140, 1997) p 198.
USE: In perfumery; manuf artificial resins; reaction medium for Grignard and Reppe reactions.

6013. Methyl Allyl Trisulfide. [34135-85-8] Methyl-2-propenyl trisulfide; allyl methyl trisulfide; methyl 2-propenyl trisulfane;

MATS. $C_4H_8S_3$; mol wt 152.30. C 31.54%, H 5.29%, S 63.16%. $CH_3SSSCH_2CH=CH_2$. Component of garlic oil which inhibits platelet aggregation. Synthesis, identification by GC: D. M. Oaks *et al.*, *Anal. Chem.* **36,** 1560 (1964). Isoln from garlic oil, effect on platelet-rich plasma: T. Ariga *et al.*, *Lancet* **1,** 150 (1981). Improved synthesis: A. W. Mott, G. Barany, *Synthesis* **1984,** 657. Use as antithrombotic agent: **JP Kokai 82 209218** (1982 to Alcon), *C.A.* **98,** 95692n (1983).

Oil, $bp_{0.05}$ 28-30°.

6014. Methylamine. [74-89-5] Methanamine; monomethylamine; aminomethane. CH_5N; mol wt 31.06. C 38.67%, H 16.23%, N 45.10%. CH_3NH_2. Occurs in herring brine, in urine of dogs after eating meat, in certain plants such as *Mentha aquatica*, in crude methanol together with di- and trimethylamine. Made by heating methyl alcohol, ammonium chloride, and zinc chloride to ~300°; by heating ammonium chloride and formaldehyde: Marvel, Jenkins, *Org. Synth.* **3,** 67 (1923); from methanol + ammonia: Smith, **US 2456599** (1948 to Comm. Solvents). Inhalation toxicity studies: L. A. Kinney *et al.*, *Inhalation Toxicol.* **2,** 29 (1990); S. N. Sarkar, M. S. Sastry, *J. Environ. Biol.* **13,** 273 (1992).

Flammable gas at ordinary temp and pressure. Fuming liq when cooled in ice and salt mixture. $d_4^{-10.8}$ 0.699. mp −93.5°. bp_{760} −6.3°; bp_{400} −19.7°; bp_{200} −32.4°; bp_{100} −43.7°; bp_{10} −73.8°. Flash pt 32.5°F (0°C). Stronger base than ammonia: pK_b (25°): 3.35. Absorption spectrum: Bielecki, Henri, *Compt. Rend.* **156,** 1861 (1913). One vol of water at 12.5° dissolves 1154 vols of the gas, and 959 vols at 25°. 100 ml of a benzene soln satd at 25° contain 10.5 g methylamine. Sol in alc; miscible with ether. LD_{50} orally in rats: 100-200 mg/kg (Kinney). LC_{50} in rats: 0.448 ml/l (Sarkar, Sastry).

Hydrochloride. Deliquescent tetragonal tablets from alcohol, mp 227-228° with sublimation. bp_{15} 225-230°. Sol in water, in abs alcohol. 100 g of boiling abs alcohol dissolve 23.01 g. Insol in chloroform, acetone, ether, ethyl acetate. *Keep well closed.* LD_{50} orally in rats: 1600-3200 mg/kg (Kinney).

Caution: Potential symptoms of overexposure are irritation of eyes, skin and respiratory system; coughing; skin and mucous membrane burns; dermatitis; conjunctivitis; direct contact with liquid may cause frostbite. *See NIOSH Pocket Guide to Chemical Hazards* (DHHS/NIOSH 97-140, 1997) p 200.

USE: Methylamine is used in tanning. Methylamine and methylamine hydrochloride are used in organic synthesis for introducing the methylamino group.

6015. 2-Methylaminoethanol. [109-83-1] Methyl(β-hydroxyethyl)amine; methylethylolamine. C_3H_9NO; mol wt 75.11. C 47.97%, H 12.08%, N 18.65%, O 21.30%. $CH_3NHCH_2CH_2OH$. *In vivo* precursor of choline; isoln from mutant of *Neurospora crassa* which has lost its ability to synthesize choline: Horowitz, *J. Biol. Chem.* **162,** 413 (1946). Prepn by mixing ethylene oxide with concd methylamine soln with external cooling: Knorr, Matthes, *Ber.* **31,** 1069 (1898); Lowe *et al.*, **GB 763434** (1956 to Oxirane Ltd.); Nikolaev *et al.*, *Zh. Obshch. Khim.* **33,** 391 (1963). Toxicity studies: R. Hartung, H. H. Cornish, *Toxicol. Appl. Pharmacol.* **12,** 486 (1968); B. Ballantyne, H.-W. Leung, *Vet. Hum. Toxicol.* **38,** 422 (1996).

Viscous liquid. Fishy odor. d^{20} 0.937. bp_{760} 155-156°; bp_{12} 64-65°. n_D^{20} 1.4385. Miscible with water, alcohol, ether. Strong base. Corrosive to cork, metals. LD_{50} in rats (g/kg): 3.36 orally, 1.33 i.p. (Hartung). LD_{50} in male, female rats (mg/kg): 1908, 1391 orally; male, female rabbits (mg/kg): 1880, 1006 dermally (Ballantyne, Leung).

Caution: Direct contact may cause skin and eye irritation, skin corrosioin. *See* Ballantyne, Leung.

6016. Methyl Aminolevulinate. [33320-16-0] 5-Amino-4-oxopentanoic acid methyl ester; P-1202. $C_6H_{11}NO_3$; mol wt 145.16. C 49.64%, H 7.64%, N 9.65%, O 33.07%. Prodrug of δ-aminolevulinic acid, *q.v.*; induces production of intracellular protoporphyrin IX. Prepn: S. I. Zav'yalov, A. G. Zavozin, *Bull. Acad. Sci. USSR Div. Chem. Sci.* **36,** 1663 (1987). Porphyrin enrichment in solar keratoses: C. Fritsch *et al.*, *Photochem. Photobiol.* **68,** 218 (1998). Clinical trial in photodynamic therapy of basal cell carcinomas: A. M. Soler *et al.*, *Br. J. Dermatol.* **145,** 467 (2001); C. Vinciullo *et al.*, *Br. J. Dermatol.* **152,** 765 (2005); in actinic kera-

tosis: R. M. Szeimies *et al.*, *J. Am. Acad. Dermatol.* **47,** 258 (2002). Review of pharmacology and clinical experience: M. A. A. Siddiqui *et al.*, *Am. J. Clin. Dermatol.* **5,** 127-137 (2004).

Hydrochloride. [79416-27-6] Metvix. $C_6H_{11}NO_3.HCl$; mol wt 181.62. mp 119-121°.

THERAP CAT: Antineoplastic (photosensitizer).

6017. *p*-Methylaminophenol Sulfate. [55-55-0] 4-(Methylamino)phenol sulfate salt (2:1); monomethyl-*p*-aminophenol sulfate; *p*-hydroxymethylaniline sulfate; Photol; Verol; Rhodol; Armol; Elon; Genol; Graphol; Photo-Rex; Pictol; Planetol; Metol. $C_{14}H_{20}N_2O_6S$; mol wt 344.38. C 48.83%, H 5.85%, N 8.13%, O 27.88%, S 9.31%.

Crystals. Discolors in air. mp ~260° with decompn. Sol in 20 parts cold, 6 parts boiling water; slightly sol in alc; insol in ether. *Keep well closed and protected from light.*

USE: Photographic developer; dyeing furs.

6018. 4-Methylaminorex. [3568-94-3] 4,5-dihydro-4-methyl-5-phenyl-2-oxazolamine; 2-amino-4-methyl-5-phenyl-2-oxazoline; 4-MAX. $C_{10}H_{12}N_2O$; mol wt 176.22. C 68.16%, H 6.86%, N 15.90%, O 9.08%. Indirect acting sympathomimetic agent related to amphetamine, *q.v.*. Exists as four isomers, (±)-*trans* and (±)-*cis;* the latter being the drug of abuse. Prepn: G. I. Poos *et al.*, *J. Med. Chem.* **6,** 266 (1963); G. I. Poos, **US 3161650** (1964 to McNeil Labs). Synthesis and chemical properties of isomers: R. F. X. Klein *et al.*, *J. Forensic Sci.* **34,** 962 (1989). Structure-activity comparison of isomers: R. A. Glennon, B. Misenheimer, *Pharmacol. Biochem. Behav.* **35,** 517 (1990). Mechanism of action study with behavioural effects: K. Batsche *et al.*, *J. Pharmacol. Exp. Ther.* **269,** 1029 (1994). Metabolism in rats: G. L. Henderson *et al.*, *J. Anal. Toxicol.* **19,** 563 (1995). Neurochemical effects: Y. Zheng *et al.*, *J. Pharm. Pharmacol.* **49,** 89 (1997).

(+)-*cis*

(±)-*cis* Form. [29493-77-4] EU4EA; U4Euh; Ice; McN-822. Crystals from benzene, mp 154.5-156° (Poos, 1963). Also reported as mp 139-142° (Glennon). $[\alpha]_D^{25}$ −244.7° for (−)-form; $[\alpha]_D^{25}$ +240.9° for (+)-form.

Note: The (±)-*cis* isomers are controlled substances (stimulant): **21 CFR,** 1308.11.

6019. Methylaniline. [100-61-8] *N*-Methylbenzenamine; monomethylaniline. C_7H_9N; mol wt 107.15. C 78.46%, H 8.47%, N 13.07%. $C_6H_5NHCH_3$. Made by heating aniline chloride and methyl alcohol under pressure. Toxicology: J. F. Treon *et al.*, *J. Ind. Hyg. Toxicol.* **31,** 1 (1949).

Colorless or slightly yellow liquid; becomes brown on exposure to air. d_4^{20} 0.989. mp −57°. bp 194-196°. $n_D^{21.2}$ 1.5702. Slightly sol in water; sol in alc, ether. LD in rabbits (g/kg): 0.28 orally; in rabbits, cats (mg/kg): 24, 24 i.v. (Treon).

Caution: Potential symptoms of overexposure are weakness, dizziness and headache; dyspnea, cyanosis; methemoglobinemia; pulmonary edema; liver and kidney damage. *See NIOSH Pocket Guide to Chemical Hazards* (DHHS/NIOSH 97-140, 1997) p 218.

6020.　Methyl Anthranilate. [134-20-3] 2-Aminobenzoic acid methyl ester; methyl 2-aminobenzoate; neroli oil (artificial). $C_8H_9NO_2$; mol wt 151.16. C 63.57%, H 6.00%, N 9.27%, O 21.17%. Occurs in neroli, ylang-ylang, bergamot, jasmine, other essential oils and in grape juice; also obtained synthetically by esterifying anthranilic acid with CH_3OH in presence of HCl.

Crystals. d 1.168. mp 24-25°. bp_{15} 135.5°. Slightly sol in water; freely sol in alcohol or ether. LD_{50} orally in rats, mice: 2910, 3900 mg/kg, P. M. Jenner *et al., Food Cosmet. Toxicol.* **2**, 327 (1964).

USE: As perfume for ointments; manuf synthetic perfumes.

6021.　2-Methylanthraquinone. [84-54-8] 2-Methyl-9,10-anthracenedione; *β*-methylanthraquinone. $C_{15}H_{10}O_2$; mol wt 222.24. C 81.07%, H 4.54%, O 14.40%. Occurs in teakwood. Prepd by oxidation of 2-methylanthracene; by formation from phthalic anhydride and toluene: Fieser, *Org. Synth.* **4**, 43 (1925); from 6- and 7-methylanthraquinone-1-carboxylic acids with powdered copper in quinoline: Fieser, Martin, *J. Am. Chem. Soc.* **58**, 1443 (1936); from 1,4-naphthoquinone and isoprene: Carothers, Berchet, *ibid.* **55**, 2813 (1933).

Needles from alcohol, mp 177°. Sublimes. Very sol in benzene, toluene, xylene; sol in alcohol, ether, glacial acetic acid, concd H_2SO_4; insol in water.

6022.　N^G-Methylarginine. [17035-90-4] N^5-[Imino(methylamino)methyl]-L-ornithine; tilarginine; targinine; N^G-monomethyl-L-arginine; L-NMA. $C_7H_{16}N_4O_2$; mol wt 188.23. C 44.67%, H 8.57%, N 29.77%, O 17.00%. Nitric oxide synthase (NOS) inhibitor; naturally occurring analog of arginine. Isoln from bovine brain and prepn: T. Nakajima *et al., Biochim. Biophys. Acta* **230**, 212 (1971). Improved prepn: J. L. Corbin, M. Reporter, *Anal. Biochem.* **57**, 310 (1974); S. Pundak, M. Wilchek, *J. Org. Chem.* **46**, 808 (1981); of acetate salt: W. Zhang *et al., Synth. Commun.* **24**, 2789 (1994). Inhibition of NO release by endothelial cells: R. M. J. Palmer *et al., Biochem. Biophys. Res. Commun.* **153**, 1251 (1988). Review of biological significance: J. Leiper, P. Vallance, *Cardiovasc. Res.* **43**, 542-548 (1999). Clinical evaluation in cardiogenic shock: G. Cotter *et al., Circulation* **101**, 1358 (2000).

Crystals from water-ethanol. $[\alpha]_D^{25}$ +26° (c = 1 in 1*N* HCl).
Acetate. [53308-83-1] $C_7H_{16}N_4O_2 \cdot C_2H_4O_2$; mol wt 248.28. White granular solid. $[\alpha]_D^{22}$ +9.5° (c = 0.10 in water). Sol in water.
USE: Reagent to inhibit nitric oxide production in biological systems.

THERAP CAT: In treatment of cardiogenic shock.

6023.　Methylbenzethonium Chloride. [25155-18-4] *N,N*-Dimethyl-*N*-[2-[2-[methyl-4-(1,1,3,3-tetramethylbutyl)phenoxy]-ethoxy]ethyl]benzenemethanaminium chloride; benzyldimethyl[2-[2-(*p*-1,1,3,3-tetramethylbutylcresoxy)ethoxy]ethyl]ammonium chloride; [2-[2-(*p*-octylcresoxy)ethoxy]ethyl]dimethylbenzyl-ammonium chloride; benzyldimethyl[2-[2-[4-(1,1,3,3-tetramethyl-butyl)tolyloxy]ethoxy]ethyl]ammonium chloride. $C_{28}H_{44}ClNO_2$; mol wt 462.11. C 72.77%, H 9.60%, Cl 7.67%, N 3.03%, O 6.92%. Quaternary ammonium salt with antimicrobial activity. Germicidal activity: F. Hart, C. L. Huyck, *J. Am. Pharm. Assoc. Sci. Ed.* **37**, 272 (1948). *In vitro* activity vs *Leishmania major:* J. El-On, G. Messer, *Am. J. Trop. Med. Hyg.* **35**, 1110 (1986). Clinical trial in combination with paromomycin, *q.v.,* in cutaneous leishmaniasis: G. Krause, A. Kroeger, *Trans. R. Soc. Trop. Med. Hyg.* **88**, 92 (1994). Review of properties, commercial uses and toxicology: *J. Am. Coll. Toxicol.* **4**, 65-106 (1985).

Monohydrate. [1320-44-1] Diaparene; Hyamine 10X. Bitter tasting crystals, mp 161-163°. Freely sol in water, alcohol, cellosolve, chloroform, hot benzene. LD_{50} in rats (mg/kg): 100 s.c. (Hart, Huyck).
USE: In cosmetics as preservative; cationic surfactant.
THERAP CAT: Antiseptic, disinfectant.

6024.　Methyl Benzoate. [93-58-3] Benzoic acid methyl ester; essence of Niobe; oil of Niobe. $C_8H_8O_2$; mol wt 136.15. C 70.57%, H 5.92%, O 23.50%. $C_6H_5COOCH_3$. Toxicity data: Smyth *et al., Arch. Ind. Hyg. Occup. Med.* **10**, 61 (1954).
Colorless, transparent liquid; pleasant odor. d_4^{15} 1.094. mp ~ −15°. bp 198-200°. n_D^{15} 1.5205. Flash pt, closed cup: 181°F (82°C). Insol in water; misc with alcohol, ether, methanol. LD_{50} orally in rats: 3.43 g/kg (Smyth).
USE: In perfumes (Peau d'Espagne).

6025.　Methyl Benzoylsalicylate. [610-60-6] 2-(Benzoyl-oxy)benzoic acid methyl ester; benzosalin. $C_{15}H_{12}O_4$; mol wt 256.25. C 70.31%, H 4.72%, O 24.97%.
Crystals. mp 85°. bp 385°. Insol in water. One gram dissolves in 35 ml alcohol; sol in benzene, chloroform, ether.

6026.　α-Methylbenzylamine. [98-84-0] α-Methylbenzene-methanamine; α-phenylethylamine; 1-phenylethylamine; α-amino-ethylbenzene. $C_8H_{11}N$; mol wt 121.18. C 79.29%, H 9.15%, N 11.56%. Prepn from acetophenone and ammonium formate: A. W. Ingersoll *et al., J. Am. Chem. Soc.* **58**, 1808 (1936); by reduction of acetophenone in liquid ammonia: J. C. Robinson, H. R. Snyder, *Org. Synth.* **coll. vol. III**, 717 (1955). Stereospecific synthesis of *R*-(+)-form: H. Takahashi *et al., Chem. Pharm. Bull.* **29**, 3387 (1981). Resolution of *(dl)*-methylbenzylamine: W. Theikecker, H.-G. Winkler, *Ber.* **87**, 690 (1954). Use of *(R)*-(+)-methylbenzylamine as resolving agent: E. J. Corey, J. Mann, *J. Am. Chem. Soc.* **95**, 6832 (1973). Use as chiral intermediate in synthesis of α-methyl-α-amino nitriles: K. Weinges *et al., Ber.* **110**, 2098 (1977); of β-amino acids: M. Furukawa *et al., Chem. Pharm. Bull.* **26**, 260 (1978). Toxicity: H. F. Smyth *et al., Arch. Ind. Hyg. Occup. Med.* **4**, 119 (1951).

dl-Form. Liquid. Aromatic odor. Absorbs CO_2 from air. d_4^{15} 0.9395. bp_{18} 80-81°. Strong base. Soly in water at 20° about 4.2%. Misc with alcohol, ether. LD_{50} orally in rats: 0.94 g/kg (Smyth).
(+)-Form. Liquid, bp 184-186°. d_4^{22} 0.950. $[\alpha]_D^{22}$ +40.3° (neat).
(−)-Form. Liquid, bp_{12} 73°. d_4^{22} 0.950. $[\alpha]_D^{22}$ −40.3° (neat).
USE: As resolving agent; chiral intermediate.

6027. 4-Methylbenzylidene Camphor. [36861-47-9] 1,7,7-Trimethyl-3-[(4-methylphenyl)methylene]bicyclo[2.2.1]heptan-2-one; 3-(4'-methylbenzylidene)camphor; 4-MBC; Eusolex 6300. $C_{18}H_{22}O$; mol wt 254.37. C 84.99%, H 8.72%, O 6.29%. Ultraviolet filter in sunscreens. Prepn: J.-C. Richer, A. Rossi, *Can. J. Chem.* **50,** 1376 (1972). TLC identification in cosmetics: D. H. Liem, L. T. H. Hilderink, *Int. J. Cosmet. Sci.* **1,** 341 (1979); electrokinetic chromatography determn of enantiomers in cosmetic formulations: B. Gómara *et al., Electrophoresis* **26,** 3952 (2005). Photostability: A. Deflandre, G. Lang, *Int. J. Cosmet. Sci.* **10,** 53 (1988); *eidem, Cosmet. Toiletries* **103,** 69 (1988). *In vivo* assessment of photostability: M. Cambon *et al., J. Cosmet. Sci.* **52,** 1 (2001). Uterotrophic activity: H. Tinwell *et al., Environ. Health Perspect.* **110,** 533 (2002). Evaluation of androgenic activity: R. Ma *et al., Toxicol. Sci.* **74,** 43 (2003).

Crystals from absolute ethanol, mp 98.5-99.5°. $[\alpha]_D^{24}$ +429° (c = 1.615 in benzene). uv max (95% ethanol): 226, 301 nm (ε 7300, 20500).

THERAP CAT: Ultraviolet screen.

6028. Methyl Blue. [28983-56-4] [[4-[Bis[4-[(sulfophenyl)amino]phenyl]methylene]-2,5-cyclohexadien-1-ylidene]amino]-benzenesulfonic acid disodium salt; sodium triphenyl-*p*-rosanilinetrisulfate; brilliant cotton blue; Helvetia blue; C.I. Acid Blue 93; C.I. 42780. $C_{37}H_{27}N_3Na_2O_9S_3$; mol wt 799.80. C 55.56%, H 3.40%, N 5.25%, Na 5.75%, O 18.00%, S 12.03%. *Do not confuse with methylene blue.* Prepn: *Colour Index* vol. 4 (3rd ed., 1971) p 4403.

Dark blue powder. Sol in water. Absorption max about 607 nm.
USE: As a coloring; dye for cotton and silk; biological stain.
THERAP CAT: Antiseptic.

6029. Methyl Bromide. [74-83-9] Bromomethane; monobromomethane; Embafume. CH_3Br; mol wt 94.94. C 12.65%, H 3.18%, Br 84.16%. Prepd industrially by the action of hydrobromic acid on methanol. Several modifications of the process, *e.g.,* sulfuric acid is added to sodium bromide and methanol, methyl bromide being removed by distillation. Acute toxicity: D. D. Irish *et al., J. Ind. Hyg. Toxicol.* **22,** 218 (1940). Atmospheric emission and potential ozone depletion from biomass burning: S. Manö, M. O. Andreae, *Science* **263,** 1255 (1994). Review of toxicology and human exposure: *Toxicological Profile for Bromomethane* (PB93-110682, 1992) 129 pp.

Colorless gas. Usually odorless; sweetish, chloroform-like odor at high concns. Burning taste. Non-flammable in air, but burns in oxygen. mp −93.66°; bp 3.56°: Egan, Kemp, *J. Am. Chem. Soc.* **60,** 2097 (1938). Vapor press. (20°): 1420 mm Hg. d_4^0 1.730. d_{gas}^{20} 3.974 g/l; n_D^{20} 1.4432. Viscosity (0°): 0.397 cP. Spec. heat at −96.6°: 0.165 cal/g/°C; at −13.0°: 1.97 cal/g/°C; at 25°: 0.107 cal/g/°C. Crit temp 194°. Soly in water (20°, 748 mm): 1.75 g/100 g of soln. Forms a cryst hydrate, $CH_3Br.20H_2O$, below 4°. Freely sol in alcohol, chloroform, ether, carbon disulfide, carbon tetrachloride, benzene. LC for rats in air (6 hrs): 514 ppm (Irish).

Caution: Potential symptoms of overexposure by inhalation are irritation of respiratory system; headache; visual disturbance; vertigo; nausea, vomiting, anorexia, abdominal pain; malaise, muscle weakness, incoordination, slurring of speech, staggering gait; hand tremor; convulsions; mental confusion; dyspnea; pulmonary edema; coma; death from respiratory or circulatory collapse. Onset of symptoms may be delayed. Direct contact may cause eye irritation, skin irritation or vesiculation; direct contact with liquid may cause frostbite. Potential occupational carcinogen. *See NIOSH Pocket Guide to Chemical Hazards* (DHHS/NIOSH 97-140, 1997) p 200; *Clinical Toxicology of Commercial Products,* R. E. Gosselin *et al.,* Eds. (Williams & Wilkins, Baltimore, 5th ed., 1984) Section III, pp 280-284.

USE: In ionization chambers. For degreasing wool. Extracting oils from nuts, seeds, flowers. Soil or space fumigant for insects, fungi, rodents. Methylating agent. Has been used as fire extinguishing agent.

6030. 2-Methyl-1-butanol. [137-32-6] Active amyl alcohol; *dl-sec*-butyl carbinol. $C_5H_{12}O$; mol wt 88.15. C 68.13%, H 13.72%, O 18.15%. $CH_3CH_2CH(CH_3)CH_2OH$. One of the minor components of fusel oil, *q.v.* Prepn: Hawthorne, *J. Org. Chem.* **23,** 1788 (1958); **GB 883375** (1961 to Continental Oil). Isoln of (−)-form by fractional distillation of fusel oil: Milburn, Truter, *J. Chem. Soc.* **1954,** 3344. Prepn of (+)-form: Carnmalm, *Chem. Ind. (London)* **1956,** 1093. Toxicity study: H. F. Smyth *et al., Am. Ind. Hyg. Assoc. J.* **23,** 95 (1962). Review of manuf by fractionation of fusel oil and *via* chlorination of pentanes, and properties: *Industrial Chemicals,* W. L. Faith *et al.,* Eds. (John Wiley, New York, 2nd ed., 1957) pp 107-114.

Liquid, bp 128°. d_4^{20} 0.816. n_D^{25} 1.4104. Flash pt, open cup: 122°F (50°C). Slightly sol in water (3.6 g/100 g at 30°); misc with alcohol, ether. LD_{50} orally in rats: 4.92 ml/kg (Smyth).

(−)-**Form.** $[\alpha]_D^{20}$ −4.75°.
(+)-**Form.** d_{20}^{20} 0.826. n_D^{20} 1.411.

6031. 3-Methyl-2-butanol. [598-75-4] *dl-sec*-Isoamyl alcohol; *sec*-isopentyl alcohol; isopropyl methyl carbinol. $C_5H_{12}O$; mol wt 88.15. C 68.13%, H 13.72%, O 18.15%. $(CH_3)_2CHCH(OH)CH_3$. Prepn: Brown, Subba Rao, *J. Am. Chem. Soc.* **81,** 6423 (1959); Cook, *J. Org. Chem.* **27,** 3873 (1962). Review of manuf by fractionation of fusel oil and *via* chlorination of pentanes, and properties: *Industrial Chemicals,* W. L. Faith *et al.,* Eds. (John Wiley, New York, 2nd ed., 1957) pp 107-114.

Liquid, bp 113-114°. bp_{742} 109.5-110.5°. d^{19} 0.819. n_D^{20} 1.4091. Flash pt, closed cup: 103°F (39°C); open cup: 95°F (35°C). Slightly sol in water (2.8 g/100 g at 30°); miscible with alcohol, ether.

Caution: Potential symptoms of overexposure are irritation of eyes, skin, nose and throat; headache, dizziness; cough, dyspnea, nausea, vomiting and diarrhea; skin cracking. *See NIOSH Pocket Guide to Chemical Hazards* (DHHS/NIOSH 97-140, 1997) p 176.

6032. Methyl *tert*-Butyl Ether. [1634-04-4] 2-Methoxy-2-methylpropane; *tert*-butyl methyl ether; MTBE. $C_5H_{12}O$; mol wt 88.15. C 68.13%, H 13.72%, O 18.15%. $(CH_3)_3C(OCH_3)$. Prepn: L. Henry, *Rec. Trav. Chim.* **23,** 324 (1904); from methanol and *t*-butyl alcohol: J. F. Norris, G. W. Rigby, *J. Am. Chem. Soc.* **54,** 2088 (1932); from methanol and isobutylene: K. R. Edlund, T. W. Evans, **US 1968601** (1934 to Shell); *eidem, Ind. Eng. Chem.* **28,** 1186 (1936); R. D. Morin, A. E. Bearse, *ibid.* **43,** 1596 (1951); from *t*-butyl alcohol and diazomethane: M. Neeman *et al., Tetrahedron* **6,** 36 (1959). Use as chromatographic eluent: C. J. Little *et al., J. Chromatogr.* **169,** 381 (1979). Experimental use to dissolve cholesterol gallstones *in vivo:* M. J. Allen *et al., Gastroenterology* **88,** 122 (1985); *eidem, N. Engl. J. Med.* **312,** 217 (1985). Method for therapeutic use in dissolving cholesterol calculi: J. L. Thistle, M. J. Allen, **US 4758596** (1988 to Research Corp.). Acute toxicity: D. F. Marsh, C. D. Leake, *Anesthesiology* **11,** 455 (1950). Reviews of toxicity: R. von Burg, *J. Appl. Toxicol.* **12,** 73-74 (1992); E. Reese, R. D. Kimbrough, *Environ. Health Perspect.* **101,** Suppl. 6, 115-131 (1993); M. G. Costantini, *ibid.* 151-160; and human exposure: *Toxicological Profile for Methyl tert-butyl ether* (PB97-121016, 1996) 268 pp.

Liquid, bp 55.2°. mp −109°. d_4^{20} 0.7404. n_D^{20} 1.3689. Vapor pressure at 25°: 245 mm Hg. Flash pt: −28°C. Ignition temp:

224°C. Soly in water: 4.8 g/100 g. Soly of water in methyl *t*-butyl ether: 1.5 g/100 g. Unstable in acid soln. Volatile; lipophilic. *Flammable.* LC$_{50}$ in mice (15 min): 1.6 mmol/liter of atmosphere (Marsh).

Caution: Potential symptoms of overexposure by inhalation are coughing, burning sensation in nose and throat, headache, nausea, vomiting, dizziness, feeling of spaciness and disorientation (PB97-121016).

USE: Octane booster in gasoline. Chromatographic eluent esp in HPLC.

THERAP CAT: Cholelitholytic agent.

6033. Methyl Butyl Ketone. [591-78-6] 2-Hexanone. C$_6$-H$_{12}$O; mol wt 100.16. C 71.95%, H 12.08%, O 15.97%. CH$_3$CO-C$_4$H$_9$. Toxicity study: H. F. Smyth *et al., Arch. Ind. Hyg. Occup. Med.* **10**, 61 (1954). Review of toxicology: P. M. J. Bos *et al., Am. J. Ind. Med.* **20**, 175-194 (1991); and human exposure: *Toxicological Profile for 2-Hexanone* (PB93-110773, 1992) 116 pp.

Colorless liquid. d 0.830. bp 127°. Slightly soluble in water; sol in alcohol, ether. LD$_{50}$ orally in rats: 2.59 g/kg (Smyth).

Caution: Potential symptoms of overexposure are irritation of eyes and nose; peripheral neuropathy; weakness, paresthesia; dermatitis; headache; drowsiness. *See NIOSH Pocket Guide to Chemical Hazards* (DHHS/NIOSH 97-140, 1997) p 164.

6034. 2-Methyl-3-butyn-2-ol. [115-19-5] 2-Hydroxy-2-methyl-3-butyne. C$_5$H$_8$O; mol wt 84.12. C 71.39%, H 9.59%, O 19.02%. Toxicity data: W. Keil *et al., Arzneim.-Forsch.* **4**, 477 (1954); K. Soehring *et al., ibid.* **5**, 161 (1955).

Liquid. d$_{20}^{20}$ 0.8672. 7.24 lbs/gal. mp 2.6°. bp$_{760}$ 104-105°; bp$_{80}$ 52°; bp$_{12}$ 20°. Flash pt 77°F (25°C). n$_D^{20}$ 1.4211. Surface tension at 25° = 23.8 dynes/cm; 5% aq soln = 41.7 dynes/cm. Miscible with water, acetone, benzene, carbon tetrachloride, Cellosolve, cyclohexanone, diethylene glycol, ethyl acetate, kerosine, methyl ethyl ketone, mineral spirits, monoethanolamine, neatsfoot oil, petr ether, soybean oil, Stoddard solvent. Azeotrope with water, bp 90.7°, contains 28.4% H$_2$O. LD$_{50}$ in mice (mg/kg): 1800 orally (Keil); 2340 s.c. (Soehring).

6035. Methyl Butyrate. [623-42-7] Butanoic acid methyl ester. C$_5$H$_{10}$O$_2$; mol wt 102.13. C 58.80%, H 9.87%, O 31.33%. CH$_3$(CH$_2$)$_2$COOCH$_3$.

Colorless liquid. d$_4^{20}$ 0.898. mp about −95°. bp 102°. Flash pt 14°C. n$_D^{20}$ 1.3879. Sol in about 60 parts water; miscible with alcohol, ether.

USE: Manuf artificial rum and fruit essences.

6036. Methyl Carbamate. [598-55-0] Urethylane; methylurethane. C$_2$H$_5$NO$_2$; mol wt 75.07. C 32.00%, H 6.71%, N 18.66%, O 42.63%. H$_2$NCOOCH$_3$. Prepn from silver or mercuricyanate with H$_2$S and methanol: Birkenbach, Kolb, *Ber.* **68**, 901 (1935). From urea and methanol: DE 753127 (1940 to I.G. Farbenind.).

White crystals, mp 52-54°. bp 177°. Freely sublimes even at room temp. Freely sol in water, alcohol.

6037. Methyl Carbitol®. [111-77-3] 2-(2-Methoxyethoxy)ethanol; diethylene glycol monomethyl ether; methyl digol. C$_5$H$_{12}$O$_3$; mol wt 120.15. C 49.98%, H 10.07%, O 39.95%. CH$_3$-OCH$_2$CH$_2$OCH$_2$CH$_2$OH. Toxicity data: Smyth *et al., J. Ind. Hyg. Toxicol.* **23**, 259 (1941).

Liquid. d$_4^{20}$ 1.035. mp <−84°. bp 193°. n$_D^{27}$ 1.4264. Flash pt, open cup: 200°F (93°C). Miscible with water, alc, glycerol, ether, acetone, DMF. LD$_{50}$ orally in rats: 9.21 g/kg (Smyth).

USE: Used in the same way as 2-ethoxyethanol where a solvent with a higher boiling point is required.

6038. Methyl Cellosolve®. [109-86-4] 2-Methoxyethanol; ethylene glycol monomethyl ether. C$_3$H$_8$O$_2$; mol wt 76.09. C 47.35%, H 10.60%, O 42.05%. HOCH$_2$CH$_2$OCH$_3$. Prepn from ethylene oxide + methanol: Finch, Hagemeyer, US 2748171 (1956 to Kodak); from ethylene glycol + diazomethane: Hesse, Majum-

dar, *Ber.* **93**, 1129 (1960). Toxicity data: Smyth, *J. Ind. Hyg. Toxicol.* **23**, 259 (1941); Werner, *ibid.* **25**, 157 (1943). Series of articles on toxicology: *Environ. Health Perspect.* **57**, 1-275 (1984).

Liquid. *Poisonous!* bp$_{760}$ 124.43°; bp$_{20}$ 34-41°. d$_4^{20}$ 0.9663. Flash pt 115°F. n$_D^{20}$ 1.4028. Miscible with water, alcohol ether, glycerol, acetone, dimethylformamide. LD$_{50}$ in rats, guinea pigs (mg/kg): 2460, 950 orally (Smyth). LC$_{50}$ (7 hr in air) in mice: 4.6 mg/l (Werner).

Caution: Potential symptoms of overexposure are irritation of eyes, nose, throat; headache, drowsiness, weakness; ataxia, tremor, somnolence; anemic pallor. *See NIOSH Pocket Guide to Chemical Hazards* (DHHS/NIOSH 97-140, 1997) p 202. Exerts principle toxic effects on brain, blood, kidneys, thymus, testes. Appreciably toxic when inhaled. Absorbed through skin; direct contact may cause skin irritation. Embryotoxic and teratogenic in exptl animals. *See Patty's Industrial Hygiene and Toxicology* vol. 2D, G. D. Clayton, F. E. Clayton, Eds. (Wiley-Interscience, New York, 4th ed., 1994) pp 2764-2776.

USE: Solvent for low-viscosity cellulose acetate, natural resins, some synthetic resins and some alcohol-soluble dyes; in dyeing leather, sealing moistureproof cellophane; in nail polishes, quick-drying varnishes and enamels, wood stains. In modified Karl Fischer reagent: Peters, Jungnickel, *Anal. Chem.* **27**, 450 (1955).

6039. Methyl Cellosolve® Acetate. [110-49-6] 2-Methoxyethanol acetate; ethylene glycol monomethyl ether acetate. C$_5$-H$_{10}$O$_3$; mol wt 118.13. C 50.84%, H 8.53%, O 40.63%. CH$_3$-OCH$_2$CH$_2$OOCCH$_3$. Toxicity data: H. F. Smyth *et al., J. Ind. Hyg. Toxicol.* **23**, 259 (1941). Series of articles on toxicology: *Environ. Health Perspect.* **57**, 1-275 (1984).

Colorless liquid. d$_{20}^{20}$ 1.0067. bp 145°. mp −65.1°. n$_D^{20}$ 1.4019. Miscible with water, most organic solvents, oils; dissolves gums, resins. LD$_{50}$ orally in rats: 3.4 g/kg (Smyth).

Caution: Potential symptoms of overexposure are kidney damage; brain damage. Direct contact may cause eye, nose and throat irritation. *See NIOSH Pocket Guide to Chemical Hazards* (DHHS/NIOSH 97-140, 1997) p 202. *See also Patty's Industrial Hygiene and Toxicology* vol. 2D, G. D. Clayton, F. E. Clayton, Eds. (Wiley-Interscience, New York, 4th ed., 1994) pp 2918-2921.

USE: Industrial solvent.

6040. Methylcellulose. [9004-67-5] Cellulose methyl ether; Methocel A; Benecel M; Celevac; Cellucon; Citrucel; Cologel; Tearisol; Tylose M. Cellulose obtained from fibrous plant material and partially etherified with methyl groups. Prepd from cellulose fibers heated with caustic solution and treated with methyl chloride. Commercial methylcellulose has a methoxyl content of 25-33% (degree of substitution 1.5 to 2.0). Review of prepns and properties: Ott, *Cellulose and Cellulose Derivatives* (Wiley-Interscience, New York, 2nd ed., 1954/55); G. K. Greminger, A. B. Savage, in *Industrial Gums*, R. L. Whistler, Ed. (Academic Press, New York, 2nd ed., 1973) pp 619-647. Clinical efficacy as laxative: J. W. Hamilton *et al., Dig. Dis. Sci.* **33**, 993 (1988). Evaluation in lens implantation surgery: J. R. Rojas *et al., Ann. Ophthalmol.* **21**, 389 (1989). Review of production and uses in the food industry: P. de Mariscal, D. A. Bell in *Handbook of Fat Replacers*, S. Roller, S. A. Jones, Eds. (CRC Press, Boca Raton FL, 1996) pp 145-159.

White granules. Odorless, tasteless. Sol in cold water. Insol in hot water. An aq soln is best prepd by dispersing the granules in hot (but not boiling) water with stirring and chilling to +5°. The soln is then stable at room temp. Presence of inorganic salts increases the viscosity. The soly is dependent upon degree of substitution. Clear films may be cast from aq soln.

USE: As a substitute for water-soluble gums; to render paper greaseproof, in adhesives, as thickening agent in cosmetics, as protective colloid in emulsions, as binder and stabilizer in foods. As fat replacer in the formulation of dietetic foods. Pharmaceutic aid (suspending agent).

THERAP CAT: Laxative; ocular lubricant.

THERAP CAT (VET): Laxative.

6041. Methyl Chloride. [74-87-3] Chloromethane; Freon 40. CH$_3$Cl; mol wt 50.49. C 23.79%, H 5.99%, Cl 70.22%. Known as early as 1835, large scale production started in 1920's. Review of mfg processes: *Faith, Keyes & Clark's Industrial Chemicals*, F. A. Lowenheim, M. K. Moran, Eds. (Wiley-Interscience,

New York, 4th ed., 1975) pp 530-538. GC-MS determn in air: D. R. Cronn, D. E. Harsch, *Anal. Lett.* **9**, 1015 (1976). X-ray emission study: D. W. Lindle *et al., Phys. Rev. A* **43**, 2353 (1991). *Review:* M. T. Holbrook in *Kirk-Othmer Encyclopedia of Chemical Technology* **vol. 5** (Wiley-Interscience, New York, 4th ed., 1993) pp 1028-1040. Review of toxicology: J. D. Repko, S. M. Lasley, *Crit. Rev. Toxicol.* **6**, 283-302 (1979); and human exposure: *Toxicological Profile for Chloromethane* (PB99-121964, 1998) 288 pp.

Colorless gas of mild odor and sweet taste. *Extremely flammable.* mp −97.7°; bp −23.7°; n_D (liq at −23.7°) 1.3712. Slightly sol in water; misc with chloroform, ether, glacial acetic acid; sol in alcohol. Soly at 20° (ml/100 ml): benzene 4723; carbon tetrachloride 3756; glacial acetic acid 3679; ethanol 3740; at 25° (g/100g): water 0.48.

Caution: Potential symptoms of overexposure are dizziness, nausea and vomiting; visual disturbance; staggering; slurred speech; convulsions, coma; liver and kidney damage; reproductive and teratogenic effects; direct contact with liquid may cause frostbite. Potential occupational carcinogen. *See NIOSH Pocket Guide to Chemical Hazards* (DHHS/NIOSH 97-140, 1997) p 202. *See also Patty's Industrial Hygiene and Toxicology* **vol. 2B**, G. D. Clayton, F. E. Clayton, Eds. (Wiley-Interscience, New York, 3rd ed., 1981) pp 3436-3442.

USE: Manuf of silicones, tetramethyleads. Solvent catalyst for butyl rubber. Has been used as a refrigerant.

6042. Methyl Chloroacetate. [96-34-4] Chloroacetic acid methyl ester. $C_3H_5ClO_2$; mol wt 108.52. C 33.20%, H 4.64%, Cl 32.67%, O 29.49%. $CH_2ClCOOCH_3$.
Colorless liquid. d_{20}^{20} 1.238. mp −33°. bp 130-132°. Insol in water; miscible with alcohol, ether.

USE: As solvent.

6043. Methyl Chlorocarbonate. [79-22-1] Carbonochloridic acid methyl ester; methyl chloroformate. $C_2H_3ClO_2$; mol wt 94.50. C 25.42%, H 3.20%, Cl 37.52%, O 33.86%. $ClCO_2CH_3$. Made from phosgene and methyl alcohol.
Clear liquid. d_4^{20} 1.223. bp 71°. Slightly sol in water and gradually dec by it; miscible with alcohol, benzene, chloroform, ether.

Caution: Vapors strongly irritating to eyes.

6044. 3-Methylcholanthrene. [56-49-5] 1,2-Dihydro-3-methylbenz[*j*]aceanthrylene; 20-methylcholanthrene; 3-MECA; 3-MC. $C_{21}H_{16}$; mol wt 268.35. C 93.99%, H 6.01%. From desoxycholic acid: Wieland, Schlichting, *Z. Physiol. Chem.* **150**, 267 (1925); Wieland, Wiedersheim, *ibid.* **186**, 229 (1930); Wieland, Dane, *ibid.* **219**, 240 (1933). From cholic acid: Cook, Haslewood, *J. Chem. Soc.* **1934**, 428; Fieser, Seligman; *J. Am. Chem. Soc.* **58**, 2482 (1936); *cf.* Bachmann, *J. Org. Chem.* **1**, 347 (1936). Methylcholanthrene has been produced also by an unusual pyrolytic degradation of cholesterol derivatives. Total synthesis: Buchta, Güllich, *Angew. Chem.* **70**, 190 (1958); P. W. Tang, C. A. Maggiulli, *J. Org. Chem.* **46**, 3429 (1981); S. A. Jacobs, R. G. Harvey, *Tetrahedron Lett.* **22**, 1093 (1981). *Review:* E. Clar, *Polycyclic Hydrocarbons* **Vol. 1 & 2** (Academic Press, 1964).

Pale yellow, slender prisms from benzene + ether, mp 179-180°. bp$_{80}$ 280°; d^{20} 1.28. Absorption spectrum: Fieser, Hershberg, *J. Am. Chem. Soc.* **60**, 940 (1938). Sol in benzene, xylene, toluene; slightly sol in amyl alcohol. Insol in water.

USE: Exptly in cancer research.

6045. Methylcobalamin. [13422-55-4] Cobinamide Comethyl deriv. dihydrogen phosphate (ester) inner salt 3′-ester with 5,6-dimethyl-1-α-D-ribofuranosyl-1*H*-benzimidazole; methyl-5,6-dimethylbenzimidazolylcobalamin; mecobalamin; methyl vitamin B$_{12}$; MeCbl; Algobaz; Hitocobamin-M; Methycobal; Methylcobaz. $C_{63}H_{91}CoN_{13}O_{14}P$; mol wt 1344.38. C 56.28%, H 6.82%, Co

4.38%, N 13.54%, O 16.66%, P 2.30%. One of the biologically active forms of vitamin B$_{12}$, *q.v.*; differing only by the substitution of a methyl for the cyano group. Coenzyme required in the biosynthesis of methionine. Identification as requirement for methionine biosynthesis by *E. coli:* R. L. Kisliuk, D. D. Woods, *Biochem. J.* **75**, 467 (1960); J. R. Guest *et al., Nature* **195**, 340 (1962). Prepn: O. Müller, G. Müller, *Biochem. Z.* **336**, 299 (1962); D. Dolphin, *Methods Enzymol.* **18**, Pt. C, 34 (1971); D. Autissier *et al., Bull. Soc. Chim. Fr.* **1980**, part 2, 192. Interrelationship with folate metabolism: B. Shane, E. L. R. Stokstad, *Annu. Rev. Nutr.* **5**, 115-141 (1985). Discussion of mechanism of action: W. S. Beck, *Am. J. Hematol.* **34**, 83-89 (1990). *Review:* "Vitamin B$_{12}$" in *Vitamins,* W. Friedrich, Ed. (de Gruyter, Berlin, 1988) pp 837-928.

Bright red crystals from water/acetone. uv max (pH 7): 522, 342, 266 nm (ε 9357, 14416, 19897); (0.1*N* HCl): 462, 304, 264 nm (ε 9599, 22855, 24737).

THERAP CAT: Vitamin (hematopoietic).

6046. Methyl Cyanoacrylate. [137-05-3] 2-Cyano-2-propenoic acid methyl ester; 2-cyanoacrylic acid methyl ester; MCA; mecrilate; mecrylate; methyl 2-cyanoacrylate; methyl α-cyanoacrylate. $C_5H_5NO_2$; mol wt 111.10. C 54.05%, H 4.54%, N 12.61%, O 28.80%. Reacts rapidly with water to form solid polymers. Preparative methods: A. E. Ardis, **US 2467927** (1949 to B. F. Goodrich); C. H. McKeever, **US 2912454** (1959 to Rohm & Haas). Prepn, polymerization and degradation: F. Leonard *et al., J. Appl. Polym. Sci.* **10**, 259 (1966). Clinical evaluation for tubal occlusion in female sterilization: *Contraception* **31**, 243 (1985). Review of chemistry and toxicology: R. Cary, *Concise Int. Chem. Assess. Doc. No. 36* (WHO, Geneva, 2001) 33 pp.

Clear, colorless liquid; strong, acrid odor; bp 48-49° (0.33-0.36 kPa). n_D^{20} 1.4459. n_D^{25} 1.443. d^{20} 1.1044. Surface tension: 37.41 dynes/cm. Vapor pressure at 25°: <0.27 kPa. Sol or partially sol in methyl ethyl ketone, toluene, DMF, acetone, nitromethane.

Polymer. [25067-29-2] Poly(methyl 2-cyanoacrylate).

Caution: Potential symptoms of overexposure are irritation of eyes, skin, nose; blurred vision, lacrimation; rhinitis. *See NIOSH Pocket Guide to Chemical Hazards* (DHHS/NIOSH 97-140, 1997) p 204.

USE: In adhesives; in mfr of plastics, electronics, scientific instruments, jewelry, sports equip; in cable joining, manicuring, dentistry, mortuaries, fingerprint development.

THERAP CAT: Tissue adhesive.

6047. Methylcyclohexane. [108-87-2] Hexahydrotoluene; cyclohexylmethane. C_7H_{14}; mol wt 98.19. C 85.62%, H 14.37%. Prepn: F. Wreden, B. Znatowicz, *Ann.* **187**, 161 (1877); E. Knoevenagel, *ibid.* **297**, 113 (1897); and physical properties: J. P. Wibaut *et al., Rec. Trav. Chim.* **58**, 12 (1939). Toxicology: J. F. Treon *et al., J. Ind. Hyg. Toxicol.* **25**, 199 (1943). Dehydrogenation to produce motor fuel: N. Gruenenfelder *et al., Proc. 20th Intersoc. Energy Convers. Eng. Conf.* **2**, 2.781 (1985). Kinetics of industrial dehydrogenation to toluene: A. Touzani *et al., Stud. Surf. Sci. Catal.* **19**, 357 (1984); use of a membrane reactor to improve process: J. K. Ali, A. Baiker, *Appl. Catal. A* **155**, 41 (1997).

Clear, fragrant liquid, mp −126.3°. bp$_{760}$ 101.2 ± 0.3°; also reported as bp$_{760}$ 103°. $n_D^{18.5}$ 1.41705; n_D^{20} 1.4230; n_D^{25} 1.42063. d$_4^{18.5}$ 0.7662; d$_4^{20}$ 0.76944; d$_4^{25}$ 0.76512. Surface tension: 23.73 dynes/cm. Insol in water at 20°.

Caution: Potential symptoms of overexposure are irritation of eyes, skin, nose and throat; lightheadedness, drowsiness. *See NIOSH Pocket Guide to Chemical Hazards* (DHHS/NIOSH 97-140, 1997) p 204.

USE: Solvent; starting material in the synthesis of toluene.

6048. **3′-Methyl-1,2-cyclopentenophenanthrene.** [549-38-2] 16,17-Dihydro-17-methyl-15H-cyclopenta[a]phenanthrene; Diels' hydrocarbon. $C_{18}H_{16}$; mol wt 232.32. C 93.06%, H 6.94%. Prepd from cholesterol, cholic acid, or suitable sapogenins: Diels, Rickert, *Ber.* **68,** 267 (1935); starting with 2-acetylphenanthrene: Gamble *et al., J. Chem. Soc.* **1935,** 443, 644.

Crystals from acetic acid, mp 126-127°. Absorption spectrum: Hillemann, *Ber.* **69,** 2610 (1936).

6049. **Methylcytisine.** [486-86-2] (1R,5S)-1,2,3,4,5,6-Hexahydro-3-methyl-1,5-methano-8H-pyrido[1,2-a][1,5]diazocin-8-one; caulophylline; 12-methylcytisine; N-methylcytisine. $C_{12}H_{16}N_2O$; mol wt 204.27. C 70.56%, H 7.89%, N 13.71%, O 7.83%. Lupine alkaloid of the quinolizidine type; occurring most abundantly in *Leguminosae.* Bioactive principle of blue cohosh, *q.v.* Isoln from *Caulophyllum thalictroides* Michx., *Berberidaceae:* F. B. Power, A. H. Salway, *J. Chem. Soc.* **103,** 191 (1913); M. S. Flom *et al., J. Pharm. Sci.* **56,** 1515 (1967); from *Baptisia australis* (L.) R. Br., *Leguminosae:* L. Marion, J. Ouellet, *J. Am. Chem. Soc.* **70,** 691 (1948). Absolute configuration: S. Okuda *et al., Chem. Pharm. Bull.* **13,** 491 (1965). Crystal structure: A. A. Freer *et al., Acta Crystallogr.* **C43,** 1119 (1987). Pharmacology: H. C. Ferguson, L. D. Edwards, *J. Am. Pharm. Assoc. Sci. Ed.* **43,** 16 (1954). Toxicity study: R. B. Barlow, L. J. McLeod, *Br. J. Pharmacol.* **35,** 161 (1969). Binding to nicotinic and muscarinic receptors: T. Schmeller *et al., J. Nat. Prod.* **57,** 1316 (1994).

Colorless, prismatic needles from benzene + light petroleum, mp 137°. $[\alpha]_D^{30}$ −224° (c = 1.05 in water). uv max: 234, 309 nm (ε 6860, 7560). Readily sol in water, alcohol, chloroform, benzene. LD_{50} in mice (mg/kg): 21 i.v.; 51 i.p. (Barlow, McLeod).

6050. **5-Methylcytosine.** [554-01-8] 4-Amino-5-methyl-2(1H)-pyrimidinone. $C_5H_7N_3O$; mol wt 125.13. C 47.99%, H 5.64%, N 33.58%, O 12.79%. Occurs in a nucleic acid obtained from tubercle bacillus. Isoln: Johnson, Coghill, *J. Am. Chem. Soc.* **47,** 2838 (1925). Synthesis from ethyl bromide addition product of thiourea and from ethyl formyl propionate: Wheeler, Johnson, *Am. Chem. J.* **29,** 492 (1903).

Prisms from water, may contain ½ mol H_2O. mp 270° (effervescence). One gram dissolves in 29 ml water.

6051. **Methyl Demeton.** [8022-00-2] Phosphorothioic acid O-[2-(ethylthio)ethyl] O,O-dimethyl ester mixt with S-[2-(ethylthio)ethyl] O,O-dimethyl phosphorothioate; demeton-methyl; methyl-mercaptophos; methyl systox; Bayer 21/116; Meta-Systox. $C_6H_{15}O_3PS_2$; mol wt 230.29. C 31.29%, H 6.57%, O 20.84%, P 13.45%, S 27.85%. Cholinesterase inhibitor. Isomeric mixture consisting of demeton-O-methyl and demeton-S-methyl (O(and S)-[2-(ethylthio)ethyl] O,O-dimethyl phosphorothioate). *Ref:* Henglein, Schrader, *Z. Naturforsch.* **10b,** 12 (1955). Prepn: GB 814332 (1959 to Bayer). Toxicology studies: M. Vandekar, *Br. J. Ind. Med.* **15,** 158 (1958); E. F. Edson, *Pharm. J.* **185,** 361 (1960).

Commercial product is a light yellow liquid. Hydrolyzed by alkali. LD_{50} in rats (mg/kg): 50-75 orally, 300-400 dermally (Edson).

Demeton-O-methyl. [867-27-6] Colorless oil, $bp_{0.15}$ 74°. d_4^{20} 1.190. n_D^{20} 1.5063. Soly in water at room temp: 330 ppm. Soluble in organic solvents.

Demeton-S-methyl. [919-86-8] Pale yellow oil, $bp_{0.15}$ 89°. d_4^{20} 1.207. n_D^{20} 1.5065. Soly in water at room temp: 3,300 ppm. Sol in organic solvents. LD_{50} in rats (mg/kg): 40 orally, 85 dermally (Edson).

Caution: Potential symptoms of overexposure are irritation of eyes, skin; aching eyes, rhinorrhea; nausea, dizziness, vomiting. *See NIOSH Pocket Guide to Chemical Hazards* (DHHS/NIOSH 97-140, 1997) p 206.

USE: Insecticide.

6052. **Methyl Dihydrojasmonate.** [24851-98-7] 3-Oxo-2-pentylcyclopentaneacetic acid methyl ester; methyl 2-pentyl-3-oxo-cyclopentyl-1-acetate; Hedione. $C_{13}H_{22}O_3$; mol wt 226.31. C 68.99%, H 9.80%, O 21.21%. Fragrance compound identified as a natural product in flowers, tea, herbs, fruits and vegetables. Synthetic commercial formulations contain a racemic, near equilibrium mixture of ~10% (±)-cis and ~90% (±)-trans forms. The (+)-(1R,2S)-form is the most organoleptically active enantiomer. Prepn: E. Demole *et al., Helv. Chim. Acta* **45,** 675, 685, 692 (1962). Fragrance monograph: *Food Chem. Toxicol.* **30,** Suppl. 1, 85S (1992). Enantioselective synthesis of (+)- and (−)-trans forms: T. Perrard *et al., Org. Lett.* **2,** 2959 (2000). Review of sensory properties of stereoisomers and enantioselective distribution in plant sources: P. Werkhoff *et al., Food Rev. Int.* **18,** 103-122 (2002).

Pale yellowish or almost colorless oil, $bp_{0.2}$ 109-112°; sweet, floral, jasmine-like odor. Flash point: >200°F (closed cup). Vapor pressure (20°): <0.001 mmHg. n^{20} 1.457-1.462. d_{20}^{20} 0.998-1.006. LD_{50} (g/kg): >5 orally in rats; >5 dermally in rabbits (*Food Chem. Toxicol.*).

(+)-(1R,2S)-Form. [39647-11-5] (+)-Methyl dihydroepijasmonate; (+)-cis-methyl dihydrojasmonate; Paradisone. Commercial formulations contain ~90% ee of the (+)-(1R,2S)-form. Enantioselective synthesis: D. A. Dobbs *et al., Angew. Chem. Int. Ed.* **39,** 1992 (2000); A. Porta *et al., J. Org. Chem.* **70,** 4876 (2005). Colorless oil; intense floral, jasmine-like, bright, fatty odor. $[\alpha]_D^{20}$ +78° (c = 1.1 in CH_2Cl_2).

(−)-(1R,2R)-Form. [2630-39-9] (−)-trans-Methyl dihydrojasmonate. Faint, slightly floral, sweet, jasmine-like odor, $bp_{0.03}$ 100°. n_D^{20} 1.4583. d_4^{21} 0.9968. $[\alpha]_D$ −33.8° (c = 2.9 in $CHCl_3$).

(+)-(1S,2S)-Form. [151716-36-8] (+)-trans-Methyl dihydrojasmonate. Colorless oil, $bp_{0.3}$ 108°. Faint, slightly floral, fatty, lemon peel-like odor. $[\alpha]_D^{20}$ +33.8° (c = 0.9 in $CHCl_3$).

USE: Fragrance ingredient in perfumes, toilette and laundry products. Flavor ingredient producing fruit, tea, tobacco, and floral flavors.

6053. **p-Methyldiphenhydramine.** [19804-27-4] N,N-Dimethyl-2-[(4-methylphenyl)phenylmethoxy]ethanamine; N,N-dimethyl-2-[(p-methyl-α-phenylbenzyl)oxy]ethylamine; β-dimethylaminoethyl 4-methylbenzhydryl ether; p-methylbenzhydryl 2-dimethylaminoethyl ether; Neo-Benodine; Toladryl. $C_{18}H_{23}NO$; mol wt 269.38. C 80.26%, H 8.61%, N 5.20%, O 5.94%. Prepn: Rieveschl, US 2527962 (1950 to Parke, Davis); GB 683483 (1952 to Fabriken Brocades-Stheeman & Pharmacia).

Hydrochloride. $C_{18}H_{23}NO.HCl$. Crystals from acetone, mp 150-152° (free base $bp_{0.1}$ 143°).

THERAP CAT: Antihistaminic.

6054. Methyldiphenylamine. [552-82-9] N-Methyl-N-phenylbenzenamine; diphenylmethylamine. $C_{13}H_{13}N$; mol wt 183.25. C 85.21%, H 7.15%, N 7.64%. $(C_6H_5)_2NCH_3$. Prepd by heating diphenylamine, methyl alcohol and HCl.

Liquid. d_4^{20} 1.0476. mp −7.6°. bp 296-297°; also given as 282-290°, 293°. n_D^{20} 1.6193. Insol in water; sol in alc, ether.

USE: Manuf dyes; as reagent similar to diphenylamine.

6055. Methyldopa. [555-30-6] 3-Hydroxy-α-methyl-L-tyrosine; L-3-(3,4-dihydroxyphenyl)-2-methylalanine; L-α-methyl-3,4-dihydroxyphenylalanine; L-2-amino-2-methyl-3-(3,4-dihydroxyphenyl)propionic acid; α-methyldopa; AMD; MK-351; Aldomet; Aldomin; Dopamet; Dopegyt; Elanpres; Equibar; Medopren; Methoplain; Sembrina; Presinol. $C_{10}H_{13}NO_4$; mol wt 211.21. C 56.87%, H 6.20%, N 6.63%, O 30.30%. Exists as the sesquihydrate. Prepn: Pfister, Stein, US 2868818 (1959 to Merck & Co.). Resolution: Jones *et al.*, US 3158648 (1964 to Merck & Co.); *cf.* Slates *et al.*, *J. Org. Chem.* **29**, 1424 (1964). Resolution and configuration: Tristram, *ibid.* 2053. Synthesis from asymmetric intermediates: Reinhold *et al.*, *J. Org. Chem.* **33**, 1209 (1968). Prepn of the ethyl ester hydrochloride: FR M2153 (1963 to Merck & Co.); of pharmaceutical dosage forms: Marcus, US 3230143 (1966 to Merck & Co.). Mode of action: Finch, Haeusler, *Br. J. Pharmacol.* **45**, 167p (1972); Day *et al.*, *ibid.* 168p. Review of pharmacology: A. Scriabine, Ed. in *Pharmacology of Antihypertensive Drugs* (Raven, New York, 1980) pp 43-54.

L-Form sesquihydrate. Crystals from water. Minute anhydr crystals from methanol, considerably hygroscopic, dec ~300°. $[\alpha]_D^{23}$ −4.0 ± 0.5° (c = 1 in 0.1N HCl). uv max: 281 nm (ε 2780). Soly in water at 25°: ~10 mg/ml. pH of satd aq soln about 5.0. (Soly of D-form in water at 25°: ~10 mg/ml, of DL-form: ~18 mg/ml) Practically insol in the common organic solvents. Sol in dil mineral acids.

Ethyl ester hydrochloride. [2508-79-4] Methyldopate hydrochloride. $C_{12}H_{18}ClNO_4$. After drying, mol wt 275.7 (1 mg = 0.77 mg of the free acid). Soluble in water to the extent of 10-300 mg/ml at pH 2-7. May be stabilized with sodium bisulfite and/or disodium EDTA.

THERAP CAT: Antihypertensive.

6056. 3-O-Methyldopa. [300-48-1] 3-Methoxy-L-tyrosine; 3-(4-hydroxy-3-methoxyphenyl)-L-alanine; L-3-methoxy-4-hydroxyphenylalanine; OM-dopa; L-3-MTO; OMD. $C_{10}H_{13}NO_4$; mol wt 211.21. C 56.87%, H 6.20%, N 6.63%, O 30.30%. A major metabolite of L-dopa in man and animals, which has a considerably longer biological half-life than L-dopa: Pletscher *et al.*, *Brain Res.* **4**, 106 (1967); Bartholini, Pletscher, *J. Pharmacol. Exp. Ther.* **161**, 14 (1968); Kuruma *et al.*, *Eur. J. Pharmacol.* **10**, 189 (1970). Proposed as a precursor of dopamine *via* its partial demethylation in the organism: Bartholini *et al.*, *Nature* **230**, 533 (1971); Chalmers *et al.*, *Br. J. Pharmacol.* **43**, 455P (1971); Bartholini *et al.*, *Life Sci.* **14**, 323 (1974). *See also* Carlsson, Waldeck, *Arch. Pharmacol.* **272**, 441 (1972); Bartholini, Pletscher, *ibid.* **274**, 404 (1972). Metabolic pathways: Bartholini *et al.*, *J. Pharmacol. Exp. Ther.* **183**, 65 (1972). Parkinsonism treatment studies: Calne *et al.*, *Clin. Pharmacol. Ther.* **14**, 386 (1973).

6057. Methyleneaminoacetonitrile. [109-82-0] α-Hydroformamine cyanide. $C_3H_4N_2$; mol wt 68.08. C 52.93%, H 5.92%, N 41.15%. $CH_2=NCH_2CN$. The actual molecular formula is $C_9H_{12}N_6$: Johnson, Rinehart, *J. Am. Chem. Soc.* **46**, 768, 1653 (1924). Prepd by the action of formaldehyde on a mixture of ammonium chloride, potassium cyanide and acetic acid: Adams, Langley, *Org. Synth.* **coll. vol. I** (2nd ed., 1941) p 355.

Trimeric form. Orthorhombic crystals from alc or acetone, mp 129°. Sol in hot water, alc; slightly sol in benzene.

6058. Methylene Azure. Azure I. A somewhat variable mixture obtained by oxidation of methylene blue, contg primarily azure A and azure B, *q.q.v.* Prepn: Bernthsen, *Ann.* **230**, 169 (1885); Kehrmann, *Ber.* **39**, 1804 (1906). *Review: H. J. Conn's Biological Stains*, R. D. Lillie, Ed. (Williams & Wilkins, Baltimore, 9th ed., 1977) pp 493-502.

Green glistening crystals. Forms blue soln in water; very sparingly sol in alcohol with a reddish brown fluorescence.

Mixture with methylene blue. Azure II; azure blue II; methylene azure II. Deep-green powder. Sol in water with blue color, less sol in alcohol, slightly sol in chloroform. Insol in ether.

Mixture with methylene blue and eosin. Azure II eosin. Chief ingredient of Giemsa stain. Green powder. Slightly sol in water; sol in alcohol, methanol, glycerol.

USE: Biological stain.

6059. 4,4'-Methylenebis[2-chloroaniline]. [101-14-4] 4,4'-Methylenebis[2-chlorobenzenamine]; 4,4'-diamino-3,3'-dichlorodiphenylmethane; di-(4-amino-3-chlorophenyl)methane; methylenebis(o-chloroaniline); MOCA; MBOCA; DACPM. $C_{13}H_{12}Cl_2N_2$; mol wt 267.15. C 58.45%, H 4.53%, Cl 26.54%, N 10.49%. Prepn: Finger, *J. Prakt. Chem.* [2] **79**, 493 (1909); Mayer, *Ber.* **47**, 1161 (1914). Acute toxicity: G. Ya. Kel'man *et al.*, *Kauch. Rezina* **26**(9), 28 (1967), *C.A.* **67**, 120013m (1967). Review of carcinogenicity studies: *IARC Monographs* **vol. 4**, 65-71 (1974); of toxicology and human exposure: *Toxicological Profile for 4,4'-Methylenebis(2-chloroaniline)* (PB95-100186, 1994) 146 p.

Flakes from alcohol, mp 110°. Slightly sol in water; sol in dil acids, ether, alcohol. LD_{50} orally in mice: 880 mg/kg (Kel'man).

Caution: Potential symptoms of overexposure are hematuria, cyanosis, nausea, methemoglobinemia, kidney irritation. *See NIOSH Pocket Guide to Chemical Hazards* (DHHS/NIOSH 97-140, 1997) p 206. This substance is reasonably anticipated to be a human carcinogen: *Report on Carcinogens, Eleventh Edition* (PB2005-104914, 2004) p III-167.

USE: Curing agent for polyurethane and epoxy resins. Research tool for studying carcinogens.

6060. Methylene Blue. [61-73-4] 3,7-Bis(dimethylamino)phenothiazin-5-ium chloride; C.I. Basic Blue 9; methylthioninium chloride; tetramethylthionine chloride; 3,7-bis(dimethylamino)phenazathionium chloride; Swiss blue; C.I. 52015; C.I. Solvent Blue 8; Urolene Blue. $C_{16}H_{18}ClN_3S$; mol wt 319.85. C 60.08%, H 5.67%, Cl 11.08%, N 13.14%, S 10.03%. First prepd by Caro in 1876. Provided technically as the zinc double chloride; used medically in a zinc free form. Prepn: H. E. Fierz-David, L. Blangey, *Fundamental Processes of Dye Chemistry* (Interscience, New York, 1949) p 311. *See also Colour Index* **vol. 4** (3rd ed., 1971) p 4470. TLC determn: G. Balansard *et al.*, *Ann. Pharm. Fr.* **46**, 129 (1988). Use as marker for reticulocytes: B. Rudensky, *Scand. J. Clin. Lab. Invest.* **57**, 291 (1997); in melanoma targeted radiotherapy: E. M. Link *et al.*, *Pigment Cell Res.* **7**, 358 (1994); P. J. Blower *et al.*, *Nucl. Med. Biol.* **24**, 305 (1997). Review of use as vital dye: P. Barbosa, T. M. Peters, *Histochem. J.* **3**, 71-93 (1971). History and properties: R. D. Lillie, P. T. Donaldson, *Stain Technol.*

54, 33-39 (1979). Review of photochemistry: E. M. Tuite, J. M. Kelly, *J. Photochem. Photobiol. B* **21,** 103-124 (1993). Review of use as cationic dye in ceramic quality control: J. E, Funk, D. R. Dinger in *Science of Whitewares,* V. E. Henkes *et al.,* Eds. (American Ceramic Society, OH, 1996) pp 21-31. Review of use in methemoglobinaemia: J. W. Harvey, A. S. Keitt, *Br. J. Haematol.* **54,** 29-41 (1983).

Trihydrate. [7220-79-3] Dark green crystals or crystalline powder with bronze luster. Odorless; stable in air. Absorption max: 668, 609 nm. Sol in water and chloroform; sparingly sol in alcohol. Deep blue soln in water or alcohol. Forms double salts.

USE: Stain in bacteriology; reagent for several chemicals; as mixed indicator; as redox colorimetric agent. Targeting agent for melanoma.

THERAP CAT: Antimethemoglobinemic; antidote (cyanide).

THERAP CAT (VET): Antiseptic; disinfectant; antidote (cyanide and nitrate).

6061. Methylene Bromide. [74-95-3] Dibromomethane. CH_2Br_2; mol wt 173.83. C 6.91%, H 1.16%, Br 91.93%. Prepn: Hartman, Dreger, *Org. Synth.* **coll. vol. I,** 357 (1941). Manuf along with bromochloromethane, from dichloromethane: Lake, Asadorian, **US 2553518** (1951 to Dow).

Liquid, bp 97°. mp $-52.7°$. d_4^{20} 2.4956. n_D^{20} 1.5419. Soly (g/1000 g water): 11.70 (15°); 11.93 (30°). Miscible with alcohol, ether, acetone.

6062. α-Methylene Butyrolactone. [547-65-9] 4,5-Dihydro-3-methylene-2(3*H*)-furanone. $C_5H_6O_2$; mol wt 98.10. C 61.22%, H 6.16%, O 32.62%. Isoln from aq extracts of *Erythronium americanum* Ker., *Liliaceae* (dogtooth violet): Cavallito, Haskell, *J. Am. Chem. Soc.* **68,** 2332 (1946).

Liquid. Polymerizes easily when heated above 70°. bp₂ 57-60°. Sol in water. pH 4 (150 mg/ml). The lactone is present in all parts of the plant and can be extracted easily with water, but not with ethanol, ether, ethyl acetate or chloroform.

Caution: Irritating to the skin.

6063. Methylene Chloride. [75-09-2] Dichloromethane; methylene dichloride; methylene bichloride. CH_2Cl_2; mol wt 84.93. C 14.14%, H 2.37%, Cl 83.49%. Prepn by chlorination of methane: Lukes *et al.,* **US 2792435** (1957 to Diamond Alkali); Pitt, Bender, **US 2979541** (1961 to Stauffer); Burks, Obrecht, **US 3126419** (1964 to Stauffer). Review of mfg processes: *Faith, Keyes & Clark's Industrial Chemicals,* F. A. Lowenheim, M. K. Moran, Eds. (Wiley-Interscience, New York, 4th ed., 1975) pp 530-538. Toxicity data: E. T. Kimura *et al., Toxicol. Appl. Pharmacol.* **19,** 699 (1971). Review of toxicology and human exposure: *Toxicological Profile for Methylene Chloride* (PB2000-108026, 2000) 313 pp.

Colorless liquid; vapor is not flammable and when mixed with air is not explosive. Soluble in ~50 parts water; miscible with alc, ether, DMF. bp₇₆₀ 39.75°. mp $-95°$. d_4^0 1.36174; d_4^{15} 1.33479; d_4^{20} 1.3255; d_4^{30} 1.30777. n_D^{20} 1.4244. LD₅₀ orally in young adult rats: 1.6 ml/kg (Kimura).

Caution: Potential symptoms of overexposure are fatigue, weakness, sleepiness, lightheadedness; numbness or tingle of limbs; nausea; irritation of eyes and skin. *See NIOSH Pocket Guide to Chemical Hazards* (DHHS/NIOSH 97-140, 1997) p 208. This substance is reasonably anticipated to be a human carcinogen:

Report on Carcinogens, Eleventh Edition (PB2005-104914, 2004) p III-91.

USE: Solvent in paint removers, for cellulose acetate; degreasing and cleaning fluids; as solvent in food processing. Extraction solvent for spice oleoresins, hops, for removal of caffeine from coffee. Pharmaceutic aid (solvent). Aerosol propellant; insecticide.

6064. Methylenedigallic Acid. [552-21-6] 2,2'-Methylenebis[3,4,5-trihydroxybenzoic acid]. $C_{15}H_{12}O_{10}$; mol wt 352.25. C 51.15%, H 3.43%, O 45.42%. Made by heating a mixture of gallic acid, formaldehyde and dil HCl on the water bath.

Crystals. Insol in cold, sparingly in hot water; sol in alcohol, alkalies.

6065. 5,5'-Methylenedisalicylic Acid. [122-25-8] 3,3'-Methylenebis[6-hydroxybenzoic acid]; 4,4'-dihydroxydiphenylmethane-3,3'-dicarboxylic acid. $C_{15}H_{12}O_6$; mol wt 288.25. C 62.50%, H 4.20%, O 33.30%. Prepd from salicylic acid and formaldehyde in the presence of sulfuric acid: Clemmensen, Heitman, *J. Am. Chem. Soc.* **33,** 737 (1911).

Wedge-like cryst from acetone + benzene. Bitter taste. Dec 238° (higher-melting material may be impure). Turns red at 180° and starts giving off CO_2. Freely sol in methanol, ethanol, ether, acetone, glacial acetic acid. Very slightly sol in hot water. Practically insol in benzene, chloroform, carbon disulfide, petr ether.

Bacitracin salt *see* Bacitracin Methylenedisalicylate.

Diacetyl deriv. $C_{15}H_{10}O_6(CH_3CO)_2$. White powder, mp 142°, practically insol in water, sol in acetone, ethanol.

6066. Methylene Iodide. [75-11-6] Diiodomethane. CH_2I_2; mol wt 267.84. C 4.48%, H 0.75%, I 94.76%. Prepd by the reduction of iodoform with sodium arsenite: Adams, Marvel, *Org. Synth.* **vol. 1,** p 57 (1921). Also by heating iodoform with sodium acetate in alcohol: Bagnara, *Eng. Min. J. Press* **116,** 51 (1923). Absorption spectrum: Lowry, Sass, *J. Chem. Soc.* **1926,** 624; Stepanov, *Acta Physicochim. URSS* **20,** 174 (1945).

Very heavy, highly refractive liq. Darkens on exposure to light, air, and moisture. d_4^{20} 3.32537. Solidifies in leaflets at 5.2° or in thin needles at 5.7°. Usually cooling to 0° is necessary to start crystn. mp 6.0°. bp₇₆₀ 181°; bp₇₀ 107°; bp₁₁ 68°. $n_D^{10.5}$ 1.7559; n_D^{15} 1.7425. Viscosity (cP): 3.35 (10°); 2.80 (20°); 2.39 (30°). Sol in about 70 parts water; miscible with alcohol, propanol, isopropanol, hexane, cyclohexane, ether, chloroform, benzene. CH_2I_2 dissolves sulfur and phosphorus (more than 1:1 at 25°).

USE: In separating mixtures of minerals. In determining the specific gravity of minerals and other substances. In the manufacture of x-ray contrast media.

6067. Methylenomycins. Members of a family of cyclopentenoid antibiotics related structurally to sarkomycins, *q.v.,* and having *in vitro* activity vs gram-positive and gram-negative organisms. Isoln from *Streptomyces violaceoruber,* physical, chemical, biological properties: M. Arai *et al.,* **JP Kokai 73 19796** (1973 to Sankyo), *C.A.* **78,** 157861 (1973); T. Haneishi *et al., J. Antibiot.* **27,** 386 (1974). Structures of methylenomycins A and B: *eidem, ibid.* 393. Crystal and molecular structure of (±)-A: B. H. Toder, A. B. Smith, *J. Cryst. Mol. Struct.* **8,** 1 (1979). Stereospecific total synthesis of (±)-A: R. M. Scarborough *et al., J. Am. Chem. Soc.* **99,** 7085 (1977); *eidem, ibid.* **102,** 3904 (1980); and absolute configuration: K. Sakai *et al., Tetrahedron Lett.* **1979,** 2365. Stereospecific total synthesis and absolute configuration of (+)-A: J.

Jernow *et al.*, *J. Org. Chem.* **44**, 4210 (1979). Revised structure and total synthesis of B: *eidem, ibid.* 4212. Concise synthesis of B: M. Mikolajczyk, R. Zurawinski, *Synlett* **8**, 575 (1991). Prepn of analogs of A and structure-activity correlations: T. Haneishi *et al.*, *J. Antibiot.* **27**, 400 (1974). Toxicity: *eidem, ibid.* 386. Methylenomycin A is the first example of an antibiotic in which all information required for synthesis is carried by a plasmid, SCP1: L. F. Wright, D. A. Hopwood, *J. Gen. Microbiol.* **95**, 96 (1976). Review of biosynthesis: U. Hornemann, D. A. Hopwood, *Antibiotics* **vol. IV**, J. W. Corcoran, Ed. (Springer-Verlag, New York, 1981) pp 123-131. General review: A. Terehara *et al.*, *Heterocycles* **13**, 353-371 (1979).

Methylenomycin A

Methylenomycin B

Methylenomycin A. [52775-76-5] [1*S*-(1α,2α,5α)]-1,5-Dimethyl-3-methylene-4-oxo-6-oxabicyclo[3.1.0]hexane-2-carboxylic acid. $C_9H_{10}O_4$; mol wt 182.17. Colorless crystals from chloroform/carbon tetrachloride, mp 115° (dec). mp of the (±)-form: 88.5-89°; after subl (70-75°, 0.025 mm Hg), 107.5-108°. $[\alpha]_D^{20}$ +42.3° (c = 1 in chloroform). uv max (methanol): 224 nm (ε 6300). Sol in benzene, chloroform, ethyl acetate, acetone, methanol, water. Slightly sol in *n*-hexane, CCl_4. pKa' 3.65. LD_{50} in mice (mg/kg): 1500 orally, 75 i.p. (Haneishi).

Methylenomycin B. [52775-77-6] 2,3-Dimethyl-5-methylene-2-cyclopenten-1-one. $C_8H_{10}O$; mol wt 122.16. Neutral colorless oil. uv max (methanol): 240 nm (ε 7650). Sol in ether, benzene, chloroform, ethyl acetate, acetone, alcohols. Slightly sol in *n*-hexane, petr ether. LD_{50} in mice (mg/kg): 260 orally, 245 i.p. (Haneishi).

6068. N-Methylephedrine. [552-79-4] α-[1-(Dimethylamino)ethyl]benzenemethanol; *erythro*-α-[1-(dimethylamino)ethyl]benzyl alcohol; 2-dimethylamino-1-phenylpropanol; *N,N*-dimethylnorephedrine. $C_{11}H_{17}NO$; mol wt 179.26. C 73.70%, H 9.56%, N 7.81%, O 8.93%. Isoln of *l*-form from *Ephedra distachya* L. (*E. vulgaris* Rich.), and allied *Gnetaceae*: Smith, *J. Chem. Soc.* **1927**, 2056; Wolfes, *Arch. Pharm.* **268**, 327 (1930). Prepn of *l*-form: Smith, *loc. cit.*; of *d*-, *l*-, and *dl*-forms, and resolution of racemic mixture: Nagai, Kanao, *Ann.* **470**, 157 (1929); of *dl*-form: Pfanz, Müller, *Arch. Pharm.* **288**, 11 (1955).

dl-**Form.** Crystals from petr ether or methanol, mp 63.5-64.5°. Readily sol in the usual solvents.

dl-**Form hydrochloride.** Metheph. Crystals from acetone, mp 207-208°.

d-**Form.** Crystals, mp 87-87.5°. $[\alpha]_D^{20}$ +29.2° (c = 4 in methanol).

d-**Form hydrochloride.** Crystals from ethyl acetate, mp 192°. $[\alpha]_D^{20}$ +30.1°.

l-**Form.** Crystals from petr ether, mp 87-88°. $[\alpha]_D$ −29.5° (c = 4.5 in methanol).

l-**Form hydrochloride.** Crystals from ethyl acetate or alcohol, mp 192°. $[\alpha]_D^{20}$ −29.8° (c = 4.6). Readily sol in water; less sol in alcohol; sparingly sol in acetone.

β-**Camphorsulfonate.** *N*-Methylephedrine camsylate; Tybraine. THERAP CAT: Analeptic.

6069. N-Methylepinephrine. [554-99-4] 4-[2-(Dimethylamino)-1-hydroxyethyl]-1,2-benzenediol; α-[(dimethylamino)methyl]-3,4-dihydroxybenzyl alcohol; α-(3,4-dihydroxyphenyl)-2-dimethylaminoethanol; α-(3,4-dihydroxyphenyl)-α-hydroxy-β-dimethylaminoethane; dimethylaminomethyl-(3,4-dihydroxyphenyl)carbinol; α-(dimethylaminomethyl)protocatechuyl alcohol; *N*-methyladrenaline. $C_{10}H_{15}NO_3$; mol wt 197.23. C 60.90%, H 7.67%, N 7.10%, O 24.34%. Prepn and resolution of racemic mixture: Manna, Campiglio, *Farmaco Ed. Sci.* **14**, 317 (1959). Configuration: Manna, Ghislandi, *ibid.* **19**, 377 (1964).

DL-Form. [6032-14-0] Methadren(e). Crystals from alcohol + ethyl acetate, mp 142-143°.

D(−)-Form. Crystals from ethyl acetate, mp 149-150°. $[\alpha]_D^{18}$ −65.1° (c = 1.41 in 0.5*N* HCl).

L(+)-Form. Crystals, mp 149-150°. $[\alpha]_D^{18}$ +62.3° (c = 1.4). THERAP CAT: Adrenergic.

6070. Methylergonovine. [113-42-8] (8*β*)-9,10-Didehydro-*N*-[(1*S*)-1-(hydroxymethyl)propyl]-6-methylergoline-8-carboxamide; *N*-[α-(hydroxymethyl)propyl]-D-lysergamide; D-lysergic acid (+)-butanolamide-(2); *d*-lysergic acid-*d*-1-hydroxybutylamide-2; methylergometrine; methylergobasine. $C_{20}H_{25}N_3O_2$; mol wt 339.43. C 70.77%, H 7.42%, N 12.38%, O 9.43%. Semisynthetic ergot alkaloid; metabolite of methysergide, *q.v.* Prepn: A. Stoll, A. Hofmann, **US 2265207** (1941 to Sandoz); *eidem, Helv. Chim. Acta* **26**, 944 (1943). HPLC determn in plasma: H. T. Smith, N. C. Molinaro, *J. Chromatogr.* **424**, 416 (1988). Clinical trial in prevention of cluster headache: L. Mueller *et al.*, *Headache* **37**, 437 (1997). Review of pharmacology and clinical use in obstetrics and gynecology: A. N. de Groot *et al.*, *Drugs* **56**, 523-535 (1998).

Shiny crystals from benzene, mp 172° (some decompn). $[\alpha]_D^{20}$ −45° (c = 0.4 in pyridine). Sparingly sol in water. Freely sol in alcohol, acetone.

Maleate. [57432-61-8] Basofortina; Methergin; Methergine; Metenarin; Methylergobrevin; Ryegonovin; Spametrin-M. $C_{20}H_{25}N_3O_2 \cdot C_4H_4O_4$; mol wt 455.50. White to pinkish-tan microcryst powder; odorless; bitter taste. Slightly sol in water, alcohol; very slightly sol in chloroform, ether. THERAP CAT: Oxytocic.

6071. Methyl Ether. [115-10-6] Oxybismethane; dimethyl ether. C_2H_6O; mol wt 46.07. C 52.14%, H 13.13%, O 34.73%. CH_3OCH_3. Prepn: J. Dumas, E. Peligot, *Ann.* **15**, 1 (1835); and thermal properties: R. M. Kennedy *et al.*, *J. Am. Chem. Soc.* **63**, 2267 (1941). Atmospheric chemistry: S. M. Japar *et al.*, *Int. J. Chem. Kinet.* **22**, 1257 (1990). Review: H. Höver in *Ullmann's Encyclopedia of Industrial Chemistry* **vol. A8** (VCH, Weinheim, 1987) pp 541-544; of use in diesel engines: A. M. Rouhi, *Chem. Eng. News* **73**, 37-39 (May 29, 1995).

Colorless, flammable gas with a slight ethereal odor. mp −141.50°. bp −24.82°. d^{25} (1 atm) 1.91855 g/l. Heat capacity at 210.51 K: 23.88 cal/deg/mole. Heat of vaporization at bp: 5141.0 cal/mole. Heat of fusion: 1179.8 cal/mole. Flash pt −41°C. One vol water takes up 37 vols gas.

USE: Aerosol propellant; alternative diesel fuel; chemical intermediate.

6072. Methyl Ethyl Ketone. [78-93-3] 2-Butanone; ethyl methyl ketone; MEK; 2-oxobutane. C_4H_8O; mol wt 72.11. C

66.62%, H 11.18%, O 22.19%. $CH_3COCH_2CH_3$. Prepn from ethyl 2-methylacetoacetate: J. Schramm, *Ann.* **398**, 242 (1913). Manuf by dehydration of 2-butanol and by catalytic oxidation of *n*-butenes: A. J. Papa, P. D. Sherman, Jr. in *Kirk-Othmer Encyclopedia of Chemical Technology* vol. **13** (Wiley-Interscience, New York, 3rd ed., 1981) pp 903-907. Toxicity: H. F. Smyth *et al.*, *Am. Ind. Hyg. Assoc. J.* **23**, 95 (1962). Review of toxicology and human exposure: *Toxicological Profile for 2-Butanone* (PB93-110708, 1992) 144 pp.

Flammable liquid; acetone-like odor. d_4^{20} 0.805. mp $-86°$. bp 79.6°. Flash pt, closed cup: 21°F ($-6°C$). n_D^{15} 1.3814. Sol in ~4 parts water (27.5%); less sol at higher temp; miscible with alcohol, ether, benzene. Constant boiling mixture with water, bp 73.4°, contains 88.7% methyl ethyl ketone. Soly of water in methyl ethyl ketone: 12.5% at 25°. LD_{50} orally in rats: 6.86 ml/kg (Smyth).

Caution: Potential symptoms of overexposure are irritation of skin, eyes and nose; dermatitis; headache; dizziness; vomiting. *See NIOSH Pocket Guide to Chemical Hazards* (DHHS/NIOSH 97-140, 1997) p 36.

USE: As solvent; in the surface coating industry; manuf smokeless powder; colorless synthetic resins.

6073. Methyleugenol. [93-15-2] 1,2-Dimethoxy-4-(2-propenyl)benzene; 4-allyl-1,2-dimethoxybenzene; 4-allylveratrole; 3,4-dimethoxyallylbenzene; eugenol methyl ether. $C_{11}H_{14}O_2$; mol wt 178.23. C 74.13%, H 7.92%, O 17.95%. Natural constituent of the volatile oils of various plants, including cinnamon, clove, nutmeg, basil, and anise. Prepn: K. U. Matsmoto, *Ber.* **11**, 122 (1878). Isoln from the bark of *Cinnamomum oliveri*: G. W. Hargreaves, *J. Chem. Soc.* **109**, 751 (1916). Raman spectroscopy: B. Susz *et al.*, *Helv. Chim. Acta* **19**, 548 (1936). Toxicity: P. M. Jenner *et al.*, *Food Cosmet. Toxicol.* **2**, 327 (1964). HPLC determn in plasma: S. W. Graves, S. Runyon, *J. Chromatogr. B* **663**, 255 (1995). GC/MS determn in basil cultivars: M. Miele *et al.*, *J. Agric. Food Chem.* **49**, 517 (2001). Biosynthesis in sweet basil: E. Lewinsohn *et al.*, *Plant Sci.* **160**, 27 (2000). Safety assessment: R. L. Smith *et al.*, *Food Chem. Toxicol.* **40**, 851 (2002).

Colorless to pale yellow liquid. bp_{30} 146-147°. bp_{760} 244°. $n_D^{?}$ 1.53432. n_D^{27} 1.5305. d_4^{20} 1.0396. LD_{50} orally in rats: 1560 mg/kg (Jenner).

Caution: This substance is reasonably anticipated to be a human carcinogen: *Report on Carcinogens, Eleventh Edition* (PB2005-104914, 2004) p III-170.

USE: Fragrance ingredient in perfumes, toiletries and detergents; flavor ingredient in baked goods.

6074. α-Methylfentanyl. [79704-88-4] *N*-[1-(1-Methyl-2-phenylethyl)-4-piperidinyl]-*N*-phenylpropanamide; *N*-[1-(α-methylphenethyl)-4-piperidyl]propionanilide; 1-(1-methyl-2-phenylethyl)-4-(*N*-propanilido)piperidine. $C_{23}H_{30}N_2O$; mol wt 350.50. C 78.81%, H 8.63%, N 7.99%, O 4.56%. Potent derivative of fentanyl, *q.v.* Prepn: P. A. J. Janssen, **FR M2430**; *idem*, **US 3164600** (1964, 1965 both to Janssen). This substance has erroneously been referred to as *"China White"*, the street term for very pure Southeast Asian heroin. Initial identification of "China White" as α-methylfentanyl: T. C. Kram *et al.*, *Anal. Chem.* **53**, 1379 A (1981). Molecular structure determn using tandem mass spectrometry: M. T. Cheng *et al.*, *ibid.* **54**, 2204 (1982). Identification and quantification in tissue: T. J. Gillespie *et al.*, *J. Anal. Toxicol.* **6**, 139 (1982). Confirmation of identity of "China White": S. Suzuki *et al.*, *Chem. Pharm. Bull.* **34**, 1340 (1986). Immunoassay for detection of use in racehorses: J. McDonald *et al.*, *Res. Commun. Chem. Pathol. Pharmacol.* **57**, 389 (1987).

Hydrochloride. [1443-44-3] $C_{23}H_{30}N_2O$.HCl. Crystals from isopropanol, mp 272.8-273.6°.

Note: This is a controlled substance (opiate): **21 CFR, 1308.11**.

6075. Methyl Fluorosulfonate. [421-20-5] Fluorosulfuric acid methyl ester; methyl fluorosulfate; methyl fluosulfonate; Magic Methyl. CH_3FO_3S; mol wt 114.10. C 10.53%, H 2.65%, F 16.65%, O 42.07%, S 28.10%. CH_3OSO_2F. Prepn from dimethyl ether and fluosulfonic acid: J. Meyer, G. Schramm, *Z. Anorg. Allg. Chem.* **206**, 24 (1932); from dimethyl sulfate and fluosulfonic acid: R. W. Alder, *Chem. Ind. (London)* **1973**, 983. Electrochemical prepn: J. P. Coleman, D. Pletcher, *Tetrahedron Lett.* **1974**, 147. Powerful methylating agent: M. G. Ahmed *et al.*, *Chem. Commun.* **1968**, 1533. Human toxicity: D. M. W. vanden Ham, D. van der Meer, *Chem. Eng. News* **54**, 5 (Aug. 30, 1976); *eidem, Chem. Ind. (London)* **1976**, 782. Toxicity study: M. Hite *et al.*, *Am. Ind. Hyg. Assoc. J.* **40**, 600 (1979).

Volatile liq, bp 92-94°, mp −95°. *Severe Poison!* d 1.412. n_D^{20} 1.3326. Good solvent for most organic compounds. Proton NMR absorption at tau 5.88. LD_{50} orally in mice: <112 mg/kg; LC_{50} 1 hr for rats: 5-6 ppm (Hite).

Caution: Extremely toxic to humans. (vanden Ham, van der Meer). Exposure can cause fatal pulmonary edema.

USE: In organic synthesis as methylating agent.

6076. *N*-Methylformamide. [123-39-7] *N*-Monomethylformamide; NMF; MMF; NSC-3051. C_2H_5NO; mol wt 59.07. C 40.67%, H 8.53%, N 23.71%, O 27.09%. HCONHCH₃. Prepn: A. Gautier, *Ann.* **151**, 239 (1869); G. F. D'Alelio, E. E. Reid, *J. Am. Chem. Soc.* **59**, 109 (1937); J. A. Marsella, G. P. Pez, *J. Mol. Catal.* **35**, 65 (1986); J. J. Cappon *et al.*, *Recl. Trav. Chim. Pays-Bas* **113**, 318 (1994). Dielectric spectrum: J. Barthel *et al.*, *Chem. Phys. Lett.* **167**, 62 (1990). Toxicology: S. P. Langdon *et al.*, *Toxicology* **34**, 173 (1985). Review of metabolism, toxicity, and pharmacology: G. L. Kennedy, Jr., *Crit. Rev. Toxicol.* **17**, 129-182 (1986). Review of antitumor activity and clinical evaluation: K. Clagett-Carr *et al.*, *J. Clin. Oncol.* **6**, 906-918 (1988).

mp −5.4°. bp 180-185°. bp_{90} 131°. d_4^{25} 0.9961. Sol in acetone, alcohol, water. LD_{50} in mice (mg/kg): 2300 i.p.; 2600 orally; 1580 i.v.; 2700 i.m. (Langdon).

USE: Solvent.

6077. Methyl Formate. [107-31-3] Formic acid methyl ester. $C_2H_4O_2$; mol wt 60.05. C 40.00%, H 6.71%, O 53.29%. HCOOCH₃.

Colorless flammable liquid, agreeable odor. d_4^{15} 0.987. bp 31.5°. n_D^{20} 1.3440. Flash pt, closed cup: −2°F (−19°C). mp ~−100°. Sol in about 3.3 parts water; miscible with alcohol.

Caution: Potential symptoms of overexposure are eye and nose irritation; chest tightness, dyspnea; visual disturbance; CNS depression. *See NIOSH Pocket Guide to Chemical Hazards* (DHHS/-NIOSH 97-140, 1997) p 210; *Patty's Industrial Hygiene and Toxicology* vol. **2A**, G. D. Clayton, F. E. Clayton, Eds. (Wiley-Interscience, New York, 3rd ed., 1981) p 2263.

USE: Fumigant and larvicide for tobacco and food crops. Fire hazard is avoided by use with CO_2.

6078. *N*-Methylglucamine. [6284-40-8] 1-Deoxy-1-(methylamino)-D-glucitol; *N*-methyl-D-glucamine; meglumine. $C_7H_{17}NO_5$; mol wt 195.21. C 43.07%, H 8.78%, N 7.18%, O 40.98%. Prepd from D-glucose and methylamine: Karrer, Herkenrath, *Helv. Chim. Acta* **20**, 83 (1937). Efficacy and toxicity in treatment of leishmaniasis: R. G. Muller *et al.*, *Arch. Inst. Cardiol. Mex.* **52**, 155 (1982); P. Bouree *et al.*, *Pathol. Biol.* **33**, 607 (1985). Antileishmanial activity in dogs: W. L. Chapman *et al.*, *Am. J. Vet. Res.* **45**, 1028 (1984).

Crystals from methanol, mp 128-129°. Does not polymerize or dehydrate unless heated above 150° for prolonged periods. $[\alpha]_D^{18}$ $-18.5°$ (Karrer); $[\alpha]_D^{20}$ $-23°$ (Rhône-Poulenc data sheet). Soly (g/100 ml): water at 25°: ~100; alcohol at 25°: 1.2; alcohol at 70°: 21. pH of 1% aq soln: 10.5. Forms salts with acids and complexes with metals. Salts with alkyl aryl sulfonic acids act as detergents.

Antimonate. [133-51-7] RP-2168; Glucantim; Glucantime; Protostib. $C_7H_{17}NO_5.HSbO_3$; mol wt 365.98. Powder. Soly in water about 35% ww. Practically insol in alcohol, ether, chloroform. pH of aq solns 6-7.

USE: In the synthesis of surface active agents, pharmaceuticals, dyes.

THERAP CAT: Antimonate as antiprotozoal (Leishmania).

6079. N-Methyl-α-L-glucosamine. [42852-95-9] 2-(Methylamino)-2-deoxy-α-L-glucopyranose. $C_7H_{15}NO_5$; mol wt 193.20. C 43.52%, H 7.83%, N 7.25%, O 41.41%. Together with streptose forms the streptobiosamine moiety of streptomycin: Kuehl *et al., J. Am. Chem. Soc.* **69**, 3032 (1947). Prepn from D-glucose by *Streptomyces griseus:* Silverman, Rieder, *J. Biol. Chem.* **235**, 1251 (1960); from the antibiotic, bluensomycin: Bannister, Argoudelis, *J. Am. Chem. Soc.* **85**, 34 (1963). *Review:* Lemieux, Wolfrom, *Adv. Carbohydr. Chem.* **3**, 337 (1948).

Glass. $[\alpha]_D^{25}$ $-62°$ (c = 1 in methanol).
Hydrochloride. $C_7H_{15}NO_5.HCl$. Needles from ethanol, mp 160-163°. Freely sol in water. Shows mutarotation. $[\alpha]_D^{25}$ $-103°$ → $-88°$ (c = 0.6).
N-Acetyl deriv. mp 165-166°. $[\alpha]_D^{25}$ $-51°$ (c = 0.4).
Pentaacetyl deriv. $C_{17}H_{25}NO_{10}$. mp 160.5-161.5°. $[\alpha]_D^{25}$ $-100°$ (c = 0.7 in chloroform).

6080. α-Methylglucoside. [97-30-3] Methyl-α-D-glucopyranoside. $C_7H_{14}O_6$; mol wt 194.18. C 43.30%, H 7.27%, O 49.44%. Prepd by refluxing finely powdered glucose with methanol-HCl: Fischer, *Ber.* **26**, 2405; **27**, 2987; **28**, 1151 (1895); Helferich, Schäfer, *Org. Synth.* **coll. vol. I**, (2nd ed., 1941) 364. Enzymatic synthesis by means of α-glucosidase from yeast: Bourquelot *et al., Compt. Rend.* **156**, 491 (1913). Prepd industrially by reacting glucose with methanol in the presence of a cation exchange material: *Chem. Eng. News* **33**, 4592 (1955). Monograph: G. N. Bollenback, *Methyl Glucoside, Preparation, Physical Constants, Derivatives* (Academic Press, New York, 1958).

Orthorhombic bisphenoidal crystals, d_4^{30} 1.46. mp 168°. $bp_{0.2}$ 200°. $[\alpha]_D^{20}$ $+158.9°$ (p = 10). pKa (25°): 13.71. Soly at 17° in water 63% (w/w); in 80% alcohol 7.3%; in 90% alcohol 1.6%. Practically insol in ether. Soly also reported at 20° as 108 g/100 g H_2O and as 5.2 g/100 g methanol.

USE: Manuf reconstituted and upgraded drying oils; tall oil esters and varnishes; fatty acid esters; plasticizers; nonionic surface active agents; fast and hard drying alkyd resins, and so-called plasticizing alkyds. In making glucoside hydroxypropyl ethers for polyurethan foam production.

6081. Methylglyoxal. [78-98-8] 2-Oxopropanal; pyruvaldehyde; 2-ketopropionaldehyde; acetylformaldehyde. $C_3H_4O_2$; mol wt 72.06. C 50.00%, H 5.60%, O 44.41%. CH_3COCHO. Physiological metabolite formed by the fragmentation of triosephosphates and by the metabolism of acetone; synthesized by microorganisms. Also occurs in a variety of foods and beverages such as coffee. Reacts with nucleic acids and proteins under physiological conditions serving as a signal for their degradation. Prepn: H. v. Pechmann, *Ber.* **20**, 3213 (1887); H. O. L. Fischer, C. Taube, *ibid.* **57**, 1502 (1924); *eidem, ibid.* **59**, 857 (1926); M. W. Kellum *et al., Anal. Biochem.* **85**, 586 (1978). GC determn in food and biological samples: S. Ohmori *et al., J. Chromatogr.* **415**, 221 (1987). Review of natural occurrance and metabolism in microorganisms: Y. Inoue, A. Kimura, *Adv. Microb. Physiol.* **37**, 177-227 (1995). Review of physiological significance and role in pathogenesis: P. J. Thornalley, *Gen. Pharmacol.* **27**, 565-573 (1996).

Clear, yellow liquid, pungent odor. bp_{760} 72°. d^{24} 1.0455. $n_D^{17.5}$ 1.4002. Hygroscopic. Polymerizes very readily, forming a brittle, resinous mass. Sol in water and alcohol, giving colorless solns.

Oxime *see* Isonitrosoacetone.

6082. Methyl Green. [14855-76-6] 4-[[4-(Dimethylamino)phenyl][4-(dimethylimino)-2,5-cyclohexadien-1-ylidene]methyl]-N-ethyl-N,N-dimethylbenzenaminium bromide chloride; C.I. 42590; ethyl green. $C_{27}H_{35}BrClN_3$; mol wt 516.94. C 62.73%, H 6.82%, Br 15.46%, Cl 6.86%, N 8.13%. Usually sold as the double salt with $ZnCl_2$. Prepn: *Colour Index* **vol. 4** (3rd ed., 1971) p 4394.

Green powder. Sol in water. Yellow soln in conc H_2SO_4, turning green on dilution.

Note: The term methyl green also applies to the trimethyl analog.

USE: Dyeing and printing textiles; as biological stain.

6083. Methylguanidine. [471-29-4] $C_2H_7N_3$; mol wt 73.10. C 32.86%, H 9.65%, N 57.48%. Isoln by Brieger in 1888 from decomposing horsemeat; described as a product of putrefaction: I. Greenwald, *J. Am. Chem. Soc.* **41**, 1109 (1919). Prepn: E. Erlenmeyer, *Ber.* **3**, 896 (1870); E. A. Werner, J. Bell, *J. Chem. Soc.* **121**, 1790 (1922); R. Phillips, H. T. Clarke, *J. Am. Chem. Soc.* **45**, 1755 (1923); E. Philippi, K. Morsch, *Ber.* **60**, 2120 (1927); T. L. Davis, E. N. Rosenquist, *J. Am. Chem. Soc.* **59**, 2112 (1937). Toxicity data: Alles, *J. Pharmacol. Exp. Ther.* **28**, 251 (1926); Führer, *Arch. Exp. Pathol. Pharmakol.* **166**, 437 (1932).

Colorless, deliquesc, strongly alkaline mass. Very sol in water; sol in alcohol. Reduces permanganate. MLD in rats (mg/kg): 250 s.c. (Alles). LD in frogs, mice (mg/kg): 170-190, 550-600 s.c. (Führer).

6084. 5-Methyl-3-heptanone. [541-85-5] Amyl ethyl ketone; ethyl amyl ketone; EAK. $C_8H_{16}O$; mol wt 128.21. C

74.94%, H 12.58%, O 12.48%. *Review:* R. F. Buller, *Ind. Eng. Chem.* **48**, 1323-1324 (1956).

Liquid. Mild fruity odor. d_{20}^{20} 0.820-0.824. One gallon weighs 6.83 lbs at 20°. bp_{760} 157-162°. Flash pt 59°C (138°F). Evaporation rate 0.3 (*n*-butyl acetate = 1.0). n_D^{15} 1.4195. Slightly miscible with water. Compatible with alcohols, ketones, ethers, many other organic solvents.

Caution: Potential symptoms of overexposure are irritation of eyes, skin, mucous membranes; headache; narcosis, coma; dermatitis. *See NIOSH Pocket Guide to Chemical Hazards* (DHHS/-NIOSH 97-140, 1997) p 210.

USE: Solvent for nitrocellulose-alkyd, nitrocellulose-maleic, and vinyl resins.

6085. Methylhexaneamine. [105-41-9] 4-Methyl-2-hexanamine; 2-amino-4-methylhexane; 1,3-dimethylamylamine; Forthane. $C_7H_{17}N$; mol wt 115.22. C 72.97%, H 14.87%, N 12.16%. Prepn: **US 2350318; US 2386273** (1944, 1945 both to Lilly).

Liquid, amine odor. d 0.7620-0.7655. n_D^{25} 1.4150-1.4175. bp_{760} 130-135°. Very slightly sol in water. Freely sol in alc, chloroform, ether, dil acids.

THERAP CAT: Adrenergic.

6086. Methylhydrazine. [60-34-4] Monomethylhydrazine; MMH. CH_6N_2; mol wt 46.07. C 26.07%, H 13.13%, N 60.81%. CH_3NHNH_2. Early prepns: *Beilstein* **4**, 546; 1st suppl., 560. Prepn of sulfate: Hatt, *Org. Synth.* **coll. vol. I**, 395 (1943); Audrieth, Diamond, *J. Am. Chem. Soc.* **76**, 4869 (1954). Manuf and properties: Knight, *Hydrocarbon Process. Petr. Refin.* **41**, 179 (1962). Toxicity and metabolism: Witkin, *Arch. Ind. Health* **13**, 34 (1956); Dost *et al., Biochem. Pharmacol.* **15**, 1325 (1966); Gregory *et al., Clin. Toxicol.* **4**, 435 (1971); Magee *et al.* in *Proc. Fifth Int. Congress Pharmacology, San Francisco, 1972* **vol. 2**, T. A. Loomis, Ed. (Karger, New York, 1973) pp 140-149.

Clear liquid, odor characteristic of short chain, organic amines. d^{25} 0.874. mp −52.4°. bp 87.5°. Heat capacity (25°): 32.25 cal/mole/°C. Flammability limits in air (%-vol): 2.5 to 97 ± 2%. Miscible with water, hydrazine, low mol wt monohydric alcohols. Sol in hydrocarbons. Mildly alkaline base. Strong reducing agent. Ignites spontaneously on contact with strong oxidizing agents such as fluorine, chlorine trifluoride, nitrogen tetroxide, fuming nitric acid. LD_{50} orally in mice, rats: 33.0, 32.5 mg/kg (Witkin); orally in rats: 70.7 mg/kg (Gregory).

Sulfate. $CH_3NHNH_2.H_2SO_4$. White plates from 80% ethanol. mp 141-142°.

Caution: Potential symptoms of overexposure to methylhydrazine are irritation of eyes, skin and respiratory system; vomiting; diarrhea; tremors and ataxia; anoxia, cyanosis; convulsions. Potential occupational carcinogen. *See NIOSH Pocket Guide to Chemical Hazards* (DHHS/NIOSH 97-140, 1997) p 210.

USE: In rocket fuel; intermediate in chemical syntheses.

6087. Methyl Iodide. [74-88-4] Iodomethane. CH_3I; mol wt 141.94. C 8.46%, H 2.13%, I 89.41%. Prepd from methyl alcohol, iodine and red phosphorus: King, *Org. Synth.* **coll. vol. II**, 399 (1943); from potassium iodide and methyl sulfate: Hartman, *ibid.* 404. Review of toxicity and carcinogenic risk: *IARC Monographs* **41**, 213-227 (1986); *ibid.* **Suppl. 7**, p 47, 52 (1987); *Evaluation of the Potential Carcinogenicity of Methyl Iodide* (PB93-196343, 1988) 17 pp.

Colorless, transparent liquid; turns brown on exposure to light. *Poisonous!* d_4^{20} 2.28. mp −66.5°. bp 42.5°; dec at 270°. n_D^{21} 1.5293. Sol in about 50 parts water; miscible with alcohol, ether. *Protect from light.* LD_{50} orally in rats: 76 mg/kg; LD_{50} s.c. in mice: 0.78 mmoles/kg (IARC, 1986).

Caution: Potential symptoms of overexposure are nausea, vomiting; vertigo, ataxia; slurred speech, drowsiness; dermatitis; direct contact may cause irritation of eyes, skin and respiratory system. *See NIOSH Pocket Guide to Chemical Hazards* (DHHS/NIOSH 97-140, 1997) p 210. *See also Patty's Industrial Hygiene and Toxicology* **vol. 2E**, G. D. Clayton, F. E. Clayton, Eds. (John Wiley & Sons, Inc., New York, 4th ed., 1994) pp 4030-4034; *Clinical Toxicology of Commercial Products*, R. E. Gosselin *et al.*, Eds. (Williams & Wilkins, Baltimore, 5th ed., 1984) Section II, pp 158-159. This substance has been listed as reasonably anticipated to be a carcinogen: *Fourth Annual Report on Carcinogens* (NTP 85-002, 1985) p 132; delisted due to IARC reevaluation as unclassifiable as to its human carcinogenicity: *Fifth Annual Report on Carcinogens* (NTP 89-239, 1989) p 340.

USE: Methylating agent; in microscopy because of its high refractive index; as imbedding material for examining diatoms; in testing for pyridine. Light sensitive etching agent for electronic circuits; component in fire extinguishers.

6088. Methyl Isobutyrate. [547-63-7] 2-Methylpropanoic acid methyl ester. $C_5H_{10}O_2$; mol wt 102.13. C 58.80%, H 9.87%, O 31.33%. $(CH_3)_2CHCOOCH_3$.

Colorless, mobile liquid. d_D^{20} 0.891. mp −85 to −84°. bp 93°. n_D^{20} 1.3840. Slightly sol in water; miscible with alcohol, ether.

6089. Methyl Isocyanate. [624-83-9] Isocyanatomethane; isocyanic acid methyl ester; MIC. C_2H_3NO; mol wt 57.05. C 42.11%, H 5.30%, N 24.55%, O 28.04%. $CH_3N=C=O$. Intermediate in the manufacture of insecticides and herbicides including carbaryl, *q.v.* Prepn via Curtius rearrangement: J. W. Boehmer, *Rec. Trav. Chim.* **55**, 379 (1933); by heating *N*,*N*-diphenyl-*N'*-methylurea: W. Siefken, *Ann.* **562**, 75 (1949); by phosgenation of bis(trimethylsilyl)methylamine: V. F. Mironov *et al., Zh. Obshch. Khim.* **39**, 2598 (1969). Used in prepn of α-aryl-β-methylureas: J. W. Boehmer, *loc. cit.*; of semicarbazides: Ch. C. P. Pacilly, *Rec. Trav. Chim.* **55**, 101 (1936); in conversion of aldoximes to nitriles: J. A. Albright, M. L. Alexander, *Org. Prep. Proced. Int.* **4**, 215 (1972). Toxicity of vapor to rats, mice, humans; physical properties: G. Kimmerle, A. Eben, *Arch. Toxicol.* **20**, 235 (1960). Uptake and distribution studies in animals: J. S. Ferguson *et al., Toxicol. Appl. Pharmacol.* **94**, 104 (1988). Acute oral toxicity: E. H. Vernot *et al., ibid.* **42**, 417 (1977).

Liquid, bp 39-40°. d^{20} 0.96. Vapor press. at 4.2°: 200 torr; at 13.5°: 300 torr; at 20.6°: 400 torr; at 31.2°: 600 torr. LD_{50} in male rats (mg/kg): 140 single oral dose (Vernot). LC_{50} in rats (4 hours exposure to vapor): 5 ppm (Kimmerle, Eben).

Note: An industrial accident during the manufacture of carbaryl in Bhopal, India on December 3, 1984 resulted in the leakage of an unknown amount of methyl isocyanate into the air. Over 2,000 people died and an estimated 200,000 were exposed to the vapor: *Chem. Eng. News* **62**, 6 (Dec. 10, 1984); *ibid.* **63**, 14 (Feb. 11, 1985). Series of articles on follow-up studies on survivors: *Indian J. Exp. Biol.* **26**, 149-176, 201-204 (1988). Review of human toxicity: P. S. Mehta *et al., J. Am. Med. Assoc.* **264**, 2781-2787 (1990).

Caution: Potential symptoms of overexposure are irritation of eyes, skin, nose and throat; respiratory sensitization; coughing, pulmonary secretions, chest pain and dyspnea; asthma; eye and skin injury. *See NIOSH Pocket Guide to Chemical Hazards* (DHHS/-NIOSH 97-140, 1997) p 212. Highly volatile. Exposure to 2 ppm for 1-5 min produced tears and irritation of the nose and throat (Kimmerle, Eben).

USE: In organic synthesis; in manufacture of carbamate pesticides.

6090. Methyl Isopropyl Ketone. [563-80-4] 3-Methyl-2-butanone; 2-acetylpropane. $C_5H_{10}O$; mol wt 86.13. C 69.72%, H 11.70%, O 18.58%. $(CH_3)_2CHCOCH_3$. Prepn: E. Frankland, B. F. Duppa, *Ann.* **138**, 328 (1866). Large scale prepn: T. W. Mears *et al., J. Res. Natl. Bur. Stand.* **44**, 299 (1950). Miscibility profile: W. M. Jackson, J. S. Drury, *Ind. Eng. Chem.* **51**, 1491 (1959). Thermodynamic properties: J. L. Hales *et al., Trans. Faraday Soc.* **63**, 1876 (1967). Acute toxicity: H. Tanii *et al., Toxicol. Lett.* **30**, 13 (1986).

Colorless, flammable liquid with an acetone-like odor. bp_{760} 94.2°. fp −94.4°. d^{20} 0.8100; d^{25} 0.8061. n_D^{20} 1.3887; n_D^{25} 1.3861. Log P (*n*-octanol/water): 0.56. LD_{50} orally in male mice: 29.86 mmol/kg (Tanii).

Caution: Potential symptoms of overexposure are irritation of eyes, skin, mucous membranes, respiratory system; cough. *See NIOSH Pocket Guide to Chemical Hazards* (DHHS/NIOSH 97-140, 1997) p 212; *Patty's Industrial Hygiene and Toxicology* **vol 2C**, G. D. Clayton, F. E. Clayton, Eds. (Wiley-Interscience, New York, 4th ed., 1994) pp 1776-1779.

USE: Solvent.

6091. Methylisothiazolinone. [2682-20-4] 2-Methyl-3-(2H)-isothiazolone; MI; MIT; Neolone 950. C_4H_5NOS; mol wt 115.15. C 41.72%, H 4.38%, N 12.16%, O 13.89%, S 27.85%. Marketed in combination with methylchloroisothiazolinone as a broad spectrum biocide. Prepn: W. D. Crow, N. J. Leonard, *Tetrahedron Lett.* **5**, 1477 (1964); *eidem, J. Org. Chem.* **30**, 2660 (1965); S. N. Lewis *et al., J. Heterocycl. Chem.* **8**, 571 (1971). HPLC determn in cosmetic products: R. Matissek, *Chromatographia* **28**, 34 (1989). *In vitro* neurotoxicity study: S. Du *et al., J. Neurosci.* **22**, 7408 (2002). Safety assessment: *J. Am. Coll. Toxicol.* **11**, 75-128 (1992). Review of epidemiology of allergic reactions: A. C. de Groot, J. W. Weyland, *J. Am. Acad. Dermatol.* **18**, 350-358 (1988) J. Fewings, T. Menné, *Contact Dermatitis* **41**, 1-13 (1999).

Colorless prisms, mp 50-51°. bp$_{0.03}$ 93°. uv max (diethyl ether): 281 nm (ε 6550). uv max (95% ethanol): 275 nm (ε 7250).

Methylchloroisothiazolinone. [26172-55-4] 5-Chloro-2-methyl-3(2H)-isothiazolone; MCI. C_4H_4ClNOS; mol wt 149.60. Crystals from ligroin (60-90°), mp 54-55°. uv max (methanol): 277 nm (log ε 3.82).

Mixture with methylchloroisothiazolinone. [55965-84-9] Kathon CG. Commercial product is supplied as a clear, light amber liquid, fp $-18°$ to $-21.5°$. d^{20} 1.19. Viscosity (23°): 5.0 ±0.2 cP. Readily misc in water, lower alcohols, glycols, other hydrophilic organic solvents. Insol in petrolatum. LD$_{50}$ (mg/kg) orally in rabbits: 30; i.p. in male, female rats: 4.6, 4.3. LC$_{50}$ (6 day) in trout, sunfish (mg/l): 0.14, 0.54. LC$_{50}$ (8 day dietary) in Bobwhite quail, Peking duck (mg/kg/day): >60, >100 (*J. Am. Coll. Toxicol.*).

USE: Antimicrobial preservative in cosmetics, hygeine products, paints, emulsions, cutting oils, paper coatings, and water storage and cooling units.

6092. Methyl Isothiocyanate. [556-61-6] Isothiocyanatomethane; methyl mustard oil; Trapex. C_2H_3NS; mol wt 73.12. C 32.85%, H 4.14%, N 19.16%, S 43.85%. $CH_3N{=}CS$. Obtained by the action of CS_2 on methylamine. Antibacterial activity: P. Klesse, P. Lukoschek, *Arzneim.-Forsch.* **5**, 505 (1955). Toxicity data: E. H. Vernot *et al., Toxicol. Appl. Pharmacol.* **42**, 417 (1977). Headspace determn in wine: N. Gandini, R. Riguzzi, *J. Agric. Food Chem.* **45**, 3092 (1997). Soil degradation study: A. Frick *et al., J. Environ. Qual.* **27**, 1158 (1998).

Crystals, mp 35-36°. bp 119°. n$_D^{37}$ 1.5258. Slightly sol in water; freely sol in alcohol, ether. LD$_{50}$ in rats, mice (mg/kg): 220, 110 orally; in rabbits (mg/kg): 33 dermally (Vernot). LD$_{50}$ s.c. in mice: 0.05 g/kg (Klesse, Lukoschek).

Caution: Highly irritating.

USE: Pesticide; soil fumigant.

6093. Methyl Isovalerate. [556-24-1] 3-Methylbutanoic acid methyl ester. $C_6H_{12}O_2$; mol wt 116.16. C 62.04%, H 10.41%, O 27.55%. $(CH_3)_2CHCH_2COOCH_3$.

Liquid; valerian odor. d$_4^{20}$ 0.881. bp 116-117°. Slightly sol in water; miscible with alcohol, ether.

6094. Methyl Lactate. [547-64-8] 2-Hydroxypropanoic acid methyl ester. $C_4H_8O_3$; mol wt 104.10. C 46.15%, H 7.75%, O 46.11%. $CH_3CH(OH)COOCH_3$. Prepd by heating 1 mole lactic acid condensation polymer with 2.5-5 moles of methanol and a small quantity of H_2SO_4 at 100° for 1-4 hours in a heavy-walled bottle: Rehberg, *Org. Synth.* **coll. vol. III**, 47-48 (1955).

Colorless, transparent liquid. d^{19} 1.09. bp 144-145°. n$_D^{16}$ 1.4156. Soluble in alcohol, ether; dec by water.

Caution: Mild irritant.

USE: Cellulose acetate solvent.

6095. Methyl Linoleate. [112-63-0] 9,12-Octadecadienoic acid methyl ester. $C_{19}H_{34}O_2$; mol wt 294.47. C 77.50%, H 11.64%, O 10.87%. $CH_3(CH_2)_4CH{=}CHCH_2CH{=}CH(CH_2)_7$-$COOCH_3$. Prepn from safflower-seed oil: Parker *et al., Biochem. Prep.* **4**, 88 (1955).

Colorless oil. d$_4^{18}$ 0.8886. mp $-35°$. bp$_{16}$ 212°; bp$_4$ 192°. n$_D^{25}$ 1.4593. Iodine value 172.4. More stable to air oxidation than linoleic acid. Miscible with dimethylformamide, fat solvents, oils.

USE: In the vitamin industry.

6096. Methyl Malonate. [108-59-8] Propanedioic acid dimethyl ester; dimethyl malonate. $C_5H_8O_4$; mol wt 132.11. C 45.46%, H 6.10%, O 48.44%. $CH_3OOCCH_2COOCH_3$.

Liquid. d$_4^{20}$ 1.154. mp $-62°$. bp 180-181°. n$_D^{17}$ 1.4149. Slightly sol in water; miscible with alcohol, ether, oils.

6097. Methyl Methanesulfonate. [66-27-3] Methanesulfonic acid methyl ester; methyl methanesulfonic acid; *as*-dimethyl sulfite; methyl mesylate; MMS. $C_2H_6O_3S$; mol wt 110.13. C 21.81%, H 5.49%, O 43.58%, S 29.12%. $CH_3SO_2OCH_3$. Prepn: A. Arbusow, P. Pischtschimuka, *Chem. Zentralbl.* **II**, 685 (1909); W. E. Bissenger *et al., J. Am. Chem. Soc.* **70**, 3940 (1948). Metabolism: E. A. Barnsley, *Biochem. J.* **106**, 18p (1968). Mutagenicity studies: U. H. Ehling *et al., Mutat. Res.* **5**, 417 (1968); J. Moutschen, *ibid.* **8**, 581 (1969). Review of carcinogenicity studies: *IARC Monographs* **7**, 253-260 (1974). Review of comparative mutagenicity of MMS and ethyl methanesulfonate, *q.v.:* S. Kondo, *Environ. Sci. Res.* **24**, 743-785 (1981).

Liquid, bp$_{753}$ 203°, bp$_{0.6}$ 59°. d$_4^{20}$ 1.2943; n$_D^{20}$ 1.4140. Soly in water about 1:5, in DMF about 1:1. Slightly sol in nonpolar solvents.

Caution: This substance is reasonably anticipated to be a human carcinogen: *Report on Carcinogens, Eleventh Edition* (PB2005-104914, 2004) p III-171.

USE: Exptly as mutagen, teratogen, brain carcinogen.

6098. S-Methylmethionine. [4727-40-6] [(3S)-3-Amino-3-carboxypropyl]dimethyl sulfonium inner salt; S-methyl-L-methionine; MeMet; vitamin U. $C_6H_{13}NO_2S$; mol wt 163.24. C 44.15%, H 8.03%, N 8.58%, O 19.60%, S 19.64%. Naturally occurring sulfonium compound found in a large number of plants. Identification of antiulcer vitamin in cabbage leaves: G. Cheney, *Calif. Med.* **77**, 248 (1952). Isoln from cabbage juice: R. A. McRorie *et al., J. Am. Chem. Soc.* **76**, 115 (1954). Activity: V. Z. Szabo, G. Vargha, *Arzneim.-Forsch.* **10**, 23 (1960). Determn in plant tissue: P. K. Macnicol, *Anal. Biochem.* **158**, 93 (1986). Review of biosynthesis and physiological role in plants: J. Giovanelli *et al.,* "Sulfur Amino Acids in Plants " in *The Biochemistry of Plants* **5**, B. J. Miflin, Ed. (Academic Press, New York, 1980) pp 453-505.

Bromide. [33515-32-1] Methylmethioninesulfonium bromide. $C_6H_{14}BrNO_2S$. White platelets from ethanol, mp 139° (dec).

DL-Form chloride. [3493-12-7]; [1115-84-0] (L-form chloride). Methylmethioninesulfonium chloride; MMSC; Cabagin-U; Vitas-U. $C_6H_{14}ClNO_2S$; mol wt 199.70. Prepn: R. O. Atkinson, F. Poppelsdorf, *J. Chem. Soc.* **1951,** 1378. HPLC determn in pharmaceutical prepns: C. P. Leung, W. K. H. Leung, *J. Chromatogr.* **479**, 361 (1989). Clinical evaluation in ulcerative colitis: A. S. Salim, *Pharmacology* **45**, 307 (1992). Crystals from hot ethanol, mp 134° (dec). Very hygroscopic; hydrolysed rapidly in alkaline media.

THERAP CAT: Antiulcerative.

6099. Methylnaltrexone Bromide. [73232-52-7]; [83387-25-1] (methylnaltrexonium). 17-(Cyclopropylmethyl)-4,5-epoxy-3,14-dihydroxy-17-methyl-6-oxo-morphinanium bromide; N-cyclopropylmethyl-noroxymorphone methobromide; naltrexone methobromide; $C_{21}H_{26}BrNO_4$; mol wt 436.34. C 57.80%, H 6.01%, Br 18.31%, N 3.21%, O 14.67%. Peripheral opioid receptor antagonist; quaternary derivative of naltrexone, *q.v.*, that does not readily cross the blood brain barrier. Prepn: L. I. Goldberg *et al., US*

4176186 (1979 to Boehringer Ing.). Determn by HPLC and solid phase extraction in plasma and urine: J. Osinski *et al., J. Chromatogr. B* **780**, 251 (2002). Clinical evaluation in methadone-induced constipation: C.-S. Yuan *et al., J. Am. Med. Assoc.* **283**, 367 (2000). Clinical pharmacokinetics: *idem et al., J. Clin. Pharmacol.* **45**, 538 (2005). Review of therapeutic potential in opioid-induced bowel dysfunction: J. F. Foss, *Am. J. Surg.* **182**, 19S-26S (2001); of preclinical and clinical experience: C.-S. Yuan, *J. Support Oncol.* **2**, 111-117 (2004).

Crystals from methanol/ether, mp 253°.

THERAP CAT: Narcotic antagonist. In treatment of opioid bowel dysfunction.

6100. Methyl Nicotinate. [93-60-7] 3-Pyridinecarboxylic acid methyl ester; nicotinic acid methyl ester; Midalgan. C_7H_7-NO_2; mol wt 137.14. C 61.31%, H 5.14%, N 10.21%, O 23.33%. Obtained by passing HCl gas into a hot methanol soln of nicotinic acid: Engler, *Ber.* **27**, 1787 (1894); by treatment with tetramethyl-ammonium hydroxide in methanol: Prelog, Piantanida, *Z. Physiol. Chem.* **244**, 56 (1936); by heating a mixture of sulfuric acid, selenium and quinoline, followed by refluxing with methanol: Kaufman, *J. Am. Chem. Soc.* **67**, 497 (1945); from nicotinyl chloride hydrochloride and methanol in pyridine: Charonnat *et al., Bull. Soc. Chim. Fr.* **1948**, 1014.

Crystals, mp 39°. bp$_{760}$ 209°; bp$_3$ 70-72°. Soluble in water, alcohol, benzene.

THERAP CAT: Rubefacient.

6101. Methyl Nitrate. [598-58-3] Nitric acid methyl ester. CH_3NO_3; mol wt 77.04. C 15.59%, H 3.93%, N 18.18%, O 62.30%. CH_3ONO_2. Prepn from methanol and nitric acid in the presence of sulfuric acid: Black, Babers, *Org. Synth.* **coll. vol. II,** 412 (1943).

Liquid. Solid at −83°. bp$_{760}$ 64.6° (explodes). d_4^{20} 1.2075. n_D^{20} 1.3748. Slightly sol in water. Sol in alcohol, ether.

USE: Has been used as rocket propellant. Does not need external oxygen for combustion.

6102. Methyl *p*-Nitrobenzenesulfonate. [6214-20-6] *p*-Nitrobenzenesulfonic acid methyl ester. $C_7H_7NO_5S$; mol wt 217.20. C 38.71%, H 3.25%, N 6.45%, O 36.83%, S 14.76%. Reagent for selective methylation of cysteine residues in chemical modification of proteins: Nakagawa, Bender, *J. Am. Chem. Soc.* **91**, 1566 (1969). Procedure: Heinrikson, *Biochem. Biophys. Res. Commun.* **41**, 967 (1970). Prepd by the general method of reacting *p*-nitrobenzene-sulfonyl chloride with alcohols. See Morgan, Cretcher, *J. Am. Chem. Soc.* **70**, 375 (1948).

White to cream crystals, mp 93-95°.

USE: Methylating agent.

6103. *N*-Methyl-*N'*-nitro-*N*-nitrosoguanidine. [70-25-7] *N*-Methyl-*N*-nitroso-*N'*-nitroguanidine; MNNG. $C_2H_5N_5O_3$; mol wt 147.09. C 16.33%, H 3.43%, N 47.61%, O 32.63%. Prepn: A. F. McKay, G. F. Wright, *J. Am. Chem. Soc.* **69**, 3028 (1947). Reviews of carcinogenicity and mutagenicity studies: *IARC Monographs* **4**, 183-195 (1974); U. Sinha, B. B. Chattoo, *J. Sci. Ind. Res.* **3**, 499-505 (1975).

Yellow crystals from methanol, mp 118° (dec). Reacts with aq KOH to form diazomethane: A. F. McKay, *J. Am. Chem. Soc.* **70**, 1974 (1948). Reacts at acid pH to give methylnitroguanidine.

Caution: This substance is reasonably anticipated to be a human carcinogen: *Report on Carcinogens, Eleventh Edition* (PB2005-104914, 2004) p III-172.

USE: Exptlly as carcinogen and mutagen. Formerly in prepn of diazomethane.

6104. Methyl Nonyl Ketone. [112-12-9] 2-Undecanone; 2-hendecanone. $C_{11}H_{22}O$; mol wt 170.29. C 77.58%, H 13.02%, O 9.40%. $CH_3(CH_2)_8COCH_3$. Primary constituent of rue oils distilled mainly from *Ruta montana* L. and *R. graveolens*. Prepn: E. v. Gorup-Besanez, F. Grimm, *Ann.* **157**, 275 (1871); V. Fiandanese *et al., Tetrahedron Lett.* **25**, 4805 (1984); T. Aoyama, T. Shioiri, *Synthesis* **1988**, 228. LC determn in formulations: R. J. Bushway, *J. Assoc. Off. Anal. Chem.* **73**, 743 (1990). Physical properties: E. Guenther, D. Althausen, *The Essential Oils* vol. 2 (D. Van Nostrand, New York, 1949) p 377. Brief review: D. L. J. Opdyke, *Food Cosmet. Toxicol.* **13**, 869-870 (1975).

Oily liquid. Strong odor. mp 12.1°. bp$_{761}$ 231.5-232.5°. bp$_7$ 99°. d_4^{20} 0.8260-0.8263. n_D^{30} 1.42527. LD$_{50}$ dermally in rabbits: >5 g/kg; LD$_{50}$ orally in rats, mice: >5, 3.88 g/kg (Opdyke).

USE: In the compounding of some synthetic essential oils. As fragrance additive in soaps, detergents, creams, lotions, and perfume. As dog and cat repellant.

6105. Methyl Orange. [547-58-0] 4-[[(4-Dimethylamino)-phenyl]azo]benzenesulfonic acid sodium salt; sodium *p*-dimethyl-aminoazobenzenesulfonate; heliantine B; C.I. Acid Orange 52; C.I. 13025; Orange III; Gold Orange; Tropaeolin D. $C_{14}H_{14}N_3NaO_3S$; mol wt 327.33. C 51.37%, H 4.31%, N 12.84%, Na 7.02%, O 14.66%, S 9.80%. Prepn from sulfanilic acid sodium nitrite + dimethylaniline: L. Gattermann, *Die Praxis des Organischen Chemikers* (de Gruyter, Berlin, 40th ed., 1961) pp 260-261. *See also Colour Index* vol. 4 (3rd ed., 1971) p 4043.

Orange-yellow powder or cryst scales. Sol in 500 parts water; more sol in hot water. Practically insol in alcohol.

USE: As indicator in 0.1% aq soln. pH: 3.1 red, 4.4 yellow. Employed for titrating most mineral acids, strong bases, estimating alkalinity of waters; useless for organic acids. In dyeing and printing of textiles.

6106. Methyl Oxalate. [553-90-2] Ethanedioic acid dimethyl ester; dimethyl oxalate. $C_4H_6O_4$; mol wt 118.09. C 40.68%, H 5.12%, O 54.19%. $CH_3OOCCOOCH_3$.

Colorless crystals. d^{54} 1.148. mp 54°. bp 163-164°. $n_D^{82.1}$ 1.379. Sol in 17 parts water, in alcohol, ether.

6107. Methylparaben. [99-76-3] 4-Hydroxybenzoic acid methyl ester; methyl *p*-hydroxybenzoate; Nipagin M; Tegosept M; Methyl Chemosept; Methyl Parasept. $C_8H_8O_3$; mol wt 152.15. C 63.15%, H 5.30%, O 31.55%. Prepn: Ladenburg, Fitz, *Ann.* **141**, 247 (1867); Zbarskii, *C.A.* **33**, 9312^3 (1939). Identification in the vaginal secretions of female dogs in estrus: M. Goodwin *et al., Science* **203**, 559 (1979).

White needles, mp 131°. bp 270-280° (dec). One gram dissolves in 400 ml water, 40 ml warm oil, about 70 ml warm glycerol; freely sol in alcohol, acetone, ether. The soly in water is also given as 0.25% w/w at 20°, and as 0.30% w/w at 25°.

USE: As preservative in foods, beverages and cosmetics.

6108. Methyl Parathion. [298-00-0] Phosphorothioic acid *O,O*-dimethyl *O*-(4-nitrophenyl) ester; *O,O*-dimethyl *O-p*-nitrophenyl phosphorothioate; *O,O*-dimethyl *O-p*-nitrophenyl thiophosphate; dimethyl parathion; parathion-methyl; metaphos; E-601; ENT-17292; Folidol-M; Metacide; Penncap M. $C_8H_{10}NO_5$-PS; mol wt 263.21. C 36.51%, H 3.83%, N 5.32%, O 30.39%, P 11.77%, S 12.18%. Cholinesterase inhibitor. Prepn: Fletcher *et al., J. Am. Chem. Soc.* **72**, 2461 (1950). Manuf: *Faith, Keyes & Clark's Industrial Chemicals*, F. A. Lowenheim, M. K. Moran, Eds. (Wiley-Interscience, New York, 4th ed., 1975) pp 552-555. Toxicity data: T. B. Gaines, *Toxicol. Appl. Pharmacol.* **14**, 515 (1969). Review of carcinogenic risk: *IARC Monographs* **30**, 131-152 (1983); of toxicology and human exposure: *Toxicological Profile for Methyl Parathion* (PB2001-109105, 2001) 267 pp.

Crystals from cold methanol, mp 37-38°. n_D^{25} 1.5367. d_4^{20} 1.358. Soly in water 50 ppm; sol in most organic solvents. LD_{50} in male, female rats (mg/kg): 14, 24 orally; 67, 67 dermally (Gaines).

Caution: Potential symptoms of overexposure are irritation of eyes and skin; nausea, vomiting, abdominal cramps, diarrhea, salivation; headache, giddiness, vertigo, weakness; rhinorrhea, chest tightness; blurred vision, miosis; cardiac irregularities; muscle fasciculations; dyspnea. *See NIOSH Pocket Guide to Chemical Hazards* (DHHS/NIOSH 97-140, 1997) p 214.

USE: Insecticide.

6109. *N*-Methylphenazonium Methosulfate. [299-11-6] 5-Methylphenazinium methyl sulfate; phenazine methosulfate. $C_{14}H_{14}N_2O_4S$; mol wt 306.34. C 54.89%, H 4.61%, N 9.14%, O 20.89%, S 10.47%. Prepn: Kehrmann, *Ber.* **46**, 341 (1913); Hillemann, *ibid.* **71**, 34 (1938); Dickens, McIlwain, *Biochem. J.* **32**, 1615 (1938). Mutagenicity study: S. Venitt, C. Crofton-Sleigh, *Mutat. Res.* **68**, 107 (1979).

Flat yellow to brown parallelepipeds from alc, mp 155-157° (Hillemann); mp 167° (Dickens). Oxidation-reduction potential at 30° and pH 7: E_h = +0.080 v.

USE: As an electron carrier in place of the flavine enzyme of Warburg in the hexosemonophosphate system: Dickens, *loc. cit.* In the prepn of succinic dehydrogenase: Green *et al., J. Biol. Chem.* **217**, 551 (1955).

6110. Methylphenidate. [113-45-1] α-Phenyl-2-piperidineacetic acid methyl ester; methyl phenidylacetate; methyl α-phenyl-α-(2-piperidyl)acetate; methylphenidan. $C_{14}H_{19}NO_2$; mol wt 233.31. C 72.07%, H 8.21%, N 6.00%, O 13.72%. Prepn: L. Panizzon, *Helv. Chim. Acta* **27**, 1748 (1944); M. Hartmann, L. Panizzon, US 2507631 (1950 to Ciba). Sepn of isomers: R. Rometsch, US 2957880 (1960 to Ciba). Toxicity data: E. N. Greenblatt, A. C. Osterberg, *J. Pharmacol. Exp. Ther.* **131**, 115 (1961).

Comprehensive description: G. R. Padmanabhan, *Anal. Profiles Drug Subs.* **10**, 473-497 (1981). Pharmacokinetics: N. R. Srinivas *et al., Pharm. Res.* **10**, 14 (1993). Clinical efficacy in attention deficit-hyperactivity disorder (ADHD): W. E. Pelham, Jr. *et al., J. Consult. Clin. Psychol.* **61**, 506 (1993); R. G. Klein, *Encephale* **19**, 89 (1993).

$bp_{0.6mm}$ 135-137°. Sol in alcohol, ethyl acetate, ether. Practically insol in water, petr ether.

Hydrochloride. [298-59-9] Ciba 4311b; Centedrin; Concerta; Equasym; Metadate; Ritalin. $C_{14}H_{19}NO_2$.HCl; mol wt 269.77. Crystals, mp 224-226°. pKa 8.9. Sol in water, alc, chloroform. A 5% aq soln is neutral to litmus. LD_{50} orally in mice: 190 mg/kg (Greenblatt, Osterberg).

***d-threo*-Form.** [40431-64-9] (αR,2R)-α-Phenyl-2-piperidineacetic acid methyl ester; dexmethylphenidate. Enantioselective synthesis: J. M. Axten *et al., J. Am. Chem. Soc.* **121**, 6511 (1999).

***d-threo*-Form hydrochloride.** [19262-68-1] Dexmethylphenidate hydrochloride; Focalin. Clinical trials in ADHD: L. E. Arnold *et al., J. Child Adolesc. Psychopharmacol.* **14**, 542 (2004); R. Silva *et al., ibid.* 555. White to off-white powder. Freely sol in water, methanol; sol in alcohol; slightly sol in chloroform, acetone.

Note: This is a controlled substance (stimulant): **21 CFR**, 1308.12.

THERAP CAT: CNS stimulant.

6111. Methylprednisolone. [83-43-2] (6α,11β)-11,17,21-Trihydroxy-6-methylpregna-1,4-diene-3,20-dione; 1-dehydro-6α-methylhydrocortisone; $Δ^1$-6α-methylhydrocortisone; 6α-methyl-11β,17α,21-triol-1,4-pregnadiene-3,20-dione; Medrate; Medrol; Medrone. $C_{22}H_{30}O_5$; mol wt 374.47. C 70.56%, H 8.07%, O 21.36%. Prepn: Spero *et al., J. Am. Chem. Soc.* **78**, 6213 (1956); Fried, *ibid.* **81**, 1235 (1959); Sebek, Spero, US 2897218 (1959 to Upjohn); Gould, US 3053832 (1962 to Schering). Review of clinical toxicology: J. D. Truwit, *Crit. Care Clin.* **7**, 639-657 (1991); of neuroprotective pharmacology: E. D. Hall, *J. Neurosurg.* **76**, 13-22 (1992); of pharmacokinetics and clinical efficacy in multiple sclerosis: O. R. Hommes *et al., Mult. Scler.* **1**, 327-328 (1996). Clinical trial in acute spinal cord injury: M. B. Bracken *et al., J. Neurosurg.* **89**, 699 (1998); in carpel tunnel syndrome: J. W. H. H. Dammers *et al., Br. Med. J.* **319**, 884 (1999).

Crystals, mp 228-237°. $[α]_D^{20}$ +83° (dioxane). uv max (95% ethanol): 243 nm ($α_M$ 14875). Sparingly sol in alcohol, dioxane, methanol; slightly sol in acetone, chloroform; very slightly sol in ether. Practically insol in water.

21-Acetate. [53-36-1] Depo-Medrol; Depo-Medrone; Vetacortyl. $C_{24}H_{32}O_6$; mol wt 416.51. Crystals, mp 205-208°. $[α]_D^{20}$ +101° (dioxane). uv max (95% ethanol): 243 nm ($α_M$ 14825). Sol in dioxane; sparingly sol in acetone, alcohol, chloroform, methanol; slightly sol in ether. Practically insol in water.

21-Succinate sodium salt. [2375-03-3] Solu-Medrol; Solu-Medrone. $C_{26}H_{33}NaO_8$; mol wt 496.53. White, or nearly white, odorless, hygrosopic, amorphous solid. Very sol in water, alcohol; very slightly sol in acetone. Insol in chloroform.

Aceponate. [86401-95-8] Advantan. $C_{27}H_{36}O_7$; mol wt 472.57.

THERAP CAT: Glucocorticoid.

THERAP CAT (VET): Glucocorticoid.

6112. Methyl Propionate. [554-12-1] Propanoic acid methyl ester. $C_4H_8O_2$; mol wt 88.11. C 54.53%, H 9.15%, O 36.32%. $CH_3CH_2COOCH_3$.

Colorless liquid. d_4^{20} 0.915. mp $-87°$. bp 79.7°. Flash pt $-2°C$. n_D^{19} 1.3769. Sol in 16 parts water; miscible with alcohol, ether.

USE: In organic synthesis.

6113. Methyl Propyl Ether. [557-17-5] 1-Methoxypropane; Neo-thyl. $C_4H_{10}O$; mol wt 74.12. C 64.82%, H 13.60%, O 21.59%. $CH_3CH_2CH_2OCH_3$. Prepd by passing a mixture of methyl and propyl alcohol through a hot layer of β-naphthalenesulfonic or benzenesulfonic acids: Krafft, *Ber.* **26**, 2832 (1893); **DE 69115**; *Frdl.* **III**, 11. Laboratory prepn from sodium propylate and methyl iodide: Chancel, *Ann.* **151**, 305 (1869); Michael, Wilson, *Ber.* **39**, 2573 (1906); Bennett, Phillip, *J. Chem. Soc.* **1928**, 1931.

Mobile, flammable liquid. d_4^0 0.7494; d_4^{13} 0.7356. bp$_{761}$ 38.8°. $n_D^{14.3}$ 1.36019. Soly in water (25°): 5 ml/100 ml H_2O. Miscible with alc, ether. Absorbs water. Oil/water coefficient 10 ± 1. Anesthetic index 2.5. Methyl propyl ether used for anesthesia usually contains 0.002 diphenylamine as stabilizer.

THERAP CAT: Anesthetic (inhalation).

6114. Methyl Propyl Ketone. [107-87-9] 2-Pentanone; ethyl acetone. $C_5H_{10}O$; mol wt 86.13. C 69.72%, H 11.70%, O 18.58%. $CH_3CH_2CH_2COCH_3$. Toxicity study: H. F. Smyth *et al., Am. Ind. Hyg. Assoc. J.* **23**, 95 (1962).

Colorless liquid. d_4^{20} 0.809. mp $-78°$. bp 102°. n_D^{20} 1.3895. Almost insol in water. Misc with alcohol, ether. LD_{50} orally in rats: 3.73 g/kg (Smyth).

Caution: Potential symptoms of overexposure are irritation of eyes, skin and mucous membranes; headache; dermatitis; narcosis, coma. *See NIOSH Pocket Guide to Chemical Hazards* (DHHS/-NIOSH 97-140, 1997) p 244.

USE: Solvent.

6115. 5-Methylpyrazole-3-carboxylic Acid. [402-61-9] $C_5H_6N_2O_2$; mol wt 126.11. C 47.62%, H 4.80%, N 22.21%, O 25.37%. Prepn: Knorr, MacDonald, *Ann.* **279**, 219 (1894); Lehninger, *J. Am. Chem. Soc.* **64**, 2507 (1942). Hypoglycemic metabolite of 3,5-dimethylpyrazole: Smith *et al., J. Med. Chem.* **8**, 350 (1965).

Crystals from water, mp 236-237°.
Methyl ester. $C_6H_8N_2O_2$. Crystals, mp 75-78°.
Ethyl ester. $C_7H_{10}N_2O_2$. Crystals, mp 83°.
Caution: A powerful hypoglycemic agent in rats (characteristic of pyrazoles).

6116. Methyl Pyridyl Ketone. [350-03-8] 1-(3-Pyridinyl)-ethanone; 3-acetylpyridine; β-acetylpyridine; methyl 3-pyridyl ketone; methyl β-pyridyl ketone. C_7H_7NO; mol wt 121.14. C 69.40%, H 5.82%, N 11.56%, O 13.21%. A nicotinic acid antagonist. Prepd in dry distillation of Ca-nicotinate with Ca-acetate. The ketone is isolated through the phenylhydrazone: Engler, Kiby, *Ber.* **22**, 597 (1889).

Liquid, bp 220°. Freely sol in acids.
Ketoxime. $NC_5H_4C(CH_3){=}NOH$. Crystals from alcohol or benzene, mp 112°.

Ketoxime hydrochloride. Crystals from alcohol, mp 204°.
Phenylhydrazone. $NC_5H_4C(CH_3){=}NNHC_6H_5$. Yellow needles from alcohol, mp 137°.

6117. 1-Methylpyrrolidone. [872-50-4] 1-Methyl-2-pyrrolidinone; N-methyl-α-pyrrolidinone; N-methyl-γ-butyrolactone; NMP; 1-methylazacyclopentan-2-one; MP; M-Pyrol. C_5H_9NO; mol wt 99.13. C 60.58%, H 9.15%, N 14.13%, O 16.14%. Dipolar aprotic solvent. Commercially prepd by condensation of butyrolactone with methylamine. Prepn: J. Tafel, O. Wassmuth, *Ber.* **40**, 2831 (1907); E. Späth, J. Lintner, *ibid.* **69**, 2727 (1936). Use in extraction of unsaturated/aromatic compounds: E. Mueller, G. Hoehfeld, *Proc. 8th World Pet. Congr.* **4** (Applied Sci. Publishers, London, 1971) pp 213-219; H. Klein, H. M. Weitz, *Hydrocarbon Process.* **47**, 135 (November, 1968); A. Sequeira *et al., ibid.* **58**, 155 (September, 1979). Physical properties and solubility: *Industrial Solvents Handbook* (3rd Ed.) 580-582 (1985). Reference guide to properties and use: *M-Pyrol®, N-Methyl-2-Pyrrolidone Handbook*, ISP (subsidiary of GAF Corp.), 1988. Acute toxicity: W. Bartsch *et al., Arzneim.-Forsch.* **26**, 1581 (1976). *Review:* E. V. Hort, L. R. Anderson in *Kirk-Othmer Encyclopedia of Chemical Technology* **vol. 19** (Wiley-Interscience, New York, 3rd ed., 1982) pp 514-520.

Clear liquid. fp $-24.4°$. bp$_{760}$ 202°. n_D^{25} 1.4690. d_4^{25} 1.027. Flash point, closed cup: 199°F; open cup: 204°F. Viscosity (25°): 1.65 cP. Surface tension at 25°: 40.7 dynes/cm. Dipole moment at 25°: 4.09 D. Dielectric constant at 25°: 32.2. Vapor pressure at 23.2°, 65°: 0.33, 5 mm Hg. Heat of combustion: 719 kcal/mol; of vaporization: 127.3 kcal/kg. Misc with water, alcohol, ether, acetone, ethyl acetate, chloroform, benzene. LD_{50} in mice, rats (ml/kg): 3.5, 2.2 i.v.; 4.3. 2.4 i.p.; 7.5, 3.8 orally (Bartsch).

USE: Industrial solvent primarily used in the extraction of aromatics from lube oils. Other applications include recovery and purification of acetylenes, olefins and diolefins, gas purification, and aromatics extraction from feedstocks. Also, used as polymer solvent.

6118. N-Methylpyrroline. [554-15-4] N-Methyl-2,5-dihydropyrrole. C_5H_9N; mol wt 83.13. C 72.24%, H 10.91%, N 16.85%. In leaves of *Nicotiana tabacum* L. and *Atropa belladonna* L. By reducing N-methylpyrrole with zinc granules in dil acetic or hydrochloric acid.

Almost colorless liquid. Unpleasant, ammonia-like odor. Fumes in air. bp 79-80°. Strong base. Miscible with water; sol in alcohol, ether, chloroform.

6119. Methyl Red. [493-52-7] 2-[[4-(Dimethylamino)-phenyl]azo]benzoic acid; C.I. Acid Red 2; C.I. 13020. $C_{15}H_{15}N_3O_2$; mol wt 269.30. C 66.90%, H 5.61%, N 15.60%, O 11.88%. Prepn by diazotization of anthranilic acid and coupling with dimethylaniline: Clarke, Kirner, *Org. Synth.* **2**, 47 (1922). *See also Colour Index* vol. 4 (3rd ed., 1971) p 4043.

Glistening, violet crystals from toluene. mp 181-182°. pKa$_1$ 2.5; pKa$_2$ 9.5; pKb 4.8. Almost insol in water; sol in alcohol and in acetic acid.

USE: As indicator in 0.1% alcoholic soln; pH: 4.4 red, 6.2 yellow. Used for titrating NH_3, weak organic bases, *e.g.*, alkaloids; not suitable for organic acids, except oxalic and picric acid. Methyl red is easily reduced, thereby losing its color, and readings should be made promptly. It is gradually being replaced by sulfonphthalein indicators, such as bromcresol green, which are more stable and exhibit a sharper change in color.

6120. Methyl Salicylate. [119-36-8] 2-Hydroxybenzoic acid methyl ester; wintergreen oil; betula oil; sweet birch oil; teaberry oil. $C_8H_8O_3$; mol wt 152.15. C 63.15%, H 5.30%, O 31.55%. Present in leaves of *Gaultheria procumbens* L., *Ericaceae*, in the bark of *Betula lenta* L., *Betulaceae;* prepd by esterification of salicylic acid with methanol. Toxicity data: P. M. Jenner *et al., Food Cosmet. Toxicol.* **2,** 327 (1964).

Colorless, yellowish or reddish, oily liq; odor and taste of gaultheria. mp −8.6°. bp 220-224°. d_{25}^{25} 1.184. d of the natural ester is ~1.180. n_D^{20} 1.535-1.538. Flash pt, closed cup: 210°F (99°C). Slightly sol in water: one gram in about 1500 ml; sol in chloroform, ether. Misc with alcohol, glacial acetic acid. LD_{50} orally in rats: 887 mg/kg (Jenner).

Caution: Potential symptoms of overexposure are hyperpnea, apathy, lassitude; anorexia, nausea, vomiting, thirst; headache, dizziness, tinitis, difficulty with hearing and vision; confusion, irritability, mania, generalized convulsions; deep coma, death due to respiratory failure or cardiovascular collapse. Direct contact may cause irritation of skin and mucous membranes. *See Clinical Toxicology of Commercial Products,* R. E. Gosselin *et al.,* Eds. (Williams & Wilkins, Baltimore, 5th ed., 1984) Section II, p 205; Section III, pp 368-375.

USE: In perfumery; for flavoring candies, etc.

THERAP CAT: Counterirritant.

THERAP CAT (VET): Counterirritant.

6121. Methyl Silicone Resins. Tympanol. Polymeric methyl silicon oxides, probably of a cross-linked siloxane structure: Rochow, Gilliam, *J. Am. Chem. Soc.* **63,** 798 (1941). Prepd by hydrolyzing dimethyldichlorosilane or its esters followed by oxidation with air and a catalyst to the desired CH_3/Si ratio: Hyde, DeLong, *ibid.* 1194; by hydrolysis of dimethyldichlorosilane mixed with methyltrichlorosilane or silicon tetrachloride followed by cocondensation of the products: Rochow, Gilliam, *loc. cit.;* by partially methylating silicon tetrachloride to the desired CH_3/Si ratio and hydrolyzing the reaction mixture: US 2258218 (1941).

Characterized by excellent thermal stability and good resistance to oxidation. Oxidize slowly in air at 300° to silica. Can be heated to 550° *in vacuo* or to 500° in hydrogen without dec or melting. CH_3/Si = 1.2. Solid. d 1.20. n_D^{20} 1.425. Hardens in 2 hours at 100°. CH_3/Si = 1.3. Solid. d 1.15. n_D^{20} 1.422. Hardens in 1.5 hours at 120°. CH_3/Si = 1.4. Solid. d 1.08. n_D^{20} 1.421. Hardens in 4 hours at 141°. CH_3/Si = 1.5. Solid. d 1.06. n_D^{20} 1.418. Hardens in 24 hours at 100°. CH_3/Si <1.2. Sticky syrups. Harden at room temp. CH_3/Si >1.5. Oily liquids. Set to a soft gel after several days or weeks at 200°.

USE: In electrical insulation; in heat-resistant paints and varnishes; in protective and decorative finishes.

6122. Methyl Sulfate. [75-93-4] Sulfuric acid monomethyl ester; methylsulfuric acid; methyl hydrogen sulfate; monomethyl sulfate; acid methyl sulfate; "Methylsäure". CH_4O_4S; mol wt 112.11. C 10.71%, H 3.60%, O 57.08%, S 28.60%. CH_3OSO_2-OH. Prepn from methanol and methyl chlorosulfonate: Levaillant, Simon, *Compt. Rend.* **169,** 855 (1919); from methanol and sulfuric acid: Dumas, Peligot, *Ann.* **15,** 40 (1835); from sulfur trioxide and

methanol below 0°: Chamberlain *et al., BIOS Final Report* **No. 1482,** pp 6 and 8 (1946). *Review:* C. M. Suter, *The Organic Chemistry of Sulfur* (John Wiley, 1944) pp 18-23.

Oily liquid; does not solidify at −30°. d_4^{15} 1.45-1.47. Freely sol in water, less sol in alcohol. Miscible with ether.

Barium salt. Barium methyl sulfate. $C_2H_6BaO_8S_2$. Dihydrate, efflorescent crystals. Sol in water, alc.

Calcium salt. Calcium methyl sulfate; calcium sulfomethylate. $C_2H_6CaO_8S_2$. Crystals. Soluble in water.

See also Dimethyl Sulfate.

USE: In sulfonation; as solvent in bromination of indigo dyes.

6123. Methyl Sulfide. [75-18-3] Thiobismethane; dimethyl sulfide. C_2H_6S; mol wt 62.13. C 38.66%, H 9.73%, S 51.61%. $(CH_3)_2S$. Metabolic product of many biosystems. Important flavor constituent in lager beer and in many cooked vegetables such as tomatoes and corn. Principal volatile sulfur compound in seawater; abundantly produced by marine algae. Prepn: V. Regnault, *Ann.* **34,** 24 (1840); and properties: D. T. McAllan *et al., J. Am. Chem. Soc.* **73,** 3627 (1951). Review of role in malting and brewing: C. J. Dickenson, *Chem. Ind.* **24,** 896-898 (1979); B. J. Anness, C. W. Bamforth, *J. Inst. Brew.* **88,** 244-252 (1982). Review of role in global sulfur cycle: P. S. Liss *et al., Philos. Trans. R. Soc. London Ser. B* **352,** 159-169 (1997). Review of gas-phase chemistry: I. Barnes *et al., Chem. Rev.* **106,** 940-975 (2006).

Flammable liquid; characteristic odor and flavor. mp −98.25°. bp 37.3°. d^{20} 0.8483 g/ml; d^{25} 0.8424 g/ml. n_D^{20} 1.4353; n_D^{25} 1.4319. Sol in alcohol, ether; sol in water at concentrations below 300 mM.

USE: Sulfiding agent.

6124. N-Methyltaurine. [107-68-6] 2-Methylaminoethanesulfonic acid; β-methylaminoethane-α-sulfonic acid. $C_3H_9NO_3S$; mol wt 139.17. C 25.89%, H 6.52%, N 10.06%, O 34.49%, S 23.04%. $CH_3NHCH_2CH_2SO_3H$. Prepn: E. Dittrich, *J. Prakt. Chem.* **18,** 63 (1878); J. W. Schick, E. F. Degering, *Ind. Eng. Chem.* **39,** 906 (1947).

Prisms, mp 241-242°. Freely sol in water. Insol in alcohol, ether.

Sodium salt. [4316-74-9] N-Methylaminoethane sodium sulfonate; sodium N-methyltaurate. $C_3H_8NNaO_3S$. Prepd as a 35% aq soln. d_4^{25} 1.21. At its freezing point (−28°) the soln becomes a suspension of crystals.

USE: Intermediate in the manuf of surface-active agents.

6125. 17-Methyltestosterone. [58-18-4] (17β)-17-Hydroxy-17-methylandrost-4-en-3-one; 17α-methyl-Δ⁴-androsten-17β-ol-3-one; Android; Metandren; Neohombreol M; Oreton Methyl; Testred. $C_{20}H_{30}O_2$; mol wt 302.45. C 79.42%, H 10.00%, O 10.58%. Prepn from 17-methyl-Δ⁵,⁶-androstene-3,17-diol: Oppenauer, *Rec. Trav. Chim.* **56,** 137 (1937); US 2384335 (1945 to Alien Property Custodian); from 17-methyl-Δ⁴-androsten-17-ol with CrO_3: Miescher, Wettstein, US 2374370; US 2374369 (both 1945 to Ciba); from androstenedione 3-enol ethyl ether: Miescher, US 2386331 (1945 to Ciba); from dehydroandrosterone: Julian *et al.,* US 2435013 (1945 to Glidden).

Crystals from hexane. mp 161-166°. Stable in air. $[\alpha]_D^{25}$ +69 to +75° (dioxane). Soluble in alcohol, methanol, ether and in other organic solvents. Sparingly sol in vegetable oils. Practically insol in water.

Note: This is a controlled substance (anabolic steroid): **21 CFR,** 1308.13, as defined in 1300.01.

THERAP CAT: Androgen.

THERAP CAT (VET): Has been used as an androgenic agent.

6126. 4-Methyl-5-thiazoleethanol. [137-00-8] 5-Hydroxyethyl-4-methylthiazole; 5-(2-hydroxyethyl)-4-methylthiazole; 4-methyl-5-(β-hydroxyethyl)thiazole. C_6H_9NOS; mol wt 143.21.

C 50.32%, H 6.33%, N 9.78%, O 11.17%, S 22.39%. The thiazole moiety of thiamine (vitamin B$_1$). Several syntheses, *e.g.*, by condensing thioformamide with bromoacetopropanol: Buchman, *J. Am. Chem. Soc.* **58**, 1803 (1936); or with γ,γ-dichloro-γ,γ-diacetodipropyl ether: Stein, Stevens, **FR 945198** and **GB 641426** (1947 and 1950 to Merck & Co.); Londergan, Schmitz, **US 2654760** (1953 to du Pont).

HO

S

H$_3$C

N

Oily, viscous liquid. d$_4^{24}$ 1.196. Characteristic disagreeable odor of thiazole compds, becoming somewhat pleasant at extreme dilutions and imparting a nut-like flavor. bp$_7$ 135°; bp$_3$ 123-124°; bp$_1$ 103°. Sol in alcohol, ether, benzene, chloroform. Very sol in water.

Hydrochloride. C$_6$H$_9$NOS.HCl. Hygroscopic crystals, sol in water, alcohol.

USE: Intermediate in the synthesis of vitamin B$_1$.

6127. Methyl Thiocyanate. [556-64-9] Methyl sulfocyanate. C$_2$H$_3$NS; mol wt 73.12. C 32.85%, H 4.14%, N 19.16%, S 43.85%. CH$_3$SC≡N. Prepd from dimethyl sulfate and aq barium thiocyanate. Toxicology: W. F. von Oettingen *et al., J. Ind. Hyg. Toxicol.* **18**, 310 (1936). Toxicity data: H. Ohkawa *et al., Pestic. Biochem. Physiol.* **2**, 85 (1972).

Colorless liquid; onion odor. d^{20} 1.068. mp −51°. bp 130-133°. n$_D^{20}$ 1.4697. Very slightly sol in water; miscible with alcohol, ether. LD$_{50}$ i.p. in mice: 315 nmoles/g (Ohkawa).

6128. Methylthiouracil. [56-04-2] 2,3-Dihydro-6-methyl-2-thioxo-4(1*H*)-pyrimidinone; 6-methyl-2-thiouracil; 4-methyl-2-thiouracil; MTU; Alkiron; Antibason; Basecil; Basethyrin; Methiacil; Methicil; Methiocil; Muracil; Prostrumyl; Strumacil; Thimecil; Thyreostat I. C$_5$H$_6$N$_2$OS; mol wt 142.18. C 42.24%, H 4.25%, N 19.70%, O 11.25%, S 22.55%. Prepn: List, *Ann.* **236**, 1 (1886). Toxicity data: Simon, *Boll. Soc. Ital. Biol. Sper.* **24**, 803 (1948).

H$_3$C

H

N

S

NH

O

Crystals, bitter taste, dec 326-331°. Sublimes readily. Very slightly sol in cold water, ether. One part dissolves in about 150 parts boiling water. Slightly sol in alcohol, acetone. Practically insol in benzene, chloroform. Freely sol in aq solns of ammonia and alkali hydroxides. A satd aq soln is neutral or slightly acid to litmus. MLD in rabbits (mg/kg): 2486 orally (Simon).

THERAP CAT: Thyroid inhibitor.

THERAP CAT (VET): Antithyroid substance to promote growth and finishing.

6129. Methyltrienolone. [965-93-5] (17β)-17-Hydroxy-17-methylestra-4,9,11-trien-3-one; 17β-hydroxy-17-methyl-19-norandrosta-4,9,11-trien-3-one; 17α-methyl-4,9,11-estratrien-17β-ol-3-one; 17α-methyl-17β-hydroxyestra-4,9,11-trien-3-one; metribolone; R-1881. C$_{19}$H$_{24}$O$_2$; mol wt 284.39. C 80.24%, H 8.51%, O 11.25%. Prepn: Velluz *et al., Compt. Rend.* **257**, 569 (1963); **NL 6401555** (1964 to Roussel-UCLAF), *C.A.* **62**, 10498d (1965).

OH

CH$_3$ CH$_3$

H

H

O

Crystals from diisopropyl ether, mp 170°. [α]$_D^{20}$ −58.7° (c = 0.5 in ethanol).

Note: This is a controlled substance (anabolic steroid): **21 CFR**, 1308.13, as defined in 1300.01.

6130. Methyltrioxorhenium. [70197-13-6] (*T*-4)-Methyltrioxorhenium; MTO. CH$_3$O$_3$Re; mol wt 249.24. C 4.82%, H 1.21%, O 19.26%, Re 74.71%. CH$_3$ReO$_3$. Acts as an oxidation catalyst by transferring an oxygen atom from one species to another; hydrogen peroxide is often the oxygen source. Prepn: I. R. Beattie, P. J. Jones, *Inorg. Chem.* **18**, 2318 (1979); W. A. Herrmann *et al., Angew. Chem. Int. Ed.* **27**, 394 (1988). Catalytic uses: *idem et al., ibid.* **30**, 1636, 1638, 1641 (1991). Photochemistry studies: H. Kunkely *et al., Organometallics* **10**, 2090 (1991); L. J. Morris *et al., ibid.* **20**, 2344 (2001). Review of catalytic chemistry: J. H. Espenson, *Chem. Commun.* **1999**, 479-488; F. E. Kühn, W. A. Herrmann, *Chemtracts Org. Chem.* **14**, 59-83 (2001).

Colorless solid, mp 110°. d^{23} 4.21. Sol in acetonitrile, benzene, chloroform, ethanol, ether. Sparingly sol in carbon disulfide, hexane. Soly at 25° (g/l): water ~50; forms a golden ppt, poly-MTO. uv max (hexane): 205, 231, 260 nm (ε 1600, 1500, 1020). uv max (aqueous): 239, 270 nm (ε 1900, 1300). Air and moisture stable, T$_{dec}$ >300°.

Poly-MTO{H$_{0.5}$[(CH$_3$)$_{0.92}$ReO$_3$]}$_n$. First known "polymeric" organometallic oxide. Formed by MTO in aqueous soln. Prepn: W. A. Herrmann, R. W. Fischer, *J. Am. Chem. Soc.* **117**, 3223 (1995). Structural study: *idem et al., ibid.* **3231**. Golden solid with graphite-like consistence and reflectance. d^{23} 4.38. Insol in practically all inorganic and organic solvents. Electric resistivity (25°): 6×10^{-3} Ω cm.

USE: Versatile organometallic catalyst active in oxidation reactions, olefin isomerization, epoxidation and metathesis.

6131. α-Methyltryptamine. [299-26-3] α-Methyl-1*H*-indole-3-ethanamine; 3-(2-aminopropyl)indole; AMT; IT-290. C$_{11}$-H$_{14}$N$_2$; mol wt 174.24. C 75.83%, H 8.10%, N 16.08%. Synthetic hallucinogen; the (*S*)-(+)-form possesses more potent bioactivity. Prepn: H. R. Synder, L. Katz, *J. Am. Chem. Soc.* **69**, 3140 (1947); A. S. F. Ash, W. R. Wragg, *J. Chem. Soc.* **1958**, 3887; A. G. Terzian *et al., Experientia* **17**, 493 (1961); D. H. Lloyd, D. E. Nichols, *J. Org. Chem.* **51**, 4294 (1986). CNS effects in animals: J. R. Vane *et al., Nature* **191**, 1068 (1961). Clinical pharmacology: H. B. Murphree *et al., Clin. Pharmacol. Ther.* **2**, 722 (1961). Synthesis and activity of enantiomers: D. B. Repke, W. J. Ferguson, *J. Heterocycl. Chem.* **13**, 775 (1976); R. A. Glennon *et al., Biochem. Pharmacol.* **32**, 1267 (1983). Case report of intoxication: H. Long *et al., Vet. Hum. Toxicol.* **45**, 149 (2003). GC-MS determn in blood and urine: T. Ishida *et al., J. Chromatogr. B* **823**, 47 (2005).

H

N

NH$_2$

CH$_3$

(*S*)-Form

White powder. Crystals from diethyl ether, mp 101-102° (Lloyd, Nichols). Also reported as mp 98-99° (Terzian).

(*S*)-**Form.** [7795-51-9] Crystals from ethyl acetate + hexane, mp 125-126°. [α]$_D^{25}$ +34.9° (c = 0.9 in methanol).

(*R*)-**Form.** [7795-52-0] mp 126-127°. [α]$_D^{25}$ −32.1° (c = 1.0 in methanol).

Note: This is a controlled substance (hallucinogen): **21 CFR**, 1308.11.

6132. α-Methyl-*m*-tyrosine. [305-96-4] 3-Hydroxy-α-methylphenylalanine; α-methyl-3-(*m*-hydroxyphenyl)alanine; α-MMT. C$_{10}$H$_{13}$NO$_3$; mol wt 195.22. C 61.52%, H 6.71%, N 7.17%, O 24.59%. Inhibitor of catecholamine synthesis. Prepn of DL-form: Stein *et al., J. Am. Chem. Soc.* **77**, 700 (1955); Pfister, Stein, **US 2868818** (1959 to Merck & Co.).

HO

COOH

H$_2$N   CH$_3$

Crystals from methanol, dec 296-297°.

6133. 6-Methyluracil. [626-48-2] 6-Methyl-2,4(1*H*,3*H*)-pyrimidinedione; 4-methyluracil. C$_5$H$_6$N$_2$O$_2$; mol wt 126.11. C 47.62%, H 4.80%, N 22.21%, O 25.37%. Prepn: Boese, **US**

2138756 (1938 to Carbide and Carbon Chem.); Gleason, **US** 2174239 (1939 to Standard Oil). Synthesis from urea and ethyl acetoacetate: J. J. Donleavy, M. A. Kise, *Org. Synth.* **coll. vol. II,** 422 (1943); by isomerization of 2-hydroxy-4-methoxy-6-methyl-pyrimidine: McOmie *et al., J. Chem. Soc.* **1957,** 1830; from urea and diketene: Khromov-Borisov, Karlinskaya, *J. Gen. Chem. USSR* **26,** 1728 (1956); **SU 101690** (1955), *C.A.* **51,** 12989f (1957).

Crystals from glacial acetic acid, dec >300°. uv max: 277 nm (log ε 3.83). pH of aq soln 13.

6134. Methyl Vinyl Ketone. [78-94-4] 3-Buten-2-one; Δ³-2-butenone; methylene acetone; acetyl ethylene; δ-oxo-α-butylene. C_4H_6O; mol wt 70.09. C 68.54%, H 8.63%, O 22.83%. CH_3-$COCH=CH_2$. Prepn by condensation of acetone and formaldehyde to 3-ketobutanol and dehydration to methyl vinyl ketone: Merling, Köhler, *J. Soc. Chem. Ind.* **29,** 1037 (1910); White, Haward, *J. Chem. Soc.* **1943,** 25. Prepn from vinylacetylene: Conaway, **US 1967225** (1934 to du Pont). For review and polymerization characteristics *see* "Vinyl Ketone Polymers" in *Encyclopedia of Polymer Science and Technology* vol. 14 (Interscience, New York, 1971) pp 617-636.

Liquid with pungent odor. bp_{760} 81.4°. n_D^{20} 1.4086. d_4^{20} 0.8636; d_4^{25} 0.8407. Easily soluble in water, methanol, ethanol, ether, acetone, glacial acetic acid. Slightly sol in hydrocarbons. Forms a binary azeotrope with water, bp_{760} 75° (12% water). uv spectrum and electric moments: Rogers, *J. Am. Chem. Soc.* **69,** 2544 (1947). Polymerizes on standing.

Caution: Readily absorbed through skin causing general poisoning of the organism. Irritating to mucous membranes and respiratory tract.

USE: Alkylating agent; commercial starting material for plastics; as intermediate in the synthesis of steroids and vitamin A.

6135. Methymycin. [497-72-3] $C_{25}H_{43}NO_7$; mol wt 469.61. C 63.94%, H 9.23%, N 2.98%, O 23.85%. Antibiotic substance produced by a streptomycete from soil near Oswego, N.Y. Has a macrolide structure (12-membered lactone ring, *compare* Picromycin). Isoln and antibacterial activity: Donin *et al., Antibiot. Annu.* **1,** 179 (1953-4). Production using *Streptomyces venezuelae* cultures: Dutcher *et al.,* **US 2916483** (1959 to Olin Mathieson). Structure: C. Djerassi, J. A. Zderic, *J. Am. Chem. Soc.* **78,** 6390 (1956). Absolute configuration: Rickards, Smith, *Tetrahedron Lett.* **1970,** 1025; Manwaring *et al., ibid.* 1029. Biosynthesis: Birch *et al., J. Chem. Soc.* **1964,** 5274. Synthesis: Masamune *et al., J. Am. Chem. Soc.* **97,** 3512 (1975). Possible mechanism of action: Wilhelm *et al., Antimicrob. Agents Chemother.* **1967,** 236.

Prisms from abs ethanol, mp 195.5-197°. $[\alpha]_D^{22}$ +61° (c = 0.7 in methanol), +74° (c = 1.1 in chloroform). Basic substance, pKb′ 5.7. uv max (methanol): 223, 322 nm (ε 10500, 47). Very slightly sol in water, hexane. Sol in methanol, acetone, chloroform, dil acids. Moderately sol in ethanol, ether.

Sulfate. $(C_{25}H_{43}NO_7)_2.H_2SO_4$. Crystals from methanol + acetone. Sol in water, methanol.

Acid sulfate. $C_{25}H_{43}NO_7.H_2SO_4$. Plates from acetone. Sol in water, methanol.

6136. Methyprylon. [125-64-8] 3,3-Diethyl-5-methyl-2,4-piperidinedione; 2,4-dioxo-3,3-diethyl-5-methylpiperidine; 3,3-diethyl-2,4-dioxo-5-methylpiperidine; Noctan; Dimerin; Noludar. $C_{10}H_{17}NO_2$; mol wt 183.25. C 65.54%, H 9.35%, N 7.64%, O 17.46%. Prepn: Frick, Lutz, **US 2680116** (1954 to Hoffmann-La Roche). *cf.* **DE 930206** (1953). Comprehensive description: B. C. Rudy, B. Z. Senkowski, *Anal. Profiles Drug Subs.* **2,** 363-382 (1973).

Crystals. Bitter taste. mp 74-77°. uv max (alcohol): 295 nm ($A_{1cm}^{1\%}$ 2.0). Sol in water, alcohol, benzene, chloroform.

Caution: This is a controlled substance (depressant): **21 CFR,** 1308.13.

THERAP CAT: Sedative, hypnotic.

6137. Methysergide. [361-37-5] (8β)-9,10-Didehydro-N-[(1S)-1-(hydroxymethyl)propyl]-1,6-dimethylergoline-8-carboxamide; N-[1-(hydroxymethyl)propyl]-1-methyl-D-lysergamide; 1-methylmethylergonovine; 1-methyl-*d*-lysergic acid butanolamide; 1-methyl-*d*-lysergic acid (+)-1-hydroxy-2-butylamide; UML-491. $C_{21}H_{27}N_3O_2$; mol wt 353.46. C 71.36%, H 7.70%, N 11.89%, O 9.05%. Serotonin receptor antagonist. Prepn: **GB 854569** (1960); A. Hofmann, F. Troxler, **US 3113133** (1963 to Sandoz). Comparative pharmacology: Z. Votava *et al., Arzneim.-Forsch.* **16,** 220 (1966); P. N. Chambers, P. B. Marshall, *J. Pharm. Pharmacol.* **19,** 65 (1967). Mechanism of action: D. A. Curran *et al., Res. Clin. Stud. Headache* **1,** 74 (1967); J. E. Hardebo *et al., Neurology* **28,** 64 (1978); S. W. J. Lamberts, R. M. Mac Leod, *Endocrinology* **103,** 287 (1978).

Crystals, mp 194-196°. $[\alpha]_D^{20}$ −45° (c = 0.5 in pyridine).

Tartrate. $C_{46}H_{60}N_6O_{10}$. Crystals, sparingly sol in water.

Dimaleate. Dec ~165°. Sol in methanol, less sol in water (1:250). Practically insol in abs ethanol.

Hydrogen maleate. [129-49-7] Methysergide maleate; Deseril; Désernil; Sansert. $C_{21}H_{27}N_3O_2.C_4H_4O_4$; mol wt 469.53.

THERAP CAT: Antimigraine.

6138. Methysticin. [495-85-2] (6R)-6-[(1E)-2-(1,3-Benzodioxol-5-yl)ethenyl]-5,6-dihydro-4-methoxy-2H-pyran-2-one; 5-hydroxy-3-methoxy-7-[3,4-(methylenedioxy)phenyl]-2,6-heptadienoic acid δ-lactone; 4-methoxy-6-[β-(3′,4′-methylenedioxyphenyl)vinyl]-5,6-dihydro-α-pyrone; 6-(3′,4′-methylenedioxystyryl)-4-methoxy-5,6-dihydro-2H-pyran-2-one; kavahin; kavatin. $C_{15}H_{14}O_5$; mol wt 274.27. C 65.69%, H 5.14%, O 29.17%. One of the active components of the intoxicating beverage Kava from the Pacific Islands. From root of *Piper methysticum* Forst., Piperaceae (kava): Pomeranz, *Monatsh. Chem.* **10,** 783 (1889); Hänsel, Beiersdorff, *Arzneim.-Forsch.* **9,** 581 (1955). Structure: Borsche *et al., Ber.* **60,** 2113 (1927). Synthesis of racemate: Klohs *et al., J. Org. Chem.* **24,** 1829 (1959). Absolute config: Snatzke, Hänsel, *Tetrahedron Lett.* **1968,** 1797. Crystal structure: P. Engel, W. Nowacki, *Z. Kristallogr.* **136,** 437 (1972). ¹³C NMR: A. Banerji *et al., Org. Magn. Reson.* **13,** 345 (1980). HPLC determn: R. M. Smith *et al., J. Chromatogr.* **283,** 303 (1984). Anticonvulsant effects: Kretzschmar, Meyer, *Arch. Int. Pharmacodyn. Ther.* **177**, 261 (1969). Neuroprotective activity: C. Backhauss, J. Krieglstein, *Eur. J. Pharmacol.* **215**, 265 (1992).

Crystals from methanol, mp 132-134°. uv max (alcohol): 226, 267, 306 nm (log ε 4.40, 4.14, 3.93). Practically insol in water. Sol in alcohol, ether, acetone.

(±)-**Dihydromethysticin.** [3155-57-5] $C_{15}H_{16}O_5$. Prisms from methanol, mp 118°. uv max (methanol): 232, 288 nm (log ε 4.18, 3.56).

6139. Metiazinic Acid. [13993-65-2] 10-Methyl-10*H*-phenothiazine-2-acetic acid; (10-methyl-2-phenothiazinyl)acetic acid; *N*-methyl-3-phenothiazinylacetic acid; methiazic acid; methiazinic acid; metiazic acid; RP-16091; Soridermal; Soripal. $C_{15}H_{13}$-NO_2S; mol wt 271.33. C 66.40%, H 4.83%, N 5.16%, O 11.79%, S 11.82%. Prepn: **FR M4163**; Farge *et al.*, **NL 6614516; US 3424748** (1966, 1967, 1969 all to Rhône-Poulenc); Messer *et al.*, *C.R. Seances Acad. Sci. Ser. C* **265** (14), 758 (1967). Series of articles on prepn, pharmacology, toxicology and metabolism: *Arzneim.-Forsch.* **19**, 1193-1221 (1969). Toxicity: L. Joulou *et al.*, *ibid.* 1198.

Crystals from benzene, mp 146°. Sol in acetone, ether, chloroform. Forms a water-sol sodium salt. uv max (0.1*N* NaOH): 253, 305 nm; min 280 nm. LD_{50} in mice, rats (mg/kg): 800, ~500 orally (Joulou).

THERAP CAT: Anti-inflammatory.

6140. Metipranolol. [22664-55-7] 4-[2-Hydroxy-3-[(1-methylethyl)amino]propoxy]-2,3,6-trimethylphenol 1-acetate; 1-(4-hydroxy-2,3,5-trimethylphenoxy)-3-(isopropylamino)-2-propanol 4-acetate; methypranol; trimepranol; VUFB-6453; Betamet; Betanol; Disorat; Glauline; Glausyn; Turoptin. $C_{17}H_{27}NO_4$; mol wt 309.40. C 65.99%, H 8.80%, N 4.53%, O 20.68%. β-Adrenergic blocker. Prepn: L. Blaha *et al.*, *CS 128471* (1968), *C.A.* **71**, 3129a (1969). Pharmacology: W. Bartsch *et al.*, *Arzneim.-Forsch.* **27**, 1022 (1977). Plasma levels and pharmacodynamics in man: O. Mayer *et al.*, *Int. J. Clin. Pharmacol. Ther. Toxicol.* **18**, 113 (1980). Metabolic effects: R. P. Faupel, R. Gotzen, *Med. Klin.* **74**, 929 (1979). Comparative effect in hypertension: K. Hayduk *et al.*, *Therapiewoche* **29**, 7528, 7530 (1979). Review of pharmacology and clinical trials in glaucoma and ocular hypertension: P. E. Battershill, E. M. Sorkin, *Drugs* **36**, 601-615 (1988). Comprehensive description: J. Dohnal *et al.*, *Anal. Profiles Drug Subs.* **19**, 367-396 (1990).

Crystals from cyclohexane, mp 105-107° (Blaha), also reported as 108.5-110.5° (Florey). uv max (methanol): 278, 274 nm ($A_{1cm}^{1\%}$ 51.3 50.5). Freely sol in 95% ethanol, chloroform, benzene; slightly sol in ether. Practically insol in water. LD_{50} in mice (mg/kg): 31 i.v. (Bartsch).

Hydrochloride. [36592-77-5] Betamann; Optipranolol. C_{17}-$H_{27}NO_4$.HCl; mol wt 345.86. Sol in water.

THERAP CAT: Antihypertensive; antiglaucoma agent.

6141. Metitepine. [20229-30-5] 1-[10,11-Dihydro-8-(methylthio)dibenzo[*b,f*]thiepin-10-yl]-4-methylpiperazine; 8-methylthio-10-(4-methylpiperazino)-10,11-dihydrodibenzo[*b,-f*]thiepine; methiothepine; methiothepin; Ro-8-6837. $C_{20}H_{24}N_2$-S_2; mol wt 356.55. C 67.37%, H 6.78%, N 7.86%, S 17.99%. Serotonin (5-HT$_2$) receptor antagonist; also exhibits affinity for 5-HT$_1$-receptors. Prepn: **NL 6608618**; M. Protiva *et al.*, **US 3379729** (1966, 1968 both to SPOFA); and pharmacology: K. Pelz *et al.*, *Collect. Czech. Chem. Commun.* **33**, 1895 (1968); J. O. Jilek *et al.*, *ibid.* **39**, 3338 (1974). Receptor-blocking study: M.-A. Monachon *et al.*, *Arch. Pharmacol.* **274**, 192 (1972). Use in classification of 5-HT receptors: P. B. Bradley *et al.*, *Neuropharmacology* **25**, 563 (1986); E. J. Mylecharane, *Clin. Exp. Pharmacol. Physiol.* **16**, 517 (1989).

Crystals from ethanol, mp 88-89°.

Maleate. [19728-88-2] $C_{20}H_{24}N_2S_2.C_4H_4O_4$. Crystals from ethanol, mp 171-173°. LD_{50} in mice (mg/kg): 51 i.v.; 94 orally (Jilek).

USE: Biochemical tool in serotonin receptor binding studies.

6142. Metobromuron. [3060-89-7] *N'*-(4-Bromophenyl)-*N*-methoxy-*N*-methylurea; 3-(*p*-bromophenyl)-1-methoxy-1-methylurea; Ciba 3126; Pattonex; Patoran. $C_9H_{11}BrN_2O_2$; mol wt 259.10. C 41.72%, H 4.28%, Br 30.84%, N 10.81%, O 12.35%. Prepd by bromination of *N*-phenyl-*N'*-methoxy-*N'*-methylurea: H. Martin *et al.*, **CH 405821**; *eidem*, **US 3288851** (both 1966 to Ciba). Toxicity study: S. Novakova, S. Dinoeva, *Egeszsegtudomany* **17**, 233 (1973), *C.A.* **80**, 56258j (1974).

Crystals from cyclohexane, mp 95-96°. Vapor pressure at 20°: 3×10^{-6} mm Hg. Soly in water at 20° = 320 ppm. Sol in methanol, ethanol, acetone, chloroform. LD_{50} orally in rats: 3875 mg/kg (Novakova, Dinoeva).

USE: Herbicide.

6143. Metoclopramide. [364-62-5] 4-Amino-5-chloro-*N*-[(2-diethylamino)ethyl]-2-methoxybenzamide; 4-amino-5-chloro-*N*-[2-(diethylamino)ethyl]-*o*-anisamide; 4-amino-5-chloro-2-methoxy-*N*-(β-diethylaminoethyl)benzamide; DEL-1267; Elieten; Eucil; Imperan; Reliveran. $C_{14}H_{22}ClN_3O_2$; mol wt 299.80. C 56.09%, H 7.40%, Cl 11.83%, N 14.02%, O 10.67%. Substituted benzamide with neuroleptic activity. Prepn: **BE 620543**; Thominet, **US 3177252** (1962, 1965 to Soc. d'Etudes Sci. Ind. de l'Ile-de-France); R. Pakula *et al.*, *Arch. Pharm.* **313**, 297 (1980). Colorimetric determn in plasma and solubility: G. Pitel, T. Luce, *Ann. Pharm. Fr.* **23**, 673 (1965). Dopamine D$_2$ receptor antagonist (adenylate cyclase independent receptors): J. W. Kebabian, D. B. Calne, *Nature* **277**, 93 (1979). Pharmacology: M. A. Smith, F. J. Salter, *Drug Intell. Clin. Pharm.* **14**, 169 (1980). Pharmacokinetics: H. Vergin *et al.*, *Arzneim.-Forsch.* **33**, 458 (1983). Review of efficacy in psychiatric disorders: E. D. Peselow, M. Stanley, *Adv. Biochem. Psychopharmacol.* **35**, 163-194 (1982); of pharmacology and clinical use: R. A. Harrington *et al.*, *Drugs* **25**, 451-494 (1983); *ibid.*, Suppl. 1, 1-88. Comprehensive description: D. Pitré, R. Stradi, *Anal. Profiles Drug Subs.* **16**, 327-361 (1987).

mp 146.5-148°. Soly at 25° (g/100 ml): water 0.02; 95% ethanol 2.30; abs ethanol 1.90; benzene 0.10; chloroform 6.60.

Dihydrochloride monohydrate. Emetid; Gastronerton; Primperan. $C_{14}H_{22}ClN_3O_2.2HCl.H_2O$; mol wt 390.73. Crystals, dec 145°. Soly at 25° (g/100 ml): water 48; ethanol (95%) 9; abs ethanol 6; benzene 0.10; chloroform 0.10. Stable in acids solns. Unstable in strongly alkaline solns.

Monohydrochloride monohydrate. [54143-57-6] AHR-3070-C; Cerucal; Clopromate; Duraclamid; Emperal; Gastrese; Gastrobid; Gastromax; Gastrosil; Gastro-Tablinen; Maxeran; Maxolon; Meclopran; Metamide; Metoclol; Metocobil; Metramid; Moriperan; Mygdalon; Parmid; Paspertin; Peraprin; Plasil; Pramiel; Reglan. $C_{14}H_{22}ClN_3O_2.HCl.H_2O$; mol wt 354.27. White crystalline powder, mp 182.5-184°. Sol in water.

THERAP CAT: Antiemetic.

6144. Metocurine Iodide. [7601-55-0] 6,6',7',12'-Tetramethoxy-2,2,2',2'-tetramethyltubocuraranium diiodide; (+)-O,O'-dimethylchondrocurarine diiodide; d-tubocurarine iodide dimethyl ether; dimethyl tubocurarine iodide; tubocurarine dimethyl ether iodide; Metubine Iodide. $C_{40}H_{48}I_2N_2O_6$; mol wt 906.63. C 52.99%, H 5.34%, I 27.99%, N 3.09%, O 10.59%. Prepd by methylation of d-tubocurarine with methyl iodide.

Crystals, dec 257-267°. $[\alpha]_D^{22}$ +148 to +158° (c = 0.25). uv max: 280 nm. $(E_{1cm}^{1\%}$ 74). Slightly soluble in water (about 300 mg/100 ml), in dil HCl, in dil NaOH. Very slightly sol in alcohol; practically insol in benzene, chloroform, ether.

Trihydrate. Large prisms from water, appreciably sol in methanol.

THERAP CAT: Neuromuscular blocking agent.

6145. Metofenazate. [388-51-2] 3,4,5-Trimethoxybenzoic acid 2-[4-[3-(2-chloro-10H-phenothiazin-10-yl)propyl]-1-piperazinyl]ethyl ester; 2-[4-[3-(2-chlorophenothiazin-10-yl)propyl]-1-piperazinyl]ethyl 3,4,5-trimethoxybenzoate; N-[β-(3,4,5-trimethoxybenzoyloxy)ethyl]-N'-[γ-(3-chloro-10-phenothiazinyl)propyl]-piperazine; methophenazine; perphenazine 3,4,5-trimethoxybenzoate. $C_{31}H_{36}ClN_3O_5S$; mol wt 598.15. C 62.25%, H 6.07%, Cl 5.93%, N 7.03%, O 13.37%, S 5.36%. Prepn: *Magy. Kem. Lapja* **17**, 169 (1962), *C.A.* **57**, 11314d (1962); Toldy et al., *Acta Chim. Acad. Sci. Hung.* **42**, 351 (1964).

Crystals from ethanol, mp 102-107°.

Difumarate. [522-23-6] Frenolon. $C_{31}H_{36}ClN_3O_5S.2C_4H_4O_4$; mol wt 830.30.

THERAP CAT: Antipsychotic.

6146. Metolachlor. [51218-45-2] 2-Chloro-N-(2-ethyl-6-methylphenyl)-N-(2-methoxy-1-methylethyl)acetamide; 2-chloro-6'-ethyl-N-(2-methoxy-1-methylethyl)acet-o-toluidide; α-chloro-2'-ethyl-6'-methyl-N-(1-methyl-2-methoxyethyl)acetanilide; metelilachlor; CGA-24705; Dual. $C_{15}H_{22}ClNO_2$; mol wt 283.79. C 63.48%, H 7.81%, Cl 12.49%, N 4.94%, O 11.28%. Selective pre-emergence herbicide. Prepn: C. Vogel, R. Aebi, **DE 2328340**; *eidem*, **US 3937730** (1973, 1976 both to Ciba-Geigy). Synthesis of stereoisomers: B. T. Cho, Y. S. Chun, *Tetrahedron: Asymmetry* **3**, 337 (1992). Metabolism: L. L. McGahen, J. M. Tiedje, *J. Agric. Food Chem.* **26**, 414 (1978). ELISA determn: T. S. Lawruk et al., *J. Agric. Food Chem.* **41**, 1426 (1993). *Review:* G. Chesters et al., *Rev. Environ. Contam. Toxicol.* **110**, 1-74 (1989); of biological activity and field trials: H. R. Gerber et al., *Proc. 12th Br. Weed Control Conf.* 787-794 (1974).

Colorless liquid. $bp_{0.001}$ 100°. n_D^{20} 1.5301. Vapor pressure at 20°: 1.3×10^{-5} mm Hg. Soly in water at 20°: 530 ppm. Sol in most organic solvents. Partition coefficient (octanol/water): 2,800. LD_{50} in rats (mg/kg): 2780 orally; >3170 dermally (Gerber).

S-Form. [87392-12-9] Dual Gold.

USE: Herbicide.

6147. Metolazone. [17560-51-9] 7-Chloro-1,2,3,4-tetrahydro-2-methyl-3-(2-methylphenyl)-4-oxo-6-quinazolinesulfonamide; 7-chloro-1,2,3,4-tetrahydro-2-methyl-4-oxo-3-o-tolyl-6-quinazolinesulfonamide; 2-methyl-3-o-tolyl-6-sulfamyl-7-chloro-1,2,3,4-tetrahydro-4-quinazolinone; SR-720-22; Metenix; Mykrox; Xuret; Zaroxolyn. $C_{16}H_{16}ClN_3O_3S$; mol wt 365.83. C 52.53%, H 4.41%, Cl 9.69%, N 11.49%, O 13.12%, S 8.77%. Prepn: B. V. Shetty, **US 3360518** (1967 to Wallace & Tiernan); B. V. Shetty et al., *J. Med. Chem.* **13**, 886 (1970). Pharmacology: E. Belair et al., *Arch. Int. Pharmacodyn. Ther.* **177**, 71 (1969); E. J. Belair, *Res. Commun. Chem. Pathol. Pharmacol.* **2**, 98 (1971). HPLC determn in urine: D. Farthing et al., *J. Chromatogr.* **534**, 228 (1990). Clinical evaluations as diuretic in chronic renal disease: R. Schoonees et al., *N. Y. State J. Med.* **71**, 566 (1971); in hypertension: C. L. Curry et al., *Clin. Ther.* **9**, 47 (1986); in congestive heart failure: A. Kiyingi et al., *Lancet* **335**, 29 (1990).

Crystals from ethanol or butanol, mp 252-254°. LD_{50} in mice (mg/kg): >5000 orally; >1500 i.p. (Shetty, 1967).

THERAP CAT: Diuretic; antihypertensive.

6148. Metomidate. [5377-20-8] 1-(1-Phenylethyl)-1H-imidazole-5-carboxylic acid methyl ester; 1-(α-methylbenzyl)imidazole-5-carboxylic acid methyl ester; methyl 1-(α-methylbenzyl)imidazole-5-carboxylate; methoxymol; methomidate. $C_{13}H_{14}N_2O_2$; mol wt 230.26. C 67.81%, H 6.13%, N 12.17%, O 13.90%. Injectable hypnotic related to etomidate, *q.v.* Prepn: **BE 662474**; E. F. Godefroi, C. A. M. van der Eijcken, **US 3354173** (1965, 1967 both to Janssen); E. F. Godefroi et al., *J. Med. Chem.* **8**, 220 (1965). Anaesthetic effect of combination with azaperone, *q.v.*: J. F. F. Callear, J. F. E. Van Gestel, *Vet. Rec.* **92**, 284 (1973); of combination with fentanyl, *q.v.*: W. Erhardt, *J. Small Anim. Pract.* **19**, 401 (1978); C. J. Green, *Lab. Anim.* **15**, 171 (1981).

Hydrochloride. R-7315; Hypnodil. $C_{13}H_{14}N_2O_2 \cdot HCl$; mol wt 266.72. Crystals from methanol-ether, mp 173-174°. LD_{50} i.v. in rats: 50 mg/kg (Godefroi).

THERAP CAT (VET): Hypnotic.

6149. Metopimazine. [14008-44-7] 1-[3-[2-(Methylsulfonyl)-10H-phenothiazin-10-yl]propyl]-4-piperidinecarboxamide; 1-[3-[2-(methylsulfonyl)phenothiazin-10-yl]propyl]isonipecotamide; 10-[3-(4-carbamoylpiperidino)propyl]-2-(methanesulfonyl)phenothiazine; 1-[3-[2-(methylsulfonyl)phenothiazin-10-yl]propyl]-4-piperidinecarboxamide; EXP-999; RP-9965; Vogalene. $C_{22}H_{27}N_3$-O_3S_2; mol wt 445.60. C 59.30%, H 6.11%, N 9.43%, S 14.39%. Prepn: Jacob, Robert, DE 1092476 (to Rhône-Poulenc), C.A. **56,** 8723h (1962). Toxicity study: E. I. Goldenthal, Toxicol. Appl. Pharmacol. **18,** 185 (1971).

Solid, mp 170-171°. LD_{50} in male rats (mg/kg): 976 orally, 1080 s.c. (Goldenthal).

THERAP CAT: Antiemetic.

6150. Metopon. [143-52-2] (5α)-4,5-Epoxy-3-hydroxy-5,17-dimethylmorphinan-6-one; methyldihydromorphinone. C_{18}-$H_{21}NO_3$; mol wt 299.36. C 72.22%, H 7.07%, N 4.68%, O 16.03%. Prepn from thebaine: Small et al., J. Am. Chem. Soc. **58,** 1457 (1936). From dihydrocodeinone enol acetate: Small et al., J. Org. Chem. **3,** 204 (1938). Structure: Stork, Bauer, J. Am. Chem. Soc. **75,** 4373 (1953).

Needles from alc; sinters 235°, mp 243-245° (evac tube). $[\alpha]_D^{24}$ $-141°$ (c = 1 in alc). Slightly sol in organic solvents.

Hydrochloride. [124-92-5] $C_{18}H_{21}NO_3 \cdot HCl$. Crystals from alc, dec 315-318° (evac tube). $[\alpha]_D^{24}$ $-105°$ (c = 1). Freely sol in water. Sparingly sol in alc. Slightly sol in chloroform. Very slightly sol in ether. Insol in benzene. A 1% aq soln has a pH of ~5.0.

Note: This is a controlled substance (opiate): 21 CFR, 1308.12.

THERAP CAT: Analgesic (narcotic).

6151. Metoprolol. [37350-58-6] 1-[4-(2-Methoxyethyl)-phenoxy]-3-[(1-methylethyl)amino]-2-propanol; (±)-1-(isopropyl-amino)-3-[p-(β-methoxyethyl)phenoxy]-2-propanol; CGP-2175; H-93/26. $C_{15}H_{25}NO_3$; mol wt 267.36. C 67.38%, H 9.42%, N 5.24%, O 17.95%. β_1-Adrenergic blocker lacking intrinsic sympathomimetic activity. Prepn: A. E. Brandstrom et al., DE 2106209; eidem, US 3998790 (1971, 1976 both to AB Hässle). Pharmacology: B. Ablad et al., Life Sci. **12,** 107 (1973); Johansson, Eur. J. Pharmacol. **24,** 194 (1973). Toxicology: N.-O. Bodin et al., Acta

Pharmacol. Toxicol. **36,** Suppl. V, 96 (1975). Clinical trials in acute myocardial infarction: L. Rydén et al., N. Engl. J. Med. **308,** 614 (1983); Drugs **29,** Suppl. 1, 2-8 (1985); in chronic heart failure: A. Hjalmarson et al., J. Am. Med. Assoc. **283,** 1295 (2000). Comprehensive description: J. R. Luch, Anal. Profiles Drug Subs. **12,** 325-356 (1983). Review of pharmacology, therapeutic efficacy: P. Benfield et al., Drugs **31,** 376-429 (1986).

Succinate. [98418-47-4] Selo-Zok; Toprol-XL. ($C_{15}H_{25}$-$NO_3)_2 \cdot C_4H_6O_4$; mol wt 652.82.

Tartrate. [56392-17-7] Beloc; Betaloc; Lopressor; Lopresor; Prelis; Seloken; Selopral. ($C_{15}H_{25}NO_3)_2 \cdot C_4H_6O_6$; mol wt 684.81. Soly (mg/ml) at 25°: water >1000; methanol >500; chloroform 496; acetone 1.1; acetonitrile 0.89; hexane 0.001. uv max (water): 223 nm (ε 23400). LD_{50} in female mice, male rats (mg/kg): 118, ~90 i.v.; 2090, 3090 orally (Bodin).

THERAP CAT: Antihypertensive; antianginal; antiarrhythmic (class II).

6152. Metoquinone. [622-91-3] $C_{20}H_{24}N_2O_4$; mol wt 356.42. C 67.40%, H 6.79%, N 7.86%, O 17.96%. [C_6H_4(OH)-NHCH$_3$]$_2 \cdot C_6H_4$(OH)$_2$. A salt-like compound of 1 mol hydroquinone and 2 mols p-monomethylaminophenol.

White crystals. mp ~135° with decompn and blackening. Sol in 100 parts water; less sol in alcohol, acetone; very slightly sol in benzene, chloroform, ether.

USE: As a photographic developer.

6153. Metralindole. [54188-38-4] 2,4,5,6-Tetrahydro-9-methoxy-4-methyl-1H-3,4,6a-triazafluoranthene; 3-methyl-8-methoxy-3H-1,2,5,6-tetrahydropyrazino[1,2,3-ab]-β-carboline. C_{15}-$H_{17}N_3O$; mol wt 255.31. C 70.57%, H 6.71%, N 16.46%, O 6.27%. Heterocyclic β-carboline derivative used as an antidepressant. Prepn: R. G. Glushkov et al., DE 2357320; eidem, US 4088647 (1974, 1978 both to All Union Khim.-Farm Instit. USSR); eidem, Khim. Farm. Zh. **16,** 1054 (1982), C.A. **98,** 53831b (1983). Psychotropic activity, toxicity: M. D. Mashkovsky et al., DE 2356091; eidem, US 3959470 (1974, 1976 both to All Union Khim.-Farm. Instit. USSR). Pharmacology: N. I. Andreeva, M. D. Mashkovsky, Farmakol. Toksikol. (Moscow) **43,** 133 (1980). Effect on the EEG of the brain cortex: L. F. Roshchina, ibid. 349. Effect on adrenergic neurotransmission: L. V. Panasiuk et al., ibid. **45,** 13 (1982). Clinical studies: M. D. Mashkovsky, N. I. Andreeva, Zh. Nevropatol. Psikhiatr. **84,** 410 (1984).

Crystals, mp 164-165°.

Hydrochloride. [53734-79-5] Incazan. $C_{15}H_{17}N_3O \cdot HCl$; mol wt 291.78. Off-white odorless powder with bitter taste. mp 305-308°. Sol in water. LD_{50} orally in mice: 445 mg/kg (Mashkovsky, 1976).

THERAP CAT: Antidepressant.

6154. Metribuzin. [21087-64-9] 4-Amino-6-(1,1-dimethyl-ethyl)-3-(methylthio)-1,2,4-triazin-5(4H)-one; 4-amino-6-tert-butyl-3-(methylthio)-as-triazin-5(4H)-one; Bay 94337; Lexone; Sencor; Sencoral. $C_8H_{14}N_4OS$; mol wt 214.29. C 44.84%, H 6.59%, N 26.15%, O 7.47%, S 14.96%. Pre- and post-emergence triazone herbicide. Prepn: BE 697083; K. Westphal et al., US 3671523 (1967, 1972 both to Bayer AG). Physicochemical properties, toxicology and herbicidal activity: L. Eue, Pflanzenschutz-Nachr. **25,** 175 (1972). Toxicity data: E. Loeser, G. Kimmerle, ibid. 186. HPLC determn in plant tissues: C. E. Parker, G. H. Degen, J. Liq. Chromatogr. **6,** 725 (1983).

White crystalline solid, mp 125-126.5°. d_4^{20} 1.28. Vapor pressure at 20°: $<10^{-5}$ mm Hg. Sol in methanol, ethanol. Soly in water: 1200 ppm. LD_{50} orally in rats: 2200 mg/kg; LC_{50} in rainbow trout: >10 ppm (Loeser, Kimmerle).

Caution: Potential symptoms of overexposure in exptl animals are CNS depression; thyroid, liver and enzyme changes. *See NIOSH Pocket Guide to Chemical Hazards* (DHHS/NIOSH 97-140, 1997) p 216.

USE: Herbicide.

6155. Metrizamide. [31112-62-6] 2-[[3-(Acetylamino)-5-(acetylmethylamino)-2,4,6-triiodobenzoyl]amino]-2-deoxy-D-glucose; 2-[3-acetamido-2,4,6-triiodo-5-(N-methylacetamido)benzamido]-2-deoxy-D-glucose; 2-[3-acetamido-2,4,6-triiodo-5-(N-methylacetamido)benzamido]-2-deoxy-D-glucopyranose; Win-39103; Amipaque. $C_{18}H_{22}I_3N_3O_8$; mol wt 789.10. C 27.40%, H 2.81%, I 48.25%, N 5.33%, O 16.22%. X-ray contrast agent related to metrizoic acid, *q.v.* Prepn: H. O. Torsten *et al., DE 2031724; eidem,* US 3701771 (1971, 1972 both to Nyegaard). Metabolism: J. G. Johansen, S. Kolmannskog, *Invest. Radiol.* 13, 93 (1978). Pharmacology: T. W. Morris *et al., ibid.* 74; G. F. Dibona, *Proc. Soc. Exp. Biol. Med.* 157, 453 (1978). Series of articles on clinical use: *Ann. Radiol.* 22, 195-206 (1979). Toxicity studies: S. Salvesen, *Radiology* 123, 241 (1977); M. Sovak *et al., ibid.* 242; P. Aspelin, *Invest. Radiol.* 11, 309 (1976). *Review:* L. Hol *et al.,* in *Pharmacological and Biochemical Properties of Drug Substances* vol. 1, M. E. Goldberg, Ed. (Am. Pharm. Assoc., Washington, DC, 1977) pp 387-412.

White crystals from isopropyl alcohol, mp 230° (dec), after drying in vacuo at room temp and 70°. $[\alpha]_D^{20}$ +18.0° (c = 10% in 0.1N HCl; equilibrated with respect to mutarotation). Very sol in water (50% w/v) at room temp. LD_{50} i.v. in mice: 15 g/kg (Torsten); 18.6 g/kg (Salveson); 11.5 g/kg (Sovak); 17.3 g/kg (Aspelin).

THERAP CAT: Diagnostic aid (radiopaque medium).

6156. Metrizoic Acid. [1949-45-7] 3-(Acetylamino)-5-(acetylmethylamino)-2,4,6-triiodobenzoic acid; 3-acetamido-2,4,6-triiodo-5-(N-methylacetamido)benzoic acid; N-methyl-3,5-diacetamido-2,4,6-triiodobenzoic acid. $C_{12}H_{11}I_3N_2O_4$; mol wt 627.94. C 22.95%, H 1.77%, I 60.63%, N 4.46%, O 10.19%. Prepn: Pitré, Fumigalli, *Farmaco Ed. Sci.* 17, 340 (1962); GB 973881 (1964 to Nyegaard), *C.A.* 62, 16139g (1965). Series of articles on use in separation of leukocytes from blood and bone marrow: A. Boyum, *Scand. J. Clin. Lab. Invest.* 21, Suppl. 97, 7-106 (1968).

Crystals, mp 281-282°.

Sodium salt. [7225-61-8] Metrizoate sodium; Isopaque; Triosil.

THERAP CAT: Diagnostic aid (radiopaque medium).

6157. Metronidazole. [443-48-1] 2-Methyl-5-nitroimidazole-1-ethanol; 1-(2-hydroxyethyl)-2-methyl-5-nitroimidazole; 1-(β-ethylol)-2-methyl-5-nitro-3-azapyrrole; Bayer 5630; RP-8823; Acea Gel; Anabact; Arilin; Clont; Deflamon; Elyzol; Flagyl; Fossyol; Klion; MetroGel; Metrolag; Metrolyl; Metrosa; Metrotop; Orvagil; Rathimed; Rosaced; Rozacrème; Rozagel; Rozex; Trichocide; Vagilen; Vagimid; Zadstat; Zidoval. $C_6H_9N_3O_3$; mol wt 171.15. C 42.11%, H 5.30%, N 24.55%, O 28.04%. Prepn: Jacob *et al.,* US 2944061 (1960 to Rhône-Poulenc); Cossar *et al., Arzneim.-Forsch.* 16, 23 (1966). Activity studies: Bock, *ibid.* 11, 587 (1961). Metabolism: Ings *et al., Biochem. Pharmacol.* 15, 515 (1966). Comprehensive description: L. L. Wearley, G. D. Anthony, *Anal. Profiles Drug Subs.* 5, 327-344 (1976). Review of activity, pharmacokinetics and use in anaerobic infection: R. N. Brogden *et al., Drugs* 16, 387-417 (1978); in rosacea: L. K. Schmadel, G. K. McEvoy, *Clin. Pharm.* 9, 94-101 (1990). *Review:* W. D. Hager, R. P. Rapp, *Obstet. Gynecol. Clin. North Am.* 19, 497-510 (1992).

Cream-colored crystals, mp 158-160°. Soly at 20° (g/100 ml): water 1.0; ethanol 0.5; ether <0.05; chloroform <0.05. Sparingly sol in DMF. Sol in dil acids. pH of satd aq soln: 5.8.

Hydrochloride. [69198-10-3] SC-326421. $C_6H_9N_3O_3$·HCl; mol wt 207.61.

Caution: Metronidazole is reasonably anticipated to be a human carcinogen: *Report on Carcinogens, Eleventh Edition* (PB2005-104914, 2004) p III-173.

THERAP CAT: Antiprotozoal (Trichomonas); antibacterial; in treatment of rosacea.

THERAP CAT (VET): Antiprotozoal (Trichomonas); antiamebic; antibacterial.

6158. Metsulfuron-methyl. [74223-64-6] 2-[[[[(4-Methoxy-6-methyl-1,3,5-triazin-2-yl)amino]carbonyl]amino]sulfonyl]benzoic acid methyl ester; N-[(4-methoxy-6-methyl-1,3,5-triazin-2-yl)aminocarbonyl]-2-methoxycarbonylbenzenesulfonamide; DPX-T6376; Ally; Allie. $C_{14}H_{15}N_5O_6S$; mol wt 381.36. C 44.09%, H 3.96%, N 18.36%, O 25.17%, S 8.41%. Sulfonyl urea used as pre- and postemergence herbicide. Prepn and herbicidal activity: G. Levitt, EP 7687 (1980 to Du Pont); *idem,* US 4383113 (1983 to Du Pont). Comparison with other herbicides in cereals: A. Aamisepp, *Weeds Weed Control* 26, 26 (1985). Efficacy in control of gorse: A. I. Popay *et al., Proc. 38th N. Z. Weed Pest Control Conf.* 1985, 94. Review of properties, herbicidal activity: P. Lefebvre, *Def. Veg.* 38, 331 (1984).

White crystals, mp 163-166°. Vapor pressure at 25°: 5.8×10^{-5} mm Hg. Soly in water: 0.27 g/l at pH 4.59; 9.5 g/l at pH 6.11. LD_{50} in male and female rats, in male and female rabbits (mg/kg): >5000, >2000 orally. LC_{50} (96 hour) in American perch, rainbow trout: 150 ppm. LD_{50} in wild ducks: 2510 mg/kg (Lefebvre).

USE: Herbicide.

6159. Metyrapone. [54-36-4] 2-Methyl-1,2-di-3-pyridyl-1-propanone; 2-methyl-1,2-bis(3-pyridyl)-1-propanone; methopyrapone; mepyrapone; metopyrone; methbipyranone; Su-4885; Metopiron(e). $C_{14}H_{14}N_2O$; mol wt 226.27. C 74.31%, H 6.24%, N 12.38%, O 7.07%. Prepn: Chart *et al., Experientia* **14,** 151 (1958); W. L. Bencze, M. J. Allen, *J. Am. Chem. Soc.* **81,** 4015 (1959); *eidem,* **US 2966493** (1960 to Ciba).

Crystals from ether and pentane, mp 50-51°.

THERAP CAT: Diagnostic aid (pituitary function).

6160. Metyridine. [114-91-0] 2-(β-Methoxyethyl)pyridine; methyridine; Dekelmin; Promintic. $C_8H_{11}NO$; mol wt 137.18. C 70.04%, H 8.08%, N 10.21%, O 11.66%. Prepn: Arnall, Greenhalgh, **GB 889748** (1962 to ICI and Midland Tar Distillers); **US 3223710** (1965).

Sweet smelling liquid, bp$_{17}$ 94-96°. d^{20} 0.988. n$_D^{20}$ 1.4975. pKa = 5.5. Very sol in water and common solvents.

Sulfate. Mintic.

Hydrochloride. mp 104-105°.

THERAP CAT (VET): Anthelmintic.

6161. Metyrosine. [672-87-7] α-Methyl-L-tyrosine; α-methyl-*p*-tyrosine; α-methyltyrosine; 4-hydroxy-α-methylphenylalanine; α-methyl-3-(*p*-hydroxyphenyl)alanine; metirosine; L-α-MT; α-MPT; MK-781; Demser. $C_{10}H_{13}NO_3$; mol wt 195.22. C 61.52%, H 6.71%, N 7.17%, O 24.59%. An inhibitor of the first and rate-limiting reaction in catecholamine biosynthesis, the hydroxylation of tyrosine to dopa. Prepn: **NL 6607757** (1966 to Merck & Co.), *C.A.* **67,** 91108p (1967). Prepn of DL-form: Stein *et al., J. Am. Chem. Soc.* **77,** 700 (1955); Potts, *J. Chem. Soc.* **1955,** 1632; Pfister, Stein, **US 2868818** (1959 to Merck & Co.); Saari, *J. Org. Chem.* **32,** 4074 (1967). Metabolism and biochemical and pharmacologic effects in man: Engelman *et al., J. Clin. Invest.* **47,** 568, 577 (1968). Review of pharmacology and clinical use: R. N. Brogden *et al., Drugs* **21,** 81-89 (1981).

Crystals, mp 310-315°.

DL-Form. [620-30-4] Crystals from water, dec 320° (Stein *et al., loc. cit.*), also reported as dec 330-332° (Potts, *loc. cit.*). Soly in water at room temp: 0.57 mg/ml.

THERAP CAT: Tyrosine hydroxylase inhibitor; as antihypertensive in pheochromocytoma.

6162. Mevaldic Acid. [541-07-1] 3-Hydroxy-3-methyl-5-oxopentanoic acid; 3-hydroxy-3-methylglutaraldehydic acid. $C_6H_{10}O_4$; mol wt 146.14. C 49.31%, H 6.90%, O 43.79%. Prepn by acid hydrolysis of 3-hydroxy-3-methyl-5,5-dimethoxypentanoic acid: Shunk *et al., J. Am. Chem. Soc.* **79,** 3294 (1957). Exists in equilibrium with *β,δ-dihydroxy-β-methyl-δ-valerolactone*.

Unstable and reactive compd. Isolated in soln only.

6163. Mevalonic Acid. [150-97-0] 3,5-Dihydroxy-3-methylpentanoic acid; 3,5-dihydroxy-3-methylvaleric acid; β,δ-dihy-

droxy-β-methylvaleric acid; hiochic acid. $C_6H_{12}O_4$; mol wt 148.16. C 48.64%, H 8.16%, O 43.19%. Precursor in the biosynthesis of cholesterol. Occurs in equilibrium with the δ-lactone. Isoln from distillers' solns: Wright *et al., J. Am. Chem. Soc.* **78,** 5273 (1956). Synthesis: Wolf *et al., ibid.* **79,** 1486 (1957); Hoffmann *et al., ibid.* 2316; Eggerer *et al., Ann.* **608,** 71 (1957); **US 2915398; US 2915531; US 2915532; US 2915533; US 2915551** (all 1959 to Merck & Co.); Shunk *et al.,* **US 3014963** (1961 to Merck & Co.); Hulcher, Hosick, **US 3119842** (1964); F. C. Huang *et al., J. Am. Chem. Soc.* **97,** 4144 (1975). Resolution: Shunk *et al., ibid.* **79,** 3294 (1957); **US 2945059** (1960 to Merck & Co.). Synthesis of the δ-lactone: R. H. Cornforth *et al., Tetrahedron* **18,** 1351 (1962); E. L. Eliel, K. Soai, *Tetrahedron Lett.* **22,** 2859 (1981); A. Banerji, G. P. Kalena, *Synth. Commun.* **12,** 225 (1982). Review of organic and biochemistry: Wagner, Folkers, *Endeavour* **20,** 177-187 (Oct. 1961). Prepn of 5-phosphate: Robinson, Wittreich, **US 3014057** (1961 to Merck & Co.). Review of role of mevalonic acid in sterol biosynthesis: G. J. Schroepfer, Jr., *Annu. Rev. Biochem.* **50,** 585-621 (1981); E. Caspi, *Tetrahedron* **42,** 3-50 (1986).

Oily liquid. Very sol in water, but also sol in organic solvents, especially polar organic solvents.

δ-Lactone. Mevalolactone; mevalonic lactone; β-hydroxy-β-methyl-δ-valerolactone. $C_6H_{10}O_3$. Hygroscopic crystals, mp 28°.

Benzhydrylamide. $C_{19}H_{23}NO_3$. Crystals from benzene + petr ether, mp 96-97°. [α]$_D^{20}$ −2.0° (c = 2 in ethanol).

6164. Mevastatin. [73573-88-3] (2*S*)-2-Methylbutanoic acid (1*S*,7*S*,8*S*,8a*R*)-1,2,3,7,8,8a-hexahydro-7-methyl-8-[2-[(2*R*,4*R*)-tetrahydro-4-hydroxy-6-oxo-2*H*-pyran-2-yl]ethyl]-1-naphthalenyl ester; 7-[1,2,6,7,8,8a-hexahydro-2-methyl-8-(methylbutyryloxy)naphthyl]-3-hydroxyheptan-5-olide; 2β-methyl-8α-(2-methyl-1-oxobutoxy)mevinic acid lactone; compactin; 6-demethylmevinolin; CS-500; ML-236 B. $C_{23}H_{34}O_5$; mol wt 390.51. C 70.74%, H 8.78%, O 20.49%. Fungal metabolite which is a potent inhibitor of HMG-CoA reductase, the rate controlling enzyme in cholesterol biosynthesis. Isoln from *Penicillium citrinum:* A. Endo *et al.,* **DE 2524355** corresp to **US 3983140** (1975, 1976 to Sankyo). Isoln from *P. brevicompactum,* crystal and molecular structure: A. G. Brown *et al., J. Chem. Soc. Perkin Trans. 1* **1976,** 1165. Inhibition of HMG-CoA reductase activity: A. Endo *et al., FEBS Lett.* **72,** 323 (1976); M. S. Brown *et al., J. Biol. Chem.* **253,** 1121 (1978). Therapeutic effects in primary hypercholesterolemia: A. Yamamoto *et al., Atherosclerosis* **35,** 259 (1980). Total synthesis: N. Y. Wang *et al., J. Am. Chem. Soc.* **103,** 6538 (1981); M. Hirama, M. Uei, *ibid.* **104,** 4251 (1982); N. N. Girotra, N. L. Wendler, *Tetrahedron Lett.* **23,** 5501 (1982); C.-T. Hsu *et al., J. Am. Chem. Soc.* **105,** 593 (1983); P. A. Grieco *et al., ibid.* 1403; D. L. J. Clive *et al., J. Am. Chem. Soc.* **110,** 6914 (1988). Review of syntheses: T. Rosen, C. H. Heathcock, *Tetrahedron* **42,** 4909-4951 (1986). Review of mevastatin and related compounds: A. Endo, *J. Med. Chem.* **28,** 401-405 (1985).

Crystals from aq ethanol, mp 152°. [α]$_D^{22}$ +283° (c = 0.48 in acetone). uv max: 230, 237, 246 nm (log ε 4.28, 4.30, 4.11).

6165. Mevinphos. [7786-34-7] 3-[(Dimethoxyphosphinyl)-oxy]-2-butenoic acid methyl ester; 3-hydroxycrotonic acid methyl ester dimethyl phosphate; 1-methoxycarbonyl-1-propen-2-yl dimethyl phosphate; methyl 3-(dimethoxyphosphinyloxy)crotonate; O,O-dimethyl 1-carbomethoxy-1-propen-2-yl phosphate; 2-carbomethoxy-1-methylvinyl dimethyl phosphate; ENT-22374; OS-2046; Phosdrin. $C_7H_{13}O_6P$; mol wt 224.15. C 37.51%, H 5.85%, O 42.83%, P 13.82%. Cholinesterase inhibitor. Prepn: A. R. Stiles, US 2685552 (1954 to Shell). Activity: R. A. Corey et al., J. Econ. Entomol. **46**, 386 (1953). Configuration of isomers: Fukuto et al., J. Org. Chem. **26**, 4620 (1961). Metabolism and degradn: K. I. Beynon et al., Residue Rev. **47**, 55 (1973). Toxicity study: T. B. Gaines, Toxicol. Appl. Pharmacol. **14**, 515 (1969).

Commercial product is a yellow liq mixture of (E)- (also referred to as cis-) and (Z)- (also referred to as trans-) isomers, the (E)-isomer being about 100 times more potent in insecticidal activity than the (Z)-isomer: Casida et al., J. Agric. Food Chem. **4**, 236 (1956). d_4^{20} 1.25. n_D^{20} 1.4494. bp_1 106-107.5°. Misc with water, acetone, benzene, carbon tetrachloride, chloroform, ethyl and isopropyl alcohols, toluene and xylene. One gram dissolves in 20 ml carbon disulfide and 20 ml kerosene. Practically insol in hexane. LD_{50} in female, male rats (mg/kg): 3.7, 6.1 orally; 4.2, 4.7 dermally (Gaines).

Caution: Potential symptoms of overexposure are miosis; rhinorrhea; headache; tight chest, wheezing, laryngeal spasm, salivation and cyanosis; anorexia, nausea, vomiting, abdominal cramps and diarrhea; paralysis; ataxia, convulsions; low blood pressure, cardiac irregularities; irritation of skin, eyes and respiratory system. *See NIOSH Pocket Guide to Chemical Hazards* (DHHS/NIOSH 97-140, 1997) p 252.

USE: Insecticide.

6166. Mexazolam. [31868-18-5] 10-Chloro-11b-(2-chlorophenyl)-2,3,7,11b-tetrahydro-3-methyloxazolo[3,2-d][1,4]benzodiazepin-6(5H)-one; 10-chloro-11b-(o-chlorophenyl)-2,3,7,11b-tetrahydro-3-methyloxazolo[3,2-d][1,4]benzodiazepin-6(5H)-one; CS-386; Melex; Melium; Sedoxil. $C_{18}H_{16}Cl_2N_2O_2$; mol wt 363.24. C 59.52%, H 4.44%, Cl 19.52%, N 7.71%, O 8.81%. Prepn from 2-amino-2',5-dichlorobenzophenone: R. Tachikawa et al., DE 1812252; eidem, US 3772371 (1969, 1973 to Sankyo). Synthesis via Schiff base, physical properties: T. Miyadera et al., J. Med. Chem. **14**, 520 (1971). Acid-base equilibrium: M. Ikeda, T. Nagai, Chem. Pharm. Bull. **30**, 3810 (1982). Effect on socially induced suppression in monkeys: T. Kamioka et al., Psychopharmacology **52**, 17 (1977). Toxicity studies: H. Masuda et al., Sankyo Kenkyusho Nempo **30**, 175 (1978), C.A. **90**, 180217d. Clinical effects on anxiety and pyschomotor performance in generalised anxiety disorder: L. Ferreira et al., Clin. Drug Invest. **23**, 235 (2003).

Crystals, mp 172-175°. pKa 6.69. LD_{50} in male, female mice; male, female rats (mg/kg): 4687, 4571, 810, 4500 orally; >6000, >6000, >4000, >4000 i.p. or s.c. (Masuda).

THERAP CAT: Anxiolytic.

6167. Mexenone. [1641-17-4] (2-Hydroxy-4-methoxyphenyl)(4-methylphenyl)methanone; 2-hydroxy-4-methoxy-4'-methylbenzophenone; benzophenone-10; Uvistat. $C_{15}H_{14}O_3$; mol wt 242.27. C 74.36%, H 5.82%, O 19.81%. Prepn: Hardy, Forster, US 2773903 (1956 to Am. Cyanamid). Reversed phase HPLC determn: L.-H. Wang, Chromatographia **50**, 565 (1999). Clinical

evaluation of skin protection efficacy: T. M. MacLeod, W. Frain-Bell, Br. J. Dermatol. **84**, 266 (1971).

THERAP CAT: Ultraviolet screen.

6168. Mexicain. [52500-59-1] A cysteine proteinase obtained from the fruit of *Pileus mexicanus* probably identical with *Leucopremna mexicana* (A.DC.) Standl., *Caricaceae:* Castaneda-Agullo et al., Science **96**, 365 (1942); J. Biol. Chem. **159**, 751 (1945). Immunological studies: Estrada-Parra et al., Rev. Latinoam. Microbiol. Parasitol. **1969**, 145, C.A. **72**, 1744u (1970). Mol wt about 31,100; lysine and alanine believed to be the N- and C-terminal amino acids resp: Soriano et al., Rev. Latinoam. Quim. **1975**, 143, C.A. **84**, 56489t (1976).

Similar to but not identical with papain. Mexicain presents some advantage over papain, since it is more stable in solns and does not require cysteine. Isoelectric pt 9.12.

6169. Mexiletine. [31828-71-4] 1-(2,6-Dimethylphenoxy)-2-propanamine; 1-(2,6-xylyloxy)-2-propylamine; 1-(2',6'-dimethylphenoxy)-2-aminopropane; 1-methyl-2-(2,6-xylyloxy)ethylamine. $C_{11}H_{17}NO$; mol wt 179.26. C 73.70%, H 9.56%, N 7.81%, O 8.93%. Prepn: FR 1551055; H. Köppe et al., US 3954872 (1968, 1976 both to Boehringer, Ing.). Pharmacology: B. N. Singh, E. M. Vaughan Williams, Br. J. Pharmacol. **44**, 1 (1972); J. D. Allen et al., ibid. **45**, 561 (1972). Characterization of metabolites by mass spec and ^{13}C-NMR: K. N. Scott et al., Drug Metab. Dispos. **1**, 506 (1973). Toxicological study: A. Kast et al., Iyakuhin Kenkyu **13**, 922 (1982), C.A. **97**, 192878q (1982). Comprehensive description: M. A. Abounassif et al., Anal. Profiles Drug Subs. **20**, 433-474 (1991). Review of pharmacology and clinical efficacy in arrhythmia: C. Y. C. Chew et al., Drugs **17**, 161-181 (1979); in diabetic neuropathy: B. Jarvis, A. J. Coukell, ibid. **56**, 691-707 (1998).

Hydrochloride. [5370-01-4] Ko-1173; Mexitil; Ritalmex. $C_{11}H_{17}NO.HCl$; mol wt 215.72. White to off-white crystals from ethanol-ether, mp 203-205°. pKa: 9.0. Slightly bitter taste. Freely sol in water, alcohol. LD_{50} in male, female rats, mice, rabbits (mg/kg): 350, 400, 310, 400, 180, 160 orally; in male, female rats, mice (mg/kg): 27, 30, 43, 50 i.v. (Kast).

THERAP CAT: Antiarrhythmic (class IB).

6170. Mezereum. Mezereon; olive spurge; dwarf bay; magell; paradise plant; spurge flax; wild pepper. Dried bark (also seed, though not official) from aerial portions of *Daphne mezereum* L., *D. gnidium* L., and *D. laureola* L., *Thymelaeaceae*. *Habit.* New England, Canada, mountainous Europe, Siberia. *Constit.* Bark: Mezerein and acrid resin, daphnin, umbelliferone, fixed oil. Seed: Fixed oil, acrid resin.

THERAP CAT: Vesicant.

6171. Mezlocillin. [51481-65-3] (2S,5R,6R)-3,3-Dimethyl-6-[[[(2R)-[[[3-(methylsulfonyl)-2-oxo-1-imidazolidinyl]carbonyl]amino]phenylacetyl]amino]-7-oxo-4-thia-1-azabicyclo[3.2.0]heptane-2-carboxylic acid; 6R-[2-[3-(methylsulfonyl)-2-oxo-1-imidazolidine carboxamido]-2-phenylacetamido]penicillanic acid; Bay f 1353. $C_{21}H_{25}N_5O_8S_2$; mol wt 539.58. C 46.74%, H 4.67%, N 12.98%, O 23.72%, S 11.89%. Semisynthetic, broad-spectrum antibiotic related to penicillins and azlocillin, q.v. Prepn: H. B. König et al., DE 2152967; eidem, US 3974142 (1973, 1976 both to Bayer). In vitro study: G. P. Bodey, T. Pan, Antimicrob. Agents Chemother. **11**, 74 (1977). Pharmacokinetics: H. Lode et al., Infection **5**, 163 (1977); S. J. Pancoast, H. C. Neu, Clin. Pharmacol.

Ther. **24,** 108 (1978). Clinical pharmacology: B. F. Issell *et al., Antimicrob. Agents Chemother.* **13,** 180 (1978). Tissue concentration and efficacy: E. Helwing *et al., Med. Klin.* **74,** 112 (1979). Series of articles on antibacterial activity, pharmacology, and clinical trials: *Arzneim.-Forsch.* **29,** 1915-2032 (1979); *Infection* **10,** Suppl. 3, S121-S266 (1982); *J. Antimicrob. Chemother.* **11,** Suppl. C, 1-108 (1983).

Sodium salt monohydrate. [59798-30-0] Baycipen; Baypen; Mezlin. $C_{21}H_{24}N_5NaO_5S_2 \cdot H_2O$; mol wt 531.58. Pale yellow cryst; sol in water, methanol, DMF. Insol in acetone and ethanol.

THERAP CAT: Antibacterial.

6172. Mianserin. [24219-97-4] 1,2,3,4,10,14b-Hexahydro-2-methyldibenzo[*cf*]pyrazino[1,2-*a*]azepine; 2-methyl-1,2,3,4,10,-14b-hexahydro-2*H*-pyrazino[1,2-*f*]morphanthridine. $C_{18}H_{20}N_2$; mol wt 264.36. C 81.78%, H 7.63%, N 10.60%. Serotonin receptor antagonist. Prepn: **NL 6603256;** van der Burg, Delobelle, **US 3534041** (1967, 1970, both to Organon); van der Burg *et al., J. Med. Chem.* **13,** 35 (1970). Pharmacology: Saxena *et al., Eur. J. Pharmacol.* **13,** 295 (1971); Vargaftig *et al., ibid.* **16,** 336 (1971); Van Riezen, *Arch. Int. Pharmacodyn. Ther.* **198,** 256 (1972). Molecular and crystal structure: van Rij, Feil, *Tetrahedron* **29,** 1891 (1973). Review of pharmacology and therapeutic efficacy in depressive illness: R. N. Brogden *et al., Drugs* **16,** 273-301 (1978). 5HT-receptor binding study: B. S. Alexander, M. D. Wood, *J. Pharm. Pharmacol.* **39,** 664 (1987). *Review:* H. van Riezen *et al., in Pharmacological and Biochemical Properties of Drug Substances* **vol. 3,** M. E. Goldberg, Ed. (Am. Pharm. Assoc., Washington, DC, 1981) pp 56-93; *Br. J. Clin. Pharmacol.* **15,** Suppl. 2, S141-S342 (1983).

Hydrochloride. [21535-47-7] GB-94; Org-GB-94; Athymil; Bolvidon; Lantanon; Norval; Tetramide; Tolvin; Tolvon. $C_{18}H_{20}$-$N_2 \cdot HCl$; mol wt 300.83. mp 282-284°. LD_{50} in male, female mice (mg/kg): 365, 390 orally; 32.5, 31.0 i.v. (van Riezen).

THERAP CAT: Antidepressant.

6173. Mibefradil. [116644-53-2] Methoxyacetic acid (1*S*,2*S*)-2-[2-[[3-(1*H*-benzimidazol-2-yl)propyl]methylamino]ethyl]-6-fluoro-1,2,3,4-tetrahydro-1-(1-methylethyl)-2-naphthalenyl ester; (1*S*,2*S*)-2-[2-[[3-(2-benzimidazolyl)propyl]methylamino]ethyl]-6-fluoro-1,2,3,4-tetrahydro-1-isopropyl-2-naphthyl methoxyacetate. $C_{29}H_{38}FN_3O_3$; mol wt 495.63. C 70.28%, H 7.73%, F 3.83%, N 8.48%, O 9.68%. Selective T-type calcium channel blocker. Prepn: Q. Branca *et al., EP 268148; eidem, US 4808605* (1988, 1989 both to Hoffmann-La Roche). Calcium channel selectivity: S. K. Mishra, K. Hermsmeyer, *Circ. Res.* **75,** 144 (1994). Metabolism in rats: H. R. Wiltshire *et al., Xenobiotica* **22,** 837 (1992). Review of pharmacology, toxicology and clinical evaluation: J.-P. Clozel *et al., Cardiovasc. Drug Rev.* **9,** 4-17 (1991); of pharmacology and pharmacokinetics: D. R. Abernethy, *Am. J. Cardiol.* **80,** 4C-11C (1997); of clinical trials in hypertension: S. Oparil, *Am. J. Hypertens.* **11,** 88S-94S (1998); in chronic stable angina pectoris: B. M. Massie, *ibid.* 95S-102S. Post-marketing safety assessment: J. Riley *et al., Int. J. Clin. Pharmacol. Ther.* **40,** 241 (2002).

Dihydrochloride. [116666-63-8] Ro-40-5967; Posicor. C_{29}-$H_{38}FN_3O_3 \cdot 2HCl$; mol wt 568.55. Bitter tasting, odorless, white crystalline powder, mp 128°. Chemically stable, light insensitive and water soluble. pKa: 4.8; 5.5. LD_{50} in mice, rats (mg/kg): 35, 23 i.v.; >800, >800 orally (Clozel).

THERAP CAT: Antihypertensive.

6174. Mibolerone. [3704-09-4] (7α,17β)-17-Hydroxy-7,17-dimethylestr-4-en-3-one; 7α,17α-dimethyl-19-nortestosterone; U-10997; Cheque. $C_{20}H_{30}O_2$; mol wt 302.45. C 79.42%, H 10.00%, O 10.58%. Synthetic anabolic steroid related to testosterone, *q.v.* Prepn: **BE 610385;** J. C. Babcock, J. A. Campbell, **US 3341557** (1962, 1967 both to Upjohn). Biological properties: J. A. Campbell *et al., Steroids* **1,** 317 (1963). Dissolution and solubility rates: W. E. Hamlin *et al., J. Pharm. Sci.* **54,** 1651 (1965). Pharmacodynamics: J. H. Sokolowski, C. W. Kasson, *Am. J. Vet. Res.* **39,** 837 (1978). Efficacy evaluation in dogs: J. H. Sokolowski, *J. Am. Vet. Med. Assoc.* **173,** 983 (1978).

Cryst solid. Soly in deionized water: 0.0454 mg/ml at 37°.

Note: This is a controlled substance (anabolic steroid): **21 CFR,** 1308.13, as defined in 1300.01.

THERAP CAT (VET): Antigonadotropic used to suppress estrus.

6175. Micafungin. [235114-32-6] 1-[(4*R*,5*R*)-4,5-Dihydroxy-*N*²-[4-[5-[4-(pentyloxy)phenyl]-3-isoxazolyl]benzoyl]-L-ornithine]-4-[(4*S*)-4-hydroxy-4-[4-hydroxy-3-(sulfooxy)phenyl]-L-threonine]pneumocandin A0. $C_{56}H_{71}N_9O_{23}S$; mol wt 1270.27. C 52.95%, H 5.63%, N 9.92%, O 28.97%, S 2.52%. Semisynthetic echinocandin antifungal; inhibits 1,3-β-glucan synthase. Prepn (stereochem unspec): H. Ohki *et al., WO 9611210; eidem, US 6107458* (1996, 2000 both to Fujisawa). Synthesis and antifungal activity: M. Tomishima *et al., J. Antibiot.* **52,** 674 (1999). Antifungal spectrum *in vitro:* S. Tawara *et al., Antimicrob. Agents Chemother.* **44,** 57 (2000). Pharmacokinetics and antifungal efficacy: V. Petraitis *et al., ibid.* **46,** 1857 (2002). Review of pharmacology and therapeutic potential: A. H. Groll, T. J. Walsh, *Curr. Opin. Anti-Infect. Invest. Drugs* **2,** 405-412 (2000); A. H. Groll *et al., Expert Opin. Invest. Drugs* **14,** 489-509 (2005).

Sodium salt. [208538-73-2] FK-463; Mycamine. $C_{56}H_{70}N_9$-$NaO_{23}S$; mol wt 1292.26. Water soluble lipopeptide.

THERAP CAT: Antifungal.

6176. Michler's Base. [101-61-1] 4,4'-Methylenebis(N,N-dimethylbenzenamine); 4,4'-methylenebis(N,N-dimethylaniline); bis(p-dimethylaminophenyl)methane; 4,4'-tetramethyldiamino-diphenylmethane; tetra-base; Arnold's base. $C_{17}H_{22}N_2$; mol wt 254.37. C 80.27%, H 8.72%, N 11.01%. Prepd by heating dimethylaniline with 40% formaldehyde and concd HCl: Mekel, **DE 1026322** (1958 to BASF); Hey, Sanderson, J. Chem. Soc. **1960**, 3203; from dimethylaniline + diacetylperoxide: Horner et al., **Ann. 626**, 1 (1959); from dimethylaniline + tert-butylperbenzoate: Sosnovsky, Yang, J. Org. Chem. **25**, 899 (1960).

Lustrous leaflets, mp 90-91°. Sublimes without decompn. bp 390°; $bp_{0.1}$ 155-157°. Insol in water. Sol in benzene, ether, carbon disulfide, acids; slightly sol in cold alcohol; more sol in hot alcohol.

Caution: This substance is reasonably anticipated to be a human carcinogen: Report on Carcinogens, Eleventh Edition (PB2005-104914, 2004) p III-168.

USE: Has been used in manufacture of dyes. As reagent for lead: Dtsch. Med. Wochenschr. **52**, 1855 (1926).

6177. Michler's Ketone. [90-94-8] Bis[4-(dimethylamino)-phenyl]methanone; 4,4'-bis(dimethylamino)benzophenone; tetramethyldiaminobenzophenone. $C_{17}H_{20}N_2O$; mol wt 268.35. C 76.09%, H 7.51%, N 10.44%, O 5.96%. Prepn from dimethylaniline + phosgene: Michler, **Ber. 9**, 716 (1876); Michler, Dupertius, ibid. 1900; from dimethylaniline, $AlCl_3$ and CCl_4: Fierz, Koechlin, Helv. Chim. Acta **1**, 218 (1918).

White to greenish leaflets, mp 172°. bp >360° with decompn. Practically insol in water. Sol in alcohol, warm benzene; very slightly sol in ether.

Caution: This substance is reasonably anticipated to be a human carcinogen: Report on Carcinogens, Eleventh Edition (PB2005-104914, 2004) p III-173.

USE: In manuf of dyes and pigments.

6178. Miconazole. [22916-47-8] 1-[2-(2,4-Dichlorophen-yl)-2-[(2,4-dichlorophenyl)methoxy]ethyl]-1H-imidazole; 1-[2,4-dichloro-β-[(2,4-dichlorobenzyl)oxy]phenethyl]imidazole. C_{18}-$H_{14}Cl_4N_2O$; mol wt 416.13. C 51.95%, H 3.39%, Cl 34.08%, N 6.73%, O 3.84%. Prepn: E. F. Godefroi et al., J. Med. Chem. **12**, 784 (1969); E. F. Godefroi, J. Heeres, **DE 1940388**; eidem, **US 3717655** (1970, 1973 to Janssen). Clinical evaluation: Brugmans et al., Arch. Dermatol. **102**, 428 (1970); Godts et al., Arzneim.-Forsch. **21**, 256 (1971). Review: P. Janssen, W. Van Bever, in Pharmacological and Biochemical Properties of Drug Substances vol. 2, M. E. Goldberg, Ed. (Am. Pharm. Assoc., Washington, DC, 1979) pp 333-354; R. C. Heel et al., Drugs **19**, 7-30 (1980).

Nitrate. [22832-87-7] R-14889; Aflorix; Albistat; Andergin; Brentan; Conoderm; Conofite; Daktar; Daktarin; Deralbine; Dermonistat; Epi-Monistat; Florid; Fungiderm; Fungisdin; Gyno-Daktarin; Gyno-Monistat; Micatin; Miconal Ecobi; Micotef; Monistat; Prilagin; Vodol. $C_{18}H_{14}Cl_4N_2O.HNO_3$; mol wt 479.14. Crystals, mp 170.5° (Godefroi, Heeres, 1970); 184-185° (Godefroi).

(+)-Form nitrate. mp 135.3°. $[\alpha]_D^{20}$ +59° (methanol).

(−)-Form nitrate. mp 135°. $[\alpha]_D^{20}$ −58° (methanol).

THERAP CAT: Antifungal (topical).

THERAP CAT (VET): Antifungal (topical).

6179. Micranthine. [36104-64-0] 6',7-Epoxy-6-methoxy-2-methyl-oxyacanthan-12'-ol. $C_{34}H_{32}N_2O_5$; mol wt 548.63. C 74.43%, H 5.88%, N 5.11%, O 14.58%. Minor alkaloid from bark of Daphnandra micrantha (Tul.) Benth., Monimiaceae. Isoln: Pyman, J. Chem. Soc. **105**, 1679 (1914). Structure: Bick, Todd, ibid. **1950**, 1606. Revised structure and stereochemistry: Bick et al., Tetrahedron Lett. **1972**, 33. Biogenesis: I. Ralph, C. Bick, Heterocycles **16**, 2105 (1981).

Needles from ethyl acetate or methanol, mp 194-196°. $[\alpha]_D^{22}$ −231° (c = 0.7 in chloroform). Sol in chloroform, ethanol; sparingly sol in methanol, ethyl acetate, benzene; practically insol in ether.

6180. Micrococcin P. [1392-46-7] Micrococcin. Antibiotic substance produced by a species of Micrococcus: cf. Br. J. Exp. Pathol. **29**, 473 (1948). Isoln of micrococcin P from B. pumilus: Heatley, Doery, Biochem. J. **50**, 247 (1951). Probable identity of micrococcin and micrococcin P: Abraham et al., Nature **178**, 44 (1956). Structure studies: Brookes et al., J. Chem. Soc. **1957**, 689; Brookes et al., ibid. **1960**, 916; Dean et al., ibid. **1961**, 3394; James, Watson, ibid. C, **1966**, 1361. The antibiotic is a mixture of two components, P_1 (major) and P_2. Proposed total structure of P_1: J. Walker et al., Chem. Commun. **1977**, 706. Revised structure of P_1 and structure of P_2: B. W. Bycroft, M. S. Gowland, ibid. **1978**, 256. Mechanism of action: E. Cundliffe, J. Thompson, Eur. J. Biochem. **118**, 47 (1981). Review: Pestka in Antibiotics vol. 3, J. W. Corcoran, F. E. Hahn, Eds. (Springer-Verlag, New York, 1975) pp 480-486.

Micrococcin P_1

Needles from ethanol, dec 222-228°. $[\alpha]_D^{21}$ +116° (c = 0.10 in 90% ethanol). uv max (ethanol): 345 nm. Sol in ethanol, chloroform, acetone, glacial acetic acid, pyridine. Insol in ether, benzene, amyl acetate, glycerol. Very slightly sol in water.

6181. Micronomicin. [52093-21-7] O-2-Amino-2,3,4,6-tetradeoxy-6-(methylamino)-α-D-$erythro$-hexopyranosyl-(1→4)-O-[3-deoxy-4-C-methyl-3-(methylamino)-β-L-arabinopyranosyl-(1→6)]-2-deoxy-D-streptamine; 6′-N-methylgentamicin C_{1a}; gentamicin C_{2b}; sagamicin (formerly); antibiotic KW-1062; KW-1062; XK-62-2. $C_{20}H_{41}N_5O_7$; mol wt 463.57. C 51.82%, H 8.91%, N 15.11%, O 24.16%. Gentamicin C complex antibiotic produced by *Micromonospora sagamiensis* var. *nonreducans:* T. Nara *et al.,* **DE 2326781** (1973 to Kyowa), *C.A.* **80**, 58389b (1974); *eidem,* **US 4045298** (1977 to Abbott). Isoln, physicochemical and antibacterial properties: R. Okachi *et al., J. Antibiot.* **27**, 793 (1974). Structure: R. S. Egan *et al., ibid.* **28**, 29 (1975). Identity with gentamicin C_{2b}: P. J. L. Daniels *et al., ibid.* **35**. Pharmacology: T. Hashimoto *et al., Jpn. J. Antibiot.* **30**, 362 (1977), *C.A.* **89**, 17113z (1978). Toxicity studies: T. Hara *et al., ibid.* 386-449, *C.A.* **89**, 209205c-8f (1978). Biosynthesis: H. Kase *et al., J. Antibiot.* **35**, 1 (1982); *eidem, Agric. Biol. Chem.* **46**, 515 (1982). Series of articles on pharmacology, metabolism and clinical studies: *Chemotherapy (Tokyo)* **25**, 1801-2287 (1977). *See also* Gentamicin.

White amorphous powder, mp 260° (dec). $[\alpha]_D^{20}$ +116° (c = 1 in water). Sol in water, methanol. Insol in chloroform, ethyl acetate, benzene, petr ether. LD$_{50}$ i.v. in mice: 93 mg/kg (Okachi).

Sulfate. 6′-N-Methylgentamicin C_{1a} hemipentasulfate; Sagamicin; Santemycin. $(C_{20}H_{41}N_5O_7)_2.5H_2SO_4$; mol wt 1417.53.

THERAP CAT: Antibacterial.

6182. Midazolam. [59467-70-8] 8-Chloro-6-(2-fluorophenyl)-1-methyl-4H-imidazo[1,5-a][1,4]benzodiazepine. $C_{18}H_{13}$-ClFN$_3$; mol wt 325.77. C 66.36%, H 4.02%, Cl 10.88%, F 5.83%, N 12.90%. Short-acting deriv of diazepam, *q.v.* Prepn: R. I. Fryer, A. Walser, **DE 2540522**; *eidem,* **US 4280957** (1976, 1981 both to Hoffmann-La Roche); A. Walser *et al., J. Org. Chem.* **43**, 936 (1978). HPLC determn in plasma: S. L. Eeckhoudt *et al., J. Chromatogr. B* **710**, 165 (1998). Toxicity data: L. Pieri *et al., Arzneim.-Forsch.* **31**, 2180 (1981). Series of articles on pharmacology, metabolism, pharmacokinetics, clinical experience: *ibid.* 2177-2288; *Br. J. Clin. Pharmacol.* **16**, Suppl. 1, 1S-199S (1983). Review of pharmacology and therapeutic use: J. W. Dundee *et al., Drugs* **28**, 519-543 (1984); in treatment of status epilepticus: D. F. Hanley, J. F. Kross, *Clin. Ther.* **20**, 1093-1105 (1998). Clinical evaluation for intranasal treatment of febrile seizures in children: E. Lahat *et al., Br. Med. J.* **321**, 83 (2000).

Colorless crystals from ether/methylene chloride/hexane, mp 158-160°. uv max (2-propanol): 220 nm (ε 30000).

Maleate. [59467-94-6] Ro-21-3981/001; Dormicum. $C_{18}H_{13}$-ClFN$_3.C_4H_4O_4$; mol wt 441.84. Crystals from ethanol/ether, mp 114-117° (solvated). LD$_{50}$ in male mice (mg/kg): 760 orally; 86 i.v. (Pieri).

Hydrochloride. [59467-96-8] Ro-21-3981/003; Hypnovel; Versed. $C_{18}H_{13}$ClFN$_3$.HCl; mol wt 362.23. Sol in aqueous solns.

Note: This is a controlled substance (depressant): **21 CFR, 1308.14.**

THERAP CAT: Anesthetic (intravenous); anticonvulsant; sedative, hypnotic.

6183. Midecamycins. Macrolide antibiotic complex produced by *Streptomyces mycarofaciens* nov. sp. Isoln and characterization of the major component, midecamycin A$_1$: T. Tsuruoka *et al.,* **JP 71 28834**; *eidem,* **US 3761588** (1971, 1973 both to Meiji); *eidem, J. Antibiot.* **24**, 319, 452 (1971). Structure: I. Shigeharu *et al., ibid.* 460. Isoln, properties, structures of the minor components, midecamycins A$_2$, A$_3$, A$_4$: T. Tsuruoka *et al., ibid.* 476, 526. Enzymatic interconversion of A$_1$ and A$_3$: Y. Matsuhashi *et al., ibid.* **32**, 777 (1979). Metabolism: T. Shomura *et al., Chem. Pharm. Bull.* **22**, 2427 (1974). Pharmacokinetics: K. Fukaya *et al., Chemotherapy (Tokyo)* **21**, 692 (1973). Pharmacology: K. Mashimo *et al., ibid.* 729. Antibacterial activity: T. Watanabe *et al., ibid.* **25**, 1624 (1977). Toxicity and teratogenicity study in mice: M. Moriguchi *et al., Jpn. J. Antibiot.* **15**, 187, 193 (1972), *C.A.* **78**, 11652a, 11653b (1973).

Midecamycin A$_1$

Midecamycin A$_1$. [35457-80-8] Leucomycin V 3,4^B-dipropanoate; espinomycin A; mydecamycin; turimycin P3; SF-837; YL-704B1; Aboren; Medemycin; Midecin; Momicine; Myoxam; Normicina; Rubimycin. $C_{41}H_{67}NO_{15}$; mol wt 813.97. Colorless needles from benzene, mp 155-156° (after drying at 80° for 8 hrs in vacuo). $[\alpha]_D^{23}$ −67° (c = 1 in ethanol). uv max (ethanol): 232 nm (E$_{1cm}^{1\%}$ 325). Weakly basic; pKa′ 6.9 in 50% aq ethanol. Sol in methanol, ethanol, acetone, chloroform, ethyl acetate, benzene, ethyl ether, acidic water. Practically insol in *n*-hexane, petr ether, water.

Midecamycin A$_3$. [36025-69-1] 9-Deoxy-9-oxoleucomycin V 3,4^B-dipropanoate; antibiotic SF-837A3. $C_{41}H_{65}NO_{15}$; mol wt 811.95. White powder, mp 122-125°. $[\alpha]_D^{22}$ −44° (c = 1 in ethanol). uv max (ethanol): 280 nm (E$_{1cm}^{1\%}$ 295). pKa′ 7.0 in 50% aq ethanol. Solubilities similar to midecamycin A$_1$.

THERAP CAT: Antibacterial.

6184. Midodrine. [42794-76-3] 2-Amino-N-[2-(2,5-dimethoxyphenyl)-2-hydroxyethyl]acetamide; 1-(2′,5′-dimethoxyphenyl)-2-glycinamidoethanol. $C_{12}H_{18}N_2O_4$; mol wt 254.28. C 56.68%, H 7.14%, N 11.02%, O 25.17%. α-Adrenergic agonist. Prepn: K. Wismayr *et al.,* **AT 241435**; *eidem,* **US 3340298** (1965, 1967 both to OSSW). Hemodynamic effects: G. Hitzenberger *et al., Int. J. Clin. Pharmacol. Ther. Toxicol.* **7**, 323 (1973). Pharmacodynamic actions: H. Pittner *et al., Arzneim.-Forsch.* **26**, 2145 (1976). Plasma levels: N. Kolassa *et al., Arch. Int. Pharmacodyn. Ther.* **238**, 96 (1979). Use in ejaculation disorders: D. Jonas *et al., Eur. Urol.* **5**, 184 (1979); in circulatory disorders: H. Sazovsky, H. Pittner, *Fortschr. Med.* **97**, 733 (1979). Synthesis of potential metabolites: T. Kappe, W. Witoszynaky, *Arch. Pharm.* **308**, 339 (1975).

Hydrochloride. [3092-17-9] ST-1085; Amatine; Gutron; Hipertan; Metligine; ProAmatine. $C_{12}H_{18}N_2O_4 \cdot HCl$; mol wt 290.74. Crystals, mp 192-193°.

THERAP CAT: Antihypotensive.

6185. Midostaurin. [120685-11-2] *N*-[(9*S*,10*R*,11*R*,13*R*)-2,3,10,11,12,13-Hexahydro-10-methoxy-9-methyl-1-oxo-9,13-epoxy-1*H*,9*H*-diindolo[1,2,3-*gh*:3′,2′,1′-*lm*]pyrrolo[3,4-*j*][1,7]benzodiazonin-11-yl]-*N*-methylbenzamide; *N*-benzoylstaurosporine; CGP-41251; PKC-412. $C_{35}H_{30}N_4O_4$; mol wt 570.64. C 73.67%, H 5.30%, N 9.82%, O 11.22%. Protein kinase C inhibitor; derivative of the naturally occurring alkaloid, staurosporine, *q.v.* Prepn: G. Caravatti, A. Fredenhagen, **EP 296110**; *eidem*, **US 5093330** (1988, 1992 both to Ciba-Geigy); G. Caravatti *et al., Bioorg. Med. Chem. Lett.* **4**, 399 (1994). HPLC determn in plasma: R. van Gijn *et al., J. Chromatogr. B* **667**, 269 (1995). Review of pharmacology: D. Fabbro *et al., Pharmacol. Ther.* **82**, 293-301 (1999); of mechanism of action and therapeutic potential: A. Gescher, *Crit. Rev. Oncol. Hematol.* **34**, 127-135 (2000). Clinical pharmacokinetics and tolerability: D. J. Propper *et al., J. Clin. Oncol.* **19**, 1485 (2001). Clinical evaluation in diabetic macular edema: P. A. Campochiaro *et al., Invest. Ophthalmol. Visual Sci.* **45**, 922 (2004); in acute myeloid leukemia: R. M. Stone *et al., Blood* **105**, 54 (2005).

mp 235-247° with darkening.

THERAP CAT: Antineoplastic.

6186. Mifepristone. [84371-65-3] (11*β*,17*β*)-11-[4-(Dimethylamino)phenyl]-17-hydroxy-17-(1-propynyl)estra-4,9-dien-3-one; 11*β*-[4-(*N*,*N*-dimethylamino)phenyl]-17*α*-(prop-1-ynyl)-Δ⁴,⁹-estradiene-17*β*-ol-3-one; RU-486; RU-38486; Mifegyne. $C_{29}H_{35}NO_2$; mol wt 429.59. C 81.08%, H 8.21%, N 3.26%, O 7.45%. Progesterone receptor antagonist with partial agonist activity. Prepn: J. G. Teutsch *et al.,* **EP 57115**; *eidem*, **US 4386085** (1982, 1983 both to Roussel-UCLAF). Pharmacology: W. Herrmann *et al., C.R. Seances Acad. Sci. Ser. 3* **294**, 933 (1982). Pituitary and adrenal responses in primates: D. L. Healy *et al., J. Clin. Endocrinol. Metab.* **57**, 863 (1983). Mechanism of action study: M. Rauch *et al., Eur. J. Biochem.* **148**, 213 (1985). Clinical study as abortifacient: B. Couzinet *et al., N. Engl. J. Med.* **315**, 1565 (1986); as postcoital contraceptive: A. Glasier *et al., ibid.* **327**, 1041 (1992). Review of mechanism of action and clinical applications: E. E. Baulieu, *Science* **245**, 1351-1357 (1989). *Reviews:* I. M. Spitz, C. W. Bardin, *N. Engl. J. Med.* **329**, 404-412 (1993); R. N. Brogden *et al., Drugs* **45**, 384-409 (1993).

mp 150°. $[\alpha]_D^{20}$ +138.5° (c = 0.5 in chloroform).

THERAP CAT: Abortifacient.

6187. Miglitol. [72432-03-2] 1,5-Dideoxy-1,5-[(2-hydroxyethyl)imino]-D-glucitol; *N*-(2-hydroxyethyl)moranoline; (2*R*,3*R*,4*R*,5*S*)-1-(2-hydroxyethyl)-2-(hydroxymethyl)-3,4,5-piperidinetriol; *N*-(*β*-hydroxyethyl)-1-deoxynojirimycin; Bay m 1099; Diastabol; Glyset. $C_8H_{17}NO_5$; mol wt 207.22. C 46.37%, H 8.27%, N 6.76%, O 38.60%. *α*-Glucosidase inhibitor; hydroxyethyl derivative of 1-deoxynojirimycin, *q.v.* Prepn: B. Junge *et al.,* **DE 2758025**; *eidem,* **US 4639436** (1979, 1987 both to Bayer AG). Inhibition of *α*-glucosidase: B. Lembcke *et al., Digestion* **31**, 120 (1985); and hypoglycemic activity: Y. Yoshikuni *et al., J. Pharmacobio-Dyn.* **11**, 356 (1988). Clinical evaluations in insulin dependent diabetes: J. Gerard *et al., Int. J. Clin. Pharmacol. Ther. Toxicol.* **25**, 483 (1987); F. P. Kennedy, J. E. Gerich, *Clin. Pharmacol. Ther.* **42**, 455 (1987). Review of pharmacology, clinical efficacy, and therapeutic potential in non-insulin dependent diabetes: L. J. Scott, C. M. Spencer, *Drugs* **59**, 521-549 (2000).

Crystals from ethanol, mp 114°. Sol in water. pKa 5.9.

THERAP CAT: Antidiabetic.

6188. Miglustat. [72599-27-0] (2*R*,3*R*,4*R*,5*S*)-1-Butyl-2-(hydroxymethyl)-3,4,5-piperidinetriol; *N*-butyldeoxynojirimycin; *N*-butylmoranoline; OGT-918; SC-48334; Zavesca. $C_{10}H_{21}NO_4$; mol wt 219.28. C 54.77%, H 9.65%, N 6.39%, O 29.19%. Amino sugar; inhibitor of glucosyltransferase, an enzyme involved in the biosynthesis of glycosphingolipids. Prepn: B. Junge *et al.,* **DE 2758025**; *see also, eidem,* **US 4639436** (1979, 1987 both to Bayer). Improved synthesis: E. W. Baxter, A. B. Reitz, *J. Org. Chem.* **59**, 3175 (1994); C. R. R. Matos *et al., Synthesis* **1999**, 571. *In vitro* efficacy vs HIV: A. Karpas *et al., Proc. Natl. Acad. Sci. USA* **85**, 9229 (1988). Inhibition of glycolipid biosynthesis: F. M. Platt *et al., J. Biol. Chem.* **269**, 8362 (1994). Clinical evaluation in Gaucher's disease: T. Cox *et al., Lancet* **355**, 1481 (2000). Review of pharmacology and clinical development in Gaucher's disease: P. L. McCormack, K. L. Goa, *Drugs* **63**, 2427-2434 (2003).

White to off-white crystalline solid, mp 125-126°. $[\alpha]_D^{25}$ −15.9° (c = 0.77 in water). Highly sol in water (>1000 mg/ml).

THERAP CAT: In treatment of inherited glycosphingolipid lysosomal storage disorders.

6189. Milbemectin. E-187; Koromite; Milbeknock. Mixture of milbemycins, *q.v*, in a 3:7 ratio of milbemycin A_3 and milbemycin A_4. Isolated from fermentation broth of *Streptomyces hygroscopicus* subsp. *aureolacrimosus* SANK60576; structurally related to the avermectins, q.v.: A. Aoki *et al.,* **DE 2329486**; *eidem,* **US 3950360** (1973, 1976 both to Sankyo); Y. Takiguchi *et al., J. Antibiot.* **33**, 1120 (1980). Synthesis of A_3: M. Hirama *et al., J. Am. Chem. Soc.* **113**, 1830 (1991); S. V. Ley *et al., Tetrahedron Lett.* **34**, 7479 (1993). Metabolism in rats: S. Sadakane *et al., J. Pestic. Sci.* **17**, 147 (1992). Review: A. Aoki *et al., ibid.* **19**, 245-247 (1994).

Milbemycin A_3 R = CH_3
Milbemycin A_4 R = CH_2CH_3

Consult the Name Index before using this section.

Stable to heat; relatively unstable under direct sunlight. Relatively unstable to acid; unstable to alkali. LD_{50} in male, female rats, mice (mg/kg): 762, 456, 324, 313 orally; in rats (mg/kg): >5000 dermally (Aoki, 1994). LC_{50} by inhalation in male, female rats (mg/l): 1.90, 2.80 (Aoki, 1994).

Milbemycin A₃. [51596-10-2] (6*R*,25*R*)-5-*O*-Demethyl-28-deoxy-6,28-epoxy-25-methylmilbemycin; milbemycin α_1; antibiotic B-41A3. $C_{31}H_{44}O_7$; mol wt 528.68. White crystalline powder, mp 212-215°. $[\alpha]_D +106°$ (c = 0.25 in acetone) (Aoki). Also reported as mp 192-194°. $[\alpha]_D^{20} +106°$ (acetone) (Hirama). uv max (ethanol): 238, 244 nm (ε 27800, 30500). Soly in water (20°): 7.2 ppm; methanol 64.8 g/l; ethanol 41.9 g/l; acetone 66.1 g/l; *n*-hexane 1.4 g/l; benzene 143.1 g/l; ethyl acetate 69.5 g/l. Vapor pressure (20°): <1 × 10¹⁰ mm Hg.

Milbemycin A₄. [51596-11-3] Milbemycin α_3; antibiotic B-41A4. $C_{32}H_{46}O_7$; mol wt 542.70. White crystalline powder, mp 212-215°. $[\alpha]_D^{20} +106°$ (c = 0.25 in acetone). uv max (ethanol): 238, 244 nm (ε 27800, 30500). Soly in water (20°): 0.88 ppm; methanol 458.8 g/l; ethanol 234.0 g/l; acetone 365.3 g/l; *n*-hexane 6.5 g/l; benzene 524.2 g/l; ethyl acetate 320.4 g/l. Vapor pressure (20°): <1 × 10¹⁰ mm Hg.

USE: Acaricide.

6190. Milbemycin Oxime. [129496-10-2] CGA-179246; Interceptor. Mixture of milbemycin oximes containing ~80% *milbemycin A₄ 5-oxime* ($C_{32}H_{45}NO_7$) and 20% *milbemycin A₃ 5-oxime* ($C_{31}H_{43}NO_7$). Prepn: J. Ide *et al.*, **EP 110667**; *eidem*, **US 4547520** (1984, 1985 both to Sankyo). Anthelmintic activity in experimentally induced infections in dogs: D. D. Bowman *et al.*, *Am. J. Vet. Res.* **49**, 1986 (1988); D. D. Bowman *et al.*, *ibid.* **52**, 64 (1991); in cats: B. L. Blagburn *et al.*, *The OVMA Newsletter* (February, 1990), 1; in naturally acquired infections in dogs: D. D. Bowman *et al.*, *Am. J. Vet. Res.* **51**, 487 (1990). Physical data and toxicity: Ciba-Geigy Material Data Safety Sheet.

Component A₃   R = CH₃
Component A₄   R = CH₂CH₃

Practically odorless white to pale yellow powder, mp 169.6-177.4°. pH of aqueous solution: 6.3. LD_{50} orally in mice: 1000-1500 mg/kg (Ciba-Geigy).

THERAP CAT (VET): Anthelmintic.

6191. Milbemycins. [51570-36-6] Antibiotic B-41. A family of novel macrolide antibiotics with insecticidal and acaricidal activity; structurally related to avermectin, *q.v.*, aglycones. Isoln from *Streptomyces hygroscopicus* subsp. *aureolacrimosus* and properties: A. Aoki *et al.*, **DE 2329486**; *eidem*, **US 3950360** (1973, 1976 both to Sankyo); of α_1-α_{10}, β_1-β_3, D-H: Y. Takiguchi *et al.*, *J. Antibiot.* **33**, 1120 (1980). Isoln and properties of D-H: Y. Takiguchi *et al.*, *J. Antibiot.* **36**, 502 (1983); of J and K: M. Ono *et al.*, *ibid.* 509. Structures of milbemycins α_1-α_{10}, β_1: M. Kurabayashi *et al.*, *18th Symp. Chem. Natural Products* (Kyoto, 1974) nos. 309-316; of β_1-β_3: H. Mishima *et al.*, *Tetrahedron Lett.* **1975**, 711; of D-H, J, K: H. Mishima *et al.*, *J. Antibiot.* **36**, 980 (1983). Total synthesis of (±)-milbemycin β_3: A. B. Smith *et al.*, *J. Am. Chem. Soc.* **104**, 4015 (1982); of the (+)-form: D. R. Williams *et al.*, *ibid.* 4708. Prepn of milbemycins from avermectins: H. Mrozik *et al.*, *Tetrahedron Lett.* **1983**, 5333. Total synthesis studies of D: M. T. Crimmins *et al.*, *ibid.* **28**, 3651 (1987). Prophylactic use of milbe-

mycin D against *Dirofilaria immitis* infection in dogs: M. Tagawa *et al.*, *Jpn. J. Vet. Sci.* **47**, 787 (1985). Toxicity data: N. Matsunuma *et al.*, *Sankyo Kenkyusho Nempo* **35**, 71 (1983), *C.A.* **101**, 32870d (1984). Review of syntheses: T. Blizzard *et al.*, in *Recent Prog. Chem. Synth. Antibiotics*, G. Lukacs, M. Ohno, Eds (Springer-Verlag, Berlin, 1990) pp 66-102. Review of structure-activity relationships: W. L. Shoop *et al.*, *Vet. Parasitol.* **59**, 139-156 (1995).

Milbemycin D

Sol in *n*-hexane, benzene, acetone, ethanol, methanol, chloroform; very slightly sol in water.

Milbemycin α_1 *see* Milbemectin.

Milbemycin β_1. [51596-16-8] 25α-Methylmilbemycin B; antibiotic B-41A1. $C_{32}H_{48}O_7$; mol wt 544.72. Amorphous solid. $[\alpha]_D^{20} +160°$ (c = 0.25 in acetone). uv max (ethanol): 245 nm (ε 26500).

Milbemycin D. [77855-81-3] (6*R*,25*R*)-5-*O*-Demethyl-28-deoxy-6,28-epoxy-25-(1-methylethyl)milbemycin B; antibiotic B-41D. $C_{33}H_{48}O_7$; mol wt 556.73. Colorless needles from hexane-ethyl acetate (20:1), mp 186-188°. $[\alpha]_D^{27} +107°$ (c = 0.25 in acetone). uv max (ethanol): 244 nm (31000).

THERAP CAT (VET): Antiparasitic.

6192. Mildiomycin. [67247-71-3] (*S*)-4-Amino-1-[4-[(2-amino-3-hydroxy-1-oxopropyl)amino]-9-[(aminoiminomethyl)amino]-6-*C*-carboxy-2,3,4,7,9-pentadeoxy-α-L-*talo*-non-2-enopyranosyl]-5-(hydroxymethyl)-2(1*H*)-pyrimidinone. $C_{19}H_{30}N_8O_9$; mol wt 514.49. C 44.36%, H 5.88%, N 21.78%, O 27.99%. A nucleoside antibiotic with anti-mildew activity and low toxicity in mammals and fish. Isoln from *Streptoverticillium rimofaciens* B-98891 and characterization: S. Harada, T. Kishi, *J. Antibiot.* **31**, 519 (1978). Taxonomy and fermentation study: T. Iwasa *et al.*, *ibid.* 511. Structure: S. Harada *et al.*, *J. Am. Chem. Soc.* **100**, 4895 (1978); *Tetrahedron* **37**, 1317 (1981). Anti-mildew spectrum: K. Suetomi, T. Kusaka, *Nippon Noyaku Gakkaishi* **4**, 349 (1979), *C.A.* **92**, 17012c (1980).

Hygroscopic solid, mp >300° (monohydrate). $[\alpha]_D^{20} +100°$ (c = 0.5 in water); +78.5° (c = 0.5 in 0.1*N* HCl). pKa': 2.8, 4.3, 7.2, >12. uv max (pH 7 and 0.1*N* NaOH): 271 nm ($E_{1cm}^{1\%}$ 164); (0.1*N* HCl): 280 nm ($E_{1cm}^{1\%}$ 247). LD_{50} in rats, mice: ~500-1000 mg/kg i.v.; ~2.5-5.0 g/kg orally (Harada, Kishi).

6193. Milk. Cow's milk. Compn and physical properties (a study of samples representing 8 million quarts of milk from 8 cities): Dahlberg, *Proc. Annu. Conv. Milk Ind. Found. Lab. Sect.* **46**, 44 (1953). *Review:* Patton, *Sci. Am.* **221** (1), 58 (July 1969).

Consult the Name Index before using this section.

White liquid. d 1.032. mp −0.54°. pH 6.62. Fat 3.82%; total solids 12.43%; protein 3.25%; lactose 4.64%; ash 0.73%. Vitamins and minerals in 100 g: Vitamin A 152 I.U.; riboflavin 0.156 mg; thiamine 0.043 mg; ascorbic acid 1.14 mg; vitamin B_{12} 0.56 γ; vitamin D 2.4 I.U.; vitamin E 0.1 mg; nicotinic acid 0.085 mg; pantothenic acid 0.35 mg; pyridoxine 0.048 mg; biotin 0.0035 mg; folic acid 0.2 γ; inositol 13 mg; choline 13 mg; essential fatty acids 99 mg; Ca 113 mg; P 90 mg; Fe 0.032 mg. Caloric value: 65 cal/100 g.

6194. Milnacipran. [92623-85-3] (1*R*,2*S*)-*rel*-2-(Aminomethyl)-*N*,*N*-diethyl-1-phenylcyclopropanecarboxamide; 1-phenyl-1-(diethylaminocarbonyl)-2-(aminomethyl)cyclopropane; midalcipran. $C_{15}H_{22}N_2O$; mol wt 246.35. C 73.13%, H 9.00%, N 11.37%, O 6.49%. Serotonin and norepinephrine reuptake inhibitor (SNRI). Prepn: G. Mouzin *et al.*, **EP 68999**; *eidem*, **US 4478836** (1983, 1984 both to Pierre Fabre); B. Bonnaud *et al.*, *J. Med. Chem.* **30**, 318 (1987). Mechanism of action study: C. Moret *et al.*, *Neuropharmacology* **24**, 1211 (1985). Clinical inhibition of monoamine uptake: C. Palmier *et al.*, *Eur. J. Clin. Pharmacol.* **37**, 235 (1989). Review of pharmacology and clinical efficacy in depression: C. M. Spencer, M. I. Wilde, *Drugs* **56**, 405-427 (1998).

Hydrochloride. [101152-94-7] F-2207; Ixel; Toledomin. $C_{15}H_{22}N_2O$·HCl; mol wt 282.81. Crystals from ethanol-ethyl ether, mp 179-181°. LD_{50} orally in mice: 237 mg/kg (Bonnaud).
THERAP CAT: Antidepressant.

6195. Milorganite®. [8049-99-8] Activated sewage sludge prepd by microbial treatment of sewage, useful as fertilizer and as a source of vitamin B_{12}: Schendel, Johnson, *J. Agric. Food Chem.* **2**, 23 (1954). Isoln of B_{12}-active product: Miner, Wolnak, **US 2646386** (1953 to Sewerage Commission of Milwaukee); **US 2941933** (1960 to UCLAF).
Caution: The dust can cause irritation of eyes, respiratory tract.

6196. Miloxacin. [37065-29-5] 5,8-Dihydro-5-methoxy-8-oxo-1,3-dioxolo[4,5-*g*]quinoline-7-carboxylic acid; 6,7-methylenedioxy-1-methoxy-4-oxo-1,4-dihydroquinoline-3-carboxylic acid; antibiotic AB 206; AB-206; Fuldazin. $C_{12}H_9NO_6$; mol wt 263.20. C 54.76%, H 3.45%, N 5.32%, O 36.47%. Quinolone antibacterial; analog of oxolinic acid, *q.v.* Prepn: T. Nakagome *et al.*, **DE 2134451**; *eidem*, **US 3799930** (1972, 1974 both to Sumitomo). Mode of action: T. Nagate *et al.*, *Antimicrob. Agents Chemother.* **17**, 763 (1980). Series of articles on antibacterial activity, absorption and excretion in animals, determn of metabolites by HPLC: *ibid.* **18**, 37-49 (1980). Reproduction studies in rats: T. Yamada *et al.*, *Oyo Yakuri* **19**, 651, 815, 833 (1980), *C.A.* **93**, 197897x, 215570s, 215571t (1980).

Colorless prisms from DMF, mp 264° (dec).
THERAP CAT: Antibacterial.

6197. Milrinone. [78415-72-2] 1,6-Dihydro-2-methyl-6-oxo-(3,4'-bipyridine)-5-carbonitrile; 1,2-dihydro-6-methyl-2-oxo-5-(4-pyridinyl)nicotinonitrile; Win-47203; Corotrope; Milrila. $C_{12}H_9N_3O$; mol wt 211.22. C 68.24%, H 4.29%, N 19.89%, O 7.57%. Selective phosphodiesterase inhibitor with vasodilating and positive inotropic activity. Prepn: G. Y. Lesher *et al.*, **BE 886336**; G. Y. Lesher, R. E. Philion, **US 4313951** (1981, 1982 both to Sterling). Improved process: B. Singh, **US 4413127** (1983 to Sterling); *idem*,

Heterocycles **23**, 1479 (1985). Pharmacological profile: A. A. Alousi *et al.*, *J. Cardiovasc. Pharmacol.* **5**, 792, 804 (1983). HPLC determn in body fluids: J. Edelson *et al.*, *J. Chromatogr.* **276**, 456 (1983). Clinical studies in congestive heart failure: C. S. Maskin *et al.*, *Circulation* **67**, 1065 (1983); L. S. Sinoway *et al.*, *J. Am. Coll. Cardiol.* **2**, 327 (1983); D. S. Baim *et al.*, *N. Engl. J. Med.* **309**, 748 (1983).

Crystals from DMF + water or from ethanol, mp >300°.
Lactate. [100286-97-3] Primacor. $C_{12}H_9N_3O$·$xC_3H_6O_3$.
THERAP CAT: Cardiotonic.

6198. Miltefosine. [58066-85-6] 2-[[(Hexadecyloxy)hydroxyphosphinyl]oxy]-*N*,*N*,*N*-trimethylethanaminium inner salt; choline phosphate hexadecyl ester, hydroxide, inner salt; hexadecyl 2-(*N*,*N*,*N*-trimethylamino)ethyl phosphate; *n*-hexadecylphosphorylcholine; hexadecylphosphocholine; HPC; D-18506; Impavido; Miltex. $C_{21}H_{46}NO_4P$; mol wt 407.57. C 61.89%, H 11.38%, N 3.44%, O 15.70%, P 7.60%. Synthetic phospholipid; affects cell-signaling pathways and membrane synthesis. Synthesis: U. Kaatze *et al.*, *Chem. Phys. Lipids* **27**, 263 (1980); W. J. Hansen *et al.*, *Lipids* **17**, 453 (1982). *See also:* H. Eibl, **EP 225608**; *idem*, **US 4837023** (1987, 1989 both to Max-Planck Ges. Wissensch.). Toxicity and anticancer properties: C. Muschiol *et al.*, *Lipids* **22**, 930 (1987). Structure-activity study: M. R. Berger *et al.*, *Cancer Treat. Rev.* **17**, 143 (1990). HPTLC determn in plasma: I. Rustenbeck, S. Lenzen, *J. Chromatogr.* **525**, 85 (1990). Clinical evaluation in topical treatment of cutaneous breast cancer metastases: C. Unger *et al.*, *Cancer Treat. Rev.* **17**, 243 (1990). Clinical trial in visceral leishmaniasis: S. Sundar *et al.*, *N. Engl. J. Med.* **347**, 1739 (2002). *Review:* H. Eibl, C. Unger, *Cancer Treat. Rev.* **17**, 233-242 (1990).

mp 232-234° (dec); discoloration at 225°. LD_{50} in rats (mg/kg): 246 orally (Muschiol).
THERAP CAT: Antineoplastic; antiprotozoal (Leishmania).

6199. Mimosine. [500-44-7] α-Amino-3-hydroxy-4-oxo-1(4*H*)-pyridinepropanoic acid; 3-hydroxy-4-oxo-1(4*H*)-pyridinealanine; β-[*N*-(3-hydroxy-4-pyridone)]-α-aminopropionic acid; leucenol; leucenine; leucaenine; leucaenol. $C_8H_{10}N_2O_4$; mol wt 198.18. C 48.48%, H 5.09%, N 14.14%, O 32.29%. A naturally occurring amino acid found in large quantities in the seeds and foliage of the legume genera *Mimosa* and *Leucena*. Isoln from *Leucena glauca* (Willd.) Benth., *Leguminosae:* Renz, *Z. Physiol. Chem.* **244**, 153 (1936); Mascré, *Compt. Rend.* **204**, 890 (1937); improved large-scale isoln: N. K. Hart *et al.*, *Heterocycles* **7**, 265 (1977). Structure: Adams, Jones, *J. Am. Chem. Soc.* **69**, 1803 (1947). Synthesis: Adams, Johnson, *ibid.* **71**, 705 (1949). Identity of mimosine and leucenol: Kleipool, Wibaut, *Rec. Trav. Chim.* **69**, 37 (1950); Wibaut, Schuhmacher, *ibid.* **71**, 1017 (1952). Crystal structure: A. Mostad *et al.*, *Acta Chem. Scand.* **27**, 164 (1973). Shown to cause inhibition of hair growth and loss of hair in mice: Crounse *et al.*, *Nature* **194**, 694 (1962). Explanation of the toxicity in animals: J. F. Thompson *et al.*, *Annu. Rev. Biochem.* **38**, 137 (1969).

dl-**Form.** Crystals from water, mp 235-236°. Slightly sol in water, much less sol in methanol and ethanol. Practically insol in the higher alcohols, in dioxane, ethyl acetate, ether, benzene, chloroform, glacial acetic acid, pyridine, Cellosolve. Sol in dil acids or bases and may be recovered from these solns by adjusting the pH so that it is just acid to bromcresol green. uv max: 282 nm (log ε 4.23).

dl-**Hemihydrate.** Crystals, darkens at 215-226°, mp 227-228°.

l-**Form.** Crystals from water, mp 225°. $[\alpha]_D^{22}$ −20°.

Hydrochloride. $C_8H_{11}ClN_2O_4$. Dec 175°, sol in water.

Hydrobromide. $C_8H_{11}BrN_2O_4$. Dec 179.5°, sol in water.

USE: Depilatory agent, Hegarty *et al.*, *Aust. J. Agric. Res.* **15**, 153 (1964), *C.A.* **60**, 16405e (1964).

6200. Minaprine. [25905-77-5] *N*-(4-Methyl-6-phenyl-3-pyridazinyl)-4-morpholineethanamine; 4-[2-[(4-methyl-6-phenyl-3-pyridazinyl)amino]ethyl]morpholine. $C_{17}H_{22}N_4O$; mol wt 298.38. C 68.43%, H 7.43%, N 18.78%, O 5.36%. Prepn: H. Laborit, DE 2229215; *idem,* US 4169158 (1973, 1979 to Centre Etudes Exper. Clin. Physio-Biologie); C.-G. Wermuth, A. Exinger, *Agressologie* **13**, 285 (1972). Pharmacology: H. Laborit *et al., ibid.* 291. Metabolism of ^{14}C-minaprine: A. G. Rico *et al., J. Pharmacol.* **9**, 170 (1978). Pharmacokinetics: J. P. Jeanniot *et al., ibid.* 169. Clinical evaluation: A. Garcia-Maffla, M. H. de Garcia, *Pharmatherapeutica* **2**, 265 (1979). Pharmacological evaluation in depression: K. Bizière *et al., Arzneim.-Forsch.* **32**, 824 (1982). Toxicologic study: A. G. Mazure *et al., Agressologie* **13**, 319 (1972).

Fine buff-colored needles from isopropanol, mp 122°. Insol in water. Slightly sol in cold ethanol, sol in hot ethanol, chloroform.

Dihydrochloride. [25953-17-7] Agr-1240; CB-30038; Brantur; Cantor. $C_{17}H_{22}N_4O.2HCl$; mol wt 371.30. Crystals from abs ethanol, mp 182°.

THERAP CAT: Antidepressant.

6201. Mineral Spirits. [64475-85-0] Petroleum spirits; white spirits; turpentine substitutes. Name applied to various types of hydrocarbon solvents, primarily petroleum distillates, which have flash points above 100°F (38°C) and distillation ranges between 300°F (149°C) and 415°F (213°C). *See: ASTM Standard Specifications D 235-83*, 71-73 (1983). Review of toxicology and human exposure: *Toxicological Profile for Stoddard Solvent* (PB95-264263, 1995) 169 pp.

Type I. [8052-41-3] Stoddard solvent; Texsolve S; Varsol 1. Regular mineral spirits. Clear liquid. Flash pt (min): 38°C (100°F). $d_{15.6}^{15.6}$ 0.754-0.820. Distillation range: initial bp (min), 149°C (300°F); 50% recovered (max), 182°C (360°F); dry pt (max), 208°C (407°F).

Type II. High flash point mineral spirits. Flash pt (min): 60°C (140°F). $d_{15.6}^{15.6}$ 0.768-0.820. Distillation range: initial bp (min), 177°C (350°F); 50% recovered (max), 196°C (385°F); dry pt (max), 211°C (412°F).

Type III. Odorless mineral spirits. Flash pt (min): 38°C (100°F). $d_{15.6}^{15.6}$ 0.775 (max). Distillation range: initial bp (min), 149°C (300°F); 50% recovered (max), 196°C (385°F); dry pt (max), 213°C (415°F).

Type IV. Texsolve S-2; Varsol 3. Low dry point mineral spirits. Flash pt (min): 38°C (100°F). $d_{15.6}^{15.6}$ 0.754-0.800. Distillation range: initial bp (min), 149°C (300°F); 50% recovered (max), 174°C (345°F); dry pt (max), 185°C (365°F).

Caution: Potential symptoms of overexposure to stoddard solvent are irritation of eyes, nose, throat; dizziness; dermatitis; aspiration of liquid may cause chemical pneumonia. *See NIOSH Pocket Guide to Chemical Hazards* (DHHS/NIOSH 97-140, 1997) p 286.

USE: Solvent; paint thinner. In the coatings and dry cleaning industries.

6202. Minocycline. [10118-90-8] [4*S*-(4α,4aα,5aα,12aα)]-4,7-Bis(dimethylamino)-1,4,4a,5,5a,6,11,12a-octahydro-3,10,12,-12a-tetrahydroxy-1,11-dioxo-2-naphthacenecarboxamide; 7-dimethylamino-6-demethyl-6-deoxytetracycline. $C_{23}H_{27}N_3O_7$; mol

wt 457.48. C 60.38%, H 5.95%, N 9.19%, O 24.48%. Second generation tetracycline antibiotic. Prepn: J. Petisi, J. H. Boothe, US 3226436 (1965 to Am. Cyanamid); M. J. Martell, J. H. Boothe, *J. Med. Chem.* **10**, 44 (1967); R. F. R. Church *et al., J. Org. Chem.* **36**, 723 (1971). HPLC determn in tissue and serum: W. R. Wrightson *et al., J. Chromatogr. B* **706**, 358 (1998). Comprehensive description: V. Zbinovsky, G. P. Chrekian, *Anal. Profiles Drug Subs.* **6**, 323-339 (1977). Series of articles on toxicology and metabolism: *Toxicol. Appl. Pharmacol.* **11**, 128-183 (1967). Review of antibacterial activity and pharmacology: M. Jonas, B. A. Cunha, *Ther. Drug Monit.* **4**, 137-145 (1982); of clinical safety and efficacy in acne: K. Freeman, *Br. J. Clin. Pract.* **43**, 112-115 (1989). Clinical evaluation in periodontal disease: R. J. Oringer *et al., J. Periodontol.* **73**, 835 (2002).

Bright yellow-orange amorphous solid. $[\alpha]_D^{25}$ −166° (c = 0.524). uv max (0.1*N* HCl): 352, 263 nm (log ε 4.16, 4.23); (0.1*N* NaOH): 380, 243 nm (log ε 4.30, 4.38).

Hydrochloride. [13614-98-7] Arestin; Dynacin; Klinomycin; Minocin; Vectrin. $C_{23}H_{27}N_3O_7.HCl$; mol wt 493.94. Yellow crystalline powder. Slightly hygroscopic; sensitive to light and to surface oxidation.

THERAP CAT: Antibacterial.

6203. Minoxidil. [38304-91-5] 6-(1-Piperidinyl)-2,4-pyrimidinediamine 3-oxide; 6-amino-1,2-dihydro-1-hydroxy-2-imino-4-piperidinopyrimidine; 2,3-dihydro-3-hydroxy-2-imino-6-(1-piperidinyl)-4-pyrimidinamine; 2,4-diamino-6-piperidinopyrimidine 3-oxide; 6-piperidino-2,4-diaminopyrimidine 3-oxide; PDP; U-10858; Alopexil; Alostil; Loniten; Lonolox; Minoximen; Normoxidil; Prexidil; Regaine; Rogaine; Tricoxidil. $C_9H_{15}N_5O$; mol wt 209.25. C 51.66%, H 7.23%, N 33.47%, O 7.65%. Prepn: NL 6615385; W. C. Anthony *et al.*, US 3382247 (1967, 1968 both to Upjohn); J. M. McCall *et al., J. Org. Chem.* **40**, 3304 (1975). *See also* W. C. Anthony, US 3644364 (1972 to Upjohn). Metabolism: R. C. Thomas *et al., J. Pharm. Sci.* **64**, 1360 (1975). Pharmacology and pharmacokinetics: D. T. Lowenthal *et al., J. Clin. Pharmacol.* **18**, 500 (1978). Percutaneous absorption and excretion: T. J. Franz, *Arch. Dermatol.* **121**, 203 (1985). Clinical studies: O. Andersson, R. Sivertsson, *Acta Med. Scand.* **205**, 213 (1979); M. Moser, *Adv. Cardiol.* **26**, 38 (1979). Clinical trial in early male pattern baldness: E. A. Olsen *et al., J. Am. Acad. Dermatol.* **13**, 185 (1985). Toxicology: R. G. Carlson, E. S. Feenstra, *Toxicol. Appl. Pharmacol.* **39**, 1 (1977). Review of pharmacology and therapeutic use: V. M. Campese, *Drugs* **22**, 257-278 (1981). Review of topical application in baldness: E. Novak *et al., Int. J. Dermatol.* **24**, 82 (1985). Comprehensive description: D. K. J. Gorecki, *Anal. Profiles Drug Subs.* **17**, 185-219 (1988).

Crystals from methanol-acetonitrile, mp 248°, dec 259-261° (Anthony, 1972). pKa 4.61. uv max (ethanol): 230, 261, 285 nm (ε 35210, 11210, 11790); (0.01*N* H_2SO_4): 232, 280 nm (ε 26350, 23850); (0.01*N* KOH): 231, 261.5, 285 nm (ε 36100, 11400, 12040). Soly (mg/ml): propylene glycol 75, methanol 44, ethanol 29, 2-propanol 6.7, dimethylsulfoxide 6.5, water 2.2, chloroform 0.5, acetone <0.5, ethylacetate <0.5, diethyl ether <0.5, benzene <0.5, acetonitrile <0.5. LD_{50} in rats, mice (mg/kg): 49, 51 i.v. (Carlson, Feenstra).

THERAP CAT: Antihypertensive. Antialopecia agent.

6204. Miokamycin. [55881-07-7] Leucomycin V 3^B,9-di-acetate 3,4^B-dipropanoate; 9,3″-diacetylmidecamycin; MOM; ponsinomycin; Miocamycin. $C_{45}H_{71}NO_{17}$; mol wt 898.04. C 60.18%, H 7.97%, N 1.56%, O 30.29%. Macrolide antibiotic; deriv of midecamycin A_1. Prepn: S. Inoue *et al., JP Kokai 74 124087; eidem,* **US 4017607** (1974, 1977 both to Meiji Seika); S. Omoto *et al., J. Antibiot.* **29,** 536 (1976); T. Nakamura *et al., Chem. Lett.* **1978,** 1293. Prepn of noncrystalline form and comparison of physico-pharmaceutical properties: T. Sato *et al., Chem. Pharm. Bull.* **29,** 2675 (1981). Antibacterial spectrum: K. Kawaharajo *et al., J. Antibiot.* **34,** 436 (1981). Metabolism: T. Shomura *et al., Chem. Pharm. Bull.* **29,** 2413 (1981). Laboratory and clinical pediatric studies: Y. Toyonaga *et al., Jpn. J. Antibiot.* **35,** 1475 (1982), *C.A.* **98,** 216y (1983). Clinical bioavailability: F. Fraschini *et al., Int. J. Clin. Pharmacol. Res.* **10,** 293 (1989).

Tasteless crystals from isopropanol, mp ~220° (with coloration). $[\alpha]_D^{25}$ −53° (c = 1.0 in chloroform). $[\alpha]_D^{20}$ −74° (c = 1 in methanol). uv max (methanol): 231 nm ($E_{1cm}^{1\%}$ 342). Sol in methanol, acetone, chloroform. Very slightly sol in water.

THERAP CAT: Antibacterial.

6205. Mipafox. [371-86-8] *N,N'*-Bis(1-methylethyl)phosphorodiamidic fluoride; *N,N'*-diisopropylphosphorodiamidic fluoride; bis(isopropylamino)fluorophosphine oxide. $C_6H_{16}FN_2OP$; mol wt 182.18. C 39.56%, H 8.85%, F 10.43%, N 15.38%, O 8.78%, P 17.00%. Prepn: Pound *et al.,* **GB 688787** (1953 to Fisons); Heath, *J. Chem. Soc.* **1956,** 3796.

Crystals, mp 65°.
Caution: Cholinesterase inhibitor.
USE: Insecticide.

6206. Miraculin. Taste-modifying protein; Miralin. A basic glycoprotein of probable mol wt 44,000. Responsible for the taste-changing properties of **Miracle fruit (agbayun)**, the red berries of *Synsepalum dulcificum* (Schum.) Daniell, *Sapotaceae* [alternate name: *Richardella dulcifica* (Schum. and Thonn) Baehni], a shrub indigenous to tropical W. Africa. Sour materials taste sweet after the tasteless mucilaginous pulp of the fruit has been applied to the tongue. First description: Daniell, *Pharm. J.* **11,** 445 (1852). Isolation studies: Inglett *et al., J. Agric. Food Chem.* **13,** 284 (1965); Kurihara, Beidler, *Science* **161,** 1241 (1968). Isoln and purif of miraculin: Brouwer *et al., Nature* **220,** 373 (1968); **NL 6911954** corresp to Brouwer *et al.,* **US 3682880** (1970, 1972 to Lever Bros.). Max sweetening effect occurs when 4×10^{-7} *M* (in 0.02 *M* citric acid) is held in the mouth for 3 mins. The protein probably binds to receptors of the taste buds and modifies their function. Mechanism of action studies: Kurihara, Beidler, *Nature* **222,** 1176 (1969). *Reviews:* Henning, *Pharm. Weekbl.* **106,** 271 (1971); Cagan, *Science* **181,** 32 (1973).

USE: Sweetening agent.

6207. Mirex. [2385-85-5] 1,1a,2,2,3,3a,4,5,5,5a,5b,6-Dodecachlorooctahydro-1,3,4-metheno-1*H*-cyclobuta[*cd*]pentalene; perchloropentacyclo[5.2.1.0^{2,6}.0^{3,9}.0^{5,8}]decane; hexachloropentadiene dimer; CG-1283; ENT-025719; Dechlorane. $C_{10}Cl_{12}$; mol wt 545.54. C 22.02%, Cl 77.98%. Prepn: Prins, *Rec. Trav. Chim.* **65,** 455 (1946); Newcomer, McBee, *J. Am. Chem. Soc.* **71,** 952

(1949); Gilbert, **US 2702305** (1955 to Allied Chem.); Johnson, **US 2724730** (1955 to Hooker Electrochem.). Structure: McBee *et al., J. Am. Chem. Soc.* **78,** 1511 (1956). Degradation in the environment to Kepone and related compds: D. A. Carlson *et al., Science* **194,** 939 (1976). Carcinogenicity study: B. M. Ullard *et al., J. Natl. Cancer Inst.* **58,** 133 (1977). Toxicity data: T. B. Gaines, *Toxicol. Appl. Pharmacol.* **14,** 515 (1969). *Reviews:* Ungnade, McBee, *Chem. Rev.* **58,** 249-320 (1958); Alley, *J. Environ. Qual.* **2,** 52-61 (1973); E. M. Waters *et al., Environ. Res.* **14,** 212-222 (1977); K. Kaiser, *Environ. Sci. Technol.* **12,** 520-528 (1978). Review of toxicology and human exposure: *Toxicological Profile for Mirex and Chlordecone* (PB95-264354, 1995) 362 pp.

Snow-white odorless crystals from benzene, dec 485°. Supports combustion. Practically insol in water. Soly at room temp: dioxane 15.3%; xylene 14.3%; benzene 12.2%; carbon tetrachloride 7.2%; methyl ethyl ketone 5.6%. Practically noncorrosive to metals. LD_{50} orally in female rats (corn oil suspension): 600 mg/kg (Gaines).

Caution: This substance is reasonably anticipated to be a human carcinogen: *Report on Carcinogens, Eleventh Edition* (PB2005-104914, 2004) p III-175.

USE: Formerly as fire retardant for plastics, rubber, paint, paper, electrical goods; insecticide for fire ants.

6208. Mirtazapine. [61337-67-5] 1,2,3,4,10,14b-Hexahydro-2-methylpyrazino[2,1-*a*]pyrido[2,3-*c*][2]benzazepine; 2-methyl-1,2,3,4,10,14b-hexahydrobenzo[*c*]pyrazino[1,2-*a*]pyrido[3,2-*f*]-azepine; 6-azamianserin; mepirzepine; Org-3770; Remeron; Zispin. $C_{17}H_{19}N_3$; mol wt 265.35. C 76.95%, H 7.22%, N 15.84%. α_2-Adrenergic blocker; analog of mianserin, *q.v.* Prepn: W. J. Van der Burg, **DE 2614406;** *idem,* **US 4062848** (1976, 1977 both to AKZO). GC determn in plasma: J. E. Paanakker, H. J. M. Van Hal, *J. Chromatogr.* **417,** 203 (1987). Pharmacology and mechanism of action study: T. De Boer *et al., Neuropharmacology* **27,** 399 (1988). Clinical comparison with amitriptyline, *q.v.:* W. T. Smith *et al., Psychopharmacol. Bull.* **26,** 191 (1990). Review of clinical experience in mood and anxiety disorders: M. J. Ostacher *et al., Expert Rev. Neurotherapeut.* **3,** 425-433 (2003); and of clinical pharmacokinetics, safety and efficacy: A. Szegedi, N. Schwertfeger, *Expert Opin. Pharmacother.* **6,** 631-641 (2005).

White crystals from petr ether, mp 114-116°. Sol in methanol and chloroform.

THERAP CAT: Antidepressant.

6209. Misch Metal. [8049-20-5] Alloy of mixed rare earth metals. Prepd by electrolysis of fused rare earth chlorides. Obtained from the lanthanide ore, **bastnaesite.** A typical composition is 48-50% cerium, 32-34% lanthanum, 13-14% neodymium, 4-5% praseodymium and 1.5% other rare earth metals. Average mol wt is 140. Uses in organic synthesis: M.-I. Lannou *et al., Tetrahedron* **59,** 10551 (2003).

Pyrophoric powder. Store under argon.

USE: In the manuf of flints for gas and cigarette lighters. Co-reductant or promoter in organic synthesis. In metallurgy: decreases microporosity and improves stress resistance, thermomalleability and heat exchange in refined steel.

6210. Misoprostol. [59122-46-2] ($11\alpha,13E$)-11,16-Dihydroxy-16-methyl-9-oxoprost-13-en-1-oic acid methyl ester; (±)-methyl-($1R,2R,3R$)-3-hydroxy-2-[(*E*)-(*4RS*)-4-hydroxy-4-methyl-1-octenyl]-5-oxocyclopentaneheptanoate; (±)-15-deoxy-(16*RS*)-16-hydroxy-16-methyl-PGE$_1$ methyl ester; SC-29333; Cytotec. $C_{22}H_{38}O_5$; mol wt 382.53. C 69.08%, H 10.01%, O 20.91%. Cytoprotective prostaglandin PGE$_1$ analog; also exhibits uterotonic and cervical-ripening actions. Double racemate comprised of the (+)- and (−)-enantiomers of the 16*R*- and 16*S*-forms. The pharmacologically active form is the (11*R*,16*S*)-enantiomer. Prepn: P. W. Collins, R. Pappo, **BE 827127**; *eidem*, **US 3965143** (1975, 1976 both to Searle); P. W. Collins *et al.*, *Tetrahedron Lett.* **48**, 4217 (1975). Prepn, activity, NMR data: P. Collins *et al.*, *J. Med. Chem.* **20**, 1152 (1977). HPLC resolution of enantiomers: D. A. Roston, R. Wijayaratne, *Anal. Chem.* **60**, 948 (1988). Mechanism of gastric secretory inhibition: D. G. Colton *et al.*, *Arch. Int. Pharmacodyn. Ther.* **236**, 86 (1978). Symposium on pharmacology and clinical efficacy: *Dig. Dis. Sci.* **30**, Suppl. 11, 114S-205S (1985). Toxicity data: F. N. Kotsonis *et al.*, *ibid.* 142S. Clinical trial in prevention of NSAID-induced ulcer: D. Y. Graham *et al.*, *Ann. Intern. Med.* **119**, 257 (1993); to induce labor: H. Fletcher *et al.*, *Obstet. Gynecol.* **83**, 244 (1994). Review of clinical experience in pregnancy: A. B. Goldberg *et al.*, *N. Engl. J. Med.* **344**, 38-47 (2001).

(11*R*, 16*S*)-Form

Light yellow oil. Sol in water. LD$_{50}$ in rats, mice (mg/kg): 40-62, 70-160 i.p.; 81-100, 27-138 orally (Kotsonis).

THERAP CAT: Antiulcerative.

6211. Mitiglinide. [145375-43-5] ($\alpha S,3aR,7aS$)-Octahydro-γ-oxo-α-(phenylmethyl)-2*H*-isoindole-2-butanoic acid; (2*S*)-2-benzyl-3-(*cis*-hexahydroisoindol-2-ylcarbonyl)propionic acid. $C_{19}H_{25}NO_3$; mol wt 315.41. C 72.35%, H 7.99%, N 4.44%, O 15.22%. Hypoglycemic agent for treatment of type 2 diabetes. Prepn: F. Sato *et al.*, **EP 507534**; *eidem*, **US 5202335** (1992, 1993 both to Kissei); T. Yamaguchi *et al.*, *Chem. Pharm. Bull.* **45**, 1518 (1997); *eidem*, *ibid.* **46**, 337 (1998). Improved synthesis: J. Liu *et al.*, *Helv. Chim. Acta* **87**, 1935 (2004). 2D-NMR conformation study: L. Lins *et al.*, *Biochem. Pharmacol.* **52**, 1155 (1996). Mechanism of action studies: F. Reimann *et al.*, *Br. J. Pharmacol.* **132**, 1542 (2001); N. Kaiser *et al.*, *ibid.* **146**, 872 (2005). Clinical evaluation in type 2 diabetes: R. Assaloni *et al.*, *Diabetologia* **48**, 1919 (2005).

Viscous oil. $[\alpha]_D^{24}$ −3.2° (c = 1.04 in methanol); $[\alpha]_D^{18}$ −3.5° (c = 1.00 in methanol).

Calcium salt dihydrate. [207844-01-7]; [145525-41-3] (anhydrous). KAD-1229; S-21403; Glufast. $C_{38}H_{48}CaN_2O_6 \cdot 2H_2O$; mol wt 704.91. Colorless crystals from 5% aqueous ethanol, mp 179-185° C. $[\alpha]_D^{18}$ +5.7° (c = 1.0 in methanol).

THERAP CAT: Antidiabetic.

6212. Mitobronitol. [488-41-5] 1,6-Dibromo-1,6-dideoxy-D-mannitol; 1,6-dideoxy-1,6-dibromo-D-mannitol; dibromomannitol; DBM; Myebrol; Myelobromol. $C_6H_{12}Br_2O_4$; mol wt 307.97. C 23.40%, H 3.93%, Br 51.89%, O 20.78%. Cytostatic agent; the first dibromohexitol introduced into clinical use. Manuf: **GB 959407** (1964 to Chinoin). Pharmaco-biochemical studies: J. Szabo *et al.*, *Neoplasma* **20**, 13 (1973). Clinical studies: D. F.

Chiuten *et al.*, *Cancer* **47**, 442 (1981). Comparative study with busulfan, *q.v.*: R. T. Silver *et al.*, *Cancer* **60**, 1442 (1987).

Crystals from methanol + dichloroethane, mp 176-178°.

THERAP CAT: Antineoplastic.

6213. Mitoguazone. [459-86-9] 2,2′-(1-Methyl-1,2-ethanediylidene)bis[hydrazinecarboximidamide]; 1,1′-[(methylethanediylidene)dinitrilo]diguanidine; methylglyoxal bis(guanylhydrazone); pyruvaldehyde bis(amidinohydrazone). $C_5H_{12}N_8$; mol wt 184.20. C 32.60%, H 6.57%, N 60.83%. Polyamine biosynthesis inhibitor. Prepn: F. Baiocchi *et al.*, *J. Med. Chem.* **6**, 431 (1963); V. T. Oliverio, C. Denham, *J. Pharm. Sci.* **52**, 202 (1963). Experimentally effective against myelogenous leukemia: Freireich *et al.*, *Cancer Chemother. Rep.* **16**, 183 (1962). HPLC determn in plasma: C.-L. Cheng *et al.*, *J. Chromatogr. B* **793**, 281 (2003). Review of clinical experience: D. D. Von Hoff, *Ann. Oncol.* **5**, 487-493 (1994).

Prepd as the hemihydrate; off-white crystals from isopropyl alcohol, dec 225°. uv max at pH 1: 283 nm (ε 38400); at pH 11: 325 nm (ε 33500). pKa: 7.63, 9.05.

Dihydrochloride. [7059-23-6] NSC-32946; Methyl-GAG. $C_5H_{12}N_8 \cdot 2HCl$; mol wt 257.12. Crystals from acetone, dec 256-257°.

THERAP CAT: Antineoplastic.

6214. Mitolactol. [10318-26-0] 1,6-Dibromo-1,6-dideoxygalactitol; 1,6-dibromo-1,6-dideoxydulcitol; dibromodulcitol; dibromodulcit; DBD; NSC-104800; Elobromol. $C_6H_{12}Br_2O_4$; mol wt 307.97. C 23.40%, H 3.93%, Br 51.89%, O 20.78%. Diastereoisomer of mitobronitol, *q.v.*, with myelosuppressive effects. Prepn and anticancer activity: **NL 6600395**; P. Horváth-Lengyel *et al.*, **US 3993781** (1966, 1976 both to Chinoin); B. Kellner *et al.*, *Nature* **213**, 402 (1967). Structure-activity correlations: L. Institoris *et al.*, *Arzneim.-Forsch.* **17**, 145 (1967). Pharmacological study: T. H. Corbett *et al.*, *Cancer* **40**, Suppl. 5, 2660 (1977). Metabolism, pharmacokinetics: I. P. Horváth *et al.*, *Eur. J. Cancer* **15**, 337 (1979). Clinical studies: W. Medina, J. M. Kirkwood, *Cancer Treat. Rep.* **66**, 195 (1982); D. C. Tormey *et al.*, *Am. J. Clin. Oncol.* **5**, 33 (1982).

Crystals from methanol, aq alc, or aq acetone, mp 187-188° (dec). LD$_{50}$ in rats (mg/kg): 1400 orally; 470 i.p. (Kellner).

THERAP CAT: Antineoplastic.

6215. Mitomycins. [1404-00-8] A group of antitumor antibiotics produced by *Streptomyces caespitosus (griseovinaceseus)*. Isoln of mitomycins A and B: T. Hata *et al.*, *J. Antibiot.* **9A**, 141 (1956). Isoln of C: S. Wakaki *et al.*, *Antibiot. Chemother.* **8**, 228 (1958); **GB 830874**; T. Hata *et al.*, **US 3660578** (1960, 1972 both to Kyowa and Kitasato Kenkyusho). Production of the complex: T.

Yamamoto, H. Umezawa, **JP 56 2898** (1956 to Nippon Antibiot. Subs. Sci. Assoc.), *C.A.* **51**, 9100 (1957). Improved method: A. Gourevitch *et al.*, **US 3042582** (1962 to Bristol-Myers). Isoln from *S. verticillatus*, constituents: D. V. Lefemine *et al.*, *J. Am. Chem. Soc.* **84**, 3184 (1962). Structures: J. S. Webb *et al.*, *ibid.* 3185, 3187. Total synthesis of mitomycins A and C: T. Fukuyama *et al.*, *Tetrahedron Lett.* **1977**, 4295. Toxicity: S. Kinoshita *et al.*, *J. Med. Chem.* **14**, 13 (1971). Review and evaluation of studies of carcinogenic action of mitomycin C in laboratory animals: *IARC Monographs* **10**, 171-179 (1976). Review of syntheses: Y. Kishi, *J. Nat. Prod.* **42**, 549-568 (1979). General review: R. W. Franck, *Fortschr. Chem. Org. Naturst.* **38**, 1-41 (1979).

Mitomycin C

Mitomycin A. [4055-39-4] $C_{16}H_{19}N_3O_6$; mol wt 349.34. The 6-methoxy analog of mitomycin C. X-ray crystallographic study: A. Tulinsky, *J. Am. Chem. Soc.* **84**, 3188 (1962); A. Tulinsky, J. H. van den Hende, *ibid.* **89**, 2905 (1967). Red-violet crystals from acetone + carbon tetrachloride, dec 159-161°. Absorption max (water): 215, 318, 530 nm ($E_{1cm}^{1\%}$ 234, 122, 118.8). Sol in water, benzene, toluene, trichloroethylene, nitrobenzene and many organic solvents. Practically insol in xylene, carbon tetrachloride, carbon disulfide, petr ether, ligroin, cyclohexane. LD_{50} i.v. in mice: 2 mg/kg (Hata, 1956; Kinoshita).

Mitomycin B. [4055-40-7] $C_{16}H_{19}N_3O_6$; mol wt 349.34. Molecular structure: R. Yahashi, I. Matsubara, *J. Antibiot.* **29**, 104 (1976); *ibid.* **31**(6), correction (1978). Violet crystals from acetone + carbon tetrachloride, dec 182-184°. Absorption max (water): 220, 320, 550 nm ($E_{1cm}^{1\%}$ 117.5, 55.0, 9.9). Sol in water and many organic solvents. Practically insol in xylene, carbon tetrachloride, carbon disulfide, petr ether, ligroin, cyclohexane, benzene, toluene, trichloroethylene, nitrobenzene. LD_{50} i.v. in mice: 10 mg/kg (Hata, 1956); also reported as 3 mg/kg (Kinoshita).

Mitomycin C. [50-07-7] [1aS-(1aα,8β,8aα,8bα)]-6-Amino-8-[[(aminocarbonyl)oxy]methyl]-1,1a,2,8,8a,8b-hexahydro-8a-methoxy-5-methylazirino[2′,3′:3,4]pyrrolo[1,2-*a*]indole-4,7-dione; MMC; Ametycine; Mitocin-C; Mutamycin. $C_{15}H_{18}N_4O_5$; mol wt 334.33. Chemistry and structure: C. L. Stevens *et al.*, *J. Med. Chem.* **8**, 1 (1965). Crystal and molecular structure: K. Ogawa *et al.*, *Bull. Chem. Soc. Jpn.* **52**, 2334 (1979). Revised absolute configuration: K. Shirahata, N. Hirayama, *J. Am. Chem. Soc.* **105**, 7199 (1983). Mechanism of action: C. Rodigheriero, *Farmaco Ed. Sci.* **33**, 651 (1978). Comprehensive description: J. H. Beijnen *et al.*, *Anal. Profiles Drug Subs.* **16**, 361-401 (1986). Blue-violet crystals, does not melt below 360°. Absorption max (methanol): 216, 360, 560 nm ($E_{1cm}^{1\%}$ 742, 742, 0.06). Sol in water, methanol, acetone, butyl acetate and cyclohexanone; slightly sol in benzene, carbon tetrachloride, ether. Practically insol in petr ether. LD_{50} i.v. in mice: 5 mg/kg (Wakaki); also reported as 9 mg/kg (Kinoshita).

N-**Methylmitomycin** C *see* Porfiromycin.

THERAP CAT: Mitomycin C as antineoplastic.

6216. Mitotane. [53-19-0] 1-Chloro-2-[2,2-dichloro-1-(4-chlorophenyl)ethyl]benzene; 1,1-dichloro-2-(*o*-chlorophenyl)-2-(*p*-chlorophenyl)ethane; 2-(2-chlorophenyl)-2-(4-chlorophenyl)-1,1-dichloroethane; 2,4′-dichlorodiphenyldichloroethane; 2,2-bis(2-chlorophenyl-4-chlorophenyl)-1,1-dichloroethane; *o,p*′-DDD; CB-313; Lysodren. $C_{14}H_{10}Cl_4$; mol wt 320.04. C 52.54%, H 3.15%, Cl 44.31%. Constituent of commercial DDD which contains about 10% of the *o,p*′-isomer. Prepn from 2,2-dichloro-1-(*o*-chlorophenyl)ethanol with chlorobenzene in presence of H_2SO_4: Haller *et al.*, *J. Am. Chem. Soc.* **67**, 1600 (1945). Isoln from technical grade DDD: Cueto, Brown, *Endocrinology* **62**, 326 (1958).

Crystals from pentane or methanol, mp 76-78°. Sol in ethanol, isooctane, carbon tetrachloride.

THERAP CAT: Antineoplastic.

6217. Mitoxantrone. [65271-80-9] 1,4-Dihydroxy-5,8-bis[[2-[(2-hydroxyethyl)amino]ethyl]amino]-9,10-anthracenedione; DHAQ; NSC-279836. $C_{22}H_{28}N_4O_6$; mol wt 444.48. C 59.45%, H 6.35%, N 12.61%, O 21.60%. Immunosuppressive and cytostatic anthracenedione. Prepn: R. K. Y. Zee-Cheng, C. C. Cheng, *J. Med. Chem.* **21**, 291 (1978); K. C. Murdock *et al.*, *ibid.* **22**, 1024 (1979); *eidem*, **DE 2835661**; K. C. Murdock, F. E. Durr, **US 4197249** (1979, 1980 both to Am. Cyanamid). Antitumor activity: R. E. Wallace *et al.*, *Cancer Res.* **39**, 1570 (1979). HPLC determn in plasma: K. T. Lin *et al.*, *J. Chromatogr.* **465**, 75 (1989). Comprehensive description: J. H. Beijnen *et al.*, *Anal. Profiles Drug Subs.* **17**, 221-258 (1988). Review of toxicology: M. McDonald *et al.*, *Drugs Exp. Clin. Res.* **10**, 745-752 (1984); of pharmacology and clinical efficacy in cancer: J. Koeller, M. Eble, *Clin. Pharm.* **7**, 574-581 (1988); of pharmacokinetics and metabolism: G. Ehninger *et al.*, *Clin. Pharmacokinet.* **18**, 365-380 (1990). Review of pharmacology and clinical efficacy in multiple sclerosis: K. K. Jain, *Expert Opin. Invest. Drugs* **9**, 1139-1149 (2000).

Crystals from ethanol/hexane, mp 160-162°. Abs max (ethanol): 244, 279, 525, 620, 660 nm (log ε 4.64, 4.31, 3.70, 4.37, 4.38). Sparingly sol in water, slightly sol in methanol. Practically insol in acetonitrile, chloroform, acetone.

Dihydrochloride. [70476-82-3] DHAD; CL-232315; NSC-301739; Novantrone; Onkotrone. $C_{22}H_{28}N_4O_6.2HCl$; mol wt 517.40. Hygroscopic blue-black solid from water/ethanol, mp 203-205°. Abs max (water): 241, 273, 608, 658 nm (ε 41000, 12000, 19200, 20900). Sparingly sol in water, slightly sol in methanol. Practically insol in acetonitrile, chloroform, acetone.

THERAP CAT: Antineoplastic; immunomodulator.

6218. Mitragynine. [4098-40-2] (16*E*,20β)-16,17-Didehydro-9,17-dimethoxycorynan-16-carboxylic acid methyl ester; (*E*)-16,17-didehydro-9,17-dimethoxy-17,18-seco-20α-yohimban-16-carboxylic acid methyl ester; 9-methoxycorynantheidine. $C_{23}H_{30}N_2O_4$; mol wt 398.50. C 69.32%, H 7.59%, N 7.03%, O 16.06%. Major alkaloid of *Mitragyna speciosa* Korth., *Rubiaceae*: Field, *J. Chem. Soc.* **119**, 887 (1921); Ing, Raison, *ibid.* **1939**, 986. Structural studies: Hendrickson, *Chem. Ind. (London)* **1961**, 713; Joshi *et al.*, *ibid.* **1963**, 573. Revised structure: Zacharias *et al.*, *Acta Crystallogr.* **18**, 1039 (1965). Pharmacology: Macko *et al.*, *Arch. Int. Pharmacodyn. Ther.* **198**, 145 (1972).

White, amorphous powder, mp 102-106°. bp$_5$ 230-240°. $[\alpha]_D$ +39° (chloroform). uv max: 226, 292 nm (ε 41,150, 6600). Soluble in alcohol, chloroform, acetic acid.

6219. Mivacurium Chloride. [106861-44-3] (1R,1'R)-2,2'-[[(4E)-1,8-Dioxo-4-octene-1,8-diyl]bis(oxy-3,1-propanediyl)]-bis[1,2,3,4-tetrahydro-6,7-dimethoxy-2-methyl-1-[(3,4,5-trimethoxyphenyl)methyl]]isoquinolinium dichloride; (R)-1,2,3,4-tetrahydro-2-(3-hydroxypropyl)-6,7-dimethoxy-2-methyl-1-(3,4,5-trimethoxybenzyl)isoquinolinium chloride, (E)-4-octenedioate (2:1); BW-B1090U; Mivacron. $C_{58}H_{80}Cl_2N_2O_{14}$; mol wt 1100.17. C 63.32%, H 7.33%, Cl 6.45%, N 2.55%, O 20.36%. Non-depolarizing neuromuscular blocking agent. Prepn: R. A. Swaringen, Jr. *et al.*, **DD 235638**; *eidem*, **US 4761418** (1986, 1988 both to Burroughs Wellcome). Clinical pharmacology: H. H. Ali *et al.*, *Br. J. Anaesth.* **61**, 541 (1988); J. J. Savarese *et al.*, *Anesthesiology* **68**, 723 (1988). *In vitro* metabolism: D. R. Cook *et al.*, *Anesth. Analg.* **68**, 452 (1989). Clinical evaluation in adults: S. Weber *et al.*, *ibid.* **67**, 495 (1988); R. P. From *et al.*, *Br. J. Anaesth.* **64**, 193 (1990); in children: J. K. Alifimoff, N. G. Goudsouzian, *ibid.* **63**, 520 (1989).

Amorphous solid. $[\alpha]_D^{20}$ −62.7° (c = 1.9 in water).
THERAP CAT: Muscle relaxant (skeletal).

6220. Mivazerol. [125472-02-8] 2-Hydroxy-3-(1H-imidazol-4-ylmethyl)benzamide; α-imidazol-4-yl-2,3-cresotamide. $C_{11}H_{11}N_3O_2$; mol wt 217.22. C 60.82%, H 5.10%, N 19.34%, O 14.73%. α$_2$-Adrenergic agonist. Prepn: E. Cossement *et al.*, **EP 341231**; *eidem*, **US 4923865** (1989, 1990 both to UCB); *idem et al.*, *J. Pharm. Belg.* **49**, 206 (1994). Specificity for α$_2$ adrenoceptors and binding studies: M. Noyer *et al.*, *Neurochem. Int.* **24**, 221 (1994). Clinical trial to improve perioperative hemodynamic stability: D. T. Mangano *et al.*, *Anesthesiology* **86**, 346 (1997). Mode of action study: M. Guyaux *et al.*, *Acta Anaesthesiol. Scand.* **42**, 238 (1998).

mp 197.6°.
Hydrochloride. [127170-73-4] UCB-22073. $C_{11}H_{11}N_3O_2$·HCl; mol wt 253.68. mp 287.8°. LD$_{50}$ i.p. in mice: 760 mg/kg (Cossement).
THERAP CAT: To reduce cardiac complications of surgery.

6221. Mizolastine. [108612-45-9] 2-[[1-[1-[(4-Fluorophenyl)methyl]-1H-benzimidazol-2-yl]-4-piperidinyl]methylamino]-4(1H)-pyrimidinone; 2-[[1-[1-(p-fluorobenzyl)-2-benzimidazolyl]-4-piperidinyl]methylamino]-4(3H)-pyrimidinone; SL-85.0324; Mizolen; Zolim. $C_{24}H_{25}FN_6O$; mol wt 432.49. C 66.65%, H 5.83%, F 4.39%, N 19.43%, O 3.70%. Nonsedating-type histamine H$_1$-receptor antagonist. Prepn: **JP Kokai 87 61979**; P. Manoury *et al.*, **US 4912219** (1987, 1990 both to Synthelabo). Receptor binding study: J. Benavides *et al.*, *Arzneim.-Forsch.* **45**, 551 (1995). HPLC determn in plasma: V. Ascalone *et al.*, *J. Chromatogr.* **619**, 275 (1993). Clinical pharmacokinetics: P. Rosenzweig *et al.*, *Ann. Allergy* **69**, 135 (1992). Effect on psychomotor performance: J. S. Kerr *et al.*, *Eur. J. Clin. Pharmacol.* **47**, 331 (1994). Clinical trial in allergic rhinitis: F. Leynadier *et al.*, *Ann. Allergy Asthma Immunol.* **76**, 163 (1996).

Crystals from ethanol, mp 217°. Sol in methanol.
THERAP CAT: Antihistaminic.

6222. Mizoribine. [50924-49-7] 5-Hydroxy-1-β-D-ribofuranosyl-1H-imidazole-4-carboxamide; 4-carbamoyl-1-β-D-ribofuranosylimidazolium-5-olate; HE-69; Bredinin. $C_9H_{13}N_3O_6$; mol wt 259.22. C 41.70%, H 5.05%, N 16.21%, O 37.03%. Nucleoside antibiotic produced by *Eupenicillium brefedianum* with cytotoxic and immunosuppressive activity. Isoln: K. Mizuno *et al.*, **BE 799805**; *eidem*, **US 3888843** (1973, 1975 to Toyo Jozo); *eidem*, *J. Antibiot.* **27**, 775 (1974). Synthesis: M. Hayashi *et al.*, *Chem. Pharm. Bull.* **23**, 245 (1975); K. Fukukuwa *et al.*, *ibid.* **32**, 1644 (1984). Prepn of the aglycone: T. Atsumi *et al.*, **JP Kokai 76 88965** (1976 to Sumitomo), *C.A.* **86**, 106582g (1977). HPLC determn in human serum: K. Takada *et al.*, *J. Chromatogr.* **222**, 156 (1981). Anti-arthritic activity: H. Iwata *et al.*, *Experientia* **33**, 502 (1977). Cytotoxic effect and comparison with aglycone: K. Sakaguchi *et al.*, *J. Antibiot.* **28**, 798 (1975). Antitumor spectrum of aglycone: N. Yoshida *et al.*, *Cancer Res.* **43**, 5851 (1983). Pharmacokinetics: K. Takada, *Eur. J. Pharmacol.* **24**, 457 (1983). Clinical trials in renal transplantation: T. Inou *et al.*, *Transplant. Proc.* **12**, 526 (1980); *eidem, ibid.* **13**, 315 (1981); A. Tajima *et al.*, *Transplantation* **38**, 116 (1984).

Crystals from methanol, mp >200° (dec). $[\alpha]_D^{27}$ −35° (c = 0.8 in H$_2$O). pKa 6.75. uv max (H$_2$O): 245, 279 nm (E 250, 580). Sol in water. Slightly sol in methanol, ethanol. Insol in most organic solvents. LD$_{50}$ in mice (g/kg): >1.5 i.v., >2.4 i.p. (Mizuno, 1975).
Aglycone. 5-Hydroxy-1H-imidazole-4-carboxamide; 4-carbamoyl-5-hydroxyimidazole; 4-carbamoylimidazolium-5-olate; SM-108. $C_4H_5N_3O_2$; mol wt 127.10.
THERAP CAT: Immunosuppressant.

6223. MMT. [12108-13-3] Tricarbonyl[(1,2,3,4,5-η)-1-methyl-2,4-cyclopentadien-1-yl]manganese; methylcyclopentadienylmanganese tricarbonyl; MCMT; tricarbonyl(η^5-methylcyclopentadienyl)manganese(I); TCMn; AK-33X. $C_9H_7MnO_3$; mol wt 218.09. C 49.56%, H 3.24%, Mn 25.19%, O 22.01%. Organometallic antiknock compound used to increase the octane quality of fuel. Prepn: J. E. Brown *et al.*, **US 2818417** (1957 to Ethyl Corp.). Evaluation of antiknock properties: R. J. Riggs *et al.*, *Proc. 37th Natural Gas Assoc. Am.* **1958**, 51. Effect on auto emissions: W. R. Pierson *et al.*, *J. Air Pollut. Control. Assoc.* **28**, 692 (1978). Use as dopant in Mn deposition: K. Hirabayashi, H. Kozawaguchi, *Jpn. J. Appl. Phys.* **25**, 711 (1986). Pyrolysis mechanism in deposition: S. Wen-bin *et al.*, *J. Cryst. Growth* **113**, 1 (1991); I. M. T. Davidson *et al.*, *J. Mater. Chem.* **4**, 13 (1994). GC determn in gasoline: W. A. Aue *et al.*, *Anal. Chem.* **62**, 2453 (1990); and in air: V. S. Gaind *et al.*, *Analyst* **117**, 161 (1992). Review as octane enhancer: J. D. Bailie, *Oil Gas J.* **74**, 69-72 (1976); D. P. Hollrah, A. M. Burns, *ibid.* **89**, 86-90 (1991). Review of toxicology: J. Stara *et al.*, *Proc. 4th*

Ann. Conf Environment. Toxicol. **AD-781 031,** 251-270 (1973); P. J. Abbott, *Sci. Total Environ.* **67,** 247-255 (1987); and environmental assessment: D. R. Lynam *et al., ibid.* **93,** 107-114 (1990.)

Yellow orange liquid, fp $-0.75°$. n_D^{20} 1.5873. d_{20}^4 1.3942. Vapor pressure ranges from 8 mm at 100° to 360.6 mm at 200°. Readily sol in hydrocarbons and the usual organic solvents including hexane, alchohols, ether, acetone, ethylene glycol, lubricating oils, and hydrocarbon fuels, such as gasoline and diesel fuel. LD_{50} orally in mice, guinea pig, rabbit: 352; 905; 95 mg/kg; orally in male, female rats: 175 ±33; 89 ±14; LC_{50} inhalation in rat: 0.22 mg/l (Stara).

USE: Antiknock fuel additive; dopant for Mn.

6224. αMNP. [63628-25-1] α-Methoxy-α-methyl-1-naphthaleneacetic acid; 2-methoxy-2-(1-naphthyl)propanoic acid. $C_{14}H_{14}O_3$; mol wt 230.26. C 73.03%, H 6.13%, O 20.85%. Chiral derivatization reagent. Prepn and application to amino acids: J. Goto *et al., Chem. Pharm. Bull.* **25,** 847 (1977); *eidem, J. Chromatogr.* **152,** 413 (1978). Resolution of enantiomers and abs config: N. Harada *et al., Tetrahedron: Asymmetry* **11,** 1249 (2000). Use in alcohol resolution: A. Ichikawa, *Chirality* **11,** 70 (1999).

(R)-(−)-form.

Colorless plates from acetone-hexane, mp 161-162°. uv max (methanol): 263, 271, 281, 287, 292 nm (log ε 3.36, 3.53, 3.57, 3.46, 3.45).

(−)-(R)-Form. [63628-26-2] Colorless plates from ether-hexane, mp 111-112°. $[\alpha]_D^{13}$ −106.3° (c = 0.16 in $CHCl_3$); $[\alpha]_D^{13}$ −128.8° (c = 0.10 in methanol).

(+)-(S)-Form. [102691-93-0] $[\alpha]_D^{26}$ +67.4° (c = 1.39 in $CHCl_3$).

Hydroxy acid. [6341-58-8] (unspecified stereo)]; [255881-88-0] (S-(+)-form). α-Hydroxy-α-methyl-1-naphthaleneacetic acid; αHNP. $C_{13}H_{12}O_3$. Prepn and abs config: A. Ichikawa *et al., Tetrahedron: Asymmetry* **10,** 4075 (1999). Colorless plates from acetone-hexane, mp 110-112°. $[\alpha]_D^{29}$ +40° (c = 0.21 in $CHCl_3$).

USE: For enantioresolution in organic syntheses.

6225. Mocimycin. [50935-71-2] Antibiotic MYC 8003; delvomycin; kirromycin; MYC-8003. $C_{43}H_{60}N_2O_{12}$; mol wt 796.94. C 64.81%, H 7.59%, N 3.52%, O 24.09%. Antibiotic produced by *Streptomyces ramocissimus.* Isoln and properties: C. Vos, J. Den Admirant, *DE 2140674; eidem, US 3927211; US 3923981* (1972, 1975, 1975 all to Gist-Brocades). Structural studies: C. Vos, P. E. J. Verwiel, *Tetrahedron Lett.* **1973,** 2823, 5173. Total structure and identity with kirromycin: H. Maehr *et al., J. Am. Chem. Soc.* **95,** 8449 (1973). Absolute stereochemistry: *eidem, ibid.* **96,** 4034 (1974). Conversion to aurodox: H. Maehr *et al., J. Antibiot.* **32,** 361 (1979). Biological studies: H. Wolf *et al., Proc. Natl. Acad. Sci. USA* **71,** 4910 (1974); J. A. M. Van De Klundeit *et al., FEBS Lett.* **81,** 303 (1977). Review of chemistry: H. Maehr *et al., Can. J. Chem.* **58,** 501-526 (1980). Review of properties and actions: A. Parmeggiani, G. Sander, *Topics in Antibiotic Chemistry* vol. 5, P. G. Sammes, Ed. (Halsted Press, New York, 1980) pp 159-221.

Yellow solid. Weakly acidic. $[\alpha]_D^{22}$ −60° (c = 1 in methanol). uv max (methanol/water): 233, 276, 286, 327 nm. Sol in chloroform, methyl isobutyl ketone, butyl acetate, ethyl acetate, acetone, methanol, alkaline soln. Slightly sol in CCl_4, benzene. Insol in diethyl ether, petr ether, water, acid soln. Stable for 4 hrs in 50% aq methanol at pH 3-12. The solid antibiotic stored at 25° and 37° and low relative humidity shows no activity loss for 5 mos. Stable for 3 mos at 25°, 100% relative humidity; for 2 mos at 37°, 100% relative humidity. LD_{50} i.p. in mice: >1000 mg/kg (DE 2140674).

1-Methyl deriv *see* Aurodox.

5,6-Dihydromocimycin. $C_{43}H_{62}N_2O_{12}$; mol wt 798.96. Isoln from *S. ramocissimus* and properties: H. Jongsma *et al., DE 2658977* (1977 to Gist-Brocades), *C.A.* **87,** 135078y (1977); *see also* C. Vos *et al., US 4062948* (1977 to Gist-Brocades). Pale yellow solid, dec begins at 123°. $[\alpha]_D^{20}$ −85° (1% methanolic soln). uv max (methanol/water): 233.5, 267, 291, 333 nm (ε 63000, 23000, 19000, 18000). Solubility similar to mocimycin in most solvents.

USE: Animal growth promotant.

6226. Moclobemide. [71320-77-9] 4-Chloro-*N*-[2-(4-morpholinyl)ethyl]benzamide; *p*-chloro-*N*-(2-morpholinoethyl)benzamide; Ro-11-1163; Aurorix; Manerix; Moclamine. $C_{13}H_{17}ClN_2O_2$; mol wt 268.74. C 58.10%, H 6.38%, Cl 13.19%, N 10.42%, O 11.91%. Reversible monoamine oxidase A (MAO-A) inhibitor. Prepn: W. Burkard, P.-C. Wyss, *DE 2706179; US 4210754* (1977, 1980 both to Hoffmann-La Roche). Gas chromatography: K. P. Maguire *et al., J. Chromatogr.* **278,** 429 (1983). Human pharmacokinetics: F. A. Wiesel *et al., Eur. J. Clin. Pharmacol.* **28,** 89 (1985). Clinical study: J. K. Larsen *et al., Acta Psychiatr. Scand.* **70,** 254 (1984). Review of pharmacology: W. P. Burkard *et al., J. Pharmacol. Exp. Ther.* **248,** 391-399 (1989); of neurochemical profile: M. DaPrada *et al., ibid.* 400-414.

Crystals from isopropanol, mp 137°. LD_{50} in rats (mg/kg): 707 orally (Burkard, Wyss).

Hydrochloride. $C_{13}H_{18}Cl_2N_2O_2$. Crystals from isopropanol, mp 208°.

THERAP CAT: Antidepressant.

6227. Modacrylic Fibers. A generic term for acrylic fibers composed of a long chain synthetic polymer containing 35-85% of acrylonitrile units such as **Dynel** and **Verel.** *See:* R. W. Moncrieff, *Man-Made Fibres* (Wiley, New York, 4th ed., 1963) p 9. *Review:* Kennedy in *Encyclopedia of Polymer Science and Technology* vol. **8,** N. M. Bikales, Ed. (Interscience, New York, 1968) pp 812-839.

USE: In pile fabrics, carpeting, paint rollers.

6228. Modafinil. [68693-11-8] 2-[(Diphenylmethyl)sulfinyl]acetamide; 2-(benzhydrylsulfinyl)acetamide; CRL-40476; Attenace; Provigil. $C_{15}H_{15}NO_2S$; mol wt 273.35. C 65.91%, H 5.53%, N 5.12%, O 11.71%, S 11.73%. α_1-Adrenergic agonist. Prepn: L. Lafon, *DE 2809625; eidem, US 4177290* (1978, 1979 both to Lab. Lafon). Effects on vigilance: F. Goldenberg, J. S. Weil, *Sleep (Stuttgart)* **8,** 343 (1988); on normal sleep: B. Saletu *et al., Int. J. Clin. Pharmacol. Res.* **9,** 183 (1989). Clinical evaluation in hypersomnia and narcolepsy: H. Bastuji, M. Jouvet, *Prog. Neuro-Psychopharmacol. Biol. Psychiatry* **12,** 695 (1988); in adult attention-deficit/hyperactivity disorder: D. C. Turner *et al., Biol. Psychiatry* **55,** 1031 (2004).

Crystals from methanol, mp 164-166°. Sparingly to slightly sol in methanol, acetone. Practically insol in water, cyclohexane.

Note: This is a controlled substance (stimulant): **21 CFR,** 1308.14.

THERAP CAT: CNS Stimulant.

6229. Moexipril. [103775-10-6] (3*S*)-2-[(2*S*)-2-[[(1*S*)-1-(Ethoxycarbonyl)-3-phenylpropyl]amino]-1-oxopropyl]-1,2,3,4-tetrahydro-6,7-dimethoxy-3-isoquinolinecarboxylic acid; RS-10085. $C_{27}H_{34}N_2O_7$; mol wt 498.57. C 65.04%, H 6.87%, N 5.62%, O 22.46%. Angiotensin converting enzyme (ACE) inhibitor; dimethoxy analog of quinapril, *q.v.* Prepn: M. L. Hoefle, S. Klutchko, **EP 49605**; *eidem,* **US 4344949** (both 1982 to Warner-Lambert); S. Klutchko *et al., J. Med. Chem.* **29,** 1953 (1986). Pharmacology: O. Edling *et al., J. Pharmacol. Exp. Ther.* **275,** 854 (1995). GC-MS determn in plasma: W. Hammes *et al., J. Chromatogr. B* **670,** 81 (1995). Clinical trials in hypertension: W. B. White *et al., J. Hum. Hypertens.* **8,** 917 (1994); M. Stimpel *et al., Cardiology* **87,** 313 (1996).

Hydrochloride. [82586-52-5] CI-925; RS-10085-197; SPM-925; Fempress; Perdix; Univasc. $C_{27}H_{34}N_2O_7 \cdot HCl$; mol wt 535.03. Crystals from ethanol + ethyl ether, mp 141-161°. $[\alpha]_D^{23}$ +34.2° (c = 1.1 in ethanol).

Diacid hydrochloride. [82586-57-0] Moexiprilat hydrochloride. $C_{25}H_{30}N_2O_7 \cdot HCl$. Prepd as the monohydrate; crystals from THF + ethanol, mp 145-170°. $[\alpha]_D^{23}$ +37.8° (c = 1.1 in methanol).

THERAP CAT: Antihypertensive.

6230. Mofarotene. [125533-88-2] 4-[2-[4-[(1*E*)-2-(5,6,7,8-Tetrahydro-5,5,8,8-tetramethyl-2-naphthalenyl)-1-propenyl]-phenoxy]ethyl]morpholine; Ro 40-8757. $C_{29}H_{39}NO_2$; mol wt 433.63. C 80.32%, H 9.07%, N 3.23%, O 7.38%. Anticancer aromatic analog of retinoic acid (arotinoid). Prepn: M. Klaus *et al.,* **EP 331983**; *eidem,* **US 4940707** (1989, 1990 both to Hoffmann-La Roche). Mode of action study: J. F. Eliason *et al., Blood* **86,** 4516 (1995). Pharmacokinetics: B. Vallès *et al., Eur. J. Drug Metab. Pharmacokinet.* **20,** 49 (1995). HPLC determn in plasma: R. Wyss *et al., J. Chromatogr. A* **729,** 315 (1996). Mechanism of growth inhibition on pancreatic cancer cells: S. Kawa *et al., Int. J. Cancer* **72,** 906 (1997). Clinical pharmacology in combination with cisplatin and etoposide: L. van Zuylen *et al., Anti-Cancer Drugs* **10,** 361 (1999).

White crystals from ethyl acetate/hexane, mp 107-109°.
THERAP CAT: Antineoplastic.

6231. Mofebutazone. [2210-63-1] 4-Butyl-1-phenyl-3,5-pyrazolidinedione; 4-butyl-1-phenyl-3,5-dioxopyrazolidine; 2-phenyl-3,5-dihydroxy-4-butylpyrazolidine; monophenylbutazone; Arcomonol Tablets; Mobutazon; Mobuzon; Mofesal; Monazan; Monobutyl; Monorheumetten; Reumatox. $C_{13}H_{16}N_2O_2$; mol wt 232.28. C 67.22%, H 6.94%, N 12.06%, O 13.78%. Prepn: Büchi *et al., Helv. Chim. Acta* **36,** 75 (1953); **GB 839057** (1960 to Comm. Farm. Milanese). Toxicity data: Schoetensack, *Arch. Exp. Pathol. Pharmakol.* **233,** 365 (1958).

Crystals from ethanol + water, mp 102-103°. uv max (ethanol): 240, 275 nm ($E_{1cm}^{1\%}$ 443, 245). LD_{50} i.v. in mice: 600 mg/kg (Schoetensack).

THERAP CAT: Anti-inflammatory.

6232. Mofezolac. [78967-07-4] 3,4-Bis(4-methoxyphenyl)-5-isoxazoleacetic acid; 3,4-di(*p*-methoxyphenyl)-5-isoxazoleacetic acid; N-22. $C_{19}H_{17}NO_5$; mol wt 339.34. C 67.25%, H 5.05%, N 4.13%, O 23.57%. Prostaglandin biosynthetase inhibitor. Prepn: R. G. Micetich *et al.,* **EP 26928**; *eidem,* **US 4327222** (1981, 1982 both to CDC Life Sci.). Physico-chemical properties: T. Ushio *et al., Iyakuhin Kenkyu* **22,** 892 (1991). HPLC determn in plasma and urine: T. Marunaka, M. Maniwa, *J. Chromatogr.* **422,** 227 (1987). Pharmacology: K. Tanaka *et al., Yakuri to Chiryo* **18,** 3347 (1990), *C.A.* **114,** 135911 (1991). Acute toxicity: K. Satoh *et al., J. Toxicol. Sci.* **15,** Suppl 2, 1 (1990).

White crystalline powder; slight characteristic odor. mp 147.5°. pKa' ~3.3. uv max (methanol): 236 nm ($\varepsilon = 1.83 \times 10^4$). Soly at 20° (w/v%): DMF 68.7; chloroform 19.5; ethyl acetate 16.5; acetone 7.32; methanol 3.93; anhydr ethanol 3.72; ether 2.90; hexane 2.90×10^{-5}; water 4.85×10^{-3}. Partition coefficient (chloroform/water): 16.6 (pH 6); 1.87 (pH 7); 0.178 (pH 8). LD_{50} in male, female mice, male, female rats (mg/kg): 1528, 1740, 920, 887 orally; 275, 321, 378, 342 i.p.; 612, 545, 572, 510 s.c. (Satoh).

THERAP CAT: Anti-inflammatory; analgesic.

6233. Molindone. [7416-34-4] 3-Ethyl-1,5,6,7-tetrahydro-2-methyl-5-(4-morpholinylmethyl)-4*H*-indol-4-one; 3-ethyl-6,7-dihydro-2-methyl-5-(morpholinomethyl)indol-4(5*H*)-one. $C_{16}H_{24}N_2O_2$; mol wt 276.37. C 69.53%, H 8.75%, N 10.14%, O 11.58%. Prepn: **BE 670798**; I. J. Pachter, K. Schoen, **US 3491093** (1966, 1970 both to Endo). Pharmacology: Sugerman, Herrmann, *Clin. Pharmacol. Ther.* **8,** 261 (1967); Claghorn, *Curr. Ther. Res.* **11,** 524 (1969); Guerrero-Figueroa *et al., ibid.* **15,** 508 (1973). Toxicity study: E. I. Goldenthal, *Toxicol. Appl. Pharmacol.* **18,** 185 (1971).

Crystals, mp 180-181°.
Hydrochloride. [15622-65-8] EN-1733A; Lidone; Moban. LD_{50} orally in rats: 261 mg/kg (Goldenthal).
THERAP CAT: Antipsychotic.

6234. Molsidomine. [25717-80-0] *N*-(Ethoxycarbonyl)-3-(4-morpholinyl)sydnone imine; *N*-carboxy-3-morpholinosydnonimine ethyl ester; morsydomine; SIN-10; Corvaton; Corvasal; Molsidolat; Morial; Motazomin. $C_9H_{14}N_4O_4$; mol wt 242.23. C 44.63%, H 5.83%, N 23.13%, O 26.42%. Coronary vasodilator;

member of a class of non-benzene aromatic, heterocyclic and meso-ionic type of compounds previously unknown in the pharmaceutical industry. Developmental work on sydnone imines: Brookes, Walker, *J. Chem. Soc.* **1957**, 4409. Prepn: K. Masuda *et al.*, **JP 70 6265**; *eidem*, US 3769283 (1970, 1973 both to Takeda); *eidem*, *Chem. Pharm. Bull.* **19**, 72 (1971). Stability studies: Asahi *et al.*, *ibid.* **19**, 1079 (1971). Pharmacological studies: Kikuchi *et al.*, *Jpn. J. Pharmacol.* **20**, 102, 187, 253 (1970); Hashimoto *et al.*, *Arzneim.-Forsch.* **21**, 1329 (1971); T. Nakaguchi *et al.*, *Toho Igakkai Zasshi* **17**, 26 (1970). Metabolism: S. Tanayama *et al.*, *Xenobiotica* **4**, 175 (1974). Pharmacokinetics: R. Bergstrand *et al.*, *Eur. J. Clin. Pharmacol.* **27**, 203 (1984). Clinical trial in angina pectoris: P. A. Majid *et al.*, *N. Engl. J. Med.* **302**, 1 (1980); in hypertension: J. Melei *et al.*, *Eur. J. Clin. Pharmacol.* **18**, 231 (1980). Synergism with penbutolol in angina pectoris: A. E. Balestrini *et al.*, *ibid.* **27**, 1 (1984). Review of pharmacology: R.-E. Nitz, V. B. Fiedler, *Pharmacotherapy* **7**, 28 (1987). *Review: Jpn. Med. Gaz.* **8**(9), 10 (1971); E. Bassenge, W. R. Kukovetz in *New Drugs Annual: Cardiovascular Drugs* Vol. 2, A. Scriabine, Ed. (Raven Press, New York, 1984) pp 177-191.

Colorless crystals or white cryst powder, practically tasteless and odorless, mp 140-141° (toluene). Freely sol in CHCl₃. Sol in dil HCl, ethanol, ethyl acetate, methanol; sparingly sol in water, acetone, benzene. Very slightly sol in ether, petr ether. pK (100°) 3.0 ± 0.1. Most stable in aq solns pH 5-7; least stable in very alkaline solns. uv max (CHCl₃): 326 nm. Sensitive to light of λ <320 mμ. LD₅₀ in male, female mice, male, female rats (mg/kg): 780, 750, 1380, 1350 s.c.; 860, 800, 830, 760 i.v.; 700, 760, 1250, 1250 i.p.; 830, 840, 1050, 1200 orally (Nakaguchi).

THERAP CAT: Antianginal.

6235. Molybdenum. [7439-98-7] Mo; at. wt 95.94; at. no. 42; valences 2,3,4,5,6. Group VIB (6). Naturally occurring isotopes: 98 (23.75%); 96 (16.5%); 95 (15.7%); 92 (15.86%); 94 (9.12%); 100 (9.62%); 97 (9.45%); artificial radioactive isotopes: 88-91; 93; 99; 101-105. Its most important ores are molybdenite, MoS₂, and wulfenite, PbMoO₄. Occurrence in the earth's crust: 1-1.5 ppm. Discovered in 1778 by Scheele; isolated in 1782 by Hjelm. Methods of preparation: L. Northcott, *Molybdenum* (Academic Press, New York, 1956) 222 pp; Hein, Herzog, in *Handbook of Preparative Inorganic Chemistry* vol. 2, G. Brauer, Ed. (Academic Press, New York, 2nd ed., 1965) pp 1401-1402. Important trace element; participates in biochemical redox reactions such as N₂-fixation: Spence, *Coord. Chem. Rev.* **4**, 475 (1969). Physical properties: Worthing, *Phys. Rev.* [2] **25**, 846 (1925); D. R. Stoll, G. C. Sinke, *Thermodynamic Properties of the Elements,* Advances in Chemistry Series **18**, (American Chemical Society, Washington, 1956) pp 23, 130-131. Review of molybdenum and its compds: Rollinson, "Chromium, Molybdenum and Tungsten" in *Comprehensive Inorganic Chemistry* vol. 3, J. C. Bailar Jr. *et al.,* Eds. (Pergamon Press, Oxford, 1973) pp 622-623, 700-742; R. Q. Barr in *Kirk-Othmer Encyclopedia of Chemical Technology* vol. 15 (Wiley-Interscience, New York, 3rd ed., 1981) pp 670-682. Biochemical review: *Bioinorg. Chem.* **II**, K. N. Raymond, Ed. (A.C.S., Washington, 1977) pp 353-430. Symposium on the chemistry and uses of molybdenum and its cmpds: *Polyhedron* **5**, 1-606 (1986).

Dark-gray or black powder with metallic luster or coherent mass of silver-white color; body-centered cubic structure. mp 2622° (Worthing). bp ~4825°. d 10.28. Spec heat 5.68 cal/g-atom/deg; heat of fusion: 6.6 kcal/g-atom; heat of vaporization: 142 kcal/g-atom (Stoll, Sinke). Fairly stable at ordinary temp; oxidized to the trioxide at a red heat; slowly oxidized by steam. Not attacked by water, by dil acids or by concd hydrochloric acid. Practically insol in alkali hydroxides or fused alkalies. Reacts with nitric acid, hot concd sulfuric acid, fused potassium chlorate or nitrate. Attacked by fluorine at ordinary temp, by chlorine or bromine at a red heat.

Caution: Potential symptoms of overexposure to Mo metal in exptl animals are irritation of eyes, nose, throat; anorexia, diarrhea, weight loss; listlessness; liver and kidney damage. Potential symptoms of overexposure to soluble Mo compds in exptl animals are irritation of eyes, nose, throat; anorexia; incoordination; dyspnea, anemia. See *NIOSH Pocket Guide to Chemical Hazards* (DHHS/-NIOSH 97-140, 1997) p 218.

USE: In the form of ferromolybdenum for manufg special steels for tools, boiler plate, rifle barrels, propeller shafts; electrical contacts, spark plugs, x-ray tubes, filaments, screens and grids for radio tubes; in the production of tungsten; glass-to-metal seals; nonferrous alloys; in colloidal form as lubricant additive.

6236. Molybdenum Disulfide. [1317-33-5] MoS₂; mol wt 160.07. Mo 59.94%, S 40.06%. Occurs as the mineral *molybdenite,* which is the principal source of molybdenum. Lab prepn: Bell, Herfert, *J. Am. Chem. Soc.* **79**, 3351 (1957).

Lead-gray, lustrous powder; the artificially prepd sulfide is black and lustrous. d₁₅¹⁵ 5.06; mp 2375°. Begins to sublime at 450°. Insol in water or dil acids.

USE: Dry lubricant and lubricant additive. Hydrogenation catalyst.

6237. Molybdenum Hexafluoride. [7783-77-9] F₆Mo; mol wt 209.93. F 54.30%, Mo 45.70%. MoF₆. Prepd by direct fluorination of powdered molybdenum: Ruff, Ascher, *Z. Anorg. Allg. Chem.* **196**, 418 (1931); from MoO₃ and SF₄: Oppengard *et al.*, *J. Am. Chem. Soc.* **82**, 3825 (1960).

Volatile, white, cubic crystals. Very hygroscopic. d₁ᵢ𝑞¹⁹ 2.543. mp 17.5°. bp 35.0°. Hydrolyzed by water. Forms blue-white clouds in moist air. Soly in anhydr HF: 1.5 moles/1000 g HF, Frlec, Hyman, *Inorg. Chem.* **6**, 1596 (1967). Should be stored in quartz ampuls.

6238. Molybdenum Sesquioxide. [1313-29-7] Mo₂O₃; mol wt 239.88. Mo 79.99%, O 20.01%.

Grayish-black powder. Very slightly sol in acids.

Combination with ferrous sulfate. Mol-Iron (obsolete).

THERAP CAT: Combination with ferrous sulfate as hematinic.

6239. Molybdenum Trioxide. [1313-27-5] Molybdenum oxide (MoO₃); molybdenum(VI) oxide; molybdic anhydride. MoO₃; mol wt 143.94. Mo 66.65%, O 33.35%. Prepn from ammonium molybdate: Schumb, Hartford, *J. Am. Chem. Soc.* **56**, 2613 (1934). Toxicity studies: L. T. Fairhall *et al.*, "The Toxicity of Molybdenum," *U.S. Public Health Service Bulletin No. 293,* Washington DC (1945) 36 pp.

White or slightly yellow to slightly bluish powder or granules. d₄²⁶ 4.696. mp 795°. Melts to dark-yellow liquid which solidifies to a yellowish-white cryst mass; sublimes at higher temp. bp 1155°. Sol in water (28°) 0.490 g/liter. Sol in concd mineral acids, in solns of alkali hydroxides, ammonia or potassium bitartrate; after strong ignition it is very slightly sol in acids.

USE: Chiefly as a reagent for chemical analysis.

6240. Molybdic(VI) Acid. [7782-91-4] H₂MoO₄; mol wt 161.95. H 1.24%, Mo 59.24%, O 39.52%. Prepd as the monohydrate from ammonium molybdate and nitric acid: Hein, Herzog in *Handbook of Preparative Inorganic Chemistry* vol. 2, G. Brauer, Ed. (Academic Press, New York, 2nd ed., 1965) pp 1412-1413.

Monohydrate. White powder. d 3.1. Sparingly soluble in cold, more in hot water; soluble in NH₄OH, H₂SO₄, fixed alkalies.

6241. Mometasone Furoate. [83919-23-7] (11β,16α)-9,21-Dichloro-17-[(2-furanylcarbonyl)oxy]-11-hydroxy-16-methylpregna-1,4-diene-3,20-dione; 9,21-dichloro-11β,17-dihydroxy-16α-methylpregna-1,4-diene-3,20-dione 17-(2-furoate); Sch-32088; Asmanex; Elocon; Nasonex. C₂₇H₃₀Cl₂O₆; mol wt 521.43. C 62.19%, H 5.80%, Cl 13.60%, O 18.41%. Topical corticosteroid. Prepn: E. L. Shapiro, **EP 57401**; *idem*, US 4472393 (1982, 1984 both to Schering Corp.); E. L. Shapiro *et al.*, *J. Med. Chem.* **30**, 1581 (1987). LC-MS-MS determn in plasma: S. Sahasranaman *et al.*, *J. Chromatogr. B* **819**, 175 (2005). Clinical trial in psoriasis: R. S. Medansky *et al.*, *Semin. Dermatol.* **6**, 94 (1987); in seasonal allergic rhinitis: D. Graft *et al.*, *J. Allergy Clin. Immunol.* **98**, 724 (1996).

Crystals from aq methanol, mp 218-220°. $[\alpha]_D^{26}$ +58.3° (dioxane). uv max (methanol): 247 nm (ε 26300). Practically insol in water. Slightly sol in octanol; moderately sol in ethyl alcohol.

THERAP CAT: Anti-inflammatory.

6242. Monacetin. [26446-35-5] 1,2,3-Propanetriol monoacetate; acetin; monoacetin; glyceryl monoacetate. $C_5H_{10}O_4$; mol wt 134.13. C 44.77%, H 7.51%, O 47.71%. $C_3H_7O_2 \cdot$OOC-CH_3. Obtained along with the di- and triacetates by heating glycerol with glacial acetic acid.

Colorless, very hygroscopic liquid; characteristic odor. The commercial product is pale yellow. d_4^{20} 1.206. bp_{17} ~158°; bp_3 129-131°. Soluble in water, alcohol, slightly in ether. Insol in benzene.

USE: In manuf of smokeless powder and dynamite; as a solvent for basic dyes; in tanning leather.

6243. Monarda. American horsemint; wild bergamot. Leaves of *Monarda punctata* L., *Labiatae*. *Habit.* New York to Florida, west to Texas and Wisconsin. *Constit.* Volatile oils: thymol, carvacrol, neryl formate, geranyl formate, cineole, γ-terpinene, α- and β-pinene. Gas chromatographic analysis of the *oil of monarda*: R. W. Scora, *J. Chromatogr.* **19**, 601 (1965).

USE: Source for thymol.

THERAP CAT: Aromatic stimulant, carminative.

6244. Monastrol. [254753-54-3] 1,2,3,4-Tetrahydro-4-(3-hydroxyphenyl)-6-methyl-2-thioxo-5-pyrimidinecarboxylic acid ethyl ester. $C_{14}H_{16}N_2O_3S$; mol wt 292.35. C 57.52%, H 5.52%, N 9.58%, O 16.42%, S 10.97%. Small molecule which inhibits mitotic kinesin motility protein, *Eg5*, thus preventing spindle assembly. Identification of activity: T. U. Mayer *et al., Science* **286**, 971 (1999). Description of preparative technique: K. Lewandowski *et al., J. Comb. Chem.* **1**, 105 (1999). X-ray structure determn and abs config: C. O. Kappe *et al., Tetrahedron* **56**, 1859 (2000). Use as probe for mitotic mechanisms: T. M. Kapoor *et al., J. Cell Biol.* **150**, 975 (2000).

Colorless crystals from ethanol-hexane, mp 184-186°. Sol in DMSO.

USE: Inhibitor of mammalian cell mitosis.

6245. Monellins. Intensely sweet principle from the fruit of the tropical plant *Dioscoreophyllum cumminsii* Diels, *Menispermaceae* ("Serendipity Berry"). First believed to consist of a single polypeptide chain of approx 91 amino acids, mol wt 10,700. Preliminary data and extraction: Inglett, May, *J. Food Sci.* **34**, 408 (1969); Van der Wel, *FEBS Lett.* **21**, 88 (1971); Van der Wel, Loeve, *ibid.* **29**, 181 (1973). Purification: Morris, Cagan, *Biochim. Biophys. Acta* **261**, 114 (1972). Characterized by scientists at the Univ. of Pennsylvania's Monell Chemical Senses Center as the first protein to elicit a sweet taste in man, a "chemostimulatory protein". *See* Morris *et al., J. Biol. Chem.* **248**, 534 (1973); Cagan, *Science* **181**, 32 (1973). Monellin is composed of two nonidentical subunits: Z. Bohak, S. Li, *Biochim. Biophys. Acta* **427**, 153 (1976); the presence of both subunits is necessary for the sweet taste to occur: B. Jirgenson, *ibid.* **446**, 255 (1976). Structure of subunit I: G. Hudson, K. Biemann, *Biochem. Biophys. Res. Commun.* **71**, 212

(1976). Complete amino acid sequence of subunits A and B consisting of 44 and 50 amino acids, resp.: G. Frank, H. Zuber, *Z. Physiol. Chem.* **357**, 585 (1976). Crystallographic studies: A. Wlodawer, K. Hodgson, *Proc. Natl. Acad. Sci. USA* **72**, 398 (1975); G. E. Tomlinson, S. H. Kim, *J. Biol. Chem.* **256**, 12476 (1981).

Water soluble. Approximately 3000 times sweeter than sucrose on a weight basis. Essentially free from carbohydrate: <5 μg/mg protein. uv max (0.01M sodium phosphate buffer): 277 nm.

USE: Potential low-calorie sweetener.

6246. Monensin. [17090-79-8] 2-[5-Ethyltetrahydro-5-[tetrahydro-3-methyl-5-[tetrahydro-6-hydroxy-6-(hydroxymethyl)-3,5-dimethyl-2H-pyran-2-yl]-2-furyl]-2-furyl]-9-hydroxy-β-methoxy-α,γ,2,8-tetramethyl-1,6-dioxaspiro[4.5]decane-7-butyric acid; monensic acid (obsolete); A-3823A. $C_{36}H_{62}O_{11}$; mol wt 670.87. C 64.45%, H 9.32%, O 26.23%. Polyether antibiotic. Major factor in antibiotic complex isolated from *Streptomyces cinnamonensis*. Discovery and isolation: Haney, Hoehn, *Antimicrob. Agents Chemother.* **1967**, 349. Production: Haney, Hoehn, US 3501568 (1970 to Lilly). Structure: Agtarap *et al., J. Am. Chem. Soc.* **89**, 5737 (1967). Crystal structure studies: Lutz *et al., Helv. Chim. Acta* **53**, 1732 (1970); *ibid.* **54**, 1103 (1971). Fermentation studies: Stark *et al., Antimicrob. Agents Chemother.* **1967**, 353. Chemistry: Agtarap, Chamberlin, *ibid.* 359. Stereocontrolled total synthesis: T. Fukuyama *et al., J. Am. Chem. Soc.* **101**, 262 (1979); D. B. Collum *et al., ibid.* **102**, 2117, 2118, 2120 (1980). ^{13}C-NMR study: J. A. Robinson, D. L. Turner, *Chem. Commun.* **1982**, 148. Biosynthesis: Day *et al., Antimicrob. Agents Chemother.* **4**, 410 (1973). *Review:* Stark, "Monensin, A New Biologically Active Compound Produced by a Fermentation Process", in *Fermentation Advances,* Pap. Int. Ferment. Symp., 3rd, **1968**, D. Perlman, Ed. (Academic Press, New York, 1969) pp 517-540.

Crystals, mp 103-105° (monohydrate). $[\alpha]_D$ +47.7°. pKa 6.6 (in 66% DMF). Very stable under alkaline conditions. Slightly sol in water; more sol in hydrocarbons; very sol in other organic solvents. LD_{50} of monensin complex in mice, chicks (mg/kg): 43.8 ± 5.2, 284 ± 47 orally (Haney, Hoehn).

Sodium salt. Coban; Romensin; Rumensin. $C_{36}H_{61}NaO_{11}$; mol wt 692.85. mp 267-269°. $[\alpha]_D$ +57.3° (methanol). Slightly sol in water; more sol in hydrocarbons; very sol in other organic solvents.

THERAP CAT (VET): Coccidiostat. Feed additive to improve feed efficiency in ruminants.

6247. Monoamine Oxidase. [9001-66-5] Amine oxidase; adrenaline oxidase; tyraminase; MAO. Since its first description by Hare in 1928 as an enzyme which catalyzed the oxidative deamination of tyramine, it has been found to be widely distributed in animals. This enzyme, which catalyzes the oxidative deamination of a variety of biogenic amines, such as serotonin, norepinephrine, epinephrine, tyramine and dopamine, deaminates compounds in which the amine group is attached to the terminal carbon group. Enzymes other than the classical amine oxidase which catalyze the oxidative deamination of amines, have been found in animals, plants and bacteria. In contrast to the classical amine oxidase, they are inhibited by carbonyl reagents and do not act on N-substituted amines. Enzymes of this group include: oxidases in microorganisms, *spermine oxidase*, *mescaline oxidase* (of rabbit liver), *plant amine oxidase*, and histaminase, *q.v.* Structural studies: Achee, *Biochemistry* **7**, 4329 (1968). Multiple forms of rat brain monoamine oxidase: M. B. H. Youdim *et al., Nature* **223**, 626 (1969). *Review:* H. Blaschko "Amine Oxidase" in *The Enzymes* **vol. 8**, P. D. Boyer *et al.,* Eds. (Academic Press, New York, 2nd ed., 1963) pp 337-351. Book: *Monoamine Oxidase: Structure, Function and*

Altered Functions, T. P. Singer *et al.,* Eds. (Academic Press, New York, 1980) 557 pp.

6248. Monobenzone. [103-16-2] 4-(Phenylmethoxy)phenol; *p*-(benzyloxy)phenol; hydroquinone monobenzyl ether; hydroquinone benzyl ether; *p*-hydroxyphenyl benzyl ether; benzyl hydroquinone; monobenzyl hydroquinone; Benoquin; Depigman; Pigmex; Benzoquin; Agerite. $C_{13}H_{12}O_2$; mol wt 200.23. C 77.98%, H 6.04%, O 15.98%. Prepd from hydroquinone and benzyl bromide in alcoholic KOH: Schiff, Pellizzari, *Ann.* **221**, 370 (1883). Clinical evaluation: S. W. Becker, Jr., M. C. Spencer, *J. Am. Med. Assoc.* **180**, 279 (1962). Toxicity study: A. Takahashi, E. A. Inglis, *Int. J. Polymer Sci. Technol.* **3**, 93 (1976).

Lustrous leaflets from water, mp 122.5°. Practically insol in cold water. Soly in boiling water ~1.0 g/100 ml. Sol in alcohol, ether, benzene. LD_{50} i.p. in mice: >600 mg/kg (Takahashi).

THERAP CAT: Depigmentor.

6249. Monobutyrin. [557-25-5] Butanoic acid 2,3-dihydroxypropyl ester; 1-butyrylglycerol; α-monobutyrin; glycerol α-monobutyrate; glyceryl 3-monobutyrate. $C_7H_{14}O_4$; mol wt 162.18. C 51.84%, H 8.70%, O 39.46%. Naturally occurring lipid that stimulates angiogenesis. Secreted by differentiating adipocytes; stimulates blood vessel formation and causes vasodilation. The *(R)*-isomer is bioactive. Prepn of optical isomers: E. Abderhalden, E. Eichwald, *Ber.* **48**, 1847 (1915); of L-form: E. Baer, H. O. L. Fischer, *J. Am. Chem. Soc.* **67**, 2031 (1945); S. Gronowitz *et al., Chem. Phys. Lipids* **14**, 174 (1975). Purification from adipocytes and identification of angiogenic activity: D. E. Dobson *et al., Cell* **61**, 223 (1990). Biosynthesis: W. O. Wilkison *et al., J. Biol. Chem.* **266**, 16886 (1991); W. O. Wilkison, B. M. Spiegelman, *ibid.* **268**, 2844 (1993). Effect on retinal circulation and probable role in pathology of diabetes: Y.-D. C. Halvorsen *et al., J. Clin. Invest.* **92**, 2872 (1993).

(R)-Form. [5309-42-2] 3-Butyryl-*sn*-glycerol; L-α-butanoyl glycerol. Cryst from pure ether at −70°. n_D^{20} 1.4493. sp wt 0.8600. $[\alpha]_D^{18}$ −0.63°; $[\alpha]_D^{25}$ −7.40° (c = 2.04 in pyridine).

6250. Monocrotaline. [315-22-0] (13α,14α)-14,19-Dihydro-12,13-dihydroxy-20-norcrotolanan-11,15-dione; crotaline; MCT; NSC-28693; NCI-C56462. $C_{16}H_{23}NO_6$; mol wt 325.36. C 59.06%, H 7.13%, N 4.30%, O 29.50%. Toxic pyrrolizidine alkaloid isolated from *Crotalaria spp.* Isoln: R. Adams, E. F. Rogers, *J. Am. Chem. Soc.* **61**, 2815 (1939); R. B. Tinker, W. M. Lauter, *Econ. Bot.* **10**, 254 (1956); C. C. J. Culvenor, L. W. Smith, *Aust. J. Chem.* **16**, 239 (1963). Structure: R. Adams *et al., J. Am. Chem. Soc.* **74**, 5612 (1952). Stereochemistry: D. J. Robins, D. H. G. Crout, *J. Chem. Soc. C* **1969**, 1386. Crystal structure: H. Stoeckli-Evans, *Acta Crystallogr.* **B35**, 231 (1979). Stereoselective synthesis: H. Niwa *et al., Tetrahedron* **48**, 10531 (1992). ELISA measurment: M. A. Bober *et al., Toxicon* **27**, 1059 (1989). Toxicology: P. M. Newberne *et al., Toxicol. Appl. Pharmacol.* **18**, 387 (1971); R. A. Roth *et al., ibid.* **60**, 193 (1981). Review of carcinogenicity studies: *IARC Monographs* **10**, 291-302, 333-342 (1976). Comprehensive reviews: L. Bull *et al., The Pyrrolizidine Alkaloids* (North-Holland, Amsterdam, 1968) 293 pp; D. J. Robins, *Fortschr. Chem. Org. Naturst.* **41**, 115-203 (1982). Review of pulmonary toxicity: D. W. Wilson *et al., Crit. Rev. Toxicol.* **22**, 307-325 (1992).

White prisms from abs ethanol, mp 197-198° (dec). $[\alpha]_D^{26}$ −54.7° (c = 5.054 in chloroform). Also reported as colorless crystals from ethanol, mp 187-190° (dec). $[\alpha]_D^{12}$ −55.0° (c = 0.16 in $CHCl_3$). uv max (96% ethanol): 217 nm (log ε 3.32), Simánek *et al., Collect. Czech. Chem. Commun.* **34**, 1832 (1969). LD_{50} orally in rats: 71 mg/kg (Newberne).

Hydrochloride. $C_{16}H_{23}NO_6 \cdot HCl$. mp 184° (dec). $[\alpha]_D^{28}$ −38.4° (c = 5.2 in water).

Methiodide. $C_{16}H_{23}NO_6 \cdot CH_3I$. mp 205° (dec). $[\alpha]_D^{28}$ +23.4° (c = 3.1 in methanol).

USE: For inducing pulmonary diseases in rats.

6251. Monocrotophos. [6923-22-4] *(E)*-Phosphoric acid dimethyl [1-methyl-3-(methylamino)-3-oxo-1-propenyl] ester; *(E)*-phosphoric acid dimethyl ester, ester with 3-hydroxy-*N*-methylcrotonamide; 3-(dimethoxyphosphinyloxy)-*N*-methyl-*cis*-crotonamide; dimethyl 2-methylcarbamoyl-1-methylvinyl phosphate; dimethyl phosphate of 3-hydroxy-*N*-methyl-*cis*-crotonamide; C-1414; ENT-27129; SD-9129; Phoskill. $C_7H_{14}NO_5P$; mol wt 223.16. C 37.67%, H 6.32%, N 6.28%, O 35.85%, P 13.88%. General prepn: Whetstone, Stiles, US **2802855**; *see also* Ward, Morales, US **3400177** (1957, 1968 both to Shell). Metabolite of dicrotophos, *q.v.*: Menzer, Casida, *J. Agric. Food Chem.* **13**, 102 (1965). Toxicity study: T. B. Gaines, *Toxicol. Appl. Pharmacol.* **14**, 515 (1969).

Crystals, mp 54-55°. Commercial product is a reddish-brown solid, mp 25-30°. Vapor pressure at 20°: 7×10^6 mm Hg. Misc with water; sol in acetone, ethanol. Practically insol in diesel oils, kerosine. LD_{50} in male, female rats (mg/kg): 17, 20 orally; 126, 112 dermally (Gaines).

Caution: Potential symptoms of overexposure are eye irritation, miosis, blurred vision; dizziness, convulsions; dyspnea; salivation, abdominal cramps, nausea, diarrhea, vomiting. *See NIOSH Pocket Guide to Chemical Hazards* (DHHS/NIOSH 97-140, 1997) p 218.

USE: Insecticide.

6252. Monoctanoin. Monooctanoin; Capmul 8210; Moctanin. Cholesterol solvent used to dissolve gallstones by direct biliary infusion. Semisynthetic mixture of mono- and di-glycerides of octanoic and decanoic acids of which glycerol 1-octanoate is the major component. Description of prepn from coconut oil and use in treatment of gallstones: V. K. Babayan, US **4205086** (1980 to Stokeley-Van Camp). Physical properties and clinical application: J. L. Thistle *et al., Gastroenterology* **78**, 1016 (1980). Factors affecting cholesterol dissolution rate: J. B. Bogardus, *J. Pharm. Sci.* **73**, 906 (1984). Clinical trial: K. R. Palmer, A. F. Hofmann, *Gut* **27**, 196 (1986). Reviews of cholelitholytic agents: G. D. Bell, *Pharmacol. Ther.* **23**, 79-108 (1983); R. J. Fitzgibbons *et al., Surg. Annu.* **21**, 237-262 (1989).

Glycerol 1-octanoate. [502-54-5] Octanoic acid 2,3-dihydroxypropyl ester; caprylic acid α-monoglyceride; α-monocaprylin. $C_{11}H_{22}O_4$; mol wt 218.29. Prepn: L. Hartman, *J. Chem. Soc.* **1959,** 4134. Crystals from light petroleum, mp 39.5-40.5°.

THERAP CAT: Cholelitholytic agent.

6253. Monorden. [12772-57-5] 8-Chloro-1a,14,15,15a-tetrahydro-9,11-dihydroxy-14-methyl-6*H*-oxireno[*e*][2]benzoxacyclotetradecin-6,12(7*H*)-dione; 5-chloro-6-(7,8-epoxy-10-hydroxy-2-oxo-3,5-undecadienyl)-β-resorcylic acid μ-lactone; radicicol. $C_{18}H_{17}ClO_6$; mol wt 364.78. C 59.27%, H 4.70%, Cl 9.72%, O 26.32%. Antibiotic substance from *Monosporium bonorden:* Delmotte, Delmotte-Plaquée, *Nature* **171,** 344 (1953). Identity with radicicol: Mirrington *et al., Tetrahedron Lett.* **1964,** 365. Structure: McCapra, Scott, *ibid.* **1964,** 869; Mirrington *et al., Aust. J. Chem.* **19,** 1265 (1966). Isoln: **NL 6506173** (1965 to Sandoz).

Crystals from chloroform, alcohol or benzene, mp 193.5°. $[\alpha]_D^{20}$ +203° (chloroform). uv max (ethanol): 264, 272 nm (ε 13200, 13100).

Diacetate. $C_{22}H_{21}ClO_8$. Crystals, mp 189°. uv max: 275 nm (ε 13000).

6254. Monosodium Glutamate. [142-47-2] L-Glutamic acid monosodium salt; sodium glutamate; Chinese seasoning; MSG; RL-50; Accent; Aji-no-moto. $C_5H_8NNaO_4$; mol wt 169.11. C 35.51%, H 4.77%, N 8.28%, Na 13.59%, O 37.84%. Prepn: K. Ikeda, S. Suzuki, **GB 9440** (1910), *C.A.* **5,** 836 (1910). Commercial prepn: P. R. Shildneck, **US 2306646** (1942 to Staley Manuf.). Determn in food by HPLC: A. T. Rhys Williams, S. A. Winfield, *Analyst* **107,** 1092 (1982); by LC: O.W. Lau, C. S. Mok, *Anal. Chim. Acta* **302,** 45 (1995). Review of use and biological effects: *Food. Technol.* **41,** 143-154 (1987). *Review:* T. Kawakita, "L-Monosodium Glutamate (MSG)" in *Kirk-Othmer Encyclopedia of Chemical Technology* **Vol. 2** (John Wiley & Sons, New York, 4th ed., 1992) pp 571-579. Review of toxicology: O. U. Eka *et al., Biokemistri* **4,** 57-73 (1994). Book: *Glutamic Acid: Advances in Biochemistry and Physiology* L. J. Filer *et al.,* Eds. (Raven Press, New York, 1979) 416 pp.

White, practically odorless, free flowing crystals often as the monohydrate, dec 225°. Below −0.8°, crystallizes as a pentahydrate which upon filtration and exposure to air becomes the monohydrate. $[\alpha]^{20}$ −3.5° (10% soln in 5° Bé HCl). $[\alpha]_D^{20}$ +25.16° (10g MSG/100ml 2*N* HCl). d^{20} (saturated water soln): 1.620. pH of 5% water soln: 6.8; of 3% soln (25°): 7.0. Soly at 20° (g/100g): 41.7 water. LD_{50} i.g. in mice: 19.9 g/kg (Eka).

USE: Flavor enhancer.

6255. Monotropein. [5945-50-6] [1*S*-(1α,4aα,7β,7aα)]-1-(β-D-Glucopyranosyloxy)-1,4a,7,7a-tetrahydro-7-hydroxy-7-(hydroxymethyl)cyclopenta[*c*]pyran-4-carboxylic acid. $C_{16}H_{22}O_{11}$; mol wt 390.34. C 49.23%, H 5.68%, O 45.09%. From herb of *Monotropa hypopitys* L., *Ericaceae:* Bridel, *Compt. Rend.* **176,** 1742 (1923); *Bull. Soc. Chim. Biol.* **5,** 722 (1923). Structure: Inouye *et al., Tetrahedron Lett.* **1963,** 1031; Bobbitt *et al., Chem. Ind. (London)* **1964,** 931. Stereochemistry: Norio *et al., Tetrahedron Lett.* **1967,** 2367. GC-mass spec studies: H. Inouye *et al., J. Chromatogr.* **118,** 201 (1976). Purgative activity: *eidem, Planta Med.* **25,** 285 (1976).

Monohydrate. Needles from water, dec 170-173°. $[\alpha]_D^{18}$ −127.7° (water). uv max: 235 nm (log ε 3.98). Soluble in water, alcohol. Practically insol in ethyl acetate.

Pentaacetate. $C_{26}H_{32}O_{16}$. Crystals, mp 173-174.5°. $[\alpha]_D^{18}$ −82.5° (ethanol).

6256. Monsel's Solution. [1310-45-8] Ferric subsulfate solution. First described in 1856 by L. Monsel. Prepd by oxidizing ferrous sulfate with nitric acid in the presence of sulfuric acid. Prepn: W. Procter, Jr., *Am. J. Pharm.* **31,** 403 (1859). Review of chemistry and mechanism of action: E. Epstein, H. I. Maibach, *Arch. Dermatol.* **90,** 226-228 (1964); of hemostatic applications: A. B. Jetmore *et al., Dis. Colon Rectum* **36,** 866-867 (1993); of history: A. P. Garrett *et al., J. Lower Genital Tract Dis.* **6,** 225-227 (2002).

Reddish-brown liquid. Almost odorless; strongly astringent taste. May be dried at >95°F to produce brilliant red scales. Sol in water, alcohol. Acid to litmus. d^{25} 1.548.

THERAP CAT: Hemostatic.

THERAP CAT (VET): Hemostatic, astringent.

6257. Montan Wax. [8002-53-7] Lignite wax. Obtained by extraction from lignite. Asphalt and resin content and physical properties vary with source of lignite. Brief review: C. S. Letcher in *Kirk-Othmer Encyclopedia of Chemical Technology* **vol. 24** (Wiley-Interscience, New York, 3rd ed., 1984) pp 471-472.

Dark-brown lumps; white or nearly white when bleached. mp 80-86°. Saponification number 88-112. Insol in water. Sol in benzene, chloroform, carbon tetrachloride, hot petr ether; incompletely sol in hot ether or boiling alcohol.

USE: Electric cable insulators; in polishes instead of carnauba wax; manuf candles, waterproof paints and varnishes.

6258. Montelukast. [158966-92-8] 1-[[[(1*R*)-1-[3-[(1*E*)-2-(7-Chloro-2-quinolinyl)ethenyl]phenyl]-3-[2-(1-hydroxy-1-methylethyl)phenyl]propyl]thio]methyl]cyclopropaneacetic acid. $C_{35}H_{36}ClNO_3S$; mol wt 586.18. C 71.71%, H 6.19%, Cl 6.05%, N 2.39%, O 8.19%, S 5.47%. Selective cysteinyl leukotriene type 1 receptor antagonist. Prepn: M. L. Belley *et al.,* **EP 480717;** *eidem,* **US 5565473** (1992, 1996 both to Merck Frosst); M. Labelle *et al., Bioorg. Med. Chem. Lett.* **5,** 283 (1995). Pharmacological profile: T. R. Jones *et al., Can. J. Physiol. Pharmacol.* **73,** 191 (1995). LC determn in human plasma: R. D. Amin *et al., J. Pharm. Biomed. Anal.* **13,** 155 (1995). Review of pharmacology and clinical efficacy in asthma: A. Markham, D. Faulds, *Drugs* **56,** 251-256 (1998). Clinical trial in pediatric asthma: B. Knorr *et al., J. Am. Med. Assoc.* **279,** 1181 (1998); with loratadine, *q.v.,* in allergic rhinitis: E. O. Meltzer *et al., J. Allergy Clin. Immunol.* **105,** 917 (2000). Comparison with cetirizine, *q.v.,* in urticaria: M. L. Pacor *et al., Clin. Exp. Allergy* **31,** 1607 (2001). Review of pharmacology and clinical experience: Z. Diamant, A. P. Sampson, *J. Drug Eval. Respir. Med.* **1,** 53-88 (2002).

Monosodium salt. [151767-02-1] MK-476; Singulair. C_{35}-$H_{35}ClNNaO_3S$; mol wt 608.17. Hygroscopic, white to off-white powder. Freely sol in ethanol, methanol, water. Practically insol in acetonitrile.

THERAP CAT: Antiasthmatic.

6259. Monteplase. [122007-85-6] 84-L-Serine-plasminogen activator (human tissue-type protein moiety reduced); E-6010; Cleactor. Genetically engineered variant of human tissue plasminogen activator (t-PA), *q.v.*, constructed with a single amino acid substitution in the epidermal growth factor domain. Prepn: E. R. Mulvihill *et al.*, **EP 293936** (1988 to ZymoGenetics; Novo; Eisai); *idem et al.*, **US 5486471** (1996 to ZymoGenetics). Thrombolytic properties: S. Suzuki *et al.*, *J. Cardiovasc. Pharmacol.* **17**, 738 (1991). Pharmacology and pharmacokinetics: *eidem, ibid.* **22**, 834 (1993). Clinical trial in treatment of myocardial infarction: C. Kawai *et al.*, *J. Am. Coll. Cardiol.* **29**, 1447 (1997); prior to angioplasty: T. Inoue *et al.*, *Am. J. Cardiol.* **95**, 506 (2005).

THERAP CAT: Thrombolytic.

6260. Montmorillonite. [1318-93-0] A clay forming the principal constituent of bentonite and fuller's earth. Approximate formula: $R_{0.33}^+(Al,Mg)_2Si_4O_{10}(OH)_2 \cdot nH_2O$ where R^+, in natural material, includes one or more of the cations Na^+, K^+, Mg^{2+}, and Ca^{2+}, and possibly others.

Caution: Inhalation of the dust can cause respiratory irritation.

USE: In industrial chromatographic technique, *e.g.*, **US 2626888** and **GB 697060** (1953 to Merck & Co.), describing the elution of vitamin B_{12}-active substances adsorbed on montmorillonite adsorbents. Widely used in the petroleum industry. Also as catalyst carrier.

6261. Monuron. [150-68-5] N'-(4-Chlorophenyl)-N,N-dimethylurea; 1,1-dimethyl-3-(p-chlorophenyl)urea; CMU; Karmex Monuron Herbicide; Telvar. $C_9H_{11}ClN_2O$; mol wt 198.65. C 54.42%, H 5.58%, Cl 17.85%, N 14.10%, O 8.05%. Prepd by reacting p-chlorophenyl isocyanate with dimethylamine: Bucha, Todd, *Science* **114**, 493 (1951); *see also* **US 2655444**; **US 2655445**; **US 2655446**; **US 2655447**. Toxicity study: G. W. Bailey, J. L. White, *Residue Rev.* **10**, 97 (1965). *Review:* McCall, *Agric. Chem.* **7**, 40 (1952).

Thin rectangular prisms from methanol, mp 170.5-171.5° (the commercial product melts at 176-177°). Vapor pressure at 25°: 5 $\times 10^{-7}$ mm; at 100°: 178 $\times 10^{-5}$ mm. Slight odor. Stable toward oxygen and moisture under ordinary conditions at neutral pH; elevated temps and more acid or alkaline conditions appreciably raise rate of hydrolysis. Very slightly sol in water and in no. 3 Diesel oil: About 230 ppm at 25°. pH of satd aq soln 6.26. Moderately sol in methanol, ethanol, acetone. Practically insol in hydrocarbon solvents. LD_{50} orally in rats: 3700 mg/kg (Bailey, White).

Trichloroacetate. Monuron TCA; Urox. $C_9H_{11}ClN_2O.C_2H$-Cl_3O_2; mol wt 362.04. Prepn: Gilbert *et al.*, **US 2782112** (1957 to Allied Chem.). Effective in control of both weeds and grasses. mp 78-81°.

Caution: Anemia and methemoglobinemia have been produced in experimental animals.

USE: Herbicide.

6262. Moore's Ketene. [29342-22-1] 2-Carbonyl-3,3-dimethylbutanenitrile; *tert*-butylcyanoketene. C_7H_9NO; mol wt 123.15. C 68.27%, H 7.37%, N 11.37%, O 12.99%. Reacts via ene insertion reactions into σ bonds. Prepn: H. W. Moore, W. Weyler, Jr., *J. Am. Chem. Soc.* **92**, 4132 (1970). Reaction with cyclopropanes: M. D. Gheorghiu *et al.*, *J. Org. Chem.* **55**, 3713 (1990). Cycloaddition reactions with vinylarenes: S. V. Sereda *et al.*, *Struct. Chem.* **4**, 333 (1993); M. D. Gheorghiu *et al.*, *Rev. Roum. Chim.* **40**, 653 (1995).

USE: Reagent in cycloaddition reactions.

6263. Moperone. [1050-79-9] 1-(4-Fluorophenyl)-4-[4-hydroxy-4-(4-methylphenyl)-1-piperidinyl]-1-butanone; *p*-fluoro-4-(4′-hydroxy-4′-*p*-tolylpiperidino)butyrophenone; *p*-fluoro-4-(4′-hydroxy-4′-*p*-methylphenylpiperidino)butyrophenone; 1-(3′-*p*-fluorobenzoylpropyl)-4-hydroxy-4-*p*-tolylpiperidine; ω-(4-hydroxy-4-*p*-tolylpiperidino)-*p*-fluorobutyrophenone; methylperidol; R-1658. $C_{22}H_{26}FNO_2$; mol wt 355.45. C 74.34%, H 7.37%, F 5.34%, N 3.94%, O 9.00%. Prepn: Janssen *et al.*, *J. Med. Pharm. Chem.* **1**, 281 (1959); Janssen, **GB 881893** (1961).

Crystals, mp 118-119.5°. uv max: 246.5 nm (ε 12200).

Hydrochloride. [3871-82-7] Luvatren. $C_{22}H_{26}FNO_2.HCl$; mol wt 391.91. Crystals from isopropyl ether, mp 216-218°.

THERAP CAT: Antipsychotic.

6264. Moprolol. [5741-22-0] 1-(2-Methoxyphenoxy)-3-[(1-methylethyl)amino]-2-propanol; 1-(isopropylamino)-3-(*o*-methoxyphenoxy)-2-propanol. $C_{13}H_{21}NO_3$; mol wt 239.31. C 65.25%, H 8.84%, N 5.85%, O 20.06%. β-Adrenergic blocker. Prepn: C. D. Lunsford *et al.*, *J. Am. Chem. Soc.* **82**, 1166 (1960); **NL 301580** corresp to A. F. Crowther, L. H. Smith, **US 3501769** (1965, 1970 both to ICI); A. F. Crowther *et al.*, *J. Med. Chem.* **12**, 638 (1969). Pharmacology: G. Croce *et al.*, *Arzneim.-Forsch.* **20**, 1074 (1970). Anti-anginal and hemodynamic effects: M. Radice *et al., ibid.* **28**, 2160 (1978). Resolution of enantiomers: G. Ferrari, V. Vecchietti, **EP 15418**; *eidem,* **US 4683245** (1980, 1987 both to Simes). Synthesis of (−)-form: K. Kan *et al.*, *Agric. Biol. Chem.* **49**, 207 (1985). Bioavailability of (−)-form in dog: A. Marzo, J. P. Desager, *Curr. Ther. Res.* **30**, 442 (1981). Pharmacokinetics of racemate and (−)-form: C. Harvengt, J. P. Desager, *Int. J. Clin. Pharmacol. Ther. Toxicol.* **20**, 57 (1982). Clinical comparison of antihypertensive activity of enantiomers: P. Ghirardi, F. Grosso, *J. Cardiovasc. Pharmacol.* **2**, 471 (1980). Clinical studies of (−)-form in hypertension: G. Vrebos *et al.*, *Curr. Ther. Res.* **29**, 654 (1981); H. Hoeffkes, *ibid.* **30**, 88 (1981).

Crystals from cyclohexane, mp 82-83°.

Hydrochloride. [27058-84-0] SD-1601; Omeral. $C_{13}H_{21}$-$NO_3.HCl$; mol wt 275.77. Crystals, mp 110-112°.

l-**Form.** [77164-20-6] Levomoprolol. Crystals from ethyl acetate, mp 78-80°. $[\alpha]$ −5.5 ±0.2° (c = 5.0 in ethanol).

l-**Form hydrochloride.** [113482-87-4] Levotensin. Crystals from ethyl acetate/95% ethanol, mp 121-123°. $[\alpha]_D^{25}$ −16.3° (c = 5.0 in ethanol).

THERAP CAT: Antihypertensive.

6265. MOPS. [1132-61-2] 4-Morpholinepropanesulfonic acid; 3-(*N*-morpholino)propanesulfonic acid; *N*-(3-sulfopropyl)-morpholine. $C_7H_{15}NO_4S$; mol wt 209.26. C 40.18%, H 7.23%, N 6.69%, O 30.58% S 15.32%. One of the zwitterionic amino acids known as "Good" buffers; active in the pH range of 6.5-8.0. Prepn: C. F. H. Allen *et al., J. Med. Pharm. Chem.* **1**, 281 (1959); N. E. Good, S. Izawa, "Hydrogen Ion Buffers," in *Methods Enzymol.* **24**, 53-65 (1972). Temperature effects on pK: M. Sankar, R. G. Bates, *Anal. Chem.* **50**, 1922 (1978); and pH: R. N. Roy *et al., Cryo-Lett.*

6, 139 (1985). Effects on "Lowry" protein determn: H. M. Himmel, W. Heller, *J. Clin. Chem. Clin. Biochem.* **25,** 909 (1987). Uses as a biological buffer: E. P. Paques *et al., Eur. J. Biochem.* **107,** 447 (1980); L. A. Sonna *et al., J. Biol. Chem.* **263,** 6625 (1988).

White powder, mp 283.5-284.5°. pKa 7.15. pKa_2 (25°): 7.184; (37°): 7.041. $\Delta pKa/°C$ −0.013. Is not completely stable when autoclaved in the presence of glucose.

USE: Biological buffer.

6266. Morantel. [20574-50-9] *(E)*-1,4,5,6-Tetrahydro-1-methyl-2-[2-(3-methyl-2-thienyl)ethenyl]pyrimidine. $C_{12}H_{16}N_2S$; mol wt 220.33. C 65.41%, H 7.32%, N 12.71%, S 14.55%. Prepn: Austin *et al.*, **GB 1120587** (1968 to Pfizer).

Crystals from chloroform + benzene, mp 239-241°.
Citrate monohydrate. Exhelm. $C_{12}H_{16}N_2S.C_6H_8O_7.H_2O$; mol wt 430.47.
Tartrate. [26155-31-7] CP-12009-18; Paratect; Suiminth. $C_{12}H_{16}N_2S.C_4H_6O_6$; mol wt 370.42.
THERAP CAT (VET): Anthelmintic.

6267. Morazone. [6536-18-1] 1,2-Dihydro-1,5-dimethyl-4-[(3-methyl-2-phenyl-4-morpholinyl)methyl]-2-phenyl-*3H*-pyrazol-3-one; 4-[(3-methyl-2-phenylmorpholino)methyl]antipyrine; 1-phenyl-2,3-dimethyl-4-(2'-phenyl-3'-methylmorpholinomethyl)-5-pyrazolone; R-445; Tarugan. $C_{23}H_{27}N_3O_2$; mol wt 377.48. C 73.18%, H 7.21%, N 11.13%, O 8.48%. Prepn: Hengen *et al., Arzneim.-Forsch.* **8,** 421 (1958); Siemer, Doppstadt, **US 2943022**; **US 3005818** (1960, 1961 both to Ravensberg Chem.). Metabolism: Cartoni *et al., J. Chromatogr.* **84,** 419 (1973).

Crystals, mp 149-150°. Freely sol in chloroform; sol in methanol, acetone; slightly sol in ether.
Hydrochloride. [50321-35-2] $C_{23}H_{27}N_3O_2.HCl$. Crystals from methanol + acetone, mp 171-172° (dec). Sol in water.
THERAP CAT: Analgesic; anti-inflammatory; antipyretic.

6268. Moricizine. [31883-05-3] [10-[3-(4-Morpholinyl)-1-oxopropyl]-10*H*-phenothiazin-2-yl]carbamic acid ethyl ester; 10-(3-morpholinopropionyl)phenothiazine-2-carbamic acid ethyl ester; ethmosine; ethmozin; moracizine; EN-313. $C_{22}H_{25}N_3O_4S$; mol wt 427.52. C 61.81%, H 5.89%, N 9.83%, O 14.97%, S 7.50%. Sodium channel blocker. Prepn: A. Gritsenko *et al.,* **DE 2014201** (1971 to Acad. Med. Sci., USSR), *C.A.* **76,** 34273a (1972); *eidem,* **US 3740395** (1973). Pharmacology and toxicity: N. V. Kaverina *et al., Russ. Pharmacol. Toxicol.* **35,** 74 (1972). Mechanism of action study: T. Yamane *et al., Br. J. Pharmacol.* **108,** 812 (1993). HPLC determn in plasma: C. C. Whitney *et al., J. Pharm. Sci.* **70,** 462 (1981). Symposium on pharmacology, pharmacokinetics, clinical safety and efficacy: *Am. J. Cardiol.* **65,** 1D-71D (1990). *Review:* C. A. Clyne *et al., N. Engl. J. Med.* **327,** 255 (1992).

Crystals, mp 156-157°. pKa 6.4.
Hydrochloride. [29560-58-5] Ethmozine. $C_{22}H_{25}N_3O_4S.$-HCl; mol wt 463.98. Crystals from dichloroethane, mp 189° (dec). Sol in water, alcohol. LD_{50} in mice, rats (mg/kg): 36, 12 i.v.; in mice (mg/kg): 131 i.p. (Kaverina).
THERAP CAT: Antiarrhythmic (class I).

6269. Morin. [480-16-0] 2-(2,4-Dihydroxyphenyl)-3,5,7-trihydroxy-*4H*-1-benzopyran-4-one; 2′,3,4′,5,7-pentahydroxyflavone; 2′-hydroxypelargidenolon 1522; C.I. Natural Yellow 8; C.I. Natural Yellow 11; C.I. 75660. $C_{15}H_{10}O_7$; mol wt 302.24. C 59.61%, H 3.33%, O 37.06%. In wood of old fustic (*Chlorophora tinctoria* (L.) Gaud., *Moraceae*), also called Cuba wood, or yellow Brazil wood. The wood of the Osage orange tree also contains morin and maclurin. Isoln: Perkin, Pate, *J. Chem. Soc.* **67,** 649 (1895); Rolland, *Teintex* **3,** 460 (1938). Synthesis by condensing phloracetophenone dimethyl ether with 2,4-dimethoxybenzaldehyde: von Kostanecki *et al., Ber.* **39,** 625, 4014, 4022 (1906). Comprehensive list of refs in *Colour Index* **vol. 4** (3rd ed., 1971) p 4636.

Crystallizes with 1 or 2 mols water. Anhydr needles from abs alcohol, dec 285-290°. One gram dissolves in 4 liters water at 20°, in 1060 ml boiling water. Freely sol in alcohol; slightly sol in ether, acetic acid. Sol in aq alkaline solns with intense yellow color which turns brown on exposure to air. Absorption spectrum: Grinbaumowna, Marchlewski, *Biochem. Z.* **290,** 261 (1937).
Calico yellow. Obtained by the action of bisulfite on fustic extract consists mainly of the bisulfite compound of morin, $C_{15}H_{10}$-O_7 + $NaHSO_3$, and is used in calico printing. The calico yellow of commerce is a good source of morin for the laboratory. The bisulfite is removed with HCl.
USE: As a spot test reagent for Al, Be, Zn, Ga, In, and Sc salts: Feigl, *Spot Tests* (New York, 1954); Beck, *Mikrochim. Acta* **2,** 287 (1937). As luminescence indicator: Kocsis, Zádor, *Z. Anal. Chem.* **124,** 42-45 (1942). As a textile dye, morin dyes wool mordanted with chromium: olive yellow; mordanted with aluminum: yellow; mordanted with tin: lemon yellow; mordanted with iron: deep olive brown.

6270. Morindin. [60450-21-7] 1,5-Dihydroxy-2-methyl-6-[(6-*O*-β-D-xylopyranosyl-β-D-glucopyranosyl)oxy]-9,10-anthracenedione; 2-[[6-*O*-(6-deoxy-α-L-mannopyranosyl)-β-D-glucopyranosyl]oxy]-1,5-dihydroxy-6-methyl-9,10-anthracenedione. C_{27}-$H_{30}O_{14}$; mol wt 578.52. C 56.05%, H 5.23%, O 38.72%. From bark of *Coprosma australis* Forst. (*C. grandifolia* Hook.), *Rubiaceae*: Briggs, Dacre, *J. Chem. Soc.* **1948,** 564. Structure: Briggs, Le Quesne, *ibid.* **1963,** 3471. On acid hydrolysis yields the aglucone *morindone*. Synthesis and structure proof: B. Vermes *et al., Phytochemistry* **19,** 119 (1980).

Yellow needles from glacial acetic acid, mp 169-171°. $[\alpha]_D^{20}$ −90.0° (c = 0.054 in dioxane). Absorption max (ethanol): 230,

261, 448 nm (log ε 4.15, 3.93, 3.57). Sol in cold water but on boiling forms a water insol form, **β-morindin**. Sol in dioxane, pyridine, acetone, methanol; slightly sol in ethanol, glacial acetic acid. Practically insol in ether, chloroform, benzene, petr ether.

6271. Moroctocog Alfa. (1-742)-(1637-1648)-Blood coagulation factor VIII (human reduced) complex with 1649-2332-blood coagulation factor VIII (human reduced); r-VIII SQ; Refacto. B-domain deleted form of factor VIII produced in Chinese hamster ovary cells by recombinant DNA technology. Prepn: A. Almstedt *et al.*, **WO 9109122** (1991 to KabiVitrum); P. Lind *et al.*, *Eur. J. Biochem.* **232**, 19 (1995). Stability of albumin-free preparation: T. Osterberg *et al.*, *Pharm. Res.* **14**, 892 (1997). Clinical pharmacokinetics: K. Fijnvandraat *et al.*, *Thromb. Haemostasis* **77**, 298 (1997). Review of development and clinical experience: E. Berntorp, *ibid.* **78**, 256-260 (1997).

THERAP CAT: Antihemophilic factor.

6272. Moroxydine. [3731-59-7] *N*-(Aminoiminomethyl)-4-morpholinecarboximidamide; 4-morpholinecarboximidoylguanidine; N^1,N^1-anhydrobis(β-hydroxyethyl)biguanide; abitilguanide; abitylguanide; ABOB; Virusmin. $C_6H_{13}N_5O$; mol wt 171.20. C 42.09%, H 7.65%, N 40.91%, O 9.35%. Prepn: **GB 776176** (1957 to AB Kabi). Proposed as influenza suppressant: Melander, *Antibiot. Chemother.* **10**, 39 (1960).

Hydrochloride. [3160-91-6] Flumidin; Virustat. $C_6H_{13}N_5$-O.HCl; mol wt 207.66. Crystals.

THERAP CAT: Antiviral.

6273. Morphazinamide. [952-54-5] *N*-(4-Morpholinylmethyl)pyrazinecarboxamide; *N*-morpholinomethylpyrazinamide; morfazinamide; morinamide; B-2310. $C_{10}H_{14}N_4O_2$; mol wt 222.24. C 54.04%, H 6.35%, N 25.21%, O 14.40%. Prepn from pyrazinamide, morpholine, and formalin: Felder, Tiepolo, **DE 1129492** (1962 to Bracco).

Crystals, mp 118.5-119.5°. uv max (ethanol): 269, 317 nm (log ε 3.95, 2.77). One gram dissolves in 3 ml water, 30 ml ethanol, 30 ml benzene, 2.5 ml chloroform.

Hydrochloride. [1473-73-0] B-2311; Piazofolina; Piazolin. $C_{10}H_{14}N_4O_2$.HCl; mol wt 258.70. Crystals, mp 196°. One gram dissolves in 2 ml water, 350 ml ethanol, 2000 ml chloroform.

THERAP CAT: Antibacterial (tuberculostatic).

6274. Morpheridine. [469-81-8] 1-[2-(Morpholinyl)ethyl]-4-phenyl-4-piperidinecarboxylic acid ethyl ester; 1-(2-morpholinoethyl)-4-phenylisonipecotic acid ethyl ester; ethyl 1-(2′-morpholinoethyl)-4-phenylpiperidine-4-carboxylate; morpholinoethyl norpethidine. $C_{20}H_{30}N_2O_3$; mol wt 346.46. C 69.33%, H 8.73%, N 8.09%, O 13.85%. Prepn: Anderson *et al.*, *J. Chem. Soc.* **1956**, 4088; Stern, Anderson, **US 2795581** (1957 to J. F. Macfarlan). HPLC determn: I. Jane, A. McKinnon, *J. Chromatogr.* **323**, 191 (1985). Analgesic activity in rats: R. A. Millar, R. P. Stephenson, *Br. J. Pharmacol.* **11**, 27 (1956). Pharmacology: A. F. Green, N. B. Ward, *ibid.* 32.

Liquid. bp$_{0.5}$ 188-192°. n_D^{18} 1.5276.

Dihydrochloride. TA-1. $C_{20}H_{30}N_2O_3$.2HCl; mol wt 419.39. Crystals from dil ethanol, mp 264-266° (dec). LD$_{50}$ in mice (mg/kg): 45 i.v. (Green, Ward); 118 i.p. (Millar, Stephenson).

Note: This is a controlled substance (opiate): **21 CFR**, 1308.11.

6275. Morphinan. [468-10-0] [4a*R*(4aα,10α,10aα)]-1,3,4,-9,10,10a-Hexahydro-2*H*-10,4a-(iminoethano)phenanthrene; 1,2,3,-9,10,10a-hexahydro-10,4a(4*H*)-iminoethanophenanthrene. C_{16}-$H_{21}N$; mol wt 227.34. C 84.53%, H 9.31%, N 6.16%. Parent substance of the morphine alkaloids, codeine, thebaine, etc. Prepd from 1-benzyl-1,2,3,4,5,6,7,8-octahydro-2-methylisoquinoline: Grewe, Mondon, *Ber.* **81**, 279 (1948); from β-cyclohexenyl-*N*-phenacylethylamine: Grewe *et al.*, *Ber.* **84**, 527 (1951).

Oily liq, bp$_{0.05}$ 115°.

Hydrochloride. Crystals from acetone + ether, dec 229°.

Sulfate. Crystals from alcohol + ether, dec 195°.

N-**Methylmorphinan.** Crystals, mp 61°.

6276. Morphine. [57-27-2]; [6009-81-0] (monohydrate). (5α,6α)-7,8-Didehydro-4,5-epoxy-17-methylmorphinan-3,6-diol; morphium; morphia. $C_{17}H_{19}NO_3$; mol wt 285.34. C 71.56%, H 6.71%, N 4.91%, O 16.82%. Principal alkaloid of opium, *q.v.*; also found endogenously in various animal tissues including brain, blood and liver. Isoln: F. W. A. Sertürner, *Trommsdorff's J. Pharm.* **13**, 234 (1805); W. Gregory, *Ann.* **7**, 261 (1833). Extraction procedure: L. B. Achor, E. M. K. Geiling, *Anal. Chem.* **26**, 1061 (1954). Structure: J. M. Gulland, R. Robinson, *J. Chem. Soc.* **123**, 980 (1923). Total synthesis: M. Gates, G. Tschudi, *J. Am. Chem. Soc.* **74**, 1109 (1952); **78**, 1380 (1956). Biogenesis: E. Leete, *J. Am. Chem. Soc.* **81**, 3948 (1959). Cystallographic study: M. Mackay, D. C. Hodgkin, *J. Chem. Soc.* **1955**, 3261. Configuration: J. Kalvoda *et al.*, *Helv. Chim. Acta* **38**, 1847 (1955). Toxicity data: M. E. Buchwald, G. S. Eadie, *J. Pharmacol. Exp. Ther.* **71**, 197 (1941). GC-MS determn in biological fluids: R. Wasels, F. Belleville, *J. Chromatogr. A* **674**, 225 (1994). Comprehensive description: F. J. Muhtadi, *Anal. Profiles Drug Subs.* **17**, 259-366 (1988). Review of syntheses: T. Hudlicky *et al.* in *Studies in Natural Products Chemistry*, Vol. 18, Atta-ur-Rahman, Ed. (Elsevier, Amsterdam, 1996) pp 43-154; J. Zezula, T. Hudlicky, *Synlett* **2005**, 388-405. Review of physiological role of endogenous morphine: G. B. Stefano *et al.*, *Trends Neurosci.* **23**, 436-442 (2000). Review of clinical experience in pain management: S. Donnelly *et al.*, *Support. Care Cancer* **10**, 13-35 (2002); of pharmacokinetics and metabolism in long term treatment: G. Andersen *et al.*, *J. Pain Symptom Manage.* **25**, 74-91 (2003).

Small rhombic prisms or needles from dil alc as the monohydrate. Becomes anhydrous at 100°, mp 253-254° with decompn. d_4^{20} 1.32. $[α]_D^{25}$ −132° (methanol). pKb at 20° = 6.13; pKa 9.85. pH of satd soln, 8.5. uv max in acid: 285 nm; in alkali: 298 nm. One gram dissolves in about 5000 ml water, 1100 ml boiling water, 210 ml alcohol, 98 ml boiling alc, 1220 ml chloroform, 6250 ml ether, 114 ml amyl alc, 10 ml boiling methanol, 525 ml ethyl acetate. Freely sol in solns of fixed alkali and alkaline earth hydroxides, in phenol, cresols; moderately sol in mixtures of chloroform with alcohols; slightly sol in ammonia, benzene.

Hydrochloride. [52-26-6] $C_{17}H_{19}NO_3 \cdot HCl$; mol wt 321.80. Occurs as the trihydrate. White flakes or crystalline powder; bitter taste. Loses its water of crystn at about 100° and usually becomes yellowish. mp about 200° (dec). $[\alpha]_D^{25}$ −113.5° (c = 2.2 in H_2O, anhydr basis). One gram dissolves in 17.5 ml water, 0.5 ml boiling water, 52 ml alc, 6 ml alc at 60°; slowly sol in glycerol. Insol in chloroform, ether. pH about 5. *Protect from light.* LD_{50} in mice (mg/kg): 226-318 i.v. (Buchwald, Eadie).

Sulfate Pentahydrate. [6211-15-0]; [64-31-3] (anhydrous). Morphine hemisulfate; Avinza; Dolcontin; Kadian; Kapanol; Morcap; Moscontin; MS Contin; MSIR; MST Continus; Oramorph; Sevredol. $2C_{17}H_{19}NO_3 \cdot H_2SO_4 \cdot 5H_2O$; mol wt 758.83. White, fine odorless crystals or powder, or cubical masses. Loses some H_2O at ordinary temp; about $3H_2O$ (7.1%) at 100°, the remainder at 130°. Discolors on exposure to light. mp ~250° with decompn when anhydr. $[\alpha]_D^{25}$ −108.7° (c = 4 in H_2O, anhydr basis). pKa 7.9. Partition coefficient (*n*-octanol/water): 1.42 (at physiological pH). One gram dissolves in 15.5 ml water at 25°, 0.7 ml water at 80°, 565 ml alcohol, 240 ml alcohol at 60°. Insol in chloroform, ether. pH about 4.8. *Keep well closed and protected from light.*

Note: This is a controlled substance (opiate): **21 CFR**, 1308.12.

THERAP CAT: Analgesic (narcotic).

THERAP CAT (VET): Analgesic (narcotic), preanesthetic, antitussive, antiperistaltic.

6277. Morpholine. [110-91-8] Tetrahydro-2*H*-1,4-oxazine; tetrahydro-1,4-oxazine; diethylene oximide; diethylene imidoxide. C_4H_9NO; mol wt 87.12. C 55.15%, H 10.41%, N 16.08%, O 18.36%. Prepd by dehydrating diethanolamine: Knorr, *Ann.* **301**, 1 (1898); Jones, Burns, *J. Am. Chem. Soc.* **47**, 2966 (1925); Hampton, Pollard, *ibid.* **58**, 2338 (1936). Toxicity study: H. F. Smyth *et al., Arch. Ind. Hyg. Occup. Med.* **10**, 61 (1954). Review of morpholine and derivatives: A. L. Wilson, *Ind. Eng. Chem.* **27**, 867-871 (1935). *Monograph:* Morpholine Technical Bulletin, Jefferson Chemical Co. (New York, 1953).

Mobile, hygroscopic liquid. Characteristic amine odor. mp −4.9°. bp_{760} 128.9°; bp_6 20.0°. d_4^{20} 1.007. n_D^{20} 1.4540. Volatile with steam. Does not form an azeotrope with water. Flash pt, open cup: 100°F (38°C). Surface tension (20°): 37.5 dynes/cm. Viscosity (20°): 2.23 cP. Dipole moment 1.58. Strong base, pKb 5.6. Immiscible with cold NaOH solns. Miscible with water with evolution of some heat, with acetone, benzene, ether, castor oil, methanol, ethanol, ethylene glycol, 2-hexanone, linseed oil, turpentine, pine oil. Will dissolve 109% dimethylamine; 34% trimethylamine; 33% methylamine; >5% naphtha; <1% paraffin oil; <5% sulfur. LD_{50} orally in female rats: 1.05 g/kg (Smyth).

Hydrochloride. $C_4H_9NO \cdot HCl$. Crystals, dec 175-176°. Sol in water.

Salicylate. [147-90-0] Retarcyl; Deposal. $C_{11}H_{15}NO_4$; mol wt 225.24. Crystals from ethanol, mp 110-111°. Soluble in water, methanol, ethanol, ethyl acetate, acetone, benzene, chloroform. Practically insol in toluene, xylene, petr ether, ether, carbon tetrachloride.

N-Methylmorpholine. $C_5H_{11}NO$; mol wt 101.15. Mobile liquid, characteristic ammonia odor. bp_{764} 116-117°; bp_{760} 115.4°. d_4^{20} 0.9168. n_D^{20} 1.4332. Miscible with water, alcohol, ether.

Caution: Potential symptoms of overexposure to morpholine are irritation of eyes, skin, nose and respiratory system; visual disturbance; coughing. *See NIOSH Pocket Guide to Chemical Hazards* (DHHS/NIOSH 97-140, 1997) p 220.

USE: Cheap solvent for resins, waxes, casein, dyes. Morpholine fatty acid salts are used as surface-active agents and emulsifiers. Other morpholine compds are used as corrosion inhibitors, antioxidants, plasticizers, viscosity improvers, insecticides, fungicides, herbicides, local anesthetics and antiseptics.

THERAP CAT: Salicylate as analgesic; antipyretic; anti-inflammatory.

6278. Mosapramine. [89419-40-9] 1′-[3-(3-Chloro-10,11-dihydro-5*H*-dibenz[b,f]azepin-5-yl)propyl]hexahydrospiro[imid-azo[1,2-a]pyridine-3(2*H*),4′-piperidin]-2-one; 1′-[3-(3-chloro-10,11-dihydro-5*H*-dibenz[b,f]azepin-5-yl)propyl]-1,2,3,5,6,7,8,8a-octahydro-2-oxoimidazo[1,2-a]-pyridine-3-spiro-4′-piperidine; 3-chloro-5-[3-(2-oxo-1,2,3,5,6,7,8,8a-octahydroimidazo[1,2-a]-pyridine-3-spiro-4′-piperidino)propyl]-10,11-dihydro-5*H*-dibenz[b,f]-azepine; clospipramine. $C_{28}H_{35}ClN_4O$; mol wt 479.06. C 70.20%, H 7.36%, Cl 7.40%, N 11.70%, O 3.34%. Dopamine receptor antagonist with adrenoceptor blocking activity; metabolite of clocapramine, *q.v.* Prepn: C. Tashiro, I. Horii, **US 4337260** (1982 to Yoshitomi); C. Tashiro *et al., Yakugaku Zasshi* **109**, 93 (1989), *C.A.* **112**, 35749j (1990). X-ray crystallographic analysis: I. Ueda, C. Tashiro, *Acta Crystallogr.* **C40**, 422 (1984). Receptor binding studies: M. Setoguchi *et al., Eur. J. Pharmacol.* **112**, 313 (1985). Pharmacokinetics and metabolism: J. Ishigooka *et al., Psychopharmacology* **97**, 303 (1989). Toxicity data: H. Horizoe *et al., Oyo Yakuri* **37**, 529 (1989); *C.A.* **111**, 167174g (1989). HPLC determn in plasma: K. Hikida *et al., Anal. Sci.* **6**, 367 (1990).

Dihydrochloride. [98043-60-8] Y-516; Cremin. $C_{28}H_{35}ClN_4O \cdot 2HCl$; mol wt 551.98. White crystals, mp 271°. LD_{50} in male and female mice (mg/kg): 1008, 1293 orally; 74, 116 i.p.; 1147, 1264 s.c. (Horizoe).

THERAP CAT: Antipsychotic.

6279. Mosapride. [112885-41-3] 4-Amino-5-chloro-2-ethoxy-*N*-[[4-[(4-fluorophenyl)methyl]-2-morpholinyl]methyl]benzamide; (±)-4-amino-5-chloro-2-ethoxy-*N*-[[4-(4-fluorobenzyl)-2-morpholinyl]methyl]benzamide. $C_{21}H_{25}ClFN_3O_3$; mol wt 421.89. C 59.78%, H 5.97%, Cl 8.40%, F 4.50%, N 9.96%, O 11.38%. Selective 5-HT$_4$ receptor agonist. Prepn: T. Kon *et al.,* **EP 243959**; *eidem,* **US 4870074** (1987, 1989 both to Dainippon); S. Kato *et al., J. Med. Chem.* **34**, 616 (1991). Pharmacology: N. Yoshida *et al., Arch. Int. Pharmacodyn. Ther.* **300**, 51 (1989). Series of articles on pharmacokinetics: *Arzneim.-Forsch.* **43**, 859-872 (1993); on pharmacology and metabolism: *ibid.* 1083-1108. HPLC determn in plasma: I. Yokoyama *et al., J. Pharm. Biomed. Anal.* **15**, 1527 (1997). Clinical evaluation in gastro-esphageal reflux disease: M. Ruth *et al., Aliment. Pharmacol. Ther.* **12**, 35 (1998). Toxicity study: S. Yatera *et al., Jpn. Pharmacol. Ther.* **21**, 21 (1993).

Crystals from ethanol, mp 151-153°.

Citrate. [112885-42-4] AS-4370; Gasmotin. $C_{21}H_{25}ClFN_3O_3 \cdot C_6H_8O_7$; mol wt 614.02. Crystals from ethanol, mp 143-145°. LD_{50} in male, female mice, rats (mg/kg): >3000, >3000, >3000, 1905 orally; >1000, 914, >1000, >1000 i.p.; all species >1000 s.c.; in male, female dogs (mg/kg): both >400 orally (Yatera).

THERAP CAT: Gastroprokinetic.

6280. Mosher's Reagent. [81655-41-6] α-Methoxy-α-(trifluoromethyl)benzeneacetic acid; (±)-Mosher's acid; MTPA; 2-methoxy-2-(trifluoromethyl)phenylacetic acid. $C_{10}H_9F_3O_3$; mol wt 234.17. C 51.29%, H 3.87%, F 24.34%, O 20.50%. Chiral derivatizing reagent. Prepn: D. L. Dull, H. S. Mosher, *J. Am. Chem. Soc.* **89**, 4230 (1967); J. A. Dale *et al., J. Org. Chem.* **34**, 2543 (1969). Microscale prepn: D. E. Ward, C. K. Rhee, *Tetrahedron Lett.* **32**, 7165 (1991). Absolute configuration: S. S. Oh *et* al., J. Org. Chem. **54,** 4499 (1989); of the acid chloride: B. S. Joshi, S. W. Pelletier, *Heterocycles* **51,** 183 (1999). Enantiomeric purity of commerical samples: W. A. König *et al., Tetrahedron Lett.* **31,** 6867 (1990). Use in determn of abs config: T. R. Hoye, M. K. Renner, *J. Org. Chem.* **61,** 2056 (1996); A. Ichikawa, *Enantiomer* **3,** 255 (1998); L. F. Tietze *et al., Eur. J. Org. Chem.* **2000,** 2247.

(R)-(+)-form

(R)-(+)-Form. [20445-31-2] bp$_{1.5\ mm}$ 116-118°. $[\alpha]_D^{25}$ +68.5 ± 1.3° (c = 1.49 in CH$_3$OH).

(S)-(−)-Form. [17257-71-5] bp$_{1.5\ mm}$ 115-117°. $[\alpha]_D^{24}$ −71.8± 0.6° (c = 3.28 in CH$_3$OH).

(R)-(−)-Acid chloride. [39637-99-5] (*R*)-MTPA-chloride. bp$_{1\ mm}$ 54-56°. $[\alpha]_D^{25}$ −10.0 ± 0.1° (neat, l = 1).

(S)-(+)-Acid chloride. [20445-33-4] bp$_{1\ mm}$ 54-56°. $[\alpha]_D^{24}$ +129.0± 0.2° (c = 5.17 in CCl$_4$).

USE: Resolution of enantiomers primarily of alcohols and amines.

6281. Motexafin Gadolinium. [246252-06-2]; [156436-89-4] (hydrate).(*PB*-7-11-233′2′4)-Bis(acetato-κ*O*)[9,10-diethyl-20,21-bis[2-[2-(2-methoxyethoxy)ethoxy]ethoxy]-4,15-dimethyl-8,11-imino-3,6:16,13-dinitrilo-1,18-benzodiazacycloeicosine-5,14-dipropanolato-κ*N*^{1},κ*N*^{18},κ*N*^{23},κ*N*^{24},κ*N*^{25}]gadolinium; 4,5-diethyl-10,23-dimethyl-9,24-bis(3-hydroxypropyl)-16,17-bis[2-[2-(2-methoxyethoxy)ethoxy]ethoxy]pentaazapentacyclo[20.2.1.1^{3,6}.-1$^{8.11}$.0^{14,19}]heptacosa-1,3,5,7,9,11(27),12,14,16,18,20,22(25),23-tridecaene gadolinium(III) complex; gadolinium texaphyrin; Gd-Tex; Gd-T2BET; NSC-695238; PCI-0120; Xcytrin. C$_{52}$H$_{72}$GdN$_5$O$_{14}$; mol wt 1148.40. C 54.38%, H 6.32%, Gd 13.69%, N 6.10%, O 19.50%. Synthetic metal-coordinating expanded porphyrin. Paramagnetic redox mediator and radiation enhancer. Prepn: J. L. Sessler *et al., US 5801229* (1998 to Board of Regents Univ. of Texas); and redox chemistry: J. L. Sessler *et al., J. Phys. Chem. A* **103,** 787 (1999). Tumor selective radiosensitizing activity and MRI characteristics: S. W. Young *et al., Proc. Natl. Acad. Sci. USA* **93,** 6610 (1996). HPLC determn in plasma: R. A. Parise *et al., J. Chromatogr. B* **749,** 145 (2000). Mechanism of action study: D. Magda *et al., Int. J. Radiat. Oncol. Biol. Phys.* **51,** 1025 (2001); S. I. Hashemy *et al., J. Biol. Chem.* **281,** 10691 (2006). Clinical pharmacokinetics: D. I. Rosenthal *et al., Clin. Cancer Res.* **5,** 739 (1999). Clinical evaluation with radiation in brain metastases: M. P. Mehta *et al., J. Clin. Oncol.* **20,** 3445 (2002); C. A. Meyers *et al., J. Clin. Oncol.* **22,** 157 (2004). Review of chemistry: T. D. Mody, J. L. Sessler, *J. Porphyr. Phthalocyan.* **5,** 134-142 (2001); of therapeutic potential in brain tumors: D. Khuntia, M. Mehta, *Expert Rev. Anticancer Ther.* **4,** 981-989 (2004).

Prepd as hemihydrate, dark green microcrystalline solid. uv max (methanol): 350, 414, 473, 739 nm (log ε 4.33, 4.67, 5.06, 4.59).

THERAP CAT: Antineoplastic adjunct (radiosensitizer).

6282. Motexafin Lutetium. [246252-04-0]; [156436-90-7] (hydrate). (*PB*-7-11-233′2′4)-Bis(acetato-κ*O*)[9,10-diethyl-20,21-bis[2-[2-(2-methoxyethoxy)ethoxy]ethoxy]-4,15-dimethyl-8,11-imino-3,6:16,13-dinitrilo-1,18-benzodiazacycloeicosine-5,14-dipropanolato-κ*N*^{1},κ*N*^{18},κ*N*^{23},κ*N*^{24},κ*N*^{25}]lutetium; 4,5-diethyl-10,23-dimethyl-9,24-bis(3-hydroxypropyl)-16,17-bis[2-[2-(2-methoxyethoxy)ethoxy]ethoxy]pentaazapentacyclo[20.2.1.1^{3,6}.1$^{8.11}$.-0^{14,19}]heptacosa-1,3,5,7,9,11(27),12,14,16,18,20,22(25),23-tridecaene lutetium(III) complex; lutetium texaphyrin; Lu-Tex; PCI-0123; Antrin; Lutrin; Optrin. C$_{52}$H$_{72}$LuN$_5$O$_{14}$; mol wt 1166.12. C 53.56%, H 6.22%, Lu 15.00%, N 6.01%, O 19.21%. Synthetic metal-coordinating expanded porphyrin. Diamagnetic photosensitizer that is activated with far-red light to generate cytotoxic singlet oxygen. Prepn: J. L. Sessler *et al., US 5801229* (1998 to Board of Regents Univ. of Texas); S. W. Young *et al., Photochem. Photobiol.* **63,** 892 (1996). Electrochemical characteristics: J. L. Sessler *et al., J. Alloys Compds.* **249,** 146 (1997); and singlet oxygen generation: L. I. Grossweiner *et al., Photochem. Photobiol.* **70,** 138 (1999). LC-MS/MS and ICP-AES determn in plasma: D. Miles *et al., AAPS PharmSci.* **5,** 1 (2003). Preclinical studies in cancer and atheromatous plaque: K. W. Woodburn *et al., J. Clin. Laser Med. Surg.* **14,** 343 (1996); in ocular angiography: M. S. Blumenkranz *et al., Am. J. Ophthalmol.* **129,** 353 (2000). Clinical evaluation in coronary arterial photodynamic therapy: D. J. Kereiakes *et al., Circulation* **108,** 1310 (2003). Review of chemistry and therapeutic potential: T. D. Mody, J. L. Sessler, *J. Porphr. Phthalocyan.* **5,** 134-142 (2001).

Prepd as hydrate, shiny green solid. Sol in water, acetonitrile, methanol, *N,N*-dimethylformamide. Aqueous solns (100 μM) stable at 2<pH<11 for several months. uv max (methanol): 354, 414, 474, 732 nm (log ε 4.33, 4.67, 5.10, 4.62).

THERAP CAT: Antiatherosclerotic, antineoplastic (photosensitizer). In treatment of age-related macular degeneration.

6283. Motilin. [52906-92-0] A gastrointestinal peptide hormone whose existence was postulated during experimental chemical stimulation of canine duodenum: J. C. Brown *et al., Gastroenterology* **50,** 333 (1966). Motilin stimulates gastric antrum, duodenum, and colon; it has been reported to be about 50 times more powerful than acetylcholine in its effects on sensitive tissue: U. Strunz *et al., ibid.* **68,** 1485 (1975). In man it is found primarily in the upper small intestine. Although its effects are not known completely, it plays a role in increasing gastric motility and stimulating pepsin output and may also be important in regulating the interdigestive myoelectric complex. *Porcine motilin,* which contains 22 amino acids, has been isolated from mucosa of hog small intestine: J. C. Brown *et al., Can. J. Physiol. Pharmacol.* **49,** 399 (1971). Purification, amino acid composition, *C*-terminal residue: *eidem, Gastroenterology* **62,** 401 (1972). Amino acid sequence: *eidem, Can. J. Biochem.* **51,** 533 (1973); revised sequence: H. Schubert, J. C. Brown, *ibid.* **52,** 7 (1974). First synthetic work: E. Wünsch *et al., Z. Naturforsch.* **28C,** 235 (1973). Synthesis of the complete docosapeptide corresponding to porcine motilin: H. Yajima *et al., Chem. Commun.* **1975,** 159. Alternate syntheses: Y. Kai *et al., Chem. Pharm. Bull.* **23,** 2346 (1975); S. Yamada *et al., J. Am. Chem. Soc.* **97,** 7174 (1975); E. Izeboud, C. H. Beyerman, *Rec. Trav. Chim.* **99,** 124 (1980). Solid phase synthesis: N. Ikota *et al., Chem. Pharm. Bull.* **28,** 3347 (1980); D. H. Coy *et al., Peptides* **3,** 137

(1982). Radioimmunoassay: J. R. Dryburgh, J. C. Brown, *Gastroenterology* **68**, 1169 (1975). Identification of motilin endocrine cells: J. M. Polak *et al.*, *Gut* **16**, 225 (1975). Rodent and canine motilin differ from porcine; human motilin has not yet been purified, although its immunologic properties suggest strong similarity to porcine motilin. The presence of a larger motilin has also been detected immunologically, *see* J. M. Polak, A. M. J. Buchan, *Gastroenterology* **76**, 1065 (1979). *Reviews:* N. D. Christofides *et al.*, "Physiology of Motilin" in *Gut Hormones*, S. R. Bloom, Ed. (Churchill Livingstone, Edinburgh, 1978) pp 343-350; S. R. Bloom, J. M. Polak, *Clin. Endocrinol. Metab.* **8**, 401-411 (1979); V. Mutt, *Vitam. Horm.* **39**, 231-426 (1982).

Phe–Val–Pro–Ile–Phe–Thr–Tyr–Gly–Glu–Leu–Gln–Arg

HO–Gln–Gly–Lys–Asn–Arg–Glu–Lys–Glu–Gln–Met

Porcine Motilin

6284. Motretinide. [56281-36-8] *(all E)-N*-Ethyl-9-(4-methoxy-2,3,6-trimethylphenyl)-3,7-dimethyl-2,4,6,8-nonatetraenamide; 9-(4-methoxy-2,3,6-trimethylphenyl)-3,7-dimethylnona-2,-4,6,8-tetraen-1-oic acid ethyl amide; Ro-11-1430; Tasmaderm. $C_{23}H_{31}NO_2$; mol wt 353.50. C 78.15%, H 8.84%, N 3.96%, O 9.05%. Aromatic analog of retinoic acid, *q.v.* Prepn: W. Bollag *et al.*, **DE 2414619**; *eidem*, **US 4215215** (1974, 1980 both to Hoffmann-La Roche). Description of properties: *idem, Chemotherapy* **21**, 236 (1975). ^{13}C-NMR study: G. Englert, *Helv. Chim. Acta* **58**, 2367 (1975). Pharmacology: L. J. Wilkoff *et al.*, *Cancer Res.* **36**, 964 (1976); S. S. Shapiro *et al.*, *ibid.* 3702. Inhibitory effect on radiation-induced neoplasms: L. Harisiades *et al.*, *Nature* **274**, 486 (1978). Use in treatment of acne: K. Nordin *et al.*, *Dermatologica* **162**, 104 (1981).

Crystals from ethanol, mp 179-180°.

THERAP CAT: Antiacne.

6285. Moveltipril. [85856-54-8] *N*-(Cyclohexylcarbonyl)-D-alanyl-(2*S*)-3-mercapto-2-methylpropanoyl-L-proline; *N*-[3-(*N*-cyclohexanecarbonyl-D-alanylthio)-2-methylpropanoyl]-L-proline; (−)-*N*-[(*S*)-[3-(*N*-cyclohexylcarbonyl-D-alanyl)thio)-2-methylpropionyl]-L-proline; altiopril. $C_{19}H_{30}N_2O_5S$; mol wt 398.52. C 57.26%, H 7.59%, N 7.03%, O 20.07%, S 8.05%. Angiotensin-converting enzyme (ACE) inhibitor; structural analog of captopril. Prepn: S. Tanaka *et al.*, **BE 893553** (1982 to Chugai), *C.A.* **98**, 215995n (1983). Pharmacology: K. Sakai *et al.*, *Tohoku J. Exp. Med.* **152**, 363 (1987). Hemodynamic effects in dogs: K. Noguchi *et al.*, *Jpn. J. Pharmacol.* **40**, 373 (1986). Antihypertensive activity: J. Aono *et al.*, *Arch. Int. Pharmacodyn.* **292**, 203 (1988). Tissue specific ACE inhibitory activity: K. Sakai *et al.*, *ibid.* **294**, 228 (1988). Determn by radioimmunoassay: Y. Hinohara *et al.*, *J. Pharmacobio-Dyn.* **11**, 411 (1988).

Solid, mp 113-116°. $[\alpha]_D$ +14.2° (c = 1.05 in methanol).
Calcium salt. [85921-53-5] MC-838; Lowpres. $C_{38}H_{58}CaN_4O_{10}S_2$; mol wt 835.10. Practically white powder, mp ~190°. Bitter taste. $[\alpha]_D^{20}$ −48 to −52° (c = 1 in methanol). Freely sol in water, methanol; sol in ethanol, chloroform. Practically insol in acetone, ethyl acetate. 10% aq soln has pH 5.5-6.5. Stable as aq soln and powder at room temp. LD_{50} in male, female mice, male, female rats (g/kg): all >10.0 orally; 2.1, 2.3, 1.3, 1.3 i.p.; 3.0, 3.8, 3.4, 3.9 s.c.; and in male, female dogs (g/kg): >6.0, >6.0 orally (Sakai).

THERAP CAT: Antihypertensive.

6286. Moxalactam. [64952-97-2] (6*R*,7*R*)-7-[[(2*R*)-Carboxy(4-hydroxyphenyl)acetyl]amino]-7-methoxy-3-[[(1-methyl-1*H*-tetrazol-5-yl)thio]methyl]-8-oxo-5-oxa-1-azabicyclo[4.2.0]oct-2-ene-2-carboxylic acid; *N*-[(6*R*,7*R*)-2-carboxy-7-methoxy-3-[[(1-methyl-1*H*-tetrazol-5-yl)thio]methyl]-8-oxo-5-oxa-1-azabicyclo[4.2.0]oct-2-en-7-yl]-2-(*p*-hydroxyphenyl)malonamic acid; 7β-[2-carboxy-2-(4-hydroxyphenyl)acetamido]-7α-methoxy-3-[[(1-methyl-1*H*-tetrazol-5-yl)thio]methyl]-1-oxa-1-dethia-3-cephem-4-carboxylic acid; lamoxactam; latamoxef. $C_{20}H_{20}N_6O_9S$; mol wt 520.47. C 46.15%, H 3.87%, N 16.15%, O 27.67%, S 6.16%. Oxa-substituted third generation cephalosporin antibiotic (oxacephalosporin). Prepn: M. Narisada, W. Nagata, **DE 2713370**; *eidem*, **US 4138486** (1977, 1979 both to Shionogi); M. Narisada *et al.*, *J. Med. Chem.* **22**, 757 (1979). Laboratory evaluation: T. Yoshida *et al.*, *Antimicrob. Agents Chemother.* **17**, 302 (1980). Mechanism of action study: Y. Komatsu, T. Nishikawa, *ibid.* 316. Pharmacokinetics: R. Wise *et al.*, *ibid.* **18**, 369 (1980). Comparative *in vitro* activity: T. O. Kurtz *et al.*, *ibid.* 645. Series of articles on pharmacology, teratology, toxicity studies: *Chemotherapy (Tokyo)* **28**, Suppl. 7, 1002-1235 (1980). Clinical evaluation in neonates and infants: U. B. Schaad *et al.*, *J. Pediatr.* **98**, 129 (1981). *Review:* *Rev. Infect. Dis.* **4**, Suppl., S489-S726 (1982).

Colorless powder, mp 117-122° (dec). $[\alpha]_D^{25}$ −15.3 ±2.6° (c = 0.216 in methanol). uv max: 276 nm (ε 10200).
Disodium salt. [64953-12-4] LY-12735; S-6059; Festamoxin; Moxalactam; Moxam; Shiomarin. $C_{20}H_{18}N_6Na_2O_9S$; mol wt 564.44. $[\alpha]_D^{22}$ −45° (water). uv max (water): 270 nm (ε 12000).

THERAP CAT: Antibacterial.

6287. Moxastine. [3572-74-5] 2-(1,1-Diphenylethoxy)-*N*,*N*-dimethylethanamine; α-methylbenzhydryl 2-dimethylaminoethyl ether; α-methyldiphenhydramine; mephenhydramine; Spofa 325; Alfadryl. $C_{18}H_{23}NO$; mol wt 269.38. C 80.26%, H 8.61%, N 5.20%, O 5.94%. Prepn: Protiva *et al.*, *Chem. Listy* **43**, 257 (1949); **CS 86516** (1957), *C.A.* **53**, 1261 (1959); Z. Vejdelek *et al.*, *Collect. Czech. Chem. Commun.* **49**, 2649 (1984).

bp$_{0.15}$ 129-136°.
Hydrochloride. $C_{18}H_{23}NO.HCl.$ mp 168°.
THERAP CAT: Antihistaminic.

6288. Moxaverine. [10539-19-2] 3-Ethyl-6,7-dimethoxy-1-(phenylmethyl)isoquinoline; 1-benzyl-3-ethyl-6,7-dimethoxyisoquinoline. $C_{20}H_{21}NO_2$; mol wt 307.39. C 78.15%, H 6.89%, N 4.56%, O 10.41%. Prepn of hydrochloride: **FR 1362765** (1964 to Orgamol, SA), *C.A.* **62**, 536f (1965). Physical properties and solution stability: E. Pawelczyk, M. Zajac, *Diss. Pharm. Pharmacol.* **24**, 5 (1972). HPLC determn in pharmaceutical formulations: E. H. Girgis, *J. Pharm. Sci.* **82**, 503 (1993).

Crystals, mp 71-72.5°. uv max (0.1 M H_2SO_4): 253 nm ($A_{1cm}^{1\%}$ 2164).

Hydrochloride. [1163-37-7] Eupaverin; Eupaverina; Kollateral. $C_{20}H_{21}NO_2 \cdot HCl$; mol wt 343.85. Crystals from ethanol, mp 208-210° (dec). Sol in hot water, hot alc, and many other organic solvents; very sparingly sol in cold water.

THERAP CAT: Antispasmodic.

6289. Moxestrol. [34816-55-2] (11β,17α)-11-Methoxy-19-nor-17-pregna-1,3,5(10)-trien-20-yne-3,17-diol; 3,17-dihydroxy-11β-methoxy-19-nor-17α-pregna-1,3,5-trien-20-yne; 17α-ethynyl-11β-methoxyestra-1,3,5(10)-triene-3,17β-diol; 11β-methoxy-17α-ethynyl-$\Delta^{1,3,5(10)}$-estratriene-3,17β-diol; 11β-methoxy-17α-ethynylestradiol; R-2858; Surestryl. $C_{21}H_{26}O_3$; mol wt 326.43. C 77.27%, H 8.03%, O 14.70%. Prepn: Bertin, Pierdet, **ZA 6703381**; *eidem*, **US 3579545**; **FR M6182**, *C.A.* **72**, 90739m (1970) (1968, 1971, 1968 all to Roussel-UCLAF); Azadian-Boulanger, Bertin, *Chim. Ther.* **8**, 451 (1973). Activity studies: Raynaud, *Steroids* **21**, 249 (1973); Raynaud *et al.*, *Mol. Pharmacol.* **9**, 520 (1973).

Crystals, mp 280°. $[\alpha]_D^{20}$ +29° (c = 0.6 in ethanol). uv max (ethanol): 280 nm ($E_{1cm}^{1\%}$ 58.4).

THERAP CAT: Estrogen.

6290. Moxidectin. [113507-06-5] (6R,23E,25S)-5-O-Demethyl-28-deoxy-25-[(1E)-1,3-dimethyl-1-butenyl]-6,28-epoxy-23-(methoxyimino)milbemycin B; 23-methyloxime LL-F282249α; (2aE,4E,5'R,6R,6'S,8E,11R,13S,15S,17aR,20R,20aR,20bS)-6'-[(E)-1,3-dimethyl-1-butenyl]-5',6,6',7,10,11,14,15,17a,20,20a,20b-dodecahydro-20,20b-dihydroxy-5',6,8,19-tetramethylspiro[11,15-methano-2H,13H,17H-furo[4,3,2-pq]benzodioxacyclooctadecin-13,2'-[2H]pyran]-4',17(3'H)-dione 4'-(E)-(O-methyloxime); CL-301423; Cydectin; Equest; Proheart 6; Quest; Vetdectin. $C_{37}H_{53}$-NO_8; mol wt 639.82. C 69.46%, H 8.35%, N 2.19%, O 20.00%. Semisynthetic macrolide antibiotic; 23-methyloxime analog of nemadectin, *q.v.*. Prepn: B. M. Bain *et al.*, **EP 237339** (1987 to Glaxo); G. Asato, D. J. France, **EP 259779** (1988 to Am. Cyanamid). Efficacy in cattle against lice: J. D. Webb *et al.*, *J. Econ. Entomol.* **84**, 1266 (1991); against gastrointestinal nematodes: G. L. Zimmerman *et al.*, *Am. J. Vet. Res.* **53**, 1409 (1992); J. C. Williams *et al.*, *Vet. Rec.* **131**, 345 (1992); against psoroptic mange: J. F. Lonneux, B. Losson, *Vet. Parasitol.* **45**, 147 (1992). Environmental effects on dung-burying beetles: G. T. Fincher, G. T. Wang, *Southwest. Entomol.* **17**, 303 (1992).

THERAP CAT (VET): Anthelmintic; antiparasitic.

6291. Moxifloxacin. [151096-09-2] 1-Cyclopropyl-6-fluoro-1,4-dihydro-8-methoxy-7-[(4aS,7aS)-octahydro-6H-pyrrolo[3,4-

b]pyridin-6-yl]-4-oxo-3-quinolinecarboxylic acid. $C_{21}H_{24}FN_3O_4$; mol wt 401.43. C 62.83%, H 6.03%, F 4.73%, N 10.47%, O 15.94%. Fluorinated quinolone antibacterial. Prepn: U. Petersen *et al.*, **EP 550903** (1993 to Bayer). Antibacterial spectrum *in vitro*: J. M. Woodcock *et al.*, *Antimicrob. Agents Chemother.* **41**, 101 (1997). Activity vs *Mycobacterium tuberculosis*: B. Ji *et al.*, *ibid.* **42**, 2066 (1998). HPLC determn in serum: C. M. Tobin *et al.*, *J. Antimicrob. Chemother.* **42**, 278 (1998). Clinical pharmacokinetics: H. Stass *et al.*, *Antimicrob. Agents Chemother.* **42**, 2060 (1998). Review of pharmacology and clinical experience: M. Miravitlles, *Expert Opin. Pharmacother.* **6**, 283-293 (2005).

mp 203-208° (dec). $[\alpha]_D^{23}$ −193°.

Hydrochloride. [186826-86-8] Bay-12-8039; Actimax; Actira; Avalox; Avelox; Octegra; Proflox; Vigamox. $C_{21}H_{24}FN_3O_4 \cdot HCl$; mol wt 437.89. Slightly yellow to yellow crystalline powder, mp 324-325° (dec). $[\alpha]_D^{25}$ −256° (c = 0.5 in water).

THERAP CAT: Antibacterial.

6292. Moxisylyte. [54-32-0] 4-[2-(Dimethylamino)ethoxy]-2-methyl-5-(1-methylethyl)phenol acetate (ester); 5-(2-dimethylaminoethoxy)carvacrol acetate; 6-acetoxythymol 2-(dimethylamino)ethyl ether; (6-acetoxythymoxy)ethyldimethylamine; 4-(2-dimethylaminoethoxy)-5-isopropyl-2-methylphenyl acetate; thymoxamine. $C_{16}H_{25}NO_3$; mol wt 279.37. C 68.79%, H 9.02%, N 5.01%, O 17.18%. α_1-Adrenergic blocker. Prepn: H. Pahlicke, **DE 905738** (1954 to Diwag), *C.A.* **52**, 16294i (1958); A. Buzas *et al.*, *Bull. Soc. Chim. Fr.* **1959**, 839. Pharmacology: K. Greeff, H. J. Schümann, *Arzneim.-Forsch.* **3**, 341 (1953); J. Mercier *et al.*, *Therapie* **26**, 785 (1971). Toxicology: J. Roquebert, J. Canellas, *ibid.* 775. α-Adrenergic antagonist activity: A. T. Birmingham, J. Szolcsanyi, *J. Pharm. Pharmacol.* **17**, 449 (1965). α_1-receptor selectivity: J. Roquebert *et al.*, *Arch. Int. Pharmacodyn.* **266**, 282 (1983). Series of articles on metabolism: K.-O. Vollmer *et al.*, *Eur. J. Drug Metab. Pharmacokinet.* **10**, 61, 71, 139 (1985). Clinical pharmacokinetics: P. Costa *et al.*, *J. Pharm. Sci.* **82**, 729, 968 (1993). HPLC determn of metabolites in plasma and urine: C. Marquer, F. Bressolle, *J. Chromatogr. B* **691**, 389 (1997). Clinical trial in Raynaud's disease and chilblains: G. V. Jaffe, J. J. Grimshaw, *Br. J. Clin. Pract.* **34**, 343 (1980). Review of clinical studies in ophthalmology: M. Wand, W. M. Grant, *Surv. Ophthalmol.* **25**, 75-84 (1980). Clinical trial in impotence: P. Costa *et al.*, *J. Urol.* **149**, 301 (1993).

Hydrochloride. [964-52-3] Arlitene; Carlytene; Erecnos; Icavex; Opilon; Uroalpha. $C_{16}H_{25}NO_3 \cdot HCl$; mol wt 315.84. Shiny beige needles from ethyl acetate/methanol, mp 208-210°. Sol in water, alcohol, chloroform. Insol in ether. LD_{50} in mice, rats (mg/kg): 265 ±19, 740 ±51 orally; 200 ±15, 190 ±19 s.c. (Roquebert, Canellas).

THERAP CAT: Vasodilator (peripheral). In treatment of male erectile dysfunction.

6293. Moxonidine. [75438-57-2] 4-Chloro-N-(4,5-dihydro-1H-imidazol-2-yl)-6-methoxy-2-methyl-5-pyrimidinamine; 4-chloro-6-methoxy-2-methyl-5-(2-imidazolin-2-yl)aminopyrimidine; BDF-5895; Cynt; Physiotens. $C_9H_{12}ClN_5O$; mol wt 241.68. C 44.73%, H 5.00%, Cl 14.67%, N 28.98%, O 6.62%. α_2-Adrenoceptor agonist. Prepn: **NL 7908192**; W. Stenzel *et al.*, **US 4323570** (1980, 1982 both to Beiersdorf AG). Series of articles on pharmacology and binding studies: *Arzneim.-Forsch.* **38**, 1426-1445 (1988). Pharmacokinetics: D. Trenk *et al.*, *J. Clin. Pharmacol.* **27**, 988 (1987); W. Kirch *et al.*, *ibid.* **30**, 1088 (1990). Clinical comparison with clonidine, *q.v.*: V. Plänitz, *ibid.* **27**, 46 (1987).

mp 217-219° (dec).

Hydrochloride. [75438-58-3] Crystals from isopropanol/ether, mp 189°.

THERAP CAT: Antihypertensive.

6294. MPTP. [28289-54-5] 1,2,3,6-Tetrahydro-1-methyl-4-phenylpyridine; 1-methyl-4-phenyl-1,2,3,6-tetrahydropyridine. $C_{12}H_{15}N$; mol wt 173.25. C 83.19%, H 8.73%, N 8.08%. Piperidine derivative which causes irreversible symptoms of parkinsonism in humans, monkeys. Prepn as hydrochloride by Grignard reaction: A. Ziering *et al.*, *J. Org. Chem.* **12**, 894 (1947). Alternative prepn: C. J. Schmidle, R. C. Mansfield, *J. Am. Chem. Soc.* **78**, 425 (1956). Identification as impurity in "synthetic heroin" and effect on drug users: J. W. Langston *et al.*, *Science* **219**, 979 (1983). Selective destruction of dopaminergic neurons in primates: R. S. Burns *et al.*, *Proc. Natl. Acad. Sci. USA* **80**, 4546 (1983). *In vitro* metabolism by rat brain monoamine oxidase to 1-methyl-4-phenylpyridinium ion (**MPP⁺**): K. Chiba *et al.*, *Biochem. Biophys. Res. Commun.* **120**, 574 (1984). Studies on mechanism of neurotoxicity: J. W. Langston *et al.*, *Science* **225**, 1480 (1984); S. P. Markey *et al.*, *Nature* **311**, 464 (1984). Binding studies in rat brain: C. M. Wieczorek *et al.*, *Eur. J. Pharmacol.* **98**, 453 (1984); B. Parsons, T. C. Rainbow, *ibid.* **102**, 375 (1984); in rat, human brain: J. A. Javitch *et al.*, *Proc. Natl. Acad. Sci. USA* **81**, 4591 (1984). Comparison of idiopathic and MPTP-induced parkinsonism in humans: R. S. Burns *et al.*, *N. Engl. J. Med.* **312**, 1418 (1985). Review: T. P. Singer *et al.*, *Trends Biochem. Sci.* **12**, 266-270 (1987); L. M. Sayre, *Toxicol. Lett.* **48**, 121-149 (1989).

Crystals from heptane, mp 40-42°. bp$_{0.8}$ 85-90°.

6295. MSH. Melanotropin; melanophore-affecting hormone; melanocyte-stimulating hormone; melanophore hormone; melanophore dilating hormone; melanophore expanding hormone; melanophore-stimulating hormone; melanotropic hormone; chromatophorotropic hormone; melanosome-dispersing hormone; pigmentation hormone. First known as *Intermedin(e)* or *B hormone*, a pituitary factor causing color changes in fish and amphibia: B. Zondek, H. Kron, *Klin. Wochenschr.* **11**, 849 (1932). Subsequently, the hormone was identified as two linear peptides designated as α- and β-MSH. γ-MSH, a third peptide has also been identified but has no significant melanocyte stimulating activity. The peptides are secreted by the pars intermedia of the pituitary gland. The brain may be a secondary site of synthesis. α-MSH derives from ACTH and β-MSH from β-lipotrophic hormone, *q.q.v.* These MSH precursors derive from two sections of pro-opiomelanocortin, *q.v.* A third portion of pro-opiomelanocortin may serve as the precursor of γ-MSH. Biosynthesis: B. G. Jenks *et al.*, *J. Endocrinol.* **98**, 19 (1983); G. J. M. Martens *et al.*, *Gen. Comp. Endocrinol.* **49**, 73 (1983). Distribution and biosynthesis in the brain: D. F. Swaab *et al.*, "The Distribution of MSH and ACTH in the Rat and Human Brain and its Relation to Pituitary Stores," in *Endogenous Peptides and Learning and Memory Processes*, J. L. Martinez, Jr. *et al.*, Eds. (Academic Press, New York, 1981) pp 7-36. The mechanism of control of MSH release from the pituitary is still being investigated. There is evidence for inhibitory control by the brain via dopaminergic neurons, inhibitory control by the peptide melanostatin (MIF-1), *q.v.* and stimulatory control by β-adrenergic agents and the peptide CRF, *q.v.*: G. Schmitt *et al.*, *Neuroendocrinology* **33**, 306 (1981); P.

G. Smelik *et al.*, "The Role of Catecholamines in the Control of the Secretion of Pro-Opiocortin-Derived Peptides from the Anterior and Intermediate Lobes and its Implications in the Response to Stress," in *The Anterior Pituitary Gland*, A. S. Bhatnagar, Ed. (Raven Press, New York, 1983) pp 113-125; L. Proulx-Ferland *et al.*, *J. Steroid Biochem.* **19**, 439 (1983). Although the role of MSH in adaptive color change in lower vertebrates in well known, its physiological significance in mammals appears to be extrapigmentary. Effects on reproduction: M. E. Celis, M. Volosin, *Prog. Clin. Biol. Res.* **87**, 113 (1982). Reviews of behavioral and neurochemical effects: P. C. Datta, M. G. King, *Neurosci. Biobehav. Rev.* **6**, 297-310 (1982); B. E. Beckwith, C. A. Sandman, *Peptides* **3**, 411-420 (1982). General reviews: Li, *Adv. Protein Chem.* **12**, 270-295 (1957); Novales, *Neuroendocrinology* **2**, 241 (1967); R. Schwyzer, *Proc. Roy. Soc. London [Biol.]* **210**, 5-20 (1980); F. L. Strand, C. M. Smith, *Pharmacol. Ther.* **11**, 509-533 (1980). Book: A. J. Thody, *The MSH Peptides* (Academic Press, New York, 1980) 162 pp.

α-Melanotropin. Contains 13 amino acids. Mammalian α-MSH is the most potent melanocyte-stimulating peptide known. Mechanism of action: T. K. Sawyer *et al.*, *Am. Zool.* **23**, 1983. Isoln from hog pituitary gland: T. H. Lee, A. B. Lerner, *J. Biol. Chem.* **221**, 943 (1956); from pig pituitary gland: Harris, Lerner, *Nature* **179**, 1346 (1957); Harris, *Biochem. J.* **71**, 451 (1959); from horse pituitary gland: Dixon, Li, *J. Am. Chem. Soc.* **82**, 4568 (1960). Structure: Lee *et al.*, *J. Biol. Chem.* **236**, 1390 (1961). Synthesis: Schwyzer *et al.*, *Helv. Chim. Acta* **44**, 159 (1961). Synthesis and biological activity of dogfish α-MSH: A. Eberle *et al.*, *Helv. Chim. Acta* **61**, 2360 (1978). Activity as centrally administered antipyretic agent: M. T. Murphy *et al.*, *Science* **221**, 192 (1983). Cardiovascular effects: D. J. Diz, D. M. Jacobowitz, *Brain Res.* **270**, 265 (1983). Review of the α-melanotropinergic system and its role in the CNS: T. L. O'Donohue, D. M. Jacobowitz in *Polypeptide Hormones*, R. F. Beers, E. G. Bassett, Eds. (Raven Press, New York, 1980) pp 203-222. $[\alpha]_D^{25}$ −58.5 ± 2.5° (c = 0.38 in 10% acetic acid).

β-Melanotropin. Contains 18-22 amino acids differing slightly from one species to another: Lee *et al.*, *J. Biol. Chem.* **236**, 1390 (1961). Isoln from hog pituitary gland: T. H. Lee, A. B. Lerner, *loc. cit.*; from pig pituitary gland: Geschwind *et al.*, *J. Am. Chem. Soc.* **78**, 4494 (1956); **79**, 620 (1957); Harris, Roos, *Biochem. J.* **71**, 434 (1959); from bovine pituitary gland: Geschwind *et al.*, *J. Am. Chem. Soc.* **79**, 6394 (1957); from human pituitary gland: Dixon, *Biochim. Biophys. Acta* **37**, 38 (1960); Harris, *Nature* **184**, 167 (1959). Synthesis of derivatives: Hofmann, *Ann. N.Y. Acad. Sci.* **88**, art. 3, p 689 (1960). Synthesis of bovine β-melanotropin: Schwyzer *et al.*, *Helv. Chim. Acta* **46**, 1975 (1963); S. Lemaire *et al.*, *J. Med. Chem.* **19**, 373 (1976). Solid-phase synthesis of human and monkey β-melanotropins: Wang *et al.*, *Int. J. Pept. Protein Res.* **5**, 33 (1973); of camel β_{c1}-MSH: Li *et al.*, *Biochemistry* **14**, 953 (1975); of camel β_{c2}-MSH: S. Lemaire *et al.*, *loc. cit.*; of dogfish β-MSH: H. Yajima *et al.*, *Chem. Pharm. Bull.* **26**, 571 (1978); of equine β-MSH: J. Izdebski *et al.*, *Int. J. Pept. Protein Res.* **19**, 327 (1982). It is probable that the human pituitary does not produce β-MSH. The substance reported as human β-MSH in early studies seems to have been an artifact formed by enzymatic degradation of β-LPH during the extraction procedure: K. Tanaka *et al.*, *J. Clin. Invest.* **62**, 94 (1978); A. J. Thody, *loc. cit.*

γ-Melanotropin. Contains 12 amino acids. Discovered during nucleotide sequencing of cloned DNA for bovine pro-opiomelanocortin: S. Nakanishi *et al.*, *Nature* **278**, 423 (1979). May be an antagonist of β-endorphin or a partial agonist/antagonist of ACTH. Synthesis and biological activity: N. Ling *et al.*, *Life Sci.* **25**, 1773 (1979); K. Okamoto *et al.*, *Chem. Pharm. Bull.* **28**, 2839 (1980); W. A. Bijl *et al.*, *Rec. Trav. Chim.* **100**, 123 (1981). Radioimmunoassay: T. Shibasaki *et al.*, *Life Sci.* **26**, 1781 (1980). Behavioral profile in rats: J. M. Van Ree *et al.*, *ibid.* **28**, 2875 (1981). Comparison with α-MSH: T. L. O'Donohue *et al.*, *Peptides* **2**, 101 (1981). *Review:* J. M. Van Ree *et al.*, *Ciba Found. Symp.* **81**, 263-276 (1981). $[\alpha]_D^{20}$ −38.0° (c 0.5 in 10% acetic acid). $[\alpha]_D^{23}$ −33.4° (c = 1.0 in 1% acetic acid).

6296. Mucins. High molecular weight glycoproteins, major constituents of saliva, gastric juice, intestinal juice, and other secretions: F. Haurowitz, *Chemistry and Biology of Proteins* (Academic Press, New York, 1950) p 199. Mucins are capable of forming viscous solutions and thereby act as lubricants or protectants in cavities of the body or on body surfaces. For prepn (*e.g.* from snails) and their biochemical role *see* P. A. Levene, *The Hexosamines and Mucoproteins* (Longmans, Green, London, 1925). Ovine submaxillary mucin consists of a single polypeptide chain with about 800 disaccharide units attached, each of which is *N*-acetylneuraminyl(2 → 6) *N*-acetylgalactosamine. Carbohydrate accounts for about 45% of the molecular weight. Structure studies: Pigman, Tanaka, *148th Am. Chem. Soc. Meet.* (Chicago, Aug.-Sept., 1964), Abstracts of Papers, p 11C; Ozeki, Yosizawa, *Arch. Biochem. Biophys.* **142**, 177 (1971); Huser *et al.*, *Z. Physiol. Chem.* **354**, 749 (1973). Glycoproteins in bovine cervical mucus: F. A. Meyer *et al.*, *Adv. Exp. Med. Biol.* **89**, 239 (1977). Review on physical and chemical properties, biosynthesis and function of mucin: several authors in *Mucus in Health and Disease*, M. Elstein, D. V. Parke, Eds. (Plenum Press, New York, 1977) pp 171-311.

Mucins are obtained as greenish-gray or yellow powders forming very viscous solns in water; generally sol in dil alkalies. Insol in acetic acid. Acidic substances with an isoelectric point between pH 3 and 5.

USE: Demulcent; adsorbent.

6297. Mucochloric Acid. [87-56-9] 2,3-Dichloro-4-oxo-2-butenoic acid; dichloromalealdehydic acid; α,β-dichloro-β-formylacrylic acid; 2,3-dichloromaleic aldehyde acid. $C_4H_2Cl_2O_3$; mol wt 168.96. C 28.43%, H 1.19%, Cl 41.97%, O 28.41%. Prepn from β,γ-dichloropyromucic acid and bromine water or dil nitric acid: Hill, Jackson, *Am. Chem. J.* **12**, 43 (1890); by heating furfural with manganese dioxide and hydrochloric acid: Simonis, *Ber.* **32**, 2085 (1899); Beattie *et al.*, *J. Chem. Soc.* **1932**, 264; Mowry, *J. Am. Chem. Soc.* **72**, 2535 (1950); by chlorination of butyne-1,4-diol: Dury, *Angew. Chem.* **72**, 864 (1960).

Monoclinic prisms from ether and ligroin, mp 127°. Slightly sol in cold water; sol in hot water; hot benzene, alc. LD_{50} in rats: 0.5-1.0 g/kg orally; 10-25 mg/kg i.p., Fassett in *Industrial Hygiene and Toxicology* **vol. II**, F. A. Patty, Ed. (Interscience, New York, 2nd ed., 1962) p 1977.

Caution: Strong irritant to skin and eyes; a potent skin sensitizer.

6298. Mucochloric Anhydride. [4412-09-3] 5,5'-Oxybis-[3,4-dichloro-2(5*H*)-furanone]; bis[3,4-dichloro-2(5)-furanonyl] ether; GC-2466. $C_8H_2Cl_4O_5$; mol wt 319.91. C 30.04%, H 0.63%, Cl 44.33%, O 25.01%. Prepd by refluxing mucochloric acid with benzenesulfonic acid in a mixture of benzene and dioxane: Mowry, *J. Am. Chem. Soc.* **72**, 2535 (1950).

Crystals from benzene + dioxane, α-isomer (racemate): mp 141-143°, β-isomer (*meso* form): mp 180°. Substantially insol in water. Sol in many organic solvents, such as acetone, xylene, cyclohexanone, methylnaphthalenes.

USE: Fungicide. *Ref:* Gilbert, *US 2861919* (1958 to Allied Chem.).

6299. Muconic Acid. [505-70-4] 2,4-Hexadienedioic acid; 1,3-butadiene-1,4-dicarboxylic acid. $C_6H_6O_4$; mol wt 142.11. C 50.71%, H 4.26%, O 45.03%. HOOCCH=CHCH=CHCOOH. Prepd by oxidation of phenol and peracetic acid: Boeseken, Engelberts, *C.A.* **26**, 2970 (1932); by treatment of ethyl 1,4-dibromoadipate with alcoholic potassium hydroxide: Guha, Sankaran, *Org. Synth.* **26**, 57 (1946); by isomerization of 3-hydroxy-4-carbomethoxybut-1-ene-1-carboxylic acid lactone: Elvidge *et al.*, *J. Chem. Soc.* **1950**, 2235; by carbonylation of acetylene: Tsuji *et al.*, *J. Am. Chem. Soc.* **86**, 2095 (1964). Configuration and separation of isomers: Boeseken, Kerkhoven, *Rec. Trav. Chim.* **51**, 964 (1932); Elvidge *et al.*, *J. Chem. Soc.* **1953**, 708.

***trans,trans*-Form.** Prisms from water, mp 301°. uv max (0.1*N* NaOH): 251, 259, 264 nm (ε 25600, 29100, 25600). One gram dissolves in about 5 liters water at 15°. Quite sol in hot alcohol and glacial acetic acid.

Dimethyl ester. $C_8H_{10}O_4$. Crystals from alcohol, mp 159°. Insol in ether.

Diethyl ester. $C_{10}H_{14}O_4$. Needles from alcohol, mp 64°; d_4^{100} 0.9829. n_{He}^{99} 1.4675.

***cis,cis*-Form.** Prisms from ethanol, mp 194-195°. uv max (0.1*N* NaOH): 251, 258, 264 nm (ε 15600, 17000, 15300). Freely sol in boiling water; sparingly sol in ether.

Dimethyl ester. $C_8H_{10}O_4$. Needles from petr ether, mp 75°. Soluble in ether.

Diethyl ester. $C_{10}H_{14}O_4$. Minute crystals from alcohol at −25°; mp 13°. Changes to the *trans-trans*-form on storage at room temp.

***cis,trans*-Form.** Needles from hot water, mp 190-191°. uv max (0.1*N* NaOH): 251, 259, 265 nm (ε 23400, 25600, 23400).

Dimethyl ester. $C_8H_{10}O_4$. Needles from aqueous methanol, mp 75°.

6300. Muira Puama. Potency wood. Wood of *Liriosma ovata* Miers, *Oleaceae*, or according to Rebourgeon, *Acanthea virilis* Wehmer, *Acanthaceae*. *Habit.* Brazil. *Constit.* Aromatic resin, muirapuamine, fat. Studies of components: Auterhoff, Pankow, *Arch. Pharm.* **301**, 481 (1968); **302**, 209 (1969). *Reviews:* Gaebler, *Dtsch. Apoth.* **22**, 94 (1970); Steinmetz, *Q. J. Crude Drug Res.* **11**, 1787 (1971).

6301. Mukaiyama Reagent. [14338-32-0] 2-Chloro-1-methylpyridinium iodide; 2-chloropyridine methiodide; 1-methyl-2-chloropyridinium iodide. C_6H_7ClIN; mol wt 255.48. C 28.21%, H 2.76%, Cl 13.88%, I 49.67%, N 5.48%. Acid-activating agent for prepn of carboxylic esters. Prepn: M. Liveris, J. Miller, *Aust. J. Chem.* **2**, 297 (1958); and reactions with hydroxide ions: G. B. Barlin, J. A. Benbow, *J. Chem. Soc. Perkin Trans.* 2 **1974**, 790. Use in synthesis of carboxylic esters: T. Mukaiyama *et al.*, *Chem. Lett.* **1975**, 1045; T. Mukaiyama, *Angew. Chem. Int. Ed.* **18**, 707 (1979). Kinetic resolution of carboxylic acids and alcohols: A. Mazón *et al.*, *Tetrahedron: Asymmetry* **3**, 1455 (1992). Kinetics of nucleophilic substitution reactions with primary and secondary amines: A. Awwal *et al.*, *Indian J. Chem.* **40B**, 32 (2001); with phenols: M. Kabir *et al.*, *ibid.* **43B**, 1779 (2004). Use in synthesis of ketenes: R. L. Funk *et al.*, *Synlett* **1989**, 36; of β-lactams: C. M. L. Delpiccolo *et al.*, *J. Comb. Chem.* **5**, 208 (2003); of esters: D. Donati *et al.*, *Tetrahedron Lett.* **46**, 2817 (2005).

Almost colorless needles, mp 207° (Liveris, Miller). Also reported as pale yellow crystals, mp 205-206° (dec) (Barlin, Benbow). uv max (pH 7.0): 213, 274 nm (log ε 3.66, 3.86).

USE: Condensation reagent for the synthesis of esters and ketenes, and for the kinetic resolution of carboxylic acids and alcohols.

6302. Mupirocin. [12650-69-0] (2*E*)-5,9-Anhydro-2,3,4,8-tetradeoxy-8-[[(2*S*,3*S*)-3-[(1*S*,2*S*)-2-hydroxy-1-methylpropyl]-oxiranyl]methyl]-3-methyl-L-*talo*-non-2-enonic acid, 8-carboxyoctyl ester; pseudomonic acid A; *trans*-pseudomonic acid; BRL-4910A; Bactoderm; Bactroban; Turixin. $C_{26}H_{44}O_9$; mol wt 500.62. C 62.38%, H 8.86%, O 28.76%. Major component of the pseudomonic acids, *q.v.*, an antibiotic complex produced by *Pseudomonas fluorescens* NCIB 10586. Isoln and characterization: A. T. Fuller *et al.*, *Nature* **234**, 416 (1971); K. D. Barrow, G. Mellows, *DE 2227739*; *eidem, US 3977943*; *eidem, US 4071536* (1973, 1976, 1978 all to Beecham). Purification: P. J. O'Hanlon *et al.*, *DE 2842358*; *eidem, US 4222942* (1979, 1980 both to Beecham). Structure: E. B. Chain, G. Mellows, *Chem. Commun.* **1974**, 847; *eidem, J. Chem. Soc. Perkin Trans. 1* **1977**, 294. Absolute configuration: R. G. Alexander *et al.*, *ibid.* **1978**, 561. Prepn from methyl pseudomonate C: *eidem, Tetrahedron Lett.* **22**, 2059 (1981). Total syntheses of (±)-form: B. B. Snider, G. B. Phillips, *J. Am. Chem. Soc.* **104**, 1113 (1982); B. B. Snider *et al.*, *J. Org. Chem.* **48**, 3003

(1983). Biosynthesis: T. C. Feline *et al., J. Chem. Soc. Perkin Trans. 1* **1977**, 309. Effect of pH on chemical stability and antibacterial activity: J. P. Clayton *et al., ibid.* **1979**, 838. Inhibition of bacterial protein synthesis: J. Hughes, G. Mellows, *J. Antibiot.* **31**, 330 (1978); of isoleucyl-tRNA synthetase: *eidem, Biochem. J.* **176**, 305 (1978); *eidem, ibid.* **191**, 209 (1980). *In vitro* antibacterial spectrum: R. Sutherland *et al., Antimicrob. Agents Chemother.* **27**, 495 (1985); M. W. Casewell, R. L. R. Hill, *J. Antimicrob. Chemother.* **15**, 523 (1985). Antimycoplasmal activity *in vitro*: R. M. Banks *et al., J. Antibiot.* **41**, 609 (1988). Clinical evaluations: G. D. Reilly, R. C. Spencer, *ibid.* **13**, 295 (1984); M. W. Casewell, R. L. R. Hill, *ibid.* **17**, 365 (1986). *Reviews:* A. Ward, D. M. Campoli-Richards, *Drugs* **32**, 425-444 (1986); M. W. Casewell, R. L. R. Hill, *J. Antimicrob. Chemother.* **19**, 1-5 (1987).

Crystals from ether, mp 77-78°. $[\alpha]_D^{20}$ −19.3° (c = 1 in methanol). uv max (ethanol): 222 nm (ε 14500).

THERAP CAT: Topical antibacterial.

THERAP CAT (VET): Topical antibacterial.

6303. Muraglitazar. [331741-94-7] *N*-[(4-Methoxyphenoxy)carbonyl]-*N*-[[4-[2-(5-methyl-2-phenyl-4-oxazolyl)ethoxy]phenyl]methyl]glycine; BMS-298585; Pargluva. $C_{29}H_{28}N_2O_7$; mol wt 516.54. C 67.43%, H 5.46%, N 5.42%, O 21.68%. Peroxisome proliferator-activated receptor (PPAR) α/γ dual agonist. Prepn: P. T. Cheng, **WO 0121602** (2001, 2002 both to Bristol-Myers Squibb); P. V. Devasthale *et al., J. Med. Chem.* **48**, 2248 (2005). Review of development and therapeutic potential: D. Barlocco, *Curr. Opin. Invest. Drugs* **6**, 427-434 (2005).

Crystals from ethanol, mp 139.1-140.2°. uv max (methanol): 224, 277 nm.

THERAP CAT: Antidiabetic.

6304. Muramic Acid. [1114-41-6] (*R*)-2-Amino-3-*O*-(1-carboxyethyl)-2-deoxy-D-glucose; 3-*O*-α-carboxyethyl-D-glucosamine. $C_9H_{17}NO_7$; mol wt 251.23. C 43.03%, H 6.82%, N 5.58%, O 44.58%. Amino sugar found (as the *N*-acetyl derivative) in *peptidoglycan*, the main skeletal component of the bacterial cell wall. Discovery: J. T. Park, *J. Biol. Chem.* **194**, 885 (1952). Isoln from spores of *Bacillus megatherium*: R. E. Strange, F. A. Dark, *Nature* **177**, 186 (1956). Identification and synthesis: R. E. Strange, L. H. Kent, *Biochem. J.* **71**, 333 (1959). Stereospecific synthesis: Y. Matsushima, J. T. Park, *J. Org. Chem.* **27**, 3581 (1962); *eidem, Biochem. Prep.* **10**, 109 (1963); T. Osawa, R. W. Jeanloz, *J. Org. Chem.* **30**, 448 (1965). Review of peptidoglycan structure: H. J. Rogers, *Ann. N.Y. Acad. Sci.* **235**, 29-51 (1974). Use to determine bacterial levels in mammalian tissues: J. Gilbart *et al., J. Microbiol. Methods* **5**, 271 (1986); in airborne dust: A. Fox *et al., Appl. Environ. Microbiol.* **59**, 4354 (1993).

Crystals from water, mp 152-154° (dec); $[\alpha]_D^{25}$ +103° (c = 0.26 in water) (Matsushima, Park). Also reported as crystals from 90% ethanol, mp 160-162° (dec); $[\alpha]_D^{22}$ +146° (6 minutes) → +116° (31 hrs) (c = 0.57 in water) (Osawa, Jeanloz).

N-Acetylmuramic acid. [10597-89-4] (*R*)-2-(Acetylamino)-3-*O*-(1-carboxyethyl)-2-deoxy-D-glucose. $C_{11}H_{19}NO_8$; mol wt 293.27. Crystals from ethyl acetate + methanol, mp 119-121°. $[\alpha]_D^{20}$ +56° (10 minutes) → +40° (24 hrs) (c = 0.68 in water).

USE: As chemical marker for the detection of bacterial contamination.

6305. Muramyl Dipeptide. [53678-77-6] *N*-(*N*-Acetylmuramoyl)-L-alanyl-D-α-glutamine; *N*-acetylmuramyl-L-alanyl-D-isoglutamine; 2-acetamido-2-deoxy-3-*O*-(D-2-propionyl-L-alanyl-D-isoglutamine)-D-glucopyranose; MDP. $C_{19}H_{32}N_4O_{11}$; mol wt 492.48. C 46.34%, H 6.55%, N 11.38%, O 35.74%. Synthetic immunoadjuvant corresponding to the smallest immunologically active glycopeptide subunit of the bacterial cell wall. Prepn: A. Adam *et al.,* **DE 2450355**; *eidem,* **US 4235771** (1975, 1980 both to Agen. Nat. Valor. Recher.); C. Merser *et al., Biochem. Biophys. Res. Commun.* **66**, 1316 (1975); P. Lefrancier *et al., Int. J. Pept. Protein Res.* **9**, 249 (1977). Structure-activity relationships: F. Ellouz *et al., Biochem. Biophys. Res. Commun.* **59**, 1317 (1974); A. Adam *et al., ibid.* **72**, 339 (1976). Review of immunoregulating activity: L. Chedid *et al., Prog. Allergy* **25**, 63-105 (1978). Tissue distribution in mice: M. Parant *et al., Int. J. Immunopharmacol.* **1**, 35 (1979). Potentiation of antitumor immunity: S. Sone *et al., J. Biol. Response Modif.* **3**, 185 (1984); A. E. Eggers, *ibid.* **7**, 229 (1988).

Crystals from methanol-acetone-ether. $[\alpha]_D^{25}$ +44° (acetic acid).

USE: Immunological adjuvant.

6306. Murexide. [3051-09-0] 5-[(Hexahydro-2,4,6-trioxo-5-pyrimidinyl)imino]-2,4,6(1*H*,3*H*,5*H*)-pyrimidinetrione monoammonium salt; 5,5′-nitrilodibarbituric acid monoammonium salt; acid ammonium purpurate; ammonium purpurate. $C_8H_8N_6O_6$; mol wt 284.19. C 33.81%, H 2.84%, N 29.57%, O 33.78%. Prepn from alloxan + NH_3: Hartley, *J. Chem. Soc.* **87**, 1791 (1905); Schwartz, Handritschk, **DD 17589** (1959), *C.A.* **55**, 3630a (1961); from alloxantin + ammonium acetate: Davidson, *J. Am. Chem. Soc.* **58**, 1821 (1936). Structure: Hartley, *J. Chem. Soc.* **87**, 1796 (1905); Winslow, *J. Am. Chem. Soc.* **61**, 2089 (1939); Schreiber, *Mitt. Dtsch. Pharm. Ges.* **28**, 20 (1958).

Purple-red crystals with green metallic luster. Absorption max in water: 520 nm. Sparingly sol in cold water, more in hot water; practically insol in alcohol, ether. The H_2O soln is deep purple and the aq NaOH soln is deep blue.

USE: Indicator for complexometric titrations.

6307. Murexine. [20284-40-6] 2-[[3-(1*H*-Imidazol-4-yl)-1-oxo-2-propenyl]oxy]-*N*,*N*,*N*-trimethylethanaminium; β-(4-imidazolyl)acrylcholine; urocanylcholine. $[C_{11}H_{18}N_3O_2]^+$. Neuromuscular blocker found, often in very large quantities, in the median zone of the hypobranchial body of *Murex trunculus* and of other related species of mollusks: Erspamer, Dordoni, *Ric. Sci. Ricostr.*

16, 1114 (1946); *Arch. Int. Pharmacodyn.* **74**, 263 (1947); Erspamer, *ibid.* **76**, 308 (1948). Isoln: *idem, Experientia* **4**, 226 (1948); M. Roseghini *et al., Eur. J. Biochem.* **12**, 468 (1970); J. E. Blankenship *et al., Comp. Biochem. Physiol.* **51C**, 129 (1975). Synthesis: Pasini *et al., Ann.* **578**, 6 (1952); Pasini, Coda, US 2956061 (1960 to Società Farmaceutici). Structure: V. Erspamer, O. Benati, *Science* **117**, 161 (1953). Effect on vertebrate and invertebrate muscles: J. C. de Freitas, *Comp. Biochem. Physiol.* **56C**, 57 (1977).

The base is instantly hydrolyzed by water; unstable both in acid or alkaline media.
Chloride. Extremely hygroscopic crystals. uv max (pH 4.5): 280-282 nm.
Chloride hydrochloride. Hygroscopic microcrystalline powder, mp 219-221° (dec); shows the same uv max as the chloride.

6308. Muromonab CD3. [140608-64-6] OKT3; Orthoclone OKT3. Murine monoclonal IgG$_{2a}$ antibody directed against the CD3 surface antigen on mature T-cells; designed as a specific T-cell inhibitor for treatment of transplant rejection. Prepn: P. C. Kung *et al., Science* **206**, 347 (1979); P. C.-S. Kung, G. Goldstein, EP 18795; *eidem*, US 4361549 (1980, 1982 both to Ortho Pharm.). Clinical study in renal transplant: G. Goldstein *et al., N. Engl. J. Med.* **313**, 337 (1985); in heart transplant: M. P. Macris *et al., J. Heart Transplant.* **8**, 281 (1989). Review of development and mechanism of action: G. Goldstein, *Transplant. Proc.* **19**, Suppl. 1, 1-6 (1987); of pharmacology and clinical use in transplantation: M. A. Hooks *et al., Pharmacotherapy* **11**, 26-37 (1991); M. I. Wilde, K. L. Goa, *Drugs* **51**, 865-894 (1996).

THERAP CAT: Immunosuppressant.

6309. Muscalure. [27519-02-4] (*Z*)-9-Tricosene; *cis*-tricos-9-ene. C$_{23}$H$_{46}$; mol wt 322.61. C 85.63%, H 14.37%. Sex pheromone of the female common house fly, *Musca domestica* L. Isoln and synthesis: Carlson *et al., Science* **174**, 76 (1971). Alternate syntheses: Eiter, *Naturwissenschaften* **59**, 468 (1972); Cargill, Rosenblum, *J. Org. Chem.* **37**, 3971 (1972); Gribble *et al., Chem. Commun.* **1973**, 735; Ho, Wong, *Can. J. Chem.* **52**, 1923 (1974); K. Abe *et al., Bull. Chem. Soc. Jpn.* **50**, 2792 (1977); V. N. Odinokov *et al., Tetrahedron Lett.* **23**, 1371 (1982). Acute toxicity study: M. Beroza *et al., Toxicol. Appl. Pharmacol.* **31**, 421 (1975).

bp$_{0.1}$ 157-158°. n_D^{26} 1.4517. LD$_{50}$ in rabbits (mg/kg): >2025 dermally; in rats (mg/kg): >23070 orally (Beroza).

USE: Insect attractant.

6310. Muscarine. [300-54-9] [2*S*-(2α,4β,5α)]-Tetrahydro-4-hydroxy-*N,N,N*,5-tetramethyl-2-furanmethanaminium. [C$_9$H$_{20}$-NO$_2$]$^+$. Alkaloid from the red variety of *Amanita muscaria* (L.) Pers., *Agaricaceae*, the fly fungus, or poisonous mushroom. Also found in some other fungi: *Inocybe patouillardi; I. fastigiata, I. umbrina; I. rimosa*. Isoln procedure for the naturally occurring L-(+)-form: Kuehl *et al., J. Am. Chem. Soc.* **77**, 6663 (1955); Eugster, *Helv. Chim. Acta* **39**, 1002 (1956). Structure and synthesis of racemate: Kögl *et al., Rec. Trav. Chim.* **76**, 109 (1957); Kögl *et al., Experientia* **13**, 137, 138 (1957); Cox *et al., Helv. Chim. Acta* **41**, 229 (1958). Alternate syntheses: GB 828395 (1960 to Hoffmann-La Roche); Matsumoto *et al., Tetrahedron* **25**, 5889 (1969); W. C. Still, J. A. Schneider, *J. Org. Chem.* **45**, 3375 (1980). Synthesis of muscarine: Whiting *et al., Can. J. Chem.* **50**, 3322 (1972); A. M. Mubarak, D. M. Brown, *Tetrahedron Lett.* **21**, 2453 (1980); *eidem, J. Chem. Soc. Perkin Trans. 1* **1982**, 809; S. Pochet, T. Huynhdinh, *J. Org. Chem.* **47**, 193 (1982). Chemistry and pharmacology: Waser, *Pharmacol. Rev.* **13**, 465-515 (1961). Toxicity study: P. J. Fraser, *Br. J. Pharmacol.* **12**, 47 (1957). *Reviews:* C. H. Eugster, *Adv. Org. Chem.* **2**, 427-455 (1960); S. Wilkinson, *Q. Rev. Chem. Soc.* **15**, 153-

171 (1961). Configurational relationship in the muscarine series: Bollinger, Eugster, *Helv. Chim. Acta* **54**, 2704 (1971).

Chloride. C$_9$H$_{20}$ClNO$_2$. Stout prisms from ethanol + acetone, mp 180-181°. Extremely hygroscopic. [α]$_D^{25}$ +8.1° (c = 3.5 in ethanol). Very sol in water, ethanol. Slightly sol in chloroform, ether, acetone. Aq solns are stable. LD$_{50}$ i.v. in mice: 0.23 mg/kg (Fraser).

Caution: Potential symptoms of toxicity following ingestion are profuse sweating, increased salivation, visual disturbances, nausea, vomiting, abdominal colic, diarrhea, headache, and bronchospasm. Very high doses may produce lacrimation, incontinence, bradycardia, hypotension and shock. *See Clinical Toxicology of Commercial Products*, R. E. Gosselin *et al.*, Eds. (Williams & Wilkins, Baltimore, 5th ed., 1984) Section II, p 247.

THERAP CAT: Cholinergic.

6311. Muscazone. [2255-39-2] α-Amino-2,3-dihydro-2-oxo-5-oxazoleacetic acid; α-amino-2-oxo-4-oxazoline-5-acetic acid. C$_5$H$_6$N$_2$O$_4$; mol wt 158.11. C 37.98%, H 3.82%, N 17.72%, O 40.48%. From *Amanita muscaria* (L.) Fr., *Agaricaceae*: Eugster *et al., Tetrahedron Lett.* **1965**, 1813. Structure: Fritz *et al., ibid.* **1965**, 2075; Reiner, Eugster, *Helv. Chim. Acta* **50**, 128 (1967). Synthesis: Göth *et al., ibid.* 137.

Crystals, decomp above 190°. uv max at pH 2-7: 212 nm (ε 8700); at pH 12: 220 nm (ε 7500).

6312. Muscimol. [2763-96-4] 5-(Aminomethyl)-3(2*H*)-isoxazolone; 5-(aminomethyl)-3-isoxazolol; 5-aminomethyl-3-hydroxyisoxazole; 3-hydroxy-5-aminomethylisoxazole; agarin; pantherine. C$_4$H$_6$N$_2$O$_2$; mol wt 114.10. C 42.11%, H 5.30%, N 24.55%, O 28.04%. Potent CNS depressant and GABA agonist isolated from *Amanita muscaria* (L.) Fr., *Agaricaceae*. Structural identity with the insecticidal substances, pantherine and agarin: Onda *et al., Chem. Pharm. Bull.* **12**, 751 (1964); Eugster *et al., Tetrahedron Lett.* **1965**, 1813; Bowden, Drysdale, *ibid.* 727. Synthesis: Gagneux *et al., ibid.* 2077; Göth *et al., Helv. Chim. Acta* **50**, 137 (1967); Bowden *et al., J. Chem. Soc. C* **1968**, 172. Improved syntheses: Nakamura, *Chem. Pharm. Bull.* **19**, 46 (1971); P. Krogsgaard-Larsen, S. B. Christensen, *Acta Chem. Scand. B* **B30**, 281 (1976); A. Barco *et al., J. Chem. Res. Synop.* **1979**, 176; B. E. McCarry, M. Savard, *Tetrahedron Lett.* **22**, 5153 (1981); V. Jager, M. Frey, *Ann.* **1982**, 817. Conformational structure: L. Brehm *et al., ibid.* **26**, 1298 (1972). Industrial patents: Hafliger, Gagneux, US 3242190, US 3397209 (1966, 1968 both to Geigy). Pharmacology: Theobald *et al., Arzneim.-Forsch.* **18**, 311 (1968). Review of pharmacology: F. V. DeFeudis, *Neurochem. Res.* **5**, 1047-1068 (1980).

Crystals, mp 175° (dec). LD$_{50}$ in mice (mg/kg): 3.8 s.c., 2.5 i.p.; in rats (mg/kg): 4.5 i.v., 45 orally (Theobald).

USE: As a molecular probe to study GABA receptors.

6313. Muscone. [541-91-3] 3-Methylcyclopentadecanone; muskone; methylexaltone. C$_{16}$H$_{30}$O; mol wt 238.41. C 80.61%, H 12.68%, O 6.71%. The odorous principle of musk. Characterization of naturally occurring (−)-form: Ruzicka, *Helv. Chim. Acta* **9**, 715 (1926). Structure: *ibid.* 1008. Synthesis of (±)-form: Ziegler, Weber, *Ann.* **512**, 164 (1934); Ruzicka, Stoll, *Helv. Chim. Acta* **17**, 1308 (1934); Hunsdiecker, *Ber.* **75B**, 1197 (1942). Review of syntheses: S. Abe *et al., Cosmet. Perfum.* **88,** 67 (1973). Recent syntheses: Stork, Macdonald, *J. Am. Chem. Soc.* **97,** 1264 (1975); H. G. Fliri *et al., Monatsh. Chem.* **110,** 245 (1979); C. Fehr *et al., Helv. Chim. Acta* **62,** 2655 (1979); K. H. Schulte-Elte *et al., ibid.* 2673; G. Cantoni *et al., J. Org. Chem.* **45,** 1906 (1980). Chiral synthesis of (*R*)-(−)- and (*S*)-(+)-forms: Q. Branca, A. Fischli, *Helv. Chim. Acta* **60,** 925 (1977).

(−)**-Form.** Oily liquid. Musk odor. bp 328°; bp$_{0.5}$ 130°. d$_4^{17}$ 0.9221. n$_D^{17}$ 1.4802. [α]$_D^{17}$ −13°. Very slightly sol in water; miscible with alc.

(±)**-Form.** Oily liquid. bp$_{0.01}$ 90°. n$_D^{26}$ 1.4767. uv max (ethanol): 285 nm (log ε 1.54).

6314. Musks. Fixatives for perfumes having a characteristic persistent musky aroma. Obtained from plant and animal sources and by chemical synthesis. Natural sources of musk include the musk glands of the male musk deer, *Moschus moschiferus,* the civet cat, *Viverra civetta,* the Louisiana muskrat, ambrette seeds, *Abelmoschus moschatus,* and angelica roots, *Angelica archangelica.* Musk odor is exhibited by several categories of chemical compounds. Natural musks are macrocyclic ketones or lactones having approximately fifteen carbons in their ring structures. Synthetic musks are of greater industrial importance and include nitro and non-nitro benzenes, indans, and tetralins; derivatives of hydrindacene, isochroman, naphthindan, and coumarin. Purification of natural and synthetic musks: Thomas, Stephens, US 3415813 (1968 to Pfizer). Review of macrocyclic musks: Berends, *Am. Perfum. Cosmet.* **80,** 35 (1965). Review of chemical studies of synthetic musks: T. F. Wood, "Chemistry of the Aromatic Musks" (Givaudan Corp., company literature).

USE: In perfumery.

6315. Mustard. Annual plant with bright yellow flowers; varieties of *Brassica* spp. (also known as *Sinapsis* spp) Cruciferae. *Habit.* Europe, Asia, naturalized in U.S. *Constit.* Sinigrin (potassium myronate), myrosin, sinapine sulfocyanate, fixed oil; erucic, behenic, and sinapolic acids. Parts used are the seeds and the oils produced from them. Only black mustard yields a volatile oil which consists almost entirely of allyl isothiocyanate, *q.v.* Brief review: S. Arctander in *Perfume and Flavor Materials of Natural Origin* (Elizabeth, NJ, 1960) pp 424-425.

Black mustard. Brown mustard; red mustard. Dried ripe seeds of *B. nigra* (L.) Koch.

White mustard. Yellow mustard. Dried ripe seeds of *B. alba* (L.) Boiss.

Fixed oil. Vegetable oil expressed from the seeds of both black and white mustard. *Constit.* Chiefly the glycerides of oleic acid and other fatty acids, including arachidic. Straw-colored or brownish-yellow, or greenish-brown liquid. d$_{15}^{15}$ 0.914-0.916. Solidif −8° to −16°. n$_D^{40}$ 1.4655-1.4670. Sapon no. 170-174. Iodine no. 92-97. Insol in water; slightly sol in alcohol; miscible with chloroform, ether, petr ether.

USE: Flavoring agent for foods. Fixed oil as cooking oil.

THERAP CAT: Counterirritant; has also been used as an emetic.

6316. Mustard Gas. [505-60-2] 1,1′-Thiobis[2-chloroethane]; bis(2-chloroethyl)sulfide; β,β′-dichloroethyl sulfide; 2,2′-dichlorodiethyl sulfide; bis(β-chloroethyl)sulfide; 1-chloro-2-(β-chloroethylthio)ethane; sulfur mustard; yellow cross liquid; Kampfstoff "Lost"; Yperite. C$_4$H$_8$Cl$_2$S; mol wt 159.08. C 30.20%, H 5.07%, Cl 44.57%, S 20.16%. (ClCH$_2$CH$_2$)$_2$S. War gas prepd by treating ethylene with sulfur chloride (Levinstein process): Mann, Pope, *J. Chem. Soc.* **121,** 594 (1922); by treating β,β′-dihydroxyethyl sulfide with HCl gas (German process): Meyer, *Ber.* **19,** 3260 (1886); *Ann.* **240,** 310 (1887); Gomberg, *J. Am. Chem. Soc.* **41,** 1427 (1919). Reactions and derivatives: Helfrich, Reid, *ibid.* **42,** 1208 (1920). Toxicity: Anslow *et al., J. Pharmacol. Exp. Ther.* **93,** 1 (1948). Review of carcinogenic risk: *IARC Monographs* **9,** 181-192 (1975); of toxicology and human

exposure: *Toxicological Profile for Mustard Gas* (PB2004-100006, 2003) 287 pp.

Oily liquid. *Deadly vesicant.* Weak, sweet, agreeable odor. On cooling it forms prisms, mp 13-14°. d^{13} 1.338 (solid); d$_4^{20}$ 1.2741 (liq). bp$_{760}$ 215-217°; bp$_{10}$ 98°. Volatile with steam. n$_D^{20}$ 1.53125. Very sparingly sol in water; sol in fat solvents, other common organic solvents. High lipid soly. Vapor pressure: 0.025 mm (0°), 0.90 mm (30°). Hydrolyzed by alkalies. Recommended neutralizing agent and inactivator: Bleaching powder, sodium hypochlorite. LD$_{50}$ in rats, mice (mg/kg): 3.3, 8.6 i.v. (Anslow).

Caution: Overexposure may cause severe irritation and tissue damage to eyes, skin, and respiratory and GI tracts; symptoms may be delayed in onset. This substance is listed as a known human carcinogen: *Report on Carcinogens, Eleventh Edition* (PB2005-104914, 2004) p III-176.

USE: Formerly in chemical warfare. In biological studies of alkylating agents.

6317. Mycaminose. [519-21-1] 3,6-Dideoxy-3-(dimethylamino)-D-glucose. C$_8$H$_{17}$NO$_4$; mol wt 191.22. C 50.25%, H 8.96%, N 7.32%, O 33.47%. Part of the carbomycin molecule. Synthesis and stereochemistry: Richardson, *Proc. Chem. Soc. London* **1961,** 430; Foster *et al., Chem. Ind. (London)* **1962,** 142. Stereochemistry: Grisebach, Hofheinz, *Angew. Chem.* **74,** 499 (1962).

Hydrochloride monohydrate. Crystals from moist isopropanol, mp 116-118°. [α]$_D$ +31° (equilib value, c = 0.96).

6318. Mycarose. [6032-92-4] 2,6-Dideoxy-3-*C*-methyl-L-*ribo*-hexose; 2,6-didesoxy-3-*C*-methyl-L-*ribo*-hexose; 2-(4,5-*cis*)-trihydroxy-4,6-dimethyltetrahydropyran. C$_7$H$_{14}$O$_4$; mol wt 162.18. C 51.84%, H 8.70%, O 39.46%. Constituent of the macrolides carbomycin A and B, spiramycin A, B and C and tylosin: Woodward, *Angew. Chem.* **69,** 50 (1957); Paul, Tchelitcheff, *Bull. Soc. Chim. Fr.* **1957,** 443; **1960,** 150; Hamill *et al., Antibiot. Chemother.* **11,** 328 (1961). Part of carbomycin molecule: Regna *et al., J. Am. Chem. Soc.* **75,** 4625 (1953). Stereochemistry: Grisebach, Hofheinz, *Angew. Chem.* **74,** 499 (1962); Foster *et al., Proc. Chem. Soc. London* **1962,** 254; Hofheinz *et al., Tetrahedron* **18,** 1265 (1962). Synthesis of DL-mycarose: Korte *et al., ibid.* 1257; Grisebach *et al., Ber.* **96,** 1823 (1963). Synthesis of L-mycarose: Lemal *et al., Tetrahedron* **18,** 1275 (1962); Koto *et al., Bull. Chem. Soc. Jpn.* **45,** 532 (1972). Synthesis of D-mycarose: Flaherty *et al., J. Chem. Soc. C* **1966,** 398. Isoln from aureolic acid: Berlin *et al., Khim. Prir. Soedin.* **8,** 535 (1972), *C.A.* **78,** 4432a (1973).

DL-Form. Crystals from acetone + petr ether, mp 110-111°.

L-Form. Needles from boiling acetone + chloroform, mp 128.5-130.5°. [α]$_D^{25}$ −31.1° (c = 4). Sol in water. Exhibits only end absorption in the ultraviolet.

3-*O*-Methylmycarose. Cladinose. C$_8$H$_{16}$O$_4$; mol wt 176.21. Constituent of erythromycin A and B. Liquid, bp$_{0.25}$ at bath temp 120-132°. [α]$_D^{25}$ −23.1° (c = 2.6 in water). Sol in water, alcohol, acetone, ether, benzene, chloroform, carbon tetrachloride; slightly sol in petr ether. Dec by strong acids.

6319. Mycelianamide. [22775-52-6] (6*S*)-3-[[4-[[(2*E*)-3,7-Dimethyl-2,6-octadienyl]oxy]phenyl]methylene]-1,4-dihydroxy-6-methyl-2,5-piperazinedione. C$_{22}$H$_{28}$N$_2$O$_5$; mol wt 400.47. C 65.98%, H 7.05%, N 7.00%, O 19.98%. Antibiotic substance found in the mycelium of *Penicillium griseofulvum:* Anslow, Raistrick, *Biochem. J.* **25,** 39 (1931); Oxford *et al., ibid.* **29,** 1102 (1935); **33,** 240 (1939); Oxford, Raistrick, *ibid.* **42,** 323 (1948). Structure:

Birch *et al., J. Chem. Soc.* **1956**, 3717; Bates, Schauble, *Tetrahedron Lett.* **1963**, 1683. Configuration: Gallina *et al., Gazz. Chim. Ital.* **94**, 1301 (1964). Partial synthesis: Brown, Meehan, *Aust. J. Chem.* **21**, 1581 (1968). Total synthesis: N. Shinmon *et al., Chem. Commun.* **1980**, 1020.

Crystals from ethyl acetate, dec 170-172°. $[\alpha]_{546}^{19}$ −217°; $[\alpha]_{579}^{19}$ −182°. Weak acid. Freely soluble in acetone, dioxane; sparingly sol in other organic solvents; sol in aq sodium carbonate solution, but not in sodium bicarbonate soln. Quickly destroyed by acids and alkalies.

6320. Mycetins. Antibiotic substances produced by *Actinomyces violaceus:* Fainshmidt, Koreniako, *Biokhimiya* **9**, 147 (1944); Krassilnikov, Koreniako, *Mikrobiologiya* **14**, 80 (1945). Chromatographic and structure studies: Yakubov *et al., ibid.* **31**, 526 (1962); Blinov *et al., J. Chromatogr.* **8**, 522 (1962); Yakubov *et al., Antibiotiki* **10**, 771 (1965).

6321. Myclobutanil. [88671-89-0] α-Butyl-α-(4-chlorophenyl)-1*H*-1,2,4-triazole-1-propanenitrile; 2-(4-chlorophenyl)-2-(1*H*-1,2,4-triazol-1-ylmethyl)hexanenitrile; RH-3866; Eagle; Laredo; Nova; Rally; Systhane. $C_{15}H_{17}ClN_4$; mol wt 288.78. C 62.39%, H 5.93%, Cl 12.28%, N 19.40%. Broad spectrum systemic triazole fungicide; ergosterol-biosynthesis inhibitor. Prepn: T. T. Fujimoto, **EP 145294** (1985 to Rohm & Haas), *C.A.* **103**, 160519z (1985). Physical properties and field trials: C. Orpin *et al., Proc. Br. Crop Prot. Conf. - Pests Dis.* **1986**, 55; A. Perrot, *Def. Veg.* **40**, 9 (1986). Antifungal activity: J. A. Quinn *et al., Pestic. Sci.* **17**, 357 (1986).

Light yellow crystals, mp 63-68°. $bp_{1.0}$ 202-208°. Vapor pressure at 25°: 1.6×10^{-6} Torr. Soly at 25°: water 142 ppm. Sol in common organic solvents such as ketones, esters, alcohols, aromatic hydrocarbons. Insol in aliphatic hydrocarbons. LD_{50} in male, female rats (mg/kg): 1600, 2229 orally; LD_{50} in rabbits (mg/kg): 7500 dermally (Orpin).

USE: Agricultural fungicide.

6322. Mycobacidin. [539-35-5] 4-Oxo-2-thiazolidine-hexanoic acid; ε-[2-(4-thiazolidone)]hexanoic acid; 4-thiazolidone-2-caproic acid; 2-(5-carboxypentyl)-4-thiazolidone; cinnamonin; actithiazic acid; acidomycin. $C_9H_{15}NO_3S$; mol wt 217.29. C 49.75%, H 6.96%, N 6.45%, O 22.09%, S 14.76%. Antibiotic substance produced by *Streptomyces lavendulae, Streptomyces virginiae* and several other *Streptomyces* spp. Isoln: Tejera *et al., Antibiot. Chemother.* **2**, 333 (1952). Production by fermentation: Grundy *et al.*, **US 2678929** (1954 to Abbott). Synthesis: McLamore *et al., J. Am. Chem. Soc.* **75**, 105 (1953); Nienburg, Friedrichsen, **DE 931651** (1955 to BASF). Toxicity studies: Miyake *et al., Pharm. Bull.* **1**, 84, 89 (1953). *Review:* Caltrider, *Antibiotics* vol. **I**, D. Gottlieb, P. D. Shaw, Eds. (Springer-Verlag, New York, 1967) pp 666-668.

l-Form. Needles from water, ethanol or ethyl acetate, mp 139-140°. $[\alpha]_D^{25}$ −54° (c = 1 in methanol); $[\alpha]_D^{25}$ −60° (c = 1 in ethanol). pK 5.1. Soluble in water, acetone, alcohol, ethylene dichloride, glacial acetic acid. Aq solns are stable over a wide pH range at room temp. Rapidly loses optical activity in dil alkali to give the racemate. Has *in vitro* activity against *Mycobacterium tuberculosis, M. ranae* and *M. phlei.* LD_{50} in mice (g/kg): 3.5 i.v., 2 s.c. (Miyake).

Methyl ester. $C_{10}H_{17}NO_3S$. Needles from ether + hexane, mp 53-54°. $[\alpha]_D^{25}$ −50.9° (methanol).

d-Form. Crystals, mp 138-139°. $[\alpha]_D^{25}$ +57° (methanol).

dl-Form. Crystals from water, mp 123°.

6323. Mycobacillin. [18524-67-9] $C_{65}H_{85}N_{13}O_{30}$; mol wt 1528.44. C 51.08%, H 5.61%, N 11.91%, O 31.40%. Antifungal polypeptide antibiotic isolated from culture filtrates of *Bacillus subtilis:* Majumdar, Bose, *Nature* **181**, 134 (1958). Structural studies: *eidem, Biochem. J.* **74**, 596 (1960); *Arch. Biochem. Biophys.* **90**, 154 (1960). Amino acid configuration: Banerjee, Bose, *Nature* **200**, 471 (1963). Nature of the peptide linkages: Sengupta *et al., Biochem. J.* **121**, 839 (1971). *Review:* Banerjee *et al., Antibiotics* vol. **II**, D. Gottlieb, P. D. Shaw, Eds. (Springer-Verlag, New York, 1967) pp 271-275, 445-446.

Ala–D-α-Asp–Pro–D-α-Asp–D-γ-Glu–Tyr
| |
| α-Asp
| |
D-α-Asp–D-γ-Glu–Leu–D-α-Asp–Ser–Tyr

Needles, mp 235-240°. uv max 277 nm in a solution of *n*-butanol-water-acetic acid-95% ethanol (10:10:2:2).

6324. Mycobactins. Growth factors for *Mycobacterium paratuberculosis (M. johnei)*, the organism responsible for Johne's disease in cattle. Mycobactins are structurally complex *siderophores* (microbial iron chelators). At least nine mycobactins, designated with the letters A, F, H, M, N, P, R, S, and T, have been isolated from various non-pathogenic species of *Mycobacterium*. Earlier studies were actually on *mycobactin P*; *see* isoln from *M. phlei:* Francis *et al., Nature* **163**, 365 (1949); *eidem, Biochem. J.* **55**, 596 (1953); structure: Snow, *ibid.* **94**, 160 (1965). Separation and identification of mycobactins: White, Snow, *ibid.* **108**, 593 (1968); **111**, 785 (1969). Chemical and biological properties: *eidem, ibid.* **115**, 1031 (1969). On saponification, mycobactin splits into *mycobactic acid* and *cobactin*. Synthetic studies: Black *et al., Aust. J. Chem.* **25**, 2155 (1972). Synthesis of mycobactin S2: P. J. Maurer, M. J. Miller, *J. Am. Chem. Soc.* **105**, 240 (1983). Review of early studies: Rose, Snow, "Mycobactin: A Growth Factor for Acid-Fast Bacilli" in G. E. W. Wolstenholme, M. P. Cameron, C. M. O'Connor, *Ciba Found. Symp. Exp. Tuberc. Bacillus Host* **1955**, 41-54. Comprehensive review: Snow, *Bacteriol. Rev.* **34**, 99 (1970).

R^2, R^3, R^5 = H or CH_3
R^1, R^4 = CH_3, CH_2CH_3 or long alkyl chain

Able to chelate with metals, showing strong selectivity toward iron. Isolated as octahedral ferric complexes in the form of red-brown glasses; purified to metal-free mycobactins as white microcrystalline powders. Characterizations, esp mass spectral studies, carried out on the aluminum complexes. Mycobactin solids have definite melting points, are stable to air and heat up to about 100°, and show apple-green fluorescence in uv light. Characteristic uv max (methanol): 250, 311 nm for mycobactins having a methyl substituent on the benzene ring; 243, 249, 304 nm for mycobactins without the methyl substituent. Very sol in chloroform; fairly sol in ethanol; less sol in other alcoholic solvents. Slightly sol in benzene, ether, aliphatic hydrocarbons. Stable to acids; easily broken down under alk. conditions.

USE: In the taxonomy of mycobacteria; in development of iron chelators for clinical use.

6325. **Mycolic Acids.** High mol wt α-branched, β-hydroxy fatty acids, components of the cell envelopes of all *Mycobacteria.* All known mycolic acids have the basic structure $R^2CH(OH)$-CHR^1COOH where R^1 is a C_{20} to C_{24} linear alkane and R^2 is a more complex structure of 30 to 60 carbon atoms that may contain various numbers of carbon-carbon double bonds and/or cyclopropane rings, methyl branches or oxygen functions such as $C=O$, $CH_3OCH=$, $COOH$. The structure of mycolic acids varies by families and species. Three principal categories are known: (1) *corynomycolic acids* ranging from C_{28} to C_{40} found mostly in *Corynebacteria;* (2) *nocardic acids,* also called *nocardomycolic acids,* ranging from C_{40} to C_{60}, produced by strains of *Nocardia;* and (3) mycobacterial mycolic acids ranging from C_{60} to C_{90}. First obtained from a human strain of *Mycobacterium tuberculosis* and studied in an impure form called "unsaponifiable wax": R. J. Anderson, *J. Biol. Chem.* **85,** 351 (1929). Isoln of the first representative of this group of acids from the human tubercle bacillus and derivation of the name "mycolic acids": F. H. Stodola *et al., ibid.* **126,** 505 (1938). Historical reviews: R. J. Anderson, *Fortschr. Chem. Org. Naturst.* **3,** 145-202 (1939); J. Asselineau, E. Lederer, *ibid.* **10,** 170-273 (1953); J. Asselineau, *The Bacterial Lipids* (Hermann-Holden Day, Paris-New York, 1962) pp 82-148; E. Lederer, *Pure Appl. Chem.* **25,** 135 (1971). Major mycolic acids of *Mycobacterium smegmatis:* M. Y. H. Wong *et al., J. Biol. Chem.* **254,** 5734 (1979); M. Y. H. Wong, G. R. Gray, *ibid.* 5741. Total synthesis of mycolic acids from *M. smegmatis:* H. C. Huang *et al., J. Org. Chem.* **47,** 4018 (1982). Evaluation as immunotherapeutic agents in the treatment of cancer in animal models: M. V. Pimm *et al., Int. J. Cancer* **24,** 780 (1979). Clinical evaluation in humans: G. J. Vosika, *Cancer* **44,** 495 (1979). Mycolic acids are acid fast. They are always isolated in the form of more or less complex mixtures. They occur in nature esterified with carbohydrates: with arabinose in the cell wall, with trehalose in cord factor, *q.q.v.*

6326. **Mycomycin.** [544-51-4] 3,5,7,8-Tridecatetraene-10,12-diynoic acid. $C_{13}H_{10}O_2$; mol wt 198.22. C 78.77%, H 5.08%, O 16.14%. $HC\equiv C-C\equiv CCH=C=CHCH=CH-CH=CHCH_2COOH$. Antibiotic substance produced by *Nocardia acidophilus:* Johnson, Burdon, *J. Bacteriol.* **54,** 281 (1947); Johnson, *Soc. Am. Bacteriologists,* 49th General Meeting (May, 1949), *Abstracts of Papers,* p 68; Celmer, Solomons, 121st *A.C.S.* Meeting (Milwaukee, 1952), *Abstracts of Papers,* p 17-J; *J. Am. Chem. Soc.* **74,** 1870, 2245 (1952); **75,** 1372 (1953). Synthesis: Bohlmann, Sucrow, *Angew. Chem.* **76,** 611 (1964).

Needles from methylene chloride at $-40°$. Very thermolabile. Complete retention of activity is possible only by storage at $-40°$ or lower. mp 7.5° (deflagrates). $[\alpha]_D^{25}$ $-130°$ (c = 0.4 in ethanol). uv max (ether): 267, 281 nm (ε 61,000, 67,000). Sol in alcohol, ether, amyl acetate, methylene chloride. Forms a water-sol sodium salt. The acid itself is sparingly sol in water and is relatively stable in extremely dil aq solns (approx 0.005 mg/ml), half-life inversely related to concn. Undergoes an unusual rearrangement in normal aq KOH at 27°, involving an allene to acetylene isomerization accompanied by migration of the existing acetylenic bonds. The rearranged acid, *isomycomycin,* has been assigned the structure *3,5-tridecadiene-7,9,11-triynoic acid,* $CH_3-C\equiv C-C\equiv C-C\equiv C-CH=CHCH=CHCH_2COOH$.

6327. **Mycophenolic Acid.** [24280-93-1] (4E)-6-(1,3-Dihydro-4-hydroxy-6-methoxy-7-methyl-3-oxo-5-isobenzofuranyl)-4-methyl-4-hexenoic acid; 6-(4-hydroxy-6-methoxy-7-methyl-3-oxo-5-phthalanyl)-4-methyl-4-hexenoic acid. $C_{17}H_{20}O_6$; mol wt 320.34. C 63.74%, H 6.29%, O 29.97%. Antibiotic produced by *Penicillium brevi-compactum, P. stoloniferum* and related spp. Selectively inhibits lymphocyte proliferation by blocking inosine

monophosphate dehydrogenase (IMPDH), an enzyme involved in the *de novo* synthesis of purine nucleotides. Isoln: C. L. Alsberg, O. F. Black, *USDA Bur. Plant Ind. Bull.* **270,** 7 (1912), *C.A.* **7,** 3992 (1913); P. W. Clutterbuck *et al., Biochem. J.* **26,** 1441 (1932); and antimicrobial activity: H. W. Florey *et al., Lancet* **1,** 46 (1946). Structure: J. H. Birkinshaw *et al., Biochem. J.* **50,** 630 (1952); W. R. Logan, G. T. Newbold, *J. Chem. Soc.* **1957,** 1946. Total synthesis: A. J. Birch, J. J. Wright, *Aust. J. Chem.* **22,** 2635 (1969). Biosynthesis: L. Canonica *et al., J. Chem. Soc. Perkin Trans. 1* **1972,** 2639. Fermentation, isoln and biological properties: R. H. Williams *et al., Antimicrob. Agents Chemother.* **1968,** 229. Immunosuppressive effect: A. Mitsui, S. Suzuki, *J. Antibiot.* **22,** 358 (1969). Mechanism of action: A. C. Allison, E. M. Eugui, *Transplant. Proc.* **26,** 3205 (1994); J. T. Ransom, *Ther. Drug Monit.* **17,** 681 (1995). HPLC determn in plasma: J. Shen *et al., J. Chromatogr. B* **817,** 207 (2005); D. Indjova *et al., ibid.* 327.

Needles from hot water, mp 141°. pKa 4.5. Partition coefficient (*n*-octanol/water): 570 (pH 2); 1.6 (pH 7.4). Almost insol in cold water. Sol in alkali. LD_{50} in mice (mg/kg): >1250 orally; 972.9±77 i.p. (Williams).

2-(4-Morpholinyl)ethyl ester. [128794-94-5] Mycophenolate mofetil; RS-61443; CellCept. $C_{23}H_{31}NO_7$; mol wt 433.49. Prepn: P. H. Nelson *et al., US 4753935* (1988 to Syntex); and bioavailability: W. A. Lee *et al., Pharm. Res.* **7,** 161 (1990). Pharmacokinetics: R. E. S. Bullingham *et al., Transplant. Proc.* **28,** 925 (1996). Clinical trial in renal transplantation: P. A. Keown *et al., Transplantation* **61,** 1029 (1996). *Reviews:* D. O. Taylor *et al., J. Heart Lung Transplant.* **13,** 571-582 (1994); J. J. Lipsky, *Lancet* **348,** 1357-1359 (1996). Review of clinical experience in inflammatory bowel disease: A. C. Ford *et al., Aliment. Pharmacol. Ther.* **17,** 1365-1369 (2003). White to off-white crystalline powder, mp 93-94°. pKa 5.6. Partition coefficient (*n*-octanol/water): 0.0085 (pH 2); 238 (pH 7.4). Sol in acetone, methanol. Slightly sol in water; sparingly sol in ethanol.

Sodium salt. [37415-62-6] Mycophenolate sodium; Myfortic. $C_{17}H_{19}NaO_6$; mol wt 342.32. Clinical trial in renal transplantation: M. Salvadori *et al., Am. J. Transplant.* **4,** 231 (2003); K. Budde *et al., ibid.* 237. Review of pharmacology and clinical development of enteric-coated formulation: *idem et al., Expert Opin. Pharmacother.* **5,** 1333-1345 (2004). LD_{50} in mice (mg/kg): 1176±151 orally; 568±53 i.p. (Williams).

THERAP CAT: Immunosuppressant.

6328. **Mycosamine.** [527-38-8] 3-Amino-3,6-dideoxymannose; 3-amino-3-deoxyrhamnose; 3,6-dideoxy-3-amino-D-mannopyranose; 3-amino-3,6-dideoxy-D-aldohexose. $C_6H_{13}NO_4$; mol wt 163.17. C 44.17%, H 8.58%, N 8.58%, O 39.22%. An amino sugar which represents the nitrogen-contg moiety of the antifungal antibiotics, nystatin and amphotericin B, *q.q.v.* Isoln and structure: Dutcher *et al., Antibiot. Annu.* **1956-1957,** 866. Walters *et al., J. Am. Chem. Soc.* **79,** 5076 (1957); Dutcher *et al., J. Org. Chem.* **28,** 995 (1963). Stereochemistry: von Saltza *et al., J. Am. Chem. Soc.* **83,** 2875 (1961); *eidem, J. Org. Chem.* **28,** 999 (1963).

N-**Acetylmycosamine.** $C_8H_{15}NO_5$. Needles from methanol + acetone, mp 195-197°. $[\alpha]_D$ $-46°$ (ethanol).

Triacetylmycosamine. $C_{12}H_{19}NO_7$. Prisms from acetone or ethanol, mp 185-187°. $[\alpha]_D^{22}$ $+85°$ (ethanol).

Tetraacetylmycosamine. $C_{14}H_{21}NO_8$. Needles from benzene, mp 159-161°. $[\alpha]_D^{23}$ $+39.3°$ (ethanol).

Hydrochloride. $C_6H_{13}NO_4$.HCl. Prismatic rods from ethanol+ether, mp 162°. $[\alpha]_D^{24}$ $-11.5°$.

6329. Mylabris. Chinese cantharides; Chinese blistering flies. Dried insect, *Mylabris sidae (Phalerata)* Pallas, *Coleoptera. Habit.* China and East India. *Constit.* Cantharidin, said to be present in larger proportions than in cantharides (1-1.2%).

Black, cylindrical body, rounded above, flattish below; smaller than cantharides; black wing cases marked with a spot at point of insertion and has three tawny bands.

Caution: Highly toxic! *See* Cantharides.

USE: Source for cantharidin.

6330. Myosin. Mol wt approx 500,000. The main protein in muscle, which, by hydrolyzing ATP, provides the energy necessary for muscular contraction. Individual molecules are rod-shaped and consist of two globular heads attached flexibly to a tail of approx 1500Å length. All muscle myosins have a similar subunit structure composed of two heavy chains and two distinct pairs of light chains. One of the light chains is involved in a Ca^{2+}-dependent regulatory process in the vertebrate skeletal muscle system. Biological prepn and review: A. G. Szent-Györgyi, *Chemistry of Muscular Contraction* (Academic Press, New York, 2nd ed., 1951) pp 38-57, 146-148. Other reviews: *idem, Adv. Enzymol. Relat. Subj. Biochem.* **16**, 313-360 (1955); A. G. Szent-Györgyi *et al.,* in *Sulfur in Proteins,* R. Benesch *et al.,* Eds. (Academic Press, New York, 1959) pp 291-295; J. Gergely, *Biochemistry of Muscle Contraction* (Little, Brown, Boston, 1964) pp 3-115; several authors in *Contractile Proteins and Muscle,* K. Laki, Ed. (Dekker, New York, 1971); several authors in *Methods Enzymol.* **85**, Part B, 55-130 (1982). Review on structure and function of myosin: W. F. Harrington, "Contractile Proteins of Muscle" in *The Proteins* vol. 4, H. Neurath, R. L. Hill, Eds. (Academic Press, New York, 1979) p 245-409. Polymorphism of mammalian myosins and distribution of isoforms in different muscle fibers reviewed by A. G. Weeds in *Plasticity of Muscle,* D. Pette, Ed. (DeGruyter, Berlin, 1980) pp 55-68. Role of myosin light chains in calcium regulation: Kendrick-Jones, *Nature* **249**, 631 (1974). Tertiary crystal structure of globular heads: I. Rayment *et al., Science* **261**, 50 (1993). *See also* Tropomyosin.

6331. β-Myrcene. [123-35-3] 7-Methyl-3-methylene-1,6-octadiene; 2-methyl-6-methylene-2,7-octadiene. $C_{10}H_{16}$; mol wt 136.24. C 88.16%, H 11.84%. Found in oil of bay, verbena, hop, and others. Isoln: Power, Kleber, *Pharm. Rundsch.* **13**, 60 (1895); *see also* Ruzicka, Stoll, *Helv. Chim. Acta* **7**, 272 (1924); Goulding, Roberts, *J. Chem. Soc.* **105**, 2614 (1914); Booker *et al., ibid.* **1940**, 1453; Kugler, Kováts, *Helv. Chim. Acta* **46**, 1480 (1963). Obtained by pyrolysis of β-pinene: Goldblatt, Palkin, *J. Am. Chem. Soc.* **63**, 3517 (1941); Rummelsburg, US 2444790 (1948 to Hercules Powder); Houlihan *et al., J. Am. Chem. Soc.* **81**, 4692 (1959). Separation of isomers: Ohloff *et al., Ann.* **675**, 83 (1964). Synthesis: O. P. Vig *et al., Indian J. Chem.* **7**, 450 (1969); **11**, 104 (1973); **13**, 1244 (1975); T. Mandai *et al., Tetrahedron Lett.* **22**, 763 (1981). Formation from isoprene: K. Takabe *et al., Synthesis* **1977**, 307.

Oil. Pleasant odor. d_4^{20} 0.794. n_D^{20} 1.4709. uv max (ethanol): 226 nm (ε 16,100). Practically insol in water. Sol in alcohol, chloroform, ether, glacial acetic acid.

α-Myrcene. 2-Methyl-6-methylene-1,7-octadiene. bp_{10} 44°. n_D^{25} 1.4661. d_4^{25} 0.7959. uv max (isooctane): 224.5 nm (ε 18,600). Not found in nature. Prepn: Mitzner *et al., J. Org. Chem.* **30**, 646 (1965); Vig *et al., J. Indian Chem. Soc.* **50**, 329 (1973).

USE: β-Myrcene as an intermediate in the manuf of perfume chemicals.

6332. Myricetin. [529-44-2] 3,5,7-Trihydroxy-2-(3,4,5-trihydroxyphenyl)-4*H*-1-benzopyran-4-one; 3,3′,4′,5,5′,7-hexahydroxyflavone; cannabiscetin; delphidenolon 1575. $C_{15}H_{10}O_8$; mol wt 318.24. C 56.61%, H 3.17%, O 40.22%. From the bark

of *Myrica nagi* Thunb., *Myriaceae:* Perkin, Hummel, *J. Chem. Soc.* **69**, 1287 (1896). Structure: Perkin, *ibid.* **81**, 203 (1902). Identity with cannabiscetin: Seshadri, Venkateswarlu, *Proc. Indian Acad. Sci.* **23A**, 296 (1946); *C.A.* **40**, 6447 (1946). Synthesis: Kalff, Robinson, *J. Chem. Soc.* **127**, 181 (1925); Rao *et al., J. Sci. Ind. Res.* **8B**, No. 6, 113 (1949). Occurrence in *Hamamelidaceae* and *Anacardiaceae:* Reznek, Egger, *Z. Naturforsch.* **15b**, 247 (1960). Metabolism: Smith, Griffiths, *Biochem. J.* **118**, 53p (1970).

Yellow needles from dil alc, mp 357°. uv max (ethanol): 375, 255 nm. Sparingly sol in boiling water; sol in alcohol. Practically insol in chloroform, acetic acid.

Hexaacetate. $C_{27}H_{22}O_{14}$. Crystals, mp 213°.

Hexaethyl ether. $C_{27}H_{34}O_8$. Needles from alcohol, mp 149-151°.

3-Rhamnoside. Myricitrin. $C_{21}H_{20}O_{12}$. Structure: Hattori, Hayashi, *Acta Phytochim.* **5**, 213 (1931), *C.A.* **26**, 990[8] (1932). Pale yellow leaflets from water, mp 199-200°. uv max (alc): 262, 352 nm. Sparingly sol in water, abs alcohol.

6333. Myristic Acid. [544-63-8] Tetradecanoic acid. C_{14}-$H_{28}O_2$; mol wt 228.37. C 73.63%, H 12.36%, O 14.01%. CH_3-$(CH_2)_{12}COOH$. Occurs in nutmeg butter *(Myristica fragrans* Houtt.) to the extent of 70-80%; predominates in the fats of the *Myristicaceae;* in palm seed fats it may comprise 20% of the total fatty acids; in milk fats between 8-12% of the total acids. Occurs in most animal and vegetable fats; has been found in considerable amounts (up to 15%) in sperm whale oil, *see* Markley, *Fatty Acids* (New York, 1947). Prepn: G. D. Beal, *Org. Synth.* **coll. vol. I**, 379 (2nd ed., 1941). Prepn from tall-oil fatty acids: Segessmann, Molnar, US 2481356 (1949); from 9-ketotetradecanoic acid: Ames *et al., J. Chem. Soc.* **1950**, 174; by electrolysis of methyl hydrogen adipate + decanoic acid: Greaves *et al., ibid.* **1950**, 3326; by Maurer oxidation of myristyl alc: Langenbeck, Richter, *Ber.* **89**, 202 (1956); from cetanol: Selwitz, US 2969380 (1961 to Gulf). Wide-line NMR spectrum: A. V. Bailey, R. A. Pittman, *J. Am. Oil Chem. Soc.* **48**, 775 (1971). Toxicity study: L. Orö, A. Wretlind, *Acta Pharmacol. Toxicol.* **18**, 141 (1961).

Crystals from methanol, mp 58.5°. bp_{100} 250.5°; bp_{16} 199°; bp_4 184°. d_4^{54} 0.8622. d_4^{70} 0.8528. d_4^{90} 0.8394. n_D^{60} 1.4305; n_D^{70} 1.4273. Soluble in abs alcohol, methanol, ether, petr ether, benzene, chloroform. Neutralization value: 245.68. Absorption spectrum: Markley, *op. cit.* LD_{50} i.v. in mice: 432.6 mg/kg (Orö, Wretlind).

Ethyl ester. Ethyl myristate. $C_{16}H_{32}O_2$. Liquid, mp 12°; bp 295°; bp_{30} 195°. d_4^{20} 0.856. Insol in water. Sol in alcohol; slightly sol in ether.

USE: As ingredient in soaps and shaving creams; in lubricants; in coatings for anodized aluminum.

6334. Myristicin. [607-91-0] 4-Methoxy-6-(2-propenyl)-1,3-benzodioxole; 5-allyl-1-methoxy-2,3-(methylenedioxy)-benzene. $C_{11}H_{12}O_3$; mol wt 192.21. C 68.74%, H 6.29%, O 24.97%. Aromatic ether extracted from nutmeg, parsley, carrots. Isoln from nutmeg, *Myristica fragrans* Houtt., *Myristicaceae* and characterization: F. B. Power, A. H. Salway, *J. Chem. Soc.* **91**, 2037 (1907); A. T. Shulgin, *Nature* **197**, 379 (1963); from carrots, *Daucus carota* L., *Umbelliferae:* S. G. Yates, R. E. England, *J. Agric. Food Chem.* **30**, 317 (1982); from parsley, *Petroselinium hortense* Hoffman, *Umbelliferae:* M. Balogh *et al., Herba Hung.* **17**, 39 (1978), *C.A.* **91**, 2543e (1979). Synthesis: V. M. Trikojus, D. E. White, *Nature* **144**, 1016 (1939); F. Dallacker, R. Sluysmans, *Monatsh. Chem.* **100**, 560 (1969). HPLC sepn: L. W. Wulf *et al., J. Chromatogr.* **161**, 271 (1978); A. W. Archer, *ibid.* **438**, 117 (1988). GC-MS study: G. M. Sammy, W. W. Nawar, *Chem. Ind.* **1968**, 1279. MS-MS study of nutmeg extract: D. V. Davis, R. G. Cooks, *J.*

Agric. Food Chem. **30**, 495 (1982). Possible psychotropic properties: A. T. Shulgin, *Nature* **210**, 380 (1966).

Colorless oil, bp$_{40}$ 173°. n_D^{20} 1.54032. d$_{20}^{20}$ 1.1437.

6335. Myristyl Alcohol. [112-72-1] 1-Tetradecanol; tetradecyl alcohol. $C_{14}H_{30}O$; mol wt 214.39. C 78.43%, H 14.10%, O 7.46%. $CH_3(CH_2)_{12}CH_2OH$. Prepn by sodium reduction of fatty acid esters: Hansley, *Ind. Eng. Chem.* **39**, 55 (1947); by LiAlH$_4$ reduction of fatty acids: Watanabe, *Bull. Chem. Soc. Jpn.* **34**, 398 (1961); from acetaldehyde + dimethylamine: Langenbeck *et al., J. Prakt. Chem.* **8**, 112 (1959).

White crystals, mp 38°. d 0.824. bp$_{15}$ 167°. Practically insol in water. Sol in ether, slightly in alcohol.

USE: As emollient for cold creams, etc., also for making the sulfated alcohol whose sodium salt is applicable as a "wetter" in textiles.

6336. Myristyltrimethylammonium Bromide. [1119-97-7] *N,N,N*-Trimethyl-1-tetradecanaminium bromide; trimethyltetradecylammonium bromide; tetradonium bromide; Morpan T; Mytab. $C_{17}H_{38}BrN$; mol wt 336.39. C 60.70%, H 11.39%, Br 23.75%, N 4.16%. $[CH_3(CH_2)_{13}N(CH_3)_3]^+Br^-$. Cationic germicidal detergent. Prepn and antibacterial activity: R. S. Shelton *et al., J. Am. Chem. Soc.* **68**, 753 (1946). Toxicity and pharmacology: B. Isomaa, K. Bjondahl, *Acta Pharmacol. Toxicol.* **47**, 17 (1980).

White powder, mp 245-250°. Sol in 5 parts water. *Corrosive!* LD$_{50}$ in mice, rats (mg/kg): 12.0, 15.0 i.v. (Issomaa, Bjondahl).

USE: Disinfectant; deodorant; laboratory reagent.

6337. Myrophine. [467-18-5] 7,8-Didehydro-4,5-epoxy-17-methyl-3-(phenylmethoxy)morphinan-6-ol tetradecanoate (ester); 3-benzylmorphine 6-myristate; benzylmorphine myristic acid ester; benzylmorphinyl myristate; myristyl benzylmorphine; 3-benzyloxy-6-myristoyloxy-*N*-methyl-4,5-epoxy-7-morphinene; 3-benzyloxy-6-myristoyloxymorphine; myrocodine; myrophinium; Leucodinine; Myricodine; Peronine myristate. $C_{38}H_{51}NO_4$; mol wt 585.82. C 77.91%, H 8.77%, N 2.39%, O 10.92%. Prepn: Jeanson, **US 2802828** (1957 to Laborec).

Solid, mp 41°.
Hydrochloride. $C_{38}H_{51}NO_4 \cdot HCl$. Solid, mp 198-199°.

Note: This is a controlled substance (opium derivative): **21 CFR**, 1308.11.

THERAP CAT: Analgesic (narcotic).

6338. Myrrh. [9000-45-7] Gum-resin myrrh. From *Commiphora abyssinica* (Berg) Eng. or from other species of *Commiphora, Burseraceae.* Yields not less than 30% alcohol-soluble extract. *Habit.* Nubia, Somaliland, Arabia. *Constit.* 20-25% resin, 57-61% gum, 7-17% volatile oil and a bitter principle.

THERAP CAT: Carminative; astringent.

6339. Myrtol. [8002-55-9] Gelomyrtol. The fraction of the volatile oil from *Myrtus communis* L., *Myrtaceae* distilling between 166-180° and consisting chiefly of eucalyptol and *dextro*-pinene with a small quantity of an undefined camphor.

Colorless or slightly yellow, strongly dextrorotatory liquid (due to *dextro*-pinene); pleasant odor resembling that of turpentine and eucalyptol. d ~0.895. $[\alpha]_D^{20}$ +10°. n_D^{20} ~1.465. Freely sol in alcohol, ether.

6340. Myxin. [13925-12-7] 6-Methoxy-1-phenazinol 5,10-dioxide; 1-hydroxy-6-methoxyphenazine 5,10-dioxide; 3C antibiotic. $C_{13}H_{10}N_2O_4$; mol wt 258.23. C 60.47%, H 3.90%, N 10.85%, O 24.78%. Potent broad-spectrum antibiotic capable of inhibiting a wide range of gram-positive and gram-negative bacteria, various fungi and yeasts. Isoln from a *Sorangium* species (strain 3C), a soil-borne myxobacter: Peterson *et al., Can. J. Microbiol.* **12**, 221 (1966). Proposed structure: Edwards, Gillespie, *Tetrahedron Lett.* **1966**, 4867. Revised structure and synthesis: Weigele, Leimgruber, *ibid.* **1967**, 715; Sigg, Toth, *Helv. Chim. Acta* **50**, 716 (1967). Activity: E. Grunberg *et al., Chemotherapia* **12**, 272 (1967). Crystal structure: Hanson, *Acta Crystallogr.* **B24**, 1084 (1968). *Review:* Edwards, Gillespie, *Proc. Int. Symp. Drug Res.* **1967**, 236; Leimgruber, Grunberg, *ibid.* 240; Baker, Vezina, *ibid.* 242.

Red needles from acetone, mp 120-130°; also reported as mp 149° (dec) (Sigg, Toth). Strongly exothermic at 149°. May explode on drying with heat: Rachlin, *Chem. Eng. News* **45**, 32 (Sept. 4, 1967). uv max (0.1 *N* HCl): 283, 340 nm (ε 97000, 5400); absorption max (0.1*N* HCl): 505 nm (ε 6500). Stable in water after 6 hours at 37° in 0.05*N* acetate buffer at pH 5.0, in 0.05*N* phosphate at pH 6.0 and 7.0, or in 0.005*N* tris-HCl at pH 8.0 and 9.0. Stable at 70° except in phosphate buffer. Acetate, methanol, or aq tris buffer solns remain stable indefinitely at 4°. LD$_{50}$ in mice (mg/kg): >2000 orally, >2000 s.c., 133 i.p. (Grunberg).

Copper(II) complex. [39238-36-3] Cuprimyxin; Ro-7-4488/1; UNITOP. $C_{26}H_{18}CuN_4O_8$; mol wt 577.99. Prepn: W. Leimgruber *et al.,* **DE 1931466**; *eidem,* **US 3586674** (1970, 1971 both to Hoffmann-La Roche). Activity studies: Maestrone *et al., Am. J. Vet. Res.* **33**, 185 (1972). Dark green, fine crystals. uv max (DMSO): 287, 300, 356 nm (ε 68500, 63200, 10000); absorption max (DMSO): 408, 610 nm (ε 10400, 9500).

THERAP CAT (VET): Antibacterial, antifungal.

N

6341. Nabam. [142-59-6] 1,2-Ethanediylbiscarbamodithioic acid disodium salt; ethylenebis[dithiocarbamic acid] disodium salt; disodium ethylenebis[dithiocarbamate]; Dithane D-14; Parzate. $C_4H_6N_2Na_2S_4$; mol wt 256.34. C 18.74%, H 2.36%, N 10.93%, Na 17.94%, S 50.04%. Prepd by treating ethylenediamine with CS_2 in the presence of NaOH: Hester, US 2317765 (1943 to Rohm & Haas); Flenner, US 2504404 (1950 to du Pont). Fluorimetric determn in water and cereals: T. Pérez-Ruiz et al., Talanta **43**, 193 (1996). Degradation study: E. Milanova et al., Pulp Paper Can. **100**, 67 (1999). Toxicology study: R. B. Smith, Jr. et al., Fed. Proc. **11**, 391 (1952).

LD_{50} orally in rats: 395 ± 12 mg/kg (Smith).
Hexahydrate. Crystals from alc. Moderately sol in water. Forms a continuous film on plant surfaces, which is said to become insol in water.

Caution: Direct contact may cause skin irritation. *See Clinical Toxicology of Commercial Products*, R. E. Gosselin et al., Eds. (Williams & Wilkins, Baltimore, 5th ed., 1984) Section II, p 312.

USE: Agricultural fungicide; biocide in pulp and paper industry.

6342. Nabilone. [51022-71-0] (6aR,10aR)-rel-3-(1,1-Dimethylheptyl)-6,6a,7,8,10,10a-hexahydro-1-hydroxy-6,6-dimethyl-9H-dibenzo[b,d]pyran-9-one; LY-109514; Cesamet. $C_{24}H_{36}O_3$; mol wt 372.54. C 77.38%, H 9.74%, O 12.88%. Synthetic cannabinoid with antiemetic, antiglaucoma, and CNS activity. Prepn: R. A. Archer, DE 2451934, idem, US 3968125 (1975, 1976 both to Lilly); R. A. Archer et al., J. Org. Chem. **42**, 2277 (1977). Pharmacology: P. Stark, R. A. Archer, Pharmacologist **17**, 210 (1975); R. M. Orzelek-O'Neil et al., Toxicol. Appl. Pharmacol. **54**, 493 (1980). Physiological disposition: A. Rubin et al., Clin. Pharmacol. Ther. **22**, 85 (1977). Pharmacokinetics: H. R. Sullivan et al., Biomed. Mass Spectrom. **5**, 296 (1978). Behavioral effects: P. Stark, P. B. Dews, J. Pharmacol. Exp. Ther. **214**, 124 (1980). Clinical studies as antiemetic in cancer patients: N. Steele et al., Cancer Treat. Rep. **64**, 219 (1980); C. J. Williams et al., Cancer Clin. Trials **3**, 363 (1980). Clinical evaluation of anxiolytic effects: L. F. Fabre et al., J. Clin. Pharmacol. **21**, Suppl 8-9, 377S (1981); R. M. Glass et al., ibid. 383S. Review of pharmacology and efficacy as antiemetic: A. Ward, B. Holmes, Drugs **30**, 127-144 (1985). Toxicity study in neonatal rats: C. L. Moss et al., Toxicol. Appl. Pharmacol. **48**, A120 (1979). Comprehensive description: R. W. Souter, Anal. Profiles Drug Subs. **10**, 499-512 (1981).

White crystals from ethyl acetate/hexane, mp 159-160°. uv max (ethanol): 207, 280 nm (ε 47000, 250). pKa in 66% DMF: 13.5.
Note: This is a controlled substance (hallucinogen): **21 CFR**, 1308.12.

THERAP CAT: Antiemetic.

6343. Nabumetone. [42924-53-8] 4-(6-Methoxy-2-naphthalenyl)-2-butanone; 4-(6-methoxy-2-naphthyl)-butan-2-one; BRL-14777; Arthaxan; Balmox; Consolan; Nabuser; Relafen; Relifex; Relifex. $C_{15}H_{16}O_2$; mol wt 228.29. C 78.92%, H 7.06%, O 14.02%. Nonacidic, lipophillic prodrug; metabolized *in vivo* to 6-methoxy-2-naphthalacetic acid which inhibits prostaglandin syn-

thesis. Prepn: A. W. Lake, C. J. Rose, DE 2442305; eidem, US 4061779 (1975, 1977 both to Beecham); A. C. Goudie et al., J. Med. Chem. **21**, 1260 (1978). Pharmacology: E. A. Boyle et al., J. Pharm. Pharmacol. **34**, 562 (1982); B. Nunn, P. D. Chamberlain, ibid. 576. Metabolism: R. E. Haddock et al., Xenobiotica **14**, 327 (1984). HPLC determn in plasma: J. E. Ray, R. O. Day, J. Chromatogr. **336**, 234 (1984). Symposia on pharmacology, pharmacokinetics and clinical efficacy: Int. Congr. Symp. Ser. - R. Soc. Med. **69**, 1-215 (1985); J. Rheumatol. **19**, Suppl. 36, 1-91 (1992). Review: S. L. Dahl, Ann. Pharmacother. **27**, 456-463 (1993).

Crystals from ethanol, mp 80°.
THERAP CAT: Anti-inflammatory; analgesic.

6344. NAD. [53-84-9] Adenosine 5'-(trihydrogen diphosphate) $P' \rightarrow 5'$-ester with 3-(aminocarbonyl)-1-β-D-ribofuranosylpyridinium inner salt; 3-carbamoyl-1-β-D-ribofuranosylpyridinium hydroxide $5' \rightarrow 5'$-ester with adenosine 5'-(trihydrogen pyrophosphate) inner salt; nicotinamide-adenine dinucleotide; diphosphopyridine nucleotide; DPN; cozymase; coenzyme I; Co I; codehydrogenase; β-NAD; NAD$^+$; nadide. $C_{21}H_{27}N_7O_{14}P_2$; mol wt 663.43. C 38.02%, H 4.10%, N 14.78%, O 33.76%, P 9.34%. One of the biologically active forms of nicotinic acid, q.v. Occurs in living cells primarily in the oxidized state. Serves as a coenzyme of the dehydrogenases, especially in the dehydrogenation of primary and secondary alcohols. NAD usually acts as a hydrogen acceptor, forming NADH which then serves as a hydrogen donor in the respiratory chain. Isoln from erythrocytes: O. Warburg, W. Christian, Biochem. Z. **287**, 291 (1936); from rabbit muscle: S. Ochoa, ibid. **292**, 68 (1937); from yeast: H. v. Euler, F. Schlenk, Z. Physiol. Chem. **246**, 64 (1937); G. A. LePage, J. Biol. Chem. **168**, 623 (1947); Biochem. Prep. **1**, 28 (1949). Manuf by fermentation: GB 1190079 (1970 to Kyowa), C.A. **73**, 54631g (1970). Synthetic approach: N. A. Hughes et al., J. Chem. Soc. **1957**, 3733. Nomenclature: M. Dixon, Science **132**, 1548 (1960). Occurs in 2 forms, α-NAD and β-NAD, distinguished by the configuration of the ribosyl nicotinamide linkage. Only the β-anomer is bioactive. Stereochemistry: R. U. Lumieux, J. W. Lown, Can. J. Chem. **41**, 889 (1963). NMR studies: N. J. Oppenheimer et al., Proc. Natl. Acad. Sci. USA **68**, 3200 (1971); R. H. Sarma, R. J. Mynott, Chem. Commun. **1972**, 977; M. Blumenstein, M. A. Raftery, Biochemistry **11**, 1643 (1972). Biosynthesis: Nutr. Rev. **30**, 139 (1972); J. W. Foster, A. G. Moat, Microbiol. Rev. **44**, 83 (1980). Combined bioluminescent assay of NAD and NADH: M. T. Karp, P. I. Vuorinen, Methods Enzymol. **122**, 147 (1986). Review: "Niacin: Nicotinic Acid, Nicotinamide, NAD(P)" in Vitamins, W. Friedrich, Ed. (Walter de Gruyter, Berlin, 1988) pp 473-542.

Very hygroscopic white powder. Freely sol in water without residue. A 1% soln has a pH of ~2. Aq solns are stable for ~1 week. $[\alpha]_D^{20}$ $-31.5°$ (c = 1.2 in water). uv max: 260 nm (ε 18100).
Reduced form. [58-68-4] NADH; DPNH; 1,4-dihydronicotinamide adenine dinucleotide. $C_{21}H_{29}N_7O_{14}P_2$. uv max: 260, 340 nm (ε 15000, 6290).

6345. Nadifloxacin. [124858-35-1] 9-Fluoro-6,7-dihydro-8-(4-hydroxy-1-piperidinyl)-5-methyl-1-oxo-1H,5H-benzo[ij]quinolizine-2-carboxylic acid; jinofloxacin; OPC-7251; Acuatim. C_{19}-

$H_{21}FN_2O_4$; mol wt 360.38. C 63.32%, H 5.87%, F 5.27%, N 7.77%, O 17.76%. Fluorinated quinolone antibacterial. Prepn: H. Ishikawa *et al.*, **BE 891046**; *eidem*, **US 4399134** (1982, 1983 both to Otsuka); *eidem*, *Chem. Pharm. Bull.* **37**, 2103 (1989). Toxicity data: K. Hashimoto *et al.*, *Iyakuhin Kenkyu* **21**, 671 (1990), *C.A.* **114**, 156625r (1991). *In vitro* antibacterial activity: K. Vogt *et al.*, *Eur. J. Clin. Microbiol. Infect. Dis.* **11**, 943 (1992). HPLC determn: M. Koike *et al.*, *J. Chromatogr.* **526**, 235 (1990). Clinical trial in treatment of acne: I. Kurokawa *et al.*, *J. Am. Acad. Dermatol.* **25**, 674 (1991).

Colorless prisms from EtOH-H_2O, mp 245-247° (dec). LD_{50} male, female mice and rats (mg/kg): 376.5, 420.6, 225.7, 240.5 i.v. (Hashimoto).

THERAP CAT: Antibacterial (topical).

6346.   Nadolol. [42200-33-9] 5-[3-[(1,1-Dimethylethyl)-amino]-2-hydroxypropoxy]-1,2,3,4-tetrahydro-2,3-naphthalenediol; 1-(*tert*-butylamino)-3-[(5,6,7,8-tetrahydro-*cis*-6,7-dihydroxy-1-naphthyl)oxy]-2-propanol; (2*R*,3*S*)-5-[3-(*tert*-butylamino)-2-hydroxypropoxy]-1,2,3,4-tetrahydronaphthalene-2,3-diol; 2,3-*cis*-1,-2,3,4-tetrahydro-5-[2-hydroxy-3-(*tert*-butylamino)propoxy]-2,3-naphthalenediol; SQ-11725; Corgard; Solgol. $C_{17}H_{27}NO_4$; mol wt 309.40. C 65.99%, H 8.80%, N 4.53%, O 20.68%. β-Adrenergic blocker. Prepn: F. P. Hauck *et al.*, **DE 2258995**; *eidem*, **US 3935267** (1973, 1976, both to Squibb). Resolution of isomers: F. P. Hauck, J. E. Sundeen, **DE 2421549** (1974 to Squibb), *C.A.* **82**, 57481e (1975). Metabolism: J. Dreyfuss *et al.*, *J. Clin. Pharmacol.* **17**, 300 (1977). Toxicology: P. L. Sibley *et al.*, *Toxicol. Appl. Pharmacol.* **44**, 379 (1978). Review of pharmacology: R. C. Heel *et al.*, *Drugs* **1**, 1-23 (1980); M. J. Antonaccio, D. B. Evans, in *Pharmacology of Antihypertensive Drugs*, A. Scriabine, Ed. (Raven Press, New York, 1980) pp 295-301. Comprehensive description: L. Slusarek, K. Florey, *Anal. Profiles Drug Subs.* **9**, 455-485 (1980). Book: *International Experience with Nadolol, a Long-Acting β-Blocking Agent*, F. Gross, Ed. (Grune & Stratton, New York, 1981) 229 pp.

Crystalline powder, mp 124-136°. uv max (methanol): 270, 278 nm ($E_{1cm}^{1\%}$ 37.5, 39.1). pKa 9.67. Freely sol in ethanol, propylene glycol; sol in hydrochloric acid; slightly sol in water, chloroform. Insol in acetone, benzene, ether, hexane. LD_{50} in mice, rats (mg/kg): 4500, 5300 orally (Antonaccio, Evans).

THERAP CAT: Antihypertensive, antianginal.

6347.   Nadoxolol. [54063-51-3] *N*,3-Dihydroxy-4-(1-naphthalenyloxy)butanimidamide; 3-hydroxy-4-(1-naphthyloxy)butyramidoxime; 4-(α-naphthyloxy)-3-hydroxybutyramidoxime. C_{14}-$H_{16}N_2O_3$; mol wt 260.29. C 64.60%, H 6.20%, N 10.76%, O 18.44%. β-Adrenergic blocker. Prepn: Lafon, **DE 2132113** corresp to **US 3819702** (1972, 1974 to Orsymonde). Pharmacology: Duteil *et al.*, *Therapie* **28**, 703 (1973). Clinical studies: Tricot *et al.*, *ibid.* 721.

Hydrochloride. [35991-93-6] LL-1530; Bradyl. $C_{14}H_{16}N_2$-O_3·HCl; mol wt 296.75. White crystalline powder from ethyl ether-methanol, mp 188°. Sol in water, methanol, ethanol. Insol in ethyl ether. LD_{50} in mice (mg/kg): 180 i.v.; 1000 orally (Lafon).

THERAP CAT: Antiarrhythmic.

6348.   NADP. [53-59-8] Adenosine 5'-(trihydrogen diphosphate) 2'-(dihydrogen phosphate) $P' \rightarrow 5'$-ester with 3-(aminocarbonyl)-1-β-D-ribofuranosylpyridinium inner salt; 3-carbamoyl-1-β-D-ribofuranosylpyridinium hydroxide $5' \rightarrow 5'$-ester with adenosine 2'-(dihydrogen phosphate) 5'-(trihydrogen pyrophosphate) inner salt; nicotinamide-adenine dinucleotide phosphate; triphosphopyridine nucleotide; TPN; coenzyme II; Co II; phosphocozymase; codehydrase II; codehydrogenase II. $C_{21}H_{28}N_7O_{17}P_3$; mol wt 743.41. C 33.93%, H 3.80%, N 13.19%, O 36.59%, P 12.50%. One of the biologically active forms of nicotinic acid, *q.v.* Differs from NAD, *q.v.*, by an additional phosphate group at the 2'-position of the adenosine moiety. Serves as a coenzyme of hydrogenases and dehydrogenases. Present in living cells primarily in the reduced form (NADPH) and is involved in synthetic reactions. Isoln from horse blood: O. Warburg *et al.*, *Biochem. Z.* **282**, 157 (1935); from hog liver by adsorption on charcoal: G. A. LePage, G. C. Mueller, *J. Biol. Chem.* **180**, 975 (1949); from sheep liver by extraction with hot water: A. Kornberg, B. L. Horecker, *Biochem. Prep.* **3**, 24 (1953); from human red blood cells by anion-exchange chromatography: G. R. Bartlett, *J. Biol. Chem.* **234**, 449, 459 (1959). Chemical and enzymatic synthesis: D. R. Walt *et al.*, *J. Am. Chem. Soc.* **106**, 234 (1984). Nomenclature: M. Dixon, *Science* **132**, 1548 (1960). Review of synthesis and metabolism: Y. Nishizuka in *Method. Chim.* vol. 11, F. Korte, Ed. (Academic Press, New York, 1977) pp 84-87. *Review:* "Niacin: Nicotinic Acid, Nicotinamide, NAD(P)" in *Vitamins*, W. Friedrich, Ed. (Walter de Gruyter, Berlin, 1988) pp 473-542.

Grayish-white powder. pKa_1 3.9; pKa_2 6.1. uv max: 260 nm (ε 18000). Sol in water, methanol. Much less sol in ethanol. Practically insol in ether, ethyl acetate.

Reduced form. [53-57-6] NADPH; $NADPH_2$; TPNH; dihydrocodehydrogenase II. $C_{21}H_{30}N_7O_{17}P_3$. uv max: 260, 340 nm (ε 18000, 6220).

6349.   Nadroparin. Tedegliparin. Low molecular weight fraction of heparin, *q.v.*, prepd from porcine mucosal heparin by selective ethanol precipitation. Mean mol wt 4500 daltons. Prepn: J.-C. Lormeau *et al.*, **DE 2944792**; *eidem*, **US 4486420**; **US 4692435** (1980, 1984, 1987 all to Choay); J. Choay *et al.*, *Thromb. Res.* **18**, 573 (1980). Comparison with unfractionated heparin: G. F. Gensini *et al.*, *Haemostasis* **14**, 466 (1984); M. D. Vandenbroek, B. Bordes, *J. Pharm. Clin.* **5**, 35 (1986); C. Doutremepuich *et al.*, *Thromb. Res.* **43**, 691 (1986). Pharmacokinetics and bioavailability in humans: J. Harenberg *et al.*, *ibid.* **44**, 549 (1986). Clinical trial in prophylaxis of postoperative thromboembolism: V. V. Kakkar, *Nouv. Rev. Fr. Hematol.* **26**, 277 (1984); V. V. Kakkar, W. J. G. Murray, *Br. J. Surg.* **72**, 786 (1985); in acute ischemic stroke: R. Kay *et al.*, *N. Engl. J. Med.* **333**, 1588 (1995).

Calcium salt. CY-216; Fraxiparine. THERAP CAT: Antithrombotic.

6350.   Nafamostat. [81525-10-2] 4-[(Aminoiminomethyl)-amino]benzoic acid 6-(aminoiminomethyl)-2-naphthalenyl ester; 6-amidino-2-naphthyl-4-guanidinobenzoate; nafamstat. $C_{19}H_{17}N_5$-O_2; mol wt 347.37. C 65.69%, H 4.93%, N 20.16%, O 9.21%. Non-peptide protease inhibitor. Prepn: S. Fujii *et al.*, **EP 48433**;

eidem, **US 4454338** (1982, 1984 both to Torii & Co.); T. Aoyama *et al., Chem. Pharm. Bull.* **33,** 1458 (1985). Inhibitory effects on trypsin, thrombin, kallikrein, plasmin and complement-mediated hemolysis: S. Fujii, Y. Hitomi, *Biochim. Biophys. Acta* **661,** 342 (1981); T. Aoyama *et al., Jpn. J. Pharmacol.* **35,** 203 (1984). Effect in experimental acute pancreatitis in rats: M. Iwaki *et al., ibid.* **41,** 155 (1986). Spectrofluorometric determn in biological material: T. Aoyama *et al., Chem. Pharm. Bull.* **33,** 2142 (1985). Clinical anti-complement activity: Y. Miyamoto *et al., Trans. Am. Soc. Artif. Intern. Organs* **31,** 508 (1985).

Dimethanesulfonate. [82956-11-4] Nafamostat mesylate; FUT-175; Futhan. $C_{19}H_{17}N_5O_2.2CH_3SO_3H$; mol wt 539.58. Crystals from ethyl ether, mp 217-220° (Fujii). Also reported as colorless powder from water, mp 260° (dec) (Aoyama).

THERAP CAT: Enzyme inhibitor (protease).

6351. Nafarelin. [76932-56-4] 6-[3-(2-Naphthalenyl)-D-alanine]luteinizing hormone-releasing factor(pig); 5-oxo-L-prolyl-L-histidyl-L-tryptophyl-L-seryl-L-tyrosyl-3-(2-naphthyl)-D-alanyl-L-leucyl-L-arginyl-L-prolylglycinamide; [6-[3-(2-naphthyl)-D-alanine]] LHRH; D-nal(2)[6]-LHRH; NAG. $C_{66}H_{83}N_{17}O_{13}$; mol wt 1322.47. C 59.94%, H 6.33%, N 18.01%, O 15.73%. Synthetic peptide agonist analog of LH-RH, *q.v.* Prepn: J. J. Nestor *et al.,* **US 4234571** (1980 to Syntex); *eidem, J. Med. Chem.* **25,** 795 (1982). Suppression of luteal and placental function in baboons: B. H. Vickery *et al., Fertil. Steril.* **36,** 664 (1981). Inhibition of ovulation in humans: J. A. Gudmundsson *et al., Contraception* **30,** 107 (1984). Radioimmunoassay in plasma and serum: C. Nerenberg *et al., Anal. Biochem.* **141,** 10 (1984). Kinetics and tissue disposition in animals: N. I. Chu *et al., Drug Metab. Dispos.* **13,** 560 (1985). Clinical evaluation in benign prostatic hyperplasia: C. A. Peters, P. C. Walsh, *N. Engl. J. Med.* **317,** 599 (1987); in endometriosis: M. R. Henzl *et al., ibid.* **318,** 485 (1988). Review of clinical studies: P. G. Hoffman *et al., J. Androl.* **8,** Suppl., S17-S22 (1987).

5-oxoPro–His–Trp–Ser–Tyr–N---C---C—Leu–Arg–Pro–GlyNH₂
                                     H   H O

Monoacetate. $C_{66}H_{83}N_{17}O_{13}.C_2H_4O_2$. mp 188-190°. $[\alpha]_D^{25}$ −27.4° (c = 0.9 in acetic acid).

Acetate hydrate. [86220-42-0] RS-94991-298; Nacenyl; Nasanyl; Synarel; Synrelina. $C_{66}H_{83}N_{17}O_{13}.xC_2H_4O_2.yH_2O$.

THERAP CAT: Treatment of endometriosis.

6352. Nafcillin. [147-52-4] (2S,5R,6R)-6-[[(2-Ethoxy-1-naphthalenyl)carbonyl]amino]-3,3-dimethyl-7-oxo-4-thia-1-azabicyclo[3.2.0]heptane-2-carboxylic acid; 6-(2-ethoxy-1-naphthamido)penicillin. $C_{21}H_{22}N_2O_5S$; mol wt 414.47. C 60.85%, H 5.35%, N 6.76%, O 19.30%, S 7.74%. Semi-synthetic antibiotic related to penicillin. Prepn: F. P. Doyle *et al.,* **GB 880400**; F. P. Doyle, J. H. C. Nayler, **US 3157639** (1961, 1964 both to Beecham). Prepn of crystalline monohydrate: D. Flitter *et al.,* **US 3506645** (1970 to American Home Prod.). HPLC determn: P. Fan-Havard, M. C. Nahata, *Ther. Drug Monit.* **11,** 105 (1989). Antibacterial activity: J. M. Steckelberg *et al., Antimicrob. Agents Chemother.* **37,** 554 (1993). Clinical efficacy: D. L. Palmer *et al., Ann. Thorac. Surg.* **59,** 626 (1995).

Sodium salt monohydrate. [7177-50-6]; [985-16-0] (anhydrous). Sodium 6-(2-ethoxy-1-naphthamido)penicillanate; Wy-3277; Nafcil; Nallpen; Unipen. $C_{21}H_{21}N_2NaO_5S.H_2O$; mol wt 454.47. Sol in water. Insol in acetone, chloroform.

THERAP CAT: Antibacterial.

THERAP CAT (VET): Antibacterial.

6353. Nafronyl. [31329-57-4] Tetrahydro-α-(1-naphthalenylmethyl)-2-furanpropanoic acid 2-(diethylamino)ethyl ester; tetrahydro-α-(1-naphthylmethyl)-2-furanpropionic acid 2-(diethylamino)ethyl ester; 3-(1-naphthyl)-2-tetrahydrofurfurylpropionic acid 2-(diethylamino)ethyl ester; α-tetrahydrofurfuryl-1-naphthalenepropionic acid 2-(diethylamino)ethyl ester; N-diethylaminoethyl β-(1-naphthyl)-β-tetrahydrofuryl isobutyrate; naftidrofuryl; Dubimax; Gevatran. $C_{24}H_{33}NO_3$; mol wt 383.52. C 75.16%, H 8.67%, N 3.65%, O 12.52%. Prepn: Szarvasi, Bayssat, **FR 1363948** corresp to **US 3334096** (1964, 1967 both to LIPHA); Szarvasi *et al., Compt. Rend.* **260,** 3095 (1965); *eidem, Bull. Soc. Chim. Fr.* **1966,** 1838. Activity studies: Fontaine *et al., C.R. Seances Acad. Sci. Ser. D* **262,** 719 (1966). Metabolism and toxicology: Fontaine *et al., Chim. Ther.* **4,** 44 (1969); Fontaine *et al., J. Eur. Toxicol.* **11,** 40 (1969). Acute toxicity: P. Bessin *et al., Eur. J. Med. Chem.* **10,** 291 (1975). Clinical studies: C. A. Clyne *et al., Br. J. Surg.* **67,** 347 (1980); R. M. Greenhalgh, *ibid.* **68,** 265 (1981).

bp$_{0.5}$ 190°. d$_4^{31}$ 1.0465. n$_D^{29}$ 1.5513. LD$_{50}$ in mice (mg/kg): 365 orally (Bessin).

Acid oxalate. [3200-06-4] EU-1806; LS-121; Citoxid; Di-Actane; Dusodril; Praxilene. $C_{24}H_{33}NO_3.C_2H_2O_4$; mol wt 473.56. Crystals from ethyl acetate, mp 110-111°. Slightly hygroscopic, sol in water.

THERAP CAT: Vasodilator.

6354. Naftalofos. [1491-41-4] 2-[(Diethoxyphosphinyl)-oxy]-1H-benz[de]isoquinoline-1,3(2H)-dione; N-hydroxynaphthalimide diethyl phosphate; O,O-diethyl O-naphthaloximide phosphate; naphthalophos; phthalophos; Bay 9002; Bayer 25820; ENT-25567; S-940; Maretin; Rametin. $C_{16}H_{16}NO_6P$; mol wt 349.28. C 55.02%, H 4.62%, N 4.01%, O 27.48%, P 8.87%. Prepn: Lorenz, Wegler, **DE 962608** and **AT 193894** (both 1957 to Bayer).

Minute crystals. The commercial product has a brown to tan color. mp 174-179°. Practically insol in water. Sparingly sol in the usual organic solvents. Fairly sol in methylene chloride.

THERAP CAT (VET): Anthelmintic.

6355. Naftifine. [65472-88-0] (*E*)-*N*-Methyl-*N*-(3-phenyl-2-propenyl)-1-naphthalenemethanamine; *(E)*-*N*-cinnamyl-*N*-methyl-1-naphthalenemethylamine; *N*-methyl-*N*-(1-naphthylmethyl)-3-phenylpropen-1-amine; naftifungin. $C_{21}H_{21}N$; mol wt 287.40. C 87.76%, H 7.36%, N 4.87%. Antimycotic allylamine. Prepn: D. Berney, **BE 853976**; *idem*, **US 4282251** (1977, 1981 both to Sandoz); A. Blade Fond, E. Mendoza-Villela, **ES 504432** (1982 to Lab. Frumtost-Prem S.A.), *C.A.* **99**, 38173r (1983); H. Loibner *et al.*, *Tetrahedron Lett.* **25**, 2535 (1984). In vitro activity against dermatophytes and *Candida* spp: A. Georgopoulos *et al.*, *Antimicrob. Agents Chemother.* **19**, 386 (1981). Morphological changes induced in *Trichophyton mentagrophytes*: J. C. Meingassner *et al.*, *J. Invest. Dermatol.* **77**, 444 (1981). Specific inhibitor of squalene epoxidase, a key enzyme in fungal ergosterol biosynthesis: F. Paltauf *et al.*, *Biochim. Biophys. Acta* **712**, 268 (1982); N. S. Ryder, *Antimicrob. Agents Chemother.* **25**, 483 (1984). HPLC determn in human plasma and urine: F. Schatz, H. Haberl, *Arzneim.-Forsch.* **36**, 1850 (1986). Clinical trials in dermatophytosis: U. Ganzinger *et al.*, *Clin. Trials J.* **19**, 342 (1982).

Colorless, viscous oil, $bp_{0.015 \text{ torr}}$ 162-167°.

Hydrochloride. [65473-14-5] AW-105-843; SN-105-843; Exoderil; Naftin; Suadian. $C_{21}H_{21}N.HCl$; mol wt 323.86. mp 177° (from propanol).

THERAP CAT: Antifungal (topical).

6356. Naftopidil. [57149-07-2] 4-(2-Methoxyphenyl)-α-[(1-naphthalenyloxy)methyl]-1-piperazineethanol; *RS*-1-[4-(2-methoxyphenyl)-1-piperazinyl]-3-(1-naphthoxy)-2-propanol; 1-(2-methoxyphenyl)-4-[3-(naphth-1-yloxy)-2-hydroxypropyl]-piperazine; KT-611; Avishot; Flivas. $C_{24}H_{28}N_2O_3$; mol wt 392.49. C 73.44%, H 7.19%, N 7.14%, O 12.23%. α₁-Adrenergic blocker and serotonin (5HT₁A) receptor agonist. Prepn: E. C. Witte *et al.*, **DE 2408804**; *eidem*, **US 3997666** (1975, 1976 both to Boehringer Mann.). Clinical pharmacodynamics: R. Kirsten *et al.*, *Eur. J. Clin. Pharmacol.* **46**, 271 (1994). Clinical pharmacokinetics: M. J. G. Farthing *et al.*, *Postgrad. Med. J.* **70**, 363 (1994). HPLC determn in human plasma: G. Niebch *et al.*, *J. Chromatogr.* **534**, 247 (1990). Clinical evaluation in BPH: K. Yasuda *et al.*, *Prostate* **25**, 46 (1994). Review of pharmacology and clinical experience: H. M. Himmel, *Cardiovasc. Drug Rev.* **12**, 32-47 (1994).

Crystals from isopropanol, mp 125-126°; also reported as colorless crystals, mp 125-129°. Insol in water. Partition coefficient (octanol/water): 75. LD_{50} in mice, rats (g/kg): 1.3, 6.4 orally (Himmel).

Dihydrochloride. [57149-08-3] $C_{24}H_{28}N_2O_3.2HCl$. Crystals from methanol/ethanol (1:2), mp 212-213°.

THERAP CAT: Antihypertensive; α-blocker in treatment of symptomatic benign prostate hypertrophy.

6357. Nalbuphine. [20594-83-6] (5α,6α)-17-(Cyclobutylmethyl)-4,5-epoxymorphinan-3,6,14-triol; *N*-cyclobutylmethyl-14-hydroxydihydronormorphine. $C_{21}H_{27}NO_4$; mol wt 357.44. C 70.56%, H 7.61%, N 3.92%, O 17.90%. Mixed opioid agonist-antagonist. Prepn: **GB 1119270** corresp to I. J. Pachter, Z. Matossian, **US 3393197** (both 1968 to Endo). Pharmacology: S. G. Holtzman *et al.*, *Probl. Drug Depend.* **1976**, 374; H. E. Shannon, S. G. Holtzman, *J. Pharmacol. Exp. Ther.* **201**, 55 (1977); G. J. Schaefer, S. G. Holtzman, *ibid.* **205**, 291 (1978). Plasma determn: S. H.

Weinstein *et al.*, *J. Pharm. Sci.* **67**, 547 (1978). Clinical study: T. Tammisto, I. Tigerstedt, *Acta Anaesthesiol. Scand.* **21**, 390 (1977). Review of pharmacology and therapeutic efficacy: J. K. Errick, R. C. Heel, *Drugs* **26**, 191-211 (1983).

Cryst from methanol-acetone, mp 230.5°.

Hydrochloride. [23277-43-2] EN-2234A; Nubain. $C_{21}H_{27}NO_4.HCl$; mol wt 393.90.

THERAP CAT: Analgesic (narcotic).

6358. Naled. [300-76-5] Phosphoric acid 1,2-dibromo-2,2-dichloroethyl dimethyl ester; dimethyl 1,2-dibromo-2,2-dichloroethyl phosphate; bromchlophos; ENT-24988; OMS-75; RE-4355; Bromex; Dibrom. $C_4H_7Br_2Cl_2O_4P$; mol wt 380.78. C 12.62%, H 1.85%, Br 41.97%, Cl 18.62%, O 16.81%, P 8.13%. Cholinesterase inhibitor. Prepn: **GB 855157**; Ospenson, Kohn, **US 2971882** (1960, 1961 both to California Res. Corp.). Toxicity study: T. B. Gaines, *Toxicol. Appl. Pharmacol.* **14**, 515 (1969).

Usually obtained as a liquid, slightly pungent odor, $bp_{0.5}$ 110°. d_4^{25} 1.96. Has been crystallized, mp 26.5-27.5°. Vapor pressure at 20° about 2×10^{-3} mm Hg. Practically insol in water. Completely hydrolyzed by water within 48 hrs. Freely sol in aromatic and chlorinated hydrocarbons, ketones, alcohols. Sparingly sol in petroleum solvents and mineral oils. LD_{50} in male rats (mg/kg): 250 orally; 800 dermally (Gaines).

Caution: Potential symptoms of overexposure are miosis, lacrimation; headache; chest tightness, wheezing and laryngeal spasm; salivation; cyanosis; anorexia, nausea, vomiting, abdominal cramps and diarrhea; weakness, twitching and paralysis; giddiness, ataxia and convulsions; low blood pressure; cardiac irregularities; irritation of skin and eyes. *See NIOSH Pocket Guide to Chemical Hazards* (DHHS/NIOSH 97-140, 1997) p 114.

USE: Insecticide; acaricide.

6359. Nalidixic Acid. [389-08-2] 1-Ethyl-1,4-dihydro-7-methyl-4-oxo-1,8-naphthyridine-3-carboxylic acid; 3-carboxy-1-ethyl-7-methyl-1,8-naphthyridin-4-one; 1-ethyl-7-methyl-1,8-naphthyridin-4-one-3-carboxylic acid; Win-18320; Betaxina; Eucistin; Innoxalon; Nalidicron; Nalitucsan; Narigix; NegGram; Negram; Nevigramon; Nicelate; Nogram; Poleon; Specifin; Uriben; Uriclar; Uralgin; Urodixin; Uroman; Uroneg; Uropan; Wintomylon. $C_{12}H_{12}N_2O_3$; mol wt 232.24. C 62.06%, H 5.21%, N 12.06%, O 20.67%. Prepn: G. Y. Lesher *et al.*, *J. Med. Pharm. Chem.* **5**, 1063 (1962); G. Y. Lesher, M. D. Gruett, **BE 612258**; *eidem*, **US 3590036** (1962, 1971 both to Sterling Drug). Mechanism of action studies: G. J. Bourguignon *et al.*, *Antimicrob. Agents Chemother.* **4**, 479 (1973); W. A. Goss, T. M. Cook, *Antibiotics* **vol. 3**, J. W. Corcoran, F. E. Hahn, Eds. (Springer-Verlag, New York, 1975) pp 174-196; A. M. Pedrini, *ibid.* **vol. 5** (pt. 1), F. E. Hahn, Ed. (1979) pp 154-175; H. T. Wright *et al.*, *Science* **213**, 455 (1981). Comprehensive description: P. E. Grubb, *Anal. Profiles Drug Subs.* **8**, 371-397 (1979).

Pale buff, crystalline powder, mp 229-230°. Soly at 23° (mg/ml): chloroform 35; toluene 1.6; methanol 1.3; ethanol 0.9; water 0.1; ether 0.1. LD$_{50}$ in mice (mg/kg): 3300 orally; 500 s.c.; 176 i.v. (Lesher, 1962).

THERAP CAT: Antibacterial.

THERAP CAT (VET): Antibacterial.

6360. Nalmefene. [55096-26-9] (5α)-17-(Cyclopropylmethyl)-4,5-epoxy-6-methylenemorphinan-3,14-diol; 6-desoxy-6-methylenenaltrexone; nalmetrene; ORF-11676. C$_{21}$H$_{25}$NO$_3$; mol wt 339.43. C 74.31%, H 7.42%, N 4.13%, O 14.14%. Structural analog of naltrexone, q.v., with opiate antagonist activity. Prepn: J. Fishman, US 3814768 (1974 to M. J. Lewenstein); E. F. Hahn et al., J. Med. Chem. **18**, 259 (1975). Improved synthesis: P. C. Meltzer, J. W. Coe, EP 140367; idem, US 4535157 (both 1985 to Key Pharm.). Comparative evaluation of efficacy in mice: R. D. Heilman et al., Res. Commun. Chem. Pathol. Pharmacol. **13**, 635 (1976). HPLC determn in human plasma: J. Hsiao, R. Dixon, ibid. **42**, 449 (1983). Receptor binding activity in rat brain: M. E. Michel et al., Methods Find. Exp. Clin. Pharmacol. **7**, 175 (1985). Clinical evaluation of narcotic antagonism: T. J. Gal, C. A. DiFazio, Anesthesiology **64**, 175 (1986). Pharmacokinetics in humans: R. Dixon et al., Clin. Pharmacol. Ther. **39**, 49 (1986); idem, J. Clin. Pharmacol. **27**, 233 (1987). Use as antagonist to opioid-induced immobilization in large animals: T. J. Kreeger et al., J. Wildl. Dis. **23**, 619 (1987). Comprehensive description: H. G. Brittain, Anal. Profiles Drug Subs. Excip. **24**, 351-395 (1996).

Crystals from ethyl acetate, mp 188-190°.

Hydrochloride. [58895-64-0] Revex. C$_{21}$H$_{25}$NO$_3$.HCl; mol wt 375.89. White to off-white crystalline powder, mp 180-185°. Soly (mg/ml): water (pH 2.25, 5.71, 6.15, 6.25, 7.85, 8.5, 9.15, 10.4): 128; 131; 133; 124; 1.09; 0.18; 0.09; 0.23; methanol 319; ethanol 86.2; acetonitrile 1.07; acetone 0.23; chloroform 0.13. log P (octanol/water): −1.125. pKa 7.63. uv max: 211, 230 nm (a$_m$ 1977, 778 litre-mol/cm).

THERAP CAT: Narcotic antagonist.

THERAP CAT (VET): Narcotic antagonist.

6361. Nalorphine. [62-67-9] (5α,6α)-7,8-Didehydro-4,5-epoxy-17-(2-propenyl)morphinan-3,6-diol; N-allylnormorphine; allorphine; antorphine; NANM. C$_{19}$H$_{21}$NO$_3$; mol wt 311.37. C 73.29%, H 6.80%, N 4.50%, O 15.42%. Prepd from normorphine: McCawley et al., J. Am. Chem. Soc. **63**, 314 (1941); amended procedure: Hart, McCawley, J. Pharmacol. **82**, 339 (1944); Weijlard, Erickson, J. Am. Chem. Soc. **64**, 869 (1942); US 2364833 (1944); Weijlard, US 2891954 (1959 to Merck & Co.). Toxicity data: E. I. Goldenthal, Toxicol. Appl. Pharmacol. **18**, 185 (1971). Comprehensive description: M. U. Zubair et al., Anal. Profiles Drug Subs. **18**, 195-219 (1989).

Crystals from ether, mp 208-209° (not 92-93° as first given by McCawley). [α]$_D^{25}$ −155.3° (c = 3 in methanol). Sparingly sol in water, ether. Sol in alc, acetone, chloroform, dil alkalies. uv max (in acid): 285 nm; (in alkali): 298 nm.

Hydrobromide. [1041-90-3] Lethidrone; Norfin. C$_{19}$H$_{21}$NO$_3$.HBr; mol wt 392.29. Crystals from alc, dec 258-259°. Sol in water.

Hydrochloride. [57-29-1] Nalline. C$_{19}$H$_{21}$NO$_3$.HCl; mol wt 347.84. Crystals from alc, mp 260-263°. Sol in water. Moderately sol in alc. uv max (water): 285 nm. IR and polarographic data: Seagers et al., J. Am. Pharm. Assoc. Sci. Ed. **41**, 640 (1952). pH of 0.5% aq soln: 5.0. LD$_{50}$ s.c. in rats: 1460 mg/kg (Goldenthal).

Note: This is a controlled substance: 21 CFR, 1308.13.

THERAP CAT: Narcotic antagonist.

THERAP CAT (VET): Narcotic antagonist.

6362. Naloxone. [465-65-6] (5α)-4,5-Epoxy-3,14-dihydroxy-17-(2-propenyl)morphinan-6-one; 17-allyl-4,5α-epoxy-3,14-dihydroxymorphinan-6-one; (−)-N-allyl-14-hydroxynordihydromorphinone; N-allylnoroxymorphone. C$_{19}$H$_{21}$NO$_4$; mol wt 327.37. C 69.71%, H 6.47%, N 4.28%, O 19.55%. Specific opioid antagonist. Prepn: H. Blumberg et al., US 3254088 (1966); R. A. Olofson et al., Tetrahedron Lett. **1977**, 1567. Clinical pharmacology and abuse potential: D. R. Jasinski et al., J. Pharmacol. Exp. Ther. **157**, 420 (1967). Metabolism: J. M. Fujimoto, Proc. Soc. Exp. Biol. Med. **133**, 317 (1970). Synthesis of (+)-form and stereospecific activity: I. Iijima et al., J. Med. Chem. **21**, 398 (1978). Clinical trial in Alzheimer's disease: B. Reisberg et al., N. Engl. J. Med. **308**, 721 (1983). Comprehensive description: M. M. A. Hasson et al., Anal. Profiles Drug Subs. **14**, 453-489 (1985). Review of pharmacology and therapeutic uses: L. F. McNicholas, W. R. Martin, Drugs **27**, 81-93 (1984); of clinical experience in Alzheimer's disease: C. Stowe, M. L. Gora, Ann. Pharmacother. **27**, 447-448 (1993); in drug overdose: J. M. Chamberlain, B. L. Klein, Am. J. Emerg. Med. **12**, 650-660 (1994).

Crystals from ethyl acetate, mp 184° (Lewenstein), 177-178° (Sankyo Co.). [α]$_D^{20}$ −194.5° (c = 0.93 in CHCl$_3$). Sol in chloroform. Practically insol in petr ether.

Hydrochloride. [357-08-4]; [51481-60-8] (dihydrate). EN-15304; Nalone; Narcan; Narcanti. C$_{19}$H$_{21}$NO$_4$.HCl; mol wt 363.84. Crystals from ethanol + ether, mp 200-205°. Sol in water, alcohol. Practically insol in ether.

THERAP CAT: Narcotic antagonist.

THERAP CAT (VET): Narcotic antagonist.

6363. Naltrexone. [16590-41-3] (5α)-17-(Cyclopropylmethyl)-4,5-epoxy-3,14-dihydroxymorphinan-6-one; N-cyclopropylmethyl-14-hydroxydihydromorphinone; UM-792. C$_{20}$H$_{23}$NO$_4$; mol wt 341.40. C 70.36%, H 6.79%, N 4.10%, O 18.75%. Nonselective opioid receptor antagonist; congener of naloxone, q.v. Prepn: H. Blumberg et al., US 3332950 (1967 to Endo). Metabolism study: E. J. Cone, Tetrahedron Lett. **1973**, 2607. Pharmacology and toxicity: R. P. Maickel et al., Ann. N.Y. Acad. Sci. **281**, 321 (1976). Clinical pharmacology: E. R. Gritz et al., Clin. Pharmacol. Ther. **19**, 773 (1976); K. Verebey et al., ibid. **20**, 315 (1976). GC determn in urine: H. E. Dayton, C. E. Inturrisi, Drug Metab. Dispos. **4**, 474 (1976). Review of pharmacokinetics and therapeutic use in opioid dependence: J. P. Gonzales, R. N. Brogden, Drugs **35**, 192-213 (1988). Clinical trials in alcoholism: B. J. Berg et al., Drug Saf. **15**, 274 (1996); R. S. Croop et al., Arch. Gen. Psychiatry **54**, 1130 (1997).

Nandinine

Crystals from acetone, mp 168-170°. LD$_{50}$ in mice (mg/kg): 586 s.c. (Maickel).

Hydrochloride. [16676-29-2] EN-1639A; Antaxone; Celupan; Nalorex; ReVia. C$_{20}$H$_{23}$NO$_4$.HCl; mol wt 377.86. Crystals from methanol, mp 274-276°.

THERAP CAT: Narcotic antagonist. In treatment of alcoholism.

6364. Nandinine. [572-76-9] (13aS)-5,8,13,13a-Tetrahydro-10-methoxy-6H-benzo[g]-1,3-benzodioxolo[5,6-a]quinolizin-9-ol; 10-methoxy-2,3-(methylenedioxy)berbin-9-ol; 5,6,13,13a-tetrahydro-9-hydroxy-10-methoxy-2,3-(methylenedioxy)-8H-dibenzo[a,g]quinolizine; (+)-tetrahydroberberrubine. C$_{19}$H$_{19}$NO$_4$; mol wt 325.36. C 70.14%, H 5.89%, N 4.30%, O 19.67%. From root bark of Nandina domestica Thunb., Berberidaceae: Eijkman, Ber. **17**, 441 (1884); Kitasato, J. Pharm. Soc. Jpn. **522**, 1 (1925). Structure: idem, Acta Phytochim. **3**, 175 (1927), C.A. **22**, 1779 (1928); Späth, Leithe, Ber. **63**, 3007 (1930). Configuration: Corrodi, Hardegger, Helv. Chim. Acta **39**, 889 (1956). Synthesis: Kametani et al., J. Chem. Soc. C **1969**, 2036; eidem, J. Chem. Soc. Perkin Trans. 1 **1977**, 1151.

Crystals from chloroform + ether, mp 195-196°.

dl-Form. [17388-17-9] Colorless needles from ethanol, mp 183-185°.

l-Form. Crystals from ether. mp 195-196°. [α]$_D^{15}$ −304° (c = 0.513 in chloroform).

6365. Nandrolone. [434-22-0] (17β)-17-Hydroxyestr-4-en-3-one; 17β-hydroxy-4-estren-3-one; 4-estren-17β-ol-3-one; 17β-hydroxy-19-nor-4-androsten-3-one; 19-nortestosterone. C$_{18}$H$_{26}$O$_2$; mol wt 274.40. C 78.79%, H 9.55%, O 11.66%. Prepd from alkyl ethers of estradiol: Birch, Q. Rev. Chem. Soc. **4**, 69 (1950); Wilds, Nelson, J. Am. Chem. Soc. **75**, 5366 (1953). Alternate syntheses: H. Ueberwasser et al., Helv. Chim. Acta **46**, 344 (1963); I. Shimizu et al., Tetrahedron Lett. **21**, 487 (1980).

Dimorphic crystals, mp 112° and 124°. [α]$_D^{22}$ +55° (c = 0.93 in chloroform). uv max (ethanol): 241 nm (ε 17000). Sol in alcohol, ether, chloroform.

Benzoate. C$_{25}$H$_{30}$O$_3$. Needles from 75% alc, mp 174-175°. [α]$_D^{20}$ +104.5° (alc).

Cyclohexanecarboxylate. [18470-94-5] 19-Nortestosterone hexahydrobenzoate; C$_{25}$H$_{36}$O$_3$; mol wt 384.55. Small, elongated prisms from petr ether, mp 88-89°, [α]$_D^{20}$ +50° (c = 0.5 in chloroform).

Decanoate. [360-70-3] 19-Nortestosterone decanoate; Deca-Durabolin; Retabolil; Retabolil. C$_{28}$H$_{44}$O$_3$; mol wt 428.65. White to yellow crystals, mp 32-35°. Practically insol in water. Freely sol in ethanol, ether, acetone, chloroform, oils.

Dodecanoate. [26490-31-3] Nandrolone laurate; Laurabolin. C$_{30}$H$_{48}$O$_3$; mol wt 456.70.

p-Hexyloxyphenylpropionate. [52279-57-9] 19-Nortestosterone-3-(p-hexyloxyphenyl)propionate. C$_{33}$H$_{46}$O$_4$; mol wt 506.72. Crystals, mp 53-55°. [α]$_D$ +45° (c = 1.0 in dioxane).

Phenpropionate. [62-90-8] 19-Nortestosterone β-phenylpropionate; Durabolin; Superanabolon; Nandrolin. C$_{27}$H$_{34}$O$_3$; mol wt 406.56. Crystals, mp 95-96°. [α]$_D$ +58° (chloroform).

Propionate. [7207-92-3] 19-Nortestosterone propionate. C$_{21}$H$_{30}$O$_3$; mol wt 330.46. Crystals from aqueous methanol or isopropyl ether, mp 55-60°. [α]$_D^{23.5}$ +58° in chloroform (Rao). uv max: 240 nm (ε 16650).

Note: This is a controlled substance (anabolic steroid): **21 CFR, 1308.13**, as defined in 1300.01.

THERAP CAT: Anabolic.

THERAP CAT (VET): Phenpropionate as anabolic steroid.

6366. Napalm. [8031-21-8] A coprecipitated aluminum soap from naphthenic acids and the fatty acids of coconut oil developed early in 1942 (Fieser, Harris, Hershberg, Morgana, Novello, Putnam) for prepn of gasoline gels for incendiary munitions: US 2606107 (1952); Herron, US 2684339 (1954 to Safety Fuel & Chem. Corp.). The name was derived from the naphthenic and palmitic acids which are its major constituents. Structure and mfg problems: Chem. Eng. News **32**, 2690 (1954). Historical account: L. F. Fieser, The Scientific Method (Reinhold, New York, 1964); Bruce, "Chemical Warfare: Flame" in Kirk-Othmer Encyclopedia of Chemical Technology (Interscience, New York, 1964) p 888.

USE: Gasoline thickener. In chemical warfare (fire bombs, flame throwers, flame land mines).

6367. Napelline. [5008-52-6] (1α,12α,15β)-21-Ethyl-4-methyl-16-methylene-7,20-cycloveatchane-1,12-15-triol; luciculine. C$_{22}$H$_{33}$NO$_3$; mol wt 359.50. C 73.50%, H 9.25%, N 3.90%, O 13.35%. Isoln from Aconitum napellus L., Ranunculaceae: Freudenberg, Rogers, J. Am. Chem. Soc. **59**, 2572 (1937); Jacobs, Craig, J. Biol. Chem. **143**, 611 (1942). The product obtained by these isoln procedures is a mixture of at least three compounds. Structure: Wiesner, Valenta, Fortschr. Chem. Org. Naturst. **16**, 53 (1958). Related stereochemical studies: Okamoto et al., Chem. Pharm. Bull. **13**, 1270 (1963). Total synthesis of racemic napelline: Wiesner et al., Can. J. Chem. **52**, 2353, 2355 (1974); S. P. Sethi et al., ibid. **58**, 1889 (1980).

Rectangular plates from ether + petr ether.

Hydrochloride. C$_{22}$H$_{34}$ClNO$_3$. Solvated crystals, dec 200-222°. [α]$_D^{22}$ −93.9° (c = 5). Sol in water.

6368. Naphazoline. [835-31-4] 4,5-Dihydro-2-(1-naphthalenylmethyl)-1H-imidazole; 2-(1-naphthylmethyl)imidazoline. C$_{14}$H$_{14}$N$_2$; mol wt 210.27. C 79.97%, H 6.71%, N 13.32%. α-Adrenergic agonist. Prepd by reacting the acetic acid anhydride of naphthoimidic acid with ethylenediamine: A. Sonn, US 2161938 (1939 to Soc. Chem. Ind. Basle); by reacting naphthylthioacetamide with ethylenediamine: DK 62889 (1944 to Lovens Kemiske), C.A. **40**, 4398 (1946). Toxicity data: J. Gylfe et al., Fed. Proc. **9**, 280 (1950). Comprehensive description: G. M. Wall, Anal. Profiles Drug Subs. Excip. **21**, 307-344 (1992).

Hydrochloride. [550-99-2] Ak-Con; Albalon; Clera; Coldan; Iridina Due; Naphcon; Niazol; Opcon; Privine; Rhinantin; Rhinoperd; Sanorin; Sanorin-Spofa; Strictylon. C$_{14}$H$_{14}$N$_2$.HCl; mol wt 246.74. Bitter crystals, mp 255-260°. uv max (ethanol): 223, 270, 280, 287, 291 nm (E$_{1cm}^{1\%}$ 3622, 239, 286, 196, 198). pKa (25°C) 10.35 ±0.02, (35°C) 10.13 ±0.02, (45°C) 9.92 ±0.03. pKa (25°C)

Consult the Name Index before using this section.

10.35 ±0.02, (35°C) 10.13 ±0.02, (45°C) 9.92 ±0.03. Freely sol in water (40 g dissolve in 100 ml) and in alcohol. Slightly sol in chloroform. Insol in benzene, ether. A 1% aq soln has a pH of ~6.2. LD_{50} s.c. in rats: 385 mg/kg (Gylfe).

THERAP CAT: Adrenergic (vasoconstrictor); decongestant.

6369. Naphthacene. [92-24-0] Tetracene; 2,3-benzanthracene; rubene; chrysogen. $C_{18}H_{12}$; mol wt 228.29. C 94.70%, H 5.30%. Occurs in coal tar. Contaminates commercial anthracene to which it imparts a yellow color. Isoln: Cook *et al., Proc. Roy. Soc. London* **B111,** 455 (1932). Isoln from crude anthracene by chromatography: Winterstein *et al., Z. Physiol. Chem.* **230,** 159 (1934). Synthesis by condensing succinic acid and phthalic anhydride in the presence of sodium acetate: Gabriel, Michael, *Ber.* **10,** 1559, 2207 (1877); **11,** 1682 (1878); Roser, *Ber.* **17,** 2744 (1884); Nathanson, *Ber.* **26,** 2582 (1893); Gabriel, Leupold, *Ber.* **31,** 1159, 1272 (1898); Wanag, *Ber.* **70,** 274 (1937); from 1-naphthol and phthalic anhydride: Deichler, Weizmann, *Ber.* **36,** 547, 719 (1903); **DE 298345** (1916); from 1,5-dihydroxynaphthalene and phthalic anhydride: Bentley *et al., J. Chem. Soc.* **91,** 411, 1588 (1907); from tetralin and phthalic anhydride: Schroeter, *Ber.* **54,** 2242 (1921); **DE 346673** (1918); *cf.* Fieser, *J. Am. Chem. Soc.* **53,** 2329 (1931). Other syntheses: Coulson, *J. Chem. Soc.* **1935,** 77; Weizmann *et al., ibid.* **1939,** 398.

Orange leaflets from xylene. d 1.35. Sublimes *in vacuo.* mp 341° (open capillary tube), mp 357° (copper block). Absorption spectrum: Clar, *Ber.* **69,** 607 (1936). Fluorescence maxima: Krishman, Seshan, *Z. Kristallogr.* **89,** 538 (1934). Difficultly sol in most solvents. Solns show slight green fluorescence in daylight. Does not form a picrate.

6370. Naphthalene. [91-20-3] Naphthalin; naphthene; tar camphor. $C_{10}H_8$; mol wt 128.17. C 93.71%, H 6.29%. Major constituent of coal tar. Dry coal tar contains about 11%. Crystallizes from the middle or "carbolic oil" fraction of the distilled tar. Purified by hot pressing, which may be followed by washing with H_2SO_4, NaOH, and water, then by fractional distillation or by sublimation. Manuf: *Faith, Keyes & Clark's Industrial Chemicals,* F. A. Lowenheim, M. K. Moran, Eds. (Wiley-Interscience, New York, 4th ed., 1975) pp 556-562. *Review:* R. M. Gaydos in *Kirk-Othmer Encyclopedia of Chemical Technology* **vol. 15** (Wiley-Interscience, New York, 3rd ed., 1981) pp 698-719. Review of toxicology and human exposure: *Toxicological Profile for Naphthalene, 1-Methylnaphthalene, and 2-Methylnaphthalene* (PB2006-100004, 2005) 347 pp.

Monoclinic prismatic plates from ether or by sublimation; also sold as white scales, powder, balls, or cakes, mp 80.2°. Odor of moth balls. Volatilizes appreciably at room temp. d_4^{20} 1.162. d_4^{100} 0.9628. Sublimes appreciably at temps above mp; volatile with steam. bp_{760} 217.9°; bp_{400} 193.2°; bp_{200} 167.7°; bp_{100} 145.5°; bp_{60} 130.2°; bp_{40} 119.3°; bp_{20} 101.7°; bp_{10} 85.8°. Flash pt, open cup 174°F (79°C); closed cup 190°F (88°C). Autoignition temp 1053°F (567°C). n_D^{100} 1.58212. Purple fluorescence in Hg light (petr ether soln). Ultraviolet absorption: Several characteristic bands between 217.5 and 320 nm in hexane. Insol in water. One gram dissolves in 13 ml methanol or ethanol, in 3.5 ml benzene or toluene, in 8 ml olive oil or turpentine, in 2 ml chloroform or carbon tetrachloride, in 1.2 ml carbon disulfide. Very sol in ether, hydronaphthalenes, in fixed and volatile oils.

Caution: Potential symptoms of overexposure are eye irritation; corneal damage, optical neuritis; dematitis; headache, confusion, excitement, malaise; nausea, vomiting, abdominal pain; bladder irritation; profuse sweating; acute intravascular hemolysis, anemia, leukocytosis, fever; jaundice; hematuria, hemoglobinuria, renal shutdown. *See NIOSH Pocket Guide to Chemical Hazards*

(DHHS/NIOSH 97-140, 1997) p 220; *Clinical Toxicology of Commercial Products,* R. E. Gosselin *et al.,* Eds. (Williams & Wilkins, Baltimore, 4th ed., 1984) Section III, pp 307-311. This substance is reasonably anticipated to be a human carcinogen: *Report on Carcinogens, Eleventh Edition* (PB2005-104914, 2004) p III-177.

USE: Manuf phthalic and anthranilic acids which are used in making indigo, indanthrene, and triphenylmethane dyes. Manuf of hydroxyl (naphthols), amino (naphthylamines), sulfonic acid and similar compds used in the dye industries. Manuf of synthetic resins, celluloid, lampblack, smokeless powder. Manuf of hydronaphthalenes (Tetralin, Decalin) which are used as solvents, in lubricants, and in motor fuels. Moth repellent and insecticide.

THERAP CAT: Has been used as antiseptic (topical and intestinal); anthelmintic (Cestodes).

THERAP CAT (VET): Has been used in dusting powders, as an insecticide and internally as an intestinal antiseptic and vermicide.

6371. 1-Naphthaleneacetic Acid. [86-87-3] α-Naphthaleneacetic acid; naphthylacetic acid; NAA; Fruitone-N; Planofix; Tre-Hold. $C_{12}H_{10}O_2$; mol wt 186.21. C 77.40%, H 5.41%, O 17.18%. Prepn from naphthalene + chloroacetic acid: Ogata, Ishiguro, *J. Am. Chem. Soc.* **72,** 4302 (1950); Southwick *et al., ibid.* **76,** 754 (1954); **US 2655531** (1953 to FMC); from naphthylacetonitrile: Wenner, **US 2489348** (1949 to Hoffmann-La Roche); *J. Org. Chem.* **15,** 548 (1950). Activity: F. E. Gardiner *et al., Science* **90,** 208 (1939). Crystal structure: S. S. Rajan, *Acta Crystallogr.* **B34,** 998 (1978). Toxicity study: G. W. Bailey, J. L. White, *Residue Rev.* **10,** 97 (1965).

Needles from water, mp 134.5-135.5°. Sol in about 30 parts alcohol; freely sol in acetone, ether, chloroform. Soly in water at 17°: 0.38 g/l. LD_{50} orally in rats: 1000 mg/kg (Bailey, White).

USE: Plant growth regulator.

6372. 1,8-Naphthalenediamine. [479-27-6] 1,8-Diaminonaphthalene. $C_{10}H_{10}N_2$; mol wt 158.20. C 75.92%, H 6.37%, N 17.71%. Prepd by reducing 1,8-dinitronaphthalene with phosphorus triiodide: Meyer, Müller, *Ber.* **30,** 775 (1897).

Crystals from dil alc, mp 66.5°. bp_{12} 205°; $n_D^{99.4}$ 1.6828; $d_4^{99.4}$ 1.1265. Sublimable. Turns brown on standing. Soluble in alcohol or ether; slightly sol in water or chloroform.

Dihydrochloride. $C_{10}H_{12}Cl_2N_2$. Leaflets, mp 280°.

USE: Antioxidant for lubricating oils. Detection of selenium and nitrites.

6373. 1,6-Naphthalenedisulfonic Acid. [525-37-1] Ewer-Pick acid. $C_{10}H_8O_6S_2$; mol wt 288.30. C 41.66%, H 2.80%, O 33.30%, S 22.24%. Prepn: Fierz-David, Hasler, *Helv. Chim. Acta* **6,** 1134 (1923).

Crystals. Very sol in water; sol in alcohol; practically insol in ether.

6374. 2,6-Naphthalenedisulfonic Acid. [581-75-9] Ebert-Merz β-acid. $C_{10}H_8O_6S_2$; mol wt 288.30. C 41.66%, H 2.80%, O

33.30%, S 22.24%. Prepn: Fierz-David, Richter, *Helv. Chim. Acta* **28**, 257 (1945).

HO₃S SO₃H structure — *(HO₃S and SO₃H substituents on naphthalene)*

Deliquesc crystals. Very sol in water, alcohol; practically insol in ether.

6375. 2,7-Naphthalenedisulfonic Acid. [92-41-1] Ebert-Merz α-acid. $C_{10}H_8O_6S_2$; mol wt 288.30. C 41.66%, H 2.80%, O 33.30%, S 22.24%. Prepn from naphthalene and concd H_2SO_4: Fierz-David, Blangey, *Fundamental Processes of Dye Chemistry* (Interscience, New York, 1949) p 209.

HO₃S SO₃H structure

Very deliquesc crystals. Very sol in water, alcohol; practically insol in ether.

USE: In dye chemistry.

6376. 1-Naphthalenesulfonic Acid. [85-47-2] α-Naphthalenesulfonic acid. $C_{10}H_8O_3S$; mol wt 208.23. C 57.68%, H 3.87%, O 23.05%, S 15.40%. Made by sulfonating naphthalene with H_2SO_4 at 0°.

SO₃H structure

Crystals. mp 90° (dihydrate). Freely sol in water or alcohol, slightly in ether.

USE: Manuf α-naphthol. The sodium salt is used for rendering phenols sol in water.

6377. 2-Naphthalenesulfonic Acid. [120-18-3] β-Naphthalenesulfonic acid. $C_{10}H_8O_3S$; mol wt 208.23. C 57.68%, H 3.87%, O 23.05%, S 15.40%. Made by sulfonating naphthalene with H_2SO_4 at 160°.

SO₃H structure

Monohydrate. White to slightly brownish, cryst leaflets; very hygroscopic. mp 124-125°. mp 91° when anhydr. Freely sol in water.

USE: Manuf β-naphthol and intermediates.

6378. 1-Naphthalenethiol. [529-36-2] α-Thionaphthol; 1-thionaphthol; 1-mercaptonaphthalene; 1-naphthyl mercaptan. $C_{10}H_8S$; mol wt 160.24. C 74.95%, H 5.03%, S 20.01%. Prepd by catalytic sulfurization of naphthalene with S, S_2Cl_2, etc., followed by hydrogenation: Lazier *et al.*; Signaigo, **US 2402645**; **US 2402686** (both 1946 to du Pont).

SH structure

Liquid, strong mercaptan odor. Solidif on cooling. d_4^0 1.1729; d_4^{20} 1.607; d_4^{23} 1.1549. bp_{760} 285°; $bp_{10.3}$ 144.8°; bp_2 138-140°. n_D^{20} 1.6802. Sol in ethanol, ether; sparingly sol in aq alkalies. Volatile with steam.

6379. 2-Naphthalenethiol. [91-60-1] β-Thionaphthol; 2-thionaphthol; 2-mercaptonapthalene; 2-naphthyl mercaptan. $C_{10}H_8S$; mol wt 160.24. C 74.95%, H 5.03%, S 20.01%. Prepd by

catalytic hydrogenation of a sulfonic acid derivative of naphthalene: Lazier, Signaigo, **US 2402641** (1946 to du Pont); by reduction of naphthalenesulfonyl chloride with zinc: Holt, **US 2216840** (1940 to du Pont).

SH structure

Crystals from ethanol, disagreeable odor. mp 81°. bp_{760} 286°; $bp_{10.3}$ 146.3°. Very sol in ethanol, ether, petr ether; sparingly sol in water. Slightly volatile with steam.

6380. Naphthalic Acid. [518-05-8] 1,8-Naphthalenedicarboxylic acid. $C_{12}H_8O_4$; mol wt 216.19. C 66.67%, H 3.73%, O 29.60%. Made by the oxidation of acenaphthene with chromic acid mixture, etc.: Graebe, Gfeller, *Ber.* **25**, 652 (1895); Ogilvie, Wilder, **US 2379032** (1945 to Allied Chem.); Karishin, Fedorenko, *Zh. Prikl. Khim.* **29**, 955 (1956), *C.A.* **50**, 14677b (1956).

HOOC COOH structure

Crystals, mp 270°. Practically insol in water; freely sol in warm alcohol, slightly in ether.

6381. 1-Naphthoic Acid. [86-55-5] 1-Naphthalenecarboxylic acid; α-naphthoic acid. $C_{11}H_8O_2$; mol wt 172.18. C 76.73%, H 4.68%, O 18.58%. Prepn from α-bromonaphthalene by Grignard reaction: Gilman *et al., Org. Synth.* **coll. vol. II**, 425 (1943); from 4-aminonaphthalenesulfonic acid by Sandmeyer reaction: Bassilios, *Bull. Soc. Chim. Fr.* **1950**, 757; from β-nitronaphthalene by von Richter reaction: Bunnett, Rauhut, *J. Org. Chem.* **21**, 934, 944 (1956); by oxidation of 1-methylnaphthalene: Aries, **US 2930802** (1960); Barker, **US 2963508** (1960 to Mid-Century).

COOH structure

Crystals from hot toluene, mp 160.5-162°. bp 300°. uv max (ethanol): 293 nm (log ε_m 3.9). Slightly sol in hot water; freely sol in hot alcohol, ether.

Caution: Moderately irritating to skin, mucous membranes.

6382. 2-Naphthoic Acid. [93-09-4] 2-Naphthalenecarboxylic acid; β-naphthoic acid; isonaphthoic acid. $C_{11}H_8O_2$; mol wt 172.18. C 76.73%, H 4.68%, O 18.58%. Prepn from β-acetylnaphthalene + NaOCl: Newman, Holmes, *Org. Synth.* **coll. vol. II**, 428 (1943); from naphthalene + octylsodium: Morton *et al., J. Am. Chem. Soc.* **64**, 2250 (1942); from 2-aminonaphthalenesulfonic acid by Sandmeyer reaction: Wahl, Bassilios, *Bull. Soc. Chim. Fr.* **1947**, 482; by carboxylation of naphthalene: Prichard, **US 2729673** (1956 to du Pont).

COOH structure

Crystals from 95% alcohol, mp 184-185°. bp >300°. uv max (ethanol): 235, 280, 335 nm (log ε_m 4.7, 3.8, 3.1). Slightly sol in hot water; sol in alcohol, ether.

Caution: Moderately irritating to skin, mucous membranes.

6383. 1-Naphthol. [90-15-3] 1-Naphthalenol; α-naphthol; alpha-naphthol; α-hydroxynaphthalene. $C_{10}H_8O$; mol wt 144.17. C 83.31%, H 5.59%, O 11.10%. Prepd by fusing the sodium salt of α-naphthalenesulfonic acid with NaOH: Tyrer, **US 2407044**; **US 2407055**; **US 2451996** (1946, 1946, 1948); by oxidation of naphthalene: Loeb, **US 3033903** (1962 to Union Carbide). Toxicity data: H. F. Smyth *et al., Am. Ind. Hyg. Assoc. J.* **23**, 95 (1962).

Prisms, mp 96°. Phenolic odor; disagreeable, burning taste. bp 288°; bp$_{40}$ 184°. d$_4^{98.7}$ 1.0954. uv max: 297, 310, 324 nm. Sublimable; volatile with steam. Darkens in light; reduces ammoniacal silver nitrate. Slightly sol in water, freely in alcohol, benzene, chloroform, ether, alkali hydroxide solns. *Protect from light.* LD$_{50}$ orally in rats: 2.59 g/kg (Smyth).

Caution: See 2-Naphthol.

USE: Manuf dyes, intermediates, synthetic perfumes; also in microscopy.

6384. 2-Naphthol. [135-19-3] 2-Naphthalenol; β-naphthol; beta-naphthol; β-hydroxynaphthalene; isonaphthol; C.I. Azoic Coupling Component 1; C.I. Developer 5; C.I. 37500. C$_{10}$H$_8$O; mol wt 144.17. C 83.31%, H 5.59%, O 11.10%. Prepn from sodium naphthalene-2-sulfonate: Schoeffel, Barton, US 2760992 (1956 to Sterling); Stevens, Harris, US 2831895 (1958 to Dow); FR 1326175 (1963 to Ciba); by oxidation of naphthalene: Simons, US 2530369 (1950 to Phillips Petroleum); from 2-bromonaphthalene + tert-butyl hydroperoxide: Lawesson, Yang, *J. Am. Chem. Soc.* **81**, 4230 (1959).

Crystals, mp 121-123°. bp 285-286°. d 1.22. Flash pt 161°C. Slight phenolic odor. Darkens with age on exposure to light. Sublimes when heated, distillable *in vacuo;* volatile with vapors of alcohol or water; reduces ammoniacal silver nitrate. uv max (95% ethanol): 226, 265, 275, 286, 320, 331 nm (ε 91,194, 3911, 4559, 3301, 1861, 2163). One gram dissolves in 1000 ml water, 80 ml boiling water, 0.8 ml alcohol, 17 ml chloroform, 1.3 ml ether; sol in glycerol, olive oil, solns of alkali hydroxides. *Protect from light. Incompat.:* Antipyrine, camphor, phenol, ferric salts, menthol, potassium permanganate and other oxidizing agents, urethane.

Sodium salt. [875-83-2] Sodium β-naphtholate; sodium naphthol; Microcidin. C$_{10}$H$_7$NaO; mol wt 166.15. Grayish-white powder; becomes reddish or brownish on exposure to light and air. Soluble in 3 parts water. *Keep well closed and protected from light.*

Caution: Potential symptoms of overexposure to 2-naphthol include crampy abdominal pain, nausea, vomiting and sometimes convulsions. Intestinal or percutaneous absorption may lead to severe nephritis, liver injury and acute hemolytic anemia. Lens opacities and retinal changes may occur. *See Clinical Toxicology of Commercial Products,* R. E. Gosselin *et al.,* Eds. (Williams & Wilkins, Baltimore, 5th ed., 1984) Section II, p 188.

USE: Manuf medicinal organics, dyes, perfumes; the largest single use is probably in making antioxidants for the synthetic rubber industry.

THERAP CAT: Formerly as anthelmintic (Nematodes).

THERAP CAT (VET): Has been used as antiseptic, anthelmintic and counter-irritant in alopecia.

6385. 1-Naphthol-8-amino-3,6-disulfonic Acid. [90-20-0] 4-Amino-5-hydroxy-2,7-naphthalenedisulfonic acid; 8-amino-1-naphthol-3,6-disulfonic acid; H acid. C$_{10}$H$_9$NO$_7$S$_2$; mol wt 319.31. C 37.61%, H 2.84%, N 4.39%, O 35.07%, S 20.08%. Prepn: Willard, *Color Trade J.* **15**, 40 (1924); Mow, US 2272272 (1942 to Allied Chem.); Hayashi, *Yamaguchi J. Sci.* **2**, 67 (1951), *C.A.* **49**, 2390f (1955); Roos *et al.*, US 2875243 (1959 to Bayer).

White crystals or gray powder. Slightly sol in water, alcohol, ether; sol in alkalies.

USE: Prepn of azo dyes.

6386. 1-Naphthol-4,8-disulfonic Acid. [117-56-6] 4-Hydroxy-1,5-naphthalenedisulfonic acid; α-naphtholdisulfonic acid S; Schöllkopf's acid. C$_{10}$H$_8$O$_7$S$_2$; mol wt 304.30. C 39.47%, H 2.65%, O 36.80%, S 21.07%. Prepd by sulfonation of 1-naphthol-8-sulfonic acid sultone: I. G. Farbenindustrie, **PB 74197,** frames 828-829.

Crystals. Soluble in water. The sodium salt is very soluble in water.

6387. 2-Naphthol-3,6-disulfonic Acid. [148-75-4] 3-Hydroxy-2,7-naphthalenedisulfonic acid; R acid. C$_{10}$H$_8$O$_7$S$_2$; mol wt 304.30. C 39.47%, H 2.65%, O 36.80%, S 21.07%. Prepn from β-naphthol and concd H$_2$SO$_4$: Fierz-David, Blangey, *Fundamental Processes of Dye Chemistry* (Interscience, New York, 1949) p 197.

Deliquesc needles. Very sol in water, alcohol. Practically insol in ether. The sodium salt is known as *R salt.*

USE: In dye chemistry.

6388. 2-Naphthol-6,8-disulfonic Acid. [118-32-1] 7-Hydroxy-1,3-naphthalenedisulfonic acid; 2-hydroxynaphthalene-6,8-disulfonic acid; G acid. C$_{10}$H$_8$O$_7$S$_2$; mol wt 304.30. C 39.47%, H 2.65%, O 36.80%, S 21.07%. Prepd by heating β-naphthol with concd H$_2$SO$_4$, 2-naphthol-3,6-disulfonic acid (R acid) being obtained as a byproduct: Fierz-David, Blangey, *Fundamental Processes of Dye Chemistry* (Interscience, New York, 1949) p 197; *see also* Forster, Keyworth, *J. Soc. Chem. Ind. London* **46**, 27T (1927).

Sodium salt. G salt. Platelets or prisms. Freely sol in water, sol in dil alcohol.

Barium salt octahydrate. C$_{10}$H$_6$BaO$_7$S$_2$.8H$_2$O. Minute prisms. Freely sol in water. Practically insol in alcohol, even when much dil with water.

USE: In the manuf of azo dyes, *see* Crossley, Resenvelt, *Ind. Eng. Chem.* **16**, 271 (1924).

6389. α-Naphtholphthalein. [596-01-0] 3,3-Bis(4-hydroxynaphthalenyl)-1(3H)-isobenzofuranone; 3,3-bis(4-hydroxy-1-naphthyl)phthalide; di-p-α-naphtholphthalide; p-α-naphtholphthalein. C$_{28}$H$_{18}$O$_4$; mol wt 418.44. C 80.37%, H 4.34%, O 15.29%. Prepn: Werner, *J. Chem. Soc.* **113**, 20 (1918). Commercial prepn contains a small amount of the isomeric 3,3-bis(2-hydroxy-1-naphthyl)phthalide.

Colorless powder when pure; usually grayish-red. mp 253-255°. Practically insol in water. Sol in alcohol.

USE: As indicator in 0.1% or 0.04% soln in alc. pH 7.3 colorless to reddish; 8.7 greenish to blue. Particularly adapted for weak acids in strong alcoholic soln.

6390. 1-Naphthol-2-sulfonic Acid. [567-18-0] 1-Hydroxy-2-naphthalenesulfonic acid; Baum's acid; Schaeffer's α-acid. $C_{10}H_8O_4S$; mol wt 224.23. C 53.56%, H 3.60%, O 28.54%, S 14.30%. Prepd by sulfonation of α-naphthol: Hodgson, Hathaway, *J. Soc. Dyers Colour.* **63**, 109 (1947).

Deliquesc crystals. Slightly sol in cold water; sol in boiling water. Practically insol in ether.

6391. 1-Naphthol-4-sulfonic Acid. [84-87-7] 4-Hydroxy-1-naphthalenesulfonic acid; Nevile and Winther's acid. $C_{10}H_8O_4S$; mol wt 224.23. C 53.56%, H 3.60%, O 28.54%, S 14.30%. Prepn from 1,4-diazonaphthalenesulfonic acid + sulfuric acid: Erdmann, *Ann.* **247**, 341 (1888); by sulfonation of α-naphthylcarbonate: Reverdin, *Ber.* **27**, 3458 (1894); from chlorosulfonic acid + α-naphthol: Gebauer-Fülnegg, *Monatsh. Chem.* **49**, 195 (1928); Baddiley *et al.*, US 1452481 (1923); from sodium naphthionate + SO_2: Binns, Lurie, US 1880701 (1933 to Virginia Smelting).

Crystals, dec 170°. K_{OH} 3×10^{-9}. Very sol in water. Salt solns give a blue color with ferric chloride.

USE: Preparation of azo dyes.

6392. 2-Naphthol-6-sulfonic Acid. [93-01-6] 6-Hydroxy-2-naphthalenesulfonic acid; Schaeffer's β-acid. $C_{10}H_8O_4S$; mol wt 224.23. C 53.56%, H 3.60%, O 28.54%, S 14.30%. Prepn from β-naphthol and concd H_2SO_4: Fierz-David, Blangey, *Fundamental Processes of Dye Chemistry* (Interscience, New York, 1949) p 194.

Leaflets. mp 125°. Very sol in water, alcohol. Practically insol in ether.

Sodium salt. Schaeffer's salt. $C_{10}H_7NaO_4S$. Light yellow to pink powder. Freely sol in water; slightly sol in alcohol.

USE: In dye chemistry.

6393. Naphthol Yellow S. [846-70-8] 8-Hydroxy-5,7-dinitro-2-naphthalenesulfonic acid disodium salt; Citronin A; Sulfur Yellow S; Acid Yellow S; FD & C Yellow no. 1; Ext. D & C Yellow no. 7; C.I. Acid Yellow 1; C.I. 10316. $C_{10}H_4N_2Na_2O_8S$; mol wt 358.19. C 33.53%, H 1.13%, N 7.82%, Na 12.84%, O 35.73%, S 8.95%. Prepn: *Colour Index* vol. **4** (3rd ed., 1971) p 4004.

Greenish yellow powder, sol in water to a yellow soln. The free acid is known as *flavianic acid*.

USE: Dye for wool, silk.

6394. 1,2-Naphthoquinone. [524-42-5] 1,2-Naphthalenedione; β-naphthoquinone. $C_{10}H_6O_2$; mol wt 158.15. C 75.94%, H 3.82%, O 20.23%. Prepd by oxidation of 1-amino-2-naphthol with ferric chloride: Fieser, *Org. Synth.* **17**, 68 (1937); by oxidation of naphthalene: Milas, US 2395638 (1946 to Research Corp.); by bacterial dissimilation of naphthalene: Murphy, Stone, *Can. J. Microbiol.* **1**, 579 (1955); from tetrachloro-*o*-benzoquinone: Horner, Dürckheimer, *Z. Naturforsch.* **14b**, 741 (1959). Structure: Hodgson, Hathaway, *Trans. Faraday Soc.* **41**, 115 (1945). Spectroscopic properties: Oliver *et al.*, *Tetrahedron* **24**, 4067 (1968).

Golden yellow needles, dec 145-147°. uv max (abs alc): 250, 340, 405 nm (log ε 4.35, 3.40, 3.40). Sol in alc, benzene, ether, 5% NaOH, 5% NaHCO₃, concd H_2SO_4 with green color. Practically insol in water.

2-Semicarbazone. [31853-38-0] Naftazone; Haemostop Injection; Mediaven; Karbinon. $C_{11}H_9N_3O_2$; mol wt 215.21.

USE: As reagent for resorcinol and thalline.

THERAP CAT: 2-Semicarbazone as hemostatic.

6395. 1,4-Naphthoquinone. [130-15-4] 1,4-Naphthalenedione; α-naphthoquinone; 1,4-dihydro-1,4-diketonaphthalene. $C_{10}H_6O_2$; mol wt 158.15. C 75.94%, H 3.82%, O 20.23%. Prepn: Fieser, *Org. Synth.* **coll. vol. I**, 383 (2nd ed., 1941); Braude, Fawcett, *ibid.* **coll. vol. IV**, 698 (1963). Substituted 1,4-naphthoquinones occur in nature, *e.g.*, phthiocol, *q.v.*, various pigments, and the vitamins K.

Yellow triclinic needles from alcohol or petr ether. Odor like that of benzoquinone. d 1.422. mp 126°. Begins to sublime below 100°. Sublimation rates: Kempf, *J. Prakt. Chem.* [2] **78**, 236, 257. Easily volatile with steam. uv spectrum: Purvis, *J. Chem. Soc.* **101**, 1318 (1912). Sparingly sol in cold water, slightly in petr ether, freely in hot alcohol, ether, benzene, chloroform, carbon bisulfide, acetic acid; sol in alkali hydroxide solns giving a reddish-brown soln.

6396. Naphthoresorcinol. [132-86-5] 1,3-Naphthalenediol; 1,3-dihydroxynaphthalene. $C_{10}H_8O_2$; mol wt 160.17. C 74.99%, H 5.03%, O 19.98%. Prepn by cyclization of ethyl phenylacetoacetate: Soliman, West, *J. Chem. Soc.* **1944**, 53; by heating 1-amino-3-hydroxy-4-naphthalenesulfonic acid in acidic soln: Meyer, Bloch, *Org. Synth.* **25**, 73 (1945); from 1,3-naphtholsulfonic acid: Kozlov, Odintsov, *J. Appl. Chem. (USSR)* **17**, 219 (1944); Kozlov *et al.*, *Zh. Prikl. Khim.* **35**, 880 (1962).

Leaflets, mp 124-125°. Freely sol in water, alcohol, ether.

USE: Reagent for sugars, oils, and for glucuronic acid in urine: Forsyth, *Nature* **161**, 239 (1948); Heyns, Kelch, *Z. Anal. Chem.* **139**, 339 (1953).

6397. 2-Naphthoxyacetic Acid. [120-23-0] 2-Naphthalenyloxyacetic acid; β-naphthoxyacetic acid; *O*-(2-naphthyl)glycolic

Consult the Name Index before using this section.

acid. $C_{12}H_{10}O_3$; mol wt 202.21. C 71.28%, H 4.98%, O 23.74%. Prepd by treating β-naphthol with chloroacetic acid in an alkaline medium: Spitzer, *Ber.* **34**, 3192 (1901); Shirley, *Organic Intermediates* (New York, 1951) p 209.

Prisms from hot water or benzene, mp 156°. Moderately sol in hot water. Soluble in alcohol, ether, acetic acid.

Ethyl ester. $C_{14}H_{14}O_3$. Leaflets from alcohol, mp 49°. Sol in alcohol, ether.

USE: As plant hormone, to promote growth of roots on clippings, to prevent fruit from falling prematurely; causes stunted growth when used in excess.

6398. 1-Naphthylamine. [134-32-7] 1-Naphthalenamine; 1-aminonaphthalene; α-naphthylamine; naphthalidine. $C_{10}H_9N$; mol wt 143.19. C 83.88%, H 6.34%, N 9.78%. Prepd by reducing α-nitronaphthalene with Fe and HCl: West, *J. Chem. Soc.* **127**, 494 (1925); from 1-naphthalenecarboxylic acid and hydroxylamine: Snyder *et al.*, *J. Am. Chem. Soc.* **75**, 2014 (1953). Review of carcinogenic risk: *IARC Monographs* **4**, 87-96 (1974).

Needles, becoming red on exposure to air, or a reddish, cryst mass; unpleasant odor. Sublimes; volatile with steam. d 1.13. mp 50°. bp 301°. Flash pt 157°C. Sol in 590 parts water; freely sol in alc, ether. Reduces warm ammoniacal silver nitrate. *Keep well closed and protected from light.*

Hydrochloride. $C_{10}H_9N\cdot HCl$. Cryst powder; becomes bluish on exposure to air and light. Sol in about 27 parts water; sol in alcohol, ether. *Protect from light.*

Sulfate dihydrate. $(C_{10}H_9N)_2\cdot H_2SO_4\cdot 2H_2O$. White to yellowish cryst powder. Slightly sol in water or alcohol.

Caution: Potential symptoms of overexposure to 1-naphthylamine are dermatitis; hemorrhagic cystitis; dyspnea, ataxia and methemoglobinemia; hematuria; dysuria. Potential occupational carcinogen. *See NIOSH Pocket Guide to Chemical Hazards* (DHHS/NIOSH 97-140, 1997) p 222.

USE: Manufacturing dyes; toning prints made with cerium salts; the hydrochloride with sulfanilic acid is a reagent for nitrate.

6399. 2-Naphthylamine. [91-59-8] 2-Naphthalenamine; 2-aminonaphthalene; β-naphthylamine. $C_{10}H_9N$; mol wt 143.19. C 83.88%, H 6.34%, N 9.78%. Prepd by heating β-naphthol with ammonium sulfite and NH_4OH at 150°: **DE 117471** (1900); *Frdl.* **6**, 190; from 2-naphthalenecarboxylic acid and hydroxylamine: Snyder *et al.*, *J. Am. Chem. Soc.* **75**, 2014 (1953). Review of carcinogenic risk: *IARC Monographs* **4**, 97-111 (1974).

White to reddish crystals; volatile with steam. d_4^{98} 1.061. mp 111-113°. bp 306°; also stated as 294°. Sol in hot water, alcohol, ether. Reduces warm ammoniacal silver nitrate.

Acetate. $C_{10}H_9N\cdot CH_3COOH$. White to yellowish scales or flakes; slight odor of acetic acid. Very sol in water or alcohol; sol in ether. *Keep well closed and protected from light.*

Caution: Potential symptoms of overexposure to 2-naphthylamine are dermatitis; hemorrhagic cystitis; dyspnea; ataxia; methemoglobinemia, hematuria; dysuria. *See NIOSH Pocket Guide to Chemical Hazards* (DHHS/NIOSH 97-140, 1997) p 222. 2-Naphthylamine is listed as a known human carcinogen: *Report on Carcinogens, Eleventh Edition* (PB2005-104914, 2004) p III-179.

USE: Formerly in manuf of dyes, as antioxidant in rubber.

6400. 1-Naphthylamine-2,7-disulfonic Acid. [486-54-4] 1-Amino-2,7-naphthalenedisulfonic acid; Kalle's acid. $C_{10}H_9$-NO_6S_2; mol wt 303.31. C 39.60%, H 2.99%, N 4.62%, O 31.65%, S 21.14%. Prepn from 1-naphthylamine-2,4,7-trisulfonic acid: **DE 62634** (1892 to Kalle); *Frdl.* **3**, 431; from 1-naphthylamine-2,5,7-trisulfonic acid: **DE 255724** (1912 to Bayer); *Frdl.* **11**, 217.

Needles.

Sodium salt. Prisms from dil alc. Solns display a blue-green fluorescence.

Barium salt. Needles. Very slightly sol in hot water.

6401. 1-Naphthylamine-4,6-disulfonic Acid. [85-74-5] 4-Amino-1,7-naphthalenedisulfonic acid; Dahl's acid II. $C_{10}H_9NO_6$-S_2; mol wt 303.31. C 39.60%, H 2.99%, N 4.62%, O 31.65%, S 21.14%. Prepn by sulfonation of α-naphthylamine and separation from mixture of sulfonic acids obtained: Erdmann, *Ann.* **275**, 192 (1893).

Crystals. Sol in 6 parts cold water; very sol in hot water; sol in alcohol.

6402. 1-Naphthylamine-4,7-disulfonic Acid. [85-75-6] 4-Amino-1,6-naphthalenedisulfonic acid; Dahl's acid III. $C_{10}H_9$-NO_6S_2; mol wt 303.31. C 39.60%, H 2.99%, N 4.62%, O 31.65%, S 21.14%. Prepn: Erdmann, *Ann.* **275**, 192 (1893).

Crystals. Sol in 145 parts cold water, in 20 parts boiling water. Practically insol in alcohol.

6403. 1-Naphthylamine-4-sulfonic Acid. [84-86-6] 4-Amino-1-naphthalenesulfonic acid; naphthionic acid; Piria's acid. $C_{10}H_9NO_3S$; mol wt 223.25. C 53.80%, H 4.06%, N 6.27%, O 21.50%, S 14.36%. Prepd on a large-scale by heating α-naphthylamine with equimolar amounts of concd H_2SO_4 at 180-200° or by heating α-naphthylamine acid sulfate: Fierz-David, Blangey, *Fundamental Processes of Dye Chemistry* (Interscience, New York, 1949).

Sesquihydrate. Shiny needles from water. d_4^{25} 1.673. Dec on heating without melting (the amide mp 206°). K at 25° = 2.1×10^{-3}. One gram dissolves in 3.45 l of water at 10°, in 3.22 l at 20°, in 1.69 l at 50°, in 438.5 ml at 100°. Very sparingly sol in alcohol, ether. Practically insol in acetic acid and acetic anhydride, but becomes sol when some pyridine is added. Sol in dil solns of alkali hydroxides or carbonates with a blue fluorescence.

Sodium salt tetrahydrate. Naphthionine; 101-E. $C_{10}H_8NNa$-$O_3S.4H_2O$; mol wt 317.29. *Ref:* Piria, *Ann.* **78,** 41 (1851). Large monoclinic prisms from water, loses 3½ mols water at 80°, anhydr at 130°. Sweet aftertaste. Freely sol in water with a blue fluorescence. Also sol in 95% alc. Practically insol in ether. Sparingly sol in concd aq and alcoholic caustic solns. pH of a 1% aq soln 6.8. Even ampuled aq solns discolor under the influence of light.

Sodium salt glucoside. Naphthionine *N*-glucoside; 101-G. $C_{16}H_{20}NNaO_8S$; mol wt 409.39. *Ref:* Estève *et al., Ann. Pharm. Fr.* **10,** 680 (1952). White powder, bitter taste. Dec 255°. $[\alpha]_D^{23.5}$ $-113°$ (c = 10). Sol in water; slightly sol in alcohol. Practically insol in ether.

USE: The sodium salt is an important dye intermediate in the manuf of Congo Red, Fast Red A, Azo Rubine, and similar azo dyes.

THERAP CAT: Sodium salt as hemostatic.

6404. 1-Naphthylamine-5-sulfonic Acid. [84-89-9] 5-Amino-1-naphthalenesulfonic acid; Laurent's acid. $C_{10}H_9NO_3S$; mol wt 223.25. C 53.80%, H 4.06%, N 6.27%, O 21.50%, S 14.36%. Prepn from 5-chloro-1-naphthalenesulfonic acid + ammonia: Oehler, *DE 72336* (1893); *Frdl.* **3,** 435; from α-naphthylamine + concd sulfuric acid: Erdmann, *Ann.* **275,** 193, 200 (1893); Sixma, *Rec. Trav. Chim.* **73,** 235 (1954); from 2-naphthylamine-8-sulfonic acid: Blangey, *Helv. Chim. Acta* **39,** 977 (1956).

White crystals. Sol in 950 parts cold water; more sol in hot water.
USE: In dye chemistry.

6405. 1-Naphthylamine-8-sulfonic Acid. [82-75-7] 8-Amino-1-naphthalenesulfonic acid; Peri acid. $C_{10}H_9NO_3S$; mol wt 223.25. C 53.80%, H 4.06%, N 6.27%, O 21.50%, S 14.36%. Prepn: Fierz, Weissenbach, *Helv. Chim. Acta* **3,** 310 (1920); Martin, *Z. Farben-Ind.* **20,** 9, 76 (1928), *C.A.* **22,** 2665 (1928); Shebuev *et al., SU 165746* (1964 to State Scientific Res. Inst. of Org. Intermediates & Dyes), *C.A.* **62,** 10392c (1965).

Needles. Sol in 4800 parts cold, 240 parts boiling water; freely sol in glacial acetic acid.
Caution: Irritating to skin.

6406. 2-Naphthylamine-1-sulfonic Acid. [81-16-3] 2-Amino-1-naphthalenesulfonic acid; Tobias acid. $C_{10}H_9NO_3S$; mol wt 223.25. C 53.80%, H 4.06%, N 6.27%, O 21.50%, S 14.36%. Prepd by sulfonation of 2-naphthylamine: Tinker, Hansen, *US 1969189* (1934 to du Pont). Utilization in viral biology study: N. Sakota *et al., J. Ferment. Technol.* **56,** 53 (1978). TLC study: J. Franc, V. Koudelkova, *J. Chromatogr.* **170,** 89 (1979).

Anhydr scales from hot water; hydrated needles from cold water. Slightly sol in cold water; more sol in hot water; very slightly sol in alcohol, ether.
Diethylammonium salt. $C_{10}H_9NO_3S.(C_2H_5)_2NH$. mp 180°.
USE: Dyestuff intermediate.

6407. 2-Naphthylamine-5-sulfonic Acid. [81-05-0] 6-Amino-1-naphthalenesulfonic acid; Dahl's acid. $C_{10}H_9NO_3S$; mol wt 223.25. C 53.80%, H 4.06%, N 6.27%, O 21.50%, S 14.36%. Prepn by reduction of 6-nitro-1-naphthalenesulfonic acid: Kappeler, *Ber.* **45,** 633 (1912); by sulfonation of β-naphthylamine and separation from mixt of sulfonic acids obtained: Green, Vakil, *J. Chem. Soc.* **113,** 35 (1918).

Needles from water. Sol in 3025 parts water at 20°. Almost insol in alcohol.
USE: Dyestuff intermediate.

6408. 2-Naphthyl Benzoate. [93-44-7] 2-Naphthalenol benzoate; betanaphthol benzoate; benzoylnaphthol; Lintrin; Haertolan. $C_{17}H_{12}O_2$; mol wt 248.28. C 82.24%, H 4.87%, O 12.89%. $C_6H_5COOC_{10}H_7$.

White, crystalline powder; darkens with age. mp 107-110°. Almost insol in water. Freely sol in hot alcohol, chloroform, glycerol, oils; slightly sol in ether.
USE: Hardening agent for paraffin.
THERAP CAT: Antiseptic (intestinal).

6409. *N*-(1-Naphthyl)ethylenediamine. [551-09-7] *N*-1-Naphthalenyl-1,2-ethanediamine; 1-amino-2-(α-naphthylamino)-ethane. $C_{12}H_{14}N_2$; mol wt 186.25. C 77.38%, H 7.58%, N 15.04%. Prepn from α-naphthylamine and bromoethylphthalimide: Bratton, Marshall, *J. Biol. Chem.* **128,** 537 (1939).

Straw-yellow, viscous liquid; bp_9 204°; bp_{760} ~320° (dec); n_D^{25} 1.6648; d^{25} 1.114. The soly in water is about 0.2 g in 100 ml at 25°; more sol in hot water. pH of satd aq soln: 10.5. Readily sol in common organic solvents except petr ether.

Dihydrochloride. $C_{12}H_{14}N_2.2HCl$. Long hexagonal prisms; mp 188-190°. Readily sol in 95% alcohol, dil hydrochloric acid, hot water; slightly sol in cold water, acetone, abs alc.
USE: Dihydrochloride in determination of sulfanilamide in body fluids; also in determination of potassium, nitrites, and sulfates.

6410. 1-Naphthylisocyanate. [86-84-0] 1-Isocyanatonaphthalene. $C_{11}H_7NO$; mol wt 169.18. C 78.09%, H 4.17%, N 8.28%, O 9.46%. $C_{10}H_7N{=}CO$.

Colorless liquid; almost odorless at ordinary temp; vapors have a pungent odor characteristic of isocyanates (*e.g.,* phenylisocyanate). d 1.181. bp 270°. Sol in chloroform, ether, petr ether, alcohol. *Keep well closed and protected from light.*

6411. 1-Naphthylisothiocyanate. [551-06-4] 1-Isothiocyanatonaphthalene; ANIT. $C_{11}H_7NS$; mol wt 185.24. C 71.32%, H 3.81%, N 7.56%, S 17.31%. $C_{10}H_7N{=}C{=}S$. Prepn: Cymerman-Craig *et al., Org. Synth.* **coll. vol. IV,** 700 (1963); Jochims, *Ber.* **101,** 1746 (1968). Has been used with pyrethrum as insecticide. Toxicity studies: Schwartz, Warren, *Public Health Rep.* **54,** 1426 (1939); Ambrose, Miller, *Fed. Proc.* **2,** 74 (1943); Becker, Plaa, *Toxicol. Appl. Pharmacol.* **7,** 804 (1965); Capizzo, Roberts, *ibid.* **17,** 262 (1970).

White needles; practically odorless and tasteless, mp 58°. Insol in water. Freely sol in ether, benzene, hot alcohol, acetone, carbon tetrachloride, olive oil, petr ether. LD_{50} orally in mice: 245 mg/kg (Becker, Plaa).
Caution: Hepatotoxic; may cause dermatitis.

6412. 2-Naphthyl Lactate. [93-43-6] 2-Hydroxypropanoic acid 2-naphthalenyl ester; lactic acid β-naphthyl ester; Lactol; Lactonaphthol. $C_{13}H_{12}O_3$; mol wt 216.23. C 72.21%, H 5.59%, O 22.20%. $CH_3CHOHCOOC_{10}H_7$. Prepd by heating equimolar amounts of β-naphthol sodium and sodium lactate to 125-130° in the presence of phosphorus oxychloride: P. Lebeau, *Traité de Pharmacie Chimique* vol. II (Masson, Paris, 1955/56) p 964.

Crystals from alcohol. Moderately sol in alcohol. Insol in water, ether.

THERAP CAT: Antiseptic (intestinal).

6413. 2-(2-Naphthyloxy)ethanol. [93-20-9] 2-(2-Naphthalenyloxy)ethanol; β-naphthoxyethanol; betanaphthoxyethanol; β-hydroxyethyl 2-naphthyl ether; 2-(β-hydroxyethoxy)naphthalene; ethylene glycol mono-2-naphthyl ether. $C_{12}H_{12}O_2$; mol wt 188.22. C 76.57%, H 6.43%, O 17.00%. Prepd by the condensation of β-naphthol with ethylene chlorohydrin: Rindfusz *et al., J. Am. Chem. Soc.* **42,** 157, 164, 165 (1920); Kirner, Richter, *ibid.* **51,** 3409 (1929); by heating β-naphthol with ethylene oxide and sodium ethoxide in alcohol: Boyd, Marle, *J. Chem. Soc.* **105,** 2117 (1914).

Crystals from benzene + petr ether, mp 76.7°. Insoluble in water. One gram dissolves in 4 g of 95% alcohol, in 2 g acetone; also sol in ether, chloroform. uv max (0.004% in chloroform): 273, 328 nm (E ~1.00, ~0.395).

THERAP CAT (VET): Formerly as anesthetic.

6414. 1-Naphthyl Salicylate. [550-97-0] 2-Hydroxybenzoic acid 1-naphthalenyl ester; α-naphthyl salicylate; α-naphthol salicylate; Alphol. $C_{17}H_{12}O_3$; mol wt 264.28. C 77.26%, H 4.58%, O 18.16%.

Crystalline powder. mp 83°. Insol in water. Freely sol in alcohol, ether, oils.

THERAP CAT: Anti-infective; anti-inflammatory.

6415. 2-Naphthyl Salicylate. [613-78-5] 2-Hydroxybenzoic acid 2-naphthalenyl ester; β-naphthol salicylate; Betol; Naphthalol; Naphthosalol; Salinaphthol. $C_{17}H_{12}O_3$; mol wt 264.28. C 77.26%, H 4.58%, O 18.16%.

White, odorless, tasteless, crystalline powder. mp 95°. Insol in water or glycerol. Sparingly sol in cold alcohol; freely sol in boiling alcohol, in benzene, ether.

THERAP CAT: Antiseptic.

6416. Napropamide. [15299-99-7] N,N-Diethyl-2-(1-naphthalenyloxy)propanamide; N,N-diethyl-2-(1-naphthyloxy)propionamide; 2-(α-naphthoxy)-N,N-diethylpropionamide; R-7465; Devrinol. $C_{17}H_{21}NO_2$; mol wt 271.35. C 75.25%, H 7.80%, N 5.16%, O 11.79%. Prepn: H. Filles *et al., US 3480671* (1969 to Stauffer). Characteristics in the soil: C. H. Wu *et al., Weed Sci.* **23,** 54 (1975). Toxicity study: T. Kawada *et al., Niigata Igakkai Zasshi* **87,** 289 (1973), *C.A.* **80,** 56257h (1974).

Light brown solid from *n*-pentane, mp 63-64° (tech, 69.5°). Solubility in water at 20°: 70 ppm. LD_{50} in mice (g/kg): >5 orally, >1 i.p., >1 s.c. (Kawada).

USE: Herbicide.

6417. Naproxen. [22204-53-1] (αS)-6-Methoxy-α-methyl-2-naphthaleneacetic acid; d-2-(6-methoxy-2-naphthyl)propionic acid; MNPA; RS-3540; Bonyl; Dysmenalgit; Equiproxen; Floginax; Laraflex; Laser; Malexin; Naixan; Napren; Naprius; Naprosyn; Naprosyne; Naprux; Naxen; Nycopren; Pranoxen; Prexan; Proxen; Proxine; Veradol; Xenar. $C_{14}H_{14}O_3$; mol wt 230.26. C 73.03%, H 6.13%, O 20.85%. Nonsteroidal anti-inflammatory. Prepn: J. H.

Fried, I. T. Harrison, **ZA 6707597**; *eidem,* **US 3904682**; *eidem,* **US 4009197** (1968, 1975, 1977 all to Syntex); I. T. Harrison *et al., J. Med. Chem.* **13,** 203 (1970). Pharmacology: Roszkowski *et al., J. Pharmacol. Exp. Ther.* **179,** 114 (1971). Activity may be due to the ability to inhibit prostaglandin biosynthesis. Mode of action studies: Tomlinson *et al., Biochem. Biophys. Res. Commun.* **46,** 552 (1972). Metabolism: Runkel *et al., J. Pharm. Sci.* **61,** 703 (1972). HPLC determn in plasma and serum: P. J. Streete, *J. Chromatogr.* **495,** 179 (1989). Stereoselective synthesis: K. T. Wan, M. E. Davis, *Nature* **370,** 449 (1994). Clinical studies: Katona *et al., Clin. Trials J.* **8,** 3 (1972); Runkel, *Chem. Pharm. Bull.* **20,** 1457 (1972). *Review: Arzneim.-Forsch.* **25,** 278-332 (1975). Review of pharmacology and therapeutic efficacy: R. N. Brogden *et al., Drugs* **18,** 241-277 (1979). Comprehensive description: F. J. Al-Shammary *et al., Anal. Profiles Drug Subs. Excip.* **21,** 345-373 (1992).

Crystals from acetone-hexane, mp 152-154°. $[\alpha]_D$ +66° (in chloroform). Sol in 25 parts ethanol (96%), 20 parts methanol, 15 parts chloroform, 40 parts ether. Practically insol in water. LD_{50} in mice (mg/kg): 435 i.v.; 1234 orally; in rats (mg/kg): 575 i.p.; 534 orally (Roszkowski).

Piperazine salt. [70981-66-7] Piproxen; Numidan. $(C_{14}H_{14}O_3)_2 \cdot C_4H_{10}N_2$; mol wt 546.65.

Sodium salt. [26159-34-2] RS-3650; Aleve; Anaprox; Antalgin; Apranax; Axer Alfa; Flanax; Gynestrel; Miranax; Naprelan; Primeral; Synflex. $C_{14}H_{13}NaO_3$; mol wt 252.24. Crystals from acetone, mp 244-246°. $[\alpha]_D$ −11° (in methanol).

THERAP CAT: Anti-inflammatory; analgesic; antipyretic.

THERAP CAT (VET): Anti-inflammatory.

6418. Naptalam. [132-66-1] 2-[(1-Naphthalenylamino)carbonyl]benzoic acid; N-1-naphthylphthalamic acid; α-naphthylphthalamic acid. $C_{18}H_{13}NO_3$; mol wt 291.30. C 74.22%, H 4.50%, N 4.81%, O 16.48%. Selective pre-emergence herbicide. Prepn: A. E. Smith, O. L. Hoffmann, **US 2556665** (1951 to U.S. Rubber). Activity: O. L. Hoffmann, A. E. Smith, *Science* **109,** 588 (1949). Mobility in soil: A. E. Smith *et al., J. Agric. Food Chem.* **5,** 748 (1957).

Crystals from ethanol, d_4^{20} 1.40. mp 203° (technical grade, mp 175-180°). Soly: <0.02 g/100 ml of water. Sol in alkaline solns, but dec above pH 9.5. Slightly sol in ethanol, acetone, benzene. Hydrolyzed by strong acids and bases.

Sodium salt. ACP-332; NPA-3; Alanap. $C_{18}H_{12}NNaO_3$; mol wt 313.28.

USE: Herbicide; as analytical reagent for thorium and zirconium.

6419. Narasin. [55134-13-9] (4S)-4-Methylsalinomycin; narasin A; Compd 79891; Antibiotic A-28086 factor A; C-7819B; Monteban. $C_{43}H_{72}O_{11}$; mol wt 765.03. C 67.51%, H 9.49%, O 23.00%. Main component of a polyether antibiotic complex produced by *Streptomyces aureofaciens* NRRL 5758 & NRRL 8092. Production: D. H. Berg *et al., DE 2525095* corresp to **US 4038384** (1975, 1977 to Lilly); L. D. Boeck *et al., Dev. Ind. Microbiol.* **18,** 471 (1976). Isoln and characterization: D. H. Berg, R. L. Hamill, *J. Antibiot.* **31,** 1 (1978). Biosynthetic studies using ^{13}C-NMR study: D. E. Dorman *et al., Helv. Chim. Acta* **59,** 2625 (1976). Structure: J. L. Occolowitz *et al., Biomed. Mass Spectrom.* **3,** 272 (1976); H. Seto *et al., J. Antibiot.* **30,** 530 (1977). Anticoccidial activity: M. D. Ruff *et al., Poult. Sci.* **59,** 2008 (1980). Total synthesis: Y. Kishi *et al., Front. Chem., Plenary Keynote Lect.*

IUPAC Congr., 28th **1981,** K. J. Laidler, Ed. (Pergamon, Oxford, 1982) pp 287-304. HPLC determn in animal feeds: M. R. La-Pointe, H. Cohen, *J. Assoc. Off. Anal. Chem.* **71,** 480 (1988).

Crystals from acetone-water, mp 98-100°; resolidif and remelts at 198-200°. uv max (ethanol): 285 nm (ε 58). $[\alpha]_D^{25}$ −54° (c = 0.2 in methanol). pKa 7.9 (80% aq DMF). Sol in alcohols, acetone, DMF, DMSO, benzene, chloroform, ethyl acetate. Insol in water. LD_{50} i.p. in mice: 7.15 mg/kg (Berg).

THERAP CAT (VET): Coccidiostat; growth stimulant.

6420. Naratriptan. [121679-13-8] *N*-Methyl-3-(1-methyl-4-piperidinyl)-1*H*-indole-5-ethanesulfonamide. $C_{17}H_{25}N_3O_2S$; mol wt 335.46. C 60.87%, H 7.51%, N 12.53%, O 9.54%, S 9.56%. Serotonin 5-HT$_{1B/1D}$ receptor agonist. Prepn: A. W. Oxford *et al., EP 303507; eidem,* **US 4997841** (1989, 1991 both to Glaxo). Pharmacology and receptor binding study: H. E. Connor *et al., Cephalalgia* **17,** 145 (1997). Determn in plasma and pharmacokinetics in rabbits: B. D. Duléry *et al., J. Pharm. Biomed. Anal.* **15,** 1009 (1997). Clinical trial in migraine: H. Havanka *et al., Clin. Ther.* **22,** 970 (2000).

Crystals from ethyl acetate, mp 170-171°.

Hydrochloride. [143388-64-1] GR-85548A; Amerge; Nara-mig. $C_{17}H_{25}N_3O_2S \cdot HCl$; mol wt 371.93. Microcrystals, mp 237-239°.

THERAP CAT: Antimigraine.

6421. Narbomycin. [6036-25-5] 12-Deoxypicromycin. $C_{28}H_{47}NO_7$; mol wt 509.68. C 65.98%, H 9.29%, N 2.75%, O 21.97%. Antibiotic substance produced by *Streptomyces narbonensis* from soil near Cannes, France: Corbaz *et al., Helv. Chim. Acta* **38,** 935 (1955). Structure: Prelog *et al., ibid.* **45,** 4 (1962). Stereochemical studies: Rickards, Smith, *Tetrahedron Lett.* **1970,** 1025; H. Ogura *et al., J. Am. Chem. Soc.* **97,** 1930 (1975); *eidem, Tetrahedron* **37,** Suppl. 1, 165 (1981). Isoln and structure of the aglycone *narbonolide*: Hori *et al., Chem. Commun.* **1971,** 304. Synthesis of narbonolide: T. Kaiho *et al., J. Org. Chem.* **47,** 1612 (1982).

Crystals from ether + petr ether, mp 113.5-115°. $[\alpha]_D^{20}$ +68.5° (c = 1.35 in chloroform). uv max (abs ethanol): 225, 286 nm (log ε 4.06, 2.23). LD_{50} s.c. in mice: 500 mg/kg (Corbaz).

6422. Narceine. [131-28-2] 6-[[6-[2-(Dimethylamino)eth-yl]-4-methoxy-1,3-benzodioxol-5-yl]acetyl]-2,3-dimethoxybenzoic acid; 6-[[6-[2-(dimethylamino)ethyl]-2-methoxy-3,4-(methylenedi-oxy)phenyl]acetyl]-*o*-veratric acid. $C_{23}H_{27}NO_8$; mol wt 445.46. C 62.01%, H 6.11%, N 3.14%, O 28.73%. Occurs in opium to the

extent of 0.1-0.5%. The separation from morphine mother liquors is tedious: Merck, *Chem. Ztg.* **13,** 525 (1889). Prepn from narcotine or gnoscopine: Roser, *Ann.* **247,** 167 (1888); Frankforter, Keller, *Ann. Chem. J.* **22,** 61 (1899); Frerichs, *Arch. Pharm.* **241,** 259 (1903); Hope, Robinson, *J. Chem. Soc.* **105,** 2100 (1914). Structure: Freund, Frankforter, *Ann.* **277,** 20 (1893); Freund, Michaels, *Ann.* **286,** 248 (1895); Freund, *Ber.* **40,** 194 (1907); Freund, Oppenheim, *Ber.* **42,** 1084 (1909); Addinall, Major, *J. Am. Chem. Soc.* **55,** 1202, 2153 (1933).

The anhydr material is very hygroscopic, mp 138°. uv max (ethanol): 270 nm (log ε 3.98). Usually the alkaloid is obtained as the trihydrate. Clusters of silky, prismatic needles from water, mp 176°. pKb (20°) = 10.7, pKa = 9.3. pH of satd soln = 5.8. One gram dissolves in 770 ml water, 220 ml boiling water. Moderately sol in hot alcohol, nearly insol in benzene, chloroform, ether, petr ether; sol in alkali hydroxide solns forming salts, also in dil mineral acids.

Ethylnarceine hydrochloride. Narcyl. $C_{25}H_{32}ClNO_8$. Plates from water, mp 208-210°. Slightly sol in cold water, sol in hot water, alcohol, chloroform; insol in ether.

THERAP CAT: Ethylnarceine hydrochloride as analgesic (narcotic); antitussive.

6423. Narcotoline. [521-40-4] (3*S*)-6,7-Dimethoxy-3-[(5*R*)-5,6,7,8-tetrahydro-4-hydroxy-6-methyl-1,3-dioxolo[4,5-*g*]-isoquinolin-5-yl]-1(3*H*)-isobenzofuranone; desmethylnarcotine. $C_{21}H_{21}NO_7$; mol wt 399.39. C 63.15%, H 5.30%, N 3.51%, O 28.04%. Found in the shell of ripe poppyseed capsules: Wrede, *Arch. Pharmacol.* **184,** 331 (1937); Baumgarten, Christ, *Pharmazie* **5,** 80 (1950); Pfeifer, Weiss, *ibid.* **10,** 658 (1955); from opium prepns: Pfeifer, *Arch. Pharm.* **290,** 209 (1957). Preliminary stereochemical studies: Battersby, Spenser, *J. Chem. Soc.* **1965,** 1087. Revised stereochemistry: Blaha *et al., Collect. Czech. Chem. Commun.* **29,** 2328 (1964); Snatzke *et al., Tetrahedron* **25,** 5059 (1969).

Rectangular rods from dil methanol, mp 202°. $[\alpha]_D^{20}$ −189° (0.1 g in 25 ml chloroform, 20 cm tube). $[\alpha]_D^{20}$ +5.8° (0.065 g in 5 ml 0.1*N* HCl in 20 cm tube). Very sparingly sol in water. Moderately sol in warm alc and ether. Freely sol in chloroform, in dil acids and in dil aq solns of KOH and NaOH. Sparingly sol in dil aq solns of Na_2CO_3.

6424. Naringenin. [480-41-1] 2,3-Dihydro-5,7-dihydroxy-2-(4-hydroxyphenyl)-4*H*-1-benzopyran-4-one; 4′,5,7-trihydroxy-flavanone; naringetol; salipurpol; pelargidanon 1602. $C_{15}H_{12}O_5$; mol wt 272.25. C 66.17%, H 4.44%, O 29.38%. The aglucon of naringin. Prepn by hydrolysis of naringin: Asahina, Inubuse, *Ber.* **61,** 1514 (1928); Haley, Bassin, *J. Am. Pharm. Assoc.* **40,** 111 (1951). From kino of *Eucalyptus maculata* Hook, *Myrtaceae:* Gell *et al., Aust. J. Chem.* **11,** 372 (1958). Synthesis: Rosenmund, Rosenmund, *Ber.* **61,** 2608 (1928); Zemplén, Bognár, *Ber.* **75,** 648

(1942). Absolute configuration: Gaffield, Waiss, *Chem. Commun.* **1968**, 29.

Needles from dilute alc, mp 251°. uv max: 226, 292 nm. Sol in alcohol, ether, benzene; almost insol in water.

Triacetylnaringenin. $C_{15}H_9(CH_3CO)_3O_5$. Crystals, mp 55°.

6425. Naringin. [10236-47-2] 7-[[2-*O*-(6-Deoxy-α-L-mannopyranosyl)-β-D-glucopyranosyl]oxy]-2,3-dihydro-5-hydroxy-2-(4-hydroxyphenyl)-4*H*-1-benzopyran-4-one; 4′,5,7-trihydroxyflavanone 7-rhamnoglucoside; naringenin-7-rhamnoglucoside; aurantiin. $C_{27}H_{32}O_{14}$; mol wt 580.53. C 55.86%, H 5.56%, O 38.58%. In the flowers of grapefruit trees *(Citrus paradisi* Macfad, *Rutaceae)*, also in fruit and rind. Most abundant in immature fruit; main bitter component of grapefruit juice. Extraction from grapefruit peel: Zoller, *Ind. Eng. Chem.* **10**, 364 (1918); Pulley, von Loesecke, *J. Am. Chem. Soc.* **61**, 175 (1939); US 2421062; US 2421063 (both 1947 to California Fruit Growers Exchange). Structure: Asahina, Inubuse, *C.A.* **23**, 3475 (1929); *cf.* also *Ber.* **61**, 1514 (1928); Horowitz, Gentili, *Tetrahedron* **19**, 773 (1963). Solubility data: G. N. Pulley, *Ind. Eng. Chem. Anal. Ed.* **8**, 360 (1936). *Review:* Kesterson, Hendrickson, *Naringin, A Bitter Principle of Grapefruit* **Bulletin no. 511** (Univ. Florida Agric. Expt. Station, Jan. 1953).

When crystallized from water, it contains 6 to 8 mols H_2O. mp ~83°. After drying at 110° to constant weight, it contains 2 mols H_2O, mp 171°. Bitter taste (1:10,000 H_2O can be tasted). $[\alpha]_D^{19}$ −82° (alcohol). One gram dissolves in 1000 ml water at 40°. At 75° one gram dissolves in 10 ml water. Sol in acetone, alcohol, warm acetic acid.

6426. Natalizumab. [189261-10-7] Anti-(human integrin α4) immunoglobulin G4 (human-mouse monoclonal AN100226 γ4-chain) disulfide with human-mouse monoclonal AN100226 light chain, dimer; Antegren; Tysabri. Recombinant humanized IgG4 monoclonal antibody directed against the leukocyte adhesion molecule VLA-4, also known as α4β1 integrin. α4-Integrin inhibitor designed to block lymphocyte activation, migration and adhesion to endothelial cells. Prepn: M. M. Bendig *et al.*, WO 9519790; *eidem*, US 5840299 (1995, 1998 both to Athena Neurosciences); O. J. P. Léger *et al.*, *Hum. Antibod.* **8**, 3 (1997). Clinical pharmacokinetics: W. A. Sheremata *et al.*, *Neurology* **52**, 1072 (1999). Clinical trial in multiple sclerosis: D. H. Miller *et al.*, *N. Engl. J. Med.* **348**, 15 (2003); in Crohn's disease: W. J. Sandborn *et al.*, *ibid.* **353**, 1912 (2005). Review of pharmacology and therapeutic potential: M. Elices, *Curr. Opin. Anti-Inflam. Immunomod. Invest. Drugs* **2**, 228-235 (2000); K. A. Keeley *et al.*, *Ann. Pharmacother.* **39**, 1833-1843 (2005).

THERAP CAT: Anti-inflammatory.

6427. Natamycin. [7681-93-8] Pimaricin; antibiotic A 5283; tennecetin; CL-12625; Mycophyt; Myprozine; Natacyn; Pimafucin; Synogil. $C_{33}H_{47}NO_{13}$; mol wt 665.73. C 59.54%, H 7.12%, N 2.10%, O 31.24%. Polyene antifungal antibiotic produced by *Streptomyces natalensis* from soil near Pietermaritzburg, South Africa and by *S. chattanoogensis.* Isoln: Struyk *et al.*,

Antibiot. Annu. **1957-1958**, 878. Prodn: GB 844289 (1960 to Koninklijke Nederlandsche Gist en Spiritus-Fabriek); GB 846933 (1960 to Am. Cyanamid). Identity with tennecetin: Divekar *et al.*, *Antibiot. Chemother.* **11**, 377 (1961). Structure: Golding *et al.*, *Tetrahedron Lett.* **1966**, 3551; Meyer, *Chem. Commun.* **1968**, 470. Configuration: Gaudiano *et al.*, *Chim. Ind. (Milan)* **48**, 1327 (1966). Revised structure: R. C. Pandey, K. L. Rinehart, *J. Antibiot.* **29**, 1035 (1976). Soly data: Marsh, Weiss, *J. Assoc. Off. Anal. Chem.* **50**, 457 (1967). Toxicology: G. J. Levinskas *et al.*, *Toxicol. Appl. Pharmacol.* **8**, 97 (1966). Comprehensive description: H. Brik, *Anal. Profiles Drug Subs. Excip.* **23**, 399-419 (1994).

Crystals from methanol + water, darkens ~200°, dec 280-300°. $[\alpha]_D^{20}$ +278° (c = 1 in CH_3COOH). Sensitive to light, but otherwise very stable in the dry state. uv max (methanol + 0.1% CH_3COOH): 220, 280, 290, 303, 318 nm (ε 21300, 26630, 52930, 83220, 76230). Soly at 20° (g/ml): 87% glycerol 0.18. Practically insol in higher alcohols, ether, esters, aromatic or aliphatic hydrocarbons, chlorinated hydrocarbons, ketones, dioxane, cyclohexanol, oils. LD_{50} orally in male, female rats (g/kg): 2.73, 4.67 (Levinskas).

THERAP CAT: Antifungal (topical).

6428. Nateglinide. [105816-04-4] *N*-[[*trans*-4-(1-Methylethyl)cyclohexyl]carbonyl]-D-phenylalanine; (−)-*N*-(*trans*-4-isopropylcyclohexyl-1-carbonyl)-D-phenylalanine; A-4166; AY-4166; SDZ-DJN-608; Fastic; Starlix; Starsis. $C_{19}H_{27}NO_3$; mol wt 317.42. C 71.89%, H 8.57%, N 4.41%, O 15.12%. Amino acid derivative that stimulates insulin secretion. Prepn: S. Toyoshima *et al.*, EP 196222; *eidem*, US 4816484 (1986, 1989 both to Ajinomoto); H. Shinkai *et al.*, *J. Med. Chem.* **32**, 1436 (1989). Effect on insulin secretion: Y. Sato *et al.*, *Diabetes Res. Clin. Pract.* **12**, 53 (1991). HPLC determn in plasma and urine: I. Ono *et al.*, *J. Chromatogr. B* **692**, 397 (1997). Series of articles on pharmacology, pharmacokinetics and toxicology: *Yakuri to Chiryo* **25**, Suppl. 1, S9-S239 (1997). Toxicity data: K. Hasegawa *et al.*, *ibid.* S5, *C.A.* **126**, 152622 (1997).

Crystals from methanol-water, mp 129-130°. $[\alpha]_D^{20}$ −9.4° (c = 1 in methanol). LD_{50} orally in rats: >2.0 g/kg (Hasegawa).

THERAP CAT: Antidiabetic.

6429. Natural Gas. American natural gas consists of about 85% methane, 9% ethane, 3% propane, 2% nitrogen, 1% butane. Northern Texas gas contains more nitrogen, also sufficient helium to warrant commercial extraction.

Caution: Narcotic in high concns. Incomplete combustion can result in production of carbon monoxide.

USE: Fuel gas, in the manuf of hydrogen, methane, ammonia.

6430. Neamine. [3947-65-7] 2-Deoxy-4-*O*-(2,6-diamino-2,6-dideoxy-α-D-glucopyranosyl)-D-streptamine; neomycin A. $C_{12}H_{26}N_4O_6$; mol wt 322.36. C 44.71%, H 8.13%, N 17.38%, O 29.78%. Component of the antibiotic complex neomycin, *q.v.* Isoln: Dutcher *et al.*, *J. Am. Chem. Soc.* **73**, 1384 (1951). Identity of neomycin A and neamine: Leach, Teeters, *ibid.* **74**, 3187 (1952). Prepn from neomycin B: Peck *et al.,* US 2691675 (1954 to Merck & Co.). Structure: Carter *et al., J. Am. Chem. Soc.* **83**, 3723 (1961); Hichens, Rinehart, *ibid.* **85**, 1547 (1963). Synthesis: Umezawa *et al., J. Antibiot.* **20A**, 53 (1967); H. Kohno *et al., Agric. Biol. Chem.* **39**, 1091 (1975); A. Harayama *et al., Bull. Chem. Soc. Jpn.* **52**, 3626 (1979).

Crystals from water or aq alc, dec 225-226°, $[\alpha]_D^{25}+112.8°$ (c = 1). IR spectrum: Leach, Teeters, *J. Am. Chem. Soc.* **73**, 2794 (1951).

Hydrochloride. $C_{12}H_{26}N_4O_6$.4HCl. Amorphous, dec 250-260°, $[\alpha]_D^{25}+83°$ (c = 1).

N-**Acetyl deriv.** $C_{12}H_{26}N_4O_6$.$(CH_3CO)_4$. Crystals from methanol, mp 334-336°. $[\alpha]_D^{25}+87°$ (c = 1).

6431. Neatsfoot Oil. Fixed oil from feet of neat (bovine) cattle.

Pale yellow liquid; peculiar odor. d 0.915. Solidif 0° to −10°. n_D^{20} 1.4695-1.4708. Sapon no. 192-203. Iodine no. 44-73.2.

USE: Waterproofing and softening leather; lubricant; oiling wool, etc.

6432. Nebivolol. [118457-14-0]; [99200-09-6] (unspecified stereo). $(\alpha R,\alpha'R,2R,2'S)$-*rel*-$\alpha,\alpha'$-[Iminobis(methylene)]bis[6-fluoro-3,4-dihydro-2*H*-1-benzopyran-2-methanol]; α,α'-(iminodimethylene)bis[6-fluoro-2-chromanmethanol]; *dl*-nebivolol; narbivolol; R-65824. $C_{22}H_{25}F_2NO_4$; mol wt 405.44. C 65.17%, H 6.22%, F 9.37%, N 3.45%, O 15.78%. β_1-Adrenergic blocker; nitric oxide-mediated vasodilator. Prepd as racemic mixture of (R,S,S,S)- and (S,R,R,R)-enantiomers. Prepn: G. R. E. Van Lommen *et al.,* EP 145067; *eidem,* US 4654362 (1985, 1987 both to Janssen); *eidem, J. Pharm. Belg.* **45**, 355 (1990). HPLC fluorescence determn in plasma: R. Woestenborghs *et al., Methodol. Surv. Biochem. Anal.* **18**, 215 (1988). Receptor binding study: P. J. Pauwels *et al., Mol. Pharmacol.* **34**, 843 (1988). Clinical study of vasodilating effects: J. R. Cockcroft *et al., J. Pharmacol. Exp. Ther.* **274**, 1067 (1995). Clinical trial in hypertension: T. J. Cleophas *et al., Clin. Ther. Res.* **62**, 451 (2001); in endothelial dysfunction with hypertension: N. Tzemos *et al., Circulation* **104**, 511 (2001). Review of pharmacology: M. Mangrella *et al., Pharmacol. Res.* **38**, 419-431 (1998); of clinical development: J. Cockcroft, *Expert Opin. Pharmacother.* **5**, 893-899 (2004).

(*S,R,R,R*)-Nebivolol (D-form)

Hydrochloride. [152520-56-4] R-67555; Lobivon; Nebilet; Nebilox. $C_{22}H_{25}F_2NO_4$.HCl; mol wt 441.90.

THERAP CAT: Antihypertensive.

6433. Nebularine. [550-33-4] 9-β-D-Ribofuranosyl-9*H*-purine. $C_{10}H_{12}N_4O_4$; mol wt 252.23. C 47.62%, H 4.80%, N 22.21%, O 25.37%. Isoln from the mushroom *Clitocybe nebularis* (Batsch.) Quel., *Agaricaceae:* Ehrenberg *et al., Sven. Kem. Tidskr.* **58**, 269 (1946); Löfgren *et al., Acta Chem. Scand.* **8**, 670 (1954); from a streptomycete: Isono, Suzuki, *J. Antibiot.* **13A**, 270 (1960). *In vitro* toxicity towards sarcoma 180 cells, mouse embryonic fibroblasts and epithelial cells: J. J. Biescle *et al., Cancer* **8**, 87 (1955). Synthesis: Brown, Weliky, *J. Biol. Chem.* **204**, 1019 (1953); Fox *et al., J. Am. Chem. Soc.* **80**, 1669 (1958); Hashizume, Iwamura, *Tetrahedron Lett.* **1966**, 643; *eidem, J. Org. Chem.* **33**, 1796 (1968). Crystal structure: T. Takeda, *Acta Crystallogr.* **30B**, 825 (1974). Alternate syntheses: V. Nair, S. G. Richardson, *Tetra-*

hedron Lett. **1979**, 1181; P. K. Gupta, D. S. Bhakuni, *Indian J. Chem.* **20B**, 534 (1981). Toxicity studies: Truant, D'Amato, *Fed. Proc.* **14**, 391 (1955).

Small rhombohedra from ethyl methyl ketone + methanol, mp 181-182°; needles from methanol, mp 182-183°. $[\alpha]_D^{25}$ −48.6° (H_2O). uv max (0.1*N* HCl): 262 nm ($E_{1cm}^{1\%}$ 232); (0.1*N* NaOH): 263 nm ($E_{1cm}^{1\%}$ 361). Considerably sol in water (about 10%). Slightly sol in cold ethanol. Very slightly sol in acetone, ether, chloroform. Aq solns may be sterilized by boiling without decompn. LD_{50} in rats, guinea pigs (mg/kg): 220, 15 s.c. (Truant, D'Amato).

6434. Nebulin. Family of giant, actin-binding proteins, varying in size from 700-900 kDa, found in the sarcomeres of vertebrate skeletal muscles; comprises ~3% of the total myofibrillar protein. Composed of small repeats of ~35 amino acid residues arranged in a 7-fold super-repeating pattern. Integral component of the cytoskeletal lattice of muscle cells (*see also* Titin). Forms inextensible filaments that are attached to the Z-line and span the length of the thin filaments. Thought to act as a "molecular ruler" that stabilizes the actin polymer and regulates thin filament length. Name derived from its histological localization in the N_2-line of the sarcomere, a nebulous striation within the I-band. Identification: K. Wang, C. L. Williamson, *Proc. Natl. Acad. Sci. USA* **77**, 3254 (1980). Distribution and organization in cytoskeletal matrix of striated muscle: K. Wang, *Adv. Exp. Med. Biol.* **170**, 285-305 (1984). Physiological role: M.-J. G. Chen *et al., J. Biol. Chem.* **268**, 20327 (1993). Quantitative determn by gel electrophoresis: H. L. M. Granzier, K. Wang, *Electrophoresis* **14**, 56 (1993). Structural study: M. Pfuhl *et al., EMBO J.* **13**, 1782 (1994). Complete primary structure: S. Labeit, B. Kolmerer, *J. Mol. Biol.* **248**, 308 (1995). *Review:* J. Trinick, *Trends Biochem. Sci.* **19**, 405-409 (1994).

6435. Neburon. [555-37-3] *N*-Butyl-*N'*-(3,4-dichlorophenyl)-*N*-methylurea; 3-(3,4-dichlorophenyl)-1-methyl-1-*n*-butylurea; Kloben Neburon. $C_{12}H_{16}Cl_2N_2O$; mol wt 275.17. C 52.38%, H 5.86%, Cl 25.77%, N 10.18%, O 5.81%. Selective pre-emergence herbicide. Prepn: Todd, US 2655444; US 2655445; US 2655446; US 2655447 (all 1953 to du Pont). Toxicity study: G. W. Bailey, J. L. White, *Residue Rev.* **10**, 97 (1965).

Crystals from dioxane + water, mp 101.5-103°. Soly in water at 24°: 48 ppm; sparingly sol in hydrocarbon solvents. Stable toward oxidation and water at ordinary temperatures. LD_{50} orally in rats: >11000 mg/kg (Bailey, White).

USE: Herbicide.

6436. Nedocromil. [69049-73-6] 9-Ethyl-6,9-dihydro-4,6-dioxo-10-propyl-4*H*-pyrano[3,2-*g*]quinoline-2,8-dicarboxylic acid; 4,6-dioxo-1-ethyl-10-propyl-4*H*,6*H*-pyrano[3,2-*g*]quinoline-2,8-dicarboxylic acid; FPL-59002. $C_{19}H_{17}NO_7$; mol wt 371.34. C 61.45%, H 4.61%, N 3.77%, O 30.16%. Mast cell stabilizer; also modulates production of cytokines by stimulated epithelial cells. Prepn and pharmacology: H. Cairns, D. Cox, BE 866622; *eidem,* US 4474787 (1978, 1984 both to Fisons); H. Cairns *et al., J. Med. Chem.* **28**, 1832 (1985). Series of articles on pharmacology, pharmacokinetics and clinical profile in allergic rhinitis: *Allergy* **51**, Suppl. 8-34 (1996). Comparative clinical trial with cromolyn sodium, *q.v.,* in asthma: H. J. Schwartz *et al., Chest* **109**, 945 (1996).

Consult the Name Index before using this section.

Yellow powder, mp 298-300° (dec).

Disodium salt. [69049-74-7] FPL-59002KP; Halamid; Irtan; Rapitil; Tilade; Tilarin; Tilavist. $C_{19}H_{15}NNa_2O_7$; mol wt 415.30. Pale yellow powder. Sol in water.

THERAP CAT: Antiallergic; antiasthmatic.

6437. Neem. Nim; Margosa tree; Indian lilac. Tropical evergreen tree, *Azadirachta indica*, A. Juss. (*Melia azadirachta* L.) *Meliaceae*. *Habit*. India, Southeast Asia, also in Indonesia, Australia, Western Africa. Key active constituent is the limonoid, azadirachtin, *q.v.* Medicinal portions are the bark, leaves, fruits, and seeds; traditionally used as anti-inflammatory, antipyretic, and anthelmintic. Series of articles on chemistry and activity of neem extracts: *Natural Pesticides from the Neem Tree*, Proc. 1st Int. Neem Conf., 1980, H. Schmutterer *et al.*, Eds. (German Agency for Technical Cooperation, Eschborn, 1981) 291 pp. Antifeedant activity of extracts against pea aphid: J. D. Stark, J. F. Walter, *J. Agric. Food Chem.* **43**, 507 (1995). Use in traditional medicinal remedies: R. N. Chopra *et al.*, *Indigenous Drugs of India* (U. N. Dhur & Sons, Calcutta, 2nd ed., 1958) pp 360-363. Cytogenetic toxicity of leaf extract: P. K. Khan, K. S. Awasthy, *Food Chem. Toxicol.* **41**, 1325 (2003). Review of biological activity of isolated compounds, medicinal use and safety: K. Biswas *et al.*, *Curr. Sci.* **82**, 1336-1345 (2002); of component and pesticide toxicity in humans and animals: S. J. Boeke *et al.*, *J. Ethnopharmacol.* **94**, 25-41 (2004); of pharmacology and use in pest management: G. Brahmachari, *Chembiochem.* **5**, 408-421 (2004); of medicinal and pharmacological activities of leaf extracts: R. Subapriya, S. Nagini, *Curr. Med. Chem. Anticancer Agents* **5**, 149-156 (2005).

Fixed oil. [8002-65-1] Oil of neem. Obtained by extraction from seeds. *Constit.* Limonoids including azadirachtin, nimbin, nimbiol, salannin; fatty acids including oleic, stearic, palmitic. Properties and constituents: J. Kumar, B. S. Parmar, *J. Agric. Food Chem.* **44**, 2137 (1996). Determn by HPLC of azadirachtin variation among seeds: O. P. Sidhu *et al.*, *J. Agric. Food Chem.* **51**, 910 (2003); by LC-MS of oils: S. Barrek, P. Paisse, *Anal. Bioanal. Chem.* **378**, 753 (2004). Toxicology of debitterized oil: N. Chinnasamy *et al.*, *Food Chem. Toxicol.* **31**, 297 (1993). Yellow oil with bitter taste and odor of garlic. d_4^{25} 0.83-0.98. n_D^{27} 1.4575-1.4675. Sol in ether, chloroform. Practically insol in alcohol, water

USE: Insect repellent, antifeedant.

6438. Nefazodone. [83366-66-9] 2-[3-[4-(3-Chlorophenyl)-1-piperazinyl]propyl]-5-ethyl-2,4-dihydro-4-(2-phenoxyethyl)-3H-1,2,4-triazol-3-one; 2-[3-[4-(3-chlorophenyl)-1-piperazinyl]-propyl]-5-ethyl-4-(2-phenoxyethyl)-2H-1,2,4-triazol-3(4H)-one. $C_{25}H_{32}ClN_5O_2$; mol wt 470.01. C 63.89%, H 6.86%, Cl 7.54%, N 14.90%, O 6.81%. Selective serotonin 5-HT$_2$ receptor antagonist. Prepn: D. L. Temple, Jr., W. G. Lobeck, Jr., US 4338317 (1982 to Mead Johnson). Synthesis and x-ray crystal structure: G. D. Madding *et al*, *J. Heterocycl. Chem.* **22**, 1121 (1985). Pharmacology: A. S. Eison *et al.*, *Psychopharmacol. Bull.* **26**, 311 (1990). HPLC determn in plasma: J. E. Franc *et al.*, *J. Chromatogr.* **570**, 129 (1991). Clinical trial in depression: M. F. D'Amico *et al.*, *Psychopharmacol. Bull.* **26**, 147 (1990); in combination with psychotherapy for chronic depression: M. B. Keller *et al.*, *N. Engl. J. Med.* **342**, 1462 (2000). *Review:* W. E. Heydorn, *Expert Opin. Invest. Drugs* **4**, 131-137 (1995).

Crystals from 2-propanol/heptane, mp 83-84°.

Hydrochloride. [82752-99-6] BMY-13754; MJ-13754-1; Dutonin; Serzone. $C_{25}H_{32}ClN_5O_2 \cdot HCl$; mol wt 506.47. Crystals from 2-propanol, with slow cooling yields a polymorph, mp 186.0-187.0°; with rapid cooling yields a polymorph, mp 181.0-182.0° (Madding). Also reported as crystals from ethanol, mp 175-177° (Temple).

THERAP CAT: Antidepressant.

6439. Nefiracetam. [77191-36-7] N-(2,6-Dimethylphenyl)-2-oxo-1-pyrrolidineacetamide; 2-(2-oxo-1-pyrrolidinyl)-N-(2,6-dimethylphenyl)acetamide; 2-oxo-1-pyrrolidineaceto-2',6'-xylidide; 2-oxo-1-pyrrolidinylacetic acid 2,6-dimethylanilide; DMMPA; DM-9384; DZL-221; Translon. $C_{14}H_{18}N_2O_2$; mol wt 246.30. C 68.27%, H 7.37%, N 11.37%, O 12.99%. Cyclic deriv of γ-aminobutyric acid. Prepn: H. Betzing *et al.*, DE 2924011; *eidem*, US 4341790 (1980, 1982 both to Nattermann). Cognition enhancing effects in rats: T. Sakurai *et al.*, *Jpn. J. Pharmacol.* **50**, 47 (1989). HPLC determn in serum and urine: Y. Fujimaki *et al.*, *J. Chromatogr.* **575**, 261 (1992). Clinical pharmacokinetics: *eidem, Xenobiotica* **23**, 61 (1993). Series of articles on pharmacology and toxicology: *Arzneim.-Forsch.* **44**, 193-259 (1994).

Crystals from water, mp 153°. LD_{50} in mice (mg/kg): 421 i.v.; 1766 orally (Betzing, 1982).

THERAP CAT: Nootropic.

6440. Nefopam. [13669-70-0] 3,4,5,6-Tetrahydro-5-methyl-1-phenyl-1H-2,5-benzoxazocine; 5-methyl-1,3,4,6-tetrahydro-5H-benz[f]-2,5-oxazocine. $C_{17}H_{19}NO$; mol wt 253.34. C 80.60%, H 7.56%, N 5.53%, O 6.32%. A cyclized analog of orphenadrine and diphenhydramine, *q.q.v.*; representative of a new class of centrally acting skeletal muscle relaxants, the benzoxazocines. Prepn: NL 6606390 (1966 to Rexall); M. W. Klohs *et al.*, US 3830803 (1974 to Riker). Pharmacology: Bassett *et al.*, *Br. J. Pharmacol.* **37**, 69 (1969); Klohs *et al.*, *Arzneim.-Forsch.* **22**, 132 (1972). Review of pharmacology and therapeutic efficacy: R. C. Heel *et al.*, *Drugs* **19**, 249-267 (1980).

Hydrochloride. [23327-57-3] Fenazoxine; R-738; Acupan; Ajan. $C_{17}H_{19}NO \cdot HCl$; mol wt 289.80. mp 238-242°. LD_{50} in mice, rats (mg/kg): 119, 178 orally; 44.5, 28 i.v. (Baltes).

THERAP CAT: Analgesic; antidepressant.

6441. Negamycin. [33404-78-3] 3,6-Diamino-2,3,4,6-tetradeoxy-L-*threo*-hexonic acid 2-(carboxymethyl)-2-methylhydrazide; 3,6-diamino-5-hydroxyhexanoic acid 2-(carboxymethyl)-2-methyl-hydrazide; [2-(3,6-diamino-5-hydroxy-1-oxohexyl)-2-methylhydrazino]acetic acid. $C_9H_{20}N_4O_4$; mol wt 248.28. C 43.54%, H 8.12%, N 22.57%, O 25.78%. Hydrazide antibiotic isolated from strains related to *Streptomyces purpeofuscus*: Hamada *et al.*, *J. Antibiot.* **23**, 170 (1970). Prepn: H. Umezawa *et al.*, ZA 7002933; *eidem*, US 3679742 (1970, 1972 both to Microbiochem. Res. Found.). Structure and partial synthesis: Kondo *et al.*, *J. Am. Chem. Soc.* **93**, 6305 (1971). Total synthesis of negamycin and its antipode: Shibahara *et al.*, *ibid.* **94**, 4353 (1972). Synthesis of racemic negamycin: W. Streicher *et al.*, *J. Antibiot.* **31**, 725 (1978); G. Pasquet *et al.*, *Tetrahedron Lett.* **21**, 931 (1980); A. Pierdet *et al.*, *Tetrahedron* **36**, 1763 (1980). Stereocontrolled synthesis of (+)-negamycin: Y. F. Wang *et al.*, *J. Am. Chem. Soc.* **104**, 6465 (1982);

S. DeBernardo *et al., Tetrahedron Lett.* **29**, 4077 (1988). Mechanism of action: Mizuno *et al., J. Antibiot.* **23**, 581 (1970); Y. Uehara *et al., Biochim. Biophys. Acta* **442**, 251 (1976).

Colorless powder, mp 110-120° (dec). $[\alpha]_D^{29}$ +2.5° (c = 2). Amphoteric compound. pKa values after treatment with HCl-methanol: 3.55, 8.10, 9.75. Sol in water. Practically insol in methanol, ethanol, butanol, ethyl acetate, chloroform and benzene. LD_{50} i.v. in mice: 400-500 mg/kg (Hameda).

THERAP CAT: Antibacterial.

6442. Nelarabine. [121032-29-9] 9-β-D-Arabinofuranosyl-6-methoxy-9H-purin-2-amine; 2-amino-9-β-D-arabinofuranosyl-6-methoxy-9H-purine; GW-506U78; 506U; Arranon. $C_{11}H_{15}N_5O_5$; mol wt 297.27. C 44.44%, H 5.09%, N 23.56%, O 26.91%. Purine nucleoside; prodrug of guanine arabinoside. Prepn: T. A. Krenitsky *et al.*, **EP 294114** (1988 to Wellcome Foundation); *idem*, D. J. T. Porter, **US 5424295** (1995 to Burroughs Wellcome); D. R. Averett *et al., Antimicrob. Agents Chemother.* **35**, 851 (1991). HPLC determn of active metabolites in leukemia cells: C. O. Rodriguez Jr. *et al., J. Chromatogr. B* **745**, 421 (2000). Mechanism of action study: *idem, et al., Blood* **102**, 1842 (2003). Clinical pharmacokinetics: D. F. Kisor *et al., J. Clin. Oncol.* **18**, 995 (2000). Clinical evaluation in T-cell malignancies: S. L. Berg *et al., ibid.* **23**, 3376 (2005). Review of pharmacology and clinical experience: D. F. Kisor, *Ann. Pharmacother.* **39**, 1056-1063 (2005).

mp 209-217° (dec). uv max (50 mM potassium phosphate buffer (pH 7.0)-ethanol (9:1, v/v)): 247.5, 279 nm (ε 9100, 9300). $[\alpha]_D^{20}$ +55.9° (c = 0.27 in DMF). Slightly sol to sol in water.

THERAP CAT: Antineoplastic.

6443. Nelfinavir. [159989-64-7] (3S,4aS,8aS)-N-(1,1-Dimethylethyl)decahydro-2-[(2R,3R)-2-hydroxy-3-[(3-hydroxy-2-methylbenzoyl)amino]-4-(phenylthio)butyl]-3-isoquinolinecarboxamide; [3S-(3R*,4aR*,8aR*,2′S*,3′S*)]-2-[2′-hydroxy-3′-phenylthiomethyl-4′-aza-5′-oxo-5′-(2″-methyl-3″-hydroxyphenyl)pentyl]decahydroisoquinoline-3-N-t-butylcarboxamide; AG-1346. $C_{32}H_{45}N_3O_4S$; mol wt 567.78. C 67.69%, H 7.99%, N 7.40%, O 11.27%, S 5.65%. HIV protease inhibitor. Prepn: B. A. Dressman *et al.*, **WO 9509843**; *eidem*, **US 5484926** (1995, 1996 both to Agouron). Physical properties: M. Longer *et al., J. Pharm. Sci.* **84**, 1090 (1995). HIV protease inhibition and antiviral activity: A. K. Patick *et al., Antimicrob. Agents Chemother.* **40**, 292 (1996). Preclinical pharmacokinetics and tissue distribution: B. V. Shetty *et al., ibid.* **110**. Review of pharmacology and clinical efficacy in HIV infection: A. Bardsley-Elliot, G. L. Plosker *et al., Drugs* **59**, 581-620 (2000).

White foam. $[\alpha]_D$ −119.23° (c = 0.26 in methanol). pKa_1 6.0; pKa_2 11.06. Log P (octanol/water): 4.1. Practically insol in water.

Methanesulfonate. [159989-65-8] Nelfinavir mesylate; AG-1343; Viracept. $C_{32}H_{45}N_3O_4S \cdot CH_3SO_3H$; mol wt 663.89. White powder. pKa −1.20. Soly (mg/ml): 4.5 in water; 2.6 in 0.1N HCl. Soly (mg/g): 70 in glycerin; >100 in propylene glycol; >200 in PEG 400. Very sol in methanol, ethanol, acetonitrile. Practically insol in soybean oil, mineral oil.

THERAP CAT: Antiviral.

6444. Nemadectin. [102130-84-7] [6R,23S,25S(E)]-5-O-Demethyl-28-deoxy-25-(1,3-dimethyl-1-butenyl)-6,28-epoxy-23-hydroxymilbemycin B; antibiotic S-541A; LL-F-28249α; F-28249α; CL-287088. $C_{36}H_{52}O_8$; mol wt 612.79. C 70.56%, H 8.55%, O 20.89%. Macrocyclic antibiotic produced by *Streptomyces cyaneogriseus* ssp. *noncyanogenus* and *Streptomyces thermoachaensis*. Structurally related to the milbemycins and the avermectins, *q.q.v.* Isoln: I. B. Wood *et al.*, **EP 170006**; I. B. Wood, J. A. Pankavich, **US 4869901** (1986, 1989 both to Am. Cyanamid). Chemical and structural characterization: G. T. Carter *et al., Chem. Commun.* **1987**, 402; G. T. Carter *et al., J. Antibiot.* **41**, 519 (1988). NMR spectroscopy: S. Rajan, G. W. Stockton, *Magn. Reson. Chem.* **27**, 437 (1989). Antiparasitic activity in horses: E. T. Lyons *et al., Am. J. Vet. Res.* **50**, 970 (1989); in dogs: M. E. Doscher *et al., Vet. Parasitol.* **34**, 255 (1989); in sheep: J. A. Pankavich *et al, Vet. Rec.* **130**, 241, (1992).

White fluffy solid from *tert*-butanol. $[\alpha]_D^{26}$ +133° (c = 0.3 in acetone). uv max (methanol): 244 nm, (log ε 4.47). Readily sol in common organic solvents. Practically insol in water.

THERAP CAT (VET): Antiparasitic.

6445. Nemifitide. [173240-15-8] 4-Fluoro-L-phenylalanyl-(4R)-4-hydroxy-L-prolyl-L-arginylglycyl-L-tryptophanamide; 4-F-Phe-4-OH-Pro-Arg-Gly-Trp-NH₂; netamifide. $C_{33}H_{43}FN_{10}O_6$; mol wt 694.76. C 57.05%, H 6.24%, F 2.73%, N 20.16%, O 13.82%. Synthetic pentapeptide produced by modification of melanocyte stimulating inhibitory factor. Prepn: H. B. Abajian, *et al.*, **WO 9530430**; *eidem*, **US 5589460** (1995, 1996 both to Innapharma). Structure activity study: J. J. Hlavka, *J. Appl. Res.* **2**, 58 (2002). Clinical pharmacokinetics: J. P. Feighner *et al., Biopharm. Drug Dispos.* **23**, 33 (2002); G. Nicolau *et al., ibid.* **26**, 379 (2005). Clinical evaluation: *eidem, Int. J. Neuropsychopharm.* **6**, 207 (2003). Review of development and therapeutic potential: J. Dingemanse, *Curr. Opin. Invest. Drugs* **4**, 859-862 (2003).

Bis(trifluoroacetate). [204992-09-6] Nemifitide ditriflutate; INN-00835. $C_{33}H_{43}FN_{10}O_6 \cdot 2C_2HF_3O_2$; mol wt 922.80.

THERAP CAT: Antidepressant.

6446. Nemonapride. [75272-39-8] *rel*-5-Chloro-2-methoxy-4-(methylamino)-*N*-[(2*R*,3*R*)-2-methyl-2-(phenylmethyl)-3-pyrrolidinyl]benzamide; (±)-*cis*-*N*-(1-benzyl-2-methyl-3-pyrrolidinyl)-5-chloro-4-(methylamino)-*o*-anisamide; *cis*-*N*-(1-benzyl-2-methylpyrrolidin-3-yl)-5-chloro-2-methoxy-4-(methylamino)-benzamide; emonapride; YM-09151-2; Emilace. $C_{21}H_{26}ClN_3O_2$; mol wt 387.90. C 65.02%, H 6.76%, Cl 9.14%, N 10.83%, O 8.25%. Selective dopamine D_2 receptor antagonist. Prepn: M. Takashima *et al.*, **JP Kokai 79 14965**; *eidem*, **US 4210660** (1979, 1980 both to Yamanouchi); S. Iwanami *et al.*, *J. Med. Chem.* **24**, 1224 (1981). Pharmacology: M. Yamamoto *et al.*, *Neuropharmacology* **21**, 945 (1982). Dopamine receptor binding study: C. W. Grewe *et al.*, *Eur. J. Pharmacol.* **81**, 149 (1982). Use as a label for D_2 receptors: A. S. Unis *et al.*, *Life Sci.* **47**, PL151 (1990). HPLC determn in plasma: T. Nagasaki *et al.*, *J. Chromatogr. B* **714**, 293 (1998). Clinical evaluation in schizophrenia: K. Satoh *et al.*, *Int. Clin. Psychopharmacol.* **11**, 279 (1996).

Colorless crystals from isopropanol, mp 152-153° (Takashima, 1980). Also reported as mp 150° (Iwanami).

THERAP CAT: Antipsychotic.

6447. Neoarsphenamine. [457-60-3] Sulfoxylic acid mono[[[5-[(3-amino-4-hydroxyphenyl)diarsenyl]-2-hydroxyphenyl]amino]methyl] ester monosodium salt; [5-[(3-amino-4-hydroxyphenyl)arseno]-2-hydroxyanilino]methanol sulfoxylate sodium; arsphenamine methylenesulfoxylic acid sodium salt; 3,3′-diamino-4,4′-dihydroxyarsenobenzenemethylenesulfoxylate sodium; Neosalvarsan; Collunovar; N.A.B.; Neo-Arsoluin; Vetarsenobillon; Novarsenobillon; Arsevan; Novarsan; Novarsenobenzol; Miarsenol. $C_{13}H_{13}As_2N_2NaO_4S$; mol wt 466.15. C 33.50%, H 2.81%, As 32.14%, N 6.01%, Na 4.93%, O 13.73%, S 6.88%. Medicinal grade contains a small amount of inert inorganic salts and some solvent. *The National Formulary* requires 19+% As. Prepn from arsphenamine + sodium formaldehydesulfoxylate: Krumwiede, *J. Am. Pharm. Assoc.* **8**, 795 (1919); Heyl, Miller, *ibid.* **11**, 432 (1922); Dohr, **US 1549465** (1925); Kober, **US 1564859** (1926); Kraft *et al.*, **SU 158388** (1962). Physicochemical properties and toxicity: H. N. Wright *et al.*, *J. Pharmacol. Exp. Ther.* **73**, 12 (1941).

Yellow powder; odorless or slight odor. Oxidizes in air, becoming darker and more toxic; higher temps accelerate the oxidation; hence marketed in air-evacuated ampuls or filled with a nonoxidizing gas. Very sol in water; sol in glycerol. Slightly sol in alcohol or acetone. Practically insol in chloroform, ether. Its aq soln is practically neutral, unlike arsphenamine, which is acid.

THERAP CAT (VET): Has been used in contagious pleuropneumonia, babesiasis, equine petechial fever, eperythrozoonosis.

6448. Neocembrene. [31570-39-5] (1*E*,5*E*,9*E*,12*R*)-1,5,9-Trimethyl-12-(1-methylethenyl)-1,5,9-cyclotetradecatriene; cembrene A; neocembrene A. $C_{20}H_{32}$; mol wt 272.47. C 88.16%, H 11.84%. Termite trail pheromone with all-*trans* configuration isolated from *Nasutitermes exitiosus* (Hill): B. P. Moore, *Nature* **211**, 746 (1966). Structure: A. J. Birch *et al.*, *J. Chem. Soc. Perkin Trans. 1* **1972**, 2653; V. D. Patil *et al.*, *Tetrahedron* **29**, 341 (1973). Synthesis: M. Kodama *et al.*, *Tetrahedron Lett.* **1975**, 3065; Y. Kitahara *et al.*, *Chem. Lett.* **1976**, 219; H. Takayanagi *et al.*, *Chem. Commun.* **1978**, 359. Synthesis of neocembrene and isomers: T. Kato *et al.*, *J. Org. Chem.* **45**, 1126 (1980).

Colorless oil, faint wax-like odor. $bp_{0.8}$ 150-152°. n_D^{30} 1.5102.

6449. Neocuproine. [484-11-7] 2,9-Dimethyl-1,10-phenanthroline; 2,9-dimethyl-*o*-phenanthroline. $C_{14}H_{12}N_2$; mol wt 208.26. C 80.74%, H 5.81%, N 13.45%. Prepn: Case, *J. Am. Chem. Soc.* **70**, 3994 (1948); O'Reilly, Plowman, *Aust. J. Chem.* **13**, 145 (1960).

Hemihydrate. $C_{14}H_{12}N_2 \cdot \frac{1}{2}H_2O$. Crystals from water or ligroin, mp 159-160°.

Dihydrate. Needles from water. Loses water over P_2O_5 or at 80°.

USE: Clinical reagent (blood glucose assay). In spectrophotometric determination of copper, Nebesar, *Anal. Chem.* **36**, 1961 (1964).

6450. Neodymium. [7440-00-8] Nd; at. wt 144.242; at. no. 60; valences 2, 3, 4. A lanthanide; belongs to the cerium group of rare earth metals. Naturally occurring isotopes (mass numbers): 142 (27.13%); 143 (12.18%); 144 (23.80%), radioactive, $T_{1/2}$ 2.1 × 10^{15} years, α-emitter; 145 (8.30%); 146 (17.19%); 148 (5.76%); 150 (5.64%). Known artificial radioactive isotopes: 127-141; 147; 149; 151; 152. Abundance in earth's crust: 24-40 ppm. Commercially important sources are the rare earth minerals monazite and bastnaesite; also found in cerite and gadolinite. Discovered by von Welsbach in 1885. Sepn from Pr: F. H. Spedding *et al.*, *J. Am. Chem. Soc.* **69**, 2786 (1947); **76**, 2557 (1954); Kauffman, Blank, *J. Chem. Educ.* **37**, 156 (1960); from other rare earths: Spedding *et al.*, *J. Am. Chem. Soc.* **69**, 2812 (1947). Metal prepd by electrolysis of the chloride: Matignon, *Compt. Rend.* **131**, 891 (1900); Sieverts, Roell, *Z. Anorg. Chem.* **150**, 261 (1926); by reduction of the chloride: Bommer, Hohmann, *ibid.* **248**, 357 (1941). Spectrum: Alberston *et al.*, *Phys. Rev.* **61**, 167 (1942). Reviews of prepn, properties and compds: *The Rare Earths*, F. H. Spedding, A. H. Daane, Eds. (Krieger, Huntington, N.Y., 1971, reprint of 1961 ed.) 641 pp; Hulet, Bode, "Separation Chemistry of the Lanthanides and Transplutonium Actinides" in *MTP Int. Rev. Sci.: Inorg. Chem., Ser. One* vol. **7**, K. W. Bagnall, Ed. (University Park Press, Baltimore, 1972) pp 1-45; Moeller, "The Lanthanides" in *Comprehensive Inorganic Chemistry* vol. **4**, J. C. Bailar Jr. *et al.*, Eds. (Pergamon Press, Oxford, 1973) pp 1-101; F. H. Spedding in *Kirk-Othmer Encyclopedia of Chemical Technology* vol. **19** (John Wiley & Sons, New York, 3rd ed., 1982) pp 833-854; *Chemistry of the Elements*, N. N. Greenwood, A. Earnshaw, Eds. (Pergamon Press, New York, 1984) pp 1423-1449. Review of toxicity: T. J. Haley, *J. Pharm. Sci.* **54**, 663-670 (1965). Brief review of properties: G. T. Seaborg, *Radiochim. Acta* **61**, 115-122 (1993).

Silver-white metal, becomes yellowish on exposure to air. Crystalline forms: hexagonal α-form, d 7.003, transforms to β-form at 868°; body-centered cubic β-form, d 6.80, exists at >868°. mp 1021°. bp 3074°. Heat of fusion: 7.134 kJ/mol. Heat of sublimation (25°): 327.6 kJ/mol. E°(aq) Nd^{3+}/Nd −2.44 V (calc). Experimental reduction potentials (referred to a normal calomel electrode): −1.870, −1.960 V: Noddack, Brukl, *Angew. Chem.* **50**, 362 (1937). Reacts slowly with cold water; rapidly on heating.

Oxide. Nd_2O_3. Commercial uses: Pings, *Colo. Sch. Mines, Miner. Ind. Bull.* **12**, no. 2 (1969) 19 pp. Blue powder, hexagonal structure, exhibits a slightly red fluorescence. Prepd by heating the hydroxide, carbonate, nitrate or oxalate. Very stable. Sol in dil acids; soly in water: 5.7×10^{-6} g-mol/l at 29°.

Hydroxide. $Nd(OH)_3$. Bluish or pink precipitate; on heating at 300-350° is converted into $2Nd_2O_3.3H_2O$, grayish-brown; on further increase in temp is converted into $Nd_2O_3.H_2O$.

Chloride. $NdCl_3$. Large purple prisms. Sol in water, in alcohol. Forms addition compds with ammonia. A hexahydrate is obtained from the aq soln; the hydrate is very sol in water (2.46 parts per 1 part of water); mp 124°. LD_{50} in mice (mg/kg): 4000 s.c., 348.3 i.p.; in male mice (mg/kg): 600 i.p., 5250 orally; in rats (mg/kg): 150-250 i.p.; in guinea pigs (mg/kg): 70 i.v., 139.6 i.p.; in rabbits (mg/kg): 200-250 i.v. (Haley).

Sulfate. $Nd_2(SO_4)_3$. Pinkish needles; prepd by heating the oxide with concd sulfuric acid. Heat of formation 57.2 kcal. Sol in water; heat of soln 36.5 kcal. Is dec at 700-800°. Forms several double salts. A penta-, an octa-, and a pentadecahydrate have been prepared.

Nitrate. $Nd(NO_3)_3$. Penta- and hexahydrates; prepd by adding the oxide to nitric acid. LD_{50} (hexahydrate) in female mice (mg/kg): 270 i.p.; in female rats (mg/kg): 270 i.p., 2750 orally, 6.4 i.v.; in male rats (mg/kg): 66.8 i.v. (Haley).

USE: Oxide as glass coloring agent; in glass filter plate laminated on color TV tubes to improve contrast and brightness; in lasers. Alloyed with iron and boron to produce powerful permanent magnets.

6451. Neoergosterol. [516-98-3] $(3\beta,22E)$-19-Norergosta-5,7,9,22-tetraen-3-ol. $C_{27}H_{40}O$; mol wt 380.61. C 85.20%, H 10.59%, O 4.20%. Prepd from ergosterol: Inhoffen, *Ann.* **497**, 130 (1932); Windaus, Deppe, *Ber.* **70**, 76 (1937); Mosettig, Scheer, *J. Org. Chem.* **17**, 764 (1952). Stereochemistry: Steele *et al., J. Am. Chem. Soc.* **85**, 1134 (1963).

Needles from methanol, mp 152-154°. $[\alpha]_D^{17} -11°$ (c = 2 in chloroform). Practically insol in water. Sol in organic solvents. Precipitated by digitonin.

Methyl ether. $C_{28}H_{42}O$. mp 94°. $[\alpha]_D^{20} -5°$ (c = 1.2 in chloroform).

6452. Neohesperidin Dihydrochalcone. [20702-77-6] 1-[4-[[2-*O*-(6-Deoxy-α-L-mannopyranosyl)-β-D-glucopyranosyl]oxy]-2,6-dihydroxyphenyl]-3-(3-hydroxy-4-methoxyphenyl)-1-propanone; 3,5-dihydroxy-4-(3-hydroxy-4-methoxyhydrocinnamoyl)phenyl-2-*O*-(6-deoxy-α-L-mannopyranosyl)-β-D-glucopyranoside; neohesperidin DHC; NHDC; Sukor. $C_{28}H_{36}O_{15}$; mol wt 612.58. C 54.90%, H 5.92%, O 39.18%. Prepn from naringen, a flavanone glycoside occurring naturally in grapefruit: Horowitz, Gentile, **US 3087821** and **US 3375242** (1963, 1968, both to U.S. Secy. Agr.); Robertson *et al., Ind. Eng. Chem. Prod. Res. Dev.* **13**, 125 (1974). Sweetening effect: Inglett *et al., J. Food Sci.* **34**, 101 (1969). Chromatography: Gentile, Horowitz, *J. Chromatogr.* **63**, 467 (1971); J. F. Fisher, *J. Agric. Food Chem.* **25**, 682 (1977). Subchronic oral toxicity study: B. A. R. Lina *et al., Food Chem. Toxicol.* **28**, 507 (1990). *Review:* P. J. Pratter, *Perfum. Flavor.* **5**, 12-18 (1981).

Crystals from acetone, mp 156-158°. 1000 to 1500 times sweeter than sucrose; 20 times sweeter than saccharin.

USE: Sweetening agent, especially in chewing gum and dentifrices.

6453. Neomethymycin. [497-73-4] (12*R*)-10-Deoxy-12-hydroxymethymycin. $C_{25}H_{43}NO_7$; mol wt 469.61. C 63.94%, H 9.23%, N 2.98%, O 23.85%. Macrolide antibiotic found in the mother liquors from methymycin, *q.v.* Differs from methymycin only in the location of one hydroxyl group, which results in marked changes in chemical behavior: Djerassi, Halpern, *J. Am. Chem. Soc.* **79**, 2022, 3926 (1957); *Tetrahedron* **3**, 255 (1958). Production from *Streptomyces venezuelae* cultures: Dutcher *et al.*, **US 2916486** (1959 to Olin Mathieson). Synthesis of the aglycone, *neomethynolide*: J. Inanago *et al., Chem. Lett.* **1981**, 1415.

Crystals from ether + hexane, mp 156-158°. $[\alpha]_D^{25} +93°$. uv max (ethanol): 227.5 nm (log ε 4.10). Solvates easily and when crystallized from dilute acetone yields 1 cm long crystals of the acetone solvate. Soluble in alcohol, acetone, chloroform, benzene, ethyl acetate, ether. Slightly sol in water, dibutyl ether. Practically insol in hexane, aliphatic hydrocarbons. *Compare also* Picromycin.

6454. Neomycin. [1404-04-2] Mycifradin; Fradiomycin; Neomin; Neolate; Neomas; Pimavecort; Vonamycin Powder V. Antibiotic complex composed of neomycins A, B and C. Produced by *Streptomyces fradiae:* Waksman, Lechevalier, *Science* **109**, 305 (1949); Waksman *et al., J. Clin. Invest.* **28**, 934 (1949); Swart *et al., ibid.* 1045; Waksman, Lechevalier, **US 2799620** (1957). Purification: Jackson, **US 2848365** (1958 to Upjohn); Haak, **US 3108996** (1963 to Upjohn). Recovery: Miller, **US 3005815** (1961 to Merck & Co.); Moses, **US 3022228** (1962 to Penick); **GB 945475** (1964 to O.W.G. Chemie). Characterization: Peck *et al., J. Am. Chem. Soc.* **71**, 2590 (1949); Regna, Murphy, *ibid.* **72**, 1045 (1950); Dutcher *et al., ibid.* **73**, 1384 (1951). Structure of neomycins B and C: K. L. Rinehart *et al., ibid.* **79**, 4567, 4568 (1957); *ibid.* **84**, 3216, 3218 (1962). Abs config of neomycin C: M. Hichens, K. L. Rinehart, *ibid.* **85**, 1547 (1963). Total synthesis of neomycin C: S. Umewaza, Y. Nishimura, *J. Antibiot.* **30**, 189 (1977); S. Umewaza *et al., Bull. Chem. Soc. Jpn.* **53**, 3259 (1980); of neomycin B: T. Usui, S. Umezawa, *J. Antibiot.* **40**, 1464 (1987). Monographs: S. A. Waksman, *Neomycin* (Rutgers Univ. Press, New Brunswick, N. J., 1953) 219 pp; K. L. Rinehart, Jr., *The Neomycins and Related Antibiotics* (Wiley, New York, 1964) 137 pp. Comprehensive description: W. F. Heyes, *Anal. Profiles Drug Subs.* **8**, 399-488 (1979).

Neomycin complex is an amorphous base sol in water, methanol and acidified alcohol. Practically insol in common organic solvents. Solns up to 250 mg/ml H_2O may be prepared.

Neomycin A *see* Neamine.

Neomycin B. [119-04-0] Antibiotique EF 185; framycetin; Enterfram; Framygen; Actilin. $C_{23}H_{46}N_6O_{13}$; mol wt 614.64. Identity of neomycin B and framycetin: K. L. Rinehart *et al., ibid.* **82,** 3938 (1960). Yields on hydrolysis neamine and *neobiosamine B*. Structure of neobiosamine B: K. L. Rinehart *et al., J. Am. Chem. Soc.* **82,** 2970 (1960).

Neomycin B hydrochloride. [25389-99-5] Amorphous white powder. $[\alpha]_D^{20}$ +57° (H_2O). Soly in mg/ml at ~28°: water 15.0; methanol 5.7; ethanol 0.65; isopropanol 0.05; isoamyl alcohol 0.33; cyclohexane 0.06; benzene 0.03. Practically insol in acetone, ether, other organic solvents. For additional soly data *see* Weiss *et al., Antibiot. Chemother.* **7,** 374 (1957).

Neomycin B sulfate. [1405-10-3] Biosol; Bykomycin; Endomixin; Fraquinol; Myacine; Neosulf; Neomix; Neobrettin; Nivemycin; Soframycin; Tuttomycin. Amorphous white powder. Practically tasteless. $[\alpha]_D^{20}$ +54° (c = 2 in H_2O). Soly in mg/ml at ~28°: water 6.3; methanol 0.225; ethanol 0.095; isopropanol 0.082; isoamyl alcohol, 0.247; cyclohexane 0.08; benzene 0.05. Practically insol in acetone, ether, chloroform. Aq solns are fairly stable at pH 2 to 9. Highly purified prepns are very stable to alkali and unstable to acids. Refluxing with barium hydroxide for 18 hrs showed no loss of activity. Boiling with mineral acids yields an aldehyde, characterized as furfural, and an organic base.

Neomycin C. [66-86-4] $C_{23}H_{46}N_6O_{13}$; mol wt 614.64. Yields on hydrolysis neamine and *neobiosamine C*. Structure of neobiosamine C: K. L. Rinehart, P. Woo, *J. Am. Chem. Soc.* **80,** 6463 (1958).

THERAP CAT: Antibacterial.

THERAP CAT (VET): Antibacterial.

6455. Neon. [7440-01-9] Ne; at. wt 20.1797; at. no. 10. Group VIIIA (18), also known as Group 0. A noble gas characterized by an electronic structure in which the outer *p* subshell is entirely filled. Naturally occurring stable isotopes (mass numbers): 20 (90.51%); 21 (0.27%); 22 (9.92%); known artificial radioactive isotopes: 16-19; 23-25. Longest-lived known isotope: 24 ($T_{1/2}$ 3.38 min, β-emitter). Abundance in igneous rock of the earth's crust: 7×10^{-5} ppm by wt; concentration in air: 18.2 ppm by vol. Obtained commercially from the atmosphere by distillation-liquefaction process. Discovered in 1898 by Travers and Ramsay: *The Discovery of the Rare Gases,* London, 1928. Monograph: *Argon, Helium and the Rare Gases* vols. **1, 2,** G. A. Cook, Ed. (Interscience, New York, 1961) 818 pp. *Reviews:* Cockett, Smith, "The Monatomic Gases" in *Comprehensive Inorganic Chemistry* vol. **1,** J. C. Bailar, Jr. *et al.,* Eds. (Pergamon Press, Oxford, 1973) pp 139-211; S.-C. Hwang, W. R. Weltmer, Jr. in *Kirk-Othmer Encyclopedia of Chemical Technology* vol. **13** (John Wiley & Sons, 4th ed., 1995) p 1-38; *Chemistry of the Elements,* N. N. Greenwood, A. Earnshaw, Eds. (Pergamon Press, New York, 1984) pp 1042-1059. Review of use in inductively coupled plasma-mass spectrometry: S. F. Durrant, *Fresenius J. Anal. Chem.* **347,** 389-392 (1993).

Colorless, odorless, tasteless, monatomic, inert gas; will form compds with highly electronegative elements such as O, F, Cl. Does not condense at the temp of liq air; solid at the temp of liq hydrogen; the solid form exists as face-centered cubic crystals at normal pressure. Soly of gas in water (20°): 10.5 cm^3/kg water. Triple pt temp 24.562 K, press 43.37 kPa. Critical temp 44.40 K, critical press 2654 kPa, critical d 483 kg/m^3. Gas: d^0 (101.3 kPa) 0.89994 kg/m^3, d (normal bp) 9.552 kg/m^3. Liquid: normal bp −246.048°, d (normal bp) 1207 kg/m^3, d (triple pt) 1247 kg/m^3, heat of vaporization (normal bp) 1.741 kJ/mol. Solid: d (triple pt) 1444 kg/m^3, heat of vaporization (triple pt) 2.139 kJ/mol, heat of fusion (triple pt) 0.335 kJ/mol. Emission spectra: T. Jacksier, R. M. Barnes, *Appl. Spectrosc.* **48,** 65 (1994).

Caution: Can act as a simple asphyxiant by displacing air. *See: Matheson Gas Data Book* (Matheson Co., Inc., 4th ed., East Rutherford, NJ, 1966) pp 359-361.

USE: Gas in neon light tubes; ingredient of gaseous fillers for antifog devices, warning signals, electrical current detectors, high-voltage indicators for high-tension electric lines, lightning arresters, wave-meter tubes; in Ne-He lasers; in mixtures with He and Ar in Geiger counters. Liquid as cryogen to produce low temps.

6456. Neopentane. [463-82-1] 2,2-Dimethylpropane; tetramethylmethane. C_5H_{12}; mol wt 72.15. C 83.23%, H 16.76%. Found in petr naphtha. Prepn from *tert*-butyl iodide and dimethyl-

zinc: Lwow, *Z. Chem.* **1870,** 520; *cf. J. Am. Chem. Soc.* **54,** 3460 (1932); from butylmagnesium iodide and dimethyl sulfate in ether: Ferrario, Fagetti, *Gaz. Chim.* **38, II,** 663 (1908); from amylene vapor and hydrogen in presence of an electric discharge: *ibid.* **62,** 621 (1932); by passing pentanes over aluminum chloride at 140°, *J. Gen. Chem. USSR* **14,** 343 (1944), *C.A.* **39,** 3783 (1945); from neopentylmagnesium chloride and water: Whitmore *et al., J. Am. Chem. Soc.* **56,** 749 (1934).

Liquid or gas. d_0^0 0.613 (liq). Solidifies to form tetragonal crystals, mp −19.8°. bp 9.5°. Insol in water.

6457. Neopentyl Alcohol. [75-84-3] 2,2-Dimethyl-1-propanol; *tert*-butyl carbinol; neoamyl alcohol; neopentanol. $C_5H_{12}O$; mol wt 88.15. C 68.13%, H 13.72%, O 18.15%. $(CH_3)_3CCH_2OH$. Prepn: Conant *et al., J. Am. Chem. Soc.* **51,** 1249 (1929). Review of manuf (by fractionation of fusel oil and via chlorination of pentanes) and properties: *Industrial Chemicals,* W. L. Faith *et al.,* Eds. (Wiley & Sons, New York, 2nd ed., 1957) pp 107-114.

Volatile crystals, peppermint odor. bp 114°. mp 53°. d_4^{20} 0.812. Vapor pressure: 16 mm at 20°; 50.5 mm at 46°; 533.5 mm at 100°. Slightly sol in water (~3.5% at 25°); miscible with alcohol, ether.

6458. Neopentyl Glycol. [126-30-7] 2,2-Dimethyl-1,3-propanediol; dimethyltrimethylene glycol. $C_5H_{12}O_2$; mol wt 104.15. C 57.66%, H 11.61%, O 30.72%. Prepd from isobutyraldehyde.

Needles from benzene, mp 127°. bp_{760} 208°. Solubility in water ~65% w/w. Freely sol in alcohol, ether.

USE: In the manuf of plasticizers, polyesters, as modifier of alkyd resins.

6459. Neophyl Chloride. [515-40-2] (2-Chloro-1,1-dimethylethyl)benzene; 1-chloro-2-methyl-2-phenylpropane; (β-chloro-*tert*-butyl)benzene. $C_{10}H_{13}Cl$; mol wt 168.66. C 71.21%, H 7.77%, Cl 21.02%. Prepn (68% yield) from benzene and methallyl chloride in the presence of concd sulfuric acid: Whitmore *et al., J. Am. Chem. Soc.* **65,** 1469 (1943); Smith, Sellas, *Org. Synth.* **coll. vol. IV,** 702 (1963).

Liquid. d_4^{25} 1.0379. bp_{741} 221° (dec); bp_{90} 111°; bp_{30} 120°; bp_{20} 105°; bp_{18} 104°; bp_{13} 97°; bp_{10} 95°; $bp_{1.0}$ 53°. n_D^{20} 1.5249; n_D^{25} 1.5228. Considerably less reactive with sodium than neopentyl chloride. Forms a Grignard reagent readily and in good yield. Salt effect in acetolysis: Fainberg, Winstein, *J. Am. Chem. Soc.* **78,** 2763 (1956).

6460. Neopine. [467-14-1] (5α,6α)-8,14-Didehydro-4,5-epoxy-3-methoxy-17-methylmorphinan-6-ol; β-codeine. $C_{18}H_{21}NO_3$; mol wt 299.36. C 72.22%, H 7.07%, N 4.68%, O 16.03%. An alkaloid from opium, isomeric with codeine. Prepn from 14-bromocodeinone: Conroy, US 2797222 (1957 to Merck & Co.); from thebaine: S. Makleit *et al., Acta Chim. Acad. Sci. Hung.* **94,** 161 (1977).

Long needles from petr ether, mp 127.5°. $[\alpha]_D^{23}$ −28° (c = 7.5 in chloroform). The absorption spectrum seems identical with that of codeine: Dobbie, Lauder, *J. Chem. Soc.* **99**, 34 (1911). Solubilities about the same as those of codeine, *q.v.*

Hydrobromide. $C_{18}H_{21}NO_3$.HBr. Prismatic crystals from water, darkens about 240°, dec 283°. $[\alpha]_D^{23}$ +17° (c = 3.7). Relatively insol in water, making possible a separation from other more sol hydrobromides of various opium alkaloids.

Note: Incorrectly called **hydroxycodeine**, *cf.* L. J. Sargent, U. Weiss, *J. Org. Chem.* **25**, 987 (1960).

6461. Neoprene. Duprene; GR-M; polychloroprene; poly(2-chloro-1,3-butadiene). Mol wt range of 100,000-300,000. An oil-resistant synthetic rubber, with predominantly *trans* configuration made by polymerization of chloroprene. Prepn: W. H. Carothers *et al., J. Am. Chem. Soc.* **53**, 4203 (1931). *Review:* P. J. Johnson in *Kirk-Othmer Encyclopedia of Chemical Technology* **vol. 8** (Wiley-Interscience, New York, 3rd ed., 1979) pp 515-534.

d^{20} approx 1.23. n_D^{20} approx 1.5512. Brittle point: −35°. Softens *ca.* 80°. Has high tensile strength, resilience and abrasion resistance.

USE: In mechanical and automotive products; as wire and cable jackets, gaskets, roof coatings, binder for fibers.

6462. Neopterin. [670-65-5] 2-Amino-6-(1,2,3-trihydroxy-propyl)-4(3H)-pteridinone; 1-(2-amino-4-hydroxy-6-pteridinyl)-1,2,3-propanetriol; 6-(1',2',3'-trihydroxy)pterin; Crithidia factor. $C_9H_{11}N_5O_4$; mol wt 253.21. C 42.69%, H 4.38%, N 27.66%, O 25.27%. Precursor in the biosynthesis of biopterin, *q.v.* Of the four possible isomers, D-*erythro*, L-*erythro*, D-*threo*, L-*threo*, two have been found in nature: the D-*erythro* form, to which the term neopterin originally referred; first isolated from the pupae of bees: Rembold, Buschmann, *Ann.* **662**, 72 (1963); the L-*threo* form, found to be the growth factor for the protozoan *Crithidia fasciculata* and isolatable from cell-free extracts of *Serratia indica*: Kobashi, Iwai, *Agric. Biol. Chem.* **35**, 47 (1971); **36**, 1685, 1695 (1972). Both natural forms found in human urine: Fukushima, Shiota, *J. Biol. Chem.* **247**, 4549 (1972). Early synthetic studies and structure: Rembold, Buschmann, *Ber.* **96**, 1406 (1963). Synthesis of L-(−)-form: Viscontini, Provenzale, *Helv. Chim. Acta* **51**, 1495 (1968). Synthesis of natural D-neopterin: Viscontini *et al., ibid.* **53**, 1202 (1970).

D-*erythro*-Neopterin

D-*erythro*-Form. [2009-64-5] $[\alpha]_D^{25}$ +45 ± 3° (c = 0.3 in 0.1N HCl).

L-*erythro*-Form. $[\alpha]_D^{25}$ −44 ± 3° (c = 0.3 in 0.1N HCl).
D-*threo*-Form. $[\alpha]_D^{25}$ −92 ± 3° (c = 0.3 in 0.1N HCl).
L-*threo*-Form. Pale yellow, spiny crystals. $[\alpha]_D^{25}$ +97 ± 3° (c = 0.3 in 0.1N HCl). uv max in 0.1N NaOH: 255, 363 nm (ε 20,900, 7050); in 0.1N HCl: 248, 323 nm (ε 11,200, 7880). Strong blue fluorescence in neutral or alkaline soln; weak fluorescence in acidic soln.

6463. Neoquassin. [76-77-7] 16-Hydroxy-2,12-dimethoxy-picrasa-2,12-diene-1,11-dione; 3a,4,5,6a,7,7a,8,11a,11b,11c-deca-hydro-5-hydroxy-2,10-dimethoxy-3,8,11a,11c-tetramethylphenan-thro[10,1-*bc*]pyran-1,11-dione. $C_{22}H_{30}O_6$; mol wt 390.47. C 67.67%, H 7.74%, O 24.58%. Found together with the quassin in the mixture of bitter constituents of the wood of *Quassia amara* L., *Simaroubaceae*, known in commerce as Surinam quassia. Forms

quassin on oxidation. Isoln: London *et al., J. Chem. Soc.* **1950**, 3431. Structure: Valenta *et al., Tetrahedron Lett.* **1960**(20), 25; Carman, Ward, *ibid.* **1961**, 317; Valenta *et al., Tetrahedron* **15**, 100 (1961).

Very bitter polymorphous crystals. Stable form, thick prisms, mp 227.5-228.5°; unstable form, long narrow plates, mp 213°. $[\alpha]_D^{20}$ +41.0° (c = 4.98 in chloroform). uv max ~255 nm (ε ~11,650). Sol in cold acetone, chloroform, pyridine, acetic acid, in warm ethyl acetate, benzene, alcohol. Sparingly sol in ether, petr ether.

6464. Neostigmine. [59-99-4] 3-[[(Dimethylamino)carbon-yl]oxy]-*N,N,N*-trimethylbenzenaminium; (3-dimethylcarbamoxy-phenyl) trimethylammonium; synstigmin; proserine. $[C_{12}H_{19}N_2-O_2]^+$. Synthesis: Aeschlimann, **US 1905990** (1933 to Hoffmann-La Roche); Yanagisawa, **JP 51 3071** (1951), *C.A.* **47**, 4908g (1953). Pharmacology and pharmacokinetics: T. N. Calvey *et al., Br. J. Clin. Pharmacol.* **7**, 149 (1979). Synergism of neostigmine toxicity by lithium: W. M. Davis, N. S. Hatoum, *Toxicology* **17**, 1 (1980). Toxicity: L. O. Randall, G. Lehmann, *J. Pharmacol. Exp. Ther.* **99**, 16 (1950). Comprehensive description: A. A. Al-Badr, M. Tariq, *Anal. Profiles Drug Subs.* **16**, 403-444 (1987). Clinical evaluation in treatment of acute colonic pseudo-obstruction: R. J. Ponec *et al., N. Engl. J. Med.* **341**, 137 (1999).

Bromide. [114-80-7] Juvastigmin (tabl.); Neoesserin; Neostig-min (tabl.); Normastigmin (tabl.); Prostigmin. $C_{12}H_{19}BrN_2O_2$; mol wt 303.20. Crystals from alcohol + ether, dec ~167°. One gram dissolves in ~1 ml water. Sol in alc.

Methyl sulfate. [51-60-5] Intrastigmina; Juvastigmin (amp.); Metastigmin; Neostigmin (inj.); Normastigmin (amp.); Prostigmin (amp.); Stiglyn. $C_{13}H_{22}N_2O_6S$; mol wt 334.39. Crystals from alc, mp 142-145°. One gram dissolves in ~10 ml water, less sol in alcohol. LD_{50} in mice (mg/kg): 0.16 i.v.; 0.42 s.c.; 7.5 orally, (Randall, Lehmann).

THERAP CAT: Cholinergic; miotic; antidote (curare).

THERAP CAT (VET): Cholinergic; antidote (curare).

6465. Neotame. [165450-17-9] *N*-(3,3-Dimethylbutyl)-L-α-aspartyl-L-phenylalanine 2-methyl ester; *N*-[*N*-(3,3-Dimethylbutyl)-L-α-aspartyl]-L-phenylalanine 1-methyl ester. $C_{20}H_{30}N_2O_5$; mol wt 378.46. C 63.47%, H 7.99%, N 7.40%, O 21.14%. Alkylated dipeptide reported to be 6000 to 10000 times sweeter than sucrose; structurally related to aspartame, *q.v.* Prepn: C. Nofre, J.-M. Tinti, **FR 2697844**; *eidem*, **US 5480668** (1994, 1996); and sweetness evaluation: I. Prakash *et al., Synth. Commun.* **29**, 4461 (1999). Crystal structure: D. J. Wink *et al., Acta Crystallogr.* **C55**, 1365 (1999). Analysis of polymorphic forms: B. E. Padden *et al., Anal. Chem.* **71**, 3325 (1999). Review of discovery, properties, and utility: C. Nofre, J.-M. Tinti, *Food Chem.* **69**, 245-257 (2000).

Occurs as the monohydrate. White crystalline powder from ethyl acetate/hexane, mp 80-83°; also reported as mp 80.9-83.4° from aq MeOH. $[\alpha]_D$ −54.84° (c = 1 in methanol); $[\alpha]_D^{20}$ −39.8° (c = 0.5 in water). pKa_1 3.01; pKa_2 8.02. pI: 5.5. Caloric value: <1.2 kJ/g. Soly in water (g/l): 10.6 (15°), 12.6 (25°), 47.5 (60°); in ethyl acetate (g/l): 43.6 (15°), 77 (25°), >1000 (60°); in abs ethanol (g/l): ~950 (25°).

USE: Non-nutritive sweetener.

6466. Neotetrazolium Chloride. [298-95-3] 3,3′-[1,1′-Biphenyl]-4,4′-diylbis[2,5-diphenyl-2H-tetrazolium] dichloride; 3,3′-[4,4′-biphenylene]bis[2,5-diphenyl-2H-tetrazolium] dichloride; 2,-2′,5,5′-tetraphenyl-3,3′-(p-diphenylene)ditetrazolium chloride; 2,2′-(p-diphenylene)-bis[3,5-diphenyl]ditetrazolium chloride; neo-tetrazolium blue; neo-T; TP; NTC. $C_{38}H_{28}Cl_2N_8$; mol wt 667.59. C 68.37%, H 4.23%, Cl 10.62%, N 16.78%. Prepn: L. J. Pannone, J. B. Rust, **US 2713581** (1955 to Montclair Res. Corp. and Ellis-Foster Co.). Purification: G. R. N. Jones, *Histochem. J.* **1,** 59 (1968). *See also* Triphenyltetrazolium chloride.

Light yellow powder, mp 297° (dec).

USE: Staining of microorganisms and plant and animal tissues. In determn of dehydrogenases in histochemical and cytochemical studies: K. Neumann, G. Koch, *Z. Physiol. Chem.* **295,** 35 (1953). In amylase determn.

6467. Neovastat®. [305838-77-1] AE-941; Naturally occurring antiangiogenic agent derived by ultrafiltration of liquid shark cartilage; composed of the molecular fraction below 500 kD. Exhibits multiple mechanisms of action: matrix metalloproteinases (MMP) inhibition, VEGF receptor binding inhibition, induction of endothelial cell apoptosis, and increased tissue-type plasminogen activator (tPA) production. Prepn from spiny dogfish (*Squalus acanthias*): E. Dupont *et al., WO 9532722; eidem,* **US 5985839** (1995, 1999 both to AEterna); and antiangiogenic activity: *eidem, J. Cutan. Med. Surg.* **2,** 146 (1998). Mechanism of action studies: R. Béliveau *et al., Clin. Cancer Res.* **8,** 1242 (2002); D. Gingras *et al., Invest. New Drugs* **22,** 17 (2004). Clinical evaluation in plaque psoriasis: D. N. Sauder *et al., J. Am. Acad. Dermatol.* **47,** 535 (2002); in lung cancer: J. Latreille *et al., Clin. Lung Cancer* **4,** 231 (2003). Purifn of tPA stimulating component: D. Boivin *et al., Arch. Biochem. Biophys.* **431,** 197 (2004). Reviews of pharmacology and clinical development: R. M. Bukowski, *Expert Opin. Invest. Drugs* **12,** 1403-1411 (2003); K. Dredge, *Curr. Opin. Invest. Drugs* **5,** 668-677 (2004).

THERAP CAT: Antineoplastic; antipsoriatic.

6468. Neovitamin A. [2052-63-3] 13-*cis*-Retinol; 2-*cis*-vitamin A. $C_{20}H_{30}O$; mol wt 286.45. C 83.86%, H 10.56%, O 5.59%. Naturally occurring, bioactive isomer of vitamin A, *q.v.* The 13-*cis*- and *all-trans*-forms come to equilibrium in solution with ~33% as 13-*cis*. Isoln from shark liver oil: C. D. Robeson, J. G. Baxter, *J. Am. Chem. Soc.* **69,** 136 (1947). Synthesis: M. Matsui *et al., J. Vitaminol.* **4,** 178 (1958). Stereoselective synthesis: J. Otera *et al., Chem. Lett.* **1985,** 1883. HPLC determn in food samples: E. Brinkmann *et al., J. Chromatogr. A* **693,** 271 (1995). Review of vitamin A compounds: W. Friedrich in *Vitamins* (Walter de Gruyter, Berlin, 1988) pp 63-140.

Pale yellow needles from ethyl formate, mp 58-60°. uv max: 328 nm (ε 41800).

6469. Nepafenac. [78281-72-8] 2-Amino-3-benzoylbenzeneacetamide; AHR-9434; AL-6515; Nevanac. $C_{15}H_{14}N_2O_2$; mol wt 254.28. C 70.85%, H 5.55%, N 11.02%, O 12.58%. Nonsteroidal anti-inflammatory with analgesic activity; selective COX-2 inhibitor. Prodrug of amfenac, *q.v.* Prepn: D. A. Walsh *et al.,* **DE 3035688** (1981 to A. H. Robins); *see also:* J. R. Shanklin, Jr. *et al.,* **US 4313949** (1982 to A. H. Robins); D. A. Walsh *et al., J. Med. Chem.* **33,** 2296 (1990). Ocular pharmacology: D. A. Gamache *et al., Inflammation* **24,** 357 (2000); T.-L. Ke *et al., ibid.* 371. Inhibition of ocular neovascularization: K. Takahashi *et al., Invest. Ophthalmol. Visual Sci.* **44,** 409 (2003). Review of clinical experience: R. Lindstrom, T. Kim, *Curr. Med. Res. Opin.* **22,** 397-404 (2006).

Yellow needles from isopropyl alcohol, mp 178.5-180.0°.

THERAP CAT: Anti-inflammatory.

6470. Nepetalactone. [490-10-8] 5,6,7,7a-Tetrahydro-4,7-dimethylcyclopenta[c]pyran-1-(4aH)-one. $C_{10}H_{14}O_2$; mol wt 166.22. C 72.26%, H 8.49%, O 19.25%. The first fully characterized methylcyclopentane monoterpenoid. Isolated from the volatile oil of catnip produced by *Nepeta cataria* L., *Labiatae:* S. M. McElvain *et al., J. Am. Chem. Soc.* **63,** 1558 (1941); J. Meinwald, *ibid.* **76,** 4571 (1954). First believed to be a single entity, it was later shown to be a mixture of the *cis-trans* and *trans-cis* isomers, the *cis-trans* isomer comprising 70-99% of the oil. Structure: S. M. McElvain, E. J. Eisenbraun, *J. Am. Chem. Soc.* **77,** 1599 (1955). Configuration of the *cis-trans* and *trans-cis* isomers: R. B. Bates *et al., ibid.* **80,** 3420 (1958). Separation and properties: R. B. Bates, C. W. Siegel, *Experientia* **19,** 564 (1963). Biosynthesis: F. E. Regnier *et al., Phytochemistry* **7,** 221 (1968). Metabolism in cats: G. R. Waller *et al., Science* **164,** 1281 (1969). Behavioral and toxicological study: J. W. Harney *et al., Lloydia* **41,** 367 (1978). Structural study of isomeric nepetalactones: E. J. Eisenbraun *et al., J. Org. Chem.* **45,** 3811 (1980).

cis-trans-Nepetalactone

Oil. Odor very attractive to cats. d_4^{25} 1.0663. $bp_{0.05}$ 71-72°. $[\alpha]_D^{23}$+3.6°. n_D^{25} 1.4859. Soluble in ether, carbon tetrachloride. When shaken with 10% NaOH yields *nepetalic acid*, crystals, mp 74°, $[\alpha]_D^{30}$ +47.6° (chloroform).

cis-trans-Form. [21651-62-7] 2-(2-Hydroxy-1-methylethenyl)-5-methylcyclopentanecarboxylic acid delta lactone. Oil, $[\alpha]_D^{21}$ +3.7° (c = 27 in chloroform). $[\alpha]_D^{27.5}$ +11.11° (chloroform). n_D^{25} 1.4878.

trans-cis-Form. mp 37-39°. $[\alpha]_D^{21}$ −24.4° (c = 6.15 in chloroform) (Eisenbraun); also reported as $[\alpha]_D^{27.5}$ +21.9° (chloroform) (Bates, Siegel). n_D^{25} 1.4878.

6471. Neptunium. [7439-99-8] Np; at. no. 93; valence 3, 4, 5, 6, 7. First man-made transuranium element; no stable nuclides. Known isotopes (mass numbers): 227-242. Discovery of isotope 239 (T½ 2.355 days, β-decay, rel. at. mass 239.0529): E. McMillan, P. Abelson, *Phys. Rev.* **57,** 1185 (1940); of isotope 237 (α-emitter, T½ 2.14 × 10⁶ years, longest-lived known isotope, rel. at. mass 237.0482): A. C. Wahl, G. T. Seaborg, *ibid.* **73,** 940 (1948). Prepn of metal: S. Fried, N. Davidson, *J. Am. Chem. Soc.* **70,** 3539 (1948); L. B. Magnusson, T. J. LaChapelle, *ibid.* 3534. Presence in nature: Seaborg, Perlman, *ibid.* **70,** 1571 (1948). Chemical properties: Seaborg, Wahl, *ibid.* 1128. *Reviews:* C. Keller, *The Chemistry of the Transactinide Elements*

(Verlag Chemie, Weinheim, English Ed., 1971) pp 253-332; W. W. Schulz, G. E. Benedict, *Neptunium-237; Production and Recovery*, AEC Critical Review Series (USAEC, Washington, D.C., 1972) 85 pp; *Comprehensive Inorganic Chemistry* **vol. 5,** J. C. Bailar, Jr. *et al.,* Eds. (Pergamon Press, Oxford, 1973) *passim;* J. A. Fahey in *The Chemistry of the Actinide Elements* **vol. 1,** J. J. Katz *et al.,* Eds. (Chapman and Hall, New York, 1986) pp 443-498; G. T. Seaborg in *Kirk-Othmer Encyclopedia of Chemical Technology* **vol. 1** (Wiley-Interscience, New York, 4th ed., 1991) pp 412-444.

Silvery metal; develops a thin oxide layer upon exposure to air for short periods. Reacts with air at high temperatures to form NpO_2. Exhibits 3 allotropic modifications: orthorhombic α-form, d 20.45, transforms to β-form at 280°; tetragonal β-form, d 19.36, transforms to γ-form at 577°; cubic γ-form transforms to liquid at mp 637°. Extrapolated bp 4174°. Np has been obtained in its five oxidation states in soln; the most stable is the pentavalent state. Tetravalent Np is readily oxidized to the hexavalent state by permanganate in the cold, or by strong oxidizing agents; on electrolytic reduction in an atmosphere of nitrogen, the trivalent form is obtained.

Caution: Radiation hazard; handling requires special equipment and shielding facilities (Katz *et al., loc. cit.* **vol. 2,** p. 1128).

USE: Source material for prodn of ^{238}U (power source).

6472. Nequinate. [13997-19-8] 6-Butyl-1,4-dihydro-4-oxo-7-(phenylmethoxy)-3-quinolinecarboxylic acid methyl ester; 7-(benzyloxy)-6-*n*-butyl-1,4-dihydro-4-oxo-3-quinolinecarboxylic acid methyl ester; 3-methoxycarbonyl-6-*n*-butyl-7-benzyloxy-4-oxoquinoline; 7-(benzyloxy)-6-*n*-butyl-4-hydroxy-3-quinolinecarboxylic acid methyl ester; 7-(benzyloxy)-6-*n*-butyl-3-methoxycarbonyl-4-quinolone; methyl benzoquate; ICI-55052; Statyl. $C_{22}H_{23}NO_4$; mol wt 365.42. C 72.31%, H 6.34%, N 3.83%, O 17.51%. Prepn: **BE 677592** and **GB 1070223** (1966 to I.C.I.), *C.A.* **68,** 68899j (1968). Coccidiostatic activity: Bowie *et al., Nature* **214,** 1349 (1967). HPLC determn in poultry feedstuffs: G. H. J. Merson *et al., Analyst* **110,** 761 (1985).

Crystals, mp 287-288°.

THERAP CAT (VET): Coccidiostat.

6473. Neridronic Acid. [79778-41-9] (6-Amino-1-hydroxyhexylidene)bisphosphonic acid. $C_6H_{17}NO_7P_2$; mol wt 277.15. C 26.00%, H 6.18%, N 5.05%, O 40.41%, P 22.35%. Bisphosphonate antiresorptive agent. Prepn: J. Jary *et al.,* **BE 885139;** *eidem,* **US 4304734** (both 1981 to Vysoka Skola Chem.-Tech.); and characterization of monosodium salt: M. Neves *et al., Nucl. Med. Biol.* **29,** 329 (2002). Crystal structure: V. M. Coiro, D. Lamba, *Acta Crystallogr.* **C45,** 446 (1989). Clinical study in Paget's disease: S. Adami *et al., Clin. Exp. Rheumatol.* **20,** 55 (2002); in osteogenesis imperfecta: *idem et al., J. Bone Miner. Res.* **18,** 126 (2003); in osteoporosis: V. Braga *et al., Bone* **33,** 342 (2003).

mp 245°.

Monosodium salt. [80729-79-9] Neridronate sodium; Nerixia. $C_6H_{16}NNaO_7P_2$; mol wt 299.13. White solid, mp 263-266° (hemihydrate).

THERAP CAT: Bone resorption inhibitor.

6474. Neriifolin. [466-07-9] (3β,5β)-3-[(6-Deoxy-3-*O*-methyl-α-L-glucopyranosyl)oxy]-14-hydroxycard-20(22)-enolide.

$C_{30}H_{46}O_8$; mol wt 534.68. C 67.39%, H 8.67%, O 23.94%. Cardiac glycoside isolated from *Thevetia neriifolia* Juss.: M. Frèrejacque, *Compt. Rend.* **221,** 645 (1945); from *Cerbera odollam* Gaertn.: S. Rangaswami, E. V. Rao, *J. Sci. Ind. Res.* **16B,** 209 (1957); from *Thevetia thevetioides* seeds: J. L. McLaughlin *et al., J. Econ. Entomol.* **73,** 39 (1980). Pharmacology: K. Mezey, *Arch. Int. Pharmacodyn. Ther.* **84,** 367 (1950); K. K. Chen *et al., ibid.* 81.

Rhombic plates from methanol, mp 218-225°. Also reported as mp 208° (Frèrejacque). $[\alpha]_D^{23} -50.2°$ (CH_3OH). uv max (CH_3-OH): 217 nm (log ε 4.1).

2'-Acetate. Cerberin; veneniferin; monoacetylneriifolin. $C_{32}H_{48}O_9$. Identity of cerberin with monoacetylneriifolin: M. Frèrejacque, *Compt. Rend.* **226,** 835 (1948); of cerberin with veneniferin: M. Frèrejacque, Durgeat, *ibid.* **228,** 1310 (1949). Coarse prisms from methanol + water, mp 212-215°. $[\alpha]_D^{19} -82°$ ($CHCl_3$). Sol in alc, $CHCl_3$, acetic acid, ether. Practically insol in water.

THERAP CAT: Cardiotonic.

6475. Nerol. [106-25-2] (*Z*)-3,7-Dimethyl-2,6-octadien-1-ol; *cis*-2,6-dimethyl-2,6-octadien-8-ol. $C_{10}H_{18}O$; mol wt 154.25. C 77.87%, H 11.76%, O 10.37%. The *cis*-isomer of geraniol, *q.v.*; found in many essential oils. Readily loses water and cyclizes forming dipentene. Isoln from neroli oil: Hesse, Zeitschel, *J. Prakt. Chem.* **66,** 502 (1902). Structure: Verley, *Bull. Soc. Chim. Fr.* **25,** 68 (1919); J. L. Simonsen, *The Terpenes* **vol. I** (University Press, Cambridge, 2nd ed., 1947) pp 52-54. Stereochemistry: Burrell *et al., Proc. Chem. Soc. London* **1959,** 263; Bates *et al., J. Org. Chem.* **28,** 1086 (1963). Synthesis: Yukawa *et al., Bull. Chem. Soc. Jpn.* **37,** 158 (1964). Stereochemistry and synthesis: Burrell *et al., J. Chem. Soc. C* **1966,** 2144; K. Takabe *et al., Chem. Lett.* **1977,** 1025.

Liquid. Odor of sweet rose. bp_{745} 224-225°; bp_{25} 125°. d^{15} 0.8813. Optically inactive. uv max: 189-194 nm (ε 18000). Sol in abs alc.

Tetrabromide. $C_{10}H_{18}Br_4O$. Crystals, mp 118°.

Allophanate. $C_{12}H_{20}N_2O_3$. Needles from petr ether, mp 84-86°.

USE: Base for manuf of perfumes.

6476. Nerolidol. [7212-44-4] 3,7,11-Trimethyl-1,6,10-dodecatrien-3-ol; peruviol. $C_{15}H_{26}O$; mol wt 222.37. C 81.02%, H 11.79%, O 7.19%. Found in essential oils from many flowers such as *Melaleuca viridiflora* Soland., *Myrtaceae* and *Myroxylon pereirae* (Royle) Klotzsch, *Leguminosae:* Naves, *Compt. Rend.* **251,** 900 (1960). Isoln: Hellyer, McKern, *J. Proc. R. Soc. N.S.W.* **89,** (Pt. 4), 188 (1955); Sutherland *et al., Aust. J. Chem.* **13,** 357 (1960). Synthesis: Nazarov *et al., Zh. Obshch. Khim.* **28,** 1444 (1958); Ofner *et al., Helv. Chim. Acta* **42,** 2577 (1959); Shvarts, Petrov, *Zh. Obshch. Khim.* **30,** 3598 (1960). Exists in two stereoisomeric forms: Bates *et al., J. Org. Chem.* **28,** 1086 (1963).

trans-form

trans-Form. [40716-66-3] Liquid. $bp_{0.15}$ 78°. n_D^{25} 1.4792.
cis-Form. [3790-78-1] Liquid. $bp_{0.10}$ 70°. n_D^{25} 1.4775.
cis/trans-Form. Liquid. bp_3 122°. n_D^{25} 1.4769. d_4^{25} 0.8720.
Sol in abs alc (still clearly sol in 3 parts of 70% alc).

6477. Nerve Growth Factor. [9061-61-4] NGF. Polypeptide factor which promotes the growth and survival of peripheral sympathetic and sensory neurons and basal forebrain cholinergic neurons. Prototype of the neurotrophins, *q.v.* Synthesized in limiting amounts by target tissues of NGF-responsive cells; anomalous sources of large amounts of NGF include mouse submaxillary gland, snake venom gland, and guinea pig prostate. Bioactive form, also referred to as *β-NGF*, is a tightly associated dimer of 2 identical polypeptide chains. Mol wt of the dimer ~26,500 Da. Initial identification as a nerve growth stimulating factor from mouse sarcoma: R. Levi-Montalcini, V. Hamburger, *J. Exp. Zool.* **116**, 321 (1951); R. Levi-Montalcini, *Ann. N.Y. Acad. Sci.* **55**, 330 (1952). Identification in snake venom: S. Cohen, *J. Biol. Chem.* **234**, 1129 (1959); in mouse submaxillary gland: *idem, Proc. Natl. Acad. Sci. USA* **46**, 302 (1960); in guinea pig prostate: G. P. Harper *et al., Nature* **279**, 160 (1979). Occurs in mouse submaxillary gland as a complex (known as 7S NGF) composed of α-, β-, and γ-subunits, of which only the β-subunit is bioactive. Characterization of subunits: S. Varon *et al., Biochemistry* **7**, 1296 (1968); A. C. Server, E. M. Shooter, *Adv. Protein Chem.* **31**, 339 (1977). Amino acid sequence of mouse NGF: R. H. Angeletti, R. A. Bradshaw, *Proc. Natl. Acad. Sci. USA* **68**, 2417 (1971). Cloning of mouse NGF: J. Scott *et al., Nature* **302**, 538 (1983); of human: A. Ullrich *et al., ibid.* **303**, 821 (1983). Crystal structure: N. Q. McDonald *et al., ibid.* **354**, 411 (1991). Review of NGF receptor: P. A. Barker, R. A. Murphy, *Mol. Cell. Biochem.* **110**, 1-15 (1992). Review of pharmacology and potential role in neurodegenerative disease: F. Hefti, P. A. Lapchak, *Adv. Pharmacol.* **24**, 239-273 (1993); in peripheral nerve regeneration: G. Raivich, G. W. Kreutzberg, *Clin. Neurol. Neurosurg.* **95** Suppl., S84-S88 (1993). *Reviews:* R. Levi-Montalcini, R. H. Angeletti, *Physiol. Rev.* **48**, 534-569 (1968); H. Thoenen, Y. A. Barde, *ibid.* **60**, 1284-1335 (1980); R. Levi-Montalcini, *Science* **237**, 1154-1162 (1987); R. A. Bradshaw *et al., Trends Biochem. Sci.* **18**, 48-52 (1993). *Book: Neurotrophic Factors* S. E. Loughlin, J. H. Fallon, Eds. (Academic Press, San Diego, 1993) 607 pp.

6478. Neticonazole. [130726-68-0] 1-[(1*E*)-2-(Methylthio)-1-[2-(pentyloxy)phenyl]ethenyl]-1*H*-imidazole. $C_{17}H_{22}N_2OS$; mol wt 302.43. C 67.51%, H 7.33%, N 9.26%, O 5.29%, S 10.60%. Antifungal that inhibits cell wall synthesis. Prepn: M. Ogawa *et al., EP 227011; eidem, US 4740601* (1987, 1988 both to SS Pharm.); and antifungal activity: M. Ogawa *et al., Chem. Pharm. Bull.* **39**, 2301 (1991). Clinical study in tinea pedis: R. Tsuboi *et al., Int. J. Dermatol.* **35**, 371 (1996).

Colorless crystals from isopropyl ether, mp 37-39°.
Hydrochloride. [130773-02-3] SS-717; Atolant. $C_{17}H_{22}N_2OS\cdot HCl$; mol wt 338.90. Colorless columns from acetonitrile, mp 145-147°.

THERAP CAT: Antifungal (synthetic).

6479. Netilmicin. [56391-56-1] *O*-3-Deoxy-4-*C*-methyl-3-(methylamino)-β-L-arabinopyranosyl-(1 → 6)-*O*-[2,6-diamino-2,3,-4,6-tetradeoxy-α-D-*glycero*-hex-4-enopyranosyl-(1 → 4)]-2-deoxy-

N^1-ethyl-D-streptamine; (2*S-cis*)-4-*O*-[3-amino-6-(aminomethyl)-3,4-dihydro-2*H*-pyran-2-yl]-2-deoxy-6-*O*-[3-deoxy-4-*C*-methyl-3-(methylamino)-β-L-arabinopyranosyl]-N^1-ethyl-D-streptamine; 1-*N*-ethylsisomicin; Sch-20569. $C_{21}H_{41}N_5O_7$; mol wt 475.58. C 53.04%, H 8.69%, N 14.73%, O 23.55%. Broad spectrum semisynthetic aminoglycoside antibiotic, related to sisomicin, *q.v.* Prepn: M. J. Weinstein *et al., DE 2437160* (1975 to Sherico); J. J. Wright, *US 4029882* (1977 to Schering); J. J. Wright *et al., US 4002742* (1977 to Schering). Structure and synthesis: J. J. Wright, *Chem. Commun.* **1976**, 206. Biological activity: G. H. Miller *et al., Antimicrob. Agents Chemother.* **10**, 827 (1976). Radioimmunoassay: A. Broughton *et al., Clin. Chem.* **24**, 717 (1978). Pharmacology: W. Raab, *Adv. Clin. Pharmacol.* **15**, 91 (1978); I. Trestman *et al., Antimicrob. Agents Chemother.* **13**, 832 (1978). Metabolism and pharmacokinetics: J. C. Pechere *et al., Clin. Pharmacol. Ther.* **23**, 677 (1978); R. E. Brummett *et al., Arch. Otolaryngol.* **104**, 579 (1978). Clinical studies: J. Klastersky *et al., Antimicrob. Agents Chemother.* **12**, 503 (1977); A. P. Panwalker *et al., ibid.* **13**, 170 (1978). Toxicity studies: L. Albiero *et al., Arch. Int. Pharmacodyn. Ther.* **233**, 343 (1978); F. C. Lust, *J. Int. Med. Res.* **6**, 286 (1978). *Review:* P. Noone, *Drugs* **27**, 548-578 (1984).

$[\alpha]_D^{26}$ +164° (c = 3 in water). LD_{50} in mice (mg/kg): 40 i.v.; 125 i.p.; 175 s.c. (Miller).
Sulfate. [56391-57-2] Certomycin; Netillin; Netilyn; Netromicine; Netromycin; Nettacin; Vectacin; Zetamicin. $(C_{21}H_{41}N_5O_7)_2 \cdot 5H_2SO_4$; mol wt 1441.55.

THERAP CAT: Antibacterial.

6480. Netobimin. [88255-01-0] 2-[[[(Methoxycarbonyl)-amino][[2-nitro-5-(propylthio)phenyl]amino]methylene]amino]ethanesulfonic acid; 2-[[[(methoxycarbonyl)amino][[2-nitro-5-(propylthio)phenyl]imino]methyl]amino]ethanesulfonic acid; methyl [*N'*-[2-nitro-5-(propylthio)phenyl]-*N*-(2-sulfoethyl)amidino]carbamate; *N*-methoxycarbonyl-*N'*-[2-nitro-5-(propylthio)phenyl]-*N''*-2-(ethylsulfonic acid)guanidine; totabin; Sch-32481; Hapadex. $C_{14}H_{20}N_4O_7S_2$; mol wt 420.46. C 39.99%, H 4.79%, N 13.33%, O 26.64%, S 15.25%. Phenylguanidine anthelmintic. Prepn: M. M. Nafissi-Varchei, *EP 50286; idem, US 4406893* (1982, 1983 both to Schering). Metabolism in animals: P. Delatour *et al., J. Vet. Pharmacol. Ther.* **9**, 230 (1986). Anthelmintic efficacy in cattle: J. C. Williams *et al., Am. J. Vet. Res.* **46**, 2188 (1985).

mp 215° (dec).
Sodium salt. $C_{14}H_{20}N_4NaO_7S_2$. Crystals, mp 150° (dec) (Nafissi-Varchei); also reported as yellow powder, mp 160° (Delatour). uv max (methanol): 225, 347 nm. Sol in water, acetone, methanol, dimethylformamide, DMSO. Insol in ether.

THERAP CAT (VET): Anthelmintic.

6481. Netropsin. [1438-30-8] 4-[[[(Aminoiminomethyl)-amino]acetyl]amino]-*N*-[5-[[(3-amino-3-iminopropyl)amino]carbonyl]-1-methyl-1*H*-pyrrol-3-yl]-1-methyl-1*H*-pyrrole-2-carboxamide; *N'*-(2-amidinoethyl)-4-(2-guanidinoacetamido)-1,1'-dimethyl-*N*,4′-bi[pyrrole-2-carboxamide]; sinanomycin; congocidine; T-1384. $C_{18}H_{26}N_{10}O_3$; mol wt 430.46. C 50.22%, H 6.09%, N 32.54%, O 11.15%. Basic oligopeptide antibiotic produced by *Streptomyces netropsis* with wide range of antimicrobial activity. Prepn and antibacterial spectrum: A. C. Finlay *et al.*, *J. Am. Chem. Soc.* **73**, 341 (1951); and trypanocidal activity: C. Cosar *et al.*, *Compt. Rend.* **234**, 1498 (1952). Antiviral activity: F. M. Schabel *et al.*, *Proc. Soc. Exp. Biol. Med.* **83**, 1 (1953). Identity with sinanomycin: K. Watanabe, *J. Antibiot.* **9A**, 102 (1956). Structural studies: M. Julia, N. Joseph, *Compt. Rend.* **243**, 961 (1956). Structure: C. W. Waller *et al.*, *J. Am. Chem. Soc.* **79**, 1265 (1957). Revised structure: M. Julia, N. Préau-Joseph, *Compt. Rend.* **257**, 1115 (1963); *eidem, Bull. Soc. Chim. Fr.* **1967**, 4348. Specific binding to DNA: Ch. Zimmer *et al.*, *J. Mol. Biol.* **58**, 329 (1971); K. Zakrzewska *et al.*, *Nucleic Acids Res.* **11**, 8825, 8841 (1983). Use in gradient separation of DNA: K. M. Tatti *et al.*, *Anal. Biochem.* **89**, 561 (1978). Selective blocking of DNAase I cleavage: Ch. Zimmer *et al.*, *Nucleic Acids Res.* **8**, 2999 (1980). Review of activity: F. E. Hahn in *Antibiotics* vol. 3, J. W. Corcoran, F. E. Hahn, Eds. (Springer-Verlag, New York, 1975) pp 79-100. Review of effect on DNA structure and function: Ch. Zimmer, *Prog. Nucleic Acid Res. Mol. Biol.* **15**, 285-318 (1975).

Disulfate. $C_{18}H_{26}N_{10}O_3 \cdot 2H_2SO_4$. Needles, mp 288°. Soly in water ~30 mg/ml at 80°, <0.5 mg/ml at 25°. Practically insol in the common organic solvents.

Dihydrochloride. $C_{18}H_{26}N_{10}O_3 \cdot 2HCl$. Prisms, mp 228°. LD_{50} in mice (mg/kg): 17 i.v.; 70 s.c.; >300 orally (Finlay).

USE: Non-intercalative DNA binding agent.

6482. Nettle. Stinging nettle. Flowering perennial herb, *Urtica dioica* L. Uricaceae. Leaves and stems are covered with bristly stinging hairs that cause a characteristic urticaria upon contact. Used in traditional medicine as a diuretic, hemostatic, and in treatment of rheumatic conditions. Medicinal portions include leaves, fruits and root. *Habit.* Widely scattered throughout the Northern hemisphere, especially in moist woods, road sides and wasteland. *Constit.* Flavonoids: glycosides of quercetin, kaempferol, isorhamnetin in the flowers; histamine, acetylcholine and serotonin in the stinging hairs; β-sitosterol, coumarin, lignans and a lectin, *U. dioica* agglutinin, in the rhizome. Botanical description: T. W. McGovern, T. M. Barkley, *Cutis* **62**, 63 (1998). Clinical evaluation of nettle sting in osteoarthritic pain: C. Randall *et al.*, *J. R. Soc. Med.* **93**, 305 (2000). Reviews of medicinal preparations: M. Wichtl, N. G. Bisset, *Herbal Drugs and Phytopharmaceuticals*, English Ed. (CRC Press, Boca Raton, 1994) pp 502-509; J. Barnes *et al.*, *Herbal Medicines* (Pharmaceutical Press, London, 2nd ed., 2002) pp 360-364.

Root extract. Bazoton; Prostaherb. Antiproliferative effects on human prostatic epithelium: J. J. Lichius *et al.*, *Pharmazie* **54**, 768 (1999). Review of clinical experience: E. Koch, *Planta Med.* **67**, 489-500 (2001).

THERAP CAT: Root extract in treatment of micturitional disorders due to benign prostatic hypertrophy.

6483. Neuraminic Acid. [114-04-5] Prehemataminic acid. $C_9H_{17}NO_8$; mol wt 267.23. C 40.45%, H 6.41%, N 5.24%, O 47.90%. Parent acid of a family of amino sugars contg 9 or more carbon atoms (sialic acids or nonulosaminic acids). May be regarded as the aldol condensation product of pyruvic acid and *N*-acetyl-D-mannosamine. Neuraminic acid has not been isolated and characterized as such, but several *N*- and *O*-substituted derivatives are widely distributed in nature. *Review:* Whelan, *Annu. Rep. Prog. Chem.* **54**, 319 (1958); A. Gottschalk, *The Chemistry and Biology of Sialic Acids and Related Substances* (Cambridge Univ. Press, 1960). *See also* Sialic Acids.

6484. Neurine. [463-88-7] *N*,*N*,*N*-Trimethylethenaminium hydroxide; trimethylvinylammonium hydroxide. $C_5H_{13}NO$; mol wt 103.16. C 58.21%, H 12.70%, N 13.58%, O 15.51%. Found in egg yolk, brain, bile, in cadavers. Formed during putrefaction by dehydration of choline: Hofmann, *Compt. Rend.* **47**, 559 (1858); Renshaw, Ware, *J. Am. Chem. Soc.* **47**, 2992 (1925). Prepn: Meyer, Hopff, *Ber.* **54**, 2277 (1921); from aq trimethylamine and acetylene: Gardner *et al.*, *J. Chem. Soc.* **1949**, 789. Separation and identification in biological fluids: E. Merlevede *et al.*, *Arch. Int. Pharmacodyn.* **122**, 474 (1959). Stereoelectronic config: *Intern. Kongr. Entomol. Verhandl., 11th, Vienna*, **1960**, No. 3, pp 87-93, *C.A.* **57**, 7749b (1962). Toxicity study: Hunt, *J. Pharmacol. Exp. Ther.* **28**, 267 (1926).

Syrupy liq. Fishy odor. *Poisonous!* Forms a crystalline trihydrate. Alkaline reaction. Readily absorbs CO_2 from the air. Sol in water, alcohol. Dec readily, forming trimethylamine. Forms an HCl salt. LD s.c. in mice: 46 mg/kg (Hunt).

6485. Neuropeptide Y. [82785-45-3] Neuropeptide tyrosine; NPY. Neuroendocrine peptide that stimulates ingestive behavior. Named for its five tyrosine (Y) residues. Member of a structurally related peptide family which includes peptide YY and pancreatic polypeptide. Most abundant known peptide in mammalian brain; widely distributed in the neurons of the central and peripheral nervous system and adrenal medullary cells. Composed of a highly conserved sequence of 36 amino acids. Exhibits wide range of physiological effects including anxiolysis, sedation, vasoconstriction, and the stimulation of food intake. Isoln from porcine brain: K. Tatemoto *et al.*, *Nature* **296**, 659 (1982). Amino acid sequence: *idem, Proc. Natl. Acad. Sci. USA* **79**, 5485 (1982). Distribution in human brain: T. E. Adrian *et al.*, *Nature* **306**, 584 (1983). Role of NPY in the antiobesity effect of the *obese* gene product (*see also* Leptin): T. W. Stephens *et al.*, *Nature* **377**, 530 (1995). Conference proceedings: *Neuropeptide Y: Karolinska Inst. Nobel Conf. Series*, V. Mutt *et al.*, Eds. (Raven Press, N.Y., 1989) 353 p. Book: *The Biology of Neuropeptide Y and Related Peptides*, W. F. Colmers, C. Wahlestedt, Eds. (Humana Press, Totowa, N. J., 1993) 564 p. Review of pharmacology: J. G. Wettstein *et al.*, *Pharmacol. Ther.* **65**, 397-414 (1995); of role as potential therapeutic target: L. Grundemar, R. Hakanson, *Trends Pharmacol. Sci.* **15**, 153-159 (1994).

6486. Neurotensin. [39379-15-2] A basic tridecapeptide, found in mammalian brain and gut, having a wide variety of hormone-like activities. Neurotensin has been shown to induce hypotension in the rat, to stimulate contraction of guinea pig ileum and rat uterus, and to cause relaxation of rat duodenum. There is also evidence that it acts as a CNS neurotransmitter. Isoln from bovine hypothalamus: R. Carraway, S. Leeman, *J. Biol. Chem.* **248**, 6854 (1973). Amino acid sequence of bovine neurotensin: *eidem, ibid.* **250**, 1907 (1975). Synthesis: *eidem, ibid.* 1912; K. Kitagawa *et al.*, *Chem. Pharm. Bull.* **24**, 2692 (1976); H. Yajima *et al.*, *Int. J. Pept. Protein Res.* **14**, 169 (1979). Isoln, amino acid sequence of chicken neurotensin: R. Carraway, Y. M. Bhatnagar, *Peptides* **1**, 167 (1980). Synthesis: H. Yajima *et al.*, *Chem. Pharm. Bull.* **29**, 2587 (1981). Radioimmunoassay and differential distribution of bovine neurotensin in CNS, small intestine, and stomach: R. Carraway, S. Leeman, *J. Biol. Chem.* **251**, 7035, 7045 (1976). CNS effects: C. B. Nemeroff *et al.*, *Brain Res.* **128**, 485 (1977). Receptor binding in brain: G. R. Uhl *et al., ibid.* **130**, 299 (1977). Pharmacokinetics and effect on gastrointestinal and pituitary hormones in man: A. M. Blackburn *et al., J. Clin. Endocrinol. Metab.* **51**, 1257 (1980). Reviews of biological activity: G. R. Uhl, S. H. Snyder, *Adv. Biochem. Psychopharmacol.* **28**, 87-106 (1981); D. R. Brown, R. J. Miller, *Annu. Rep. Med. Chem.* **17**, 271-280 (1982). Book: *Ann. N.Y. Acad. Sci.* **400**, entitled "Neurotensin, a Brain and Gastrointestinal Peptide", C. B. Nemeroff, A. J. Prange, Eds. (1982) pp 1-444.

5-oxoPro–Leu–Tyr–Glu–Asn–Lys–Pro–Arg–Arg–Pro– Tyr–Ile–LeuOH

Bovine Neurotensin

Bovine neurotensin triacetate hexahydrate. Neurotensin (ox) triacetate (salt). $C_{84}H_{133}N_{21}O_{26}.6H_2O$. Fluffy white powder. $[\alpha]_D^{23}$ −65.6° (c = 0.5 in water).

6487. Neurotrophins. Family of highly conserved, target-derived, secretory proteins that promote the differentiation, growth, and survival of neurons in the peripheral and central nervous systems. Produced in limiting amounts by innervated tissues to enhance neuronal differentiation and survival. Five closely related factors have been identified: nerve growth factor (NGF), *q.v.*, brain-derived neurotrophic factor (BDNF), neurotrophin-3 (NT-3), NT-4, and NT-5. Neurotrophins differ in their sites of synthesis, developmental patterns of expression, and neuronal targets. Amino acid sequences are highly homologous. Most of the sequence differences are contained in 4 specific regions which are presumed to be responsible for the biological specificities of the factors. Purification of BDNF from pig brain: Y.-A. Barde *et al., EMBO J.* **1**, 549 (1982). Cloning and expression of BDNF: J. Leibrock *et al., Nature* **341**, 149 (1989). Identification of rat NT-3: P. C. Maisonpierre *et al., Science* **247**, 1446 (1990); of human NT-3: Y. Kaisho *et al., FEBS Lett.* **266**, 187 (1990); A. Rosenthal *et al., Neuron* **4**, 767 (1990). Isolation of NT-4 from *Xenopus laevis*: F. Hallböök *et al., ibid.* **6**, 845 (1991). Identification of NT-5 in rat and human: L. R. Berkemeier *et al., ibid.* **7**, 857 (1991). Proposed identity of NT-5 as the mammalian homolog of Xenopus NT-4: N. Y. Ip *et al., Proc. Natl. Acad. Sci. USA* **89**, 3060 (1992). Comparison of neurotrophins and other neurotrophic factors: H. Thoenen, *Trends Neurosci.* **14**, 165 (1991). Discussion of neurotrophin receptors: S. O. Meakin, E. M. Shooter, *ibid.* **15**, 323 (1992). Review of amino acid sequences and molecular structure: T. Ebendal, *J. Neurosci. Res.* **32**, 461-470 (1992). Review of bioactivity and distribution in the nervous system: G. Vantini, *Psychoneuroendocrinology* **17**, 401-410 (1992); of bioactivity and therapeutic potential in neurologic disease: F. F. Eide *et al., Exp. Neurol.* **121**, 200-214 (1993).

Brain-derived neurotrophic factor. BDNF. 119 Amino acid peptide; mol wt ~13.5 kDa. pI ~9.99. Localized primarily, but not exclusively, in CNS. Amino acid sequence identical in human, pig, mouse and rat. Exhibits ~50% sequence homology with NGF.

Neurotrophin-3. [130939-66-1] NT-3; HDNF; hippocampal-derived neurotrophic factor; nerve growth factor-2; NGF-2; neuronotrophin-3. 119 Amino acid peptide; mol wt ~13.5 kDa. pI ~9.5. Produced primarily in peripheral tissues; also produced in the CNS. Amino acid sequence identical in human, mouse and rat. Exhibits ~57% sequence homology with NGF; ~58% homology with BDNF.

6488. Neutral Red. [553-24-2]; [366-13-2] (free base). N^8,-N^8,3-Trimethyl-2,8-phenazinediamine monohydrochloride; C.I. Basic Red 5; 3-amino-7-dimethylamino-2-methylphenazine hydrochloride; toluylene red; neutral red chloride; nuclear fast red (basic dye); aminodimethylaminotoluaminozine hydrochloride; C.I. 50040; Kernechtrot; Michrome no. 226. $C_{15}H_{17}ClN_4$; mol wt 288.78. C 62.39%, H 5.93%, Cl 12.28%, N 19.40%. Prepn from *N,N*-dimethyl-*p*-nitrosoaniline hydrochloride + toluene-2,4-diamine: Witt, *Ber.* **12**, 931 (1879); **DE 15272** (1880), *Frdl.* **1**, 274; Bernthsen, Schweitzer, *Ann.* **236**, 332 (1886); Pokorny, *J. Soc. Dyers Colour.* **42**, 347 (1926). Toxicity data: F. Stolarsky, T. J. Haley, *Fed. Proc.* **10**, 337 (1951). Brief review: *H. J. Conn's Biological Stains*, R. D. Lillie, Ed. (Williams & Wilkins, Baltimore, 9th ed., 1977) pp 377-380, 596. *See also: Colour Index* vol. 4 (3rd ed., 1971) p 4446.

Dark green powder. Absorption max (50% alc): 533 nm. pKa 6.7. Soluble in water or alcohol with red color. Soly in water 4.0%, in abs alcohol 1.8%, in Cellosolve 3.75%, in ethylene glycol 3.0%. Practically insol in xylene. LD_{50} in mice, rats, rabbits (mg/kg): 142, 112, 97 i.v. (Stolarsky, Haley).

Note: Not to be confused with *Nuclear Fast Red (acid dye)* which is *C.I. 60760*.

USE: As indicator (0.1% in 60% alcohol) for alkalinity of water, urea, nitrite, etc. pH: 6.8 red; 8.0 yellow. Also used for preparing neutral-red paper. As biological stain (study of the Golgi apparatus in cells).

6489. Neutral Spirits. Distilled from suitable raw materials, is 95% ethanol (v/v) meaning that it is at least 190 proof when distilled. Used for blending with straight whisky (*see* Whisky) and for making gin, cordials, liqueurs and vodka. It may be made from grain or molasses or by redistillation of other beverages, such as brandy or rum, and is almost colorless and contains no extraneous flavoring.

6490. Nevirapine. [129618-40-2] 11-Cyclopropyl-5,11-dihydro-4-methyl-6*H*-dipyrido[3,2-*b*:2′,3′-*e*][1,4]diazepin-6-one; BI-RG-587; Viramune. $C_{15}H_{14}N_4O$; mol wt 266.30. C 67.65%, H 5.30%, N 21.04%, O 6.01%. Non-nucleoside reverse transcriptase inhibitor (NNRTI) of the dipyridodiazepinone class. Prepn: K. D. Hargrave *et al.*, **EP 429987** (1991 to Boehringer, Ing; Thomae); *eidem*, **US 5366972** (1994 to Boehringer, Ing.); *eidem, J. Med. Chem.* **34**, 2231 (1991). Inhibition of HIV-1 reverse transcriptase: V. J. Merluzzi *et al., Science* **250**, 1411 (1990). Studies of structure-activity and binding site: P. M. Grob *et al., AIDS Res. Hum. Retroviruses* **8**, 145 (1992). HPLC determn in serum: R. M. Lopez *et al., J. Chromatogr. B* **751**, 371 (2001). Clinical pharmacokinetics: S. H. Cheeseman *et al., Antimicrob. Agents Chemother.* **37**, 178 (1993). Review of clinical experience: A. Carr, D. A. Cooper, *Adv. Exp. Med. Biol.* **394**, 299-304 (1996); of safety profile: R. B. Pollard *et al., Clin. Ther.* **20**, 1071-1092 (1998). Clinical trial in prevention of perinatal HIV-1 transmission: L. A. Guay *et al., Lancet* **354**, 795 (1999).

Crystals from pyridine + water, mp 247-249°. pKa 2.8. Lipophilic. Soly in water ~0.1 mg/ml at neutral pH; highly sol at pH<3.

THERAP CAT: Antiviral.

6491. Nialamide. [51-12-7] 4-Pyridinecarboxylic acid 2-[3-oxo-3-[(phenylmethyl)amino]propyl]hydrazide; 1-[2-(benzylcarbamoyl)ethyl]-2-isonicotinoylhydrazide; *N*-[2-(benzylcarbamyl)ethylamino]isonicotinamide; *N*-benzyl-β-(isonicotinoylhydrazino)propionamide; *N*-isonicotinoyl-*N*′-[β-(*N*-benzylcarboxamido)ethyl]hydrazide; isonicotinic acid 2-[2-(benzylcarbamoyl)ethyl]hydrazide; Espril; Niamid; Niamidal; Niaquitil; Nuredal; Nyazin. C_{16}-$H_{18}N_4O_2$; mol wt 298.34. C 64.41%, H 6.08%, N 18.78%, O 10.73%. Monoamine oxidase (MAO) inhibitor. Prepn: Bloom, Carnahan, **US 2894972**; **US 3040061** (1959, 1962 both to Pfizer). Toxicology study: C. S. Delahunt, J. M. Pepin, *Toxicol. Appl. Pharmacol.* **1**, 524 (1959).

Slightly bitter crystals from ethyl acetate, mp 151.1-152.1°. Sparingly sol in water; freely sol in acidic solvents. LD_{50} in mice, rats (mg/kg): 1000, 1700 orally; 742, 760 i.p. (Delahunt).

THERAP CAT: Antidepressant.

6492. Niaprazine. [27367-90-4] N-[3-[4-(4-Fluorophenyl)-1-piperazinyl]-1-methylpropyl]-3-pyridinecarboxamide; N-[3-[4-(p-fluorophenyl)-1-piperazinyl]-1-methylpropyl]nicotinamide; Nopron. $C_{20}H_{25}FN_4O$; mol wt 356.44. C 67.39%, H 7.07%, F 5.33%, N 15.72%, O 4.49%. Prepn: R. Y. Mauvernay, **DE 1957371** corresp to **US 3712893** (1970, 1973 both to CERM). Pharmacology: P. Duchene-Marrullaz et al., Therapie **26**, 1203 (1971). Psycholeptic effects in mice: J. Hache, J. Tachon, J. Pharmacol. **7**, 469 (1976). Brain catecholamine depletion: P. E. Keane, M. S. Benedetti, Neuropharmacology **18**, 595 (1979).

Cryst from ethyl acetate, mp 131°. Photosensitive. LD_{50} in mice (mg/kg): 890 orally, 145 i.v. (Mauvernay).

THERAP CAT: Sedative; hypnotic.

6493. Nicaraven. [79455-30-4] N,N'-(1-Methyl-1,2-ethanediyl)bis-3-pyridinecarboxamide; 1,2-bis(nicotinamido)propane; (±)-N,N'-propylenedinicotinamide; AVS; Antevas. $C_{15}H_{16}N_4O_2$; mol wt 284.31. C 63.37%, H 5.67%, N 19.71%, O 11.25%. Hydroxyl radical scavenger. Prepn: T. Mori et al., **EP 29602**; eidem, **US 4366161** (1981, 1982 both to Chugai); T. Doi et al., Synlett **1999**, 1751. Effect on human platelet aggregation: T. Komiya et al., Clin. Neuropharmacol. **22**, 11 (1999). Clinical trial in subarachnoid hemorrhage: T. Asano et al., J. Neurosurg. **84**, 792 (1996). Review: K. K. Jain, Expert Opin. Invest. Drugs **9**, 859-870 (2000).

Crystals from ethyl acetate, mp 156-157°. Sol in water.

THERAP CAT: In treatment of vasospasm following subarachnoid hemorrhage.

6494. Nicarbazin. [330-95-0] N,N'-Bis(4-nitrophenyl)urea, compd with 4,6-dimethyl-2(1H)-pyrimidinone (1:1); 4,4'-dinitrocarbanilide compd with 4,6-dimethyl-2-pyrimidinol (1:1); Nicarb; Nicoxin; Nicrazin. $C_{19}H_{18}N_6O_6$; mol wt 426.38. C 53.52%, H 4.26%, N 19.71%, O 22.51%. Prepn: Cuckler et al., Science **122**, 244 (1955); Basso, O'Neill, **US 2731382**; **US 2731383**; **US 2731384** (all 1956 to Merck & Co.). Effect on nutritional encephalopathy in chicks: I. Bartov, P. Budowski, Poult. Sci. **58**, 597 (1979).

Crystals, dec 265-275°. uv max (concd H_2SO_4): 298 nm ($A_{1cm}^{1\%}$ 670). Practically insol in water. Complex is slowly dec by tritu-

ration with water, or more rapidly by dil aq acids. The dry crystals are strongly electrostatic and present some dry-mixing problems.

THERAP CAT (VET): Coccidiostat.

6495. Nicardipine. [55985-32-5] 1,4-Dihydro-2,6-dimethyl-4-(3-nitrophenyl)-3,5-pyridinedicarboxylic acid methyl 2-[methyl(phenylmethyl)amino]ethyl ester. $C_{26}H_{29}N_3O_6$; mol wt 479.52. C 65.12%, H 6.10%, N 8.76%, O 20.02%. Dihydropyridine calcium channel blocker. Prepn: M. Murakami et al., **BE 811324**; eidem, **US 3985758** (1974, 1976 both to Yamanouchi); M. Iwanami et al., Chem. Pharm. Bull. **27**, 1426 (1979). Vasodilator profile: T. Takenaka et al., Arzneim.-Forsch. **26**, 2172 (1976). Absorption, excretion, metabolism: S. Higuchi et al., Xenobiotica **7**, 469 (1977). Clinical pharmacology: T. Seki, T. Takenaka, Int. J. Clin. Pharmacol. Biopharm. **15**, 267 (1977). Mechanism of action: K. Satoh et al., Clin. Exp. Pharmacol. Physiol. **7**, 249 (1980). Acute toxicity study: Y. Odani, T. Sado, Oyo Yakuri **18**, 301 (1979), C.A. **92**, 104384u (1980). Symposium: Br. J. Clin. Pharmacol. **20**, Suppl. 1, 1S-208S (1985). Clinical synergy with captopril, q.v.: K. A. Conrad et al., Clin. Pharmacol. Ther. **42**, 113 (1987). Review of pharmacodynamics, pharmacokinetics and therapeutic efficacy: E. M. Sorkin, S. P. Clissold, Drugs **33**, 296-345 (1987).

Hydrochloride. [54527-84-3] RS-69216; YC-93; Antagonil; Barizin; Bionicard; Cardene; Dacarel; Lecibral; Lescodil; Loxen; Nerdipina; Nicant; Nicardal; Nicarpin; Nicapress; Nicodel; Nimicor; Perdipina; Perdipine; Ranvil; Ridene; Rycarden; Rydene; Vasodin; Vasonase. $C_{26}H_{29}N_3O_6$·HCl; mol wt 515.99. Isolated in two crystalline forms from acetone. α-form: mp 179-181°; β-form: mp 168-170°. The forms also have different IR and x-ray diffraction patterns. LD_{50} in male, female rats (mg/kg): 634, 557 orally; 18.1, 25.0 i.v.; in male, female mice: 634, 650 orally; 20.7, 19.9 i.v. (Odani, Sado).

THERAP CAT: Antianginal; antihypertensive.

6496. Nicergoline. [27848-84-6] (8β)-10-Methoxy-1,6-dimethylergoline-8-methanol 5-bromo-3-pyridinecarboxylate (ester); 1-methyllumilysergol 8-(5-bromonicotinate) 10-methyl ether; 4,6,6a,7,8,9,10,10a-octahydro-10aα-methoxy-4,7-dimethylindolo[4,3-fg]quinoline-9-methanol 5-bromonicotinate; 8β-[(5-bromonicotinoyloxy)methyl]-1,6-dimethyl-10α-methoxyergoline; nicotergoline; nimergoline; MNE; FI-6714; Cergodum; Circo-Maren; Dilasenil; Duracebrol; Ergotop; Ergobel; Memoq; Nicergolent; Sermion; Vasospan. $C_{24}H_{26}BrN_3O_3$; mol wt 484.39. C 59.51%, H 5.41%, Br 16.50%, N 8.67%, O 9.91%. Prepn: Bernardi et al., **US 3228943**; Temperilli, **DE 2112273** (1966, 1971, both to Farmitalia); Arcari et al., Experientia **28**, 819 (1972). Series of articles on pharmacology, clinical studies, tolerability: Arzneim.-Forsch. **29**, 1213-1316 (1979). Toxicity study: B. W. Neumann, F. Lauschner, ibid. 1206. Hemodynamic effects in the dog: ibid. **31**, 1693 (1981). Use in acute myocardial infarction with diastolic hypertension: E. Triulzi et al., Farmaco Ed. Prat. **36**, 449 (1981).

mp 136-138°. LD$_{50}$ in male mice, rats (mg/kg): 860, 2800 orally; 46, 43 i.v. (Neumann, Lauschner).

THERAP CAT: Vasodilator (cerebral, peripheral).

6497. Niceritrol. [5868-05-3] 3-Pyridinecarboxylic acid 2,2-bis[[(3-pyridinylcarbonyl)oxy]methyl]-1,3-propanediyl ester; nicotinic acid neopentanetetrayl ester; pentaerythritol tetranicotinate; 8-AL; Perycit; Bufor. C$_{29}$H$_{24}$N$_4$O$_8$; mol wt 556.52. C 62.59%, H 4.35%, N 10.07%, O 23.00%. Prepn: FR M2046 (1963 to Soc. d'Etudes et de Recherches Pharmacotechniques), *C.A.* **60**, 10656e (1964); GB 1022880; GB 1053689 (1966, 1967 to Aktiebolag Bofors), *C.A.* **64**, 19708d (1966), *C.A.* **66**, 104907e (1967); Kuriyama, Kudo, JP 67 2359 (1967 to Yoshitomi), *C.A.* **66**, 115935p (1967). Acute toxicity data: T. Sugawara *et al., Oyo Yakuri* **14**, 741 (1977), *C.A.* **88**, 131005v (1977).

Crystals, mp reported as 160-162° and as 163-164°. LD$_{50}$ in mice, rats (g/kg): >20, >20 orally; >5, >5 s.c.; >5, >5 i.p.; in rabbits (g/kg): >10 orally; >5 i.p. (Sugawara).

THERAP CAT: Antilipemic.

6498. Nickel. [7440-02-0] Ni; at. wt 58.6934; at. no. 28; valence 2; seldom 1, 3, 4. Group VIII (10). Naturally occurring isotopes (mass numbers): 58 (68.27%), 60 (26.10%), 61 (1.13%), 62 (3.59%), 64 (0.91%); known artificial radioactive isotopes: 53, 55-57, 59 (longest-lived known isotope, T$_{1/2}$ 7.5 × 10^4 years, decay by electron capture), 63, 65-67. Abundance in earth's crust 99 ppm. Discovered by Cronstedt in 1754: Cronstedt, *Mineralogie* (Stockholm, 1758) p 218. Isoln: Berthier, *Ann. Chim. Phys.* [2] **14**, 52 (1820); **25**, 94 (1824). Occurs free in meteorites. Found in many ores as sulfides, arsenides, antimonides and oxides or silicates; chief sources include chalcopyrite, *q.v.,* pyrrhotite, *pentlandite* [(Fe,Ni)$_9$-S$_8$] and *garnierite* [3(Mg,Ni)O.2SiO$_2$.2H$_2$O]; other ores include *niccolite* (NiAs) and *millerite* (NiS). Methods of extraction and purification: Mackiw, *Can. J. Chem. Eng.* **46**, 3 (1968); Houot, *Ann. Mines* **1969** (April), 9; Queneau, *J. Met.* **22**, 44-48 (1970). Prepn of high purity nickel: Wise, Schaefer, *Metals Alloys* **16**, 424 (1924); from NiO and H$_2$: Glemser in *Handbook of Preparative Inorganic Chemistry* vol. 2, G. Brauer, Ed. (Academic Press, New York, 2nd ed., 1965) pp 1543-1544; by electrolysis: Vu Quang Kinh, Nardin, *C.R. Seances Acad. Sci. Ser. C* **266**, 307 (1968). Comprehensive reviews: *Gmelins, Nickel* (8th ed.) **57**, 5 vols, about 3500 pp (1965-1967); Nicholls in *Comprehensive Inorganic Chemistry* vol. 3, J. C. Bailar, Jr. *et al.,* Eds. (Pergamon Press, Oxford, 1973) pp 1109-1161; J. K. Tien, T. E. Howson in *Kirk-Othmer Encyclopedia of Chemical Technology* vol. 15 (Wiley-Interscience, New York, 3rd ed., 1981) pp 787-801; *Chemistry of the Elements* N. N. Greenwood, A. Earnshaw, Eds. (Pergamon Press, New York, 1984) pp 1328-1363. Book: *Nickel Toxicology,* S. S. Brown, F. W. Sunderman, Eds. (Academic Press, New York, 1980) 193 pp. Review of carcinogenic risk: *IARC Monographs* **11**, 75-112 (1976); of toxicology and human exposure: *Toxicological Profile for Nickel* (PB2006-100005, 2005) 397 pp.

Lustrous white, hard, ferromagnetic metal; face-centered cubic crystals. mp 1453°. bp (calc) 2732°. Also reported as bp (calc) 2837° (3110 K): D. R. Stull, G. C. Sinke, *Thermodynamic Properties of the Elements,* Advances in Chemistry Series **18** (A.C.S., Washington, 1956). d 8.908. Heat capacity (25°) 6.23 cal/g-atom/°C. Mohs' hardness 3.8. Latent heat of fusion 73 cal/g. Electrical resistivity (20°): 6.844 μohms-cm. E°(aq) Ni/Ni^{2+} 0.250 V. Stable in air at ordinary temp; burns in oxygen, forming NiO; not affected by water; decomposes steam at a red heat. Slowly attacked by dil hydrochloric or sulfuric acid; readily attacked by nitric acid. Not attacked by fused alkali hydroxides.

Caution: Potential symptoms of overexposure are sensitization dermatitis, allergic asthma, pneumonitis. *See NIOSH Pocket Guide to Chemical Hazards* (DHHS/NIOSH 97-140, 1997) p 224. *See also Patty's Industrial Hygiene and Toxicology* vol. 2C, G. D. Clayton, F. E. Clayton, Eds. (John Wiley & Sons, New York, 4th ed., 1994) 2157-2173. Metallic nickel is reasonably anticipated to be a human carcinogen; nickel compounds are listed as known human carcinogens: *Report on Carcinogens, Eleventh Edition* (PB2005-104914, 2004) p III-181.

USE: Nickel-plating; for various alloys such as new silver, Chinese silver, German silver; for coins, electrotypes, storage batteries; magnets, lightning-rod tips, electrical contacts and electrodes, spark plugs, machinery parts; catalyst for hydrogenation of oils and other organic substances. *See also* Raney nickel. Manuf of Monel metal, stainless steels, heat resistant steels, heat and corrosion resistant alloys, nickel-chrome resistance wire; in alloys for electronic and space applications.

6499. Nickel Acetate. [373-02-4] C$_4$H$_6$NiO$_4$; mol wt 176.78. C 27.18%, H 3.42%, Ni 33.20%, O 36.20%. Ni(CH$_3$-CO$_2$)$_2$. Review of toxicology and human exposure: *Toxicological Profile for Nickel* (PB2006-100005, 2005) 397 pp.

Tetrahydrate. Green, cryst mass or powder; acetic odor. d 1.744. Sol in 6 parts water, in alcohol. *Keep well closed.*

Caution: Nickel compounds are listed as known human carcinogens: *Report on Carcinogens, Eleventh Edition* (PB2005-104914, 2004) p III-181.

USE: Catalyst; mordant for textiles.

6500. Nickel Acetylacetonate. [3264-82-2] Bis(2,4-pentanedionato-*O,O'*)nickel; bisacetylacetonatonickel(II); bis(2,4-pentanediono)nickel(II); 2,4-pentanedione nickel complex. C$_{10}$H$_{14}$-NiO$_4$; mol wt 256.91. C 46.75%, H 5.49%, Ni 22.85%, O 24.91%. Ni(CH$_3$COCHCOCH$_3$)$_2$. Also Ni(acac)$_2$ or Ni(AA)$_2$. Prepn from acetylacetone and Ni(OH)$_2$: Gach, *Monatsh. Chem.* **21**, 103 (1900); from acetylacetone and NiCl$_2$.6H$_2$O: Charles, Pawlikowski, *J. Phys. Chem.* **62**, 440 (1958); from 4-diethylamino-3-pentene-2-one and NiCl$_2$.6H$_2$O: Gash, *Can. J. Chem.* **45**, 2109 (1967). *See also* Fernelius, Bryant, *Inorg. Synth.* **5**, 105 (1957). Exists as a trimer in the solid state: Bullen, *Nature* **177**, 537 (1956); Bullen *et al., Inorg. Chem.* **4**, 456 (1965); as a monomer in the vapor phase: Fackler *et al., J. Phys. Chem.* **72**, 4631 (1972). Structure of dihydrate: Montgomery, Lingafelter, *Acta Crystallogr.* **17**, 1481 (1964).

Emerald-green orthorhombic crystals. mp 229-230°. bp$_{11}$ 220-235°. d^{17} 1.455. uv max (10^{-4}M in CHCl$_3$): 298, 265 nm (log ε 4.34, 4.44). Sol in water, alcohol, chloroform, benzene. Insol in ether, ligroin.

USE: Catalyst.

6501. Nickel Ammonium Sulfate. [15699-18-0] Sulfuric acid ammonium nickel(2+) salt (2:2:1); ammonium nickel sulfate; diammonium nickel disulfate; H$_8$N$_2$NiO$_8$S$_2$; mol wt 286.90. H 2.81%, N 9.76%, Ni 20.46%, O 44.61%, S 22.35%. Ni(NH$_4$)$_2$-(SO$_4$)$_2$. Physical properties of aqueous solns: J. W. Mullin, M. M. Osman, *J. Chem. Eng. Data* **12**, 516 (1967); and crystal growth rates: *eidem, ibid.* **18**, 353 (1973). Toxicity study: E. L. Reagan, *J. Am. Coll. Toxicol.* **11**, 694 (1992). Crystal structure of hexahydrate: T. H. Tahirov, T.-H. Lu, *Acta Crystallogr.* **C50**, 668 (1994); and thermo-stability and optical transmission properties: G. Su *et al., J. Phys. D: Appl. Phys.* **35**, 2652 (2002). Review of toxicology and human exposure: *Toxicological Profile for Nickel* (PB2006-100005, 2005) 397 pp.

Hexahydrate. [7785-20-8] Deep-green crystalline powder. d 1.923. d^{20} (satd soln): 1.050. Viscosity of satd soln: 1.2×10^{-3} N sec/m^2. Soly in water (g anhydrous salt/100 g water) at 10°: 5.19; at 25°: 7.52; at 40°: 10.9. Insol in alcohol. LD$_{50}$ orally in rats: 418 mg/kg (Reagan).

USE: Formerly in electroplating metals.

6502. Nickel Bromide. [13462-88-9] Nickel dibromide. Br$_2$Ni; mol wt 218.50. Br 73.14%, Ni 26.86%. NiBr$_2$.

Trihydrate. Yellowish-green, very deliquesc crystals; loses its water at about 200°, the anhydr salt is a golden-yellow color and sublimable in absence of air. Sol in one part water, in alcohol. *Keep well closed.*

6503. Nickel Carbonate Hydroxide. [12607-70-4] CH_4-Ni_3O_7; mol wt 304.12. C 3.95%, H 1.33%, Ni 57.90%, O 36.83%. $NiCO_3 \cdot 2Ni(OH)_2$. Tetrahydrate occurs in nature as the mineral *zaratite*. Review of toxicology and human exposure: *Toxicological Profile for Nickel* (PB2006-100005, 2005) 397 pp.

Tetrahydrate. Green, odorless powder. Insol in water. Sol in ammonia and in dil acids with effervescence.

Caution: Nickel compounds are listed as known human carcinogens: *Report on Carcinogens, Eleventh Edition* (PB2005-104914, 2004) p III-181.

USE: Nickel-plating; catalyst for hardening of fats; in ceramic colors and glazes.

6504. Nickel Carbonyl. [13463-39-3] Nickel tetracarbonyl. C_4NiO_4; mol wt 170.73. C 28.14%, Ni 34.38%, O 37.48%. $Ni(CO)_4$. Intermediate in nickel refining. Made by passing carbon monoxide over finely divided nickel: Mond *et al., J. Chem. Soc.* **57**, 749 (1890); Gilliland, Blanchard, *Inorg. Synth.* **2**, 234 (1946). Use of nickel carbonyl in organic synthesis: G. Wilke *et al., Angew. Chem. Int. Ed.* **5**, 151 (1966); M. F. Semmelhack in *Organic Reactions* **vol. 19** (Wiley, New York, 1972) p 115; E. J. Corey, H. A. Kirst, *J. Am. Chem. Soc.* **94**, 667 (1972). Kinetic studies: D. H. Stedman *et al., Science* **208**, 1029 (1980). Toxicity study: Hackett, Sunderman, *Arch. Environ. Health* **14**, 604 (1967). *Review:* Nicholls in *Comprehensive Inorganic Chemistry* **vol. 3**, J. C. Bailar, Jr. *et al.,* Eds. (Pergamon Press, Oxford, 1973) pp 1115-1119.

Colorless, volatile liquid. *Poisonous!* Oxidizes in the air: explodes at about 60°. d^{17} 1.318. bp 43°. mp −19.3°. Crit temp about 200°. Crit pressure about 30 atm. Sol in about 5000 parts water free from air; sol in alcohol, benzene, chloroform, acetone, carbon tetrachloride. LD_{50} in rats (mg/kg): 39 i.p.; 63 s.c.; 66 i.v. (Hackett, Sunderman).

Caution: Potential symptoms of overexposure are headache, vertigo; nausea, vomiting, epigastric pain; substernal pain; cough, hyperpnea; cyanosis; weakness; leukocytosis; pneumonitis; delirium; convulsions. See *NIOSH Pocket Guide to Chemical Hazards* (DHHS/NIOSH 97-140, 1997) p 222. *See also Clinical Toxicology of Commercial Products,* R. E. Gosselin *et al.,* Eds. (Williams & Wilkins, Baltimore, 5th ed., 1984) Section II, p. 145. Nickel compounds are listed as known human carcinogens: *Report on Carcinogens, Eleventh Edition* (PB2005-104914, 2004) p III-181.

USE: In organic synthesis; production of high-purity nickel powder and continuous nickel coatings on steel and other metals.

6505. Nickel Chloride. [7718-54-9] Nickel dichloride. Cl_2Ni; mol wt 129.60. Cl 54.71%, Ni 45.29%. $NiCl_2$. Evaluation of carcinogenic risk: *IARC Monographs* **49**, 257-445 (1990). Review of toxicology and human exposure: *Toxicological Profile for Nickel* (PB2006-100005, 2005) 397 pp.

Yellow deliquescent scales. Soly in water (g/l): 642 (20°), 876 (100°). Sol in ethanol, ammonium hydroxide. Insol in nitric acid. Sublimable in absence of air and readily absorbs NH_3. The aq soln is acid; pH about 4. *Keep well closed.* LD_{50} in mice, rats (mg/kg): 48, 11 i.p. (IARC).

Hexahydrate. [7791-20-0] Green, deliquesc crystals or cryst powder. Monoclinic. Structure reported to be *trans*-$[NiCl_2(H_2O)_4] \cdot 2H_2O$: Mizuno, *J. Phys. Soc. Jpn.* **16**, 1574 (1960), *C.A.* **55**, 26605g (1961). Sol in about one part water, in alcohol.

Caution: Nickel compounds are listed as known human carcinogens: *Report on Carcinogens, Eleventh Edition* (PB2005-104914, 2004) p III-181.

USE: Anhydr salt as absorbent for NH_3 in gas masks. Hexahydrate for nickel electroplating; manuf nickel catalysts.

6506. Nickel Cyanide. [557-19-7] C_2N_2Ni; mol wt 110.73. C 21.69%, N 25.30%, Ni 53.01%. $Ni(CN)_2$. Prepn of yellow-brown anhydr salt: Aynsley, Campbell, *J. Chem. Soc.* **1958**, 1723. The commercial salt usually contains 20-25% water. Review of toxicology and human exposure: *Toxicological Profile for Nickel* (PB2006-100005, 2005) 397 pp.

Tetrahydrate. Apple-green powder. *Poison!* Insol in water. Slightly sol in dil acids, freely in alkali cyanides, in ammonia, and in ammonium carbonate.

USE: In nickel-plating.

6507. Nickel Dimethylglyoxime. [13478-93-8] Bis[(2,3-butanedione dioximato)(1−)-*N,N'*]nickel; bis(dimethylglyoximato)nickel. $C_8H_{14}N_4NiO_4$; mol wt 288.91. C 33.26%, H 4.88%, N 19.39%, Ni 20.32%, O 22.15%. Prepn: Banks *et al., J. Am. Chem. Soc.* **77**, 324 (1955); F. J. Welcher, *Organic Analytical Reagents* **vol. 3** (Van Nostrand, New York, 1947) pp 165-179; Thabet *et al., Inorg. Nucl. Chem. Lett.* **8**, 211 (1972). Structure: Godycki, Rundle, *Acta Crystallogr.* **6**, 487 (1953); Merritt, *Anal. Chem.* **25**, 718 (1953).

Scarlet-red, cryst powder. Sublimes at 250°. Insol in water, acetic acid, ammonia. Sol in dil mineral acids and appreciably sol in abs alcohol.

USE: As sun-fast pigment in paints, lacquers, cellulose compounds and cosmetics.

6508. Nickel Fluoride. [10028-18-9] Nickel difluoride; nickelous fluoride. F_2Ni; mol wt 96.69. F 39.30%, Ni 60.70%. NiF_2. Prepn: Henkel, Klemm, *Z. Anorg. Allg. Chem.* **222**, 74 (1935); Priest, *Inorg. Synth.* **3**, 173 (1950); Rochow, Kukin, *J. Am. Chem. Soc.* **74**, 1615 (1952); Haendler *et al., ibid.* 3167. Book: *Medical and Biologic Effects of Environmental Pollutants: Nickel* (National Acad. Sci., Washington DC, 1975) 277 pp.

Yellowish to green tetragonal crystals (rutile type). d 4.72. Sublimes in HF stream above 1000°. Slightly sol in water (4 g/100 ml at 25°). Aq solns are dec by boiling. Insol in alcohol, ether. LD_{50} i.v. in mice: 130 mg/kg (Nat. Acad. Sci.).

Caution: Chronic exposure may cause mottling of teeth, changes in bones.

6509. Nickel Formate. [3349-06-2] $C_2H_2NiO_4$; mol wt 148.73. C 16.15%, H 1.36%, Ni 39.46%, O 43.03%. $Ni(HCOO)_2$. Prepd by reaction of formic acid with Ni: Johnson, **US 2576072** (1951 to Harshaw Chemical); with $NiCO_3$: Bircumshaw, Edwards, *J. Chem. Soc.* **1950**, 1800.

Dihydrate. Fine, green, monoclinic crystals. Becomes anhydr on careful heating to 130-140°; decomposes at 180-200° yielding Ni, CO, CO_2, H_2, H_2O, CH_4. $d^{20.2}$ 2.154. Moderately sol in water. Practically insol in alc, formic acid.

USE: Manuf of Ni; prepn of Ni catalysts for organic reactions, particularly hydrogenation catalysts.

6510. Nickel Hydroxide. [12054-48-7] "Green nickel oxide". H_2NiO_2; mol wt 92.71. H 2.17%, Ni 63.31%, O 34.51%. $Ni(OH)_2$.

Monohydrate. Apple-green powder. Decomp above 200° to form NiO and H_2O. Insol in water. Sol in dil acids, in ammonia.

Caution: Nickel compounds are listed as known human carcinogens: *Report on Carcinogens, Eleventh Edition* (PB2005-104914, 2004) p III-181.

6511. Nickel Iodide. [13462-90-3] Nickel diiodide. I_2Ni; mol wt 312.50. I 81.22%, Ni 18.78%. NiI_2.

Iron-black color. Sublimes in absence of air. Hexahydrate, bluish-green very deliquesc crystals. Very sol in water or alcohol. *Keep well closed.*

6512. Nickel Monoxide. [1313-99-1] Nickel oxide (NiO); nickel(II) oxide; nickelous oxide; nickel protoxide. NiO; mol wt 74.69. Ni 78.58%, O 21.42%. Occurs as the mineral *bunsenite*. Review of toxicology and human exposure: *Toxicological Profile for Nickel* (PB2006-100005, 2005) 397 pp.

Green powder; yellow when hot. Insol in water. Sol in acids.

Caution: Nickel compounds are listed as known human carcinogens: *Report on Carcinogens, Eleventh Edition* (PB2005-104914, 2004) p III-181.

USE: Painting on porcelain.

6513. Nickel Nitrate. [13138-45-9] N_2NiO_6; mol wt 182.70. N 15.33%, Ni 32.13%, O 52.54%. $Ni(NO_3)_2$. Toxicity study: H. F. Smyth *et al., Am. Ind. Hyg. Assoc. J.* **30**, 470 (1969).

Review of toxicology and human exposure: *Toxicological Profile for Nickel* (PB2006-100005, 2005) 397 pp.

Hexahydrate. Green, deliquesc crystals. d 2.05. mp 56.7°. bp 137°. Sol in 0.4 part water, in alcohol. The aq soln is acid; pH about 4. *Keep well closed.* LD$_{50}$ orally in rats: 1.62 g/kg (Smyth).

USE: Nickel-plating; manuf brown ceramic colors.

6514. Nickel Oxalate. [547-67-1] C$_2$NiO$_4$; mol wt 146.71. C 16.37%, Ni 40.01%, O 43.62%. NiC$_2$O$_4$.

Dihydrate, light green powder. Insol in water; sol in mineral acids, in solns of ammonium chloride, nitrate, or sulfate.

6515. Nickel Phosphate. [10381-36-9] Ni$_3$O$_8$P$_2$; mol wt 366.02. Ni 48.11%, O 34.97%, P 16.92%. Ni$_3$(PO$_4$)$_2$.

Octahydrate, light green powder. Insol in water; sol in acids, ammonia.

USE: On ignition yields "nickel yellow"—a pigment used in oil and water colors.

6516. Nickel Sesquioxide. [1314-06-3] Nickelic oxide; black nickel oxide. Ni$_2$O$_3$; mol wt 165.39. Ni 70.98%, O 29.02%. Contains a variable quantity of water.

Gray-black powder. Dec at ~600° into NiO and oxygen. Insol in water; very slightly sol in cold acid; dissolved by hot HCl with evolution of Cl, and by hot H$_2$SO$_4$ or HNO$_3$ with evolution of oxygen.

6517. Nickel Sulfate. [7786-81-4] Sulfuric acid nickel(2+) salt (1:1). NiO$_4$S; mol wt 154.76. Ni 37.93%, O 41.35%, S 20.72%. NiSO$_4$. Soly study: F. C. Vilbrandt, J. A. Bender, *Ind. Eng. Chem.* **15**, 967 (1923). Specific gravity, viscosity, and soly of aqueous solns of α-hexahydrate: V. R. Phillips, *J. Chem. Eng. Data* **17**, 357 (1972). Thermal dehydration study of α-hexahydrate: N. Koga, H. Tanaka, *J. Phys. Chem.* **98**, 10521 (1994). Acute toxicity data: E. L. Reagan, *J. Am. Coll. Toxicol.* **1**, 685 (1992). Evaluation of carcinogenic risk: *IARC Monographs* **49**, 257-445 (1990); *Toxicology and Carcinogenesis Studies* (NTP TR-454, NIH 96-3370, 1996) 379 pp. Use in patch testing for nickel allergies: V. Simonetti *et al.*, *Contact Dermatitis* **39**, 187 (1998). Review of toxicology and human exposure: *Toxicological Profile for Nickel* (PB2006-100005, 2005) 397 pp.

Pale green to yellow crystals; dec at 848°. Soly at 20° (g/l): water 293. Insol in ethanol, diethyl ether.

Hexahydrate. [10101-97-0] Two known phases. α-Form, blue to blue-green tetragonal crystals; transition to β-form at 53.3°. β-Form, green transparent crystals. α-Form is more stable; commercially available. d 2.07. Soly in water of α-form (g anhydrous salt/100 g water) at 50.00°: 52.267; of β-form at 60.11°: 55.557. Sol in ethanol. pH of 5% soln at 25°: 3.8. LD$_{50}$ in male, female rats (mg/kg): 335, 264 orally (Reagan).

Heptahydrate. [10101-98-1] Green, orthorhombic crystals; efflorescent. Soly in water (g anhydrous salt/100 g water) at 0.00°: 26.189; at 25.00°: 40.469. Sol in ethanol.

Caution: Nickel compounds are listed as known human carcinogens: *Report on Carcinogens, Eleventh Edition* (PB2005-104914, 2004) p III-181.

USE: In electrolytic and electroless nickel-plating; as mordant in dyeing; in catalyst mfr; in prepn of other nickel compds.

THERAP CAT: Diagnostic aid (contact allergen).

6518. Niclofolan. [10331-57-4] 5,5'-Dichloro-3,3'-dinitro-[1,1'-biphenyl]-2,2'-diol; 4,4'-dichloro-6,6'-dinitro-*o,o*'-biphenol; 5,5'-dichloro-2,2'-dihydroxy-3,3'-dinitrobiphenyl; menichlopholan; Bayer 9015; ME-3625; Bilevon-M. C$_{12}$H$_6$Cl$_2$N$_2$O$_6$; mol wt 345.09. C 41.77%, H 1.75%, Cl 20.55%, N 8.12%, O 27.82%. Anthelmintic activity: Meiser, Federmann, US 3082151 (1963 to Bayer); P. J. Lane, J. M. Stewart, *Vet. Rec.* **80**, 702 (1967). Pharmacokinetics in desert sheep: B. H. Ali *et al.*, *J. Vet. Pharmacol. Ther.* **13**, 217 (1990).

THERAP CAT (VET): Anthelmintic (fasciolicide).

6519. Niclosamide. [50-65-7] 5-Chloro-*N*-(2-chloro-4-nitrophenyl)-2-hydroxybenzamide; 2',5-dichloro-4'-nitrosalicylanilide; 5-chloro-*N*-(2'-chloro-4'-nitrophenyl)salicylamide; 5-chlorosalicyloyl-(*o*-chloro-*p*-nitranilide); *N*-(2'-chloro-4'-nitrophenyl)-5-chlorosalicylamide; Bayer 2353; Cestocide; Niclocide; Ruby; Trédémine; Yomesan. C$_{13}$H$_8$Cl$_2$N$_2$O$_4$; mol wt 327.12. C 47.73%, H 2.47%, Cl 21.68%, N 8.56%, O 19.56%. Prepn: **GB 824345** (1959 to Bayer), *C.A.* **54**, 15822b (1960). *See also:* E. Schraufstätter, R. Gönnert, US 3079297; R. Strufe *et al.*, US 3113067 (both 1963 to Bayer); Bekhli *et al.*, *Med. Prom. SSSR* **1965**, 25.

Pale yellow crystals, mp 225-230°. Practically insol in water. Sparingly sol in ethanol, chloroform, ether.

Ethanolamine salt. [1420-04-8] Clonitrilide; Bayluscid. C$_{13}$H$_8$Cl$_2$N$_2$O$_4$.C$_2$H$_7$NO; mol wt 388.20. Yellow-brown solid, mp 204°.

USE: The ethanolamine salt as a molluscicide.

THERAP CAT: Anthelmintic (Cestodes).

THERAP CAT (VET): Anthelmintic (Cestodes).

6520. Nicomorphine. [639-48-5] (5α,6α)-7,8-Didehydro-4,5-epoxy-17-methylmorphinan-3,6-diol di-3-pyridinecarboxylate (ester); morphine ester with nicotinic acid; morphine bis(nicotinate); morphine bis(pyridine-3-carboxylate); nicotinic acid morphine ester; morphine dinicotinate; Gewalan; Vilan. C$_{29}$H$_{25}$N$_3$O$_5$; mol wt 495.53. C 70.29%, H 5.09%, N 8.48%, O 16.14%. Prepn: Pongratz, Zirm, *Monatsh. Chem.* **88**, 330 (1957); **GB 807115** (1959 to Lannacher Heilmittel).

Crystals, mp 178-178.5° (corr.). Practically insol in water. Sol in ethanol.

Hydrochloride. C$_{29}$H$_{25}$N$_3$O$_5$.HCl. Dec 248°. Sol in water with neutral reaction.

Note: This is a controlled substance (opium derivative): 21 CFR, 1308.11.

THERAP CAT: Analgesic (narcotic).

6521. Nicorandil. [65141-46-0] *N*-[2-(Nitrooxy)ethyl]-3-pyridinecarboxamide; *N*-(2-hydroxyethyl)nicotinamide nitrate (ester); SG-75; Adancor; Ikorel; Perisalol; Sigmart. C$_8$H$_9$N$_3$O$_4$; mol wt 211.17. C 45.50%, H 4.30%, N 19.90%, O 30.31%. Nicotinamide derivative; exhibits dual mechanism of action as vasodilator and potassium channel activator. Prepn: H. Nagano *et al.*, **DE 2714713**; *eidem*, US 4200640 (1977, 1980 both to Chugai). Pharmacology: N. Taira *et al.*, *Clin. Exp. Pharmacol. Physiol.* **6**, 301 (1979). Mechanism of action: F. Yoneyama *et al.*, *Cardiovasc. Drugs Ther.* **4**, 1119 (1990). Symposia on pharmacology and clinical efficacy: *Am. J. Cardiol.* **63**, Suppl, 1J-85J (1989); *J. Cardiovasc. Pharmacol.* **20**, Suppl. 3, S1-S108 (1992). Review of clinical potential in ischemic heart disease: H. Purcell, K. Fox, *Br. J. Clin. Pract.* **47**, 150-154 (1993). Clinical prevention of coronary events in patients with angina: IONA Study Group, *Lancet* **359**, 1269 (2002).

Colorless needles from ether/ethanol, mp 92-93°. LD_{50} in rats (mg/kg): 1200-1300 orally; 800-1000 i.v. (Nagano).

THERAP CAT: Antianginal.

6522. Nicosulfuron. [111991-09-4] 2-[[[[(4,6-Dimethoxy-2-pyrimidinyl)amino]carbonyl]amino]sulfonyl]-*N*,*N*-dimethyl-3-pyridinecarboxamide; SL-950; MU-495; DPX-V9360; Accent; Nostoc. $C_{15}H_{18}N_6O_6S$; mol wt 410.41. C 43.90%, H 4.42%, N 20.48%, O 23.39%, S 7.81%. Post-emergence sulfonylurea herbicide. Prepn: F. Kimura *et al.*, EP 232067 (1987 to Ishihara Sangyo Kaisha); M. A. Hanagan, US 4789393 (1988 to DuPont); and structure-activity study: S. Murai *et al.*, *ACS Symp. Ser.* **504**, 43 (1992). Activity in soil: T. C. Mueller *et al.*, *Tenn. Farm Home Sci.* **167**, 17 (1993). Adsorption on clay minerals: L. Ukrainczyk, N. Rashid, *J. Agric. Food Chem.* **43**, 855 (1995). Field trial for johnsongrass in corn and effect on yield: N. G. Gubbiga *et al.*, *Weed Technol.* **9**, 574 (1995).

Colorless white solid, mp 169-173°. Vapor pressure at 25°: 1.2 × 10⁻¹⁶ mm Hg. pKa (25°): 4.6. Soly in water (ppm): 44 (pH 3.5); 22000 (pH 7).

USE: Herbicide.

6523. Nicotinamide. [98-92-0] 3-Pyridinecarboxamide; niacinamide; nicotinic acid amide; Nicobion; Papulex. $C_6H_6N_2O$; mol wt 122.12. C 59.01%, H 4.95%, N 22.94%, O 13.10%. Precursor of the coenzymes NAD and NADP, *q.q.v.* The terms *niacin*, *Vitamin B₃*, and *Vitamin PP* have been used to refer to both nicotinamide and nicotinic acid, *q.v.* Isolation: H. v. Euler *et al.*, *Z. Physiol. Chem.* **258**, 212 (1939); P. Karrer, H. Keller, *Helv. Chim. Acta* **22**, 1292 (1939). Prepn from 3-cyanopyridine: E. J. Gasson, D. J. Hadley, US 2904552 (1959 to Distillers). Alternately prepd by passing NH_3 gas into molten nicotinic acid: A. Truchan, J. B. Davidson, US 2993051 (1961 to Cowles Chem.). Isoln and analysis by liquid chromatography: C. Bernofsky, *Methods Enzymol.* **66**, 23 (1980). Extraction from cereal products: R. B. Roy, J. J. Merten, *J. Assoc. Off. Anal. Chem.* **66**, 291 (1983). Toxicity data: F. G. Brazda, R. A. Coulson, *Proc. Soc. Exp. Biol. Med.* **62**, 19 (1946). Clinical trial in acne: A. R. Shalita *et al.*, *Int. J. Dermatol.* **34**, 434 (1995); to preserve beta cell function in diabetes: P. Pozzilli *et al.*, *Diabetologia* **38**, 848 (1995). *Review:* Niacin: Nicotinic Acid, Nicotinamide, NAD(P)" in *Vitamins*, W. Friedrich, Ed. (Walter de Gruyter, Berlin, 1988) pp 473-542. Comprehensive description: E. M. Abdel Moety *et al.*, *Anal. Profiles Drug Subs.* **20**, 475-555 (1991).

Needles from benzene, mp 128-131°. Distills at 150-160° at 5×10⁻⁴ mm Hg. Absorption spectrum: Kuhn, Vetter, *Ber.* **68**, 2374 (1935). uv max: 261 nm ($A_{1cm}^{1\%}$ 451). pK (20°C): 3.3. One gram dissolves in about one ml water, in about 1.5 ml alcohol, in 10 ml glycerol. A 10% w/v soln in water is neutral to litmus. Forms

cryst salts with acids. LD_{50} s.c. in rats: 1.68 g/kg (Brazda, Coulson).

Compd with ascorbic acid. [1987-71-9] Nicotinamide ascorbate; nicoscorbine. $C_{12}H_{14}N_2O_7$. Prepn: W. Wenner, *J. Org. Chem.* **14**, 22 (1949). Yellow crystals, mp 141-145°. $[\alpha]_D^{20}$ +27.5° (c = 8 in H_2O). pH of 5% aq soln ~4.0. Soly (20°): water 40%; abs ethanol 2.4%; methanol 10%. Sparingly sol in acetone. Practically insol in benzene, ether.

THERAP CAT: Antiacne; vitamin (enzyme cofactor).

THERAP CAT (VET): Vitamin (enzyme cofactor).

6524. Nicotine. [54-11-5] 3-[(2*S*)-1-Methyl-2-pyrrolidinyl]pyridine; 1-methyl-2-(3-pyridyl)pyrrolidine; β-pyridyl-α-*N*-methylpyrrolidine; Habitrol; Nicabate; Nicoderm CQ; Nicolan; Nicopatch; Nicotinell; NiQuitin CQ; Tabazur. $C_{10}H_{14}N_2$; mol wt 162.23. C 74.04%, H 8.70%, N 17.27%. From the dried leaves of *Nicotiana tabacum* and *N. rustica* where it occurs to the extent of 2 to 8%, combined with citric and malic acids. Extraction procedure: Gattermann, Wieland, *Laboratory Methods of Organic Chemistry* (New York, 24th ed., 1937); Schwyzer, *Die Fabrikation pharmazeutischer und chemisch-technischer Produkte* (Berlin, 1931). Purification: Ratz, *Monatsh. Chem.* **26**, 1241 (1905). Structure and synthesis: Pinner, *Ber.* **26**, 294 (1893); Pictet, Rotschy, *Ber.* **37**, 1225 (1904); Craig, *J. Am. Chem. Soc.* **55**, 2854 (1933); M. Nakane, C. R. Hutchinson, *J. Org. Chem.* **43**, 3922 (1978). Conformation in soln: T. P. Pitner *et al.*, *J. Am. Chem. Soc.* **100**, 246 (1978). HPLC determn in plasma: M. Harlharan *et al.*, *Clin. Chem.* **34**, 724 (1988). Toxicity data: R. B. Barlow, L. J. McLeod, *Br. J. Pharmacol.* **35**, 161 (1969). Review and bibliography: Jackson, *Chem. Rev.* **29**, 123 (1941). Review of pharmacology: R. W. Ryall in *Neuropoisons: Their Pathophysiological Actions* vol. 2, L. L. Simpson, D. R. Curtis, Eds. (Plenum, New York, 1974) pp 61-97; N. L. Benowitz, *Annu. Rev. Med.* **37**, 21-32 (1986). Clinical trial of long-term efficacy in smoking cessation: T. Blondal *et al.*, *Br. Med. J.* **318**, 285 (1999). Review of clinical experience in Tourette syndrome: A. A. Silver *et al.*, *CNS Spectrums* **4**, 68-76 (1999).

Colorless to pale yellow, oily liq; very hygroscopic; turns brown on exposure to air or light. Acrid burning taste. Develops odor of pyridine. bp_{745} 247° (partial decomp); bp_{17} 123-125°. Volatile with steam. n_D^{20} 1.5282. d_4^{20} 1.00925. $[\alpha]_D^{20}$ −169.3° (neat); $[\alpha]_{5461}$ −204.1°. pK_1 (15°) 6.16; pK_2 10.96. pH of 0.05*M* soln: 10.2. Forms salts with almost any acid and double salts with many metals and acids. Absorption spectrum: Purvis, *J. Chem. Soc.* **97**, 1035 (1910); Dobbie, Fox, *ibid.* **103**, 1194 (1913). Optical rotatory properties: T. M. Lowry, W. V. Lloyd, *J. Chem. Soc.* **1929**, 1771. Misc with water below 60°; on mixing nicotine with water the volume contracts. Very sol in alc, chloroform, ether, petr ether, kerosene, oils. Distribution of nicotine between water and petroleum oils: Norton, *Ind. Eng. Chem., Ind. Ed.* **32**, 241 (1940). LD_{50} in mice (mg/kg): 0.3 i.v.; 9.5 i.p.; 230 orally (Barlow, McLeod).

Hydrochloride. [21361-93-3] $C_{10}H_{14}N_2$.HCl. Deliquesc crystals. $[\alpha]_D^{20}$ +104° (p = 10).

Dihydrochloride. [6019-02-9] $C_{10}H_{14}N_2$.2HCl. Deliquesc crystals, very sol in water and alcohol. Nearly insol in ether.

Sulfate. [65-30-5] Nicotine neutral sulfate. $(C_{10}H_{14}N_2)_2$.H_2SO_4. Six-sided tablets. $[\alpha]_D^{20}$ +88° (p = 70). Sol in water, alcohol.

Bitartrate. [65-31-6] Nicotine tartrate. $C_{10}H_{14}N_2$.$2C_4H_6O_6$. Dihydrate, crystals. mp 90°. $[\alpha]_D^{20}$ +26° (c = 10). Very sol in water or alcohol.

Zinc chloride double salt monohydrate. $C_{10}H_{16}Cl_4N_2Zn$.H_2O. Also with $4H_2O$. Very sol in water; sparingly sol in abs alcohol and ether.

Salicylate. [29790-52-1] Eudermol. $C_{17}H_{20}N_2O_3$; mol wt 300.35. Six-sided plates, mp 118°. $[\alpha]_D^{20}$ +13° (c = 9). Freely sol in water or alcohol.

Polacrilex. [96055-45-7] Nicorette. Prepn: S. Lichtneckert *et al.*, DE 2136119; *eidem*, US 3901248 (1972, 1975 both to AB Leo). Review of efficacy in smoking cessation: K. O. Fagerström, *Prog. Clin. Biol. Res.* **261**, 109-128 (1988).

Caution: Nicotine can be absorbed through the alimentary canal, respiratory tract and intact skin. Potential symptoms of overexposure are nausea, salivation, abdominal pain, vomiting, diarrhea; headache, dizziness, auditory and visual disturbances; confusion, weakness, incoordination; paroxysmal atrial fibrillation; convulsions, dyspnea. Death may result from paralysis of respiratory muscles. *See NIOSH Pocket Guide to Chemical Hazards* (DHHS/-NIOSH 97-140, 1997) p 224; *Clinical Toxicology of Commercial Products,* R. E. Gosselin *et al.,* Eds. (Williams & Wilkins, Baltimore, 5th ed., 1984) Section III, pp 311-314.

USE: Insecticide; fumigant. In the U.S. a 40% soln of nicotine sulfate, **Black Leaf 40**, was the commonly used form. As a contact poison it is most effective as soap, *i.e.,* as the laurate, oleate, or naphthenate. As a stomach poison a combination with bentonite has come into use.

THERAP CAT: Treatment of smoking withdrawal syndrome.

THERAP CAT (VET): Ectoparasiticide. Has been used as an anthelmintic.

6525. Nicotinic Acid. [59-67-6] 3-Pyridinecarboxylic acid; pyridine-β-carboxylic acid; P. P. factor; pellagra preventive factor; antipellagra vitamin; niacin; Niacor; Niaspan; Nicangin; Nicobid; Nicolar; Niconacid. $C_6H_5NO_2$; mol wt 123.11. C 58.54%, H 4.09%, N 11.38%, O 25.99%. Precursor of the coenzymes NAD and NADP, *q.q.v.* Widely distributed in nature; appreciable amounts are found in liver, fish, yeast and cereal grains. Dietary deficiency is associated with pellagra. The term "niacin" has also been applied to nicotinamide, *q.v.,* or to other derivatives exhibiting the biological activity of nicotinic acid. Prepn by oxidation of alkyl β-substituted pyridines: A. Ladenburg, *Ann.* **301**, 152 (1898). Synthesis from pyridine: S. M. McElvain, M. A. Goese, *J. Am. Chem. Soc.* **63**, 2283 (1941). Prepn by oxidation of nicotine: S. M. McElvain, *Org. Synth.* **coll. vol. I**, 385 (1941); C. F. Woodward *et al., Ind. Eng. Chem.* **36**, 540, 544 (1944). Toxicity study: F. G. Brazda, R. A. Coulson, *Proc. Soc. Exp. Biol. Med.* **62**, 19 (1946). LC determn in foods: G. W. Chase, Jr. *et al., J. AOAC Int.* **76**, 390 (1993). Lipid-modifying effect in diabetic patients: M. B. Elam *et al., J. Am. Med. Assoc.* **284**, 1263 (2000). Review of nutritional requirements, bioavailability and relationship with tryptophan: W. J. Darby *et al., Nutr. Rev.* **33**, 289-297 (1975); of biosynthesis, metabolism and physiological effects: L. M. Henderson, *Annu. Rev. Nutr.* **3**, 289-307 (1983); of pharmacology and therapeutic uses: J. R. DiPalma, W. S. Thayer, *ibid.* **11**, 169-187 (1991). *Review:* "Niacin: Nicotinic Acid, Nicotinamide, NAD(P)" in *Vitamins,* W. Friedrich, Ed. (Walter de Gruyter, Berlin, 1988) pp 473-542.

Needles from alcohol or water, mp 236.6°. Nonhygroscopic and stable in air. Sublimes without decompn. pKa 4.85. pH of satd aq soln 2.7. uv max: 263 nm, Hünecke, *Ber.* **60**, 1451 (1927). One gram dissolves in 60 ml water. Freely sol in boiling water and in boiling alcohol, in alkali hydroxides and carbonates; sol in propylene glycol. Insol in ether. LD_{50} s.c. in rats: 5 g/kg (Brazda, Coulson).

N-Oxide *see* Oxiniacic Acid.

Sodium salt sesquihydrate. Direktan. $C_6H_4NNaO_2 \cdot 1\frac{1}{2}H_2O$; mol wt 154.10. White crystals or crystalline powder; stable in air. One gram dissolves in ~1.4 ml water, in ~60 ml alc, in 10 ml glycerol. Insol in ether. pH of aq soln: ~7.

THERAP CAT: Antilipemic; vitamin (enzyme cofactor).

THERAP CAT (VET): Vitamin (enzyme cofactor).

6526. Nicotinic Acid Benzyl Ester. [94-44-0] 3-Pyridinecarboxylic acid phenylmethyl ester; pyridine-β-carboxylic acid benzyl ester; benzyl nicotinate; Rubiment; Pycaril; Pykaryl. $C_{13}H_{11}NO_2$; mol wt 213.23. C 73.23%, H 5.20%, N 6.57%, O 15.01%. Prepn: **GB 817103** (1959 to Nordmark-Werke).

Liquid, bp_{3-4} 170°.

THERAP CAT: Rubefacient.

6527. Nicotinyl Alcohol. [100-55-0] 3-Pyridinemethanol; β-pyridylcarbinol; 3-hydroxymethylpyridine; nicotinic alcohol; Nu-2121; Roniacol; Ronicol. C_6H_7NO; mol wt 109.13. C 66.04%, H 6.47%, N 12.83%, O 14.66%. Prepd by catalytic hydrogenation of 3-pyridinecarboxaldehyde: Panizzon, *Helv. Chim. Acta* **24**, supplemental issue in honor of Gadient Engi, p 26E (1941); by lithium aluminum hydride reduction of ethyl nicotinate: Rosenmund, Zymalkowski, *Ber.* **85**, 156 (1952); Cohen, **US 2520037** (1950); Mosher, Tessieri, *J. Am. Chem. Soc.* **73**, 4926 (1951); of methyl nicotinate: Bohlmann, *Ber.* **86**, 1423 (1953). From 3-cyanopyridine: Chase, **US 2615896** (1952 to Hoffmann-La Roche); from 3-aminomethylpyridine: Schläpfer, **US 2547048** (1951 to Hoffmann-La Roche); from thionicotinic acid *S*-methyl ester: Ruzicka, Prelog, **US 2509171** (1950 to Ciba).

Very hygroscopic liquid. bp_{28} 154°; bp_{16} 144-145°; bp_{12} 114°; $bp_{0.1}$ 110°. Freely sol in water, ether. Sparingly sol in petr ether.

d-Tartrate. [6164-87-0] Roniacol Tartrate; Radecol; Niltuvin. $C_6H_7NO \cdot C_4H_6O_6$; mol wt 259.21. Crystals, sour taste, mp 147-148°. Sol in ether, water, alcohol.

USE: Solubilizer for riboflavin: **US 2458430** (1949).

THERAP CAT: Vasodilator (peripheral).

6528. Nifedipine. [21829-25-4] 1,4-Dihydro-2,6-dimethyl-4-(2-nitrophenyl)-3,5-pyridinedicarboxylic acid dimethyl ester; 4-(2′-nitrophenyl)-2,6-dimethyl-3,5-dicarbomethoxy-1,4-dihydropyridine; Bay a 1040; Adalat(e); Adipine; Aldipin; Anifed; Aprical; Cardilate; Chronadalate; Coracten; Cordicant; Cordilan; Corotrend; Duranifin; Ecodipin; Fortipine; Hexadilat; Nifedicor; Nifelan; Nifelat; Nifensar; Orix; Pidilat; Procardia; Sepamit; Tensipine; Zenusin. $C_{17}H_{18}N_2O_6$; mol wt 346.33. C 58.96%, H 5.24%, N 8.09%, O 27.72%. Dihydropyridine calcium channel blocker. Prepn: Bossert, Vater, **ZA 6801482**; *eidem,* **US 3485847** (1968, 1969 both to Bayer). Series of articles on pharmacology, pharmacokinetics, biotransformation, clinical studies: *Arzneim.-Forsch.* **22**, 1-56, 330-388 (1972). Toxicity data: Vater *et al., ibid.* 1. Comprehensive description: S. L. Ali, *Anal. Profiles Drug Subs.* **18**, 221-288 (1989). Review of analytical methods in biological fluids: P. A. Soons *et al., J. Pharm. Biomed. Anal.* **9**, 475-484 (1991). Review of clinical efficacy in hypertension and Raynaud's phenomenon: W. Kiowski *et al., Cardiovasc. Drugs Ther.* **4**, 935-940 (1990); in hypertension and angina: J. G. Tijssen, P. G. Hugenholtz, *Eur. Heart J.* **17**, 1152-1157 (1996). Comparative clinical trial in prevention of complications from hypertension: M. J. Brown *et al., Lancet* **356**, 366 (2000).

Yellow crystals, mp 172-174°. uv max (methanol): 340, 235 nm (ε 5010, 21590); (0.1*N* HCl): 338, 238 nm (ε 5740, 20600); (0.1*N* NaOH): 340, 238 nm (ε 5740, 20510). Soly at 20° (g/L): acetone 250, methylene chloride 160, chloroform 140, ethyl acetate 50, methanol 26, ethanol 17. Very light sensitive in soln. LD_{50} in mice, rats (mg/kg): 494, 1022 orally; 4.2, 15.5 i.v. (Vater).

THERAP CAT: Antianginal; antihypertensive.

6529. Nifekalant. [130636-43-0] 6-[[2-[(2-Hydroxyethyl)[3-(4-nitrophenyl)propyl]amino]ethyl]amino]-1,3-dimethyl-2,-4(1*H*,3*H*)-pyrimidinedione. $C_{19}H_{27}N_5O_5$; mol wt 405.45. C 56.28%, H 6.71%, N 17.27%, O 19.73%. Nonselective potassium channel blocker. Prepn: T. Katakami *et al.*, **EP 369627**; *eidem*, **US 5008267** (1990, 1991 both to Mitsui Toatsu Chem.); *eidem, J. Med. Chem.* **35**, 3325 (1992). Pharmacology: J. Kamiya *et al.*, *Drug Dev. Res.* **30**, 37 (1993). Clinical experience: M. Igawa *et al.*, *J. Cardiovasc. Pharmacol.* **40**, 735 (2002); T. Minami *et al.*, *Pacing Clin. Electrophysiol.* **27**, 212 (2004). Review of pharmacology: H. Nakaya, H. Uemura, *Cardiovasc. Drug Rev.* **16**, 133-144 (1998); of development and therapeutic potential: A. Zaza, *Curr. Opin. Cardiovasc. Pulm. Renal Invest. Drugs* **2**, 86-94 (2000). Clinical evaluation in ventricular tachyarrhythmias: T. Katoh *et al., Circ. J.* **69**, 1237 (2005); T. Washizuka *et al., ibid.* 1508; in shock-refractory ventricular fibrillation: Y. Tahara *et al., ibid.* **70**, 442 (2006).

Crystals from ethanol, mp 117.5-118.5°. Also reported as mp 125-126° (Katakami, 1992).

Hydrochloride. [130656-51-8] MS-551; Shinbit. $C_{19}H_{27}N_5$-O_5.HCl; mol wt 441.91. Light yellow to yellow crystals from methanol, mp 172-174°. Very sol in water, slightly sol in methanol, very slightly sol in ethanol. Practically insol in ether. pH 4.0 - 5.5 (5 mg/ml saline soln). pKa 7.05.

THERAP CAT: Antiarrhythmic (class III).

6530. Nifenalol. [7413-36-7] α-[[(1-Methylethyl)amino]-methyl]-4-nitrobenzenemethanol; α-[(isopropylamino)methyl]-*p*-nitrobenzyl alcohol; 1-(4-nitrophenyl)-2-(isopropylamino)ethanol; isophenethanol; INPEA. $C_{11}H_{16}N_2O_3$; mol wt 224.26. C 58.91%, H 7.19%, N 12.49%, O 21.40%. β-Adrenergic blocker. Prepn: Teotino *et al., Farmaco Ed. Sci.* **17**, 252 (1962); *eidem,* **GB 950682** (1964 to Selvi), *C.A.* **60**, 13184h (1964). Pharmacology: Somani, Lum, *J. Pharmacol. Exp. Ther.* **147**, 194 (1965); Almirante *et al., Farmaco Ed. Sci.* **21**, 637 (1966). Prepn of the optical isomers: Almirante, Murmann, *J. Med. Chem.* **9**, 650 (1966); *eidem,* **BE 673273** (1966 to Selvi), *C.A.* **66**, 65278d (1967).

mp 98°.

Hydrochloride. [5704-60-9] Inpea. $C_{11}H_{16}N_2O_3$.HCl; mol wt 260.72. mp 181°.

THERAP CAT: Antianginal; antiarrhythmic.

6531. Niflumic Acid. [4394-00-7] 2-[[3-(Trifluoromethyl)-phenyl]amino]-3-pyridinecarboxylic acid; 2-(α,α,α-trifluoro-*m*-toluidino)nicotinic acid; 2-[3-(trifluoromethyl)anilino]nicotinic acid; UP-83; Actol; Forenol; Landruma; Nifluril. $C_{13}H_9F_3N_2O_2$; mol wt 282.22. C 55.33%, H 3.21%, F 20.20%, N 9.93%, O 11.34%. Prepn: **NL 6414717**; C. Hoffmann, A. Faure, **US 3415834** (1965, 1968 both to Lab. U.P.S.A.); *eidem, Bull. Soc. Chim. Fr.* **1966**, 2316. Pharmacological and metabolic studies: Glasson *et al., Biochem. Pharmacol.* **18**, 633 (1969); Boissier *et al., Therapie* **26**, 211 (1971). Toxicity data: J. R. J. Sorenson, *J. Med. Chem.* **19**, 135 (1976). Determn in human plasma by GLC: G. Houin *et al., J. Chromatogr.* **223**, 351 (1981).

Crystals from ethanol, mp 204°. LD_{50} in rats (mg/kg): 370 orally; 155 i.p. (Sorenson).

β-Morpholinoethyl ester. [65847-85-0] Morniflumate; Flomax; Nifluril (suppositories). $C_{19}H_{20}F_3N_3O_3$; mol wt 395.38.

Prepn of the ester HCl: Hoffmann, **DE 1802777**; *idem,* **US 3708481** (1969, 1973 both to Hexachimie).

Phthalidyl ester *see* Talniflumate.

THERAP CAT: Anti-inflammatory.

6532. Nifuratel. [4936-47-4] 5-[(Methylthio)methyl]-3-[[(5-nitro-2-furanyl)methylene]amino]-2-oxazolidinone; 5-[(methylthio)methyl]-3-[(5-nitrofurfurylidene)amino]-2-oxazolidinone; 5-(methylmercaptomethyl)-3-(5-nitro-2-furfurylideneamino)-2-oxazolidinone; methylmercadone; Inimur; Macmiror; Magmilor; Omnes; Polmiror; Tydantil. $C_{10}H_{11}N_3O_5S$; mol wt 285.28. C 42.10%, H 3.89%, N 14.73%, O 28.04%, S 11.24%. Prepn: **BE 635608** (1963 to Polichimica SAP), *C.A.* **61**, 16069c (1964), corresp to **GB 969126**.

Crystals from acetic acid, mp 182°.

THERAP CAT: Antibacterial; antifungal; antiprotozoal (Trichomonas).

6533. Nifurfoline. [3363-58-4] 3-(4-Morpholinylmethyl)-1-[[(5-nitro-2-furanyl)methylene]amino]-2,4-imidazolidinedione; 3-(morpholinomethyl)-1-[(5-nitrofurfurylidene)amino]hydantoin; Urbac. $C_{13}H_{15}N_5O_6$; mol wt 337.29. C 46.29%, H 4.48%, N 20.76%, O 28.46%. Prepn: J. A. Bofill-Auge, J. M. Espinos-Taya, **ES 297087** (1964), *C.A.* **63**, 11572e (1966); **GB 1245095** (1971 to Esteve), *C.A.* **75**, 121382h (1971).

Yellow cryst, mp 206°; also reported as mp 194-196°, J. Klosa, H. Starke, **DD 508615** (1966), *C.A.* **66**, 65501w (1967).

THERAP CAT: Antibacterial.

6534. Nifuroquine. [57474-29-0] 4-(5-Nitro-2-furanyl)-2-quinolinecarboxylic acid 1-oxide; 2-carboxy-4-[2'-(5'-nitrofuryl)]-quinoline 1-oxide; 4-(5-nitro-2-furyl)quinaldic acid 1-oxide; quinaldofur; Abimasten 100. $C_{14}H_8N_2O_6$; mol wt 300.22. C 56.01%, H 2.69%, N 9.33%, O 31.98%. Prepn: R. R. G. Haber, E. Schoenberger, **ZA 6703320** corresp to **US 4217456** and **US 4224448** (1967, 1980, 1980). Use in bovine mastitis: R. R. G. Haber *et al.*, **DE 2612250** corresp to **US 4070469** (1977, 1978 both to ABIC). *In vitro* study: G. Ziv *et al., Zentralbl. Veterinaermed. (B)* **23**, 301 (1976). Pharmacology: G. Ziv, A. Saran, *ibid.* 310. Activity under anaerobic conditions: G. M. Maluszynska, L. Bassalik-Chabielska, *Pr. Mater. Zootech.* **23**, 63 (1980), *C.A.* **93**, 143793 (1980).

Yellow cryst powder, mp 190° (dec). Practically insol in water.

THERAP CAT (VET): Antibacterial.

6535. Nifuroxazide. [965-52-6] 4-Hydroxybenzoic acid [(5-nitro-2-furanyl)methylene]hydrazide; *p*-hydroxybenzoic acid (5-nitrofurfurylidene)hydrazide; 1-(*p*-hydroxybenzoyl)-2-(5-nitrofurfurylidene)hydrazine; 5-nitro-2-furaldehyde *p*-hydroxybenzoylhydrazone; RC-27109; Adral; Bacifurane; Diarlidan; Dicoferin; Ercefurol; Ercefuryl; Pentofuryl. $C_{12}H_9N_3O_5$; mol wt 275.22. C 52.37%, H 3.30%, N 15.27%, O 29.07%. Prepn: **FR 1327840** (1963 to Robert et Carriere), *C.A.* **59**, 12763b (1963); M. C. E. Carron, **GB 962706**; *idem,* **US 3290213** (1964, 1966 both to Robert et Carriere). Antiseptic and antibacterial properties: M. C. E. Carron *et al., Ann. Pharm. Fr.* **21,** 287 (1963). *In vitro* study of activity spectrum: A. Thabaut, J. L. Durosoir, *Gaz. Med. Fr.* **85,** 4516 (1978), *C.A.* **90,** 1487 (1979).

Crystals from pyridine, mp 298°. Practically insol in water.
THERAP CAT: Intestinal antiseptic.

6536. Nifuroxime. [6236-05-1] 5-Nitro-2-furancarboxaldehyde oxime; *anti*-5-nitro-2-furaldoxime; Micofur. $C_5H_4N_2O_4$; mol wt 156.10. C 38.47%, H 2.58%, N 17.95%, O 41.00%. Prepd by treating 5-nitrofurfural with hydroxylamine in alcohol: Ikeda, *C.A.* **50,** 10701 (1956). Claimed in Stillman *et al.,* **US 2319481** (1943 to Norwich Pharmacal).

Tasteless, pale yellow or greenish crystals from ethanol. Darkens on exposure to light. mp 156° (Ikeda); mp 163-164° (Stillman *et al.*). Soly at 25° in water: ~1 g/l, in methanol: 89.0 g/l, in 95% ethanol: 39.0 g/l.
THERAP CAT: Topical anti-infective; antiprotozoal (Trichomonas).

6537. Nifurpirinol. [13411-16-0] 6-[2-(5-Nitro-2-furanyl)-ethenyl]-2-pyridinemethanol; 6-[2-(5-nitro-2-furyl)vinyl]-2-pyridinemethanol; 6-(hydroxymethyl)-2-[2-(5-nitro-2-furyl)vinyl]pyridine; furpirinol; furpyrinol; P-7138; Furanace. $C_{12}H_{10}N_2O_4$; mol wt 246.22. C 58.54%, H 4.09%, N 11.38%, O 25.99%. Prepn: Fujita *et al., J. Pharm. Soc. Jpn.* **86,** 1014 (1966); **GB 1053730** (1967 to Dainippon), *C.A.* **66,** 115605f (1967); Murakami, Iwanami, **JP 70 14072** (1970 to Yamanouchi), *C.A.* **73,** 45364v (1970). Antibacterial activity: Shimizu, Takase, *Prog. Antimicrob. Anticancer Chemother., Proc. 6th Int. Congr. Chemother.* **2,** 388 (1970); D. F. Amend, A. J. Ross, *Prog. Fish Cult.* **32,** 19 (1970); A. J. Ross, *ibid.* **34,** 18 (1972); Y. Takase *et al., Chem. Pharm. Bull.* **21,** 144 (1973).

Yellow needles from acetone or methanol, mp 170-171°.
THERAP CAT: Antibacterial.
THERAP CAT (VET): Antibacterial in fish diseases.

6538. Nifurtimox. [23256-30-6] 3-Methyl-*N*-[(5-nitro-2-furanyl)methylene]-4-thiomorpholinamine 1,1-dioxide; 4-[(5-nitrofurfurylidene)amino]-3-methylthiomorpholine-1,1-dioxide; tetrahydro-3-methyl-4-[(5-nitrofurfurylidene)amino]-2*H*-1,4-thiazine 1,1-dioxide; 1-[(5-nitrofurfurylidene)amino]-2-methyltetrahydro-1,4-thiazine 4,4-dioxide; Bay 2502; Lampit. $C_{10}H_{13}N_3O_5S$; mol wt 287.29. C 41.81%, H 4.56%, N 14.63%, O 27.85%, S 11.16%. Prepn from 5-nitrofurfural and 4-amino-3-methyltetrahydro-1,4-thiazine 1,1-dioxide: Herlinger *et al.,* **DE 1170957** corresp to **US 3262930** (1964 and 1966 to Bayer). Series of articles on pharmacology and clinical findings: *Arzneim.-Forsch.* **22,** 1563-1642 (1972). Toxicity data: K. Hoffmann, *ibid.* 1590.

Orange-red crystals from dil acetic acid, mp 180-182°. LD_{50} in mice, rats (mg/kg): 3720, 4050 by gavage (Hoffmann).
THERAP CAT: Antiprotozoal (Trypanosoma).

6539. Nifurtoinol. [1088-92-2] 3-(Hydroxymethyl)-1-[[(5-nitro-2-furanyl)methylene]amino]-2,4-imidazolidinedione; 3-(hydroxymethyl)-1-[(5-nitrofurfurylidene)amino]hydantoin; 1-[(5-nitrofurfurylidene)amino]-3-(hydroxymethyl)hydantoin; Urfadyn. $C_9H_8N_4O_6$; mol wt 268.18. C 40.31%, H 3.01%, N 20.89%, O 35.80%. Prepn: Michels, **BE 611941** corresp to **US 3446802** (1962, 1969 to Norwich Pharmacal); Spencer, Michels, *J. Org. Chem.* **29,** 3416 (1964).

Yellow crystals from aq formaldehyde. When heated on a melting-point block, loses formaldehyde, then further decomposes at same temp as nitrofurantoin. uv max (2% in dimethylformamide): 367.5, 265 nm (ε 17900, 12800).
THERAP CAT: Antibacterial.

6540. Nifurzide. [39978-42-2] 5-Nitro-2-thiophenecarboxylic acid [3-(5-nitro-2-furanyl)-2-propenylidene]hydrazide; N^1-(5-nitro-2-furylacrylidene)-N^2-(5-nitro-2-thenoyl)hydrazine; 5-nitro-2-thiophenecarboxylic acid [3-(5-nitro-2-furyl)allylidene]hydrazide; Ricridene. $C_{12}H_8N_4O_6S$; mol wt 336.28. C 42.86%, H 2.40%, N 16.66%, O 28.55%, S 9.54%. Bactericidal agent related to nitrofurazone, *q.v.* Prepn: E. Szarvasi, L. Fontaine, **DE 2200375**; *eidem,* **US 3847911** (1972, 1974 both to Lipha); E. Szarvasi *et al., J. Med. Chem.* **16,** 281 (1973). Mode of action study: A. Delsarte *et al., Antimicrob. Agents Chemother.* **19,** 477 (1981).

trans-form

Yellow crystals from DMF/ether, mp 235-236°. LD_{50} orally in mice: 3200 mg/kg (Szarvasi, Fontaine, 1972).
THERAP CAT: Anti-infective.

6541. Nigericin. [28380-24-7] Antibiotic K 178; antibiotic X-464; azalomycin M; helixin C; polyetherin A. $C_{40}H_{68}O_{11}$; mol wt 724.96. C 66.27%, H 9.45%, O 24.28%. Polyether antibiotic which affects ion transport and ATPase activity in mitochondria; produced by *Streptomyces hygroscopicus* E-749 and structurally related to monensin, *q.v.* Isoln, characterization, production: R. L. Harned *et al., Antibiot. Chemother.* **1,** 594 (1951); J. Berger *et al., J. Am. Chem. Soc.* **73,** 5295 (1951); J. Shoji *et al., J. Antibiot.* **21,** 402 (1968). Structure: L. K. Steinrauf *et al., Biochem. Biophys. Res. Commun.* **33,** 29 (1968); T. Kubota *et al., Chem. Commun.* **1968,** 1541; T. Kubota, S. Matsutani, *J. Chem. Soc. C* **1970,** 695. Use in coccidiosis: M. Gorman, R. L. Hamill, **US 3555150** (1971 to Lilly). Effect on calcium uptake and membrane potential in mitochondria: H. Rottenberg, A. Scarpa, *Biochemistry* **13,** 4811 (1974). Stimulation of ATPase activity: H. Sze, *Proc. Natl. Acad. Sci. USA* **77,** 5904 (1980). Approach to synthesis: C. P. Holmes, P. A. Bartlett, *J. Org. Chem.* **54,** 98 (1989).

Colorless needles, mp 183.5-185°. $[\alpha]_D^{24}$ +36.2° (c = 0.842 in $CHCl_3$). Sol in alcohols, acetone, ethyl acetate, chloroform, benzene, ether; slightly sol in satd hydrocarbons. Practically insol in water. LD_{50} in mice (mg/kg): 10-15 i.p. (Shoji); also reported as 2.5 i.p. (Harned).

Sodium salt. $C_{40}H_{67}NaO_{11}$. Crystals, mp 245-255° (dec). Sol in chloroform. Practically insol in water.

6542. Nihydrazone. [67-28-7] Acetic acid [(5-nitro-2-furanyl)methylene]hydrazide; acetic acid 5-(nitrofurfurylidene)hydrazide; 5-nitro-2-furaldehyde acetylhydrazone; N-acetyl-5-nitro-2-furaldehyde hydrazide; 1-(5-nitro-2-furfurylidene)-2-acetylhydrazine; 1-acetyl-2-(5-nitro-2-furfurylidene)hydrazide; NF-64; HC-064; Furiton; Nidrafur. $C_7H_7N_3O_4$; mol wt 197.15. C 42.65%, H 3.58%, N 21.31%, O 32.46%. Prepn: Stillman, Scott, **US 2416234** and **US 2416236** (1947 to Eaton Labs).

Yellow crystals from acetic acid + ethanol, dec 230-235°. uv max (water): 253, 364 nm (log ε 4.11, 4.23). Soly in water 1:20,000.

THERAP CAT (VET): Antibacterial, antiprotozoal.

6543. Nikethamide. [59-26-7] N,N-Diethyl-3-pyridinecarboxamide; N,N-diethylnicotinamide; pyridine-3-carboxylic acid diethylamide; nicotinic acid diethylamide; Anacardone; Astrocar; Carbamidal; Cardamine; Cardiamid; Cardimon; Coracon; Coractiv N; Coramine; Cordiamin; Corediol; Cormed; Cormid; Corvitol; Corvotone; Dynacoryl; Eucoran; Inicardio; Niamine; Nicamide; Nicor; Nicorine; Nikardin; Pyricardyl; Salvacard; Stimulin; Ventramine. $C_{10}H_{14}N_2O$; mol wt 178.23. C 67.39%, H 7.92%, N 15.72%, O 8.98%. Prepd by the action of thionyl chloride on nicotinic acid, followed by treatment with diethylamine hydrochloride; also formed by heating nicotinic acid or quinolinic acid anhydride with diethylamine: Hartmann, Seiberth, **US 1403117** (1922); from nicotinic acid + benzenesulfonyldiethyl amide: Oxley et al., J. Chem. Soc. **1946**, 763. Toxicity data: E. I. Goldenthal, Toxicol. Appl. Pharmacol. **18**, 185 (1971).

Slightly viscous liquid or cryst solid. Faintly bitter taste followed by a faint sensation of warmth. d_4^{25} 1.058-1.066 (liq). mp 24-26°. bp760 296-300° (some decompn); bp10 158-159°; bp3 128-129°; bp0.4 115°. n_D^{20} 1.525-1.526; n_D^{25} 1.522-1.524. Misc with water, ether, chloroform, acetone, alc. Usually marketed as a 25% w/v aq soln, pH 6.0-6.5. Incompatible with Na_2CO_3 solns which cause precipitation; tannates produce an amorph ppt. LD50 i.p. in rats: 272 mg/kg (Goldenthal).

THERAP CAT: CNS and respiratory stimulant.

THERAP CAT (VET): Respiratory stimulant.

6544. Nilutamide. [63612-50-0] 5,5-Dimethyl-3-[4-nitro-3-(trifluoromethyl)phenyl]-2,4-imidazolidinedione; 1-(3'-trifluoromethyl-4'-nitrophenyl)-4,4-dimethylimidazoline-2,5-dione; RU-23908; Anandron; Nilandron. $C_{12}H_{10}F_3N_3O_4$; mol wt 317.22. C 45.43%, H 3.18%, F 17.97%, N 13.25%, O 20.17%. Nonsteroidal antiandrogen. Prepn: J. Perronnet et al., **DE 2649925**; idem, **US 4097578** (1977, 1978 both to Roussel-UCLAF). Pharmacology: J.-P. Raynaud et al., J. Steroid Biochem. **11**, 93 (1979). Review of kinetics, metabolism and clinical studies: idem et al., Prog. Clin. Biol. Res. **185A**, 99-120 (1985); of therapeutic efficacy in prostate cancer: M. G. Harris et al., Drugs Aging **3**, 9-25 (1993).

Crystals from ethanol, mp 149°. Freely sol in ethyl acetate, acetone, chloroform, ethanol, dichloromethane, methanol. Soly in water at 25°: < 0.1%.

THERAP CAT: Antineoplastic (hormonal).

6545. Nilvadipine. [75530-68-6] 2-Cyano-1,4-dihydro-6-methyl-4-(3-nitrophenyl)-3,5-pyridinedicarboxylic acid 3-methyl 5-(1-methylethyl) ester; 5-isopropyl-3-methyl-2-cyano-1,4-dihydro-6-methyl-4-(m-nitrophenyl)-3,5-pyridinedicarboxylate; isopropyl 6-cyano-5-methoxycarbonyl-2-methyl-4-(3-nitrophenyl)-1,4-dihydropyridine-3-carboxylate; nivadipine; nivaldipine; FR-34235; FK-235; SKF-102362; Escor; Nivadil. $C_{19}H_{19}N_3O_6$; mol wt 385.37. C 59.22%, H 4.97%, N 10.90%, O 24.91%. Dihydropyridine calcium channel blocker. Prepn: Y. Sato, **BE 879263**; idem, **US 4338322** (1980, 1982 both to Fujisawa). Structural studies: A. Miyamae et al., Chem. Pharm. Bull. **34**, 3071 (1986). Determn in plasma and urine: Y. Tokuma et al., J. Chromatogr. **415**, 156 (1987). Preliminary pharmacokinetics and resolution of enantiomers: idem, J. Pharm. Sci. **76**, 310 (1987). Pharmacokinetics in rabbits: Y. Nezasa et al., Kankyo Igaku Kenkyusho Nenpo **38**, 200 (1987), C.A. **107**, 89273q (1987). Mode of action: P. A. Molyvdas, N. Sperelakis, J. Cardiovasc. Pharmacol. **8**, 449 (1986). Cardiovascular effects: G. J. Gross et al., Gen. Pharmacol. **14**, 677 (1983). Clinical evaluation in hypertension: K. Mizuno et al., Res. Commun. Chem. Pathol. Pharmacol. **52**, 3 (1986).

Yellow prisms from ethanol, mp 148-150°.
(+)-Form. $[\alpha]_D^{20}$ +222.42° (c = 1 in methanol).
(−)-Form. $[\alpha]_D^{20}$ −219.62° (c = 1 in methanol).

THERAP CAT: Antihypertensive; antianginal.

6546. Nimbin. [5945-86-8] $(4\alpha,5\alpha,6\alpha,7\alpha,15\beta,17\alpha)$-6-(Acetyloxy)-7,15:21,23-diepoxy-4,8-dimethyl-1-oxo-18,24-dinor-11,12-secochola-2,13,20,22-tetraene-4,11-dicarboxylic acid dimethyl ester; 5-(acetyloxy)-2-(3-furanyl)-3,3a,4a,5,5a,6,9,9a,10,10a-decahydro-6-(methoxycarbonyl)-1,6,9a,10a-tetramethyl-9-oxo-2H-cyclopenta[b]naphtho[2,3-d]furan-10-acetic acid. $C_{30}H_{36}O_9$; mol wt 540.60. C 66.65%, H 6.71%, O 26.64%. Bitter principle from various parts of the neem tree, Azadirachta indica A. Juss. (Melia azadirachta L.), Meliaceae: Siddiqui, Curr. Sci. **11**, 278 (1942). Structure: C. R. Narayanan et al., Chem. Ind. (London) **1964**, 322; C. R. Narayanan, R. V. Pachapurkar, Tetrahedron Lett. **1965**, 4333. Stereochemistry: eidem, J. Org. Chem. **31**, 2691 (1966); Harris et al., Tetrahedron **24**, 1517 (1968). Crystal structure of dihydronimbin: C. R. Narayanan et al., Acta Crystallogr. **B36**, 486 (1980).

Crystals from methanol, mp 205°. $[\alpha]_D^{24}$ +170° (abs ethanol). uv max (95% ethanol): 210, 330 nm (ε 32700; 66). Practically insol in water. Sol in ether, abs alcohol.

Dihydronimbin. $C_{30}H_{38}O_9$. Crystals from methanol, mp 215-216°. $[\alpha]_D$ +167.5° (chloroform). uv max (95% ethanol): 210, 298 nm (ε 16200; 29).

6547. Nimbiol. [561-95-5] (4aS-trans)-2,3,4,4a,10,10a-Hexahydro-6-hydroxy-1,1,4a,7-tetramethyl-9(1H)-phenanthrenone; 6-hydroxy-7-methyl-9-oxopodocarpane. $C_{18}H_{24}O_2$; mol wt 272.38. C 79.37%, H 8.88%, O 11.75%. (+)-Form found in the bark of the neem tree, Azadirachta indica A. Juss. (Melia azadir-

achta L.), *Meliaceae:* P. Sengupta *et al., Chem. Ind. (London)* **1958**, 861. Structure: P. Sengupta *et al., Tetrahedron* **10**, 45 (1960). Also obtained by conversion of podocarpic acid: Bible, *ibid.* **11**, 22 (1960); Wenkert *et al., J. Am. Chem. Soc.* **83**, 2320 (1961). Total synthesis of (±)-form: W. L. Meyer *et al., J. Org. Chem.* **40**, 3686 (1975). Synthesis of (±)-methyl ether: Ramachandran, Dutta, *J. Chem. Soc.* **1960**, 4766; Delobelle, Fétizon, *Bull. Soc. Chim. Fr.* **1961**, 1900; Nasipuri, Roy, *J. Indian Chem. Soc.* **40**, 327 (1963).

Crystals from dilute methanol or platelets by high vac sublimation. mp 248-252°. $[\alpha]_D^{25}$ +33° (chloroform). uv max (abs alcohol): 234, 283 nm (log ε 4.13, 4.10).

Methyl ether. $C_{19}H_{26}O_2$. Crystals, mp 143°. $[\alpha]_D^{25}$ +43.7° (chloroform). uv max (alcohol): 207, 232, 279 nm (log ε 4.18, 4.15, 4.12).

(±)-Form. White needles from CH_3OH, mp 237.0-237.5°.

(±)-Methyl ether. $C_{19}H_{26}O_2$. Crystals from hexane. mp 112-113°. uv max (alcohol): 207, 232, 279 nm (log ε 4.13, 4.13, 4.11) (Delobelle, Fétizon). Also reported as needles from CH_3OH, mp 117-118° (Nasipuri, Roy).

6548. Nimesulide. [51803-78-2] *N*-(4-Nitro-2-phenoxyphenyl)methanesulfonamide; 4-nitro-2-phenoxymethanesulfonanilide; R-805; Aulin; Fansidol; Flogovital; Mesulid; Nide; Nidol; Nisulid. $C_{13}H_{12}N_2O_5S$; mol wt 308.31. C 50.64%, H 3.92%, N 9.09%, O 25.95%, S 10.40%. Prostaglandin synthetase and platelet aggregation inhibitor. Prepn and anti-inflammatory activity: **BE 801812**; G. G. I. Moore, J. K. Harrington, **US 3840597** (both 1974 to Riker). Activity, comparison with other non-steroidal anti-inflammatories: K. F. Swingle *et al., Arch. Int. Pharmacodyn. Ther.* **221**, 132 (1976). Mechanism of action: R. L. Vigdahl, R. H. Tukey, *Biochem. Pharmacol.* **26**, 307 (1977). Chromatographic determn in plasma: S. F. Chang *et al., J. Pharm. Sci.* **66**, 1700 (1977). Pharmacology: K. F. Swingle, G. G. I. Moore, *Drugs Exp. Clin. Res.* **10**, 587 (1984). Clinical trials in rheumatic disorders: R. Weissenbach, *J. Int. Med. Res.* **9**, 349 (1981); in osteoarthritis: M. Reiner, *ibid.* **10**, 92 (1982); in acute inflammation: J. M. Pais, F. M. Rosteiro, *ibid.* **11**, 149 (1983); C. Milvio, *ibid.* **12**, 327 (1984); M. E. Nouri, *Clin. Ther.* **6**, 142 (1984).

Light tan crystals from ethanol, mp 143-144.5°. LD_{50} orally in rats: 324 mg/kg (Swingle, Moore).

THERAP CAT: Anti-inflammatory.

THERAP CAT (VET): Anti-inflammatory.

6549. Nimetazepam. [2011-67-8] 1,3-Dihydro-1-methyl-7-nitro-5-phenyl-2*H*-1,4-benzodiazepin-2-one; 1-methyl-5-phenyl-7-nitro-1,3-dihydro-2*H*-1,4-benzodiazepin-2-one; 1-methylnitrazepam; S-1530; Erimin. $C_{16}H_{13}N_3O_3$; mol wt 295.29. C 65.08%, H 4.44%, N 14.23%, O 16.25%. The desmethyl derivative of nitrazepam, *q.v.* Prepn: L. H. Sternbach *et al., J. Med. Chem.* **6**, 261 (1963); E. Reeder, L. H. Sternbach, **US 3109843**; **US 3144439**; **US 3141890**; **US 3243427** (1963, 1964, 1964, 1966 all to Hoffmann-La Roche); O. Keller *et al.,* **US 3121114**; **US 3203990** (1964, 1965 to Hoffmann-La Roche); Sorrentino, **ZA 6706791** (1968 to Dumex), *C.A.* **70**, 57916c (1969); Yamamoto *et al.,* **DE 1816046** (1970 to Sumitomo), *C.A.* **73**, 120690d (1970); Inaba *et al., Chem. Pharm.*

Bull. **19**, 722 (1971). Pharmacology: S. Sakai *et al., Arzneim.-Forsch.* **22**, 534 (1972).

Pale yellow plates from ethanol, mp 156.5-157.5°. uv max (methanol): 259, 308 nm (ε 15800, 9600). LD_{50} in male, female mice, rats (mg/kg): 910, 750, 1150, 970 orally; 970, 840, 970, 980 i.p.; 1500, 1500, 1000, 1000 s.c. (Sakai).

Note: This is a controlled substance (depressant): **21 CFR, 1308.14.**

THERAP CAT: Sedative, hypnotic.

6550. Nimidane. [50435-25-1] 4-Chloro-*N*-1,3-dithietan-2-ylidene-2-methylbenzeneamine; cyclic methylene (4-chloro-*o*-tolyl)dithioimidocarbonate; AC-84633; ENT-29106; Abequito. $C_9H_8ClNS_2$; mol wt 229.75. C 47.05%, H 3.51%, Cl 15.43%, N 6.10%, S 27.91%. Prepn: R. W. Addor, S. Kantor, **DE 2305517** (1973 to Am. Cyanamid), *C.A.* **79**, 115553f (1973); W. W. Brand, M. W. Bullock, **US 3842096** (1974 to Am. Cyanamid). Tickicidal activity: N. K. Amaral *et al., J. Econ. Entomol.* **67**, 387 (1974).

White solid, mp 43-46°.

THERAP CAT (VET): Acaricide.

6551. Nimodipine. [66085-59-4] 1,4-Dihydro-2,6-dimethyl-4-(3-nitrophenyl)-3,5-pyridinedicarboxylic acid 2-methoxyethyl 1-methylethyl ester; 2-methoxyethyl 1,4-dihydro-5-(isopropoxycarbonyl)-2,6-dimethyl-4-(3-nitrophenyl)-3-pyridinecarboxylate; isopropyl 2-methoxyethyl 1,4-dihydro-2,6-dimethyl-4-(3-nitrophenyl)-3,5-pyridinedicarboxylate; 2,6-dimethyl-4-(3'-nitrophenyl)-1,4-dihydropyridine-3,5-dicarboxylic acid 3-β-methoxyethyl ester 5-isopropyl ester; Bay e 9736; Admon; Nimotop; Periplum. $C_{21}H_{26}N_2O_7$; mol wt 418.44. C 60.28%, H 6.26%, N 6.69%, O 26.77%. Dihydropyridine calcium channel blocker. Prepn: H. Meyer *et al.,* **DE 2117571**; *eidem,* **US 3799934** (1972, 1974 to Bayer). Pharmacology: R. Towart, S. Kazda, *Br. J. Pharmacol.* **67**, 409P (1979); K. Tanaka *et al., Arzneim.-Forsch.* **30**, 1494 (1980); L. M. Auer, *ibid.* **31**, 1423 (1981). Prepn of isomers and pharmacological comparison with racemate: R. Towart *et al., ibid.* **32**, 338 (1982). Use as cerebral vasodilator: H. Meyer *et al.,* **GB 2018134**; *eidem,* **US 4406906** (1979, 1983 to Bayer). Effect on associative learning in aging rabbits: R. A. Deyo *et al., Science* **243**, 809 (1989). GC and LC determns in biological fluids: G. J. Krol *et al., J. Chromatogr.* **305**, 105 (1984). Clinical trial in prophylaxis of cerebral vasospasm: G. S. Allen *et al., N. Engl. J. Med.* **308**, 619 (1983). Toxicology: H. Schlüter, *Arzneim.-Forsch.* **36**, 1733 (1986). Series of articles on clinical pharmacology and therapeutic use: *Am. J. Cardiol.* **55**(3), 139B-153B (1985).

Crystals from petr ether/acetic ester, mp 125°. LD_{50} in mice, rats (mg/kg): 3562, 6599 orally; 33, 16 i.v. (Schlüter).

(+)-**Form.** $[\alpha]_D^{20}$ +7.9° (c = 0.439 in dioxane).
(−)-**Form.** $[\alpha]_D^{20}$ −7.93° (c = 0.374 in dioxane).
THERAP CAT: Vasodilator (cerebral).

6552. Nimorazole. [6506-37-2] 4-[2-(5-Nitro-1H-imidazol-1-yl)ethyl]morpholine; N-2-morpholinoethyl-5-nitroimidazole; 1-(2-N-morpholinylethyl)-5-nitroimidazole; nitrimidazine; K-1900; Esclama; Naxofem; Naxogin. $C_9H_{14}N_4O_3$; mol wt 226.23. C 47.78%, H 6.24%, N 24.77%, O 21.22%. Prepn: **BE 667262**; Giraldi, Mariotti, **US 3399193** (1965, 1968 both to Carlo Erba); **NL 6609552; NL 6609553**; Gal and Carlson *et al.*, **US 3458528** and **US 3646027** (1967, 1967, 1969, 1972, all to Merck & Co.). Synthesis and biological activity studies: Giraldi *et al.*, *Arzneim.-Forsch.* **20**, 52 (1970). Pharmacology and toxicology: de Carneri *et al.*, *Progr. Antimicrob. Anticancer Chemother., Proc. 6th Int. Congr. Chemother.* **vol. I**, Tokyo, 1969 (Univ. of Tokyo Press, 1970, Tokyo) pp 149-154. Clinical results: Emanueli, de Carneri, *ibid.* **vol. II**, pp 369-372; Evans, Catterall, *Br. Med. J.* **IV**, 146 (1971). Metabolic studies: Giraldi, *Biochem. Pharmacol.* **20**, 339 (1971). Acute toxicity data: B. Cavalleri *et al.*, *J. Med. Chem.* **21**, 781 (1978).

Crystals from water, mp 110-111°. Slightly sol in water at room temp; sol in alcohols, acetone, chloroform. LD_{50} orally in mice: 1530 mg/kg (Cavalleri).
THERAP CAT: Antiprotozoal (Trichomonas).

6553. Nimustine. [42471-28-3] N'-[(4-Amino-2-methyl-5-pyrimidinyl)methyl]-N-(2-chloroethyl)-N-nitrosourea. C_9H_{13}-ClN_6O_2; mol wt 272.69. C 39.64%, H 4.81%, Cl 13.00%, N 30.82%, O 11.73%. Chloroethylnitrosourea derivative with antitumor activity. Prepn: H. Nakao *et al.*, **DE 2257360**; *eidem*, **US 4003901** (1973, 1977 both to Sankyo); *eidem*, *Yakugaku Zasshi* **94**, 1932 (1974), *C.A.* **82**, 43263y (1975). Effects on macrophage cytostatic activity in rats: N. Saijo *et al.*, *Br. J. Cancer* **42**, 162 (1980). Distribution, excretion, metabolism in mice: M. Tanaka *et al.*, *Cancer Treat. Rep.* **64**, 575 (1980). Exptl and clinical effect: N. Saijo *et al.*, *Cancer Chemother. Pharmacol.* **4**, 165 (1980). Acute toxicity: H. Masuda *et al.*, *Sankyo Kenkyusho Nempo* **29**, 118 (1977), *C.A.* **88**, 146298s (1978).

Pale yellow crystals from ethanol, dec 125°.
Hydrochloride. [55661-38-6] NSC-245382; ACNU; Nidran. $C_9H_{13}ClN_6O_2 \cdot HCl$; mol wt 309.15. White to light yellow cryst powder. uv max (0.04N HCl): 245 nm ($E_{1cm}^{1\%}$ 480-510). Sol in methanol, slightly sol in abs ethanol, n-butanol. Practically insol in ethyl acetate, ether, chloroform, benzene, n-hexane. Gradually develops greenish yellow color in light; decomposes slowly in humid air. LD_{50} in mice, rats (mg/kg): 62, 46 i.v. (Masuda).
THERAP CAT: Antineoplastic.

6554. Ninhydrin. [485-47-2] 2,2-Dihydroxy-1H-indene-1,3(2H)-dione; 2,2-dihydroxy-1,3-indanedione; 1,2,3-indantrione monohydrate; triketohydrinden hydrate. $C_9H_6O_4$; mol wt 178.14. C 60.68%, H 3.39%, O 35.93%. Prepn: Ruhemann, *J. Chem. Soc.* **97**, 1438 (1910); Teeters, Shriner, *J. Am. Chem. Soc.* **55**, 3026 (1933); Wanag, Lode, *Ber.* **71**, 1267 (1938). Improved syntheses: L. F. Fieser, *Experiments in Organic Chemistry* (Boston, 3rd ed., 1955) p 123; Becker, Russell, *J. Org. Chem.* **28**, 1896 (1963). Absorption spectrum: Polonovski *et al.*, *Bull. Soc. Chim.* [5] **6**, 1557 (1939). Poisonous action on bacteria, mice, guinea pigs: O. Loew, *Biochem. Z.* **69**, 111 (1915). Acute toxicity study: J. C. Breton *et al.*, *C.R. Seances Soc. Biol. Ses Fil.* **151**, 719 (1957).

Monograph: Henri Plagnol, *Influence de la Structure des Composés Aminés dans leur Reaction avec la Ninhydrine* (Bordeaux, 1962) 156 pp. *Reviews:* J. C. Breton, *Etudes Chimiques et Biologiques sur la Ninhydrine, Réactif des Aminoacides* (Imprimerie E. Drouillard, Bordeaux, 1958) 285 pp; McCaldin, *Chem. Rev.* **60**, 39 (1960); A. Schoenberg, E. Singer, *Tetrahedron* **34**, 1285-1300 (1978).

Monohydrate. Pale yellow prisms from water or alcohol. Reddens at 125°, swells at 139°, dec 241°. Freely sol in water. LD_{50} i.p. in mice: 78 mg/kg (Breton, 1957).
USE: Reagent for the detection of free amino and carboxyl groups in proteins and peptides, yielding a blue color under the proper conditions.

6555. Ninopterin. [2179-16-0] N-[4-[[1-(2-Amino-1,4-dihydro-4-oxo-6-pteridinyl)ethyl]amino]benzoyl]-L-glutamic acid; 9-methylpteroylglutamic acid; 9-methylfolic acid; Bremfol. C_{20}-$H_{21}N_7O_6$; mol wt 455.42. C 52.75%, H 4.65%, N 21.53%, O 21.08%. Folic acid analog. Prepn: Hultquist *et al.*, *J. Am. Chem. Soc.* **71**, 619 (1949); Hultquist, Smith, **GB 667098** (1952 to Am. Cyanamid). Clinical study in neoplastic diseases: J. C. Wright *et al.*, *J. Natl. Med. Assoc.* **43**, 211 (1951). *In vitro* evaluation as folic acid antagonist: S. Waxman *et al.*, *Chemotherapy (Basel)* **28**, 402 (1982).

uv max in 0.1N NaOH: 255, 283, 365 nm (ε 26, 30, 8 × 10³); in 0.1N HCl: 297 nm (ε 18 × 10³).
THERAP CAT: Experimental antineoplastic.

6556. Niobium. [7440-03-1] Columbium. Nb; at. wt 92.90638; at. no. 41; valence 2, 3, 4, 5; usually pentavalent. Group VB (5). One naturally occurring isotope: ⁹³Nb; artificial, radioactive isotopes: 88-92; 94-101. Approximately as abundant as nickel. Occurs in nature together with tantalum in the minerals *columbite* [(Fe,Mn)(Nb,Ta)$_2O_6$], *pyrochlore* (NaCaNb$_2O_6$F) and *tantalite* [(Fe,Mn)(Ta,Nb)$_2O_6$]. Discovered by Hatchett in 1801, isolated by Blomstrand in 1866, named after Niobe, daughter of Tantalos. Extracted from columbite which is mined largely in Nigeria and Zaire. Less than 10% of niobium-bearing ores come from the US, Canada, and Norway. Reviews of niobium and its compds: *Technology of Columbium (Niobium)* B. W. Gonser, E. M. Sherwood, Eds. (Wiley, New York, 1958); G. L. Miller, *Tantalum and Niobium* (Academic Press, New York, 1959) 767 pp; Brown, "The Chemistry of Niobium and Tantalum" in *Comprehensive Inorganic Chemistry* **Vol. 3**, J. C. Bailar, Jr. *et al.*, Eds. (Pergamon Press, Oxford, 1973) pp 553-622; P. H. Payton in *Kirk-Othmer Encyclopedia of Chemical Technology* **vol. 15** (Wiley-Interscience, New York, 3rd ed., 1981) pp 820-840.

Steel-gray, lustrous metal. Ductile and malleable when pure. Lattice structure: body-centered cube, lattice constant: 3.294 Å. d 8.57. mp 2468°. bp 4927°. Sp ht: 6.012 cal/g-atom/°C. Heat of sublimation: 170.9 kcal/g-atom; heat of combustion: 2379 cal/g. Coefficient of linear expansion per °C: 7.1 × 10⁻⁶. Electrical resistivity (20°): 13.2 μohm-cm. Temp coefficient of electrical resistivity per °C: 0.00395. Electron work function: 4.01 ev. Ionization potential: 6.77 V. Inert toward HCl, HNO_3 or aqua regia, but attacked by fusion with akali hydroxides or oxidizing agents.

USE: In ferrous metallurgy: Ferroniobium (produced by silicon reduction of columbite) is used to alloy stainless steels and metals for welding rods. In niobium base alloys for high temps and nuclear reactions. Niobium has some use as a getter in electronic vacuum tubes.

6557. Niobium Pentachloride. [10026-12-7] Niobium chloride ($NbCl_5$); columbium pentachloride; niobium(V) chloride. Cl_5Nb; mol wt 270.17. Cl 65.61%, Nb 34.39%. $NbCl_5$. Exists as dimeric units in the solid state. Prepn: Epperson *et al.*, *Inorg. Synth.* **7**, 163 (1963); *cf.* Rolsten, *J. Am. Chem. Soc.* **80**, 2952 (1958). Toxicity studies: T. J. Haley *et al.*, *Toxicol. Appl. Pharmacol.* **4**, 385 (1962); N. A. Zhilova, A. A. Kasparov, *Hyg. Sanit.* **31**, 328 (1966). Review of niobium halides: Fairbrother in *Halogen Chemistry* **Vol. 3**, V. Gutmann, Ed. (Academic Press, New York, 1967) pp 123-178. Review of applications in organic synthesis: C. K. Z. Andrade, *Curr. Org. Synth.* **1**, 333-353 (2004).

Yellow, very deliquesc, monoclinic crystals; dec in moist air with evolution of HCl. d 2.75. mp 204.7-209.5°; bp ~250°, but begins to sublime at 125°. Sol in HCl, carbon tetrachloride. LD_{50} in mice (mg/kg): 61 i.p., 940 orally (Haley). LD_{50} in mice, rats (mg/kg): 829, 1400 orally (Zhilova, Kasparov).

USE: Lewis acid catalyst in organic synthesis.

6558. Niobium Pentafluoride. [7783-68-8] Columbium pentafluoride. F_5Nb; mol wt 187.90. F 50.55%, Nb 49.44%. NbF_5. Prepn from $NbCl_5$ + HF: Ruff, Zedner, *Ber.* **42**, 492 (1909); Ruff, Schiller, *Z. Anorg. Allg. Chem.* **72**, 329 (1911); Kwasnik in *Handbook of Preparative Inorganic Chemistry* **Vol. 1**, G. Brauer, Ed. (Academic Press, New York, 2nd ed., 1963) p 254. Prepn from the elements: Fairbrother, Frith, *J. Chem. Soc.* **1951**, 3051; Junkins *et al.*, *J. Am. Chem. Soc.* **74**, 3464 (1952). Review of transition metal pentafluorides: Peacock, *Adv. Fluorine Chem.* **7**, 113-145 (1973).

Strongly refractive, deliquescent, monoclinic crystals, d_4^{80} 2.6955. mp 80.0°; bp 234.9°. Appreciable vapor pressure at 50°. Hydrolyzes in water, alc, caustic solns. Sparingly sol in carbon disulfide, chloroform. More sol in concd H_2SO_4 than TaF_5. Forms complexes with Lewis bases.

6559. Niobium Pentoxide. [1313-96-8] Niobium oxide (Nb_2O_5); columbium pentoxide; niobium(V) oxide. Nb_2O_5; mol wt 265.81. Nb 69.90%, O 30.10%. Separation: Münchow, *Chem. Ztg.* **84**, 490, 527 (1960). Review of polymorphism: Schäfer *et al.*, *Angew. Chem. Int. Ed.* **5**, 40-52 (1966).

White, orthorhombic crystals. Becomes yellow on heating. d 4.6. mp 1520°. Insol in water; sol in HF, hot H_2SO_4.

6560. Nioxime. [492-99-9] 1,2-Cyclohexanedione dioxime. $C_6H_{10}N_2O_2$; mol wt 142.16. C 50.69%, H 7.09%, N 19.71%, O 22.51%. Prepn: Hach *et al.*, *Org. Synth.* **32**, 35 (1952); Boyer, Ellzey, *J. Am. Chem. Soc.* **82**, 2525 (1960); Borger *et al.*, *Bull. Soc. Chim. Belg.* **73**, 73 (1964); Arthur, **FR 1339224** (1963 to du Pont).

Crystals, mp 185-188° (darkening at 170°).
USE: Analytical reagent for nickel and palladium.

6561. Nipecotic Acid. [498-95-3] 3-Piperidinecarboxylic acid; hexahydronicotinic acid. $C_6H_{11}NO_2$; mol wt 129.16. C 55.79%, H 8.58%, N 10.84%, O 24.77%. Prepd by hydrogenation of nicotinic acid with platinum oxide catalyst: McElvain, Adams, *J. Am. Chem. Soc.* **45**, 2738 (1923); with rhodium on alumina catalyst: Freifelder, *J. Org. Chem.* **28**, 1135 (1963); *idem*, **US 3159639** (1964 to Abbott).

Crystals, mp 261° (dec). Freely sol in water. Practically insol in abs alcohol and ether.

Hydrochloride. $C_6H_{11}NO_2$·HCl. mp 240-242°. Very sol in water; slightly sol in alc (also reported as freely sol in alc); slightly sol in chloroform. Practically insol in ether, benzene, and acetone.

6562. Nipradilol. [81486-22-8] 3,4-Dihydro-8-[2-hydroxy-3-[(1-methylethyl)amino]propoxy]-2*H*-1-benzopyran-3-ol 3-nitrate; 3,4-dihydro-8-(2-hydroxy-3-isopropylamino)propoxy-3-nitroxy-2*H*-1-benzopyran; 8-[2-hydroxy-3-(isopropylamino)propoxy]-3-chromanol 3-nitrate; nipradolol; K-351; Hypadil. $C_{15}H_{22}N_2O_6$; mol wt 326.34. C 55.21%, H 6.79%, N 8.58%, O 29.42%. β-Adrenergic blocker with vasodilating activity. Prepn: M. Shiratsuchi *et al.*, **EP 42299**; *eidem*, **US 4394382** (1981, 1983 both to Kowa). Synthesis: M. Shiratsuchi *et al.*, *Chem. Pharm. Bull.* **35**, 632 (1987). Resolution of isomers: M. Shiratsuchi *et al.*, **EP 154511**; *eidem*, **US 4727085** (1985, 1988 both to Kowa). Synthesis and activity of isomers: M. Shiratsuchi *et al.*, *Chem. Pharm. Bull.* **35**, 3691 (1987). Pharmacology: Y. Uchida *et al.*, *Arch. Int. Pharmacodyn.* **262**, 132 (1983). Hemodynamic effects in dogs: H. Hisa *et al.*, *ibid.* **271**, 169 (1984). Effects on cardiac function in dogs: M. Sakanashi *et al.*, *ibid.* **274**, 47 (1985); M. Fujii *et al.*, *Jpn. Heart J.* **27**, 233 (1986). Pharmacokinetics and metabolism in rats: S. Kabuto *et al.*, *Arzneim.-Forsch.* **35**, 1674 (1985); H. Kimata *et al.*, *ibid.* 1680. Metabolic fate in dog and man: M. Yoshimura *et al.*, *Chem. Pharm. Bull.* **33**, 3456 (1985). Clinical evaluation in angina: H. Kishida *et al.*, *Jpn. Heart J.* **29**, 309 (1988).

Colorless needles, mp 107-116° (Shiratsuchi, 1983); also reported as mp 110-122° (Shiratsuchi, 1987). LD_{50} i.v. in mice, rats: 74.0, 73.0 mg/kg; orally in mice: 540 mg/kg (Shiratsuchi, 1988).
THERAP CAT: Antianginal; antihypertensive.

6563. Niridazole. [61-57-4] 1-(5-Nitro-2-thiazolyl)-2-imidazolidinone; 1-(5-nitro-2-thiazolyl)-2-oxotetrahydroimidazole; nitrothiamidazol; Ba-32644; Ciba 32644-Ba; Ambilhar. $C_6H_6N_4O_3S$; mol wt 214.20. C 33.64%, H 2.82%, N 26.16%, O 22.41%, S 14.97%. Prepn: **BE 632989** (1963 to Ciba), *C.A.* **61**, 1873d (1964), corresp to **GB 986562**; Lambert *et al.*, *Experientia* **20**, 452 (1964).

Yellow crystals from dimethylformamide, mp 260-262°.
THERAP CAT: Anthelmintic (Schistosoma).

6564. Nisin. [1414-45-5] Nisin A; Nisaplin; Novasin. $C_{143}H_{230}N_{42}O_{37}S_7$; mol wt 3354.07. C 51.21%, H 6.91%, N 17.54%, O 17.65%, S 6.69%. Ribosomally synthesized antimicrobial peptide produced by *Lactococcus lactis* (formerly *Streptococcus lactis*); name derived from "group N inhibitory substance". Member of the class I bacteriocins known as lantibiotics; structure contains 34 amino acid residues, eight of which are rarely found in nature, including lanthionine, *q.v.*, and β-methyllanthionine. Isoln and antibacterial activity: A. T. R. Mattick, A. Hirsch, *Nature* **154**, 551 (1944); *eidem*, *Lancet* **250**, 417 (1946); **253**, 5 (1947). Purification and nature of nisin: N. J. Berridge *et al.*, *Biochem. J.* **52**, 529 (1952). Production: H. B. Hawley, R. H. Hall, **US 2935503** (1960 to Aplin & Barrett). Structure: E. Gross, J. L. Morrell, *J. Am. Chem. Soc.* **93**, 4634 (1971). Confirmation of structure of nisin and its major degradation product: M. Barber *et al.*, *Experientia* **44**, 266 (1988). Partial synthesis: K. Fukase *et al.*, *Bull. Chem. Soc. Jpn.* **59**, 2505 (1986). Total synthesis: K. Fukase *et al.*, *Tetrahedron Lett.* **29**, 795 (1988). Biosynthetic study: G. W. Buchman *et al.*, *J. Biol. Chem.* **263**, 16260 (1988). Review of properties and commercial applications: A. Hurst, D. G. Hoover, *Food Sci. Technol.* **57**, 369-394 (1993); J. Delves-Broughton *et al., Antonie van Leeuwenhoek* **69**, 193-202 (1996); of biosynthesis: C.-I. Cheigh, Y.-R. Pyun, *Biotechnol. Lett.* **27**, 1641-1648 (2005); of biosynthesis, mode of action and comparison with other lantibiotics: C. Chatterjee *et al., Chem. Rev.* **105**, 633-683 (2005).

Abu = α-aminobutyric acid
Dha = dehydroalanine
Dhb = dehydrobutyrine

Crystals from ethanol. Soly in dilute HCl: 12% (pH 2.5); 4% (pH 5.0). Stable to boiling in acid soln.

Nisin Z. [137061-46-2] 27-L-Asparagine-nisin. $C_{141}H_{229}N_{41}$-$O_{38}S_7$; mol wt 3331.03. Naturally occurring nisin variant. Identification: J. W. Mulders *et al., Eur. J. Biochem.* **201**, 581 (1991).

USE: Food preservative, esp. for cheese and other dairy products, canned vegetables, and some baked goods.

6565. Nisoldipine. [63675-72-9] 1,4-Dihydro-2,6-dimethyl-4-(2-nitrophenyl)-3,5-pyridinedicarboxylic acid methyl 2-methylpropyl ester; isobutyl methyl 1,4-dihydro-2,6-dimethyl-4-(*o*-nitrophenyl)-3,5-pyridinedicarboxylate; isobutyl 1,4-dihydro-5-methoxycarbonyl-2,6-dimethyl-4-(2-nitrophenyl)-3-pyridinecarboxylate; 2,6-dimethyl-3-carbomethoxy-4-(2-nitrophenyl)-5-carbisobutoxy-1,4-dihydropyridine; Bay k 5552; Baymycard; Sular; Syscor; Zadipina. $C_{20}H_{24}N_2O_6$; mol wt 388.41. C 61.85%, H 6.23%, N 7.21%, O 24.72%. Dihydropyridine calcium channel blocker. Prepn: E. Wehinger *et al.,* DE **2549568**; *eidem,* US **4154839** (1977, 1979 both to Bayer). Pharmacology: S. Kazda *et al., Arzneim.-Forsch.* **30**, 2144 (1980). Hemodynamics: A. Vogt *et al., ibid.* **2162**. Series of articles on pharmacokinetics: *ibid.* **38**, 1093-1110 (1988). Reviews of pharmacology and clinical efficacy: H. A. Friedel, E. M. Sorkin, *Drugs* **36**, 682-731 (1988); J. Mitchell *et al., J. Clin. Pharmacol.* **33**, 46-52 (1993).

Crystals from ethanol, mp 151-152°.
THERAP CAT: Antihypertensive; antianginal.

6566. Nitarsone. [98-72-6] 4-Nitrophenylarsonic acid; *p*-nitrobenzenearsonic acid. $C_6H_6AsNO_5$; mol wt 247.04. C 29.17%, H 2.45%, As 30.33%, N 5.67%, O 32.38%. Prepn: Jacobs *et al., J. Am. Chem. Soc.* **40**, 1580 (1918); Doak, Freedman, US **2653160** (1953 to the U.S.A. as represented by the Administrator of the Federal Security Agency); Ruddy, Starkey, *Org. Synth.* **coll. vol. III**, 665 (1955).

Pale yellow leaflets from water, dec 298-300°. Very slightly sol in cold water, cold alcohol; readily sol in warm water, warm alcohol.
THERAP CAT (VET): Antihistomonad.

6567. Nitazoxanide. [55981-09-4] 2-(Acetyloxy)-*N*-(5-nitro-2-thiazolyl)benzamide; *N*-(5-nitro-2-thiazolyl)salicylamide acetate (ester); 2-(2′-acetoxy)benzamido-5-nitrothiazole; PH-5776; Alinia; Cryptaz. $C_{12}H_9N_3O_5S$; mol wt 307.28. C 46.90%, H 2.95%, N 13.67%, O 26.03%, S 10.44%. Broad spectrum antiparasitic agent; inhibits pyruvate ferredoxin oxidoreductase. Prepn: J. F. Rossignol, R. Cavier, DE **2438037**; *eidem,* US **3950351** (1975, 1976 both to S.P.R.L. Phavic); and antiparasitic activity: R. Cavier *et al., Eur. J. Med. Chem. - Chim. Ther.* **13**, 539 (1978). Antibacterial spectrum *in vitro:* L Dubreuil *et al., Antimicrob. Agents Chemother.* **40**, 2266 (1996). Toxicology: J. R. Murphy, J.-C. Friedmann, *J. Appl. Toxicol.* **5**, 49 (1985). Clinical pharmacokinetics: A. Stockis *et al., Int. J. Clin. Pharmacol. Ther.* **34**, 349 (1996). Clinical trial in intestinal protozoan and helminthic infections: H. Abaza *et al., Curr. Ther. Res.* **59**, 116 (1998). Review of mechanism of action and clinical experience: H. M. Gilles, P. S. Hoffman, *Trends Parasitol.* **18**, 95-97 (2002).

Light yellow crystalline powder. Crystals from methanol, mp 202°. Poorly sol in ethanol. Practically insol in water. LD_{50} orally in male, female mice: 1350, 1380 mg/kg; in rats: >10 g/kg (Murphy, Friedmann).
THERAP CAT: Anthelmintic (cestodes); antiprotozoal (Cryptosporidium).

6568. Nitenpyram. [150824-47-8] (1*E*)-*N*-[(6-Chloro-3-pyridinyl)methyl]-*N*-ethyl-*N′*-methyl-2-nitro-1,1-ethenediamine; 1-[*N*-(6-chloro-3-pyridylmethyl)-*N*-ethylamino-2-nitroethylene; TI-304; Bestguard; Capstar. $C_{11}H_{15}ClN_4O_2$; mol wt 270.72. C 48.80%, H 5.58%, Cl 13.10%, N 20.70%, O 11.82%. Chloronicotinyl insecticide; orally administered flea adulticide. Prepn: I. Minamida *et al.,* EP **302389**; *eidem,* US **5849768** (1989, 1998 both to Takeda); and insecticidal activity: *eidem, J. Pestic. Sci.* **18**, 41 (1993). Physical and biological properties: Y. Kashiwada, *Agrochem. Jpn.* **68**, 18 (1996). Effects on neuronal nicotinic acetylcholine receptor channel in rat cells: K. Nagata *et al., J. Pestic. Sci.* **24**, 143 (1999). Efficacy study in flea infested dogs: M.-C. Cadiergues *et al., Am. J. Vet. Res.* **60**, 1122 (1999). LC-MS determn in fruits and vegetables: D. Zywitz *et al., Deutsche Lebens.-Rundschau* **99**, 188 (2003).

White crystals, mp 83-84°; also reported as pale yellow solid. Vapor pressure: 8.3×10^{-12} mmHg. Soly at 25° (g/l): water 840; chloroform 700; acetone 290; methanol 670; ethanol 89. Log P (octanol/water): −0.64. LD_{50} in male, female rats, male, female mice (mg/kg): 1680, 1575, 867, 1281 orally; in male, female rats (mg/kg): >2000, >2000 dermally. LC_{50} (48 hr) in carp, water fleas (ppm): >1000, >10000 (Kashiwada).
THERAP CAT (VET): Ectoparasiticide.

6569. Nithiazide. [139-94-6] *N*-Ethyl-*N′*-(5-nitro-2-thiazolyl)urea; Hepzide. $C_6H_8N_4O_3S$; mol wt 216.22. C 33.33%, H 3.73%, N 25.91%, O 22.20%, S 14.83%. Prepd by the condensation of ethyl isocyanate with 2-amino-5-nitrothiazole in toluene: Cuckler *et al., Proc. Soc. Exp. Biol. Med.* **92**, 483 (1956); O'Neill *et al.,* US **2755285** (1956 to Merck & Co.).

Crystals, dec 228°. pKa 7.3. Practically insol in water: 3 mg/100 ml.

Sodium salt. Orange plates. Soly in water: 8 g/100 ml. Aq solns are alkaline and unstable.

Potassium salt. Crystals. Soly in water: 3 g/l00 ml. Aq solns are more stable than those of the Na salt.

THERAP CAT (VET): Antiprotozoal.

6570. Nitisinone. [104206-65-7] 2-[2-Nitro-4-(trifluoromethyl)benzoyl]-1,3-cyclohexanedione; NTBC; Orfadin. $C_{14}H_{10}$-F_3NO_5; mol wt 329.23. C 51.07%, H 3.06%, F 17.31%, N 4.25%, O 24.30%. Herbicidal triketone that inhibits 4-hydroxyphenyl-pyruvate dioxygenase (HPPD), an enzyme involved in plastoquinone biosynthesis in plants and in tyrosine catabolism in mammals. Prepn: C. G. Carter, **EP 186118** (1986 to Stauffer); *idem,* **US 5006158** (1991 to ICI). Inhibition of HPPD in plants: M. P. Prisbylla *et al., Brighton Crop Prot. Conf. - Weeds* **1993,** 731; in rats: M. K. Ellis *et al., Toxicol. Appl. Pharmacol.* **133,** 12 (1995). LC determn in plasma: M. Bielenstein *et al., J. Chromatogr. B* **730,** 177 (1999). Clinical evaluation in hereditary tyrosinemia type I: S. Lindstedt *et al., Lancet* **340,** 813 (1992). Review of toxicology and therapeutic development: E. A. Lock *et al, J. Inherited Metab. Dis.* **21,** 498-506 (1998); of clinical experience: E. Holme, S. Lindstedt, *ibid.* 507-517.

Solid, mp 88-94°.

THERAP CAT: In treatment of inherited tyrosinemia type I.

6571. Nitracrine. [4533-39-5] *N,N*-Dimethyl-*N′*-(1-nitro-9-acridinyl)-1,3-propanediamine; 9-[[3-(dimethylamino)propyl]amino]-1-nitroacridine. $C_{18}H_{20}N_4O_2$; mol wt 324.38. C 66.65%, H 6.21%, N 17.27%, O 9.86%. Deriv of acridine, *q.v.,* with cytostatic and cytotoxic properties. Prepn: **FR 1458183** (1966 to Polfa), *C.A.* **68,** 39493s (1968); A. Ledochowski, B. Stefanska, *Rocz. Chem.* **40,** 301 (1966), *C.A.* **65,** 2219b (1966). Pharmacological studies: J. Gieldanowski *et al., Arch. Immunol. Ther. Exp.* **20,** 399 (1972); *eidem, ibid.* 419. Mechanism of action: J. Konopa *et al., Mater. Med. Pol.* **8,** 258 (1976). Cytotoxicity study: I. Szumiel, M. Walicka, *Neoplasma* **27,** 697 (1980). DNA binding activity: L. Szmigiero, M. Gniazdowski, *Arzneim.-Forsch.* **31,** 1875 (1981). Comprehensive review: M. Gniazdowski *et al.* in *Antibiotics* **Vol. V,** part 2, F. E. Hahn, Ed. (Springer-Verlag, New York, 1979) pp 275-297.

Crystals from benzene/petr ether, mp 134-135°. Practically insol in water. Sol in most organic solvents. pKa_1 6.45; pKa_2 8.8.

Dihydrochloride monohydrate. [55429-45-3] C-283; Ledakrin. $C_{18}H_{20}N_4O_2 \cdot 2HCl \cdot H_2O$; mol wt 415.31. Orange crystals, mp 223-224°. Sol in water, methanol, ethanol, slightly sol in benzene, diethyl ether. Conc water solns are acidic (pH 4). LD_{50} in rats, mice (mg/kg): 1, 0.72 i.v.; 34, 26 i.g. (Gniazdowski).

THERAP CAT: Antineoplastic.

6572. Nitramide. [7782-94-7] $H_2N_2O_2$; mol wt 62.03. H 3.25%, N 45.16%, O 51.59%. H_2NNO_2. Prepd from potassium nitrocarbamate: Thiele, Lachmann, *Ber.* **27,** 1909 (1894); *Ann.* **288,** 267 (1895); Marlies, La Mer, *J. Am. Chem. Soc.* **57,** 2008 (1935); Marlies *et al., Inorg. Synth.* **1,** 68 (1939).

Unstable, shiny, white leaflets from ether + petr ether, mp 72-75° (dec). Dipole moment 3.7. Should be freshly prepd when needed. Does not explode under ordinary conditions. *Handle in glass or platinum!* Sol in ether, alcohol, acetone, water. Slightly sol in benzene. Practically insol in petr ether, chloroform.

6573. Nitramine. [479-45-8] *N*-Methyl-*N*,2,4,6-tetranitrobenzenamine; *N*-methyl-*N*,2,4,6-tetranitroaniline; picrylmethylnitramine; picrylnitromethylamine; Tetralite; Tetryl. C_7H_5-N_5O_8; mol wt 287.14. C 29.28%, H 1.76%, N 24.39%, O 44.58%. Review of toxicology and human exposure: *Toxicological Profile for Tetryl* (PB95-264271, 1995) 133 pp.

Yellow crystals. d 1.57. mp 130-132°; explodes at about 180-190°. Insol in water. Sol in alc, ether, benzene, glacial acetic acid. *Keep soln in the dark.* Causes yellow staining to skin and hair.

Caution: Potential symptoms of overexposure are sensitization dermatitis, itching, erythema; edema on nasal folds, cheeks and neck; keratitis; sneezing; anemia; fatigue; coughing, coryza; irritability; malaise, headache, lassitude and insomnia; nausea, vomiting; liver and kidney damage. *See NIOSH Pocket Guide to Chemical Hazards* (DHHS/NIOSH 97-140, 1997) p 304.

USE: As indicator, 0.1 g in 60 ml alcohol with water to make 100 ml. pH: 10.8 colorless, 13.0 reddish-brown. One to five drops of soln required for 10 ml liquid. Salt error said to be small. Also used in explosives.

6574. Nitrapyrin. [1929-82-4] 2-Chloro-6-(trichloromethyl)pyridine; α,α,α,6-tetrachloro-2-picoline; N-Serve. $C_6H_3Cl_4N$; mol wt 230.91. C 31.21%, H 1.31%, Cl 61.41%, N 6.07%. Prepn: Johnston *et al., GB 957276, BE 624800* (1964, 1963 to Dow), *C.A.* **61,** 1841b (1964).

Crystals, mp 62.5-62.9° (CH_2Cl_2-pentane). bp_{11} 136-137.5°.

USE: Fertilizer additive to control nitrification and prevent loss of soil nitrogen.

6575. Nitrazepam. [146-22-5] 1,3-Dihydro-7-nitro-5-phenyl-2*H*-1,4-benzodiazepin-2-one; LA-1; Ro-4-5360; Benzalin; Calsmin; Eatan; Eunoctin; Imeson; Mogadan; Mogadon; Nelbon; Nitrados; Radedorm; Remnos; Somnased; Somnibel; Somnite; Surem; Unisomnia. $C_{15}H_{11}N_3O_3$; mol wt 281.27. C 64.05%, H 3.94%, O 14.94%, N 17.06%. Prepn: Sternbach *et al., J. Med. Chem.* **6,** 261 (1963); O. Keller *et al., US 3121076* (1964 to Hoffmann-La Roche). Crystal structure: G. Gilli *et al., Acta Crystallogr.* **33B,** 2664 (1977). Pharmacokinetic studies: Rieder, *Arzneim.-Forsch.* **23,** 212 (1973); L. Kangas, *Acta Pharmacol. Toxicol.* **45,** 16 (1979). Toxicity data: Randall *et al., Schweiz. Med. Wochenschr.* **95,** 334 (1965). *Review:* Rieder, Wendt in *Benzodiazepines,* S. Garattini *et al.,* Eds. (Raven Press, New York, 1973) pp 99-127. Comprehensive description: H. Y. Aboul-Enein *et al., Anal. Profiles Drug Subs.* **9,** 487-517 (1980).

Yellow crystals from ethanol, mp 224-226°. uv max (0.1*N* H$_2$-SO$_4$): 277.5 nm (E$_{1cm}^{1\%}$ 1500). Sol in alc, acetone, chloroform, ethyl acetate. Practically insol in water, ether, benzene, hexane. LD$_{50}$ orally in rats: 825 ±80 mg/kg (Randall).

Note: This is a controlled substance (depressant): **21 CFR,** 1308.14.

THERAP CAT: Anticonvulsant; hypnotic.

6576. Nitrendipine. [39562-70-4] 1,4-Dihydro-2,6-dimethyl-4-(3-nitrophenyl)-3,5-pyridinedicarboxylic acid ethyl methyl ester; ethyl 1,4-dihydro-5-(acetoxycarbonyl)-2,6-dimethyl-4-(3-nitrophenyl)-3-pyridinecarboxylate; 3-ethyl-5-methyl-1,4-dihydro-2,6-dimethyl-4-(3-nitrophenyl)-3,5-pyridinedicarboxylate; Bay e 5009; Bayotensin; Baypress; Bylotensin; Deiten; Nidrel. C$_{18}$H$_{20}$N$_2$O$_6$; mol wt 360.36. C 59.99%, H 5.59%, N 7.77%, O 26.64%. Dihydropyridine calcium channel blocker. Prepn: H. Meyer *et al., DE* **2117571**; *eidem,* **US 3799934** (1972, 1974 both to Bayer); *eidem, Arzneim.-Forsch.* **31,** 407 (1981). Series of articles on pharmacology: *ibid.* 2056-2067. Hemodynamic effects: H. O. Ventura *et al., Am. J. Cardiol.* **51,** 783 (1983). Pharmacokinetics: L. Hansson *et al., Hypertension* **5,** Suppl. II, II-25 (1983). HPLC determn in human serum: R. A. Janis *et al., J. Clin. Pharmacol.* **23,** 266 (1983). Double-blind, controlled clinical trial: U. Brugmann *et al., Herz* **10,** 53 (1985). Symposium on pharmacology and clinical efficacy: *J. Cardiovasc. Pharmacol.* **6** Suppl. 7, S929-S1113 (1984). Toxicology studies: K. Hoffmann, "Toxicological Studies with Nitrendipine" in *Nitrendipine,* A. Scriabine *et al.,* Eds. (Urban & Schwarzenberg, Baltimore, 1984) pp 25-32. *Review:* A. Scriabine *et al.,* "Nitrendipine" in *New Drugs Annual: Cardiovascular Drugs* Vol. 2, A. Scriabine, Ed. (Raven Press, New York, 1984) pp 37-49.

Crystals from ethanol, mp 158°. Relatively insol in water. LD$_{50}$ in mice, rats (mg/kg): 39, 12.6 i.v.; 2540, >10000 orally (Hoffmann).

THERAP CAT: Antihypertensive.

6577. Nitric Acid. [7697-37-2] Aqua fortis; azotic acid; Salpetersäure (German). HNO$_3$; mol wt 63.01. H 1.60%, N 22.23%, O 76.18%. Strong monobasic acid and oxidizing agent. Usually produced by the catalytic oxidation of ammonia. Reviews of industrial processes: F. D. Miles, *Nitric Acid, Manufacture and Uses* (Oxford Univ. Press, 1961, 1963); W. Sommer in *Ullmanns Encyklopädie der technischen Chemie* vol. 15, pp 3-67 (3rd ed., 1964). Pure acid prepd by distillation of concd nitric acid with concd sulfuric acid; by treating sodium or potassium nitrate with 100% H$_2$SO$_4$ and removing HNO$_3$ by distillation; by fractional crystallization of concd HNO$_3$. Review of preparation and properties of pure HNO$_3$: S. A. Stern *et al., Chem. Rev.* **60,** 185-207 (1960); S. S. Pannu, *J. Chem. Educ.* **61,** 174-176 (1984). *Reviews: Mellor's* Vol. VIII, supplement II, *Nitrogen* (part 2), 278-352 (1967); Jones in *Comprehensive Inorganic Chemistry* vol. 2, J. C. Bailar, Jr. *et al.,* Eds. (Pergamon Press, Oxford, 1973) pp 375-388; D. J. Newman in *Kirk-Othmer Encyclopedia of Chemical Technology* vol. 15 (Wiley-Interscience, New York, 1981) pp 853-871. Review of photochemistry: J. R. Huber, *Chem. Phys. Chem.* **5,** 1663-1669 (2004).

Colorless liquid. Fumes in moist air. Characteristic choking odor. d$_4^4$ 1.51. mp −41.59°. bp$_{760}$ 86.2°. Forms white, monoclinic crystals; d$^{-41.6}$ (solid) 1.895. Heat of fusion: 2.503 kcal/mole. Heat of infinite dilution (298.1 K): −7971 cal/mole. Forms an azeotrope with water, so-called constant boiling acid at 68% HNO$_3$, bp 120.5°, d$_4^{20}$ 1.41. Develops yellow color in the presence of light due to nitrogen oxide formation. Stains woolen fabrics and animal tissue a bright yellow. Reacts violently with combustible or readily oxidizable materials such as alcohols, tur-

pentine, charcoal, organic refuse. Reacts with most metals to release hydrogen gas.

Nitric acid, concentrated. Defined as an aqueous solution containing approx 70% HNO$_3$. Density of aq solns: d$_4^{20}$ 1.0036 (1% HNO$_3$ w/w); 1.0543 (10%); 1.1150 (20%); 1.1800 (30%); 1.2463 (40%); 1.3100 (50%); 1.3667 (60%); 1.4134 (70%); 1.4521 (80%); 1.4826 (90%); 1.5129 (100%): *International Critical Tables* **III,** 58 (1928).

Nitric acid, fuming. Concentrated nitric acid containing dissolved nitrogen dioxide. May be prepared from concd nitric acid by passing nitrogen dioxide into it or by adding a small amount of organic reducing agent, such as formaldehyde. Yellow to brownish-red, clear, strongly fuming, very corrosive liq; evolves suffocating, poisonous, yellowish-red fumes of nitrogen dioxide and nitrogen tetroxide. The density increases as the free NO$_2$ content increases: concd HNO$_3$ with 7.5% NO$_2$ added d$_4^{20}$ = 1.526; with 12.7% NO$_2$ d$_4^{20}$ = 1.544. Miscible with water. *Handle with extreme care.*

Caution: Potential symptoms of overexposure are irritation of eyes, mucous membranes and skin; delayed pulmonary edema, pneumonitis and bronchitis; dental erosion. *See NIOSH Pocket Guide to Chemical Hazards* (DHHS/NIOSH 97-140, 1997) p 224. *See also Clinical Toxicology of Commercial Products,* R. E. Gosselin *et al.,* Eds. (Williams & Wilkins, Baltimore, 5th ed., 1984) Section III, pp 8-11.

USE: Manufacture of inorganic and organic nitrates and nitro compounds for fertilizers, dye intermediates, explosives, rocket fuels. As laboratory reagent, in photoengraving, metal etching. Pharmaceutic aid (acidifier).

6578. Nitric Oxide. [10102-43-9] Nitrogen oxide (NO); mononitrogen monoxide; nitrogen monoxide; endothium-derived relaxing factor; EDRF. NO; mol wt 30.01. N 46.67%, O 53.31%. Highly reactive, potentially toxic gas produced by the partial oxidation of atmospheric nitrogen. Major air pollutant along with its oxidative by-products (NO$_x$) resulting from incomplete combustion of fossil fuels. Also found ubiquitously in animals; generated *in vivo* from arginine, *q.v.,* by *nitric oxide synthase* (NOS). Increases guanylate cyclase activity to produce cyclic GMP, *q.v.* Involved in a wide range of physiological functions, including vasodilation, neurotransmission, cytotoxicity of macrophages, and inhibition of platelet aggregation. Laboratory prepn: Blanchard, *Inorg. Synth.* **2,** 126 (1946); Schenk in *Handbook of Preparative Inorganic Chemistry* vol. 1, G. Brauer, Ed. (Academic Press, New York, 2nd ed., 1963) pp 485-487. General reviews: Beattie, "Nitric Oxide" in *Mellor's* Vol. VIII, supplement II, *Nitrogen* (part 2) 216-240 (1967); Jones in *Comprehensive Inorganic Chemistry* vol. 2, J. C. Bailar, Jr. *et al.,* Eds. (Pergamon Press, Oxford, 1973) pp 323-334. Role in cGMP production: W. P. Arnold *et al., Proc. Natl. Acad. Sci. USA* **74,** 3203 (1977). Identification of endothelium dependent vasorelaxation: R. F. Furchgott, J. V. Zawadzki, *Nature* **288,** 373 (1980). Identity of NO and EDRF: L. J. Ignarro *et al., Proc. Natl. Acad. Sci. USA* **84,** 9265 (1987). Reviews of physiological role: S. Moncada *et al., Pharmacol. Rev.* **43,** 109-142 (1991); A. R. Butler, D. L. H. Williams, *Chem. Soc. Rev.* **22,** 233-242 (1993). Role in airway function: R. J. Martin *et al., Semin. Perinatol.* **26,** 432 (2002). Clinical trial of inhaled NO in neonatal respiratory failure: G. M. Sokol, R. A. Ehrenkranz, *ibid.* **27,** 311 (2003). Review of pharmacology and therapeutic potential of inhaled NO: F. Ichinose *et al., Circulation* **109,** 3106-3111 (2004). Review of chemistry: D. L. H. Williams, *Org. Biomol. Chem.* **1,** 441-449 (2003); of coordination chemistry in bio-inorganic systems: J. A. McCleverty, *Chem. Rev.* **104,** 403-418 (2004).

Colorless gas. Burns only when heated with hydrogen. triple tp −163.6°. bp −151.8°. d$^{-150.2}$ (liq) 1.27. Relative d (gas) 1.036 (air = 1). Absolute d (gas) 1.227 (air = 1). n$_D^{25}$ 1.0002697. Trouton constant 27.1. Contains an odd number of electrons and is paramagnetic. Crit temp −92.9°. Crit press. 64.6 atm. Heat of formation (18°): −21.5 kcal/mole. Heat of vaporization (bp): 3.293 kcal/mole. Ionization potential: 9.26 eV. Electron affinity: 0.024 eV. Solubility in water (ml/100 ml; 1 atm): 7.38 (0°); 4.6 (20°); 2.37 (60°). Combines with oxygen to form NO$_2$ and with chlorine and bromine to form the nitrosyl halides, such as NOCl, *see* N. V. Sidgwick, *Chemical Elements and Their Compounds* vol. I (Oxford, 1950) p 683.

Caution: Potential symptoms of overexposure are irritation of eyes, wet skin, nose and throat; drowsiness; unconsciousness; methemoglobinemia. *See NIOSH Pocket Guide to Chemical Hazards* (DHHS/NIOSH 97-140, 1997) p 224. On contact with air, nitric oxide is converted to the highly poisonous nitrogen dioxide, *q.v.* Respiratory protection and adequate ventilation should be used to avoid overexposure. *See Patty's Industrial Hygiene and Toxicology* **vol. 2F,** G. D Clayton, F. E. Clayton, Eds. (John Wiley & Sons, New York, 4th ed., 1994) pp 4566-4591.

USE: Manuf of nitric acid; in the bleaching of rayon; as stabilizer (to prevent free-radical decompn) for propylene, methyl ether, etc.

THERAP CAT: Vasodilator (pulmonary); in treatment of neonatal cardiorespiratory failure.

6579. Nitrilotriacetic Acid. [139-13-9] *N,N*-Bis(carboxy-methyl)glycine; triglycollamic acid; α,α',α''-trimethylaminetricar-boxylic acid; tri(carboxymethyl)amine; triglycine; NTA. $C_6H_9N-O_6$; mol wt 191.14. C 37.70%, H 4.75%, N 7.33%, O 50.22%. N-$(CH_2COOH)_3$. Prepn: Heintz, *Ann.* **122,** 260 (1862); Michaelis, Schubert, *J. Biol. Chem.* **106,** 331 (1934); Martell, Bersworth, *J. Org. Chem.* **15,** 46 (1950); Singer, Weisberg, US 2855428 and US 3061628 (1958 and 1962, both to Hampshire Chem.). IR studies: Nakamoto *et al., J. Am. Chem. Soc.* **84,** 2081 (1962); Chapman *et al., Proc. Chem. Soc. London* **1962,** 336. Solubility data: Bird, *J. Soc. Dyers Colour.* **56,** 473 (1940). Toxicity data: *Soap Chem. Spec.* **42,** 58 (1966). pK data: Schwarzenbach *et al., Helv. Chim. Acta* **28,** 828 (1945). Review: Souchay, Graizon, *Bull. Soc. Chim. Fr.* **1952,** 34.

Prismatic crystals from hot water, mp 230-235° dec (Michaelis, Schubert). mp 241.5° (dec). 1.28 g dissolves in 1 liter of water at 22.5°, pH of satd aq soln is 2.3 (Bird). At 20° pK 3.03, pK$_2$ 3.07, pK$_3$ 10.70.

Sodium salt. NTANa$_3$; Trilon A. $C_6H_6NNa_3O_6$; mol wt 257.08. MLD orally in rats >4,000 mg/kg (*Soap Chem. Spec.*).

Caution: Nitrilotriacetic acid is reasonably anticipated to be a human carcinogen: *Report on Carcinogens, Eleventh Edition* (PB-2005-104914, 2004) p III-184.

USE: Chelating and sequestering agent; builder in synthetic detergents.

6580. Nitrin. [553-74-2] 2-Aminobenzaldehyde phenyl-hydrazone. $C_{13}H_{13}N_3$; mol wt 211.26. C 73.91%, H 6.20%, N 19.89%. Prepd by refluxing 2-nitrobenzaldehyde with phenylhydrazine: Knöpfer, *Monatsh. Chem.* **31,** 97 (1910).

Needles from acetone, mp 227-229° (dec). Sol in acetone. Sparingly sol in cold alcohol, ether, chloroform, benzene. A soln in alcohol or acetone develops a red color with nitrites upon addn of acid.

USE: Detection of nitrites, colibacilli in urine: Pfeiffer, *Muench. Med. Wochenschr.* **92,** 1315 (1950).

6581. Nitroacetanilide. $C_8H_8N_2O_3$; mol wt 180.16. C 53.33%, H 4.48%, N 15.55%, O 26.64%.

m-**Nitroacetanilide.** [122-28-1] *N*-(3-Nitrophenyl)acetamide. Leaflets. mp 151-153°. Sparingly sol in hot water; freely sol in chloroform, nitrobenzene. Practically insol in ether.

o-**Nitroacetanilide.** [552-32-9] Yellow leaflets, d 1.42. mp 93-94°. Moderately sol in cold water, freely in boiling water, in cold fixed alkali hydroxide solns; sol in chloroform, alcohol, ether.

p-**Nitroacetanilide.** [104-04-1] Prisms. mp 214-216°. Almost insol in cold water. Sol in hot water, alcohol, ether; sol in KOH with orange color.

6582. *m*-Nitroaniline. [99-09-2] 3-Nitrobenzenamine; *m*-nitraniline. $C_6H_6N_2O_2$; mol wt 138.12. C 52.18%, H 4.38%, N 20.28%, O 23.17%. Prepn by nitration of aniline: Holleman *et al., Ber.* **44,** 704 (1911); by reduction of *m*-dinitrobenzene: Brady *et al., J. Chem. Soc.* **1929,** 2266; Kubota *et al., J. Pharm. Soc. Jpn.* **76,** 801 (1956); Kuhn, US 2768209 (1956 to Ringwood); from *m*-nitrobenzoic acid: Snyder *et al., J. Am. Chem. Soc.* **75,** 2014 (1953).

Yellow crystals from water, mp 114°. Calc bp 306°. d_4^{25} 0.9011. One gram dissolves in 880 ml water, about 20 ml alcohol, 18 ml ether, 11.5 ml methanol. Forms water-sol salts with mineral acids.

Caution: Highly toxic; absorbed through skin. Avoid breathing dust; avoid contact with skin, eyes, clothing. In case of contact, immediately flush skin or eyes with plenty of water for at least 15 minutes; for eyes, get medical attention. Wash clothing before reusing. Acute exposure can cause methemoglobinemia, cyanosis. Chronic exposure may cause liver damage.

USE: Dyestuff intermediate.

6583. *o*-Nitroaniline. [88-74-4] *o*-Nitraniline. $C_6H_6N_2O_2$; mol wt 138.12. C 52.18%, H 4.38%, N 20.28%, O 23.17%. Prepn from *o*-dinitrobenzene: Meisenheimer, Hesse, *Ber.* **52,** 1166 (1919); from *o*-nitroaniline-*p*-sulfonic acid: Ehrenfeld, Puterbaugh, *Org. Synth.* **coll. vol. I,** 388 (1941); from ψ-*o*-dinitrosobenzene: Boyer *et al., J. Am. Chem. Soc.* **77,** 5688 (1955).

Orange-yellow crystals from boiling water, mp 69-71°. Calc bp 284°. d_4^{25} 0.9015. Slightly sol in cold water; sol in hot water, alcohol, chloroform. Forms water soluble salts with mineral acids.

Caution: See m-Nitroaniline.

USE: Dyestuff intermediate.

6584. *p*-Nitroaniline. [100-01-6] *p*-Nitraniline. $C_6H_6N_2-O_2$; mol wt 138.12. C 52.18%, H 4.38%, N 20.28%, O 23.17%. Prepn from acetanilide: Bart, US 2406578 (1946 to Am. Cyanamid); by Schmidt reaction: Stockel, Hall, *Nature* **197,** 787 (1963).

Bright yellow powder, mp 146°. Calc bp 332°. One gram dissolves in 1250 ml water, 45 ml boiling water, 25 ml alcohol, 30 ml ether; sol in benzene, methanol. Forms water soluble salts with mineral acids.

Caution: Potential symptoms of overexposure are irritation of nose and throat; cyanosis, ataxia; tachycardia, tachypnea; dyspnea; irritability; vomiting, diarrhea; convulsions; respiratory arrest; anemia; methemoglobinemia; jaundice. *See NIOSH Pocket Guide to Chemical Hazards* (DHHS/NIOSH 97-140, 1997) p 226.

USE: Dyestuff intermediate.

6585. Nitroanisole. Methoxynitrobenzene; nitrophenyl methyl ether. $C_7H_7NO_3$; mol wt 153.14. C 54.90%, H 4.61%, N 9.15%, O 31.34%.

5-Nitrobarbituric Acid

***m*-Nitroanisole.** [555-03-3] Crystals. d 1.373. mp 38-39°. bp 258°. Volatile with steam. Insol in water; sol in alc.

***o*-Nitroanisole.** [91-23-6] Colorless to yellowish liquid. d_4^{20} 1.254. mp 9.4°. bp 277°; also stated as 272-273°. n_D^{20} 1.5620. Volatile with steam. Insol in water; sol in alc, ether.

***p*-Nitroanisole.** [100-17-4] Crystals. d 1.233. mp 54°. bp 260°; also stated as 274°. Insol in water; freely sol in alc, ether, boiling petr ether; slightly sol in cold petr ether.

Caution: *o*-Nitroanisole is reasonably anticipated to be a human carcinogen: *Report on Carcinogens, Eleventh Edition* (PB2005-104914, 2004) p III-185.

USE: *o*-Isomer as dye intermediate; in organic syntheses.

6586. 5-Nitrobarbituric Acid. [480-68-2] 5-Nitro-2,4,-6(1*H*,3*H*,5*H*)-pyrimidinetrione; dilituric acid. $C_4H_3N_3O_5$; mol wt 173.08. C 27.76%, H 1.75%, N 24.28%, O 46.22%.

Trihydrate. Prisms and leaflets from water. mp 176° with decompn, when anhydr. Soluble in ~1200 parts cold water; more sol in hot water; sol in alcohol, in sodium hydroxide soln. Insol in ether.

USE: As a microreagent for potassium with which it forms a characteristic precipitate.

6587. Nitrobenzaldehyde. $C_7H_5NO_3$; mol wt 151.12. C 55.63%, H 3.33%, N 9.27%, O 31.76%.

***m*-Nitrobenzaldehyde.** Yellowish, cryst powder. mp 58°. bp_{23} 164°. Volatile with steam. Almost insol in water; sol in alcohol, chloroform, ether.

***o*-Nitrobenzaldehyde.** Light yellow needles. mp 42-44°. bp_{23} 153°. Volatile with steam. Slightly sol in water, freely in alcohol, benzene, ether.

***p*-Nitrobenzaldehyde.** White to yellow crystals, mp 106-107°. Sublimes; slightly volatile with steam. Slightly sol in water or ether; sol in alc, benzene, glacial acetic acid.

USE: *o*-Nitrobenzaldehyde as reagent for isopropyl alcohol and acetone.

6588. Nitrobenzene. [98-95-3] Nitrobenzol; essence of mirbane; oil of mirbane. $C_6H_5NO_2$; mol wt 123.11. C 58.54%, H 4.09%, N 11.38%, O 25.99%. Industrial prepn: *Faith, Keyes & Clark's Industrial Chemicals,* F. A. Lowenheim, M. K. Moran, Eds. (Wiley-Interscience, New York, 4th ed., 1975) p 571. Crystal structure: R. Boese *et al., Struct. Chem.* **3**, 363 (1992). Vibrational spectra: V. A. Shlyapochnikov *et al., J. Mol. Struct.* **326**, 1 (1994). HPLC determn of metabolite in urine: A. Astier, *J. Chromatogr.* **573**, 318 (1992). Review of toxicology and human exposure: *Toxicological Profile for Nitrobenzene* (PB91-180398, 1990) 117 pp; of carcinogenic risk: *IARC Monographs* **65**, 381-408 (1996). *Review:* R. L. Adkins in *Kirk-Othmer Encyclopedia of Chemical Technology* vol. 17 (Wiley-Interscience, New York, 4th ed., 1996) pp 133-152.

Colorless to pale yellow, oily liquid; odor of volatile oil almond. *Poisonous!* Use only with adequate ventilation. d_4^{15} 1.205. mp 6°.

bp 210-211°. Flash pt, closed cup: 190°F (88°C). n_D^{20} 1.5529. Volatile with steam. Sol in ~500 parts water; freely sol in alcohol, benzene, ether, oils. LD_{50} orally in rats: 600 mg/kg (PB91-108398).

Caution: Potential symptoms of overexposure are irritation of skin and eyes; anoxia; dermatitis; anemia; methemoglobinemia. *See NIOSH Pocket Guide to Chemical Hazards* (DHHS/NIOSH 97-140, 1997) p 226. This substance is reasonably anticipated to be a human carcinogen: *Report on Carcinogens, Eleventh Edition* (PB2005-104914) p III-190.

USE: For the manuf of aniline; in soaps, shoe polishes; for refining lubricating oils; manuf pyroxylin compds.

6589. Nitrobenzoic Acid. $C_7H_5NO_4$; mol wt 167.12. C 50.31%, H 3.02%, N 8.38%, O 38.29%. Prepn of *m*-isomer: O. Kamm, J. B. Segur, *Org. Synth.* **coll. vol. I** (2nd ed., 1964) p 391; of *p*-isomer: O. Kamm, A. O. Matthews, *ibid.* p 392.

***m*-Nitrobenzoic acid.** Monoclinic leaflets from water. Bitter taste. d 1.494. mp 142°. Melts in hot water. K (25°) = 3.48 × 10^{-4}. Absorption spectrum: Purvis, *J. Chem. Soc.* **107**, 971 (1915). One gram dissolves in 320 ml water, 3 ml alc, 4 ml ether, 18 ml chloroform, ~2 ml methanol, 2.5 ml acetone; very slightly sol in benzene, carbon disulfide, petr ether.

***o*-Nitrobenzoic acid.** Yellowish-white, intensely sweet crystals. d 1.58. mp 147-148°. One gram dissolves in 146 ml water, 3 ml alcohol, 220 ml chloroform, 4.5 ml ether, 2.5 ml acetone, 2.5 ml methanol; very slightly sol in benzene, carbon disulfide, petr ether.

***p*-Nitrobenzoic acid.** Monoclinic leaflets, plates from benzene. d 1.58. mp 242.4°. Sublimes. One gram dissolves in 2380 ml water, 110 ml alcohol, 12 ml methanol, 150 ml chloroform, 45 ml ether, 20 ml acetone; slightly sol in benzene, carbon disulfide; insol in petr ether.

USE: Manuf intermediates; also as a reagent for alkaloids and thorium.

6590. 4-Nitrobenzoyl Chloride. [122-04-3] $C_7H_4ClNO_3$; mol wt 185.56. C 45.31%, H 2.17%, Cl 19.11%, N 7.55%, O 25.87%. $NO_2C_6H_4COCl$. Prepd by the action of phosphorus pentachloride on *p*-nitrobenzoic acid: Adams, Jenkins, *Org. Synth.* **3**, 75 (1923).

Bright yellow needles from petr ether. Pungent odor. mp 75°. bp_{105} 205°; bp_{12} 154°. Decomposed by water and alcohol; sol in ether. *Keep well closed.*

6591. *p*-Nitrobenzyl Cyanide. [555-21-5] 4-Nitrobenzene-acetonitrile; *p*-nitrophenylacetonitrile; *p*-nitro-α-toluinitrile. C_8H_6-N_2O_2; mol wt 162.15. C 59.26%, H 3.73%, N 17.28%, O 19.73%. $NO_2C_6H_4CH_2CN$. Prepd by the action of concd nitric acid on benzyl cyanide: Robertson, *Org. Synth.* **2**, 57 (1922).

Elongated prisms from alcohol. mp 117°. Insol in water; sol in alcohol, ether.

USE: In the prepn of *p*-nitrophenylacetic acid.

6592. *o*-Nitrobiphenyl. [86-00-0] 2-Nitro-1,1'-biphenyl; *o*-nitrodiphenyl; ONB. $C_{12}H_9NO_2$; mol wt 199.21. C 72.35%, H 4.55%, N 7.03%, O 16.06%. Prepn from diazotized *o*-nitroaniline and benzene by a modified Gomberg reaction: Elks *et al., J. Chem. Soc.* **1940**, 1284. Prepd industrially by direct nitration of biphenyl (yields ~50% para, 35% ortho).

Orthorhombic bipyramidal plates from ethanol. Characteristic sweetish odor. mp 36.7°. d_4^{25} 1.44. $d_{15.5}^{40}$ (liq) 1.189. The technical liq weighs ~10 lbs/gal. bp_{760} 325°; bp_{30} 205°; bp_{13} 170°; bp_4 166°. n_D^{25} (tech liq) 1.613. Flash pt 179°C (354°F). uv max: 325

Consult the Name Index before using this section.

nm. Dipole moment: 3.79. Viscosity of tech liquid (cP): 12 (45°); 38 (25°). Insol in water. Sol in methanol, ethanol, tetrahydrofurfuryl alcohol, acetone, DMF, carbon tetrachloride, perchlorethylene, mineral spirits, turpentine, glacial acetic acid.

USE: Plasticizer for resins, cellulose acetate and nitrate, polystyrenes; fungicide for textiles; wood preservative; dye intermediate.

6593. p-Nitrobiphenyl. [92-93-3] 4-Nitro-1,1'-biphenyl; 4-nitrobiphenyl; p-nitrodiphenyl; PNB. $C_{12}H_9NO_2$; mol wt 199.21. C 72.35%, H 4.55%, N 7.03%, O 16.06%. Prepn: G. Schultz, Ann. **174**, 210 (1874); O. Kühling, Ber. **28**, 42 (1895); E. Bamberger, ibid. 404; R. L. Jenkins et al., Ind. Eng. Chem. **22** (1), 31 (1930); K. Dimroth et al., Ber. **101**, 2215 (1968). Crystal structure: M. Prasad et al., J. Indian Chem. Soc. **13**, 519 (1936), C.A. **31**, 1271[5] (1937). Review of carcinogenic risk: IARC Monographs **vol. 4**, 113-117 (1974).

Needles from alcohol, mp 113.7°. bp_{760} 340°; bp_{30} 223.7-224.1°. Insol in water. Slightly sol in cold alc; more readily sol in hot alc; sol in chloroform, ether. uv spectrum: D. F. DeTor, H. J. Scheifele, J. Am. Chem. Soc. **73**, 1442 (1951).
Caution: Potential symptoms of overexposure are headache, drowsiness and dizziness; dyspnea; ataxia, lassitude; methemoglobinemia; urinary burning; acute hemorrhagic cystitis. Potential occupational carcinogen. See NIOSH Pocket Guide to Chemical Hazards (DHHS/NIOSH PB2003-100121, 2003) p 226.
USE: Formerly in prepn of p-biphenylamine, q.v.

6594. Nitrocefin. [41906-86-9] (6R,7R)-3-[(1E)-2-(2,4-Dinitrophenyl)ethenyl]-8-oxo-7-[(2-thienylacetyl)amino]-5-thia-1-azabicyclo[4.2.0]oct-2-ene-2-carboxylic acid; 3-(2,4-dinitrostyryl)-(6R,7R)-7-(2-thienylacetamido)-ceph-3-em-4-carboxylic acid, E-isomer; 87/312. $C_{21}H_{16}N_4O_8S_2$; mol wt 516.50. C 48.83%, H 3.12%, N 10.85%, O 24.78%, S 12.42%. Chromogenic cephalosporin. Prepd (not claimed): C. H. O'Callaghan et al., US 3830700 (1974 to Glaxo). Characterization and use in detection of β-lactamases: idem et al., Antimicrob. Agents Chemother. **1**, 283 (1972). Synthesis: N. C. M. Barendse et al., Synthesis **1998**, 145. Improved synthesis: M. Lee et al., J. Org. Chem. **70**, 367 (2005). Review of commercially available nitrocefin-based β-lactamase tests: A. T. Meszaros et al., Am. Clin. Lab. **14**, 20-22 (1995).

Orange solid, mp 103-113° (dec) (O'Callaghan, 1974); also reported as crystals from methanol, mp 167-169° (dec) (Lee). $[\alpha]_D^{20}$ −224° (c = 1.0 in dioxane). Absorption max (ethanol): 231, 289, 386 nm (ε 24300, 10300, 18000). Absorption max (0.1M pH 6 phosphate buffer): 233, 290, 391 nm (ε 22200, 12200, 17400). Undergoes a color change from yellow to pink or red upon exposure to β-lactamases.
USE: In determn of β-lactamase activity in biological samples.

6595. m-Nitrocinnamic Acid. [555-68-0] 3-(3-Nitrophenyl)-2-propenoic acid. $C_9H_7NO_4$; mol wt 193.16. C 55.96%, H 3.65%, N 7.25%, O 33.13%. $NO_2C_6H_4CH=CHCOOH$. Prepd by heating a mixture of m-nitrobenzaldehyde, sodium acetate and acetic anhydride: Thayer, Org. Synth. **5**, 83 (1925). From m-nitrobenzaldehyde and malonic acid in the presence of glycine in a little water at 100°: Dakin, J. Biol. Chem. **7**, 54 (1909-1910).
trans-Form. Prepd by the above methods. White needles from benzene or alcohol. mp 200-201°. Can be sublimed or distilled at atmospheric press. with very little decompn. Absorption spectrum: Purvis, J. Chem. Soc. **107**, 971 (1906). One gram dissolves in ~100 ml alcohol at 25°.

cis-Form. Prepd by ultraviolet irradiation of a soln in water-alcohol-ammonia giving a 22% yield: Wollring, Ber. **47**, 112 (1914). Minute needles from toluene + methanol, mp 158°. By reirradiation of a chloroform soln containing a trace of bromine, the more stable trans-form is regenerated.

6596. Nitrodan. [962-02-7] 3-Methyl-5-[(4-nitrophenyl)-azo]-2-thioxo-4-thiazolidinone; 3-methyl-5-[(p-nitrophenyl)azo]-rhodanine; 3-methyl-5-[(p-nitrophenyl)azo]-2-thio-2,4-thiazolidinedione; CTR-6110; Nidanthel; Everfree. $C_{10}H_8N_4O_3S_2$; mol wt 296.33. C 40.53%, H 2.72%, N 18.91%, O 16.20%, S 21.64%. Prepn: Benghiat, Howard, US 2952673 (1960 to Stauffer); BE 637282 (1964 to Cooper, Tinsley Labs.).

Yellow powder, mp 267-268°. Sparingly sol in water.
THERAP CAT (VET): Anthelmintic.

6597. Nitroethane. [79-24-3] $C_2H_5NO_2$; mol wt 75.07. C 32.00%, H 6.71%, N 18.66%, O 42.63%. $CH_3CH_2NO_2$. Obtained by vapor phase nitration of ethane with HNO_3: Reidel, Oil Gas J. **54**, no. 36, 110-114 (1956). Laboratory prepn by treating 1.5 moles sodium nitrite with 1 mole sodium ethyl sulfate at 125-130° in the presence of 0.0625 moles potassium carbonate: Desseigne, Giral, Mem. Poudres **34**, 49-53 (1952), C.A. **49**, 836 (1955). Similar procedure according to the equation $EtOSO_2OEt + NaNO_2 \rightarrow EtOSO_2ONa + EtNO_2$: McCombie et al., J. Chem. Soc. **1944**, 24.
Oily liquid; pleasant odor. d_{25}^{25} 1.041; d_{20}^{20} 1.052. Flash pt, open cup: 106°F (41.11°C). mp ~−50°. bp 114-115°. Undergoes thermal decompn at 335-382°. Heating value (liq): 7,720 Btu/lb. Lower limit of flammability in air = 4.0% by volume. Viscosity (25°): 0.661 cP. n_D^{20} 1.3917; $n_D^{24.3}$ 1.39007. Soly in water: 4.5 ml/100 ml H_2O at 20°. Miscible with methanol, ethanol, ether. Sol in chloroform, aq solns of alkalies. Has high heat of absorption. Sudden absorption of the anhydr liq or gas on activated carbon or Hopcalite may result in flames: Chem. Eng. News **30**, 2344 (1952).
Caution: Potential symptom of overexposure by direct contact is dermatitis. See NIOSH Pocket Guide to Chemical Hazards (DHHS/NIOSH 97-140, 1997) p 228. Potential symptom of overexposure by ingestion is methemoglobinemia. See G. Shepherd et al., Clin. Toxicol. **36**, 613 (1998).
USE: Solvent, artificial fingernail glue remover; in organic syntheses. Experimentally as liq propellant.

6598. Nitrofen. [1836-75-5] 2,4-Dichloro-1-(4-nitrophenoxy)benzene; 2,4-dichlorophenyl-p-nitrophenyl ether; nitraphen; nitrophen; nitrofene; FW-925; TOK. $C_{12}H_7Cl_2NO_3$; mol wt 284.09. C 50.73%, H 2.48%, Cl 24.96%, N 4.93%, O 16.90%. Selective pre- and post-emergence herbicide. Prepn: H. F. Wilson, H. M. Dougal, US 3080225 (1963 to Rohm & Haas). Toxicity studies: A. M. Ambrose et al., Toxicol. Appl. Pharmacol. **19**, 263 (1971). Carcinogenicity studies: J. F. Robens, Vet. Hum. Toxicol. **22**, 328 (1980). Review of carcinogenic risk: IARC Monographs **30**, 271-282 (1983).

Crystalline solid, mp 70-71°. Vapor pressure at 40°: 8×10^{-6} mm Hg. Soly in water at 22°: 0.7-1.2 ppm. LD_{50} orally in rats: 3.58 g/kg (Ambrose).
Caution: This substance is reasonably anticipated to be a human carcinogen: Report on Carcinogens, Eleventh Edition (PB2005-104914, 2004) p III-192.
USE: Formerly as herbicide.

6599. Nitrofurantoin. [67-20-9] 1-[[(5-Nitro-2-furanyl)-methylene]amino]-2,4-imidazolidinedione; N-(5-nitro-2-furfurylidene)-1-aminohydantoin; 1-(5-nitro-2-furfurylideneamino)hydantoin; Berkfurin; Chemiofuran; Cyantin; Cystit; Fua-Med; Furachel; Furalan; Furadantin; Furadantine MC; Furadoin; Furantoina; Furobactina; Furophen T-Caps; Ituran; Macrodantin; Parfuran; Trantoin; Urantoin; Urizept; Urodin; Urolong; Uro-Tablinen; Welfurin. C_8-$H_6N_4O_5$; mol wt 238.16. C 40.34%, H 2.54%, N 23.52%, O 33.59%. Prepn from 1-aminohydantoin sulfate and 5-nitro-2-furaldehyde diacetate: K. J. Hayes, US 2610181 (1952 to Eaton Labs.); Swirska *et al., Przem. Chem.* **11** (34), 306 (1955), *C.A.* **52**, 14079b (1958). Alternate routes: J. G. Michels, US 2898335; G. Gever, C. J. O'Keefe, US 2927110 (1959, 1960 both to Norwich Pharmacal). LC-MS/MS determn of residues in meat: P. Mottier *et al., J. Chromatogr. A* **1067**, 85 (2005). Clinical trial in urinary tract infection: R. G. Rogers *et al., Am. J. Obstet. Gynecol.* **191**, 182 (2004). Comprehensive description: D. E. Cadwallader, H. W. Jun, *Anal. Profiles Drug Subs.* **5**, 345-373 (1976).

Orange-yellow needles from dil acetic acid, dec 270-272°. pKa 7.2. uv max: 370 nm ($E_{1cm}^{1\%}$ 776). Soly (mg/100 ml): water (pH 7) 19.0; 95% ethanol 51.0; acetone 510; DMF 8000; peanut oil 2.1; glycerol 60; polyethylene glycol 1500.

Monohydrate. [17140-81-7] Macrobid.

THERAP CAT: Antibacterial.

THERAP CAT (VET): Antibacterial.

6600. Nitrofurazone. [59-87-0] 2-[(5-Nitro-2-furanyl)methylene]hydrazinecarboxamide; 5-nitro-2-furaldehyde semicarbazone; Amifur; Furacin; Chemofuran; Furesol; Nifuzon; Nitrofural; Nitrozone; Furacinetten; Furacoccid; Furazol W; Mammex; Furaplast; Coxistat; Aldomycin; Nefco; Vabrocid. $C_6H_6N_4O_4$; mol wt 198.14. C 36.37%, H 3.05%, N 28.28%, O 32.30%. Prepd from 2-formyl-5-nitrofuran and semicarbazide hydrochloride: Stillman, Scott, US 2416234 (1947 to Eaton Labs.). Alternate route: Gever, O'Keefe, US 2927110 (1960 to Norwich Pharmacal). LC-MS/MS determn of residues in meat: P. Mottier *et al., J. Chromatogr. A* **1067**, 85 (2005). Toxicity: J. Godwin *et al., J. Am. Med. Assoc.* **133**, 299 (1947). Tumorigenic activity: Morris *et al., Cancer Res.* **29**, 2145 (1969); Ertürk *et al., ibid.* **30**, 1409 (1970).

Pale yellow needles, dec 236-240°. Bitter aftertaste. Darkens on prolonged exposure to light. uv max: 260, 375 nm. Very slightly sol in water (1:4200); slightly sol in alcohol (1:590), in propylene glycol (1:350). Sol in alkaline solns with dark orange color. Insol in ether. pH of satd water soln 6.0 to 6.5. LD_{50} in rats (g/kg): 0.59 orally; 3.0 s.c. (Godwin).

THERAP CAT: Anti-infective (topical).

THERAP CAT (VET): Antimicrobial.

6601. Nitrogen. [7727-37-9] N; at. wt 14.00674; at. no. 7; valences 3, 5; elemental state: N_2. Group VA (15). Two naturally occurring isotopes: 14 (99.635%); 15 (0.365%); five short-lived, artificial, radioactive isotopes: 12; 13; 16-18. Discovered in 1772 by Daniel Rutherford and independently by Scheele and Cavendish. Constitutes about 75.5% by weight or 78.06% by volume of the atmosphere; found frequently in volcanic or mine gases, gases from springs and gases occluded in minerals and rocks; an essential constituent of all living organisms; fixed or combined nitrogen is present in many mineral deposits. Prepn from sodium (and alkaline earth) azides by heating the azide: Tiede, *Ber.* **46**, 4100 (1913); **49**, 1745 (1916); Justi, *Ann. Phys.* [5] **10**, 985 (1931). Prepd industrially by fractional distln of liquid air; by removal of oxygen by combustion; by reduction of ammonia. Purification of nitrogen furnished in steel cylinders: Kautsky, Thiele, *Z. Anorg. Allg. Chem.* **152**, 342 (1926); Kendall, *Science* **73**, 395 (1931); Schenk

in *Handbook of Preparative Inorganic Chemistry* vol. **1**, G. Brauer, Ed. (Academic Press, New York, 2nd ed., 1963) pp 458-460. Review of nitrogen and nitrogen compounds: Jones in *Comprehensive Inorganic Chemistry* vol. **2**, J. C. Bailar, Jr. *et al.*, Eds. (Pergamon Press, Oxford, 1973) pp 147-388; R. W. Schroeder in *Kirk-Othmer Encyclopedia of Chemical Technology* vol. **15** (Wiley-Interscience, New York, 3rd ed., 1981) pp 932-941. Books: W. L. Jolly, *The Inorganic Chemistry of Nitrogen* (Benjamin, New York, 1964) 124 pp; *Mellor's* Vol. **VIII**, Supplements I, II, *Nitrogen,* part 1 (1964) 619 pp; part 2 (1967) 676 pp; M. Sittig, *Nitrogen in Industry* (Van Nostrand, Princeton, 1965) 278 pp.

Odorless gas; condenses to a liq, bp −195.79° (77.36 K); solidifies to a snow-white mass, mp −210.01° (63.14 K). d^{gas} (0°, 1 atm) 1.25046 g/l. Critical temp: −147.1°; critical press: 33.5 atm; critical density: 0.311 g/cm³. Sparingly sol in water: 100 volumes of water absorbs 2.4 volumes of gas at 0°, 1.6 volumes at 20°. Soly in water at 50, 75 and 100° from 25 to 1000 atmospheres: Wiebe *et al., J. Am. Chem. Soc.* **55**, 947 (1933). Soly in liq ammonia: Wiebe *et al., ibid.* 975. Soly in alc: one volume of alcohol dissolves 0.1124 volume of nitrogen at 20°. Liquid oxygen at −195.5° absorbs 50.7% of its weight of gaseous nitrogen. Heat of dissociation of the nitrogen molecule (N_2): 225.1 kcal/mole. Combines with oxygen and hydrogen on sparking, forming nitric oxide and ammonia, respectively. Combines directly with lithium, and at a red heat with calcium, strontium, and barium to form nitrides. Forms cyanides when heated with carbon in presence of alkalies or barium oxide.

Caution: In high concns it is a simple asphyxiant.

USE: In manuf of ammonia, nitric acid, nitrates, cyanides, etc.; in manuf explosives; in filling high-temp thermometers, incandescent bulbs; to form an inert atm for preservation of materials, for use in dry boxes or glove bags. Liquid nitrogen in food-freezing processes; in the laboratory as a coolant. Pharmaceutic aid (air displacement).

6602. Nitrogen Chloride. [10025-85-1] Nitrogen trichloride; chlorine nitride; trichlorine nitride; Agene. Cl_3N; mol wt 120.37. Cl 88.36%, N 11.64%. NCl_3. Prepared by the action of chlorine gas or hypochlorous acid on ammonium salts: Dulong, *Ann. Chim. Phys.* [1] **86**, 37 (1813); Balard, *ibid.* [2] **57**, 258 (1834); Hentschel, *Ber.* **30**, 1792, 2642 (1897); Noyes, *J. Am. Chem. Soc.* **42**, 2173 (1920); by reaction of anhydr ammonia and anhydr chlorine: Noyes, Haw, *ibid.* 2167; industrially by electrolyzing an acidified soln of ammonium chloride: US 2118903 (1938); DE 641816 (1937); GB 494188 (1938); for bleaching flour by blowing an air stream containing hydrogen chloride gas through a bed of finely powdered ammonium chloride and potassium hypochlorite distributed on an inert carrier to form a gas mixture of chlorine dioxide and nitrogen chloride: GB 597199 (1948). *Review:* Richards in *Mellor's* Vol. **VIII**, supplement II, *Nitrogen* (part 2), 411-415 (1967).

Yellow, thick, oily liq, d 1.653, pungent odor, evaporates rapidly in air, very unstable. Dec in light, vapor pressure at room temp is ~150 mm Hg. Explodes when heated to 93°, subjected to a flash of direct sunlight or magnesium light, sealed in glass containers at 60° after 13 seconds, frozen in liq air and thawed *in vacuo,* in contact with ozone, nitric oxide, grease, and several organic substances. Insol in water. Dec in water after 24 hours, sol in carbon disulfide, phosphorus trichloride, benzene, carbon tetrachloride, chloroform.

USE: Bleaching of flour; wastage control of citrus fruit.

6603. Nitrogen Dioxide. [10102-44-0] NO_2; mol wt 46.01. N 30.44%, O 69.55%. Damaging component of photochemical smog. Prepd industrially from nitric oxide and air. Convenient lab prepn from lead nitrate: Schenk in *Handbook of Preparative Inorganic Chemistry* vol. **1**, G. Brauer, Ed. (Academic Press, New York, 1963) pp 488-489. Ultrapure NO_2 from N_2O_5: Hackspill, Besson, *Bull. Soc. Chim. Fr. Mem.* [5] **16**, 479 (1949). *Reviews:* Beattie, "Nitrogen Dioxide and Dinitrogen Tetroxide" in *Mellor's* Vol. **VIII**, supplement II, *Nitrogen* (part 2) 246-268 (1967); Jones in *Comprehensive Inorganic Chemistry* vol. **2**, J. C. Bailar, Jr. *et al.*, Eds. (Pergamon Press, Oxford, 1973) pp 340-356. Symposium on chemistry and toxicology: *Toxicology* **89**, 1-312 (1994).

Reddish-brown gas. Liquid below 21.15°. Irritating odor. *Deadly poison!* The commercial brown liq under pressure is called **nitrogen tetroxide**. Actually this is an equilibrium mixture of NO_2 and the colorless N_2O_4. d_4^{20} (liq) 1.448; d (gas) 1.58 (air = 1); $d_{gas}^{21.3}$

3.3 g/liter. mp −9.3°. bp 21.15°. Crit temp 158.2°. Crit press. 99.96 atm. Heat of vaporization (bp) 9.110 kcal/mole. Does not burn, but supports the combustion of carbon, phosphorus, sulfur. Sol in concd sulfuric and nitric acids. Dec in water forming nitric acid and nitric oxide, reacts with alkalies to form nitrates and nitrites. Corrosive to steel when wet, but may be stored in steel cylinders when moisture content is 0.1% or less.

Caution: Potential symptoms of overexposure are coughing, mucoid frothy sputum, decreased pulmonary function, chronic bronchitis, dyspnea; chest pain; pulmonary edema, cyanosis, tachypnea and tachycardia; eye, nose and throat irritation. *See NIOSH Pocket Guide to Chemical Hazards* (DHHS/NIOSH 97-140, 1997) p 228. One of the most insidious gases. Inflammation of lungs may cause only slight pain or pass unnoticed, but the resulting edema several days later may cause death. 100 ppm is dangerous for even a short exposure, and 200 ppm may be fatal: Y. Henderson, H. W. Haggard, *Noxious Gases,* A.C.S. Monograph Series, no. 35 (Reinhold, New York, 2nd ed., 1943) pp 134-137, 141. *See also Clinical Toxicology of Commercial Products,* R. E. Gosselin *et al.,* Eds. (Williams & Wilkins, Baltimore, 5th ed., 1984) Section III, pp 319-326.

USE: Intermediate in nitric and sulfuric acid production. Used in the nitration of organic compds and explosives, in the manuf of oxidized cellulose compds (hemostatic cotton). Has been used to bleach flour. Proposed as oxidizing agent in rocket propulsion. *See also:* Sisler, "Reactions in Liquid Dinitrogen Tetroxide," *J. Chem. Educ.* **34,** 555 (1957).

6604. Nitrogen Fluoride. [7783-54-2] Nitrogen trifluoride. F_3N; mol wt 71.00. F 80.27%, N 19.73%. NF_3. Prepd by electrolysis of melted ammonium acid fluoride, NH_4F_2H: Ruff *et al., Z. Anorg. Allg. Chem.* **172,** 417 (1928); Ruff, *ibid.* **197,** 273 (1931); Ruff, Staub, *ibid.* **198,** 32 (1931); Kwasnik in *Handbook of Preparative Inorganic Chemistry* **vol. 1,** G. Brauer, Ed. (Academic Press, New York, 2nd ed., 1963) pp 181-183. Reviews of prepn and chemistry: Hoffman, Neville, *Chem. Rev.* **62,** 1-18 (1962); Kemmitt, Sharp, *Adv. Fluorine Chem.* **4,** 189-190 (1965).

Colorless gas. Moldy odor. mp −208.5°. bp −129°. d (liq at bp) 1.885. Trouton const 19.9. Insoluble in water. Rather inert chemically. Does not attack glass, mercury. Decomposed by electric sparks.

Caution: Potential symptoms of overexposure in exptl animals are anoxia, cyanosis; methemoglobinemia; weakness, dizziness, headache; liver, kidney injury. *See NIOSH Pocket Guide to Chemical Hazards* (DHHS/NIOSH 97-140, 1997) p 228.

6605. Nitrogen Pentoxide. [10102-03-1] Dinitrogen pentoxide; nitric anhydride. N_2O_5; mol wt 108.01. N 25.94%, O 74.06%. Usually prepd by dehydration of nitric acid by means of phosphorus pentoxide: Gruenhut *et al., Inorg. Synth.* **3,** 78 (1950). *Reviews:* Beattie, "Dinitrogen Pentoxide" in *Mellor's* **Vol. VIII,** supplement II, *Nitrogen* (part 2), 269-277 (1967); Jones in *Comprehensive Inorganic Chemistry* **vol. 2,** J. C. Bailar, Jr. *et al.,* Eds. (Pergamon Press, Oxford, 1973) pp 356-360.

Colorless hexagonal crystals. mp 30°. Sublimes at 32.4° but undergoes moderately fast decompn into O_2 and the NO_2/N_2O_4 equilibrium mixture at temps above −10°. d^{15} 2.05. bp_{760} 47.0°; bp_{100} 7.0°; bp_{10} −20°. Dipole moment 1.39. Freely sol in chloroform without appreciable decomposition. Less sol in carbon tetrachloride. Chloroform solns may be stored at −20° for as long as one week without excessive decompn.

USE: As nitrating agent in chloroform soln.

6606. Nitrogen Selenide. [12033-88-4] Selenium nitride. N_4Se_4; mol wt 371.87. N 15.07%, Se 84.93%. Prepd by passing dry ammonia over selenium tetrachloride: Wöhler, *Bull. Soc. Chim.* [1] **1,** 25 (1859); by treating a dil soln of selenium oxychloride in benzene with dry ammonia and washing the precipitate with water and potassium cyanide: Lenher, Wolesensky, *J. Am. Chem. Soc.* **29,** 215 (1907); by the action of dry ammonia on a dilute soln of selenium monochloride in carbon disulfide: van Valkenburg, Bailar, *ibid.* **47,** 2134 (1925); by the action of dry ammonia on diethyl selenite or dimethyl selenite dissolved in benzene and washing with potassium cyanide: Strecker, Schwarzkopf, *Z. Anorg. Chem.* **221,** 193 (1934); by reacting anhydr, liquid ammonia with selenium dioxide: Jander, Doetsch, *Ber.* **93,** 561 (1960). Crystal structure:

Baernighausen *et al., Acta Crystallogr.* **15,** 615 (1962); **21,** 571 (1966).

Orange-red, amorphous powder or monoclinic crystals. d 4.2. Very hygroscopic. *Explosive.* Sparingly sol in carbon disulfide, benzene, acetic acid; insol in water, ether, abs alc.

6607. Nitroglycerin. [55-63-0] 1,2,3-Propanetriol trinitrate; glyceryl trinitrate; glycerol nitric acid triester; nitroglycerol; trinitroglycerol; glonoin; trinitrin; blasting gelatin; blasting oil; S.N.G.; Adesitrin; Anginine; Aquo-Trinitrosan; Cordipatch; Corditrine; Deponit; Diafusor; Discotrine; Lenitral; Millisrol; Minitran; Nitradisc; Nitro-Bid; Nitrocine; Nitrocontin; Nitroderm; Nitro-Dur; Nitrogard; Nitroglin; Nitroglyn; Nitrolingual; Nitromex; Nitronal; Nitrong; Nitrostat; Nitrosylon; Percutol; Perlinganit; Rectogesic; Suscard; Sustac; Transderm-Nitro; Transiderm-Nitro; Tridil; Trinitrosan. $C_3H_5N_3O_9$; mol wt 227.09. C 15.87%, H 2.22%, N 18.50%, O 63.41%. Nitric oxide donor that induces vasodilation. Prepn: Sobrero, *Ann.* **64,** 398 (1847); Williamson, *Ann.* **92,** 305 (1854). Review of the early literature: J. W. Lawrie, *Glycerol and the Glycols* (New York, 1928). Review of chemistry and biochemistry: F. J. DiCarlo, *Drug Metab. Rev.* **4,** 1-38 (1975). Review of mechanism of action: S. F. Vatner, G. R. Heyndrickx, *Handb. Exp. Pharmakol.* **40,** 131-161 (1975). Molecular mechanism of nitric oxide release: Z. Chen *et al., Proc. Natl. Acad. Sci. USA* **99,** 8306 (2002). Review of the first hundred years: J. R. Parratt, *J. Pharm. Pharmacol.* **31,** 801-809 (1979). Comprehensive description: E. F. McNiff *et al., Anal. Profiles Drug Subs.* **9,** 519-541 (1980). Symposium on nitroglycerin therapy, perspectives and mechanisms: *Am. J. Med.* **74,** no. 6B, 1-94 (1983). Review of pharmacology and clinical studies of intravenous administration in heart disease: E. M. Sorkin *et al., Drugs* **27,** 45 (1984). Clinical trial in treatment of anal fissures: J. H. Scholefield *et al., Gut* **52,** 264 (2005).

Pale yellow, oily liquid. Sweet burning taste. Produces headache on tasting. Explodes on rapid heating or on concussion. Crystallizes in 2 forms: labile form, mp 2.8°; stable form, mp 13.5°. d_{15}^{15} 1.599; d_4^4 1.6144; d_4^{15} 1.6009; d_{25}^{25} 1.5918. n_D^{15} 1.474. Begins to dec at 50-60°, appreciably volatile at 100°, evolves nitrous yellow vapors at 135°, explodes at 218°. Vapor pressure at 20°: 0.00026 mm; at 93°: 0.31 mm. One gram dissolves in 800 ml water, in 4 g ethanol, in 18 g methanol, in 120 g carbon disulfide. Misc with ether, acetone, glacial acetic acid, ethyl acetate, benzene, nitrobenzene, pyridine, chloroform, ethylene bromide, dichloroethylene. Sparingly sol in petr ether, liq petrolatum, glycerol. Heat of combustion: 1580 cal/g. On explosion harmless gases are produced: $4C_3H_5(ONO_2)_3 \rightarrow 12CO_2 + 10H_2O + 6N_2 + O_2$.

Spirit of Glyceryl Trinitrate. Spirit of nitroglycerin; spirit of glonoin. An alcoholic soln contg 1.0-1.1% glyceryl trinitrate. Colorless, clear liquid. d 0.814-0.820. Miscible with alcohol, chloroform, ether; 1 ml dissolves in 6 ml almond oil; very slightly sol in water; miscible with chloroform, ether.

Caution: Potential symptoms of overexposure by percutaneous or respiratory absorption are throbbing headache, dizziness, nausea, vomiting, abdominal pain; hypotension; flushing; palpitations; methemoglobinemia; delerium, CNS depression; angina; cyanosis; coma. Direct contact may cause skin irritation. *See NIOSH Pocket Guide to Chemical Hazards* (DHHS/NIOSH 97-140, 1997) p 228; *Patty's Industrial Hygiene and Toxicology* **vol. 2B,** G. D. Clayton, F. E. Clayton, Eds. (Wiley-Interscience, New York, 4th ed., 1994) pp 1064-1067.

USE: Manuf of *dynamite* (75% nitroglycerol, 24.5% diatomaceous earth, 0.5% sodium carbonate), smokeless powders and blasting gelatin; in rocket propellants.

THERAP CAT: Antianginal; vasodilator (coronary). Topically in treatment of anal fissures.

6608. Nitroguanidine. [556-88-7] $CH_4N_4O_2$; mol wt 104.07. C 11.54%, H 3.87%, N 53.84%, O 30.75%. H_2NC-(NH)NHNO$_2$. Prepd by the action of concd H_2SO_4 on guanidine nitrate: Davis, *Org. Synth.* **7,** 68 (1927).

α-Form. (The usual stable form): Needles, prisms from water, dec 225-250° (depending on speed of heating) giving off NH₃ fumes. Absorption spectrum: Riegel, Buchwald, *J. Am. Chem. Soc.* **51**, 491 (1929). One liter of water dissolves 4.4 g at 25°; 82.5 g at 100°. Slightly soluble in methanol (<0.5%), alcohol; practically insol in ether. Sol in concd acids from which it is precipitated by water. Sol in cold solns of alkalies (not of carbonates) with slow decompn.

β-Form. Prepd by the nitration of guanidine sulfate with fuming HNO₃. Is converted into the α-form by dissolving in concd H₂SO₄ and pouring into ice water: Davis *et al.*, *J. Am. Chem. Soc.* **47**, 1065 (1925).

USE: Explosive of moderate power. Can be exploded only with a detonator. Intermediate in the synthesis of pharmaceuticals.

6609. Nitrohydrochloric Acid. [8007-56-5] Aqua regia; nitromuriatic acid; chloronitrous acid; chloroazotic acid. Made by mixing 18 ml HNO₃, 82 ml HCl. In addition to the free acids, it contains nitrosyl chloride (NOCl) and some free chlorine.

Yellow, fuming, corrosive, volatile liq; suffocating odor; attacks all metals including gold and platinum. Miscible with water. *Keep in well-closed, glass-stoppered bottles in a cool place and protected from light.*

Caution: Undiluted form is a strong irritant, corrosive.

6610. Nitromersol. [133-58-4] [2-Methyl-5-nitrophenol-ato(2−)-C^6,O^1]mercury; 5-methyl-2-nitro-7-oxa-8-mercurabicyclo[4.2.0]octa-1,3,5-triene; 3-(hydroxymercuri)-4-nitro-*o*-cresol inner salt; Metaphen. C₇H₅HgNO₃; mol wt 351.71. C 23.90%, H 1.43%, Hg 57.03%, N 3.98%, O 13.65%. According to the National Formulary this compd is the anhydride of 4-nitro-3-hydroxymercuri-*o*-cresol. Prepd by treating 4-nitro-*o*-cresol with mercuric acetate: US 1544293; US RE 17563 (1925).

Yellow, odorless, tasteless powder or granules. Insol in water; almost insol in acetone, alcohol, ether, aq soln of sodium carbonate. Sol in solns of alkalies and of ammonia by opening the anhydride ring and the formation of a salt. Also sol in boiling glacial acetic acid.

THERAP CAT: Antiseptic.

THERAP CAT (VET): Disinfectant (topical).

6611. Nitromethane. [75-52-5] Nitrocarbol. CH₃NO₂; mol wt 61.04. C 19.68%, H 4.95%, N 22.95%, O 52.42%. Prepd by the interaction of sodium nitrite and sodium chloroacetate: Whitmore, *Org. Synth.* **3**, 83 (1923). Monograph: *Am. Ind. Hyg. Assoc. J.* **22**, 518 (1961). Toxicity study: Weatherby, *Arch. Ind. Health* **11**, 102 (1955).

Oily liquid with a moderately strong, somewhat disagreeable odor. d_4^{25} 1.1322. One gallon weighs 9.5 lbs. Flash pt 112°F. mp −29°. bp₇₆₀ 101.2°; bp₁₀₀ 46.6°; bp₄₀ 27.5°; bp₂₀ 14.1°; bp₁₀ 2.8°; bp₅ −7.9°; bp₁.₀ −29°. n_D^{22} 1.38056. Absorption spectrum: Hantzsch, Voigt, *Ber.* **45**, 106 (1912). Slightly sol in water (9.5% by vol at 20°); sol in alc, ether, DMF. Water solns are acid to litmus. pH of 0.01*M* aq soln 6.12. Forms an explosive sodium salt which bursts into flame on contact with water. LC (in air) in guinea pigs: 1000 ppm; LD₅₀ orally in mice: 1.44 g/kg (Weatherby).

Caution: Potential symptom of overexposure is dermatitis. *See NIOSH Pocket Guide to Chemical Hazards* (DHHS/NIOSH 97-140, 1997) p 230. This substance is reasonably anticipated to be a human carcinogen: *Report on Carcinogens, Eleventh Edition* (PB-2005-104914, 2004) p III-193.

USE: Rocket fuel; solvent for zein. Used in the coating industry.

6612. Nitromide. [121-81-3] 3,5-Dinitrobenzamide. C₇-H₅N₃O₅; mol wt 211.13. C 39.82%, H 2.39%, N 19.90%, O 37.89%. Prepd from 3,5-dinitrobenzoyl chloride and ammonium acetate: Finan, Fothergill, *J. Chem. Soc.* **1962**, 2824.

Leaflets from water, mp 183°. Slightly sol in cold water, somewhat more sol in hot water.

Note: An ingredient of *Tristat, Unistat, Unistat-3.*

THERAP CAT (VET): Antibacterial, coccidiostat (for poultry).

6613. Nitron. [2218-94-2] 1,4-Diphenyl-3-(phenylamino)-1*H*-1,2,4-triazolium inner salt. C₂₀H₁₆N₄; mol wt 312.37. C 76.90%, H 5.16%, N 17.94%. Orginally represented as *3,5,6-triphenyl-2,3,5,6-tetraazabicyclo[2.1.1]hex-1-ene.* Prepn: **DE 159692** (1904 to E. Merck); M. Busch, *Ber.* **38**, 856 (1905). Corrected structure determn as meso-ionic compound: W. Baker, W. D. Ollis, *Q. Rev. Chem. Soc.* **11**, 15 (1957); G. A. Olah, *J. Inorg. Nucl. Chem.* **16**, 225 (1961). Mass spectrum: W. D. Ollis, C. A. Ramsden, *J. Chem. Soc. Perkin Trans. 1* **1974**, 645. NMR study: W. Bocian *et al.*, *Magn. Reson. Chem.* **33**, 134 (1995). Use in determn of metals: N. Gantchev, A. Dimitrova, *Mikrochim. Acta* **1971**, 476; T. J. Koralewski, G. A. Parker, *Anal. Chim. Acta* **113**, 389 (1980); H. Chen *et al. Acta Chim. Sin.* **1989**, 412. In determn of nitrate: A. Hulanicki, M. Maj, *Talanta* **22**, 767 (1975); A. Hioki *et al. Anal. Sci.* **6**, 757 (1990). Chemical sensor of stratospheric nitric acid: K. Meadows, V. R. Morris, *Proc. NOBCChE* **25**, 1 (1998).

Intensely yellow leaflets from alcohol, solvated needles from chloroform, dec ~189°. Insol in nitrates, water. Sol in alcohol, benzene, slightly sol acetone, chloroform, ethyl acetate; sparingly sol in ether. The alc soln undergoes partial decompn, indicated by a red color. Dipole moment in benzene: 7.2. pKa 10.34 ± 0.02

USE: Determination of boron, nitrate, perchlorate, rhenium, tungsten, molybdenum.

6614. 1-Nitronaphthalene. [86-57-7] α-Nitronaphthalene. C₁₀H₇NO₂; mol wt 173.17. C 69.36%, H 4.07%, N 8.09%, O 18.48%. Prepd from napthalene and a mixture of nitric and sulfuric acids at 50°.

Yellow crystals. d 1.331. mp 59-61°. bp 304°. Insol in water; sol in alcohol, freely in chloroform, ether, carbon disulfide. Gives a dark red soln with concd H₂SO₄.

USE: Deblooming petr oils, 2-3 parts suffice for 1000 parts oil; manuf dyes and intermediates.

6615. 1-Nitro-2-naphthol. [550-60-7] 1-Nitro-2-naphthalenol; α-nitro-β-naphthol; 1-nitro-2-hydroxynaphthalene. C₁₀H₇-NO₃; mol wt 189.17. C 63.49%, H 3.73%, N 7.40%, O 25.37%.

Yellow needles or platelets, mp 103°. Insol in water. Sol in alcohol, ether, glacial acetic acid, in alkali hydroxide solns.

USE: As a reagent for the determination of cobalt with which it gives a precipitate.

6616.   3-Nitropentane. [551-88-2] $C_5H_{11}NO_2$; mol wt 117.15. C 51.26%, H 9.46%, N 11.96%, O 27.31%. CH_3CH_2-$CH(NO_2)CH_2CH_3$.

Colorless liquid; fusel oil odor. d_4^0 0.957. bp 153-155°. Insol in water; sol in alcohol, ether.

6617.   5-Nitro-*o*-phenetidine. [136-79-8] 2-Ethoxy-5-nitro-benzenamine; 5-nitro-2-ethoxyaniline; 1-ethoxy-2-amino-4-nitro-benzene; 1-nitro-3-amino-4-phenyl ethyl ether; 4-nitro-2-amino-phenetole; Neo-Douxan. $C_8H_{10}N_2O_3$; mol wt 182.18. C 52.74%, H 5.53%, N 15.38%, O 26.35%. Prepn: Verkade *et al.*, *Rec. Trav. Chim.* **65**, 346 (1946). Toxicology: Grupp, Bilger, *Arzneim.-Forsch.* **1**, 326 (1951).

Brown-yellow crystals from benzene, mp 97.5-98.5°. 950 times as sweet as cane sugar, claimed to have no aftertaste.

USE: Sweetening agent.

6618.   Nitrophenide. [537-91-7] Bis(3-nitrophenyl)disul-fide; *m,m'*-dinitrodiphenyl disulfide; NP; Megasul. $C_{12}H_8N_2O_4S_2$; mol wt 308.33. C 46.74%, H 2.62%, N 9.09%, O 20.76%, S 20.80%. Prepd by the reduction of *m*-nitrobenzenesulfonylchloride with hydriodic acid: Ekbom, *Ber.* **24**, 336 (1891); Foss *et al.*, *J. Am. Chem. Soc.* **60**, 2729 (1938). Anticoccidial activity: Waletzky *et al.*, *Ann. N.Y. Acad. Sci.* **52**, 543 (1949).

Yellow rhomboid crystals, mp 83°. Freely sol in ether, less sol in alcohol. Insol in water.

THERAP CAT (VET): Coccidiostat.

6619.   *m*-Nitrophenol. [554-84-7] 3-Nitrophenol. C_6H_5-NO_3; mol wt 139.11. C 51.80%, H 3.62%, N 10.07%, O 34.50%. Prepn by boiling diazotized *m*-nitroaniline with water and H_2SO_4: Adams, Wilson, *Org. Synth.* **3**, 87 (1923); Bachmann, Rottschaefer, *ibid.* **18**, 88 (1938); Manske, *ibid.* **coll. vol. I**, 404 (2nd ed., 1941).

Monoclinic prisms from ether or dil HCl. d_4^{20} 1.485; d_4^{100} 1.2797. mp 97°. bp_{70} 194°. Dec when distilled at ordinary pressure. pK (18°) 8.34. Absorption spectrum: Baly *et al.*, *J. Chem. Soc.* **97**, 586 (1910); Marchlewski, Moroz, *Bull. Soc. Chim.* [4] **35**, 476 (1924). An aq soln satd at 40° contains 3.02 g in 100 g soln; at 98.7°, 40.9 g: Sidgwick *et al.*, *J. Chem. Soc.* **107**, 1202 (1915). Soly (g/100 g solvent) in acetone: 169.35 (0.2°); 1305.9 (84°); in alcohol: 116.9 (1°); 1105.25 (85°); in ether: 105.9 (0.2°); 1065.8 (83°): Carrick, *J. Phys. Chem.* **25**, 635 (1921). Sol in hot and dil acids, in caustic solns. Insol in petr ether. LD_{50} orally in mice, rats: 1414, 933 mg/kg, K. C. Back *et al.*, *Reclassification of Materials Listed as Transportation Health Hazards* (TSA-20-72-3; PB214-270, 1972).

USE: As indicator in 0.3% soln in 50% alc. pH: 6.8 colorless, 8.6 yellow.

6620.   *o*-Nitrophenol. [88-75-5] 2-Nitrophenol. $C_6H_5NO_3$; mol wt 139.11. C 51.80%, H 3.62%, N 10.07%, O 34.50%. Prepd by the nitration of phenol; separated by steam distillation. Review of toxicology and human exposure: *Toxicological Profile for Nitro-*

phenols: 2-Nitrophenol and 4-Nitrophenol (PB93-110823, 1992) 131 pp.

Light yellow needles or prisms; peculiar, aromatic odor. d 1.495. mp 44-45°. bp 214-216°. Volatile with steam. Slightly sol in cold water, freely in hot water, in alcohol, benzene, ether, carbon disul-fide, alkali hydroxides. LD_{50} orally in mice, rats: 1.297, 2.828 g/kg, K. C. Back *et al.*, *Reclassification of Materials Listed as Transportation Health Hazards* (TSA-20-72-3; PB214-270, 1972).

USE: Manuf dyes, paint colorings, rubber chemicals, and fungi-cides. Indicator in 2% alc soln. pH: 5.0 colorless, 7.0 yellow, but the color change is not sharp and cannot be used where CO_2 is present; as reagent for glucose.

6621.   *p*-Nitrophenol. [100-02-7] 4-Nitrophenol. C_6H_5-NO_3; mol wt 139.11. C 51.80%, H 3.62%, N 10.07%, O 34.50%. Review of toxicology and human exposure: *Toxicological Profile for Nitrophenols: 2-Nitrophenol and 4-Nitrophenol* (PB93-110823, 1992) 131 pp.

Colorless to slightly yellow, odorless crystals; sweetish, then burning taste. d_4^{120} 1.270. mp 113-114°. Sublimes; slightly vol-atile with steam. Moderately sol in cold water, freely in alcohol, chloroform, ether; also sol in solns of fixed alkali hydroxides and carbonates. LD_{50} orally in mice, rats: 467, 616 mg/kg, K.C. Back *et al.*, *Reclassification of Materials Listed as Transportation Health Hazards* (TSA-20-72-3; PB214-270, 1972).

USE: Manuf of pharmaceuticals, fungicides, dyes. Indicator in 0.1% alcohol soln. pH: 5.6 colorless, 7.6 yellow.

6622.   *p*-Nitrophenylacetic Acid. [104-03-0] 4-Nitroben-zeneacetic acid; *p*-nitro-α-toluic acid. $C_8H_7NO_4$; mol wt 181.15. C 53.04%, H 3.89%, N 7.73%, O 35.33%. $NO_2C_6H_4CH_2COOH$. Prepd by hydrolysis of *p*-nitrobenzyl cyanide with 50% H_2SO_4: Robertson, *Org. Synth.* **2**, 59 (1922); **coll. vol. I**, 406 (2nd ed., 1941).

Long, pale yellow needles from water. mp 153°. pK (25)° 3.98. Absorption spectrum: Hewitt *et al.*, *J. Chem. Soc.* **101**, 1774 (1912). Sparingly sol in cold water; sol in alcohol, ether, benzene.

Methyl ester. $C_9H_9NO_4$. mp 54°.

Benzyl ester. $C_{15}H_{13}NO_4$. mp 92°.

Nitrile see *p*-Nitrobenzyl Cyanide.

6623.   4-Nitro-*o*-phenylenediamine. [99-56-9] 4-Nitro-1,2-benzenediamine; 1,2-diamino-4-nitrobenzene; 4-nitro-1,2-diamino-benzene; 4-nitro-1,2-phenylenediamine. $C_6H_7N_3O_2$; mol wt 153.14. C 47.06%, H 4.61%, N 27.44%, O 20.90%. Prepd by the reduction of 2,4-dinitroaniline using H_2S in ammonia water: Kehrmann, *Ber.* **28**, 1707 (1895); Griffin, Peterson, *Org. Synth.* **coll. vol. III**, 242 (1955). Use as reagent for α-keto acids: Hockenhull, Floodgate, *Biochem. J.* **52**, 38 (1952); Taylor, Smith, *Analyst* **80**, 607 (1955). Toxicity study: C. Burnett *et al.*, *J. Toxicol. Environ. Health* **2**, 657 (1977).

Dark red needles from hot water. mp 201°. Sparingly sol in water. Sol in aq solns of hydrochloric acid. LD_{50} in rats (mg/kg): 3720 orally; >1600 i.p. (Burnett).

USE: Reagent for α-keto acids.

6624. (4-Nitrophenyl)hydrazine. [100-16-3] $C_6H_7N_3O_2$; mol wt 153.14. C 47.06%, H 4.61%, N 27.44%, O 20.90%.

Orange-red leaflets or needles. mp ~157° with dec. Slightly sol in cold water; sol in hot water or hot benzene, alcohol, chloroform, ether, ethyl acetate.

USE: As reagent for ketones, aliphatic aldehydes.

6625. o-Nitrophenylpropiolic Acid. [530-85-8] 3-(2-Nitrophenyl)-2-propynoic acid. $C_9H_5NO_4$; mol wt 191.14. C 56.55%, H 2.64%, N 7.33%, O 33.48%.

Yellowish to light brown scales or crystals. mp ~157° with decompn and may explode. Moderately sol in cold water, more in hot water or alcohol, very slightly in chloroform. Almost insol in carbon disulfide and petr ether.

USE: As a reagent for alkaloids and glucose.

6626. (4-Nitrophenyl)urea. [556-10-5] $C_7H_7N_3O_3$; mol wt 181.15. C 46.41%, H 3.89%, N 23.20%, O 26.50%. Prepn from N-substituted S-phenylthiocarbamates: Crosby, Niemann, *J. Am. Chem. Soc.* **76**, 4458 (1954).

Prisms from abs ethanol, needles from dil ethanol, mp 238°. Practically insol in cold water. Sol in boiling water, methanol, ethanol, dimethylformamide. Sparingly sol in ether, benzene.

6627. 1-Nitropropane. [108-03-2] $C_3H_7NO_2$; mol wt 89.09. C 40.44%, H 7.92%, N 15.72%, O 35.92%. $CH_3CH_2CH_2$-NO_2. Prepd by vapor-phase nitration of propane: Hass *et al.*, **US 1967667** (1934 to Purdue Res. Found.); *Ind. Eng. Chem.* **28**, 339 (1936); from natural gas: Bachman, Pollack, *ibid.* **46**, 713 (1954).

Liquid. d_4^{25} 0.9934. wt 8.4 lb/U.S. gal. mp −108°. bp$_{760}$ 131.6°; bp$_{728}$ 130°; bp$_{401}$ 110°; bp$_{94}$ 70°; bp$_{7.5}$ 20°; bp$_4$ 10°. n_D^{20} 1.4018. Flash pt 34°C (93°F). Heat of formation −40.05 kcal/mole at 25°; heat of combustion 481.33 kcal/mole at 25°. Latent heat of vaporization 10.37 kcal/mole at 25°. Slightly insol in water (1.4 ml/100 ml); 0.5 ml water dissolves in 100 ml of 1-nitropropane. Miscible with many organic solvents.

Caution: Potential symptoms of overexposure are eye irritation, headache, nausea, vomiting and diarrhea. See *NIOSH Pocket Guide to Chemical Hazards* (DHHS/NIOSH 97-140, 1997) p 230.

USE: Solvent for cellulose acetate, vinyl resins, lacquers, synthetic rubbers, fats, oils, dyes, other organic materials; as intermediate, propellant.

6628. 2-Nitropropane. [79-46-9] $C_3H_7NO_2$; mol wt 89.09. C 40.44%, H 7.92%, N 15.72%, O 35.92%. $CH_3CH(NO_2)CH_3$. Prepn: Hass *et al.*, **US 1967667** (1934 to Purdue Res. Found.); *Ind. Eng. Chem.* **28**, 339 (1936); from natural gas: Bachman, Pollack, *ibid.* **46**, 713 (1954). Toxicity and carcinogenicity study: T. R. Lewis *et al.*, *J. Environ. Pathol. Toxicol.* **2**, 233 (1979). Health hazard alert: *Am. Ind. Hyg. Assoc. J.* **41**, 18 (1980).

Liquid. d_4^{25} 0.9821. wt 8.4 lb/U.S. gal. mp −93°. bp$_{760}$ 120.3°; bp$_{564}$ 110°; bp$_{300}$ 90°; bp$_{95}$ 60°; bp$_7$ 10°. n_D^{20} 1.3944. Flash pt 24°C (75°F). Heat of formn −43.78 kcal/mole at 25°; heat of combustion 477.60 kcal/mole at 25°. Latent heat of vaporization 9.88 kcal/mole at 25°. Slightly sol in water (1.7 ml/100 ml); 0.6 ml water dissolves in 100 ml of 2-nitropropane. Misc with many organic solvents.

Caution: Potential symptoms of overexposure are headache, anorexia, nausea, vomiting, diarrhea; irritation of eyes, skin, nose

and respiratory system; kidney and liver damage. See *NIOSH Pocket Guide to Chemical Hazards* (DHHS/NIOSH 97-140, 1997) p 230. This substance is reasonably anticipated to be a human carcinogen: *Report on Carcinogens, Eleventh Edition* (PB2005-104914, 2004) p III-194.

USE: Solvent in inks, paints, adhesives, varnishes, polymers, synthetic material; as chemical intermediate.

6629. 5′-Nitro-2′-propoxyacetanilide. [553-20-8] N-(5-Nitro-2-propoxyphenyl)acetamide; 1-propoxy-2-acetamino-4-nitrobenzene; Falimint. $C_{11}H_{14}N_2O_4$; mol wt 238.24. C 55.46%, H 5.92%, N 11.76%, O 26.86%. Prepd by reacting 1-chloro-2,4-dinitrobenzene with sodium alkoxide, followed by partial reduction and treatment with acetic anhydride: Profft, *Chem. Tech. (Leipzig)* **5**, 393 (1953), *C.A.* **47**, 12757a (1953); by nitration of 1-propoxy-2-acetylaminobenzene: Verkade *et al.*, *Rec. Trav. Chim.* **66**, 374 (1947); also **GB 597835** (1948 to N. V. Polak & Schwarz's Essencefabrieken).

Crystals from propanol, mp 102.5-103.5°. Flat taste.

THERAP CAT: Antipyretic, analgesic.

6630. 5-Nitro-2-propoxyaniline. [553-79-7] 5-Nitro-2-propoxybenzenamine; 2-amino-4-nitro-1-propoxybenzene; 1-propoxy-2-amino-4-nitrobenzene; P-4000; Ultrasüss. $C_9H_{12}N_2O_3$; mol wt 196.20. C 55.09%, H 6.16%, N 14.28%, O 24.46%. A substance which is 4000 times sweeter than sugar, with no bitter aftertaste. Prepn: Verkade *et al.*, *Rec. Trav. Chim.* **65**, 346-360 (1946); **NL 6514769** (1967 to N. V. Koffie en Theehandel), *C.A.* **67**, 108430n (1967); A. J. de Koning, *J. Chem. Educ.* **53**, 521 (1976); J. McK. Woollard, *ibid.* **57**, 464 (1980). Toxicity studies: Fitzhugh *et al.*, *J. Am. Pharm. Assoc.* **46**, 583 (1951).

Orange crystals from n-propanol + petr ether. mp 47.5-48.5°. Soly in water at 20°: 136 mg/liter. Stable in boiling water and in dil acids.

6631. 3-Nitrosalicylic Acid. [85-38-1] 2-Hydroxy-3-nitrobenzoic acid. $C_7H_5NO_5$; mol wt 183.12. C 45.91%, H 2.75%, N 7.65%, O 43.69%. The 3- and 5-nitrosalicylic acids are formed by the nitration of salicylic acid with H_2SO_4 and HNO_3.

Monohydrate. Yellowish crystals. mp 123°; mp 148° when anhydr. Slightly sol in water; freely sol in alcohol, benzene, chloroform, ether.

USE: In dye chemistry.

6632. 5-Nitrosalicylic Acid. [96-97-9] 2-Hydroxy-5-nitrobenzoic acid; anilotic acid. $C_7H_5NO_5$; mol wt 183.12. C 45.91%, H 2.75%, N 7.65%, O 43.69%.

Yellowish crystals. d 1.65. mp 228-230°. One gram dissolves in 1475 ml water; more sol in hot water; freely sol in alcohol, ether.

6633. Nitroscanate. [19881-18-6] 1-Isothiocyanato-4-(4-nitrophenoxy)benzene; isothiocyanic acid p-(p-nitrophenoxy)-phenyl ester; p-(p-nitrophenoxy)phenyl isothiocyanate; 1-(4-isothiocyanatophenoxy)-4-nitrobenzene; 4-nitro-4'-isothiocyanodiphenyl ether; cantrodifene (obsolete); CGA-23654; GS-23654; Lopatol; Skanitrol. $C_{13}H_8N_2O_3S$; mol wt 272.28. C 57.35%, H 2.96%, N 10.29%, O 17.63%, S 11.78%. Prepn: **FR 1491477** (1967 to Agripat); F. Paltauf *et al.*, **US 3697555** (1972 to Ciba-Geigy); A. Martvon, K. Antos, *Chem. Zvesti* **23**, 181 (1969). Activity in dogs: M. A. Gemmell, G. Oudemans, *Res. Vet. Sci.* **19**, 217 (1975).

Crystals, mp 107-113° (Martvon, Antos); also reported as 124-125° (Paltauf). Insol in water. Sol in organic solvents.

THERAP CAT (VET): Anthelmintic.

6634. 3-Nitrosobenzamide. [144189-66-2] NOBA. $C_7H_6N_2O_2$; mol wt 150.13. C 56.00%, H 4.03%, N 18.66%, O 21.31%. Antiretroviral zinc ejecting agent. Prepn: E. Kun *et al.*, **WO 9108902** (1991 to Octamer). Tumoricidal activity: W. G. Rice *et al.*, *Proc. Natl. Acad. Sci. USA* **89**, 7703 (1992). Inhibition of HIV-1 infectivity: W. G. Rice *et al.*, *Nature* **361**, 473 (1993); and site of action: *eidem, Proc. Natl. Acad. Sci. USA* **90**, 9721 (1993); of SIV: A. J. Chuang *et al.*, *FEBS Lett.* **326**, 140 (1993).

Light yellow solid. Darkens above 135°, softens with polymerization 150-160°; mp 240-250° (dec). In solution the compound is dark green. uv/vis max (absol. ethanol): 218, 304, 750nm (ε 1.5 × 10^4, 5.35 × 10^3, 37.6).

6635. N-Nitrosodiethanolamine. [1116-54-7] 2,2'-(Nitrosoimino)bisethanol; 2,2'-nitrosiminodiethanol; di-(2-hydroxyethyl)nitrosamine; NDELA. $C_4H_{10}N_2O_3$; mol wt 134.13. C 35.82%, H 7.51%, N 20.89%, O 35.78%. $(HOCH_2CH_2)_2NNO$. Formed by the action of nitrites on di- or triethanolamine. Prepn: E. R. H. Jones, W. Wilson, *J. Chem. Soc.* **1949**, 547; R. Preussmann, *Ber.* **95**, 1571 (1962); W. Lijinsky *et al.*, *J. Natl. Cancer Inst.* **49**, 1239 (1972). Carcinogenicity study: H. Druckery *et al.*, *Z. Krebsforsch.* **69**, 103 (1967). Impurity in cutting fluids: T. Y. Fan *et al.*, *Science* **196**, 70 (1977); in cosmetics: *eidem, Food Cosmet. Toxicol.* **15**, 423 (1977). Mutagenicity study: A. Hesbert *et al.*, *Mutat. Res.* **68**, 207 (1979).

Light yellow oil, bp$_{0.01}$ 125°. n_D^{20} 1.4849.

Caution: This substance is reasonably anticipated to be a human carcinogen: *Report on Carcinogens, Eleventh Edition* (PB2005-104914, 2004) p III-197.

6636. N-Nitrosodiethylamine. [55-18-5] N-Ethyl-N-nitrosoethanamine; diethylnitrosamine; DEN; DENA; NDEA. $C_4H_{10}N_2O$; mol wt 102.14. C 47.04%, H 9.87%, N 27.43%, O 15.66%. $(C_2H_5)_2NNO$. Detected in trace amounts in tobacco smoke: Druckney, Preussman, *Naturwissenschaften* **49**, 498 (1962) and in various processed foods: Hedler, Marquardt, *Food Cosmet. Toxicol.* **6**, 341 (1968); Friemuth, Glaeser, *Nahrung* **14**, 357 (1970). Formed by the interaction of nitrite with diethylamine and by the action of nitrate-reducing bacteria. Industrial prepn: Reilly, **DE 1085166** (1960 to du Pont), *C.A.* **56**, 4594h (1962); Levering, Maury, **US 3090786** (1963 to Hercules Powder); Minisci, Galli, *Chim. Ind. (Milan)* **46**, 173 (1964). Hepatotoxicity and carcinogenicity studies: Schmaehl *et al.*, *Naturwissenschaften* **54**, 341 (1967); Grover, Fischer, *Eur. J. Cancer* **7**, 77 (1971); Bader *et al.*, *Arch. Geschwulstforsch.* **37**, 327 (1971). General review: Magee, Barnes, *Adv. Cancer Res.* **10**, 163-246 (1967).

Slightly yellow liq. d_4^{20} 0.9422. bp 175-177°. bp$_5$ 47°. n_D^{20} 1.4388. Sol in water, alc, ether.

Caution: This substance is reasonably anticipated to be a human carcinogen: *Report on Carcinogens, Eleventh Edition* (PB2005-104914, 2004) p III-198.

USE: Gasoline and lubricant additive; antioxidant; stabilizer in plastics.

6637. N-Nitrosodimethylamine. [62-75-9] N-Methyl-N-nitrosomethanamine; dimethylnitrosamine; DMN; DMNA. $C_2H_6N_2O$; mol wt 74.08. C 32.43%, H 8.16%, N 37.82%, O 21.60%. $(CH_3)_2NNO$. Reportedly found in trace amounts in tobacco smoke condensates: Rhoades, Johnson, *Nature* **236**, 307 (1972); in cured meat products, notably bacon: Sen *et al., ibid.* **241**, 473 (1973); in smoked and salted fish: Fazio *et al., J. Agric. Food Chem.* **19**, 250 (1971); Fong, Chan, *Nature* **243**, 421 (1973). Formed by the interaction of nitrite with dimethylamine and by the action of nitrate-reducing bacteria. Industrial prepn: **GB 772331** (1957 to Olin Mathieson), *C.A.* **51**, 14783a (1957); Ioffe, *Zh. Obshch. Khim.* **28**, 1296 (1958); Norris, *J. Am. Chem. Soc.* **81**, 3346 (1959); Campbell, **US 2981752** (1961 to C.S.C.); Datin, Elliott, **US 3136821** (1964 to Allied Chem.). Chemistry: Layne *et al., J. Am. Chem. Soc.* **85**, 435, 1816 (1963). Metabolism and toxicity: Magee, Vandekar; Magee, *Biochem. J.* **70**, 600, 606 (1958); Heath, *ibid.* **85**, 72 (1962). Carcinogenicity studies: Magee, Barnes, *Br. J. Cancer* **10**, 114 (1956); *see also eidem, Adv. Cancer Res.* **10**, 163-246 (1967). Review of toxicology and human exposure: *Toxicological Profile for N-Nitrosodimethylamine* (PB90-182130, 1989) 132 pp.

Yellow liquid. bp 151-153°. bp$_{40}$ 67.1°. d_4^{20} 1.0048. n_D^{20} 1.4368. Very sol in water, alcohol, ether. LD$_{50}$ i.p. in rats: 34 mg/kg (Heath).

Caution: Potential symptoms of overexposure are nausea, vomiting, diarrhea and abdominal cramps; headache; fever; enlarged liver, jaundice; reduced function of liver, kidneys and lungs. *See NIOSH Pocket Guide to Chemical Hazards* (DHHS/NIOSH 97-140. 1997) p 232. This substance is reasonably anticipated to be a human carcinogen: *Report on Carcinogens, Eleventh Edition* (PB-2005-104914, 2004) p III-199.

USE: Formerly in the prodn of rocket fuels; antioxidant; additive for lubricants; softener of copolymers.

6638. p-Nitroso-N,N-dimethylaniline. [138-89-6] N,N-Dimethyl-4-nitrosobenzenamine; Accelerine. $C_8H_{10}N_2O$; mol wt 150.18. C 63.98%, H 6.71%, N 18.65%, O 10.65%. Prepd in the cold from NaNO$_2$ and a soln of dimethylaniline in HCl.

Green plates or leaflets. mp 92.5-93.5°; also stated as 87-88°. Volatile with steam. Insol in water. Sol in alcohol, ether.

USE: Manuf organic compds; accelerator in vulcanizing; in printing fabrics.

6639. p-Nitrosodiphenylamine. [156-10-5] 4-Nitroso-N-phenylbenzenamine. $C_{12}H_{10}N_2O$; mol wt 198.22. C 72.71%, H 5.08%, N 14.13%, O 8.07%. $C_6H_5NHC_6H_4NO$. Review of toxicology and human exposure: *Toxicological Profile for N-Nitrosodiphenylamine* (PB93-182509, 1993) 114 pp.

Green plates with bluish luster (from benzene) or steel-blue prisms or plates (from ether + water). mp 144-145°. Slightly sol in water or petr ether; freely sol in alcohol, ether, chloroform, benzene. Dissolves in H_2SO_4 with a red color, which suddenly changes to violet on warming.

Note: This substance was formerly anticipated to be a carcinogen: *Fifth Annual Report on Carcinogens* (NTP 89-239, 1989) p 212; delisted for insufficient evidence of carcinogenicity: *Sixth Annual Report on Carcinogens* (PB92-120666, 1991) p 13.

USE: Has been used as retardant in vulcanizing rubber.

6640. N-Nitrosomorpholine. [59-89-2] 4-Nitrosomorpholine; NMOR. $C_4H_8N_2O_2$; mol wt 116.12. C 41.37%, H 6.94%, N 24.12%, O 27.56%. Prepn: L. Knorr, *Ann.* **301**, 1 (1898); F. Chapman, *J. Chem. Soc.* **1949**, 1631; G. Oláh *et al., Ber.* **89**, 2374 (1956). Metabolism: B. W. Stewart, P. N. Magee, *Biochem. J.* **126**, 21P (1972). Carcinogenicity studies: H. Druckrey *et al., Naturwissenschaften* **48**, 134 (1961); P. Bannasch, H.-A. Müller, *Arzneim.-Forsch.* **14**, 805 (1964); *IARC Monographs* **17**, 263 (1978).

Yellow crystals, mp 29°. bp$_{25}$ 139-140°; bp$_{747}$ 224-224.5°. Sol in water. LD$_{50}$ orally in rats: 282 mg/kg (Druckrey).

Caution: This substance is reasonably anticipated to be a human carcinogen: *Report on Carcinogens, Eleventh Edition* (PB2005-104914, 2004) p III-205.

6641. 1-Nitroso-2-naphthol. [131-91-9] 1-Nitroso-2-naphthalenol; nitroso-β-naphthol. $C_{10}H_7NO_2$; mol wt 173.17. C 69.36%, H 4.07%, N 8.09%, O 18.48%. Prepared by the addition of H_2SO_4 to a mixture of β-naphthol dissolved in aq NaOH and NaNO$_2$: C. S. Marvel, P. K. Porter, *Org. Synth.* **coll. vol. I,** 411 (2nd ed., 1941).

Yellowish-brown needles from petr ether, mp 109-110°. Sol in 1000 parts water, 35 parts alcohol; also sol in hot alcohol, benzene, ether, carbon disulfide, caustic alkali solns, glacial acetic acid; slightly sol in cold petr ether.

USE: To prevent gum formation in gasoline; in analytical chemistry in the determination of cobalt (to separate it from nickel).

6642. 4-Nitrosophenol. [104-91-6] Quinone oxime; quinone monoxime. $C_6H_5NO_2$; mol wt 123.11. C 58.54%, H 4.09%, N 11.38%, O 25.99%.

Pale yellow orthorhombic needles, browns at 126° (dec 144°). *Explodes on contact with concentrated acid, alkali, or fire. A technical grade exploded on storage.* Ka at 25° = 3.3 × 10^{-7}. Moderately sol in water. Sol in dil alkalies giving green to brownish green solns. Sol in alc, ether, acetone.

6643. *N*-Nitrosopyrrolidine. [930-55-2] 1-Nitrosopyrrolidine; NPYR; NO-PYR. $C_4H_8N_2O$; mol wt 100.12. C 47.99%, H 8.05%, N 27.98%, O 15.98%. Cyclic nitrosamine that occurs in food products and tobacco smoke. Prepn: F. C. Peterson, *Ber.* **21,** 290 (1888). Carcinogenicity studies: H. Druckrey *et al., Z. Krebsforsch.* **69,** 103 (1967); M. Greenblatt *et al., J. Natl. Cancer Inst.* **48,** 1687 (1972); *IARC Monographs* **17,** 313 (1978). Mechanism of mutagenicity: L. I. Hecker *et al., Mutat. Res.* **62,** 213 (1979). Metabolism: R. C. Cottrell *et al., Adv. Exp. Med. Biol.* **136B,** 1165 (1982).

Yellow liquid, bp$_{20}$ 104-106°. Sol in water. LD$_{50}$ orally in rats: 900 mg/kg (Druckrey).
Caution: This substance is reasonably anticipated to be a human carcinogen: *Report on Carcinogens, Eleventh Edition* (PB2005-104914, 2004) p III-207.

6644. Nitroso-R Salt. [525-05-3] 3-Hydroxy-4-nitroso-2,7-naphthalenedisulfonic acid disodium salt; sodium salt of 1-nitroso-2-hydroxynaphthalene-3,6-disulfonic acid. $C_{10}H_5NNa_2O_8S_2$; mol wt 377.26. C 31.84%, H 1.34%, N 3.71%, Na 12.19%, O 33.93%, S 17.00%.

Golden-yellow, fan-shaped crystals. Sol in ~40 parts water; more sol in hot water; slightly sol in methyl or ethyl alcohol.
USE: As a reagent for cobalt and potassium.

6645. 2-Nitro-4-sulfobenzoic Acid. [552-23-8] $C_7H_5NO_7$-S; mol wt 247.18. C 34.01%, H 2.04%, N 5.67%, O 45.31%, S 12.97%. Prepn by sulfonation of *o*-nitrotoluene and oxidation of the resulting 2-nitro-4-toluenesulfonic acid with potassium permanganate: Hart, *Am. Chem. J.* **1,** 352 (1879-80).

Needles from hydrochloric acid. Stable in air under ordinary conditions.
USE: Alkalimetric standard.

6646. Nitrosyl Chloride. [2696-92-6] ClNO; mol wt 65.46. Cl 54.16%, N 21.40%, O 24.44%. NOCl. Best prepared from nitrosylsulfuric acid and dry HCl: Coleman *et al., Inorg. Synth.* **1,** 55 (1939).
Non-explosive, very corrosive, reddish-yellow gas; liquid at −5.5°; solid at −61.5°. Decomposed by water. Sol in fuming H_2SO_4. Critical temp 167°; crit press. 92.4 atm. The orange color of aqua regia is produced by nitrosyl chloride.
Caution: Intensely irritating to eyes, skin, mucous membranes. Inhalation may cause pulmonary edema, hemorrhage.

6647. Nitrosyl Fluoride. [7789-25-5] Nitrogen oxyfluoride. FNO; mol wt 49.00. F 38.77%, N 28.59%, O 32.65%. Preparation: Ruff *et al., Z. Anorg. Allg. Chem.* **208,** 293 (1932); Balz, Mailänder, *ibid.* **217,** 166 (1934); Faloon, Kenna, *J. Am. Chem. Soc.* **73,** 2937 (1951); Kwasnik in *Handbook of Preparative Inorganic Chemistry* **vol. 1,** G. Brauer, Ed. (Academic Press, New York, 2nd ed., 1963) pp 184-185. *Reviews:* Hoffman, Neville, *Chem. Rev.* **62,** 1-18 (1962); Kemmitt, Sharp, *Adv. Fluorine Chem.* **4,** 194-195 (1965); Woolf, *ibid.* **5,** 1-30 (1965); Schmutzler, *Angew. Chem. Int. Ed.* **7,** 440-455 (1968).
Colorless gas. Often bluish because of impurities. Vigorous reaction with glass, corroding action on quartz. May be kept in quartz ampuls if cooled in liq oxygen. mp −132.5°. bp −59.9°. d (liq at bp) 1.326. d (solid) 1.719. Trouton const. 21.3. Reacts with water to form NO, HNO$_3$ and HF.
Caution: Highly irritating to skin, eyes, mucous membranes. *See also* Fluorine.
USE: Oxidizer in rocket propellants; stabilizing agent for liquid SO$_3$; fluorinating agent.

6648. Nitrosylsulfuric Acid. [7782-78-7] Sulfuric acid monoanhydride with nitrous acid; nitrosyl sulfate; chamber crystals; nitrososulfuric acid; nitroxylsulfuric acid; nitrosulfonic acid; nitrosyl hydrogen sulfate; nitro acid sulfite; Nitrose. HNO$_5$S; mol wt 127.08. H 0.79%, N 11.02%, O 62.95%, S 25.23%. Formed as an intermediate in the lead chamber process for sulfuric acid by the reaction of sulfur dioxide, nitrogen trioxide, oxygen, and water: Clément, Désormes, *Ann. Chim. Phys.* [1] **59,** 329 (1806); Lunge, *J. Chem. Soc.* **47,** 470 (1885). Prepd from sulfur trioxide, nitrogen oxides and water: Döbereiner, *Schweigger's Journ.* **8,** 239 (1812); de Claubry, *Ann. Chim. Phys.* [2] **45,** 284 (1832); Kuhlmann, *ibid.* [3] **1,** 116 (1843); from silver acid sulfate and nitrosyl bromide: Berl *et al., Z. Anorg. Allg. Chem.* **209,** 264 (1932). *See also* US **1909557** and US **1909558.** The formation of crystals of nitrosylsulfuric acid may be observed by igniting a mixture of 1 part sulfur and 2 or 3 parts potassium nitrate under a bell jar.

Prisms, dec 73.5°. In moist air the crystals dec with the formation of sulfuric and nitric acids and above 50° nitric oxide and nitrogen dioxide are evolved. Sol in sulfuric acid, dec in water.
USE: For bleaching cereal milling products.

6649. Nitrosyl Tetrafluoroborate. [14635-75-7] Nitrosonium tetrafluoroborate; nitrosyl borofluoride; nitrosyl fluoborate.

BF_4NO; mol wt 116.81. B 9.26%, F 65.06%, N 11.99%, O 13.70%. $NOBF_4$. Prepd according to the equation: $2 HBF_4 + N_2O_3 \rightarrow 2 NOBF_4 + H_2O$: Wilke-Dörfurt, Balz, *Z. Anorg. Allg. Chem.* **159**, 219 (1927); Balz, Mailänder, *ibid.* **217**, 162 (1934); H. S. Booth, D. R. Martin, *Boron Trifluoride and Its Derivatives* (New York, 1949) p 133 sqq. Review of tetrafluoroborates: Sharp, *Adv. Fluorine Chem.* **1**, 68-128 (1960).

Birefringent, orthorhombic, hygroscopic platelets. d_4^{25} 2.185. Sublimes at 0.01 mm and 250° without decompn. Decomposed by water. May be stored in glass bottles if absolutely dry.

USE: In the prepn of diazonium fluoborates.

6650. Nitrotoluene. Methylnitrobenzene. $C_7H_7NO_2$; mol wt 137.14. C 61.31%, H 5.14%, N 10.21%, O 23.33%. Nitration of toluol by a mixture of HNO_3 and H_2SO_4 yields principally *o*- and *p*-nitrotoluol. Prepn of *m*-nitrotoluene from 3-nitro-4-amino-toluene and $NaNO_2$: Clark, Taylor, *Org. Synth.* **3**, 91 (1923).

m-**Nitrotoluene.** [99-08-1] 3-Nitrotoluene. Liquid. d_4^{15} 1.1630; d_4^{20} 1.1581; d_4^{59} 1.124; d_4^{121} 1.063. Solidifies in an ice and salt cooling mixture; mp 15°. bp_{760} 232°; bp_{100} 156.9°; bp_{40} 130.7°; bp_{20} 112.8°; bp_{10} 96.0°; bp_5 81.0°; $bp_{1.0}$ 50.2°. n_D^{30} 1.5426. Absorption spectrum: Marchlewski, Mayer, *Bull. Acad. Polon.* [A] **1929**, 188. Miscible with alcohol and ether. Sol in benzene. Soly in water at 30° (mg/l): 498. Log P (octanol/water): 2.40.

o-**Nitrotoluene.** [88-72-2] 2-Nitrotoluene. Technical report: *NTP Technical Report on the Toxicology and Carcinogenesis Studies of o-Nitrotoluene* (NTP TR-504/NIH 02-4438, 2002) 368 pp. Yellowish liquid at ordinary temp. d_{15}^{19} 1.1622. mp −9.3°. bp 220.4°. n_D^{20} 1.5472. Soly in water at 30° (mg/l): 652. Sol in alcohol, benzene, petr ether. Log P (octanol/water): 2.30.

p-**Nitrotoluene.** [99-99-0] 4-Nitrotoluene. Technical report: *NTP Technical Report on the Toxicology and Carcinogenesis Studies of p-Nitrotoluene* (NTP TR-498/NIH 02-4432, 2002) 277 pp. Yellowish crystals. d 1.286. mp 51.7°. bp 238.3°. Flash pt 106°C. Soly in water at 30° (mg/l): 442. Sol in alcohol, benzene, ether, chloroform, acetone. Log P (octanol/water): 2.37.

Caution: Potential symptoms of overexposure are anoxia, cyanosis; headache, lassitude, dizziness; ataxia; dyspnea; tachycardia; nausea, vomiting. *See NIOSH Pocket Guide to Chemical Hazards* (DHHS/NIOSH 97-140, 2003) p 232.

USE: Manuf of dyes, toluidines, nitrobenzoic acids, agricultural and rubber chemicals.

6651. Nitrourea. [556-89-8] *N*-Nitrocarbamide. $CH_3N_3-O_3$; mol wt 105.05. C 11.43%, H 2.88%, N 40.00%, O 45.69%. $NH_2CONHNO_2$. Prepd by the action of concd sulfuric acid upon urea nitrate: Thiele, Lachman, *Ann.* **288**, 281 (1895); Ingersoll, Armendt, *Org. Synth.* **5**, 85 (1925). By dropwise addition of HCl to a cooled mixture of silver cyanate and nitramide in water: Davis, Blanchard, *J. Am. Chem. Soc.* **51**, 1794 (1929).

Platelets from alcohol + petr ether dec 158.4-158.8°. pK (20°) 2.15. Absorption spectrum: Baly, Desch, *J. Chem. Soc.* **93**, 1753 (1908). Soluble in hot water, but water solns are unstable. Decompn in aq alkaline solns is almost instantaneous. Freely sol in acetone, alcohol, acetic acid. Sparingly sol in petr ether, chloroform, benzene. Stable to oxidizing agents. Can be detonated, but is not sensitive to percussion or heating.

6652. Nitrous Acid. [7782-77-6] HNO_2; mol wt 47.01. H 2.14%, N 29.80%, O 68.07%. Formed by the action of strong acids on inorganic nitrites. *Review:* Block, "Nitrous Acid, Hyponitrous Acid and their Salts" in *Mellor's* Vol. **VIII**, supplement II, *Nitrogen* (part 2) 353-408 (1967).

Known only in soln (pale blue in color). Weak acid. pK (25°) 3.35. In water it changes quickly into nitric oxide and nitric acid. Forms stable, water-sol nitrites with Li, Na, K, Ca, Sr, Ba, Ag. Does not form salts with weak polyvalent cations like Al or Be. Forms stable esters with alcohols.

6653. Nitrous Oxide. [10024-97-2] Dinitrogen monoxide; laughing gas; hyponitrous acid anhydride; factitious air. N_2O; mol wt 44.01. N 63.65%, O 36.35%. Constituent of the earth's atm, about 0.00005% by volume: Slobod, Krogh, *J. Am. Chem. Soc.* **72**, 1175 (1950). Prepd by thermal decompn of ammonium nitrate: E. H. Archibald, *The Preparation of Pure Inorganic Substances* (Wiley, New York, 1932) p 246; Castner, Kirst, US 2111276 (1938 to du Pont). Preparation and purification: Schenk in *Handbook of Preparative Inorganic Chemistry* vol. **1**, G. Brauer, Ed. (Academic Press, New York, 2nd ed., 1963) pp 484-485. The chief impurity of the commercial product is N_2, although NO_2, N, O_2, and CO_2 may also be present. Teratogenicity study: G. A. Lane *et al.*, *Science* **210**, 899 (1980). *Reviews:* Beattie, "Nitrous Oxide" in *Mellor's* Vol. **VIII**, suppl II, *Nitrogen* (part 2) 189-215 (1967); Jones in *Comprehensive Inorganic Chemistry* vol. **2**, J. C. Bailar, Jr. *et al.*, Eds. (Pergamon Press, Oxford, 1973) pp 316-323.

Colorless gas. *Asphyxiant.* Slightly sweetish odor and taste. Supports combustion. Very stable and rather inert chemically at room temperatures. Dissociation begins above 300° when the gas becomes a strong oxidizing agent. mp −90.81°; bp_{760} −88.46°; Trouton constant 21.4: Hoge, *J. Res. Natl. Bur. Stand.* **34**, 281 (1945). Dipole moment 0.166. d^{-89} (liq) 1.226; d(S.T.P.) 1.967; d(gas) 1.53 (air = 1). Critical temp 36.5°; crit press. 71.7 atm. Heat of vaporization (bp): 3.956 kcal/mole. While in the steel cylinder nitrous oxide is compressed to the form of gas over liq and has a pressure of ~800 lbs/sq. in. at room temp. At 20° and 2 atm one liter of the gas dissolves in 1.5 liters of water. Freely sol in sulfuric acid. Sol in alcohol, ether, oils.

Caution: Potential symptoms of overexposure are dyspnea; drowsiness, headache; asphyxia; reproductive effects; direct contact with liquid may cause frostbite. *See NIOSH Pocket Guide to Chemical Hazards* (DHHS/NIOSH 97-140, 1997) p 234.

USE: To oxidize organic compds at temps >300°; to make nitrites from alkali metals at their boiling points; in rocket fuel formulations (with carbon disulfide); in the prepn of whipped cream.

THERAP CAT: Anesthetic (inhalation); analgesic.

6654. Nitrovin. [804-36-4] 2-[3-(5-Nitro-2-furanyl)-1-[2-(5-nitro-2-furanyl)ethenyl]-2-propenylidene]hydrazinecarboximidamide; [[3-(5-nitro-2-furyl)-1-[2-(5-nitro-2-furyl)vinyl]allylidene]-amino]guanidine; *sym*-bis(5-nitro-2-furfurylidene)acetone guanylhydrazone; 1,5-bis(5-nitro-2-furyl)-3-pentadienone guanylhydrazone; 1,5-bis(5-nitro-2-furyl)-3-pentadienone amidinohydrazone; Panazon; Payzone. $C_{14}H_{12}N_6O_6$; mol wt 360.28. C 46.67%, H 3.36%, N 23.33%, O 26.64%. Prepn: Uota *et al.*, JP 52 2673 (1952 to Toyama), *C.A.* **48**, 2115h (1954); Uoda, Tanizaki, JP 64 4479 (1964 to Fukuju Pharm.), *C.A.* **62**, 10412f (1965).

Blackish violet crystals from ethyl alcohol, mp 217° (dec).

Hydrochloride. mp 280° (dec).

THERAP CAT (VET): Growth promoter; antibacterial.

6655. Nitroxoline. [4008-48-4] 5-Nitro-8-quinolinol; 5-nitro-8-hydroxyquinoline; Enterocol; Nibiol; Noxibiol; Uritrol; Urocoli. $C_9H_6N_2O_3$; mol wt 190.16. C 56.84%, H 3.18%, N 14.73%, O 25.24%. Prepn: Kostanecki, *Ber.* **24**, 154 (1891); Petrow, Sturgeon, *J. Chem. Soc.* **1954**, 570; Pratt, Duke, *J. Am. Chem. Soc.* **82**, 1155 (1960). *In vitro* antibacterial and antifungal activity: A. Desvignes, P. Leguen, *Ann. Pharm. Fr.* **21**, 803 (1963); M. Medic-Saric *et al.*, *Chemotherapy* **26**, 263 (1980). Toxicological study: O. Angelova *et al.*, *Adv. Antimicrob. Antineoplast. Chemother.*, *Proc. 7th Int. Congr. Chemother.* **1**, 507 (1972). Clinical pharmacokinetics: A. Mrhar *et al.*, *Int. J. Clin. Pharmacol. Biopharm.* **17**, 476 (1979). HPLC determn in plasma and urine: R. H. A. Sorel *et al.*, *J. Chromatogr.* **222**, 241 (1981). Clinical evaluation in urinary tract infections: M. R. Jacobs *et al.*, *S. Afr. Med. J.* **54**, 959 (1978); B. Cancet, A. Amgar, *Pathol. Biol.* **35**, 879 (1987).

Yellow needles from alcohol or acetic acid, mp 179.5-181.5°. Freely sol in alkali and hot HCl; sparingly sol in alcohol, ether.

Hydrochloride. $C_9H_7ClN_2O_3$. Yellow needles from alcohol, mp 258°.

THERAP CAT: Antibacterial.

6656. Nitroxynil. [1689-89-0] 4-Hydroxy-3-iodo-5-nitrobenzonitrile; Dovenix. $C_7H_3IN_2O_3$; mol wt 290.01. C 28.99%, H 1.04%, I 43.76%, N 9.66%, O 16.55%. Prepn: **NL 6516359** corresp to Collins *et al.*, **US 3331738** (1966, 1967 both to May & Baker).

Yellow crystals from benzene, mp 137-138°. Sparingly sol in water; moderately sol in most organic solvents.

D-N-Methylglucamine salt. [36508-79-9] Nitroxynil meglumine; 4-hydroxy-3-iodo-5-nitrobenzonitrile compd with D-1-deoxy-1-(methylamino)glucitol (1:1). $C_{14}H_{20}IN_3O_8$. Solid, mp 85-90°.

N-Ethylglucamine. [27917-82-4] Nitroxynil eglumine; 4-hydroxy-3-iodo-5-nitrobenzonitrile compd with 1-deoxy-1-(ethylamino)glucitol (1:1); Trodax. $C_{15}H_{22}IN_3O_8$; mol wt 499.25. Readily sol in water with a yellow, odorless and substantially neutral soln. Aq soln is very stable but contamination with calcium and certain other salts can result in pptn of an insol salt of nitroxynil.

THERAP CAT (VET): Anthelmintic (fasciolicide).

6657. Nitryl Chloride. [13444-90-1] Nitroxyl chloride. $ClNO_2$; mol wt 81.46. Cl 43.52%, N 17.19%, O 39.28%. NO_2Cl. Conveniently prepd by the addn of chlorosulfonic acid to nitric acid: Dachlauer, **DE 509405** (1929 to I. G. Farben); Kaplan, Schechter, *Inorg. Synth.* **4**, 52 (1953); Collis *et al.*, *J. Chem. Soc.* **1958**, 438. Corrosive, toxic, colorless gas. Chlorine-like odor. Vapor density (100°): 2.81 g/l. Dec >120°. bp -14.3°. mp -145°. d^0_{liq} 1.37; d^{16}_{liq} 1.33. Even the purest liquid may have a pale yellow color. Solns in polar solvents are always yellow. The gas or liquid may attack organic matter with explosive violence.

Caution: Strong irritant, corrosive.

USE: Nitrating and chlorinating agent in organic syntheses.

6658. Nitryl Fluoride. [10022-50-1] FNO_2; mol wt 65.00. F 29.23%, N 21.55%, O 49.23%. Credit for original prepn by the spontaneous combustion of nitric oxide in an atm of fluorine is given to Moissan, Lebeau, *Compt. Rend.* **140**, 1573, 1621 (1905); more easily prepd by mixing nitrogen dioxide and fluorine: Ruff *et al.*, *Z. Anorg. Allg. Chem.* **208**, 298 (1932); Faloon, Kenna, *J. Am. Chem. Soc.* **73**, 2937 (1951). Reviews of prepn and chemistry: Hoffman, Neville, *Chem. Rev.* **62**, 1-18 (1962); Kwasnik in *Handbook of Preparative Inorganic Chemistry* **vol. 1**, G. Brauer, Ed. (Academic Press, New York, 2nd ed., 1963) pp 186-187; Kemmitt, Sharp, *Adv. Fluorine Chem.* **4**, 195-196 (1965); Woolf, *ibid.* **5**, 1-30 (1965); Schmutzler, *Angew. Chem. Int. Ed.* **7**, 440-455 (1968).

Colorless gas. Pungent odor. Attacks mucous membranes. mp -166.0°. bp -72.4°. d (liq at bp) 1.796. d (solid) 1.924. Trouton const 21.2. May be stored in quartz ampuls if cooled in liq oxygen. Purification can be accomplished by fractional distillation at reduced press. in dry glass or quartz apparatus. Rapidly hydrolyzed in water to form nitric and hydrofluoric acids. Powerful oxidizing agent, with fluorinating powers; slightly weaker than fluorine. Absorbs mercury completely. Spontaneously ignites iodine, selenium, phosphorus (red and white), arsenic, antimony,

boron, silicon, thorium, molybdenum. On mild warming attacks lead, bismuth, chromium, manganese, iron, nickel, tungsten, sulfur, charcoal. Does not react readily with hydrogen in the cold. Converts ethanol to ethyl nitrate; benzene to nitrobenzene.

Caution: See Fluorine.

USE: Oxidizer in rocket propellants; fluorinating agent.

6659. Nivalenol. [23282-20-4] $(3\alpha,4\beta,7\alpha)$-12,13-Epoxy-3,-4,7,15-tetrahydroxytrichothec-9-en-8-one; $3\alpha,4\beta,7\alpha,15$-tetrahydroxyscirp-9-en-8-one. $C_{15}H_{20}O_7$; mol wt 312.32. C 57.68%, H 6.45%, O 35.86%. *Trichothecene mycotoxin* isolated from *Fusarium nivale*: T. Tatsuno *et al.*, *Chem. Pharm. Bull.* **16**, 2519 (1968). Structure: *eidem*, *Tetrahedron Lett.* **1969**, 2823. Toxicology: T. Tatsuno, *Cancer Res.* **28**, 2393 (1968). Implicated as a chemical warfare agent in Southeast Asia with T-2 toxin, *q.v.*: N. Wade, *Science* **214**, 34 (1981); R. T. Rosen, J. D. Rosen, *Biomed. Mass Spectrom.* **9**, 443 (1982).

Crystals, mp 222-223° (dec). $[\alpha]^{24}_D$ +21.54° (c = 1.3 in ethanol). uv max (methanol): 218 nm (ε 6300). Slightly sol in water; sol in polar organic solvents. LD_{50} i.p. in mice: 40 μg/10 g (Tatsuno).

Caution: Potential symptoms of overexposure include fever, nausea, vomiting, diarrhea, leukopenia, bleeding, sepsis; necrotic lesions of skin and mucosa. *See* M. J. Ellenhorn, D. G. Barceloux in *Medical Toxicology: Diagnosis and Treatment of Human Poisoning* (Elsevier, New York, 1988) pp. 1312-1314.

6660. Nizatidine. [76963-41-2] N-[2-[[[2-1-(Dimethylamino)methyl]-4-thiazolyl]methyl]thio]ethyl]-N'-methyl-2-nitro-1,1-ethenediamine; N-[4-(6-methylamino-7-nitro-2-thia-5-aza-6-heptene-1-yl)-2-thiazolylmethyl]-N,N-dimethylamine; LY-139037; ZE-101; ZL-101; Axid; Calmaxid; Cronizat; Distaxid; Gastrax; Nizax; Nizaxid. $C_{12}H_{21}N_5O_2S_2$; mol wt 331.46. C 43.48%, H 6.39%, N 21.13%, O 9.65%, S 19.35%. Histamine H_2-receptor antagonist related to ranitidine, *q.v.* Prepn: R. P. Pioch, **EP 49618**; *idem*, **US 4375547** (1982, 1983 both to Eli Lilly). General pharmacology in animals: K. Bemis *et al.*, *Arzneim.-Forsch.* **39**, 240 (1989). Pharmacokinetics and gastric acid suppression in humans: J. T. Callaghan *et al.*, *Clin. Pharmacol. Ther.* **37**, 162 (1985). Study of effect on hepatic drug metabolism in humans: J. W. Secor *et al.*, *Br. J. Clin. Pharmacol.* **20**, 710 (1985). Disposition and metabolism in humans: M. P. Knadler *et al.*, *Drug Metab. Dispos.* **14**, 175 (1986). Symposium on pharmacology and clinical studies: *Scand. J. Gastroenterol.* **22**, Suppl. 136, 1-88 (1987). Comprehensive description: T. J. Wozniak, *Anal. Profiles Drug Subs.* **19**, 397-427 (1990).

Crystals from ethanol-ethyl acetate, mp 130-132°. uv max (methanol): 240, 325 nm (ε 8400, 19600); (water): 260, 314 nm (ε 11820, 15790). pKa_1 2.1; pKa_2 6.8. Partition coefficient (octanol/water): 0.3 (pH 7.4). Soly (mg/ml): chloroform >100; methanol 50.0-100.0; water 10.0-33.3; isopropanol 3.33-5.0; ethyl acetate 1.0-2.0; benzene, diethyl ether, octanol <0.5. LD_{50} in mice, rats (mg/kg): 265, >300 i.v.; 1685, 1680 orally (Pioch).

THERAP CAT: Antiulcerative.

6661. Nizofenone. [54533-85-6] (2-Chlorophenyl)[2-[2-[(diethylamino)methyl]-1H-imidazol-1-yl]-5-nitrophenyl]methanone; 2'-chloro-2-[2-[(diethylamino)methyl]imidazol-1-yl]-5-nitrobenzophenone; 1-[2-(2-chlorobenzoyl)-4-nitrophenyl]-2-(diethylaminomethyl)imidazole. $C_{21}H_{21}ClN_4O_3$; mol wt 412.87. C

61.09%, H 5.13%, Cl 8.59%, N 13.57%, O 11.63%. Imidazole derivative exhibiting protective activity against cerebral anoxia or ischemia. Prepn: M. Nakanishi *et al.*, **DE 2403416**; *eidem*, **US 3915981** (1974, 1975 both to Yoshitomi). Antianoxic effect in animal models: H. Yasuda *et al.*, *Arch. Int. Pharmacodyn.* **233**, 136 (1978). Mechanism of action: *eidem, ibid.* **242**, 77 (1979). Multicenter clinical studies: I. Saito *et al.*, *Neurol. Res.* **5**, 29 (1983); T. Ohta *et al.*, *J. Neurosurg.* **64**, 420 (1986). Toxicity studies: H. Horizoe *et al.*, *Oyo Yakuri* **30**, 627 (1985), *C.A.* **104**, 61754m (1986); K. Okumura *et al., ibid.* 633, *C.A.* **104**, 61755 (1986).

Pale yellow crystals from isopropyl ether, mp 75-76°.

Fumarate. [54533-86-7] Midafenone; Y-9179; Ekonal. $C_{21}H_{21}ClN_4O_3.C_4H_4O_4$; mol wt 528.94. Pale yellow crystals from isopropyl ether, mp 157-158°. LD_{50} in male, female mice, male, female rats (mg/kg): 495, 504, 1711, 1580 orally; 62, 70, 63, 65 i.v.; 270, 278, 1830, 1629 s.c. (Horizoe).

THERAP CAT: Nootropic.

6662. NMDA. [6384-92-5] *N*-Methyl-D-aspartic acid; *N*-methyl-D-aspartate; *N*-methyl-D-asparaginsaure (German). C_5H_9-NO_4; mol wt 147.13. C 40.82%, H 6.17%, N 9.52%, O 43.50%. Excitotoxic amino acid used to identify a specific subset of excitatory amino acid receptors; consequently the receptors are known as NMDA receptors. *See also* quisqualic acid, kainic acid. Prepn: O. Lutz, *Z. Physiol. Chem.* **70**, 256 (1909); O. Lutz, Br. Jirgensons, *Ber.* **63**, 448 (1930). Isoln from the blood shell, *Scapharca broughtonii*: M. Sato *et al., Biochem. J.* **241**, 309 (1987). Identification as a neuroexcitant: D. R. Curtis, J. C. Watkins, *J. Physiol.* **166**, 1 (1963); of neurotoxic properties: J. W. Olney *et al., Life Sci.* **25**, 537 (1979); R. Zaczek *et al., Neurosci. Lett.* **24**, 181 (1981); M. V. Sofroniew, R. C. A. Pearson, *Brain Res.* **339**, 186 (1985). Receptor binding studies: C. K. Mitchell, D. A. Redburn, *Neurosci. Lett.* **28**, 241 (1982); D. T. Monaghan, C. W. Cotman, *J. Neurosci.* **5**, 2909 (1985); J. M. M. Olson *et al., Neuroscience* **22**, 913 (1987). Review of NMDA and its receptor: J. C. Watkin, R. H. Evans, *Annu. Rev. Pharmacol. Toxicol.* **21**, 165-204 (1981); T. W. Stone, N. R. Burton, *Prog. Neurobiol.* **30**, 333-368 (1988).

6663. NMN. [1094-61-7] 3-(Aminocarbonyl)-1-(5-*O*-phos-phono-β-D-ribofuranosyl)pyridinium inner salt; 3-carbamoyl-1-β-D-ribofuranosylpyridinium hydroxide 5'-(dihydrogen phosphate) inner salt; nicotinamide mononucleotide. $C_{11}H_{15}N_2O_8P$; mol wt 334.22. C 39.53%, H 4.52%, N 8.38%, O 38.30%, P 9.27%. Prepd by incubation of NAD with potato pyrophosphatase in a non-phosphate buffer and in the presence of fluoride: Plaut, Plaut, *Arch. Biochem. Biophys.* **48**, 189 (1954); *Biochem. Prep.* **5**, 55 (1957). Enzymatic synthesis from nicotinamide by human erythrocytes and hemolyzates: Preiss, Handler, *J. Biol. Chem.* **225**, 759 (1957). Prepn by hydrolysis of NAD by a yeast enzyme: Takei, *Agric. Biol. Chem.* **34**, 23 (1970); by cleavage of NAD with crude rattlesnake venom: Apps, *FEBS Lett.* **15**, 277 (1971); R. Jeck, C. Wönckhaus, *Methods Enzymol.* **66**, 62 (1980). NMR studies and conformation of α- and β-nicotinamide nucleotide: N. J. Oppenheimer, N. O. Kaplan, *Biochemistry* **15**, 3981 (1976).

Can be precipitated from slightly acidic aq soln by a large vol of acetone. Freely sol in water, practically insol in acetone. More stable when stored frozen in soln, than when in dry form.

6664. Nobelium. [10028-14-5] No; at. no. 102; valence 2, 3. Man-made radioactive element. No stable nuclides; known isotopes (mass numbers): 250-259. Longest-lived known isotope: 259 ($T_{1/2}$ 1.00 hours, α-emitter, rel. at. mass 259.1011). Discovery of element 102 first claimed by P. R. Fields *et al., Phys. Rev.* **107**, 1460 (1957); later experiments failed to confirm these results. Prepn of isotope originally assigned mass 254, later identified as ^{252}No ($T_{1/2}$ 2.3 sec, α-emitter) by $^{244}Cm(^{12}C,4n)$ reaction: A. Ghiorso *et al., Phys. Rev. Lett.* **1**, 18 (1958). Prepn of ^{259}No by bombardment of ^{248}Cm with ^{18}O ions: Silva *et al., Nucl. Phys. A* **216**, 97 (1973), *C.A.* **80**, 43040g (1974). *Reviews:* G. T. Seaborg, *J. Chem. Educ.* **36**, 38-44 (1959); A. Ghiorso, T. Sikkeland, *Phys. Today* **20** (9), 25-32 (1967); G. N. Flerov, *U.S. Atomic Energy Commission* **JINR-D7-3444** (1967) 36 pp, *C.A.* **68**, 34658q (1968); C. Keller, *The Chemistry of the Transuranium Elements* (Verlag Chemie, Weinheim, English Ed., 1971) pp 601-607; Silva, "Trans-Curium Elements" in *MTP Int. Rev. Sci.: Inorg. Chem., Ser. One* **vol. 8**, A. G. Maddock, Ed. (University Park Press, Baltimore, 1972) pp 71-105; *Comprehensive Inorganic Chemistry* **vol. 5**, J. C. Bailar, Jr., *et al.*, Eds. (Pergamon Press, Oxford, 1973) *passim;* Ghiorso, *Handb. Exp. Pharmakol.* **36**, 691-715 (1973); Taylor, *ibid.* 717-738 (1973); R. J. Silva in *The Chemistry of the Actinide Elements* **vol. 2**, J. J. Katz *et al.*, Eds. (Chapman and Hall, New York, 1986) pp 1096-1099; *The Elements Beyond Uranium*, G. T. Seaborg, W. D. Loveland, Eds. (John Wiley & Sons, Inc., New York, 1990) pp 46-49.

Caution: Radiation hazard; handling requires special equipment and shielding facilities (Katz *et al., loc. cit.* **vol. 2**, p. 1128).

6665. Nocardamin. [26605-16-3] 1,12,23-Trihydroxy-1,6,-12,17,23,28-hexaazacyclotritriacontane-2,5,13,16,24,27-hexone. $C_{27}H_{48}N_6O_9$; mol wt 600.70. C 53.99%, H 8.05%, N 13.99%, O 23.97%. Antibiotic substance produced by a *Nocardia* isolated from old bee-honeycombs: Stoll *et al., Schweiz. Z. Pathol. Bakteriol.* **14**, 225 (1951); *Helv. Chim. Acta* **34**, 862 (1951). Structure: Keller-Schierlein, Prelog, *ibid.* **44**, 1981 (1961).

Needles from hot methanol, mp 192-195°. Optically inactive. Has no basic properties. Soluble in hot water, methanol. An 0.5% aq soln at room temp has a pH of 4.55.

Triacetate. $C_{33}H_{54}N_6O_{12}$. Crystals, mp 115-117°.

6666. Nocardicin(s). Monocyclic β-lactam antibiotics with antimicrobial activity which inhibit bacterial cell wall biosynthesis. Nocardicins A, B, C, D, E, F, G have been identified. All are produced by *Nocardia uniformis* subsp. *tsuyamenensis*, A being the most important component. Prodn: H. Aoki *et al.*, **DE 2242699** (1973 to Fujisawa), *C.A.* **78**, 134496k (1973); **US 3923977** (1975 to Fujisawa). Isoln and characterization of A: H. Aoki *et al., J. Antibiot.* **29**, 492 (1976); of B: M. Kurita *et al., ibid.* 1243. Nocardicin A has also been produced by *Actinosynnema mirum*: K. Watanabe *et al., ibid.* **36**, 321 (1983). Structural determination of A and B: M. Hashimoto *et al., J. Am. Chem. Soc.* **98**, 3023 (1976), *J. Antibiot.* **29**, 890 (1976). Isoln, characterization, and structures of C, D, E, F, G: J. Hosoda *et al., Agric. Biol. Chem.* **41**, 2013 (1977). Total synthesis of A: G. A. Koppel *et al., J. Am. Chem. Soc.* **100**, 3933 (1978); W. V. Curran *et al., J. Antibiot.* **35**, 329 (1981); of A and D: T. Kamiya *et al., Tetrahedron* **1979**, 323; of A and B: H. P. Isenring, W. Hofheinz, *Tetrahedron* **1983**, 2591. Biosynthetic studies of A: J. Hosada *et al., Agric. Biol. Chem.* **41**, 2007 (1977); C. A. Townsend *et al., J. Am. Chem. Soc.* **105**, 919 (1983). Series of articles on antimicrobial activity of A: *J. Antibiot.* **30**, 917-944 (1977).

Nocardicin A

Nocardicin A. [39391-39-4] (α*R*,3*S*)-3-[[(2*Z*)-[4-[(3*R*)-3-Amino-3-carboxypropoxy]phenyl](hydroxyimino)acetyl]amino]-α-(4-hydroxyphenyl)-2-oxo-1-azetidineacetic acid. $C_{23}H_{24}N_4O_9$; mol wt 500.46. Colorless needles from acidic water, mp 214-216° (dec). $[\alpha]_D^{25}$ −135° (for the sodium salt). uv max (1/15*M* phosphate buffer): 272 nm ($E_{1cm}^{1\%}$ 310); (0.1*N* NaOH): 244, 283 nm ($E_{1cm}^{1\%}$ 460, 270). Sol in alkaline solns, slightly sol in methanol. Insol in chloroform, ethyl acetate, ethyl ether. LD_{50} in male mice, rats (mg/kg): >8000 orally; >2000 i.v.; 2500, 2600 i.p. (Aoki).

Nocardicin B. [60134-71-6] The *E*-isomer of nocardicin A. Colorless needles, mp 262-264° (dec). $[\alpha]_D^{25}$ −162° (for the sodium salt). uv max (ethanol/water): 224, 270 nm (ε 24600, 9700); (ethanol/0.1*N* NaOH): 245, 280 nm (ε 26000, 11100).

6667. Nociceptin. [170713-75-4] Orphanin FQ (swine); orphanin FQ; OFQ. $C_{79}H_{129}N_{27}O_{22}$; mol wt 1809.04. C 52.45%, H 7.19%, N 20.91%, O 19.46%. Seventeen amino acid neuropeptide identified as the endogenous ligand of the orphan opioid receptor, ORL-1. Shows a wide variety of pharmacological effects. Structurally related to the opioids, but does not bind to opiate receptors. Isoln from rat brain: J.-C. Meunier *et al., Nature* **377**, 532 (1995); from porcine hypothalmus: R. K. Reinscheid *et al., Science* **270**, 792 (1995). Distribution and localization of binding with opioid peptides: S. Schulz *et al., NeuroReport* **7**, 3021 (1996). Binding affinity: I. D. Adapa, L. Toll, *Neuropeptides* **31**, 403 (1997). *Review:* J.-C. Meunier, *Eur. J. Pharmacol.* **340**, 1-15 (1997). Review of pharmacology and structure-activity: G. Henderson, A. T. McKnight, *Trends Pharmacol. Sci.* **18**, 293-300 (1997).

Phe—Gly—Gly—Phe—Thr—Gly—Ala—Arg—Lys—Ser—Ala—Arg—Lys—Leu—Ala—Asn—Gln

6668. Nodakenin. [495-31-8] 2-[1-(β-D-Glucopyranosyloxy)-1-methylethyl]-2,3-dihydro-7*H*-furo[3,2-*g*][1]benzopyran-7-one; nodakenetin glucoside. $C_{20}H_{24}O_9$; mol wt 408.40. C 58.82%, H 5.92%, O 35.26%. From root of *Peucedanum decursivum* Maxim., *Umbelliferae:* Arima, *Bull. Chem. Soc. Jpn.* **4**, 16, 113 (1929); Späth, Kainrath, *Ber.* **69**, 2062 (1936). Structure: Späth, Tyray, *ibid.* **72**, 2089 (1939).

Thin leaflets from alc, dec 218-219°. From dil alc or water it crystallizes with one mol H_2O in form of yellow prisms, melting at 216°. $[\alpha]_D^{30}$ +56.6°. Sol in hot water or alcohol.

Tetraacetate. $C_{28}H_{32}O_{13}$. Crystals from methanol, mp 195-196°.

6669. Nodulisporic acid. [163120-03-4] (2*E*,4*E*)-5-[(3*S*,-4*S*,4a*R*,6a*S*,12a*R*,13*S*,15*S*,16b*S*,16c*S*)-2,3,4,4a,5,6,6a,7,10,12,12a,-13,14,15,16b,16c-Hexadecahydro-3,13-dihydroxy-4,10,10,12,12,-16b,16c-heptamethyl-15-(1-methylethenyl)-14-oxo-1*H*-benz[6,7]-indeno[1,2-*b*]pyrano[3′,4′:4,5]cyclopenta[1,2-*f*]pyrrolo[3,2,1-*hi*]indol-4-yl]-2-methyl-2,4-pentadienoic acid; nodulisporic acid A; NsA A. $C_{43}H_{53}NO_6$; mol wt 679.88. C 75.96%, H 7.86%, N 2.06%, O 14.12%. Indole diterpene alkaloid which activates glutamate-gated chloride channels. Isolated from the fungus *Nodulisporium* sp.; it occurs naturally as the (+)-form. Isoln: A. W. Dombrowski *et al.,* US 5399582 (1995 to Merck & Co.); structure determination and insecticidal activity: J. G. Ondeyka *et al., J. Am. Chem. Soc.* **119**, 8809 (1997). Mode of action: M. M. Smith *et al., Biochemistry* **39**, 5543 (2000). Synthetic studies: A. B. Smith, III *et al., Org. Lett.* **3**, 3967, 3971 (2001). Biosynthesis: K. M. Byrne *et al., J. Am. Chem. Soc.* **124**, 7055 (2002). Systemic efficacy against fleas on dogs: W. L. Shoop *et al., J. Parasitol.* **87**, 419 (2001). Review of chemical and biological properties: P. T. Meinke *et al., Curr. Top. Med. Chem.* **2**, 655-674 (2002).

Yellow powder, mp 250-255°. $[\alpha]_D^{22}$ +13° (c = 0.4 in $CHCl_3$). uv max (methanol): 241, 265, 385 nm (ε 43900, 49800, 7360).

USE: Insecticide.

6670. Noformicin. [155-38-4] 5-Amino-*N*-(3-amino-3-iminopropyl)-3,4-dihydro-2*H*-pyrrole-2-carboxamide; *N*-(2-amidinoethyl)-5-imino-2-pyrrolidinecarboxamide; 2-[*N*-(2-amidinoethyl)carbamoyl]-5-iminopyrrolidine; β-(5-imino-2-pyrrolidinecarboxamido)propamidine; noformycin. $C_8H_{15}N_5O$; mol wt 197.24. C 48.72%, H 7.67%, N 35.51%, O 8.11%. Antiviral agent produced by *Nocardia formica,* culture no. N.R.R.L. 2470: Peck *et al.,* US 2804463 (1957 to Merck & Co.); Gray, *Phytopathology* **45**, 281 (1955). Activity studies: Furusawa *et al., Proc. Soc. Exp. Biol. Med.* **116**, 938 (1964); *eidem, Med. Pharmacol. Exp.* **12**, 259 (1965). Synthesis of (+)- and (±)-forms: Diana, *J. Med. Chem.* **16**, 857 (1973).

(+)-Form dihydrochloride. $C_8H_{17}Cl_2N_5O$. The biologically active form. Crystals from methanol, dec 263-264°. $[\alpha]_D^{25}$ +8.8° (methanol). Sol in water. Somewhat sol in organic solvents. pKa 9.4.

(±)-Form dihydrochloride. mp 252-254°.

6671. Nogalamycin. [1404-15-5] [2*R*-(2α,3β,4α,5β,6α,-11β,13α,14α)]-11-[(6-Deoxy-3-*C*-methyl-2,3,4-tri-*O*-methyl-α-L-mannopyranosyl)oxy]-4-(dimethylamino)-3,4,5,6,9,11,12,13,14,-16-decahydro-3,5,8,10,13-pentahydroxy-6,13-dimethyl-9,16-dioxo-2,6-epoxy-2*H*-naphthaceno[1,2-*b*]oxocin-14-carboxylic acid methyl ester; U-15167; NSC-70845. $C_{39}H_{49}NO_{16}$; mol wt 787.80. C 59.46%, H 6.27%, N 1.78%, O 32.49%. Antitumor antibiotic isolated from *Streptomyces nogalater* var. *nogalater:* B. K. Bhuyan, A. Dietz, *Antimicrob. Agents Chemother.* **1965**, 836; B. K. Bhuyan *et al.,* US 3183157 (1965 to Upjohn). Characterization: P. F. Wiley *et al., Tetrahedron Lett.* **1968**, 663. Structure: *eidem, J. Am. Chem. Soc.* **99**, 542 (1977). Stereochemistry: *eidem, J. Org. Chem.* **44**, 4030 (1979). Biosynthesis: *eidem, ibid.* **43**, 3457 (1978). Synthesis of *L-nogalose,* sugar component: L. Valente *et al., Tetrahedron Lett.* **1979**, 1153; J. Yoshimura *et al., Chem. Lett.* **1979**, 687. Partial stereospecific synthesis: R. P. Joyce *et al., Tetrahedron Lett.* **27**, 4885 (1986). Molecular structure, absolute stereochemistry and interactions with DNA: S. K. Arora, *J. Am. Chem. Soc.* **105**, 1328 (1983). Toxicity data: Z. Hadidian, *PB Report* 173334 (1966). Review of pharmacology: B. K. Bhuyan, C. G. Smith, *Handb. Exp. Pharmacol.* **38** (pt. 2), 623-632 (1975).

Orange-red solid from methanol, mp 195-196° (dec). $[\alpha]_D^{25}$ +425° (c = 0.11 in CHCl$_3$). pKa′ 7.45 (60% ethanol). uv max (ethanol): 236, 258, 292 nm (ε 52360, 24755, 9890). Sol in methylene chloride, acetone, chloroform, ethyl acetate. Insol in water, methanol, ethanol. LD$_{50}$ in mice (mg/kg): 11.75 i.v., 4.79 i.p. (Hadidian).

6672. Nolatrexed. [147149-76-6] 2-Amino-6-methyl-5-(4-pyridinylthio)-4(1*H*)-quinazolinone; 2-amino-3,4-dihydro-6-methyl-4-oxo-5-(4-pyridylthio)quinazoline; 2-amino-6-methyl-5-(pyridin-4-ylsulfanyl)-3*H*-quinazolin-4-one. C$_{14}$H$_{12}$N$_4$OS; mol wt 284.34. C 59.14%, H 4.25%, N 19.70%, O 5.63%, S 11.28%. Antifolate thymidylate synthase inhibitor. Prepn: S. E. Webber *et al.*, **WO 9320055**; *eidem*, **US 5707992** (1993, 1998 both to Agouron); S. E. Webber *et al., J. Med. Chem.* **36**, 733 (1993). Solid-state properties: A. K. Dash, P. Tyle, *J. Pharm. Sci.* **85**, 1123 (1996). Pharmacology: S. Webber *et al., Cancer Chemother. Pharmacol.* **37**, 509 (1996). Clinical pharmacokinetics: I. Rafi *et al., Clin. Cancer Res.* **1**, 1275 (1995). Clinical evaluation in hepatocellular carcinoma: K. Stuart *et al., Cancer* **86**, 410 (1999).

Tan solid, mp 301-302°.
Dihydrochloride. [152946-68-4] AG-337; Thymitaq. C$_{14}$H$_{12}$N$_4$OS.2HCl; mol wt 357.26. Hygroscopic; occurs as a dihydrate. Sol in water. pKa 4.1; 5.9; 9.8. Partition coefficient (octanol/water) at 25°: 1.9. Upon heating, dehydrates and forms metastable, plate-like crystals, mp 213°. Recrystallizes at 261° into stable, needle-like crystals, mp 312° (dec).
THERAP CAT: Antineoplastic.

6673. Nomifensine. [24526-64-5] 1,2,3,4-Tetrahydro-2-methyl-4-phenyl-8-isoquinolinamine; 8-amino-1,2,3,4-tetrahydro-2-methyl-4-phenylisoquinoline. C$_{16}$H$_{18}$N$_2$; mol wt 238.33. C 80.63%, H 7.61%, N 11.75%. Novel antidepressant distinguished from existing tricyclic and tetracyclic antidepressants by its bicyclic structure. Prepn: **GB 1164192** corresp to G. Ehrhart *et al.*, **US 3577424** (1969, 1971, both to Farbwerke Hoechst); I. Hoffmann *et al., Arzneim.-Forsch.* **21**, 1045 (1971). Pharmacology: I. Hoffmann, *ibid.* **23**, 45 (1973); P. Hunt *et al., J. Pharm. Pharmacol.* **26**, 370 (1974); B. Costall *et al., Psychopharmacologia* **41**, 153 (1975). Pharmacokinetics: L. Vereczkey *et al., ibid.* **45**, 225 (1975). Study on abuse potential in humans: C. Spyraki, H. C. Fibiger, *Science* **212**, 1167 (1981). *Review: Br. J. Clin. Pharmacol.* **4**, Suppl. 2 (1977) pp 1S-248S; *Int. Pharmacopsychiatry* **17**, Suppl. 1 (1982) pp 1-148.

mp 179-181°.
Maleate. [32795-47-4] HOE-984; Alival; Hostalival; Merital; Neurolene; Psicronizer. C$_{16}$H$_{18}$N$_2$.C$_4$H$_4$O$_4$; mol wt 354.40. Crystals from ethanol, mp 199-201°. LD$_{50}$ in mice, rats (mg/kg): 400, 430 orally; 90, 72 i.v.; in mice (mg/kg): 410 s.c. (Hoffman, 1973).
THERAP CAT: Antidepressant.

6674. Nomilin. [1063-77-0] 1-(Acetyloxy)-1,2-dihydroobacunoic acid ε-lactone; 1-(3-furyl)decahydro-11-hydroxy-4b,7,-7-11a,13a-pentamethyloxireno(4,4a)-2-benzopyrano[6,5-g](2)benzoxepin-3,5,9(3a*H*,4b*H*,6*H*)-trione acetate. C$_{28}$H$_{34}$O$_9$; mol wt 514.56. C 65.36%, H 6.66%, O 27.98%. Bitter principle from citrus juice, seeds. Isoln: O. H. Emerson, *J. Am. Chem. Soc.* **70**, 545 (1948). Structure elucidation: D. L. Dreyer, *Tetrahedron* **21**, 75 (1965); *idem, ibid.* **24**, 3273 (1968). Distribution in citrus seeds: S. Hasegawa *et al., J. Agric. Food Chem.* **28**, 922 (1980); R. L. Rouseff, S. Nagy, *Phytochemistry* **21**, 85 (1982). Identification in grapefruit juice: R. L. Rouseff, *J. Agric. Food Chem.* **30**, 504 (1982). Reduction of nomilin bitterness by *Arthrobacter globiformis* cells: S. Hasegawa, V. A. Pelton, *ibid.* **31**, 178 (1983); by *Cornebacterium fascians*: S. Hasegawa *et al., ibid.* **32**, 457 (1984); *eidem, J. Food Sci.* **50**, 330 (1985). Antifeedant effect against *Spodoptera frugiperda*: M. A. Altieri *et al., Prot. Ecol.* **6**, 91 (1984). Biosynthetic pathways: S. Hasegawa *et al., Phytochemistry* **23**, 1601 (1984).

Needles from methanol, mp 278-279°. Slightly sol in 2-propanol, ethyl acetate. $[\alpha]_D^{23}$ −95.7°.

6675. Nonactin. [6833-84-7] (1*R*,2*R*,5*R*,7*R*,10*S*,11*S*,14*S*,-16*S*,19*R*,20*R*,23*R*,25*R*,28*S*,29*S*,32*S*,34*S*)-2,5,11,14,20,23,29,32-Octamethyl-4,13,22,31,37,38,39,40-octaoxapentacyclo-[32.2.1.1^{7,10}.1^{16,19}.1^{25,28}]tetracontane-3,12,21,30-tetrone. C$_{40}$H$_{64}$O$_{12}$; mol wt 736.93. C 65.19%, H 8.75%, O 26.05%. Macrotetrolide antibiotic. Produced by several *Streptomyces* spp.: Corbaz *et al., Helv. Chim. Acta* **38**, 1445 (1955); Wallhäusser *et al., Arzneim.-Forsch.* **14**, 356 (1964). Structure: Dominguez *et al., Helv. Chim. Acta* **45**, 129 (1962). Crystal structure: Dobler, *ibid.* **55**, 1371 (1972). Stereoselective syntheses of *nonactic acid*, building block of nonactin: Gerlach, Wetter, *ibid.* **57**, 2306 (1974); R. E. Ireland, J.-P. Vevert, *J. Org. Chem.* **45**, 4260 (1980). Total synthesis of (+)- and (−)-nonactic acids: *eidem, Can. J. Chem.* **59**, 572 (1981). Synthesis of nonactin: Gombos *et al., Monatsh. Chem.* **106**, 1043 (1975); *eidem, Tetrahedron Lett.* **1975**, 3391; Gerlach *et al., Helv. Chim. Acta* **58**, 2036 (1975); U. Schmidt *et al., Ber.* **109**, 2628 (1976). Three homologs, *monactin*, C$_{41}$H$_{66}$O$_{12}$, *dinactin*, C$_{42}$H$_{68}$O$_{12}$, and *trinactin*, C$_{43}$H$_{70}$O$_{12}$ are known: Beck *et al., Helv. Chim. Acta* **45**, 620 (1962); Gerlach, Prelog, *Ann.* **669**, 121 (1963). Activity of nonactin and its homologues: Meyers *et al., J. Antibiot.* **18A**, 128 (1965). Biosynthesis study: J. E. Cox, N. D. Priestley, *J. Am. Chem. Soc.* **127**, 7976 (2005).

Needles from methanol, mp 147-148°. uv max (ethanol): slight peak at 264 nm (log ε 1.5). Remarkably inert to chemical compds.

6676. 2-Nonenal. [18829-56-6] (*E*)-2-Nonenal; *trans*-2-nonenaldehyde. $C_9H_{16}O$; mol wt 140.22. C 77.09%, H 11.50%, O 11.41%. Widely distributed in nature; found in beer, coffee, cucumbers, watermelon, palm oil, potatoes, carrots etc. Prepn: R. Delaby, S. Guillot-Allègre, *Bull. Soc. Chim. Fr.* **53**, 301 (1933); J. Braun *et al., Ber.* **67**, 269 (1934); J. Ficini, H. Normant, *Bull. Soc. Chim. Fr.* **1964**, 1294; J. Ficini *et al., Tetrahedron Lett.* **1977**, 3589; M. Wado *et al., Chem. Lett.* **1977**, 345. Insecticidal activity: P. M. Guerin, M. F. Ryan, *Experientia* **36**, 1387 (1980). Cockroach repellant activity: T. H. Maugh, *Science* **218**, 278 (1982).

Liquid, bp$_{16}$ 100-102°. n_D^{18} 1.4403.

USE: As flavoring agent.

6677. Nonoxynol. [26027-38-3] α-(4-Nonylphenyl)-ω-hydroxypoly(oxy-1,2-ethanediyl); polyethyleneglycols mono(nonylphenyl) ether; macrogol nonylphenyl ether; nonoxinol; polyoxyethylene(*n*)nonylphenyl ether; nonylphenyl polyethyleneglycol ether; nonylphenoxypolyethoxyethanol. Nonionic surfactant mixtures prepd by reacting nonylphenol with ethylene oxide. Prepn of polyoxyethylated alkyl phenols: A. Steindorff *et al.*, US 2213477 (1940 to GAF). Average number of ethylene oxide units (*n*) per molecule is indicated by number following nonoxynol (e.g. nonoxynol-15 for n = 15). Trademarks for nonoxynol series include *Conco NI*, *Dowfax 9N*, *Igepal CO*, *Makon*, *Neutronyx 600's*, *Nonipol NO*, *Polytergent B*, *Renex 600's*, *Solar NP*, *Sterox*, *Surfonic N*, *T-DET-N*, *Tergitol NP*, *Triton N*. Individual members of series indicated by numerical suffixes. Toxicology study: H. F. Smyth Jr., J. C. Calandra, *Toxicol. Appl. Pharmacol.* **14**, 315 (1969). Inactivation of HIV *in vitro* by nonoxynol-9: M. Malkovsky *et al., Lancet* **1**, 645 (1988). Clinical evaluation of nonoxynol-9 in sexually transmitted diseases: W. C. Louv *et al., J. Infect. Dis.* **158**, 518 (1988). Review: C. R. Enyeart, "Polyoxyethylene Alkylphenols" in *Nonionic Surfactants*, M. J. Schick, Ed. (Dekker, New York, 1967) pp 44-85.

Nonoxynol-9

Highly stable compounds. Lower adducts (n <15) are yellow to almost colorless liquids; higher adducts (n >20) are pale yellow to off-white pastes or waxes. Lower adducts (n <6) sol in oil; higher ones sol in water. Review of physical properties: Enyeart, *loc. cit.*

Nonoxynol-9. C-Film; Conco NI-90; Dowfax 9N9; Encare; Gynol II; Igepal CO-630; Intercept; Neutronyx 611; Semicid; Staycept; Tergitol TP-9. Av. mol wt 617. A component of *Conceptrol*, *Delfen*, *Gentersal*, *Ortho-creme*. Almost colorless liquid. For Igepal CO-630: d_4^{25} 1.06; solidif pt 26 ±2°F; pour point 37 ±2°F; flash point 535-555°F; cloud point (1% aq soln) 126-133°F; viscosity (25°): 175-250 cP. Sol in water, ethanol, ethylene glycol, ethylene dichloride, xylene, corn oil. Insoluble in Stoddard solvent, deodorized kerosene, low viscosity white mineral oil.

Nonoxynol-11. Duragel; Duracreme.

USE: Nonionic surfactants used as detergents, emulsifiers, wetting agents, dispersants, stabilizers, intermediates in synthesis of anionic surfactants, defoaming agents. Nonoxynols-9, 11 as spermaticide. Nonoxynols-4, 15, 30 as pharmaceutical aids (surfactants).

6678. n-Nonyl Acetate. [143-13-5] Acetic acid *n*-nonyl ester; *n*-nonyl ethanoate; nonanol acetate; Acetate C-9. $C_{11}H_{22}O_2$; mol wt 186.29. C 70.92%, H 11.90%, O 17.18%. CH_3-$COO(CH_2)_8CH_3$.

Liquid. Pungent odor, suggestive of mushrooms, resembles odor of gardenias when dil. d_4^{15} 0.8785 (commercial grade, d_{25}^{25} 0.864-0.868). bp 208-212°. n_D^{20} 1.4328 (commercial grade, n_D^{20} 1.422-1.426). Insoluble in water. Freely sol in abs alcohol and ether; 33 ml dissolve in 100 ml of 80% ethanol.

Note: The nonyl acetate of commerce may be the above compound or any of its isomers such as diisobutylcarbinyl acetate.

USE: In perfumery.

6679. n-Nonyl Alcohol. [143-08-8] 1-Nonanol; nonalol. $C_9H_{20}O$; mol wt 144.25. C 74.94%, H 13.97%, O 11.09%. CH_3(CH_2)$_7CH_2$OH. Occurs in oil of orange. Prepn by reduction of ethyl Δ^1-nonylenate: Harding, Weizmann, *J. Chem. Soc.* **97**, 304 (1910); by reduction of pelargonic aldehyde: Tomecko, Adams, *J. Am. Chem. Soc.* **49**, 529 (1927); by oxo process: Russum, Hengstebeck, US 2638487 (1953 to Standard Oil of Indiana); by reductive cleavage of oleic acid ozonide: Sousa, Bluhm, *J. Org. Chem.* **25**, 108 (1960); from diborane and propylene trimer: Marshall, Smith, GB 879242 (1961 to I.C.I.).

Colorless to yellowish liquid; odor of citronella oil. bp$_{760}$ 215°; bp$_{15}$ 107.5°; bp$_{7.5}$ 95.6°. d_4^{20} 0.8279. n_D^{20} 1.4338. Practically insol in water. Miscible with alcohol, ether.

USE: In manufacture of artificial lemon oil.

6680. 2-Nonyldioxolane. [4353-06-4] 2-Nonyl-1,3-dioxolane; SEPA. $C_{12}H_{24}O_2$; mol wt 200.32. C 71.95%, H 12.08%, O 15.97%. Dermal penetration enhancer. Prepn: S. S. Nigam, B. C. L. Weedon, *J. Chem. Soc.* **1956**, 4049; B. B. Michniak *et al., Drug Delivery* **2**, 117 (1995). Use as transdermal enhancer: C. M. Samour, S. Daskalakis, *EP 268460; eidem,* US 4861764 (1988, 1989 both to MacroChem). GC-MS determn in serum: W. Z. Zhong *et al., J. Chromatogr. B* **705**, 39 (1998). Pharmacology: R. W. Pelham, C. M. Samour, *Proc. Int. Symp. Controlled Release Bioact. Mater.* **22**, 694 (1995). Clinical evaluation for topical delivery of prostaglandin E_1: K. T. McVary *et al., J. Urol.* **162**, 726 (1999).

Clear oil, bp$_{0.55\text{ torr}}$ 90-93°. bp$_{0.01\text{mm}}$ 68-70°. n_D^{20} 1.4390.

USE: Pharmaceutic aid (excipient).

6681. Nonyl Phenol. [25154-52-3] Approx mol wt 215. A technical grade mixture of monoalkyl phenols, predominantly *para* substituted. The side chains are isomeric branched-alkyl radicals. Manuf of *p*-nonylphenol: *Faith, Keyes & Clark's Industrial Chemicals*, F. A. Lowenheim, M. K. Moran, Eds. (Wiley-Interscience, New York, 4th ed., 1975) pp 575-578.

Pale yellow liquid. Slight characteristic phenolic odor. Comparatively high viscosity. Hydroxyl no. 253. d_4^{20} 0.950. bp 293-297°. n_D^{20} 1.513. Flash pt (open cup) 300°F. Practically insol in water or dil aq NaOH. Sol in benzene, chlorinated solvents, aniline, heptane, aliphatic alcohols, ethylene glycol.

USE: In the prepn of lubricating oil additives, resins, plasticizers, surface active agents.

6682. (p-Nonylphenoxy)acetic Acid. [3115-49-9] $C_{17}H_{26}$-O_3; mol wt 278.39. C 73.34%, H 9.41%, O 17.24%. Prepd by the reaction of sodium chloroacetate with nonyl phenol in alkaline medium: Preston, GB 812938 and Preston, Taylor, GB 831883 (1959, 1960, to I.C.I.).

Liquid. d_4^{20} 1.010-1.025. Viscosity (30°): 5200 cP. Flow pt 5°. Practically insol in water. Miscible with benzene, mineral oil, kerosene, petr ether.

USE: Corrosion inhibitor and antifoaming agent in gasoline and cutting oils.

6683. Nopol. [35836-73-8]; [128-50-7] ((±)-form). (1R,5S)-6,6-Dimethylbicyclo[3.1.1]hept-2-ene-2-ethanol. $C_{11}H_{18}$-O; mol wt 166.26. C 79.46%, H 10.91%, O 9.62%. Bicyclic primary alcohol found in carrot root oil; synthesized from β-pinene, q.v. Prepn: J. P. Bain, *J. Am. Chem. Soc.* **68**, 638 (1946). Thermal isomerization: *idem et al., ibid.* **74**, 4292 (1952). Isoln from carrot root oil: D. M. Alabran *et al., J. Agric. Food Chem.* **23**, 229 (1975). Applications as a polymer substrate: J. V. Crivello, S. S. Liu, *J. Polym. Sci. A* **37**, 1199 (1999). Improved syntheses: U. R. Pillai, E. Sahle-Demessie, *Chem. Commun.* **2004**, 826; A. L. Villa de P *et al., Catal. Today* **107-108**, 942 (2005).

bp$_{10}$ 110.5°. n_D^{25} 1.4920. d$_4^{25}$ 0.9647. [α]$_D^{25}$ −36.5°.

USE: In the synthesis of pesticides, soaps, detergents and other household products.

6684. Noprylsulfamide. [576-97-6] 1-[[4-(Aminosulfonyl)phenyl]amino]-3-phenyl-1,3-propanedisulfonic acid disodium salt; 1-phenyl-3-p-sulfamoylanilino-1,3-propanedisulfonic acid disodium salt; N^4-(disodium 1,3-disulfo-3-phenylpropyl)sulfanilamide; disodium 1-phenyl-3-p-sulfamoylanilino-1,3-propanedisulfonate; disodium p-(γ-phenylpropylamino)benzenesulfonamide-α,γ-disulfonate; RP-40; Solucin; Soluseptasine; Soluseptazine; Solusetazine; Sulphasolucin; Sulphasolutin. $C_{15}H_{16}N_2Na_2O_8S_3$; mol wt 494.47. C 36.44%, H 3.26%, N 5.67%, Na 9.30%, O 25.89%, S 19.45%. Prepd by the action of sodium bisulfite on N^4-cinnamylidenesulfanilamide (prepd from cinnamic aldehyde and sulfanilamide): Despois, **US 2262544** (1941 to Rhône-Poulenc).

Crystals. One gram dissolves in 5 ml water. Neutral reaction. Breaks down in the body with the liberation of free sulfanilamide.

THERAP CAT: Antibacterial.

6685. Noracymethadol. [1477-39-0] α-Ethyl-β-[2-(methylamino)propyl]-β-phenylbenzeneethanol acetate; α-dl-6-(methylamino)-4,4-diphenyl-3-heptanol acetate; α-dl-3-acetoxy-4,4-diphenyl-6-methylaminoheptane; α-dl-3-acetoxy-6-methylamino-4,4-diphenylheptane; α-dl-4,4-diphenyl-6-methylamino-3-heptanol acetate. $C_{22}H_{29}NO_2$; mol wt 339.47. C 77.84%, H 8.61%, N 4.13%, O 9.43%. Metabolite of methadyl acetate, q.v. Prepn: A. Pohland, **US 3021360** (1962 to Lilly). Metabolism: G. L. Henderson *et al., Drug Metab. Dispos.* **5**, 321 (1977); M. Man *et al., ibid.* **8**, 55 (1980). HPLC determn: C.-H. Kiang *et al., J. Chromatogr.* **222**, 81 (1981).

Hydrochloride. [5633-25-0] NIH-7667. $C_{22}H_{29}NO_2$·HCl; mol wt 375.93. Crystals from acetone + ether, mp ∼216-217°.

Note: This is a controlled substance (opiate): **21 CFR,** 1308.11.

6686. Norbolethone. [1235-15-0] (17α)-(±)-13-Ethyl-17-hydroxy-18,19-dinorpregn-4-en-3-one; dl-13β,17α-diethyl-17β-hydroxygon-4-en-3-one; Wy-3475. $C_{21}H_{32}O_2$; mol wt 316.48. C 79.70%, H 10.19%, O 10.11%. 19-nor anabolic steroid. Prepn

of dl-, d-, and l-forms: Smith *et al., J. Chem. Soc.* **1964**, 4472. Biological activities of dl-, d-, and l-forms: Edgren *et al., Steroids* **2**, 731 (1963). Toxicity study: E. I Goldenthal, *Toxicol. Appl. Pharmacol.* **18**, 185 (1971). GC/MS determn in athletes' urine: D. H. Catlin *et al., Rapid Commun. Mass Spectrom.* **16**, 1273 (2002).

Crystals from alcohol, mp 144-145°. uv max: 241 nm (ε 16500). LD$_{50}$ orally in mice: >5010 mg/kg (Goldenthal).

d-Form. [28439-19-2] Crystals from acetone + hexane, mp 175-176°. [α]$_D$ +20.7° (in chloroform).

l-Form. Crystals from acetone + hexane, mp 172-175.5°. [α]$_D$ −18.1° (in chloroform).

Note: This is a controlled substance (anabolic steroid): **21 CFR,** 1308.13, as defined in 1300.01.

6687. Norbormide. [991-42-4] 3a,4,7,7a-Tetrahydro-5-(hydroxyphenyl-2-pyridinylmethyl)-8-(phenyl-2-pyridinylmethylene)-4,7-methano-1H-isoindole-1,3(2H)-dione; 5-(α-hydroxy-α-2-pyridylbenzyl)-7-(α-2-pyridylbenzylidene)-5-norbornene-2,3-dicarboximide; McN-1025; Raticate; Shoxin. $C_{33}H_{25}N_3O_3$; mol wt 511.57. C 77.48%, H 4.93%, N 8.21%, O 9.38%. Prepn: A. P. Roszkowski *et al., Science* **144**, 412 (1964); R. J. Mohrbacher *et al.,* **BE 659610**; *eidem,* **US 3378566** (1965, 1968 both to McNeil). Stereoisomerism: *idem et al., J. Org. Chem.* **31**, 2141 (1966); S. Abrahamsson, B. Nilsson, *ibid.* 3631. Structure-activity studies: G. I. Poos *et al., J. Med. Chem.* **9,** 537 (1966). Toxicity data: A. P. Roszkowski, *J. Pharmacol. Exp. Ther.* **149**, 288 (1965).

Crystals from methylene chloride + ether, mp 190-198°. uv max (methanol): 250 nm (ε 17500). LD$_{50}$ in rats (mg/kg): 5.3 orally; 0.65 i.v. (Roszkowski). Practically insol in water unless pH is below 4.

USE: Rodenticide.

6688. Norcarane. [286-08-8] Bicyclo[4.1.0]heptane; 1,2-methylenecyclohexane. C_7H_{12}; mol wt 96.17. C 87.42%, H 12.58%. Prepd by distilling the barium salt of norcaranecarboxylic acid with ZnO + BaO: Ebel *et al., Helv. Chim. Acta* **12**, 19 (1929); by the action of methylene iodide and zinc-copper couple on cyclohexene: Smith, Simmons, *Org. Synth.* **41**, 72 (1961); Simmons, **US 3074984** (1963 to du Pont); from cyclohexene + diazomethane + zinc iodide: Applequist, Badad, *J. Org. Chem.* **27**, 288 (1962); from methylene chloride + cyclohexyl lithium: Closs, *J. Am. Chem. Soc.* **84**, 809 (1962).

Liquid. bp 116-117°. n_D^{25} 1.4546.

6689. Norcholanic Acid. [511-18-2] (5β)-24-Norcholan-23-oic acid. $C_{23}H_{38}O_2$; mol wt 346.55. C 79.71%, H 11.05%, O

9.23%. Prepn from ethyl cholanate: Wieland *et al., Z. Physiol. Chem.* **161**, 80 (1926); from 3,7-diketonorcholanic acid: Windaus, van Schoor, *ibid.* **173**, 312 (1928); from 12-ketonorcholanic acid: Cook, Haslewood, *J. Chem. Soc.* **1934**, 428; from 3α,23-dihydroxy-cholanic acid: Yanuka *et al., Tetrahedron Lett.* **1968**, 1725.

Needles from acetic acid, mp 177°.
Methyl ester. $C_{24}H_{40}O_2$. Needles from methanol, mp 74°.
Ethyl ester. $C_{25}H_{42}O_2$. Prisms from alcohol, mp 67°.

6690. Norcodeine. [467-15-2] (5α,6α)-7,8-Didehydro-4,5-epoxy-3-methoxymorphinan-6-ol; *N*-desmethylcodeine; normorphine 3-methyl ether. $C_{17}H_{19}NO_3$; mol wt 285.34. C 71.56%, H 6.71%, N 4.91%, O 16.82%. Prepn from acetylcodeine: von Braun, *Ber.* **47**, 2312 (1914); **DE 286743** (1914); *Chem. Zentralbl.* **1915**, II, 862; *Frdl.* **12**, 741; *Houben* **4**, 588; cf. **DE 289273** (1914); from codeine N-oxide: Diels, Fischer, *Ber.* **49**, 1723 (1916); from codeine: Speyer, Walther, *Ber.* **63**, 822 (1930).

Plates or needles from acetone or ethyl acetate, mp 185°. Sparingly sol in water, ether. Moderately sol in acetone. Freely sol in hot methanol, ethanol.
Hydrochloride trihydrate. $C_{17}H_{19}NO_3 \cdot HCl \cdot 3H_2O$. Needles from water. When anhyd, dec 309°. Sparingly sol in cold water, more sol in hot water. Freely sol in methanol, ethanol. Almost insol in acetone.
Sulfate. $2C_{17}H_{19}NO_3 \cdot H_2SO_4$. Crystals, freely sol in water.
Acetate (salt). $C_{17}H_{19}NO_3 \cdot C_2H_4O_2$. Crystals, freely sol in water.

6691. Nordazepam. [1088-11-5] 7-Chloro-1,3-dihydro-5-phenyl-2*H*-1,4-benzodiazepin-2-one; desmethyldiazepam; nordiazepam; DMDZ; A-101; Ro-5-2180; Calmday; Madar; Nordaz; Praxadium; Stilny. $C_{15}H_{11}ClN_2O$; mol wt 270.71. C 66.55%, H 4.10%, Cl 13.10%, N 10.35%, O 5.91%. Desmethyl analog and principal metabolite of diazepam, *q.v.* Prepn: L. H. Sternbach, E. Reeder, *J. Org. Chem.* **26**, 4936 (1961); E. Reeder *et al.,* **DE 1136709**; E. Reeder, L. Sternbach, **US 3051701** (both 1962 to Hoffmann-La Roche); A. Stempel, **BE 620020**; *idem,* **US 3202699** (1963, 1965, both to Hoffmann-La Roche); S. C. Bell *et al., J. Org. Chem.* **27**, 562 (1962); A. Stempel, G. W. Landgraf, *ibid.* 4675. Pharmacology: U. Traversa *et al., J. Pharm. Pharmacol.* **29**, 504 (1977); M. Babbini *et al., Pharmacology* **17**, 121 (1978). Metabolism: U. Klotz *et al., Br. J. Clin. Pharmacol.* **7**, 119 (1979). Pharmacokinetics: M. Konishi, *J. Pharm. Sci.* **67**, 1777 (1978). Clinical study: V. Andreoli *et al., Arzneim.-Forsch.* **27**, 436 (1977). Toxicity study: L. O. Randall *et al., Curr. Ther. Res.* **7**, 590 (1965). Teratogenicity study: R. P. Miller *et al., Toxicol. Appl. Pharmacol.* **25**, 453 (1973).

White or pale yellow crystalline powder from acetone, mp 216-217°. uv max (chloroform): 313 nm ($E_{1cm}^{1\%}$ 82). Slightly sol in alc, chloroform. Practically insol in water. LD_{50} in mice (mg/kg): 2750 orally, >400 i.p. (Randall). Also reported as LD_{50} in mice, rats (mg/kg): 1300, >5200 orally (company communication).
Note: This is a controlled substance (depressant): **21 CFR,** 1308.14.
THERAP CAT: Anxiolytic.

6692. Nordefrin. [6539-57-7] (unspecified stereo); [74812-63-8] (*R*,S**-(±)-form). 4-(2-Amino-1-hydroxypropyl)-1,2-benzenediol; α-(1-aminoethyl)-3,4-dihydroxybenzyl alcohol; 3,4-dihydroxynorephedrine; 3,4-dihydroxyphenylpropanolamine; 3,4-dihydroxyphenylaminopropanol; α-(α-aminoethyl)protocatechuyl alcohol; α-methylnoradrenaline; α-methylnorepinephrine; norhomoepinephrine; isoadrenaline; aminopropanolpyrocatechol; homoarterenol. $C_9H_{13}NO_3$; mol wt 183.20. C 59.00%, H 7.15%, N 7.65%, O 26.20%. α-Adrenergic agonist. Prepn: **DE 254438** (1912 to Bayer); W. H. Hartung *et al., J. Am. Chem. Soc.* **53**, 4149 (1931); M. Bockmühl *et al.,* **US 1948162** (1934 to Winthrop); Bruckner *et al., Ber.* **76B**, 466 (1943). Configuration: Fodor *et al., Monatsh. Chem.* **83**, 1146 (1952). Prepn of optical isomers: **DE 269327** (1913 to Bayer); Bockmühl, Gorr, **DE 639126** (1936 to I. G. Farbenind.). Pharmacology: F. P. Luduena *et al., J. Dent. Res.* **37**, 206 (1958). HPLC determn in plasma: D. A. Jenner *et al., J. Chromatogr.* **224**, 507 (1981). Effect on toxicity of local anesthetics: S. E. Taylor, R. L. Dorris, *Anesth. Prog.* **36**, 79 (1989). Review of use in local anesthesia: T. M. Hensley *et al., J. Foot Surg.* **26**, 504-510 (1987).

Hydrochloride. [138-61-4] (unspecified stereo); [61-96-1] (*R*,S**-(±)-form). Corbasil; Cobefrin. $C_9H_{13}NO_3 \cdot HCl$; mol wt 219.67. Crystals, dec 178-179°. One gram dissolves in about 1.5 ml water, 15 ml alcohol. Practically insol in ether. Solns are neutral and are easily destroyed by traces of alkali.
(−)-Form. [829-74-3] Corbadrine; levonordefrin; Neo-Cobefrin. Crystals, dec 212-215°. $[\alpha]_D^{25}$ −31.0° (c = 0.5 in 0.01N HCl). uv max (dil HCl): 278 nm. Practically insol in water. Freely sol in aq solns of mineral acids. Very slightly sol in acetone, chloroform, ethanol, ether. LD_{50} in mice (mg/kg): 12.6 i.v. (Luduena).
THERAP CAT: Vasoconstrictor.

6693. Nordihydroguaiaretic Acid. [27686-84-6] (*meso*-form); [500-38-9] (unspecified stereo). (*R*,S**)-4,4′-(2,3-Dimethyl-1,4-butanediyl)bis[1,2-benzenediol]; *meso*-4,4′-(2,3-dimethyltetramethylene)dipyrocatechol; 2,3-bis(3,4-dihydroxybenzyl)butane; β,γ-dimethyl-α,δ-bis(3,4-dihydroxyphenyl)butane; NDGA; masoprocol; CHX-100; Actinex. $C_{18}H_{22}O_4$; mol wt 302.36. C 71.50%, H 7.33%, O 21.17%. Lipoxygenase inhibitor; occurs as the *meso*-form in the resinous exudate of the creosote bush, *Larrea divaricata, Zygophyllaceae (Covillea tridentata).* Isoln: C. W. Waller, O. Gisvold, *J. Am. Pharm. Assoc.* **34**, 78 (1945). Prepn from guaiaretic acid dimethyl ether: G. Schroeter *et al., Ber.* **51**, 1587 (1918); R. D. Haworth *et al., J. Chem. Soc.* **1934**, 1423. Synthesis: S. V. Lieberman *et al., J. Am. Chem. Soc.* **69**, 1540 (1947); and configuration of naturally occurring form: C. W. Perry *et al., J. Org. Chem.* **37**, 4371 (1972). Use as antioxidant: W. M. Lauer, **US 2373192** (1945 to U. S. Secr'y of Agriculture). Antiproliferative effect on cultured keratinocytes: D. I. Wilkinson, E. K. Orenberg, *Int. J. Dermatol.* **26**, 660 (1987); on cultured glioma cells: D. E. Wilson *et al., J. Neurosurg.* **71**, 551 (1989). Clinical trial in actinic keratoses: E. A. Olsen *et al., J. Am. Acad. Dermatol.* **24**, 738 (1991).

Crystals from acetic acid, mp 185-186°. uv max (methanol): 283, 218 nm (ε 6660, 13400). Sol in ethanol, methanol, ether, concd

H_2SO_4; slightly sol in hot water, chloroform; sol in dil alkalies, developing a deep red color. Practically insol in petr ether, benzene, toluene, dil HCl.

USE: As antioxidant for fats and oils in foods.

THERAP CAT: Antineoplastic.

6694. Norelgestromin. [53016-31-2] (17α)-13-Ethyl-17-hydroxy-18,19-dinorpregn-4-en-20-yn-3-one oxime; 17-deacetyl-norgestimate; 18-methylnorethindrone oxime; levonorgestrel 3-oxime; RWJ-10553. $C_{21}H_{29}NO_2$; mol wt 327.46. C 77.02%, H 8.93%, N 4.28%, O 9.77%. Bioactive metabolite of norgestimate, q.v. Prepd as intermediate of norgestrel, q.v.: NL 7306609 (1973 to Richter Gedeon). Prepn and identification as norgestimate metabolite: S. F. Sisenwine et al., Contraception 15, 25 (1977). Pharmacology: J. L. McGuire et al., Am. J. Obstet. Gynecol. 163, 2127 (1990). Use as contraceptive patch: J. Jona et al., WO 9640355; eidem, US 5876746 (1996, 1999 both to Cygnus). Clinical pharmacokinetics: L. S. Abrams et al., Br. J. Clin. Pharmacol. 53, 141 (2002). Review of clinical pharmacology and efficacy: R. T. Burkman, Int. J. Fertil. 47, 69-76 (2002); B. L. Sicat, Pharmacotherapy 23, 472-480 (2003).

Crystals, mp 112°.

Combination with ethinyl estradiol. [396715-57-4] Evra; Ortho Evra.

THERAP CAT: Progestogen; in combination with estrogen as transdermal contraceptive.

6695. Norepinephrine. [51-41-2] 4-[(1R)-2-Amino-1-hydroxyethyl]-1,2-benzenediol; (−)-α-(aminomethyl)-3,4-dihydroxybenzyl alcohol; l-3,4-dihydroxyphenylethanolamine; noradrenaline; levarterenol; Adrenor; Levophed. $C_8H_{11}NO_3$; mol wt 169.18. C 56.79%, H 6.55%, N 8.28%, O 28.37%. Demethylated precursor of epinephrine, q.v. Occurs in animals and man, and is a sympathomimetic hormone of both adrenal origin and adrenergic orthosympathetic postganglionic origin in man. Physiologic review: Malmejac, Physiol. Rev. 44, 186 (1964). It has also been found in plants, e.g., Portulaca olerocea L., Portulacaceae: Fing et al., Nature 191, 1108 (1961). Synthesis of dl-form: Payne, Ind. Chem. 37, 523 (1961). Historic review of synthesis: Loewe, Arzneim.-Forsch. 4, 583 (1954). Resolution of dl-form: Tullar, J. Am. Chem. Soc. 70, 2067 (1948); idem, US 2774789 (1956 to Sterling Drug). Configuration: Pratesi et al., J. Chem. Soc. 1959, 4062. Comprehensive description: C. F. Schwender, Anal. Profiles Drug Subs. 1, 149-173 (1972); T. D. Wilson, ibid. 11, 555-586 (1982).

Microcrystals, dec 216.5-218°. $[\alpha]_D^{25}$ −37.3° (c = 5 in water with 1 equiv HCl).

Hydrochloride. [329-56-6] Arterenol. $C_8H_{11}NO_3 \cdot HCl$; mol wt 205.64. Crystals, mp 145.2-146.4°. $[\alpha]_D^{25}$ −40° (c = 6). Freely sol in water. Solns slowly oxidize under the influence of light and oxygen in a manner comparable to epinephrine hydrochloride.

d-Bitartrate. [69815-49-2] Levarterenol bitartrate; Aktamin; Binodrenal. $C_8H_{11}NO_3 \cdot C_4H_6O_6$; mol wt 319.26. Obtained as the monohydrate, crystals, mp 102-104°. $[\alpha]_D^{25}$ −10.7° (c = 1.6 in H_2O). When anhydr, mp 158-159° (some decompn). Freely sol in water.

dl-Form. Crystals, dec 191°. Sparingly sol in water; very slightly sol in alc, ether; readily sol in dilute acids, caustic.

THERAP CAT: Adrenergic (vasopressor); antihypotensive.

THERAP CAT (VET): Sympathomimetic; vasopressor in shock.

6696. Norethandrolone. [52-78-8] (17α)-17-Hydroxy-19-norpregn-4-en-3-one; 17α-ethyl-19-nortestosterone; 17α-ethyl-17-hydroxy-4-norandrosten-3-one; 17α-ethyl-17-hydroxy-19-norandrost-4-en-3-one; Nilevar; Solevar. $C_{20}H_{30}O_2$; mol wt 302.45. C 79.42%, H 10.00%, O 10.58%. Prepn by catalytic hydrogenation of 17α-ethynyl-19-nortestosterone: Colton, US 2721871 (1955 to Searle); J. Am. Chem. Soc. 79, 1123 (1957).

Crystals from methanol, mp 140-141°. uv max: 240 nm (ε 16500). Sol in alcohol, benzene, ether, ethyl acetate. Insol in water.

Note: This is a controlled substance (anabolic steroid): 21 CFR, 1308.13, as defined in 1300.01.

THERAP CAT: Androgen.

6697. Norethindrone. [68-22-4] (17α)-17-Hydroxy-19-norpregn-4-en-20-yn-3-one; 19-nor-17α-ethynyltestosterone; 17α-ethynyl-19-nortestosterone; 19-nor-17α-ethynyl-17β-hydroxy-4-androsten-3-one; 19-nor-17α-ethynylandrosten-17β-ol-3-one; anhydrohydroxynorprogesterone; 19-norethisterone; norpregneninolone; "mini-pill"; Camila; Conludag; Menzol; Micronor; Micronovum; Mini-Pe; Norcolut; Noriday; Primolut N; Utovlan. $C_{20}H_{26}O_2$; mol wt 298.42. C 80.50%, H 8.78%, O 10.72%. Prepn from 19-nor-4-androstene-3,17-dione: Djerassi et al., J. Am. Chem. Soc. 76, 4092 (1954); US 2744122 (1956 to Syntex); De Ruggieri, US 2849462 (1958). Pharmacokinetics: H. Singh et al., Am. J. Obstet. Gynecol. 135, 409 (1979); M. Humpel, Contraception 26, 83 (1982). Double-blind, comparative clinical trial: S. Koetsawang et al., ibid. 25, 231 (1982); A. Sheth et al., ibid. 243. Multicenter trial of combination with ethinyl estradiol: M. Toews et al., Curr. Ther. Res. 41, 509 (1987). Review of carcinogenicity studies: IARC Monographs 21, 441-460 (1979). Comprehensive description: A. P. Schroff, E. S. Moyer, Anal. Profiles Drug Subs. 4, 268-293 (1975).

Crystals from ethyl acetate, mp 203-204°. $[\alpha]_D^{20}$ −31.7° (chloroform). First reported as $[\alpha]_D^{20}$ −25° (chloroform). uv max (ethanol): 240 nm (log ε 4.24).

Mixture with ethinyl estradiol. Binovum; Brevicon; Estrostep; Modicon; Neocon 1/35; Norimin; Norinyl 1+35; Ortho-Novum; Ovcon; Ovysmen; Tri-Norinyl; Trinovum.

Mixture with mestranol. Norinyl-1+50; Ortho-Novin 1/50; Ortho-Novum 1/50.

Acetate. [51-98-9] Aygestin; Milligynon; Norlutate; Primolut-Nor. $C_{22}H_{28}O_3$; mol wt 340.46. Prepn: O. Engelfried et al., US 2964537 (1960 to Schering AG). Crystals from methylene chloride + hexane, mp 161-162°. uv max: 240 nm (ε 18690).

Acetate, mixture with ethinyl estradiol. Etalontin; Primosiston; Anovlar; Gynovlar; Loestrin; Minovlar; Norlestrin.

Enanthate. Noristerat. $C_{27}H_{38}O_3$; mol wt 410.59. Clinical trial as injectable contraceptive: S. K. Banerjee et al., Contraception 30, 561 (1984).

Caution: Norethindrone is reasonably anticipated to be a human carcinogen: Report on Carcinogens, Eleventh Edition (PB2005-104914, 2004) p III-208.

THERAP CAT: Progestogen. Norethindrone and acetate in combination with estrogen as contraceptive (oral). Enanthate as contraceptive (injectable).

6698. Norethynodrel. [68-23-5] (17α)-17-Hydroxy-19-norpregn-5(10)-en-20-yn-3-one; 17α-ethynyl-17-hydroxy-5(10)-estren-3-one; 13-methyl-17-ethynyl-17-hydroxy-1,2,3,4,6,7,8,9,11,-12,13,14,16,17-tetradecahydro-15*H*-cyclopenta[*a*]phenanthren-3-one. $C_{20}H_{26}O_2$; mol wt 298.42. C 80.50%, H 8.78%, O 10.72%. Prepn: Colton, US 2691028, US 2725389 (1954, 1955 to Searle). Metabolism studies in mice: Freudenthal *et al., Toxicol. Appl. Pharmacol.* **24**, 125 (1973).

Crystals from aq methanol, mp 169-170°. $[\alpha]_D$ +108° (1% chloroform).

Mixture with mestranol. [8015-30-3] Conovid E; Enavid; Enovid.

THERAP CAT: Progestogen. In combination with estrogen as contraceptive (oral).

6699. Norfenefrine. [536-21-0] α-(Aminomethyl)-3-hydroxybenzene methanol; α-(aminomethyl)-*m*-hydroxybenzyl alcohol; 1-(*m*-hydroxyphenyl)-2-aminoethanol; *m*-hydroxyphenylethanolamine; norphenylephrine. $C_8H_{11}NO_2$; mol wt 153.18. C 62.73%, H 7.24%, N 9.14%, O 20.89%. Chem synthesis: Sachs, **FR 866569** (1941), *C.A.* **43**, 5043c (1949); Legerlotz, **US 2312916** (1943 to Ciba); Credner, Neugebauer, *Arzneim.-Forsch.* **3**, 462 (1953); Bretschneider, Hörmann, *Monatsh. Chem.* **84**, 1021 (1953). Synthesis and resolution: D'Amico *et al., Chim. Ind. (Milan)* **38**, 93 (1956). Biosynthesis: Hartman *et al., J. Am. Chem. Soc.* **77**, 816 (1955). Activity studies: Gersmeyer, Albrecht, *Med. Welt* **1966**, 657. Metabolism: Barac, *C.R. Seances Soc. Biol. Ses Fil.* **155**, 1598 (1961).

***dl*-Form hydrochloride.** [15308-34-6] Coritat; Depot-Novadral; Energona; Esbuphon; Molycor-R; Novadral; Stagural; Tonolift; Vingsal; Zondel. $C_8H_{11}NO_2 \cdot HCl$; mol wt 189.64. Crystals, mp 159-160°. uv max: 274 nm ($E_{1cm}^{1\%}$ 91.21). Freely soluble in water.

THERAP CAT: Adrenergic.

6700. Norfloxacin. [70458-96-7] 1-Ethyl-6-fluoro-1,4-dihydro-4-oxo-7-(1-piperazinyl)-3-quinolinecarboxylic acid; AM-715; MK-366; Baccidal; Barazan; Chibroxin(e); Chibroxol; Floxacin; Fulgram; Gonorcin; Lexinor; Noflo; Nolicin; Noracin; Norocin; Noroxin(e); Norxacin; Sebercim; Uroxacin; Utinor; Zoroxin. $C_{16}H_{18}FN_3O_3$; mol wt 319.33. C 60.18%, H 5.68%, F 5.95%, N 13.16%, O 15.03%. Fluorinated quinolone antibacterial. Prepn: T. Irikura, **BE 863429**; *eidem,* **US 4146719** (1978, 1979 both to Kyorin); M. Pesson, **DE 2840910**; *eidem,* **US 4292317** (1979, 1981 both to Roger Bellon/Dainippon); H. Koga *et al., J. Med. Chem.* **23**, 1358 (1980). Comparative antibacterial activity: K. Hirai *et al., Antimicrob. Agents Chemother.* **19**, 188 (1981); M. Y. Khan *et al., ibid.* 265; H. H. Gadebusch *et al., Infection* **10**, 41 (1982). Series of articles on *in vivo* and *in vitro* activity, pharmacology, pharmacokinetics, metabolism, early clinical studies, toxicology: *Chemotherapy (Tokyo)* **29**, Suppl. 4, 1-1000 (1981). Acute toxicity data: T. Irikura *et al., ibid.* 783. *In vitro* activity vs gentamicin-resistant *P. aeruginosa:* J. Downs *et al., Antimicrob. Agents Chemother.* **21**, 670 (1982). Treatment of lower urinary tract infection: H. Giamarellou *et al., Eur. J. Clin. Microbiol.* **2**, 266 (1983); of penicillin-resistant gonorrhea: S. R. Crider *et al., N. Engl. J. Med.* **311**, 137 (1984). Review of pharmacokinetics, antibacterial activity, clinical trials: B. Holmes *et al., Drugs* **30**, 482-513 (1985); R. C. Rowen *et al., Pharmacotherapy* **7**, 92-110 (1987). Symposium on clinical experience: *Scand. J. Infect. Dis.* Suppl. 48, 1-91 (1986). Comprehensive description: C. Mazuel, *Anal. Profiles Drug Subs.* **20**, 557-600 (1991).

White to light-yellow crystalline powder, mp 220-221°. uv max (0.1*N* NaOH): ~274, 325, 336 nm ($A_{1cm}^{1\%}$ ~1109, 437, 425). pKa_1 6.34; pKa_2 8.75. Partition coefficient (octanol/water): 0.46. Soly at 25° (mg/ml): water 0.28; methanol 0.98; ethanol 1.9; acetone 5.1; chloroform 5.5; diethyl ether 0.01; benzene 0.15; ethyl acetate 0.94; octyl alcohol 5.1; glacial acetic acid 340. Solubility in water is pH dependent, increasing sharply at pH <5 or at pH >10. Hygroscopic in air, forms a hemihydrate. LD_{50} in mice, rats (mg/kg): >4000 orally (both species); 1500 s.c. (both species); 470, >500 i.m.; 220, 270 i.v. (Irikura).

THERAP CAT: Antibacterial.

6701. Norflurazon. [27314-13-2] 4-Chloro-5-(methylamino)-2-[3-(trifluoromethyl)phenyl]-3(2*H*)-pyridazinone; 4-chloro-5-(methylamino)-2-(α,α,α-trifluoro-*m*-tolyl)-3(2*H*)-pyridazinone; 1-(3-trifluoromethylphenyl)-4-methylamino-5-chloropyridazone; SAN-9789; Solicam; Zorial. $C_{12}H_9ClF_3N_3O$; mol wt 303.67. C 47.46%, H 2.99%, Cl 11.67%, F 18.77%, N 13.84%, O 5.27%. Selective pre-emergent herbicide which inhibits carotenoid biosynthesis in susceptible species. Prepn: C. Ebner, M. Schuler, **BE 712832**; *eidem,* **US 3644355** (1968, 1972 both to Sandoz). Absorption and metabolism: R. H. Strang, R. L. Rogers, *J. Agric. Food Chem.* **22**, 1119 (1974). Mechanism of action: G. Sandmann *et al., Pestic. Biochem. Physiol.* **14**, 185 (1980). HPLC determn in edible crops: W. M. Draper, J. C. Street, *J. Agric. Food Chem.* **29**, 724 (1981). Comprehensive description: E. Ummel *et al., Proc. Brit. Weed Contr. Conf.* **13**, 313 (1976).

Crystals from alcohol, mp 183-185°. Soly in water (25°): 28 ppm. LD_{50} orally in rats: 9300 mg/kg (Ummel).

USE: Herbicide.

6702. Norgesterone. [13563-60-5] (17α)-17-Hydroxy-19-norpregna-5(10),20-dien-3-one; 17β-hydroxy-17α-vinylestr-5(10)-en-3-one; 17α-vinyl-5(10)-estren-17β-ol-3-one; norvinodrel; vinylestrenolone. $C_{20}H_{28}O_2$; mol wt 300.44. C 79.95%, H 9.39%, O 10.65%. Prepn: Ruggieri, Ferrari, **US 2983735** (1961 to Richter); *eidem,* **US 3062713** (1962). Synthesis of racemic form: Hiscock, Whitehurst, *J. Chem. Soc.* **1965**, 5772. Biological properties: Ruggieri *et al., Steroids* **5**, 73 (1965).

Crystals from diethyl ether-hexane, mp 142-143°. $[\alpha]_D$ +161° (chloroform).

Mixture with ethinyl estradiol. [8064-75-3] Vestalin.

THERAP CAT: Progestogen.

6703. Norgestimate. [35189-28-7] (17α)-17-(Acetyloxy)-13-ethyl-18,19-dinorpregn-4-en-20-yn-3-one 3-oxime; (+)-13-ethyl-17-hydroxy-18,19-dinor-17α-pregn-4-en-20-yn-3-one oxime acetate (ester); 17α-acetoxy-13-ethyl-17-ethynylgon-4-en-3-one oxime; dexnorgestrel acetime; D-138; ORF-10131. $C_{23}H_{31}NO_3$; mol wt 369.50. C 74.76%, H 8.46%, N 3.79%, O 12.99%. Acetate oxime of D-norgestrel, *q.v.* Prepn: A. P. Shroff, **DE 2633210**; *idem*, **US 4027019** (both 1977 to Ortho). HPLC determn: P. A. Lane *et al.*, *J. Pharm. Sci.* **76**, 44 (1987). Pharmacology: D. W. Hahn *et al.*, *Contraception* **16**, 541 (1977); J. Killinger *et al.*, *ibid.* **32**, 311 (1985). Pharmacodynamics: H. S. Weintraub *et al.*, *J. Pharm. Sci.* **67**, 1406 (1978). Metabolism in female monkeys: S. F. Sisenwine *et al.*, *Contraception* **15**, 25 (1977); in women: K. B. Alton *et al.*, *ibid.* **29**, 19 (1984). Clinical trial as a contraceptive in combination with ethinyl estradiol: B. Rubio-Lotvin, R. Gonzales-Ansorena, *Acta Eur. Fertil.* **9**, 1 (1978).

Crystals from methylene chloride, mp 214-218°. $[\alpha]_D^{25}$ +110°.
Mixture with ethinyl estradiol. [79871-54-8] Cilest; Ortho Cyclen; Ortho Tri-Cyclen; Ortrel; TriCilest.
THERAP CAT: Progestogen. In combination with estrogen as oral contraceptive.

6704. Norgestrel. [6533-00-2] (17α)-(±)-13-Ethyl-17-hydroxy-18,19-dinorpregn-4-en-20-yn-3-one; Wy-3707; Neogest; Ovrette. $C_{21}H_{28}O_2$; mol wt 312.45. C 80.72%, H 9.03%, O 10.24%. The bioactive enantiomer is levorotatory. Prepn: H. Smith, **BE 623844** (1963), *C.A.* **61**, 4427c (1964); G. A. Hughes, H. Smith, **US 3959322** (1976 to Herchel Smith); H. Smith *et al.*, *Experientia* **19**, 394 (1963); *eidem*, *J. Chem. Soc.* **1964**, 4472; M. Rosenberger *et al.*, *Helv. Chim. Acta* **54**, 2857 (1971). Comprehensive description: A. M. Sopirak, L. F. Cullen, *Anal. Profiles Drug Subs.* **4**, 294-318 (1975).

(−)-form

Crystals from methanol, mp 205-207°. uv max (ethanol): 241 nm (ε 16700).
Mixture with ethinyl estradiol. [8056-51-7] Lo/Ovral; Ovral; Stédiril. Clinical efficacy as oral contraceptive: T. R. Dunson *et al.*, *Contraception* **48**, 109 (1993)
(+)-**Form.** [797-64-8] (8α,9β,10α,13α,14β)-13-Ethyl-17-hydroxy-18,19-dinorpregn-4-en-20-yn-3-one; dextronorgestrel. Crystal structure determn: N. J. DeAngelis *et al.*, *Acta Crystallogr.* **31B**, 2040 (1975). Crystals, mp 238-242°. $[\alpha]_D^{25}$ +40.7° (CHCl₃).
(−)-**Form.** [797-63-7] 17-Ethynyl-18-methyl-19-nortestosterone; 13β-ethyl-17α-ethynyl-17β-hydroxygon-4-en-3-one; levonorgestrel; D-norgestrel; dexnorgestrel (obsolete); Levonelle; Levonova; Microlut; Microval; Mirena; Norgeston; Norlevo; Norplant. Prepn: C. Rufer *et al.*, *Ann.* **702**, 141 (1967); H. Baier *et al.*, *Helv. Chim. Acta* **68**, 1054 (1985). Metabolism: F. Z. Stanczyk, S. Roy, *Contraception* **42**, 67 (1990). Comparative clinical trial with mifepristone, *q.v.*, in emergency contraception: H. von Hertzen *et al.*, *Lancet* **360**, 1803 (2002). Review of clinical pharmacokinetics: K. Fotherby, *Clin. Pharmacokinet.* **28**, 203-215 (1995); of clinical efficacy of subdermal implant: A. J. Coukell, J. A. Balfour, *Drugs* **55**, 861-887 (1998); of intrauterine implant: P. Lähteenmäki *et al.*, *Steroids* **65**, 693-697 (2000); T. Luukkainen, *ibid.* **699-702**. Crystals from methanol, mp 235-237°. $[\alpha]_D^{20}$ −32.4° (c = 0.496 in CHCl₃). uv max (methanol): 241 nm (ε 16770).
Mixture of levonorgestrel with ethinyl estradiol. [39366-37-5] Levlen; Logynon; Microgynon; Nordette; Ovran; Ovranette; Tetra-

gynon; Tri-Levlen; Trinordiol; Triphasil. Clinical trial in acne treatment: L. J. Diaz-Sandoval *et al.*, *Fertil. Steril.* **76**, 461 (2001).
THERAP CAT: Progestogen; oral contraceptive; as contraceptive implant.

6705. Norgestrienone. [848-21-5] (17α)-17-Hydroxy-19-norpregna-4,9,11-trien-20-yn-3-one; 17α-ethynyl-4,9,11-estratrien-17β-ol-3-one; 17α-ethynyl-17β-hydroxy-3-oxo-4,9,11-estratriene; 17α-ethynyl-13β-methyl-Δ^{4,9,11}-gonatriene-17β-ol-3-one; Ogyline. $C_{20}H_{22}O_2$; mol wt 294.39. C 81.60%, H 7.53%, O 10.87%. Prepn: **NL 6401555**, corresp to Nominé *et al.*, **US 3257278** (1964 and 1966, both to Roussel-UCLAF); Nominé *et al.*, *Compt. Rend.* **260**, 4545 (1965); **FR M3060** and **NL 6517141** (1965 and 1966, both to Roussel-UCLAF), *C.A.* **63**, 8449b (1965) and **65**, 15470b (1966).

Pale yellow needles from diisopropyl ether, mp 169°. $[\alpha]_D^{20}$ +63° (c = 0.5 in alc). uv max: 342, 238 nm (ε 29100, 5920). Sol in alcohols, ether, acetone, benzene, chloroform; practically insol in water, dil aq acids and alkalies.
THERAP CAT: Progestogen.

6706. Norleucine. [327-57-1] 2-Aminohexanoic acid; α-aminocaproic acid; glycoleucine; caprine. $C_6H_{13}NO_2$; mol wt 131.17. C 54.94%, H 9.99%, N 10.68%, O 24.39%. $CH_3(CH_2)_3-CH(NH_2)COOH$. An amino acid classified as nonessential with respect to its growth effect in rats. Several syntheses: prepn from α-bromo-*n*-caproic acid by action of 25% ammonia at 50-55°: Marvel, du Vigneaud, *Org. Synth.* **4**, 3 (1925).
DL-Form. Lustrous leaflets from water. d 1.172. Dec 327°. pK₁ 2.39; pK₂ 9.76. Soly in water: 11.49 g/l at 25°, 17.27 g/l at 50°, 28.61 g/l at 75°, 52.0 g/l at 100°. Sparingly sol in alcohol: 0.42 g/100 g at 25°. Sol in acids.
L(+)-Form. Slightly sweet, shiny leaflets from water. mp 301° (partial decompn). Sublimes partially at 275-280°. [M]_D +32.1° (5N HCl); +47.9° (glacial acetic acid). $[\alpha]_D^{20}$ +21.3° (c = 4.25 in 6N HCl); +6.26° (c = 0.70 in water).
D(−)-Form. Bitter, shiny leaflets from water. mp 301° (partial decompn). Sublimes partially at 275-280°. $[\alpha]_D^{20}$ −22.4° (c = 4.69 in 6N HCl); −4.49° (c = 0.96 in water).

6707. Norlevorphanol. [1531-12-0] Morphinan-3-ol; (−)-3-hydroxymorphinan; 1,3,4,9,10,10a-hexahydro-6-hydroxy-2H-10,4a-iminoethanophenanthrene; 1,3,4,9,10,10a-hexahydro-2H-10,4a-iminoethanophenanthren-6-ol; NIH-7539. $C_{16}H_{21}NO$; mol wt 243.34. C 78.97%, H 8.70%, N 5.76%, O 6.57%. Prepn: Schnider, Grüssner, *Helv. Chim. Acta* **34**, 2211 (1951); Hellerbach, *et al.*, *ibid.* **39**, 429 (1956); **GB 765920** (1957 to Hoffmann-La Roche).

Crystals from acetone + methanol, mp 270-272°. $[\alpha]_D^{21}$ −42 ±2° (c = 1 in methanol).
Hydrochloride. $C_{16}H_{21}NO\cdot HCl$. Crystals from water, mp 320°.
Hydrobromide. $C_{16}H_{21}NO\cdot HBr$. Crystals from water, mp 222-224°.
Note: This is a controlled substance (opiate): 21 CFR, 1308.11.
THERAP CAT: Analgesic (narcotic).

6708. Normetanephrine. [97-31-4] α-(Aminomethyl)-4-hydroxy-3-methoxybenzenemethanol; α-(aminomethyl)vanillyl alcohol; 4-hydroxy-3-methoxy-α-(aminomethyl)benzyl alcohol; 1-(4-hydroxy-3-methoxyphenyl)-2-aminoethanol; 3-*O*-methylarterenol; 3-*O*-methylnoradrenaline; 3-*O*-methylnorepinephrine. $C_9H_{13}NO_3$; mol wt 183.20. C 59.00%, H 7.15%, N 7.65%, O 26.20%. A naturally occurring derivative of epinephrine, found together with metanephrine in urine and in certain tissues. Prepn: Fodor *et al., Acta Chim. Acad. Sci. Hung.* **1,** 395 (1951), *C.A.* **49,** 897 (1955); Axelrod *et al., J. Biol. Chem.* **233,** 697 (1958); Heacock, Hutzinger, *Chem. Ind. (London)* **1961,** 595.

dl-**Form hydrochloride.** $C_9H_{13}NO_3 \cdot HCl$. Prisms from abs ethanol, dec 206-207°. uv max (abs ethanol): 232, 282 nm (ε 7100, 2970).

6709. Normethadone. [467-85-6] 6-(Dimethylamino)-4,4-diphenyl-3-hexanone; 1-dimethylamino-3,3-diphenyl-4-hexanone; 1,1-diphenyl-1-(2-dimethylaminoethyl)-2-butanone; isoamidone I; desmethylmethadone; phenyldimazone; Hoechst 10582. $C_{20}H_{25}$-NO; mol wt 295.42. C 81.31%, H 8.53%, N 4.74%, O 5.42%. Prepn from 4-bromo-2,2-diphenylbutanenitrile and dimethylamine: Bockmühl, Ehrhart, *Ann.* **561,** 72 (1948); Easton *et al., J. Am. Chem. Soc.* **74,** 5772 (1952). Toxicity data: Eddy *et al., J. Pharmacol. Exp. Ther.* **98,** 121 (1950).

Oily liquid, bp$_3$ 164-167°. Alkaline reaction.

Hydrochloride. [847-84-7] Ticarda. $C_{20}H_{25}NO \cdot HCl$; mol wt 331.88. Crystals from acetone, mp 174-175°. Sol in water, alcohol. pH of 1% aq soln ~5. LD_{50} in mice: 90 mg/kg (Eddy).

Note: This is a controlled substance (opiate): **21 CFR,** 1308.11.

THERAP CAT: Antitussive; analgesic (narcotic).

6710. Normethandrone. [514-61-4] (17β)-17-Hydroxy-17-methylestr-4-en-3-one; 17α-methyl-19-nortestosterone; methylestrenolone; normethandrolone; normetandrone; methylnortestosterone; Orgasteron; Metalutin; Methalutin. $C_{19}H_{28}O_2$; mol wt 288.42. C 79.12%, H 9.79%, O 11.09%. Prepn: Djerassi *et al., US* **2744122** and US **2774777** (1956 to Syntex); *J. Am. Chem. Soc.* **76,** 4092 (1956); De Ruggieri, **US 2849461** (1958).

Crystals from ether-hexane, mp 156-158° (Kofler). [α]$_D$ +33°. uv max (ethanol): 240 nm (log ε 4.23).

Note: This is a controlled substance (anabolic steroid): **21 CFR,** 1308.13, as defined in 1300.01.

THERAP CAT: Androgen.

6711. Normorphine. [466-97-7] (5α,6α)-7,8-Didehydro-4,5-epoxymorphinan-3,6-diol; desmethylmorphine. $C_{16}H_{17}NO_3$; mol wt 271.31. C 70.83%, H 6.32%, N 5.16%, O 17.69%. Prepd by hydrolysis of cyanonormorphine: von Braun, *Ber.* **47,** 2312 (1914); Speyer, Walther, *Ber.* **63,** 852 (1930); Weijlard, Erickson, *J. Am. Chem. Soc.* **64,** 869 (1942); Rapoport, Look, **US 2890221** (1959 to U.S.A.E.C.).

Sesquihydrate. Crystals from water, mp 273°; when anhydr, mp 276-277°. Sparingly sol in hot water, alcohol. Insol in ether, chloroform.

Hydrochloride monohydrate. Cryst from water, dec 305°.

Note: This is a controlled substance (opium derivative): **21 CFR,** 1308.11.

THERAP CAT: Analgesic (narcotic).

6712. Nornicotine. [494-97-3] 3-(2-Pyrrolidinyl)pyridine; 2-(3-pyridyl)pyrrolidine. $C_9H_{12}N_2$; mol wt 148.20. C 72.94%, H 8.16%, N 18.90%. Occurs in ordinary tobacco, in other species of *Nicotiana*, and also in *Duboisia hopwoodii* F. Muell., *Solanaceae.* Synthesis: Mizogruchi, *Chem. Pharm. Bull.* **9,** 818 (1961); M. Nakane, C. R. Hutchinson, *J. Org. Chem.* **43,** 3922 (1978). Pharmacology: P. S. Larson, H. B. Haag, *J. Pharmacol. Exp. Ther.* **77,** 343 (1943). Toxicity: P. S. Larson *et al., Proc. Soc. Exp. Biol. Med.* **58,** 231 (1945). *Review:* Markwood, *U.S. Dept. Agr. Bur. Entomol. Plant Quarantine* E-561 (1942), Supplement by Roark, **E-645** (1945).

Hygroscopic, somewhat viscous liquid, develops a slight amine odor, less pungent than that of nicotine. bp 270°; bp$_{11}$ 131°; bp$_3$ 105-107°. Hardly volatile with steam (difference from nicotine which is readily volatile). d_4^{20} 1.0737. [α]$_D^{22}$ −89° (c = 100). n_D^{20} 1.5378. Miscible with water. Very sol in alcohol, chloroform, ether, petr ether, kerosene, oils. Less volatile and less easily oxidized than nicotine. LD_{50} in mice, rabbits (mg/kg): 21.7, >13.7 i.p.; 3.4, 3.0 i.v. (Larson *et al.*).

USE: Agricultural or horticultural insecticide.

6713. Norphenazone. [89-25-8] 2,4-Dihydro-5-methyl-2-phenyl-3*H*-pyrazol-3-one; 3-methyl-1-phenyl-2-pyrazolin-5-one; 1-phenyl-3-methyl-5-pyrazolone; C.I. Developer 1; developer Z; norantipyrine; MCI-186. $C_{10}H_{10}N_2O$; mol wt 174.20. C 68.95%, H 5.79%, N 16.08%, O 9.18%. Free radical scavenger; metabolite of antipyrine, *q.v.* Prepn: L. Knorr, *Ann.* **238,** 137 (1887). Structural determn by NMR and IR: R. Jones *et al., Tetrahedron* **19,** 1497 (1963); F.-D. Höppner *et al., J. Prakt. Chem.* **318,** 555 (1976). Crystal structure: F. Bechtel *et al., Cryst. Struct. Commun.* **3,** 469 (1973). HPLC determn in urine: M. A. Mikati *et al., J. Chromatogr.* **433,** 305 (1988). Anti-ischemic and radical scavenging actions: T. Watanabe *et al., J. Pharmacol. Exp. Ther.* **268,** 1597 (1994).

White crystals from benzene, mp 129-130°. Also reported as mp 127° (Knorr). bp$_{265}$ 287°.

THERAP CAT: In treatment of stroke.

6714. Norpseudoephedrine. [492-39-7] (αS)-α-[(1S)-1-Aminoethyl]benzenemethanol; D-*threo*-2-amino-1-hydroxy-1-phenylpropane; (1S,2S)-2-amino-1-phenylpropan-1-ol; nor-*d*-ψ-ephedrine; *d*-ψ-norephedrine; *d*-norisoephedrine; cathine; katine.

$C_9H_{13}NO$; mol wt 151.21. C 71.49%, H 8.67%, N 9.26%, O 10.58%. Sympathomimetic amine naturally occurring in the leaves of the khat plant, *Catha edulis* Forsk. (Celastraceae) and in several species of *Ephedra* (Ephedraceae) known in traditional medicine as Ma Huang. Isoln from *C. edulis*: A. Beitter, *Arch. Pharm.* **239**, 17 (1901); O. Wolfes, *ibid.* **268**, 81 (1930); from Ma Huang: S. Smith, *J. Chem. Soc.* **1928**, 51. Physical measurements: C. S. Gibson, B. Levin, *ibid.* **1929**, 2754. Synthesis: W. N. Nagai, S. Kanao, *Ann.* **470**, 157 (1929); J. Sicher, M. Pankova, *Collect. Czech. Chem. Commun.* **20**, 1409 (1955). Pharmacology: H. Hofmann *et al.*, *Arzneim.-Forsch.* **5**, 367 (1955). Clinical pharmacokinetics: F. Frosch, *ibid.* **27**, 665, 1076 (1977). Clinical evaluation for weight reduction: H. Muth, G. Issmeier, *Ther. Ggw.* **119**, 1173 (1980). HPLC determn in urine: P. J. van der Merwe *et al., J. Chromatogr. B* **661**, 357 (1994).

Prisms from benzene, mp 77.5-78°. $[\alpha]_{546}^{20}$ +37.9° (c = 3 in methanol). pKa 8.92. Sol in alcohol, chloroform, ether, dil acids.
Hydrochloride. [2153-98-2] Amorphan; Adiposetten; Exponcit N; Fasupond; Minusin. $C_9H_{13}NO.HCl$; mol wt 187.67. Prisms from alcohol, mp 180-181°. $[\alpha]_D^{20}$ +42.53°. Sol in water.
Note: This is a controlled substance (stimulant): **21 CFR**, 1308.14.
USE: In the optical resolution of externally compensated acids.
THERAP CAT: Anorexic.

6715. Nortriptyline. [72-69-5] 3-(10,11-Dihydro-5*H*-dibenzo[*a,d*]cyclohepten-5-ylidene)-*N*-methyl-1-propanamine; 10,11-dihydro-*N*-methyl-5*H*-dibenzo[*a,d*]cycloheptene-Δ$^{5,\gamma}$-propylamine; 5-(α-methylaminopropylidene)dibenzo[*a,d*]cyclohepta[1,4]diene; 3-(10,11-dihydro-5*H*-dibenzo[*a,d*]cyclohepten-5-ylidene)-*N*-methylpropylamine; 10,11-dihydro-5-(3-methylaminopropylidene)-5*H*-dibenzo[*a,d*][1,4]cycloheptene; desitriptilina; desmethylamitriptyline; Avantyl; Aventyl; Noritren; Ateben; Psychostyl; Sensaval. $C_{19}H_{21}N$; mol wt 263.38. C 86.64%, H 8.04%, N 5.32%. Tricyclic antidepressant. Prepn: Hoffsommer *et al., J. Org. Chem.* **27**, 4134 (1962); **NL 6408512**; E. I. Engelhardt, **US 3922305** (1965, 1975 both to Merck & Co.). Alternative process: N. L. Wendler, **US 3442949** (1969 to Merck & Co.). GC determn in plasma: J. E. Burch, *J. Chromatogr.* **308**, 165 (1984). Determn in plasma or serum by radioimmunoassay: J. F. Sayegh, *Neurochem. Res.* **11**, 193 (1986). Pharmacokinetics: E. H. Rubin *et al., J. Clin. Psychiatry* **46**, 418 (1985). Clinical trial in post-stroke depression: J. R. Lipsey *et al., Lancet* **1**, 297 (1984). Anticholinergic effect and clinical efficacy in urinary dysfunction: I. Nissenkorn *et al., Eur. Urol.* **12**, 109 (1986). Comprehensive description: J. L. Hale, *Anal. Profiles Drug Subs.* **1**, 233-247 (1972).

Hydrochloride. [894-71-3] Acetexa; Allegron; Nortrilen; Norzepine; Pamelor; Sensival; Vividyl. $C_{19}H_{21}N.HCl$; mol wt 299.84. Crystals from ether + ethanol, mp 213-215°. Sol in ethanol, water, chloroform. Practically insol in ether, acetone, benzene. uv max (methanol): 240 nm (ε 13900).
THERAP CAT: Antidepressant.

6716. Norvaline. [6600-40-4] 2-Aminovaleric acid; α-aminovaleric acid; 2-aminopentanoic acid. $C_5H_{11}NO_2$; mol wt 117.15. C 51.26%, H 9.46%, N 11.96%, O 27.31%. $CH_3(CH_2)_2$-$CH(NH_2)COOH$. Prepd by treating butyraldehyde ammonia with HCN and HCl: Slimmer, *Ber.* **35**, 404 (1902); from 2-acetylvaleric acid ethyl ester: Hamlin, Hartung, *J. Biol. Chem.* **145**, 349 (1942); from acetamidomalonic acid diethyl ester: Archer, Albertson, **US**

2445817 (1948 to Winthrop-Stearns); from 1-nitrobutane: Stiles, Finkbeiner, *J. Am. Chem. Soc.* **85**, 616 (1963); **US 3055936** (1962 to Res. Corp.). Prepn of optically active forms: Abderhalden, Kurton, *Fermentf.* **4**, 328; *Chem. Zentralbl.* **1921, III**, 296.
DL-Form. Minute leaflets from alcohol or water, mp 303° (closed capillary). pK$_1$' 2.36; pK$_2$' 9.72. Sublimes without decompn. One gram dissolves in 10 ml water at 18°. Freely sol in hot water; practically insol in alcohol, ether, chloroform, ethyl acetate, petr ether.
L(+)-Form. Crystals from dil alc. mp ~305° (closed capillary). $[M]_D$ +29.2° (5*N* HCl); $[M]_D$ +41.0° (glacial acetic acid). $[\alpha]_D^{20}$ +23.0° (c = 10 in 20% HCl). Freely sol in hot water; insol in alcohol, ether, chloroform, ethyl acetate, petr ether.
D(−)-Form. Minute leaflets. mp ~307°. $[\alpha]_D^{20}$ −24.2° (c = 10 in 20% HCl). Freely sol in hot water; insol in alcohol, ether, chloroform, ethyl acetate, petr ether.

6717. Norvinisterone. [6795-60-4] (17α)-17-Hydroxy-19-norpregna-4,20-dien-3-one; 17-hydroxy-17α-vinyl-4-estren-3-one; 17-hydroxy-13-methyl-17α-vinyl-1,2,3,6,7,8,9,10,11,12,13,14,16,-17-tetradecahydro-15*H*-cyclopenta[*a*]phenanthren-3-one; 17α-vinyl-19-nortestosterone; Nor-Progestelea. $C_{20}H_{28}O_2$; mol wt 300.44. C 79.95%, H 9.39%, O 10.65%. Prepn: Colton, **US 2655518; US 2802015** (both 1953 to Searle).

Crystals from ethyl acetate + petr ether, mp 169-171°. $[\alpha]_D$ +36°.
THERAP CAT: Progestogen.

6718. Noscapine. [128-62-1] (3*S*)-6,7-Dimethoxy-3-[(5*R*)-5,6,7,8-tetrahydro-4-methoxy-6-methyl-1,3-dioxolo[4,5-*g*]isoquinolin-5-yl]-1(3*H*)-isobenzofuranone; narcotine; *l*-α-narcotine; *l*-α-2-methyl-8-methoxy-6,7-methylenedioxy-1-(6,7-dimethoxy-3-phthalidyl)-1,2,3,4-tetrahydroisoquinoline; narcosine; methoxyhydrastine; opian; opianine; NSC-5366; Nipaxon. $C_{22}H_{23}NO_7$; mol wt 413.42. C 63.91%, H 5.61%, N 3.39%, O 27.09%. An opium alkaloid, isolated from the plant *Papaver somniferum* L. Papaveraceae. Present in amounts up to 11% depending on season and locality. First isoln: Robiquet, *Ann. Chim. Phys.* [2] **5**, 275 (1817). Extractable from the water-insoluble residue remaining from the processing of opium for the manufacture of morphine. Racemization to gnoscopine: Rabe, McMillian, *Ann.* **377**, 233 (1910); and structural studies: Perkin, Robinson, *J. Chem. Soc.* **99**, 775 (1911); Marshall *et al., ibid.* **1934**, 1318. Preliminary stereochemical studies: Ohta *et al., Tetrahedron Lett.* **1963**, 1857; Battersby, Spenser, *J. Chem. Soc.* **1965**, 1087. Revised stereochemistry: Blaha *et al., Collect. Czech. Chem. Commun.* **29**, 2328 (1964); Snatzke *et al., Tetrahedron* **25**, 5059 (1969). Synthesis of racemate: Kerekes, Bognar, *J. Prakt. Chem.* **313**, 923 (1971). Biosynthesis: Battersby, Hirst, *Tetrahedron Lett.* **1965**, 669. Metabolism: N. Tsunoda, Y. Yoshimura, *Xenobiotica* **9**, 181 (1979); *eidem, ibid.* **11**, 23 (1981). Pharmacokinetics: B. Dhalstroem *et al., Eur. J. Clin. Pharmacol.* **22**, 535 (1982). Clinical evaluation as antitussive: D. W. Empey *et al., ibid.* **16**, 393 (1979). HPLC determn in serum: K. M. Jensen, *J. Chromatogr.* **274**, 381 (1983). Comprehensive description: M. A. Al-Yahya, M. M. A. Hassan, *Anal. Profiles Drug Subs.* **11**, 407-461 (1982).

Orthorhombic bisphenoidal prisms, tablets from diacetone. Triboluminescent. d 1.395. mp 176°. Sublimes at 150-160° under 11 mm pressure at 2 mm distance. Very weak base forming unstable salts with acids and strong bases. pK 7.8. uv max (ethanol): 209, 291, 309-310 nm (log ε 4.86, 3.60, 3.69). Practically insol in vegetable oils. Slightly sol in NH_4OH, hot solns of KOH and NaOH, forming salts. Salts formed with acids are dextrorotatory and unstable in water.

Hydrochloride. [912-60-7] Capval. $C_{22}H_{23}NO_7 \cdot HCl$; mol wt 449.88. Hemihydrate to tetrahydrate, crystals, very sol in water forming basic salts.

Camphorsulfonate. [25333-79-3] Tulisan. $C_{22}H_{23}NO_7 \cdot C_{10}H_{16}O_4S$; mol wt 645.72. Contains 35.97% camphosulfonic acid. Prepn: Maillard, **US 3108106** (1963 to Jacques Logeais). Crystals, mp 188-191°. $[\alpha]_D^{33}$ +32.7° (c = 4.56 in water). Freely sol in water. Sol in methanol, ethanol. Slightly sol in ethyl acetate. Practically insol in ether.

***dl*-Form.** [6035-40-1] *dl*-Narcotine; gnoscopine. Long needles from methanol, mp 232° (dec). pK 7.8. Freely sol in carbon disulfide, hot chloroform; sol in ~1500 parts alcohol; sparingly sol in benzene, water.

THERAP CAT: Antitussive.

6719. Nosiheptide. [56377-79-8] Multhiomycin; RP-9671; Primofax. $C_{51}H_{43}N_{13}O_{12}S_6$; mol wt 1222.36. C 50.11%, H 3.55%, N 14.90%, O 15.71%, S 15.74%. Polythiazole antibiotic produced by *Streptomyces actuosus*. Isoln and characterization: S. Pinnert *et al.*, *FR 1392453*; *eidem*, **US 3155581** (1961, 1964 both to Rhône-Poulenc); F. Benazet *et al.*, *Experientia* **36**, 414 (1980). NMR determination of mol wt and elemental formula: H. Depaire *et al.*, *Tetrahedron Lett.* **1977**, 1397, 1401. Structure and configuration: T. Prange *et al.*, *Nature* **265**, 189 (1977); C. Pascard *et al.*, *J. Am. Chem. Soc.* **99**, 6418 (1977). Biosynthetic study: D. P. Houck *et al.*, *ibid.* **109**, 1250 (1987). Identity with multhiomycin: T. Endo, H. Yonehara, *J. Antibiot.* **31**, 623 (1978). Mode of action: E. Cundliffe, J. Thompson, *J. Gen. Microbiol.* **126**, 185 (1981). *Review:* F. Benazet *et al.*, *Experientia* **36**, 414-416 (1980).

Yellow needles, mp 310-320° (dec). $[\alpha]_D^{20}$ +38° (c = 1 in pyridine). uv max (water/DMF): 242, 322 nm ($E_{1cm}^{1\%}$ 525, 229). Sol in chloroform, dioxane, pyridine, DMF, DMSO; slightly sol in methanol, ethanol, ethyl acetate, benzene. Insol in water and petr ether.

THERAP CAT (VET): Antibacterial; growth promotant.

6720. Novaluron. [116714-46-6] *N*-[[[3-Chloro-4-[1,1,2-trifluoro-2-(trifluoromethoxy)ethoxy]phenyl]amino]carbonyl]-2,6-difluorobenzamide; 1-[3-chloro-4-(1,1,2-trifluoro-2-trifluoromethoxyethoxy)phenyl]-3-(2,6-difluorobenzoyl)urea; MCW-275; Pedestal; Rimon. $C_{17}H_9ClF_8N_2O_4$; mol wt 492.70. C 41.44%, H

1.84%, Cl 7.20%, F 30.85%, N 5.69%, O 12.99%. Insect growth regulator. Prepn: P. Massardo *et al.*, **EP 271923**; *eidem*, **US 4980376** (1988, 1990 both to Ist. Guido Donegani); F. Rama *et al.*, *Pestic. Sci.* **35**, 145 (1992). Greenhouse trials vs beet armyworm and greenhouse whitefly: I. Ishaaya *et al.*, *Brighton Crop Prot. Conf. - Pests Dis.* **1998**, 49.

mp 172-174°.
USE: Insecticide.

6721. Noviflumuron. [121451-02-3] *N*-[[[3,5-Dichloro-2-fluoro-4-(1,1,2,3,3,3-hexafluoropropoxy)phenyl]amino]carbonyl]-2,6-difluorobenzamide; *N*-[3,5-dichloro-2-fluoro-4-(1,1,2,3,3,3-hexafluoropropoxy)phenyl]-*N'*-(2,6-difluorobenzoyl)urea; XDE-007; X-550007; Recruit III; Recruit IV. $C_{17}H_7Cl_2F_9N_2O_3$; mol wt 529.14. C 38.59%, H 1.33%, Cl 13.40%, F 32.31%, N 5.29%, O 9.07%. Chitin synthesis inhibitor. Prepn: J. Drabek, **DE 3827133** (1989 to Ciba-Geigy). *See also*: R. J. Sbragia *et al.*, **US 5886221** (1999 to Dow AgroSciences). Laboratory performance and pharmacokinetics in eastern subterranean termites: L. L. Karr *et al.*, *J. Econ. Entomol.* **97**, 593 (2004).

White crystalline powder, mp 153-154° (Drabek). Also reported as light tan solid, mp 156-157° (Sbragia). Vapor pressure (20°): 2.20×10^{-10} mm Hg. Log P (octanol/water): 4.94 (20°). Relative density: 1.88 g/cm³. Soly in water (20°): 0.194 mg/l. Soly at 19° (g/l): acetone 425.0, acetonitrile 44.9, 1,2-dichloroethane 20.7, ethyl acetate 290.0, heptane 0.068, methanol 48.9, 1-octanol 8.1, *p*-xylene 93.3.

USE: Insecticide for control of termites.

6722. Novobiocin. [303-81-1] *N*-[7-[[3-*O*-(Aminocarbonyl)-6-deoxy-5-*C*-methyl-4-*O*-methyl-β-L-*lyxo*-hexopyranosyl]oxy]-4-hydroxy-8-methyl-2-oxo-2*H*-1-benzopyran-3-yl]-4-hydroxy-3-(3-methyl-2-butenyl)benzamide; crystallinic acid; streptonivicin; PA-93; U-6591. $C_{31}H_{36}N_2O_{11}$; mol wt 612.62. C 60.78%, H 5.92%, N 4.57%, O 28.73%. Antibiotic substance produced by *Streptomyces spheroides*: Kaczka *et al.*, *J. Am. Chem. Soc.* **77**, 6404 (1955); Wolf, **US 3000873** (1961 to Merck & Co.); Stammer, Miller; Miller; Wallick, **US 3049475**; **US 3049476**; **US 3049534** (all 1962 to Merck & Co.). By *Streptomyces niveus:* Hoeksema *et al.*, *J. Am. Chem. Soc.* **77**, 6710 (1955); *Antibiot. Chemother.* **6**, 143 (1956); French, **US 3068221** (1962 to Upjohn). Structure: Shunk *et al.*, *J. Am. Chem. Soc.* **78**, 1770 (1956); Hoeksema *et al.*, *ibid.* 2019; Walton *et al.*, *ibid.* **82**, 1489 (1960). Conformation: Golding, Richards, *Chem. Ind. (London)* **1963**, 1081. Revised configuration: O. Achmatowicz *et al.*, *Tetrahedron* **32**, 1051 (1976). Synthesis: Stammer, **US 2925411** (1960); Walton, Spencer, **US 2966484** (1960 to Merck & Co.); Vaterlaus *et al.*, *Helv. Chim. Acta* **47**, 390 (1964). Conversion of *isonovobiocin* to novobiocin: Caron *et al.*, **US 2983723** (1961 to Upjohn). Antiviral activity: Chang, Weinstein, *Antimicrob. Agents Chemother.* **1970**, 165. Efficacy in canine respiratory infections: B. W. Maxey, *Vet. Med. Small Anim. Clin.* **75**, 89 (1980). Mechanism of action studies: Smith, Davis, *J. Bacteriol.* **93**, 71 (1967); H. T. Wright *et al.*, *Science* **213**, 455 (1981); I. W. Althaus *et al.*, *J. Antibiot.* **41**, 373 (1988). *Review:* Brock in *Antibiotics* vol. 1, R. Gottlieb, P. Shaw, Eds. (Springer-Verlag, New York, 1967) pp 651-665; M. J. Ryan, *ibid.* vol. 5(pt. 1), F. E. Hahn, Ed. (1979) pp 214-234.

Pale yellow orthorhombic crystals from ethanol. *Sensitive to light*. d 1.3448. Dec at 152-156° (a rarer modification dec 174-178°). Acid reaction: pKa$_1$ 4.3; pKa$_2$ 9.1. $[\alpha]_D^{24}$ −63.0° (c = 1 in ethanol). uv max (0.1N NaOH; 0.1N methanolic HCl; pH 7 phosphate buffer): 307; 324; 390 nm (E$_{1cm}^{1\%}$ 600, 390, 350 resp.). Sol in aq soln above pH 7.5. Practically insol in more acidic solns. Sol in acetone, ethyl acetate, amyl acetate, lower alcohols, pyridine. Additional soly data: Weiss *et al.*, *Antibiot. Chemother.* **7**, 374 (1957).

Monosodium salt. [1476-53-5] Albamycin. C$_{31}$H$_{35}$N$_2$NaO$_{11}$; mol wt 634.61. Minute crystals, dec 220°. $[\alpha]_D^{24}$ −38° (c = 2.5 in 95% ethanol); $[\alpha]_D^{24}$ −33° (c = 2.5 in water). Freely sol in water. A 100 mg/ml soln has a pH of 7.5 and a half-life of ~30 days at 25° and several months at 4°. Soly data: Weiss *et al.*, *loc. cit.* Properties: Birlova, Traktenberg, *Antibiotiki* **13**, 997 (1968).

THERAP CAT: Antibacterial.

THERAP CAT (VET): Antimicrobial.

6723. Novoldiamine. [140-80-7] N^1,N^1-Diethyl-1,4-pentanediamine; 1-diethylamino-4-aminopentane; 4-amino-1-diethylaminopentane; 2-amino-5-diethylaminopentane; δ-diethylamino-α-methylbutylamine; δ-diethylaminoisopentylamine. C$_9$H$_{22}$N$_2$; mol wt 158.28. C 68.29%, H 14.01%, N 17.70%. Prepd commercially from 2-diethylaminoethanol and ethyl acetoacetate. 2-Chlorotriethylamine (formed by the action of thionyl chloride on the alcohol) is condensed with the sodium derivative of ethyl acetoacetate to yield an intermediate ester, which is hydrolyzed and decarboxylated to *novol ketone* (5-diethylamino-2-pentanone). This is hydrogenated in the presence of ammonia to yield novoldiamine. Several other prepns, i.e., from 1,4-pentanediol and diethylamine: Kyrides, US 2365825 (1944 to Monsanto). Purification procedure: Jones, US 2400934 (1946 to Lilly).

Liquid. Amine odor. d$_{26}^{20}$ 0.819. bp$_{753}$ 200-200.5°. n$_D^{26}$ 1.4403. Sol in water, alcohol, ether.

USE: Manuf quinacrine and other antimalarials having the same basic side chain.

6724. Noxythiolin. [15599-39-0] N-(Hydroxymethyl)-N'-methylthiourea; 1-(hydroxymethyl)-3-methyl-2-thiourea; noxytiolin; Noxyflex-S. C$_3$H$_8$N$_2$OS; mol wt 120.17. C 29.98%, H 6.71%, N 23.31%, O 13.31%, S 26.68%. Prepn: A. Aebi, E. Hafstetter, GB 970414 (1964 to Ed. Geistlich Söhne), *C.A.* **61**, 15981e (1964). Antibacterial activity *in vitro*: D. Horsfield, *Clin. Trials J.* **4**, 625 (1967); J. I. Blenkharn, *J. Pharm. Pharmacol.* **42**, 589 (1990). Inhibition of bacterial adherence *in vitro*: S. P. Gorman *et al.*, *J. Appl. Bacteriol.* **60**, 311 (1986). Clinical evaluation in peritonitis: F. Antos, *Clin. Trials J.* **17**, 159 (1980); in urinary tract sepsis: M. A. Jones, A. Hasan, *Br. J. Urol.* **62**, 311 (1988).

Crystals. mp 88-90°. Sol in water (10% w/v), ethanol (4% w/v). pH of 2.5% soln: 6.31-7.0. LD$_{50}$ orally in mice: >3 g/kg (Aebi, Hafstetter).

THERAP CAT: Antiseptic.

6725. NPPB. [107254-86-4] 5-Nitro-2-[(3-phenylpropyl)-amino]benzoic acid; HOE-144. C$_{16}$H$_{16}$N$_2$O$_4$; mol wt 300.31. C 63.99%, H 5.37%, N 9.33%, O 21.31%. Inhibits efflux of ion

channels; specificity is cell type dependent. Prepn: H. C. Englert *et al.*, DE 3528048; *eidem*, US 4994493 (1987, 1991 both to Hoechst). Synthesis and characterization as potassium channel blocker: K. R. Giles *et al.*, *Bioorg. Med. Chem. Lett.* **13**, 293 (2003). Blocking kinetics of chloride channels: J. Dreinhöfer *et al.*, *Biochim. Biophys. Acta* **946**, 135 (1988). Effect on chloride ion transport: B. R. Branchini *et al.*, *Biochem. Biophys. Res. Commun.* **176**, 459 (1991); *eidem*, *Arch. Biochem. Biophys.* **318**, 221 (1995); J.-A. Kim *et al.*, *Biochem. Biophys. Res. Commun.* **309**, 291 (2003).

Yellow crystals from isopropanol, mp 178-180°. Soly (mg/ml): 25 DMSO, 10 ethanol.

USE: Biochemical probe primarily as a Cl$^-$ channel blocker.

6726. Nucleocidin. [24751-69-7] 4'-C-Fluoroadenosine 5'-sulfamate; 9-(4-fluoro-5-O-sulfamoylpentofuranosyl)adenine; 4'-fluoro-5'-O-sulfamoyladenosine. C$_{10}$H$_{13}$FN$_6$O$_6$S; mol wt 364.31. C 32.97%, H 3.60%, F 5.21%, N 23.07%, O 26.35%, S 8.80%. Antitrypanosomal antibiotic produced by *Streptomyces calvus*. The first naturally occurring derivative of a fluoro sugar. Isoln and activity studies: Thomas *et al.*, *Antibiot. Annu.* **1956-1957**, 716; Hewitt *et al.*, *ibid.* 722. Partial structure: Waller *et al.*, *J. Am. Chem. Soc.* **79**, 1011 (1957). Revised formula and structure: Morton *et al.*, *ibid.* **91**, 1535 (1969). Synthesis: Jenkins *et al.*, *ibid.* **93**, 4323 (1971).

As the monohydrate, crystalline, weakly alkaline substance. mp >190° (dec). uv max (methanol): 259 nm (ε 15000). LD$_{50}$ i.p. in mice: ~0.2 mg/kg (Thomas).

6727. Nupharidine. [468-89-3] [1R-(1α,4β,5α,7β,9aα)]-4-(3-Furanyl)octahydro-1,7-dimethyl-2H-quinolizine 5-oxide. C$_{15}$H$_{23}$NO$_2$; mol wt 249.35. C 72.25%, H 9.30%, N 5.62%, O 12.83%. From rhizome of *Nuphar luteum* (L.) Sibth. & Sm. (*Nymphaea lutea* L.), Nymphaeaceae: Goris, Crété, *Bull. Sci. Pharmacol.* **17**, 13 (1910). Isoln from *N. japonicum* DC., Nymphaeaceae and structure: Kotake *et al.*, *Ann.* **606**, 148 (1957). Total synthesis: Kotake *et al.*, *Bull. Chem. Soc. Jpn.* **35**, 698 (1962). Abs configuration: Kawasaki *et al.*, *ibid.* **41**, 1264 (1968); La Londe *et al.*, *J. Am. Chem. Soc.* **93**, 2501 (1971). Determn of crystal structure, abs config and stereochemistry by x-ray diffraction methods: J. Ohrt *et al.*, *J. Cryst. Mol. Struct.* **3**, 3 (1973).

Crystals, mp 221°. $[\alpha]_D$ +15°. Soluble in alcohol, chloroform, ether, acetone, amyl alcohol, dil acids. The base is tasteless, the salts bitter.

Consult the Name Index before using this section.

6728. Nutgall. Galla; galls; Aleppo-galls; Turkey-galls; Mecca-galls. Excrescence from the young twigs of *Quercus infectoria* Oliv. and other allied species of *Quercus, Fagaceae. Habit.* Asia Minor (Levant). *Constit.* 50-60% tannic acid, 2-4% gallic acid, ellagic acids, resin.

Chinese nutgall. Is the excrescence on the leaf or leafstalk of *Rhus semialata* Murr., *Anacardiaceae.* Contains about 70% tannin. *Incompat:* Alkalies, alkaloids; salts of Cu, Fe, Pb, Zn; $AgNO_3$; opium in soln.

Caution: Irritating to mucous membranes.

USE: Manuf tannin and ink; dyeing; tanning.

THERAP CAT: Astringent.

THERAP CAT (VET): Has been used as a topical astringent.

6729. Nutmeg. Myristica. Large tropical tree, *Myristica fragrans* Houtt., *Myristicaceae,* with fleshy edible fruit. The dried ripe seeds are widely used in cooking and in traditional medicine. The spice prepared from the seed's lacy red covering (aril) is known as **mace**. *Habit.* Molucca Islands; cultivated in Indonesia, West Indies. *Constit.* Seeds: 25-40% fixed oil; 5-15% volatile oils; triterpene saponins; sterols. Description of constituents: A. T. Weil, *Econ. Bot.* **19,** 194 (1965). Extraction of oils with liquid CO_2: C. B. Spricigo *et al., J. Supercrit. Fluids* **15,** 253 (1999). Toxicity data: P. M. Jenner *et al., Food Cosmet. Toxicol.* **2,** 327 (1964). Review of ethnobotany: C. Van Gils, P. A. Cox, *J. Ethnopharmacol.* **42,** 117-124 (1994); of constituents and uses: A. Y. Leung, S. Foster, *Encyclopedia of Common Natural Ingredients,* (Wiley-Interscience, Hoboken, 2nd Ed., 2003) pp 385-387; J. Gruenwald *et al., PDR for Herbal Medicines* (Medical Economics, Montvale, 3rd Ed., 2004) pp 594-595. Comprehensive description: B. Krishnamoorthy, J. Rema in *Handbook of Herbs and Spices,* K. V. Peter, Ed., (CRC Press, Boca Raton, 2001) pp 238-243.

Fixed oil. Nutmeg butter. Obtained by expressing the crushed seeds or by extracting with solvents. *Constit.* Trimyristin (84%), oleic acid (3.5%), resins (2.3%), linolenic acid (0.6%), other fatty acids. Orange-red to reddish-brown, soft solid. mp 45-51°. Odor and taste of nutmeg. d 0.990-0.995. Sapon no. 172-179. Iodine no. 40-52. Acid no. 17-23. Partly sol in cold alcohol, almost completely sol in hot alcohol; freely sol in chloroform, ether.

Volatile oil. [8008-45-5] Oil of nutmeg. Obtained by steam distillation from the dried kernals of the ripe seed. *Constit.* Monoterpene hydrocarbons (~88%) including camphene, pinene, sabinene; monoterpene alcohols; myristicin (4-8%); elemicin; safrole. Colorless or pale yellow liquid; odor and taste of nutmeg. East Indian oil: d_{25}^{25} 0.880-0.910; n_D^{20} 1.4740-1.4880; angular rotation between +8° and +30°. Sol in 3 vols 90% alcohol. West Indian oil: d_{25}^{25} 0.854-0.880; n_D^{20} 1.469-1.476; angular rotation between +25° and +45°. Sol in 4 vols 90% alcohol. *Keep well closed, cool and protected from light.* LD_{50} orally in rats: 2620 mg/kg (Jenner).

Caution: Ingestion of large quantities may cause intense thirst, nausea, anxiety, drowsiness, hallucinations, stupor, death (Gruenwald).

USE: As a cooking spice, flavoring in food and beverages. Nutmeg oil as fragrance in soaps, detergents, creams, lotions, perfumes. Fixed oil in candles.

THERAP CAT: Carminative.

6730. Nux Vomica. Quaker buttons; bachelor's buttons; poison nut; dog buttons; vomit nut. Dried, ripe seeds of *Strychnos nux-vomica* L., *Loganiaceae. Habit.* Southern Asia, Northern Australia. *Constit.* 1-1.4% strychnine, about an equal amount of brucine; strychnicine, loganin, caffeotannic (igasuric) acid, proteins. Nux vomica from Saigon contains 1.6-2% strychnine.

Caution: Extremely poisonous.

THERAP CAT: Formerly as bitter tonic.

THERAP CAT (VET): Has been used as a bitter tonic.

6731. Nybomycin. [30408-30-1] 8-(Hydroxymethyl)-6,11-dimethyl-2*H*,4*H*-oxazolo[5,4,3-*ij*]pyrido[3,2-*g*]quinoline-4,10(11*H*)-dione; 6,11-dimethyl-8-(hydroxymethyl)pyrido[3,2-*g*]-oxazolo[5,4,3-*ij*]quinoline-4,10(2*H*,11*H*)-dione. $C_{16}H_{14}N_2O_4$; mol wt 298.29. C 64.42%, H 4.73%, N 9.39%, O 21.45%. Antibiotic substance produced by *Streptomycete* A 717 isolated from Missouri soil: Strelitz *et al., Proc. Natl. Acad. Sci. USA* **41,** 620 (1955); Eble *et al., Antibiot. Chemother.* **8,** 627 (1958); Brock, Sokolski, *ibid.* 631. Structure: Rinehart, Renfroe, *J. Am. Chem.*

Soc. **83,** 3729 (1961). Revised structure: Rinehart *et al., ibid.* **92,** 6994 (1970). Total synthesis of *deoxynybomycin*: Forbis, Rinehart, *ibid.* 6995. Total synthesis of nybomycin: *eidem, J. Antibiot.* **24,** 326 (1971); *eidem, J. Am. Chem. Soc.* **95,** 5003 (1973).

Needles from acetic acid, mp 325-330°. Sublimes at 250° (15 mm). Optically inactive. uv max (ethanol): 266, 285 nm. Soluble in concd acids. Very slightly sol in water, alkalies, and common organic solvents. Shows antiphage and antibacterial properties. LD_{50} i.p. in mice: 650 mg/kg (Brock, Sokolski). ^{13}C NMR spectrum: A. M. Nadzan, K. L. Rinehart, *J. Am. Chem. Soc.* **99,** 4647 (1977).

Acetate. $C_{18}H_{16}N_2O_5$. Crystals from chloroform + ethanol, mp 236-237°.

Succinate. $C_{20}H_{19}N_2O_7$. Crystals from dimethylformamide. Practically insol in water.

6732. Nylidrin. [447-41-6] 4-Hydroxy-α-[1-[(1-methyl-3-phenylpropyl)amino]ethyl]benzenemethanol; *p*-hydroxy-α-[1-[(1-methyl-3-phenylpropyl)amino]ethyl]benzyl alcohol; *p*-hydroxy-*N*-(1-methyl-3-phenylpropyl)norephedrine; buphenine; 1-(*p*-hydroxyphenyl)-2-(1′-methyl-3′-phenylpropylamino)-1-propanol; phenyl-*sec*-butyl norsuprifen. $C_{19}H_{25}NO_2$; mol wt 299.41. C 76.22%, H 8.42%, N 4.68%, O 10.69%. Prepn: **FR 968273** (1950 to Troponwerke Dinklage); **GB 669574; GB 669575** (1952); *Chem. Eng. News* **33,** 2896 (1955); Külz, Schöpf, **US 2661372; US 2661373** (1953). Pharmacology: T. T. Yen, D. V. Pearson, *Res. Commun. Chem. Pathol. Pharmacol.* **23,** 11 (1979); B. Fichtl, W. Felix, *Eur. J. Pharmacol.* **65,** 333 (1980).

Crystals from methanol, mp 111-112°.

Hydrochloride. [849-55-8] SKF-1700-A; Arlidin; Bufedon; Buphedrin; Dilatal; Dilatol; Dilatropon; Dilydrin; Opino; Penitardon; Perdilatal; Rudilin; Rydrin; Tocodilydrin; Tocodrin. $C_{19}H_{25}$-NO_2.HCl; mol wt 335.87. Crystals. Sparingly sol in water; slightly sol in alcohol. Practically insol in ether, chloroform, benzene.

THERAP CAT: Vasodilator (peripheral).

6733. Nylon. Polyamide. Generic term used to describe "a manufactured fiber in which fiber-forming substances are any long-chain synthetic polyamide having recurring polyamide groups (—CONH—) as an integral part of the polymer chain". Formed from various combinations of diacids, diamines, and amino acids. May be formed also by addition polymerization. The linear polyamides have achieved the greatest commercial success. Shorthand nomenclature of nylons involves the use of numbers: a single numeral indicating the number of carbon atoms in a monomer, e.g. nylon 6; two numbers indicating a polymer formed from diamines and dibasic acids, the first numeral indicating the number of carbon atoms separating the nitrogen atoms of the diamine, the second indicating the number of straight-chain carbon atoms in the dibasic acid, e.g. nylon 6,6. First produced by E. I. du Pont de Nemours & Co. according to patents of W. H. Carothers. The name **nylon** was dedicated to public domain on Oct. 27, 1938 at the Herald Tribune Forum where the product itself was announced. *Reviews:* R. W. Moncrieff, *Man-Made Fibres* (John Wiley, New York, 1963) pp 335-355; Snider, Richardson, "Polyamide Fibers" in *Encyclopedia of Polymer Science and Technology* **vol. 10** (Interscience, New York, 1969) pp 347-460; J. H. Saunders, "Polyamides (Fibers)" in *Kirk-Othmer Encyclopedia of Chemical Technology* vol. **18** (Wiley-Interscience, New York, 3rd ed., 1982) pp 372-405. *Book: Nylon Plastics,* M. I. Kohan, Ed. (Wiley-Interscience, New York, 1973).

Crystalline solids characterized by low specific gravity, high strength, durability, high flexibility, and high tensile strength. Soluble in phenol, cresols (especially *m*-cresol), xylenol, formic acid. Insoluble in alcohols, esters, ketones, hydrocarbons. Hydrolysis and degradation occur at higher temperatures, esp in the melt. Stable to aqueous alkali. Degrades rapidly in aqueous acids. Undergoes photodegradation.

USE: In production of synthetic fibers for various textile and domestic uses. Surgical aid (nonabsorbable suture).

6734. Nylon 6. [25038-54-4] Poly[imino(1-oxo-1,6-hexanediyl)]; poly(iminocarbonylpentamethylene); Caprolan; Enkalon; Grilon; Kapron; Mirlon; Perlon; Phrilon; Amilan. Linear polymer obtained by polymerization of ε-caprolactam, *q.v.:* Schlack, US **2241321** (1941 to I. G. Farbenind.). The importance of this fiber increased with the discovery that caprolactam can be produced by the nitrosation of cyclohexanecarboxylic acid: Muench *et al., US* **3022291** and US **3108096** (1962, 1963, both to Snia Viscosa). *Review:* R. W. Moncrieff, *Man-Made Fibres* (John Wiley & Sons, New York, 1963) pp 335-355; H. K. Reimschuessel, *J. Polym. Sci. Macromol. Rev.* **12,** 65-139 (1977).

n = approx 200

Softens at 210°. mp 223°. Can withstand a temp of 100° for long periods of time. d_4^{20} 1.14. Moisture regain is about 4%. Swelling is low; if steeped in water and then centrifuged its volume increases by about 13-14%. Immune to microbiological attack. Resistant to most org chemicals, but dissolved by phenol, cresol, and strong acids.

USE: Tire cord; fishing lines; tow ropes; hose manuf; woven fabrics.

6735. Nylon 46. [50327-22-5] Poly[imino-1,4-butanediylimino(1,6-dioxo-1,6-hexanediyl)]; poly(tetramethyleneadipamide); Stanyl. Symmetrical polyamide with higher melting point and greater tensile strength than nylon 66 or nylon 6, *q.v.* Prepn from 1,4-diaminobutane and adipic acid: W. H. Carothers, US **2130948** (1938 to Du Pont). Improved process: E. H. J. P. Bour, J. M. M. Warnier, EP **77106** corresp to US **4463166** (1983, 1984 both to Stamicarbon). Account of prepn by melt polymerization, physical properties: R. J. Gaymans *et al., J. Polym. Sci. Polym. Chem. Ed.* **15,** 537 (1977). Brief account: D. O'Sullivan, *Chem. Eng. News* **62,** 33 (May 21, 1984).

Clear polymer, mol wt 22,000-45,000. mp 283-319°. d 1.20 (solution-cast film). Insol in most solvents. Sol in formic acid. Slightly sol in trifluoroacetic acid.

USE: Industrial fiber; fiber-reinforced rubber products.

6736. Nystatin. [1400-61-9] Fungicidin; Biofanal; Diastatin; Candex; Candio-Hermal; Mycostatin; Moronal; Nystan; O-V

Statin. Polyene antifungal antibiotic complex containing 3 biologically active components, A_1, A_2, A_3. Produced by *Streptomyces noursei, S. aureus* and other *Streptomyces* spp: Hazen, Brown, *Science* **112,** 423 (1950); *Proc. Soc. Exp. Biol. Med.* **76,** 93 (1951); Raubitscheck *et al., Antibiot. Chemother.* **2,** 179 (1952); Cohen, Webb, *Arch. Pediatr.* **69,** 414 (1952); Dutcher *et al., Antibiot. Annu.* **1953-1954,** 191; *eidem, Therapy of Fungus Diseases* (Little, Brown, Boston, 1955) p 168. Review of early literature: Brown, Hazen, *Trans. N.Y. Acad. Sci.* **19** (1956-1957) pp 447-456. Purification: Vandeputte, US **2832719** (1958 to Olin Mathieson); Renella, US **3517100** (1970 to Am. Cyanamid). Chemistry and partial structure: Birch *et al., Tetrahedron Lett.* **1964,** 1491; of nystatin A_1 and A_2: Shenin *et al., Antibiotiki* **13,** 387 (1968). Structure of the aglycone: Manwaring *et al., ibid.* **1969,** 5319. Complete structure of A_1: Chong, Rickards, *ibid.* **1970,** 5145; Borowski *et al., ibid.* **1971,** 685. Revised structure: R. C. Pandey, K. L. Rinehart, *J. Antibiot.* **29,** 1035 (1976). Stereochemical study of A_1: J. M. Lancelin *et al., Tetrahedron Lett.* **29,** 2827 (1988). Structure of A_3: J. Zielinski *et al., J. Antibiot.* **41,** 1289 (1988). Mechanism of action: R. W. Holz in *Antibiotics* vol. 5, pt. 2, F. E. Hahn, Ed. (Springer-Verlag, New York, 1979) pp 313-340. Toxicity study: H. Seneca, *Antibiot. Annu.* **1955-1956,** 697. Comprehensive description: G. W. Michel, *Anal. Profiles Drug Subs.* **6,** 341-421 (1977).

Nystatin A₁

Light yellow powder. Gradually decomposes above 160° without melting by 250°. $[\alpha]_D^{25}$ −10° (glacial acetic acid); +21° (pyridine); +12° (DMF); −7° (0.1*N* HCl in methanol). uv max (ethanol): 290, 307, 322 nm. Exhibits strong reducing properties. Solubilities determined by Weiss *et al., Antibiot. Chemother.* **7,** 374 (1957) in mg/ml at about 28°: water 4.0; methanol 11.2; carbon tetrachloride 1.23; chloroform 0.48; benzene 0.28; ethylene glycol 8.75. Solns and aq suspensions begin to lose activity soon after prepn. Aq suspensions are stable for 10 minutes on heating to 100° at pH 7.0; also stable in moderately alkaline media, but labile at pH 9 and pH 2. Heat, light, and oxygen accelerate decompn. Activity not diminished by blood or serum. LD_{50} i.p. in mice: ~200 mg/kg (Seneca).

Nystatin A₁. [34786-70-4] $C_{47}H_{75}NO_{17}$; mol wt 926.09.

THERAP CAT: Antifungal.

THERAP CAT (VET): Antifungal; growth promotant.

6737. Nysted Reagent. [41114-59-4] Cyclo-dibromodi-μ-methylene[μ-(tetrahydrofuran)]trizinc. $C_6H_{12}Br_2OZn_3$; mol wt 456.19. C 15.80%, H 2.65%, Br 35.03%, O 3.51%, Zn 43.01%. Olefination reagent with two *gem*-dimetallic subunits. Prepn: GB **1304465**; L. N. Nysted, US **3865848** (1973, 1975 both to G. D. Searle). Methylenation of carbonyl compounds: S. Matsubara, *et al., Synlett* **1998,** 313.

Commercial product is a white suspension in THF. Low soly in ether, THF, and other aprotic solvents.

USE: Reagent for the methylenation of ketones and aldehydes.

O

6738. Obidoxime Chloride. [114-90-9] 1,1'-[Oxybis(methylene)]bis[4-(hydroxyimino)methyl]pyridinium dichloride; 1,1'-(oxydimethylene)bis[4-formylpyridinium]dichloride dioxime; *N,N*-dimethyleneoxidebis(pyridinium-4-aldoxime) dichloride; bis(4-hydroxyiminomethylpyridinium-1-methyl) ether dichloride; bis(isonicotinaldoxime 1-methyl) ether dichloride; BH-6; LüH6; Toksobidin; Toxogonin. $C_{14}H_{16}Cl_2N_4O_3$; mol wt 359.21. C 46.81%, H 4.49%, Cl 19.74%, N 15.60%, O 13.36%. Cholinesterase reactivator. Prepn from pyridine aldoxime and α,α'-dichlorodimethyl ether: GB 3137702; Lüttringhaus *et al.*, US 3137702 (1963, 1964 to E. Merck); Lüttringhaus, Hagedorn, *Arzneim.-Forsch.* **14**, 1 (1964). Pharmacology and toxicology: W. D. Erdman, H. Engelhard, *ibid.* 5; Mayer, Michalek, *Biochem. Pharmacol.* **20**, 3029 (1971); Bajgar *et al.*, *Eur. J. Pharmacol.* **19**, 199 (1972). Hydrolysis studies: Christenson, *Acta Pharm. Suec.* **9**, 309 (1972).

Occurs in two interchangeable isomeric forms (*syn* and *anti*). Crystals from HCl contg 70% alcohol, dec 225°. Also reported as *syn*, mp 235-236°; *anti*, mp 218-220° [Leitis *et al.*, *C.A.* **71**, 81098d (1969)]. Freely sol in water, stable in 1-10% aq solns. LD$_{50}$ in mice, rats (mg/kg): 70, 133 i.v.; 150, 225 i.p.; >2240, >4000 orally; in mice (mg/kg): 172 i.m. (Erdman, Engelhard).

Dibromide. $C_{14}H_{16}Br_2N_4O_3$. Dec 202-203°.

THERAP CAT: Antidote (organophosphate insecticide poisoning).

6739. Oblimersen Sodium. [190977-41-4] d(P-thio)(T-C-T-C-C-C-A-G-C-G-T-G-C-G-C-C-A-T)DNA; augmerosen; G-3139; Genasense. Synthetic 18 base phosphorothioate antisense oligonucleotide (AS ON); designed to bind to human *bcl-2* oncogene, resulting in the down-regulation of an apoptosis-inhibiting protein Bcl-2. Prepn: J. C. Reed, WO 9508350 (1995); *idem*, US 5831066 (1998 to Univ. of Penn.). LC/MS determn in plasma and urine: G. Dai *et al.*, *J. Chromatogr. B* **825**, 201 (2005). Pharmacokinetics: F. I. Raynaud *et al.*, *J. Pharmacol. Exp. Ther.* **281**, 420 (1997). Mechanism of action study: L. Benimetskaya *et al.*, *Oligonucleotides* **15**, 206 (2005). Clinical evaluations in malignant melanoma: B. Jansen *et al.*, *Lancet* **356**, 1728 (2000); in non-Hodgkin's lymphoma: J. S. Waters *et al.*, *J. Clin. Oncol.* **18**, 1812 (2000); in prostate cancer: K. N. Chi *et al.*, *Clin. Cancer Res.* **7**, 3920 (2001). Review of pharmacology, preclinical and clinical development: R. J. Klasa *et al.*, *Antisense Nucleic Acid Drug Dev.* **12**, 193-213 (2002). Review of therapeutic potential in lung cancer: R. S. Herbst, S. R. Frankel, *Clin. Cancer Res.* **10**, 4245s-4248s (2004); in prostate cancer: K. N. Chi, *World J. Urol.* **23**, 33-37 (2005).

THERAP CAT: Antineoplastic.

6740. Ochratoxins. Toxic metabolites from *Aspergillus ochraceus* Wilh.: Scott, *Mycopathol. Mycol. Appl.* **25**, 213 (1965); *A. sulphureus* and *A. melleus*: Lai *et al.*, *Appl. Microbiol.* **19**, 542 (1970); and *Penicillium viridicatum* Westling: van Walbeek *et al.*, *Can. J. Microbiol.* **15**, 1281 (1969). As these molds occur widely, some toxins have been found as natural contaminants on corn, peanuts, storage grains, cottonseed and other decaying vegetation. Isolns: van Walbeek *et al.*, *ibid.* **14**, 131 (1968); Shotwell *et al.*, *Appl. Microbiol.* **17**, 765 (1969); Nesheim, *J. Assoc. Off. Anal. Chem.* **52**, 975 (1969); Natori *et al.*, *Chem. Pharm. Bull.* **18**, 2259 (1970). Structure and stereochemistry: van der Merwe *et al.*, *J. Chem. Soc.* **1965**, 7083; *Nature* **205**, 1112 (1965). Synthesis of ochratoxins A, B and ester deriv: Steyn, Holzapfel, *Tetrahedron* **23**, 4449 (1967); Nesheim, *loc. cit.*; Roberts, Woolven, *J. Chem. Soc. C* **1970**, 278. Facile synthesis of A: G. A. Kraus, *J. Org. Chem.* **46**, 201 (1981). Toxicity study: Purchase, Theron, *Food Cosmet. Tox-*

icol. **6**, 479 (1968). Physicochemical data: A. E. Pohland *et al.*, *Pure Appl. Chem.* **54**, 2220 (1982). Comprehensive reviews: Steyn, "Ochratoxin and other Dihydroisocoumarins" in *Microbial Toxins* vol. VI, A. Ciegler, *et al.*, Eds. (Academic Press, New York, 1971) p 179-205; F. S. Chu, *Crit. Rev. Toxicol.* **2**, 499-524 (1974); P. Krogh in *Natural Toxins*, D. Eaker, P. Wadström, Eds. (Pergamon, New York, 1980) pp 673-680; A. E. Pohland *et al.*, *Pure Appl. Chem.* **64**, 1029-1046 (1992).

Ochratoxin A

Ochratoxin A. [303-47-9] (*R*)-*N*-[(5-Chloro-3,4-dihydro-8-hydroxy-3-methyl-1-oxo-1*H*-2-benzopyran-7-yl)carbonyl]-L-phenylalanine. $C_{20}H_{18}ClNO_6$; mol wt 403.81. The major ochratoxin component. Crystals from xylene, mp 169°. Exhibits green fluorescence. $[\alpha]_D$ −118° (c = 1.1 in CHCl$_3$). uv max (ethanol): 215, 333 nm (ϵ 34000; 2400) (van der Merwe). Also frequently reported as mp 90° from benzene (one mole of benzene of crystallization). uv max: 213, 332 nm (ϵ 36800; 6400) (Steyn, Holzapfel). LD$_{50}$ orally in rats: 20-22 mg/kg (Purchase, Theron).

Ochratoxin B. [4825-86-9] (*R*)-*N*-[(3,4-Dihydro-8-hydroxy-3-methyl-1-oxo-1*H*-2-benzopyran-7-yl)carbonyl]-L-phenylalanine. $C_{20}H_{19}NO_6$; mol wt 369.37. The less toxic dechloro deriv of ochratoxin A. Crystals from methanol, mp 221° (van der Merwe); also reported as 208-209° (Nesheim). Exhibits blue fluorescence. $[\alpha]_D$ −35° (c = 0.15 in ethanol). uv max: 218, 318 nm (ϵ 37200, 6900).

Ochratoxin C. [4865-85-4] (*R*)-*N*-[(5-Chloro-3,4-dihydro-8-hydroxy-3-methyl-1-oxo-1*H*-2-benzopyran-7-yl)carbonyl]-L-phenylalanine ethyl ester. $C_{22}H_{22}ClNO_6$; mol wt 431.87. The equally toxic amorphous ethyl ester of ochratoxin A: Steyn, Holzapfel, *J. S. Afr. Chem. Inst.* **20**, 186 (1967), *C.A.* **69**, 2797p (1968). uv max (ethanol): 333 nm (ϵ 6500).

Caution: Ochratoxin A is reasonably anticipated to be a human carcinogen: *Report on Carcinogens, Eleventh Edition* (PB2005-104914, 2004) p III-209.

USE: Exptlly as teratogen and carcinogen.

6741. Ocimene. [29714-87-2] $C_{10}H_{16}$; mol wt 136.23. C 88.16%, H 11.84%. From the leaves of *Ocimum basilicum* L., *Labiatae*; *Baronia dentigeroides* Cheel, *Rutaceae*; *Litsea zeylanica* C. & T. Nees, *Lauraceae*; *Homoranthus flavescens* A. Cunn., *Myrtaceae*. From the fruits of *Evodia rutaecarpa* (Juss.) Hook. f. & Thoms., *Rutaceae*. Exists in two modifications: α-form, *3,7-dimethyl-1,3,7-octatriene*; and β-form, *3,7-dimethyl-1,3,6-octatriene*. *Cis* and *trans* refers to the stereochemistry at the double bond between positions 3 and 4. Isoln and structure: van Romburgh, *Proc. K. Ned. Akad. Wet.* **3**, 454 (1900); Enklaar, *Rec. Trav. Chim.* **26**, 157 (1907); **27**, 422 (1908); **36**, 215 (1917); **45**, 337 (1926). Structure: Sutherland, *J. Am. Chem. Soc.* **74**, 2688 (1952). Separation of isomers: Ohloff *et al.*, *Ann.* **675**, 83 (1964). Synthesis of *trans*-α-form: O. P. Vig *et al.*, *Indian J. Chem.* **7**, 1111 (1969). Stereospecific synthesis: O. P. Vig *et al.*, *ibid.* **15B**, 25 (1977).

trans-β-Ocimene

Oil. Pleasant odor. Mixture of isomers. bp$_{70}$ 100°. d$_4^{20}$ 0.8006. n_D^{20} 1.4862. uv max (methanol): 233 nm (ϵ 26,200). Practically insol in water. Sol in alcohol, chloroform, ether, glacial acetic acid.

trans-β-**Form.** [3779-61-1] d$_4^{20}$ 0.799. n_D^{20} 1.4893. uv max (ethanol): 232 nm (ϵ 27,600).

cis-β-**Form.** d$_4^{20}$ 0.799. n_D^{20} 1.4877. uv max (ethanol): 237.5 nm (ϵ 21,000).

***trans*-α-Form.** d_4^{20} 0.793. n_D^{20} 1.4802. uv max (ethanol): 231 nm (ε 27,300).

***cis*-α-Form.** d_4^{20} 0.794. n_D^{20} 1.4789. uv max (ethanol): 234.5 nm (ε 21,600).

6742. Octabenzone. [1843-05-6] [2-Hydroxy-4-(octyloxy)-phenyl]phenylmethanone; 2-hydroxy-4-(octyloxy)benzophenone; benzophenone-12; Spectra-Sorb UV 531. $C_{21}H_{26}O_3$; mol wt 326.43. C 77.27%, H 8.03%, O 14.70%. Prepn: Armitage *et al.*, US 3098842 (1963 to du Pont).

Crystals, mp 45-46°.

USE: To stabilize polyethylene against deterioration by ultraviolet light.

THERAP CAT: Ultraviolet screen.

6743. Octacaine. [13912-77-1] 3-(Diethylamino)-*N*-phenylbutanamide; 3-diethylaminobutyranilide. $C_{14}H_{22}N_2O$; mol wt 234.34. C 71.75%, H 9.46%, N 11.95%, O 6.83%. Prepn: Hofstetter, Wilder Smith, *Helv. Chim. Acta* **36**, 1698 (1953); Hofstetter, US 2851393 (1958 to E. Geistlich Söhne).

Crystals from petr ether, mp 46-47°. bp₁ 200°. Easily sol in stoichiometric amount of HCl, in ether, alc, benzene.

Hydrochloride. [59727-70-7] Amplicain. $C_{14}H_{22}N_2O.HCl$; mol wt 270.80. mp 132-134°. Sol in water.

THERAP CAT: Anesthetic (local).

6744. Octacosanol. [557-61-9] 1-Octacosanol; *n*-octacosanol; octacosyl alcohol. $C_{28}H_{58}O$; mol wt 410.76. C 81.87%, H 14.23%, O 3.90%. $CH_3(CH_2)_{26}CH_2OH$. Constituent of vegetable waxes. Isoln from the wax found on green blades of wheat: Pollard *et al.*, *Biochem. J.* **27**, 1889 (1933); from carnauba wax: Koonce, Brown, *Oil Soap (Chicago)* **21**, 231 (1944). Synthesis starting with behenic acid: Bleyberg, Ulrich, *Ber.* **64**, 2504 (1931); Francis *et al.*, *Proc. Roy. Soc. (London)* A **158**, 691 (1937).

Crystals from much acetone, mp 83.4°. Insol in water. Sol in carbon disulfide, other fat solvents, oils.

6745. Octafluorocyclobutane. [115-25-3] Perfluorocyclobutane; Freon C318. C_4F_8; mol wt 200.03. C 24.02%, F 75.98%. Prepd by pyrolysis of chlorodifluoromethane: Downing *et al.*, US 2384821 (1945 to Kinetic Chem.); US 2551573; US 2615926 (1951; 1952 to du Pont). Thermodynamic studies: Furukawa *et al.*, *J. Res. Natl. Bur. Stand.* **52**, 11 (1954); Duus, *Ind. Eng. Chem.* **47**, 1445 (1955).

Nonflammable, nontoxic gas. d_{vapor}^{27} 8.2. mp −41.4°. bp −6.04° (also reported bp −5°). Heat of formation at 25° = 352 kcal. Heat of combustion 1359 ±39 cal/g.

USE: Refrigerant; heat-transfer medium.

6746. 2,2,3,3,4,4,5,5-Octafluoro-1-pentanol. [355-80-6] 1*H*,1*H*,5*H*-Octafluoropentanol. $C_5H_4F_8O$; mol wt 232.07. C 25.88%, H 1.74%, F 65.49%, O 6.89%. $CHF_2(CF_2)_3CH_2OH$. Prepd by free radical telomerization of tetrafluoroethylene in meth-

anol: Hanford, Joyce, US 2562547 and Joyce, US 2559625 (both 1951 to du Pont).

Liquid. d_4^{20} 1.6647. bp₇₆₀ 140-141°. n_D^{20} 1.3178. Surface tension at 20° = 27.6 dynes/cm.

USE: To introduce fluoroalkyl groups into an organic molecule: Kramer, Gilbert, US 2963526 (1960 to Esso). Proposed intermediate for plastics, surface-active agents, lubricants, elastomers.

6747. Octamethylcyclotetrasiloxane. [556-67-2] C_8H_{24}-O_4Si_4; mol wt 296.62. C 32.39%, H 8.16%, O 21.58%, Si 37.87%. Isolated from the hydrolysis product of dimethyldichlorosilane: Patnode, Wilcock, *J. Am. Chem. Soc.* **68**, 358 (1946).

Oily liquid. mp 17.5°. bp 175°. bp₂₀ 74°. d 0.9558. n_D^{20} 1.3968.

USE: Preparation of methyl silicon oils.

6748. Octamethyltrisiloxane. [107-51-7] $C_8H_{24}O_2Si_3$; mol wt 236.53. C 40.62%, H 10.23%, O 13.53%, Si 35.62%. Prepn: Patnode, Wilcock, *J. Am. Chem. Soc.* **68**, 358 (1946).

$(H_3C)_3Si$ — O — $\underset{\underset{CH_3}{|}}{\overset{\overset{CH_3}{|}}{Si}}$ — O — $Si(CH_3)_3$

Liquid. bp 153°. d 0.8200. n_D^{20} 1.3848. mp ∼−80°. Stable. Inert to most chemical reagents and rubber. Maintains about the same viscosity over a wide temp range. Sol in benzene and the lighter hydrocarbons; slightly sol in alcohol and heavy hydrocarbons.

USE: As a basis for silicone oils or fluids designed to withstand extremes of temp; as a foam suppressant in petroleum lubricating oil.

6749. Octane. [111-65-9] C_8H_{18}; mol wt 114.23. C 84.12%, H 15.88%. $CH_3(CH_2)_6CH_3$. Found in petroleum.

Flammable liquid. mp −56.8°. d_4^{20} 0.7028. bp₇₆₀ 125.6°. n_D^{20} 1.39764. Flash pt, open cup: 72°F (22°C). Insol in water. Slightly sol in alcohol; sol in ether; miscible with benzene, petr ether, gasoline. The term "octane rating" is explained under Gasoline.

Caution: Potential symptoms of overexposure are irritation of eyes and nose; drowsiness; dermatitis; aspiration of liquid may cause chemical pneumonia. *See NIOSH Pocket Guide to Chemical Hazards* (DHHS/NIOSH 97-140, 1997) p 236.

6750. Octanohydroxamic Acid. [7377-03-9] *N*-Hydroxyoctanamide; caprylohydroxamic acid; Oct HA; Taselin. C_8H_{17}-NO_2; mol wt 159.23. C 60.34%, H 10.76%, N 8.80%, O 20.10%. $CH_3(CH_2)_6CONHOH$. Prepn and chemical study: Inoue, Yukawa, *J. Agric. Chem. Soc. Jpn.* **16**, 504 (1940); Ichim *et al.*, *Igiena* **9**, 319 (1960), *C.A.* **55**, 16662a (1961). Activity as a urease inhibitor: Kobashi *et al.*, *Biochim. Biophys. Acta* **65**, 380 (1962); **227**, 429 (1971); as an antimicrobial: Hase *et al.*, *Chem. Pharm. Bull.* **19**, 363 (1971).

White plates from benzene, mp 78.5-79°. Water soluble. Practically insol in petr ether.

THERAP CAT (VET): Antimicrobial; growth promotant.

6751. 1-Octanol. [111-87-5] Caprylic alcohol. $C_8H_{18}O$; mol wt 130.23. C 73.78%, H 13.93%, O 12.29%. $CH_3(CH_2)_6$-CH_2OH. Occurs in the form of esters in some essential oils. Prepd from the esterified products of coconut oil, the methyl caprylate being reduced by Na and alcohol.

Colorless liquid; penetrating, aromatic odor. d_4^{20} 0.827. mp −17 to −16°. bp 194-195°. n_D^{20} 1.430. Insol in water. Miscible with alcohol, chloroform, ether.

USE: Manuf of perfumes and esters.

6752. 2-Octanol. [123-96-6] Secondary caprylic alcohol; methyl hexyl carbinol; hexylmethylcarbinol. $C_8H_{18}O$; mol wt 130.23. C 73.78%, H 13.93%, O 12.29%. $CH_3(CH_2)_5CH$-$(OH)CH_3$. Prepd by heating sodium ricinoleate with caustic soda in a copper vessel and distilling: Adams, Marvel, *Org. Synth.* **1**, 61 (1921); Kenyon, *ibid.* **6**, 68 (1926); Ellis, Reid, *J. Am. Chem. Soc.* **54**, 1678 (1932).

dl-**Form.** Oily, refractive liquid. Aromatic, yet somewhat unpleasant odor, particularly on heating. d_4^{20} 0.8193. mp $-38.6°$. bp_{760} 178.5°; bp_{60} 107.4°; bp_{20} 83.3°; bp_{10} 70.0°; bp_5 57.6°; $bp_{1.0}$ 32.8°. n_D^{20} 1.42025 [Béhal, *Bull. Soc. Chim.* [4] **25**, 482 (1919)]. Flash pt ~140°F (60°C). Soly in water: 0.096 ml/100 ml. Miscible with alc, ether.

d-**Form.** bp_{20} 86°. $[\alpha]_D^{17}$ +9.9°. d_4^{20} 0.8216.

l-**Form.** bp_{20} 86°. $[\alpha]_D^{17}$ −9.9°.

USE: In the manuf of perfumes; in disinfectant soaps. To prevent foaming. Solvent for fats and waxes.

6753. 3-Octanone. [106-68-3] Ethyl *n*-amyl ketone. C_8-$H_{16}O$; mol wt 128.21. C 74.94%, H 12.58%, O 12.48%. Volatile chemical found fungi; constituent of lavender oil. Mediates interactions between plants, herbivores, and their natural enemies. Isoln from bituminous tar: J. Herzenberg, E. v. Winterfeld, *Ber.* **64**, 1025 (1931); from the essential oil of *Rosmarinus officinalis* L: A. Koedam, M. J. M. Gijbels, *Z. Naturforsch.* **33C**, 144 (1978). Prepn: Y. R. Naves, *Helv. Chim. Acta* **26**, 1034 (1943); P. G. Gassman, G. D. Richmond, *J. Org. Chem.* **31**, 2355 (1966). Oxidation potential and uv spectrum: R. A. Day, Jr. *et al., J. Am. Chem. Soc.* **72**, 1379 (1950). Role as an alarm pheromone in carpenter ants: R. M. Duffield, M. S. Blum, *Comp. Biochem. Physiol.* **51B**, 281 (1975); in herbivore and parasitoid response profiles: R. Ramachandran *et al., J. Agric. Food Chem.* **39**, 2310 (1991). Colorimetric determn: D. H. E. Tattje, C. Scholtens, *Pharm. Weekbl.* **94**, 137 (1959). GC determn in lavender oil: P. A. Stadler, *Helv. Chim. Acta* **43**, 1601 (1960). Extraction from king oyster mushrooms: J.-L. Mau *et al., J. Agric. Food Chem.* **46**, 4587 (1998).

Colorless to slightly yellow liquid; sharp, pungent, somewhat fruity odor. bp 162-165°. bp_{30} 76-77°. $bp_{1.5}$ 55-58°. n_D^{20} 1.4153-1.4154 (Naves); also reported as n_D^{21} 1.4179 (Stadler). d^{21} 0.8260. uv max (methanol): 278 nm (ε 23.7).

USE: Ingredient in lavender perfumes; mushroom and pungent cheese flavors.

6754. Octenidine. [71251-02-0] N,N'-(1,10-Decanediyldi-1(4H)-pyridinyl-4-ylidene)bis[1-octanamine]; 1,10-bis-[4-(octylamino)-1-pyridinium]decane; Win-41464. $C_{36}H_{62}N_4$; mol wt 550.90. C 78.49%, H 11.34%, N 10.17%. Prepn: D. M. Bailey, **BE 851807**; *idem*, **US 4206215** (1977, 1980 both to Sterling); D. M. Bailey *et al., J. Med. Chem.* **27**, 1457 (1984). Structure-activity study: A. M. Slee *et al., Antimicrob. Agents Chemother.* **23**, 531 (1983). Antiplaque activity: A. M. Slee, J. R. O'Connor, *ibid.* 379; microbiocidal activity: D. M. Sedlock, D. M. Bailey, *ibid.* **28**, 786 (1985). Antimycotic effects: M. A. Ghannoum *et al., J. Antimicrob. Chemother.* **25**, 237 (1990). Clinical evaluation as topical disinfectant: B. Christiansen, *Z. Bakteriol. Mikrobiol. Hyg.* **186**, 368 (1988). Clinical trials in prevention of plaque and gingivitis: M. R. Patters *et al., J. Periodontal Res.* **21**, 154 (1986); B. B. Beiswanger *et al., J. Dent. Res.* **69**, 454 (1990).

$CH_3(CH_2)_7N$ [structure] $N-(CH_2)_{10}-N$ [structure] $N(CH_2)_7CH_3$

Dihydrochloride. [70775-75-6] Win-41464-2; Neo Kodan; Octeniderm; Octenisept. $C_{36}H_{62}N_2 \cdot 2HCl$; mol wt 595.81. Solid from ether, mp 215-217°.

Disaccharin. [86767-75-1] Win-41464-6. $C_{36}H_{62}N_2 \cdot 2C_7H_5$-$NO_3S$; mol wt 889.26.

THERAP CAT: Antiseptic (topical).

6755. Octhilinone. [26530-20-1] 2-Octyl-3(2H)-isothiazolone; 2-octyl-4-isothiazolin-3-one; RH-893; Kathon. $C_{11}H_{19}NOS$;

mol wt 213.34. C 61.93%, H 8.98%, N 6.57%, O 7.50%, S 15.03%. Prepn: S. N. Lewis *et al.,* **FR 1555416** corresp to **US 3761488** (1969, 1973 to Rohm & Haas); *eidem, J. Heterocycl. Chem.* **8**, 571 (1971).

[chemical structure]

Liquid, $bp_{0.01}$ 120°. uv max (methanol): 280 nm (log ε 3.88). USE: Fungicide. Biocide in cooling-tower water, paints, cutting oils, cosmetics and shampoo; for leather preservation.

6756. Octocrylene. [6197-30-4] 2-Cyano-3,3-diphenyl-2-propenoic acid 2-ethylhexyl ester; 2-ethylhexyl-2-cyano-3,3-diphenylacrylate; Eusolex OCR; Neo Heliopan 303; Uvinul 3039. $C_{24}H_{27}NO_2$; mol wt 361.48. C 79.74%, H 7.53%, N 3.87%, O 8.85%. Photostable UV-B filter in sunscreens and cosmetics. Prepn: A. F. Strobel, S. C. Catino, **BE 619809**; *eidem*, **US 3215724** (1962, 1965 both to General Aniline & Film Corp.). Toxicity study: M. R. Odio *et al., Fundam. Appl. Toxicol.* **22**, 355 (1994). HPTLC determn in sun protection lotions: J. Fisher, J. Sherma, *J. Planar Chromatogr. Mod. TLC* **13**, 388 (2000).

[chemical structure]

Clear yellow viscous liquid, $bp_{0.9}$ 205-209°. fp −10°. d^{25} 1.05. uv max: 303 nm. Miscible in methanol, *n*-butanol, ethyl acetate, mineral oil, hexane, toluene. Immiscible in water.

USE: Solvent for solid sunscreens. UV absorber for plastics and paints.

THERAP CAT: Ultraviolet screen.

6757. Octodrine. [543-82-8] 6-Methyl-2-heptanamine; 6-methyl-2-heptylamine; 2-methyl-6-aminoheptane; 6-amino-2-methylheptane; 2-amino-6-methylheptane; α,ε-dimethylhexylamine; 1,5-dimethylhexylamine; SKF-51; Vaporpac. $C_8H_{19}N$; mol wt 129.24. C 74.35%, H 14.82%, N 10.84%. α-Adrenergic agonist. Prepd from the corresponding saturated ketone: Rohrmann, Shonle, *J. Am. Chem. Soc.* **66**, 1516 (1944). Pharmacology: E. J. Fellows, *J. Pharmacol. Exp. Ther.* **90**, 351 (1947).

[chemical structure]

dl-**Form.** Viscous liquid, fishy odor, bp 154-156°. n_D^{24} 1.4200.

Hydrochloride. $C_8H_{19}N \cdot HCl$. Crystals, sol in water. LD_{50} in mice, rats (mg/kg): 59, 41.5 i.p. (Fellows).

Sulfate. $(C_8H_{19}N)_2 \cdot H_2SO_4$. Crystals, sol in water.

THERAP CAT: Decongestant.

6758. Octogen. [2691-41-0] Octahydro-1,3,5,7-tetranitro-1,3,5,7-tetrazocine; 1,3,5,7-tetranitro-1,3,5,7-tetrazacyclooctane; cyclotetramethylene tetranitramine; HMX. $C_4H_8N_8O_8$; mol wt 296.16. C 16.22%, H 2.72%, N 37.84%, O 43.22%. Prepn: H. Fischer, *Ber.* **82**, 192 (1949); A. F. McKay *et al., Can. J. Res.* **27**, 462 (1949). Determn in explosives by infrared: W. Selig, *U.S. Atomic Energy Commission* **UCRL-7873** (part II), 29 (1965); by HPLC: P. Vouros *et al., Anal. Chem.* **49**, 1039 (1977). Mass spec: E. P. Burrows, *Org. Mass Spectrom.* **26**, 1027 (1991). Thermal analysis of phases using x-ray diffraction: M. Herrmann *et al., Z. Kristallogr.* **204**, 121 (1993). ^{14}N-NMR: M. Kony *et al., J. Org. Chem.* **59**, 5623 (1994). Review of syntheses and properties: B. Singh *et al., Def. Sci. J.* **28**, 41-50 (1978); of thermal behavior: T. L. Boggs, *Prog. Astronaut. Aeronaut.* **90**, 121-175 (1984). Review of toxicology and human exposure: *Toxicological Profile for HMX* (PB98-101058, 1997) 130 pp.

Highly explosive! White crystalline solid, mp 281°. Non-hygroscopic. Four polymorphic forms: α, β, γ and δ. Stability at 300 K: $\beta > \alpha > \gamma > \delta$. β is stable at room temp; α at 115-156°C; γ at 156°C; δ at ~170-279°C. Density (g/cm^3): β=1.903; α=1.87; γ=1.82; δ=1.78. Practically insol in water.

USE: In solid propellants and explosives.

6759. Octopamine. [104-14-3] α-(Aminomethyl)-4-hydroxybenzenemethanol; α-(aminomethyl)-*p*-hydroxybenzyl alcohol; 1-(*p*-hydroxyphenyl)-2-aminoethanol; norsympatol; norsynephrine; *p*-hydroxyphenylethanolamine; WV-569. $C_8H_{11}NO_2$; mol wt 153.18. C 62.73%, H 7.24%, N 9.14%, O 20.89%. A biogenic amine that is the phenol analog of noradrenaline (norepinephrine, *q.v.*). It is a neurosecretory product found in several vertebrates and invertebrates. Formed by β-hydroxylation of tyramine by the enzyme dopamine β-hydroxylase: Pisano *et al.*, *Biochim. Biophys. Acta* **43**, 566 (1960). Identification: Erspamer, *Nature* **169**, 375 (1952). Found in the salivary glands of *Octopus vulgaris, O. macropus,* and of *Eledone moschata: idem, Arzneim.-Forsch.* **2**, 253 (1952); in mammalian nerves: Molinoff, Axelrod, *Science* **164**, 428 (1969); in cockroach nervous system: Nathanson, Greengard, *ibid.* **180**, 308 (1973). Prepd synthetically: Asscher, US 2585988 (1952). The natural D(−) form is 3 times more potent than the L(+) form in producing cardiovascular adrenergic responses in anesthetized dogs and cats: Korol, Soffer, *Pharmacologist* **5**, 247 (1963). Prepn of D- and L-forms: Kappe, Armstrong, *J. Med. Chem.* **7**, 569 (1964). In invertebrate nervous systems octopamine may function as a neurotransmitter: Saavedra *et al.*, *Science* **185**, 364 (1974). Effects on neuromuscular transmission in crustacean muscle: C. A. Breen, H. L. Atwood, *Nature* **303**, 716 (1983).

D(−)-Form. [876-04-0] Crystals from hot water which change at about 160° to a compd which melts above 250° (dec). $[\alpha]_D^{25}$ −56.0° (0.1*N* HCl); −37.4° (H$_2$O).

DL-Form hydrochloride. [770-05-8] Epirenor; Norden; Norfen; Norphen (ampules). $C_8H_{11}NO_2 \cdot HCl$; mol wt 189.64. Crystals, dec 170°. Freely sol in water.

THERAP CAT: Adrenergic.

6760. Octotiamine. [137-86-0] 6-(Acetylthio)-8-[[2-[[(4-amino-2-methyl-5-pyrimidinyl)methyl]formylamino]-1-(2-hydroxyethyl)-1-propenyl]dithio]octanoic acid methyl ester; 8-[[2-[*N*-[(4-amino-2-methyl-5-pyrimidinyl)methyl]formamido]-1-(2-hydroxyethyl)propenyl]dithio]-6-mercaptooctanoic acid methyl ester *S*(or 6)-acetate; *S*-(3-acetylthio-7-carbomethoxyheptylthio)thiamine; thiamine 8-(methyl 6-acetyldihydrothioctate) disulfide; Gerostop; Neuvitan; TATD. $C_{23}H_{36}N_4O_5S_3$; mol wt 544.75. C 50.71%, H 6.66%, N 10.28%, O 14.69%, S 17.66%. Prepn: Ohara *et al.*, US 3098856 (1963 to Fujisawa).

E-form

Crystals, mp 106-109°. uv max: 234, 277 nm (ε 16200, 5820).

Hydrochloride. $C_{23}H_{36}N_4O_5S_3 \cdot HCl$. Crystals from ether + abs ethanol, mp 134.5-135°. uv max: 233 nm (ε 23000).

THERAP CAT: Vitamin (enzyme cofactor).

6761. Octoxynol. [9002-93-1] α-[4-(1,1,3,3,-Tetramethylbutyl)phenyl]-ω-hydroxypoly(oxy-1,2-ethanediyl); octylphenoxy polyethoxyethanol; polyethylene glycol *p*-isooctylphenyl ether. Prepd by reacting isooctylphenol with ethylene oxide. Average number of ethylene oxide units (n) per molecule is indicated by number following octoxynol. *See also* nonoxynol. Trademarks for series of octoxynols include *Igepal CA, Polytergent G, Triton X*.

n = 5 to 15

Mixture in which n ranges from about 5 to 15. Pale yellow, viscous liquid. d_4^{25} 1.0595. n_D^{25} 1.4894. Miscible with water, alcohol, acetone. Sol in benzene, toluene. Insol in petr ether. pH of 5% aq soln: 7-9. *Octoxynol-9*, average comp. (n = 9): $C_{34}H_{62}O_{11}$; av mol wt 647. Trademarks of products where n = 9 to 10: *Conco NIX-100, Igepal CA-630, Neutronyx 605, Triton X-100*. Ingredient of *Preceptin*.

USE: Nonionic detergent, emulsifier, dispersing agent. Octoxynol-9 as spermaticide.

6762. Octreotide. [83150-76-9] D-Phenylalanyl-L-cysteinyl-L-phenylalanyl-D-tryptophyl-L-lysyl-L-threonyl-*N*-[2-hydroxy-1-(hydroxymethyl)propyl]-L-cysteinamide cyclic (2 → 7)-disulfide; 1,2-dithia-5,8,11,14,17-pentaazacycloeicosane cyclic peptide deriv; SMS-201-995. $C_{49}H_{66}N_{10}O_{10}S_2$; mol wt 1019.24. C 57.74%, H 6.53%, N 13.74%, O 15.70%, S 6.29%. Octapeptide analog of somatostatin, *q.v.* Prepn: W. Bauer, J. Pless, EP 29579; *eidem,* US 4395403 (1981, 1983 both to Sandoz); and pharmacology: W. Bauer *et al.*, *Life Sci.* **31**, 1133 (1982). Opiate antagonist properties: R. Maurer *et al.*, *Proc. Natl. Acad. Sci. USA* **79**, 4815 (1982). Inhibitory effect on human gastroenteropancreatic hormone secretion: M. E. Kraenzlin *et al.*, *Experientia* **41**, 738 (1985). Endocrine profile in humans: E. del Pozo *et al.*, *Acta Endocrinol.* **111**, 433 (1986). Clinical evaluation in acromegaly: G. Plewe *et al.*, *Lancet* **2**, 782 (1984); in autonomic neuropathy: R. D. Hoeldtke *et al.*, *ibid.* **2**, 602 (1986). Symposium on chemistry, pharmacology and clinical trials: *Scand. J. Gastroenterol.* **21**, Suppl. 119, 1-274 (1986); on clinical evaluation in gastrointestinal endocrine tumors: *Am. J. Med.* **82**, Suppl. 5B, 1-99 (1987).

D-Phe—Cys—Phe—D-Trp—Lys—Thr—Cys—NH

Acetate. [79517-01-4] SMS-201-995ac; Longastatin; Sandostatin. $C_{49}H_{66}N_{10}O_{10}S_2 \cdot xC_2H_4O_2$. $[\alpha]_D^{20}$ −42° (c = 0.5 in 95% acetic acid).

THERAP CAT: Gastric antisecretory agent. Treatment of acromegaly.

6763. Octyl Acetate. [103-09-3] Acetic acid 2-ethylhexyl ester; 2-ethylhexyl acetate. $C_{10}H_{20}O_2$; mol wt 172.26. C 69.72%, H 11.70%, O 18.58%. $CH_3(CH_2)_3CH(C_2H_5)CH_2OOCCH_3$. Toxicity data: H. F. Smyth, C. P. Carpenter, *J. Ind. Hyg. Toxicol.* **26**, 269 (1944).

Liquid. d_{20}^{20} 0.873. bp 199°. mp ~ −80°. n_D^{20} 1.4204. Flash pt, open cup: 190°F (88°C); closed cup: 56°F (13°C). Very slightly sol in water; misc with alcohol, oils, and other organic liquids. LD_{50} orally in rats: 3.0 g/kg (Smyth, Carpenter).

USE: Solvent for nitrocellulose, some resins, waxes, and oils.

6764. *n*-Octyl Bromide. [111-83-1] 1-Bromooctane. $C_8H_{17}Br$; mol wt 193.12. C 49.75%, H 8.87%, Br 41.38%. $CH_3(CH_2)_6CH_2Br$. Prepd from hydrobromic acid and *n*-octanol: O. Kamm, C. S. Marvel, *Org. Synth.* **coll. vol. I**, 30 (2nd ed., 1941); *cf.* Norris *et al.*, *J. Am. Chem. Soc.* **38**, 1076 (1916); Whitmore *et al.*, *ibid.* **67**, 2059 (1945); from PBr$_3$ and *n*-octanol: Coulson *et al.*, *J. Chem. Soc.* **1965**, 2364. Toxicity study: H. F. Smyth *et al.*, *Am. Ind. Hyg. Assoc. J.* **30**, 470 (1969).

Colorless liquid. d_4^{25} 1.108. bp 198-200°. mp −55°. n_D^{25} 1.4503. Insol in water. Miscible with alcohol, ether. LD_{50} orally in rats: 4.49 ml/kg (Smyth).

USE: In organic syntheses.

6765.   *sec*-Octyl Bromide. [557-35-7] 2-Bromooctane. C_8-$H_{17}Br$; mol wt 193.12. C 49.75%, H 8.87%, Br 41.38%. CH_3-$CHBr(CH_2)_5CH_3$. Prepd by the action of PBr_3 on *sec*-octyl alcohol: Hsueh, Marvel, *J. Am. Chem. Soc.* **50,** 856 (1928); Reynolds, Adkins, *ibid.* **51,** 279 (1929); Shriner, Young, *ibid.* **52,** 3332 (1930); Ellis, Reid, *ibid.* **54,** 1680 (1932); Coulson *et al., J. Chem. Soc.* **1965,** 2364.

***dl*-Form.** d_4^{25} 1.0878. bp_{14} 72°. bp_6 66°. bp_3 61°. n_D^{25} 1.4442. Insol in water, miscible with alcohol, ether.

***l*-Form.** d_4^{25} 1.0982. bp_{18} 73°. bp_{14} 71°. bp_3 60°. n_D^{25} 1.4475. α_D^{20} −44.91°.

***d*-Form.** d_4^{25} 1.0982. bp_{18} 77°. bp_{14} 71°. bp_3 60°. n_D^{25} 1.4475.

6766.   Octyl Cyanoacrylate. [6701-17-3] 2-Cyano-2-propenoic acid octyl ester; ocrilate; ocrylate; *n*-octyl α-cyanoacrylate; capryl α-cyanoacrylate; octyl 2-cyanoacrylate; Dermabond; Nexaband; Soothe-N-Seal. $C_{12}H_{19}NO_2$; mol wt 209.28. C 68.87%, H 9.15%, N 6.69%, O 15.29%. Biodegradable, topical surgical glue; upon contact with tissue anions, monomer rapidly polymerizes to form a strong adhesive. Preparative method: A. E. Ardis, **US 2467927** (1949 to B. F. Goodrich). Prepn, polymerization and degradation: F. Leonard *et al., J. Appl. Polym. Sci.* **10,** 259 (1966). Biocompatibility, histomorphology, and clinical characteristics: A. Nitsch *et al., Aesth. Plast. Surg.* **29,** 53 (2005). Clinical trial for closure of lacerations: J. Quinn *et al, J. Am. Med. Assoc.* **277,** 1527 (1997); of lacerations and incisions: A. J. Singer *et al., Surgery* **131,** 270 (2002); for repair of inguinal hernia: G. Miyano *et al., J. Pediatr. Surg.* **39,** 1867 (2004).

$bp_{1.8}$ 117°; d^{20} 0.931; n_D^{20} 1.4489. Surface tension: 29.18 dynes/cm.

Polymer. [26877-34-9] Poly(octyl cyanoacrylate).

THERAP CAT: Tissue adhesive.

THERAP CAT (VET): Tissue adhesive.

6767.   *n*-Octyl-β-D-glucoside. [29836-26-8] Octyl-β-D-glucopyranoside; *n*-octylglucoside; OG. $C_{14}H_{28}O_6$; mol wt 292.37. C 57.51%, H 9.65%, O 32.83%. Nonionic detergent primarily used for solubilizing membrane-bound proteins. Prepn: C. R. Noller, C. W. Rockwell, *J. Am. Chem. Soc.* **60,** 2076 (1938). Partition behavior between water and membrane phases: M. Ueno, *Biochemistry* **28,** 5631 (1989); thermodynamics and structural impact: M. R. Wenk *et al., Biophys. J.* **72,** 1719 (1997). Solubilzation and reconstitution of liposomes: O. López *et al., J. Phys. Chem. B* **105,** 9879 (2001). Solubilization of lipid vesicles: A. Meister, A. Blume, *Phys. Chem. Chem. Phys.* **6,** 1551 (2004). Micelle formation: A. Walter *et al., Biochim. Biophys. Acta* **1508,** 20 (2000); in mixed systems: A. Lainez *et al., Langmuir* **20,** 5745 (2004).

White solid, mp 65-99°. $[\alpha]_D^{25}$ −30.3° (methanol). Critical micelle concentration: 20-25 mM.

USE: Detergent and surfactant for biological systems.

6768.   *sec*-Octyl Iodide. [557-36-8] 2-Iodooctane. $C_8H_{17}I$; mol wt 240.13. C 40.01%, H 7.14%, I 52.85%. CH_3CHI-$(CH_2)_5CH_3$. Prepn: Coulson *et al., J. Chem. Soc.* **1965,** 2364.

***dl*-Form.** Oily liquid; discolors in light. d_{15}^{18} 1.318. bp about 210° with decompn; also stated as 190°. *Protect from air and light.*

***l*-Form.** α_D^{20} −64.63°.

6769.   Octyl Methoxycinnamate. [5466-77-3] 3-(4-Methoxyphenyl)-2-propenoic acid 2-ethylhexyl ester; 2-ethylhexyl *p*-methoxycinnamate; octinoxate; Eusolex 2292; Neo Heliopan AV; Parsol MCX; Uvinul MC 80. $C_{18}H_{26}O_3$; mol wt 290.40. C 74.45%, H 9.02%, O 16.53%. UV-B blocker. Manuf process and purification: P. Schudel *et al.,* **US 4713473** (1987 to Givaudan). Use in sunscreen preparations: D. H. Liem, L. T. H. Hilderink, *Int. J. Cosmet. Sci.* **1,** 341 (1979). Assessment of photostability: R. Aberturas *et al., Boll. Chim. Farm.* **126,** 208 (1987); A. Deflandre, G. Lang, *Int. J. Cosmet. Sci.* **10,** 53 (1988). HPLC determn in cosmetics: L. Gagliardi *et al., J. Chromatogr.* **408,** 409 (1987). Effect of reflectance of light on protection of skin: G. J. Smith *et al., Photochem. Photobiol.* **75,** 122 (2002).

bp at 1 mbar: 185-195°; bp at 0.1 mbar: 140-150°.

THERAP CAT: Ultraviolet screen.

6770.   Octyl Salicylate. [118-60-5] 2-Hydroxybenzoic acid 2-ethylhexyl ester; 2-ethylhexyl salicylate; octisalate; Eusolex OS; Neo Heliopan OS. $C_{15}H_{22}O_3$; mol wt 250.33. C 71.97%, H 8.86%, O 19.17%. UV-B filter in sunscreens and cosmetics. Prepn: F. H. McMillan, J. A. King, *J. Am. Chem. Soc.* **67,** 2271 (1945). *In vitro* skin penetration studies: K. A. Walters *et al., Food Chem. Toxicol.* **35,** 1219 (1997); R. Jiang *et al., J. Pharm. Sci.* **86,** 791 (1997). Determn in sun protection lotions by GC-MS: K. W. Ro *et al., J. Chromatogr. A* **688,** 375 (1994); by HPTLC: E. Westgate, J. Sherma, *Am. Lab.* **32,** 13 (2000).

Colorless to pale yellow liquid, bp_{21} 189-190°. n_D^{25} 1.5018. Misc with cosmetic oils, silicone oils.

USE: Solvent for solid sunscreens.

THERAP CAT: Ultraviolet screen.

6771.   Ofloxacin. [82419-36-1] 9-Fluoro-2,3-dihydro-3-methyl-10-(4-methyl-1-piperazinyl)-7-oxo-7*H*-pyrido[1,2,3-*de*]-1,4-benzoxazine-6-carboxylic acid; ofloxacine; DL-8280; HOE-280; Exocin; Flobacin; Floxil; Floxin; Monoflocet; Oculflox; Oflocet; Oflocin; Tarivid. $C_{18}H_{20}FN_3O_4$; mol wt 361.37. C 59.83%, H 5.58%, F 5.26%, N 11.63%, O 17.71%. Broad spectrum, fluorinated quinolone antibacterial. Prepn: I. Hayakawa *et al.,* **EP 47005;** *eidem,* **US 4382892** (1982, 1983 both to Daiichi). Total synthesis: H. Egawa *et al., Chem. Pharm. Bull.* **34,** 4098 (1986). Synthesis and activity of optical isomers: S. Atarashi *et al., ibid.* **35,** 1896 (1987). Antibacterial spectrum of racemate: K. Sato *et al., Antimicrob. Agents Chemother.* **22,** 548 (1982). Mechanism of differential activity of enantiomers: I. Morrissey *et al., ibid.* **40,** 1775 (1996). Toxicity data: H. Ohno *et al., Chemotherapy (Tokyo)* **32,** Suppl. 1, 1084 (1984). Pharmacology and clinical efficacy: *Infection* **14,** Suppl. 1, S1-S109 (1986). Symposium on pharmacokinetics and therapeutic use: *Scand. J. Infect. Dis.* **Suppl. 68,** 1-69 (1990). Review of antibacterial spectrum, pharmacology, and clinical efficacy: J. P. Monk, D. M. Campoli-Richards, *Drugs* **33,** 346-391 (1987); of mechanism of action: K. Drlica, *Curr. Opin. Microbiol.* **2,** 504-508 (1999).

Colorless needles from ethanol, mp 250-257° (dec). LD_{50} in male, female mice, male, female rats (mg/kg): 5450, 5290, 3590,

3750 orally; 208, 233, 273, 276 i.v.; >10000, >10000, 7070, 9000 s.c. (Ohno).

S-(−)-Form. [100986-85-4]; [138199-71-0] (hemihydrate). Levofloxacin; DR-3355; Cravit; Levaquin; Tavanic; Quixin. Toxicity study: M. Kato *et al.*, *Arzneim.-Forsch.* **42**, 365 (1992). Series of articles on pharmacology and toxicology: *ibid.*, 368-418. Clinical study in bacterial conjunctivitis: D. G. Hwang *et al.*, *Br. J. Ophthalmol.* **87**, 1004 (2003). *Review:* D. S. North *et al.*, *Pharmacotherapy* **18**, 915-935 (1998). Prepd as the hemihydrate; needles from ethanol + ethyl ether, mp 225-227° (dec). $[\alpha]_D^{23}$ −76.9° (c = 0.385 in 0.5N NaOH). Freely sol in glacial acetic acid, chloroform; sparingly sol in water. LD_{50} in male, female mice, male, female rats (mg/kg): 1881, 1803, 1478, 1507 orally (Kato).

THERAP CAT: Antibacterial.

6772. Oil Anise, Japanese. Volatile oil from fruit of *Illicium anisatum* L., *Magnoliaceae* (Japanese star anise). *Constit.* Chiefly anethole; also safrol, eugenol.

Colorless to slightly yellow liquid. d about 1.006. Solidifies at −10° to −15°. α_D^{20} about −8°.

THERAP CAT: Carminative; expectorant.

6773. Oil Bergamot. Volatile oil expressed from rind of fresh fruit of *Citrus aurantium L.*, var. *bergamia* Wight & Arn., *Rutaceae.* *Constit.* 36-45% *l*-linalyl acetate, about 6% *l*-linalool; *d*-limonene, dipentene, bergaptene.

Yellowish-green liquid; agreeable odor. d_{25}^{25} 0.875-0.880. α_D^{25} +8 to +24°. n_D^{20} 1.464-1.467. Acid no. 1-4. Almost insol in water. Sol in 0.5 vol 95% alcohol, 2 vols 80% alcohol. *Keep well closed in a cool place, protected from light.*

USE: For masking many disagreeable odors, such as iodoform, naphthalene, etc. In perfumery, hair oils, pomades.

6774. Oil of Balm. Oil of melissa balm; oil of lemon balm. Volatile oil from leaves and tops of *Melissa officinalis* L., *Labiatae.* Chiefly citral. Composition studies: Hefendehl, *Arch. Pharm.* **303**, 345 (1970).

Yellow to yellowish-green liquid. d_{15}^{15} 0.89-0.925. Practically insol in water. Sol in alcohol. *Keep well closed, cool, and protected from light.*

6775. Oil of Basil. Volatile oil from leaves of *Ocimum basilicum* L., *Labiatae* (sweet basil). *Constit.* Methylchavicol, eucalyptol, linalool, estragol.

Yellowish to greenish liquid; aromatic odor. d_{20}^{20} 0.905-0.930. α_D^{20} −6 to −22°. Almost insol in water. Sol in 2 vols 80% alc; miscible with ether, chloroform. *Keep well closed, cool and protected from light.*

6776. Oil of Bay. Oil of Myrcia. Volatile oil distilled from leaves of *Pimenta (Myrcia) acris* Kostel., *Myrtaceae.* *Constit.* 40-55% eugenol; myrcene, chavicol, methyleugenol, methylchavicol, citral, *l*-phellandrene; total phenols, 50-65% by volume.

Yellow to brownish-yellow liq; pleasant odor; sharp, spicy taste; becomes brown on exposure to air. d_{25}^{25} 0.962-0.990. α_D^{25} −3°. n_D^{20} 1.500-1.520. Insoluble in water. Very sol in alcohol, carbon disulfide, glacial acetic acid.

USE: Pharmaceutic aid (aromatic). Manuf bay rum.

6777. Oil of Bitter Almond. Volatile oil from dried ripe kernels of bitter almonds or from other kernels containing amygdalin, such as apricots, cherries, plums, and especially peaches. Obtained by macerating with water, then steam distilling. *Constit.* Not less than 95% benzaldehyde; 2-4% HCN and phenoxyacetonitrile.

Colorless to yellow, very refractive liq; characteristic odor and taste of benzaldehyde. d_{25}^{25} 1.038-1.060. n_D^{20} 1.5428-1.5439. Slightly sol in water; miscible with alcohol, ether, oils. *Keep cool and protected from light.*

Caution: Hydrogen cyanide, *q.v.*, component responsible for highly toxic properties. *Very poisonous!*

USE: Only the oil *free from HCN* may be used for liqueurs and foods.

THERAP CAT: Formerly as topical antipruritic.

6778. Oil of Bitter Orange. Volatile oil expressed from fresh peel of *Citrus aurantium* L., *Rutaceae.* *Constit.* About 90% *d*-

limonene; citral, decyl aldehyde, methyl anthranilate, linalool, terpineol.

Pale yellow liquid; bitter taste. d_{25}^{25} 0.842-0.848. α_D^{25} +88 to +98°. Very slightly sol in water; miscible with abs alcohol; sol in 4 vols alcohol, in 1 vol glacial acetic acid. *Keep well closed, cool, and protected from light.*

USE: As flavoring; in perfumery.

6779. Oil of Cajeput. Cajuput oil; cajeputi oil. Volatile oil from fresh leaves and twigs of several varieties of *Melaleuca leucadendron* L., and other species of *Melaleuca, Myrtaceae.* *Constit.* 50-60% eucalyptol (cineol); *l*-pinene, terpineol; valeric, butyric, benzoic and other aldehydes. Toxicity: P. M. Jenner *et al.*, *Food Cosmet. Toxicol.* **2**, 327 (1964).

Colorless or yellowish liquid, agreeable aromatic odor, and bitter aromatic taste. d 0.912-0.925. α_D^{20} <−4°. n_D^{20} 1.4660-1.4710. Very slightly sol in water; sol in 1 vol 80% alcohol. Misc with alcohol, chloroform, ether, carbon disulfide. *Keep well closed, cool, and protected from light.* LD_{50} orally in rats: 3870 mg/kg (Jenner).

THERAP CAT: Expectorant, counterirritant, scabicide.

THERAP CAT (VET): Rubefacient, topical antimycotic.

6780. Oil of Camphor, Rectified. Formosa oil of camphor; Japanese oil of camphor; white oil of camphor; light oil of camphor. Volatile oil from *Cinnamomum camphora* T. Nees & Eberm., *Lauraceae.* *Constit.* Safrol, acetaldehyde, camphor, terpineol, eugenol, cineol, *d*-pinene, phellandrene, dipentene, cadinene.

Colorless or yellowish liquid; camphor odor. d_{20}^{20} 0.875-0.900. α_D^{20} +9 to +24°. n_D^{20} 1.465-1.470. Insol in water. Sol in chloroform, ether, oils, in about 3 vols alcohol. *Keep well closed, cool, and protected from light.*

USE: As solvent in paint and lacquer industry; in perfuming of soaps and detergents; in technical odor masking.

THERAP CAT: Rubefacient.

6781. Oil of Cashew Nut Shell. From *Anacardium occidentale* L., *Anacardiaceae* (Southern India). Consists mostly (90%) of anacardic acid, *q.v.* Review and bibliography: Sanyal, Das, *Indian Pharm.* **10**, 272-283 (1955).

Wijs iodine no. over 250. Polymerizes easily when heated with acid.

USE: In insulating varnishes, typewriter rolls, coldsetting cements, floor tile, brake linings; molding compounds from polymers: Harvey, US **2767150** (1956 to The Harvel Corp.).

6782. Oil of Cedar Wood. Volatile oil from wood of *Juniperus virginiana* L., *Cupressaceae,* and other species of cedar. *Constit.* Chiefly cedrene (a terpene), and cedral (cedar camphor).

Colorless or slightly yellow, somewhat viscid liquid. d_{20}^{20} 0.940-0.950. α_D^{20} −25 to −46°. n_D^{20} 1.495-1.510. Insol in water. Sol in 10-20 vols 90% alcohol; sol in ether. *Keep well closed, cool, and protected from light.*

USE: In perfumery; as insect repellent; the thickened oil is used in microscopy as a clearing agent and for use with immersion lenses.

6783. Oil of Celery. Volatile oil from celery seed, *Apium graveolens* L., *Umbelliferae.* *Constit.* *d*-Limonene, phenols, sedanolide, sedanoic acid.

Colorless liquid; celery odor. d 0.870-0.895. α_D^{20} +67 to +79°. Slightly sol in water; very sol in alcohol. *Keep well closed, cool, and protected from light.*

USE: As flavor for soft drinks, unpleasant medicaments.

6784. Oil of Champaca. Volatile oil from flowers of *Michelia champaca* L., *Magnoliaceae.* *Constit.* Esters of benzoic acid, benzaldehyde, benzyl alcohol, isoeugenol.

Light yellow or reddish-yellow to brownish liquid. d_{15}^{15} 0.906-0.935. α_D −12 to −52°. Sapon no. ~77. Slightly sol in water; sol in chloroform, ether; sparingly sol in alcohol. *Keep well closed, cool and protected from light.*

USE: In perfumes.

6785. Oil of Chenopodium. Oil of American wormseed; Chenopodiol; Chenoposan; Chenoposetten. Volatile oil from fresh, aboveground parts of flowering and fruiting plant of *American wormseed, Chenopodium ambrosioides* L. var. *anthelminticum* (L.) Aellen, *Chenopodiaceae* also known as *Mexican tea, Spanish tea, Jerusalem tea, ambrosia.* Habit. Central America, U.S.,

Canada. Oil contains 60-70% ascaridole, the principal active constituent; *p*-cymene, α-terpinene, *l*-limonene, methadiene.

Colorless or pale yellow liquid; characteristic disagreeable odor and taste. d$_{25}^{25}$ 0.950-0.980. α$_D^{20}$ −4 to −8°. n$_D^{20}$ 1.4723-1.4790. Insoluble in water. Sol in 8 vols 70% alcohol; partly sol in glacial acetic acid. *Keep well closed, cool and protected from light.*

THERAP CAT: Anthelmintic.

THERAP CAT (VET): Anthelmintic.

6786. Oil of Cherry Laurel. Volatile oil from leaves of *Prunus laurocerasus* L., *Rosaceae. Constit.* HCN, benzaldehyde, benzaldehyde cyanhydrin, benzyl alcohol.

Pale yellow liquid; odor and taste similar to oil of bitter almond. *Very poisonous!* d$_{20}^{20}$ 1.054-1.066. Slightly sol in water; sol in 2 vols 70% alcohol, in benzene, chloroform, ether. *Keep well closed, cool and protected from light.*

Caution: Hydrogen cyanide, *q.v.*, component responsible for highly toxic properties.

6787. Oil of Citronella. Volatile oil from fresh grass of *Cymbopogon (Andropogon) nardus* (L.) Rendle, *Gramineae. Constit.* Ceylon: about 60% geraniol, about 15% citronellal, 10-15% camphene and dipentene, small quantities of linalool, borneol. Java: 25-50% citronellal, 25-45% geraniol.

Almost colorless to pale yellow liq; gradually becomes reddish; pleasant odor. d Ceylon, 0.897-0.912; Java, 0.885-0.900. α$_D^{20}$: Ceylon, −6 to −14°; Java, −2 to −5°. n$_D^{20}$ Ceylon 1.479-1.485; Java, 1.468-1.473. Slightly sol in water; sol in 10 vols 80% alcohol. *Keep well closed, cool and protected from light.*

USE: As perfume; insect repellent.

6788. Oil of Cumin. Volatile oil from fruit of *Cuminum cyminum* L., *Umbelliferae. Constit.* 30-40% cuminaldehyde; *p*-cymene, β-pinene, dipentene.

Colorless to yellow liquid. d$_{25}^{25}$ 0.900-0.935. α$_D^{20}$ +4 to +8°. n$_D^{20}$ 1.4950-1.5090. Almost insol in water; sol in 10 vols 80% alcohol; more sol in stronger alcohol; very sol in chloroform, ether. *Keep well closed, cool and protected from light.*

USE: Flavoring in Indian curry powder.

6789. Oil of Cypress. Volatile oil from leaves and young branches of *Cupressus sempervirens* L., *Pinaceae. Constit.* Furfural, *d*-pinene, *d*-camphene, cymene, *d*-terpineol, *l*-cadinene, sylvestrene, cypress camphor.

Yellowish liquid. d 0.88-0.89. α$_D^{20}$ +4 to +18°. Slightly sol in water; sol in 2-6 vols 90% alcohol. *Keep well closed, cool and protected from light.*

USE: In perfumery.

6790. Oil of Dill. Dill seed oil; dill fruit oil. Volatile oil from dried ripe fruit of *Anethum graveolens* L., *Umbelliferae. Constit.* About 50% carvone *d*-limonene, phellandrene and other terpenes.

Colorless or pale yellow liquid; characteristic odor. d$_{15}^{15}$ 0.900-0.915. α$_D^{20}$ +70 to +80°. n$_D^{20}$ 1.481-1.492. Insol in water; sol in 1 vol 90% alcohol. *Keep well closed, cool and protected from light.*

THERAP CAT: Aromatic carminative.

6791. Oil of Dwarf Pine Needles. Oil of mountain pine; Pinus Montana oil; Pinus pumilio oil. Volatile oil from fresh leaves of *Pinus montana* Mill. (*P. pumilio* Haenke), *Pinaceae. Constit. l*-Pinene, *l*-phellandrene, sylvestrene, dipentene, cadinene, 5-7% bornyl acetate.

Colorless or faintly yellow liq; pleasant odor; bitter taste. d$_{25}^{25}$ 0.853-0.869. α$_D^{25}$ −5 to −12°. n$_D^{20}$ 1.4750-1.4800. Insol in water. Sol in 4.5-8 vols 90% alcohol; very sol in chloroform, ether. *Keep well closed, cool and protected from light.*

USE: Pharmaceutic aid (flavor and perfume).

THERAP CAT: Expectorant.

6792. Oil of Fir. Oil of silver pine; oil of silver fir. Volatile oil from needles and young twigs of *Abies alba* Mill. (*A. picea* Lindl., *A. pectinata* DC.), *Pinaceae. Constit. l*-Pinene, *l*-limonene, *l*-bornyl acetate.

Colorless, clear liquid; balsamic odor; terebinthinate taste. d$_{15}^{15}$ 0.869-0.875. α$_D^{20}$ −20 to −59°. Insol in water. Sol in 5 vols 90% alc, in ether. *Keep well closed, cool and protected from light.*

USE: Pharmaceutic aid (flavor and perfume).

THERAP CAT: Expectorant.

6793. Oil of Fir —Siberian. Oil of pine; oleum abietis; Siberian pine needle oil. Volatile oil from fresh leaves of *Abies sibirica* Ledeb., *Pinaceae. Constit.* About 40% esters calculated as bornyl acetate; pinene, camphene, dipentene, and phellandrene.

Colorless or pale yellow liquid; aromatic odor; pungent taste. d$_{15}^{15}$ 0.905-0.925. α$_D^{20}$ −32 to −45°. n$_D^{20}$ 1.466-1.476. Sol in an equal vol 90% alcohol. *Keep well closed, cool and protected from light.*

USE: Pharmaceutic aid (flavor and perfume).

THERAP CAT: Expectorant.

6794. Oil of Fleabane. Oil of Canada fleabane; oil of erigeron. Volatile oil from fresh flowering herb of *Conyza canadensis* (L.) Cron. (*Erigeron canadensis* L., *Leptilon canadense* (L.)) Britt., *Compositae. Constit. d*-Limonene, aldehydes.

Pale yellow liquid; becomes darker and thicker with age and on exposure to air; peculiar odor; aromatic, slightly pungent taste. d$_{25}^{25}$ 0.845-0.865. α$_D^{20}$ ~+45°. Slightly sol in water; sol in 1 vol alcohol; very sol in chloroform, ether. *Keep well closed, cool and protected from light.*

6795. Oil of Geranium. Oil of pelargonium geranium; oil of rose geranium. Volatile oil from leaves of *Pelargonium odoratissimum* Ait. and allied species, *Geraniaceae. Constit.* Geraniol esters, calculated as geranyl tiglate, 21-30% in Algerian or French oil, 25-35% in Bourbon oil; citronellol; some linalool.

Colorless, greenish or brownish liquid. d$_{15}^{15}$ 0.894-0.905. α$_D^{20}$ −7 to −11°. n$_D^{20}$ 1.4650-1.470. Slightly sol in water; sol in 3 vols 10% alcohol; more sol in stronger alcohol; very sol in chloroform, ether. *Keep well closed, cool and protected from light.*

USE: In perfumery; as odorant for tooth and dusting powders, ointments, etc. In manuf of rhodinol, *q.v.*

6796. Oil of Geranium —East Indian. Turkish geranium oil; palmarosa oil; Indian grass oil; rusa oil. Volatile oil from *Andropogon schoenanthus* L., *Gramineae*, and allied species grown in India (not Turkey). *Constit.* 85-95% geraniol; citronellol, dipentene; it is practically devoid of esters.

Colorless or light yellow liquid; pleasant rose odor. d$_{15}^{15}$ 0.885-0.896. α$_D$ +1.67 to −2°. n$_D^{20}$ 1.476-1.4085.

6797. Oil of Hyssop. Volatile oil from *Hyssopus officinalis* L., *Labiatae. Constit.* About 50% pinene, small quantities of aromatic alcohol, probably also sesquiterpenes.

Colorless or greenish-yellow liquid; sharp, camphor-like taste. d$_{15}^{15}$ 0.925-0.940. α$_D^{20}$ −17 to −23°. bp ~200°. Almost insol in water; sol in 2 to 4 vols 80% alcohol. *Keep well closed and protected from light.*

6798. Oil of Lemon. Cedro oil. Volatile oil expressed from fresh peel of *Citrus limonum* (L.) Risso (*C. medica* var. *limon* L.), *Rutaceae. Constit.* About 90% of limonene, terpinene, phellandrene, and pinene combined; 4-6% aldehydes calculated as citral, some citronellal, geranyl acetate, sesquiterpenes.

Pale yellow or greenish-yellow liquid. d$_{25}^{25}$ 0.849-0.855. α$_D^{25}$ +57 to +65.6°. n$_D^{20}$ 1.4742-1.4755. Slightly sol in water; sol in 3 vols alcohol; miscible with carbon disulfide, glacial acetic acid. *Keep cool, in well-filled and well-closed bottles, protected from light.*

USE: For flavoring medicaments; as a flavor in liqueurs, pastry, foods, beverages; also in perfumes.

6799. Oil of Lemon Grass. Indian oil of verbena; Indian melissa oil. Volatile oil from *Cymbopogon (Andropogon) citratus* (DC.) Stapf, and of *C. flexuosus* (Nees) Stapf, *Gramineae. Constit.* 75-85% citral; methylheptenone, citronellal, geraniol, limonene, dipentene.

Reddish-yellow or brownish-red liquid; strong odor of verbena. d$_{15}^{15}$ 0.895-0.908 (0.878-0.882 of West Indian oil). α$_D$ −3°. n$_D^{20}$ 1.483-1.489. Slightly sol in water; sol in 3 vols 70% alcohol; sol in chloroform, ether. *Keep well closed, cool and protected from light.*

USE: As source of citral (synthesis of vitamin A) and in perfumery.

6800. Oil of Levant Wormseed. Volatile oil from the flowers of *Artemisia maritima* var *stechmanniana* Bess (*A. pauciflora* Weber), *Compositae. Constit.* Largely eucalyptol (cineol).

Pale yellow to yellowish-green liquid. d$_{20}^{20}$ 0.915-0.940. Insol in water; sol in alcohol, ether. *Keep well closed, cool and protected from light.*

THERAP CAT: Anthelmintic.

6801. Oil of Linaloe. Volatile oil distilled from a Mexican wood *(Bursera delpechiana* Poiss. and probably other species of *Bursera, Burseraceae). Constit.* Linalool, geraniol, methyl-heptenone.

Colorless to yellowish liquid; pleasant odor. d_{15}^{15} 0.875-0.890. α_D −5 to −12°. n_D^{20} 1.4638. Slightly sol in water; sol in 2 vols 70% alcohol; sol in ether, chloroform. *Keep well closed, cool and protected from light.*

USE: In perfumery.

6802. Oil of Marjoram. Volatile oil from *Origanum marjorana* L., *Labiatae. Constit.* About 40% terpenes, chiefly terpinene; *d*-terpineol.

Yellow or greenish-yellow liquid. d_{15}^{15} 0.888-0.912. α_D^{20} +13 to +18°. Insol in water; sol in 2 vols 80% alcohol; sol in chloroform, ether.

USE: In perfumes and microscopy.

6803. Oil of Myrtle. Volatile oil from leaves of *Myrtus communis* L., *Myrtaceae. Constit. d*-Pinene, eucalyptol, dipentene, camphor.

Yellow to greenish liquid; fragrant odor. d_{15}^{15} 0.890-0.915. α_D +10 to +30°. Insol in water; sol in alcohol, chloroform, ether.

6804. Oil of Niaouli. Volatile oil from leaves of *Melaleuca viridiflora* (Soland.) Gaertn., *Myrtaceae. Constit.* About 65% cineol, about 30% terpineol, limonene and *d*-pinene combined.

Slightly yellow liquid; aromatic odor; pungent, refreshing peppermint-like taste. d_{15}^{15} 0.908-0.932. Insol in water or glycerol; sol in alcohol, benzene, ether.

THERAP CAT: Anthelmintic.

6805. Oil of Orange. Oil sweet orange. Volatile oil expressed from fresh peel of ripe fruit of the orange *(Citrus aurantium* var *sinensis* L., *Rutaceae). Constit.* About 90% *d*-limonene; citral, decyl aldehyde, methyl anthranilate, linalool, terpineol.

Yellow to deep orange liquid; characteristic orange taste and odor. d_{25}^{25} 0.842-0.846. α_D^{25} +94 to +99°. n_D^{20} 1.4723-1.4737. Slightly sol in water; sol in 2 vols 90% alcohol, in 1 vol glacial acetic acid; miscible with abs alcohol, carbon disulfide. *Keep well closed, cool and protected from light.*

USE: Chiefly as flavor and perfume. Pharmaceutical aid (flavor).

THERAP CAT: Expectorant.

6806. Oil of Orange Flowers. Oil of neroli. Volatile oil distilled from fresh orange flowers. *Constit.* Limonene, *l*-linalool, geraniol, 7-18% linalyl acetate; some methyl anthranilate, nerol and neroli camphor.

Yellowish, fluorescent liquid; very intense and pleasant odor; becomes brown on exposure to light. d_{25}^{25} 0.86-0.88. $[\alpha]_D^{25}$ +1.50 to +9.13°. n_D^{20} 1.475. Slightly sol in water; sol in 1.5-2 vols 80% alcohol with fine violet fluorescence. *Keep well closed, cool and protected from light.*

USE: As perfume and flavor.

6807. Oil of Origanum. Oil of wild marjoram. Volatile oil from flowering tops of *Origanum vulgare* L., *Labiatae. Constit.* Carvacrol, terpenes.

Light yellow liquid. d_{15}^{15} 0.870-0.910. α_D ~ −34°. Very slightly sol in water; very sol in alcohol. *Keep well closed, cool and protected from light.*

USE: In perfumery.

6808. Oil of Patchouli. Patchouli oil. Essential oil from leaves of several *Labiatae* species. The commercial oil is obtained from the cultivated species, *Pogostemon cablin* (Blanco) Benth. (*P. patchouly* Pellet. var *suavis* Hook. f.), *Labiatae.* Major constituent is patchouli alcohol, *q.v.,* minor constituents include patchoulene, azulene, eugenol, and several unidentified sesquiterpenes: Pfau, Plattner, *Helv. Chim. Acta* **19**, 874 (1936); Naoko *et al., Bull. Chem. Soc. Jpn.* **40,** 597 (1967). *Review:* E. Guenther, *The Essential Oils* **vol. III** (Van Nostrand, New York, 1949) pp 552-575.

Yellowish or greenish to dark brown oil, intense and persistent fragrant odor. Can be stored indefinitely. Odor seems to improve with age. d_{15}^{15} 0.975-0.987. $[\alpha]_D$ −54 to −65.3°. n_D^{20} 1.5099 to 1.5111. Saponif no. 3.3 to 9.3. Ester no. after acetylation: 17.7 to 22.4. Practically insol in water. Soluble in ether.

USE: In perfume formulations to impart a lasting oriental fragrance, in incense, soaps, cosmetics. To scent fine Indian fabrics and shawls.

6809. Oil of Pettigrain. Volatile oil from leaves, twigs and unripe fruit of *Citrus vulgaris* Risso (*C. bigaradia* Loisel.), *Rutaceae. Constit.* 40-80% linalyl acetate; geraniol, geranyl acetate, limonene.

Yellow liquid. d_{15}^{15} 0.887-0.900. α_D^{20} +3.72 to −1.37°. n_D^{20} 1.4623. Slightly sol in water; sol in 2 vols 80% alcohol. *Keep well closed, cool and protected from light.*

USE: In perfumes.

6810. Oil of Pine Needles. Oil of Scotch fir; fir-wood oil. Volatile oil from *Pinus sylvestris* L., *Pinaceae. Constit.* Dipentene, pinene, sylvestrene, cadinene, 3-3.5% bornyl acetate.

Yellowish liquid. d_{15}^{15} 0.884-0.886. α_D^{20} +7.05 to +10°. Insol in water. Sol in 10 vols 90% alcohol. *Keep well closed, cool and protected from light.*

USE: Pharmaceutical aid (flavor and perfume).

THERAP CAT: Expectorant.

6811. Oil of Rose. Otto of rose; essence of rose; attar of rose. Volatile oil from fresh flowers of *Rosa gallica* L. and *R. damascena* Mill. and varieties of these species *(Rosaceae). Constit.* 70-75% free geraniol and citronellol; small amounts of their esters; terpenes.

Colorless to pale yellow liquid; viscous at 25°; highly fragrant, rose odor. d_{15}^{30} 0.848-0.863. Congeals at 18-22° to a translucent, cryst mass. α_D^{25} −1 to −4°. n_D^{30} 1.457-1.463. Very slightly sol in water, sparingly sol in alcohol; sol in fatty oils, chloroform. *Keep cool in well-closed and well-filled containers and protected from light.*

USE: Largely in perfumery; for flavoring lozenges, ointments, and toilet prepns.

6812. Oil of Rue. Volatile oil from *Ruta graveolens* L., Rutaceae. *Constit.* About 90% methyl nonyl ketone, methyl anthranilate.

Pale yellow liquid; characteristic, sharp, unpleasant odor, but odor is pleasant on dilution. d_{15}^{15} 0.832-0.845. Solidif +8° to +10°. Optically inactive or slightly dextrorotatory. n_D^{20} 1.430-1.440. Almost insol in water; sol in 3 vols 70% alcohol. *Keep well closed, cool and protected from light.*

Caution: Frequent dermal contact produces erythema, vesication. Ingestion of large quantities causes epigastric pain, nausea, vomiting, confusion, convulsions, death; may cause abortion.

USE: Flavoring agent in food.

6813. Oil of Sweet Almond. Expressed almond oil. Fixed oil from kernels of varieties of *Prunus amygdalus* Stokes (*Amygdalus communis* L.), *Rosaceae. Constit.* Chiefly glyceryl oleate with small amounts of glycerides of linolic, etc., acids. Stated to contain no stearic acid.

Colorless or pale yellow, almost odorless, oily liq; bland taste. d_{25}^{25} 0.910-0.915. It is clear at −10°; congeals near −20°. n_D^{40} 1.4593-1.4646. Sapon no. 191-200. Iodine no. 93-100. Insol in water. Slightly sol in alcohol; miscible with benzene, chloroform, ether, petr ether. *Keep well closed, cool and protected from light.*

USE: In perfumery, manuf fine soaps; as lubricant for delicate mechanisms such as watches, firearms, etc. Emollient.

THERAP CAT: Cathartic.

6814. Oil of Tansy. Volatile oil from leaves and tops of *Tanacetum vulgare* L., *Compositae. Constit.* Thujone, borneol, camphor.

Yellow liq; becomes brown on exposure to air and light. *Poisonous!* d_{15}^{15} 0.925-0.950. α_D +30 to +45°. Almost insol in water; sol in alcohol, chloroform, ether. *Keep cool in well-filled and well-closed containers, protected from light.*

6815. Oil of Thyme. Volatile oil distilled from flowering plant *Thymus vulgaris* L., *Labiatae. Constit.* 20-40% by vol of thymol and carvacrol; cymene, pinene, linalool, bornyl acetate.

Colorless to reddish-brown liq; pleasant thymol odor; sharp taste. d_{25}^{25} 0.894-0.930. α_D <−4°. n_D^{20} 1.4830-1.5100. Very slightly sol in water; sol in 2 vols 80% alcohol. *Keep well closed, cool and protected from light.*

Note: Often misnamed "oil of origanum."

THERAP CAT: Rubefacient, counterirritant, antiseptic, carminative.

6816. Oil of Vetiver. Vetiver oil; oleum Andropogonis muricati; vetyver oil; khas khas oil; khus oil; cus cus oil; vetivert oil; vetiver oil Java; vetiver oil Haiti; vetiver oil Reunion (Bourbon). Distilled from roots of vetiver grass *Vetiveria zizanioides* Stapf., (*Andropogon muricatus* Retz., *Anatherum zizanioides* (L.) Hitch. & Chase, *Gramineae*), grown chiefly in Java, India, Reunion Island and Haiti. The constituents of vetiver oil vary according to the place of origin. Java and Reunion vetiver oils may contain 8-35% (usually 15-27%) sesquiterpene ketones of which α- and β-vetivones, *q.v.* have been isolated. The content of vetivenols (vetiverols, vetiver alcohols) varies from 45 to 65%. Other isolated components are vetivenyl vetivenate, vetivenic acid ($C_{15}H_{22}O_2$), palmitic acid, benzoic acid, and vetivene ($C_{15}H_{24}$). Major constituents of Indian vetiver oil are khusol, khusitol, khusinol. Review of chemical studies: Anh, Fetizon, *Am. Perfum. Cosmet.* **80**, 40 (1965). Biogenetically significant components: Kaiser, Naegeli, *Tetrahedron Lett.* **1972**, 2009; Paknikar *et al., ibid.* **1975**, 2973. Isoln and synthesis of **zizanal** and **epizizanal**, two insect repellent constituents, from Javanese vetiver oil: S. C. Jain *et al., Tetrahedron Lett.* **23**, 4639 (1982).

Brown to reddish-brown viscous oil. Aromatic to harsh, woody odor which improves on aging. d_{15}^{15} 0.990-1.040. n_D^{20} 1.5200-1.5280. $[\alpha]_D^{20}$ +15 to +45°. Ester value after acetylation 110-165. Soluble in 1-3 volumes of 80% alcohol, becoming slightly turbid upon further dilution. Sol in all proportions in most fixed oils, diethyl phthalate, benzyl benzoate, mineral oil (slight turbidity). Practically insol in glycerol and propylene glycol. Fairly stable to dilute acids and weak alkalies; unstable to strong acids and alkalies. Should be stored in a cool place and protected from light. *Refs:* Kretchmar, Pictet, *Chimia* **8**, 123 (1954); Pfau, Plattner, *Helv. Chim. Acta* **22**, 640 (1939); Guenther, *The Essential Oils* **vol. IV** (Van Nostrand, New York, 1950) p 156.

USE: In soap and perfumery formulations.

6817. Oil of Wine, "Heavy". An oily liq obtained by distilling alcohol or ether (or both) with sulfuric acid. *Constit.* Etherin and etherol ($C_2H_4)_n$, polymers of ethylene; ethyl sulfate and ethyl sulfovinate.

Colorless to slightly yellow liq; penetrating odor; sharp, bitter taste. d_{15}^{15} 1.095-1.130. Almost insol in water; miscible with alcohol, ether.

USE: For making ethereal oil which is used in making Hoffman's anodyne; sometimes for flavoring brandy.

6818. Oil Palm. African oil palm. Tropical tree, *Elaeis guineensis* Jacq., *Arecaceae* (alt. *Palmae*), bearing large bunches of plum-sized fruit. Grown primarily for the edible oils obtained from the fruit and seed. *Habit.* West Africa, Malaysia. The closely related **American oil palm**, *E. oleifera* (Kunth) Cortés, is grown in Central and South America and is also used. Review of cultivation, oil production, characteristics and uses: J. A. Cornelius, *Prog. Chem. Fats Other Lipids* **15**, 5-27 (1977); Y. Basiron, *J. Oleo Sci.* **50**, 295-303 (2001). Review of safety assessment of oils: W. Johnson, Jr., *Int. J. Toxicol.* **19**, Suppl. 2, 7-28 (2000).

Palm oil. [8002-75-3] Obtained from the fleshy orange-red mesocarp of the fruit. *Constit.* Fatty acids, primarily palmitic (44%), oleic (39%), and linoleic (10%); carotenoids, esp. α- and β-carotene; tocopherols, esp. γ-tocotrienol; sterols, esp. β-sitosterol. May be refined to remove color and odor components and separated into olein and stearin fractions. Review of biochemistry, toxicology and role in nutrition: D. O. Edem, *Plant Foods Human Nutr.* **57**, 319-341 (2002). Crude oil is deep orange in color with characteristic sweetish odor. Semisolid at 21-27°; mp 27-50°. d_{25}^{50} 0.89-0.92. n_D^{40} 1.453-1.459. Sapon. no. 196-209. Iodine no. 46-60.

Palm olein. Liquid oil, mp 21.6°. d^{50} 0.91-0.92. *n* 1.47. Sapon. no. 189-198.0. Iodine no. 55.0-61.54.

Palm stearin. Solid, mp 44.5-56.2°. d^{50} 0.88-0.89. *n* 1.45. Sapon. no. 193-206. Iodine no. 21.6-49.4.

Palm kernel oil. [8023-79-8] Obtained from seed by mechanical expression or solvent extraction. *Constit.* Fatty acids, primarily lauric (48%), myristic (16%) and oleic (15%); sterols, esp. β-sitosterol; triterpene alcohols; hydrocarbons. Review of properties and uses: T. P. Pantzaris, M. J. Ahmed, *Palm Oil Devel.* **35**, 1123

(2001). Colorless to brownish yellow oil, solidifying to a white to yellowish fat. Crude oil has a strong, characteristic taste and odor and is most often refined before use. mp 25-30°. d_{25}^{40} 0.900-0.913. n_D^{40} 1.4495-1.4515. Sapon. no. 244-254. Iodine no. 14-20.

USE: Cooking and frying oil. In margarines, shortenings, non-dairy creamers, whipping creams; as cocoa butter substitute. In manuf of soaps, oleochemicals. In cosmetics, personal care products as skin conditioner, viscosity increasing agent, solvent.

6819. Okadaic Acid. [78111-17-8] 9,10-Deepithio-9,10-didehydroacanthifolicin; halochondrine A. $C_{44}H_{68}O_{13}$; mol wt 805.00. C 65.65%, H 8.51%, O 25.84%. First ionophoric polyether identified in marine organisms; isolated from marine black sponges, *Halichondria (okadai* or *melanodocia*). Tumor promoting cytotoxin associated with diarrhetic seafood poisoning. Isoln: K. Tachibana *et al., J. Am. Chem. Soc.* **103**, 2469 (1981). Total synthesis: M. Isobe *et al., Tetrahedron* **43**, 4767 (1987). Contractile effects: S. Shibata *et al., J. Pharmacol. Exp. Ther.* **223**, 135 (1982). Inhibition of protein phosphatases: A. Takai *et al., FEBS Lett.* **217**, 81 (1987); C. Bialojan, A. Takai, *Biochem. J.* **256**, 283 (1988). Tumor promoting activity: M. Suganuma *et al., Proc. Natl. Acad. Sci. USA* **85**, 1768 (1988). Review of mechanism of action and use as a probe for cellular regulation: P. Cohen *et al., Trends Biochem. Sci.* **15**, 98-102 (1990); A. Schönthal, *New Biol.* **4**, 16-21 (1992). Review of tumor promoting activity: H. Fujiki, M. Suganuma, *J. Biochem.* **115**, 1-5 (1994).

Crystals from dichloromethane/hexane, mp 171-175°. $[\alpha]_D^{20}$ +21° (c = 0.33 in $CHCl_3$). Also reported as crystals from benzene-$CHCl_3$, mp 164-166°. $[\alpha]_D^{25}$ +25.4° (c = 0.24 in $CHCl_3$). LD_{50} i.p. in mice: 192 μg/kg (Shibata).

USE: Biochemical tool as tumor promoter and probe of cellular regulation.

6820. Olaflur. [6818-37-7] 2,2′-[[3-[(2-Hydroxyethyl)-octadecylamino]propyl]imino]bisethanol dihydrofluoride; AmF 297; amine fluoride 297; N-(diethanolaminopropyl)-N-(ethanol)-octadecylamine dihydrofluoride; N,N,N′-tris(2-hydroxyethyl)-N′-octadecyl-1,3-diaminopropane dihydrofluoride; SKF-38095; RonaCare. $C_{27}H_{58}N_2O_3$.2HF; mol wt 498.77. C 65.02%, H 12.13%, N 5.62%, O 9.62%, F 7.62%. Anticariogenic organic amine fluoride; often used in combination with stannous fluoride or sodium fluoride, *q.q.v.* Reduces surface tension of saliva, forming a protective film on tooth surfaces. Prepn: H. Schmid, H. R. Mühlemann, US 3083143 (1963 to GABA). In vitro antimicrobial activity: H. M. Kay, M. Wilson, *J. Periodontol.* **59**, 266 (1988). Adsorption and desorption to hydroxyapatite: J. Sefton *et al., Biomaterials* **17**, 37 (1996). Clinical evaluation of caries inhibition in children: T. M. Marthaler, *Br. Dent. J.* **119**, 153 (1965); of effects on plaque and gingivitis in adults: L. Shapira *et al., J. Int. Acad. Periodontol.* **4**, 117 (1999); of reduction of erosion in enamel and dentine: C. Ganss *et al., Caries Res.* **38**, 561 (2004).

Sol in water, ethanol, methanol. Aq soln foams. Slightly acidic pH.

USE: Dental caries prophylactic.

6821. Olah's Reagent. [62778-11-4] Hydrofluoric acid homopolymer compd with pyridine; pyridinium poly(hydrogen fluoride); PPHF. $(C_5H_5N)_x(HF)_y$. Nucleophilic fluorinating agent; acts as a stabilized, less volatile form of hydrogen fluoride, *q.v.* Consists of approx 30% pyridine and 70% hydrogen fluoride (w/w) in equilibrium with a small amount of free hydrogen fluoride. Use in fluorination of steroids: C. G. Bergstrom *et al., J. Org. Chem.* **28**,

2633 (1963). Prepn and use as an organic fluorinating reagent: G. A. Olah *et al.*, *Synthesis* **1973**, 779; *idem et al.*, *J. Org. Chem.* **44**, 3872 (1979). Peptide deprotection: S. Matsuura *et al.*, *J. Chem. Soc. Chem. Commun.* **1976**, 451. Review of use in organic synthesis: G. A. Olah *et al.*, *J. Fluorine Chem.* **33**, 377-396 (1986).

Liquid, stable to 55°.

USE: Fluorinating reagent; deprotecting reagent in peptide chemistry.

6822. Olanzapine. [132539-06-1] 2-Methyl-4-(4-methyl-1-piperazinyl)-10*H*-thieno[2,3-*b*][1,5]benzodiazepine; LY-170053; Zyprexa. $C_{17}H_{20}N_4S$; mol wt 312.43. C 65.35%, H 6.45%, N 17.93%, S 10.26%. Serotonin (5-HT$_2$) and dopamine (D$_1$/D$_2$) receptor antagonist with anticholinergic activity. Prepn: J. K. Chakrabarti *et al.*, *EP 454436*; *eidem*, *US 5229382* (1991, 1993 both to Lilly). Comparative pharmacology: N. A. Moore *et al.*, *Curr. Opin. Invest. Drugs* **2**, 281 (1993). HPLC determn in human plasma: J. T. Catlow *et al.*, *J. Chromatogr. B* **668**, 85 (1995). Clinical evaluation in schizophrenia: D. S. Baldwin, S. A. Montgomery, *Int. Clin. Psychopharmacol.* **10**, 239 (1995); in mania of bipolar disorder: M. Tohen *et al.*, *Am. J. Psychiatry* **156**, 702 (1999). Review of pharmacology and clinical experience: B. C. Lund, P. J. Perry, *Expert Opin. Pharmacother.* **1**, 305-323 (2000).

Crystals from acetonitrile, mp 195°. Practically insol in water.

THERAP CAT: Antipsychotic.

6823. Olaquindox. [23696-28-8] *N*-(2-Hydroxyethyl)-3-methyl-2-quinoxalinecarboxamide 1,4-dioxide; Bay Va 9391; Bay-o-nox; Fedan. $C_{12}H_{13}N_3O_4$; mol wt 263.25. C 54.75%, H 4.98%, N 15.96%, O 24.31%. Prepn: *FR 1594628*; K. Ley *et al.*, *US 3908008* (1970, 1975 to Bayer). Growth promotant activity for pigs: R. S. Barber *et al.*, *Anim. Feed Sci. Technol.* **4**, 117 (1979). HPLC analysis: G. F. Bories, *J. Chromatogr.* **172**, 505 (1979). LC determn in animal feeds: F. J. dos Ramos *et al.*, *ibid.* **558**, 125 (1991).

Pale yellow crystals, mp 209° (dec). Slightly sol in water. Insol in most organic solvents.

THERAP CAT (VET): Growth stimulant.

6824. Old Yellow Enzyme. [9001-68-7] Reduced nicotinamide adenine dinucleotide phosphate dehydrogenase; dihydronicotinamide adenine dinucleotide phosphate diaphorase; NADPH$_2$ diaphorase; OYE. Mol wt 102,000-106,000. Flavoprotein which catalyzes the oxidation of reduced triphosphopyridine nucleotide by oxygen or ferricytochrome c. When the oxidizing agent is molecular oxygen, OYE functions as a true hydrogen carrier, whereas when ferricytochrome c is the oxidizing agent, only electrons are passed on to the cytochrome, the protons being liberated as free hydrogen ions. Shows diaphorase activity as well as low cytochrome c reductase activity. Isoln from dried brewer's bottom yeast: Warburg, Christian, *Biochem. Z.* **266**, 377 (1933); Theorell, Akeson, *Biochem. Prep.* **6**, 54 (1958). Each molecule contains two flavin mononucleotide groups: Ehrenberg, *Acta Chem. Scand.* **11**, 1257 (1957). *Review:* Akeson *et al.*, *The Enzymes* vol. 7, P. D. Boyer *et al.*, Eds. (Academic Press, New York, 1963) pp 477-494.

6825. Oleandomycin. [3922-90-5] PA-105; Amimycin; Landomycin; Romicil. $C_{35}H_{61}NO_{12}$; mol wt 687.86. C 61.11%, H 8.94%, N 2.04%, O 27.91%. Antibiotic substance produced by *Streptomyces antibioticus* no. ATCC 11891: Sobin *et al.*; Ratajak, Nubel, *US 2757123*; *US 2842481* (1956, 1958 to Pfizer). Structure: Hochstein *et al.*, *J. Am. Chem. Soc.* **82**, 3225 (1960). Absolute configuration: Celmer, *ibid.* **87**, 1797 (1965); Celmer, Hobbs, *Carbohydr. Res.* **1**, 137 (1965); S. Omura *et al.*, *Tetrahedron Lett.* **1975**, 2939. Synthetic study: K. Tatsuta *et al.*, *ibid.* **29**, 3975 (1988). Activity: Hahn, *Antibiotics* **1**, 378, 755 (1967). For a review of macrolide antibiotics *see* Keller-Schierlein, *Fortschr. Chem. Org. Naturst.* **30**, 313-460 (1973). Toxicity: H. Sous *et al.*, *Arzneim.-Forsch.* **8**, 386 (1958).

White amorphous powder. uv max (methanol): 286-289 nm. Moderately sol in water. Sol in dil acids. Freely sol in methanol, ethanol, butanol, acetone. Practically insol in hexane, carbon tetrachloride, dibutyl ether.

Hydrochloride. [6696-47-5] $C_{35}H_{61}NO_{12}$.HCl. Long needles from ethyl acetate, mp 134-135°. $[\alpha]_D^{25}$ −54° (methanol). Freely sol in water. Forms various cryst hydrates. LD$_{50}$ in mice, rats (mg/kg): 8200, >10000 orally; 600, 400 i.v. (Sous).

Phosphate. [7060-74-4] Matromycin. $C_{35}H_{61}NO_{12}$.H$_3$PO$_4$; mol wt 785.85.

Triacetyl deriv *see* Troleandomycin.

THERAP CAT: Antibacterial.

THERAP CAT (VET): Antibacterial.

6826. Oleandrin. [465-16-7] (3β,5β,16β)-16-(Acetyloxy)-3-[(2,6-dideoxy-3-*O*-methyl-α-L-*arabino*-hexopyranosyl)oxy]-14-hydroxycard-20(22)-enolide; neriolin; Corrigen; Folinerin. $C_{32}H_{48}O_9$; mol wt 576.72. C 66.64%, H 8.39%, O 24.97%. Cytotoxic glycoside from the leaves of *Nerium oleander* L., Apocynaceae (Laurier rose). Component of the commercial oleander extract, **Anvirzel**. Isoln: Tanret, *Compt. Rend.* **194**, 914 (1932); Neumann, *Ber.* **70**, 1547 (1937). Prepn by enzymic hydrolysis of urechitoxin: Hassall, *J. Chem. Soc.* **1951**, 3193. Structure: Tschesche, *Ber.* **70**, 1554 (1937); Krasso *et al.*, *Helv. Chim. Acta* **46**, 1691 (1963). LC/MS/MS determn in tissues and biological fluids: E. R. Tor *et al.*, *J. Agric. Food Chem.* **53**, 4322 (2005). Apoptotic activity study: Y. Sreenivasan *et al.*, *Biochem. Pharmacol.* **66**, 2223 (2003). Pharmacology: D. Ni *et al.*, *J. Exp. Ther. Oncol.* **2**, 278 (2002). Review of toxicity: S. D. Langford, P. J. Boor, *Toxicology* **109**, 1-13 (1996).

Crystals from dil methanol, mp 250°. $[\alpha]_D^{25}$ −48.0° (c = 1.3 in methanol). uv max: 220 nm (log ε 4.20). Practically insol in water. Sol in alcohol, chloroform.

Desacetyloleandrin. [36190-93-9] $C_{30}H_{46}O_8$. Leaflets from alcohol, mp 238-240°. $[\alpha]_D^{18}$ −24.9°.

THERAP CAT: Cardiotonic; diuretic.

6827. Oleanolic Acid. [508-02-1] (3β)-3-Hydroxyolean-12-en-28-oic acid; oleanol; caryophyllin. $C_{30}H_{48}O_3$; mol wt 456.70. C 78.90%, H 10.59%, O 10.51%. Occurs in the free state in leaves of *Olea europaea, Oleaceae,* in leaves of *Viscum album* L., *Loranthaceae,* in buds of *Syzygium aromaticum* (L.) Merr. & Perry, *Myrtaceae* (cloves), in *Swertia japonica* (Maxim.) Makino, and in *Centaurium umbellatum* Gilib. (*Erythraea centaurium* (L.) Pers.), *Gentianaceae;* as acetate in birch bark, as glycoside in many saponins. Isoln procedures (from cloves): Winterstein, Stein, *Z. Physiol. Chem.* **202**, 222 (1931); Ruzicka, Hofmann, *Helv. Chim. Acta* **19**, 114 (1936); Picard *et al., J. Chem. Soc.* **1939**, 1047. Structure: Ruzicka *et al., Helv. Chim. Acta* **29**, 210 (1946). *Review:* J. Simonsen, W. C. T. Ross, *The Terpenes* **vol. 5** (University Press, Cambridge, 1957) pp 221-285. *Cf.* α- and β-amyrin.

Fine, solvated needles from alc. After drying, mp 310°. $[\alpha]_D^{20}$ +83.3° (c = 0.6 in chloroform). pK 2.52. Insol in water. Sol in 65 parts ether, 106 parts 95% alcohol, 35 parts boiling 95% alcohol, 118 parts chloroform, 180 parts acetone, 235 parts methanol.

Acetate. $C_{32}H_{50}O_4$. Needles from methanol, mp 268°. $[\alpha]_D^{17}$ +74.5° (c = 0.6 in CHCl₃).

Methyl ester. $C_{31}H_{50}O_3$. mp 201°. $[\alpha]_D^{20}$ +75° (c = 0.6 in CHCl₃).

Acetate of methyl ester. $C_{33}H_{52}O_4$. Needles from alcohol, mp 223°. $[\alpha]_D^{20}$ +70° (c = 0.6 in CHCl₃).

6828. Oleic Acid. [112-80-1] (Z)-9-Octadecenoic acid. $C_{18}H_{34}O_2$; mol wt 282.46. C 76.54%, H 12.13%, O 11.33%. Obtained by the hydrolysis of various animal and vegetable fats and oils. Prepn from olive oil: *Biochem. Prep.* **2**, 100 (1952). Separation from olive oil by double fractionation via urea adducts: Rubin, Paisley, *Biochem. Prep.* **9**, 113 (1962). Stereochemistry: Thieme, *Ann.* **343**, 354 (1905). Synthesis: Robinson, Robinson, *J. Chem. Soc.* **127**, 175 (1925). ^{13}C-NMR studies: W. Stoffel *et al., Z. Physiol. Chem.* **353**, 1962 (1972); J. G. Batchelor *et al., J. Org. Chem.* **39**, 1698 (1974). Toxicity data: L. Orö, A. Wretlind, *Acta Pharmacol. Toxicol.* **18**, 141 (1961). Exptl use of ^{131}I-labelled oleic acid in myocardial imaging: F. J. Bonte *et al., Radiology* **108**, 195 (1973). Review of diagnostic use of ^3H-oleic acid in pancreatic function: N. T. Pedersen, *Digestion* **37**, Suppl. 1, 25-34 (1987).

Pure oleic acid is a colorless or nearly colorless liq (above 5-7°). d_{25}^{25} ~0.895. Solidifies to cryst mass, mp 4°. bp_{100} 286°. At atm pressure it dec when heated at 80-100°. n_D^{18} 1.463; n_D^{26} 1.4585. Iodine no. 89.9; acid value 198.6. On exposure to air, especially when impure, it oxidizes and acquires a yellow to brown color and rancid odor. Practically insol in water. Sol in alcohol, benzene, chloroform, ether, fixed and volatile oils. *Keep well closed, protected from light.* LD₅₀ i.v. in mice: 230±18 mg/kg (Orö, Wretlind). Several grades of the acid are available in commerce, varying in color from pale yellow to red-brown and, depending on the amount of saturated acid present, becoming turbid at 8-16°. The acid of commerce usually contains 7-12% saturated acids, e.g., stearic, palmitic; also some linoleic, etc., unsaturated acids.

Methyl ester. Methyl oleate. $C_{19}H_{36}O_2$. Prepd by refluxing oleic acid with *p*-toluene sulfonic acid in methanol: Rubin, Paisley, *loc. cit.* Iodine no. 85.6. d_4^{18} 0.879. n_D^{26} 1.4510. bp_2 168-170°. Miscible with anhyd ethanol, ether.

Ethyl ester. Ethyl oleate; (Z)-9-octadecenoic acid ethyl ester. $C_{20}H_{38}O_2$. Yellowish, oily liquid. d 0.87. bp 205-208° (some dec). Insol in water. Misc with alcohol, ether.

Barium salt. Barium oleate. $C_{36}H_{66}BaO_4$. Yellowish-white, granular masses. *Poisonous!* Practically insol in water. Slightly sol in boiling alcohol.

Sodium salt. [143-19-1] Eunatrol. $C_{18}H_{33}NaO_2$; mol wt 304.44. White powder, slight tallow-like odor. Sol in ~10 parts water, ~20 parts alcohol. Generally contains small quantities of the sodium salts of stearic, etc. acids. Alkaline in aq solns due to hydrolysis but not in alcohol solns.

Caution: Mildly irritating to skin, mucous membranes.

USE: Prepn of Turkey red oil, soft soap and other oleates; in polishing compds; waterproofing textiles, oiling wool; manuf driers; thickening lubricating oils. Pharmaceutic aid (solvent). The barium salt in rodent extermination.

THERAP CAT: Diagnostic aid (pancreatic function).

6829. Oleocanthal. [289030-99-5] (3S,4E)-4-Formyl-3-(2-oxoethyl)-4-hexenoic acid 2-(4-hydroxyphenyl)ethyl ester; deacetoxy ligstroside aglycon. $C_{17}H_{20}O_5$; mol wt 304.34. C 67.09%, H 6.62%, O 26.29%. Secoiridoid found in virgin olive oil; induces a characteristic burning sensation in the throat when tasted. Isoln and proposed formation from ligstroside: G. Montedoro *et al., J. Agric. Food Chem.* **41**, 2228 (1993). Antioxidant activity: R. W. Owen *et al., Food Chem. Toxicol.* **38**, 647 (2000). Identification as key contributor to pungency of olive oil: P. Andrewes *et al., J. Agric. Food Chem.* **51**, 1415 (2003). Inhibitory effect on cyclooxygenase: G. K. Beauchamp *et al., Nature* **437**, 45 (2005). Synthesis and abs config: A. B. Smith, III *et al., Org. Lett.* **7**, 5075 (2005).

$[\alpha]_D^{25}$ −0.78° (c = 0.9 in chloroform). uv max (chloroform): 242, 277, 283 sh, 325 nm.

6830. Oleuropein. [32619-42-4] [2S-(2α,3E,4β)]-3-Ethyl-idene-2-(β-D-glucopyranosyloxy)-3,4-dihydro-5-(methoxycarbonyl)-2H-pyran-4-acetic acid 2-(3,4-dihydroxyphenyl)ethyl ester. $C_{25}H_{32}O_{13}$; mol wt 540.51. C 55.55%, H 5.97%, O 38.48%. Bitter glucoside; first *secoiridoid* to be isolated. Isolation from olives and the leaves and bark of the olive tree, *Olea europaea* L., *Oleaceae* and structural studies: Panizzi *et al., Gazz. Chim. Ital.* **90**, 1449 (1960); Beyerman *et al., Bull. Soc. Chim. Fr.* **1961**, 1821; Shasha, Leibowitz, *J. Org. Chem.* **26**, 1948 (1961). Isoln from the ripe fruits of *Ligustrum lucidum* and *L. japonicum* Thunb, *Oleaceae:* Inouye, Nishioka, *Tetrahedron* **28**, 4231 (1972). Revised structure and stereochemistry: Inouye *et al., Tetrahedron Lett.* **1970**, 2459. Pharmacology: Petkov, Manolov, *Arzneim.-Forsch.* **22**, 1476 (1972). Partial synthesis: A. Bianco *et al., J. Nat. Prod.* **55**, 760 (1992).

O—β-D-glucopyranose

Minute crystals from ethyl acetate, mp 87-89°. Hygroscopic. $[\alpha]_D^{20}$ −147° (H_2O, alcohol, or acetone). Shows mutarotation $[\alpha]_D^{20}$ −127° after 9 hrs (H_2O). Freely sol in acetone, ethanol, methanol, pyridine, glacial acetic acid, 5% aq NaOH soln. Moderately sol in water, dioxane, butanol, ethyl acetate, butyl acetate. Practically insol in ether, petr ether, chloroform, benzene, carbon tetrachloride.

6831. Oleyl Alcohol. [143-28-2] (Z)-9-Octadecen-1-ol; *cis*-9-octadecen-1-ol; Ocenol. $C_{18}H_{36}O$; mol wt 268.48. C 80.52%, H 13.52%, O 5.96%. $CH_3(CH_2)_7CH=CH(CH_2)_7CH_2OH$. Found in fish oils. Usually obtained as a mixture of C_{16} and C_{18} unsaturated alcohols with C_{18} predominating. Prepd from butyl oleate by a Bouveault-Blanc reduction with sodium and butyl alcohol; or from triolein by hydrogenation in the presence of zinc chromite: Noller, Bannerot, *J. Am. Chem. Soc.* **56**, 1563 (1934); Reid *et al.*, *Org. Synth.* **15**, 72 (1935); Adkins, Gillespie, *ibid.* coll. vol. III, 671 (1955). Purification by fractional crystallization at −40° from acetone, followed by distillation: Swern *et al.*, *Oil Soap (Chicago)* **21**, 113 (1944); Loev, Dawson, *J. Am. Chem. Soc.* **78**, 1182 (1956).

Oily liquid. Usually pale yellow. Gives off acrid fumes when heated. d_4^{20} 0.850. mp 13-19°. bp_8 195°. $bp_{1.5}$ 182-184°. (Distilling range at 760 mm: 305-370°.) $n_D^{27.5}$ 1.4582. Insol in water; sol in alcohol, ether.

USE: Chiefly in the manuf of its sulfuric esters which are detergents and wetting agents, as an antifoam agent; metal cutting lubricant; in carbon paper, stencil paper, printing ink; as a plasticizer; for softening and lubricating textile fabrics; carrier for medicaments.

6832. Olibanum. [8050-07-5] Frankincense; gum thus. Gum resin from *Boswellia carterii* Birdwood and other species of *Boswellia (Burseraceae)*. *Habit.* Ethiopia, Egypt, Arabia, Somaliland. *Constit.* 3-8% volatile oil (pinene, dipentene, etc.); about 60% resins; 20% gum (polysaccharide fraction); 6-8% bassorin; bitter principle. Discussion of polysaccharides present: F. Smith, R. Montgomery, *The Chemistry of Plant Gums and Mucilages* (Reinhold, New York, 1959) pp 312-313.

6833. Oligomycins. Macrolide antibiotic complex produced by an actinomycete similar to *Streptomyces diastatochromogenes*: Smith *et al.*, *Antibiot. Chemother.* **4**, 962 (1954); McCoy, Peterson, **US 2927057** (1960 to Wisconsin Alumni Res. Foundation). Complex of several closely related compounds: Masamune *et al.*, *J. Am. Chem. Soc.* **80**, 6092 (1958). Separation of oligomycins A, B and C: Marty, McCoy, *Antibiot. Chemother.* **9**, 286 (1959). Isoln and activity of D from *Streptomyces rutgersensis*: R. Q. Thompson *et al.*, *Antimicrob. Agents Chemother.* **1961**, 474. Partial structure of B: Prouty *et al.*, *Biochem. Biophys. Res. Commun.* **44**, 619 (1971); total structure of B: Glehn *et al.*, *FEBS Lett.* **20**, 267 (1972). Structures of A and C: G. T. Carter, *Diss. Abstr. Int. B* **37**, 766 (1976); of D: C. Merienne, T. Staron, *Chem. Commun.* **1978**, 318. Review: P. D. Shaw in *Antibiotics* **vol. l**, D. Gottlieb, P. D. Shaw, Eds. (Springer-Verlag, New York, 1967) pp 585-610.

Oligomycin A

Oligomycin A. [579-13-5] $C_{45}H_{74}O_{11}$; mol wt 791.06. Two crystalline modifications, mp 140-141° and mp 150-151° (hexagonal crystals, melting with rapid decompn). uv max (abs ethanol): 225 nm (ε about 20,000). Solys at 25° (g/100 ml solvent): water 0.002; ether 28; benzene 6; Skellysolve B 0.02; abs ethanol 25; glacial acetic acid 37.5; acetone 85.

Oligomycin B. [11050-94-5] 28-Oxooligomycin A. $C_{45}H_{72}$-O_{12}; mol wt 805.05. Potent inhibitor of oxidative phosphorylation: Lardy *et al.*, *Arch. Biochem. Biophys.* **78**, 587 (1958).

Oligomycin C. [11052-72-5] 12-Deoxyoligomycin A. C_{45}-$H_{74}O_{10}$; mol wt 775.06.

Oligomycin D. [1404-59-7] 26-Demethyloligomycin A; rutamycin; A-272; RR-32705. $C_{44}H_{72}O_{11}$; mol wt 777.04. mp 116-119°. $[\alpha]_D^{20}$ −62° (c = 1.36 in $CHCl_3$).

THERAP CAT: Oligomycin D as antifungal.

6834. Olivacine. [484-49-1] 1,5-Dimethyl-6*H*-pyrido[4,3-*b*]carbazole; guatambuinine. $C_{17}H_{14}N_2$; mol wt 246.31. C 82.90%, H 5.73%, N 11.37%. Isolated from the bark and stem of *Aspidosperma olivaceum* Müll. Arg., *A. australe* Müll. Arg., *A. longepetiolatum* Kuhlm., *Apocynaceae*: Schmutz, Hunziger, *Pharm. Acta Helv.* **33**, 341 (1958). Identity with guatambuinine: Marini-Bettolo, Carvalho-Ferreira, *Ann. Chim.* **49**, 869 (1959). Structure: Marini-Bettolo, Schmutz, *Helv. Chim. Acta* **42**, 2146 (1959); Ondetti, Deulofeu, *Tetrahedron* **15**, 160 (1961). Synthesis: Schmutz, Wittwer, *Helv. Chim. Acta* **43**, 793 (1960); Wenkert, Dave, *J. Am. Chem. Soc.* **84**, 94 (1962); Mosher *et al.*, *J. Med. Chem.* **9**, 237 (1966); R. Besselievre, H. Husson, *Tetrahedron Lett.* **1976**, 1873; J. Bergman, R. Carlsson, *ibid.* **1978**, 4055; J. P. Kutney *et al.*, *Heterocycles* **16**, 1469 (1981).

Fine yellow needles from dilute methanol, yellow prisms from undiluted methanol, mp 317-325°. Fluoresces in dilute alcoholic soln. uv max (ethanol): 224, 238, 276, 287, 292, 314, 329, 375 nm (log ε 4.39, 4.33, 4.70, 4.85, 4.83, 3.66, 3.80, 3.66). Soly in methanol, acetone, chloroform, carbon tetrachloride, carbon disulfide, tetrahydrofuran, dioxane less than 1%.

6835. Olivanic Acids. A family of naturally occurring carbapenem β-lactamase inhibitors with antibacterial activity, produced by *Streptomyces olivaceus*: D. Butterworth, G. N. Rolinson, **DE 2146400**; *eidem* **US 3919415** (1972, 1975 both to Beecham). Isoln: A. G. Brown *et al.*, *J. Antibiot.* **29**, 668 (1976). The family contains seven members, all containing the 7-oxo-1-azabicyclo[3.2.0]hept-2-ene ring system. Compounds **MM 4550**, **MM 13902**, and **MM 17880** are sulfated and are predominant when *S. olivaceus* is grown with glucose in sulfate-containing media. **MM 22380**, **MM 22381**, **MM 22382**, **MM 22383** are non-sulfated hydroxy analogs and are produced in sulfate-free media or by mutants of *S. olivaceus* unable to complete the sulfation process. Detection, properties, fermentation of the sulfated members: D. Butterworth *et al.*, *ibid.* **32**, 287 (1979); isoln, characterization: J. D. Hood *et al.*, *ibid.* 295. Fermentation, isoln, characterization of the non-sulfated members: S. J. Box *et al.*, *ibid.* 1239. Structures of MM 4550, MM 13902: A. G. Brown *et al.*, *Chem. Commun.* **1977**, 523; of MM 17880: D. F. Corbett *et al.*, *ibid.* 953. Structures of MM 22380-3: A. G. Brown *et al.*, *J. Antibiot.* **32**, 963 (1979). Total synthesis of racemic MM 22383: R. J. Ponsford, R. Southgate, *Chem. Commun.* **1980**, 1085. Comparative antibacterial activity *in vitro*: M. J. Basker *et al.*, *J. Antibiot.* **33**, 878 (1980). MM 22380, MM 22382, MM 22381, MM 22383, MM 13902, and MM 17880 are identical to **epithienamycins** A through F, respectively, *cf.* E. O. Stapley *et al.*, *ibid.* **34**, 628 (1981); P. J. Cassidy *et al.*, *ibid.* 637. Synthetic study on epithienamycins: T. Kametani *et al.*, *J. Chem. Soc. Perkin Trans. 1* **1981**, 3048.

MM 4550	R = –S–CH=CH–NHCOCH₃	(E)
MM 13902	R = –S–CH=CH–NHCOCH₃	(E)
MM 17880	R = –S–CH₂CH₂NHCOCH₃	

MM 4550, MM 13902, MM 17880 are isolated as disodium salts. Sol in water, methanol, DMF, DMSO. Practically insol in other organic solvents. uv max (water): of MM 4550: 240, 287 nm ($E_{1cm}^{1\%}$ 268); MM 13902: 227, 307 nm ($E_{1cm}^{1\%}$ 356); MM 17880: 298 nm ($E_{1cm}^{1\%}$ 192). The antibiotics are unstable in aq soln outside a narrow pH range; in acids, degradation leads to changes in uv spectra. Addition of hydroxylamine or cysteine to neutral solns results in rapid degradation.

6836. Olive Oil. A fixed oil obtained from ripe olives, the fruit of the cultivated olive tree *Olea europaea* L., *Oleaceae*. Produced almost exclusively in the countries adjoining the Mediterranean Sea, Spain being the largest producer. Whole olives are crushed in edge runner mills and the oil is expressed in open hydraulic presses. *Constit.* Mixed glycerides of oleic acid 83.5%, of palmitic acid 9.4%, of linoleic acid 4.0%, of stearic acid 2.0%, of arachidic acid 0.9%. Minor constitutents are squalene, up to 0.7%, phytosterol and tocopherols about 0.2%. *Reviews and bibliographies:* José M. de Soroa y Pineda, *El aceite de oliva* (Dossat, Madrid, 1944); R. F. Simari, G. B. Martinenghi, *Olivicoltura e Oleificio* (Hoepli, Milano, 1950); P. G. Garoglio, *Technologia de los Aceites Vegetales* (Mendoza, Argentina, 1951); E. W. Eckey, *Vegetable Fats and Oils* (Reinhold, New York, 1954).

Pale yellow or light greenish-yellow oil with a pleasing delicate flavor. Becomes rancid on exposure to air. Begins to get turbid at +5 to +10°, below 0° it forms a whitish, granular mass. Flash pt 437°F (225°C). Ignition temp 650°F (343°C). d_4^{15} 0.914-0.919; d_{25}^{25} 0.909-0.915. n_D^{25} 1.466-1.468; n_D^{40} 1.460-1.464. Titer 17-26°. Acid value 0.2-2.8. Saponification value 187-196. Iodine value 79-90. Thiocyanogen value 75-83. Hydroxyl value 4-12. Reichert-Meissl value 0.2-1.0. Unsaponifiable 0.5-1.3%. Slightly sol in alcohol. Miscible with ether, chloroform, carbon disulfide.

USE: As food in salads, with sardines, for cooking and baking. In the manuf of soaps, textile lubricants, sulfonated oils, cosmetics and pharmaceutical preparations. Emollient.

THERAP CAT (VET): Laxative, emollient.

6837. Olivil. [2955-23-9] [2*S*-(2α,3β,4α)]-Tetrahydro-4-hydroxy-2-(4-hydroxy-3-methoxyphenyl)-4-[(4-hydroxy-3-methoxyphenyl)methyl]-3-furanmethanol. $C_{20}H_{24}O_7$; mol wt 376.40. C 63.82%, H 6.43%, O 29.75%. From gum-resin of *Olea europaea* L., *Oleaceae*. Isoln: Pelletier, *Ann. Chim. Phys.* **51**, 196 (1833). Structure: Traverso, *Gazz. Chim. Ital.* **90**, 792 (1960); Smith, *Tetrahedron Lett.* **1963**, 991. Revised structure: Ayres, Mhasalkar, *ibid.* **1964**, 335; *eidem, J. Chem. Soc.* **1965**, 3586.

Monohydrate. Crystals. mp 118-120°; when anhydr, mp 142-143°. $[\alpha]_D^{12}$ −127°. Sol in hot water, alcohol, acetic acid, fatty oils.

6838. Olivomycins. A mixture of antibiotics produced by *Streptomyces olivoreticuli:* Gauze *et al., Antibiotiki* **7**, 34 (1962); Brazhnikova *et al., ibid.* 39. Similar to the chromomycins, *q.v.:* Berlin *et al., Tetrahedron Lett.* **1966**, 1643. Prepn: Gauze, **GB 1152748**; **FR 1554600** (1969, both to Sci. Res. Inst. Antibiot.), *C.A.* **71**, 37490b, 128693m (1969). Composed of olivomycins A (major component), B, C, and D. Separation: Berlin *et al., Khim. Prir. Soedin.* **1967**, 331, *C.A.* **68**, 40017w (1968). Structural elucidation of the aglycone, *olivin*, and the carbohydrate moieties: Berlin *et al., Tetrahedron Lett.* **1964**, 1323; **1966**, 1431; Berlin *et al., Khim. Prir. Soedin.* **1969**, 567, *C.A.* **73**, 25823r (1970). Stereochemistry: Bakhaeva *et al., Chem. Commun.* **1967**, 10; Berlin *et al., Khim. Prir. Soedin.* **1972**, 519. Revised structure: J. Thiem, B. Meyer, *Tetrahedron* **37**, 551 (1981). Synthetic studies: J. H. Dodd, S. M. Weinreb, *Tetrahedron Lett.* **1979**, 3593; J. H. Dodd *et al., J. Org. Chem.* **47**, 4045 (1982). Series of articles on pharmacology: *Antibiotiki* **17** (1972). Toxicity data: M. Slavik, S. K. Carter, *Adv.*

Pharmacol. Chemother. **12**, 1 (1975). *Review:* J. D. Skarbek, M. K. Speedie, in *Antitumor Compounds of Natural Origin* **vol. 1**, A. Aszalos, Ed. (CRC Press, Boca Raton, 1981) pp 191-235.

Olivomycin A

Olivomycin A. [6988-58-5] 3^D-*O*-[2,6-Dideoxy-3-*C*-methyl-4-*O*-(2-methyl-1-oxopropyl)-α-L-*arabino*-hexopyranosyl]olivomycin D. $C_{58}H_{84}O_{26}$; mol wt 1197.27. Formerly known as olivomycin and variant I. Yellow crystals from ethanol-hexane, mp 160-165°. $[\alpha]_D^{20}$ −36° (c = 0.5 in ethanol). uv max (ethanol): 228, 277, 318, 406 nm (log ε 4.39, 4.67, 3.81, 4.05). Sol in alc, ether, chloroform. Insol in benzene, carbon tetrachloride, petr ether, water. LD$_{50}$ i.v. in mice: 13.75 mg/kg (Slavik, Carter).

THERAP CAT: Antineoplastic.

6839. Olmesartan. [144689-63-4] 4-(1-Hydroxy-1-methylethyl)-2-propyl-1-[[2′-(1*H*-tetrazol-5-yl)[1,1′-biphenyl]-4-yl]methyl]-1*H*-imidazole-5-carboxylic acid (5-methyl-2-oxo-1,3-dioxol-4-yl)methyl ester; (5-methyl-2-oxo-1,3-dioxolen-4-yl)methyl 4-(1-hydroxy-1-methylethyl)-2-propyl-1-[4-[2-(tetrazol-5-yl)phenyl]phenyl]methylimidazole-5-carboxylate; olmesartan medoxomil; CS-866; Benicar; Olmetec. $C_{29}H_{30}N_6O_6$; mol wt 558.59. C 62.36%, H 5.41%, N 15.05%, O 17.19%. Angiotensin II receptor antagonist. Prepn: H. Yanagisawa *et al.,* **EP 503785**; *eidem,* **US 5616599** (1992, 1997 both to Sankyo); *eidem, J. Med. Chem.* **39**, 323 (1996). Clinical evaluation in hypertension: K. Püchler *et al., J. Hypertens.* **15**, 1809 (1997). *Review:* M. Elisaf, *Curr. Opin. Cardiovasc. Pulm. Renal Invest. Drugs* **2**, 378-383 (2000).

Monoclinic crystals from ethanol, mp 180-182° (dec). Practically insol in water. Sparingly sol in methanol.

THERAP CAT: Antihypertensive.

6840. Olopatadine. [113806-05-6] (11*Z*)-11-[3-(Dimethylamino)propylidene]-6,11-dihydrodibenz[*b,e*]oxepin-2-acetic acid. $C_{21}H_{23}NO_3$; mol wt 337.41. C 74.75%, H 6.87%, N 4.15%, O 14.23%. Dual acting histamine H$_1$-receptor antagonist and mast cell stabilizer. Prepn: E. Oshima *et al.,* **EP 235796**; *eidem,* **US 5116863** (1987, 1992 both to Kyowa); *eidem, J. Med. Chem.* **35**, 2074 (1992). Pharmacology: C. Kamei *et al., Arzneim.-Forsch.* **45**, 1005 (1995); J. M. Yanni *et al., J. Ocul. Pharmacol. Ther.* **12**, 389 (1996). Receptor binding profile: N. A. Sharif *et al., J. Pharmacol. Exp. Ther.* **278**, 1252 (1996). Clinical trial in allergic conjunctivitis: M. B. Abelson, L. Spitalny, *Am. J. Ophthalmol.* **125**, 797 (1998).

Crystallized as the hemihydrate from 2-propanol + water, mp 188-189.5°.

Hydrochloride. [140462-76-6] AL-4943A; KW-4679; Opatanol; Patanol. $C_{21}H_{23}NO_3 \cdot HCl$; mol wt 373.87. Crystals from acetone-water, mp 248° (dec). Sol in water.

THERAP CAT: Antiallergic; antihistaminic.

6841. Olsalazine. [15722-48-2] 3,3'-Azobis(6-hydroxybenzoic acid); C.I. Mordant Yellow 5; 3,3'-dicarboxy-4,4'-dihydroxyazobenzene; 5,5'-azobis(salicylic acid); azodisal. $C_{14}H_{10}N_2O_6$; mol wt 302.24. C 55.63%, H 3.33%, N 9.27%, O 31.76%. Dimer of mesalamine, *q.v.*, originally used as a mordant dye. Prepn: **DE 278613**; C. Mettler, **US 1157169** (1914, 1915 both to J. R. Geigy). Improved prepn: K. H. Agback, A. S. Nygren, **EP 36636**; *idem*, **US 4528367** (1981, 1985 both to Pharmacia AB). HPLC determn in biological samples: R. A. van Hogezand *et al., J. Chromatogr.* **305**, 470 (1984). *In vitro* effect on fecal bacteria: H. Sandberg-Gertzen *et al., Scand. J. Gastroenterol.* **20**, 607 (1985). Clinical pharmacokinetics and metabolism: C. P. Willoughby *et al., Gut* **23**, 1081 (1982). Clinical trial in ulcerative colitis: H. Sandberg-Gertzen *et al., Gastroenterology* **90**, 1024 (1986). Review of clinical experience in inflammatory bowel disease: A. N. Wadworth, A. Fitton, *Drugs* **41**, 647-664 (1991).

Disodium salt. [6054-98-4] Azodisal sodium; disodium azodisalicylate; C.I. 14130; CJ-91B; Dipentum. $C_{14}H_8N_2Na_2O_6$; mol wt 346.20. Yellow crystalline powder, mp 240° (dec). Sol in water, DMSO. Practically insol in ethanol, chloroform, ether.

USE: Mordant dye for wool.

THERAP CAT: Anti-inflammatory (gastrointestinal).

6842. Omalizumab. [242138-07-4] Anti-(human immunoglobulin E Fc region) immunoglobulin G (human-mouse monoclonal E25 clone pSVIE26 γ-chain) disulfide with human-mouse monoclonal E25 clone pSVIE26 κ-chain, dimer; olizumab; rhuMAb-E25; CGP-51901; Xolair. Humanized monoclonal antibody directed against human immunoglobulin E (IgE). Complexes with circulating IgE to prevent the IgE-mediated degranulation of mast cells during an allergic reaction. Prepn: L. G. Presta *et al., J. Immunol.* **151**, 2623 (1993). Pharmacokinetics and effect on circulating IgE levels in allergy patients: J. Corne *et al., J. Clin. Invest.* **99**, 879 (1997). Clinical trial in allergic asthma: H. Milgrom *et al., N. Engl. J. Med.* **341**, 1966 (1999); in allergic rhinitis: T. B. Casale *et al., J. Am. Med. Assoc.* **286**, 2956 (2001). Reviews of clinical efficacy in allergic asthma: S. Holgate *et al., Curr. Med. Res. Opin.* **17**, 233-240 (2001); G. D'Amato, *Expert Opin. Biol. Ther.* **3**, 371-376 (2003).

THERAP CAT: Antiallergic; antiasthmatic.

6843. Omapatrilat. [167305-00-2] (4S,7S,10aS)-Octahydro-4-[[(2S)-2-mercapto-1-oxo-3-phenylpropyl]amino]-5-oxo-7H-pyrido[2,1-b][1,3]thiazepine-7-carboxylic acid; BMS-186716; Vanlev. $C_{19}H_{24}N_2O_4S_2$; mol wt 408.53. C 55.86%, H 5.92%, N 6.86%, O 15.67%, S 15.70%. Dual metalloprotease inhibitor of neutral endopeptidase (NEP) and angiotensin converting enzyme (ACE). Prepn: J. A. Robl *et al., EP 629627*; *idem*, **US 5508272** (1994, 1996 both to Bristol-Myers Squibb); and pharmacological evaluation: *idem et al., J. Med. Chem.* **40**, 1570 (1997). HPLC-MS determn in rat plasma: M. Jemal, D. J. Hawthorne, *J. Chromatogr.*

B **698**, 123 (1997). Antihypertensive activity in rats: N. C. Trippodo *et al., Am. J. Hypertens.* **11**, 363 (1998). Clinical pharmacodynamics: C. Massien *et al., Clin. Pharmacol. Ther.* **65**, 448 (1999). Review of pharmacology and clinical use: M. Weber, *Am. J. Hypertens.* **12**, 139S-147S (1999). Clinical trial in heart failure: J. L. Rouleau *et al., Lancet* **356**, 615 (2000).

Fine, white solid, mp 218-220°. $[\alpha]_D$ −78.9° (c = 0.46 in DMF).

THERAP CAT: Antihypertensive.

6844. Omega-3 Acid Ethyl Esters. [308081-97-2] Omega-3 polyunsaturated fatty acids ethyl esters; Omacor. Mixture of ethyl esters of long-chain omega-3 fatty acids extracted from fish oil, primarily docosahexaenoic and eicosapentaenoic acids, *q.q.v.* Purification from crude fish oil: H. Breivik *et al., US 5656667* (1997 to Norsk Hydro). Clinical effect on lipid profile in hyperlipidemia: L. Calabresi *et al., Atherosclerosis* **148**, 387 (2000); in combination with simvastatin: P. N. Durrington *et al., Heart* **85**, 544 (2001). Clinical trial to prevent sudden death following myocardial infarction: A. Macchia *et al., Eur. J. Heart Fail.* **7**, 904 (2005).

Light yellow liquid with slight fish-like odor. Practically insol in water. Very sol in acetone, dehydrated alcohol, heptane, methanol.

THERAP CAT: Antilipemic.

6845. Omeprazole. [73590-58-6] 5-Methoxy-2-[[(4-methoxy-3,5-dimethyl-2-pyridinyl)methyl]sulfinyl]-1H-benzimidazole; H-168/68; Gastrogard; Losec; Mopral; OmeLich; Omelind; Omepral; Omeprazen; Osiren; Parizac; Pepticum; Prilosec; Zegerid; Zoltum. $C_{17}H_{19}N_3O_3S$; mol wt 345.42. C 59.11%, H 5.54%, N 12.16%, O 13.90%, S 9.28%. Gastric proton-pump inhibitor. Prepn: U. K. Junggren, S. E. Sjostrand, **EP 5129**; *idem*, **US 4255431** (1979, 1981 both to AB Hässle). Resolution and activity of enantiomers: P. Erlandsson *et al., J. Chromatogr.* **532**, 305 (1990). Manuf process for optically pure salts: S. Von Unge, **US 5693818** (1997 to Astra). Pharmacology: P. Muller *et al., Arzneim.-Forsch.* **33**, 1685 (1983). Mechanism of action study: B. Wallmark *et al., Biochim. Biophys. Acta* **778**, 549 (1984). LC determn in plasma and urine: P. Lagerstrom, B. Persson, *J. Chromatogr.* **309**, 347 (1984). Survey of preclinical data: *Scand. J. Gastroenterol.* **20**, Suppl 108, 1-120 (1985). Toxicological studies: L. Ekman *et al., ibid.* 53. Clinical trial in Zollinger-Ellison syndrome: C. B. H. W. Lamers *et al., N. Engl. J. Med.* **310**, 758 (1984); in duodenal ulcer: K. Lauritsen *et al., ibid.* **312**, 958 (1985). Veterinary trial in race horses: M. J. Murray *et al., Equine Vet. J.* **29**, 425 (1997). Review of pharmacology and clinical efficacy: H. D. Langtry, M. I. Wilde, *Drugs* **56**, 447-486 (1998).

Crystals from acetonitrile, mp 156°. Freely sol in ethanol, methanol; slightly sol in acetone, isopropanol; very slightly sol in water. LD$_{50}$ in mice, rats (g/kg): 0.08, >0.05 i.v.; >4, >4 orally (Ekman).

Magnesium salt. [95382-33-5] Antra; Gastracid; Gastroloc; Omebeta; Omep; Ome-Puren. $C_{34}H_{36}MgN_6O_6S_2$; mol wt 713.12.

S-Form. [119141-88-7] Esomeprazole; perprazole; H-199/18. LC-MS determn in plasma: H. Stenhoff *et al., J. Chromatogr. B* **734**, 191 (1999). Colorless syrup. $[\alpha]_D^{20}$ −155° (c = 0.5 in chloroform).

S-Form magnesium salt. [161973-10-0] (T-4)-Bis[5-methoxy-2-[(S)-[(4-methoxy-3,5-dimethyl-2-pyridinyl)methyl]sulfinyl]-1Hbenzimidazolato]magnesium; esomeprazole magnesium; Nexium. Review of clinical experience in acid disorders: D. A. Johnson, *Expert Opin. Pharmacother.* **4**, 253-264 (2003). White powder. $[\alpha]_D^{20}$ -128.2° (c = 1 in methanol).

THERAP CAT: Antiulcerative; in treatment of Zollinger-Ellison syndrome.

THERAP CAT (VET): Antiulcerative.

6846. Omoconazole. [74512-12-2] 1-[(1*Z*)-2-[2-(4-Chlorophenoxy)ethoxy]-2-(2,4-dichlorophenyl)-1-methylethenyl]-1*H*-imidazole; (*Z*)-1-[2,4-dichloro-β-[2-(*p*-chlorophenoxy)ethoxy]-α-methylstyryl]imidazole; CM-8282. $C_{20}H_{17}Cl_3N_2O_2$; mol wt 423.72. C 56.69%, H 4.04%, Cl 25.10%, N 6.61%, O 7.55%. Prepn: L. Zirngibl *et al.*, **DE 2839388**; *eidem*, **US 4210657** (both 1980 to Siegfried); and crystal structure: K. Thiele *et al., Helv. Chim. Acta* **70**, 441 (1987). Stereospecific synthesis: L. Zirngibl, K. Thiele, **US 4554356** (1985 to Siegfried). *In vitro* fungistatic activity: M. Mosse *et al., Pathol. Biol.* **34**, 684 (1986).

Crystals from ethyl acetate/hexane (1:4), mp 89-90°.

Nitrate. [83621-06-1] Sgd-12878; Afongan; Azameno; Fungisan; Fongamil. $C_{20}H_{17}Cl_3N_2O_2 \cdot HNO_3$; mol wt 486.73. Crystals from ethyl acetate/ethanol, mp 118-120° (Büchi), 122.5° (Mettler).

THERAP CAT: Antifungal (topical).

6847. Onapristone. [96346-61-1] (11β,13α,17α)-11-[4-(Dimethylamino)phenyl]-17-hydroxy-17-(3-hydroxypropyl)estra-4,9-dien-3-one; 11β-(4-dimethylaminophenyl)-17α-hydroxy-17β-(3-hydroxypropyl)-13α-methyl-4,9-gonadien-3-one; ZK-98299. $C_{29}H_{39}NO_3$; mol wt 449.62. C 77.47%, H 8.74%, N 3.12%, O 10.68%. Progesterone receptor antagonist. Prepn: G. Neef *et al.*, **EP 129499**; *eidem*, **US 4780461** (1984, 1988 both to Schering AG); *idem et al., Steroids* **44**, 349 (1984). HPLC determn in plasma and serum: C. Zurth, F. Kagels, *J. Chromatogr.* **532**, 115 (1990). *In vitro* effect on breast cancer cells: S. Classen *et al., J. Steroid Biochem. Mol. Biol.* **45**, 315 (1993). Mechanism of action study: D. P. Edwards *et al., ibid.* **53**, 449 (1995). Clinical antifolliculotrophic effect: H. B. Croxatto *et al., Hum. Reprod.* **9**, 1442 (1994).

Amorphous glass. $[\alpha]_D^{25}$ +446.2° (c = 0.51 in chloroform).

THERAP CAT: Antiprogestin; antineoplastic (hormonal).

6848. Ondansetron. [99614-02-5] 1,2,3,9-Tetrahydro-9-methyl-3-[(2-methyl-1*H*-imidazol-1-yl)methyl]-4*H*-carbazol-4-one. $C_{18}H_{19}N_3O$; mol wt 293.36. C 73.70%, H 6.53%, N 14.32%, O 5.45%. Specific serotonin (5HT$_3$) receptor antagonist. Prepn: I. H. Coates *et al.*, **EP 191562**; *eidem*, **US 4695578** (1986, 1987 both to Glaxo). Pharmacology: A. Butler *et al., Br. J. Pharmacol.* **94**, 397 (1988). Clinical trials in cancer chemotherapy-induced nausea and vomiting: M. G. Kris *et al., J. Clin. Oncol.* **6**, 659 (1988); L. Cubeddu *et al., N. Engl. J. Med.* **322**, 810 (1990); M. Marty *et al., ibid.* 816. Clinical evaluation in treatment of bulimia: P. L. Faris *et al., Lancet* **355**, 792 (2000); in early onset alcoholism: B. A. Johnson *et al., J. Am. Med. Assoc.* **284**, 963 (2000). Review of pharmacology and therapeutic use: A. Markham, E. M. Sorkin, *Drugs* **45**, 931-952 (1993); of clinical pharmacokinetics: K. H. Simpson, F. M. Hicks, *J. Pharm. Pharmacol.* **48**, 774-781 (1996).

Crystals from methanol, mp 231-232°.

Hydrochloride dihydrate. [99614-01-4] GR-38032F; GR-C507/75; SN-307; Zofran; Zophren. $C_{18}H_{19}N_3O \cdot HCl \cdot 2H_2O$; mol wt 365.85. White crystalline solid from water/isopropanol, mp 178.5-179.5°. pKa 7.4.

3*S*-Form. $[\alpha]_D^{25}$ -14° (c = 0.19 in methanol).

3*R*-Form. $[\alpha]_D^{24}$ +16° (c = 0.34 in methanol).

THERAP CAT: Antiemetic.

6849. Onion Oil. Obtained from crushed onion seeds, the seeds of *Allium cepa* L., *Liliaceae:* Loew, *Ind. Quim.* **10**, 5 (1948); Phadnis *et al., J. Univ. Bombay* **17A**, no. 24, 62 (1948). Contains allylpropyl bisulfide, *S*-(1-propenyl)cysteine sulfoxide and 1-propenylsulfenic acid which is thought to be the lacrimator in onions: Virtanen, Sprare, *Suom. Kemistil.* **35B**, 28, 29 (1962); *Chem. Ztg.* **86**, 816 (1962).

Pale yellow oil. Strong odor of onions. d_4^{15} 0.9289. Solidifies at -15°. n_D^{25} 1.4730. $[\alpha]_D^{20}$ -1.5°. Sol in ether, chloroform, carbon disulfide.

6850. Oosporein. [475-54-7] 2,2',5,5'-Tetrahydroxy-4,4'-dimethyl[bi-1,4-cyclohexadien-1-yl]-3,3',6,6'-tetrone; 3,3',6,6'-tetrahydroxy-5,5'-dimethyl-2,2'-bi-*p*-benzoquinone; chaetomidin; iso-oosporein. $C_{14}H_{10}O_8$; mol wt 306.22. C 54.91%, H 3.29%, O 41.80%. Fungal pigment isolated from *Oospora colorans* van Beyma.: Kögl, van Wessem, *Rec. Trav. Chim.* **63**, 5 (1944); from *Chaetonium aureum* Chivers and identity with chaetomidin: Lloyd *et al., J. Chem. Soc.* **1955**, 2163; from *Acremonium* spp: Divekar *et al., Can. J. Chem.* **37**, 2097 (1959); from *Beauveria bassiana* (Bals.) Vuill.: Vining *et al., Can. J. Microbiol.* **8**, 931 (1962). Identity with iso-oosporein: Smith, Thomson, *Tetrahedron* **10**, 148 (1960). Synthesis: J. Kalamar *et al., Helv. Chim. Acta* **57**, 2368 (1974). Biosynthesis: E. Steiner *et al., ibid.* 2377.

Bronze plates from aq methanol, mp 290-295°. uv max (ethanol): 216, 287 nm (log ε 3.51, 4.67).

Tetraacetate. $C_{22}H_{28}O_{12}$. Yellow needles from methanol, mp 190°. uv max (ethanol): 262 nm (log ε 4.41).

Tetramethyl ether. $C_{18}H_{18}O_8$. Orange needles from aq methanol, mp 123°. uv max (ethanol): 285.5, 394 nm (log ε 4.40, 2.98).

6851. Opianic Acid. [519-05-1] 6-Formyl-2,3-dimethoxybenzoic acid; 5,6-dimethoxyphthalaldehydic acid. $C_{10}H_{10}O_5$; mol wt 210.18. C 57.14%, H 4.80%, O 38.06%. Obtained (together with cotarnine) by heating narcotine with dil HNO_3. Prepn: Wilson *et al., J. Org. Chem.* **16**, 792 (1951); Blair, *J. Chem. Soc.* **1955**, 708. NMR studies: Buu-Hoi *et al., Bull. Soc. Chim. Fr.* **1970**, 137.

Needles from water, mp 150°. Sol in 400 parts cold, 60 parts boiling water; sol in alcohol, ether. uv max: 215, 284 nm (ε 20,700, 6500).

6852. Opiniazide. [2779-55-7] 4-Pyridinecarboxylic acid [(2-carboxy-3,4-dimethoxyphenyl)methylene]hydrazide; 5,6-dimethoxyphthalaldehydic acid isonicotinoylhydrazone; 1-(2-carboxy-3,4-dimethoxybenzylidene)-2-isonicotinoylhydrazine; 2-carboxy-3,4-dimethoxybenzal isonicotinylhydrazone; saluside; saliuzid; saluzid. $C_{16}H_{15}N_3O_5$; mol wt 329.31. C 58.36%, H 4.59%, N 12.76%, O 24.29%. Description: G. N. Pershin, S.A. Vichkanova, *C.A.* **51,** 10747e (1957); *C.A.* **52,** 1485-1486 (1958); V. A. Buskina, *C.A.* **54,** 744f (1960). Bioavailability: A. F. Zaeko, V. G. Perkova, *Farmatsiya (Moscow)* **28,** 28 (1979), *C.A.* **92,** 185805g (1980). Toxicity study: R. A. Akhundov, *Mater. Nauchn. Konf. Azgosmedinstituta* **1975,** 137, *C.A.* **86,** 50678y (1977).

LD$_{50}$ i.v. in guinea pigs: 1.634 g/kg (Akhundov).

THERAP CAT: Antibacterial (tuberculostatic).

6853. Opipramol. [315-72-0] 4-[3-(5H-Dibenz[b,f]azepin-5-yl)propyl]-1-piperazineethanol; 5-[γ-[4-(β-hydroxyethyl)piperazino]propyl]dibenzo[b,f]azepine; N-[3-[4-(2-hydroxyethyl)piperazino]propyl]iminostilbene; 4-[3-(5H-dibenzo[b,f]azepin-5-yl)propyl]-1-(2-hydroxyethyl)piperazine. $C_{23}H_{29}N_3O$; mol wt 363.50. C 76.00%, H 8.04%, N 11.56%, O 4.40%. Prepn: **FR M209** (1961 to Rhône-Poulenc), *C.A.* **58,** 3442f (1963); Schindler, **DE 1133729; CH 359143; CH 360061** (all 1962 to Geigy), *C.A.* **58,** 10219a, 10218f, 10218h (1963).

Crystals, mp 100-101°.

Dihydrochloride. [909-39-7] Dinsidon; Ensidon; Insidon. $C_{23}H_{29}N_3O.2HCl$; mol wt 436.42. Crystals from ethanol, mp 210° (**FR M209**); mp 228-230° (**DE 1133729**). Sol in water, alcohol; sparingly sol in acetone.

THERAP CAT: Antidepressant; antipsychotic.

6854. Opium. Gum opium; crude opium. Air-dried, milky exudation from incised, unripe capsules of *Papaver somniferum* L., or *P. album* Mill., *Papaveraceae. Habit.* of the plant: Asia Minor, Persia, China, Africa, India; cultivated in the Balkan States, Hungary, Southern Russia. In Japan the strain cultivated from the production of opium is called "Ikkanshu." Appearance and sources: *Chem. Eng. News* **32,** 2701 (1954). *Constit.* About 20 alkaloids, constituting about 25% of the opium; meconic acid, some lactic and sulfuric acids, sugar, resinous and waxy-like substances; 12-25% water. Morphine is the most important alkaloid and occurs to the extent of 10-16%, noscapine 4-8%, codeine 0.8-2.5%, papaverine 0.5-2.5%, thebaine 0.5-2%.

Deodorized opium. "Denarcotized" opium. Powdered opium freed from its odor and nauseating substances by treatment with petr ether. Contains 10-10.5% anhyd morphine.

Granulated opium. Opium dried at not above 70°, reduced to a 16-50 mesh powder and adjusted with lactose or other inert diluent to contain 10-10.5% anhyd morphine.

Powdered opium. Opium dried at a temp not above 70°, finely powdered amd adjusted with lactose or other inert diluent to contain 10-10.5% anhyd morphine.

Note: This is a controlled substance: **21 CFR,** 1308.12.

USE: Largely for the manuf of morphine, codeine and other opium alkaloids.

THERAP CAT: Analgesic (narcotic). Hypnotic.

THERAP CAT (VET): Analgesic (narcotic); antidiarrheal; antitussive.

6855. Opromazine. [969-99-3] 2-Chloro-N,N-dimethyl-10H-phenothiazine-10-propanamine 5-oxide; 2-chloro-10-[3-(dimethylamino)propyl]phenothiazine 5-oxide; 10-(γ-dimethylaminopropyl)-3-chlorphenothiazine 9-oxide; 5-oxychlorpromazine; chlorpromazine sulfoxide; Secotil. $C_{17}H_{19}ClN_2OS$; mol wt 334.86. C 60.98%, H 5.72%, Cl 10.59%, N 8.37%, O 4.78%, S 9.58%. Metabolite of chlorpromazine, *q.v.:* Salzman, Brodie, *J. Pharmacol. Exp. Ther.* **118,** 46 (1956). Preparation by enzymatic oxidation of chlorpromazine: Gillette, Kamm, *ibid.* **130,** 262 (1960). Synthesis: **FR 1167653** (1958 to Rhône-Poulenc). Toxicity data: Minami, Yoshimoto, *Nara Igaku Zasshi* **8,** 50 (1957), *C.A.* **51,** 16966a (1957).

Crystals, mp 115°. LD$_{50}$ s.c. in mice: 102 mg/kg (Minami, Yoshimoto).

6856. Opsins. Broad class of species-specific proteins which form the basis of the visual pigments and of bacteriorhodopsin, *q.v.* Structurally integrated into the rods and cones of the retina of the eye or into the photoreceptor membranes of certain bacteria. Each of these cell types produces a genetically specified opsin which has been classified on the basis of cellular source: **scotopsins** (rods), **photopsins** (cones), and **bacteriopsins** (bacteria). Methods for purification, prepn and assay: R. Hubbard *et al., Methods Enzymol.* **18,** 615-653 (1971). Series of articles on photoreceptor biosynthesis: *ibid.* **81,** 763-815 (1982). Review of biosynthetic process: D. S. Papermaster, B. G. Schneider in *Cell Biology of the Eye,* D. McDevitt, Ed. (Academic Press, New York, 1982) p 475. The photoreceptor activity of visual pigments is due to a carotenoid chromophore, retinal or 3-dehydroretinal, *q.q.v.,* bound as a protonated Schiff base to a lysine moiety in the opsin portion of the molecule: A. R. Osenoff, R. Callender, *Biochemistry* **13,** 4243 (1974). Each pigment has unique physicochemical properties. The most significant is the absorption spectrum which is regulated by electrostatic interactions between the chromophore and the charged or dipolar groups on the opsin: R. Hubbard, L. Sperling, *Exp. Eye Res.* **17,** 581 (1973); B. Honig *et al., J. Am. Chem. Soc.* **101,** 7084 (1979). A visual system, a set of pigments spanning the light sensitivity range of a particular species, is generally based on one type of chromophore combined with various opsins. Visual systems based on retinal are the most widespread in nature. The 11-cis isomer is utilized by rhodopsin, *q.v.,* the most common pigment of rod cells, and by the corresponding trichromatic cone pigments (*see* Iodopsin). Bacteriorhodopsin is composed of bacterioopsin and *trans* retinal. Visual systems based on 3-dehydroretinal, exemplified by the pigments porphyropsin and cyanopsin, *q.q.v.,* have been found to occur only in certain fish and amphibians. Visual pigments utilizing both types of chromophore have been found to coexist in the retina of some of these species: T. E. Reuter *et al., J. Gen. Physiol.* **58,** 351 (1971). Exposure to light initiates the bleaching of the pigment through a series of distinct intermediates involving the isomerization and ultimate dissociation of the chromophore from the opsin: R. Hubbard, A. Kropf, *Proc. Natl. Acad. Sci. USA* **44,** 140 (1958); B. Honig *et al., ibid.* **76,** 2503 (1979). This process initiates the mechanism of energy transduction and visual excitation: T. G. Ebrey, B. Honig, *Q. Rev. Biophys.* **8,** 129-184 (1975); B. Honig, *Annu. Rev. Phys. Chem.* **29,** 31-57 (1978); R. Uhl, E. W. Abrahamson, *Chem. Rev.* **81,** 291 (1981). Review of energy transduction in invertebrate photoreceptors: P. Hillman *et al., Physiol. Rev.* **63,** 668-772 (1983); in bacteriorhodopsin: H. V. Westerhoff, Z. Dancshazy, *Trends Biochem. Sci.* **9,** 112 (1984). General reviews: G. Wald, *Science* **162,** 230-239 (1968); D. F. O'Brien, *ibid.* **218,** 961-966 (1982); A. Maeda, T. Yoshizawa, *Photochem. Photobiol.* **35,** 891-898 (1983); P. S. Zurer, *Chem. Eng. News* **61,** 24-35 (Nov. 28, 1983). *See also: Methods Enzymol.* **88,** 1-836 (1982).

6857. Orange I. [523-44-4] 4-[(4-Hydroxy-1-naphthalen-yl)azo]benzenesulfonic acid monosodium salt; Tropaeolin OOO no. 1; C.I. Acid Orange 20; FD & C Orange I; Ext. D & C Orange 3; C.I. 14600; α-naphthol orange; sodium azo-α-naphtholsulfanilate. $C_{16}H_{11}N_2NaO_4S$; mol wt 350.32. C 54.86%, H 3.16%, N 8.00%, Na 6.56%, O 18.27%, S 9.15%. Prepared by coupling diazotized sulfanilic acid with α-naphthol: *Colour Index* **vol. 4** (3rd ed., 1971) p 4065.

Reddish-brown powder. Sol in water to orange-red soln, in alcohol to orange soln. Acids ppt the aq soln. Sodium hydroxide intensifies the red color of the aq soln. pH: 7.6 brownish-yellow; 8.9 purple.

6858. Orange II. [633-96-5] 4-[(2-Hydroxy-1-naphthalen-yl)azo]benzenesulfonic acid monosodium salt; C.I. Acid Orange 7; β-naphthol orange; D & C Orange No. 4; C.I. 15510; Mandarin G; Tropaeolin OOO no. 2. $C_{16}H_{11}N_2NaO_4S$; mol wt 350.32. C 54.86%, H 3.16%, N 8.00%, Na 6.56%, O 18.27%, S 9.15%. Anionic azo dye. Prepd by coupling β-naphthol, *q.v.*, with diazotized sulfanilic acid, *q.v.*, in alkaline soln, *cf. Org. Synth.* **coll. vol. II**, 36 (1943); *Colour Index* **vol. 4** (3rd ed., 1971) p 4078. *Review:* H. J. *Conn's Biological Stains*, R. D. Lillie, Ed. (Williams & Wilkins, Baltimore, 9th ed., 1977) pp 112-113, 573.

Orange-brown powder. Indicator color transitions: amber to orange pH 7.4-8.6; orange to red pH 10.2-11.8. Soly (mg/ml): water 130 mg/ml; ethanol 4 mg/ml. Absorption max (water): 483 nm.

Pentahydrate. Orange needles from water. One gram dissolves in 20 ml water. Sol in alc. Absorption max 484.4 nm.

USE: Dye; biological stain; external colorant. Limited use as an indicator.

6859. Orange B. [15139-76-1] 4,5-Dihydro-5-oxo-4-[(4-sulfo-1-naphthalenyl)azo]-1-(4-sulfophenyl)-1H-pyrazole-3-carboxylic acid 3-ethyl ester disodium salt; 5-oxo-4-[(4-sulfo-1-naph-thyl)azo]-1-(p-sulfophenyl)-2-pyrazoline-3-carboxylic acid 3-ethyl ester disodium salt; 5-hydroxy-4-[(4-sulfo-1-naphthalenyl)azo]-1-(4-sulfophenyl)-1H-pyrazole-3-carboxylic acid 3-ethyl ester disodium salt; 1-(4-sulfophenyl)-3-ethylcarboxyl-4-(4-sulfonaphthylazo)-5-hydroxypyrazole disodium salt; C.I. Acid Orange 137; C.I. 19235. $C_{22}H_{16}N_4Na_2O_9S_2$; mol wt 590.49. C 44.75%, H 2.73%, N 9.49%, Na 7.79%, O 24.39%, S 10.86%. Prepn: W. H. Kretlow *et al.*, **US 3285906** (1966 to Stange Co.). *Review: Fed. Regist.* **43**, 45611 (1978). *See also Colour Index* **vol. 4** (3rd ed., 1971) p 4134.

Dull orange crystals. Absorption max (0.04N ammonium acetate): 442 nm. Soly in water at 77°: 220 g/l. Violet soln in conc H_2SO_4, changing to fuchsia then red on dilution. Red soln in conc HCl. Yellowish soln in 10% NaOH, changing to brownish yellow on dilution.

USE: In coloring sausage and frankfurter casings.

6860. Orange Peel. Rind of the fruit of *Citrus aurantium* L., *Rutaceae. Habit.* N. India; cultivated near Mediterranean Sea, Spain, W. Indies, Florida, California. Review: A. Y. Leung, *Encyclopedia of Common Natural Ingredients* (John Wiley & Sons, New York, 1980) pp 248-252.

Bitter orange peel. Dried rind of unripe fruit. *Constit.* Volatile oil, hesperidine, naringin, aurantiamarin, acrid resin, gum, tannin.

Sweet orange peel. Fresh rind of ripe fruit of *C. aurantium*, var *sinensis* (also known as *C. sinensis*). *Constit.* Volatile oil, hesperidine, fixed oil, resin, gum, tannin. Closely resembles bitter orange peel, but has an orange-yellow color; sweetish, fragrant odor; aromatic and only slightly bitter taste.

USE: Flavoring agent.

6861. Orazamide. [2574-78-9] 1,2,3,6-Tetrahydro-2,6-di-oxo-4-pyrimidinecarboxylic acid compd with 5-amino-1H-imida-zole-4-carboxamide (1:1); 5-aminoimidazole-4-carboxamide oro-tate; orotic acid compd with 5(or 4)-aminoimidazole-4(or 5)-car-boxamide (1:1); 4-amino-5-imidazolecarboxamide orotate; AICA orotate; Aicamin; Aicorat. $C_9H_{10}N_6O_5$; mol wt 282.21. C 38.30%, H 3.57%, N 29.78%, O 28.35%. Prepn: **FR 1351141**; Haraoka, Kamiya, **US 3271398** (1964, 1966 both to Fujisawa). Pharmacology and toxicology: Tamura, Shibayama, *Yakugaku Kenkyu* **35**, 94 (1963), *C.A.* **64**, 2652h (1966); Hashimoto, *J. Vita-minol.* **13**, 9, 19 (1967).

Dihydrate. Crystals, dec 284-285°. LD_{50} in mice (g/kg): 0.6 i.p.; >4.0 orally (Tamura, Shibayama).

THERAP CAT: Hepatoprotectant.

6862. Orbifloxacin. [113617-63-3] *rel*-1-Cyclopropyl-7-[(3R,5S)-3,5-dimethyl-1-piperazinyl]-5,6,8-trifluoro-1,4-dihydro-4-oxo-3-quinolinecarboxylic acid ; 1-cyclopropyl-5,6,8-trifluoro-(cis-3,5-dimethyl-1-piperazinyl)-1,4-dihydro-4-oxoquinoline-3-carbox-ylic acid; CP-104594; Orbax. $C_{19}H_{20}F_3N_3O_3$; mol wt 395.38. C 57.72%, H 5.10%, F 14.42%, N 10.63%, O 12.14%. Fluorinated quinoline antibacterial. Prepn: J. Matsumoto *et al.*, **EP 242789**; *eidem*, **US 4886810** (1987, 1989 both to Dainippon). *In vitro* activity vs *Staphylococcus intermedius*: J.-P. Ganière *et al., Res. Vet. Sci.* **77**, 67 (2004). Photodegradation kinetics: T. Morimura *et al., Chem. Pharm. Bull.* **43**, 1000 (1995). Pharmacokinetics in mares: G. R. Haines *et al., Can. J. Vet. Res.* **65**, 181 (2001). HPLC determn in rabbit plasma: M. A. Garcia *et al., J. Chromatogr. Sci.* **37**, 199 (1999); LC/fluorescence/MS determn in eggs: M. J. Schneider, D. J. Donoghue, *Anal. Chim. Acta* **483**, 39 (2003). Localization of drug to diseased skin: P. A. Kay-Mugford *et al., Vet. Ther.* **3**, 1 (2002). Review of veterinary use in Japan: S. Nakamura, *Drugs* **49**, Suppl. 2, 152-158 (1995); of use in companion animals: R. D. Walker, *Aust. Vet. J.* **78**, 84-90 (2000).

Crystals from chlororform-ethanol, mp 259-260°. pKa_1: 5.60; pKa_2 8.90.

THERAP CAT (VET): Antibacterial.

6863. Orcein. [1400-62-0] A dye first prepared from lichens (cudbear, *q.v.*, or *archil*). Prepn by oxidation of orcinol with H_2O_2 in the presence of ammonia water: Zulkowski, Peters, *Monatsh. Chem.* **11**, 227 (1890). Can be separated into 14 dyes by distribution chromatography: Musso, *Ber.* **89**, 1659 (1956). The eight compds depicted are the major components of orcein; β- and γcomponents are *cis-trans* isomers of the same compd. Structure studies: Beecken *et al., Angew. Chem.* **73**, 665 (1961). Brief review: *H. J. Conn's Biological Stains*, R. D. Lillie, Ed. (Williams & Wilkins, Baltimore, 9th ed., 1977) pp 400-403. Review of use as textile dye and histological stain for elastin: H. Puchter, S. N. Meloan, *Histochemistry* **64**, 119 (1979).

	R_1	R_2	R_3
α-Aminoorcein	H	O	NH_2
α-Hydroxyorcein	H	O	OH
β- and γ-Aminoorcein	orcinol	O	NH_2
β- and γ-Hydroxyorcein	orcinol	O	OH
β- and γ-Aminoorceimine	orcinol	NH	NH_2

Brownish-red microcryst powder. Practically insol in water, benzene, chloroform, ether, carbon disulfide. Sol in alcohol, acetone or acetic acid with red color, in dil aq alkali with bluish-violet color.

USE: Biological stain.

6864. Orcinol. [504-15-4] 5-Methyl-1,3-benzenediol; 5-methylresorcinol; orcin; 3,5-dihydroxytoluene. $C_7H_8O_2$; mol wt 124.14. C 67.73%, H 6.50%, O 25.78%. Occurs in many species of lichens: Sastry, Rao, *Curr. Sci.* **10**, 437 (1941). Prepn: Anker, Cook, *J. Chem. Soc.* **1945**, 311; Kisteneva, Rozhdestvenskii, *Zh. Prikl. Khim.* **22**, 1108 (1949); Stevens, US 2603662 (1952 to Gulf); Zimmer, US 3028410 (1962 to Hooker Chem.). Toxicity studies: I. Veldre *et al., Vopr. Gig. Tr. Prof. Patol. Est. SSR* **2**, 160 (1970), *C.A.* **74**, 51746h (1971).

Monohydrate. Crystals; sweet but unpleasant taste; reddens on exposure to air due to oxidation. mp about 58°; 107° when anhydr. bp 290°; bp$_{14-20}$ 165-170°; bp$_5$ 147°. Freely sol in water, alcohol, ether; less sol in benzene; slightly sol in chloroform or carbon disulfide. *Keep well closed and protected from light.* LD$_{50}$ in mice, rats, rabbits, guinea pigs (mg/kg): 772, 844, 2400, 1678 orally (Veldre).

USE: As a reagent for pentoses, lignin, beet sugar, saccharoses, arabinose, diastase.

6865. Oregovomab. [213327-37-8] Anti-(human CA125-(carbohydrate antigen)) immunoglobulin G1(mouse monoclonal B43.13 γ$_1$-chain) disulfide with mouse monoclonal B43.13 κ-chain dimer; OvaRex. Murine monoclonal antibody directed against the ovarian tumor associated antigen CA-125; induces tumor specific cellular immune response. Prepn: M. J. Krantz *et al., J. Cell Biochem.* Suppl. 12E, 139 (1988). Preparative method as radioimmunodiagnostic: V. Capstick *et al., Int. J. Biol. Markers* **6**, 129 (1991). Clinical experience in antiidiotype induction therapy: R. Madiyalakan *et al., Hybridoma* **14**, 199 (1995). Clinical pharmacokinetics: S. A. McQuarrie *et al., Nucl. Med. Commun.* **18**, 878 (1997). Immunopharmacology: B. C. Schultes *et al., Hybridoma* **18**, 47 (1999); A. A. Noujaim *et al., Cancer Biother. Radiopharm.* **16**, 187 (2001). Assay to monitor immune response: B. C. Schultes, T. L. Whiteside, *J. Immunol. Methods* **279**, 1 (2003). Clinical evaluation in ovarian cancer: J. S. Berek *et al., J. Clin. Oncol.* **22**, 3507 (2004); combined with chemotherapy: A. N. Gordon *et al., Gynecol. Oncol.* **94**, 340 (2004). Reviews of development and therapeutic potential: I. Bruckner, *IDrugs* **4**, 457-462 (2001); J. S. Berek *Expert Opin. Biol. Ther.* **4**, 1159-1165 (2004).

THERAP CAT: Antineoplastic, immunomodulator.

6866. Orexins. Hypocretins. Neuropeptides produced in the hypothalamus that are involved in the regulation of feeding behavior and the sleep-wake cycle. Name derived from the Greek word, orexis, meaning appetite. Fasting increases orexin production; administration of exogenous orexin stimulates feeding. Also implicated in the pathophysiology of narcolepsy. Two forms are known (orexins A and B); both are derived from the same precursor protein. Two orexin receptors (OX$_1$R and OX$_2$R) have been identified in mammalian brain. OX$_1$R binds only orexin A while OX$_2$R is a nonselective receptor for both A and B. Identification of the orexin precursor: L. De Lecea *et al., Proc. Natl. Acad. Sci. USA* **95**, 322 (1998). Purification and biological activity of orexins: T. Sakurai *et al., Cell* **92**, 573 (1998). Immunohistochemical localization in rat brain: Y. Date *et al., Proc. Natl. Acad. Sci. USA* **96**, 748 (1999). Association of canine narcolepsy with OX$_2$R defect: L. Lin *et al., Cell* **98**, 365 (1999); of sleep disorder in orexin knockout mice: R. M. Chemelli *et al., ibid.* 437. Clinical determn of orexin deficiency in CSF of narcoleptic patients: S. Nishino *et al., Lancet* **355**, 39 (2000). Review of structure, tissue distribution and role in feeding behavior: T. Sakurai, *Regul. Pept.* **85**, 25-30 (1999). Review of role in narcolepsy and potential therapeutic application: J. M. Siegel, *Cell* **98**, 409-412 (1999).

Orexin A. [205599-75-3] Hypocretin-1. Cyclic, 33-amino acid peptide; mol wt 3562 Da. Sequence is completely conserved in human, rat, mouse, cow and pig.

Orexin B. [205599-76-4] Hypocretin-2. Linear, 28-amino acid peptide; mol wt 2937 Da. Sequence is 46% homologous with orexin A. Human and rodent forms differ by 2 amino acid substitutions.

6867. Oripavine. [467-04-9] (5α)-6,7,8,14-Tetrahydro-4,5-epoxy-6-methoxy-17-methylmorphinan-3-ol; O^3-demethylthebaine. $C_{18}H_{19}NO_3$; mol wt 297.35. C 72.71%, H 6.44%, N 4.71%, O 16.14%. From *Papaver orientale* L., and *P. bracteatum* Lindl., *Papaveraceae:* Junusov *et al., Ber.* **68**, 2158 (1935); Kiselev, Konovalova, *J. Gen. Chem. USSR* **18**, 142 (1948). Identity of *O*-methyl derivative with thebaine: *eidem, Zh. Obshch. Khim.* **18**, 855 (1948). Biosynthesis: Gross, Dawson, *Biochemistry* **2**, 186 (1963). *Reviews:* H. L. Holmes in *The Alkaloids* vol. II, Manske, Holmes, Eds. (Academic Press, New York, 1952) p 167; K. W. Bentley, *The Chemistry of the Morphine Alkaloids* (Oxford, 1954) pp 192-196. Synthesis from morphine: Barber, Rapoport, *J. Med. Chem.* **18**, 1074 (1975).

Crystals, mp 200-201°. $[\alpha]_D^{20}$ −211.8°.

Hydrochloride. $C_{18}H_{19}NO_3$·HCl. Crystals, dec 244-245°.

Methiodide. $C_{18}H_{19}NO_3$·CH$_3$I. Crystals, dec 207-208°.

6868. Oritavancin. [171099-57-3] (4″R)-22-O-(3-Amino-2,3,6-trideoxy-3-C-methyl-α-L-*arabino*-hexopyranosyl)-$N^{3''}$-[(4′-chloro[1,1′-biphenyl]-4-yl)methyl]vancomycin; LY-333328. C_{86}-$H_{97}Cl_3N_{10}O_{26}$; mol wt 1793.10. C 57.61%, H 5.45%, Cl 5.93%, N 7.81%, O 23.20%. Semisynthetic glycopeptide antibiotic. Prepn: R. D. G. Cooper *et al.*, WO 9630401; *eidem* US 5840684 (1996, 1998 both to Eli Lilly). *In vitro* antibacterial activity: F. Biavasco *et al., Antimicrob. Agents Chemother.* **41**, 2165 (1997). Mechanism of action: N. E. Allen, T. I. Nicas, *FEMS Microbiol. Rev.* **26**, 511 (2003). Clinical pharmacokinetics: S. M. Bhavnani *et al., Diagn. Microbiol. Infect. Dis.* **50**, 95 (2004); G. J. Fetterly *et al., Antimicrob. Agents Chemother.* **49**, 148 (2005). Clinical evaluation in *Staphylococcus aureus* bacteremia: S. M. Bhavnani *et al., ibid.* **50**, 994 (2006). Review of pharmacology and clinical development: D. R. P. Guay, *Pharmacotherapy* **24**, 58-68 (2004).

Diphosphate. [192564-14-0] $C_{86}H_{97}Cl_3N_{10}O_{26}\cdot2H_3PO_4$; mol wt 1989.09. Sol in water.

THERAP CAT: Antibacterial.

6869. Orlistat. [96829-58-2] N-Formyl-L-leucine (1S)-1-[[(2S,3S)-3-hexyl-4-oxo-2-oxetanyl]methyl]dodecyl ester; N-formyl-L-leucine ester with (3S,4S)-3-hexyl-4-[(2S)-2-hydroxytridecyl]-2-oxetanone; (−)-tetrahydrolipstatin; orlipastat; Ro-18-0647; Xenical. $C_{29}H_{53}NO_5$; mol wt 495.73. C 70.26%, H 10.78%, N 2.83%, O 16.14%. Isoln from fermentation broth of *Streptomyces toxytricini:* P. Hadvary *et al., EP 129748*; eidem, *US 4598089* (1985, 1986 both to Hoffmann-LaRoche). Structural elucidation: E. Hochuli *et al., J. Antibiot.* **40,** 1086 (1987). Synthesis and absolute configuration: P. Barbier, F. Schneider, *Helv. Chim. Acta* **70,** 196 (1987). Total synthesis: S. Hanessian *et al., J. Org. Chem.* **58,** 7768 (1993). Mechanism of action: B. Borgström, *Biochim. Biophys. Acta* **962,** 308 (1988). Clinical pharmacology: J. B. Hauptman *et al., Am. J. Clin. Nutr.* **55,** 309S (1992). Clinical trial: M. H. Davidson *et al., J. Am. Med. Assoc.* **281,** 235 (1999). Review of pharmacology and clinical efficacy in treatment of obesity: W. McNeely, P. Benfield, *Drugs* **56,** 241-249 (1998). Evaluation of long-term efficacy and tolerability: J. Hauptman *et al., Arch. Fam. Med.* **9,** 160 (2000).

Crystals, mp 43°. $[\alpha]_D^{20}$ −32.0° (c = 1 in chloroform).

THERAP CAT: Antiobesity agent.

6870. Orlon®. Polyacrylonitrile; Fiber A. Obtained by polymerizing acrylonitrile. Review of prepn, properties, and uses: R. W. Moncrieff, *Man-Made Fibres* (John Wiley, New York, 1963) pp 446-467.

White fiber. Sticks at 235°. Ironing temps above 160° may cause yellowing. Sp gr 1.17. Flammability similar to that of rayon and cotton. Generally has very good resistance to mineral acids; excellent resistance to common solvents, oils, greases, neutral salts, sunlight; fairly good resistance to weak alkalies but is degraded by strong alkalies. Resists attack by molds, mildew, insects. 100% polyacrylonitrile fibers rarely used commercially due to difficulty in dyeing.

USE: Fiber suitable for outdoor furnishings (awnings, tents, outdoor furniture), indoor furnishings, anode bags in electroplating, knitwear, rugs.

6871. Ormosinine. [14350-67-5] 21-Ormosanin-20-yl panamine. $C_{40}H_{66}N_6$; mol wt 630.99. C 76.14%, H 10.54%, N 13.32%. From seed of *Ormosia dasycarpa* Jacks., *Leguminosae:* Hess, Merck, *Ber.* **52,** 1976 (1919); from *O. panamensis* Benth., *Leguminosae:* Lloyd, Horning, *J. Am. Chem. Soc.* **80,** 1506 (1958). Structural studies: Wilson, *Chem. Ind. (London)* **1965,** 472; *Tetrahedron* **21,** 2561 (1965). Composed of one molecule of **panamine** and one molecule of **ormosanine**; NMR elucidation of structure: N. S. Bhacca *et al., J. Am. Chem. Soc.* **105,** 2538 (1983).

Needles from ethyl acetate, mp 219-220°. $[\alpha]_{436}^{25}$ +16.0°. $[\alpha]_{589}^{25}$ +8.9° (c = 1.29 in chloroform). Sol in chloroform; slightly sol in ether. Practically insol in water, alcohol. Sublimes to panamine.

6872. Ornidazole. [16773-42-5] α-(Chloromethyl)-2-methyl-5-nitro-1H-imidazole-1-ethanol; 1-(3-chloro-2-hydroxypropyl)-2-methyl-5-nitroimidazole; Ro-7-0207; Madelen; Ornidal; Tiberal. $C_7H_{10}ClN_3O_3$; mol wt 219.63. C 38.28%, H 4.59%, Cl 16.14%, N 19.13%, O 21.85%. Prepn: **NL 6606853**; M. Hoffer, **US 3435049** and **US 3493582** (1966, 1969 and 1970, all to Hoffmann-La Roche). Activity studies: E. Grunberg *et al., Proc. Soc. Exp. Biol. Med.* **133,** 490 (1970). Synthesis and antiprotozoal activity: M. Hoffer, E. Grunberg, *J. Med. Chem.* **17,** 1019 (1974). Pharmacokinetics: D. E. Schwartz, F. Jeunet, *Chemotherapy* **22,** 19 (1976).

Crystals from toluene, mp 77-78°. uv max (2-propanol): 288, 312 nm (ε 3720, 9150). pKa: 2.4 ± 0.1. LD_{50} in rats, mice (mg/kg): 1780, 1420 orally (Grunberg). Also reported as LD_{50} in mice (mg/kg): >2000 orally, >2000 i.p. (Hoffer, Grunberg).

THERAP CAT: Anti-infective.

6873. Ornipressin. [3397-23-7] 8-L-Ornithinevasopressin; orn(8)-vasopressin; POR-8. $C_{45}H_{63}N_{13}O_{12}S_2$; mol wt 1042.19. C 51.86%, H 6.09%, N 17.47%, O 18.42%, S 6.15%. Synthetic analog of vasopressin, q.v., in which L-ornithine replaces L-arginine. Prepn: R. L. Huguenin, R. A. Boissonnas, *Helv. Chim. Acta* **46,** 1669 (1963); *eidem,* **FR 1396607** corresp to **US 3299036** (1965, 1967 both to Sandoz). Separation by reversed-phase HPLC: K. Krummen, R. W. Frei, *J. Chromatogr.* **132,** 27 (1977). Pharmacologic properties: B. Berde *et al., Experientia* **20,** 42 (1964). Pharmacodynamics: S. Keppens, H. de Wulf, *Biochim. Biophys. Acta* **588,** 63 (1979). Comparison of hemostatic and cardiovascular effects: L. Saarnivaara, P. Leander, *Anaesthesist* **26,** 144 (1977). Clinical study: D. J. Adendorff, D. Davies, *S. Afr. Med. J.* **51,** 131 (1977).

Cys-Tyr-Phe-Gln-Asn-Cys-Pro-Orn-GlyNH₂

THERAP CAT: Vasoconstrictor.

6874. Ornithine. [70-26-8] L-Ornithine; α,δ-diaminovaleric acid; 2,5-diaminopentanoic acid. $C_5H_{12}N_2O_2$; mol wt 132.16. C 45.44%, H 9.15%, N 21.20%, O 24.21%. Non-essential amino acid for human development but is required intermediate in arginine biosynthesis. Found in virtually all vertebrate tissues as well as incorporated into proteins, such as tyrocidine, *q.v.* Isolation from chicken excreta: M. Jaffe, *Ber.* **10**, 1925 (1877). Early chemistry and biochemistry: J. P. Greenstein, M. Winitz, *Chemistry of the Amino Acids* (John Wiley and Sons, Inc., New York, 1961) pp. 2477-2491, *passim.* Review of synthesis: R. Yoshida, *Synth. Prod. Util. Amino Acids*, T. Kaneko *et al.*, Eds (Kodansha Ltd, Tokyo, Japan, 1974) pp 166-170; of biosynthesis in plants: P. D. Shargool *et al.*, *Phytochemistry* **27**, 1571-1574 (1988). Brief historical review: H. A. Akers, E. V. Dromgoole, *Trends Biochem. Sci.* **7**, 156-157 (1982). Review of metabolism: V. E. Shih, *Enzyme* **26**, 254-258 (1981); of role in CNS functions: N. Seiler, G. Daune-Anglard, *Metab. Brain Dis.* **8**, 151-179 (1993).

Colorless crystals. $[\alpha]_D^{25}$ +11.5° (c = 6.5). Aq solns are alkaline. pK_1' 1.94; pK_2' 8.65; pK_3' 10.76. Freely sol in water, alc; sparingly sol in ether.

L-Form aspartate. [3230-94-2] L-Ornithine-L-aspartate; Hepa-Merz. Crystal structure: D. M. Salunke, M. Vijayan, *Int. J. Pept. Protein Res.* **22**, 154 (1983). Clinical trial in hyperammonemia: J. Fehér *et al.*, *Med. Sci. Monit.* **3**, 669 (1997); S. Stauch *et al.*, *J. Hepatol.* **28**, 856 (1998).

DL-Form. [616-07-9] Crystals from water. Sparingly sol in alcohol.

THERAP CAT: In treatment of hyperammonemia.

6875. Ornoprostil. [70667-26-4] (1*R*,2*R*,3*R*)-3-Hydroxy-2-[(1*E*,3*S*,5*S*)-3-hydroxy-5-methyl-1-nonenyl]-ε,5-dioxocyclopentaneheptanoic acid; (11α,13*E*,15*S*,17*S*)-11,15-dihydroxy-17,20-dimethyl-6,9-dioxoprost-13-en-1-oic acid methyl ester; 17*S*,20-dimethyl-6-oxoprostaglandin E_1 methyl ester; 6-oxo-17*S*,20-dimethyl-PGE$_1$ methyl ester; ronoprost; ONO-1308; OU-1308; Alloca; Ronok. $C_{23}H_{38}O_6$; mol wt 410.54. C 67.29%, H 9.33%, O 23.38%. Analog of prostaglandin E_1, *q.v.* Prepn: M. Hayashi *et al.*, **DE 2840032**; *eidem*, **US 4278688** (1979, 1981 both to Ono). Effect on gastric mucosal lesions in rats: H. Kuwata *et al.*, *Nippon Shokakibyo Gakkai Zasshi* **82**, 1858 (1985), *C.A.* **104**, 15709c (1986); *eidem*, *Curr. Clin. Pract. Ser.* **36**, 243 (1986); on experimental esophagitis: S. Inoue *et al.*, *Gendai Iryo* **19**, 1348 (1987), *C.A.* **107**, 626m (1987).

THERAP CAT: Antiulcerative.

6876. Orotic Acid. [65-86-1] 1,2,3,6-Tetrahydro-2,6-dioxo-4-pyrimidinecarboxylic acid; uracil-6-carboxylic acid; whey factor; animal galactose factor; Oropur; Orotyl. $C_5H_4N_2O_4$; mol wt 156.10. C 38.47%, H 2.58%, N 17.95%, O 41.00%. A pyrimidine precursor in animal organisms, found in milk: Bachstez, *Ber.* **64**, 2683 (1931); Hilbert, *J. Am. Chem. Soc.* **54**, 2082 (1932); Johnson, Schroeder, *ibid.* 2942. Synthesis from aspartic acid: Nye, Mitchell, *ibid.* **69**, 1382 (1947). Prepn by condensation of urea with monoethyl ester of oxalacetic acid in methanol: Scriabine, **US 2937175** (1960 to Rhône-Poulenc). Older syntheses from urea and oxalacetic ester: Müller, *J. Prakt. Chem.* **56**, 488 (1897); Behrend, Struve, *Ann.* **378**, 165 (1910). Microbial process by a pyrimidine-requiring *Micrococcus glutamicus* mutant: Kinoshita *et al.*, **US 3086917** (1963 to Kyowa). Classed as a vitamin: Moruzzi *et al.*, *Biochem. Z.* **333**, 318 (1960). Relationship to *vitamin B$_{13}$*: Manna, Hauge, *J. Biol. Chem.* **202**, 91 (1953).

Crystals from water, mp 345-346°.

Monohydrate. [50887-69-9] Lactinium; Oroturic. Crystals, mp 334°. uv max: 282 nm; min: 255 nm. Sol in water ~1.7 mg/ml.

Methyl ester. [6153-44-2] $C_6H_6N_2O_4$. Crystals, mp 249°.

Ethyl ester. [1747-53-1] $C_7H_8N_2O_4$. Crystals, mp 188-189°.

Choline salt. [24381-49-5] Choline orotate; Cholergol. $C_5H_4N_2O_4 \cdot C_5H_{14}NO$; mol wt 260.27.

USE: Has been proposed as feed supplement in combination with methionine to aid growth of calves.

THERAP CAT: Uricosuric.

6877. Orotidine. [314-50-1] 1,2,3,6-Tetrahydro-2,6-dioxo-3-β-D-ribofuranosyl-4-pyrimidinecarboxylic acid; 3-β-D-ribofuranosylorotic acid; 6-carboxyuridine. $C_{10}H_{12}N_2O_8$; mol wt 288.21. C 41.67%, H 4.20%, N 9.72%, O 44.41%. An orotic acid riboside obtained from cultures of *Neurospora crassa* mutants: Michelson *et al.*, *Proc. Natl. Acad. Sci. USA* **37**, 396 (1951). Isoln: Mitchell, Michelson, **US 2788346** (1957 to California Inst. Res. Found.). Structure: Fox *et al.*, *Biochim. Biophys. Acta* **23**, 295 (1957). Synthesis: Curran, Angier, *J. Org. Chem.* **31**, 201 (1966); **US 3282919** (1966 to Am. Cyanamid). Synthesis of orotidine 5'-phosphate: Moffatt, *J. Am. Chem. Soc.* **85**, 1118 (1963).

Needles from methanol + benzene. Turned brown near 200° but failed to melt at 400°. uv max (methanol): 268 nm (ε 8900); in 0.1*N* HCl: 267 nm (ε 9570); in 0.1*N* methanolic NaOH: 265 nm (ε 8960). Soluble in hot water, lower aliphatic alcohols and aq solns of such alcohols.

Cyclohexamine salt. $C_{16}H_{25}N_3O_8$. Crystals from ethanol + benzene, mp 183-184°. $[\alpha]_D$ +15° (c = 1). Also isolated as the lead salt.

Orotidine 5'-phosphate trisodium salt trihydrate. $C_{10}H_{10}N_2O_{11}PNa_3 \cdot 3H_2O$. uv max (0.1*N* HCl): 267 nm (ε 9430). Soluble in water.

N^3-Methylorotidine methyl ester. $C_{12}H_{16}N_2O_8$. Stout crystals from isopropanol, mp 135-137°. uv max (methanol): 271 nm (ε 7620).

6878. Oroxylin A. [480-11-5] 5,7-Dihydroxy-6-methoxy-2-phenyl-4*H*-1-benzopyran-4-one; 5,7-dihydroxy-6-methoxyflavone; oroxylin. $C_{16}H_{12}O_5$; mol wt 284.26. C 67.60%, H 4.26%, O 28.14%. From root bark of *Oroxylum indicum* Vent., *Bignoniaceae:* Naylor, Chaplin, *Pharm. J.* **20**, 257 (1890); Naylor, Dyer, *J. Chem. Soc.* **79**, 954 (1901); Row *et al.*, *Proc. Indian Acad. Sci.* **28A**, 189 (1948). Structure: Shah *et al.*, *J. Chem. Soc.* **1936**, 591; **1938**, 1555. Synthesis: Murti, Seshadri, *Proc. Indian Acad. Sci.* **29A**, 1 (1949); Sarin, Seshadri, *J. Sci. Ind. Res.* **19B**, 117 (1960); Molho, Gerphagnon, *Bull. Soc. Chim. Fr.* **1963**, 607; Varady, *Tetrahedron Lett.* **1965**, 4281.

Yellow plates from ethanol, mp 231-232°. Sol in alc, acetone, hot benzene, ether, alkalies, glacial acetic acid; sparingly sol in chloroform; practically insol in water.

Diacetyl oroxylin. $C_{20}H_{16}O_7$. Needles from alcohol, mp 131-132°.

6879. Orphenadrine. [83-98-7] *N,N*-Dimethyl-2-[(2-methylphenyl)phenylmethoxy]ethanamine; *N,N*-dimethyl-2-(*o*-methyl-α-phenylbenzyloxy)ethylamine; *o*-methyldiphenhydramine; *o*-monomethyldiphenhydramine; 2-(phenyl-*o*-tolylmethoxy)ethyldimethylamine; phenyl-*o*-tolylmethyl dimethylaminoethyl ether; β-dimethylaminoethyl 2-methylbenzhydryl ether; BS-5930; Biorphen; Brocasipal. $C_{18}H_{23}NO$; mol wt 269.38. C 80.26%, H 8.61%, N 5.20%, O 5.94%. Prepd by the action of 2-methylbenzhydryl chloride on dimethylaminoethanol: Bijlsma *et al., Arzneim.-Forsch.* **5,** 72 (1955); Harms, Nauta, *J. Med. Pharm. Chem.* **2,** 57 (1960). Covered, but not described in Rieveschl, **US 2567351** (1951 to Parke, Davis). Resolution of optical isomers: van der Stelt *et al., Arzneim.-Forsch.* **19,** 2010 (1969). Synthesis and pharmacological study of metabolites: Den Besten *et al., ibid.* **20,** 538 (1970). Prepn of dosage forms: Harms, **US 2991225** (1961 to Brocades-Stheeman).

Liquid. bp$_{12}$ 195°.

Hydrochloride. Disipal; Mephenamin. $C_{18}H_{23}NO.HCl$; mol wt 305.84. Crystals, mp 156-157°. Sol in water, alcohol, chloroform. Sparingly sol in acetone, benzene. Practically insol in ether. pH of aq soln about 5.5.

Citrate. [4682-36-4] Banflex; Norflex; X-Otag. $C_{18}H_{23}$-$NO.C_6H_8O_7$; mol wt 461.50.

THERAP CAT: Muscle relaxant (skeletal); antihistaminic.

6880. Orris. White flag. Rhizome of *Iris florentina* L., *I. pallida* Lam. or *I. germanica* L., *Iridaceae. Habit.* Northern Italy, Germany, France. *Constit.* Iridin, irone, ionone, resin, starch, volatile oil (butter of orris). *Review:* W. A. Poucher, *Perfumes, Cosmetics and Soaps* vol. 1 (Chapman & Hall, London, 1974) pp 287-290.

Oil. Orris root oil. *Constit.* About 85% myristic acid; the odorous principle irone; methyl myristate, oleic aldehyde. Yellowish-white to yellow, semisolid fatty substance; violet-like odor. mp 44-50°. Slightly dextrorotatory. Acid no. 213-222. Sapon no. 2-6.

USE: In perfumes and soaps. As dusting powder.

6881. *o*-Orsellinic Acid. [480-64-8] 2,4-Dihydroxy-6-methylbenzoic acid; 6-methyl-β-resorcylic acid; 4,6-dihydroxy-*o*-toluic acid; 2,4-dihydroxy-6-methylbenzenecarboxylic acid; orcinolcarboxylic acid. $C_8H_8O_4$; mol wt 168.15. C 57.14%, H 4.80%, O 38.06%. Found in conjugated form or in depside form in *Roccella* and *Lecanora* lichens, postulated to arise by autocondensation of acetoacetic acid. Isoln from the fungus *Chaetomium cochliodes:* Mosback, *Z. Naturforsch.* **14B,** 69 (1959). Synthesis: Sonn, *Ber.* **61,** 926 (1928); Kloss, Clayton, *J. Org. Chem.* **30,** 3566 (1965).

Needles from acetone, mp 176° (effervescence). pK (25°) 3.90. uv max (0.1*N* HCl): 214, 260, 296 nm; in 0.1*N* NaOH: 272 nm. Sol in water, alcohol, glycerol. Soly in ether at 20° = 15.7%. Slightly sol in benzene.

Monohydrate. Needles from water, mp 186-189°.
Methyl ester. $C_9H_{10}O_4$. Crystals, mp 140°.
Ethyl ester. $C_{10}H_{12}O_4$. Crystals, mp 132°.

6882. Orthanilic Acid. [88-21-1] 2-Aminobenzenesulfonic acid; *o*-sulfanilic acid; *o*-anilinesulfonic acid. $C_6H_7NO_3S$; mol wt 173.19. C 41.61%, H 4.07%, N 8.09%, O 27.71%, S 18.51%. Prepn from *o*-nitrobenzenesulfonyl chloride: Wertheim, *Org. Synth.* **coll. vol. II,** 271 (1943).

Minute hexagonal plates, dec ~325°. Slow crystallization from water below 13.5° may yield a hemihydrate. pK (25°) 2.48. Slowly and sparingly sol in water.

6883. Orthocaine. [536-25-4] 3-Amino-4-hydroxybenzoic acid methyl ester; methyl 3-amino-4-hydroxybenzoate; Orthoform; Orthoform New. $C_8H_9NO_3$; mol wt 167.16. C 57.48%, H 5.43%, N 8.38%, O 28.71%. Prepd by dissolving 3-amino-4-hydroxybenzoic acid in methanol, saturating with HCl gas: Einhorn, Pfyl, *Ann.* **311,** 46 (1900); **DE 97333;** *Chem. Zentralbl.* **1898, II,** 525. Also prepd by reduction of methyl 3-nitro-4-hydroxybenzoate with aluminum amalgam: Auwers, Röhrig, *Ber.* **30,** 991 (1897); with tin and HCl or with stannous chloride and alcoholic HCl: **DE 97334;** *Chem. Zentralbl.* **1898, II,** 526.

Needles from benzene, mp 143°. When crystallized from chloroform it sometimes assumes an allotropic form, mp 111°, which on melting changes to the normal form and after solidifying always melts at 143°. Odorless and tasteless. Neutral reaction. Almost insol in cold water. Moderately sol in hot water with gradual decompn forming 3-amino-4-hydroxybenzoic acid and methanol. One gram dissolves in 6 ml alcohol, 50 ml ether; readily dissolves in aq NaOH. Forms water sol salts with HCl and HBr.

Note: The name Orthoform was applied originally to the methyl ester of 4-amino-3-hydroxybenzoic acid which was also used as a local anesthetic. This compd now is designated as Orthoform Old.

THERAP CAT: Anesthetic (topical).
THERAP CAT (VET): Anesthetic (topical).

6884. Orthoformic Acid. [463-78-5] Methanetriol; trihydroxymethane. CH_4O_3; mol wt 64.04. C 18.75%, H 6.30%, O 74.95%. Hypothetical compd, illustrated for nomenclature purposes only. The hydrogens of the hydroxyl groups are replaceable with alkyl groups giving rise to orthoformic esters, which are real compds (produced by various syntheses, e.g. from sodium alcoholates and chloroform). Monograph: H. W. Post, *The Chemistry of the Aliphatic Orthoesters* (Reinhold, New York, 1943), 188 pp.

Orthoformic Acid   Methyl Orthoformate

Trimethyl ester. [149-73-5] Trimethoxymethane; methyl orthoformate. $C_4H_{10}O_3$. Prepd from chloroform and methanol in presence of sodium: Sah, Ma, *J. Am. Chem. Soc.* **54,** 2965 (1932). Liquid. d_4^{20} 0.9676; d_4^{25} 0.9623. bp$_{760}$ 100.6°. n_D^{25} 1.3773.

Triethyl ester. [122-51-0] 1,1',1''-[Methylidynetris(oxy)]-tris[ethane]; ethyl orthoformate; triethoxymethane; triethyl orthoformate; Aethone. $C_7H_{16}O_3$; mol wt 148.20. Prepd from chloroform and ethanol in presence of sodium: Chu, Shen, *C.A.* **38,** 2930[7]

(1944). Toxicity study: H. F. Smyth *et al., Arch. Ind. Hyg. Occup. Med.* **4**, 119 (1951). Liquid, sweetish odor resembling that of pine needles. d_4^{20} 0.8909; d_4^{25} 0.8858. bp$_{765}$ 143°. mp < −18°. n_D^{25} 1.3900. Slightly sol in water with decompn; misc with alcohol, ether. LD$_{50}$ orally in rats: 7.06 g/kg (Smyth).

6885. Oryzalin. [19044-88-3] 4-(Dipropylamino)-3,5-dinitrobenzenesulfonamide; 3,5-dinitro-N^4,N^4-dipropylsulfanilamide; EL-119; Surflan. $C_{12}H_{18}N_4O_6S$; mol wt 346.36. C 41.61%, H 5.24%, N 16.18%, O 27.72%, S 9.26%. Selective pre-emergence herbicide. Prepn: Q. F. Soper, **US 3367949** (1968 to Lilly). Soil degradation: T. Golab *et al., Pestic. Biochem. Physiol.* **5**, 196 (1975); E. W. Stoller, L. M. Wax, *J. Environ. Qual.* **6**, 124 (1977). *Review:* O. D. Decker, W. S. Johnson, *Anal. Methods Pestic. Plant Growth Regul.* **8**, 433 (1976).

Yellow-orange crystals, mp 137-138° (tech, 141-142°). Soly in water at 25°: 2.5 ppm. Sol in acetone, ethanol, methanol, acetonitrile; slightly sol in benzene. Practically insol in hexane. Vapor pressure at 30°: <1 × 10^{-7} mm Hg. LD$_{50}$ orally in rats: >10 g/kg (Decker, Johnson).

USE: Herbicide.

6886. γ-Oryzanol. [11042-64-1] OZ; γ-OZ; γ-orizanol; Caclate; Gammajust 50; Gamma-OZ; Gammariza; Gammatsul; Guntrin; Hi-Z; Maspiron; Oliver; Oryvita; Oryzaal; Thiaminogen. Mixture of ferulic acid esters of sterols (campestrol, stigmasterol, β-sitosterol) and triterpene alcohols (cycloartanol, cycloartenol, 24-methylenecycloartanol, cyclobranol) extracted from rice bran, corn and barley oils. Isoln from rice bran oil: R. Kaneko, T. Tsuchiya, *J. Chem. Soc. Jpn. Ind. Chem. Sect.* **57**, 526 (1954); T. Tsuchiya *et al.,* **JP 56 7182** (1956 to Agcy Ind. Sci. Technol.), *C.A.* **52**, 15848b (1958); *eidem,* **JP 57 4895** (1957 to Bureau Ind. Technics), *C.A.* **52**, 5758i (1958); from corn oil: T. Tsuchiya, O. Okubo, **JP 60 2945** (1960 to Bureau Ind. Technics), *C.A.* **54**, 25609g (1960). Extraction from rice bran, corn and barley oils and purification: T. Yamamoto, **DE 1301002** (1969 to Toyo Koatsu), *C.A.* **71**, 128704r (1969). Separation of 3 major components designated oryzanols A, B and C: M. Shimizu *et al., Chem. Pharm. Bull.* **5**, 36 (1957). Structure of A: G. Ohta, M. Shimizu, *ibid.* 40; of C: *eidem, ibid.* **6**, 325 (1958); G. Ohta, *ibid.* **8**, 5, 9 (1960). Oryzanol B was subsequently found to be a mixture of A and C: M. Shimizu, G. Ohta, *ibid.* 108. Separation and properties of the seven components of γ-oryzanol: T. Endo *et al., Yukagaku* **17**, 344 (1968), *C.A.* **69**, 37319m (1968); *eidem, ibid.* **18**, 63 (1969), *C.A.* **70**, 89042f (1969). General pharmacology: Y. Yamaji *et al., Oyo Yakuri* **25**, 947 (1983), *C.A.* **99**, 151730h (1983). Antioxidant activity in cytochrome model systems: K. Tajima *et al., Biochem. Biophys. Res. Commun.* **115**, 1002 (1983). Effect on lipid metabolism in rats: M. Shinomiya, *Tohoku J. Exp. Med.* **141**, 191 (1983). Antiulcerative effect on gastric lesions in mice: Y. Ichimaru *et al., Nippon Yakurigaku Zasshi* **84**, 537 (1984), *C.A.* **102**, 55922g (1985). Clinical evaluation in chronic gastritis: T. Arai, *Kitakanto Igaku* **30**, 71, 85 (1980); in hyperlipidemia: G. Yoshino *et al., Curr. Ther. Res.* **45**, 543 (1989).

Oryzanol A

White or slightly yellowish, tasteless powder with little or no odor. Crystals from acetone, mp 135-137°. uv max (heptane): 216, 231, 291, 315 nm.

Oryzanol A. [21238-33-5] (3β)-9,19-Cyclolanost-24-en-3-ol 3-(4-hydroxy-3-methoxyphenyl)-2-propenoate; cycloartenyl ferulate. $C_{40}H_{58}O_4$; mol wt 602.89. Prepd as the monohydrate, mp 150-151.5°. [α]$_D$ +40° (c = 0.68). uv max (heptane): 231, 290, 315 nm (log ε 4.15, 4.24, 4.34).

Oryzanol C. [469-36-3] (3β)-24-Methylene-9,19-cyclolanostan-3-ol 3-(4-hydroxy-3-methoxyphenyl)-2-propenoate; 24-methylenecycloartanyl ferulate. $C_{41}H_{60}O_4$; mol wt 616.91.

THERAP CAT: Antiulcerative; antilipemic. Also used in treatment of menopausal syndrome.

6887. Osalmid. [526-18-1] 2-Hydroxy-*N*-(4-hydroxyphenyl)benzamide; 4'-hydroxysalicylanilide; *N*-(*p*-hydroxyphenyl)-salicylamide; *N*-salicoylaminophenol; oksafenamide; oxaphenamide; Driol; Jestmin; Kanochol; Saryuvain; Yoshicol. $C_{13}H_{11}NO_3$; mol wt 229.23. C 68.11%, H 4.84%, N 6.11%, O 20.94%. Prepn: Weizmann *et al., J. Org. Chem.* **13**, 796 (1948). Description: *Subsidia Med.* **8**, 103 (1956). HPLC determn in plasma: T. Sadanaga *et al., J. Chromatogr.* **223**, 243 (1981).

Crystals, mp 179°. Practically insol in cold water, acetic acid. Slightly sol in warm water, benzene, toluene. Freely sol in methanol, ethanol, ether, acetone.

Diacetate. $C_{17}H_{15}NO_5$. Needles from alcohol, mp 151°.
THERAP CAT: Choleretic.

6888. Osaterone. [105149-04-0] 6-Chloro-17-hydroxy-2-oxapregna-4,6-diene-3,20-dione. $C_{20}H_{25}ClO_4$; mol wt 364.86. C 65.84%, H 6.91%, Cl 9.72%, O 17.54%. Androgen receptor antagonist. Prepn: K. Shibata *et al.,* **EP 193871**; *eidem,* **US 4785103** (1986, 1988 both to Teikoku Hormone); K. Shibata *et al., Chem. Pharm. Bull.* **40**, 935 (1992). Pharmacology: M. Murakoshi *et al., Acta Pathol. Jpn.* **42**, 151 (1992); T. Ichikawa *et al., Endocr. J.* **40**, 425 (1993); M. Murakoshi *et al., ibid.* 479.

Colorless prisms from acetone/hexane, mp 218-221°.
Acetate ester. [105149-00-6] 2-Oxachlormadinone acetate; TZP-4238. $C_{22}H_{27}ClO_5$; mol wt 406.90. Colorless prisms from acetone/hexane, mp 253-255°.

THERAP CAT: Treatment of benign prostatic hypertrophy; antiandrogen.

6889. Oseltamivir. [196618-13-0] (3R,4R,5S)-4-(Acetylamino)-5-amino-3-(1-ethylpropoxy)-1-cyclohexene-1-carboxylic acid ethyl ester. $C_{16}H_{28}N_2O_4$; mol wt 312.40. C 61.51%, H 9.03%, N 8.97%, O 20.49%. Orally active inhibitor of influenza virus neuraminidase; converted *in vivo* to the active acid metabolite, **GS-4071**. Prepn: N. W. Bischofberger *et al.,* **US 5763483** (1998 to Gilead Sci.). Degradation kinetics: R. Oliyai *et al., Pharm. Res.* **15**, 1300 (1998). Bioavailability and pharmacokinetics: W. Li *et al., Antimicrob. Agents Chemother.* **42**, 647 (1998). Review of structure-activity studies and clinical development: C. U. Kim, *Med. Chem. Res.* **8**, 392-399 (1998). Clinical trial in prevention of influenza: F. G. Hayden *et al., N. Engl. J. Med.* **341**, 1336 (1999); in treatment of acute influenza: J. J. Treanor *et al., J. Am. Med. Assoc.* **283**, 1016 (2000). Review of potential use in influenza pandemic: P. Ward *et al., J. Antimicrob. Chemother.* **55**, Suppl. S1, i5-i21 (2005).

Pale solid. pKa 7.7 (25°); 6.6 (70°).

Phosphate. [204255-11-8] GS-4104; Tamiflu. $C_{16}H_{28}N_2O_4 \cdot H_3PO_4$; mol wt 410.40. White crystalline solid.

THERAP CAT: Antiviral (influenza).

6890. Osmaron B. [8031-66-1] Composed of benzoates of primary aliphatic fatty amines obtained from palm kernel oil and corn oil as starting materials. Preponderantly dodecylammonium benzoate and tetradecylammonium benzoate. Total nitrogen 4.15% by analysis; average benzoic acid content 27.6% by analysis. Yellowish-brown, thick oil. mp −4 to −3°. n_D^{40} 1.4855-1.4885. Vapors of Osmaron B turn wet litmus paper blue and turmeric paper brown. Soluble in methanol, ethanol, ethylene glycol, glycerol, acetone, ethyl acetate, carbon disulfide, formic acid, acetic acid, and lactic acid. Forms turbid solns with ether, gasoline, benzene and its homologs and chlorinated hydrocarbons which become clear upon deposition of the fine precipitate on standing. *Ref:* E. Benk, *Chem. Ztg.* **75**, 351 (1951).

USE: Disinfectant; cationic surface-active agent; in udder ointments used with milking machines.

6891. Osmium. [7440-04-2] Os; at. wt 190.23; at. no. 76; valences 1-8; most common states 3, 4, 6. Group VIII (8). Seven naturally occurring isotopes: 184 (0.02%); 186 (1.6%); 187 (1.6%); 188 (13.3%); 189 (16.1%); 190 (26.4%); 192 (41.0%); artificial radioactive isotopes: 181-183; 185; 191; 193-195. Occurrence in earth's crust ∼0.001 ppm. Found in the mineral osmiridium and in all platinum ores. Discovered by Tennant in 1804. Prepn: Berzelius *et al.,* cited by Mellor, *A Comprehensive Treatise on Inorganic and Theoretical Chemistry* **15**, 687 (1936). Reviews of prepn, properties and chemistry of osmium and other platinum metals: Gilchrist, *Chem. Rev.* **32**, 277-372 (1943); Beamish *et al.* in *Rare Metals Handbook,* C. A. Hampel, Ed. (Reinhold, New York, 1956) pp 291-328; Griffith, *Q. Rev. Chem. Soc.* **19**, 254-273 (1965); *idem, The Chemistry of the Rarer Platinum Metals* (John Wiley, New York, 1967) pp 1-125; Livingstone in *Comprehensive Inorganic Chemistry* vol. 3, J. C. Bailar, Jr. *et al.,* Eds. (Pergamon Press, Oxford, 1973) pp 1163-1189, 1209-1233.

Bluish-white, lustrous metal; close-packed hexagonal structure. d_4^{20} 22.61; long believed to be the densest element; x-ray data show it to be slightly less dense than iridium. mp ∼2700°. bp ∼5500°. Sp heat (0°) 0.0309 cal/g/°C. Hardness 7.0 on Mohs' scale. Electrical resistivity (0°) 8.12 μohms-cm. Stable in air in the cold; when finely divided, is slowly oxidized by air even at ordinary temp to form tetroxide. Attacked by fluorine above 100°; by dry chlorine on heating; not attacked by bromine or iodine. Attacked by aqua regia, by oxidizing acids over a long period of time; barely affected by HCl, H_2SO_4. Burns in vapor of phosphorus to form a phosphide, in vapor of sulfur to form a sulfide. Attacked by molten alkali hydrosulfates, by potassium hydroxide and oxidizing agents. Finely divided osmium absorbs a considerable amount of hydrogen.

Osmarins. High-molecular weight polymers of carbohydrate and osmium. Potential use in the treatment of arthritis: *Chem. Eng. News* **60**, 8 (April 5, 1982).

USE: As alloy with iridium for pen points and fine machine bearings; as catalyst in the synthesis of ammonia; as catalyst in hydrogenation of organic compounds.

6892. Osmium Hexafluoride. [13768-38-2] F_6Os; mol wt 304.22. F 37.47%, Os 62.53%. OsF_6. Prepd by fluorination of osmium metal: Weinstock, Malm, *J. Am. Chem. Soc.* **80**, 4466 (1958); Hargreaves, Peacock, *Proc. Chem. Soc. London* **1959**, 85. Previously thought to be *osmium octafluoride*: Ruff, Tschirch, *Ber.* **46**, 929 (1913).

Pale yellow, volatile solid. *Highly poisonous! Very corrosive to skin!* mp 32.1°; bp 45.9°. Also reported: mp 33.4°; bp 47.5°, Cady, Hargreaves, *J. Chem. Soc.* **1961**, 1563. Hydrolyzed on ex-

posure to moisture; forms white corrosive fumes which soon turn bluish. May be stored in quartz ampuls.

6893. Osmium Tetroxide. [20816-12-0] Osmic acid. O_4Os; mol wt 254.23. O 25.17%, Os 74.83%. OsO_4. Prepd by heating (at 300-400°) finely divided osmium metal in a stream of air or oxygen. Lab prepn: Grube in *Handbook of Preparative Inorganic Chemistry* vol. 2, G. Brauer, Ed. (Academic Press, New York, 2nd ed., 1965) pp 1603-1604. Use in treatment of arthritis: M. Nissilä *et al., Scand. J. Rheumatol.* **5**, 111 (1977); A. S. Hendricson *et al., Acta Orthop. Scand.* **52**, 17 (1982). Review of chemistry and biochemistry: W. P. Griffith, *Platinum Met. Rev.* **18**, 94-96 (1974); of toxicity: E. Browning, *Toxicity of Industrial Metals* (Appleton-Century-Crofts, New York, 2nd ed., 1969) pp 261-266.

Pale yellow solid; monoclinic crystals. *Vapor poisonous! Safeguards necessary when opening container.* Acrid, chlorine-like odor. Minimum perceptible concn 0.02 mg/liter of air. mp 40.6°. d 5.10 (calc): Ueki *et al., Acta Crystallogr.* **19**, 157 (1965). bp$_{760}$ 130.0°; bp$_{400}$ 109.3°; bp$_{200}$ 89.5°; bp$_{100}$ 71.5°; bp$_{60}$ 59.4°. Begins to sublime and distil well below the boiling point. Vapor press at 27°: 11 mm. Critical temp 405°; crit press. 170 atm. Sol in benzene. Soly at 25° (g/100 g): water 7.24; carbon tetrachloride 375: Anderson, Yost, *J. Am. Chem. Soc.* **60**, 1822 (1938). Also sol in alc, ether, ammonium hydroxide, phosphorus oxychloride.

Caution: Potential symptoms of overexposure are irritation of eyes and respiratory system; lacrimation, visual disturbance; conjunctivitis; headache; coughing; dyspnea; dermatitis. *See NIOSH Pocket Guide to Chemical Hazards* (DHHS/NIOSH 97-140, 1997) p 238.

USE: Oxidizing agent, particularly for converting olefins to glycols. Catalyzes chlorate, peroxide, periodate, and other oxidations: P. N. Rylander, *Organic Syntheses with Noble Metal Catalysts* (Academic Press, New York, 1973) pp 121-144. As fixing and staining agent for cell and tissue studies.

6894. Osteocalcin. [75757-02-7] (human reduced) Bone Gla protein; BGP. Abundant noncollageous, calcium-binding protein of bone; constitutes ∼1-2% of the total bone matrix. Also found in tooth dentin and cementum. Contains 46-50 amino acid residues (human: 49); mol wt ∼5800 daltons. Amino acid sequence is highly conserved across species. Characterized by 3 residues of the vitamin K-dependent amino acid, γ-carboxyglutamic acid (Gla), *q.v.* Synthesized by osteoblasts and odontoblasts; modulated by calcitriol, *q.v.* Detectable in serum as an indicator of bone metabolism. Identification in chicken bone: P. V. Hauschka *et al., Proc. Natl. Acad. Sci. USA* **72**, 3925 (1975). Characterization of calf BGP: P. A. Price *et al. ibid.* **73**, 1447 (1976). Biosynthesis in bone cell culture: S. K. Nishimoto, P. A. Price, *J. Biol. Chem.* **254**, 437 (1979). RIA determn in plasma: P. A. Price *et al., J. Clin. Invest.* **66**, 878 (1980). Review of isoln and characterization: C. M. Gundberg *et al., Methods Enzymol.* **107B**, 516-544 (1984). Review of hydroxyapatite binding characteristics: P. V. Hauschka, F. H. Wians, Jr. *Anat. Rec.* **224**, 180-188 (1989). Comprehensive review: P. V. Hauschka *et al., Physiol. Rev.* **69**, 990-1047 (1989). Review of diagnostic methods and clinical applications: M. J. Power, P. F. Fottrell, *Crit. Rev. Clin. Lab. Sci.* **28**, 287-335 (1991). Immunohistochemical study and potential role in bone mineralization and resorption: H. I. Roach, *Cell Biol. Int.* **18**, 617-628 (1994).

Very acidic, pI 4.0. Selective affinity for insoluble Ca^{2+} salts; binds tightly to hydroxyapatite.

6895. Osthole. [484-12-8] 7-Methoxy-8-(3-methyl-2-butenyl)-2H-1-benzopyran-2-one; 7-methoxy-8-(3-methyl-2-butenyl)-coumarin; 8-(3-methyl-2-butenyl)herniarin. $C_{15}H_{16}O_3$; mol wt 244.29. C 73.75%, H 6.60%, O 19.65%. From rhizome of *Peucedanum ostruthium* (L.) Koch (*Imperatoria ostruthium* L.) *Umbelliferae:* Herzog, Krohn, *Arch. Pharm.* **247**, 553 (1909); Butenandt, Marten, *Ann.* **495**, 187 (1932); from *Prangos pabularia* Lindl., *Umbelliferae:* Pigulevskii, Kuznetsova, *Dokl. Akad. Nauk SSSR* **61**, 309 (1948), *C.A.* **43**, 3416d (1949); from *Flindersia bennettiana* F. Muell., *Rutaceae:* Galbraith *et al., Aust. J. Chem.* **13**, 427 (1960). Structure: Späth, Pesta, *Ber.* **66**, 754 (1933). Synthesis: Späth, Holzen, *ibid.* **67**, 264 (1934); Murayama *et al., Chem. Pharm. Bull.* **20**, 741 (1972).

Prisms from ether. mp 83-84°. uv max: 322, 258 nm (ε 8000, 4300). Practically insol in water; sol in aq alkalies, alcohol, chloroform, acetone, boiling petr ether.

6896. Ostruthin. [148-83-4] *(E)*-6-(3,7-Dimethyl-2,6-octadienyl)-7-hydroxy-2*H*-1-benzopyran-2-one; *(E)*-6-(3,7-dimethyl-2,6-octadienyl)-7-hydroxycoumarin; 6-(3,7-dimethyl-2,6-octadienyl)umbelliferone. $C_{19}H_{22}O_3$; mol wt 298.38. C 76.48%, H 7.43%, O 16.09%. From the root of *Peucedanum ostruthium* (L.) Koch *(Imperatoria ostruthium* L.), *Umbelliferae:* Butenandt, Marten, *Ann.* **495**, 187 (1932); from *Eriostemon tomentellus, Rutaceae:* Duffield, Jeffries, *Aust. J. Chem.* **16**, 123 (1963). Structure: Späth, Klager, *Ber.* **67**, 859 (1934); Späth, Kainrath, *ibid.* **70**, 2272 (1937).

Crystals from alcohol, mp 117-119°. Practically insol in water, petr ether. Sol in chloroform, ethyl acetate, hot alc.

Acetate. $C_{21}H_{24}O_4$. Leaflets from alcohol, mp 81°. Practically insol in water. Sol in alc, ether, benzene, chloroform.

6897. Ostruthol. [642-08-0] *(2Z)*-2-Methyl-2-butenoic acid *(1R)*-2-hydroxy-2-methyl-1-[[(7-oxo-7*H*-furo[3,2-*g*][1]benzopyran-4-yl)oxy]methyl]propyl ester. $C_{21}H_{22}O_7$; mol wt 386.40. C 65.28%, H 5.74%, O 28.98%. From rhizome of *Peucedanum ostruthium* L. Koch *(Imperatoria ostruthium* L.), *Umbelliferae:* Herzog, Koch, *Arch. Pharm.* **247**, 553 (1909). Structure: Späth, Christiani, *Ber.* **66**, 1150 (1933). Synthesis: Chatterjee, Dutta, *Sci. Cult.* **34**, 460 (1968).

Silky needles from benzene, mp 136-137°. $[\alpha]_D^{15}$ −18.3° (pyridine). Slightly sol in water or in ether; sol in hot alcohol, benzene, toluene, pyridine.

6898. Otilonium Bromide. [26095-59-0] *N,N*-Diethyl-*N*-methyl-2-[[4-[[2-(octyloxy)benzoyl]amino]benzoyl]oxy]ethanaminium bromide; octylonium bromide; SP-63; Doralin; Menoctyl; Pasminox; Spasen; Spasmoctyl; Spasmomen. $C_{29}H_{43}BrN_2O_4$; mol wt 563.57. C 61.80%, H 7.69%, Br 14.18%, N 4.97%, O 11.36%. Quaternary ammonium salt with gastrointestinal spasmolytic activity. Prepn: **BE 704269**; M. Ghelardoni *et al.*, **US 3536723** (1968, 1970 both to Menarini); *idem et al., J. Med. Chem.* **16**, 1063 (1973). Determn of finished pharmaceutical forms by HPLC: C. Mannucci *et al., J. Pharm. Sci.* **82**, 367 (1993); by CE: S. Furlanetto *et al., Analyst* **126**, 1700 (2001). Receptor binding study: S. Lindqvust *et al., Br. J. Pharmacol.* **137**, 1134 (2002). Clinical trial in irritable bowel syndrome: G. Battaglia *et al., Aliment. Pharmacol. Ther.* **12**, 1003 (1998). Review of pharmacology and clinical efficacy: S. Evangelista, *J. Int. Med. Res.* **27**,

207-222 (1999); comparative review of clinical studies: *idem, Curr. Pharm. Des.* **10**, 3561-3568 (2004).

Crystals from ethanol, mp 166-168°. LD_{50} in mice (mg/kg) 87.0 i.p. (Ghelardoni, 1973).

THERAP CAT: Antispasmodic.

6899. Otobain. [3738-01-0] *(7S,8R,9R)*-9-(1,3-Benzodioxol-5-yl)-6,7,8,9-tetrahydro-7,8-dimethylnaphtho[1,2-*d*]-1,3-dioxole; 5,6-methylenedioxy-2,3-dimethyl-4-(3′,4′-methylenedioxyphenyl)-1,2,3,4-tetrahydronaphthalene; otobite. $C_{20}H_{20}O_4$; mol wt 324.37. C 74.06%, H 6.21%, O 19.73%. Lignan isolated from otoba butter, the fat expressed from the fruit of *Myristica otoba* Humb. & Bonpl., *Myristicaceae*. Isoln: W. F. Baughman *et al., J. Am. Chem. Soc.* **43**, 199 (1921). Structure: T. Gilchrist *et al., J. Chem. Soc.* **1962**, 1780; N. S. Bhacca, R. Stevenson, *J. Org. Chem.* **28**, 1638 (1963). Absolute configuration: W. Klyne *et al., J. Chem. Soc. C* **1966**, 893. Synthesis of (±)-form: I. Maclean, R. Stevenson, *ibid.* 1717; T. B. H. McMurry, H. K. Kennedy-Skipton, *Tetrahedron Lett.* **1966**, 975.

Needles from ethanol, mp 137-138°. $[\alpha]_D$ −40.5° (c = 3.2 in chloroform). uv max (ethanol): 234, 287 nm (ε 9300, 6700). Sol in ether, hot alcohol. Practically insol in water.

6900. Ouabagenin. [508-52-1] (1β,3β,5β,11α)-1,3,5,11,-14,19-Hexahydroxycard-20(22)-enolide; G-strophanthidin. $C_{23}H_{34}O_8$; mol wt 438.51. C 63.00%, H 7.82%, O 29.19%. Prepn from ouabain with HCl in cold acetone: Mannich, Siewert, *Ber.* **75**, 737 (1942). Review of structure: Reichstein, Reich, *Annu. Rev. Biochem.* **15**, 155 (1946). Proof of this structure: Tamm *et al., Helv. Chim. Acta* **40**, 1469 (1957), *cf. Experientia* **13**, 185 (1957); Turner, Meschino, *J. Am. Chem. Soc.* **80**, 4862 (1958); Volpp, Tamm, *Helv. Chim. Acta* **42**, 1408, 1418 (1959).

Monohydrate. Clusters of needles from water, mp 235-238°. One gram dissolves in about 10 ml boiling water. At room temp the soly in water is <1%. Also sol in dil alcohol. Practically insol in abs alcohol, ether, and chloroform. Becomes anhydr at 100° *in vacuo* over P_2O_5. The anhydr compd is hygroscopic, mp 255-256°. $[\alpha]_D^{17}$ +11.3° (c = 1.27).

Tetraacetylouabagenin trihydrate. $C_{31}H_{42}O_{12}.3H_2O$. Needles from 10% alcohol, mp 282-285°.

Dihydroouabagenin. $C_{23}H_{36}O_8.CH_3OH$. Solvated crystals from methanol + ether contg 1 mol methanol, mp 261°.

6901. Ouabain. [630-60-4] $(1\beta,3\beta,5\beta,11\alpha)$-3-[(6-Deoxy-$\alpha$-L-mannopyranosyl)oxy]-1,5,11,14,19-pentahydroxycard-20(22)-enolide; G-strophanthin; Gratus strophanthin; acocantherin. $C_{29}H_{44}O_{12}$; mol wt 584.65. C 59.58%, H 7.59%, O 32.84%. Obtained from the seeds of *Strophanthus gratus* (Wall. & Hock.) Baill.; also occurs in *Acokanthera ouabaio* Cathel and other *A.* spp, *Apocynaceae.* Isoln: Schwartze *et al., J. Pharmacol.* **36,** 481 (1929). Hydrolysis yields one mol ouabagenin and one mol rhamnose: Jacobs, Bigelow, *J. Biol. Chem.* **96,** 647 (1932). Toxicity study: Small *et al., Toxicol. Appl. Pharmacol.* **20,** 44 (1971). *See also* Fieser, Fieser, *Steroids* (1959, Reinhold, New York; Chapman & Hall, London) pp 768, 772; Reichstein, Reich, *Annu. Rev. Biochem.* **15,** 155 (1946).

Octahydrate. Purostrophan; Strodival; Strophoperm. Shiny plates (from water) which give up their water of crystn at 130°. When anhydr dec about 190°. $[\alpha]_D^{25}$ -31 to $-32.5°$ (c = 1 calcd as anhydr). Stable in air, but affected by light. One gram dissolves in about 75 ml water, in 5 ml boiling water, in 100 ml alcohol, in 8 ml boiling alcohol. Also sol in amyl alcohol, dioxane. Slightly sol in ether, chloroform, ethyl acetate. Aq solns are neutral to litmus. LD_{50} i.v. in rats: 14 mg/kg (Small).

THERAP CAT: Cardiotonic.

THERAP CAT (VET): Cardiotonic, diuretic.

6902. Ovalbumin. Egg albumin. The major protein constituent (75%) of egg white from hen's eggs. Mol wt about 45,000. Produced under hormonal control by the bird oviduct. May be isolated and crystallized readily from the filtrate of an acidified mixture of egg white and an equal volume of satd. ammonium sulfate: Sorensen, Hoyrup, *C.R. Trav. Lab. Carlsberg* **12,** 12 (1917). Alternate method: Kekwick, Cannan, *Biochem. J.* **30,** 227 (1936). Can be separated by electrophoresis and chromatography from about ten other minor components including avidin, lysozyme, conalbumin, *q.q.v.,* and ovomucoid. Structure is a complex protein consisting of a single polypeptide chain of about 400 residues (about half of which are hydrophobic), a maximum of two phosphate residues per mole, and an oligosaccharide side chain composed of only mannose and glucosamine residues. Sequences of *N*- and *C*-terminal segments: Narita, Ishii, *J. Biochem.* **52,** 367 (1962); Thompson *et al., Aust. J. Biol. Sci.* **24,** 525 (1971). *Reviews:* R. C. Warner in Neurath-Bailey, *The Proteins* **vol. II,** part A (New York, 1954) p 443 sqq; Taborsky, *Adv. Protein Chem.* **28,** 34-50 (1974).

Needles or elongated prisms, frequently forming rosettes. The crystals usually contain 2 mols protein and 3 mols H_2SO_4. $[\alpha]_D^{20}$ $-30.7°$. Coagulation temp 56°. Sol in electrolyte-free water. Combines with salts, acids, and bases. Denaturation can be induced by heating to 56°, by vigorous shaking, by electric current, and by various chemicals, such as acids, ammonia salts, heavy metal salts, and alcohols. All methods produce complete and irreversible denaturation. Isoelectric point: 4.63.

6903. Oxaceprol. [33996-33-7] (4*R*)-1-Acetyl-4-hydroxy-L-proline; 4-hydroxy-*N*-acetylproline; 1-acetyl-4-hydroxy-2-pyrrol-idinecarboxylic acid; CO-61; AHP-200; Jonctum. $C_7H_{11}NO_4$; mol wt 173.17. C 48.55%, H 6.40%, N 8.09%, O 36.96%. Derivative of hydroxyproline having anti-inflammatory activity. Prepn: R. L. M. Synge, *Biochem. J.* **33,** 1924 (1939); J. J. Kolb, G. Toennies, *J. Biol. Chem.* **144,** 193 (1942); O. Leonardo *et al.,* **DE 2301358** corresp to **US 3860607** (1973, 1975 to Richardson-Merrell). Elucidation of cyclic conformation and *cis/trans* isomerism about the amide bond: T. Prange *et al., Biochem. Biophys. Res. Commun.* **61,** 104 (1974). Crystal structure: M. Hospital *et al., Biopolymers* **18,** 1141 (1979). In crystals, the acetyl group is in the *trans* conformation and the ring is puckered. The *trans* form is more stable than the *cis* form in solutions: W. A. Thomas, M. K. Williams, *J. Chem. Soc. Chem. Commun.* **1972,** 994. Anti-inflammatory and wound-healing activity in animals: P. Coirre, B. Coirre, **GB 1246141** (1971) related to P. Coirre *et al.,* **US 3891765** and **US 3932638** (1975, 1976 both to Franco Chimie). Clinical studies of use in several rheumatic conditions: P. Grellat, *Rhumatologie* **27,** 223 (1975); in degenerative joint disease, R. Schubotz, L. Hausmann, *Therapiewoche* **27,** 4248 (1977); in treatment of burns, tumors and other wounds (applied locally): Y. Privat, *Gaz. Med. Fr.* **84,** 618 (1977).

Crystals from acetone, mp 133-134° (Synge); also reported as mp 126-128° (Leonardo). $[\alpha]_D^{20}$ $-116.5°$ (c = 3.2); $[\alpha]_D^{18}$ $-119.5°$ (c = 3.75). Very sol in alcohol. Sol in water, methanol. Insol in ether, chloroform.

Monohydrate. $C_7H_{13}NO_5$. Crystals from moist ethyl acetate or acetone, mp 74-76°.

Zinc salt. $C_{14}H_{20}N_2O_8Zn$. mp 120°.

THERAP CAT: Anti-inflammatory; vulnerary.

6904. Oxacillin. [66-79-5] (2*S*,5*R*,6*R*)-3,3-Dimethyl-6-[[(5-methyl-3-phenyl-4-isoxazolyl)carbonyl]amino]-7-oxo-4-thia-1-azabicyclo[3.2.0]heptane-2-carboxylic acid; 5-methyl-3-phenyl-4-isoxazolylpenicillin; 6-(5-methyl-3-phenyl-2-isoxazoline-4-carboxamido)penicillanic acid; oxazocilline. $C_{19}H_{19}N_3O_5S$; mol wt 401.44. C 56.85%, H 4.77%, N 10.47%, O 19.93%, S 7.99%. Semi-synthetic antibiotic related to penicillin. Prepn: Doyle, Nayler, **US 2996501** (1961); Doyle *et al., Nature* **192,** 1183 (1961). Toxicity: E. I. Goldenthal, *Toxicol. Appl. Pharmacol.* **18,** 185 (1971).

Sodium salt monohydrate. [7240-38-2] Penicillin P-12; sodium oxacillin; BRL-1400; Bactocill; Bristopen; Crypticillin; Micropenin; Penstapho; Prostaphlin; Stapenor. $C_{19}H_{18}N_3NaO_5S.H_2O$; mol wt 441.43. Crystals from isopropanol mp 188° (dec). $[\alpha]_D^{20}$ $+201°$ (c = 1 in water). LD_{50} orally in rats: >8000 mg/kg (Goldenthal).

THERAP CAT: Antibacterial.

THERAP CAT (VET): Antibacterial.

6905. Oxadiargyl. [39807-15-3] 3-[2,4-Dichloro-5-(2-propynyloxy)phenyl]-5-(1,1-dimethylethyl)-1,3,4-oxadiazol-2(3*H*)-one; 5-*tert*-butyl-3-(2,4-dichloro-5-propargyloxyphenyl)-1,3,4-oxadiazol-2-(3*H*)-one; Raft; Topstar. $C_{15}H_{14}Cl_2N_2O_3$; mol wt 341.19. C 52.80%, H 4.14%, Cl 20.78%, N 8.21%, O 14.07%. Protoporphyrinogen IX oxidase inhibitor; pre-emergence herbicide for use in rice and other food crops. Prepn: R. Boesch, **DE 2227012**; *idem,* **US 3818026** (1972, 1974 both to Rhone-Poulenc). Properties and field trials: R. Dickmann *et al., Brighton Crop Prot. Conf. - Weeds* **1997,** 51; G. Tracchi *et al., ibid.* 885.

Odorless, white powder with little agglomerates, mp 131°. Soly in water (20°): 0.37 mg/l. LD$_{50}$ in rats (mg/kg): >5000 orally; >2000 dermally; LC$_{50}$ (4 hr) in rats: >5.16 mg/l (Dickmann).

USE: Herbicide.

6906. 1,3,4-Oxadiazole. [288-99-3] C$_2$H$_2$N$_2$O; mol wt 70.05. C 34.29%, H 2.88%, N 39.99%, O 22.84%. Prepn: Ainsworth, *J. Am. Chem. Soc.* **87**, 5800 (1965).

Liquid. bp 150°. Thermally stable.

6907. Oxadiazon. [19666-30-9] 3-[2,4-Dichloro-5-(1-methylethoxy)phenyl]-5-(1,1-dimethylethyl)-1,3,4-oxadiazol-2(3*H*)-one; 2-*tert*-butyl-4-(2,4-dichloro-5-isopropoxyphenyl)-Δ^2-1,3,4-oxadiazolin-5-one; 5-*tert*-butyl-3-(2,4-dichloro-5-isopropoxyphenyl)-1,3,4-oxadiazolin-2-one; RP-17623; Ronstar. C$_{15}$H$_{18}$Cl$_2$-N$_2$O$_3$; mol wt 345.22. C 52.19%, H 5.26%, Cl 20.54%, N 8.11%, O 13.90%. Selective pre-emergence herbicide. Prepn: J. Metivier, R. Boesch, US 3385862 (1968 to Rhône Poulenc). Metabolism: A. Guardigli *et al., Arch. Environ. Contam. Toxicol.* **4**, 145 (1976). Persistence in soil: D. Ambrosi *et al., J. Agric. Food Chem.* **25**, 868 (1977). Efficacy and phytotoxicity: G. W. Knox, *Proc. Fla. State Hort. Soc.* **99**, 270 (1986). Weed control: S. S. Lim, *Proc. Nat. Semin. Workshop Rice Field Weed Mgmt.* **1988**, 169.

White, odorless, non-hygroscopic crystals, mp 88-90°. Vapor pressure at 20°: <1 × 10^{-6} mm Hg. Soly at 20° (g/l): water ~0.0007; ethanol, methanol ~100; cyclohexanone ~200; acetone, acetophenone, anisole carbon tetrachloride, isophorone, methylethylketone ~600; benzene, chloroform, methylene chloride, toluene ~1000. LD$_{50}$ orally in rats, bobwhite quail, mallard duck: 8000, 6000, 1000 mg/kg (Lim).

USE: Herbicide.

6908. Oxadixyl. [77732-09-3] N-(2,6-Dimethylphenyl)-2-methoxy-N-(2-oxo-3-oxazolidinyl)acetamide; 2-methoxy-N-(2-oxo-1,3-oxazolidin-3-yl)acet-2′,6′-xylidide; SAN-371F; Sandofan. C$_{14}$H$_{18}$N$_2$O$_4$; mol wt 278.30. C 60.42%, H 6.52%, N 10.07%, O 23.00%. Systemic fungicide belonging to the oxazolidinones. Prepn: J. Harr *et al.,* BE 884661; R. Sandmeier, H. Schelling, US 4457937 (1981, 1984 both to Sandoz). Description of physical properties, biological properties, and activity: U. Gisi *et al., Meded. Fac. Landbouwwet. Univ. Gent* **48**, 541-549 (1983). Field trial of synergistic mixture with cymoxanil and mancozeb: M. R. Redbond *et al., Brighton Crop Prot. Conf. - Pests Dis.* **1990**, 1115. GC determn in cucumber: W.-O. Lee, S.-K. Wong, *Analyst* **120**, 2475 (1995). Soil degradation: N. D. Anan'yeva *et al., Eurasian Soil Sci.* **28**, 157 (1996).

Colorless crystals from ethanol, mp 104-105°. Soly (% w/w) at 25°: water 0.34, ethanol 11.2, ethanol 5.0, acetone 34.4, DMSO

39.0. LD$_{50}$ in female rats (mg/kg): 1860 orally; >2000 dermally (Gisi).

USE: Fungicide.

6909. Oxalacetic Acid. [328-42-7] Oxobutanedioic acid; oxosuccinic acid; ketosuccinic acid. C$_4$H$_4$O$_5$; mol wt 132.07. C 36.38%, H 3.05%, O 60.57%. HOOCCOCH$_2$COOH. Prepd by hydrolyzing sodium diethyloxalacetate with concd HCl: Heidelberger, Hurlbert, *J. Am. Chem. Soc.* **72**, 4704 (1950). Prepn of *cis*-enol form: Heidelberger, *Biochem. Prep.* **3**, 59 (1953).

Diethyl ester see Ethyl Oxalacetate.

***trans*-enol Form.** Hydroxyfumaric acid. Crystals from acetone + benzene, mp 184°. K at 17° = 2.76 × 10^{-3}. Soluble in water, ethanol, ether. Can be converted into the lower-melting *cis*-form, mp 152°, by dissolving the acid in water and re-isolating it as rapidly as possible.

***cis*-enol Form.** Hydroxymaleic acid. Crystals from ethyl acetate + carbon tetrachloride, mp 152°. K at 17° = 2.505 × 10^{-3}. Sol in ethanol, acetone, ethyl acetate. Sparingly sol in ether. Insol in benzene, chloroform, ligroin.

6910. Oxalenediuramidoxime. [580-52-9] N,N″-Bis(aminocarbonyl)-N′,N‴-dihydroxyethanediimidamide. C$_4$H$_8$N$_6$O$_4$; mol wt 204.14. C 23.53%, H 3.95%, N 41.17%, O 31.35%. Prepn: Zinkeisen, *Ber.* **1889**, 2952.

Needles from dil alcohol. mp 191-192° (dec). Insol in cold water, in ether, chloroform, benzene, petr ether. Very sol in alcohol, acids, alkalies.

USE: As a reagent for the determination of nickel, with which it gives an orange ppt in dil ammoniacal soln.

6911. Oxalic Acid. [144-62-7] Ethanedioic acid. C$_2$H$_2$O$_4$; mol wt 90.03. C 26.68%, H 2.24%, O 71.08%. (COOH)$_2$. Present in many plants and vegetables, notably in those of the *Oxalis* and *Rumex* families, where it occurs in the cell sap of the plant as the potassium or calcium salt. It is a product of the metabolism of many molds. Several species of *Penicillium* and *Aspergillus* convert sugar into calcium oxalate with 90% yields under optimum conditions. Oxalic acid was formerly manuf by fusion of cellulose matter, e.g. sawdust, with NaOH or by oxidation with HNO$_3$; it is now made by passing carbon monoxide into concd NaOH or by heating sodium formate in the presence of NaOH or Na$_2$CO$_3$: Wallace, US 1602802 (1926); Beckman, US 2687433 (1951 to Allied Chem.). Efficient laboratory prepn of anhydrous form: H. T. Clarke, A. W. Davis, *Org. Synth.* coll. vol. I, 421 (2nd ed., 1941). Toxicity study: E. H. Vernot *et al., Toxicol. Appl. Pharmacol.* **42**, 417 (1977). *Review:* Wilson, "Miscellaneous *Aspergillus* Toxins" in *Microbial Toxins* vol. VI, A. Ciegler *et al.,* Eds. (Academic Press, New York, 1971) pp 268-273; C. A. Bernales in *Kirk-Othmer Encyclopedia of Chemical Technology* vol. **16** (Wiley-Interscience, New York, 3rd ed., 1981) pp 618-636.

Dihydrate. Monoclinic tablets, prisms, granules. *Poisonous!* d$_4^{18.5}$ 1.653. mp 101-102° giving off water of crystn and starting to sublime. pK$_1$ 1.27; pK$_2$ 4.28. pH of 0.1*M* soln 1.3. One gram dissolves in about 7 ml water, 2 ml boiling water; 2.5 ml alcohol, 1.8 ml boiling alcohol, 100 ml ether, 5.5 ml glycerol. Practically insol in benzene, chloroform, petr ether. d$_4^{17.5}$ of aq solns: 1% (w/w) 1.0035; 3% 1.0105; 5% 1.0175; 10% 1.0350; 13% 1.0455. Oxalic acid can be dehydrated by careful drying at 100°, but considerable loss occurs through sublimation; this, moreover, is harmful to the oven. LD$_{50}$ orally in rats (5% solution): 9.5 ml/kg (Vernot).

Anhydr oxalic acid. Crystallized from glacial acetic acid, is orthorhombic, the crystals being pyramidal or elongated octahedra. Hygroscopic, mp 189.5° (dec). Sublimes best at 157°. At higher temps dec into CO$_2$, CO, formic acid, and H$_2$O. d$_4^{17}$ 1.90. 100 g of aq soln satd at 15° contain 6.71 g, at 20° 8.34 g, at 25° 9.81 g.

Caution: Potential symptoms of overexposure by ingestion are corrosion of alimentary tract mucosa; localized pain; vomiting, shock, hypotension, cardiovascular collapse; headache, muscle cramps, tatany; convulsions, stupor, coma; kidney damage. Direct contact may cause eye, skin and mucous membrane irritation; eye burns. *See NIOSH Pocket Guide to Chemical Hazards* (DHHS/NIOSH 97-140, 1997) p 238; *Clinical Toxicology of Commercial Products*, R. E. Gosselin *et al.*, Ed. (Williams & Wilkins, Baltimore, 5th ed., 1984) Section III, pp 326-328.

USE: As analytical reagent; in calico printing and dyeing; for bleaching straw (hats) and leather; removing paint or varnish, rust or ink stains; cleaning wood; manuf oxalates; blue ink; celluloid; intermediates and dyes; in metal polishes; in indigo dyeing; in purifying methanol; for decolorizing crude glycerol; for stabilizing hydrocyanic acid. As a general reducing agent; in ceramics and pigments; in metallurgy as cleanser; in the paper industry; in photography; in process engraving; in the rubber industry; in making glucose from starch; as condensing agent in organic chemistry. *In vitro* blood specimen anticoagulant.

THERAP CAT (VET): In 5% solution with 5% malonic acid as hemostatic agent.

6912. Oxaliplatin. [61825-94-3] (SP-4-2)-[(1R,2R)-1,2-Cyclohexanediamine-$\kappa N,\kappa N'$][ethanedioato(2−)-$\kappa O^1,\kappa O^2$]platinum; [(1R,2R)-1,2-cyclohexanediamine-N,N'][oxalato (2−)-O,-O']platinum; oxalato (1R,2R-cyclohexanediamine)platinum(II); Pt(oxalato)(*trans-l*-dach); oxalato (*trans-l*-1,2-diaminocyclohexane)platinum (II); oxalatoplatinum; *l*-OHP; RP-54780; NSC-266046; Eloxatin; Elplat. $C_8H_{14}N_2O_4Pt$; mol wt 397.29. C 24.19%, H 3.55%, N 7.05%, O 16.11%, Pt 49.10%. Third generation platinum complex. Prepn and antitumor activity: Y. Kidani *et al.*, *J. Med. Chem.* **21**, 1315 (1978); Y. Kidani *et al.*, *Gann* **71**, 637 (1980). Crystal structure: M. A. Bruck *et al.*, *Inorg. Chim. Acta* **92**, 279 (1984). FAB and LAMMA MS analysis: J. Claereboudt *et al.*, *J. Pharm. Biomed. Anal.* **7**, 1599 (1989). Pharmacokinetics: R. Kizu *et al.*, *Cancer Chemother. Pharmacol.* **31**, 475 (1993). Clinical evaluation in colorectal cancer: F. Levi *et al.*, *Eur. J. Cancer* **29A**, 1280 (1993). Brief review of antitumor and clinical activity: G. Mathé *et al.*, *Biomed. Pharmacother.* **43**, 237-250 (1989). Review of clinical experience in combination therapy for colorectal cancer: D. Simpson *et al.*, *Drugs* **63**, 2127-2156 (2003).

Colorless, thin triangular plates with truncated vertices. Sol in water 7.9 mg/ml.
THERAP CAT: Antineoplastic.

6913. Oxalomolybdic Acid. [53450-33-2] [Ethanedioato-(2−)-O,O']trioxomolybdate(2−) dihydrogen; [ethanedioato(1−)-O]hydroxydioxomolybdenum; hydrogen trioxooxalatomolybdate-(VI). $C_2H_2MoO_7$; mol wt 233.97. C 10.27%, H 0.86%, Mo 41.01%, O 47.87%. $H_2[MoO_3(C_3O_4)]$. Usually contains 1 or 2 H_2O.
Colorless crystals, sol in water.
USE: In invisible inks.

6914. Oxalyl Chloride. [79-37-8] Ethanedioyl dichloride. $C_2Cl_2O_2$; mol wt 126.93. C 18.92%, Cl 55.86%, O 25.21%. (COCl)$_2$. Obtained from oxalic acid and PCl$_5$.
Colorless, fuming liquid; penetrating odor. *Poisonous!* d_4^{13} 1.488. mp −12°. bp 63-64°. n_D^{13} 1.4340. Violently dec by water, also by alcohol.
Caution: Severely irritating to skin, eyes, respiratory tract.

6915. Oxamarin. [15301-80-1] 6,7-Bis[2-(diethylamino)ethoxy]-4-methyl-2H-1-benzopyran-2-one; 6,7-bis[2-(diethylamino)ethoxy]-4-methylcoumarin. $C_{22}H_{34}N_2O_4$; mol wt 390.52. C 67.66%, H 8.78%, N 7.17%, O 16.39%. Deriv of α-pyrone, related structurally to sulmarin, *q.v.* Prepn: E. Massarani, *Farmaco Ed. Sci.* **12**, 691 (1957); G. Cavallini, E. Massarani, US 2895963 (1959 to Maggioni); E. Massarani *et al.*, *J. Med. Pharm. Chem.* **3**, 231 (1961). Comparative study in treatment of varicose syndrome: G. Frantoli *et al.*, *Panminerva Med.* **14**, 290 (1972), *C.A.* **78**, 92741

(1973). Transcutaneous absorption: G. Ciaceri, P. Marini, *Boll. Chim. Farm.* **111**, 321 (1972). Cardiovascular, intestinal smooth muscle effects: *eidem, G. Ital. Patol. Sci. Affini* **19**, 11 (1972), *C.A.* **81**, 130823 (1974). Anti-inflammatory action: *eidem, ibid.* 1, *C.A.* **81**, 130952 (1974).

Oil, bp$_{0.5}$ 195°.
Dihydrochloride. [6830-17-7] MG-652; Idro P$_3$. $C_{22}H_{34}N_2O_4$.2HCl; mol wt 463.44. Crystals from ethanol, mp 224-226° (Massarani, 1957); also reported as mp 234-236° (Massarani *et al.*, 1961).
THERAP CAT: Hemostatic.

6916. Oxametacine. [27035-30-9] 1-(4-Chlorobenzoyl)-N-hydroxy-5-methoxy-2-methyl-1H-indole-3-acetamide; 1-(*p*-chlorobenzoyl)-5-methoxy-2-methylindole-3-acetohydroxamic acid; indoxamic acid; Dinulcid; Flogar. $C_{19}H_{17}ClN_2O_4$; mol wt 372.80. C 61.21%, H 4.60%, Cl 9.51%, N 7.51%, O 17.17%. Deriv of indomethacin, *q.v.* Prepn: R. Aries, FR 1599495 (1969), *C.A.* **73**, 3797h (1970); F. De Martiis, DE 2008332 (both 1971 to ABC); *eidem, Boll. Chim. Farm.* **114**, 309 (1975). Pharmaco-toxicological evaluation: *eidem, ibid.* 319. Disposition in rats: L. F. Elsom *et al.*, *Arzneim.-Forsch.* **29**, 1155 (1979). Pharmacokinetics: P. Dittrich *et al.*, *ibid.* **31**, 518 (1981). Effect on prostaglandin biosynthesis: J. S. Franzone *et al.*, *Farmaco Ed. Sci.* **35**, 498 (1980). Clinical study: J. Polderman, M. Colon, *J. Int. Med. Res.* **8**, 156 (1980).

Cryst from dioxane, mp 181-182° (dec). Sol in most organic solvents at elevated temperatures. In strong alkali it is hydrolyzed quickly to the debenzoylated product. LD$_{50}$ orally in rats: 96 mg/kg (De Martiis, U.S. patent).
THERAP CAT: Anti-inflammatory.

6917. Oxamic Acid. [471-47-6] Aminooxoacetic acid; oxamidic acid. $C_2H_3NO_3$; mol wt 89.05. C 26.98%, H 3.40%, N 15.73%, O 53.90%. $H_2NCOCOOH$. Prepd by heating oxamide in water with ammonia, followed by neutralization of resulting ammonium salt: Toussaint, *Ann.* **120**, 237 (1861).
Cryst powder from water, or prisms from alcohol, dec about 210 or 214°. Sparingly sol in water. Practically insol in abs alcohol, ether.
Ammonium salt. $H_2NCOCOONH_4$. Monoclinic prisms, dec about 226°. Very slightly sol in cold water, alcohol.

6918. Oxamide. [471-46-5] Ethanediamide; oxalamide; oxalic acid diamide; ethanedioic acid diamide. $C_2H_4N_2O_2$; mol wt 88.07. C 27.28%, H 4.58%, N 31.81%, O 36.33%. $H_2NCOCONH_2$. Prepd from formamide by glow-discharge electrolysis: Brown *et al.*, *J. Org. Chem.* **27**, 3698 (1962). Crystal structure: G. De With, S. Harkema, *Acta Crystallogr.* **33B**, 2367 (1977). Metabolized in body to form oxalic acid.
Triclinic needles, dec 350°. d_4^{20} 1.667. Sparingly sol in hot water, alcohol.

6919. Oxamniquine. [21738-42-1] 1,2,3,4-Tetrahydro-2-[[(1-methylethyl)amino]methyl]-7-nitro-6-quinolinemethanol; 1,2,-3,4-tetrahydro-2-[(isopropylamino)methyl]-7-nitro-6-quinolinemethanol; 6-hydroxymethyl-2-isopropylaminomethyl-7-nitro-1,2,-3,4-tetrahydroquinoline; UK-4271; Mansil; Vansil. $C_{14}H_{21}N_3O_3$; mol wt 279.33. C 60.20%, H 7.58%, N 15.04%, O 17.18%. Prepn: H. C. Richards, **ZA 6803636**; *idem*, **US 3821228** (1967, 1974 both to Pfizer). Discovery of schistosomicidal activity: H. C. Richards, R. Foster, *Nature* **222**, 581 (1969). Metabolism: N. M. Woolhouse, B. Kaye, *Parasitology* **15**, 111 (1977). Genetic activity: T. M. Ong, *Mutat. Res.* **55**, 43 (1978). *In vitro* activity: C. J. Chavasse *et al.*, *Ann. Trop. Med. Parasitol.* **72**, 293 (1978). Mutagenicity study: R. P. Batzinger, E. Bueding, *J. Pharmacol. Exp. Ther.* **200**, 1 (1977). Pharmacology: R. Foster, *Rev. Inst. Med. Trop. Sao Paulo* **15**, Suppl. 1, 189 (1973), *C.A.* **83**, 188417g (1975). Clinical study: R. J. Pitchford, M. Lewis, *S. Afr. Med. J.* **53**, 677 (1978). HPLC determn in biological fluids: H. W. Jun, M. A. Radwan, *Anal. Lett.* **18**, 1345 (1985). Comprehensive description: I. Ahmad, *et al.*, *Anal. Profiles Drug Subs.* **20**, 601-625 (1991).

Pale yellow crystals from isopropanol, mp 147-149°. Sol in acetone, chloroform and methanol. Sol in about 3300 parts of water at 27°C. pH of a 1% soln 8.0-10.0. uv max (methanol) 205.5, 249.5, 389.5 nm ($A_{1cm}^{1\%}$ 486, 695, 62.5). LD_{50} in mice, rabbits (mg/kg): >2000, >1000 i.m., 1300, 800 orally (Foster).

THERAP CAT: Anthelmintic (Schistosoma).

6920. Oxamyl. [23135-22-0] 2-(Dimethylamino)-*N*-[[(methylamino)carbonyl]oxy]-2-oxoethanimidothioic acid methyl ester; *N'*,*N'*-dimethyl-*N*-[(methylcarbamoyl)oxy]-1-thiooxamimidic acid methyl ester; *N*,*N*-dimethyl-α-methylcarbamoyloxyimino-α-(methylthio)acetamide; methyl 1-(dimethylcarbamoyl)-*N*-(methylcarbamoyloxy)thioformimidate; thioxamyl; DPX-1410; Vydate. $C_7H_{13}N_3O_3S$; mol wt 219.26. C 38.34%, H 5.98%, N 19.16%, O 21.89%, S 14.62%. Prepn: J. B. Buchanan, **ZA 6803629**; *eidem*, **US 3530220**, and **US 3658870** (1968, 1970, 1972 all to du Pont). Decompn: J. Harvey, Jr., J. Han, *J. Agric. Food Chem.* **26**, 536 (1978). Metabolism: *eidem, ibid.* 902; J. Harvey, Jr. *et al.*, *ibid.* 529. Toxicity study: M. Fahmy *et al.*, *J. Agric. Food Chem.* **26**, 550 (1978).

Crystalline solid, slight sulfurous odor. mp 100-102°, changing to a different crystalline form, mp 108-110°. Soly in g/100 ml at 25°: water 28; acetone 67; ethanol 33; 2-propanol 11; methanol 144; toluene 1. LD_{50} orally in rats: 5 mg/kg (Fahmy).

Caution: Toxic to wildlife, fish, bees.

USE: Insecticide, nematocide, acaricide.

6921. Oxandrolone. [53-39-4] (4a*S*,4b*S*,6a*S*,7*S*,9a*S*,9b*R*,-11a*S*)-Tetradecahydro-7-hydroxy-4a,6a,7-trimethylcyclopenta[5,-6]naphtho[1,2-c]pyran-2(1*H*)-one; 17β-hydroxy-17α-methyl-2-oxa-5α-androstan-3-one; dodecahydro-3-hydroxy-6-(hydroxymethyl)-3,3a,6-trimethyl-1*H*-benz[e]indene-7-acetic acid δ-lactone; Anavar; Lonavar; Provitar; Vasorome. $C_{19}H_{30}O_3$; mol wt 306.44. C 74.47%, H 9.87%, O 15.66%. Prepn: R. Pappo, C. J. Jung, *Tetrahedron Lett.* **9**, 365 (1962); R. Pappo, **US 3128283** (1964 to Searle).

Crystals, mp 235-238°. $[\alpha]_D^{25}$ −23° (c = approx 1% in chloroform).

Note: This is a controlled substance (anabolic steroid): **21 CFR**, 1308.13, as defined in 1300.01.

THERAP CAT: Androgen.

6922. Oxantel. [36531-26-7] (*E*)-3-[2-(1,4,5,6-Tetrahydro-1-methyl-2-pyrimidinyl)ethenyl]phenol; (*E*)-*m*-[2-(1,4,5,6-tetrahydro-1-methyl-2-pyrimidinyl)vinyl]phenol; 1-methyl-1,4,5,6-tetrahydro-2-[2-(3-hydroxyphenyl)vinyl]pyrimidine; CP-14445. C_{13}-$H_{16}N_2O$; mol wt 216.28. C 72.19%, H 7.46%, N 12.95%, O 7.40%. Analog of pyrantel, *q.v.*, with activity vs whipworms (*Trichuris* spp.). Prepn: J. W. Mc Farland, **ZA 6804589** corresp to **US 3579510** and **US 3708584** (1968, 1971, 1973 all to Pfizer). Synthesis and evaluation in whipworm control: J. W. Mc Farland, H. L. Howes *J. Med. Chem.* **15**, 365 (1972). Evaluation vs *Trichuris* in dogs: H. L. Howes, *Proc. Soc. Exp. Biol. Med.* **139**, 394 (1972). Efficacy vs *T. trichiuris* in humans: E. L. Lee *et al.*, *Am. J. Trop. Med. Hyg.* **25**, 563 (1976); vs *T. suis* in swine: M. Robinson, *Vet. Parasitol.* **5**, 223 (1979). Anthelmintic effects of combination with pyrantel pamoate: B. Sinniah, D. Sinniah, *Ann. Trop. Med. Parasitol.* **75**, 315 (1981).

Hydrochloride. $C_{13}H_{16}N_2O \cdot HCl$. Crystals from ethanol, mp 207-208°. uv max (water): 231, 274 nm (ε 12700, 20100).

Pamoate. [68813-55-8] Oxantel embonate; CP-14445-16; Telopar. $C_{13}H_{16}N_2O \cdot C_{23}H_{16}O_6$; mol wt 604.65.

Mixture with pyrantel pamoate (1:1) *see* Pyrantel.

THERAP CAT: Anthelmintic (Nematodes).

THERAP CAT (VET): Anthelmintic (Nematodes).

6923. Oxapropanium Iodide. [541-66-2] *N*,*N*,*N*-Trimethyl-1,3-dioxolane-4-methanaminium iodide; (1,3-dioxolan-4-yl-methyl)trimethylammonium iodide; 4-(dimethylaminomethyl)-1,3-dioxacyclopentane methiodide; 1-dimethylamino-2,3-dioxamethyl-enepropane methiodide; vasodilatateur 2249F; 2249-F; Dilvasene. $C_7H_{16}INO_2$; mol wt 273.11. C 30.78%, H 5.90%, I 46.47%, N 5.13%, O 11.72%. Prepd by the reaction of a cyclic acetal of an α-monohalohydrin of glycerol with dimethylamine which on treatment with methyl iodide results in a quaternary ammonium salt: Fourneau, **US 2445393** (1948 to Rhône-Poulenc).

Crystals, mp 158-160° (the free base bp$_{21}$ 68°). Freely sol in water. Sol in boiling alcohol (about 40% w/v). Sparingly sol in cold alcohol, ether, chloroform, benzene.

THERAP CAT: Cholinergic.

6924. Oxaprozin. [21256-18-8] 4,5-Diphenyl-2-oxazole-propanoic acid; β-(4,5-diphenyloxazol-2-yl)propionic acid; Wy-21743; Alvo; Daypro. $C_{18}H_{15}NO_3$; mol wt 293.32. C 73.71%, H 5.15%, N 4.78%, O 16.36%. First description of anti-inflammatory properties: K. Brown *et al.*, *Nature* **219**, 164 (1968). Prepn: **FR 2001036** (1969 to Inst. Farm. Serono), *C.A.* **72**, 66930w (1970); K. Brown, **GB 1206403** and **US 3578671** (1970, 1971 both to Wyeth). Biochemical properties: M. W. Whitehouse *et al.*, *Biochem. Pharmacol.* **20**, 2309 (1971). Metabolism: F. W. Janssen *et al.*, *Drug Metab. Dispos.* **6**, 465 (1978). Pharmacology: D. A. Shriver *et al.*, *Toxicol. Appl. Pharmacol.* **42**, 75 (1977); F. Awouters *et al.*, *J. Pharm. Pharmacol.* **30**, 41 (1978). Clinical studies: R. Jamar, J. Dequeker, *Curr. Med. Res. Opin.* **5**, 433 (1978); J. A. Hubsher *et al.*, *J. Int. Med. Res.* **7**, 69 (1979); *eidem, Arthritis Rheum.* **25**, S117 (1982). Protein binding and clearance: C. A. Homon *et al.*, *Agents Actions* **12**, 211 (1982). Symposium on pharmacology and clinical efficacy: *Semin. Arthritis Rheum.* **15**, Suppl. 3, 1-107 (1986). Review of mechanism of action and clinical efficacy: F. Dallegri *et. al.*, *Expert Opin. Pharmacother.* **6**, 777-785 (2005).

Crystals from methanol, mp 160.5-161.5°. Slightly sol in alcohol. Insol in water. Partition coefficient (octanol/water): 4.8 (pH 7.4). pKa 4.3.

THERAP CAT: Anti-inflammatory.

6925. Oxatomide. [60607-34-3] 1-[3-[4-(Diphenylmethyl)-1-piperazinyl]propyl]-1,3-dihydro-2H-benzimidazol-2-one; 1-[3-[4-(diphenylmethyl)-1-piperazinyl]propyl]-2-benzimidazolinone; R-35443; Celtect; Cobiona; Dasten; Tinset. $C_{27}H_{30}N_4O$; mol wt 426.55. C 76.03%, H 7.09%, N 13.13%, O 3.75%. Orally active anti-allergic agent, related structurally to cinnarizine, q.v., and having a novel biphasic mode of action. Prepn: J. Vandenberk et al., **DE 2714437**; eidem, **US 4250176** (1977, 1981 both to Janssen). Inhibition of release and effects of allergic mediators: F. Awouters et al., Experientia **33**, 1657 (1977). In vitro study of inhibition and stimulation of histamine release: M. K. Church et al., Agents Actions **10**, 4 (1980). In vivo study: S. Gatti et al., Br. J. Dermatol. **103**, 671 (1980). Clinical studies: S. W. Barham, F. Moran, Br. J. Clin. Pract. **34**, 323 (1980); E. F. Juniper et al., Clin. Allergy **11**, 61 (1981); W. Peremans et al., Dermatologia **162**, 42 (1981). Review of pharmacological and clinical studies: D. M. Richards et al., Drugs **27**, 210 (1984).

White powder, mp 153.6°. LD_{50} in guinea pigs, mice, rats (mg/kg): 320, >2560, >2560 orally; 23, 27, 30 i.v. (Richards).

THERAP CAT: Antiallergic; antiasthmatic.

6926. Oxazepam. [604-75-1] 7-Chloro-1,3-dihydro-3-hydroxy-5-phenyl-2H-1,4-benzodiazepin-2-one; 7-chloro-3-hydroxy-5-phenyl-1,3-dihydro-2H-1,4-benzodiazepin-2-one; Wy-3498; Adumbran; Azutranquil; Durazepam; Hilong; Limbial; Noctazepam; Praxiten; Serax; Serenid; Serepax; Séresta; Serpax; Sobril; Uskan. $C_{15}H_{11}ClN_2O_2$; mol wt 286.71. C 62.84%, H 3.87%, Cl 12.37%, N 9.77%, O 11.16%. Prepn: Bell, Childress, J. Org. Chem. **27**, 1691 (1962); **NL 298071**; S. C. Bell, **US 3296249** (1965, 1967 both to American Home Prod.). Crystal and molecular structure: G. Gilli et al., Acta Crystallogr. **B34**, 2826 (1978). Metabolic studies: Sisenwine et al., Arzneim.-Forsch. **22**, 682 (1972); Knowles, Ruelius, ibid. 687. Pharmacokinetics: D. J. Greenblatt, Clin. Pharmacokinet. **6**, 89 (1981). Toxicity data: E. I. Goldenthal, Toxicol. Appl. Pharmacol. **18**, 185 (1971). Comprehensive description: C. M. Shearer, C. R. Pilla, Anal. Profiles Drug Subs. **3**, 441-464 (1974). Review: Acta Psychiatr. Scand. Suppl. **274**, R. Chinnery, A. Sundwall, Eds. (1978) 128 pp.

Crystals from alcohol, mp 205-206°. Sol in alcohol, chloroform, dioxane. Practically insol in water. LD_{50} in mice, rats (mg/kg): >5010, >5010 orally (Goldenthal).

Note: This is a controlled substance (depressant): **21 CFR, 1308.14.**

THERAP CAT: Anxiolytic.

6927. Oxazolam. [27167-30-2] 10-Chloro-2,3,7,11b-tetrahydro-2-methyl-11b-phenyloxazolo[3,2-d][1,4]benzodiazepin-6(5H)-one; 10-chloro-2,3,5,6,7,11b-hexahydro-2-methyl-11b-phenylbenzo[6,7]-1,4-diazepino[5,4-b]oxazol-6-one; oxazolazepam; Hializan; Serenal; Tranquit. $C_{18}H_{17}ClN_2O_2$; mol wt 328.79. C 65.75%, H 5.21%, Cl 10.78%, N 8.52%, O 9.73%. Prepn: Tachikawa et al., **DE 1812252**; eidem, **US 3772371** (1969, 1973 to Sankyo). Synthesis and pharmacology: Miyadera et al., J. Med. Chem. **14**, 520 (1971). Metabolism studies: Shindo et al., Chem. Pharm. Bull. **19**, 60 (1971); Yasumura et al., ibid. 1929.

Crystals, mp 186-188°. Sol in chloroform; slightly sol in ethanol. Practically insol in water.

Note: This is a controlled substance (depressant): **21 CFR, 1308.14.**

THERAP CAT: Anxiolytic.

6928. Ox Bile Extract. Purified oxgall; sodium choleate; Bi-Ketolan; Bilein; Bilicholan; Cholatol; Crescefel; Desicol; Doxychol; Panoxolin; Plebilin. One gram = 8 g ox bile. Constit. Chiefly the sodium salts of glycocholic and taurocholic acids; also cholesterol, lecithin, glycocol and choline compounds.

Yellowish-green, soft solid; peculiar odor; partly sweet, partly bitter, disagreeable taste. Very sol in water or alc.

THERAP CAT: Choleretic.

THERAP CAT (VET): Has been used as a choleretic.

6929. Oxcarbazepine. [28721-07-5] 10,11-Dihydro-10-oxo-5H-dibenz[b,f]azepine-5-carboxamide; oxacarbazepine; GP-47680; Trileptal. $C_{15}H_{12}N_2O_2$; mol wt 252.27. C 71.42%, H 4.79%, N 11.10%, O 12.68%. Ketoderivative of carbamazepine, q.v. Prepn: W. Schindler, **DE 2011087** (1970 to Geigy); idem, **US 3642775** (1972 to Ciba-Geigy). Improved prepn: D. Kaufmann et al., Tetrahedron Lett. **45**, 5275 (2004). Metabolism: H. Schütz et al., Xenobiotica **16**, 769 (1986). Hyponatremic effects: O. A. Nielsen et al., Epilepsy Res. **2**, 269 (1988). Determn of oxcarbazepine and main metabolites by GC in plasma: G. E. Von Unruh, W. D. Paar, J. Chromatogr. **345**, 67 (1985); by HPLC: A. A. Elyas, V. D. Goldberg, ibid. **528**, 473 (1990). Clinical evaluation in treatment of epilepsy: M. Dam et al., Epilepsy Res. **3**, 70 (1989); in management of trigeminal neuralgia: J. M. Zakrzewska, P. N. Patsalos, J. Neurol. Neurosurg. Psychiatry **52**, 472 (1989). Review of pharmacology and therapeutic efficacy: A. Beydoun, E. Kutluay, Expert Opin. Pharmacother. **3**, 59-71 (2001).

Crystals from ethanol, mp 215-216°.

THERAP CAT: Anticonvulsant.

6930. Oxeladin. [468-61-1] α,α-Diethylbenzeneacetic acid 2-[2-(diethylamino)ethoxy]ethyl ester; 2-ethyl-2-phenylbutyric acid 2-(2-diethylaminoethoxy)ethyl ester; 2-(2-diethylaminoethoxy)ethyl α,α-diethylphenylacetate; α,α-diethylphenylacetic acid 2-(2-di-ethylaminoethoxy)ethyl ester. $C_{20}H_{33}NO_3$; mol wt 335.48. C 71.60%, H 9.91%, N 4.18%, O 14.31%. Prepn: V. Petrow *et al.*, *J. Pharm. Pharmacol.* **10**, 40 (1958); *eidem*, US 2885404 (1959 to Brit. Drug Houses).

Yellow oil with an acrid odor and bitter taste. bp$_{0.5}$ 150°; bp$_{0.1}$ 140°. Soluble in dil HCl, ethanol, acetone, ether, toluene; practically insol in water. Stable in acids, unstable in alkalies. Non-hygroscopic.

Citrate. [52432-72-1] Pectamol; Pectamon; Paxeladine. C_{20}-$H_{33}NO_3 \cdot C_6H_8O_7$; mol wt 527.60. Small needles from ethyl acetate, mp 90-91°. Sol in water.

THERAP CAT: Antitussive.

6931. Oxendolone. [33765-68-3] (16β,17β)-16-Ethyl-17-hydroxyestr-4-en-3-one; 16β-ethyl-19-nortestosterone; TSAA-291; Prostetin. $C_{20}H_{30}O_2$; mol wt 302.45. C 79.42%, H 10.00%, O 10.58%. Prepn: K. Hiraga *et al.*, DE 2100319; *eidem*, US 3856829 (1971, 1974 both to Takeda); K. Yoshioka *et al.*, *Chem. Pharm. Bull.* **23**, 3203 (1975). Stereoselective synthesis and NMR study: G. Goto *et al.*, *ibid.* **25**, 1295 (1977). Synthesis and anti-androgenic activity: *eidem*, *ibid.* **26**, 1718 (1978). Physico-chemical properties and stabilities: K. Itakura *et al.*, *Takeda Kenkyushoho* **37**, 297 (1978), *C.A.* **91**, 20879 (1979). Disposition and metabolism: S. Tanayama *et al.*, *Steroids* **33**, 65 (1979). Series of articles on pharmacology, mechanism of action, anti-androgen effects: *Acta Endocrinol.* **92** (Suppl 2), 1-107 (1979).

Crystals from ether, mp 152-153°. [α]$_D$ +41° (c = 1.0 in ethanol). uv max (ethanol): 240 nm (ε 15800). Stable against heat, humidity, indoor light. Converted to the 16α- and 17α-epimers in sunlight. LD$_{50}$ in rats, mice (g/kg): >10 orally; 5-10 i.m. and i.p. (Hiraga, 1971).

THERAP CAT: Anti-androgen; in treatment of benign prostatic hypertrophy.

6932. Oxenin. [3230-75-9] 11,12-Didehydro-7,10-dihydro-10-hydroxyretinol; 3,7-dimethyl-9-(2,6,6-trimethyl-1-cyclohexen-1-yl)nona-2,7-dien-4-yne-1,6-diol. $C_{20}H_{30}O_2$; mol wt 302.45. C 79.42%, H 10.00%, O 10.58%. Intermediate in the vitamin A synthesis. Prepn: Isler *et al.*, *Helv. Chim. Acta* **30**, 1911 (1947); Isler, US 2451739 (1948 to Hoffmann-La Roche); Kardys, US 3046310 (1962 to Pfizer).

Very viscous yellow oil. d$_4^{27}$ 0.9984; n$_D^{22}$ 1.5344. Has been crystallized, mp 58.5-59°.

6933. Oxethazaine. [126-27-2] 2,2'-[(2-Hydroxyethyl)imino]bis[N-(1,1-dimethyl-2-phenylethyl)-N-methylacetamide]; N,N-bis[N-methyl-N-phenyl-*tert*-butylacetamido]-β-hydroxyethylamine; oxetacaine; oxethazine; Wy-806; Storocain; Topicain. $C_{28}H_{41}$-

N_3O_3; mol wt 467.64. C 71.91%, H 8.84%, N 8.99%, O 10.26%. Prepn: Seifter *et al.*, US 2780646 (1957 to Am. Home Prods.); Salomon, IL 10062 (1957), *C.A.* **52**, 15569 (1958). Pharmacology: Axerio Agnessetti, *An. R. Acad. Farm.* **35**, 183 (1969), *C.A.* **71**, 122082q (1969). Toxicity studies: J. M. Glassman *et al.*, *Toxicol. Appl. Pharmacol.* **5**, 184 (1963). Clinical trial of combination with antacid in ulcer pain: F. T. M. Cordeiro *et al.*, *Curr. Ther. Res.* **19**, 230 (1976); A. Zanni *et al.*, *Curr. Med. Res. Opin.* **10**, 128 (1986). Evaluation as dental anesthetic: P. A. Brennan, J. D. Langdon, *Br. J. Oral Maxillofac. Surg.* **28**, 26 (1990).

Crystals from benzene + hexane, mp 104-104.5°. Insol in water. Sol in dil acids.

Hydrochloride. [13930-31-9] Emoren. $C_{28}H_{41}N_3O_3 \cdot HCl$; mol wt 504.10. mp 146-147°. Easily sol in water. LD$_{50}$ (calculated as base) in mice, rats (mg/kg): 399.9, 625.9 orally; 247.2, 502.3 i.m.; 3.6, 1.3 i.v.; LD$_{50}$ (calculated as base) in rabbits (mg/kg): 0.54 i.v. (Glassman).

Combination with aluminum and magnesium hydroxides. Mutesa; Muthesa; Oxaine M; Tepilta.

THERAP CAT: Anesthetic (local).

6934. Oxetorone. [26020-55-3] 3-Benzofuro[3,2-c][1]benzoxepin-6(12H)-ylidene-N,N-dimethyl-1-propanamine; N,N-dimethylbenzofuro[3,2-c][1]benzoxepin-Δ$^{6(12H),γ}$-propylamine; 6-(3-dimethylaminopropylidene)benzo[b]benzofurano[2,3-e]oxepine. $C_{21}H_{21}NO_2$; mol wt 319.40. C 78.97%, H 6.63%, N 4.39%, O 10.02%. Novel serotonin and histamine antagonist with antimigraine activity. Prepn: F. Binon, M. Descamps, DE 1963205 corresp to US 3651051 (1970, 1972 both to Labaz). Metabolism *in vitro:* E. Rossi *et al.*, *J. Chromatogr.* **152**, 228 (1978). Use in treatment of migraine: J. J. Dufresne, *Praxis* **67**, 1148 (1978); J. Florence, *ibid.* 1323; in chronic headache: U. Thoden, *Therapiewoche* **30**, 492 (1980).

Fumarate. [34522-46-8] L-6257; Nocertone; Oxedix. C_{25}-$H_{25}NO_6$; mol wt 435.47. Cryst from isopropanol, mp 160°.

THERAP CAT: Analgesic (specific in migraine).

6935. Oxfendazole. [53716-50-0] [5-(Phenylsulfinyl)-1H-benzimidazol-2-yl]carbamic acid methyl ester; methyl-5-(phenylsulfinyl)-2-benzimidazolecarbamate; 5-phenylsulfinyl-2-carbomethoxyaminobenzimidazole; RS-8858; Autoworm; Benzelmin; Synanthic; Systamex. $C_{15}H_{13}N_3O_3S$; mol wt 315.35. C 57.13%, H 4.16%, N 13.32%, O 15.22%, S 10.17%. Prepn: C. Beard *et al.*, DE 2363351; *eidem*, US 3929821 (1974, 1975, both to Syntex); E. A. Averkin *et al.*, *J. Med. Chem.* **18**, 1164 (1975). Metabolism: J. P. Bell, R. V. Tomlinson, *Fed. Proc.* **35**, 487 (1976). Radioimmunoassay: C. Nerenberg *et al.*, *J. Pharm. Sci.* **67**, 1553 (1978). Efficacy evaluations: J. L. Duncan, J. G. Reid, *Vet. Rec.* **103**, 332 (1978); N. F. Baker *et al.*, *Am. J. Vet. Res.* **39**, 1258 (1978).

Crystals from chloroform-methanol, mp 253° (dec). LD$_{50}$ in dogs, rats, mice: >1600, >6400, >6400 mg/kg (Averkin).

THERAP CAT (VET): Anthelmintic.

6936. Oxibendazole. [20559-55-1] (5-Propoxy-1*H*-benzimidazol-2-yl)carbamic acid methyl ester; 5-propoxy-2-benzimidazolecarbamic acid methyl ester; 5-propoxy-2-(carbomethoxyamino)benzimidazole; SKF-30310; Anthelcide EQ; Equitac. C$_{12}$-H$_{15}$N$_3$O$_3$; mol wt 249.27. C 57.82%, H 6.07%, N 16.86%, O 19.26%. Prepn: **GB 1123317** corresp to P. P. Actor, J. F. Pagano, **US 3574845** (1968, 1971 both to SK & F). Comparative anthelmintic effects in mice: C. S. Karunakaran, D. A. Denham, *J. Parasitol.* **66,** 929 (1980). Clinical studies in foals and horses: J. H. Drudge *et al., Am. J. Vet. Res.* **42,** 526 (1981); E. T. Lyons *et al., ibid.* 685; D. K. Hass *et al., ibid.* **43,** 534 (1982).

Cryst, mp 230-230.5°.

THERAP CAT (VET): Anthelmintic.

6937. Oxiconazole Nitrate. [64211-46-7] (*Z*)-1-(2,4-Dichlorophenyl)-2-(1*H*-imidazol-1-yl)ethanone *O*-[(2,4-dichlorophenyl)methyl]oxime mononitrate; 2′,4′-dichloro-2-(imidazol-1-yl)acetophenone *O*-(2,4-dichlorobenzyl)oxime nitrate; Sgd-301-76; Ro-13-8996; Gyno-Myfungar; Myfungar; Oceral; Oxistat. C$_{18}$-H$_{14}$Cl$_4$N$_4$O$_4$; mol wt 492.14. C 43.93%, H 2.87%, Cl 28.82%, N 11.38%, O 13.00%. Broad spectrum topical antimycotic agent. Prepn: G. Mixich *et al., DE 2657578; eidem, US 4124767* (1977, 1978 both to Siegfried). Stereospecific synthesis of *(E)-, (Z)*-isomers, ^{1}H NMR study: G. Mixich, K. Thiele, *Arzneim.-Forsch.* **29,** 1510 (1979). GLC determn in plasma: M. Zell, L. Herzfeld, *J. Chromatogr.* **229,** 111 (1982). *In vitro* and *in vivo* antifungal activity: A. Polak, *Arzneim.-Forsch.* **32,** 17 (1982). Study of skin, nail penetration: G. Stueltgen, E. Bauer, *Mykosen* **25,** 74 (1982). Comparison of antifungal imidazoles: W. H. Beggs, *IRCS Med. Sci.* **11,** 677 (1983).

Crystals from ethanol, mp 137-138°.

THERAP CAT: Antifungal.

6938. Oxidimethiin. [55290-64-7] 2,3-Dihydro-5,6-dimethyl-1,4-dithiin 1,1,4,4-tetraoxide; tetrathiin; UBI-N252; Harvade. C$_6$H$_{10}$O$_4$S$_2$; mol wt 210.27. C 34.27%, H 4.79%, O 30.44%, S 30.50%. Prepn: A. D. Brewer *et al., FR 2228429* corresp to **US 3920438** (1974, 1975 to Uniroyal). Activity: R. W. Neidermyer *et al., Proc. 12th Br. Weed Control Conf.* **3,** 959 (1974). Crystal structure: S. K. Arora *et al., Acta Crystallogr.* **B34,** 2918 (1978).

Long white needles from water, mp 166-168°.

USE: Plant growth regulator.

6939. Oxidized Cellulose. Absorbable cellulose; cellulosic acid; polyanhydroglucuronic acid; Oxycel; Hemo-Pak. A cellulose of varied carboxyl content retaining the fibrous structure. Prepd by oxidizing cellulose with nitrogen dioxide: Yackel, Kenyon, *J. Am. Chem. Soc.* **64,** 121 (1942).

The degree of oxidation is sufficiently high to make the product sol in dil alk solns. Insol in water or acidic solns.

THERAP CAT: Hemostatic (local).

THERAP CAT (VET): Hemostatic (local).

6940. Oxidronic Acid. [15468-10-7] (Hydroxymethylene)bisphosphonic acid; (hydroxymethylene)diphosphonic acid; HDP; HMDP. CH$_6$O$_7$P$_2$; mol wt 192.00. C 6.26%, H 3.15%, O 58.33%, P 32.26%. Bisphosphonate similar to etidronic acid, *q.v.* Prepn: O. T. Quimby, **FR 1506840;** *idem,* **US 3422137** (1967, 1969 both to Procter & Gamble); of sodium salt: *idem et al., J. Org. Chem.* **32,** 4111 (1967). Prepn of ^{99m}Tc-complex: J. A. Bevan, **EP 7676;** *idem,* **US 4247534** (1980, 1981 both to Procter & Gamble); and osteotropic properties: T. S. T. Wang *et al., J. Nucl. Med.* **21,** 767 (1980). Biodistribution: J. A. Bevan *et al., ibid.* 961. Radiochemical purity: W. Majewski *et al., J. Nucl. Med. Technol.* **11,** 23 (1983). Clinical evaluation as skeletal imaging agent: P. A. Domstad *et al., Radiology* **136,** 209 (1980). Diagnostic use in Paget's disease: A. Evans *et al., Eur. J. Nucl. Med.* **18,** 757 (1991); for localization of bone metastases: F. Tenenbaum *et al., ibid.* **20,** 1168 (1993).

Sodium salt. [14255-61-9] Disodium monohydroxy methylene diphosphonate; oxidronate sodium. CH$_4$Na$_2$O$_7$P$_2$. Crystals from methanol/water (6/1), mp 297-300°.

[99m]Tc-complex. [72945-61-0] Technetium ^{99m}Tc oxidronate; TechneScan HDP; Osteoscan-HDP.

THERAP CAT: ^{99m}Tc-complex as diagnostic aid (radioactive imaging agent).

6941. Oxiniacic Acid. [2398-81-4] 3-Pyridinecarboxylic acid 1-oxide; nicotinic acid 1-oxide; 3-carboxypyridine *N*-oxide. C$_6$H$_5$NO$_3$; mol wt 139.11. C 51.80%, H 3.62%, N 10.07%, O 34.50%. Prepn: Clemo, Koenig, *J. Chem. Soc.* **1949,** S231; Taylor, Crovetti, *J. Org. Chem.* **19,** 1633 (1954). Mass spectrum: Bild, Hesse, *Helv. Chim. Acta* **50,** 1885 (1967). Therapeutic effect: Debay, Thery, **BE 618968** (1962), *C.A.* **58,** 12375e (1963).

Needles, mp 254-255° (dec). Slightly soluble in cold water, more sol in hot water, hot glacial acetic acid, hot methanol, less sol in ethanol. Insol in light petroleum, benzene, chloroform. uv max (0.1*N* H$_2$SO$_4$): 220, 260 nm (ε 22400, 10200).

Ethanolamine salt. [36296-31-8] Ethanolamine oxiniacate; Novacyl. C$_6$H$_5$NO$_3$.C$_2$H$_7$NO; mol wt 200.19.

THERAP CAT: Antilipemic.

6942. Oxiracetam. [62613-82-5] 4-Hydroxy-2-oxo-1-pyrrolidineacetamide; 2-(4-hydroxypyrrolidin-2-on-1-yl)acetamide; hydroxypiracetam; CT-848; ISF-2522; Neuractiv; Neuromet. C$_6$-H$_{10}$N$_2$O$_3$; mol wt 158.16. C 45.56%, H 6.37%, N 17.71%, O 30.35%. Analog of piracetam, *q.v.,* with psychostimulant activity. Prepn: G. Pifferi, M. Pinza, **DE 2635853;** *eidem,* **US 4118396** (1977, 1978 both to I.S.F.); *eidem, Farmaco Ed. Sci.* **32,** 602 (1977). Effect on learning and memory in animals and prepn of enantiomers: S. Banfi *et al., ibid.* **39,** 16 (1984). Effect in animals with cerebral impairment: S. Banfi *et al., Pharmacol. Res. Commun.* **16,** 67 (1984). Pharmacokinetics in humans: E. Perucca *et* *al., Eur. J. Drug Metab. Pharmacokinet.* **9,** 267 (1984). Clinical evaluation in organic brain syndrome: B. Saletu *et al., Neuropsychobiology* **13,** 44 (1985).

White, microcrystalline powder from methanol, mp 165-168°.
(R)-Form. Crystals from acetone + water, mp 135-136°. $[\alpha]_D$ +36.2° (c = 1.00 in water).
(S)-Form. Crystals from acetone + water, mp 135-136°. $[\alpha]_D$ −36.0° (c = 1.00 in water).
THERAP CAT: Nootropic.

6943. Oxitropium Bromide. [30286-75-0] [7(S)-(1α,2β,-4β,5α,7β)]-9-Ethyl-7-(3-hydroxy-1-oxo-2-phenylpropoxy)-9-methyl-3-oxa-9-azoniatricyclo[3.3.1.0^{2,4}]nonane bromide; (8r)-6β,7β-epoxy-8-ethyl-3α-hydroxy-1αH,5αH-tropanium bromide (−)-tropate; (−)-N-ethylnorscopolamine methobromide; Ba-253; Ba-253-BR-L; Oxivent; Tersigat; Ventilat. C$_{19}$H$_{26}$BrNO$_4$; mol wt 412.32. C 55.35%, H 6.36%, Br 19.38%, N 3.40%, O 15.52%. Anticholinergic bronchodilating agent. Prepn: K. Zeile *et al.,* US 3472861 (1969 to Boehringer, Ing.). Comparison with fenoterol, *q.v.:* D. Nolte, *Respiration* **36,** 32 (1978); with ipratropium bromide, *q.v.:* J. Lulling *et al., ibid.* **42,** 188 (1981). Efficacy in bronchial asthma: H. M. Beumer *et al., Int. J. Clin. Pharmacol. Ther. Toxicol.* **19,** 168 (1981); in exercise-induced asthma: K. Larsson, *Respiration* **43,** 57 (1982).

Crystals, mp 203-204° (dec). $[\alpha]_D^{21}$ −25° (c = 2.0 in water).
THERAP CAT: Bronchodilator.

6944. Oxolamine. [959-14-8] *N,N*-Diethyl-3-phenyl-1,2,4-oxadiazole-5-ethanamine; 5-(2-diethylaminoethyl)-3-phenyl-1,2,4-oxadiazole; 3-phenyl-5-(β-diethylaminoethyl)-1,2,4-oxadiazole; 683-M. C$_{14}$H$_{19}$N$_3$O; mol wt 245.32. C 68.54%, H 7.81%, N 17.13%, O 6.52%. Prepn: DE 1097998 (1961 to Angelini Francesco), *C.A.* **56,** 11598h (1962). Teratogenicity studies of oxolamine citrate: L. Nilsson, *Arzneim.-Forsch.* **17,** 781 (1967).

Liquid, bp$_{0.4}$ 127°.
Hydrochloride. [1219-20-1] C$_{14}$H$_{19}$N$_3$O.HCl. Crystals, mp 153-154°.
Citrate. [1949-20-8] AF-438; Bredon; Broncatar; Perebron; Prilon; Flogobron; Oxarmin. C$_{14}$H$_{19}$N$_3$O.C$_6$H$_8$O$_7$; mol wt 437.44. Crystals, slightly sol in water, alcohol. uv max (aq soln): 239 nm (ε 260), 273, 283 nm.
THERAP CAT: In inflammatory conditions of respiratory tract.

6945. Oxolinic Acid. [14698-29-4] 5-Ethyl-5,8-dihydro-8-oxo-1,3-dioxolo[4,5-g]quinoline-7-carboxylic acid; 1-ethyl-1,4-dihydro-6,7-methylenedioxy-4-oxo-3-quinolinecarboxylic acid; 1-ethyl-6,7-methylenedioxy-4-quinolone-3-carboxylic acid; W-4565; Inoxyl; Nidantin; Uritrate; Urotrate. C$_{13}$H$_{11}$NO$_5$; mol wt 261.23. C 59.77%, H 4.24%, N 5.36%, O 30.62%. Quinolone antibacterial. Prepn: Kaminsky, Meltzer, US 3287458 (1966 to Warner-Lambert); *eidem, J. Med. Chem.* **11,** 160 (1968). Pharmacology: Turner *et al., Antimicrob. Agents Chemother.* **1967,** 475 sqq. Metabolism studies: DiCarlo *et al., Arch. Biochem. Biophys.* **127,** 503 (1968); Crew *et al., Xenobiotica* **1,** 193 (1971). Use in urinary tract infections: S. Kalowski *et al., Med. J. Aust.* **21,** 345 (1979); E. Anza *et al., Minerva Med.* **70,** 2333 (1979). Mechanism of action study: H. T. Wright *et al., Science* **213,** 455 (1981). Brief review of therapeutic use: R. Glickman *et al., Am. J. Hosp. Pharm.* **36,** 1077-1079 (1979).

Crystals from DMF, mp 314-316° (dec). LD$_{50}$ in mice, rats (mg/kg): >6000, >2000 orally (Turner).
THERAP CAT: Antibacterial.
THERAP CAT (VET): Antibacterial.

6946. Oxomemazine. [3689-50-7] *N,N,β*-Trimethyl-10*H*-phenothiazine-10-propanamine 5,5-dioxide; 10-(3-dimethylamino-2-methylpropyl)phenothiazine 5,5-dioxide; 3-(9,9-dioxo-10-phenothiazinyl)-2-methyl-1-dimethylaminopropane; RP-6847; Dysedon. C$_{18}$H$_{22}$N$_2$O$_2$S; mol wt 330.44. C 65.43%, H 6.71%, N 8.48%, O 9.68%, S 9.70%. Prepn: Jacob, Robert, US 2972612 (1961 to Rhône-Poulenc).

Crystals from heptane, mp 115°.
Hydrochloride. Doxergan; Imakol. C$_{18}$H$_{22}$N$_2$O$_2$S.HCl; mol wt 366.91. Crystals from ethanol + isopropanol, mp 250°.

6947. Oxonic Acid. [937-13-3] 1,4,5,6-Tetrahydro-4,6-dioxo-1,3,5-triazine-2-carboxylic acid; allantoxanic acid; 5-azaorotic acid; *s*-triazine-2,4-dione-6-carboxylic acid; 2,4-dioxo-1,2,3,4-tetrahydro-1,3,5-triazine-6-carboxylic acid. C$_4$H$_3$N$_3$O$_4$; mol wt 157.08. C 30.58%, H 1.93%, N 26.75%, O 40.74%. Formed during alkaline oxidation of uric acid with H$_2$O$_2$ or KMnO$_4$. Prepn and structure: Brandenberger, *Helv. Chim. Acta* **37,** 641 (1954); Brandenberger, Brandenberger, *ibid.* **37,** 2207 (1954); Piskala, Gut, *Collect. Czech. Chem. Commun.* **27,** 1572 (1962). Metabolism: Chelbova *et al., Biochem. Pharmacol.* **19,** 2785 (1970); Cihak, Sorm, *ibid.* **21,** 607 (1972).

Free acid is very unstable; can be isolated as the monopotassium salt. uv max (pH 9): 255 nm (ε 6800); (pH 12): 252 nm (ε 4600).
Oxonic acid amide. C$_4$H$_4$N$_4$O$_3$. Microcrystalline substance. Practically insol in organic solvents, sparingly sol in boiling water. Does not melt below 350°, darkens above 300°.

6948. Oxophenarsine Hydrochloride. [538-03-4] 2-Amino-4-arsenosophenol hydrochloride; 3-amino-4-hydroxyphenyl arsinoxide hydrochloride; Ehrlich 5; Arseno 39; Arsenoxide; Mapharsen; Mapharside; Mapharsal; Fontarsan; Arsenosan; Oxiarsolan. $C_6H_7AsClNO_2$; mol wt 235.50. C 30.60%, H 3.00%, As 31.81%, Cl 15.05%, N 5.95%, O 13.59%. *Ref:* G. W. Raiziss, J. L. Gavron, *Organic Arsenical Compounds* (Chem. Catalog Co., New York, 1923), pp 136-137; Scott, Tullar, *CA* 405532 (1942 to Parke, Davis).

Hygroscopic, white or nearly white, powder contg ½ mole ethanol. Readily sol in water, methanol, ethanol, in solns of alkali hydroxides and carbonates, in dil mineral acids. Sparingly sol in glacial acetic acid. Practically insol in acetone, ether. The aq soln is acid to litmus or methyl red, but alkaline to Congo red. Solns darken on exposure to air. Usually marketed mixed with buffering agents to render its soln physiologically compatible with human blood.

THERAP CAT: Antiprotozoal (Trypanosoma).

THERAP CAT (VET): Has been used as an antirickettsial.

6949. Oxophenylarsine. [637-03-6] Arsenosobenzene; phenyl arsenoxide; phenylarsine oxide; Arzene. C_6H_5AsO; mol wt 168.02. C 42.89%, H 3.00%, As 44.59%, O 9.52%. Prepn: Blicke, Smith, *J. Am. Chem. Soc.* **51**, 3479 (1929); **52**, 2946 (1930).

Crystals, mp 144-146° (also reported as mp 119-120°).

USE: Pesticide.

THERAP CAT (VET): Coccidiostat (poultry).

6950. L-2-Oxo-4-thiazolidinecarboxylic acid. [19771-63-2] (4R)-2-Oxo-4-thiazolidinecarboxylic acid; OTCA; OTC; Procysteine. $C_4H_5NO_3S$; mol wt 147.15. C 32.65%, H 3.42%, N 9.52%, O 32.62%, S 21.79%. Cysteine prodrug. Prepn: J. A. Maclaren, *Aust. J. Chem.* **21**, 1891 (1968); T. Kömives, *Org. Prep. Proced. Int.* **21**, 251 (1989). Crystal structure: N. Ramasubbu, R. Parthasarathy, *Int. J. Pept. Protein Res.* **34**, 153 (1989). Precursor for cysteine and use as glutathione biosynthesis stimulant: J. M. Williamson *et al., Proc. Natl. Acad. Sci. USA* **79**, 6246 (1982); in chicks: T. K. Chung *et al., J. Nutr.* **120**, 158 (1990). Toxicity: R. D. White *et al., Acute Toxic. Data* **1**, 164 (1992); R. D. White *et al., Toxicol. Lett.* **69**, 15 (1993). Clinical evaluation in HIV infection: G. Giorgi *et al., Curr. Ther. Res.* **52**, 461 (1992); in asymptomatic HIV infection: R. C. Kalayjian *et al., J. Acquired Immune Defic. Syndr.* **7**, 369 (1994). HPLC determn in plasma: L. W. Webb *et al., J. Chromatogr. B* **654**, 257 (1994).

Colorless cubes, mp 171-173° (dec) (Maclaren). Also reported as white crystals, mp 173-174° (Kömives). pKa (22°): 3.32. $[\alpha]_D^{20}$ −59.4° (c = 2). Readily sol in alcohol. Insol in benzene and ethyl acetate.

6951. Oxotremorine. [70-22-4] 1-[4-(1-Pyrrolidinyl)-2-butynyl]-2-pyrrolidinone; 1-(2-oxo-1-pyrrolidinyl)-4-(1-pyrrolidinyl)-2-butyne. $C_{12}H_{18}N_2O$; mol wt 206.28. C 69.87%, H 8.80%, N 13.58%, O 7.76%. Active metabolite of tremorine, *q.v.:* Cho *et al., Biochem. Biophys. Res. Commun.* **5**, 276 (1961). Synthesis: Bebbington, Shakeshaft, *J. Med. Chem.* **8**, 274 (1965); Nau, **US 3444185** (1969 to Soc. Civile Auguil). Cholinergic agent, used experimen-

tally as convulsant in study of parkinsonism: Cho *et al., Proc. 2nd Int. Pharmacol. Meet.* **2**, 75 (1964).

Pale yellow liquid. bp$_{0.6}$ 150-155°; bp$_{0.1}$ 124°. n_D^{25} 1.5156.

Picrolonate. $C_{22}H_{26}N_6O_6$. Crystals from acetone, mp 157-159°.

USE: Pharmacological tool.

6952. Oxprenolol. [6452-71-7] 1-[(1-Methylethyl)amino]-3-[2-(2-propenyloxy)phenoxy]-2-propanol; 1-[o-(allyloxy)phenoxy]-3-(isopropylamino)-2-propanol; 1-(isopropylamino)-2-hydroxy-3-[o-(allyloxy)phenoxy]propane. $C_{15}H_{23}NO_3$; mol wt 265.35. C 67.90%, H 8.74%, N 5.28%, O 18.09%. β-Adrenergic blocker. Prepn: **BE 669402** (1966 to Ciba), *C.A.* **65**, 5402d (1966), corresp to **GB 1077603**. Metabolic studies: Garteiz, *J. Pharmacol. Exp. Ther.* **179**, 354 (1971). Crystal structure of hydrochloride: J. M. Leger *et al., Acta Crystallogr.* **33B**, 2156 (1977). Long-term prevention study in coronary heart disease: S. H. Taylor *et al., N. Engl. J. Med.* **307**, 1293 (1982).

Crystals from hexane, mp 78-80°.

Hydrochloride. [6452-73-9] Ba-39089; Coretal; Laracor; Paritane; Trasicor; Trasacor. $C_{15}H_{23}NO_3 \cdot HCl$; mol wt 301.81. Crystals, mp 107-109°.

THERAP CAT: Antihypertensive, antianginal, antiarrhythmic.

6953. Oxyacanthine. [548-40-3] 6,6′,7-Trimethoxy-2,2′-dimethyloxyacanthan-12′-ol; vinetine. $C_{37}H_{40}N_2O_6$; mol wt 608.72. C 73.00%, H 6.62%, N 4.60%, O 15.77%. From root of *Berberis vulgaris* L., Berberidaceae: Rüdel, *Arch. Pharm.* **229**, 631 (1891); Späth, Kolbe, *Ber.* **58**, 2280 (1925). Structure: v. Bruchhausen *et al., Ann.* **507**, 144 (1933); Fujita, *J. Pharm. Soc. Jpn.* **72**, 213 (1952), *C.A.* **47**, 6429b (1953).

White, cryst, bitter powder. mp 216-217°. $[\alpha]_D^{20}$ +131.5° (chloroform). Practically insol in water; sol in alcohol, chloroform, ether, dil acids.

Dihydrochloride. $C_{37}H_{40}N_2O_6 \cdot 2HCl$. mp 270-271°. $[\alpha]_D$ +185.5°. Sol in water.

6954. Oxybenzone. [131-57-7] (2-Hydroxy-4-methoxyphenyl)phenylmethanone; 2-hydroxy-4-methoxybenzophenone; 4-methoxy-2-hydroxybenzophenone; benzophenone-3; MOB; Cyasorb UV 9; Eusolex 4360; Neo Heliopan BB; Uvinul M-40. $C_{14}H_{12}O_3$; mol wt 228.24. C 73.67%, H 5.30%, O 21.03%. UV-A/B absorber in cosmetics and sunscreens. Prepn: König, v. Kostanecki, *Ber.* **39**, 4027 (1906); Hardy, Forster, **US 2773903** (1956 to Am. Cyanamid); Stanley *et al.,* **US 2861104; US 2861105; US 3073866** (1958, 1958, 1963 all to General Aniline & Film). Toxicity study: H. -J. Lewerenz *et al., Food Cosmet. Toxicol.* **10**, 41 (1972).

Crystals from isopropanol, mp 66°. Readily sol in most organic solvents. LD$_{50}$ orally in rats: >12.8 g/kg (Lewerenz).

USE: Ultraviolet light absorber and stabilizer, esp in plastics and paints.

THERAP CAT: Ultraviolet screen.

6955. Oxybutynin. [5633-20-5] α-Cyclohexyl-α-hydroxy-benzeneacetic acid 4-(diethylamino)-2-butynyl ester; α-phenyl-cyclohexaneglycolic acid 4-(diethylamino)-2-butynyl ester; 4-diethylamino-2-butynyl phenylcyclohexylglycolate; oxibutinina. C$_{22}$H$_{31}$NO$_3$; mol wt 357.49. C 73.91%, H 8.74%, N 3.92%, O 13.43%. Muscarinic receptor antagonist. Prepn: **GB 940540** (1963 to Mead Johnson). Physico-chemical properties: E. Miyamoto *et al., Analyst* **119,** 1489 (1994). GC-MS determn in plasma: K. S. Patrick *et al., J. Chromatogr.* **487,** 91 (1989). Toxicity: E. I. Goldenthal, *Toxicol. Appl. Pharmacol.* **18,** 185 (1971). Review of pharmacodynamics and therapeutic use: Y. E. Yarker *et al., Drugs Aging* **6,** 243-262 (1995).

pKa 8.04. Log P (*n*-octanol/water): 2.9 (pH 6). Soly in water (mg/ml): 77 (pH 1); 0.8 (pH 6); 0.012 (pH >9.6).

Hydrochloride. [1508-65-2] Oxybutynin chloride; MJ-4309-1; Cystrin; Ditropan; Dridase; Kentera; Pollakisu; Tropax. C$_{22}$H$_{31}$NO$_3$·HCl; mol wt 393.95. Crystals, mp 129-130°. Sol in water, acids. Practically insol in alkali. LD$_{50}$ orally in rats: 1220 mg/kg (Goldenthal).

THERAP CAT: In treatment of urinary incontinence.

6956. Oxychlorosene. [8031-14-9] Monoxychlorosene; Clorpactin; Clorpactin XCB. C$_{20}$H$_{35}$ClO$_4$S; mol wt 407.01. C 59.02%, H 8.67%, Cl 8.71%, O 15.72%, S 7.88%. C$_{20}$H$_{34}$O$_3$·S.HOCl. Described as a buffered organic hypochlorous acid derivative with slightly acid pH. Contains a long chain hydrocarbon (surface-active agent). The chain (14 carbons) may be branched or straight but actually consists of a constant mixture having predominantly the straight chain. The hydrocarbon chain also has a phenyl substituent which in turn holds a sulfonic acid group. The complex corresponds to a formula: HO$_3$S—C$_6$H$_4$—(C$_{14}$H$_{29}$).HOCl.

Aq solns are unstable and should be freshly prepd; the solid may be stored in properly stoppered bottles.

Sodium salt. [52906-84-0] Clorpactin WCS.

THERAP CAT: Antiseptic.

6957. Oxycinchophen. [485-89-2] 3-Hydroxy-2-phenyl-4-quinolinecarboxylic acid; 3-hydroxy-2-phenylcinchoninic acid; 3-hydroxycinchophen; HPC; Fenidrone; Magnofenyl; Magnophenyl; Oxinofen; Reumalon. C$_{16}$H$_{11}$NO$_3$; mol wt 265.26. C 72.45%, H 4.18%, N 5.28%, O 18.09%. Prepn: Berlingozzi, Capuano, *Atti Accad. Lincei* [V] **33,** II, 91 (1924); John, Fränkel, *J. Prakt. Chem.* **133,** 259 (1932); improved procedure: Marshall, Blanchard, *J. Pharmacol.* **95,** 186 (1949); Kreysa, **US 2776290** (1957 to Chemo Puro).

Minute, deep yellow prisms from alc, dec 206-207°. Sol in acetic acid, alkalies, hot alc, benzene. Sparingly sol in water, ether. Forms an alkaline, water-sol sodium salt.

THERAP CAT: Antidiuretic; uricosuric.

6958. Oxyclozanide. [2277-92-1] 2,3,5-Trichloro-N-(3,5-dichloro-2-hydroxyphenyl)-6-hydroxybenzamide; 3,3′,5,5′,6-pentachloro-2′-hydroxysalicylanilide; 3,3′,5,5′,6-pentachloro-2,2′-dihy-

droxybenzanilide; Zanil. C$_{13}$H$_6$Cl$_5$NO$_3$; mol wt 401.46. C 38.89%, H 1.51%, Cl 44.16%, N 3.49%, O 11.96%. Prepn: **NL 6409325** corresp to Broome *et al.,* **US 3349090** (1965, 1967, both to I.C.I.).

Crystals, mp 209-211°.

THERAP CAT (VET): Anthelmintic (Trematodes).

6959. Oxycodone. [76-42-6] (5α)-4,5-Epoxy-14-hydroxy-3-methoxy-17-methylmorphinan-6-one; 6-deoxy-7,8-dihydro-14-hydroxy-3-O-methyl-6-oxomorphine; dihydrohydroxycodeinone; 14-hydroxydihydrocodeinone; Dihydrone. C$_{18}$H$_{21}$NO$_4$; mol wt 315.36. C 68.55%, H 6.71%, N 4.44%, O 20.29%. μ-Opioid receptor agonist. Prepn from thebaine: M. Freund, E. Speyer, *J. Prakt. Chem.* **94,** 135 (1916); R. Krassnig *et al., Arch. Pharm.* **329,** 325 (1996); from codeine: A. J. Walker, N. C. Bruce, *Tetrahedron* **60,** 561 (2004). Bibliography: Small, Lutz, "Chemistry of the Opium Alkaloids," Suppl. No. 103 to Public Health Reports, Washington (1932); K. W. Bentley, The Chemistry of the Morphine Alkaloids (Oxford, 1954). *In vitro* liposolubility and protein binding: R. Pöyhiä, T. Seppälä, *Pharmacol. Toxicol.* **74,** 23 (1994). HPLC determn in serum: A. W. E. Wright *et al., J. Chromatogr. B* **712,** 169 (1998). Review of pharmacokinetics and clinical experience: E. Kalso, *J. Pain Symptom Manage.* **29,** S47-S56 (2005); of abuse potential: T. J. Cicero *et al., J. Pain* **6,** 662-672 (2005).

Long rods from alc, mp 218-220°. pKa 8.53. Sol in alcohol, chloroform. Nearly insol in ether, water, KOH, NaOH, NH$_4$OH.

Hydrochloride. [124-90-3] Dinarkon; Eubine; Eukodal; Oxy-Contin; Oxygesic; Oxynorm; Supeudol. C$_{18}$H$_{21}$NO$_4$·HCl; mol wt 351.82. Component of *Percocet* and *Percodan.* Long rods from water, dec 270-272°. [α]$_D^{20}$ −125° (c = 2.5). Partition coefficient (octanol/water): 0.7. One gram dissolves in 6-7 ml water. Slightly sol in alcohol.

Pectinate. [9012-92-4] Proladone. Used for prolonged action.

Note: This is a controlled substance (opiate): **21 CFR,** 1308.12.

THERAP CAT: Analgesic (narcotic).

6960. 4,4′-Oxydi-2-butanol. [821-33-0] 4,4′-Oxybis[2-butanol]; 3,3′-dihydroxydibutyl ether; bis[3-hydroxybutyl] ether; DHBE; Diskin; Dyskinébyl; Dis-Cinil; Colenormol. C$_8$H$_{18}$O$_3$; mol wt 162.23. C 59.23%, H 11.18%, O 29.59%. CH$_3$-CH(OH)CH$_2$CH$_2$OCH$_2$CH$_2$CH(OH)CH$_3$. Prepn: Joulty, **FR 1267084** (1960). Action on bile flow: Bornmann, *Arzneim.-Forsch.* **2,** 122 (1952). Use as choleretic and antispasmodic: Albot, Toulet, *Presse Med.* **67,** 2053 (1959). General pharmacological properties: Fregnan, Porta, *Arzneim.-Forsch.* **26,** 2116 (1976).

Clear, almost colorless, bitter fluid. Miscible with water.

THERAP CAT: Choleretic.

6961. 10,10′-Oxydiphenoxarsine. [58-36-6] 10,10′-Oxy-bis-10H-phenoxarsine; bis(phenoxarsin-10-yl)ether; bis(10-phenoxarsyl)oxide; bis(10-phenoxarsinyl)oxide; OBPA; Vinyzene. C$_{24}$H$_{16}$As$_2$O$_3$; mol wt 502.23. C 57.40%, H 3.21%, As 29.84%, O 9.56%. Prepn: W. L. Lewis *et al., J. Am. Chem. Soc.* **43,** 891 (1921). Synthesis: K. D. Shvetsova-Shilovskaya *et al., J. Gen. Chem. USSR* **31,** 776 (1961). Use in control of plant growth: M. L. Joseph, J. L. Hardy, **US 3069252** (1962 to Dow Chemical); as bactericide in plastics: C. C. Yeager, **US 3288674** (1966 to Scientific Chemicals). Toxicity study: D. G. Clark, *Toxicol. Appl. Pharmacol.* **21**, 315 (1972).

Colorless monoclinic prisms, mp 184-185°. dec. 380°. sp. gr. 1.40-1.42. Sol in alcohol, chloroform, methylene chloride. Practically insol in water (5 ppm at 20°) and alkali. LD$_{50}$ in male rats: 35-50 mg/kg (Ventron, company data sheet).

USE: Primarily for fungicidal and bactericidal protection of plastics.

6962. Oxyfedrine. [15687-41-9] 3-[[(1*S*,2*R*)-2-Hydroxy-1-methyl-2-phenylethyl]amino]-1-(3-methoxyphenyl)-1-propanone; L-3-[(β-hydroxy-α-methylphenethyl)amino]-3'-methoxypropiophenone; L-(1-hydroxy-1-phenyl-2-propylamino)-1-(*m*-methoxyphenyl)-1-propanone; oxyphedrine. C$_{19}$H$_{23}$NO$_3$; mol wt 313.39. C 72.82%, H 7.40%, N 4.47%, O 15.32%. Partial β-adrenergic agonist with coronary vasodilating and positive inotropic effects. Prepn: K. Thiele, **BE 630296**; *idem*, **US 3225095** (1963, 1965 both to Degussa). K. Thiele *et al., Arzneim.-Forsch.* **16**, 1064 (1966). Absolute configuration determined by circular dichroism: J. Engel *et al., Chem. Ztg.* **105**, 85 (1981). TLC determn: Musumarra, *J. Chromatogr.* **350**, 151 (1985). Pharmacology: H. Hueller *et al., Pharmazie* **27**, 242 (1972). Mode of action: P. Mentz, W. Forster, *Arzneim.-Forsch.* **34**, 1739 (1984); N. Sternitzke, *Z. Kardiol.* **73**, 586 (1984). In prevention of experimental myocardial necrosis in rats: S. D. Seth *et al., Arzneim.-Forsch.* **34**, 678 (1984). Comparison with atenolol, *q.v.*, in angina pectoris: L. Fananapazir, C. Bray, *Br. J. Clin. Pharmacol.* **20**, 405 (1985).

L-**Form hydrochloride.** [16777-42-7] D-563; Ildamen; Modacor. C$_{19}$H$_{23}$NO$_3$.HCl; mol wt 349.85. Crystals from methanol, mp 192-194°. LD$_{50}$ in mice (mg/kg): 29 i.v. (Hueller).

DL-**Form hydrochloride.** [16648-69-4] mp 173-175°. LD$_{50}$ in mice (mg/kg): 34 i.v. (Hueller).

THERAP CAT: Antianginal. Treatment of coronary insufficiency.

6963. Oxyfluorfen. [42874-03-3] 2-Chloro-1-(3-ethoxy-4-nitrophenoxy)-4-(trifluoromethyl)benzene; 2-chloro-α,α,α-trifluoro-*p*-tolyl-3-ethoxy-4-nitrophenyl ether; RH-2915; Delta Goal; Goal. C$_{15}$H$_{11}$ClF$_3$NO$_4$; mol wt 361.70. C 49.81%, H 3.07%, Cl 9.80%, F 15.76%, N 3.87%, O 17.69%. Selective pre- and post-emergence herbicide. Prepn: **NL 7303590**; H. O. Bayer *et al., US 3798276* (1973, 1974 both to Rohm & Haas). Activity: R. Y. Yih, C. Swithenbank, *J. Agric. Food Chem.* **23**, 592 (1975). Metabolism: I. L. Adler *et al., ibid.* **25**, 1339 (1977).

Orange crystalline solid, mp 83-84°. Soly in water: 0.1 ppm. Sol in most organic solvents. LD$_{50}$ orally in male albino rats: >5000 mg/kg (Yih, Swithenbank).

USE: Herbicide.

6964. Oxygen. [7782-44-7] O; at. wt 15.9994; at. no. 8; valence 2. Group VIA (16). Occurs normally as the diatomic gas O$_2$, also as ozone O$_3$. Atomic oxygen (O) can be prepd. Three naturally occurring isotopes: 16 (99.759%); 17 (0.037%); 18 (0.204%); artificial radioactive isotopes: 13-15; 19; 20. The most abundant element on earth; makes up 46.6% of earth's crust; 20.95% by vol of dry air. Obtained on a large scale by liquefaction of air. First obtained by Scheele in 1771 and independently by Priestley in 1774. Monograph: M. Ardon, *Oxygen: Elementary Forms and Hydrogen Peroxide* (Benjamin, New York, 1965) 106 pp. Review of oxygen and its compounds: Ebsworth *et al., in Comprehensive Inorganic Chemistry* vol. 2, J. C. Bailar, Jr. *et al.,* Eds. (Pergamon Press, Oxford, 1973) pp 685-794; A. H. Taylor in *Kirk-Othmer Encyclopedia of Chemical Technology* vol. 16 (Wiley-Interscience, New York, 3rd ed., 1981) pp 653-673.

Colorless, odorless, tasteless, neutral gas; supports combustion. d^0 (gas) 1.429 g/l; d^{-183} (liquid) 1.14 g/ml. mp $-218.4°$. bp $-182.96°$. Critical temp $-118.95°$. Critical press. 50.14 atm. Heat of vaporization ($-183°$): 50.9 cal/g. Usually marketed under pressure in metal cylinders. One vol gas dissolves in 32 vols water at 20°; in 7 vols alcohol at 20°; also sol in other organic liquids and usually to a greater extent than in water. *Caution:* Avoid smoking, flames, electric sparks; explosion hazard.

USE: In oxyhydrogen or oxyacetylene flame for welding metals and for lighting (calcium light, etc); submarine work by divers, propellant for rockets. In the production of synthesis gas which can be used in the Fischer-Tropsch process for liquid fuels.

THERAP CAT: Medicinal gas to relieve hypoxia; at hyperbaric pressures in cardiac and other surgery, anaerobic infections, carbon monoxide poisoning; in cryotherapy (liq form).

THERAP CAT (VET): In hypoxia and in conjunction with volatile anesthetics.

6965. Oxymesterone. [145-12-0] (17β)-4,17-Dihydroxy-17-methylandrost-4-en-3-one; 4,17β-dihydroxy-17α-methyl-3-oxoandrost-4-ene; 4-hydroxy-17α-methyltestosterone; 17α-methyl-4-androstene-4,17β-diol-3-one; oxymestrone; Anamidol; Oranabol; Theranabol. C$_{20}$H$_{30}$O$_3$; mol wt 318.45. C 75.43%, H 9.50%, O 15.07%. Prepn: **GB 848288**; Camerino *et al., US 3060201* (1960, 1962 to Farmitalia).

Crystals, mp 169-171°. [α]$_D^{20}$ +69° (ethanol). uv max (ethanol): 278 nm (E$_{1cm}^{1\%}$ 406). Practically insol in water. Sol in chloroform, acetone, alcohol.

Note: This is a controlled substance (anabolic steroid): **21 CFR**, 1308.13, as defined in 1300.01.

THERAP CAT: Androgen; anabolic.

6966. Oxymetazoline. [1491-59-4] 3-[(4,5-Dihydro-1*H*-imidazol-2-yl)methyl]-6-(1,1-dimethylethyl)-2,4-dimethylphenol; 6-*tert*-butyl-3-(2-imidazolin-2-ylmethyl)-2,4-dimethylphenol; 2-(4-*tert*-butyl-2,6-dimethyl-3-hydroxybenzyl)-2-imidazoline; H-990; Navisin; Hazol; Rhinofrenol; Rhinolitan; Sinerol; Nezeril. C$_{16}$H$_{24}$N$_2$O; mol wt 260.37. C 73.81%, H 9.29%, N 10.76%, O 6.14%. Prepd from (4-*tert*-butyl-2,6-dimethyl-3-hydroxyphenyl)acetonitrile and ethylenediamine: Fruhstorfer, Mueller-Calgan, **DE 1117588** (1961 to E. Merck), *C.A.* **57**, 4674a (1962). Toxicity data: Hotovy *et al., Arzneim.-Forsch.* **11**, 1016 (1961).

Crystals from benzene, mp 181-183°.

Hydrochloride. [2315-02-8] Afrazine; Afrin; Iliadin; Nafrine; Nasivin; Oxilin; Sinex. $C_{16}H_{24}N_2O.HCl$; mol wt 296.84. Crystals, dec 300-303°. Freely sol in water, alcohol. Practically insol in ether, chloroform, benzene. LD_{50} orally in mice: 10 mg/kg (Hotovy).

Note: Ingredient of *Drixin*.

THERAP CAT: Adrenergic (vasoconstrictor); nasal decongestant.

6967. Oxymetholone. [434-07-1] $(5\alpha,17\beta)$-17-Hydroxy-2-(hydroxymethylene)-17-methylandrostan-3-one; 2-hydroxymethylene-17α-methyldihydrotestosterone; 4,5α-dihydro-2-hydroxymethylene-17α-methyltestosterone; 2-hydroxymethylene-17α-methyl-17β-hydroxy-5α-androstan-3-one; 2-hydroxymethylene-17α-methylandrostan-17β-ol-3-one; anasterone; Adroyd; Anapolon; Anadrol; Pardroyd; Plenastril; Protanabol; Nastenon; Synasteron. $C_{21}H_{32}$-O_3; mol wt 332.48. C 75.86%, H 9.70%, O 14.44%. Anabolic steroid. Prepn: Ringold *et al.*, *J. Am. Chem. Soc.* **81,** 427 (1959); Ringold, Rosenkranz, **DE 1070632** (1959 to Syntex).

Crystals from ethyl acetate, mp 178-180°. $[\alpha]_D$ +38°. uv max: 285 nm (log ε 3.99).

Enol acetate. $C_{23}H_{34}O_4$. Crystals from hexane, mp 144-148°. $[\alpha]_D$ +27° (ethanol). uv max: 255 nm (log ε 4.09).

Enol propionate. $C_{24}H_{36}O_4$. Crystals from hexane, mp 135°. $[\alpha]_D$ +26° (ethanol). uv max: 257 nm (log ε 4.11).

Enol benzoate. $C_{28}H_{36}O_4$. Crystals from acetone + water, mp 188-190°. uv max: 230 nm (log ε 4.19).

Caution: Oxymetholone is reasonably anticipated to be a human carcinogen: *Report on Carcinogens, Eleventh Edition* (PB2005-104914, 2004) p III-211. This is a controlled substance (anabolic steroid): **21 CFR,** 1308.13, as defined in 1300.01.

THERAP CAT: Androgen.

THERAP CAT (VET): Anabolic steroid for small animals.

6968. Oxymethurea. [140-95-4] N,N'-Bis(hydroxymethyl)urea; N,N'-dihydroxymethylurea; Methural. $C_3H_8N_2O_3$; mol wt 120.11. C 30.00%, H 6.71%, N 23.32%, O 39.96%. $(HOCH_2$-$NH)_2CO$. Prepn: Einhorn, Hamburger, *Ber.* **41,** 26 (1908); Walter, **US 1863426** (1927); **US 2436355** (1946 to du Pont).

Crystals from alcohol, mp 137-139°. Very sol in cold water, hot ethyl alcohol, methanol.

USE: In the textile industry in cotton crease- and shrink-proofing, finishing, drying, sizing; in tanning; pesticides; in photographic developers.

THERAP CAT: Antiseptic.

6969. Oxymorphone. [76-41-5] (5α)-4,5-Epoxy-3,14-dihydroxy-17-methylmorphinan-6-one; dihydrohydroxymorphinone; dihydro-14-hydroxymorphinone; 14-hydroxydihydromorphinone. $C_{17}H_{19}NO_4$; mol wt 301.34. C 67.76%, H 6.36%, N 4.65%, O 21.24%. Obtained from dihydrohydroxycodeinone by boiling with concd aq hydrobromic acid: Weiss, *J. Am. Chem. Soc.* **77,** 5891 (1955); Lewenstein, Weiss, **US 2806033** (1957).

Crystals from boiling ethanol, ethyl acetate or benzene. mp 248-249° (dec). Levorotatory. Sol in boiling acetone and chloroform;

readily sol in aq alkalies; moderately sol in boiling ethanol; sparingly sol in benzene.

Hydrochloride. [357-07-3] Numorphan. $C_{17}H_{19}NO_4.HCl$; mol wt 337.80. Crystals.

Note: This is a controlled substance (opiate): **21 CFR,** 1308.12.

THERAP CAT: Analgesic (narcotic).

THERAP CAT (VET): Analgesic (narcotic).

6970. Oxypendyl. [5585-93-3] 4-[3-(10H-Pyrido[3,2-b]-[1,4]benzothiazin-10-yl)propyl]-1-piperazineethanol; 10-[3-[4-(2-hydroxyethyl)-1-piperazinyl]propyl]-10H-pyrido[3,2-b][1,4]benzothiazine; 10-[3-(1-hydroxyethyl-4-piperazinyl)propyl]-4-azaphenothiazine; oxipendyl; D-706. $C_{20}H_{26}N_4OS$; mol wt 370.51. C 64.83%, H 7.07%, N 15.12%, O 4.32%, S 8.65%. Prepn: Schuler, Klebe, *Ann.* **653,** 172 (1962).

bp$_1$ 260-265°, bp$_6$ 280-300°.

Dihydrochloride. [17297-82-4] Pervetral. $C_{20}H_{26}N_4OS$.-2HCl; mol wt 443.43. Crystals, mp 218-220°.

THERAP CAT: Antiemetic.

6971. Oxypertine. [153-87-7] 5,6-Dimethoxy-2-methyl-3-[2-(4-phenyl-1-piperazinyl)ethyl]-1H-indole; 1-[2-(5,6-dimethoxy-2-methyl-3-indolyl)ethyl]-4-phenylpiperazine; Win-18501-2; Equipertine; Forit; Integrin (formerly). $C_{23}H_{29}N_3O_2$; mol wt 379.50. C 72.79%, H 7.70%, N 11.07%, O 8.43%. Prepn: Archer *et al.*, *J. Am. Chem. Soc.* **84,** 1306 (1962).

THERAP CAT: Antidepressant.

6972. Oxyphenbutazone. [129-20-4] 4-Butyl-1-(4-hydroxyphenyl)-2-phenyl-3,5-pyrazolidinedione; 4-butyl-2-(*p*-hydroxyphenyl)-1-phenyl-3,5-pyrazolidinedione; 1-phenyl-2-(*p*-hydroxyphenyl)-3,5-dioxo-4-*n*-butylpyrazolidine; 1-(*p*-hydroxyphenyl)-2-phenyl-4-butylpyrazolidine-3,5-dione; *p*-hydroxyphenyl-butazone; G-27202; Califonit; Crovaril; Flogitolo; Flogoril; Frabel; Neo-Farmadol; Oxalid; Rapostan; Tandearil; Visubutina. $C_{19}H_{20}$-N_2O_3; mol wt 324.37. C 70.35%, H 6.21%, N 8.64%, O 14.80%. Prepn: Hafliger, **US 2745783** (1956 to Geigy); Pfister, Hafliger, *Helv. Chim. Acta* **40,** 395 (1957).

Monohydrate. [7081-38-1] Imbun; Phlogistol; Phlogase; Phlogont. Crystals, mp 96°. Anhyd crystals from ether + petr ether, mp 124-125°. Acidic reaction. Soluble in ethanol, methanol, chloroform, benzene, ether. Forms a water-soluble sodium salt.

THERAP CAT: Anti-inflammatory.

6973. Oxyphencyclimine. [125-53-1] α-Cyclohexyl-α-hydroxybenzeneacetic acid (1,4,5,6-tetrahydro-1-methyl-2-pyrimidinyl)methyl ester; 1,4,5,6-tetrahydro-1-methyl-2-pyrimidinylmethyl α-phenylcyclohexaneglycolate; α-phenylcyclohexaneglycolic acid 1-methyl-2-tetrahydroxypyrimidylmethyl ester; 1-methyl-1,4,5,6-tetrahydro-2-pyrimidylmethyl α-cyclohexyl-α-phenylglycolate; Antulcus; Caridan; Daricol; Setrol; Vio-Thene; Daricon; Naridan; Zamanil. $C_{20}H_{28}N_2O_3$; mol wt 344.45. C 69.74%, H 8.19%, N 8.13%, O 13.93%. Anticholinergic. Prepn: **GB 795758** (1958 to Pfizer); Faust *et al., J. Am. Chem. Soc.* **81**, 2214 (1959).

Hydrochloride. [125-52-0] $C_{20}H_{28}N_2O_3$·HCl. Crystals, dec 231-232°. Solubility in water: 1.2 g/100 ml.
THERAP CAT: Antispasmodic.

6974. Oxyphenisatin Acetate. [115-33-3] 3,3-Bis[4-(acetyloxy)phenyl]-1,3-dihydro-2*H*-indol-2-one; 3,3-bis(*p*-acetoxyphenyl)oxindole; acetphenolisatin; endophenolphthalein; diacetyldiphenolisatin; diacetyldihydroxydiphenylisatin; diacetylhydroxyphenylisatin; diacetoxydiphenylisatin; di(acetoxyphenyl)oxindole; diphesatin; diacetyldioxyphenylisatin; Isacen; Isocrin; Isaphen; Laxo-Isatin; Promassolax; Sanapert; Bydolax; Cirotyl; Lisagal; Contax; Prulet; Purgaceen; Bisatin. $C_{24}H_{19}NO_5$; mol wt 401.41. C 71.81%, H 4.77%, N 3.49%, O 19.93%. Prepd from isatin by treatment with phenol followed by acetylation in the presence of H_2SO_4 at temps below 100°: Baeyer, Lazarus, *Ber.* **18**, 2641 (1885); Hoffmann-La Roche, **CH 100806**; **DE 406210** (1923); **US 1624675** (1927); **DE 482435** (1929); Mizuno, Turuga, **JP 129200** (1939).

Tasteless crystals, mp 242°. Practically insol in water, ether, dilute HCl. Slightly sol in alcohol.
THERAP CAT: Cathartic.

6975. Oxyphenonium Bromide. [50-10-2] 2-[(Cyclohexylhydroxyphenylacetyl)oxy]-*N,N*-diethyl-*N*-methylethanaminium bromide; diethyl(2-hydroxyethyl)methylammonium α-phenylcyclohexaneglycolate bromide; α-phenylcyclohexaneglycolic acid ester diethyl(2-hydroxyethyl)methylammonium bromide; diethylaminoethyl α-phenylcyclohexaneglycolate methylbromide; 2-diethylaminoethyl α-cyclohexyl-α-phenylglycolate methobromide; cyclohexylhydroxyphenylacetic acid diethylmethylaminoethyl ester bromide; phenylcyclohexyloxyacetic acid diethylaminoethyl ester bromomethylate; Ba-5473; C-5473; Antrenyl; Spasmophen. $C_{21}H_{34}BrNO_3$; mol wt 428.40. C 58.88%, H 8.00%, Br 18.65%, N 3.27%, O 11.20%. Anticholinergic. Prepn: **CH 259948** (1949 to Ciba).

Crystals, mp 189-194° from ethyl acetate + alc. Freely sol in water. Sparingly sol in alc. Aq solns are neutral.
THERAP CAT: Antispasmodic.

6976. Oxytetracycline. [79-57-2] [4S-(4α,4aα,5α,5aα,6β,-12aα)]-4-(Dimethylamino)-1,4,4a,5,5a,6,11,12a-octahydro-3,5,6,-10,12,12a-hexahydroxy-6-methyl-1,11-dioxo-2-naphthacenecarboxamide; glomycin; riomitsin; hydroxytetracycline. $C_{22}H_{24}N_2O_9$; mol wt 460.43. C 57.39%, H 5.25%, N 6.08%, O 31.27%. Antibiotic substance isolated from the elaboration products of the actinomycete, *Streptomyces rimosus,* grown on a suitable medium: Finlay *et al., Science* **111**, 85 (1950). Isoln: Regna, Solomons, *Ann. N.Y. Acad. Sci.* **53**, 221 (1950); Regna *et al., J. Am. Chem. Soc.* **73**, 4211 (1951). Production from *Streptomyces rimosus:* Sobin *et al.,* **US 2516080** (1950 to Pfizer). Isoln from *S. xanthophaeus:* Brockmann, Musso, *Naturwissenschaften* **41**, 451 (1954); Brockmann *et al.,* **DE 913687** (1954 to Bayer), *C.A.* **53**, 4662h (1959). Solubility data: Weiss *et al., Antibiot. Chemother.* **7**, 374 (1957). Structure: Hochstein *et al., J. Am. Chem. Soc.* **74**, 3708 (1952). Abs config: Dobrynin *et al., Tetrahedron Lett.* **1962**, 901. Stereochemistry: Schach von Wittenau *et al., J. Am. Chem. Soc.* **87**, 134 (1965). Total synthesis of the *dl*-form: H. Muxfeldt *et al., ibid.* **101**, 689 (1979).

Stability: Oxytetracycline crystals show no loss in potency on heating for 4 days at 100°, the hydrochloride crystals show <5% inactivation after 4 mos at 56°. Aq solns of the hydrochloride at pH 1.0 to 2.5 are stable for at least 30 days at 25°. Solns at pH 3.0 to 9.0 show no detectable loss in potency on storage at 5° for at least 30 days. Half-life in hours of aq oxytetracycline solns at 37°: pH 1.0 = 114; pH 2.5 = 134; pH 4.6 = 45; pH 5.5 = 45; pH 7.0 = 26; pH 8.5 = 33; pH 10.0 = 14.

Dihydrate. Alamycin; Imperacin; Liquamycin; Terralon; Terramycin; Tetradure. Needles from water or methanol, dec 181-182°. $[\alpha]_D^{25}$ −196.6° (0.1*N* HCl); $[\alpha]_D^{25}$ −2.1° (0.1*N* NaOH); $[\alpha]_D^{25}$ +26.5° (methanol). uv max (pH 4.5 phosphate buffer 0.1*M*): 249, 276, 353 nm ($E_{1cm}^{1\%}$ 240, 322, 301). Soly in water at 23°: pH 1.2 = 31,400 μg/ml, pH 2.0 = 4600 μg/ml; pH 3.0 = 1400 μg/ml; pH 5.0 = 500 μg/ml, pH 6.0 = 700 μg/ml, pH 7.0 = 1100 μg/ml, pH 9.0 = 38,600 μg/ml. Soly in abs ethanol 12,000 μg/ml, in 95% ethanol 200 μg/ml.

Hydrochloride. [2058-46-0] Berkmycin; Duphacycline; Engemycin; Geomycin; Oxy-Mycin; Oxytetrin; Posicycline; Tetra-Tablinen; Toxinal. Yellow platelets from water. Very soluble in water (1 g/ml). Concd aq solns at neutral pH hydrolyze on standing and deposit crystals of oxytetracycline. Soly in abs ethanol: 12,000 μg/ml, in 95% ethanol: 33,000 μg/ml.

Disodium salt dihydrate. $C_{22}H_{22}N_2Na_2O_9$·2H_2O. Yellow crystals; darkens on standing. Soly in abs alc: 8,000 μg/ml, in methanol: 1500 μg/ml.

USE: To treat lethal yellowing in palm trees.
THERAP CAT: Antibacterial.
THERAP CAT (VET): Antibacterial.

6977. Oxythiamine. [582-36-5] 3-[(1,4-Dihydro-2-methyl-4-oxo-5-pyrimidinyl)methyl]-5-(2-hydroxyethyl)-4-methylthiazolium chloride; 5-(2-hydroxyethyl)-3-[(4-hydroxy-2-methyl-5-pyrimidinyl)methyl]-4-methylthiazolium chloride. $C_{12}H_{16}ClN_3O_2S$; mol wt 301.79. C 47.76%, H 5.34%, Cl 11.75%, N 13.92%, O 10.60%, S 10.62%. Prepn: F. Bergel, A. R. Todd, *J. Chem. Soc.* **1937**, 1504; M. Soodak, L. R. Cerecedo, *J. Am. Chem. Soc.* **66**, 1988 (1944). Improved prepn: H. N. Rydon, *Biochem. J.* **48**, 383 (1951). Thiamine antagonist activity: A. J. Eusebi, L. R. Cerecedo, *Science* **110**, 162 (1949); L. J. Daniel, L. C. Norris, *Proc. Soc. Exp. Biol. Med.* **72**, 165 (1949); and distribution in tissues: C. J. Gubler, D. S. Murdock, *J. Nutr. Sci. Vitaminol.* **28**, 217 (1982).

Proposed mechanism of action: S. A. Strumilo *et al., Biomed. Biochim. Acta* **43**, 159 (1984). Determn by HPLC: B. C. Hemming, C. J. Gubler, *J. Liq. Chromatogr.* **3**, 1697 (1980).

Hydrochloride. $C_{12}H_{16}ClN_3O_2S$.HCl. Flat needles grouped in rosettes, dec 195°. uv max (acid soln): 265, 258, 228, 223 nm; (alkaline soln): 268, 260, 228, 221 nm. Does not give the thiochrome reaction.

Diphosphate. Crystals, mp 127-129°.

Monophosphoric acid ester. Hygroscopic crystals, dec 185-186°.

Triphosphoric acid ester. Minute crystals, dec 245-255°.

6978. Oxythioquinox. [2439-01-2] 6-Methyl-1,3-dithiolo-[4,5-*b*]quinoxalin-2-one; dithiocarbonic acid cyclic *S,S*-(6-methyl-2,3-quinoxalinediyl) ester; 6-methyl-2,3-quinoxalinedithiol cyclic *S,S*-dithiocarbonate; 6-methyl-2-oxo-1,3-dithio[4,5-*b*]quinoxaline; chinomethionat(e); quinomethionate; Bayer 36205; Forstan; Morestan. $C_{10}H_6N_2OS_2$; mol wt 234.30. C 51.26%, H 2.58%, N 11.96%, O 6.83%, S 27.37%. Prepn and review of chemical and fungicidal properties and toxicology: F. Grewe, H. Kaspers, *Pflanzenschutz-Nachr. Bayer (Engl. Ed.)* **18** (1), 1-23 (1965). Toxicity study: T. B. Gaines, *Toxicol. Appl. Pharmacol.* **14**, 515 (1969).

Yellow crystals from benzene, mp 172°. Practically insol in water. Freely sol in DMF. Sol in hot benzene, toluene, dioxane. Slightly sol in methanol, ethanol, acetone. LD_{50} in male, female rats (mg/kg): 1800, 1100 orally (Gaines).

USE: Acaricide; agricultural fungicide.

6979. Oxytocin. [50-56-6] Alpha-hypophamine; ocytocin; Intertocine-S; Perlacton; Pitocin; Syntocinon; Orasthin; Partocon; Synpitan; Uteracon. $C_{43}H_{66}N_{12}O_{12}S_2$; mol wt 1007.19. C 51.28%, H 6.60%, N 16.69%, O 19.06%, S 6.37%. The principal uterus-contracting and lactation-stimulating hormone of the posterior pituitary gland. Isoln: Pierce *et al., J. Biol. Chem.* **199**, 929 (1952). Structure and synthesis: Tuppy, Michl, *Monatsh. Chem.* **84**, 1011 (1953); Tuppy, *Biochim. Biophys. Acta* **11**, 449 (1953); du Vigneaud *et al., J. Am. Chem. Soc.* **75**, 4879 (1953); **76**, 3115 (1954); Bodanszky, du Vigneaud, *ibid.* **81**, 2504 (1959); Cash *et al., J. Med. Pharm. Chem.* **5**, 413 (1962); Sakakibara *et al., Bull. Chem. Soc. Jpn.* **38**, 120 (1965). Solid phase synthesis: Bayer, Hagenmaier, *Tetrahedron Lett.* **1968**, 2037; Ives, *Can. J. Chem.* **46**, 2318 (1968). Synthesis of D-oxytocin: Flouret, du Vigneaud, *J. Am. Chem. Soc.* **87**, 3775 (1965). Description of commercial process: Velluz *et al., US 2938891* and *US 3076797* (1960, 1963, both to Roussel-UCLAF). Radioimmunoassay: T. Chard, *Clin. Biochem. Anal.* **5**, 209 (1977). *Review:* du Vigneaud, *Experientia Suppl.* **II** (14th Intl. Congr. Pure and Appl. Chem.), 9-26 (1955); R. Caldeyro-Barcia, H. Heller, *Proc. Intl. Symp. on Oxytocin* (Montevideo 1959) 443 pp; several authors, *Adv. Exp. Med. Biol.* **2**, 53-104 (1968); C. R. W. Edwards in *Hormones in Blood* vol. 2, C. H. Gray, V. James, Ed. (Academic Press, New York, 3rd ed., 1979) pp 401-421. Review of role in parturition: A.-R. Fuchs, F. Fuchs, *Adv. Exp. Med.* **1980**, 403-428. Comprehensive description: F. Nachtmann *et al., Anal. Profiles Drug Subs.* **10**, 563-600 (1981). Book: *Oxytocin: Cellular and Molecular Approaches in Medicine and Research*, R. Ivell, J. A. Russell, Eds. (Plenum Press, New York, 1995) 673 pp.

Cys-Tyr-Ile-Gln-Asn-Cys-Pro-Leu-GlyNH$_2$

White powder. $[\alpha]_D^{22}$ $-26.2°$ (c = 0.53). Sol in water, 1-butanol, 2-butanol.

THERAP CAT: Oxytocic.

THERAP CAT (VET): Stimulates milk let-down, uterine contraction.

6980. Ozagrel. [82571-53-7] (2*E*)-3-[4-(1*H*-Imidazol-1-yl-methyl)phenyl]-2-propenoic acid; *(E)*-4-(imidazol-1-ylmethyl)cinnamic acid; OKY-046. $C_{13}H_{12}N_2O_2$; mol wt 228.25. C 68.41%, H 5.30%, N 12.27%, O 14.02%. Prepn: K. Iizuka *et al.,* **DE 2923815**; *eidem,* **US 4226878** (both 1980 to Ono; Kissei). Synthesis and thromboxane synthetase inhibitory activity: K. Iizuka *et al., J. Med. Chem.* **24**, 1139 (1981). Pharmacology: S. Hiraku *et al., Jpn. J. Pharmacol.* **41**, 393 (1986). Pulmonary vascular effects: R. Garcia-Szabo *et al., Prostaglandins* **28**, 851 (1984). Metabolism in animals: M. Shimizu *et al., Iyakuhin Kenkyu* **17**, 289 (1986), *C.A.* **105**, 72012q (1986). HPLC determn in biological fluids: *eidem, ibid.* 298, *C.A.* **105**, 72013r (1986). Clinical pharmacology and evaluation in myocardial infarction: T. Ito *et al., Biomed. Biochim. Acta* **43**, S125 (1984). Clinical evaluation in prevention of cerebral vasospasm: S. Suzuki *et al., Acta Neurochir.* **77**, 133 (1985); in coronary artery disease: M. Shikano *et al., Jpn. Heart J.* **28**, 663 (1987). Toxicity data: T. Nishigake *et al., Clin. Rep.* **20**, 2671 (1986). Series of articles on pharmacology: *Pharmacometrics* **31**, 527-565 (1986), *C.A.* **105**, 35349-35352 (1986).

Prisms from ethanol-ether, mp 223-224°.

Hydrochloride. [78712-43-3] $C_{13}H_{12}N_2O_2$.HCl. Crystals from ethanol-ether, mp 214-217°.

Sodium salt. Cataclot; Xanbon. $C_{13}H_{11}N_2NaO_2$; mol wt 250.23. LD_{50} in male, female mice, male, female rats (mg/kg): 1940, 1580, 1150, 1300 i.v.; 3800, 3600, 5900, 5700 orally; 2450, 2100, 2300, 2250 s.c. (Nishigake).

THERAP CAT: Antithrombotic; antianginal.

6981. Ozone. [10028-15-6] Triatomic oxygen. O_3; mol wt 48.00. Found in the atm in varying proportions (about 0.05 ppm at sea level), since it is produced continuously in the outer layers of the atm by the action of solar uv radiation on the oxygen of the air. So-called sterilizing lamps operate on the same principle. In the laboratory ozone is prepd by passing dry air between two plate electrodes connected to an alternating current source of several thousand volts. The reaction is reversible, and after a little ozone has been produced it is dec at the same rate as it is generated. Obtained in pure form by cooling ozonized air to $-180°$ when it separates as a dark blue liquid. *See also* C. E. Thorp, *Bibliography of Ozone Technology* (Armour Res. Found., Chicago). Lab prepn: *Org. Synth.* **coll. vol. III**, 673 (1955). Conference proceedings: *Adv. Chem. Ser.* **21**, entitled "Ozone Chemistry and Technology," H. A. Leedy, Ed. (ACS, Washington D.C., 1959) 465 pp. *Review:* C. Nebel in *Kirk-Othmer Encyclopedia of Chemical Technology* vol. **16** (Wiley-Interscience, New York, 3rd ed., 1981) pp 683-713.

Bluish, explosive gas or blue liquid. Pleasant, characteristic odor in concns of less than 2 ppm. Irritating and injurious in higher concns. Powerful oxidizing agent. d^0 (gas): 2.144 g/l; $d^{-195.4}$ (liq) 1.614 g/ml. mp $-193°$. bp $-111.9°$. Critical temp $-12.1°$. Critical press. 53.8 atm. Heat of formation 34.4 kcal/mole at 25°. Intense absorption band beginning at about 290 nm. Unstable. Solutions contg ozone explode on warming. Prepn of ozone solns in liq oxygen: Cook, **US 3008902** (1961 to Union Carbide). Although the stability of ozone in aq solns decreases as alkalinity rises, this effect is reversed at high concns. For example, the half life of ozone is 2 min in 1*N* NaOH; it is increased to 83 hrs in 20*N* NaOH: Heidt, Landi, *J. Chem. Phys.* **41**, 176 (1964).

Caution: Potential symptoms of overexposure are irritation of eyes and mucous membranes; pulmonary edema; chronic respiratory disease. *See NIOSH Pocket Guide to Chemical Hazards* (DHHS/NIOSH 97-140, 1997) p 238.

USE: As disinfectant for air and water by virtue of its oxidizing power. For bleaching waxes, textiles, oils. In organic syntheses. Forms ozonides which are sometimes useful oxidizing compds.

P

Controlled Rel. **109**, 120-126 (2005); M. Man, H. Rugo, *IDrugs* **8**, 739-754 (2005).

6982. Paclitaxel. [33069-62-4] ($\alpha R,\beta S$)-β-(Benzoylamino)-α-hydroxybenzenepropanoic acid (2aR,4S,4aS,6R,9S,11S,12S,-12aR,12bS)-6,12b-bis(acetyloxy)-12-(benzoyloxy)-2a,3,4,4a,5,6,9,-10,11,12,12a,12b-dodecahydro-4,11-dihydroxy-4a,8,13,13-tetramethyl-5-oxo-7,11-methano-1H-cyclodeca[3,4]benz[1,2-b]oxet-9-yl ester; 5β,20-epoxy-1,2α,4,7β,10β,13α-hexahydroxytax-11-en-9-one 4,10-diacetate 2-benzoate 13-ester with (2R,3S)-N-benzoyl-3-phenylisoserine; taxol A; NSC-125973; Anzatax; Paxene; Taxol. $C_{47}H_{51}NO_{14}$; mol wt 853.91. C 66.11%, H 6.02%, N 1.64%, O 26.23%. Antiproliferative agent first isolated, as the l-form, from the bark of the Pacific yew tree, *Taxus brevifolia, Taxaceae;* promotes the assembly of microtubules and inhibits the tubulin disassembly process. Isoln and structure: M. C. Wani *et al., J. Am. Chem. Soc.* **93**, 2325 (1971). *In vitro* promotion of microtubule assembly: P. B. Schiff *et al., Nature* **277**, 665 (1979). Isoln from *Taxus baccala* L. and *in vitro* inhibition of depolymerization of microtubules into tubulin: G. Chauviere *et al., C.R. Seances Acad. Sci. Ser. 2* **293**, 501 (1981). Total synthesis of *taxusin*, which contains the entire ring skeleton: R. A. Holton *et al., J. Am. Chem. Soc.* **110**, 6558 (1988). Total stereosynthesis: R. A. Holton *et al., ibid.* **116**, 1597, 1599 (1994); K. C. Nicolaou *et al., Nature* **367**, 630 (1994). Production by *Taxomyces andreanae*, an endophytic fungus associated with *T. brevifolia*: A. Stierle *et al., Science* **260**, 214 (1993). Review of mechanism of action: J. J. Manfredi, S. B. Horwitz, *Pharmacol. Ther.* **25**, 83-125 (1984); S. B. Horwitz *et al., Ann. N.Y. Acad. Sci.* **466**, 733-744 (1986); S. B. Horwitz, *Trends Pharmacol. Sci.* **13**, 134-136 (1992). Symposium on clinical toxicology, pharmacology and efficacy: *Semin. Oncol.* **20**, Suppl. 3, 1-60 (1993). Review of clinical experience in cancer therapy: T. M. Mekhail, M. Markman, *Expert. Opin. Pharmacother.* **3**, 755-766 (2002). Clinical trial in prevention of coronary artery restenosis: G. W. Stone *et al., N. Engl. J. Med.* **350**, 221 (2004).

Needles from aq methanol, mp 213-216° (dec). $[\alpha]_D^{20}$ −49° (methanol). uv max (methanol): 227, 273 nm (ε 29800, 1700).

USE: Tool in study of structure and function of microtubules.

THERAP CAT: Antineoplastic; antirestenotic.

6983. Paclitaxel Poliglumex. [263351-82-2] (1R,2S)-2-(Benzoylamino)-1-[[[(2aR,4S,4aS,6R,9S,11S,12S,12aR,12bS)-6,12b-bis(acetyloxy)-12-(benzoyloxy)-2a,3,4,4a,5,6,9,10,11,12,-12a,12b-dodecahydro-4,11-dihydroxy-4a,8,13,13-tetramethyl-5-oxo-7,11-methano-1H-cyclodeca[3,4]benz[1,2-b]oxet-9-yl]oxy]-carbonyl]-2-phenylethyl ester L-glutamic acid homopolymer; L-polyglutamic paclitaxel; PG-TXL; CT-2103; Xyotax. Biodegradable polymer drug conjugate resulting from the random condensation of L-polyglutamic acid and paclitaxel, *q.v.*, which has on average 10.4 monomeric glutamic acid units per paclitaxel-glutamate conjugate unit. Mol wt 48 kDa. Prepn: C. Li *et al., Cancer Res.* **58**, 2404 (1998). *See also: eidem,* US **5977163** (1999 to PG-TXL Co.). *In vitro* activities in comparison with paclitaxel: A. S. Multani *et al., Anticancer Res.* **17**, 4269 (1997); E. A. Oldham *et al., Int. J. Oncol.* **16**, 125 (2000). Irradiation enhanced tumor specificity: C. Li *et al., Clin. Cancer Res.* **6**, 2829 (2000); L. Milas *et al., Int. J. Radiat. Oncol. Biol. Phys.* **55**, 707 (2003). Review of properties and preclinical characterization: J. W. Singer *et al., Adv. Exp. Med. Biol.* **519**, 81-99 (2003); of clinical development: J. W. Singer, *J.*

White to off-white powder. Insol in ether; practically insol in 0.1M HCl and acetonitrile. Sol in 0.1M NaOH, 0.1M Na_2HPO_4 (pH 6.5); slightly sol in methanol, DMSO, dimethylformamide.

THERAP CAT: Antineoplastic.

6984. Paclobutrazol. [76738-62-0] ($\alpha R,\beta R$)-*rel*-β-[(4-Chlorophenyl)methyl]-α-(1,1-dimethylethyl)-1H-1,2,4-triazole-1-ethanol; 1-*tert*-butyl-2-(p-chlorobenzyl)-2-(1,2,4-triazol-1-yl)ethanol; (2RS,3RS)-1-(4-chlorophenyl)-4,4-dimethyl-2-(1H-1,2,4-triazol-1-yl)pentan-3-ol; ICI-PP-333; PP-333; Bonzi; Cultar; Parlay; Trimmit. $C_{15}H_{20}ClN_3O$; mol wt 293.79. C 61.32%, H 6.86%, Cl 12.07%, N 14.30%, O 5.45%. Plant growth regulator with fungicidal activity. Prepn: B. C. Baldwin *et al.,* DE **2734426**; S. Balasubramanyan, M. C. Shephard, US **4243405** (1978, 1981 both to ICI). Physical properties and biological activity: B. G. Lever *et al., Proc. Br. Crop Prot. Conf. - Weeds* **1982**, 3. Resolution and activity of isomers: B. Sugavanam, *Pestic. Sci.* **15**, 296 (1984). GC determn in plant tissue: E. A. Stahly, D. A. Buchanan, *HortScience* **21**, 534 (1986). Comparison with daminozide, *q.v.*, of effect on apple trees: G. R. Stinchcombe *et al., J. Hortic. Sci.* **59**, 323 (1984).

White crystalline solid, mp 165-166°. d 1.22. Vapor pressure at 20°: 1×10^{-6} Pa. Soly: water 35 mg/l, methanol 15%, propylene glycol 5%, acetone 11%, cyclohexanone 18%, methylene dichloride 10%, hexane 1%, xylene 6%.

USE: Plant growth regulator.

6985. Pactamycin. [23668-11-3] 2-Hydroxy-6-methylbenzoic acid [(1S,2R,3R,4S,5S)-5-[(3-acetylphenyl)amino]-4-amino-3-[[(dimethylamino)carbonyl]amino]-1,2-dihydroxy-3-[(1S)-1-hydroxyethyl]-2-methylcyclopentyl]methyl ester; NSC-52947; U-15800. $C_{28}H_{38}N_4O_8$; mol wt 558.62. C 60.20%, H 6.86%, N 10.03%, O 22.91%. Antitumor antibiotic produced by *Streptomyces pactum* var *pactum*. Discovery and biological properties: Bhuyan *et al., Antimicrob. Agents Chemother.* **1961**, 184. Isoln and characterization: Argoudelis *et al., ibid.* 191. Manuf: GB **980346** (1965 to Upjohn), *C.A.* **62**, 11115f (1965). Structure: Wiley *et al., J. Org. Chem.* **35**, 1420 (1970). Revised structure: D. J. Duchamp, *Am. Crystallogr. Assn.* (Winter Mtg., Albuquerque, 1972) p 23. Mechanism of action: T. A. Beerman *et al., Adv. Enzyme Regul.* **14**, 207 (1976). ^{13}C-NMR study: D. D. Weller *et al., J. Antibiot.* **30**, 997 (1978). Biosynthesis: D. D. Weller, K. L. Rinehart, *J. Am.*

Chem. Soc. **100,** 6757 (1978). *Review:* Goldberg in *Antibiotics* **vol. 3,** J. W. Corcoran, F. E. Hahn, Eds. (Springer-Verlag, New York, 1975) pp 498-515.

$[\alpha]_D^{25}$ +79° (ethanol) changing to +23° on standing. $[\alpha]$ changes in acetone on standing from +25° to +76° in 24 hours. Amphoteric. Sol in ethanol, chloroform, methylene chloride, benzene, ether, in solns <pH 5 and >9.5. Insol in Skellysolve B, cyclohexane; insol at isoelectric pt, pH 8.3. Unstable in solution. LD_{50} in mice (mg/kg): 10.7 orally; 15.6 i.v.; in rats (mg/kg): 1.4 i.v. (Bhuyan).

6986. Palifermin. [162394-19-6] 24-163-Keratinocyte growth factor (human); 24-163-fibroblast growth factor 7 (human); rHuKGF; Kepivance. Recombinant epithelial tissue growth factor of 141 amino acid residues; N-terminal truncated form of endogenous KGF. Mol wt approx 16.3 kDa. Prepn: D. J. Gospodarowicz, F. R. Masiarz, **WO 9501434;** *idem,* **US 5677278** (1995, 1997 both to Chiron). *In vivo* radioprotective effect: C. L. Farrell *et al., Cancer Res.* **58,** 933 (1998). Clinical study in mucositis associated with myelosuppressive therapy: R. Spielberger *et al., N. Engl. J. Med.* **351,** 2590 (2004). Review of therapeutic potential in oral mucositis: M. A. A. Siddiqui, K. Wellington, *Drugs* **65,** 2139-2146 (2005); M. L. Radtke, J. M. Kolesar, *J. Oncol. Pharm. Pract.* **11,** 121-125 (2005).

THERAP CAT: Radioprotective agent.

6987. Palitantin. [15265-28-8] $(2R,3S,5R,6R)$-*rel*-3-(1*E*,3*E*)-1,3-Heptadienyl-5,6-dihydroxy-2-(hydroxymethyl)cyclohexanone. $C_{14}H_{22}O_4$; mol wt 254.32. C 66.12%, H 8.72%, O 25.16%. Metabolic product of *Penicillium palitans* Westling. Isoln: J. H. Birkinshaw, H. Raistrick, *Biochem. J.* **30,** 801 (1936). Derivs and degradation products: J. H. Birkinshaw, *ibid.* **51,** 271 (1952). Structure: K. Bowden *et al., J. Chem. Soc.* **1959,** 1662. Biosynthesis: P. Chaplen, R. Thomas, *Biochem. J.* **77,** 91 (1960); A. J. Birch, M. Kocor, *J. Chem. Soc.* **1960,** 866. Reactivity studies: A. T. Austin, B. Pearson, *Chem. Ind. (London)* **1966,** 1228. Stereoselective synthesis of (±)-form: A. Ichihara *et al., Tetrahedron Lett.* **1977,** 3473; *idem, Tetrahedron* **36,** 1547 (1980).

Needles from hot water, mp 165°. $[\alpha]_{5461}^{23}$ +4.4° (c = 0.8 in $CHCl_3$). uv max (ethanol): 323 nm (ε 34,000). Sol in hot water, alc, chloroform; slightly sol in cold water, ether.

6988. Palivizumab. [188039-54-5] Anti-(respiratory syncytial virus protein F) immunoglobulin G1 (human-mouse monoclonal MEDI-493 γ_1-chain) disulfide with human-mouse monoclonal MEDI-493 κ-chain, dimer; MEDI-493; Synagis. Humanized monoclonal antibody directed to a neutralizing epitope on the F glycoprotein of respiratory syncytial virus (RSV). Mol wt ~148 kDa. Consists of ~95% human and ~5% murine antibody sequences. Prepn and neutralizing activity: L. S. Johnson, **WO 9605229;** *idem,* **US 5824307** (1996, 1998 both to MedImmune); S. Johnson *et al., J. Infect. Dis.* **176,** 1215 (1997). Clinical pharmacokinetics and safety: X. Sáez-Llorens *et al., Pediatr. Infect. Dis. J.* **17,** 787 (1998). Clinical trial in high risk infants: Impact-RSV Study

Group, *Pediatrics* **103,** 531 (1998). *Review:* H. C. Meissner *et al., Pediatr. Infect. Dis. J.* **18,** 223-231 (1999).

THERAP CAT: Antiviral (in prophylaxis of RSV infection).

6989. Palladium. [7440-05-3] Pd; at. wt 106.42; at. no. 46; valences 2, 4. Group VIII (10). Six naturally occurring isotopes: 102 (1.0%); 104 (11.0%); 105 (22.2%); 106 (27.3%); 108 (26.7%); 110 (11.8%); artificial, radioactive isotopes: 98-101, 103; 107; 109; 111-115. Abundance in earth's crust 0.001-0.01 ppm. Discovered in 1803 by Wollaston. Belongs to the platinum group of metals. Occurs in nature alloyed with platinum or gold and as a selenide; found in nickel sulfide ores; found in the minerals stibiopalladinite, braggite, porpezite. Isoln: Vauquelin *et al.,* cited by Mellor, *A Comprehensive Treatise on Inorganic and Theoretical Chemistry* **15,** 595 (1936). Reviews of prepn, properties and chemistry of palladium and other platinum metals: Gilchrist, *Chem. Rev.* **32,** 277-372 (1943); Beamish *et al.,* in *Rare Metals Handbook,* C. A. Hampel, Ed. (Reinhold, New York, 1956) pp 291-328; Livingstone in *Comprehensive Inorganic Chemistry* vol. 3, J. C. Bailar, Jr. *et al.,* Eds. (Pergamon Press, Oxford, 1973) pp 1163-1189, 1274-1329. Review of uses: E. M. Wise, *Palladium, Recovery, Properties, Uses* (Academic Press, New York, 1968) 187 pp. Use of organic palladium derivatives in synthesis: P. M. Maitlis, *The Organic Chemistry of Palladium* (Academic Press, New York, 1971); J. Tsuji, *Top. Curr. Chem.* **91,** 29 (1980); B. M. Trost, *Tetrahedron* **33,** 2615 (1977); *idem, Acc. Chem. Res.* **13,** 385 (1980).

Silver-white metal, face-centered cubic structure; occurs also as black powder and as spongy masses which can be compressed to a compact mass. mp 1555°. bp 3167°. d_4^{20} 12.02. Hardness on Mohs' scale 4.8, Brinell hardness 61.0. Spec heat 0.0584 cal/g at 0°C. Electrical resistivity at 0° = 10.0 microohms-cm. Appreciably volatile at high temps. At a red heat is converted into the monoxide. Forms dihalides with fluorine or chlorine at a red heat. Reacts with nitric acid, sulfuric acid, a mixture of hydrochloric and chloric acids. Reacts slightly with concd HCl; more readily in the presence of air or free chlorine. Forms a sulfide when heated with sulfur, a phosphide when heated with phosphorus. Absorbs a considerable amount of hydrogen.

USE: In form of gold, silver, and copper alloys in dentistry; for alloy bearings, springs, balance wheels of watches; for mirrors in astronomical instruments; as catalyzer in manuf of sulfuric acid and in other oxidizing processes; in powder form as catalyst in hydrogenation and in ignition of hydrogen or hydrocarbons with oxygen; the spongy form is used in gas analysis for separating hydrogen from mixtures of gases.

6990. Palladium Chloride. [7647-10-1] Palladous chloride. Cl_2Pd; mol wt 177.33. Cl 39.99%, Pd 60.01%. $PdCl_2$. Prepn: Krustinsons, *Z. Elektrochem.* **44,** 537 (1938). Toxicity study: Orestano, *Boll. Soc. Ital. Biol. Sper.* **8,** 1154 (1933). Review of $PdCl_2$ and other halides: J. H. Canterford, R. Colton, *Halides of the Second and Third Row Transition Metals* (John Wiley, New York, 1968) pp 358-389.

Red crystals. mp 678-680°. Dec at high temp to palladium and chlorine. MLD i.v. in rabbits: 0.0186 g/kg (Orestano).

Dihydrate. Dark brown crystals. Sol in water, alcohol, acetone. Reduced in soln by hydrogen or CO to metal. *Keep tightly closed.*

USE: In photography, for preparing pictures to be transferred to porcelain; toning solutions; electroplating parts of clocks and watches; manuf indelible ink; for the prepn of the metal for use as a catalyst; $PdCl_2$ paper is used for detecting CO, to find leaks in buried gas pipes. Prepn of palladium catalysts using $PdCl_2$: Mozingo, *Org. Synth.* coll. vol. III, 685 (1955).

6991. Palladium Diacetate. [19807-27-3] Acetic acid palladium salt; bis(acetato)palladium; diacetatopalladium(II); palladium(II) acetate. $C_4H_6O_4Pd$; mol wt 224.51. C 21.40%, H 2.69%, O 28.51%, Pd 47.40%. $(CH_3COO)_2Pd$. Prepn from palladium sponge or palladium nitrate and glacial acetic acid: Morehouse *et al., Chem. Ind. (London)* **1964,** 544; Stephenson *et al., J. Chem. Soc.* **1965,** 3632; from hydrated palladium oxide and acetic acid: Hausman *et al.,* **FR 1403398** corresp to **US 3318891** (1965, 1967 to Engelhard). Crystal structure of trimeric palladium acetate: Skapski, Smart, *Chem. Commun.* **1970,** 658.

Orange-brown crystals; mp 205° (dec). Shown to be trimeric by osmometric determn of mol wt in benzene (37°); monomeric by ebullioscopic measurement in benzene (80°). Crystals are trimeric. Sol in chloroform, methylene dichloride, acetone, acetonitrile, diethyl ether; sol with dec in aq HCl, aq KI solutions. Insol in water, aq NaCl, NaNO₃, NaOAc solns, petroleum, alcohols. Dec when warmed with alcohols.

USE: Catalyst.

6992. Palladium Nitrate. [10102-05-3] Palladous nitrate. N₂O₆Pd; mol wt 230.43. N 12.16%, O 41.66%, Pd 46.18%. Pd(NO₃)₂. Prepn from palladium and nitric acid: *Gmelins, Palladium* (8th ed.) **65**, 269 (1942). Reported to be the dihydrate: Gatehouse *et al., J. Chem. Soc.* **1957**, 4222.

Brown, deliquesc crystals. Sol in water with turbidity; with much water a brown basic salt precipitates; completely sol in dil HNO₃. *Keep well closed, protected from light.*

USE: Sepn of Cl₂ and I₂; catalyst in organic syntheses.

6993. Palladium Oxide. [1314-08-5] Palladium monoxide; palladous oxide. OPd; mol wt 122.42. O 13.07%, Pd 86.93%. PdO. Prepn: Shriner, Adams, *J. Am. Chem. Soc.* **46**, 1685 (1924).

Black powder. d 8.3. Insol in water, acids; slightly sol in aqua regia; sol in 48% HBr. Dec when strongly heated; also in the presence of H₂.

USE: Reduction catalyst in synthesis of organic compds.

6994. Palmatine. [3486-67-7] 5,6-Dihydro-2,3,9,10-tetramethoxydibenzo[*a,g*]quinolizinium; 7,8,13,13a-tetradehydro-2,3,9,10-tetramethoxyberbinium; calystigine. [C₂₁H₂₂NO₄]⁺. Obtained only in form of its salts. First isolated from Calumba root *(Jateorhiza palmata* (DC.) Miers, *Menispermaceae)*. Now found in many other genera. Palmatine and tetrahydropalmatine, *q.v.* are probably the most widely distributed Berberis alkaloids. Extraction procedure: Feist, Dschu, *Arch. Pharm.* **263**, 301 (1925). Structure: Feist, Sandstede, *ibid.* **256**, 2, 5 (1918); Späth, Lang, *Ber.* **54**, 3064, 3068 (1921); Späth, Böhm, *Ber.* **55**, 2988 (1922); Späth, Meinhard, *Ber.* **75**, 400 (1942). Synthesis: Späth, Quientensky, *Ber.* **54**, 2267 (1925); R. D. Haworth *et al., J. Chem. Soc.* **1927**, 548; Z. Kiparissides *et al., Can. J. Chem.* **58**, 2770 (1980). Identity with calystigine, alkaloid of the Chinese drug Chi-Kuo-Lan: Huang, Chen, *C.A.* **52**, 15827i (1958).

Palmatine forms addn products with acetone and chloroform, as does berberine.

Iodide. (C₂₁H₂₂NO₄)I. Yellow needles from water, dec 239°; also a dihydrate. Sparingly sol in hot water and alc.

Nitrate. (C₂₁H₂₂NO₄)NO₃. Sesqui- or dihydrate, yellow needles, dec 239°. Freely sol in most solvents.

Chloride trihydrate. (C₂₁H₂₂NO₄)Cl.3H₂O. Yellowish-green needles from water. Freely sol in hot water and alc.

Sulfate pentahydrate. (C₂₁H₂₂NO₄)₂SO₄.5H₂O. Yellow needles, mp 250°. Very sol in alc, sol in water.

6995. Palmidrol. [544-31-0] *N*-(2-Hydroxyethyl)hexadecanamide; *N*-(2-hydroxyethyl)palmitamide. C₁₈H₃₇NO₂; mol wt 299.49. C 72.19%, H 12.45%, N 4.68%, O 10.68%. CH₃(CH₂)₁₄-CONHCH₂CH₂OH. A naturally occurring anti-inflammatory agent. Isolated from soybean lecithin, egg yolk, and peanut meal: Kuehl *et al., J. Am. Chem. Soc.* **79**, 5577 (1957). Synthesis by refluxing ethanolamine with palmitic acid: Roe *et al., ibid.* **74**, 3442 (1952).

Crystals from 95% ethanol or cyclohexane, mp 98-99°.

6996. Palmitic Acid. [57-10-3] Hexadecanoic acid; hexadecylic acid; cetylic acid. C₁₆H₃₂O₂; mol wt 256.42. C 74.94%, H 12.58%, O 12.48%. CH₃(CH₂)₁₄COOH. Occurs as the glyceryl ester in many oils and fats. Obtained from palm oil, Japan wax, or

Chinese vegetable tallow. Purification: Magne *et al.,* US **2791596** (1957 to Secretary of Agriculture). Toxicity study: L. Orö, A. Wretlind, *Acta Pharmacol. Toxicol.* **18**, 141 (1961).

White, crystalline scales. d₄⁶² 0.853. mp 63-64°. bp₁₅ 215°. n_D⁸⁰ 1.4273. Insol in water. Sparingly sol in cold alcohol or in petr ether; freely sol in hot alcohol, in ether, propyl alcohol, chloroform. LD₅₀ i.v. in mice: 57±3.4 mg/kg (Orö, Wretlind).

6997. Palonosetron. [135729-61-2] (3a*S*)-2-(3*S*)-1-Azabicyclo[2.2.2]oct-3-yl-2,3,3a,4,5,6-hexahydro-1*H*-benz[*de*]isoquinolin-1-one. C₁₉H₂₄N₂O; mol wt 296.41. C 76.99%, H 8.16%, N 9.45%, O 5.40%. Serotonin 5-HT₃ receptor antagonist. Prepn: J. Berger *et al.,* EP **430190**; *eidem,* US **5202333** (1991, 1993 both to Syntex); R. D. Clark *et al., J. Med. Chem.* **36**, 2645 (1993). Improved synthesis: B. A. Kowalczyk, *Heterocycles* **43**, 1439 (1996). Receptor binding study: E. H. F. Wong *et al., Br. J. Pharmacol.* **114**, 851 (1995). Pharmacology: R. M. Eglen *et al., ibid.* 860. Clinical efficacy and pharmacokinetics: P. Eisenberg *et al., Ann. Oncol.* **15**, 330 (2004). Clinical trial in prevention of chemotherapy-induced nausea and vomiting: R. Gralla *et al., Ann. Oncol.* **14**, 1570 (2003). Review of pharmacology and clinical experience: S. M. Grunberg, J. M. Koeller, *Expert. Opin. Pharmacother.* **4**, 2297-2303 (2003); M. A. A. Siddiqui, L. J. Scott, *Drugs* **64**, 1125-1132 (2004).

mp 87-88°. [α]_D −136° (c = 0.25 in chloroform).

Hydrochloride. [135729-62-3] RS-25259-197; Aloxi; Onicit. C₁₉H₂₄N₂O.HCl; mol wt 332.87. Crystals from ethanol, mp >290°. [α]_D²⁵ −94.1° (c = 0.4 in water). Freely sol in water; sol in propylene glycol; slightly sol in ethanol, 2-propanol.

THERAP CAT: Antiemetic.

6998. Palustric Acid. [1945-53-5] [1*R*-(1α,4aβ,10aα)]-1,2,-3,4,4a,5,6,9,10,10a-Decahydro-1,4a-dimethyl-7-(1-methylethyl)-1-phenanthrenecarboxylic acid; 13-isopropylpodocarpa-8,13-dien-15-oic acid. C₂₀H₃₀O₂; mol wt 302.45. C 79.42%, H 10.00%, O 10.58%. Isoln from gum rosin: Loeblich *et al., J. Am. Chem. Soc.* **77**, 2823 (1955); Joye *et al., J. Org. Chem.* **30**, 654 (1965). Structure: Shuller *et al., J. Am. Chem. Soc.* **82**, 1734 (1960). Prepn of the 4-*epi*-form: Tabacik, Poisson, *Bull. Soc. Chim. Fr.* **1969**, 3264.

Crystals from methanol, mp 162-167°. [α]_D +71.6°. uv max (0.01*N* NaOH): 265-266 nm.

Methyl ester. C₂₁H₃₂O₂. Crystals from methanol, mp 25-27°. [α]_D +67.7°. uv max: 265-266 nm.

6999. Palytoxin. [77734-91-9] Palytoxin (C51-55 hemiacetal); PTX. C₁₂₉H₂₂₃N₃O₅₄; mol wt 2680.14. C 57.81%, H 8.39%, N 1.57%, O 32.24%. Potent toxin isolated from zoanthid coral of the genus *Palythoa* that is the most poisonous non-proteinaceous substance known. Isoln from "Limu-make-o-Hana", the Hawaiian name for the highly toxic coelenterate *Palythoa toxica:* R. E. Moore, P. J. Scheuer, *Science* **172**, 495 (1971). Structure: R. E.

Moore, G. Bartolini, *J. Am. Chem. Soc.* **103,** 2491 (1981). Structure of palytoxin from *P. tuberculosa* of Okinawa (differs from palytoxin from *P. toxica* at two positions): D. Uemura *et al., Tetrahedron Lett.* **22,** 2781 (1981). Proposed absolute configuration of 60 of the 64 chiral centers: R. E. Moore *et al., J. Am. Chem. Soc.* **104,** 3776 (1982). Structure and stereochemistry: J. K. Cha *et al., ibid.* 7369. Discussion of the structural elucidation, *see* Y. Shimizu, *Nature* **302,** 212 (1983); review: R. E. Moore, *Prog. Chem. Org. Nat. Prod.* **48,** 82-202 (1985). Synthetic studies: Y. Kishi, *Chem. Scr.* **27,** 573 (1987). Pharmacological study: P. N. Kaul *et al., Proc. West. Pharmacol. Soc.* **17,** 294 (1974). Mechanism of action and treatment of palytoxin poisoning: J. A. Vick *et al., Toxicol. Appl. Pharmacol.* **34,** 214 (1975). Mode of contractile action on vascular smooth muscle: K. Ito *et al., Eur. J. Pharmacol.* **46,** 9 (1977). Depolarizing action on frog spinal cord: Y. Kudo, S. Shibata, *Br. J. Pharmacol.* **71,** 575 (1980). Toxicology and toxicity studies: J. S. Wiles *et al., Toxicon* **12,** 427 (1974); K. Ito *et al., Arch. Int. Pharmacodyn. Ther.* **258,** 146 (1982). Brief review of biology: P. J. Scheuer, *Acc. Chem. Res.* **10,** 33-39 (1977). Review of synthetic studies and conformational analysis: Y. Kishi, *Pure Appl. Chem.* **61,** 313-324 (1989).

= R1

= R2

White amorphous hygroscopic solid. No definite mp; chars when heated to 300°. $[\alpha]_D^{25}$ +26° (water). Insol in chloroform, ether, acetone. Sparingly sol in methanol, ethanol. Sol in pyridine, DMSO, water. LD$_{50}$ in mice: 0.45 μg/kg i.v. (Wiles); 50-100 ng/kg i.p. (Kaul).

Caution: Palytoxin is an intense vasoconstrictor. In intact dogs, doses of >0.06 μg/kg i.v. caused a transient rise in arterial pressure followed by rapid hypotension and resulted in death within 5 minutes (Ito, 1982).

USE: As a physiological tool to evaluate anti-anginal chemotherapeutic agents.

7000. Pamabrom. [606-04-2] 8-Bromo-3,7-dihydro-1,3-dimethyl-1*H*-purine-2,6-dione compd with 2-amino-2-methyl-1-pro-

panol (1:1); 8-bromotheophylline compd with 2-amino-2-methyl-1-propanol (1:1); 2-amino-2-methyl-2-propanol 8-bromotheophyllinate. $C_{11}H_{18}BrN_5O_3$; mol wt 348.20. C 37.94%, H 5.21%, Br 22.95%, N 20.11%, O 13.78%. Prepn from 2-amino-2-methyl-1-propanol and 8-bromotheophylline: J. M. Holbert, I. W. Grote, **US 2711411** (1955 to Chattanooga Med.). Prepn and diuretic activity: J. M. Holbert *et al., J. Am. Pharm. Assoc. Sci. Ed.* **44,** 355 (1955).

Fine white powder, dec 300°. Soly in water >30 g/100 ml at 25°. pH of satd aq soln 8.0-8.5.

Mixture with acetaminophen and pyrilamine maleate. Midol PMS; Premsyn PMS; Sunril.

THERAP CAT: Diuretic.

7001. Pamaquine. [491-92-9] N^1,N^1-Diethyl-N^4-(6-methoxy-8-quinolinyl)-1,4-pentanediamine; 8-[[4-(diethylamino)-1-methylbutyl]amino]-6-methoxyquinoline. $C_{19}H_{29}N_3O$; mol wt 315.45. C 72.34%, H 9.27%, N 13.32%, O 5.07%. Prepn: **GB 295656** (1927 to I. G. Farbenind); K. H. Slotta, *Grundriss der modernen Arzneistoff-Synthese* (Stuttgart, 1931); Elderfield *et al., J. Am. Chem. Soc.* **70,** 40 (1948). *Review:* Cooper, *Public Health Rep.* **64,** 717 (1949). HPLC determn in plasma: Y. S. Endoh *et al., J. Chromatogr.* **579,** 123 (1992). Historical review: D. Greenwood, *J. Antimicrob. Chemother.* **36,** 857-872 (1995).

Dark yellow oil. bp$_{0.3}$ 175-180°; bp$_1$ 182-194°.

Pamoate. [635-05-2] Pamaquine embonate; pamaquine naphthoate; Aminoquin; Plasmochin; Plasmoquine; Praequine. $C_{19}H_{29}N_3O \cdot C_{23}H_{16}O_6$; mol wt 703.82. Yellow to orange-yellow odorless, almost tasteless powder. Numbs the tongue. Insol in water. Sol in alcohol, acetone. *Protect from light.*

THERAP CAT: Antimalarial.

7002. Pamicogrel. [101001-34-7] 2-[4,5-Bis(4-methoxyphenyl)-2-thiazolyl]-1*H*-pyrrole-1-acetic acid ethyl ester; ethyl 2-[4,5-bis(*p*-methoxyphenyl)-2-thiazolyl]pyrrole-1-acetate; KB-3022; KBT-3022. $C_{25}H_{24}N_2O_4S$; mol wt 448.53. C 66.94%, H 5.39%, N 6.25%, O 14.27%, S 7.15%. Cyclooxygenase inhibitor. Prepn: K. Yoshino *et al.,* **EP 159677**; *eidem,* **US 4659726** (1985, 1987 both to Kanebo). HPLC determn in plasma and urine: Y. Nakada *et al., Chem. Pharm. Bull.* **38,** 1093 (1990). Pharmacokinetics: Y. Nakada *et al., Yakuzaigaku* **53,** 210 (1993), *C.A.* **120,** 315100 (1993). Activity as antithrombotic: K. Yokoto *et al., Jpn. J. Pharmacol.* **68,** 201 (1995); as platelet aggregation inhibitor: K. Yokoto *et al., J. Pharm. Pharmacol.* **47,** 768 (1995). Evaluation of cerebral protective effects: N. Yamamoto *et al., Jpn. J. Pharmacol.* **69,** 421 (1995); *eidem, Eur. J. Pharmacol.* **297,** 225 (1996).

Crystals from ligroin, mp 132.5-135.5°. LD$_{50}$ orally in male mice: >3000 mg/kg (Yoshino).

THERAP CAT: Antithrombotic.

7003. Pamidronic Acid. [40391-99-9] (3-Amino-1-hydroxypropylidene)bisphosphonic acid; 3-amino-1-hydroxypropane-1,1-diphosphonic acid; ADP; AHPrBP. C$_3$H$_{11}$NO$_7$P$_2$; mol wt 235.07. C 15.33%, H 4.72%, N 5.96%, O 47.64%, P 26.35%. Bisphosphonate antiresorptive agent. Prepn: F. Krueger et al., **DE 2130794** (1973 to Benckiser), C.A. **78**, 84528z (1973); K.-H. Worms et al., Z. Anorg. Allg. Chem. **457**, 214 (1979). Improved process: H. Blum, K.-H. Worms, **US 4327039** (1982 to Henkel). Mechanism of action study: P. M. Boonekamp et al., Bone Miner. **1**, 27 (1986). HPLC determn in serum and plasma: R. W. Sparidans et al., J. Chromatogr. B **705**, 331 (1998). Clinical trial to prevent postmenopausal bone loss: B. Lees et al., Osteoporos. Int. **6**, 480 (1996). Review of pharmacology and therapeutic use in resorptive bone disease: A. Fitton, D. McTavish, Drugs **41**, 289-318 (1991); A. J. Coukell, A. Markham, Drugs Aging **12**, 149-168 (1998).

Disodium salt. [57248-88-1] Pamidronate disodium; GCP-23339A; Aminomux; Aredia. C$_3$H$_9$NNa$_2$O$_7$P$_2$; mol wt 279.03.

THERAP CAT: Bone resorption inhibitor.

7004. Pamiteplase. 275-L-Glutamic acid (1-91)-(174-527)-plasminogen activator (human tissue-type protein moiety); YM-866; Solinase. Genetically engineered variant of human tissue plasminogen activator (t-PA), q.v. Derived by deletion of the first kringle domain and the substitution of glutamic acid for arginine at position 275. Prepn: Y. Kawauchi et al., **WO 8903874**; eidem, **US 5556621** (1989, 1996 both to Yamanouchi). Thrombolytic activity: T. Kawasaki et al., Jpn. J. Pharmacol. **63**, 9 (1993); M. Suzuki et al., Curr. Ther. Res. **61**, 7 (2000). Toxicology: A. Ishikawa et al., J. Toxicol. Sci. **22**, 117 (1997). Review of thrombolytic agents: M. Verstraete, Am. J. Med. **109**, 52-58 (2000).

THERAP CAT: Thrombolytic.

7005. Pamoic Acid. [130-85-8] 4,4'-Methylenebis[3-hydroxy-2-naphthalenecarboxylic acid]; 4,4'-methylenebis(3-hydroxy-2-naphthoic acid); 4,4'-methylenedi(3-hydroxy-2-naphthoic acid); 2,2'-dihydroxy-1,1'-dinaphthylmethane-3,3'-dicarboxylic acid; embonic acid. C$_{23}$H$_{16}$O$_6$; mol wt 388.37. C 71.13%, H 4.15%, O 24.72%. Prepn from 2-hydroxy-3-naphthoic acid + formaldehyde: Strohback, Ber. **34**, 4162 (1901); Brass, Sommer, ibid. **61**, 993 (1928); Barber, Gaimster, J. Appl. Chem. **2**, 565 (1952). Prepn of salts: Puetzer, **US 2397903** (1946 to Vick Chem.); Barber, **US 2641610** (1953 to May & Baker).

Crystals from dil pyridine, dec above 280° without melting. Practically insoluble in water, alcohol, ether, benzene, acetic acid. Sparingly sol in chloroform; sol in nitrobenzene, pyridine.

Methyl ether. C$_{24}$H$_{18}$O$_6$. Yellow crystals from dil methanol, dec 277-282°.

7006. Pancreatic Extract. Pancreas powder; Creon; Ku-Zyme; Pancrease; Pancrex-Vet; Panzytrat; Ultrase; Viokase. Substance prepd from fresh or frozen mammalian pancreas, usually from swine, that contains various enzymes having proteolytic, lipolytic and amylolytic activities. Pharmacopeial specifications differ on the quantity of amylase, lipase and protease required; most commercial formulations are of higher digestive power. Method of

production from cow or pig pancreas: S. Hoek, **US 3223594** (1965 to N. American Philips). Clinical pharmacology and comparison of formulations: Y. W. Cho, D. M. Aviado, J. Clin. Pharmacol. **21**, 224 (1981). Analysis of pharmaceutical preparations: C. L. Case et al., Pancreas **30**, 180 (2005). Clinical trial in weight loss prevention in pancreatic cancer: M. J. Bruno et al., Gut **42**, 92 (1998); in cystic fibrosis: R. C. Stern et al., Am. J. Gastroenterol. **95**, 1932 (2000); C. J. Patchell et al., J. Cyst. Fibr. **1**, 287 (2002).

Slightly brown, amorphous powder. Partly sol in water. Practically insol in alcohol, ether.

Pancreatin. [8049-47-6] Pancreatic enzyme concentrate containing not less than 2 USP units of lipase, 25 of amylase and 25 of protease activities per mg. British Pharmacopeia specifies not less than 20 FIP units of lipase, 24 of amylase and 1.4 of protease activities per mg.

Pancrelipase. [53608-75-6] Porcine pancreatic enzyme concentrate containing not less than 24 USP units of lipase, 100 of amylase and 100 of protease activities per mg.

THERAP CAT: Enzyme replacement therapy (pancreatic exocrine insufficiency).

THERAP CAT (VET): Enzyme replacement therapy in pancreatic enzyme deficiency.

7007. Pancuronium Bromide. [15500-66-0] 1,1'-[(2β,3α,-5α,16β,17β)-3,17-Bis(acetyloxy)androstane-2,16-diyl]bis[1-methylpiperidinium] dibromide; 1,1'-(3α,17β-dihydroxy-5α-androstan-2β,16β-ylene)bis[1-methylpiperidinium] dibromide diacetate; 3α,17β-diacetoxy-2β,16β-dipiperidino-5α-androstane dimethobromide; 2β,16β-dipiperidino-5α-androstane-3α,17β-diol diacetate dimethobromide; poncuronium bromide (rescinded USAN); NA-97; Org-NA-97; Mioblock; Pavulon. C$_{35}$H$_{60}$Br$_2$N$_2$O$_4$; mol wt 732.67. C 57.38%, H 8.25%, Br 21.81%, N 3.82%, O 8.73%. Aminosteroid, competitive neuromuscular blocker. Prepn: W. R. Buckett et al., Chim. Ther. **2**, 186 (1967); eidem, J. Med. Chem. **16**, 1116 (1973). Structural studies: Savage et al., J. Chem. Soc. B **1971**, 410. Structure-activity correlation: Waser, Anaesthesist **20**, 23 (1971). Pharmacology: W. R. Buckett, I. L. Bonta, Fed. Proc. **25**, 718 (1966); W. R. Buckett et al., Br. J. Pharmacol. Chemother. **32**, 671 (1968); I. L. Bonta et al., Eur. J. Pharmacol. **4**, 83, 303 (1968). Comparative study of neuromuscular blocking and vagolytic effect: S. L. Son et al., Anesthesiology **55**, 12 (1981). Review: Speight, Avery, Drugs **4**, 163-226 (1972).

Odorless crystals with bitter taste, mp 215°. One gram dissolves in 30 parts chloroform, one part water (20°). LD$_{50}$ in mice (mg/kg): 0.047 i.v.; 0.152 i.p.; 0.167 s.c.; 21.9 orally; in rats, rabbits: 0.153, 0.016 i.v. (Buckett, 1968).

THERAP CAT: Neuromuscular blocking agent.

THERAP CAT (VET): Neuromuscular blocking agent.

7008. Pangamic Acid. Controversial mixture of compounds erroneously labeled as *vitamin B$_{15}$*. Allegedly isolated from apricot kernel: E. T. Krebs, Sr. et al., Int. Rec. Med. **164**, 18 (1951). Originally named pangamic acid because of its supposed ubiquity in seeds. There is no clear chemical identity for pangamic acid. An historical review by J. C. Micheau et al., in Chim. Ther. **7**, 103 (1972) contains structural studies, analyses, syntheses and discussion of various components of pangamic acid. Products sold as pangamic acid in the U.S. vary considerably in their composition. Some are mixtures of calcium gluconate and N,N-dimethylglycine, q.q.v.; others contain diisopropylamine dichloroacetate, q.v.: FDA Drug Bulletin vol. **8**(6), Dec. 1978-Jan. 1979. Ref.: V. Herbert,

Am. J. Clin. Nutr. **32,** 1534 (1979); V. Herbert, R. Herbert, in *Controversies in Nutrition,* L. Ellenbogen, Ed. (Churchill-Livingstone, New York, 1981) pp 159-170.

7009. Panipenem. [87726-17-8] (5*R*,6*S*)-6-[(1*R*)-1-Hydroxyethyl]-3-[[(3*S*)-1-(1-iminoethyl)-3-pyrrolidinyl]thio]-7-oxo-1-azabicyclo[3.2.0]hept-2-ene-2-carboxylic acid; (5*R*,6*S*)-6-[(*R*)-1-hydroxyethyl]-2-[(*S*)-1-acetimidoylpyrrolidin-3-ylthio]-1-carbapen-2-em-3-carboxylic acid; (+)-(5*R*,6*S*)-3-[[(*S*)-1-acetimidoyl-3-pyrrolidinyl]thio]-6-[(*R*)-1-hydroxyethyl]-7-oxo-1-azabicyclo[3.2.0]hept-2-ene-2-carboxylic acid; CS-533; RS-533. $C_{15}H_{21}$-N_3O_4S; mol wt 339.41. C 53.08%, H 6.24%, N 12.38%, O 18.86%, S 9.45%. Carbapenem antibiotic. Prepn: T. Miyadera *et al., J. Antibiot.* **36,** 1034 (1983). Manufacturing process: A. Yoshida, K. Oda, **EP 587436** (1994 to Sankyo). Antibacterial spectrum *in vitro:* H. C. Neu *et al., Antimicrob. Agents Chemother.* **30,** 828 (1986). Series of articles on pharmacology and clinical efficacy in combination with betamipron, *q.v: Chemotherapy (Tokyo)* **39** Suppl 3, 1-813 (1991). Toxicology: K. Kimura *et al., ibid.* 140.

Prepd as the hemihydrate; colorless fine prisms, mp 198-200° (dec). uv max (water): 298 nm (ε 10400). Approx LD_{50} in male, female mice (mg/kg): 1700-2200, 1300-1700 i.v. (Kimura).

Mixture with betamipron. [138240-65-0] CS-976; Carbenin.

THERAP CAT: Antibacterial.

7010. Panitumumab. [339177-26-3] Anti-(human epidermal growth factor receptor) immunoglobulin (human monoclonal ABX-EGF heavy chain) disulfide with human monoclonal ABX-EGF light chain, dimer; ABX-EGF. Fully human monoclonal antibody secreted by the E7.6.3 hybridoma; directed against human epidermal growth factor receptor (EGFr), a transmembrane cell-surface glycoprotein overexpressed in a variety of cancers. Prepn: A. Jakobovits *et al.,* **WO 9850433**; *eidem,* **US 6235883** (1998, 2001 both to Abgenix); and *in vivo* antitumor activity: X.-D. Yang *et al., Cancer Res.* **59,** 1236 (1999). Clinical pharmacokinetics: E. K. Rowinsky *et al., J. Clin. Oncol.* **22,** 3003 (2004). Review of preclinical and clinical evaluations: K. A. Foon *et al., Int. J. Radiat. Oncol. Biol. Phys.* **58,** 984-990 (2004).

THERAP CAT: Antineoplastic.

7011. Pantetheine. [496-65-1] 2,4-Dihydroxy-*N*-[3-[(2-mercaptoethyl)amino]-3-oxopropyl]-3,3-dimethylbutanamide; 2,4-dihydroxy-*N*-[2-[(2-mercaptoethyl)carbamoyl]ethyl]-3,3-dimethyl-butyramide; *N*-(pantothenyl)-β-aminoethanethiol; α,γ-dihydroxy-β,β-dimethylbutyryl-β-alanyl-β-aminoethanethiol. $C_{11}H_{22}N_2O_4S$; mol wt 278.37. C 47.46%, H 7.97%, N 10.06%, O 22.99%, S 11.52%. Growth factor for *Lactobacillus bulgaricus:* Williams *et al., J. Biol. Chem.* **177,** 933 (1949). Intermediate in the pathway of coenzyme A, *q.v.,* formation in mammalian liver and in some microorganisms. Synthesis: Schwyzer, *Helv. Chim. Acta* **35,** 1903 (1952); Baddiley, Thain, *J. Chem. Soc.* **1952,** 800; King *et al., J. Am. Chem. Soc.* **75,** 1290 (1953); Walton *et al., ibid.* **76,** 1146 (1954); Walton, **US 2744119** and **US 2835704** (1956, 1958, both to Merck & Co.). *Reviews:* Snell, Brown, *Adv. Enzymol.* **14,** 49 (1953); Snell, Wittle, *Methods Enzymol.* **3,** 918 (1957).

Syrup or glass. $[\alpha]_D^{20}$ +12.9° (c = 4.5 in water). Microbiological activity: 20,000 LBF units/mg. An LBF unit is that amount of the growth factor contained in one mg of Basamine-Busch, a standard yeast extract manuf by Anheuser-Busch, Inc.

Silver mercaptide. $C_{11}H_{21}AgN_2O_4S$. Yellow noncryst solid. $[\alpha]_D^{25}$ +8° (c = 4.27 in 0.9*N* NaCl). Very sol in water. 11,000 LBF units/mg.

Mercuric mercaptide. $C_{22}H_{42}HgN_4O_8S_2.C_3H_6O$. Crystals from acetone, mp 96-98°. $[\alpha]_D^{27}$ +9.6° (c = 4 in water). 15,500 LBF units/mg. uv max: 260-265 nm (ε 1000). Sol in water, methanol.

***S*-Benzoylpantetheine.** $C_{18}H_{26}N_2O_5S$. Crystals from ethyl acetate, mp 116°. $[\alpha]_D^{27}$ +31° (ethanol). Sol in water, ethyl acetate, chloroform.

***S*-Acetylpantetheine.** $C_{13}H_{24}N_2O_5S$. Thick syrup. $[\alpha]_D^{27}$ +39° (c = 0.8 in ethanol).

7012. Pantethine. [16816-67-4] *N,N'*-[Dithiobis[2,1-ethanediylimino(3-oxo-3,1-propanediyl)]]bis[2,4-dihydroxy-3,3-dimethylbutanamide]; *N,N'*-[dithiobis(ethyleneiminocarbonyl-ethylene)]bis(2,4-dihydroxy-3,3-dimethylbutyramide; D-bis(*N*-pantothenyl-β-aminoethyl) disulfide; Lipodel; Pantetina; Panthecin; Pantomin; Pantosin. $C_{22}H_{42}N_4O_8S_2$; mol wt 554.72. C 47.63%, H 7.63%, N 10.10%, O 23.07%, S 11.56%. [$HOCH_2C(CH_3)_2$-$CHOHCONHCH_2CH_2CONHCH_2CH_2S]_2$. Disulfide dimer of pantetheine, *q.v.* Growth factor for *Lactobacillus bulgaricus:* Williams *et al., J. Biol. Chem.* **177,** 933 (1949). Formed by oxidation of pantetheine: Brown, Snell, *J. Biol. Chem.* **198,** 375 (1952). Structure: Snell *et al., J. Am. Chem. Soc.* **72,** 5349 (1950). Synthesis: Wieland, Bokelmann, *Naturwissenschaften* **38,** 384 (1951); Wittle *et al., J. Am. Chem. Soc.* **75,** 1694 (1953); Viscontini *et al., Helv. Chim. Acta* **37,** 375 (1954); Bowman, Cavalla, *J. Chem. Soc.* **1954,** 1171; Shimizu *et al., Chem. Pharm. Bull.* **13,** 180 (1965). Clinical trial in hyperlipoproteinemia: A. Gaddi *et al., Atherosclerosis* **50,** 73 (1984).

Glassy, colorless to light yellow substance. $[\alpha]_D^{27}$ +13.5° (c = 3.75 in water). Freely sol in water; less sol in ethanol. Practically insol in ether, acetone, ethyl acetate, benzene, chloroform.

THERAP CAT: Antilipemic.

7013. Pantolactone. [599-04-2] Dihydro-3-hydroxy-4*H*-dimethyl-2(3*H*)-furanone; pantoic acid γ-lactone; pantoyl lactone; pantoic lactone; 2,4-dihydroxy-3,3-dimethylbutyric acid γ-lactone; α-hydroxy-β,β-dimethyl-γ-butyrolactone. $C_6H_{10}O_3$; mol wt 130.14. C 55.37%, H 7.75%, O 36.88%. A degradation product of pantothenic acid from liver: Williams, Major, *Science* **91,** 246 (1940). Important intermediate in the synthesis of pantothenic acid. May be prepd by condensing isobutyraldehyde with formaldehyde yielding α,α-dimethyl-β-hydroxypropionaldehyde which is condensed with hydrocyanic acid in the presence of calcium chloride to form racemic pantolactone. Various modifications of this procedure exist: Glaser, *Monatsh. Chem.* **25,** 46 (1904); Stiller *et al., J. Am. Chem. Soc.* **62,** 1785 (1940); Reichstein, Grüssner, *Helv. Chim. Acta* **23,** 650 (1940); Carter, Ney, *J. Am. Chem. Soc.* **63,** 312 (1941). Vast patent literature, *e.g.,* Beckmann *et al.;* Klein, **US 2967869** and **US 3024250** (1961, 1962, both to Nopco).

D(−)-Form. Hygroscopic crystals from benzene + petr ether, mp 92°. $[\alpha]_D^{25}$ −50.7° (c = 2.05 in H_2O). Can be purified by microsublimation.

L(+)-Form. Hygroscopic crystals from benzene, mp 91°. $[\alpha]_D^{25}$ +50.1° (c = 2 in H_2O).

DL-Form. Hygroscopic rosettes or prisms, mp 80°, bp_{18} 130°. Freely sol in water. Sol in ether, benzene, chloroform, alcohol, carbon disulfide.

7014. Pantoprazole. [102625-70-7] 5-(Difluoromethoxy)-2-[[(3,4-dimethoxy-2-pyridinyl)methyl]sulfinyl]-1*H*-benzimidazole; SKF-96022; BY-1023. $C_{16}H_{15}F_2N_3O_4S$; mol wt 383.37. C 50.13%, H 3.94%, F 9.91%, N 10.96%, O 16.69%, S 8.36%. Gastric proton pump inhibitor. Prepn: B. Kohl *et al.,* **EP 166287**; *eidem,* **US 4758579** (1986, 1988 both to Byk Gulden); *eidem, J. Med. Chem.* **35,** 1049 (1992). Mechanism of action: W. A. Simon *et al., Biochem. Pharmacol.* **39,** 1799 (1990).

HPLC determn in plasma and serum: R. Huber *et al.*, *J. Chromatogr.* **529**, 389 (1990). Clinical pharmacokinetics: B. Simon *et al.*, *Z. Gastroenterol.* **28**, 443 (1990). Clinical trial in duodenal ulcer: P. Müller *et al., ibid.* **30**, 771 (1992); in Zollinger-Ellison syndrome: E. A. Lew *et al.*, *Gastroenterology* **118**, 696 (2000). Review of pharmacology and clinical experience: P. Poole, *Am. J. Health-Syst. Pharm.* **58**, 999-1008 (2001).

Off-white solid, mp 139-140° (dec). pKa_1 3.92; pKa_2 8.19.

Sodium salt. [138786-67-1] Eupantol; Pantecta; Pantozol; Pantopan; Pantorc; Peptazol; Protium; Protonix; Somac. $C_{16}H_{14}F_2N_3$-NaO_4S; mol wt 405.35. Prepd as the sesquihydrate. White to off-white crystalline powder, dec >130°. uv max (methanol): 289 (ε 1.64 × 10^4). Freely sol in water; very slightly sol in phosphate buffer (pH 7.4). Practically insol in *n*-hexane.

THERAP CAT: Antiulcerative; in treatment of Zollinger-Ellison syndrome.

7015. Pantothenic Acid. [79-83-4] *N*-[(2*R*)-2,4-Dihydroxy-3,3-dimethyl-1-oxobutyl]-β-alanine; D(+)-*N*-(2,4-dihydroxy-3,3-dimethylbutyryl)-β-alanine; chick antidermatitis factor; vitamin B$_5$. $C_9H_{17}NO_5$; mol wt 219.23. C 49.31%, H 7.82%, N 6.39%, O 36.49%. A member of the B complex vitamins; essential vitamin for the biosynthesis of coenzyme A in mammalian cells. Occurs ubiquitously in all animal and plant tissue. The richest common source is liver, but jelly of the queen bee contains 6 times as much as liver. Rice bran and molasses are other good sources. Isoln from liver: R. J. Williams *et al.*, *J. Am. Chem. Soc.* **60**, 2719 (1938). Synthesis: E. T. Stiller *et al., ibid.* **62**, 1785 (1940); Reichstein, Grüssner, *Helv. Chim. Acta* **23**, 650 (1940); Grüssner *et al., ibid.* 1276. Absolute configuration: Hill, Chan, *Biochem. Biophys. Res. Commun.* **38**, 181 (1970). Only the natural, dextrorotatory form has vitamin activity. Review of chemistry, biochemistry and pharmacology: W. Friedrich, *Vitamins* (de Gruyter, Berlin, 1988) pp 809-835; of metabolism: A. G. Tahiliani, C. J. Beinlich, *Vitam. Horm.* **46**, 165-228 (1991).

Unstable, viscous oil. Extremely hygroscopic. Easily destroyed by acids, bases, heat. $[\alpha]_D^{25}$ +37.5°. Freely sol in water, ethyl acetate, dioxane, glacial acetic acid; moderately sol in ether, amyl alcohol. Practically insol in benzene, chloroform.

Sodium salt. [867-81-2] $C_9H_{16}NNaO_5$. Very hygroscopic crystals. $[\alpha]_D^{25}$ +27.1° (c = 2). Can be stored in sealed ampuls only.

Calcium salt. [137-08-6] Calpanate; Pantholin. $C_{18}H_{32}CaN_2$-O_{10}; mol wt 476.53. Prepn: Wehrmeister, US 2780645 (1957 to Commercial Solvents); Kagan, US 2845456 (1958 to Upjohn). Minute needles from CH_3OH. Sweetish taste with slightly bitter aftertaste. Dec 195-196°. Moderately hygroscopic. $[\alpha]_D^{25}$ +28.2° (c = 5). One gram dissolves in 2.8 ml H_2O. Sol in glycerol; slightly sol in alcohol, acetone. pH of 5% aq soln: 7.2-8.0; pH in CO_2-free water: 8.7.

THERAP CAT: Vitamin.

THERAP CAT (VET): Nutritional factor: dietary essential except in horses, ruminants.

7016. Papain. [9001-73-4] Papayotin; vegetable pepsin; Arbuz; Nematolyt; Summetrin; Tromasin; Velardon; Vermizym. First recognized member of the class of proteolytic enzymes that needs a free sulfhydryl group for activity. Isolated from the latex of the green fruit and leaves of *Carica papaya* L., *Caricaceae*. Initial isolation and crystallization: Balls *et al.*, *Science* **86**, 379 (1937); Balls, Lineweaver, *J. Biol. Chem.* **130**, 669 (1939). Prepn from commercial dried papaya latex and physical properties: Kimmel,

Smith, *ibid.* **207**, 515 (1954); *see also ibid.* 533-573; Becker, *Econ. Bot.* **12**, 62 (1958). Purification: Gibian, Bratfisch, US 2950227 (1960 to Schering AG); Lesuk, US 3011952 (1961 to Sterling Drug); Blumberg *et al.*, *Eur. J. Biochem.* **15**, 97 (1970). The papain molecule consists of one folded polypeptide chain of 212 residues, mol wt ~23,400. Complete amino acid sequence: Drenth *et al.*, *Nature* **218**, 929 (1968); Mitchel *et al., J. Biol. Chem.* **245**, 3485 (1970). Mechanism of action studies: Morihara, *J. Biochem.* **62**, 250 (1967). Use in treatment of contact lenses to prolong wearing time in keratoconic patients with papillary conjunctivitis: D. R. Korb *et al.*, *Arch. Ophthalmol.* **101**, 48 (1983). *Reviews:* Kimmel, Smith in *Adv. Enzymol. Relat. Subj. Biochem.* **19**, 267-334 (1957); Glazer, Smith in *The Enzymes* vol. **III**, P. D. Boyer, Ed. (Academic Press, New York, 3rd ed., 1971) pp 501-537; *see also* Drenth *et al., ibid.* 485-498 and *eidem, Adv. Protein Chem.* **25**, 79-115 (1971) for a comprehensive review of the structural elucidation.

White or grayish-white, slightly hygroscopic powder. uv max: 278 nm (A$_{1cm}^{1\%}$ 25.0). Incompletely sol in water, glycerol. Practically insol in most organic solvents. *Keep well closed.* Potency varies according to process of prepn, etc. with the usual grade digesting ~35 times its wt of lean meat. Best grades render sol 200-300 times their wt of coagulated egg albumin in alkaline media. A temp. range of 60-90° is favorable for the digestive process with 65° the optimum point. Best pH is 5.0, but it functions also in neutral or alkaline media. Activated by reduction (HCN, H_2S etc.) and inactivated by oxidation (H_2O_2, iodoacetate).

Note: The term papain is currently applied to both the crude dried latex and the crystalline proteolytic enzyme.

USE: For tenderizing meats; for clearing beverages; for bating skins.

THERAP CAT: Enzyme (proteolytic). Debriding agent; digestive aid. Has been used to prevent adhesions; as anthelmintic (Nematodes).

7017. Papaveraldine. [522-57-6] (6,7-Dimethoxy-1-isoquinolinyl)(3,4-dimethoxyphenyl)methanone; 6,7-dimethoxy-1-isoquinolyl 3,4-dimethoxyphenyl ketone; 6,7-dimethoxy-1-veratroylisoquinoline; xanthaline. $C_{20}H_{19}NO_5$; mol wt 353.37. C 67.98%, H 5.42%, N 3.96%, O 22.64%. The old name papaveraldine is retained to avoid confusion. From opium; whether papaveraldine occurs as such in the poppy plant, or is formed during the process of extraction, has not been investigated. Oxidation of papaverine to papaveraldine by SeO_2: Menon, *Proc. Indian Acad. Sci.* **19A**, 21 (1944). For older references *see:* Small, Lutz, "Chemistry of the Opium Alkaloids," in *U.S. Public Health Reports* **Suppl. No. 103** (Washington, 1932). Synthesis from Reissert compds: Popp, McEwen, *J. Am. Chem. Soc.* **79**, 3773 (1957).

Crystals from abs ethanol, mp 208-209°. Sol in benzene, chloroform; slightly sol in alcohol, ether, petr ether; nearly insol in water, alkalies or carbonates.

Hydrochloride. $C_{20}H_{19}NO_5$·HCl. Yellow crystals from abs alcohol, mp 200°.

7018. Papaveretum. [8002-76-4] "Concentrated opium"; Omnopon; Pantopon. A mixture of the hydrochlorides of the opium alkaloids in their approximate natural proportions. Contains approx 50% morphine, 3% codeine, 20% noscapine, and 5% papaverine. Exhibits biological action of morphine and other alkaloids present in opium. Clinical evaluation in intravenous analgesia: J. A. Catling *et al.*, *Br. Med. J.* **281**, 478 (1980).

Yellowish-gray, cryst powder. Freely sol in water.

Note: This is a controlled substance (opium derivative): 21 **CFR**, 1308.12.

THERAP CAT: Analgesic (narcotic).

7019. Papaverine. [58-74-2] 1-[(3,4-Dimethoxyphenyl)-methyl]-6,7-dimethoxyisoquinoline; 6,7-dimethoxy-1-veratryl-

Consult the Name Index before using this section.

isoquinoline. $C_{20}H_{21}NO_4$; mol wt 339.39. C 70.78%, H 6.24%, N 4.13%, O 18.86%. Smooth muscle relaxant found in opium (0.8-1.0%). Synthesis: Pictet, Gams, *Compt. Rend.* **149**, 210 (1909); *Ber.* **42**, 2943 (1909). Review of commercial syntheses: Goldberg, *Chem. Prod. Chem. News* **17**, 371 (1954). Improved synthetic procedures: Braz, Chizhov, *Soviet Pharmaceutical Research* **3**, 90-93 (New York, 1958). Biosynthetic studies: Battersby, Harper, *J. Chem. Soc.* **1962**, 3526; Brochmann-Hanssen *et al., J. Pharm. Sci.* **60**, 1672 (1971). Pharmacology and toxicology: Preininger in *The Alkaloids* vol. **15**, R. H. F. Manske, Ed. (Academic Press, New York, 1975) pp 209-223. Toxicity: S. Levis *et al., Arch. Int. Pharmacodyn.* **123**, 264 (1960). Clinical effect on cerebral blood flow: H. L. Karpman, J. J. Sheppard, *Angiology* **26**, 592 (1975). Clinical evaluation in intermittent claudication: Y. Sheino *et al., ibid.* **34**, 257 (1983). Comprehensive description: M. S. Hifnawy, F. J. Muhtadi, *Anal. Profiles Drug Subs.* **17**, 367-447 (1988).

Triboluminescent, orthorhombic prisms from alcohol + ether, mp 147°. Sublimes at 135-140° at 11 mm pressure and 2 mm distance. d_4^{20} 1.337. pK (25°) 8.07. uv max (ethanol): 239, 278-280, 314, 327 nm (log ε 4.83, 3.86, 3.60, 3.67). Almost insol in water. Sol in hot benzene, glacial acetic acid, acetone; slightly sol in chloroform, carbon tetrachloride, petr ether. Optimal pH for storage of papaverine solns: 2.0-2.8.

Hydrochloride. [61-25-6] Artegodan; Cepaverin; Cerebid; Cerespan; Dynovas; Optenyl; Pameion; Panergon; Papital T.R.; Pavabid; Pavacen; Pavadel; Pavagen; Pavakey; Pavased; Spasmo-Nit; Therapav; Vasal; Vasospan. $C_{20}H_{21}NO_4 \cdot HCl$; mol wt 375.85. Monoclinic rods from water, mp 220-225°. uv max (ethanol): 249-250, 280-282, 311 nm (log ε 4.69, 3.80, 3.82). One gram dissolves in about 40 ml water. Sol in alcohol and chloroform. Practically insol in ether. pH of 0.05 molar soln 3.9; pH of 2% aq soln 3.3. LD_{50} in mice, rats (mg/kg): 27.5, 20 i.v.; 150, 370 s.c. (Levis).

Nitrite. [132-40-1] $C_{20}H_{21}NO_4 \cdot HNO_2$. Light yellow, crystalline powder. Slightly soluble in water or alcohol; freely sol in chloroform, acetone.

THERAP CAT: Vasodilator (cerebral).

7020. Papaya. Papaw; Carica; melon tree. Fruit of *Carica papaya* L., *Caricaceae. Habit.* Tropical America and Asia, Florida. *Constit.* Papain, the dried and purified latex of the fruit; carpaine; carposide (a glucoside).

USE: Manufacture of papain.

7021. Papuamine. [112455-84-2] (4aS,5aR,10aR,11aS,-15aR,15bS,16E,18E,19aS,19bR)-2,3,4,4a,5,5a,6,7,8,9,10,10a,11,-11a,12,13,14,15,15a,15b,19a,19b-Docosahydro-1H-diindeno[2,1-f:1',2'-1][1,5]diazacyclotridecine. $C_{25}H_{40}N_2$; mol wt 368.60. C 81.46%, H 10.94%, N 7.60%. Alkaloid originally isolated from *Haliclona sp.*, a marine sponge found in Papua, New Guinea. Exhibits antifungal and antimicrobial activity. Isoln and characterization: B. J. Baker *et al., J. Am. Chem. Soc.* **110**, 965 (1988). Total synthesis: R. M. Borzilleri *et al., ibid.* **116**, 9789 (1994).

White solid, mp 167.5-169°. $[\alpha]_D$ −150° (c = 1.5 in methanol).

Dihydrochloride. [112347-74-7] White solid, mp 230° (dec). $[\alpha]_D$ −140° (c = 1.3 in CH_3OH). uv max (methanol): 241 nm (ε 3000).

7022. Parabanic Acid. [120-89-8] Imidazolidinetrione; imidazoletrione; oxalylurea. $C_3H_2N_2O_3$; mol wt 114.06. C 31.59%, H 1.77%, N 24.56%, O 42.08%. Prepd by the condensation of urea with diethyl oxalate in a methanol soln of sodium methoxide: Murray, *Org. Synth.* **37**, 71 (1957).

Crystals, mp about 230°; also stated as 243° with decomposition. Sublimes at 100°. Soluble in about 20 parts water, in alcohol. Its salts are unstable.

7023. Paraffin. Paraffin wax; hard paraffin. A mixture of solid hydrocarbons having the general formula C_nH_{2n+2}, obtained from petroleum.

Colorless or white, somewhat translucent, odorless mass; greasy feel; burns with a luminous flame. d about 0.90. mp 50-57°; also available with higher and lower melting ranges. Insol in water or alcohol. Sol in benzene, chloroform, ether, carbon disulfide, oils; miscible when melted with wax, spermaceti, fats.

Caution: Potential symptoms of overexposure to fumes are irritation of eyes, skin, respiratory system; discomfort and nausea. See *NIOSH Pocket Guide to Chemical Hazards* (DHHS/NIOSH 97-140, 1997) p 240.

USE: For raising mp of ointments. Manuf paraffin paper and candles (so-called wax paper or candles); for fixing drawings, etc., on muslin; water-proofing wood, cork, paper, leather; manuf varnishes; to render wooden vessels impermeable to water or alcohol; in lubricants; to cover food products; in floor polishes, cosmetics, electrical insulators; for extracting perfumes from flowers. Pharmaceutic aid (stiffening agent).

7024. Paraffin Chlorinated. Chlorcosane; Cereclor. Prepared by chlorinating a liquid paraffin. Contains about 50% Cl.

Light yellow to amber, thick, oily liq; odorless and stable in air. d 1.00-1.07. Insol in water. Slightly sol in alc; miscible with benzene, chloroform, ether, carbon tetrachloride.

Caution: Chlorinated paraffins (C_{12}, 60% Cl) are reasonably anticipated to be human carcinogens: *Report on Carcinogens, Eleventh Edition* (PB2005-104914, 2004) p III-51.

USE: As solvent for dichloramine-T, dissolving about 8%.

7025. Paraformaldehyde. [30525-89-4] Polyoxymethylene; Paraform; Formagene. Also erroneously referred to as *Triformol* or as *"trioxymethylene"*. Polymerized formaldehyde, $(CH_2O)_n$. Obtained by concentrating formaldehyde soln. Use in mummifying dental pulp: I. Curson, *Br. Dent. J.* **121**, 519 (1966); P. Hobson, *ibid.* **128**, 275 (1970).

White, cryst powder, having an odor of formaldehyde. Slowly sol in cold, more readily in hot water, with evolution of formaldehyde; insol in alcohol, ether; sol in fixed alkali hydroxide solns. *Keep tightly closed.*

USE: For disinfecting sickrooms, clothing, linen, and sickroom utensils. Active ingredient of contraceptive creams. Also used as fumigant; in dentistry; in manuf synthetic resins and artificial horn or ivory.

7026. Paraherquamide. [77392-58-6] (−)-Paraherquamide; [1'R-(1'α,5'aβ,7'β,8'aβ,9'aβ)]-2',3',8'a,9'-tetrahydro-1'-hydroxy-1',4,4,8',8',11'-hexamethylspiro[4H,8H-[1,4]dioxepino[2,3-g]indole-8,7'(8'H)-[5H,6H-5a,9a](iminomethano)[1H]cyclopent[f]indolizine]-9,10'(10H)-dione. $C_{28}H_{35}N_3O_5$; mol wt 493.59. C 68.13%, H 7.15%, N 8.51%, O 16.21%. Oxindole alkaloid fungal metabolite. Isolation from *Penicillium paraherquei* and structure: M. Yamazaki *et al., Maikotokishin* **10**, 27 (1980), *C.A.* **95**, 19321p (1981); M. Yamazaki *et al., Tetrahedron Lett.* **22**, 135 (1981); from *P. charlesii* and nematocidal activity: J. G. Ondeyka *et al., J. Antibiot.* **43**, 1375 (1990). Absolute stereochemistry: T. A. Blizzard *et al., J. Org. Chem.* **54**, 2657 (1989). Approach to synthesis: R. M. Williams, T. D. Cushing, *Tetrahedron Lett.* **31**, 6325 (1990). Anthelmintic activity in sheep: W. L. Shoop *et al., J. Parasitol.* **76**, 349 (1990); in dogs: W. L. Shoop *et al., Vet.*

Parasitol. **40,** 339 (1991). Toxicity: *eidem, Am. J. Vet. Res.* **53,** 2032 (1992). Mode of action: J. M. Schaeffer *et al., Biochem. Pharmacol.* **43,** 679 (1992).

Colorless prisms, mp 244-247° (dec). $[\alpha]_D^{22}$ −28° (c = 0.43 in methanol). uv max (ethanol): 226, 260, 290nm (ε 32400, 6100, 1600). Sol in methanol, ethyl acetate, acetone, DMSO. Practically insol in water.

THERAP CAT (VET): Anthelmintic.

7027. Paraldehyde. [123-63-7] 2,4,6-Trimethyl-1,3,5-tri-oxane; paracetaldehyde; Paral. $C_6H_{12}O_3$; mol wt 132.16. C 54.53%, H 9.15%, O 36.32%. A polymer of acetaldehyde. Prepd by the polymerization of acetaldehyde catalyzed by HCl and H_2SO_4 at medium to high temp: Kekulé, Zincke, *Ann.* **162,** 125 (1872); Baer, Mahan, **US 2864827** (1958 to Phillips). Toxicity data: Figot *et al., Acta Pharmacol. Toxicol.* **8,** 290 (1952).

Liquid, characteristic aromatic odor and warm, but disagreeable taste. d_{25}^{25} ~0.994. bp ~124°. mp 12°. n_D^{20} 1.4049. Sol in 8 parts water at 25°, in 17 parts boiling water; miscible with alc, chloroform, ether, oils. Gives acetaldehyde on heating with dil HCl or on warming with several drops concd H_2SO_4. LD_{50} orally in rats: 1.65 g/kg (Figot).

Note: This is a controlled substance (depressant): **21 CFR,** 1308.14.

USE: Manuf organic compounds.

THERAP CAT: Sedative; hypnotic.

7028. Paramethadione. [115-67-3] 5-Ethyl-3,5-dimethyl-2,4-oxazolidinedione; 3,5-dimethyl-5-ethyloxazolidine-2,4-dione; Paradione. $C_7H_{11}NO_3$; mol wt 157.17. C 53.49%, H 7.05%, N 8.91%, O 30.54%. Prepn: Spielman, **US 2575693** (1951 to Abbott).

Liquid. Fruity, esterlike odor. d_4^{25} 1.1180-1.1240. n_D^{25} 1.449. Slightly sol in water. Freely sol in alcohol, benzene, chloroform, ether.

THERAP CAT: Anticonvulsant.

7029. Paramethasone. [53-33-8] (6α,11β,16α)-6-Fluoro-11,17,21-trihydroxy-16-methylpregna-1,4-diene-3,20-dione; 6α-fluoro-16α-methylprednisolone; 16α-methyl-6α-fluoroprednisolone. $C_{22}H_{29}FO_5$; mol wt 392.46. C 67.33%, H 7.45%, F 4.84%, O 20.38%. Prepn: Edwards *et al., J. Am. Chem. Soc.* **82,** 2318 (1960). Toxicity study: E. I. Goldenthal, *Toxicol. Appl. Pharmacol.* **18,** 185 (1971).

21-Acetate. [1597-82-6] Cortidene; Dilar; Dillar; Haldrate; Haldrone; Metilar; Monocortin; Paramezone; Syntecort; Stemex. $C_{24}H_{31}FO_6$; mol wt 434.50. mp 228-241° (dec). $[\alpha]_D$ +85°. uv max (ethanol): 243 nm (log ε 4.16). Sol in ethanol, acetone; slightly sol in water. LD_{50} i.p. in female rats: 392±23 mg/kg (Goldenthal).

Disodium phosphate. Soludillar.

Mixture of 21-acetate and disodium phosphate. Triniol.

THERAP CAT: Glucocorticoid.

7030. Paraoxon. [311-45-5] Phosphoric acid diethyl 4-nitrophenyl ester; diethyl *p*-nitrophenyl phosphate; phosphacol; E-600; Ester 25; Eticol; Fosfakol; Mintacol; Miotisal A; Soluglaucit. $C_{10}H_{14}NO_6P$; mol wt 275.20. C 43.64%, H 5.13%, N 5.09%, O 34.88%, P 11.26%. Prepd by the action of diethyl chlorophosphate on sodium *p*-nitrophenolate or by nitration of diethyl phenyl phosphate: Schrader, *BIOS Final Report* **No. 714,** 52 (1947); *Angew. Chem.* **62,** 471 (1950); **CH 257649** (1949); Fagerlind *et al., Sven. Farm. Tidskr.* **56,** 303, *C.A.* **46,** 9259. Physical properties: E. F. Williams, *Ind. Eng. Chem.* **43,** 950 (1951). Formation from parathion on citrus foliage and soil surface: R. C. Spear *et al., J. Agric. Food Chem.* **23,** 808 (1975); W. F. Spencer *et al., Bull. Environ. Contam. Toxicol.* **14,** 265 (1975). Toxicity study: W. R. Pickering, J. C. Malone, *Biochem. Pharmacol.* **16,** 1183 (1967). Brief review: G. Schrader, *Die Entwicklung neuer insektizider Phosphorsäure-Ester* (Verlag Chemie, Weinheim, 1963) pp 259-272.

Oily liq. Slight odor. *Poisonous!* $bp_{1.0}$ 169-170°. d_4^{25} 1.2683. n_D^{20} 1.50959. uv max: 274 nm (ε 8.9×10³). Soly in water (25°): 2400 μg/mL. Freely sol in ether, other organic solvents. Aq solns are stable up to pH 7. Roughly 300 times more stable to hydrolysis than tetraethyl pyrophosphate. The uncatalyzed reaction with water is very small and the overall velocity constant is K = 0.52[OH] + 1×10^{-6} min⁻¹. *See:* Coates, *Ann. Appl. Biol.* **36,** 158 (1949). LD_{50} orally in rats: 1.8 mg/kg (Pickering, Malone).

Caution: Cholinesterase inhibitor. For symptoms *see* Parathion.

USE: Insecticide.

7031. Paraquat. [4685-14-7] 1,1'-Dimethyl-4,4'-bipyridinium; *N,N'*-dimethyl-γ,γ'-dipyridylium; methyl viologen (2+). $[C_{12}H_{14}N_2]^{2+}$. Non-selective contact herbicide. Prepn of dichloride and bismethyl sulfate derivs: L. Michaelis, E. S. Hill, *J. Am. Chem. Soc.* **55,** 1481 (1933); R. C. Brian *et al.,* **GB 813531** (1959 to ICI). Activity: R. F. Homer *et al., J. Sci. Food Agric.* **11,** 309 (1960); A. D. Dodge, *Endeavour* **30,** 130 (1971). Degradation: A. Calderbank, P. Slade, *Outlook Agric.* **5,** 55 (1966); A. Calderbank, T. E. Tomlinson, *ibid.* 252 (1968); A. Calderbank, *ibid.* **6,** 128 (1970). Toxicity studies: D. G. Clark *et al., Br. J. Ind. Med.* **23,** 126 (1966); D. M. Conning *et al., Br. Med. Bull.* **25,** 245 (1969); R. D. Kimbrough, T. B. Gaines, *Toxicol. Appl. Pharmacol.* **17,** 679 (1970); J. F. Dasta, *Am. J. Hosp. Pharm.* **35,** 1368 (1978). Controversial use on marijuana plants: R. J. Smith, *Science* **199,** 861 (1978). *Review:* A. A. Akhavein, D. L. Linscott, *Residue Rev.* **23,** 97-145 (1968); A. Calderbank, P. Slade in *Herbicides: Chemistry, Degradation and Mode of Action,* P. C. Kearney, D. Kaufman, Eds. (Dekker, New York, 2nd ed., 1976) pp 501-540.

Dichloride. [1910-42-5] PP-148; Gramoxone. $C_{12}H_{14}Cl_2N_2$; mol wt 257.16. Colorless crystals, mp 300° (dec). Very sol in water, slightly sol in lower alcohols. Insol in hydrocarbons. Hydrolyzed by alkali. Inactivated by inert clays and anionic surfactants. Corrosive to metal. Non-volatile. Normal potential at 30°: −0.446 volts. LD_{50} orally in rats: 125 mg/kg (Conning).

Bismethyl sulfate. [2074-50-2] Paraquat I; PP-910. $C_{14}H_{20}$-$N_2O_8S_2$; mol wt 408.45. Yellow solid. LD_{50} orally in male rats: 100 mg/kg (Kimbrough, Gaines).

Caution: Potential symptoms of overexposure to paraquat dichloride are irritation of eyes, skin, nose, throat, respiratory system; epistaxis; dermatitis; fingernail damage; irritation of GI tract; heart, liver, kidney damage. *See NIOSH Pocket Guide to Chemical Hazards* (DHHS/NIOSH 97-140, 1997) p 240.

USE: Herbicide. Dichloride as biological oxidation-reduction indicator.

7032. Parasorbic Acid. [10048-32-5] (6*S*)-5,6-Dihydro-6-methyl-2*H*-pyran-2-one; 5-hydroxy-2-hexenoic acid lactone; δ-$\Delta^{\alpha,\beta}$-hexenolactone; 2-hexen-5,1-olide; sorbic oil. $C_6H_8O_2$; mol wt 112.13. C 64.27%, H 7.19%, O 28.54%. The sole constituent of "Vogelbeeröl", an oil obtained by steam distillation of the acidified juice of the ripe berries of the mountain ash, *Sorbus aucuparia* L., *Rosaceae:* Hofmann, *Ann.* **110,** 129 (1859); Doebner, *Ber.* **27,** 344 (1894); Kuhn, Jerchel, *Ber.* **76,** 413 (1943). Structure: *eidem, ibid.* Synthesis: Haynes, Jones, *J. Chem. Soc.* **1946,** 954; Lamberti *et al., Recl. Trav. Chim. Pays-Bas* **86,** 504 (1967). Pharmacology and acute toxicity: H. J. Meyer, R. Kretzschmar, *Arzneim.-Forsch.* **19,** 617 (1969).

Oily liquid, sweet aromatic odor. bp_{14} 104-105°; bp_{22} 119-123°. n_D^{25} 1.4682. d_4^{18} 1.079. $[\alpha]_D^{18}$ +49.3°; $[\alpha]_D^{19}$ +210° (c = 2 in alc). Soluble in water; freely sol in alcohol, ether. Aq solns are neutral and turn acid on storage. LD_{50} in mice (mg/kg): 420 ±6.3 i.p.; 195 ±13.6 i.v. (Meyer, Kretzschmar).

7033. Parathion. [56-38-2] Phosphorothioic acid *O,O*-diethyl *O*-(4-nitrophenyl) ester; *O,O*-diethyl *O-p*-nitrophenyl phosphorothioate; diethyl-*p*-nitrophenyl monothiophosphate; DNTP; S.N.P.; E-605; AC-3422; ENT-15108; Alkron; Folidol; Fostox E; Rhodiatox; Thiophos. $C_{10}H_{14}NO_5PS$; mol wt 291.26. C 41.24%, H 4.84%, N 4.81%, O 27.47%, P 10.63%, S 11.01%. Non-systemic contact and stomach insecticide and acaricide; cholinesterase inhibitor. Prepn: Thurston, *FIAT Report* **949** (1946); Coates, Topley, *BIOS Final Report* **1808** (1947). See also Fletcher *et al., J. Am. Chem. Soc.* **70,** 3943 (1948). Conversion to toxic oxygen analogs: *See* Paraoxon. Toxicity study: T. B. Gaines, *Toxicol. Appl. Pharmacol.* **14,** 515 (1969). *Review:* Hall in *Adv. Chem. Ser.* **1,** entitled "Agricultural Control Chemicals" (ACS, Washington DC, 1950) p 150. Review of industrial syntheses: Chadwick, Watt, "Thiophosphates" in *Phosphorus and Its Compounds* vol. 2, J. R. Van Wazer, Ed. (Interscience, New York, 1961) pp 1257-1262. Review of distribution, transport and fate in the environment: M. S. Mulla *et al., Residue Rev.* **81,** 1-159 (1981); of carcinogenic risk: *IARC Monographs* **30,** 153-181 (1983).

Pale yellow liquid. bp_{760} 375°; $bp_{0.6}$ 157-162°. mp 6°. n_D^{25} 1.5370. d_4^{25} 1.26. Vapor pressure at 20°: 3.78×10^{-5} mm Hg. Surface tension at 25°: 39.2 dynes/cm. Viscosity (25°): 15.30 cP. Absorption spectra: Williams, *Ind. Eng. Chem.* **43,** 950 (1951). Freely sol in alcohols, esters, ethers, ketones, aromatic hydrocarbons. Practically insol in water (20 ppm), petr ether, kerosene, and the usual spray oils. Incompatible with substances having a pH higher than 7.5. LD_{50} in female, male rats (mg/kg): 3.6, 13 orally; 6.8, 21 dermally (Gaines).

Caution: Potential symptoms of overexposure are miosis; rhinorrhea; headache; tight chest, wheezing, laryngeal spasm, salivation and cyanosis; anorexia, nausea, vomiting, abdominal cramps and diarrhea; sweating; muscle fasciculation, weakness and paralysis; giddiness, confusion and ataxia; convulsions, coma; low blood pressure; cardiac irregularities; skin, eye and respiratory system irritation. *See NIOSH Pocket Guide to Chemical Hazards* (DHHS/NIOSH 97-140, 1997) p 240; *Clinical Toxicology of Commercial Products*, R. E. Gosselin *et al.,* Eds. (Williams & Wilkins, Baltimore, 5th ed., 1984) Section III, pp 336-343.

USE: Insecticide; acaricide.

7034. Parathyroid Hormone. [9002-64-6] Parathormone; PTH. Regulatory factor in the homeostatic control of calcium and phosphate metabolism, its principal sites of activity being the skeleton, kidneys, and gastrointestinal tract. Prime function is to raise plasma calcium concns. Acts synergistically with vitamin D_3, *q.v.* except in the kidneys where the latter causes phosphate retention. Secretion from the parathyroid gland varies inversely with serum Ca^{2+} concentrations, unlike calcitonin, *q.v.,* which is secreted in direct proportion to serum calcium levels. Structure consists of a single-chain polypeptide of 84 amino acid residues. Sequence varies slightly among mammalian species. Sequence of bovine PTH: Niall *et al., Z. Physiol. Chem.* **351,** 1586 (1970); Brewer, Ronan, *Proc. Natl. Acad. Sci. USA* **67,** 1862 (1970). Sequence of porcine PTH: O'Riordan *et al., Proc. R. Soc. Med.* **64,** 1263 (1971). Isoln of human PTH from parathyroid adenomas: O'Riordan *et al., Endocrinology* **89,** 234 (1971). Fragment exhibiting full biological activity consists of about 35 amino acid residues from the *N*-terminal: Potts *et al.* in *Parathyroid Hormone and Thyrocalcitonin (Calcitonin)*, R. V. Talmage, L. F. Belanger, Eds. (Excerpta Medica, New York, 1968) p 44; *see* in entirety for review and special studies. Synthesis of active bovine fragment: Potts *et al., Proc. Natl. Acad. Sci. USA* **68,** 63 (1971); of human PTH (1-38): S. Funakoshi *et al., Pept. Chem.* **18,** 223 (1980). Reviews of early literature: Potts *et al., Recent Prog. Horm. Res.* **22,** 101 (1966); Arnaud *et al., Annu. Rev. Physiol.* **29,** 349 (1967). *Reviews:* Behrens, Grinnan, *Annu. Rev. Biochem.* **38,** 83 (1969); Auerbach *et al., Recent Prog. Horm. Res.* **28,** 353 (1972); Parsons, Potts, "Physiology and Chemistry of Parathyroid Hormone" in *Clinics in Endocrinology and Metabolism* I. MacIntyre, Ed. (Saunders, Philadelphia, 1972) pp 33-78. Biosynthetic review: J. F. Habener *et al., Recent Prog. Horm. Res.* **33,** 249 (1977).

Note: Aqueous solns of the active principles of bovine parathyroid gland have been used under the names: *Parathorm, Parathor-mone, Paroidin.*

THERAP CAT: Blood calcium regulator.

7035. Parbendazole. [14255-87-9] (5-Butyl-1*H*-benzimidazol-2-yl)carbamic acid methyl ester; methyl 5-butyl-2-benzimidazolecarbamate; 5-butyl-2-(carbomethoxyamino)benzimidazole; SKF-29044; Helmatac; Verminum; Worm Guard. $C_{13}H_{17}N_3O_2$; mol wt 247.29. C 63.14%, H 6.93%, N 16.99%, O 12.94%. Prepd from 4-butyl-*o*-phenylenediamine and carbomethoxycyanamide: Actor *et al., Nature* **215,** 321 (1967); **GB 1123317** and Stedman; Actor, Pagano, **US 3480642; US 3574845** (1968, 1969, 1971 all to SKF). Activity: Ostmann, Scheidy, *Prog. Antimicrob. Anticancer Chemother., Proc. 6th Int. Congr. Chemother.* **1,** 159 (1970). Identification of metabolites: Dunn *et al., J. Med. Chem.* **16,** 996 (1973).

Crystals from aq ethanol, mp 225-227° (dec). uv max (95% ethanol/1*N* HCl): 282, 288 nm (ε 16200, 20000). Practically insol in water. LD_{50} in mice, rats (g/kg): >4 orally, both species (Actor).

THERAP CAT (VET): Anthelmintic.

7036. Parecoxib. [198470-84-7] *N*-[[4-(5-Methyl-3-phenyl-4-isoxazolyl)phenyl]sulfonyl]propanamide. $C_{19}H_{18}N_2O_4S$; mol wt 370.42. C 61.61%, H 4.90%, N 7.56%, O 17.28%, S

8.66%. Injectable prodrug of valdecoxib, *q.v.*, a selective cyclo-oxygenase-2 (COX-2) inhibitor. Prepn: J. J. Talley *et al.,* **WO 9738986;** *eidem,* **US 5932598** (1997, 1999 both to Searle); *eidem, J. Med. Chem.* **43,** 1661 (2000). Clinical pharmacokinetics: A. Karim *et al., J. Clin. Pharmacol.* **41,** 1111 (2001). Pharmacological profile: S. S. V. Padi *et al., Eur. J. Pharmacol.* **491,** 69 (2004). Clinical evaluation in post-surgical pain: N. A. Nussmeier *et al., Anesthesiology* **104,** 518 (2006). Comparison of GI effects with ketorolac: R. R. Stoltz *et al., Am. J. Gastroenterol.* **97,** 65 (2002). Review of pharmacology and clinical experience: S. M. Cheer, K. L. Goa, *Drugs* **61,** 1133-1141 (2001).

mp 148.9-151°.

Sodium salt. [198470-85-8] SC-69124A; Dynastat. $C_{19}H_{17}N_2NaO_4S$; mol wt 392.40. mp 271.5-272.7°.

THERAP CAT: Anti-inflammatory; analgesic.

7037. Pareira. Pareira brava. Dried root of *Chondodendron platiphyllum* (A. St. Hil.) Miers, *C. microphyllum* (Eichl.) Mold., and *C. tomentosum* Ruiz et Pavon, *Menispermaceae. Habit.* Brazil. *Constit.* Bebeerine, chondrodine, fatty acids, tannin.

THERAP CAT: Diuretic, anti-infective (urinary).

7038. Pargyline. [555-57-7] *N*-Methyl-*N*-2-propynylbenzenemethanamine; *N*-methyl-*N*-2-propynylbenzylamine; *N*-benzyl-*N*-methyl-2-propynylamine; *N*-methyl-*N*-propargylbenzylamine; MO-911; A-19120; Eudatin; Supirdyl. $C_{11}H_{13}N$; mol wt 159.23. C 82.97%, H 8.23%, N 8.80%. Monoamine oxidase inhibitor. Prepd from propargyl bromide and benzylmethylamine: **GB 906245;** Martin, **US 3155584** (1962 and 1964, both to Abbott). Activity as a glucuronyl transferase inducer: Yeh, Mitchell, *Experientia* **28,** 298 (1972).

Free base, bp$_{11}$ 96-97°.

Hydrochloride. [306-07-0] Eutonyl. $C_{11}H_{13}N \cdot HCl$; mol wt 195.69. Crystals from ethanol + ether, mp 154-155°. Readily sol in water. Aq solns are unstable.

THERAP CAT: Antihypertensive.

7039. Paricalcitol. [131918-61-1] $(1\alpha,3\beta,7E,22E)$-19-Nor-9,10-secoergosta-5,7,22-triene-1,3,25-triol; 19-nor-1α,25-dihydroxyvitamin D_2; Zemplar. $C_{27}H_{44}O_3$; mol wt 416.64. C 77.83%, H 10.64%, O 11.52%. Synthetic analog of vitamin D. Prepn: H. F. DeLuca *et al.,* **EP 387077;** *eidem,* **US 5587497** (1990, 1996 both to Wisconsin Alum. Res.). Series of articles on pharmacology and clinical experience in secondary hyperparathyroidism: *Am. J. Kidney Dis.* **32,** Suppl. 2, S40-S66 (1998). *Review:* M. M. Goldenberg, *Clin. Ther.* **21,** 432-441 (1999).

THERAP CAT: Antihyperparathyroid.

7040. Park Nucleotide. [18836-50-5] (L-lysyl form); [120010-32-4] (pimelate form). UDP-MurNAc-L-Ala-γ-D-Glu-X-D-Ala-D-Ala; stem peptide. Glyco-pentapeptide; key intermediate in bacterial cell-wall synthesis. Residue 3 varies from species to species; it is usually L-Lys in Gram positive bacteria and mesodiaminopimelate in Gram negative bacteria. Identification and isolation from *Staphylococcus aureus:* J. T. Park, *J. Biol. Chem.* **194,** 885 (1952). Total synthesis: S. A. Hitchcock *et al., J. Am. Chem. Soc.* **120,** 1916 (1998); of radioiodinated analog: C. N. Eid *et al., J. Labelled Compd. Radiopharm.* **41,** 705 (1998).

L-Lysyl Form

USE: Tool for antibacterial screen development.

7041. Paromomycin. [7542-37-2] *O*-2-Amino-2-deoxy-α-D-glucopyranosyl-(1 → 4)-*O*-[*O*-2,6-diamino-2,6-dideoxy-β-L-idopyranosyl-(1 → 3)-β-D-ribofuranosyl-(1 → 5)]-2-deoxy-D-streptamine; *O*-2,6-diamino-2,6-dideoxy-β-L-idopyranosyl-(1 → 3)-*O*-β-D-ribofuranosyl-(1 → 5)-*O*-[2-amino-2-deoxy-α-D-glucopyranosyl-(1 → 4)]-2-deoxystreptamine; paromomycin I; amminosidin; catenulin; crestomycin; estomycin; hydroxymycin; monomycin A; neomycin E; paucimycin; R-400. $C_{23}H_{45}N_5O_{14}$; mol wt 615.63. C 44.87%, H 7.37%, N 11.38%, O 36.38%. Oligosaccharide-type antibiotic isolated from various *Streptomyces.* From *S. rimosus* forma *paromomycinus:* Frohardt *et al.,* **US 2916485** (1959 to Parke, Davis); from *S. catenulae:* Davisson, Finlay, **US 2895876** (1959 to Pfizer); from *S. chrestomyceticus:* Canevazzi, Scotti, *G. Microbiol.* **7,** 242 (1959); Arcamone *et al., ibid.* 251. Identity of paromomycin, catenulin, hydroxymycin and aminosidine: Schillings, Schaffner, *Antimicrob. Agents Chemother.* **1961,** 274. Structure: Haskell *et al., J. Am. Chem. Soc.* **81,** 3480, 3482 (1959); Rinehart *et al., ibid.* **84,** 3218 (1962); Hichens, Rinehart, *ibid.* **85,** 1547 (1963). Probable identity with *zygomycin A:* Horii, *J. Antibiot.* **15A,** 187 (1962). Identity with monomycin A: Konstantinova, Brazhnikova, *Antibiotiki* **10**(1), 34 (1965); with neomycin E: Hessler *et al., J. Antibiot.* **23,** 464 (1970). Toxicity data: A. DiMarco, C. Bertazzoli, *Antibiot. Chemother.* **11,** 2 (1963). Review of antimicrobial activity: G. L. Coffey *et al., ibid.* **9,** 730 (1959). Review of pharmacology: Gasparini, Pignatelli, *Veterinaria (Milan)* **21,** 7 (1972).

Amorphous white powder. $[\alpha]_D^{25}$ +65 ±3°. Soluble in water; moderately sol in methanol; sparingly sol in abs ethanol. LD$_{50}$ in rats, mice (mg/kg): >1625, >2275 orally; >650, 423 s.c.; 156, 90 i.v. (Coffey).

Sulfate. [1263-89-4] 1600 Antibiotic; FI-5853; Aminoxidin; Aminosidine; Farmiglucin; Farminosidin; Gabbromicina; Gabbromycin; Gabbroral; Humagel; Humatin; Pargonyl; Paramicina; Paricina; Sinosid. $C_{23}H_{45}N_5O_{14}.H_2SO_4$; mol wt 713.71. $[\alpha]_D^{25}$ +50.5° (c = 1.5 in water pH 6). LD_{50} in mice (mg/kg): ~15,000 orally; 700 s.c.; 110 i.v. (Di Marco, Bertazzoli).

THERAP CAT: Antibacterial; antiamebic.

THERAP CAT (VET): Antiamebic.

7042. Parotin. [1392-81-0] Salivary gland hormone; protein of globulin nature having an isoelectric point of pH 5.7. Produced by the parotid gland. Structure studies: Ito *et al., Endocrinol. Jpn.* **12**, 249 (1966); Shimasaki *et al., ibid.* **14**, 11 (1967). Generally acts on the mesenchymal tissues, esp the hard and connective tissues, to promote their development and growth. Also has a protein-anabolic function. Hypocalcemic and leukocytosis-promoting activities: Ito *et al., ibid.* **12**, 298 (1966). *Reviews:* Yosoji Ito, *J. Jpn. Biochem. Soc.* **25**, 143-164 (1953); *Ann. N.Y. Acad. Sci.* **85**, art. 1, 228-310 (1960).

7043. Paroxetine. [61869-08-7] (3S-*trans*)-3-[(1,3-Benzodioxol-5-yloxy)methyl]-4-(4-fluorophenyl)piperidine; (−)-*trans*-4-(*p*-fluorophenyl)-3-[[3,4-(methylenedioxy)phenoxy]methyl]piperidine; FG-7051; BRL-29060. $C_{19}H_{20}FNO_3$; mol wt 329.37. C 69.28%, H 6.12%, F 5.77%, N 4.25%, O 14.57%. Selective serotonin (5-HT) reuptake inhibitor (SSRI). Prepn: J. A. Christensen, R. F. Squires, **DE 2404113**; *eidem*, **US 3912743**; **US 4007196** (1974, 1975, 1977 all to Ferrosan); of crystalline hydrochloride hemihydrate: R. D. B. Barnes *et al.*, **EP 223403**; **US 4721723** (1987, 1988 both to Beecham). Characterization of serotonin inhibition: J. Buus Lassen, *Eur. J. Pharmacol.* **47**, 351 (1978). Binding to serotonin transporter complex: E. Habert *et al., ibid.* **118**, 107 (1985). Clinical pharmacokinetics: J. Lund *et al., Acta Pharmacol. Toxicol.* **51**, 351 (1982). HPLC determn in plasma: M. A. Brett *et al., J. Chromatogr.* **419**, 438 (1987). Clinical trial in obsessive-compulsive disorder: J. Zohar *et al., Br. J. Psychiatry* **169**, 468 (1996); in social phobia: M. B. Stein *et al., J. Am. Med. Assoc.* **280**, 708 (1998). Review of pharmacology and clinical use in depression: K. L. Dechant, S. P. Clissold, *Drugs* **41**, 225-253 (1991); of clinical experience: D. Dunner, R. Kumar, *Pharmacopsychiatry* **31**, 89-101 (1998); of use in generalized social anxiety disorder: M. Van Ameringen *et al., Expert Opin. Pharmacother.* **6**, 819-830 (2005).

Hydrochloride hemihydrate. [110429-35-1]; [78246-49-8] (hydrochloride). Aropax; Deroxat; Paxil; Seroxat. $C_{19}H_{20}FNO_3$.-$HCl.\frac{1}{2}H_2O$; mol wt 374.83. Crystals, mp 129-131°. Soly in water: 5.4 mg/ml.

Maleate. [64006-44-6] Crystals from ethanol-ether, mp 136-138°. $[\alpha]_D$ −87° (c = 5 in ethanol). LD_{50} in mice (mg/kg): 845 s.c.; 500 orally (Christensen, Squires, 1977).

THERAP CAT: Antidepressant; antiobsessional.

7044. Paroxypropione. [70-70-2] 1-(4-Hydroxyphenyl)-1-propanone; 4'-hydroxypropiophenone; *p*-hydroxypropiophenone; paraoxypropiophenone; *p*-propionylphenol; ethyl *p*-hydroxyphenyl ketone; P.O.P.; B-360; H-365; Profenone; Frenantol; Frenohypon; Paroxon; Possipione; Hypostat. $C_9H_{10}O_2$; mol wt 150.17. C 71.98%, H 6.71%, O 21.31%. Prepn: Perkin, *J. Chem. Soc.* **55**, 546 (1889); Goldzweig, Kaiser, *J. Prakt. Chem.* [2] **43**, 86 (1891); Cox, *J. Am. Chem. Soc.* **49**, 1028 (1927); Hartung *et al., ibid.* **53**, 4153 (1931); Farinholt, *ibid.* **55**, 3386 (1933); Miller, Hartung, *Org. Synth.* **coll. vol. II** (1943) p 543. Derivatives: Buu-Hoi, *Rec. Trav. Chim.* **68**, 759 (1949).

Needles or prisms from water. mp 149°. One part dissolves in 2896 parts of water at 15°, in 30 parts at 100°. Freely sol in alcohol or ether.

THERAP CAT: Pituitary gonadotropic hormone inhibitor.

7045. Parsalmide. [30653-83-9] 5-Amino-N-butyl-2-(2-propynyloxy)benzamide; 5-amino-O-propynyl-N-butylsalicylamide; 2-propargyloxy-5-amino-N-butylbenzamide; MY-41-6; Sinovial; Parsal. $C_{14}H_{18}N_2O_2$; mol wt 246.30. C 68.27%, H 7.37%, N 11.37%, O 12.99%. Prepn: B. Gradnik *et al.*, **DE 2029991**; *eidem*, **US 3739030** (1970, 1973 both to Soc. Etude Recher. Sci. Med.). Synthesis and pharmacology: A. Pedrazzoli *et al., Boll. Chim. Farm.* **115**, 125 (1976). Effect on gastric secretion in laboratory animals: G. Bertaccini *et al., Farmaco Ed. Prat.* **34**, 482 (1979). Inhibition of platelet aggregation: R. Fantasia *et al., Arzneim.-Forsch.* **32**, 1312 (1982). Clinical comparison with phenylbutazone, *q.v.*, in management of joint pain: A. Bajardi, S. Fantato, *Minerva Med.* **67**, 3371 (1976); S. Menci *et al., ibid.* 3403. Series of articles on anti-inflammatory activity, pharmacology and toxicology: *Boll. Chim. Farm.* **115**, 135-230 (1976), *C.A.* **85**, 13981-13986 (1976).

Crystals from ethanol, mp 83-85°. pKa (aq soln, 20°) 4.6 ±0.03. uv max (abs alcohol): 220 ±1, 327 ±2 nm; (water, pH 2): 284 nm (log ε 3.39); (water, pH 8.5): 313 nm (log ε 3.40). Very soluble in alcohol, chloroform, acetone, ethyl acetate, dioxane; slightly sol in water. Practically insol in petr ether, cyclohexane.

THERAP CAT: Anti-inflammatory; analgesic.

7046. Parsley. Biennial herb, *Petroselinum crispum* (Mill.) Nyman, *Umbelliferae*; also known as *P. sativum* Hoffm. *Habit.* Mediterranean region; cultivated worldwide. *Constit.* Flavonoids, esp. apiin, luteolin; furocoumarins, incl. bergapten (0.02%), oxypeucedanin (0.01%); volatile oils (0.05% in leaf, 2-7% in seed); fixed oil, protein, carbohydrate, vitamins, esp. A and C. GC-MS determn of volatile components: M. G. López *et al., J. Agric. Food Chem.* **47**, 3292 (1999). Comprehensive description and medicinal uses: J. Barnes *et al., Herbal Medicines* (Pharmaceutical Press, London, 2nd Ed., 2002) pp 365-367.

Parsley seed oil. [8000-68-8] Obtained by steam distillation of the ripe seed. *Constit.* Apiole, myristicin, tetramethoxyallylbenzene. Review of toxicology: *Food Cosmet. Toxicol.* **15**, 897-898 (1975). Yellow to light brown liquid with herbal-like odor. d_{25}^{25} 1.040-1.080. n_D^{20} 1.513-1.522. Saponification value between 2 and 10. Acid value not more than 4.0. Very slightly sol in water; slightly sol in propylene glycol; sol in 6 vols 80% alcohol. Insol in glycerin.

USE: Flavoring in foods and pharmaceuticals.

THERAP CAT: In treatment of urinary tract inflammation and kidney stones; carminative.

7047. Parthenin. [508-59-8] [3aS-(3aα,6β,6aα,9aβ,9bα)]-3,3a,4,5,6,6a,9a,9b-Octahydro-6a-hydroxy-6,9a-dimethyl-3-methyleneazuleno[4,5-b]furan-2,9-dione; 1,6β-dihydroxy-4-oxo-10αH-ambrosa-2,11(13)-dien-12-oic acid γ-lactone; parthenicin. $C_{15}H_{18}O_4$; mol wt 262.30. C 68.68%, H 6.92%, O 24.40%. From herb of *Parthenium hysterophorus* L., *Compositae*. Parthenin is the substance largely responsible for the allergic contact dermatitis caused by *P. hysterophorus*. Isoln: Arny, *Am. J. Pharm.* **69**, 169 (1897). Isoln and structure: Herz *et al., Tetrahedron Lett.* **1961**, 82; Herz *et al., J. Am. Chem. Soc.* **84**, 2601 (1962). Abs config: Emerson *et al., Tetrahedron Lett.* **1966**, 6151. Total synthesis of (±)-form: P. Kok *et al., Bull. Soc. Chim. Belg.* **87,** 615 (1978); C. H. Heathcock *et al., J. Am. Chem. Soc.* **104,** 6081 (1982).

Crystals from water, mp 163-166°. $[\alpha]_D^{25}$ +7.02° (c = 2.71 in chloroform). uv max: 215, 340 nm (ε 15,100; 22). Practically insol in water. Sol in alcohol, chloroform, ether, ethyl acetate.

7048. Parthenolide. [20554-84-1] (1a*R*,4*E*,7a*S*,10a*S*,-10b*S*)-2,3,6,7,7a,8,10a,10b-Octahydro-1a,5-dimethyl-8-methyl-eneoxireno[9,10]cyclodeca[1,2-*b*]furan-9(1a*H*)-one; 4,5α-epoxy-6β-hydroxy-germacra-1(10),11(13)-dien-12-oic acid γ-lactone. $C_{15}H_{20}O_3$; mol wt 248.32. C 72.55%, H 8.12%, O 19.33%. Sesquiterpene lactone found in feverfew, *q.v.,* and in other plants. Isolation from *Chrysanthemum parthenium* (L.) Bernh. *Compositae* and characterization: V. Herout *et al., Chem. Ind. (London)* **1959,** 1069; M. Soucek *et al., Collect. Czech. Chem. Commun.* **26,** 803 (1961); from *Magnolia grandiflora* L., *Magnoliaceae:* F. S. El-Feraly, Y.-M. Chan, *J. Pharm. Sci.* **67,** 347 (1978). Revised structure and spectral analysis: T. R. Govindachari *et al., Tetrahedron* **21,** 1509 (1965). Absolute configuration: A. S. Bawdekar *et al., Tetrahedron Lett.* **1966,** 1225. Crystal structure: A. Quick, D. Rogers, *J. Chem. Soc. Perkin Trans. 2* **4,** 465 (1976). HPLC determn: D. Strack *et al., Z. Naturforsch.* **35,** 915 (1980). Cytotoxicity: K.-H. Lee *et al., Cancer Res.* **31,** 1649 (1971); L. A. J. O'Neill *et al., Br. J. Clin. Pharmacol.* **23,** 81 (1987).

Colorless plates, mp 115-116°. $[\alpha]_D^{20}$ −81.4° (c = 1.04 in chloroform); $[\alpha]_D^{22}$ −71.4° (c = 0.220 in CH_2Cl_2). uv max: 214 nm (log ε 4.22).

7049. Partricin. [11096-49-4] Ayfactin; SPA-S-132; Heptaene macrolide antibiotic complex produced by *Streptomyces aureofaciens* NRRL 3878. Isoln: T. Bruzzese, R. Ferrari, **US 3773925** (1973 to SPA). Recovery and purification process: S. Magnaghi *et al.,* **GB 1462442** (1977 to SPA), *C.A.* **87,** 66588a (1977). *In vitro* activity: W. Ritzerfeld, *Farmaco Ed. Sci.* **27,** 235 (1972); G. A. Meloni *et al., ibid.* **34,** 183 (1979). Use in treatment of benign prostatic hypertrophy: T. Bruzzese, L. Ferrari, **US 4237117** (1980 to SPA). Separation, characterization and structure of components A and B: R. C. Tweit *et al., J. Antibiot.* **35,** 997 (1982).

Partricin A   R′ = CH_3
Partricin B   R′ = H

Partricin A. $C_{59}H_{86}N_2O_{19}\cdot 4H_2O$; mol wt 1199.38. Greenish-yellow powder, mp >300° (dec). uv max (75% methanol in DMF): 232, 240, 247, 288, 342, 358, 378, 400 nm (ε 33476, 32237, 22936,

15493, 58282, 76883, 102308, 89280). pKa's (70% aq DMF): 6.07, 8.91.

Partricin B. $C_{58}H_{84}N_2O_{19}\cdot 2\frac{1}{2}H_2O$; mol wt 1158.33. Brownish-yellow powder, mp >300° (dec). uv max (75% methanol in DMF): 232, 240, 247, 288, 342, 358, 378, 400 nm (ε 34761, 32826, 23174, 20594, 50207, 73392, 100425, 87558). pKa's (70% aq DMF): 6.31, 8.95. $[\alpha]_D^{26}$ +87.2° (c = 0.06 in DMF).

Complex. Amphoteric yellow crystals. uv max (ethanol): 401, 379, 359, 341 nm. Sol in DMF, DMSO, dimethyl acetamide, pyridine. Practically insol in water, common organic solvents. LD_{50} in mice (mg/kg): 300 orally; 0.5 i.p. (Bruzzese).

Methyl ester *see* Mepartricin.

7050. Parvaquone. [4042-30-2] 2-Cyclohexyl-3-hydroxy-1,4-naphthalenedione; 2-cyclohexyl-3-hydroxy-1,4-naphthoquinone; 2-hydroxy-3-cyclohexyl-1,4-naphthoquinone; BW-993C; Clexon. $C_{16}H_{16}O_3$; mol wt 256.30. C 74.98%, H 6.29%, O 18.73%. Prepn: L. F. Fieser, *J. Am. Chem. Soc.* **70,** 3165 (1948); L. F. Fieser, M. T. Leffler, **US 2553648** (1951 to Research Corp.). Antimalarial activity: L. F. Fieser, A. P. Richardson, *J. Am. Chem. Soc.* **70,** 3156 (1948). Electron transport inhibition: A. L. Tappel, *Biochem. Pharmacol.* **3,** 289 (1960); by uncoupling: J. L. Howland, *Biochim. Biophys. Acta* **131,** 247 (1967). *In vitro* and *in vivo* antiprotozoal activity: A. T. Hudson *et al., Parasitology* **90,** 45 (1985). Bioassay in serum: N. McHardy, J. Mercer, *Kenya Vet.* **8**(2), 9 (1984). Treatment of East Coast fever in cattle: T. T. Dolan *et al., Vet. Parasitol.* **15,** 103 (1984); of *Theileria annulata* in calves: N. McHardy, D. W. Morgan, *Res. Vet. Sci.* **39,** 1 (1985). Field comparison of antitheilarial activity with buparvaquone, *q.v.:* N. McHardy *et al., ibid.* 39.

Bright yellow needles, mp 135-136°.
THERAP CAT (VET): Antiprotozoal (Theileria).

7051. Passiflora. Passion flower; passion vine; May pops. Dried flowering and fruiting tops of *Passiflora incarnata* L., *Passifloraceae. Habit.* Southeastern U.S. *Constit.* Harman.
THERAP CAT: Sedative, analgesic.

7052. Patchouli Alcohol. [5986-55-0] [1*R*-(1α,4β,4aα,6β,-8aα)]-Octahydro-4,8a,9,9-tetramethyl-1,6-methanonaphthalen-1(2*H*)-ol; patchouli camphor. $C_{15}H_{26}O$; mol wt 222.37. C 81.02%, H 11.79%, O 7.19%. A tricyclic sesquiterpene alcohol isolated from oil of patchouli: Gadamer, Amenomiya, *Arch. Pharm.* **241,** 39 (1903). Proposed structure: Treibs, *Ann.* **564,** 141 (1949). Revised structure: Dobler *et al., Proc. Chem. Soc. London* **1963,** 383. Structural studies: Büchi *et al., J. Am. Chem. Soc.* **78,** 1262 (1956); **83,** 927 (1961); **84,** 3205 (1962); **86,** 4438 (1964). Synthesis of *dl*-form: Danishevsky, Dumas, *Chem. Commun.* **1968,** 1287; Mirrington, Schmalzl, *J. Org. Chem.* **37,** 2871 (1972); K. Yamada *et al., Tetrahedron* **35,** 293 (1979). Stereoselective total synthesis of racemic form: F. Näf, G. Ohloff, *Helv. Chim. Acta* **57,** 1868 (1974); of natural, racemic and (+)-forms: F. Näf *et al., ibid.* **64,** 1387 (1981). *Review:* Walker, *Manuf. Chem. Aerosol News* **39,** no. 7, 27 (1968).

Large crystals (hexagonal-trapezohedral) from the higher boiling fractions of oil of patchouli or from petr ether, mp 56°. mp (racemate) 39-40° (Danishevsky, Dumas); also reported as mp 46-47° (Mirrington, Schmalzl). bp_8 140°. d_4^{20} 1.0284. $[\alpha]_D^{20}$ −97.4° (c = 24 in chloroform). n_D^{65} 1.5029. Practically insol in water. Sol in alcohol, ether, common organic solvents.

7053. Patulin. [149-29-1] 4-Hydroxy-4*H*-furo[3,2-*c*]pyran-2(6*H*)-one; clavacin; clavatin; claviformin; expansine; mycoin C₃; penicidin; C₇H₆O₄; mol wt 154.12. C 54.55%, H 3.92%, O 41.52%. An antibiotic derived from the metabolites of a number of fungi, e.g., *Aspergillus clavatus, A. claviforme, A. giganteus, A. terreus, Penicillium patulum, P. expansum, P. melinii, P. leucopus, P. urticae* and *Gymnoascus* spp. Isoln and antibacterial activity: Birkinshaw *et al., Lancet* **245,** 625 (1943); Birkinshaw, Michael, **US 2417584** (1947 to Therap. Res. Corp. of Great Britain); cf. Waksman *et al., Science* **96,** 202 (1942); Brack, *Helv. Chim. Acta* **30,** 1 (1947); Norstadt, McCalla, *Appl. Microbiol.* **17,** 193 (1969). Structure: Birkinshaw, *loc. cit.;* Bergel *et al., J. Chem. Soc.* **1944,** 415; Woodward, Singh, *J. Am. Chem. Soc.* **71,** 758 (1949); Shemyakin, Khokhlov, *Dokl. Akad. Nauk SSSR* **75,** 47 (1950). Synthesis: Woodward, Singh, *J. Am. Chem. Soc.* **72,** 1428 (1950). Biosynthesis: Bu'Lock, Ryan, *Proc. Chem. Soc. London* **1958,** 222; Tanenbaum, Bassett, *J. Biol. Chem.* **234,** 1861 (1959). Inhibition of K⁺ ion uptake in erythrocytes: Kahn, *J. Pharmacol. Exp. Ther.* **121,** 234 (1957). Physicochemical data: A. E. Pohland *et al., Pure Appl. Chem.* **54,** 2219 (1982). Has carcinogenic activity attributable to α,β-unsaturation together with an external conjugated double bond attached to 4 position of the γ-lactone ring: Dickens, *Br. Med. Bull.* **20,** 96 (1964). Toxicity: R. Kinosita, T. Shikata, "On Toxic Moldy Rice" in *Mycotoxins in Foodstuffs,* G. N. Wogan, Ed. (The M.I.T. Press, Cambridge, 1965) pp 117-119. Review and evaluation of studies of carcinogenic action in laboratory animals: *IARC Monographs* **10,** 205-210 (1976). *Review:* Ciegler *et al.,* "Patulin, Penicillic Acid and Other Carcinogenic Lactones" in *Microbial Toxins* **vol. VI,** A. Ciegler *et al.,* Eds. (Academic Press, New York, 1971) p 409-414.

Compact prisms or thick plates from ether or chloroform, mp 111.0°; also reported as 105-108° (Pohland). [α]$_D^{21}$ −6.2° (chloroform). uv max: 276.5 nm (Bergel). Sol in water and the common organic solvents except petr ether; very sol in ethyl or amyl acetate. Unstable in alkali with loss of biological activity. LD₅₀ s.c. in mice: 10-15 mg/kg (Kinosita, Shikata).

Acetylpatulin. C₉H₈O₅. Prisms from 50% alcohol, mp 118-120°.

7054. Pavoninins. Shark repellent compounds isolated from the defense secretion of the Pacific sole, *Pardachirus pavoninus.* Series of ichthyotoxic and hemolytic steroid amine glycosides; pavoninin-5 is the most abundant. Isoln, structure determn and evaluation of pavoninins 1-6 as shark repellents: K. Tachibana *et al., Science* **226,** 703 (1984); and ¹³C- and ¹H-NMR studies: *eidem, Tetrahedron* **41,** 1027 (1985). Synthesis of pavoninin-1: Y. Ohnishi, K. Tachibana, *Bioorg. Med. Chem.* **5,** 2251 (1997); of pavoninin-4: J. R. Williams *et al., J. Org. Chem.* **70,** 10732 (2005).

Pavoninin-5

Pavoninin-1. [94426-01-4] (7α,25*R*)-7-[[2-(Acetylamino)-2-deoxy-β-D-glucopyranosyl]oxy]-26-(acetyloxy)cholest-4-en-3-one. C₃₇H₅₉NO₉; mol wt 661.87. [α]$_D^{20}$ +19° (c = 1.1 in chloroform). uv max (methanol): 244 nm (Log ε 4.1).

Pavoninin-4. [94359-66-7] (3α,5α,15α,25*R*)-26-(Acetyloxy)-3-hydroxycholestan-15-yl 2-(acetylamino)-2-deoxy-β-D-glucopyra-

noside. C₃₇H₆₃NO₉; mol wt 665.90. White solid, mp 134-136°. [α]$_D^{20}$ +28° (c = 0.4 in ethanol).

Pavoninin-5. [94480-49-6] (3β,15α,25*R*)-26-(Acetyloxy)-3-hydroxycholest-5-en-15-yl 2-(acetylamino)-2-deoxy-β-D-glucopyranoside. C₃₇H₆₁NO₉; mol wt 663.88. Sol in ethyl acetate. [α]$_D^{29}$ +21° (c = 0.7 in ethanol).

7055. Pazufloxacin. [127045-41-4] (3*S*)-10-(1-Aminocyclopropyl)-9-fluoro-2,3-dihydro-3-methyl-7-oxo-7*H*-pyrido[1,2,3-*de*]-1,4-benzoxazine-6-carboxylic acid; T-3761. C₁₆H₁₅FN₂O₄; mol wt 318.30. C 60.37%, H 4.75%, F 5.97%, N 8.80%, O 20.11%. Fluorinated quinolone. Prepn: H. Narita *et al.,* **DE 3913245;** *eidem,* **US 4990508** (1989, 1991 both to Toyama). Synthesis: Y. Todo *et al., Chem. Pharm. Bull.* **42,** 2569 (1994). Antimicrobial activity: Y. Fukuoka *et al., Antimicrob. Agents Chemother.* **37,** 384 (1993).

Crystals, mp 269-271.5°. [α]$_D^{25}$ −88.0° (c = 0.5 in 0.05*N* aq NaOH). LD₅₀ i.v. in male mice: >500 mg/kg (Todo).

Methanesulfonate. [163680-77-1] Pazufloxacin mesylate; T-3762. C₁₆H₁₅FN₂O₄·CH₃SO₃H; mol wt 414.41. Colorless prisms, mp 258-259°(dec). [α]$_D^{20}$ −64.2° (c = 1 in 1.0*N* NaOH). Soly (25°) in water >200 mg/ml.

THERAP CAT: Antibacterial.

7056. PBN. [3376-24-7] 2-Methyl-*N*-(phenylmethylene)-2-propanamine *N*-oxide; benzylidene-*tert*-butylamine oxide; *N*-tert-butyl-α-phenylnitrone. C₁₁H₁₅NO; mol wt 177.24. C 74.54%, H 8.53%, N 7.90%, O 9.03%. Spin trapping agent for short-lived radicals in biological systems. Prepn: W. D. Emmons, *J. Am. Chem. Soc.* **79,** 5739 (1957); R. W. Murray *et al., J. Org. Chem.* **61,** 8099 (1996). Effects on ischemia in brain: J. W. Phillis, C. Clough-Helfman, *Med. Sci. Res.* **18,** 403 (1990); K. Pahlmark, B. K. Siesjö, *Acta Physiol. Scand.* **157,** 41 (1996). Review of chemical properties and biological applications: G. Chen *et al.* in *The Oxygen Paradox, PBN and Its Applications in Biology,* K. J. A. Davies, F. Ursini, Eds. (Cleup Press, Italy, 1995) pp. 789-800.

Crystals, mp 72-74°. Stored at ambient temperature, it is stable for one year unopened. Sensitive to light, especially in solution. Easily sol in medium polar organic solvents such as methanol, ethanol, acetonitrile, toluene, benzene and chloroform. Soly: 2.9% (water); 2.3% (saline); >5% (chloroform). uv max (ethanol): 293.5, 224 nm (ε 17700, 7240); (CH₃CN): 298 nm (ε 17716).

USE: Spin trap reagent for carbon- or oxygen- or nitrogen-centered free radicals.

7057. Peach Oil, Expressed. Persic oil. Fixed oil from seed of *Prunus persica* (L.) Stokes and allied spp., *Rosaceae.*

Light yellow liquid; closely resembles expressed oil of almond. d$_{15}^{15}$ 0.917-0.921. Solidif not above −15°. n$_D^{40}$ 1.464-1.465. Sapon no. 189-193. Iodine no. 100-110. Acid no. about 8. Sol in chloroform, ether, petr ether, slightly sol in alcohol.

USE: Emollient.

7058. Peanut. Groundnut; earthnut. Ripe, underground pods with seeds of *Arachis hypogaea* L., *Leguminosae. Habit.* Parana River Valley in Paraguay, Brazil and Argentina. Cultivated in the reasonably warm regions of all continents, e.g., through the southern U.S.A. *Composition:* pericarp (shell) 21-29%, episperm (skin) 1.95-3.2%, kernel (+ germ) 71-75%. Botanically the peanut is kin to peas and beans, but its constituents are more like those of true nuts. *Constit.* of kernels (roasted with skin): proteins 26.2%, oil 48.7%, water 1.8%, carbohydrates 20.6%, ash 2.7%. The chief proteins are arachin (25% in oil-free meal) and conarchin (8%). Both are globulins of different solv: Johns, Jones, *J. Biol. Chem.* **28**, 77 (1916). The vitamin content of peanuts is moderate, the largest portion being in the episperm. Trace mineral content of kernels: iron 20 mg/kg; manganese 8.51 mg/kg; copper 6.8 mg/kg; zinc 16 mg/kg. *Reviews:* J. Adam, *Les Plantes a Matiere Grasse*, **vol. 3**, *L'Arachide* (Paris, 1947); N. J. Morris, F. G. Dollear, *Abstract Bibliography of the Chemistry and Technology of Peanuts*, Southern Regional Res. Lab. (New Orleans, 1949); J. G. Woodruff, C. T. Young in *Kirk-Othmer Encyclopedia of Chemical Technology* **vol. 14** (Interscience, New York, 1967) p 122.

USE: In peanut butter, candy; as salted peanuts; for fodder and seeding; crushed for oil. Peanut proteins have been used to produce a fiber, **Sarelon**. The shells are used in the manuf of furfural, xylose, cellulose, plastics, mucilage, also in fertilizers and cattle feed.

7059. Peanut Oil. Arachis oil; groundnut oil; earthnut oil; katchung oil. Prepd by pressing the shelled and skinned seeds of *Arachis hypogaea* L., *Leguminosae:* N. J. Morris, F. G. Dollear, *Abstract Bibliography of the Chemistry and Technology of Peanuts* (Southern Regional Res. Lab., New Orleans, 1949); E. W. Eckey, *Vegetable Fats and Oils* (Reinhold, New York, 1954). *Constits.* of cold pressed oil: glycerides of the following fatty acids: palmitic 8.3%, stearic 3.1%, arachidic 2.4%, behenic 3.1%, lignoceric 1.1%, oleic 56.0%, linoleic 26.0%. Traces of capric and lauric acids have been reported. Unsaponifiable matter 0.8% (includes tocopherols 0.022 to 0.059%, sterols 0.19 to 0.25%, squalene 0.027% and other hydrocarbons).

Greenish-yellow or almost colorless oil. Mild, pleasant odor; bland taste. d_{15}^{15} 0.917-0.921. d_{25}^{25} 0.910-0.915. Clouds at low room temp. Solidifies at ~-5°. A.S.T.M. cloud point +4.5°; A.S.T.M. pour point +1°. Titer 26 to 32°. Flash pt 540°F (283°C); ignition temp 833°F (443°C). n_D^{25} 1.466-1.470; n_D^{40} 1.4605-1.4645. Acid value 0.08-6; saponification value 188-195; iodine value 84-102; thiocyanogen value 67-73; hydroxyl value 2.5-9.5; Reichert-Meissl value 0.2-1.0; Polenske value 0.2-0.7. Very slowly thickens and becomes rancid on prolonged exposure to air. Miscible with ether, petr ether, chloroform, carbon disulfide. Sol in benzene, carbon tetrachloride, oils; very slightly sol in alc.

USE: Edible oil: for salad oil as is; in hydrogenated state as shortening, in mayonnaise, in confections. For the manuf of margarine, soaps, paints. In pharmacy as vehicle for i.m. medication, in the laboratory as heat transfer medium in melting point apparatus. Pharmaceutic aid (solvent).

THERAP CAT (VET): Has been used in control of pasture bloat.

7060. Pearlman's Catalyst. [12135-22-7] Palladium hydroxide (Pd(OH)₂); palladium hydroxide on carbon. H₂O₂Pd; mol wt 140.43. H 1.44%, O 22.79%, Pd 75.78%. Pd(OH)₂/C. Commercial product contains 20 wt % Pd(OH)₂ on carbon. Prepn: W. M. Pearlman, *Tetrahedron Lett.* **8**, 1663 (1967); and catalytic activity study: R. J. Card *et al., J. Catal.* **79**, 13 (1983). Catalytic applications in debenzylating amines: R. C. Bernotas, R. V. Cube, *Synth. Commun.* **20**, 1209 (1990); in Nef-type reactions: T. Capecchi *et al., J. Chem. Soc. Perkin Trans. 1* **2000**, 2681; in Pd-catalyzed coupling reactions: Y. Mori, M. Seki, *J. Org. Chem.* **68**, 1571 (2003); in oxidation of silyl enol ethers: J.-Q. Yu *et al., Org. Lett.* **7**, 1415 (2005).

USE: Nonpyrophoric catalyst for hydrogenolysis of benzyl-nitrogen and benzyl-oxygen bonds.

7061. Pebulate. [1114-71-2] Butylethylcarbamothioic acid *S*-propyl ester; *S*-propyl butylethylthiocarbamate; propyl-*n*-butylthiolcarbamate; PEBC; Stauffer 2061; Tillam. C₁₀H₂₁NOS; mol wt 203.34. C 59.07%, H 10.41%, N 6.89%, O 7.87%, S 15.77%. Prepn: Campbell, Klingman, **US 2983747** (1961 to Stauffer). Toxicity data: G. W. Bailey, J. L. White, *Residue Rev.* **10**, 97 (1965).

Liquid, bp₂₀ 142°. n_D^{30} 1.4752. d_4^{30} 0.9458. Slightly sol in water; miscible with acetone, benzene, isopropanol, methanol, xylene. LD₅₀ orally in rats: 1.12 g/kg (Bailey, White).

USE: Selective herbicide.

7062. Pecilocin. [19504-77-9] 1-[(2E,4E,6E,8R)-8-Hydroxy-6-methyl-1-oxo-2,4,6-dodecatrienyl]-2-pyrrolidinone; Supral; Variotin. C₁₇H₂₅NO₃; mol wt 291.39. C 70.07%, H 8.65%, N 4.81%, O 16.47%. Antifungal antibiotic isolated from *Paecilomyces varioti* Bainier var. *antibioticus:* S. Takeuchi *et al., J. Antibiot.* **12A**, 109, 195 (1959); Sumiki *et al.,* **GB 866425** (1961 to Japan. Antibiot. Res. Assoc. and Nippon Kayaku). Structure: S. Takeuchi *et al., J. Antibiot.* **17A**, 267 (1964). Stereochemistry: S. Takeuchi, H. Yonehara, *Tetrahedron Lett.* **1966**, 5197. Revised structure and stereochemistry (E,Z,E to E,E,E): *eidem, J. Antibiot.* **22**, 179 (1969). Synthesis of the *dl*-form: A. Ishida, T. Mukaiyama, *Chem. Lett.* **1977**, 467; *eidem, Bull. Chem. Soc. Jpn.* **51**, 2077 (1978).

Neutral oil with ester-like odor. Does not show definite boiling or dec pt. $[\alpha]_D^{28}$ -5.68° (methanol). Freely sol in methanol, ethanol, acetone, ethyl acetate, benzene, ether, chloroform, pyridine, dioxane, acetic acid; slightly sol in water, petr ether, ligroin. uv max (methanol): *ca.* 318, 324 nm (E₁cm^1% 1198). Unstable and gradually loses antifungal activity in desiccator, though it is fairly stable in organic solvents. Unstable under alkaline conditions.

Monohydrate. Needles from ethyl acetate + petr ether, mp 41.5-42.5°. uv max: 320 nm (ε 46,000).

THERAP CAT: Antifungal.

7063. Pectin. [9000-69-5] Polysaccharide substance present in cell walls of all plant tissues which functions as an intercellular cementing material. One of the richest sources of pectin is lemon or orange rind which contains about 30% of this polysaccharide. Occurs naturally as the partial methyl ester of α-(1 → 4) linked D-polygalacturonate sequences interrupted with (1 → 2)-L-rhamnose residues. Neutral sugars: D-galactose, L-arabinose, D-xylose and L-fucose form side chains on the pectin molecule. Structure studies: D. A. Rees, A. W. Wight, *J. Chem. Soc. B* **1971**, 1366. Secondary and tertiary structure in solution and in gels: D. A. Rees, E. J. Welsh, *Angew. Chem. Int. Ed.* **16**, 214 (1977). Review and bibliography: Towle, Christensen, in *Industrial Gums*, R. L. Whistler, Ed. (Academic Press, New York, 2nd ed., 1973) p 429-461. Book: Z. I. Kertesz, *The Pectic Substances* (Interscience, New York, 1951).

Occurs as a coarse or fine powder, yellowish-white in color, practically odorless, and with a mucilaginous taste. Almost completely sol in 20 parts water, forming a viscous soln contg negatively charged, very much hydrated particles. Acid to litmus. Insol in alcohol or in diluted alcohol, and in other organic solvents. Dissolves more readily in water, if first moistened with alcohol, glycerol or sugar syrup, or if first mixed with 3 or more parts of sucrose. Stable under mildly acidic conditions; more strongly acidic or basic conditions cause depolymerization.

USE: In the preparation of jellies and similar food products: Owens *et al.,* "Factors Influencing Gelation with Pectin" in *Natural Plant Hydrocolloids, Advances in Chemistry Series* (ACS, Washington, 1954) pp 10-15.

THERAP CAT (VET): Antidiarrheal.

7064. Pectolinarigenin. [520-12-7] 5,7-Dihydroxy-6-methoxy-2-(4-methoxyphenyl)-4H-1-benzopyran-4-one; 5,7-dihydroxy-4',6-dimethoxyflavone; 6-methoxyacacetin; 6-hydroxypelargidenon-6,4'-dimethyl ether 1467. C₁₇H₁₄O₆; mol wt 314.29. C 64.97%, H 4.49%, O 30.54%. From leaves of *Linaria vulgaris* Mill., *Scrophulariaceae:* Schmid, Rumpel, *Monatsh. Chem.* **57**, 421 (1931); Merz, Wu, *Arch. Pharm.* **274**, 126 (1936). Structure: Schmid, Rumpel, *Monatsh. Chem.* **60**, 8 (1932). Synthesis: Wessely, Moser, *ibid.* **56**, 97 (1930); Zemplén, Farkas, *Ber.* **76**, 937 (1943); Murti, Seshadri, *Proc. Indian Acad. Sci.* **30A**, 78

(1949), *C.A.* **44,** 3987d (1950); Farkas, Strelisky, *Tetrahedron Lett.* **1970,** 187.

Yellow needles from methanol, mp 220-223°. uv max (methanol): 275, 335 nm. Sol in alcohol, acetone, ether, ethyl acetate. Practically insol in water, benzene, chloroform, petr ether.

Diacetate. $C_{21}H_{18}O_8$. Needles from 96% alcohol, mp 151°.

7-Rutinoside. Pectolinarin; neolinarin. $C_{29}H_{34}O_{15}$. From leaves of *L. vulgaris* Mill., *Scrophulariaceae:* Klobb, *Compt. Rend.* **145,** 331 (1907); Zemplén *et al., Ber.* **75,** 489 (1942); from *Cirsium oleraceum* Scop., *Compositae:* Wagner *et al., Arch. Pharm.* **293,** 1053 (1960). Structure: Zemplén, Bognár, *Ber.* **74,** 1818 (1941). Yellow crystals from methanol, mp 275°. uv max (methanol): 275, 330 nm (log ε 4.256, 4.365).

7065. Pederin. [27973-72-4] (1*S*)-2,6-Anhydro-3,5,7-trideoxy-1-*C*-[[(2*S*)-hydroxy[(2*R*,5*R*,6*R*)-tetrahydro-2-methoxy-5,6-dimethyl-4-methylene-2*H*-pyran-2-yl]acetyl]amino]-5,5-dimethyl-1,8,9-tri-*O*-methyl-D-*manno*-nonitol; *N*-[[6-(2,3-dimethoxypropyl)tetrahydro-4-hydroxy-5,5-dimethyl-2*H*-pyran-2-yl]methoxymethyl]tetrahydro-2-methoxy-5,6-dimethyl-4-methylene-2*H*-pyran-2-glycolamide; pederine; paederine. $C_{25}H_{45}NO_9$; mol wt 503.63. C 59.62%, H 9.01%, N 2.78%, O 28.59%. The toxic principle isolated from blister beetles, *Paederus fuscipes* Curt.: Pavan, Bo, *Physiol. Comp. Oecol.* **3,** 307 (1953), *C.A.* **48,** 10217g (1954); **GB 932875** (1963 to Farmitalia). Powerful inhibitor of protein biosynthesis and mitosis. Structure: Cardani *et al., Gazz. Chim. Ital.* **96,** 3 (1966). Revised structure: Matsumoto *et al., Tetrahedron Lett.* **1968,** 6297. Biosynthesis: Cardani *et al., ibid.* **1973,** 2815. Total synthesis: F. Matsuda *et al., Tetrahedron Lett.* **23,** 4043 (1982); **24,** 1277 (1983).

Crystals from hexane, benzene + hexane, ether + hexane. mp 112-112.5°. Slightly sol in water, hexane. Sol in methanol, ethanol, carbon disulfide, chloroform, carbon tetrachloride, benzene, and acids. Practically insol in petr ether, NH_4OH, NaOH.

Pseudopederin. [10352-73-5] *N*-[[6-(2,3-Dimethoxypropyl)tetrahydro-4-hydroxy-5,5-dimethyl-2*H*-pyran-2-yl]methoxymethyl]tetrahydro-α,2-dihydroxy-5,6-dimethyl-4-methylene-2*H*-pyran-2-acetamide; ψ-paederine; ψ-pederine; pseudopaederine. $C_{24}H_{43}NO_9$; mol wt 489.60. Isoln from blister beetles, *Paederus fuscipes:* Quilico *et al., Chem. Ind. (Milan)* **43,** 1434 (1961), *cf.* Cardani *et al., Tetrahedron Lett.* **1965,** 2537; **GB 932875** (1963 to Farmitalia). Crystals from benzene, mp 133°.

7066. Pefloxacin. [70458-92-3] 1-Ethyl-6-fluoro-1,4-dihydro-7-(4-methyl-1-piperazinyl)-4-oxo-3-quinolinecarboxylic acid; pefloxacine; EU-5306; 1589RB; AM-725. $C_{17}H_{20}FN_3O_3$; mol wt 333.36. C 61.25%, H 6.05%, F 5.70%, N 12.61%, O 14.40%. Fluorinated quinolone antibacterial; analog of norfloxacin, *q.v.* Prepn: M. Pesson, **DE 2840910**; *idem,* **US 4292317** (1979, 1981 to Roger Bellon/Dainippon). Pharmacology and antibacterial spectrum: Y. Goueffon *et al., C.R. Seances Acad. Sci. Ser. 3* **292,** 37 (1981). Pharmacokinetics: J. Barre *et al., J. Pharm. Sci.* **73,** 1379 (1984). Bioavailability and metabolism: A. Contrepois *et al., J. Antimicrob. Chemother.* **14,** 51 (1984); G. Montay *et al., Antimicrob. Agents Chemother.* **25,** 463 (1984). HPLC determn in urine and plasma: *idem, J. Chromatogr.* **272,** 359 (1983). Adsorptive stripping voltammetry determn in bulk form, tablets and serum: A. M.

Beltagi, *J. Pharm. Biomed. Anal.* **31,** 1079 (2003). Symposium on pharmacokinetics, clinical efficacy and safety: *J. Antimicrob. Chemother.* **26,** Suppl. B, 1-229 (1990).

Crystals from DMF, mp 270-272° (dec). Slightly sol in water; sol in alkaline and acidic solutions. LD_{50} in mice (mg/kg): 225 i.v., 1000 orally; in rats (g/kg): 1.5 i.p., 2.5 orally (Goueffon).

Methanesulfonate dihydrate. [149676-40-4]; [70458-95-6] (methanesulfonate). Pefloxacin mesylate; 1589mRB; Peflacine; Peflox. $C_{17}H_{20}FN_3O_3 \cdot CH_3SO_3H.2H_2O$; mol wt 465.49.

THERAP CAT: Antibacterial.

7067. Pefurazoate. [101903-30-4] 2-[(2-Furanylmethyl)(1-*H*-imidazol-1-ylcarbonyl)amino]butanoic acid 4-pentenyl ester; pent-4-enyl-*N*-furfuryl-*N*-imidazol-1-ylcarbonyl-DL-homoalaninate; UR-0003; UHF-8615; Healthied. $C_{18}H_{23}N_3O_4$; mol wt 345.39. C 62.59%, H 6.71%, N 12.17%, O 18.53%. Ergosterol biosynthesis inhibitor which acts as a rice seed disinfectant. Prepn: Y. Hirota *et al.,* **JP 60260572**; *eidem,* **CA 1324608** (1985, 1993 both to Ube); and fungicidal activity: M. Takenaka *et al., J. Pestic. Sci.* **18,** 15 (1993). Soil degradation and adsorption: *idem et al.,* **16,** 631 (1991). Metabolism in rice seedlings: S. Sakai *et al., ibid.* **18,** 217 (1993). Review of properties and use as disinfectant: M. Takenaka, I. Yamane, *Jpn. Pestic. Inf.* **57,** 33-36 (1990); T. Wada *et al., J. Pestic. Sci.* **24,** 238-240 (1999).

Pale brownish liquid, dec at 235°. $n_D^{24.4}$ 1.5140. d_4^{20} 1.152. Vapor pressure (23°): 6.48×10^{-4} Pa. Soly at 25° (g/l): water 0.443; *n*-Hexane 12.0; cyclohexane 36.9; DMSO >1000; ethanol >1000; acetone >1000; acetonitrile >1000; chloroform >1000; ethyl acetate >1000; toluene >1000. Log P (octanol/water): 3.00. LD_{50} in male, female rats, male, female mice (mg/kg): 981, 1051, 1299, 946 orally; in rats (mg/kg): >2000 dermally. LC_{50} in rats (mg/m³): >3450 by inhalation. LC_{50} (48 hr) in carp, rainbow trout, bluegill sunfish (ppm): 16.9, 4.0, 12.0 (Takenaka, 1990).

USE: Fungicide.

7068. Pegaptanib Sodium. [222716-86-1] PEG-t44-OMe; EYE-001; NX-1838; Macugen. 2′-Fluoropyrimidine RNA aptamer to human VEGF$_{165}$; composed of 28-mer oligonucleotide conjugated to 40 kDa polyethylene glycol moiety. Prepn: N. Janjic *et al.,* **WO 9818480**; *eidem,* **US 6168778** (1998, 2001 both to NeXstar Pharm.); and binding affinity studies: J. Ruckman *et al., J. Biol. Chem.* **273,** 20556 (1998). Inhibition of *in vitro* VEGF-mediated responses: C. Bell *et al., In Vitro Cell. Dev. Biol. Animal* **35,** 533 (1999). HPLC determn in plasma: C. E. Tucker *et al., J. Chromatogr. B* **732,** 203 (1999). Pharmacokinetics: D. W. Drolet *et al., Pharm. Res.* **17,** 1503 (2000). Pharmacology and clinical safety study: Eyetech Study Group, *Retina* **22,** 143 (2002). Clinical study in age-related macular degeneration: E. S. Gragoudas *et al., N. Engl. J. Med.* **351,** 2805 (2004). Review of development and therapeutic potential: S. A. Vinores, *Curr. Opin. Mol. Ther.* **5,** 673-679 (2003); of clinical experience and safety in macular degeneration: A. A. Moshfeghi, C. A. Puliafito, *Expert Opin. Invest. Drugs* **14,** 671-682 (2005).

THERAP CAT: In treatment of age-related macular degeneration and diabetic macular edema.

7069. Pegvisomant. [218620-50-9] Pegylated somatotropin [18-aspartic acid, 21-asparagine, 120-lysine, 167-asparagine, 168-alanine, 171-serine, 172-arginine, 174-serine, 179-threonine] (human); B2036-PEG; Somavert. Growth hormone receptor antagonist. Genetically engineered analog of human growth hormone conjugated to polyethylene glycol (PEG), *q.v.*, to improve bioavailability. Prepn: B. C. Cunningham *et al.*, **WO 9711178**; *eidem*, **US 5849535** (1997, 1998 both to Genentech). Receptor binding and effects of pegylation on structure and function: R. J. M. Ross *et al. J. Clin. Endocrinol. Metab.* **86**, 1716 (2001). Clinical pharmacology: M. O. Thorner *et al., ibid.* **84**, 2098 (1999). Clinical trial in acromegaly: P. J. Trainer *et al., N. Engl. J. Med.* **342**, 1171 (2000); A. J. van der Lely *et al., Lancet* **358**, 1754 (2001). Review of clinical experience: C. Parkinson, P. J. Trainer, *Expert Opin. Invest. Drugs* **10**, 1725-1735 (2001); of structure and function: S. Pradhananga *et al., J. Mol. Endocrinol.* **29**, 11-14 (2002); of preclinical and clinical development: V. Goffin, P. Touraine, *Curr. Opin. Invest. Drugs* **5**, 463-468 (2003).

THERAP CAT: In treatment of acromegaly.

7070. Pelargonic Acid. [112-05-0] Nonanoic acid; nonylic acid; nonoic acid. $C_9H_{18}O_2$; mol wt 158.24. C 68.31%, H 11.47%, O 20.22%. $CH_3(CH_2)_7COOH$. Occurs as an ester in oil of pelargonium: Redtenbacher, *Ann.* **59**, 41, 52, 54 (1846). Prepn from unsaturated hydrocarbons by the oxo process: Hill, **US 2815355** (1957 to Standard Oil of Indiana); from tall oil unsaturated fatty acids: Maggiolo, **US 2865937** (1958 to Welsbach); by oxidation of oleic acid: Mackenzie, Morgan, **US 2820046** (1958 to Celanese); from rice bran oil fatty acid: Mihara *et al.*, **US 3060211** (1962 to Toya Koatsu Ind.). Purification: Port, Riser, **US 2890230** (1959 to U.S.D.A.). Toxicity study: L. Orö, A. Wretlind, *Acta Pharmacol. Toxicol.* **18**, 141 (1961).

Colorless, oily liquid at ordinary temp; crystallizes when cooled; characteristic odor. d_4^{20} 0.907. mp 12.5°. bp_{756} 252-253°; bp_{14} 143-145°; $bp_{6.3}$ 132-133°. n_D^{20} 1.4330; n_D^{40} 1.4245. Practically insol in water. Sol in alcohol, chloroform, ether. LD_{50} i.v. in mice: 224±4.6 mg/kg (Orö, Wretlind).

Caution: Strong irritant.

USE: In the production of hydrotropic salts (hydrotropic salts form aq solns which dissolve sparingly sol substances to a greater extent than water); in the manuf of lacquers, plastics.

7071. Pelargonidin. [134-04-3] 3,5,7-Trihydroxy-2-(4-hydroxyphenyl)-1-benzopyrylium chloride; 3,4′,5,7-tetrahydroxyflavylium chloride; 3,4′,5,7-tetrahydroxy-2-phenylbenzopyrylium chloride. $C_{15}H_{11}ClO_5$; mol wt 306.70. C 58.74%, H 3.62%, Cl 11.56%, O 26.08%. The aglucone of pelargonin: Willstätter, Bolton, *Ann.* **408**, 42 (1914). Synthesis: Malkin, Robinson, *J. Chem. Soc.* **127**, 1190 (1925); Robertson *et al.*, **1928**, 1533. Prepn from kaempferol: Mirza, Robinson, *Nature* **166**, 997 (1950); King, White, *J. Chem. Soc.* **1957**, 3901.

Reddish-brown prisms from 2% HCl or from alcoholic HCl. Not melted at 350°. Absorption max (ethanol + 0.01% HCl): 530 nm (ε 32,000). Sol in alcohol, methanol; moderately sol in water; slightly sol in chloroform.

3,5-Diglucoside. [17334-58-6] 3,5-Bis(β-D-glucopyranosyloxy)-7-hydroxy-2-(4-hydroxyphenyl)-1-benzopyrylium chloride; pelargonin; monardin; salvinin; punicin. $C_{27}H_{31}ClO_{15}$; mol wt 630.98. From flowers of *Pelargonium zonale* Ait. var. meteor, *Geraniaceae:* Willstätter, Bolton, *loc. cit.;* from scarlet roses: Harborne, *Experientia* **17**, 72 (1961). Identity with monardin and salvinin: Robinson, Todd, *J. Chem. Soc.* **1932**, 2488. Identity with punicin: Karrer, Widmer, *Helv. Chim. Acta* **10**, 67 (1927). Structure: Leon *et al., J. Chem. Soc.* **1931**, 2672. Red needles with green luster from methanol + HCl, dec 175-180°. $[\alpha]_D$ −291°. Absorption max (methanol + HCl): 269, 505 nm. Sol in water, alc.

3-Glucoside. [18466-51-8] 3-(β-D-Glucopyranosyloxy)-5,7-dihydroxy-2-(4-hydroxyphenyl)-1-benzopyrylium chloride; callistephin. $C_{21}H_{21}ClO_{10}$; mol wt 468.84. From purple-red aster *(Callistephus chinensis* (L.) Nees, *Compositae):* Willstätter, Burdick, *Ann.* **412**, 149 (1916); from strawberries: Sondheimer, Kertesz, *J. Am. Chem. Soc.* **70**, 3476 (1948). Structure and synthesis: Robertson, Robinson, *J. Chem. Soc.* **1928**, 1460. Dark brownish-red needles with bronze luster. Absorption max (ethanol + HCl): 515 nm (ε 13,000). Sol in water, methanol, ethanol, 0.5-7% aq HCl; moderately sol in 10% HCl.

7072. Pelletierine. [4396-01-4] 1-(2-Piperidinyl)-2-propanone; 2-acetonylpiperidine; punicine. $C_8H_{15}NO$; mol wt 141.21. C 68.04%, H 10.71%, N 9.92%, O 11.33%. From the rootbark of the pomegranate tree, *Punica granatum* L., *Punicaceae.* Isoln: Tanret, *Compt. Rend.* **86**, 1270 (1878). Structure: Gilman, Marion, *Bull. Soc. Chim. Fr.* **1961**, 1993; Drillien, Viel, *ibid.* **1963**, 2393. Abs config: H. C. Beyerman *et al., Rec. Trav. Chim.* **86**, 80 (1967). Synthesis: Anet *et al., Nature* **164**, 501 (1949); T. Nagasaka *et al., Heterocycles* **29**, 155 (1989).

Isopelletierine. [539-00-4] (±)-Pelletierine. Slightly colored oily liq; bp 195°; bp_{11} 102-107°. d_4^{20} 0.988. Sol in alc, ether, chloroform. One gram dissolves in 20 ml water. Should be stored under nitrogen.

Hydrochloride. [5984-61-2] $C_8H_{15}NO.HCl$. Crystals from alcohol + ether, mp 145°. Soluble in water and alcohol.

N-methylpelletierine. $C_9H_{17}NO$. Oily liquid. d_4^{20} 0.948. bp_{13} 96-98°. n_D^{20} 1.46737. Sol in water, petr ether.

Note: In the early literature the names pelletierine and isopelletierine were used interchangeably.

THERAP CAT: Anthelmintic (Cestodes).

7073. Pellitorine. [18836-52-7] (2*E*,4*E*)-*N*-(2-Methylpropyl)-2,4-decadienamide; (*E,E*)-*N*-isobutyl-2,4-decadienamide. $C_{14}H_{25}NO$; mol wt 223.35. C 75.29%, H 11.28%, N 6.27%, O 7.16%. Pungent principle isolated from *Anacyclus pyrethrum* DC., *Compositae:* J. M. Gulland, G. U. Hopton, *J. Chem. Soc.* **1930**, 6. Structure: M. Jacobson, *J. Am. Chem. Soc.* **71**, 366 (1949). Synthesis: *idem, ibid.* **75**, 2584 (1953); L. Crombie, *J. Chem. Soc.* **1955**, 1007; J. Tsuji *et al., Tetrahedron Lett.* **1977**, 1917; J. Nokami *et al., ibid.* **21**, 4455 (1980); T. Mandai *et al., Chem. Lett.* **1980**, 313. Stereoselective synthesis: R. Bloch, D. Hassangonzales, *Tetrahedron* **42**, 4975 (1986). Insecticidal activity: R. T. Lalonde *et al., J. Chem. Ecol.* **6**, 35 (1980).

Needles from petr ether. mp 90°. uv max (abs ethanol): 258 nm ($E_{1cm}^{1\%}$ 1330). Sol in organic solvents; sparingly sol in water. Practically insol in dil acid or alkalies.

7074. Pellotine. [83-14-7] 1,2,3,4-Tetrahydro-6,7-dimethoxy-1,2-dimethyl-8-isoquinolinol; *N*-methylanhalonidine; 8-hydroxy-6,7-dimethoxy-1,2-dimethyl-1,2,3,4-tetrahydroisoquinoline. $C_{13}H_{19}NO_3$; mol wt 237.29. C 65.80%, H 8.07%, N 5.90%, O 20.23%. From the mescal buttons (pellote) of *Lophophora williamsii* (Lemaire) Coult., *Cactaceae.* Structure: Späth *et al., Ber.* **65**, 1771 (1932). Synthesis: Brossi *et al., Helv. Chim. Acta* **47**, 2089 (1964); **49**, 403 (1966); Takido *et al., J. Pharm. Sci.* **59**, 271 (1970). Biosynthetic studies: Battersby *et al., Tetrahedron Lett.* **1967**, 563; **1968**, 6111.

Plates from petr ether, mp 112°. Alkaline reaction. Freely sol in alc, acetone, ether, chloroform; sparingly sol in water.

Hydrochloride. $C_{13}H_{19}NO_3 \cdot HCl$. Prisms, freely sol in water; sparingly in alcohol.

Hydriodide. $C_{13}H_{19}NO_3 \cdot HI$. Prisms, mp 130°, sol in water, alcohol, almost insol in ether.

7075. α-Peltatin. [568-53-6] [5R-(5α,5aβ,8aα)]-5,8,8a,9-Tetrahydro-10-hydroxy-5-(4-hydroxy-3,5-dimethoxyphenyl)-furo[3′,4′:6,7]naphtho[2,3-d]-1,3-dioxol-6(5aH)-one; 8-hydroxy-2-hydroxymethyl-6,7-methylenedioxy-4-(4′-hydroxy-3′,5′-dimethoxyphenyl)-1,2,3,4-tetrahydronaphthalene-3-carboxylic acid lactone. $C_{21}H_{20}O_8$; mol wt 400.38. C 63.00%, H 5.03%, O 31.97%. Exists as a glucoside in the rhizomes of *Podophyllum peltatum* L., *Berberidaceae*: von Wartburg *et al., Helv. Chim. Acta* **40**, 1331 (1957). Isoln from resin podophyllum: Hartwell, Detty, *J. Am. Chem. Soc.* **72**, 246 (1950).

Prismatic leaflets from abs ethanol. Begins to sinter at 236°. Dec 242-246°. $[\alpha]_D^{20} -124.8°$ (c = 0.5 in chloroform). Soly in water at 20°: ~30 mg/liter. Fairly sol in chloroform, hot ethanol, acetic acid, acetone, dilute caustic; less sol in benzene, ether, carbon tetrachloride, propylene glycol. Practically insol in petr ether.

α-Peltatin-β-D-glucoside. $C_{27}H_{30}O_{13}$. Prismatic needles from acetone, mp 168-171°. $[\alpha]_D^{20} -128.9°$ (c = 0.590 in methanol); $[\alpha]_D^{20} -174.4°$ (c = 0.579 in pyridine).
Caution: Irritates the skin.

7076. β-Peltatin. [518-29-6] [5R-(5α,5aβ,8aα)]-5,8,8a,9-Tetrahydro-10-hydroxy-5-(3,4,5-trimethoxyphenyl)furo[3′,4′:6,7]-naphtho[2,3-d]-1,3-dioxol-6(5aH)-one; 8-hydroxy-2-hydroxymethyl-6,7-methylenedioxy-4-(3′,4′,5′-trimethoxyphenyl)-1,2,3,4-tetrahydronaphthalene-3-carboxylic acid lactone; β-peltatin A. $C_{22}H_{22}O_8$; mol wt 414.41. C 63.76%, H 5.35%, O 30.89%. Exists as a glucoside in the rhizomes of *Podophyllum peltatum* L., *Berberidaceae*: von Wartburg *et al., Helv. Chim. Acta* **40**, 1331 (1957). Isoln from resin podophyllum: Hartwell, Detty, *J. Am. Chem. Soc.* **70**, 2833 (1948); **72**, 246 (1950); from *Hyptis verticillata* Jacq., *Labiatae*: German, *J. Pharm. Sci.* **60**, 649 (1971).

Prisms from abs ethanol. Dec 238-241° (slight sintering begins at 234°). $[\alpha]_D^{20} -122.9°$ (c = 0.578 in chloroform). Somewhat less sol than α-peltatin. Soly in water at 23°: 13 mg/liter. Fairly sol in chloroform, hot ethanol, acetic acid, acetone, dil caustic; less sol in benzene, ether, carbon tetrachloride, propylene glycol. Practically insol in petr ether.

β-Peltatin-β-D-glucoside. $C_{28}H_{32}O_{13}$. White amorph powder from acetone + ether, dec 156-159°. $[\alpha]_D^{20} -122.7°$ (c = 0.587 in methanol); $[\alpha]_D^{20} -169.2°$ (c = 0.556 in pyridine).
Caution: Irritates the skin.

7077. Pemetrexed. [137281-23-3] N-[4-[2-(2-Amino-4,7-dihydro-4-oxo-1H-pyrrolo[2,3-d]pyrimidin-5-yl)ethyl]benzoyl]-L-glutamic acid. $C_{20}H_{21}N_5O_6$; mol wt 427.41. C 56.20%, H 4.95%, N 16.39%, O 22.46%. Multitargeted antifolate; inhibits thymidylate synthase as well as other folate dependent enzymes. Prepn: E. C. Taylor *et al., EP 432677; idem, US 5344932* (1991, 1994 both to Trustees Princeton Univ.); *idem et al., J. Med. Chem.* **35**, 4450 (1992). Profile of enzyme inhibition: C. Shih *et al., Adv. Enzyme Regul.* **38**, 135 (1998). HPLC determn in plasma: C. L. Hamilton, J. A. Kirkwood, *J. Chromatogr. B* **654**, 297 (1994). Clinical pharmacokinetics in cancer patients: A. C. McDonald *et al., Clin. Cancer Res.* **4**, 605 (1998). Clinical evaluation in colorectal carcinoma: W. John *et al., Cancer* **88**, 1807 (2000); in pancreatic cancer: K. D. Miller *et al., Ann. Oncol.* **11**, 101 (2000).

Crystals from 50% methanol/methylene chloride.
Sodium salt. [150399-23-8] Pemetrexed disodium; LY-231514; Alimta. $C_{20}H_{19}N_5Na_2O_6$; mol wt 471.37.
THERAP CAT: Antineoplastic.

7078. Pemirolast. [69372-19-6] 9-Methyl-3-(1H-tetrazol-5-yl)-4H-pyrido[1,2-a]pyrimidin-4-one. $C_{10}H_8N_6O$; mol wt 228.21. C 52.63%, H 3.53%, N 36.83%, O 7.01%. Inhibitor of chemical mediator release from tissue mast cells. Prepn: P. F. Juby, **US 4122274** (1978 to Bristol-Myers). LC determn in plasma: H. Cheng *et al., J. Pharm. Sci.* **76**, 918 (1987). Immunopharmacology and mechanism of action studies: Y. Yanagihara *et al., Jpn. J. Pharmacol.* **48**, 91, 103 (1988). Clinical evaluation in allergic rhinitis: D. G. Tinkelman, R. B. Berkowitz, *Ann. Allergy* **66**, 162 (1991).

Crystals from DMF, mp 310-311° (dec).
Potassium salt. [100299-08-9] BMY-26517; TBX; Pemilaston. $C_{10}H_7KN_6O$; mol wt 266.30. Yellowish-white crystalline powder. Highly soluble in water.
THERAP CAT: Antiallergic.

7079. Pemoline. [2152-34-3] 2-Amino-5-phenyl-4(5H)-oxazolone; phenoxazole; phenylisohydantoin; phenylpseudohydantoin; azoxodone; PIO; LA-956; YH-1; Cylert; Tradon. $C_9H_8N_2O_2$; mol wt 176.17. C 61.36%, H 4.58%, N 15.90%, O 18.16%. Prepn: W. Traube, R. Ascher, *Ber.* **46**, 2077 (1913); L. Schmidt, H. Scheffler, **US 2892753** (1959 to Boehringer, Ing.). Prepn of magnesium hydroxide mixture, originally thought to be a chelate complex: W. E. Lange *et al., J. Pharm. Sci.* **51**, 477 (1962); B. H. Candon, M. Chessin, **US 3108045** (1963 to Purdue Frederick). CNS stimulant activity: L. Schmidt, *Arzneim.-Forsch.* **6**, 423 (1956). Efficacy in minimal brain dysfunction in hyperkinetic children: C. K. Connors *et al., Psychopharmacologia* **26**, 321 (1972); J. G. Page *et al., J. Learn. Disabil.* **7**, 498 (1974). Toxicity data: E. W. Schafer, *Toxicol. Appl. Pharmacol.* **21**, 315 (1972). *Review:* A. T. Dren, R. S. Janicki, in *Pharmacological and Biochemical Properties of Drug Substances* **vol. 1**, M. E. Goldberg, Ed. (Am. Pharm. Assoc., Washington, DC, 1977) pp 33-65.

Crystals, mp 256-257° (dec). Practically insol in water, ether, acetone, dil hydrochloric acid. Sol in propylene glycol (1%); in hot alcohol. LD_{50} orally in rats: 500 mg/kg (Schafer).

Magnesium hydroxide mixture. [18968-99-5] Magnesium pemoline; Abbott 30400

Note: This is a controlled substance (stimulant): **21 CFR,** 1308.14.

THERAP CAT: CNS stimulant.

7080. Pempidine. [79-55-0] 1,2,2,6,6-Pentamethylpiperidine. $C_{10}H_{21}N$; mol wt 155.28. C 77.35%, H 13.63%, N 9.02%. Ganglion blocking agent. Prepn by methylation of 2,2,6,-6-tetramethylpiperidine: Leonard, Hauck, *J. Am. Chem. Soc.* **79,** 5289 (1957); Hall, *ibid.* 5447. Description: Spinks, Young, *Nature* **181,** 1397 (1958); Lee *et al., ibid.* 1717.

Liquid. pK at 30° = 11.25. Extremely basic reaction for a tertiary amine. bp_{760} 147°. n_D^{21} 1.4550.

p-**Toluenesulfonate.** $C_{17}H_{19}NO_3S$. Crystals from ethyl acetate + ethanol, mp 162-163°.

Tartrate. [546-48-5] M & B 4486; Pempidil; Pempiten; Perolysen; Tenormal; Tensinol; Tensoral. $C_{10}H_{21}N.C_4H_6O_6$; mol wt 305.37. Crystals, mp 160°. Sol in alcohol, moderately sol in water.

Hydrochloride. $C_{10}H_{21}N.HCl$. Crystals, sol in water, alc.

THERAP CAT: Tartrate as antihypertensive.

7081. Penamecillin. [983-85-7] (2*S*,5*R*,6*R*)-3,3-Dimethyl-7-oxo-6-[(phenylacetyl)amino]-4-thia-1-azabicyclo[3.2.0]heptane-2-carboxylic acid (acetyloxy)methyl ester; penicillin G hydroxymethyl ester acetate; acetoxymethyl benzylpenicillinate; benzylpenicillin acetoxymethyl ester; Wy-20788; Havapen; Maripen. $C_{19}H_{22}N_2O_6S$; mol wt 406.45. C 56.15%, H 5.46%, N 6.89%, O 23.62%, S 7.89%. Semi-synthetic antibiotic related to penicillin. Prepn: A. B. A. Jansen, T. J. Russell, *J. Chem. Soc.* **1965,** 2127; *eidem,* **GB 1003479** (1965 to John Wyeth & Brother); *eidem,* **US 3250679** (1966 to Am. Home).

Crystals from isopropanol + ethanol, mp 106-108°. $[\alpha]_D^{20}$ +154°. Not inactivated by gastric acid.

THERAP CAT: Antibacterial.

7082. Penbutolol. [38363-40-5] (2*S*)-1-(2-Cyclopentylphenoxy)-3-[(1,1-dimethylethyl)amino]-2-propanol; (*S*)-1-(*tert*-butylamino)-3-(*o*-cyclopentylphenoxy)-2-propanol; (−)-1-*tert*-butylamino-2-hydroxy-3-(2′-cyclopentylphenoxy)propane. $C_{18}H_{29}$-NO_2; mol wt 291.43. C 74.18%, H 10.03%, N 4.81%, O 10.98%. β-Adrenergic blocker. Prepn: H. Ruschig *et al.,* **ZA 6807915**; *eidem,* **US 3551493** (1969, 1970 both to Hoechst). Preliminary chemistry and pharmacology: G. Härtfelder *et al., Arzneim.-Forsch.* **22,** 930 (1972). Physicochemical and analytical study: P. Hajdu, D. Damm, *ibid.* **29,** 602 (1979). Pharmacology: J. Kaiser

et al., ibid. **30,** 420 (1980). Action specificity: J. Kaiser *ibid.* 427. Crystallographic study: J. M. Leger *et al., Mol. Pharmacol.* **17,** 339 (1980). Hemodynamic effects: P. Lund-Johansen, *Eur. J. Clin. Pharmacol.* **16,** 149 (1979). Clinical study in hypertension: J. L. Cangiano *et al., J. Clin. Pharmacol.* **19,** 384 (1979). HPLC determn in plasma: R. K. Bhamra *et al., Biomed. Chromatogr.* **1,** 140 (1986). Review of pharmacology and therapeutic efficacy: R. C. Heel *et al., Drugs* **22,** 1-25 (1981).

Crystals, mp 68-72°. $[\alpha]_D^{20}$ −11.5° (c = 1 in methanol). pKa 9.3 (1.5 mmol/l in 25% ethanol). Sol in methanol, ethanol, chloroform.

Sulfate. [38363-32-5] HOE-893d; HOE-39-893d; Betapressin; Levatol; Paginol. $(C_{18}H_{29}NO_2)_2.H_2SO_4$; mol wt 680.94. Crystals, mp 216-218° (dec). $[\alpha]_D^{20}$ −24.6° (c = 1 in methanol).

THERAP CAT: Antihypertensive; antianginal; antiarrhythmic.

7083. Penciclovir. [39809-25-1] 2-Amino-1,9-dihydro-9-[4-hydroxy-3-(hydroxymethyl)butyl]-6*H*-purin-6-one; 9-[4-hydroxy-3-(hydroxymethyl)but-1-yl]guanine; PCV; BRL-39123; Denavir; Vectavir. $C_{10}H_{15}N_5O_3$; mol wt 253.26. C 47.42%, H 5.97%, N 27.65%, O 18.95%. Carba analog of ganciclovir, *q.v.,* active against several herpes viruses. Prepn: U. K. Pandit *et al., Synth. Commun.* **2,** 345 (1972); R. L. Jarvest, M. R. Harnden, **US 5075445** (1991 to Beecham). Synthesis: M. R. Harnden *et al., J. Med. Chem.* **30,** 1636 (1987); J. Hannah *et al., J. Heterocycl. Chem.* **26,** 1261 (1989). Crystal and molecular structures: M. R. Harnden *et al., Nucleosides Nucleotides* **9,** 499 (1990). *In vitro* activity of enantiomers in comparison with acyclovir, *q.v.:* G. Abele *et al., Antiviral Chem. Chemother.* **2,** 163 (1991); against herpes simplex viruses: A. Weinberg *et al., Antimicrob. Agents Chemother.* **36,** 2037 (1992). Clinical pharmacokinetics: S. E. Fowles *et al., Eur. J. Clin. Pharmacol.* **43,** 513 (1992). HPLC determn in plasma and urine: J. R. McMeekin *et al., Anal. Proc.* **29,** 178 (1992). Review of development and antiviral activity: M. R. Harnden, *Drugs Future* **14,** 347-358 (1989).

White crystalline solid from water, (monohydrate), mp 275-277°; also reported as colorless matted needles, mp 272-275°. uv max (in water): 253 nm (ε 11500). uv max (aq 0.01*N* NaOH): 215, 268 nm (ε 18140, 10710). Sol in water (20°): 1.7 mg/ml, pH 7.

Sodium salt. BRL-39123A. Occurs as monohydrate, stable crystalline solid. Sol in water (20°): >200 mg/ml. 30 mg/ml soln has pH 11.

THERAP CAT: Antiviral.

7084. Pendimethalin. [40487-42-1] *N*-(1-Ethylpropyl)-3,4-dimethyl-2,6-dinitrobenzenamine; *N*-(1-ethylpropyl)-2,6-dinitro-3,4-xylidine; *N*-(1-ethylpropyl)-3,4-dimethyl-2,6-dinitroaniline; penoxalin; AC-92553; Herbadox; Pendimax; Prowl; Stomp. $C_{13}H_{19}$-N_3O_4; mol wt 281.31. C 55.50%, H 6.81%, N 14.94%, O 22.75%. Pre-emergence and pre-planting herbicide. Prepn: R. H. Kupelian, **DE 2232263** *C.A.* **78,** 84010z (1973) and A. W. Lutz, R. E. Diehl, **DE 2241408** *C.A.* **78,** 135858s (1973) (both 1973 to Am. Cyanamid). Activity: H. A. Roberts, W. Bond, *Proc. 12th Br. Weed Control Conf.* **1,** 387 (1974). Persistence in soil: A. Walker, W. Bond, *Pestic. Sci.* **8,** 359 (1977).

Orange-yellow cryst solid, mp 56-57°. Vapor press at 25°: 3×10^{-5} mm Hg. Soly in water at 20°: 0.3 mg/l. Sol in most organic solvents.

USE: Herbicide.

7085. Penethamate Hydriodide. [808-71-9] (2S,5R,6R)-3,3-Dimethyl-7-oxo-6-[(phenylacetyl)amino]-4-thia-1-azabicyclo[3.2.0]heptane-2-carboxylic acid 2-(diethylamino)ethyl ester monohydriodide; penicillin G 2-diethylaminoethyl ester hydriodide; benzylpenicillin β-diethylaminoethyl ester hydriodide; β-diethylaminoethyl benzylpenicillinate hydriodide; ephicillin hydriodide; penethecillin; Bronchocillin; Estopen; Leocillin; Mamyzin; Neo-Penil. $C_{22}H_{32}IN_3O_4S$; mol wt 561.48. C 47.06%, H 5.74%, I 22.60%, N 7.48%, O 11.40%, S 5.71%. Prepn: K. A. Jensen *et al.*, *Ugeskr. Laeg.* **112**, 1043, 1075 (1950); E. K. Frederiksen, E. J. Nielsen, US 2694061; A. B. A. Jansen, J. C. Hamlet, US 2880203 (1954, 1959 both to Lövens). Selective concentration in lung: A. G. S. Heathcote, E. Nassau, *Lancet* **260**, 1255 (1951). Properties: W. A. Woodard, *J. Pharm. Pharmacol.* **4**, 1009 (1952). Veterinary trial in cows: G. Ziv, M. Storper, *J. Vet. Pharmacol. Ther.* **8**, 276 (1985).

Crystals, mp 178-179°. Slightly soluble in water (0.96% at 20°). pH of satd aq soln 4.5-5.2. Aq solns are unstable, the ester is hydrolyzed to free penicillin and diethylaminoethanol, the velocity of the reaction increasing with rise in temperature and pH.

THERAP CAT: Antibacterial.

THERAP CAT (VET): Antibacterial.

7086. Penetratin. [188842-14-0] Penetratin-1. $C_{104}H_{168}$-$N_{34}O_{20}S$; mol wt 2246.73. C 55.60%, H 7.54%, N 21.20%, O 14.24%, S 1.43%. Nuclear transport protein capable of delivering bioactive molecules to the cytoplasm and nucleus of living cells by an energy-independent mechanism. Consists of a 16 amino acid segment of the DNA-binding domain (homeodomain) of Antennapedia, a transcription factor found in *Drosophila*. Prepn: D. Derossi *et al.*, *J. Biol. Chem.* **269**, 10444 (1994). Study of translocation mechanism: *idem et al.*, *ibid.* **271**, 18188 (1996). Use to deliver antigens to target cells: M.-P. Schutze-Redelmeier *et al.*, *J. Immunol.* **157**, 650 (1996). *Review*: A. Prochiantz, *Curr. Opin. Neurobiol.* **6**, 629-634 (1996); D. Derossi *et al.*, *Trends Cell Biol.* **8**, 84-87 (1998).

Arg–Gln–Ile–Lys–Ile–Trp–Phe–Gln–Asn–Arg–Arg–Met–Lys–Trp–Lys–Lys

USE: Internalization vector for peptides and oligonucleotides into living cells.

7087. Penfluridol. [26864-56-2] 1-[4,4-Bis(4-fluorophenyl)butyl]-4-[4-chloro-3-(trifluoromethyl)phenyl]-4-piperidinol; 1-[4,4-bis(*p*-fluorophenyl)butyl]-4-(4-chloro-α,α,α-trifluoro-*m*-tolyl)-4-piperidinol; 1-(4,4-bis(4-fluorophenyl)butyl)-4-hydroxy-4-(3-trifluoromethyl-4-chlorophenyl)piperidine; R-16341; Semap. C_{28}-$H_{27}ClF_5NO$; mol wt 523.97. C 64.18%, H 5.19%, Cl 6.77%, F 18.13%, N 2.67%, O 3.05%. Prepn: H. K. F. Hermans, C. J. E. Niemegeers, DE 2040231; *eidem*, US 3575990 (both 1971 to Janssen); Sindelár *et al.*, *Collect. Czech. Chem. Commun.* **38**, 3879 (1973). Pharmacology and toxicology: Janssen *et al.*, *Eur. J. Pharmacol.* **11**, 139 (1970). Crystal structure: Koch, *Acta Crystallogr.* **29B**, 1538 (1973).

White, microcrystals, mp 105-107°. Slightly sol in water, dil HCl (<0.5 mg/ml). LD_{50} orally in mice (day 7): 86.8 mg/kg (Janssen).

THERAP CAT: Antipsychotic.

7088. Penicillamine. [52-67-5] 3-Mercapto-D-valine; (*S*)-3,3-dimethylcysteine; α-amino-β-methyl-β-mercaptobutyric acid; DMC; β-thiovaline; D-penicillamine; Cuprimine; Cupripen; Depen; D-Penamine; Distamine; Mercaptyl; Metalcaptase; Reumacillin; Sufortan; Trisorcin; Trolovol. $C_5H_{11}NO_2S$; mol wt 149.21. C 40.25%, H 7.43%, N 9.39%, O 21.45%, S 21.49%. Characteristic degradation product of penicillin type antibiotics. Active as copper chelating agent and as a disease modifying antirheumatic drug (DMARD). Prepn by hydrolysis of penicillins: E. P. Abraham *et al.*, *Nature* **151**, 107 (1943). Review of syntheses of DL-form and enantiomers: H. M. Crooks in *The Chemistry of Penicillin*, H. T. Clarke *et al.*, Eds. (Princeton Univ. Press, 1949) pp 455-472; W. M. Weigert *et al.*, *Angew. Chem. Int. Ed.* **14**, 330 (1975). Polymorphism of D-form: J. A. G. Vidler, *J. Pharm. Pharmacol.* **28**, 662 (1976). Toxicity data: Veis *et al.*, *Antibiotiki* **14**, 837 (1969). General reviews: I. A. Jaffe in *Pharmacological and Biochemical Properties of Drug Substances* Vol. 2, M. E. Goldberg, Ed. (Am. Pharm. Assoc., Washington, DC, 1979) pp 465-478; C. C. Chiu, L. T. Grady, *Anal. Profiles Drug Subs.* **10**, 601-637 (1981). Review of assay methods: N. Kucharczyk, S. Shahiniam, *J. Rheumatol.* **8**, Suppl. 7, 28-34 (1981); of metabolism and pharmacology: D. Perrett, *ibid.* 41-50; of clinical pharmacokinetics: D. A. Joyce, *Pharmacol. Ther.* **42**, 405-427 (1989). Clinical trial in Wilson's disease: A. Czlonkowska *et al.*, *J. Neurol.* **243**, 269 (1996). Review of clinical experience in rheumatoid arthritis: R. Munro, H. A. Capell, *Br. J. Rheumatol.* **36**, 104-109 (1997).

White or practically white, crystalline powder. mp 202-206° (Weigert). $[\alpha]_D^{25}$ −63° (c = 0.1 in pyridine). Freely sol in water; slightly sol in alcohol. Insol in ether, acetone, benzene, carbon tetrachloride. LD_{50} in rats (mg/kg): >10000 orally, >660 i.p. (Jaffe).

Hydrochloride. [2219-30-9] Pemine. $C_5H_{11}NO_2S.HCl$; mol wt 185.67. Hygroscopic crystals, dec 177.5°. $[\alpha]_D^{25}$ −63° (1N NaOH). Freely sol in water, sol in ethanol. Aq solns are comparatively stable at pH 2-4. LD_{50} i.v. in mice: 2289 mg/kg (Veis).

DL-Form. [52-66-4] Crystals, dec 201°. pK: 1.8 (carboxyl); 7.9 (α-amino); 10.5 (β-thiol). LD_{50} orally in rats: 365 mg/kg (Jaffe).

DL-Form hydrochloride. [22572-05-0] Crystals, dec 145-148°.

L-Form. [1113-41-3] Crystals, mp 190-194°. $[\alpha]_D^{25}$ +63° (in 1N NaOH). LD_{50} i.p. in rats: 350 mg/kg (Jaffe).

THERAP CAT: Antirheumatic. Chelating agent (copper); Wilson's Disease treatment.

7089. Penicillamine Cysteine Disulfide. [18840-45-4] 3-[[(2R)-2-Amino-2-carboxyethyl]dithio]-D-valine; 3,3-dimethyl-3-3'-dithiodialanine; 1,6-diamino-5-5-dimethyl-3,4-dithiahexane-1,6-dicarboxylic acid. $C_8H_{16}N_2O_4S_2$; mol wt 268.35. C 35.81%, H 6.01%, N 10.44%, O 23.85%, S 23.90%. Prepn: Tabachnick *et al.*, *Nature* **174**, 701 (1954); Schöberl *et al.*, *Angew. Chem.* **68**, 213 (1956); Schöberl, Grafje, *Ann.* **617**, 71 (1958); Levine, *Nature* **187**, 940 (1960).

Crystals, mp 195°.

7090. Penicillamine Disulfide. [312-10-7] 3,3′-Dithio-bisvaline; 3,3′-dithiodivaline; 3,3,3′,3′-tetramethylcystine. $C_{10}H_{20}$-$N_2O_4S_2$; mol wt 296.41. C 40.52%, H 6.80%, N 9.45%, O 21.59%, S 21.64%. Prepn: Süs, *Ann.* **561,** 31 (1948); Berg *et al.*, **GB 621915** (1949 to Merck & Co.); Butenandt *et al., Z. Physiol. Chem.* **285,** 238 (1950).

DL-Form. [21174-80-1] Crystals, mp 181-183°.
D-Form. [20902-45-8] Crystals, mp 204-205°. $[\alpha]_D^{23}$ +27° (c = 1.46 in 1*N* HCl).
L-Form. [113626-33-8] Crystals, mp 207°. $[\alpha]_D^{22}$ −26° (1*N* HCl).

7091. Penicillanic Acid. [87-53-6] (2*S*,5*R*)-3,3-Dimethyl-7-oxo-4-thia-1-azabicyclo[3.2.0]heptane-2-carboxylic acid. Building block of penicillin, devoid of significant antibacterial activity: Sheehan *et al., J. Am. Chem. Soc.* **75,** 3292 (1953); **81,** 5838 (1959). Separation from its esters and other penicillins by gas chromatog: Evard *et al., Nature* **201,** 1124 (1964). *See also* 6-Amino-penicillanic Acid.

7092. Penicillic Acid. [90-65-3] 3-Methoxy-5-methyl-4-oxo-2,5-hexadienoic acid; γ-keto-β-methoxy-δ-methylene-Δ$^\alpha$-hexenoic acid. $C_8H_{10}O_4$; mol wt 170.16. C 56.47%, H 5.92%, O 37.61%. Antibiotic mycotoxin produced by the following fungi: *Penicillium puberulum, P. cyclopium, P. thomii, P. suaveolens, P. baarnense, Aspergillus ochraceus, A. melleus.* Isoln: Alsberg, Black, *USDA Bur. Plant Ind. Bull.* **270,** (1913); Birkinshaw *et al., Biochem. J.* **30,** 394 (1936); Oxford *et al., Chem. Ind. (London)* **20,** 22 (1942); Karow *et al., Arch. Biochem.* **5,** 279 (1944); Burton, *Nature* **165,** 274 (1950); Natori *et al., Chem. Pharm. Bull.* **18,** 2259 (1970). Activity studies: Suzuki *et al., Agric. Biol. Chem.* **35,** 287 (1971). Acid in tautomeric equilibrium with its lactone. Structure: Birkinshaw *et al., loc. cit.* Physical properties: Kovac, Solcaniova, *Tetrahedron* **25,** 3617 (1969). Synthesis: Raphael, *Nature* **160,** 261 (1947); *J. Chem. Soc.* **1948,** 1508; C. L. Yeh *et al., Tetrahedron Lett.* **1978,** 3987. Biosynthesis: Birch *et al., J. Chem. Soc.* **1958,** 4582; Bentley, Keil, *J. Biol. Chem.* **237,** 867 (1962). Physicochemical data: A. E. Pohland *et al., Pure Appl. Chem.* **54,** 2219 (1982). Toxicity studies: P. K. Chan *et al., Toxicol. Appl. Pharmacol.* **52,** 1 (1980); P. K. Chan, A. W. Hayes, *J. Toxicol. Environ. Health* **7,** 169 (1981). Evaluation of carcinogenic risk: *IARC Monographs* **10,** 211-216 (1976). *Review:* Ciegler *et al.,* "Patulin, Penicillic Acid and Other Carcinogenic Lactones" in *Microbial Toxins* **vol. VI,** A. Ciegler *et al.,* Eds. (Academic Press, New York, 1971) p 414.

Needles from petr ether, mp 83-84°. uv max: about 220 nm. Acid reaction, turns Congo red paper blue. Moderately sol in cold water (2 g/100 ml); freely sol in hot water, alcohol, ether, benzene,

chloroform; slightly sol in hot petr ether. Practically insol in pentane-hexane. LD_{50} i.p. in mice: 90.00 mg/kg (Chan *et al.*).
Monohydrate. Large transparent monoclinic or triclinic, rhombic crystals from water, mp 58-64°.

7093. Penicillinase. [9001-74-5] β-Lactamase; Neutrapen. Mol wt about 50,000. Enzymes found in many bacteria which destroy penicillins and cephalosporins by catalyzing the hydrolysis of the amide bond in the β-lactam ring. Good penicillinase producers are *Bact. coli,* the *Bacillus subtilis-mesentericus* group, *Bacillus anthracis* and *Staphylococci.* Both intra- and extracellular penicillinase are of protein nature. There are probably as many different penicillinases as there are bacteria producing them. Ion-exchange procedures for the purification of penicillinase: Puetzer, Boschetti, **US 2982696** (1961 to Schenley). Amino acid sequence studies: Ambler, Meadway, *Nature* **222,** 24 (1969). Therapeutic use in penicillin allergy: Y. P. Borodin, *Allerg. Asthma* **14,** 43 (1968). *Reviews:* Chain *et al.* in *Antibiotics* **vol. 2,** Flory *et al.,* Eds. (Oxford, 1949) p 1090; Rothe, *Pharmazie* **5,** 25 (1950); Citri, Pollock, *Adv. Enzymol.* **28,** 237 (1966); Citri in *The Enzymes* P. D. Boyer, Ed. (Academic Press, New York, 3rd ed., 1971) pp 23-46.

USE: In culture media to antagonize antibacterial activity of penicillin.

THERAP CAT: Has been used in the treatment of allergic reactions to penicillin.

7094. Penicillin G. [61-33-6] (2*S*,5*R*,6*R*)-3,3-Dimethyl-7-oxo-6-[(phenylacetyl)amino]-4-thia-1-azabicyclo[3.2.0]heptane-2-carboxylic acid; benzylpenicillin; benzylpenicillinic acid; penicillin II. $C_{16}H_{18}N_2O_4S$; mol wt 334.39. C 57.47%, H 5.43%, N 8.38%, O 19.14%, S 9.59%. Discovery of antibiotic substance produced by *Penicillium* sp: A. Fleming, *Br. J. Exp. Pathol.* **10,** 226 (1929). Preliminary isoln: P. W. Clutterbuck *et al., Biochem. J.* **26,** 1907 (1932); and chemotherapeutic properties: E. Chain *et al., Lancet* **2,** 226 (1940); E. P. Abraham *et al., ibid.* **2,** 177 (1941). Review of early studies: E. Chain, *Annu. Rev. Biochem.* **17,** 657-704 (1948); H. T. Clarke *et al., The Chemistry of Penicillin* (Princeton Univ. Press, 1949) 1094 pp. Crystal structure: D. C. Hodgkin, *Adv. Sci.* **6,** 85 (1949). Fermentation process: A. L. Demain, N. L. Somerson, **US 3024169** (1962 to Merck & Co.). Total synthesis: J. C. Sheehan, K. R. Henery-Logan, *J. Am. Chem. Soc.* **81,** 5838 (1959); R. A. Firestone *et al., J. Org. Chem.* **39,** 437 (1974). Review of clinical pharmacokinetics of penicillins: M. Barza, L. Weinstein, *Clin. Pharmacokinet.* **1,** 297 (1976). Comprehensive description of the potassium salt: J. Kirschbaum, *Anal. Profiles Drug Subs.* **15,** 427-507 (1987).

Amorphous white powder. $[\alpha]_D$ +282° (ethanol). Sparingly sol in water. Sol in methanol, ethanol, ether, ethyl acetate, benzene, chloroform, acetone. Insol in petr ether.
Sodium salt. [69-57-8] Crystapen; Penilevel. $C_{16}H_{17}N_2$-NaO_4S; mol wt 356.37. Crystals from methanol + ethyl acetate. $[\alpha]_D^{24.8}$ +301° (c = 2.0 in water). uv max (water): 252, 257.5, 264 nm (E_M about 300, 240, 180). Freely sol in water, isotonic saline, glucose solns. Sol in methanol; less sol in ethanol. Practically insol in acetone, chloroform, ether, ethyl acetate, fixed oils, liq paraffin.
Potassium salt. [113-98-4] Cristapen; Falapen; Megacillin (tabl.); Pentids; Pfizerpen. $C_{16}H_{17}KN_2O_4S$; mol wt 372.48. Crystals from aq butanol, mp 214-217° (dec). Moderately hygroscopic. $[\alpha]_D^{22}$ +285° (c = 0.748 in water). Freely sol in water, isotonic saline, glucose solns; sparingly sol in ethanol. Practically insol in chloroform, ether, fixed oils, liq paraffin. pH of 6% aq soln 5.0 to 7.5.
Mixture with clemizole. [6011-39-8] Clemizole-penicillin; Neopenyl. $C_{19}H_{20}ClN_3.C_{16}H_{18}N_2O_4S$; mol wt 660.23. Repository form of penicillin. Prepn: H. Mückter *et al., Arzneim.-Forsch.* **4,** 487 (1954). White powder, mp 144-145°. $[\alpha]_D^{24}$ +144.5° (c = 10

in DMF). Sol in methanol, ethanol, DMF; slightly sol in water, acetone, dioxane.

THERAP CAT: Antibacterial.

THERAP CAT (VET): Antibacterial.

7095. Penicillin G Benethamine. [751-84-8] (2*S*,5*R*,6*R*)-3,3-Dimethyl-7-oxo-6-[(phenylacetyl)amino]-4-thia-1-azabicyclo[3.2.0]heptane-2-carboxylic acid compd with *N*-(phenylmethyl)-benzeneethanamine (1:1); benzylpenicillinic acid *N*-benzyl-β-phenylethylamine salt; benethamine penicillin G. $C_{31}H_{35}N_3O_4S$; mol wt 545.69. C 68.23%, H 6.46%, N 7.70%, O 11.73%, S 5.88%. Repository form of penicillin G. Prepn: Jansen, Hems, **GB 732559** (1955 to Glaxo). Clinical studies: Nelson *et al.*, *Br. Med. J.* **II**, 339 (1954); Boger *et al.*, *Antibiot. Annu.* **1954-55**, 123.

Crystals, mp 146-147°. Slight, characteristic, amine taste. Very slightly sol in water (0.1 w/v at 40°).

THERAP CAT: Antibacterial.

7096. Penicillin G Benzathine. [1538-09-6] (2*S*,5*R*,6*R*)-3,3-Dimethyl-7-oxo-6-[(phenylacetyl)amino]-4-thia-1-azabicyclo[3.2.0]heptane-2-carboxylic acid compd with *N*,*N*′-bis(phenylmethyl)-1,2-ethanediamine (2:1); penicillin G *N*,*N*′-dibenzylethylenediamine salt; *N*,*N*′-dibenzylethylenediamine bis[benzylpenicillin]; dibenzylethylenediamine dipenicillin G; benzethacil; benzathine penicillin G; DBED-penicillin; Beacillin; Bicillin L-A; Cepacilina; Extencilline; Lentopenil; Megacillin (susp.); Penidural; Permapen; Tardocillin. $C_{48}H_{56}N_6O_8S_2$; mol wt 909.12. C 63.41%, H 6.21%, N 9.24%, O 14.08%, S 7.05%. Repository form of penicillin. Prepn: J. L. Szabo *et al.*, *Antibiot. Chemother.* **1**, 499 (1951); J. L. Szabo, W. F. Bruce, **US 2627491** (1953 to Wyeth). Comprehensive description: F. Kreuzig, *Anal. Profiles Drug Subs.* **11**, 463-482 (1982). Review of clinical efficacy in syphilis: E. W. Hook, III, *Rev. Infect. Dis.* **11**, Suppl. 6, S1511-S1517 (1989); in prophylaxis of rheumatic fever: B. J. Currie, *Pediatrics* **97**, 989 (1996).

Crystals from formamide, mp 123-124°. $[\alpha]_D^{25}$ +206° (c = 0.105 in formamide). Soly at 23° (mg/ml): water 0.15; benzene 0.38; alc 5.2; acetone 1.5; formamide 28.0. pH of satd aq soln about 6. Solubilities determined by Weiss *et al.*, *Antibiot. Chemother.* **7**, 374 (1957) in mg/ml: water 0.315; methanol 16.9; ethanol 15.4.

THERAP CAT: Antibacterial.

THERAP CAT (VET): Antibacterial.

7097. Penicillin G Procaine. [6130-64-9] (2*S*,5*R*,6*R*)-3,3-Dimethyl-7-oxo-6-[(phenylacetyl)amino]-4-thia-1-azabicyclo[3.2.0]heptane-2-carboxylic acid compd with 2-(diethylamino)-ethyl 4-aminobenzoate (1:1) monohydrate; penicillin G compd with 2-(diethylamino)ethyl *p*-aminobenzoate monohydrate; benzylpenicillin procaine; procaine benzylpenicillinate; procaine penicillin G; Abbocillin; Cilicaine; Crysticillin; Duracillin; Farmaproina; Mammacillin; Monocillin; Pfizerpen-AS; Wycillin. $C_{29}H_{38}N_4O_6$-S.H_2O; mol wt 588.72. C 59.16%, H 6.85%, N 9.52%, O 19.02%, S 5.45%. Semi-synthetic antibiotic. Prepn: N. P. Sullivan *et al.*, *Science* **107**, 169 (1948); C. J. Sullivan *et al.*, *J. Am. Chem. Soc.* **70**, 1287 (1948); H. W. Rhodehamel, Jr., **US 2515898** (1950 to Eli Lilly). Crystal structure: Rose, *Anal. Chem.* **27**, 1841 (1955). Toxicity: K. Soehring *et al.*, *Arzneim.-Forsch.* **1**, 28 (1951). Soly profile: P. J. Weiss *et al.*, *Antibiot. Chemother.* **7**, 374 (1957). Pharmacokinetics in horses: S. M. Stover *et al.*, *Am. J. Vet. Res.* **42**, 629 (1981); in humans: B. T. Goh *et al.*, *Br. J. Vener. Dis.* **60**, 371 (1984). Review of use in syphilis: M. W. Adler, *Br. Med. J.* **288**, 551-553 (1984).

Monoclinic hemimorphic crystals from methanol-water, mp 106-110° (with decompn). d 1.255-1.256. Not appreciably affected by air or light. Aq solns are dextrorotatory. The pH of a satd aq soln is between 5 and 7.5. Soly in mg/ml at about 28°: water 6.8; methanol >20; isopropanol 6.5; benzene 0.075; toluene 1.05; petr ether 0.12; isooctane 0.0; carbon tetrachloride 0.12; ethyl acetate 3.35. LD50 s.c. in mice: 2.3 g/kg (Soehring).

THERAP CAT: Antibacterial.

THERAP CAT (VET): Antibacterial.

7098. Penicillin N. [525-94-0] (2*S*,5*R*,6*R*)-6-[[(5*R*)-5-Amino-5-carboxy-1-oxopentyl]amino]-3,3-dimethyl-7-oxo-4-thia-1-azabicyclo[3.2.0]heptane-2-carboxylic acid; 6-(D-5-amino-5-carboxyvaleramido)-3,3-dimethyl-7-oxo-4-thia-1-azabicyclo[3.2.0]-

heptane-2-carboxylic acid; (D-4-amino-4-carboxybutyl)penicillinic acid; cephalosporin N; adicillin; Synnematin B. $C_{14}H_{21}N_3O_6S$; mol wt 359.40. C 46.79%, H 5.89%, N 11.69%, O 26.71%, S 8.92%. Antibiotic substance produced by *Cephalosporium* spp found in sewage outpours: Gottshall *et al.*, *Proc. Soc. Exp. Biol. Med.* **76**, 307 (1951); Abraham *et al.*, *Nature* **171**, 343 (1953); **176**, 551 (1955). Produced also by *Paecilomyces persicimus*: Pisano *et al.*, *Antimicrob. Agents Annu.* **1960** (Plenum Press, New York, 1961) pp 41, 48; by *Penicillium chrysogenum*: Flynn *et al.*, *J. Am. Chem. Soc.* **84**, 4594 (1962). Structure: Abraham, Newton, *Biochem. J.* **58**, 103 (1954). Production: Miller *et al.*, **US 2831797** (1958). Purification: Goodall, Sutcliffe, **US 2899425** (1959 to ICI).

Soluble in water. Dextrorotatory. Inactivated by penicillinase as is penicillin G, but differs from the common peni-cillin by its anti-bacterial activity and hydrophilic character. When an aq soln is kept at pH 2.7 and 37° for 2 hrs, there is a loss of antibacterial activity and an increase in dextrorotation. Active against *Sarcina lutea*, *Proteus vulgaris*, *Salmonella typhimurium*, *Diplococcus pneumoniae*. Shows practically no activity against *B. subtilis* and *Staph. aureus*. The toxicity is somewhat less than that of penicillin G, although penicillin N is excreted more slowly.

Barium salt. White powder. $[\alpha]_D^{20}$ +187° (c = 0.6). Freely sol in water, sparingly sol in methanol. Practically insol in ethanol.

THERAP CAT: Antibacterial.

7099. Penicillin O. [87-09-2] (2*S*,5*R*,6*R*)-3,3-Dimethyl-7-oxo-6-[[(2-propenylthio)acetyl]amino]-4-thia-1-azabicyclo[3.2.0]-heptane-2-carboxylic acid; [(allylthio)methyl] penicillin; allylmercaptomethylpenicillin; allylmercaptomethylpenicillinic acid; penicillin AT. $C_{13}H_{18}N_2O_4S_2$; mol wt 330.42. C 47.25%, H 5.49%, N 8.48%, O 19.37%, S 19.41%. Antibiotic produced by *Penicillium chrysogenum*. Biosynthesis of salts: Behrens *et al.*, *J. Biol. Chem.* **175**, 793 (1948); Rhodehamel, Behrens *et al.*, **US 2528175** and **US 2623876** (1950, 1952, both to Lilly); Ford *et al.*, *Antibiot. Chemother.* **3**, 1149 (1953); Ford, **US 2647894** (1953 to Upjohn); Palecková, Slechta, *C.A.* **50**, 17309g (1956).

2-Chloroprocaine salt monohydrate. Chloroprocaine penicillin O; penicillin O 2-chloroprocaine; Depo-Cer-O-Cillin Chloroprocaine. $C_{26}H_{37}ClN_4O_6S_2.H_2O$; mol wt 619.19. Slender needles from hot water, mp 79-81°. Practically insol in cold water. Stable in dry form at room temp. Aq suspensions are stable at room temp for 1 week, at refrigerator temps for 3 weeks. Calculated activity: 949 units/mg. Solubilities: Weiss *et al.*, *Antibiot. Chemother.* **7**, 374 (1957).

Potassium salt. [897-61-0] Potassium penicillin O; penicillin O potassium. $C_{13}H_{17}KN_2O_4S_2$. Crystals from acetone. Soluble in water. Stable in dry form at room temp for at least 3 years. Requires no refrigeration when dry. Aq solns may be kept for 3 days at +10° without significant loss of activity. Behrens' prepn assayed 1630 units/mg. Less toxic than benzylpenicillin in exptl animals.

Procaine salt. $C_{26}H_{38}N_4O_6S_2$. Crystals from water.

Sodium salt. [7177-54-0] Cer-O-Cillin Sodium. $C_{13}H_{17}N_2$-NaO$_4S_2$; mol wt 352.40. Crystals from acetone.

THERAP CAT: Antibacterial.

7100. Penicillin V. [87-08-1] (2*S*,5*R*,6*R*)-3,3-Dimethyl-7-oxo-6-[(phenoxyacetyl)amino]-4-thia-1-azabicyclo[3.2.0]heptane-

2-carboxylic acid; 6-phenoxyacetamidopenicillanic acid; penicillin phenoxymethyl; phenoxymethylpenicillin; phenoxymethylpenicillinic acid; Fenospen; Oracilline; V-Cillin. $C_{16}H_{18}N_2O_5S$; mol wt 350.39. C 54.84%, H 5.18%, N 7.99%, O 22.83%, S 9.15%. Obtained by adding 2-phenoxyethanol to the *Penicillium* culture using yeast autolyzate as source of nitrogen: Brandl *et al., Wien. Med. Wochenschr.* **1953**, 602; Brandl, Margreiter, *Oesterr. Chem.-Ztg.* **55**, 11-21 (1954), *C.A.* **48**, 10296 (1954). Purification: Parker *et al., J. Pharm. Pharmacol.* **7**, 683 (1953). Total synthesis: Sheehan, Henery-Logan, *J. Am. Chem. Soc.* **79**, 1262 (1957); **81**, 3089 (1959); **84**, 2983 (1962). Prepn from 6-aminopenicillanic acid: Glambitza, *Ann.* **673**, 166 (1964). Soly data: Weiss *et al., Antibiot. Chemother.* **7**, 374 (1957). The biologically active form is the dextrorotatory D-form; the DL-form is half as active. L-Penicillin V has little, if any, antibiotic activity. Toxicity data: E. I. Goldenthal, *Toxicol. Appl. Pharmacol.* **18**, 185 (1971). Comprehensive description of the potassium salt: J. M. Dunham in *Anal. Profiles Drug Subs.* **1**, 249-300 (1972); D. H. Sieh, *ibid.* **17**, 677-748 (1988).

Crystals, dec 120-128°. Stable in air up to 37°; relatively stable to acid. uv max: 268, 274 nm (ε 1330, 1100). Soly in water at pH 1.8 (acidified with HCl) = 25 mg/100 ml. Sol in polar organic solvents. Practically insol in vegetable oils and in liq petrolatum.

Potassium salt. [132-98-9] Antibiocin; Calciopen; Cliacil; Fenoxypen; Milcopen; Ospen; Pen-Vee K; Primcillin; Veetids; Vepicombin; V-Pen; V-Tablopen. $C_{16}H_{17}KN_2O_5S$; mol wt 388.48. Soluble in water. $[\alpha]_D^{25}$ +223° (c = 0.2). LD_{50} orally in rats: >1040 mg/kg (Goldenthal).

Calcium salt. [147-48-8] Arcasin; Calcipen; Isocillin; Ispenoral; Megacillin. $C_{32}H_{34}CaN_4O_{10}S_2$; mol wt 738.84.

Compd with dibenzylethylenediamine. [5928-84-7] Penicillin V benzathine; penicillin V DBED; benzathine penicillin V; phenoxymethylpenicillin benzathine; benzathine benzylpenicillin. $(C_{16}H_{18}N_2O_5S)_2 \cdot C_{16}H_{20}N_2$; mol wt 941.12. Prepn: R. Brunner *et al., US 2820789* (1958 to American Home Products). Practically white powder having a characteristic odor, mp 105-109°. Soly at ~28° (mg/ml): water 0.321; ethanol 14.6.

THERAP CAT: Antibacterial.

THERAP CAT (VET): Antibacterial.

7101. Penicilloyl Polylysine. [53608-77-8] Benzylpenicilloyl polylysine; PPL; Cilligen; Pre-Pen; Testarpen. Prepn from polylysine and a penicillenic acid: Parker *et al., J. Exp. Med.* **115**, 803 (1962). Prepn and use as diagnostic aid: M. A. Stahmann, S. S. Wagle, *GB 1226773; eidem, US 3979508* (1971, 1976 both to Kremers-Urban Co.). Intradermal test for penicillin sensitivity: Brown *et al., J. Am. Med. Assoc.* **189**, 599 (1964); Van Arsdale, *ibid.* **191**, 238 (1965); T. J. Sullivan, *J. Allergy Clin. Immunol.* **68**, 171 (1981).

THERAP CAT: Diagnostic aid (penicillin sensitivity).

7102. Pennyroyal. European pennyroyal. Perennial herb, *Mentha pulegium*, L., *Labiatae*. Medicinal portions are the fresh or dried leaves and flowering tops and the essential oil; traditionally used as an emmenagogue and abortifacient. *Habit.* Mediterranean region. *Constit.* Volatile oil (1-2%); tannins such as rosmaric acid; flavonoids incl. diosmin, hesperidin. Also used is the closely related **American pennyroyal**, *Hedeoma pulegioides* (L.) Pers., *Labiatae*. Fragrance monograph: D. L. J. Opdyke, *Food Cosmet. Toxicol.* **12**, 949 (1974). Extraction processes and composition of oil: N. Aghel *et al., Talanta* **62**, 407 (2004). Review of toxicology: I. B. Anderson *et al., Ann. Intern. Med.* **124**, 726-734 (1996); of components and pharmacology: J. Barnes *et al., Herbal Medicines* (Pharmaceutical Press, London, 2nd Ed., 2002) pp 372-373; J. Gruenwald *et al., PDR for Herbal Medicines* (Medical Economics, Montvale, 3rd Ed., 2004) pp 627-628.

Pennyroyal oil. [8013-99-8] Oil of pennyroyal; oil of pulegium. Volatile oil obtained by steam distillation of the fresh or

partially dried plant. *Constit.* Pulegone (60-90%), menthone, isomenthone, piperitone. Light yellow to yellow liquid; aromatic mint-like odor; aromatic taste. d_{25}^{25} 0.928-0.940. n_D^{20} 1.483-1.488. Rotation: +18° to +25°. Sol in most fixed oils, propylene glycol, in 2 vols 70% alcohol, with cloudiness in mineral oil. Practically insol in glycerin. LD_{50} orally in rats: 0.4 g/kg; dermally in rabbits: 4.2 g/kg (Opdyke). *Keep well closed, cool and protected from light.*

American pennyroyal oil. [8007-44-1] Oil of hedeoma. Volatile oil from leaves and flowering tops of *H. pulegioides. Constit.* Chiefly pulegone, menthone, isomenthone, acetic, formic, butyric, salicylic acids. Pale yellow liquid; herbaceous, mint-like odor; bitter, slightly burning taste. d_{15}^{15} 0.925-0.940. Rotation: +18° to +35°. n_D^{20} 1.482. Slightly sol in water; sol in 2 vols 70% alcohol; very sol in chloroform, ether.

Caution: Hepatotoxic. Ingestion of large quantities may cause vomiting, blood pressure elevation, anesthetic-like paralysis, death through respiratory failure (Gruenwald).

USE: Fragrance component in soaps, perfumes; flavoring agent; insect repellent.

7103. Penoxsulam. [219714-96-2] 2-(2,2-Difluoroethoxy)-*N*-(5,8-dimethoxy[1,2,4]triazolo[1,5-*c*]pyrimidin-2-yl)-6-(trifluoromethyl)benzenesulfonamide; DE-638; Granite; Grasp; Viper. C_{16}-$H_{14}F_5N_5O_5S$; mol wt 483.37. C 39.76%, H 2.92%, F 19.65%, N 14.49%, O 16.55%, S 6.63%. Triazolopyrimidine sulfonamide herbicide for weed control in rice; inhibits acetolactate synthase (ALS). Prepn: T. C. Johnson *et al., US 5858924* (1999 to Dow AgroSciences). Dissipation study in rice fields: D. W. Roberts *et al., Proc. 12th Symp. Pestic. Chem.* **2003**, 349. Comprehensive review: D. Larelle *et al., BCPC Int. Congr. - Crop Sci. Technol.* **2003**, 75-80.

Tan solid, mp 223-224°. Vapor pressure (mm Hg): 7.16×10^{-16} at 25°, 1.87×10^{-16} at 20°. pKa 5.1. Soly in water at 20° (mg/l): 5.7 pH 5, 408 pH 7, 1460 pH 9. Log P (octanol/water): -0.354 (19°, unbuffered water). LD_{50} (mg/kg): >5000 orally in rats; >5000 dermally in rabbits. LC_{50} (8 day) in bobwhite quail, mallard duck (ppm): >4411, >4310. LC_{50} (96 hr) in rainbow trout, bluegill sunfish, common carp (mg/l): >102, >103, >101 (Larelle).

USE: Herbicide.

7104. Pentaborane(9). [19624-22-7] Pentaboron nonahydride. B_5H_9; mol wt 63.13. B 85.62%, H 14.37%. Prepd from diborane: Stock, Mathing, *Ber.* **69B**, 1456 (1936); Schlesinger, Burg, *J. Am. Chem. Soc.* **53**, 4321 (1931); **55**, 4009 (1933). Molecular structure determination by rotational spectroscopy: D. Schwoch *et al., Inorg. Chem.* **16**, 3219 (1977). Review of toxicity: *see* Decaborane(14). *Review:* Greenwood in *Comprehensive Inorganic Chemistry* vol. 1, J. C. Bailar, Jr. *et al.,* Eds. (Pergamon Press, Oxford, 1973) pp 792-801.

Liquid. mp $-46.6°$; bp 60°. d_4^0 0.61; vp 66 mm Hg at 0°. Dec very slowly at 150°. Ignites spontaneously in air. Hydrolyzes in water after long heating. Reacts with ammonia to form a diammoniate.

Caution: Potential symptoms of overexposure are dizziness, headache, drowsiness and lightheadedness; incoordination, tremor, convulsions, behavioral changes; tonic spasms of face, neck, abdomen and limbs; irritation of eyes and skin. *See NIOSH Pocket Guide to Chemical Hazards* (DHHS/NIOSH 97-140, 1997) p 242.

7105. Pentaborane(11). [18433-84-6] Dihydropentaborane(9); pentaboron undecahydride. B_5H_{11}; mol wt 65.14. B 82.98%, H 17.02%. Prepd from diborane: Burg, Schlesinger, *J. Am. Chem. Soc.* **55**, 4009 (1933).

Liquid. mp $-123°$. bp 63°; bp_{53} 0°. Unstable. When heated or allowed to stand for long periods of time, it produces diborane, tetraborane, hydrogen, pentaborane, decaborane and brown nonvolatile liqs and solids. Ignites spontaneously in air. Hydrolyzes in water to boric acid and hydrogen. Reacts with ammonia to form a tetraammoniate.

7106. Pentabromoacetone. [79-49-2] 1,1,1,3,3-Penta-bromo-2-propanone. C_3HBr_5O; mol wt 452.56. C 7.96%, H 0.22%, Br 88.28%, O 3.54%. $CBr_3COCHBr_2$. Prepd by the addition of 12 parts bromine to 1 part acetone: Mulder, *Jahresber. Fortschr. Chem.* **1864,** 330.

Orthorhombic needles or prisms from alcohol or ether. Penetrating odor. mp 76° (sublimes above mp). Volatile with steam. Practically insol in water. Freely sol in organic solvents. Forms bromoform under the influence of alkalies.

7107. Pentacene. [135-48-8] Benzo[*b*]naphthacene; 2,3,6,-7-dibenzoanthracene; *lin*-naphthoanthracene. $C_{22}H_{14}$; mol wt 278.35. C 94.93%, H 5.07%. Synthesis from *m*-xylene or from 4-benzyl-1,3-dimethylbenzene and benzoyl chloride in presence of aluminum chloride or from terephthalyl chloride and *o*-tolyl-magnesium bromide: Clar, John, *Ber.* **62,** 940 (1929); **63,** 2967 (1930); **64,** 981 (1931). Synthesis by reduction of 6,13-pentacene-quinone: Bruckner *et al., Tetrahedron Lett.* **1960,** no. 1, 5; Bruckner, Tomasz, *Acta Chim. Acad. Sci. Hung.* **28**(4), 405 (1961). Structure: Campbell *et al., Acta Crystallogr.* **14,** 705 (1961).

Deep blue needles with violet luster from hot nitrobenzene. Sublimes in CO_2 stream under reduced pressure at ~300° (Clar, John, *loc. cit.).* In presence of air dec >300°. Practically insol in water; sparingly sol in organic solvents. *Note:* Anthracene (3 linear rings) is colorless; naphthacene (4 linear rings) is orange; pentacene (5 linear rings) is blue; hexacene (6 linear rings) is green.

7108. Pentachloroethane. [76-01-7] Pentalin. C_2HCl_5; mol wt 202.29. C 11.87%, H 0.50%, Cl 87.63%. CCl_3CHCl_2. Toxicity data: G. S. Barsoum, K. Saad, *Q. J. Pharm. Pharmacol.* **7,** 205 (1934).

Liquid; chloroform-like odor. d_4^{25} 1.6712; bp 161-162°. mp −29°. n_D^{15} 1.5054. Insol in water. Miscible with alcohol, ether. MLD (mg/kg) in dogs: 1750 orally; 100 i.v.; in rabbits: 700 s.c. (Barsoum, Saad).

Caution: Potential symptoms of overexposure in exptl animals are irritation of eyes, skin; weakness, restlessness, irregular respiration, muscle incoordination; liver, kidney, lung changes. *See NIOSH Pocket Guide to Chemical Hazards* (DHHS/NIOSH 97-140, 1997) p 242.

7109. Pentachlorophenol. [87-86-5] Penta; PCP; penchlorol; Santophen 20. C_6HCl_5O; mol wt 266.34. C 27.06%, H 0.38%, Cl 66.56%, O 6.01%. Prepd by the chlorination of phenol in the presence of a catalyst. Toxicity study: T. B. Gaines, *Toxicol. Appl. Pharmacol.* **14,** 515 (1969). Review of toxicology and human exposure: *Toxicological Profile for Pentachlorophenol* (PB2001-109106, 2001) 316 pp.

Needle-like crystals, mp 190-191°; bp ~309-310° (dec). d_4^{22} 1.978. Very pungent odor only when hot. Sublimes in needles. Almost insol in water (8 mg in 100 ml). Freely sol in alc, ether; sol in benzene; slightly sol in cold petr ether. LD_{50} in male, female rats (mg/kg): 146, 175 orally (Gaines).

Sodium salt. Sodium pentachlorophenate; sodium pentachlorophenoxide; Santobrite; Dowicide G. Sol in water.

Caution: Potential symptoms of overexposure are irritation of eyes, nose, throat; sneezing, cough; weakness, anorexia, weight loss; sweating; headache, dizziness; nausea, vomiting; dyspnea, chest pain; high fever. Direct contact may cause dermatitis. *See NIOSH Pocket Guide to Chemical Hazards* (DHHS/NIOSH 97-140, 1997) p 242; *Patty's Industrial Hygiene and Toxicology* **vol. 2B,** G. D. Clayton, F. E. Clayton, Eds. (Wiley-Interscience, New York, 1994) pp 1603-1613.

USE: Insecticide for termite control; pre-harvest defoliant; general herbicide. Antimicrobial preservative and fungicide for wood, wood products, starches, textiles, paints, adhesives, leather, pulp, paper, industrial waste systems, building materials. Surface disinfectant.

7110. 3-Pentadecylcatechol. [492-89-7] 3-Pentadecyl-1,2-benzenediol; 3-pentadecylpyrocatechol; tetrahydrourushiol; hydrourushiol; dihydrorhengol; 3-PDC. $C_{21}H_{36}O_2$; mol wt 320.51. C 78.69%, H 11.32%, O 9.98%. Constituent of the irritant oil of poison ivy (*Toxicodendron radicans* (L.) Kuntze) and other *Toxicodendron* spp. *(Anacardiaceae).* Prepn by hydrogenation of extracts from fruits of *Semecarpus heterophylla:* Backer, Haack, *Rec. Trav. Chim.* **57,** 225 (1938). Synthesis from 2,3-dimethoxybenzaldehyde and tetradecyl chloride: Mason, *J. Am. Chem. Soc.* **67,** 1538 (1945); from *o*-veratraldehyde: Backer, Haack, *loc. cit.;* Dawson *et al., J. Am. Chem. Soc.* **68,** 534 (1946); Keil *et al., US 2451955* (1948); from 2,3-dibenzyloxybenzaldehyde: Loev, Dawson, *J. Org. Chem.* **24,** 980 (1959); from furan derivs: Boehme, *J. Am. Chem. Soc.* **82,** 499 (1960); from catechol: Hanafusa, Yukawa, *Chem. Ind. (London)* **1961,** 23. Criticism of reported syntheses and synthesis of dimethyl deriv: Byck, Dawson, *J. Org. Chem.* **32,** 1084 (1967). Total synthesis: E. Wenkert *et al., J. Am. Chem. Soc.* **105,** 2021 (1983). Evaluation of diagnostic patch test: M. V. Dahl *et al., Arch. Dermatol.* **120,** 1022 (1984).

Short needles from toluene or petr ether, mp 59-60°. Can be purified by molecular distn. uv max: 277 nm. Sol in alc, ether, benzene, toluene. Sparingly sol in petr ether.

THERAP CAT: Diagnostic aid (contact allergen).

7111. Pentaerythritol. [115-77-5] 2,2-Bis(hydroxymethyl)-1,3-propanediol; tetrakis(hydroxymethyl)methane; tetramethylolmethane; Metab-Auxil; Penetek; Pentek. $C_5H_{12}O_4$; mol wt 136.15. C 44.11%, H 8.88%, O 47.01%. Prepd by treating acetaldehyde with formaldehyde in an aq soln of calcium hydroxide: H. B. J. Schurink, *Org. Synth.* **coll. vol. I,** 425 (2nd ed., 1941); Fieser, Fieser, *Organic Chemistry* (2nd ed, 1950) p 133. Review of mfg processes: P. W. Sherwood, *Petroleum Refiner* **Nov. 1956,** p 171-179; *Faith, Keyes & Clark's Industrial Chemicals,* F. A. Lowenheim, M. K. Moran, Eds. (Wiley-Interscience, New York, 4th ed., 1975) pp 598-603. Monograph: E. Berlow *et al., The Pentaerythritols,* ACS Monograph Series no. **136** (Reinhold, New York, 1958).

Ditetragonal crystals from dil HCl, mp 260°. One gram dissolves in 18 ml water at 15°. Sol in ethanol, glycerol, ethylene glycol, formamide. Insol in acetone, benzene, paraffin, ether, carbon tetrachloride.

Tetraacetate. [597-71-7] 2,2-Bis[(acetyloxy)methyl]-1,3-propanediol diacetate; tetra-*O*-acetylpentaerythritol; pentaerythrityl tetraacetate. $C_{13}H_{20}O_8$; mol wt 304.29. Prepn: Wolfrom *et al., J. Am. Chem. Soc.* **73,** 874 (1951); Bonner *et al., J. Chem. Soc.* **1960,** 2914. Crystals, mp 83-84°.

Trinitrate see Pentrinitrol.

Caution: Potential symptoms of overexposure to pentaerythritol are irritation of eyes and respiratory system. *See NIOSH Pocket Guide to Chemical Hazards* (DHHS/NIOSH 97-140, 1997) p 244.

USE: In synthetic resins, in paint and varnish industries.

7112.   Pentaerythritol Tetranitrate. [78-11-5] 2,2-Bis[(nitrooxy)methyl]-1,3-propanediol dinitrate (ester); pentaerythrityl tetranitrate; 2,2-bisdihydroxymethyl-1,3-propanediol tetranitrate; PETN; nitropentaerythritol; penthrit; niperyt; Lentrat; Hasethrol; Peritrate; Mycardol; Nitropenton; Pentral 80; Dilcoran-80; Terpate; Pentrite; Perityl; Pentanitrine; Prevangor; Subicard; Pentryate; Vasodiatol; Neo-Corovas; Pentafin; Quintrate; Pergitral; Pentitrate; Metranil; Cardiacap; Angitet; Nitropenta. $C_5H_8N_4O_{12}$; mol wt 316.14. C 19.00%, H 2.55%, N 17.72%, O 60.73%. Prepn: Acken, Vyverberg, **US 2370437** (1945 to Du Pont). GC/MS analysis in post-explosion residues: T. Tamiri *et al.* in *Adv. Anal. Detect. Explosives*, J. Yinon, Ed. (Kluwer, Netherlands, 1993) pp 323-334.

ONO₂ ONO₂ O₂NO ONO₂ (structure)

Tetragonal holohedra from acetone + alcohol, mp 140°. d_4^{20} 1.773. Soluble in acetone. Practically insoluble in water (1.5 γ/ml). Sparingly sol in alcohol, ether. Does not reduce Fehling's soln (difference from erythrityl tetranitrate). *Explodes on percussion.* More sensitive to shock than TNT. For medicinal purposes it is dil with an inert ingredient, usually lactose, to prevent accidental explosions.

USE: Mainly in the manuf of detonating fuse (Primacord), a waterproof textile filled with powdered PETN.

THERAP CAT: Vasodilator (coronary).

7113.   Pentagastrin. [5534-95-2] *N*-[(1,1-Dimethylethoxy)carbonyl]-β-alanyl-L-tryptophyl-L-methionyl-L-α-aspartyl-L-phenylalaninamide; *N*-carboxy-β-alanyl-L-tryptophyl-L-methionyl-L-aspartylphenyl-L-alaninamide *N-tert*-butyl ester; *N*-(α-carbamoylphenethyl)-3-[2-[2-[3-(carboxyamino)propionamido]-3-indol-3-yl-propionamido]-4-(methylthio)butyramido]succinamic acid *N-tert*-butyl ester; *N*-[*N*-[*N*-[*N*-(*N-tert*-butoxycarbonyl-β-alanyl)-L-tryptophanyl]-L-methionyl]-L-aspartyl]-L-phenylalaninamide; Boc-β-Ala-Trp-Met-Asp-Phe(NH₂); AY-6608; ICI-50123; Gastrodiagnost; Peptavlon. $C_{37}H_{49}N_7O_9S$; mol wt 767.89. C 57.87%, H 6.43%, N 12.77%, O 18.75%, S 4.18%. Prepn: P. M. Hardy *et al.*, **BE 665591**; *eidem*, **US 3896103** (1965, 1975 to I.C.I.); Davey *et al.*, *J. Chem. Soc. C* **1966**, 555; Sakakibara *et al.*, *Bull. Chem. Soc. Jpn.* **41**, 438 (1968). Structure-function relationship studies: Morley *et al.*, *Nature* **207**, 1356 (1965). Formulation and pharmacological studies: Wai *et al.*, *J. Pharm. Pharmacol.* **22**, 923 (1970). *Reviews:* Makhlouf, *Fed. Proc.* **27**, 1322 (1968); Sanders, Schimmel, *Am. J. Med.* **49**, 380 (1970).

H₃C / H₃C—O / H₃C (Boc structure) TrpMetAspPheNH₂

Fine, colorless needle-shaped crystals from 2-ethoxyethanol + water; mp 229-230° (dec). $[\alpha]_D^{22}$ -28.8 ±0.5° (DMF). uv max (2N NH₄OH): 280, 289 nm (ε 5340, 4590). Sol in DMF, DMSO. Almost insol in water, ethanol, ether, benzene.

THERAP CAT: Diagnostic aid (gastric secretion stimulant).

7114.   Pentagestrone. [7001-56-1] 3-(Cyclopentyloxy)-17-hydroxypregna-3,5-dien-20-one; 17α-hydroxyprogesterone 3-cyclopentyl enol ether. $C_{26}H_{38}O_3$; mol wt 398.58. C 78.35%, H 9.61%, O 12.04%. Prepn of acetate: Ercoli, Gardi, *J. Am. Chem. Soc.* **82**, 746 (1960); of free alcohol and acetate: Ercoli, **US 3019241** (1962).

(steroid structure)

Solid, mp 184.5-186.5°. $[\alpha]_D$ -115° (dioxane).
Acetate. [1178-60-5] 17α-Acetoxyprogesterone 3-cyclopentyl enol ether; Gestovis. $C_{28}H_{40}O_4$; mol wt 440.61. Solid, mp 137-

138°; also reported as 157-158°, Ercoli, **GB 893315** (1962 to Vismara). $[\alpha]_D$ -147° (dioxane).

THERAP CAT: Progestogen.

7115.   Pentamidine. [100-33-4] 4,4'-[1,5-Pentanediyl-bis(oxy)]bisbenzenecarboximidamide; 4,4'-(pentamethylenedioxy)-dibenzamidine; 4,4'-diamidino-α,ω-diphenoxypentane. $C_{19}H_{24}N_4$-O_2; mol wt 340.42. C 67.04%, H 7.11%, N 16.46%, O 9.40%. Prepn: A. J. Ewins, **GB 507565** (1939); J. N. Ashley *et al.*, *J. Chem. Soc.* **1942**, 103; of isethionate: G. Newbery, A. P. T. Easson, **US 2394003** (1946 to May & Baker). Trypanocidal activity: E. M. Lourie, W. Yorke, *Ann. Trop. Med. Parasitol.* **33**, 289 (1939). Preliminary pharmacological studies in animals: R. Wien, *ibid.* **37**, 1 (1943). Activity in fibrinolytic systems: J. D. Geratz, *Thromb. Diath. Haemorrh.* **29**, 154 (1973). Pharmacodynamics in men and mice: T. P. Waalkes *et al.*, *Clin. Pharmacol. Ther.* **11**, 505 (1970). *In vitro* activity against *Pneumocystis carinii:* E. L. Pesanti, C. Cox, *Infect. Immun.* **34**, 908 (1981). Uptake and distribution of aerosolized form in animals: R. J. Debs *et al.*, *Am. Rev. Respir. Dis.* **135**, 731 (1987). *In vivo* efficacy of aerosolized form in rats: *eidem, Antimicrob. Agents Chemother.* **31**, 37 (1987). Determn in plasma, urine and tissues: T. P. Waalkes, V. T. DeVita, *J. Lab. Clin. Med.* **75**, 871 (1970); by HPLC: C. M. Dickinson *et al.*, *J. Chromatogr.* **345**, 91 (1985). Preliminary clinical evaluation in *P. carinii* pneumonia: V. T. DeVita *et al.*, *N. Engl. J. Med.* **280**, 287 (1968). Comparison with sulfamethoxazole-trimethoprim mixture in *P. carinii* pneumonia in AIDS: J. M. Wharton *et al.*, *Ann. Intern. Med.* **105**, 37 (1986). Early review of pharmacology, mode of action and clinical applications: E. B. Schoenbach, E. M. Greenspan, *Medicine* **27**, 327-377 (1948). *Review:* S. Drake *et al.*, *Clin. Pharm.* **4**, 507-516 (1985); M. Sands *et al.*, *Rev. Infect. Dis.* **7**, 625-634 (1985); of activity, pharmacokinetics and therapeutic use: K. L. Goa, D. M. Campoli-Richards, *Drugs* **33**, 242-258 (1987).

(structure)

Crystallizes as colorless plates from water. Dec 186°.
Dihydrochloride. [50357-45-4] $C_{19}H_{24}N_4O_2 \cdot 2HCl$. Fine needles from dil HCl, mp 232-234°. LD_{50} in mice (mg/g): 0.028 i.v.; 0.064 s.c. (Wein).
Isethionate. [140-64-7] M & B 800; RP-2512; NebuPent; Pentacarinat; Pentam. $C_{19}H_{24}N_4O_2 \cdot 2C_2H_6O_4S$; mol wt 592.68. Hygroscopic, very bitter crystals, mp ~180°. Slight butyric odor. Sol in water (~1 in 10 at 25°, ~1 in 4 at 100°); sol in glycerol, more readily on warming; slightly sol in alcohol. Insol in ether, acetone, chloroform, liq petr. pH of a 5% w/v soln in water: 4.5 to 6.5.
Dimethanesulfonate. [6823-79-6] Pentamidine mesylate. $C_{19}H_{24}N_4O_2 \cdot 2CH_3SO_3H$; mol wt 532.63. White powder.

THERAP CAT: Antiprotozoal (Trypanosoma, Leishmania); antipneumocystic.

THERAP CAT (VET): Antiprotozoal (Babesia, Leishmania).

7116.   Pentane. [109-66-0] *n*-Pentane. C_5H_{12}; mol wt 72.15. C 83.23%, H 16.76%. $CH_3CH_2CH_2CH_2CH_3$. Occurs in petroleum; it is a constituent of petr ether. Sepn from natural gasoline: Love, *Pet. Eng.* **12**, no. 10, 130 sqq (1941), *C.A.* **35**, 7162 (1941); from virgin naphthas: Tongberg *et al.*, *Ind. Eng. Chem.* **30**, 166 (1938). Prepd by dehydration and subsequent hydrogenation of 2- and 3-pentanol: Mair, *Bur. Stand. J. Res.* **9**, 457 (1932); from 2-bromopentane by Grignard reaction: Noller, *Org. Synth.* **11**, 84 (1931). Toxicity data: Fühner, *Biochem. Z.* **115**, 235 (1921).

Flammable liq. d_4^0 0.64529; d_4^{20} 0.62638; d_4^{30} 0.6163; mp -129.7°. bp₇₆₀ 36.1°; bp₄₀₀ 18.5°; bp₂₀₀ 1.9°; bp₁₀₀ -12.6°; bp₆₀ -22.2°; bp₄₀ -29.2°; bp₂₀ -40.2°; bp₁₀ -50.1°; bp₅ -62.5°; bp₁.₀ -76.6°; n_D^{20} 1.35768. Flash pt, closed cup: <-40°F (-40°C). Explosive limits, % by vol in air: lower 1.4; upper 8.0. Autoignition temp +588°F (+309°C). Soly in water at 16°: 0.36 g/l. Miscible with alc, ether, many organic solvents. LC (in air) in mice: 377 mg/l (Fühner).

Caution: Potential symptoms of overexposure are drowsiness; irritation of eyes, skin, nose. Direct contact may cause dermatitis;

aspiration of liquid may cause chemical pneumonia. *See NIOSH Pocket Guide to Chemical Hazards* (DHHS/NIOSH 97-140, 1997) p 244.

7117. 1,5-Pentanediol. [111-29-5] Pentamethylene glycol; 1,5-dihydroxypentane. $C_5H_{12}O_2$; mol wt 104.15. C 57.66%, H 11.61%, O 30.72%. HOCH$_2$(CH$_2$)$_3$CH$_2$OH. Prepd by hydrogenolysis of tetrahydrofurfuryl alcohol in the presence of copper chromite: Connor, Adkins, *J. Am. Chem. Soc.* **54**, 4678 (1932); D. Kaufman, W. Reeve, *Org. Synth.* **coll. vol. III,** 693 (1955). Toxicity study: H. F. Smyth *et al., Am. Ind. Hyg. Assoc. J.* **23,** 95 (1962).

Viscous, oily liquid. Bitter taste. d^{20} 0.9941. mp $-18°$. bp$_{760}$ 239°, bp$_{3.0}$ 120°. n_D^{20} 1.4499. Flash pt 125°C (275°F). Miscible with water, methanol, alc, acetone, ethyl acetate. Soly in ether (25°): 11% w/w. Limited soly in benzene, trichloroethylene, methylene chloride, petr ether, heptane. LD$_{50}$ orally in rats: 5.89 g/kg (Smyth).

USE: As plasticizer in cellulose products and adhesives, in brake fluid compositions. Forms esters and polyesters which can be used as plasticizers, emulsifying agents and resin intermediates.

7118. 1-Pentanol. [71-41-0] Pentyl alcohol; *n*-amyl alcohol; *n*-butyl carbinol. $C_5H_{12}O$; mol wt 88.15. C 68.13%, H 13.72%, O 18.15%. CH$_3$(CH$_2$)$_4$OH. Prepn from 1-pentene: Brown, Rao, *J. Am. Chem. Soc.* **81,** 6434 (1959); Brown, US 2925437 (1960). Toxicity study: P. M. Jenner *et al., Food Cosmet. Toxicol.* **2,** 327 (1964). Review of manuf by fractionation of fusel oil and via chlorination of pentanes, and properties: *Industrial Chemicals,* W. L. Faith *et al.,* Eds. (John Wiley, New York, 2nd ed., 1957) pp 107-114.

Liquid, mild characteristic odor. bp 137.5°. mp $-79°$. d^{20} 0.8146; d^{25} 0.8110. n_D^{20} 1.4103: Mumford, Phillips, *J. Chem. Soc.* **1950,** 75. Flash pt, closed cup: 100°F (38°C). Slightly sol in water (2.7 g/100 ml at 22°); misc with alc, ether. LD$_{50}$ orally in rats: 3030 mg/kg (Jenner).

Caution: Irritating to eyes, respiratory passages. Narcotic: E. Browning, *Toxicity and Metabolism of Industrial Solvents* (Elsevier, New York, 1965) pp 356-367.

USE: In organic syntheses; as solvent.

7119. 2-Pentanol. [6032-29-7] *dl-sec*-Amyl alcohol; methyl propyl carbinol. $C_5H_{12}O$; mol wt 88.15. C 68.13%, H 13.72%, O 18.15%. CH$_3$CH$_2$CH$_2$CH(OH)CH$_3$. Prepn: Brown, Nakagawa, *J. Am. Chem. Soc.* **77,** 3614 (1955); Brown, Wheeler, *ibid.* **78,** 2199 (1956). Sepn of optical isomers: Adembri, *Ann. Chim. (Rome)* **46,** 62 (1956). Review of manuf by fractionation of fusel oil and via chlorination of pentanes, and properties: *Industrial Chemicals,* W. L. Faith *et al.,* Eds. (John Wiley, New York, 2nd ed., 1957) pp 107-114.

Liquid, characteristic odor. bp 119.3°. bp$_{745}$ 118°. d^{20} 0.8098. n_D^{25} 1.4041, n_D^{20} 1.406. Flash pt (open cup) 105°F. Slightly sol in water (16.6 g/100 ml at 20°). Miscible with alcohol, ether.

Caution: See 1-Pentanol.

7120. 3-Pentanol. [584-02-1] Diethyl carbinol. $C_5H_{12}O$; mol wt 88.15. C 68.13%, H 13.72%, O 18.15%. CH$_3$CH$_2$CH(OH)CH$_2$CH$_3$. Prepn: Brown, Nakagawa, *J. Am. Chem. Soc.* **77,** 3614 (1955). Toxicity study: H. F. Smyth *et al., Arch. Ind. Hyg. Occup. Med.* **10,** 61 (1954). Review of manuf and properties: *Industrial Chemicals,* W. L. Faith *et al.,* Eds. (John Wiley, New York, 2nd ed., 1957) pp 107-114.

Liquid, characteristic odor. bp 115.6°, bp$_{738}$ 113.5-113.7°. d^{25} 0.815; n_D^{25} 1.4077, n_D^{20} 1.4097. Slightly sol in water (5.5 g/100 g at 30°); sol in alcohol, ether. LD$_{50}$ orally in rats: 1.87 g/kg (Smyth).

Caution: See 1-Pentanol.

USE: Flotation agent; solvent in organic synthesis.

7121. Pentazocine. [359-83-1] (2*R*,6*R*,11*R*)-*rel*-1,2,3,4,5,6-Hexahydro-6,11-dimethyl-3-(3-methyl-2-butenyl)-2,6-methano-3-benzazocin-8-ol; 2-dimethylallyl-5,9-dimethyl-2′-hydroxybenzomorphan; 3-(3-methyl-2-butenyl)-1,2,3,4,5,6-hexahydro-6,11-dimethyl-2,6-methano-3-benzazocin-8-ol; NSC-107430; Win-20228; Fortralin. $C_{19}H_{27}NO$; mol wt 285.42. C 79.95%, H 9.53%, N 4.91%, O 5.61%. Mixed opioid agonist-antagonist. Prepn: Archer, BE 611000 (1962 to Sterling Drug), *C.A.* **58,** 2440b (1963); Archer *et al., J. Med. Chem.* **7,** 123 (1964). Review of pharmacology: Brogden *et al., Drugs* **5,** 6-91 (1973). Clinical study in postoperative pain: F. Camu, *Eur. J. Clin. Pharmacol.* **19,** 259 (1981).

HPLC analysis in blood and plasma: R. D. Anderson *et al., J. Chromatogr.* **227,** 239 (1982). Toxicity data: E. I. Goldenthal, *Toxicol. Appl. Pharmacol.* **18,** 185 (1971).

Crystals from methanol + water, mp 145.4-147.2°. LD$_{50}$ s.c. in male rats: 175±36 mg/kg (Goldenthal).

Hydrochloride. [64024-15-3] Fortalgesic (tabl.); Fortral (tabl.). $C_{19}H_{27}NO.HCl$; mol wt 321.88.

Lactate. [17146-95-1] Liticon; Pentagin; Sosegon; Talwin. $C_{19}H_{27}NO.C_3H_6O_3$; mol wt 375.50.

Note: This is a controlled substance: **21 CFR,** 1308.14.

THERAP CAT: Analgesic (narcotic).

THERAP CAT (VET): Analgesic (narcotic).

7122. 1-Pentene. [109-67-1] Propylethylene; *α-n*-amylene. C_5H_{10}; mol wt 70.13. C 85.63%, H 14.37%. CH$_3$(CH$_2$)$_2$-CH=CH$_2$. Occurs in coal tar. Prepd from allyl bromide and ethylmagnesium bromide in ether or better in dipropyl ether: Meisenheimer, Casper, *Ber.* **54,** 1663 (1921); Norris, Joubert, *J. Am. Chem. Soc.* **49,** 885 (1927); Kirrmann, *Compt. Rend.* **184,** 1178 (1927).

Liquid. d_4^0 0.6429; bp$_{760}$ 30.1°; n_D^{20} 1.3714. Insol in water. Miscible with alcohol, ether, benzene.

7123. 2-Pentene. [109-68-2] *β-n*-Amylene; *sym*-methylethylethylene. C_5H_{10}; mol wt 70.13. C 85.63%, H 14.37%. CH$_3$-CH$_2$CH=CHCH$_3$. Prepn of mixture of *cis* and *trans* isomers by dehydration of 2-pentanol: Norris, *Org. Synth.* **coll. vol. I,** (2nd ed., 1941) p 430. Prepn of the geometrical isomers from *cis*- and *trans*-α-methyl-β-ethylacrylic acids: Lucas, Prater, *J. Am. Chem. Soc.* **59,** 1682 (1937). Prepn of the *cis* form from 1-ethyl-2-iodobutyric acid with quinoline, of the *trans* form from 1-ethyl-2-iodobutyric acid with sodium carbonate: Sherrill, Matlak, *ibid.* 2134; prepn of both isomers from *sec*-amyl alcohol with H$_2$SO$_4$ and diatomaceous earth at 90-110° for 3 hrs: Lucas *et al., ibid.* **63,** 22 (1941). Absorption spectra: Carr, Stücklen, *ibid.* **59,** 2138 (1937).

cis-**Form.** Liquid. d_4^{20} 0.6503; d_4^{80} 0.5824; d_4^{30} 0.6392; d_4^0 0.6710. mp -180 to $-178°$. bp$_{760}$ 37.0°. n_D^{20} 1.38130.

trans-**Form.** Liquid. d_4^{20} 0.6482; d_4^{80} 0.5814; d_4^{30} 0.6381; d_4^0 0.6675. mp -136 to $-135°$. bp$_{760}$ 35.85°. n_D^{20} 1.37921.

7124. Pentetate Calcium Trisodium. [12111-24-9] [*N*-[2-[Bis(carboxy-*κO*)methyl]amino-*κN*]ethyl]-*N*-[2-[[(carboxy-*κO*)methyl](carboxymethyl)amino-*κN*]ethyl]glycinato(5−)-*κN*-calciate(3−) trisodium; [*N,N*-bis[2-[bis(carboxymethyl)amino]ethyl]glycinato(5−)]calciate(3−) trisodium; calcium trisodium pentetate; sodium[[[(carboxymethyl)imino]bis(ethylenenitrilo)]tetraacetato]calciate; [[(carboxymethyl)imino]bis(ethylenenitrilo)]tetraacetic acid calcium complex trisodium salt; trisodium calcium diethylenetriaminepentaacetate; pentacin; Calcium Chel 330; Ditripentat; Penthamil. $C_{14}H_{18}CaN_3Na_3O_{10}$; mol wt 497.35. C 33.81%, H 3.65%, Ca 8.06%, N 8.45%, Na 13.87%, O 32.17%. Prepn: Rubin, Dexter, US 3062719 (1962 to Geigy). Effects in uranium poisoning in rats: R. Dagirmanjian *et al., J. Pharmacol. Exp. Ther.* **117,** 20 (1956); in mixed fusion products poisoning: K. Kostial *et al., J. Appl. Toxicol.* **3,** 291 (1983).

Solid. Sol in water. Practically insol in alcohol. Used in aq soln. LD$_{50}$ i.p. in rats: 3.8 g/kg (Dagirmanjian).

THERAP CAT: Chelating agent (plutonium and other transuranium elements).

7125. Pentetic Acid. [67-43-6] *N,N*-Bis[2-[bis(carboxymethyl)amino]ethyl]glycine; [[(carboxymethyl)imino]bis(ethylenenitrilo)]tetraacetic acid; pentacarboxymethyl diethylenetriamine; diethylenetriamine pentaacetic acid; DTPA. $C_{14}H_{23}N_3O_{10}$; mol wt 393.35. C 42.75%, H 5.89%, N 10.68%, O 40.67%. Prepn of the acid: Curme *et al., US **2384816** (1945 to Carbide and Carbon Chem.); Samoilova, Yashunskii, **SU 144479** (1962), *C.A.* **57,** 12326d (1962); of Na salt: **GB 601816**; **GB 601817** (both 1948 to Carbide and Carbon Chem.). Structure and infrared spectrum: Nakamoto *et al., J. Am. Chem. Soc.* **85,** 309 (1963).

Trisodium calcium salt *see* Pentetate Calcium Trisodium.
USE: Chelating agent.
THERAP CAT: Chelating agent (iron).

7126. Pentetreotide. [138661-02-6] *N*-[2-[[2-[Bis(carboxymethyl)amino]ethyl](carboxymethyl)amino]ethyl]-*N*-(carboxymethyl)glycyl-D-phenylalanyl-L-cysteinyl-L-phenylalanyl-D-tryptophyl-L-lysyl-L-threonyl-*N*-[(1*R*,2*R*)-2-hydroxy-1-(hydroxymethyl)propyl]-L-cysteinamide cyclic (3 → 8)-disulfide; [DTPA-D-Phe^1]-octreotide; DTPA-SMS; SDZ-215-811. $C_{63}H_{87}N_{13}O_{19}S_2$; mol wt 1394.57. C 54.26%, H 6.29%, N 13.06%, O 21.80%, S 4.60%. Octapeptide analog of somatostatin, *q.v.* Prepn of compd and chelate, and binding characteristics: W. H. Bakker *et al., Life Sci.* **49,** 1583 (1991). Synthesis, biological activity and somatostatin receptor-positive tumor imaging: R. Albert *et al., Actual. Chim. Ther.* **21,** 111 (1994). Clinical metabolism and scintigraphic studies: E. P. Krenning *et al., J. Nucl. Med.* **33,** 652 (1992). Diagnostic imaging: E. Bombardieri *et al., Eur. J. Cancer* **31A,** 184 (1995); F. Jamar *et al., J. Nucl. Med.* **36,** 542 (1995); G. Kahaly *et al., ibid.* 550. Review of diagnostic use in neuroendocrine tumors: C. A. Hoefnagel, *Eur. J. Nucl. Med.* **21,** 561-581 (1994); of mechanism of action: E. P. Krenning *et al., Semin. Oncol.* **21,** Suppl. 13, 6-14 (1994).

^{111}In chelate. [139096-04-1] ^{111}In pentetreotide; [^{111}In-DTPA-D-Phe^1]-octreotide; MP-1727; OctreoScan. $C_{63}H_{84}$^{111}InN$_{13}$O$_{19}$S$_2$.
THERAP CAT: ^{111}In chelate as diagnostic aid (radioactive imaging agent).

7127. Pentifylline. [1028-33-7] 1-Hexyl-3,7-dihydro-3,7-dimethyl-1*H*-purine-2,6-dione; 1-hexyltheobromine; 1-hexyl-3,7-dimethylxanthine; 3,7-dimethyl-1-hexyl-1*H*,3*H*-purin-2,6-dione; SK-7; Cosaldon. $C_{13}H_{20}N_4O_2$; mol wt 264.32. C 59.07%, H 7.63%, N 21.20%, O 12.11%. Prepn from theobromine and hexyl halide: Eidebenz, Schuh, **DE 860217** (1952 to Chem. Werke Albert); Serchi, *Chimica* **40,** 451 (1964); Chkhikvadze *et al., SU* 202152 (1967), *C.A.* **69,** 19368x (1968). Pharmacology: Cugurra, Echinard-Garin, *Arch. Int. Pharmacodyn. Ther.* **123,** 481 (1960); Ramos *et al., ibid.* **153,** 430 (1965); Mohler *et al., Arzneim.-Forsch.* **16,** 1524 (1966). Metabolic studies: Mohler *et al., Arch. Pharm.* **299,** 448 (1966).

Crystals, mp 82-83°.
USE: Stabilizer of vitamin preparations: Nook, Eidebenz, **DE 1810705** (1970 to Chem. Werke Albert).
THERAP CAT: Vasodilator.

7128. Pentigetide. [62087-72-3] N^2-[1-[*N*-(*N*-L-α-Aspartyl-L-seryl)-L-α-aspartyl]-L-prolyl]-L-arginine; human IgE pentapeptide; HEPP; Pentyde. $C_{22}H_{36}N_8O_{11}$; mol wt 588.57. C 44.89%, H 6.17%, N 19.04%, O 29.90%. Synthetic pentapeptide with antiallergic activity. Structure corresponds to amino acids 320-324 of the epsilon chain of human immunoglobulin E (IgE). Prepn: R. N. Hamburger, **DE 2602443**; *idem, US **4171299** (1976, 1979 both to Univ. California). Inhibition of IgE-mediated immediate hypersensitivity response: *idem, Science* **189,** 389 (1975). Stimulation of peritoneal macrophages: E. Tzehoval *et al., Proc. Natl. Acad. Sci. USA* **75,** 3400 (1978). Mechanism of action study: R. N. Hamburger, *Immunology* **38,** 781 (1979). Clinical evaluations in allergic rhinitis: G. A. Cohen *et al., Ann. Allergy* **52,** 83 (1984); B. M. Prenner, *ibid.* **58,** 332 (1987).

Asp–Ser–Asp–Pro–Arg

$[\alpha]_D^{20}$ −78.6° (c = 1 in water).
THERAP CAT: Antiallergic.

7129. Pentisomide. [78833-03-1] α-[2-[Bis(1-methylethyl)amino]ethyl]-α-(2-methylpropyl)-2-pyridineacetamide; 2-[2-(diisopropylamino)ethyl]-4-methyl-2-(2-pyridyl)pentanamide; propisomide; penticainide; CM-7857; ME-3202. $C_{19}H_{33}N_3O$; mol wt 319.48. C 71.43%, H 10.41%, N 13.15%, O 5.01%. Sodium channel blocker; derivative of disopyramide, *q.v.* Prepn: H. Demarne *et al., EP 27412; eidem, US **4356177** (1981, 1982 both to C. M. Industries); C. A. Bernhart *et al., J. Med. Chem.* **26,** 451 (1983). Electrophysiological study: V. Kühlkamp *et al., Int. J. Cardiol.* **36,** 69 (1992). HPLC determn in plasma, urine, and tissues: T. A. Plomp, M. J. H. Buijs, *J. Chromatogr.* **612,** 123 (1993). Clinical evaluation: S. G. Priori *et al., Am. J. Cardiol.* **60,** 1068 (1987); S. G. Mangini *et al., Eur. Heart J.* **12,** 712 (1991). *Review:* S. Yuan, S. B. Olsson, *Cardiovasc. Drug Rev.* **11,** 74-93 (1993).

White crystals from diisopropyl ether, mp 108-109°. Sol in water.
THERAP CAT: Antiarrhythmic (class I).

7130. Pentobarbital. [76-74-4] 5-Ethyl-5-(1-methylbutyl)-2,4,6(1*H*,3*H*,5*H*)-pyrimidinetrione; 5-ethyl-5-(1-methylbutyl)barbituric acid; mebumbital; pentobarbitone; Neodorm. $C_{11}H_{18}N_2O_3$; mol wt 226.27. C 58.39%, H 8.02%, N 12.38%, O 21.21%. Prepn: **DE 293163** (1916 to Bayer), *Frdl.* **13,** 799 (1923); and hypnotic activity: E. H. Volwiler, D. L. Tabern, *J. Am. Chem. Soc.* **52,** 1676 (1930). Toxicity data: E. W. Schafer, *Toxicol. Appl. Pharmacol.* **21,** 315 (1972). HPLC determn in plasma: M. J. Avram, T. C. Krejcie, *J. Chromatogr.* **414,** 484 (1986). Use in clinical management of elevated intracranial pressure: P. S. Woster, K. L. LeBlanc, *Clin. Pharm.* **9,** 762 (1990); for euthanasia: A. T. Evans *et al., J. Am. Vet. Med. Assoc.* **203,** 664 (1993).

Crystals from alcohol, mp 129-130°.
Sodium salt. [57-33-0] Pentobarbital sodium; soluble pentobarbital; Carbrital; Narcoren; Nembutal; Pentone; Praecicalm; Sopental. $C_{11}H_{17}N_2NaO_3$; mol wt 248.25. White powder; slightly

bitter taste. Dec ~127°. Freely sol in water, alc. Practically insol in benzene, ether. Aq solns are unstable. LD_{50} orally in rats: 118 mg/kg (Schafer).

Calcium salt. [7563-42-0] Pentobarbital calcium; Repocal. $C_{22}H_{34}CaN_4O_6$; mol wt 490.61.

Note: This is a controlled substance (depressant): **21 CFR,** 1308.12 and 1308.13.

THERAP CAT: Sedative, hypnotic.

THERAP CAT (VET): Anesthetic (intravenous); for euthanasia.

7131. 1-Pentol. [105-29-3] 3-Methyl-2-penten-4-yn-1-ol; 1-hydroxy-3-methyl-2-penten-4-yne. C_6H_8O; mol wt 96.13. C 74.97%, H 8.39%, O 16.64%. Prepd by allylic rearrangement of methylvinylethynyl carbinol with moderately strong acid at 80°: Oroshnik, *J. Am. Chem. Soc.* **78,** 2651 (1956).

trans - Isomer

cis-Form. 1'-Pentol. Oily liquid. $bp_{9.4}$ 65°. n_D^{20} 1.4820. uv max (ethanol): 223 nm (ε 11,000).

cis-Form p-nitrobenzoate. mp 61-62°.

trans-Form. 1″-Pentol. Oily liquid. $bp_{9.4}$ 73°. n_D^{20} 1.4934. uv max (ethanol): 224 nm (ε 13,100).

trans-Form p-nitrobenzoate. mp 63-64°.

Caution: Both isomers tend to polymerize and will explode when heated above 120° in a sealed bomb tube.

USE: Intermediate in vitamin A synthesis.

7132. Pentolinium Tartrate. [52-62-0] 1,1'-(1,5-Pentane-diyl)bis[1-methylpyrrolidinium] salt with (2R,3R)-2,3-dihydroxy-butanedioic acid (1:2); pentamethylene-1,5-bis(1-methylpyrrolidinium) hydrogen tartrate; pentamethylpyrrolidinium bitartrate; pentolonium bitartrate; M & B 2050A; Ansolysen Tartrate; Ansolysen Bitartrate; Pentilium. $C_{23}H_{42}N_2O_{12}$; mol wt 538.59. C 51.29%, H 7.86%, N 5.20%, O 35.65%. General procedure of prepn: Libman *et al., J. Chem. Soc.* **1952,** 2305. Ganglionic blocking agent.

$2C_4H_5O_6^-$

Crystals, dec 203°. Non-hygroscopic. Acid taste. Freely sol in water or in 25% aq polyvinylpyrrolidone soln. One gram dissolves in 0.4 ml water, in 810 ml ethanol. Insol in ether, chloroform. A 10% aq soln has a pH of about 3.5.

THERAP CAT: Antihypertensive.

7133. Pentorex. [434-43-5] α,α,β-Trimethylbenzeneethan-amine; α,α,β-trimethylphenethylamine; 1,1-dimethyl-2-phenylpropylamine; DL-2-phenyl-3-methyl-3-butylamine; phenpentermine. $C_{11}H_{17}N$; mol wt 163.26. C 80.92%, H 10.50%, N 8.58%. Prepn: **FR M2594** (1964 to Nordmark), *C.A.* **61,** 16013f (1964). GC determn in plasma and urine: F. T. Delbeke, M. Debackere, *J. Chromatogr.* **273,** 141 (1983).

bp_{20} 109-111°.

Hydrochloride. [5585-52-4] $C_{11}H_{17}N\cdot HCl$. Crystals, mp 164-166°.

Hydrogen D-tartrate. [22232-55-9] Liprodène; Modatrop. $C_{11}H_{17}N\cdot C_4H_6O_6$; mol wt 313.35. Crystals, mp 160-162°. $[\alpha]_D$ +13.4° (c = 0.8 in water).

D-Form hydrogen D-tartrate. Crystals, mp 167-169°. $[\alpha]_D^{20}$ +17.9°.

L-Form hydrogen D-tartrate. Crystals, mp 164-166°. $[\alpha]_D^{20}$ +3.45°.

THERAP CAT: Anorexic.

7134. Pentosan Polysulfate. [37300-21-3] Xylan hydrogen sulfate; xylan polysulfate; CB-8061; Semi-synthetic sulfated poly-anion composed of β-D-xylopyranose residues with properties similar to heparin, *q.v.* Mol wt ranges from 1500 to 5000. Prepn: **CH 293566** (1953 to Wander), *C.A.* **49,** 1787h (1955). Anticoagulant activity: B. Paramelle, *Therapie* **17,** 719 (1962); J.-B., Dureux *et al., ibid.* **19,** 879 (1964). Pharmacokinetics: R. Taugner *et al., Arch. Int. Pharmacodyn.* **189,** 250 (1971). Effects on aggregation of human blood platelets: G. Kindness *et al., Thromb. Res.* **16,** 97 (1979). Comparison of pentosan polysulfate with heparin: C. Soria *et al., ibid.* **19,** 455 (1980); M. Ryde *et al., ibid.* **23,** 435 (1981); A.-M. Fischer *et al., Thromb. Haemostasis* **47,** 104, 109 (1982). Mechanism of antiadherence activity in urinary bladder: C. L. Parsons *et al., Science* **208,** 605 (1980); *eidem, Infect. Immun.* **27,** 876 (1980). Clinical trials in interstitial cystitis: A. Fritjofsson *et al., J. Urol.* **138,** 508 (1987); S. G. Mulholland *et al., Urology* **6,** 552 (1990).

Sodium salt. [37319-17-8] Sodium pentosan polysulfate; sodium xylan polysulfate; Cartrophen; Elmiron; Fibrase; Fibrezym; Hémoclar; SP-54; Thrombocid. White odorless powder, slightly hygroscopic. $[\alpha]_D^{20}$ −57°. pH of 10% aq soln ~6.0. n_D^{20} of 10% aq soln: 1.344. Sol in water.

THERAP CAT: In treatment of interstitial cystitis; antithrombotic.

THERAP CAT (VET): Anti-inflammatory.

7135. Pentostatin. [53910-25-1] (8R)-3-(2-Deoxy-β-D-*erythro*-pentofuranosyl)-3,4,7,8-tetrahydroimidazo[4,5-*d*][1,3]-diazepin-8-ol; 2'-deoxycoformycin; DCF; 2'-dCF; CL-67310465; NSC-218321; CI-825; Nipent. $C_{11}H_{16}N_4O_4$; mol wt 268.27. C 49.25%, H 6.01%, N 20.88%, O 23.86%. Adenosine deaminase inhibitor. Isoln from *Streptomyces antibioticus* and structure determn: P. W. K. Woo *et al., J. Heterocycl. Chem.* **11,** 641 (1974). Isoln and purification: A. Ryder *et al.,* **DE 2517596;** *eidem,* **US 3923785** (both 1975 to Parke-Davis). Total synthesis: E. Chan *et al., J. Org. Chem.* **47,** 3457 (1982). Preliminary biosynthetic study: J. C. Hanvey *et al., Biochemistry* **27,** 5790 (1988). Inhibition of deaminases *in vitro:* T. Rogler-Brown *et al., Biochem. Pharmacol.* **27,** 2289 (1978); C. Frieden *et al., Biochem. Biophys. Res. Commun.* **91,** 278 (1979); *in vivo:* W. Plunkett *et al., Biochem. Pharmacol.* **28,** 201 (1979). Toxicology study: J. F. Smyth *et al., Cancer Chemother. Pharmacol.* **1,** 49 (1978). Clinical pharmacology: J. F. Smyth *et al., ibid.* **5,** 93 (1980); P. P. Major *et al., Blood* **58,** 91 (1981); F. J. Cummings *et al., Clin. Pharmacol. Ther.* **44,** 501 (1988). Enzymatic determn in biological fluids: M. M. Chassin *et al., Biochem. Pharmacol.* **28,** 1849 (1979); A. E. Staubus *et al., ibid.* **33,** 1633 (1984). Clinical evaluation in hairy cell leukemia: J. B. Johnston *et al., J. Natl. Cancer Inst.* **80,** 765 (1988). Brief review: P. O'Dwyer *et al., Ann. Intern. Med.* **108,** 733 (1988). Review of clinical pharmacology and immunosuppressive effects: M. Higman *et al., Expert Opin. Pharmacother.* **5,** 2605-2613 (2004).

White crystals from methanol/water, mp 220-225° (Woo), also reported as 204-209.5° with darkening at >150° (Chan). uv max (water, pH 7): 282 nm (ε 8000); (pH 11): 283 nm (ε 7970); (pH 2): 273 nm (ε 7570 initially, 3143 after 6.5 hrs). $[\alpha]_D^{25}$ +76.4° (c = 1 in water); $[\alpha]_D^{23}$ +73.0° (c = 1, pH 7 buffer). pKa 5.2 in water. Freely sol in distilled water.

THERAP CAT: Antineoplastic.

7136. Pentoxifylline. [6493-05-6] 3,7-Dihydro-3,7-dimethyl-1-(5-oxohexyl)-1*H*-purine-2,6-dione; 1-(5-oxohexyl)theobromine; 1-(5-oxohexyl)-3,7-dimethylxanthine; 3,7-dimethyl-1-(5-oxohexyl)-1*H*,3*H*-purin-2,6-dione; oxpentifylline; vazofirin; BL-191; Azupentat; Durapental; Rentylin; Torental; Trental. $C_{13}H_{18}$-N_4O_3; mol wt 278.31. C 56.10%, H 6.52%, N 20.13%, O 17.25%. Methylxanthine derivative that improves blood flow by decreasing blood viscosity. Identity as a metabolite of pentifylline, *q.v.*: Mohler *et al., Arch. Pharm.* **299,** 448 (1966); Mohler *et al., Arzneim.-Forsch.* **16,** 1524 (1966). Prepn: NL 6511581; Mohler *et al.,* DE 1235320; *eidem,* US 3422107 (1966, 1967, 1969 all to Chem. Werke Albert). Series of articles on chemistry, pharmacology and clinical trials: *Arzneim.-Forsch.* **21,** 1159-1177 (1971). Toxicity data: K. Popendiker *et al., ibid.* 1160. Review of hemorheologic properties and use in cerebrovascular disease: R. Müller, F. Lehrach, *Curr. Med. Res. Opin.* **7,** 253-263 (1981); of pharmacology and therapeutic uses: A. Ward, S. P. Clissold, *Drugs* **34,** 50-97 (1987); C. P. Samlaska, E. A. Winfield, *J. Am. Acad. Dermatol.* **30,** 603-621 (1994).

Bitter tasting, colorless needles from methanol, mp 105°. uv max: 273, 208 nm ($E_{1cm}^{1\%}$ 365, 935). Soly in water: 77 mg/ml at 25°, 191 mg/ml at 37°; in benzene: 11 g/100 ml. LD_{50} orally in mice: 1385 mg/kg (Popendiker).

THERAP CAT: Hemorheologic agent.

7137. Pentoxyl. [147-61-5] 5-Hydroxymethyl-6-methyl-2,-4(1*H*,3*H*)-pyrimidinedione; 5-hydroxymethyl-6-methyluracil; 5-hydroxymethyl-4-methyluracil; 4-methyl-5-hydroxymethyluracil. $C_6H_8N_2O_3$; mol wt 156.14. C 46.15%, H 5.16%, N 17.94%, O 30.74%. Prepn: Endicott, Johnson, *J. Am. Chem. Soc.* **63,** 2063 (1941).

Crystals from boiling water, dec 314-315°.

THERAP CAT: Leukopoietic stimulant.

7138. Pentrinitrol. [1607-17-6] 2,2-Bis[(nitrooxy)methyl]-1,3-propanediol mononitrate (ester); pentaerythritol trinitrate; W-2197; Petrin. $C_5H_9N_3O_{10}$; mol wt 271.14. C 22.15%, H 3.35%, N 15.50%, O 59.01%. Coronary vasodilator related to pentaerythritol tetranitrate, *q.v.* Prepn (no data given): DE 638422; DE 638423 (both 1936 to Westfälisch-Anhaltisch Sprengstoff), *C.A.* **31,** 1212² (1937); N. J. Marans *et al., J. Am. Chem. Soc.* **76,** 1304 (1954); A. T. Camp *et al., ibid.* **77,** 751 (1955); J. Simecek, *Collect. Czech. Chem. Commun.* **27,** 362 (1962). Use in coronary insufficiency: F. J. DiCarlo, US 3419571 (1968 to Warner-Lambert). Electrical moment and molecular rotation: A. R. Lawrence, A. J. Matuszko, *J. Phys. Chem.* **65,** 1903 (1961). Chromatographic determn: I. W. F. Davidson *et al., J. Chromatogr.* **57,** 345 (1971). Metabolism: F. J. DiCarlo *et al., Clin. Pharmacol. Ther.* **22,** 309 (1977). Comparative duration of action: J. Vohra *et al., Aust. N.Z. J. Med.* **9,** 554 (1979).

Viscous liq. n_D^{20} 1.4941. d_4^{20} 1.554. Viscosity (cSt): 166.8 (40°); 77.8 (50°). Soly in water: 0.705 g/100 ml at 20°; in benzene: 21.40 g/100 ml at 20°. Very sol in ethanol, ether. Forms a cryst hydrate, mp 32°, when washed with water and allowed to stand overnight at 20°; returns to unhydrated form when allowed to stand at 60° for 2 hrs. When used medicinally it is usually diluted with lactose or mannitol to reduce explosive liability, *see* pentaerythritol tetranitrate.

THERAP CAT: Vasodilator (coronary).

7139. Pentryl. [4481-55-4] 2-[Nitro(2,4,6-trinitrophenyl)-amino]ethanol nitrate (ester); 2-(*N*,2,4,6-tetranitroanilino)ethanol nitrate; *sym*-trinitrophenylnitroaminoethyl nitrate. $C_8H_6N_6O_{11}$; mol wt 362.17. C 26.53%, H 1.67%, N 23.20%, O 48.59%. Prepd by nitration of 2,4-dinitrophenylaminoethanol: Clark, *Ind. Eng. Chem.* **25,** 1385 (1933); Desseigne, *Mem. Poudres* **33,** 255 (1951); B. T. Fedoroff *et al., Encyclopedia of Explosives and Related Items* vol. **I** (Picatinny Arsenal, Dover, New Jersey, 1960) pp A425-429.

Small, cream-colored crystals from chloroform, mp 129° (slight decompn). d 1.82. Explodes when heated to 235°. Heat of combustion: 911.6 kcal/mole; heat of explosion: 372.4 kcal/mole; heat of formation: 43.4 kcal/mole. Soly (w/w) at 25° in benzene: 0.70; carbon tetrachloride: trace; chloroform: 0.07; ethanol: 0.11; ether: 0.16; ethylene dichloride: 0.72; methanol: 0.67; nitroglycerol: freely sol; toluene: 0.63; water: trace.

USE: High explosive. Base charge in detonators.

7140. *tert*-Pentyl Alcohol. [75-85-4] 2-Methyl-2-butanol; *tert*-amyl alcohol; dimethyl ethyl carbinol; ethyl dimethyl carbinol; *tert*-pentanol; amylene hydrate. $C_5H_{12}O$; mol wt 88.15. C 68.13%, H 13.72%, O 18.15%. $(CH_3)_2C(OH)CH_2CH_3$. Prepd from 2-methyl-2-butene alone and mixed with 2-methyl-1-butene: Fenske, Jones, US 2858331 (1958 to Esso); Odioso *et al., Ind. Eng. Chem.* **53,** 209 (1961). Review of manuf by fractionation of fusel oil and *via* chlorination of pentanes, and properties: *Industrial Chemicals,* W. L. Faith *et al.,* Eds. (John Wiley, New York, 2nd ed., 1957) pp 107-114. Toxicity: Schaffarzick, Brown, *Science* **116,** 663 (1952).

Volatile liquid; characteristic odor, burning taste. bp_{765} 102.5°. mp −9.0°. d^{20} 0.8084: Costello, Bowden, *Rec. Trav. Chim.* **77,** 36 (1958). n_D^{20} 1.4052. Flash pt, closed cup: 67°F (19°C); open cup: 70°F (21°C). Sol in 8 parts water; miscible with alcohol, ether, benzene, chloroform, glycerol, oils. *Keep tightly closed and protected from light.* LD_{50} orally in rats: 1.0 g/kg (Schaffarzick, Brown).

Caution: Moderately irritating to mucous membranes. Narcotic in high concns. *See also* 1-Pentanol.

THERAP CAT: Hypnotic.

7141. Pentylenetetrazole. [54-95-5] 6,7,8,9-Tetrahydro-5*H*-tetrazolo[1,5-*a*]azepine; α,β-cyclopentamethylenetetrazole; 1,5-pentamethylenetetrazole; 6,7,8,9-tetrahydro-5-azepotetrazole; 1,2,3,3a-tetrazacyclohepta-8a,2-cyclopentadiene; 7,8,9,10-tetrazabicyclo[5.3.0]-8,10-decadiene; pentetrazol; Cardiazol; Cenalene-M; Cenazol; Coranormol; Corazole; Corvasol; Deumacard; Gewazol; Korazol; Metrazol; Phrenazol; Ventrazol. $C_6H_{10}N_4$; mol wt 138.17. C 52.16%, H 7.29%, N 40.55%. Prepd by the addition of cyclohexanone to a benzene or Tetralin soln of hydrazoic acid: Schmidt, *Ber.* **57,** 704 (1924); US 1564631 (1925); US 1599493 (1926); Prochazka, CS 92456 (1959), *C.A.* **56,** 4776e (1962). Synthesis from caprolactam: Glushkov, Golovchinskaya, *Zh. Prikl. Khim.* **32,** 920 (1959); *Med. Prom. SSSR* **14,** no. 1, 12 (1960). Toxicity study: E. I. Goldenthal, *Toxicol. Appl. Pharmacol.* **18,** 185 (1971).

Slightly pungent, bitter crystals, mp 57-60°. Freely sol in water, most organic solvents. Aq solns are neutral to litmus. Very stable, not easily attacked by other substances. LD_{50} in rats (mg/kg): 85±2 s.c., 62 i.p. (Goldenthal).

THERAP CAT: CNS stimulant.

THERAP CAT (VET): CNS stimulant; narcotic antagonist.

7142. p-tert-Pentylphenol. [80-46-6] 4-(1,1-Dimethylpropyl)phenol; p-tert-amylphenol; 2-methyl-2-p-hydroxyphenylbutane; Pentaphen. $C_{11}H_{16}O$; mol wt 164.24. C 80.44%, H 9.82%, O 9.74%. Prepd by condensation of tert-pentanol or 2-methyl-3-butanol with phenol in the presence of aluminum chloride: Huston, Hsieh, J. Am. Chem. Soc. **58**, 439 (1936); Huston et al., ibid. **67**, 899 (1945). Physical properties: Pardee, Weinrich, Ind. Eng. Chem. **36**, 595 (1944). Toxicity study: H. F. Smyth et al., Am. Ind. Hyg. Assoc. J. **23**, 95 (1962).

Crystals, mp 94-95°. bp 262.5°. bp_{740} 248-250°, bp_{15} 138.5°, bp_3 112-120°. d_4^{20} 0.962. Practically insol in water. Sol in alcohol, ether, benzene, chloroform. LD_{50} orally in rats: 3.08 g/kg (Smyth).

USE: In the manuf of oil-soluble resins; has been recommended as a germicide and fumigant; intermediate for organic mercury germicides, for pesticides, for chemicals used in rubber and petroleum industries.

7143. Peonidin. [134-01-0] 3,5,7-Trihydroxy-2-(4-hydroxy-3-methoxyphenyl)-1-benzopyrylium chloride; 3,4',5,7-tetrahydroxy-3'-methoxyflavylium chloride; 3,4',5,7-tetrahydroxy-3'-methoxy-2-phenylbenzopyrylium chloride. $C_{16}H_{13}ClO_6$; mol wt 336.72. C 57.07%, H 3.89%, Cl 10.53%, O 28.51%. The aglucon of peonin: R. Willstätter, Ann. **408**, 136 (1915). Structure and synthesis: T. J. Nolan et al., J. Chem. Soc. **1926**, 1968; S. Murakami, R. Robinson, ibid. **1928**, 1537.

Monohydrate. Reddish-brown needles from aq 20% hydrochloric acid soln. Moderately sol in water giving a reddish-brown soln. Sol in alc giving a purplish-red soln.

3,5-Diglucoside. 3,5-Bis(β-D-glucopyranosyloxy)-7-hydroxy-2-(4-hydroxy-3-methoxyphenyl)-1-benzopyrylium chloride; peonin. $C_{28}H_{33}ClO_{16}$. From deep violet-red peonies: R. Willstätter, T. J. Nolan, loc. cit. Synthesis: R. Robinson, A. R. Todd, J. Chem. Soc. **1932**, 2488. Deep purple needles with water of crystn from dil HCl, mp 165-167° (dec).

7144. Peplomycin. [68247-85-8] N^1-[3-[[(1S)-1-Phenylethyl]amino]propyl]bleomycinamide; N^1-[3-[[(S)-α-methylbenzyl]amino]propyl]bleomycinamide; pepleomycin; NK-631. $C_{61}H_{88}N_{18}O_{21}S_2$; mol wt 1473.59. C 49.72%, H 6.02%, N 17.11%, O 22.80%, S 4.35%. Deriv of bleomycin, q.v. with cytostatic activity and less pulmonary toxicity than the natural bleomycin mixture. Prepn of the (R,S)-form: H. Umezawa et al., US 3846400 (1974 to Microbiochem. Res. Found.); of the (S)-form: T. Takita et al., DE 2828933; eidem, US 4195018 (1979, 1980 both to Nippon Kayaku); W. Tanaka et al., Heterocycles **13**, 469 (1979). Biological study of degradation products: K. Takahashi et al., J. Antibiot. **32**, 36 (1979). General pharmacology: Y. Ishii et al., Jpn. J. Antibiot. **31**, 886 (1978), C.A. **91**, 215c (1979). Absorption, distribution, excretion, metabolism: H. Takayama et al., ibid. 895, C.A. **91**, 32580j (1979). Properties and stability: A. Fuji et al., Iyakuhin

Kenkyu **10**, 197 (1979), C.A. **91**, 9408a (1979). Effect in prostatic cancer: T. Niijima, K. Koiso, Scand. J. Respir. Dis. **Suppl. 55**, 177 (1980). Relative pulmonary toxicity: B. I. Sikic et al., Cancer Treat. Rep. **64**, 659 (1980). Acute toxicity study: K. Ito et al., Jpn. J. Antibiot. **31**, 719 (1978), C.A. **91**, 68461k (1979). Review of clinical studies: S. Oko, Recent Results Cancer Res. **74**, 163 (1980).

Sulfate salt. [70384-29-1] Pepleo Injection. $C_{61}H_{88}N_{18}O_{21}S_2.H_2SO_4$; mol wt 1571.67. Pale yellow amorphous powder, mp 196-198°. $[\alpha]_{436}^{25}$ -2.0° (c = 1 in water). pKa 2.9, 4.8, 7.4, 9.0. Sol in water, methanol, acetic acid, DMSO, DMF. Slightly sol in dioxane. Insol in ethyl acetate, acetone, ether, benzene. Stable at 37° for 3 months, 50° for 6 weeks, room temp for 30 months in a sealed container. LD_{50} in male rats, mice (mg/kg): 234, 88 s.c.; 208, 85 i.p.; 245, 51 i.v. (Ito).

THERAP CAT: Antineoplastic.

7145. Peppermint. Brandy mint; lamb mint. Perennial herb, Mentha piperita L., Labiatae. Habit. Asia, Europe, North America; cultivated in gardens. Medicinal parts are the essential oil, dried leaves and flowering tops, or the fresh flowering plant. Constit. Volatile oil (1-3%), flavonoids incl. luteolin, rutin, hesperidin; phenolic acids incl. caffeic, chlorogenic and rosmarinic acids; triterpenes. GC determn of menthol components in oil: J. P. Sang, J. Chromatogr. **253**, 109 (1982); in pharmaceutical preparations: D. Y.-H. Yeung et al., J. Pharm. Biomed. Anal. **30**, 1469 (2003). HPLC determn of phenolic compounds in leaves: F. M. Areias et al., Food Chem. **73**, 307 (2001). Review of constituents and medicinal uses: P. R. Bradley, British Herbal Compendium (British Herbal Medicines Association, Dorset, 1992) pp 174-176. Series of articles on pharmacology and clinical experience in irritable bowel syndrome: H.-G. Grigoleit, P. Grigoleit, Phytomedicine **12**, 601-616 (2005).

Volatile oil. [8006-90-4] Oil of peppermint; Colpermin; Mintec. Steam-distilled from fresh leaves and flowering tops. Constit. Chiefly menthol (35-55%), menthone (10-40%), menthyl acetate (1-10%), menthofuran (1-10%), cineol (2-13%), limonene, (+)-isomenthone, viridoflorol, dimethyl sulfide. Colorless to pale yellow liquid; strong, penetrating peppermint odor and pungent taste. d_{25}^{25} 0.896-0.908. n_D^{20} 1.459-1.465. Rotation between -18 and -32. Very slightly sol in water; sol in 3 vols 70% alcohol. Insol in propylene glycol.

Spirit of Peppermint. An alcoholic soln contg per liter 100 ml oil of peppermint and the alcohol-soluble principles from 10 g of powdered peppermint previously macerated with water.

USE: Flavoring agent in pharmaceuticals, foods, liqueurs, confectionary. In hair tonics, stimulating shampoos, conditioners. Leaves in herbal teas.

THERAP CAT: Carminative; antispasmodic.

7146. Pepsin. [9001-75-6] Puerzym. Principle digestive enzyme of gastric juice; controls the degradation of proteins to proteoses and peptones. Distinctive among enzymes for having a very low isoelectric point and a very low pH optimum. Hydrolyzes only peptide linkages. The N.F. grade digests not less than 3000 or more than 3500 times its wt of freshly coagulated and disintegrated egg albumin in 2½ hours at 52° in water acidulated with HCl. Isoln from gastric juice of swine and beef: Northrup, J. Gen. Physiol. **13**, 739 (1930); **16**, 615 (1933); from salmon and tuna:

Norris, Edam, *J. Biol. Chem.* **134**, 443 (1940); **204**, 673 (1953). Amino acid composition: Brand in *Crystalline Enzymes*, J. H. Northrup *et al.* (Columbia Univ. Press, New York, 2nd ed., 1948) p 26. Active site: Herriott, *J. Gen. Physiol.* **45**, Suppl., 57 (1962). *Review:* Bovey, Yanari in *The Enzymes* vol. 4, P. D. Boyer *et al.*, Eds. (Academic Press, New York, 1960) pp 63-92.

White or yellowish-white translucent scales or granules, or an amorphous slightly hygroscopic powder, or spongy masses. It has a slightly acid or saline taste. $[\alpha]_D^{26}$ $-64.5°$ (water pH 4.6). Isoelectric point <pH 1.0. Freely sol in water with more or less opalescence. Practically insol in alc, chloroform, ether. Very stable to acid. The activity of pepsin in solns is destroyed by heating above 70°, or by alkalies; dry pepsin is not injured by heating to 100°. *Incompat.* Alc, tannin, alkaline substances and salts of heavy metals. *Note:* Pepsin of an activity of 4000, 5000, 6000, 10,000, 15,000, and 20,000 is likewise available, and it has also been obtained in pure crystalline form.

THERAP CAT: Enzyme (digestive).

THERAP CAT (VET): Has been used as a digestive aid in deficiency of pepsin secretion.

7147. Pepstatin. [26305-03-3] *N*-(3-methyl-1-oxobutyl)-L-valyl-L-valyl-(3*S*,4*S*)-4-amino-3-hydroxy-6-methylheptanoyl-*N*-[(1*S*)-1-[(1*S*)-2-carboxy-1-hydroxyethyl]-3-methylbutyl]-L-alaninamide; Pepstatin A; *N*-isovaleryl-L-valyl-L-valyl-3-hydroxy-6-methyl-γ-aminoheptanoyl-L-alanyl-3-hydroxy-6-methyl-γ-aminoheptanoic acid. $C_{34}H_{63}N_5O_9$; mol wt 685.89. C 59.54%, H 9.26%, N 10.21%, O 20.99%. A pentapeptide pepsin inhibitor, isolated from cultured broths of *Streptomyces testaceus* Hamada *et* Okami and *Streptomyces argenteolus* var. *toyonakensis:* H. Umezawa *et al., J. Antibiot.* **23**, 259 (1970). Prepn: H. Umezawa *et al.*, **DE 2028403** (1971 to Microbiochemical Res. Found.), *C.A.* **74**, 75201c (1971). Structure: H. Morishima *et al., J. Antibiot.* **23**, 263 (1970). Synthesis: H. Morishima *et al.*, *ibid.* **25**, 551 (1972). Biological properties: T. Aoyagi *et al., ibid.* **24**, 687 (1971). *N-n-*Caproyl and *N-iso*-caproyl derivatives, *pepstatin B* and *pepstatin C*, also isolated from pepstatin-producing *Streptomyces*, as minor components of crude preparations: T. Miyano *et al., ibid.* **25**, 489 (1972). Mechanism of pepsin inhibition: S. Kunimoto *et al.*, *ibid.* 251; **27**, 413 (1974); J. Marciniszyn *et al., Adv. Exp. Med. Biol.* **95**, 199 (1977); D. H. Rich, E. T. O. Sun, *Biochem. Pharmacol.* **29**, 2205 (1980); of other acid protease inhibition: D. H. Rich *et al., Biochemistry* **24**, 3165 (1985). Tissue distribution in rats: D. A. W. Grant *et al., Biochem. Pharmacol.* **31**, 2302 (1982). Effect on gastric ulcers in man: O. Bonnevie *et al., Gut* **20**, 624 (1979); L. B. Svendsen *et al., Scand. J. Gastroenterol.* **14**, 929 (1979).

Colorless needles, mp 228-229° (dec). $[\alpha]_D^{27}$ $-90.3°$ (c = 0.288 in methanol). Sol in methanol, ethanol, acetic acid DMSO. Practically insol in benzene, chloroform, ether, and water. LD_{50} in mice, rats, rabbits, dogs (mg/kg): 1090, 875, 820, 450 i.p.; all >2000 orally (Umezawa, 1970).

7148. Peptide T. [106362-32-7] $C_{35}H_{55}N_9O_{16}$; mol wt 857.86. C 49.00%, H 6.46%, N 14.69%, O 29.84%. Octapeptide segment of the human immunodeficiency virus (HIV) envelope glycoprotein (gp 120); named peptide T because of its high threonine content. Has been reported to block the *in vitro* binding of HIV envelope to human leukocyte receptor CD4. Isolation, neuropharmacology and anti-HIV activity of peptide and analogs: C. B. Pert *et al., Proc. Natl. Acad. Sci. USA* **83**, 9254 (1986). Characterization of active core structure, T[4-8], and chemotactic effects: C. B. Pert, M. R. Ruff, *Clin. Neuropharmacol.* **9**, Suppl. 4, 482 (1986). Chemotactic effects and structural homology with vasoactive intestinal peptide (VIP), *q.v.:* M. R. Ruff *et al., FEBS Lett.* **211**, 17 (1987). Competitive binding studies at VIP receptor: T. D. Nguyen, *Peptides* **9**, 425 (1988). Structural homology with thymosin α_1, *q.v.:* T. D. Nguyen, L. A. Scheving, *Biochem. Biophys. Res. Commun.* **145**, 884 (1987). Evaluation of anti-HIV activity: J. Sodroski *et al., Lancet* **1**, 1428 (1987). Clinical evaluation in treatment of AIDS:

L. Wetterberg *et al., ibid.* 159. Chromatographic purification of *[D-ala¹] peptide T amide*, a metabolically stable and more potent analog of peptide T: T. R. Burke, M. Knight, *J. Chromatogr.* **411**, 431 (1987). Blood to brain transport of the amide in mice: C. M. Barrera *et al., Brain Res. Bull.* **19**, 629 (1987). Brief review of debate over effectiveness of peptide T: D. M. Barnes, *Science* **237**, 128 (1987).

Ala–Ser–Thr–Thr–Thr–Asn–Tyr–Thr

7149. Peptide YY. [106388-42-5] (unspecified source); [118997-30-1] (human); [81858-94-8] (porcine). Peptide tyrosine-tyrosine; PYY_{1-36}. 36 amino acid peptide hormone named for its N- and C-terminal tyrosine (Y) residues. Evolutionarily related to pancreatic polypeptide and neuropeptide Y, *q.v.*. Regulates gut motility and secretion of gastric fluids. The two main endogenous circulating forms, PYY_{1-36} and PYY_{3-36}, are released from endocrine L-cells in response to caloric intake. Abnormalities in intestinal PYY are linked to many gastrointestinal disorders including obesity and diabetes. Isoln and characterization of porcine form: K. Tatemoto, V. Mutt, *Nature* **285**, 417 (1980); K. Tatemoto, *Proc. Natl. Acad. Sci. USA* **79**, 2514 (1982); of human form: *idem et al., Biochem. Biophys. Res. Commun.* **157**, 713 (1988). Structural characterization of human PYY_{3-36} and PYY_{1-36}: G. A. Eberlein *et al., Peptides* **10**, 797 (1989). CD and NMR soln structure studies: D. A. Keire *et al., Biochemistry* **39**, 9935 (2000). Review of physiologic role in digestion: F. L. C. Hill *et al., Steroids* **56**, 77-82 (1991). Series of articles on physiological roles and clinical potential: *Peptides* **23**, 249-407 (2002). Review of potential role in appetite regulation and obesity therapy: B. M. C. McGowan, S. R. Bloom, *Curr. Opin. Pharmacol.* **4**, 583-588 (2004); D. Renshaw, R. L. Batterham, *Curr. Drug Targets* **6**, 171-179 (2005).

Tyr–Pro–Ile–Lys–Pro–Glu–Ala–Pro–Gly–Glu–Asp–Ala–Ser–Pro–Glu–Glu–Leu–Asn
|
Arg
|
NH₂–Tyr–Arg–Gln–Arg–Thr–Val–Leu–Asn–Leu–Tyr–His–Arg–Leu–Ser–Ala–Tyr–Tyr

Human Form

Peptide YY (3-36). [126339-09-1] (porcine) PYY_{3-36}. Produced by cleavage of the two N-terminal amino acids by dipeptidyl peptidase IV. Inhibition of food intake in rats: R. L. Batterham *et al., Nature* **418**, 650 (2002); in mice: B. G. Challis *et al., Biochem. Biophys. Res. Commun.* **311**, 915 (2003).

7150. Peracetic Acid. [79-21-0] Ethaneperoxoic acid; peroxyacetic acid; acetyl hydroperoxide; Proxitane. $C_2H_4O_3$; mol wt 76.05. C 31.59%, H 5.30%, O 63.11%. CH_3COOOH. Commercial product is an equilib soln of peracetic acid, hydrogen peroxide, acetic acid and water, *q.q.v.* Prepn: J. D'Ans, **DE 251802** (1911); J. D'Ans, W. Frey, *Ber.* **45**, 1845 (1912); using solid superacid catalysts: M. S. Saha *et al., Tetrahedron Lett.* **44**, 5535 (2003). Decomposition study: E. Koubek *et al., J. Am. Chem. Soc.* **85**, 2263 (1963). HPLC Determn: U. Pinkernell *et al., Anal. Chem.* **66**, 2599 (1994); *idem et al., J. Chromatogr. A* **730**, 203 (1996). Biocidal properties and water treatment applications: J. F. Kramer, *Mater. Perform.* **36**, 42 (1997). Review of of use in pharmaceutical synthesis: H. Feigenbaum, *Spec. Chem.* **17**, 80-84 (1997); of prepn and properties: B. B. Klopotek, *Chim. Oggi* **16**, 33-37 (1998); of use as a bleaching agent: R. B. Chavan *et al., Colourage* **47**, 15-20 (2000).

Liquid, acrid odor. mp 0°. $bp_{1.6\ hPa}$ 25°. d_4^{20} 1.0375. n_D^{20} 1.3974. Flash pt: 133°F (56°C). pKa 8.2. Explodes violently on heating to 110°. Freely sol in water, alcohol, ether, H_2SO_4. Stable in dil aq soln. Strong oxidizing agent. LD_{50} (mg/kg) in rats: 1540 orally; in rabbits: 1410 dermally. LC_{50} in rats (mg/m³): 450 by inhalation (Klopotek).

Caution: Strongly irritating to skin and eyes.

USE: Environmentally friendly biocide; disinfectant in the food and beverage industry; bleaching agent for textiles and paper. Oxidizing agent in organic synthesis.

7151. Perazine. [84-97-9] 10-[3-(4-Methyl-1-piperazinyl)-propyl]-10*H*-phenothiazine; *N*-methylpiperazinyl-*N*'-propyl-phenothiazine; 10-(γ-methylpiperazinopropyl)phenothiazine; P-725; Taxilan. $C_{20}H_{25}N_3S$; mol wt 339.50. C 70.76%, H 7.42%,

N 12.38%, S 9.44%. Prepn: Hromatka *et al., Monatsh. Chem.* **88,** 56, 193 (1957); **91,** 107 (1960); Horclois, **GB 780193** (1957 to Rhône-Poulenc).

Crystals, mp 51-53°. bp$_{0.001}$ 160-170° (air bath temp).
Dihydrochloride. C$_{20}$H$_{27}$Cl$_2$N$_3$S. Hygroscopic needles, dec 228-230°.
Dihydrochloride hemihydrate. Platelets from ethanol, mp 225-227°.
Dimaleate. C$_{28}$H$_{33}$N$_3$O$_8$S. Crystals from water, mp 210°.
THERAP CAT: Antipsychotic.

7152. Perbenzoic Acid. [93-59-4] Benzenecarboperoxoic acid; peroxybenzoic acid; benzoyl hydroperoxide. C$_7$H$_6$O$_3$; mol wt 138.12. C 60.87%, H 4.38%, O 34.75%. C$_6$H$_5$COOOH. Prepd from dibenzoyl peroxide by treatment with a soln of sodium methoxide in methanol at 0°: Braun, *Org. Synth.* **13,** 86 (1933); *cf.* Bergmann, Witte, **DE 409779;** *Chem. Zentralbl.* **1925, I,** 1911.
Leaflets from benzene. Acrid odor. mp 41-43°. Very volatile. Sublimes in desiccator. bp$_{15}$ 100-110° (partial decomposition). Volatile with steam. Very sparingly sol in water, but turns liquid upon contact with water; sparingly sol in petr ether; freely sol in other organic solvents. Stability of solns with chloroform, carbon tetrachloride, ether, benzene: Prileshajew, *Chem. Zentralbl.* **1911, I,** 1280; Kolthoff *et al., J. Polym. Sci.* **2,** 199 (1947), *C.A.* **41,** 4960 (1947). Forms an unstable acid sodium salt, and a somewhat more stable neutral sodium salt.
USE: To convert ethylenic compounds into oxides; in analysis of unsatd compounds, to determine the number of double bonds.

7153. Perchloric Acid. [7601-90-3] ClHO$_4$; mol wt 100.46. Cl 35.29%, H 1.00%, O 63.70%. HClO$_4$. Prepd from potassium perchlorate and sulfuric acid: Schmeisser in *Handbook of Preparative Inorganic Chemistry* vol. **1,** G. Brauer, Ed. (Academic Press, New York, 2nd ed., 1963) pp 318-320. Comprehensive monograph: J. C. Schumacher, *Perchlorates* (Reinhold, New York, 1960).
The anhyd acid is a colorless, volatile, very hygroscopic liquid. d^{22} 1.768; bp$_{11}$ 19°. Dec when distilled at atmospheric pressure, sometimes with explosive violence. mp −112°. Combines vigorously with water with evolution of heat. Undergoes spontaneous and explosive decompn, hence it is marketed only in mixture with water contg 60-70% HClO$_4$, density 1.5 and 1.6, respectively. The aq acid is very caustic and may deflagrate in contact with oxidizable substances. Density of aq solns at 15°: 1% = 1.0050; 10% = 1.0597; 20% = 1.1279; 30% = 1.2067; 40% = 1.2991; 50% = 1.4103; 60% = 1.5389; 70% = 1.6736. Density of aq solns at 25°: 65.0% = 1.597; 70.0% = 1.664; 75.0% = 1.731.
Caution: Corrosive to skin, mucous membranes.
USE: The acid in analytical chemistry as an oxidizer and for separation of potassium from sodium. Its salts for explosives and for plating of metals.

7154. Perchloryl Fluoride. [7616-94-6] ClFO$_3$; mol wt 102.45. Cl 34.61%, F 18.54%, O 46.85%. *Reviews:* Downs, Adams in *Comprehensive Inorganic Chemistry* vol. **2,** J. C. Bailar, Jr. *et al.,* Eds. (Pergamon Press, Oxford, 1973) pp 1391-1393; Christe, Schack in *Adv. Inorg. Chem. Radiochem.* **18,** 319-398.

Characteristic sweet odor. Usually stored in cylinders as liq under pressure. mp −147.7°. bp −46.7°. d^{20} (liq) 1.434. Critical temp 95.2°. Crit pressure 53 atm. Crit density: 0.637. Heat of vaporization 4.6 kcal/mol. Trouton constant: 20.4. Dipole moment 0.03. Heat of formation of gas at 25° −5.12 kcal/mol. Sp heat of liq: 0.229 cal/g/°C at −40°; 0.290 at +50°. Does not

corrode base metals when anhydr. Shows the greatest resistance to electrical breakdown known for any gas. *Handle with care.* Do not bring in direct contact with reducing agents, alcohols, etc.: *Chem. Eng. News* **37,** 60 (1959). Explosions have occurred.
Caution: Potential symptom of overexposure is respiratory system irritation; direct contact with liquid may cause frostbite. *See NIOSH Pocket Guide to Chemical Hazards* (DHHS/NIOSH 97-140, 1997) p 246. May cause methemoglobinemia, cyanosis, alveolar edema, bronchopneumonia. *See Patty's Industrial Hygiene and Toxicology* vol. **2F,** G. D. Clayton, F. E. Clayton, Eds. (John Wiley & Sons, New York, 4th ed., 1994) p 4478.
USE: In organic synthesis to introduce fluorine atoms into organic molecules. As oxidizing agent; insulator for high voltage systems.

7155. Perezone. [3600-95-1] 2-[(1R)-1,5-Dimethyl-4-hexenyl]-3-hydroxy-5-methyl-2,5-cyclohexadiene-1,4-dione; 2-(1,5-dimethyl-4-hexenyl)-3-hydroxy-5-methyl-*p*-benzoquinone; pipitzahoic acid. C$_{15}$H$_{20}$O$_3$; mol wt 248.32. C 72.55%, H 8.12%, O 19.33%. From roots of *Trixis pipitzahuac* Shaffner *(Perezia adnata* Gr., *Compositae):* Weld, *Ann.* **95,** 188 (1855); from roots of *Radix pereziae:* Mylius, *Ber.* **18,** 463, 480, 937 (1885); Anschütz, *Ber.* **18,** 709 (1885); Fichter *et al., Ann.* **395,** 1, 15 (1913). Structure: Archer, Thomson, *Chem. Commun.* **1965,** 354; Bates *et al., Chem. Ind. (London)* **1965,** 1793.

Yellow plates from water or alcohol, mp 103-104°. [α]$_D^{20}$ −17° (ether).

7156. Perflubron. [423-55-2] 1-Bromo-1,1,2,2,3,3,4,4,5,5,-6,6,7,7,8,8,8-heptadecafluorooctane; bromoperfluorooctane; perfluoroctyl bromide; PFOB; L-1913; Imagent; LiquiVent; Oxygent. C$_8$BrF$_{17}$; mol wt 498.96. C 19.26%, Br 16.01%, F 64.73%. CF$_3$-(CF$_2$)$_6$CF$_2$Br. Synthetic second generation brominated fluorocarbon. Prepd not claimed: **FR 1512068;** L. A. Loree, **US 3456024** (1968, 1969 both to Dow Corning). Radiopacity and toxicology: D. M. Long *et al., Radiology* **105,** 323 (1972). Biodistribution and determn in plasma and tissue: F. H. Lee *et al., J. Pharm. Sci.* **67,** 1038 (1978). Clinical trial in abdominal imaging: R. F. Mattrey, *Radiology* **191,** 841 (1994). Toxicity studies: A. R. Burgan *et al., Biomater. Artif. Cells Artif. Organs* **16,** 681 (1988). Review of physicochemical properties and therapeutic potential: D. M. Long *et al., ibid.* 411-420; of oxygen delivery characteristics: J. G. Riess, *ibid.* **20,** 183-202 (1992).
Liquid, bp$_{760}$ 141°. d^{25} 1.928. Vapor pressure (37.5°) 14 torr. Surface tension 18.2 dynes/cm. Insol in water. LD$_{50}$ i.v. in female rats: 41 g/kg (Burgan).
THERAP CAT: Diagnostic aid (contrast agent).

7157. Perfluorohexane. [355-42-0] Tetradecafluorohexane; perfluoro-*n*-hexane; Imavist. C$_6$F$_{14}$; mol wt 338.04. C 21.32%, F 78.68%. CF$_3$(CF$_2$)$_4$CF$_3$. Commercial grade perfluorohexanes contain a mixture of five acyclic C$_6$F$_{14}$ isomers and two C$_6$F$_{12}$ perfluorinated cyclic alkanes. Discovery: J. H. Simons, L. P. Block, *J. Am. Chem. Soc.* **59,** 1407 (1937). Prepn and physical properties: V. E. Stiles, G. H. Cady, *ibid.* **74,** 3771 (1952); R. D. Dunlap *et al., ibid.* **80,** 83 (1958). Critical properties and virial coefficients: Z. L. Taylor, Jr., T. M. Reed, III, *AIChE J.* **16,** 738 (1970). Conformational analysis: P. Piaggio *et al., J. Mol. Struct.* **26,** 421 (1975). ^{19}F-NMR characterization of commercial product: T. A. Kestner, *J. Fluorine Chem.* **36,** 77 (1987). Use as a solvent in bromination reactions: S. M. Pereira *et al., Synth. Commun.* **25,** 1023 (1995). Evaluation in acute lung injury in rabbits: M. Hübler *et al., Crit. Care Med.* **30,** 422 (2002).
Coarse, transparent, needle-like crystals, mp −82.26 ±0.01°. bp 57.23°. d^0 1.7560. d^{25} 1.66970 (air satd, 1 atm). d^{25} 1.6717 (degassed, equilib vapor pressure). n$_D^{22}$ 1.2515. Viscosity at 0°: 9.79 mP. Heat of fusion: 1580 ±90 cal/mol. Molar heat of vaporization (cal) at bp: 7307; at 20°: 7793.

USE: In the electronics industry as a coolant and test bath medium. Non-toxic, non-ozone-depleting, inert reaction medium.

THERAP CAT: Diagnostic aid (Ultrasound contrast agent).

7158. Perfluoropropane. [76-19-7] Octafluoropropane; 1,-1,1,2,2,3,3,3-octafluoropropane; perflutren; K-218; PFC-218; R-218; Ispan. C_3F_8; mol wt 188.02. C 19.16%, F 80.84%. Non-ozone depleting fluorocarbon; formulated for surgical and diagnostic use. Prepn: J. H. Simons, L. P. Block, *J. Am. Chem. Soc.* **61**, 2962 (1939). *See also:* J. H. Simons, US 2456027 (1948 to Minnesota Mining Manuf). Physical properties: J. A. Brown, *J. Chem. Eng. Data* **8**, 106 (1963). Thermophysical properties: D. R. Defibaugh, M. R. Moldover, *ibid.* **42**, 160 (1997). Clinical experience in repair of retinal detachment: N. R. Sabates *et al., Retina* **16**, 7 (1996). Review of properties and description: *Matheson Gas Data Book*, W. Braker, A. L. Mossman, Eds. (Matheson, Lyndhurst, NJ, 6th ed., 1980) p 590-595; of electron interactions for modeling behavior: L. G. Christophorou, J. K. Oltoff, *J. Phys. Chem. Ref. Data* **27**, 889-913 (1998).

Colorless, nonflammable gas. mp −183°. bp −36.7°. d^{20} (liq) 1.352. Critical temp 71.9°. Critical press 25.45 atm. Critical density 0.629.

Human albumin microsphere suspension. FS-069; Optison. Clinical study as echocardiographic contrast agent: J. L. Cohen *et al., J. Am. Coll. Cardiol.* **32**, 746 (1998). Toxicology and safety study: Y. Greener *et al., Int. J. Toxicol.* **17**, 631 (1998). Physical and biochemical stability: S. Podell *et al., Biotechnol. Appl. Biochem.* **30**, 213 (1999). Review of diagnostic use: L. N. Clark, H. C. Dittrich, *Am. J. Cardiol.* **86**, Suppl., 14G-18G (2000). Mean microsphere particle diameter: 3.0 - 4.5 μm.

Lipid microsphere suspension. DMP-115; DMX-115; MRX-115; Definity. Preparative method: E. C. Inger, US 5874062 (1999 to ImaRx Pharm.). Clinical evaluation in echocardiography: D. W. Kitzman *et al., Am. J. Cardiol.* **86**, 669 (2000). Mean microsphere particle diameter: 1.1 - 3.3 μm.

USE: High voltage insulating gas; refrigerant when combined with chlorofluoro hydrocarbons; plasma processing gas; fire protection agent.

THERAP CAT: Diagnostic aid (ultrasound contrast agent). Adjunct in repair of retinal detachment.

7159. Perforin. Cytolysin; pore-forming protein; PFP; C9-related protein. Complement-like protein produced by cytotoxic T-lymphocytes (CTLs) and natural killer (NK) cells; released from cytoplasmic granules during the cytolytic process. Perforates the membrane of target cells by forming transmembrane pores that perturb membrane permeability and result in cell lysis. Pore-formation is mediated by the Ca^{2+}-dependent polymerization of perforin within the target cell membrane. Also thought to act as a conduit for the endocytosis of *granzymes*, serine proteinases produced by cytotoxic lymphocytes, that initiate nuclear disintegration. Glycoprotein; mol wt 66-70 kDa. Identification of pore-forming tubular complexes produced by NK cells: E. R. Podack, G. Dennert, *Nature* **302**, 442 (1983). Partial purification of protein: E. R. Podack, P. J. Konigsberg, *J. Exp. Med.* **160**, 695 (1984). Cloning and amino acid sequence of human perforin: M. G. Lichtenheld *et al., Nature* **335**, 448 (1988); of murine: D. M. Lowrey *et al., Proc. Natl. Acad. Sci. USA* **86**, 247 (1989). Confirmation of biological activity: D. Kägi *et al., Nature* **369**, 31 (1994). Review of structure and function: E. R. Podack, *Curr. Top. Microbiol. Immunol.* **178**, 175-184 (1992); C-C. Liu *et al., Immunol. Today* **16**, 194-201 (1995).

7160. Performic Acid. [107-32-4] Methaneperoxoic acid; peroxyformic acid; permethanoic acid; formyl hydroperoxide. CH_2O_3; mol wt 62.02. C 19.37%, H 3.25%, O 77.39%. HCOOOH. A strong oxidizing agent. A 90% soln is obtained when a mixture of 20 g formic acid, 25 g 100% H_2O_2 and 6.5 g H_2SO_4 is allowed to interact for 2 hrs and is then distilled: D'Ans, Kneip, *Ber.* **48**, 1137 (1915); Greenspan, *J. Am. Chem. Soc.* **68**, 907 (1946).

The 90% soln is a colorless liq. *Prone to explode on contact with metals, their oxides, reducing substances, or on distillation.* Has lower vapor pressure than formic acid. Miscible with water, alc, ether. Sol in benzene, chloroform. Solns are unstable, gassing being noticeable after a few hours, and the effective concn showing a definite decline in 2 hrs.

Caution: Irritant.

USE: For oxidation, epoxidation and hydroxylation reactions.

7161. Perfosfamide. [62435-42-1]; [39800-16-3] (unspecified stereo). *rel*-(2*R*,4*R*)-2-[Bis(2-chloroethyl)amino]tetrahydro-2*H*-1,3,2-oxazaphosphorin-4-yl hydroperoxide *P*-oxide; *cis*-(±)-2-[bis(2-chloroethyl)amino]-4-hydroperoxytetrahydro-2*H*-1,3,2-oxazaphosphorine 2-oxide; *cis*-4-hydroperoxycyclophosphamide; 4-HC; NSC-181815; Pergamid. $C_7H_{15}Cl_2N_2O_4P$; mol wt 293.08. C 28.69%, H 5.16%, Cl 24.19%, N 9.56%, O 21.84%, P 10.57%. Prepn (stereochem. unspecified): NL 7208895; A. Takamizawa, T. Iwata, US 3808297 (1972, 1974 both to Shionogi); *idem et al., J. Am. Chem. Soc.* **95**, 985 (1973). Structural study: A. Camerman *et al., Acta Crystallogr.* **B33**, 678 (1977). Cytostatic activity: A. Takamizawa *et al., J. Med. Chem.* **18**, 376 (1975). Clinical use: D. Biggs *et al., Prog. Clin. Biol. Res.* **389**, 9 (1994). Review of use as purging agent in autologous bone marrow transplantation: A. M. Yeager *et al., Am. J. Pediatr. Hematol. Oncol.* **12**, 245-256 (1990); R. J. Jones, *J. Hematother.* **1**, 343-348 (1992).

White crystals from acetone/ether (unspecified form). mp 107-108°. LD_{50} in rats, mice (mg/kg): 115, 235 i.v.; 131, 181 i.p. (Takamizawa, 1975).

THERAP CAT: Antineoplastic; bone marrow purging agent.

7162. Pergolide. [66104-22-1] (8β)-8-[(Methylthio)methyl]-6-propylergoline; D-6-*n*-propyl-8β-methylmercaptomethylergoline; LY-141B. $C_{19}H_{26}N_2S$; mol wt 314.49. C 72.56%, H 8.33%, N 8.91%, S 10.20%. D_1/D_2 dopaminergic agonist that also decreases plasma prolactin concentrations. Prepn: E. C. Kornfeld, N. J. Bach, US 4166182 (1979 to Lilly). Industrial synthesis: W. Cabri *et al., Org. Process Res. Dev.* **10**, 198 (2006). Dopaminergic effects in rats: R. W. Fuller *et al., Life Sci.* **24**, 375 (1979); T. T. Yen *et al., ibid.* **25**, 209 (1979). Clinical pharmacology: L. Lemberger, R. E. Crabtree, *Science* **205**, 1151 (1979). Pharmacological evaluation as antiparkinson agent: W. C. Koller, *Neuropharmacology* **19**, 831 (1980). Clinical study in galactorrhea: J. T. Callaghan *et al., Life Sci.* **28**, 95 (1981); in hyperprolactinemia: S. Francks *et al., Lancet* **2**, 659 (1981); in treatment of pituitary tumors secreting prolactin or growth hormone: D. L. Kleinberg *et al., N. Engl. J. Med.* **309**, 704 (1983). Clinical studies in Parkinson's disease: J. Jankovic, J. Orman, *Adv. Neurol.* **45**, 551 (1986); C. W. Olanow, M. J. Alberts, *ibid.* 555; in restless legs syndrome: C. Trenkwalder *et al., Neurology* **62**, 1391 (2004). Comprehensive description: D. J. Sprankle, E. C. Jensen, *Anal. Profiles Drug Subs. Excip.* **21**, 375-413 (1992). Review of clinical experience in Parkinson's disease: U. Bonuccelli *et al., Clin. Neuropharmacol.* **25**, 1-10 (2002).

Solid, mp 217.5°.

Mesylate. [66104-23-2] LY-127809; Celance; Permax; Nopar. $C_{19}H_{26}N_2S.CH_3SO_3H$; mol wt 410.59. Crystals, mp 258-260°

(dec) (Sprankle, Jensen); also reported as mp 267.4° (Cabri). uv max (water): 279 nm (ε 6385); (methanol): 280 nm (ε 6980); (dehydrated ethanol): 281 nm (ε 6993). α_D^{20} between −18.0° and −23.0° (c = 10 mg/ml in DMF). pKa (66% DMF) 7.8. Sparingly sol in DMF, methanol; slightly sol in water, 0.01N HCl, chloroform, acetonitrile, dichloromethane, dehydrated ethanol; very slightly sol in acetone. Practically insol in 0.1N NaOH, 0.1N HCl, ether. Partition coefficient at 25° (chloroform/water): 6.14 (pH 2.19); 119.6 (pH 4.02).

THERAP CAT: Antiparkinsonian.

7163. Perhexiline. [6621-47-2] 2-(2,2-Dicyclohexylethyl)-piperidine; 1,1-dicyclohexyl-2-(2-piperidyl)ethane; perhexilene. $C_{19}H_{35}N$; mol wt 277.49. C 82.24%, H 12.71%, N 5.05%. Calcium blocking agent. Prepn: **GB 1025578** (1966 to Richardson-Merrell), *C.A.* **65**, 2229f (1966). Pharmacology: Hudak *et al., J. Pharmacol. Exp. Ther.* **173**, 371 (1970). Clinical studies: Winsor, *Clin. Pharmacol. Ther.* **11**, 85 (1970). Toxicity study: Causa, Perri, *Arzneim.-Forsch.* **21**, 114 (1971). Series of articles: *Postgrad. Med. J. Suppl.* **49**, 8-132 (1973). Book: *Antiarrhythmic Action and the Puzzle of Perhexiline*, E. M. Vaughan Williams, Ed. (Academic Press, New York, 1980) 143 pp.

Maleate. [6724-53-4] Pexid. $C_{19}H_{35}N.C_4H_4O_4$; mol wt 393.56. mp 188.5-191°. LD_{50} in rats, mice (g/kg): >7, 4.37 orally (Causa, Perri).

Hydrochloride. $C_{19}H_{35}N.HCl$. White crystalline powder, mp 243-245.5° (dec).

THERAP CAT: Vasodilator (coronary); diuretic.

7164. Pericyazine. [2622-26-6] 10-[3-(4-Hydroxy-1-piperidinyl)propyl]-10H-phenothiazine-2-carbonitrile; 2-cyano-10-[3-(4-hydroxypiperidino)propyl]phenothiazine; periciazine; propericiazine; RP-8908; Aolept; Neulactil; Neuleptil. $C_{21}H_{23}N_3OS$; mol wt 365.49. C 69.01%, H 6.34%, N 11.50%, O 4.38%, S 8.77%. Psychotherapeutic phenothiazine. Prepn: Robert, Jacques, **FR 1212031** (1960 to Rhône-Poulenc). Hypotensive action in dogs: K. P. Singh *et al., Indian J. Med. Res.* **58**, 1467 (1970). GLC determn in human urine: A. P. De Leenheer, *J. Pharm. Sci.* **63**, 389 (1974). Clinical studies in psychiatric patients: U. Spiegelberg, G. Kleu, *Arzneim.-Forsch.* **17**, 159 (1967); J. C. Barker, M. Miller, *Br. J. Psychiatry* **115**, 169 (1969). Toxicity and metabolism: L. Julou *et al., Proc. Eur. Soc. Study Drug Toxic.* **9**, 11 (1968). Toxicity data: Schafer, *Toxicol. Appl. Pharmacol.* **21**, 315 (1972). Use in spectrophotometry: H. Gowda *et al., Anal. Chem.* **55**, 1816 (1983); A. T. Gowda *et al., Anal. Chim. Acta* **154**, 347 (1983).

Crystals, mp 116-117°. uv max: 232.5, 271.5 nm (log ε 4319, 4503). LD_{50} orally in rats: 395 mg/kg (Schafer).

USE: Spectrophotometric reagent for palladium and ruthenium.

THERAP CAT: Antipsychotic.

7165. Perifosine. [157716-52-4] 4-[[Hydroxy(octadecyloxy)phosphinyl]oxy]-1,1-dimethylpiperidinium inner salt; octadecyl-(1,1-dimethylpiperidinio-4-yl)phosphate; D-21266; KRX-0401; NSC-639966. $C_{25}H_{52}NO_4P$; mol wt 461.66. C 65.04%, H 11.35%, N 3.03%, O 13.86%, P 6.71%. Synthetic alkylphosphocholine anticancer agent. Inhibits the phosphatidylinositol 3-kinase

regulated Akt/PKB survival pathway and induces apoptosis. Prepn: G. Nössner *et al.,* **DE 4222910**; *eidem,* **US 6172050** (1994, 2001 both to Asta Medica). Mechanism of action study: G. A. Ruiter *et al., Anti-Cancer Drugs* **14**, 167 (2003). LC-ESI-MS determn in plasma: E. W. Woo *et al., J. Chromatogr. B* **759**, 247 (2001). Biodistribution and tumor uptake: S. R. Vink *et al., Invest. New Drugs* **23**, 279 (2005). Clinical pharmacokinetics: M. Crul *et al., Eur. J. Cancer* **38**, 1615 (2002); evalution in advanced cancer: L. Van Ummersen *et al., Clin. Cancer Res.* **10**, 7450 (2004).

Crystals from methyl ethyl ketone, mp 271-272° (dec).

THERAP CAT: Antineoplastic.

7166. Perilla Ketone. [553-84-4] 1-(3-Furanyl)-4-methyl-1-pentanone; 1-(3-furyl)-4-methyl-1-pentanone; β-furyl isoamyl ketone. $C_{10}H_{14}O_2$; mol wt 166.22. C 72.26%, H 8.49%, O 19.25%. Potent pulmonary edematogenic agent. Isoln from the mint plant, *Perilla frutescens* Britton, *Labiatae,* and structure: R. Goto, *J. Pharm. Soc. Jpn.* **57**, 77 (1937). Synthesis: T. Matsuura, *Bull. Chem. Soc. Jpn.* **30**, 430 (1957); K. Kondo, M. Matsumoto, *Tetrahedron Lett.* **1976**, 4363; T. Kitamura *et al., Synth. Commun.* **7**, 521 (1977); K. Inomata *et al., Chem. Lett.* **1979**, 709. Potent lung toxin implicated in emphysema of grazing cattle: B. J. Wilson *et al., Science* **197**, 573 (1977).

Colorless oil, bp 196°. n_D^{20} 1.4781; d_{15}^{15} 0.9920. uv max (ethanol): 207, 253 nm (ε 14100, 5800). Sensitive to oxygen; becomes reddish-orange on standing. LD_{50} in female, male mice, male rats (mg/kg): 2.5, 6, 10 i.p. (Wilson).

7167. Perillaldehyde. [2111-75-3] 4-(1-Methylethenyl)-1-cyclohexene-1-carboxaldehyde; 4-isopropenyl-1-cyclohexene-1-carboxaldehyde. $C_{10}H_{14}O$; mol wt 150.22. C 79.95%, H 9.39%, O 10.65%. Isoln from *Perilla arguta* Benth., *Labiatae:* Semmler, Zaar, *Ber.* **44**, 52, 815 (1911); from essential oil of *Sium latifolium* L., *Umbelliferae:* Parczewski, *Diss. Pharm.* **12**, 223 (1960), *C.A.* **55**, 7765c (1961); from mandarin peel oil (*Citrus reticulata* Blanco, *Rutaceae):* Kugler, Kováts, *Helv. Chim. Acta* **46**, 1480 (1963). Prepn by chromic oxidation of perilla alcohol: Naves, *ibid.* **29**, 553 (1946); Ritter, Ginsburg, *J. Am. Chem. Soc.* **72**, 2381 (1950); Kergomard, Philibert-Bigou, *Bull. Soc. Chim. Fr.* **1958**, 393, 1174; Naves, Grampoloff, *ibid.* **1960**, 37. Brief review: *Food Chem. Toxicol.* **20**, Suppl. I-IV, 799-800 (1982).

LD_{50} in mice (g/kg): 1.72 orally; in guinea pigs (g/kg): >5 dermally (*Food Chem. Toxicol.*).

d-**Form.** Liquid. bp_{745} 237°; bp_7 98-100°. d_4^{20} 0.953. n_D^{20} 1.5058. $[\alpha]_D^{20}$ +127° (c = 13.1 in carbon tetrachloride).

l-**Form.** Liquid. bp_{10} 104-105°. d_4^{20} 0.9645. n_D^{20} 1.5069. $[\alpha]_D^{20}$ −146°.

Oxime. [138-91-0] *l*-Perillaldehyde α-*syn*-oxime; perillartine; "perilla sugar". $C_{10}H_{15}NO$. Previously referred to as *l-perillal-*

dehyde α-anti-oxime. Synthesis: Andô *et al., Science (Tokyo)* **17**, 241 (1947), *C.A.* **45**, 1976d (1951). Clarification of structure: Acton *et al., Experientia* **26**, 473 (1970). Needles, mp 102°. uv max (alc): 232 nm (ε 21800). About 2000 times as sweet as sucrose: Furukawa, *Koryo* **No. 11**, 11, 40 (1950), *C.A.* **44**, 6083g (1950).

USE: The oxime is used as sweetening agent in Japan.

7168. Perimethazine. [13093-88-4] 1-[3-(2-Methoxy-10*H*-phenothiazin-10-yl)-2-methylpropyl]-4-piperidinol; 2-methoxy-10-[2-methyl-3-(4-hydroxypiperidino)propyl]phenothiazine; 3-methoxy-10-[3-(4-hydroxypiperidyl)-2-methylpropyl]phenothiazine; perimetazine; RP-9159; AN-1317; Leptryl. $C_{22}H_{28}N_2O_2S$; mol wt 384.53. C 68.72%, H 7.34%, N 7.29%, O 8.32%, S 8.34%. Prepn: **GB 904210**; Jacob, Robert, **US 3075976** (1962, 1963 both to Rhône-Poulenc). Pharmacology: L. Julon *et al., C.R. Seances Soc. Biol. Ses Fil.* **160**, 1852 (1966). Clinical evaluation as antipsychotic: M. Bourgeois, A.-M. Sicart, *Bordeaux Med.* **3**, 515 (1970).

Crystalline powder from benzene:cyclohexane (15:85), mp 137-138°.

Hydrochloride. $C_{22}H_{28}N_2O_2S \cdot HCl$. LD_{50} in mice (mg/kg): 115 i.v.; 140 i.p.; 330 s.c.; 310 orally (Julon).

THERAP CAT: Antipsychotic.

7169. Perimycin. [11016-07-2] Aminomycin; fungimycin; WX-2412; NC-1968; Polyene antifungal antibiotic complex produced by *Streptomyces coelicolor* var. *aminophilus* NRRL 2390: W. E. Wooldridge, **US 2956925** (1960); R. R. Mohan *et al., Antimicrob. Agents Chemother.* **1963**, 462; L. E. McDaniel *et al., US 3182004** (1965 to Warner-Lambert). Purification: E. Borowski *et al., Antimicrob. Agents Annu.* **1960**, 532. Found to be a mixture of three active components, perimycin A (major), B, and C. Mechanism of action with succinyl adduct: E. Borowski, B. Cybulska, *Nature* **213**, 1034 (1967). Ionophoric and hemolytic activities: B. Cybulska *et al., Biochem. Pharmacol.* **38**, 1755 (1989). Isoln of perimycins A, B, C and structural elucidation of A: P. Kolodziejczyk *et al., Tetrahedron Lett.* **1976**, 3603. Stereochemistry and revised structure: J. Pawlak *et al., J. Antibiot.* **48**, 1034 (1995).

Perimycin A

Amorphous, golden-yellow solid. Has no definite mp but dec slowly with darkening upon heating. uv max (methanol): 383 nm ($E_{1cm}^{1\%}$ 1000). Sol in the following solvents in the presence of water: lower alcohols, pyridine, tetrahydrofuran, acetone, dioxane. Sol in warm methanol, DMF, dimethylsulfoxide, and the lower fatty acids. Practically insol in water, petr ether, ethyl acetate, benzene.

Perimycin A. [62327-61-1] 4'-Amino-3'-deamino-18-decarboxy-40-demethyl-4'-deoxy-3,7-dideoxo-3,3',7-trihydroxy-*N*47,-18,dimethyl-5-oxocandicidin D cyclic 15,19-hemiacetal. $C_{59}H_{88}$-N_2O_{17}; mol wt 1097.33. uv max: 380 nm (E_1^1 1000).

THERAP CAT: Antifungal.

7170. Perindopril. [82834-16-0] (2*S*,3a*S*,7a*S*)-1-[(2*S*)-2-[[(1*S*)-1-(Ethoxycarbonyl)butyl]amino]-1-oxopropyl]octahydro-

1*H*-indole-2-carboxylic acid; (2*S*,3a*S*,7a*S*)-1-[(*S*)-*N*-[(*S*)-1-carboxybutyl]alanyl]hexahydro-2-indolinecarboxylic acid 1-ethyl ester; (2*S*)-2-[(1*S*)-1-carbethoxybutylamino]-1-oxopropyl-(2*S*,3a*S*,7a*S*)-perhydroindole-2-carboxylic acid; S-9490; McN-A-2833. $C_{19}H_{32}$-N_2O_5; mol wt 368.47. C 61.93%, H 8.75%, N 7.60%, O 21.71%. Angiotensin-converting enzyme (ACE) inhibitor. Hydrolyzed *in vivo* to the active diacid metabolite. Prepn: G. Remond *et al., EP 49658** (1982 to Sci. Union et Cie. - Soc. Franc. Rech. Med.); M. Vincent *et al., US 4508729** (1985 to ADIR). Stereoselective synthesis: M. Vincent *et al., Tetrahedron Lett.* **23**, 1677 (1982). NMR study: N. Platzer *et al., Magn. Reson. Chem.* **26**, 296 (1988). Hemodynamic effects in humans: K. R. Lees, J. L. Reid, *Br. J. Clin. Pharmacol.* **23**, 159 (1987). Clinical evaluation in essential hypertension: T. Morgan *et al., J. Cardiovasc. Pharmacol.* **10**, Suppl. 7, S116 (1987). Pharmacokinetics, pharmacodynamics of the diacid: K. R. Lees, J. L. Reid, *ibid.* **10**, 129 (1987). Review of pharmacology and clinical use: P. A. Todd, A. Fitton, *Drugs* **42**, 90-114 (1991). Symposium on clinical efficacy in cardiovascular disease: *Am. J. Cardiol.* **88**, Suppl. 1, 1-40 (2001).

***tert*-Butylamine.** [107133-36-8] Perindopril erbumine; S-9490-3; McN-A-2833-109; Aceon; Coversum; Coversyl; Procaptan. $C_{19}H_{32}N_2O_5 \cdot C_4H_{11}N$; mol wt 441.60.

Diacid form. [95153-31-4] Perindoprilat; S-9780. $C_{17}H_{28}N_2$-O_5; mol wt 340.41.

THERAP CAT: Antihypertensive.

7171. Periodic Acid. [10450-60-9] H_5IO_6; mol wt 227.94. H 2.21%, I 55.67%, O 42.11%. Prepd by electrolytic oxidation of iodic acid or from barium periodate and nitric acid: Willard, *Inorg. Synth.* **1**, 172 (1939). Chemistry of periodic acid and periodates: H. Siebert, *Fortschr. Chem. Forsch.* **8**, 470 (1967). Periodic acid and periodates in organic and bioorganic chemistry: A. J. Fatiadi, *Synthesis* **1974**, 229. Book: G. Dryhurst, *Periodate Oxidation of Diol and Other Functional Groups* (Pergamon Press, New York, 1970).

Monoclinic, hygroscopic crystals. mp 122°; dec 130-140° forming I_2O_5, H_2O, and O_2. Freely sol in water. A 38% w/w soln had d_4^{17} 1.3875. Sol in alcohol, slightly in ether. Soly in nitric acid (d 1.42) at 26° = 7.82 g/100 ml. When aq solns are evapd at room temp the "ortho" acid H_5IO_6 crystallizes out. If this is heated in a vacuum at 100° and 12 mm it loses water and is converted to the "meta" acid HIO_4, an intermediate $H_4I_2O_9$ being formed at 80°. Periodic acid is a dibasic acid, much weaker than perchloric acid. K_1 at 25° = 2.3×10^{-2}; $K_2 = 2 \times 10^{-6}$. Very easily reduced to iodic acid by nitrous or sulfurous acids and even by hydrochloric and sulfuric acids. Oxidizes organic material.

USE: In organic synthesis.

7172. Periodyl. [53586-99-5] 12-Hydroxy-9,10-diiodo-9-octadecenoic acid; diiodoricinstearolic acid; ricinstearolic acid diiodide; 8,9-diiodo-11-hydroxy-8-heptadecene-1-carboxylic acid; Diiodyl; Joristen. $C_{18}H_{32}I_2O_3$; mol wt 550.25. C 39.29%, H 5.86%, I 46.13%, O 8.72%. $CH_3(CH_2)_5CHOHCH_2CI=CI(C$-$H_2)_7COOH$. Prepn: Mühle, *Ber.* **46**, 2091 (1913); **DE 296495** (to Riedel).

Tasteless needles from dil alcohol, mp 62°. Practically insol in water, acids; sol in dil alkalies, alcohol, ether, chloroform; slightly sol in benzene.

THERAP CAT: Iodine source.

7173. Periplanones. Sex pheromones of the American cockroach, *Periplaneta americana* L., found primarily in the alimentary tract and excreta of the insect. They act as close proximity sex-excitants and function over relatively short distances compared to long range insect sex-attractants. Isoln: D. R. A. Wharton *et al., Science* **137**, 1062 (1962). Improved isolns, identification and proposed structures of periplanone B: C. J. Persoons *et al., Tetrahedron Lett.* **1976**, 2055; E. Talman *et al., Isr. J. Chem.* **17**, 227

(1978); C. J. Persoons *et al., J. Chem. Ecol.* **5**, 221 (1979). Total synthesis and structure of (±) periplanone B: W. C. Still, *J. Am. Chem. Soc.* **101**, 2493 (1979); H. Hauptmann, G. Muhlbauer, *Tetrahedron Lett.* **27**, 1315 (1986); of the (−)-form: T. Kihara *et al., ibid.* 1343. Absolute configuration of B: M. A. Adams *et al., J. Am. Chem. Soc.* **101**, 2495 (1979). Structural and stereochemical studies of periplanone A: C. J. Persoons *et al., J. Chem. Ecol.* **8**, 439 (1982); H. Hauptmann, G. Muhlbauer, *Tetrahedron Lett.* **27**, 6189 (1986); Y. Shizuri *et al., ibid.* **28**, 1791, 1795 (1987); L. MacDonald *et al., Heterocycles* **25**, 305 (1987). Short synthesis of periplanone A: Y. Shizuri *et al., Tetrahedron Lett.* **29**, 1971 (1988). Use in insecticidal formulations: W. J. Bell *et al., Environ. Entomol.* **13**, 448 (1984); W. J. Bell *et al., Pest Control* **54**, 40 (1986).

Periplanone B

Periplanone A. [112709-47-4] (3*S*,6*S*,7*E*,11*Z*)-9-Methylene-6-(1-methylethyl)-1-oxaspiro[2.9]dodeca-7,11-dien-4-one. $C_{15}H_{20}$-O_2; mol wt 232.32. Found primarily in excreta of *P. americana,* it is unstable and gradually rearranges to a biologically inactive compound. uv max (hexane): 220 nm (log ε 4.18).

Periplanone B. [61228-92-0] (1*R*,2*R*,5*S*,6*E*,10*R*)-8-Methylene-5-(1-methylethyl)spiro[11-oxabicyclo[8.1.0]undec-6-ene-2,2'-oxiran]-3-one; (−)-periplanone B. $C_{15}H_{20}O_3$; mol wt 248.32. More stable and more active than periplanone A, it is found in both the alimentary tract and excreta of *P. americana.* The ratio of A to B in excreta is 1:10. Crystals, mp 47-50°. $[α]_D^{22}$ −667° (c = 0.13 in *n*-hexane).

(±)-Periplanone B. [70613-99-9] Crystals, mp 48-50°. uv max (hexane): 226 nm.

7174. Periplocin. [13137-64-9] 3β-[(2,6-Dideoxy-4-*O*-β-D-glucopyranosyl-β-D-*ribo*-hexopyranosyl)oxy]-5β,14-dihydroxycard-20(22)-enolide; glucoperiplocymarin; periplocoside. $C_{36}H_{56}$-O_{13}; mol wt 696.82. C 62.05%, H 8.10%, O 29.85%. Isoln from *Periploca graeca* L., *Asclepiadaceae:* Lehmann, *Arch. Pharm.* **235**, 157 (1897); W. A. Jacobs, A. Hoffmann, *J. Biol. Chem.* **79**, 519 (1928); from *Strophanthus preussii* Engl. and Pax., *Apocynaceae:* Ruppol, Trukovic, *J. Pharm. Belg.* **10**, 221 (1955), *C.A.* **50**, 12089d (1956). Structure: Stoll, Renz, *Helv. Chim. Acta* **22**, 1193 (1939). Pharmacology and toxicity: M. H. MacKeith, *J. Pharmacol. Exp. Ther.* **27**, 449 (1926).

Amorphous yellowish powder. Readily sol in water. Acid hydrolysis yields periplogenin, *q.v.,* and periplobiose (cymarose + glucose, $C_{13}H_{24}O_9$, $[α]_D^{20}$ +32°). Enzymatic hydrolysis with strophanthobiase splits off glucose, yielding periplocymarin. The biose is attached to the hydroxyl group at C-3 of the aglycon. LD in rabbits, rats (mg/kg): 10, 480 s.c. (MacKeith).

Dihydrate. Fine needles from water. Becomes anhyd after drying for one hour in high vacuum at 105°. mp 224° when bath is preheated to 200°. $[α]_D^{20}$ +23° (c = 0.7 in alcohol). One gram dissolves in ~20 ml boiling water, at 25° the soly is ~1:2500. Freely sol in alcohol. Almost insol in ether, chloroform.

Tetraacetylperiplocin. $C_{44}H_{64}O_{17}$. Six-sided prisms from alcohol, mp 195°. $[α]_D^{20}$ +20° (c = 0.5 in alcohol). Sol in alcohol, chloroform; very slightly sol in water.

7175. Periplocymarin. [32476-67-8] (2,6-Dideoxy-3-*O*-methyl-β-D-*ribo*-hexopyranosyl)oxy-5,14-dihydroxy-card-20(22)-enolide. $C_{30}H_{46}O_8$; mol wt 534.68. C 67.39%, H 8.67%, O 23.94%. By extracting bark and wood of *Periploca graeca* L., *Asclepiadaceae* with 70% alcohol and treating with the enzyme strophanthobiase from seeds of *Strophanthus courmonti* Sacleux, *Apocynaceae:* Jacobs, Hoffmann, *J. Biol. Chem.* **79**, 519 (1928); Katz, Reichstein, *Pharm. Acta Helv.* **19**, 231 (1944); from *S. hypoleucus* Stapf: von Euw, Reichstein, *Helv. Chim. Acta* **33**, 544 (1950); from *S. ledienii* Stein: Lichti *et al., ibid.* **39**, 1914 (1956); from *S. eminii* Asch. et Pax.: Zelnik, Schindler, *ibid.* **40**,

2110 (1957). Structure: von Euw, Reichstein, *ibid.* **31**, 883 (1948). Acid hydrolysis yields one mol periplogenin and one mol cymarose, *q.q.v..* The cymarose is attached to the hydroxyl group at C-3 of the aglycon.

Lustrous needles from methanol contg approx one mol CH_3OH of crystn. Bitter taste, but not nearly so marked as that of cymarin. Becomes solvent-free at 100° *in vacuo.* Sinters at 138°. mp 148°. $[α]_D^{27}$ +29° (c = 0.94 in 95% alcohol for the anhydr substance). Readily sol in alcohol, chloroform, acetone; less readily in methanol; very sparingly sol in water and practically insol in ether. Readily hydrolyzed in the cold.

7176. Periplogenin. [514-39-6] (3β,5β)-3,5,14-Trihydroxycard-20(22)-enolide; desoxostrophanthidin. $C_{23}H_{34}O_5$; mol wt 390.51. C 70.74%, H 8.78%, O 20.49%. The aglycon of periplocin and periplocymarin; accompanies strophanthidin in *Strophanthus eminii* Asch. et Pax., *Apocynaceae.* Isoln: Lehmann, *Arch. Pharm.* **235**, 157 (1897); Jacobs, Hoffmann, *J. Biol. Chem.* **79**, 519 (1928); Stoll, Renz, *Helv. Chim. Acta* **22**, 1193 (1939); Lardon, *ibid.* **33**, 639 (1950). Structure: Speiser, Reichstein, *Experientia* **3**, 323 (1947); *eidem, Helv. Chim. Acta* **30**, 2143 (1947); **31**, 622 (1948). Synthesis: Deghenghi, Gaudry, *Tetrahedron Lett.* **1963**, 2045; Kamano *et al., J. Org. Chem.* **39**, 2319 (1974).

Solvated prisms from methanol which contain an undetermined amount of methanol, sinter at 140°, mp 235°. $[α]_D^{27}$ +31.5° (c = 1.04 in alcohol). Sol in alcohol and chloroform; slightly sol in ether, water (1:2500); practically insol in benzene, petr ether. pH of aq solns ~7. Strong positive Legal test.

Monobenzoate. $C_{30}H_{38}O_6$. Stout glistening wedges from 95% alcohol, mp 235°.

Dihydroperiplogenin. $C_{23}H_{36}O_5$. Stout prisms from 25% alcohol, mp 204° (slight preliminary softening).

3-*O*-Acetylperiplogenin. $C_{25}H_{36}O_6$. Crystals, mp 242-244°, $[α]_D^{22}$ +46.9° (c = 0.32 in chloroform).

7177. Perisoxal. [2055-44-9] α-(5-Phenyl-3-isoxazolyl)-1-piperidineethanol; 3-(2-piperidino-1-hydroxyethyl)-5-phenylisoxazole. $C_{16}H_{20}N_2O_2$; mol wt 272.34. C 70.56%, H 7.40%, N 10.29%, O 11.75%. Prepn: **NL 6408694**; H. Kano *et al.,* **US 3321475** (1965, 1967 both to Shionogi); *eidem, J. Med. Chem.* **10**, 411 (1967). Series of articles on pharmacological properties: *Oyo Yakuri* **6**, 1285-1338 (1972), *C.A.* **79**, 49117h-49179k (1973). Studies on physical dependence in rats: K. Yamamoto *et al., ibid.* **16**, 871 (1978), *C.A.* **90**, 180250w (1979). Absorption, excretion, distribution, metabolism: J. Watanabe *et al., Chem. Pharm. Bull.* **27**, 1075 (1979). Toxicity study: H. Kano *et al., J. Med. Chem.* **10**, 411 (1967).

Colorless plates from 50% aq ethanol, mp 107-108°.

Citrate. [2139-25-5] S-31252; Isoxal. $(C_{16}H_{20}N_2O_2)_2 \cdot C_6H_8$-$O_7$; mol wt 736.81. Colorless prisms from ethanol/acetone, mp 143-145°. LD_{50} s.c. in mice: 416 mg/kg (Kano).

THERAP CAT: Anti-inflammatory; analgesic.

7178. Perivine. [2673-40-7] 4-Demethyl-3-oxovobasan-17-oic acid methyl ester. $C_{20}H_{22}N_2O_3$; mol wt 338.40. C 70.99%, H 6.55%, N 8.28%, O 14.18%. Indole alkaloid from *Vinca rosea* Linn., *Apocynaceae:* G. Svoboda, *J. Am. Pharm. Assoc.* **47**, 834 (1958); G. Svoboda *et al., ibid.* **48**, 659 (1959). Structure: Gorman, Sweeny, *Tetrahedron Lett.* **1964**, 3105. Cytotoxicity: D. G. I. Kingston, *J. Pharm. Sci.* **67**, 272 (1978).

Prisms from methanol, dec 218-221°. Also reported as 180-181° (Svoboda 1959). $[\alpha]_D^{26}$ −121.4° (chloroform). pKa in 66% DMF: 7.5. uv max (ethanol): 314 nm ($E_{1cm}^{1\%}$ 2.67).

7179. Perlapine. [1977-11-3] 6-(4-Methyl-1-piperazinyl)-11*H*-dibenz[*b,e*]azepine; 6-(4-methyl-1-piperazinyl)morphanthridine; AW-14'2333; HF-2333; MP-11; Hypnodin. $C_{19}H_{21}N_3$; mol wt 291.39. C 78.32%, H 7.26%, N 14.42%. Prepn: **GB 1006156**; J. Schmutz, F. Hunziker, **US 3389139** (1965, 1968 both to Wander); Hunziker *et al., Helv. Chim. Acta* **49**, 1433 (1966). Pharmacology: Y. Take *et al., J. Takeda Res. Lab.* **29**, 416 (1970); G. Stille *et al., Psychopharmacologia* **28**, 325 (1973). Toxicology study: H. Yokotani *et al., J. Takeda Res. Lab.* **29**, 441 (1970).

Yellow, prismatic crystals from acetone-petrol ether, mp 136-138°. LD_{50} in male, female mice, rats (mg/kg): 61, 61, 60, 66 i.v.; 250, 300, 480, 420 s.c., 270, 280, 660, 720 orally (Yokotani).

THERAP CAT: Hypnotic.

7180. Permethrin. [52645-53-1] 3-(2,2-Dichloroethenyl)-2,2-dimethylcyclopropanecarboxylic acid (3-phenoxyphenyl)methyl ester; 3-(phenoxyphenyl)methyl (±)-*cis,trans*-3-(2,2-dichloroethenyl)-2,2-dimethylcyclopropanecarboxylate; *m*-phenoxybenzyl (±)-*cis,trans*-3-(2,2-dichlorovinyl)-2,2-dimethylcyclopropanecarboxylate; FMC-33297; NIA-33297; NRDC-143; PP-557; SBP-1513; S-3151; Ambush; Coopex; Dragnet; Ectiban; Eksmin; Elimite; Nix; Perigen; Pounce; Permasect; Ridect. $C_{21}H_{20}Cl_2O_3$; mol wt 391.29. C 64.46%, H 5.15%, Cl 18.12%, O 12.27%. Synthetic pyrethroid insecticide, more stable to light and at least as active as the natural pyrethrins and with low mammalian toxicity: M. Elliott *et al., Nature* **246**, 169 (1973). Of the four possible isomers, the (1*R,trans*)- and the (1*R,cis*)-isomers are the two esters primarily responsible for insecticidal activity: P. E. Burt *et al., Pestic. Sci.* **5**, 791 (1974). Prepn of the racemic mixture: T. Mizutani *et al.*, **DE 2437882** (1975 to Sumitomo); F. Mori *et al.*, **DE 2544150**; *eidem*, **US 4113968** (1976, 1978, both to Kuraray). Metabolism: M. Elliott *et al., J. Agric. Food Chem.* **24**, 270 (1976); L. C. Gaughan *et al., ibid.* **26**, 613 (1978). Photodecompn: R. L. Holmstead *et al., ibid.* 590. Analysis: H. Swaine, M. J. Tandy, *Anal. Methods Pestic. Plant Growth Regul.* **13**, 103-120 (1984). Field evaluation to control flies and ticks in cows: S. S. Quisenberry, D. R. Strohbehn, *J. Econ. Entomol.* **77**, 422 (1984); R. B. Davey, E. H. Ahrens, *Am. J. Vet. Res.* **45**, 1008 (1984). Clinical trial in pediatric pediculosis: E. Ares Mazas *et al., Int. J. Dermatol.* **24**, 603 (1985). Toxicity studies in mammals: L. Metker *et al., U.S. NTIS AD Rep.* **1977**, AD-

AO47284, 70 pp; F. Cantalamessa, *Arch. Toxicol.* **67**, 510 (1993). *Review:* C. N. E. Ruscoe, *Pestic. Sci.* **8**, 236 (1977). Review of toxicology and human exposure: *Toxicological Profile for Pyrethrins and Pyrethroids* (PB2004-100004, 2003) 332 pp.

(*1R-cis*)-form

Technical material is a mixture of ~60% *trans*- and 40% *cis*-isomers: Colorless crystals to a pale yellow viscous liquid, mp ~35°. bp$_{0.05}$ 220°. d^{20} 1.190-1.272. Vapor pressure at 50° <1 × 10^{-6} mm Hg. Soly in water: <1 ppm. Sol or miscible with org solvents except ethylene glycol. LD_{50} orally in female rats: 3801 mg/kg (Metker). LD_{50} in 8 day old rats, male adult rats (mg/kg): 340.5, 1500.0 orally (Cantalamessa). Toxic to bees and fish.

Caution: Mild irritant to skin and eyes (Metker).

USE: Insecticide.

THERAP CAT: Ectoparasiticide.

THERAP CAT (VET): Ectoparasiticide.

7181. Pernambuco. Fernambuco; Brazil wood; Nicaragua wood; Lima wood; redwood. Wood of *Caesalpinia echinata* Lam., *Leguminosae. Habit.* Brazil. *Constit.* Brazilin.

USE: Dyeing red; manuf of a red lake pigment. With alkalies = purplish-red; with acids = yellow.

7182. Perospirone. [150915-41-6] (3a*R*,7a*S*)-*rel*-2-[4-[4-(1,2-Benzisothiazol-3-yl)-1-piperazinyl]butyl]hexahydro-1*H*-isoindole-1,3(2*H*)-dione; *cis-N*-[4-[4-(1,2-benzisothiazol-3-yl)-1-piperazinyl]butyl]-1,2-cyclohexanedicarboximide. $C_{23}H_{30}N_4O_2S$; mol wt 426.57. C 64.76%, H 7.09%, N 13.13%, O 7.50%, S 7.52%. Serotonin (5-HT$_2$) and dopamine (D$_2$) antagonist (SDA). Prepn (stereochem unspec): K. Ishizumi *et al.*, **EP 196096**; *eidem*, **US 4745117** (1986, 1988 both to Sumitomo). Prepn of *cis*-form: *eidem, Chem. Pharm. Bull.* **43**, 2139 (1995). Receptor binding profile in rat brain: T. Kato *et al., Jpn. J. Pharmacol.* **54**, 478 (1990). Pharmacology: H. Sakamoto *et al., Pharmacol. Biochem. Behav.* **60**, 873 (1998). Clinical trial in schizophrenia: M. Murasaki *et al., Clin. Eval.* **24**, 159 (1996). Review of pharmacological profile: Y. Ohno *et al., Pol. J. Pharmacol.* **49**, 213-219 (1997); and clinical experience: S. V. Onrust, K. McClellan, *CNS Drugs* **15**, 329-337 (2001).

Hydrochloride. [129273-38-7] SM-9018; Lullan. $C_{23}H_{30}N_4$-$O_2S·HCl$; mol wt 463.04. Prepd as dihydrate, mp 192-193°.

THERAP CAT: Antipsychotic.

7183. Perphenazine. [58-39-9] 4-[3-(2-Chloro-10*H*-phenothiazin-10-yl)propyl]-1-piperazineethanol; 2-chloro-10-[3-[1-(2-hydroxyethyl)-4-piperazinyl]propyl]phenothiazine; 1-(2-hydroxyethyl)-4-[3-(2-chloro-10-phenothiazinyl)propyl]piperazine; chlorpiprazine; chlorpiprozine; PZC; Sch-3940; Trilafon; Trilifan; Decentan; Fentazin; Perphenan. $C_{21}H_{26}ClN_3OS$; mol wt 403.97. C 62.44%, H 6.49%, Cl 8.78%, N 10.40%, O 3.96%, S 7.94%. Prepn: Cusic, **US 2766235** (1956); Sherlock, Sperber, **US 2860138** (1958 to Schering). Metabolism: U. Breyer, H. J. Gaertner, *Adv. Biochem. Psychopharmacol.* **9**, 167 (1974); H. J. Gaertner *et al., Drug Metab. Dispos.* **3**, 437 (1975). Crystal structure: J. J. H. McDowell, *Acta Crystallogr.* **B34**, 686 (1978).

Crystals. Sensitive to light. mp 94-100°. bp$_{0.15}$ 214-218°; bp$_1$ 278-281°. Practically insol in water. Soly (mg/ml): ethanol 153; acetone 82. Practically insol in sesame oil.

Dihydrochloride. C$_{21}$H$_{28}$Cl$_3$N$_3$OS. Crystals from alcohol, mp 225-226°.

THERAP CAT: Antipsychotic.

THERAP CAT (VET): Tranquilizer, pre-anesthetic agent.

7184. Perylene. [198-55-0] Dibenz[de,kl]anthracene; peri-dinaphthalene. C$_{20}$H$_{12}$; mol wt 252.31. C 95.21%, H 4.79%. Occurs in coal tar. Isoln from pitch distillate: Cook et al., J. Chem. Soc. **1933**, 395. From 2,2'-dihydroxy-1,1'-dinaphthyl: Zinke et al., Monatsh. Chem. **64**, 415 (1934). From the reaction of phenanthrene with acrolein in anhyd HF: Weinmayr, US 2145905 (1939); cf. J. Am. Chem. Soc. **61**, 949 (1939).

Yellow to colorless crystals from toluene. mp 273-274°. Sublimes 350-400°. d 1.35. Absorption spectrum: Clar, Ber. **65**, 848 (1932). Freely sol in CS$_2$, chloroform; moderately sol in benzene; slightly in ether, alcohol, acetone; very sparingly sol in petr ether. Insol in water.

Monopicrate. C$_{26}$H$_{15}$N$_3$O$_7$. Dark violet-blue needles, mp 223-225°.

7185. Petrolatum. Petroleum jelly; paraffin jelly; vasoliment; Cosmoline; Saxoline; Stanolene; Vaseline. Purified mixture of semisolid hydrocarbons, chiefly of the methane series of the general formula C$_n$H$_{2n+2}$. Actually, petrolatum is a colloidal system of nonstraight-chain solid hydrocarbons and high-boiling liq hydrocarbons, in which most of the liq hydrocarbons are held inside the micelles. Detailed historical account including chemistry and modern mfg methods: Schindler, Drug Cosmet. Ind. **89**, 36-37, 76, 78-80, 82 (1961).

Yellowish to light amber or white, semisolid, unctuous mass; practically odorless and tasteless. d$_{25}^{60}$ 0.820-0.865. mp 38-54°. n$_D^{60}$ 1.460-1.474. White petrolatum is transparent in thin layers even at 0°. Practically insol in water, glycerol, alcohol. Sol in benzene, chloroform, ether, petr ether, carbon disulfide, oils.

USE: As ointment base in pharmaceuticals and cosmetics. Lubricating firearms and machinery, leather grease, shoe polish, rust preventives, modeling clays.

7186. Petrolatum, Liquid. Liquid paraffin; mineral oil; white mineral oil; paraffin oil; Clearteck; Drakeol; Hevyteck; Kremol; Kaydol; Alboline; Nujol; Paroleine; Saxol; Adepsine oil; Glymol. A mixture of liquid hydrocarbons from petroleum.

Colorless, oily liquid; practically tasteless and odorless even when warmed. The density of the "light" oil is usually 0.83-0.860; the "heavy" 0.875-0.905. Surface tension at 25° slightly below 35 dynes/cm. Insol in water, alc. Sol in benzene, chloroform, ether, carbon disulfide, petr ether, oils.

USE: Lubricant. Pharmaceutic aid (vehicle, solvent). As formulation aid in foods. In cosmetics as emollient.

THERAP CAT: Cathartic.

THERAP CAT (VET): Laxative, externally as a protectant, lubricant.

7187. Petroleum. Crude oil; mineral oil; rock oil; coal oil; seneca oil. Consists of a mixture of hydrocarbons from C$_2$H$_6$ and

up —chiefly of the paraffins, cycloparaffins, or of cyclic aromatic hydrocarbons, with small amounts of benzene hydrocarbons, sulfur, and oxygenated compounds. Occurrence: U.S., Mexico, Iran, Russia, Roumania, Poland, Dutch East Indies, etc.

Dark yellow to brown or greenish-black, oily liquid. Insol in water and only a small portion of it may dissolve in alcohol; sol in benzene, chloroform, ether.

USE: Source of gasoline, petr ether, liq and solid petrolatum, fuel and lubricating oils, butane, isopropyl alcohol, etc.

7188. Petroleum Benzin. [8030-30-6] Naphtha; benzin; petroleum naphtha. Term that has been applied to low boiling fractions of petroleum, consisting chiefly of hydrocarbons of the methane series, principally pentanes and hexanes.

Clear, colorless, nonfluorescent, highly flammable, volatile liq; characteristic odor; does not solidify in the cold. The vapors mixed with air explode if ignited. Keep tightly closed in a cool place and away from fire. d 0.625-0.660; bp between 35-80°. Insol in water. Miscible with abs alc, benzene, chloroform, ether, carbon disulfide, carbon tetrachloride, and oils except castor oil.

Caution: Potential symptoms of overexposure are lightheadedness, drowsiness; irritation of eyes, nose and skin; dermatitis. See NIOSH Pocket Guide to Chemical Hazards (DHHS/NIOSH 97-140, 1997) p 220.

USE: Pharmaceutic aid (solvent).

THERAP CAT: Counterirritant.

7189. Petroselinic Acid. [593-39-5] cis-6-Octadecenoic acid; petroselic acid; 5-heptadecylene-1-carboxylic acid; Δ^5-octadecylenic acid. C$_{18}$H$_{34}$O$_2$; mol wt 282.46. C 76.54%, H 12.13%, O 11.33%. CH$_3$(CH$_2$)$_{10}$CH=CH(CH$_2$)$_4$COOH. Isoln from parsley seed oil, the oil extracted from dried ripe seed of Petroselinum hortense Hoffm., Umbelliferae: Fore et al., J. Am. Oil Chem. Soc. **37**, 490 (1960).

Leaflets from petr ether, mp 29.5-30.1°. bp$_{18}$ 237-238°; d$_4^{40}$ 0.8700. n$_D^{40}$ 1.4533. Low temp solubilities: Heptane at $-10°$ = 0.50 g/100 g solution; methanol at $-20°$ = 0.48 g/100 g; ethyl acetate at $-20°$ = 0.73 g/100 g; ether at $-20°$ = 3.52 g/100 g. Ozonolysis yields 85% of adipic acid. Neutralization equivalent: 282.45; iodine value 89.87%.

Methyl ester. C$_{19}$H$_{36}$O$_2$. Liq, d$_4^{20}$ 0.8767; n$_D^{20}$ 1.4501; bp$_{10}$ 208-210°.

Glyceryl triester. Glyceryl tripetroselinate; tripetroselin. C$_{57}$-H$_{104}$O$_6$. Solidifies at 16.5°. n$_D^{40}$ 1.4619.

Amide. C$_{18}$H$_{35}$NO. Needles, mp 76°.

7190. Petunidin. [1429-30-7] 2-(3,4-Dihydroxy-5-methoxyphenyl)-3,5,7-trihydroxy-1-benzopyrylium chloride; 3,3',4',5,7-pentahydroxy-5'-methoxyflavylium chloride; petunidol. C$_{16}$H$_{13}$-ClO$_7$; mol wt 352.72. C 54.48%, H 3.71%, Cl 10.05%, O 31.75%. The aglucone of petunin: Willstätter, Burdick, Ann. **412**, 217 (1917). Synthesis: Bradley et al., J. Chem. Soc. **1930**, 793; Robinson, Robinson, Biochem. J. **25**, 1687 (1931). Chromatographic separation: Spaeth, Rosenblatt, Anal. Chem. **22**, 1321 (1950).

Gray-brown leaflets or prisms from dil HCl.

3,5-Diglucoside. [25846-73-5] 2-(3,4-Dihydroxy-5-methoxyphenyl)-3,5-bis(β-D-glucopyranosyloxy)-7-hydroxy-1-benzopyrylium chloride; petunin. C$_{28}$H$_{33}$ClO$_{17}$; mol wt 677.00. From Petunia hybrida Hort., Solanaceae: Willstätter, Burdick, loc. cit. Synthesis: Bell, Robinson, J. Chem. Soc. **1934**, 1604. Violet plates with a coppery luster from dil HCl, mp ~178°. Absorption max (methanolic HCl): 540 nm.

7191. Peucedanin. [133-26-6] 3-Methoxy-2-(1-methylethyl)-7H-furo[3,2-g][1]benzopyran-7-one; 6-hydroxy-2-isopropyl-3-methoxy-5-benzofuranacrylic acid δ-lactone; 4-methoxy-5-isopropylfuro[2,3:6,7]coumarin; oreoselone methyl ether. $C_{15}H_{14}$-O_4; mol wt 258.27. C 69.76%, H 5.46%, O 24.78%. Coumarin deriv obtained from rhizome of *Peucedanum officinale* L., *Umbelliferae:* Schlatter, *Ann.* **5**, 201 (1833); Hlasiwetz, Weidel, *ibid.* **174**, 67 (1874); A. Jassoy, P. Haensel, *Arch. Pharm.* **236**, 662 (1898); Popper, *Monatsh. Chem.* **19**, 268 (1898); from *Peucedanum morisonii*, Bess., *Umbelliferae:* G. K. Nikonov, A. A. Ivashenko, *Zh. Obshch. Khim.* **33**, 2740 (1963). Fluorescence spectrum: R. H. Goodwin, F. Kavanagh, *Arch. Biochem.* **27**, 182 (1950). Antitumor activity and toxicity studies: E. M. Vermel, S. A. Kruglyak-Syrkina, *Vopr. Onkol.* **5**, 43 (1959), *C.A.* **53**, 19162h (1959). Structure: E. Späth *et al., Ber.* **64**, 2203 (1931); E. Späth, K. Klager, *ibid.* **66**, 749 (1933). Synthesis: H. Schmid, A. Ebnöther, *Helv. Chim. Acta* **34**, 1982 (1951).

Colorless needles from ether/petr ether, mp 84-87°; also reported as mp 95-97° (Schmid, Ebnöther); from ligroin, mp 102.5° (Nikonov, Ivashenko). uv max (methanol): 255, 295, 340 nm (log ε 4.40, 4.05, 3.70). Practically insol in water. Freely sol in chloroform, CS_2; sol in hot alcohol, ether, acetic acid; sparingly sol in benzene, petr ether. LD_{50} orally in mice: 315 mg/kg (Vermel, Kruglyak-Syrkina).

7192. Pexelizumab. [219685-93-5] Anti-(human complement C5 α-chain) immunoglobulin (human-mouse monoclonal 5G1.1-SC single chain); h5G1.1-scFv. Single-chain fragment of humanized monoclonal antibody directed against complement component C5; designed to prevent complement-mediated inflammation and tissue injury. Prepn: M. J. Evans *et al.*, **WO 9529697**; *eidem*, **US 6355245** (1995, 2002 both to Alexion); and complement inhibition study: T. C. Thomas *et al., Mol. Immunol.* **33**, 1389 (1996). Clinical pharmacology: J. C. K. Fitch *et al., Circulation* **100**, 2499 (1999). Clinical studies in acute myocardial infarction: K. W. Mahaffey *et al., ibid.* **108**, 1176 (2003), C. B. Granger *et al., ibid.* 1184; in coronary artery bypass graft surgery: E. D. Verrier *et al., J. Am. Med. Assoc.* **291**, 2319 (2004). Review of development and therapeutic potential: P. A. Whiss, *Curr. Opin. Invest. Drugs* **3**, 870-877 (2002); A. J. Fleisig, E. D. Verrier, *Expert Opin. Biol. Ther.* **5**, 833-839 (2005).

THERAP CAT: Anti-inflammatory.

7193. Pexiganan. [147664-63-9] 7-L-Lysine-8-L-lysine-10-L-lysine-18-L-lysine-19-*de*-L-glutamic acid-21-L-leucine-23-L-lysinamide magainin I. $C_{122}H_{210}N_{32}O_{22}$; mol wt 2477.17. C 59.15%, H 8.54%, N 18.09%, O 14.21%. Synthetic, 22 amino acid peptide; analog of the magainins, *q.v.* Prepn: B. Berkowitz, L. Jacob, **WO 9301723** (1993 to Magainin). *In vitro* antibacterial spectrum: Y. Ge *et al., Diagn. Microbiol. Infect. Dis.* **35**, 45 (1999). Review of development: L. Jacob, M. Zasloff, *Ciba Found. Symp.* **186**, 197-216 (1994); of structure-activity studies: W. L. Maloy, U. P. Kari, *Biopolymers* **37**, 105-122 (1995); of pharmacology and clinical trials in diabetic foot ulcers: H. M. Lamb, L. R. Wiseman, *Drugs* **56**, 1047-1052 (1998).

Gly–Ile–Gly–Lys–Phe–Leu–Lys–Lys–Ala–Lys–Lys
|
H₂N-Lys–Lys–Leu–Ile–Lys–Val–Phe–Ala–Lys–Gly–Phe

Acetate. [172820-23-4] MSI-78; Locilex. $C_{122}H_{210}N_{32}O_{22}$·$xC_2H_4O_2$
THERAP CAT: Antibacterial.

7194. Pfeiffer's Substance. [8015-18-7] 5,5-Diethyl-2,4,-6(1H,3H,5H)-pyrimidinetrione mixture with 4-(dimethylamino)-1,2-dihydro-1,5-dimethyl-2-phenyl-3H-pyrazol-3-one; 4-(Dimethylamino)antipyrine compd with 5,5-diethylbarbituric acid (1:1); corps de Pfeiffer. $C_{21}H_{29}N_5O_4$; mol wt 415.49. C 60.71%, H

7.04%, N 16.86%, O 15.40%. A molecular compd of aminopyrine and barbital, prepd by repeated crystn of stoichiometric amounts of the components from a minimum of hot water: Pfeiffer, *Z. Physiol. Chem.* **146**, 98 (1925).

Silky needles, mp 113-115°. At 115° the melt is turbid, but turns into a clear liquid at 140°. Freely sol in water. The aminopyrine moiety dissolves in benzene, while the barbital moiety precipitates out.

7195. P-Glycoprotein. Glycoprotein-P; P-gp; P-170; permeability glycoprotein. Highly conserved cell-surface glycoprotein of M_r 170,000 daltons; protein product of the mammalian multidrug resistance (*mdr*) gene. Present in selective human tissues where it functions as an energy-dependent efflux pump. Increased expression in mammalian tumor cells is associated with multidrug resistance (MDR) to cancer chemotherapy agents. Identification and isolation from colchicine-resistant Chinese hamster ovary (CHO) cells: R. J. Juliano, V. Ling, *Biochim. Biophys. Acta* **455**, 152 (1976). Purification from plasma membrane of CHO cells: J. R. Riordan, V. Ling, *J. Biol. Chem.* **254**, 12701 (1979). MDR associated with P-glycoprotein in mammalian cell lines: N. Kartner *et al., Science* **221**, 1285 (1983); N. Kartner *et al., Cancer Res.* **43**, 4413 (1983). Deduced amino acid sequence from mouse *mdr* cDNA: P. Gros *et al., Cell* **47**, 371 (1986); from human *mdr*1 cDNA: C.-j. Chen *et al., ibid.* 381. Transfection and expression of human *mdr*1 gene in cell culture: K. Ueda *et al., Proc. Natl. Acad. Sci. USA* **84**, 3004 (1987). Characterization of ATPase activity: H. Hamada, T. Tsuruo, *Cancer Res.* **48**, 4926 (1988). Detection in normal human tissues: F. Thiebaut *et al., Proc. Natl. Acad. Sci. USA* **84**, 7735 (1987); R. N. Hitchins *et al., Eur. J. Cancer Clin. Oncol.* **24**, 449 (1988); and in human tumor cells: D. R. Bell *et al., J. Clin. Oncol.* **3**, 311 (1985); W. S. Dalton *et al., Blood* **73**, 747 (1989). Review of role in MDR in human cancer: I. Pastan, M. Gottesman, *N. Engl. J. Med.* **316**, 1388 (1987); of biochemistry of MDR: J. A. Endicott, V. Ling, *Annu. Rev. Biochem.* **58**, 137-171 (1989); of mechanism of action: S. Ruetz, P. Gros, *Trends Pharmacol. Sci.* **15**, 260-263 (1994).

7196. Phalloidin. [17466-45-4] Phalloidine. $C_{35}H_{48}N_8$-$O_{11}S$; mol wt 788.87. C 53.29%, H 6.13%, N 14.20%, O 22.31%, S 4.06%. Best known of the toxins isolated from the poisonous green fungus *Amanita phalloides* (Fr.) Seer., *Agaricaceae*, known as "the green death cap" or "deadly agaric": Lynen, Wieland, *Ann.* **533**, 93 (1938). Structure: Wieland, Schön, *ibid.* **593**, 157 (1955); Wieland, Schöpf, *ibid.* **626**, 174 (1959); Wieland, Schnabel, *ibid.* **657**, 225 (1962). Differs from amanitin in rapidity of action; at high dose levels, death of mice or rats occurs within 1 or 2 hours. Phalloidin acts by binding actin, *q.v.*, an essential internal structural protein. Ultrastructural pathology: M. A. Russo *et al., Am. J. Pathol.* **109**, 133 (1982). Toxicity study: Vogt, *Arch. Exp. Pathol. Pharmakol.* **190**, 406 (1938). Review of the chemistry and toxicology of the toxins of *Amanita phalloides:* Wieland, Wieland, *Pharmacol. Rev.* **11**, 87-107 (1959); *see also* T. Wieland, *Fortschr. Chem. Org. Naturst.* **25**, 214-250 (1967); T. Wieland, H. Faulstich, *Crit. Rev. Biochem.* **5**, 185-260 (1978).

Hexahydrate, needles from water, mp 280-282°. uv max (water): 295 nm ($E_{1cm}^{1\%}$ 0.597). Soly in water (0°): 0.5%; much more sol in hot water; freely sol in methanol, ethanol, butanol, pyridine. LD_{50} i.m. in albino mice: 3.3 μg/g (Vogt). LD_{50} i.p. in mice: 2 mg/kg (Wieland, Wieland).

Caution: See Amanitin.

7197. Phanquinone. [84-12-8] 4,7-Phenanthroline-5,6-dione; 4,7-phenanthroline-5,6-quinone; 5,6-dioxo-5,6-dihydro-4,7-phenanthroline; phanchinone; phanquone; Ciba 11925; Entobex. $C_{12}H_6N_2O_2$; mol wt 210.19. C 68.57%, H 2.88%, N 13.33%, O 15.22%. Prepd from 5,(6)-methoxy-4,7-phenanthroline: Druey, Schmidt, *Helv. Chim. Acta* **33**, 1080 (1950); **GB 688802** (1953 to Ciba).

Crystals from methanol, mp 295° (dec). Sparingly sol in water, alcohol; sol in dil mineral acids.

THERAP CAT: Antiamebic.

7198. Phaseolin. [13401-40-6] (6b*R-cis*)-6b,12b-Dihydro-3,3-dimethyl-3*H*,7*H*-furo[3,2-*c*:5,4-*f'*]bis[1]benzopyran-10-ol; phaseollin. $C_{20}H_{18}O_4$; mol wt 322.35. C 74.52%, H 5.63%, O 19.85%. Antifungal phytoalexin isolated from French bean (*Phaseolus vulgaris* L., *Leguminosae):* I. A. M. Cruickshank, D. R. Perrin, *Life Sci.* **2**, 680 (1963). Structure: D. R. Perrin, *Tetrahedron Lett.* **1964**, 29; D. R. Perrin *et al., ibid.* **1972**, 1673. Crystal structure: C. DeMartinis *et al., Tetrahedron* **34**, 1849 (1978). Biosynthesis: S. L. Hess *et al., Phytopathology* **61**, 79 (1971); P. M. Dewick, M. J. Steele, *Phytochemistry* **21**, 1599 (1982). Total synthesis: S. E. N. Mohamed *et al., J. Chem. Soc. Perkin Trans. 1* **1987**, 431. Mode of action: F. D. Van Etten, D. F. Bateman, *Phytopathology* **61**, 1363 (1971). Antifungal properties: I. A. M. Cruickshank, D. R. Perrin, *Phytopathol. Z.* **70**, 209 (1971); M. A. Gordon *et al., Antimicrob. Agents Chemother.* **17**, 120 (1980).

Crystals, mp 177-178°. $[\alpha]_{578}$ -145°. pKa 9.13. uv max (ethanol): 207, 230, 280, 286 nm (log ε 4.68, 4.40, 3.97, 3.90).

7199. Phasin. [1392-87-6] Poisonous agglutinin from beans. A polypeptide composed of glutamic acid, aspartic acid, serine, alanine, tyrosine, lysine and arginine: Piekarski, *Diss. Pharm.* **9**, 255 (1957), *C.A.* **52**, 6456i (1958). Prepn: Wienhaus, *Biochem. Z.* **18**, 228 (1909), *C.A.* **3**, 2471 (1909); Piekarski, *loc. cit.*

Amorphous powder. Its toxicity and agglutination properties are destroyed by heating.

7200. α-Phellandrene. [99-83-2] 2-Methyl-5-(1-methylethyl)-1,3-cyclohexadiene; *p*-mentha-1,5-diene; 5-isopropyl-2-methyl-1,3-cyclohexadiene; 4-isopropyl-1-methyl-1,5-cyclohexadiene. $C_{10}H_{16}$; mol wt 136.23. C 88.16%, H 11.84%. Isoln of *l*-form from essential oils of *Eucalyptus dives* Schau. and *E. phellandra* Baker & Smith, *Myrtaceae:* Smith *et al., J. Chem. Soc.* **123**, 1657 (1923). Isoln of *d*-form from oil of bitter fennel (*Foeniculum vulgare* Mill., *Umbelliferae):* Wallach, *Ann.* **336**, 9 (1904). Structure: Semmler, *Ber.* **36**, 1749 (1903). Synthesis of *dl*-form: Read, Storey, *J. Chem. Soc.* **1930**, 2770; B. Singaram, J. Verghese, *Indian J. Chem.* **14B**, 1003 (1976). Configuration: Burgstahler *et al., J. Am. Chem. Soc.* **83**, 4460 (1961). Circular dichroism: G. Snatzke *et al., Tetrahedron Lett.* **1966**, 4551. *Review:* J. L. Simonsen, *The Terpenes* vol. 1 (Univ. Press, Cambridge, 2nd ed., 1947) pp 193-204; B. Singaram, J. Verghese, *Perfum. Flavor.* **2**, 33-38 (1978).

l-**Form.** [4221-98-1] Mobile oil. bp_{758} 171-172°; bp_{16} 58-59°. d_4^{20} 0.8410. n_D^{20} 1.4709. $[\alpha]_D^{20}$ -217°. Practically insol in water; sol in ether.

d-**Form.** [2243-33-6] Mobile oil. bp_{16} 66-68°. d_4^{25} 0.8463. n_D^{25} 1.4777. $[\alpha]_D^{16}$ +86.4°. Practically insol in water; sol in ether.

Caution: Can be irritating to, and absorbed through, skin. Ingestion can cause vomiting, diarrhea.

USE: In fragrances.

7201. β-Phellandrene. [555-10-2] 3-Methylene-6-(1-methylethyl)cyclohexene; *p*-mentha-1(7),2-diene; 3-isopropyl-6-methylene-1-cyclohexene; 4-isopropyl-1-methylene-2-cyclohexene. $C_{10}H_{16}$; mol wt 136.23. C 88.16%, H 11.84%. Isoln of *d*-form from oil of water fennel (*Phellandrium aquaticum* L., *Umbelliferae):* Berry *et al., J. Chem. Soc.* **1937**, 1448. Isoln of *l*-form from Canada balsam oil: Macbeth *et al., ibid.* **1938**, 119. Structure: Wallach, *Ann.* **343**, 28 (1905). Synthesis of *dl*-form: Deorha, Sareen, *Rec. Trav. Chim.* **82**, 137 (1965); B. Singaram, J. Verghese, *Indian J. Chem.* **14B**, 1003 (1976).

d-**Form.** [6153-16-8] Mobile oil. bp_{760} 171-172°; bp_{11} 57°. d_4^{20} 0.8520. n_D^{20} 1.4788. $[\alpha]_D^{20}$ +65.2°. Practically insol in water; sol in ether.

l-**Form.** [6153-17-9] Mobile oil. bp_{758} 178-179°; bp_{12} 53°. d_{15}^{15} 0.8497. n_D^{20} 1.4800. $[\alpha]_D^{20}$ -51.9°. Practically insol in water, alcohol; sol in ether.

7202. Phenacaine Hydrochloride. [620-99-5] *N,N'*-Bis(4-ethoxyphenyl)ethanimidamide monohydrochloride; N^1,N^2-bis(*p*-ethoxyphenyl)acetamidine hydrochloride; Holocaine Hydrochloride. $C_{18}H_{23}ClN_2O_2$; mol wt 334.84. C 64.57%, H 6.92%, Cl 10.59%, N 8.37%, O 9.56%. Prepn: **DE 79868; DE 80568.**

Monohydrate. [6153-19-1] Faintly bitter crystals producing transient numbness of the tongue. Stable in air. When anhydr, mp 190-192°. One gram dissolves in 50 ml water. Freely sol in boiling water, alcohol, chloroform. Insol in ether. Incompatible with alkalies and their carbonates and the usual alkaloidal reagents. Aq solns are stable and are not dec by boiling.

THERAP CAT: Topical anesthetic (ophthalmic).

THERAP CAT (VET): Ocular anesthetic.

7203. Phenacemide. [63-98-9] *N*-(Aminocarbonyl)benzeneacetamide; (phenylacetyl)urea; phenacetylurea; Epiclase; Phacetur; Phenurone; Phetylureum; $C_9H_{10}N_2O_2$; mol wt 178.19. C 60.66%, H 5.66%, N 15.72%, O 17.96%. $C_6H_5CH_2CONH\cdot CONH_2$. Prepd by the action of aq NH_3 on phenacetylurethan: Basterfield, Greig, *Can. J. Res.* **8**, 454 (1933); of phenacetyl chloride on urea: Spielman *et al., J. Am. Chem. Soc.* **70**, 4189 (1948). Toxicity study: K. Nakamura *et al., Arzneim.-Forsch.* **18**, 524 (1968).

Crystals from alcohol, mp 212-216°. Very slightly sol in water; slightly sol in alcohol, benzene, chloroform, ether. LD_{50} in mice, rats (mmol/kg): 5.54, >10 orally (Nakamura).

THERAP CAT: Anticonvulsant.

7204. Phenacetin. [62-44-2] N-(4-Ethoxyphenyl)acetamide; p-acetophenetidide; p-ethoxyacetanilide; acetophenetidin; *para*-acetphenetidin; acet-p-phenetidin; p-acetophenetide. $C_{10}H_{13}$-NO_2; mol wt 179.22. C 67.02%, H 7.31%, N 7.82%, O 17.85%. Prepn: *Beilstein* **vol. XIII,** 461. Improved process: Eaker, Campbell, **US 2887513** (1959 to Monsanto). *Monograph:* P. K. Smith, *Acetophenetidin* (Interscience, New York, 1958) 180 pp. Toxicity: Boyd, *Toxicol. Appl. Pharmacol.* **1,** 240 (1959). Review of toxicity and metabolism studies: L. Fishbein, *IARC Sci. Publ.* **40,** 287-310 (1981). Epidemiologic study of renal morbidity and mortality: U. C. Dubach *et al., N. Engl. J. Med.* **308,** 357 (1983). Evaluation of renal effects: D. P. Sandler *et al., ibid.* **320,** 1238 (1989).

Slightly bitter, cryst scales or powder. mp 134-135°. One gram dissolves in 1310 ml cold water, 82 ml boiling water; 15 ml cold alcohol, 2.8 ml boiling alcohol; 14 ml chloroform, 90 ml ether; sol in glycerol. Gives a pasty mass with phenol, chloral hydrate or pyrocatechol, strong acids or alkalies, salicylic acid, oxidizers, iodine, spirit nitrous ether. LD_{50} orally in rats: 1.65 g/kg (Boyd).

Note: Component of **APC** tablets, analgesic mixture also containing aspirin and caffeine.

Caution: Phenacetin is reasonably anticipated to be a human carcinogen; analgesic mixtures containing phenacetin are listed as known human carcinogens: *Report on Carcinogens, Eleventh Edition* (PB2005-104914, 2004) p III-212.

THERAP CAT: Analgesic, antipyretic.

THERAP CAT (VET): Analgesic, antipyretic.

7205. Phenacetolin. [1340-26-7] Degener's indicator. Reaction product of concd H_2SO_4 and glacial acetic acid on phenol.

Yellowish-brown powder. Slightly sol in water; sol in alc.

USE: Has been employed as indicator, particularly for mixtures of alkali hydroxides and carbonates; the yellow color changes to red when hydroxide is neutralized, and again to yellow when carbonate is fully dec by acid; was also used for determining alkalinity of water. The indicator soln is prepd by digesting 1 g with 100 ml warm alcohol and filtering after cooling; 2-3 drops used for 100 ml liquid.

7206. Phenacylamine. [613-89-8] 2-Amino-1-phenylethanone; 2-aminoacetophenone; α-aminoacetophenone; ω-aminoacetophenone. C_8H_9NO; mol wt 135.16. C 71.09%, H 6.71%, N 10.36%, O 11.84%. Prepn from α-phenylethylamine: H. E. Baumgarten, J. M. Petersen, *J. Am. Chem. Soc.* **82,** 459 (1960); *eidem, Org. Synth.* **coll. vol. V,** 909 (1973).

Hydrochloride. $C_8H_9NO.HCl$. Crystals from isopropanol + HCl, dec 188.5°.

7207. Phenadoxone. [467-84-5] 6-(4-Morpholinyl)-4,4-diphenyl-3-heptanone; 6-tetrahydrooxazine-4,4-diphenyl-3-heptanone; heptazone; morphodone. $C_{23}H_{29}NO_2$; mol wt 351.48. C 78.60%, H 8.32%, N 3.99%, O 9.10%. Prepn: M. Bockmühl, G. Ehrhart, *Ann.* **561,** 52 (1948). Comparison with other analgesics: C. A. Winter, L. Flataker, *J. Pharmacol. Exp. Ther.* **98,** 305 (1950). HPLC determn: I. Jane *et al., J. Chromatogr.* **323,** 191 (1985).

mp 75-76°.

Hydrochloride. [545-91-5] Hoechst 10600; CB-11; Hepagin; Heptalgin; Heptalin; Heptone; Supralgin. $C_{23}H_{29}NO_2.HCl$; mol wt 387.94. Crystals, mp 224-225° (some decompn). pKa (25°): 6.7 in 40% alcohol. pH of 1% aq soln 4.1; of 5% aq soln 3.7. The free base begins to precipitate when the pH is raised to 5.5. uv max (abs alcohol): 260, 295 nm. Soly (g/100 ml) in water: 10 at 25°; 80 at the bp; in methanol: 27; in abs ethanol: 24; in chloroform: 50. Slightly sol in acetone. Almost insol in benzene, ethyl acetate. LD_{50} i.v. in mice: 47.5 mg/kg (Winter, Flataker).

Note: This is a controlled substance (opiate): **21 CFR,** 1308.11.

THERAP CAT: Analgesic (narcotic).

7208. Phenamidine. [101-62-2] 4,4'-Oxybisbenzenecarboximidamide; 4,4'-oxydibenzamidine; 4,4'-diamidinodiphenyl ether. $C_{14}H_{14}N_4O$; mol wt 254.29. C 66.13%, H 5.55%, N 22.03%, O 6.29%. Prepn: A. J. Ewins *et al.,* **GB 507565** (1939 to May & Baker); J. N. Ashley *et al., J. Chem. Soc.* **1942,** 103; of isethionate: G. Newbery, A. P. T. Easson, **US 2410796** (1946 to May & Baker). Trypanocidal activity: E. M. Lourie, W. Yorke, *Ann. Trop. Med. Parasitol.* **33,** 289 (1939). Preliminary pharmacology: R. Wien, *ibid.* **37,** 1 (1943). Use in treatment of Babesia infections in dogs: M. D. Ruff *et al., Am. J. Vet. Res.* **34,** 641 (1973); R. Gothe *et al., Kleintier-Praxis* **32,** 97 (1987). Early review of pharmacology, mode of action and clinical applications: E. M. Schoenbach, E. M. Greenspan, *Medicine* **27,** 327-377 (1948).

Irregular plates from water, mp 215-216°.

Isethionate. [620-90-6] M & B 736; Lomadine. $C_{14}H_{14}N_4$-$O.2C_2H_6O_4S$; mol wt 506.55. Crystals, mp 225° (dec). One part is sol in 1.4 parts water; 300 parts alcohol. Practically insol in ether, chloroform.

THERAP CAT (VET): Antiprotozoal (Babesia).

7209. Phenampromid(e). [129-83-9] N-[1-Methyl-2-(1-piperidinyl)ethyl]-N-phenylpropanamide; N-(1-methyl-2-piperidinoethyl)propionanilide; 1-piperidino-2-(N-propionylanilino)propane. $C_{17}H_{26}N_2O$; mol wt 274.40. C 74.41%, H 9.55%, N 10.21%, O 5.83%. Prepn and analgesic activity: W. B. Wright, Jr. *et al., J. Am. Chem. Soc.* **81,** 1518 (1959); W. B. Wright, Jr., H. J. Brabander, **US 3016382** (1962 to Am. Cyanamid). (−)-Phenampromid(e), the more active enantiomer, has the R-configuration. Absolute configuration: Portoghese, *J. Med. Chem.* **8,** 147 (1965). Pharmacology: Kikuchi *et al., Nippon Yakurigaku Zasshi* **57,** 585 (1961), *C.A.* **59,** 2082b (1963). Determn by HPLC: I. Jane, A. McKinnon, *J. Chromatogr.* **323,** 191 (1985).

(−)-Phenampromid(e)

Liquid, $bp_{0.2}$ 124-128°. n_D^{28} 1.518.

(−)-Hydrochloride. $C_{17}H_{27}ClN_2O$. Crystals from alcoholic HCl + ether, mp 201-202°.

Note: This is a controlled substance (opiate): **21 CFR,** 1308.11.

7210. Phenazopyridine. [94-78-0] 3-(Phenylazo)-2,6-pyridinediamine; 2,6-diamino-3-phenylazopyridine; β-phenylazo-α,α'-diaminopyridine. $C_{11}H_{11}N_5$; mol wt 213.24. C 61.96%, H 5.20%, N 32.84%. Azo dye used in treatment of urinary tract infections. Prepn: A. E. Chichibabin, O. A. Zeide, *J. Russ. Phys. Chem. Soc.* **46**, 1216 (1914); *Chem. Zentralbl.* **1915, I,** 1064; I. Ostromislensky, **US 1680109** (1928 to Pyridium); and bacteriostatic properties: R. N. Shreve *et al., J. Am. Chem. Soc.* **65**, 2241 (1943). Physical characteristics: G. W. Collins, *J. Am. Pharm. Assoc.* **20**, 455 (1931). Toxicity data: B. A. Becker, J. G. Swift, *Toxicol. Appl. Pharmacol.* **1**, 42 (1959). Comprehensive description: K. W. Blessel *et al., Anal. Profiles Drug Subs.* **3**, 465-482 (1974). LC-MS determn in plasma and pharmacokinetics: E. Shang *et al., Anal. Bioanal. Chem.* **382**, 216 (2005). Review of clinical experience in urinary tract infections: S. A. Zelenitsky, G. G. Zhanel, *Ann. Pharmacother.* **30**, 866-868 (1996).

mp 136-137°.

Hydrochloride. [136-40-3] Prodium; Pyridium; Pyridacil; Sedural. $C_{11}H_{11}N_5$·HCl; mol wt 249.70. Brick-red microcrystals, slight violet luster. Slightly bitter taste. Slightly sol in cold water, about 1 part in 300; sol in boiling water, about 1 part in 20. One part is sol in about 100 parts glycerol. Sol in ethylene and propylene glycols. Slightly sol in alc, lanolin; sol in acetic acid. Insol in acetone, benzene, chloroform, ether, toluene. Aq solns are yellow to brick-red and slightly acid. Forms supersatd solns easily. Will precipitate out of a 2% soln at 25° after about 2 days, out of a 1% soln only after months. Aq solns may be stabilized by the addn of 10% glucose. LD_{50} orally in rats: 403 mg/kg (Becker, Swift).

Caution: Phenazopyridine hydrochloride is reasonably anticipated to be a human carcinogen: *Report on Carcinogens, Eleventh Edition* (PB2005-104914, 2004) p III-213.

THERAP CAT: Analgesic (urinary tract).

THERAP CAT (VET): Analgesic (urinary tract).

7211. Phenothrin. [26002-80-2] 2,2-Dimethyl-3-(2-methyl-1-propenyl)cyclopropanecarboxylic acid (3-phenoxyphenyl)methyl ester; 2,2-dimethyl-3-(2-methylpropenyl)cyclopropanecarboxylic acid *m*-phenoxybenzyl ester; 3-phenoxybenzyl *cis,trans*-chrysanthemate; S-2539; Sumithrin. $C_{23}H_{26}O_3$; mol wt 350.45. C 78.83%, H 7.48%, O 13.70%. Synthetic pyrethroid insecticide. Prepn of racemic mixture: N. Itaya *et al.,* **DE 1926433** corresp to **US 3666789** (1969, 1972 to Sumitomo). Comparative activity of isomers: K. Fujimoto *et al., Agric. Biol. Chem.* **37**, 2681 (1973); Y. Okuno *et al.,* **DE 2348930** corresp to **US 3934023** (1973, 1976 to Sumitomo). Analysis: Y. Takimoto *et al., Anal. Methods Pestic. Plant Growth Regul.* **13**, 133-146 (1984). Review of toxicology and human exposure: *Toxicological Profile for Pyrethrins and Pyrethroids* (PB2004-100004, 2003) 332 pp.

(1*R-trans*)-form

The commercial product is a mixture of isomers. Colorless liquid. d_{25}^{25} 1.06; n_D^{25} 1.5483. Sol in acetone, xylene. Insol in water.

USE: Insecticide.

7212. Phenanthrene. [85-01-8] $C_{14}H_{10}$; mol wt 178.23. C 94.34%, H 5.66%. Isomeric with anthracene. Occurs in coal tar, *q.v.,* and in products of incomplete combustion. Isoln: Ostermayer, Fittig, *Ber.* **5**, 933 (1872); Glaser, *ibid.* 982. Purification (from contaminating carbazole and anthracene): Clar, *Ber.* **65**, 852 (1932). Formation from toluene, bibenzil, 9-methylfluorene or

stilbene by passage through red-hot tube: Graebe, *Ber.* **7**, 48 (1874); *Ann.* **167**, 161 (1879); *Ber.* **37**, 4145 (1904). Also from coumarone and benzene: Kraemer, Spilker, *Ber.* **23**, 85 (1890). Pschorr synthesis from *o*-nitrobenzaldehyde and phenylacetic acid: *Ber.* **29**, 500 (1896). From diphenylethylene: Cook, Hewett, *J. Chem. Soc.* **1933**, 1098. Diene synthesis from 1-vinylnaphthalene and maleic anhydride: Cohen, Warren, *ibid.* **1937**, 1315. From *o*-phenylbenzoic acid: Schönberg, Warren, *Chem. Ind. (London)* **58**, 199 (1939). By irradiation of stilbene: Mallory *et al., J. Am. Chem. Soc.* **84**, 4361 (1962). Synthesis by double succinoylation of benzene: Rahman *et al., J. Org. Chem.* **28**, 3571 (1963). Structure: Trotter, *Acta Crystallogr.* **16**, 605 (1963). Review of carcinogenic risk: *IARC Monographs* **32**, 419-430 (1983); of toxicology and human exposure: *Toxicological Profile for Polycyclic Aromatic Hydrocarbons* (PB95-264370, 1995) 487 pp.

Monoclinic plates from alcohol. d^{25} 1.179; mp 100°; bp 340°. Sublimes in high vacuum. Absorption spectrum: Clar, Lombardi, *Ber.* **65**, 1412 (1932); Mayneord, Roe, *Proc. Roy. Soc. London* A **152**, 317 (1935). Practically insol in water. Sol in organic solvents, especially in aromatic hydrocarbons. One gram dissolves in 60 ml cold, 10 ml boiling 95% alcohol, 25 ml abs alcohol, 2.4 ml toluene or carbon tetrachloride, 2 ml benzene, 1 ml carbon disulfide, 3.3 ml anhydr ether. Soluble in glacial acetic acid. Solns exhibit a blue fluorescence. Forms molecular compds with picric acid, picryl chloride, dinitrobenzene and similar nitro compounds. LD_{50} i.p. in mice: 700 mg/kg (IARC).

Caution: Can cause photosensitization of skin.

7213. Phenanthrenequinone. [84-11-7] 9,10-Phenanthrenedione; 9,10-phenanthraquinone. $C_{14}H_8O_2$; mol wt 208.21. C 80.76%, H 3.87%, O 15.37%. Prepn by oxidation of phenanthrene: Curtis *et al.,* **US 2956065** (1960 to U.S. Steel); Binder, Koch, **DE 1166176** (1964).

Orange-red crysts. mp 206-207°. bp ~360°. d 1.405. Sublimes. Practically insol in water; sol in benzene, ether, glacial acetic acid, hot alc. With concd H_2SO_4 gives a dark green color.

7214. *o*-Phenanthroline. [66-71-7] 1,10-Phenanthroline; 4,5-phenanthroline. $C_{12}H_8N_2$; mol wt 180.21. C 79.98%, H 4.47%, N 15.54%. Metal chelator. Prepn: F. Blau, *Monatsh. Chem.* **19**, 666 (1898); K. Madeja, *J. Prakt. Chem.* **17**, 104 (1962). Solubilities: J. Burgess, R. I. Haines, *J. Chem. Eng. Data* **23**, 196 (1978). Crystal and molecular structure: S. Nishigaki *et al., Acta Crystallogr.* **B34**, 875 (1978). Review of analytical uses: F. Vydra, M. Kopanica, *Chemist-Analyst* **52**, 88-94 (1963); of chemistry and reactivity: L. A. Summers, *Adv. Heterocycl. Chem.* **22**, 1-69 (1978); W. Sliwa, *Heterocycles* **12**, 1207-1237 (1979); P. G. Sammes, G. Yahioglu, *Chem. Soc. Rev.* **1994**, 327-334; of chiral derivatives used in asymmetric catalysis: E. Schoffers, *Eur. J. Org. Chem.* **2003**, 1145-1152.

White, cryst powder. mp 117°. pKa_1: 4.8-5.2. uv max (water): 265 nm (ε 29510). Soly at 298.2 K (mol/dm³): water 0.0149; ethanol 2.78.

USE: As an analytical reagent for determn of metals in chemical and biological systems through complex formation. As an indicator (*"Ferroin"*) in combination with ferrous ions for oxidation/reduction reactions. In organic syntheses as an activator.

7215. Phenarsazine Chloride. [578-94-9] 10-Chloro-5,10-dihydrophenarsazine; 5-aza-10-arsenaanthracene chloride; 10-chloro-5,10-dihydroarsacridine; diphenylaminechlorarsine; phenazarsine chloride; adamsite; DM. $C_{12}H_9AsClN$; mol wt 277.58. C 51.92%, H 3.27%, As 26.99%, Cl 12.77%, N 5.05%. Prepd by heating diphenylamine with arsenic trichloride: **DE 281049** (1914 to I. G. Farben.); Wieland, Reinheimer, *Ann.* **423**, 12 (1921); Lewis, Hamilton, *J. Am. Chem. Soc.* **43**, 2222 (1921); Burton, Gibson, *J. Chem. Soc.* **1926**, 450.

Canary-yellow crystals from carbon tetrachloride. *Poisonous.* Dimorphous. The stable form occurs as orthorhombic crystals; d 1.65; mp 195°; bp 410° (decompn). Sublimes readily. Vapor press. at 20° = 2×10^{-13} mm; volatility 0.02 mg/cu m; heat of volatilization 54.8 cal; spec heat 0.268 cal. Practically insol in water. Slightly sol in benzene, xylene, carbon tetrachloride. Corrodes iron, bronze, brass. (The metastable form melts at 186° if monoclinic, and at 182° if triclinic.)

Caution: Irritating to skin and respiratory tract. Causes profuse watery nasal discharge; severe pain in nose, sinuses, chest; sneezing, coughing, nausea, vomiting, marked depression, weakness. Sensory disturbances may occur later.

USE: As war gas, dispersed in air in the form of minute particles. For riots in combination with tear gas (chloroacetophenone). In the formulation of wood-treating solns, against marine borers and similar pests.

7216. Phenatine. [139-68-4] *N*-(1-Methyl-2-phenylethyl)-3-pyridinecarboxamide; *N*-(α-methylphenethyl)nicotinamide; nicotinic acid β-phenylisopropylamide; nicotinoyl-β-phenylisopropylamine; fenatin; perviton. $C_{15}H_{16}N_2O$; mol wt 240.30. C 74.97%, H 6.71%, N 11.66%, O 6.66%. Synthesis from nicotinoyl chloride and $C_6H_5CH_2CH(CH_3)NH_2$: Arbuzov *et al.*, *Sb. Statei Obshch. Khim.* **1**, 714 (1953), *C.A.* **49**, 1072 (1955). Pharmacology: Arbuzov, *Farmakol. Toksikol.* **31**, 373 (1968). Analysis: P. P. Suprun, *Farm. Zh. (Kiev)* **30**, 49 (1975); O. N. Shcherbina *et al.*, *ibid.* **1979**, 49.

Crystals from benzene, mp 99-100°.
Phosphate. $C_{15}H_{16}N_2O.2H_3PO_4$. Crystals from alcohol + ether, mp 162°. Sol in water, warm alcohol. Insol in ether. Aq solns may be boiled for 3 hrs without decompn.

7217. Phenazine. [92-82-0] Dibenzopyrazine; dibenzoparadiazine; azophenylene. $C_{12}H_8N_2$; mol wt 180.21. C 79.98%, H 4.47%, N 15.54%. Obtained (with other products) by passing aniline vapor through a red-hot tube: Bernthsen, *Ber.* **19**, 3257 (1886); by heating aniline with nitrobenzene and sodium hydroxide to 140°: Wohl, Aue, *Ber.* **34**, 2446 (1901); Wohl, *Ber.* **36**, 4135 (1903); by heating o-phenylenediamine with pyrocatechol in sealed tube: Ris, *Ber.* **19**, 2206 (1886); Hinsberg, Garfunkel, *Ann.* **292**, 258 (1896); upon distilling 2-aminodiphenylamine with lead monoxide: Fischer, Heiler, *Ber.* **26**, 383 (1893); by heating 2-aminodiphenylamine with 2-nitrodiphenylamine in the presence of sodium acetate: Kehrmann, Havas, *Ber.* **46**, 342 (1913); by heating nitrobenzene with barium oxide: Zerewitinoff, Ostromisslensky, *Ber.* **44**, 2402 (1911); by boiling 2,2'-dinitrodiphenylamine with stannous chloride

in hydrochloric and acetic acids, followed by oxidation with hydrogen peroxide: Eckert, Steiner, *Monatsh. Chem.* **35**, 1154 (1914).

Pale yellow needles from alcohol or by sublimation. Colorless needles from dilute alcohol. mp 171°; bp above 360°. Practically insol in water. One part dissolves in 50 parts alcohol. Moderately sol in ether, benzene; sol in mineral acids giving yellow to red solns.

7218. Phenazocine. [127-35-5] 1,2,3,4,5,6-Hexahydro-6,11-dimethyl-3-(2-phenethyl)-2,6-methano-3-benzazocin-8-ol; 2'-hydroxy-2-(*N,β*-phenethyl)-5,9-dimethyl-6,7-benzomorphan; 2'-hydroxy-5,9-dimethyl-2-phenethyl-6,7-benzmorphan; phenethylazocine; phenobenzorphan. $C_{22}H_{27}NO$; mol wt 321.46. C 82.20%, H 8.47%, N 4.36%, O 4.98%. Prepn: E. L. May, N. B. Eddy, *J. Org. Chem.* **24**, 294, 1435 (1959); Ager, May, *ibid.* **25**, 984 (1960); Gordon *et al.*, **US 2959594** (1960 to SK&F).

(±)-**Form.** Rods from methanol, mp 181-182°.
(−)-**Form.** Needles from methanol, mp 159-159.5°. $[\alpha]_D^{20}$ −122° (c = 0.74 in 95% ethanol).
(±)-**Hydrobromide.** [1239-04-9] NIH-7519; SKF-6574; Narphen; Prinadol; Xenagol. $C_{22}H_{27}NO.HBr$; mol wt 402.37. Rods from acetone or abs alc + ether, mp 166-170°. LD$_{50}$ s.c. in mice: 332 mg/kg (May, Eddy).
(−)-**Hydrobromide.** Crystals, mp 284-287°. $[\alpha]_D^{20}$ −84.1° (c = 1.12 in 95% ethanol). LD$_{50}$ s.c. in mice: 147 mg/kg (May, Eddy).
Note: This is a controlled substance (opiate): **21 CFR**, 1308.12.
THERAP CAT: Analgesic (narcotic).

7219. Phencyclidine. [77-10-1] 1-(1-Phenylcyclohexyl)-piperidine; angel dust; HOG; PCP; CI-395. $C_{17}H_{25}N$; mol wt 243.39. C 83.89%, H 10.35%, N 5.75%. Prepn: **GB 836083** and Godefroi *et al.*, **US 3097136** (1960, 1963 to Parke, Davis); V. H. Maddox *et al.*, *J. Med. Chem.* **8**, 230 (1965). Pharmacology: G. Chen *et al.*, *J. Pharmacol. Exp. Ther.* **127**, 241 (1959); J. C. Munch, *Bull. Narc.* **26**, 9 (1974). Human metabolism: L. K. Wong, K. Biemann, *Biomed. Mass Spectrom.* **2**, 204 (1975). Toxicity: K. Bailey *et al.*, *J. Pharm. Pharmacol.* **28**, 713 (1976). Extensive bibliography: R. L. Balster, R. S. Pross, *J. Psychedelic Drugs* **10**, 1-15 (1978). *Review:* R. E. Garey, *ibid.* **11**, 265-275 (1979). Review of neuropharmacology: K. M. Johnson, S. M. Jones, *Annu. Rev. Pharmacol. Toxicol.* **30**, 707-750 (1990).

Colorless crystals, mp 46-46.5°. bp$_{1.0}$ 135-137°. uv max (0.1N HCl): 252, 257.5, 262, 268.5 nm (E$_{1cm}^{1\%}$ 7.9, 11.2, 13.0, 9.7).
Hydrochloride. [956-90-1] Sernyl; Sernylan. $C_{17}H_{25}N.HCl$; mol wt 279.85. Crystals from 2-propanol, mp 233-235°. uv max (ethanol): 254, 258, 262.5, 269 nm (E$_{1cm}^{1\%}$ 7.9, 10.8, 12.7, 10.0). LD$_{50}$ orally in mice: 76.5 mg/kg (Bailey).
Hydrobromide. Crystals, mp 214-218°.
Caution: This is a controlled substance (depressant): **21 CFR**, 1308.12. The ethylamine, pyrrolidine and thiophene analogs are controlled substances (hallucinogens): **21 CFR**, 1308.11.
THERAP CAT: Anesthetic (intravenous).
THERAP CAT (VET): Analgesic; anesthetic.

7220. Phendimetrazine. [634-03-7] 3,4-Dimethyl-2-phenylmorpholine; *d*-2-phenyl-3,4-dimethylmorpholine; 3,4-dimethyl-2-phenyltetrahydro-1,4-oxazine. $C_{12}H_{17}NO$; mol wt 191.27. C 75.35%, H 8.96%, N 7.32%, O 8.36%. Prepn from ethylene chlorohydrin and *l*-ephedrine: Otto, *Angew. Chem.* **68**, 181 (1956); from 2-phenyl-2-hydroxy-3,4-dimethylmorpholine: Boehringer *et al.*, **GB 791416** (1958); **GB 862198** (1961). Stereochemistry: Dvornik, Schilling, *J. Med. Chem.* **8**, 466 (1965). Toxicity data: Stegen *et al.*, *Toxicol. Appl. Pharmacol.* **2**, 589 (1960).

bp$_8$ 122-124°; bp$_{12}$ 134-135°.

Bitartrate. [50-58-8] Adphen; Bacarate; Neo-Nilorex; Obepar; Phenazine; Plegine; Statobex; Symetra; Trimstat; Trimtabs.

Hydrochloride. [7635-51-0] Antapentan. $C_{12}H_{17}NO.HCl$; mol wt 227.73. mp 191° (Otto), 208° (Boehringer). $[\alpha]_D^{20}$ +35.7°. LD$_{50}$ in rats (mg/kg): 455 orally; 245 i.p. (Stegen).

Pamoate. [27922-80-1] Fringanor. $(C_{12}H_{17}NO)_2.C_{23}H_{16}O_6$; mol wt 770.91.

Note: This is a controlled substance (stimulant): **21 CFR**, 1308.13.

THERAP CAT: Anorexic.

7221. Phenelzine. [51-71-8] (2-Phenylethyl)hydrazine; *β*-phenylethylhydrazine; phenalzine. $C_8H_{12}N_2$; mol wt 136.19. C 70.55%, H 8.88%, N 20.57%. $C_6H_5CH_2CH_2NHNH_2$. Monoamine oxidase inhibitor. Prepn: Votocek, Leminger, *Collect. Czech. Chem. Commun.* **4**, 271 (1932); *C.A.* **26**, 5294 (1932); Biel *et al.*, *J. Am. Chem. Soc.* **81**, 2805 (1959); Biel, **US 3000903** (1959 to Lakeside). Toxicity: J. A. Gylys *et al.*, *Ann. N.Y. Acad. Sci.* **107**, 899 (1963). Comprehensive description: R. E. Daly, *Anal. Profiles Drug Subs.* **2**, 383-407 (1973).

Liquid. bp$_{0.1}$ 74°. n_D^{20} 1.5494.

Acid sulfate. [156-51-4] W-1544a; Nardelzine; Nardil. $C_8H_{12}N_2.H_2SO_4$; mol wt 234.27. White powder, sol in water. LD$_{50}$ orally in rats: 156 mg/kg (Gylys).

Hydrochloride. $C_8H_{12}N_2.HCl$. Crystals, mp 174°.

THERAP CAT: Antidepressant.

7222. Phenetharbital. [357-67-5] 5,5-Diethyl-1-phenyl-2,-4,6(1*H*,3*H*,5*H*)-pyrimidinetrione; 5,5-diethyl-1-phenylbarbituric acid; 5,5-diethyl-2,4,6-trioxo-1-phenylhexahydropyrimidine; 1-phenyl-5,5-diethylbarbituric acid; *N*-phenylbarbital; phenidiemal; Fedibaretta; Pyrictal. $C_{14}H_{16}N_2O_3$; mol wt 260.29. C 64.60%, H 6.20%, N 10,76%, O 18.44%. Prepd from ethyl diethylmalonate and phenylurea: Fischer, Dilthey, *Ann.* **335**, 334 (1904); Buck, *J. Am. Chem. Soc.* **58**, 1284 (1936).

Small, thick, glittering plates, mp 178°. Freely sol in hot alcohol, alkali.

Note: This is a controlled substance (depressant): **21 CFR**, 1308.13.

THERAP CAT: Anticonvulsant.

7223. Phenethicillin Potassium. [132-93-4] (2*S*,5*R*,6*R*)-3,3-Dimethyl-7-oxo-6-[(1-oxo-2-phenoxypropyl)amino]-4-thia-1-azabicyclo[3.2.0]heptane-2-carboxylic acid monopotassium salt; (*α*-phenoxyethyl)penicillin potassium; *α*-phenoxyethylpenicillinic acid potassium salt; 6-(*α*-phenoxypropionamido)penicillanic acid potas-

sium salt; penicillin-152; penicillin MV; penicillin-152 potassium; potassium phenethicillin; Maxipen; Syncillin. $C_{17}H_{19}KN_2O_5S$; mol wt 402.51. C 50.73%, H 4.76%, K 9.71%, N 6.96%, O 19.87%, S 7.97%. Semi-synthetic antibiotic related to penicillin. Prepn from 6-aminopenicillanic acid: Perron *et al.*, *Antibiot. Annu.* **1959-1960**, 107; *J. Am. Chem. Soc.* **82**, 3934 (1960); Glombitza, *Ann.* **673**, 166 (1964).

dl-**Form.** Crystals from acetone, dec 230-232°. Much less hygroscopic than benzylpenicillin sodium. Freely sol in water.

l-**Form.** Epiphenethicillin potassium. Crystals from 20% butanol, dec 238-239°. $[\alpha]_D^{24}$ +218° (c = 0.01 in water).

THERAP CAT: Antibacterial.

7224. Phenethyl Alcohol. [60-12-8] Benzeneethanol; 2-phenylethanol; *β*-phenylethyl alcohol; benzyl carbinol; *β*-hydroxyethylbenzene. $C_8H_{10}O$; mol wt 122.16. C 78.66%, H 8.25%, O 13.10%. Found in a number of natural essential oils, such as rose, carnation, hyacinth, Aleppo pine, orange blossom, geranium Bourbon, neroli and in the essential oil of champaca. Prepd by reduction of ethyl phenylacetate with sodium in abs alcohol: Bouveault, Blanc, *Bull. Soc. Chim.* [3] **31**, 672 (1904); Leonard, *J. Am. Chem. Soc.* **47**, 1778 (1925); by hydrogenation of phenylacetaldehyde in the presence of nickel catalyst: Skita, Ritter, *Ber.* **43**, 3398 (1910); v. Braun, Kochendörfer, *Ber.* **56**, 2176 (1923); Milligan, Reid, *J. Am. Chem. Soc.* **44**, 204 (1922). Isoln from the fungus *Gibberella fujikuroi*: Cross *et al.*, *J. Chem. Soc.* **1963**, 2937. Antibacterial activity: R. M. E. Richards *et al.*, *J. Pharm. Pharmacol.* **21**, 681 (1969). Use as preservative in ophthalmic solutions: R. M. E. Richards, R. J. McBride, *ibid.* **24**, 145 (1972). Toxicity: Jenner *et al.*, *Food Cosmet. Toxicol.* **2**, 327 (1964).

Liquid. Floral odor, rose character. mp −27°. d$_{25}^{25}$ 1.017 to 1.019. bp$_{750}$ 219-221°; bp$_{14}$ 104°; bp$_{12}$ 98-100°. n_D^{20} 1.530 to 1.533. Two ml dissolve in 100 ml water after thorough shaking. One part is clearly sol in 1 part of 50% alc. Miscible with alcohol, ether. LD$_{50}$ orally in rats: 1790 mg/kg (Jenner).

USE: Pharmaceutic aid (antimicrobial). In flavors and perfumery (esp rose perfumes).

7225. Phenethylamine. [64-04-0] Benzeneethanamine; *β*-phenylethylamine; 1-amino-2-phenylethane; *β*-aminoethylbenzene; PEA. $C_8H_{11}N$; mol wt 121.18. C 79.29%, H 9.15%, N 11.56%. $C_6H_5CH_2CH_2NH_2$. Endogenous amine related structurally and pharmacologically to amphetamine: P. Mantegazza, M. Riva, *J. Pharm. Pharmacol.* **15**, 472 (1963). Present in oil of bitter almonds. Found in normal human urine (about 30 μg/liter). Prepn: Johnson, Guest, *Am. Chem. J.* **42**, 346 (1909); Robinson, Snyder, *Org. Synth.* **coll. vol. III**, 720 (1955). Elevated levels in urine due to paranoid chronic schizophrenia: S. G. Potkin *et al.*, *Science* **206**, 470 (1979); due to stress: M. A. Paulos, R. E. Tessel, *ibid.* **215**, 1127 (1982).

Liquid. Fishy odor. Absorbs CO$_2$ from air. Does not solidify when cooled in an ice-salt mixture. Strong base. d$_4^{25}$ 0.9640; bp 194.5-195°. Sol in water. Freely sol in alc, ether.

Hydrochloride. $C_8H_{11}N.HCl$. Orthorhombic bipyramidal platelets from abs alcohol, mp 217°. Freely sol in water (100 parts H_2O will dissolve 80 parts at 15°). Sol in alc. Insol in ether. LD$_{50}$ s.c. in mice: 470 mg/kg (Mantegazza, Riva).

Caution: Skin irritant and possible sensitizer.

7226. Phenethyl Isothiocyanate. [2257-09-2] (2-Isothiocyanatoethyl)benzene; 2-phenylethyl isothiocyanate; PEITC. C_9H_9NS; mol wt 163.24. C 66.22%, H 5.56%, N 8.58%, S 19.64%. Chemopreventive agent found in cruciferous vegetables; produced by hydrolysis of **gluconasturtiin**. Prepn: J. v. Braun, H. Deutsch, *Ber.* **45**, 2188 (1912); E. Schmidt *et al., Ann.* **612**, 11 (1958); and isoln from turnips: E. P. Lichtenstein *et al., J. Agric. Food Chem.* **10**, 30 (1962). Isoln from cabbage and watercress seeds: N. Kaoulla *et al., Phytochemistry* **19**, 1053 (1980). LC/MS determn in plasma and urine: Y. Ji, M. E. Morris, *Anal. Biochem.* **323**, 39 (2003). Chemopreventive studies in animal models: G. D. Stoner, *Curr. Top. Plant Physiol.* **15**, 78 (1995); A. Nishikawa *et al., Curr. Cancer Drug Targets* **4**, 373 (2004). Mechanistic studies of anticancer activity and induction of apoptosis: Y.-R. Chen *et al., J. Biol. Chem.* **277**, 39334 (2002); R. Hu *et al., Carcinogenesis* **24**, 1361 (2003); D. Xiao *et al., Clin. Cancer Res.* **11**, 2670 (2005).

Colorless to pale yellow liquid; bp_{11} 139-140°. $bp_{1.4-1.5}$ 102-103°. n_D^{20} 1.5904. d_4^{20} 1.0942. LD_{50} in mice (mg/kg): 700 orally; 150 s.c.; 50 i.v. (Lichtenstein).

USE: Flavor ingredient; provides the hot or burning sensation in horseradish.

7227. o-Phenetidine. [94-70-2] 2-Ethoxybenzenamine; 2-aminophenetole. $C_8H_{11}NO$; mol wt 137.18. C 70.04%, H 8.08%, N 10.21%, O 11.66%.
Oily liquid; rapidly becomes brown on exposure to light and air. mp < −20°. bp 228-230°. Insol in water. Sol in alcohol.
Caution: Absorbed through skin; vapor hazardous.
USE: Manuf of dyes.

7228. p-Phenetidine. [156-43-4] 4-Ethoxybenzenamine; 4-aminophenetole; 4-ethoxyaniline; *p*-aminophenyl ethyl ether. $C_8H_{11}NO$; mol wt 137.18. C 70.04%, H 8.08%, N 10.21%, O 11.66%. Prepn by reduction of *p*-nitrophenetole: West, *J. Chem. Soc.* **127**, 494 (1925). Prepn from nitrobenzene, ethanol, Mg, and sulfuric acid: Yukawa, *J. Chem. Soc. Jpn.* **71**, 547 (1950).

Colorless liquid; becomes red to brown on exposure to air and light. d_4^{16} 1.0652; mp about 3°; bp 253-255°. Practically insol in water. Sol in alcohol. *Keep well closed and protected from light.*
Citrate. Citrophen. $C_8H_{11}NO.C_6H_8O_7$; mol wt 329.30. Crystalline powder, mp 186-188°. Slightly acid taste. Sol in about 40 parts water.
Caution: Absorbed through skin; vapor hazardous.
USE: Manuf acetophenetidine, phenocoll, dulcin, dyes.

7229. Phenetole. [103-73-1] Ethoxybenzene; ethyl phenyl ether; phenyl ethyl ether. $C_8H_{10}O$; mol wt 122.16. C 78.66%, H 8.25%, O 13.10%. $C_6H_5OC_2H_5$. Prepd from phenol or its salts by the use of the ethylating agent ethyl chloride: Wohl, *Ber.* **39**, 1953 (1906); ethyl bromide: White *et al., J. Am. Chem. Soc.* **46**, 965 (1924); ethyl *p*-toluenesulfonate: Finzi, *Ann. Chim. Appl.* **15**, 41 (1925); diethyl sulfate or triethyl phosphate: Noller, Dutton, *J. Am. Chem. Soc.* **55**, 424 (1933). Toxicity data: Binet, *Rev. Med. Suisse Romande* **15**, 561 (1895).
Oily liquid. d_4^{20} 0.967; mp −30°; bp 171-173°; n_D^{20} 1.507. Practically insol in water. Freely sol in alcohol, ether. MLD in rats (mg/kg): 3500-4000 s.c. (Binet).

7230. Pheneturide. [90-49-3] *N*-(Aminocarbonyl)-α-ethylbenzeneacetamide; (2-phenylbutyryl)urea; α-phenyl-α-ethylacetylurea; *N*-(α-phenylbutyryl)urea; α-ethyl-α-phenylacetylurea; ethylphenacemide; EPA; PBU; Benuride. $C_{11}H_{14}N_2O_2$; mol wt 206.24. C 64.06%, H 6.84%, N 13.58%, O 15.52%. Prepd by heating α-phenylbutyric acid chloride with urea: DE 249241 (1912 to Bayer); *Chem. Zentralbl.* **1912**, II, 396; *Frdl.* **10**, 1165. From α-phenylbutyric acid chloride, urea, and antipyrine: Gold-Aubert,

Helv. Chim. Acta **41**, 1512 (1958); **CH 374644** (1964 to Labs. Sapos). Pharmacokinetics: R. L. Galeazzi *et al., J. Pharmacokinet. Biopharm.* **7**, 453 (1979). Toxicity: M. J. Orloff *et al., Neurology* **1**, 377 (1951). Clinical studies: J. C. Bowe, *Br. J. Clin. Pract.* **27**, 174 (1973); F. B. Gibberd *et al., J. Neurol. Neurosurg. Psychiatry* **45**, 1113 (1982).

***dl*-Form.** Needles from ethanol, mp 149-150°.
***d*-Form.** Needles from ethanol, mp 168-169°. $[\alpha]_D^{17}$ +54.0° (c = 1 in ethanol); $[\alpha]_D^{22}$ +53.8° (c = 1 in acetone); +48.2° (c = 1 in dioxane).
***l*-Form.** Crystals from 50% ethanol, mp 162-163°. $[\alpha]_D^{30}$ −51.6° (c = 1 in ethanol).
THERAP CAT: Anticonvulsant.

7231. Phenformin. [114-86-3] *N*-(2-Phenylethyl)imidodicarbonimidic diamide; 1-phenylbiguanide; phenethyldiguanide; *N'*-β-phenethylformamidinyliminourea; fenformin; fenormin; β-PEBG; PEDG. $C_{10}H_{15}N_5$; mol wt 205.26. C 58.51%, H 7.37%, N 34.12%. Prepn: Shapiro *et al., J. Am. Chem. Soc.* **81**, 2220 (1959); Shapiro, Freedman, US 2961377; US 3057780 (1960, 1962 both to U.S.V.). Metabolism: R. Beckmann, *Diabetologia* **3**, 368 (1967). Association with lactic acidosis in diabetic patients: R. I. Misbin, *Ann. Intern. Med.* **87**, 591 (1977). Toxicity study: G. Proske *et al., Arzneim.-Forsch.* **12**, 314 (1962). Comprehensive description: J. E. Moody, *Anal. Profiles Drug Subs.* **4**, 319-332 (1975). Review of phenformin-induced lactic acidosis: M. E. McGuinness, R. L. Talbert, *Ann. Pharmacother.* **27**, 1183-1187 (1993).

Hydrochloride. [834-28-6] Insoral. $C_{10}H_{15}N_5.HCl$; mol wt 241.72. Crystals from isopropanol, mp 175-178°. Sol in water; pH (0.1*M* aq soln): 6.7. LD_{50} in mice (mg/kg): 19 i.v., 450 orally; in rats: 1050 orally; in guinea pigs: 47 orally, 19 s.c. (Proske).
THERAP CAT: Antidiabetic.

7232. Phenicin. [128-68-7] 2,2'-Dihydroxy-4,4'-dimethyl-[bi-1,4-cyclohexadien-1-yl]-3,3',6,6'-tetrone; 3,3'-dihydroxy-5,5'-dimethyl-2,2'-bi-*p*-benzoquinone; phoenicin. $C_{14}H_{10}O_6$; mol wt 274.23. C 61.32%, H 3.68%, O 35.01%. Fungal pigment produced by *Penicillium phoeniceum* and *P. rubrum:* Friedheim, *Helv. Chim. Acta* **21**, 1464 (1938); Charollais *et al., Arch. Sci.* **16**, 474 (1963). Synthesis: Posternak *et al., Helv. Chim. Acta* **26**, 2031 (1943); Musso, Beecken, *Ber.* **92**, 1416 (1959); J. Kalamar *et al., Helv. Chim. Acta* **57**, 2368 (1974). Biosynthesis: E. Steiner *et al., ibid.* 2377.

Yellowish-brown crystals from alc, mp 230-231°. uv max (chloroform): 268, 406 nm (log ε 4.52, 3.36). Sparingly sol in water; freely sol in chloroform, acetic acid, hot alcohol. Very acidic solns are yellow, turning red at pH 1.6-3.6 and violet at pH 4.9-6.

7233. Phenindamine. [82-88-2] 2,3,4,9-Tetrahydro-2-methyl-9-phenyl-1*H*-indeno[2,1-*c*]pyridine; 2-methyl-9-phenyl-2,3,4,9-tetrahydro-1-pyridindene; 1,2,3,4-tetrahydro-2-methyl-9-phenyl-2-azafluorene; Nu-1504. $C_{19}H_{19}N$; mol wt 261.36. C 87.31%, H 7.33%, N 5.36%. Prepn: J. T. Plati, W. Wenner, US 2470108 (1949 to Hoffmann-La Roche). Pharmacology: G. Lehmann, *J. Pharmacol. Exp. Ther.* **92**, 249 (1948); W. Schallek, *ibid.* **105**, 291 (1952).

Crystals from ether, mp 90-91°, d 1.17.

Hydrogen tartrate. [569-59-5] Pernovin; Thephorin. $C_{19}H_{19}$-N.$C_4H_6O_6$; mol wt 411.45. Crystals, mp 160°. Soly: about 2.5% in water; sparingly sol in propylene glycol. Insol in 95% ethanol, glycerol, ether. LD_{50} in mice (mg/kg): 27 i.v., 170 i.p., 265 orally (Schallek).

Hydrochloride. [5503-08-2] $C_{19}H_{19}N.HCl$. Crystals, sol in water. LD_{50} in mice (mg/kg): 88 ±11 i.p., 22.5 ±2.5 i.v., 255 ±21 orally, 270 ±60 s.c.; in rats (mg/kg): 280 ±50 orally; in guinea pigs (mg/kg): 140 ±42 i.p.; in rabbits (mg/kg): 15 ±2.4 i.v., 500 orally; in dogs (mg/kg): 33 i.v. (Lehmann).

Note: Thephorin was formerly used to designate theobromine sodium formate.

THERAP CAT: Tartrate as antihistaminic.

7234. Phenindione. [83-12-5] 2-Phenyl-1*H*-indene-1,3(2*H*)-dione; 2-phenyl-1,3-indandione; 2-phenyl-1,3-diketohydrindene; PID; Pindione; Bindan; Dindevan; Dineval; Hemolidione; Indon; Indema; Fenilin; Fenhydren; Rectadione; Cronodione; Thrombasal. $C_{15}H_{10}O_2$; mol wt 222.24. C 81.07%, H 4.54%, O 14.40%. By heating phthalide with benzaldehyde and sodium ethylate soln: Dieckmann, *Ber.* **47**, 1439 (1914).

Leaflets from alcohol, mp 149-151°. Practically insol in cold water. Slightly sol in warm water. pH of satd soln at 25° = 4.5. Readily sol in alkaline solns. Soluble in methanol, ethanol, ether, acetone, benzene, chloroform. Solns in alkalies are red, in concd H_2SO_4 blue.

THERAP CAT: Anticoagulant.

7235. Pheniramine. [86-21-5] *N,N*-Dimethyl-γ-phenyl-2-pyridinepropanamine; 2-[α-(2-dimethylaminoethyl)benzyl]pyridine; 1-phenyl-1-(2-pyridyl)-3-dimethylaminopropane; 3-phenyl-3-(2-pyridyl)-*N,N*-dimethylpropylamine; prophenpyridamine; propheniramine. $C_{16}H_{20}N_2$; mol wt 240.34. C 79.96%, H 8.39%, N 11.66%. Synthesis: Sperber *et al.*, **US 2567245** and **US 2676964** (1951, 1954, both to Schering).

Oily liq. Slightly yellow color. Characteristic amine-like odor. d 1.0081; bp_{13} 181°; bp_2 142°; $bp_{0.5}$ 135°; n_D^{25} 1.5519 to 1.5521. Insol in water. Sol in dil acids, alcohol, benzene, chloroform, ether.

Maleate. [132-20-7] Avil; Daneral; Inhiston; Trimeton. $C_{16}H_{20}N_2.C_4H_4O_4$; mol wt 356.42. Crystals from amyl alcohol, faint amine-like odor, mp 107°. Freely sol in water, alcohol. Slightly sol in ether, benzene. pH of 1% aq soln between 4.3 and 4.9.

p-**Aminosalicylate.** [3269-83-8] $C_{16}H_{20}N_2.C_7H_7NO_3$. Small needles from acetone + ethyl acetate, large octahedra from water, dec 142°. One gram dissolves in 10 ml water, freely sol in alcohol. Sparingly sol in ethyl acetate, ether, acetone.

THERAP CAT: Antihistaminic.

7236. Phenmedipham. [13684-63-4] 3-(Methylphenyl)-carbamic acid 3-[(methoxycarbonyl)amino]phenyl ester; *m*-hy-droxycarbanilic acid methyl ester *m*-methylcarbanilate; methyl 3-(*m*-tolylcarbamoyloxy)phenylcarbamate; Schering 38584; Betanal. $C_{16}H_{16}N_2O_4$; mol wt 300.31. C 63.99%, H 5.37%, N 9.33%, O 21.31%. Prepn: **NL 6604363** (1966 to Schering AG), *C.A.* **66**, 104813w (1967). Persistence in the soil: K. Kossmann, *Weed Res.* **10**, 349 (1970).

Colorless crystals, mp 139-142° (tech, 143-144°). Soly in water at room temp: <10 ppm.

USE: Herbicide.

7237. Phenmetrazine. [134-49-6] 3-Methyl-2-phenyl-morpholine; 3-methyl-2-phenyltetrahydro-2*H*-1,4-oxazine; 2-phenyl-3-methyltetrahydro-1,4-oxazine; A-66. $C_{11}H_{15}NO$; mol wt 177.24. C 74.54%, H 8.53%, N 7.90%, O 9.03%. Prepn: Thomae, Wick, **US 2835669** (1958 to Boehringer, Ing.); Siemer, Hengen, **US 3018222** (1962 to Ravensberg Chem.); Clark, *J. Org. Chem.* **27**, 3251 (1962); Klosa, *J. Prakt. Chem.* **21**, 12 (1963).

Liquid. bp_{12} 138-140°; bp_1 104°.

Hydrochloride. [1707-14-8] Marsin; Neo-Zine; Preludin. $C_{11}H_{15}NO.HCl$; mol wt 213.70. Crystals from ethanol + ether, mp 182°. One gram dissolves in 0.4 ml water, in 2.0 ml 95% alc, in 2.0 ml chloroform. Sparingly sol in ether.

Note: This is a controlled substance (stimulant): **21 CFR**, 1308.12.

THERAP CAT: Anorexic.

7238. Phenobarbital. [50-06-6] 5-Ethyl-5-phenyl-2,4,-6(1*H*,3*H*,5*H*)-pyrimidinetrione; 5-ethyl-5-phenylbarbituric acid; phenylethylmalonylurea; phenobarbitone; Agrypnal; Barbiphenyl; Barbipil; Gardenal; Luminal; Phenobal. $C_{12}H_{12}N_2O_3$; mol wt 232.24. C 62.06%, H 5.21%, N 12.06%, O 20.67%. Prepn: **DE 247912** (1911 to Bayer); Hoerlein, **US 1025872** (1912), *Frdl.* **11**, 926; *Chem. Zentralbl.* **1912, II,** 212; Chamberlain *et al.*, *J. Am. Chem. Soc.* **57**, 352 (1935); Inman, Bitler, **US 2358072** (1944 to Kay-Fries Chem.); J. T. Pinhey, B. A. Rowe, *Tetrahedron Lett.* **21**, 965 (1980). Toxicity data: Schaffarzick, Brown, *Science* **116**, 663 (1952); E. I. Goldenthal, *Toxicol. Appl. Pharmacol.* **18**, 185 (1971). Series of articles on pharmacology and mechanism of antiepileptic action: *Adv. Neurol.* **27**, 473-562 (1980). Clinical evaluation in febrile convulsions: R. W. Newton, *Arch. Dis. Child.* **63**, 1189 (1988). Comprehensive description: M. K. C. Chao *et al., Anal. Profiles Drug Subs.* **7**, 359-399 (1978).

Crystals (3 different phases), mp 174-178°. uv max (pH 10 buffer): 240 nm ($A_{1cm}^{1\%}$ 431); (0.1*N* NaOH): 256 nm ($A_{1cm}^{1\%}$ 314). Slightly bitter taste. One gram dissolves in about one liter of water, 8 ml alc, 40 ml chloroform, 13 ml ether, about 700 ml benzene. Soluble in alkali hydroxides and carbonates. A satd aq soln is acid to litmus. pK_1 7.3, pK_2 11.8. LD_{50} orally in rats: 162 ±14 mg/kg (Goldenthal).

Sodium salt. [57-30-7] Sol phenobarbital; sol phenobarbitone. $C_{12}H_{11}N_2NaO_3$. Bitter, slightly hygroscopic crystals or white powder. One gram dissolves in about 1 ml water, about 10 ml alcohol. Insol in ether or chloroform. Aq solns are alkaline to litmus and phenolphthalein, pH ~9.3. LD$_{50}$ orally in rats: 660 mg/kg (Schaffarzick, Brown).

Note: This is a controlled substance (depressant): **21 CFR, 1308.14.**

THERAP CAT: Anticonvulsant; sedative; hypnotic.

THERAP CAT (VET): Anticonvulsant; sedative.

7239. Phenocoll. [103-97-9] 2-Amino-*N*-(4-ethoxyphenyl)-acetamide; 2-amino-*p*-acetophenetidide; α-amino-*p*-acetophenetide; aminoacetophenetidine; 4-glycylaminophenol ethyl ether; glycine *p*-phenetidide; 4-glycylaminophenetol; glycocoll-*p*-phenetidide; phenokoll; Phenamine. C$_{10}$H$_{14}$N$_2$O$_2$; mol wt 194.23. C 61.84%, H 7.27%, N 14.42%, O 16.47%. Prepn: Majert, **DE 59121**; **DE 59874** (1891 to Schering), *Frdl.* **3**, 915, 918; **DE 346809** (1921 to Schering), *Frdl.* **13**, 1066; Karrer, Haebler, *Helv. Chim. Acta* **7**, 534 (1924).

Crystals, mp 100.5°.

Monohydrate. Crystals, mp 95°.

Hydrochloride. [539-10-6] C$_{10}$H$_{14}$N$_2$O$_2$.HCl. Cryst powder. Sol in 20 parts water, in alcohol. More sol in hot water; slightly sol in benzene, chloroform, ether. Aq soln is neutral. *Incompat.* Alkali hydroxides or carbonates.

Salicylate. [140-47-6] Salocoll. C$_{10}$H$_{14}$N$_2$O$_2$.C$_7$H$_6$O$_3$; mol wt 332.35. Fine needles. Sweetish taste. Sol in 200 parts cold, 20 parts hot water. *Incompat.* As for the hydrochloride; with substances incompat with salicylates.

THERAP CAT: Antipyretic, analgesic.

7240. Phenoctide. [78-05-7] *N,N*-Diethyl-*N*-[2-[4-(1,1,3,3-tetramethylbutyl)phenoxy]ethyl]benzenemethanaminium chloride; benzyldiethyl-2-[(*p*-1,1,3,3-tetramethylbutyl)phenoxy]ethylammonium chloride; β-*p-tert*-octylphenoxyethyldiethylbenzylammonium chloride; Octaphen. C$_{27}$H$_{42}$ClNO; mol wt 432.08. C 75.05%, H 9.80%, Cl 8.21%, N 3.24%, O 3.70%. Prepn: Goldberg, Besly, **GB 703477** (1954 to Ward Blenkinsop); Erekaev, *C.A.* **54**, 12483i (1960).

Crystals from ethyl acetate. mp 112-114° (Goldberg, Besly); mp 95° (Erekaev).

USE: Orthophosphate as lubricant: Semmens, Summers-Smith, **GB 790056** (1958 to I.C.I.).

THERAP CAT: Anti-infective (topical).

7241. Phenol. [108-95-2] Carbolic acid; phenic acid; phenylic acid; phenyl hydroxide; hydroxybenzene; oxybenzene. C$_6$H$_6$O; mol wt 94.11. C 76.57%, H 6.43%, O 17.00%. Obtained from coal tar, or made by fusing sodium benzenesulfonate with NaOH, or by heating monochlorobenzene with aq NaOH under high pressure. The crystalline article of commerce contains at least 98% phenol. Review of mfg processes: A. Dierichs, R. Kubicka, *Phenole und Basen, Vorkommen und Gewinnung* (Akademie-Verlag, Berlin, 1958) 472 pp; *Faith, Keyes & Clark's Industrial Chemicals,* F. A. Lowenheim, M. K. Moran, Eds. (Wiley-Interscience, New York, 4th ed., 1975) pp 612-623. Use in treatment of spasticity: D. E. Garland *et al., Clin. Orthop.* **165**, 217 (1982); *eidem, Arch. Phys. Med. Rehabil.* **65**, 243 (1984). Toxicity study: W. B. Deichmann, S. Witherup, *J. Pharmacol. Exp. Ther.* **80**, 233 (1944). Review of use in pain relief: K. M. Wood, *Pain* **5**, 205-229 (1978). *Review:* C. Thurman in *Kirk-Othmer Encyclopedia of Chemical Technology* **vol. 17** (Wiley-Interscience, New York, 3rd ed., 1982) pp 373-384. Review of toxicology: H. Babich, D. L. Davis, *Regul. Toxicol. Pharmacol.* **1**, 90-109 (1981); and human exposure: *Toxicological Profile for Phenol* (PB99-122012, 1998) 241 pp.

Colorless, acicular crystals or white, crystalline mass. Characteristic odor, somewhat sickeningly sweet and acrid with a sharp and burning taste. *Poisonous and caustic!* Prone to redden on exposure to air and light, hastened by presence of alkalinity. d 1.071. When free from water and cresols it congeals at 41° and melts at 43°. Ultrapure material mp 40.85°. The commercial product contains an impurity which raises the mp. bp 182°. Flash pt, closed cup: 175°F (79°C). n_D^{41} 1.5425. pKa at 25° = 10.0. pH of aq solns ~6.0. It is liquefied by mixing with ~8% water. One gram dissolves in ~15 ml water, 12 ml benzene; very sol in alcohol, chloroform, ether, glycerol, carbon disulfide, petrolatum, volatile and fixed oils, aq alkali hydroxides. Almost insol in petr ether. LD$_{50}$ orally in rats: 530 mg/kg (Deichmann, Witherup). *Keep well closed and protected from light. Do not handle with bare hands.*

Ammonium salt. [5973-17-1] Ammonium phenate; ammonium carbolate. C$_6$H$_6$O.NH$_3$. White to pink crystalline masses. Sol in water.

Sodium salt. [139-02-6] Phenol sodium; sodium carbolate; sodium phenolate; sodium phenoxide. C$_6$H$_5$NaO. Crystal structure and reactivity study: M. Kunert *et al., Ber./Recl.* **130**, 1461 (1997). Colorless crystals, mp 380°. Very sol in water; sol in alcohol. The aq soln is caustic.

Caution: Potential symptoms of acute overexposure are steatorous breathing, mucous rales, froth at mouth and nose, frank pulmonary edema; cyanosis; tremor, convulsions, twitching; death due to respiratory failure. Chronic overexposure may result in vomiting, difficulty swallowing, excess salivation, diarrhea, anorexia, weight loss; headache, fainting, vertigo, mental disturbances; muscle aches and pain, weakness; damage to liver and kidney, dark urine. Ingestion may cause burning of mouth and throat; white necrotic lesions in mouth, esophagus and stomach; abdominal pain. Direct contact may cause irritation of eyes, nose and throat; skin burns; dermatitis; ochronosis. *See NIOSH Pocket Guide to Chemical Hazards* (DHHS/NIOSH 2003-100121, 2003) p 248; *Clinical Toxicology of Commercial Products,* R. E. Gosselin *et al.,* Eds. (Williams & Wilkins, Baltimore, 5th ed., 1984) Section III, p344-348; *Patty's Industrial Hygiene and Toxicology* **vol. 2B**, G. D. Clayton, F. E. Clayton, Eds. (Wiley-Interscience, New York, 4th ed., 1994) p 1567-1584.

USE: As a general disinfectant, either in soln or mixed with slaked lime, etc., for toilets, stables, cesspools, floors, drains, etc.; for the manuf of colorless or light-colored artificial resins, many medical and industrial organic compds and dyes; as a reagent in chemical analysis. Pharmaceutic aid (preservative).

THERAP CAT: Aqueous soln as topical anesthetic; topical antiseptic; topical antipruritic.

THERAP CAT (VET): Antiseptic caustic. Topical anesthetic in pruritic skin conditions. Has been used internally and externally as an antiseptic.

7242. Phenoldisulfonic Acid. [96-77-5] 4-Hydroxy-1,3-benzenedisulfonic acid; 4-hydroxy-*m*-benzenedisulfonic acid; 1-phenol-2,4-disulfonic acid. C$_6$H$_6$O$_7$S$_2$; mol wt 254.24. C 28.34%, H 2.38%, O 44.05%, S 25.22%. Conveniently prepd by hydrolysis of the dichloride which is obtained by the action of chlorosulfonic acid on phenol at room temp: Pollak *et al., Monatsh. Chem.* **46**, 395 (1925). Monograph: E. E. Gilbert, *Sulfonation and Related Reactions* (Interscience, New York, 1965) 529 pp.

Deliquescent needles, vague melting range from 89° to 100°. Decomp above 100°. Freely sol in water, methanol. Practically insol in ether, petr ether.

USE: In the manuf of aminophenoldisulfonic acids which are intermediates in the dye industry.

7243. Phenolphthalein. [77-09-8] 3,3-Bis(4-hydroxyphenyl)-1(3*H*)-isobenzofuranone; 3,3-bis(*p*-hydroxyphenyl)phthalide; α-(*p*-hydroxyphenyl)-α-(4-oxo-2,5-cyclohexadien-1-ylidine)-*o*-toluic acid; white phenolphthalein. $C_{20}H_{14}O_4$; mol wt 318.32. C 75.46%, H 4.43%, O 20.10%. Prepn: A. Baeyer, *Ber.* **4**, 658 (1871); *idem, Ann.* **202**, 36 (1880); M. Hubacher, US 2192485 (1940 to Ex Lax). Reactions at various pH values: G. Wittke, *J. Chem. Educ.* **60**, 239 (1983). Polarographic analysis in aqueous soln: M. M. Ellaithy *et al., Farmaco Ed. Prat.* **41**, 326 (1986). Subchronic toxicity studies: D. D. Dietz *et al., Fundam. Appl. Toxicol.* **18**, 48 (1992). Toxicology and carcinogenicity studies: *NTP Technical Report 465* (PB97-3390) 348 pp. Comprehensive description of properties, clinical and laboratory uses: F. J. Al-Shammary *et al., Anal. Profiles Drug Subs.* **20**, 627-664 (1991).

White or yellowish white minute, triclinic crystals, often twinned. mp 258-262°. d 1.299. Sol in 95% alcohol and ether, slightly sol in chloroform. One gram dissolves in 12 ml alcohol, in ~100 ml ether. Almost insol in water. Sol in dil solns of alkali hydroxides and hot solns of alkali carbonates forming a red soln. pKa (25°C): 9.7. uv max (methanol): 205, 229, 276 nm (ε 27261.147, 14692.144, 2006.369). Log P (octanol/pH 7.4): 2.4. Shows color change from colorless in acid range to purple at pH 8-9.

Yellow Phenolphthalein. [8053-05-2] Produced in the mfg process prior to final purification of white phenolphthalein. Contains yellow bodies which impart characteristic color. Review of chemistry and use as a laxative: M. H. Hubacher, S. Doernberg, *J. Am. Pharm. Assoc. Sci. Ed.* **37**, 261 (1948). d_4^{20} 1.290-1.296. mp 255-260°. One gram dissolves in 12 ml alcohol, in 102 ml ether. Solns show a slight greenish fluorescence.

Caution: Phenolphthalein is reasonably anticipated to be a human carcinogen: *Report on Carcinogens, Eleventh Edition* (PB2005-104914, 2004) p III-214.

USE: A 1% alcoholic soln as an indicator in titrations of mineral and organic acids and most alkalies.

THERAP CAT: Cathartic.

THERAP CAT (VET): Has been used as a laxative.

7244. Phenolphthalin. [81-90-3] 2-[Bis(4-hydroxyphenyl)-methyl]benzoic acid; decolorized phenolphthalein; phthalin; 4′,4″-dihydroxytriphenylmethane-2-carboxylic acid. $C_{20}H_{16}O_4$; mol wt 320.34. C 74.99%, H 5.03%, O 19.98%. Made by boiling phenolphthalein with zinc dust in alkaline soln. Called *"Kastle-Meyer reagent"* when in soln. Prepd by dissolving 2 g phenolphthalin + 20 g KOH in a desired amt of doubly distd H_2O and diluting with an equal vol of 95% ethanol. Detailed directions for prepn of test soln and its use: Lecoq, *Bull. Soc. Chim. Belg.* **54**, 186-202 (1945), *C.A.* **41**, 2346i (1947).

Colorless crystals, mp 237°. Insol in water; sol in alcohol, ether, aq alkali. The alkaline solns gradually become pink on exposure to air or other oxidizing substances.

USE: As a reagent for oxidases, blood, HCN, peroxides, copper.

7245. Phenolphthalol. [81-92-5] 2-[Bis(4-hydroxyphenyl)-methyl]benzenemethanol; *o*-[bis(*p*-hydroxyphenyl)methyl]benzyl alcohol; dihydroxyphenylmethenylbenzyl alcohol; 2-(4,4′-dihydroxybenzhydryl)benzyl alcohol; bis(4-hydroxyphenyl)-(2-hydroxymethylphenyl)methane; Egmol; Regolax. $C_{20}H_{18}O_3$; mol wt 306.36. C 78.41%, H 5.92%, O 15.67%. Prepn: Hubacher, *J. Am. Chem. Soc.* **74**, 5216 (1952); Schultz, Geller, *Arch. Pharm.* **288**, 234 (1955); Bulcsu, DE 1141293 (1962 to Iromedica), *C.A.* **59**, 1535b (1963).

Crystals from dil alcohol, mp 201-202°.

Monoacetate. $C_{22}H_{20}O_4$. Crystals from benzene or chloroform, mp 171-174°. Soluble in dil NaOH.

Triacetate. $C_{26}H_{24}O_6$. Crystals from methanol or ethanol, mp 104-106°. Practically insol in dil alkali.

THERAP CAT: Cathartic.

7246. *p*-Phenolsulfonic Acid. [98-67-9] 4-Hydroxybenzenesulfonic acid; sulfocarbolic acid. $C_6H_6O_4S$; mol wt 174.17. C 41.38%, H 3.47%, O 36.74%, S 18.41%. Commercially available as a 65% soln. Prepn by hydrolysis of *p*-chloro- or *p*-bromobenzenesulfonic acid: Zollinger, Roehling, US 1321271 (1920); by sulfonation of phenol: Davidson, Byrne, GB 820659 (1959 to Hardman & Holden). Prepn of ammonium salt: Oxley *et al., J. Chem. Soc.* **1948**, 303.

Deliquescent needles. Miscible with water, alcohol.

Ammonium salt. Ammonium *p*-phenolsulfonate. $C_6H_9NO_4S$. Plates from water, dec 270-271°.

Barium salt. Barium *p*-phenolsulfonate. $C_{12}H_{10}BaO_8S_2$. Monohydrate, powder. *Poisonous!* Sol in water; slightly sol in alcohol.

Caution: Irritating to skin.

USE: Intermediate in mfg of pharmaceuticals, dyestuffs. In the Ferrostan process of tin plating (U.S. Steel).

7247. Phenolsulfonphthalein. [143-74-8] 4,4′-(3*H*-2,1-Benzoxathiol-3-ylidene)bisphenol *S,S*-dioxide; α-hydroxy-α,α-bis(*p*-hydroxyphenyl)-*o*-toluenesulfonic acid γ-sultone; 3,3-bis(*p*-hydroxyphenyl)-3*H*-2,1-benzoxathiole 1,1-dioxide; phenol red; P.S.P.; Sulfonphthal. $C_{19}H_{14}O_5S$; mol wt 354.38. C 64.40%, H 3.98%, O 22.57%, S 9.05%. Prepd by the action of *o*-sulfobenzoic anhydride or of *o*-sulfobenzoyl chloride on phenol: Kekulé, Barbaglia, *Ber.* **5**, 876 (1872); Kekulé, *Ber.* **6**, 943 (1873); Heumann, Kochlin, *Ber.* **15**, 1118 (1882); DE 142116; *Chem. Zentralbl.* **II**, 79 (1903); Orndorff, Sherwood, *J. Am. Chem. Assoc.* **45**, 486 (1923). Diagnostic use: G. Dunea, P. Freedman, *J. Am. Med. Assoc.* **204**, 159 (1968); R. D. Wilkes *et al., Vet. Med. Small Anim. Clin.* **76**, 289 (1981). Molecular structure: K. Yamaguchi *et al., Anal. Sci.* **13**, 521 (1997).

Bright red to dark red crystals. Stable in air. pK = 7.9. d 1.445 Mg m^{-3}. One gram dissolves in ~1300 ml water, in ~350 ml alc, in 500 ml acetone. Almost insol in chloroform, ether. Readily sol in aq alkali hydroxides or carbonates with red color, which is discharged by boiling with zinc dust.

USE: As indicator in 0.02-0.05% alcohol soln. pH 6.8 yellow, 8.4 red.

THERAP CAT: Diagnostic aid (renal function).

THERAP CAT (VET): Diagnostic aid (renal function).

7248. Phenoltetrachlorophthalein. [639-44-1] 4,5,6,7-Tetrachloro-3,3-bis(4-hydroxyphenyl)-1(3H)-isobenzofuranone; 3,-4,5,6-tetrachlorophenolphthalein. $C_{20}H_{10}Cl_4O_4$; mol wt 456.10. C 52.67%, H 2.21%, Cl 31.09%, O 14.03%. Prepd by condensation of phenol and tetrachlorophthalic acid or its anhydride: W. R. Orndorff, J. A. Black, *Am. Chem. J.* **41,** 349 (1909); Zalkind, Belikova, *Zh. Prikl. Khim.* **8,** 1210 (1935). Metabolism and hepatic chromosecretion of phthalein dyes: P. Hykes, J. Jirsa, *Acta Univ. Carol. Med.* **25,** 135 (1979), *C.A.* **95,** 111282z (1981).

White powder, dec >300°. Almost insol in water, chloroform, benzene. Sol in alcohol, ether, acetone, glacial acetic acid; sol in aq alkali hydroxides or carbonates with deep purple color when concd, violet-red when dil, and bluish when very dil.

Disodium salt. [128-71-2] Chlor-Tetragnost. $C_{20}H_8Cl_4Na_2$-O_4; mol wt 500.07. Dihydrate, violet crystals. Freely sol in water. Dec on exposure to air.

THERAP CAT: Cathartic; disodium salt as diagnostic aid (hepatic function).

7249. Phenomorphan. [468-07-5] 17-(2-Phenylethyl)-morphinan-3-ol; 3-hydroxy-N-(2-phenylethyl)morphinan; (−)-1,3,-4,9,10,10a-hexahydro-11-phenethyl-2H-10,4a-iminoethanophenan-thren-6-ol; NIH-7274. $C_{24}H_{29}NO$; mol wt 347.49. C 82.95%, H 8.41%, N 4.03%, O 4.60%. Prepn: Grüssner *et al., Helv. Chim. Acta* **40,** 1232 (1957).

Crystals from dimethylformamide, mp 243-245°.

Hydrobromide. $C_{24}H_{30}BrNO$. Crystals from dil alc, mp 300-301°. $[\alpha]_D^{20}$ −63.12° (c = 3.27 in alc).

D-Tartrate monohydrate. $C_{28}H_{35}NO_7 \cdot H_2O$. Crystals from isopropanol, mp 125-126°. $[\alpha]_D^{20}$ −42.75° (c = 0.983 in water).

Methyl bromide. $C_{25}H_{32}BrNO$. Crystals from alcohol, mp 239-240°. $[\alpha]_D^{20}$ −42.81° (c = 1.155 in methanol).

Note: This is a controlled substance (opiate): **21 CFR,** 1308.11.

7250. Phenoperidine. [562-26-5] 1-(3-Hydroxy-3-phenyl-propyl)-4-phenyl-4-piperidinecarboxylic acid ethyl ester; 1-(3-hy-droxy-3-phenylpropyl)-4-phenylisonipecotic acid ethyl ester; 1-[γ-hydroxy-γ-phenylpropyl]-4-phenyl-4-carbethoxypiperidine; 3-(4-carbethoxy-4-phenylpiperidino)-1-phenyl-1-propanol; 1-phenyl-3-[(4'-phenyl-4'-carbethoxy)piperidino]-1-propanol; phenoperidin. $C_{23}H_{29}NO_3$; mol wt 367.48. C 75.17%, H 7.95%, N 3.81%, O 13.06%. Prepn: Janssen, Eddy, *J. Med. Pharm. Chem.* **2,** 31 (1960); Pohland, **US 2951080** (1960 to Lilly); Cutler, Fisher, **US 2962501** (1960 to Merck & Co.).

Hydrochloride. [3627-49-4] Lealgin; Operidine. $C_{23}H_{29}$-$NO_3 \cdot HCl$; mol wt 403.94. Crystals from ethyl acetate + methanol, or ethanol, mp 200-202°. Soluble in water.

Note: This is a controlled substance (opiate): **21 CFR,** 1308.11.

THERAP CAT: Analgesic (narcotic).

7251. Phenosafranin. [81-93-6] 3,7-Diamino-5-phenyl-phenazinium chloride; C.I. 50200; Safranin B Extra. $C_{18}H_{15}ClN_4$; mol wt 322.79. C 66.98%, H 4.68%, Cl 10.98%, N 17.36%. Prepd by dichromate oxidation of 1 mol p-phenylenediamine hydrochloride and 2 mols aniline hydrochloride: Witt, *Ber.* **12,** 939 (1879); **19,** 3121 (1886). *See also Colour Index* **vol. 4** (3rd ed., 1971) p 4449.

Green, lustrous needles from dil HCl. Freely sol in water, also sol in alc. Aq and alcoholic solns are purplish-red and have a greenish-yellow fluorescence. Absorption max ~530 nm.

USE: Biological stain.

7252. Phenothiazine. [92-84-2] 10H-Phenothiazine; thio-diphenylamine; dibenzothiazine; AFI-Tiazin; Antiverm; Fentiazin; Helmetina; Lethelmin; Nemazine; Orimon; Phénégic; Phenoverm; Phenovis; Phenoxur; Reconox; Souframine; Vermitin. $C_{12}H_9NS$; mol wt 199.27. C 72.33%, H 4.55%, N 7.03%, S 16.09%. Prepd by fusing diphenylamine with sulfur: Bernthsen, *Ber.* **16,** 2896 (1883); *Ann.* **230,** 73 (1885); **DE 25150** (1883), *Frdl.* **1,** 252. Improved yields with iodine as catalyst: Knoevenagel, *J. Prakt. Chem.* [2] **89,** 11 (1914); Mitchell, Webb, **US 2415363** (1947 to Koppers). Purification: Vierling, **US 2887482** (1959); Rigby, **US 3000887** (1961 to Shell Oil). Crystal structure: J. D. Bell *et al., Chem. Commun.* **1968,** 1656.

Yellow, rhombic leaflets or diamond-shaped plates from toluene or butanol, mp 185.1°. Sublimes at 130° at 1 mm. bp$_{760}$ 371°; bp$_{40}$ 290°. Freely sol in benzene; sol in ether, in hot acetic acid; slightly sol in alcohol and in mineral oils. Practically insol in petr ether, chloroform, water. Readily oxidized by sunlight or when in presence of a finely divided inert carrier, acquiring a greenish-brown tint. This can be prevented by the admixture of 0.3-1.0% methen-amine.

Caution: Potential symptoms of overexposure are itching, irritation and reddening skin; hepatitis, hemolytic anemia, abdominal cramps, tachycardia; kidney damage; skin sensitization and photophobia. *See NIOSH Pocket Guide to Chemical Hazards* (DHHS/-NIOSH 97-140, 1997) p 248.

USE: Insecticide; manuf pharmaceuticals.

THERAP CAT (VET): Anthelmintic.

7253. Phenoxazine. [135-67-1] Phenazoxine. $C_{12}H_9NO$; mol wt 183.21. C 78.67%, H 4.95%, N 7.65%, O 8.73%. Prepn from 2-aminophenol and 2-aminophenol-HCl: Kehrmann, Neil, *Ber.* **47,** 3107 (1903); de Antoni, *Bull. Soc. Chim. Fr.* **1963,** 2871; by heating 2-amino-2'-hydroxydiphenyl ether in a sealed tube at 270-280° for 40 hrs: Cullinane *et al., J. Chem. Soc.* **1934,** 718.

Leaflets from alc, mp 156°. Freely sol in abs methanol, ethanol, ether, CHCl₃, benzene. Sparingly sol in petr ether.

10-Acetylphenoxazine. $C_{14}H_{11}NO_2$. Prisms, mp 142°. Sparingly sol in hot water; sol in alc; freely sol in glacial acetic acid.

7254. Phenoxyacetic Acid. [122-59-8] Phenoxyethanoic acid; *O*-phenylglycolic acid; phenyl ether glycolic acid; Phenylium. $C_8H_8O_3$; mol wt 152.15. C 63.15%, H 5.30%, O 31.55%. Prepd from phenol and monochloroacetic acid: Giacosa, *J. Prakt. Chem.* [2] **19**, 396 (1879); van Alphen, *Rec. Trav. Chim.* **46**, 148 (1927).

Needles from water, mp 98°; bp 285° (some decompn). pK (25°) 3.12. One gram dissolves in ~75 ml water. Freely sol in alcohol, ether, benzene, carbon disulfide, glacial acetic acid.

Caution: Mild irritant.

USE: Fungicide; keratin exfoliative (to relieve and to soften calluses, corns, and other hard skin surfaces; applied as plasters, pads or in liquids).

7255. Phenoxyacetyl Cellulose. [68332-77-4] Cellulose phenoxyacetate; Enzorb-A. Support used to immobilize proteins, enzymes and microsomes by hydrophobic adsorption. The attractive forces between the hydrophobic phenoxyacetate groups of the support and the hydrophobic surface areas of protein molecules arise from the common repulsion of the aqueous medium. Prepn and properties: L. G. Butler, *Arch. Biochem. Biophys.* **171**, 645 (1975). Applications: J. Dixon *et al., Biotechnol. Bioeng.* **21**, 2113 (1979).

Stable in dry form; slowly hydrolyzed in aq media above pH 8. Resistant to enzymatic hydrolysis.

USE: In enzyme immobilization.

7256. Phenoxybenzamine. [59-96-1] *N*-(2-Chloroethyl)-*N*-(1-methyl-2-phenoxyethyl)benzenemethanamine; *N*-(2-chloroethyl)-*N*-(1-methyl-2-phenoxyethyl)benzylamine; *N*-phenoxy-isopropyl-*N*-benzyl-β-chloroethylamine; bensylyt; 688-A. $C_{18}H_{22}$-ClNO; mol wt 303.83. C 71.16%, H 7.30%, Cl 11.67%, N 4.61%, O 5.27%. Prepn: Kerwin, Ullyot, **US 2599000** (1952 to SK&F).

Crystals from petr ether, mp 38-40°. Sol in benzene.

Hydrochloride. [63-92-3] Dibenyline; Dibenzyline; Dibenzyran. $C_{18}H_{22}$ClNO.HCl; mol wt 340.29. Crystals from alcohol + ether, mp 137.5-140°. Sol in alcohol, propylene glycol. Very sparingly sol in water. Solutions in propylene glycol should be sterilized by filtration.

Caution: Phenoxybenzamine hydrochloride is reasonably anticipated to be a human carcinogen: *Report on Carcinogens, Eleventh Edition* (PB2005-104914, 2004) p III-216.

THERAP CAT: Antihypertensive.

7257. 2-Phenoxyethanol. [122-99-6] 1-Hydroxy-2-phenoxyethane; ethylene glycol monophenyl ether; β-hydroxyethyl phenyl ether; Phenoxethol; Phenoxetol; Phenyl Cellosolve. C_8H_{10}-O_2; mol wt 138.16. C 69.55%, H 7.30%, O 23.16%. $C_6H_5OCH_2$-CH_2OH. Obtained by treating phenol with ethylene oxide in an alkaline medium: Becker, Barthell, *Monatsh. Chem.* **77**, 80 (1947); *see also* Roithner, *ibid.* **15**, 674, 678 (1894); Rindfusz, *J. Am. Chem. Soc.* **41**, 669 (1919). Toxicity study: H. F. Smyth *et al., J. Ind. Hyg. Toxicol.* **23**, 259 (1941).

Oily liquid. Faint aromatic odor. Burning taste. d_{20}^{20} 1.1094; d_{20}^{22} 1.102; mp 14°; bp_{760} 245.2°; bp_{80} 165°; bp_{25} 137°; bp_{20} 128-130°; n_D^{20} 1.534. Flash pt 250°F. Soly in water: 2.67 g/100 ml. Freely

sol in alcohol, ether, NaOH solns. LD_{50} orally in rats: 1.26 g/kg (Smyth).

Acetate. $C_{10}H_{12}O_3$. Liquid, bp 243°.

USE: Fixative for perfumes, in org synthesis; as bactericide in conjunction with quaternary ammonium compds; as insect repellent.

THERAP CAT: Antiseptic (topical).

7258. Phenprobamate. [673-31-4] Benzenepropanol carbamate; carbamic acid 3-phenylpropyl ester; 1-carbamoyloxy-3-phenylpropane; γ-phenylpropyl carbamate; proformiphen; MH-532; Extacol; Spantol; Gamaquil. $C_{10}H_{13}NO_2$; mol wt 179.22. C 67.02%, H 7.31%, N 7.82%, O 17.85%. $H_2NCOOCH_2CH_2$-C_6H_5. Prepn: **GB 837718** (1960 to Siegfried AG). Pharmacology: G. Stille, *Arzneim.-Forsch.* **12**, 340 (1962). HPLC determn in plasma: J. X. S. Sun *et al., Biopharm. Drug Dispos.* **8**, 341 (1987). Clinical pharmacokinetics: F. C. Tulunay *et al., Arzneim.-Forsch.* **48**, 1068 (1998).

Shiny leaflets from aq ethanol, mp 101-104°. Slightly bitter, somewhat burning taste. Numbs the tongue slightly afterwards. Soluble in abs ethanol, chloroform, propylene glycol, ethylenediamine, dimethylformamide; sparingly sol in ether, 50% ethanol. Practically insol in water. LD_{50} orally in mice: 840 mg/kg (Stille).

THERAP CAT: Muscle relaxant (skeletal).

7259. Phenprocoumon. [435-97-2] 4-Hydroxy-3-(1-phenylpropyl)-2*H*-1-benzopyran-2-one; 3-(α-ethylbenzyl)-4-hydroxycoumarin; 3-(1-phenylpropyl)-4-hydroxycoumarin; Marcoumar; Marcumar; Liquamar. $C_{18}H_{16}O_3$; mol wt 280.32. C 77.12%, H 5.75%, O 17.12%. Prepn: Grüssner, Balthasar, **US 2723276** (1955 to Hoffmann-La Roche); Junek, Ziegler, *Monatsh. Chem.* **87**, 218 (1956); Schroeder, Link, *J. Am. Chem. Soc.* **79**, 3291 (1957); **US 2872457** (1959 to Wisconsin Alumni Res. Found.); **GB 805748** (1958 to Geigy); L. R. Pohl, *J. Med. Chem.* **18**, 513 (1975). Resolution: Preis *et al.*, **US 3239529** (1966 to Wisconsin Alumni Res. Found.). Conformation in soln: E. J. Valente *et al., J. Med. Chem.* **21**, 141, 231 (1978).

Crystals or prisms from dil methanol, mp 179-180°.

THERAP CAT: Anticoagulant.

7260. Phenserine. [101246-66-6]; [159652-53-6] (racemate). (3a*S*,8a*R*)-1,2,3,3a,8,8a-Hexahydro-1,3a,8-trimethylpyrrolo[2,3-*b*]indol-5-ol phenylcarbamate (ester); (−)-eseroline phenylcarbamate. $C_{20}H_{23}N_3O_2$; mol wt 337.42. C 71.19%, H 6.87%, N 12.45%, O 9.48%. Physostigmine, *q.v.*, analog; acetylcholinesterase inhibitor that reduces β-amyloid precursor protein (β-APP) formation. Prepn: M. Polonovski, *Bull. Soc. Chim. Fr.* **19**, 46 (1916). *See also:* M. Pomponi *et al.*, **EP 154864**; M. Brufani *et al.*, **US 5306825** (1985, 1994 both to Consig. Naz. Delle Ricerche). Anticholinesterase activity: M. Brzostowska *et al., Med. Chem. Res.* **2**, 238 (1992). Pharmacology: S. Iijima *et al., Psychopharmacology* **112**, 415 (1993). Pharmacokinetics: N. H. Greig *et al., Acta Neurol. Scand.* Suppl. **176**, 74 (2000). Mode of action study for regulating β-APP expression: K. T. Y. Shaw *et al., Proc. Natl. Acad. Sci. USA* **98**, 7605 (2001). Review of total synthesis and biological activity: N. H. Greig *et al., Med. Res. Rev.* **15**, 3-31 (1995); A. Brossi *et al., Aust. J. Chem.* **49**, 171-181 (1996). Review of development and therapeutic potential: U. Thatte, *IDrugs* **3**, 1222-1228 (2000).

mp 150°. $[\alpha]_D$ −80° (in ethanol).

Tartrate. [156910-61-1] $C_{20}H_{23}N_3O_2.C_4H_6O_6$; mol wt 487.50. mp 142-145°. $[\alpha]_D$ −58.7° (c = 0.75 in methanol). Highly sol in water.

THERAP CAT: In treatment of Alzheimer's disease. Cholinesterase inhibitor.

7261. Phensuximide. [86-34-0] 1-Methyl-3-phenyl-2,5-pyrrolidinedione; N-methyl-2-phenylsuccinimide; N-methyl-α-phenylsuccinimide; Milontin. $C_{11}H_{11}NO_2$; mol wt 189.21. C 69.83%, H 5.86%, N 7.40%, O 16.91%. Prepd by the action of methylamine on phenylsuccinic acid: Miller, Long, *J. Am. Chem. Soc.* **73**, 4895 (1951); US 2643258 (1953 to Parke, Davis). Toxicity study: Chen, Ensor, *J. Lab. Clin. Med.* **41**, 78 (1953).

Fine crystals from hot 95% ethanol, mp 71-73°. Slightly sol in water (about 4.2 mg/ml at 25°). Readily sol in methanol, ethanol. Aq solns are fairly stable at pH 2-8, but hydrolysis sets in under more alkaline conditions. LD_{50} orally in mice: 960 mg/kg (Chen, Ensor).

THERAP CAT: Anticonvulsant.

7262. Phentermine. [122-09-8] α,α-Dimethylbenzeneethanamine; α,α-dimethylphenethylamine; phenyl-*tert*-butylamine; α-benzylisopropylamine. $C_{10}H_{15}N$; mol wt 149.23. C 80.48%, H 10.13%, N 9.39%. Prepn: Shelton, Van Campen, US 2408345 (1946 to Wm. S. Merrell); Abell *et al.*, US 2590079 (1952 to Wyeth).

Oily liquid. bp_{750} 205°; bp_{21} 100°.
Hydrochloride. [1197-21-3] Adipex-P; Fastin; Wilpo. $C_{10}H_{15}N.HCl$; mol wt 185.69. Crystals, mp 198°.
Ion exchange resin complex. Duromine; Ionamin; Linyl; Mirapront; Omnibex.
Note: This is a controlled substance (stimulant): **21 CFR,** 1308.14.

THERAP CAT: Anorexic.

7263. Phentetiothalein Sodium. [18265-54-8] 4,5,6,7-Tetraiodophenolphthalein sodium; 3,3-bis(4-hydroxyphenyl)-4,5,6,-7-tetraiodo-1(3*H*)-isobenzofuranone disodium salt; 3,4,5,6-tetraiodophenolphthalein disodium salt; phenoltetraiodophthalein sodium; Iso-Iodeikon. $C_{20}H_8I_4Na_2O_4$; mol wt 865.87. C 27.74%, H 0.93%, I 58.63%, Na 5.31%, O 7.39%. Prepd by the condensation of phenol and tetraiodophthalic acid or its anhydride: Orndorff, Black, *Am. Chem. J.* **41**, 349 (1909); Zalkind, Belikova, *Zh. Prikl. Khim.* **8**, 1210 (1935). Isomeric with iodophthalein sodium, *q.v.*

Bronze-purple, odorless, slightly hygroscopic granules. Dec on exposure becoming incompletely sol. Sol in water, alcohol. *Keep tightly closed.*

THERAP CAT: Diagnostic aid (radiopaque medium—cholecystography and hepatic function).

7264. Phentolamine. [50-60-2] 3-[[(4,5-Dihydro-1*H*-imidazol-2-yl)methyl](4-methylphenyl)amino]phenol; 2-[N-(*m*-hy-droxyphenyl)-*p*-toluidinomethyl]imidazoline; 2-(*m*-hydroxy-N-*p*-tolylanilinomethyl)-2-imidazoline; 2-(N'-*p*-tolyl-N'-*m*-hydroxyphenylaminomethyl)-2-imidazoline; C-7337. $C_{17}H_{19}N_3O$; mol wt 281.35. C 72.57%, H 6.81%, N 14.94%, O 5.69%. α-Adrenergic blocker. Prepn: K. Miescher *et al.*, US 2503059 (1950 to Ciba); E. Urech *et al.*, *Helv. Chim. Acta* **33**, 1386 (1950). Pharmacology and toxicity: R. Meier *et al.*, *Proc. Soc. Exp. Biol. Med.* **71**, 70 (1949). HPLC determn in biological samples: B. D. Kerger *et al.*, *Anal. Biochem.* **170**, 145 (1988). Diagnostic use: G. Spergel *et al.*, *J. Am. Med. Assoc.* **211**, 266 (1970). Review of pharmacology and therapeutic applications: L. Gould, C. V. R. Reddy, *Am. Heart J.* **92**, 397-402 (1976). Clinical efficacy of combination with papaverine in impotence: A. Bechara *et al.*, *J. Urol.* **157**, 2132 (1997).

Crystals, mp 174-175°.
Hydrochloride. [73-05-2] $C_{17}H_{19}N_3O.HCl$. Bitter crystals, mp 239-240°. One gram dissolves in 50 ml water, in 70 ml alcohol. Very slightly sol in chloroform. Practically insol in acetone, ethyl acetate. pH of 1% aq soln 4.5-5.5. Aq solns cannot be stored. LD_{50} in rats (mg/kg): 75 i.v.; 275 s.c.; 1250 orally (Meier).
Methanesulfonate. [65-28-1] Phentolamine mesylate; Regitine; Rogitine. $C_{17}H_{19}N_3O.CH_3SO_3H$; mol wt 377.46. Crystals, mp 177-181°. One gram dissolves in 50 ml water, 23 ml alcohol, 660 ml chloroform. pH of 1% aq soln 4.5-5.5. Aq solns cannot be stored.

THERAP CAT: Antihypertensive in treatment of pheochromocytoma; diagnostic aid (pheochromocytoma). In treatment of male erectile dysfunction.

7265. Phenylacetaldehyde. [122-78-1] Benzeneacetaldehyde; α-toluic aldehyde; α-tolualdehyde; Hyacinthin. C_8H_8O; mol wt 120.15. C 79.97%, H 6.71%, O 13.32%. $C_6H_5CH_2CHO$. Prepd by oxidizing phenylethyl alcohol with chromic acid. High-yield synthesis from styrene oxide or styrene glycol: G. Paparatto, G. Gregorio, *Tetrahedron Lett.* **29**, 1471 (1988).

Oily, colorless liq which polymerizes and grows more viscous on standing. Odor reminiscent of lilac and hyacinth. (Has been crystallized, mp 33-34°.) d_{25}^{25} 1.023-1.030; bp_{760} 195°; bp_{18} 88°; bp_{10} 78°; n_D^{20} 1.524-1.528. Slightly sol in water. Soluble in alcohol, ether. One part is sol in 2 parts of 80% alc forming a clear solution.

USE: In perfumery; intermediate in organic synthesis.

7266. α-Phenylacetamide. [103-81-1] Benzeneacetamide; α-toluamide. C_8H_9NO; mol wt 135.16. C 71.09%, H 6.71%, N 10.36%, O 11.84%. The amide of phenylacetic acid, not to be confused with N-phenylacetamide which is acetanilide. Prepd by Willgerodt reaction from acetophenone or from styrene. Review and lab procedures: Carmack, Spielman in *Org. React.* II (New York, 1946) p 83. Has also been prepd by heating the ammonium salt of phenylacetic acid: Menschutkin, *Ber.* **31**, 1429 (1898). Lab procedure from benzyl cyanide: Wenner, *Org. Synth.* **coll. vol. IV**, 760 (1963).

Bimorphous plates, leaflets. mp 155°. Distils *in vacuo*. Freely sol in alc. Slightly sol in water, ether, benzene.

USE: In manuf of penicillin G.

7267. Phenyl Acetate. [122-79-2] Acetic acid phenyl ester; acetylphenol. $C_8H_8O_2$; mol wt 136.15. C 70.57%, H 5.92%, O 23.50%. $C_6H_5OOCCH_3$. Prepd from phenol and acetyl chloride.

Colorless, mobile, highly refractive liquid; phenolic odor. d_4^{20} 1.073; bp 195-196°. n_D^{20} 1.5030 (almost the same as glass). Practically insol in water. Miscible with alc, chloroform, ether; sol in glacial acetic acid. LD_{50} orally in rats: 1.63 ml/kg, H. F. Smyth *et al., Am. Ind. Hyg. Assoc. J.* **30**, 470 (1969).

7268. Phenylacetic Acid. [103-82-2] Benzeneacetic acid; α-toluic acid. $C_8H_8O_2$; mol wt 136.15. C 70.57%, H 5.92%, O 23.50%. $C_6H_5CH_2COOH$. Made by refluxing benzyl cyanide with dil H_2SO_4 or HCl: Adams, Thal, *Org. Synth.* **2**, 63 (1922). Absorption spectrum: Baly, Tryhorn, *J. Chem. Soc.* **107**, 1065 (1915).

Leaflets on distillation *in vacuo;* plates, tablets from petr ether; mp 76.5°. bp_{760} 265.5°; bp_{100} 198.2°; bp_{40} 173.6°; bp_5 127°; $bp_{1.0}$ 97°. d_4^{77} 1.091. pK (25°): 4.25. Slightly sol in cold, freely in hot water. The aq soln satd at 25° is 0.131*N*. Sol in alcohol, ether. Soly at 25° in chloroform (moles/l): 4.422; in carbon tetrachloride: 1.842; in acetylene tetrachloride: 4.513; in trichlorethylene: 3.299; in tetrachlorethylene: 1.558; in pentachloroethane: 3.252.

Methyl ester. $C_9H_{10}O_2$. Liquid, bp 215°.

Ethyl ester *see* Ethyl phenylacetate.

USE: Starting material in manuf synthetic perfumes, condensation products with aldehydes.

7269. Phenylacetone. [103-79-7] 1-Phenyl-2-propanone; benzyl methyl ketone. $C_9H_{10}O$; mol wt 134.18. C 80.56%, H 7.51%, O 11.92%. $C_6H_5CH_2COCH_3$. Prepn from phenylacetic and acetic acids: R. H. Pickard, J. Kenyon, *J. Chem. Soc.* **105**, 1124 (1914); R. M. Herbst, R. H. Manske, *Org. Synth.* **coll. vol. II**, 389 (1943); from α-phenylacetoacetonitrile: P. L. Julian, J. J. Oliver, *ibid.* 391; from α-methyl-α-phenylethylene oxide: S. Danilow, E. Venus-Danilowa, *Ber.* **60**, 1050 (1927); from diethyl malonate: H. G. Walker, C. R. Hauser, *J. Am. Chem. Soc.* **68**, 1386 (1946). Conformational calculations: M. Hirota *et al., Tetrahedron* **39**, 3091 (1983). Use as prochiral ketone in enantioselective hydrosilylation: H. Brenner *et al., Ber.* **117**, 1330 (1984).

Oil, mp −16 to −15°. bp_{760} 214°; bp_{14} 100-101°. d_4^{20} 1.0157. n_D 1.5174. uv max (ethanol): 258, 283 nm (ε 255, 150).

Note: This is a controlled substance: (immediate precursor) **21 CFR,** 1308.12.

USE: In organic synthesis; production of benzyl radicals by photolysis.

7270. Phenyl Acetylsalicylate. [134-55-4] 2-(Acetyloxy)benzoic acid phenyl ester; acetylphenylsalicylate; Acetylsalol; Spiroform; Vesipyrin. $C_{15}H_{12}O_4$; mol wt 256.25. C 70.31%, H 4.72%, O 24.97%. $CH_3COOC_6H_4COOC_6H_5$.

White, crystalline powder. mp 97°; bp_{11} 198°. Insol in water. Sol in alcohol, ether.

THERAP CAT: Analgesic, antipyretic, anti-inflammatory.

7271. Phenylalanine. [63-91-2] L-Phenylalanine; Phe; F; β-phenylalanine; α-aminohydrocinnamic acid; (*S*)-2-amino-3-phenylpropanoic acid; α-amino-β-phenylpropionic acid. $C_9H_{11}NO_2$; mol wt 165.19. C 65.44%, H 6.71%, N 8.48%, O 19.37%. Essential amino acid for human development. Originally isolated from the sprouts of lupine: E. Schulze, J. Barbieri, *Ber.* **12**, 1924 (1879). Early chemistry and biochemistry: *Amino Acids and Proteins*, D. M. Greenberg, Ed. (Charles C. Thomas, Springfield, Ill., 1951) 950 pp. *passim;* J. P. Greenstein, M. Winitz, *Chemistry of the Amino Acids* **vols 1-3** (John Wiley and Sons, Inc., New York, 1961) pp. 2156-2177, *passim.* Synthesis from L-tyrosine: V. Viswanatha, V. J. Hruby, *J. Org. Chem.* **45**, 2010 (1980). Colorimetric determn in blood: R. S. Campbell *et al., Ann. Clin. Biochem.* **31**, 140 (1994). Effects on food intake: G. H. Anderson, L. A. Leiter, *Appetite* **11**, Suppl. 48 (1988); P. J. Rogers, J. E. Blundell, *Physiol. Behav.* **56**, 247 (1994). Clinical trial in vitiligo: C. Antoniou *et al., Int. J. Dermatol.* **28**, 545 (1989); A. H. Siddiqui *et al., Dermatology* **188**, 215 (1994). Review of metabolism: H. N. Munro, *J. Toxicol. Environ. Health* **2**, 189-206 (1976). Review of role in phenylketonuria: S. P. Bessman, *Nutr. Rev.* **37**, 209-220 (1979); F. Güttler, *Acta Paediatr. Scand.* **73**, 705-716 (1984). Review of microbial production: T. K. Maiti, S. P. Chatterjee, *Hind. Antibiot. Bull.* **32**, 3-26 (1990).

Monoclinic plates, leaflets from warm concd aq solns. Hydrated needles from dil solns. Dec 283°. Sublimes *in vacuo.* $[\alpha]_D^{20}$ −35.1° (c = 1.94). pK_1 1.83; pK_2 9.13. Soly in water (g/l): 19.8 at 0°; 29.6 at 25°; 44.3 at 50°; 66.2 at 75°; 99.0 at 100°. Very slightly sol in methanol, ethanol.

D-Form. [673-06-5] (*R*)-Phenylalanine; Sabiden. Occurs naturally in microbial products such as tyrocidine, *q.v.:* A. H. Gordon *et al., Biochem. J.* **37**, 313 (1943). May be used as a source for L-form in man. Biotransformation: S. Tokuhisa *et al., Chem. Pharm. Bull.* **29**, 514 (1981). Evaluation of D-form in multiple sclerosis: A. Winter, *Neurol. Orthopaed. J. Med. Surg.* **5**, 39 (1984). Leaflets from water, dec 285°. $[\alpha]_D^{20}$ +35.0° (c = 2.04); $[\alpha]_D^{20}$ +7.1° (c = 3.8 in 18% HCl). One gram dissolves in 35.5 ml water at 16°. Sparingly sol in methanol.

DL-Form. [150-30-1] Monoclinic leaflets or prisms from water or alcohol, sweetish taste. Dec 271-273°. Sublimes *in vacuo.* pK_1 2.58; pK_2 9.24. Soly in water (g/l): 9.97 at 0°; 14.11 at 25°; 21.87 at 50°; 37.08 at 75°; 68.9 at 100°.

USE: Component of the artificial sweetner aspartame, *q.v.;* nutrient.

7272. Phenyl Aminosalicylate. [133-11-9] 4-Amino-2-hydroxybenzoic acid phenyl ester; *p*-aminosalicylic acid phenyl ester; phenyl *p*-aminosalicylic acid; *p*-aminosalol; fenamisal; Phenyl PAS; Pheny-PAS-Tebamin; Tebamin; Tebanyl. $C_{13}H_{11}NO_3$; mol wt 229.23. C 68.11%, H 4.84%, N 6.11%, O 20.94%. Description of properties: Meyer, *Antibiot. Annu.* **1957-1958**, 614. Prepd by Raney nickel reduction of the corresp nitro ester in ethyl acetate: Friere, **US 2604488** (1952 to Rhône-Poulenc).

Crystals from isopropanol, mp 153°. Soly in water: 0.7 mg/100 ml; in serum: 12 mg/100 ml. One gram of phenyl PAS is equivalent to 0.67 g PAS.

THERAP CAT: Antibacterial (tuberculostatic).

7273. *N*-Phenylanthranilic Acid. [91-40-7] 2-(Phenylamino)benzoic acid; 2-anilinobenzoic acid; diphenylamine-2-carboxylic acid. $C_{13}H_{11}NO_2$; mol wt 213.23. C 73.23%, H 5.20%, N 6.57%, O 15.01%. Prepd from *o*-chlorobenzoic acid and aniline: Ullmann, Dieterle, *Ann.* **365**, 322 (1907); Ullmann, *Ber.* **36**, 2382 (1907); from 2-iodobenzoic acid and phenylhydroxylamine: Wieland, Roseeu, *Ber.* **48**, 1120 (1915). Use: Adamovich, Zagorulko, *Zavod. Lab.* **9**, 465 (1940), *C.A.* **37**, 1346 (1943).

Leaflets from alcohol, dec 183-184°. Sol in hot alcohol. Very slightly sol in hot water, hot benzene, ether.

USE: Detection of vanadium in steel.

7274. 2-Phenyl-1*H*-benzimidazole. [716-79-0] *N,N'*-Benzenyl-*o*-phenylenediamine; phenzidole; Gainex. $C_{13}H_{10}N_2$; mol wt 194.23. C 80.39%, H 5.19%, N 14.42%. Prepn from *N*-benzoyl-*o*-phenylenediamine: v. Auwers, Frese, *Ber.* **59**, 548 (1926); from *o*-phenylenediamine and benzonitrile: Hölljes, Wagner, *J. Org. Chem.* **9**, 31 (1944). Anthelmintic in sheep: Forsyth, *Aust. Vet. J.* **38**, 398 (1962).

Needles from benzene, plates from water, mp 291°. Sol in methanol, abs ethanol. Sparingly sol in water, benzene, chloroform.

Hydrochloride. $C_{13}H_{10}N_2$.HCl. Needles from alcohol, dec 328°. Freely sol in water.

THERAP CAT (VET): Has been used as an anthelmintic.

7275.   Phenyl Benzoate. [93-99-2] Benzoic acid phenyl ester. $C_{13}H_{10}O_2$; mol wt 198.22. C 78.77%, H 5.08%, O 16.14%. $C_6H_5COOC_6H_5$.

Monoclinic prisms; geranium odor. d 1.235; mp 70°; bp 314°. Insoluble in water. Freely sol in hot alcohol; slightly sol in cold alcohol or ether.

7276.   Phenyl Biguanide. [102-02-3] *N*-Phenylimidodicarbonimidic diamide; phenyl diguanide; 1-phenylbiguanide; *N*-phenyl-*N'*-guanylguanidine; $C_8H_{11}N_5$; mol wt 177.21. C 54.22%, H 6.26%, N 39.52%. Prepd by reacting aniline hydrochloride and dicyandiamide in water: Cohn, *J. Prakt. Chem.* [2] **84**, 396; from aniline, dicyandiamide in pyridine contg HCl: Jacobs, Jolles, **GB 587907** (1947 to ICI).

Crystals from water or toluene. Sharp, somewhat bitter taste. mp 144-146°. pK_1 10.76, pK_2 2.13. Freely sol in water and in alcohol.

Hydrochloride. $C_8H_{11}N_5$.HCl. Prisms, mp 237°. Sol in about 115 parts of water at 32°.

Nitrate. $C_8H_{11}N_5$.HNO$_3$. Crystals, mp 208-209°.

7277.   Phenylbutazone. [50-33-9] 4-Butyl-1,2-diphenyl-3,5-pyrazolidinedione; 4-butyl-1,2-diphenyl-3,5-dioxopyrazolidine; 3,5-dioxo-1,2-diphenyl-4-*n*-butylpyrazolidine; flexazone; diphebuzol; fenibutazona; G-13871; R-3-ZON; Ambene; Artrizin; Azolid; Bizolin; Butacote; Butadion; Butapirazol; Butadiona; Butatron; Butoz; Butazolidin; Buzon; Ecobutazone; Equipalazone; Exrheudon N; Fenibutol; Intrabutazone; Intrazone; Mepha-Butazon; Phenyzene; Robizone-V; Tevcodyne; Uzone. $C_{19}H_{20}N_2O_2$; mol wt 308.37. C 74.00%, H 6.54%, N 9.08%, O 10.38%. Prepn: Stenzl, **US 2562830** (1951 to Geigy); *cf.* **GB 812449** (1959 to Geigy). Review of synthesis: *Ullmanns Encyklopädie der technischen Chemie* vol. **13**, 298 (1962). Physical properties and pharmacology: v. Rechenberg, *Phenylbutazone* (Edward Arnold, London, 1962) 197 pp. Acute toxicity: T. B. Gaines, R. E. Linder, *Fundam. Appl. Toxicol.* **7**, 299 (1986). Soly data: Pulver *et al., Schweiz. Med. Wochenschr.* **86**, 1080 (1956). Comprehensive description: S. L. Ali, *Anal. Profiles Drug Subs.* **11**, 483-521 (1982). Review of hematological effects: G. A. Faich, *Pharmacotherapy* **7**, 25 (1987).

Crystals from ethanol, mp 105°. Soly in water at 22.5°: 0.7 mg/ml (also reported as 2.2 mg/ml). pK 4.5 (from uv in water), pK 4.89 (titration in 50% ethanol), pK 5.25 (titration in 80% 2-methoxyethanol). uv max (acid methanol): 239.5 nm (log ε 4.19).

Sodium salt. [129-18-0] GP-26872; Elmedal. $C_{19}H_{19}N_2$-NaO$_2$; mol wt 330.36. Crystals, freely sol in water. pH of aq solns ~8.2.

Calcium salt. Ticinil Calcico. $C_{38}H_{36}CaN_4O_4$; mol wt 652.79. LD_{50} in adult male, female rats (mg/kg): 1311, 647 orally (Gaines, Linder).

Piperazine salt. Pyrazinobutazone; pyrasanone; Carudol. C_{19}-$H_{20}N_2O_2$.$C_4H_{10}N_2$; mol wt 394.51. mp 140-141° (solidifies and remelts at ~180°).

2-Amino-2-thiazoline salt. [54749-86-9] 4-Butyl-1,2-diphenyl-3,5-pyrazolidinedione compd with 4,5-dihydro-2-thiazolamine (1:1); thiazolinobutazone; TZB; LAS-11871; Fordonal. $C_{22}H_{26}N_4$-O_2S; mol wt 410.53. C 64.36%, H 6.38%, N 13.65%, O 7.79%, S 7.81%. Prepn: J. Moragues *et al., Arzneim.-Forsch.* **24**, 1785 (1974). Pharmacology: M. Márquez, D. J. Roberts, *ibid.* 1786, 1790; M. Colombo *et al., ibid.* **26**, 1347 (1976). White crystals, mp 164-166°. LD_{50} orally in rats, mice: 1425, 1650 mg/kg (Colombo).

THERAP CAT: Anti-inflammatory.

THERAP CAT (VET): Analgesic; anti-inflammatory.

7278.   Phenyl Carbonate. [102-09-0] Carbonic acid diphenyl ester; diphenyl carbonate. $C_{13}H_{10}O_3$; mol wt 214.22. C 72.89%, H 4.71%, O 22.41%. $C_6H_5OCOOC_6H_5$. Prepn: Eckenroth, *Ber.* **27**, 3410 (1894); Bischoff, *ibid.* **35**, 3434 (1902); Gomberg, Snow, *J. Am. Chem. Soc.* **47**, 198 (1925).

Lustrous needles, mp 80-81°. bp 302-306°; bp$_{15}$ 168°. Practically insol in water. Sol in hot alcohol, benzene, ether, glacial acetic acid.

USE: In the molten state as solvent for nitrocellulose.

7279.   2-Phenyl-6-chlorophenol. [85-97-2] 3-Chloro[1,1'-biphenyl]-2-ol; 6-chlororthoxenol. $C_{12}H_9ClO$; mol wt 204.65. C 70.43%, H 4.43%, Cl 17.32%, O 7.82%.

Pale yellow, viscous liquid. Slight, characteristic odor. d_4^{25} about 1.24; mp 6°; bp 317-318° (dec). n_D^{30} 1.6237. Insoluble in water. Sol in fixed alkali hydroxide solns and in most organic solvents.

USE: Germicide; fungicide.

7280.   4-Phenyl-2-chlorophenol. [92-04-6] 3-Chloro-(1,1'-biphenyl)-4-ol. $C_{12}H_9ClO$; mol wt 204.65. C 70.43%, H 4.43%, Cl 17.32%, O 7.82%.

Pale yellow crystals. mp ~77°. bp$_7$ ~160-162°. Soly and use as for 2-phenyl-6-chlorophenol, *q.v.*

7281.   α-Phenylcinnamic Acid. [3368-16-9] α-(Phenylmethylene)benzeneacetic acid; 2,3-diphenylacrylic acid; 2,3-diphenylpropenoic acid; stilbene-α-carboxylic acid. $C_{15}H_{12}O_2$; mol wt 224.25. C 80.34%, H 5.39%, O 14.27%. Prepn of *cis*-form: Buckles, Hausman, *J. Am. Chem. Soc.* **70**, 415 (1948); Buckles, *J. Chem. Educ.* **27**, 210 (1950); Buckles, Bremer, *Org. Synth.* **coll. vol. IV**, 777 (1963); B. H. Patwardhan, G. Bagavant, *Indian J. Chem.* **10**, 59 (1972). Prepn of *cis*- and *trans*-forms: L. F. Fieser, *Experiments in Organic Chemistry* (Heath, Boston, 3rd ed., 1955) p 182. Isomerization studies: S. V. Kessar *et al., Indian J. Chem.* **20B**, 4 (1981).

cis-form

cis-**Form.** [91-47-4] Silky needles from ether + petr ether, mp 174°. pKa 6.1 in 60% ethanol. uv max (ethanol): 223, 280 nm (ε 32100, 19500). Sol in hot water, methanol, ethanol, isopropanol, ether, benzene.

trans-**Form.** [91-48-5] Stout prisms from ether + petr ether, mp 138-139°. Less stable than the *cis*-form. pKa 4.8 in 60% ethanol. uv max (ethanol): 222, 289 nm (ε 14500, 22500). More sol than the *cis*-form.

7282.   Phenyl Dichlorophosphate. [770-12-7] Phosphorodichloridic acid phenyl ester; PCDP. $C_6H_5Cl_2O_2P$; mol wt 210.98.

C 34.16%, H 2.39%, Cl 33.61%, O 15.17%, P 14.68%. Phosphorylation reagent. Prepn: G. Jacobsen, *Ber.* **8**, 1519 (1875); R. Anschütz, W. O Emery, *Ann.* **253**, 105 (1889). Activation of carboxyl groups: H.-J. Liu, S. I. Sabesan, *Can. J. Chem.* **58**, 2645 (1980); for lactam synthesis: J. M. Aizpurua *et al.*, *Tetrahedron Lett.* **25**, 3905 (1984); L. Banfi, G. Guanti, *ibid.* **43**, 7427 (2002). Oxidative rearrangements: H.-J. Liu, J. M. Nyangulu, *ibid.* **30**, 5097 (1989); J. P. Jeyadevan *et al.*, *J. Med. Chem.* **47**, 1290 (2004). Brief review: A. K. Adak, *Synlett* **2004**, 1651-1652.

Liquid, bp$_{9mmHg}$ 103-106°; bp$_{13-14mm}$ 116°. d$_4^{20}$ 1.41214.

USE: In organic synthesis for preparation of lactams, phosphate diesters and for oxidation reactions.

7283. m-Phenylenediamine. [108-45-2] 1,3-Benzenediamine; *m*-diaminobenzene. C$_6$H$_8$N$_2$; mol wt 108.14. C 66.64%, H 7.46%, N 25.90%. Prepd by the reduction of *m*-dinitrobenzene: Kuhn, US 2768209 (1956 to Ringwood); Faust, *J. Prakt. Chem.* **6**, 14 (1958); Neilson *et al.*, *J. Chem. Soc.* **1962**, 371; Tallee, Peltier, *Compt. Rend.* **259**, 400 (1964). Toxicity study: C. Burnett *et al.*, *J. Toxicol. Environ. Health* **2**, 657 (1977).

White crystals becoming red on exposure to air. d 1.139; mp 62-63°; bp 284-287°; dipole moment 1.79. Fire point: 175°. Sol in water, methanol, ethanol, chloroform, acetone, dimethylformamide, methyl ethyl ketone, dioxane. Slightly sol in ether, carbon tetrachloride, dibutyl phthalate, isopropanol. Very slightly sol in benzene, toluene, xylene, butanol. *Keep well closed and protected from light.* LD$_{50}$ in rats (mg/kg): 650 orally; 283 i.p. (Burnett).

Hydrochloride. White or slightly red, crystalline powder; becomes darker on exposure to air. Freely sol in water; sol in alcohol.

USE: Manuf dyes; rubber curing agents, ion exchange resins, decolorizing resins, formaldehyde condensates, resinous polyamides, block polymers, textile fibers, urethanes, petroleum additives, rubber chemicals, corrosion inhibitors; in photography; as reagent for gold and bromine. The hydrochloride chiefly as a reagent for nitrite.

7284. o-Phenylenediamine. [95-54-5] 1,2-Benzenediamine; *o*-diaminobenzene. C$_6$H$_8$N$_2$; mol wt 108.14. C 66.64%, H 7.46%, N 25.90%. Made by reducing *o*-nitroaniline with Zn and NaOH.

Brownish-yellow crystals. mp 103-104°. bp 256-258°. Slightly sol in water; freely sol in alcohol, chloroform, ether. LD$_{50}$ in rats (mg/kg): 1070 orally; 516 i.p., C. Burnett *et al.*, *J. Toxicol. Environ. Health* **2**, 657 (1977).

USE: Manufacture of dyes.

7285. p-Phenylenediamine. [106-50-3] 1,4-Benzenediamine; *p*-diaminobenzene; *p*-aminoaniline; orsin; C.I. 76076; Ursol D. C$_6$H$_8$N$_2$; mol wt 108.14. C 66.64%, H 7.46%, N 25.90%. Prepn: A. Rinne, T. Zincke, *Ber.* **7**, 869 (1874); **DE 202170** (1907 to BASF), *C.A.* **3**, 382 (1909); A. J. Quick, *J. Am. Chem. Soc.* **42**, 1033 (1920); J. F. Norris, E. O. Cummings, *Beilstein* **17**, 305 (1925). *See also: Beilstein* **XIII**, 61 (1930). Crystal structure: A. Domenicano *et al.*, *Acta Crystallogr.* **B33**, 1664 (1977). Mutagenicity studies: B. N. Ames *et al.*, *Proc. Natl. Acad. Sci. USA* **72**, 2423

(1975); W. G. H. Blijleven, *Mutat. Res.* **48**, 181 (1977). Toxicity study: C. Burnett *et al.*, *J. Toxicol. Environ. Health* **2**, 657 (1977).

White to slightly red crystals; darkens on exposure to air. mp 145-147°. bp 267°. Sol in 100 parts cold water; sol in alcohol, chloroform, ether. A black color is developed with 3% H$_2$O$_2$; brown with 5% FeCl$_3$ soln. *Keep well closed and protected from light.* LD$_{50}$ in rats (mg/kg): 80 orally, 37 i.p. (Burnett).

Hydrochloride. White to slightly reddish crystals. Freely sol in water, slightly in alcohol, ether.

Caution: Potential symptoms of overexposure are irritation of pharynx and larynx; bronchial asthma; sensitization dermatitis. See *NIOSH Pocket Guide to Chemical Hazards* (DHHS/NIOSH 97-140, 1997) p 248.

USE: Dyeing furs; also in photochemical measurements, accelerating vulcanization; manuf azo dyes, etc. The hydrochloride as reagent for blood, H$_2$S, amyl alcohol; in testing of milk.

7286. Phenylephrine. [59-42-7] (*αR*)-3-Hydroxy-α-[(methylamino)methyl]benzenemethanol; (−)-*m*-hydroxy-α-[(methylamino)methyl]benzyl alcohol; *l*-1-(*m*-hydroxyphenyl)-2-methylaminoethanol; *l*-α-hydroxy-β-methylamino-3-hydroxy-1-ethylbenzene; *m*-methylaminoethanolphenol; metaoxedrin. C$_9$H$_{13}$NO$_2$; mol wt 167.21. C 64.65%, H 7.84%, N 8.38%, O 19.14%. α-Adrenergic agonist. Prepn: H. Legerlotz, **US 1932347** (1933 to Frederick Stearns); E. D. Bergmann, M. Sulzbacher, *J. Org. Chem.* **16**, 84 (1951); M. K. Gurjar *et al.*, *Org. Process Res. Dev.* **2**, 422 (1998). Spectrophotometric determn: S. A. Shama, *J. Pharm. Biomed. Anal.* **30**, 1385 (2002). Toxicity data: M. R. Warren, H. W. Werner, *J. Pharmacol. Exp. Ther.* **86**, 284 (1946). Clinical efficacy in mydriasis: V. Tanner, A. G. Casswell, *Eye* **10**, 95 (1996). Clinical evaluation in fecal incontinence: M. J. Cheetham *et al.*, *Gut* **48**, 356 (2001). Comprehensive description: C. A. Gaglia, Jr., *Anal. Profiles Drug Subs.* **3**, 483-512 (1974). Review of ophthalmologic uses: S. M. Meyer, F. T. Fraunfelder, *Ophthalmology* **87**, 1177-1180 (1980); of clinical trials vs ephedrine, *q.v.*, in treatment of hypotension during cesarean delivery: A. Lee *et al.*, *Anesth. Analg.* **94**, 920-926 (2002).

mp 170-171°.

Hydrochloride. [61-76-7] Ak-Dilate; Ak-Nefrin; Alconefrin; Incostop; Mydfrin; Neo-Synephrine; Nostril; Prefrin; Rhinall. C$_9$-H$_{13}$NO$_2$.HCl; mol wt 203.67. Bitter crystals. mp 140-145°. [α]$_D$ −44.0° (c = 2.16 in H$_2$O). pK$_1$ 8.77; pK$_2$ 9.84. uv max (0.05 *N* HCl): 216, 274, 279 nm (ε × 10^{-3} 5.91, 1.81, 1.65). uv max (0.05 *N* NaOH): 239, 292.5 (ε × 10^{-3} 8.95, 3.04). Freely sol in water or alcohol. LD$_{50}$ in rats (mg/kg): 17 ±1.1 i.p.; 33 ±2.0 s.c. (Warren, Werner).

THERAP CAT: Mydriatic; decongestant; in treatment of fecal incontinence.

7287. Phenylethanolamine. [7568-93-6] α-(Aminomethyl)benzenemethanol; α-(aminomethyl)benzyl alcohol; β-hydroxyphenethylamine. C$_8$H$_{11}$NO; mol wt 137.18. C 70.04%, H 8.08%, N 10.21%, O 11.66%. Prepn: Dornow, Theidel, *Ber.* **88**, 1267 (1955).

Pale yellow crystals, mp 56-57°. bp$_{17}$ 157-160°. Freely sol in water. Gives an alkaline reaction in water and forms salts with acids under mild conditions.

Sulfate. [613-82-1] dl-α-Phenyl-β-aminoethanol sulfate; Apophedrin. $(C_8H_{11}NO)_2.H_2SO_4$; mol wt 372.44. Prepn: Roth, *Arch. Pharm.* **292,** 76 (1959). Crystals, mp 275-276° (Kofler). Soluble in water.

USE: Free base as a stopping agent during polymerization of styrene-butadiene rubber; in the hardening of waxes. Intermediate in the manuf of pressor amines.

THERAP CAT: Sulfate as topical vasoconstrictor.

7288. Phenyl Ether. [101-84-8] 1,1'-Oxybisbenzene; diphenyl ether; diphenyl oxide. $C_{12}H_{10}O$; mol wt 170.21. C 84.68%, H 5.92%, O 9.40%. $C_6H_5OC_6H_5$. Prepd by heating sodium phenolate with chlorobenzene.

Liquid; characteristic odor. d^{20} 1.075 (liq); mp 28°, and remains liq at lower temp; bp 259°. Flash pt 115°C. Insol in water; sol in alcohol, benzene, ether, glacial acetic acid.

Caution: Potential symptoms of overexposure to vapor are nausea; irritation of eyes, nose and skin. *See NIOSH Pocket Guide to Chemical Hazards* (DHHS/NIOSH 97-140, 1997) p 248.

USE: As heat transfer medium; in perfuming soaps; in organic syntheses.

7289. 5-(α-Phenylethyl)semioxamazide. [93-95-8] Oxo-[(1-phenylethyl)amino]acetic acid hydrazide; 5-(α-methylbenzyl)-semioxamazide. $C_{10}H_{13}N_3O_2$; mol wt 207.23. C 57.96%, H 6.32%, N 20.28%, O 15.44%. Prepd from α-phenylethylamine, ethyl oxalate, and hydrazine: Leonard, Boyer, *J. Org. Chem.* **15,** 42 (1950).

dl-Form. Fine needles from ethanol, mp 157°.
d-Form. Crystals, mp 167-168°. $[\alpha]_D^{25}$ +102.0° (c = 1.04 in chloroform).
l-Form. Crystals, mp 167-168°. $[\alpha]_D^{25}$ −102.5° (c = 0.625 in chloroform).

USE: The racemic form as reagent for the characterization of aldehydes and ketones. The optically active forms as resolving agents for carbonyl compds possessing asymmetric carbon atoms.

7290. Phenylglyceryl Ether. [538-43-2] 3-Phenoxy-1,2-propanediol; Antodyne. $C_9H_{12}O_3$; mol wt 168.19. C 64.27%, H 7.19%, O 28.54%. $C_6H_5OCH_2CH(OH)CH_2OH$. Prepd from phenol and 3-chloro-1,2-propylene carbonate: Smith, *US 2967892* (1961 to Dow). Toxicity study: Hine *et al., J. Pharmacol. Exp. Ther.* **97,** 414 (1949).

Crystals, mp 50-52°, bp$_{0.6}$ 129-142°. Sol in water, alcohol. LD$_{50}$ i.p. in mice: 1280 mg/kg (Hine).

7291. α-Phenylglycine. [69-91-0] α-Aminobenzeneacetic acid; α-aminophenylacetic acid; α-amino-α-toluic acid; C-phenylglycine. $C_8H_9NO_2$; mol wt 151.16. C 63.57%, H 6.00%, N 9.27%, O 21.17%. $C_6H_5CH(NH_2)COOH$. Prepd by hydrolysis of α-aminophenylacetonitrile with dil hydrochloric acid: Marvel, Noyes, *J. Am. Chem. Soc.* **42,** 2264 (1920); R. E. Steiger, *Org. Synth.* **coll. vol. III,** 84 (1955).

dl-Form. Lustrous platelets. Sublimes without melting at ~255°. Slightly sol in the usual organic solvents. Sol in alkalies.
Methyl ester. $C_9H_{11}NO_2$. Needles from petr ether, mp 32°. Sol in alcohol, ether, benzene.
Ethyl ester. $C_{10}H_{13}NO_2$. Liquid, bp 257°; bp$_{16}$ 149°; bp$_5$ 114-115°; n_D^{25} 1.500.
l-Form. Needles from dil alc, mp 305-310°. $[\alpha]_D^{20}$ −157.8° (dil HCl).
d-Form. Crystals. $[\alpha]_D^{20}$ +156° (dil HCl).

7292. N-Phenylglycine. [103-01-5] Anilinoacetic acid. $C_8H_9NO_2$; mol wt 151.16. C 63.57%, H 6.00%, N 9.27%, O 21.17%. $C_6H_5NHCH_2COOH$. Prepd from aniline and chloroacetic acid: Curtius, *J. Prakt. Chem.* **38,** 436 (1888); Thorpe, Wood, *J. Chem. Soc.* **103,** 1606 (1913).

Crystals, mp 127-128°. pK (25°): 5.42. Moderately sol in water. Less sol in alc. Sparingly sol in ether. Forms water-sol salts with alkali hydroxides.

Ethyl ester. $C_{10}H_{13}NO_2$. Leaflets, mp 58°. Sol in alc, ether.

USE: In the Heumann synthesis of indigo.

7293. Phenylhydrazine. [100-63-0] Hydrazinobenzene. $C_6H_8N_2$; mol wt 108.14. C 66.64%, H 7.46%, N 25.90%. C_6H_5-NHNH$_2$. Prepd by diazotizing aniline with NaNO$_2$ and HCl, then treating the soln with Na$_2$SO$_3$ followed by NaOH: Fischer, *Anleitung zur Darstellung organischer Präparate* (Braunschweig, 10th ed., 1922) p 23; Coleman, *Org. Synth.* **2,** 71 (1922), **coll. vol. I** (2nd ed., 1941) p 442. Mechanism of oxidative hemolysis of erythrocytes: B. Goldberg, A. Stern, *Mol. Pharmacol.* **13,** 832 (1977); B. Vilsen, H. Nielsen, *Biochem. Pharmacol.* **33,** 2739 (1984). Review of interaction with hemoglobin: M. D. Shetlar, H. A. O. Hill, *Environ. Health Perspect.* **64,** 265-281 (1985).

Monoclinic prisms or oil. Turns yellow to dark red on exposure to air and light. Faint aromatic odor. d_4^{20} 1.0978; mp 19.5°; bp$_{760}$ 243.5° (dec); bp$_{100}$ 173.5°; bp$_{40}$ 148.2°; bp$_{20}$ 131.5°; bp$_{10}$ 115.8°; bp$_5$ 101.6°; bp$_{1.0}$ 71.8°; $n_D^{20.3}$ 1.60813. Weak base, pK (15°): 8.79. Miscible with alcohol, ether, chloroform, benzene. Sparingly sol in water, petr ether; sol in dil acids. Forms a hemihydrate, mp 24°. *Keep well closed and protected from light.*

Hydrochloride. [59-88-1] $C_6H_8N_2$.HCl. Prepn: Fischer, *Ann.* **190,** 83 (1878); Brunner, Eiermann, *Ber.* **31,** 1406 (1898); Rüetschi, Trümpler, *Helv. Chim. Acta* **36,** 1649 (1953); Hupfer, **DE 1143825** (1963 to Hoechst). Leaflets from alc, mp 243-246° (slight browning). Sublimes. Freely sol in water; sol in alcohol. Practically insol in ether.

Caution: Potential symptoms of overexposure are skin sensitization, hemolytic anemia, dyspnea and cyanosis; jaundice; kidney damage; vascular thrombosis. Potential occupational carcinogen. *See NIOSH Pocket Guide to Chemical Hazards* (DHHS/NIOSH 97-140, 1997) p 250. *See also Patty's Industrial Hygiene and Toxicology* vol. 2A, G. D. Clayton, R. E. Clayton, Eds. (Wiley-Interscience, New York, 3rd ed., 1981) pp 2792-2795, 2804-2805.

USE: Manuf dyes, antipyrine, nitron (a stabilizer for explosives); reagent for sugars, aldehydes, ketones.

THERAP CAT: Hemolytic.

7294. Phenylhydroxylamine. [100-65-2] N-Hydroxybenzenamine; β-phenylhydroxylamine; N-phenylhydroxylamine. C_6H_7NO; mol wt 109.13. C 66.04%, H 6.47%, N 12.83%, O 14.66%. C_6H_5NHOH. Prepd by zinc reduction of nitrobenzene in ammonium chloride soln: Kamm, *Org. Synth.* **4,** 57 (1925).

Needles from satd NaCl soln. mp 82°. *Deteriorates on storage and should be used promptly.* Sol in 50 parts cold, in 10 parts hot water. Freely sol in alcohol, ether, carbon disulfide, chloroform, hot benzene, dil mineral acids, acetic acid. Slightly sol in petr ether. The oxalate is more stable.

USE: Manufacture of cupferron.

7295. Phenyliodine(III) Bis(trifluoroacetate). [2712-78-9] Phenylbis(trifluoroacetato-κO)iodine; bis(trifluoroacetoxy)iodobenzene; iodobenzene ditrifluoroacetate; PIFA. Hypervalent iodine(III) reagent. Prepn: N. W. Alcock, T. C. Waddington, *J. Chem. Soc.* **1963,** 4103; I. I. Maletina *et al., J. Org. Chem. USSR* **10,** 294 (1974). Structural study: N. W. Alcock *et al., J. Chem. Soc. Dalton Trans.* **1984,** 1709. Use as a one-electron oxidant: L. Eberson *et al., Acta Chem. Scand.* **49,** 640 (1995). Review of applications in organic synthesis: G. Pohnert, *J. Prakt. Chem.* **342,** 731-734 (2000).

Crystals from chloroform + petroleum ether, mp 120-121°.

USE: In oxidation, cyclization, dehydrogenation, and dearomatization reactions.

7296. Phenyl Isocyanate. [103-71-9] Isocyanatobenzene; carbanil; phenylcarbimide. C_7H_5NO; mol wt 119.12. C 70.58%,

H 4.23%, N 11.76%, O 13.43%. C_6H_5N=C=O. Prepd by passing carbonyl chloride into a hot soln of aniline in toluene, saturated with HCl: Hardy, *J. Chem. Soc.* **1934**, 2011.

Liquid, with acrid odor. $d_4^{11.6}$ 1.101; d_4^{15} 1.092; $d_4^{19.6}$ 1.0956; $d_4^{25.9}$ 1.08870. bp 158-168°; bp_{18-20} 58.2-59.5°; bp_{13} 55°. $n_D^{19.6}$ 1.53684; $n_D^{25.9}$ 1.53412.

Caution: Irritating to eyes.

7297. Phenyl Isothiocyanate. [103-72-0] Isothiocyanatobenzene; isothiocyanic acid phenyl ester; phenyl mustard oil; thiocarbanil. C_7H_5NS; mol wt 135.19. C 62.19%, H 3.73%, N 10.36%, S 23.72%. C_6H_5N=C=S. Prepd from ammonium phenyldithiocarbamate by the action of lead nitrate: Dains *et al., Org. Synth.* **coll. vol. I** (2nd ed., 1941) p 447.

Liquid. mp −21°. d_4^{25} 1.1288; d_4^{35} 1.1202; d_4^{50} 1.1061. bp_{760} 221°; bp_{33} 117.1°; bp_{12} 95°. Distills with water without dec. $n_D^{23.4}$ 1.64918. Insol in water. Sol in alcohol, ether.

USE: Derivatizing agent for primary, secondary amines. In sequencing of peptides by Edman degradation. In amino acid analyses by HPLC (Pico-Tag).

7298. Phenylmagnesium Chloride. [100-59-4] Chlorophenylmagnesium. C_6H_5ClMg; mol wt 136.86. C 52.66%, H 3.68%, Cl 25.90%, Mg 17.76%. C_6H_5MgCl. One of the Grignard reagents. Prepd by reacting chlorobenzene with magnesium at reflux temperatures in the presence of catalytic amounts of an organic nitrate: Ramsden, US **2816937** (1957 to M. & T. Corp.).

Sol in ether (ethyl ether, other ethers may be used as solvents). A solution which is about 3 molar has an approx strength of 48%, and a d_4^{20} of ~1.15. Reacts with water, steam or acids to produce toxic and flammable vapors with evolution of heat.

USE: In organic synthesis, especially in the production of hydrocarbons, alcohols, ketones, organic acids, amines, silicones, boranes.

7299. *N*-Phenylmaleimide. [941-69-5] 1-Phenyl-1*H*-pyrrole-2,5-dione. $C_{10}H_7NO_2$; mol wt 173.17. C 69.36%, H 4.07%, N 8.09%, O 18.48%. Prepn from maleanilic acid: Cava *et al., Org. Synth.* **41**, 93 (1961).

Canary-yellow needles from cyclohexane, mp 89-89.8°.

USE: Dienophile in the Diels-Alder reaction. Usually gives cryst adducts.

7300. Phenylmercuric Acetate. [62-38-4] (Acetato)phenylmercury; acetoxyphenylmercury; phenylmercury acetate; PMA; PMAC; PMAS; Agrosan; Ceresan; Mergamma; Unisan. C_8H_8-HgO_2; mol wt 336.74. C 28.53%, H 2.39%, Hg 59.57%, O 9.50%. $C_6H_5HgOOCCH_3$. Prepn: E. Dreher, R. Otto, *Ann.* **154**, 93 (1870); F. C. Whitmore, *Organic Compounds of Mercury* (Chemical Catalog Co., New York, 1921) pp 175; Grave *et al., J. Am. Pharm. Assoc.* **25**, 752 (1936). Control of crabgrass: J. A. DeFrance, *Greenkeepers Rep.* **15**, 30 (1947). Metabolism in animals: V. L. Miller *et al., Toxicol. Appl. Pharmacol.* **2**, 344 (1960). GC determn in air: M. G. Rosell *et al., Pergamon Ser. Environ. Sci.* **7**, 299 (1982).

Small, lustrous prisms from ethanol, mp 149°. Sol in ~600 parts water; sol in alcohol, benzene, acetone.

USE: Herbicide; fungicide.

7301. Phenylmercuric Chloride. [100-56-1] Chlorophenylmercury; phenylmercury chloride. C_6H_5ClHg; mol wt 313.15. C 23.01%, H 1.61%, Cl 11.32%, Hg 64.06%. C_6H_5HgCl. Antibacterial activity: H. L. Friedman, *Ann. N.Y. Acad. Sci.* **65**, 461 (1957). Use as fungicide: U. Prota, *Phytopathol. Mediterr.* **8**, 87 (1970), *C.A.* **72**, 42138t (1970); M. Makes, Z. Lokaj, *Agrochemia* **16**, 181 (1976), *C.A.* **85**, 187602t (1976). Toxicity: M. Umeda *et al., Jpn. J. Exp. Med.* **39**, 47 (1969).

White satiny leaflets, mp 250-252°. Sol in ~20,000 parts cold water; in benzene, ether, pyridine; slightly sol in hot alcohol. LD_{50} s.c. in rats: 30 mg/kg (Umeda).

USE: Has been used as an agricultural fungicide.

7302. Phenylmercuric Nitrate. [55-68-5] (Nitrato-*O*)phenylmercury; merphenyl nitrate; Phe-Mer-Nite; Phenmerzyl nitrate. $C_6H_5HgNO_3$; mol wt 339.70. C 21.21%, H 1.48%, Hg 59.05%, N 4.12%, O 14.13%. Prepn: R. Otto *J. Prakt. Chem.* **1**, 179 (1870); F. L. Pyman, H. A. Stevenson, *Pharm. J.* **133**, 269 (1934); T. B. Grave *et al., J. Am. Pharm. Assoc.* **25**, 752 (1936). Toxicity of basic salt: R. Wien, *Q. J. Pharm. Pharmacol.* **12**, 212 (1939). HPLC determn in pharmaceuticals: M. Larroque, L. Vian, *J. Pharm. Biomed. Anal.* **11**, 173 (1993).

Needles or plates from dry chloroform, mp 130-132°.

Basic salt. [8003-05-2] Hydroxyphenylmercury mixt with (nitrato-*O*)phenylmercury; basic phenylmercuric nitrate. C_6H_5-$HgOH.C_6H_5HgNO_3$; mol wt 634.40. Pearly lustrous scales, mp 187-190° (dec). Soluble in ~1250 parts water; slightly sol in alcohol, moderately in glycerol. Practically insol in other usual organic solvents. LD_{50} in mice (mg/g): 0.045 s.c.; 0.027 i.v. (Wien).

USE: Pharmaceutical aid (antimicrobial). Tree wound dressing.

THERAP CAT (VET): Antiseptic.

7303. Phenylmercury Borate. [102-98-7] [Orthoborato-(3−)-*O*]phenylmercurate(2−) dihydrogen; (dihydrogen borato)phenylmercury; phenylmercuric borate; Famosept; Merfen. C_6H_7-$BHgO_3$; mol wt 338.52. C 21.29%, H 2.08%, B 3.19%, Hg 59.25%, O 14.18%. Prepn: Christiansen, US **2196384** (1950 to Lever Bros.).

Crystalline powder, mp 112-113°. Sol in water, alcohol, glycerol.

Note: Product of commerce may be an equimolar composition of phenylmercuriborate and phenylmercurihydroxide.

THERAP CAT: Antiseptic (topical).

7304. *o*-Phenylphenol. [90-43-7] (1,1'-Biphenyl)-2-ol; 2-biphenylol; orthoxenol; *o*-hydroxydiphenyl; 2-hydroxydiphenyl; Dowicide 1. $C_{12}H_{10}O$; mol wt 170.21. C 84.68%, H 5.92%, O 9.40%. Prepn from phenyl ether: Lüttringhaus, Sääf, *Ann.* **542**, 241 (1939); from dibenzofuran: Gilman, Esmay, *J. Am. Chem. Soc.* **75**, 2947 (1953); Müller, US **2862035** (1958 to Bayer). Purification: Widiger, US **3087969** (1963 to Dow). Toxicity data: Hodge *et al., J. Pharmacol. Exp. Ther.* **104**, 202 (1952). Review of carcinogenic risk: *IARC Monographs* **30**, 329-344 (1983).

White, flaky crystals. Mild, characteristic odor. mp 55.5-57.5°; bp 280-284°; bp_{15} 152-154°. Practically insol in water. Sol in fixed alkali hydroxide solns and most organic solvents. LD_{50} orally in rats: 2.48 g/kg (Hodge).

Sodium salt. [132-27-4] Natriphene; sodium *o*-phenylphenate; sodium 2-phenylphenoxide; Dowicide A. $C_{12}H_9NaO$; mol wt 192.19. White flakes. Soly at 25° (g/100 g solvent): water 120; acetone 330; methanol 468; propylene glycol >200. Practically insol in petroleum fractions, pine oil. pH of satd water soln at 25° = 12.0-13.5.

Caution: Toxic symptoms similar to phenol, *q.v. See Clinical Toxicology of Commercial Products,* R. E. Gosselin *et al.,* Eds. (Williams & Wilkins, Baltimore, 5th ed., 1984) Section II, p 316.

USE: Antimicrobial additive in the mfr of adhesives, leather, metalworking fluids, and textiles; preservative in automotive polishes, ceramic glazes, laundry starch, inks, floor wax emulsions; agricultural fungicide.

7305. *p*-Phenylphenol. [92-69-3] (1,1'-Biphenyl)-4-ol; 4-hydroxydiphenyl; Paraxenol.

mp 164-165°; bp 305-308°. Possesses approx the soly of the ortho compd.

USE: As intermediate in the manuf of resins; also in the rubber industry.

7306. Phenyl Phthalate. [84-62-8] 1,2-Benzenedicarboxylic acid diphenyl ester; diphenyl phthalate. $C_{20}H_{14}O_4$; mol wt 318.32. C 75.46%, H 4.43%, O 20.10%. $C_6H_4(COOC_6H_5)_2$. Prepd from phenol and phthalic anhydride.

White odorless crystals. d^{74} 1.572; mp 70-73°; bp_{14} ~255°. Insol in water; sol in acetone and other ketones, in liquid esters and chlorinated hydrocarbons.

USE: Plasticizer in nitrocellulose lacquers.

7307. Phenylpropanolamine. [14838-15-4] (αS)-rel-α-[(1R)-1-Aminoethyl]benzenemethanol; (1RS,2SR)-2-amino-1-phenyl-1-propanol; erythro-2-amino-1-phenyl-1-propanol; dl-norephedrine. $C_9H_{13}NO$; mol wt 151.21. C 71.49%, H 8.67%, N 9.26%, O 10.58%. Sympathomimetic amine; racemic mixture of d- and l- norephedrine. Prepn: F. W. Calliess, Arch. Pharm. **250**, 141 (1912); P. Rabe, Ber. **45**, 2163 (1912); F. W. Hoover, H. B. Hass, J. Org. Chem. **12**, 506 (1947); and prepn of enantiomers: W. N. Nagai, S. Kanao, Ann. **470**, 157 (1929); C. Jarowski, W. H. Hartung, J. Org. Chem. **8**, 564 (1943). Crystal structure: A. Podder et al., Indian J. Phys. **53A**, 652 (1979). HPLC determn in plasma and urine: K. Yamashita et al., J. Chromatogr. **527**, 103 (1990). Clinical studies of decongestant activity: O. K. Haugeto et al., J. Otolaryngol. **10**, 359 (1981); M. Bende et al., Rhinology **23**, 43 (1985); in stress incontinence: E. Fossberg et al., Urol. Int. **38**, 293 (1983); in weight loss: D. E. Schteingart, Int. J. Obes. **16**, 487 (1992). Toxicity: E. I. Goldenthal, Toxicol. Appl. Pharmacol. **18**, 185 (1971). Comprehensive description: I. Kanfer et al., Anal. Profiles Drug Subs. **12**, 357-383 (1983). Review of anorexic effects: P. J. Wellman, Neurosci. Biobehav. Rev. **14**, 339-355 (1990); of toxicology: R. Hanzlick, G. Davis, Am. J. Forensic Med. Pathol. **13**, 37-41 (1992). Evaluation of risk of hemorrhagic stroke: W. N. Kernan et al., N. Engl. J. Med. **343**, 1826 (2000).

(+)-Form

mp 101-101.5°.

Hydrochloride. [154-41-6] Boxogetten; Kontexin; Monydrin; Proin; Propalin; UriCon. Crystals, mp 190-194°. Odor resembling that of crude benzoic acid. pKa 9.44±0.04. Freely sol in water, alcohol. Practically insol in ether, chloroform, benzene. The aq soln is neutral to litmus. LD_{50} orally in rats: 1490 mg/kg (Goldenthal).

(+)-Form hydrochloride. $[\alpha]_D^{25}$ +32° (water). mp 171-172°.

D-threo-Form see Norpseudoephedrine.

THERAP CAT: Decongestant (nasal); anorexic; in treatment of urinary incontinence.

THERAP CAT (VET): In treatment of urinary incontinence in dogs and cats; decongestant (nasal).

7308. Phenylpropylmethylamine. [93-88-9] N,β-Dimethylbenzeneethanamine; dl-N,β-dimethylphenethylamine; dl-N-methyl-2-phenylpropylamine; 1-methylamino-2-phenylpropane; phenpromethamine; 1-methylamino-2-methyl-2-phenylethane; Vonedrine. $C_{10}H_{15}N$; mol wt 149.23. C 80.48%, H 10.13%, N 9.39%. Synthesis starting with the condensation of chlorobenzene with allyl chloride, followed by ammonolysis: Patrick et al., J. Am. Chem. Soc. **68**, 1009 (1946).

Volatile liquid. d_2^{25} 0.915-0.925; bp_{760} 205-210°; bp_{15} 95-96°; n_D^{20} 1.5102. Slightly sol in water (1.2 g/100 ml). Freely sol in alcohol, ether, benzene. Aq solns are strongly alkaline; pH of a soln of 2 drops (~0.1 ml) dil with 10 ml H_2O is ~10.5.

Hydrochloride. $C_{10}H_{15}N.HCl$. mp 144-148°.

THERAP CAT: Adrenergic.

7309. 1-Phenyl-3-pyrazolidinone. [92-43-3] 1-Phenyl-3-pyrazolidone; Phenidone. $C_9H_{10}N_2O$; mol wt 162.19. C 66.65%, H 6.21%, N 17.27%, O 9.86%. Prepd by heating phenylhydrazine with β-chloropropionic acid: **DE 53834** (1889); by acid hydrolysis of 3-amino-1-phenylpyrazoline: Kendall, Duffin, **GB 650911** and **GB 669591** (1951, 1952, both to Ilford). Review: Kendall, Br. J. Photogr. **100**, 56 (1953).

Leaflets or needles from benzene, mp 121°. One gram dissolves in 10 ml boiling water, in 10 ml hot alcohol, in 37.5 ml boiling benzene. Practically insol in ether, petr ether. Freely sol in dil aq solns of acids and alkalies. Pharmacological tests indicate low oral toxicity. No cases of dermatitis have occurred.

USE: Non-staining, high contrast photographic developer. The amount required is about one-fifth to one-tenth that of Metol.

7310. Phenyl Salicylate. [118-55-8] 2-Hydroxybenzoic acid phenyl ester; Salol. $C_{13}H_{10}O_3$; mol wt 214.22. C 72.89%, H 4.71%, O 22.41%. Made by the action of phosphorus oxychloride on a mixture of phenol and salicylic acid.

White, small crystals or crystalline powder; pleasant aromatic odor and taste. d 1.25; mp 41-43°; bp_{12} 173°. One gram dissolves in 6670 ml water, 6 ml alcohol, 1.5 ml benzene, 5 ml amyl alcohol, 10 ml liq paraffin, 4 ml almond oil. Sol in acetone, chloroform, ether, oils; very slightly sol in glycerol. Solubility at 25° in g/100 g: absolute ethanol 53; ethyl acetate 470; methyl ethyl ketone 620; toluene 460; Stoddard solvent 88; water less than 0.1%. Incompat. Bromine water, ferric salts; camphor, monobromated camphor, phenol, chloral hydrate, thymol or urethan in trituration.

USE: In the manuf of various polymers for the plastics industry, also in lacquers, adhesives, waxes, polishes. In suntan oils and cremes. As light absorber to prevent discoloration of plastics. Has some plasticizer properties.

THERAP CAT: Analgesic, antipyretic, anti-inflammatory.

THERAP CAT (VET): Has been used externally as a disinfectant, internally as an intestinal antiseptic and antipyretic.

7311. Phenylselenotrimethylsilane. [33861-17-5] Trimethyl(phenylseleno)silane; trimethylsilyl phenyl selenide; PSTMS. $C_9H_{14}SeSi$; mol wt 229.25. C 47.15%, H 6.16%, Se 34.44%, Si 12.25%. Organoselenium compound for the introduction of selenium into molecules. Prepn: N. Y. Derkach et al., Zh. Org. Khim. **7**, 1543 (1971); and use: D. Liotta et al., Tetrahedron Lett. **1978**, 5091. Improved synthesis: N. Miyoshi et al., Synthesis **1979**, 300. Synthetic applications: S. D. Rychnovsky, D. J. Skalitzky, Synlett **1995**, 555; H. Abe et al., Chem. Pharm. Bull. **46**, 1311 (1998); M. W. DeGroot, J. F. Corrigan, Dalton **2000**, 1235. Brief review: M. David, Synlett **2001**, 445.

Colorless mobile liquid with a very unpleasant odor, slowly decomposes on exposure to air. $bp_{9-10\ mm}$ 93-95°; $bp_{5\ mm}$ 86.5°. mp −14-−9°. d_{20}^{20} 1.1960. n_D^{20} 1.5525.

USE: Selenating reagent.

7312. 4-Phenylsemicarbazide. [537-47-3] *N*-Phenylhydrazinecarboxamide; anilinoformylhydrazine. $C_7H_9N_3O$; mol wt 151.17. C 55.62%, H 6.00%, N 27.80%, O 10.58%. C_6H_5-NHCONHNH₂. Prepd by the action of hydrazine hydrate on phenylurea: Curtius, *J. Prakt. Chem.* [2] **58**, 216 (1898); Wheeler, *Org. Synth.* **coll. vol. I** (2nd ed., 1941) p 450.

Orthorhombic plates from water, mp 122°. Insol in ether, difficultly sol in hot water. Freely sol in alcohol, chloroform, dil acids and alkalies.

Hydrochloride. $C_7H_9N_3O.HCl$. Prisms, mp 215°; freely sol in water and alcohol.

7313. *N*-Phenylsulfanilic Acid. [101-57-5] 4-(Phenylamino)benzenesulfonic acid; 4-diphenylaminesulfonic acid; *p*-anilinobenzenesulfonic acid. $C_{12}H_{11}NO_3S$; mol wt 249.29. C 57.82%, H 4.45%, N 5.62%, O 19.25%, S 12.86%. Prepd by acetylation followed by sulfonation of diphenylamine: Merz, Weith, *Ber.* **6**, 1512 (1873); Gnehm, Werdenberg, *Z. Angew. Chem.* **12**, 1027 (1899); Sarver, Kolthoff, *J. Am. Chem. Soc.* **53**, 1902 (1931).

Leaves. Becomes blue on exposure to light. Soluble in water, in alcohol. Insol in ether. Dec into diphenylamine and sulfuric acid when heated above 200° with water contg hydrochloric acid.

Sodium salt. $C_{12}H_{10}NNaO_3S$. Very sol in water.

Potassium salt. $C_{12}H_{10}KNO_3S$. Leaves; slightly sol in alcohol, very sol in water.

Barium salt. $(C_{12}H_{10}NO_3S)_2Ba$. Leaflets; slightly sol in water. *Poisonous!*

USE: Colorimetric determination of nitrates; oxidation-reduction indicator; detection of oxidizing substances.

7314. Phenyl Sulfide. [139-66-2] 1,1′-Thiobis[benzene]; diphenylsulfide. $C_{12}H_{10}S$; mol wt 186.27. C 77.38%, H 5.41%, S 17.21%. $(C_6H_5)_2S$. Willard, Hall, *J. Am. Chem. Soc.* **44**, 2219 (1922). Toxicity study: H. F. Smyth *et al., Am. Ind. Hyg. Assoc. J.* **23**, 95 (1962).

Colorless, almost odorless liquid. d_{15}^{15} 1.118; mp about −40°; bp 295-297°; n_D^{18} 1.6350. Insol in water. Sol in hot alcohol; misc with benzene, ether, carbon disulfide. LD_{50} orally in rats: 0.49 ml/kg (Smyth).

7315. Phenylthiourea. [103-85-5] Phenylthiocarbamide. $C_7H_8N_2S$; mol wt 152.22. C 55.23%, H 5.30%, N 18.40%, S 21.06%. C_6H_5NHCSNH₂. Prepd by evaporating an aq soln of aniline hydrochloride and ammonium thiocyanate and carefully heating the residue. Toxicity data: Scheline *et al., J. Med. Pharm. Chem.* **4**, 109 (1961).

Bitter or tasteless needles, depending upon heredity of taster. d 1.3. mp 154°. Soluble in 400 parts cold water, 17 parts boiling water; soluble in alcohol. LD_{50} in rats, rabbits (mg/kg): 3, 40 orally (Scheline).

USE: In medical genetics.

7316. Phenyltoloxamine. [92-12-6] *N,N*-Dimethyl-2-[2-(phenylmethyl)phenoxy]ethanamine; *N,N*-dimethyl-2-(α-phenyl-*o*-tolyloxy)ethylamine; *N,N*-dimethyl-2-(α-phenyl-*o*-toloxy)ethylamine; 2-(2-dimethylaminoethoxy)diphenylmethane; 2-benzhydryl β-dimethylaminoethyl ether; 2-benzylphenyl β-dimethylaminoethyl ether; PRN; bistrimin; C-5581H; Antin; Phenoxadrine. $C_{17}H_{21}NO$; mol wt 255.35. C 79.96%, H 8.29%, N 5.49%, O 6.27%. Prepn: Cheney *et al., J. Am. Chem. Soc.* **71**, 60 (1949); Binkley, Cheney, **US 2703324** (1955 to Bristol Labs.).

Oily liquid, bp 141-144° (at <0.1 mm Hg).

Dihydrogen citrate. $C_{17}H_{21}NO.C_6H_8O_7$. Crystals from water or methanol, mp 138-140°. Soluble in water.

Hydrochloride. $C_{17}H_{21}NO.HCl$. Crystals from methyl isobutyl ketone, mp 119-121°. Soluble in water.

THERAP CAT: Dihydrogen citrate as antihistaminic.

7317. Phenyl Tolyl Ketone. $C_{14}H_{12}O$; mol wt 196.24. C 85.69%, H 6.16%, O 8.15%. *o*-Isomer made from benzene and *o*-toluic acid chloride in the presence of $AlCl_3$. *p*-Isomer made from benzoyl chloride and toluene in presence of $AlCl_3$.

o-**Phenyl tolyl ketone.** (2-Methylphenyl)phenylmethanone; 2-methylbenzophenone. Oily liquid. mp below −18°. bp 309-311°. Insol in water. Freely sol in alcohol, oils, most organic solvents.

p-**Phenyl tolyl ketone.** (4-Methylphenyl)phenylmethanone; 4-methylbenzophenone. Crystals, mp 59-60°. bp_{720} 311-312°. Insol in water. Sol in alcohol; easily sol in benzene, ether, oils.

USE: As fixative in perfumery.

7318. Phenyltrimethylammonium Iodide. [98-04-4] *N,N,N*-Trimethylbenzaminium iodide. $C_9H_{14}IN$; mol wt 263.12. C 41.08%, H 5.36%, I 48.23%, N 5.32%. $C_6H_5(CH_3)_3NI$. *Ref:* Pass, Ward, *Analyst* **58**, 667 (1933).

White, cryst powder. mp 175°. Sol in water or alcohol.

USE: For the detection and determination of cadmium.

7319. Phenylurea. [64-10-8] Phenylcarbamide. $C_7H_8N_2$-O; mol wt 136.15. C 61.75%, H 5.92%, N 20.58%, O 11.75%. C_6H_5NHCONH₂. Obtained with carbanilide as byproduct by refluxing aniline hydrochloride and urea in water: Davis, Blanchard, *Org. Synth.* **3**, 95 (1923).

Monoclinic prisms from water or alcohol. d 1.302; mp 147° (dec); bp 238°. On slow cooling separates in needles several centimeters in length. Soluble in hot water, hot alcohol, ether, ethyl acetate, glacial acetic acid.

7320. Phenylurethan(e). [101-99-5] Phenylcarbamic acid ethyl ester; ethyl phenylcarbamate; ethyl carbanilate. $C_9H_{11}NO_2$; mol wt 165.19. C 65.44%, H 6.71%, N 8.48%, O 19.37%. C_6H_5-NHCOOC₂H₅. Made by the action of aniline on ethyl chloroformate.

White, acicular crystals. d 1.106; mp 52-53°; bp 238° with slight decompn; n_D^{20} 1.5376. Slightly sol in water, freely in alcohol, ether; scarcely attacked by boiling for a short time with HCl or NaOH.

7321. Phenyramidol. [553-69-5] α-[(2-Pyridinylamino)methyl]benzenemethanol; 2-(β-hydroxyphenethylamino)pyridine; fenyramidol. $C_{13}H_{14}N_2O$; mol wt 214.26. C 72.87%, H 6.59%, N 13.07%, O 7.47%. Prepn from 2-mandelamidopyridine or 2-aminopyridine: Gray *et al., J. Am. Chem. Soc.* **81**, 4347, 4351 (1959).

Crystals from dil methanol, mp 82-85°. uv max (95% ethanol): 243, 303 nm (log ε 4.24, 3.63). pKa 5.85.

Hydrochloride. [326-43-2] IN-511; MJ-505; NSC-17777; Cabral. $C_{13}H_{14}N_2O.HCl$; mol wt 250.72. Crystals from ethanol + ether, mp 140-142°. Soluble in water. Aq solns are slightly acid and stable in ampuls.

Methiodide. $C_{13}H_{14}N_2O.CH_3I$. Crystals from ethanol + ether, mp 164-166°.

THERAP CAT: Analgesic.

7322. Phenytoin. [57-41-0] 5,5-Diphenyl-2,4-imidazolidinedione; diphenylhydantoin; Di-Hydan; Dilantin; Hydantin; Hydantol; Lehydan; Zentropil. $C_{15}H_{12}N_2O_2$; mol wt 252.27. C 71.42%, H 4.79%, N 11.10%, O 12.68%. Prepn from benzophenone: H. R. Henze, US 2409754 (1946 to Parke, Davis); of sodium salt from benzil, urea and NaOH: Biltz, *Ber.* **41**, 1391 (1908); **44**, 411 (1911). Pharmacology: Gillis *et al., J. Pharmacol. Exp. Ther.* **179**, 599 (1971). Toxicity of base: G. Stille, I. Brunckow, *Arzneim.-Forsch.* **4**, 723 (1954); of sodium salt: G. B. Fink, E. A. Swinyard, *J. Pharmacol. Exp. Ther.* **127**, 318 (1959). *Reviews:* Damato, *Prog. Cardiovasc. Dis.* **12**, 1-15 (1969); Dreifus, Watanabe, *Am. Heart J.* **80**, 709-713 (1970). Review of carcinogenicity studies: *IARC Monographs* **13**, 201-225 (1977). Comprehensive description: J. Philip *et al., Anal. Profiles Drug Subs.* **13**, 417-445 (1984).

Powder, mp 295-298°. Practically insol in water. One gram dissolves in about 60 ml alcohol, about 30 ml acetone. Sol in alkali hydroxides. LD_{50} in mice (mg/kg): 92 i.v.; 110 s.c. (Stille, Brunckow).

Sodium salt. [630-93-3] Phenytoin soluble; sodium 5,5-diphenyl hydantoinate; Aurantin; Dintoina; Epanutin; Phenhydan; Pyoredol; Tacosal. $C_{15}H_{11}N_2NaO_2$; mol wt 274.25. White powder; bitter, soapy taste. Somewhat hygroscopic. Easily dissociated even by weak acids (incl CO_2 absorbed on exposure to air) regenerating phenytoin. One gram dissolves in 10.5 ml alc; in ~66 ml water (aq soln turbid unless pH adjusted to >11.7, the pH of a satd soln). Insol in ether, chloroform. LD_{50} orally in mice: 490 mg/kg (Fink, Swinyard).

Caution: Phenytoin is reasonably anticipated to be a human carcinogen: *Report on Carcinogens, Eleventh Edition* (PB2005-104914, 2004) p III-216.

THERAP CAT: Anticonvulsant; antiepileptic.

THERAP CAT (VET): Anticonvulsant.

7323. Phillyrin. [487-41-2] [1S-(1α,3aα,4β,6aα)]-4-[4-(3,4-Dimethoxyphenyl)tetrahydro-1H,3H-furo[3,4-c]furan-1-yl]-2-methoxyphenyl-β-D-glucopyranoside; phyllyrin; phillyroside; forsythin. $C_{27}H_{34}O_{11}$; mol wt 534.55. C 60.67%, H 6.41%, O 32.92%. From bark of *Phillyrea latifolia* L., and allied *Oleaceae:* Campona, *Ann.* **24**, 242 (1837); Eijkman, *Rec. Trav. Chim.* **5**, 127 (1886); Kramer, *Compt. Rend.* **196**, 814 (1933); Sosa, *Bull. Soc. Chim. Biol.* **29**, 918 (1947). Structure: Kaku *et al., J. Pharm. Soc. Jpn.* **59**, 248 (1939); M. Chiba *et al., Chem. Pharm. Bull.* **25**, 3435 (1977).

α-Form. Needles from dil alc, mp 154-155°. $[α]_D$ +48.4° (alcohol).

β-Form. Needles, mp 184-185°. $[α]_D$ +48.5° (alcohol).

7324. PhIP. [105650-23-5] 1-Methyl-6-phenyl-1H-imidazo[4,5-b]pyridin-2-amine; 2-amino-1-methyl-6-phenylimidazo-[4,5-b]pyridine. $C_{13}H_{12}N_4$; mol wt 224.26. C 69.62%, H 5.39%, N 24.98%. Most abundant of the mutagenic heterocyclic amines found in well-cooked meat and fish. Isoln from fried ground beef: J. S. Felton *et al., Carcinogenesis* **7**, 1081 (1986). Synthesis: M. G. Knize, J. S. Felton, *Heterocycles* **24**, 1815 (1986); T. Choshi *et al., J. Org. Chem.* **58**, 7952 (1993); F. S. Bavetta *et al., Tetrahedron Lett.* **44**, 7793 (1997). Mutagenicity in Chinese hamster ovary cells: L. H. Thompson *et al., Mutagenesis* **2**, 483 (1987). Evaluation of carcinogenic risk: *IARC Monographs* **56**, 229-242 (1993). Review of bioavailability, content in foods, metabolism: N. J. Gooderham *et al., Br. J. Clin. Pharmacol.* **42**, 91-98 (1996). Correlation of dietary intake with breast cancer risk: R. Sinha *et al., J. Natl. Cancer Inst.* **92**, 1352 (2000).

Gray-white crystals, mp 327-328°. uv max (methanol): 225, 273, 316 nm (log ε 4.46, 4.00, 4.46). Sol in methanol, DMSO.

Caution: This substance is reasonably anticipated to be a human carcinogen: *Report on Carcinogens, Eleventh Edition* (PB2005-104914, 2004) p III-135.

7325. Phloionic Acid. [23843-52-9] (9R,10R)-rel-9,10-Dihydroxyoctadecanedioic acid; floionic acid. $C_{18}H_{34}O_6$; mol wt 346.46. C 62.40%, H 9.89%, O 27.71%. Isoln from cork: Guillemonat, Cesaire, *Bull. Soc. Chim. Fr.* **1949**, 792; Ribas, Seoane, *An. R. Soc. Esp. Fis. Quim.* **50B**, 963 (1954), *C.A.* **50**, 806f (1956); Brown, Rosen, US 2872464 (1959 to Crown Cork). Structure: Duhamel, *Bull. Soc. Chim. Fr.* **1965**, 399. Synthesis: Ruzicka *et al., Helv. Chim. Acta* **25**, 1086 (1942); Gensler, Schlein, *J. Am. Chem. Soc.* **77**, 4846 (1955). Resolution of isomers: Gender, Mahadevan, *ibid.* **78**, 169 (1956); Alvarez-Varquez, Ribas-Marques, *An. Quim.* **64**, 783 (1968). Synthesis of (±), (+), and (−) forms: McGhie *et al., Chem. Ind. (London)* **1972**, 536.

Crystals from ethanol + water, mp 126°.

Dimethyl ester. $C_{20}H_{38}O_6$. Crystals from ethanol, mp 77.5-78°.

7326. Phloretin. [60-82-2] 3-(4-Hydroxyphenyl)-1-(2,4,6-trihydroxyphenyl)-1-propanone; 2′,4′,6′-trihydroxy-3-(p-hydroxyphenyl)propiophenone; β-(p-hydroxyphenyl)phloropropiophenone; β-(p-hydroxyphenyl)-2,4,6-trihydroxypropiophenone. $C_{15}H_{14}O_5$; mol wt 274.27. C 65.69%, H 5.14%, O 29.17%. The aglucon of phlorizin, q.v. From root bark of apple trees: Rochleder, *J. Prakt. Chem.* **98**, 205 (1866). Structure: Seshadri, *Annu. Rev. Biochem.* **20**, 495 (1951). Synthesis: Fischer, Nouri, *Ber.* **50**, 611 (1917); Rosenmund, Rosenmund, *ibid.* **61B**, 2608 (1928); Shinoda *et al., J. Pharm. Soc. Jpn.* **49**, 797 (1929); Johnston, US 2789995 (1957 to Union Carbide).

Needles from dil alcohol, dec 262°. Absorption spectrum: Lambrechts, *Arch. Int. Physiol.* **44**, Suppl., 1-39 (1937). Freely sol in alc, methanol, acetone; sol in alkalies in hot glacial acetic acid; very sparingly sol in benzene, chloroform. Practically insol in water, ether, the soly being increased by addition of alcohol.

7327. Phloridzin. [60-81-1] 1-[2-(β-D-Glucopyranosyl-oxy)-4,6-dihydroxyphenyl]-3-(4-hydroxyphenyl)-1-propanone; phlorhizin; phlorizin; phlorrhizen; phloretin-2′-β-glucoside; 4,6-di-hydroxy-2-(β-D-glucosido)-β-(p-hydroxyphenyl)propiophenone. $C_{21}H_{24}O_{10}$; mol wt 436.41. C 57.80%, H 5.54%, O 36.66%. A dihydrochalcone occurring in all parts of the apple tree except the mature fruit. Once thought to occur in pear, plum, cherry trees and other *Rosaceae:* A. H. Williams in *Comparative Phytochemistry,* T. Swain, Ed. (Academic Press, New York, 1966) pp 297-307. Isoln from root bark: De Koninck, *Ann.* **15**, 75, 258 (1835); Stass, *Ann.* **30**, 192 (1839); Bridel, Kramer, *Bull. Soc. Chim. Biol.* **15**, 544 (1933). Hydrolysis by dil mineral acids yields phloretin and glu-cose. Procedure for acid hydrolysis: Wessely, Sturm, *Monatsh. Chem.* **53-54**, 557 (1929); Müller, Robertson, *J. Chem. Soc.* **1933**, 1170. The energy of activation required for the hydrolysis is much less than for other glucosides and approaches that for γ-fructosides (sucrose, raffinose). Is hydrolyzed by saccharase at pH 4.45, by enzymes of *Aspergillus niger* and other enzymes found in inverte-brates: Kobert, *Pfluegers Arch. Gesamte Physiol. Menschen Tiere* **99**, 116 (1903); Moelwyn-Hughes, *J. Gen. Physiol.* **13**, 807 (1930); *cf. Trans. Faraday Soc.* **25**, 81 (1929). Synthesis: Zemplen, Bog-nár, *Ber.* **75B**, 1040 (1942); *cf. ibid.* 645 and **76B**, 386 (1943).

Dihydrate. Long needles from water, mp 110°. Sweet, with bitter aftertaste. $[\alpha]_D^{25}$ −52° (0.16 g in 5 ml of 96% alcohol). One gram dissolves in about one liter of water at 22°, in 64 ml at 60°, in 22 ml at 70°. Freely sol in boiling water; in about 4 parts alcohol, in methanol, amyl alcohol, acetone, ethyl acetate, pyridine, aniline, quinoline and other organic bases; in aq alkaline solns and in glacial acetic acid. Practically insol in ether, chloroform, benzene.

USE: Experimentally to produce glycosuria in animals.

7328. Phloroglucinol. [108-73-6] 1,3,5-Benzenetriol; 1,3,5-trihydroxybenzene; phloroglucin. $C_6H_6O_3$; mol wt 126.11. C 57.14%, H 4.80%, O 38.06%. Isolation as dimer from phloretin, *q.v.*: H. Hlasiwetz, *Ann.* **96**, 118 (1855). Prepn: J. R. Hwu, S.-C. Tsay, *J. Org. Chem.* **55**, 5987 (1990). GC-MS determn in human plasma: C. Lartigue-Mattei *et al., J. Chromatogr.* **617**, 140 (1993). Clinical evaluation: G. Cargill *et al., Presse Med.* **21**, 19 (1992). Toxicology: R. Cahen *et al., Therapie* **17**, 1349 (1962); *J. Am. Coll. Toxicol.* **14**, 468 (1995). Review: G. Leston in *Kirk-Othmer En-cyclopedia of Chemical Technology* **vol. 19** (Wiley-Interscience, New York, 4th ed., 1996) pp 792-812. Biosynthesis study: J. Achkar *et al., J. Am. Chem. Soc.* **127**, 5332 (2005).

White micro crystals, mp 217-219° with quick heating; 200-209° with slow heating. Sweet taste. Discolors in light. Sol in ether, benzene, pyrimidine, pyridine. Soluble in 10 parts methanol, 10 parts ethanol, 100 parts water (25°). LD$_{50}$ in mice, rats (g/kg): 4.7, 4.0 i.g. (Cahen).

Dihydrate. [6099-90-7] Spasfon-Lyoc; Spassirex. Colorless, odorless white rhombic crystals, mp 113-116° with quick heating; 116.5-117.0° with slow heating. Loses water of crystallization at 110°.

USE: In diazo-type printing, textile dyeing. In cosmetics, as antioxidant; hair colorant. As reagent for detection of aldehydes, carbohydrates including lignin, and HCl. Cloud seeding. Rooting medium for woody plants.

THERAP CAT: Antispasmodic.

7329. Pholcodine. [509-67-1] (5α,6α)-7,8-Didehydro-4,5-epoxy-17-methyl-3-[2-(4-morpholinyl)ethoxy]morphinan-6-ol; 3-[2-(4-morpholinyl)ethyl]morphine; tetrahydro-1,4-oxazinyl-methylcodeine; 3-(2-morpholinoethyl)morphine; β-morpholinyleth-ylmorphine; homocodeine; Ethnine; Galenphol; Galphol; Memine; Codylin; Pectolin; Weifacodine. $C_{23}H_{30}N_2O_4$; mol wt 398.50. C 69.32%, H 7.59%, N 7.03%, O 16.06%. Prepn: Chabrier *et al.*, **US 2619485** (1952 to Dausse). Description: *Ann. Pharm. Fr.* **8**, 261 (1950). Toxicity data: B. Kelentey *et al., Arzneim.-Forsch.* **8**, 325 (1958).

Monohydrate. Crystals, mp 91°. Bitter taste. $[\alpha]_D^{20}$ −95.3° (c = 2 in ethanol). Slightly sol in water (2% w/v), ether. Sol in alc (1:3), chloroform, benzene. pH of 2% aq soln 9.5 to 9.8. LD$_{50}$ s.c. in mice: 0.540 g/kg (Kelentey).

Note: This is a controlled substance (opium derivative): **21 CFR**, 1308.11.

THERAP CAT: Antitussive.

7330. Pholedrine. [370-14-9] 4-[2-(Methylamino)pro-pyl]phenol; p-hydroxy-N,α-dimethylphenethylamine; β-(p-hydroxy-phenyl)isopropylmethylamine; α-(p-hydroxyphenyl)-β-methylami-nopropane; p-hydroxy-N-methylbenzedrine; Knoll H$_{75}$. $C_{10}H_{15}$-NO; mol wt 165.23. C 72.69%, H 9.15%, N 8.48%, O 9.68%. α-Adrenergic agonist. Prepd from p-methoxybenzyl methyl ketone: **FR 822422**, **GB 482414**, **DE 674753** (1937, 1938 and 1939 to Knoll); Hildebrandt and Hildebrandt, Freese, **DE 665793** and **DE 767161** (1938 and 1951 to Knoll). Synthesis: Savitskii, Makh-nenko, *J. Gen. Chem. USSR* **10**, 1819 (1940); Buzas, Dufour, *Bull. Soc. Chim. Fr.* **1950**, 139. Toxicity data: Lindner, *Arch. Exp. Pathol. Pharmakol.* **188**, 675 (1938).

Crystals from methanol, mp 162-163°. Acrid, burning taste. Alkaline reactions. Slightly sol in water. Sol in alcohol, ether; readily sol in dil acids.

Sulfate. [6114-26-7] Paredrinol; Pulsotyl; Veritol. ($C_{10}H_{15}$-NO)$_2$.H$_2$SO$_4$; mol wt 428.54. Crystals, dec 320-323°. Sol in water. LD s.c. in rats: 500 mg/kg (Lindner).

THERAP CAT: Antihypotensive.

THERAP CAT (VET): Circulatory stimulant.

7331. Phorate. [298-02-2] Phosphorodithioic acid O,O-di-ethyl S-[(ethylthio)methyl] ester; O,O-diethyl S-(ethylthio)methyl phosphorodithioate; O,O-diethyl S-ethylmercaptomethyl dithio-phosphate; AC-3911; EI-3911; ENT-24042; Rampart; Thimet. C_7-$H_{17}O_2PS_3$; mol wt 260.38. C 32.29%, H 6.58%, O 12.29%, P 11.90%, S 36.94%. Cholinesterase inhibitor. Prepn: Schrader, Lorenz, **US 2759010**; **GB 797307** (1956, 1958 both to Bayer). Metabolism: J. B. Bowman, J. E. Casida, *J. Agric. Food Chem.* **5**, 192 (1957). Persistence in soil: D. L. Suett, *Pestic. Sci.* **6**, 385 (1975). Toxicity study: T. B. Gaines, *Toxicol. Appl. Pharmacol.* **14**, 515 (1969).

Clear liquid, $bp_{0.1}$ 75-78°, $bp_{0.8}$ 118-120°, $bp_{2.0}$ 125-127°. d_4^{25} 1.156. n_D^{25} 1.5329. Vapor pressure at 20°: 8.4×10^{-4} mm Hg. Soly: 50 ppm in water. Misc with xylene, carbon tetrachloride, dioxane, methyl cellosolve, dibutyl phthalate, vegetable oils. Stable at room temp. Hydrolyzed in the presence of water and alkali. LD_{50} in female, male rats (mg/kg): 1.1, 2.3 orally; 2.5, 6.2 dermally (Gaines).

Caution: Potential symptoms of overexposure are irritation of eyes, skin, respiratory system; miosis; rhinorrhea; headache, chest tightness, wheezing, laryngeal spasms, salivation, cyanosis; anorexia, nausea, vomiting, abdominal cramps, diarrhea; sweating; muscle fasciculations, weakness, paralysis; giddiness, confusion, ataxia; convulsions, coma; low blood pressure; cardiac irregularities. *See NIOSH Pocket Guide to Chemical Hazards* (DHHS/-NIOSH 97-140, 1997) p 252.

USE: Insecticide.

7332. Phorbol. [17673-25-5] [1a*R*-(1aα,1bβ,4aβ,7aα,7bα,-8α,9β,9aα)]-1,1a,1b,4,4a,7a,7b,8,9,9a-Decahydro-4a,7b,9,9a-tetrahydroxy-3-(hydroxymethyl)-1,1,6,8-tetramethyl-5*H*-cyclopropa[3,-4]benz[1,2-*e*]azulen-5-one. $C_{20}H_{28}O_6$; mol wt 364.43. C 65.91%, H 7.74%, O 26.34%. Parent alcohol of the tumor promoting compounds in croton oil, *q.v.*, the oil expressed from the seeds of *Croton tiglium* L., *Euphorbiaceae*. Phorbol has a structural skeleton based on cyclopropabenzazulene. Isoln: Flaschenträger, Wigner, *Helv. Chim. Acta* **25**, 569 (1942); Kauffmann, Neumann, *Ber.* **92**, 1715 (1959); S. Tseng *et al.*, *J. Org. Chem.* **42**, 3645 (1977). Structure and stereochemistry: Hecker *et al.*, *Tetrahedron Lett.* **1967**, 3165; Pettersen, Ferguson, *Chem. Commun.* **1967**, 716. Unlike its diesters, phorbol does not appear to be co-carcinogenic or enhance chemically-induced mutagenesis: C. J. Soper, F. J. Evans, *Cancer Res.* **37**, 2487 (1977). Mechanism of action study on phorbol esters: A. S. Kraft, W. B. Anderson, *Nature* **301**, 621 (1983). Comprehensive review of phorbol and its esters: Hecker, Schmidt, *Fortschr. Chem. Org. Naturst.* **31**, 377-467 (1974); P. M. Blumberg, *Crit. Rev. Toxicol.* **8**, 199-234 (1981).

Anhydr crystals, dec 250-251°. Two forms of solvated crystals from ethyl acetate: mp 162-163° and 233-234°. Solvated crystals from methanol or ethanol; mp 249-250°. $[\alpha]_D^{24}$ +102° (water). $[\alpha]_D^{20}$ +118° (c = 0.4 in dioxane). uv max (ethanol): 235, 334 nm (ε 5200, 70). Quite sol in polar solvents, including water.

12-Myristate 13-acetate diester. 12-*O*-Tetradecanoylphorbol-13-acetate; TPA; croton oil factor A_1. $C_{36}H_{56}O_8$. uv max (ethanol): 232, 333 nm (ε 5400, 73). Differentiation of human leukemia cells: J. B. Weinberg, *Science* **213**, 655 (1981).

7333. Phorone. [504-20-1] 2,6-Dimethyl-2,5-heptadien-4-one; diisopropylideneacetone. $C_9H_{14}O$; mol wt 138.21. C 78.21%, H 10.21%, O 11.58%. $(CH_3)_2C\!=\!CHCOCH\!=\!C(CH_3)_2$. Prepn from isobutenyllithium + CO_2: Braude, Timmons, *J. Chem. Soc.* **1950**, 2000; from acetone: Dolgov, Samsonova, *Zh. Obshch. Khim.* **22**, 632 (1952); Joseph, Blumenthal, *J. Org. Chem.* **24**, 1371 (1959); Tsmur, *Zh. Prikl. Khim.* **34**, 1628 (1961); M. Konieczny, G. Sosnovsky, *Z. Naturforsch.* **33B**, 454 (1978).

Yellow liquid or yellowish-green prisms, mp 28°. bp 198-199°; bp_{17} 88°. d_4^{20} 0.885. n_D^{21} 1.4968.

7334. Phosalone. [2310-17-0] Phosphorodithioic acid *S*-[(6-chloro-2-oxo-3(2*H*)-benzoxazolyl)methyl] *O,O*-diethyl ester; phosphorodithioic acid, *O,O*-diethyl ester, *S*-ester with 6-chloro-3-(mercaptomethyl)-2-benzoxazolinone; 3-(*O,O*-diethyldithiophosphorylmethyl)-6-chlorobenzoxazolinone; 6-chloro-3-(*O,O*-diethyldithiophosphorylmethyl)benzoxazolone; *S*-(6-chloro-2-oxobenzox-

azolin-3-yl)methyl diethyl phosphorothiolothionate; RP-11974; Zolone. $C_{12}H_{15}ClNO_4PS_2$; mol wt 367.81. C 39.19%, H 4.11%, Cl 9.64%, N 3.81%, O 17.40%, P 8.42%, S 17.44%. Organophosphorous pesticide; cholinesterase inhibitor. Prepn: **GB 1005372** (1965 to Rhône-Poulenc). Toxicology, metabolism, insecticidal properties: D. L. Colinese, H. J. Terry, *Chem. Ind. (London)* **1968**, 1507. Use as molluscicide: Cessac, **FR 1453989** (1966 to Rhône-Poulenc).

Crystals, mp 47.5-48°. Sol in ketones, alcohols and most aromatic solvents. Practically insol in water and aliphatic hydrocarbons. LD_{50} in mice, female, male rats, guinea pigs (mg/kg): 180-205, 135-170, 120, 82-150 orally; female rats (mg/kg): 390 dermally (Colinese, Terry).

USE: Insecticide, acaricide.

7335. Phosgene. [75-44-5] Carbonic dichloride; carbonyl chloride; chloroformyl chloride. CCl_2O; mol wt 98.92. C 12.14%, Cl 71.68%, O 16.17%. $Cl_2C\!=\!O$. Prepn from chlorine + carbon monoxide: Whitehouse, **US 1231226** (1917); Peacock, **US 1360312** (1921); Bradner, **US 1457493** (1923); Douthitt, **US 2847470** (1958 to Texas Co.); from carbon monoxide + nitrosyl chloride: Williams, **US 1746506** (1930 to du Pont Ammonia Corp.); from carbon tetrachloride + oleum: Murphy, Reuter, *Aust. Chem. Inst. J. Proc.* **15**, 144 (1948). Toxicology: S. A. Cucinell, *Arch. Environ. Health* **28**, 272 (1974). *Review:* E. E. Hardy in *Kirk-Othmer Encyclopedia of Chemical Technology* vol. 17 (Wiley-Interscience, New York, 3rd ed., 1982) pp 416-425.

Colorless, highly toxic gas; suffocating odor; when much diluted with air there is an odor reminiscent of moldy hay. Condenses at ~0° to a clear, colorless, fuming liquid. d_4^0 1.432. mp −118°. bp_{760} 8.2°. Vapor press at 20°: 1215 mm. Slightly sol in water and slowly hydrolyzed by it; freely sol in benzene, toluene, glacial acetic acid and most liq hydrocarbons.

Caution: Severe pulmonary irritant, although not immediately irritating even in potentially lethal exposures. Potential symptoms of overexposure by inhalation may initially be mild and transient and include burning of eyes, cough, dry burning throat, dyspnea, foamy sputum, chest pain, vomiting. Delayed symptoms include peribronchial edema, pulmonary congestion, alveolar edema, cyanosis, anoxia. Direct contact with liquid may cause frostbite. *See Clinical Toxicology of Commercial Products*, R. E. Gosselin *et al.*, Eds. (Williams & Wilkins, Baltimore, 5th ed., 1984) Section II, p 96; *NIOSH Pocket Guide to Chemical Hazards* (DHHS/NIOSH, 97-140, 1997) p 252; *Patty's Industrial Hygiene and Toxicology* vol. 2F, G. D. Clayton, F. E. Clayton, Eds. (Wiley-Interscience, New York, 4th ed., 1994) pp 4557-4563.

Note: Paper soaked in alcoholic or carbon tetrachloride soln contg 10% of a mixture of equal parts of *p*-dimethylaminobenzaldehyde and colorless diphenylamine, then dried, will turn from yellow to deep orange in the presence of approx the max allowable concn of phosgene, and should always be used where the generation of this gas is possible or suspected.

USE: For the prepn of many organic chemicals; as a war gas.

7336. Phosmet. [732-11-6] Phosphorodithioic acid *S*-[(1,3-dihydro-1,3-dioxo-2*H*-isoindol-2-yl)methyl] *O,O*-dimethyl ester; phosphorodithioic acid *O,O*-dimethyl ester *S*-ester with *N*-(mercaptomethyl)phthalimide; *O,O*-dimethyl *S*-phthalimidomethyl phosphorothioate; *N*-(mercaptomethyl)phthalimide *S*-(*O,O*-dimethyl phosphorodithioate); phthalophos (USSR); ENT-25705; R-1504; Imidan; Prolate. $C_{11}H_{12}NO_4PS_2$; mol wt 317.32. C 41.64%, H 3.81%, N 4.41%, O 20.17%, P 9.76%, S 20.21%. Prepn: Fancher, **US 2767194** (1956 to Stauffer). Activity: B. A. Butt, J. C. Keller, *J. Econ. Entomol.* **54**, 813 (1961). GC determn in produce: M. A. Luke *et al.*, *J. Assoc. Off. Anal. Chem.* **64**, 1187 (1981). Toxicity study: T. B. Gaines, *Toxicol. Appl. Pharmacol.* **14**, 515 (1969).

Off-white, crystalline solid, mp 71.9°. Tech product (95-98% pure), mp 66.5-69.5°. Dec below its boiling point. Vapor pressure at 50°: 1×10^{-3} mm Hg. Soly in water at 25°: 25 ppm. LD_{50} in male, female rats (mg/kg): 113, 160 orally (Gaines).

USE: Insecticide, acaricide.

7337. Phosphamidon. [13171-21-6] Phosphoric acid 2-chloro-3-(diethylamino)-1-methyl-3-oxo-1-propenyl dimethyl ester; phosphoric acid dimethyl ester, ester with 2-chloro-N,N-diethyl-3-hydroxycrotonamide; 2-chloro-2-diethylcarbamoyl-1-methyl-vinyl dimethyl phosphate; Ciba 570; ENT-25515; Kinadon. C_{10}-$H_{19}ClNO_5P$; mol wt 299.69. C 40.08%, H 6.39%, Cl 11.83%, N 4.67%, O 26.69%, P 10.34%. Cholinesterase inhibitor. Commercial product consists of 73/27 mixture of cis (Z)/ trans (E) isomers. Prepn: Beriger, Sallmann, US 2908605 (1959 to Ciba); Anliker et al., Helv. Chim. Acta **44**, 1622 (1961). GC determn: W. E. West-lake et al., J. Agric. Food Chem. **21**, 846 (1973). Toxicity data: T. B. Gaines, Toxicol. Appl. Pharmacol. **14**, 515 (1969). Review: Residue Rev. **37**, 1-202 (1971).

Z-isomer

Oil. d_4^{25} 1.2132. n_D^{25} 1.4718. $bp_{1.5}$ 162°; $bp_{0.001}$ 120°. mp −45°. Vapor pressure at 20°: 2.5×10^{-5} mm Hg. Misc with water and most organic solvents except saturated hydrocarbons. One gram dissolves in ~30 g hexane. Stable in neutral or acid media; hydrolyzed by alkali. LD_{50} orally in rats: 24 mg/kg (Gaines).

Caution: See Parathion.
USE: Insecticide.

7338. Phosphine. [7803-51-2] H_3P; mol wt 34.00. H 8.89%, P 91.10%. PH_3. Formed in small quantity in the putrefaction of organic matter contg phosphorus. Prepd from white phosphorus and aq alkali hydroxide; also by treatment of PH_4I with KOH: Klement in Handbook of Preparative Inorganic Chemistry vol. **1**, G. Brauer, Ed. (Academic Press, New York, 2nd ed., 1963) pp 525-530; by pyrolysis of phosphorous acid: Gokhale, Jolly, Inorg. Synth. **9**, 56 (1967); by hydrolysis of a metal phosphide such as calcium phosphide: Klement, loc. cit.; Baudler et al., Z. Anorg. Allg. Chem. **353**, 122 (1967). Review of human exposure and toxicity: N. Brautbar, J. Howard, Toxicol. Ind. Health **18**, 71-75 (2002).

Gas. Poisonous! Odor of decaying fish; bp −87.7°. mp −133°. Spontaneously flammable in air if there is a trace of P_2H_4 present; burns with a luminous flame. Slightly sol in water (0.26 vol. at 20°). Combines violently with oxygen and the halogens. Liberates hydrogen and forms the phosphide when passed over heated metal. Forms phosphonium salts when brought in contact with the halogen acids.

Caution: Potential symptoms of overexposure are nausea, vomiting, abdominal pain, diarrhea; thirst; chest tightness, dyspnea; muscle pain, chills; stupor or syncope; pulmonary edema. Direct contact with liquid may cause frostbite. See NIOSH Pocket Guide to Chemical Hazards (DHHS/NIOSH 97-140, 1997) p 254. See also Clinical Toxicology of Commercial Products, R. E. Gosselin et al., Eds. (Williams & Wilkins, Baltimore, 5th ed., 1984) Section II, p 119.

7339. Phosphinothricin. [35597-44-5] (2S)-2-Amino-4-(hydroxymethylphosphinyl)butanoic acid; 2-ammonio-4-methylphosphinicobutyrate; L-PPT. $C_5H_{12}NO_4P$; mol wt 181.13. C 33.15%, H 6.68%, N 7.73%, O 35.33%, P 17.10%. First natural L-amino acid containing a phosphinic acid group. Isolated from the tripeptide antibiotic, **bialaphos**; inhibits glutamine synthetase. Isoln from S. viridochromogenes and synthesis of DL-form: E. Bayer et al., Helv. Chim. Acta **55**, 224 (1972). Synthesis of DL-form: H. Gross, T. Gnauk, J. Prakt. Chem. **318**, 157 (1976); of enantiomers: N. Minowa et al., Tetrahedron Lett. **25**, 1147 (1984). Crystal structure: E. F. Paulus, S. Grabley, Z. Kristallogr. **160**, 63 (1982). Determn in biological fluids: A. Suzuki, M. Kawana, Bull. Environ. Contam. Toxicol. **43**, 17 (1989). Environmental impact in lakes: M. J. Faber et al., Environ. Toxicol. Chem. **17**, 1291 (1998). Field trial in orchards and vineyards as herbicide: P. Langelüddeke et al., Meded. Fac. Landbouwwet. Rijksuniv. Gent **47**, 95 (1982); on seed potato as desiccant: H. M. Lawson, J. S. Wiseman, Brighton Crop Prot. Conf. - Weeds **1991**, 233. Review of syntheses, activities and uses: G. Hoerlein, Rev. Environ. Contam. Toxicol. **138**, 73-145 (1994).

$[\alpha]_D^{25}$ +13.4° (c = 1 in water).
D-Form. [73679-07-9] $[\alpha]_D^{25}$ −12.4° (c = 1 in water).
DL-Form. [51276-47-2] Glufosinate. mp 229-231° (dec).
DL-Form monoammonium salt. [77182-82-2] Glufosinate-ammonium; ammonium DL-homoalanine-4-yl(methyl)phosphinate; HOE-661; HOE-39866; Basta; Liberty; Rely. $C_5H_{15}N_2O_4P$; mol wt 198.16. Sol in water. LD_{50} in male, female mice, male, female rats (mg/kg): 431, 416, 2000, 1620 orally (Langelüddeke).

USE: Postemergent herbicide; desiccant.

7340. Phosphocreatine. [67-07-2] N-[Imino(phosphono-amino)methyl]-N-methylglycine; N-(phosphonoamidino)sarcosine; creatine phosphate; creatinephosphoric acid; PC. $C_4H_{10}N_3O_5P$; mol wt 211.11. C 22.76%, H 4.77%, N 19.90%, O 37.89%, P 14.67%. Phosphorylated form of creatine, q.v. Occurs primarily in skeletal muscle; also found in heart and brain. Involved in the transfer of high energy phosphate to ADP. Isoln from frog muscle: Eggleton, Biochem. J. **21**, 190 (1927); from cat muscle: Fiske, Subbarow, J. Biol. Chem. **81**, 629 (1929). Synthesis by phosphorylation of creatine: Zeile, Fawaz, Z. Physiol. Chem. **256**, 193 (1938); Ennor, Stocken, Biochem. J. **43**, 190 (1948). Enzymic determn in skeletal muscle: K. Yoshikawa et al., Anal. Biochem. **159**, 303 (1986). HPLC determn in cardiac muscle: T. Teerlink et al., Anal. Biochem. **214**, 278 (1993). Clinical trial as cardioprotective: M. L. Semenovsky et al., J. Thorac. Cardiovasc. Surg. **94**, 762 (1987); as antiarrhythmic: M. Y. Ruda et al., Am. Heart J. **116**, 393 (1988). Review of role in energy metabolism: S. P. Bessman, C. L. Carpenter, Annu. Rev. Biochem. **54**, 831-862 (1985).

Sodium salt. Creatergyl; Neoton. $C_4H_8N_3Na_2O_5P$; mol wt 255.08. Occurs as the hexahydrate, platelets from water + ethanol. Very sol in water. (Free acid, pKa_2 is 4.6).
Calcium salt tetrahydrate. $C_4H_8CaN_3O_5P.4H_2O$. Hygroscopic crystals. Sol in water; sparingly sol in alcohol.
Note: The term **phosphagen**, originally a synonym for phosphocreatine, has since been used to describe any naturally occurring phosphorylated guanidine compd.

THERAP CAT: Cardioprotective.

7341. Phosphocysteamine. [5746-40-7] 2-Aminoethanethiol dihydrogen phosphate (ester); phosphorothioic acid S-(2-aminoethyl) ester; cysteamine-S-phosphate; MEAP. $C_2H_8NO_3PS$; mol wt 157.12. C 15.29%, H 5.13%, N 8.91%, O 30.55%, P 19.71%, S 20.41%. $H_2NCH_2CH_2SPO_3H_2$. Radioprotectant. Prepn of sodium salt: S. Åkerfeldt, Acta Chem. Scand. **13**, 1479 (1959); of free acid: idem, ibid. **14**, 1980 (1960). Radioprotective effect: B. Hansen, B. Sörbo, Acta Radiol. **56**, 141 (1961); A. Vacek et al., Folia Biol. (Prague) **17**, 340 (1971). Mechanism of action: B.

Shapiro *et al.*, *Radiat. Res.* **44**, 421 (1970). Radiobiological and biochemical profile: J. W. Harris, T. L. Phillips, *ibid.* **46**, 362 (1971). Photoreactivity: S. A. Grachev *et al.*, *Radiochem. Radioanal. Lett.* **19**, 283 (1974); H. Neumann, M. Sokolovsky, *Biochim. Biophys. Acta* **381**, 292 (1975). Clinical evaluation in cystinosis: L. A. Smolin *et al.*, *Pediatr. Res.* **23**, 616 (1988); D. S. Theodoropoulos *et al.*, *J. Am. Med. Assoc.* **270**, 2200 (1993).

Crystals from glacial acetic acid, mp 156°. pKa: 2.2, 5.0, 10.3.

Sodium salt. [3724-89-8] Sodium hydrogen-*S*-(2-aminoethyl)-phosphorothioate; cystafos; cystaphos; WR-638. $C_2H_7NNaO_3PS$; mol wt 179.11. White crystalline water soluble powder. LD_{50} i.p. in male mice: 0.93 ±0.03 g/kg (Hansen).

USE: Research radioprotective agent.

THERAP CAT: Treatment of cystinosis.

7342. Phosphomolybdic Acid. [11104-88-4] Molybdophosphoric acid; dodecamolybdophosphoric acid. Formula approx $24MoO_3.P_2O_5.xH_2O$. Prepn: Wu, *J. Biol. Chem.* **43**, 189 (1920); Hastings, Frediani, *Anal. Chem.* **20**, 382 (1948). Formula also reported to be $20MoO_3.P_2O_5.51H_2O$: *U.S.P.* **XXI**, 1398. Review of phosphomolybdic acids: *Mellor's* **Vol. XI**, pp 659-672 (1931).

Bright yellow crystals. Sol in less than 0.4 part water; very sol in alcohol, ether.

USE: Weighting silks; as reagent for alkaloids, uric acid, xanthine, creatinine, some metals, with hematoxylin as nerve stain in microscopy.

7343. Phosphonium Iodide. [12125-09-6] H_4IP; mol wt 161.91. H 2.49%, I 78.38%, P 19.13%. PH_4I. Prepd by hydrolysis of a mixture of diphosphorus tetraiodide and white phosphorus: Work, *Inorg. Synth.* **2**, 141 (1946). Improved apparatus for its prepn: Beredjick, *ibid.* **6**, 91 (1960).

Large, transparent, colorless crystals (usually cubes). Tetragonal system. Sublimes at room temp. *Store in sealed ampuls in refrigerator!* Vapor pressure: 50 mm at 20°; 760 mm at 62.5°. mp 18.5° under its own vapor pressure. Heat of fusion 12,680 cal/mol. *Caution:* Heat or traces of moisture or alcohol cause decompn into PH_3 and HI. Will detonate if heated rapidly.

USE: In the laboratory prepn of phosphine.

7344. Phosphoric Acid. [7664-38-2] Orthophosphoric acid. H_3O_4P; mol wt 98.00. H 3.09%, O 65.30%, P 31.61%. H_3PO_4. Obtained commercially from phosphate rock deposits in Florida, Tennessee, and the Western United States. Phosphate rock is essentially tricalcium phosphate and one of the large scale processes is based on the equation: $Ca_3(PO_4)_2 + 3H_2SO_4 + 6H_2O \rightarrow 2H_3PO_4 + 3(CaSO_4.2H_2O)$. Description of various processes: W. H. Waggaman, *Phosphoric Acid, Phosphates and Phosphatic Fertilizers* (Reinhold, New York, 1952); *Phosphoric Acid* **Vol. 1**, parts I, II, A. V. Slack, Ed. (Dekker, New York, 1968) 1159 pp; *Faith, Keyes & Clark's Industrial Chemicals*, F. A. Lowenheim, M. K. Moran, Eds. (Wiley-Interscience, New York, 4th ed., 1975) pp 628-639. Prepn of ultrapure, cryst H_3PO_4: Simon, Schulze, *Z. Anorg. Allg. Chem.* **242**, 322 (1939); Weber, King, *Inorg. Synth.* **1**, 101 (1939). Reviews: J. R. Van Wazer, *Phosphorus and Its Compounds* **Vol. 1**, *Chemistry* (Interscience, New York, 1958) pp 479-491; R. B. Hudson *et al.*, "Phosphoric Acids and Phosphates" in *Kirk-Othmer Encyclopedia of Chemical Technology* **Vol. 17** (Wiley-Interscience, New York, 3rd ed., 1982) pp 426-472.

$$HO-\underset{\underset{OH}{|}}{\overset{\overset{O}{||}}{P}}-OH$$

Unstable, orthorhombic crystals, mp 42.35°, or clear, syrupy liquid; easily supercooled into a glass. Pleasing acid taste when suitably diluted. An acid containing ~88% H_3PO_4 will frequently crystallize on prolonged cooling; forms hemihydrate, mp 29.32°. Becomes anhydr at 150°, gradually changes to pyrophosphoric acid at ~200°, and changes to metaphosphoric acid when heated above 300°. The hot concd acid attacks porcelain and granite ware. May be stored in suitable stainless steel containers. Tribasic acid: pK_1: 2.15; pK_2: 7.09; pK_3: 12.32. Other reported values of dissociation constants and viscosity data reviewed by Van Wazer. The pH of a 0.1*N* aq soln is 1.5. Heat of formation (crystals): −306.2 kcal/mole. Heat of soln: +2.79 kcal/mole. Sol in water, alc; sol in

8 vols of a 3:1 ether: alcohol mixture. Properties of phosphoric acid solns. d^{25} 1.8741 (100% soln); 1.6850 (85% soln); 1.3334 (50% soln); 1.0523 (10% soln). Density measurements: Christensen, Reed, *Ind. Eng. Chem.* **47**, 1277 (1950); Egan, Luff, *ibid.* 1280. $n_D^{17.5}$ 1.34203 (10% soln); 1.35032 (20% soln); 1.35846 (30% soln). Spec heat (21.3°): 0.4359 (88% soln).

Caution: Potential symptoms of overexposure are irritation of upper respiratory system, eyes and skin; burns skin and eyes; dermatitis. *See NIOSH Pocket Guide to Chemical Hazards* (DHHS/NIOSH 97-140, 1997) p 254.

USE: In the manuf of superphosphates for fertilizers, other phosphate salts, polyphosphates, detergents. Acid catalyst in making ethylene, purifying hydrogen peroxide. As acidulant and flavor, synergistic antioxidant and sequestrant in food. Pharmaceutic aid (solvent). In dental cements; process engraving; rustproofing of metals before painting; coagulating rubber latex; as analytical reagent.

THERAP CAT (VET): Has been used in lead poisoning.

7345. Phosphoric Acid, Meta. [37267-86-0] Metaphosphoric acid; glacial phosphoric acid. $(HPO_3)_n$; H 1.26%, O 60.01%, P 38.73%.

Transparent, glass-like solid or soft silky masses; hygroscopic. Volatilizes at red heat. Very slowly sol in cold water, slowly changing to H_3PO_4, the change is hastened by boiling; sol in alcohol. *Keep tightly closed.* For greater convenience it is also marketed in form of rods made by the addition of sodium phosphate.

USE: In dentistry for making zinc oxyphosphate cement; as reagent in chemical analysis.

7346. Phosphorous Acid. [13598-36-2] Phosphonic acid. H_3O_3P; mol wt 82.00. H 3.69%, O 58.53%, P 37.77%. Prepd by hydrolysis of PCl_3 according to the equation $PCl_3 + 3H_2O \rightarrow H_3PO_3 + 3HCl$, the rather violent reaction can be slowed down by the initial presence of concd HCl: Milobedzki, Friedmann, *Chem. Pol.* **15**, 76 (1917); *Chem. Z.* **1918**, I, 933; Simon, Fehér, *Z. Anorg. Allg. Chem.* **230**, 298 (1937). Alternate procedure carrying out the reaction in carbon tetrachloride: Voight, Gallais, *Inorg. Synth.* **4**, 55 (1953). *Review:* Ohashi, "Lower Oxo Acids of Phosphorus and Their Salts" in *Topics in Phosphorus Chemistry* **Vol. 1**, M. Grayson, E. J. Griffith, Eds. (Interscience, New York, 1964) pp 113-187.

$$HO-\underset{\underset{HO}{|}}{\overset{\overset{O}{||}}{P}}-H$$

White, very hygroscopic and deliquesc, crystalline mass; garlic-like taste; slowly oxidized by oxygen (air) to H_3PO_4. d_4^{21} 1.65; d_4^{76} liq 1.597. mp ~73°; above 180° is dec into PH_3 and H_3PO_4. Very sol in water, alcohol. pK_1 1.29; pK_2 6.74. Usually marketed as a 20% aq soln.

7347. Phosphorus. [7723-14-0] P; at. wt 30.973762; at. no. 15; valences 3, 5. Group VA (15). One naturally occurring isotope: ^{31}P; artificial, radioactive isotopes: 28-30; 32-34. Abundance in earth's crust: about 0.12%. Does not occur free in nature; found in the form of phosphates in the minerals *chlorapatite* [$3Ca_2(PO_4)_2.$-$CaCl_2$], *fluorapatite* [$3Ca(PO_4)_2.CaF_2$], vivianite, wavellite and "phosphate rock" or phosphorite; occurs in small quantities in granite rocks; occurs in all fertile soil; an essential constituent of protoplasm, nervous tissue and bones. Discovered in 1669 by Brandt. Prepn: Ullmann, *Enzyklopädie der Technischen Chemie* **8**, 362 (1931); DeWitt, Skolnik, *J. Am. Chem. Soc.* **68**, 2305 (1946); Skolnik *et al.*, *ibid.* 2310. Lab prepn and purification: Klement in *Handbook of Preparative Inorganic Chemistry* **vol. 1**, G. Brauer, Ed. (Academic Press, New York, 2nd ed., 1963) pp 518-525. *Reviews:* J. R. Van Waser, *Phosphorus and Its Compounds* 2 vols. (Interscience, New York, 1958, 1961) 2046 pp; Corbridge, "The Structural Chemistry of Phosphorus Compounds" in *Topics in Phosphorus Chemistry* **Vol. 3**, E. J. Griffith, M. Grayson, Eds. (Interscience, New York, 1966) pp 57-394; Toy, "Phosphorus" in *Comprehensive Inorganic Chemistry* **Vol. 2**, J. C. Bailar, Jr. *et al.*, Eds. (Pergamon Press, Oxford, 1973) pp 389-545; J. R. Van Wazer in *Kirk-Othmer Encyclopedia of Chemical Technology* **vol. 17** (Wiley-Interscience, New York, 3rd ed., 1982) pp 473-490. Review of toxicology and human exposure: *Toxicological Profile for White Phosphorous* (PB98-101090, 1997) 248 pp.

Phosphorus exists in three main allotropic forms: white, black, and red. The same liquid is obtained on melting. *Caution:* Avoid contact with $KClO_3$, $KMnO_4$, peroxides and other oxidizing agents; explosions may result on contact or friction. Phosphorus atoms exist as symmetrical, tetrahedral P_4 molecules in the liquid phase and in the vapor phase below 800°; molecules dissociate to P_2 above 800°.

White phosphorus. Colorless or white, transparent, cryst solid; waxy appearance; darkens on exposure to light. Sometimes called yellow phosphorus; color due to impurities. Two allotropic modifications: α-form exists at room temp; cubic crystals containing P_4 molecules; d 1.83. β-Form prepd by conversion of α-form at −79.6°; hexagonal crystals; d 1.88. mp 44.1° (vapor press. 0.181 mm); bp 280°. Volatile; sublimes *in vacuo* at ordinary temp when exposed to light. When exposed to air in the dark, emits a greenish light and gives off white fumes. Solubilities in water: one part/300,000 parts water; in abs alc: one g/400 ml; in abs ether: one g/102 ml; in $CHCl_3$: one g/40 ml; in benzene: one g/35 ml; in CS_2: one g/0.8 ml. Soly in oils: one gram phosphorus dissolves in 80 ml olive oil, 60 ml oil of turpentine, ~100 ml almond oil. Ignites at about 30° in moist air; the ignition temp is higher when the air is dry. *Handle with forceps. Keep under water. Poisonous.* Combines directly with the halogens to form tri- or pentahalides; combines with sulfur to form sulfides. Reacts with several metals to form phosphides. Yields orthophosphoric acid when treated with nitric acid. Reacts with alkali hydroxides with formation of phosphine and sodium hypophosphite.

Black Phosphorus. Polymorphic. Orthorhombic crystalline form: stable in air; resembles graphite in texture; produced from the white modification under high pressures: Bridgman, *J. Am. Chem. Soc.* **36**, 1344 (1914); Jacobs, *J. Chem. Phys.* **5**, 945 (1937); Krebs, *Inorg. Synth.* **7**, 60 (1963). d 2.691. Does not catch fire spontaneously. Insol in organic solvents. Amorphous form prepd at lower pressures: Jacobs, *loc. cit.* At higher pressure the orthorhombic form undergoes reversible transition to a rhombohedral structure, d 3.56, and a cubic structure, d 3.83: Jamieson, *Science* **139**, 1291 (1963).

Red phosphorus. Polymorphism: Roth *et al.*, *J. Am. Chem. Soc.* **69**, 2881 (1947); Corbridge, *loc. cit.* Crystal structure of one form, *Hittorf's phosphorus:* Thurn, Krebs, *Acta Crystallogr.* **25B**, 125 (1969). Red to violet powder. The properties of red phosphorus are intermediate between those of the white and black forms. Sublimes at 416°, triple point 589.5° under 43.1 atm. d 2.34. Insol in organic solvents. Sol in phosphorus tribromide. Less active than the white form; reacts only at high temp. Yields the white modification when distilled at 290°. Catches fire when heated in air to about 260° and burns with formation of the pentoxide. Burns when heated in an atmosphere of chlorine.

Caution: Potential symptoms of acute poisoning by ingestion of white (or yellow) phosphorous are burning pain in throat and abdomen; intense thirst; nausea, vomiting, diarrhea; garlic breath; luminescent vomitus and feces. Direct contact may cause eye and skin burns. May be followed by symptoms of systemic poisoning, including hematemesis; hepatomegaly, jaundice; hemorrhages into skin, mucous membranes, viscera; oliguria, hematuria, albuminuria; cardiovascular collapse; convulsions, confusion, coma. Potential symptoms of chronic poisoning from inhalation or ingestion are cachexia, anemia, bronchitis. general debility, necrosis of mandible. *See Clinical Toxicology of Commercial Products,* R. E. Gosselin *et al.*, Eds. (Williams & Wilkins, Baltimore, 5th ed., 1984) Section III, pp 348-352; *NIOSH Pocket Guide to Chemical Hazards* (DHHS/-NIOSH 97-140, 1997) p 254.

USE: White phosphorus: manuf rat poisons; for smoke screens, gas analysis. Red phosphorus: pyrotechnics; manuf safety matches; in organic synthesis; manuf phosphoric acid, phosphine, phosphoric anhydride, phosphorus pentachloride, phosphorus trichloride; manuf fertilizers, pesticides, incendiary shells, smoke bombs, tracer bullets.

7348. Phosphorus Oxybromide. [7789-59-5] Phosphoryl bromide; phosphoryl tribromide. Br_3OP; mol wt 286.69. Br 83.61%, O 5.58%, P 10.80%. $POBr_3$. Prepd according to the equation: $3PBr_5 + P_2O_5 \rightarrow 5POBr_3$: Hönigschmid, Hirschbold-

Wittner, *Z. Anorg. Allg. Chem.* **243**, 355 (1940); Johnson, Nunn, *J. Am. Chem. Soc.* **63**, 141 (1941); Booth, Seegmiller, *Inorg. Synth.* **2**, 151 (1946).

Thin plates, faint orange tint, d 2.822. mp 56° (in hot water). bp_{758} 193° (dec). Slowly hydrolyzes in water forming H_3PO_4 and HBr. Sol in ether, benzene, chloroform, carbon disulfide, concd H_2SO_4. *Store in sealed glass ampuls!*

7349. Phosphorus Oxychloride. [10025-87-3] Phosphoryl chloride; phosphorus chloride. Cl_3OP; mol wt 153.33. Cl 69.37%, O 10.43%, P 20.20%. $POCl_3$. Manuf: *Faith, Keyes & Clark's Industrial Chemicals,* F. A. Lowenheim, M. K. Moran, Eds. (Wiley-Interscience, New York, 4th ed., 1975) pp 646-649.

Colorless, clear, strongly fuming liquid; pungent odor. d^{25} 1.645. bp 105.8°; mp 1.25°: J. R. Van Wazer, *Phosphorus and Its Compounds* vol. 1 (Interscience, New York, 1958) p 254. Reacts exothermically with water, alc. *Keep in tightly closed containers.*

Caution: Potential symptoms of overexposure are irritation of eyes, skin, respiratory system; eye, skin burns; dyspnea, cough, lung edema; dizziness, headache, weakness; abdominal pain, nausea, vomiting; nephritis. *See NIOSH Pocket Guide to Chemical Hazards* (DHHS/NIOSH 97-140, 1997) p 254.

USE: As chlorinating agent, especially to replace oxygen in organic compounds; as solvent in cryoscopy.

7350. Phosphorus Pentabromide. [7789-69-7] Phosphoric bromide; phosphorus perbromide. Br_5P; mol wt 430.49. Br 92.81%, P 7.20%. PBr_5. *Review:* Payne, "The Chemistry of Phosphorus Halides" in *Topics in Phosphorus Chemistry* **Vol. 4**, M. Grayson, E. J. Griffith, Eds. (Interscience, New York, 1967) pp 85-155.

Yellow, cryst mass. mp >100° with decompn. Dec by water or alcohol; sol in carbon disulfide or tetrachloride. *Keep tightly closed. Corrosive.*

USE: Brominating agent for converting organic acids to acyl bromides.

7351. Phosphorus Pentachloride. [10026-13-8] Phosphoric chloride; phosphorus perchloride. Cl_5P; mol wt 208.24. Cl 85.13%, P 14.87%. PCl_5. Prepn: Maxson, *Inorg. Synth.* **1**, 99 (1939). *Review:* Payne, "The Chemistry of Phosphorus Halides" in *Topics in Phosphorus Chemistry* **Vol. 4**, M. Grayson, E. J. Griffith, Eds. (Interscience, New York, 1967) pp 85-155.

White to pale yellow, fuming, deliquesc, cryst mass; pungent, unpleasant odor; attacks the eyes and mucous membranes. mp 148° under pressure; sublimes at about 100° without melting. bp 160°. Hydrolyzed by water to form phosphoric acid and hydrogen chloride. Reacts with alcohols (ROH) to form the corresponding chloride (RCl). Sol in carbon disulfide or tetrachloride. *Keep in tightly closed containers and handle with caution. Corrosive.*

Caution: Potential symptoms of overexposure are irritation of eyes, skin and respiratory system; bronchitis; dermatitis. *See NIOSH Pocket Guide to Chemical Hazards* (DHHS/NIOSH 97-140, 1997) p 256.

USE: As catalyst in manuf acetylcellulose; for replacing hydroxyl groups by Cl, particularly for converting acids into acid chlorides.

7352. Phosphorus Pentafluoride. [7647-19-0] F_5P; mol wt 125.97. F 75.41%, P 24.59%. PF_5. Prepd by treating PF_3 with bromine to form PF_3Br which then disproportionates to PF_5 and PBr_5: Moissan, *C.R. Hebd. Seances Acad. Sci.* **100**, 1348; **101**, 1490 (1885); by heating P_2O_5 with CaF_2: Lucas, Ewing, *J. Am. Chem. Soc.* **49**, 1270 (1927); Booth, Bozarth, *ibid.* **55**, 3890 (1933); from PCl_5 and AsF_3: Thorpe, *Ann.* **182**, 201 (1876); *Proc. Roy. Soc.* **25**, 122 (1877); O. Ruff, *Die Chemie des Fluors* (Berlin, 1920), p 29; Kwasnik in *Handbook of Preparative Inorganic Chemistry* **vol. 1**, G. Brauer, Ed. (Academic Press, New York, 2nd ed., 1963) pp 190-191; from PCl_3 and CaF_2: Muetterties *et al.*, *J. Inorg. Nucl. Chem.* **16**, 52 (1960); from phosphoryl fluoride, hydrogen fluoride and sulfur trioxide: Wiesboeck, **US 3584999**; **US 3592594** (1971 to U.S. Steel). *Reviews:* Burg in *Fluorine Chemistry* vol. 1, J. H. Simons, Ed. (Academic Press, New York, 1950) pp 97-98; Kemmitt, Sharp, *Adv. Fluorine Chem.* **4**, 197-198 (1965); Schmutzler, *ibid.* **5**, 32-285 (1965).

Colorless gas. Fumes strongly in air. d (gas) 5.805 g/l. mp −93.8°. bp −84.6°. Trouton constant 21.8. Dipole moment:

zero. High thermal stability. Does not attack dry glass even at 250°, but a slight trace of moisture leads to formation of POF_3 and HF. Water hydrolysis ultimately yields phosphoric acid; intermediates are oxyfluophosphates. Lewis acid; forms complexes with amines, ethers, nitrates, sulfoxides, organic bases. Forms a cryst addn product $PF_5 \cdot NO_2$ at $-10°$ which dissociates on warming. May be stored in steel cylinders.

Caution: Intensely irritating to skin, eyes, mucous membranes. Inhalation may cause pulmonary edema.

USE: Catalyst in ionic polymerization reactions.

7353. Phosphorus Pentaselenide. [1314-82-5] P_2Se_5; mol wt 456.75. P 13.56%, Se 86.44%. Prepd by melting a mixture of phosphorus and selenium in an atm of CO_2 or N_2: Carius, Bogen, *Ann.* **124**, 57 (1862); Kudchadker *et al., Can. J. Chem.* **46**, 1415 (1968).

Amorphous, glass, black-purple solid. Dec in steam and boiling water. Reacts with CCl_4; insol in carbon disulfide.

7354. Phosphorus Pentasulfide. [1314-80-3] Phosphoric sulfide; thiophosphoric anhydride; phosphorus persulfide. P_2S_5; mol wt 222.27. P 27.87%, S 72.13%. Exists as P_4S_{10}. Conveniently prepd by fusing red phosphorus with sulfur: Stock, Herscovici, *Ber.* **43**, 1223 (1910); Klement in *Handbook of Preparative Inorganic Chemistry* vol. **1**, G. Brauer, Ed. (Academic Press, New York, 2nd ed., 1963) p 567. Manuf: *Faith, Keyes & Clark's Industrial Chemicals*, F. A. Lowenheim, M. K. Moran, Eds. (Wiley-Interscience, New York, 4th ed., 1975) pp 650-653.

Light yellow, triclinic crystals; peculiar odor. d 2.09. mp 286-290°; bp 513-515°. Dec by water forming H_3PO_4 and H_2S; sol in carbon disulfide, in aq soln of alkali hydroxides. *Keep tightly closed.*

Caution: Potential symptoms of overexposure are irritation of eyes, skin and respiratory system; apnea, coma and convulsions; conjunctival pain, lacrimation, photophobia, kerato-conjunctivitis and corneal vesiculation; dizziness; headache; fatigue; irritability, insomnia; GI disturbance. *See NIOSH Pocket Guide to Chemical Hazards* (DHHS/NIOSH 97-140, 1997) p 256.

USE: In manuf of lube oil additives and pesticides. Manuf safety matches, ignition compds, and for introducing sulfur into organic compds.

7355. Phosphorus Pentoxide. [1314-56-3] Phosphorous oxide (P_2O_5); phosphoric anhydride; diphosphorus pentoxide. O_5P_2; mol wt 141.94. O 56.36%, P 43.64%. P_2O_5. Exists as P_4O_{10}. Prepd commercially by burning phosphorus in a current of dry air. Purification: Manley, *J. Chem. Soc.* **121**, 331 (1922); de Decker, McGillavry, *Rec. Trav. Chim.* **60**, 153, 413 (1941). Review of phosphorus oxides: J. R. Van Waser, *Phosphorus and Its Compounds* vol. **1** (Interscience, New York, 1958) pp 267-286.

Very deliquescent crystals. *Corrosive.* Several crystalline and amorphous modifications. Commercial form; hexagonal; d 2.30. mp 340°. Sublimation temperature 360°. Nonflammable. Does not support combustion. Heat of formation: -365.83 kcal/mole. Sp heat: 0.170 cal/g/°C. Heat of fusion: 8.2 kcal/mole. Heat of volatilization: 22.7 kcal/mole of P_4O_{10}. Readily absorbs moisture from the air. Exothermic hydrolysis by water to form phosphoric acid. The reaction with alcohol is similar.

Caution: Strong irritant; corrosive to skin, mucous membranes and eyes.

USE: Drying and dehydrating agent. Condensing agent in organic synthesis.

7356. Phosphorus Sulfochloride. [3982-91-0] Thiophosphoryl chloride. Cl_3PS; mol wt 169.40. Cl 62.79%, P 18.28%, S 18.93%. $PSCl_3$. Prepd from $P_2S_5 + PCl_5$: Martin, Duvall, *Inorg. Synth.* **4**, 73 (1953). Alternate procedure from PCl_3, $AlCl_3$ and S: Moeller *et al., ibid.* 71.

Fuming liq, crystallizes as α-form at $-40.8°$ or as β-form at $-36.2°$. bp_{760} 125°. n_D^{25} 1.635. Sol in benzene, carbon tetrachloride, carbon disulfide, chloroform. Hydrolyzes slowly in water, rapidly in alkaline solns. In water the hydrolysis products are orthophosphoric acid, hydrochloric acid, and hydrogen sulfide.

Caution: Strong irritant.

7357. Phosphorus Tribromide. [7789-60-8] Phosphorous bromide. Br_3P; mol wt 270.69. Br 88.56%, P 11.44%. PBr_3. Prepn: Gray, Maxson, *Inorg. Synth.* **2**, 147 (1946). *Review:*

Payne, "The Chemistry of Phosphorus Halides" in *Topics in Phosphorus Chemistry* vol. **4**, M. Grayson, E. J. Griffith, Eds. (Interscience, New York, 1967) pp 85-155.

Colorless, fuming liquid; very penetrating odor. d^{15} 2.85. mp $-41.5°$. bp 173.2°. Vapor pressure: 10 mm (48°). Dissolved and dec by water or alc; sol in acetone, carbon disulfide. *Keep tightly closed. Corrosive.*

7358. Phosphorus Trichloride. [7719-12-2] Phosphorous chloride. Cl_3P; mol wt 137.33. Cl 77.45%, P 22.55%. PCl_3. Prepd from red phosphorus and dry chlorine in the presence of refluxing PCl_3: Forbes *et al., Inorg. Synth.* **2**, 145 (1946). Manuf: *Faith, Keyes & Clark's Industrial Chemicals*, F. A. Lowenheim, M. K. Moran, Eds. (Wiley-Interscience, New York, 4th ed., 1975) pp 654-657. *Review:* Payne, "Chemistry of Phosphorus Halides" in *Topics in Phosphorus Chemistry* vol. **4**, M. Grayson, E. J. Griffith, Eds. (Interscience, New York, 1967) pp 85-155.

Colorless, clear, fuming liquid. d_4^{21} 1.574. mp $-112°$. bp 76°. Vapor pressure: 100 mm (21°). Decomposed by water or alc. Sol in benzene, chloroform, ether, carbon disulfide. *Keep in tightly closed containers and handle with caution.*

Caution: Potential symptoms of overexposure are irritation of eyes, skin, nose and throat; pulmonary edema; burns eyes and skin. *See NIOSH Pocket Guide to Chemical Hazards* (DHHS/NIOSH 97-140, 1997) p 256.

USE: As of phosphorus oxychloride; manuf $POCl_3$, PCl_5; producing iridescent metallic deposits.

7359. Phosphorus Trifluoride. [7783-55-3] F_3P; mol wt 87.97. F 64.79%, P 35.21%. PF_3. Prepd by halogen exchange between PCl_3 and AsF_3: Moissan, *Compt. Rend.* **100**, 272 (1885); Hoffman, *Inorg. Synth.* **4**, 149 (1953); between PCl_3 and ZnF_2: Williams, *ibid.* **5**, 95 (1957); between PCl_3 and CaF_2 or SbF_3: Booth, Bozarth, *J. Am. Chem. Soc.* **61**, 2927 (1939); Muetterties *et al., J. Inorg. Nucl. Chem.* **16**, 52 (1960); between PCl_3 and HF: Kwasnik in *Handbook of Preparative Inorganic Chemistry* vol. **1**, G. Brauer, Ed. (Academic Press, New York, 2nd ed., 1963) pp 189-190. *Reviews:* Burg in *Fluorine Chemistry* vol. **1**, J. H. Simons, Ed. (Academic Press, New York, 1950) pp 98-100; Kemmitt, Sharp, *Adv. Fluorine Chem.* **4**, 198-199 (1965); Schmutzler, *ibid.* **5**, 32-285 (1965).

Colorless gas. Does not fume in air. Does not attack glass except at high temps. *Poisonous!* d (gas) 3.907 g/l. mp $-151.30°$. bp $-101.38°$. Critical temp $-2.05°$; critical press. 42.69 atm. May be stored in steel cylinders or in glass, also in a gasometer over Hg. Slowly hydrolyzed by water. Absorbed by aq bases at a rate increasing with pH, producing a fluophosphite which boiling aq HNO_3 does not convert to phosphate. Anhyd KOH may be used to dry PF_3 with little loss. Dry NH_3 forms a solid addn product. Aq oxidizers such as chromic acid, permanganate, or bromine rapidly destroy PF_3, and alcohols convert it to alkyl phosphite. Phosphides and fluorides are formed upon reaction with hot metals.

Caution: See Phosphorus Pentafluoride.

7360. Phosphorus Trioxide. [1314-24-5] Diphosphorus trioxide. O_3P_2; mol wt 109.95. O 43.65%, P 56.34%. P_2O_3. Exists as P_4O_6. Prepd by treating PCl_3 with tetramethylammonium sulfite in liq SO_2: Jander *et al., Ber.* **77**, 689 (1944). Alternate prepn from the elements: Thorpe, Tutton, *J. Chem. Soc.* **57**, 545 (1890); Miller, *ibid.* **1928**, 1847; **1929**, 1823; Wolf, Schmager, *Ber.* **62**, 779 (1929). Chemistry: Riess, Van Wazer, *Inorg. Chem.* **5**, 178 (1966).

Transparent monoclinic crystals or colorless liquid. *Very poisonous!* d_4^{21} 2.135. mp 23.8°. bp 173.1° in nitrogen atm. Disproportionates into red P and P_2O_4 when heated above 210°. Sol in benzene, carbon disulfide. When placed in cold water, H_3PO_3 is formed slowly. Hot water produces a violent reaction with the formation of red phosphorus, phosphine, and H_3PO_4.

7361. Phosphorus Triselenide. [1314-86-9] Tetraphosphorus triselenide. P_4Se_3; mol wt 360.78. P 34.34%, Se 65.66%. Prepn: Meyer, *Z. Anorg. Chem.* **30**, 258 (1902); **61B**, 1807 (1928); Irgolic *et al., Inorg. Chem.* **4**, 1421 (1965).

Orange-red crystals. Irritating odor. mp 245-246°. d 1.31. bp 360-400°. Phosphoresces at 160°. Flammable when heated in air. Dec in moist air. Sol in carbon tetrachloride, carbon disulfide, chloroform, benzene, toluene, acetone, acetylene dichloride, acetylene trichloride.

7362. Phosphorylcholine. [107-73-3] *N,N,N*-Trimethyl-2-(phosphonooxy)ethanaminium chloride; choline chloride dihydrogen phosphate; (2-hydroxyethyl)trimethylammonium chloride phosphate; phosphorylcholine chloride; choline phosphate chloride; choline chloride phosphate; choline phosphoric acid ester (chloride). $C_5H_{15}ClNO_4P$; mol wt 219.60. C 27.35%, H 6.88%, Cl 16.14%, N 6.38%, O 29.14%, P 14.10%. $[(CH_3)_3^+NCH_2CH_2OPO_3^-$H_2]Cl^-$. Prepd by phosphorylation of choline chloride with diphenylphosphoryl chloride: Baer, McArthur, *J. Biol. Chem.* **154**, 451 (1944); Baer, *J. Am. Chem. Soc.* **69**, 1253 (1947); *Biochem. Prep.* **2**, 96 (1952); by heating choline or choline chloride with pyrophosphoric or polyphosphoric acid: Cherbuliez, Rabinowitz, *Helv. Chim. Acta* **42**, 1154 (1959).

Barium salt. [6484-71-5] $C_5H_{13}BaClNO_4P$. Hydrated glistening leaflets from water + alcohol. Must be dried *in vacuo* (0.5 mm) over P_2O_5 at 100° for 16 hrs. Freely sol in water, practically insol in abs ethanol, ether.

Calcium salt. [4826-71-5] Colifos; Epafosforil; Fosfocolina; Isocolin. $C_5H_{13}CaClNO_4P$; mol wt 257.67.

Magnesium salt. [17032-39-2] Heparexine. $C_5H_{13}ClMgNO_4P$; mol wt 241.89.

THERAP CAT: Hepatobiliary dysfunction.

7363. Phosphoserine. [407-41-0] Serine dihydrogen phosphate (ester); serine phosphate; *O*-phospho-DL-serine. $C_3H_8NO_6P$; mol wt 185.07. C 19.47%, H 4.36%, N 7.57%, O 51.87%, P 16.74%. Prepn: Neuhaus, Korkes, *Biochem. Prep.* **6**, 75 (1958); D. M. Theodoropoulos, *J. Chem. Soc.* **1960**, 5257. Other methods of prepn and isoln from protein hydrolysates: Greenstein, Winitz, *Chemistry of the Amino Acids* (Wiley, New York, 1961), *passim.* Crystal structure: G. H. McCallum, *Nature* **184**, 1863 (1959).

Crystals from ethanol + ether, mp 166-167° (dec).

Note: Used in combination with L-glutamine and vitamin B_{12} as a roborant: *Fosforina B_{12}, Vitasprint B_{12}.*

7364. Phosphotungstic Acid. [12067-99-1] Tungstophosphoric acid. Approx composition $24WO_3.2H_3PO_4.48H_2O$. The H_2O content may vary appreciably. Prepn: Bailar, *Inorg. Synth.* **1**, 132 (1939).

White or slightly yellowish-green, slightly efflorescent crystals or cryst powder. Sol in about 0.5 part water. Also sol in alcohol and in ether.

USE: As reagent for alkaloids and many other nitrogen bases, for phenols, albumin, peptone, amino acids, uric acid, urea, blood, carbohydrates; as biological stain.

7365. Phosvitin. [9008-96-2] A phosphoprotein of mol wt about 40,000. Isoln from egg yolk: Mecham, Olcott, *J. Am. Chem. Soc.* **71**, 3670 (1949); *Biochem. Prep.* **2**, 15 (1952); Joubert, Cook, *Can. J. Biochem. Physiol.* **36**, 399 (1958); from roe: Mano, Yoshida, *J. Biochem. (Tokyo)* **66**, 105 (1969). Represents about 7% of the total yolk protein; high in phosphorus content and a ratio of serine to all other amino acid residues of 6:4. *In vitro* synthesis in hens liver: Heald, McLachlan, *Biochem. J.* **94**, 32 (1965); Rudack, Wallace, *Biochim. Biophys. Acta* **155**, 299 (1968). Estradiol-induced synthesis in roosters: Veuving, Gruber, *ibid.* **232**, 524, 529 (1971); Jailkhani, Talwar, *Nature New Biol.* **236**, 239 (1972). Amino acid sequence: Belitz, *Angew. Chem.* **76**, 574 (1964); Shainkin, Perlmann, *J. Biol. Chem.* **246**, 2278 (1971). Conformation: Grizzuti, Perlmann, *ibid.* **245**, 2573 (1970). Anticlotting activity studies: Sato *et al., Am. J. Physiol.* **203**, 1170 (1962). *Review:* Taborsky, *Adv. Protein Chem.* **28**, 50-78 (1974).

THERAP CAT: Anticoagulant.

7366. Phoxim. [14816-18-3] 4-Ethoxy-7-phenyl-3,5-dioxa-6-aza-4-phosphaoct-6-ene-8-nitrile 4-sulfide; phenylglyoxylonitrile oxime *O,O*-diethyl phosphorothioate; *O,O*-diethyl *O*-(α-cyano-

benzylideneamino)phosphorothioate; α-[[(diethoxyphosphinothioyl)oxy]imino]benzeneacetonitrile; Bay 5621; Bay 77488; Baythion; Sebacil; Volaton. $C_{12}H_{15}N_2O_3PS$; mol wt 298.30. C 48.32%, H 5.07%, N 9.39%, O 16.09%, P 10.38%, S 10.75%. Prepn: **NL 6605907**; W. Lorenz *et al.*, **US 3591662** (1966, 1971 both to Bayer). Activity: C. R. Harris, *J. Econ. Entomol.* **63**, 782 (1970); D. C. Read, *ibid.* **69**, 429 (1976). Toxicity studies: J. H. Vinopal, T. R. Fukuto, *Pestic. Biochem. Physiol.* **1**, 44 (1971). Degradation in soil: G. Dräger, *Pflanzenschutz-Nachr.* **30**, 28 (1977).

Pale yellow oil, bp$_{0.01}$ 102°. n_D^{20} 1.5405. d_4^{20} 1.176. Sol in alc, ketones, aromatic hydrocarbons. LD$_{50}$ orally in mice: >2000 mg/kg (Vinopal, Fukuto).

USE: Insecticide.

7367. Phrenosin. [586-02-7] (2*R*)-*N*-[(1*S*,2*R*,3*E*)-1-[(β-D-Galactopyranosyloxy)methyl]-2-hydroxy-3-heptadecenyl]-2-hydroxytetracosanamide; $C_{48}H_{93}NO_9$; mol wt 828.25. C 69.61%, H 11.32%, N 1.69%, O 17.39%. Cerebroside easily separated from a commercially available beef spinal cord lipid concentrate or from nerve tissue. A large proportion of its fatty acid content (25%) is 2-hydroxystearic acid, the rest is cerebronic (2-hydroxylignoceric) acid. Isoln: Radin *et al., J. Biol. Chem.* **219**, 977 (1956); Skipski *et al., Arch. Biochem. Biophys.* **82**, 487 (1959). Synthesis: Shapiro, Flowers, *J. Am. Chem. Soc.* **83**, 3327 (1961).

Cryst from pyridine + acetone, methanol + chloroform, toluene + alcohol (1:1) or chloroform + alcohol + water, [α] +4.5° (c = 2 in pyridine). IR spectrum: H. P. Schwarz *et al., Ann. N.Y. Acad. Sci.* **69**, 116 (1957). Sol in hot dioxane, 1,1-dichloro-1-nitroethane, butanol and acetonitrile + chloroform.

7368. *o*-Phthalaldehyde. [643-79-8] 1,2-Benzenedicarboxaldehyde; *o*-phthaldialdehyde; Cidex OPA. $C_8H_6O_2$; mol wt 134.13. C 71.64%, H 4.51%, O 23.86%. Alternative to glutaraldehyde, *q.v.* for high-level disinfection. Prepn: A. Colson, H. Gautier, *Bull. Soc. Chim.* **45**, 509 (1886); J. Thiele, O. Günther, *Ann.* **347**, 106 (1906); T. C. Chaudhuri, *J. Am. Chem. Soc.* **64**, 315 (1942). Polarographic determn: N. H. Furman, D. R. Norton, *Anal. Chem.* **26**, 1111 (1954). Use in fluorogenic determn of peptides: M. Roth, *ibid.* **43**, 880 (1971); T. M. Joys, H. Kim, *Anal. Biochem.* **94**, 371 (1979); of biological thiols: K. Mopper, D. Delmas, *Anal. Chem.* **56**, 2557 (1984). Biocidal properties: S. E. Walsh *et al., J. Appl. Microbiol.* **86**, 1039 (1999). Mechanism of antibacterial action: *idem et al., ibid.* **87**, 702 (1999). Bactericidal efficacy study: J. C. N. Shackelford *et al., J. Antimicrob. Chemother.* **57**, 335 (2006). Hospital disinfection of endoscopes: S. M. Hession, *Gastroenterol. Nurs.* **26**, 110 (2003). Review of reactivity with nucleophiles: P. Zuman, *Chem. Rev.* **104**, 3217-3238 (2004).

Long, pale yellow needles from petroleum ether mp 56-56.5° (Thiele, Günther). Also reported as colorless powder, mp 54° (Chaudhuri).

USE: Disinfectant. Reagent in fluorometric determn of primary amines and thiols.

7369. Phthalamide. [88-96-0] 1,2-Benzenedicarboxamide; phthalic acid diamide. $C_8H_8N_2O_2$; mol wt 164.16. C 58.53%, H 4.91%, N 17.06%, O 19.49%. Prepd from phthalic anhydride and anhyd ammonia in benzene: Dominikiewcz, *Arch. Chem. Farm.* **3**, 141 (1937).

Minute crystals, mp 228° (commercial grades mp 221- 223°). Melts with decomposition to NH_3 and phthalimide. Slightly sol in cold water, methanol. More sol in hot solvents. Heat of combustion 921.7 cal/mol. Boiling of aq or alcoholic solns produces NH_3 and phthalimide. The presence of acids accelerates decompn.

7370. Phthalazine. [253-52-1] 2,3-Benzodiazine; benzo-[*d*]pyridazine; β-phenodiazine. $C_8H_6N_2$; mol wt 130.15. C 73.83%, H 4.65%, N 21.52%. Prepd by reduction of 1-chlorophthalazine with hydriodic acid and red phosphorus: Gabriel, Eschenbach, *Ber.* **30**, 3024 (1897); Paul, *Ber.* **32**, 2015 (1899); by redn of 1-hydrazinophthalazine: Armarego, *J. Appl. Chem.* **11**, 70 (1961); from *o*-phthalaldehyde + hydrazine sulfate: Smith, Otremba, *J. Org. Chem.* **27**, 879 (1962); from 1,2-benzodinitrile: Carter, Cheeseman, *Org. Prep. Proced. Int.* **6**, 67 (1974).

Pale yellow needles from ether, mp 90-91°. bp 315-317° (dec); bp$_{29}$ 189°; bp$_{17}$ 175°. uv max (water): 218, 261, 292, 305 nm (log ε 4.83, 3.53, 3.18, 3.11). Freely sol in water; sol in ethanol, methanol, benzene, ethyl acetate; less sol in ether. Practically insol in ligroin.

Hydrochloride. $C_8H_6N_2$·HCl. Needles from ether, mp 231° (efferv).

7371. Phthalic Acid. [88-99-3] 1,2-Benzenedicarboxylic acid. $C_8H_6O_4$; mol wt 166.13. C 57.84%, H 3.64%, O 38.52%. Manufactured by catalytic oxidation of *o*-toluic acid and oxidation of xylene: Taylor, Dean, **US 3064046** (1962 to I.C.I.); Cier, **US 3088974** (1963 to Esso Res. & Eng.). Isoln from the fungus, *Gibberella fujikuroi:* Cross *et al., J. Chem. Soc.* **1963**, 2937. Toxicity studies: C. B. Shaffer *et al., J. Ind. Hyg. Toxicol.* **27**, 130 (1945); A. R. Singh *et al., J. Pharm. Sci.* **61**, 59 (1972). Review of toxicology: A. M. Api, *Food Chem. Toxicol.* **39**, 97-108 (2001).

Crystals, mp ~230° when rapidly heated, forming phthalic anhydride and water. One gram dissolves in 160 ml water, 10 ml alc, 205 ml ether, 5.3 ml methanol. Practically insol in chloroform. LD_{50} orally in rats: 7.9 g/kg (Shaffer).

Ethyl ester. [84-66-2] Ethyl phthalate; diethyl phthalate; Neantine; Palatinol A. $C_{12}H_{14}O_4$; mol wt 222.24. Review of toxicology and human exposure: *Toxicological Profile for Diethyl Phthalate* (PB95-264214, 1995) 159 pp. Colorless, practically odorless, oily liq; bitter disagreeable taste. d$_4^{14}$ 1.232. bp 295°. Flash pt 140°C. n$_D^{14}$ 1.5049. Insol in water. Misc with alcohol, ether and many other organic solvents. LD_{50} i.p. in rats: 5.06 ml/kg (Singh).

Caution: Potential symptoms of overexposure to diethyl phthalate are irritation of eyes, skin, nose, throat; headache, dizziness,

nausea; lacrimation; polyneuritis, vestibular dysfunction; pain, numbness, weakness, spasms in arms and legs. *See NIOSH Pocket Guide to Chemical Hazards* (DHHS/NIOSH 97-140, 1997) p 108.

USE: Ethyl phthalate used in manuf celluloid; solvent for cellulose acetate in manuf varnishes and dopes; denaturing alc. Vehicle for fragrance and cosmetic ingredients.

7372. Phthalic Anhydride. [85-44-9] 1,3-Isobenzofuran-dione. $C_8H_4O_3$; mol wt 148.12. C 64.87%, H 2.72%, O 32.40%. Prepd from naphthalene by oxidation with a mixture of $HgSO_4$ and $CuSO_4$ in presence of H_2SO_4; by passing naphthalene and oxygen over a suitable catalyst at 400-500°. Review of mfg processes: *Faith, Keyes & Clark's Industrial Chemicals,* F. A. Lowenheim, M. K. Moran, Eds (Wiley-Interscience, New York, 4th ed., 1975) pp 658-665.

White, lustrous needles. d 1.53; mp 130.8°; bp 295°. Sublimes. Sol in 162 parts water, more in hot water with conversion into phthalic acid, in 125 parts carbon disulfide; sol in alcohol, sparingly in ether.

Caution: Potential symptoms of overexposure are irritation of eyes, skin and upper respiratory system; conjunctivitis; nasal ulcer bleeding; bronchitis, bronchial asthma; dermatitis. *See NIOSH Pocket Guide to Chemical Hazards* (DHHS/NIOSH 97-140, 1997) p 256.

USE: Manuf phthaleins, phthalates, benzoic acid, synthetic indigo, artificial resins (glyptal).

7373. Phthalimide. [85-41-6] 1*H*-Isoindole-1,3(2*H*)-dione. $C_8H_5NO_2$; mol wt 147.13. C 65.31%, H 3.43%, N 9.52%, O 21.75%. Prepd from phthalic anhydride and NH_4OH or $(NH_4)_2$-CO_3: W. A. Noyes, P. K. Porter, *Org. Synth.* **coll. vol. I**, 457 (2nd ed., 1941). Teratogenicity study: K. Fickentscher *et al., Pharmazie* **31**, 172 (1976).

Monoclinic prisms from water or by sublimation. mp 238°. Has slightly acidic properties, Ka = 5 × 10^{-9}. Absorption spectrum: Hartley, Hedley, *J. Chem. Soc.* **91**, 317 (1907). Slightly soluble in water. A satd aq soln contains 0.036 g at 25°; 0.07 g at 40°; about 0.4 g at the bp. 100 g of boiling alcohol dissolves 5 g phthalimide. Almost insol in benzene, petr ether; fairly sol in boiling acetic acid; freely sol in aq alkali hydroxides.

7374. Phthalofyne. [131-67-9] 1,2-Benzenedicarboxylic acid mono(1-ethyl-1-methyl-2-propynyl) ester; phthalic acid 1-ethyl-1-methyl-2-propynyl ester; 1-ethyl-1-methyl-2-propynyl acid phthalate; 3-methyl-1-pentyn-3-yl acid phthalate; ftalofyne; NSC-25614; Whipcide. $C_{14}H_{14}O_4$; mol wt 246.26. C 68.28%, H 5.73%, O 25.99%. Prepn: Sugimoto, Okumura, **JP 54 1833** (1954 to Tanabe), *C.A.* **49**, 11711e (1955); **GB 736993** (1955 to Schering).

Crystals from benzene or hexane, mp 96-98°. Weak acid. Slightly sol in water. Unstable in strong alkali.

THERAP CAT (VET): Anthelmintic.

7375. Phthaloyl Chloride. [88-95-9] 1,2-Benzenedicarbonyl dichloride. $C_8H_4Cl_2O_2$; mol wt 203.02. C 47.33%, H 1.99%, Cl 34.93%, O 15.76%. Obtained by the action of PCl_5 on phthalic anhydride.

Colorless, oily liquid. d^{20} 1.409. Solidif +12°; mp 15-16°; bp 280-282°; n_D^{20} 1.5692. Dec by water or alcohol; sol in ether. *Keep tightly closed.*

7376. Phthalylsulfacetamide. [131-69-1] 2-[[[4-[(Acetylamino)sulfonyl]phenyl]amino]carbonyl]benzoic acid; 4'-(acetylsulfamyl)phthalanilic acid; phthalylsulfacetimide; N^1-acetyl-N^4-phthaloylsulfanilamide; N^1-acetyl-N^4-phthalylsulfanilamide; phthaloylsulfacetamide; ftalicetimida; N-[p-(o-carboxybenzamido)benzenesulfonyl]acetamide; N-(o-carboxybenzoyl)sulfacetamide; Enterocid; Enterosulfamid; Enterosulfon; Talecid; Thalamyd; Rabalan; Sterathal. $C_{16}H_{14}N_2O_6S$; mol wt 362.36. C 53.03%, H 3.89%, N 7.73%, O 26.49%, S 8.85%. Prepn: Basu, *J. Indian Chem. Soc.* **26**, 130 (1949).

Needles from dil alcohol, mp 196°. Soluble in alcohol. Very sparingly sol in water. Forms a water-sol sodium salt.

THERAP CAT: Antibacterial.

THERAP CAT (VET): Antibacterial.

7377. Phthalylsulfathiazole. [85-73-4] 2-[[[4-[(2-Thiazolylamino)sulfonyl]phenyl]amino]carbonyl]benzoic acid; 4'-(2-thiazolylsulfamyl)phthalanilic acid; 2-(N⁴-phthalylaminobenzenesulfonamido)thiazole; 2-(N⁴-phthalylsulfanilamido)thiazole; phthalylsulfonazole; Estreptocarbocaftiazol; Thalazole. $C_{17}H_{13}N_3O_5S_2$; mol wt 403.43. C 50.61%, H 3.25%, N 10.42%, O 19.83%, S 15.90%. May be prepd by condensing sulfathiazole with phthalic anhydride: M. L. Moore, **US 2324013**; **US 2324015** (1943 to Sharp & Dohme). Prepn of 8-hydroxyquinoline salt: **DE 1008296** (1957 to Geistlich Söhne). Toxicity data: P. A. Mattis *et al., J. Pharmacol. Exp. Ther.* **81**, 116 (1944).

Crystals. Slightly bitter taste. Darkens on prolonged exposure to light. Effervesces at 244° to 250°. mp 272-277° (dec) when the melting point bath is preheated to 220-225°. Slightly sol in alcohol; very slightly sol in ether; readily sol in NaOH or KOH soln, ammonia water and concd HCl. Practically insol in chloroform and water. LD_{50} i.p. in mice: 920 mg/kg (Mattis).

8-Hydroxyquinoline salt. Yellow crystals from dil methanol, dec above 220°. Split into its components by dil acids.

THERAP CAT: Antibacterial.

THERAP CAT (VET): Antibacterial.

7378. Phthiocol. [483-55-6] 2-Hydroxy-3-methyl-1,4-naphthalenedione; 2-hydroxy-3-methyl-1,4-naphthoquinone. $C_{11}H_8O_3$; mol wt 188.18. C 70.21%, H 4.29%, O 25.51%. Antibiotic substance produced by *Mycobacterium tuberculosis:* Terni, *Boll. Soc. Ital. Biol. Sper.* **25**, 60 (1949), *C.A.* **45**, 2054f (1951). Possesses some vitamin K activity. Isoln and synthesis: Anderson,

Newman, *J. Biol. Chem.* **101**, 773 (1933); **103**, 197, 405 (1933); L. F. Fieser, *ibid.* **133**, 391 (1940); Tarbell *et al., J. Am. Chem. Soc.* **72**, 379 (1950); Burton, Praill, *J. Chem. Soc.* **1952**, 755; Eistert, Müller, *Ber.* **92**, 2071 (1959); H. Kallmayer, *Arch. Pharm.* **307**, 806 (1974); K. Maruyama, S. Arakawa, *J. Org. Chem.* **42**, 3793 (1977).

Yellow prisms from ether-petr ether, mp 173-174°. Sublimes. Volatile with steam. Slightly sol in water; sol in the usual organic solvents except petr ether. Forms deep red water-sol salts. E_0^{alc} 0.299 volts.

Acetate. $C_{13}H_{10}O_4$. Pale yellow crystals, mp 101-102°.

7379. Phycobiliproteins. Deeply colored, highly fluorescent photoreceptor pigments found in blue-green, red and cryptomonad algae that contain a linear tetrapyrrole as the prosthetic group. They are composed of a bile pigment or *phycobilin* and an apoprotein. Phycobiliproteins are classified according to uv-vis absorption maxima as *phycocyanins* (blue pigment), *phycoerythrins* (red pigment), and *allophycocyanins* (pale blue pigment). Phycocyanins and phycoerythrins occur as large mol wt aggregates called *phycobilisomes* that are attached to the photosynthetic membranes. They are closely linked to the chlorophyll containing system for efficient energy transfer. *Phytochrome* is a similar biliprotein that functions in plant photomorphogenesis. It is widely distributed in plants but only in trace amounts. It exists in two forms that are interconverted upon alternate exposure to red and far-red light. *Reviews:* H. W. Siegelman *et al., Biochem. Soc. Symp.* **28**, 107-120 (1968); P. O'Carra, C. O'hEocha in *Chemistry and Biochemistry of Plant Pigments* vol. 1, T. W. Goodwin, Ed. (Academic, New York, 2nd ed., 1976) pp 328-376; A. Bennett, H. W. Siegelman in *Porphyrins* vol. 6, D. Dolphin, Ed. (Academic, New York, 1979) pp 493-520.

7380. Phylloquinone. [84-80-0] 2-Methyl-3-[(2E,7R,11R)-3,7,11,15-tetramethyl-2-hexadecenyl]-1,4-naphthalenedione; 2-methyl-3-phytyl-1,4-naphthoquinone; 3-phytylmenadione; phytomenadione; phytonadione; vitamin K₁; AquaMephyton; Konakion; Mephyton; Mono-Kay; Veda-K₁; Veta-K₁. $C_{31}H_{46}O_2$; mol wt 450.70. C 82.61%, H 10.29%, O 7.10%. Photosynthetic electron carrier; occurs widely in green plants, algae, photosynthetic bacteria. Major dietary source of vitamin K, *q.v.* Isoln from alfalfa: H. Dam *et al., Helv. Chim. Acta* **22**, 310 (1939). Structure: D. W. MacCorquodale *et al., J. Biol. Chem.* **131**, 357 (1939); L. F. Fieser, *J. Am. Chem. Soc.* **61**, 3467 (1939). Partial syntheses from menadione and phytol: H. J. Almquist, A. A. Klose, *ibid.* 2557; S. B. Binkley *et al., ibid.* 2558; L. F. Fieser, *ibid.* 2559. Stereochemistry and total synthesis: H. Mayer *et al., Helv. Chim. Acta* **47**, 221 (1964); L. M. Jackman *et al., ibid.* **48**, 1332 (1965). Synthesis using a π-allylic nickel(I) complex: Sato *et al., J. Chem. Soc. Perkin Trans. 1* **1973**, 2289. Alternate synthesis: Y. Tachibana, *Chem. Lett.* **1977**, 901. Metabolic studies: M. J. Shearer *et al., Br. J. Haematol.* **18**, 297 (1970); **22**, 579 (1972). The *cis* isomer is not bioactive: J. T. Matschiner *et al., J. Nutr.* **102**, 625 (1972). Isoln from chloroplasts: E. Interschick-Niebler, H. K. Lichtenthaler, *Z. Naturforsch.* **36C** 276 (1981). Role in photosystem I: K. Brettel *et al., FEBS Lett.* **203**, 220 (1986). Conversion *in vivo* to menaquinone-4, *q.v.*: H. H. W. Thijssen, M. J. Drittij-Reijnders, *Br. J. Nutr.* **72**, 415 (1994). HPLC determn in foods: S. L. Booth *et al., J. Agric. Food Chem.* **42**, 295 (1994). Clinical efficacy in hemorrhagic disease of newborn: P. M. Loughnan, P. N. McDougall, *J. Paediatr. Child Health* **29**, 171 (1993). Comprehensive description: M. M. A. Hassan *et al., Anal. Profiles Drug Subs.* **17**, 449-531 (1988).

Yellow viscous oil. $[\alpha]_D^{25}$ $-0.28°$ (dioxane). n_D^{20} 1.5263. uv max (petr ether): 242, 248, 260, 269, 325 nm ($E_{1cm}^{1\%}$ 396, 419, 383, 387, 68). Insol in water. Sparingly sol in methanol; sol in ethanol, acetone, benzene, petr ether, hexane, dioxane, chloroform, ether, other fat solvents and in vegetable oils. Stable to air and moisture, but dec in sunlight. Unaffected by dil acids, but destroyed by solns of alkali hydroxides and by reducing agents. *Keep well closed and protected from light.*

Dihydro form. [572-96-3] Phytonadiol; dihydrovitamin K_1; α-phyllohydroquinone. Waxy mass. Freely sol in ether; sparingly sol in petr ether. Insol in water.

Dihydro form sodium diphosphate. [5988-22-7] Phytonadiol sodium diphosphate; Kayhydrin. $C_{31}H_{48}Na_2O_8P_2$. mp 138°. Sol in water and methanol.

2,3-Epoxide. [25486-55-9] Vitamin K_1 epoxide; vitamin K_1 oxide. $C_{31}H_{46}O_3$. Prepn: Fieser *et al., J. Am. Chem. Soc.* **61**, 3216 (1939). Colorless oil. uv max (95% alc): 259, 305 nm (log E_M 3.79, 3.31). Insol in water.

THERAP CAT: Vitamin (prothrombogenic).

THERAP CAT (VET): Vitamin (prothrombogenic); antidote for dicoumarol poisoning.

7381. Physalaemin. [2507-24-6] Physalemin. $C_{58}H_{84}N_{14}$-$O_{16}S$; mol wt 1265.44. C 55.05%, H 6.69%, N 15.50%, O 20.23%, S 2.53%. An undecapeptide belonging to the group of proteins named tachykinins. Found in skin of the amphibian *Physalaemus fuscumaculatus:* Erspamer *et al., Experientia* **18**, 562 (1962). Structure: Erspamer *et al., ibid.* **20**, 489 (1964); Anastasi *et al., Arch. Biochem. Biophys.* **108**, 341 (1964). Synthesis: Bernardi *et al., Experientia* **20**, 490 (1964); Nakamura *et al.,* **JP 71 25384** (1971 to Dainippon), *C.A.* **75**, 152083r (1971). Solid-phase synthesis: W. Voelter *et al., Tetrahedron* **28**, 5963 (1972). Biological activities similar to the tachykinins eledoisin and substance P, *q.q.v.* Exerts a powerful hypotensive action, stimulates salivary secretion, intestinal contraction, and vasodilation. Occurrence in other *Physalaemus* spp. and pharmacology: G. Bertaccini *et al., Br. J. Pharmacol.* **25**, 363 (1965); G. Bertaccini, *Pharmacol. Rev.* **28**, 127 (1976). Differentiation of physalaemin and substance P: Geipert *et al., Arch. Pharmacol.* **265**, 225 (1969). Immunoreactivity study in human lung small-cell carcinoma: L. H. Lazarus *et al., Science* **219**, 79 (1983).

5-oxo-Pro–Ala–Asp–Pro–Asn–Lys–Phe–Tyr–Gly–Leu–MetNH$_2$

Trifluoroacetate dihydrate. $C_{58}H_{84}N_{14}O_{16}S.CF_3COOH.2H_2$-O. Dec 180°. $[\alpha]_D^{20}$ $-56°$ (c = 0.2 in ethanol). uv max: 278 nm (ε 1780). Slowly loses activity when incubated in blood. Inactivated by liver and kidney homogenates.

Hydrochloride trihydrate. $C_{58}H_{84}N_{14}O_{16}S.HCl.3H_2O$. Dec about 185°. $[\alpha]_D^{}$ $-43°$ (c = 1 in 95% acetic acid).

7382. Physodic Acid. [84-24-2] 3,8-Dihydroxy-11-oxo-1-(2-oxoheptyl)-6-pentyl-11*H*-dibenzo[*b,e*][1,4]dioxepin-7-carboxylic acid; 4,4′,6′-trihydroxy-6-(2-oxoheptyl)-2′-pentyl-2,3′-oxydibenzoic acid-ε-lactone; physodalin. $C_{26}H_{30}O_8$; mol wt 470.51. C 66.37%, H 6.43%, O 27.20%. From the lichens *Parmelia physodes* (L.) Ach.: Hesse, *Ber.* **30**, 1983 (1897); Klosa, *Pharm. Ind.* **15**, 46 (1953); and *Cetraria ciliaris* Ach.: Culberson, *Science* **143**, 255 (1964). Structure: Asahina, Nogami, *Ber.* **67**, 805 (1934); **68**, 77 (1935).

Needles from methanol, mp 205°. uv max (95% ethanol): 256 nm (log ε 4.2). Sol in ether, acetone, hot methanol; somewhat sol in cold ethanol, methanol, hot chloroform; practically insol in benzene, petr ether, carbon disulfide.

Diacetate. $C_{30}H_{34}O_{10}$. Plates from acetone + carbon disulfide, mp 153-155.5°.

Methyl ester. $C_{27}H_{32}O_8$. Prisms from 80% alcohol, mp 156-157°.

7383. Physostigma. Calabar bean; ordeal bean; chop nut; split nut. Dried ripe seed of *Physostigma venenosum* Balf., *Leguminosae. Poisonous! Habit.* West Africa (near mouths of Niger and Old Calabar Rivers); introduced into India and Brazil. *Constit.* 0.15-0.3% alkaloids consisting of physostigmine (eserine), physovenine, eseridine, eseramine, phytosterol.

7384. Physostigmine. [57-47-6] (3a*S-cis*)-1,2,3,3a,8,8a-Hexahydro-1,3a,8-trimethylpyrrolo[2,3-*b*]indol-5-ol methylcarbamate (ester); eserine; Synapton. $C_{15}H_{21}N_3O_2$; mol wt 275.35. C 65.43%, H 7.69%, N 15.26%, O 11.62%. Acetylcholinesterase inhibitor. From Calabar beans, the seeds of the vine *Physostigma venenosum* Balf., *Leguminosae:* Jobst, Hesse, *Ann.* **129**, 115 (1864); Hesse, *ibid.* **141**, 82 (1867). Extraction procedure: Schwyzer, *Die Fabrikation pharmazeutischer und chemisch-technischer Produkte* (Berlin, 1931) p 338; Chemnitius, *J. Prakt. Chem.* **116**, 59 (1927). Structure: Stedman, Barger, *J. Chem. Soc.* **127**, 247 (1925). Absolute configuration: R. B. Longmore, B. Robinson, *Chem. Ind. (London)* **1969**, 622. Crystal structure: Petcher, Pauling, *Nature* **241**, 277 (1973). Synthesis: Julian, Pikl, *J. Am. Chem. Soc.* **57**, 755 (1935); Harley-Mason, Jackson, *J. Chem. Soc.* **1954**, 3651; J. Wijnberg, W. N. Speckamp, *Tetrahedron* **34**, 2399 (1978). Cholinesterase inhibitor: Engelhart, Loewi, *Arch. Exp. Pathol. Pharmakol.* **150**, 1 (1930); Matthes, *J. Physiol.* **70**, 338 (1930). Toxicity data: W. T. Lynch, J. M. Coon, *Toxicol. Appl. Pharmacol.* **21**, 53 (1972); R D. Sofia, L. C. Knabloch, *ibid.* **28**, 227 (1974). Improvement of long-term memory: K. L. Davis *et al., Science* **201**, 272 (1978). Memory enhancement in Alzheimer's disease: L. J. Thal *et al., N. Engl. J. Med.* **308**, 720 (1983); *eidem, Ann. Neurol.* **13**, 491 (1983); L. Gustafson *et al., Psychopharmacology* **93**, 31 (1987). Review: B. Robinson in *The Alkaloids* **Vol. XIII**, R. H. F. Manske, Ed. (Academic Press, New York, 1971) pp 213-226. Comprehensive description: F. J. Muhtadi, S. S. El-Hawary, *Anal. Profiles Drug Subs.* **18**, 289-350 (1989).

Orthorhombic sphenoidal prisms or clusters of leaflets from ether or benzene. mp 105-106° (also an unstable, low-melting form, mp 86-87°). $[\alpha]_D^{17}$ $-76°$ (c = 1.3 in chloroform); $[\alpha]_D^{25}$ $-120°$ (benzene). pKa_1 6.12; pKa_2 12.24. Slightly sol in water; sol in alc, benzene, chloroform, oils. Solid and solns turn red on exposure to heat, light, air, and on contact with traces of metals. Under certain conditions the oxidation may proceed to yield *eserine blue*, C_{26}-$H_{31}N_5O_2$. LD_{50} orally in mice: 4.5 mg/kg (Lynch, Coon).

Salicylate. [57-64-7] Antilirium. $C_{22}H_{27}N_3O_5$; mol wt 413.47. Acicular crystals, mp 185-187°. uv max (methanol): 239, 252, 303 nm (log ε 4.09, 4.04, 3.78). One gram dissolves in 75 ml water at 25° (pH of 0.5% aq soln 5.8); in 16 ml water at 80°; in 16 ml alcohol, 5 ml boiling alcohol, in 6 ml chloroform, 250 ml ether. *Solns should be kept well closed in light-resistant, alkali-free glass containers and used within a week.* Turns red and loses effectiveness on exposure to heat, light, air. LD_{50} i.p. in mice: 0.64 mg/kg (Sofia, Knabloch).

Sulfate. [64-47-1] $(C_{15}H_{21}N_3O_2)_2.H_2SO_4$. Deliquescent scales, mp 140° (after drying at 100°). One gram dissolves in 0.4 ml alcohol, 4 ml water (pH of 0.05*M* soln 4.7), 1200 ml ether. The solns are more prone to change color than those of the salicylate.

Sulfite. $(C_{15}H_{21}N_3O_2)_2.H_2SO_3$. White powder, freely sol in water, alcohol. The aq soln is stated to remain colorless for a long time.

THERAP CAT: Cholinergic; miotic.

THERAP CAT (VET): Cholinergic; miotic.

7385. Physovenine. [6091-05-0] (3aS-cis)-3,3a,8,8a-Tetrahydro-3a,8-dimethyl-2H-furo[2,3-b]indol-5-ol methylcarbamate (ester). $C_{14}H_{18}N_2O_3$; mol wt 262.30. C 64.11%, H 6.92%, N 10.68%, O 18.30%. From seed of *Physostigma venenosum* Balf., *Leguminosae:* Salway, *J. Chem. Soc.* **99**, 2148 (1911). Structure: Robinson, *ibid.* **1964**, 1503. Synthesis: Longmore, Robinson, *Chem. Ind. (London)* **1965**, 1297. Abs config: *eidem, ibid.* **1969**, 622.

Plates from ether, mp 124-125°. $[\alpha]_D^{22.5}$ −92° (ethanol). uv max (ethanol): 252, 310 nm (ε 13200, 3300). Sol in alcohol, benzene, chloroform; slightly sol in ether. Practically insol in water, petr ether.

7386. Phytantriol. [74563-64-7] 3,7,11,15-Tetramethyl-1,2,3-hexadecanetriol; phytane-1,2,3-triol. $C_{20}H_{42}O_3$; mol wt 330.55. C 72.67%, H 12.81%, O 14.52%. Cosmetic ingredient; improves moisture retention properties of hair and skin; acts as a penetration enhancer to increase the effects of panthenol, vitamins, and amino acids. Prepn: W. Guex *et al.*, **DE 1149700** (1963 to F. Hoffmann-La Roche); T. C. Jain, R. J. Striha, *Can. J. Chem.* **47**, 4359 (1969). Cosmetic uses: E. Wagner, *Parfuem. Kosmet.* **75**, 260 (1994). Aqueous phase behavior: J. Barauskas, T. Landh, *Langmuir* **19**, 9562 (2003).

Light yellow oil, bp$_{0.01}$ 130° (Guex); also reported as white crystals from acetone-acetonitrile, mp 56-57° (Jain).

USE: Penetration enhancer in hair and skin care products.

7387. Phytic Acid. [83-86-3] *myo*-Inositol hexakis(dihydrogen phosphate); inositolhexaphosphoric acid; 1,2,3,4,5,6-cyclohexanehexolphosphoric acid; cyclohexanehexyl hexaphosphate; Alkalovert. $C_6H_{18}O_{24}P_6$; mol wt 660.04. C 10.92%, H 2.75%, O 58.18%, P 28.16%. $C_6H_6[OPO(OH)_2]_6$. Major phosphorus compound in plants; particularly abundant in oil seeds, legumes and cereal grains. Forms insoluble complexes with di- and trivalent cations. Prepn: S. Posternak, **US 1313014** (1919 to Ciba); *idem, Helv. Chim. Acta* **4**, 155 (1921); M. J. Thomas, **US 2718523** (1955 to Staley Mfg.); D. S. Bolley *et al.*, **US 2732395** (1956 to Natl. Lead Co.); A. R. Baldwin *et al.*, **US 2815360** (1957 to Corn Prods. Ref.). HPLC determn in plants: E. Graf, F. R. Dintzis, *Anal. Biochem.* **119**, 413 (1982); in foods and biological samples: B.E. Knuckles *et al., J. Food Sci.* **47**, 1257 (1982). Review of effect of dietary phytate on zinc metabolism: *Nutr. Rev.* **41**, 64-66 (1983); on mineral bioavailability: J. L. Kelsay, *Am. J. Gastroenterol.* **82**, 983-986 (1987).

Syrupy, straw-colored liquid. Dec on heating. Acid reaction; the pH of a 10% aq soln has been reported as 0.86. Miscible with water, 95% alc, glycerol; sol in water contg alcohol-ether mixtures; very slightly sol in abs alc, methanol. Practically insol in anhydr ether, benzene, chloroform.

Calcium iron salt. Obtained in the processing of corn. Grayish powder contg 20% Ca, 14% P, and 2% Fe. Sparingly sol in water, dil mineral acids.

Calcium magnesium salt. [3615-82-5] Phytin. White, odorless powder. Poor soly in water. Sol in dil acids.

Sodium salt. [7205-52-9] Sodium phytate; Phytat D.B.; Rencal. $C_6H_9Na_9O_{24}P_6$; mol wt 857.87. Soluble in water with neutral reaction.

USE: Complexing agent for the removal of traces of heavy metal ions (also employed as the sodium salt). Starting material in manufacture of inositol. Fermentation nutrient.

THERAP CAT: Sodium salt as hypocalcemic.

7388. Phytochlorin. [19660-77-6] 18-Carboxy-20-(carboxymethyl)-8-ethenyl-13-ethyl-2,3-dihydro-3,7,12,17-tetramethyl-21H,23H-porphine-2-propanoic acid; chlorin e_6; phytochlorin e. $C_{34}H_{36}N_4O_6$; mol wt 596.67. C 68.44%, H 6.08%, N 9.39%, O 16.09%. Prepn from broccoli-leaf extract: Wall, **US 2555583** (1951 to U.S.D.A.). *Review:* H. Fischer, A. Stern, *Die Chemie des Pyrrols* vol. **II**, 2 (Leipzig, 1940) pp 91-94; *The Chlorophylls*, L. P. Vernon, G. R. Seely, Eds. (Academic Press, New York, 1966) pp 9, 12, 71, 90, 95, 98, 142.

Greenish-brown rectangular plates. May contain one mol water. $[\alpha]_D^{20}$ −141° in acetone. Ether solns are olive-green with deep red fluorescence. Sparingly sol in ethanol, ether, acetone. Freely sol in pyridine.

7389. Phytofluene. [540-05-6] 7,7',8,8',11,12-Hexahydro-ψ,ψ-carotene; 5,6,7,8,9,10,10',9',8',7',6',5'-dodecahydrolycopene; *all-trans*-phytofluene. $C_{40}H_{68}$; mol wt 548.97. C 87.51%, H 12.49%. Polyene hydrocarbon widespread in the vegetable kingdom where it has been observed in chlorophyll-free tissues which contain considerable amounts of carotenoid pigments. Extracted from *Diospyros kaki* L.f., *Ebenaceae, Arbutus unedo* L., *Ericaceae, Pyracantha angustifolia* (Franch.) Schneid., *Rosaceae,* and tomatoes: Zechmeister, Sandonal, *J. Am. Chem. Soc.* **68**, 197 (1946); Wallace, Porter, *Arch. Biochem. Biophys.* **36**, 468 (1952); from the basidiomycete, *Dacromyces stillatus*: Goodwin, *Biochem. J.* **53**, 538 (1953). Structure: Porter, Lincoln, *Arch. Biochem. Biophys.* **27**, 390 (1950); Zechmeister, *Experientia* **10**, 1 (1954).

Pale orange, viscous oil which solidifies upon cooling, forming a glassy mass without apparent crystal structure. bp$_{0.0001}$ 140-185° (bath temp). uv max (petr ether): 367, 348, 332 nm. Freely sol in petr ether, ether, benzene. Practically insol in water, methanol, ethanol. Strong green fluorescence in ultraviolet spectra.

7390. Phytol. [150-86-7] (2E,7R,11R)-3,7,11,15-Tetramethyl-2-hexadecen-1-ol; 2,6,10,14-tetramethylhexadec-14-en-16-ol. $C_{20}H_{40}O$; mol wt 296.53. C 81.01%, H 13.60%, O 5.40%. Decompn product of chlorophyll: Willstätter, *Ann.* **354**, 205 (1907); **371**, 1 (1909); **378**, 1, 73 (1911); **418**, 121 (1918). Synthesis: Fischer, Löwenberg, *Ann.* **475**, 183 (1929); Karrer, Ringier, *Helv. Chim. Acta* **22**, 610 (1939); Karrer *et al., ibid.* **26**, 1741 (1943); from ethyl levulinate: Lukes, Zobacova, *Chem. Listy* **51**, 330 (1957); from acetone: Sato *et al., J. Org. Chem.* **32**, 177 (1967). Stereochemistry: Burrell *et al., Proc. Chem. Soc. London* **1959**, 263. Abs config: Crabbe *et al., ibid.* **1959**, 264. Stereochemistry and synthesis: Burrell *et al., J. Chem. Soc. C* **1966**, 2144. Stereoselective total synthesis of natural phytol: T. Fujisawa *et al., Tetrahedron Lett.* **22**, 4823 (1981); M. Schmid *et al., Helv. Chim. Acta* **65**, 684 (1982). *Review:* J. Simonsen, D. H. R. Barton, *The Terpenes* vol. **III** (Cambridge University Press, Cambridge, 1952) pp 345-349.

Oily liquid. d_4^{25} 0.8497. n_D^{25} 1.4595. bp$_{10}$ 203-204°; bp$_{0.03}$ 145°. uv max (abs alcohol): 212 nm (log ε 3.04), Bader, *Helv. Chim. Acta* **34**, 1632 (1951). Practically insol in water; sol in the usual organic solvents.

USE: Preparation of vitamins E and K$_1$.

7391. Phytolacca. Poke root; garget; pocan; American night-shade root; scoke. Dried root of *Phytolacca americana* L. (*P. decandra* L.), *Phytolaccaceae* (berries also used). *Habit*. North America; naturalized in Southern Europe. *Constit*. Resin, tannin, about 10% sugar; phytolaccine, phytolaccic acid, asparagine.

THERAP CAT: Antirheumatic; emetic; ectoparasiticide.

7392. Piberaline. [39640-15-8] 1-(Phenylmethyl)-4-(2-pyr-idinylcarbonyl)piperazine; 1-benzyl-4-picolinoylpiperazine; EGYT-475; Trelibet. C$_{17}$H$_{19}$N$_3$O; mol wt 281.35. C 72.57%, H 6.81%, N 14.94%, O 5.69%. Prepn: J. Körösi *et al.*, **BE 781494**; *eidem*, **US 3865828** (1972, 1975 both to EGYT). Alternate prepns: Z. Budai *et al.*, **DE 2828888** *C.A.* **90**, 168643u (1979); *eidem*, **HU 17182** *C.A.* **92**, 215463p (1980) (both 1979 to EGYT); *eidem*, *Acta Chim. Acad. Sci. Hung.* **105**, 241 (1980), *C.A.* **94**, 192275d (1981). HPLC separation: J. Borda *et al.*, *J. Chromatogr.* **258**, 271 (1983). Effect on avoidance behavior in rats: G. Telegdy *et al.*, *Arch. Int. Pharmacodyn. Ther.* **266**, 50 (1983). Metabolism in animals and humans: K. Magyar, *Pol. J. Pharmacol. Pharm.* **39**, 107 (1987). Mechanism of action study: K. Tekes *et al.*, *ibid.* 203.

Dihydrochloride. C$_{17}$H$_{19}$N$_3$O.2HCl. Crystals from ethanol, mp 214-215°.

Maleate. C$_{17}$H$_{19}$N$_3$O.C$_4$H$_4$O$_4$. Crystals, mp 169-170°.

Fumarate. C$_{17}$H$_{19}$N$_3$O.C$_4$H$_4$O$_4$. Crystals, mp 165°.

THERAP CAT: Antidepressant.

7393. Piboserod. [152811-62-6] *N*-[(1-Butyl-4-piperidin-yl)methyl]-3,4-dihydro-2*H*-[1,3]oxazino[3,2-*a*]indole-10-carboxamide; SB-207266. C$_{22}$H$_{31}$N$_3$O$_2$; mol wt 369.50. C 71.51%, H 8.46%, N 11.37%, O 8.66%. Selective 5-HT$_4$ receptor antagonist. Prepn: L. M. Gaster, P. A. Wyman, **WO 9318036**; *eidem*, **US 5852014** (1993, 1998 both to SKB). *In vitro* and *in vivo* studies of bioavailability, pharmacokinetics, and duration: K. A. Wardle *et al.*, *Br. J. Pharmacol.* **118**, 665 (1996). Effect on gastrointestinal function: G. J. Sanger *et al.*, *Neurogastroenterol. Motil.* **10**, 271 (1998); *idem et al.*, *Br. J. Pharmacol.* **130**, 706 (2000). Clinical evaluation in irritable bowel syndrome: L. A. Houghton *et al.*, *Aliment. Pharmacol. Ther.* **13**, 1437 (1999).

White solid from ether, mp 110-113°.

Hydrochloride. [178273-87-5] SB-207266A. C$_{22}$H$_{31}$N$_3$O$_2$.-HCl; mol wt 405.96. White crystals from ETOH/petrol, mp 254-256° (dec).

THERAP CAT: Gastroprokinetic

7394. Picaridin. [119515-38-7] 2-(2-Hydroxyethyl)-1-piperidinecarboxylic acid 1-methylpropyl ester; icaridin; 1-methyl-propyl 2-(2-hydroxyethyl)piperidine-1-carboxylate; hydroxyethyl isobutyl piperidine carboxylate; KBR 3023; Bayrepel. C$_{12}$H$_{23}$-NO$_3$; mol wt 229.32. C 62.85%, H 10.11%, N 6.11%, O 20.93%. Acts on certain olfactory receptor cell types to reduce the activating or attracting effect of odor sources. Prepn: B.-W. Krüger *et al.*, **EP 289842**; *eidem*, **US 4900834** (1988, 1990 both to Bayer). Synthesis and mode of action: J. Boeckh *et al.*, *Pestic. Sci.* **48**, 359 (1996).

Field trials in mosquito repellency: H. H. Yap *et al.*, *J. Vector Ecol.* **23**, 62 (1998); A. Badolo *et al.*, *Trop. Med. Int. Health* **9**, 330 (2004). Physical, chemical and toxicological properties: *WHO Interim Specification for Icaridin* (WHO/IS/TC/668/2001) 16 pp. MS characterization: T. P. Knepper, *J. Chromatogr. A* **1046**, 159 (2004).

Colorless, nearly odorless liquid. mp <−170°. bp$_{1013 \text{ hPa}}$ 280°. d^{20} 1.07. n_D^{20} 1.4717. Flash pt: 142°C. Log P (octanol/water) at 20°: 2.11 (unbuffered), 2.23 (pH 4-9). Vapor pressure (hPa): 3.4×10^{-4} at 20°; 5.9×10^{-4} at 25°; 7.1×10^{-3} at 50°. Soly at 20° (g/l): water 8.2 (pH 4-9), 8.6 (unbuffered); acetone 7250. Viscosity at 20°: 135.5 mPa s. LD$_{50}$ in rats (mg/kg): 4743 orally; >2000 dermally (Yap). LC$_{50}$ in rainbow trout (96 hr): 173 mg/l; in bobwhite quail (5 day diet): >5000 ppm a.i. in diet (WHO).

USE: Insect repellent.

7395. Picein. [530-14-3] 1-[4-(β-D-Glucopyranosyloxy)-phenyl]ethanone; *p*-(acetylphenyl)-β-D-glucopyranoside; 4′-(β-D-glucopyranosyloxy)acetophenone; *p*-hydroxyacetophenone-D-glucoside; piceoside; salinigrin; salicinerein; ameliaroside. C$_{14}$H$_{18}$-O$_7$; mol wt 298.29. C 56.37%, H 6.08%, O 37.55%. In needles and sprouts of *Pinus picea* L., *Picea excelsa* Link., *Picea glehnii* Mast., *Coniferae*: Tanret, *Bull. Soc. Chim.* [3] **11**, 944 (1894); Kariyone *et al.*, *Yakugaku Zasshi* **79**, 394 (1959), *C.A.* **53**, 14096i (1953). In various willow barks, especially in bark of *Salix discolor* Muhl., *S. nigra* Marsh., *Salicaceae*: Jowett, *J. Chem. Soc.* **77**, 707 (1900); Nonomura, *J. Pharm. Soc. Jpn.* **75**, 80 (1955). In English mistletoe, *Amelanchier vulgaris* Moench., *Rosaceae*: Bridel *et al.*, *Compt. Rend.* **187**, 56 (1928). Synthesis: Mauthner, *J. Prakt. Chem.* [2] **85**, 564 (1912).

Needles or prisms from methanol; mp 195-196°. $[\alpha]_D^{23}$ −88° (c = 1). One gram dissolves in 50 ml water at 15°, in 1 ml boiling water, in ∼650 ml abs alc at 15°, in ∼40 ml boiling abs alc, in 140 ml ethyl acetate at 15°. Sol in hot glacial acetic acid. Practically insol in ether, chloroform. Hydrolysis with dil mineral acids or with emulsin yields D-glucose and *p*-hydroxyacetophenone (**Piceol**). Alkaline hydrolysis yields levoglucosan and *p*-hydroxyaceto-phenone: Montgomery *et al.*, *J. Org. Chem.* **10**, 194 (1945).

7396. Picene. [213-46-7] 3,4-Benzchrysene; 1,2,7,8-di-benzphenanthrene; dibenzo[*a,i*]phenanthrene; β,β-binaphthylene-ethene. C$_{22}$H$_{14}$; mol wt 278.35. C 94.93%, H 5.07%. Found in tar oils from soft coal: Burg, *Ber.* **13**, 1834 (1880); Lang *et al.*, *ibid.* **97**, 494 (1964); in petroleum residues from the cracking process: Meyer, Hofmann, *Monatsh. Chem.* **37**, 681 (1916). Synthesis from cholic acid by selenium dehydrogenation: Ruzicka *et al.*, *Helv. Chim. Acta* **17**, 200 (1934); from *o*-xylylenedicyanide with *o*-nitro-benzaldehyde by a double Pschorr synthesis: Waldmann, Pitschak, *Ann.* **527**, 183 (1937); by a diene synthesis with tetrahydro-dinaphthyl and maleic anhydride: Weidlich, *Ber.* **71**, 1203 (1938); from 9,10-dihydrophenanthrene: Phillips, *J. Am. Chem. Soc.* **75**, 3223 (1953); from ethyl 4,6-dioxoheptane-1,5-dicarboxyl-ate: Nasipuri, *Chem. Ind. (London)* **1956**, 795.

Fluorescent plates from ethyl acetate, mp 366-367°. bp 518-520°. Absorption spectrum: Mayneord, Roe, *Proc. Roy. Soc. Lon-*

don **A152,** 319 (1935). Difficultly sol in most solvents. Somewhat sol in boiling benzene, chloroform, glacial acetic acid; more sol in cumene (isopropylbenzene).

7397. Picloram. [1918-02-1] 4-Amino-3,5,6-trichloro-2-pyridinecarboxylic acid; 4-amino-3,5,6-trichloropicolinic acid; Pinene; Tordon. $C_6H_3Cl_3N_2O_2$; mol wt 241.46. C 29.85%, H 1.25%, Cl 44.05%, N 11.60%, O 13.25%. Plant growth regulator. Prepn: H. Johnston, M. S. Tomita, **BE 628487;** *eidem,* **US 3285925** (1963, 1966 both to Dow). Activity: J. W. Hamaker *et al., Science* **141,** 363 (1963). Carcinogenicity study: M. D. Reuber, *J. Toxicol. Environ. Health* **7,** 207 (1981). Review of properties and analytical methods: J. R. Ramsey, *Anal. Methods Pestic. Plant Growth Regul. Food Addit.* **5,** 507-525 (1967); of toxicology and environmental fate: W. R. Mullison, *Proc. West. Soc. Weed Sci.* **38,** 21-92 (1985).

White powder, mp 218-219° with decomp starting at 190°. Readily sublimes at 190° under 12 mm Hg. Vapor pressure at 45°: 1.07×10^{-6} mm Hg. pKa 4.1. Soly at 25° (ppm): acetone 19800; ethanol 10500; acetonitrile 1600; ethyl ether 1200; water 430; benzene 200; carbon disulfide 50. LD_{50} in rats, mice, rabbits, guinea pig, chickens, sheep, cattle (mg/kg): 8200, 2000-4000, 2000, 3000, 6000, >1000, >750 orally (Mullison).

Caution: Potential symptoms of overexposure are irritation of eyes, skin, respiratory system; nausea. *See NIOSH Pocket Guide to Chemical Hazards* (DHHS/NIOSH 97-140, 1997) p 258.

USE: Herbicide.

7398. Picloxydine. [5636-92-0] *N,N''*-Bis[[(4-chlorophenyl)amino]iminomethyl]-1,4-piperazine dicarboximidamide; *N,N''*-bis[(*p*-chlorophenyl)amidino]-1,4-piperazinedicarboxamidine; 1,4-bis(*N*⁴'-*p*-chlorophenylamidinoamidinyl)piperazine; 1,1'-[1,4-piperazinediylbis(imidocarbonyl)]bis[3-(*p*-chlorophenyl)guanidine]. $C_{20}H_{24}Cl_2N_{10}$; mol wt 475.38. C 50.53%, H 5.09%, Cl 14.92%, N 29.46%. Heterocyclic biguanide with antibacterial activity. Prepn: J. W. James, L. F. Wiggins, **GB 855017;** *eidem,* **US 3101336** (1960, 1963 both to Aspro-Nicholas). Prepn and antibacterial spectrum: J. W. James *et al., J. Med. Chem.* **11,** 942 (1968). Bactericidal effect in disinfectant formulations: A. M. Gordon, *J. Clin. Pathol.* **22,** 496 (1969). Mode of action study: B. D. Rawal, J. V. Hardy, *Microbios* **14,** 135 (1974). *In vitro* activity vs *Chlamydia trachomatis:* D. Thomas *et al., Pathol. Biol.* **32,** 544 (1984).

Dihydrochloride. [19803-62-4] Vitabact. $C_{20}H_{24}Cl_2N_{10} \cdot 2 \cdot HCl$; mol wt 548.30. Crystals from water, mp 274°. LD_{50} in mice (mg/kg): 150 i.p. (James).

THERAP CAT: Antibacterial (topical).

7399. Picolinafen. [137641-05-5] *N*-(4-Fluorophenyl)-6-[3-(trifluoromethyl)phenoxy]-2-pyridinecarboxamide; 4'-fluoro-6-[(α,α,α-trifluoro-*m*-tolyl)oxy]picolinanilide; AC-900001; Pico. $C_{19}H_{12}F_4N_2O_2$; mol wt 376.30. C 60.64%, H 3.21%, F 20.19%, N 7.44%, O 8.50%. Aryloxypicolinamide herbicide for use in barley and wheat. Inhibits phytoene desaturase, an enzyme involved in carotenoid biosynthesis. Prepn: C. J. Foster *et al., EP 447004;* *eidem,* **US 5294597** (1991, 1994 both to Shell). Comprehensive description of properties and field trials: R. H. White *et al., Brighton Crop Prot. Conf. - Weeds* **1999,** 47-52.

White to chalky-white, finely crystalline solid, mp 107.2-107.6°. Vapor pressure (20°): 1.66×10^{-7} Pa (est.). Log P (octanol/water): 5.36-5.43 (pH 5-9). Soly in water (20°): $3.8-4.7 \times 10^{-5}$ g/l. LD_{50} in rats (mg/kg): >5000 orally; >4000 dermally. LC_{50} in rats (mg/l): >5.9 by inhalation. LC_{50} in rainbow trout (96 hr): 0.281 mg/l (White).

USE: Herbicide.

7400. α-Picoline. [109-06-8] 2-Methylpyridine. C_6H_7N; mol wt 93.13. C 77.38%, H 7.58%, N 15.04%. Found in coal tar and in bone oil. Synthesis (40-50% yield) from cyclohexylamine with excess ammonia and zinc chloride at 350°: Nordt, *PB Report 704* (1941). Prepn from ethylene-mercuric acetate adduct and ammonia water (70% yield): Gumboldt, Feichtinger, *Z. Naturforsch.* **4b,** 123 (1949). Toxicity study: H. F. Smyth *et al., Arch. Ind. Hyg. Occup. Med.* **4,** 119 (1951). Physical properties: Biddiscombe *et al., J. Chem. Soc.* **1954,** 1957. Review of the various methods of condensing aldehydes, ketones, ethylene, butadiene, etc., with ammonia: F. Brody, P. R. Ruby in A. Weissberger, *The Chemistry of Heterocyclic Compounds* vol. **14,** part I (New York, 1960) pp 99-589. Contains 1851 references.

Colorless liquid; strong unpleasant odor. mp −70°. bp 128-129°. d_4^{15} 0.950; n_D^{20} 1.501. Freely sol in water; miscible with alcohol, ether. LD_{50} orally in rats: 1.41 g/kg (Smyth).

Caution: Irritating to respiratory tract.

USE: Solvent; intermediate in the dye and resins industries.

7401. β-Picoline. [108-99-6] 3-Methylpyridine. C_6H_7N; mol wt 93.13. C 77.38%, H 7.58%, N 15.04%.

Colorless liq; sweetish, not unpleasant odor. d_4^{15} 0.9613; bp 143-144°; n_D^{24} 1.5043. Miscible with water, alcohol, ether.

USE: Solvent; intermediate in the dye and resins industries; in the manuf of insecticides, waterproofing agents, niacin, and niacinamide.

7402. γ-Picoline. [108-89-4] 4-Methylpyridine; 4-picoline. C_6H_7N; mol wt 93.13. C 77.38%, H 7.58%, N 15.04%. Found in coal tar, in bone oil, in urine of horses. Isoln from technical picolines: Flaschner, *J. Chem. Soc.* **95,** 669 (1909). Toxicity study: H. F. Smyth *et al., Arch. Ind. Hyg. Occup. Med.* **10,** 61 (1954).

Flammable liquid. Obnoxious, sweetish odor. Turns brown if not very pure. d_4^{15} 0.9571. bp_{760} 145°. n_D^{17} 1.5064. Kb at 25° = 1.1×10^{-8}. Sol in water, alcohol, ether. LD_{50} orally in rats: 1.29 g/kg (Smyth).

USE: Manuf isonicotinic acid and derivatives. In waterproofing agents for fabrics. As solvent for resins.

7403. Picolinic Acid. [98-98-6] 2-Pyridinecarboxylic acid; *o*-pyridinecarboxylic acid. $C_6H_5NO_2$; mol wt 123.11. C 58.54%, H 4.09%, N 11.38%, O 25.99%. Naturally occuring isomer of nicotinic acid; by-product of tryptophan catabolism. Prepn: Singer, McElvain, *Org. Synth.* **coll. vol. III,** 740 (1955). *Review:* Oliveto, "Pyridinecarboxylic Acids" in *Pyridine and Its Derivatives* **Part 3,** E. Klingsberg, Ed. (Interscience, New York, 1962) p 179. Review of immunobiology and effect on macrophage activation: G. Melillo *et al., Adv. Exp. Med. Biol.* **398,** 135-141 (1996). HPLC determn in biological fluids: C. Dazzi *et al., J. Chromatogr. B* **751,** 61 (2001).

Needles from water, alcohol or benzene, mp 134-136°. pK 5.4. Sublimes. Very sol in glacial acetic acid; practically insol in ether, chloroform, carbon disulfide.

Hydrochloride. Crystals from abs ethanol/ether, mp 210-212° (slow heating).

7404. Picoperine. [21755-66-8] *N*-Phenyl-*N*-[2-(1-piperidinyl)ethyl]-2-pyridinemethanamine; 1-[2-[*N*-(2-pyridylmethyl)-anilino]ethyl]piperidine; *N*-(2-pyridylmethyl)-*N*-phenyl-*N*-(2-piperidinoethyl)amine; 1-[2-[phenyl(2-pyridylmethyl)amino]ethyl]piperidine; *N*-(2-picolyl)-*N*-phenyl-*N*-(2-piperidinoethyl)amine; *N*-(2-piperidinoethyl)-*N*-(2-pyridylmethyl)aniline; *N*-phenyl-*N*-(2-pyridylmethyl)-2-piperidinoethylamine; picoperidamine; TAT-3. $C_{19}H_{25}N_3$; mol wt 295.42. C 77.25%, H 8.53%, N 14.22%. Prepn: **FR 1511398** and **US 3471501** (1968 and 1969 to Takeda); Miyano *et al.*, *J. Med. Chem.* **13**, 704 (1970). Prepn of salts: Sawa *et al.*, *Takeda Kenkyusho* **29**(2), 275 (1970), *C.A.* **73**, 98758h (1970); Masuda *et al.*, *DE 1935172* (1970 to Takeda), *C.A.* **73**, 98818c (1970). Pharmacology: Y. Kasé *et al.*, *Arzneim.-Forsch.* **19**, 1916 (1969); *eidem, ibid.* **20**, 37 (1970). *Review: Jpn. Med. Gaz.* **8**(11), 9 (1971).

Pale yellow liquid, bp_4 195-196°.

Hydrochloride. [24699-40-9] Coben. $C_{19}H_{25}N_3 \cdot HCl$; mol wt 331.88. Water-soluble white crystalline powder, odorless with slightly bitter taste, mp 183-185°. Freely sol in ethanol and chloroform. Slightly sol in acetone, dioxane, benzene. Practically insol in hexane, ether. LD_{50} in mice (mg/kg): 210 s.c.; 85 i.p.; 17 i.v.; 240 orally (Kasé, 1969).

Tripalmitate. [24656-22-2] Coben P. $C_{19}H_{25}N_3 \cdot 3C_{16}H_{32}O_2$; mol wt 1064.69. White, tasteless, odorless crystalline powder, mp 57-60°. Freely sol in ethanol, chloroform; slightly sol in dioxane, acetone, benzene. Practically insol in hexane, water. LD_{50} orally in mice: 1900 mg/kg (Kasé, 1969).

THERAP CAT: Antitussive.

7405. Picoplatin. [181630-15-9] (*SP*-4-3)-Amminedichloro(2-methylpyridine)platinum; *cis*-amminedichloro(2-methylpyridine)platinum(II); AMD-473; JM-473; NX-473; ZD-473. $C_6H_{10}Cl_2N_2Pt$; mol wt 376.15. C 19.16%, H 2.68%, Cl 18.85%, N 7.45%, Pt 51.86%. Third generation, sterically hindered Pt-complex that exhibits reduced reactivity with sulfur ligands such as glutathione, *q.v.*; designed to overcome acquired Pt-chemotherapy resistance. Prepn: B. A. Murrer, **EP 727430** (1996 to AnorMED; Inst. of Cancer Research); *idem*, **US 5665771** (1997 to Johnson Matthey). Pharmacology and pharmacokinetics: F. I. Raynaud *et al.*, *Clin. Cancer Res.* **3**, 2063 (1997). Cytotoxicity and DNA binding activity: J. Holford *et al.*, *Anti-Cancer Drug Design* **13**, 1 (1998). *In vitro* circumvention of cisplatin resistance: *idem, et al,. Br. J. Cancer* **77**, 366 (1998); of radiosensitizing activity: G. P. Raaphorst *et al.*, *Anticancer Res.* **24**, 613 (2004). LC/MS determn in plasma: T. Oe *et al.*, *Anal. Chem.* **74**, 591 (2002); in urine: *eidem, J. Chromatogr. B* **792**, 217 (2003). Series of articles on clinical evaluations: *Eur. J. Cancer* **38**, Suppl. S1-S31 (2002). Review of early development: L. R. Kelland *et al.*, *J. Inorg. Biochem.* **77**, 111-115 (1999); and therapeutic potential: M. P. Hay, *Curr. Opin. Invest. Drugs* **1**, 263-266 (2000).

Pale yellow solid. *Sensitive to light.* uv max (0.15*M* sodium chloride): 268 nm. $A_{250}/A_{268} = 0.62$. LD_{50} in mice (mg/kg): 43 i.p., 560 orally (Murrer).

THERAP CAT: Antineoplastic.

7406. Picosulfate Sodium. [10040-45-6] 4,4'-(2-Pyridinylmethylene)bisphenol bis(hydrogen sulfate) (ester) disodium salt; 4,4'-(2-pyridylmethyl)diphenolbis(hydrogen sulfate) (ester) disodium salt; 4,4'-(2-picolidene)bis(phenylsulfuric acid) disodium salt; 2-picolylidenebis(*p*-phenyl sodium sulfate); disodium 4,4'-disulfoxydiphenyl-(2-pyridyl)methane; picosulfol; sodium picosulfate; Guttalax-Fher; Laxoberal; Laxoberon; Neopax; Pico-Salax. $C_{18}H_{13}NNa_2O_8S_2$; mol wt 481.41. C 44.91%, H 2.72%, N 2.91%, Na 9.55%, O 26.59%, S 13.32%. Prepn: Pala, **FR M5832** and **US 3528986**, **US 3558643** (1968, 1970, 1971 all to Ist. de Angeli); Seeger, Machleidt, **DE 1904322** (1970 to Thomae). Synthesis and physical-chemical data: Pala *et al.*, *Helv. Chim. Acta* **51**, 1164 (1968). Pharmacology: Pala *et al.*, *Arch. Int. Pharmacodyn. Ther.* **164**, 356 (1966). Metabolism: Perego *et al.*, *Arzneim.-Forsch.* **19**, 1889 (1969).

White crystalline solid from ethanol or methanol, mp 272-275° (dec). uv max (H2O): 218, 262 nm (ε 20450, 6075). Readily sol in water; slightly sol in alcohol. Practically insol in most organic solvents.

THERAP CAT: Cathartic.

7407. Picotamide. [32828-81-2] 4-Methoxy-*N,N'*-bis(3-pyridinylmethyl)-1,3-benzenedicarboxamide; 4-methoxy-*N,N'*-bis(3-pyridylmethyl)isophthalamide; *N,N'*-bis(3-picolyl)-4-methoxyisophthalamide; G-137. $C_{21}H_{20}N_4O_3$; mol wt 376.41. C 67.01%, H 5.36%, N 14.88%, O 12.75%. Prepn: R. Selleri *et al.*, *Chim. Ther.* **6**, 203 (1971); G. Orzalesi, R. Selleri, **FR 2100850** *C.A.* **77**, 164502f (1972); prepn and use as inhibitor of blood platelet aggregation: *eidem*, **US 3973026** (1972, 1976 both to Soc. Italo-Brit. L. Manetti-H. Roberts). Crystal structure of monohydrate: E. Foresti *et al.*, *Acta Crystallogr.* **C42**, 220 (1986). Mechanism of action study: M. Berrettini *et al.*, *Boll. Soc. Ital. Biol. Sper.* **59**, 309 (1983). Clinical studies: R. Schmutzler *et al.*, *Age Ageing* **7**, 246 (1978); V. Coto *et al.*, *Minerva Cardioangiol.* **34**, 601 (1986).

Crystalline powder from benzene, mp 124°. LD_{50} i.p. in male mice: 1205 mg/kg (Orzalesi, Selleri, 1976).

Monohydrate. [80530-63-8] Plactidil. $C_{21}H_{20}N_4O_3 \cdot H_2O$; mol wt 394.42.

THERAP CAT: Antithrombotic; fibrinolytic; anticoagulant.

7408. Picoxystrobin. [117428-22-5] (*αE*)-α-(Methoxymethylene)-2-[[[6-(trifluoromethyl)-2-pyridinyl]oxy]methyl]benzeneacetic acid methyl ester; methyl (*E*)-2-[2-[6-(trifluoromethyl)pyridin-2-yloxymethyl]phenyl]-3-methoxyacrylate; ZA-1963; Acanto. $C_{18}H_{16}F_3NO_4$; mol wt 367.32. C 58.86%, H 4.39%, F 15.52%, N 3.81%, O 17.42%. Strobilurin fungicide for use in cereal crops. Prepn: J. M. Clough *et al.*, **EP 278595**; *eidem*, **US 5021581** (1988, 1991 both to ICI). Comprehensive description: J. R. Godwin *et al.*, *Brighton Crop Prot. Conf. - Pests Dis.* **2000**, 533-540; M. Hiemer *et al.*, *Gesunde Pflanz.* **53**, 191-195 (2001).

Consult the Name Index before using this section.

Solid, mp 75°. d^{20} 1.4. Vapor pressure at 20°: 5.5×10^{-9} kPa. Log P (n-octanol/water) at 20°: 3.6. Soly in water (20°): 3.1 mg/l. MLD in rats (mg/kg): >5000 orally; >2000 dermally; MLC in rats (mg/l): 2.12 by inhalation (Godwin).

USE: Agricultural fungicide.

7409. Picramic Acid. [96-91-3] 2-Amino-4,6-dinitrophenol; 4,6-dinitro-2-aminophenol. $C_6H_5N_3O_5$; mol wt 199.12. C 36.19%, H 2.53%, N 21.10%, O 40.18%. Prepd from picric acid, concd NH_4OH, and H_2S followed by acetic acid neutralization of ammonium salt: Egerer, *J. Biol. Chem.* **35**, 565 (1918). Prepn of ammonium salt from picric acid, aqueous NH_3-soln, and ammonium sulfide: Dehn, **US 1472791** (1924).

Dark red needles from alcohol, prisms from chloroform. mp 169-170°. At 22-25°, 0.065 g dissolves in 100 ml H_2O; not much more sol in hot water. Sparingly sol in ether, chloroform; moderately sol in alcohol; sol in benzene, glacial acetic acid, aniline. Flashes at 210°; in contact with open flame in glass tube or beaker, ignites rapidly and burns relatively fast: Blinov, *Khim. Prom.* **1959**, 419, *C.A.* **55**, 6866d (1961).

Caution: Toxic symptoms similar to 2,4-dinitrophenol, *q.v.*

USE: Manuf of azo dyes; rarely as indicator (yellow with acids, red with alkalies); reagent for albumin.

7410. Picric Acid. [88-89-1] 2,4,6-Trinitrophenol; picronitric acid; carbazotic acid; nitroxanthic acid. $C_6H_3N_3O_7$; mol wt 229.10. C 31.46%, H 1.32%, N 18.34%, O 48.89%. Prepd by sulfonating phenol then treating with nitric acid: Olsen, Goldstein, *Ind. Eng. Chem.* **16**, 66 (1924); by treating benzene with nitric acid and mercuric nitrate: Teeters, Mueller, **US 2455322** (1948 to Allied Chem.); by nitration of 2-*tert*-butyl-4,6-dinitropenol: Ley, Müller, *Ber.* **89**, 1402 (1956). Crystal structure: E. N. Duesler *et al.*, *Cryst. Struct. Commun.* **7**, 449 (1978).

Pale yellow, odorless, intensely bitter crystals. d 1.763. mp 122-123°. Explodes above 300°. One gram dissolves in 78 ml water, 15 ml boiling water, 12 ml alc, 10 ml benzene, 35 ml chloroform, 65 ml ether. *Keep in a cool place and remote from fire. Explodes when rapidly heated or by percussion! Note:* For safety in transportation, 10-20% water is usually added.

Caution: Potential symptoms of overexposure are irritation of eyes, skin; sensitization dermatitis; yellow stained hair, skin; weakness, myalgia, anuria, polyuria; bitter taste, GI disturbances; hepatitis; hematuria, albuminuria, nephritis. *See NIOSH Pocket Guide to Chemical Hazards* (DHHS/NIOSH 97-140, 1997) p 258; *Clinical Toxicology of Commercial Products*, R. E. Gosselin *et al.*, Eds. (Williams & Wilkins, Baltimore, 5th ed., 1984) Section II, p 197.

USE: Explosives; matches; in leather industry; electric batteries; etching copper; manuf colored glass; textile mordant; also as reagent.

7411. Picrocrocin. [138-55-6] (4R)-4-(β-D-Glucopyranosyloxy)-2,6,6-trimethyl-1-cyclohexene-1-carboxaldehyde; saffronbitter. $C_{16}H_{26}O_7$; mol wt 330.37. C 58.17%, H 7.93%, O 33.90%. From stigmas of *Crocus sativus* L., *Iridaceae*. Isoln: Kayser, *Ber.* **17**, 2228 (1884). Structure: Kuhn, Winterstein, *Ber.* **67**, 344 (1934). Exerts sex-determining influences in the plant organism: Kuhn, *Angew. Chem.* **53**, 1 (1940). Its moieties are glucose and safranal, *q.q.v.* Abs config: Buchecker, Eugster, *Helv. Chim. Acta* **56**, 1121 (1973). Synthesis: H. Mayer, J.-M. Santer, *Helv. Chim. Acta* **63**, 1463 (1980).

Crystals, mp 154-156°. $[\alpha]_D^{20}$ −58° (c = 0.6). Bitter taste. Alkali unstable. Sol in water, alcohol; slightly sol in chloroform, ether. Practically insol in petr ether, benzene.

7412. Picrolonic Acid. [550-74-3] 2,4-Dihydro-5-methyl-4-nitro-2-(4-nitrophenyl)-3H-pyrazol-3-one; 3-methyl-4-nitro-1-(p-nitrophenyl)-2-pyrazolin-5-one. $C_{10}H_8N_4O_5$; mol wt 264.19. C 45.46%, H 3.05%, N 21.21%, O 30.28%.

Yellow leaflets, mp 116-117°; dec at 125°. Sparingly sol in water; sol in alcohol.

USE: As reagent for alkaloids, tryptophan, phenylalanine, and for the detection and estimation of calcium.

7413. Picromycin. [19721-56-3] (E)-14-Ethyl-13-hydroxy-3,5,7,9,13-pentamethyl-6-[[3,4,6-trideoxy-3-(dimethylamino)-β-D-xylo-hexopyranoside]oxy]oxacyclotetradec-11-ene-2,4,10-trione; pikromycin; albomycetin; amaromycin. $C_{28}H_{47}NO_8$; mol wt 525.67. C 63.98%, H 9.01%, N 2.66%, O 24.35%. First macrolide antibiotic isolated. Isoln from *Actinomyces* spp by Lindenbein and Bauer, *see* Brockmann, Henkel, *Naturwissenschaften* **37**, 138 (1950); *Ber.* **84**, 284 (1951); Brockmann, Bohne, **US 2693433** (1954 to Schenley). Structure: Brockmann, Oster, *Ber.* **90**, 605 (1957); Anliker, Gubler, *Helv. Chim. Acta* **40**, 119, 1768 (1957). Studies in stereochemistry: Djerassi, Halpern, *J. Am. Chem. Soc.* **79**, 3926 (1957); Ogura *et al.*, *ibid.* **97**, 1930 (1975); *eidem*, *Tetrahedron* **37**, Suppl. 1, 165 (1981). Revised structure: Rickards, Smith, *Chem. Commun.* **1968**, 1049; Muxfeldt *et al.*, *J. Am. Chem. Soc.* **90**, 4748 (1968). Synthesis from narbonolide: Maezawa *et al.*, *J. Antibiot.* **26**, 771 (1973).

Very bitter, rectangular platelets from methanol, mp 169.5-170°. Stable to heat. $[\alpha]_D^{24}$ +8.2° (c = 3.5 in ethanol); $[\alpha]_D^{20}$ −33.5° (c = 2.07 in chloroform); $[\alpha]_D^{24}$ −50.2° (c = 6.3 in chloroform). uv max (ethanol): 225 nm (log ε 3.97). Rotary dispersion data: Djerassi, Halpern, *Tetrahedron* **3**, 268 (1958). Very sparingly sol in water, petr ether, carbon disulfide. Soly in ethanol: 3.5 g/100 ml at 20°. Freely sol in acetone, benzene, chloroform, ethyl acetate, dioxane. Moderately sol in ether, methanol.

7414. Picrotin. [21416-53-5] (1a*R*,2a*R*,3*S*,6*R*,6a*S*,8a*S*,-8b*R*,9*S*)-Hexahydro-2a-hydroxy-9-(1-hydroxy-1-methylethyl)-8b-methyl-3,6-methano-8*H*-1,5,7-trioxacyclopenta[*ij*]cycloprop[*a*]azulene-4,8(3*H*)-dione. $C_{15}H_{18}O_7$; mol wt 310.30. C 58.06%, H 5.85%, O 36.09%. Nontoxic component of picrotoxin. Prepn from picrotoxin: Meyer, Bruges, *Ber.* **31**, 2958 (1898). Structure studies: Bensted *et al., J. Chem. Soc.* **1952**, 1042; Slater, Wilson, *ibid.* 1597; Holker *et al., ibid.* **1958**, 2987. Total synthesis: E. J. Corey, H. L. Pearce, *Tetrahedron Lett.* **21**, 1823 (1980). Toxicity data: C. H. Jarboe *et al., J. Med. Chem.* **11**, 729 (1968). *Review:* Porter, *Chem. Rev.* **67**, 441 (1967).

Fine needles from water; thick, shiny prisms from aq alc soln, mp 248-250°. $[\alpha]_D$ −64.7° (c = 2.31 in abs alc). Freely sol in abs alc, acetic acid, boiling water. Slightly sol in cold water. Practically insol in ether, chloroform, benzene. LD_{50} i.p. in mice: 135 mg/kg (Jarboe).

7415. Picrotoxin. [124-87-8] Cocculin. $C_{30}H_{34}O_{13}$; mol wt 602.58. C 59.80%, H 5.69%, O 34.52%. Bitter principle isolated from the seed of *Anamirta cocculus* L. Wight & Arn., *Menispermaceae*, also found in *Tinomiscium philippinense* Diels. Molecular compd of one mole picrotoxinin and one mole picrotin, *q.q.v.*, into which it is readily separated. Extraction procedure: Clark, *J. Am. Chem. Soc.* **57**, 1111 (1935). Chemical bibliography: *Helv. Chim. Acta* **32**, 1859 (1949). Crystal and molecular structure: L. Dupont *et al., Acta Crystallogr.* **B32**, 2987 (1976). Toxicity study: I. Setnikar *et al., J. Pharmacol. Exp. Ther.* **128**, 176 (1960).

Intensely bitter shiny rhomboid leaflets, mp 203°. *Very poisonous!* $[\alpha]_D^{16}$ −29.3° (c = 4 in abs ethanol). One gram dissolves in ~350 ml water, in ~5 ml boiling water, in 13.5 ml 95% ethanol, in ~3 ml boiling alcohol. Sparingly sol in ether, chloroform. Readily sol in strong ammonia water, in aq solns of NaOH. Highly toxic to fish. LD_{50} i.p. in mice: 7.2 mg/kg (Setnikar).

THERAP CAT: CNS and respiratory stimulant.

THERAP CAT (VET): CNS stimulant, antidote to barbiturates.

7416. Picrotoxinin. [17617-45-7] (1a*R*,2a*R*,3*S*,6*R*,6a*S*,-8a*S*,8b*R*,9*R*)-Hexahydro-2a-hydroxy-8b-methyl-9-(1-methylethenyl)-3,6-methano-8*H*-1,5,7-trioxacyclopenta[*ij*]cycloprop[*a*]azulene-4,8(3*H*)-dione. $C_{15}H_{16}O_6$; mol wt 292.28. C 61.64%, H 5.52%, O 32.84%. Toxic component of picrotoxin, *q.v.* Prepn from picrotoxin: Horrmann, *Ber.* **45**, 2090 (1912). Structure: Conroy, *J. Am. Chem. Soc.* **73**, 1889 (1951); **79**, 5550 (1957); Craven, *Tetrahedron Lett.* no. 19, 21 (1960). Total synthesis: E. J. Corey, H. L. Pearce, *J. Am. Chem. Soc.* **101**, 5841 (1979). Structure-activity relationship: C. H. Jarboe *et al., J. Med. Chem.* **11**, 729 (1968). *Review:* Porter, *Chem. Rev.* **67**, 441 (1967).

Very bitter large prisms or small crystals contg water, mp 209.5°. $[\alpha]_D^{17}$ +4.4° (c = 4.28 in abs alc), +3.49° (c = 7.57 in acetone). Soluble in hot common organic solvents, in cold alcohol and chloroform. LD_{50} i.p. in mice: 3 mg/kg (Jarboe).

7417. Picryl Chloride. [88-88-0] 2-Chloro-1,3,5-trinitrobenzene. $C_6H_2ClN_3O_6$; mol wt 247.55. C 29.11%, H 0.81%, Cl 14.32%, N 16.97%, O 38.78%.

Almost white needles. d 1.797. mp 83°. Insol in water; freely sol in benzene, hot chloroform, boiling alcohol, slightly in ether or petr ether.

7418. Picumast. [39577-19-0] 7-[3-[4-[(4-Chlorophenyl)methyl]-1-piperazinyl]propoxy]-3,4-dimethyl-2*H*-1-benzopyran-2-one; 7-[3-[4-(*p*-chlorobenzyl)-1-piperazinyl]propoxy]-3,4-dimethylcoumarin; 1-(4-chlorobenzyl)-4-[3-(3,4-dimethylcoumarin-7-yl-oxy)propyl]piperazine. $C_{25}H_{29}ClN_2O_3$; mol wt 440.96. C 68.09%, H 6.63%, Cl 8.04%, N 6.35%, O 10.88%. Mast cell degranulation inhibitor with histamine antagonist activity. Prepn: E. C. Witte *et al.,* **DE 2123924**; *eidem,* **US 3810898** (1972, 1974 both to Boehringer, Mann.); E. C. Witte, *Arzneim.-Forsch.* **39**, 1309 (1989). Mechanism of action studies: O. H. Wilhelms, *Int. Arch. Allergy Appl. Immunol.* **82**, 544, 547 (1987). Series of articles on pharmacology, pharmacokinetics, and clinical trials: *Arzneim.-Forsch.* **39**, 1307-1376 (1989).

Crystals from isopropanol, mp 112-114° (Witte, 1974); also reported as mp 115-117° (Witte, 1989).

Dihydrochloride. [39577-20-3] BM-15100; Auteral. $C_{25}H_{29}ClN_2O_3.2HCl$; mol wt 513.88. Crystals from aq ethanol, mp 266-268°.

THERAP CAT: Antiallergic.

7419. Pidotimod. [121808-62-6] (4*R*)-3-[[(2*S*)-5-Oxo-2-pyrrolidinyl]carbonyl]-4-thiazolidinecarboxylic acid; 3-L-pyroglutamyl-L-thiazolidine-4-carboxylic acid; (*R*)-3-[(*S*)-5-oxoprolyl]-4-thiazolidinecarboxylic acid; PGT/1A; Axil; Onaka; Pigitil; Polimod. $C_9H_{12}N_2O_4S$; mol wt 244.27. C 44.25%, H 4.95%, N 11.47%, O 26.20%, S 13.13%. Peptide-like biological response modifier. Prepn: S. Poli, **EP 276752**; *idem,* **US 4839387** (1988, 1989 both to Poli). Immunostimulant effect in mice: A. Vacca *et al., Int. J. Immunother.* **9**, 85 (1993); on human peripheral blood monocytes: M. O. Borghi *et al., ibid.* **10**, 35 (1994). HPLC determn in plasma and urine: G. Coppi, M. Barchielli, *J. Chromatogr.* **563**, 385 (1991). Clinical trial in recurrent acute tonsillitis: P. Careddu *et al., Adv. Otorhinolaryngol.* **47**, 328 (1992). Toxicity study: G. Coppi *et al., Arzneim.-Forsch.* **44**, 1448 (1994). Series of articles on chemistry, pharmacology, toxicology and clinical experience: *ibid.,* 1399-1530.

White or slightly ivory, odorless microcrystalline powder, mp 194-198° (dec). Also reported as white crystals from water, mp 192-194° (Poli). $[\alpha]_D^{25}$ −150° (c = 2 in 5*N* HCl). pKa 3.03. Soly (g/l): water 37.8; methanol 13.8; ethanol 4.4; DMF 72.4. Practically insol in chloroform, hexane. LD_{50} in mice and rats (mg/kg): >4000 i.v.; >4000 i.m.; >8000 i.p.; >8000 orally (Coppi).

THERAP CAT: Immunomodulator.

7420. Pifarnine. [56208-01-6] 1-(1,3-Benzodioxol-5-ylmethyl)-4-(3,7,11-trimethyl-2,6,10-dodecatrienyl)piperazine; 1-piperonyl-4-(3,7,11-trimethyl-2,6,10-dodecatrienyl)piperazine; U-27; Pifazin. $C_{27}H_{40}N_2O_2$; mol wt 424.62. C 76.37%, H 9.49%, N 6.60%, O 7.54%. Non-anticholinergic gastric anti-secretory agent.

Prepn: S. Tricerri *et al.*, **DE 2310044** corresp to **US 3875163** (1973, 1975 both to Pierrel); *eidem, Eur. J. Med. Chem.* **9**, 555 (1974). Pifarnine is a mixture of four stereoisomers: *ZZ, EZ, ZE, EE*. Separation does not give compounds with significantly different activity/toxicity ratios from the mixture. Stereochemistry and pharmacology of the four isomers: G. Guadagnini *et al., ibid.* **10**, 585 (1975). Pharmacological study of pifarnine: A. Bianchetti *et al., Arzneim.-Forsch.* **25**, 580 (1975). Physical-chemical and analytical studies: G. Guadagnini *et al., Pharm. Ind.* **38**, 296 (1976). Absorption, distribution, excretion: M. Riva *et al., Farmaco Ed. Prat.* **34**, 542 (1979). Clinical studies: A. Porro *et al., ibid.* 85; M. Petrillo *et al., Curr. Ther. Res.* **25**, 457 (1979).

(E,E)-isomer

Light yellow viscous liq with a slight odor and bitter taste. uv max (ethanol): 287 nm ($E_{1cm}^{1\%}$ 94.6). n_D^{20} 1.5235. Relative density at 20°: 1.013-1.015. pK_1 4.10; pK_2 3.25. Readily sol in most org solvents. Slightly sol in aq solns of organic acids. Practically insol in alkali, water. LD_{50} in mice, rats (mg/kg): 2175, 2610 orally; 40.6, 33.3 i.v. (Bianchetti). Approx LD_{50} i.p. in mice: 500 mg/kg (Tricerri, 1974).

THERAP CAT: Antiulcerative.

7421. Pifithrin-α. [63208-82-2] 1-(4-Methylphenyl)-2-(4,-5,6,7-tetrahydro-2-imino-3(2*H*)-benzothiazolyl)ethanone monohydrobromide; 2-(2-imino-4,5,6,7-tetrahydrobenzothiazol-3-yl)-1-*p*-tolylethanone hydrobromide; PFT-α. $C_{16}H_{18}N_2OS.HBr$; mol wt 367.30. C 52.32%, H 5.21%, N 7.63%, O 4.36%, S 8.73%, Br 21.75%. Small molecule inhibitor of p53-mediated gene activation and apoptosis; the name pifithrin is an abbreviation for p-fifty three inhibitor. Converted *in vitro* to the planar tricyclic condensation product, pifithrin-β. Prepn: A. Singh *et al., Indian J. Chem.* **14B**, 997 (1976). Identification of p53 inhibition: P. G. Komarov *et al., Science* **285**, 1733 (1999). Synthesis and neuroprotective activity: X. Zhu *et al., J. Med. Chem.* **45**, 5090 (2002). Inhibition of heat shock and glucocorticoid signal transduction pathways: E. A. Komarova *et al., J. Biol. Chem.* **278**, 15465 (2003). Characterization as an aryl hydrocarbon receptor agonist: M. S. Hoagland *et al., J. Pharmacol. Exp. Ther.* **314**, 603 (2005). Conversion to pifithrin-β: R. K. Gary, D. A. Jensen, *Mol. Pharm.* **2**, 462 (2005).

mp 182°. pKa 9.11. Sol in water, DMSO.
Pifithrin-β. [60477-34-1]; [511296-88-1] (hydrobromide). 5,-6,7,8-Tetrahydro-2-(4-methylphenyl)imidazo[2,1-*b*]benzothiazole; 2-(4-methylphenyl)imidazo[2,1*b*]-5,6,7,8-tetrahydrobenzothiazole; 2-*p*-tolyl-5,6,7,8-tetrahydrobenzo[*d*]imidazo[2,1-*b*]thiazole; cyclic pifithrin-α. $C_{16}H_{16}N_2S$; mol wt 268.38. Crystal structure: W. Clegg, C. Jamieson, *Acta Crystallogr.* **E61**, o1486 (2005). Crystals from methanol. mp 185°. pKa 4.36. Log P (octanol/water): 4.26. Crystal density: 1.318 Mg/m³.

USE: Biochemical tool in studies of p53 function and apoptosis.

7422. Piketoprofen. [60576-13-8] 3-Benzoyl-α-methyl-*N*-(4-methyl-2-pyridinyl)benzeneacetamide; *m*-benzoyl-*N*-(4-methyl-2-pyridyl)hydratropamide; 2-(3-benzoylphenyl)-*N*-(4-methyl-2-pyridyl)propionamide; Calmatel (aerosol). $C_{22}H_{20}N_2O_2$; mol wt 344.41. C 76.72%, H 5.85%, N 8.13%, O 9.29%. Derivative of ketoprofen, *q.v.* used topically as cream or aerosol. Prepn: R. G. W. Spickett *et al.*, **GB 1436502** (1976 to Antonio Gallardo, S.A.). Pharmacology and clinical efficacy: E. Tarrus *et al., 2nd Eur. Congr. Biopharm. Pharmacokinet.* **1**, 483 (1984).

Oil, sol in methylene chloride, ethanol. Insol in water.
Hydrochloride. [59512-37-7] Calmatel (cream). $C_{22}H_{20}N_2$-$O_2.HCl$; mol wt 380.87. mp 180-182°.

THERAP CAT: Anti-inflammatory (topical).

7423. Pildralazine. [64000-73-3] 6-[(2-Hydroxypropyl)-methylamino]-3(2*H*)-pyridazinone hydrazone; 3-hydrazino-6-[(2-hydroxypropyl)methylamino]pyridazine; (±)-1-[(6-hydrazino-3-pyridazinyl)methylamino]-2-propanol; propyldazine; propildazine. $C_8H_{15}N_5O$; mol wt 197.24. C 48.72%, H 7.67%, N 35.51%, O 8.11%. Peripheral vasodilator with hypotensive activity; related to hydralazine, *q.v.* Prepn: G. Pifferi, **DE 2154245**; *idem*, **US 3769278** (1972, 1973 both to I.S.F.); G. Pifferi *et al., J. Med. Chem.* **18**, 741 (1975). Pharmacology in animals: L. Dorigotti *et al., Pharmacol. Res. Commun.* **8**, 295 (1976); L. Dorigotti *et al., Arzneim.-Forsch.* **34**, 876 (1984); in humans: L. Terzoli *et al., Boll. Soc. Ital. Cardiol.* **22**, 1053 (1977). GLC determn in plasma: P. Ventura *et al., J. Chromatogr.* **161**, 237 (1978). Clinical evaluation in essential hypertension: R. Pellegrini, G. Abbondati, *Farmaco Ed. Prat.* **32**, 19 (1977). Pharmacokinetics and tissue binding: E. Noack *et al., Arzneim.-Forsch.* **37**, 407 (1987).

Dihydrochloride. [56393-22-7] ISF-2123; Atensil. $C_8H_{15}N_5$-$O.2HCl$; mol wt 270.16. Crystals from ethanol, mp 206-209° (dec). LD_{50} in mice, rats (mg/kg): 357, 355 i.p.; 1170, 1230 orally (Dorigotti, 1976).

THERAP CAT: Antihypertensive.

7424. Pilocarpine. [92-13-7] (3*S-cis*)-3-Ethyldihydro-4-[(1-methyl-1*H*-imidazol-5-yl)methyl]-2(3*H*)-furanone; Ocusert Pilo. $C_{11}H_{16}N_2O_2$; mol wt 208.26. C 63.44%, H 7.74%, N 13.45%, O 15.36%. Cholinergic principle from *Pilocarpus jaborandi* Holmes, *Rutaceae*. Isoln: Petit, Polanovski, *Bull. Soc. Chim.* [3] **17**, 557, 702 (1897). Structure: Jowett, *J. Chem. Soc.* **77**, 473, 851 (1900); **83**, 438 (1903). Stereoisomeric with isopilocarpine: Polonovski, Polonovski, *Bull. Soc. Chim.* [4] **31**, 1314 (1922). Has the *cis* configuration; isopilocarpine is *trans*: Zav'yalov, *Dokl. Akad. Nauk SSSR* **82**, 257 (1952). Absolute configuration: Hill, Barcza, *Tetrahedron* **22**, 2889 (1966). Synthesis: Preobrashenski *et al., Ber.* **66**, 1187 (1933); Samokhvalov, *Med. Prom. SSSR* **11**, no. 2, 10 (1957); DeGraw, *Tetrahedron* **28**, 967 (1972); Link, Bernauer, *Helv. Chim. Acta* **55**, 1053 (1972). Stereoselective synthesis: A. Noordam *et al., Rec. Trav. Chim.* **98**, 467 (1979). Review: Langenbeck, *Angew. Chem.* **60**, 297 (1948); van Rossum *et al., Experientia* **16**, 373 (1960). Toxicity studies: Beccari, *Boll. Chim. Farm.* **106**, 8 (1967). Comprehensive description: A. A. Al-Badr, H. Y. Aboul-Enein, *Anal. Profiles Drug Subs.* **12**, 385-432 (1983). Clinical trial in Sjögren's syndrome: F. B. Vivino *et al., Arch. Intern. Med.* **159**, 174 (1999); in radiation-induced xerostomia: J.-C. Horiot *et al., Radiother. Oncol.* **55**, 233 (2000).

Oil or crystals, mp 34°. bp₅ 260° (partial conversion to isopilocarpine). $[\alpha]_D^{18}$ +106° (c = 2). pK_1 (20°) 7.15; pK_2 (20°) 12.57.

Sol in water, alcohol, chloroform; sparingly sol in ether, benzene. Almost insol in petr ether.

Hydrochloride. [54-71-7] Akarpine; Almocarpine; Isopto Carpine; Pilogel; Pilopine HS; Pilostat; Salagen. $C_{11}H_{16}N_2O_2 \cdot HCl$; mol wt 244.72. Hygroscopic crystals from alcohol, mp 204-205°. $[\alpha]_D^{18}$ +91° (c = 2). Freely sol in water, alcohol. Practically insol in ether, chloroform. *Keep well closed and protected from light.*

Nitrate. [148-72-1] Chibro Pilocarpine; Licarpin; Pilo; Pilofrin; Pilagan. $C_{11}H_{16}N_2O_2 \cdot HNO_3$; mol wt 271.27. mp 173.5-174.0° (dec). *Poisonous!* $[\alpha]_D$ +77 to +83° (c = 10). One gram dissolves in 4 ml water, 75 ml alcohol. Insol in chloroform, ether. *Incompat.* Silver nitrate, mercury bichloride, iodides, gold salts, tannin, calomel, $KMnO_4$, alkalies.

Isopilocarpine. β-Pilocarpine. Hygroscopic oily liquid or prisms. bp_{10} 261°. $[\alpha]_D^{18}$ +50° (c = 2). pK_1 (18°) 7.17. Miscible with water and alcohol; very sol in chloroform; less sol in benzene, ether. Almost insol in petr ether.

Isopilocarpine hydrochloride hemihydrate. $C_{11}H_{16}N_2O_2 \cdot HCl \cdot \frac{1}{2}H_2O$. Scales from alcohol + ether, mp 127°; when anhydr, mp 161°. $[\alpha]_D^{18}$ +39° (c = 5). Sol in 0.27 part water; 2.1 parts alcohol.

Isopilocarpine nitrate. $C_{11}H_{16}N_2O_2 \cdot HNO_3$. Prisms from water, scales from alcohol, mp 159°. $[\alpha]_D^{18}$ +39° (c = 2). Sol in 8.4 parts water, in 350 parts abs alcohol.

THERAP CAT: Antiglaucoma agent; miotic; sialogogue.

THERAP CAT (VET): Parasympathomimetic; miotic; gastric secretory stimulant.

7425. Pilocarpus. Jaborandi. Leaves of *Pilocarpus jaborandi* Holmes (Pernambuco jaborandi), or of *P. microphyllus* Stapf (Maranhao jaborandi), *Rutaceae. Habit.* Brazil, Paraguay. *Constit.* About 1% alkaloids of which about 0.5% is pilocarpine; pilocarpidine, isopilocarpine, jaborine, jaboridine, jaboric acid, pilocarpic acid.

THERAP CAT: Sudorific; miotic.

7426. Piloty's Acid. [599-71-3] N-Hydroxybenzenesulfonamide; benzenesulfohydroxamic acid; N-(phenylsulfonyl)hydroxylamine. $C_6H_7NO_3S$; mol wt 173.19. C 41.61%, H 4.07%, N 8.09%, O 27.71%, S 18.51%. Decomposes to produce nitroxyl (HNO). Prepn: O. Piloty, *Ber.* **29**, 1559 (1896). Reaction with aldehydes: A. Hassner *et al., J. Org. Chem.* **35**, 1962 (1970). Crystal structure: J. N. Scholz *et al., Tetrahedron* **45**, 7695 (1989). Decompn study: F. T. Bonner, Y. Ko, *Inorg. Chem.* **31**, 2514 (1992).

mp 126° (Piloty). Also reported as crystals from water, mp 109-110° (Scholz). pKa 9.29. Sol in alcohol, ether, ethyl acetate, acetone, warm water. Slightly sol in toluene, benzene, chloroform.

USE: HNO/NO^- donor in biochemical model studies. In the Angeli-Rimini test for aldehydes.

7427. Pilsicainide. [88069-67-4] N-(2,6-Dimethylphenyl)-tetrahydro-1H-pyrrolizine-7a(5H)-acetamide; tetrahydro-1H-pyrrolizine-7a(5H)-aceto-2′,6′-xylidide; N-(2,6-dimethylphenyl)-8-pyrrolizidineacetamide. $C_{17}H_{24}N_2O$; mol wt 272.39. C 74.96%, H 8.88%, N 10.28%, O 5.87%. Structural analog of lidocaine, *q.v.* Prepn: S. Miyano *et al.,* **EP 89061**; *eidem,* **US 4564624** (1983, 1986 both to Suntory); *eidem, J. Med. Chem.* **28**, 714 (1985). Pharmacology: K. Aisaka *et al., Arzneim.-Forsch.* **35**, 1239 (1985); T. Hidaka *et al., ibid.* 1381. Clinical evaluation in supraventricular tachycardia: T. Terazawa *et al., Am. Heart J.* **121**, 1437 (1991).

Hydrochloride hemihydrate. [88069-49-2] SUN-1165; Sunrythm. $C_{17}H_{24}N_2O \cdot HCl \cdot \frac{1}{2}H_2O$; mol wt 317.85. Crystals from ethanol-ether, mp 212-214°. LD_{50} in mice (mg/kg): 410 s.c. (Miyano, 1985).

THERAP CAT: Antiarrhythmic.

7428. Pimaric Acid. [127-27-5] [1R-(1α,4aβ,4bα,7β,-10aα)]-7-Ethenyl-1,2,3,4,4a,4b,5,6,7,9,10,10a-dodecahydro-1,4a,7-trimethyl-1-phenanthrenecarboxylic acid; 13α-methyl-13-vinyl-podocarp-8(14)-ene-15-oic acid; dextropimaric acid; d-pimaric acid; α-pimaric acid. $C_{20}H_{30}O_2$; mol wt 302.45. C 79.42%, H 10.00%, O 10.58%. Isoln from American rosin: Rimbach, *Ber. Dtsch. Pharm. Ges.* **6**, 61 (1896); from French galipot from *Pinus maritima* Mill, *Pinaceae:* Ruzicka, Balas, *Helv. Chim. Acta* **6**, 677 (1923); Ruzicka *et al., ibid.* **15**, 915 (1932). Structure: Ruzicka, Sternbach, *ibid.* **23**, 124 (1940); Fleck, *J. Am. Chem. Soc.* **62**, 2044 (1940); Harris, Sanderson, *ibid.* **70**, 2081 (1948). Stereochemistry: Wenkert, Chamberlin, *ibid.* **81**, 688 (1959).

Orthorhombic, bisphenoidal crystals from acetone or acetic acid, mp 217-219°; bp_{18} 282°; $[\alpha]_D^{18}$ +74.7° (c = 0.4 in chloroform); $[\alpha]_D^{20}$ +87.3° (in chloroform).

Hydrochloride. $C_{20}H_{31}O_2Cl$. Dec 184°. $[\alpha]_D^{20}$ +13.6° (c = 0.5 in alcohol). Can be reconverted by heating with quinoline at 250°.

Quinidine salt. $C_{40}H_{54}N_2O_4$. mp 90°.

Methyl ester. $C_{21}H_{32}O_2$. mp 69°.

7429. Pimecrolimus. [137071-32-0] (3S,4R,5S,8R,9E,12S,-14S,15R,16S,18R,19R,26aS)-3-[(1E)-2-[(1R,3R,4S)-4-Chloro-3-methoxycyclohexyl]-1-methylethenyl]-8-ethyl-5,6,8,11,12,13,14,-15,16,17,18,19,24,25,26,26a-hexadecahydro-5,19-dihydroxy-14,16-dimethoxy-4,10,12,18-tetramethyl-15,19-epoxy-3H-pyrido[2,1-c][1,4]oxaazacyclotricosine-1,7,20,21(4H,23H)-tetrone; 33-epi-chloro-33-desoxyascomycin; SDZ-ASM-981; Elidel. $C_{43}H_{68}ClNO_{11}$; mol wt 810.45. C 63.73%, H 8.46%, Cl 4.37%, N 1.73%, O 21.72%. Macrolactam ascomycin derivative; inhibits production of pro-inflammatory cytokines by T cells and mast cells. Prepn: K. Baumann, G. Emmer, **EP 427680** (1991 to Sandoz); *eidem,* **US 5912238** (1999 to Novartis). *In vitro* pharmacology: M. Gassberger *et al., Br. J. Dermatol.* **141**, 264 (1999). Clinical evaluation in psoriasis: U. Mrowietz *et al., ibid.* **139**, 992 (1998); in contact dermatitis: C. Queille-Roussel *et al., Contact Dermatitis* **42**, 349 (2000).

THERAP CAT: Immunosuppressant.

7430. Pimefylline. [10001-43-1] 3,7-Dihydro-1,3-dimethyl-7-[2-[(3-pyridinylmethyl)amino]ethyl]-1*H*-purine-2,6-dione; 7-[2-[(3-pyridylmethyl)amino]ethyl]theophylline; 7-(β-3′-picolyl-aminoethyl)theophylline; pimephylline; ES-771. $C_{15}H_{18}N_6O_2$; mol wt 314.34. C 57.31%, H 5.77%, N 26.74%, O 10.18%. Prepn: **NL 6600250**; Suter, Zutter, **US 3350400** (1966, 1967 both to Eprova). Structure determn, properties and chemistry: *eidem, Pharm. Acta Helv.* **48**, 133 (1973). Pharmacology: Ciaceri, Attaguile, *Gazz. Med. Ital.* **132**, 36, 108 (1973). Metabolism: Pitrè, *Farmaco Ed. Prat.* **29**, 46 (1974).

Crystals from isopropyl acetate, mp 111-112°. uv max (water): 270 nm. Readily sol in cold water, chloroform; sol in acetone, ethanol. LD_{50} in mice (mg/kg): 1900 orally, 402 i.v. (Suter, Zutter, 1973).

Nicotinate. [10058-07-8] ES-902; Teonicon. $C_{15}H_{18}N_6O_2$·$C_6H_5NO_2$; mol wt 437.45. Colorless, odorless powder from ethanol, mp 159-160°. uv max (water): 267 nm. Very sol in water (40% soln can be prepd); slightly sol in methanol; very slightly sol in acetone, chloroform. LD_{50} in mice (mg/kg): 2530 orally, 470 i.v. (Suter, Zutter, 1973).

THERAP CAT: Vasodilator (coronary).

7431. Pimelic Acid. [111-16-0] Heptanedioic acid; 1,5-pentanedicarboxylic acid. $C_7H_{12}O_4$; mol wt 160.17. C 52.49%, H 7.55%, O 39.96%. HOOC(CH₂)₅COOH. Prepn starting with cyclohexanone and ethyl oxalate: Snyder *et al., Org. Synth.* **coll. vol. II**, p 531 (1943); by the action of sodium and isoamyl alcohol on salicylic acid: Müller, *ibid.* p 535.

Monoclinic prisms from benzene, mp 105.7-105.8°. Tends to sublime. bp_{100} 272°; bp_{50} 251.5°; bp_{15} 223°; bp_{10} 212°. 2.52 parts dissolve in 100 parts water at 13.5°; 5 parts dissolve in 100 parts water at 20°. Freely sol in alcohol, ether. Practically insol in cold benzene.

Diethyl ester. $C_{11}H_{20}O_4$. Liquid, d_4^{20} 0.99448; bp_{748} 254°; bp_{24} 155°; bp_{15} 140°. Sol in alcohol, ether, ethyl acetate.

7432. Pimenta. Jamaica pepper. Small, evergreen tree, *Pimenta dioica* L. (syn. *P. officinalis* Lindl.), Myrtaceae, bearing deep purple or glossy black berries. The dried unripe fruits resemble peppercorns and are known as *allspice*. Flavor similar to a combination of clove, cinnamon and nutmeg. *Habit.* West Indies, Central America, Mexico. *Constit.* Volatile oil (4%), quercetin glycosides, catechins, proanthocyanidins, protein, lipid, fixed oil, sugar, vitamins, minerals. *Reviews:* A. Y. Leung, S. Foster, *Encyclopedia of Common Natural Ingredients,* (Wiley-Interscience, Hoboken, 2nd Ed., 2003) pp 20-22; B. Krishnamoorthy, J. Rema in *Handbook of Herbs and Spices,* **Vol. 2**, K. V. Peter, Ed., (CRC Press, Boca Raton, 2004) pp 117-139.

Pimenta berry oil. [8006-77-7] Oil of pimenta; pimento oil; allspice berry oil. Volatile oil obtained by distillation of dried immature berries. *Constit.* Complex mixture of components, chiefly eugenol (60-80%), methyl eugenol, β-caryophyllene, humulene, terpinen-4-ol, 4,5-cineole, α-phellandrene, 1,8-cineole. Yellow to brownish-yellow liquid with warm spicy sweet odor. d_{25}^{25} 1.018-1.048. n_D^{20} 1.527-1.540. Rotation between −4° and 0°. Sol in propylene glycol, most vegetable oils, in 2 vols 70% alcohol. *Keep well closed, cool and protected from light.*

Pimenta leaf oil. Volatile oil obtained by distillation of fresh or dried leaves. *Constit.* Eugenol (up to 96%) and other terpenes. Brownish-yellow liquid becoming darker with age; woody, spicy aromatic odor. d_{25}^{25} 1.037-1.050. n_D^{20} 1.531-1.536. Rotation between −2° and +0.5°. Sol in propylene glycol, in most fixed oils with slight opalescence, in 2 vols 70% alcohol. Insol in glycerin, mineral oil. *Keep well closed, cool and protected from light.*

USE: Spice in cooking; component of Caribbean jerk seasoning. Fragrance component of cosmetics, perfumes, soaps.

THERAP CAT: Carminative.

7433. Piminodine. [13495-09-5] 4-Phenyl-1-[3-(phenylamino)propyl]-4-piperidinecarboxylic acid ethyl ester; 1-(3-anilinopropyl)-4-phenylisonipecotic acid ethyl ester; ethyl 4-phenyl-1-[(3-phenylamino)propyl]-4-piperidinecarboxylate; ethyl 4-phenyl-1-(3-anilinopropyl)-4-phenylisonipecotate. $C_{23}H_{30}N_2O_2$; mol wt 366.50. C 75.37%, H 8.25%, N 7.64%, O 8.73%. Prepn: Elpern *et al., J. Am. Chem. Soc.* **81**, 3784 (1959).

Dihydrochloride. $C_{23}H_{30}N_2O_2$·2HCl. Crystals, mp 219.4-222.2°.

Ethanesulfonate. [7081-52-9] NIH-7590; Win-14098; Alvodine; Pimadin. $C_{25}H_{36}N_2O_5S$; mol wt 476.63.

Note: This is a controlled substance (opiate): **21 CFR**, 1308.12.

THERAP CAT: Analgesic (narcotic).

7434. Pimobendan. [74150-27-9] 4,5-Dihydro-6-[2-(4-methoxyphenyl)-1*H*-benzimidazol-5-yl]-5-methyl-3(2*H*)-pyridazinone; UD-CG 115; UD-CG 115 BS; 2-(4-methoxyphenyl)-5(6)-(5-methyl-3-oxo-4,5-dihydro-2*H*-6-pyridazinyl)benzimidazole. $C_{19}H_{18}N_4O_2$; mol wt 334.37. C 68.25%, H 5.43%, N 16.76%, O 9.57%. Positive inotropic agent. Prepn: V. Austel *et al.,* **DE 2837161**; *eidem,* **US 4361563** (1980, 1982 both to Thomae). Cardiovascular effects: J. C. A. von Meel, *Arzneim.-Forsch.* **35**, 284 (1985); P. D. Verdouw *et al., Eur. J. Pharmacol.* **126**, 21 (1986). Comparison of enantiomer activity: K. Fujino *et al., J. Pharmacol. Exp. Ther.* **247**, 519 (1988). Clinical trial in congestive heart failure: F. Hagemeijer, *Am. Heart J.* **122**, 517 (1991); S. D. Katz *et al., ibid.* **123**, 95 (1992).

Hydrochloride. [77469-98-8] $C_{19}H_{18}N_4O_2$·HCl. Crystals from methanol and ethereal HCl, mp 311°(dec). LD_{50} orally in mice: ~600 mg/kg (Austel, 1982).

THERAP CAT: Cardiotonic.

7435. Pimozide. [2062-78-4] 1-[1-[4,4-Bis(4-fluorophenyl)butyl]-4-piperidinyl]-1,3-dihydro-2*H*-benzimidazol-2-one; 1-[1-[4,4-bis(*p*-fluorophenyl)butyl]-4-piperidyl]-2-benzimidazolinone; 1-[4,4-di-(4-fluorophenyl)butyl]-4-(2-oxo-1-benzimidazolinyl)-piperidine; R-6238; Orap; Opiran. $C_{28}H_{29}F_2N_3O$; mol wt 461.55. C 72.86%, H 6.33%, F 8.23%, N 9.10%, O 3.47%. Prepn: Janssen, **FR M3695** (1965 to Janssen), *C.A.* **66**, 115709t (1967). Pharmacological studies: Janssen *et al., Arzneim.-Forsch.* **18**, 261, 279, 282 (1968). Metabolism in rats: Soudijn, Wijngaarden, *Life Sci.* **8**, 291 (1969). Clinical experience: Poldinger, *Curr. Ther. Res.* **13**, 23 (1971). Pimozide blocks establishment but not expression of amphetamine-produced environment-specific conditioning: R. J. Beninger, B. L. Hahn, *Science* **220**, 1304 (1983). Use in treatment of acute schizophrenia: B. Shopsin, G. Selzer, *Curr. Ther. Res.* **21**, 755 (1977); in treatment of chronic schizophrenia: F. Kline *et al., ibid.* 768. In management of Gilles de la Tourette's syndrome: M. S. Ross, H. Moldofsky, *Lancet* **1**, 103 (1977); A. K. Shapiro, E. Shapiro, *Am. J. Psychiatry* **140**, 1235 (1983); *eidem, J. Am. Acad. Child Psychiatry* **23**, 161 (1984).

Microcrystals, mp 214-218°. Weak base, pKa 7.32. Almost insol in water (<0.01 mg/ml). Very slightly sol in dil aq solns of organic and mineral acids (<5 mg/ml).

THERAP CAT: Antipsychotic.

7436. Pimpinella. Pimpernel; brunet saxifrage; small saxifrage. Root of *Pimpinella saxifraga* L. or *P. magna* L. *Umbelliferae.* Habit. Europe; adventitious in U.S. Constit. Volatile oil, resin, benzoic acid, pimpinellin.

THERAP CAT: Aromatic carminative.

7437. Pimpinellin. [131-12-4] 5,6-Dimethoxy-2H-furo[2,-3-h]-1-benzopyran-2-one; 4-hydroxy-6,7-dimethoxy-5-benzofuranacrylic acid δ-lactone. $C_{13}H_{10}O_5$; mol wt 246.22. C 63.41%, H 4.09%, O 32.49%. Found in *Pimpinella saxifraga* L., *Heracleum spondylium* L., *H. lanatum* Michx., and *H. panaces* L., *Umbelliferae.* Isoln: Heut, *Arch. Pharm.* **236**, 162 (1898); Herzog, Hancu, ibid. **246**, 402 (1908); Wessely, Kallab, *Monatsh. Chem.* **59**, 161 (1932); Späth, Simon, ibid. **67**, 344 (1936); Fujita, Furuya, *J. Pharm. Soc. Jpn.* **74**, 795 (1954); **76**, 535 (1956); Svendsen, Ottestad, *Pharm. Acta Helv.* **32**, 457 (1957); Svendsen, *C.A.* **52**, 2173g (1958); Svendsen *et al., Planta Med.* **7**, 113 (1959); *Pharm. Acta Helv.* **34**, 33 (1959); Jastrzebski, *C.A.* **54**, 1205b (1960). Synthesis: M. W. Reed, H. W. Moore, *J. Org. Chem.* **53**, 4166 (1988).

Off-white needles from methylene chloride/hexane, mp 119°. Practically insol in water. Sol in alcohol. Absorption spectrum: Wessely, Koltan, *Monatsh. Chem.* **86**, 430 (1955).

7438. Pinacidil. [60560-33-0] N-Cyano-N'-4-pyridinyl-N''-(1,2,2-trimethylpropyl)guanidine; P-1134. $C_{13}H_{19}N_5$; mol wt 245.32. C 63.65%, H 7.81%, N 28.55%. Potassium channel opening vasodilator. Prepn: H. J. Petersen, DE 2557438; idem, US 4057636 (1976, 1977 both to Leo Pharm.); H. J. Petersen *et al., J. Med. Chem.* **21**, 773 (1978). Mechanism of action: E. Arrigoni-Martelli *et al., Experientia* **36**, 445 (1980); K. M. Bray *et al., Br. J. Pharmacol.* **91**, 421 (1987). Metabolism: E. Eilertsen *et al., Xenobiotica* **12**, 187 (1982). Bioavailability: eidem, ibid. 177. Determn in plasma: M. Hamilton *et al., J. Chromatogr.* **375**, 359 (1986). Pharmacokinetics and hypotensive effects: J. W. Ward *et al., Eur. J. Clin. Pharmacol.* **26**, 603 (1984). Clinical comparison with hydralazine, *q.v.:* R. L. Byyny *et al., Clin. Pharmacol. Ther.* **42**, 50 (1987). Review of pharmacology and mechanism of action: M. L. Cohen: *Drug Dev. Res.* **9**, 249-258 (1986).

Monohydrate. [85371-64-8] Pindac. $C_{13}H_{19}N_5 \cdot H_2O$; mol wt 263.34. Crystals, mp 164-165°. LD_{50} in mice, rats (mg/kg): 600, 570 orally (Petersen, 1978).

THERAP CAT: Antihypertensive.

7439. Pinacol. [76-09-5] 2,3-Dimethyl-2,3-butanediol; pinacone; tetramethylethylene glycol. $C_6H_{14}O_2$; mol wt 118.17. C 60.98%, H 11.94%, O 27.08%. Prepd by the reduction of acetone: Holleman, *Rec. Trav. Chim.* **25**, 206 (1906); R. Adams, E. W. Adams, *Org. Synth.* coll. vol. I, 459 (2nd ed., 1941); DE 233894 in *Frdl.* **10**, 1000. Convenient lab procedure: L. F. Fieser, *Experiments in Organic Chemistry* (Boston, 3rd ed., 1955) p 101. Crystal structure: G. A. Jeffrey, A. Robbins, *Acta Crystallogr.* **B34**, 3817 (1978).

Hexahydrate. $C_6H_{14}O_2 \cdot 6H_2O$. Four-sided plates from water. mp 45.4°; d^{15} 0.967 (supercooled liquid). The anhydr compd crystallizes in needles from alc or ether, mp 41.1°; bp_{760} 174.4°. Freely sol in hot water, in alc, in ether; slightly sol in cold water, carbon disulfide.

Dimethyl ether. $C_8H_{18}O_2$. Liquid. Agreeable odor. bp 144°.

7440. Pinacolone. [75-97-8] 3,3-Dimethyl-2-butanone; tert-butyl methyl ketone; pinacolin. $C_6H_{12}O$; mol wt 100.16. C 71.95%, H 12.08%, O 15.97%. Prepd by distillation of pinacol hydrate with dil H_2SO_4: Fittig, *Ann.* **114**, 56 (1860); Hill, Flosdorf, *Org. Synth.* coll. vol. I (2nd ed., 1941) p 462; L. F. Fieser, K. L. Williamson, *Organic Experiments* (D. C. Heath and Co., Lexington, Mass., 5th ed., 1983) p 332. Almost quantitative yields are obtained when 56.5 g pinacol hydrate is boiled for 3 hrs with 0.5 liter 25% H_2SO_4 and the product is steam distilled: Boeseken, van Tonningen, *Rec. Trav. Chim.* **39**, 189 (1920).

Liquid. Peppermint or camphor-like odor. d_{25}^{25} 0.7250. mp −52.5°. bp_{760} 106.2°. n_D^{25} 1.3939. Volatile in steam. Moderately sol in water (2.44% at 15°). Soluble in alcohol, ether, acetone.

Oxime. $C_6H_{13}NO$. Needles from aq alcohol. mp 78°. bp_{748} 171.6°. Sol in alc, ether, petr ether, benzene, chloroform.

7441. Pinaverium Bromide. [53251-94-8] 4-[(2-Bromo-4,5-dimethoxyphenyl)methyl]-4-[2-[2-(6,6-dimethylbicyclo[3.1.1]-hept-2-yl)ethoxy]ethyl]morpholinium bromide; 4-(6-bromo-veratryl)-4-[2-[2-(6,6-dimethyl-2-norpinyl)ethoxy]ethyl]morpholinium bromide; LAT-1717; Dicetel. $C_{26}H_{41}Br_2NO_4$; mol wt 591.42. C 52.80%, H 6.99%, Br 27.02%, N 2.37%, O 10.82%. Spasmolytic agent with low incidence of anticholinergic effects. Prepn: BE 769469; R. Baronnet, US 3845048 (1971, 1974 both to Societe Berri-Balzac). Synthesis and pharmacology: R. Baronnet *et al., Eur. J. Med. Chem.* **9**, 182 (1974). Pharmacodynamics: J. Bretaudeau *et al., Therapie* **30**, 919 (1975). Synthesis of ${}^{14}C$ pinaverium bromide and pharmacokinetics: C. Jacquot *et al., Eur. J. Med. Chem.* **13**, 61 (1978). Mechanism of action: J. Bretaudeau, O. Foussard-Blanpin, *J. Pharmacol.* **11**, 233 (1980). Inhibition of gastrointestinal contractile activity in dogs: Z. Itoh, T. Takahashi, *Arzneim.-Forsch.* **31**, 1450 (1981). Effects in humans on gastric emptying and transit time: J. Bertrand *et al., Therapie* **36**, 555 (1981).

Crystals from methyl ethyl ketone, mp 181°; also reported as mp ~170° (Baronnet, 1974). LD_{50} in mice (mg/kg): 1400 orally; 66 i.v. (Baronnet, 1974); also reported as LD_{50} i.v. in mice: 37 ±2.4 mg/kg (Baronnet *et al.*).

THERAP CAT: Antispasmodic.

7442. Pinazepam. [52463-83-9] 7-Chloro-1,3-dihydro-5-phenyl-1-(2-propynyl)-2H-1,4-benzodiazepin-2-one; 7-chloro-1-propargyl-5-phenyl-3H-1,4-benzodiazepin-2(1H)-one; Z-905; Domar; Duna. $C_{18}H_{13}ClN_2O$; mol wt 308.76. C 70.02%, H 4.24%, Cl 11.48%, N 9.07%, O 5.18%. Prepn: F. Tenconi *et al.*, **DE 2339790** (1974 to Zambeletti), *C.A.* **80,** 133492k (1974); C. Podesva, K. Vagi, **US 3842094** (1974 to Delmar). Metabolism study: A. Trebbi *et al., J. Chromatogr.* **110,** 309 (1975). Pharmacological and toxicological studies: F. Scrollini *et al., Arzneim.-Forsch.* **25,** 934 (1975). Pharmacokinetics: P. M. Boselli, F. Scrollini, *Boll. Chim. Farm.* **116,** 363 (1977). Psychopharmacological properties: F. Scrollini *et al., Arzneim.-Forsch.* **28,** 423 (1978). Physico-chemical profile: G. Filipi, A Trebbi, *Boll. Chim. Farm.* **118,** 105 (1979). Clinical study: V. Bertoncelli *et al., Clin. Ter.* **94,** 641 (1980).

Cryst from methanol/water, mp 140-142°. LD$_{50}$ in mice, rats (mg/kg): 1355, 5819 orally; 266, 622 i.p. (Scrollini, 1975). Also reported as LD$_{50}$ in mice (mg/kg): 670 orally (Podesva, Vagi).

Note: This is a controlled substance (depressant): **21 CFR,** 1308.14.

THERAP CAT: Anxiolytic.

7443. Pindolol. [13523-86-9] 1-(1H-Indol-4-yloxy)-3-[(1-methylethyl)amino]-2-propanol; 4-[2-hydroxy-3-(isopropylamino)-propoxy]indole; prinodolol; LB-46; Betapindol; Blocklin L; Decreten; Pectobloc; Pinbetol; Pindoptan; Visken. $C_{14}H_{20}N_2O_2$; mol wt 248.32. C 67.71%, H 8.12%, N 11.28%, O 12.89%. Mixed β-adrenergic blocker and serotonin 5HT$_{1A}$-receptor antagonist. Prepn: **NL 6601040;** F. Troxler, A. Hofmann, **US 3471515** (1966, 1969 both to Sandoz). HPLC determn in plasma: H. Smith, *J. Chromatogr.* **415,** 95 (1987). Symposia on cardiovascular pharmacology and clinical studies: *Am. Heart J.* **104,** Suppl. 2, pt. 2, 333-520 (1982); *Br. J. Clin. Pharmacol.* **13,** Suppl. 2, 143S-450S (1982). Effect on serotonin levels in rat brain: L. J. Dreshfield *et al., Neurochem. Res.* **21,** 557 (1996). Clinical trial with fluoxetine, *q.v.,* in depression: V. Pérez *et al., Lancet* **349,** 1594 (1997).

Crystals from ethanol, mp 171-173°.

THERAP CAT: Antihypertensive; antianginal; antiarrhythmic; antiglaucoma.

7444. Pindone. [83-26-1] 2-(2,2-Dimethyl-1-oxopropyl)-1H-indene-1,3(2H)-dione; 2-pivaloyl-1,3-indandione; 2-pivalyl-1,3-indandione; 2-trimethylacetyl-1,3-indandione; pivalyl indandione; pivaldione; Pival; Pivalyl Valone; Tri-Ban. $C_{14}H_{14}O_3$; mol wt 230.26. C 73.03%, H 6.13%, O 20.85%. Prepn: Kilgore *et al., Ind. Eng. Chem.* **34,** 494 (1942); Zelmens, Vanags, *C.A.* **53,** 21830d (1959). Toxicity study: T. B. Gaines, *Toxicol. Appl. Pharmacol.* **14,** 515 (1969).

Bright yellow crystals from ethanol, mp 108-110°. LD$_{50}$ orally in male rats: 280 mg/kg (Gaines).

Sodium salt. Pivalyn. Bright yellow crystals, mp 205-210°. Schwarz, **US 2880132** (1959 to Morton Chem.). Sol in water.

Caution: Potential symptoms of overexposure are epistaxis, excess bleeding from minor cuts and bruises; smoky urine, black tarry stools; abdominal and back pain. *See NIOSH Pocket Guide to Chemical Hazards* (DHHS/NIOSH 97-140, 1997) p 258.

USE: Rodenticide; insecticide.

7445. α-Pinene. [80-56-8] 2,6,6-Trimethylbicyclo[3.1.1]-hept-2-ene; 2-pinene; pinene. $C_{10}H_{16}$; mol wt 136.23. C 88.16%, H 11.84%. Obtained from oil of turpentine which contains 58-65% α-pinene along with 30% β-pinene, *q.v.*: E. Gildemeister, F. Hoffmann, *Die ätherischen Ole* **Band IV** (Akademie-Verlag, Berlin, 4th ed., 1956) p 39. α-Pinene in North American oils is dextrorotatory, in most European oils it is levorotatory. Constituent of many volatile oils. Isoln of *d*-α-pinene from Port Oxford cedar wood oil *(Chamaecyparis lawsoniana* Parl., *Pinaceae):* Thurber, Roll, *Ind. Eng. Chem.* **19,** 739 (1927). Isoln of *l*-α-pinene from mandarin peel oil *(Citrus reticulata* Blando, *Rutaceae):* Kugler, Kováts, *Helv. Chim. Acta* **46,** 1480 (1963). Total synthesis of α- and β-forms: Komppa, *Ann. Acad. Sci. Fenn.* **A59,** 3 (1943), *C.A.* **41,** 425 (1947); Thomas, Fallis, *Tetrahedron Lett.* **1973,** 4687; *eidem, J. Am. Chem. Soc.* **98,** 1227 (1976). *Review:* Palmer, *Ind. Eng. Chem.* **34,** 1028 (1942); J. L. Simonsen, *The Terpenes* **vol. II** (Cambridge Univ. Press, 2nd ed., 1949) pp 105-191; D. V. Banthorpe, D. Whittaker, *Chem. Rev.* **66,** 643-654 (1966); *Food Cosmet. Toxicol.* **16,** Suppl. I, 853-857 (1978).

dl-Form. Liquid, characteristic odor of turpentine. bp$_{760}$ 155-156°; bp$_{20}$ 52.5°. d$_D^{20}$ 0.8592. n_D^{20} 1.4664. Practically insol in water. Sol in alc, chloroform, ether, glacial acetic acid.

Hydrochloride. $C_{10}H_{17}Cl$. mp 132°.

d-Form. bp$_{760}$ 155-156°. d$_4^{20}$ 0.8591. n_D^{20} 1.4663. $[\alpha]_D^{20}$ +51.14°.

Hydrochloride. mp 132°. $[\alpha]_D^{20}$ +33.52° (alcohol).

l-Form. bp$_{760}$ 155-156°. d$_4^{20}$ 0.8590. n_D^{20} 1.4662. $[\alpha]_D^{20}$ -51.28°.

Hydrochloride. mp 132°. $[\alpha]_D^{20}$ -33.24° (alcohol).

Caution: Toxic effects similar to turpentine, *q.v.*

USE: Manufacture of camphor, insecticides, solvents, plasticizers, perfume bases, synthetic pine oil.

7446. β-Pinene. [127-91-3] 6,6-Dimethyl-2-methylenebicyclo[3.1.1]heptane; nopinene. $C_{10}H_{16}$; mol wt 136.23. C 88.16%, H 11.84%. Found in most essential oils which contain α-pinene, but in far smaller proportions; the *l*-form occurs most commonly. Initial identification: A. von Baeyer, *Ber.* **29,** 25 (1896). Isoln of the *d*-form from *Ferula galbaniflua* Boiss. et Buhse, *Umbelliferae:* B. N. Rutovski, I. V. Vinogradova, *J. Prakt. Chem.* **120,** 41 (1928); from *Cynomarathrum nuttallii* A. Gray, *Umbelliferae:* E. K. Nelson, *J. Am. Chem. Soc.* **55,** 3400 (1933). Irreversible isomerization of β-pinene to α-pinene occurs on shaking with platinum black satd with hydrogen: F. Richter, W. Wolff, *Ber.* **59,** 1733 (1926). Synthesis: G. Bonnet, *Bull. Inst. Pin* **1938,** 217; **1939,** 1, *C.A.* **33,** 4223[4] (1939); K. J. Crowley, *Proc. Chem. Soc. London* **1962,** 245; *Tetrahedron* **21,** 1001 (1965); L. M. Harwood, M. Julia, *Synthesis* **1980,** 456. For general refs *see* α-pinene.

dl-Form. bp$_{760}$ 165-166°.

d-Form. bp$_{760}$ 164-166°. d$_{20}^{20}$ 0.8654. n_D^{20} 1.4739. $[\alpha]_D$ +28.59° (Nelson). Also reported as bp$_{760}$ 162-163°. d$_{20}^{20}$ 0.8662. n_D^{20} 1.4745. $[\alpha]_D$ +20.75° (Rutovski, Vinogradova).

l-Form. bp$_{760}$ 162-163°. d^{15} 0.874. n_D^{15} 1.4872, $[\alpha]_D$ -22.4°.

7447. Pine Oil. Yarmor. An oil from *Pinus palustris* Mill. and certain other species of pines, *Pinaceae*. It is obtained from pitch-soaked pine wood by steam distillation or solvent extraction followed by steam distillation and also by destructive distillation. It consists mainly of isomeric tertiary and secondary, cyclic terpene alcohols.

Colorless to pale yellow liquid, turpentine-like odor. d about 0.9; bp 200-220°. Insol in water. Sol in the usual organic solvents.

Caution: Irritating to skin, mucous membranes. Large doses may cause CNS depression.

USE: Pharmaceutic aid (flavor and perfume). Manuf terpin hydrate and other terpin products; as a solvent, disinfectant and deodorant; in textile scouring; for flotation of lead and zinc ores.

7448. Pine Tar. A product obtained by destructive distillation of wood of *Pinus palustris* Mill., or other species of pine, *Pinaceae*.

Blackish-brown, viscous liquid; heavier than water; empyreumatic odor and sharp taste. Slightly sol in water; sol in alc, chloroform, ether, acetone, glacial acetic acid, fixed and volatile oils, and in solns of caustic alkalies. Principal constituents: turpentine, resin, guaiacol, creosol, methylcreosol, phenol, phlorol, toluene, xylene, and other hydrocarbons.

THERAP CAT: Topical antieczematic; rubefacient.

THERAP CAT (VET): Mild irritant, antiseptic in chronic skin conditions. Expectorant.

7449. Pinguinain. [37288-97-4] A proteolytic enzyme obtained from the juice of the fruit of *Bromelia pinguin* Plum. ex L., *Bromeliaceae* (pineapple family): Asenjo, *Science* **95**, 48 (1942); Bloch, Messing, **US 2977287** (1961 to Ethicon). Immunochemical studies: E. Toro-Goyco, I. Rodriguez-Costas, *Arch. Biochem. Biophys.* **175**, 359 (1976). Structure studies: E. Toro-Goyco *et al., Biochim. Biophys. Acta* **622**, 151 (1980).

Aq solns are capable of digesting necrotic tissue, but do not attack viable tissue. Optimum proteolytic activity is at pH 5.2 to 5.5 and also at pH 7.3. Inactivated at temps above 80°.

7450. Pinolenic Acid. [16833-54-8] (5Z,9Z,12Z)-5,9,12-Octadecatrienoic acid. $C_{18}H_{30}O_2$; mol wt 278.43. C 77.65%, H 10.86%, O 11.49%. Characteristic fatty acid of the seed oils of *Pinus* spp., *Pinaceae*. Positional isomer of γ-linolenic acid, *q.v.* Isoln from tall oil: E. Elomaa *et al., Suom. Kemistil. B* **36**, 52 (1963); A. Hase *et al., J. Am. Oil Chem. Soc.* **69**, 832 (1992). Review of occurrence in the genus *Pinus*: R. L. Wolff *et al., Lipids* **35**, 1-22 (2000). Effect of pinolenic acid-enriched pine nut oil on fatty acid metabolism in rats: M. Sugano *et al., Br. J. Nutr.* **72**, 775 (1994); on LDL-receptor activity: J.-W. Lee *et al., Lipids* **39**, 383 (2004).

n_D^{20} 1.4804. Acid no. 201.8. Iodine no. 268.

THERAP CAT: Nutritional supplement.

7451. Pinosylvin. [22139-77-1] (*E*)-5-(2-Phenylethenyl)-1,3-benzenediol; *E*-3,5-stilbenediol; 5-styrylresorcinol; *trans*-3,5-dihydroxystilbene. $C_{14}H_{12}O_2$; mol wt 212.24. C 79.23%, H 5.70%, O 15.08%. Occurs together with its monomethyl and dimethyl ethers in the heartwood of pine and other woody plants. Naturally occurring pinosylvins have the *trans* configuration. Isoln from *Pinus sylvestris* L., *Pinaceae*: H. Erdtman, *Ann.* **539**, 116 (1939); from other *Pinus* species: G. Lindstedt, *Acta Chem. Scand.* **3**, 755-772 (1949); J. C. Alvarez-Novoa *et al., ibid.* **4**, 444 (1950); from *Alnus sieboldiana, Betulaceae:* Y. Asakawa, *Bull. Chem. Soc. Jpn.* **44**, 2761 (1971); from *Polygonum nodosum, Polygonaceae:* M. Kuroyanagi *et al., Chem. Pharm. Bull.* **30**, 1602 (1982). Synthesis of pinosylvin: E. Späth, F. Liebherr, *Ber.* **74**, 869 (1941); of monomethyl ether: E. Späth, K. Kromp, *ibid.* 1424; of dimethyl ether: G. Aulin-Erdtman, H. Erdtman, *ibid.* 50; of pinosylvin and derivatives: A. A. Loman, L. R. Snowdon, *Can. J. Chem.* **48**, 1554 (1970). Biosynthesis: Birch, *Fortschr. Chem. Org. Naturst.* **14**, 186 (1957). Toxicological study: K. O. Frykholm, *Nature* **155**, 454 (1945). Use as antimicrobial agent: E. H. Sheers, **DE 1952451**; *idem,* **US 3577230** (1970, 1971 both to Arizona Chem. Co.). Deterrent to feeding behavior of snowshoe hare: J. P. Bryant *et al., Science* **222**, 1023 (1983).

Fine needles from glacial acetic acid, mp 155.5-156°. uv max (ethanol): 305 nm (log ε 4.49). Practically insol in water. Sol in benzene, acetone, chloroform, glacial acetic acid.

Monomethyl ether. $C_{15}H_{14}O_2$. Crystals, mp 122-123°. uv max (ethanol): 303 nm (log ε 4.26). More sol in benzene than pinosylvin. Also sol in methanol, glacial acetic acid.

Dimethyl ether. $C_{16}H_{16}O_2$. Crystals from methanol-water, mp 55-56°. uv max (ethanol): 305 nm (log ε 4.39).

7452. Pioglitazone. [111025-46-8] 5-[[4-[2-(5-Ethyl-2-pyridinyl)ethoxy]phenyl]methyl]-2,4-thiazolidinedione; (±)-5-[*p*-[2-(ethyl-2-pyridyl)ethoxy]benzyl]-2,4-thiazolidinedione; AD-4833. $C_{19}H_{20}N_2O_3S$; mol wt 356.44. C 64.02%, H 5.66%, N 7.86%, O 13.47%, S 9.00%. Insulin sensitizer. Prepn: K. Meguro, T. Fujita, **EP 193256**; *eidem,* **US 4687777** (1986, 1987 both to Takeda); T. Sohda *et al., Arzneim.-Forsch.* **40**, 37 (1990). Pharmacology: H. Ikeda *et al., ibid.* 156. HPLC determn in serum: W. Z. Zhong, D. B. Lakings, *J. Chromatogr.* **490**, 377 (1989). Mechanism of action: C. Hofmann *et al., Endocrinology* **129**, 1915 (1991); M. Kobayashi *et al., Diabetes* **41**, 476 (1992). Effect on adipocyte differentiation: T. Sandouk *et al., Am. J. Physiol.* **264**, C1600 (1993). Clinical evaluation in noninsulin-dependent diabetes: R. Kawamori *et al., Diabetes Res. Clin. Pract.* **41**, 35 (1998).

Colorless needles from DMF + water, mp 183-184°.

Hydrochloride. [112529-15-4] U-72107A; Actos. $C_{19}H_{20}N_2$-$O_3S.HCl$; mol wt 392.90. Colorless prisms from ethanol, mp 193-194°. Sol in DMF; slightly sol in ethanol; very slightly sol in acetone, acetonitrile. Practically insol in water; insol in ether.

THERAP CAT: Antidiabetic.

7453. Pipacycline. [1110-80-1] [4S-(4α,4aα,5aα,6β,12aα)]-4-(Dimethylamino)-1,4,4a,5,5a,6,11,12a-octahydro-3,6,10,12,12a-pentahydroxy-*N*-[[4-(2-hydroxyethyl)-1-piperazinyl]methyl]-6-methyl-1,11-dioxo-2-naphthacenecarboxamide; *N*-[[4-(2-hydroxyethyl)-1-piperazinyl]methyl]tetracycline; *N*-[4-(β-hydroxyethyl)-diethylenediamino-1-methyl]tetracycline; mepicycline; mepiciclina; Ambra-Vena; Sieromicin; Valtomicina. $C_{29}H_{38}N_4O_9$; mol wt 586.63. C 59.37%, H 6.53%, N 9.55%, O 24.55%. Semisynthetic broad spectrum antibiotic related to tetracycline. Prepn: Pedrazzoli *et al., Boll. Chim. Farm.* **98**, 516 (1959), *C.A.* **54**, 3856a (1960); Gradnik *et al.,* **GB 888968** corresp to **US 3149114** (1962 and 1964 to E.R.A.S.M.E.). Properties: *eidem, Pharm. Acta Helv.* **35**, 529 (1960). Pharmacokinetic studies: A. Scalvini, A. Delmonte, *Gazz. Med. Ital.* **131**, 1 (1972).

Yellow cryst powder, dec 162-163°. $[\alpha]_D^{20}$ −195° (c = 0.5). $[\alpha]_D^{20}$ −175° (c = 0.5 in methanol). uv max (10 γ/ml 0.1*N* HCl): 286, 355 nm. pH of 2% aq soln, 7.2-7.4. Freely sol in water, methanol, formamide; slightly sol in ethanol, isopropanol. Practically insol in ether, benzene, chloroform. Sensitive to light, heat, and air. LD$_{50}$ i.v. in white mice: 188 mg/kg (Scalvini, Delmonte).

THERAP CAT: Antibacterial.

7454. Pipamazine. [84-04-8] 1-[3-(2-Chloro-10*H*-phenothiazin-10-yl)propyl]-4-piperidinecarboxamide; 1-[3-(2-chlorophenothiazin-10-yl)propyl]isonipecotamide; 10-[3-(4-carbamoylpiperidin-1-yl)propyl]-2-chlorophenothiazine; 2-chloro-10-[3-(4-carbamoylpiperidinyl)propyl]phenothiazine; 10-[3-(4-carbamoylpiperidino)propyl]-2-chlorophenothiazine; SC-9387; Nausidol; Mornidine. $C_{21}H_{24}ClN_3OS$; mol wt 401.95. C 62.75%, H 6.02%, Cl 8.82%, N 10.45%, O 3.98%, S 7.98%. Prepn: Cusic *et al.*, **US 2957870** (1960 to Searle).

Crystals from 2-propanol + petr ether, mp about 139°.
Hydrochloride. Crystals, mp about 196-197° with formation of bubbles.
THERAP CAT: Antiemetic.

7455. Pipamperone. [1893-33-0] 1'-[4-(4-Fluorophenyl)-4-oxobutyl]-[1,4'-bipiperidine]-4'-carboxamide; 1'-[3-(*p*-fluorobenzoyl)propyl]-[1,4'-bipiperidine]-4'-carboxamide; 1-(*p*-fluorophenyl)-4-(4-piperidino-4-carbamoylpiperidino)-1-butanone; 1-[γ-(4-fluorobenzoyl)propyl]-4-piperidinopiperidine-4-carboxamide; 4'-fluoro-4-[*N*-[4-(*N*-piperidino)-4-carbamido]piperidino]butyrophenone; floropipamide; R-3345. $C_{21}H_{30}FN_3O_2$; mol wt 375.48. C 67.17%, H 8.05%, F 5.06%, N 11.19%, O 8.52%. Prepn of the dihydrochloride by reaction of γ-chloro-4-fluorobutyrophenone and 4-piperidinopiperidine-4-carboxamide: Janssen, **BE 610830** (1962 to Janssen), *C.A.* **57,** 13740b (1962).

Dihydrochloride. [2448-68-2] Dipiperon; Piperonil; Propitan. $C_{21}H_{30}FN_3O_2 \cdot 2HCl$; mol wt 448.40. Crystals, mp 124.5-126.0°.
THERAP CAT: Antipsychotic.

7456. Pipazethate. [2167-85-3] 10*H*-Pyrido[3,2-*b*][1,4]benzothiadiazine-10-carboxylic acid 2-(2-piperidinoethoxy)ethyl ester; 2-(2-piperidinoethoxy)ethyl 10*H*-pyrido[3,2-*b*][1,4]benzothiadiazine-10-carboxylate; thiophenylpyridylamino-10-carboxylic acid piperidinoethoxyethyl ester; 2-(2-piperidinoethoxy)ethyl 10-thia-1,9-diazaanthracene-10-carboxylate; 1-azaphenothiazine-10-carboxylic acid 2-(2-piperidinoethoxy)ethyl ester; D-254. $C_{21}H_{25}$-N_3O_3S; mol wt 399.51. C 63.13%, H 6.31%, N 10.52%, O 12.01%, S 8.03%. Prepn: Schuler *et al.*, *Ann.* **673,** 102 (1964); Schuler, **US 2989529** (1961 to Degussa).

Hydrochloride. [6056-11-7] Lenopect; Selvigon; Selvjgon; Theratuss. $C_{21}H_{25}N_3O_3S \cdot HCl$; mol wt 435.97. Pale yellow crystals from isopropanol, mp 160-161°. Soluble in water, methanol. Practically insol in acetone, petr ether. LD_{50} orally in rats: 560 mg/kg (Schuler).
THERAP CAT: Antitussive.

7457. Pipebuzone. [27315-91-9] 4-Butyl-4-[(4-methyl-1-piperazinyl)methyl]-1,2-diphenyl-3,5-pyrazolidinedione; 1,2-diphenyl-3,5-dioxo-4-[(4-methyl-1-piperazinyl)methyl]-4-butylpyrazolidine; LD-4644; Elarzone. $C_{25}H_{32}N_4O_2$; mol wt 420.55. C 71.40%, H 7.67%, N 13.32%, O 7.61%. The 4-[(4-methyl-1-piperazinyl)methyl]- deriv of phenylbutazone, *q.v.* Prepn: **DE 1958722** and **FR M7914** (both 1970 to Dausse), *C.A.* **73,** 25460v (1970); **76,** 140797j (1972).

Crystals from isopropanol, mp 129°.
THERAP CAT: Anti-inflammatory; antipyretic; analgesic.

7458. Pipecolic Acid. [535-75-1] 2-Piperidinecarboxylic acid; pipecolinic acid; hexahydropicolinic acid; homoproline; dihydrobaikiaine. $C_6H_{11}NO_2$; mol wt 129.16. C 55.79%, H 8.58%, N 10.84%, O 24.77%. The *l*-form occurs in plants: Phillips, *Chem. Ind. (London)* **1953,** 127. Prepn: A. Ladenburg, *Ber.* **24,** 640 (1891); Stevens, Ellman, *J. Biol. Chem.* **182,** 75 (1950); V. Asher *et al., Tetrahedron Lett.* **22,** 141 (1981). Synthesis of L-pipecolic acid from L-lysine: Fujii, Miyoshi, *Bull. Chem. Soc. Jpn.* **48,** 1341 (1975). Synthesis of racemate: R. T. Shuman *et al., J. Org. Chem.* **55,** 738 (1990).

*l***-Form.** Needles by sublimation, mp 270°. $[\alpha]_D^{25}$ −34.9°. Sol in water, dil alcohol. Sparingly sol in abs alcohol, acetone, chloroform. Insol in ether.
*d***-Form.** Platelets from alcohol, mp 270°. $[\alpha]_D^{25}$ +35.7°. Sol in water. Somewhat sol in alcohol.
*dl***-Form.** Leaflets from water, mp 264°. Sol in water, boiling alcohol.
*dl***-Hydrochloride.** $C_6H_{11}NO_2 \cdot HCl$. Crystals (warts) from alcohol + benzene, mp 258-262°.

7459. Pipecurium Bromide. [52212-02-9] 4,4'-[(2β,3α,-5α,16β,17β)-3,17-Bis(acetyloxy)androstane-2,16-diyl]bis(1,1-dimethylpiperazinium)dibromide; 4,4'-(3α,17β-dihydroxy-5α-androstan-2β,16β-ylene)bis(1,1-dimethylpiperazinium)dibromide diacetate; pipecuronium bromide; RGH-1106; Arduan. $C_{35}H_{62}Br_2N_4$-O_4; mol wt 762.70. C 55.12%, H 8.19%, Br 20.95%, N 7.35%, O 8.39%. Aminosteroid, competitive neuromuscular blocker. Prepn: Z. Tuba *et al.*, **DE 2337882** (1974 to Gedeon Richter), *C.A.* **80,** 121210d (1974); Z. Tuba, *Arzneim.-Forsch.* **30,** 342 (1980). Toxicity study: E. Kárpáti, K. Biro, *ibid.* 346. Series of articles on pharmacology, properties, disposition, pharmacokinetics, safety tests, clinical studies: *ibid.* 346-394. Determn in human serum: G. Szabo, E. Tassonyi, *ibid.* **31,** 1013 (1981).

Crystals from methylene dichloride/acetone, mp 262-264° (dec). $[\alpha]_D^{25}$ +8.1° (c = 1 in water). LD_{50} in mice, rats (mg/kg): 29.7, 172.6 i.v.; 70.6, 449.6 i.p.; 60.5, 455.8 s.c. (Kárpáti, Biro).

THERAP CAT: Neuromuscular blocking agent.

7460.   Pipemidic Acid. [51940-44-4] 8-Ethyl-5,8-dihydro-5-oxo-2-(1-piperazinyl)pyrido[2,3-d]pyrimidine-6-carboxylic acid; piperamic acid; 1489-RB; Filtrax; Memento 400; Pi-Coli; Pipeacid; Pipedac; Pipemid; Pipurin; Tractur; Uropimid; Urosten; Uroval. $C_{14}H_{17}N_5O_3$; mol wt 303.32. C 55.44%, H 5.65%, N 23.09%, O 15.82%. Quinolone antibacterial. Prepn: S. Minami et al., **DE 2341146**; eidem, **US 3887557** (1974, 1975 both to Dainippon Pharm.); Pesson et al., C.R. Seances Acad. Sci. Ser. C **278**, 1169 (1974); De Lajudie et al., ibid. Ser. D **279**, 1931 (1974); Matsumoto, Minami, J. Med. Chem. **18**, 74 (1975). Characterization: Ficicchia, Farmaco Ed. Prat. **30**, 207 (1974). Antibacterial activity: Ficicchia, De Lajudie, ibid. 252. Pharmacology: Shimizu et al., Antimicrob. Agents Chemother. **7**, 441 (1975).

Yellowish-white, odorless, bitter-tasting crystals, mp 253-255°. Hygroscopic. Yellows slowly in light. Sol in acid soln and alkaline. Very slightly sol in water, alcohol; slightly sol in chloroform (0.5%), methanol (0.4%). Practically insol in ether, benzene. LD_{50} in mice (mg/kg): 4000 orally; 1000 i.p., 50 i.v. (Ficicchia).

Trihydrate. [72571-82-5] Deblaston; Dolcol; Pipram; Solupemid. Nearly colorless needles, mp 253-255°.

THERAP CAT: Antibacterial.

THERAP CAT (VET): Antibacterial.

7461.   Pipenzolate Bromide. [125-51-9] 1-Ethyl-3-[(hydroxydiphenylacetyl)oxy]-1-methylpiperidinium bromide; 1-ethyl-3-hydroxy-1-methylpiperidinium bromide benzilate; benzilic acid 1-ethyl-3-piperidyl ester methyl bromide; N-ethyl-3-piperidyl benzilate methobromide; pipenzolate methylbromide; pipenzolone bromide; JB-323; Piptal. $C_{22}H_{28}BrNO_3$; mol wt 434.37. C 60.83%, H 6.50%, Br 18.40%, N 3.22%, O 11.05%. Anticholinergic. Prepn from N-ethyl-3-chloropiperidine and benzilic acid: Biel et al., J. Am. Chem. Soc. **74**, 1485 (1952); **US 2918406** (1959 to Lakeside).

Crystals from methyl ethyl ketone, mp 179-180°. Soluble in water.

Note: N-Ethyl-3-piperidyl benzilate is a controlled substance (hallucinogen): **21 CFR**, 1308.11.

THERAP CAT: Antispasmodic.

7462.   Piperacetazine. [3819-00-9] 1-[10-[3-[4-(2-Hydroxyethyl)-1-piperidinyl]propyl]-10H-phenothiazin-2-yl]ethanone; 10-[3-[4-(2-hydroxyethyl)piperidino]propyl]phenothiazin-2-yl methyl ketone; 2-acetyl-10-[3-[4-(β-hydroxyethyl)piperidino]-propyl]phenothiazine; 2-acetyl-10-[3-[4-(γ-2-hydroxyethyl)piperi-dino]propyl]phenothiazine; PC-1421; Quide. $C_{24}H_{30}N_2O_2S$; mol wt 410.57. C 70.21%, H 7.36%, N 6.82%, O 7.79%, S 7.81%. Prepn: **GB 861807** (1961 to Searle). Clinical trial in schizophrenia: R. T. Rada, P. T. Donlon, Curr. Ther. Res. **16**, 124 (1974).

Hydrochloride. mp 100-110°.

THERAP CAT: Antipsychotic.

7463.   Piperacillin. [61477-96-1](2S,5R,6R)-6-[[(2R)-[[(4-Ethyl-2,3-dioxo-1-piperazinyl)carbonyl]amino]phenylacetyl]amino]-3,3-dimethyl-7-oxo-4-thia-1-azabicyclo[3.2.0]heptane-2-car-boxylicacid;(2S,5R,6R)-6-[(R)-2-(4-ethyl-2,3-dioxo-1-piperazine-carboxamido)-2-phenylacetamido]-3,3-dimethyl-7-oxo-4-thia-1-azabicyclo[3.2.0]heptane-2-carboxylicacid;6-D(−)-α-(4-ethyl-2,3-dioxo-1-piperazinylcarbonylamino)-α-phenylacetamido-penicillanic acid; 4-ethyl-2,3-dioxopiperazine carbonyl ampicillin. $C_{23}H_{27}N_5O_7S$; mol wt 517.55. C 53.38%, H 5.26%, N 13.53%, O 21.64%, S 6.20%. Broad spectrum semi-synthetic antibiotic related to pencillin. Prepn: I. Saikawa et al., **DE 2519400**; eidem, **US 4087424** (1976, 1978 both to Toyama). In vitro studies: G. P. Bodey, B. LeBlanc, Antimicrob. Agents Chemother. **14**, 78 (1978); R. Wise et al., ibid. 549. In vitro and in vivo: N. A. Kuck, G. S. Redin, J. Antibiot. **31**, 1175 (1978). Pharmacokinetics: M. A. Evans et al., J. Antimicrob. Chemother. **4**, 255 (1978). Metabolism: K. Iida et al., Antimicrob. Agents Chemother. **14**, 257 (1978). Clinical study: T. Saito, Y. Yamada, Jpn. J. Antibiot. **30**, 835 (1977). Toxicity study: A. Takai et al., Chemotherapy (Tokyo) **25**, 816 (1977). Review of antibacterial activity, pharmacokinetics: G. L. Mandell, Clin. Ther. **7**, Suppl. B, 28-35 (1985). Review of clinical experience in urinary tract infections: S. J. Childs, ibid. 36-45. Series of articles on antibacterial activity and clinical use: Chemotherapy (Tokyo) **36**, Suppl. 7, 1-85 (1988).

Sodium salt. [59703-84-3] CL-227193; T-1220; Isipen; Pentcillin; Pipracil; Pipril. $C_{23}H_{26}N_5NaO_7S$; mol wt 539.54. mp 183-185° (dec). LD_{50} in mice, rats, dogs, monkeys (g/kg): 5, 2.7, >6, >4 i.v. (Takai).

THERAP CAT: Antibacterial.

7464.   Piperazine. [110-85-0] Hexahydropyrazine; pipera-zidine; diethylenediamine. $C_4H_{10}N_2$; mol wt 86.14. C 55.77%, H 11.70%, N 32.52%. Prepn: Cloez, Jahresber. **1853**, 468; Wolff, Ber. **26**, 724 (1893); Kyrides, **US 2267686** (1941); Martin, Martell, J. Am. Chem. Soc. **70**, 1817 (1948); MacKenzie, Turbin, **US 2901482** (1959 to Dow); Moss, Godfrey, **US 3037023** (1962 to Jefferson Chem.). Prepn of salts: Hefferren et al., J. Am. Pharm. Assoc. **44**, 678 (1955). Determn in animal feeds: J. D. McLean, O. L. Daniels, J. Assoc. Off. Anal. Chem. **54**, 555 (1971). Veterinary trial in combination with levamisole: J. H. Drudge et al., Am. J. Vet. Res. **35**, 67 (1974). Clinical efficacy in roundworm infection: A. S. Nanivadekar et al., J. Postgrad. Med. **30**, 144 (1984).

Leaflets from alc, mp 106°. Salty taste. bp$_{760}$ 146°. Strong base: pKa: 4.19, absorbs water and CO_2 from air. Absorption spectrum: Purvis, *J. Chem. Soc.* **103**, 2286, 2293 (1913). Freely sol in water, glycerol, glycols; one gram dissolves in 2 ml of 95% alcohol. Insol in ether. pH of a 10% aq soln 10.8-11.8. Forms a sol compd with theophylline. *Keep tightly closed and protect from light.*

Hexahydrate. Dietelmin; Helmifren; Parid; Paravermin; Tasnon (elixir); Upixon; Uvilon. $C_4H_{10}N_2.6H_2O$; mol wt 194.23. Crystals from water (contg 44.34% anhydr piperazine), mp 44°. bp 125-130°. The piperazine of commerce is usually this hydrate. Freely sol in water; sol in alc (~1:2). Practically insol in ether. pH of a 10% aq soln 10.8-11.8.

Citrate. [144-29-6] Tripiperazine dicitrate; Helmezine; Oxucide; Parazine; Pinozan; Pipizan Citrate; Pipracid (syrup); Rhomex; Ta-Verm; Worm Away. $3C_4H_{10}N_2.2C_6H_8O_7$; mol wt 642.65. Crystals, dec 182-187°. Freely sol in water. Practically insol in alcohol, ether, chloroform. pH of a 10% aq soln 5.0-6.0.

Edetate calcium. [12002-30-1] Piperazine calcium edathamil; Perin. $C_{14}H_{24}CaN_4O_8$; mol wt 416.44. Prepn: Schlesinger *et al.*, **US 2834782** (1958 to Endo). Occurs as the dihydrate. Crystals; slightly salty taste. Freely sol in water. Very slightly sol in alcohol, chloroform. Practically insol in ether. pH of 20% aq soln 4.3-5.4.

Phosphate. Antepar; Pinrou; Piperverm; Piperazate; Tasnon (tabl.). $C_4H_{10}N_2.H_3PO_4$; mol wt 184.13. Minute crystals. Very slightly sol in water. pH of saturated aq soln, 6.5.

Tartrate. [133-36-8] Noxiurotan; Piperate. $C_4H_{10}N_2.C_4H_6$-O_6; mol wt 236.22. Crystals, dec 258-263°. Soly in g/100 ml at 25°: water 26; alcohol 0.01; chloroform 0.01. pH of 1% soln: 4.8.

N^1,N^4-**Dibenzoylpiperazine.** $C_{18}H_{18}N_2O_2$. Prepd from piperazine and benzoyl chloride in dil NaOH. Crystals from alc, mp 191°.

THERAP CAT: Anthelmintic (Nematodes).

THERAP CAT (VET): Anthelmintic (Nematodes).

7465. Piperazine Adipate. [142-88-1] Hexanedioic acid compd with piperazine (1:1); Entacyl; Oxyzin (tabl.); Vermicompren (tabl.); Nometan; Oxypaat; Pipadox; Oxurasin. $C_{10}H_{20}N_2O_4$; mol wt 232.28. C 51.71%, H 8.68%, N 12.06%, O 27.55%. C_4-$H_{10}N_2.C_6H_{10}O_4$. The neutral salt of piperazine and adipic acid: Davies *et al.*, *J. Pharm. Pharmacol.* **6**, 707 (1954). Prepn in methanolic medium: Forrest, Petrow, **US 2799617** (1957 to British Drug Houses); **GB 767826**. Pharmacology: B. G. Cross *et al.*, *J. Pharm. Pharmacol.* **6**, 711 (1954).

Prisms, mp 256-257°. Stable to heat and air. Pleasant, slightly acid taste. Dissolves slowly. Soly in 100 ml water at 20°: 5.53 g, at 30°: 6.61 g, at 56.3°: 10.14 g; in 100 g methanol at 25°: 0.02 g. Practically insol in abs ethanol, isopropanol, dioxane. Aq solns of 0.2-0.01M have pH 5.45 which is only slightly affected by increases in ionic strength caused by the addition of simple neutral salts. LD$_{50}$ in mice, rats (g/kg): 11.4, 7.9 orally (Cross).

THERAP CAT: Anthelmintic (Nematodes).

THERAP CAT (VET): Anthelmintic (Nematodes).

7466. 2,5-Piperazinedione. [106-57-0] Glycine anhydride; cycloglycylglycine; α,γ-diacipiperazine; glycylglycine lactam; diglycolyldiamide; 2,5-diketopiperazine; 2,5-dioxopiperazine. C_4-$H_6N_2O_2$; mol wt 114.10. C 42.11%, H 5.30%, N 24.55%, O 28.04%. Can exist in 5 enol forms: Richardson *et al.*, *J. Am. Chem. Soc.* **51**, 3074 (1929). Prepn from glycine ethyl ester hydrochloride: Fischer, *Ber.* **39**, 2930 (1906).

Platelets from water, needles by sublimation. Dec 311-312° (begins to sublime at 260° and sinters at 305°). Sparingly sol in water; sol in HCl (d 1.19) from which it can be precipitated by the addition of alcohol. Acts as a weak base. Hydrolyzed to glycylglycine by acids and alkalies.

Hydrochloride. $C_4H_6N_2O_2.HCl$. Crystals, mp 129-130°.

7467. Piperic Acid. [5285-18-7] 5-(1,3-Benzodioxol-5-yl)-2,4-pentadienoic acid; 5-(3,4-methylenedioxyphenyl)-2,4-pentadienoic acid. $C_{12}H_{10}O_4$; mol wt 218.21. C 66.05%, H 4.62%, O 29.33%. Early literature treats the title compound without specifying stereochemistry; however, four isomers exist: piperinic acid *(E,E)*; isochavicinic acid *(E,Z)*; isopiperinic acid *(Z,E)*; chavicinic acid *(Z,Z)*. Physical constants given in early references for piperic acid agree with those of piperinic acid. *See Beilstein* **19**, 281; suppl. II, 300. Synthesis of *(E,E)*-form: L. von Babo, E. Keller, *J. Prakt. Chem.* **72**, 53 (1857); A. Ladenburg, M. Sholtz, *Ber.* **27**, 2958 (1894); of *(E,Z)*-form: H. Lohaus, H. Gall, *Ann.* **517**, 278 (1935); of *(Z,Z)*-form: E. Ott, F. Eichler, *Ber.* **55**, 2653 (1922); of *(Z,Z)*-form: *idem, loc. cit.*; H. Lohaus, H. Gall, *loc. cit.*; of all isomers: R. Grewe *et al.*, *Ber.* **103**, 3752 (1970); R. De Cleyn, A. Verzele, *Bull. Soc. Chim. Belg.* **81**, 529 (1972).

(E,E)-form

(E,E)-**Form.** [136-72-1] Piperinic acid; piperinsäure (German). Needles from alc. Colorless when freshly prepd, rapidly turns yellow on exposure to light. mp 216-217°. Sublimes as yellow needles with partial decompn. uv max (methanol): 340 nm (ε 28800). Sol in 50 parts boiling alcohol, 275 parts abs alcohol at 25°. Practically insol in water, ether, benzene, carbon disulfide.

(E,Z)-**Form.** [495-87-4] Isochavicinic acid. Yellow crystals from methanol/water, sublimes as needles. mp 134-136° (Lohaus, Gall); 143° (Grewe). uv max (methanol): 335 nm (ε 14500). Sol in methanol, benzene.

(Z,E)-**Form.** [495-88-5] Isopiperinic acid. Needles from benzene. mp 145° (Ott, Eichler); 153° (Grewe); 138° (DeCleyn, Verzele). uv max (methanol): 328 nm (ε 22000). Sol in benzene.

(Z,Z)-**Form.** [495-89-6] Chavicinic acid. Amorphous yellow granules from benzene. Wide disparities in mp have been reported: 200-202° (Ott, Eichler); 130° (Grewe); 120° (De Cleyn, Verzele). uv max (methanol): 335 nm (ε 17500). 0.55 g sol in 16 g boiling 95% alcohol, and in 65 g boiling benzene.

7468. Piperidine. [110-89-4] Hexahydropyridine. C_5H_{11}-N; mol wt 85.15. C 70.53%, H 13.02%, N 16.45%. Found in small quantities in *Piper nigrum* L., *Piperaceae* (black pepper). May be obtained from piperine by heating with alcoholic KOH, or from 1,5-diaminopentane hydrochloride by cyclization. Usually prepd by electrolytic reduction of pyridine. Forms complexes with salts of heavy metals. Because of its reactivity, piperidine is useful in the prepn of cryst derivatives of aromatic nitro compds contg nuclear halogen atoms: Seikel, *J. Am. Chem. Soc.* **62**, 750 (1940). Toxicity study: H. F. Smyth *et al.*, *Am. Ind. Hyg. Assoc. J.* **23**, 95 (1962). Review of physical constants of piperidine and *N*-alkyl piperidines: Magnusson, Schierz, *Univ. Wyo. Publ.* **7**, 1 (1940).

Liquid. Characteristic odor. Soapy feel. Solidifies −13° to −17°; mp −7°; bp$_{760}$ 106°; bp$_{20}$ 18°; d$_4^{20}$ 0.8622; n_D^{20} 1.4534. Infrared absorption spectrum: Freymann, *Compt. Rend.* **205**, 852 (1937); *Ann. Chim.* **11**, 11 (1939). Ultraviolet and Raman spectra: Lecomte, *Compt. Rend.* **207**, 395 (1938). Strong base: pK (25°): 2.80. Misc with water. Sol in alcohol, benzene, chloroform. LD$_{50}$ orally in rats: 0.52 ml/kg (Smyth).

Hydrochloride. $C_5H_{11}N.HCl$. Orthorhombic prisms from alcohol, mp 247°. Freely sol in water, alcohol.

Nitrate. $C_5H_{11}N.HNO_3$. Hygroscopic plates, sublimes 75° (10 mm), mp 110°. Freely sol in water, alcohol, ether. Absorption spectrum: Harper, Macbech, *J. Chem. Soc.* **107**, 91 (1915).

Bitartrate. $C_5H_{11}N.C_4H_6O_6$. Crystals, freely sol in water.

Aurichloride. $C_5H_{11}N.HAuCl_4$. Yellow crystals, mp 219°.

Platinichloride. $2C_5H_{11}N.H_2PtCl_6$. Yellow monoclinic prisms from water, mp 202°. Freely sol in water, slightly in alcohol.

N-Benzoylpiperidine. Long needles, mp 44-48°. *Ref: Org. Synth.* coll. vol. I (2nd ed., 1941) p 99.

Phosphate. [767-21-5] Prepn from piperidine + phosphoric acid: Abood, **US 3035977** (1962). Crystals, mp 204-206°.

7469. Piperidione. [77-03-2] 3,3-Diethyl-2,4-piperidine-dione; 3,3-diethyl-2,4-dioxopiperidine; dihyprylone; Sedulon; Tusseval. $C_9H_{15}NO_2$; mol wt 169.22. C 63.88%, H 8.93%, N 8.28%, O 18.91%. Prepn: Tsukita, *J. Pharm. Soc. Jpn.* **69**, 194 (1949).

Crystals, mp 102-107°. Bitter taste. Freely sol in water, alcohol, chloroform.

THERAP CAT: Sedative, antitussive.

7470. Piperidolate. [82-98-4] α-Phenylbenzeneacetic acid 1-ethyl-3-piperidinyl ester; diphenylacetic acid 1-ethyl-3-piperidyl ester; *N*-ethyl-3-piperidyl diphenylacetate; JB-305. $C_{21}H_{25}NO_2$; mol wt 323.43. C 77.98%, H 7.79%, N 4.33%, O 9.89%. Anticholinergic. Prepd from diphenylacetyl chloride and *N*-ethyl-3-hydroxypiperidine: Biel *et al., J. Am. Chem. Soc.* **74**, 1485 (1952); **US 2918407** (1959 to Lakeside Labs.).

Liquid. $bp_{0.18}$ 191-192°.

Hydrochloride. [129-77-1] Crapinon; Dactil. $C_{21}H_{25}NO_2\cdot$HCl; mol wt 359.89. Crystals, mp 195-196°. Soluble in water.

THERAP CAT: Antispasmodic.

7471. Piperilate. [4546-39-8] α-Hydroxy-α-phenylbenzeneacetic acid 2-(1-piperidinyl)ethyl ester; β-piperidylethyl benzilate; pipethanate; benzilic acid 1-piperidineethanol ester; 1-piperidineethanol benzilate; 2-(1-piperidino)ethyl benzilate. $C_{21}H_{25}NO_3$; mol wt 339.43. C 74.31%, H 7.42%, N 4.13%, O 14.14%. Anticholinergic. Prepn: Ford-Moore, Ing, *J. Chem. Soc.* **1947**, 55.

Hydrochloride. [4544-15-4] Daipisate; Norticon; Pensanate; Pipenale. $C_{21}H_{25}NO_3\cdot$HCl; mol wt 375.89. Crystals from acetone or ethanol, mp 170-171°.

Ethyl bromide. Panpurol. $C_{23}H_{30}BrNO_3$; mol wt 448.39.

THERAP CAT: Antispasmodic.

7472. Piperine. [94-62-2] 1-[(2*E*,4*E*)-5-(1,3-Benzodioxol-5-yl)-1-oxo-2,4-pentadienyl]piperidine; (*E,E*)-1-piperoylpiperidine. $C_{17}H_{19}NO_3$; mol wt 285.34. C 71.56%, H 6.71%, N 4.91%, O 16.82%. Isolated from black pepper (*Piper nigrum* L.); also in *P. longum* L., *P. retrofractum* Vahl. (*P. officinarum* C.D.C.), and *P. clusii* C.D.C.; in root bark of *Piper geniculatum* Sw., *Piperaceae.* Extraction procedure: Cazeneuve, Caillot, *Bull. Soc. Chim.* [2] **27**, 291 (1877). Synthesis: Rugheimer, *Ber.* **15**, 1390 (1882); Newman, *Chem. Prod.* **16**, 379 (1953); Normant, Feugeas, *Compt. Rend.* **258**, 2846 (1964). Spectroscopic structural elucidation and prepa-

rative separation of piperine and its stereoisomers isopiperine, isochavicine and chavicine, *q.v.:* R. De Cleyn, M. Verzele, *Bull. Soc. Chim. Belg.* **84**, 435 (1975). Synthesis of isomers: R. Grewe *et al., Ber.* **103**, 3752 (1970); of piperine and isochavicine: S. Tsuboi *et al., Tetrahedron Lett.* **1979**, 1043. Stereoselective synthesis of piperine: R. A. Olsen, G. O. Spessard, *J. Agric. Food Chem.* **29**, 942 (1981). More toxic to houseflies than pyrethrum: Harvill *et al., Contrib. Boyce Thompson Inst.* **13**, 87 (1943).

Monoclinic prisms from alcohol, mp 130°. Tasteless at first, but burning aftertaste. Neutral to litmus. pK (18°): 12.22. Almost insol in water (40 mg/liter at 18°), in petr ether. One gram dissolves in 15 ml alcohol, 1.7 ml chloroform, 36 ml ether. Sol in benzene, acetic acid.

(*E,Z*)-Form. Isochavicine. Crystals from chloroform + hexane, mp 89° (Grewe), 103° (De Cleyn). uv max (methanol): 333 nm (ε 16300).

(*Z,E*)-Form. Isopiperine. Crystals from chloroform + hexane, mp 110° (Grewe), 86° (De Cleyn). uv max (methanol): 332 nm (ε 21800).

USE: To impart pungent taste to brandy. As insecticide.

7473. Piperitone. [89-81-6] 3-Methyl-6-(1-methylethyl)-2-cyclohexen-1-one; *p*-menth-1-en-3-one; 4-isopropyl-1-methyl-1-cyclohexen-3-one. $C_{10}H_{16}O$; mol wt 152.23. C 78.90%, H 10.59%, O 10.51%. Isoln of *d*-form from oil of *Cymbopogon sennaarensis* Chiov., *Gramineae:* Roberts, *J. Chem. Soc.* **107**, 1465 (1915); from oil of *Andropogon iwarancusa* Jones: Simonsen, *ibid.* **119**, 1644 (1921); from oil of *Mentha* spp., *Labiatae:* Reitsma, *J. Am. Pharm. Assoc.* **47**, 265, 267 (1958). Isoln of *l*-form from Sitka spruce oil: von Rudloff, *Can. J. Chem.* **42**, 1057 (1964). Isoln of *dl*-form from oil of *Eucalyptus dives* Schau., *Myrtaceae:* Read, Smith, *J. Chem. Soc.* **119**, 779 (1921); from peppermint oil: Katsuragi, *Koryo* No. 24, 16 (1953). Synthesis of *dl*-form: Misrock, Church, *Ind. Eng. Chem.* **49**, 822 (1957); Bain *et al.*, **US 2972632** (1961 to Glidden); Wiemann, Dubois, *Bull. Soc. Chim. Fr.* **1962**, 1813; Stepanov, Myrsina, *Zh. Obshch. Khim.* **34**, 3092 (1964).

d-Form. Liquid. Peppermint odor. bp 232-235°; bp_{20} 116-118.5°. d_4^{20} 0.9344. $[\alpha]_D^{20}$ +49.13°. n_D^{20} 1.4848.

l-Form. Liquid. bp_{15} 109.5-110.5°. d_4^{20} 0.9324. $[\alpha]_D^{20}$ −15.9°. n_D^{20} 1.4823. Practically insol in water. Sol in alcohol, oils.

dl-Form. Liquid. bp_{769} 232-233°; bp_{16} 116-118°. d_4^{20} 0.9331. n_D^{24} 1.4823. uv max (ethanol): 232.5 nm (ε 13350).

USE: In masking odors in dentifrices.

7474. Piperocaine. [136-82-3] 2-Methyl-1-piperidinepropanol benzoate; γ-(2-methylpiperidyl)propyl benzoate; (2-methylpiperidino)propyl benzoate; 3-benzoxy-1-(2-methylpiperidino)-propane; benzoyl-γ-(2-methylpiperidino)propanol. $C_{16}H_{23}NO_2$; mol wt 261.36. C 73.53%, H 8.87%, N 5.36%, O 12.24%. Prepn of the hydrochloride: S. M. McElvain, **US 1784903** (1930). Pharmacology: K. H. Beyer, A. R. Latven, *J. Pharmacol. Exp. Ther.* **106**, 37 (1952). Structure activity study: P. P. Koelzer, K. H. Wehr, *Arzneim.-Forsch.* **8**, 708 (1958).

LD$_{50}$ i.v. in rabbits: 18 ±6 mg/kg (Beyer, Latven).

Hydrochloride. [533-28-8] C$_{16}$H$_{23}$NO$_2$.HCl. Crystals from alc-ether, mp 167-169°. Stable in air. One gram dissolves in 1.5 ml water, 4.5 ml alcohol. Sol in alc, chloroform. Practically insol in ether, fixed oils. LD$_{50}$ in mice (mg/20g): 9 s.c.; in rats (mg/kg): 129 i.p. (Koelzer).

THERAP CAT: Anesthetic (local).

THERAP CAT (VET): Anesthetic (local).

7475. Piperonal. [120-57-0] 1,3-Benzodioxole-5-carboxaldehyde; 3,4-(methylenedioxy)benzaldehyde; heliotropin; piperonylaldehyde; dioxymethyleneprotocatechuic aldehyde. C$_8$H$_6$O$_3$; mol wt 150.13. C 64.00%, H 4.03%, O 31.97%. Prepn: Blair, **US 2916499** (1959 to Welsbach Corp.); Holum, *J. Org. Chem.* **26,** 4814 (1961); Feugeas, *Bull. Soc. Chim. Fr.* **1964,** 1892. Toxicity: Hagan *et al., Toxicol. Appl. Pharmacol.* **7,** 18 (1965).

Colorless, lustrous crystals, mp 37°. Heliotrope odor. bp ~263°; bp$_{0.5}$ 88°. Sol in 500 parts water; freely sol in alcohol, ether. *Keep in cool place protected from light.* LD$_{50}$ orally in rats: 2700 mg/kg (Hagan).

USE: In perfumery, in cherry and vanilla flavors, in organic syntheses.

THERAP CAT: Has been used as pediculicide.

7476. Piperonyl Butoxide. [51-03-6] 5-[[2-(2-Butoxyethoxy)ethoxy]methyl]-6-propyl-1,3-benzodioxole; α-[2-(2-butoxyethoxy)ethoxy]-4,5-methylenedioxy-2-propyltoluene; [3,4-(methylenedioxy)-6-propylbenzyl] butyl diethyleneglycol ether; 6-propylpiperonyl butyl diethylene glycol ether; butylcarbityl (6-propylpiperonyl) ether; ENT-14250; Butacide. C$_{19}$H$_{30}$O$_5$; mol wt 338.44. C 67.43%, H 8.93%, O 23.64%. Prepn: H. Wachs, **US 2485681; US 2550737** (1949, 1951 both to U.S. Industrial Chemicals); *idem, Science* **105,** 530 (1947). Toxicity: T. B. Gaines, *Toxicol. Appl. Pharmacol.* **14,** 515 (1969). Review of carcinogenic risk: *IARC Monographs* **30,** 183-195 (1983).

Liquid. d 1.04-1.07. bp$_{1.0}$ 180°. n_D^{20} 1.50. Flash pt 340°F. Miscible with methanol, ethanol, benzene, Freons, Geons, other organic solvents, oils. LD$_{50}$ orally in female, male rats: 6150, 7500 mg/kg (Gaines).

Mixture with synthetic pyrethroids. Derringer; Duracide; Grovex; Prentox; Scourge.

In combination with rotenone. PB-NOX; Chem-Fish; Rotacide.

Caution: Large doses have caused vomiting, diarrhea: Sarles *et al., Am. J. Trop. Med.* **29,** 151 (1949).

USE: Insecticide synergist, especially for pyrethroids and rotenone.

7477. Piperonylic Acid. [94-53-1] 1,3-Benzodioxole-5-carboxylic acid; 3,4-methylenedioxybenzoic acid; protocatechuic acid methylene ether. C$_8$H$_6$O$_4$; mol wt 166.13. C 57.84%, H 3.64%, O 38.52%. Occurs in Paracoto bark. Prepd by permanganate oxidation of piperonal: Shriner, Kleiderer, *Org. Synth.* **10,** 82 (1930).

Prisms (by sublimation), needles from alc, feathery crystals from water. mp 229°. Sublimes around 210°. Slightly sol in water, chloroform, cold alcohol, ether. Absorption spectrum: Dobbie, Lauder, *J. Chem. Soc.* **83,** 621 (1903).

Methyl ester. C$_9$H$_8$O$_4$. mp 53°. Sublimes easily. Volatile in steam. Freely sol in alcohol, ether.

7478. Piperoxan. [59-39-2] 1-[(2,3-Dihydro-1,4-benzodioxin-2-yl)methyl]piperidine; 2-piperidinomethyl-1,4-benzodioxan; 2-(1-piperidylmethyl)-1,4-benzodioxan; benzodioxane; Benodaine. C$_{14}$H$_{19}$NO$_2$; mol wt 233.31. C 72.07%, H 8.21%, N 6.00%, O 13.72%. α-Adrenergic blocker. Prepn: Fourneau, **US 2056046** (1936 to Rhône-Poulenc).

bp$_{17}$ 193°.

***dl*-Form hydrochloride.** Compd 933F; Fourneau 933. C$_{14}$H$_{19}$NO$_2$.HCl; mol wt 269.77. Crystals, mp 232-234° (darkens at 220°). uv max: 275 nm (E$_{1cm}^{1\%}$ 82); min: 240 nm (E$_{1cm}^{1\%}$ <5). Freely sol in water, pH of 1% soln ~5. Alkalies liberate the water-insol base. Soluble in acid solns. Soly in isopropanol: ~10.8 mg/g at 25°. Crystals are not hygroscopic and are stable to light, air, and normal storage temps. An aq soln at its own pH (5) is stable to autoclaving and to many months of storage at room temp.

THERAP CAT: Antihypertensive. Diagnostic aid (pheochromocytoma).

7479. PIPES. [5625-37-6] 1,4-Piperazinediethanesulfonic acid; piperazine-N,N'-bis(2-ethanesulfonic acid); 1,4-piperazinebis(ethanesulfonic acid). C$_8$H$_{18}$N$_2$O$_6$S$_2$; mol wt 302.37. C 31.78%, H 6.00%, N 9.26%, O 31.75%, S 21.21%. One of the zwitterionic N-substituted aminosulfonic acids known as "Good" buffers; active in the pH range 6-8.5. Prepn: N. Good *et al., Biochemistry* **5,** 467 (1966). Interference with Lowry protein determn: H. M. Himmel, W. Heller, *J. Clin. Chem. Clin. Biochem.* **25,** 909 (1987). Use as biological buffer: R. Salema, I. Brandao, *J. Submicrosc. Cytol.* **5,** 79 (1973); S. Haviernick *et al., J. Microsc.* **135,** 83 (1984).

Monosodium salt. [10010-67-0] C$_8$H$_{17}$N$_2$NaO$_6$S$_2$. Crystals from water and alcohol, mp >300° (dec). pKa$_1$ ~3, pKa$_2$ (20°): 6.82 (0.1*M*); 6.82 (0.2*M*); 6.96 (0.01*M*). ΔpKa/°C −0.0085.

Disodium salt. [76836-02-7] Sodium pipesate. C$_8$H$_{16}$N$_2$Na$_2$O$_6$S$_2$.

USE: Biological buffer.

7480. Pipobroman. [54-91-1] 1,4-Bis-(3-bromo-1-oxopropyl)piperazine; 1,4-bis(3-bromopropionyl)piperazine; A-8103; NSC-25154; Amedel; Vercyte. C$_{10}$H$_{16}$Br$_2$N$_2$O$_2$; mol wt 356.05. C 33.73%, H 4.53%, Br 44.88%, N 7.87%, O 8.99%. Prepn: Horrom, Carbon, **DE 1138781** (1962 to Abbott), *C.A.* **58,** 7955c (1963); Groszkowski, *Rocz. Chem.* **38,** 229 (1964), *C.A.* **60,** 14506a (1964). Structure-cytostatic effect studies: Groszkowski *et al., J. Med. Chem.* **11,** 621 (1968); Oteleanu, Retezeanu, *Farmacia (Bucharest)* **16,** 279 (1968), *C.A.* **69,** 33591w (1968).

Crystals, mp 106-107°.

THERAP CAT: Antineoplastic.

7481. Piposulfan. [2608-24-0] 1,4-Bis[3-[(methylsulfonyl)oxy]-1-oxopropyl]piperazine; 1,4-dihydracryloylpiperazine dimethanesulfonate; 1,4-bis(3-hydroxypropionyl)piperazine dimethanesulfonate; N,N'-bis(3-methanesulfonyloxypropionyl)piperazine; N,N'-bis(3-methylsulfonyloxypropionyl)piperazine; A-20968; NSC-47774; Ancyte. C$_{12}$H$_{22}$N$_2$O$_8$S$_2$; mol wt 386.44. C 37.30%, H 5.74%, N 7.25%, O 33.12%, S 16.60%. Prepn: Horrom, Carbon, **DE 1177162** (1964 to Abbott), *C.A.* **61,** 13329a (1964).

Crystals from water, mp 175-177°.
THERAP CAT: Antineoplastic.

7482. Pipotiazine. [39860-99-6] 10-[3-[4-(2-Hydroxyeth-yl)-1-piperidinyl]propyl]-*N*,*N*-dimethyl-10*H*-phenothiazine-2-sulfonamide; 2-[1-[3-[2-[(dimethylamino)sulfonyl]-10*H*-phenothia-zin-10-yl]propyl]-4-piperidinyl]ethanol; pipothiazine; RP-19366; Piportil. $C_{24}H_{33}N_3O_3S_2$; mol wt 475.67. C 60.60%, H 6.99%, N 8.83%, O 10.09%, S 13.48%. Prepn: **FR M7835** (1970 to Rhône-Poulenc), *C.A.* **78**, 43499x (1973). Pharmacokinetics: P. J. De Schepper *et al., Arzneim.-Forsch.* **29**, 1056 (1979); and HPLC determn in plasma: D. A. Ogden *et al., J. Pharm. Biomed. Anal.* **7**, 1273 (1989). Series of articles on pharmacology and clinical use: *Acta Psychiat. Scand.,* Suppl. 241, 9-138 (1973). Toxicity: L. Julou *et al., ibid.* 9.

LD$_{50}$ in mice (mg/kg): 108 i.p.; 360 s.c.; 440 orally (Julou).
Palmitic ester. [37517-26-3] Pipotiazine palmitate; RP-19552; Piportil L4. $C_{40}H_{63}N_3O_4S_2$; mol wt 714.08.
Undecylenic ester. [22178-11-6] Pipotiazine undecylenate; RP-19551; Piportil M2. $C_{35}H_{51}N_3O_4S_2$; mol wt 641.93.
THERAP CAT: Antipsychotic.

7483. Pipoxolan Hydrochloride. [18174-58-8] 5,5-Di-phenyl-2-[2-(1-piperidinyl)ethyl]-1,3-dioxolan-4-one hydrochloride; 2-(β-*N*-piperidylethyl)-4,4-diphenyl-1,3-dioxolan-5-one hydrochloride; BR-18; Rowapraxin. $C_{22}H_{26}ClNO_3$; mol wt 387.90. C 68.12%, H 6.76%, Cl 9.14%, N 3.61%, O 12.37%. Prepn: M. Pailer *et al., Monatsh. Chem.* **99**, 891 (1968); **GB 1109959** and **BE 719230** (1968, 1969 to Rowa-Wagner). Pharmacology and acute toxicity: K. Morsdorf, H. Wengenroth, *Pharmacology* **3**, 193 (1970).

• HCl

Crystals from isopropyl alc, mp 207-209°. Soluble in water; stable to mild attack by acids or bases. LD$_{50}$ in rats, mice (mg/kg): 1500, 700 orally; 60, 35 i.v.; 130, 130 i.p.; in rats (mg/kg): >300 s.c. (Morsdorf).
THERAP CAT: Antispasmodic.

7484. Pipradrol. [467-60-7] α,α-Diphenyl-2-piperidine-methanol; α-(2-piperidyl)benzhydrol; alpha-pipradrol; pipradol; MRD-108. $C_{18}H_{21}NO$; mol wt 267.37. C 80.86%, H 7.92%, N 5.24%, O 5.98%. Prepd by hydrogenation of α,α-diphenyl-2-pyridinemethanol: Tilford *et al., J. Am. Chem. Soc.* **70**, 4001 (1948); Werner, Tilford, **US 2624739** (1953 to Merrell).

Hydrochloride. [71-78-3] Meratran; Stimolag. $C_{18}H_{21}$-NO.HCl; mol wt 303.83. Crystals from butanone, dec 308-309°. Slightly bitter taste. One gram dissolves in 60 ml of hot water.
Note: This is a controlled substance (stimulant): **21 CFR,** 1308.14.
THERAP CAT: CNS stimulant.

7485. Piprozolin. [17243-64-0] [3-Ethyl-4-oxo-5-(1-piper-idinyl)-2-thiazolidinylidene]acetic acid ethyl ester; 3-ethyl-4-oxo-5-piperidino-$\Delta^{2,\alpha}$-thiazolidineacetic acid ethyl ester; Gö-919; W-3699; Coleflux; Epsyl; Probilin; Secrebil. $C_{14}H_{22}N_2O_3S$; mol wt 298.40. C 56.35%, H 7.43%, N 9.39%, O 16.09%, S 10.75%. Prepn: G. Satzinger, *Ann.* **665**, 150 (1963); G. Satzinger *et al.,* **DE 2414345** (1975 to Goedecke), corresp to **US 3971794** (1976 to Warner-Lambert). Metabolism and pharmacokinetics: K. O. Vollmer, F. W. Koss, *Arch. Int. Pharmacodyn. Ther.* **198**, 312 (1972). Mechanism of action: F. W. Koss *et al., ibid.* 333. Series of articles on synthesis, pharmacology, toxicology and clinical studies: *Arzneim.-Forsch.* **27**, 463-526 (1977). Toxicity data: M. Herrmann *et al., ibid.* 467.

Colorless cryst, mp 86-87°. Practically insol in water. Sol in dil aq acids and most organic solvents. uv max (methanol): 245, 285 nm (ε 8200, 20000) (Vollmer). LD$_{50}$ in mice, rats (mg/kg): 1070, 3256 orally (Herrmann).
THERAP CAT: Choleretic.

7486. Pipsyl Chloride. [98-61-3] 4-Iodobenzenesulfonyl chloride; *p*-iodophenyl sulfonyl chloride. Usually prepd from iodide ion and *p*-diazobenzenesulfonic acid, followed by treatment with phosphorus pentachloride. A 5-10-fold excess reacts quantitatively with amino acids as indicated by the disappearance of amino nitrogen. Radioactive pipsyl chloride is used in the analysis of proteins: Keston *et al., J. Am. Chem. Soc.* **68**, 1390 (1946).

7487. Piracetam. [7491-74-9] 2-Oxo-1-pyrrolidineacet-amide; 2-pyrrolidoneacetamide; 2-pyrrolidinoneacetamide; 2-keto-pyrrolidine-1-ylacetamide; 1-acetamido-2-pyrrolidinone; UCB-6215; Avigilen; Axonyl; Cerebroforte; Encetrop; Gabacet; Geram; Nootrop; Nootropil; Nootropyl; Norzetam; Normabraïn; Piracebral; Piracetrop; Sinapsan. $C_6H_{10}N_2O_2$; mol wt 142.16. C 50.69%, H 7.09%, N 19.71%, O 22.51%. Prepn: H. Morren, **NL 6509994**; *eidem,* **US 3459738** (1966, 1969 both to U.C.B.). Pharmacology: Giurgea *et al., Arch. Int. Pharmacodyn. Ther.* **166**, 238 (1967); Giurgea, Moyersoons, *ibid.* **188**, 401 (1970); Giurgea *et al., Psychopharmacologia* **20**, 160 (1971). Metabolism and biochemical studies: Gobert, *J. Pharm. Belg.* **27**, 281 (1972). Clinical studies: W. J. Oosterveld, *Arzneim.-Forsch.* **30**, 1947 (1980); G. Chouinard *et al., Psychopharmacol. Bull.* **17**, 129 (1981); in dyslexia: M. Di Ianni *et al., J. Clin. Psychopharmacol.* **5**, 272 (1985).

Crystals from isopropanol, mp 151.5-152.5°.
THERAP CAT: Nootropic.

7488. Pirarubicin. [72496-41-4] (8*S*,10*S*)-10-[[3-Amino-2,3,6-trideoxy-4-*O*-[(2*S*)-tetrahydro-2*H*-pyran-2-yl]-α-L-*lyxo*-hexopyranosyl]oxy]-7,8,9,10-tetrahydro-6,8,11-trihydroxy-8-(hydroxyacetyl)-1-methoxy-5,12-naphthacenedione; 4′-*O*-tetrahydropyranyl doxorubicin; (2″*R*)-4′-*O*-tetrahydropyranyladriamycin; tepirubicin; THP; THP-ADM; THP-adriamycin; 1609-RB; Theprubicin. $C_{32}H_{37}NO_{12}$; mol wt 627.64. C 61.24%, H 5.94%, N 2.23%, O 30.59%. Structural analog of doxorubicin, *q.v.* Prepn of (2″*R*) and (2″*S*)-diastereomers: H. Umezawa *et al., J. Antibiot.* **32**, 1082 (1979); *idem et al.,* **EP 14853**; *eidem,* **US 4303785** (1980, 1981 both to Microbiochem. Res. Found. Japan). Absolute configuration: *idem et al., J. Antibiot.* **37**, 1094 (1984). HPLC determn in biological fluids: Y. Matsushita *et al., ibid.* **36**, 880 (1983). Cellular uptake and inhibition of DNA synthesis: S. Kunimoto *et al., ibid.* 312 (1983). Mechanism of action study: K.-I. Kiyomiya *et al., Int. J. Oncol.* **21**, 1081 (2002). Clinical pharmacokinetics and toxicity: A. A. Miller, C. G. Schmidt, *Cancer Res.* **47**, 1461 (1987). Overview of clinical experience: H. Majima, K. Ohta, *Biomed. Pharmacother.* **41**, 237-243 (1987). Clinical evaluation in metastatic colon cancer: D. Fallik *et al., Ann. Oncol.* **14**, 856 (2003)

Red solid, mp 188-192° (dec). $[\alpha]_D^{25}$ +175 ±25° (c = 0.2 in CHCl₃). uv and visible max (methanol): 234, 252, 290, 498, 531.5, 580 nm ($E_{1cm}^{1\%}$ 480, 350, 110, 140, 100, 45). Sol in ethyl acetate, chloroform, and ethanol; slightly sol in water, *n*-hexane, petr ether. Ethanolic and acidic solutions are red in color; give a positive ninhydrin reaction and do not reduce Fehling's solution. LD_{50} i.v. in mice: 27.8 mg/kg (Umezawa, 1979).

Hydrochloride. [95343-20-7] Pinorubin; Therarubicin. $C_{32}H_{37}NO_{12} \cdot HCl$; mol wt 664.10. Red crystalline solid. Sol in water and methanol.

THERAP CAT: Antineoplastic.

7489. Pirbuterol. [38677-81-5] α^6-[[(1,1-Dimethylethyl)amino]methyl]-3-hydroxy-2,6-pyridinedimethanol; 2-hydroxymethyl-3-hydroxy-6-(1-hydroxy-2-*tert*-butylaminoethyl)pyridine. $C_{12}H_{20}N_2O_3$; mol wt 240.30. C 59.98%, H 8.39%, N 11.66%, O 19.97%. Analog of albuterol, *q.v.*, with β_2-adrenergic stimulating activity. Prepn: W. E. Barth, **DE 2204195**; *idem,* **US 3700681** (both 1972 to Pfizer). Stability study: P. C. Bansal, D. C. Monkhouse, *J. Pharm. Sci.* **66**, 819 (1977). Biotransformation: H. M. McIlhenny, M. S. D. Ghaly, *Fed. Proc.* **38**, 1130 (1979). Pharmacokinetics and cardiopulmonary effects in dogs: J. W. Constantine *et al., J. Pharmacol. Exp. Ther.* **208**, 371 (1979). Comparative study in respiratory disease: A. J. Dyson, A. D. Mackay, *Br. J. Dis. Chest* **74**, 70 (1980). Use in treatment of cardiac failure: N. A. Awan *et al., Clin. Res.* **28**, 17A (1980); W. S. Colucci *et al., N. Engl. J. Med.* **305**, 185 (1981); G. I. Nelson *et al., Eur. Heart J.* **3**, 238 (1982); K. T. Weber *et al., Circulation* **66**, 1262 (1982). Review of pharmacology and efficacy in bronchospastic disease: D. M. Richards, R. N. Brogden, *Drugs* **30**, 6-21 (1985).

Dihydrochloride. [38029-10-6] CP-24314-1. $C_{12}H_{22}Cl_2N_2O_3$; mol wt 313.22. Crystals from ethanol/isopropyl ether, mp 182° (dec).

Monoacetate. Maxair; Spirolair. $C_{14}H_{24}N_2O_5$; mol wt 300.35. Freely sol in water.

THERAP CAT: Bronchodilator.

7490. Pirenoxine. [1043-21-6] 1-Hydroxy-5-oxo-5*H*-pyrido[3,2-*a*]phenoxazine-3-carboxylic acid; 1-hydroxy-5*H*-pyrido[3,2-*a*]phenoxazin-5-one-3-carboxylic acid; 1-hydroxy-3-carboxy-5*H*-pyrido[3,2-*a*]phenoxazin-5-one; pirfenoxone; Catalin. $C_{16}H_8N_2O_5$; mol wt 308.25. C 62.34%, H 2.62%, N 9.09%, O 25.95%. Prepn: S. Ogino, **JP 59 2227**, *C.A.* **54**, 11058i (1960); S. Ishii, **JP 61 1782**, *C.A.* **55**, 21494e (1961) (1959, 1961 both to Chizu Drug); of the sodium salt: S. Ishii, K. Ogata, **JP 73 2672** (1973 to Senju), *C.A.* **80**, 6959t (1974). Pharmacological studies: F. Ikemoto *et al., Oyo Yakuri* **8**, 937 (1974), *C.A.* **83**, 71663t (1975). Toxicological studies: *eidem, ibid.* 911, 923, *C.A.* **82**, 51617g, 68262k (1975). Influence on carbohydrate metabolism in the lens: I. Korte *et al., Ophthalmic Res.* **7**, 282 (1975). Effect on NADH, NADPH: *eidem, ibid.* 440. Effect on senile cataracts: T. Murata, *Folia Ophthalmol. Jpn.* **31**, 1217 (1980). Clinical trial in treatment of cataracts: S. K. Angra *et al., Indian J. Ophthalmol.* **31**, 5 (1983).

Orange-yellow powder, mp 247-248° (dec).

Sodium salt. [51410-30-1] Clarvisan. $C_{16}H_7N_2NaO_5$; mol wt 330.23. Very sol in water. LD_{50} in mice (mg/kg): >10000 orally; >5000 s.c.; 2120-2250 i.p.; LD_{50} i.p. in rats (mg/kg): 2400 (males); 1460 (females) (Ikemoto).

THERAP CAT: Treatment of cataracts.

7491. Pirenzepine. [28797-61-7] 5,11-Dihydro-11-[(4-methyl-1-piperazinyl)acetyl]-6*H*-pyrido[2,3-*b*][1,4]benzodiazepin-6-one; LS-519. $C_{19}H_{21}N_5O_2$; mol wt 351.40. C 64.94%, H 6.02%, N 19.93%, O 9.11%. Tricyclic gastric-acid inhibitor. Prepn: **FR 1505795** (1967 to Thomae), *C.A.* **70**, 4154w (1969). Pharmacology: W. Eberlein *et al., Arzneim.-Forsch.* **27**, 356 (1977). Pharmacokinetics: R. Hammes *et al., ibid.* 928. Mechanism of action: G. Heller *et al., Verh. Dtsch. Ges. Inn. Med.* **84**, 991 (1978), *C.A.* **90**, 132984s (1979). Human pharmacology: H. Brunner *et al., Arzneim.-Forsch.* **27**, 684 (1977). Multicenter controlled clinical trial: *Scand. J. Gastroenterol.* **17**, Suppl. 81, 1-42 (1982). Radioimmunoassay determn in human plasma and urine: C. A. Homon *et al., Ther. Drug Monit.* **9**, 236 (1987). Symposium: *ibid.* Suppl. 72, 1-273. Review of pharmacology and therapeutic efficacy: A. A. Carmine, R. N. Brogden, *Drugs* **30**, 85-126 (1985). Comprehensive description: H. A. El-Obeid *et al., Anal. Profiles Drug Subs.* **16**, 445-506 (1987).

Dihydrochloride. [29868-97-1] LS-519-Cl2; Duogastral; Durapirenz; Gasteril; Gastrozepin; Leblon; Maghen; Renzepin; Tabe; Ulcuforton; Ulcosan. $C_{19}H_{21}N_5O_2 \cdot 2HCl$; mol wt 424.32. Sol in water, slightly sol in methanol. Practically insol in ether.

THERAP CAT: Antiulcerative.

7492. Piretanide. [55837-27-9] 3-(Aminosulfonyl)-4-phenoxy-5-(1-pyrrolidinyl)benzoic acid; 4-phenoxy-3-(1-pyrrolidinyl)-5-sulfamoylbenzoic acid; HOE-118; S-73-4118; Diumax; Eurelix; Tauliz. $C_{17}H_{18}N_2O_5S$; mol wt 362.40. C 56.34%, H 5.01%, N 7.73%, O 22.07%, S 8.85%. High-ceiling loop diuretic, structurally related to bumetanide, *q.v.* Prepn: D. Bormann *et al.,* **DE 2419970**; *eidem,* **US 4010273** (1975, 1977 both to Hoechst). Chemistry and pharmacology: W. Merkel *et al., Eur. J. Med.*

Chem. **11,** 399 (1976). Diuretic activity in man: N. Pozet *et al.,* *Br. J. Clin. Pharmacol.* **9,** 577 (1980); T. Saruta, E. Kato, *Arzneim.-Forsch.* **30,** 1807 (1980). Vascular effects of piretanide: E. Klaus *et al., ibid.* **33,** 1273 (1983); renal effects: M. Omosu *et al., ibid.* 1277. Review of pharmacology and therapeutic efficacy: S. P. Clissold, R. N. Brogden, *Drugs* **29,** 489-530 (1985).

Pale yellow platelets from methanol/water, mp 225-227°. Exhibits intense light blue fluorescence at 366 nm. LD_{50} in rats, mice (mg/kg): 5601, 3672 orally (Merkel).

Monosodium salt. [112132-09-9] Arelix. $C_{17}H_{17}N_2NaO_5S$; mol wt 384.38.

THERAP CAT: Diuretic.

7493. Piribedil. [3605-01-4] 2-[4-(1,3-Benzodioxol-5-yl-methyl)-1-piperazinyl]pyrimidine; 2-(4-piperonyl-1-piperazinyl)-pyrimidine; 2-[4-(3,4-methylenedioxybenzyl)piperazino]pyrimidine; 1-(2-pyrimidyl)-4-piperonylpiperazine; 1-(2″-pyrimidyl)-4-(methylene-3′,4′-dioxybenzyl)piperazine; ET-495; EU-4200; Trivastal. $C_{16}H_{18}N_4O_2$; mol wt 298.34. C 64.41%, H 6.08%, N 18.78%, O 10.73%. Central dopaminergic agonist. Prepn: **NL 6413349;** G. Regnier *et al.,* **US 3299067;** *eidem,* **GB 1101425** (1965, 1967, 1968 all to Sci. Union et Cie-Soc. Franc. Rech. Med.); G. Regnier *et al., J. Med. Chem.* **11,** 1151 (1968). Activity in man: R. Royer, *Proc. 3rd Int. Pharmacol. Meet.* **3,** R. K. Richards, Ed. (Pergamon Press, New York, 1968) pp 45-55. Pharmacology: M. Laubie *et al., Eur. J. Pharmacol.* **6,** 75 (1969). Metabolism: D. B. Campbell *et al., Adv. Neurol.* **3,** 199 (1973). Review of mechanism of action: P. Jenner, *J. Neurol.* **239,** Suppl. 1, S2-S8 (1992).

Crystals from anhydr ethanol, mp 98°. LD_{50} in mice (mg/kg): 88 i.v., 690 i.p., 1460 orally (Laubie).

THERAP CAT: Vasodilator (peripheral).

7494. Piridocaine. [87-21-8] 2-Piperidineethanol 2-amino-benzoate (ester); anthranilic acid 2-(2-piperidyl)ethyl ester; 2-piperidineethanol anthranilate; β-(2-piperidyl)ethyl *o*-aminobenzoate; PT-14; Lucaine. $C_{14}H_{20}N_2O_2$; mol wt 248.32. C 67.71%, H 8.12%, N 11.28%, O 12.89%. Prepn: Walter, Fosbinder, *J. Am. Chem. Soc.* **61,** 1713 (1939); **US 2229533** (1941 to Maltbie Chem.).

Hydrochloride. $C_{14}H_{21}ClN_2O_2$. Crystals from abs alcohol, mp 209-211°.

THERAP CAT: Anesthetic (local).

7495. Pirifibrate. [55285-45-5] 2-(4-Chlorophenoxy)-2-methylpropanoic acid [6-(hydroxymethyl)-2-pyridinyl]methyl ester; 2,6-pyridinedimethanol mono-*p*-chlorophenoxyisobutyrate; EL-466; Bratenol. $C_{17}H_{18}ClNO_4$; mol wt 335.78. C 60.81%, H 5.40%, Cl 10.56%, N 4.17%, O 19.06%. Hypolipemic agent related structurally to clofibrate, *q.v.* Prepn: D. Humbert, R. Ratouis, **DE 2432322;** *eidem,* **US 3971798** (1975, 1976 both to Roussel). Multi-center study in hyperlipoproteinemias: A. J. Domingo *et al., Clin. Ther.* **3,** 219 (1980).

Crystals from isopropyl ether, mp 46°. LD_{50} in mice (mg/kg): 915-1098 i.p. (Humbert, Ratouis, 1975).

Hydrochloride. $C_{17}H_{18}ClNO_4 \cdot HCl$. Crystals, mp 110°. LD_{50} (calculated as base) in mice (mg/kg): 1098-1281 i.p. (Humbert, Ratouis, 1975).

THERAP CAT: Antilipemic.

7496. Pirimicarb. [23103-98-2] Dimethylcarbamic acid 2-(dimethylamino)-5,6-dimethyl-4-pyrimidinyl ester; 2-(dimethylamino)-5,6-dimethyl-4-pyrimidinyl dimethylcarbamate; 5,6-di-methyl-2-dimethylamino-4-dimethylcarbamoyloxypyrimidine; PP-062; ENT-27766; Aphox; Fernos; Pirimor. $C_{11}H_{18}N_4O_2$; mol wt 238.29. C 55.44%, H 7.61%, N 23.51%, O 13.43%. Selective aphicide. Prepn: F. L. C. Baranyovits *et al.,* **ZA 6701588;** *eidem,* **US 3493574** (1968, 1970 to ICI). Activity: F. L. C. Baranyovits, R. Ghosh, *Chem. Ind. (London)* **1969,** 1018. Degradn in soil: I. R. Hill, *ACS Symp. Ser.* **29,** 358 (1976). GLC analysis: P. D. Bland, *J. Assoc. Off. Anal. Chem.* **64,** 1315 (1981).

Crystalline solid, mp 90.5°. Vapor pressure at 30°: 3×10^{-5} mm Hg. Soly in water at 25°: 2.7 g/l. Sol in most organic solvents. Dec by prolonged boiling with acids or alkali. Aq solns are unstable to light. LD_{50} orally in female rats: 147 (mg/kg) (Baranyovits, Ghosh).

USE: Insecticide.

7497. Pirimiphos-ethyl. [23505-41-1] *O*-[2-(Diethylami-no)-6-methyl-4-pyrimidinyl]phosphorothioic acid *O,O*-diethyl ester; *O,O*-diethyl *O*-[2-(diethylamino)-6-methyl-4-pyrimidinyl]-phosphorothioate; PP-211; Primicid. $C_{13}H_{24}N_3O_3PS$; mol wt 333.39. C 46.83%, H 7.26%, N 12.60%, O 14.40%, P 9.29%, S 9.62%. Broad spectrum contact and fumigant insecticide. Prepn: B. K. Snell, S. P. Sharpe, **GB 1205000** (1970 to ICI), *C.A.* **74,** 52482f (1971). Efficacy against wireworms: C. E. Lilly, *J. Econ. Entomol.* **66,** 1205 (1973). Persistence and degradn in soil: D. L. Suett, *Pestic. Sci.* **6,** 385 (1975). Review of properties and analytical methods: D. J. W. Bullock, *Anal. Methods Pestic. Plant Growth Regul.* **8,** 171-184 (1976).

Straw-colored liquid, dec >130°. d^{20} 1.14; n_D^{25} 1.520. Vapor pressure at 25°: 2.9×10^{-4} mm Hg. Miscible with most organic solvents. Soly in water (30°): 1 ppm. Weakly basic. uv max (methanol): 248 nm (ε 21300). LD_{50} in rats, mice, guinea pigs (mg/kg); 140-200, 105, 50-150 orally; dermally in rats: 1000-2000 mg/kg (Bullock).

O,O-Dimethyl analog. [29232-93-7] Pirimiphos-methyl; PP-511; Actellic; Actellifog; Blex; Dominator; Silosan. $C_{11}H_{20}N_3O_3$-PS; mol wt 305.33. Straw-colored liquid, d^{30} 1.157; n_D^{25} 1.527.

Vapor press at 30°: $\sim 1 \times 10^{-4}$ mm Hg. Soly in water at 30°: 5 mg/l.

USE: Insecticide.

THERAP CAT (VET): Ectoparasiticide.

7498. Piritramide. [302-41-0] 1'-(3-Cyano-3,3-diphenyl-propyl)-[1,4'-bipiperidine]-4'-carboxamide; 1-(3,3-diphenyl-3-cyanopropyl)-4-piperidino-4-piperidinecarboxamide; 2,2-diphenyl-4-(4-piperidino-4-carbamoylpiperidino)butyronitrile; pirinitramide; A-65; R-3365; Dipidolor; Piridolan. $C_{27}H_{34}N_4O$; mol wt 430.59. C 75.31%, H 7.96%, N 13.01%, O 3.72%. Prepn: **BE 606850**; P. A. J. Janssen, **US 3080366** (1961, 1963 both to Janssen). Crystal structure: C. Humblet *et al., Acta Crystallogr.* **B33**, 1615 (1977).

Crystals from acetone, mp 149-150°.

Note: This is a controlled substance (opiate): **21 CFR,** 1308.11.

THERAP CAT: Analgesic (narcotic).

7499. Piritrexim. [72732-56-0] 6-[(2,5-Dimethoxyphenyl)-methyl]-5-methylpyrido[2,3-*d*]pyrimidine-2,4-diamine; 2,4-diamino-6-(2,5-dimethoxybenzyl)-5-methylpyrido[2,3-*d*]pyrimidine; BW-301U; NSC-351521. $C_{17}H_{19}N_5O_2$; mol wt 325.37. C 62.75%, H 5.89%, N 21.52%, O 9.83%. Lipid soluble dihydrofolate reductase inhibitor. Prepn: E. M. Grivsky *et al., J. Med. Chem.* **23**, 327 (1980); E. M. Grivsky *et al.,* **EP 21292** (1981 to Wellcome); E. M. Grivsky, **US 4959474** (1990 to Burroughs Wellcome). Biochemistry and antitumor activity: D. S. Duch *et al., Cancer Res.* **42**, 3987 (1982). Cytotoxicity: I. W. Taylor *et al., ibid.* **45**, 978 (1985). Pharmacology and toxicology: C. W. Sigel *et al., NCI Monogr.* **5**, 111 (1987). Antipneumocystis and antitoxoplasma activities: J. A. Kovacs *et al., Antimicrob. Agents Chemother.* **32**, 430 (1988). HPLC determn in plasma: R. G. Foss, C. W. Sigel, *J. Pharm. Sci.* **71**, 1176 (1982). Determn by protein binding assay in plasma: J. L. Woolley, Jr., *et al., ibid.* **78**, 749 (1989). Crystal structure and conformational analysis: P. A. Sutton, V. Cody, *J. Am. Chem. Soc.* **110**, 6219 (1988). Clinical pharmacology in children: P. C. Adamson *et al., Cancer Res.* **50**, 4464 (1990). Clinical evaluation in lung cancer: M. G. Kris *et al., Cancer Treat. Rep.* **71**, 763 (1987); in advanced squamous head and neck cancer: W.-C. Uen *et al., Cancer* **69**, 1008 (1992).

Yellow powder from ethanol/water, mp 252-254°. log P (octanol/water): 1.74.

Isethionate. [79483-69-5] $C_{17}H_{19}N_5O_2 \cdot C_2H_6O_4S$. LD_{50} orally in rats: 1168 mg/kg (Sigel).

THERAP CAT: Antineoplastic.

7500. Pirlimycin. [79548-73-5] (2S-*cis*)-Methyl 7-chloro-6,7,8-trideoxy-6-[[(4-ethyl-2-piperidinyl)carbonyl]amino]-1-thio-L-*threo*-α-D-galactooctopyranoside. $C_{17}H_{31}ClN_2O_5S$; mol wt 410.96. C 49.68%, H 7.60%, Cl 8.63%, N 6.82%, O 19.47%, S 7.80%. Semi-synthetic lincosaminide antibiotic; structural analog of clindamycin, *q.v.* Prepn: R. D. Birkenmeyer, **DE 3043502**; *idem*, **US 4278789** (both 1981 to Upjohn); R. D. Birkenmeyer *et al., J. Med. Chem.* **27**, 216 (1984). *In vitro* activity vs aerobic bacteria: V. I. Ahonkhai *et al., Antimicrob. Agents Chemother.* **21**, 902 (1982); vs anaerobic bacteria: S. M. H. Qadri *et al., J. Antibiot.* **36**, 42 (1983). HPLC determn in biological fluids: J. A.

Shah, D. J. Weber, *J. Chromatogr.* **309**, 95 (1984). Ion-pairing LC determn in pharmaceutic prepns: D. L. Theis, *ibid.* **402**, 335 (1987). Metabolism and residue studies in dairy cows: R. E. Hornish *et al., ACS Symp. Ser.* **503**, 132-147 (1992). Evaluation in bovine mastitis: W. E. Owens *et al., Agri-Pract.* **15**, 19 (1994).

Hydrochloride. [78822-40-9] U-57903E; Pirsue. Crystals from water, mp 222-224°. $[\alpha]_D^{25}$ +176° (**US 4278789**). Also reported as mp 210-212°. $[\alpha]_D^{25}$ +181°. LD_{50} i.p. in mice: 600 mg/kg (Birkenmeyer, 1984).

THERAP CAT (VET): Antibacterial.

7501. Pirmenol. [68252-19-7] *cis*-(±)-α-[3-(2,6-Dimethyl-1-piperidinyl)propyl]-α-phenyl-2-pyridinemethanol; (±)-*cis*-2,6-dimethyl-α-phenyl-α-2-pyridyl-1-piperidinebutanol; (±)-1-phenyl-1-(2-pyridyl)-4-(*cis*-2,6-dimethyl-1-piperidyl)butanol. $C_{22}H_{30}N_2O$; mol wt 338.49. C 78.06%, H 8.93%, N 8.28%, O 4.73%. Prepn: R. W. Fleming, **DE 2806654**; *idem*, **US 4112103** (both 1978 to Parke, Davis). Anti-arrhythmic profile in dogs: T. E. Mertz, T. J. Steffe, *J. Cardiovasc. Pharmacol.* **2**, 527 (1980). Toxicology study: J. L. Schardein *et al., Toxicol. Appl. Pharmacol.* **56**, 294 (1980). HPLC determn in biological fluids: E. L. Johnson, L. A. Pachla, *J. Pharm. Sci.* **73**, 754 (1984). Pharmacokinetics in humans: S. C. Hammill *et al., Circulation* **65**, 369 (1982); S. W. Sanders *et al., J. Clin. Pharmacol.* **23**, 113 (1983). Hemodynamic effects in cardiac patients: M. S. Nieminen *et al., Eur. Heart J.* **7**, 150 (1986). Clinical evaluations in ventricular arrhythmias: L. K. Toivonen *et al., J. Cardiovasc. Pharmacol.* **8**, 156 (1986); E. M. Hampton *et al., Eur. J. Clin. Pharmacol.* **31**, 15 (1986). Chronic toxicity study: J. R. Watkins *et al., Drug Invest.* **3**, 141 (1991). Evaluation of carcinogenicity: G. E. Macallum *et al., ibid.* 278. Symposium on pharmacology and clinical efficacy: *Am. J. Cardiol.* **59**, Suppl., 1H-57H (1987).

Crystals from petroleum ether, mp 70-71°.

Monohydrochloride. CI-845. $C_{22}H_{30}N_2O \cdot HCl$; mol wt 374.95. mp 171-172°. LD_{50} in mice, rats, dogs (mg/kg): 20.8, 23.6, >7.0 i.v.; 215.5, 359.9, >40.0 orally (Schardein).

THERAP CAT: Antiarrhythmic (class IA).

7502. Piroctone. [50650-76-5] 1-Hydroxy-4-methyl-6-(2,4,4-trimethylpentyl)-2(1*H*)-pyridinone. $C_{14}H_{23}NO_2$; mol wt 237.34. C 70.85%, H 9.77%, N 5.90%, O 13.48%. Pyridone deriv related structurally to ciclopirox, *q.v.* Prepn: G. Lohaus, W. Dittmar, **DE 2, DE 214608** corresp to **US 3972888** (1973, 1976 both to Hoechst); *eidem, Arzneim.-Forsch.* **31**, 1311 (1981). Evaluation of efficacy as anti-dandruff agent: E. Futterer, *J. Soc. Cosmet. Chem.* **32**, 327 (1981).

Crystals, mp 108°.

Ethanolamine salt (1:1). [68890-66-4] Octopirox. $C_{16}H_{30}N_2O_3$; mol wt 298.42.

THERAP CAT: Antiseborrheic.

7503. Piroheptine. [16378-21-5] 3-(10,11-Dihydro-5*H*-dibenzo[*a,d*]cyclohepten-5-ylidene)-1-ethyl-2-methylpyrrolidine. $C_{22}H_{25}N$; mol wt 303.44. C 87.08%, H 8.30%, N 4.62%. Prepn: NL **6609280**; Y. Deguchi *et al.*, US **3454595** (1967, 1969 both to Fujisawa). Crystal structure: Y. Tokuma *et al., Bull. Chem. Soc. Jpn.* **44**, 2665 (1971). Pharmacological studies: M. Hitomi *et al., Arzneim.-Forsch.* **22**, 953, 961 (1972). *In vitro* study: T. Ohashi *et al., ibid.* 966. Metabolism: Y. Tokuma *et al., Bull. Chem. Soc. Jpn.* **48**, 294 (1975). Clinical pharmacology: A. Barbeau, *Annu. Rev. Pharmacol.* **14**, 91 (1974). Toxicity study: M. Hitomi *et al., Arzneim.-Forsch.* **22**, 961 (1972).

Liquid, bp$_4$ 167°. uv max (95% ethanol): 240 nm (ε 12100).

Hydrochloride. [16378-22-6] Trimol. $C_{22}H_{25}N.HCl$; mol wt 339.90. Crystals, mp 250-253°. LD$_{50}$ in male mice, rats (mg/kg): 153, 600 orally; 19, 17 i.v.; 95, 110 i.p.; 109, 330 s.c. (Hitomi).

THERAP CAT: Antiparkinsonian.

7504. Piromen. [9008-99-5] Desacchromin dispersion; Pyromen. Pyrogenic *pseudomonas* polysaccharide-nucleic acid complex. Prepd by proteolyzing the bacterial organism and separating the complex from inactive material by dialyzing: N. M. Nesset, L. G. Ginger, GB **699663** (1953 to Baxter Labs.), *C.A.* **48**, 6083 (1954). Contains deoxyribonucleic acid, ribonucleic acid, and hexosamine, the pyrogenic reducing sugar: N. M. Nesset *et al., J. Am. Pharm. Assoc.* **39**, 456 (1950). Use in detn of bone marrow granulocyte reserves: B. C. Korbitz *et al., Curr. Ther. Res.* **11**, 491 (1969). Effects on spinal cord regeneration: M. A. Matthews *et al., Neuropathol. Appl. Neurobiol.* **5**, 161 (1979); *eidem, Acta Neurobiol. Exp.* **40**, 489 (1980).

7505. Piromidic Acid. [19562-30-2] 8-Ethyl-5,8-dihydro-5-oxo-2-(1-pyrrolidinyl)pyrido[2,3-*d*]pyrimidine-6-carboxylic acid; 5,8-dihydro-8-ethyl-5-oxo-2-pyrrolidinopyrido[2,3-*d*]pyrimidine-6-carboxylic acid; PD-93; Bactramyl; Enterol; Gastrurol; Panacid; Pirodal; Purim; Reelon; Septural; Uropir. $C_{14}H_{16}N_4O_3$; mol wt 288.30. C 58.32%, H 5.59%, N 19.43%, O 16.65%. Quinolone antibacterial. Prepn: S. Minami *et al.*, JP **67 25912**; *eidem*, GB **1129358** (1967, 1968 both to Dainippon Pharm.); *eidem, Chem. Pharm. Bull.* **19**, 1426 (1971). Activity studies: M. Shimizu *et al., Antimicrob. Agents Chemother.* **1970**, 117. Metabolism: *eidem, ibid.* 123.

Crystals from ethanol-chloroform, mp 314-316°. LD$_{50}$ in male, female mice, male, female rats (mg/kg): 287, 268, 177, 158 i.v.; all >4000 orally, s.c. and i.p. (Shimizu).

THERAP CAT: Antibacterial.

7506. Piroxicam. [36322-90-4] 4-Hydroxy-2-methyl-*N*-2-pyridinyl-2*H*-1,2-benzothiazine-3-carboxamide 1,1-dioxide; 3,4-dihydro-2-methyl-4-oxo-*N*-2-pyridyl-2*H*-1,2-benzothiazine-3-carboxamide 1,1-dioxide; CP-16171; Artroxicam; Baxo; Bruxicam; Caliment; Erazon; Feldene; Flogobene; Geldene; Improntal; Larapam; Pirkam; Piroflex; Reudene; Riacen; Roxicam; Roxiden; Sasu-

len; Solocalm; Zunden. $C_{15}H_{13}N_3O_4S$; mol wt 331.35. C 54.37%, H 3.95%, N 12.68%, O 19.31%, S 9.68%. Non-steroidal anti-inflammatory with long half-life. Prepn (keto form): J. Lombardino, DE **1943265**; *idem*, US **3591584** (1970, 1971 to Pfizer). Synthesis and biological properties: J. Lombardino, E. Wiseman, *J. Med. Chem.* **15**, 848 (1972); J. Lombardino *et al., ibid.* **16**, 493 (1973). Pharmacology: E. Wiseman *et al., Arzneim.-Forsch.* **26**, 1300 (1976). Evaluation of ulcerogenic effects: G. Palacios *et al., Methods Find. Exp. Clin. Pharmacol.* **9**, 353 (1987). Clinical pharmacology: L. Martinez *et al., ibid.* **10**, 729 (1988). *Review: eidem*, in *Pharmacological and Biochemical Properties of Drug Substances* vol. 3, M. E. Goldberg, Ed. (Am. Pharm. Assoc., Washington, DC, 1981) pp 324-346. Review of pharmacology and therapeutic efficacy: R. N. Brogden *et al., Drugs* **22**, 165-187 (1981); *eidem, ibid.* **28**, 292-323 (1984). Symposium on clinical efficacy and safety: *Am. J. Med.* **81**, Suppl. 5B, 1-55 (1986). Comprehensive description: M. Mihalic *et al., Anal. Profiles Drug Subs.* **15**, 509-531 (1986).

Crystals from methanol, mp 198-200°. pKa 6.3 (2:1 dioxane-water). LD$_{50}$ orally in mice: 360 mg/kg (Wiseman).

Cinnamic acid ester. [87234-24-0] Piroxicam cinnamate; cinnoxicam; SPA-S-510; Sinartrol; Zelis; Zen. $C_{24}H_{19}N_3O_5S$; mol wt 461.49.

Compd with β-cyclodextrin. [121696-62-6] Brexin; Cicladol; Cycladol. $C_{57}H_{83}N_3O_{39}S$; mol wt 1466.33.

THERAP CAT: Anti-inflammatory.

7507. Pirozadil. [54110-25-7] 3,4,5-Trimethoxybenzoic acid 2,6-pyridinediylbis(methylene)ester; 2,6-pyridinedimethanol bis(3,4,5-trimethoxybenzoate); 722 D; Pemix. $C_{27}H_{29}NO_{10}$; mol wt 527.52. C 61.47%, H 5.54%, N 2.66%, O 30.33%. Hypolipidemic agent that inhibits platelet aggregation. Prepn: J. P. Cochs, DE **2411902** (1974 to Inst. Int. Ter.), *C.A.* **82**, 4136q (1975). Effect on cerebral metabolic blood flow in rabbits: J. Balasch, L. Palacios, *Arch. Farmacol. Toxicol.* **3**, 137 (1977). Efficacy in exptl atherosclerosis: M. R. Parwaresch *et al., Atherosclerosis* **31**, 395 (1978). Toxicological and histopathological study: J. Roca *et al., Arch. Farmacol. Toxicol.* **6**, 41 (1980). Clinical trials in hyperlipoproteinemia: M. Shinomiya *et al., Arzneim.-Forsch.* **37**, 1069 (1987); R. Tapounet, I. Marti Ragué, *Drugs Exp. Clin. Res.* **13**, 447 (1987).

White cryst powder, mp 119-126°. Very sol in chloroform; sol in dioxane, acetonitrile. Practically insol in ether, water.

THERAP CAT: Antilipemic.

7508. Pitavastatin. [147511-69-1] (3*R*,5*S*,6*E*)-7-[2-Cyclopropyl-4-(4-fluorophenyl)-3-quinolinyl]-3,5-dihydroxy-6-heptenoic acid; itavastatin; nisvastatin. $C_{25}H_{24}FNO_4$; mol wt 421.46. C 71.24%, H 5.74%, F 4.51%, N 3.32%, O 15.18%. HMG CoA reductase inhibitor. Prepn: Y. Fujikawa *et al.*, EP **304063**; *eidem*, US **5011930** (1989, 1991 both to Nissan Chem. Ind.). Prepn of lactone: S. Takano *et al., Tetrahedron: Asymmetry* **4**, 201 (1993). Chiral synthesis: M. Suzuki *et al., Bioorg. Med. Chem. Lett.* **9**, 2977 (1999). Structure-activity study: *idem et al., Bioorg. Med. Chem.* **9**, 2727 (2001). Pharmacology: T. Aoki *et al., Arzneim.-Forsch.* **47**, 904 (1997). HPLC determn in plasma: J. Kojima *et al., J. Chromatogr. B* **724**, 173 (1999). Metabolism: I. Yamada *et al., Xenobiotica* **33**, 789 (2003). Clinical comparison with pravastatin: Y. Saito *et al., Atherosclerosis* **162**, 373 (2002). Clinical evaluation in hypercholesterolemia: S. Park *et al., Clin. Ther.* **27**, 1074 (2005). Review of pharmacokinetics and clinical experience: K. Kajinami *et al., Cardiovasc. Drug Rev.* **21**, 199-215 (2003); R. Y. A. Mukhtar *et al., Int. J. Clin Pract.* **59**, 239-252 (2005).

Calcium salt. [147526-32-7] Monocalcium bis[(3*R*,5*S*,6*E*)-7-[2-cyclopropyl-4-(4-fluorophenyl)-3-quinolinyl]-3,5-dihydroxy-6-heptenoate]; NK-104; Livalo. $C_{50}H_{46}CaF_2N_2O_8$; mol wt 880.98. Lipophilic. $[\alpha]_D^{20}$ +23.1° (c = 1.00 in acetonitrile/water).

Lactone. [141750-63-2] (4*R*,6*S*)-6-[(1*E*)-2-[2-Cyclopropyl-4-(4-fluorophenyl)-3-quinolinyl]ethenyl]tetrahydro-4-hydroxy-2*H*-pyran-2-one. $C_{25}H_{22}FNO_3$; mol wt 403.45. mp 138-139°. $[\alpha]_D^{32}$ +8.84° (c = 0.92 in chloroform).

THERAP CAT: Antilipemic.

7509. Pithecolobine. [22368-82-7] 19-Heptyl-10-hydroxy-1,5,10,14-tetraazacyclononadecan-15-one. $C_{22}H_{46}N_4O_2$; mol wt 398.63. C 66.29%, H 11.63%, N 14.05%, O 8.03%. Occurs in the bark of *Samanea saman* Merr. (formerly *Pithecolobium saman* Benth.), bark and seed of *P. bigeminum* Mart. and *P. lobatum* Benth., *Leguminosae*. Isoln: Greshoff, *Ber.* **23**, 3541 (1890); K. Wiesner *et al., Can. J. Chem.* **30**, 761 (1952). Structure: *eidem, J. Am. Chem. Soc.* **75**, 6348 (1953); D. E. Orr, K. Wiesner, *Chem. Ind. (London)* **1959**, 672; K. Wiesner, D. E. Orr, *Tetrahedron Letters* no. 16, 11 (1960); K. Wiesner *et al., Can. J. Chem.* **46**, 1886, 3617 (1968).

Crystals, mp 67-69° or oily liquid, $bp_{0.007}$ 230°. Sublimes at 135° at 0.007 mm pressure. Sol in water, alcohol, chloroform, ether, petr ether.

7510. Pituitary, Posterior. Pituamin; Di-Sipidin; Pituitrin. Desiccated hypophysis. The cleaned, dried, and powdered posterior lobe of pituitary body of domesticated animals used for food by man. Contains both oxytocin and vasopressin, *q.q.v.*

Yellowish or grayish, amorphous powder; characteristic odor. Partially sol in water. *Keep well closed and in a cool place.*

THERAP CAT: Oxytocic; antidiuretic.

THERAP CAT (VET): Oxytocic; antidiuretic.

7511. Pivalic Acid. [75-98-9] 2,2-Dimethylpropanoic acid; α,α-dimethylpropionic acid; trimethylacetic acid. $C_5H_{10}O_2$; mol wt 102.13. C 58.80%, H 9.87%, O 31.33%. HOOCC(CH₃)₃. Prepd by the reaction of *tert*-butylmagnesium chloride and carbon dioxide: Bouveault, *Compt. Rend.* **138**, 1108 (1904); Puntambeker, Zoellner, *Org. Synth.* **8**, 104 (1928); other methods: *ibid.* 108. Forms higher esters (e.g., isobutyl ester) only with difficulty.

Needles, mp 35.5°. bp_{760} 163.8°; d^{50} 0.905; $n_D^{36.5}$ 1.3931. pKa (25°): 5.01. One gram dissolves in 40 ml water. Freely sol in alcohol, ether.

Ethyl ester. $C_7H_{14}O_2$. Liquid. d_4^{18} 0.8580; bp 118.2°; n_D^{18} 1.3922.

7512. Pivampicillin. [33817-20-8] (2*S*,5*R*,6*R*)-6-[[(2*R*)-Aminophenylacetyl]amino]-3,3-dimethyl-7-oxo-4-thia-1-azabicyclo[3.2.0]heptane-2-carboxylic acid (2,2-dimethyl-1-oxopropoxy)-methyl ester; hydroxymethyl 6-(2-amino-2-phenylacetamido)-3,3-dimethyl-7-oxo-4-thia-1-azabicyclo[3.2.0]heptane-2-carboxylate pivalate (ester); 6-[D-α-aminophenylacetamido]penicillanic acid pivaloyloxymethyl ester; pivaloyloxymethyl D-α-aminobenzyl-

penicillinate; ampicillin pivaloyloxymethyl ester; pivaloyloxy-methyl ampicillinate; MK-191. $C_{22}H_{29}N_3O_6S$; mol wt 463.55. C 57.00%, H 6.31%, N 9.06%, O 20.71%, S 6.92%. Semi-synthetic antibiotic related to penicillin. Prepn: E. K. Frederiksen, W. O. Godtfredsen, **ZA 6805952**; *eidem*, **US 3660575** (1969, 1972 to Lövens Kemiske Fabrik); von Daehne *et al., J. Med. Chem.* **13**, 607 (1970). Pharmacology: *eidem, loc. cit.;* Jordan *et al., Antimicrob. Agents Chemother.* **1970**, 438; Foltz *et al., ibid.* 442. Pharmacokinetics in man: M. Ehrnebo *et al., J. Pharmacokinet. Biopharm.* **7**, 429 (1979). Toxicity: von Daehne *et al., Antimicrob. Agents Chemother.* **1970**, 430.

Hydrochloride. [26309-95-5] Pondocil; Pondocillin; Pondocillina; Sanguicillin. $C_{22}H_{29}N_3O_6S.HCl$; mol wt 500.01. Microcrystalline powder, mp 155-156° (decomp). $[\alpha]_D^{20}$ +196° (c = 1 in water). Weak uv max (water): 268, 262, 256 nm ($E_{1cm}^{1\%}$ ~3.9, 5.7, 6.3). pKa ~7.0. Relatively stable in acid soln; ester hydrolyzes slowly in neutral soln. pH of 0.5 g/100 ml water: ~4.5. Very sol in water and chloroform; freely sol in ethanol; sparingly sol in *n*-propanol, *tert*-butanol, and ethyl ether. LD₅₀ in mice, rats (g/kg): 3.34, 5.00 orally; 3.60, 4.50 s.c. (von Daehne).

THERAP CAT: Antibacterial.

7513. Pivcefalexin. [63836-75-9] (6*R*,7*R*)-7-[[(2*R*)-Amino-phenylacetyl]amino]-3-methyl-8-oxo-5-thia-1-azabicyclo[4.2.0]-oct-2-ene-2-carboxylic acid (2,2-dimethyl-1-oxopropoxy)methyl ester; 7-(D-2-amino-2-phenylacetamido)desacetoxycephalosporanic acid pivaloyloxymethyl ester; pivcephalexin. $C_{22}H_{27}N_3O_6S$; mol wt 461.53. C 57.25%, H 5.90%, N 9.10%, O 20.80%, S 6.95%. Orally active semi-synthetic cephalosporin antibiotic; deriv of cephalexin, *q.v.* Prepn: W. O. Godtfredsen, E. T. Binderup, **DE 1951012** (1970 to Lövens Kemiske Fabrik), *C.A.* **72**, 132761v (1970). Pharmacology: P. Foresta *et al., Arzneim.-Forsch.* **27**, 819 (1977). Absorption and excretion: E. Trabucchi *et al., Clin. Ther.* **81**, 299 (1977). Clinical trial: C. Vittorini *et al., Arzneim.-Forsch.* **31**, 1163 (1981).

Hydrochloride. [27726-31-4] ST-21; Ausocef; Bencef; Cefalen; Cefalex; Pivacef; Sigmacef. $C_{22}H_{27}N_3O_6S.HCl$; mol wt 497.99.

THERAP CAT: Antibacterial.

7514. Pixantrone. [144510-96-3] 6,9-Bis[(2-aminoethyl)-amino]benz[*g*]isoquinoline-5,10-dione; $C_{17}H_{19}N_5O_2$; mol wt 325.37. C 62.75%, H 5.89%, N 21.52%, O 9.83%. Second generation aza-anthracenedione analog which intercalates DNA and inhibits topoisomerase II; structurally similar to mitoxantrone, *q.v.* Prepn: P. A. Krapcho, **EP 503537** (1992 to Univ. of Vermont); *idem et al., J. Med. Chem.* **37**, 828 (1994). Solid-state characterization: A. Marini *et al., J. Pharm. Sci.* **92**, 577 (2003). Antitumor spectrum and evaluation of cardiotoxic potential: G. Beggiolin *et al., Tumori* **87**, 407 (2001). Immunosuppressant activity: G. Cavaletti *et al., J. Neuroimmunol.* **151**, 55 (2004). Clinical pharmacokinetics: S. Faivre *et al., Clin. Cancer Res.* **7**, 43 (2001). Clinical evaluation in non-Hodgkin's lymphoma: P. Borchmann *et al., Haematologica* **88**, 888 (2003). Review of development and therapeutic potential: P. Borchmann, R. Schnell, *Expert Opin. Invest. Drugs* **14**, 1055-1061 (2005).

Dimalate salt. [144675-97-8] BBR-2778. $C_{17}H_{19}N_5O_2 \cdot 2C_4H_{14}O_4$; mol wt 577.67. Blue solid from ethanol and ether, mp 192° (dec). Moderately sol in physiological saline.

Hydrochloride. [175989-38-5] $C_{17}H_{19}N_5O_2 \cdot HCl$; mol wt 361.83. Dark blue hygroscopic solid from chloroform, mp 209-212°.

THERAP CAT: Antineoplastic.

7515. Pizotyline. [15574-96-6] 4-(9,10-Dihydro-4*H*-benzo-[4,5]cyclohepta[1,2-*b*]thien-4-ylidene)-1-methylpiperidine; 4-(1-methyl-4-piperidylidene)-9,10-dihydro-4*H*-benzo[4,5]cyclohepta[1,2-*b*]thiophene; pizotifen; pizotyl; pizotifan; BC-105. $C_{19}H_{21}NS$; mol wt 295.44. C 77.24%, H 7.16%, N 4.74%, S 10.85%. Serotonin antagonist structurally related to cyproheptadine, *q.v.* Prepn: Jucker *et al.*, **BE 636717** and **US 3272826** (1964, 1966 to Sandoz); Bastian *et al.*, *Helv. Chim. Acta* **49**, 214 (1966). Toxicity data: Bagdon, Dorado, *Pharmacologist* **12**, No. 2, 297 (1970). Mechanism of action study: E. Müller-Schweinitzer, *J. Cardiovasc. Pharmacol.* **8**, 805 (1986). Clinical trial in migraine: D. Crowder, W. P. Maclay, *Curr. Med. Res. Opin.* **9**, 280 (1984). Review of pharmacology and therapeutic efficacy: Speight, Avery, *Drugs* **3**, 159-203 (1972).

Hydrochloride. [73391-87-4] Crystals from isopropanol-ether, mp 261-263° (dec).

Malate. [5189-11-7] Litec; Sandomigran; Sanmigran; Sanomigran; Mosegor. $C_{19}H_{21}NS \cdot C_4H_6O_5$; mol wt 429.53. Crystals from methanol, mp 185-186° (dec).

THERAP CAT: Antimigraine; appetite stimulant.

7516. Plafibride. [63394-05-8] 2-(4-Chlorophenoxy)-2-methyl-*N*-[[(4-morpholinylmethyl)amino]carbonyl]propanamide; *N*-2-(*p*-chlorophenoxy)isobutyryl-*N'*-morpholinomethylurea; ITA-104; Idonor; Perifunal. $C_{16}H_{22}ClN_3O_4$; mol wt 355.82. C 54.01%, H 6.23%, Cl 9.96%, N 11.81%, O 17.99%. Analog of clofibrate, *q.v.* Prepn: J. Iniesta-Pons, **DE 2716374** (1977 to Investigacion Tecnica y Aplicada), *C.A.* **88**, 37810g (1978). Toxicity data: J. Zapatero, L. Brugeghini, *Arch. Farmacol. Toxicol.* **4**, 137 (1978). Series of articles on antiplatelet aggregation activity, hypolipemic activity, pharmacology, and toxicology: *ibid.*, 132-142.

Crystals, mp 100-102°. Sol in acetone. Slightly sol in alcohol. Practically insol in water, petr ether. LD_{50} in mice, rats, guinea pigs (mg/kg): 3569, >4000, 2168 orally (Zapatero, Brugeghini).

THERAP CAT: Antithrombotic.

7517. Plantago Seed. Psyllium seed; plantain seed; flea seed. Seed from *Plantago ovata* Forsk., *Plantaginaceae,* known as blond or Indian plantago seed, *P. psyllium* L. known as Spanish psyllium

seed, or *P. indica* L. (*P. arenaria* Waldst. & Kit.) known as French psyllium seed. Habit. Mediterranean countries, India. Cultivated in India, Pakistan, France. *Psyllium husk* is the epidermis from seeds of any of the above plantago species; *Ispaghula husk* refers specifically to the epidermis of *P. ovata* seeds. The husk contains a water-soluble mucilage consisting of a highly branched, acidic arabinoxylan: J. F. Kennedy *et al., Carbohydr. Res.* **75**, 265 (1979). Use in chronic constipation: M. Borgia *et al., J. Int. Med. Res.* **11**, 124 (1983). *Review:* J. N. BeMiller in *Industrial Gums,* R. L. Whistler, Ed. (Academic Press, New York, 2nd ed., 1973) pp 345-354. Review of therapeutic potential in reducing blood cholesterol: H. Lipsky *et al., J. Clin. Pharmacol.* **30**, 699-703 (1990).

Small, dark reddish-brown, odorless, almost tasteless seeds. Mixed with an equal bulk of water, forms a mucilaginous mass.

Ispaghula husk. Fibrolax; Fybozest; Fybogel; Isogel; Regulan.

Psyllium hydrophilic mucilloid. [8063-16-9] Psyllium hydrocolloid; psyllium seed gum; Effer-Syllium; Fiberall; Metamucil; Perdiem Fiber; Serutan. Obtained from epidermis of *P. ovata* seeds. White to cream-colored, slightly granular powder. Slightly acid taste; little or no odor.

THERAP CAT: Laxative.

7518. Plantisul. [1407-93-8] Banabins. Orally effective antidiabetic principle contained in aq extracts from the leaves and fruits of the banaba tree, *Lagerstroemia speciosa* (L.) Pers., *Lythraceae.* Extraction procedure: Faustino Garcia, *Philipp. J. Sci.* **76**, no. 3, 3-21 (1944); *J. Philipp. Med. Assoc.* **31**, 216-224 and 276-282 (1955). *Constit.* of banaba extracts: Carew, Chin, *Nature* **190**, 1108 (1961).

7519. Plasmalogens. Aldehydogenic lipids characteristic of the animal kingdom; references to their existence in plants and bacteria are rare. Plasmalogens contain an aldehydogenic chain linked to glycerol as an α,β-unsaturated ether. Although most are aldehydogenic phosphatides, nonphosphatide or neutral plasmalogens have been detected in animal tissues. "Native plasmalogens", when deacylated, yield lysoderivatives, *lysoplasmalogens,* contg the aldehydogenic chain linked to glycerol as an α,β-unsaturated ether. The nomenclature *"phosphatidal ethanolamine", "phosphatidal choline",* etc. has been proposed for native plasmalogen phosphatides, and *"lysophosphatidal ethanolamine", "lysophosphatidal choline",* etc. for corresponding deacylated derivatives. This nomenclature minimizes the confusion arising from less precise terms, such as "plasmalogen" or *"ethanolamine plasmalogen", "choline plasmalogen",* etc. to designate either native compds, lysoderivatives, or other structures which may occur (molecules with two α,β-unsaturated ether chains or with one saturated ether and one α,β-unsaturated ether chain, and true cyclic glyceryl acetal derivatives). First isoln of a pure native plasmalogen (phosphatidal choline): Gottfried, Rapport, *Fed. Proc.* **20**, 278 (1961); *eidem, J. Biol. Chem.* **237**, 329 (1962). *Ref:* Rapport, Norton, *Annu. Rev. Biochem.* **31**, 103 (1962). Synthesis: Piantadosi *et al., J. Org. Chem.* **28**, 2425 (1963); Chacko *et al., ibid.* **32**, 3698 (1967); Slotboom *et al., Chem. Phys. Lipids* **1**, 192 (1967); Gigg, Gigg, *J. Chem. Soc. C* **1968**, 16, 2030; Vtorov *et al., Tetrahedron Lett.* **1971**, 4605. *Reviews:* E. Klenk, H. Debuch, "Plasmalogens" in Holman *et al., Progr. Chem. Fats Lipids* vol. 6, (Macmillan, New York, 1963) pp 1-29; Piantadosi, Snyder, *J. Pharm. Sci.* **59**, 283-297 (1970).

7520. Plasmin. [9001-90-5] Fibrinolysin; serum tryptase; Actase; Thrombolysin. Mol wt about 90,000. Trypsin-like proteolytic enzyme which cleaves fibrin, fibrinogen, *q.q.v.,* and other plasma proteins. Component of the mammalian fibrinolytic system specifically responsible for the dissolution of fibrin clots. Exists in plasma as an inactive precursor, plasminogen, *q.v.* Converted to the active enzyme at the clot site by tissue plasminogen activator, *q.v.* Also activated by streptokinase and urokinase, *q.q.v.* Rapidly inactivated in plasma by α_2-*antiplasmin,* a glyceroprotein with high specific binding affinity for plasmin. Prepn: Christensen, MacLeod, *J. Gen. Physiol.* **28**, 599 (1945); E. C. Loomis, **US 2624691** (1953 to Parke, Davis); J. H. Hink, J. K. McDonald, **US 3234106** (1966 to Cutter Labs); K. C. Robbins, L. Summaria, *J. Biol. Chem.* **238**, 952 (1963). Converted from plasminogen by proteolysis of a single arg-val bond: K. C. Robbins *et al., ibid.* **242**, 2333, 4279 (1967). Structure consists of two polypeptide chains connected by

two disulfide bonds. The heavy (A) chain (MW ~65,000) origi-nates from the amino-terminal portion of plasminogen and contains the binding sites. The light (B) chain (MW ~25,000) originates from the carboxy-terminus and contains the active site. Isolation and characterization of heavy and light chains: L. Summaria *et al., J. Biol. Chem.* **242**, 5046 (1967); *eidem, ibid.* **246**, 2143 (1971). Amino acid sequence studies: W. R. Groskopf *et al., ibid.* **244**, 3590 (1969); Hartley, *Philos. Trans. R. Soc. London Ser. B* **257**, 77 (1970); S. Nagasawa, T. Suzuki, *Biochem. Biophys. Res. Commun.* **41**, 562 (1970). Amino acid sequence of active site: K. C. Robbins *et al., J. Biol. Chem.* **248**, 1631 (1973). Review of structural studies: F. J. Castellino, *Semin. Thromb. Hemostasis* **10**, 18-23 (1984). Enzyme specificity for lysine and arginine peptide bonds: W. Troll *et al., J. Biol. Chem.* **208**, 85 (1954). Review of biochemis-try: D. Ogston, *J. Clin. Pathol.* **33**, Suppl. 14, 5-9 (1980). *Reviews:* D. Collen, *Thromb. Haemostasis* **43**, 77-89 (1980); K. C. Robbins *et al., Methods Enzymol.* **80**, 379-387 (1981); K. K. Kane, *Ann. Clin. Lab. Sci.* **14**, 443-449 (1984).
THERAP CAT: Thrombolytic enzyme.

7521. Plasminogen. [9001-91-6] Profibrinolysin; plasma trypsinogen. Mol wt ~90,000. The circulating plasma precursor (zymogen) or inactive form of plasmin, *q.v.* Prepn from blood plasma: Loomis *et al., Arch. Biochem.* **12**, 1 (1947); Oncley *et al., J. Am. Chem. Soc.* **71**, 541 (1949). Purification: Christensen, Smith, *Proc. Soc. Exp. Biol. Med.* **74**, 840 (1950); Kline, *J. Biol. Chem.* **204**, 949 (1953); Hagan *et al., ibid.* **235**, 1005 (1960); Hagan *et al., US 3066079* (1962 to Am. Cyanamid); Derechin *et al., Bio-chem. J.* **84**, 336 (1962); Mertz, Chan, *Can. J. Biochem. Physiol.* **41**, 1811 (1963); D. G. Deutsch, E. T. Mertz, *Science* **170**, 1095 (1970). Physical properties: Davies, Englert, *J. Biol. Chem.* **235**, 1011 (1960). Converted to plasmin by natural activators such as strepto-kinase, urokinase, or tissue plasminogen activator, *q.q.v.,* through the cleavage of a single arg-val bond. Mechanism of activation: K. C. Robbins *et al., ibid.* **242**, 2333, 4279 (1967). Native plasmino-gen is a single chain glycopeptide. Two major molecular forms exist, differing in carbohydrate content and separable by affinity chromatography. Mol wt studies: Barlow *et al., ibid.* **244**, 1138 (1969). Sequence studies: K. C. Robbins *et al., ibid.* **247**, 6757 (1972); F. J. Castellino *et al., Biochem. Biophys. Res. Commun.* **53**, 845 (1973). Carbohydrate comp: M. L. Hayes, F. J. Castellino, *J. Biol. Chem.* **254**, 8768, 8772, 8777 (1979). Amino acid sequence and biochemistry: F. J. Castellino, *Semin. Thromb. Hemostasis* **10**, 18 (1984). Biosynthesis and secretion by cultured hepatocytes: J. F. Bohmfalk, G. M. Fuller, *Science* **209**, 408 (1980). Therapeutic use with streptokinase: I. D. Walker *et al., Thromb. Haemostasis* **51**, 204 (1984). Review of fibrinolytic system: D. Collen, *ibid.* **43**, 77-89 (1980). *Reviews: Fibrinolysis,* D. L. Kline, K. N. N. Reddy, Eds. (CRC, Boca Raton, 1980) 256 pp; F. J. Castellino, *Chem. Rev.* **81**, 431-446 (1981).
Soluble below pH 5 and above pH 9 and only sparingly sol at intermediate pH values. Resistant to heat below pH 5. Displays maximum stability at pH 2-3.

7522. Plasmocid. [551-01-9] *N,N*-Diethyl-*N'*-(6-methoxy-8-quinolinyl)-1,3-propanediamine; 8-(3-diethylaminopropyl-amino)-6-methoxyquinoline; 6-methoxy-8-(3-diethylaminopropyl-amino)quinoline; 710-F; SN-3115; Fourneau 710; Antimalarine; Rhodoquine. $C_{17}H_{25}N_3O$; mol wt 287.40. C 71.04%, H 8.77%, N 14.62%, O 5.57%. Prepn: Fourneau *et al., Ann. Inst. Pasteur* **44**, 503 (1930); **46**, 514 (1931); **50**, 731 (1933); Magidson, Strukov, *Arch. Pharm.* **271**, 359 (1933); Strukov, *SU 39105* (1934), *C.A.* **30**, 3445 (1936); Magidson *et al., J. Appl. Chem. USSR* **9**, 304 (1936); Giral, *Ciencia (Mexico City)* **6**, 253 (1945), *C.A.* **40**, 3563 (1946); Yanko *et al., J. Am. Chem. Soc.* **67**, 664 (1945).

Oily liquid, d_4^{24} 1.0569. bp$_{1.0}$ 182°. n_D^{24} 1.5855.
Dihydrochloride. $C_{17}H_{27}Cl_2N_3O$. Yellow crystals, mp 218-220°. Slightly sol in water, alcohol.

Diphosphate. Yellow crystals, mp 169-171°. Slightly sol in water, alcohol.
Note: The name Rhodoquine was first applied to 8-(3-dimethyl-aminopropylamino)-6-methoxyquinoline.
THERAP CAT: Antimalarial.

7523. Plastoquinones. PQs. Family of lipid-soluble benzo-quinone derivatives involved in photosynthetic electron transport. Structurally and functionally analogous to the ubiquinones, *q.v.* Structures are characterized by a side chain of repeating isoprenoid units with 9 units being the most common. Originally discovered by Kofler in 1946. Isoln of PQ-9 from alfalfa: F. L. Crane, *Plant Physiol.* **34**, 546 (1959). Localization in chloroplasts and role in photosynthesis: N. I. Bishop, *Proc. Natl. Acad. Sci. USA* **45**, 1696 (1959). Structure: M. Kofler *et al., Helv. Chim. Acta* **42**, 2252 (1959); N. R. Trenner *et al., J. Am. Chem. Soc.* **81**, 2026 (1959). Synthesis: C. H. Shunk *et al., ibid.* 5000. Identification of plasto-quinone analogs B and C: L. P. Kegel *et al., Biochem. Biophys. Res. Commun.* **8**, 294 (1962). Review of role in photosynthetic electron flow: U. Siggel, *Bioelectrochem. Bioenerg.* **3**, 302-318 (1976); A. Trebst in *Coenzyme Q,* G. Lenaz, Ed. (John Wiley & Sons, Chi-chester, 1985) pp 257-284.

Plastoquinone 9

Plastoquinone 9. [4299-57-4] (*all-E*)-2,3-Dimethyl-5-(3,7,11,-15,19,23,27,31,35-nonamethyl-2,6,10,14,18,22,26,30,34-hexatria-contanonaenyl)-2,5-cyclohexadiene-1,4-dione; 2,3-dimethyl-5-sol-anesyl-1,4-benzoquinone; Kofler's quinone; plastoquinone A; plas-toquinone 45; Q-254; PQ-9. $C_{53}H_{80}O_2$; mol wt 749.20. Yellow crystals, mp 48-49°. uv max (isooctane): 254, 262 nm (E $_{1cm}^{1\%}$ 247, 226).

7524. Platelet Activating Factor. [65154-06-5] PAF; 1-*O*-alkyl-2-acetyl-*sn*-glycero-3-phosphorylcholine; acetyl glyceryl ether phosphorylcholine; AGEPC; PAF-acether; antihypertensive polar renomedullary lipid; APRL. Phospholipid mediator of plate-let aggregation, inflammation, and anaphylaxis. Produced in re-sponse to specific stimuli by a variety of cell types, including neutrophils, basophils, platelets, and endothelial cells. Several mo-lecular species of PAF have been identified which vary in the length of the *O*-alkyl side chain. *In vitro* identification of a soluble platelet activating factor produced by antigen stimulated leukocytes: P. M. Henson, *J. Exp. Med.* **131**, 287 (1970). Isoln from rabbit basophils, characterization of PAF response and potential role in immune complex disease: J. Benveniste *et al., ibid.* **136**, 1356 (1972). Isoln from human leukocytes: J. Benveniste, *Nature* **249**, 581 (1974). Release of PAF *in vivo* during anaphylaxis: R. N. Pinckard *et al., J. Immunol.* **123**, 1847 (1979). Structural study: J. Benve-niste *et al., Nature* **269**, 170 (1977); and synthetic approaches: J. Benveniste *et al., C.R. Seances Acad. Sci. Ser. D* **289**, 1037 (1979); C. A. Demopoulos *et al., J. Biol. Chem.* **254**, 9355 (1979). Identity with APRL and antihypertensive activity: M. L. Blank *et al., Bio-chem. Biophys. Res. Commun.* **90**, 1194 (1979). Structures of 1-*O*-octadecyl- and 1-*O*-hexadecyl-PAF, two of the predominant molec-ular forms: D. J. Hanahan *et al., ibid.* **255**, 5514 (1980). Total synthesis of 1-*O*-octadecyl-PAF: J. Godfroid *et al., FEBS Lett.* **116**, 161 (1980). Enantiomeric synthesis of C_{16}- and C_{18}-PAF: M. Ohno *et al., Chem. Pharm. Bull.* **33**, 572 (1985). Molecular heter-ogeneity of naturally occurring PAF: R. N. Pinckard *et al., Bio-chem. Biophys. Res. Commun.* **122**, 325 (1984); H. W. Mueller *et al., J. Biol. Chem.* **259**, 14554 (1984). Ulcerogenic effects: A.-C. Rosam *et al., Nature* **319**, 54 (1986). Effects on human pulmonary and cardiovascular function: F. M. Cuss *et al., Lancet* **2**, 189 (1986). Review of isoln and analytical methods: D. J. Hanahan, S. T. Weintraub, *Methods Biochem. Anal.* **31**, 195-219 (1985); of chemical and biochemical characteristics: D. J. Hanahan, R. Ku-mar, *Prog. Lipid Res.* **26**, 1-28 (1987). Reviews of biosynthesis, biological activities and PAF antagonists: P. Braquet *et al., Phar-*

macol. Rev. **39**, 97-145 (1987); P. J. Barnes et al., J. Allergy Clin. Immunol. **81**, 919-934 (1988). Books: *Platelet-Activating Factor and Related Lipid Mediators*, F. Snyder, Ed. (Plenum Press, New York, 1987) 471 pp; *Prog. Biochem. Pharmacol.* **22** entitled "Biologically Active Ether Lipids" by P. Braquet et al., Eds. (Karger, Basel, 1988).

n usually represents 15 or 17

1-O-Hexadecyl PAF. (R)-7-(Acetyloxy)-4-hydroxy-N,N,N-trimethyl-3,5,9-trioxa-4-phosphapentacosan-1-aminium hydroxide inner salt 4-oxide; C_{16}-PAF. $C_{26}H_{54}NO_7P$. White, amorphous solid, mp 247° (dec). $[\alpha]_D^{21}$ −3.66° (c = 0.71 in chloroform).

1-O-Octadecyl-PAF. (R)-7-(Acetyloxy)-4-hydroxy-N,N,N-trimethyl-3,5,9-trioxa-4-phosphaheptacosan-1-aminium hydroxide inner salt 4-oxide; C_{18}-PAF. $C_{28}H_{58}NO_7P$. mp 212-215° (dec). $[\alpha]_D^{20}$ −4.00° (c = 0.71 in chloroform).

7525. Platelet-Derived Growth Factor. PDGF. Cationic glycoprotein; mol wt ~30 kDa. Chemoattractant and mitogen for fibroblasts, smooth muscle cells and glial cells. Involved in both normal and pathologic processes such as wound healing, atherosclerosis, and neoplasia. Composed of two disulfide-linked polypeptide chains, A and B, which may be assembled as a heterodimer or as AA or BB homodimers. PDGF-AB is the most abundant. Originally isolated from platelets, subsequently found to be secreted by a number of cell types including macrophages, fibroblasts, and endothelial cells. Identification: R. Ross et al., Proc. Natl. Acad. Sci. USA **71**, 1207 (1974); N. Kohler, A. Lipton, Exp. Cell Res. **87**, 297 (1974). Isoln: H. N. Antoniades et al., Proc. Natl. Acad. Sci. USA **72**, 2635 (1975). Purification: H. N. Antoniades et al., ibid. **76**, 1809 (1979); C.-H. Heldin et al., ibid. 3722. Structure: A. Johnsson et al., Biochem. Biophys. Res. Commun. **104**, 66 (1982); A. Hammacher et al., J. Biol. Chem. **263**, 16493 (1988). PDGF-B is structurally homologous to *p28sis*, the transforming protein of the simian sarcoma virus: M. D. Waterfield et al., Nature **304**, 35 (1983); R. F. Doolittle et al., Science **221**, 275 (1983). Comparison of biological properties and transforming potential of A and B chains: M. P. Beckmann et al., Science **241**, 1346 (1988). Identification of PDGF receptor: C.-H. Heldin et al., Proc. Natl. Acad. Sci. USA **78**, 3664 (1981). Molecular mechanisms of action: L. T. Williams, Science **243**, 1564 (1989). Review of role in atherosclerosis: R. Ross, N. Engl. J. Med. **314**, 488-500 (1986); in wound healing: G. F. Pierce et al., J. Cell. Biochem. **45**, 319-326 (1991). Reviews: R. Ross, Annu. Rev. Med. **38**, 71-79 (1987); B. Westermark et al., Ciba Found. Symp. **150**, 6-22 (1990); K. C. Hart et al., Genet. Eng. (NY) **17**, 181-208 (1995); W. Meyer-Ingold, W. Eichner, Cell Biol. Int. **19**, 389-398 (1995).

Becaplermin. [165101-51-9] rhPDGF-BB; RWJ-60235; Regranex. Recombinant protein corresponding to endogenous human PDGF-BB homodimer. Clinical trial in treatment of diabetic foot ulcers: D. L. Steed et al., J. Am. Coll. Surg. **183**, 61 (1996).

THERAP CAT: Vulnerary.

7526. Platinic Chloride. [16941-12-1] Hydrogen hexachloroplatinate(IV); acid platinic chloride; hexachloroplatinic(IV) acid; chloroplatinic acid. Cl_6H_2Pt; mol wt 409.82. Cl 51.91%, H 0.49%, Pt 47.60%. H_2PtCl_6. Exists as hexahydrate.

Hexahydrate, brownish-yellow, very deliquesc, cryst mass. d 2.431; mp 60°. Easily sol in water, alcohol. *Keep tightly closed, protected from light.*

Caution: May cause asthma or dermatitis, E. Browning, *Toxicity of Industrial Metals* (Appleton-Century-Crofts, New York, 2nd ed., 1969) pp 270-275.

USE: In platinum plating, photography, platinum mirrors, platinum luster on glass and porcelain, platinized carbon for acetic acid manuf; platinizing pumice stone or asbestos, as catalyst in manuf of

SO_3; indelible ink; relief etching of zinc for artistic and commercial purposes; fixing microscopic prepns, etc.

7527. Platinic Oxide. [1314-15-4] Platinum dioxide; Adams' catalyst. O_2Pt; mol wt 227.08. O 14.09%, Pt 85.91%. PtO_2. Prepd by the interaction of platinic chloride and excess NaOH: Wöhler, Z. Anorg. Chem. **40**, 434 (1904); Bellucci ibid. **44**, 171 (1905); by the reduction of chloroplatinic acid with formaldehyde: Willstätter, Waldschmidt-Leitz, Ber. **54**, 113 (1921); Feulgen, ibid. 360; by fusing chloroplatinic acid with sodium nitrate: Adams et al., Org. Synth. **8**, 92 (1928). Determination of orthorhombic ($CaCl_2$) crystal structure of β-PtO_2: Siegel et al., J. Inorg. Nucl. Chem. **31**, 3803 (1969).

Several hydrates have been reported; the compd generally used for catalysis is the monohydrate. Black powder. When freshly pptd it is sol in concd acids, also in dil H_3PO_4, esp when warmed. Easily sol in dilute solns of potassium hydroxide.

USE: As catalyst in hydrogenations. The actual catalyst is platinum black which is formed *in situ* by reduction of the PtO_2 by the hydrogen used for the hydrogenation. Especially useful for reduction at room temp and hydrogen pressures up to 4 atmospheres. Suitable for the reduction of double and triple bonds, aromatic nuclei, carbonyl groups, nitro groups, and nitriles.

7528. Platinous Chloride. [10025-65-7] Cl_2Pt; mol wt 265.99. Cl 26.66%, Pt 73.34%. $PtCl_2$. Prepn from hexachloroplatinic acid, $H_2PtCl_6.6H_2O$: Cohen, Inorg. Synth. **6**, 209 (1960).

Grayish-green to brown powder. d 5.87. Insol in water, alcohol, ether. Sol in hydrochloric acid. Combines with PCl_3 to form a compd sol in benzene or chloroform.

7529. Platinum. [7440-06-4] Pt; at. wt 195.084; at. no. 78; valences 2,4; seldom 1, 5, 6. Group VIII (10). Six naturally occurring isotopes: 190 (0.01%); 192 (0.8%); 194 (32.9%); 195 (33.8%); 196 (25.2%); 198 (7.2%); 190 is radioactive: $T_{1/2}$ 6.9 × 10^{11} years. Artificial, radioactive isotopes: 173-189; 191; 193; 197; 199-201. Abundance in earth's crust about 0.01 ppm. Believed to be mentioned by Pliny under the name *"alutiae"*. Has been known and used in South America as "platina del Pinto". Reported by Ulloa in 1735; brought to Europe by Wood, and described by Watson in 1741. Occurs native alloyed with one or more members of its group (iridium, osmium, palladium, rhodium, and ruthenium) in gravels and sands. Prepn: Wichers et al., Trans. Am. Inst. Min. Metall. Eng. **76**, 602 (1928). Reviews of prepn, properties and chemistry of platinum and other platinum metals: Gilchrist, Chem. Rev. **32**, 277-372 (1943); Beamish et al., in Rare Metals Handbook, C. A. Hampel, Ed. (Reinhold, New York, 1956) pp 291-328; Livingstone in Comprehensive Inorganic Chemistry Vol. 3, J. C. Bailar, Jr. et al., Eds. (Pergamon Press, Oxford, 1973) pp 1163-1189, 1330-1370; F. R. Hartley, The Chemistry of Platinum and Palladium with Particular Reference to Complexes of the Elements (Halsted Press, New York, 1973).

Silver-gray, lustrous, malleable and ductile metal; face-centered cubic structure. Also prepd in the form of a black powder (platinum black) and as spongy masses (platinum sponge). mp 1773.5 ± 1°; Roeser et al., Natl. Bur. Stand. J. Res. **6**, 1119 (1931); bp about 3827°. d 21.447 (calcd). Brinell hardness: 55. Sp heat 0.0314 cal/g at 0°. Electrical resistivity (20°) 10.6 μohm-cm. Does not tarnish on exposure to air. Absorbs hydrogen at a red heat and retains it tenaciously at ord. temp, gives off the gas at a red heat in vacuo. Occludes carbon monoxide, carbon dioxide, nitrogen. Volatilizes considerably when heated in air at 1500°. The heated metal absorbs oxygen; gives it off on cooling. Not affected by water or by single mineral acids. Reacts with boiling aqua regia with formation of chloroplatinic acid, also with molten alkali cyanides. Attacked by halogens, by fusion with caustic alkalies, alkali nitrates, alkali peroxides; by arsenates and phosphates in presence of reducing agents.

Caution: Potential symptoms of overexposure to Pt metal are irritation of eyes, skin, respiratory system; dermatitis. Potential symptoms of overexposure to soluble Pt salts are irritation of eyes, nose; cough, dyspnea, wheezing, cyanosis; dermatitis, skin sensitization; lymphocytosis. See NIOSH Pocket Guide to Chemical Hazards (DHHS/NIOSH 97-140, 1997) p 260. See also E. Browning, Toxicity of Industrial Metals (Appleton-Century-Crofts, New York, 2nd ed., 1969) pp 270-275.

USE: Manuf apparatus for laboratory and industrial use, thermocouples, platinum resistance thermometers, acidproof containers, electrodes, etc. In dentistry; jewelry; electroplating. As oxidation catalyst in manuf acetic acid, nitric acid from ammonia, manuf sulfuric acid; control of automotive emissions.

7530. Platonin. [3571-88-8] 2,2'-[3-[(3-Heptyl-4-methyl-2(3H)-thiazolylidene)ethylidene]-1-propene-1,3-diyl]bis(3-heptyl-4-methylthiazolium) diiodide; 4,4',4''-trimethyl-3,3',3''-triheptyl-8-(2''-thiazolyl)-2,2'-pentamethinethiazolocyanine3,3''-diiodide; 3,3',3''-triheptyl-4,4',4''-trimethyl-7-(2''-methylthiazolyl-2,2'-trimethine)thiazolcyanine 3,3''-diiodide; platonin J; NK-19; Kankohso 101; Photosensitizer 101. $C_{38}H_{61}I_2N_3S_3$; mol wt 909.91. C 50.16%, H 6.76%, I 27.89%, N 4.62%, S 10.57%. Photosensitizing cyanine dye with antimicrobial and immunomodulating activities. General prepn and use in rheumatoid arthritis: I. Yamamoto, **BE 894635**; *idem*, **US 4464383** (1983, 1984). Antifungal properties: K. Ito, P. K. Kuroda, *Bull. Pharm. Res. Inst. Osaka Med. Coll.* **3**, 20 (1952), *C.A.* **47**, 11335f (1953). Effect on experimentally induced leukopenia: H. Iwata *et al.*, *Folia Pharmacol. Jpn.* **50**, 169 (1954), *C.A.* **49**, 10518b (1955). Immunomodulating effect in animals: H. Ichihashi, T. Kondo, *Gann* **58**, 529 (1967); Y. Oyanagui, *Arch. Int. Pharmacodyn. Ther.* **266**, 162 (1983). Enzyme immunoassay in plasma: I. Yamamoto, K. Morishita, *J. Immunoassay* **7**, 17 (1986). Toxicity study: T. Kimoto, K. Nishitani, *Kanko Shikiso* **85**, 43 (1977), *C.A.* **86**, 84374m (1977).

$2 I^-$

Brilliant green crystalline powder, mp 204°. Sol in water, alcohol. LD_{50} in male, female mice (mg/kg): 46.9, 50.5 i.p.; in male, female rats (mg/kg): 1539, 1571 orally (Kimoto, Nishitani).

THERAP CAT: Immunomodulator.

7531. Platyphylline. [480-78-4] (1α)-1,2-Dihydro-12-hydroxysenecionan-11,16-dione; platifillin. $C_{18}H_{27}NO_5$; mol wt 337.41. C 64.07%, H 8.07%, N 4.15%, O 23.71%. Toxic pyrrolizidine alkaloid from *Senecio platyphyllus* DC. and other *Senecio* spp., *Compositae*: Orékhov, Tiedebel, *Ber.* **68**, 650 (1935); Orékhov *et al.*, *ibid.* 1886; Konovalova, Orékhov, *ibid.* **69**, 1908 (1936); *Bull. Soc. Chim. Fr.* [5] **4**, 2037 (1937); Allen, *Am. J. Pharm.* **117**, 110 (1945). Structure: Dry *et al.*, *J. Chem. Soc.* **1955**, 63. Comprehensive reviews of platyphylline and other pyrrolizidine alkaloids: L. Bull *et al.*, *The Pyrrolizidine Alkaloids* (North-Holland, Amsterdam, 1968) 293 pp; F. L. Warren in *The Alkaloids* **vol. 12**, R. H. F. Manske, Ed. (Academic Press, New York, 1970) pp 245-331.

Crystals, mp 129°. [α]$_D^{20}$ −56.4° (c = 0.7 in chloroform). Practically insol in water. Sol in alcohol, chloroform, ether, dil acids.

Bitartrate. $C_{18}H_{27}NO_5 \cdot C_4H_6O_6$. Crystals, mp 199°. [α]$_D^{25}$ −40° (c = 2). Sol in 10 parts of water, in 5 parts of hot water. Sparingly sol in alc, in 42 parts of boiling alc. Nearly insol in chloroform, ether.

7532. Plaunotol. [64218-02-6] (2Z,6E)-2-[(3E)-4,8-Dimethyl-3,7-nonadienyl]-6-methyl-2,6-octadiene-1,8-diol; (E,Z,E)-7-hydroxymethyl-3,11,15-trimethyl-2,6,10,14-hexadecatetraen-1-ol; CS-684; Kelnac. $C_{20}H_{34}O_2$; mol wt 306.48. C 78.38%, H 11.18%, O 10.44%. Acyclic diterpene alcohol isolated from a Thai medicinal plant identified as *Croton sublyratus* Kurz, *Euphorbiaceae*. Isoln, synthesis and anti-ulcer activity: H. Mishima *et al.*, **JP Kokai 77 62213**; *idem*, **US 4059641** (both 1977 to Sankyo); A. Ogiso *et al.*, *Chem. Pharm. Bull.* **26**, 3117 (1978). Pharmacology: S. Kobayashi *et al.*, *Oyo Yakuri* **24**, 599 (1982).

Light yellow oil. Aromatic odor, bitter taste. Sol in benzene, acetone, alcohols, ethers. Insol in water. LD_{50} in male, female mice, rats (μl/kg): 8800, 8100, 10900, 11200 orally (Kobayashi).

THERAP CAT: Antiulcerative.

7533. Pleconaril. [153168-05-9] 3-[3,5-Dimethyl-4-[3-(3-methyl-5-isoxazolyl)propoxy]phenyl]-5-(trifluoromethyl)-1,2,4-oxadiazole; 5-[3-[2,6-dimethyl-4-[5-(trifluoromethyl)-1,2,4-oxadiazol-3-yl]phenoxy]propyl]-3-methylisoxazole; VP-63843; Win-63843. $C_{18}H_{18}F_3N_3O_3$; mol wt 381.35. C 56.69%, H 4.76%, F 14.95%, N 11.02%, O 12.59%. Picornavirus replication inhibitor. Prepn: G. D. Diana, T. J. Nitz, **EP 566199**; *eidem*, **US 5464848** (1993, 1995 both to Sterling Winthrop). Stability and HPLC determn of degradation products: A. B. C. Yu *et al.*, *Drug Dev. Ind. Pharm.* **21**, 1827 (1995). Activity spectrum vs enteroviruses: D. C. Pevear *et al.*, *Antimicrob. Agents Chemother.* **43**, 2109 (1999). Clinical pharmacokinetics in children: G. L. Kearns *et al.*, *ibid.* 634; in adults: S. M. Abdel-Rahman, G. L. Kearns, *J. Clin. Pharmacol.* **39**, 613 (1999). Clinical trial in induced respiratory infection: G. M. Schiff, J. R. Sherwood, *J. Infect. Dis.* **181**, 20 (2000).

White solid, mp 61-62°. Soly at 25° (ng/ml): water < 20. Sol in safflower seed oil, corn oil or corn oil-ethanol solutions.

THERAP CAT: Antiviral.

7534. Pleuromutilin. [125-65-5] Hydroxyacetic acid (3aS,-4R,5S,6S,8R,9R,9aR,10R)-6-ethenyldecahydro-5-hydroxy-4,6,9,10-tetramethyl-1-oxo-3a,9-propano-3aH-cyclopentacycloocten-8-yl ester; glycolic acid 8-ester with octahydro-5,8-dihydroxy-4,6,9,10-tetramethyl-6-vinyl-3a,9-propano-3aH-cyclopentacycloocten-1(4H)-one; drosophilin B; BC-757. $C_{22}H_{34}O_5$; mol wt 378.50. C 69.81%, H 9.05%, O 21.14%. Antibiotic substance produced by the basidiomycetes *Pleurotus mutilus* (Fr.) Sacc. and *P. passeckerianus* Pilat.: Kavanagh *et al.*, *Proc. Natl. Acad. Sci. USA* **37**, 570 (1951); **38**, 555 (1952). Isoln procedure: Anchel, *J. Biol. Chem.* **199**, 133 (1952). Structure: D. Arigoni, *Gazz. Chim. Ital.* **92**, 884 (1962); A. J. Birch *et al.*, *Chem. Ind. (London)* **1963**, 374; *Tetrahedron* **Suppl. 8**, 359 (1966). Stereochemistry: D. Arigoni, *Pure Appl. Chem.* **17**, 331 (1968). Fermentation and biosynthetic study: F. Knauseder, E. Brandl, *J. Antibiot.* **29**, 125 (1976). Mechanism of action: G. Hoegenauer, *Antibiotics* **vol. 5**, pt. 1, F. E. Hahn, Ed. (Springer-Verlag, New York, 1979) p 344. Synthetic studies: E. G. Gibbons, *J. Org. Chem.* **45**, 1540 (1980); M. Kahn, *Tetrahedron Lett.* **21**, 4547 (1980). Total synthesis: E. G. Gibbons, *J. Am. Chem. Soc.* **104**, 1767 (1982).

Crystals from ethyl acetate + Skellysolve B, mp 170-171°. $[\alpha]_D^{24}$ +20° (c = 3 in abs ethanol). uv max (5 mg/ml in 95% ethanol): 290 nm. Soluble in methanol, ethanol, ethyl acetate, chloroform. LD_{50} in mice: >60 mg/kg (Kavanagh, 1952).

Diacetate. $C_{26}H_{38}O_7$. Crystals from abs ethanol, mp 145.5°.

7535. Pleurotin(e). [1404-23-5] (2aα,4aβ,5β,6β,8aα,12bβ,-12cβ,12dβ)-(−)-2a,3,4,4a,5,6,7,8a,12b,12c-Decahydro-6-methyl-2H-5,12d-ethanofuro[4′,3′,2′:4,10]anthra[9,1-bc]oxepin-2,9,12-trione. $C_{21}H_{22}O_5$; mol wt 354.40. C 71.17%, H 6.26%, O 22.57%. Antibiotic substance produced by the fungus *Pleurotus griseus:* Robbins *et al., Bull. Torrey Bot. Club* **72**, 165 (1945). Isoln: Robbins *et al., Proc. Natl. Acad. Sci. USA* **33**, 171 (1947). Partial structure: Huls, *Publ. Univ. Congo Elisabethville* **4**, 109 (1962), *C.A.* 3894f (1965). Structure and stereochemistry: J. Grandjean, R. Huls, *Tetrahedron Lett.* **1974**, 1893. Synthesis of racemate: D. J. Hart, H.-C. Huang, *J. Am. Chem. Soc.* **110**, 1634 (1988).

Amber crystals from ether + chloroform, mp 200-215°. $[\alpha]_D^{23}$ −20° (chloroform). Neutral reaction. Sparingly sol in water which inactivates it. More stable at acid pH, but still loses ~50% of its activity when boiled for 10 min at pH 3. Aq solns also are inactivated on exposure to light. Moderately sol in alcohol, ether. Freely sol in chloroform.

7536. Plicamycin. [18378-89-7] Mithramycin; aureolic acid; mithracin; mitramycin; aurelic acid; antibiotic LA-7017. C_{52}-$H_{76}O_{24}$; mol wt 1085.15. C 57.55%, H 7.06%, O 35.39%. Oligosaccharide antibiotic produced by *Streptomyces argillaceus* n. sp. and *S. tanashiensis.* Isoln: Grundy *et al., Antibiot. Chemother.* **3**, 1215 (1953); Philip, Schenck, *ibid.* 1218; Rao *et al., ibid.* **12**, 182 (1962). Identity of aureolic acid with mithramycin: Berlin *et al., Nature* **218**, 193 (1968). Prepn: Gado *et al.,* **HU 155679** (1969 to Gyogyszerkutato Intezet), *C.A.* **70**, 118093f (1969). Similar to the chromomycins and olivomycins, *q.q.v.* Structural elucidation of the aglycone, **chromomycinone**, and the carbohydrate moieties: Bakhaeva *et al., Tetrahedron Lett.* **1968**, 3595; Berlin *et al., Khim. Prir. Soedin.* **1972**, 537, 542, *C.A.* **78**, 16436t, 16443t (1973). Revised structure: J. Thiem, B. Meyer, *Tetrahedron* **37**, 551 (1981). NMR and fluorometric characterization: N. R. Krishna *et al., J. Antibiot.* **43**, 1543 (1990). Metabolic studies: Kennedy *et al., Cancer Res.* **27**, 1534 (1967). Mode of action studies: Kushch *et al., Antibiotiki* **17**, 504 (1972). Toxicity study: M. Slavik, S. K. Carter, *Adv. Pharmacol. Chemother.* **12**, 1 (1975). *Review:* J. D. Skarbek, M. K. Speedie in *Antitumor Compounds of Natural Origin* **vol. 1**, A. Aszalos, Ed. (CRC Press, Boca Raton, 1981) pp 191-235.

Yellow solid, mp 180-183°. $[\alpha]_D^{20}$ −51° (c = 0.4 in ethanol). Sol in lower alcohols, acetone, ethyl acetate, water. Moderately sol in chloroform. Slightly sol in ether, benzene. LD_{50} in mice, rats (mg/kg): 2.14, 1.74 i.v. (Slavik, Carter).

THERAP CAT: Antineoplastic.

7537. Plicatic Acid. [16462-65-0] (1S,2S,3R)-1-(3,4-Dihydroxy-5-methoxyphenyl)-1,2,3,4-tetrahydro-2,3,7-trihydroxy-3-(hydroxymethyl)-6-methoxy-2-naphthalenecarboxylic acid. C_{20}-$H_{22}O_{10}$; mol wt 422.38. C 56.87%, H 5.25%, O 37.88%. Coloring constituent and agent associated with western red cedar asthma. Low-molecular weight lignan which occurs as the (-)-form. Isolation from the heartwood of western red cedar, *Thuja plicata* Donn: J. A. F. Gardner *et al., Can. J. Chem.* **37**, 1703 (1959). Structure determn: *idem et al., ibid.* **44**, 52 (1966). Absolute configuration: R. J. Swan *et al., ibid.* **45**, 319 (1967). Chromatographic analysis: B. F. MacDonald, E. P. Swan, *J. Chromatogr.* **51**, 553 (1970). Identification as coloring material: Y. Kai, E. P. Swan, *Mokuzai Gakkaishi* **36**, 218 (1990). Role in asthma: M. Chan-Yeung *et al., Am. Rev. Respir. Dis.* **108**, 1094 (1973); *eidem, J. Allergy Clin. Immunol.* **79**, 792 (1987). Mechanism of action study: M. Chan-Yeung, *Am. J. Ind. Med.* **25**, 13 (1994).

Light tan powder. $[\alpha]_D^{21}$ −9.99° (water). uv max (water): 281 nm (log ε 3.58). pKa: 3.0. Very sol in water; sol in absolute acetone and ethanol; very slightly sol in ethyl acetate and ether.

7538. Plumbagin. [481-42-5] 5-Hydroxy-2-methyl-1,4-naphthalenedione; 5-hydroxy-2-methyl-1,4-naphthoquinone. C_{11}-H_8O_3; mol wt 188.18. C 70.21%, H 4.29%, O 25.51%. Found in the roots of *Plumbago europaea* L., *P. zeylanica, P. rosea* L., *Plumbaginaceae.* Isoln: Dulong d'Astafort, *J. Pharm. Chim.* **14**, 441 (1828); Wefers-Bettink, *Rec. Trav. Chim.* **8**, 319 (1889); Ray, Dutt, *J. Indian Chem. Soc.* **5**, 419 (1928). Structure and synthesis: Fieser, Dunn, *J. Am. Chem. Soc.* **58**, 572 (1936). Biosynthesis: Durand, Zenk, *Tetrahedron Lett.* **1971**, 3009. Chemotherapeutic properties: Vichkanova *et al., C.A.* **78**, 66906s (1973). Efficient syntheses: A. Ichihara, *Agric. Biol. Chem.* **44**, 211 (1980); G. Wurm *et al., Arch. Pharm.* **314**, 861, 1055 (1981); H. Möhrle, H. Foltmann, *ibid.* **321**, 259 (1988). Toxicity data: M. Debray *et al., Plant Med. Phytother.* **7**, 77 (1973), *C.A.* **79**, 14255e (1973).

Yellow needles from dil alcohol, mp 78-79°. Sublimes. Volatile with steam. Slightly sol in hot water; sol in alc, acetone, chloroform, benzene, acetic acid. LD_{50} i.p. in mice: ~0.015 g/kg (Debray).

7539. Plumericin. [77-16-7] (3E,3aS,4aR,7aS,9aS,9bS)-3-Ethylidene-3,3a,7a,9b-tetrahydro-2-oxo-2H,4aH-1,4,5-trioxadicyclopent[a,hi]indene-7-carboxylic acid methyl ester. $C_{15}H_{14}O_6$; mol wt 290.27. C 62.07%, H 4.86%, O 33.07%. A sesquiterpenoid, exhibiting *in vitro* activity against fungi, some bacteria including *Mycobacterium tuberculosis* 607. Isoln from roots of *Plumeria multiflora* Muell.-Arg., *Apocynaceae,* also from roots of *P. rubra* var. *alba:* J. E. Little, D. B. Johnstone, *Arch. Biochem.* **30**, 445 (1951); from *Allamanda cathartica* Linn., *Apocynaceae:* B. R. Pai *et al., Indian J. Chem.* **8**, 851 (1970). Structure, physical properties and IR, ¹HNMR spectra: G. Albers-Schönberg, H. Schmid, *Helv. Chim. Acta* **44**, 1447 (1961). Synthetic approach: J. K. Whitesell *et al., Synth. Commun.* **7**, 355 (1977). Biomimetic total synthesis of (±)-form: B. M. Trost *et al., J. Am. Chem. Soc.* **105**, 6755 (1983); *eidem, ibid.* **108**, 4974 (1986). Alternate synthesis of (±)-form: *eidem, ibid.* 4965; K. E. B. Parkes, G. Pattenden, *J. Chem. Soc. Perkin Trans. 1* **1988**, 1119.

Narrow, rectangular plates from alc, toluene or methylene chloride + ether, dec 211.5-212.5°. Sublimes in high vacuum at 160-180°. $[\alpha]_D^{25}$ +197.5 ±2° (c = 0.982 in chloroform). uv max (ethanol): 214-215 nm (log ε 4.24). Sol in chloroform; slightly sol in methanol, alc, ether, acetone, benzene. Practically insol in petr ether, water.

7540. Plumieride. [511-89-7] (1*S*,2'*R*,4a*S*,7a*S*)-1-(β-D-Glucopyranosyloxy)-4a,7a-dihydro-4'-[(1*S*)-1-hydroxyethyl]-5'-oxospiro[cyclopenta[*c*]pyran-7(1*H*),2'(5'*H*)-furan]-4-carboxylic acid methyl ester; agoniadin. $C_{21}H_{26}O_{12}$; mol wt 470.42. C 53.62%, H 5.57%, O 40.81%. Found in bark of *Plumeria lancifolia* Muell.-Arg., *Apocynaceae,* also in *P. acutifolia* and *P. rubra* var. *alba:* Peckolt, *Arch. Pharm.* [2] **142**, 40 (1870); *E. Merck's Jahresber.* **1895**, 11; Boorsma, *Mededeel. Lands Plant.* **13**, 27 (1894); **31**, 132 (1899); Franchimont, *Rec. Trav. Chim.* **18**, 334, 477 (1899); **19**, 350 (1900); Halpern, Schmid, *Helv. Chim. Acta* **41**, 1109 (1958). Structure: Albers-Schönberg, Schmid, *ibid.* **44**, 1447 (1961). Biosynthesis: D. A. Yeowell, H. Schmid, *Experientia* **20**, 250 (1964); K. Inoue *et al., Chem. Pharm. Bull.* **27**, 3115 (1979).

Monohydrate, bitter crystals, mp 156-158°. When anhydrous, mp 224-225°. $[\alpha]_D^{20}$ −114°; $[\alpha]_D^{20}$ −80° (methanol). Broad uv absorption: 217-238 nm. Sol in water, alcohol, ethyl acetate.

7541. Plutonium. [7440-07-5] Pu; at. no. 94; valences 3, 4, 5, 6, 7. No stable nuclides, known isotopes (mass numbers): 232-246. Longest-lived known isotopes: ^{242}Pu ($T_{1/2}$ 3.76 × 10^5 years, α-emitter, rel. at. mass 242.0587), 244 ($T_{1/2}$ 8.26 × 10^7 years, α-emitter, rel. at. mass 244.0642). Commercially useful isotopes: ^{238}Pu ($T_{1/2}$ 87.74 years; α-emitter, rel. at. mass 238.0496); ^{239}Pu ($T_{1/2}$ 2.41 × 10^4 years; α-emitter, rel. at. mass 239.0522). Occurrence in the earth's crust: 10^{-22}%. Discovery of isotope ^{238}Pu: G. T. Seaborg *et al., Phys. Rev.* **69**, 366, 367 (1946); of isotope ^{239}Pu: J. W. Kennedy *et al., ibid.* **70**, 555 (1946). Isoln of ^{239}Pu from pitchblende: G. T. Seaborg, M. L. Perlman, *J. Am. Chem. Soc.* **70**, 1571 (1948). Prepn of metal: B. B. Cunningham, L. B. Werner, *ibid.* **71**, 1521 (1949). Chemical properties: Seaborg, Wahl, *ibid.* 1128; Harvey *et al., J. Chem. Soc.* **1947**, 1010. *Reviews:* J. M. Cleveland, *The Chemistry of Plutonium* (Gordon & Breach, New York, 1970) 653 pp; C. Keller, *The Chemistry of the Transuranium Elements* (Verlag Chemie, Weinheim, English Ed., 1971) pp 333-484; *Comprehensive Inorganic Chemistry* vol. 5, J. C. Bailar, Jr. *et al.,* Eds. (Pergamon Press, Oxford, 1973) *passim; Handb. Exp. Pharmakol.* **36**, 307-688 (1973); F. Weigel in *Kirk-Othmer Encyclopedia of Chemical Technology* vol. 18 (Wiley-Interscience, New York, 3rd ed., 1982) pp 278-301; *Plutonium Chemistry,* W. T. Car-

nall, G. R. Choppin, Eds. (Am. Chem. Soc., Washington, D.C., 1983) 484 pp; F. Weigel *et al.* in *The Chemistry of the Actinide Elements* vol. 1, J. J. Katz *et al.,* Eds. (Chapman and Hall, New York, 1986) pp 499-886. Review of toxicology: W. J. Bair, R. C. Thompson, *Science* **183**, 715-722 (1974); and health effects: *Toxicological Profile for Plutonium* (PB91-180406, 1990) 206 pp.

Silvery-white metal. Highly reactive. Oxidizes readily in dry air and oxygen, rate increases in presence of moisture. Six allotropic forms: simple monoclinic α-form, d^{21} 19.86, transforms to β-form at 122 ±4°; body-centered monoclinic β-form, d^{190} 17.70, transforms to γ-form at 207 ±5°; face-centered orthorhombic γ-form, d^{235} 17.14, transforms to δ-form at 315 ±3°; face-centered cubic δ-form, d^{320} 15.92, transforms to δ'-form at 457 ±2°; body-centered tetragonal δ'-form, d^{405} 16.00, transforms to ε-form at 479 ±4°; body-centered cubic ε-form, d^{490} 16.51, transforms to liquid at mp 640 ±2°.

Trivalent plutonium. Weak reducing agent. Stable in soln in absence of air. Slowly oxidized to the tetravalent plutonium by atmospheric oxygen, by permanganate in acid soln in the cold; oxidized to the hexavalent form by permanganate at 60°. Trivalent salts are blue; form complexes very readily; form a series of double sulfates. Crystal structure of the complex and double salts: Zachariasen, *J. Am. Chem. Soc.* **70**, 2147 (1948).

Tetravalent plutonium. Reduced in aq soln to the trivalent form by sulfur dioxide, hydroxylamine hydrochloride, hydrazine hydrochloride, the uranous ion, the iodide ion; by shaking with mercury in chloride soln; electrolytically at a platinum cathode. Tetravalent salts are pink or greenish; form complexes very readily.

Hexavalent plutonium. Obtained by the action of strong oxidizing agents (ceric salts, dichromates, permanganates, or hot bromate soln containing nitric acid) on the tri- or tetravalent form. Reduced to tri- or tetravalent plutonium by sulfur dioxide or ferrocyanide.

Caution: Radiation hazard; handling requires special equipment and shielding facilities. Animal studies have indicated that inhaled ^{239}Pu as particulate matter may remain in the lungs, or move to the bones, liver or other body organs, and over a period of time may give rise to neoplasms due to its α-emitting radioactive decay. *See* Katz *et al., loc. cit.* vol. 2, p. 1128, 1182-1188. Max permissible concn of ^{238}Pu in air: 7 × 10^{-13} μCurie/cc; of ^{239}Pu in air: 6 × 10^{-13} μCurie/cc: *Natl. Bur. Stand. Handb.* **69**, 87 (1959). *See also Handb. Exp. Pharmakol. loc. cit.*

USE: ^{238}Pu as heat source; as radioisotope thermoelectric generator; in radionuclide batteries for pacemakers. ^{239}Pu as fuel in atomic weapons and nuclear power reactors.

7542. PMSF. [329-98-6] Benzenemethanesulfonyl fluoride; phenylmethanesulfonyl fluoride; α-toluenesulfonyl fluoride. $C_7H_7FO_2S$; mol wt 174.19. C 48.27%, H 4.05%, F 10.91%, O 18.37%, S 18.41%. Serine and cysteine protease inhibitor. Prepn: W. Davies, J. H. Dick, *J. Chem. Soc.* **1932**, 483; and protease inhibition study: D. E. Fahrney, A. M. Gold, *J. Am. Chem. Soc.* **85**, 997 (1963). Stability studies: G. T. James, *Anal. Biochem.* **86**, 574 (1978). Analgesic effects and toxicity in rodents: C. Pinsky *et al., Life Sci.* **31**, 1193 (1982). Neuropathologic effects in organophosphorus ester-induced delayed neuropathy in hens: C. Massicotte *et al., Neurotoxicology* **20**, 749 (1999).

Colorless needles from light petroleum, mp 90-91°. LD$_{50}$ (24 hr) in mice (mg/kg): 215 ±55 i.p. (Pinsky).

USE: Standard protease inhibitor in biological research; in protein purification to prevent proteolytic degradation.

7543. Podocarpic Acid. [5947-49-9] [1*S*-(1α,4aα,10aβ)]-1,2,3,4,4a,9,10,10a-Octahydro-6-hydroxy-1,4a-dimethyl-1-phenanthrenecarboxylic acid; 12-hydroxypodocarpa-8,11,13-trien-16-oic acid. $C_{17}H_{22}O_3$; mol wt 274.35. C 74.42%, H 8.08%, O 17.50%. Chief acidic constituent of the resin of the Javanese *Podocarpus cupressina* (L'Hérit.) Pers., *Coniferae,* esp. in var. *imbricata.* Also in New Zealand kahikatea resin (from *Podocarpus dacrydioides*) and in rimu resin *(Dacrydium cupressinum).* A related component, nimbiol, *q.v.,* occurs in the nim tree, *Azadirachta indica* Juss. *(Melia azadirachta* L.), *Meliaceae.* Isoln from *Podo-*

carpus cupressina: A. C. Oudemans, *Ber.* **6**, 1122 (1873); from *Dacrydium cupressinum:* I. R. Sherwood, W. F. Short, *J. Chem. Soc.* **1938**, 1008. Structure: Campbell, Todd, *J. Am. Chem. Soc.* **64**, 928 (1942). Conversion to nimbiol as proof of structure: Bible, *Tetrahedron* **11**, 22 (1960). Synthesis from desoxypodocarpic acid: Wenkert, Jackson, *J. Am. Chem. Soc.* **80**, 217 (1958). Total synthesis of *dl*-form: Meyer, Maheshwari, *Tetrahedron Lett.* **1964**, 2175; P. R. Kanjilal *et al., Synth. Commun.* **11**, 795 (1981). Synthesis: Pelletier *et al., Tetrahedron Lett.* **1971**, 4179.

Platelets from dil alcohol, mp 193.5°. $[\alpha]_{546}^{20}$ +165° (c = 4 in abs ethanol). Sol in methanol, ethanol, ether, acetic acid. Practically insol in water, chloroform, benzene, carbon disulfide.

Methyl ester. $C_{18}H_{24}O_3$. Crystals from alcohol, mp 208°.

7544. Pododacric Acid. [32630-75-4] [1S-(1α,4aα,10aβ)]-1,2,3,4,4a,9,10,10a-Octahydro-6-hydroxy-7-[2-hydroxy-1-(hydroxymethyl)ethyl]-1,4a-dimethyl-1-phenanthrenecarboxylic acid; 12-hydroxy-13-[2-hydroxy-1-(hydroxymethyl)ethyl]podocarpa-8,11,13-trien-16-oic acid. $C_{20}H_{28}O_5$; mol wt 348.43. C 68.94%, H 8.10%, O 22.96%. From heartwood of *Podocarpus dacrydioides; P. totara:* Briggs *et al., Tetrahedron* **7**, 270 (1959); Cambie, Mander, *ibid.* **18**, 465 (1962). Structure: Cambie, Mathai, *Chem. Commun.* **1971**, 154.

Colorless needles from 30% methanol, mp 213-214°. $[\alpha]_D^{25}$ +118° (c = 0.9 in 5:1 chloroform-methanol). uv max: 225, 284 nm (ε 5500, 3100). pK 8.44 (in methyl cellosolve system).

7545. Podophyllic Acids. $C_{22}H_{24}O_9$; mol wt 432.42. C 61.11%, H 5.59%, O 33.30%. Since the prepn of a "podophyllic acid", mp 145-150° (crude), 163-165° (pure), by Borsche, Niemann, *Ann.* **494**, 126 (1932), studies have been made of two isomers: the 2,3-*trans*-hydroxy acid and the 2,3-*cis*-hydroxy acid. Prepn of the *trans*-acid: Kuhn, Wartburg, *Experientia* **19**, 391 (1963); NL **6405480** (1964 to Sandoz), *C.A.* **62**, 9083c (1965); and *cis*-acid: Renz *et al., Ann.* **681**, 207 (1965). Prepn of a DL-stereoisomer: Gensler *et al., J. Am. Chem. Soc.* **76**, 315 (1954). Configuration and nomenclature: Rutschmann, Renz, *Helv. Chim. Acta* **42**, 890 (1959).

Podophyllinic Acid

2,3-*trans*-Hydroxy acid. [1853-37-8] Podophyllinic acid. Crystals from acetone + ether, mp 164-168°. $[\alpha]_D^{20}$ −199.9° (c = 0.463 in ethanol), −292.6° (c = 0.671 in pyridine).

2,3-*cis*-Hydroxy acid. [477-67-8] Picropodophyllic acid. Needles from methanol + ether, double mp 150-155° and 200-232°. $[\alpha]_D^{21}$ −100.4° (c = 0.615 in ethanol), −185° (c = 0.746 in pyridine).

2,3-*trans*-Hydroxy acid hydrazide. [78178-41-3] Podophyllinic acid hydrazide. Prepn and properties: Rutschmann, US **2977359** (1961 to Sandoz). Prisms from methanol, mp 198-199°. $[\alpha]_D$ −202° (c = 0.4 in ethanol).

***trans*-2-Ethylhydrazide.** [1508-45-8] Podophyllinic acid 2-ethylhydrazide; SP-I. Prepn: Rutschmann, US **3054802** (1962 to Sandoz). Amorphous powder, pptd from chloroform + petr ether. $[\alpha]_D$ −154° (c = 0.5 in chloroform).

7546. Podophyllotoxin. [518-28-5] (5R,5aR,8aR,9R)-5,8,-8a,9-Tetrahydro-9-hydroxy-5-(3,4,5-trimethoxyphenyl)furo[3′,-4′:6,7]naphtho[2,3-d]-1,3-dioxol-6(5aH)-one; 1-hydroxy-2-hydroxymethyl-6,7-methylenedioxy-4-(3′,4′,5′-trimethoxyphenyl)-1,2,-3,4-tetrahydronaphthalene-3-carboxylic acid lactone; podophyllinic acid lactone; podofilox; Condyline; Condylox; Wartec; Warticon. $C_{22}H_{22}O_8$; mol wt 414.41. C 63.76%, H 5.35%, O 30.89%. Precursor of antineoplastics etoposide, teniposide, q.q.v. Found in the rhizomes of North American *Podophyllum peltatum* L., *Podophyllaceae:* V. Podwyssotski, *Arch. Exp. Pathol. Pharmakol.* **13**, 29 (1880); also in *P. emodi* Wall.: von Wartburg *et al., Helv. Chim. Acta* **40**, 1331 (1957); in *Juniperus virginiana* L., *Cupressaceae:* Kupchan *et al., J. Pharm. Sci.* **54**, 659 (1965). Structure and absolute configuration: Schrecker, Hartwell, *J. Org. Chem.* **21**, 381 (1956). Crystal structure: T. J. Petcher *et al., J. Chem. Soc. Perkin Trans. 2* **1973**, 288. Synthesis: Gensler, Gatsonis, *J. Am. Chem. Soc.* **84**, 1748 (1962); T. Kaneko, H. Wong, *Tetrahedron Lett.* **28**, 517 (1987). Asymmetric total synthesis: R. C. Andrews *et al., J. Am. Chem. Soc.* **110**, 7854 (1988); E. J. Bush, D. W. Jones, *Chem. Commun.* **1993**, 1200. Toxicity data: F. S. Phillips *et al., Fed. Proc.* **7**, 249 (1948). ELISA determn in plants: K.-J. Yoo, J. R. Porter, *J. Nat. Prod.* **56**, 715 (1993). Clinical evaluation for treatment of genital warts: A. Lassus, *Lancet* **2**, 513 (1987); K. R. Beutner *et al., ibid.* **1**, 831 (1989). Review of early literature: Hartwell, Schrecker in *Fortschr. Chem. Org. Naturst.* **15**, 98-121 (1958). Review of chemistry and antineoplastic activity: I. Jardine, *Anticancer Agents Based on Natural Product Models,* J. M. Cassady, J. D. Douros, Eds. (Academic Press, New York, 1980) pp 319-351. Review of syntheses: R. S. Ward, *Synthesis* **1992**, 719-730. Review: D. L. Sackett, *Pharmacol. Ther.* **59**, 163-228 (1993).

Solvated crystals. mp 114-118° (effervescence). Several polymorphic modifications. After drying: mp 183.3-184.0°. $[\alpha]_D^{20}$ −132.7° (chloroform). Soly in water at 23°: 120 mg/l. Sol in alcohol, chloroform, acetone, warm benzene, glacial acetic acid. LD_{50} in rats (mg/kg): 8.7 i.v.; 15 i.p. (Phillips).

Podophyllotoxin-β-D-glucoside. $C_{28}H_{32}O_{13}$. Hygroscopic amorphous white flakes, mp 152-154°. $[\alpha]_D^{20}$ −76.4° (c = 0.576 in methanol); $[\alpha]_D^{20}$ −117.0° (c = 0.668 in pyridine).

Picropodophyllin. [477-47-4] Picropodophyllinic acid lactone. $C_{22}H_{22}O_8$; mol wt 414.41. C 63.76%, H 5.35%, O 30.89%. Found in resin podophyllum, a dried alcoholic extract of *Podophyllum peltatum* L., *Berberidaceae* but not in the fresh plant. 5aS-Isomer of podophyllotoxin. Isoln from resin podophyllum: Späth *et al., Ber.* **65**, 1545 (1932). Structure: Schrecker, Hartwell, *J. Am. Chem. Soc.* **76**, 752 (1954). Synthesis: Gensler, Wang, *J. Am. Chem. Soc.* **76**, 5890 (1954); Gensler *et al., ibid.* **82**, 1714 (1960). Crystals from acetone. Irritates the skin. mp 214°. Higher-melting modification from abs ethanol, mp 228°. $[\alpha]_D^{20}$ +9.4° (c = 0.7 in chloroform). Soly in water at 25° ~100 mg/l. Fairly sol in chloroform, hot ethanol, acetic acid, acetone, dil caustic; less sol in benzene, ether, carbon tetrachloride, propylene glycol. Practically insol in petr ether.

THERAP CAT: Antiviral (topical).

7547. Podophyllum. Genus of perennial flowering plants of the family *Podophyllaceae*, formerly, *Berberidaceae*; represented in traditional medicine by two species: *Podophyllum peltatum* L., known as American podophyllum, and *P. hexandrum* R., syn. *P. emodi* Wall., known as Indian podophyllum. Medicinal portions are the dried rhizome and the resin extracted from it. Has been used as a cathartic, emetic and cholagogue and externally as a caustic. Constituents are similar in both species, but vary in concentration. The antimitotic lignin, podophyllotoxin, *q.v.*, is the principal active component. History, isoln procedures, structures: J. L. Hartwell, A. W. Schrecker, *Fortschr. Chem. Org. Naturst.* **15**, 83-166 (1958); and review of medicinal uses: J. Singh, N. C. Shah, *Curr. Res. Med. Aromat. Plants* **16**, 53-83 (1994). HPLC determn of constituents in plant extracts: J. K. Bastos *et al., Phytochem. Anal.* **6**, 101 (1995). Production of cytotoxic lignins by cell culture: M. Petersen, A. W. Alfermann, *Appl. Microbiol. Biotechnol.* **55**, 135 (2001).

American podophyllum. Mayapple; American mandrake; Indian apple; vegetable calomel. *Habit.* North America. *Constit.* Chiefly podophyllotoxin (0.25-1.0%), *α*- and *β*-peltatins, quercetin, kaempferol.

Indian podophyllum. Papra; ban-kakari. *Habit.* Himalayas, east Asia. *Constit.* Chiefly podophyllotoxin (1.0-4.0%), 4'-demethylpodophyllotoxin, podophyllotoxone, quercetin, kaempferol.

Podophyllin. [9000-55-9] Podophyllum resin. Dried ethanolic extract obtained from the dried rhizomes and roots. Description, pharmacology and comparison with podophyllotoxin in treatment of anogenital warts: E. Longstaff, G. von Krogh, *Regul. Toxicol. Pharmacol.* **33**, 117-137 (2001). Light brown to greenish-yellow powder, darkens on exposure to light. *Irritating to skin and mucous membranes.*

THERAP CAT: Caustic.

7548. Poi. The root of the taro plant, *Colocasia esculenta* (L.) Schott, *Araceae*. Used as a cereal substitute, particularly in allergy cases and potentially allergic infants.

THERAP CAT: Nutrient.

7549. Poison Ivy. Poison vine; markweed. *Toxicodendron radicans* (L.) Kuntze, *Anacardiaceae*. Erroneously called poison oak. Vigorous woody vine, shrub, or subshrub with trifoliate, alternate leaves. *Habit.* All states of the United States east of the Cascade Mountains, the Great Basin, and the Mojave Desert (absent in Nevada); all states of Mexico except in the Yucatan Peninsula and northern Baja California. Its southern limit is Huehuetenango Department of Guatemala and its northern limit is the 52nd parallel of latitude. It is found in Bermuda and several islands in the Bahamas, in Japan, and in the middle elevations in the mountains of Taiwan and of central and western China. *Review:* Gillis in J. M. Kingsbury, *Poisonous Plants of the United States and Canada* (Prentice-Hall, Englewood Cliffs, N. J., 1964) pp 209-214. *Constit.* Toxic constituent: urushiol, *q.v.:* Dawson, *Trans. N.Y. Acad. Sci.* **18**, 427 (1956).

Caution: Can cause severe allergic dermatitis.

THERAP CAT: Extract as antiallergic (hyposensitization therapy).

7550. Poison Oak. Western poison oak. *Toxicodendron diversilobum* (T. & G.) Greene, *Anacardiaceae*. Similar to poison ivy in that it has three leaflets, grows as a shrub or vine and produces dermatitis in man. Interbreeds with poison ivy. *Habit.* Western North America from southern British Columbia to northern Baja California. *Constit.* Poisons presumably closely related if not identical to those in poison ivy.

Eastern poison oak. *Toxicodendron quercifolium* (Michx.) Greene, *Anacardiaceae*. Differs significantly from poison ivy. Never climbs or produces aerial roots and rarely hybridizes with poison ivy. *Habit.* Southern New Jersey to Florida, west to eastern Texas and Kansas. *Constit.* Poisons may be the same as in poison ivy or Western poison oak.

Extract of *T. quercifolium.* Anergex.

Caution: Direct contact can cause severe allergic dermatitis. *See* M.J. Ellenhorn, D.G. Barceloux, *Medical Toxicology: Diagnosis and Treatment of Human Poisoning* (Elsevier, New York, 1988) pp 1301-1306.

THERAP CAT: Extract as antiallergic (hyposensitization therapy).

7551. Poison Sumac. Poison elder. *Toxicodendron vernix* (L.) Kuntze, *Anacardiaceae*. Tall, rangy shrub with leaves com-

pounded with seven to eleven leaflets. Rachis is bright red and leaflets have no teeth on their margins, thus differing from non-poisonous sumacs. *Habit.* Southern Quebec to central Florida predominantly east of Mississippi River. Found only in bogs, swamps and wet bottom lands.

Caution: Can cause severe allergic dermatitis.

THERAP CAT: Extract as antiallergic (hyposensitization therapy).

7552. Polaprezinc. [107667-60-7] [*N*-*β*-Alanyl-L-histidinato(2−)-*N,N^N,O^α*]zinc; *catena-(S)*-[*μ*-[*N^α*-(3-aminopropionyl)-L-histidinato(2−)-*N^1,N^2,O:N^τ*]zinc]; zinc L-carnosine; *β*-alanyl-L-histidinato zinc; *N*-(3-aminopropionyl)-L-histidinato zinc; Z-103; Promac. Polymeric zinc(II) complex with L-carnosine, corresponding to the formula, $(C_9H_{12}N_4O_3Zn)_n$. Exhibits antioxidant and gastroprotective properties. Prepn of crystalline complex: T. Matsukura *et al.,* **EP 303380**; *eidem,* **US 4981846** (1989, 1991 both to Hamari). Prepn and structure elucidation: T. Matsukura *et al., Chem. Pharm. Bull.* **38**, 3140 (1990). Pharmacology: T. Arakawa *et al., Dig. Dis. Sci.* **35**, 559 (1990). Mechanism of action study: T. Yoshikawa *et al., Biochim. Biophys. Acta* **1115**, 15 (1991). Series of articles on metabolism: *Arzneim.-Forsch.* **41**, 965-995 (1991); on toxicology: *ibid.* 1033-1057. Acute toxicity: K. Matsuda *et al., ibid.* 1033.

White or pale yellow crystalline powder. Insol in water and common organic solvents. LD_{50} in male, female mice, rats (mg/kg): 220, 165, 405, 422 i.p.; 758, 874, >5000, >5000 s.c.; 1269, 1331, 8441, 7375 orally (Matsuda).

THERAP CAT: Antiulcerative.

7553. Polar® Yellow. [6372-96-9] 5-Chloro-2-[4,5-dihydro-3-methyl-4-[[4-[[(4-methylphenyl)sulfonyl]oxy]phenyl]azo]-5-oxo-1*H*-pyrazol-1-yl]benzenesulfonic acid monosodium salt; 4-*p*-hydroxybenzeneazo-1-*p*-chloro-*o*-sulfophenyl-3-methyl-5-hydroxypyrazole toluene-*p*-sulfonyl ester sodium salt; C.I. Acid Yellow 40; C.I. 18950. $C_{23}H_{18}ClN_4O_7S_2$; mol wt 584.98. C 47.22%, H 3.10%, Cl 6.06%, N 9.58%, Na 3.93%, O 19.15%, S 10.96%. Prepn from diazotized *p*-aminophenol and 1-(*o*-sulfo-*p*-chlorophenyl)-3-methyl-5-pyrazolone: B. Richard, **US 1067881** (Geigy). *See also: Colour Index* **vol. 4** (3rd ed., 1971) p 4128.

Yellowish-brown powder. Sol in water giving a pure yellow soln; in alcohol (yellow color); in alkalies; in concd sulfuric acid. Slightly sol in ethanol, acetone. Insol in other org solvents. Precipitated by dil acids.

USE: To dye wool. In the isoln of polymyxin.

7554. Poldine Methylsulfate. [545-80-2] 2-[[(Hydroxydiphenylacetyl)oxy]methyl]-1,1-dimethylpyrrolidinium methyl sulfate (salt); 2-hydroxymethyl-1,1-dimethylpyrrolidinium methyl sulfate benzilate; 2-benziloyloxymethyl-1,1-dimethylpyrrolidinium methyl sulfate; (1-methyl-2-pyrrolidinyl)methyl benzilate methylmethosulfate; IS-499; McN-R-726-47; Nacton; Nactate. $C_{22}H_{29}$-NO_7S; mol wt 451.53. C 58.52%, H 6.47%, N 3.10%, O 24.80%, S 7.10%. Anticholinergic. Prepn: Doyle *et al., J. Chem. Soc.* **1958**, 4458. Prepn of the base: Blicke, Lu, *J. Am. Chem. Soc.* **79**, 29 (1955).

Needles from methyl ethyl ketone + ethanol + ether, mp 154-155°. Soluble in water.

THERAP CAT: Antispasmodic.

7555. Policosanol. [142583-61-7] Sugar cane wax alcohols; Ateromixol; Lipex; Mercol; Phytocor; PPG. Mixture of higher (C_{24} to C_{34}) primary aliphatic alcohols purified from wax of sugar cane, *Saccharum officinarum* L., *Gramineae*. Composed of octacosanol (60-70%), triacontanol (10-15%), dotriacontanol (5-10%), hexacosanol (3-8%), heptacosanol, nonacosanol, tetratriacontanol, and tetracosanol. Prepn: L. Granja *et al.*, **WO 9407830**; *eidem*, **US 5856316** (1994, 1999 both to Dalmar). Clinical pharmacology: I. Gouni-Berthold, H. K. Berthold, *Am. Heart J.* **143**, 356 (2002). Antiplatelet effects: M. L. Arruzazabala *et al.*, *Clin. Exp. Pharmacol. Physiol.* **29**, 891 (2002). Review of clinical studies: M. Janikula, *Altern. Med. Rev.* **7**, 203-217 (2002); and comparison with plant sterols and stanols: J. T. Chen *et al.*, *Pharmacotherapy* **25**, 171-183 (2005).

Off-white, odorless crystalline powder. mp 78-82°. Insol in water, hexane, methanol, ethanol. Slightly sol in chloroform.

THERAP CAT: Antilipemic.

7556. Policresulen. [9011-02-3] Hydroxymethylbenzenesulfonic acid polymer with formaldehyde; methylenebis(hydroxytoluenesulfonic acid) polymer; dihydroxydimethyldiphenylmethanedisulfonic acid polymer; Albocresil; Albothyl; Negatol. Condensation product prepd by reacting *m*-cresolsulfonic acid and formaldehyde, e.g. the product obtained by Thuau, *CA* **417272** (1943 to Lilly), *C.A.* **38**, 1077 (1944).

Sol in water, forming colloidal solns.

THERAP CAT: Antiseptic.

THERAP CAT (VET): Antiseptic.

7557. Polidexide. [9064-92-0] Sephadex 2-(diethylamino)-ethyl ether; dextran 2-(diethylamino)ethyl 2-[[2-(diethylamino)ethyl]diethylammonio]ethyl ether chloride hydrochloride epichlorohydrin crosslinked; poly[2-(diethylamino)ethyl] polyglycerylene dextran hydrochloride; PDX chloride; Secholex; DEAE-Sephadex. Anion exchange resin containing quaternary ammonium groups. Bile acid sequestrant that has been used to reduce serum cholesterol. Prepn: **GB 1013585** (1965 to Pharmacia AB). Clinical evaluation in hyperlipidemia: R. J. C. Evans *et al.*, *Angiology* **24**, 22 (1973); S. Ritland *et al.*, *Scand. J. Gastroenterol.* **10**, 791 (1975). Review of use in chromatographic purification of proteins: D. M. Bollag, *Methods Mol. Biol.* **36**, 11-22 (1994).

Tasteless powder; forms gel in water.

USE: Ion exchange resin.

THERAP CAT: Antilipemic.

7558. Polidocanol. [9002-92-0] α-Dodecyl-ω-hydroxypoly(oxy-1,2-ethanediyl); polyethylene glycol (9) monododecyl

ether; dodecyl alcohol polyoxyethylene ether; hydroxypolyethoxydodecane; laureth 9; polyoxyethylene lauryl ether; Aethoxysklerol; Aetoxisclerol; Atlas G-4829; Hetoxol L-9. $C_{12}H_{25}(OCH_2CH_2)_n$-OH. Contains an average of nine ethylene oxide units and has an average mol wt ~600. Prepd by reaction of ethylene oxide and dodecyl alcohol: Pertsemlides, Soehring, *Arzneim.-Forsch.* **10**, 990 (1960). Toxicology: H. S. Zipf *et al.*, *ibid.* **7**, 162 (1957). Review of clinical experience: P. M. Goldman, *J. Dermatol. Surg. Oncol.* **15**, 204-209 (1989).

Sol in water, ethanol, toluene. Miscible with hot mineral, natural and synthetic oils; with fats and fatty alcohols. LD_{50} in mice (mg/kg): 1170 orally, 125 i.v. (Zipf).

USE: Solvent; nonionic emulsifier; pharmaceutic aid (surfactant); spermaticide.

THERAP CAT: Anesthetic (topical); antipruritic; sclerosing agent.

7559. Polifeprosan. [90409-78-2] Decanedioic acid polymer with 4,4′-[1,3-propanediylbis(oxy)]bis[benzoic acid]; 1,3-bis(*p*-carboxyphenoxy)propane-sebacic acid copolymer; poly[1,3-bis(*p*-carboxyphenoxy)propane-sebacic acid]; PCPP-SA. Biodegradable, hydrophobic polymers developed for use as implantable drug delivery systems. Prepn of various copolymers: K. W. Leong *et al.*, *Polym. Prepr.* **25**, 201 (1984); *eidem*, *J. Biomed. Mater. Res.* **19**, 941 (1985). Toxicology and biocompatibility studies: C. T. Laurencin *et al.*, *Clin. Lab. Med.* **10**, 549 (1990). Review of polymer design, synthesis and physical properties: J. Tamada, R. Langer, *J. Biomater. Sci. Polym. Ed.* **3**, 315-353 (1992).

Polifeprosan 20   *m* = 20   *n* = 80

Polifeprosan 20. High mol wt polymer consisting of bis(*p*-carboxyphenoxy)propane and sebacic acid in a 20:80 ratio. Mol wt 20,000-200,000. Prepn: A. J. Domb, R. S. Langer, **EP 266603**; *eidem*, **US 4757128** (both 1988 to MIT); *eidem*, *J. Polym. Sci.* **25**, 3373 (1987). White solid, mp 68°. Viscosity (in chloroform at 23°): 0.92 dl/g. Soly (g/100ml): >20 in chloroform; <1 in hexane.

Gliadel. Polifeprosan 20 combined with carmustine, *q.v.*, in an implantable wafer. Prepn and characterization of polymer-drug matrix: W. Dang *et al.*, *Pharm. Res.* **13**, 683 (1996); A. J. Domb *et al.*, *ibid.* **16**, 762 (1999). Clinical trial of surgically implanted wafer for malignant gliomas: H. Brem *et al.*, *Lancet* **345**, 1008 (1995); S. Valtonen *et al.*, *Neurosurgery* **41**, 44 (1997).

USE: Pharmaceutic aid for controlled release drug delivery.

7560. Polihexanide. [32289-58-0]; [28757-47-3] (base). Poly(iminocarbonimidoyliminocarbonimidoylimino-1,6-hexanediyl) hydrochloride; polyaminopropylbiguanide; polyhexamethylene biguanide hydrochloride; polyhexanide; PHMB; Cosmocil CQ; Lavasept; Vantocil. $(C_8H_{17}N_5)_n$.xHCl. Broad spectrum antimicrobial polymer; binds and disrupts cytoplasmic membranes. Prepn: F. L. Rose, G. Swain, **US 2643232** (1953 to ICI). Antibacterial action: A. Davies *et al.*, *J. Appl. Bacteriol.* **31**, 448 (1968). Synthesis and characterization of solution behavior: G. C. East *et al.*, *Polymer* **38**, 3973 (1997). Interactions with phospholipid membranes: P. Broxton *et al.*, *J. Appl. Bacteriol.* **57**, 115 (1984); T. Ikeda *et al.*, *Bull. Chem. Soc. Jpn.* **58**, 705 (1985). Mechanism of action study: W. Khunkitti *et al.*, *J. Appl. Microbiol.* **82**, 107 (1997). Titrimetric determn of biguanide groups: T. Hattori *et al.*, *Anal. Sci.* **19**, 1525 (2003). Clinical evaluation of mouthrinse formulations on bacterial count and plaque growth: M. Rosin *et al.*, *J. Clin. Periodontol.* **28**, 1121 (2001); **29**, 392 (2002).

Sol in water.

USE: Biocide in personal hygiene products, contact lens solutions, industrial disinfectants, textiles, and household products; preservative in cosmetics.

THERAP CAT: Antiseptic; disinfectant.

7561. Polonium. [7440-08-6] Po; at. no. 84; valence 4, occasionally 2, rarely 6. No stable nuclides. Isotopes range in mass number from 193-218; all are radioactive; 210 is naturally occurring. The first radioactive substance discovered by Mme. Curie in 1898. A product of disintegration of radium; one gram is contained in ~25,000 tons of pitchblende or in 7.5 kg radium that is more than 30 years old. Separated in form of a deposit on a bismuth plate immersed in a soln of the chloride: Marckwald, *Ber.* **35**, 2285 (1902); using a silver, gold or nickel plate: Curie, Joliot, *J. Chim. Phys.* **28**, 201 (1931); Haissinsky, *ibid.* **33**, 97 (1936); Rollier, *Gazz. Chim. Ital.* **66**, 797 (1936); Ziv, *C. R. Acad. Sci. URSS* **25**, 743 (1939). Obtained in the metallic form by volatilization from nickel on a collodion film: Rollier *et al., J. Chim. Phys.* **4**, 648 (1936). The only readily accessible isotope is the penultimate member of the radium decay series, $^{210}_{84}$Po, also called *Radium F* (Ra-F). Decays by α-emission (T½ 138.4 days, rel. at. mass 209.9828) to $^{206}_{82}$Pb. Comprehensive reviews: K. W. Bagnall, *Chemistry of the Rare Radioelements* (Butterworths, London, 1957); *idem, Endeavour* **22**(86), 61 (May 1963); *idem,* "Selenium, Tellurium and Polonium" in *Comprehensive Inorganic Chemistry* vol. 2, J. C. Bailar, Jr., et al., Eds. (Pergamon Press, Oxford, 1973) pp 935-1008.

Two allotropic forms; coexist between 18° and 54°; d (α-form) 9.196; d (β-form) 9.398. mp 254°; bp 962°. Latent heat of vaporization: 24.597 kcal/mole. Resistivity: α-Po = 42 μohm-cm at 0°; β-Po = 44 μohm-cm at 0°. Physical properties: Maxwell, *J. Chem. Phys.* **17**, 1288 (1949). Chemically resembles tellurium and bismuth. Forms a volatile, unstable hydride, PoH$_2$. Forms a polonide, Na$_2$Po; a carbonyl PoCO; a hydroxide Po(OH)$_4$.

Caution: Radiation hazard; alpha emitter. Sol compds hazard to kidneys, spleen; insol, airborne compds hazard to lungs. Max permissible concn of insol $^{210}_{84}$Po in air: 7×10^{-11} μ-Curie/cc, *Natl. Bur. Stand. Handb.* **69**, 79 (1959).

7562. Poloxamers. [106392-12-5] Methyloxirane block polymer with oxirane; polyethylene glycol-polypropylene glycol block copolymer; α-hydro-ω-hydroxypoly(oxyethylene)poly-(oxypropylene)poly(oxyethylene) block copolymer. Series of nonionic surfactants with the structure HO(CH$_2$CH$_2$O)$_a$(CH(CH$_3$)-CH$_2$O)$_b$(CH$_2$CH$_2$O)$_c$H where b is at least 15, a and c are approximately equal and the polyoxyethylene content is 10 to 80% of the total polymer weight. Mol wt ranges from 1000 to >16,000. The polyoxypropylene segment is hydrophobic; the polyoxyethylene segment hydrophilic. Prepn: L. G. Lundsted, US 2674619 (1954 to Wyandotte). Comprehensive description of manufacture and properties: I. R. Schmolka in *Nonionic Surfactants*, M. Schick, Ed. (Dekker, New York, 1967) pp 300-371; I. F. Paterson *et al.* in *Handbook of Engineering Polymeric Materials*, N. P. Cheremisinoff, Ed. (Marcel Dekker, New York, 1997) pp 765-774. Review of chemistry and medical applications: L. E. Reeve in *Handbook of Biodegradable Polymers*, A. J. Domb *et al.*, Eds. (Gordon & Breach, New York, 1997) pp 231-249.

Mobile liquids, pastes or flakeable solids. Relatively nonhygroscopic. Vary from water-insol to very water-sol compds; more sol in cold than hot water. Low-foaming properties. Stable to acids, alkalies, metallic ions.

Poloxalene. [9003-11-6] SKF-18667; Bloat Guard; Therabloat. a = 12, b = 34, c = 12; av. mol wt 3000. Use in treatment of ruminant bloat: E. E. Bartley, G. C. Scott, US 3465083 (1969 to Kansas State Univ. and SKF). Comparative field trial in cattle: W. Majak *et al., J. Anim. Sci.* **73**, 1493 (1995).

Poloxamer 182. Pluronic L62. a = 8, b = 30, c = 8; av. mol wt 2500. Liquid, mp −4°. d$^{25}_{25}$ 1.03. Brookfield viscosity (25°): 450 cP; cloud pt (10% aq soln): 24°. Sol in water, ethanol, toluene. Insol in kerosene, ethylene glycol.

Poloxamer 188. Exocorpol; Pluronic F68; Synperonic PE/F68. a = 75, b = 30, c = 75; av. mol wt 8400. Flakeable solid. mp 52°. Brookfield viscosity (77°): 1000 cP; cloud pt (10% aq soln): >100°. Sol in water, ethanol; partially sol in toluene. Insol in kerosene, ethylene glycol.

Poloxamer 331. Pluronic L101. a = 7, b = 54, c = 7; av. mol wt 3800. Liquid, mp −23°. d$^{25}_{25}$ 1.018; Brookfield viscosity (25°): 800 cP; cloud pt (10% aq soln): 11°. Sol in ethanol, toluene. Insol in water, kerosene, ethylene glycol.

Purified Poloxamer 188. Flocor. Highly purified pharmaceutical grade for intravenous use; lowers blood viscosity and improves blood flow. Pharmacology: R. M. Emanuele, *Expert Opin. Invest. Drugs* **7**, 1193-1200 (1998). Clinical trial in sickle cell disease: E. P. Orringer *et al., J. Am. Med. Assoc.* **286**, 2099 (2001).

USE: Pharmaceutic aids; food additives; defoamers; antistatic agents; demulsifiers; detergents, wetting agents, gelling agents; emulsifiers; foam controllers; dispersants; dye levelers.

THERAP CAT: Poloxamer 188 as hemorheologic agent.

THERAP CAT (VET): Poloxalene in prevention of bloat in cattle.

7563. Polybrominated Biphenyls. PBBs; brominated biphenyls; polybromobiphenyls. Mixtures of isomers and congeners with structures similar to polychlorinated biphenyls, *q.v.*, where each X = H or Br. Once widely used commercially. Prepn: H. Hahn *et al.*, **DE 1161547** (1964 to Chem. Fabrik Kalb); G. A. Burk, **US 3733366** (1973 to Dow); L. C. Mitchell, D. R. Breckenridge, **US 3763248** and **US 3833674** (1973, 1974 both to Ethyl Corp.). Persistence in soils: L. W. Jacobs *et al., J. Agric. Food Chem.* **24**, 1198 (1976). Photodegradation: L. O. Ruzo *et al., ibid.* 1062. Reviews of environmental hazards: K. Kay, *Environ. Res.* **13**, 74-93 (1977); F. J. DiCarlo *et al., Environ. Health Perspect.* **23**, 351-365 (1978); of toxicology and mechanism of action: S. Safe, *Crit. Rev. Toxicol.* **13**, 319-395 (1984); of carcinogenicity: E. M. Silberhorn *et al., ibid.* **20**, 439-496 (1990); of toxicology and human exposure: *Toxicological Profile for Polybrominated Biphenyls and Polybrominated Diphenyl Ethers* (PB2004-107334, 2004) 624 pp.

Firemaster BP-6. Major component is *2,2′,4,4′,5,5′-hexabromobiphenyl*. Softens at 72°; dec >300°. Low vapor pressure; degraded by uv light. Very sol in benzene, toluene. Insol in water.

Caution: The 1973 "Michigan Incident" in which BP-6 was accidentally added to animal feed, and resulted in the contamination of the food chain and wide-spread destruction of contaminated farm animals, led to the removal of BP-6 from the market: L. J. Carter, *Science* **192**, 240 (1976). Reported symptoms of overexposure include impaired immune system; hypothyroidism; neurological effects, headache, joint stiffness, memory loss; chloracne-like lesions (Safe). *See also Patty's Industrial Hygiene and Toxicology* vol. 2D, G. D. Clayton, F. E. Clayton, Eds. (John Wiley & Sons, New York, 4th ed., 1994) p 2433-2504. These substances are reasonably anticipated to be human carcinogens: *Report on Carcinogens, Eleventh Edition* (PB2005-104914, 2004) p III-217.

USE: Formerly as flame retardant.

7564. Polychlorinated Biphenyls. PCBs; chlorinated biphenyls; chlorobiphenyls; Aroclor; Clophen; Fenclor; Kanechlor; Pyralene. Once widely used industrial chemicals whose high stability contributed to both their commercial usefulness and their long-term deleterious environmental and health effects. Synthesis: H. Schmidt, G. Schulz, *Ann.* **207**, 338 (1881). Commercially available since 1930: C. Penning, *Ind. Eng. Chem.* **22**, 1180 (1930). Commercial PCBs are mixtures of various isomers and congeners. The Aroclors are characterized by four digit numbers. The first two digits indicate that the mixture contains biphenyls (12), triphenyls (54) or both (25, 44); the last two digits give the weight percent of chlorine in the mixture (e.g. Aroclor 1242 contains biphenyls with ~42% chlorine). Accumulation of airborne PCBs in foliage: E. H. Buckley, *Science* **216**, 520 (1982). *Reviews:* H. L. Hubbard in *Kirk-Othmer Encyclopedia of Chemical Technology* vol. 5 (Interscience, New York, 2nd ed., 1964) pp 289-297; O. Hutzinger *et al., The Chemistry of PCBs* (CRC Press, Cleveland, Ohio, 1974) 269 pp; J. W. Lloyd *et al., J. Occup. Med.* **18**, 109-113 (1976). Reviews of environmental impact and toxicity: L. Fishbein, *Annu. Rev. Pharmacol.* **14**, 139-156 (1974); *National Conference on Polychlorinated Biphenyls*, Nov. 19-21, 1975 (EPA-560/6-75-004, 1976) 487 pp; R. D. Kimbrough, *Crit. Rev. Toxicol.* **2**, 445-498 (1974); S. H. Safe, *ibid.* **24**, 87-149 (1994). Reviews of carcinogenicity: *IARC Mono-*

graphs **18**, 43-103 (1978); E. M. Silberhorn *et al.*, *Crit. Rev. Toxicol.* **20**, 439-496 (1990); of toxicology and mechanism of action: S. Safe, *ibid.* **13**, 319-395 (1984); of toxicology and human exposure: *Toxicological Profile for Polychlorinated Biphenyls* (PB2000-108027, 2000) 948 pp.

X = H or Cl

Aroclor 1242. Clear, mobile liquid; av. number Cl/molecule: 3.10. d_4^{25} 1.381, $d_4^{15.5}$ 1.392. Distillation range 325-366°. Flash point (open cup) 348-356°F. n_D^{20} 1.627-1.629. Dielectric constant (1000 cycles) 5.6 (25°), 4.9 (100°).

Aroclor 1254. Light yellow, viscous liquid; av. number Cl/molecule: 4.96. d_4^{65} 1.495; $d_4^{15.5}$ 1.505. Distillation range 365-390°. No open cup flash point to boiling. n_D^{20} 1.629-1.641. Dielectric constant (1000 cycles) 5.0 (25°), 4.3 (100°). LD_{50} orally in weanling rats: 1295 mg/kg (Kimbrough).

Aroclor 1260. Light yellow, soft, sticky resin; av. number Cl/molecule: 6.30. d_4^{90} 1.555; $d_4^{15.5}$ 1.566. Distillation range 385-420. No open cup flash point to boiling. n_D^{20} 1.647-1.649. Dielectric constant (1000 cycles) 4.3 (25°); 3.7 (100°). LD_{50} orally in weanling rats: 1315 mg/kg (Kimbrough).

Caution: In Japan, 1968, oral intoxication to humans due to accidental contamination of rice bran oil with Kanechlor 400 led to an outbreak of what became known as "Yusho disease". Symptoms of oral intoxication in humans included nausea, lethargy, chloracne, brown pigmentation of skin and nails, subcutaneous edema of the face, distinctive hair follicles, excessive eye discharge, swelling of eyelids, visual disturbances, GI disturbances and jaundice. *See* M. Kuratsune *et al.*, (EPA-560/6-75-004, 1976) p 14. Potential symptoms of occupational overexposure are chloracne, dermal lesions; hepatic injury; decreased pulmonary function; decreased birth weight in offspring of exposed mothers; eye irritation (Safe, 1994). *See also Patty's Industrial Hygiene and Toxicology* **vol. 2D**, G. D. Clayton, F. E. Clayton, Eds. (John Wiley & Sons, Inc., New York, 4th ed., 1994) 2433-2504. These substances are reasonably anticipated to be human carcinogens: *Report on Carcinogens, Eleventh Edition* (PB2005-104914, 2004) p III-218.

USE: In electrical capacitors, electrical transformers, gas-transmission turbines, vacuum pumps. Formerly used in U.S. as hydraulic fluids, plasticizers, adhesives, fire retardants, wax extenders, dedusting agents, pesticide extenders, inks, lubricants, cutting oils, in heat transfer systems, carbonless reproducing paper.

7565. Polydextrose. [68424-04-4] Litesse. Randomly bonded condensation polymer of dextrose with small amounts of bound sorbitol and citric acid. Functions to replace the bulk and mouthfeel of sugar and/or fat in reduced calorie foods. Prepn: H. H. Rennhard, US 3766165 (1973 to Pfizer). Improved process: D. B. Guzek *et al.*, EP 473333 (1992 to Pfizer); *C.A.* **116**, 237725s (1992). Reviews of physical properties and applications in foods: A. Torres, R. D. Thomas, *Food Technol.* **35**, 44-49 (1981); F. K. Moppett in *Food Sci. Technol.* **48**, entitled "Alternative Sweeteners", L. O. Nabors, R. C. Gelardi, Eds. (1991) pp 401-421.

White to light tan, amorphous powder, mp >130°. Bland, nonsweet taste. Hygroscopic. pH of 10% w/w aq soln: 2.5-3.5. Viscosity of 50% aq soln: 35 cP. Very sol in water (to ~80%). Partially sol in glycerin, propylene glycol. Insol in ethanol. Caloric utilization value in humans: 1 kcal/g.

USE: Bulking agent for reduced calorie foods.

7566. Polyestradiol Phosphate. [28014-46-2] Estradiol phosphate polymer; PEP; Estradurin. Polymeric ester of phosphoric acid and estradiol. Mol wt ~26,000. Prepn: Diczfalusy, *Endocrinology* **54**, 471 (1954); Fernö *et al.*, *Acta Chem. Scand.* **12**, 1675 (1958); Diczfalusy *et al.*, US 2928849 (1960 to AB Leo). Clinical pharmacology: P. O. Gunnarsson, B. J. Norlén, *Prostate*

13, 299 (1988). Clinical trial in prostatic carcinoma: J. Aro, *ibid.* **18**, 131 (1991).

n is approx. 80

Solid, mp 195-202°. Very sol in aq pyridine; sol in aq alkali; very slightly sol in ethanol, ethanol + water (1:1), water, dioxane, acetone, chloroform. Intrinsic viscosity [η] in 0.25M NaCl soln at pH 7.5 = 0.04.

THERAP CAT: Antineoplastic (hormonal).

7567. Polyethylene. [9002-88-4] Ethene homopolymer; Agilene; Alathon; Alkathene; Courlene; Lupolen; Platilon; Polythene; Pylen; Reevon. Mol wt about 1500-100,000. C 85.7%, H 14.3%. Prepd by polymerization of liq ethylene at high temps and high or low pressure. *Reviews:* Aggarwal, Sweeting, *Chem. Rev.* **57**, 665-742 (1957); Raff, Allison, *Polyethylene* **vol. XI** of High Polymers series (Interscience, New York, 1956); Faith *et al.*, *Industrial Chemicals* (Wiley, New York, 3rd ed., 1965) pp 624-630.

$$*\left[CH_2-CH_2\right]*$$

Plastic solid of milky transparency. d_4^{20} 0.92. Tough and flexible at room temps, mp 85-110°. Breaks with cryst fracture at −50°. Good electrical insulator. Surface resistivity: 10^{14} ohms. Will burn, but hardly supports combustion. Stable to water, non-oxidizing acids and alkalies, alcohols, ethers, ketones, esters at ordinary temps. Attacked by oxidizing acids such as nitric acid and perchloric acid, free halogens, benzene, petr ether, gasoline and lubricating oils, aromatic and chlorinated hydrocarbons.

USE: Laboratory tubing; in making prostheses; electrical insulation; packaging materials; kitchenware; tank and pipe linings; paper coatings; textile stiffeners.

7568. Polyethylene Glycol. [25322-68-3] α-Hydro-ω-hydroxypoly(oxy-1,2-ethanediyl); macrogol; PEG; Carbowax; Pluracol E; Poly-G; Polyglycol E. Liquid and solid polymers of the general formula $H(OCH_2CH_2)_nOH$, where n is greater than or equal to 4. In general, each PEG is followed by a number which corresponds to its average mol wt. Synthesis: Fordyce, Hibbert, *J. Am. Chem. Soc.* **61**, 1905, 1910 (1939). Polyethylene glycols are compds of low toxicity: Smyth *et al.*, *J. Am. Pharm. Assoc. Sci. Ed.* **39**, 349 (1950). Toxicity data (PEG 400): W. Bartsch *et al.*, *Arzneim.-Forsch.* **26**, 1581 (1976). *Reviews: Glycols*, G. O. Curme, F. Johnston, Eds. (Reinhold, New York, 1952) pp 176-202; Kastens in *High Polymers*, H. Mark *et al.*, Eds., **vol. 13** entitled *Polyethers*, **part 1** (Interscience, New York, 1963) pp 169-189, 274-291; G. M. Powell, III in *Handbook of Water-Soluble Gums & Resins*, R. L. Davidson, Ed. (McGraw-Hill, New York, 1980) pp 18/1-18/31. *Book: Poly(Ethylene Glycol) Chemistry: Biotechnical and Biomedical Applications*, J. M. Harris, Ed. (Plenum Press, New York, 1992) 385 pp. Series of articles on pegylation to enhance delivery of protein drugs: *Adv. Drug Delivery Rev.* **54**, 453-609 (2002). Clinical evaluation as laxative: S. Chaussade, M. Minic, *Aliment. Pharmacol. Ther.* **17**, 165 (2003).

Clear, viscous liquids or white solids which dissolve in water forming transparent solns. Sol in many organic solvents. Readily sol in aromatic hydrocarbons. Only slightly sol in aliphatic hydrocarbons. Do not hydrolyze or deteriorate on storage, will not support mold growth. Solvent action on some plastics.

Polyethylene glycol 200. Average value of n is 4, mol wt range 190-210. Viscous, hygroscopic liq; slight characteristic odor; d_{25}^{25} 1.127. Viscosity (210°F): 4.3 cSt. Supercools upon freezing.

Polyethylene glycol 400. Average value of n between 8.2 and 9.1, mol wt range 380-420. Viscous, slightly hygroscopic liq; slight characteristic odor; d_{25}^{25} 1.128. mp 4-8°. Viscosity (210°F): 7.3 cSt. LD_{50} orally in rats: 30 ml/kg (Bartsch).

Polyethylene glycol 600. Average value of n between 12.5 and 13.9, mol wt range 570-630. Viscous, slightly hygroscopic liq; characteristic odor; d_{25}^{25} 1.128. mp 20-25°. Viscosity (210°F): 10.5 cSt.

Polyethylene glycol 1500. Average value of n between 29 and 36, mol wt range 1300-1600. White, free-flowing powder; d_{25}^{25} 1.210. mp 44-48°. Viscosity (210°F): 25-32 cSt.

Polyethylene glycol 4000. Forlax; Idrolax. Average value of n between 68 and 84, mol wt range 3000-3700. White, free-flowing powder or creamy-white flakes; d_{25}^{25} 1.212. mp 54-58°. Viscosity (210°F): 76-110 cSt. LD_{50} orally in rats (divided doses): 59 g/kg (Smyth).

Polyethylene glycol 6000. Average value of n between 158 and 204, mol wt range 7000-9000. Powder or creamy-white flakes; d_{25}^{25} 1.21. mp 56-63°. Viscosity (210°F): 470-900 cSt. LD_{50} orally in rats: >50 g/kg (Smyth).

USE: Pharmaceutic aid (ointment and suppository base; tablet excipient). As water-soluble lubricants for rubber molds, textile fibers, and metal-forming operations. In food and food packaging. In hair prepns, in cosmetics in general. As a stationary phase in gas chromatography. Also in water paints, paper coatings, polishes and in the ceramics industry.

THERAP CAT: Laxative.

7569. Polyethylene Terephthalates. PET. Fiber forming polyesters prepd from terephthalic acid, q.v. or its esters and ethylene glycol: Whinfield, Dickson, US 2465319 (1949 to du Pont). Review of structures, definition of trade names: R. W. Moncrieff, *Man-Made Fibres* (John Wiley & Sons, New York, 4th ed., 1963) pp 361-389, 707-723.

R = OH, **Dacron**, **Amilar**, **Fiber V**. Solid, dec at approx 250°. Sp gr 1.38. Sol in hot *m*-cresol, trifluoroacetic acid, *o*-chlorophenol, a mixture of 7 parts of trichlorophenol and 10 parts (by wt) of phenol, a mixture of 2 parts of tetrachloroethane and 3 parts (by wt) of phenol. Fiber has good resistance to weak acids even at boiling temp, to strong acids in the cold, to weak alkalies, to bleaches, to most alcohols, ketones, soaps, detergents, and dry cleaning agents. Fabric has good resistance to creasing, abrasion, heat aging, and sunlight when behind glass. When "heat-set", fabric will not shrink in either boiling water or boiling drycleaning solvent. Fabric burns, but local melting generally prevents spread of fire. Insects cannot thrive on the fiber, but some can cut through it. Molds, mildew, and fungi may grow on applied finishes, but do not attack fiber. R = OCH_3, **Terylene**. For physical properties, *see* Dacron above. Other similar products: **Diolen, Enkalene, Fortrel, Tergal, Terital, Terlenka, Trevira, Mylar**.

USE: In fabric manufacture; as films; as base for magnetic coatings. Surgical aid (arterial grafts).

7570. Polygodial. [6754-20-7] (1R,4aS,8aS)-1,4,4a,5,6,7,-8,8a-Octahydro-5,5,8a-trimethyl-1,2-naphthalenedicarboxalde-hyde; tadeonal. $C_{15}H_{22}O_2$; mol wt 234.33. C 76.88%, H 9.46%, O 13.66%. Widely distributed drimane sesquiterpene with insect antifeedant properties; naturally occurring as the (−)-form. Isoln from *Polygonum hydropiper* L., *Polygonaceae* (Australia) and structure: C. S. Barnes, J. W. Loder, *Aust. J. Chem.* **15**, 322 (1962); from the bark of *Warburgia stuhlmanni* Engl. or *W. ugandensis*, *Canellacceae* (E. Africa): I. Kubo *et al., Chem. Commun.* **1976**, 1013; from nudibranch *Dendrodons limbata* (Mediterranean): G. Cimino *et al., Science* **219**, 1237 (1983); from nudibranchs *D. nigra, D.*

tuberculosa (Hawaii) and *D. krebsii* (Mexico): R. K. Okuda *et al., J. Org. Chem.* **48**, 1866 (1983). Relationship between structure and antifeedant-activity: K. Nakanishi, I. Kubo, *Isr. J. Chem.* **16**, 28 (1977); M. D'Ischia *et al., Tetrahedron Lett.* **1982**, 3295. Synthesis of racemate: T. Kato *et al., Tetrahedron Lett.* **1971**, 1961; S. C. Howell *et al., Chem. Commun.* **1981**, 507. Synthesis of (−)-form: I. Razmilic *et al., Synth. Commun.* **17**, 95 (1987).

Colorless needles from petroleum (40-60°), mp 57° (Barnes, Loder). $[\alpha]_D^{24}$ −131° (c = 0.96 in ethanol). uv max (ethanol): 231, 295 nm (ε 11800, 76).

(±)-**Form.** mp 93-94° (Tanis, Nakanishi).

7571. Polylysine. [25104-18-1] L-Lysine, homopolymer. A lysine polypeptide or homopolymer, the chain length of which varies with the method of prepn. Prepn: Katchalski *et al., J. Am. Chem. Soc.* **69**, 2564 (1947); **70**, 2094 (1948); Fasman *et al., ibid.* **83**, 709 (1961); Sela *et al., Biopolymers* **1**, 517 (1963); Strojny, White, US 3215684 (1965 to Dow). For structure *see* Lysine.

L-**Form hydriodide.** Average dp (or n) = 32. Transparent, solid, film-like polymer. Readily sol in water; practically insol in the usual organic solvents. Transition of high-mol-wt poly-L-lysine (dp 1500) in aq soln from a helical to a randomly coiled conformation under the influence of decreasing pH or increasing temp: Applequist, Doty, C.A. **58**, 6925b (1963).

7572. Polymerized Pyridoxylated Hemoglobin. Poly SFH-P; PolyHeme. Acellular oxygen carrier consisting of pyridoxylated, stroma-free hemoglobin polymerized with glutaraldehyde. Average mol wt 150 kDa. Prepn and oxygen-carrying capacity: L. R. Sehgal *et al., Prog. Clin. Biol. Res.* **122**, 19 (1983); *eidem, Surgery* **95**, 433 (1984). Pharmacology: S. A. Gould *et al., Ann. Emerg. Med.* **15**, 1416 (1986). Clinical trial in acute blood loss: *idem et al., J. Am. Coll. Surg.* **187**, 113 (1998). Review of clinical development: S. A. Gould, G. S. Moss, *World J. Surg.* **20**, 1200-1207 (1996).

Prepd as solution containing 12-14 g hemoglobin/dl. Oxygen-carrying capacity: 16-19 vol%. Binding coefficient (ml O_2/g Hb): 1.30. Colloid osmotic pressure: 20-25 mm Hg.

THERAP CAT: Blood substitute.

7573. Polymyxin. [1406-11-7] Antibiotic complex produced by *Bacillus polymyxa*: Brownlee, Jones, *Biochem. J.* **43**, XXV (1948). Prepn: Ainsworth, Pope, US 2565057 (1951 to Burroughs Wellcome); Petty, US 2595605 (1952 to Am. Cyanamid); Benedict, Stodola, US 2771397 (1956 to USDA). Purification: Hastings *et al.,* GB 782926 (1957 to Distillers Co.). Polymyxins A, B, C, D, E, F, K, M, P, S and T have been identified. Isoln of polymyxins A, B, C and E: Few, Schulman, *Biochem. J.* **54**, 171 (1953); of *polymyxin D*: Stansley *et al., Bull. Johns Hopkins Hosp.* **81**, 43 (1947); of *polymyxin F*: W. L. Parker *et al, J. Antibiot.* **30**, 767 (1977); of *polymyxin K*: Kimura, JP 71 16152 (1971), *C.A.* **75**, 62180r (1971); of *polymyxin M*: Khokhlov *et al., C.A.* **55**, 5653h (1961); of *polymyxin P*: Kimura *et al., J. Antibiot.* **22**, 449 (1969); of *polymyxin S*$_1$ and *polymyxin T*$_1$: J. Shoji *et al., ibid.* **30**, 1029 (1977). Resolution of polymyxin B into B$_1$ and B$_2$: Hausmann, Craig, *J. Am. Chem. Soc.* **76**, 4892 (1954). Structure and synthesis of polymyxin B$_1$: Wilkinson, Lowe, *Nature* **202**, 1211 (1964); Vogler *et al., Helv. Chim. Acta* **48**, 1161 (1965). Structure of polymyxin B$_2$: Wilkinson, Lowe, *Nature* **204**, 993 (1964). Separation of polymyxin D into D$_1$ and D$_2$ and structures: Hayashi *et al., Experientia* **22**, 354 (1966). Structure of polymyxin S$_1$: J. Shoji *et al., J. Antibiot.* **30**, 1035 (1977); of polymyxin T$_1$: *eidem, ibid.* 1042. *Review:* Vogler, Studer, *Experientia* **22**, 345-354 (1966); Paulus, "Polymyxins" in *Antibiotics* **II**, D. Gottlieb, P. Shaw, Eds. (Springer-Verlag, New York, 1967) pp 254-267.

DAB = L-α,γ-diaminobutyric acid

Sol in water.
USE: Pharmaceutic aid (adjuvant).
THERAP CAT: Immunomodulator.

Polymyxin B₁	R = (+)-6-methyloctanoyl	X = Phe	Y = Leu	Z = DAB

Polymyxin B₁   R = (+)-6-methyloctanoyl   X = Phe   Y = Leu   Z = DAB
          B₂   R = 6-methylheptanoyl   X = Phe   Y = Leu   Z = DAB
          D₁   R = (+)-6-methyloctanoyl   X = Leu   Y = Thr   Z = D-Ser
          D₂   R = 6-methylheptanoyl   X = Leu   Y = Thr   Z = D-Ser

Obtained as the hydrochloride. Nearly colorless powder, dec 228-230°. $[\alpha]_D^{23}$ −40° (c = 1.05). The hydrochloride is very sol (more than 40%) in water and methanol. The soly decreases in the higher alcs. Practically insol in the usual ethers, esters, ketones, hydrocarbons, and the chlorinated solvents. Forms water insol salts with a number of ppts such as picric acid, helianthic acid, Reinecke salt. The free base is slightly sol in water; almost insol in alc.

Polymyxin B. [1404-26-8] Mixture of polymyxins B₁ and B₂. $[\alpha]_{5461}$ −106.3° (1N HCl).

Polymyxin B sulfate. [1405-20-5] Aerosporin; Mastimyxin. Solubilities: Weiss et al., Antibiot. Chemother. **7**, 374 (1957).

Polymyxin B sulfate mixture with trimethoprim. Polytrim.

Polymyxin B₁. [4135-11-9] $C_{56}H_{98}N_{16}O_{13}$; mol wt 1203.48.

Polymyxin B₁ pentahydrochloride. $C_{56}H_{98}N_{16}O_{13}$.5HCl. White powder. $[\alpha]_D^{25}$ −85.11° (c = 2.33 in 75% ethanol).

Polymyxin B₂. [34503-87-2] $C_{55}H_{96}N_{16}O_{13}$; mol wt 1189.45. $[\alpha]_{5461}^{22}$ −112.4° (2% Acetic acid).

Polymyxin D₁. [10072-50-1] $C_{50}H_{93}N_{15}O_{15}$; mol wt 1144.36.

Polymyxin D₂. [34167-45-8] $C_{49}H_{91}N_{15}O_{15}$; mol wt 1130.34.

Polymyxin E see Colistin.

THERAP CAT: Antibacterial.
THERAP CAT (VET): Antibacterial.

7574. Polynoxylin. Anaflex; Larex; Ponoxylan. Alkali condensation product of formaldehyde and urea. Prepn: D. Haler, A. Aebi, Nature **190**, 734 (1961); GB 905195 (1962 to Ed. Geistlich Soehne). Antimicrobial activity and toxicity study: H. Brodhage, A. R. Stofer, Antibiot. Chemother. **11**, 205 (1961). Mechanism of action study: J. I. Blenkharn, J. Clin. Hosp. Pharm. **10**, 367 (1985).

Amorphous powder, dec 200° (without melting). Soly in water: 0.28-0.31%.

THERAP CAT: Antiseptic.

7575. Polyoxidonium. Synpol. Immunostimulant copolymer of N-oxidized 1,4-ethylenepiperazine and (N-carboxyethyl)-1,4-ethylenepiperazine bromide; mol wt 60-100 kDa. Prepn: R. V. Petrov et al., WO 9507100; A. V. Nekrasov et al., US 5503830 (1995, 1996 both to Petrovax). Adjuvant activity in mice: K. S. Nandakumar, V. R. Muthukkaruppan, Scand. J. Immunol. **50**, 188 (1999). Effect on human peripheral blood leukocytes: V. A. Dyakonova et al., Int. Immunopharmacol. **4**, 1615 (2004). Review of development and use in influenza vaccine: V. A. Kabanov, Pure Appl. Chem. **76**, 1659-1677 (2004).

7576. Polyoxins. [11113-80-7] Agricultural antifungal antibiotic complex produced by Streptomyces cacaoi var asoensis and S. piomogenus. Polyoxins A through O are known, all except C and I having specific activity against phytopathogenic fungi by inhibiting cell wall chitin synthesis. Isoln and characterization of polyoxin A: S. Suzuki et al., J. Antibiot. **18A**, 131 (1965); of A and B: K. Isono et al., Agric. Biol. Chem. **29**, 848 (1965); S. Suzuki et al., JP 66 15520; of C through L: K. Isono et al., Agric. Biol. Chem. **30**, 817 (1966); **31**, 190 (1967); **32**, 792 (1968); of M: K. Isono, S. Suzuki, Tetrahedron Lett. **1970**, 425. Isoln of polyoxins N and O: S. Suzuki et al., JP Kokai 72 23596 (to Inst. Phys. Chem. Res., and Hokko Chem. Ind.), C.A. **78**, 41566t (1973); production of N and O: eidem, JP 77 20555 (1977 to Inst. Phys. Chem. Res.), C.A. **87**, 150183x (1977). Isoln and structure of N: M. Uramoto et al., Nucleic Acids Res. Spec. Publ. **5**, 327 (1978). Structural elucidation of polyoxins A through L: K. Isono et al., J. Am. Chem. Soc. **91**, 7490 (1969). Revised structure of A: S. Hanessian et al., Tetrahedron Lett. **34**, 4153 (1993). Total synthesis of J: H. Kuzuhara et al., ibid. **1973**, 5055. Biosynthetic studies: K. Isono et al., Biochemistry **14**, 2992 (1975); S. Funayama, K. Isono, ibid. 5568; K. Isono, R. J. Suhadolnick, Arch. Biochem. Biophys. **173**, 141 (1976); S. Funayama, K. Isono, Biochemistry **16**, 3121 (1977); K. Isono et al., J. Am. Chem. Soc. **100**, 3937 (1978). Mode of action: N. Ohta et al., Agric. Biol. Chem. **34**, 1224 (1970); M. Hori et al., ibid. **35**, 1280 (1971); **38**, 691, 699 (1974). Review: R. J. Suhadolnick, Nucleoside Antibiotics (Wiley-Interscience, New York, 1970) pp 218-234; K. Isono, S. Suzuki, Heterocycles **13**, 333-351 (1979).

Polyoxin A

Polyoxin A. [19396-03-3] [S-(Z)]-1-[5-[[2-Amino-5-O-(aminocarbonyl)-2-deoxy-L-xylonoyl]amino]-1,5-dideoxy-1-[3,4-dihydro-5-(hydroxymethyl)2,4-dioxo-1(2H)-pyrimidinyl]-β-D-allofuranuronoyl]-3-ethylidene-2-azetidinecarboxylic acid. $C_{23}H_{32}N_6O_{14}$; mol wt 616.53. Colorless needles from aq ethanol, dec >180°. $[\alpha]_D$ −30°. uv max (0.05N HCl): 262 nm (log ε 3.94); (0.05N NaOH): 264 nm (log ε 3.80).

Polyoxin B. [19396-06-6] 5-[[2-Amino-5-O-(aminocarbonyl)-2-deoxy-L-xylonoyl]amino]-1,5-dideoxy-1-[3,4-dihydro-5-(hydroxymethyl)-2,4-dioxo-1(2H)-pyrimidinyl]-β-D-allofuranuronic acid; Polyoxin AL. $C_{17}H_{25}N_5O_{13}$; mol wt 507.41. Amorphous powder from aq ethanol. $[\alpha]_D^{20}$ +34°. uv max (0.05N HCl): 262 nm (log ε 3.94); (0.05N NaOH): 264 nm (log ε 3.82).

USE: Fungicide, esp for Alternaria leaf spot of many agricultural products.

7577. Polyoxyethylene Alcohols. Polyethylene glycol fatty alcohol ethers; ethoxylated fatty alcohols; macrogol fatty alcohol ethers; alcohol ethoxylates; POE alcohol ethers. Nonionic surfactants prepared by ethoxylation of fatty alcohols with ethylene oxide. Of the general structure $R(OCH_2CH_2)_nOH$ where R is a long chain alkyl group or mixture of alkyl groups. Prepn and reaction mechanism: J. D. Malkemus, *J. Am. Oil Chem. Soc.* **33**, 571 (1956); W. Satkowski, C. G. Hsu, *Ind. Eng. Chem.* **49**, 1875 (1957); R. D. Fine, *J. Am. Oil Chem. Soc.* **35**, 542 (1958). Compounds with a broad range of properties can be prepared by varying the fatty alcohol (lipophile) used and the degree of polymerization of the polyethylene glycol (hydrophile) segment. CFTA-assigned names based on fatty alcohol segment include *ceteth* (cetyl alc), *laureth* (lauryl alc), *myreth* (myristyl alc), *oleth* (oleyl alc), *steareth* (stearyl alc), *trideth* (tridecyl alc). The average number of ethylene oxide units in the polyethylene glycol segment is indicated by an appended number (e.g. ceteth-20). Additional products prepared from fatty alcohol mixtures include *ceteareth* (cetyl/stearyl alcs), *laneth* (lanolin alcs). Trademarks for some commercially available series of compounds: *Alfonic*, *Bio Soft* (E, EA, EN), *Brij*, *Dehydol*, *Ethosperse*, *Eumulgin* (B, O), *Hetoxol*, *Lipocol*, *Macol* (LA, SA, TD), *Polychol*, *Rhodasurf*, *Tergitol* (S, TMN), *Trycol*, *Volpo*. Comprehensive description: W. B. Satkowski *et al.,* "Polyoxyethylene Alcohols" in *Nonionic Surfactants* M. J. Schick, Ed. (Dekker, New York, 1967) pp 86-141. Effects of structure on properties: T. Kuwamura, *ACS Symp. Ser.* **253**, 27-47 (1984). Review of properties and uses in household cleaning products: K. W. Dillan *et al., Household Pers. Prod. Ind.* **23**, 32 (1986).

Liquids to waxy solids. Compds with one to five moles ethylene oxide are sol in oil and many hydrocarbons. Water soly increases with increasing ethylene oxide content. Properties of Brij surfactants: G. King, *Drug Cosmet. Ind.* **90**, 24 (1962).

Laureth 9 *see* Polidocanol.

Ceteth 20. Polyoxyethylene (20) cetyl ether; Brij 58; Hetoxol CS-20; Lipocol C-20. $C_{16}H_{33}(OCH_2CH_2)_nOH$ where the average value of n is 20. Waxy solid. Pour point ~39°; cloud point ~45°. Sol in water; 2% ethanol.

USE: Used as emulsifiers, wetting agents, antistats, solubilizers, defoamers, detergents, lubricants in pharmaceutical, cosmetic and other industrial applications.

7578. Polyoxyethylene Fatty Acid Esters. Polyethylene glycol esters of fatty acids; PEG fatty acid esters; POE fatty acid esters; ethoxylated fatty acid esters; macrogol fatty acid esters. Nonionic surfactants prepared commercially by esterification of fatty acids with ethylene oxide or with polyethylene glycol. Of the general structure $RCOO(CH_2CH_2O)_nH$ or $RCOO(CH_2CH_2O)_n$-OCR where R is a long chain alkyl group or mixture of alkyl groups. Wide range of properties achieved by changing the hydrophobic fatty acid segment and/or varying the degree of polymerization of the hydrophilic polyoxyethylene segment. Trademarks for some commercially available series of compounds include *Emerest* (2600, 2700 series), *Emulsynt*, *Ethofat*, *Lipopeg*, *Mapeg*, *Myrj*, *Nopalcol*, *Pegosperse*, *Renex 20*, *Varonic LI*. Review of prepn, properties and uses: W. B. Satkowski *et al.,* "Polyoxyethylene Esters of Fatty Acids" in *Nonionic Surfactants*, M. J. Schick, Ed. (Dekker, New York, 1967) pp 142-174.

Liquids, soft solids, solids or flakes. Solubility properties depend on length of polyoxyethylene (POE) segment added to a specific fatty acid. Sol in oil and hydrocarbon solvents when <8 ethylene oxide units are added. Soly in water begins when 12-15 ethylene oxide units are added. Specific gravity and viscosity increase with increasing ethylene oxide content.

Polyoxyl 8 stearate. Polyethylene glycol 400 monostearate; PEG-400 monostearate; POE (8) stearate; macrogol ester 400; Emerest 2711; Lipopeg 4-S; Myrj 45; Mapeg 400 MS; Pegosperse 400-MS. $C_{17}H_{35}COO(CH_2CH_2)_nH$ where the average value of n is 8. Prepn and properties: R. L. Birkmeier, J. D. Brandner, *J. Agric. Food Chem.* **6**, 471 (1958).

Polyoxyl 40 stearate. Polyoxyethylene (40) stearate; POE (40) monostearate; Myrj 52; Myrj 52S; Pegosperse 1750-MS. The average number of oxyethylene units is 40. Waxy, white to light tan solid; odorless or faint fat-like odor. Sol in water, alc, ether, acetone. Insol in mineral oil, vegetable oils.

USE: As antistats, emulsifiers, defoamers, wetting agents, solubilizers, conditioning agents, lubricants, detergents. Have wide range of cosmetic, pharmaceutical and other industrial applications. Polyoxyl 8 and 40 stearates as pharmaceutic aid (surfactant).

7579. Polyphosphazenes. Polymers containing an inorganic backbone of alternating nitrogen and phosphorus atoms substituted with very long chains of skeletal atoms. They exist as glasses, flexible solids, or rubbery solids with a low tendency for crystallization; non-flammable and more elastic than carbon-backbone polymers. Prepn of the first polyphosphazene, hexachlorocyclotriphosphazene: J. Liebig, *Ann.* **11**, 139 (1834). Improved synthesis and basis of modern mfg methods: R. Schenck, G. Römer, *Ber.* **57B**, 1343 (1924). Review of syntheses, properties, chemistry and applications: H. R. Allcock, *Science* **193**, 1214-1219 (1976); idem, *Angew. Chem. Int. Ed.* **16**, 147-156 (1977); E. N. Peters, "Inorganic High Polymers", in *Kirk-Othmer Encyclopedia of Chemical Technology* vol. **13** (Wiley-Interscience, New York, 3rd ed., 1981) pp 398-413.

USE: In waterproofing; as flame retardants; in gaskets, o-rings, hydrocarbon fuel hoses.

7580. Polyphosphoric Acid. Phospholeum; tetraphosphoric acid. May be prepd by heating H_3PO_4 with sufficient phosphoric anhydride to give the resulting product an 82-85% P_2O_5 content: Bell, *Ind. Eng. Chem.* **40**, 1464 (1949); Van Wazer, Holst, *J. Am. Chem. Soc.* **72**, 639 (1950); Kennard, *Org. Chem. Bull.* **29**, no. 1 (1957). Consists of about 55% tripolyphosphoric acid, the remainder being H_3PO_4 and other polyphosphoric acids. Typical analysis: 83.0% P_2O_5; ortho equivalent 115.0%.

Viscous liquid at room temps. Conveniently fluid at 60°. Solidifies to a glass at low temps. Sol in water with evolution of heat and hydrolysis to H_3PO_4.

Caution: In strong concns moderately irritating to skin, mucous membranes.

USE: In organic synthesis for cyclizations and acylations.

7581. Polypropylene. [9003-07-0] 1-Propene homopolymer; propylene polymer. Class of compounds also known as olefins. Three forms are possible. *Isotactic* (fiber-forming): methyl groups are all on same side of plane of zig-zag carbon atom chain. *Syndiotactic:* methyl groups are on alternate sides of plane of carbon atom chain. *Atactic* (not fiber-forming, amorphous): methyl groups are in a random arrangement with respect to plane of carbon atom chain. Early synthesis of isotactic form with Ziegler catalyst and comparison with atactic form: Natta *et al., J. Chem. Soc.* **77**, 1708 (1955); Natta, *J. Polym. Sci.* **16**, 143 (1955). *Reviews:* N. G. Gaylord, H. F. Mark, *Linear and Stereoregular Addition Polymers* (Interscience, New York, 1959) pp 54-65; R. W. Moncrieff, *Man-Made Fibres* (Wiley, New York, 4th ed., 1963) pp 500-510; J. G. Cook, *Handbook of Textile Fibres* (Merrow Publishing Co., England, 3rd ed., 1964) pp 369-379; G. Crespi, L. Luciani, "Olefin Polymers (Polypropylene)" in *Kirk-Othmer Encyclopedia of Chemical Technology* Vol. **16** (Wiley-Interscience, New York, 3rd ed., 1981) pp 453-469. Review of thermal decomposition and toxicity: V. Purohit, R. A. Orzel, *J. Am. Coll. Toxicol.* **7**, 221-242 (1988).

Isotactic form. Amco; Amerfil; Beamette; Courlene PY; DLP; Gerfil; Herculon; Lambeth; Meraklon; Moplen; Olane; Prolene; Tuff-Lite; Ulstron. Solid material, softens at ~155°, mp ~165°. Low flammability comparable to that of wool. Keeps strength down to −100°. d 0.90-0.92. Practically insol in cold org solvents. Sol in hot decalin, hot tetralin, boiling tetrachloroethane. Shrinks in boiling trichloroethylene. Resistant to acids, alkalies; attacked by strong oxidizing agents, *e.g.*, hydrogen peroxide. Good resistance to abrasion ("pilling"). Tendency to develop static charges. Unstabilized material has poor resistance to sunlight. Difficult to dye, lacks dye-attracting polar groups in structure.

USE: Isotactic form: for fishing gear, ropes, filter cloths, laundry bags, protective clothing, blankets, fabrics, carpets, yarns, etc.

7582. Polysorbates. Polyoxyethylene sorbitan esters; POE sorbitan esters. Nonionic surfactants derived from sorbitan esters, q.v. Comprehensive description: P. Becher, "Polyol Surfactants" in *Nonionic Surfactants,* M. J. Schick, Ed. (Dekker, New York, 1967) pp 247-299. Description of prepn and uses: L. R. Chislett, J. Walford, *Int. Flavours Food Addit.* **7,** 61 (1976). Pharmacology of polysorbate 80: R. K. Varma *et al., Arzneim.-Forsch.* **35,** 804 (1985). Determn in foods: H. Kato *et al., J. Assoc. Off. Anal. Chem.* **72,** 27 (1989).

HO(CH₂CH₂O)ᵥᵥ   (OCH₂CH₂)ₓOH
                  (OCH₂CH₂)ᵧOH
                  (OCH₂CH₂)ᵤ—O C₁₇H₃₃

Polysorbate 80
(Sum of w, x, y, and z is 20)

Polysorbate 80. [9005-65-6] Polyoxyethylene (20) sorbitan monooleate; POE (20) sorbitan monooleate; Emsorb 6900; Liposorb O-20; Monitan; Sorlate; T-Maz 80; Tween 80. Lemon- to amber-colored, oily liquid. d 1.06-1.09. Viscosity (25°): 300-500 cSt. Very sol in water; sol in alcohol, cottonseed oil, corn oil, ethyl acetate, methanol, toluene. Insol in mineral oil. pH of 5% aq soln between 6 and 8. LD₅₀ in mice, rats (ml/kg): 7.5, 6.3 i.p. (Varma).

USE: As emulsifiers and dispersing agents in medicinal products; as defoamers and emulsifiers in foods. Pharmaceutic aid (surfactant).

7583. Polytetrafluoroethylene. [9002-84-0] Tetrafluoroethene homopolymer; tetrafluoroethylene polymer; polytetrafluoroethylene resin; polytef; PTFE; Fluon; Teflon; Tetran. A highly stable thermoplastic tetrafluoroethylene, q.v., homopolymer. Composed of at least 20,000 C₂F₄ monomer units linked into very long unbranched chains. Prepd by polymerization of tetrafluoroethylene: Plunkett, **US 2230654** (1941 to Kinetic Chem.); Brubaker, **US 2393967**; Joyce, **US 2394243** (both 1946 to du Pont); Hanford, Joyce, *J. Am. Chem. Soc.* **68,** 2082 (1946); Renfrew, **US 2534058** (1950 to du Pont); C. E. Schildknecht, *Vinyl and Related Polymers* (Wiley, New York, 1952) pp 483-494. Account of discovery by Roy J. Plunkett: A. B. Garrett, *J. Chem. Educ.* **39,** 288 (1962). *Reviews:* M. M. Renfrew, E. E. Lewis, *Ind. Eng. Chem.* **38,** 870-877 (1946); R. W. Moncrieff, *Man-Made Fibres* (John Wiley, New York, 4th ed., 1963) pp 512-517; McCane in *Encyclopedia of Polymer Science and Technology* **vol. 13,** N. M. Bikales, Ed. (Interscience, New York, 1970) pp 623-654; S. V. Gangal in *Kirk-Othmer Encyclopedia of Chemical Technology* **vol. 11** (Wiley-Interscience, New York, 4th ed., 1994) pp 621-644.

F F
| |
—C—C—
| |
F F

Nonflammable, high polymer. White translucent to opaque solid (depending on thickness). Very inert chemically. Useful temp range from cryogenic to +260°. Melts to an extremely viscous gel at 327° and reverts to the gaseous monomer at temperatures above 400°. d 2.2. Shore hardness 55-56. Tensile strength 3500-4500 psi. Flexural modulus ~80,000-90,000 psi at room temp. Brittle point below −80°. Dielectric constant (at 60 to 3 × 10⁹ cycles) 2.0-2.05. Not affected by water, aqua regia, chlorosulfonic acid, acetyl chloride, boron fluoride, hot nitric acid, boiling solns of sodium hydroxide, and organic solvents. Not wetted by water. No substance has been found which will dissolve the polymer at moderate temperatures, but prolonged contact with fluorine, hot plasticizers and polymeric waxes is not recommended. Is subject to cold flow at high pressure. Because of its high melt viscosity molding

and sintering techniques similar to those used in powder metallurgy are normally used for fabrication.

Caution: Potential symptom of overexposure by inhalation to the heated polymer is polymer fume fever, characterized by dizziness, headache, nausea, chills, weakness, cough, chest tightness, sore throat, pyrexia. *See Clinical Toxicology of Commercial Products,* R. E. Gosselin *et al.,* Eds. (Williams & Wilkins, Baltimore, 5th ed., 1984) Section II, p 412; *Patty's Industrial Hygiene and Toxicology* **vol. 2E,** G. D. Clayton, F. E. Clayton, Eds. (John Wiley & Sons, New York, 4th ed., 1994) 3791-3793.

USE: For hookup and hookup-type wire in electronic equipment; in computer wire, electrical tape, electrical components, spaghetti tubing. Seals and piston rings, basic shapes, bearings, mechanical tapes, coated glass fabrics. As tubing and sheets for chemical laboratory and process work; for lining reaction vessels; for gaskets and pump packings, sometimes mixed with graphite or glass fibers; as electrical insulator esp in high frequency applications; filtration fabrics; protective clothing. Prosthetic aid.

7584. Polythiazide. [346-18-9] 6-Chloro-3,4-dihydro-2-methyl-3-[[(2,2,2-trifluoroethyl)thio]methyl]-2H-1,2,4-benzothiadiazine-7-sulfonamide 1,1-dioxide; 2-methyl-3-(β,β,β-trifluoroethylthiomethyl)-6-chloro-7-sulfamyl-3,4-dihydro-1,2,4-benzothiadiazine 1,1-dioxide; 6-chloro-3,4-dihydro-2-methyl-7-sulphamoyl-3-(2,2,2-trifluoroethylthiomethyl)-2H-benzo-1,2,4-thiadiazine 1,1-dioxide; Drenusil; Nephril; Renese. C₁₁H₁₃ClF₃N₃O₄S₃; mol wt 439.88. C 30.03%, H 2.98%, Cl 8.06%, F 12.96%, N 9.55%, O 14.55%, S 21.87%. Prepn: J. M. McManus, **US 3009911** (1961 to Pfizer). Comprehensive description: T. Negendra Varo Prasad, *Anal. Profiles Drug Subs.* **20,** 665-692 (1991).

Crystals from isopropanol, mp 202.5°. Sol in methanol and acetone. Practically insol in water and chloroform. Sol in aq solns made alkaline with carbonates or hydroxides of the alkali metals. Rate of decompn increases with increase in pH.

THERAP CAT: Diuretic, antihypertensive.

7585. Polyvinyl Alcohol. [9002-89-5] Ethenol homopolymer; PVA; Akwa Tears; Elvanol; Gelvatol; Liquifilm; Mowiol; Polyviol; Sno Tears; Vinarol; Vinol. A polymer prepd from polyvinyl acetates by replacement of the acetate groups with hydroxyl groups. The alcoholysis proceeds most rapidly in a methanol + methyl acetate mixture in the presence of catalytic amounts of alkali or mineral acids: Hermann, Haehnel, *Ber.* **60,** 1658 (1927). *Monograph:* C. E. Schildknecht, *Vinyl and Related Polymers* (Wiley, New York, 1952). The head-to-tail or 1,3-glycol structure is favored: Staudinger *et al., Ber.* **60,** 1782 (1927); *J. Prakt. Chem.* **155,** 261 (1940); Marvel, Denoon, *J. Am. Chem. Soc.* **60,** 1045 (1938); McDowell, Kenyon, *ibid.* **62,** 415 (1940); Marvel, Inskeep, *ibid.* **65,** 1710 (1943). *Reviews:* M. Leeds in *Kirk-Othmer Encyclopedia of Chemical Technology* **vol. 21** (Wiley-Interscience, New York, 2nd ed., 1970) pp 353-368; *Polyvinyl Alcohol,* A. C. Finch, Ed. (Wiley, New York, 1973) 640 pp; A. S. Dunn, *Chem. Ind. (London)* **1980,** 801-806. Vinyl alcohol monomer has not been isolated. *Review:* R. B. Seymour, G. B. Kauffman, *J. Chem. Educ.* **71,** 582 (1994). Comprehensive description: D. Wong, J. Parasrampuria, *Anal. Profiles Drug Subs. Excip.* **24,** 397-441 (1996).

H
|
—CH₂—C—
|
OH

Dry, unplasticized polyvinyl alcohol powders are white to cream colored, soften at about 200° with decompn. Commercial polyvinyl alcohols have different contents of residual acetyl groups and therefore different viscosity characteristics. The first code number following the trade name indicates the degree of hydrolysis, while the second set of numbers indicates the approx viscosity in cP (4% aq soln at 20°). Polyvinyl alcohols are essentially sol in hot and cold water, but those coded 20-105 require alcohol-water mixtures. Aq solns are colloidal and compatible with lower alcohols. Pure aq solns are neutral or faintly acid and subject to mold growth. Insol in petroleum solvents.

USE: In the plastics industry in molding compds, surface coatings, films resistant to gasoline, textile sizes and finishing compositions; can be compounded to yield elastomers to be used in manuf artificial sponges, fuel hoses, etc., also in printing inks for plastics and glass, in pharmaceutical finishing, cosmetics, water-sol film and sheeting. Pharmaceutic aid (viscosity increasing agent); ophthalmic lubricant.

7586. Polyvinyl Chloride. [9002-86-2] Chloroethene homopolymer; chloroethylene polymer; PVC; Geon; Breon; Welvic; Movyl; Tevilon; Koroseal; Marvinol. Polyvinyl chloride fibers are marketed under the names: *Rhovyl, Fibravyl, Thermovyl, Isovyl, Retractyl, Crinovyl, Envilon, Nip.* Average mol wt ~60,000 to 150,000. Prepn: Baumann, *Ann.* **163**, 308 (1872); Schoenfeld, **US 2168808** (1937 to B. F. Goodrich). Structure: Natta, Rigamonti, *Atti Accad. Naz. Lincei Cl. Sci. Fis. Mat. Nat. Rend.* **24**, 381 (1936); *C.A.* **31**, 4563[9] (1937); Marvel *et al., J. Am. Chem. Soc.* **61**, 3241 (1939). *Reviews:* C. E. Schildknecht, *Vinyl and Related Polymers* (Wiley, New York, 1952) pp 392-442. Technology: W. S. Penn, *PVC Technology* (Maclaren, London, 1962); J. A. Davidson, K. L. Gardner, "Vinyl Polymers (PVC)" in *Kirk-Othmer Encyclopedia of Chemical Technology* vol. 23 (Wiley-Interscience, New York, 3rd ed., 1983) pp 886-936. Book: Sarvetnick, *Polyvinyl Chloride* (Van Nostrand, Reinhold, New York, 1969).

$$*\text{---}CH_2\text{---}CH\text{---}*$$
$$|$$
$$Cl$$

Plastic solid. d 1.406; n 1.54. Stabilizers are necessary to prevent discoloration from exposure to light or heat. Solvents for unmodified polyvinyl chloride of high mol wt: cyclohexanone, methyl cyclohexanone, dimethyl formamide, nitrobenzene, tetrahydrofuran, isophorone, mesityl oxide. Solvents for lower polymers: dipropyl ketone, methyl amyl ketone, methyl isobutyl ketone, acetonylacetone, methyl ethyl ketone, dioxane, methylene chloride.

USE: Rubber substitutes, electric wire and cable-coverings, pliable thin sheeting, film finishes for textiles, non-flammable upholstery, raincoats, tubing, belting, gaskets, shoe soles.

7587. Pomegranate. Granatum. Dried bark of stem or root of *Punica granatum* L., *Punicaceae. Habit.* Mediterranean region; Eastern, Western, and Southern Asia; cultivated in subtropical countries. *Constit.* 0.5-1% alkaloids consisting of pelletierine, methylpelletierine, pseudopelletierine (granatonine), and isopelletierine; mannite, about 20% tannin. Rind of fruit contains about 30% tannin.

THERAP CAT: Formerly as teniafuge.

7588. Ponasterone A. [13408-56-5] $(2\beta,3\beta,5\beta,22R)$-2,3,-14,20,22-Pentahydroxycholest-7-en-6-one; 25-deoxyecdysterone; 25-deoxy-20-hydroxyecdysone. $C_{27}H_{44}O_6$; mol wt 464.63. C 69.80%, H 9.55%, O 20.66%. Polyhydroxylated steroid with strong moulting hormone activity; first phytoecdysteroid to be isolated. Isoln with ponasterones B, C, D, from plant source, *Podocarpus nakaii* Hay., *Podocarpaceae* and structure determn: K. Nakanishi *et al., Chem. Commun.* **1966**, 915; isoln from various Japanese ferns: T. Takemoto *et al., Chem. Pharm. Bull.* **21**, 2336 (1973). Isoln from crustaceans: J. F. McCarthy, *Steroids* **34**, 799 (1979). Stereochemical elucidation: H. Moriyama, K. Nakanishi, *Tetrahedron Lett.* **1968**, 1111; using ^{13}C-NMR: H. Hikino *et al., Chem. Pharm. Bull.* **23**, 125 (1975). Chromatographic sepn: M. Hori, *Steroids* **14**, 33 (1969). HPLC analysis: I. D. Wilson *et al., J. Chromatogr.* **238**, 97 (1982); R. E. Isaac *et al., ibid.* **246**, 317 (1982). Synthesis: G. Hüppi, J. B. Siddall, *Tetrahedron Lett.* **1968**, 1113. Moulting hormone activity on houseflies, silkworms: M. Kobayashi *et al., Steroids* **9**, 529 (1967); on various insects: W. E. Robbins *et al., ibid.* **16**, 105 (1970). Hormonal regulation to increase yield from silkworms: T. Okauchi *et al., US 3941879* (1976 to Takeda). Used

to characterize ecdysteroid receptors in *Drosophilia* cells: P. Maroy *et al., Proc. Natl. Acad. Sci. USA* **75**, 6035 (1978); B. A. Sage *et al., J. Biol. Chem.* **257**, 6373 (1982). *Review of ponasterones:* K. Nakanishi, *Bull. Soc. Chim. Fr.* **1969**, 3475. *See also* Ecdysteroids.

Crystals from ethanol, mp 259-260° (dec). $[\alpha]_D^{15}$ +90° (methanol). uv max (methanol): 244, 326 nm (ε 12400, 130).

7589. Ponazuril. [69004-04-2] 1-Methyl-3-[3-methyl-4-[4-[(trifluoromethyl)sulfonyl]phenoxy]phenyl]-1,3,5-triazine-2,4,-6(1H,3H,5H)-trione; toltrazuril sulfone; Bay Vi 9143; Marquis. $C_{18}H_{14}F_3N_3O_6S$; mol wt 457.38. C 47.27%, H 3.09%, F 12.46%, N 9.19%, O 20.99%, S 7.01%. Metabolite of toltrazuril, *q.v.*; triazine trione antiprotozoal. Prepn: A. Haberkorn *et al.,* **DE 2718799**; *eidem,* **US 4219552** (1978, 1980 both to Bayer). Stereoselective generation by microsomes: E. Benoit *et al., Biochem. Pharmacol.* **46**, 2337 (1993). LC/MS determn in meat and eggs: V. Hormazábal *et al., J. Liq. Chromatogr. Relat. Technol.* **26**, 791 (2003). Activity vs *Sarcocystis neurona,* the causative agent of EPM: D. S. Lindsay *et al., Vet. Parasitol.* **92**, 165 (2000); R. P. Franklin *et al., ibid.* **114**, 123 (2003); vs *Neospora canium*: A. K. Darius *et al., Parasitol. Res.* **92**, 453, 520 (2004).

mp 242°.

THERAP CAT (VET): Antiprotozoal. In treatment of equine protozoal myeloencephalitis (EPM).

7590. Ponceau 3R. [3564-09-8] 3-Hydroxy-4-[(2,4,5-trimethylphenyl)azo]-2,7-naphthalenedisulfonic acid disodium salt; sodium cumeneazo-β-naphthol disulfonate; C.I. Food Red 6; C.I. 16155; FD & C Red no. 1; Ext. D & C Red no. 15. $C_{19}H_{16}N_2$-$Na_2O_7S_2$; mol wt 494.45. C 46.15%, H 3.26%, N 5.67%, Na 9.30%, O 22.65%, S 12.97%. Prepn: *Colour Index* vol. 4 (3rd ed., 1971) p 4092. Toxicity studies: Hansen *et al., Toxicol. Appl. Pharmacol.* **5**, 105 (1963).

Dark red powder. Soluble in water with cherry-red color, slightly in alcohol. Addition of HCl to its aq soln does not change the color, but NaOH produces a yellow ppt. It dissolves in concd H_2SO_4 to a cherry-red soln which does not change color on dilution.

USE: Dyeing wool. Colorant in food, drugs and cosmetics.

7591. Ponceau SX. [4548-53-2] 3-[(2,4-Dimethyl-5-sulfophenyl)azo]-4-hydroxy-1-naphthalenesulfonic acid disodium salt;

FD & C Red No. 4; C.I. Food Red 1; C.I. 14700. $C_{18}H_{14}N_2Na_2$-O_7S_2; mol wt 480.42. C 45.00%, H 2.94%, N 5.83%, Na 9.57%, O 23.31%, S 13.35%. Azo dye. Prepn: E. Nölting, O. Kohn, *Ber.* **19**, 137 (1886). Metabolism: J. L. Radomski, T. J. Mellinger, *J. Pharmacol. Exp. Ther.* **136**, 259 (1962). Toxicity studies: F. C. Lu, A. Lavalle, *Can. Pharm. J.* **97**, 30 (1964); K. J. Davis *et al., Toxicol. Appl. Pharmacol.* **8**, 306 (1966). Determn in maraschino cherries: R. E. Draper, *J. Assoc. Off. Anal. Chem.* **56**, 703 (1973); HPLC determn in lipstick: L. Gagliardi *et al., J. Chromatogr.* **394**, 345 (1987). *Review: IARC Monographs* **8**, 207-214 (1975). *See also: Colour Index* **vol. 4** (3rd ed., 1971) p 4068.

Red crystals. Absorption max (0.02 N CH$_3$COONH$_4$): 500 nm. Sol in water; slightly sol in ethanol. Insol in vegetable oils. Deep red soln in conc H_2SO_4, changing to red ppt on dilution. Orange soln in conc HNO_3, turning yellow. LD$_{50}$ orally in rats: >2 g/kg (Lu, Lavalle).

USE: Dye in externally applied drugs, cosmetics; food colorant in maraschino cherries.

7592. Poppy Capsules. Poppy heads. Fully grown, dried capsules of *Papaver somniferum* L., *Papaveraceae*. *Habit.* Europe, Asia. *Constit.* Capsules: 0.15-0.5% morphine and small amounts of other opium alkaloids. Seed: Fixed oil (poppy oil), albuminoids.

USE: For preparing emulsions — only the white seeds should be used. Seeds are chiefly used for making the oil, and in baking; the bluish-black variety is generally used in the US for baking.

7593. Poppy Oil. Poppy-seed oil. Expressed from poppy seeds. Contains no morphine or other opium alkaloids. *See also* Ethiodized Oil; Iodized Oil.

Pale yellow, drying oil; pleasant odor and taste. d 0.924-0.927. Solidif about $-18°$. n_D^{20} 1.4766-1.4774. Sapon. no. 189-197. Iodine no. 133-158.

USE: Manuf paints, varnishes, and soaps. Edible grades are marketed in Europe and Asia.

7594. Populin. [99-17-2] 2-(Hydroxymethyl)phenyl-β-D-glucopyranoside 6-benzoate; populoside; salicin benzoate. C_{20}-$H_{22}O_8$; mol wt 390.38. C 61.53%, H 5.68%, O 32.79%. In bark and leaves of *Populus tremula* L., *P. nigra* L., *P. nigra* L. var. *italica* Duroi, *P. canadensis* Moench., *P. grandidentate* Michx., and *P. tremuloides* Michx., *Salicaceae*, perhaps also in *Salix helix, Salix purpurea* L. var *helix* (L.) Koch. Isoln: Pearl *et al., J. Org. Chem.* **27**, 2685 (1962). May be made from salicin by melting with benzoic anhydride, or from salicin and benzoyl chloride in presence of potassium hydroxide: Richtmyer, Yeakel, *J. Am. Chem. Soc.* **56**, 2495 (1934). Alkaline cleavage produces benzoic acid and salicin. Enzymatic hydrolysis using taka-diastase, *q.v.*, gives salicyl alcohol and benzoyl glucose: Kitasato, *Biochem. Z.* **190**, 109 (1927).

Dihydrate. Needles from water, sweet taste, like licorice. Becomes anhyd at 100°. mp 179°. $[\alpha]_D^{20}$ $-2.0°$ (c = 5 in pyridine); $[\alpha]_D^{25}$ $-29.7°$ (c = 5 in acetone). One gram dissolves in about 2 liters water, in 42 ml boiling water, in about 100 ml alcohol. Practically insol in ether.

7595. Poractant Alfa. [129069-19-8] PLS; Curosurf. Porcine lung extract composed of 99% polar lipids and 1% apoproteins.

The phospholipid component consists primarily of phosphatidylcholine and its derivatives. Differs from other pulmonary surfactants in its 9.9% sphingomyelin content. Isolation: T. Curstedt *et al., Eur. J. Biochem.* **168**, 255 (1987). Characterization of phospholipid content: E. Redenti *et al., Farmaco* **49**, 285 (1994). Evaluation as surfactant replacement in rabbit: B. Robertson *et al., Eur. J. Pediatr.* **147**, 168 (1988); in comparison with synthetic surfactants: S. Bongrani *et al., Biol. Neonate* **65**, 406 (1994). Multicenter clinical trial in RDS in infants: Collab. Eur. Multicent. Study Group, *Pediatrics* **82**, 683 (1988); H. L. Halliday *et al., Arch. Dis. Child.* **69**, 276 (1993).

THERAP CAT: Pulmonary surfactant; in treatment of respiratory distress syndrome.

7596. Porfimer Sodium. [87806-31-3] CL-184116; Photofrin. Light sensitive polyporphyrin oligomer linked via ethers and esters; purification product of hematoporphyrin derivative. Forms aggregates with combined mol wt ~10000. Prepn: T. J. Dougherty *et al.,* "Photoradiation Therapy - Clinical and Drug Advances" in *Porphyrin Photosensitization,* D. Kessel, T. J. Dougherty, Eds. (Plenum Press, New York, 1983) pp 3-13; T. J. Dougherty *et al.,* US **4649151** (1987 to Health Res.). Structural studies: *idem, Photochem. Photobiol.* **46**, 569 (1987); R. K. Pandey *et al., Biomed. Environ. Mass Spectrom.* **19**, 405 (1990). Photobleaching: J. Moan, D. Kessel, *J. Photochem. Photobiol. B* **1**, 429 (1988); J. D. Spikes, *Photochem. Photobiol.* **55**, 797 (1992). Pharmacokinetics in mice: D. A. Bellnier *et al., ibid.* **50**, 221 (1989). Clinical evaluation in treatment of esophageal cancer: T. Okunaka *et al., Surg. Endosc.* **4**, 150 (1990). Imaging study for premalignant lesions: C. Liebow *et al., Proc. Natl. Acad. Sci. USA* **90**, 1897 (1993). Clinical use as imaging agent for lung cancer: S. Lam *et al., Chest* **97**, 333 (1990).

Orange red color.

USE: Fluorescent imaging of malignancies.

THERAP CAT: Antineoplastic (photosensitizer).

7597. Porfiromycin. [801-52-5] [1a*S*-(1aα,8β,8aα,8bα)]-6-Amino-8-[[(aminocarbonyl)oxy]methyl]-1,1a,2,8,8a,8b-hexahydro-8a-methoxy-1,5-dimethylazirino[2′,3′:3,4]pyrrolo[1,2-*a*]indole-4,7-dione; *N*-methylmitomycin C; U-14743. $C_{16}H_{20}N_4O_5$; mol wt 348.35. C 55.17%, H 5.79%, N 16.08%, O 22.96%. Antibiotic substance isolated from a *Streptomyces ardus* fermentation broth: Herr *et al., Antimicrob. Agents Annu.* **1960**, 23. Isoln from *S. verticillatus* and structure: Webb *et al., J. Am. Chem. Soc.* **84**, 3185, 3187 (1962). Production process: Bohonos *et al.,* US **3219530** (1965 to Am. Cyanamid). Synthesis of (±)-form: F. Nakatsubo *et al., J. Am. Chem. Soc.* **99**, 8115 (1977). For stereochemistry and other synthetic studies, *see* Mitomycins.

Dark purple triclinic crystals, dec 201-201.5°. $[\alpha]_D^{25}$ +275 ±55° (c = 0.1% in methanol); $[\alpha]_D^{25}$ +242 ±100° (c = 0.045% in methanol). uv max (methanol): 217, 360, 555 nm (ε 24600, 23000, 209). Slightly sol in water, moderately sol in polar organic solvents. Practically insol in hydrocarbon solvents.

THERAP CAT: Antibacterial; antineoplastic.

7598. Porofor® BSH. [80-17-1] Benzenesulfonic acid hydrazide; benzenesulfohydrazide; phenylsulfohydrazide. $C_6H_8N_2$-O_2S; mol wt 172.20. C 41.85%, H 4.68%, N 16.27%, O 18.58%, S 18.62%. $C_6H_5SO_2NHNH_2$. *Ref:* Lober, *Angew. Chem.* **64**, 65 (1952).

Crystals, dec 103-104° with the evolution of nitrogen. May be stored indefinitely at temps up to 80°. Sensitive to moist oxidizing agents.

USE: Gas generating agent for use in making foam rubber and foam plastics.

Consult the Name Index before using this section.

7599. Porphine. [101-60-0] $21H,23H$-Porphine; porphin. $C_{20}H_{14}N_4$; mol wt 310.35. C 77.40%, H 4.55%, N 18.05%. Parent substance of the *porphyrins*, a group of compounds found in all living matter which are the basis of respiratory pigments in animals and plants. In porphyrins, side chains are substituted for the hydrogens in the porphine pyrrole rings. *Chlorins* are dihydroporphyrins. *See also:* chlorophyll, hemoglobin, vitamin B_{12}, hematin. Prepn of porphine: Fischer, Gleim, *Ann.* **521**, 157 (1935); Rothemund, *J. Am. Chem. Soc.* **58**, 625 (1936); Krol, *J. Org. Chem.* **24**, 2065 (1959). Study of porphyrin analogs: C. L. Honeybourne *et al., Tetrahedron* **36**, 1833 (1980). Review of biosyntheses of porphyrins and chlorins: A. R. Battersby, E. McDonald in *Porphyrins Metalloporphyrins*, K. M. Smith, Ed. (Elsevier, New York, 1975) pp 61-122. Review of porphyrin syntheses: R. P. Evstigneeva, *Pure Appl. Chem.* **53**, 1129-1140 (1981). Comprehensive seven volume treatise: *The Porphyrins*, D. Dolphin, Ed. (Academic Press, New York, 1978).

Dark red, shiny leaflets from chloroform-methanol. Darkens at 360° but does not melt. The absorption bands are those characteristic of the substituted porphyrins, details in Fischer-Orth, *Die Chemie des Pyrrols* **vol. II**, 1, 175 (1937). Sol in pyridine, dioxane, and phenol; slightly sol in chloroform, bromoform, glacial acetic acid. Almost insol in acetone, methanol, ether. HCl number: 1.7 (Fischer); 3.3 (Rothemund).

Iron salt. $C_{20}H_{12}N_4$.FeCl. Brown cubes from ether.
Magnesium salt. $C_{20}H_{12}MgN_4$. Red needles.
Copper salt. $C_{20}H_{12}N_4$Cu. Brown needles.

7600. Porphobilinogen. [487-90-1] 5-(Aminomethyl)-4-(carboxymethyl)-1H-pyrrole-3-propanoic acid; 2-aminomethyl-pyrrol-3-acetic acid 4-propionic acid. $C_{10}H_{14}N_2O_4$; mol wt 226.23. C 53.09%, H 6.24%, N 12.38%, O 28.29%. An intermediate in the biosynthesis of heme, *q.v.*, found in the urine of patients with acute porphyria: Westall, *Nature* **170**, 614 (1952). Isoln and structure: Cookson, Rimington, *Biochem. J.* **57**, 476 (1954). Synthesis: Jackson, MacDonald, *Can. J. Chem.* **35**, 715 (1957). Chemistry of conversion into porphyrins: Mathewson, Corwin, *J. Am. Chem. Soc.* **83**, 135 (1961).

Monohydrate. Minute pink crystals from dil ammonium acetate soln at pH 4. Dec 172-175°. $pK' = 3.70$; 4.95; 10.1. Slightly sol in water. Converted to uroporphyrins by hot dil HCl or by blood hemolyzates.
Hydrochloride monohydrate. Fine triclinic needles from dil HCl, dec 165-170°. Soluble in water.

7601. Porphyropsin. [9009-58-9] Photoreceptor protein found in the retinal rod cells of fresh water and migrating fish, lampreys, and certain amphibians. Absorption maximum approx 520-530 nm. Composed of the chromophore, 11-*cis*-3-dehydroretinal, *q.v.*, bound to scotopsin, the specific protein component of rod pigments (see Opsins). Biological activity is similar to that of rhodopsin, *q.v.* Isoln from retinas: G. Wald, *Nature* **139**, 1017 (1937); *idem, J. Gen. Physiol.* **22**, 775 (1939). Prepn from 3-dehydroretinal and opsin: *idem, Annu. Rev. Biochem.* **22**, 497 (1953). Methods of purification, prepn and assay: R. Hubbard *et al., Methods Enzymol.* **18**, 615-653 (1971). Exposure to light initiates the conversion of porphyropsin through a series of distinct intermediates to yield opsin and *trans*-3-dehydroretinal. Bleaching kinetics and photochemistry: T. Yoshizawa in *Handbook of Sensory Physiology* **Vol. VII**(2), H. J. A. Dartnall, Ed. (Springer-Verlag, New York, 1972) pp 146-179. Porphyropsin may co-exist with rhodopsin in the retinas of certain amphibians and fish: T. E. Reuter *et al., J. Gen. Physiol.* **58**, 351 (1971). Environmental effect on visual pigment formation and interconversion: P. Witkovsky *et al., ibid.* **72**, 821 (1978); A. T. C. Tsin, D. D. Beatty, *Exp. Eye Res.* **30**, 143 (1980). *Review:* G. Wald, *Science* **162**, 230-239 (1968).

7602. Posaconazole. [171228-49-2] 2,5-Anhydro-1,3,4-trideoxy-2-C-(2,4-difluorophenyl)-4-[[4-[4-[4-[1-[(1S,2S)-1-ethyl-2-hydroxypropyl]-1,5-dihydro-5-oxo-4H-1,2,4-triazol-4-yl]phenyl]-1-piperazinyl]phenoxy]methyl]-1-(1H-1,2,4-triazol-1-yl)-D-*threo*-pentitol; (3R-*cis*)-4-[4-[4-[4-[5-(2,4-difluorophenyl)-5-(1,2,4-triazol-1-ylmethyl)tetrahydrofuran-3-ylmethoxy]phenyl]piperazin-1-yl]phenyl]-2-[1(S)-ethyl-2(S)-hydroxypropyl]-3,4-dihydro-2H-1,2,4-triazol-3-one; Sch-56592; Noxafil. $C_{37}H_{42}F_2N_8O_4$; mol wt 700.78. C 63.41%, H 6.04%, F 5.42%, N 15.99%, O 9.13%. Orally active triazole antifungal. Prepn: A. K. Saksena *et al.,* **WO 9517407**; *eidem,* **US 5661151** (1995, 1997 both to Schering); *eidem, Tetrahedron Lett.* **37**, 5657 (1996). Comparative antifungal spectrum: A. Cacciapuoti *et al., Antimicrob. Agents Chemother.* **44**, 2017 (2000). Pharmacokinetics, safety and tolerability: R. Courtney *et al., ibid.* **47**, 2788 (2003). HPLC determn in serum: H. Kim *et al., J. Chromatogr. B* **738**, 93 (2000). Review of development: A. K. Saksena *et al.* in *Anti-Infectives: Recent Advances in Chemistry and Structure Activity Relationships* (Royal Soc. Chem., Cambridge, 1997) pp 180-199; and clinical efficacy in fungal infections: R. Herbrecht, *Int. J. Clin. Pract.* **58**, 612-624 (2004).

White solid, mp 170-172°.
THERAP CAT: Antifungal.

7603. Posatirelin. [78664-73-0] N-[(6-oxo-2-piperidinyl)-carbonyl]-L-leucyl-L-prolinamide; (2S)-N-[(1S)-1-[[(2S)-2-carbamoyl-1-pyrrolidinyl]carbonyl]-3-methylbutyl]-6-oxopipecolamide; L-6-ketopiperidine-2-carbonyl-L-leucyl-L-proline amide; RGH-2202; Pyladox. $C_{17}H_{28}N_4O_4$; mol wt 352.43. C 57.94%, H 8.01%, N 15.90%, O 18.16%. Thyrotropin releasing hormone analog. Prepn: L. Kisfaludy *et al.,* **DE 3024256** (1981 to Gedeon Richter); *eidem,* **US 4386073** (1983 to Patentbureau Danubia); T. Szirtes *et al., J. Med. Chem.* **29**, 1654 (1986). Pharmacology: M. Oka *et al., Arzneim.-Forsch.* **39**, 297 (1989). Clinical efficacy in Alzheimer's disease: L. Parnetti *et al., Acta Neurol. Scand.* **92**, 135 (1995).

White crystals from ethanol/diethyl ether, mp 214-216°. $[\alpha]_D^{25}$ −80.2° (c = 1 in acetic acid).
THERAP CAT: Nootropic.

7604. Potassium. [7440-09-7] Kalium. K; at. wt 39.0983; at. no. 19; valence 1. Group IA (1). Alkali metal. Occurrence in earth's crust: 2.59% by wt. Naturally occurring isotopes: 39 (93.26%); 40 (0.012%); 41 (6.73%); ^{40}K is radioactive: $T_{1/2}$ 1.27 × 10⁹ years; known isotopes range in mass number from 35 to 54. Found mainly as the chloride (sylvite); also in the aluminosilicates *orthoclase*, and *microcline* (KAlSi₃O₈), and as *carnallite* (KCl.-MgCl₂.6H₂O). Major essential element for plant growth. First prepd in free form by Davy in 1807 by electrolysis of fused potassium hydroxide. Produced industrially by chemical reduction. Prepns: Hackspill, *Helv. Chim. Acta* **11**, 1003 (1928); Jackson, Werner, **US 2480655** (1949 to Mine Safety Appliances Co.). NMR spectrum of potassium anion (K⁻): P. P. Edwards *et al.*, *Nature* **317**, 242 (1985). *Reviews:* Whaley, "Sodium, Potassium, Rubidium, Cesium, and Francium" in *Comprehensive Inorganic Chemistry* vol. 1, J. C. Bailar, Jr. *et al.*, Eds. (Pergamon Press, Oxford, 1973) pp 369-529; *Chemistry of the Elements* N. N. Greenwood, A. Earnshaw, Eds. (Pergamon Press, New York, 1984) pp 75-116; K.-W. Chiu in *Kirk-Othmer Encyclopedia of Chemical Technology* vol. 19 (Wiley-Interscience, New York, 4th ed., 1996) pp 1047-1057.

Soft, silvery-white metal; body-centered cubic structure; tarnishes on exposure to air; becomes brittle at low temps; mp 63.2°. bp 765.5°. d^{20} 0.856. Specific heat (0°): 0.176 cal/g deg. Thermal conductivity (cal/sec °C cm): 0.23 (21°); 0.956 (400°). Sol in liq ammonia, ethylenediamine, aniline; sol in several metals; forms liquid alloys with other alkali metals. Emits characteristic violet color (766.5 nm) in flame. One of the most active metals; E^0 (aq) K/K^+ 2.922 V. Reacts vigorously with oxygen; with water even at −100°; with acids; with the halogens, igniting with bromine and iodine. Molten metal reacts with sulfur; with hydrogen sulfide. Reacts with hydrogen slowly at 200°, rapidly at 350-400°. Reacts slowly with anhydr hydrogen halides at room temp; molten metal ignites in the reaction. Reduces silicates, sulfates, nitrates, carbonates, phosphates, oxides and hydroxides of the heavy metals, often with the separation of the metal. Reacts with organic compds containing active groups. Inert to saturated aliphatic and to aromatic hydrocarbons. *Keep under liquid containing no oxygen*, e.g., liquid petrolatum, petroleum, etc.

Caution: Direct contact with metal may be corrosive and cause skin and eye burns. *See: Fire Protection Guide to Hazardous Materials* (National Fire Protection Assoc., Quincy, MA, 12th ed., 1997) Section 49, p 109.

USE: In synthesis of inorganic potassium compds; in organic syntheses involving condensation, dehalogenation, reduction, and polymerization reactions. As heat transfer medium together with sodium: *Chem. Eng. News* **33**, 648 (1955). Radioactive decay of ⁴⁰K to ⁴⁰Ar used as tool for geological dating.

7605. Potassium Acetate. [127-08-2] $C_2H_3KO_2$; mol wt 98.14. C 24.48%, H 3.08%, K 39.84%, O 32.61%. CH_3COOK.
Colorless, lustrous, rapidly deliquesc crystals or white cryst powder or flakes. d^{25} 1.57. mp 292°. One gram dissolves in 0.5 ml water, 0.2 ml boiling water, 2.9 ml alcohol. The aq soln is alkaline to litmus. pH of 0.1 molar aq soln 9.7. *Keep tightly closed.* LD_{50} orally in rats: 3.25 g/kg, H. F. Smyth *et al., Am. Ind. Hyg. Assoc. J.* **30**, 470 (1969).
THERAP CAT: Electrolyte replenisher; potassium supplement.

7606. Potassium p-Aminobenzoate. [138-84-1] *p*-Aminobenzoic acid potassium salt; potassium *para*-aminobenzoate; KPABA; Potaba. $C_7H_6KNO_2$; mol wt 175.23. C 47.98%, H 3.45%, K 22.31%, N 7.99%, O 18.26%. Prepn: E. A. Meyers *et al., J. Am. Chem. Soc.* **89**, 3565 (1967). Crystal structure: G. S. Ciminago, *C.R. Seances Acad. Sci. Ser. C* **267**, 1402 (1968). Antifibrotic efficacy in idiopathic pulmonary fibrosis: U. H. Cegla *et al., Pneumonologie* **152**, 75 (1975); in Peyronie's disease: A. J. Riley, *Br. J. Sex. Med.* **6**, 29 (1970); G. Williams, N. A. Green, *Br. J. Urol.* **52**, 392 (1980).

Crystals from alcohol. Saline taste. Slightly alkaline to litmus. pH of 1% soln about 7. Very freely sol in water, less sol in alc. Practically insol in ether. Reported to cause less gastric irritation than the free acid or the sodium salt.
USE: Catalyst in the manuf of condensation polymers of polyglycol ethers.
THERAP CAT: Antifibrotic.

7607. Potassium Arsenate. [7784-41-0] Potassium acid arsenate; potassium dihydrogen arsenate; Macquer's salt. AsH_2KO_4; mol wt 180.03. As 41.62%, H 1.12%, K 21.72%, O 35.55%. KH_2AsO_4.
Colorless crystals or white, cryst mass or powder. *Poisonous!* d 2.8. Sol in 5.5 parts cold, more sol in hot water, slowly in 1.6 parts glycerol. Insol in alcohol.
USE: In the textile, tanning, and paper industries. In insecticidal formulations (especially fly paper).

7608. Potassium Arsenite. [13464-35-2] Commercial material prepd as variable composition; approx $KH(AsO_2)_2.H_2O$. Toxicity data: A. J. Lehman, *Q. Bull. Assoc. Food Drug Off. U.S.* **15**, 122 (1951). Evaluation of carcinogenic risk: *IARC Monographs* **2**, 48-73 (1973); *Comm. Eur. Communities, Toxicol. Chem.* **3**, 53-58 (1991).
White, hygroscopic powder; gradually dec on exposure to air (by the CO_2). *Very poisonous!* Sol in water. *Keep well closed.* LD_{50} orally in rats: 14 mg/kg (Lehman).
Potassium arsenite solution. [1332-10-1] Fowler's solution; arsenical solution. Prepd by dissolving arsenic trioxide in aq potassium bicarbonate and ethanol. Toxicity study: H. Tinwell *et al., Environ. Health Perspect.* **95**, 205 (1991).
USE: In manuf of mirrors to reduce the silver salt to metallic silver.
THERAP CAT: Fowler's soln formerly as antineoplastic, dermatologic.
THERAP CAT (VET): Fowler's soln has been used as an alterative or tonic, in pulmonary emphysema, chronic coughs, anemias, chronic skin diseases.

7609. Potassium Bicarbonate. [298-14-6] Potassium acid carbonate; K-Lyte. $CHKO_3$; mol wt 100.12. C 12.00%, H 1.01%, K 39.05%, O 47.94%. $KHCO_3$. Contains not less than 99% $KHCO_3$.
Colorless, transparent crystals, white granules or powder. Sol in 2.8 parts water, 2 parts water at 50°. Almost insol in alcohol. pH: 8.2 (in 0.1 molar concn).
USE: In baking powders, effervescent salts.
THERAP CAT: Potassium supplement.

7610. Potassium Bifluoride. [7789-29-9] Potassium acid fluoride; potassium hydrogen fluoride. F_2HK; mol wt 78.10. F 48.65%, H 1.29%, K 50.06%. KF.HF. Prepd according to the eq $KOH + 2HF = KHF_2 + H_2O$: Lange, Eichler, *Z. Phys. Chem.* **129**, 285 (1927); Kwasnik in *Handbook of Preparative Inorganic Chemistry* vol. 1, G. Brauer, Ed. (Academic Press, New York, 2nd ed., 1963) p 237. Made commercially from potassium carbonate and hydrofluoric acid.
Tetragonal crystals. *Poisonous!* d 2.37. mp 238.7°. Transformation pt 195°. Soly in water (g/100 ml): 30.1 (10°); 39.2 (20°); 114.0 (80°). Sol in dil alc. Insol in abs alc.
Caution: Corrosive and irritating to skin, mucous membranes.
USE: In the prepn of pure potassium fluoride; as an electrolyte in the manuf of fluorine; frosting glass; treating coal to prevent slag formation; flux for silver solders; catalyst in the alkylation of benzene with olefins.

7611. Potassium Binoxalate. [127-95-7] Potassium acid oxalate; salt of sorrel; sal acetosella. C_2HKO_4; mol wt 128.13. C 18.75%, H 0.79%, K 30.51%, O 49.95%. KOOCCOOH. Incorrectly *salt of lemon*. The same synonyms apply to potassium tetraoxalate.
Monohydrate. White, odorless crystals. *Poisonous!* d 2.0. Sol in 40 parts cold, 6 parts boiling water, slightly in alcohol. pH of 0.1 molar aq soln: 2.7.
USE: Removing ink stains; scouring metals, cleaning wood; photography; as mordant in dyeing; bleaching stearic acids.

7612. Potassium Biphthalate. [877-24-7] Phthalic acid potassium acid salt; potassium acid phthalate; potassium hydrogen phthalate; acid potassium phthalate. $C_8H_5KO_4$; mol wt 204.22. C 47.05%, H 2.47%, K 19.15%, O 31.34%. $HOOCC_6H_4COOK$. Prepd by half-neutralization of a phthalic anhydride soln: F. J. Welcher, *Organic Analytical Reagents* vol. 2 (Van Nostrand, New York, 1947) pp 75-79.

Consult the Name Index before using this section.

Orthorhombic crystals, stable in air. d_4^{25} 1.636. Acid reaction; pH of $0.05M$ aq soln at $25° = 4.005$ (glass electrode). Sol in about 12 parts cold water, 3 parts boiling water; slightly sol in alcohol.

USE: As primary standard for preparing volumetric alkali solns, also as a buffer in pH determinations.

7613. Potassium Bisulfate. [7646-93-7] Potassium acid sulfate; potassium hydrogen sulfate; sal enixum. HKO_4S; mol wt 136.17. H 0.74%, K 28.71%, O 47.00%, S 23.55%. $KHSO_4$.

White, deliquesc crystals, pieces, or granules. d 2.24. mp 197°; at higher temp loses water and is converted into pyrosulfate. Sol in 1.8 parts water, 0.85 part boiling water. *Keep well closed.*

USE: As flux in analysis of ores and siliceous compds.

THERAP CAT: Cathartic.

7614. Potassium Bisulfide. [1310-61-8] Potassium hydrosulfide; potassium hydrogen sulfide; potassium sulfhydrate. HKS; mol wt 72.17. H 1.40%, K 54.18%, S 44.43%. KHS. Prepd industrially from $Ca(HS)_2$ and K_2SO_4: Hene, **DE 380385** (1922); from H_2S and K_2S: Bassett, **US 1662735** (1925); Strosacker, Jones, **US 1771384** (1926 to Dow). Prepn of pure material by the action of dry H_2S upon potassium metal dissolved in abs ethanol: Rule, *J. Chem. Soc.* **99**, 558, 564 (1911); West, *Z. Kristallogr.* **88**, 102 (1934).

Colorless, deliquescent crystals or white, strongly hygroscopic, cryst mass. Usually present as the hemihydrate. Trigonal system. d 1.70. Rapidly becomes yellow on exposure to air with formation of polysulfides and H_2S. Becomes anhydr at 175-200°. mp 450-510° forming a dark red liquid. Heat of formation: +62.5 kcal. Heat of soln at 17°: +0.77 kcal, for hemihydrate at 16°: +0.62 kcal. Freely sol in water, alcohol.

7615. Potassium Bitartrate. [868-14-4] Potassium acid tartrate; acid potassium tartrate; potassium hydrogen tartrate; cream of tartar; cremor tartari; faecula; faecla. $C_4H_5KO_6$; mol wt 188.18. C 25.53%, H 2.68%, K 20.78%, O 51.01%. $KHC_4H_4O_6$. Obtained from the sediments in the manuf of wine, known as argols or wine lees. The salt is at least 99.5% pure. *See also* Argol and Tartaric Acid.

Colorless crystals or white, cryst powder; pleasant acidulous taste. One gram dissolves in 162 ml water, in 16 ml boiling water, 8820 ml alcohol; readily sol in dil mineral acids, in solns of alkalies or borax. Soly in water also given as about 0.4% at 10° to about 6% at 100°.

USE: Largely in baking powders; coloring metals; galvanic tinning of metals; reducer of CrO_3 in mordants for wool.

THERAP CAT: Cathartic.

THERAP CAT (VET): Laxative, diuretic.

7616. Potassium Borohydride. [13762-51-1] Potassium tetrahydroborate. BH_4K; mol wt 53.94. B 20.04%, H 7.47%, K 72.48%. KBH_4. Prepn: H. I. Schlesinger *et al., J. Am. Chem. Soc.* **75**, 199 (1953). Commercial process: M. D. Banus *et al., ibid.* **76**, 3848 (1954). NMR relaxation study: T. Tsang, T. C. Farrar, *J. Chem. Phys.* **50**, 3498 (1969); IR and Raman spectra: K. B. Harvey, N. R. McQuaker, *Can. J. Chem.* **49**, 3272 (1971). Use as reducing agent in protein labelling: E. K. J. Pauwels *et al., Nucl. Med. Biol.* **20**, 825 (1993); in simple reductions: C. Than *et al., J. Labelled Compd. Radiopharm.* **38**, 693 (1996); J. C. Briggs *et al., Tetrahedron* **53**, 3943 (1997). Review of potassium and other metal tetrahydroborates: B. D. James, M. G. H. Wallbridge, *Prog. Inorg. Chem.* **11**, 99-231 (1970).

Non-hygroscopic crystals. Stable to air. d 1.11. n_D 1.490. Dec commences at about 500°. Supports combustion. Negative heat of soln in H_2O = 6.3 kcal/mol. Soly (w/w) in water at 25°: 19%; liq ammonia at 25°: 20%; ethylenediamine at 75°: 3.9%; methanol at 20°: 0.7%; DMF at 20°: 15.0%. 0.25 g dissolves in 100 g of 95% ethanol at 25°. Soly in a 4:1 water-methanol mixture: 13 g/100 g. Insol (< 0.01%) in isopropylamine, benzene, hexane, ether, dioxane, tetrahydrofuran and acetonitrile. Alkaline aq solutions are stable.

USE: Reducing agent; source of H^-.

7617. Potassium Bromate. [7758-01-2] $BrKO_3$; mol wt 167.00. Br 47.85%, K 23.41%, O 28.74%. $KBrO_3$.

White crystals or granules. d 3.27. mp about 350°, decomposing at about 370° with evolution of oxygen. Sol in 12.5 parts water, 2 parts boiling water. Almost insol in alc.

Caution: Ingestion may cause vomiting, diarrhea, methemoglobinemia, renal injury.

USE: Bread- and flour-improving agent; in analytical chemistry.

7618. Potassium Bromide. [7758-02-3] BrK; mol wt 119.00. Br 67.15%, K 32.86%. KBr. Continuous electrolytic process of prepn: Maylott, Elkins, **US 2989450** (1961 to Dow).

Colorless crystals or white granules or powder. d 2.75. mp 730°. One gram dissolves in 1.5 ml water, 1 ml boiling water, 250 ml alc, 4.6 ml glycerol. The aq soln is neutral.

Caution: Large doses cause CNS depression. Prolonged intake may cause mental deterioration, acneform skin eruptions.

USE: Manuf photographic papers and plates; process engraving.

THERAP CAT: Sedative, anticonvulsant.

THERAP CAT (VET): Sedative.

7619. Potassium Carbonate. [584-08-7] Salt of tartar; pearl ash. CK_2O_3; mol wt 138.21. C 8.69%, K 56.58%, O 34.73%. K_2CO_3.

Hygroscopic, odorless granules or granular powder. d 2.29; mp 891°. Sol in 1 part cold, 0.7 part boiling water. Practically insol in alcohol. Its aq soln is strongly alkaline. pH 11.6. *Keep tightly closed.* LD_{50} orally in rats: 1.87 g/kg, H. F. Smyth *et al., Am. Ind. Hyg. Assoc. J.* **30**, 470 (1969).

Sesquihydrate. Small granular crystals. When it contains the full amount of water (16.36%) it is not hygroscopic. Sol in less than 1 part water. Practically insol in alcohol. The aq soln is strongly alkaline.

Caution: Irritant, caustic.

USE: Manuf soap, glass, pottery, smalts and many potassium salts; in process engraving and lithography; tanning and finishing leather; liq shampoos; for removal of water from organic liqs; in anal. chemistry. Pharmaceutic aid (alkalizer).

7620. Potassium Chlorate. [3811-04-9] Potcrate. $ClKO_3$; mol wt 122.55. Cl 28.93%, K 31.90%, O 39.17%. $KClO_3$. Contains at least 99% $KClO_3$.

Colorless, lustrous crystals, or white granules or powder. d 2.32. mp 368°; above this temp it dec into perchlorate and oxygen. One gram dissolves slowly in 16.5 ml water, 1.8 ml boiling water, about 50 ml glycerol. Almost insol in alcohol. *Keep out of contact with organic matter or other oxidizable substances. Caution:* Explodes with sulfuric acid; inflames with explosion if triturated with any organic substances, sulfur, phosphorus, sulfite, hypophosphite, and other oxidizable substances. *Incompat.* Iodides, tartaric acid.

Caution: Irritating to G.I. tract, kidney; can cause hemolysis of red blood cells and methemoglobinemia: *Clinical Toxicology of Commercial Products,* R. E. Gosselin *et al.,* Eds. (Williams & Wilkins, Baltimore, 5th ed., 1984) Section II, p 112; Section III, pp 74-77.

USE: Explosives; fireworks; matches; printing and dyeing cotton and wool black; manuf aniline black and other dyes; source of oxygen; in chemical analyses.

THERAP CAT: Formerly as topical antiseptic.

THERAP CAT (VET): In dilute soln as antiseptic mouthwash.

7621. Potassium Chloride. [7447-40-7] Diffu-K; Kaleorid; Kalitabs; Kaon-Cl; Kay-Cee-L; K-Contin; K-Dur; Lento-Kalium; Potassiject; Slow-K; Span-K. ClK; mol wt 74.55. Cl 47.56%, K 52.45%. KCl. Occurs in nature as the mineral *sylvine* or *sylvite.* Industrial prepns: *Faith, Keyes & Clark's Industrial Chemicals,* F. A. Lowenheim, M. K. Moran, Eds. (Wiley-Interscience, New York, 4th ed., 1975) pp 666-673.

White crystals or crystalline powder. d 1.98. mp 773°. One gram dissolves in 2.8 ml water, 1.8 ml boiling water, 14 ml glycerol, about 250 ml alcohol. Insol in ether, acetone. Hydrochloric acid, sodium or magnesium chlorides diminish its soly in water. d of saturated aq soln at 15° is 1.172. pH: about 7.

Caution: Large doses by mouth can cause G.I. irritation, purging, weakness and circulatory disturbances.

USE: In photography. In buffer solns, electrode cells.

THERAP CAT: Electrolyte replenisher.

THERAP CAT (VET): Potassium supplement.

7622. Potassium Chromate(VI). [7789-00-6] Neutral potassium chromate. CrK_2O_4; mol wt 194.19. Cr 26.78%, K 40.27%, O 32.96%. K_2CrO_4.

Lemon-yellow crystals; d 2.73; mp 975°. Sol in 1.6 parts cold, 1.2 parts boiling water. Insol in alcohol. The aq soln is alkaline to litmus or phenolphthalein.

USE: Has a limited application in enamels, finishing leather, rustproofing of metals, being replaced by the sodium salt; as reagent in analytical chemistry.

7623. Potassium Citrate. [866-84-2] 2-Hydroxy-1,2,3-propanetricarboxylic acid tripotassium salt; tripotassium citrate. $C_6H_5K_3O_7$; mol wt 306.39. C 23.52%, H 1.64%, K 38.28%, O 36.55%. $K_3C_6H_5O_7$. Manufacturing process: G. Kominek, US 3819696 (1974 to Jungbunzlauer). Effect on urinary chemistry and crystallization of stone forming salts: K. Sakhaee et al., *Kidney Int.* **24**, 348 (1983). Use in oral rehydration solutions: M. R. Islam, *Arch. Dis. Child.* **60**, 852 (1985). Clinical trial in nephrolithiasis: C. Y. C. Pak et al., *J. Urol.* **134**, 11 (1985); following shockwave lithotripsy: T. Soygür et al., *J. Endourol.* **16**, 149 (2002).

Monohydrate. [6100-05-6] K-CIT-V; Urocit-K. $C_6H_5K_3O_7 \cdot H_2O$; mol wt 324.41. White crystals, granules or powder; odorless with cooling, salty taste. Loses its water at 180°. One gram dissolves in 0.65 ml water; very slowly in 2.5 ml glycerol. Practically insol in alcohol. The aq soln is alkaline to litmus; pH about 8.5.

USE: In foods and beverages as buffering, sequestering or emulsifying agent.

THERAP CAT: Alkalinizing agent; antiurolithic.

THERAP CAT (VET): Alkalinizing agent; antiurolithic.

7624. Potassium Citrate, Monobasic. [866-83-1] Monopotassium citrate. $C_6H_7KO_7$; mol wt 230.21. C 31.30%, H 3.06%, K 16.98%, O 48.65%. $KH_2C_6H_5O_7$.

White, cryst powder. Sol in water; the soln is subject to molding.

USE: A 0.05 molal solution as standard for pH scale (at 25° 3.776): Staples, Bates, *J. Res. Natl. Bur. Stand.* **73A**, 37 (1969).

7625. Potassium Cyanate. [590-28-3] CKNO; mol wt 81.12. C 14.81%, K 48.20%, N 17.27%, O 19.72%. Inhibitor of sickling of erythrocytes *in vitro:* Cerami, Manning, *Proc. Natl. Acad. Sci. USA* **68**, 1180 (1971). *See also* Sodium Cyanate. Pharmacology: A. Cerami et al., *J. Pharmacol. Exp. Ther.* **185**, 653 (1973). Brief review: *Dangerous Prop. Ind. Mater. Rep.* **13**, 408-415 (1993).

White, cryst powder. d 2.05. Sol in water, very slightly in alcohol. LD_{50} i.p. in mice: 320 mg/kg (Cerami).

7626. Potassium Cyanide. [151-50-8] CKN; mol wt 65.12. C 18.44%, K 60.04%, N 21.51%. KCN. Article of commerce contains about 95% KCN. Toxicity study: Hayes, *Toxicol. Appl. Pharmacol.* **11**, 327 (1967). Review of toxicology and human exposure: *Toxicological Profile for Cyanide* (PB98-101207, 1997) 291 pp.

White, deliquesc, granular powder or fused pieces; odor of HCN. *Violent poison!* On exposure to air it is gradually dec by CO_2 and moisture. d 1.52; mp 634°. Sol in 2 parts cold, 1 part boiling water, 2 parts glycerol, 100 parts alcohol, 25 parts methanol. The aq soln is strongly alkaline and rapidly dec. pH of 0.1N aq soln: 11.0. *Keep tightly closed and protected from light.* LD_{50} orally in rats: 10 mg/kg (Hayes).

Caution: Potential symptoms of overexposure are irritation of eyes, skin and upper respiratory system; weakness, headache and confusion; nausea, vomiting; increased rate of respiration; slow gasping respiration; asphyxia; thyroid and blood changes. *See NIOSH Pocket Guide to Chemical Hazards* (DHHS/NIOSH 97-140, 1997) p 262.

USE: Extracting gold and silver from ores; electroplating baths; silver plating; case hardening steel by liquid nitriding; reagent in analytical chemistry.

7627. Potassium Dichromate(VI). [7778-50-9] Potassium bichromate. $Cr_2K_2O_7$; mol wt 294.18. Cr 35.35%, K 26.58%, O 38.07%. $K_2Cr_2O_7$. In the U.S.A. it is usually prepared by the reaction of potassium chloride on sodium dichromate: Vetter in *Kirk-Othmer Encyclopedia of Chemical Technology* **vol. 3** (Interscience, New York, 1949) p 951; Hartford, Copson, *ibid.* **vol. 5** (2nd ed., 1964) pp 484-488. In Germany it is obtained from potassium chromate produced by roasting the chrome ore with KOH. *Ref:* Müller, Glissmann in *Ullmanns Encyklopädie der technischen Chemie* **vol. 5** (Munich, 3rd ed., 1954) p 580.

Bright orange-red crystals. Not hygroscopic or deliquescent (difference from sodium dichromate). Crystal habit: prismatic. Crystal system: triclinic pinacoidal, transition to monoclinic at 241.6°. d_4^{25} 2.676. Bulk density: 100 lbs/cu ft. mp 398°. Dec at about 500°. Heat of fusion 29.8 cal/g. Heat of soln −62.5 cal/g. Specific heat 0.186 at 16° −98°. Soluble in water. A satd aq soln contains at 0°: 4.3%, at 20°: 11.7%, at 40°: 20.9%, at 60°: 31.3%, at 80°: 42.0%, at 100°: 50.2%. Acid reaction: A 1% aq soln has a pH of 4.04 and a 10% soln has a pH of 3.57.

Caution: Corrosive poison if ingested. Industrial contact may result in ulceration of hands, destruction of mucous membranes and perforation of nasal septum. *See* E. Browning, *Toxicity of Industrial Metals* (Appleton-Century Crofts, New York, 2nd ed., 1969) pp 119-131. *See also* Chromium.

USE: In tanning leather, dyeing, painting, decorating porcelain, printing, photolithography, pigment-prints, staining wood, pyrotechnics, safety matches; for bleaching palm oil, wax, and sponges; waterproofing fabrics; as oxidizer in the manuf of organic chemicals; in electric batteries; as depolarizer for dry cells. As corrosion inhibitor in preference to sodium dichromate where lower soly is advantageous. Pharmaceutic aid (oxidizing agent).

THERAP CAT (VET): Caustic.

7628. Potassium Dicyanoaurate(I). [13967-50-5] Gold potassium cyanide; potassium aurocyanide. C_2AuKN_2; mol wt 288.10. C 8.34%, Au 68.37%, K 13.57%, N 9.72%. $KAu(CN)_2$. Prepd by electrolysis of Au in KCN: Glassford, Napier, *Philos. Mag.* **25**, 61 (1844).

Dihydrate. Cryst powder. One gram dissolves in 7 ml water, 0.5 ml boiling water; slightly sol in alcohol. Practically insol in ether.

USE: For electroplating.

7629. Potassium Diformate. [20642-05-1] Formic acid potassium salt (2:1); potassium hydrogen diformate; Formi. $C_2H_3KO_4$; mol wt 130.14. C 18.46%, H 2.32%, K 30.04%, O 49.18%. $KH(HCOO)_2$. Conjugated salt of potassium formate and formic acid. Feed additive for pigs; promotes growth and controls microbial activity by decreasing the pH of the digestive tract. Prepn: E. Groschuff, *Ber.* **36**, 1783 (1903). X-ray crystal structure: G. Larsson, I. Nahringbauer, *Acta Crystallogr.* **B24**, 666 (1968). Electron density study: K. Hermansson, R. Tellgren, *ibid.* **B45**, 252 (1989). Growth-promoting effects in pigs: B. R. Paulicks et al., *Agribiol. Res.* **49**, 318 (1996); M. Kirchgessner et al., *ibid.* **50**, 1 (1997). Antimicrobial effects in pig digestive tracts: N. Canibe et al., *J. Anim. Sci.* **79**, 2123 (2001).

Crystals from ethanol, mp 108.6°.

THERAP CAT (VET): Antimicrobial; growth promotant.

7630. Potassium Ferricyanide. [13746-66-2] Tripotassium hexakis(cyano-C)ferrate(3−); potassium hexacyanoferrate(III); red prussiate of potash. $C_6FeK_3N_6$; mol wt 329.24. C 21.89%, Fe 16.96%, K 35.63%, N 25.53%. $K_3Fe(CN)_6$.

Ruby-red crystals. d 1.89. Slowly sol in 2.5 parts cold water, in 1.3 parts boiling water; slightly sol in alc; dec by acids. The aq soln dec slowly on standing. *Protect from light.*

USE: Chiefly for blueprints; in photography; also for staining wood, dyeing wool, calico printing, as etching liquid (Mercer's liquor), tempering iron and steel; in electroplating; as a mild oxidizing agent in organic synthesis; in analytical chemistry.

7631. Potassium Ferrocyanide. [13943-58-3] Tetrapotassium hexakis(cyano-C)ferrate(4−); potassium hexacyanoferrate(II); yellow prussiate of potash. $C_6FeK_4N_6$; mol wt 368.34. C 19.56%, Fe 15.16%, K 42.46%, N 22.82%. $K_4Fe(CN)_6$. Review of properties, chemistry and syntheses: *The Chemistry of Ferrocyanides,* American Cyanamid Co. (Beacon Press, New York, 1953) 112 p.

Trihydrate. Soft, slightly efflorescent crystals; begins to lose water at 60°, becomes anhydr at 100°. d 1.85.

7632. Potassium Fluoride. [7789-23-3] FK; mol wt 58.10. F 32.70%, K 67.29%. KF. Prepd by thermal decompn of KHF_2 or by neutralizing HF with K_2CO_3: Lange, Eichler, *Z. Phys. Chem.* **129**, 285, 286 (1927); Kwasnik in *Handbook of Preparative Inorganic Chemistry* **vol. 1**, G. Brauer, Ed. (Academic Press, New York, 2nd ed., 1963) p 236. Toxicity data: Simonin, *C.R. Seances Soc. Biol. Ses Fil.* **124**, 133 (1937).

Cubic crystals (NaCl lattice). Usually obtained as white, deliquesc powder or solid. *Poisonous!* d 2.481. mp 859.9°. bp 1505°. Soly in water (g/100 ml): 92.3 (18°); 96.4 (21°). Very freely sol in boiling water. Also sol in aq HF, liq NH_3. Insol in alcohol unless water is present. May be stored in aluminum containers. Attracts moisture from the air. Aq solns corrode glass and porcelain. MLD in guinea pigs (mg/kg): 250 orally, 350 s.c.; in frogs (mg/kg): 375 s.c. (Simonin).

Dihydrate. Monoclinic crystals, mp 41°. Soly in water (18°): 349.3 g/100 ml.

Tetrahydrate. Crystals, mp 19.3°.

Caution: Irritating to skin, eyes, mucous membranes.

USE: In the fluorination of organic compds; in flux for hard solder; to prevent unwanted fermentations; in insecticide formulations; for frosting glass.

7633. Potassium Formate. [590-29-4] Formic acid potassium salt. $CHKO_2$; mol wt 84.12. C 14.28%, H 1.20%, K 46.48%, O 38.04%. HCOOK. Environmentally friendly, biodegradable source of potassium ion. Prepn: E. Groschuff, *Ber.* **36**, 1783 (1903); and complex formation with formic acid: J. Kendall, H. Adler, *J. Am. Chem. Soc.* **43**, 1470 (1921). Crystal structure: B. F. Mentzen, Y. Oddon, *Inorg. Chim. Acta* **43**, 237 (1980); J. W. Bats, H. Fuess, *Acta Crystallogr.* **B36**, 1940 (1980). Properties and applications as a secondary refrigerant: A. Aittomäki, A. Lahti, *Int. J. Refrig.* **20**, 276 (1997).

mp 157° (Groschuff); also reported as mp 167.5 ±0.5° (Kendall). d^{18} 1.95. Very sol in water. The aq soln is practically neutral. Exceedingly hygroscopic.

USE: Reducing agent; secondary refrigerant; anti-oxidant in oil drilling applications.

7634. Potassium Guaiacolsulfonate. [1321-14-8] 3-Hydroxy-4-methoxybenzenesulfonic acid monopotassium salt mixt with monopotassium 4-hydroxy-3-methoxybenzenesulfonate; sulfogaiacol; Thiocol; Orthocoll. $C_7H_7KO_5S$; mol wt 242.29. C 34.70%, H 2.91%, K 16.14%, O 33.02%, S 13.23%. A mixture of the potassium salts of 4- and 5-guaiacolsulfonic acid.

White, odorless crystals or cryst powder; faint bitter taste. Gradually turns pink on exposure to air and light. Soluble in 7.5 parts water. Almost insol in alcohol. Insol in ether. The aq soln is neutral to litmus. *Keep well closed and protected from light.*

THERAP CAT: Expectorant.

7635. Potassium Hexachloroosmate(IV). [16871-60-6] Osmium potassium chloride. Cl_6K_2Os; mol wt 481.14. Cl 44.21%, K 16.25%, Os 39.54%. $K_2[OsCl_6]$. Preparation: Turner *et al., Anal. Chem.* **30**, 1708 (1958).

Dark red to almost black, cubic crystals. Freely sol in water; sparingly sol in alcohol.

7636. Potassium Hexachloroplatinate(IV). [16921-30-5] Platinic potassium chloride; potassium platinic chloride; potassium chloroplatinate. Cl_6K_2Pt; mol wt 486.00. Cl 43.77%, K 16.09%, Pt 40.14%. $K_2[PtCl_6]$.

Orange-yellow crystals or yellow powder. d 3.50. Slightly sol in cold water; sol in hot water. Almost insol in alcohol.

USE: In photography.

7637. Potassium Hexacyanocobaltate(III). [13963-58-1] Tripotassium hexakis(cyano-*C*)cobaltate(3−); potassium cyanocobaltate(III); potassium cobalticyanide; potassium cobaltihexacyanide; cobalt potassium cyanide. $C_6CoK_3N_6$; mol wt 332.33. C 21.68%, Co 17.73%, K 35.29%, N 25.29%. $K_3[Co(CN)_6]$. Prepd by reacting cobalt acetate or cyanide with potassium cyanide, followed by air-oxidation of the cobaltocyanide formed: Biltz, Biltz, *Z. Anorg. Allg. Chem.* **50**, 108 (1906); Grube, *Z. Elektrochem.* **32**, 561 (1926); Benedetti-Pichler, *Z. Anal. Chem.* **70**, 258 (1927); Bigelow, *Inorg. Synth.* **2**, 225 (1946).

Faintly yellow, monoclinic crystals from water. d 1.906. Melts with decompn forming an olive-green mass. Freely sol in water, acetic acid solns. Insol in alcohol. Very slightly sol in liq ammonia. Dec by strong mineral acids. Aq solns are slightly yellow and are regarded as non-poisonous when freshly prepd: Zwenger, *Ann.* **62**, 178 (1847). An odor of HCN develops after about one week's standing in the dark. Exposure to light causes rapid development of a yellow color, but hydrolysis is slight.

7638. Potassium Hexafluorosilicate. [16871-90-2] Potassium fluosilicate; potassium silicofluoride. F_6K_2Si; mol wt 220.27. F 51.75%, K 35.50%, Si 12.75%. $K_2[SiF_6]$.

White, fine powder or crystals. d 2.27. Slightly sol in cold water. Insol in alcohol. In hot water it hydrolyzes to KF, HF, and silicic acid. pH of 1% aq soln 3.4.

Caution: Strong irritant. Ingestion can cause vomiting, diarrhea.

USE: In the manuf of opalescent glass, in porcelain enamels, in insecticides. Also used in aluminum metallurgy.

7639. Potassium Hexafluorozirconate(IV). [16923-95-8] Potassium zirconium fluoride; zirconium potassium fluoride. F_6K_2Zr; mol wt 283.41. F 40.22%, K 27.59%, Zr 32.19%. $K_2[ZrF_6]$.

Crystals. Slightly sol in cold water, sol in hot water.

USE: For manuf of metallic zirconium.

7640. Potassium Hydroxide. [1310-58-3] Potassium hydrate; caustic potash; potassa. HKO; mol wt 56.11. H 1.80%, K 69.68%, O 28.51%. KOH. Prepd industrially by electrolysis of potassium chloride: *Faith, Keyes & Clark's Industrial Chemicals*, F. A. Lowenheim, M. K. Moran, Eds. (Wiley-Interscience, New York, 4th ed., 1975) pp 674-678. Toxicity: H. F. Smyth *et al., Am. Ind. Hyg. Assoc. J.* **30**, 470 (1969).

White or slightly yellow lumps, rods, pellets. Rapidly absorbs moisture and CO_2 from the air and deliquesces. mp about 360°; mp 380° when anhydr. Sol in 0.9 part water, about 0.6 part boiling water, 3 parts alcohol, 2.5 parts glycerol. When dissolved in water or alcohol or when the soln is treated with an acid, much heat is generated. *Keep tightly closed and do not handle with bare hands.* A $0.1M$ aq soln has a pH of 13.5. LD_{50} orally in rats: 1.23 g/kg (Smyth).

Caution: Extremely corrosive. Potential symptoms of overexposure are irritation of eyes, skin, respiratory system; eye and skin burns; cough, sneezing; vomiting, diarrhea. Direct contact may cause painful burns and liquefaction necrosis. See *NIOSH Pocket Guide to Chemical Hazards* (DHHS/NIOSH 97-140, 1997) p 262; *Clinical Toxicology of Commercial Products*, R. E. Gosselin *et al.*, Eds. (Williams & Wilkins, Baltimore, 5th ed., 1984) Section III, pp 245-252.

USE: Manuf liq soap; mordant for wood; absorbing CO_2; mercerizing cotton; paint and varnish removers; electroplating, photoengraving and lithography; printing inks; in analytical chemistry and in organic syntheses. Pharmaceutic aid (alkalizer).

THERAP CAT (VET): Caustic. In disbudding calves' horns. In aq solution to dissolve scales and hair in skin scrapings.

7641. Potassium Hypophosphite. [7782-87-8] H_2KO_2P; mol wt 104.09. H 1.94%, K 37.56%, O 30.74%, P 29.76%. KH_2PO_2.

White crystals or granular, deliquesc powder. Odorless; pungent, saline taste. When strongly heated it dec with evolution of phosphine which ignites spontaneously in air. *It explodes when triturated with chlorates or other oxidizing agents.* One gram dissolves in 0.6 ml water, 9 ml alc, 5 ml boiling alc. The aq soln is neutral or slightly alkaline. *Keep well closed.*

7642. Potassium Iodate. [7758-05-6] IKO_3; mol wt 214.00. I 59.30%, K 18.27%, O 22.43%. KIO_3.

White, odorless crystals or cryst powder. d 3.89. mp 560° with partial decompn. Slowly sol in 12 parts water, in 3.1 parts boiling water. Insol in alcohol.

USE: Oxidizing agent in volumetric chemical analysis; as maturing agent and dough conditioner.

THERAP CAT: Topical antiseptic (mucous membrane).

THERAP CAT (VET): In feeds as a source of iodine.

7643. Potassium Iodide. [7681-11-0] Jodid; Thyroblock; Thyrojod. IK; mol wt 166.00. I 76.45%, K 23.55%. KI. Potassium iodide of commerce contains about 99.5% KI. Prepd from HI and $KHCO_3$. Purification by melting in dry hydrogen: Lingane, Kolthoff, *Inorg. Synth.* **1**, 163 (1939). Continuous electrolytic process for large scale industrial prepn: Morylott, Elkins, US 2989450 (1961 to Dow). Toxicity data: Hildebrandt, *Arch. Exp. Pathol. Pharmakol.* **96**, 292 (1923). Use in the treatment of radiation poisoning resulting from a nuclear accident: W. K. Waterfall, *Br. Med. J.* **281**, 988 (1980); *Bull. N.Y. Acad. Med.* **57**, 395 (1981).

Consult the Name Index before using this section.

Colorless or white, cubical crystals, white granules, or powder. Slightly deliquescent in moist air; on long exposure to air becomes yellow due to liberation of iodine, and small quantities of iodate may be formed; light and moisture accelerate the decomp. Aq solns also become yellow in time due to oxidation, but a small amount of alkali prevents it. d 3.12. mp 680° (volatilizes at higher temp). One gram dissolves in 0.7 ml water, 0.5 ml boiling water, 22 ml alcohol, 8 ml boiling alcohol, 51 ml abs alcohol, 8 ml methanol, 75 ml acetone, 2 ml glycerol, about 2.5 ml glycol. Potassium iodide solns readily dissolve elemental iodine. The aq soln is neutral or, usually, slightly alkaline. pH: 7-9. 30 g KI with 21 ml water gives 30 ml of a saturated soln at 25°. Approx LD i.v. in rats: 285 mg/kg (Hildebrandt). *Incompat.* Alkaloidal salts, chloral hydrate, tartaric and other acids, calomel, potassium chlorate, metallic salts.

USE: Manuf photographic emulsions; in animal and poultry feeds to the extent of 10-30 parts per million; in table salt as a source of iodine and in some drinking water; also in anal. chemistry.

THERAP CAT: Antifungal; expectorant; iodine supplement.

THERAP CAT (VET): In actinobacillosis, actinomycosis. For simple goiter. As expectorant. In iodine deficiency and in chronic poisoning with lead or mercury. Orally only, not by injection. Externally for treatment of bursal enlargements.

7644. Potassium Manganate(VI). [10294-64-1] K_2MnO_4; mol wt 197.13. K 39.67%, Mn 27.87%, O 32.46%. Prepn: Scholder, Waterstradt, *Z. Anorg. Allg. Chem.* **277**, 172 (1954).

Dark green crystals; dec at 190°. Sol in water. Sol and stable in KOH solns. It is an oxidizing agent. With HCl it gives free chlorine.

7645. Potassium Metabisulfite. [16731-55-8] Potassium pyrosulfite. $K_2O_5S_2$; mol wt 222.32. K 35.17%, O 35.98%, S 28.85%. $K_2S_2O_5$. The article of commerce contains ~95% $K_2S_2O_5$.

White crystals or cryst powder; sulfur dioxide odor; acid reaction; liberates SO_2 with acids; oxidizes in air to sulfate, more readily in presence of moisture. It may catch fire if much heat develops in powdering it. Freely sol in water; insol in alcohol. *Keep dry and well closed.*

USE: As antifermentative in breweries and wineries; bleaching straw; preservative for fruits and vegetables.

7646. Potassium Metaphosphate. [7790-53-6] Potassium Kurrol's salt; potassium polymetaphosphate; potassium polyphosphate. $(KPO_3)_x$. High mol wt polymer; degree of polymerization dependent upon preparative conditions. Prepd by dehydration of KH_2PO_4: Pfansteil, Iler, *J. Am. Chem. Soc.* **74**, 6059 (1952). Structural studies: Jost, *Acta Crystallogr.* **16**, 623 (1963); Jost, Schulze, *ibid.* **25B**, 1110 (1969); *eidem, ibid.* **27B**, 1345 (1971). Reviews of metaphosphates: J. R. Van Wazer, *Phosphorus and Its Compounds* vol 1 (Interscience, New York, 1958) pp 601-678; Thilo, *Adv. Inorg. Chem. Radiochem.* **4**, 1-75 (1962).

White, monoclinic crystals. d^{20} 2.45. Insol in pure water. Sol in aq solns of alkali metal (except potassium) salts.

7647. Potassium Molybdate(VI). [13446-49-6] K_2MoO_4; mol wt 238.13. K 32.84%, Mo 40.29%, O 26.88%.

Pentahydrate. White, deliquesc, cryst powder. d 2.3; mp 919°. Sol in 0.6 part water; insol in alc. *Keep well closed.*

7648. Potassium Nitrate. [7757-79-1] Nitric acid potassium salt. KNO_3; mol wt 101.10. K 38.67%, N 13.85%, O 47.48%. Occurs in nature as the mineral **saltpeter** or **niter**. Polymorphism: F. C. Kracek, *J. Phys. Chem.* **34**, 225 (1930). Prepn from potassium chloride: D. L. Reed, K. G. Clark, *Ind. Eng. Chem.* **29**, 333 (1937); by molten salt technique: R. W. Pfeiffer *et al., J. Agric. Food Chem.* **15**, 949 (1967); by solvent separation of strong acids: A. Eyal *et al., Ind. Eng. Chem. Process Des. Dev.* **24**, 387 (1985). Viscosity: R. E. Wellman *et al., J. Chem. Eng. Data* **11**, 156 (1966). Heat capacity: E. W. Dewing, *ibid.* **20**, 221 (1975). Clinical evaluations in tooth hypersensitivity: M. Hodosh, *J. Am. Dent. Assoc.* **88**, 831 (1974); T. Nagata *et al., J. Clin. Periodontol.* **21**, 217 (1994); S. C. Frechoso *et al., ibid.* **30**, (2003).

Colorless transparent prisms, white granular or cryst powder; cooling, saline, pungent taste. d 2.11; mp 333°; dec at 400° with evolution of O_2. One gram dissolves in 2.8 ml water, 0.5 ml boiling water, 620 ml alc. Sol in glycerol; insol in abs alc. Dissolves in

water with a lowering of the temp. pH ~7. LD_{50} orally in rabbits: 1.166 g anion/kg, Dollahite, Rowe, *Southwest. Vet.* **27**, 246 (1974).

Caution: Ingestion of large quantities may cause violent gastroenteritis. Prolonged exposure to small amts may produce anemia, methemoglobinemia, nephritis.

USE: In fireworks, fluxes, pickling meats; production of nitric acid; manuf glass, matches, gunpowder; freezing mixtures. Agricultural fertilizer. Preservative in foods. In dentrifices to reduce tooth hypersensitivity.

THERAP CAT: Diuretic.

7649. Potassium Nitrite. [7758-09-0] KNO_2; mol wt 85.10. K 45.94%, N 16.46%, O 37.60%. The nitrite of commerce usually contains ~85% KNO_2, the remainder consisting chiefly of nitrate.

White or slightly yellow, deliquesc granules or rods. Dec even by weak acids with evolution of brown fumes of nitrous anhydride. d 1.915; mp 441° (decompn starts at 350°). Sol in 0.35 part water, slightly in alc. The aq soln is alkaline. *Keep well closed.* LD_{50} orally in rabbits: 108 mg anion/kg, Dollahite, Rowe, *Southwest. Vet.* **27**, 246 (1974).

USE: In analytical chemistry.

THERAP CAT: Vasodilator; antidote (cyanide poisoning).

7650. Potassium Oleate. [143-18-0] Oleic acid potassium salt. Approx $C_{18}H_{33}KO_2$.

Yellowish or brownish, soft mass. Sol in water, alc. The aq soln is alkaline to phenolphthalein.

USE: Detergent.

7651. Potassium Oxalate. [583-52-8] $C_2K_2O_4$; mol wt 166.22. C 14.45%, K 47.04%, O 38.50%. $K_2C_2O_4$.

Occurs as the monohydrate, colorless, odorless crystals; efflorescent in warm dry air. *Poisonous!* d 2.13. Loses its water at ~160°; when ignited is converted into carbonate without appreciable charring. Sol in 3 parts water.

USE: Cleaning and bleaching straw, removing stains in photography; *in vitro* blood anticoagulant; also in analytical chemistry.

7652. Potassium Percarbonate. [589-97-9] $C_2K_2O_6$; mol wt 198.21. C 12.12%, K 39.45%, O 48.43%. $K_2C_2O_6$. Prepn of practically anhyd compd: Partington, Fathallah, *J. Chem. Soc.* **1950**, 1934.

Monohydrate. White, granular mass. Sol in water with evolution of oxygen. One part potassium percarbonate is sol in 15 parts of cold water; dec in boiling water; 100 parts water dissolve 6.5 parts potassium percarbonate at ordinary temp. *Keep dry and protected from light.*

Caution: Strong irritant. Causes vomiting if swallowed. Large quantities can be fatal.

USE: Has been used in microscopy for detecting tubercle bacilli stained with fuchsin in smears; in photography under the name *Antihypo*, to remove last traces of sodium thiosulfate; also as oxidizing agent in chem analyses, but is no longer favored.

7653. Potassium Perchlorate. [7778-74-7] Peroidin; Perchloracap. $ClKO_4$; mol wt 138.55. Cl 25.59%, K 28.22%, O 46.19%. $KClO_4$.

Colorless crystals or white, cryst powder. Dec at 400°; also dec by organic matter, oxidizable substances and on concussion, but is less reactive than the chlorate. d 2.52. Sol in 65 parts cold water, 15 parts boiling water; practically insol in alcohol.

USE: In explosives, pyrotechnics and photography, in analytical chemistry.

7654. Potassium Periodate. [7790-21-8] Potassium metaperiodate. IKO_4; mol wt 230.00. I 55.18%, K 17.00%, O 27.83%. KIO_4. Prepd by oxidizing potassium iodate with chlorine in alkaline soln: Hill, *J. Am. Chem. Soc.* **50**, 2678 (1928); *Inorg. Synth.* **1**, 171 (1939).

Colorless tetragonal crystals, d_4^{15} 3.618. mp 582°. Soly in water (g/100 g H_2O): 0.168 at 0°; 0.42 at 20°; 0.93 at 40°; 2.16 at 60°; 4.44 at 80°; 7.87 at 100°; also given as 0.66 at 13°. Sparingly sol in aq KOH.

Caution: Highly irritating to skin, eyes, mucous membranes.

USE: Powerful oxidizer in acid soln, oxidizing manganese compds to permanganate; used for this purpose in analytical chemistry (colorimetric estimation of Mn), also for the oxidation of some organic compds.

7655. Potassium Permanganate. [7722-64-7] Permanganic acid potassium salt; chameleon mineral. $KMnO_4$; mol wt 158.03. K 24.74%, Mn 34.76% O 40.50%. Prepn from manganese ore by electrolytic oxidation: *Faith, Keyes & Clark's Industrial Chemicals*, F. A. Lowenheim, M. K. Moran, Eds. (Wiley-Interscience, New York, 4th ed., 1975) pp 679-683. Toxicity study: H. F. Smyth *et al., Am. Ind. Hyg. Assoc. J.* **30**, 470 (1969).

Dark purple or bronze-like, odorless crystals. Almost opaque by transmitted light and of a blue metallic luster by reflected light. Sweet with astringent aftertaste; stable in air. Dec ~240° with evolution of oxygen. d 2.7. Soluble in 14.2 parts cold, 3.5 parts boiling water. Dec by alc and many other organic solvents, also by concd acids with liberation of oxygen; with HCl, chlorine is liberated. Readily dec by many reducing substances, such as ferrous salts, iodides, oxalates, etc., especially in the presence of an acid. *Take great care in handling as explosions may occur if it is brought into contact with organic or other readily oxidizable substances, either in soln or in the dry state. Incompat.* Alcohol, arsenites, bromides, iodides, hydrochloric acid, charcoal; organic substances generally; ferrous or mercurous salts, hypophosphites, hyposulfites, sulfites, peroxides, oxalates. LD_{50} orally in rats: 1.09 g/kg (Smyth).

Caution: Dilute solns are mildly irritating and high concns are caustic.

USE: Bleaching resins, waxes, fats, oils, straw, cotton, silk and other fibers and chamois skins; dyeing wood brown; printing fabrics; washing CO_2 in manuf mineral waters; exterminating *Oidium tuckeri;* photography; tanning leathers; purifying water; with formaldehyde soln to expel formaldehyde gas for disinfecting; as an important reagent in analytical and synthetic organic chemistry.

THERAP CAT: Anti-infective (topical).

THERAP CAT (VET): Antiseptic (topical), astringent, deodorant.

7656. Potassium Persulfate. [7727-21-1] $K_2O_8S_2$; mol wt 270.32. K 28.93%, O 47.35%, S 23.72%. $K_2S_2O_8$. The article of commerce contains 93-97% $K_2S_2O_8$.

Colorless or white, odorless crystals. Gradually dec, losing available oxygen; dec more quickly at higher temps; completely dec ~100°. A powerful oxidizing agent. Sol in ~50 parts water, 25 parts water at 40°; insol in alc; the aq soln dec at ordinary temp and more rapidly on warming. The aq soln is acid. *Keep well closed, in a cool place.*

USE: Bleaching fabrics, soaps; in photography under the name **Anthion** to remove last traces of thiosulfate from plates and paper; in analytical chemistry.

7657. Potassium Phenoxide. [100-67-4] Phenol potassium salt; potassium phenate; potassium phenylate; potassium carbolate. C_6H_5KO; mol wt 132.20. C 54.51%, H 3.81%, K 29.58%, O 12.10%. C_6H_5OK. Prepd from phenol and KOH in dil methanol: Kornblum, Lurie, *J. Am. Chem. Soc.* **81**, 2710 (1959).

White to reddish, hygroscopic, cryst lumps. Very sol in water; sol in alcohol. The aq soln is strongly alkaline. *Keep tightly closed.*

7658. Potassium Phosphate, Dibasic. [7758-11-4] Dipotassium phosphate; dikalium phosphate; DKP; dipotassium hydrogen phosphate. HK_2O_4P; mol wt 174.18. H 0.58%, K 44.89%, O 36.74%, P 17.78%. K_2HPO_4.

White, somewhat hygroscopic granules. Very sol in water, slightly in alcohol. 100 g will dissolve rapidly and completely in 67 g of cold water. Converted into pyrophosphate by ignition. The aq soln is slightly alkaline to phenolphthalein. *Keep well closed.*

USE: Buffering agent in antifreeze solns; nutrient in the culturing of antibiotics; ingredient of instant fertilizers; as sequestrant in the prepn of non-dairy powdered coffee creams.

THERAP CAT: Cathartic.

7659. Potassium Phosphate, Monobasic. [7778-77-0] Potassium biphosphate; potassium acid phosphate; potassium dihydrogen phosphate; monopotassium phosphate; Sörensen's potassium phosphate. H_2KO_4P; mol wt 136.09. H 1.48%, K 28.73%, O 47.03%, P 22.76%. KH_2PO_4.

Colorless crystals or white, granular powder; permanent in air; at 400° loses H_2O, forming metaphosphate. d 2.34. Sol in ~4.5 parts water. Insol in alcohol. pH 4.4-4.7.

USE: In buffers for determination of pH. Pharmaceutic aid (buffering agent).

7660. Potassium Phosphate, Tribasic. [7778-53-2] Tripotassium phosphate. K_3O_4P; mol wt 212.27. K 55.26%, O 30.15%, P 14.59%. K_3PO_4. Purification: Jänecke, *Z. Phys. Chem.* **127**, 75 (1927); Simon, Schulze, *Z. Anorg. Allg. Chem.* **242**, 331 (1939).

Deliquescent, orthorhombic crystals. d_4^{17} 2.564. mp 1340°. Soly in water: 43.7% at 0°; 50.8% at 25°; 59.7% at 45.1°. Insol in alcohol. Aq solns are strongly alkaline.

Octahydrate. Flat, rectangular platelets, mp 45.1°.

7661. Potassium Phosphite. [13492-26-7] HK_2O_3P; mol wt 158.18. H 0.64%, K 49.44%, O 30.34%, P 19.58%. K_2HPO_3.

White, deliquesc powder. Slowly oxidizes in the air to phosphate; dec by heat. Very sol in water; insol in alcohol. *Keep well closed.*

7662. Potassium Pyroantimonate, Acid. [10090-54-7] Potassium antimonate(V). Approx $K_2H_2Sb_2O_7.4H_2O$.

White granules or cryst powder. Moderately sol in cold water; insol in alcohol.

USE: Formerly used for detection of sodium.

7663. Potassium Pyrophosphate. [7320-34-5] Diphosphoric acid tetrapotassium salt. $K_4O_7P_2$; mol wt 330.34. K 47.34%, O 33.90%, P 18.75%. $K_4P_2O_7$. Manuf: *Faith, Keyes & Clark's Industrial Chemicals*, F. A. Lowenheim, M. K. Moran, Eds. (Wiley-Interscience, New York, 4th ed., 1975) pp 684-687.

Trihydrate. Colorless, deliquesc granules or cryst mass; freely sol in water; insol in alcohol. The aq soln is alkaline.

USE: In detergents and surfactants; in water treatment; in drilling muds as a clay thinner.

7664. Potassium Pyrosulfate. [7790-62-7] Disulfuric acid dipotassium salt; "anhydrous" potassium sulfate. $K_2O_7S_2$; mol wt 254.32. K 30.75%, O 44.04%, S 25.22%. $K_2S_2O_7$.

Colorless, fused pieces. d 2.28. mp ~325°. Sol in water. The aq soln is strongly acid.

7665. Potassium Salicylate. [578-36-9] $C_7H_5KO_3$; mol wt 176.21. C 47.71%, H 2.86%, K 22.19%, O 27.24%. HOC_6H_4-COOK.

White, odorless powder. Becomes pink on exposure to light. Very sol in water, alcohol. One gram dissolves in 0.85 ml H_2O. A satd aq soln contains 55.82% w/w at 28.5°. *See* Sidgwick, Ewbank, *J. Chem. Soc.* **121**, 1847, 1850 (1922). The aq soln is neutral or slightly acid to litmus. *Keep well closed and protected from light.*

7666. Potassium Selenate. [7790-59-2] K_2O_4Se; mol wt 221.15. K 35.36%, O 28.94%, Se 35.70%. K_2SeO_4.

Colorless crystals or white powder. d 3.07. Sol in about one part water.

USE: Reagent.

7667. Potassium Selenide. [1312-74-9] K_2Se; mol wt 157.16. K 49.76%, Se 50.24%. Prepd by heating selenium with excess potassium: Fonzes-Diacon, *Contribution a l'Etudes des Séléniures Métalliques,* Montpellier (1901); by adding selenium to a soln of potassium in liq ammonia: Hugot, *Recherches sur l'Action du Sodammonium et du Potassammonium sur Quelque Métalloides,* Paris (1900); Feher in *Handbook of Preparative Inorganic Chemistry* **vol. 1**, G. Brauer, Ed. (Academic Press, New York, 2nd ed., 1963) p 421; by igniting potassium selenite or selenate in an atm of hydrogen: Berzelius, cited in *Mellor's* **vol. 10**, 767 (1930).

Crystalline mass. d 2.29. Reddens on exposure to air. Turns brownish-black when heated. Deliquescent. Forms potassium selenite with selenious acid. Forms potassium hydroselenide with hydrogen selenide. Sol in water; insol in ammonia.

Nonahydrate. Needle-like cryst. Freely sol in water.

7668. Potassium Silicate. [1312-76-1] Soluble potash glass; soluble potash water glass. Variable composition: $K_2Si_2O_5$ to $K_2Si_3O_7$; may also contain water.

Consult the Name Index before using this section.

Colorless or yellowish, translucent to transparent, hygroscopic, glass-like pieces; strong alkaline reaction. Usually very slowly sol in cold water, or depending on the composition, almost insol. More readily sol in water when heated with it under pressure. Insol in alcohol; dec by acids with precipitation of silica. *Keep well closed.*

USE: As binder (*e.g.*, in carbon electrodes, lead pencils, protective coatings, insol pigments); detergent, in glass and ceramics manuf.

7669. Potassium Silver Cyanide. [506-61-6] Potassium bis(cyano-*κC*)argentate(1−); potassium dicyanoargentate. C_2-AgKN$_2$; mol wt 199.00. C 12.07%, Ag 54.21%, K 19.65%, N 14.08%. KAg(CN)$_2$. Review of toxicology and human exposure: *Toxicological Profile for Cyanide* (PB98-101207, 1997) 291 pp.

White crystals; sensitive to light. *Poisonous!* Sol in water; acids ppt silver cyanide from the soln. *Protect from light.*

USE: In silver plating.

7670. Potassium Sodium Tartrate. [304-59-6] Rochelle salt; Seignette salt. $C_4H_4KNaO_6$; mol wt 210.16. C 22.86%, H 1.92%, K 18.60%, Na 10.94%, O 45.68%. KNaC$_4$H$_4$O$_6$.

Tetrahydrate. Translucent crystals or white, cryst powder; cooling saline taste. Slightly effloresces in warm air. d 1.79; mp 70-80°; at 100° loses 3H$_2$O; becomes anhyd at 130-140°; at 220° begins to dec. Sol in 0.9 part water. Almost insol in alcohol. The aq soln is slightly alkaline to litmus. pH 7-8. *Incompat.* Acids, calcium or lead salts, magnesium sulfate, silver nitrate.

USE: Manuf of mirrors; as a constituent of Fehling's soln. For the control of radio frequencies, and wherever piezoelectric crystals are used.

THERAP CAT: Cathartic.

7671. Potassium Sorbate. [24634-61-5] 2,4-Hexadienoic acid potassium salt; sorbic acid potassium salt; potassium 2,4-hexadienoate; BB powder. $C_6H_7KO_2$; mol wt 150.22. C 47.97%, H 4.70%, K 26.03%, O 21.30%. CH$_3$CH=CHCH=CHCOOK. Prepd from sorbic acid and KOH: Probst, Oehme, **US 3173948** (1965 to Hoechst).

Crystals, d$_{20}^{25}$ 1.363. Dec above 270°. Soly in water at 20°: 58.2%; in alc: 6.5%.

USE: As mold and yeast inhibitor, like sorbic acid, esp where greater soly in water is desirable.

7672. Potassium Stannate(IV). [12142-33-5] K$_2$O$_3$Sn; mol wt 244.90. K 31.93%, O 19.60%, Sn 48.47%.

Trihydrate. Colorless crystals. d 3.197. Sol in one part water. Insol in alcohol. The aq soln is alkaline.

USE: In textile dyeing and printing, in tin plating.

7673. Potassium Stearate. [593-29-3] Stearic acid potassium salt. Approx KC$_{18}$H$_{35}$O$_2$. The article of commerce contains a considerable proportion of palmitate.

White powder; usually with slight odor of fat. Slowly sol in cold, readily in hot water or alcohol. The aq soln is strongly alkaline to litmus or phenolphthalein, but the alcoholic soln is only slightly alkaline to phenolphthalein.

USE: In the manuf of textile softeners.

7674. Potassium Sulfate. [7778-80-5] Sal polychrestum; arcanum duplicatum; tartarus vitriolatus. K$_2$O$_4$S; mol wt 174.26. K 44.87%, O 36.73%, S 18.40%. K$_2$SO$_4$. Contains at least 99% K$_2$SO$_4$.

Colorless or white, odorless, hard, bitter crystals, or white granules or powder; permanent in air. d 2.66; mp 1067°. One gram dissolves in 8.3 ml water, 4 ml boiling water, 75 ml glycerol. Insol in alcohol. Its soly in water is decreased by KCl or (NH$_4$)$_2$SO$_4$ and is practically insol in a saturated soln of the latter. The aq soln is neutral. pH about 7.

Caution: Swallowing large doses causes severe G.I. irritation.

USE: Technical grades are used in fertilizers for manuf of potassium alum, potassium carbonate and glass; the reagent grade is used in the Kjeldahl determination of nitrogen.

THERAP CAT: Cathartic.

7675. Potassium Sulfide. [1312-73-8] Potassium monosulfide. K$_2$S; mol wt 110.26. K 70.92%, S 29.08%. Best prepd from the elements in liq ammonia: Klemm *et al.*, *Z. Anorg. Allg. Chem.* **241**, 281 (1939); Feher in *Handbook of Preparative Inorganic*

Chemistry **vol. 1,** G. Brauer, Ed. (Academic Press, New York, 2nd ed., 1963) pp 360-361.

White, cubic crystals or fused plates. Discolors in air. Very hygroscopic. Unstable. May explode on percussion or rapid heating. d 1.74. mp 912°. Freely sol in water. Aq solns are strongly alkaline.

Pentahydrate. Colorless rhombs. Odor of hydrogen sulfide. Discolors upon exposure to light and air (yellow to yellowish red). mp 60°. Freely sol in water, alc, glycerol. Insol in ether. Densities of aq solutions at 25° (calcd as % K$_2$S.5H$_2$O): 1.82%: 1.009; 10.90%: 1.049; 21.80%: 1.100; 29.07%: 1.136; 39.97%: 1.192; 50.88%: 1.250; 81.77%: 1.432. Aq solns are very caustic and prone to decompn. *See* the hydrolysis reactions *under* Sodium Sulfide.

7676. Potassium Sulfite. [10117-38-1] K$_2$O$_3$S; mol wt 158.26. K 49.41%, O 30.33%, S 20.26%. K$_2$SO$_3$. The sulfite of commerce is 90-95% pure.

Dihydrate. White crystals or cryst powder; gradually oxidizes in the air to sulfate. Soluble in about 3.5 parts water, slightly in alcohol; dec by dil acids with evolution of sulfur dioxide. pH about 8. *Keep well closed in a cool place.*

USE: In photographic developers.

THERAP CAT: Cathartic, diuretic.

7677. Potassium Tartrate. [921-53-9] Soluble tartar. C_4-H$_4$K$_2$O$_6$; mol wt 226.27. C 21.23%, H 1.78%, K 34.56%, O 42.43%.

Hemihydrate. White crystals or granular powder; loses its water at about 150°. d 1.98. Sol in about 0.5 part water. Almost insol in alc. The aq soln is slightly alkaline to litmus; pH 7-8.

THERAP CAT: Cathartic.

7678. Potassium Tellurate(IV). [7790-58-1] Potassium tellurite. K$_2$O$_3$Te; mol wt 253.79. K 30.81%, O 18.91%, Te 50.28%. K$_2$TeO$_3$.

White, granular powder. Sol in water to an alkaline soln.

USE: In 1:50,000 soln for detecting presence of living pathogenic bacteria in sera and vaccines, such organisms forming characteristic black reduction compds.

7679. Potassium Tellurate(VI). [15571-91-2] K$_2$O$_4$Te; mol wt 269.79. K 28.98%, O 23.72%, Te 47.30%. K$_2$TeO$_4$. Crystallizes with 3 or 5H$_2$O.

Trihydrate. White, cryst powder. Sol in 4 parts water.

USE: Anhidrotic.

7680. Potassium Tetraborate. [1332-77-0] Potassium biborate; potassium borate. B$_4$K$_2$O$_7$; mol wt 233.44. B 18.52%, K 33.50%, O 47.98%. K$_2$B$_4$O$_7$.

Pentahydrate. White, cryst powder. Sol in 4 parts water, slightly in alc.

7681. Potassium Tetrachloroaurate(III). [13682-61-6] Gold potassium chloride; potassium aurichloride. AuCl$_4$K; mol wt 377.88. Au 52.12%, Cl 37.53%, K 10.35%.

Dihydrate. Yellow, monoclinic crystals. Sol in water. *Protect from light.*

USE: Photography, painting on porcelain and glass; prepn of several other gold compds.

7682. Potassium Tetrachloroplatinate(II). [10025-99-7] Platinous potassium chloride; potassium platinochloride; potassium chloroplatinate. Cl$_4$K$_2$Pt; mol wt 415.09. Cl 34.16%, K 18.84%, Pt 47.00%. K$_2$[PtCl$_4$].

Ruby-red crystals. Sol in water.

USE: In photography, in acid toning baths.

7683. Potassium Tetracyanomercurate(II). [591-89-9] Dipotassium tetrakis(cyano-*C*)mercurate(2−); mercuric potassium cyanide. C$_4$HgK$_2$N$_4$; mol wt 382.86. C 12.55%, Hg 52.39%, K 20.42%, N 14.63%. K$_2$[Hg(CN)$_4$].

Colorless or white crystals. Sol in water. *Violent poison!*

USE: In manuf of mirrors to prevent the silver coating from becoming yellow; as reagent in testing for free acids.

7684. Potassium Tetracyanonickelate(II). [14220-17-8] Dipotassium tetrakis(cyano-*C*)nickelate(2−); nickel potassium cyanide. $C_4K_2N_4Ni$; mol wt 240.96. C 19.94%, K 32.45%, N 23.25%, Ni 24.36%. $K_2[Ni(CN)_4]$.

Monohydrate. Orange-yellow, cryst powder. *Poison!* Loses H_2O at about 100°. Sol in water.

7685. Potassium Tetracyanoplatinate(II). [562-76-5] Dipotassium tetrakis(cyano-C)platinate(2−); platinous potassium cyanide; potassium platinocyanide. $C_4K_2N_4Pt$; mol wt 377.35. C 12.73%, K 20.72%, N 14.85%, Pt 51.70%. $K_2[Pt(CN)_4]$. Crystallizes as a tri- or a dodecahydrate.

Trihydrate. Almost colorless, rhombic prisms; blue in direction of principal axis. Sol in hot water.

7686. Potassium Tetrafluoroborate. [14075-53-7] Potassium borofluoride; potassium fluoborate; avogadrite. BF_4K; mol wt 125.90. B 8.59%, F 60.36%, K 31.06%. KBF_4. Prepared according to the eq $H_3BO_3 + 4HF + KOH = KBF_4 + 4H_2O$: Vorländer *et al., Ber.* **65**, 535 (1932); Kwasnik in *Handbook of Preparative Inorganic Chemistry* **vol. 1**, G. Brauer, Ed. (Academic Press, New York, 2nd ed., 1963) p 223. For other methods of prepn *see* H. S. Booth, D. R. Martin, *Boron Trifluoride and Its Derivatives* (New York, 1949) pp 99-106.

Orthorhombic bipyramidal or cubic crystals. d_4^{20} 2.505. mp 530°. Soly in water (g/100 g): 0.3 (3°); 0.448 (20°); 0.55 (25°); 1.4 (40°); 6.27 (100°). Index of refraction of solns is lower than that of water. A satd soln (0.6%) on heating gives color effects, if excess crystals are added. With a 10% aq soln a transparent blue color appears at 100°, turning green at 90°, and yellow at 60°. In a concd fluoboric acid soln these phenomena occur with variations in room temp. Aq solns of KBF_4 are at first neutral to litmus, but upon standing, diluting, or heating become acidic without etching their glass containers. Slightly sol in boiling alc.

USE: Has been proposed as a flux for soldering and brazing; filler in resin-bonded grinding wheels.

7687. Potassium Tetraiodocadmate. [584-10-1] Dipotassium tetraiodocadmate(2−); cadmium potassium iodide; potassium cadmium iodide; potassium iodocadmate; Marme's reagent. CdI_4K_2; mol wt 698.23. Cd 16.10%, I 72.70%, K 11.20%. $K_2[CdI_4]$. Dihydrate prepd from aq solns of stoichiometric amounts of CdI_2 and KI; must be recrystallized from water at low temps: Croft, *Philos. Mag.* **21**, 355 (1842); *J. Prakt. Chem.* **58**, 399 (1856); Hittorf, *Pogg. Ann.* **106**, 525 (1859); Eder, *Photogr. Mitt.* **13**, 67 (1867); Rimbach, *Ber.* **38**, 1562 (1905).

Dihydrate. Large, water-clear, somewhat distorted octahedra. Deliquesc upon standing in air. Turns yellow with age. d_4^{21} 3.359. One part (w/w) dissolves at 15° in 0.73 part water, in 1.4 part alcohol, in 24.5 parts ether, in 4.5 parts of a 1:1 alcohol-ether mixture; also sol in ethyl acetate.

USE: In testing for alkaloids, amines, imines, heterocyclic nitrogens, peroxides in ether. In chelatometric quantitative organic analysis: *Chim. Anal. (Paris)* **43**, 449 (1961).

7688. Potassium Tetraiodomercurate(II). [7783-33-7] Mercuric potassium iodide. HgI_4K_2; mol wt 786.40. Hg 25.51%, I 64.55%, K 9.94%. Also crystallizes with 1-2 mols H_2O.

Sulfur-yellow crystals; deliquesc in moist air. *Poison!* Very sol in water; sol in alcohol, ether, acetone. *Keep well closed.*

THERAP CAT: Anti-infective (topical); disinfectant.

THERAP CAT (VET): Antiseptic (topical); disinfectant.

7689. Potassium Tetroxalate. [127-96-8] Potassium quadroxalate; sal acetosella; salt of sorrel. $C_4H_3KO_8$; mol wt 218.16. C 22.02%, H 1.39%, K 17.92%, O 58.67%. $KHC_2O_4 \cdot H_2C_2O_4$. Incorrectly called *essential salt of lemons.*

Dihydrate. Colorless or white crystals; permanent in air. Sol in 60 parts cold, 12 parts boiling water; slightly sol in alcohol.

USE: Removing rust and ink spots; in metal polishes; in analytical chemistry.

7690. Potassium Thiocarbonate. [26750-66-3] Potassium sulfocarbonate; potassium trithiocarbonate. CK_2S_3; mol wt 186.40. C 6.44%, K 41.95%, S 51.61%. K_2CS_3. Monograph: K. N. Johri, *Chemical Analysis without H_2S using Potassium Trithiocarbonate* (Asia Pub., New York, 1963) 107 pp.

Yellowish-red, deliquesc granules or crystals. Very sol in water. The aq soln is strongly alkaline. *Keep tightly closed.*

Caution: Irritant, caustic.

USE: In analytical chemistry.

7691. Potassium Thiocyanate. [333-20-0] Potassium sulfocyanate; potassium rhodanide; Rhocya. CKNS; mol wt 97.18. C 12.36%, K 40.23%, N 14.41%, S 33.00%. KSCN.

Colorless, deliquesc crystals. d 1.89; mp ~173°, the fused salt turning brown, then green, blue, and white again on cooling. One gram dissolves in 0.5 ml water, 12 ml alcohol, 8 ml boiling alcohol. When dissolved in its own wt of water, the temp drops about 30°. The aq soln is neutral. *Keep well closed.* LD_{50} orally in mice, rats: 594, 854 mg/kg, Andersen, Chen, *J. Am. Pharm. Assoc.* **29**, 152 (1940).

Caution: May cause skin eruptions, psychosis.

USE: Manuf artificial mustard oil; printing and dyeing textiles; in photography as intensifier; in analytical chemistry. The sodium salt now is replacing it for most of these uses.

THERAP CAT: Hypotensive.

7692. Potassium Thiosulfate. [10294-66-3] Potassium hyposulfite. $K_2O_3S_2$; mol wt 190.32. K 41.09%, O 25.22%, S 33.70%. $K_2S_2O_3$.

Colorless, hygroscopic crystals. Sol in water. Insol in alcohol. May crystallize with 0.33 to 1.5 mol H_2O. *Keep well closed.*

7693. Potassium Titanyl Oxalate. [14402-67-6] Dipotassium bis[ethanedioato(2−)-O,O']oxotitanate(2−); titanium potassium oxalate; titanyl potassium oxalate. $C_4K_2O_9Ti$; mol wt 318.10. C 15.10%, K 24.58%, O 45.27%, Ti 15.05%. $K_2TiO(C_2O_4)_2$.

Crystals or cryst powder. Very sol in water.

Dihydrate. Potassium oxodioxalatodiaquotitanate(IV).

USE: As mordant in dyeing cotton and leather.

7694. Potassium Tungstate(VI). [7790-60-5] K_2O_4W; mol wt 326.03. K 23.98%, O 19.63%, W 56.39%. K_2WO_4. Crystallizes also with $2H_2O$.

Heavy, deliquesc, cryst powder. d 3.12. mp 921°. Sol in about 2 parts cold, about 0.7 part boiling water. Insol in alcohol. *Keep well closed.*

7695. Potassium Uranate(VI). [7790-63-8] Potassium diuranate; uranium oxide orange. $K_2O_7U_2$; mol wt 666.25. K 11.74%, O 16.81%, U 71.45%. $K_2U_2O_7$.

Orange powder. Insol in water; sol in acids.

USE: Painting on porcelain.

7696. Potassium Xanthogenate. [140-89-6] Carbonodithioic acid O-ethyl ester potassium salt; ethylxanthic acid potassium salt; potassium ethyldithiocarbonate; potassium ethylxanthogenate; potassium ethylxanthate. $C_3H_5KOS_2$; mol wt 160.30. C 22.48%, H 3.14%, K 24.39%, O 9.98%, S 40.01%. $C_2H_5OCS_2K$. Made by treating an alcoholic soln of CS_2 with alcoholic KOH. Usually contains 8-10% H_2O.

White to pale yellow crystals or cryst powder. Very sol in water; sol in alcohol. The aq soln is strongly alkaline. *Keep well closed and protected from light.*

USE: As reagent in analytical chemistry.

7697. Povidone. [9003-39-8] 1-Ethenyl-2-pyrrolidinone homopolymer; 1-vinyl-2-pyrrolidinone polymers; poly[1-(2-oxo-1-pyrrolidinyl)ethylene]; polyvinylpyrrolidone; polyvidone; PVP; Kollidon; Luviskol; Periston; Plasdone; Protagent. Homopolymer of N-vinyl-2-pyrrolidone, produced commercially as a series of products having mean mol wts ranging from 2,500 to 1,000,000. Prepd by free radical polymerization of the monomer. *See* J. W. Reppe, *Acetylene Chemistry* (PB Report 18852-s, U.S. Dept. Commerce, 1949) pp 68-72. Review of clinical use and early literature: W. Wessel *et al., Arzneim.-Forsch.* **21**, 1468-1482 (1971); of synthesis and physical properties: H. Warson, *Polym. Paint Colour J.* **161**, 637-644 (1972); F. Haaf *et al., Polym. J.* **17**, 143-152 (1985); of use in cosmetics: F. G. M. Vogel, *Soap Cosmet. Chem. Spec.* **65**, 42-47, 128 (1989). Book: *PVP: A Critical Review of the Kinetics and Toxicology of Polyvinylpyrrolidone (Povidone)*, B. V. Robinson *et al.,* Eds. (Lewis Publishers, Chelsea, MI, 1990) 209 pp. Comprehensive description: C. M. Adeyeye, E. Barabas, *Anal. Profiles Drug Subs. Excip.* **22**, 555-685 (1993). Size exclusion chromatography: C. Wu *et al., Chromatogr. Sci. Ser.* **69**, 311 (1995).

White, hygroscopic powder. Sol in water, alcohol, chloroform, formic acid, acetic acid, N-methylpyrrolidone, methylcyclohexanone, dichloromethane, ethylenediamine, glycerol, diethyleneglycol, PEG 400. Insol in xylene, toluene, diethylether, ethylacetate, acetone, cyclohexanone, chlorobenzene, dioxane, carbon tetrachloride, mineral oil.

Crospovidone. Polyvinylpolypyrrolidone; PVPP; Divergan; Kollidon CL; Polyclar; Polyplasdone XL. Crosslinked insoluble homopolymer of NVP. Review of properties and applications: A. H. Bronnsack in *Proc. Intl. Symp. Povidone*, G. A. Digenis, J. Ansell, Eds. (Univ. Kentucky, Coll. Pharmacy, Lexington, 1983) pp 471-490. Comprehensive description: E. S. Barabas, C. M. Adeyeye, *Anal. Profiles Drug Subs. Excip.* **24**, 87-163 (1996). Free flowing, white, almost tasteless powder. Hygroscopic; swells on contact with water. Insol in water, strong mineral acids, caustic solns, and common organic solvents.

Monomer. [88-12-0] 1-Ethenyl-2-pyrrolidinone; N-vinyl-2-pyrrolidinone; NVP. C_6H_9NO; mol wt 111.14. Clear to light straw colored liquid. bp_{14} 96°, bp_{400} 193°. Freezing pt 13.5°. d_4^{24} 1.04. n_D^{25} 1.511. Flash pt (open cup) 100.5°C (213°F). Viscosity (25°): 2.07 cP. Sol in water and many organic solvents.

Complex with iodine *see* Povidone-Iodine.

USE: Povidone as pharmaceutic aid (dispersing, suspending and viscosity-increasing agent; tablet coating and binder). Thickener, dispersant, lubricant, film-forming agent and binder in cosmetics. Stabilizer, diluent, and dye dispersant in food. Dye dispersant in paper and textiles. Adhesive; paper coating. Coating and processing aid in photographic products. Manuf of plastics and rubber. Cryoprotectant for biological samples. Crospovidone as pharmaceutic aid (tablet binder and disintegrant); clarifying and stabilizing agent in beverages. Monomer as dispersant and wetting agent in pigments.

THERAP CAT: Povidone formerly as a synthetic blood plasma expander. Crospovidone as antidiarrheal.

7698. Povidone-Iodine. [25655-41-8] 1-Ethenyl-2-pyrrolidinone homopolymer compd with iodine; 1-vinyl-2-pyrrolidinone polymers, iodine complex; iodine-polyvinylpyrrolidone complex; polyvinylpyrrolidone-iodine complex; PVP-I; Betadine; Betaisodona; Braunol; Braunosan H; Disadine D.P.; Efodine; Isodine; Proviodine; Traumasept. An iodophor, *q.v.*, prepd by Beller, Hosmer, **US 2706701**; Hosmer, **US 2826532**; Siggia, **US 2900305** (1955, 1958, and 1959, all to GAF). Prepn, history and use: Shelanski, Shelanski, *J. Int. Coll. Surg.* **25**, 727 (1956).

Yellowish-brown, amorphous powder with slight characteristic odor. Aq solns have a pH near 2 and may be made more neutral (but less stable) by the addition of sodium bicarbonate. Sol in alc, water. Practically insol in chloroform, carbon tetrachloride, ether, solvent hexane, acetone. Solns do not give the familiar starch test when freshly prepared.

THERAP CAT: Anti-infective (topical).

THERAP CAT (VET): Anti-infective (topical).

7699. PPACK. [71142-71-7] D-Phenylalanyl-N-[4-[(amino-iminomethyl)amino]-1-(chloroacetyl)butyl]-L-prolinamide; D-phenylalanyl-prolyl-arginine chloromethyl ketone; FPRMeCl. $C_{21}H_{31}ClN_6O_3$; mol wt 450.96. C 55.93%, H 6.93%, Cl 7.86%, N 18.64%, O 10.64%. Selective irreversible inhibitor of thrombin: C. A. Kettner, E. N. Shaw, *Thromb. Res.* **14**, 969 (1979). Synthesis: E. N. Shaw, C. A. Kettner, **US 4318904** (1982 to Research Corp.). Anticoagulant and antithrombotic activity: J. Hauptman, F. Markwardt, *Thromb. Res.* **20**, 347 (1980). *In vivo* studies: D. Collen *et al.*, *J. Lab. Clin. Med.* **99**, 76 (1982).

D-Phe–Pro–ArgCH₂Cl

Note: Commercially available as the dihydrochloride.

USE: As a research tool; as a clinical reagent to measure the level of thrombin in blood.

7700. Practolol. [6673-35-4] N-[4-[2-Hydroxy-3-[(1-methylethyl)amino]propoxy]phenyl]acetamide; 4′-[2-hydroxy-3-(isopropylamino)propoxy]acetanilide; 1-(4-acetamidophenoxy)-3-isopropylamino-2-propanol; AY-21011; ICI-50172; Dalzic; Eraldin. $C_{14}H_{22}N_2O_3$; mol wt 266.34. C 63.13%, H 8.33%, N 10.52%, O 18.02%. β-Adrenergic blocker. Prepn: Howe, Smith, **NL 6512676**; *eidem*, **US 3408387** (1966, 1968, to I.C.I.). Synthesis of *R(+)*-form: Danilewicz, Kemp, *J. Med. Chem.* **16**, 168 (1973). Pharmacological studies: Dunlop, Shanks, *Br. J. Pharmacol. Chemother.* **32**, 201 (1968); Barrett, *Postgrad. Med. J. Suppl.* **47**, 7 (1971). Metabolic studies: Scales, Cosgrove, *J. Pharmacol. Exp. Ther.* **175**, 338 (1970).

mp 134-136° (BuOAc). Sol in warm isopropanol.

Hydrochloride monohydrate. mp 140-142°.

R(+)-Form. Crystals from dioxane, mp 130-131.5°. $[\alpha]_{365}^{25}$ +4.3°, $[\alpha]_{578}^{25}$ +3.5° (ethanol).

R(+)-Hydrochloride. $[\alpha]_{436}^{25}$+26.0°, $[\alpha]_{578}^{25}$ +14.0°.

THERAP CAT: Antiarrhythmic.

7701. Pradofloxacin. [195532-12-8] 8-Cyano-1-cyclopropyl-6-fluoro-1,4-dihydro-7-[(4aS,7aS)-octahydro-6H-pyrrolo[3,4-b]pyridin-6-yl]-4-oxo-3-quinolinecarboxylic acid; 8-cyano-1-cyclopropyl-7-((1S,6S)-2,8-diazabicyclo[4.3.0]nonan-8-yl)-6-fluoro-1,4-dihydro-4-oxo-3-quinolinecarboxylic acid. $C_{21}H_{21}FN_4O_3$; mol wt 396.41. C 63.63%, H 5.34%, F 4.79%, N 14.13%, O 12.11%. Cyanofluorinated quinoline antibiotic. Prepn: S. Bartel *et al.*, **WO 9731001**; *eidem*, **US 6323213** (1997, 2001 both to Bayer). LC/MS/MS determn in biological fluids: R. Krebber, *J. Vet. Pharmacol. Ther.* **26**, Suppl 1, 102 (2003). Bioavailability: M. A. Bregante *et al.*, *ibid.* 87; K. Fraatz *et al.*, *ibid.* 88. Clinical trial in dogs in comparison with amoxicillin and clavulanic acid, *q.q.v.*: B. Stephan *et al.*, *ibid.* 217.

mp 246-248° (dec).

THERAP CAT (VET): Antibacterial.

7702. Prajmaline. [35080-11-6] (17R,21α)-17,21-Dihydroxy-4-propylajmalanium; N^4-propylajmalinium; prajmalium; N-propylajmaline. $[C_{23}H_{33}N_2O_2]^+$. Prepn: J. Keck, *Z. Naturforsch.* **18b**, 177 (1963); A. Bonati, E. Bombardelli, *Farmaco Ed. Sci.* **18**, 851 (1963); J. Keck, **DE 1154120** (1963 to Thomae); *idem*, **US 3414577** (1968 to Boehringer, Ing.). Pharmacology: R. Koch, *Arzneim.-Forsch.* **22**, 2079 (1972); H. M. Mertens *et al.*, *ibid.* **23**, 642 (1973); K.-W. Diederich, D. Boyksen, *ibid.* 1302. Toxicology: G. Von Philipsborn, B. Stalder, *ibid.* **22**, 2085 (1972). Pharmacokinetics: A. T. Trompler *et al.*, *ibid.* **33**, 436 (1983). Mechanism of action: H. Langenfeld *et al.*, *J. Cardiovasc. Pharmacol.* **15**, 338 (1990). GC/MS determn in urine: H. H. Maurer, *Arch. Toxicol.* **64**, 218 (1990). Clinical comparison with tocainide, *q.v.*: B. Schwartzkopff *et al.*, *Arzneim.-Forsch.* **33**, 153 (1983).

Hydrogen tartrate. [2589-47-1] Prajmaline bitartrate; NPAB; GT-1012; Neo-Gilurytmal. $C_{23}H_{33}N_2O_2.C_4H_5O_6$; mol wt 518.60. White crystals from ethanol + ether, mp 149-152°. LD_{50} in mice (mg/kg): 43 orally; 1.7 i.v. (Von Philipsborn, Stalder).

THERAP CAT: Antiarrhythmic.

7703. Pralidoxime Chloride. [51-15-0] 2-[(Hydroxyimino)methyl]-1-methylpyridinium chloride; 2-formyl-1-methylpyridinium chloride oxime; 1-methyl-2-formylpyridinium chloride oxime; N-methylpyridinium-2-aldoxime chloride; 2-pyridine aldoxime methyl chloride; 2-PAM chloride; Protopam. $C_7H_9ClN_2O$; mol wt 172.61. C 48.71%, H 5.26%, Cl 20.54%, O 9.27%. Cholinesterase reactivator. Prepn of salts: I. B. Wilson et al., US 2816113 (1957 to U.S. Sec'y of Army); A. A. Kondritzer et al., J. Pharm. Sci. 50, 109 (1961). Manufacturing processes: R. I. Ellin et al., US 3140289 (1964 to U.S. Dept. of the Army); McDowell, US 3155674 (1964 to Olin Mathieson). Commercial prepn: R. I. Ellin, Ind. Eng. Chem. Prod. Res. Dev. 3 (1), 20 (1964). HPLC determn in serum: P. Houzé et al., J. Chromatogr. B 814, 149 (2005). Toxicology: Christensen, Richter, Arch. Environ. Health 15, 599 (1967). Toxicity data: Fleisher et al., Toxicol. Appl. Pharmacol. 16, 40 (1970); R. I. Ellin, J. H. Wills, J. Pharm. Sci. 53, 1143 (1964). Comprehensive description: U. V. Banakar, U. N. Patel, Anal. Profiles Drug Subs. 17, 533-569 (1988).

Crystals from alcohol + ether, mp 235-238° (dec). Soly (g/100 ml) 25°: acetone 0, isopropanol 0.09, ethanol 0.89, methanol 8.5, water 65.5. LD_{50} in rats (mg/kg): 96 i.v. (Fleisher). LD_{50} in rabbits (mg/kg): 95 i.v.; LD_{50} in mice (mg/kg): 115 i.v., 205 i.p., 4100 orally (Ellin, Wills).

Pralidoxime iodide. [94-63-3] 2-Pyridine aldoxime methiodide; 2-PAM. $C_7H_9IN_2O$; mol wt 264.06. Yellow crystals from alcohol, mp 225-226°. Soly at 25°: 48 mg/ml. Very sol in water, fairly sol in hot alcohol, poorly sol in cold alcohol. Insol in ether, acetone. LD_{50} in mice (mg/kg): 140-178 i.v., 136-260 i.p., 290-340 s.c., 1500-4000 orally (Ellin, Wills).

Pralidoxime mesylate. [154-97-2] Contrathion. $C_8H_{12}N_2O_4$-S; mol wt 232.26. Very hygroscopic crystals from ethanol, mp 155°. pKa 8.0. Soly in water: 1 g in 2 ml. LD_{50} in mice (mg/kg): 118-122 i.v., 216 i.p., 3700 orally; in rats (mg/kg): 109 i.v., 262 i.p. (Ellis, Wills).

THERAP CAT: Antidote (nerve gases and organophosphate insecticide poisoning.)

7704. Prallethrin. [23031-36-9] 2,2-Dimethyl-3-(2-methyl-1-propenyl)cyclopropanecarboxylic acid 2-methyl-4-oxo-3-(2-propynyl)-2-cyclopenten-1-yl ester; (S)-2-methyl-4-oxo-3-(2-propynyl)cyclopent-2-enyl (1R)-cis-chrysanthemate; S-4068; S-4068SF; Etoc. $C_{19}H_{24}O_3$; mol wt 300.39. C 75.97%, H 8.05%, O 15.98%. Synthetic pyrethroid; propynyl analog of allethrin. The commercial product is a mixture of the ester of the (4S)-alcohol with the (1R)-cis/trans-chrysanthemic acids; the trans isomer is the most bioactive. Initial report: W. A. Gersdorff, P. G. Piquett, J. Econ. Entomol. 54, 1250 (1961). Synthesis and resolution of labelled commerical isomers: H. Kanamaru et al., J. Labelled Compd. Radiopharm. 23, 995 (1986). Pharmacology: T. Segawa et al., Oyo Yakuri 34, 181 (1987). Insecticidal activity: T. Matsunaga et al., Jpn. J. Sanit. Zool. 38, 219 (1987). Efficacy against mosquitoes: R. L. Groves et al., J. Am. Mosq. Control Assoc. 13, 184 (1997). Review of biological activity: Y. Abe et al., Brighton Crop Prot. Conf. - Pests Dis. 1994, 1023. Brief review of structure-activity: N. Matsuo, Pestic. Sci. 52, 21-28 (1998).

Yellow to yellow brown liquid (commerical product). d_4^{20} 1.03. Vapor pressure (20°): 3.5×10^{-5}; (30°) 1.0×10^{-4} mm Hg. Sol in most organic solvents. Soly in water (25°): 8.51 ppm.

USE: Insecticide.

7705. Pramipexole. [104632-26-0] (S)-4,5,6,7-Tetrahydro-N^6-propyl-2,6-benzothiazolediamine; (S)-2-amino-4,5,6,7-tetrahydro-6-(propylamino)benzothiazole. $C_{10}H_{17}N_3S$; mol wt 211.33. C 56.83%, H 8.11%, N 19.88%, S 15.17%. Dopamine D_2-receptor agonist. Prepn of racemate: G. Griss et al., EP 186087; eidem, US 4886812 (1986, 1989 both to Thomae); of enantiomers: C. S. Schneider, J. Mierau, J. Med. Chem. 30, 494 (1987). Pharmacology: J. Mierau, G. Schingnitz, Eur. J. Pharmacol. 215, 161 (1992). Clinical safety and pharmacodynamics: J. C. Schilling et al., Clin. Pharmacol. Ther. 51, 541 (1992). Clinical trial in Parkinson's disease: K. Kieburtz et al., J. Am. Med. Assoc. 278, 125 (1997).

Dihydrochloride monohydrate. [191217-81-9]; [104632-25-9] (dihydrochloride). SND-919; Mirapex; Mirapexin; Sifrol. C_{10}-$H_{17}N_3S.2HCl.H_2O$; mol wt 302.26. White to off-white powder, mp 296-301° (dec). $[\alpha]_D^{20}$ −67.2° (c = 1 in methanol). Soly: water >20%; methanol ~8%; ethanol ~0.5%. Practically insol in dichloromethane.

THERAP CAT: Antiparkinsonian.

7706. Pramiracetam. [68497-62-1] N-[2-[Bis(1-methylethyl)amino]ethyl]-2-oxo-1-pyrrolidineacetamide; N-[2-(diisopropylamino)ethyl]-2-oxo-1-pyrrolidineacetamide; amacetam. C_{14}-$H_{27}N_3O_2$; mol wt 269.38. C 62.42%, H 10.10%, N 15.60%, O 11.88%. Cognition enhancer structurally related to piracetam, q.v. Prepn: Y. J. L'Italien, I. C. Nordin, DE 2808067; eidem, US 4145347 (1978, 1979 both to Parke, Davis); D. E. Butler et al., J. Med. Chem. 27, 684 (1984). Pharmacology: B. P. H. Poschel et al., Drugs Exp. Clin. Res. 9, 853 (1983). GC determn in plasma: T. Chang, R. M. Young, J. Chromatogr. 274, 346 (1983). Clinical pharmacokinetics: T. Chang et al., J. Clin. Pharmacol. 25, 291 (1985). Clinical evaluation in Alzheimer's disease: R. J. Branconnier et al., Psychopharmacol. Bull. 19, 726 (1983); in various cognitive disorders: R. Dejong, Curr. Ther. Res. 41, 254 (1987).

$bp_{0.15}$ 162-164°. Monohydrate, mp 47-48°.

Sulfate. [72869-16-0] CI-879. $C_{14}H_{27}N_3O_2.H_2SO_4$; mol wt 367.46. LD_{50} in male, female mice (mg/kg): 5434, 4355 orally (Poschel).

THERAP CAT: Nootropic.

7707. Pramiverin. [14334-40-8] N-(1-Methylethyl)-4,4-diphenylcyclohexanamine; N-isopropyl-4,4-diphenylcyclohexylamine; pramiverine; primaverine; propaminodiphen. $C_{21}H_{27}N$; mol wt 293.45. C 85.95%, H 9.27%, N 4.77%. Prepn: NL 6515046; R. Unger et al., US 3376312 (1966, 1968 both to E. Merck). Pharmacology: H. J. Enenkel et al., Arzneim.-Forsch. 26, 690 (1976). Toxicological study: M. Von Eberstein et al., ibid., 703. Series of articles on pharmacology, pharmacokinetics, GC determn, clinical studies: ibid., 686-752. Use in management of labor: G. LoDico et al., Minerva Ginecol. 31, 683 (1979).

Liq, bp$_{0.05}$ 164-165°; also reported as a solid, mp 70° (Enenkel).

Hydrochloride. [14334-41-9] EMD-9806; HSP-2986; Monoverin; Sistalgin. $C_{21}H_{27}N.HCl$; mol wt 329.91. Off-white crystalline powder, mp 230°; also reported as 234-237° (Enenkel). Soly at 25° (g/100 ml): in water 0.3; in ethanol 4; in chloroform 5. Practically insol in ether. LD$_{50}$ (after 14 days) in mice, rats (mg/kg): 346, 623 orally; 25, 26 i.v. (Von Eberstein).

THERAP CAT: Antispasmodic.

7708. Pramlintide. [151126-32-8] 25-L-Proline-28-L-proline-29-L-proline-amylin (human); tripro-amylin; AC-137; Symlin. $C_{171}H_{267}N_{51}O_{53}S_2$; mol wt 3949.39. C 52.00%, H 6.81%, N 18.09%, O 21.47%, S 1.62%. Analog of human amylin, *q.v.* Prepn: L. S. L. Gaeta *et al.,* **WO 9310146**; *eidem,* **US 5686411** (1993, 1997 both to Amylin Pharm.). Pharmacology: A. A. Young *et al., Drug Dev. Res.* **37,** 231 (1996). Clinical pharmacokinetics, pharmacodynamics: W. A. Colburn *et al., J. Clin. Pharmacol.* **36,** 13 (1996). Clinical evaluation in insulin-dependent diabetes: O. G. Kolterman *et al., Diabetologia* **39,** 492 (1996).

Lys–Cys–Asn–Thr–Ala–Thr–Cys–Ala–Thr–Gln–Arg–Leu–Ala–Asn–Phe–Leu–Val–His
                                        Ser
                                        Ser
H$_2$N–Tyr–Thr–Asn–Ser–Gly–Val–Asn–Thr–Pro–Pro–Leu–Ile–Pro–Gly–Phe–Asn–Asn

THERAP CAT: In treatment of insulin-dependent diabetes.

7709. Pramoxine. [140-65-8] 4-[3-(4-Butoxyphenoxy)propyl]morpholine; *p*-butoxyphenyl γ-morpholinopropyl ether; γ-morpholinopropyl 4-*n*-butoxyphenyl ether; pramocaine; proxazocain. $C_{17}H_{27}NO_3$; mol wt 293.40. C 69.59%, H 9.28%, N 4.77%, O 16.36%. Prepn: Wright, Moore, *J. Am. Chem. Soc.* **73,** 2281 (1951); **76,** 4396 (1954); **US 2870151** (1959 to Abbott). Pharmacology: O. Blanpin, *Anesth. Analg. Reanimat.* **14,** 225 (1957). Toxicity studies: J. L. Schmidt *et al., Toxicol. Appl. Pharmacol.* **1,** 454 (1959); S. Monash, D. Gibbs, *Anesth. Analg.* **38,** 265 (1959).

bp$_6$ 196°; bp$_{2.8}$ 183-184°. LD$_{50}$ in mice (mg/kg): 300 i.p., 900 s.c. (Monash, Gibbs).

Hydrochloride. [637-58-1] Proctofoam-NS; Tronolane; Tronothane. $C_{17}H_{27}NO_3.HCl$; mol wt 329.86. Crystals, mp 181-183°. Sol in water. LD$_{50}$ i.v. in mice: 79.5 ±2.7 mg/kg (Schmidt). LD$_{50}$ in mice (mg/kg): 300 i.p., 750 s.c. (Monash, Gibbs).

THERAP CAT: Anesthetic (local).

7710. Pranlukast. [103177-37-3] *N*-[4-Oxo-2-(1*H*-tetrazol-5-yl)-4*H*-1-benzopyran-8-yl]-4-(4-phenylbutoxy)benzamide; 8-[4-(4-phenylbutoxy)benzamido]-2-(tetrazol-5-yl)-4*H*-1-benzopyran-4-one; 8-[*p*-(4-phenylbutoxy)benzoyl]amino-2-(5-tetrazolyl)-4-oxo-4*H*-1-benzopyran; ONO-1078; ONO-RS-411; Onon. $C_{27}H_{23}N_5O_4$; mol wt 481.50. C 67.35%, H 4.81%, N 14.54%, O 13.29%. Leukotriene antagonist. Prepn: M. Toda *et al.,* **EP 173516**; *eidem,* **US 4780469** (1986, 1988 both to Ono); H. Nakai *et al., J. Med. Chem.* **31,** 84 (1988). Pharmacology: T. Obata *et al., Adv. Prostaglandin Thromboxane Leukotriene Res.* **15,** 229 (1985); *idem et al., ibid.* **17,** 540 (1987). Clinical evaluations in asthma: Y. Taniguchi *et al., J. Allergy Clin. Immunol.* **92,** 507 (1993); H. Yamamoto *et al. Am. J. Respir. Crit. Care Med.* **150,** 254 (1994).

Occurs as the hemihydrate. Crystals, mp 244-245°. LD$_{50}$ in male mice (mg/kg): >1000 i.v. (Toda).

THERAP CAT: Antiasthmatic.

7711. Pranoprofen. [52549-17-4] α-Methyl-5*H*-[1]benzopyrano[2,3-*b*]pyridine-7-acetic acid; 2-(5*H*-[1]benzopyrano[2,3-*b*]-pyridin-7-yl)propionic acid; Y-8004; Niflan. $C_{15}H_{13}NO_3$; mol wt 255.27. C 70.58%, H 5.13%, N 5.49%, O 18.80%. Prepn: M. Nakanishi *et al.,* **DE 2337052**; *eidem,* **US 3931205** (1974, 1976 both to Yoshitomi); *eidem, Yakugaku Zasshi* **96,** 99 (1976), *C.A.* **84,** 135515b (1976). Physicochemical properties: M. Nobutoki, Y. Ota, *Iyakuhin Kenkyu* **7,** 200 (1976), *C.A.* **88,** 110468h (1978). Absorption, metabolism, distribution, excretion: Y. Kato *et al., Yakuri to Chiryo* **4,** 1473 (1976), *C.A.* **88,** 130710j (1978). Pharmacological study: Y. Maruyama *et al., Nippon Yakurigaku Zasshi* **73,** 113 (1977), *C.A.* **88,** 276m (1978). Toxicity study: M. Edanaga *et al., Iyakuhin Kenkyu* **7,** 211 (1976), *C.A.* **88,** 131015y (1978).

Cryst from aq dioxane, mp 182-183°. LD$_{50}$ in male mice, rats (mg/kg): 447.3, 87.3 orally (Edanaga).

THERAP CAT: Anti-inflammatory.

7712. Praseodymium. [7440-10-0] Pr; at. wt 140.90765; at. no. 59; valences 3, 4. A lanthanide; belongs to the cerium group of rare earth metals. Naturally occurring isotope (mass number): 141; known artificial radioactive isotopes: 126, 129-140; 142-152. Prepn of radioactive isotopes by bombardment: Seaborg, *Chem. Rev.* **27,** 199 (1940); Huber *et al., Helv. Phys. Acta* **18,** 221 (1945). Abundance in earth's crust 5.5-9.1 ppm; found in rare earth minerals. Reported in 1843 by Mosander as *didymium* which was a mixture of Pr and Nd; separated in 1885 by von Welsbach. Separated from other rare earth elements by fractional crystn. Also by ion exchange: Spedding *et al., J. Am. Chem. Soc.* **69,** 2786, 2812 (1947). Prepn of metal by electrolysis: Muthmann, Weiss, *Ann.* **331,** 1 (1904); Canneri, Rossi, *Gazz. Chim. Ital.* **62,** 1160 (1932); Mazza, *Atti X Congr. Int. Chim.* **3,** 604 (1939); Trombe, Mahn, *Compt. Rend.* **220,** 778 (1945). Toxicity study: Haley *et al., Toxicol. Appl. Pharmacol.* **6,** 614 (1964). Reviews of prepn, properties and compds: *The Rare Earths,* F. H. Spedding, A. H. Daane, Eds. (Krieger, Huntington, N.Y., 1971, reprint of 1961 ed.) 641 pp; Hulet, Bode, "Separation Chemistry of the Lanthanides and Transplutonium Actinides" in *MTP Int. Rev. Sci.: Inorg. Chem., Ser. One* Vol. 7, K. W. Bagnall, Ed. (Univ. Park Press, Baltimore, 1972) pp 1-45; Moeller, "The Lanthanides", *Comprehensive Inorganic Chemistry* Vol. 4, J. C. Bailar, Jr. *et al.,* Eds. (Pergamon Press, Oxford, 1973) pp 1-101; F. H. Spedding in *Kirk-Othmer Encyclopedia of Chemical Technology* vol. 19 (John Wiley & Sons, New York, 3rd ed., 1982) pp 833-854; *Chemistry of the Elements,* N. N. Greenwood, A. Earnshaw, Eds. (Pergamon Press, New York, 1984) pp 1423-1449. Brief review of properties: G. T. Seaborg, *Radiochim. Acta* **61,** 115-122 (1993).

Yellowish metal, forms oxide film on exposure to moist air. Two crystalline forms: hexagonal α-form, d 6.475, transforms to β-form at 798°; body-centered cubic β-form, d 6.64, exists at >798°. mp 935°. bp 3020°; also reported as bp 3520° (Spedding). E^0 (aq) Pr^{3+}/Pr -2.47 V (calc). Experimental reduction potentials (referred to a normal calomel electrode): -1.875, -1.990 V: Noddack, Brukl, *Angew. Chem.* **50,** 362 (1937). Heat of sublimation (25°): 355.6 kJ/mol. Heat of fusion: 6.912 kJ/mol (Spedding, 1982). Also reported as heat of fusion: 11.3 ±2.1 kJ/mol (Greenwood, Earnshaw).

Oxide. Pr_2O_3. d 7.07, prepd by reducing with hydrogen the oxides PrO_2 or Pr_6O_{11}. Oxidizes to Pr_6O_{11} on heating in air; forms the dioxide, PrO_2, on fusing with potassium chlorate.

Hydroxide. $Pr(OH)_3$. A gelatinous pale green precipitate, obtained by the action of alkali hydroxide on a soln of a praseodymium salt; a purple powder when obtained by the action of water on praseodymium carbide.

Chloride. $PrCl_3$. Heptahydrate, green crystals; mp in its water of crystn at 111°; on partial dehydration yields the hexa-, tri-, or

Consult the Name Index before using this section.

monohydrate; on heating to 180-200° in a stream of hydrogen chloride yields the anhydr chloride, green needles, mp 769-782°, sol in water, alcohol. LD$_{50}$ in mice: 600 mg/kg i.p.; 4.5 g/kg orally (Haley).

Sulfate. Pr$_2$(SO$_4$)$_3$. Light green crystals, prepd by evaporating a soln of the oxide in H$_2$SO$_4$ and cooling the resulting product over phosphorus pentoxide. Several hydrates and double sulfates are known.

7713. Pratensein. [2284-31-3] 5,7-Dihydroxy-3-(3-hydroxy-4-methoxyphenyl)-4H-1-benzopyran-4-one; 3′,5,7-trihydroxy-4′-methoxyisoflavone. C$_{16}$H$_{12}$O$_6$; mol wt 300.26. C 64.00%, H 4.03%, O 31.97%. Isoln from red clover (*Trifolium pratense* L., *Leguminosae*), structure and synthesis: E. Wong, *J. Org. Chem.* **28,** 2336 (1963). Alternate syntheses: A. C. Jain, P. K. Bambab, *Indian J. Chem.* **26B,** 488 (1987).

Needles from ethanol, mp 272-273°. uv max (ethanol): 263 nm (log ε 4.53).

Triacetylpratensein. C$_{22}$H$_{18}$O$_9$. White needles from chloroform, mp 175-177°.

7714. Pravastatin Sodium. [81131-70-6] (βR,δR,1S,2S,-6S,8S,8aR)-1,2,6,7,8,8a-Hexahydro-β,δ,6-trihydroxy-2-methyl-8-[(2S)-2-methyl-1-oxobutoxy]-1-naphthaleneheptanoic acid monosodium salt; sodium (+)-(3R,5R)-3,5-dihydroxy-7-[(1S,2S,6S,8S,-8aR)-6-hydroxy-2-methyl-8-[(S)-2-methylbutyryloxy]-1,2,6,7,8,8a-hexahydro-1-naphthyl]heptanoate; eptastatin sodium; 3β-hydroxycompactin sodium salt; CS-514; SQ-31000; Elisor; Lipostat; Liprevil; Mevalotin; Oliprevin; Pravachol; Pravaselect; Pravasin; Selectin; Selipran; Vasten. C$_{23}$H$_{35}$NaO$_7$; mol wt 446.51. C 61.87%, H 7.90%, Na 5.15%, O 25.08%. HMG-CoA reductase inhibitor; bioactive metabolite of mevastatin, *q.v.* Prepn by microbial hydroxylation: A. Terahara, M. Tanaka, **DE 3122499**; *eidem,* **US 4346227** (1981, 1982 both to Sankyo); N. Serizawa *et al., J. Antibiot.* **36,** 604 (1983). Structure elucidation: H. Haruyama *et al., Chem. Pharm. Bull.* **34,** 1459 (1986). HPLC determn in biological fluids: S. Bauer *et al., J. Chromatogr. B* **818,** 257 (2005). Effect on serum lipid concentration: N. Nakaya *et al., Atherosclerosis* **61,** 125 (1986); on hepatic metabolism of cholesterol: E. Reihnér *et al., N. Engl. J. Med.* **323,** 224 (1990). Clinical comparison with probucol, *q.v.:* G. Yoshino *et al., Lancet* **2,** 740 (1986). Clinical reduction of risk of major cardiovascular events in patients with coronary heart disease: LIPID Study Group, *N. Engl. J. Med.* **339,** 1349 (1998). Clinical effect on risk of stroke: H. D. White *et al., ibid.* **343,** 317 (2000).

Odorless, white to off-white, fine or crystalline powder. uv max (methanol): 230, 237, 245 nm. Sol in methanol, water; slightly sol in isopropanol. Practically insol in acetone, acetonitrile, chloroform, ether.

Lactone. C$_{23}$H$_{34}$O$_6$. Colorless plate crystals, mp 138-142°. [α]$_D^{22}$ +194.0° (c = 0.51 in methanol). uv max (methanol): 230, 237, 245 nm.

THERAP CAT: Antilipemic.

7715. Prazepam. [2955-38-6] 7-Chloro-1-(cyclopropylmethyl)-1,3-dihydro-5-phenyl-2H-1,4-benzodiazepin-2-one; 1-(cyclopropylmethyl)-5-phenyl-7-chloro-1H-1,4-benzodiazepin-2(3H)-one; W-4020; Centrax; Demetrin; Lysanxia; Prazene; Sedapran; Trepidan. C$_{19}$H$_{17}$ClN$_2$O; mol wt 324.80. C 70.26%, H 5.28%, Cl 10.92%, N 8.62%, O 4.93%. Prepn: McMillan, Pattison, **FR 1394287**, corresp to **US 3192199** (both 1965 to Warner-Lambert); Wuest, **US 3192200** (1965); Inaba *et al., Chem. Pharm. Bull.* **17,** 1263 (1969). Pharmacology: Robichaud *et al., Arch. Int. Pharmacodyn. Ther.* **185,** 213 (1970). Metabolism: DiCarlo *et al., J. Pharm. Sci.* **58,** 960 (1969).

Crystals from methanol, mp 145-146°.

Note: This is a controlled substance (depressant): **21 CFR,** 1308.14.

THERAP CAT: Anxiolytic.

7716. Praziquantel. [55268-74-1] 2-(Cyclohexylcarbonyl)-1,2,3,6,7,11b-hexahydro-4H-pyrazino[2,1-a]isoquinolin-4-one; EMBAY 8440; Biltricide; Cesol; Droncit. C$_{19}$H$_{24}$N$_2$O$_2$; mol wt 312.41. C 73.05%, H 7.74%, N 8.97%, O 10.24%. Prepn: J. Seubert *et al.,* **DE 2362539**; *eidem,* **US 4001411** (1975, 1977, both to E. Merck, W. Ger.); D. Frehel *et al., Heterocycles* **20,** 1731 (1983). Properties: J. Seubert *et al., Experientia* **33,** 1036 (1977). *In vitro* study: C. J. Chavasse *et al., Z. Parasitenkd.* **58,** 169 (1979). Effect on ultrastructure of trematodes: H. Mehlhorn *et al., Arzneim.-Forsch.* **33,** 91 (1983). Pharmacodynamics: G. C. Coles, *J. Helminthol.* **53,** 31 (1979). Ovicidal activity in *Echinococcus:* A. S. Thakur *et al., Exp. Parasitol.* **47,** 131 (1979). Clinical pharmacology: G. Leopold *et al., Eur. J. Clin. Pharmacol.* **14,** 281 (1978). Efficacy in dogs: F. L. Anderson *et al., Am. J. Vet. Res.* **40,** 700 (1979). Mutagenicity study: H. Bartsch *et al., Mutat. Res.* **58,** 133 (1978). Tolerance study: P. Muermann *et al., Vet. Med. Rev.* **1976** (2), 142. Symposium on African schistosomiasis: *Arzneim.-Forsch.* **31,** 535-618 (1981). Clinical studies (human schistosomiasis): T. E. Nash *et al., Am. J. Trop. Med. Hyg.* **31,** 977 (1982); R. N. H. Pugh, C. H. Teesdale, *Br. Med. J.* **286,** 429 (1983); C. H. Schutte *et al., S. Afr. Med. J.* **64,** 7 (1983). Clinical trial in human parenchymal brain cysticercosis: J. Sotelo *et al., N. Engl. J. Med.* **310,** 1001 (1984).

Crystals, mp 136-138°. Soly (g/100 ml): ethanol 9.7; chloroform 56.7; water 0.04. LD$_{50}$ in mice, rats (mg/kg): 2000-3000 orally; >3000 s.c. (Muermann).

THERAP CAT: Anthelmintic (Schistosoma).

THERAP CAT (VET): Anthelmintic.

7717. Prazosin. [19216-56-9] 1-(4-Amino-6,7-dimethoxy-2-quinolinyl)-4-(2-furanylcarbonyl)piperazine; 2-[4-(2-furoyl)-piperazin-1-yl]-4-amino-6,7-dimethoxyquinazoline; furazosin. C$_{19}$H$_{21}$N$_5$O$_4$; mol wt 383.40. C 59.52%, H 5.52%, N 18.27%, O 16.69%. α$_1$-Adrenergic blocker. Prepn: **GB 1156973**; Hess, **US 3511836** (1969, 1970 both to Pfizer); **NL 7206067** (1972 to Brocades-Stheeman), *C.A.* **78,** 72180s (1973); E. Honkanen *et al., J. Heterocycl. Chem.* **17,** 797 (1980). Pharmacology and clinical data: Scriabine *et al., Experientia* **24,** 1150 (1968); Cohen, *J. Clin. Pharmacol. J. New Drugs* **10,** 408 (1970). Pharmacokinetics: P. Jaillon, *Clin. Pharmacokinet.* **5,** 365 (1980). HPLC determn in biological fluids: R. K. Bhamra *et al.*, *J. Chromatogr.* **380**, 216 (1986). Clinical evaluation in Raynaud's phenomenon: I. J. Russell, J. A Lessard, *J. Rheumatol.* **12**, 94 (1985); in dysuria with benign prostatic hypertrophy: A. LeDuc *et al.*, *Urol. Int.* **45**, Suppl. 1, 56 (1990). Book: *Prazosin: Pharmacology, Hypertension and Congestive Heart Failure*, M. D. Rawlins, Ed. (Grune & Stratton, New York, 1981) 143 pp. Review of pharmacology and therapeutic use: W. F. Stanaszek *et al.*, *Drugs* **25**, 339-384 (1983); J. L. Reid, J. Vincent, *Cardiology* **73**, 164-174 (1986). Comprehensive description: L. J. Kostek, *Anal. Profiles Drug Subs.* **18**, 351-378 (1989).

Crystals, mp 278-280°.

Hydrochloride. [19237-84-4] CP-12299-1; Alpress LP; Duramipress; Eurex; Hypovase; Minipress; Peripress; Sinetens. $C_{19}H_{21}$-N_5O_4.HCl; mol wt 419.86. uv max (methanolic 0.01*N* HCl): 246, 329 nm (a_M 137 ±3, 27.6 ±0.3). Soly at ambient temp (mg/ml): acetone 0.0072, methanol 6.4, ethanol 0.84, dimethylformamide 1.3, dimethylacetamide 1.2, water (pH~3.5) 1.4, chloroform 0.041.

THERAP CAT: Antihypertensive.

7718. Precocenes. Anti-JH. Anti-juvenile hormones found in plants that induce reversible precocious metamorphosis and sterilization in insects by suppressing the function of the corpora allata gland: W. S. Bowers *et al.*, *Science* **193**, 542 (1976); W. S. Bowers, R. Martinez-Pardo, *ibid.* **197**, 1369 (1977). Isoln from *Ageratum mexicanum* Sw., *Compositae* and structure: A. R. Alertsen, *Acta Chem. Scand.* **9**, 1725 (1955). Synthesis of precocene I: R. Livingstone, R. B. Watson, *J. Chem. Soc.* **1957**, 1509; of precocene II: R. Huls, *Bull. Soc. Chim. Belg.* **66**, 409 (1957); **67**, 22 (1958); of I and II: J. R. Hlubucek *et al.*, *Aust. J. Chem.* **24**, 2347 (1971); A. Banerji, N. C. Goomer, *Indian J. Chem.* **20B**, 144 (1981); V. K. Ahluwalia *et al.*, *Chem. Ind. (London)* **1982**, 369. Biosynthesis: A. V. Vyas, N. B. Mulchandani, *Phytochemistry* **19**, 2597 (1980). Metabolism studies: D. M. Soderlund *et al.*, *J. Agric. Food Chem.* **1980**, 724; B. J. Bergot *et al.*, *Pestic. Biochem. Physiol.* **13**, 95 (1980). Mechanism of action: W. S. Bowers, *Am. Zool.* **21**, 737 (1981).

Precocene I   R = H
Precocene II   R = OCH₃

Precocene I. 7-Methoxy-2,2-dimethyl-2*H*-1-benzopyran; 7-methoxy-2,2-dimethylchromene; 6-demethoxyageratochromene. $C_{12}H_{14}O_2$; mol wt 190.24. Oil, bp₆ 120°. n_D^{21} 1.5548. uv max (ethanol): 280, 304 nm (ε 6644, 5844).

Precocene II. 6,7-Dimethoxy-2,2-dimethyl-2*H*-1-benzopyran; 6,7-dimethoxy-2,2-dimethylchromene; ageratochromene. $C_{13}H_{16}$-O_3; mol wt 220.26. Crystals, mp 47.5°, bp₆ 136°. uv max (ethanol): 280, 323 nm (ε 5500, 9200).

7719. Prednicarbate. [73771-04-7] (11β)-17-[(Ethoxycarbonyl)oxy]-11-hydroxy-21-(1-oxopropoxy)pregna-1,4-diene-3,20-dione; 11β,17,21-trihydroxypregna-1,4-diene-3,20-dione 17-(ethyl carbonate) 21-propionate; prednisolone 17-ethylcarbonate 21-propionate; HOE-777; S-77-0777; Dermatop; Prednitop; Regenit. C_{27}-$H_{36}O_8$; mol wt 488.57. C 66.38%, H 7.43%, O 26.20%. Topical anti-inflammatory agent. Prepn: U. Stache *et al.*, **DE 2735110**; *eidem*, **US 4242334** (1979, 1980 both to Hoechst AG); U. Stache *et al.*, *Arzneim.-Forsch.* **35**, 1753 (1985). Topical and systemic activ-

ity in rats: H. G. Alpermann *et al.*, *ibid.* **32**, 633 (1982). Series of articles on pharmacology, pharmacokinetics and clinical efficacy: *Z. Hautkrankhr.* **61**, Suppl. 1, 1-96 (1986).

Crystals from ethanol + diethylether, mp 110-112°; second crystalline form, mp 183°. uv max (ethanol): 241 nm (ε 15000). $[\alpha]_D^{20}$ +63° (c = 0.1 in ethanol). Practically insol in water. Freely sol in ethanol.

THERAP CAT: Glucocorticoid.

7720. Prednimustine. [29069-24-7] (11β)-21-[4-[4-[Bis(2-chloroethyl)amino]phenyl]-1-oxobutoxy]-11,17-dihydroxypregna-1,4-diene-3,20-dione; 11β,17,21-trihydroxypregna-1,4-diene-3,20-dione 21-[4-[p-[bis(2-chloroethyl)amino]phenyl]butyrate]; prednisolone 21-[4-[p-[bis(2-chloroethyl)amino]phenyl]butyrate]; Leo-1031; Sterecyt; Stereocyt. $C_{35}H_{45}Cl_2NO_6$; mol wt 646.64. C 65.01%, H 7.01%, Cl 10.97%, N 2.17%, O 14.85%. Prednisolone ester of chlorambucil, *q.v.* Prepn: H. F. Fex *et al.*, **DE 2001305** corresp to **US 3732260** (1970, 1973 both to AB Leo). *In vitro* study: A. H. Evenaar *et al.*, *Eur. J. Cancer* **9**, 773 (1973). Metabolism: R. Y. Kirdani *et al.*, *Oncology* **35**, 47 (1978). Clinical studies: L. Hakarsson *et al.*, *ibid.* 103; J. E. Johnsson *et al.*, *Cancer Treat. Rep.* **63**, 421 (1970). Toxicity and antitumor activity study: K. R. Harrap *et al.*, *Eur. J. Cancer* **13**, 873 (1977). Series of articles on pharmacology, toxicology and clinical efficacy: *Semin. Oncol.* **13**, Suppl. 1, 1-44 (1986).

Crystals from methanol-water, mp 163-164°. $[\alpha]_D^{24}$ +92.9° (c = 1.06 in chloroform).

THERAP CAT: Antineoplastic.

7721. Prednisolone. [50-24-8] (11β)-11,17,21-Trihydroxypregna-1,4-diene-3,20-dione; 1,4-pregnadiene-3,20-dione-11β,-17α,21-triol; 1,4-pregnadiene-11β,17α,21-triol-3,20-dione; 3,20-dioxo-11β,17α,21-trihydroxy-1,4-pregnadiene; metacortandralone; delta F; Δ¹-dehydrocortisol; Δ¹-hydrocortisone; Δ¹-dehydrohydrocortisone; hydroretrocortine; Codelcortone; Decaprednil; Decortin H; Deltacortril; Klismacort; Meticortelone; Precortisyl; Prednicen; Predonine; Solone. $C_{21}H_{28}O_5$; mol wt 360.44. C 69.98%, H 7.83%, O 22.19%. Synthetic corticosteroid; metabolically interconvertible with prednisone, *q.v.* Prepn: A. Nobile *et al.*, *J. Am. Chem. Soc.* **77**, 4184 (1955); A. Nobile, **US 2837464**; **US 3134718** (1958, 1964, both to Schering); Herzog *et al.*, *Tetrahedron* **18**, 581 (1962). HPLC determn in urine: B. M. Frey, F. J. Frey, *J. Chromatogr.* **229**, 283 (1982). Clinical use in advanced cancer: R. G. Twycross, D. Guppy, *Practitioner* **229**, 57 (1985); in inflammatory bowel disease: C. J. Hawkey, *Neth. J. Med.* **35** Suppl 1, S21-S26 (1989). Review of clinical pharmacology: W. J. Jusko, J. Q. Rose, *Ther. Drug Monit.* **2**, 169-176 (1980); of pharmacokinetics and metabolism: B. M. Frey, F. J. Frey, *Clin. Pharmacokinet.* **19**, 126-146 (1990). Comprehensive description: S. L. Ali, *Anal. Profiles Drug Subs. Excip.* **21**, 415-500 (1992).

Crystals, dec 240-241°. $[\alpha]_D^{25}$ +102° (dioxane). uv max (methanol): 242 nm (ε 15000; $A_{1cm}^{1\%}$ 414). Very slightly sol in water. One gram dissolves in about 30 ml of alcohol, in about 180 ml of chloroform, in about 50 ml of acetone. Sol in methanol, dioxane.

21-Acetate. [52-21-1] Ak-Tate; Deltastab; Inflanefran; Pred Forte; Pred Mild; Scherisolon; Sterane. $C_{23}H_{30}O_6$; mol wt 402.48. Crystals, decomp 237-239°. $[\alpha]_D^{25}$ +116° (dioxane).

21-tert-Butylacetate. [7681-14-3] Prednisolone tebutate; Codelcortone-T.B.A.. $C_{27}H_{38}O_6$; mol wt 458.59. Prepn: Sarett, **US 2736734** (1956 to Merck & Co.). Crystals from ethanol, mp 266-273°.

21-Disodium Phosphate. [125-02-0] Prednisolone sodium phosphate; Codelsol; Colicort; Hefasolon i.v.; Inflamase; Orapred; Predsol; Solucort. $C_{21}H_{27}Na_2O_8P$; mol wt 484.39. C 52.07%, H 5.62%, Na 9.49%, O 26.42%, P 6.39%. Prepn: Sarett, **US 2789117** (1957 to Merck & Co.). Alternate synthesis: Poos *et al., Chem. Ind. (London)* **1958**, 1260; Elks, Phillips, **US 2936313** (1960 to Glaxo). White powder. Slightly hygroscopic. Stable at room temp. $[\alpha]_D^{25}$ +102.5°. uv max (methanol): 243 nm ($A_{1cm}^{1\%}$ 308). Sol in water, methanol, ethanol. pH of 1% aq soln 7.5 to 8.5.

21-Succinate sodium salt. [1715-33-9] Prednisolone sodium succinate; Meticortelone Soluble; Solu-Decortin-H. $C_{25}H_{31}NaO_8$; mol wt 482.50. Prepn: Shull, Kita, **DE 1045400** (1958 to Pfizer), *C.A.* **55**, 2746f (1961).

21-Stearoylglycolate. [5060-55-9] Prednisolone steaglate; Sintisone. $C_{41}H_{64}O_8$; mol wt 684.94. Prepn: Giraldi, Nannini, **US 3171846** (1965 to Carlo Erba); Giraldi *et al., Arzneim.-Forsch.* **16**, 162 (1966). Crystals from dilute alcohol or butyl ether, mp 105-107°. uv max (methanol): 242 nm ($E_{1cm}^{1\%}$ 212 ±10). $[\alpha]_D^{20}$ +57-63°.

21-m-Sulfobenzoate sodium salt. [630-67-1] (11β)-11,17-Dihydroxy-21-[(3-sulfobenzoyl)oxy]pregna-1,4-diene-3,20-dione monosodium salt; prednisolone sodium metasulfobenzoate; Predenema; Predfoam; Solupred. $C_{28}H_{31}NaO_9S$; mol wt 566.60. Prepn: Allais, Girault, **US 3032568**; Joly, Warnant, **US 3037034** (both 1962 to Roussel-UCLAF). Crystals from water, dec 293-295°. $[\alpha]_D^{20}$ +170° (water).

21-Trimethylacetate. [1107-99-9] Prednisolone 21-pivalate; Ultracortenol. $C_{26}H_{36}O_6$; mol wt 444.56. Prepn: Vischer *et al., Helv. Chim. Acta* **38**, 1502 (1955); Joly, Warnant, **US 3037034** (1962 to Roussel-UCLAF). Crystals from acetone, mp 233-236°. $[\alpha]_D^{26}$ +103° (c = 1.208 in chloroform); $[\alpha]_D^{20}$ +97.5° (c = 1 in chloroform). uv max: 244 nm (ε 14700).

THERAP CAT: Glucocorticoid.

THERAP CAT (VET): Glucocorticoid.

7722. Prednisone. [53-03-2] 17,21-Dihydroxypregna-1,4-diene-3,11,20-trione; 1,4-pregnadiene-17α,21-diol-3,11,20-trione; Δ^1-dehydrocortisone; Δ^1-cortisone; deltacortisone; delta E; metacortandracin; retrocortine; NSC-10023; Colisone; Cortancyl; Dacortin; Decortin; Deltacortene; Deltacortone; Deltasone; Deltison; Di-Adreson; Encorton; Hostacortin; Meticorten; Orasone; Rectodelt; Sone; Ultracorten. $C_{21}H_{26}O_5$; mol wt 358.43. C 70.37%, H 7.31%, O 22.32%. Prepn: Oliveto, Gould, **US 2897216** (1959 to Schering). Microbiological prepn: Nobile *et al., J. Am. Chem. Soc.* **77**, 4184 (1955); Nobile, **US 2837464** and **US 3134718** (1958, 1964 both to Schering); Herzog *et al., Tetrahedron* **18**, 581 (1962). Structure: Herzog *et al., Science* **121**, 176 (1955); *cf.* Djerassi *et al.*, **US 2579479** (1951 to Syntex).

Crystals, dec 233-235°. $[\alpha]_D^{25}$ +172° (dioxane). uv max (methanol): 238 nm (ε 15500). Very slightly sol in water. One gram dissolves in about 150 ml alcohol, in about 200 ml chloroform. Slightly sol in methanol, dioxane.

21-Acetate. [125-10-0] $C_{23}H_{28}O_6$. Crystals, dec 226-232°. $[\alpha]_D^{25}$ +186° (dioxane). uv max (ethanol): 238 nm (ε 16100).

THERAP CAT: Glucocorticoid.

THERAP CAT (VET): Adrenocortical steroid. Glucocorticoid, anti-inflammatory.

7723. Prednival. [15180-00-4] (11β)-11,21-Dihydroxy-17-[(1-oxopentyl)oxy]pregna-1,4-diene-3,20-dione; 11β,17,21-trihydroxypregna-1,4-diene-3,20-dione 17-valerate; prednisolone 17-valerate; W-4869. $C_{26}H_{36}O_6$; mol wt 444.56. C 70.24%, H 8.16%, O 21.59%. Prepn: Vitali, Ercoli, *Tetrahedron Lett.* **1961**, 448; Ercoli, Gardi, **US 3152154** (1964 to Vismara).

Crystals from aq methanol, mp 210-213°. $[\alpha]_D$ +3.5° (dioxane).

21-Acetate. Acepreval. $C_{28}H_{38}O_7$; mol wt 486.60.

THERAP CAT: Glucocorticoid.

7724. Prednylidene. [599-33-7] (11β)-11,17,21-Trihydroxy-16-methylenepregna-1,4-diene-3,20-dione; $\Delta^{1,4}$-pregnadiene-16-methylene-11β,17α,21-triol-3,20-dione; 16-methylene-11β,17α,21-trihydroxypregna-1,4-diene-3,20-dione; 16-methyleneprednisolone; Dacortilen; Decortilen. $C_{22}H_{28}O_5$; mol wt 372.45. C 70.95%, H 7.58%, O 21.48%. Prepn: Mannhardt *et al., Tetrahedron Lett.* no. 16, 21 (1960). Prepn of the 21-diethylaminoacetate: *idem et al.*, **DE 1134074** (1962 to E. Merck), *C.A.* **58**, 568a (1963).

Solid, mp 233-235°. $[\alpha]_D^{23}$ +31° (dioxane). uv max: 243 nm (ε 15900).

21-Diethylaminoacetate hydrochloride. [22887-42-9] Decortilen soluble. $C_{28}H_{39}NO_6 \cdot HCl$; mol wt 522.07. Solid, mp 245-246°. $[\alpha]_D$ +45° (water). uv max (water): 246-247 nm ($E_{1cm}^{1\%}$ 300).

THERAP CAT: Glucocorticoid.

7725. Pregabalin. [148553-50-8] (3S)-3-(Aminomethyl)-5-methylhexanoic acid; (S)-(+)-4-amino-3-(2-methylpropyl)butanoic acid; (S)-(+)-3-isobutyl-γ-aminobutyric acid; CI-1008; PD-144723; Lyrica. $C_8H_{17}NO_2$; mol wt 159.23. C 60.34%, H 10.76%, N 8.80%, O 20.10%. Structural analog of γ-aminobutyric acid, *q.v.*; ligand at $\alpha_2\delta$ subunit of voltage-gated calcium channels. Prepn of racemate: R. Andruszkiewicz, R. B. Silverman, *Synthesis* **1989**, 953. Enantioselective synthesis: P. Yuen *et al., Bioorg. Med. Chem. Lett.* **4**, 823 (1994). Manufacturing process: M. S. Hoekstra *et al., Org. Process Res. Dev.* **1**, 26 (1997). HPLC determn in biological fluids: B. L. Windsor, L. L. Radulovic, *J. Chromatogr. B* **674**, 143 (1995). Clinical trial in post-herpetic neuralgia: R. Sabatowski *et al., Pain* **109**, 26 (2004). Overview of mechanism and pharmacology: S. M. Stahl, *J. Clin. Psychiatry* **65**, 596, 1033 (2004). Review of pharmacology and clinical experience: B. A. Lauria-Horner, R. B. Pohl, *Expert Opin. Invest. Drugs* **12**, 663-672 (2003); R. Huckle, *Curr. Opin. Invest. Drugs* **5**, 82-89 (2004).

White crystalline solid, mp 186-188°. $[\alpha]_D^{23}$ +10.52° (c = 1.06 in water).

THERAP CAT: Anticonvulsant; anxiolytic; analgesic in treatment of peripheral neuropathic pain.

7726. Pregnane. [481-26-5] 5β-Pregnane; 17β-ethyletiocholane. $C_{21}H_{36}$; mol wt 288.51. C 87.42%, H 12.58%. Prepd by reduction of etiocholyl methyl ketone or of pregnanedione: Butenandt, *Ber.* **64,** 2529 (1931); Marker *et al., J. Am. Chem. Soc.* **60,** 1067 (1938); Steiger, Reichstein, *Helv. Chim. Acta* **21,** 161 (1938).

Monoclinic scales, plates from methanol; mp 83.5°. d_4^{15} 1.032. $[\alpha]_D^{19}$ +20° (c = 2 in chloroform).

7727. Pregnanediol. [80-92-2] (3α,5β,20S)-Pregnane-3,20-diol. $C_{21}H_{36}O_2$; mol wt 320.51. C 78.69%, H 11.32%, O 9.98%. A metabolite of progesterone, present in large amounts in pregnancy urine. Isoln from pregnancy urine of women: Marrian, *Biochem. J.* **23,** 1090 (1929), Butenandt, *Ber.* **63,** 659 (1930); of cows, mares, and chimpanzees: Fish *et al., J. Biol. Chem.* **143,** 716 (1942). Prepn by reduction of pregn-16-ene-3,20-dione: Marker *et al.,* US 2352852 (1944 to Parke, Davis). Conversion to progesterone: Butenandt, Schmidt, *Ber.* **67,** 1893, 1901 (1934). Conversion to 3α-hydroxypregnan-20-one: Marker, US 2223377 (1940 to Parke, Davis). Prepn of the 3-acetate: Hirschmann, *J. Biol. Chem.* **140,** 797 (1941); Ralls *et al., ibid.* **210,** 709 (1954). Prepn of the 20-acetate: Hirschmann, *loc. cit.* Prepn of the diacetate: Johnson *et al., J. Chem. Soc.* **1954,** 1302. Crystal structure: Haner, Norton, *Acta Crystallogr.* **16,** 707 (1963). Review of metabolism, bioactivity and assay during pregnancy: P. J. Keller, *Contrib. Gynecol. Obstet.* **2,** 75-91 (1976).

Crystals from acetone or ethanol, mp 239°. $[\alpha]_D^{20}$ +27.4° (c = 0.7 in alc). Sparingly sol in organic solvents. Not precipitated by digitonin.

3-Acetate. 3α-Acetoxypregnan-20α-ol. $C_{23}H_{38}O_3$. Crystals, mp 132°. $[\alpha]_D^{25}$ +45° (CHCl₃).

20-Acetate. 20α-Acetoxypregnan-3α-ol. $C_{23}H_{38}O_3$. Crystals, mp 174°.

Diacetate. 3α,20α-Diacetoxypregnane. $C_{25}H_{40}O_4$. Crystals from light petroleum, mp 180°, also reported as mp 182-183°. $[\alpha]_D^{15}$ +35° (c = 1.1 in CHCl₃).

USE: In manuf of progesterone.

7728. 3,20-Pregnanedione. [128-23-4] (5β)-Pregnane-3,20-dione. $C_{21}H_{32}O_2$; mol wt 316.48. C 79.70%, H 10.19%, O 10.11%. From pregnancy urine of mares. Prepn from other steroids: Butenandt, *Ber.* **63,** 659 (1930); Butenandt, Fleischer, *Ber.* **68,** 2094 (1935); Marker *et al., J. Am. Chem. Soc.* **59,** 1595 (1937); Shoppee, Reichstein, *Helv. Chim. Acta* **24,** 356 (1941); US 2160719; US 2352852; US 2323276; US 2229818.

Needles from dil alc, mp 123°. Insol in water. Freely sol in the usual organic solvents.

Dioxime. $C_{21}H_{34}N_2O_2$. Dec above 250°.

7729. Pregnan-3α-ol-20-one. [128-20-1] (3α,5β)-3-Hydroxypregnan-20-one; 3α-hydroxy-5β-pregnan-20-one; pregnanolone; eltanolone; KABI 2213. $C_{21}H_{34}O_2$; mol wt 318.49. C 79.19%, H 10.76%, O 10.05%. Naturally occurring metabolite of progesterone, *q.v.* Isoln from urine of pregnant women: R. E. Marker, O. Kamm, *J. Am. Chem. Soc.* **59,** 1373 (1937); from bile of pregnant cows: W. H. Pearlman, E. Cerceo, *J. Biol. Chem.* **176,** 847 (1948). Prepn: R. E. Marker *et al., J. Am. Chem. Soc.* **59,** 1841 (1937); L. Gyermek *et al., J. Med. Chem.* **11,** 117 (1968); T. L. G. Lemos, J. D. McChesney, *J. Nat. Prod.* **53,** 152 (1990). Pharmacokinetics and pharmacodynamics: P. Carl *et al., Acta Anaesthesiol. Scand.* **38,** 734 (1994). Comparative clinical evaluation: J. Van Hemelrijck *et al., Anesthesiology* **80,** 36 (1994); H. Eriksson *et al., Acta Anaesthesiol. Scand.* **39,** 479 (1995). Hemodynamic effects in humans: J. W. Sear *et al., J. Clin. Anesth.* **7,** 126 (1995).

Needles from aq methanol, mp 148-148.5° (Pearlman, Cerceo); also reported as cryst from hexane, mp 131-132° (Lemos, McChesney). $[\alpha]_D^{23}$ +59.6° (c = 0.3 in chloroform). $[\alpha]_D^{26}$ +108.5 ±1° (c = 9.23 mg/1.23 ml abs ethanol). LD_{50} in mice, rats (mg/kg): 66 ± 10, 27.5 ± 2.4 i.v. (Gyermek).

THERAP CAT: Anesthetic (local).

7730. 4-Pregnene-11β,17α,20β,21-tetrol-3-one. [116-58-5] 11β,17,20β,21-Tetrahydroxypregn-4-en-3-one; 17-(1,2-dihydroxyethyl)androsten-3-one-11,17-diol; Reichstein's substance E. $C_{21}H_{32}O_5$; mol wt 364.48. C 69.20%, H 8.85%, O 21.95%. Occurs in adrenal cortex. Isoln: Reichstein, *Helv. Chim. Acta* **19,** 29 (1936); **20,** 953 (1937); Reichstein, von Euw, *ibid.* **24,** 247E (1941).

Hydrated crystals from dil acetone, dec 125°. $[\alpha]_D^{20}$ +87° (alc). $[M]_D$ +317°. uv max: 240 nm.

20,21-Diacetate. Crystals, dec 229-230°. $[\alpha]_D^{20}$ +162.7°. $[M]_D$ +730° (acetone).

7731. 4-Pregnene-17α,20β,21-triol-3,11-dione. [116-59-6] (20R)-17,20,21-Trihydroxypregn-4-ene-3,11-dione; Reichstein's substance U. $C_{21}H_{30}O_5$; mol wt 362.46. C 69.59%, H 8.34%, O 22.07%. Isoln from adrenal glands: Reichstein, von Euw, *Helv. Chim. Acta* **24,** 247E (1941).

Clusters of needles from acetone + ether, mp 208-209°.

20,21-Diacetate. $C_{25}H_{34}O_7$. Pointed needles from acetone + ether or chloroform + ether, mp 253°. $[\alpha]_D^{21}$ +178.5° (c = 0.924 in acetone). uv max (alc): 239 nm (log ε 4.1). Less sol than the 20,21-diacetate of 4-pregnene-11β,17α,20,21-tetrol-3-one.

7732. 4-Pregnene-17α,20β,21-triol-3-one. [128-19-8] (20R)-17,20,21-Trihydroxypregn-4-en-3-one; 17-(1,2-dihydroxy-ethyl)-Δ⁴-androsten-3-on-17α-ol; 17α-pregnenetriolone. $C_{21}H_{32}$-O_4; mol wt 348.48. C 72.38%, H 9.26%, O 18.36%. Prepd from 17-ethynyltestosterone by hydrogenation with palladium in pyridine, allylic rearrangement, and hydroxylation with osmium tetroxide: Ruzicka, Müller, *Helv. Chim. Acta* **22**, 755 (1939); Logemann, *Naturwissenschaften* **27**, 196 (1939); from a 3-enol ester of a 17,21-diacyloxyprogesterone by reduction followed by saponification: CH 207496 (1940), *C.A.* **36**, 3636 (1942).

Crystals from methanol. mp 190°. Sol in dioxane, chloroform, methanol. $[\alpha]_D$ +63° (c = 1 in dioxane). uv max: 240 nm (log ε 4.1).

20,21-Diacetate. $C_{25}H_{36}O_6$. Crystals from acetone + ether. Polymorphic; mp 170° and 194°; $[\alpha]_D^{20}$ +125° (dioxane). Reaction with zinc in toluene yields 17-isodesoxycorticosterone acetate.

7733. Pregnenolone. [145-13-1] (3β)-3-Hydroxypregn-5-en-20-one; Δ⁵-pregnen-3β-ol-20-one; 17β-(1-ketoethyl)-Δ⁵-androsten-3β-ol. $C_{21}H_{32}O_2$; mol wt 316.48. C 79.70%, H 10.19%, O 10.11%. Prepn from stigmasterol: Butenandt *et al., Ber.* **67**, 1611 (1934); Butenandt, Fleischer, *Ber.* **70**, 96 (1937); from androstenolone: H. Butenandt, J. Schmidt-thome, *Ber.* **72**, 182 (1939); S. Danishefsky *et al., J. Org. Chem.* **40**, 1989 (1975); from Δ⁵-3-acetoxyetiocholenic acid chloride: Wettstein, *Helv. Chim. Acta* **23**, 1373 (1940); from diosgenin: Marker, Krueger, *J. Am. Chem. Soc.* **62**, 3349 (1940); Marker *et al., ibid.* **69**, 2173 (1947); from nologenin: *eidem, ibid.* 2395; by treating a 21-halo-Δ⁵-pregnen-3-ol-20-one with a reducing agent: CH 215139 (1941), *C.A.* **42**, 3144 (1948). Crystal structure: J. Bordner *et al., Cryst. Struct. Commun.* **7**, 513 (1978).

Needles from dil alc, mp 193°. $[\alpha]_D^{20}$ +28° (alc). Very sparingly sol in water. Soly (g/100 ml of soln): carbon tetrachloride 0.5; petr ether 0.1; ethyl acetate 1.1; acetone 0.6; chloroform 17.0; ethanol 1.9; benzene 0.9; isopropanol 1.5. Soly (g/100 ml of solvent): propylene glycol 1.0; dioxane 3.1; benzyl alcohol 8.1. On refluxing with methyl alcohol yields the 17-isopregnenolone, mp 172-173°, $[\alpha]_D^{20}$ −140.5° (alcohol).

Acetate. $C_{23}H_{34}O_3$. Needles from alcohol, mp 149-151°. $[\alpha]_D^{20}$ +22° (alcohol). Soly (g/100 ml of soln): carbon tetrachloride 5.0; petr ether 1.0; ethyl acetate 7.9; acetone 2.7; chloroform 55.0; ethanol 2.5; benzene 26.0; isopropanol 2.0. Soly (g/100 ml of solvent): propylene glycol 0.1; dioxane 20.2; benzyl alcohol 11.1; benzyl benzoate 9.1.

Methyl ether. [511-26-2] $C_{22}H_{34}O_2$. Crystals from abs or dil methanol, mp 123.5°. $[\alpha]_D^{18}$ +18° (c = 1.085 in chloroform).

7734. Prelog-Djerassi Lactone. [69056-12-8] (αR,2S,3S,-5R)-Tetrahydro-α,3,5-trimethyl-6-oxo-2H-pyran-2-acetic acid; (+)-Prelog-Djerassi lactonic acid; 6-(1-carboxyethyl)-3,4,5,6-tetrahydro-3,5-dimethyl-2-pyranone. $C_{10}H_{16}O_4$; mol wt 200.23. C 59.98%, H 8.05%, O 31.96%. Intermediate in the synthesis of macrolide antibiotics. Isoln as degradation product of narbomycin, *q.v.*: R. Anliker *et al., Helv. Chim. Acta* **39**, 1785 (1956); of methymycin, *q.v.*: C. Djerassi, J. A. Zderic, *J. Am. Chem. Soc.* **78**, 6390 (1956). Abs config: R. W. Rickards, R. M. Smith, *Tetrahedron Lett.* **1970**, 1025. Synthesis: P. A. Grieco *et al., J. Am. Chem. Soc.* **101**, 4749 (1979); D. A. Evans, J. Bartroli, *Tetrahedron Lett.* **23**, 807 (1982). Synthesis of (±)-form: S. Masamune *et al., J. Am. Chem. Soc.* **97**, 3512 (1975); C. Santelli-Rouvier *et al., Tetrahedron Lett.* **35**, 6101 (1994). Review of stereoselective syntheses: S. F. Martin, D. E. Guinn, *Synthesis* **1991**, 245.

Crystals, mp 124-125°. $[\alpha]_D$ +33° (c = 0.797 in CHCl₃).

7735. Prenalterol. [57526-81-5] 4-[(2S)-2-Hydroxy-3-[(1-methylethyl)amino]propoxy]phenol; (−)-(S)-1-(p-hydroxyphenoxy)-3-(isopropylamino)-2-propanol. $C_{12}H_{19}NO_3$; mol wt 225.28. C 63.98%, H 8.50%, N 6.22%, O 21.31%. A β₁-adrenergic agonist. Prepn: K. A. Jaeggi *et al.*, DE 2503968 corresp to US 3978041 and US 4049797 (1974, 1976, 1977, all to Ciba-Geigy). Pharmacologic study: E. Carlsson *et al., Arch. Pharmacol.* **300**, 101 (1977). Metabolism, hemodynamic effects, pharmacokinetics in man: O. Rönn *et al., Eur. J. Clin. Pharmacol.* **17**, 81 (1980). Cardiovascular effects: D. H. Scott *et al., Br. J. Clin. Pharmacol.* **7**, 365 (1979). Clinical study in coronary heart disease: I. Hutton *et al., Br. Heart J.* **43**, 134 (1980). *See also* T. P. Kenakin, D. Beek, *J. Pharmacol. Exp. Ther.* **213**, 406 (1980) for a discussion of the selectivity of action. Prepns of the racemic mixture: NL 6409883 corresp to H. Köppe *et al.*, US 3637852 (1965, 1972 both to Boehringer, Ing.); NL 301580 corresp to A. F. Crowther, L. H. Smith, US 3501769 (1965, 1970 both to ICI); A. F. Crowther *et al., J. Med. Chem.* **12**, 638 (1969). Symposium: *Acta Med. Scand.* **Suppl. 659**, 1-325 (1982).

Crystals from ethyl acetate, mp 127-128°. $[\alpha]_D^{20}$ −1 ±1°; $[\alpha]_{Hg}^{20}$ +2 ±1° (c = 0.940 in methanol).

Hydrochloride. [61260-05-7] H-133/22; CGP-7760B; (−)H-80/62; Hyprenan. $C_{12}H_{19}NO_3$·HCl; mol wt 261.75.

THERAP CAT: Cardiotonic.

7736. Prenoxdiazine Hydrochloride. [982-43-4] 1-[2-[3-(2,2-Diphenylethyl)-1,2,4-oxadiazol-5-yl]ethyl]piperidine monohydrochloride; 3-(β,β-diphenylethyl)-5-(β-piperidinoethyl)-1,2,4-oxadiazole hydrochloride; HK-256; Libexin; Lompacet; Tibexin. $C_{23}H_{28}ClN_3O$; mol wt 397.94. C 69.42%, H 7.09%, Cl 8.91%, N 10.56%, O 4.02%. Prepn: K. Harsanyi *et al.*, HU 151748 (1964 to Chinoin), *C.A.* **62**, 11821f (1965). Pharmacology: L. Tardos, I. Erdély, *Arzneim.-Forsch.* **16**, 617 (1966). Stability study: E. Pandula *et al., Acta Pharm. Hung.* **38**, 68 (1968). Review of pharmacology and clinical studies: K. Harsanyi *et al., Boll. Chim. Farm.* **112**, 691 (1973).

• HCl

Crystals from ethanol, mp 192-193°. LD_{50} in mice, rats (mg/kg): 920, >2000 orally; 34, 32 i.v. (Tardos, Erdély).

THERAP CAT: Antitussive.

7737. Prenylamine. [390-64-7] N-(1-Methyl-2-phenylethyl)-γ-phenylbenzenepropanamine; N-(3,3-diphenylpropyl)-α-methylphenethylamine; N-(3'-phenyl-2'-propyl)-1,1-diphenyl-3-propylamine; 1-phenyl-2-[1',1'-diphenylpropyl-3'-amino]propane; B-436; Elecor. $C_{24}H_{27}N$; mol wt 329.48. C 87.49%, H 8.26%, N 4.25%. Prepn: G. Ehrhart et al., **DE 1100031** C.A. **56**, 3413h (1962) and **DE 1111642** corresp to **US 3152173** (1961, 1961, 1964 all to Hoechst); G. Erhart, Arch. Pharm. **295**, 196 (1962). Series of articles on pharmacology and chemistry: Arzneim.-Forsch. **10**, 569-588 (1960). Metabolism: M. Volz, ibid. **21**, 1320 (1971). Review: J. E. Murphy, J. Int. Med. Res. **1**, 204-209 (1973).

mp 36.5-37.5°.

Lactate. [69-43-2] Angormin; Bismetin; Carditin-Same; Coredamin; Corontin; Crepasin; Daxauten; Hostaginan; Incoran; Irrorin; Lactamin; Plactamin; Reocorin; Roinin; Seccidin; Sedolatan; Segontin; Synadrin. $C_{27}H_{33}NO_3$; mol wt 419.56. mp 140-142°. Sparingly sol in water (~0.5%); sol in organic solvents. uv max (chloroform): 260 nm ($E_{1cm}^{1\%}$ 170).

THERAP CAT: Vasodilator (coronary).

7738. Prephenic Acid. [126-49-8] 1-Carboxy-4-hydroxy-α-oxo-2,5-cyclohexadiene-1-propanoic acid; 1-carboxy-4-hydroxy-2,5-cyclohexadiene-1-pyruvic acid. $C_{10}H_{10}O_6$; mol wt 226.18. C 53.10%, H 4.46%, O 42.44%. Non-aromatic biosynthetic intermediate that represents a secondary branch-point in the pathway from chorismic acid to phenylalanine and tyrosine, q.q.v., in many organisms. Isoln from cultures of mutant Escherichia coli: B. D. Davis, Science **118**, 251 (1953). Characterized as cryst Ba salt: U. Weiss et al., ibid. **119**, 774 (1954); R. L. Metzenberg, H. K. Mitchell, Arch. Biochem. Biophys. **64**, 51 (1956). Structure: H. Plieninger, G. Keilich, Z. Naturforsch. **16b**, 81 (1961). Synthetic approaches: H. Plieninger, Angew. Chem. Int. Ed. **1**, 367 (1962). Total synthesis of disodium salt: S. Danishevsky, M. Hirama, J. Am. Chem. Soc. **99**, 7740 (1977); S. Danishevsky et al., ibid. **101**, 7013 (1979); W. Gramlich, H. Plieninger, Ber. **112**, 1571 (1979). Review: U. Weiss, J. M. Edwards, The Biosynthesis of Aromatic Compounds (Wiley, New York, 1980) pp 144-184. See also shikimic acid.

Barium salt monohydrate. $C_{10}H_8BaO_6.H_2O$. Crystals from water + methanol or water + pyridine.

7739. Presenilins. Integral membrane proteins required for the proteolytic processing of the *amyloid precursor protein* (APP) to yield amyloid-β peptide (Aβ), q.v. Missense mutations in the presenilin genes result in the production of an abnormal form of Aβ which is the major component of the amyloid plaques deposited in the brains of patients with Alzheimer's disease (AD). Highly hydrophobic, *presenilin 1* (*PS1*) and its homolog *presenilin 2* (*PS2*), consist of 463 and 448 amino acid residues, respectively. PS1 is believed to be a catalytic subunit of γ-*secretase*. Thought to have 7 or 8 transmembrane domains that span the membranes of the endoplasmic reticulum, nuclear envelope and Golgi apparatus. Identification of the gene for PS1: R. Sherrington et al., Nature **375**, 754 (1995); for PS2: E. I. Rogaev et al., ibid. **376**, 775 (1995). Characterization of PS1 and distribution in human and rodent brain: G. A. Elder et al., J. Neurosci. Res. **45**, 308 (1996). Structural study: N. N. Dewji et al., Proc. Natl. Acad. Sci. USA **101**, 1057 (2004). Review of structure, possible physiological functions, and role in Alzheimer's disease: C. Haass, B. De Strooper, Science **286**, 916-919 (1999); P. E. Fraser et al., Biochim. Biophys. Acta **1502**, 1-15 (2000).

7740. Pretilachlor. [51218-49-6] 2-Chloro-N-(2,6-diethylphenyl)-N-(2-propoxyethyl)acetamide; N-propoxyethyl-N-chloroacetyl-2,6-diethylaniline; 2,6-diethyl-N-(2'-n-propoxyethyl)chloroacetanilide; CGA-26423; CG-113; Rifit. $C_{17}H_{26}ClNO_2$; mol wt 311.85. C 65.47%, H 8.40%, Cl 11.37%, N 4.49%, O 10.26%. Selective herbicide for control of perennial weeds in transplanted rice. Prepn, herbicidal properties: **NL 7307584**; C. Vogel, R. Aebi, **US 4168965** (1973, 1979 both to Ciba-Geigy). Residue analysis, stability: H. Egli, J. Agric. Food Chem. **30**, 861 (1982). Effect on leaf elongation in rice, use in combination with a safening agent (CGA 123,407): R. A. Christ, Weed Res. **25**, 193 (1985). Brief account: J. Rufener, M. Quadranti, Proc. 10th Conf. Int. Congr. Plant Prot. **1**, 332 (1983).

Colorless liquid, $bp_{0.001}$ 135°. Vapor pressure at 20°: 1×10^{-6} mm Hg. Almost insol in water (50 mg/l at 20°). Sol in most organic solvents. n_D^{20} 1.5204. LD_{50} in rats (mg/kg): 6099 orally; >3100 dermally (Rufener, Quadranti). LC_{50} in rainbow trout, carp, catfish: 3.0, 3.0, 2.6 ppm (Vogel, Aebi).

USE: Herbicide for use in rice paddys.

7741. Pridinol. [511-45-5] α,α-Diphenyl-1-piperidinepropanol; 1,1-diphenyl-3-piperidino-1-propanol; 3-piperidino-1,1-diphenyl-1-propanol; 1,1-diphenyl-3-(1-piperidyl)-1-propanol; 3-(N-piperidyl)-1,1-diphenyl-1-propanol; ridinol; C-238. $C_{20}H_{25}NO$; mol wt 295.42. C 81.31%, H 8.53%, N 4.74%, O 5.42%. May be prepd from ethyl 1-piperidinepropionate and phenylmagnesium bromide: Adamson, **GB 624118** (1949 to Wellcome Found.). Toxicity study: R. W. Cunningham et al., J. Pharmacol. Exp. Ther. **96**, 151 (1949).

Crystals, mp 120-121°. Soluble in acetone.

Hydrochloride. [968-58-1] Parks 12. $C_{20}H_{25}NO.HCl$; mol wt 331.88. Crystals, dec 238°. Sol in alc. LD_{50} in mice, rats (mg/kg): 35, 33 i.v.; 131, 91 i.p. (Cunningham).

Methanesulfonate. [6856-31-1] Pridinol mesylate; Konlax; Loxeen; Lyseen; Myoson. $C_{20}H_{25}NO.CH_3SO_3H$; mol wt 391.52. Crystals, mp 152.5-155.0°. Sparingly sol in water.

THERAP CAT: Antiparkinsonian; muscle relaxant (skeletal).

7742. Prifinium Bromide. [4630-95-9] 3-(Diphenylmethylene)-1,1-diethyl-2-methylpyrrolidinium bromide; 3-(diphenylmethylene)-1-ethyl-2-methylpyrrolidine ethyl bromide; pyrodifenium bromide; Padrin; Riabal. $C_{22}H_{28}BrN$; mol wt 386.37. C 68.39%, H 7.30%, Br 20.68%, N 3.63%. Prepn: Sadao Oki, **JP 65 22462** (1965), *C.A.* **64**, 3489a (1966); of the free base: *idem,* **JP 65 17015** (1965), *C.A.* **63**, 18034b (1965). Ganglion blocking agent. Metabolism: Nakai *et al., Arzneim.-Forsch.* **20**, 1112 (1970). Toxicity studies: Kumada *et al., ibid.* **22**, 706 (1972).

Crystals, mp 216-218°. (Free base, $bp_{0.15}$ 183-185°). LD_{50} in male mice (mg/kg): 11 i.v.; 43 i.p.; 30 s.c.; 330 orally (Kumada).
THERAP CAT: Antispasmodic.

7743. Prilocaine. [721-50-6] *N*-(2-Methylphenyl)-2-(propylamino)propanamide; 2-(propylamino)-*o*-propionotoluidide; *N*-(α-propylaminopropionyl)-*o*-toluidine; α-propylamino-2-methylpropionanilide; propitocaine. $C_{13}H_{20}N_2O$; mol wt 220.31. C 70.87%, H 9.15%, N 12.72%, O 7.26%. Prepn: N. Löfgren, C. Tegner, *Acta Chem. Scand.* **14**, 486 (1960); **GB 839943**; N. Löfgren, C. Tegner, **US 3160662** (1960, 1964 both to Astra).

Needles, mp 37-38°. $bp_{0.1}$ 159-162°. n_D^{20} 1.5298.
Hydrochloride. [1786-81-8] L-67; Citanest; Xylonest. $C_{13}H_{20}N_2O.HCl$; mol wt 256.77. Crystals from ethanol + isopropyl ether, mp 167-168°. Readily sol in water.
THERAP CAT: Anesthetic (local).

7744. Primaquine. [90-34-6] N^4-(6-Methoxy-8-quinolinyl)-1,4-pentanediamine; 8-(4-amino-1-methylbutylamino)-6-methoxyquinoline; SN-13272. $C_{15}H_{21}N_3O$; mol wt 259.35. C 69.47%, H 8.16%, N 16.20%, O 6.17%. Prepn following the synthesis of pamaquine: Elderfield *et al., J. Am. Chem. Soc.* **68**, 1525 (1946); improved procedure: Elderfield *et al., ibid.* **77**, 4816 (1955). *Review:* Olenick in *Antibiotics* vol. 3, J. W. Corcoran, F. E. Hahn, Eds. (Springer-Verlag, New York, 1975) pp 516-520.

Viscous liquid, $bp_{0.2}$ 175-179°. Soluble in ether.
Diphosphate. [63-45-6] $C_{15}H_{21}N_3O.2H_3PO_4$. Yellow crystals from 90% ethanol, mp 197-198°. Moderately sol in water.
Oxalate. $C_{15}H_{21}N_3O.C_2H_2O_4$. Yellow crystals from 80% ethanol, mp 182.5-185°.
THERAP CAT: Antimalarial.

7745. Primeverose. [26531-85-1] 6-*O*-β-D-Xylopyranosyl-D-glucose; 6-(β-D-xylosido)-D-glucose. $C_{11}H_{20}O_{10}$; mol wt 312.27. C 42.31%, H 6.46%, O 51.24%. By enzymatic hydrolysis of gaultherin (monotropitoside), primeverin, rhamnicoside and other glycosides: Goris, Vischniac, *Compt. Rend.* **169**, 871 (1919); Bridel, *ibid.* **179**, 991 (1924); Bridel, Charaux, *ibid.* **180**, 857 (1925); Richter, *J. Chem. Soc.* **1936**, 1701. Synthesis: Helferich, Rauch, *Ber.* **59**, 2655 (1926); *Ann.* **455**, 168 (1927); McCloskey, Coleman, *J. Am. Chem. Soc.* **65**, 1778 (1943).

Crystals from methanol or 80% alcohol. Darkens at 190°, mp 209-210° (copper block). Shows mutarotation. $[α]_D^{20}$ +23° → −3.2° (c = 5 in water). Sol in water, methanol, 80% alcohol. Is hydrolyzed to 1 mol D-glucose and 1 mol D-xylose by boiling 2% H_2SO_4 for 5 hrs. Reduces Fehling's soln slowly in the cold, instantly when hot.

7746. Primidone. [125-33-7] 5-Ethyldihydro-5-phenyl-4,-6(1*H*,5*H*)-pyrimidinedione; 5-ethyl-5-phenylhexahydropyrimidine-4,6-dione; 2-desoxyphenobarbital; Liskantin; Mylepsinum; Mysoline; Resimatil; Sertan. $C_{12}H_{14}N_2O_2$; mol wt 218.25. C 66.04%, H 6.47%, N 12.84%, O 14.66%. Prepd by electrolytic reduction of phenobarbital or by catalytic desulfuration of the corresp 2-thiobarbituric acid: Boon *et al.,* **GB 666027** (1952 to I.C.I.); Bogue, Carrington, *Br. J. Pharmacol.* **8**, 230 (1953). Comprehensive description: R. D. Daley in *Anal. Profiles Drug Subs.* **2**, 409-437 (1973); A. A. Al-Badr, H. A. El-Obeid, *ibid.* **17**, 749-795 (1988). HPLC determn in urine: V. Ferranti *et al., J. Chromatogr. B* **718**, 199 (1998). Clinical trial in essential tremor: M. Serrano-Dueñas, *Parkinsonism Relat. Disord.* **10**, 29 (2003).

Crystals, mp 281-282°. Practically tasteless. Has no acidic properties. Sparingly sol in water (0.6 g/l at 37°); in most organic solvents.
THERAP CAT: Anticonvulsant.
THERAP CAT (VET): Anticonvulsant. Chiefly to control epileptiform seizures.

7747. Primisulfuron-methyl. [86209-51-0] 2-[[[[[4,6-Bis-(difluoromethoxy)-2-pyrimidinyl]amino]carbonyl]amino]sulfonyl]-benzoic acid methyl ester; 2-[3-(4,6-bis(difluoromethoxy)pyrimidin-2-yl)ureidosulfonyl]benzoic acid methyl ester; *N*-(2-methoxycarbonylphenylsulfonyl)-*N* '-[4,6-bis(difluoromethoxy)pyrimidin-2-yl]urea; CGA-136872; Beacon; Tell. $C_{15}H_{12}F_4N_4O_7S$; mol wt 468.34. C 38.47%, H 2.58%, F 16.23%, N 11.96%, O 23.91%, S 6.85%. Post-emergence sulfonylurea herbicide. Prepn: W. Meyer *et al.,* **EP 84020**; *eidem,* **US 4478635** (1983, 1984 both to Ciba-Geigy). Comprehensive description: W. Maurer *et al., Proc. Br. Crop Prot. Conf. - Weeds* **1987**, 41-48. Field trial in corn: C. L. Foy, H. L. Witt, *Weed Technol.* **4**, 615 (1990).

Colorless crystals, mp 203.1° (Maurer); also reported as mp 186-188° (Meyer). Vapor pressure (20°): $<7.5 \times 10^{-12}$ mm Hg. Soly in water (pH 7): 0.07 g/l at 20°. LD_{50} in rats (mg/kg): >4000 orally; >2000 dermally (Maurer).
USE: Herbicide.

7748. Primocarcin. [3750-26-3] 5-(Acetylamino)-4-oxo-5-hexenamide; 4-acetamido-4-penten-3-one-1-carboxamide. C_8H_{12}-

N_2O_3; mol wt 184.19. C 52.17%, H 6.57%, N 15.21%, O 26.06%. Antineoplastic antibiotic produced by the actinomycete, *Nocardia fukaya.* Isoln: Y. Sumiki *et al., J. Antibiot.* **13A,** 416 (1960); Isono, Suzuki, *ibid.* **15A,** 77 (1962). Isoln from *Streptomyces diastatochromogens* var. *luteus:* H. Abe *et al., ibid.* **20A,** 167 (1967). Structure: Isono, *ibid.* **15A,** 80 (1962). Synthesis: Bowman *et al., J. Chem. Soc.* **1965,** 470.

Needles from hot methanol, mp 130-131°. Sol in water, lower alcohols, acetone, pyridine; slightly sol in most other organic solvents. Aq soln stable from pH 5-8. uv max (water): 253 nm (ε 3420); in 0.1*N* NaOH: 215, 347 nm (ε 3230, 304). LD_{50} in mice (mg/kg): 50-60 i.p.; 300 i.v. (Isono, Suzuki).

Dihydroprimocarcin. $C_8H_{14}N_2O_3$. Plates from acetone, mp 137-141°.

Tetrahydroprimocarcin. $C_8H_{16}N_2O_3$. Needles from methanol + acetone, mp 183°.

7749. Primulaverin. [154-61-0] $C_{20}H_{28}O_{13}$; mol wt 476.43. C 50.42%, H 5.92%, O 43.66%. Isoln from species of *Primulaceae:* Thieme, Winkler, *Pharmazie* **26,** 434 (1971). Synthesis: Chaudhury *et al., J. Chem. Soc.* **1948,** 2220.

Dihydrate. Star-shaped clusters from ethyl acetate, needles from alc, mp 163°. $[\alpha]_D^{20}$ −67°. Sol in water, alc, acetone.

7750. Primycin. Macrolide antibiotic complex of more than 20 components produced by actinomycetes found in the intestinal tract of the wax moth *(Galeria melonella).* Nine primary components, in 3 major groups designated A, B, and C, represent 90% of the total material. Originally thought to be a single entity which was subseqently identified as the major component, primycin A_1. Isoln from cultures of *Streptomyces primycini:* Vályi-Nagy *et al., Nature* **174,** 1105 (1954); **HU 146332** and **HU 151197** (1962, 1964 both to Hung. Acad. Sci.). Production by *Thermopolyspora galeriensis* (also designated *Micromonospora galeriensis):* T. Vályi-Nagy *et al.,* **HU 153593;** *eidem,* **US 3498884** (1967, 1970 both to Chinoin). Structure of A_1: J. Aberhart *et al., J. Am. Chem. Soc.* **92,** 5816 (1970); *eidem, J. Chem. Soc. Perkin Trans. 1* **1974,** 816, 836. TLC sepn of components: I. Szilagyi *et al., J. Chromatogr.* **295,** 141 (1984). Structures of the nine primary components: J. Frank *et al., Tetrahedron Lett.* **28,** 2759 (1987). Antibacterial activity and toxicity: T. Vályi-Nagy *et al., Pharmazie* **11,** 304 (1956). Antifungal activity *in vitro:* J. V. Uri, P. Actor, *J. Antibiot.* **32,** 1207 (1979). Mode of action: I. Horvath *et al., Arch. Microbiol.* **121,** 135 (1979). Clinical studies in dermatological infections: C. Mészáros, K. Vezekényi, *Ther. Hung.* **35,** 77 (1987); J. Biro, V. Várkonyi, *ibid.* 136; G. Bálint, *ibid.* 140. *Review:* J. V. Uri, *Acta Microbiol. Hung.* **33,** 141 (1986).

Primycin A_1

Sulfate. mp 192-195° (dec) (Aberhart, 1974); also reported as 202-206° (dec) (Uri, 1986). Infrared and ultraviolet spectra: Szilágyi *et al., Nature* **193,** 243 (1962). Fairly soluble in methanol (2.5%), less sol in the higher alcohols, sparingly sol in pyridine, glacial acetic acid, water. LD_{50} in mice, guinea pigs, rats, rabbits (mg/kg): 2.5, 5.0, 10.0, 10.0 i.p. (Vályi-Nagy, 1956).

THERAP CAT: Antibacterial (topical).

7751. Prinomastat. [192329-42-3] (3*S*)-*N*-Hydroxy-2,2-dimethyl-4-[[4-(4-pyridinyloxy)phenyl]sulfonyl]-3-thiomorpholinecarboxamide; 3(*S*)-*N*-hydroxy-4-((4-((pyrid-4-yl)oxy)benzenesulfonyl)-2,2-dimethyl)tetrahydro-2*H*-1,4-thiazine-3-carboxamide; AG-3340. $C_{18}H_{21}N_3O_5S_2$; mol wt 423.51. C 51.05%, H 5.00%, N 9.92%, O 18.89%, S 15.14%. Selective matrix metalloproteinase inhibitor with antiangiogenic activity. Prepn: S. E. Zook *et al.,* **WO 9720824;** S. L. Bender, M. J. Melnick, **US 5753653** (1997, 1998 both to Agouron). Pharmacokinetic and antitumor efficacy in rats: O. Santos *et al., Clin. Exp. Metastasis* **15,** 499 (1997). Review of pharmacology: D. R. Shalinsky *et al., Ann. N.Y. Acad. Sci.* **878,** 236-270 (1999); and clinical experiences: R. Scatena, *Expert Opin. Invest. Drugs* **9,** 2159-2165 (2000).

White powder, mp 149.8°. Also reported as 184-186° with gas evolution. Water soluble.

THERAP CAT: Antineoplastic.

7752. Pristane. [1921-70-6] 2,6,10,14-Tetramethylpentadecane; norphytane; Robuoy. $C_{19}H_{40}$; mol wt 268.52. C 84.99%, H 15.01%. Isoprenoid alkane obtained from the unsaponifiable fraction of shark liver oil where it occurs to an extent of 14%: Tsujimoto, *J. Soc. Chem. Ind.* **51,** 317T (1932); Sörensen, Mehllum, *Acta Chem. Scand.* **2,** 140 (1948). Identity with norphytane: Pliva, Sörensen, *ibid.* **4,** 846 (1950). Isoln from petroleum crude oils: Bendoraitis *et al., Anal. Chem.* **34,** 49 (1962); from wool wax: Mold *et al., Nature* **199,** 283 (1963). Synthesis from phytol: Sörensen, Sörensen, *Acta Chem. Scand.* **3,** 939 (1949). Metabolism: McKenna, Kallio, *Proc. Natl. Acad. Sci. USA* **68,** 1552 (1971). Use in inducing murine plasmacytomas: P. N. Anderson, M. Potter, *Nature* **222,** 994 (1969). Effect on ascites tumor formation and monoclonal antibody production: N. J. Hoogenraad, C. J. Wraight, *Methods Enzymol.* **121,** 375 (1986).

Mobile, transparent, stable liq. d_4^{20} 0.78267. Congealing point −100°. bp_{760} 296°; bp_{10} 158°; $bp_{0.001}$ 68° (bath temp). n_D^{20} 1.43848. Acid no. 0-5. Iodine no. 0-7.5. Sapon no. 0-5. Viscosity at 25°: 5 cP. Soluble in ether, petr ether, benzene, chloroform, carbon tetrachloride.

USE: Lubricant; transformer oil. Anti-corrosion agent. Biological marker. In experimental systems to induce plasmacytomas; in production of monoclonal antibodies.

7753. Pristinamycin. [270076-60-3] RP-7293; Pyostacine. One of the streptogramins, *q.v.,* produced by *Streptomyces pristinaespiralis* (NRRL 2958). The two major components are IA and IIA. Isoln: W. D. Celmer, B. A. Sobin, *Antibiot. Annu.* **1955-1956,** 437; D. I. Mancy *et al., eidem,* **US 3154475** (1962, 1964 both to Rhône-Poulenc); J. Preud'homme *et al., Compt. Rend.* **260,** 1309 (1965). Isoln and characterization of constituents: *idem et al., Bull. Soc. Chim. Fr.* **1968,** 585. HPLC determn of major components in plasma: C. Koechlin *et al., J. Chromatogr.* **425,** 197 (1988). Total synthesis of IIB: P. Breuilles, D. Uguen, *Tetrahedron Lett.* **39,** 3149 (1998). Pharmacokinetics: C. Koechlin *et al., J. Antimicrob. Chemother.* **25,** 651 (1990). Clinical trial in pneumonia: R. Poirier, *Presse Med.* **28,** Suppl. 1, 13 (1999).

on mechanism of action, clinical efficacy and safety: *Am. J. Cardiol.* **57**, 1H-54H (1986). Clinical trial to prevent restenosis following angioplasty: J.-C. Tardif *et al.*, *N. Engl. J. Med.* **337**, 365 (1997).

White crystalline solid from ethanol, mp 124.5-126°; fine, yellow crystals from isopropanol, mp 125-126.5°.

THERAP CAT: Antilipemic.

7756. Procainamide Hydrochloride. [614-39-1] 4-Amino-*N*-[2-(diethylamino)ethyl]benzamide monohydrochloride; procaine amide hydrochloride; Amisalin; Novocamid; Procamide; Procanbid; Procan-SR; Procapan; Pronestyl. $C_{13}H_{22}ClN_3O$; mol wt 271.79. C 57.45%, H 8.16%, Cl 13.04%, N 15.46%, O 5.89%. Prepn: M. Yamazaki *et al.*, *J. Pharm. Soc. Jpn.* **73**, 294 (1953); Y. Tashika, M. Kuranari, *ibid.* 1069. Comprehensive description: R. B. Poet, H. Kadin, *Anal. Profiles Drug Subs.* **4**, 333-383 (1975).

Crystals, mp 165-169°. uv max: 278 nm. Freely sol in water. Sol in alc; slightly sol in chloroform; very sparingly sol in benzene, ether. The pH of a 10% aq soln is 5.5.

THERAP CAT: Antiarrhythmic (class IA).

7757. Procaine. [59-46-1] 4-Aminobenzoic acid 2-(diethylamino)ethyl ester; *p*-aminobenzoyldiethylaminoethanol; 2-diethylaminoethyl *p*-aminobenzoate. $C_{13}H_{20}N_2O_2$; mol wt 236.31. C 66.07%, H 8.53%, N 11.85%, O 13.54%. Benzoic acid derivative with anesthetic activity. Prepn: A. Einhorn, **US 812554** (1906); *idem, Ann.* **371**, 125 (1909); A. Einhorn, E. Uhlfelder, *ibid.* 131. CNS effects: C. G. Peterson, *Anesthesiology* **16**, 976 (1955). Intravenous pharmacokinetics in humans: A. B. Seifen *et al.*, *Anesth. Analg.* **58**, 382 (1979). Clinical evaluation as anti-arrhythmic and cough suppressant during anesthesia: D. S. Thompson *et al.*, *Am. J. Surg.* **138**, 798 (1979). Stabilization of vascular smooth muscle *in vitro*: K. Kitamura *et al.*, *Drugs Exp. Clin. Res.* **12**, 773 (1986). Toxicity data: W. C. North, K. F. Urbach, *J. Am. Pharm. Assoc. Sci. Ed.* **45**, 382 (1956); E. I. Goldenthal, *Toxicol. Appl. Pharmacol.* **18**, 185 (1971).

Hygroscopic, anhydr plates, tablets from ligroin or ether, mp 61°. When freshly precipitated, one gram dissolves in 200 ml water. Sol in alc, ether, benzene, chloroform. LD₅₀ in mice (mg/kg): 195 i.p.; 45 i.v. (North, Urbach).

Dihydrate. [6192-89-8] Needles from aq alc, mp 51°. Slightly bitter taste; applied to the tongue causes transitory numbing sensation.

Nitrate. [6192-92-3] $C_{13}H_{20}N_2O_2.HNO_3$. Crystals, mp 100-102°. Sol in water, alcohol. The aq soln is neutral. Particularly useful with silver nitrate because no precipitate forms.

Butyrate. [136-55-0] Probutylin. $C_{13}H_{20}N_2O_2.C_4H_8O_2$; mol wt 324.42. Hygroscopic crystals. Soluble in water, alcohol, vegetable oils.

Hydrochloride. [51-05-8] Anestil; Enpro; Gero; Jenacaine; Medaject; Naucaine; Neocaine; Novocain; Omnicain; Planocaine; Rocain; Syntocain. $C_{13}H_{20}N_2O_2.HCl$; mol wt 272.77. Crystals.

Pristinamycin IA

Pristinamycin IA. [3131-03-1] Streptogramin B; mikamycin IA; ostreogrycin B; vernamycin Bα. $C_{45}H_{54}N_8O_{10}$; mol wt 866.96. Acid-base properties: M. Largeron, M. B. Fleury, *J. Pharm. Sci.* **81**, 565 (1992). Biosynthesis: V. de Crècy-Lagard *et al.*, *Antimicrob. Agents Chemother.* **41**, 1904 (1997). White microcrystalline powder from methanol, mp 198°. $[\alpha]_D^{22}$ −57.5° (c = 0.25 in ethanol). uv max (ethanol): 243, 260, 281, 303 nm ($E_{1cm}^{1\%}$ 140, 213, 60, 104).

Pristinamycin IIA *see* Virginiamycin M1.

THERAP CAT: Antibacterial.

7754. Probenecid. [57-66-9] 4-[(Dipropylamino)sulfonyl]-benzoic acid; *p*-(dipropylsulfamoyl)benzoic acid; *p*-(dipropylsulfamyl)benzoic acid; Benemid; Probecid; Proben. $C_{13}H_{19}NO_4$-S; mol wt 285.36. C 54.72%, H 6.71%, N 4.91%, O 22.43%, S 11.24%. Prepn from *p*-carboxybenzenesulfonyl chloride and dipropylamine: C. S. Miller, **US 2608507** (1952 to Sharp & Dohme). Study of metabolites: Z. H. Israili *et al.*, *J. Med. Chem.* **15**, 709 (1972). Clinical pharmacokinetics: R. F. Cunningham *et al.*, *Clin. Pharmacokinet.* **6**, 135 (1981). Toxicology studies: S. E. McKinney *et al.*, *J. Pharmacol. Exp. Ther.* **102**, 208 (1951); *NTP Technical Report 395* (PB92-129584, 1991) 220 pp. Comprehensive description: A. A. Al-Badr, H. A. El-Obeid, *Anal. Profiles Drug Subs.* **10**, 639-663 (1981).

Crystals from dilute alcohol, mp 194-196°. uv max (0.1*N* NaOH): 242.5 nm. pKa 5.8. Slightly bitter taste, pleasant aftertaste. Sol in chloroform, in dil solns of NaOH buffered to pH 7.4. Nearly insol in water.

Sodium salt. [23795-03-1] $C_{13}H_{18}NNaO_4S$. LD₅₀ in mice (mg/kg): 458 i.v., 1156 s.c., 1666 orally; in rats (mg/kg): 394 i.p., 611 s.c., 1604 orally (McKinney).

THERAP CAT: Uricosuric.

7755. Probucol. [23288-49-5] 4,4′-[(1-Methylethylidene)-bis(thio)]bis[2,6-bis(1,1-dimethylethyl)phenol]; 4,4′-(isopropylidenedithio)bis[2,6-di-*tert*-butylphenol]; acetone bis(3,5-di-*tert*-butyl-4-hydroxyphenyl)mercaptole; DH-581; Lorelco; Lurselle; Sinlestal. $C_{31}H_{48}O_2S_2$; mol wt 516.84. C 72.04%, H 9.36%, O 6.19%, S 12.41%. Lipid-lowering antioxidant. Prepn: M. B. Neuworth, **FR 1561853**; *idem*, **US 3576883** (1969, 1971 both to Consolidation Coal Co.); and use as a cholesterol-lowering agent: J. W. Barnhart, P. J. Shea, **US 3862332** (1975 to Dow). Prepn and activity studies: M. B. Neuworth *et al.*, *J. Med. Chem.* **13**, 722 (1970). Review of pharmacology and therapeutic use in hyperlipidemia: R. C. Heel *et al.*, *Drugs* **15**, 409-428 (1978). Symposium

Procarbazine

Six-sided plates, monoclinic or triclinic. mp 153-156°. Numbing taste. Stable in air. One gram dissolves in 1 ml water and in 30 ml alcohol. Slightly sol in chloroform. Almost insol in ether. The pH of a 0.1M aq soln is 6.0. Aq solns may be sterilized by boiling. LD_{50} in mice (mg/kg): 660 ± 60 s.c. (Goldenthal).

THERAP CAT: Anesthetic (local).

THERAP CAT (VET): Anesthetic (local).

7758. Procarbazine. [671-16-9] N-(1-Methylethyl)-4-[(2-methylhydrazino)methyl]benzamide; N-isopropyl-α-(2-methylhydrazino)-p-toluamide; N-4-isopropylcarbamoylbenzyl-N'-methylhydrazine; p-(N^l-methylhydrazinomethyl)-N-isopropylbenzamide; ibenzmethyzin; MIH; Ro-4-6467. $C_{12}H_{19}N_3O$; mol wt 221.30. C 65.13%, H 8.65%, N 18.99%, O 7.23%. Alkylating agent. Prepn: **BE 618638**; W. Bollag *et al.*, **US 3520926** (1962, 1970 to Hoffmann-La Roche). Toxicity studies: E. I. Goldenthal, *Toxicol. Appl. Pharmacol.* **18**, 185 (1971). Comprehensive description: R. J. Rucki, *Anal. Profiles Drug Subs.* **5**, 403-427 (1976). HPLC determn in plasma: X. He *et al.*, *J. Chromatogr. B* **799**, 281 (2004). Review of clinical experience in hematological malignancies: M. Massoud *et al.*, *Eur. J. Cancer* **40**, 1924-1927 (2004).

Hydrochloride. [366-70-1] Matulane; Natulan. $C_{12}H_{19}N_3$O.HCl; mol wt 257.76. Crystals from methanol, mp 223-226°. LD_{50} orally in rats: 785 ±34 mg/kg (Goldenthal).

Hydrobromide. $C_{12}H_{19}N_3$O.HBr. Crystals from methanol + ether, dec 216-217°.

Caution: Procarbazine hydrochloride is reasonably anticipated to be a human carcinogen: *Report on Carcinogens, Eleventh Edition* (PB2005-104914, 2004) p III-222.

THERAP CAT: Antineoplastic.

7759. Procaterol. [72332-33-3] *rel*-8-Hydroxy-5-[(1R,2S)-1-hydroxy-2-[(1-methylethyl)amino]butyl]-2(1H)-quinolinone; (±)-*erythro*-8-hydroxy-5-[1-hydroxy-2-(isopropylamino)butyl]carbostyril. $C_{16}H_{22}N_2O_3$; mol wt 290.36. C 66.18%, H 7.64%, N 9.65%, O 16.53%. Sympathomimetic amine with selective β_2-adrenergic agonist activity. Prepn: K. Nakagawa *et al.*, **BE 823841**; *eidem*, **US 4026897** (1975, 1977 both to Otsuka); S. Yoshizaki *et al.*, *J. Med. Chem.* **19**, 1138 (1976). Prepn of optical isomers: *eidem, ibid.* **20**, 1103 (1977). Assessment of selective action: H. Himori, N. Taira, *Br. J. Pharmacol.* **61**, 9 (1977). Metabolism: Y. Yasuda *et al.*, *Arzneim.-Forsch.* **29**, 261 (1979). Pharmacokinetics: M. Ishigami *et al., ibid.* 266. Series of reproduction studies: *Iyakuhin Kenkyu* **10**, 68-111 (1979), *C.A.* **90**, 197728f-30a (1979). Antigenicity test: N. Nakagiri, S. Tei, *Oyo Yakuri* **17**, 363 (1979), *C.A.* **91**, 186577a (1979).

Hydrochloride hemihydrate. [81262-93-3] OPC-2009; Lontermin; Masacin; Meptin; Onsukil; Procadil; Promaxol; Propulm. $C_{16}H_{22}N_2O_3$.HCl.½H_2O; mol wt 335.83. Off-white crystalline powder, mp 193-197° (dec). Sol in methanol; slightly sol in ethanol. Practically insol in acetone, ether, ethyl acetate, chloroform, benzene. Colors on exposure to light. LD_{50} of the hydrochloride in male rats (mg/kg): 2600 orally, 80 i.v. (Nakagawa).

THERAP CAT: Bronchodilator.

7760. Prochloraz. [67747-09-5] N-Propyl-N-[2-(2,4,6-trichlorophenoxy)ethyl]-1H-imidazole-1-carboxamide; 1-[N-propyl-

N-[2-(2,4,6-trichlorophenoxy)ethyl]carbamoyl]imidazole; BTS-40542; Sportak. $C_{15}H_{16}Cl_3N_3O_2$; mol wt 376.67. C 47.83%, H 4.28%, Cl 28.24%, N 11.16%, O 8.50%. Broad spectrum fungicide for use on cereal crops, fruit and vegetables. Prepn from imidazole: R. F. Brookes *et al.*, **DE 2429523**; *eidem*, **US 3991071** (1975, 1976 both to Boots). Fungicidal properties: R. J. Birchmore *et al.*, *Proc. Br. Crop Prot. Conf. - Pests Dis.* **1977**, 593; R. G. Harris *et al., ibid.* **1979**, 53. Efficacy against cereal powdery mildew: D. M. Weighton *et al., ibid.* **1977**, 25. Protective effect against blotch in winter wheat and barley: R. G. Harris, G. Barnes, *ibid.* **1981**, 267. Effect on cytochrome P-450 and sterol biosynthesis in Japanese quail: J.-L. Riviere *et al.*, *Pestic. Sci.* **15**, 317 (1984). HPLC/MS determn in rainbow trout: L. Debrauwer *et al., J. Agric. Food Chem.* **49**, 3821 (2001). *Review:* A. de Saint-Blanquat, J. My, *Def. Veg.* **37**, 121 (1983).

White crystalline solid, mp 38.5-41°. Technical product is pale yellow viscous oil. Vapor pressure at 20°: 0.57×10^{-9} torr. Almost insol in water (0.0055 g/l). Soln in chloroform, diethyl ether, toluene, xylene: 2500 g/l; in acetone: 3500 g/l. LD_{50} in rats (mg/kg): 1600 orally; >5000 s.c.; 400-800 i.p.; LC_{50} (96 hour) in rainbow trout, bluegill (mg/l): 1, 2.2 (de Saint-Blanquat, My). Relatively non-toxic to bees.

USE: Fungicide.

7761. Prochlorperazine. [58-38-8] 2-Chloro-10-[3-(4-methyl-1-piperazinyl)propyl]-10H-phenothiazine; 3-chloro-10-[3-(4-methyl-1-piperazinyl)propyl]phenothiazine; 2-chloro-10-[3-(1-methyl-4-piperazinyl)propyl]phenothiazine; N-[γ-(4'-methyl-piperazinyl-1')propyl]-3-chlorophenothiazine; chlormeprazine; prochlorpemazine; proclorperazine; Bayer A 173; RP-6140; SKF-4657. $C_{20}H_{24}ClN_3S$; mol wt 373.94. C 64.24%, H 6.47%, Cl 9.48%, N 11.24%, S 8.57%. Prepn: R. J. Horclois, **GB 780193**; **FR 1167627**; **US 2902484** (1957, 1958, 1959 all to Rhône-Poulenc). Pharmacology and toxicity: S. Courvoisier *et al., C.R. Seances Soc. Biol. Ses Fil.* **152**, 1371 (1958). Pharmacokinetics: W. B. Taylor, D. N. Bateman, *Br. J. Clin. Pharmacol.* **23**, 137 (1987). Clinical efficacy as antiemetic and antipsychotic: J. Lapierre *et al., Can. Psychiatr. Assoc. J.* **14**, 267 (1969). Clinical trial in treatment of nausea, dizziness and vertigo: A. E. Ward, *Br. J. Clin. Pract.* **42**, 228 (1988).

Dimaleate. [84-02-6] Buccastem; Compazine; Meterazine; Stemetil; Vertigon. $C_{20}H_{24}ClN_3S.2C_4H_4O_4$; mol wt 606.09. Minute crystals, mp 228°. Very slightly sol in water (<0.1% at 20°). Slightly sol in methanol, ethanol. Practically insol in ether, benzene, chloroform. LD_{50} in mice (mg/kg): 400 s.c.; 120 i.p.; 90 i.v., 400 orally (Courvoisier).

Dimethanesulfonate. [51888-09-6] Prochlorperazine mesylate; Novamin; Tementil. $C_{20}H_{24}ClN_3S.2CH_4O_3S$; mol wt 566.15.

THERAP CAT: Antiemetic; antipsychotic. In treatment of vertigo.

THERAP CAT (VET): Antiemetic.

7762. Procodazole. [23249-97-0] 1H-Benzimidazole-2-propanoic acid; β-(2-benzimidazolyl)propionic acid; 2-(2-carboxyethyl)benzimidazole; propazol; AL-1241; Estimulocel. $C_{10}H_{10}N_2O_2$; mol wt 190.20. C 63.15%, H 5.30%, N 14.73%, O 16.82%. Non-specific, active immunoprotective agent against viral and bac-

Consult the Name Index before using this section.

terial infections. Prepn: J. Maier, *Ann.* **327,** 17 (1903); R. Meyers, H. Lüders, *ibid.* **415,** 29 (1918); B. Chatterjee, *J. Chem. Soc.* **1929,** 2966; **ES 407882** (1972 to Lafarquim). Pharmacological studies: C. Fernández *et al., Rev. Clin. Esp.* **135,** 539 (1974); *eidem, ibid.* **141,** 51 (1976). Clinical studies: M. Pérez Tascon, J. M. Monturio, *Med. Klin.* **181,** 78 (1976).

Silky white needles from water, mp 228° (dec). Sol in alc, warm water. Practically insol in ether, benzene. The water soln is extremely sweet-tasting.

THERAP CAT: Immunopotentiator (non-specific).

7763. Procyclidine. [77-37-2] α-Cyclohexyl-α-phenyl-1-pyrrolidinepropanol; 1-cyclohexyl-1-phenyl-3-(1-pyrrolidinyl)-1-propanol; 1-cyclohexyl-1-phenyl-3-pyrrolidino-1-propanol. C_{19}-$H_{29}NO$; mol wt 287.44. C 79.39%, H 10.17%, N 4.87%, O 5.57%. Anticholinergic. Prepn of free base and hydrochloride: Adamson *et al., J. Chem. Soc.* **1951,** 52; Adamson, **US 2891890** (1959 to Burroughs Wellcome). Prepn of methochloride: Bottorff, **US 2826590** (1958 to Lilly); Harfenist, Magnien, **US 2842555** (1958 to Burroughs Wellcome).

Crystals from petr ether, mp 85.5-86.5°. uv max (0.17% in ethanol): 258.5 nm (ε 233).

Hydrochloride. [1508-76-5] Arpicolin; Kemadrin; Osnervan. $C_{19}H_{29}NO.HCl$; mol wt 323.90. Crystals from ethanol + ethyl acetate, dec 226-227°. Moderately sol in water (about 3.0 g/100 ml); more sol in alcohol, chloroform; very slightly sol in ether.

Methochloride. 1-(3-Cyclohexyl-3-hydroxy-3-phenylpropyl)-1-methylpyrrolidinium chloride; tricyclamol chloride; Lergine. $C_{19}H_{29}NO.CH_3Cl$; mol wt 337.93. Crystals from nitroethane, mp 159-164°. Moderately sol in water, alcohol. Practically insol in ether.

Methosulfate. $C_{21}H_{35}NO_5S$. Crystals, mp ~100°. Soluble in water (about 2% at 25°), alcohol. Practically insol in ether.

THERAP CAT: Antiparkinsonian.

7764. Procymate. [13931-64-1] α-Ethylcyclohexanemethanol carbamate; carbamic acid 1-cyclohexylpropyl ester; 1-cyclohexylpropyl carbamate; T-3033; Equipax. $C_{10}H_{19}NO_2$; mol wt 185.26. C 64.83%, H 10.34%, N 7.56%, O 17.27%. Prepn: Swierkot, **GB 979236** (1960 to Comp. Franc. Matières Colorantes).

Crystals, mp 128-129°.
THERAP CAT: Tranquilizer.

7765. Procymidone. [32809-16-8] 3-(3,5-Dichlorophenyl)-1,5-dimethyl-3-azabicyclo[3.1.0]hexane-2,4-dione; *N*-(3,5-dichlorophenyl)-1,2-dimethyl-1,2-cyclopropanedicarboximide; dicyclidine; S-7131; Sumisclex; Sumilex. $C_{13}H_{11}Cl_2NO_2$; mol wt 284.14. C 54.95%, H 3.90%, Cl 24.95%, N 4.93%, O 11.26%. Dicarboximide fungicide systemically active against *Botrytis* and *Sclerotinia spp.* on fruits and vegetables. Prepn: **NL 7003836**; A. Fujinami *et al.,* **US 3903090** (1970, 1975 both to Sumitomo). Antimicrobial spectrum and systemic activity: Y. Hisada *et al., J. Pestic. Sci.* **1,** 145 (1976). Mechanism of action: A. C. Pappas, D. J. Fisher, *Pestic. Sci.* **10,** 239 (1979). Field evaluation: I. F. Jack-

son, B. N. Smith, *Proc. 32nd N.Z. Weed Pest Control Conf.* 278 (1979). HPLC determn in wine musts and extracts: P. Cabras *et al., J. Chromatogr.* **256,** 176 (1983). *Review:* N. Mikami, J. Miyamoto, *Rev. Plant Prot. Res.* **14,** 85-95 (1981).

Crystalline solid, mp 165-167°. d^{25} 1.42-1.46. Vapor pressure: 1.32×10^{-4} mm Hg. uv max: 207.5, 275 nm (ε 4.2×10^4, 4.1×10^2). Soly in water (25°): 4.5 ppm. Highly sol in acetonitrile, acetone, ether, chloroform. Moderately sol in benzene, toluene. Stable in solvents. Unstable in alkaline media. LD_{50} in male rats (mg/kg): 6800 orally, >10000 dermally (Jackson). Also reported as LD_{50} in male, female rats (g/kg): 7.8, 9.1 orally (Mikami).

USE: Systemic agricultural fungicide.

7766. Prodiamine. [29091-21-2] 2,4-Dinitro-N^3,N^3-dipropyl-6-(trifluoromethyl)-1,3-benzenediamine; α,α,α-trifluoro-3,5-dinitro-N^4,N^4-dipropyltoluene-2,4-diamine; 5-dipropylamino-α,α,α-trifluoro-4,6-dinitro-*o*-toluidine; 2,6-dinitro-N^1,N^1-dipropyl-4-trifluoromethyl-*m*-phenylenediamine; N^3,N^3-di-*n*-propyl-2,4-dinitro-6-trifluoromethyl-1,3-phenylenediamine; USB-3153; CN-11-2936; Barricade; Endurance; Factor. $C_{13}H_{17}F_3N_4O_4$; mol wt 350.29. C 44.57%, H 4.89%, F 16.27%, N 15.99%, O 18.27%. Broad-spectrum, pre-emergence dinitroaniline herbicide. Prepn: D. L. Hunter *et al., DE 2013510; eidem, US 3764623* (1970, 1973 both to U.S. Borax and Chemical Corp.). Weed control in container grown plants: T. A. Fretz, W. J. Sheppard, *HortScience* **15,** 489 (1980); S. A. Duray, F. T. Davies, *J. Environ. Hort.* **5,** 82 (1987). Field studies: M. G. Sybouts, *Proc. West. Soc. Weed Sci.* **40,** 169 (1987). Evaluation of herbicidal activity: W. Bond, *Crop Prot.* **7,** 75 (1988). Review of herbicidal activity: S. J. Bowe, *Proc. West. Soc. Weed Sci.* **39,** 216-218 (1986).

Orange needles from 95% ethanol, mp 124-125°.
USE: Herbicide.

7767. Prodigiosin. [82-89-3] 4-Methoxy-5-[(5-methyl-4-pentyl-2*H*-pyrrol-2-ylidene)methyl]-2,2′-bi-1*H*-pyrrole; 2,2′-[3-methoxy-4′-amyl-5′-methyl-5-(2″-pyrryl]dipyrrylmethene; prodigiosine. $C_{20}H_{25}N_3O$; mol wt 323.43. C 74.27%, H 7.79%, N 12.99%, O 4.95%. Antibiotic pigment produced by *Chromobacterium prodigiosum (Serratia marcescens)*. Exhibits antimicrobial and cytotoxic properties. Isoln: Wrede, Hettche, *Ber.* **62,** 2678 (1929); Lasseur, Georges, *Trav. Lab. Microbiol. Fac. Pharm. Nancy* **9,** 47 (1936); Lasseur, Melcion, *ibid.* **13,** 192 (1944). Purification: Morgan, Tanner, *J. Chem. Soc.* **1955,** 3305. Structure: Wrede, Rothhaas, *Z. Physiol. Chem.* **226,** 95 (1934). Revised structure and synthesis: H. H. Wasserman *et al., J. Am. Chem. Soc.* **82,** 506 (1960); H. Rapoport, K. G. Holden, *ibid.* **84,** 635 (1962); A. J. Castro *et al., J. Org. Chem.* **28,** 857 (1963). Total synthesis and *in vitro* cytotoxic activity: D. L. Boger, M. Patel, *Tetrahedron Lett.* **28,** 2499 (1987); *eidem, J. Org. Chem.* **53,** 1405 (1988). NMR studies: R. J. Cushley *et al., Can. J. Chem.* **53,** 148 (1975). Antimalarial activity: A. J. Castro, *Nature* **213,** 903 (1967). *Review:* R. P. Williams, W. R. Hearn in *Antibiotics* vol. 2, D. Gottlieb, P. D. Shaw, Eds. (Springer-Verlag, New York, 1967) pp 410-432, 449-451. Review of synthesis: A. H. Jackson, K. M. Smith, in *The Total Synthesis of Natural Products* vol. 1, J. ApSimon, Ed. (Wiley-Interscience, New York, 1973) pp 227-232; of biological activity and production: V. Alonzo, *Ig. Mod.* **81,** 557-564 (1984), *C.A.* **101,** 126398h (1984).

Lustrous square pyramids (dark red with green reflex) from petr ether, mp 151-152°. Almost insol in water. Moderately sol in alcohol, ether; freely sol in chloroform, bromoform, benzene. Alkaline or neutral solns are orange-yellow, acid solns are red. Absorption max (isopropanol): 466 nm (ε 43000); 336, 280 nm.

Hydrochloride. [112373-40-7] $C_{20}H_{26}ClN_3O$. Magenta crystals from benzene + petr ether, dec 148.5-150°. Absorption max (isopropanol): 540, 294 nm (ε 70700, 10800).

7768. Prodipine. [31314-38-2] 1-(1-Methylethyl)-4,4-diphenylpiperidine; 1-isopropyl-4,4-diphenylpiperidine. $C_{20}H_{25}N$; mol wt 279.42. C 85.97%, H 9.02%, N 5.01%. CNS stimulating agent with antidepressant and antiparkinson properties. Prepn: H. G. Menge, J. Klosa, **DE 1936452**; *eidem*, **US 4016280** (1971, 1977 both to Byk Gulden). Evaluation of MAO-inhibitory properties *in vivo* and *in vitro*: G. Planz *et al.*, *Arzneim.-Forsch.* **23**, 281 (1973). Effects on 5-hydroxytryptamine uptake in platelets: M. Eltze *et al.*, *ibid.* **30**, 1129 (1980). Comparative study of effects in Parkinson's disease: E. Gründig, F. Gerstenbrand, *Wien. Klin. Wochenschr.* **92**, 868 (1980).

Oil, bp$_{0.01}$ 117-125°.

Hydrochloride. [31314-39-3] Anthen. $C_{20}H_{25}N.HCl$; mol wt 315.88. Crystals from isopropanol, mp 267°.

THERAP CAT: Antiparkinsonian.

7769. Prodlure. [50767-79-8] (9Z,11E)-9,11-Tetradecadien-1-ol acetate; *cis*-9,*trans*-11-tetradecadienyl acetate; *cis*-9,*trans*-11-TDDA; litlure A. $C_{16}H_{28}O_2$; mol wt 252.39. C 76.14%, H 11.18%, O 12.68%. Major component of sex pheromone of female *spodoptera litura* (F.) and Egyptian cotton leafworm, *S. littoralis* (Boisd.). Isoln and prepn: Y. Tamaki *et al.*, *Appl. Entomol. Zool.* **8**, 200 (1973); B. F. Nesbitt *et al.*, *Nature New Biol.* **244**, 208 (1973). Prepn: T. Yushimo *et al.*, **DE 2406259** (1974 to Natl. Inst. Agr. Sci.), *C.A.* **82**, 97681b (1975). Stereoselective synthesis: D. R. Hall *et al.*, *Chem. Ind. (London)* **1975**, 216; G. Goto *et al.*, *Chem. Lett.* **1975**, 103; G. Decodts *et al.*, *Synthesis* **7**, 510 (1979). Activity studies in presence of minor component, *(Z,E)-9,12-tetradecadien-1-ol acetate*: S. Neumark *et al.*, *Environ. Lett.* **6**, 219 (1974); Y. Tamaki, T. Yushima *et al.*, *J. Insect Physiol.* **20**, 1005 (1974); M. Kehat *et al.*, *Appl. Entomol. Zool.* **11**, 45 (1976).

Colorless liquid, bp$_{0.2}$ 147-148°, bp$_{0.003}$ 85-86°. uv max (hexane): 232 nm (ε 27300).

USE: Insect attractant.

7770. Profenofos. [41198-08-7] *O*-(4-Bromo-2-chlorophenyl)phosphorothioic acid *O*-ethyl *S*-propyl ester; CGA-15324; OMS-2004; Curacron; Sanofos; Selecron. $C_{11}H_{15}BrClO_3PS$; mol wt 373.63. C 35.36%, H 4.05%, Br 21.39%, Cl 9.49%, O 12.85%, P 8.29%, S 8.58%. Organophosphorus insecticide for use in cotton and vegetables. Prepn: E. Beriger, J. Drabek, **BE 789937**; *eidem*, **US 3992533** (1973, 1976 both to Ciba-Geigy). Resolution and biological activity of chiral isomers: H. Leader, J. E. Casida, *J. Agric. Food Chem.* **30**, 546 (1982). Persistence and biochemical effects of residue in potatoes: R. A. Habiba *et al.*, *ibid.* **40**, 1852 (1992); in tomatoes: S. M. M. Ismail *et al.*, *ibid.* **41**, 610 (1993).

Effect on microbial flora of soil: A. Y. Abdel-Mallek *et al.*, *Microbiol. Res.* **149**, 167 (1994). Toxicity to eastern rainbow fish: A Kumar, J. C. Chapman, *Environ. Toxicol. Chem.* **17**, 1799 (1998). Review of physical properties and field trials: F. Buholzer, *Proc. 8th Br. Insectic. Fungic. Conf.* **1975**, 659-665.

Slightly yellowish liquid. bp$_{0.001}$ 110°. d^{20} 1.455 g/cc. Soly in water at 20°: 20 ppm. Misc with methanol, dichloromethane, benzene, hexane. Vapor pressure at 20°: ~10^{-5} mm Hg. n$_D^{20}$ 1.5466. LD$_{50}$ in rat (mg/kg): 358-400 orally; ~3300 dermally; LC$_{50}$ (4 hr) in rat (mg/m^3): ~3000 by inhalation (Buholzer). LC$_{50}$ (96 hr) in rainbow fish: 0.91 mg/l (Kumar, Chapman).

USE: Insecticide; acaricide.

7771. Proflavine. [92-62-6] 3,6-Acridinediamine; 3,6-diaminoacridine; 2,8-diaminoacridine. $C_{13}H_{11}N_3$; mol wt 209.25. C 74.62%, H 5.30%, N 20.08%. Prepn: M. Schöpff, *Ber.* **27**, 2320 (1894); **DE 230412** (1910 to Cassella), *C.A.* **5**, 2734 (1911); W. P. Thompson, **GB 137214** (1919 to Poulenc Frères), *C.A.* **14**, 1445 (1920); A. Albert, *J. Chem. Soc.* **1941**, 121, 484; **1947**, 244. Toxicity study: S. D. Rubbo, *Br. J. Exp. Pathol.* **28**, 1 (1947). *Review: The Acridines*, A. Albert, Ed. (St. Martin's Press, New York, 2nd ed., 1966) pp 300-302; *Acridines*, R. M. Acheson, Ed. (Interscience, New York, 1956) pp 341-344.

Yellow needles from alc, mp 281° (Schöpff), mp 288° (Albert). Sol in water, ethanol. Practically insol in benzene, ether. pKa 9.7. Solns are brownish and when diluted are fluorescent. *Solns should be discarded when they become turbid.* LD$_{50}$ s.c. in mice: 0.14 g/kg (Rubbo).

Dihydrochloride. [531-73-7] $C_{13}H_{11}N_3.2HCl$. Orange-yellow needles. pH of 0.1% soln 2.5-3.0.

Sulfate. [553-30-0] Proflavine hemisulfate; neutral proflavine sulfate. $C_{13}H_{11}N_3.H_2SO_4$. Occurs as the hydrate. Red needles, hygroscopic. Sol in 300 parts cold water, in 1 part boiling water; slightly sol in alc. Practically insol in ether, CHCl$_3$. pH of satd soln is 6-8. pH of 0.1% soln is 2.5.

Mixture with 3,6-diamino-10-methylacridinium chloride *see* Acriflavine.

THERAP CAT: Topical antiseptic.

THERAP CAT (VET): Topical antiseptic.

7772. Progabide. [62666-20-0] 4-[[(4-Chlorophenyl)(5-fluoro-2-hydroxyphenyl)methylene]amino]butanamide; 4-[[α-(p-chlorophenyl)-5-fluorosalicylidene]amino]butyramide; 4-[[α-(p-chlorophenyl)-5-fluoro-2-hydroxybenzylidene]amino]butyramide; halogabide; SL-76.002; Gabren(e). $C_{17}H_{16}ClFN_2O_2$; mol wt 334.77. C 60.99%, H 4.82%, Cl 10.59%, F 5.68%, N 8.37%, O 9.56%. Gamma-aminobutyric acid (GABA) antagonist with antiepileptic activity. Prepn: J.-P. Kaplan *et al.*, **DE 2634288**; *eidem*, **US 4094992** (1977, 1978 to Synthelabo); *eidem*, *J. Med. Chem.* **23**, 702 (1980). Use as analgesic: J.-P. Kaplan, **US 4361583** (1982 to Synthelabo). Pharmacokinetics: I. Johno *et al.*, *J. Pharm. Sci.* **71**, 633 (1982). HPLC determn in biological fluids: P. Padovani *et al.*, *J. Chromatogr.* **308**, 229 (1984). Double-blind clinical trial in therapy resistant epilepsy: P. Loiseau *et al.*, *Epilepsia* **24**, 703 (1983); in spasticity: K. Mondrup, E. Pedersen, *Acta Neurol. Scand.* **69**, 200 (1984).

Crystals from cyclohexane and toluene, mp 133-135°; possible second crystalline form, mp 142.5° (Kaplan, *J. Med. Chem.*). uv max in methanol: 332, 250, 210 (ε 4200, 10800, 24000). LD_{50} i.p. in mice: 900 mg/kg (Kaplan).

THERAP CAT: Anticonvulsant.

7773. Progesterone. [57-83-0] Pregn-4-ene-3,20-dione; Δ^4-pregnene-3,20-dione; corpus luteum hormone; luteohormone; Crinone; Cyclogest; Estima; Gestone; Menaelle; Progestasert; Progestogel; Progeston; Proluton; Utrogestan. $C_{21}H_{30}O_2$; mol wt 314.46. C 80.21%, H 9.62%, O 10.18%. Active principle of the corpus luteum, secreted during the latter half of the menstrual cycle. If pregnancy ensues, secretion continues. Exerts an antiovulatory effect when administered during days 5 to 25 of the normal menstrual cycle. Isoln from corpus luteum of pregnant sows: Butenandt, Westphal, *Ber.* **67**, 1440 (1934); Wintersteiner, Allen, *J. Biol. Chem.* **107**, 321 (1934). Structure: Butenandt *et al., Ber.* **67**, 1611 (1934). Synthesis of DL-form: Johnson *et al., J. Am. Chem. Soc.* **93**, 4332 (1971). Prepn from other steroids in review by W. H. Strain in Gilman's *Organic Chemistry* **vol. II** (Wiley, New York, 2nd ed., 1943) pp 1487-1489. Numerous patents, e.g., **US 2379832**; **US 2232438**; **US 2314185**. Anesthetic effect and toxicity: H. Selye, *Proc. Soc. Exp. Biol. Med.* **46**, 116 (1941). Review of physiology: Csapo, *Sci. Am.* **198**, 40-46 (April, 1958); Rothchild, *Vitam. Horm.* **23**, 209-327 (1965). Book: *Progesterone and Progestins*, C. W. Bardin *et al.*, Eds. (Raven Press, New York, 1982) 462 pp.

Exists in two cryst forms of equal physiologic activity and which are readily interconverted. The α-form is orthorhombic (prisms from dil alc) with a:b:c = 0.750:1:0.905. Crystals show (011), (110), (010). Poor (011) cleavage. d^{23} 1.166. mp 127-131°. The β-form is orthorhombic (needles) with a:b:c = 0.563:1:0.275. Crystals acicular with parallel extinction and negative elongation. Cleavage on (001) and (110). d^{20} 1.171. mp 121°. $[\alpha]_D^{20}$ +172 to +182° (c = 2 in dioxane). uv max: 240 nm. Insol in water. Sol in alcohol, acetone, dioxane, concd H_2SO_4. Sparingly sol in vegetable oils. 1 mg = 1 I.U.

Caution: This substance is reasonably anticipated to be a human carcinogen: *Report on Carcinogens, Eleventh Edition* (PB2005-104914, 2004) p III-223.

THERAP CAT: Progestogen.

THERAP CAT (VET): Progestogen. Has been used to control habitual abortion, to suppress or synchronize estrus.

7774. Proglumetacin. [57132-53-3] 1-(4-Chlorobenzoyl)-5-methoxy-2-methyl-1*H*-indole-3-acetic acid 2-[4-[3-[[4-(benzoylamino)-5-(dipropylamino)-1,5-dioxopentyl]oxy]propyl]-1-piperazinyl]ethyl ester; ($\pm$)-*N*-[2-[1-(*p*-chlorobenzoyl)-5-methoxy-2-methyl-3-indolylacetoxy]ethyl]-*N*'-[3-(*N*-benzoyl-*N*',*N*'-di-*n*-propyl-DL-isoglutaminoyl)oxypropyl]piperazine. $C_{46}H_{58}ClN_5O_8$; mol wt 844.43. C 65.43%, H 6.92%, Cl 4.20%, N 8.29%, O 15.16%. Deriv of indomethacin, *q.v.* Prepn: F. Makovec *et al.*, **DE 2535799** corresp to **US 3985878** (both 1976 to Rotta). Series of articles on pharmacology, mechanism of action, safety: *Arzneim.-Forsch.* **29**, 1116-1129 (1979). Bioavailability study: A. A. Bignamini, P. L. Casula, *Curr. Med. Res. Opin.* **6**, 299 (1979). Clinical evaluation: J. Münzenberg, S. Tachibana, *Pharmatherapeutica* **2**, 279 (1980); P. Loizzi *et al., ibid.* 285. Mutagenicity study: R. Vidal y Plana *et al., Farmaco Ed. Prat.* **33**, 543 (1978). Toxicity data for dimaleate: A. L. Rovati *et al., Arzneim.-Forsch.* **29**, 1116 (1979).

Dimaleate. [59209-40-4] Protacine; CR-604; Afloxan; Miridacin; Protaxon; Proxil. $C_{46}H_{58}ClN_5O_8 \cdot 2C_4H_4O_4$; mol wt 1076.58. Crystals from ethanol, mp 146-148°. LD_{50} in male mice, rats (mg/kg): 262, 450 orally (Rovati).

THERAP CAT: Anti-inflammatory.

7775. Proglumide. [6620-60-6] 4-(Benzoylamino)-5-(dipropylamino)-5-oxopentanoic acid; DL-4-benzamido-*N*,*N*-dipropylglutaramic acid; *N*-benzoyl-*N*',*N*'-di-*n*-propyl-DL-isoglutamine; xylamide; CR-242; W-5219; Milid; Milide; Promid. $C_{18}H_{26}N_2O_4$; mol wt 334.41. C 64.65%, H 7.84%, N 8.38%, O 19.14%. Prepn: **NL 6510006**; **ZA 6504065** (both 1966 to Rotta), *C.A.* **65**, 3793b (1966). Pharmacological activity: A. L. Rovati *et al., Minerva Med.* **58**, 3653 (1967); T. Umetzu *et al., Eur. J. Pharmacol.* **64**, 69 (1980). Pharmacokinetic study: A. A. Bignamini *et al., Arzneim.-Forsch.* **29**, 639 (1979). Clinical study in duodenal ulcer: W. Bergemann *et al., Med. Klin.* **76**, 226 (1981). Cholecystokinin receptor antagonist activity: W. F. Hahne *et al., Proc. Natl. Acad. Sci. USA* **78**, 6304 (1981). Selective blockade of cholecystokinin CNS effects: L. A. Chiodo, B. S. Bunney, *Science* **219**, 1449 (1983).

Crystals, mp 142-145°. LD_{50} in mice (mg/kg): 2211-2649 i.v.; 7350-8861 orally (Rovati).

THERAP CAT: Anticholinergic.

7776. Proheptazine. [77-14-5] Hexahydro-1,3-dimethyl-4-phenyl-1*H*-azepin-4-ol propanoate (ester); DL-α-1,3-dimethyl-4-phenyl-4-propionoxyazacycloheptane; 1,3-dimethyl-4-phenyl-4-propionoxyhexamethylenimine; 4-phenyl-4-propionoxy-1,3-dimethylazacycloheptane; 4-propionoxy-1,3-dimethyl-4-phenylhexamethylenimine; dimepheprimine; Wy-757. $C_{17}H_{25}NO_2$; mol wt 275.39. C 74.14%, H 9.15%, N 5.09%, O 11.62%. Prepn: Diamond, Bruce, **US 2775589** (1956 to American Home Prod.). Structure and synthesis: Diamond *et al., J. Med. Chem.* **7**, 57 (1964).

Liquid, $bp_{0.3}$ 126°. n_D^{28} 1.5182. n_D^{21} 1.5215.

Hydrobromide. $C_{17}H_{26}BrNO_2$. Crystals from acetone + methanol, dec 207-207.5°. Soly in water at 25°: 1-2%.

Hydrochloride. $C_{17}H_{26}ClNO_2$. Crystals, dec 207°.

Note: This is a controlled substance (opiate): **21 CFR**, 1308.11.

THERAP CAT: Analgesic (narcotic).

7777. Prohexadione. [88805-35-0] 3,5-Dioxo-4-(1-oxopropyl)cyclohexanecarboxylic acid; 3,5-dioxo-4-propionylcyclohexanecarboxylic acid. $C_{10}H_{12}O_5$; mol wt 212.20. C 56.60%, H 5.70%, O 37.70%. Gibberellin biosynthesis inhibitor. Prepn: K. Motojima *et al.*, **EP 123001**; *eidem*, **US 4678496** (1984, 1987 both to Kumiai). Review of properties and field trials: T. Miyazawa *et al., Brighton Crop Prot. Conf. - Weeds* **1991**, 967-972.

mp 98-99°.

Calcium salt. [127277-53-6] BX-112; KIM-112; KUH-833; Medax; Viviful. $C_{10}H_{10}CaO_5$; mol wt 250.26. Fine white powder, mp >360°. Vapor pressure (20°): 1.335×10^{-5} Pa. Soly at 20° (mg/l): water 174.2; methanol 1.11. LD_{50} in rats (mg/kg): >5000 orally; >2000 dermally; LC_{50} in carp, bluegill sunfish, rainbow trout (mg/l): >150, >100, >100 (Miyazawa).

USE: Plant growth regulator.

7778. Proinsulin. [9035-68-1] Single chain insulin precursor consisting of the insulin A and B chains and a connecting polypeptide (C-peptide), which contains 30-35 amino acids; the number and sequence of these amino acids are species dependent. Its presence was discovered in a human islet cell adenoma: D. F. Steiner, P. E. Oyer, *Proc. Natl. Acad. Sci. USA* **57**, 473 (1967). Conversion of proinsulin to insulin has a half-time of about 1 hour in rat islets *in vitro;* it is postulated that proteolytic enzymes cleave proinsulin at the sites where two amino acids connect the C-peptide to the insulin chain. This cleavage results in the production of insulin and the C-peptide, both of which are retained in the secretory granules of the beta cells and discharged in equimolar amounts during exocytosis of the granules. *See* W. Kemmler, D. F. Steiner, *Biochem. Biophys. Res. Commun.* **41**, 1223 (1970). *In vitro* conversion of proinsulin to insulin with trypsin and carboxypeptidase B: W. Kemmler *et al., J. Biol. Chem.* **246**, 6786(1971), **248**, 4544 (1973). Isoln of bovine proinsulin: D. F. Steiner *et al., Diabetes* **17**, 725 (1968). Structural studies on mammalian proinsulin: R. E. Chance *et al., Science* **161**, 165 (1968) (porcine); C. Nolan *et al., J. Biol. Chem.* **246**, 2780 (1971) (bovine); P. E. Oyer *et al., ibid.* 1365 (human, monkey); J. D. Petersen *et al., ibid.* **247**, 4866 (1972) (monkey, sheep, dog); H. S. Tager, D. F. Steiner, *ibid.* 7936 (rat, horse); D. E. Massey, D. G. Smyth, *ibid.* **250**, 628 (1975) (guinea pig). Proposed three-dimensional structure: C. R. Snell, D. G. Smyth, *ibid.* 6291. Syntheses of C-peptides and human proinsulin: N. Yanaihara *et al., Diabetes* **27**(Suppl. 1), 149 (1978). Synthesis of rat proinsulin in bacteria: L. Villa-Komaroff *et al.,* in *Polypeptide Hormones,* R. F. Beers, E. G. Bassett, Eds. (Raven Press, New York, 1980) pp 49-65. *Reviews:* D. F. Steiner *et al.* in *Diabetes, 8th Proc. Congr. Int. Diabetes Fed.,* W. J. Malaisse, J. Pirart, Eds. (Excerpta Med., Amsterdam, 1974) pp 119-133; A. H. Rubenstein *et al.,* in *Recent Progr. Horm. Res.* **33**, R. O. Greep, Ed. (Academic Press, New York, 1977) pp 435-475; A. E. Kitabshi, *Metabolism* **26**, 547-587 (1977). Book: *Proinsulin, Insulin, C-Peptides,* S. Baba *et al.,* Eds. (Excerpta Medica, Amsterdam, 1979) 468 pp.

7779. Prolactin. [9002-62-4] Pituitary lactogenic hormone; adenohypophysial luteotropin; anterior pituitary luteotropin; lactogen; galactin; mammotropin; luteotropic hormone; luteotropin; LTH; Ferolactan. Polypeptide hormone of mol wt about 23,000; active principle of adenohypophysial gland essential in the induction of lactation in mammals at parturition. Its synergistic action with estrogen promotes mammary gland proliferation. Also brings about the release of progesterone, *q.v.* from lutein cells which renders the uterine mucosa suited for the imbedding of the ovum, should fertilization occur. Isoln procedures from adenohypophyseal tissue or whole pituitary glands of ox, sheep, and swine: Lyons, *Cold Spring Harbor Symp. Quant. Biol.* **5**, 198 (1937); Li *et al., J. Biol. Chem.* **146**, 627 (1942); White *et al., ibid.* **143**, 447 (1942). Isoln from sheep pituitaries: Reisfeld *et al., J. Am. Chem. Soc.* **83**, 3719 (1961); from other mammalian pituitaries: Nelson; Eppstein, US **3265580** and US **3317392** (1966, 1967, both to Upjohn); from human pituitaries: Lewis *et al., Biochem. Biophys. Res. Commun.* **44**, 1169 (1971). Amino acid sequence of ovine prolactin: Li *et al., Nature* **224**, 695 (1969); Li, Dixon, *Arch. Biochem. Biophys.* **146**, 233 (1971). Review of structural studies of human prolactin and relationship to somatotropin, *q.v.:* H. D. Niall *et al., Recent Prog. Horm. Res.* **29**, 387 (1973). Amino acid sequence of human prolactin: B. Shome, A. F. Parlow, *J. Clin. Endocrinol. Metab.* **45**, 1112 (1977). Effects of prolactin on the murine immune system: E. Nagy *et al., Acta Endocrinol.* **102**, 351 (1983). Symposium on clinical endocrinology: *Horm. Res.* **22**, 129-252 (1985). General reviews: Li, Evans, *Hormones* **1**, 631 (1948); White, *Vitam. Horm.* **7**, 253 (1949); Voss, *Arzneim.-Forsch.* **4**, 467 (1954); Apostalakis, *Vitam. Horm.* **26**, 197 (1968). Books: *Prolactin* vols. **1-8**, D. F. Horrobin, Ed. (Eden Press, Quebec, 1973-1981); *Prolactin: Physiology, Pharmacology and Clinical Findings,* O. Hutzinger *et al.,*

Eds. (Springer-Verlag, New York, 1982) 224 pp; *Prolactin and Prolactinomas,* G. Tolis *et al.,* Eds. (Raven Press, New York, 1983) 478 pp.

Crystals. Isoelectric point 5.73. $[\alpha]_D^{25}$ $-40.5°$ (c = 1 in phosphate buffer of pH 7). Practically insol in water (0.102 g/l) unless electrolytes are present. Forms a water-soluble hydrochloride. Sol in abs methanol or ethanol, if a small amount of acid is present. These data apply to prolactin obtained from ox glands. Prolactin from sheep glands is slightly different: In $0.357M$ NaCl at pH 2.25 the sheep hormone has a soly of 0.506 g/l, while the soly of the ox hormone is only 0.316 g. In citrate buffer ($1M$, pH 6.36) and in alcohol the ox protein is more sol than the sheep protein. In the absence of salt, prolactin shows little loss of potency after boiling for one hour at pH 8.0 or at 60° for 5 hours; in the presence of salts complete destruction may occur. An 0.04% soln was stable in a boiling water bath for 15 minutes at pH 1 to 9, but lost activity rapidly at pH 11 and 13. As a rule the hormone is more stable in acid than in alkaline solns. 1 mg = 30 I.U.

THERAP CAT: Lactation stimulating hormone.

7780. Proline. [147-85-3] L-Proline; Pro; P; (S)-2-pyrrolidinecarboxylic acid. $C_5H_9NO_2$; mol wt 115.13. C 52.16%, H 7.88%, N 12.17%, O 27.79%. Non-essential amino acid for human development. Only imino acid of the 20 amino acids commonly found in proteins. Shows *cis-trans* isomerism. First synthesized: R. Willstätter, *Ber.* **33**, 1160 (1900); prior to identification in casein: E. Fischer, *Ber.* **34**, 454 (1901). Named in 1904 by Fischer. Early chemistry and biochemistry: *Amino Acids and Proteins,* D. M. Greenberg, Ed. (Charles C. Thomas, Springfield, IL, 1951) 950 pp., *passim;* J. P. Greenstein, M. Winitz, *Chemistry of the Amino Acids* vols. **1-3** (John Wiley and Sons, Inc., New York, 1961) pp. 2178-2201, *passim.* Stereospecific synthesis: S. L. Titouani *et al., Tetrahedron* **36**, 2961 (1980). HPLC determn: A. Carisano, *J. Chromatogr.* **318**, 132 (1985). HPLC separation of *cis-trans* isomers of peptides: S. Friebe *et al., ibid. A* **661**, 7 (1994). Review of biosynthesis and degradation: E. Adams, L. Frank, *Annu. Rev. Biochem.* **49**, 1005-1061 (1980). Review of effects on protein structure and biological function: A. Yaron, F. Naider, *Crit. Rev. Biochem. Mol. Biol.* **28**, 31-81 (1993); G. Vanhoof *et al., FASEB J.* **9**, 736-744 (1995).

Flat needles from alcohol + ether, prisms from water, dec 220-222°. $[\alpha]_D^{23.4}$ $-85.0°$; $[\alpha]_D^{20}$ $-52.6°$ (c = 0.57 in $0.50N$ HCl); $[\alpha]_D^{20}$ $-93.0°$ (c = 2.42 in $0.6N$ KOH). pI 6.30. pK_1 1.99; pK_2 10.60. Soly in 100 ml water: 127.4 g at 0°; 162.3 g at 25°; 206.7 g at 50°; 239 g at 65°. Sol in alcohol 1.55% at 35°. Insol in ether, butanol, isopropanol.

DL-Form. [609-36-9] Monohydrate, crystals, mp 190° (when anhydr, dec 205°). Sol in water, alc; sparingly sol in acetone, chloroform, benzene; insol in ether.

7781. Prolintane. [493-92-5] 1-[1-(Phenylmethyl)butyl]-pyrrolidine; 1-(α-propylphenethyl)pyrrolidine; 1-phenyl-2-pyrrolidylpentane; phenylpyrrolidinopentane; SP-732. $C_{15}H_{23}N$; mol wt 217.35. C 82.89%, H 10.67%, N 6.44%. Prepn: **GB 807835**; Seeger, Kottler, **DE 1093799** (1959, 1960 both to Thomae), *C.A.* **55**, 19950c (1961). Pharmacological studies: R. Kadatz, E. Pötzsch, *Arzneim.-Forsch.* **7**, 344 (1957); K. Takagi *et al., Oyo Yakuri* **5**, 5 (1971), *C.A.* **76**, 94575k (1972).

bp$_{0.5}$ 105°; bp$_{16}$ 153°.

Hydrochloride. [1211-28-5] Katovit; Promotil. $C_{15}H_{23}$-N.HCl; mol wt 253.81. Crystals from methyl ether, mp 133-134°. LD_{50} orally in mice: 257 mg/kg (Kadatz, Pötzsch).

THERAP CAT: CNS stimulant; antidepressant.

7782. Prolonium Iodide. [123-47-7] 2-Hydroxy-*N,N,N,-N',N',N'*-hexamethyl-1,3-propanediaminium diiodide; (2-hydroxy-trimethylene)bis[trimethylammonium] iodide; 1,3-bis(trimethyl-amino)-2-propanol diiodide; hexamethyldiaminoisopropanol diiodide; di(iodohexamethyl)diaminoisopropanol; iodisan; Endojodin. $C_9H_{24}I_2N_2O$; mol wt 430.11. C 25.13%, H 5.62%, I 59.01%, N 6.51%, O 3.72%. Prepn: Callsen, **US 1526627** (1925).

White, crystalline powder. mp ~275° with decompn, but becomes brown at 240°. Freely sol in water, slightly in alcohol. Practically insol in ether, acetone.

THERAP CAT: Iodine source.

7783. Promazine. [58-40-2] *N,N*-Dimethyl-10*H*-phenothiazine-10-propanamine; 10-(3-dimethylaminopropyl)phenothiazine; RP-3276; Wy-1094; A-145. $C_{17}H_{20}N_2S$; mol wt 284.42. C 71.79%, H 7.09%, N 9.85%, S 11.27%. Prepd by heating a xylene soln of phenothiazine and 3-dimethylamino-1-chloropropane in the presence of sodamide: Charpentier, **US 2519886** (1950 to Rhône-Poulenc).

Oily liq. Amine odor. Alkaline reaction. $bp_{0.3}$ 203-210°.

Hydrochloride. [53-60-1] Liranol; Promwill; Prazine; Protactyl; Sparine; Talofen. $C_{17}H_{20}N_2S.HCl$; mol wt 320.88. White to slightly yellow crystals, dec 181° (microblock). Oxidizes upon prolonged exposure to air and acquires a blue or pink color. Hygroscopic. One gram dissolves in about 3 ml water. Sol in methanol, ethanol, chloroform. Practically insol in ether, benzene. Aq solns are slightly acid to litmus. Incompatible with alkalies, oxidizing agents, heavy metals.

THERAP CAT: Antipsychotic.

THERAP CAT (VET): Tranquilizer.

7784. Promedol. [64-39-1] 1,2,5-Trimethyl-4-phenyl-4-piperidinol propanoate (ester); 1,2,5-trimethyl-4-phenyl-4-propionyloxypiperidine; 1,2,5-trimethyl-4-phenyl-4-piperidyl propionate; dimethylmeperidine. $C_{17}H_{25}NO_2$; mol wt 275.39. C 74.14%, H 9.15%, N 5.09%, O 11.62%. Prepn: Nazarov *et al., J. Gen. Chem. USSR* **26**, 3117 (1956); Nazarov, Shvestov, *ibid.* 3533. Conformation studies: Prostakov, Mikheeva, *ibid.* **31**, 108 (1961); **33**, 2931 (1963); *eidem, Russ. Chem. Rev.* **31**, 556 (1962). Of the four possible isomers α and γ are shown.

α-isomer　　　γ-isomer

α-Isomer hydrochloride. α-Promedol. $C_{17}H_{25}NO_2.HCl$. Crystals from benzene, mp 153-154°. Has been also reported as mp 106-107° or 126-131° (Prostakov, Mikheeva, 1961).

β-Isomer hydrochloride. Isopromedol. Crystals, mp 183-184°, Nazarov, Shvestov, *Bull. Acad. Sci. USSR Phys. Ser.* **1959**, 2059.

γ-Isomer hydrochloride. Trimeperidine; γ-promedol. Crystals from acetone, mp 222-223°.

Note: This is a controlled substance (opiate): **21 CFR,** 1308.11.

THERAP CAT: Analgesic (narcotic).

7785. Promegestone. [34184-77-5] (17β)-17-Methyl-17-(1-oxopropyl)estra-4,9-dien-3-one; 17α-methyl-17-propionylestra-4,9-dien-3-one; 17α-methyl-17β-propionyl-19-nor-4,9-androsta-dien-3-one; 17α,21-dimethyl-19-norpregna-4,9-diene-3,20-dione; R-5020; RU-5020; Surgestone. $C_{22}H_{30}O_2$; mol wt 326.47. C 80.94%, H 9.26%, O 9.80%. Synthetic progestin with no androgenic activity and with high affinity for the progesterone receptor. Prepn: J. Warnant, A. Farcilli, **BE 763099**; *eidem*, **US 3679714, US 3761591** (1971, 1972, 1973 all to Roussel-UCLAF). Inhibition of gonadotropin secretion and lack of androgenic activity: F. Labrie *et al., Fertil. Steril.* **28**, 1104 (1977). Binding studies in mouse uterus: D. Philibert, J.-P. Raynaud, *Steroids* **22**, 89 (1973); *eidem, Endocrinology* **94**, 627 (1974). Binding to human endometrium: *eidem, Contraception* **10**, 457 (1974); M. Haukkamaa, T. Luukkainen, *J. Steroid Biochem.* **5**, 447 (1974). Review and possible use in treatment of hormone-dependent breast cancer: J.-P. Raynaud, T. Ojasoo, *J. Gynecol. Obstet. Biol. Reprod.* **12**, 697 (1983).

Colorless crystals from isopropyl ether, mp 152°. Sol in acetone, benzene. Insol in water. $[\alpha]_D^{20}$ −262° (c = 0.5 in ethanol). uv max in ethanol: 215, 305 nm ($E_{1cm}^{1\%}$ 202, 648).

USE: As radioligand for the progestin receptor.

THERAP CAT: Progestogen.

7786. Promethazine. [60-87-7] *N,N,α*-Trimethyl-10*H*-phenothiazine-10-ethanamine; 10-(2-dimethylaminopropyl)phenothiazine; 10-(2-dimethylamino-2-methylethyl)phenothiazine; *N*-(2'-dimethylamino-2'-methyl)ethylphenothiazine; proazamine; RP-3277; Fargan. $C_{17}H_{20}N_2S$; mol wt 284.42. C 71.79%, H 7.09%, N 9.85%, S 11.27%. Prepn from 10-phenothiazinepropyl chloride and dimethylamine in presence of Cu: Charpentier, *Compt. Rend.* **225**, 306 (1947); **US 2530451** (1950 to Rhône-Poulenc); from Grignard complexes of dimethylaminopropyl halide and phenothiazine: Berg, Ashley, **US 2607773** (1952 to Rhône-Poulenc). Structure and isomerism: Edge, Wragg, *J. Pharm. Pharmacol.* **5**, 279 (1953). Metabolic studies: Huang *et al., J. Pharm. Sci.* **59**, 772 (1970). Toxicity: Rajsner, *Collect. Czech. Chem. Commun.* **34**, 1019 (1969). Comprehensive description: C. M. Shearer, S. M. Miller, *Anal. Profiles Drug Subs.* **5**, 429-465 (1976).

Crystals, mp 60°. bp_3 190-192°.

Hydrochloride. [58-33-3] RP-3389; Atosil; Farganesse; Fenazil; Hiberna; Lergigan; Phenergan; Prothazin. $C_{17}H_{20}N_2S.HCl$; mol wt 320.88. Crystals from ethylene dichloride, mp 230-232° (some dec). Turns blue on prolonged exposure to air and moisture. uv max (water): 249, 297 nm (ε 28770, 3400). pH of 10% aq soln 5.3. Freely sol in water. Sol in alcohol, chloroform. Practically insol in acetone, ether, ethyl acetate. LD_{50} i.v. in mice: 55.0 mg/kg (Rajsner).

Compd with 8-chlorotheophylline. [17693-51-5] Promethazine teoclate; Avomine. $C_{17}H_{20}N_2S.C_7H_7ClN_4O_2$; mol wt 499.03.

THERAP CAT: Antihistaminic.

THERAP CAT (VET): Antihistaminic, antiemetic, CNS depressant.

7787. Promethium. [7440-12-2] Pm; at. no. 61; valence 3. No stable nuclides, known radioactive isotopes (mass numbers): 132-155. Longest-lived known isotope: 145 (rel. at. mass 144.9127, $T_{1/2}$ 17.7 years, α-emitter). Most available isotope: 147 (rel. at. mass 146.9151, $T_{1/2}$ 2.6234 years, β-emitter). Abundance in the earth's crust reported as 4.5×10^{-20} ppm; present at low levels in uranium ores. Independent discovery in rare earth concentrate claimed by: J. A. Harris, B. S. Hopkins, *J. Am. Chem. Soc.* **48**, 1585 (1926); J. A. Harris *et al., ibid.* 1594; and by: L. Rolla, L. Fernandez, *Gazz. Chim. Ital.* **56**, 435 (1926). Synthetic prepn: H. B. Law *et al., Phys. Rev.* **59**, 936 (1941). Positive identification from fission products of ^{235}U by ion-exchange chromatography: J. A. Marinsky *et al., J. Am. Chem. Soc.* **69**, 2781 (1947). Metal prepd by reduction of halides: Weigel, *Angew. Chem. Int. Ed.* **2**, 326 (1963); E. J. Wheelwright, *J. Phys. Chem.* **73**, 2867 (1969). Review of prepn, properties and compds: Boyd, *J. Chem. Educ.* **36**, 3-14 (1959); Weigel, *Fortschr. Chem. Forsch.* **12**, 539-621 (1969); F. H. Spedding in *Kirk-Othmer Encyclopedia of Chemical Technology* vol. **19** (John Wiley & Sons, New York, 3rd ed., 1982) pp 833-854; *Chemistry of the Elements*, N. N. Greenwood, A. Earnshaw, Eds. (Pergamon Press, New York, 1984) pp 1423-1449. Review of chemistry, toxicology and industrial uses: *Promethium Technology*, E. J. Wheelwright, Ed. (American Nuclear Society, Hindsdale, IL, 1973) 395 pp. Brief review of properties: G. T. Seaborg, *Radiochim. Acta* **61**, 115-122 (1993).

^{147}Pm, metallic solid; d 7.22. mp 1080° (Weigel); also reported as 1169° (Wheelwright). A number of salts have been prepared including the trihalides (PmX₃), the sesquioxide (Pm₂O₃), the hydroxide [Pm(OH)₃] and the nitrate [Pm(NO₃)₃.xH₂O].

USE: ^{147}Pm as energy source for nuclear powered batteries, β-particle source for thickness gauges; in the prepn of self-luminous compds; as portable x-ray sources.

7788. Prometon. [1610-18-0] 6-Methoxy-*N,N'*-bis(1-methylethyl)-1,3,5-triazine-2,4-diamine; 2,4-bis(isopropylamino)-6-methoxy-*s*-triazine; 2-methoxy-4,6-bis(isopropylamino)-*s*-triazine; methoxypropazine; prometone; G-31435; Gesafram; Pramitol. C₁₀H₁₉N₅O; mol wt 225.29. C 53.31%, H 8.50%, N 31.09%, O 7.10%. Nonselective pre- and post-emergent herbicide for use on noncrop land. General preparative information and use as herbicide: H. Gysin, E. Knüsli, **US 2909420** (1959 to Geigy); *see also:* M. A. Priola, **US 3713806** (1973 to Ciba-Geigy). Alternate process: H. V. Lemaster, **US 3663542** (1972 to Geigy). Comparison with other triazine herbicides: H. Gysin, E. Knüsli, *Adv. Pest Contr. Res.* **3**, 289 (1960). Metabolism in rats: J. E. Bakke *et al., J. Agric. Food Chem.* **15**, 628 (1967). GC determn in human urine: *ibid.* **27**, 740 (1979). Toxicology study in sheep and cattle: A. E. Johnson *et al., Am. J. Vet. Res.* **33**, 1433 (1972). Review of properties and analytical methods: B. G. Tweedy, R. A. Kahrs, *Anal. Methods Pestic. Plant Growth Regul.* **10**, 493 (1978).

Crystalline solid, mp 91-92°. Soly in water (20°): 750 ppm. Very sol in organic solvents. Vapor pressure at 20°: 2.3×10⁻⁶ Torr. LD₅₀ in mice, rats (mg/kg): 2160, 2980 orally (Gysin, Knüsli, 1960). LC₅₀ (96 hour) in bluegill sunfish, rainbow trout (ppm): >32, 20 (Tweedy, Kahrs).

USE: Nonselective herbicide.

7789. Prometryn. [7287-19-6] *N,N'*-Bis(1-methylethyl)-6-methylthio-1,3,5-triazine-2,4-diamine; 2,4-bis(isopropylamino)-6-(methylthio)-*s*-triazine; 2-methylthio-4,6-bis(isopropylamino)-*s*-triazine; G-34161; Gesagard; Caparol. C₁₀H₁₉N₅S; mol wt 241.36. C 49.76%, H 7.93% N 29.02%, S 13.29%. Selective pre- and post-emergence herbicide. General preparative information and use as herbicide: H. Gysin, E. Knüsli, **CH 337019**; *eidem,* **US 2909420** (both 1959 to Geigy). See also: M. A. Priola, **US 3713806** (1973 to Ciba-Geigy). Alternative process: **FR 1372089**; E. Knüsli, W. Stammbach, **US 3207756** (1964, 1965 both to Geigy). Activity: H. Gysin, *Chem. Ind. (London)* **1962**, 1393. Metabolism in rats and rabbits: C. Böhme, F. Bär, *Food Cosmet. Toxicol.* **5**, 23 (1967). Toxicity: Geigy, *Toxicology Data on Prometryne* July, 1964. Review of properties and analytical methods: B. G. Tweedy, R. A. Kahrs, *Anal. Methods Pestic. Plant Growth Regul.* **10**, 493 (1978).

Crystals, mp 118-120°. Vapor pressure at 20°: 1×10⁻⁶ mm Hg. Soly in water at 20°: 48 ppm. Readily sol in org solvents. Stable in neutral or slightly acid or alkaline media. Hydrolyzed under stronger acidic or basic conditions. LD₅₀ orally in rats: 3.75 g/kg (Geigy). LC₅₀ (96 hour) in bluegill sunfish, rainbow trout (ppm): 10.0, 2.5 (Tweedy, Kahrs).

USE: Herbicide.

7790. Pronethalol. [54-80-8] α-[[(1-Methylethyl)amino]-methyl]-2-naphthalenemethanol; α-[(isopropylamino)methyl]-2-naphthalenemethanol; [2-hydroxy-2-(2-naphthyl)ethyl]isopropyl-amine; 2-isopropylamino-1-(2-naphthyl)ethanol; 1-(2'-naphthyl)-2-isopropylaminoethanol; nethalide. C₁₅H₁₉NO; mol wt 229.32. C 78.56%, H 8.35%, N 6.11%, O 6.98%. β-Adrenergic blocker. Prepd by reduction of 2-naphthacyl bromide with NaBH₄ followed by reaction with isopropylamine: Stephenson, **GB 909357** (1962 to ICI). Pharmacology: Black *et al., Br. J. Pharmacol. Chemother.* **25**, 577 (1965). Carcinogenicity in mice: R. Howe, *Nature* **207**, 594 (1965). Metabolism: W. G. Stillwell, M. G. Horning, *Res. Commun. Chem. Pathol. Pharmacol.* **9**, 601 (1974).

Crystals, mp 108°.

Hydrochloride. [51-02-5] ICI-38174; Alderlin. C₁₅H₁₉NO.-HCl; mol wt 265.78. Crystals, mp 184°. LD₅₀ in mice (mg/kg): 512 orally, 46 i.v. (Black).

THERAP CAT: Antianginal; antiarrhythmic; antihypertensive.

7791. Pro-opiomelanocortin. [66796-54-1] Proopiocortin; ACTH-β-lipotropin common precursor; precursor to ACTH-LPH-β-endorphin; 31K-precursor; POMC. A precursor protein of mol wt ~30,000, synthesized in the hypothalamus, pituitary gland, brain, and several peripheral tissues that incorporates the amino acid sequences of the pituitary hormones ACTH and β-lipotropin. These two hormones, in turn, contain biologically active component peptides: α-MSH, *corticotropin-like intermediate lobe peptide* (*CLIP*), α-LPH, β-MSH, endorphins, and met-enkephalin. First description of the presence of ACTH and LPH in the same molecule: P. J. Lowry *et al., Int. Congr. Ser. - Excerpta Med.* **402**, 71 (1976). Confirmation of the common precursor by radioimmunoassay: R. E. Mains *et al., Proc. Natl. Acad. Sci. USA* **74**, 3014 (1977); J. L. Roberts, E. Herbert, *ibid.* 4826, 5300. Isoln of rat pro-opiomelanocortin: M. Rubenstein *et al., ibid.* **75**, 669 (1978). Partial sequence analysis using cDNA from mouse: J. L. Roberts *et al., ibid.* **76**, 2153 (1979). Complete sequence of bovine POMC using cloned cDNA: S. Nakanishi *et al., Nature* **278**, 423 (1979). The precursor has also been found in human ACTH ectopic tumor: X. Bertagna *et al., Proc. Natl. Acad. Sci. USA* **75**, 5160 (1978). Primary structure of the NH₂-terminal glycopeptide of human pituitary POMC: N. G. Seidah *et al., J. Biol. Chem.* **256**, 7977 (1981). *Reviews:* M. Chrétien, N. G. Seidah, *Mol. Cell. Biochem.* **34**, 101-127 (1981); D. De Wied, J. Jolles, *Physiol. Rev.* **62**, 976-1059 (1982); Y. P. Loh *et al., Peptides* **3**, 397-404 (1982).

7792. Propacetamol. [66532-85-2] *N,N*-Diethylglycine 4-(acetylamino)phenyl ester; *N,N*-diethylglycine ester with 4'-hydroxyacetanilide; 4-acetamidophenyl (diethylamino)acetate. C₁₄H₂₀N₂O₃; mol wt 264.32. C 63.62%, H 7.63%, N 10.60%, O 18.16%. Injectable prodrug of acetaminophen, *q.v.* Prepn and pharmacology: J. C. Cognacq, **BE 854376**; *idem,* **US 4127671** (1977, 1978 both to Hexachimie). Clinical comparison with injectable aspirin: R. De Marneffe, L. Mokassa, *C. R. Ther. Pharmacol.*

Clin. **3,** 23 (1985). Clinical studies: P. Delacroix *et al., Sem. Hop.* **61,** 2739 (1985); J. Modai, *ibid.* **62,** 587 (1986).

Thick oil.

Hydrochloride. [66532-86-3] UP-34101; Pro-Dafalgan. C_{14}-$H_{20}N_2O_3$·HCl; mol wt 300.78. mp 228°. Sol in water.

THERAP CAT: Analgesic; antipyretic.

7793. Propachlor. [1918-16-7] 2-Chloro-*N*-(1-methylethyl)-*N*-phenylacetamide; 2-chloro-*N*-isopropylacetanilide; *N*-isopropyl-α-chloroacetanilide; CP-31393; Ramrod. $C_{11}H_{14}ClNO$; mol wt 211.69. C 62.41%, H 6.67%, Cl 16.75%, N 6.62%, O 7.56%. Selective pre-emergence herbicide. Prepn: P. C. Hamm, A. J. Speziale, **US 2863752** (1958 to Monsanto). Activity studies: Duke, *Diss. Abstr. B* **28,** 1315 (1967); Jaworski, *J. Agric. Food Chem.* **17,** 165 (1969); Lamoureaux *et al., ibid.* **19,** 346 (1971); Dhillon, Anderson, *Weed Res.* **12,** 182 (1972). Metabolism: J. E. Bakke *et al., Science* **210,** 433 (1980). Toxicity data: E. E. Kenaga, *Down Earth* **35,** 25 (1979).

Light tan solid, mp 67-76°. Vapor pressure at 110°: 0.03 mm Hg. Soly in water at 20°: 700 mg/l. Sol in common organic solvents except aliphatic hydrocarbons. LD_{50} orally in rats: 710 mg/kg (Kenaga).

USE: Herbicide.

7794. Propafenone. [54063-53-5] 1-[2-[2-Hydroxy-3-(propylamino)propoxy]phenyl]-3-phenyl-1-propanone; 2′-[2-hydroxy-3-(propylamino)propoxy]-3-phenylpropiophenone; SA-79. C_{21}-$H_{27}NO_3$; mol wt 341.44. C 73.87%, H 7.97%, N 4.10%, O 14.06%. Sodium channel blocker. Prepn: R. Sachse, **DE 2001431** (1971 to Helopharm), *C.A.* **75,** 151538f (1971). Pharmacology: H.-J. Hapke, E. Prigge, *Arzneim.-Forsch.* **26,** 1849 (1976). Pharmacokinetics: M. Hollmann *et al., ibid.* **33,** 763 (1983). HPLC determn in plasma and urine: U. Hofmann *et al., J. Chromatogr. B* **748,** 113 (2000). Review of pharmacology and therapeutic efficacy: H. M. Bryson *et al., Drugs* **45,** 85-130 (1993). Review of clinical trials in supraventricular arrhythmias and atrial fibrillation: A. P. Rae, *Am. J. Cardiol.* **82,** 59N-65N (1998); S. C. Reimold *et al., ibid.* 66N-71N.

Hydrochloride. [34183-22-7] Arythmol; Pronon; Rythmol; Rytmonorm. $C_{21}H_{27}NO_3$·HCl; mol wt 377.90. Fine white crystals. Slightly bitter taste. Sol in basic lower aliphatic alcohols, CCl_4, hot water; slightly sol in cold water. Insol in ether. LD_{50} in rats (mg/kg): 18.8 i.v.; 700 orally (Hapke, Prigge).

THERAP CAT: Antiarrhythmic (class IC).

7795. Propagermanium. [12758-40-6] 3,3′-(1,3-Dioxo-1,3-digermoxanediyl)bispropanoic acid; 2-(carboxyethyl)germanium sesquioxide; 3-oxygermylpropionic acid polymer; poly-*trans*-[(2-carboxyethyl)germasesquioxane]; proxigermanium; repagermanium; GE-132; SK-818; Serocion. $C_6H_{10}Ge_2O_7$; mol wt 339.42. C 21.23%, H 2.97%, Ge 42.80%, O 33.00%. $(GeCH_2CH_2$-$COOH)_2O_3$. Biologic response modifier. Polymeric organoger-

manium compound. Orginally synthesized at Asai Germanium Institute in 1967. Prepn and crystal structure: M. Tsutsui *et al., J. Am. Chem. Soc.* **98,** 8287 (1976). Toxicology and clinical pharmacokinetics: K. Miyao *et al., Curr. Chemother. Infect. Dis.* **2,** 1527 (1979). TLC quantitation: X. Peishan *et al., J. Planar Chromatogr. Mod. TLC* **3,** 141 (1990). Electrochemical behavior and determn: K. Hasebe *et al., Electroanalysis* **6,** 779 (1994). Antiviral activity: Y. Ishiwata *et al., Arzneim.-Forsch.* **44,** 357 (1994). Review of biological activities and mechanism of antitumor action: R. R. Brutkiewicz, F. Suzuki, *In Vivo* **1,** 189-204 (1987). *Review:* K. Miyao, N. Tanaka, *Drugs Future* **13,** 441-453 (1988). Review of clinical use as an immunostimulant: H. Fukazawa *et al., Head Neck* **16,** 30-38 (1994).

Colorless, monoclinic crystals or crystalline powder having no odor but a slightly acidic taste. mp 270° (dec). pKa 3.6. Sol in water at 1.09% at 20°. Insol or very slightly sol in almost all organic solvents. Very sol in water under alkaline conditions; >10% at pH 7.4. Aq solns exhibit acid reactions. Stable at pH 2-12, especially at pH 7.4 especially where decomposition does not occur at 110° for 5 min. LD_{50} i.p. in mice: 2.8 g/kg (Brutkiewicz).

THERAP CAT: Antineoplastic; immunostimulant.

7796. Propallylonal. [545-93-7] 5-(2-Bromo-2-propenyl)-5-(1-methylethyl)-2,4,6(1*H*,3*H*,5*H*)pyrimidinetrione; 5-(2-bromoallyl)-5-isopropylbarbituric acid; Noctal. $C_{10}H_{13}BrN_2O_3$; mol wt 289.13. C 41.54%, H 4.53%, Br 27.64%, N 9.69%, O 16.60%. Prepn: **US 1622129** (1927); *cf.* Herzog, *Arch. Pharm.* **263,** 216 (1925). Acute toxicity: Maloney, *J. Pharmacol. Exp. Ther.* **42,** 267 (1931).

Crystals. mp 177-179°. Slightly bitter taste. Slightly sol in water; freely sol in alcohol, glacial acetic acid, acetone, alkalies. Sparingly sol in ether, chloroform, benzene. MLD orally in rabbits: 300-350 mg/kg (Maloney).

Note: This is a controlled substance (depressant): **21 CFR,** 1308.13.

THERAP CAT: Sedative, hypnotic.

7797. Propamidine. [104-32-5] 4,4′-[1,3-Propanediylbis-(oxy)]bisbenzenecarboximidamide; 4,4′-(trimethylenedioxy)dibenzamidine; 4,4′-diamidino-α,ω-diphenoxypropane. $C_{17}H_{20}N_4O_2$; mol wt 312.37. C 65.37%, H 6.45%, N 17.94%, O 10.24%. Prepn: A. J. Ewins *et al.,* **GB 507565** (1939 to May & Baker); J. N. Ashley *et al., J. Chem. Soc.* **1942,** 103; of isethionate: G. Newbery, A. P. T. Easson: **US 2394003** (1946 to May & Baker). Trypanocidal activity: E. M. Lourie, W. Yorke, *Ann. Trop. Med. Parasitol.* **33,** 289 (1939). Preliminary pharmacology: R. Wien, *ibid.* **37,** 1 (1943). Determn in biological fluids: D. P. Jackson *et al., J. Biol. Chem.* **167,** 377 (1947). Mode of action: M. J. Pine, *Biochem. Pharmacol.* **17,** 75 (1968). Activity in fibrinolytic systems: J. D. Geratz, *Thromb. Diath. Haemorrh.* **29,** 154 (1973). Clinical use in treatment of *Acanthamoeba* keratitis: D. L. Easty, *Br. Med. J.* **296,** 228 (1988); J. J. Wiens, W. B. Jackson, *Can. J. Ophthalmol.* **23,** 107 (1988). Early review of pharmacology, mode of action and clinical applications: E. B. Schoenbach, E. M. Greenspan, *Medicine* **27,** 327-377 (1948).

Isethionate. [140-63-6] M & B 782; Brolene Drops. $C_{21}H_{32}$-$N_4O_{10}S_2$; mol wt 564.63. Hygroscopic, very bitter crystals or granular powder, mp ~235°. Soluble in water (~1 in 5), glycerol, 95% alcohol (~1 in 33). Practically insol in ether, chloroform, fixed oils, liq petrolatum. pH of a 5% w/v soln in water = 4.5 to 6.5.

THERAP CAT: Antiprotozoal (Trypanosoma); antiamebic.

THERAP CAT (VET): Anti-infective (topical). Formerly used as antiprotozoal (Trypanosoma, Babesia).

7798. Propamocarb. [24579-73-5] [3-(Dimethylamino)-propyl]carbamic acid propyl ester; propyl-(3-dimethylaminopropyl) carbamate. $C_9H_{20}N_2O_2$; mol wt 188.27. C 57.42%, H 10.71%, N 14.88%, O 17.00%. Systemic carbamate fungicide. Prepn: **BE 708057** (1968 to Schering AG). Prepn of salts: G.-A. Hoyer, E. A. Pieroh, **US 3649674** (1972 to Schering AG). Properties and activity: E. A. Pieroh *et al., Meded. Fac. Landbouwwet. Rijksuniv. Gent* **43,** 933 (1978). Metabolic fate in bluegills and catfish: C. Gray, C. O. Knowles, *Chemosphere* **10,** 469 (1981). Efficacy vs late blight fungus on potato: Y. Samoucha, Y. Cohen, *Phytoparasitica* **18,** 27 (1990). GC determn in food products: T. Nagayama *et al., J. AOAC Int.* **79,** 769 (1996). Uptake and redistribution in potato and grapevine: R. I. Harris, *Brighton Crop Prot. Conf. - Pests Dis.* **1996,** 281.

bp$_{18mm}$ 139-141°. n_D^{20} 1.4490.

Hydrochloride. [25606-41-1] SN-66752; AE-B066752; HOE-102791; Banol; Previcur; Proplant. $C_9H_{20}N_2O_2 \cdot HCl$; mol wt 224.73. Colorless, odorless crystals, mp 45-55°. Soly at 25° (g/100ml): water >70; dichloromethane >43; methanol >50. Vapor pressure at 25°: 6×10^{-6} torr. LD$_{50}$ orally in rats: 8600 mg/kg. LC$_{50}$ (96 hr) in rainbow trout, sunfish, carp (ppm): 616, 415, 234 (Pieroh).

USE: Agricultural fungicide.

7799. Propane. [74-98-6] Dimethylmethane; propyl hydride. C_3H_8; mol wt 44.10. C 81.71%, H 18.28%. $CH_3CH_2CH_3$. Constituent of natural gas and of crude petroleum. Obtained by the so-called "stabilization process" using fractional distillation under pressure: Francis, Robbins, *J. Am. Chem. Soc.* **55,** 4339 (1933). Many syntheses, e.g., by using butyronitrile and sodium: Timmermans, *J. Chim. Phys.* **18,** 133 (1920).

Gas. Odorless when pure. Burns with a luminous, smoky flame. Explosive limits, % by vol in air: 2.37-9.5. Heavier than air. One liter weighs 2.0200 g at 0° and 760 mm; 1.8324 g at 25° and 760 mm. Liquefies at −42°; solid at −187.7°. bp (1 atm) −42.1°; bp (2 atm) −25.6°; bp (5 atm) 1.4°; bp (10 atm) 26.9°; bp (20 atm) 58.1°; bp (30 atm) 78.7°; bp (40 atm) 94.8°. Crit temp 96.81°; crit press. 42.01 atm. Heat of combustion (const vol) 528.4 cal, (const pressure) 553.5 cal. 100 vols water dissolve 6.5 vols at 17.8° and 753 mm pressure; 100 vols abs alc dissolve 790 vols at 16.6° and 754 mm pressure; 100 vols ether dissolve 926 vols at 16.6° and 757 mm pressure; 100 vols chloroform dissolve 1299 vols at 21.6° and 757 mm pressure; 100 vols benzene dissolve 1452 vols at 21.5° and 757 mm pressure; 100 vols turpentine dissolve 1587 vols at 17.7° and 757 mm pressure.

Caution: Potential symptoms of overexposure are dizziness, confusion, excitation, asphyxia; direct contact with liquid may cause frostbite. *See NIOSH Pocket Guide to Chemical Hazards* (DHHS/-NIOSH 97-140, 1997) p 262.

USE: As fuel gas, sometimes mixed with butane. In organic syntheses. As refrigerant.

7800. 1-Propanearsonic Acid. [107-34-6] *n*-Propylarsonic acid. $C_3H_9AsO_3$; mol wt 168.02. C 21.45%, H 5.40%, As 44.59%, O 28.57%. $C_3H_7AsO(OH)_2$.

White needles, mp 125°. Freely sol in water; sol in alcohol. Insol in ether.

USE: For the determination of zirconium.

7801. 1,3-Propanedithiol. [109-80-8] 1,3-Dimercaptopropane; trimethylenedithioglycol; dithiotrimethyleneglycol; trimethylenedimercaptan. $C_3H_8S_2$; mol wt 108.23. C 33.29%, H 7.45%, S 59.25%. $HSCH_2CH_2CH_2SH$. Prepd by alkaline hydrolysis of propylene-1,3-diisothiuronium dihydrochloride: Grogan *et al., J. Org. Chem.* **20,** 50 (1955).

Oil. Disagreeable odor. d_4^{20} 1.0772. bp$_{760}$ 169-170°; bp$_{759}$ 170-171°; bp$_{56}$ 92-98°. n_D^{20} 1.5392. Volatile with steam. Slightly sol in water. Miscible with alcohol, ether, chloroform and benzene.

7802. Propanethial *S*-Oxide. [32157-29-2] Thiopropionaldehyde *S*-oxide; thiopropanal *S*-oxide. C_3H_6OS; mol wt 90.14. C 39.97%, H 6.71%, O 17.75%, S 35.57%. $CH_3CH_2CH = SO$. Lachrymatory factor of the onion, *Allium cepa L.*, found as a 95% *cis*- and 5% *trans*- mixture. Early structure studies: W. D. Niegisch, W. H. Stahl, *Food Res.* **21,** 657 (1956); C. G. Spare, A. I. Virtanen, *Acta Chem. Scand.* **17,** 641 (1963). Structure: M. H. Brodnitz, J. V. Pascale, *J. Agric. Food Chem.* **19,** 269 (1971). Stereochemistry: E. Block *et al., J. Am. Chem. Soc.* **101,** 2200 (1979); *eidem, Tetrahedron Lett.* **21,** 1277 (1980). Chemistry: *eidem, J. Am. Chem. Soc.* **102,** 2490 (1980).

7803. Propanidid. [1421-14-3] 4-[2-(Diethylamino)-2-oxoethoxy]-3-methoxybenzeneacetic acid propyl ester; [4-[(diethylcarbamoyl)methoxy]-3-methoxyphenyl]acetic acid propyl ester; [3-methoxy-4-[(*N,N*-diethylcarbamido)methoxy]phenyl]acetic acid *n*-propyl ester; propyl 4-[(diethylcarbamoyl)methoxy]-3-methoxyphenyl]acetate; Bayer 1420; FBA-1420; Epontol; Sombrevin. $C_{18}H_{27}NO_5$; mol wt 337.41. C 64.07%, H 8.07%, N 4.15%, O 23.71%. Prepn: R. Hiltmann *et al., DE 1134981; US 3086978* (1962, 1963 both to Bayer). Toxicity study: E. I. Goldenthal, *Toxicol. Appl. Pharmacol.* **18,** 185 (1971).

Pale yellow oil, bp$_{0.7}$ 210-212°. Practically insol in water; sol in alcohol, chloroform. LD$_{50}$ orally in rats: >10,000 mg/kg (Goldenthal).

THERAP CAT: Anesthetic (intravenous).

7804. Propanil. [709-98-8] *N*-(3,4-Dichlorophenyl)propanamide; 3′,4′-dichloropropionanilide; *N*-(3,4-dichlorophenyl)propionamide; DPA; FW-734; Stam; Stampede. $C_9H_9Cl_2NO$; mol wt 218.08. C 49.57%, H 4.16%, Cl 32.51%, N 6.42%, O 7.34%. Selective contact herbicide. Prepn: W. Schäfer *et al., DE 1039779* (1958 to Bayer), *C.A.* **54,** 20060i (1960); Huffman, Allen, *J. Agric. Food Chem.* **8,** 298 (1960). Use in nematocide formulations: Fielding, Stoddard, **US 3108038** (1963 to du Pont). Toxicity study: G. W. Bailey, J. L. White, *Residue Rev.* **10,** 97 (1965).

White crystalline solid, mp 91-93°. Soly in water at room temp: 225 ppm. LD$_{50}$ orally in rats: 1384 mg/kg (Bailey, White).

USE: Herbicide.

7805. Propantheline Bromide. [50-34-0] *N*-Methyl-*N*-(1-methylethyl)-*N*-[2-[(9*H*-xanthen-9-ylcarbonyl)oxy]ethyl]-2-propanaminium bromide; (2-hydroxyethyl)diisopropylmethylammonium bromide xanthene-9-carboxylate; β-diisopropylaminoethyl 9-xanthenecarboxylate methobromide; Corrigast; Ercotina; Pro-Banthine; Neo-Metantyl; Pantheline. $C_{23}H_{30}BrNO_3$; mol wt 448.39. C 61.61%, H 6.74%, Br 17.82%, N 3.12%, O 10.70%. Synthetic quaternary ammonium anticholinergic. Prepn: Cusic, Robinson, *J. Org. Chem.* **16,** 1921 (1951); **US 2659732** (1953 to Searle). Metabolic studies: Beermann *et al., Clin. Pharmacol. Ther.* **13,** 212 (1972).

Crystals from isopropanol + ether, mp 159-161°. Very soluble in water, alcohol, chloroform. Practically insol in ether, benzene.

THERAP CAT: Antispasmodic; in treatment of urinary incontinence.

7806. Propaquizafop. [111479-05-1] (R)-2-[4-[(6-Chloro-2-quinoxalinyl)oxy]phenoxy]propanoic acid 2-[[(1-methylethylidene)amino]oxy]ethyl ester; 2-isopropylideneaminooxyethyl (R)-2-[4-(6-chloroquinoxalin-2-yloxy)phenoxy]propionate; Ro-17-3664; Prilan. $C_{22}H_{22}ClN_3O_5$; mol wt 443.88. C 59.53%, H 5.00%, Cl 7.99%, N 9.47%, O 18.02%. Post-emergence graminicide for use in broadleaf crops. Prepn: G. Frater et al., **US 4687849** (1987 to Hoffmann-La Roche); R. Klaus et al., ACS Symp. Ser. **443,** 226-235 (1991). Comprehensive description: P. F. Bocion et al., Proc. Br. Crop Prot. Conf. - Weeds **1987,** 55-62. Review of comparative field trials: J. D. A. Wevers, Meded. Fac. Landbouwwet. Rijksuniv. Gent **56,** 611-615 (1991).

Crystals from ether/hexane, mp 62-64°. $[\alpha]_D^{20}$ +29.7° (c = 0.93% in chloroform). d^{20} 1.29. Vapor pressure (20°): 1.3×10^{-8} Pa. Log P (n-octanol/water at pH 7): 3.5. Soly in water (25°): 2 ppm (pH 7). LD_{50} in rats (mg/kg): >5000 orally; >2000 dermally (Bocion).

USE: Herbicide.

7807. Proparacaine. [499-67-2] 3-Amino-4-propoxybenzoic acid 2-(diethylamino)ethyl ester; 2-(diethylamino)ethyl 3-amino-4-propoxybenzoate; proxymetacaine. $C_{16}H_{26}N_2O_3$; mol wt 294.39. C 65.28%, H 8.90%, N 9.52%, O 16.30%. Prepn of the hydrochloride: Clinton et al., J. Am. Chem. Soc. **74,** 592 (1952). Pharmacology: McIntyre, Sievers, J. Pharmacol. Exp. Ther. **63,** 369 (1938). Comprehensive description: D. B. Whigan, Anal. Profiles Drug Subs. **6,** 423-456 (1977).

Hydrochloride. [5875-06-9] Ak-Taine; Alcaine; Ophthaine; Ophthetic. $C_{16}H_{26}N_2O_3 \cdot HCl$; mol wt 330.85. Prisms from abs alcohol + ethyl acetate, mp 182.0-183.3°. uv max (methanol): 225, 270, 300 nm. Sol in water, warm alcohol, methanol. Insol in ether, benzene. Solns are neutral to litmus. pKa 3.2.

THERAP CAT: Topical anesthetic (ophthalmic).

THERAP CAT (VET): Anesthetic (local).

7808. Propargite. [2312-35-8] Sulfurous acid 2-[4-(1,1-dimethylethyl)phenoxy]cyclohexyl 2-propynyl ester; sulfurous acid 2-(p-tert-butylphenoxy)cyclohexyl 2-propynyl ester; 2-(p-tert-butylphenoxy)cyclohexyl propargyl sulfite; cyclosulfyne; propargil; BPPS; ENT-27226; DO-14; Omite; Comite. $C_{19}H_{26}O_4S$; mol wt 350.47. C 65.11%, H 7.48%, O 18.26%, S 9.15%. Acaricide for control of mites on crops. Prepn and insecticidal properties: R. A. Covey et al., **US 3272854** (1966 to U.S. Rubber). Field tests, comparison with other acaricides in control of Pacific spider mite: E. M. Stafford, J. Econ. Entomol. **61,** 1641 (1968). Efficacy against citrus red mite: L. R. Jeppson et al., ibid. **62,** 531 (1969). Residue determn: J. M. Devine, H. R. Sisken, J. Agric. Food Chem. **20,** 59 (1972). Brief account of properties, analysis: G. M. Stone, Anal. Methods Pestic. Plant Growth Regul. **7,** 355 (1973). Toxicity studies: T. B. Gaines, Toxicol. Appl. Pharmacol. **14,** 515 (1969).

Viscous liquid, distils with decomp, stabilized by adding 0.5-1.0% propylene oxide. Soluble in most organic solvents. Practically insoluble in water (10.5 ppm). LD_{50} in male, female rats (mg/kg): 1480, 1480 orally; 250, 680 dermally (Gaines). LC_{50} in rainbow trout, bluegill sunfish (ppb): >100, 31 (Stone).

USE: Acaricide.

7809. Propargyl Alcohol. [107-19-7] 2-Propyn-1-ol. C_3H_4O; mol wt 56.06. C 64.27%, H 7.19%, O 28.54%. $HC \equiv CCH_2$-OH. Prepd by heating β-bromoallyl alcohol with conc KOH: Henry, Ber. **5,** 456, 569 (1872); **6,** 729 (1873); **14,** 404 (1881); from formaldehyde and sodium acetylide: Henne, Greenlee, J. Am. Chem. Soc. **67,** 484 (1945); from epichlorohydrin + sodium: Eglinton et al., J. Chem. Soc. **1952,** 2873; from acetylene and formaldehyde: Reppe, Ann. **596,** 1 (1955). Toxicity study: W. Guilian, B. Naibin, Chemosphere **36,** 1475 (1998).

Moderately volatile liquid. Mild geranium odor. d_4^{20} 0.9715. mp −52 to −48°. bp_{760} 114-115°; $bp_{490.3}$ 100°; $bp_{147.6}$ 70°; $bp_{35.4}$ 40°; $bp_{20.6}$ 30°; $bp_{11.6}$ 20°. n_D^{20} 1.43064. Viscosity at 20° = 1.68 cP. Flash pt 33°C. Spec heat: 0.616 cal/g. Misc with water, benzene, chloroform, 1,2-dichloroethane, ethanol, ether, acetone, dioxane, tetrahydrofuran, pyridine. Appreciable heat is evolved on mixing with pyridine. Moderately sol in carbon tetrachloride. Immiscible with aliphatic hydrocarbons. With water, propargyl alcohol forms an azeotrope, bp 97.5°. This mixture has a composition of 39.5 parts by weight of propargyl alcohol and 60.5 parts of water. Polymerized by heat or caustic. Acidified aq solns are resistant to polymerization. LD_{50} in rats, mice (mg/kg): 20, 50 orally (Guilian, Naibin).

Caution: Potential symptoms of overexposure are irritation of skin, mucous membranes; CNS depression. See NIOSH Pocket Guide to Chemical Hazards (DHHS/NIOSH 97-140, 1997) p 264.

7810. Propargyl Chloride. [624-65-7] 3-Chloro-1-propyne. C_3H_3Cl; mol wt 74.51. C 48.36%, H 4.06%, Cl 47.58%. Prepd by treating propargyl alcohol with phosphorus trichloride: Henry, Ber. **7,** 761 (1874); **8,** 398 (1875); Kirsmann, Bull. Soc. Chim. Fr. [4] **39,** 698 (1926).

Liquid. d_4^{25} 1.0306. mp −78°. bp_{760} 57°. Flash pt <60°F. Practically insol in water, glycerol. Miscible with benzene, carbon tetrachloride, ethanol, ethylene glycol, ether, ethyl acetate. Reacts with hydroxy compds to form ethers; with sulfides, ammonia, amines or metal hypoiodites to give the corresp propargyl compds; with aldehydes and ketones to give β-acetylenic alcohols. Undergoes isomerization.

USE: Intermediate in organic synthesis.

7811. Propatyl Nitrate. [2921-92-8] 2-Ethyl-2-[(nitrooxy)-methyl]-1,3-propanediol dinitrate (ester); 2-ethyl-2-(hydroxymethyl)-1,3-propanediol trinitrate; 1,1,1-tris(nitratomethyl)propane; ethyltrimethylolmethane trinitrate; trimethylolethylmethane trinitrate; 2,2-bis(hydroxymethyl)-1-butanol trinitrate; 1-hydroxy-2,2-bis(hydroxymethyl)butane trinitrate; etriol trinitrate; ETTN; Win-9317; Atrilon 5; Etrynit; Gina; Ginapect; Vasangor. $C_6H_{11}N_3O_9$; mol wt 269.17. C 26.77%, H 4.12%, N 15.61%, O 53.50%. $(O_2NOCH_2)_3CCH_2CH_3$. Prepn: Médard, Mem. Poudres **35,** 113 (1953); Bourjol, ibid. **36,** 79 (1954); Hensinger, **FR 1103113** (1955).

White powder, mp 51-52°. d 1.49. Readily sol in acetone, alcohol. Practically insol in water. Lowest explosive temp: 220°. Heat of combustion 829.2 kcal/mol. Explosive but only slightly sensitive to shock.

THERAP CAT: Vasodilator (coronary).

7812. Propazine. [139-40-2] 6-Chloro-N,N'-bis(1-methylethyl)-1,3,5-triazine-2,4-diamine; 2-chloro-4,6-bis(isopropylamino)-s-triazine; 2,4-bis(isopropylamino)-6-chloro-s-triazine; G-30028; Prozinex. $C_9H_{16}ClN_5$; mol wt 229.71. C 47.06%, H 7.02%, Cl 15.43%, N 30.49%. Selective pre-emergence herbicide. Prepn: Gysin, Knüsli, **CH 342784; CH 342785** (both 1960 to Geigy). Toxicity study: G. W. Bailey, J. L. White, Residue Rev. **10,** 97 (1965).

Crystals, mp 213°. Solubility in water at 20° = 8.6 ppm; diffi-cultly sol in organic solvents. LD$_{50}$ orally in rats: >5000 mg/kg (Bailey, White).

USE: Herbicide.

7813. Propentofylline. [55242-55-2] 3,7-Dihydro-3-meth-yl-1-(5-oxohexyl)-7-propyl-1H-purine-2,6-dione; 3-methyl-1-(5-oxohexyl)-7-propylxanthine; 1-(5'-oxohexyl)-3-methyl-7-propyl-xanthine; HWA-285; Albert-285; HOE-285; Hextol; Karsivan. C$_{15}$H$_{22}$N$_4$O$_3$; mol wt 306.36. C 58.81%, H 7.24%, N 18.29%, O 15.67%. Peripheral vasodilator which inhibits cyclic AMP phos-phodiesterase. Prepn: W. Mohler et al., **DE 2330742**; eidem, **US 4289776** (1975, 1981 both to Hoechst). Cardiovascular effects in animals: O. Hudlicka et al., Br. J. Pharmacol. **72**, 723 (1981). Effect on cAMP phosphodiesterase: K. Nagata et al., Arzneim.-Forsch. **35**, 1034 (1985). Inhibition of adenosine uptake: B. B. Fredholm, K. Lindström, Acta Pharmacol. Toxicol. **58**, 187 (1986). Cerebrovascular effects in animals: J. J. Grome et al., Drug Dev. Res. **5**, 111 (1985). Effect on postischemic brain edema: B. B. Mrsulja et al., ibid. **6**, 339 (1985). Effect on cognitive function in humans: I. Hindmarch, Z. Subhan, ibid. **5**, 379 (1985). Acute toxicity: M. Inazu et al., Oyo Yakuri **31**, 357 (1986), C.A. **104**, 218960a (1986).

Crystals from diisopropyl ether, mp 69-70°. Soly in water at 25°: 3.2%; in ethanol: >10%; in DMSO: >10%. LD$_{50}$ in male, female mice, male, female rats (mg/kg): 900, 780, 1150, 940 orally; 168, 170, 180, 195 i.v.; 375, 346, 199, 196 i.p.; 450, 508, 400, 338 s.c. (Inazu).

THERAP CAT: Nootropic.

THERAP CAT (VET): Vasodilator (peripheral and cerebral).

7814. Properdin. [11016-39-0] A highly basic serum pro-tein believed to be a factor in natural immunity against germ and virus diseases, perhaps also against cancer: L. Pillemer et al., Science **120**, 279 (1954). Combines with zymosan, q.v., the insol cell wall residue from yeast: L. Pillemer, O. A. Ross, ibid. **121**, 732 (1955). Participates also in a nonspecific manner in a variety of immunological reactions of normal serum. Isoln from human se-rum: L. Pillemer et al., J. Exp. Med. **103**, 1 (1956). Purification: Spicer et al., **US 3038838** (1962 to Merck & Co.). Characterization of highly purified human properdin: J. Pensky et al., J. Immunol. **100**, 142 (1968). Activity studies: O. Götze, H. J. Müller-Eber-hard, J. Exp. Med. **139**, 44 (1974). The human properdin system has been studied extensively; it was the subject of long years of scien-tific controversy. Components of the human properdin system that have been identified and characterized are: properdin, factor B, factor D and C3. Comprehensive review of L. Pillemer's work and history of the properdin system discovery: I. H. Lepow, J. Immunol. **125**, 471 (1980). The rabbit properdin system: G. B. Naff, ibid. **124**, 2625 (1980).

7815. Propetamphos. [31218-83-4] (E)-3-[[(Ethylamino)-methoxyphosphinothioyl]oxy]-2-butenoic acid 1-methylethyl ester; (E)-3-hydroxycrotonic acid isopropyl ester O-ester with O-methyl ethylphosphoramidothioate; (E)-1-methylethyl 3-[[(ethylamino)-methoxyphosphinothioyl]oxy]-2-butenoate; (E)-O-2-isopropoxy-carbonyl-1-methylvinyl O-methyl ethylphosphoramidothioate; SAN-322I; Catalyst. C$_{10}$H$_{20}$NO$_4$PS; mol wt 281.31. C 42.70%, H 7.17%, N 4.98%, O 22.75%, P 11.01%, S 11.40%. Prepn: J. P. Leber, K. Lutz, **DE 2035103** corresp to **US 3758645** (1971, 1973 to Sandoz). Activity: W. Berg, R. Gothe, Proc. Br. Crop Prot. Conf. - Pests Dis. **1979**, 517.

Yellowish liquid, bp$_{0.005}$ 87-89°. n$_D^{20}$ 1.495. d$_4^{20}$ 1.1294. Soly in water at 24°: 110 mg/l. Sol in most organic solvents. LD$_{50}$ orally in male rats: 82 mg/kg (Berg, Gothe).

USE: Insecticide.

THERAP CAT (VET): Ectoparasiticide.

7816. Propham. [122-42-9] Phenylcarbamic acid 1-meth-ylethyl ester; carbanilic acid isopropyl ester; N-phenyl isopropyl carbamate; isopropyl carbanilate; O-isopropyl N-phenyl carbamate; INPC; IPC; isoPPC. C$_{10}$H$_{13}$NO$_2$; mol wt 179.22. C 67.02%, H 7.31%, N 7.82%, O 17.85%. Prepn: Allen, **US 2615916** (1952 to Columbia-Southern Chem. Corp.); Kovalenko, Zh. Obshch. Khim. **24**, 1041 (1954); J. L. Hermanson, R. Olson, Trans. Kans. Acad. Sci. **64**, 231 (1961). Acute toxicity: T. B. Gaines, R. E. Linder, Fun-dam. Appl. Toxicol. **7**, 299 (1986).

Crystals, mp 90°. Practically insol in water. Sol in most organic solvents. LD$_{50}$ in male, female rats (mg/kg): 3724, 4315 orally (Gaines, Linder).

USE: Herbicide, applied as a spray to the soil.

7817. Propicillin. [551-27-9] (2S,5R,6R)-3,3-Dimethyl-7-oxo-6-[(1-oxo-2-phenoxybutyl)amino]-4-thia-1-azabicyclo[3.2.0]-heptane-2-carboxylic acid; 6-(α-phenoxybutyramido)penicillanic acid; α-phenoxypropylpenicillin; levopropylcillin. C$_{18}$H$_{22}$N$_2$O$_5$S; mol wt 378.44. C 57.13%, H 5.86%, N 7.40%, O 21.14%, S 8.47%. Semi-synthetic antibiotic related to penicillin. Prepn from 6-aminopenicillanic acid: **GB 877120** (1961 to Beecham); of salts: Perron et al., J. Am. Chem. Soc. **82**, 3934 (1960); Glombitza, Ann. **673**, 166 (1964). Metabolism in humans: M. Cole et al., Anti-microb. Agents Chemother. **3**, 463 (1973). TLC determn: S. Hen-drickx et al., J. Chromatogr. **291**, 211 (1984).

Potassium salt. [1245-44-9] BRL-284; PA-248; Baycillin; Brocillin; Cetacillin; Oricillin; Trescillin; Ultrapen. C$_{18}$H$_{21}$KN$_2$-O$_5$S; mol wt 416.53. Crystals, dec 195-197°. Soluble at 20° in 1.2 parts water, 23 parts 95% (w/v) alcohol. pH of 1% w/v soln: 5-7.5.

THERAP CAT: Antibacterial.

7818. Propiconazole. [60207-90-1] 1-[[2-(2,4-Dichloro-phenyl)-4-propyl-1,3-dioxolan-2-yl]methyl]-1H-1,2,4-triazole; pro-conazole; CGA-64250; Banner; Orbit; PropiMax; Tilt. C$_{15}$H$_{17}$Cl$_2$-N$_3$O$_2$; mol wt 342.22. C 52.64%, H 5.01%, Cl 20.72%, N 12.28%, O 9.35%. Systemic foliar fungicide. Prepn: G. Van Reet et al., **DE 2551560**; eidem, **US 4079062** (1976, 1978 both to Janssen). Physicochemical properties, toxicity and antifungal activity: P. A. Urech et al., Proc. Br. Crop Prot. Conf. - Pests Dis. **1979**, 508. Efficacy vs cereal diseases: G. Eyries, Phytiatr.-Phytopharm. **30**, 37 (1981). GC determn in soil, water, plant material: B. Büttler, J. Agric. Food Chem. **31**, 762 (1983).

Yellowish, viscous liquid. bp$_{0.1mm}$ 180°. Vapor pressure at 20°: <3 × 10^{-6} mm Hg. Soly in water at 20°: 110 mg/l. Sol in most organic solvents. LD$_{50}$ orally in rats: 1517 mg/kg (Urech).

USE: Agricultural fungicide.

Consult the Name Index before using this section.

7819. Propineb. [12071-83-9] [[(1-Methyl-1,2-ethanediyl)-bis[carbamodithioato]](2−)]zinc; [propylenebis(dithiocarbamato)]zinc; zinc 1,2-propylene bisdithiocarbamate; mezineb; methylzineb; Bayer 46131; Antracol. $C_5H_8N_2S_4Zn$; mol wt 289.80. C 20.72%, H 2.78%, N 9.67%, S 44.26%, Zn 22.57%. Prepn and use as fungicide: **IT 611046** (1960 to Montecatini); Lehmann *et al.*, **BE 611960** and **BE 628114** (1962 and 1963 to Bayer). Chemistry, biological activity and toxicology: Grewe, *Pflanzenschutz-Nachr.* **20**, 581 (1967). Fungicidal activity: A. G. Channon, *Ann. Appl. Biol.* **65**, 481 (1965); E. J. S. Reddy *et al.*, *Pesticides* **19**, 67 (1985). Distribution and degradation in soil: W. Mittelstaedt, F. Fuhr, *Landwirtsch. Forsch.* **30**, 221 (1977); in fruit: K. Vogeler *et al.*, *Pflanzenschutz-Nachr.* **30**, 72 (1977).

White to yellowish powder, practically odorless. Decomposes and turns brown above 160°. Decomposes in strongly acid or alkaline media. Practically insol in all conventional solvents. LD_{50} in male rats, rabbits, cats (mg/kg): 8500, >2500, >2500 orally (Grewe).

USE: Agricultural fungicide.

7820. β-Propiolactone. [57-57-8] 2-Oxetanone; hydracrylic acid β-lactone; β-propionolactone; propanolide; NSC-21626; Betaprone. $C_3H_4O_2$; mol wt 72.06. C 50.00%, H 5.60%, O 44.41%. Prepd by the condensation of ketene with formaldehyde: Küng, **US 2356459** (1941). Purification: Gresham, Jansen, **US 2602802** (1952 to B. F. Goodrich). Use in Diels-Alder diene synthesis: Gresham *et al.*, *J. Am. Chem. Soc.* **76**, 609 (1954). Review of carcinogenic risk: *IARC Monographs* **4**, 259-269 (1974).

Liquid. d_4^{20} 1.1460; d_4^{25} 1.1420; d_2^{20} 1.1490. mp −33.4°. bp_{760} 162° (dec); bp_{750} 150° (dec); bp_{20} 61°; bp_{10} 51°. Flash pt 70°C (158°F). n_D^{20} 1.4131; n_D^{25} 1.4110. Dipole moment 3.8. Slowly hydrolyzed to hydracrylic acid. Stable when stored at 5° in glass containers. Soly in water: 37% v/v. Misc with alcohol, acetone, ether, chloroform.

Caution: Potential symptoms of overexposure are skin irritation, blistering and burns; corneal opacity; frequent urination; dysuria; hematuria. *See NIOSH Pocket Guide to Chemical Hazards* (DHHS/NIOSH 97-140, 1997) p 264. This substance is reasonably anticipated to be a human carcinogen: *Report on Carcinogens, Eleventh Edition* (PB2005-104914, 2004) p III-225.

USE: Versatile intermediate in organic synthesis.

THERAP CAT: Disinfectant.

7821. Propiolic Acid. [471-25-0] 2-Propynoic acid; acetylenecarboxylic acid; propargylic acid. $C_3H_2O_2$; mol wt 70.05. C 51.44%, H 2.88%, O 45.68%. CH≡CCOOH. Prepn: Wilson, Wenzke, *J. Am. Chem. Soc.* **57**, 1265 (1935); Owen, Sultanbawa, *J. Chem. Soc.* **1949**, 3109; Wolf, *Ber.* **86**, 735 (1953); **87**, 668 (1954). Manuf: Wolf, **US 2786022** (1957); Pachter, **US 2799703** (1957 to Ethyl Corp.). Review on its occurrence and biological activity: Reisch, *Pharmazie* **20**, 194 (1965).

Liquid at room temp (crystals from carbon disulfide, mp 9°). bp 144° (dec), $bp_{10.5}$ 54-55°; bp_{50} 70-75°. d_4^{15} 1.1435, d_4^{20} 1.1380, d_4^{25} 1.1325. $n_D^{20.4}$ 1.4302. Dipole moment at 25°, 2.08D (in dioxane): Wilson, Wenzke, *loc. cit.*

7822. Propiomazine. [362-29-8] 1-[10-[2-(Dimethylamino)propyl]-10H-phenothiazin-2-yl]-1-propanone; 10-dimethylaminoisopropyl-2-propionylphenothiazine; propionylpromethazine; Wy-1359. $C_{20}H_{24}N_2OS$; mol wt 340.48. C 70.55%, H 7.10%, N 8.23%, O 4.70%, S 9.42%. Prepn: Schmitt *et al.*, *Bull. Soc. Chim. Fr.* **1957**, 1474; Schmitt, **FR addn. 71342** (addn. to **FR 1176919** to Clin-Byla). Comprehensive description of the hydrochloride: K.

B. Crombie, L. F. Cullen, *Anal. Profiles Drug Subs.* **2**, 439-466 (1973). GC determn in plasma and urine: U. Ahs, G. Wickström, *J. Chromatogr.* **183**, 229 (1980). Clinical use as sedative: W. F. Powell *et al.*, *Anesth. Analg.* **49**, 132 (1970); as hypnotic: M. Viukari, P. Miettinen, *Neuropsychobiology* **12**, 134 (1984).

$bp_{0.5}$ 235-245°.

Maleate. CB-1678; Indorm; Propavan. $C_{20}H_{24}N_2OS.C_4H_4O_4$; mol wt 456.55. Crystals from isopropanol, mp 160-161°.

Hydrochloride. [1240-15-9] Largon. $C_{20}H_{24}N_2OS.HCl$; mol wt 376.94. Yellow, practically odorless powder. Very soluble in water; freely sol in alcohol. Insol in benzene.

THERAP CAT: Sedative, hypnotic.

THERAP CAT (VET): Tranquilizer.

7823. Propionaldehyde. [123-38-6] Propanal; methylacetaldehyde; propylaldehyde. C_3H_6O; mol wt 58.08. C 62.04%, H 10.41%, O 27.55%. CH_3CH_2CHO. Prepd by treating propyl alcohol with a bichromate oxidizing mixture: C. D. Hurd, R. N. Meinert, *Org. Synth.* **coll. vol. II**, 541 (1943); by passing propyl alcohol vapor over copper at high temp: Sabatier, Senderens, *Compt. Rend.* **136**, 923 (1903); Willimott, *Analyst* **50**, 13; *Chem. Zentralbl.* **1925, I**, 2097. Toxicity study: H. F. Smyth *et al.*, *Arch. Ind. Hyg. Occup. Med.* **4**, 119 (1951).

Liq. Suffocating odor. d_4^0 0.8432; $d_4^{9.7}$ 0.8192; d_4^{20} 0.8071; d_4^{33} 0.7898. mp −81°. bp_{760} 49°; bp_{740} 47°; bp_{687} 45°. n_{580}^{16} 1.3695; n_D^{19} 1.36460. Flash pt, open cup: <20°F (<−6°C). Absorption spectrum: Kwiecinski, Marchlewski, *Bull. Soc. Chim.* [4] **45**, 608 (1929). Sol in 5 vols water at 20°. Misc with alc and ether. LD_{50} orally in rats: 1.4 g/kg; LC for rats in air: 8000 ppm (Smyth).

7824. Propionamide. [79-05-0] Propanamide; propionic acid amide. C_3H_7NO; mol wt 73.09. C 49.30%, H 9.65%, N 19.16%, O 21.89%. Prepd by heating ammonium propionate under pressure: Hofmann, *Ber.* **15**, 981 (1882); by dropping propionyl chloride into cooled ammonia water: Aschan, *Ber.* **31**, 2347 (1898).

Orthorhombic platelets from benzene. d_4^{20} 1.0335; d_4^{80} 0.9597; mp 79°; bp 222.2°. Volatile with steam. n_D^{110} 1.4160. Freely sol in water, alcohol, ether, chloroform.

7825. Propionic Acid. [79-09-4] Propanoic acid; methylacetic acid; ethylformic acid. $C_3H_6O_2$; mol wt 74.08. C 48.64%, H 8.16%, O 43.19%. CH_3CH_2COOH. Occurs in dairy products in small amounts. Can be obtained from wood pulp waste liquor by a fermentation process using bacteria of the genus *Propionibacterium*: Wayman *et al.*, **US 3067107** (1962 to Columbia Cellulose). Prepn from ethylene, carbon monoxide and steam: Reppe, *Angew. Chem.* **1956**, 46; Larson, **US 2448375** (1948 to du Pont); from ethanol and carbon monoxide using a boron trifluoride catalyst: Loder, **US 2135448**; **US 2135451**; **US 2135453** (all 1939 to du Pont); by oxidation of propionaldehyde: Hasche, **US 2294984** (1942 to Kodak); from natural gas by the Fischer-Tropsch process; as a byproduct in the pyrolysis of wood; by the action of microorganisms on a variety of materials in small yields. Very pure propionic acid can be obtained from propionitrile. Toxicity study: H. F. Smyth *et al.*, *Am. Ind. Hyg. Assoc. J.* **23**, 95 (1962).

Oily liquid. Slightly pungent, disagreeable, rancid odor. d_4^{20} 0.99336. mp −21.5°. bp_{760} 141.1°; bp_{400} 122.0°; bp_{100} 85.8°; $bp_{1.0}$ 4.6°. n_D^{25} 1.3848. Flash pt, open cup: 136°F (58°C). Viscosity (cP) at 15°: 1.175; at 25°: 1.020; at 30°: 0.956; at 60°: 0.668; at 90°: 0.495. Surface tension in dynes/cm at 15°: 27.21. Ka at 25°: 1.34×10^{-5}. Misc with water. Can be salted out of water solns by the addn of $CaCl_2$ or other salts. Sol in alcohol, ether, chloroform. Azeotrope with water, bp 99.98°, contains 17.7% acid; with toluene, bp 110.45°, contains 3% acid; with o-xylene, bp 135.4°, contains 43% acid; with ethylbenzene, bp 131.1°, contains 28% acid. LD$_{50}$ orally in rats: 4.29 g/kg (Smyth).

Barium salt monohydrate. Barium propionate. C$_6$H$_{10}$BaO$_4$.-H$_2$O. Powder, usually with slight odor. *Poisonous!* Freely sol in water; slightly sol in alcohol.

Caution: Potential symptoms of overexposure to propionic acid are irritation of eyes, skin, nose, throat; blurred vision, corneal burns; skin burns; abdominal pain, nausea, vomiting. *See NIOSH Pocket Guide to Chemical Hazards* (DHHS/NIOSH 97-140, 1997) p 266.

USE: Esterifying agent; in the production of cellulose propionate (thermoplastic) and other propionates, e.g., calcium propionate, used as mold inhibitors and preservatives; in the manuf of ester solvents, fruit flavors, and perfume bases.

THERAP CAT: Antifungal.

7826. Propionic Anhydride. [123-62-6] Propanoic acid anhydride; propanoic anhydride; methylacetic anhydride. C$_6$H$_{10}$O$_3$; mol wt 130.14. C 55.37%, H 7.75%, O 36.88%. (CH$_3$CH$_2$CO)$_2$O. Obtained by dehydration of the acid or by carbonylation of its esters: Reppe, Friederich, **US 2730546** (1956 to Badische Anilin- & Soda-Fabrik); from propionaldehyde by air oxidation in the presence of cobalt and copper acetate catalysts: McFarlane, **US 2491572** (1949 to Celanese). Other syntheses, e.g., from ethanol and carbon monoxide. Toxicity study: H. F. Smyth *et al., Arch. Ind. Hyg. Occup. Med.* **10,** 61 (1954).

Liquid. Odor more pungent than that of the acid. d$_4^0$ 1.0336; d$_4^{15}$ 1.0169; d$_4^{20}$ 1.0125; d$_4^{40}$ 0.98974; d$_4^{50}$ 0.97913. 8.4 lbs/gal at 20°. mp −45°. bp$_{760}$ 167.0°; bp$_{400}$ 146.0°; bp$_{200}$ 127.8°; bp$_{100}$ 107.2°; bp$_{60}$ 94.5°; bp$_{40}$ 85.6°; bp$_{20}$ 70.4°; bp$_{10}$ 57.7°; bp$_5$ 45.3°; bp$_{1.0}$ 20.6°. Flash pt, open cup: 165°F (74°C). n$_D^{17}$ 1.4041; n$_D^{20}$ 1.4038. Viscosity (cP): 1.144 at 20°; 0.978 at 30°; 0.853 at 40°; 0.7511 at 50°. Dec by water. Sol in methanol, ethanol, ether, chloroform. LD$_{50}$ orally in rats: 2.36 g/kg (Smyth).

USE: Esterifying agent for certain perfume oils, fats, oils, and especially cellulose. In the production of alkyd resins, dyestuffs and drugs. Has been used as a dehydrating agent in some sulfonations and nitrations.

7827. Propionitrile. [107-12-0] Propanenitrile; ethyl cyanide. C$_3$H$_5$N; mol wt 55.08. C 65.42%, H 9.15%, N 25.43%. CH$_3$CH$_2$CN. Prepd by dehydration of propionamide (or propionic acid + NH$_3$) or by distilling ethyl sulfate and concd aq KCN, also by reduction of acrylonitrile. Studies as duodenal ulcerogen in rats: S. Szabo *et al., Res. Commun. Chem. Pathol. Pharmacol.* **16,** 311 (1977); L. M. Lichtenberger *et al., Gastroenterology* **73,** 1305 (1977). Toxicity study: H. F. Smyth *et al., Arch. Ind. Hyg. Occup. Med.* **4,** 119 (1951).

Liquid. *Poisonous when heated to decompn or on contact with acids.* Pleasant, ethereal, sweetish odor. d$_4^0$ 0.8020; d$_4^{20}$ 0.7818; d$_4^{30}$ 0.7716; d$_4^{56}$ 0.7515; d$_4^{70.2}$ 0.7291. mp −91.8°. bp$_{760}$ 97.2°; bp$_{400}$ 77.7°; bp$_{200}$ 58.2°; bp$_{100}$ 41.4°; bp$_{60}$ 30.1°; bp$_{40}$ 22.0°; bp$_{20}$ 8.8°; bp$_{10}$ −3.0°; bp$_5$ −13.6°; bp$_{1.0}$ −35.0°. n$_D^{15}$ 1.36812; n$_D^{20}$ 1.36585; n$_D^{30}$ 1.36132. Soly in water at 40° = 11.9 g/100 g H$_2$O; at 100° = 29 g/100 g H$_2$O. Misc with alcohol, ether, DMF. LD$_{50}$ orally in rats: 39 mg/kg (Smyth).

Caution: Potential symptoms of overexposure are irritation of eyes, skin, respiratory system; nausea, vomiting; chest pains; weakness, stupor, convulsions. *See NIOSH Pocket Guide to Chemical Hazards* (DHHS/NIOSH 97-140, 1997) p 266.

7828. Propionyl Chloride. [79-03-8] Propanoyl chloride. C$_3$H$_5$ClO; mol wt 92.52. C 38.95%, H 5.45%, Cl 38.32%, O 17.29%.

Liquid, pungent odor. d$_4^{20}$ 1.065; mp −94°; bp 80°; n$_D^{20}$ 1.4051. Vigorously dec and dissolved by water or alcohol.

7829. Propionylpromazine. [3568-24-9] 1-[10-[3-(Dimethylamino)propyl]-10*H*-phenothiazin-2-yl]-1-propanone; 3-propionyl-10-(γ-dimethylaminopropyl)phenothiazine; 10-(3-dimethylaminopropyl)-2-propionylphenothiazine; propiopromazine; 1497-CB. C$_{20}$H$_{24}$N$_2$OS; mol wt 340.48. C 70.55%, H 7.10%, N 8.23%, O 4.70%, S 9.42%. Prepn: Schmitt *et al., Bull. Soc. Chim. Fr.* **1957,** 938, 1474; Schmitt, **FR addn. 71342** (1956 to Clin-Byla), *C.A.* **56,** 3486h (1962).

Crystals, mp 69-70°.

Hydrochloride. Tranvet. C$_{20}$H$_{24}$N$_2$OS.HCl; mol wt 376.94.

Maleate. C$_{20}$H$_{24}$N$_2$OS.C$_4$H$_4$O$_4$. Crystals from acetone, mp 135°.

Methiodide. C$_{20}$H$_{24}$N$_2$OS.CH$_3$I. Yellow crystals from isopropanol, mp 79-80°.

THERAP CAT (VET): Tranquilizer.

7830. Propiophenone. [93-55-0] 1-Phenyl-1-propanone; ethyl phenyl ketone; propionylbenzene; phenyl ethyl ketone. C$_9$-H$_{10}$O; mol wt 134.18. C 80.56%, H 7.51%, O 11.92%. Prepared from propionyl chloride and benzene in the presence of anhydr aluminum chloride: Read, *J. Am. Chem. Soc.* **44,** 1751 (1922).

Leaflets or tabular crystals. Strong, persistent, agreeable, flowery odor. Usually supplied as a liquid. d$_4^0$ (solid) 1.157; d$_4^{20}$ (liq) 1.0105; d$_{20}^{20}$ 1.0118; d$_{25}^{25}$ 1.0087; d$_4^{41.8}$ 0.9934; d$_4^{61.2}$ 0.9776; d$_4^{85.5}$ 0.9572. mp 21°. Typical freezing point: 18.6°. bp$_{760}$ 218.0°; bp$_{400}$ 194.2°; bp$_{200}$ 170.2°; bp$_{100}$ 149.3°; bp$_{60}$ 135.0°; bp$_{40}$ 124.3°; bp$_{20}$ 107.6°; bp$_{10}$ 92.2°; bp$_5$ 77.9°. n$_D^{15.9}$ 1.5290; n$_D^{20}$ 1.5269. uv max (hexane): 250, 280, 323 nm. Dipole moment: 2.7. Parachor 328.7. Flash pt 99°C (210°F). Misc with methanol, anhydr ethanol, ether, benzene, toluene. Insol in water, glycerol, ethylene glycol, propylene glycol.

USE: In perfumery; in the synthesis of ephedrine and related compds.

7831. Propiram. [15686-91-6] *N*-[1-Methyl-2-(1-piperidinyl)ethyl]-*N*-2-pyridinylpropanamide; *N*-(1-methyl-2-piperidinoethyl)-*N*-2-pyridylpropionamide; *N*-propionyl-2-(1-piperidinoisopropyl)aminopyridine; *N*-propionyl-*N*-(2-pyridyl)-1-piperidino-2-aminopropane. C$_{16}$H$_{25}$N$_3$O; mol wt 275.39. C 69.78%, H 9.15%, N 15.26%, O 5.81%. Prepn: Hiltmann *et al.,* **GB 939947** corresp to **US 3163654**; **FR M 2283** (1963, 1964, 1964 all to Bayer). Resolution of isomers: **NL 6610362**; Wollweber *et al.,* **US 3594477** (1967, 1971 both to Bayer). Pharmacology: Jasinski *et al., Clin. Pharmacol. Ther.* **12,** 613 (1971). Series of articles on chemistry, pharmacology, toxicology, pharmacokinetics, clinical trials: *Arzneim.-Forsch.* **24,** 581-722 (1974). Toxicity data: D. Tettenborn, *ibid.* 624. Absolute configuration and analgesic activity of enantiomers: W. Wollweber, *Eur. J. Med. Chem. -Chim. Ther.* **17,** 125 (1982).

bp 162-163°.

Fumarate. [13717-04-9] FBA-4503; Bay 4503; Algeril. C$_{20}$-H$_{29}$N$_3$O$_5$; mol wt 391.46. LD$_{50}$ in mice, rats (mg/kg): 874, 1657 orally (Tettenborn).

Note: This is a controlled substance (opiate): **21 CFR,** 1308.11.

THERAP CAT: Analgesic (narcotic).

7832. Propiverine. [60569-19-9] α-Phenyl-α-propoxybenzeneacetic acid 1-methyl-4-piperidinyl ester; α,α-diphenyl-α-propoxyacetic acid 1-methyl-4-piperidyl ester; 1-methyl-4-piperidyl diphenylpropoxyacetate. C$_{23}$H$_{29}$NO$_3$; mol wt 367.48. C

75.17%, H 7.95%, N 3.81%, O 13.06%. Prepn: C. Starke *et al.*, **DD 106643** (1974), *C.A.* **82**, 155841s (1975). GC-MS determn in plasma and urine: T. Marunaka *et al., J. Chromatogr.* **420**, 43 (1987). Pharmacology: A. Haruno, *Arzneim.-Forsch.* **42**, 815, 1459 (1992). Acute toxicity: K. Yamashita *et al., J. Toxicol. Sci.* **14**, Suppl. 2, 1 (1989), *C.A.* **112**, 172060 (1990). Clinical pharmacokinetics: C. Müller *et al., Eur. J. Drug Metab. Pharmacokinet.* **18**, 265 (1993). Clinical trial in urinary incontinence: D. Mazur *et al., Urologe* **A33**, 447 (1994).

Hydrochloride. [54556-98-8] P-4; Detrunorm; Mictonorm; Mictonetten. $C_{23}H_{29}NO_3 \cdot HCl$; mol wt 403.94. mp 216-218°. Sparingly sol in water and ethanol. LD_{50} in male, female mice, male, female rats (mg/kg): 36, 36, 22, 25 i.v.; 223, 283, 1632, 1411 s.c.; 410, 323, 1000, 1092 orally (Yamashita).

THERAP CAT: In treatment of urinary incontinence.

7833. Propizepine. [10321-12-7] 6-[2-(Dimethylamino)-propyl]-1,6-dihydro-5*H*-pyrido[2,3-*b*][1,5]benzodiazepin-5-one; 6,11-dihydro-6-[2-(dimethylamino)-2-methylethyl]-5*H*-pyrido[2,3-*b*][1,5]benzodiazepin-5-one. $C_{17}H_{20}N_4O$; mol wt 296.37. C 68.89%, H 6.80%, N 18.90%, O 5.40%. Prepn: **NL 6600065** (1966 to Labs. U.P.S.A.); Hoffmann, Faure, *Bull. Soc. Chim. Fr.* **1966**, 2316. Psychopharmacology: Lwoff *et al., Therapie* **26**, 451 (1971).

Hydrochloride. [14559-79-6] UP-106; Vagran. $C_{17}H_{20}N_4O \cdot HCl$; mol wt 332.83. mp 235°.

THERAP CAT: Antidepressant.

7834. Propofol. [2078-54-8] 2,6-Bis(1-methylethyl)phenol; 2,6-diisopropylphenol; disoprofol; ICI-35868; Ansiven; Diprivan; Disoprivan; Rapinovet. $C_{12}H_{18}O$; mol wt 178.27. C 80.85%, H 10.18%, O 8.97%. Prepn: A. J. Kolka *et al., J. Org. Chem.* **21**, 712 (1956); **22**, 642 (1957); G. G. Ecke, A. J. Kolka, **US 2831898** (1958 to Ethyl Corp.); T. J. Kealy, D. D. Coffman, *J. Org. Chem.* **26**, 987 (1961); B. E. Firth, T. J. Rosen, **US 4447657** (1984 to Universal Oil Products). Chromatographic study: J. K. Carlton, W. C. Bradbury, *J. Am. Chem. Soc.* **78**, 1069 (1956). Animal studies: J. B. Glen, *Br. J. Anaesth.* **52**, 731 (1980). Pharmacokinetics: H. K. Adam *et al., ibid.* 743; *idem, ibid.* **55**, 97 (1983). Determn in blood: *eidem, J. Chromatogr.* **223**, 232 (1981). Comparative studies vs other injectable anesthetics: B. Kay, D. K. Stephenson, *Anaesthesia* **35**, 1182 (1980); D. V. Rutter *et al., ibid.* 1188. Use in i.v. anesthesia: E. Major *et al., ibid.* **37**, 541 (1982). Cardiovascular effects: D. Al-Khudhairi *et al., ibid.* 1007. Pharmacology of emulsion formulation: J. B. Glen, S. C. Hunter, *Br. J. Anaesth.* **56**, 617 (1984). Series of articles on pharmacology and clinical experience: *Postgrad. Med. J.* **61**, Suppl. 3, 1-169 (1985).

bp_{30} 136°. bp_{17} 126°. mp 19°. n_D^{20} 1.5134. n_D^{25} 1.5111. d_{20} 0.955.

THERAP CAT: Anesthetic (intravenous).

THERAP CAT (VET): Intravenous anesthetic (dogs and cats).

7835. Propolis. Bee glue. Resinous substance of complex composition produced by bees for use in construction and protection of hives. Used in traditional folk medicine for its broad spectrum biological activities. *Constit.* 50% resin and vegetable balsam, 30% wax, 10% essential and aromatic oils, 5% pollen, and 5% other substances, including organic debris. Analysis by LC-MS: K. Midorikawa *et al., Phytochem. Anal.* **12**, 366 (2001). Review of the origin, chemical constituents and therapeutic activity: M. H. Haydak, *State of Iowa, Repts. State Apiarist 1953*, p 74-87; M. Vanhaelen, R.Vanhaelen-Fastre, *J. Pharm. Belg.* **34**, 253 (1979); of composition and toxicology: G. A. Burdock, *Food Chem. Toxicol.* **36**, 347-363 (1998); of plant sources and chemical constituents: V. S. Bankova *et al., Apidologie* **31**, 3-15 (2000). Review of biological activities and therapeutic use: S. L. De Castro, *ARBS Annu. Rev. Biomed. Sci.* **3**, 49-83 (2001); of pharmacology and mechanism of action: A. H. Banskota *et al., Phytother. Res.* **15**, 561-571 (2001).

Yellow-green to dark brown material. Aromatic odor. Hard and brittle when cold; soft and sticky when warm. Extraction with alcohol yields the insol ***propolis wax*** and alcohol sol ***propolis balsam***.

7836. Propoxur. [114-26-1] 2-(1-Methylethoxy)phenol methylcarbamate; *o*-isopropoxyphenyl *N*-methylcarbamate; aprocarb; Bay 39007; Bay 9010; Baygon; Bifex; Blattanex; Propyon; Suncide; Unden. $C_{11}H_{15}NO_3$; mol wt 209.24. C 63.14%, H 7.23%, N 6.69%, O 22.94%. Prepn: **US 3111539** (1963 to Bayer; Chemagro Corp.). Properties: W. Behrenz, E. Boecker, *Pflanzenschutz-Nachr. Bayer (Ger. Ed.)* **18**, 53 (1965). Toxicity data: T. B. Gaines, *Toxicol. Appl. Pharmacol.* **14**, 515 (1969). Efficacy vs fleas and ticks in domestic animal collars: R. G. Hughes, *Vet. Med. Rev.* **1**, 80 (1985). Teratogenicity study: K. D. Courtney *et al., J. Environ. Sci. Health* **B20**, 373 (1985). Environmental fate and LC/MS determn: L. Sun, H. K. Lee, *J. Chromatogr. A* **1014**, 153 (2003).

Minute crystals, mp 91.5°. Dec at high temp forming methyl isocyanate. Sol in methanol, acetone and many organic solvents, but only slightly sol in cold hydrocarbons. Water soly about 0.2% at 20°. Unstable in highly alkaline media. LD_{50} orally in male, female rats: 83, 86 mg/kg (Gaines).

Caution: Potential symptoms of overexposure are miosis, blurred vision; sweating, salivation; abdominal cramps, nausea, diarrhea, vomiting, headache, weakness, muscle twitching. *See NIOSH Pocket Guide to Chemical Hazards* (DHHS/NIOSH 97-140, 1997) p 266.

USE: Insecticide.

7837. Propoxycaine Hydrochloride. [550-83-4] 4-Amino-2-propoxybenzoic acid 2-diethylaminoethyl ester hydrochloride; 2-diethylaminoethyl 4-amino-2-propoxybenzoate hydrochloride; 2-diethylaminoethyl 2-propoxy-4-aminobenzoate hydrochloride; Ravocaine Hydrochloride; Blockain Hydrochloride. $C_{16}H_{27}ClN_2O_3$; mol wt 330.85. C 58.08%, H 8.23%, Cl 10.72%, N 8.47%, O 14.51%. Prepn: Clinton, Laskowski, **US 2689248** (1954 to Sterling Drug).

White, odorless crystals, mp 148-150°. Discolors upon prolonged exposure to light and to air. Very sol in water; slightly sol in alcohol, chloroform. Practically insol in ether. pH of a 2% aq soln 5.4.

THERAP CAT: Anesthetic (local).

7838. Propoxycarbazone. [145026-81-9] 2-[[[(4,5-Dihydro-4-methyl-5-oxo-3-propoxy-1H-1,2,4-triazol-1-yl)carbonyl]amino]sulfonyl]benzoic acid methyl ester; methyl 2-[[[(4-methyl-5-oxo-3-propoxy-4,5-dihydro-1H-1,2,4-triazol-1-yl)carbonyl]amino]sulfonyl]benzoate. $C_{15}H_{18}N_4O_7S$; mol wt 398.39. C 45.22%, H 4.55%, N 14.06%, O 28.11%, S 8.05%. Triazolinone graminicide for use in cereal crops; acetolactate synthase inhibitor. Prepn: K.-H. Müller et al., EP 507171; eidem, US 5534486 (1992, 1996 both to Bayer). Review of properties and field trials: D. Feucht et al., Brighton Crop Prot. Conf. - Weeds 1999, 53-58. Absorption and fate in weeds: L. Fandrich et al., Weed Sci. 49, 717 (2001).

mp 141°. pKa: 2.1.

Sodium salt. [181274-15-7] BAY MKH 6561; Attribut; Olympus. $C_{15}H_{17}N_4NaO_7S$; mol wt 420.37. Colorless crystalline powder, mp 230-240° (dec). Vapor pressure (20°): <1 × 10⁻⁸ Pa. Log P (octanol/water) at 20°: −0.30 (pH 4); −1.55 (pH 7); −1.59 (pH 9). Soly in water at 20° (g/l): 2.9 (pH 4); 42.0 (pH 7, pH 9). LD_{50} in rats (mg/kg): >5000 orally; >5000 dermally. LC_{50} in rats (mg/m³): >5030 in air by inhalation. LC_{50} (96 hr) in bluegill sunfish, rainbow trout (mg/l): >94.7; >77.6 (Feucht).

USE: Herbicide.

7839. Propoxyphene. [469-62-5] (αS)-α-[(1R)-2-(Dimethylamino)-1-methylethyl]-α-phenylbenzeneethanol propanoate (ester); α-d-4-dimethylamino-3-methyl-1,2-diphenyl-2-butanol propionate; (+)-1,2-diphenyl-2-propionoxy-3-methyl-4-dimethylaminobutane; (+)-4-dimethylamino-1,2-diphenyl-3-methyl-2-propionyloxybutane; α-d-propoxyphene; dextropropoxyphene. $C_{22}H_{29}NO_2$; mol wt 339.47. C 77.84%, H 8.61%, N 4.13%, O 9.43%. Prepn of racemate: Pohland, Sullivan, J. Am. Chem. Soc. 75, 4458 (1953); Pohland, US 2728779 (1955 to Lilly). Prepn of (+)-form: Pohland, Sullivan, J. Am. Chem. Soc. 77, 3400 (1955). Stereochemistry: Sullivan et al., J. Org. Chem. 28, 2381 (1963); Casy, Myers, J. Pharm. Pharmacol. 16, 455 (1964). Stereospecific synthesis: Pohland et al., J. Org. Chem. 28, 2483 (1963). Metabolism: S. L. Due et al., Biomed. Mass Spectrom. 3, 217 (1976). The α-dl- and d-diastereoisomers possess marked analgesic activity in contrast to the β-diastereoisomers which are substantially inactive. Toxicity: E. I. Goldenthal, Toxicol. Appl. Pharmacol. 18, 185 (1971); J. L. Emerson et al., ibid. 19, 445 (1971). Comprehensive description: B. McEwan, Anal. Profiles Drug Subs. 1, 301-318 (1972). Symposium on pharmacology, toxicology, and clinical efficacy of propoxyphene alone and in combination with acetaminophen: Hum. Toxicol. 3, Suppl., 1S-238S (1984).

Crystals from petr ether, mp 75-76°. $[\alpha]_D^{25}$ +67.3° (c = 0.6 in chloroform).

Hydrochloride. [1639-60-7] Darvon; Deprancol; Develin. $C_{22}H_{29}NO_2 \cdot HCl$; mol wt 375.93. Bitter crystals from methanol +

ethyl acetate, mp 163-168.5°. $[\alpha]_D^{25}$ +59.8° (c = 0.6 in water). Sol in water, alc, chloroform, acetone. Practically insol in benzene, ether. LD_{50} in mice, rats (mg/kg): 28, 15 i.v.; 111, 58 i.p.; 211, 134 s.c.; 282, 230 orally (Emerson).

Napsylate monohydrate. [26570-10-5] Darvon-N. $C_{22}H_{29}-NO_2 \cdot C_{10}H_8O_3S \cdot H_2O$; mol wt 565.72. Odorless, white crystalline powder; bitter taste. Sol in methanol, ethanol, chloroform, acetone; very slightly sol in water. LD_{50} orally in female rats: 990 mg/kg (Goldenthal).

α-l-Form see Levopropoxyphene.

α-dl-Form. Racemic propoxyphene; diméprotane.

α-dl-Form hydrochloride. Crystals from methanol + ethyl acetate, mp 170-171°. Soluble in water, alcohol, chloroform. Practically insol in benzene, ether.

β-dl-Form. Crystals from acetone + ether. mp 187-188°. More soluble than the α-form.

Note: Bulk dextropropoxyphene (non-dosage forms) is a controlled substance (opiate): **21 CFR,** 1308.12; dextropropoxyphene is a controlled substance (narcotic): **21 CFR,** 1308.14.

THERAP CAT: Analgesic (narcotic).

7840. Propranolol. [525-66-6] 1-[(1-Methylethyl)amino]-3-(1-naphthalenyloxy)-2-propanol; 1-(isopropylamino)-3-(1-naphthyloxy)-2-propanol; Avlocardyl; Euprovasin. $C_{16}H_{21}NO_2$; mol wt 259.34. C 74.10%, H 8.16%, N 5.40%, O 12.34%. β-Adrenergic blocker. Prepn: BE 640312 and BE 640313; Crowther, Smith, US 3337628 and US 3520919 (1964, 1964, 1967, 1970 all to I.C.I.). Description of optical isomers: Howe, Shanks, Nature 210, 1336 (1966). Biological studies: Barrett, Cullum, Br. J. Pharmacol. 34, 43 (1968). Metabolism: Bond, Nature 213, 721 (1967). Multicenter clinical trial in myocardial infarction: V. Hansteen et al., Br. Med. J. 284, 155 (1982). Use as migraine prophylactic: S. Diamond, E. Millstein, J. Clin. Pharmacol. 28, 193 (1988); S. Diamond et al., Headache 27, 70 (1987). Toxicity data: M. Martin, P. Linee, Eur. J. Med. Chem. 9, 563 (1974). Review of pharmacokinetics: P. A. Routledge, D. G. Shand, Appl. Pharmacokinet. 1980, 464-485; of pharmacology: J. D. Fitzgerald in Pharmacology of Antihypertensive Drugs, A. Scriabine, Ed. (Raven Press, New York, 1980) pp 195-208. Series of articles on use in hypertension: Drugs 37, Suppl. 2, 42-76 (1989).

Crystals from cyclohexane, mp 96°.

Hydrochloride. [318-98-9] AY-64043; ICI-45520; NSC-91523; Angilol; Apsolol; Bedranol; Beprane; Berkolol; Beta-Tablinen; Beta-Timelets; Cardinol; Deralin; Dociton; Duranol; Efektolol; Elbrol; Frekven; Inderal; Kemi S; Oposim; Propabloc; Prophylux; Propranur; Rapynogen; Sumial; Tesnol. $C_{16}H_{21}NO_2 \cdot HCl$; mol wt 295.80. Crystals from n-propanol, mp 163-164°. Sol in water, alc. Practically insol in ether, benzene, ethyl acetate. LD_{50} in mice (mg/kg): 565 orally; 22 i.v.; 107 i.p. (Martin, Linee).

THERAP CAT: Antihypertensive; antianginal; antiarrhythmic (class II).

7841. Propyl Acetate. [109-60-4] Acetic acid n-propyl ester. $C_5H_{10}O_2$; mol wt 102.13. C 58.80%, H 9.87%, O 31.33%. $CH_3COOCH_2CH_2CH_3$. Prepn from acetic acid and n-propyl alcohol: Wagner, J. Chem. Educ. 27, 245 (1950). Manuf from acetic acid and mixture of propene + propane in the presence of $ZnCl_2$ catalyst: Biller, GB 872876 (1961). Toxicity study: P. M. Jenner et al., Food Cosmet. Toxicol. 2, 327 (1964).

Liquid, odor of pears, bp 101.6°. mp −92°. d_4^{20} 0.836, d_{20}^{20} 0.887. n_D^{20} 1.3844. Flash pt, closed cup: 58°F (14°C). Soly in water at 16°: 1.6:100. Misc with alcohol, ether. LD_{50} in rats, mice (mg/kg): 9370, 8300 orally (Jenner).

Caution: Potential symptoms of overexposure in exptl animals are irritation of eyes, nose and throat; narcosis; dermatitis. See NIOSH Pocket Guide to Chemical Hazards (DHHS/NIOSH 97-140, 1997) p 266.

USE: Mfg flavors, perfumes. Solvent for resins, cellulose derivatives, plastics.

7842. n-Propyl Alcohol. [71-23-8] 1-Propanol; propylic alcohol; Optal. C_3H_8O; mol wt 60.10. C 59.95%, H 13.42%, O 26.62%. $CH_3CH_2CH_2OH$. Discovered by Chancel in 1853 in crude fusel oil and obtained therefrom by fractionation; available as a byproduct of the reaction between carbon monoxide and hydrogen. Toxicity study: Smyth *et al.*, *Arch. Ind. Hyg. Occup. Med.* **10**, 61 (1954).
Liquid; alcoholic and slightly stupefying odor. mp $-127°$. bp 97.2°. d_4^{20} 0.8053; d_4^{25} 0.8016: Mumford, Phillips, *J. Chem. Soc.* **1950**, 75. Flash pt 22°C. n_D^{20} 1.3862. Miscible with water, alcohol, ether. LD_{50} orally in rats: 1.87 g/kg (Smyth).
Caution: Potential symptoms of overexposure are irritation of eyes, nose and throat; dry cracking skin; drowsiness, headache; ataxia, GI pain; abdominable cramps; nausea, vomiting and diarrhea. *See NIOSH Pocket Guide to Chemical Hazards* (DHHS/NIOSH 97-140, 1997) p 268.
USE: As a solvent for resins and cellulose esters, etc.

7843. Propylamine. [107-10-8] 1-Propanamine; 1-aminopropane. C_3H_9N; mol wt 59.11. C 60.96%, H 15.35%, N 23.70%. $CH_3CH_2CH_2NH_2$. Prepn from propionaldehyde + ammonia with a Raney nickel catalyst: Olin, Schwoegler, US 2373705 (1945 to Sharples); by low pressure catalytic hydrogenation of nitropropane: Iffland, Cassis, *J. Am. Chem. Soc.* **74**, 6284 (1952); by catalytic hydrogenation of propionitrile: Rylander, Kaplan, US 3117162 (1964 to Englehard). Toxicity study: H. F. Smyth *et al.*, *Am. Ind. Hyg. Assoc. J.* **23**, 95 (1962).
Colorless, alkaline liq; strong ammonia odor. d_{20}^{20} 0.719; mp $-83°$; bp 48-49°; n_D^{20} 1.389. Flash pt, closed cup: 10°F ($-12°C$). Misc with water, alcohol, ether. *Keep tightly closed.* LD_{50} orally in rats: 0.57 g/kg (Smyth).
Hydrochloride. $C_3H_9N·HCl$. Deliquesc crystals, mp 157-158°. Soluble in 0.4 part water, 1.5 parts chloroform. *Keep well closed.*
Caution: Strong irritant, possible skin sensitizer.

7844. n-Propylbenzene. [103-65-1] 1-Phenylpropane. C_9H_{12}; mol wt 120.19. C 89.94%, H 10.06%. $C_6H_5CH_2CH_2CH_3$. Prepd by the action of diethyl sulfate on benzylmagnesium chloride: H. Gilman, W. E. Catlin, *Org. Synth.* **coll. vol. I**, 471 (2nd ed., 1941). Toxicity study: P. M. Jenner *et al.*, *Food Cosmet. Toxicol.* **2**, 327 (1964).
Liquid. d_4^{20} 0.8621. mp $-99.2°$. bp_{760} 159.2°; bp_{400} 135.7°; bp_{200} 113.5°; bp_{100} 94°; bp_{40} 71.6°; bp_{20} 56.8°; bp_{10} 43.4°; bp_5 31.3°; $bp_{1.0}$ 6.3°. n_D^{20} 1.4919. Very slightly sol in water (0.06 g/l); sol in alcohol, ether. LD_{50} orally in rats: 6040 mg/kg (Jenner).
USE: In textile dyeing and printing; as solvent for cellulose acetate.

7845. Propyl Bromide. [106-94-5] 1-Bromopropane. C_3H_7Br; mol wt 122.99. C 29.30%, H 5.74%, Br 64.97%. $CH_3CH_2CH_2Br$. Review of human reproductive risks: *NTP-CERHR Monograph* (NIH Publ. No. 04-4479, 2003) 88 pp.
Colorless liquid. d_{20}^{20} 1.353; mp $-110°$; bp 71°; n_D^{20} 1.4341. Sol in 400 parts water; miscible with alcohol, etc.
USE: Solvent for fats, waxes and resins; intermediate in synthesis of pharmaceuticals, insecticides and other compds; in spray adhesives; degreaser; cleaner for metal and precision electronic components.

7846. Propyl Butyrate. [105-66-8] Butanoic acid propyl ester. $C_7H_{14}O_2$; mol wt 130.18. C 64.58%, H 10.84%, O 24.58%. $CH_3CH_2CH_2COOC_3H_7$.
Colorless liquid. d_4^{15} 0.879; mp $-95°$; bp 143°; n_D^{20} 1.4005. Slightly sol in water; misc with alcohol, ether. LD_{50} orally in rats: 15,000 mg/kg, P. M. Jenner *et al.*, *Food Cosmet. Toxicol.* **2**, 327 (1964).

7847. Propyl Chloride. [540-54-5] 1-Chloropropane. C_3H_7Cl; mol wt 78.54. C 45.88%, H 8.98%, Cl 45.14%. $CH_3CH_2CH_2Cl$. Prepd from propyl alc and PCl_3 in the presence of $ZnCl_2$.
Colorless liquid. d_{20}^{20} 0.890; mp -123 to $-122°$; bp 46-47°; n_D^{20} 1.3886. Sol in ~300 parts water; miscible with alcohol, ether.

7848. Propyl Chlorocarbonate. [109-61-5] Carbonochloridic acid propyl ester; propyl chloroformate. $C_4H_7ClO_2$; mol wt 122.55. C 39.20%, H 5.76%, Cl 28.93%, O 26.11%. C_3H_7-OCOCl.
Colorless liquid. d^{20} 1.090; bp 114-116°. Gradually dec by water or alc; miscible with benzene, chloroform, ether.
Caution: Vapors strongly irritating to eyes and mucous membranes.

7849. Propylene. [115-07-1] 1-Propene; methylethylene; methylethene. C_3H_6; mol wt 42.08. C 85.63%, H 14.37%. H_2-C=CHCH₃. Obtained from petr oils during the refining of gasoline. Catalytic or thermal cracking of hydrocarbons always yields propylene. Can be obtained by catalytic dehydrogenation of propane. Chronic toxicity studies: J. A. Quest *et al.*, *Toxicol. Appl. Pharmacol.* **76**, 288 (1984). *Reviews:* R. F. Goldstein, *The Petroleum Chemicals Industry* (New York-London, 1949) p 114 sqq.; Sherwood, *Ind. Chem.* **1960**, 542-546; *Chim. Ind. (Paris)* **1961**, 576-587; Haney, "Ethylene, Propylene and 1-Butene" in *Vinyl and Diene Monomers*, E. C. Leonard, Ed. (Interscience, New York, 1971) pp 577-689; M. R. Schoenberg *et al.*, in *Kirk-Othmer Encyclopedia of Chemical Technology* vol. **19** (Wiley-Interscience, New York, 3rd ed., 1982) pp 228-246. Review of carcinogenic risk: *IARC Monographs* **60**, 161-180 (1994).
Flammable gas. Burns with yellow sooty flame. d 1.49 (air = 1.0). mp (triple pt) $-185°$. bp_{760} $-48°$. Critical temp 91.8°. Critical pressure 45.6 atm. Heat of fusion 717.6 cal/mol. Liquefies at 7-8 atm. d_4^0 (liq) 0.5139. Flammable limits in air: 2.4-10.3% (by volume). Latent heat of vaporization at bp: 104.62 cal/g. Dipole moment 0.35. n_D^{-40} 1.3567. Surface tension at 90°: 16.70 dynes/cm. Shipped as a liquefied gas in low pressure steel cylinders under its own vapor pressure of ~136 pounds per square inch. Contaminants are propane, ethane, carbon dioxide.
Caution: Gas may act as a simple asphyxiant and mild anesthetic. Direct contact with liquid may cause skin burns. *See Patty's Industrial Hygiene and Toxicology* Vol. **2B**, G. D. Clayton, F. E. Clayton, Eds. (John Wiley & Sons, Inc., New York, 4th ed., 1994) p 1244-1245.
USE: In polymerized form as polypropylene for plastics and carpet fibers. Chemical intermediate in the manuf of acetone, isopropylbenzene, isopropanol, isopropyl halides, propylene oxide, acrylonitrile, cumene.

7850. Propylene Chlorohydrin. [78-89-7] 2-Chloro-1-propanol; 2-chloropropyl alcohol. C_3H_7ClO; mol wt 94.54. C 38.11%, H 7.46%, Cl 37.50%, O 16.92%. $CH_3CHClCH_2OH$.
Colorless liquid; pleasant odor. d^{20} 1.103; bp 133-134°; n_D^{20} 1.4362. Sol in water, alcohol, etc. LD_{50} orally in rats: 0.22 ml/kg; by skin penetration in rabbits: 0.48 ml/kg, Smyth *et al.*, *Am. Ind. Hyg. Assoc. J.* **30**, 470 (1969).
USE: In prepn of propylene oxide, *q.v.*

7851. sec-Propylene Chlorohydrin. [127-00-4] 1-Chloro-2-propanol; 1-chloroisopropyl alcohol. C_3H_7ClO; mol wt 94.54. C 38.11%, H 7.46%, Cl 37.50%, O 16.92%. $ClCH_2CH(OH)CH_3$.
Colorless liquid. d^{20} 1.115; bp 126-127°; n_D^{20} 1.4392. Sol in water, alcohol, etc.

7852. Propylenediamine. [78-90-0] 1,2-Propanediamine. $C_3H_{10}N_2$; mol wt 74.12. C 48.61%, H 13.60%, N 37.79%. CH_3-$CH(NH_2)CH_2NH_2$. Prepd from propylene dibromide and alcoholic ammonia at 100°.
Extremely hygroscopic, strongly alkaline liq. Rapidly absorbs moisture to form a hemihydrate. d^{15} 0.878 in anhyd form. bp 119-120°. Very sol in water. *Keep tightly closed.*
USE: In conjunction with cupric sulfate it is a very sensitive reagent for mercury.

7853. Propylene Dibromide. [78-75-1] 1,2-Dibromopropane. $C_3H_6Br_2$; mol wt 201.89. C 17.85%, H 3.00%, Br 79.16%. $CH_3CHBrCH_2Br$. Prepd from propyl bromide and Br in the presence of $AlCl_3$ or $AlBr_3$.
Colorless liquid. mp $-55°$; bp 140-142°; n_D^{20} 1.5203; d^{20} 1.933. Slightly sol in water; miscible with organic solvents.

7854. Propylene Dichloride. [78-87-5] 1,2-Dichloropropane. $C_3H_6Cl_2$; mol wt 112.99. C 31.89%, H 5.35%, Cl

62.75%. $CH_3CHClCH_2Cl$. Prepd from propyl chloride and Sb_2-Cl_5. Toxicity data: H. F. Smyth *et al., Am. Ind. Hyg. Assoc. J.* **30**, 470 (1969). Review of toxicology and human exposure: *Toxicological Profile for 1,2-Dichloropropane* (PB90-182122, 1989) 131 pp.

Flammable, mobile liq. Odor of chloroform. d_{25}^{25} 1.159; bp 95-96°. Solidifies below $-70°$. n_D^{20} 1.4388. Flash point (ASTM open cup) 21°C (70°F). Despite the low flash pt it does not catch fire readily in industrial applications. Fire pt 38°. Slightly sol in water; miscible with organic solvents. LD_{50} orally in rats: 1.19 ml/kg (Smyth).

Caution: Potential symptoms of overexposure are eye, skin and respiratory system irritation; drowsiness, lightheadedness; liver and kidney damage. Potential occupational carcinogen. *See NIOSH Pocket Guide to Chemical Hazards* (DHHS/NIOSH 97-140, 1997) p 268.

USE: Solvent for oils, fats, resins, waxes, rubber; in ion exchange manuf; in photographic film prodn; paper coating; petroleum catalyst regeneration. Has been used as a soil fumigant.

7855. Propylene Glycol. [57-55-6] 1,2-Propanediol; methyl glycol; 1,2-dihydroxypropane. $C_3H_8O_2$; mol wt 76.09. C 47.35%, H 10.60%, O 42.05%. $CH_3CHOHCH_2OH$. Prepn from glycerol: Raschig, Prahl, *Ber.* **61**, 185 (1928). Prepn of levorotatory propylene glycol from hydroxyacetone by yeast reduction: Levene, Walti, *Org. Synth.* **coll. vol. II**, 545 (1943). Synthesis of S-(+)-form: C. Melchiorre, *Chem. Ind. (London)* **1976**, 218. Manuf from propylene oxide by hydration: *Faith, Keyes & Clark's Industrial Chemicals*, F. A. Lowenheim, M. K. Moran, Eds. (Wiley-Interscience, New York, 4th ed., 1975) pp 688-691. Toxicity data: W. Bartsch *et al., Arzneim.-Forsch.* **26**, 1581 (1976). GC/MS determn in plasma: C. Giachetti *et al., Biomed. Environ. Mass Spectrom.* **18**, 592 (1989). Review of toxicity, metabolism and biochemistry: Ruddick, *Toxicol. Appl. Pharmacol.* **21**, 102 (1972); of toxicology and human exposure: *Toxicological Profile for Ethylene Glycol and Propylene Glycol* (US DHHS, PB98-101109, 1997) 250 pp.

dl-Form. Hygroscopic, viscous liquid. Slightly acrid taste. d_4^{25} 1.036. mp $-59°$. bp_{760} 188.2°; bp_{400} 168.1°; bp_{200} 149.7°; bp_{100} 132.0°; bp_{60} 119.9°; bp_{40} 111.2°; bp_{20} 96.4°; bp_{10} 83.2°; bp_5 70.8°; $bp_{1.0}$ 45.5°. Flash pt, open cup: 210°F (99°C). Miscible with water, acetone, chloroform. Sol in ether. Will dissolve many essential oils, but is immiscible with fixed oils. It is a good solvent for rosin. Under ordinary conditions propylene glycol is stable, but at high temps it tends to oxidize giving rise to products such as propionaldehyde, lactic acid, pyruvic acid and acetic acid. LD_{50} orally in rats: 25 ml/kg (Bartsch).

l-Form. bp_{12} 88-90°, bp_{760} 187-189°. $[\alpha]_D^{20}$ $-15.0°$.

d-Form. bp_{14} 94-96°. $[\alpha]_D^{20}$ +15.84° (neat). d^{25} 1.04.

USE: Nontoxic antifreeze in breweries and dairy establishments. Substitute for ethylene glycol and glycerol. In the manuf of synthetic resins and de-icing solutions. Emulsifier in foods; solvent for food colors and flavors. Pharmaceutic aid (humectant, solvent). As mist to disinfect air; to create artificial smoke and mist for theatrical use.

THERAP CAT (VET): Glucogenic (orally) in ruminants.

7856. Propylene Oxide. [75-56-9] Methyloxirane; propene oxide. C_3H_6O; mol wt 58.08. C 62.04%, H 10.41%, O 27.55%. Results from the action of KOH (aq) on propylene chlorohydrin. Toxicity: H. F. Smyth *et al., J. Ind. Hyg. Toxicol.* **23**, 259 (1941). Toxicological comparison with ethylene oxide, *q.v.*: E. Agurell *et al., Mutat. Res.* **250**, 229 (1991). *Reviews:* Holden in *Glycols*, G. O. Curme, F. Johnston, Eds. (Reinhold, New York, 1952) pp 250-261; *Faith, Keyes & Clark's Industrial Chemicals*, F. A. Lowenheim, M. K. Moran, Eds. (Wiley-Interscience, New York, 4th ed., 1975) pp 692-697; R. O. Kirk, T. J. Dempsey in *Kirk-Othmer Encyclopedia of Chemical Technology* vol. **19** (Wiley-Interscience, New York, 3rd ed., 1982) pp 246-274. Review of manufacturing processes: *Chem. Eng. News* **70**, 9-12 (Mar. 2, 1992); of carcinogenic risk: *IARC Monographs* **60**, 181-213 (1994).

Colorless ethereal liquid. *Extremely flammable.* d_4^0 0.859. mp $-112.13°$. bp 34.23°. Flash pt, closed cup: $-31°F$ ($-35°C$). Soly in water (20°): 40.5% by wt; soly of water in propylene oxide: 12.8% by wt; miscible with alcohol, ether. LD_{50} orally in rats: 1.14 g/kg (Smyth).

Caution: Potential symptoms of overexposure are irritation of eyes, skin and respiratory system; blistering and burns. *See NIOSH Pocket Guide to Chemical Hazards* (DHHS/NIOSH 97-140, 1997) p 270. This substance is reasonably anticipated to be a human carcinogen: *Report on Carcinogens, Eleventh Edition* (PB2005-104914, 2004) p III-226.

USE: Chemical intermediate in prepn of polyethers to form polyurethanes; in prepn of urethane polyols and propylene and dipropylene glycols; in prepn of lubricants, surfactants, oil demulsifiers. As solvent; fumigant; soil sterilant.

7857. Propyl Ether. [111-43-3] 1,1'-Oxybispropane; dipropyl ether. $C_6H_{14}O$; mol wt 102.17. C 70.53%, H 13.81%, O 15.66%. $C_3H_7OC_3H_7$. Obtained by heating propyl alcohol with benzenesulfonic acid.

Mobile liquid. Extremely flammable. d_4^{20} 0.7360; mp $-122°$; bp 89-91°; n_D^{20} 1.3807. Flash pt, open cup: $-5°F$ ($-20°C$). Slightly sol in water; sol in alcohol, ether. Highly volatile. Tends to form explosive peroxides, esp when anhydr. Do not allow to evaporate to near dryness.

7858. Propyl Formate. [110-74-7] Formic acid propyl ester. $C_4H_8O_2$; mol wt 88.11. C 54.53%, H 9.15%, O 36.32%. $HCOOC_3H_7$.

Colorless liquid; pleasant odor. d^{20} 0.901; mp $-93°$; bp 81-82°. Flash pt, closed cup: 27°F ($-3°C$). n_D^{20} 1.3771. Sol in 45 parts water; misc with alcohol, ether. LD_{50} orally in rats: 3980 mg/kg, P. M. Jenner *et al., Food Cosmet. Toxicol.* **2**, 327 (1964).

7859. Propyl Gallate. [121-79-9] 3,4,5-Trihydroxybenzoic acid propyl ester; *n*-propyl gallate; gallic acid propyl ester; PG; Progallin P; Tenox PG. $C_{10}H_{12}O_5$; mol wt 212.20. C 56.60%, H 5.70%, O 37.70%. Spectrophotometric determn: C. S. Sastry *et al., Talanta* **29**, 917 (1982). Effects on survival of *Saccharomyces cerevisiae:* V. L. Eubanks, L. R. Beuchat, *J. Food Prot.* **46**, 29 (1983). Antioxidant effectiveness: M. A. Augustin, S. K. Berry, *J. Am. Oil Chem. Soc.* **60**, 105 (1983). Comprehensive review of biological effects and toxicology: *J. Am. Coll. Toxicol.* **4**, 23-64 (1985).

Crystals, mp 150°. Soly at 25° in water = 0.35 g/100 ml; in alcohol = 103 g/100 g; in ether = 83 g/100 g. Soly in cottonseed oil at 30° = 1.23 g/100 g; in lard at 45° = 1.14 g/100 g. Darkens in the presence of iron and iron salts. Synergic with acids, BHA, BHT. pKa 8.11. Partition coefficient (oleyl alcohol:water) 17. Partition coefficient (octanol:water) 32. pH (0.05% aq soln) 6.3; (0.1% aq soln) 5.9; (0.2% aq soln) 5.7. LD_{50} in mice, rats, hamsters, rabbits (g/kg): 1.70-3.50, 2.1-7, 2.48, 2.75 orally; LD_{50} i.p. in rats: 0.38 g/kg (*J. Am. Coll. Toxicol.*).

USE: Antioxidant for cosmetics, foods, fats, oils, ethers, emulsions, waxes, transformer oils.

7860. Propylhexedrine. [101-40-6] N,α-Dimethylcyclohexaneethanamine; 1-cyclohexyl-2-methylaminopropane; hexahydrodesoxyephedrine; Benzedrex. $C_{10}H_{21}N$; mol wt 155.28. C 77.35%, H 13.63%, N 9.02%. Prepd by catalytic hydrogenation of the phenyl analog using Adams platinum catalyst and glacial acetic acid as the solvent: Zenitz *et al., J. Am. Chem. Soc.* **69**, 1117 (1947); Ullyot, **US 2454746** (1948 to SK & F).

dl-Form. [3595-11-7] Oily liq, d_4^{25} 0.8501, amine odor, bp$_{760}$ 205°; bp$_{20}$ 92-93°; volatilizes slowly at room temp. n_D^{20} 1.4600. Very slightly sol in water. Absorbs carbon dioxide from air and its aq solns are alkaline to litmus. Miscible with alcohol, chloroform, ether.

dl-Form hydrochloride. [6192-95-6] $C_{10}H_{21}N.HCl$. Crystals, dec 127-128°. Sol in water.

d-Form. [6556-29-2] Oily liq, bp$_{10}$ 82-83°; n_D^{20} 1.4588.

d-Form hydrochloride. [6192-96-7] Crystals, dec 138-139°; $[\alpha]_D^{26}$ +14.73°. Sol in water.

l-Form. [6192-97-8] Oily liq, bp$_9$ 80-81°. n_D^{20} 1.4590.

l-Form ethylphenylbarbiturate. [4388-82-3] l-1-Cyclohexyl-2-(methylamino)propane ethylphenylbarbiturate; phenobarbital compd with 1-propylhexedrine; barbexaclone; Maliasin. $C_{22}H_{33}N_3O_3$; mol wt 387.52.

l-Form hydrochloride. [6192-98-9] Crystals, dec 138-139°; $[\alpha]_D^{26}$ −14.74°. Sol in water.

THERAP CAT: Adrenergic (vasoconstrictor); decongestant (nasal).

7861. Propylidene Chloride. [78-99-9] 1,1-Dichloropropane. $C_3H_6Cl_2$; mol wt 112.99. C 31.89%, H 5.35%, Cl 62.75%. $CH_3CH_2CHCl_2$. Obtained by the action of PCl_5 on propionaldehyde. Toxicity data: Smyth *et al., Arch. Ind. Hyg. Occup. Med.* **10**, 61 (1954).

Liquid. d^{10} 1.143; bp 87°. Very slightly sol in water; sol in many organic solvents. LD$_{50}$ orally in rats: 6.5 g/kg (Smyth *et al.*).

7862. Propyl Iodide. [107-08-4] 1-Iodopropane. C_3H_7I; mol wt 169.99. C 21.20%, H 4.15%, I 74.65%. $CH_3CH_2CH_2I$. Prepd by heating propyl alcohol with iodine and red phosphorus.

Colorless or slightly yellow liquid. d_4^{20} 1.747; mp ~−98°; bp 102-103°; n_D^{20} 1.5051. Sol in 575 parts water; miscible with alcohol, ether.

7863. Propyliodone. [587-61-1] 3,5-Diiodo-4-oxo-1(4H)-pyridineacetic acid propyl ester; 3,5-diiodo-4-pyridone-N-acetic acid propyl ester; propyl 3,5-diiodo-4-pyridone-N-acetate; propiodone; Dionosil. $C_{10}H_{11}I_2NO_3$; mol wt 447.01. C 26.87%, H 2.48%, I 56.78%, N 3.13%, O 10.74%. Prepn: Branscombe, **GB 517382** (1940 to I.C.I.). Description: Tomich *et al., Br. J. Pharmacol.* **8**, 166 (1953).

Crystals, dec 186-187°. Slightly sol in saline, serum. Solubility in water at 15°: 0.014 g/100 ml; at 35°: 0.020 g/100 ml; at 95°: 0.020 g/100 ml. LD$_{50}$ i.v. in mice: 300 mg/kg (Tomich).

THERAP CAT: Diagnostic aid (radiopaque medium).

7864. n-Propyl Nitrate. [627-13-4] Nitric acid propyl ester. $C_3H_7NO_3$; mol wt 105.09. C 34.29%, H 6.71%, N 13.33%, O 45.67%. $CH_3CH_2CH_2ONO_2$. Prepd by nitration of propanol with nitric acid, usually in the presence of urea and ammonium nitrate or sulfuric acid: Vogel, *J. Chem. Soc.* **1948**, 1847.

Pale yellow liquid. Sweet, sickly odor. d_4^{20} 1.0538. bp$_{762}$ 110°. *Heating may cause it to explode.* n_D^{20} 1.3979. Dipole moment: 2.98. Azeotrope with water contg 75% $C_3H_7NO_3$, bp$_{760}$ 84.8°. Very slightly sol in water. Sol in alcohol, ether. Physical data concerning combustion and propulsion: Penner, Ducarme, *The Chemistry of Propellants* (Pergamon Press, 1960).

Caution: Potential symptoms of overexposure in exptl animals are irritation of eyes and skin; methemoglobinemia, anoxia, cyanosis; dyspnea, weakness, dizziness, headache. *See NIOSH Pocket Guide to Chemical Hazards* (DHHS/NIOSH 97-140, 1997) p 270.

USE: Fuel ignition promoter, in rocket fuel formulations, as organic intermediate.

7865. n-Propyl Nitrite. [543-67-9] Nitrous acid n-propyl ester. $C_3H_7NO_2$; mol wt 89.09. C 40.44%, H 7.92%, N 15.72%, O 35.92%. $CH_3CH_2CH_2ONO$. Prepd from silver nitrite and n-propyl bromide: Reynolds, Adkins, *J. Am. Chem. Soc.* **51**, 279 (1929);

from n-propanol, sodium nitrite, and dil sulfuric acid: Cowley, Partington, *J. Chem. Soc.* **1933**, 1252.

Liquid. d_4^{20} 0.8864. bp$_{760}$ 46-48°. n_D^{20} 1.3592; also reported as n_D^{20} 1.3613. Soluble in alcohol, ether.

Caution: Inhalation causes vasodilation, smooth muscle relaxation, hypotension.

USE: Jet propellant.

7866. Propylparaben. [94-13-3] 4-Hydroxybenzoic acid propyl ester; propyl p-hydroxybenzoate; Nipasol M; Solbrol P; Propyl Parasept. $C_{10}H_{12}O_3$; mol wt 180.20. C 66.65%, H 6.71%, O 26.64%. Prepn: Stohmann, *J. Prakt. Chem.* **36**, 368 (1887); L. Nobli, *Giorn. Farm. Chim.* **84**, 168 (1935), *C.A.* **30**, 3423^9 (1936). Review of safety assessment: M. G. Soni *et al., Food Chem. Toxicol.* **39**, 513-532 (2002).

White crystals, mp 96-97°. Sol in 2000 parts water; freely sol in alcohol, ether; slightly sol in boiling water.

USE: Pharmaceutic aid (antifungal). Antimicrobial preservative in foods and cosmetics.

7867. Propyl Propionate. [106-36-5] Propanoic acid propyl ester. $C_6H_{12}O_2$; mol wt 116.16. C 62.04%, H 10.41%, O 27.55%. $CH_3CH_2COOC_3H_7$.

Liquid. d^{20} 0.883; mp −76°; bp 122-124°; n_D^{20} 1.3935. Sol in 200 parts water; miscible with alcohol, ether.

7868. Propyl Sulfide. [111-47-7] 1,1'-Thiobispropane; dipropyl sulfide. $C_6H_{14}S$; mol wt 118.24. C 60.95%, H 11.93%, S 27.12%. $C_3H_7SC_3H_7$. Prepd from propyl bromide and an alcoholic soln of Na_2S.

Colorless liquid. d^{17} 0.814; mp ~−102°; bp 142°. Insol in water; sol in alcohol, ether.

7869. Propylthiouracil. [51-52-5] 2,3-Dihydro-6-propyl-2-thioxo-4(1H)pyrimidinone; 6-propyl-2-thiouracil; 2-thio-4-oxo-6-propyl-1,3-pyrimidine; 2-thio-6-propyl-1,3-pyrimidin-4-one; Propacil; Propycil; Propyl-Thyracil; Thyreostat II. $C_7H_{10}N_2OS$; mol wt 170.23. C 49.39%, H 5.92%, N 16.46%, O 9.40%, S 18.84%. Prepd by the condensation of ethyl β-oxocaproate with thiourea: Anderson *et al., J. Am. Chem. Soc.* **67**, 2197 (1945). Comprehensive description: H. Y. Aboul-Enein, *Anal. Profiles Drug Subs.* **6**, 457-486 (1977). Review of pharmacology and clinical experience: D. S. Cooper *et al., N. Engl. J. Med.* **311**, 1353-1362 (1984).

White, bitter cryst powder of starch-like appearance to the eye and to the touch, mp 219-221°. uv max (methanol): 275, 214 nm (ε 15800, 15600); (methanolic KOH): 315.5, 260, 207.5 nm (ε 10900, 10700, 15400). One part dissolves in ~900 parts water at 20°, in 100 parts boiling water, in 60 parts ethyl alcohol, in 60 parts acetone. Practically insol in ether, chloroform, benzene. Freely sol in aq solns of ammonia and alkali hydroxides. A satd aq soln is neutral or slightly acid to litmus.

Caution: This substance is reasonably anticipated to be a human carcinogen: *Report on Carcinogens, Eleventh Edition* (PB2005-104914, 2004) p III-227.

THERAP CAT: Antihyperthyroid.

THERAP CAT (VET): Antihyperthyroid. Has been used to promote fattening.

7870. Propylure. [10297-61-7] (E)-10-Propyl-5,9-tridecadien-1-ol acetate; trans-1-acetoxy-10-(n-propyl)trideca-5,9-diene; 10-propyl-trans-5,9-tridecadienyl acetate. $C_{18}H_{32}O_2$; mol wt 280.45. C 77.09%, H 11.50%, O 11.41%. Once thought to be the sex pheromone of the pink bollworm moth, *Pectinophora gossypiella* (Saunders), a destructive cotton pest: H. E. Hummel *et al., Science* **181,** 873 (1973), cf. Gossyplure. Reported as the first known natural product possessing di-*n*-propyl branching. Isoln, structure, and synthesis: Jones *et al., Science* **152,** 1516 (1966). Improved total syntheses: Pattenden, *J. Chem. Soc. C* **1968,** 2385; Meyers, Collington, *Tetrahedron* **27,** 5979 (1971); Vig *et al., J. Indian Chem. Soc.* **50,** 39 (1973); K. Utimoto *et al., Tetrahedron Lett.* **1975,** 4233. Photochemical synthesis: Kossanyi *et al., ibid.* **1973,** 3459. Stereoselective synthesis: A. Alexakis *et al., ibid.* **1978,** 2027. *trans*-Propylure is rendered inactive by the presence of >15% of the *cis*-isomer: Jacobson, *Science* **163,** 190 (1969).

Colorless liquid having no detectable odor. bp$_{0.1}$ 135°. n_D^{25} 1.4635. Strong IR band at 970 cm^{-1}.

USE: Insect attractant.

7871. Propyphenazone. [479-92-5] 1,2-Dihydro-1,5-dimethyl-4-(1-methylethyl)-2-phenyl-3*H*-pyrazol-3-one; 4-isopropylantipyrine; 4-isopropyl-2,3-dimethyl-1-phenyl-3-pyrazolin-5-one; 2,3-dimethyl-1-phenyl-4-isopropylpyrazolone; isopropylphenazone; Budirol; Causyth; Eufibron; Isoprochin P. C$_{14}$H$_{18}$N$_2$O; mol wt 230.31. C 73.01%, H 7.88%, N 12.16%, O 6.95%. Prepn: Stenz, US 1972036 (1934 to Hoffmann-La Roche); Sawa, *J. Pharm. Soc. Jpn.* **57,** 953 (1937), *C.A.* **32,** 2533 (1938).

Slightly bitter crystals, mp 103°. Readily sol in alcohol, ether. Soly in water: 0.24 g/100 ml at 16.5°.

THERAP CAT: Analgesic; antipyretic; anti-inflammatory.

7872. Propyzamide. [23950-58-5] 3,5-Dichloro-*N*-(1,1-dimethyl-2-propynyl)benzamide; pronamid; RH-315; Kerb. C$_{12}$H$_{11}$-Cl$_2$NO; mol wt 256.13. C 56.27%, H 4.33%, Cl 27.68%, N 5.47%, O 6.25%. Selective pre-emergence herbicide. Prepn: B. W. Horrom *et al.,* ZA 6800090; *eidem,* US 3534098; US 3640699 (1969, 1970, 1972 all to Rohm & Haas). Activity: K. L. Viste *et al., Science* **167,** 280 (1970); C. Swithenbank *et al., J. Agric. Food Chem.* **19,** 417 (1971). Metabolism: R. Y. Yih *et al., Weed Sci.* **18,** 604 (1970); R. Y. Yih, C. Swithenbank, *J. Agric. Food Chem.* **19,** 314, 320 (1971); J. D. Fisher, *ibid.* **22,** 606 (1974). Carcinogenicity study: M. D. Reuber, *Environ. Res.* **23,** 1 (1980).

White solid, mp 155-156°. Soly in water at 25°: 15 ppm. Sol in aliphatic, aromatic solvents. Vapor pressure at 25°: 8.5 × 10^{-5} mm Hg. LD$_{50}$ in male, female rats (mg/kg): 8350, 5620 orally (Viste).

USE: Herbicide.

7873. Proquazone. [22760-18-5] 7-Methyl-1-(1-methylethyl)-4-phenyl-2(1*H*)-quinazolinone; 1-isopropyl-7-methyl-4-

phenyl-2(1*H*)-quinazolinone; RU-43-715; Sandoz 43-715; Biarison. C$_{18}$H$_{18}$N$_2$O; mol wt 278.35. C 77.67%, H 6.52%, N 10.06%, O 5.75%. Prepn: H. Ott, M. Denzer, DE 1805501 corresp to US 3845128 and US 3925548 (1969, 1974 and 1975, all to Sandoz); R. V. Coombs *et al., J. Med. Chem.* **16,** 1237 (1973). Metabolism: M. B. Zucker, *Proc. Soc. Exp. Biol. Med.* **156,** 209 (1977); H. Ott, J. Meier, *Scand. J. Rheumatol. Suppl.* **21,** 12 (1978). Pharmacology: H. U. Gubler, M. Baggiolini, *ibid.* 8; H. Ott, *ibid.* 5. Clinical studies: P. Sfikakis, P. Tsachalos, *Ther. Umsch.* **34,** 730 (1977); series of articles in *Scand. J. Rheumatol. Suppl.* **21,** 15-39 (1978). Review of pharmacodynamics, pharmacokinetics and therapeutic efficacy: S. P. Clissold, R. Beresford, *Drugs* **33,** 478-502 (1987).

Yellow crystals from ethyl acetate, mp 137-138°. Sol in chloroform. Insol in water.

THERAP CAT: Anti-inflammatory.

7874. Proscillaridin. [466-06-8] (3β)-3-[(6-Deoxy-α-L-mannopyranosyl)oxy]-14-hydroxybufa-4,20,22-trienolide; 14-hydroxy-3β-(rhamnosyloxy)bufa-4,20,22-trienolide; 3β-rhamnosido-14β-hydroxy-Δ^{4,20,22}-bufatrienolide; proscillaridin A; desglucotransvaaline; scillarenin 3β-rhamnoside; Caradrin; Proscillan; Purosin-TC; Stellarid; Talusin. C$_{30}$H$_{42}$O$_8$; mol wt 530.65. C 67.90%, H 7.98%, O 24.12%. Prepn by acid cleavage of scillaren A: Stoll *et al., Helv. Chim. Acta* **16,** 703 (1933); by enzymic decompn of glucoscillaren A with strophanthobiase: Stoll *et al., ibid.* **35,** 2495 (1952); from *Urginea burkei* Baker, *Liliaceae:* Zoller, Tamm, *ibid.* **36,** 1744 (1953); from *U. (Scilla) maritima* (L.) Baker, *Liliaceae:* Görlich, *Arzneim.-Forsch.* **10,** 770 (1960). Structure: Stoll *et al., Helv. Chim. Acta* **35,** 1934 (1952). Pharmacology: Lenke, Brock, *Arzneim.-Forsch.* **20,** 1 (1970). Metabolic studies: Davis *et al., Arch. Int. Pharmacodyn.* **177,** 231 (1969); Nakano *et al., ibid.* **183,** 199 (1970). Clinical studies: Several authors, *Minerva Med.* **58,** 4243-4322 (1967). Toxicity study: E. I. Goldenthal, *Toxicol. Appl. Pharmacol.* **18,** 185 (1971). Series of articles on prepn, pharmacology, toxicology, pharmacokinetics, metabolism of 4′-methyl ether: *Arzneim.-Forsch.* **28,** 493-573 (1978).

Prisms from methanol, mp 219-222°. [α]$_D^{20}$ −91.5° (CH$_3$OH). LD$_{50}$ in male, female rats (mg/kg): 56, 76 orally (Goldenthal).

Proscillaridin-4-methyl ether. [33396-37-1] Meproscillarin; Clift. C$_{31}$H$_{44}$O$_8$; mol wt 544.68. mp 213-217°. [α]$_D^{20}$ −94° (CH$_3$OH). uv max (CH$_3$OH): 297 nm (log ε 3.79), (1*N* KOH/CH$_3$-OH): 355 nm (log ε 4.65). Sol in methanol, ethanol, THF, dioxane;

slightly sol in $CHCl_3$, CH_2Cl_2, acetone. Practically insol in water, nonpolar organics.

THERAP CAT: Cardiotonic.

7875. Prostacyclin. [35121-78-9] (5*Z*,9*α*,11*α*,13*E*,15*S*)-6,9-Epoxy-11,15-dihydroxyprosta-5,13-dien-1-oic acid; (5*Z*)-9-deoxy-6,9*α*-epoxy-Δ⁵-PGF$_{1α}$; epoprostenol; prostaglandin I₂; prostaglandin X; PGI₂; PGX; U-53217. $C_{20}H_{32}O_5$; mol wt 352.47. C 68.15%, H 9.15%, O 22.70%. A prostaglandin produced by enzymatic transformation of prostaglandin endoperoxides (**PGG₂, PGH₂**), which dilates blood vessels and is approximately 30 times more potent than prostaglandin E₁, *q.v.*, in inhibiting platelet aggregation. Evidence for its occurrence during biosynthetic conversion of arachidonic acid by rat stomach homogenates: C. Pace-Asciak, L. S. Wolfe, *Biochemistry* **10**, 3657 (1971). Isoln from microsomes of pig and rabbit aorta by J. R. Vane and co-workers: S. Moncada *et al., Nature* **263**, 663 (1976). Prepn: S. Moncada, N. Whittaker, **DE 2720999**; S. Moncada, **US 4539333** (1977, 1985 both to Wellcome Found.). PGI₂ is also synthesized in bovine coronary arteries as well as human arteries and veins: *eidem, Lancet* **1**, 18 (1977); G. J. Dusting *et al., Prostaglandins* **13**, 3 (1977); by cultured human and bovine endothelial cells: B. B. Weksler *et al., Proc. Natl. Acad. Sci. USA* **74**, 3922 (1977); by pig aortic endothelial cells: D. E. Mac-Intyre *et al., Nature* **271**, 549 (1978). It has been suggested that endoperoxides released by platelets can be converted to PGI₂ by vascular tissue and that a balance between formation of PGI₂ and release of thromboxane A₂, *q.v.*, which induces platelet aggregation, controls the formation of thrombi in blood vessels. It has also been postulated that PGI₂ acts to stimulate platelet adenylate cyclase and to prevent the action of thrombi on phospholipid breakdown as well as platelet aggregation. Structure: R. A. Johnson *et al., Prostaglandins* **12**, 915 (1976). Synthesis: E. J. Corey *et al., J. Am. Chem. Soc.* **99**, 3006 (1977); of sodium salt and stereochemistry: R. A. Johnson *et al., ibid.* 4182. Additional syntheses: I. Tomoskozi *et al., Tetrahedron Lett.* **1977**, 2627; N. Whittaker, *ibid.* 2805; K. Nicolaou, *Chem. Commun.* **1977**, 630. Synthesis of the 5*E*-isomer: E. J. Corey *et al., Tetrahedron Lett.* **1977**, 3529. Chemical stability in aq solns: M. J. Cho, M. A. Allen, *Prostaglandins* **15**, 943 (1978). Biosynthetic study: V. Tomasi *et al., Nature* **273**, 670 (1978). Biological properties: R. J. Gryglewski *et al., Prostaglandins* **12**, 685 (1976). Preliminary clinical study: A. E. S. Gimson *et al., Lancet* **1**, 173 (1980). Antimetastatic effects: K. V. Honn *et al., Science* **212**, 1270 (1981); *eidem, ibid.* **217** 542 (1982). Preliminary study of effect of PGX infusion in patients with acute myocardial infarction: O. Edhag *et al., N. Engl. J. Med.* **308**, 1032 (1983). Review of biological properties: S. Moncada, J. R. Vane, *Clin. Sci.* **61**, 369-372 (1981); of therapeutic potential: *eidem, Pharmacol. Ther.* **4**, 215-233 (1982); of physiological role: J. R. Vane *et al., Int. Rev. Exp. Pathol.* **23**, 161-207 (1982). General reviews: S. Moncada, J. R. Vane, *Fed. Proc.* **38**, 66-71 (1979); J. C. McGiff, *Annu. Rev. Pharmacol.* **21**, 479-509 (1981); S. Moncada *et al., Adv. Pharmacol. Ther.* **6**, 39-47 (1982). Books: *Prostacyclin*, J. R. Vane, S. Bergstrom, Eds. (Raven Press, New York, 1979) 453 pp; *Prostaglandins in Cardiovascular and Renal Function*, A. Scriabine *et al.*, Eds. (Spectrum Publications, New York, 1980) 498 pp.

Chemically unstable in aq soln. Hydrolyzes to 6-oxo-PGF$_{1α}$. Half-life at 4° is approx 14.5 min when total phosphate is 0.165 *M*. Anti-aggregating activity disappears within 0.25 min on boiling or within 10 min at 37°.

Sodium salt. [61849-14-7] U-53217A; Flolan. $C_{20}H_{31}NaO_5$; mol wt 374.45. Hygroscopic, free-flowing white powder. Stable for 2 months if kept dry at −30°.

THERAP CAT: Platelet aggregation inhibitor.

7876. Prostaglandin E₁. [745-65-3] (11*α*,13*E*,15*S*)-11,15-Dihydroxy-9-oxoprost-13-en-1-oic acid; 3-hydroxy-2-(3-hydroxy-1-octenyl)-5-oxocyclopentaneheptanoic acid; alprostadil; PGE₁; U-10136; Caverject; Edex; Liple; Liprostin; Minprog; Muse; Palux; Prostandin; Prostin VR; Prostivas. $C_{20}H_{34}O_5$; mol wt 354.48. C 67.77%, H 9.67%, O 22.57%. A primary prostaglandin; easily crystallized from purified biological extracts. Isoln from sheep seminal vesicle tissue, and structure: Bergstrom *et al., Acta Chem. Scand.* **16**, 501 (1962); *eidem, J. Biol. Chem.* **238**, 3555 (1963). Enzymic conversion from 8,11,14-eicosatrienoic acid: Nugteren *et al., Rec. Trav. Chim.* **85**, 405 (1966). Synthesis of the *dl*-form: Corey *et al., J. Am. Chem. Soc.* **90**, 3245, 3247 (1968); Schneider *et al., ibid.* 5895; **91**, 5372 (1969); Axen *et al., Chem. Commun.* **1969**, 303; Taub *et al., ibid.* **1970**, 1258; Slates *et al., ibid.* **1972**, 304; Kuo *et al., Tetrahedron Lett.* **1972**, 5317; Taub *et al., Tetrahedron* **29**, 1447 (1973); Miyano, Stealey, *Chem. Commun.* **1973**, 180; Finch *et al., J. Org. Chem.* **38**, 4412 (1973). Synthesis of natural form: Corey *et al., J. Am. Chem. Soc.* **91**, 535 (1969); **92**, 2586 (1970); Sih *et al., ibid.* **94**, 3643 (1972); **95**, 1676 (1973); Schaaf, Corey, *J. Org. Chem.* **37**, 2921 (1974); Slates *et al., Tetrahedron* **30**, 819 (1974). Metabolism in guinea pigs: Anggard, Samuelsson, *J. Biol. Chem.* **239**, 4097 (1964). Metabolism in humans: Hamberg, Samuelsson, *ibid.* **246**, 6713 (1971). Review of biological activities: Berti *et al., Prog. Biochem. Pharmacol.* **3**, 110 (1967). Comparative pharmacology with respect to other prostaglandins: Weeks, *Annu. Rev. Pharmacol.* **12**, 317 (1972). Clinical use in neonates with cyanotic congenital heart disease: P. M. Olley *et al., Adv. Prostaglandin Thromboxane Res.* **7**, 913 (1980). Use in non-atherosclerotic vasculopathy: D. L. Wooster *et al., J. Am. Med. Assoc.* **245**, 1846 (1981). Clinical trials in impotence: O. I. Linet, F. G. Ogrinc, *N. Engl. J. Med.* **334**, 873 (1996); H. Padma-Nathan *et al., ibid.* **336**, 1 (1997).

Crystals from ethyl acetate + heptane, mp 115-116°. [*α*]$_{578}$ −61.6° (c = 0.56 in tetrahydrofuran). Soly at 35°: 8000 *μ*g/100 ml double distilled water. Easily dehydrated in soln at pHs <4 or >8.

THERAP CAT: Vasodilator (peripheral). In treatment of male erectile dysfunction.

7877. Prostaglandin E₂. [363-24-6] (5*Z*,11*α*,13*E*,15*S*)-11,15-Dihydroxy-9-oxoprosta-5,13-dien-1-oic acid; 7-[3-hydroxy-2-(3-hydroxy-1-octenyl)-5-oxocyclopentyl]-5-heptenoic acid; dinoprostone; PGE₂; U-12062; Minprostin E₂; Prepidil; Propess; Prostin E₂. $C_{20}H_{32}O_5$; mol wt 352.47. C 68.15%, H 9.15%, O 22.70%. The most common and most biologically potent of mammalian prostaglandins. Isoln from sheep prostate: S. Bergström, J. Sjövall, **GB 851827**; *eidem*, **US 3598858** (1960, 1971); from sheep seminal vesicle tissue: S. Bergström *et al., Acta Chem. Scand.* **16**, 501 (1962). Total synthesis of the *dl*-form: W. P. Schneider, *Chem. Commun.* **1969**, 304; E. J. Corey *et al., J. Am. Chem. Soc.* **91**, 5675 (1969); E. J. Corey *et al., Tetrahedron Lett.* **1970**, 307; W. P. Schneider, **DE 2011969** (1970 to Upjohn), *C.A.* **74**, 87486n (1971); J. Fried *et al., J. Am. Chem. Soc.* **94**, 4342 (1972). Synthesis of naturally occurring form: E. J. Corey *et al., ibid.* **92**, 397, 2586 (1970); J. B. Heather *et al., Tetrahedron Lett.* **1973**, 2313; from *Plexaura homomalla* prostaglandin intermediates: G. L. Bundy *et al., J. Am. Chem. Soc.* **94**, 2123 (1972); W. P. Schneider *et al., Chem. Commun.* **1973**, 254. Biosynthesis: D. A. Van Dorp *et al., Biochim. Biophys. Acta* **90**, 204 (1964); S. Bergström *et al., ibid.* 207; **NL 6505799** (1965 to Unilever), *C.A.* **65**, 7584h (1966). Metabolism: E. Anggard, B. Samuelsson, *Mem. Soc. Endocrinol.*, no. 14, 107 (1966); M. Hamberg, B. Samuelsson, *J. Biol. Chem.* **246**, 6713 (1971). Several reviews in *Prostaglandin Symp. Worcester Found. Exp. Biol.*, P. Ramwell, Ed. (Interscience, New York, 1968). For general refs *see* Prostaglandins.

Prostaglandin $F_{2\alpha}$

Natural form, colorless crystals. mp 66-68°. $[\alpha]_D^{26}$ −61° (c = 1 in tetrahydrofuran). Easily dehydrated in soln at pHs <4 or >8.

THERAP CAT: Oxytocic; abortifacient.

7878. Prostaglandin $F_{2\alpha}$. [551-11-1] (5Z,9α,11α,13E,15S)-9,11,15-Trihydroxyprosta-5,13-dien-1-oic acid; 7-[3,5-dihydroxy-2-(3-hydroxy-1-octenyl)cyclopentyl]-5-heptenoic acid; dinoprost; $PGF_{2\alpha}$; U-14583; Enzaprost F; Prostarmon F. $C_{20}H_{34}O_5$; mol wt 354.48. C 67.77%, H 9.67%, O 22.57%. One of the most biologically studied of the primary prostaglandins. Closely related to prostaglandin E_2 (PGE_2) in that both prostaglandins are biosynthesized from the same precursors and that $PGF_{2\alpha}$ is the synthetic reduction product of PGE_2. For refs to synthesis of dl and natural forms see Prostaglandin E_2. Prepn of the tromethamine salt: W. Morozowich, **DE 2126127**; *idem*, **US 3657327** (1971, 1972 both to Upjohn). Alternate synthesis of natural $PGF_{2\alpha}$: Schneider, Murray, *J. Org. Chem.* **38**, 397 (1973); R. B. Woodward *et al., J. Am. Chem. Soc.* **95**, 6853 (1973); G. Stork *et al., ibid.* **100**, 8272 (1978); K. Kondo *et al., Tetrahedron Lett.* **1978**, 3927; N. R. A. Beeley *et al., Tetrahedron* **37**, Suppl. 9, 411 (1981); R. J. Cave *et al., J. Chem. Soc. Perkin Trans. 1* **1981**, 646. Causes vasocontraction and exhibits luteolytic activity; is most commonly associated with its role in pregnancy: Karim *et al., J. Obstet. Gynaecol. Brit. Commonw.* **78**, 172 (1971). Metabolism in female subjects: Granstrom, Samuelsson, *J. Biol. Chem.* **246**, 5254 (1971). Toxicity data: T. Fujita *et al., Iyakuhin Kenkyu* **9**, 261 (1978), *C.A.* **89**, 71399k (1978). For general refs see Prostaglandins.

Natural form, crystals, mp 25-35°. $[\alpha]_D^{25}$ +23.5° (c = 1 in tetrahydrofuran). Freely sol in methanol, abs ethanol, ethyl acetate, chloroform; slightly sol in water. Stable for two years in light resistant containers at 5-15°. Degrades in one week when exposed to sunlight or in three months at 40°. LD_{50} in rabbits (mg/kg): 2.5-5.0 i.v.; 2.5-5.0 i.m. (Fujita).

Tromethamine salt. [38562-01-5] In-Synch; Lutalyse. $C_{20}H_{34}O_5 \cdot C_4H_{11}NO_3$; mol wt 475.62. White or off-white cystalline powder, mp 100-101°. Readily sol in water to at least 200 mg/ml.

THERAP CAT: Oxytocic; abortifacient.

THERAP CAT (VET): Oxytocic.

7879. Prostaglandin(s). A family of biologically potent lipid acids first discovered in seminal fluid and extracts of accessory genital glands of man and sheep: von Euler, *Arch. Exp. Pathol. Pharmakol.* **175**, 78 (1934); *Klin. Wochenschr.* **14**, 1182 (1935). Isoln: Bergstrom, Sjovall, **US 3069322** and **US 3598858** (1962, 1971); Samuelsson, *J. Biol. Chem.* **238**, 3229 (1963). Also found in lower concns in other organs: *idem, Biochim. Biophys. Acta* **84**, 707 (1964). The single non-mammalian source of prostaglandin intermediates, or *syntons*, is the gorgonian sea whip or sea fan, *Plexaura homomalla:* Weinheimer, Spraggins, *Tetrahedron Lett.* **1969**, 5185; Schneider *et al., J. Am. Chem. Soc.* **94**, 2122 (1972). Prostaglandins are named as derivatives of ***prostanoic acid***. Prostaglandins are divided into the types E, F, A, B, C, and D based on functions in the cyclopentane ring. Numerical subscripts refer to the number of unsaturations in the side chains; α or β subscripts refer to the configuration of substituents in the ring. Six naturally occurring prostaglandins, E_1, E_2, E_3, $F_{1\alpha}$, $F_{2\alpha}$, $F_{3\alpha}$, are considered primary in that no one is derived from another in the living organism. First structural and stereochemical elucidations: Bergstrom *et al., Acta Chem. Scand.* **16**, 501 (1962); *eidem, J. Biol. Chem.* **238**, 3555

(1963). Absolute config: Nugteren *et al., Nature* **212**, 38 (1966). First total synthesis of racemic PGE_1 and $PGF_{1\alpha}$: Corey *et al., J. Am. Chem. Soc.* **90**, 3245 (1968). Review of synthetic studies: Pike, *Fortschr. Chem. Org. Naturst.* **28**, 313 (1970); Axen *et al.*, in *The Total Synthesis of Natural Products* vol. 1, J. ApSimon, Ed. (Wiley-Interscience, New York, 1973) pp 81-143; Clarkson in *Progress in Organic Chemistry* vol. 8, W. Carruthers, J. K. Sutherland, Eds. (Wiley, New York, 1973) pp 1-28. Book: J. S. Bindra, R. Bindra, *Prostaglandin Synthesis* (Academic Press, New York, 1977). Biosynthesis occurs by enzymatic conversion of unsaturated twenty-carbon fatty acids. Review of biosynthetic studies: Samuelsson, *Prog. Biochem. Pharmacol.* **5**, 109 (1969). Review of metabolism: Samuelsson *et al., Ann. N.Y. Acad. Sci.* **180**, 138 (1971). Biological activities include stimulation of smooth muscle, dilation of small arteries, bronchial dilation, lowering of blood pressure, inhibition of gastric secretion, of lipolysis, and of platelet aggregation, induction of labor, abortion, and menstruation, and increase in ocular pressure. Implicated also in dysmenorrhea, inflammatory reactions, nasal vasoconstriction, kidney function, and in autonomic neurotransmission. Reviews of pharmacological and biochemical aspects: Horton, *Experientia* **21**, 113 (1965); Weeks, *Annu. Rev. Pharmacol.* **12**, 317 (1972); Hinman, *Annu. Rev. Biochem.* **41**, 161 (1972). Review of biological activities of synthetic prostaglandins: Ramwell *et al., Nature* **221**, 1251 (1969). Review of analytical and preparative techniques: "Prostaglandins and Arachidonate Metabolites" in *Methods Enzymol.* **86**, 705, (1982). General reviews: Bergstrom, *Science* **157**, 382 (1967); Bergstrom *et al., Pharmacol. Rev.* **20**, 1 (1968); Ramwell, Shaw, *Recent Prog. Horm. Res.* **26**, 139 (1970); Pike, *Sci. Am.* **225**, 84 (Nov., 1971); Bindra, Bindra, *Progress in Drug Research* vol. 17 (Birkhäuser Verlag, Basel, 1973) pp 410-487. Books: *The Prostaglandins* vols. 1, 2, P. Ramwell, Ed. (Plenum Press, New York, 1973, 1974); *Prostaglandins in Cardiovascular and Renal Function*, A. Scriabine *et al.*, Eds. (Spectrum Publications, New York, 1980) 498 pp; *Cardiovascular Pharmacology of the Prostaglandins*, A. Herman, Ed. (Raven Press, New York, 1982) 472 pp.

Prostanoic acid

7880. Prostalene. [54120-61-5] (9α,11α,13E,15R)-(±)-9,11,15-Trihydroxy-15-methylprosta-4,5,13-trien-1-oic acid methyl ester; (±)-methyl-7-[3,5-dihydroxy-2-[(E)-3-hydroxy-3-methyl-1-octenyl]cyclopentyl]-4,5-heptadienoate; RS-9390; Synchrocept. $C_{22}H_{36}O_5$; mol wt 380.52. C 69.44%, H 9.54%, O 21.02%. Synthetic analog of prostaglandin $F_{2\alpha}$, *q.v.* Prepn: P. Crabbé, J. H. Fried, **DE 2258668** corresp to **US 3879438** (1973, 1975 both to Syntex). Use in induction of parturition in sows: W. Holtz *et al., J. Anim. Sci.* **49**, 367 (1979). Pharmacodynamics in mares: R. G. Loy *et al., J. Reprod. Fertil. Suppl.* **27**, 229 (1979).

THERAP CAT (VET): Luteolytic.

7881. Prosulfuron. [94125-34-5] *N*-[[(4-Methoxy-6-methyl-1,3,5-triazin-2-yl)amino]carbonyl]-2-(3,3,3-trifluoropropyl)-benzenesulfonamide; 1-(4-methoxy-6-methyl-1,3,5-triazin-2-yl)-3-[2-(3,3,3-trifluoropropyl)phenylsulfonyl]urea; 1-[2-(3,3,3-trifluoropropyl)phenylsulfonyl]-3-(4-methoxy-6-methyl-1,3,5-triazin-2-yl)-urea; CGA-152005; Peak. $C_{15}H_{16}F_3N_5O_4S$; mol wt 419.38. C 42.96%, H 3.85%, F 13.59%, N 16.70%, O 15.26%, S 7.65%. Post-emergence sulfonylurea herbicide for use in maize; acetolactate synthase inhibitor. Prepn: W. Meyer, K. Oertle, **EP 120814**; *idem*, **US 4671819** (1984, 1987 both to Ciba-Geigy); J. G. Dingwall,

Consult the Name Index before using this section.

Pestic. Sci. **41,** 259 (1994). Comprehensive description: M. Schulte *et al., Brighton Crop Prot. Conf. - Weeds* **1993,** 53-59.

Colorless, odorless crystals, mp 155° (dec). Vapor pressure (25°): <3.5 × 10⁻⁶ Pa. Soly in water (25°): 4000 mg/l (pH 6.8). Log P (*n*-octanol/water): −0.21 (pH 6.9). LD_{50} orally in rats: 986 mg/kg; dermally in rabbits: >2000 mg/kg. LC_{50} (4 hr) by inhalation in rats: >5000 mg/m³ (Schulte).

USE: Herbicide.

7882. Prosultiamine. [59-58-5] *N*-[(4-Amino-2-methyl-5-pyrimidinyl)methyl]-*N*-[4-hydroxy-1-methyl-2-(propyldithio)-1-butenyl]formamide; 2-(2-methyl-4-aminopyrimidin-5-yl)methyl-formamido-5-hydroxy-2-penten-3-yl propyl disulfide; vitamin B₁ propyl disulfide; thiamine propyl disulfide; dithiopropylthiamine; DTPT; TPD; Alinamin; Binova. $C_{15}H_{24}N_4O_2S_2$; mol wt 356.51. C 50.53%, H 6.79%, N 15.72%, O 8.98%, S 17.99%. Synthesis: Matsukawa, Kawasuki, *J. Pharm. Soc. Jpn.* **73,** 216 (1953), *C.A.* **48,** 2071 (1954); Matsukawa *et al., J. Vitaminol.* **1,** 13 (1954); Fujiwara *et al., US 2833768* (1958 to Takeda), *cf. FR 1068459* (1954 to Takeda). Structural studies: Nishikawa *et al., Chem. Pharm. Bull.* **17,** 932 (1969). Metabolism: Suzuoki-Ziro *et al., J. Biochem.* **58,** 279 (1965); Nishikawa *et al., J. Pharmacol. Exp. Ther.* **157,** 589 (1967).

E-form

Prisms from benzene, dec 128-129°. Sparingly soluble in water. Sol in organic solvents and lipids. Better absorbed upon oral ingestion by man, than thiamine hydrochloride.

Hydrochloride. [973-99-9] $C_{15}H_{24}N_4O_2S_2$·HCl. Crystals, dec 160-161°.

THERAP CAT: Vitamin (enzyme co-factor).

7883. Protactinium. [7440-13-3] Protoactinium. Pa; at. no. 91; at. wt 231.03588 (characteristic naturally occurring isotopic mixture); valences 3, 4, 5. No stable nuclides; known isotopes (mass numbers): 216, 222-238; naturally occurring isotopes: 231, 234m, 234. First isotope discovered, ²³⁴ᵐPa (T₁ 1.17 minutes); called *brevium*, *uranium X₂* or *UX₂*, natural decay product of ²³⁸U. Modes of decay: γ by isomeric transition to yield ²³⁴Pa; β⁻ to yield ²³⁴U. Longest-lived isotope, ²³¹Pa (T₁ 3.276 × 10⁴ years, rel. at. mass 231.0359); natural decay product of ²³⁵U. Decays by α emission; parent of ²²⁷Ac. ²³⁴Pa (T₁ 6.75 hrs); called *Uranium Z* or *UZ*; natural decay product of ²³⁸U. Decays by β⁻ emission. Discovery of ᵐ²³⁴Pa: K. Fajans, O. H. Göhring, *Naturwissenschaften* **1,** 339 (1913), *C.A.* **7,** 3916 (1913); *eidem, Phys. Z.* **14,** 877 (1913), *C.A.* **7,** 297 (1913); of ²³¹Pa: O. Hahn, L. Meitner, *ibid.* **19,** 208 (1918); and independently by F. Soddy, J. A. Cranston, *Proc. Roy. Soc.* **94A,** 384 (1918); of ²³⁴Pa: O. Hahn, *Ber.* **54B,** 1131 (1921). Prepn of metal: A. V. Grosse, M. Agrass, *J. Am. Chem. Soc.* **56,** 2200 (1934). Review of discovery: K. Fajans, D. F. C. Morris, *Nature* **244,** 137-138 (1973); of use in nuclear fuel cycle: O. L. Keller, *Radiochim. Acta* **25,** 211-223 (1978). *Reviews: Comprehensive Inorganic Chemistry* **vol. 5,** J. C. Bailar, Jr. *et al.,* Eds. (Pergamon Press, Oxford, 1973) *passim*; H. W. Kirby in *The Chemistry of the Actinide Elements* **vol. 1,** J. J. Katz *et al.,* Eds. (Chapman and Hall, New York, 1986) pp 102-168.

Shiny, silvery, malleable, ductile metal. Body-centered tetragonal crystal structure. Easily tarnished in air to an undetermined oxide. mp 1560°; also reported as 1575° (Bailar). bp 4227°. d^{25}

15.37. Reacts with H₂ at 250-300° to form PaH₃. In dil solns of HF, is deposited (10-96%) on Be, Al, Mn, Zn, and Pl; gives small deposits on Cr, Ta, Fe, Cd, Ni, Cu, Hg, W: Camarcat *et al., J. Chim. Phys.* **46,** 153-157 (1949).

Caution: Radiation hazard; handling requires special equipment and shielding facilities (Katz *et al., loc. cit.* **vol 2,** p 1128). Inhalation hazard in insol form; general hazard if absorbed systemically. Max permissible concn of insoluble form in air: 4 × 10⁻¹¹ μCi/cc; of sol form in air: 4 × 10⁻¹³ μCi/cc; *Natl. Bur. Stand. Handb.* **69,** 83 (1959).

USE: ²³³Pa as intermediate in production of fissile ²³³U in thorium breeder reactors.

7884. Protein C. [60202-16-6] Blood-coagulation factor XIV. Vitamin K-dependent plasma protein involved in the regulation of hemostasis. Two-chain, multi-domain glycoprotein, mol wt ~62,000. Circulates as a zymogen; activated by thrombin complexed with thrombomodulin, *q.v.* Activated protein C is a serine protease that controls coagulation by the selective inactivation of factors Va and VIIIa. This activity is potentiated by factor V and by **Protein S,** a vitamin K-dependent protein unrelated to the serine proteases. Identification of **autoprothrombin II-A,** an anticoagulant obtained from purified prothrombin complex: E. F. Mammen *et al., Thromb. Diath. Haemorrh.* **5,** 218 (1960). Purification: W. H. Seegers *et al., Thromb. Res.* **1,** 443 (1972). Characterization: J. Stenflo, *J. Biol. Chem.* **251,** 355 (1976). Identity with autoprothrombin II-A: W. H. Seegers *et al., Thromb. Res.* **8,** 543 (1976). Isoln from human plasma: W. Kisiel, *J. Clin. Invest.* **64,** 761 (1979). Amino acid sequence of bovine protein C: P. Fernlund, J. Stenflo, *J. Biol. Chem.* **257,** 12170, 12180 (1982). Review of role in hemostasis: L. H. Clouse, P. C. Comp, *N. Engl. J. Med.* **314,** 1298-1304 (1986); C. T. Esmon, *J. Biol. Chem.* **264,** 4743-4746 (1989); of preparative methods and mechanism of activation: C. T. Esmon *et al., Methods Enzymol.* **222,** 359-385 (1993). Review of protein C system and role in thromboembolic disease: B. Dahlbäck, *Thromb. Res.* **77,** 1-43 (1995).

Drotrecogin alfa. [98530-76-8] Recombinant human activated protein C; rhAPC; Xigris; Zovant. Prepn: S. C. B. Yan *et al., Biotechnology* **8,** 655-661 (1990). Review of development and clinical potential: S. B. Yan, B. W. Grinnell, *Perspect. Drug Discovery Des.* **1,** 503-520 (1993). Clinical trial in severe sepsis: G. R. Bernard *et al., N. Engl. J. Med.* **344,** 699 (2001).

THERAP CAT: In treatment of severe sepsis.

7885. Protein Hydrolysates. Aminosol; Dekamin; Parentamin; Travamin. Sterile solution of amino acids and short-chain peptides which represent the approx nutritive equivalent of the casein, lactalbumin, plasma, fibrin or other suitable protein from which it is derived by acid, enzymatic or other method of hydrolysis. It may be modified by partial removal and restoration or addn of one or more amino acids. It may contain alcohol, dextrose, or other carbohydrate suitable for i.v. infusion. Not <50% of the total nitrogen present is in the form of α-amino nitrogen.

THERAP CAT: Parenteral nutrient.

THERAP CAT (VET): Parenteral nutrient.

7886. Protheobromine. [50-39-5] 3,7-Dihydro-1-(2-hydroxypropyl)-3,7-dimethyl-1*H*-purine-2,6-dione; 1-(2-hydroxypropyl)theobromine; Tebe; Bonicor. $C_{10}H_{14}N_4O_3$; mol wt 238.24. C 50.41%, H 5.92%, N 23.52%, O 20.15%. Prepn: Rojahn, Fegler, *Arch. Pharm.* **268,** 570 (1930); *GB 816299* (1959 to Chemiewerk Homburg), *cf. DE 1067025.* Improved procedure: Carstens, Donat, *DD 26757* (1964). Pharmacology: Giertz *et al., Arzneim.-Forsch.* **6,** 457 (1956). Toxicity study: R. Taugner *et al., Arzneim.-Forsch.* **6,** 601 (1956).

Crystals from isopropanol, mp 140-142°. Freely sol in water at neutral or slightly acid pH. Sol in chloroform, hot ethanol, warm

Prothioconazole

glycerol. Practically insol in ether. LD$_{50}$ s.c. in mice: 580 mg/kg (Taugner).

THERAP CAT: Diuretic.

7887. Prothioconazole. [178928-70-6] 2-[2-[(1-Chloro-cyclopropyl)-3-(2-chlorophenyl)-2-hydroxypropyl]-1,2-dihydro-3H-1,2,4-triazole-3-thione; 2-(1-chlorocyclopropyl)-1-(2-chloro-phenyl)-3-(5-mercapto-1,2,4-triazol-1-yl)propan-2-ol; JAU-6476; Proline; Redigo. C$_{14}$H$_{15}$Cl$_2$N$_3$OS; mol wt 344.26. C 48.84%, H 4.39%, Cl 20.60%, N 12.21%, O 4.65%, S 9.31%. Fungal sterol demethylation inhibitor. Prepn: M. Jautelat *et al.,* **DE 19528046**; *eidem,* **US 5789430** (1996, 1998 both to Bayer). Comprehensive description: A. Mauler-Machnik *et al., BCPC Conf. - Pests Dis.* **2002**, 389-394.

White to light beige crystalline powder. mp 139.1-144.5°. Vapor pressure (20°): < 4×10^{-7} Pa. pKa: 6.9. Log P (octanol/water): 4.05 (unbuffered at 20°). Soly in water (20°): 0.3 g/l. LD$_{50}$ in rats (mg/kg): > 6200 orally; > 2000 dermally. LC$_{50}$ in rats (mg/m^3): > 4990 by inhalation. LC$_{50}$ (96 hr) in rainbow trout: 1.83 mg/l (Mauler-Machnik).

USE: Agricultural fungicide.

7888. Prothipendyl. [303-69-5] *N,N*-Dimethyl-10*H*-pyrido[3,2-*b*][1,4]benzothiazine-10-propanamine; 10-(3-dimethyl-aminopropyl)-10*H*-pyrido[3,2-*b*][1,4]benzothiazine; 10-(γ-dimeth-ylaminopropyl)-1-azaphenothiazine; *N*-(3-dimethylaminopropyl)-thiophenylpyridylamine; 2,3-pyridino-(5′,6′)-5,6-benzo-4-(3″-di-methylaminopropyl)-1,4-thiazine. C$_{16}$H$_{19}$N$_3$S; mol wt 285.41. C 67.33%, H 6.71%, N 14.72%, S 11.23%. Prepn: Yale, Bernstein, **US 2943086** (1960 to Olin Mathieson); von Schlichtegroll, *Proc. 1st Int. Congr. Neuro-Pharm.* **1958**, 408 (1959), *C.A.* **54**, 13400g (1960); **FR 1173134** (1959 to Rhône-Poulenc).

Liquid, bp$_{0.7}$ 217-219°; bp$_{0.5}$ 195-198°.

Hydrochloride. [1225-65-6] D-206; Dominal; Tolnate. C$_{16}$-H$_{19}$N$_3$S.HCl; mol wt 321.87. mp 177-178° with sintering ~176°. Monohydrate as crystals, mp 108-112°. Freely sol in water, methanol. Practically insol in ether, petr ether.

Dihydrochloride. C$_{16}$H$_{19}$N$_3$S.2HCl. Crystals from acetonitrile, mp 205-207°.

THERAP CAT: Antipsychotic.

7889. Prothrombin. [9001-26-7] Blood-coagulation factor II; Factor II; prothrombase; serozyme; thrombogen. Mol wt 69,000-74,000. Coagulation proenzyme present in highest concentration in blood. Prothrombin is one of the vitamin-K dependent blood coagulation factors. It is converted to thrombin by the action of factor X$_a$, factor V and phospholipid in the presence of Ca^{2+} ions. Accounts for < 0.2% of total plasma protein. Prepn of human and bovine prothrombin: Goldstein *et al., J. Biol. Chem.* **234**, 2857 (1959); Lanchantin *et al., ibid.* **238**, 238 (1963). Chemistry of activation: Magnussen, *Biochem. J.* **115**, 2P (1969). Synthesized normally by liver parenchymal cells in a cyclic asynchronous manner. Dicoumarol derivatives halt the synthesis, while vitamin K$_1$ stimulates synchronized activity of all the liver parenchymal cells: Barnhart, Anderson, *Biochem. Pharmacol.* **9**, 23 (1962). The glycoprotein structure probably consists of a single polypeptide chain

containing between 8 and 10% carbohydrate: Magnussen, *Thromb. Diath. Haemorrh.* **suppl. 54**, 31 (1973). *Reviews:* W. H. Seegers, *Prothrombin* (Harvard Univ. Press, 1962) 728 pp; Magnussen "Prothrombin and Thrombin," in *The Enzymes* **Vol. III**, P. D. Boyer, Ed. (Academic Press, New York, 3rd ed., 1971) pp 277-321; K. G. Mann, *Methods Enzymol.* **45B**, 123-156 (1976). Review on prothrombin activation: several authors in *Ann. N.Y. Acad. Sci.* **370**, 336-528 (1981).

Most stable within the range pH 4-9.5. Isoelec pt pH 4.2. Very sol in water but pptd at pH 4.2-4.5. Solns tend to activate spontaneously. There is little loss of activity when drying from the frozen state but the dry material alters in a few months. Drying with organic solvents destroys activity.

7890. Protiofate. [58416-00-5] 3,4-Dihydroxy-2,5-thio-phenedicarboxylic acid dipropyl ester; dipropyl 3,4-dihydroxy-2,5-thiophenedicarboxylate; Atrimycon. C$_{12}$H$_{16}$O$_6$S; mol wt 288.32. C 49.99%, H 5.59%, O 33.30%, S 11.12%. Thiophene derivative with antimycotic activity: L. Riviera *et al., Chemioterapia* **3**, 116 (1984). Prepn: **FR 2255063** (1975 to Bioindustria), *C.A.* **84**, 89986f (1976).

Crystals from ethanol-water, mp 96-97°.

THERAP CAT: Topical fungicide.

7891. Protionamide. [14222-60-7] 2-Propyl-4-pyridinecar-bothioamide; 2-propylthioisonicotinamide; prothionamide; 2-pro-pyl-4-thiocarbamoylpyridine; Ektebin; Peteha; Trevintix. C$_9$H$_{12}$-N$_2$S; mol wt 180.27. C 59.96%, H 6.71%, N 15.54%, S 17.79%. Prepn: D. Liberman *et al., Compt. Rend.* **242**, 2409 (1956); **GB 800250**, D. Liberman, **US 2901488** (1958, 1959 both to Chimie et Atomistique); L. N. Yakhontov *et al., Khim. Farm. Zh.* **10**, 96 (1976), *C.A.* **85**, 32787h (1976). Pharmacology: A. M. Il'in, *Farmakol. Toksikol.* **38**, 471 (1975).

Crystals, mp 142°. Sol in ethanol, methanol; slightly sol in ether, chloroform. Practically insol in water. LD$_{50}$ in mice, rats (g/kg): 1.0, 1.32 orally (Il'in).

THERAP CAT: Antibacterial (tuberculostatic).

7892. Protoanemonin. [108-28-1] 5-Methylene-2(5*H*)-fu-ranone; 4-hydroxy-2,4-pentadienoic acid γ-lactone; 5-methylene-2-oxodihydrofuran; Isomycin. C$_5$H$_4$O$_2$; mol wt 96.08. C 62.50%, H 4.20%, O 33.30%. An antibacterial principle of *Anemone pulsatilla* L., *Ranunculaceae:* Seegal, Holden, *Science* **101**, 413 (1945). Exists as a glucoside, *ranunculin*, in the intact plant, and is released by an enzymatic process on maceration of the plant tissue: R. Hill, R. van Heyningen, *Biochem. J.* **49**, 332 (1951). Isoln: Asahina, Fujita, *Acta Phytochim.* **1**, 1 (1922); Baer *et al., J. Biol. Chem.* **162**, 65 (1946). Structure and synthesis: Asahina, Fujita, *loc. cit.;* Muskat *et al., J. Am. Chem. Soc.* **52**, 326 (1930); Fox, Jr., *Proc. Soc. Exp. Biol.* **51**, 102 (1942); Shaw, *J. Am. Chem. Soc.* **68**, 2510 (1946). Industrial prepns: Seegal, **GB 759999** (1956 to Olin Mathieson), *C.A.* **51**, 9678f (1957); Reicheneder *et al.,* **DE 1088047** (BASF), *C.A.* **56**, 14086i (1962); Sakuma, Hirano, **US 3203863** (1965 to Lion Dentifrice).

Pale yellow oil; volatile with steam. bp$_{1.5}$ 45°. Sol in ethylene dichloride, chloroform. Solubility in water ~1%. Stable in water.

When pure the compd turns to a hard polymer which, when ground and extracted with boiling ethyl acetate, yields anemonin, *q.v.*

THERAP CAT: Antibacterial.

7893. Protocatechualdehyde. [139-85-5] 3,4-Dihydroxy-benzaldehyde; 3,4-dihydroxybenzenecarbonal; protocatechuic aldehyde; rancinamycin IV. $C_7H_6O_3$; mol wt 138.12. C 60.87%, H 4.38%, O 34.75%. Prepn from catechol: Reimer, Tiemann, *Ber.* **9**, 1268 (1876); Tiemann, Koppe, *ibid.* **14**, 2015 (1881); from vanillin: Tiemann, Haarmann, *ibid.* **7**, 620 (1874); from veratric aldehyde: Dreyfus, *DE 193958*; *Frdl.* **9**, 161 (1908-10); from piperonal: Hoering, Baum, *Ber.* **41**, 1914 (1908); Barger, *J. Chem. Soc.* **93**, 563 (1908); Buck, Zimmerman, *Org. Synth.* **coll. vol. II**, 549 (1943).

Platelets from water or toluene. Dimorphic. Dec 153-154°. pK (25°) 7.55. Soly in water (g/100 ml): 5 (20°); 33 (99°); in ethanol: 79 (78°). Freely sol in ether.

7894. Protocatechuic Acid. [99-50-3] 3,4-Dihydroxy-benzoic acid. $C_7H_6O_4$; mol wt 154.12. C 54.55%, H 3.92%, O 41.52%. Minute amounts are found in wheat grains, in wheat seedlings, and in many other plants: L. Hörhammer, A. Scherm, *Arch. Pharm.* **288**, 441 (1955). Prepd by the alkaline fusion of vanillin: Tiemann, Haarmann, *Ber.* **7**, 617 (1874); Pearl, *J. Am. Chem. Soc.* **68**, 2180 (1946); *Org. Synth.* **coll. vol. III**, 745 (1955).

White to brownish, cryst powder; discolors in air. d 1.54. mp ~200° with decompn. Sol in 50 parts water; sol in alcohol, ether. *Keep well closed.*

7895. Protokylol. [136-70-9] 4-[2-[[2-(1,3-Benzodioxol-5-yl)-1-methylethyl]amino]-1-hydroxyethyl]-1,2-benzenediol; α-[(α-methyl-3,4-methylenedioxyphenethylamino)methyl]protocatechuyl alcohol; α-(3,4-dihydroxyphenyl)-β-[2-(3,4-methylenedioxyphenyl)isopropylamino]ethanol; 1-(3,4-dihydroxyphenyl)-2-(α-methyl-3,4-methylenedioxyphenethylamino)ethanol; *N*-[β-(3,4-methylene-dioxyphenyl)isopropyl]-β-(3,4-dihydroxyphenyl)-β-hydroxyethyl-amine; *N*-[2-(3,4-methylenedioxyphenylisopropyl)]norepinephrine. $C_{18}H_{21}NO_5$; mol wt 331.36. C 65.24%, H 6.39%, N 4.23%, O 24.14%. β-Adrenergic agonist. Prepn: Biel *et al., J. Am. Chem. Soc.* **76**, 3149 (1954); Biel, *US 2900415* (1959 to Lakeside Labs.). Toxicity: E. I. Goldenthal, *Toxicol. Appl. Pharmacol.* **18**, 185 (1971).

Hydrochloride. [136-69-6] JB-251; Caytine; Ventaire. $C_{18}H_{21}NO_5 \cdot HCl$; mol wt 367.82. Crystals from isopropanol, mp 126-127°. Sol in water. LD_{50} orally in rats: 938 ±96 mg/kg (Goldenthal).

THERAP CAT: Bronchodilator.

THERAP CAT (VET): Bronchodilator.

7896. Protopine. [130-86-9] 4,6,7,14-Tetrahydro-5-methylbis[1,3]benzodioxolo[4,5-c:5',6'-g]azecin-13(5H)-one; 7-methyl-2,3:9,10-bis(methylenedioxy)-7,13a-secoberbin-13a-one; fumarine;

macleyine. $C_{20}H_{19}NO_5$; mol wt 353.37. C 67.98%, H 5.42%, N 3.96%, O 22.64%. From opium: Hesse, *Ber.* **4**, 693 (1871); also from the herb *Fumaria officinalis* L., *Chelidonium majus* L., and many other *Papaveraceae* and *Fumariaceae:* Manske in *The Alkaloids* **vol. IV**, R. H. F. Manske, H. L. Holmes, Eds. (Academic Press, New York, 1954) pp 157-159. Structure: Perkin, Jr., *J. Chem. Soc.* **109**, 815 (1916); Gadamer, Bruchhausen, *Arch. Pharm.* **260**, 97 (1922); Mottus *et al., Can. J. Chem.* **31**, 1144 (1953); Anet, Marion, *ibid.* **32**, 452 (1954). Synthesis: Haworth, Perkin, *J. Chem. Soc.* **1926**, 1769. Crystal structure: Hall, Ahmed, *Acta Crystallogr.* **24B**, 337 (1968).

Monoclinic prisms from alcohol + chloroform, mp 208°. d 1.399 (calc). uv max (95% ethanol): 293 nm (log ε 3.93). Sol in 15 parts chloroform, 900 parts alc, 1000 parts ether. Slightly sol in ethyl acetate, carbon disulfide, benzene, petr ether. Practically insol in water.

Hydrochloride. $C_{20}H_{19}NO_5 \cdot HCl$. Prisms from alcohol, sol in 143 parts water at 13°, sol in alcohol. Also a hexahydrate, needles from water.

Methiodide. $C_{20}H_{19}NO_5 \cdot CH_3I$. Twinned crystals from methanol, dec 217°.

7897. Protoporphyrin IX. [553-12-8] 7,12-Diethenyl-3,8,-13,17-tetramethyl-21H,23H-porphine-2,18-dipropanoic acid; 3,7,-12,17-tetramethyl-8,13-divinyl-2,18-porphinedipropionic acid; 1,-3,5,8-tetramethyl-2,4-divinylporphine-6,7-dipropionic acid; ooporphyrin; Kammerer's porphyrin. $C_{34}H_{34}N_4O_4$; mol wt 562.66. C 72.58%, H 6.09%, N 9.96%, O 11.37%. Biological precursor of blood and plant pigments. Prepd from hemin: Fischer-Orth, *Die Chemie des Pyrrols* **II**, 1, 396 (Leipzig, 1937); Ramsey, *Biochem. Prep.* **3**, 39 (1953). Structure: Sparatore, Mauzerall, *J. Org. Chem.* **25**, 1073 (1960). Synthesis: Carr *et al., J. Chem. Soc. C* **1971**, 487. Crystal and molecular structure: W. S. Caughey, J. A. Ibers, *J. Am. Chem. Soc.* **99**, 6639 (1977). Chelates with metals, esp iron, in the ferrous state to form heme, *q.v.,* in the ferric state to form hematin, *q.v. Review:* Rimington, Kennedy, in M. Florkin, H. S. Mason, *Comparative Biochemistry* (Academic Press, New York, 1962) pp 557-614.

Monoclinic, brownish-yellow prisms from ether. Absorption max (25% HCl): 602.4, 582.2, 557.2 nm. Freely sol in chloroform, glacial acetic acid, alcohol contg HCl, ether contg some glacial acetic acid, hydrochloric acid. Somewhat sol in dil alkalies, aniline, pyridine. Forms sparingly sol disodium and dipotassium salts.

Disodium salt. [50865-01-5] Depocolin-S. $C_{34}H_{32}N_4Na_2O_4$; mol wt 606.62.

Dimethyl ester. [5522-66-7] $C_{36}H_{38}N_4O_4$. Crystals from chloroform + methanol, mp 228-230°. Absorption max (25% HCl): 601, 556, 409 nm. Soluble in chloroform, slightly sol in methanol. Insol in sodium carbonate solns.

THERAP CAT: In liver disease.

7898. Protostephanine. [549-28-0] 6,7,8,9-Tetrahydro-2,-3,10,12-tetramethoxy-7-methyl-5*H*-dibenz[*d,f*]azonine. $C_{21}H_{27}$-NO_4; mol wt 357.44. C 70.56%, H 7.61%, N 3.92%, O 17.90%. A member of the hasubanan alkaloids. First alkaloid known to possess the unique dibenz[*d,f*]azonine structure. Isoln from *Stephania japonica*, Miers, *Menispermaceae*: H. Kondo, T. Sanada, *J. Pharm. Soc. Jpn.* **541**, 177 (1927), *C.A.* **21**, 2700[4] (1927); H. Kondo, T. Watanabe, *ibid.* **58**, 268 (1938), *C.A.* **32**, 5403[5] (1938). Structure: K. Takeda, *Bull. Agric. Chem. Soc. Jpn.* **20**, 165 (1956). Synthesis: *idem, C.A.* **60**, 5570f (1964); B. Pecherer, A. Brossi, *J. Org. Chem.* **32**, 1053 (1967); A. R. Battersby *et al., J. Chem. Soc. Perkin Trans. 1* **1981**, 2002. Biosynthesis: *eidem, ibid.* 2010, 2016, 2030.

White crystalline solid from benzene, mp 84-86° (Pecherer). Also reported as mp 75° (Kondo).

7899. Protoveratrines. From the rhizome of *Veratrum album* L., *Liliaceae*: Salzberger, *Arch. Pharm.* **228**, 462 (1890); Poethke, *ibid.* **275**, 357 (1937); Craig, Jacobs, *J. Biol. Chem.* **143**, 427 (1942); **149**, 271 (1943). Mixture of protoveratrines A and B: Glen *et al., Nature* **170**, 932 (1952); Klohs *et al., J. Am. Chem. Soc.* **74**, 5107 (1952); Nash, Brooker, *ibid.* **75**, 1942 (1953); Stoll, Seebeck, *Helv. Chim. Acta* **36**, 718 (1953); Nash, Brooker, **US 2929812** (1960 to Allied Labs). Structure of protoveratrines A and B: Kupchan, Ayres, *J. Am. Chem. Soc.* **82**, 2252 (1960). Comparative toxicity: O. Krayer *et al., J. Pharmacol. Exp. Ther.* **82**, 167 (1944); K. Tanaka, *ibid.* **113**, 89 (1955).

Protoveratrine A R = H
Protoveratrine B R = OH

Slightly bitter, sternutative crystals from alc, dec 266-267°. $[\alpha]_D^{25}$ −38.6° (pyridine). $[\alpha]_D^{25}$ −8.5° (c = 1.99 in chloroform). Soluble in chloroform; dil aq acidic solns; slightly sol in ether. Practically insol in water, petr ether. LD_{50} i.v. in mice: 0.048 mg/kg (Krayer).

Protoveratrine A. [143-57-7] [3β(*S*),4α,6α,7α,15α(*R*),16β]-4,9-Epoxycevane-3,4,6,7,14,15,16,20-octol 6,7-diacetate 3-(2-hydroxy-2-methylbutanoate) 15-(2-methylbutanoate); Protalba. C_{41}-$H_{63}NO_{14}$; mol wt 793.94. Crystals from acetone, dec 267-269°. $[\alpha]_D^{25}$ −40.5° (pyridine); $[\alpha]_D^{25}$ −10.5° (chloroform). Soluble in chloroform, pyridine, hot alcohol. LD_{50} s.c. in male mice: 0.29 mg/kg (Tanaka).

Protoveratrine B. [124-97-0] [3β(2*R*,3*R*),4α,6α,7α,15α(*R*),-16β]-4,9-Epoxycevane-3,4,6,7,14,15,16,20-octol 6,7-diacetate 3-(2,3-dihydroxy-2-methylbutanoate) 15-(2-methylbutanoate); veratetrine; neoprotoveratrine. $C_{41}H_{63}NO_{15}$; mol wt 809.94. Crystals from acetone, dec 268-270°. $[\alpha]_D^{25}$ −37° (pyridine); $[\alpha]_D^{25}$ −3.5°

(chloroform). Soluble in chloroform, pyridine, hot alcohol. LD_{50} s.c. in male mice: 0.21 mg/kg (Tanaka).
Mixture of protoveratrine A and B. Provell; Tensatrin.
THERAP CAT: Antihypertensive.

7900. Protoverine. [76-45-9] (3β,4α,6α,7α,15α,16β)-4,9-Epoxycevane-3,4,6,7,14,15,16,20-octol. $C_{27}H_{43}NO_9$; mol wt 525.63. C 61.70%, H 8.25%, N 2.66%, O 27.39%. Obtained by alkaline hydrolysis of protoveratrine A: Poethke, *Arch. Pharm.* **275**, 571 (1937); Stoll, Seebeck, *Helv. Chim. Acta* **36**, 718 (1953). Structure: Kupchan *et al., Chem. Ind. (London)* **1958**, 1626; *J. Am. Chem. Soc.* **81**, 1009 (1959); **82**, 2242 (1960). Comparative toxicity: O. Krayer *et al., J. Pharmacol. Exp. Ther.* **82**, 167 (1944); K. Tanaka, *ibid.* **113**, 89 (1955).

Fine needles from methanol, dec 220-222°. $[\alpha]_D^{20}$ −15.7° (c = 1.1 in pyridine). Sol in $CHCl_3$, methanol, pyridine. LD_{50} i.v. in mice: 194.0 mg/kg (Krayer). LD_{50} s.c. in male mice: 520 mg/kg (Tanaka).

7901. Protriptyline. [438-60-8] *N*-Methyl-5*H*-dibenzo[*a,d*]cycloheptene-5-propanamine; 5-(3-methylaminopropyl)-5*H*-dibenzo[*a,d*]cycloheptene; 7-(3-methylaminopropyl)-1,2:5,6-dibenzocycloheptatriene; amimetilina. $C_{19}H_{21}N$; mol wt 263.38. C 86.64%, H 8.04%, N 5.32%. Prepn: Engelhardt, Christy, **BE 617967** (1962 to Merck & Co.), *C.A.* **59**, 517f (1963); Tishler *et al.*, **US 3244748** and **US 3271451** (both 1966 to Merck & Co.); Engelhardt *et al., J. Med. Chem.* **11**, 325 (1968). Metabolism in man, pig and dog: Sisenwine *et al., J. Pharmacol. Exp. Ther.* **175**, 51 (1970). Use in treatment of sleep apnea: R. W. Clark *et al., Neurology* **29**, 1287 (1979); L. G. Brownell *et al., N. Engl. J. Med.* **307**, 1037 (1982).

Hydrochloride. [1225-55-4] MK-240; Concordin; Triptil; Vivactil. $C_{19}H_{21}N.HCl$; mol wt 299.84. Crystals from isopropanol-ethyl ether, mp 169-171°. uv max: 290 nm (ε 13311). Freely sol in water. pKa 8.2.
THERAP CAT: Antidepressant.

7902. Pro-Urokinase. [82657-92-9] Prourokinase (enzyme-activating); single-chain urokinase-type plasminogen activator; single-chain pro-urokinase; scu-PA; pro-UK; pro u-PA; PUK; Sandolase; Thombolyse; Tomieze. Single-chain proenzyme form of urokinase, *q.v.* Produced by the kidney; present in urine and blood. Consists of 411 amino acid residues, mol wt ~54,000 daltons. Converted by plasmin or kallikrein to active two-chain urokinase by proteolytic cleavage of the Lys 158 - Ile 159 peptide bond. Identification of proenzyme activity from cultured human kidney cells: M. B. Bernik, *J. Clin. Invest.* **52**, 823 (1973). Isoln from culture media: C. Nolan *et al., Biochim. Biophys. Acta* **496**, 384 (1977). Purification from human plasma: T.-C. Wun *et al., J. Biol. Chem.* **257**, 3276 (1982); from human urine: S. S. Husain *et al., Arch. Biochem. Biophys.* **220**, 31 (1983). Amino acid sequence and cleavage site: S. Kasai *et al., J. Biol. Chem.* **260**, 12382 (1985). Clot-specific activity: V. Gurewich *et al., J. Clin. Invest.* **73**, 1731 (1984). Clinical pharmacology: G. Trübestein *et al., Haemostasis* **17**, 238 (1987). Clinical trials in acute myocardial infarction: C. Bode *et al., Am. J. Cardiol.* **61**, 971 (1988); in combination with t-PA: V. Gurewich, *J. Am. Coll. Cardiol.* **10**, 16B (1987). Review of mechanism of action studies: V. Gurewich, R. Pannell, *Semin. Thromb. Hemostasis* **13**, 146-151 (1987); and physicochemical properties: V. Gurewich, *ibid.* **14**, 110-115 (1988).

Saruplase. [99149-95-8] Prourokinase (enzyme-activating) (human clone pUK4/pUK18 protein moiety reduced); CG-4509. Nonglycosylated human prourokinase produced in *E. coli* by recombinant DNA technology. Prepn: H. L. Heyneker *et al.,* **EP 92182**; *eidem,* **US 5112755** (1983, 1992 both to Genentech); W. E. Holmes *et al., Biotechnology* **3**, 923 (1985). Series of articles on thrombolytic activity: *Thromb. Haemostasis* **52**, 19-33 (1984). Pharmacokinetics: A. de Boer *et al., ibid.* **70**, 320 (1993). Clinical trial: PRIMI Trial Study Group, *Lancet* **1**, 863 (1989); J. Schofer *et al., Eur. Heart J.* **14**, 958 (1993).

THERAP CAT: Thrombolytic.

7903. Proxazole. [5696-09-3] *N,N*-Diethyl-3-(1-phenylpropyl)-1,2,4-oxadiazole-5-ethanamine; 5-[2-(diethylamino)ethyl]-3-(α-ethylbenzyl)-1,2,4-oxadiazole; propaxoline. $C_{17}H_{25}N_3O$; mol wt 287.40. C 71.04%, H 8.77%, N 14.62%, O 5.57%. Smooth muscle relaxant. Prepn: **GB 924608**; Palazzo, Silvestrini, **US 3141019** (1963, 1964 both to Angelini Francesco). Pharmacology: Silvestrini, Pozzatti, *Arzneim.-Forsch.* **13**, 798 (1963). Separation and pharmacology of the enantiomers: De Feo *et al., Farmaco Ed. Sci.* **26**, 370 (1971). Clinical trial in cerebrovascular insufficiency: G. Esposito, M. De Gregorio, *Arzneim.-Forsch.* **24**, 1692 (1974).

bp$_{0.2}$ 132°.

Citrate. [132-35-4] AF-634; Flou; Pirecin; Toness. $C_{17}H_{25}N_3O\cdot C_6H_8O_7$; mol wt 479.52. LD$_{50}$ in rats (mg/kg): 39 i.p., 60 orally (Silvestrini, Pozzatti).

Nitrate. Crystals, mp 127-128°.

THERAP CAT: Antispasmodic.

THERAP CAT (VET): Antispasmodic.

7904. Proxibarbal. [2537-29-3] 5-(2-Hydroxypropyl)-5-(2-propenyl)-2,4,6(1*H*,3*H*,5*H*)-pyrimidinetrione; 5-allyl-5-(2-hydroxypropyl)barbituric acid; 5-allyl-5-(β-hydroxypropyl)barbituric acid; 5-allyl-5-(β-hydroxypropyl)malonylurea; proxibarbital; HH-184; Axeen; Centralgol; Centralgyl; Ipronal. $C_{10}H_{14}N_2O_4$; mol wt 226.23. C 53.09%, H 6.24%, N 12.38%, O 28.29%. Prepn: Bobranski *et al., Rocz. Chem.* **30**, 175 (1956), *C.A.* **51**, 438f (1957); **GB 953387** (1964 to Hommel A.G.), *C.A.* **61**, 3123a (1964); Smissman *et al., J. Med. Chem.* **14**, 853 (1971). Metabolism: Bobranski *et al., Arch. Immunol. Ther. Exp.* **10**, 895 (1962); B. Lambrey *et al., Eur. J. Med. Chem. - Chim. Ther.* **15**, 463 (1980). Pharmacokinetics: *eidem, ibid.* **12**, 565 (1977).

Crystals from benzene + ethanol, mp 157-158°; also reported as mp 166.5-168.5° from acetone + chloroform (Smissman). Moderately sol in water.

Note: This is a controlled substance (depressant): **21 CFR**, 1308.13.

THERAP CAT: Sedative, hypnotic.

7905. Proxyphylline. [603-00-9] 3,7-Dihydro-7-(2-hydroxypropyl)-1,3-dimethyl-1*H*-purine-2,6-dione; 7-(2-hydroxypropyl)theophylline; Brontyl; Spasmolysin; Theon. $C_{10}H_{14}N_4O_3$; mol wt 238.24. C 50.41%, H 5.92%, N 23.52%, O 20.15%. Smooth muscle relaxant. Prepd by refluxing 1-chloro-2-propanol with theophylline in an alkaline medium: Rice, **US 2715125** (1955 to Gane's Chem. Works).

Crystals from abs ethanol, mp 135-136°. One gram dissolves in about 1 ml water, in 14 ml abs ethanol. More sol in boiling ethanol. pH of a 5% aq soln 5.5 to 7.0. Solns may be sterilized by heating.

THERAP CAT: Bronchodilator; vasodilator.

7906. Prozapine. [3426-08-2] 1-(3,3-Diphenylpropyl)-hexahydro-1*H*-azepine; 1-(3,3-diphenylpropyl)hexamethylenimine; 1,1-diphenyl-3-hexamethyleneiminopropane; hexadiphane. $C_{21}H_{27}N$; mol wt 293.45. C 85.95%, H 9.27%, N 4.77%. Prepn: Janssen, de Jongh, **US 2881165** (1959 to N. V. Nederland. Comb. Chem. Ind.).

bp$_1$ 170-174°.

Mixture of hydrochloride with sorbitol. Norbiline.

THERAP CAT: Antispasmodic.

7907. Prucalopride. [179474-81-8] 4-Amino-5-chloro-2,3-dihydro-*N*-[1-(3-methoxypropyl)-4-piperidinyl]-7-benzofuran-carboxamide; R-93877; Resolor. $C_{18}H_{26}ClN_3O_3$; mol wt 367.87. C 58.77%, H 7.12%, Cl 9.64%, N 11.42%, O 13.05%. Benzofuran derivative; specific serotonin 5-HT$_4$ receptor agonist. Prepn: G. H. P. Van Daele *et al.,* **WO 9616060**; *eidem,* **US 5854260** (1996, 1998 both to Janssen). Effect on isolated gastrointestinal muscle: N. H. Prins *et al., Br. J. Pharmacol.* **127**, 1431 (1999). Clinical stimulation of colonic transit: E. P. Bouras *et al., Gut* **44**, 682 (1999).

Monohydrate, mp 90.7°.

THERAP CAT: Gastroprokinetic.

7908. Prulifloxacin. [123447-62-1] 6-Fluoro-1-methyl-7-[4-[(5-methyl-2-oxo-1,3-dioxol-4-yl)methyl]-1-piperazinyl]-4-oxo-1*H*,4*H*-[1,3]thiazeto[3,2-*a*]quinoline-3-carboxylic acid; NM-441; Quisnon; Sword; Unidrox. $C_{21}H_{20}FN_3O_6S$; mol wt 461.46. C 54.66%, H 4.37%, F 4.12%, N 9.11%, O 20.80%, S 6.95%. Fluoroquinolone antibacterial; prodrug for active metabolite, *ulifloxacin*. Prepn: M. Kise *et al.,* **EP 315828**; *eidem,* **US 5086049** (1989, 1992 both to Nippon Shinyaku); J. Segawa *et al., J. Med. Chem.* **35**, 4727 (1992). Comparative *in vivo* activity: M. Ozaki *et al., Antimicrob. Agents Chemother.* **35**, 2496 (1991). Clinical pharmacokinetics: M. Nakashima *et al., J. Clin. Pharmacol.* **34**, 930 (1994). Clinical comparison with ciprofloxacin in chronic bronchitis: C. Grassi *et al., Respiration* **69**, 217 (2002). Review of pharmacology: M. G.

Matera, *Pulm. Pharmacol. Ther.* **19,** 20-29 (2006); of clinical development: M. Cazzola *et al., ibid.* 30-37.

Pale yellow powder from acetonitrile, mp 220° (dec).
THERAP CAT: Antibacterial.

7909. Prunetin. [552-59-0] 5-Hydroxy-3-(4-hydroxyphenyl)-7-methoxy-4*H*-1-benzopyran-4-one; 4′,5-dihydroxy-7-methoxyisoflavone; prunusetin. $C_{16}H_{12}O_5$; mol wt 284.26. C 67.60%, H 4.26%, O 28.14%. Isoln from *Prunus* spp., *Rosaceae:* Hasegawa, Shirato, *J. Am. Chem. Soc.* **79,** 450 (1957); Hasegawa, *ibid.* 1738; Goel, Seshadri, *Tetrahedron* **5,** 91 (1959); Plouvier, *Compt. Rend.* **250,** 594 (1960). Identity with prunusetin: King, Jurd, *J. Chem. Soc.* **1952,** 3211. Structure: Shrimer, Hull, *J. Org. Chem.* **10,** 288 (1945). Synthesis: Bradbury, White, *J. Chem. Soc.* **1953,** 871.

Needles from ethanol, mp 240°.
Diacetate. $C_{20}H_{16}O_7$. Rods from methanol, mp 222.5°.
4′-Glucoside. Prunitrin. $C_{22}H_{22}O_{10}$. Isoln: Finnemore, *Pharm. J.* **31,** 604 (1910). Structure and synthesis: Zemplén, Farkas, *Ber.* **90,** 836 (1957). Needles, mp 235-236°. Sol in hot water, ethyl acetate.

7910. Prussian Blue. [14038-43-8]; [12240-15-2] (unspecified formula). (*OC*-6-11)-Iron(3+) (3:4) hexakis(cyano-*κC*) ferrate(4−); ferric ferrocyanide; ferric hexacyanoferrate(II); iron(III) hexacyanoferrate(4−); C.I. 77510; Berlin blue; Chinese blue; Hamburg blue; insoluble Prussian blue; Iron blue; Milori blue; Paris blue; Radiogardase. $C_{18}Fe_7N_{18}$; mol wt 859.23. C 25.16%, Fe 45.50%, N 29.34%. $Fe_4[Fe(CN)_6]_3$. Discovered by Diesbach in 1704; one of the first synthetic coordination compounds and modern colors. The structure consists of alternating ferric and ferrous ions on face centered cubic lattice sites; the remaining charge is balanced by potassium or ferric ions. Early characterization: J. Brown, *Philos. Trans.* **33,** 17 (1724). Prepn: *Colour Index* vol. 4 (3rd ed, 1971) p 4673. Structural study: J. F. Keggin, F. D. Miles, *Nature* **137,** 577 (1936). Crystal structure: H. J. Buser *et al., Inorg. Chem.* **16,** 2704 (1977). Physicochemical properties and efficacy in thallium poisoning: J. Kravzov *et al., J. Appl. Toxicol.* **13,** 213 (1993). Review of toxicology: J. Pearce, *Food Chem. Toxicol.* **32,** 577-582 (1994); of clinical efficacy in radiocesium poisioning: D. F. Thompson, C. O. Church, *Pharmacotherapy* **21,** 1364-1367 (2001); of use in chemical and biological sensors: R. Koncki, *Crit. Rev. Anal. Chem.* **32,** 79-96 (2002).

Purple powder. d 1.75-1.81. Soly (mg/ml): water 6; ethanol 20. Slightly sol in most organic solvents. Sol in oxalic acid; precipitates on exposure to light. Absorption max (water): 694 nm.
Ammonium Ferric Hexacyanoferrate. [25869-00-5] Ferric ammonium ferrocyanide. $C_6H_4Fe_2N_7$; mol wt 285.83. NH_4-$Fe[Fe(CN)_6]$. LD$_{50}$ orally in mice: >5 g/kg (Pearce).
Potassium Ferric Ferrocyanide. [25869-98-1] C.I. 77520; C.I. Pigment Blue 27; iron(III) potassium hexacyanoferrate(4−); soluble Prussian blue. $C_6Fe_2KN_6$; mol wt 306.89. $KFe[Fe(CN)_6]$.

USE: As pigment in printing inks, paints, alkyd resin enamels, linoleum, leathercloth, carbon papers, typewriter ribbons, plastics, artists' colors; in chemical and biological sensors.

THERAP CAT: Antidote (radioactive cesium and thallium poisoning).

7911. Pseudobaptigenin. [90-29-9] 3-(1,3-Benzodioxol-5-yl)-7-hydroxy-4*H*-1-benzopyran-4-one; 7-hydroxy-3′,4′-(methylenedioxy)isoflavone. $C_{16}H_{10}O_5$; mol wt 282.25. C 68.09%, H 3.57%, O 28.34%. The aglycon of pseudobaptisin. Prepn by hydrolysis of natural pseudobaptisin: Gorter, *Arch. Pharm.* **235,** 494 (1897). Structure: Späth, Schmidt, *Monatsh. Chem.* **53,** 454 (1929). Syntheses: Späth, Lederer, *Ber.* **63,** 743 (1930); Mahal *et al., J. Chem. Soc.* **1934,** 1771; Baker *et al., ibid.* **1937,** 805; **1953,** 1852; Farkas, *Ber.* **91,** 2858 (1958); Dhoubhadel, Joshi, *J. Indian Chem. Soc.* **52,** 440 (1975).

Long, felted needles from alc, dec 296-298°. Sublimes in high vacuum at ~220°. Sparingly sol in the usual solvents.
7-Rhamnoglucoside trihydrate. Pseudobaptisin. $C_{28}H_{30}$-$O_{14}\cdot3H_2O$. Crystals, becomes anhydr at 120°. mp 148-150° (evac tube). If heating is continued, it resolidif at 180-210° and melts again at 249-251°. $[\alpha]_D^{14}$ −98.1° (c = 1.1 in methanol). Freely sol in methanol, hot water, hot acetone.

7912. Pseudococaine. [478-73-9] [1*R*-(2-*endo*,3-*exo*)]-3-(Benzoyloxy)-8-methyl-8-azabicyclo[3.2.1]octane-2-carboxylic acid methyl ester; 3β-hydroxy-1α*H*,5α*H*-tropane-2α-carboxylic acid methyl ester benzoate; 2α-carbomethoxy-3β-benzoxytropane; depsococaine; dextrocaine; isococaine; Delcaine. $C_{17}H_{21}NO_4$; mol wt 303.35. C 67.31%, H 6.98%, N 4.62%, O 21.10%. Cocaine diastereomer with greater local anesthetic activity than the natural substance. Synthesis: Einhorn, Marquardt, *Ber.* **23,** 468, 981 (1890); Willstätter, Bode, *Ann.* **326,** 42 (1903); Willstätter, Bommer, *ibid.* **422,** 34 (1921); Willstätter *et al., ibid.* **434,** 138 (1923); **GB 210050** (1923 to E. Merck). Configuration: S. P. Findlay, *J. Am. Chem. Soc.* **76,** 2855 (1954). Conformational analysis and ^{1}H, ^{13}C NMR studies: F. I. Carroll *et al., J. Org. Chem.* **1982,** 13. Pharmacokinetics: A. L. Misra *et al., Experientia* **32,** 895 (1976). Interaction with sodium channels: J C. Matthews, A. Collins, *Biochem. Pharmacol.* **32,** 455 (1983). Pharmacology of cocaine and pseudococaine: G. Schmidt *et al., Arch. Exp. Pathol. Pharmakol.* **240,** 523 (1961).

Prisms, mp 47°. $[\alpha]_D^{20}$ +42° (c = 5 in chloroform). Freely sol in ether, chloroform, benzene, petr ether. Slightly sol in water.
Hydrochloride. [6363-57-1] $C_{17}H_{21}NO_4\cdot HCl$. Crystals from alcohol, mp 210°. $[\alpha]_D^{20}$ +41° (c = 5), less sol in water than cocaine hydrochloride.
Tartrate. [1176-03-0] Psicaine. $C_{17}H_{21}NO_4\cdot C_4H_6O_6$; mol wt 453.44. Crystals, mp 139°. $[\alpha]_D^{20}$ +43° (c = 5 in water). Sol in 4 parts water, in alcohol. The aq soln is stable and may be sterilized by boiling, without decompn. pH about 3.7 (2% soln).
Sodium tartrate. Psicaine N. More sol in water than the tartrate; esp useful where a neutral soln is desired.
n-**Propyl ester analog.** [55608-72-5] Neopsicaine. $C_{19}H_{25}$-NO_4; mol wt 331.41.

THERAP CAT: Formerly as anesthetic (local).

7913. Pseudocodeine. [466-96-6] (5α,8β)-6,7-Didehydro-4,5-epoxy-3-methoxy-17-methylmorphinan-8-ol; ψ-codeine; neoisocodeine. $C_{18}H_{21}NO_3$; mol wt 299.36. C 72.22%, H 7.07%, N 4.68%, O 16.03%. An isomer of codeine. Review and bibliography: K. W. Bentley, *The Chemistry of the Morphine Alkaloids* (Oxford, 1954).

White needles, mp 181-182°. $[\alpha]_D$ −96.6° (alc). Slightly sol in water; sol in alcohol.

7914. Pseudoconhydrine. [140-55-6] (3S-*trans*)-6-Propyl-3-piperidinol; 5-hydroxy-2-propylpiperidine; 5-hydroxyconiine. $C_8H_{17}NO$; mol wt 143.23. C 67.08%, H 11.96%, N 9.78%, O 11.17%. In *Conium maculatum* L., *Umbelliferae* (hemlock). Extraction procedure: Ladenburg *et al., Ber.* **24**, 1671 (1891); Braun, *Ber.* **38**, 3108 (1905); Löffler, *Ber.* **42**, 116 (1909). Structure: E. Späth *et al., Ber.* **66**, 591 (1933). Stereochemistry: R. K. Hill, *J. Am. Chem. Soc.* **80**, 1611 (1958); K. Tadano *et al., J. Carbohydr. Chem.* **4**, 129 (1985).

Hygroscopic needles from abs ether, mp 106° (monohydrate, scales, mp 60° from moist ether). bp 236°. $[\alpha]_D^{20}$ +11° (c = 10 in alc). pK (18°): 3.70. Soluble in water and most organic solvents. **Hydrochloride.** $C_8H_{17}NO.HCl$. Crystals from alcohol, mp 213°. Freely sol in water, sparingly sol in alcohol, acetone.

7915. Pseudocumene. [95-63-6] 1,2,4-Trimethylbenzene; pseudocumol; asymmetrical trimethylbenzene. C_9H_{12}; mol wt 120.19. C 89.94%, H 10.06%. Occurs in coal tar and in many petroleums. Physical properties: Hirschler, Falconer, *J. Am. Chem. Soc.* **68**, 210 (1946). Metabolism study: J. Huo *et al., Xenobiotica* **19**, 161 (1989). GC/MS determn in serum: E. Kenndler *et al., J. Anal. Toxicol.* **13**, 211 (1989). Neurotoxic effects of inhalation exposure: Z. Korsak, K. Rydzynski, *Int. J. Occup. Med. Environ. Health* **9**, 341 (1996). Genotoxicity study: E. Janik-Spiechowicz *et al., Mutat. Res.* **412**, 299 (1998).

Liquid. d_4^{20} 0.8761. bp 169-171°. mp −43.78° (Hirschler, Falconer). n_D^{21} 1.5044. Practically insol in water. Sol in alc, benzene, ether. Oxidation yields trimellitic anhydride. LD_{50} i.p. in male, female mice (mg/kg): 5000, 4100 (Janik-Spiechowicz).

Caution: Potential symptoms of overexposure are irritation of eyes, skin, nose, throat, respiratory system; bronchitis; hypochromic anemia; headache, drowsiness, fatigue, dizziness, nausea, incoordination; vomiting, confusion; aspiration of liquid may cause chemical pneumonia. *See NIOSH Pocket Guide to Chemical Hazards* (DHHS/NIOSH 97-140, 1997) p 320.

USE: Sterilizing catgut by heating one hour at 160°; solvent in manuf dyes, perfumes and resins. Solvent for liquid scintillation counting solns.

7916. Pseudoephedrine. [90-82-4] (αS)-α-[(1S)-1-(Methylamino)ethyl]benzenemethanol; (1S,2S)-2-methylamino-1-phenyl-propan-1-ol; d-ψ-ephedrine; d-isoephedrine. $C_{10}H_{15}NO$; mol wt 165.23. C 72.69%, H 9.15%, N 8.48%, O 9.68%. Sympathomimetic amine found in plants of the genus *Ephedra (Ephedraceae)* known in traditional medicine as Ma Huang. α-Adrenergic agonist; (+)-*threo*-isomer of ephedrine, *q.v.* Isoln from *E. vulgaris*: A. Ladenburg, C. Oelschlägel, *Ber.* **22**, 1823 (1889). Synthesis: E. Späth, R. Göhring, *Monatsh. Chem.* **41**, 319 (1920). HPLC determn in Ma Huang: B. J. Gurley *et al., J. Pharm. Sci.* **87**, 1547 (1998); in plasma: P. Guo *et al., Biomed. Chromatogr.* **13**, 61 (1999). Tox-

icity: M. D. Fairchild, G. A. Alles, *J. Pharmacol. Exp. Ther.* **158**, 135 (1967). Comprehensive description: S. A. Benezra, J. W. McRae, *Anal. Profiles Drug Subs.* **8**, 489-507 (1979). Review of clinical pharmacology: D. T. D. Hughes *et al., J. Clin. Hosp. Pharm.* **8**, 315-321 (1983). Clinical trial for prevention of otic barotrauma: J. S. Jones *et al., Am. J. Emerg. Med.* **16**, 262 (1998); in nasal congestion: D. Taverner *et al., Clin. Otolaryngol.* **24**, 47 (1999).

Crystals from ether, mp 118-118.7°. $[\alpha]_D^{20}$ +51.2° (in ethanol). Sparingly sol in water. Freely sol in alc or ether.
Hydrochloride. [345-78-8] Galpseud; Novafed; Rhinalair; Otrinol; Sudafed. Needles, mp 182.5-183.5°. $[\alpha]_D^{20}$ +62.05°. uv max (ethanol): 208, 251, 257, 264 nm (ε 8300, 161, 201, 161). pKa 9.22. Soly at 25° (g/ml): water 2.0; chloroform 0.011; ethanol 0.278. Partition coefficient (25°): 0.010 (*n*-octanol/water, pH 1.2); 0.049 (*n*-octanol/water, pH 6.0). LD_{50} i.p. in mice: 1.0 mmole/kg (Fairchild, Alles).
Sulfate. [7460-12-0] Afrinol.
THERAP CAT: Decongestant (nasal).

7917. Pseudoionone. [141-10-6] 6,10-Dimethyl-3,5,9-un-decatriene-2-one; citrylideneacetone; 2,6-dimethylhendeca-2,6,8-trien-10-one. $C_{13}H_{20}O$; mol wt 192.30. C 81.20%, H 10.48%, O 8.32%. Intermediate in the synthesis of α- and β-ionone. Prepn from citral and acetone: Tiemann, Krüger, *Ber.* **26**, 2692 (1893); Stiehl, *J. Prakt. Chem.* [2] **58**, 84 (1898); Tiemann, *Ber.* **32**, 115 (1899); Hibbert, Cannon, *J. Am. Chem. Soc.* **46**, 119 (1924); A. Russel, R. L. Kenyon, *Org. Synth.* **coll. vol. III**, 747 (1955). A less pure product is obtained by the treatment of oil of lemon grass and acetone with bleaching powder, cobalt nitrate, and alcohol: Ziegler, *J. Prakt. Chem.* [2] **57**, 493 (1898); Tiemann, *Ber.* **31**, 2313 (1898); Haarmann, Reimer & Co., **DE 73089**; *Frdl.* **3**, 889. Synthesis: T. Onishi *et al., Synthesis* **1980**, 651.

Pale yellow oil, bp_2 114-116°; bp_4 124-126°; bp_{12} 143-145°; d^{20} 0.8984; n_D^{20} 1.53346.

7918. Pseudomonic Acids. A group of antibacterial antibiotics produced by *Pseudomonas fluorescens* NCIB 10586 that have unusual structural features. Four members of the group are known: *pseudomonic acid A*, the major component; *pseudomonic acid B*, the 3,4,5-trihydroxy analog of A (also referred to as *pseudomonic acid I*); *pseudomonic acid D*, the 4-nonenoic acid analog of A; and *pseudomonic acid C*, in which the epoxide oxygen is replaced by a double bond. Isoln and characterization of A and B: A. T. Fuller *et al., Nature* **234**, 416 (1971); K. D. Barrow, G. Mellows, **DE 2227739**; *eidem,* **US 3977943** (1973, 1976 both to Beecham). Structure of B: E. B. Chain, G. Mellows, *J. Chem. Soc. Perkin Trans. 1* **1977**, 318. Prepn of C: N. H. Rogers, P. J. O'Hanlon, **EP 3069**; *eidem,* **US 4205002** (1979, 1980 both to Beecham). Isoln, structure, configuration of C: J. P. Clayton *et al., Tetrahedron Lett.* **21**, 881 (1980). Total syntheses of naturally occurring (+)-form of C: A. P. Kozikowski *et al., J. Am. Chem. Soc.* **102**, 6577 (1980); in high yield: C. Mckay *et al., Chem. Commun.* **2000**, 1109; of racemic A or C: B. B. Snider, G. B. Phillips, *J. Am. Chem. Soc.* **104**, 1113 (1982); B. B. Snider *et al., J. Org. Chem.* **48**, 3003 (1983). Prepn of D: P. J. O'Hanlon, **EP 68680** (1983 to Beecham), *C.A.* **98**, 159135t (1983); P. J. O'Hanlon *et al., J. Chem. Soc. Perkin Trans. 1* **1983**, 2655. Antimycoplasmal activity in vitro: R. M. Banks *et al., J. Antibiot.* **41**, 609 (1988).

Pseudomonic Acid C

Isolated as a mixture of sodium salts. Can be stored at 0° for several months with no activity loss. Stable within pH 4-9 at 37° for 24 hrs. Hemolytic; inactivated by serum at conc >50%.

Pseudomonic Acid A *see* Mupirocin.

Pseudomonic Acid C. [71980-98-8] (2E)-5,9-Anhydro-2,3,4,-8-tetradeoxy-8-[(2E,4R,5S)-5-hydroxy-4-methyl-2-hexenyl]-3-methyl-L-*talo*-non-2-enonic acid 8-carboxyoctyl ester. $C_{26}H_{44}O_8$; mol wt 484.62. $[\alpha]_D^{25}$ +7.64° (c = 0.78 in chloroform). uv max (ethanol): 222 nm (ε 14100).

Pseudomonic Acid D. [85248-93-7] (2E)-5,9-Anhydro-2,3,4,-8-tetradeoxy-8-[[(2S,3S)-3-[(1S,2S)-2-hydroxy-1-methylpropyl]-oxiranyl]methyl]-L-*talo*-non-2-enoic acid (5E)-8-carboxy-5-octenyl ester. $C_{26}H_{42}O_9$; mol wt 498.61. Oil. uv max (ethanol): 220 nm (ε 15499).

7919.   Pseudomorphine. [125-24-6] (5'α,6'α)-7,7',8,8'-Tetradehydro-4,5:4',5'-diepoxy-17,17'-dimethyl-[2,2'-bimorphinan]-3,3',6,6'-tetrol; 2,2'-bimorphine; pseudomorphine (C34 alkaloid). $C_{34}H_{36}N_2O_6$; mol wt 568.66. C 71.81%, H 6.38%, N 4.93%, O 16.88%. A dimolecular base formed by the gentle oxidation of morphine in alkaline soln. *Refs:* Broockmann, Polstorff, *Ber.* **13**, 88 (1880); Bentley, Dyke, *J. Chem. Soc.* **1959**, 2574. Review and bibliography: K. W. Bentley, *The Chemistry of the Morphine Alkaloids* (Oxford, 1954) p 54.

Trihydrate. Crystalline powder; levorotatory in acid soln. Becomes anhydr at 150° and dec at about 327°. Insol in cold water, alcohol, ether, dil H_2SO_4. Slightly sol in cold, more sol in hot ammonia; sol in fixed alkali hydroxide solns, in pyridine, aniline, benzyl alcohol, guaiacol.

Note: Name pseudomorphine is also used for the C17 alkaloid base.

7920.   Pseudopelletierine. [552-70-5] 9-Methyl-9-azabicyclo[3.3.1]nonan-3-one; 9-methyl-3-granatanone; pseudopunicine. $C_9H_{15}NO$; mol wt 153.22. C 70.55%, H 9.87%, N 9.14%, O 10.44%. In root bark of *Punica granatum* L., *Punicaceae*. Extraction procedure: Hess, Eichel, *Ber.* **50**, 380, 1391, 1395 (1917); *ibid.* **52**, 1012 (1919). Synthesis under physiological conditions from calcium acetonedicarboxylate, glutardialdehyde, and methylamine: Menzies, Robinson, *J. Chem. Soc.* **1924**, 2163; *cf.* Schöpf, *Angew. Chem.* **50**, 779, 797 (1937). Alternate syntheses: Cope *et al., Org. Synth.* **37**, 73 (1957); Robinson, Hunt, *J. Pharm. Pharmacol.* **22**, 29S (1970); Bottini, Gal, *J. Org. Chem.* **36**, 1718 (1971). Conformation: Chen, LeFevre, *J. Chem. Soc. B* **1966**, 539.

Orthorhombic prisms from petr ether, mp 54°; bp 246°. Volatile. Strong base. One gram dissolves in about 2.5 ml water, 10 ml ether. Freely sol in alcohol and chloroform; sparingly sol in petr ether.

Dihydrate. Plates from water.

Hydrochloride. $C_9H_{15}NO.HCl$. Rhombohedra. One gram dissolves in about 1 ml water.

Sulfate tetrahydrate. $2C_9H_{15}NO.H_2SO_4.4H_2O$. Crystals, sol in water.

7921.   Pseudotropine. [135-97-7] *exo*-8-Methyl-8-azabicyclo[3.2.1]octan-3-ol; 1αH,5αH-tropan-3β-ol; 3β-tropanol; ψ-tropine; 3-pseudotropanol. $C_8H_{15}NO$; mol wt 141.21. C 68.04%, H 10.71%, N 9.92%, O 11.33%. Stereoisomeric with tropine. Prepn, structure, separation from tropine, and stereochemical configuration: *See* Tropine. Stereochemical synthesis: J. J. Tufariello *et al., J. Am. Chem. Soc.* **101**, 2435 (1979).

Orthorhombic, bipyramidal crystals from petr ether + benzene. mp 109°; bp 241°; pK (15°): 3.80. pH of 0.05 M soln 11.5. Freely sol in water, alcohol, benzene.

Hydrochloride. $C_8H_{15}NO.HCl$. Needles from alcohol, dec 282°. Soluble in water, hot alcohol.

Tropate. $C_8H_{15}NO.C_9H_8O_2$. Cryst from benzene, mp 132°.

7922.   Pseudoyohimbine. [84-37-7] (3β,16α,17α)-17-Hydroxyyohimban-16-carboxylic acid methyl ester. $C_{21}H_{26}N_2O_3$; mol wt 354.44. C 71.16%, H 7.39%, N 7.90%, O 13.54%. Present in the bark of *Corynanthe johimbe* K. Schum., *Rubiaceae*. Obtained from the residues of commercial isoln procedures for the manuf of yohimbine: Karrer, Salomon, *Helv. Chim. Acta* **9**, 1059 (1926). Structure and stereochemistry: Janot *et al., Bull. Soc. Chim. Fr.* **1952**, 1085; **1961**, 637. Synthesis: van Tamelen *et al., J. Am. Chem. Soc.* **80**, 5006 (1958); **91**, 7315 (1969); Stork, Guthikonda, *ibid.* **94**, 5109 (1972).

Rhombic platelets, mp 293° (corr, Maquenne block), mp 268° (open capillary), browns at 250°. Also reported as crystals from methanol, mp 252-256° (van Tamelen). $[\alpha]_D^{19}$ +27° (pyridine). uv max (methanol): 225, 281, 290 nm (log ε 4.54, 3.86, 3.80).

Hydrochloride. $C_{21}H_{26}N_2O_3.HCl$. Needles from alcohol + ether, dec 258°. $[\alpha]_D^{20}$ −10° (c = 1 in water).

7923.   Psicofuranine. [1874-54-0] 9-β-D-Psicofuranosyl-9H-purin-6-amine; 9β-D-psicofuranosyladenine; 6-amino-9-D-psicofuranosylpurine; angustmycin C; U-9586. $C_{11}H_{15}N_5O_5$; mol wt 297.27. C 44.44%, H 5.09%, N 23.56%, O 26.91%. Nucleoside antibiotic produced by *Streptomyces hygroscopicus* var. *decoyicus*: Eble *et al., Antibiot. Chemother.* **9**, 419 (1959); Yüntsen, *J. Antibiot.* **11A**, 244 (1958); Eble, Lewis, **US 3020274** (1962 to Upjohn). Antibacterial and antitumor activity: N. Tanaka *et al., J. Antibiot.* **14A**, 98 (1961). Structure: Schroeder, Hoeksema, *J. Am. Chem. Soc.* **81**, 1767 (1959); Garrett, *ibid.* **82**, 827 (1960). Synthesis: Farkas, Sorm, *Collect. Czech. Chem. Commun.* **28**, 882 (1963); L. A. Aleksandrova, F. W. Lichtenthaler, *Nucleic Acids Symp. Ser.* **9**, 263 (1981). Biosynthesis: Sugimori, Suhadolnik, *J. Am. Chem. Soc.* **87**, 1136 (1965). Inhibits the conversion of xanthosine-5'-phosphate to guanosine-5'-phosphate: Slechta, *Biochem. Pharmacol.* **5**, 96 (1960).

Crystals, dec 212-214°. $[\alpha]_D^{25}$ −68° (dimethylformamide). uv max (0.01N acid): 259 nm ($E_{1cm}^{1\%}$ 508); in 0.01N base: 261 nm ($E_{1cm}^{1\%}$ 527). Soly at 25° (mg/ml): water 8; methanol 8; ethanol 6; butanol 2; ethyl acetate 0.23.

7924. D-Psicose. [551-68-8] D-*ribo*-2-Ketohexose; D-ribo-hexulose; D-allulose; D-erythrohexulose; pseudofructose. $C_6H_{12}O_6$; mol wt 180.16. C 40.00%, H 6.71%, O 53.28%. Occurrence and identification as a non-fermentable substance in cane molasses: Zerban, Sattler, *Ind. Eng. Chem.* **34**, 1180 (1942). Structure: Ohle, Just, *Ber.* **68**, 601 (1935). Prepn starting with D-ribono-γ-lactone: Wolfrom *et al., J. Am. Chem. Soc.* **67**, 1793 (1945); from D-allose: Steiger, Reichstein, *Helv. Chim. Acta* **19**, 184 (1937); from D-glucose: Hough *et al., J. Chem. Soc.* **1953**, 2005.

Sweet syrupy liquid. $[\alpha]_D^{25}$ +4.7° (c = 4.3 in water; no detectable mutarotation). Soluble in water, methanol, ethanol. Practically insol in acetone.

Phenylosazone. $C_{18}H_{22}N_4O_4$. Yellow crystals from water, mp about 162-163° (dec); also reported mp 178°.

7925. Psilocin. [520-53-6] 3-[2-(Dimethylamino)ethyl]-1*H*-indol-4-ol; 4-hydroxy-*N,N*-dimethyltryptamine; psilocyn. $C_{12}H_{16}N_2O$; mol wt 204.27. C 70.56%, H 7.89%, N 13.71%, O 7.83%. The minor hallucinogenic component of Teonanácatl, the sacred mushroom of Mexico. Isolated in trace amounts from the fruiting bodies of *Psilocybe mexicana* Heim, *Agaricaceae:* Hofmann *et al., Experientia* **14**, 107 (1958); Heim *et al., Helv. Chim. Acta* **42**, 1557 (1959). Prepn: Heim *et al.,* **DE 1087321** (1960 to Sandoz). Synthetic precursor of psilocybin: Hofmann, Troxler, **US 3075992** (1963 to Sandoz). Psilocin, the 4-hydroxy analog of psilocybin, is formed by metabolic dephosphorylation of psilocybin and is the active species in the central nervous system: Horita, Weber, *Toxicol. Appl. Pharmacol.* **4**, 730 (1962). Crystal structure: T. J. Petcher, H. P. Weber, *J. Chem. Soc. Perkin Trans. 2* **1974**, 946. *Review:* Hofmann, *Bull. Narc.* **23**, 3 (1971).

Plates from methanol, mp 173-176°. Amphoteric substance. Unstable in soln, esp. akaline soln. Very slightly sol in water. uv max: 222, 260, 267, 283, 293 nm (log ε 4.6, 3.7, 3.8, 3.7, 3.6).
Note: This is a controlled substance (hallucinogen): **21 CFR,** 1308.11.

7926. Psilocybin. [520-52-5] 3-[2-(Dimethylamino)ethyl]-1*H*-indol-4-ol dihydrogen phosphate ester; *O*-phosphoryl-4-hydroxy-*N,N*-dimethyltryptamine; Indocybin. $C_{12}H_{17}N_2O_4P$; mol wt 284.25. C 50.70%, H 6.03%, N 9.86%, O 22.51%, P 10.90%. The major of two hallucinogenic components of Teonanácatl, the sacred mushroom of Mexico, the other component being psilocin, *q.v.* from the fruiting bodies of *Psilocybe mexicana* Heim, *Agaricaceae:* Hofmann *et al., Experientia* **14**, 107 (1958); Heim *et al., Helv. Chim. Acta* **42**, 1557 (1959); Heim *et al.,* **DE 1087321** (1960 to Sandoz). Structure: Hofmann *et al., Experientia* **14**, 397 (1958). Synthesis: Hofmann, Troxler, **US 3075992** (1963 to Sandoz). Crystal structure: H. P. Weber, T. J. Petcher, *J. Chem. Soc. Perkin Trans. 2* **1974**, 942. Converted to psilocin *in vivo.* Toxicity data: E. Usdin, D. H. Efron, *Psychotropic Drugs and Related Compounds* (National Institute of Mental Health, Rockville, Md., 2nd ed., 1972) p 138. *Reviews:* Hofmann, *Proc. 1st Int. Congr. Neuro-Pharmacol.* **1958**, 446; Cerletti, *Dtsch. Med. Wochenschr.* **84**, 2317 (1959); Hofmann, *Bull. Narc.* **23**, 3 (1971).

Crystals from boiling water, mp 220-228°; from boiling methanol, mp 185-195°. uv max (methanol): 220, 267, 290 nm (log ε 4.6, 3.8, 3.6). pH 5.2 in 50% aq ethanol. Sol in 20 parts boiling water, 120 parts boiling methanol; difficultly sol in ethanol. Practically insol in chloroform, benzene. LD_{50} in mice, rats, rabbits (mg/kg): 285, 280, 12.5 i.v. (Usdin, Efron).
Note: This is a controlled substance (hallucinogen): **21 CFR,** 1308.11.
THERAP CAT: Psychomimetic.

7927. PSK®. [66455-27-4] KRESTIN. Protein-bound polysaccharide; biological response modifier having immunostimulant and anticancer properties. Isolated from a basidiomycete, *Coriolus versicolor* (Fr.) Quel.: S. Otsuka *et al.,* **JP 73 8489** (1973 to Kureha), *C.A.* **80**, 41025g (1974). Antitumor activity: S. Tsukagoshi *et al., Prog. Chemother. (Antibacterial, Antiviral, Antineoplast.), Proc. Int. Congr. Chemother., 8th, Athens 1973* **vol. 3,** G. K. Daikos, Ed. (Hellen. Soc. Chemother., Athens, 1974) pp 799-803. Clinical studies as postoperative immunotherapy: M. Torisu *et al., Cancer Immunol. Immunother.* **31**, 261 (1990); Y. Kuroda *et al., Int. J. Clin. Oncol.* **3**, 311 (1998). *Review:* S. Tsukagoshi *et al., Cancer Treat. Rev.* **11**, 131-155 (1984). Review of antimicrobial and biological activity: H. Sakagami, M. Takeda in *Mushroom Biology and Mushroom Products* (Chinese Univ. Press, Hong Kong, 1993) p 237-245; antimetastatic effects: H. Kobayashi *et al., Cancer Epidemiol. Biomarkers Prev.* **4**, 275-281 (1995).

Brownish powder. Tasteless, but has a slight odor. Sol in water. Practically insol in methanol, pyridine, chloroform, benzene, hexane. pH of 1% soln is 6.6-7.2.
THERAP CAT: Antineoplastic.

7928. Psoralen. [66-97-7] 7*H*-Furo[3,2-*g*][1]benzopyran-7-one; 6-hydroxy-5-benzofuranacrylic acid δ-lactone; furo[3,2-*g*]coumarin; ficusin. $C_{11}H_6O_3$; mol wt 186.16. C 70.97%, H 3.25%, O 25.78%. One of a group of furocoumarins occurring naturally in more than two dozen plant sources, including *Rutaceae* (*e.g.* bergamot, limes, cloves), *Umbelliferae* (*e.g.* celery, parsnips), *Leguminosae* (*e.g. Psoralen coryfolia*), and *Moraceae* (*e.g.* figs). Isoln: H. S. Jois *et al., J. Indian Chem. Soc.* **10**, 41 (1933); A. Stoll *et al., Helv. Chim. Acta* **33**, 1637 (1950); F. E. King *et al., J. Chem. Soc.* **1954**, 1392. Synthesis: E. Späth *et al., Ber.* **69**, 1087 (1936); R. C. Esse, B. E. Christensen, *J. Org. Chem.* **25**, 1565 (1960); O. Dann, D. Volz, *Arch. Pharm.* **308**, 121 (1975); V. K. Ahluwalia *et al., Monatsh. Chem.* **111**, 877 (1980). Psoralens are **phytoalexins**; they are used by plants in a defensive response to attacks by fungi and insects: M. Berenbaum, P. Feeny, *Science* **212**, 927 (1981). They have also shown photosensitizing and phototoxic effects in animals and humans and have been used in photochemotherapy for management of vitiligo, psoriasis, and mycosis fungoides, *cf.* T. F. Anderson, J. J. Voorhees, *Annu. Rev. Pharmacol. Toxicol.* **20**, 235 (1980); A. Kornhauser *et al., Science* **217**, 733 (1982). Review of psoralen photochemistry: B. J. Parsons, *Photochem. Photobiol.* **32**, 813-821 (1980). Review of genetic toxicity of psoralen and uv radiation in human cells: *Acta Derm. Venereol.* **Suppl. 104**, 4-40 (1982). *See* Methoxsalen, Trioxsalen, Bergapten for additional refs.

Crystals from ether, mp 163-164°; 169-179° (Späth). Absorption spectra: Wessely, Kaltan, *Monatsh. Chem.* **86**, 430 (1955).
USE: As photochemical probe in biological systems: P.-S. Song, C.-N. Ou, *Ann. N.Y. Acad. Sci.* **346**, 355 (1980).

7929. Psychotrine. [7633-29-6] 1′,15-Didehydro-7′,10,11-trimethoxyemetan-6′-ol. $C_{28}H_{36}N_2O_4$; mol wt 464.60. C 72.38%,

H 7.81%, N 6.03%, O 13.77%. Minor alkaloid found in ipecac, the ground roots of *Uragoga ipecacuanha* (Brot.) Baill. [*Cephaelis ipecacuanha* (Brot.) A. Rich.], *Rubiaceae:* F. H. Carr, F. L. Pyman, *J. Chem. Soc.* **105**, 1591 (1914); O. Hesse, *Ann.* **405**, 1 (1914). Structure and stereochemistry: A. R. Battersby *et al., J. Chem. Soc.* **1959**, 2704, 3512. Mass spectrum: H. Budzikiewicz *et al., Tetrahedron* **20**, 399 (1964); ^{1}H,^{13}C-NMR of *O*-methylpsychotrine: T. Fujii *et al., Chem. Pharm. Bull.* **30**, 598 (1982); ^{13}C-NMR of psychotrine: *eidem, ibid.* **31**, 2583 (1983). Proposed alternate structure with exocyclic double bond: E. E. van Tamelen *et al., J. Am. Chem. Soc.* **79**, 4817 (1957); C. Schuij *et al., J. Chem. Soc. Perkin Trans. 1* **1979**, 970. *Review:* M. Janot in Manske, Holmes, *The Alkaloids* vol. 3 (Academic Press, New York, 1953) pp 363-394.

Tetrahydrate. Yellow prisms with blue fluorescence from dil acetone or alcohol. *Very bitter taste, produces nausea instantly.* The anhydr material sinters at 120°, becomes transparent at 120-126° and melts completely at 128°. $[\alpha]_D^{15}$ +69.3° (c = 2 in alcohol, calcd as the tetrahydrate). Sparingly sol in water, benzene, petr ether, ether. More sol in alcohol, acetone, chloroform. uv max (0.1*N* HCl): 240, 288, 306, 356 nm (ε 13900, 5700, 6250, 6800).

Sulfate trihydrate. $C_{28}H_{36}N_2O_4 \cdot H_2SO_4 \cdot 3H_2O$. Pale yellow scales from water, dec 214-217° when anhydr. $[\alpha]_D^{20}$ +39.2°.

O-Methylpsychotrine. Has a methoxy group in place of the hydroxyl group. mp 123-124°. $[\alpha]_D^{20}$ +43.2° (alc). uv max (water) pH 1: 241.5, 288.5, 305, 354 (log ε 4.26, 3.86, 3.92, 3.91); pH 13: 226, 278.5, 307 (log ε 4.43, 3.96, 3.77).

7930. Ptaquiloside. [87625-62-5] 7′a-(β-D-Glucopyranosyloxy)-1′,3′a,4′,7′a-tetrahydro-4′-hydroxy-2′,4′,6′-trimethyl-(2′*R*,3′a*R*,4′*S*,7′a*R*)-spiro[cyclopropane-1,5′-[5*H*]inden]-3′(2′*H*)-one; braxin C; PT. $C_{20}H_{30}O_8$; mol wt 398.45. C 60.29%, H 7.59%, O 32.12%. Norsequiterpene glucoside identified as the carcinogenic prinicple of the bracken ferns, *Pteridium spp.* Isoln from *P. aquilinum* var. *latiusculum:* H. Niwa *et al., Tetrahedron Lett.* **24**, 4117 (1983). Structure elucidation: *eidem, ibid.* 5371. HPLC determn in ferns: M. P. Agnew, D. R. Lauren, *J. Chromatogr.* **538**, 462 (1991). Mechanism of carcinogenesis: M. Ojika *et al., Tetrahedron* **43**, 5261 (1987); A. S. Prakash *et al., Nat. Toxins* **4**, 221 (1996). Levels in cow's milk and health implications: M. E. Alonso-Amelot *et al., Lait* **78**, 413 (1998). Review of chemistry and carcinogenic mechanisms: K. Yamada *et al., Angew. Chem. Int. Ed.* **37**, 1818-1826 (1998); of biological activity: M. Shahin *et al., Mutat. Res.* **443**, 69-79 (1999).

Colorless, hygroscopic, amorphous compound. $[\alpha]_D^{22}$ −188° (c = 1 in methanol). Sol in water, methanol and ethyl acetate.

7931. Pteridine. [91-18-9] Pyrazino[2,3-*d*]pyrimidine; pyrimido[4,5-*b*]pyrazine; pyrimidine-4′,5′:2,3-pyrazine; 1,3,5,8-

tetraazanaphthalene; azinepurine; benzotetrazine. $C_6H_4N_4$; mol wt 132.12. C 54.54%, H 3.05%, N 42.41%. Prepn from 4,5-diaminopyrimidine and polyglyoxal or glyoxal sodium bisulfite: Albert *et al., J. Chem. Soc.* **1951**, 474.

Yellow crystals from benzene, mp 138-138.5°. uv max (water): 298, 309 nm (log ε 3.87, 3.83). Sol in 7.2 parts water at 20-25°.

Caution: Related to folic acid antagonists.

7932. Pterocarpin. [524-97-0] (6a*R-cis*)-6a,12a-Dihydro-3-methoxy-6*H*-[1,3]dioxolo[5,6]benzofuro[3,2-*c*][1]benzopyran. $C_{17}H_{14}O_5$; mol wt 298.29. C 68.45%, H 4.73%, O 26.82%. From red sandalwood *(Pterocarpus santalinus* L.f., *Leguminosae):* Cazeneuve, Hugouneng, *Compt. Rend.* **104**, 1722 (1887); **107**, 737 (1888); Leonhardt, Fay, *Arch. Pharm.* **273**, 53 (1935); McGookin *et al., J. Chem. Soc.* **1940**, 787; from *Pterocarpus* spp: King *et al., ibid.* **1953**, 3693. Structure: Bredenberg, Shoolery, *Tetrahedron Lett.* **1961**, 285. Synthesis of the *dl*-form: Fukui, Nakayama, *ibid.* **1966**, 1805; *eidem, Bull. Chem. Soc. Jpn.* **42**, 1408 (1969); Uchiyama, Matsui, *Agric. Biol. Chem.* **31**, 1490 (1967). Stereochemistry: Ito *et al., Chem. Commun.* **1965**, 595; Pachler, Underwood, *Tetrahedron* **23**, 1817 (1967).

Crystalline plates from petr ether or from ethanol, mp 164.5°. $[\alpha]_D$ −214.5° and $[\alpha]_{5461}^{20.5}$ −207.5° (c = 0.53 in chloroform). Practically insol in water, cold alcohol or ether. Sol in hot alcohol, chloroform.

7933. Pteroic Acid. [119-24-4] 4-[[(2-Amino-1,4-dihydro-4-oxo-6-pteridinyl)methyl]amino]benzoic acid; *p*-[(2-amino-4-hydroxy-6-pteridylmethyl)amino]benzoic acid. $C_{14}H_{12}N_6O_3$; mol wt 312.28. C 53.85%, H 3.87%, N 26.91%, O 15.37%. Intermediate in the synthesis of folic acids. Prepn: Waller *et al., J. Am. Chem. Soc.* **70**, 19 (1948); *cf.* Hultquist *et al., ibid.* 23; Boothe, **US 2472462** (1949 to Am. Cyanamid); C. Temple *et al., J. Org. Chem.* **46**, 3666 (1981). Synthesis: M. G. Nair *et al., ibid.* 3152.

Crystals from dil HCl. Sol in aq NaOH solns.

7934. Pteropterin. [89-38-3] *N*-[*N*-[*N*-[4-[[(2-Amino-1,4-dihydro-4-oxo-6-pteridinyl)methyl]amino]benzoyl]-L-γ-glutamyl]-L-glutamyl]-L-glutamic acid; *N*-[*N*-(*N*-pteroyl-γ-glutamyl)-γ-glutamyl]glutamic acid; fermentation L. casei Factor; pteroyl-γ-glutamyl-γ-glutamylglutamic acid; pteroyldi-γ-glutamylglutamic acid; pteroyltriglutamic acid; PTGA; Teropterin. $C_{29}H_{33}N_9O_{12}$; mol wt 699.63. C 49.78%, H 4.75%, N 18.02%, O 27.44%. Isoln from aerobic culture of *Corynebacterium:* Hutchings *et al., J. Am. Chem. Soc.* **70**, 1 (1948). Identification, structure and synthesis: Boothe *et al., ibid.* 1099; *ibid.* **71**, 2304 (1949). Prepn: Cosulich, **US 2563707** (1951 to Am. Cyanamid).

Forms a crystalline barium salt.

Monohydrate. Crystals from water adjusted to pH 2.8 with HCl and contg some NaCl. Has the general properties of a polypeptide. Absorption spectrum, Hutchings, *loc. cit.* Soly in water at 5°: 0.10 mg/ml; at 80°: 3.00 mg/ml. Sol in NaOH solns.

Methyl ester. Crystals from methanol contg NaCl. Soly in water at 5°: 0.12 mg/ml; at 80°: 1.00 mg/ml; in methanol at −5°: 0.30 mg/ml; at 60°: 5.00 mg/ml.

THERAP CAT: Formerly as antineoplastic.

7935. Pteroylhexaglutamylglutamic Acid. [6484-74-8] Pteroylheptaglutamic acid; vitamin Bc conjugate; Bc conjugate; PHGA. $C_{49}H_{61}N_{13}O_{24}$; mol wt 1216.08. C 48.40%, H 5.06%, N 14.97%, O 31.58%. One of the naturally occurring polyglutamates of folic acid. Isoln from yeast: Pfiffner *et al., Science* **102**, 228 (1945); *J. Am. Chem. Soc.* **68**, 1392 (1946). Solid phase synthesis: C. L. Krumdieck, C. M. Baugh, *Biochemistry* **8**, 1568 (1969); *eidem, Methods Enzymol.* **66**, 523 (1980). Chain length characterization of pteroylpolyglutamates: D. G. Priest *et al., Anal. Biochem.* **115**, 163 (1981).

Rosettes of minute needles from 5% NaCl soln. Has no definite mp. When heated on the hot stage it begins to darken from about 200° and partially melts at 230-260°, and remains partially melted up to 360°. The ultraviolet absorption curves are practically identical with those of folic acid. Sparingly sol in water contg NaCl. Sol in dil NaOH soln.

7936. Pukateine. [81-67-4] (7aR)-6,7,7a,8-Tetrahydro-7-methyl-5H-benzo[g]-1,3-benzodioxolo[6,5,4-de]quinolin-12-ol; 1,2-(methylenedioxy)-6aβ-aporphin-11-ol. $C_{18}H_{17}NO_3$; mol wt 295.33. C 73.20%, H 5.80%, N 4.74%, O 16.25%. From bark of *Laurelia novaezelandiae* A. Cunn, *Lauraceae*. Isoln: Aston, *J. Chem. Soc.* **97**, 1381 (1910); Bernauer, *Helv. Chim. Acta* **50**, 1583 (1967). Structure: Barger, Giradet, *ibid.* **14**, 481, 504 (1931); Barger, Schlittler, *ibid.* **15**, 381 (1932). Total synthesis: Zymalkowski, Happel, *Tetrahedron Lett.* **1969**, 219; *Ber.* **102**, 2959 (1969); Kametani *et al., J. Chem. Soc. Perkin Trans. I* **1972**, 1435.

Crystals from alcohol, mp 208-212°. $[\alpha]_D^{25}$ −240° (c = 0.097 in alcohol). Practically insol in water. Sol in alc, ether, chloroform, pyridine; slightly sol in petr ether.

dl-Form. Crystals from absolute alcohol, mp 232-233°.

7937. Pulegone. [89-82-7] (5R)-5-Methyl-2-(1-methylethylidene)cyclohexanone; R-(+)-p-menth-4(8)-en-3-one; 1-methyl-4-isopropylidene-3-cyclohexanone. $C_{10}H_{16}O$; mol wt 152.23. C 78.90%, H 10.59%, O 10.51%. Found in oils derived from plants of the *Labiatae* family as (+)-form. Readily isolated in quantity from the pennyroyal oils from *Mentha pulegium* L., *M. longifolia* (L.) Huds., and *Hedeoma pulegioides* (L.) Pers., *Labiatae*: Gildemeister, Hoffmann, *Die ätherischen Ole* Vol. I, p 560 (1928); Simonsen, *The Terpenes* Vol. I (2nd ed, 1947) p 370. Synthesis: Kuhn, Schinz, *Helv. Chim. Acta* **36**, 161 (1953). Synthesis of the

(±)-form: Black *et al., J. Chem. Soc.* **1956**, 2971; Wolinsky *et al., J. Org. Chem.* **30**, 3207 (1965); of the S(−)-form: E. J. Corey *et al., ibid.* **41**, 380 (1976). Improved synthesis of the R(+)-form: T. Sato *et al., Tetrahedron Lett.* **1980**, 3377. Conversion of the R(+) to the S(−)-form: H. E. Ensley, R. V. C. Carr, *ibid.* **1977**, 513. Biosynthetic study: A. Akhila, D. V. Banthorpe, *Z. Pflanzenphysiol.* **99**, 277 (1980), *C.A.* **94**, 2073r (1981).

Oil. Pleasant odor, midway between peppermint and camphor. d_4^{15} 0.9346. bp_{760} 224°; bp_{100} 151-153°; bp_{17} 103°; bp_6 84°. $[\alpha]_D^{20}$ +21°; $[\alpha]_{546}^{20}$ +28.2°. n_D^{20} 1.4894. Practically insol in water. Miscible with alcohol, ether, chloroform.

(±)-Form. Liquid. bp_7 78-80°. n_D^{16} 1.4856. uv max (alc): 253.3 nm (log ε 3.86).

(−)-Form. Liquid. bp_{20} 104-108°. $[\alpha]_D^{23}$ −22.5° (neat).

7938. Pulsatilla. Pasque flower; wind flower; meadow anemone; Easter flower. Dried herb of *Anemone pulsatilla* L. (*Pulsatilla vulgaris* Mill.), *A. pratensis* L. (*P. pratensis* (L.) Mill.), or *A. patens* L. (*P. patens* (L.) Mill.), *Ranunculaceae*. Habit. Europe, Asia. *Constit.* Anemone camphor, volatile oil, tannin.

7939. Pumactant. ALEC; Zofac. Artificial lung expanding compound composed of **dipalmitoylphosphatidylcholine** (DPPC) and egg **phosphatidylglycerol** in a 7:3 (w/w) ratio. Description of prepn and clinical evaluation in premature babies: C. J. Morley *et al., Lancet* **1**, 64 (1981). Clinical trials in premature babies: Ten Centre Study Group, *Br. Med. J.* **294**, 991 (1987). Review of physical properties and design of mixture: A. D. Bangham *et al., Easy Breathing and the Design of Artificial Lung Expanding Compounds* (ALEC) in *Topics in Lipid Research*, R. Klein, B. Schmitz, Eds (Royal Society of Chemistry, London, Great Britain, 1986) 268-275; of various surfactant treatments: C. J. Morley, in *Surfactant Replacement Therapy*, D. L. Shapiro, R. H. Notter, Eds (Alan R. Liss, Inc., NY, NY, 1989) 219-234. Clinical trial in treatment of asthma: K. S. Babu *et al., Eur. Resp. J.* **21**, 1046 (2003).

Fine crystalline powder.

THERAP CAT: Pulmonary surfactant.

7940. Pumice. Light, hard, rough, porous, gray masses or a gritty, gray-colored powder of volcanic origin. Found chiefly in the Lipari islands and in the Greek archipelagos. Consists mainly of complex silicates of Al, K, and Na. It is insol in water and is not attacked by acids.

USE: Abrasive in metal polishes; in fireproofing and insulating compds; also as a carrier for metal catalysts. In pharmacy as filtering medium and dispersant. In cosmetics for removing rough skin.

7941. Pumpkin Seed. Pepo. Dried ripe seeds of cultivated varities of *Cucurbita pepo* L., *Cucurbitaceae*. Habit. Southern Asia, Europe, America. *Constit.* Fixed oil, acrid resin, myosin, vitellin, sugar.

THERAP CAT: Anthelmintic.

7942. 1H-Purine. [120-73-0] 7H-Imidazo[4,5-d]pyrimidine. $C_5H_4N_4$; mol wt 120.11. C 50.00%, H 3.36%, N 46.65%. Prepd by heating 4,5-diaminopyrimidine with anhyd formic acid in a current of carbon dioxide: Isay, *Ber.* **39**, 251 (1906); by boiling 2,6-diiodopurine with zinc dust and water under carbon dioxide: Fischer, *ibid.* **31**, 2551, 2564 (1898).

Needles from toluene or alcohol, mp 216-217° (partial sublimation on rapid heating). Freely sol in water, hot alcohol. Slightly sol in hot ethyl acetate, acetone. Practically insol in ether, chloroform. Aq solns are neutral to litmus. Forms salts with acids and bases.

7943. Puromycin. [53-79-2] 3′-[[(2S)-2-Amino-3-(4-methoxyphenyl)-1-oxopropyl]amino]-3′-deoxy-N,N-dimethyladenosine; L-3′-(α-amino-p-methoxyhydrocinnamamido)-3′-deoxy-N,N-dimethyladenosine; 6-dimethylamino-9-[3-deoxy-3-(p-methoxy-L-phenylalanylamino)-β,D-ribofuranosyl]-β-purine; 6-dimethylamino-9-[3′-(p-methoxy-L-phenylalanylamino)-3′-deoxy-β,D-ribofuranosyl]purine; stylomycin; CL-13900; P-638; 3123-L. $C_{22}H_{29}N_7$-O_5; mol wt 471.51. C 56.04%, H 6.20%, N 20.79%, O 16.97%. Aminonucleoside antibiotic produced by the soil actinomycete *Streptomyces alboniger*. Structural analog of aminoacyl-tRNA; inhibits protein synthesis. Isoln: J. N. Porter *et al.*, *Antibiot. Chemother.* **2**, 409 (1952); *eidem*, US 2763642 (1956 to Am. Cyanamid). Structure: C. W. Waller *et al.*, *J. Am. Chem. Soc.* **75**, 2025 (1953); P. W. Fryth *et al.*, *ibid.* **80**, 2736 (1958). Synthesis: B. R. Baker *et al.*, *ibid.* **76**, 4044 (1954); **77**, 12 (1955); M. J. Robins *et al.*, *J. Org. Chem.* **66**, 8204 (2001). Conformation: O. Jardetzky, *J. Am. Chem. Soc.* **85**, 1823 (1963). Effect on protein synthesis: D. Nathans, *Proc. Natl. Acad. Sci. USA* **51**, 585 (1964). Use in gene transfer studies: S. de la Luna *et al.*, *Gene* **62**, 121 (1988). *Review:* D. Nathans in *Antibiotics* **vol. I**, D. Gottlieb, P. D. Shaw, Eds. (Springer-Verlag, New York, 1967) pp 259-277.

Crystals from water, mp 175.5-177°. $[\alpha]_D^{25}$ −11° (ethanol). uv max (0.1N NaOH): 275 nm (ε 20300); in 0.1N HCl: 267.5 nm (ε 19500). pKa: 6.8, 7.2. Sparingly sol in water, organic solvents. LD_{50} in mice (mg/kg): 350 i.v.; 525 i.p.; 675 orally (Porter, 1952).
Dihydrochloride. [58-58-2] $C_{22}H_{29}N_7O_5$.2HCl; mol wt 544.43. White crystals or powder. Prepd as the dihydrate, mp 174° (dec). Sol in water.
USE: Research tool for studying protein synthesis; cell line selection agent in gene transfer experiments.

7944. Purothionin. [9009-72-7] A low mol wt wheat protein composed of α_1-, α_2- and β-purothionins. Contains about 20% cystine, 10% arginine and 10% lysine. Isoln from unbleached patent flour: A. K. Balls, W. S. Hale, *Cereal Chem.* **17**, 243 (1940); A. K. Balls *et al.*, *ibid.* **19**, 279 (1942). Inhibits the growth of bacteria and yeasts: L. S. Stuart, T. H. Harris, *ibid.* 288. Toxic effects in animals: E. J. Coulson *et al.*, *ibid.* 301. Sepn and characterization of α- and β-purothionin: D. G. Redman, N. Fisher, *J. Sci. Food Agric.* **19**, 651 (1968); C. C. Nimmo *et al.*, *ibid.* **25**, 607 (1974). Amino acid sequences of α_1- and β-purothionin: S. Ohtani *et al.*, *Agric. Biol. Chem.* **39**, 2269 (1975); *eidem*, *J. Biochem.* **82**, 753 (1977); of β-purothionin: A. S. Mak, B. L. Jones, *Can. J. Chem.* **54**, 835 (1976); of α_1 and α_2-purothionin: B. L. Jones, A. S. Mak, *Cereal Chem.* **54**, 511 (1977). *Review:* D. D. Kasarda *et al.*, "Wheat Proteins" in *Advances in Cereal Science and Technology* **vol. 1** (Am. Cereal Chem., St. Paul, 1976) pp 208-210.
Forms a cryst hydrochloride. Freely sol in water. Easily digested by proteolytic enzymes including cryst chymotrypsin, chymopapain, papain.
α_1-**Purothionin.** 5-L-Arginine-27-glycine-33-L-isoleucine-34-L-serine-42-glycine-purothionin A I (reduced); purothionin A II. $C_{198}H_{340}N_{68}O_{56}S_8$; mol wt 4825.76.
α_2-**Purothionin.** 5-L-Arginine-6-L-threonine-18-L-serine-26-L-serine-27-L-threonine-42-glycine-purothionin A I (reduced). C_{202}-$H_{348}N_{68}O_{59}S_8$; mol wt 4929.86.

β-Purothionin. Purothionin A I. $C_{203}H_{339}N_{67}O_{59}S_8$; mol wt 4918.80.

7945. Purpurin. [81-54-9] 1,2,4-Trihydroxy-9,10-anthracenedione; 1,2,4-trihydroxyanthraquinone; C.I. Natural Red 8; C.I. Natural Red 16; C.I. 58205; C.I. 75410. $C_{14}H_8O_5$; mol wt 256.21. C 65.63%, H 3.15%, O 31.22%. Occurs as glycoside in the madder root *(Rubia tinctorum* L., *Rubiaceae)* of commerce. Is formed during storage; no appreciable amount in the fresh root: Hill, Richter, *J. Chem. Soc.* **1936**, 1714. Although a dye itself, it is usually considered as an undesirable contaminant of alizarin extracted from madder. May be prepd from alizarin by oxidation with ammonium persulfate: Wacker, *J. Prakt. Chem.* [2] **54**, 90 (1896); also by Friedel-Crafts condensation of hydroxyhydroquinone with phthalic anhydride: Dimroth, Fick, *Ann.* **411**, 321 (1916).

Long orange needles with 1 H_2O from dil alcohol, anhydr at 100°. Anhydr red needles from abs alcohol or by sublimation around 150° in high vacuum (less than 2 mm Hg). mp 257°. Absorption spectrum: Meek, *J. Chem. Soc.* **111**, 969 (1917); Ezaby, *ibid. (B)* **1970**, 1293. More sol in boiling water than alizarin (yellow color with yellowish hue). Freely sol in alcohol (red), in ether (intensely yellow with fluorescence). Soluble in benzene, toluene, xylene (dark yellow), in boiling alum soln (red).
2-Methyl ether. $C_{15}H_{10}O_5$. Orange crystals from benzene, mp 240°.
2,4-Dimethyl ether. $C_{16}H_{12}O_5$. Orange needles, mp 186-189°.
USE: Forms colored "lakes" with various metal salts and is a fast dye for cotton printing. Now used mostly in the manuf of acid and chrome dyes. Reagent for the detection of boron; for detection of insol calcium salts in the cell contents of histological material and as a nuclear stain.

7946. Purpurogallin. [569-77-7] 2,3,4,6-Tetrahydroxy-5H-benzocyclohepten-5-one. $C_{11}H_8O_5$; mol wt 220.18. C 60.00%, H 3.66%, O 36.33%. The aglycone of several glycosides from various nutgalls. Prepn by oxidation of pyrogallol: Perkin, Steven, *J. Chem. Soc.* **83**, 192 (1903); Perkin, *ibid.* **101**, 803 (1912); Nierenstein, Spiers, *Ber.* **46**, 3151 (1913); Evans, Dehn, *J. Am. Chem. Soc.* **52**, 3647 (1930). Structure: Willstätter, Heiss, *Ann.* **433**, 17 (1923); Barltrop, Nicholson, *J. Chem. Soc.* **1948**, 116. Synthesis: Caunt *et al.*, *ibid.* **1950**, 1631; **1951**, 1313.

Deep red needles from glacial acetic acid, dec 274-275°. Sparingly sol in most solvents.
Diglucoside. Dryophantin. $C_{23}H_{28}O_{15}$. Coloring matter of "red pea" gall produced by *Dryophanta divisa* Ald. on *Quercus pedunculata* Ehrh., *Fagaceae:* Nierenstein, *J. Chem. Soc.* **115**, 1328 (1919); Nierenstein, Swanton, *Biochem. J.* **38**, 373 (1944). Dark red needles with bronze luster, mp 220-221°. Slightly sol in water, cold alcohol; sol in boiling alcohol; in methanol, acetone.
USE: As an additive to edible or inedible fats or oils, hydrocarbon fuels or lubricants, retards oxidation or metal contamination: Thompson, US 2770545 (1956 to Universal Oil Prod.).

7947. Putrescine. [110-60-1] 1,4-Butanediamine; tetramethylenediamine. $C_4H_{12}N_2$; mol wt 88.15. C 54.50%, H 13.72%, N 31.78%. $NH_2(CH_2)_4NH_2$. Biogenic polyamine and precursor of spermidine, *q.v.*, initially detected in decaying animal tissues, but now known to be present in all cells and certain bacterial cultures. It is essential for both normal and neoplastic tissue growth. Formed via decarboxylation of ornithine or by decarboxylation of arginine, followed by hydrolysis. Prepn: A. Ladenburg, *Ber.* **19**, 780 (1886); G. Ciamician, C. U. Zanetti, *ibid.* **22**, 1970 (1889); R. Willstätter, W. Heubner, *ibid.* **40**, 3871 (1907); of the dihydrochloride: *Org. Synth.* **coll. vol. IV** (1963) p 819. Role in cell growth processes: C. W. Tabor, H. Tabor, *Annu. Rev. Biochem.* **45**, 285 (1976); J. Janne *et al., Biochim. Biophys. Acta* **473**, 241 (1978). Formation and interconversion of putrescine and spermidine in mammalian cells: A. E. Pegg *et al., Adv. Enzyme Regul.* **19**, 427 (1980). Biosynthetic study in fungi: L. Stevens, *Med. Biol.* **59**, 308 (1981). Regulation of tRNA methyl transferase activity: M. Mach *et al., Biochem. J.* **202**, 153 (1982). Alteration of DNA conformation in rat brain tumor cells by depletion of intracellular putrescine: D. T. Hung *et al., Science* **221**, 368 (1983). Use of labeled putrescine as a positron-emission tomographic tracer in brain tumors: N. Volkow *et al., ibid.* 673. Reviews of early literature: M. Guggenheim, *Die biogenen Amine* (S. Karger, Basel, 1951, 4th ed.) 619 pp; H. Tabor *et al., Annu. Rev. Biochem.* **30**, 579-604 (1961). Review of formation of GABA, the major inhibitory neurotransmitter in vertebrate brains, from putrescine: N. Seiler, *Physiol. Chem. Phys.* **12**, 411-429 (1980). Review of metabolism: T. L. Sourkes, K. Missala, *Agents Actions* **11**, 20-27 (1981). Book: *Polyamines in Biology and Medicine*, D. R. Morris, L. J. Marton, Eds. (Dekker, New York, 1981) 512 pp.

Colorless oil, bp 158-160°. Cryst on cooling, mp 23-24°. Strong piperidine-like odor. Very sol in water.

Dihydrochloride. $C_4H_{12}N_2 \cdot 2HCl$. Cryst from 85% alc, mp >275°.

USE: As a tool in biochemical research.

7948. PVNO. [26715-00-4] 4-Ethenylpyridine 1-oxide homopolymer; poly(4-vinylpyridine-*N*-oxide); PVPNO. $(C_7H_7NO)_x$. Prepn and thermal properties: P. Ranganathan *et al., J. Polym. Sci. A* **28**, 2711 (1990). Viscosity and light scattering: C.-M. Lee *et al., Polymer* **37**, 4283 (1996); fluorescence and metal-ion complexation: Y. Okamoto *et al., Macromolecules* **31**, 9201 (1998). Interaction with sodium dodecyl sulfate, *q.v.*: P. Bahadur *et al., Langmuir* **11**, 1951 (1995). Use as a dye transfer inhibitor: R. K. Panandiker *et al.*, **WO 9513354**; *idem*, **US 5466802** (both 1995 to Proctor & Gamble); as adsorbent stabilizer for metal catalysis: A. B. R. Mayer, J. E. Mark, *J. Macromol. Sci. Pure Appl. Chem.* **A34**, 2151 (1997); T. Balakrishnan, V. Rajendran, *J. Appl. Polym. Sci.* **78**, 2075 (2000). GC/MS determn in laundry detergents: T. Uchiyama *et al., J. Anal. Appl. Pyrolysis* **45**, 111 (1998).

Crystallized as white solid monomer from benzene-hexane. mp 122°. Polymerizes at 100-125° under vacuum in a sealed tube; decomposes 290°. uv max (water): 257 nm (ε 19844). Sol in water and acidic media. Insol in most organic solvents including DMSO, dimethylacetamide, THF, and acetone.

USE: Dye transfer inhibitor used in laundry detergents. Support for metal catalysts.

7949. Pygeum Africanum Extract. [85865-74-3] Tadenan. Extract from the bark of the tree *Pygeum africanum* Hook, also known as *Prunus africana* (Hook) F. Kalkm (Rosaceae-Amygdaleae), which is native to tropical Asia and Africa. Prepn: J. Debat, **FR 1578711**; *idem*, **FR M6703**; *idem*, **US 3856946** (1969, 1969, 1974 all to Labs. du Debat). Pharmacology: L. Thieblot *et al., Therapie* **26**, 575 (1971). Identification of 1-docosanol, *q.v.*, as active principle: *idem et al., ibid.* **32**, 99 (1977). Characterization of components: R. Longo, S. Tira, *Farmaco Ed. Prat.* **38**, 287 (1983); E. M. Martinelli *et al., J. High Resolut. Chromatogr. Chromatogr. Commun.* **9**, 106 (1986). Clinical study in BPH: A. Barlet *et al., Wien. Klin. Wochenschr.* **102**, 667 (1990). Review of clinical experience: A. Ishani *et al., Am. J. Med.* **109**, 654-664 (2000).

THERAP CAT: In treatment of micturitional disorders due to benign prostatic hypertrophy.

7950. Pymetrozine. [123312-89-0] *(E)*-4,5-Dihydro-6-methyl-4-[(3-pyridinylmethylene)amino]-1,2,4-triazin-3(2H)-one; CGA-215944; Plenum; Fulfill. $C_{10}H_{11}N_5O$; mol wt 217.23. C 55.29%, H 5.10%, N 32.24%, O 7.37%. Pyridine azomethine antifeedant. Prepn: H. Kristinsson, **EP 314615**; *idem*, **US 4931439** (1989, 1990 both to Ciba-Geigy). Comprehensive description: C. R. Flückiger *et al., Brighton Crop Prot. Conf. - Pests Dis.* **1992**, 43-50. Field trials against aphids and white flies: *idem et al., ibid.* 1187. Historical account of discovery, synthesis, and development: H. Kristinsson, *Spec. Publ. - R. Soc. Chem.* **147**, 85-102 (1994).

Crystalline, mp 234.4°. Vapor pressure at 20°: $< 9.7 \times 10^{-8}$ Pa. Soly at 20° (g/l): water 0.270; ethanol 2.25; hexane <0.001. Partition coefficient (*n*-octanol/water): 0.2. LD_{50} orally in rats: 5820 mg/kg (Flückiger).

USE: Insecticide.

7951. Pyocyanine. [85-66-5] 5-Methyl-1(5H)-phenazinone. $C_{13}H_{10}N_2O$; mol wt 210.23. C 74.27%, H 4.79%, N 13.33%, O 7.61%. Blue redox pigment produced by *Pseudomonas aeruginosa*. Important virulence factor in pseudomonal infection. Isoln: Wrede, Strack, *Z. Physiol. Chem.* **140**, 1 (1924); Schoental, *Br. J. Exp. Pathol.* **22**, 137 (1941). Synthesis: Wrede, Strack, *Z. Physiol. Chem.* **181**, 58 (1929); *Ber.* **62**, 2051 (1929); Surrey, *Org. Synth.* **26**, 86 (1946); **coll. vol. III**, 753 (1955). HPLC determn in sputum: R. Wilson *et al., Infect. Immun.* **56**, 2515 (1988). Review of biosynthesis and role in pathogenesis: G. W. Lau *et al., Trends Mol. Med.* **10**, 599-606 (2004).

Dark blue needles from water (usually with 1 H_2O which is lost at 50° over P_2O_5 *in vacuo*). mp 133°. Upon further heating it sublimes with decompn. Absorption spectrum: Nitzsche, *Ber.* **77**, 337 (1944). Freely sol in chloroform. Sol in nitrobenzene, pyridine, phenol, acetic acid, hot water, hot alcohol. Slightly sol in cold water and benzene. The blue water soln, made alkaline with Na_2CO_3, is easily rendered colorless by reduction with glucose or sodium hydrosulfite. Acidic $KMnO_4$ solns are decolorized by pyocyanine. An alkaline water soln of pyocyanine acquires a maroon color upon heating.

7952. Py-Phe. [199612-75-0] *N*-[1-Oxo-4-(1-pyrenyl)butyl]-L-phenylalanine; *N*-(1-phenylalanine)-4-(1-pyrene)butyramide. $C_{29}H_{25}NO_3$; mol wt 435.51. C 79.98%, H 5.79%, N 3.22%, O 11.02%. Photoactivated chemical protease. Prepn: C. V. Kumar, A. Buranaprapuk, *Angew. Chem. Int. Ed.* **36**, 2085 (1997). Site specificity: *idem et al., Proc. Natl. Acad. Sci. USA* **95**, 10361 (1998).

ε 42600 $M^{-1}cm^{-1}$ at 343 nm.

USE: Photocleavage probe.

7953. Pyraclostrobin. [175013-18-0] [2-[[[1-(4-Chlorophenyl)-1*H*-pyrazol-3-yl]oxy]methyl]phenyl]methoxycarbamic acid methyl ester; methyl *N*-[2-[[1-(4-chlorophenyl)-1*H*-pyrazol-3-yl]oxymethyl]phenyl]-*N*-methoxycarbamate; BAS-500F; Cabrio; Comet; Headline. $C_{19}H_{18}ClN_3O_4$; mol wt 387.82. C 58.84%, H 4.68%, Cl 9.14%, N 10.83%, O 16.50%. Strobilurin fungicide for use in seed grass and food crops. Prepn: B. Müller *et al., DE 4423612; eidem, US 5869517* (1996, 1999 both to BASF). Comprehensive description: E. Ammermann *et al., Brighton Crop Prot. Conf. - Pests Dis.* **2000**, 541-548. Review of activity and field trials: R. Stierl *et al., ibid.* 859-864.

White or light beige crystalline solid, mp 63.7-65.2°. Vapor pressure at 20°: 2.6×10^{-8} Pa. Log P (*n*-octanol/water) at 22°: 3.99. Soly in water (20°): 1.9 mg/l. LD_{50} in rats (mg/kg): >5000 orally; >2000 dermally; LC_{50} in rainbow trout: 0.006 mg/l (Ammermann).

USE: Agricultural fungicide.

7954. Pyranine. [6358-69-6]; [27928-00-3] (free acid). 8-Hydroxy-1,3,6-pyrenetrisulfonic acid trisodium salt; C.I. 59040; C.I. Solvent Green 7; HPTS. $C_{16}H_7Na_3O_{10}S_3$; mol wt 524.39. C 36.65%, H 1.35%, Na 13.15%, O 30.51%, S 18.34%. Fluorescent dye with pH-sensitive spectral properties. Prepn: E. Tietze, O. Bayer, *Ann.* **540**, 189 (1939). Use as a pH probe for liposome interiors: K. Kano, J. H. Fendler, *Biochim. Biophys. Acta* **509**, 289 (1978); for phospholipid vesicles: N. R. Clement, J. M. Gould, *Biochemistry* **20**, 1534 (1981); in yeast cells: A. Peña *et al., J. Bacteriol.* **177**, 1017 (1995); in organelles: C. C. Overly *et al., Proc. Natl. Acad. Sci. USA* **92**, 3156 (1995); in cytosol: B. S. Gan *et al., Am. J. Physiol. Cell Physiol.* **275**, 1158 (1998). Effects of salt and polyethylene glycol concentration on pKa: Y. Avnir, Y. Barenholz, *Anal. Biochem.* **347**, 34 (2005). Review of use as a biological stain: *Conn's Biological Stains*, R. W. Horobin, J. A. Kiernan, Eds. (BIOS Scientific Publishers Ltd, Oxford, UK, 10th ed., 2002) 399-400.

Crystals from aq acetone. pKa 7.22 ± 0.04. Changes from blue to green at pH 6.5-7.5. Highly sol in water; slightly sol in glacial acetic acid. Absorption max (acidic aq soln): 403 nm. Absorption max (aq alkali soln): 454 nm. Emission max (aq alkali soln): 511 nm.

USE: Fluorescent pH indicator for biological systems. Biological stain; dye for solvents, cosmetics and pharmaceuticals.

7955. Pyrantel. [15686-83-6] (*E*)-1,4,5,6-Tetrahydro-1-methyl-2-[2-(2-thienyl)ethenyl]pyrimidine. $C_{11}H_{14}N_2S$; mol wt 206.31. C 64.04%, H 6.84%, N 13.58%, S 15.54%. Prepn: **BE 658987** (1965 to Pfizer), *C.A.* **64**, 8192c (1966); Austin *et al., Nature* **212**, 1273 (1966); Kasubrick, McFarland, **ZA 6800516**; *eidem,* **US 3502661** (1968, 1970 both to Pfizer). Structure-activity studies: McFarland *et al., J. Med. Chem.* **12**, 1066 (1969). Pharmacology and animal trials: Cornwell, *Vet. Rec.* **79**, 590 (1966); Howes, Lynch, *J. Parasitol.* **53**, 1085 (1967); Eyre, *J. Pharm. Pharmacol.* **22**, 26 (1970).

Crystals from methanol, mp 178-179°.

Tartrate. [33401-94-4] CP-10423-18; Banminth; Strongid. $C_{11}H_{14}N_2 \cdot C_4H_6O_6$; mol wt 356.39. White crystals from hot methanol, mp 148-150°. uv max (water): 312 nm (log ε 4.27).

Pamoate. [22204-24-6] Pyrantel embonate; CP-10423-16; Cobantril; Combantrin; Helmex; Helmintox; Nemex. $C_{11}H_{14}N_2 \cdot C_{23}H_{16}O_6$; mol wt 594.68. Tasteless, yellow crystalline powder. Insol in water.

THERAP CAT: Anthelmintic (Nematodes).

THERAP CAT (VET): Anthelmintic (Nematodes).

7956. Pyrazinamide. [98-96-4] Pyrazinecarboxamide; pyrazinoic acid amide; pyrazine carboxylamide; D-50; Pezetamid; Pyrafat; Pirilène; Piraldina; Tebrazid; Unipyranamide; Zinamide. $C_5H_5N_3O$; mol wt 123.11. C 48.78%, H 4.09%, N 34.13%, O 13.00%. Prepn: O. Dalmer, E. Walter, **DE 632257** (1936 to E. Merck); *eidem,* **US 2149279** (1939 to Merck & Co.); S. A. Hall, P. E. Spoerri, *J. Am. Chem. Soc.* **62**, 664 (1940). Structure-activity study: S. Kushner *et al., ibid.* **74**, 3617 (1952). Pharmacology: I. M. Weiner, J. P. Tinker, *J. Pharmacol. Exp. Ther.* **180**, 411 (1972). HPLC determn in biological samples: J. E. Conte, Jr. *et al., J. Chromatogr. Sci.* **38**, 33 (2000). Clinical pharmacokinetics: C. A. Peloquin *et al., Pharmacotherapy* **18**, 1205 (1998). Clinical trial in combination with rifampicin and isoniazid, *q.q.v.:* S. K. Teo, *Int. J. Tuberc. Lung Dis.* **3**, 126 (1999); in prevention of tuberculosis: F. Gordin *et al., J. Am. Med. Assoc.* **283**, 1445 (2000). Comprehensive description: E. Feldner, D. Pitre, *Anal. Profiles Drug Subs.* **12**, 433-462 (1983). Review of clinical experience: M. A. Steele, R. M. Des Prez, *Chest* **94**, 845-850 (1988).

Crystals from water or alcohol, mp 189-191°. Begins to sublime at 60°. pKa 0.5. uv max: 269 nm ($E_{1cm}^{1\%}$ 660). Soly (mg/ml): water 15; methanol 13.8; abs ethanol 5.7; isopropanol 3.8; ether 1.0; isooctane 0.01; chloroform 7.4. Aq solns are neutral.

THERAP CAT: Antibacterial (tuberculostatic).

7957. Pyrazine. [290-37-9] 1,4-Diazine; paradiazine. $C_4H_4N_2$; mol wt 80.09. C 59.99%, H 5.03%, N 34.98%. Prepn: S. Gabriel, G. Pinkus, *Ber.* **26**, 2197 (1893); P. Brandes, C. Stoehr, *J. Prakt. Chem.* [2] **54**, 481 (1896). *See also: Beilstein* **XXIII**, 91 (1936). Crystal structure: G. De With *et al., Acta Crystallogr.* **B32**, 3178 (1976).

Crystals or wax-like solid. Strong pyridine-like odor. d_4^{61} 1.031; mp 53°; bp 115-118°; n_D^{61} 1.4953. Freely sol in water, alcohol, ether. Volatile with steam.

7958. 2,3-Pyrazinedicarboxylic Acid. [89-01-0] $C_6H_4N_2O_4$; mol wt 168.11. C 42.87%, H 2.40%, N 16.66%, O 38.07%. Prepd by permanganate oxidation of quinoxaline: Gabriel, Sonn, *Ber.* **40**, 4850 (1907); Sausville, Spoerri, *J. Am. Chem. Soc.* **63**, 3153 (1941); Jones, McLaughlin, *Org. Synth.* **30**, 86 (1950).

Dihydrate. Prisms from water. Becomes anhydr at 100°, then melts at 183-185° (with evolution of CO_2). The dry dust provokes sneezing. Freely sol in water. Soluble in methanol, acetone, ethyl acetate. Slightly sol in ethanol, ether, chloroform, benzene, petr ether.

Dimethyl ester. $C_8H_8N_2O_4$. Crystals, mp 50°. Sol in water, acetone. Insol in benzene, petr ether.

Diamide. $C_6H_6N_4O_2$. Crystals, dec 240°. Sol in boiling water.

7959. Pyrazinoic Acid. [98-97-5] Pyrazinecarboxylic acid; pyrazinemonocarboxylic acid. $C_5H_4N_2O_2$; mol wt 124.10. C 48.39%, H 3.25%, N 22.57%, O 25.78%. Prepn by thermal decompn of 2,3-pyrazinedicarboxylic acid: Hall, Spoerri, *J. Am. Chem. Soc.* **62**, 664 (1940); by oxidation of alkylpyrazines: Gainer, *J. Org. Chem.* **24**, 691 (1959).

Fine white needles from water, dec 225-229°. Sublimes. pK (25°) 2.92. Slightly sol in cold water, more sol in hot water. One gram dissolves in 120 g abs ethanol at 25°. Practically insol in ether, chloroform, benzene.

Methyl ester. Crystals from ether, mp 59°.

Amide see Pyrazinamide.

7960. Pyrazole. [288-13-1] 1,2-Diazole. $C_3H_4N_2$; mol wt 68.08. C 52.93%, H 5.92%, N 41.15%. Prepn from acetylene and diazomethane: H. v. Pechmann, *Ber.* **31**, 2950 (1898). Two tautomeric forms. ^{1}H-NMR: J. F. K. Wilshire, *Aust. J. Chem.* **19**, 1935 (1966); ^{13}C-NMR: W. M. Litchman, *J. Am. Chem. Soc.* **101**, 545 (1979); ^{15}N-NMR: I. I. Schuster *et al., J. Org. Chem.* **44**, 1765 (1979). Spectral studies: D. Dumanovic *et al., Talanta* **22**, 819 (1975). Inhibition of alcohol dehydrogenase: W. K. Lelbach, *Experientia* **25**, 816 (1969). Induction of thyroid necrosis: S. Szabo *et al., Science* **199**, 1209 (1979). Toxicity: G. Magnussen *et al., Experientia* **28**, 1198 (1972).

Needles or prisms from petr ether; pyridine-like odor, bitter taste. mp 69.5-70°. bp$_{757.9}$ 186-188°. pK (25°) 11.52. uv max (12M H_2SO_4): 215 nm (log ε 3.76); at pH 6.1: 310 nm (log ε 3.61). Sol in water, alcohol, ether, benzene. LD$_{50}$ (24 hr) in rats, mice (mmol/kg): 19, 21 i.v.; 21, 22 orally (Magnussen).

USE: Chelating agent; in organic synthesis.

7961. 2-Pyrazoline. [109-98-8] 4,5-Dihydro-1H-pyrazole. $C_3H_6N_2$; mol wt 70.09. C 51.41%, H 8.63%, N 39.97%. Prepn from ethylene and diazomethane: Azzarello, *Atti Accad. Lincei* [5] **14**, II, 285 (1905).

Liquid. Faint amine odor. An odor resembling chocolate has been detected in some prepns. d$_4^{17}$ 1.0200. bp$_{760}$ 144°. Volatile with steam. $n_{587}^{17.2}$ 1.4796. Miscible with water, alc.

7962. Pyrazophos. [13457-18-6] 2-[(Diethoxyphosphinothioyl)oxy]-5-methylpyrazolo[1,5-a]pyrimidine-6-carboxylic acid ethyl ester; 2-hydroxy-5-methylpyrazolo[1,5-a]pyrimidine-6-carboxylic acid ethyl ester, O-ester with O,O-diethyl phosphorothioate; HOE-2873; Afugan; Curamil. $C_{14}H_{20}N_3O_5PS$; mol wt 373.36. C 45.04%, H 5.40%, N 11.25%, O 21.43%, P 8.30%, S 8.59%. Systemic fungicide. Prepn: NL 6602131; O. Scherer, H. Mildenberger, US 3632757 (1966, 1972 both to Hoechst). Account of fungicidal properties and toxicity: F. M. Smit, *Meded. Rijksfac. Landbouwwet. Gent* **34**, 763 (1969), *C.A.* **73**, 76038w (1970). In control of rusty spot on peaches: R. H. Daines, *Plant Dis. Res.* **58**, 254 (1974). Effectiveness against powdery mildew: D. J. Butt *et al., Ann. Appl. Biol.* **75**, 217 (1973); F. O. Riordain, *Plant Dis. Rep.* **58**, 12 (1974); R. T. Burchill, M. E. Cook, *Plant Pathol.* **24**, 194

(1975). Enzymatic detection by TLC: G. F. Ernst, F. Schuring, *J. Chromatogr.* **49**, 325 (1970). Absorption and metabolism by plants: S. Gorbach *et al., Environ. Qual. Saf. Suppl.* **3**, 840 (1975).

Yellow oil, mp 38-40°C. LD$_{50}$ in rats, marmots, rabbits (mg/kg): 140, 184, 435 orally (Smit).

USE: Fungicide.

7963. Pyrene. [129-00-0] Benzo[def]phenanthrene. $C_{16}H_{10}$; mol wt 202.25. C 95.02%, H 4.98%. Occurs in coal tar, q.v. Isoln: Kruber, *Ber.* **64**, 84 (1931). Also obtained by the destructive hydrogenation of hard coal: I. G. Farben., **DE 639240; DE 640580; DE 654201**. Purification by chromatography: Winterstein *et al., Z. Physiol. Chem.* **230**, 162 (1934). Synthesis from o,o'-ditolyl: Weitzenböck, *Monatsh. Chem.* **34**, 193 (1913). From peri-trimethylenenaphthalene and malonyl chloride with AlCl₃: Fleischer, Retze, *Ber.* **55**, 3280 (1922). From α-tetralone: Braun, Rath, *Ber.* **61**, 956 (1928). From 4-keto-1,2,3,4-tetrahydrophenanthrene by a Reformatsky reaction: Cook, Hewett, *J. Chem. Soc.* **1934**, 366. Review of toxicology and human exposure: *Toxicological Profile for Polycyclic Aromatic Hydrocarbons* (PB95-264370, 1995) 487 pp.

Monoclinic prismatic tablets from alcohol or by sublimation. d^{23} 1.271. Pure pyrene is colorless, the usual contaminant which gives it a yellow color is tetracene. Solid and solns have slight blue fluorescence. mp 156°. bp 404°. Absorption spectrum: Clar, *Ber.* **69**, 1677 (1936); Seshan, *Proc. Indian Acad. Sci.* **A3**, 148 (1936). Fluorescence maxima: Sannié, Poremski, *Bull. Soc. Chim.* [5] **3**, 1139 (1936). Insol in water. Fairly sol in organic solvents.

7964. Pyrethrins. Active insecticidal constituents of pyrethrum flowers. Isoln: Staudinger, Ruzicka, *Helv. Chim. Acta* **7**, 177 (1924). Prepn by reconstitution from pyrethrolone and chrysanthemic acid: Elliott, Janes, *Chem. Ind. (London)* **1969**, 270. Structure: Crombie *et al., J. Chem. Soc.* **1956**, 3963; Godin *et al., ibid. (C)* **1966**, 332. Stereochemistry: Begley *et al., Chem. Commun.* **1972**, 1276. Biosynthesis: Crowley *et al., Biochim. Biophys. Acta* **60**, 312 (1962). *Review:* Crombie, Elliott, *Fortschr. Chem. Org. Naturst.* **19**, 120 (1961). Review of toxicology and human exposure: *Toxicological Profile for Pyrethrins and Pyrethroids* (PB-2004-100004, 2003) 332 pp.

Pyrethrin I   R = CH₃
Pyrethrin II   R = COOCH₃

Pyrethrin I. [121-21-1] (1R,3R)-2,2-Dimethyl-3-(2-methyl-1-propenyl)cyclopropanecarboxylic acid (1S)-2-methyl-4-oxo-3-(2Z)-2,4-pentadienyl-2-cyclopenten-1-yl ester; chrysanthemummonocarboxylic acid pyrethrolone ester. $C_{21}H_{28}O_3$; mol wt 328.45. Viscous liquid. bp$_{0.0005}$ 146-150°. n_D^{20} 1.5242. [α]$_D^{20}$ −14° (isooctane). uv max (95% ethanol): 225 nm (ε 36400). Oxidizes readily and becomes inactive in air. *Should be refrigerated and stored in darkness.* Stability data of pyrethrins I and II: Godin, *Pyrethrum*

Post **9**, 17 (1968), *C.A.* **71**, 12031q (1969). Practically insol in water. Sol in alcohol, petr ether, kerosene, carbon tetrachloride, ethylene dichloride, nitromethane.

Pyrethrin II. [121-29-9] (1*R*,3*R*)-3-[(1*E*)-3-Methoxy-2-methyl-3-oxo-1-propenyl]-2,2-dimethylcyclopropanecarboxylic acid (1*S*)-2-methyl-4-oxo-3-(2*Z*)-2,4-pentadienyl-2-cyclopenten-1-yl ester; chrysanthemumdicarboxylic acid monomethyl ester pyrethrolone ester. $C_{22}H_{28}O_5$; mol wt 372.45. Viscous liquid. Oxidizes rapidly and becomes inactive in air. $bp_{0.007}$ 192-193°. n_D^{20} 1.5355. $[\alpha]_D^{19}$ +14.7° (isooctane-ether). uv max (95% ethanol): 229 nm (ε 45850). Practically insol in water. Sol in alc, petr ether (less sol than pyrethrin I), kerosene, carbon tetrachloride, ethylene dichloride, nitromethane.

Caution: Direct skin contact or inhalation may cause severe allergic attacks in sensitive people. Potential symptoms of overexposure are erythema, dermatitis, papules, pruritus; asthma, sneezing, vasomotor rhinitis, anaphylactic reactions; numbness of lips and tongue, sneezing, vomiting, diarrhea; tinnitus, headache, restlessness, incoordination, clonic convulsions, stupor, prostration; death due to respiratory paralysis. *See: Clinical Toxicology of Commercial Products*, R. E. Gosselin *et al.*, Eds. (Williams & Wilkins, Baltimore, 5th ed., 1984) Section III, pp 352-355; *NIOSH Pocket Guide to Chemical Hazards* (DHHS/NIOSH 97-140, 1997) p 270.

USE: Insecticide.

7965. Pyrethrosin. [28272-18-6] (1a*R*,4*E*,6*R*,6a*R*,9a*S*,-10a*R*)-6-(Acetyloxy)-1a,3,6,6a,7,9a,10,10a-octahydro-4,10a-dimethyl-7-methyleneoxireno[8,9]cyclodeca[1,2-*b*]furan-8(2*H*)-one; 1,10-epoxy-6,8-dihydroxygermacra-4,11(13)-dien-12-oic acid 12,8-lactone acetate. $C_{17}H_{22}O_5$; mol wt 306.35. C 66.65%, H 7.24%, O 26.11%. From flowers of *Chrysanthemum cinerariaefolium* Vis., *Compositae*. Isoln: Thoms, *Pharm. Ztg.* **1891**, 503. Structure: Barton, de Mayo, *J. Chem. Soc.* **1957**, 150; Barton *et al., ibid.* **1960**, 2263. Revised structure: S. Iriuchijima, S. Tamura, *Agric. Biol. Chem.* **34**, 204 (1970); E. J. Gabe *et al., Chem. Commun.* **1971**, 559.

Crystals from ethanol, ethyl acetate or benzene + light petroleum, mp 198-200°. $[\alpha]_D$ −31° (c = 1.73 in chloroform). uv max: 204, 210, 220, 230 nm (ε 14,600; 12,200; 6000; 1700). Practically insol in water. Sol in hot alcohol, chloroform; slightly sol in ether or petr ether.

7966. Pyrethrum Flowers. Dalmatian insect powder; Persian insect powder. Flowers of *Chrysanthemum (Pyrethrum) cinerariaefolium* Vis., and of *C. coccineum* Willd. (*C. roseum* Adam), *Compositae*. *Habit*. Dalmatia, Montenegro, Western Asia. *Constit*. About 1-1.5% volatile oil; pyrethrin, pyretol, pyrethrotoxic acid, pyrethrosin, chrysanthemine, chrysathemumic acid.

USE: In insecticide prepns.

THERAP CAT: Scabicide.

THERAP CAT (VET): Ectoparaciticide.

7967. Pyridaben. [96489-71-3] 4-Chloro-2-(1,1-dimethylethyl)-5-[[[4-(1,1-dimethylethyl)phenyl]methyl]thio]-3(2*H*)-pyridazinone; 2-*tert*-butyl-5-(4-*tert*-butylbenzylthio)-4-chloropyridazin-3(2*H*)-one; NC-129; NCI-129; Sanmite; Nexter. $C_{19}H_{25}ClN_2OS$; mol wt 364.93. C 62.53%, H 6.91%, Cl 9.72%, N 7.68%, O 4.38%, S 8.79%. Pyridazinone derivative. Prepn: **JP Kokai 85 4173**; M. Taniguchi *et al., US 4877787* (1985, 1989 both to Nissan). Chemical and biological properties: K. Hirata *et al., Brighton Crop Prot. Conf. - Pests Dis.* **1988**, 41; K. Hirata *et al., J. Pestic. Sci.* **20**, 177 (1995). HPLC determn in soil: C. Y. Deng *et al., Fenxi Huaxue* **23**, 1357 (1995); *C.A.* **124**, 7749 (1995). Field trials against mites: G. Sterk, C. Versmissen, *Meded. Fac. Landbouwwet. Univ. Gent* **57**, 941 (1992). Review of field trials: G. Sterk, *Brighton Crop Prot. Conf. - Pests Dis.* **1994**, 559-568.

Odorless, white crystalline solid, mp 111-112°. d_4^{20}: 1.2. Vapor pressure (20°): 1.9×10^{-6} mm Hg. Soly at 20° (g/100ml): acetone 46, corn oil 4.2, ethanol 5.7, methyl cellosolve 11, xylene 39, benzene 11, cyclohexane 32, hexane 1.0, *n*-octanol 6.3, water 1.2 $\times 10^{-6}$. Stable in water at pH 4, 7, 9. Stable in most organic solvents. Stable to heat at 50° for 3 months. LD_{50} in male, female rats, bobwhite quail, mallard ducks (mg/kg): 435, 358, >2250, >2500 orally (Hirata). LD_{50} in male, female rabbits (mg/kg): >2000, >2000 dermally (Hirata).

USE: Acaricide.

7968. Pyridate. [55512-33-9] *O*-(6-Chloro-3-phenyl-4-pyridazinyl)carbonothioic acid *S*-octyl ester; fenpyrate; CL-11344; Lentagran. $C_{19}H_{23}ClN_2O_2S$; mol wt 378.92. C 60.22%, H 6.12%, Cl 9.36%, N 7.39%, O 8.44%, S 8.46%. Contact herbicide for control of weeds in cereals. Prepn: **BE 816574**; R. Schonbeck *et al., US 3953445* (1974, 1976 to Chemie Linz). Description: A. Diskus *et al., Proc. Br. Crop Prot. Conf. - Weeds* **1976**, 717; M. Chéroux, J.-M. Moncorge, *Def. Veg.* **38**, 310 (1984). Residue analysis by HPLC: W. Lindner, H. Ruckendorfer, *Int. J. Environ. Anal. Chem.* **16**, 205 (1983).

Oily brown liquid, $bp_{0.1}$ 220°. mp 27°. n_D^{20} 1.568. d^{20} 1.555. Flash pt (open cup): 200°C. Almost insol in water (90 ppm). Sol in organic solvents. LD_{50} in male rats, female rats, mice (mg/kg): 1970, 2400, >10,000 orally; in rabbits (mg/kg): >3450 dermally. LC_{50} (96 hr) in carp, trout: >100, 81 mg/l (Chéroux, Moncorge).

USE: Herbicide.

7969. Pyridazine. [289-80-5] 1,2-Diazine; orthodiazine; oizine. $C_4H_4N_2$; mol wt 80.09. C 59.99%, H 5.03%, N 34.98%. Prepd from maleic hydrazide: Mizzoni, Spoerri, *J. Am. Chem. Soc.* **73**, 1873 (1951). Resonance energy and position of double bonds: Maccoll, *J. Chem. Soc.* **1946**, 671.

Liquid. d_4^{18} 1.107; $d_4^{23.5}$ 1.1035. mp −8°. bp_{760} 208°; bp_{14} 87°; $bp_{1.0}$ 48°. $n_D^{23.5}$ 1.52311. Dipole moment in dioxane at 35° = 3.94. uv max: 338 nm. Resonance energy: 22 kcal. Miscible with water, benzene, DMF. Freely sol in methanol, ethanol, ether. Practically insol in petr ether.

Hydrochloride. $C_4H_4N_2$·HCl. Yellow solid, mp 161-163°.

7970. Pyridine. [110-86-1] C_5H_5N; mol wt 79.10. C 75.92%, H 6.37%, N 17.71%. Discovered in coal tar: T. Anderson, *Ann.* **60**, 86 (1846). Physical data: B. A. Middleton, J. R. Partington, *Nature* **141**, 516 (1938). Acute toxicity study: H. F. Smyth Jr. *et al., Arch. Ind. Hyg. Occup. Med.* **4**, 119 (1951). Books: H. Maier-Bode, *Das Pyridin und Seine Derivate in Wissenschaft und Technik* (Edwards Bros., Ann Arbor, Mich., 1943); Hill in *Chemistry of Coal Utilization* vol 2, H. H. Lowry, Ed. (Wiley, New York, 1945), Chapter 27; *The Chemistry of Heterocyclic Compounds* **vol. 14**, a series of books entitled "Pyridine and its Derivatives": Parts 1-4, E. Klingsberg, Ed. (1960-1964); Suppl. Parts 1-4, R. A. Abramovitch, Ed. (1974-1975); Part 5, G. R. Newkome, Ed. (1984) (Wiley-

Interscience, New York). *Review:* G. L. Goe in *Kirk-Othmer Encyclopedia of Chemical Technology* **vol. 19** (Wiley-Interscience, New York, 3rd ed., 1982) pp 454-483. Review of commercial synthesis and uses of pyridine and derivatives: D. J. Berry, *Spec. Chem.* **3**, 13 (1983); of occurrence of pyridine and derivatives in foods, tobacco and essential oils: G. Vernin, *Perfum. Flavor.* **7**, 23-26 (1982); of use in the study of surface properties of transition metal oxides: M. C. Kung, H. H. Kung, *Catal. Rev. Sci. Eng.* **27**, 425-460 (1985). Review of toxicology and environmental fate: A. Jori *et al.*, *Ecotoxicol. Environ. Saf.* **7**, 251 (1983); and human exposure: *Toxicological Profile for Pyridine* (PB93-110831, 1992) 108 pp.

Flammable, colorless liq; characteristic disagreeable odor; sharp taste. d_4^{20} 0.98272. Flash pt, closed cup: 68°F (20°C). mp −41.6°. bp 115.2-115.3°. n_D^{20} 1.50920. Dipole moment in benzene: 2.26. Forms an azeotropic mixture with 3 mols water, boiling at 92-93°. Volatile with steam. Miscible with water, alcohol, ether, petr ether, oils and many other organic liquids. Good solvent for many organic and inorganic compds. Weak base; forms salts with strong acids. pKa 5.19. pH of 0.2 molar soln in H_2O: 8.5. LD_{50} orally in rats: 1.58 g/kg (Smyth).

Caution: Potential symptoms of overexposure are headache, nervousness, dizziness and insomnia; nausea, anorexia; eye irritation; dermatitis; liver and kidney damage. *See NIOSH Pocket Guide to Chemical Hazards* (DHHS/NIOSH 97-140, 1997) p 272.

USE: As solvent for anhydr mineral salts. Synthetic intermediate in laboratory and industry.

7971. 3-Pyridineacetic Acid. [501-81-5] Lioxone; 3PAA; Minedil. $C_7H_7NO_2$; mol wt 137.14. C 61.31%, H 5.14%, N 10.21%, O 23.33%. Metabolite of nicotine, *q.v.* Prepn: K. Miescher, H. Kägi, *Helv. Chim. Acta* **24**, 1471 (1941); S. Carboni, *Gazz. Chim. Ital.* **85**, 1194 (1955). Manuf. process: M. Hartmann *et al.*, US 2408020 (1946 to Ciba). Pharmacology: E. Ginoulhiac, L. T. Tenconi, *Minerva Med.* **51**, 1166 (1960). Clinical evaluation as hypocholesteremic: F. Pupita, *ibid.* 1140. Thermal and photodecarboxylation: F. R. Stermitz, W. H. Huang, *J. Am. Chem. Soc.* **93**, 3427 (1971). Determn in biological fluids by HPLC: G. A. Kyerematen *et al.*, *J. Chromatogr.* **419**, 191 (1987); by thermospray LC-MS: K. T. McManus *et al.*, *J. Chromatogr. Sci.* **28**, 510 (1990).

Crystals from ethyl acetate or alcohol, mp 144°.

Note: Often confused with homonicotinic acid, (4-methyl-3-pyridinecarboxylic acid), in early literature.

THERAP CAT: Antilipemic.

7972. Pyridine 1-Oxide. [694-59-7] Pyridine *N*-oxide. C_5-H_5NO; mol wt 95.10. C 63.15%, H 5.30%, N 14.73%, O 16.82%. Prepd industrially by heating pyridine in glacial acetic acid at 80° with 30% hydrogen peroxide. The acid is neutralized and the oxide recovered by distillation: Katritzky *et al.*, *J. Chem. Soc.* **1957**, 1769. Laboratory procedure using peracetic acid: H. S. Mosher *et al.*, *Org. Synth.* **coll. vol. IV**, 828 (1963).

Deliquescent crystals, mp 66°; $bp_{1.0}$ 100-105°.

Hydrochloride. $C_5H_5NO.HCl$. Crystals from isopropanol, mp 179.5-181°.

USE: Synthetic intermediate.

7973. Pyridinium Bromide Perbromide. [39416-48-3] Hydrogen tribromide compd with pyridine (1:1). $C_5H_6Br_3N$; mol wt 319.82. C 18.78%, H 1.89%, Br 74.95%, N 4.38%. C_5H_5-$N^+HBr_3^-$. Prepd from pyridine, hydrobromic acid, and bromine: L. F. Fieser, M. Fieser, *Reagents for Organic Chemistry* **vol. 1** (John Wiley, New York, 1967) p 967.

Orange-needles from acetic acid. Odorless. Nonvolatile. Sparingly sol in acetic acid. Dissociates in the presence of a bromine acceptor, such as an alkene, to liberate one mole of bromine.

USE: In small-scale brominations, where it is much more convenient and agreeable to measure and use than elemental bromine.

7974. Pyridinium Chlorochromate. [26299-14-9] Chlorotrioxochromate(1−), hydrogen, compd with pyridine (1:1); PCC. $C_5H_6ClCrNO_3$; mol wt 215.56. C 27.86%, H 2.81%, Cl 16.45%, Cr 24.12%, N 6.50%, O 22.27%. Oxidizing agent for the efficient conversion of primary or secondary alcohols to carbonyl compounds. Prepn: R. J. Meyer, H. Best, *Z. Anorg. Allg. Chem.* **22**, 192 (1899); J. Bernard, M. Camelot, *C.R. Hebd. Seances Acad. Sci.* **258**, 5881 (1964); and use as an oxidant: E. J. Corey, J. W. Suggs, *Tetrahedron Lett.* **1975**, 2647. Improved prepn: S. Agarwal *et al.*, *Tetrahedron* **46**, 4417 (1990). Oxidation, ring enlargement of furans to pyranones: G. Piancatelli *et al.*, *Tetrahedron Lett.* **1977**, 2199; oxidation of tertiary allylic alcohols: W. G. Dauben, D. M. Michno, *J. Org. Chem.* **42**, 682 (1977). Role in oxidative cationic cyclization: E. J. Corey, D. L. Boger, *Tetrahedron Lett.* **1978**, 2461. *Review:* G. Piancatelli *et al.*, *Synthesis* **1982**, 245-258.

$\bullet\ CrO_3Cl^-$

Orange-yellow solid, mp 205° (dec). Insol in dichloromethane.

USE: Oxidizing agent in organic synthesis.

7975. Pyridinol Carbamate. [1882-26-4] 2,6-Pyridinedimethanol bis(methylcarbamate) (ester); 2,6-pyridinylenebis[methyl-*N*-methylcarbamate]; pyricarbate; H-3749; Anginin; Angioxine; Aterosan; Atover; Cicloven; Colesterinex; Duvaline; Movecil; Prodectin; Ravenil; Sospitan; Vasagin; Vasocil; Vasoverin. $C_{11}H_{15}N_3$-O_4; mol wt 253.25. C 52.17%, H 5.97%, N 16.59%, O 25.27%. Prepd by the reaction of methylamine with 2,6-pyridinedimethanol bis[phenylcarbonate] in methanol: Matsumoto, JP 66 22185 (1966 to Banyu), *C.A.* **66**, 75907x (1967). Pharmacology and clinical evaluation: T. Shimamoto *et al.*, *Am. Heart J.* **71**, 297 (1966). Metabolism: Mallein *et al.*, *Therapie* **28**, 115 (1973). Effects on lipid metabolism and antiatherogenic effect in animals: V. Orbetzova *et al.*, *Artery* **8**, 560 (1980). HPLC determn in biological fluids: A. Suenaga *et al.*, *Acta Pharm. Suec.* **23**, 245 (1986).

Needles from methanol or acetone, mp 136-137°. uv max (methanol): 264-265 nm. Sparingly sol in cold water; freely sol in hot water. LD_{50} in mice, rats, rabbits, dogs (mg/kg): 4500, 3400, 5200, 1000 orally (Shimamoto).

THERAP CAT: Antiarteriosclerotic.

7976. Pyridomycin. [18791-21-4] 3-Hydroxy-*N*-[(2Z,5R,-6S,9S,10S,11R)-10-hydroxy-5,11-dimethyl-2-(1-methylpropylidene)-3,7,12-trioxo-9-(3-pyridinylmethyl)-1,4-dioxa-8-azacyclododec-6-yl]-2-pyridinecarboxamide. $C_{27}H_{32}N_4O_8$; mol wt 540.56. C 59.99%, H 5.97%, N 10.36%, O 23.68%. Antimycobacterial antibiotic substance produced by *Streptomyces albidofuscus* Okami et Umezawa, nov sp., renamed *S. pyridomyceticus*. Isoln: Maeda *et al.*, *J. Antibiot.* **6A**, 140 (1953); K. Yagishita, *ibid.* **7A**, 143 (1954). Degradation studies: Maeda, *ibid.* **10A**, 94 (1957). Structure: Koyama *et al.*, *Tetrahedron Lett.* **1967**, 3587; H. Ogawara *et al.*, *Chem. Pharm. Bull.* **16**, 679 (1968). Synthetic study: M. Kinoshita, M. Awamura, *Bull. Chem. Soc. Jpn.* **51**, 869 (1978); M. Kinoshita *et al., ibid.* 3595. Production: **JP 54 7048**; **JP 55 1349**; **JP 56 9566** (1954, 1955, 1956 all to Nippon Antibiotic Subst. Sci. Assoc.).

Crystals from ethanol, mp 222°. uv max (ethanol): 303 nm ($E_{1cm}^{1\%}$ 209). Soluble in lower alcohols, ethyl or butyl acetate, benzene, acetone, dioxane, tetrahydrofuran. Practically insol in water.

Hydrochloride. Crystals, mp 194-196°. Freely sol in water. $[\alpha]_D^{16}$ −53.2° (water). pH of aq solns about 2.0. LD_{50} i.p. in mice: >2100 mg/kg (Yagishita).

7977. Pyridostigmine Bromide. [101-26-8] 3-[[(Dimethyl-amino)carbonyl]oxy]-1-methylpyridinium bromide; 3-hydroxy-1-methylpyridinium bromide dimethylcarbamate; 1-methyl-3-hydroxypyridinium bromide dimethylcarbamate; 3-(dimethyl-carbamyloxy)-1-methylpyridinium bromide; Ro-1-5130; Kalymin; Mestinon; Regonol. $C_9H_{13}BrN_2O_2$; mol wt 261.12. C 41.40%, H 5.02%, Br 30.60%, N 10.73%, O 12.25%. Reversible inhibitor of acetylcholinesterase. Prepn: Urban, **US 2572579** (1951 to Hoffmann-La Roche). Mechanism of protective effect in soman poisoning: X. Deyi *et al., Fundam. Appl. Toxicol.* **1**, 217 (1981). Evaluation of effect on neuromuscular function: M. Glikson *et al., ibid.* **16**, 288 (1991). Evaluation of side effects profile under desert conditions: J. E. Cook *et al., Mil. Med.* **157**, 250 (1992). Review of prophylactic effect in nerve agent poisoning: R. M. Dawson, *J. Appl. Toxicol.* **14**, 317 (1994).

Shiny, hygroscopic crystals from abs ethanol, mp 152-154°. Freely sol in water, alcohol. Practically insol in ether, acetone, benzene. Aq solns may be sterilized by autoclaving with steam.

THERAP CAT: Cholinergic; in treatment of myasthenia gravis. Pre-exposure antidote to chemical warfare agents.

7978. Pyridoxal. [66-72-8] 3-Hydroxy-5-(hydroxymethyl)-2-methyl-4-pyridinecarboxaldehyde; 3-hydroxy-5-(hydroxymethyl)-2-methylisonicotinaldehyde; 2-methyl-3-hydroxy-4-formyl-5-hydroxymethylpyridine. $C_8H_9NO_3$; mol wt 167.16. C 57.48%, H 5.43%, N 8.38%, O 28.71%. Synthesis and structure: Harris *et al., J. Biol. Chem.* **154**, 315 (1944); *J. Am. Chem. Soc.* **66**, 2088 (1944).

Hydrochloride. $C_8H_9NO_3 \cdot HCl$. Rhombic crystals, mp approx 165° with decompn. Soluble in water (1 g/2 ml); sol in 95% ethanol (1.7 g/100 ml); pH of 1% water soln = 2.65. The water solns are

sensitive to heat. uv max: 292.5 nm (E mol 7600). Can be reduced to pyridoxine hydrochloride (mp 206-208°).

Monoethylacetal hydrochloride. 1,3-Dihydro-1-ethoxy-6-methylfuro[3,4-*c*]pyridin-7-ol hydrochloride. $C_{10}H_{14}ClNO_3$. Crystals from alcohol and ether, mp 142-143°.

7979. Pyridoxal 5-Phosphate. [54-47-7] 3-Hydroxy-2-methyl-5-[(phosphonooxy)methyl]-4-pyridinecarboxaldehyde; pyridoxal 5-monophosphoric acid ester; 3-hydroxy-5-(hydroxymethyl)-2-methylisonicotinaldehyde 5-phosphate; codecarboxylase; Pyromijin; Sechvitan; Vitazechs. $C_8H_{10}NO_6P$; mol wt 247.14. C 38.88%, H 4.08%, N 5.67%, O 38.84%, P 12.53%. Prepn by the action of adenosine triphosphate on pyridoxal: Gunsalus *et al., J. Biol. Chem.* **155**, 685 (1944); by the action of phosphorus oxychloride on pyridoxal in aq soln: Gunsalus *et al., ibid.* **161**, 743 (1945); Umbreit *et al., Arch. Biochem.* **7**, 189 (1945); by phosphorylation of pyridoxamine with 100% H_3PO_4 followed by oxidation: Wilson, Harris, *J. Am. Chem. Soc.* **73**, 4693 (1951). Alternate route: Schorre, **US 3124587** (1964 to E. Merck). Isoln in pure form as the oxime and as the *O*-methyl oxime and structure: Heyl *et al., J. Am. Chem. Soc.* **73**, 3430 (1951). Activity as a cotransaminase in the synthesis of amino acids: Lichstein *et al., J. Biol. Chem.* **161**, 311 (1945). Activity of natural and synthetic material: Umbreit *et al., loc. cit.*

Colorless in acid soln, bright-yellow in alkaline soln. uv max (alkaline soln): 390 nm (E_m 3.7); in acid soln: 295 nm (E_m 5.1). Gives a negative 2,6-dichloroquinone chlorimide test. On oxidation with H_2O_2 in alkaline solution yields [(2-methyl-3,4-dihydroxy-5-pyridyl)methyl]phosphoric acid.

Oxime. [634-25-3] $C_8H_{11}N_2O_6P$. Crystals, dec 229-230°. Practically insol in water, alcohol, ether.

O-Methyloxime. [20905-71-9] $C_9H_{13}N_2O_6P$. Crystals, dec 212-213°. Practically insol in water, alcohol, ether.

Calcium salt. [29956-24-9] Aderoxal. Yellow precipitate. Practically insol in water, alcohol or ether.

THERAP CAT: Vitamin (enzyme co-factor).

7980. Pyridoxamine Dihydrochloride. [524-36-7] 4-(Aminomethyl)-5-hydroxy-6-methyl-3-pyridinemethanol dihydrochloride; 2-methyl-3-hydroxy-4-aminomethyl-5-hydroxymethyl-pyridine dihydrochloride. $C_8H_{14}Cl_2N_2O_2$; mol wt 241.11. C 39.85%, H 5.85%, Cl 29.41%, N 11.62%, O 13.27%. Synthesis and structure: Harris *et al., J. Biol. Chem.* **154**, 315 (1944); *J. Am. Chem. Soc.* **66**, 2088 (1944).

Platelets, mp 226-227° with dec. Soluble in water (approx 1 g/2 ml); sol in 95% alc (0.65 g/100 ml). Reasonably stable at room temp; shows no decompn in a few days at 60°. Liquefies on exposure to 80% relative humidity. pH of a 1% water soln 2.4. uv max (pH 1.94): 287.5 nm (E mol 91,000).

Free base. Crystals from alc; mp 193-193.5°; sol in alc.

Pyridoxamine phosphate. 2-Methyl-3-hydroxy-4-aminomethyl-5-pyridylmethylphosphoric acid. $C_8H_{13}N_2O_5P$. Prepn in soln by autoclaving codecarboxylase with glutamic acid: McNutt, Snell, *J. Biol. Chem.* **182**, 557 (1950); prepn by direct phosphorylation of pyridoxamine in aq soln with phosphorus oxychloride: Heyl *et al., J. Am. Chem. Soc.* **73**, 3430 (1951).

7981. 4-Pyridoxic Acid. [82-82-6] 3-Hydroxy-5-(hydroxy-methyl)-2-methyl-4-pyridinecarboxylic acid; 3-hydroxy-5-(hydroxymethyl)-2-methylisonicotinic acid; 2-methyl-3-hydroxy-4-

carboxy-5-hydroxymethylpyridine. $C_8H_9NO_4$; mol wt 183.16. C 52.46%, H 4.95%, N 7.65%, O 34.94%. Occurs in urine. It is the chief metabolic product of pyridoxine, pyridoxal, and pyridoxamine. Isoln from human urine: Singal, Sydenstricker, *Science* **78**, 545 (1941). Isoln and synthesis: Huff, Perlzweig, *J. Biol. Chem.* **155**, 345 (1944).

Wedge-shaped crystals, mp 247-248°. Slightly sol in water, alcohol, pyridine. Insoluble in ether and in aq acid soln, but completely sol in aq alkaline soln. Possesses two acidic groups, one a phenolic and the other a carboxyl having pK values of 9.75 and 5.50, respectively. Characteristic blue fluorescence, max at pH 3 to 4. The fluorescence disappears on reduction with hydrosulfite and is restored to the original intensity with H_2O_2. Is adsorbed on zeolite from aq solns at pH 4 to 5 and can be eluted with 25% KCl; butanol extracts of neutral eluates also show characteristic blue fluorescence which is increased by a trace of acetic acid. Stable to boiling with dil alkali (1N); but upon being heated with 0.5N acid for a few minutes it is converted to the lactone.

Lactone. β-Pyracine. $C_8H_7NO_3$. mp 263-265°, exhibits much stronger fluorescence. Is more easily followed in the course of biochemical investigations.

7982. Pyridoxine Hydrochloride. [58-56-0] 5-Hydroxy-6-methyl-3,4-pyridinedimethanol hydrochloride; pyridoxol hydrochloride; vitamin B_6 hydrochloride; pyridoxinium chloride; adermine hydrochloride; 2-methyl-3-hydroxy-4,5-bis(hydroxymethyl)-pyridine hydrochloride; 5-hydroxy-6-methyl-3,4-pyridinedicarbinol hydrochloride; 3-hydroxy-4,5-dimethylol-α-picoline hydrochloride; Bonasanit; Hexabione hydrochloride; Hexabetalin; Hexavibex; Pyridipca; Pyridox; Bécilan; Benadon; Hexermin; Campoviton 6; Hexobion. $C_8H_{12}ClNO_3$; mol wt 205.64. C 46.73%, H 5.88%, Cl 17.24%, N 6.81%, O 23.34%. One of the vitamins of the B_6 complex; *see also* Codecarboxylase; Pyridoxal; Pyridoxamine Dihydrochloride. Present in many foodstuffs; esp good sources are yeast, liver and cereals. Isoln: Keresztesy, Stevens, *Proc. Soc. Exp. Biol. Med.* **38**, 64 (1938); György, *J. Am. Chem. Soc.* **60**, 983 (1938); Kuhn, Wendt, *Ber.* **71**, 780, 1118 (1938). Structure: E. T. Stiller *et al., J. Am. Chem. Soc.* **61**, 1237 (1939); R. Kuhn *et al., Ber.* **72**, 305 sqq. (1939). uv absorption spectrum: E. A. Peterson, H. A. Sober, *J. Am. Chem. Soc.* **76**, 169 (1954). Synthesis: Harris, Folkers, *J. Am. Chem. Soc.* **61**, 1242, 1245, 3307 (1939); P. G. Stevens, **US 2680743** and **US 2734063** (1954, 1956 both to Gen. Aniline); P. I. Pollak, **US 2904551, US 3024244, US 3024245** (1959, 1962, 1962 all to Merck & Co.); E. E. Harris *et al., J. Org. Chem.* **27**, 2705 (1962); W. Böll, H. König, *Ann.* **1979**, 1657; T. Shono *et al., Chem. Lett.* **1981**, 1121. Biosynthesis: Hiel, Spenser, *Science* **169**, 773 (1970). *Review: The Vitamins* vol. 2, W. H. Sebrell, R. S. Harris, Eds. (Academic, New York, 2nd ed., 1968) pp 1-117.

Platelets or thick, birefringent rods from alcohol + acetone. Reasonably stable to light and air. Dec 205-212°. Sublimes. (Free base, mp 160°.) uv max (0.1N HCl): 290 nm (ε 8400); (phosphate buffer, pH 7): 253, 325 nm (ε 3700, 7100). One gram dissolves in about 4.5 ml water, 90 ml alcohol. Sol in propylene glycol. Sparingly sol in acetone. Insol in ether, chloroform. pH of a 10% w/v soln in water: 3.2. Acidic aq solns are stable and may be heated for 30 min at 120° without decompn.

THERAP CAT: Vitamin (enzyme cofactor).
THERAP CAT (VET): Nutritional factor.

7983. Pyrifenox. [88283-41-4] 1-(2,4-Dichlorophenyl)-2-(3-pyridinyl)ethanone O-methyloxime; 2',4'-dichloro-2-(3-pyridyl)-acetophenone O-methyloxime; ACR-3453A; Ro-15-1297; Dorado.

$C_{14}H_{12}Cl_2N_2O$; mol wt 295.16. C 56.97%, H 4.10%, Cl 24.02%, N 9.49%, O 5.42%. Ergosterol biosynthesis inhibitor for use on crops. Prepn: F. Dorn, **DE 3310148**; *idem*, **US 4605656** (1983, 1986 both to Hoffmann-La Roche). Review of physical properties, toxicity and bioactivity: P. Zobrist *et al., Proc. Br. Crop Prot. Conf. - Pests Dis.* **1986**, 47-53; of field trials: G. Neumann *et al., Meded. Fac. Landbouwwet. Rijksuniv. Gent* **54**, 635-642 (1989).

Slightly viscous, tan liquid with mild aromatic odor. $bp_{0.1}$ >150°. vapor pressure at 25°: 1.4×10^{-5} torr. Soly (at 20°) in water at pH 7: 115 mg/l; in hexane: <1 g/l; in acetone, ethyl acetate, chloroform, diethyl ether, DMF, isopropyl alcohol, toluene: >250 g/l. LD_{50} in rats (mg/kg): 950 i.p.; 2900 orally; >5000 dermally; LC_{50} by inhalation in rats: >2.05 mg/l (Zobrist).

USE: Agricultural fungicide.

7984. Pyrilamine. [91-84-9] N-[(4-Methoxyphenyl)methyl]-N',N'-dimethyl-N-2-pyridinyl-1,2-ethanediamine; 2-[(2-dimethylaminoethyl)(p-methoxybenzyl)amino]pyridine; N-p-methoxybenzyl-N',N'-dimethyl-N-α-pyridylethylenediamine; mepyramine; pyranisamine; RP-2786. $C_{17}H_{23}N_3O$; mol wt 285.38. C 71.55%, H 8.12%, N 14.72%, O 5.61%. Prepn: Bovet *et al., C.R. Seances Soc. Biol. Ses Fil.* **138**, 99 (1944); Huttrer *et al., J. Am. Chem. Soc.* **68**, 1999 (1946); Viaud, *Prod. Pharm.* **2**, 53 (1947); Horclois, **US 2502151** (1950 to Rhône-Poulenc). Toxicity: A. von Schlichtergroll, *Arzneim.-Forsch.* **7**, 237 (1957); of the maleate: F. Hunziker *et al., ibid.* **13**, 324 (1963).

Oily liquid. bp_5 201°; $bp_{0.06}$ 168-172°. n_D^{25} 1.5760-1.5765. LD_{50} orally in mice: 312 mg/kg (Schlichtergroll).

Hydrochloride. $C_{17}H_{23}N_3O \cdot HCl$. Crystals, mp 143-143.5°. Very sol in water.

Maleate. [59-33-6] Antamine; Anthisan; Dorantamin; Enrumay; Histalon; Histan; Histapyran; Histatex; Neo-Antergan; Paraminyl; Parmal; Pyramal; Stamine; Stangen; Thylogen. Crystals. Bitter saline taste. Stable in air. mp 100-101°. uv max: 244 nm ($E_{1cm}^{1\%}$ 420). One gram dissolves in about 0.4 ml water, in about 15 ml abs alc. pH of 10% soln ~5.1. On raising the pH to 7.5 or 8.0 pptn of the oily, free base begins. Slightly sol in benzene, ether. LD_{50} in mice: 338 mg/kg (Hunziker).

THERAP CAT: Antihistaminic.
THERAP CAT (VET): Antihistaminic.

7985. Pyrimethamine. [58-14-0] 5-(4-Chlorophenyl)-6-ethyl-2,4-pyrimidinediamine; 2,4-diamino-5-(p-chlorophenyl)-6-ethylpyrimidine; RP-4753; Daraprim; Malocide. $C_{12}H_{13}ClN_4$; mol wt 248.71. C 57.95%, H 5.27%, Cl 14.25%, N 22.53%. Dihydrofolate reductase inhibitor; generally used in combination with other antimicrobial agents. Prepn: P. B. Russell, G. H. Hitchings, *J. Am. Chem. Soc.* **73**, 3763 (1951); G. H. Hitchings *et al.,* **US 2576939** (1951 to Burroughs Wellcome); W. Logemann *et al., Ber.* **87**, 435 (1954); R. M. Jacob, **US 2680740** (1954 to Rhône-Poulenc). Review of antimicrobial activity and mechanism of action: Burchall in *Antibiotics* **vol. 3**, J. W. Corcoran, F. E. Hahn, Eds. (Springer-Verlag, New York, 1975) pp 312-320. Comprehensive description: M. A. Loutfy, H. Y. Aboul-Enein, *Anal. Profiles Drug Subs.* **12**, 463-482 (1983). LC-MS determn in plasma: B. A. Sinnaeve *et al., J. Chromatogr. A* **1076**, 97 (2005). Clinical evaluations in toxoplasmosis in AIDS patients: C. Leport *et al., Am. J. Med.* **84**, 94 (1988);

B. Dannemann *et al., Ann. Intern. Med.* **116**, 33 (1992). Review of clinical experience in malaria: H. M. McIntosh *et al., Ann. Trop. Med. Parasitol.* **93**, 265-270 (1998); C. V. Plowe *et al., Br. Med. J.* **328**, 545 (2004).

Crystals, mp 233-234° (capillary); mp 240-242° (copper block). Practically insol in water. Slightly sol in ethanol, (about 9 g/l), in dil HCl (about 5 g/l); sol in boiling ethanol (about 25 g/l). Very sparingly sol in propylene glycol and dimethylacetamide at 70°.
Combination with sulfadoxine. [37338-39-9] Fansidar.
THERAP CAT: Antiprotozoal (Toxoplasma); antimalarial.
THERAP CAT (VET): Antiprotozoal (Toxoplasma).

7986. Pyrimethanil. [53112-28-0] 4,6-Dimethyl-*N*-phenyl-2-pyrimidinamine; 2-anilino-4,6-dimethylpyrimidine; *N*-(4,6-dimethylpyrimidin-2-yl)aniline; Scala. $C_{12}H_{13}N_3$; mol wt 199.25. C 72.34%, H 6.58%, N 21.09%. Anilino-pyrimidine fungicide for control of *Botrytis* and *Venturia* spp. in food crops; inhibits secretion of cell wall degrading enzymes required for fungal infection. Prepn: S. Angerstein, *Ber.* **34**, 3956 (1901). Mode of action studies: A. Daniels *et al., Brighton Crop Prot. Conf. - Pests Dis.* **1994**, 525; A. Daniels, J. A. Lucas, *Pestic. Sci.* **45**, 33 (1995); R. J. Milling, C. J. Richardson, *ibid.* 43. Degradation study: A. Agüera *et al., Environ. Sci. Technol.* **34**, 1563 (2000). Determn in soil by headspace solid-phase microextraction and GC/MS: A. Navalón *et al., Anal. Bioanal. Chem.* **379**, 1100 (2004). Comprehensive review: G. L. Neumann *et al., Brighton Crop Prot. Conf. - Pests Dis.* **1992**, 395-402.

White crystalline solid, mp 96.3°. Soly in water (25°): 0.121 g/l. Sol in most organic solvents. Log P (*n*-octanol/water): 2.48. Vapor pressure (25°): 2.2×10^{-3} Pa. LD_{50} (mg/kg): 4061-5358 orally in mice; 4150-5971 orally in rats; >5000 dermally in rats. LC_{50} (96 hr) in mirror carp, rainbow trout (mg/l): 35.36, 10.56 (Neumann).
USE: Fungicide.

7987. Pyrimidine. [289-95-2] 1,3-Diazine; metadiazine; miazine. $C_4H_4N_2$; mol wt 80.09. C 59.99%, H 5.03%, N 34.98%. Prepd by reducing 2,4,6-trichloropyrimidine with zinc dust: Gabriel, *Ber.* **33**, 3666 (1900); by reducing tetrachloropyrimidine: Emery, *ibid.* **34**, 4180 (1901); by reducing 2,4-dichloropyrimidine with magnesium oxide and palladium-charcoal: Wittaker, *J. Chem. Soc.* **1953**, 1646.

Liquid or cryst mass; penetrating odor. mp 20-22°. bp_{762} 123-124°. uv max (water): 240 nm (ε 2400). Soluble in water, alcohol, ether.
Methiodide. $C_4H_4N_2 \cdot CH_3I$. Yellow plates from ethanol, mp 136-137°.

7988. Pyriminil. [53558-25-1] *N*-(4-Nitrophenyl)-*N'*-(3-pyridinylmethyl)urea; *N*-3-pyridylmethyl-*N'*-*p*-nitrophenylurea; pyrinuron; RH-787; DLP-787; Vacor. $C_{13}H_{12}N_4O_3$; mol wt 272.26. C 57.35%, H 4.44%, N 20.58%, O 17.63%. Prepn: J. E. Ware *et al.,* **DE 2409686** (1974 to Rohm & Haas). Evaluation as rodenticide: D. L. Peardon, *Pest Control* **42**, 14, 16, 18, 27 (1974); J. E. Brooks, P. T. Htun, *J. Hyg.* **80**, 401 (1978). Mode of action: D. L. Peardon, J. E. Ware, *Pest Control* **45**, 49 (1977).

mp 223-225° (dec). LD_{50} orally in male, female rats: 6.2, 7.2 mg/kg (Brooks, Htun).
USE: Rodenticide.

7989. Pyrinoline. [1740-22-3] α-[3-(Di-2-pyridinylmethyl-ene)-1,4-cyclopentadien-1-yl]-α-2-pyridinyl-2-pyridinemethanol; 3-(di-2-pyridylmethylene)-α,α-di-2-pyridyl-1,4-cyclopentadiene-1-methanol; di-2-pyridyl-(6,6-di-2-pyridylfulven-2-yl)methanol; McN-1210; Surexin. $C_{27}H_{20}N_4O$; mol wt 416.47. C 77.87%, H 4.84%, N 13.45%, O 3.84%. Prepn: **GB 1009012** (1965 to McNeil).

Crystals, mp 146.5-147.5°.
THERAP CAT: Antiarrhythmic (cardiac depressant).

7990. Pyriproxyfen. [95737-68-1] 2-[1-Methyl-2-(4-phen-oxyphenoxy)ethoxy]pyridine; 4-phenoxyphenyl *(RS)*-2-(2-pyridyloxy)propyl ether; S-9318; S-31183; Sumilarv. $C_{20}H_{19}NO_3$; mol wt 321.37. C 74.75%, H 5.96%, N 4.36%, O 14.94%. Juvenile hormone mimic. Prepn: S. Nishida *et al.,* **GB 2140010**; *eidem,* **US 4751225** (1984, 1988 both to Sumitomo). Ovicidal activity: K. R. S. Ascher, M. Eliyahu, *Phytoparasitica* **16**, 15 (1988). Environmental persistence study: C. H. Schaefer *et al., Ecotoxicol. Environ. Saf.* **21**, 207 (1991). Field trial to control tsetse flies: J. W. Hargrove, P. A. Langley, *Bull. Entomol. Res.* **83**, 361 (1993).

Pale yellow liquid. $n_D^{20.5}$ 1.5823. Solidifies upon standing to give crystals, mp 49.7°.
USE: Insecticide.
THERAP CAT (VET): Ectoparasiticide.

7991. Pyrisuccideanol. [33605-94-6] Butanedioic acid 2-(dimethylamino)ethyl [5-hydroxy-4-(hydroxymethyl)-6-methyl-3-pyridinyl]methyl ester; pyridoxol 3-[2-(dimethylamino)ethyl succinate]; 2-(dimethylamino)ethyl [5-hydroxy-4-(hydroxymethyl)-6-methyl-3-pyridyl]succinic acid methyl ester; pirisudanol. $C_{16}H_{24}N_2O_6$; mol wt 340.37. C 56.46%, H 7.11%, N 8.23%, O 28.20%. Prepn: Esanu, **DE 2102831** (1971 to Soc. d'Etudes de Prods. Chim.) corresp to **US 3717636** (1973). Activity studies: Hugelin *et al., C.R. Seances Soc. Biol. Ses Fil.* **166**, 1435 (1972).

Dimaleate. [53659-00-0] Mentium; Nadex; Stivane. $C_{16}H_{24}N_2O_6 \cdot 2C_4H_4O_4$; mol wt 572.52. mp 134°.
THERAP CAT: Antidepressant.

7992. Pyrithiamine. [534-64-5] 1-[(4-Amino-2-methyl-5-pyrimidinyl)methyl]-3-(2-hydroxyethyl)-2-methylpyridinium bromide monohydrobromide; 1-(2-methyl-4-amino-5-pyrimidyl)methyl-2-methyl-3-hydroxyethylpyridinium bromide hydrobromide;

neopyrithiamine. $C_{14}H_{20}Br_2N_4O$; mol wt 420.14. C 40.02%, H 4.80%, Br 38.04%, N 13.34%, O 3.81%. Thiamine antagonist prepd by condensation of 2-methyl-3-(β-hydroxyethyl)pyridine with the pyrimidine moiety of vitamin B_1: Tracy, Elderfield, *J. Org. Chem.* **6**, 54 (1941); improved procedure: Wilson, Harris, *J. Am. Chem. Soc.* **71**, 2231 (1949); US 2587262 (1952 to Merck & Co.). *Cf.* Woolley, *J. Am. Chem. Soc.* **72**, 5763 (1950).

Crystals from acetone, dec 218-220°. uv max (water): 238, 271 nm. Sol in water.

Chloride hydrochloride. $C_{14}H_{20}Cl_2N_4O$. Dec 234-236°. uv max (water): 235, 273 nm. Sol in water.

7993. Pyrithiobac. [123342-93-8] 2-Chloro-6-[(4,6-dimethoxy-2-pyrimidinyl)thio]benzoic acid; KIH-8921. $C_{13}H_{11}-ClN_2O_4S$; mol wt 326.76. C 47.78%, H 3.39%, Cl 10.85%, N 8.57%, O 19.59%, S 9.81%. Pyrimidinylsalicylic acid herbicide for use in cotton; acetolactate synthase inhibitor. Prepn: Y. Saito *et al., EP 315889; eidem,* US 4923501 (1989, 1990 both to Kumiai Chem. Ind.; Ihara Chem. Ind.). Field trials in cotton: J. W. Keeling *et al. Weed Technol.* **7**, 930 (1993). Mechanism of action: T. Shimizu *et al., J. Pestic. Sci.* **19**, 59 (1994). Comprehensive description: S. Takahashi *et al., Brighton Crop Prot. Conf. - Weeds* **1991**, 57-62.

Ochre powder, mp 148-151°.

Sodium salt. [123343-16-8] KIH-2031; DPX-PE350; Staple. $C_{13}H_{10}ClN_2NaO_4S$; mol wt 348.74. White solid, mp 247.7° (dec). Soly in water (10°): 760 g/l. LD_{50} in male, female rats (mg/kg): 1000-3000, 3000-5000 orally. LD_{50} in rats (mg/kg): >2000 dermally (Takahashi).

USE: Herbicide.

7994. Pyrithione. [1121-30-8] 1-Hydroxy-2(1H)-pyridinethione; 2-pyridinethiol 1-oxide; 2-mercaptopyridine 1-oxide; PTO; Omadine. C_5H_5NOS; mol wt 127.16. C 47.23%, H 3.96%, N 11.02%, O 12.58%, S 25.22%. Prepn: Shaw *et al., J. Am. Chem. Soc.* **72**, 4362 (1950); Semenoff, Dolliver, US 2745826 (1956 to Olin Mathieson).

Sodium salt. Fonderma. C_5H_4NNaOS; mol wt 149.15.

Zinc derivative. [13463-41-7] Zinc pyrithione; zinc pyridinethione; bis(2-pyridylthio)zinc 1,1'-dioxide; bis-(1-hydroxy-2(1H)-pyridinethionato-O,S)zinc; Desquaman. $C_{10}H_8N_2O_2S_2Zn$; mol wt 317.72. Prepn: GB 761171 (1956 to Olin Mathieson). Activity: Karsten *et al.,* US 3236733; Judge *et al.,* US 3281366 (both 1966 to Procter and Gamble).

Dimer. Dipyrithione; 2,2'-dithiobispyridine 1,1'-dioxide; OMDS; Omadine Disulfide. $C_{10}H_8N_2O_2S_2$; mol wt 252.31.

USE: Fungicide, bactericide.

THERAP CAT: Antibacterial; antifungal. Zinc deriv also as antiseborrheic.

7995. Pyrithyldione. [77-04-3] 3,3-Diethyl-2,4-(1H,-3H)pyridinedione; 3,3-diethyl-2,4-dioxotetrahydropyridine; 2,4-di-oxo-3,3-diethyltetrahydropyridine; 2,4-dioxo-3,3-diethyl-1,2,3,4-tetrahydropyridine; Presidon; Persedon; Tetridin; Benedorm. $C_9-H_{13}NO_2$; mol wt 167.21. C 64.65%, H 7.84%, N 8.38%, O 19.14%. Prepn: Schnider, *Festschr. Emil Barell* **1936**, 195; Preiswerk, Schnider, US 2090068 (1937 to Hoffmann-La Roche); Strukov *et al., Med. Prom. SSSR* **13**, no. 9, 9 (1959). Alternate procedure: Rechen *et al.,* US 3019230 (1962 to Hoffmann-La Roche).

Exists in three cryst modifications: I, mp 92-93°; II, mp 97-98°; III, mp 81-86° [Scheibl, Wachter, *Arch. Toxikol.* **18**, 253 (1960)]. bp_{14} 187-189°. Moderately sol in water; freely sol in the usual organic solvents except petr solvents. Aq solns are just acid to litmus.

THERAP CAT: Sedative, hypnotic.

7996. Pyritinol. [1098-97-1] 3,3'-[Dithiobis(methylene)]-bis[5-hydroxy-6-methyl-4-pyridinemethanol]; bis(4-hydroxymethyl-5-hydroxy-6-methyl-3-pyridylmethyl) disulfide; bis[(3-hydroxy-4-hydroxymethyl-2-methyl-5-pyridyl)methyl] disulfide; dipyridoxolyldisulfide; pyridoxine-5-disulfide; pyrithioxin. $C_{16}H_{20}N_2O_4S_2$; mol wt 368.47. C 52.15%, H 5.47%, N 7.60%, O 17.37%, S 17.40%. Prepn: Zima, Schorre, US 3010966 (1961 to E. Merck); Iwanami *et al., Bitamin* **36**, 122 (1967); *J. Vitaminol.* **14**, 321, 326 (1968). HPLC determn in urine: K. Kitao *et al., Chem. Pharm. Bull.* **25**, 1335 (1977). Pharmacokinetics and metabolism: Darge *et al., Arzneim.-Forsch.* **19**, 5, 9, (1969); Nowak, Schorre, *ibid.* 11. Clinical trial in dementia: S. Hoyer *et al., ibid.* **27**, 671 (1977); A. J. Cooper, R. V. Magnus, *Pharmacotherapeutica* **2**, 317 (1980); in cerebrovascular disorders: Y. Tazaki *et al., J. Int. Med. Res.* **8**, 118 (1980).

Crystals, mp 218-220°.

Dihydrochloride monohydrate. Biocefalin; Bonifen; Enbol; Encephabol; Enerbol; Epocan; Life. $C_{16}H_{20}N_2O_4S_2.2HCl.H_2O$; mol wt 459.41. mp 184°. *Note:* Has no vitamin B_6 activity.

THERAP CAT: Nootropic.

7997. Pyrocalciferol. [128-27-8] (3β,10α,22E)-Ergosta-5,7,22-trien-3-ol; 9α-lumisterol; 9α-lumista-5,7,22-trien-3β-ol. $C_{28}H_{44}O$; mol wt 396.65. C 84.78%, H 11.18%, O 4.03%. Differs from ergosterol in the steric configuration at C-9 and C-10. Formation via isopyrocalciferol: Askew *et al., Proc. Roy. Soc. London* **B109**, 488 (1932); Windaus *et al., Nachr. Ges. Wiss. Goettingen Math.-Phys. Kl.* **1932**, 150. Dehydrogenation with selenium gives Diel's hydrocarbon (3'-methyl-1,2-cyclopentenophenanthrene). Fieser, Fieser, *Steroids* (New York, 1959) pp 136-143, argue the configuration at C-9 and C-10. *See also* Castells *et al., J. Chem. Soc.* **1959**, 1159. Critical examination and comparison with other un-natural steroids: Castells *et al., ibid.* **1962**, 2907.

Needles from methanol, mp 93-95°. $[\alpha]_D^{20}$ +512°, $[\alpha]_{546}^{20}$ +624° (c = 0.15 in alcohol). uv max: 274, 294 nm (Askew).

Acetate. $C_{30}H_{46}O_2$. mp 81-82°, $[\alpha]_D$ +403° (chloroform).

3,5-Dinitrobenzoate. $C_{35}H_{46}N_2O_6$. mp 168-170°. $[\alpha]_D^{21}$ +195°, $[\alpha]_{546}^{20}$ +249° (both c = 2 in chloroform).

7998. Pyrocarbonic Acid Diethyl Ester. [1609-47-8] Dicarbonic acid diethyl ester; oxydiformic acid diethyl ester; diethyl pyrocarbonate; diethyl oxydiformate; DEPC; Ue-5908; Baycovin. $C_6H_{10}O_5$; mol wt 162.14. C 44.45%, H 6.22%, O 49.34%. $C_2H_5OOCOCOOC_2H_5$. Prepd according to the equation $R_1OOCCl + NaOCOOR_2 \rightarrow R_1OOCOCOOR_2 + NaCl$: Kovalenko, *Zh. Obshch. Khim.* **22**, 1546 (1952); Thoma, Rinke, *Ann.* **624**, 30 (1959); alternate method: Degering *et al.*, *J. Am. Pharm. Assoc. Sci. Ed.* **39**, 626 (1950). *Review: Handbook of Food Additives*, T. A. Furia, Ed. (Chemical Rubber Co., Cleveland, 1968) pp 181-185.

Viscous liquid. Fruity odor. d_4^{20} 1.12. Viscosity at 20° = 1.97 cP. Soluble in alcohols, esters, ketones, hydrocarbons. A 50% w/w soln in ethanol may be prepd. Slowly sol in water with hydrolytic decompn yielding ethanol and CO_2.

Caution: Concd DEPC is irritating to eyes, mucous membranes and skin.

USE: Gentle esterifying agent. Preservative for wines, soft drinks, fruit juices.

7999. Pyrocatechol. [120-80-9] 1,2-Benzenediol; pyrocatechin; catechol; 1,2-dihydroxybenzene. $C_6H_6O_2$; mol wt 110.11. C 65.45%, H 5.49%, O 29.06%. Prepd by treating salicylaldehyde with hydrogen peroxide, or from its monomethyl ether (guaiacol) by treatment with hydrobromic acid: Dakin, *Org. Synth.* **coll. vol. I**, 149 (2nd ed., 1941). Toxicity data: A. J. Lehman *et al.*, *Adv. Food Res.* **3**, 197 (1951). Carcinogenicity study: M. Hirose *et al.*, *Carcinogenesis* **14**, 525 (1993). *Review:* J. Varagnat, "Hydroquinone, Resorcinol, and Catechol", in *Kirk-Othmer Encyclopedia of Chemical Technology* vol. 13 (Wiley-Interscience, New York, 3rd ed., 1981) pp 39-69.

Monoclinic tablets, prisms from toluene. Discolors in air and light. d 1.344; mp 105°; bp_{760} 245.5°; bp_{400} 221.5°; bp_{200} 197.7°; bp_{100} 176°; bp_{60} 161.7°; bp_{40} 150.6°; bp_{20} 134°; bp_{10} 118.3°; bp_5 104°. Sublimes. Volatile with steam. pK (18°) 9.48. Sol in 2.3 parts water, in alcohol, benzene, chloroform, ether; very sol in pyridine, aq alkalies. Its aq solns soon turn brown. LD_{50} in mice (mg/kg): 260 orally; 190 i.p. (Lehman).

Note: Catechol also refers to catechin, *q.v.*

Caution: Potential symptoms of overexposure are irritation of eyes, skin, respiratory system; lacrimation, eye burns; convulsions, increased blood pressure. Direct contact may cause skin sensitization and dermatitis. Systemic effects similar to phenol, *q.v. See NIOSH Pocket Guide to Chemical Hazards* (DHHS/NIOSH 97-140, 1997) p 56; *Patty's Industrial Hygiene and Toxicology* vol. 2B, G. D. Clayton, F. E. Clayton, Eds. (Wiley-Interscience, New York, 4th ed., 1994) pp 1584-1586.

USE: In photography; dyeing fur; as reagent.

THERAP CAT: Antiseptic.

8000. Pyrogallol. [87-66-1] 1,2,3-Benzenetriol; 1,2,3-trihydroxybenzene; pyrogallic acid. $C_6H_6O_3$; mol wt 126.11. C 57.14%, H 4.80%, O 38.06%. Observed by Scheele in 1786; prepd by Braconot in 1818. Prepn from gallic acid: Marsh, **GB 144897** (1919); Rinderknecht, Niemann, *J. Am. Chem. Soc.* **70**, 2605 (1948); from *p-tert*-butylphenol: Stevens, **US 2603662** (1952 to Gulf). Synthesis from aliphatic sources: Shipchandler *et al.*, *J. Chem. Soc. Perkin Trans. 1* **1975**, 1400. Isoln from *Penicillium patulum*: Tanenbaum, Bassett, *Biochim. Biophys. Acta* **28**, 21 (1958). Acute toxicity: J. W. Dollahite *et al.*, *Am. J. Vet. Res.* **23**, 1264 (1962).

White, odorless crystals, mp 131-133°. Becomes grayish on exposure to air and light. *Poisonous!* d 1.45; bp 309°. Sublimes when slowly heated. One gram dissolves in 1.7 ml water, 1.3 ml alc, 1.6 ml ether; slightly sol in benzene, chloroform, carbon disulfide. The aq soln darkens on exposure to air, quite rapidly when alkaline. *Keep well closed and protected from light.* Incompat. Alkalies, ammonium hydroxide, antipyrine, camphor, phenol, menthol. LD_{50} orally in rabbits: 1.6 g/kg (Dollahite).

Monoacetate. [1330-51-4] Eugallol. $C_8H_8O_4$; mol wt 168.15. White or brownish liquid, bp_{23} ~185°. Sol in water, alcohol, chloroform, ether, acetone and castor oil. Marketed as a 67% soln in acetone.

Triacetate. [525-52-0] Acetpyrogall; Lenigallol. $C_{12}H_{12}O_6$; mol wt 252.22. White, crystalline powder, mp 165°. Slightly sol in water; sol in alcohol. Dec by alkali hydroxide solns.

Caution: Potential symptoms of overexposure are vomiting, hypothermia, fine tremors, weakness, muscle incoordination, diarrhea, loss of reflexes, coma, asphyxia. Direct contact may cause skin irritation and sensitization. *See Patty's Industrial Hygiene and Toxicology* Vol. 2B, G. D. Clayton, F. E. Clayton, Eds. (Wiley Interscience, New York, 4th ed., 1994) p 1595-1597.

USE: Developer in photography; making colloidal solns of metals; as mordant for wool, staining leather, process engraving; manuf various dyes; dyeing furs, hair, etc.; in analytical chemistry as a reagent for antimony and bismuth; as an active reducer for gold, silver and mercury salts; especially for absorption of oxygen in gas analysis.

THERAP CAT: Has been used as antipsoriatic.

8001. L-Pyroglutamic Acid. [98-79-3] 5-Oxo-L-proline; 5-oxo-2-pyrrolidinecarboxylic acid; 2-pyrrolidone-5-carboxylic acid; glutimic acid; glutiminic acid; α-aminoglutaric acid lactam; glutamic acid lactam; pyroGlu. $C_5H_7NO_3$; mol wt 129.11. C 46.51%, H 5.46%, N 10.85%, O 37.18%. Cyclized internal amide of L-glutamic acid found in vegetables, fruits, grasses, and molasses. Easily prepd from L-glutamic acid by autoclaving with an equal wt of water at 135-140°: Dearborn, Stekol, **US 2738267**; purification: Blish, **US 2738353** (1950, 1956, both to International Minerals and Chem.). *Review:* Orlowski, Meister, in *The Enzymes* vol. 4, P. D. Boyer, Ed. (Academic Press, New York, 3rd ed., 1971) pp 123-151; C. Moret, M. Briley, *Trends Pharmacol. Sci.* **9**, 278-279 (1988).

Orthorhombic bisphenoidal crystals from alcohol + petr ether. mp 162-163°. $[\alpha]_D^{20}$ −11.9° (c = 2); $[\alpha]_D^{25}$ −23.6° (c = 5 at pH 7). Sol in water, alcohol, acetone.

USE: In the resolution of racemic amines.

8002. Pyrolan. [87-47-8] Dimethylcarbamic acid 3-methyl-1-phenyl-1*H*-pyrazol-5-yl ester; 1-phenyl-3-methyl-5-pyrazolyl dimethylcarbamate; 3-methyl-1-phenyl-5-pyrazolyl dimethylcarbamate; ENT-17588; G-22008. $C_{13}H_{15}N_3O_2$; mol wt 245.28. C 63.66%, H 6.16%, N 17.13%, O 13.05%. Prepn from 1-phenyl-3-methyl-5-pyrazolone and dimethylcarbamoyl chloride: **CH 279553** (1952 to Geigy); **GB 681376**. Anticholinesterase activity: Pulver, Domenjoz, *Experientia* **7**, 306 (1951); Ferguson, Alexander, *J. Agric. Food Chem.* **1**, 888 (1953); Müller, Spindler, *Experientia* **10**, 91 (1954). Toxicity study: E. W. Schafer, *Toxicol. Appl. Pharmacol.* **21**, 315 (1972).

Crystals, mp 50°. $bp_{0.2}$ 160-162°. Possesses water and lipid solubility. LD_{50} orally in rats: 62 mg/kg (Schafer).

Caution: Cholinesterase inhibitor.

USE: Insecticide.

8003. Pyroligneous Acid. [8030-97-5] Wood vinegar; pyroligneous vinegar. Obtained by destructive distillation of wood.

Yellowish, acid liquid; empyreumatic odor; contains about 6% acetic acid. Miscible with water, alcohol.

USE: Largely for smoking meats.

8004. Pyromellitic Acid. [89-05-4] 1,2,4,5-Benzenetetracarboxylic acid. $C_{10}H_6O_8$; mol wt 254.15. C 47.26%, H 2.38%, O 50.36%. Prepd by heating mellitic (benzenehexacarboxylic) acid with $KHSO_4$ and H_2SO_4: Silberrad, *J. Chem. Soc.* **89,** 1795 (1906) (actually the dianhydride, mp 286°, is obtained by this method). Laboratory prepn from pine or spruce charcoal: Philippi, Thelen, *Org. Synth.* **coll. vol. II,** 551 (1943); by oxidation of benzene derivatives contg substituents in the 1,2,4,5 positions: Jacobsen, *Ber.* **17,** 2516 (1884).

HOOC—[benzene ring]—COOH / HOOC—[ring]—COOH

Dihydrate. Triclinic plates from water. When anhydr, mp 276°. Distills with anhydride formation. 1.5 g (anhydr) dissolves in 100 ml water. Freely sol in alc.

Tetramethyl ester. $C_{14}H_{14}O_8$. Leaflets from alc, mp 141.5°.

8005. Pyronaridine. [74847-35-1] 4-[(7-Chloro-2-methoxybenzo[*b*]-1,5-naphthyridin-10-yl)amino]-2,6-bis(1-pyrrolidinylmethyl)phenol; malaridine. $C_{29}H_{32}ClN_5O_2$; mol wt 518.05. C 67.23%, H 6.23%, Cl 6.84%, N 13.52%, O 6.18%. Prepn: X.-Y. Zheng *et al., Yao Hsueh Hsueh Pao* **14,** 736 (1979), *C.A.* **93,** 132397 (1980). HPLC determn in blood and urine: S. A. Wages *et al., J. Chromatogr.* **527,** 115 (1990). *In vitro* activity vs drug resistant malaria: E. I. Elueze *et al., J. Antimicrob. Chemother.* **37,** 511 (1996). Clinical trial: P. Ringwald *et al., Lancet* **347,** 24 (1996). *Reviews:* B. Shao, *Chin. Med. J.* **103,** 428-434 (1990); C. Chang *et al., Trans. R. Soc. Trop. Med. Hyg.* **86,** 7-10 (1992).

Tetraphosphate. [76748-86-2] $C_{29}H_{32}ClN_5O_2 \cdot 4H_3PO_4$. Hygroscopic, yellow needles, mp 233-236° (dec). Odorless; slightly bitter taste. Sol in water; very sparingly sol in ethanol. Insol in choroform, ether, and other organic solvents. LD_{50} in mice (mg/kg): 251 ±33 i.m.; 1368 ±239 orally (Shao).

THERAP CAT: Antimalarial.

8006. Pyronine B. [2150-48-3] 3,6-Bis(diethylamino)xanthylium chloride; [6-(diethylamino)-3*H*-xanthen-3-ylidene]diethylammonium chloride; C.I. 45010. $C_{21}H_{27}ClN_2O$; mol wt 358.90. C 70.28%, H 7.58%, Cl 9.88%, N 7.81%, O 4.46%. Prepn of metallic complex: **DE 54190** (1889 to Bayer); **DE 59003** (1891 to A. Leonhardt); Biehringer, *Ber.* **27,** 3299 (1894); *J. Prakt. Chem.* **54,** 217 (1896); Albert, *J. Chem. Soc.* **1947,** 244. Structure: Chamberlin *et al., J. Org. Chem.* **27,** 2263 (1962). The commercial product is a complex with iron as depicted below.

Ferric chloride complex. Green metallic needles, mp 176-178°. Absorption max (50% ethanol): 555 nm ($E_{1cm}^{1\%}$ 2324).

USE: Stain for bacteria, molds, ribonucleic acids.

8007. Pyronine Y. [92-32-0] 3,6-Bis(dimethylamino)xanthylium chloride; *N*-[6-(dimethylamino)-3*H*-xanthene-3-ylidene]-*N*-methylmethanaminium chloride; [6-(dimethylamino)-3*H*-xanthen-3-ylidene]dimethylammonium chloride; tetramethyldiaminoxanthylium chloride; C.I. 45005; pyronine G. $C_{17}H_{19}ClN_2O$; mol wt 302.80. C 67.43%, H 6.32%, Cl 11.71%, N 9.25%, O 5.28%. Prepn from dimethyl-*m*-aminophenol: Mohlau, Koch, *Ber.* **27,** 2887 (1894); **DE 58955**; **DE 59003**; **DE 63081** (1892 to Leonhardt); *Frdl.* **3,** 92-94. *See also: Colour Index* **vol. 4** (3rd ed., 1971) p 4417.

Ferric chloride complex, lustrous green crystals from alc. Soly in water at 26°: 8.96% giving a red soln. Soly in alc at 26°: 0.60%. Solns show a yellowish fluorescence. Absorption max about 552 nm; curves: Stotz *et al., Stain Technol.* **25,** 57 (1950).

USE: Bacterial and biological stain.

8008. Pyrophosphoric Acid. [2466-09-3] Diphosphoric acid. $H_4O_7P_2$; mol wt 177.98. H 2.27%, O 62.93%, P 34.81%. Prepd according to the equation $5H_3PO_4 + POCl_3 \rightarrow 3H_4P_2O_7 + 3HCl$: Geuther, *J. Prakt. Chem.* [2] **8,** 359 (1874); Partington, Wallsom, *Chem. News* **136,** 97 (1928); by heating H_3PO_4: Bell, *Ind. Eng. Chem.* **40,** 1464 (1948).

Hygroscopic glass, seldom acicular crystals, mp 61°. K_1 at 18° = 0.14; $K_2 = 0.011$; $K_3 = 2.1 \times 10^{-7}$; $K_4 = 4.1 \times 10^{-10}$. Forms normal salts, such as $Na_4P_2O_7$, and dihydrogen salts, such as $Na_2H_2P_2O_7$. Solubility in water (23°): 709 g/100 ml. Quickly converted to phosphoric acid when dissolved in hot water. Sol in alcohol and ether.

8009. Pyrosulfuric Acid. [7783-05-3] Disulfuric acid. $H_2O_7S_2$; mol wt 178.14. H 1.13%, O 62.87%, S 36.00%. $H_2S_2O_7$. Colorless to slightly yellow, very hygroscopic crystals, fuming strongly in air. d 1.89; mp 35°. Very sol in water with violent hissing and liberation of much heat. *Keep tightly closed and handle with caution.*

8010. Pyrovalerone. [3563-49-3] 1-(4-Methylphenyl)-2-(1-pyrrolidinyl)-1-pentanone; 4′-methyl-2-(1-pyrrolidinyl)valerophenone; α-pyrrolidino-*p*-methylvalerophenone; 1-(1-pyrrolidinyl)butyl *p*-tolyl ketone; 1-(*p*-tolyl)-1-oxo-2-pyrrolidino-*n*-pentane; 1-(*p*-tolyl)-2-pyrrolidino-1-pentanone. $C_{16}H_{23}NO$; mol wt 245.36. C 78.32%, H 9.45%, N 5.71%, O 6.52%. Prepn: **GB 927475** (1963 to Wander); **GB 933507**; E. Seeger, **US 3314970** (1963, 1967 both to Thomae); Heffe, *Helv. Chim. Acta* **47,** 1289 (1964). Pharmacology: Stille *et al., Arzneim.-Forsch.* **13,** 871 (1963). Metabolism: Michaelis *et al., J. Med. Chem.* **13,** 497 (1970).

$bp_{0.08}$ 104°.

Hydrochloride. [1147-62-2] F-1983; Centroton; Thymergix. $C_{16}H_{23}NO \cdot HCl$; mol wt 281.82. Crystals from 2-butanone or from methanol + acetone + diethyl ether, mp 178°. LD_{50} orally in mice: 350 mg/kg (Stille).

Note: This is a controlled substance (stimulant): **21 CFR,** 1308.15.

THERAP CAT: CNS stimulant.

8011. Pyroxylin. [9004-70-0] Cellulose nitrate; nitrocellulose; collodion cotton; soluble gun cotton; collodion wool; colloxylin; xyloidin; celloidin; Parlodion. Variable mixture which consists chiefly of cellulose tetranitrate. *Review:* R. T. Bogan *et al.* in *Kirk-Othmer Encyclopedia of Chemical Technology* **vol. 5** (Wiley-Interscience, New York, 3rd ed., 1979) pp 129-143.

Yellowish-white, matted mass of filaments, having the appearance of raw cotton. *Highly flammable;* pyroxlin with higher nitrogen content *may explode!* When kept in well-closed containers and exposed to light it dec. Sol in 25 parts of a mixture of 1 vol alcohol and 3 vols ether; also sol in methanol, acetone, glacial acetic acid, amyl acetate. *Keep loosely packed in cartons and protected from light and moisture.* Can be shipped with safety only when wet with 25-30% water or alcohol.

USE: In manuf of collodions; in lacquer coatings, inks, adhesives. Cellulose hexanitrate is used in explosives and propellants. Celloidin is used for embedding sections in microscopy; in electrotechnics, photography, galvanoplasty.

THERAP CAT: Topical protectant.

8012. Pyrrobutamine. [91-82-7] 1-[4-(4-Chlorophenyl)-3-phenyl-2-butenyl]pyrrolidine; 1-[γ-*p*-(chlorobenzyl)cinnamyl]pyrrolidine; 1-*p*-chlorophenyl-2-phenyl-4-pyrrolidyl-2-butene; Pyronil. $C_{20}H_{22}ClN$; mol wt 311.85. C 77.03%, H 7.11%, Cl 11.37%, N 4.49%. Prepn: J. Mills, **US 2655509** (1953 to Eli Lilly). Pharmacology and toxicity: H. M. Lee *et al., Proc. Soc. Exp. Biol. Med.* **80,** 458 (1952). Pharmacology and physical properties: N. G. Lordi, J. E. Christian, *J. Am. Pharm. Assoc.* **45,** 300 (1956). Structure-activity and stereochemical study: A. F. Casy, R. R. Ison, *J. Pharm. Pharmacol.* **22,** 270 (1970). GC-MS determn in urine: H. Maurer, K. Pfleger, *J. Chromatogr.* **430,** 31 (1988).

Oily liquid, $bp_{0.3}$ 190-195°. On standing gives crystals, mp 48-49°. d^{25} 1.1052. uv max (95% ethanol): 360, 243 nm (α 112, 9500), (c = 0.538, 0.00538 mg/ml).

Diphosphate. [135-31-9] $C_{20}H_{28}ClNO_8P_2$. Crystals from alcohol + ether, mp 129.5-130°. pKa_1 8.77, pka_2 5.23. Sol in warm water to the extent of 10%. Soly in alcohol at 25° about 5%. Soly at pH 7.4 (37.5°): 0.00087 M/l. Practically insol in chloroform, ether. LD$_{50}$ in mice, guinea pigs (mg/kg): 1270 ±156, 1241 ±165 s.c.; 836.8 ±95, 625.6 ±41.9 i.m.; 1116 ±73, 992.6 ±107 orally; in mice (mg/kg): 53.53 ±1.61 i.v. (Lee).

Hydrochloride. $C_{20}H_{22}ClN.HCl$. Crystals from alcohol + ether, mp 227-228°.

Hydrobromide. $C_{20}H_{22}ClN.HBr$. Crystals from alcohol + ether, mp 228-229°.

THERAP CAT: Antihistaminic.

8013. Pyrrocaine. [2210-77-7] *N*-(2,6-Dimethylphenyl)-1-pyrrolidineacetamide; 1-pyrrolidineaceto-2′,6′-xylidide; 2-(1-pyrrolidinyl)-2′,6′-acetoxylidide; 1-pyrrolidinoaceto-2,6-dimethylanilide; EN-1010; NSC-52644; Endocaine; Dynacaine. $C_{14}H_{20}N_2O$; mol wt 232.32. C 72.38%, H 8.68%, N 12.06%, O 6.89%. Prepn: Schlesinger, Gordon, **US 2813861** (1957 to Endo); Löfgren *et al., Acta Chem. Scand.* **11,** 1724 (1957).

Crysts from hexane or petr ether + dibutyl ether, mp 83°.

Hydrochloride. [2210-64-2] $C_{14}H_{20}N_2O.HCl$. Crystals from isopropanol, mp 205°. Soluble in water, alcohol, isopropyl alcohol. Practically insol in chloroform, ether.

THERAP CAT: Anesthetic (local).

8014. 1*H*-Pyrrole. [109-97-7] Azole; imidole; divinylenimine. C_4H_5N; mol wt 67.09. C 71.61%, H 7.51%, N 20.88%. A constituent of coal tar and bone oil: Runge, *Ann. Phys.* **31,** 67 (1834). Prepd industrially by fractional distillation of bone oil, or by the thermal decompn of ammonium mucate with glycerol or mineral oil: McElvain, Bolliger, *Org. Synth.* **coll. vol. I** (2nd ed., 1941) p 473; Blicke, Powers, *Ind. Eng. Chem.* **19,** 1334 (1927). Also formed on heating of albumin; on heating sheep's wool with aq barium hydroxide soln; by pyrolysis of gelatin. Alternate prepns from acetaldehyde and ammonia: Tschitschibabin, *Chem. Zentralbl.* **1916,** I, 920; from succinaldehyde with ammonia and acetic acid: Harries, *Ber.* **34,** 1496 (1901); **35,** 1183 (1902); distilling succinimide with zinc or sodium: Bell, Bernthsen, *Ber.* **13,** 877, 1049 (1880). Purification and physical properties: R. V. Helm *et al., J. Phys. Chem.* **62,** 858 (1958). *Review:* Fischer-Orth, *Die Chemie des Pyrrols* (Leipzig, 1934-1940); E. Vittort, L. R. Anderson in *Kirk-Othmer Encyclopedia of Chemical Technology* **vol. 19** (Wiley-Interscience, New York, 3rd ed., 1982) pp 499-520.

Liquid. Agreeable empyreumatic odor resembling that of chloroform. Colorless when freshly distilled, darkens unless every trace of oxygen is removed. d_4^{20} 0.9691. bp_{760} 129.8°. Best distilled *in vacuo.* n_D^{20} 1.5085. Flash pt, closed cup: 102°F (39.0°C). Absorption spectrum: Menczel, *Phys. Chem.* **125,** 161; *Chem. Zentralbl.* **1927,** I, 2510. Sparingly sol in water; freely sol in alcohol, benzene, ether. Insol in aq alkalies. Sol in dil acids with decompn. Solns in dil HCl yield pyrrole red, an amorphous, orange-colored substance; also polymerization takes place under the influence of acids and glycols.

8015. Pyrrolidine. [123-75-1] Tetrahydropyrrole. C_4H_9N; mol wt 71.12. C 67.55%, H 12.76%, N 19.69%. Found in tobacco and carrot leaves. Probable biosynthesis from ornithine and putrescine. Usually prepd by reduction of pyrrole.

Almost colorless liquid; unpleasant ammonia-like odor. Fumes in air. bp 88.5-89°. $d_4^{22.5}$ 0.8520. n_D^{28} 1.4402. Strong base. pK (25°) 2.89. Miscible with water. Soluble in alcohol, ether, chloroform.

8016. 2-Pyrrolidone. [616-45-5] 2-Pyrrolidinone; 2-oxopyrrolidine; α-pyrrolidone; 2-ketopyrrolidine. C_4H_7NO; mol wt 85.10. C 56.45%, H 8.29%, N 16.46%, O 18.80%. Prepd on a large scale from butyrolactone by a Reppe process: **DE 1085525** (to BASF). Other prepns: Metzger, Seelert, *Angew. Chem.* **75,** 919 (1963); Copenhaver, Ney, **US 3095423** (1963 to Minnesota Mining & Manuf); Lidov, **US 3109005** (1963 to Halcon International).

Liquid above 25°. bp_{760} 245°; $bp_{9.2}$ 113-114°; $bp_{0.2}$ 76°. d_4^{25} 1.116. Flash pt, open cup: 265°F (129°C). Viscosity at 25° = 13.3 cP. Dipole moment: 2.3. In the presence of the stoichiometric amount of water a cryst monohydrate, mp 30°, can be formed. Noncorrosive. Good chemical stability. Miscible with water, ethanol, ether, chloroform, benzene, ethyl acetate, carbon disulfide.

USE: Intermediate in the manuf of polyvinylpyrrolidone and polypyrrolidone (a polymer, formed in the presence of alkaline catalysts). Also used as high-boiling solvent in petroleum processing, acrylonitrile manuf. Industrial solvent for polymers, chlordane, DDT, sorbitol, glycerol, iodine, sugars. In specialty printers inks. As plasticizer and coalescing agent for acrylic-styrene emulsion-type floor polishes.

8017. 3-Pyrroline. [109-96-6] 2,5-Dihydro-1*H*-pyrrole. C_4H_7N; mol wt 69.11. C 69.52%, H 10.21%, N 20.27%. Prepd by reduction of pyrrole with zinc and glacial acetic or hydrochloric acid.

Almost colorless liquid. Unpleasant, ammonia-like odor. Fumes in air. Very hygroscopic, also absorbs CO_2. bp_{748} 90-91°; d_4^{20} 0.9097; n_D^{20} 1.4664. Strong base. Miscible with water. Sol in alcohol, ether, chloroform.

8018. Pyrrolnitrin. [1018-71-9] 3-Chloro-4-(3-chloro-2-nitrophenyl)pyrrole; 3-chloro-4-(2'-nitro-3'-chlorophenyl)pyrrole; PN; Pyroace. $C_{10}H_6Cl_2N_2O_2$; mol wt 257.07. C 46.72%, H 2.35%, Cl 27.58%, N 10.90%, O 12.45%. Antifungal antibiotic isolated from *Pseudomonas pyrrocinia* n. sp.: K. Arima *et al.*, *Agric. Biol. Chem.* **28**, 575 (1964); *eidem, J. Antibiot.* **18**, 201 (1965). Structure: Imanaka *et al., ibid.* 207. Synthesis: S. Umio *et al.*, **BE 670427**; *eidem,* **US 3428648** (1964, 1969 both to Fujisawa); Nakano *et al., Tetrahedron Lett.* **1966,** 737; S. Umio *et al.* (10 publications) *Chem. Pharm. Bull.* **17,** 559-628 (1969); Gosteli, *Helv. Chim. Acta* **55**, 451 (1972). Pharmacological studies: M. Nishida *et al., J. Antibiot.* **18**, 211 (1965).

Pale yellow crystals from hot cyclohexane, mp 124.5°. Gradually changes to a red or brown color on exposure to sunlight and loses antibiotic activity. uv max: 252 nm (ε 7500). Slightly sol in water, petr ether, cyclohexane; sol in methanol, ethanol, butanol, acetone, ethyl acetate, benzene, ether, chloroform, carbon tetrachloride, pyridine, acetic acid. LD_{50} in rats, rabbits (mg/kg): 68, 105 i.p. (Nishida).

THERAP CAT: Antifungal.

8019. Pyrrolysine. [448235-52-7] N^6-[(3*R*)-1,5-Didehydro-3-methyl-D-prolyl]-L-lysine; L-pyrrolysine. $C_{12}H_{21}N_3O_3$; mol wt 255.31. C 56.45%, H 8.29%, N 16.46%, O 18.80%. Naturally occurring, genetically encoded amino acid found in certain methanogenic Archaea; originally described as L-lysine ε-amide linked to (4*R*,5*R*)-4-substituted-1-pyrroline-5-carboxylate. Identification of pyrrolysine-specific tRNA in *Methanosarcina barkeri*: G. Srinivasan *et al., Science* **296**, 1459 (2002). Identification as UAG-encoded residue in monomethylamine methyltransferase: B. Hao *et al., ibid.* 1462. Identification of C_4-substituent as a methyl group, synthesis and properties: *idem et al., Chem Biol.* **11**, 1317 (2004). MS analysis: J. A. Soares *et al., J. Biol. Chem.* **280**, 36962 (2005). *Reviews:* C. Fenske *et al., Angew. Chem. Int. Ed.* **42**, 606-610 (2003); J. A. Krzycki, *Curr. Opin. Microbiol.* **8**, 706-712 (2005).

Lithium salt. $C_{12}H_{20}LiN_3O_3$; mol wt 261.25. White solid. $[\alpha]_D^{20}$ -2.1° (c = 0.25 in CH_3OH). uv max (methanol): 310 nm (sh) (ε 35.4).

8020. Pyruvate Decarboxylase. [9001-04-1] Pyruvic decarboxylase; pyruvic carboxylase; α-carboxylase; 2-oxo-acid carboxylyase. An enzyme found in yeast, in plants, in wheat germ and

bacteria: Neuberg, Rosenthal, *Biochem. Z.* **51**, 142 (1913); Holzer *et al., ibid.* **327**, 331 (1956); Singer, Pensky, *J. Biol. Chem.* **196**, 375 (1952); King, Chelelin, *ibid.* **208**, 821 (1954); Howells, Lindstrom, *J. Bacteriol.* **75**, 305 (1958). Cofactors: Diphosphothiamine, divalent metal ions. Catalyzes decarboxylation of α-ketoacids to aldehydes + CO_2: Juni, *J. Biol. Chem.* **236**, 2302 (1961). Structure and mechanism of action of the yeast enzyme: Schellenberger, *Angew. Chem. Int. Ed.* **6**, 1024 (1967). *Review:* Utter, *The Enzymes* **vol. 5**, P. D. Boyer *et al.,* Eds. (Academic Press, New York, 2nd ed., 1961) pp 320-323.

8021. Pyruvic Acid. [127-17-3] 2-Oxopropanoic acid; α-ketopropionic acid; acetylformic acid; pyroracemic acid; brenztraubensäure (German). $C_3H_4O_3$; mol wt 88.06. C 40.92%, H 4.58%, O 54.51%. $CH_3COCOOH$. Intermediate in sugar metabolism and in enzymatic carbohydrate degradation (alcoholic fermentation) where it is converted to acetaldehyde and CO_2 by carboxylase, *see* Nord, *Chem. Rev.* **26**, 423 (1940). In muscle, pyruvic acid (derived from glycogen) is reduced to lactic acid during exertion, which is reoxidized and partially retransformed to glycogen during rest. The liver can convert pyruvic acid to alanine by amination. Pyruvic acid has been isolated from cane sugar fermentation broth by fixation with β-naphthylamine giving α-methyl-β-naphthocinchonic acid: Grab, *Biochem. Z.* **123**, 84 (1921). The most practical method of preparing pyruvic acid is by distillation of tartaric acid in presence of potassium acid sulfate as dehydrating agent. The distillate must be fractionated under reduced pressure: Erlenmeyer, *Ber.* **14**, 321 (1881); Döbner, *Ann.* **242**, 269 (1887); Howard, Fraser, *Org. Synth.* **coll. vol. I** (2nd ed., 1941) p 475.

Liquid. Odor resembling that of acetic acid. d_4^{15} 1.267; mp 11.8°; bp_{760} 165° (dec); bp_{100} 106.5°; bp_{40} 85.3°; bp_{20} 70.8°; bp_{10} 57.9°; bp_5 45.8°; $bp_{1.0}$ 21.4°; n_D^{20} 1.4138. Absorption spectrum: Henri, Fromageot, *Bull. Soc. Chim.* [4] **37**, 846 (1925). pK (25°) 2.49. Miscible with water, alcohol, ether. Polymerizes and dec on standing unless pure and kept in container with airtight closure.

Methyl ester. $C_4H_6O_3$. Liquid, bp_{760} 134-137°.

Ethyl ester. $C_5H_8O_3$. Liquid, bp_{760} 155°; bp_{750} 147.5°; bp_{42} 69-71°; bp_{20} 66° also 56°. Prepn from ethyl lactate by oxidation with $KMnO_4$: Cornforth, *Org. Synth.* **coll. vol. IV**, 467 (1963).

8022. Pyrvinium Pamoate. [3546-41-6] 6-(Dimethylamino)-2-[2-(2,5-dimethyl-1-phenyl-1*H*-pyrrol-3-yl)ethenyl]-1-methylquinolinium salt with 4,4'-methylenebis[3-hydroxy-2-naphthalenecarboxylic acid] (2:1); bis[6-(dimethylamino)-2-[2-(2,5-dimethyl-1-phenylpyrrol-3-yl)vinyl]-1-methylquinolinium] 4,4'-methylenebis(3-hydroxy-2-naphthoate); 6-(dimethylamino)-2-[2-(2,5-dimethyl-1-phenyl-3-pyrryl)vinyl]-1-methylquinolinium salt of 2,2'-dihydroxy-1,1'-dinaphthylmethane-3,3'-dicarboxylic acid; pyrvinium embonate; viprynium embonate; Molevac; Povanyl; Pyrcon; Vanquin. $C_{75}H_{70}N_6O_6$; mol wt 1151.39. C 78.24%, H 6.13%, N 7.30%, O 8.34%. Cyanine dye. Prepn: E. F. Elslager, D. F. Worth, **US 2925417** (1960 to Parke, Davis). Determn in pharmaceutical prepn: H. D. Beckstead, S. J. Smith, *J. Pharm. Sci.* **56**, 390 (1967); by HPLC: U. G. G. Hennig *et al., Arch. Toxicol.* **60**, 278 (1987). Clinical trial: R. A. Buchanan *et al., Clin. Pharmacol. Ther.* **16**, 716 (1974). Clinical pharmacology: T. C. Smith *et al., ibid.* **19**, 802 (1976). Review of use in *Enterobius vermicularis* infections: G. C. Cook, *Gut* **35**, 1159-1162 (1994).

Bright orange or orange-red to almost black precipitate, mp 210-215° (softens at 190°). Absorption max: 236, 356, 503 nm. Stable to heat, light and air. Slightly sol in chloroform, methoxyethanol; very slightly sol in alcohol. Practically insol in water, ether.

Pyrvinium chloride. [548-84-5] Viprynium chloride; SN-4395. $C_{26}H_{28}ClN_3$; mol wt 417.97. Prepn: E. Van Lare, L. G. S. Brooker, **US 2515912** (1950 to Eastman Kodak). May occur as dihydrate, deep-red powder, dec 249-251°. Sparingly sol in water.

THERAP CAT: Anthelmintic (Nematodes).

Q

8023. Q-Enzyme. [9001-97-2] α-Glucan branching glycosyltransferase; potato branching enzyme; enzyme Q; branching factor; glucosan transglycosylase. A widely distributed enzyme which transfers part of a 1,4-glucosan chain from a 4- to a 6-position in polysaccharides. Isoln from potatoes: Barker *et al., J. Chem. Soc.* **1949,** 1705. Crystallization: Gilbert, Patrick, *Biochem. J.* **51,** 181 (1952). Improved isoln procedure: Griffen, Wu, *Biochemistry* **7,** 3063 (1968). Although Q-enzyme is unstable in aq soln, it can be stored for long periods without appreciable loss in activity when it is freeze-dried. *Review:* Barker, Bourne, *Q. Rev. Chem. Soc.* **7,** 65-68 (1953); Dixon, Webb, *Enzymes* (Academic Press, New York, 1958) *passim.*

8024. Quantum Dye. $C_{38}H_{36}EuN_8S_2$; mol wt 820.84. C 55.60%, H 4.42%, Eu 18.51%, N 13.65%, S 7.81%. Macrocyclic europium-chelate fluorimetric tracer. Prepn and optical properties: L. M. Vallarino *et al., Proc. SPIE Int. Soc. Opt. Eng.* **1885,** 376 (1993). Quantification of Eu^{3+} in dye: K. Saito *et al., Anal. Biochem.* **258,** 311 (1998). Use as quantitative fluorescent label for glycoproteins: Y. C. Lee *et al, Glycobiology* **8,** 849 (1998); I. L. Deras *et al., Carbohydr. Res.* **306,** 469 (1998).

R = H₂C— [benzene ring] —N=C=S

R is attached at (a or b) and (c or d).

White crystalline solid. Water soluble. Absorption max: 360 nm (excitation); 615 nm (emission).

USE: Fluorescent probe especially for glycoproteins.

8025. Quassia. Bitter wood; bitter ash. The wood of *Picrasma excelsa* (Sw.) Planch, or of *Quassia amara* L., Simaroubaceae. The first is known in commerce as Jamaica quassia, the second as Surinam quassia. *Habit. Picrasma excelsa* inhabits Jamaica and the Caribbean Islands; *Quassia amara* is a native of Brazil and Guiana and is cultivated in Colombia, Panama, and the West Indies. Quassin and neoquassin are the bitter principles of Surinam quassia; picrasmin, that of Jamaica quassia. These bitter pinciples are obtained in yields of 0.1-0.2% and appear commercially under the name of quassin.

Unground quassia occurs usually in chips, raspings, or shavings, occasionally in billets; yellowish-white to bright yellow with a few light gray pieces; coarsely grained, fibrous. Slight odor; very bitter taste. The powdered form is pale yellow in color.

USE: The extract is used for fly poison on flypaper; to imitate hops.

THERAP CAT: Anthelmintic.

THERAP CAT (VET): Has been used as a bitter, as an anthelmintic.

8026. Quassin. [76-78-8] 2,12-Dimethoxypicrasa-2,12-diene-1,11,16-trione; 3αβ,6αβ,7,7aα,8,11a,11bα,11c-octahydro-2,10-dimethoxy-3,8α,11aβ,11cβ-tetramethylphenanthro[10,1-*bc*]pyran-1,5,11(4*H*)-trione; nigakilactone D. $C_{22}H_{28}O_6$; mol wt 388.45. C 68.02%, H 7.27%, O 24.71%. One of the bitter constituents of the wood of *Quassia amara* L., Simaroubaceae known in commerce as Surinam quassia. Obtained by the resolution of the mixture of bitter constituents of quassia wood: E. P. Clark, *J. Am. Chem. Soc.* **59,** 927 (1937); London *et al., J. Chem. Soc.* **1950,** 3431. Structure:

Valenta *et al., Tetrahedron Lett.* no. **20,** 25 (1960); Carman, Ward, *ibid.* **1961,** 317; Valenta *et al., Tetrahedron* **15,** 100 (1961). Stereochemistry: Valenta *et al., ibid.* **18,** 1433 (1962). Identity with nigakilactone D: Murae *et al., ibid.* **27,** 1545 (1971). Synthetic approach: Stojanac *et al., Can. J. Chem.* **53,** 619 (1975); P. A. Grieco *et al., Tetrahedron Lett.* **21,** 1619 (1980). Total synthesis of *dl*-form: eidem, *J. Am. Chem. Soc.* **102,** 7586 (1980).

Very bitter rectangular plates from dilute methanol, mp 222°. $[\alpha]_D^{20}$ +34.5° (c = 5.09 in $CHCl_3$). uv max: ~255 nm (ε ~11,650). Sol in benzene, alc, acetone, chloroform, pyridine, acetic acid, hot ethyl acetate. Sparingly sol in ether, petr ether. Bitterness threshold 1:60,000.

8027. Quaternium-15. [4080-31-3] 1-(3-Chloro-2-propenyl)-3,5,7-triaza-1-azoniatricyclo[3.3.1.1³,⁷]decane chloride; 1-(3-chloroallyl)-3,5,7-triaza-1-azoniaadamantane chloride; *N*-(3-chloroallyl)hexaminium chloride; CTAC; Dowicil 75. $C_9H_{16}Cl_2N_4$; mol wt 251.16. C 43.04%, H 6.42%, Cl 28.23%, N 22.31%. Microbiocide. Prepn and antibacterial activity: C. R. Scott, P. A. Wolf, *Appl. Microbiol.* **10,** 211 (1962). Cosmetic ingredient review: *J. Am. Coll. Toxicol.* **5,** 61-101 (1986).

cis-Form

Cream colored powder with pungent odor. Dec above 60°. Soly at 25° (g/100 g): mineral oil <0.1, isopropanol <0.1, ethanol 2.4, methanol 20.8, glycerine 12.6, propylene glycol 18.7, water 127.2. LD_{50} (as 50% aq soln) in female rats, rabbits (mg/kg): 1552, 78.5 orally; in female rabbits (mg/kg): 565 dermally (cosmetic ingredient review). *Keep dry and cool.*

*cis***-Form.** [51229-78-8] Dowicil 200; CoSept 200. Off-white powder with slight amine odor. Bulk density (25°): 0.44 g/cc. Vapor pressure (25°): 1×10^{-9} mm Hg. Miscible with water. *Flammable, keep dry and cool.*

USE: Preservative in cosmetics, hair care products, soaps, adhesives.

8028. Quatrimycin. [79-85-6] [4*R*-(4α,4aβ,5aβ,6α,12aβ)]-4-(Dimethylamino)-1,4,4a,5,5a,6,11,12a-octahydro-3,6,10,12,12a-pentahydroxy-6-methyl-1,11-dioxo-2-naphthacenecarboxamide; epitetracycline. $C_{22}H_{24}N_2O_8$; mol wt 444.43. C 59.45%, H 5.44%, N 6.30%, O 28.80%. Prepn by epimerization of tetracycline: McCormick *et al., J. Am. Chem. Soc.* **79,** 2849 (1957); Kaplan *et al., Antibiot. Chemother.* **7,** 569 (1957); Remmers *et al., J. Pharm. Sci.* **52,** 752 (1963). Acute toxicity: L. Kung, H. Sun, *Yao Hsueh Hsueh Pao* **13,** 244 (1966); *C.A.* **65,** 7869e (1966).

Monohydrate. Crystals, mp 178° dec. $[\alpha]_D^{25}$ −335° (c = 0.5 in 0.03*N* HCl). uv max (0.01*N* H_2SO_4): 216, 255, 270, 355 (ε 13,900, 16,400, 15,200, 14,700). LD_{50} i.v. in mice: 85.8 mg/kg (Kung, Sun).

Ammonium salt monohydrate. $C_{22}H_{27}N_3O_8 \cdot H_2O$. Yellow crystals, mp 170° dec. $[\alpha]_D^{25}$ −321° (c = 0.5 in 0.03N HCl). Soly in water >50 mg/kg.

Hydrochloride. $C_{22}H_{25}ClN_2O_8$. Amorphous yellow solid. $[\alpha]_D^{25}$ −325° (c = 0.58 in 0.2N HCl). Soly in water >100 mg/ml.

Methiodide. $C_{23}H_{27}IN_2O_8$. Crystals, mp 161-162°. $[\alpha]_D^{25}$ −265° (c = 0.5 in 0.03N HCl).

8029. Quazepam. [36735-22-5] 7-Chloro-5-(2-fluorophenyl)-1,3-dihydro-1-(2,2,2-trifluoroethyl)-2H-1,4-benzodiazepine-2-thione; Sch-16134; Doral; Dormalin; Oniria; Prosedar; Quazium; Selepam. $C_{17}H_{11}ClF_4N_2S$; mol wt 386.79. C 52.79%, H 2.87%, Cl 9.17%, F 19.65%, N 7.24%, S 8.29%. Benzodiazepine hypnotic. Prepn: M. Steinman, DE 2138773; idem, US 3845039 (1972, 1974 both to Schering Corp.); M. Steinman et al., J. Med. Chem. 16, 1354 (1973). Pharmacology: A. Barnett et al., Arzneim.-Forsch. 32, 1452 (1982); E. Ongini et al., ibid. 1456. GC determn in plasma: J. M. Hilbert et al., J. Pharm. Sci. 73, 516 (1984). Pharmacokinetics: M. Chung et al., Clin. Pharm. Ther. 35, 520 (1984). Metabolism: N. Zampaglione et al., Drug Metab. Dispos. 13, 25 (1985). Clinical trials in insomnia: J. W. Goethe, G. Kader, Curr. Ther. Res. 32, 150 (1982); M. Mamelak et al., J. Clin. Pharmacol. 24, 65 (1984). Toxicology: H. E. Black et al., Arzneim.-Forsch. 37, 906 (1987).

Crystals from methylene chloride-hexane, mp 137.5-139°. LD_{50} in mice (mg/kg): >1370 i.v., >5000 orally (Orgini). LD_{50} in male, female mice, rats (mg/kg): 845, 921, 3072, 2749 i.p. (Black).

Note: This is a controlled substance (depressant): **21 CFR,** 1308.14.

THERAP CAT: Sedative, hypnotic.

8030. Quebrachamine. [4850-21-9] 7-Ethyl-1,4,5,6,7,8,9,-10-octahydro-2H-3,7-methanoazacycloundecino[5,4-b]indole; kamassin. $C_{19}H_{26}N_2$; mol wt 282.42. C 80.80%, H 9.28%, N 9.92%. From bark of *Aspidosperma quebracho blanco* Schlecht., *Apocynaceae:* Hesse, Ann. 211, 249 (1882); Field, J. Chem. Soc. 125, 1444 (1924). Identity with kamassin: Gellert, Witkop, Helv. Chim. Acta 35, 114 (1952). Structure: Witkop, J. Am. Chem. Soc. 79, 3193 (1957); Kny, Witkop, J. Org. Chem. 25, 635 (1960); Biemann, Spiteller, J. Am. Chem. Soc. 84, 4578 (1962). Crystal structure: C. Puglisi et al., Acta Crystallogr. B32, 1900 (1976). Total synthesis of dl-form: Stork, Dolfini, J. Am. Chem. Soc. 85, 2872 (1963); Ziegler et al., ibid. 91, 2342 (1969); Kutney et al., ibid. 92, 1727 (1970); V. S. Giri et al., J. Heterocycl. Chem. 17, 1133 (1980); S. Takano et al., Heterocycles 16, 247 (1981). Enantioselective synthesis: eidem, Chem. Commun. 1980, 616; 1981, 1153.

Bitter leaflets, mp 145-147°. $[\alpha]_D^{20}$ −109 to −110° (acetone). uv max (methanol): 230, 287, 293 nm (log ε 4.55, 3.85, 3.84). Sol in acetone, alc, chloroform, ether, dil acids.

8031. Quebracho Colorado. Red quebracho. Wood of *Loxopterygium lorentzii* Griseb., *Anacardiaceae.* Habit. Argentine Republic. *Constit.* Tannin, coloring matter, loxopterygine.

USE: In dyeing and tanning.

8032. Queen Substance. [334-20-3] (E)-9-Oxo-2-decenoic acid. $C_{10}H_{16}O_3$; mol wt 184.23. C 65.19%, H 8.75%, O 26.05%.

Secreted in the mandibular gland of queen honey bees *(Apis mellifera, A. florea, A. cerana, A. dorsata);* inhibits the development of ovaries in worker bees, prevents queen cell formation and attracts male bees (drones) to virgin queens for the purpose of mating: Butler, Experientia 13, 256 (1957); Sannasi, Rajulu, Life Sci. 10, part 2, 195 (1971). Similarity with the ovary inhibiting hormone of prawns *(Leander serratus):* Carlisle, Butler, Nature 177, 276 (1956). Extraction and purification: Carlisle, Butler, loc. cit.; Butler et al., Nature 184, 1871 (1959). Synthesis: Barbier et al., Compt. Rend. 251, 1133 (1960); Jaeger, Robinson, Tetrahedron 14, 320 (1961); Y. Naoshima et al., Agric. Biol. Chem. 48, 2151 (1984); U. P. Dhokte, A. S. Rao, Synth. Commun. 17, 355 (1987).

Transparent elongated plates from ether + petr ether or aq methanol, mp 54.5-55.5°. Stable to heat, acids, less stable to alkalies. Sol in acetone, alcohol. IR spectrum: Butler et al., loc. cit.

8033. Quercetagetin. [90-18-6] 2-(3,4-Dihydroxyphenyl)-3,5,6,7-tetrahydroxy-4H-1-benzopyran-4-one; 3,3',4',5,6,7-hexahydroxyflavone; 6-hydroxycyanidenolon 1555. $C_{15}H_{10}O_8$; mol wt 318.24. C 56.61%, H 3.17%, O 40.22%. From flowers of French marigold, *Tagetes patula* Linn., *Compositae:* Perkin, J. Chem. Soc. 103, 209 (1913). Synthesis: Baker et al., ibid. 1929, 74; Rao, Seshadri, Proc. Indian Acad. Sci. 23A, 23 (1946), C.A. 40, 5052[2] (1946).

Dihydrate. Pale yellow needles from dil alcohol, mp 318°. uv max (alc): 259, 361 nm (log ε 4.23, 4.34). Sol in hot alcohol; sparingly sol in boiling water.

Hexaacetate. $C_{27}H_{22}O_{14}$. Needles from alcohol + acetic acid, mp 209-211°. Sparingly sol in alc.

7-Glucoside. Quercetagitrin. $C_{21}H_{20}O_{13}$. From flowers of the African marigold, *Tagetes erecta* L., *Compositae:* Rao, Seshadri, Proc. Indian Acad. Sci. 14A, 289 (1941), C.A. 36, 2555[3] (1942); from *Chrysanthemum coronarium* L., *Compositae:* Anyas, Steelink, Arch. Biochem. Biophys. 90, 63 (1960). Structure: Rajagopalan, Seshadri, Proc. Indian Acad. Sci. 28A, 31 (1948), C.A. 43, 4265b (1949). Crystals from aqueous pyridine, dec 236-238°. uv max (95% ethanol): 260, 272, 362 nm.

8034. Quercetin. [117-39-5] 2-(3,4-Dihydroxyphenyl)-3,5,7-trihydroxy-4H-1-benzopyran-4-one; 3,3',4',5,7-pentahydroxyflavone; meletin; sophoretin; cyanidenolon 1522. $C_{15}H_{10}O_7$; mol wt 302.24. C 59.61%, H 3.33%, O 37.06%. The aglucon of quercitrin, of rutin, and of other glycosides. Widely distributed in the plant kingdom, esp in rinds and barks, in clover blossoms and in ragweed pollen. Isoln from *Rhododendron cinnabarinum* Hook, *Ericaceae:* Rangaswami et al., Proc. Indian Acad. Sci. 56A, 239 (1962), C.A. 58, 9414a (1963). Structure: Underhill et al., Can. J. Biochem. Physiol. 35, 219 (1957). Biosynthesis: Watkin et al., ibid. 229; Grisebach, Biochem. J. 85, 3p (1962); Patschke et al., Z. Naturforsch. 21b, 201 (1966). Synthesis: Shakhova et al., Zh. Obshch. Khim. 32, 390 (1962), C.A. 58, 1426f (1963). Metabolism: Nakagawa et al., Biochim. Biophys. Acta 97, 233 (1965). Toxicity data: M. Sullivan et al., Proc. Soc. Exp. Biol. Med. 77, 269 (1951). *See also* Bioflavonoids.

Dihydrate. [6151-25-3] Yellow needles from dil alcohol. Becomes anhydr at 95-97°. When anhydr dec 314°. uv max (alc): 258, 375 nm (log ε 2.75, 2.75). One gram dissolves in 290 ml abs alc, in 23 ml boiling alc. Soluble in glacial acetic acid; in aq alkaline solns with yellow color. Practically insol in water. Alcoholic solns taste very bitter. LD_{50} orally in mice: 160 mg/kg (Sullivan).

Pentabenzyl ether. [13157-90-9] 3,3′,4′,5,7-Pentakis(benzyloxy)flavone; penta-*O*-benzylquercetin; Parietrope. $C_{50}H_{40}O_7$; mol wt 752.85. Prepn: Chopin, Chadenson, *C.R. Seances Acad. Sci. Ser. C* **263**, 729 (1966); Binovic, **DE 2122514** (1972 to Biosedra), *C.A.* **76**, 113072n (1972). Crystals, mp 123-125°. uv max (chloroform): 249, 343 nm (log ε 4.43, 4.14).

3-β-D-Galactoside hemipentahydrate. Hyperin; hyperoside. $C_{21}H_{20}O_{12}.2\frac{1}{2}H_2O$. From *Acacia melanoxylon* R. Br., *Leguminosae:* Falco, de Vries, *Naturwissenschaften* **51**, 462 (1964). Yellow needles from ethanol, dec 227-230°. $[\alpha]_D^{20}$ -83° (c = 0.2 in pyridine). uv max: 259, 364 nm (log ε 4.31, 4.39).

THERAP CAT: Capillary protectant.

8035. Quercimeritrin. [491-50-9] 2-(3,4-Dihydroxyphenyl)-7-(β-D-glucopyranosyloxy)-3,5-dihydroxy-4*H*-1-benzopyran-4-one; quercetin-7-D-glucoside; 3,3′,4′,5,7-pentahydroxyflavone-7-D-glucoside. $C_{21}H_{20}O_{12}$; mol wt 464.38. C 54.31%, H 4.34%, O 41.34%. Found in flowers of *Gossypium herbaceum* L., *Malvaceae:* Perkin, *J. Chem. Soc.* **95**, 2181 (1909); from leaves of *Chrysanthemum ségetum* L. and *C. coronarium* L., *Compositae:* Geissman, Steelink, *J. Org. Chem.* **22**, 946 (1957); Anyas, Steelink, *Arch. Biochem. Biophys.* **90**, 63 (1960). In the mother liquor from quercimeritrin the glucosides gossypitrin and isoquercitrin, *q.v.*, are also found. Structure: Attree, Perkin, *J. Chem. Soc.* **1927**, 234; Rao, Seshadri, *Proc. Indian Acad. Sci.* **9A**, 365 (1939), *C.A.* **34**, 107¹ (1940); Pacheco, Grouiller, *Compt. Rend.* **253**, 1178 (1961).

Trihydrate. Yellow plates from aq pyridine. The water of crystn is given up at 100°, the anhydr material is hygroscopic, mp 247-249°. uv max (ethanol): 372, 257 nm (log ε 4.33, 4.38). Practically insol in cold water, more sol in hot water; sol in methanol. Sol in aq alkaline solns with deep yellow color. Is hydrolyzed by 7% H_2SO_4 yielding 1 mol quercetin and 1 mol D-glucose.

Gossypitrin. $C_{21}H_{20}O_{13}$; mol wt 480.38. Orange-yellow needles melting at 200-202°; slightly sol in alcohol and acetic acid.

8036. d-Quercitol. [488-73-3] 2-Deoxy-D-*chiro*-inositol; D-1-deoxy-*muco*-inositol; "acorn sugar"; (+)-protoquercitol; 1,2,3,4,-5-cyclohexanepentol. $C_6H_{12}O_5$; mol wt 164.16. C 43.90%, H 7.37%, O 48.73%. Found in the acorns of various spp of *Quercus, Fagaceae:* Prunier, *Ann. Chim. Phys.* **15**, 1 (1878); from leaves of the European palm (*Chaemerops humilis):* Muller, *J. Chem. Soc.* **91**, 1766 (1907). Configuration: Posternak, *Helv. Chim. Acta* **19**, 1007 (1936). Synthesis: G. E. McCasland *et al., J. Org. Chem.* **33**, 4220 (1968).

Sweet crystals. mp 234-235°. $[\alpha]_D^{20}$ +24 to +26°. Sol in water; slightly sol in hot, almost insol in cold alcohol; practically insol in ether.

8037. Quercitrin. [522-12-3] 3-[(6-Deoxy-α-L-mannopyranosyl)oxy]-2-(3,4-dihydroxyphenyl)-5,7-dihydroxy-4*H*-1-benzopyran-4-one; quercitroside; quercimelin; quercetin-3-L-rhamnoside; thujin. $C_{21}H_{20}O_{11}$; mol wt 448.38. C 56.25%, H 4.50%, O 39.25%. From *Aesculus hippocastanum* L., *Hippocastanaceae:* Hörhammer *et al., Arch. Pharm.* **292**, 113 (1959). Structure: Zemplén *et al., Ber.* **61**, 2486 (1928); Marchlewski, Skarzynski, *Biochem. Z.* **297**, 56 (1938); Wolfrom, Thompson in R. L. Whistler, M. L. Wolfrom, *Methods in Carbohydrate Chemistry* vol. 1 (Academic Press, New York, 1962) p 202.

Yellow crystals from dil methanol or ethanol, mp 176-179°; from water, mp 167°. uv max (ethanol): 350, 258 nm (log ε 4.18, 4.30). Practically insol in cold water, ether; sol in alc; moderately sol in hot water; sol in aq alkaline solns with intense yellow color which is oxidized by air to brown.

USE: Has been used as textile dye. *Flavine yellow shade* is prepared by extracting quercitron bark with high pressure steam and consists mainly of quercitrin: Tisdale, *Can. Text. J.* **57**, 44 (1941).

8038. Quercus. White oak. Dried inner bark of trunk and branches of *Quercus alba* L., *Fagaceae.* Habit. Eastern U.S. and Canada. *Constit.* Tannic acid, oak-red, resin, pectin, levulin, quercitol.

THERAP CAT: Astringent.

8039. Quetiapine. [111974-69-7] 2-[2-(4-Dibenzo[*b,f*][1,-4]thiazepin-11-yl-1-piperazinyl)ethoxy]ethanol; 11-[4-[2-(2-hydroxyethoxy)ethyl]-1-piperazinyl]dibenzo[*b,f*][1,4]thiazepine. $C_{21}H_{25}N_3O_2S$; mol wt 383.51. C 65.77%, H 6.57%, N 10.96%, O 8.34%, S 8.36%. Combined serotonin ($5HT_2$) and dopamine (D_2) receptor antagonist. Prepn: E. J. Warawa, B. M. Migler, **EP 240228**; *eidem,* **US 4879288** (1987, 1989 both to ICI). HPLC and GC/MS determn in plasma: R. H. Pullen *et al., J. Chromatogr.* **573**, 49 (1992). Series of articles on pharmacology: *Psychopharmacology* **112**, 285-307 (1993). Clinical evaluation in schizophrenia: H. Wetzel *et al., ibid.* **119**, 231 (1995). Review of clinical experience: B. Green, *Curr. Med. Res. Opin.* **15**, 145-151 (1999).

Hemifumarate. [111974-72-2] ICI-204636; Seroquel. $(C_{21}-H_{25}N_3O_2S)_2.C_4H_4O_4$; mol wt 883.09. Crystals from ethanol, mp 172-173°.

THERAP CAT: Antipsychotic.

8040. Quillaja. Soap bark; quillay bark; Panama bark; China bark; Murillo bark. Inner dried bark of *Quillaja saponaria* Molina, *Rosaceae. Habit.* South America (Peru, Chile); cultivated in Northern Hindustan. *Constit.* Quillaic acid, quillajasaponin, sucrose, tannin.

USE: Manuf of saponin; in mineral water industry, shampoo liquids, etc.; as foam producer.

8041. Quillaja Saponin. The saponin of quillay bark. Isolation: Kobert, *Arch. Exp. Pathol. Pharmakol.* **23**, 233 (1887); Pachorukow, *Arbeiten des Pharmakologischen Instituts zu Dorpat* **I**, 5 (1888); Cofman-Nicoresti, *Pharm. J.* **111**, 103 (1923), found the total saponin content of quillay bark to be ~9 or 10%. The saponin is built from quillaic acid, a sugar and possibly other substances.

Amorphous, deliquescent powder which causes sneezing when dispersed in the air. Freely sol in dil alc. Foams easily when shaken with water, the foam being relatively stable.

8042. Quin2. [73630-23-6] (salt); [83014-44-2] (acid). *N*-[2-[[8-[Bis(carboxymethyl)amino]-6-methoxy-2-quinolinyl]methoxy]-4-methylphenyl]-*N*-(carboxymethyl)glycine tetrapotassium salt; 2-[[2-[bis(carboxymethyl)amino]-5-methylphenoxy]methyl]-6-methoxy-8-[bis(carboxymethyl)amino]quinoline; quin-2. $C_{26}-H_{23}K_4N_3O_{10}$; mol wt 693.87. C 45.01%, H 3.34%, K 22.54%, N 6.06%, O 23.06%. Fluorescent indicator dye which is primarily used for measuring changes in intracellular Ca^{2+}. Increases in ion concn results in increased fluorescence without a shift in wavelengths. Prepn: R. Y. Tsien, *Biochemistry* **19**, 2396 (1980). Use in measuring Ca^{2+} flow: J. N. Crofts, G. J. Barritt, *Biochem. J.* **264**, 61 (1989); Zn^{2+}-protein interactions: J. R. Jefferson *et al., Anal. Biochem.* **187**, 328 (1990); in fluorescent lifetime imaging of cells: J. R. Lakowicz *et al., Cell Calcium* **15**, 7 (1994). Fluorescent properties of acetoxymethyl ester: N. Miyoshi *et al., Appl. Fluoresc. Technol.* **4**, 3 (1992). Dissociation parameters for Ca^{2+} and Mg^{2+} complexes: D. T. W. Bryant, *Biochem. J.* **226**, 613 (1985); and photophysics: V. Van Den Bergh *et al., Photochem. Photobiol.* **61**, 442 (1995). Review of use in measurement of Ca^{2+}: R. Y. Tsien, T. Pozzan, *Methods Enzymol.* **172**, 230-232 (1989).

uv max absorption (0.1M KCl): 261, 354 nm (ε 37000, 5000) free dye; 240, 332 nm (ε 36000, 5000) Ca^{2+} complex.

Acetoxymethyl ester. [83104-85-2] Quin-2AM. $C_{38}H_{43}N_3$-O_{18}.

USE: Fluorescent probe for measurement of calcium in biological systems and for selected divalent cations.

8043. Quinacillin. [1596-63-0] (2S,5R,6R)-6-[[(3-Carboxy-2-quinoxalinyl)carbonyl]amino]-3,3-dimethyl-7-oxo-4-thia-1-aza-bicyclo[3.2.0]heptane-2-carboxylic acid; 3-carboxy-2-quinoxalinyl-penicillin. $C_{18}H_{16}N_4O_6S$; mol wt 416.41. C 51.92%, H 3.87%, N 13.45%, O 23.05%, S 7.70%. Semi-synthetic antibiotic related to penicillin. Prepd by condensation of quinoxaline-2,3-dicarboxylic anhydride with 6-aminopenicillanic acid: Richards et al., Nature **199,** 354 (1963).

Disodium salt. [985-32-0] $C_{18}H_{14}N_4Na_2O_6S$. Crystals, dec 261-262°. [α]$_D^{23}$ +183.5° (water). Very hygroscopic. uv max (containing 9.2% water): 242, 326 nm (ε 32,100; 7280). Acquires a bright yellow color on exposure to strong sunlight but is stable at 100° for at least 3 months. Freely sol in water; a 25% aq soln is stable for 2 months at 0°. Antimicrobial activity is highest against *Staphylococcus aureus*.

Bistriethylammonium salt monohydrate. $C_{30}H_{46}N_6O_6S.H_2$-O. Crystals from acetone, dec 135-137°. [α]$_D^{20}$ +142° (c = 0.376 in water).

THERAP CAT: Antibacterial.

8044. Quinacrine. [83-89-6] N^4-(6-Chloro-2-methoxy-9-acridinyl)-N^1,N^1-diethyl-1,4-pentanediamine; 6-chloro-9-[[4-(di-ethylamino)-1-methylbutyl]amino]-2-methoxyacridine; 3-chloro-7-methoxy-9-(1-methyl-4-diethyl aminobutylamino)acridine; 2-chlo-ro-5-(ω-diethylamino-α-methylbutylamino)-7-methoxyacridine; mepacrine. $C_{23}H_{30}ClN_3O$; mol wt 399.96. C 69.07%, H 7.56%, Cl 8.86%, N 10.51%, O 4.00%. Prepd by condensing 1-diethyl-amino-4-aminopentane with 3,9-dichloro-7-methoxyacridine: F. Mietzsch, H. Mauss, DE **553072**; DE **571499** (1934); eidem, US **2113357** (1938 to Winthrop Chemical); cf. Drosdov, Cherutzov, J. Gen. Chem. USSR **5,** 1576, 1736 (1935); **8,** 1192 (1938); Magidson, Grigorovskii, Khim. Farm. Prom. **1933,** 187; Jensch, Eisleb, US **1782727** (1930); Schulemann et al., US **1889704** (1932). Review of quinacrine and other acridines: A. O. Wolfe in Antibiotics vol. 3, J. W. Corcoran, F. E. Hahn, Eds. (Springer-Verlag, New York, 1975) pp 203-233.

Dihydrochloride dihydrate. [6151-30-0] RP-866; SN-390; Atabrine hydrochloride. $C_{23}H_{30}ClN_3O.2HCl.2H_2O$; mol wt

508.91. Bitter, bright yellow crystals. Dec 248-250° (mp poorly discernible). One gram dissolves in ~35 ml water. Much more sol in hot water. Slightly sol in ethanol, somewhat more sol in meth-anol. Insol in ether, benzene, acetone. pH of a 1% aq soln ~4.5. Under uv light the yellow aq solns exhibit a vivid fluorescence which is detectable in a dilution of 1:5,000,000.

Methanesulfonate monohydrate. [6598-46-5] $C_{25}H_{38}ClN_3$-$O_7S_2.H_2O$. Bitter, bright yellow crystals. One part dissolves in 3 parts water at 15.5°, in 36 parts 95% alcohol at 15.5°. pH of 2.0% w/v soln in water 3.0-5.0.

THERAP CAT: Anthelmintic (Cestodes); antimalarial.

THERAP CAT (VET): Antiprotozoal, teniacide.

8045. Quinagolide. [87056-78-5] (3R,4aR,10aS)-rel-N,N-Diethyl-N'-(1,2,3,4,4a,5,10,10a-octahydro-6-hydroxy-1-propyl-benzo[g]quinolin-3-yl)sulfamide; ($\pm$)-1-n-propyl-3α-diethylsulfa-moylamino-6-hydroxy-1,2,3,4,4aα,5,10,10aβ-octahydrobenzo[g]-quinoline. $C_{20}H_{33}N_3O_3S$; mol wt 395.56. C 60.73%, H 8.41%, N 10.62%, O 12.13%, S 8.11%. Nonergot dopamine D$_2$-receptor agonist. Prepn: R. Nordmann, T. J. Petcher, EP **77754**; eidem, US **4565818** (1983, 1986 both to Sandoz); eidem, J. Med. Chem. **28,** 367 (1985). Receptor binding study in vivo: A. Closse et al., Brain Res. **440,** 123 (1988). Clinical pharmacology: R. C. Gaillard, J. Brownell, Life Sci. **43,** 1355 (1988). Clinical evaluation in hyper-prolactinemia: C. Rasmussen et al., Acta Endocrinol. **125,** 170 (1991).

Beige powder, mp 122.5-124°.

Hydrochloride. [94424-50-7] CV-205-502; SDZ-205-502; Norprolac. $C_{20}H_{33}N_3O_3S.HCl$; mol wt 432.02. Crystals from methylene chloride + methanol, mp 234-236°.

THERAP CAT: Prolactin inhibitor.

8046. Quinaldic Acid. [93-10-7] 2-Quinolinecarboxylic acid; quinaldinic acid. $C_{10}H_7NO_2$; mol wt 173.17. C 69.36%, H 4.07%, N 8.09%, O 18.48%.

Dihydrate, crystals. mp 155-157° (anhydr). Moderately sol in water; sol in alcohol and in alkali solns.

USE: For the determination of copper, zinc and uranium with which it forms insol salts.

8047. Quinaldine. [91-63-4] 2-Methylquinoline. $C_{10}H_9N$; mol wt 143.19. C 83.88%, H 6.34%, N 9.78%. Occurs in coal tar; made from aniline, acetaldehyde and HCl. Lab procedure: A. I. Vogel, Practical Organic Chemistry (Longmans, London, 3rd ed., 1959) p 831; Gattermann-Wieland, Praxis des Organischen Chem-ikers (de Gruyter, Berlin, 40th ed., 1961) p 318. Pharmacology: Brown et al., Comp. Biochem. Physiol. **42A,** 223 (1972). Toxicity data: Smyth et al., Arch. Ind. Hyg. Occup. Med. **4,** 119 (1951); L. L. Marking, Invest. Fish Control **23,** 3 (1969).

Colorless, oily liquid; quinoline odor; becomes reddish-brown on exposure to air. d ~1.06. bp 246-247°. Practically insol in water. Sol in chloroform, ether. *Keep tightly closed and protected from light.* LD$_{50}$ orally in rats: 1.23 g/kg (Smyth).

Sulfate. [655-76-5] $C_{10}H_9N.H_2SO_4$. Prepn: S. Hoogewerff, W. A. Van Dorp, Rec. Trav. Chim. **3,** 345 (1884); J. L. Allen, J. B.

Sills, *Invest. Fish Control* **47**, 3 (1973). Efficacy as anesthetic in fish: P. A. Gilderhus *et al., ibid.* **49**, 3 (1973); G. C. Blasiola Jr., *J. Fish Biol.* **10**, 113 (1977). Toxicity: L. L. Marking, V. K. Dawson, *Invest. Fish Control* **48**, 3 (1973). Light yellow crystalline powder, mp 211-214°. uv max (0.1N H_2SO_4): 236, 317 nm. Soly (g/100 ml) in water 104.05, in methanol 7.44, in ethanol 2.27, in acetone 0.08. Practically insol in ether, benzene, hexane. LC_{50} (96 hour) in largemouth bass: 6.80 mg/l; in carp: 72.5 mg/l (Marking, Dawson).

USE: As anesthetic in transport and handling of fish.

8048. Quinaldine Blue. [2768-90-3] 1-Ethyl-2-[3-(1-ethyl-2(1H)-quinolinylidene)-1-propenyl]quinolinium chloride; bis[1-eth-ylquinoline-(2)]trimethinecyanine chloride; 1,1'-diethyl-2,2'-tri-methinequinocyanine chloride; pinacyanol chloride; Vernitest Reagent. $C_{25}H_{25}ClN_2$; mol wt 388.93. C 77.20%, H 6.48%, Cl 9.12%, N 7.20%. Prepn: Fischer, *J. Prakt. Chem.* **98**, 204 (1918). Properties and use as histological stain: F. Proescher, *Proc. Soc. Exp. Biol. Med.* **31**, 79 (1933); H. P. Klinger *et al., Stain Technol.* **46**, 43 (1971); R. K. J. Narayan, *ibid.* **55**, 9 (1980).

Bright blue-green alcohol-containing prisms or needles from alcohol. Drying at 110° expels alcohol of crystn. Dec at ~263°. Moderately sol in water with a violet-red color, in alcohol with a blue color. Solns are dichroic.

USE: Histological stain (chromosomes).

8049. Quinaldine Red. [117-92-0] 2-[2-[4-(Dimethylami-no)phenyl]ethenyl]-1-ethylquinolinium iodide; 2-[p-(dimethylami-no)styryl]-1-ethylquinolinium iodide; 2-(p-dimethylaminostyryl)-quinoline ethiodide; α-(p-dimethylaminophenylethylene)quinoline ethiodide; Eastman no. 1361. $C_{21}H_{23}IN_2$; mol wt 430.33. C 58.61%, H 5.39%, I 29.49%, N 6.51%. Prepd by condensing quinaldine ethyliodide and p-dimethylaminobenzaldehyde in alc in the presence of piperidine: König, *J. Prakt. Chem.* [2] **86**, 172 (1912); DE 294744; Frdl. **14**, 735.

Very dark red powder. Sparingly sol in water. Freely sol in alcohol, giving a dark red soln. Solns are slowly dec by light. pKb 11.25. Colorless at pH 1.4; red at pH 3.2. In the presence of chlorides the transition interval is from pH 1.2 to pH 3.0.

USE: As an indicator.

8050. Quinalizarin. [81-61-8] 1,2,5,8-Tetrahydroxy-9,10-anthracenedione; 1,2,5,8-tetrahydroxyanthraquinone; alizarin bordeaux B; C.I. Mordant Violet 26; C.I. 58500. $C_{14}H_8O_6$; mol wt 272.21. C 61.77%, H 2.96%, O 35.27%. From hemipic (hemipinic) acid and hydroquinone with H_2SO_4: Liebermann, Kostanecki, *Ann.* **240**, 245 (1887); Liebermann, Wense, *Ber.* **20**, 862 (1887). From alizarin or quinizarin by treatment with 80% oleum, then boiling with caustic: Gattermann, *J. Prakt. Chem.* [2] **43**, 246 (1891); Schmidt, *ibid.* **237**, 242 (1891); *Bull. Soc. Ind. Mulhouse* **84**, 409 (1914). *See also: Colour Index* vol. 4 (3rd ed., 1971) p 4519.

Red needles with green metallic luster from acetic acid or from nitrobenzene or by sublimation *in vacuo*. mp >275°. Absorption spectrum: Meek, Watson, *J. Chem. Soc.* **109**, 544 (1916); Meek, *ibid.* **111**, 969 (1917). Insol in water. Very slightly sol in most other solvents. Dissolves in aq solns of alkalies with reddish-violet, in acetic acid with yellow, in sulfuric acid with blue-violet color.

USE: Dyes cotton mordanted with Al salts dark red, cotton mordanted with Cr salts bluish-violet. No longer used as a dye, except occasionally in printing cotton.

8051. Quinapril. [85441-61-8] (3S)-2-[(2S)-2-[[(1S)-1-(Ethoxycarbonyl)-3-phenylpropyl]amino]-1-oxopropyl]-1,2,3,4-tetrahydro-3-isoquinolinecarboxylic acid; (S)-2-[(S)-N-[(S)-1-car-boxy-3-phenylpropyl]alanyl]-1,2,3,4-tetrahydro-3-isoquinolinecar-boxylic acid 1-ethyl ester. $C_{25}H_{30}N_2O_5$; mol wt 438.52. C 68.47%, H 6.90%, N 6.39%, O 18.24%. Angiotensin converting enzyme (ACE) inhibitor. Prepn: M. L. Hoefle, S. Klutchko, **EP 49605**; *eidem,* US **4344949** (both 1982 to Warner-Lambert); S. Klutchko *et al., J. Med. Chem.* **29**, 1953 (1986). Synthesis of purified crystalline form: O. P. Goel, U. Krolls, US **4761479** (1988 to Warner-Lambert). Pharmacology: H. R. Kaplan *et al., Fed. Proc.* **43**, 1326 (1984); M. J. Ryan *et al., ibid.* 1330. HPLC determn of quinapril and quinaprilat in plasma and urine: H. Hengy, M. Most, *J. Liq. Chromatogr.* **11**, 517 (1988). Toxicity data: H. R. Kaplan *et al., Angiology* **40**, 335 (1989). Review of pharmacology, pharmacokinetics and clinical experience in congestive heart failure and hypertension: C. R. Culy, B. Jarvis, *Drugs* **62**, 339-385 (2002).

Hydrochloride. [82586-55-8] CI-906; PD-109452-2; Accupril; Accupro; Acequin; Acuitel; Korec; Quinazil. $C_{25}H_{30}N_2O_5 \cdot HCl$; mol wt 474.98. Crystals from ethyl acetate-toluene, mp 120-130°. $[\alpha]_D^{23}$ +14.5° (c = 1.2 in ethanol) (Klutchko). Also reported as white crystalline solid from acetonitrile, mp 119-121.5°. $[\alpha]_D^{25}$ +15.4° (c = 2 in methanol) (Goel, Krolls). Freely sol in aq solvents. LD_{50} in male, female mice, rats (mg/kg): 1739, 1840, 4280, 3541 orally; 504, 523, 158, 107 i.v. (Kaplan, 1989).

Diacid. [82768-85-2] Quinaprilat; CI-928; Accupril. $C_{23}H_{26}$-N_2O_5; mol wt 410.46. Active metabolite. Hydrate, crystals from methanol-ethyl ether, mp 166-168°. $[\alpha]_D^{23}$ +20.9° (c = 1 in methanol).

Mixture with hydrochlorothiazide. Accuretic; Acequide; Ko-retic.

THERAP CAT: Antihypertensive. In treatment of congestive heart failure.

8052. Quinapyramine. [20493-41-8] 4-Amino-6-[(2-ami-no-1,6-dimethyl-4(1H)-pyrimidinylidene)amino]-1,2-dimethyl-quinolinium conjugate monoacid; 4-amino-6-[(2-amino-6-methyl-4-pyrimidinyl)amino]-1-methylquinaldinium methosalts; 4-amino-6-[(2-amino-1,6-dimethyl-4-pyrimidinyl)amino]-1,2-dimethylquin-oline salts; 4-amino-6-(2-amino-6-methyl-4-pyrimidylamino)quin-aldine-1,1'-dimethosalts; M-7555; Antrycide. Prepn: F. H. S. Curd, D. G. Davey, *Br. J. Pharmacol.* **5**, 25 (1950); Curd, US **2585917** (1952 to I.C.I.); Ainley *et al., J. Chem. Soc.* **1953**, 59.

Dimethosulfate. $C_{19}H_{28}N_6O_8S_2$. Creamy white crystals from aq methanol, mp 265-266°. Freely sol in water. LD_{50} i.v. in mice: 10-15 mg/kg (Curd, Davey).

Diiodide. Pale cream needles, mp 312-313° (dec). Sparingly sol in water.

Dichloride. Crystals from water, mp 316-317° (dec). Sparingly sol in water. LD_{50} i.v. in mice: 10-15 mg/kg (Curd, Davey).

THERAP CAT: Antiprotozoal (Trypanosoma).

8053. Quinazoline. [253-82-7] 1,3-Benzodiazine; benzo-[*a*]pyrimidine; 5,6-benzopyrimidine; phenmiazine. $C_8H_6N_2$; mol wt 130.15. C 73.83%, H 4.65%, N 21.52%. Prepn from 2-nitrobenzylidenebis(formamide): Riedel, **DE 174941**; *Chem. Zentralbl.* **1906, II**, 1372; *Frdl.* **8**, 1238; Bogert, McColm, *J. Am. Chem. Soc.* **49**, 2650 (1927).

Leaflets from petr ether; odor of quinoline. Slightly bitter taste. mp 48.0-48.5°. $bp_{772.5}$ 243°; bp_{764} 241.5°. Freely sol in water. Neutral reaction. Sol in many organic solvents.

8054. Quince Seed. Gum quince seed; semen cydonia; golden apple seed; cydonia seed. Seed of *Cydonia oblonga* Mill. (*C. vulgaris* Pers.), *Rosaceae*. *Habit.* Southern Asia, Europe; widely cultivated. *Constit.* Amygdalin, emulsin, about 15% fatty oil, about 20% of a mucilage named cydonin. Brief review of seed and gum uses: BeMiller in *Industrial Gums*, R. L. Whistler, Ed. (Academic Press, New York, 2nd ed., 1973) pp 339-345.

USE: Gum from the seeds as suspending agent, stabilizer; in hair and cosmetic prepns.

8055. Quinestrol. [152-43-2] (17α)-3-(Cyclopentyloxy)-19-norpregna-1,3,5(10)-trien-20-yn-17-ol; 17α-ethinylestradiol 3-cyclopentyl ether; W-3566; Estrovis. $C_{25}H_{32}O_2$; mol wt 364.52. C 82.37%, H 8.85%, O 8.78%. Prepn: Ercoli, Gardi, *Chem. Ind. (London)* **1961**, 1037; Ercoli, **US 3159543**; Ercoli *et al.*, **US 3231567** (1964, 1966, both to Vismara).

Crystals, mp 107-108°. $[\alpha]_D^{25}$ +5° (c = 0.5 in dioxane).

THERAP CAT: Estrogen.

8056. Quinethazone. [73-49-4] 7-Chloro-2-ethyl-1,2,3,4-tetrahydro-4-oxo-6-quinazolinesulfonamide; 7-chloro-2-ethyl-6-sulfamoyl-1,2,3,4-tetrahydro-4-quinazolinone; 7-chloro-2-ethyl-1,2,3,4-tetrahydro-4-oxo-6-sulfamoylquinazoline; CL-36010; Hydromox; Aquamox. $C_{10}H_{12}ClN_3O_3S$; mol wt 289.74. C 41.45%, H 4.17%, Cl 12.24%, N 14.50%, O 16.57%, S 11.07%. Prepn: Cohen *et al.*, *J. Am. Chem. Soc.* **82**, 2731 (1960); Cohen, Vaughan, Jr., **US 2976289** (1961 to Am. Cyanamid).

Fibrous crystals from 50% acetone, mp 250-252°. Sol in acetone, alcohol.

THERAP CAT: Diuretic, antihypertensive.

8057. Quinfamide. [62265-68-3] 2-Furancarboxylic acid 1-(dichloroacetyl)-1,2,3,4-tetrahydro-6-quinolinyl ester; 2-furoic acid ester with 1-(dichloroacetyl)-1,2,3,4-tetrahydro-6-quinolinol; 1-(dichloroacetyl)-6-(2-furoyloxy)-1,2,3,4-tetrahydroquinoline; Win-40014; Amenox; Amenide. $C_{16}H_{13}Cl_2NO_4$; mol wt 354.18. C 54.26%, H 3.70%, Cl 20.02%, N 3.95%, O 18.07%. Prepn: D. M. Bailey, **US 3997542** (1976 to Sterling); D. M. Bailey *et al.*, *J. Med.*

Chem. **22**, 600 (1979). Amebicidal activity and toxicological evaluation: R. G. Slighter *et al.*, *Parasitology* **81**, 157 (1980). Distribution and metabolism in rats: J. F. Baker, *Arch. Int. Pharmacodyn.* **258**, 29 (1982). HPLC determn in biological samples: J. M. Morales *et al.*, *J. Chromatogr. B* **746**, 133 (2000). Clinical evaluation in adults with chronic amebiasis: L. Guevara *et al.*, *Clin. Ther.* **6**, 43 (1983); in children: F. A. Rojas *et al., ibid.* 47.

Crystals from ethyl acetate, mp 150.5-151°.

THERAP CAT: Antiamebic.

8058. Quinhydrone. [106-34-3] 2,5-Cyclohexadiene-1,4-dione compd with 1,4-benzenediol (1:1); green hydroquinone. $C_{12}H_{10}O_4$; mol wt 218.21. C 66.05%, H 4.62%, O 29.33%. An addn compd of one mol hydroquinone and one mol quinone. Prepn from hydroquinone and quinone: Gattermann-Wieland, *Praxis des Organischen Chemikers* (de Gruyter, Berlin, 40th ed., 1961) p 270. Alternate prepn by the action of ferric ammonium sulfate on hydroquinone: A. I. Vogel, *Practical Organic Chemistry* (Longmans, London, 3rd ed., 1959) p 747. Toxicity study: Woodward *et al., Fed. Proc.* **8**, 348 (1949).

Green crystals with metallic luster; reddish-brown by transmitted light. d 1.40. mp 171°; sublimes with partial decompn. Slightly sol in cold water; sol in hot water, ammonia, alc, ether. Insol in petr ether. LD_{50} orally in rats: 225 mg/kg (Woodward).

USE: In pH determinations (quinhydrone electrode).

8059. Quinic Acid. [77-95-2] (1α,3R,4α,5R)-1,3,4,5-Tetrahydroxycyclohexanecarboxylic acid; chinic acid; kinic acid; (−)-hexahydro-1,3,4,5-tetrahydroxybenzoic acid. $C_7H_{12}O_6$; mol wt 192.17. C 43.75%, H 6.29%, O 49.95%. Found in cinchona bark, particularly in South American barks; also in many other plants, such as tobacco leaves, carrot leaves, apples, peaches, pears, plums, etc. Structure and configuration: Fischer, Dangschat, *Ber.* **65**, 1009 (1932). Total synthesis: Grewe *et al., ibid.* **87**, 793 (1954); Smissman, Oxman, *J. Am. Chem. Soc.* **85**, 2184 (1963). Stereospecific synthesis: Wolinsky *et al., J. Org. Chem.* **29**, 3596 (1964). *Review:* Bohm, *Chem. Rev.* **65**, 435 (1965).

White crystals; strong acid taste. d 1.64. mp 162-163°; at higher temps forms a lactone. $[\alpha]_D^{20}$ −42 to −44° in water. Sol in 2.5 parts water, in alcohol, glacial acetic acid.

8060. Quinidine. [56-54-2] (9*S*)-6′-Methoxycinchonan-9-ol; α-(6-methoxy-4-quinolyl)-5-vinyl-2-quinuclidinemethanol; conquinine; pitayine; β-quinine. $C_{20}H_{24}N_2O_2$; mol wt 324.42. C 74.04%, H 7.46%, N 8.63%, O 9.86%. A dextrorotatory stereoisomer of quinine, *q.v.* Present in cinchona barks to the extent of 0.25-3.0%. Found in quinine sulfate mother liquors. Review of structural elucidation and early synthetic studies: R. B. Turner, R.

B. Woodward, in *The Alkaloids* vol. 3, 1-63 (1953). Configuration: Prelog, Zalán, *Helv. Chim. Acta* **27**, 535 (1944); Prelog, Häfliger, *ibid.* **33**, 2021 (1950); Roth, *Pharmazie* **16**, 257 (1961). Crystal and molecular structure: R. Doherty *et al., J. Pharm. Sci.* **67**, 1698 (1978). Rotatory dispersion studies: Lyle, Gaffield, *Tetrahedron Lett.* **1963**, 1371. Prepn by isomerization of quinine: W. E. Doering *et al., J. Am. Chem. Soc.* **69**, 1700 (1949). Total synthesis: J. Gutzwiller, M. Uskokovic, *ibid.* **92**, 204 (1970); *eidem, Helv. Chim. Acta* **56**, 1494 (1973); *eidem, J. Am. Chem. Soc.* **100**, 576 (1978). Toxicity data: C. Turba *et al., Arzneim.-Forsch.* **18**, 1127 (1968); K. Dietmann *et al., ibid.* **27**, 589 (1977). Comprehensive description of the sulfate: M. A. Loutfy *et al., Anal. Profiles Drug Subs.* **12**, 483-546 (1983). Clinical evaluation in severe malaria: R. E. Phillips *et al., N. Engl. J. Med.* **312**, 1273 (1985). Review of pharmacology and clinical efficacy in cardiac arrhythmias: J. W. Mason, L. M. Hondeghem, *Ann. N.Y. Acad. Sci.* **432**, 162-176 (1984); A. R. Leon, J. D. Merlino, *Heart Dis. Stroke*, **2**, 407-413 (1993).

Triboluminescent. mp 174-175° after drying of solvated crystals. $[\alpha]_D^{15}$ +230° (c = 1.8 in chloroform), $[\alpha]_D^{17}$ +258° (alc), $[\alpha]_D^{17}$ +322° (c = 1.6 in 2*M* HCl). pK$_1$ (20°) 5.4; pK$_2$ 10.0. Blue fluorescence in dil H$_2$SO$_4$. The uv absorption spectrum is identical with that of quinine. One gram dissolves in about 2000 ml cold, 800 ml boiling water, 36 ml alcohol, 56 ml ether, 1.6 ml chloroform; very sol in methanol. Practically insol in petr ether. LD$_{50}$ in rats (mg/kg): 30 i.v., orally (Dietmann).

Hemipentahydrate. Prisms from dil alcohol, loses ½ H$_2$O in air, mp ~168°.

Hydrogen sulfate tetrahydrate. [6151-39-9] Quinidine bisulfate; Chinidin-Duriles; Kiditard; Kinichron; Kinidin Durules; Quiniduran. C$_{20}$H$_{24}$N$_2$O$_2$.H$_2$SO$_4$.4H$_2$O; mol wt 494.56. Rods, sol in 8 parts water with blue fluorescence.

Sulfate dihydrate. [6591-63-5]; [50-54-4] (anhydrous). Cin-Quin; Quinidex Extentabs; Quinicardine; Quinora. (C$_{20}$H$_{24}$N$_2$-O$_2$)$_2$.H$_2$SO$_4$.2H$_2$O; mol wt 782.94. White, very bitter, odorless, fine crystals, frequently cohering in masses. Darkens on exposure to light. Does not lose all of its water below 120°. $[\alpha]_D^{25}$ ~+212° (95% alcohol); ~+260° (dil HCl). pKa 4.2, 8.8. pH (1% aq soln): 6.0-6.8. One gram dissolves in about 90 ml water, 15 ml boiling water, 10 ml alcohol, 3 ml methanol, 12 ml chloroform. Insol in ether, benzene. *Protect from light.* LD$_{50}$ in mice, rats (mg/kg): 700, 455.8 orally; 83, 56 i.v. (Turba).

Gluconate. [7054-25-3] Gluconic acid quinidine salt; Duraquin; Quinaglute. C$_{26}$H$_{36}$N$_2$O$_9$; mol wt 520.57. Crystals, mp 175-176.5°. Sol in 9 parts water, 60 parts alcohol.

Polygalacturonate. [7681-28-9] Cardioquin; Galactoquin; Naticardina. (C$_{20}$H$_{24}$N$_2$O$_2$.C$_6$H$_{10}$O$_7$.H$_2$O)$_x$. Prepn: A. Halpern *et al., Am. J. Pharm.* **130**, 190 (1958). Pharmacology: A. Halpern *et al., Antibiot. Chemother.* **9**, 97 (1959). Amorphous powder, mp 180° (dec). Anhydr product is insol in methanol, ethanol, chloroform, ether, acetone, dioxane. Soly in hot 40% methanol or ethanol: 12%; in water at 25°: ~2%. LD$_{50}$ in rats, mice (mg/kg): 3200 ± 350, 2680 ± 210 orally (Halpern, 1959).

THERAP CAT: Antiarrhythmic (class IA); antimalarial.

THERAP CAT (VET): Antiarrhythmic.

8061. Quinine. [130-95-0] (8α,9*R*)-6'-Methoxycinchonan-9-ol. C$_{20}$H$_{24}$N$_2$O$_2$; mol wt 324.42. C 74.04%, H 7.46%, N 8.63%, O 9.86%. Primary alkaloid of various species of *Cinchona* (Rubiaceae), *see* Cinchona. Representative samples of dried bark contain ~0.8 to 4% quinine. Optical isomer of quinidine, *q.v.* Isoln: Pelletier, Caventau, *Ann. Chem. Phys.* [2], **15**, 291 (1820). Extraction procedure: Jucker, Stoll, in *Ullmanns Encyklopädie der technischen Chemie* vol. 3, 213-218 (1953). Configuration: Pre-

log, Zalán, *Helv. Chim. Acta* **27**, 535 (1944); Prelog, Häfliger, *ibid.* **33**, 2021 (1950); Roth, *Pharmazie* **16**, 257 (1961). Synthesis: Woodward, Doering, *J. Am. Chem. Soc.* **66**, 849 (1944); **67**, 860 (1945); Taylor, Martin, *ibid.* **94**, 6218 (1972); Gutzwiller, Uskokovic, *ibid.* **100**, 576 (1978); G. Grethe *et al., ibid.* 589; T. Imanishi *et al., Chem. Pharm. Bull.* **30**, 1925 (1982). Review of structural elucidation and early synthetic studies: R. B. Turner, R. B. Woodward in *The Alkaloids* vol. 3, 1-63 (1953); of bioactivity: F. E. Hahn, Ed. in *Antibiotics* vol. 5 (pt. 2) (Springer-Verlag, New York, 1979) pp 353-362. Comprehensive description of the hydrochloride: F. J. Muhtadi *et al., Anal. Profiles Drug Subs.* **12**, 547-621 (1983). LC determn in soft drinks: L. P. Valenti, *J. Assoc. Off. Anal. Chem.* **68**, 782 (1985). HPLC determn in blood: V. K. Dua *et al. J. Chromatogr.* **614**, 87 (1993). Clinical evaluation to relieve nocturnal leg cramps: P. S. Connolly *et al., Arch. Intern. Med.* **152**, 1877 (1992). Clinical efficacy in malaria: P. G. Kremsner *et al., J. Infect. Dis.* **169**, 467-470 (1994). Review of historical importance and total syntheses: T. S. Kaufman, E. A. Ruveda, *Angew. Chem. Int. Ed.* **44**, 854-885 (2005).

Triboluminescent, orthorhombic needles from abs alcohol, mp 177° (some decompn). Sublimes in high vacuum at 170-180°. $[\alpha]_D^{15}$ −169° (c = 2 in 97% alcohol), $[\alpha]_D^{17}$ −117° (c = 1.5 in chloroform), $[\alpha]_D^{15}$ −285° (c = 0.4*M* in 0.1*N* H$_2$SO$_4$). pK$_1$ (18°) 5.07; pK$_2$ 9.7. pH of satd aq soln 8.8. Absorption spectra: Dobbie, Lauder, *J. Chem. Soc.* **99**, 1260 (1911); Dobbie, Fox, *ibid.* **101**, 78 (1912). Fluorescence: Rabe, Marschall, *Ann.* **382**, 362 (1911). The blue fluorescence is especially strong in dil H$_2$SO$_4$. One gram dissolves in 1900 ml water, 760 ml boiling water, 0.8 ml alcohol, 80 ml benzene (in 18 ml benzene at 50°), in 1.2 ml chloroform; 250 ml dry ether, 20 ml glycerol, 1900 ml of 10% ammonia water. Almost insol in petr ether.

Trihydrate. Microcrystalline powder, mp 57°, efflorescent, loses one H$_2$O in air, two H$_2$O over H$_2$SO$_4$, anhydr at 125°.

Bisulfate heptahydrate. [6183-68-2]; [549-56-4] (anhydrous). Biquinate. C$_{20}$H$_{24}$N$_2$O$_2$.H$_2$SO$_4$.7H$_2$O; mol wt 548.60. Very bitter crystals or cryst powder; efflorescent on exposure to air and darkens on exposure to light. One gram dissolves in 9 ml water, 0.7 ml boiling water, 23 ml alcohol, 0.7 ml alcohol at 60°, 625 ml chloroform, 2500 ml ether, 15 ml glycerol. pH: 3.5.

Dihydrochloride. [60-93-5] Quinine dichloride; quinine bimuriate; acid quinine hydrochloride. C$_{20}$H$_{24}$N$_2$O$_2$.2HCl. Very bitter powder or crystals. One gram dissolves in about 0.6 ml water, in about 12 ml alcohol. Slightly sol in chloroform, very slightly sol in ether. Aq solns are strongly acid to litmus paper (pH about 2.6).

Hydrochloride dihydrate. [6119-47-7]; [130-89-2] (anhydrous). C$_{20}$H$_{24}$N$_2$O$_2$.HCl.2H$_2$O. Bitter, silky needles. Effloresces on exposure to warm air. Does not lose all its water below 120°. One gram dissolves in 16 ml water, in 0.5 ml boiling water, in 1.0 ml alcohol, in about 7.0 ml glycerol, in about 1 ml chloroform, in about 350 ml ether. pH (1% aq soln): 6.0-7.0. Bitterness threshold 1:30000. *Protect from light.*

Sulfate dihydrate. [6119-70-6]; [804-63-7]. Quinamm; Quinate. (C$_{20}$H$_{24}$N$_2$O$_2$)$_2$.H$_2$SO$_4$.2H$_2$O; mol wt 782.94. Dull needles or rods, making a light and readily compressible mass. Becomes brownish on exposure to light. Loses its water of crystn at about 100°. $[\alpha]_D^{15}$ −220° (5% soln in about 0.5*N* HCl). One gram dissolves in 810 ml water, 32 ml boiling water, 120 ml alcohol, 10 ml alcohol at 78°. Slightly sol in chloroform, ether, but freely sol in a mixture of 2 vols chloroform and 1 vol abs alcohol. Aq solns are neutral to litmus, pH of satd soln 6.2.

USE: Flavor in carbonated beverages.

THERAP CAT: Antimalarial; muscle relaxant (skeletal).

THERAP CAT (VET): Antiprotozoal for fish.

8062. Quininic Acid. [86-68-0] 6-Methoxy-4-quinolinecarboxylic acid; 6-methoxycinchoninic acid. $C_{11}H_9NO_3$; mol wt 203.19. C 65.02%, H 4.46%, N 6.89%, O 23.62%.

Pale yellow crystals. mp about 280° with dec. Slightly sol in water, cold alcohol or ether; sol in about 80 parts boiling abs alcohol; sol in aq alkalies.

8063. Quininone. [84-31-1] (8α)-6'-Methoxycinchonan-9-one. $C_{20}H_{22}N_2O_2$; mol wt 322.40. C 74.51%, H 6.88%, N 8.69%, O 9.93%. By careful oxidation of quinine or quinidine: Rabe, Kuliga, *Ann.* **364**, 346, 349 (1909); Woodward *et al., J. Am. Chem. Soc.* **67**, 1425 (1945). Alternate procedure: Rabe, Kindler, *Ber.* **51**, 466 (1918). Prepn of amorphous epimeric mixture of quininone and quinidinone from quinotoxine: Gutzwiller, Uskokovic, *Helv. Chim. Acta* **56**, 1494 (1973).

Crystals from ether, mp 108° (rapid heating). Shows mutarotation, final $[\alpha]_D^{20}$ +76° (c = 2 in alcohol). Alkaline reaction to litmus. Freely sol in alcohol, ether, chloroform, benzene. Almost insol in water and petr ether.

Hydrochloride. $C_{20}H_{22}N_2O_2$·HCl. Hygroscopic crystals, mp 212°. Final $[\alpha]_D^{18}$ +59° (c = 2 in abs alcohol).

8064. Quinizarin. [81-64-1] 1,4-Dihydroxy-9,10-anthracenedione; 1,4-dihydroxyanthraquinone; C.I. 58050. $C_{14}H_8O_4$; mol wt 240.21. C 70.00%, H 3.36%, O 26.64%. Prepn from *p*-chlorophenol and phthalic anhydride: Reynolds, Bigelow, *J. Am. Chem. Soc.* **48**, 420 (1926); **US 1845632**, *C.A.* **26**, 2203; *Org. Synth.* coll. vol. **I**, 476 (New York, 1941). Prepn from hydroquinone: Gattermann-Wieland, *Praxis des Organischen Chemikers* (de Gruyter, Berlin, 40th ed., 1961) p 299. Also prepd from diazotized *p*-chloroaniline and phthalic anhydride: **GB 373999**, *C.A.* **27**, 3946 (1933); by treating anthraquinone with ammonium persulfate in sulfuric acid: Wacker, *J. Prakt. Chem.* [2] **54**, 90 (1896). Purification from contaminating purpurin: *Org. Synth.* (*loc. cit.*). See also: *Colour Index* vol. **4** (3rd ed., 1971) p 4515.

Orange crystals from acetic acid, mp 200-203° (*Org. Syn.*). Orange plates from ether. Deep red needles from alcohol, benzene, toluene, xylene. mp 196°. Sublimes in high vacuum. Absorption spectrum: Meek, Watson, *J. Chem. Soc.* **109**, 544 (1916); Meek, *ibid.* **111**, 969 (1917). pK (18°) 9.51. Moderately sol in alcohol with red color. Sol in ether with brown color and yellow fluorescence. Sol with violet color in aq alkalies and in ammonia. Black precipitate with CO_2. One gram dissolves in about 13 g of boiling glacial acetic acid.

Dimethyl ether. $C_{16}H_{12}O_4$. mp 177°.

8065. Quinizarin Green SS. [128-80-3] 1,4-Bis[(4-methylphenyl)amino]-9,10-anthracenedione; 1,4-di-*p*-toluidinoanthraqui-

none; D & C Green No. 6; C.I. Solvent Green 3; C.I. 61565. $C_{28}H_{22}N_2O_2$; mol wt 418.49. C 80.36%, H 5.30%, N 6.69%, O 7.65%. Discovered by R. E. Schmidt in 1894: *Colour Index* vol. **4** (3rd ed., 1971) p 4541.

Dark violet needles, mp 218°. Blue soln in conc H_2SO_4 giving a blue-green ppt on dilution.

USE: For sutures: *Fed. Regist.* **40**, 18167 (1975). Permitted for use in externally applied drugs and cosmetics: *ibid.* **47**, 14138 (1982).

8066. Quinmerac. [90717-03-6] 7-Chloro-3-methyl-8-quinolinecarboxylic acid; BAS-518; BAS-518H. $C_{11}H_8ClNO_2$; mol wt 221.64. C 59.61%, H 3.64%, Cl 16.00%, N 6.32%, O 14.44%. Auxin-type herbicide. Prepn: H. Hagen *et al.*, **DE 3233089**; *eidem*, **US 4715889** (1984, 1987 both to BASF). ELISA determn in cereals: R. A. Baumann, V. M. 't Hart-De Kleijn, *Meded. Fac. Landbouwwet. Univ. Gent* **58**, 173 (1993). Mode of action study: K. Grossman, F. Scheltrup, *Pestic. Sci.* **52**, 111 (1998). Field trials in cereals, rapeseed and sugarbeets: W. Nuyken *et al., Proc. Br. Crop Prot. Conf. - Weeds* **1985**, 71. Review: B. Wuerzer *et al., ibid.* 63-70.

Colorless, odorless crystalline solid from DMF, mp 244°. Soly at 20° (g/100g solvent): water 2.1×10^{-3}, olive oil <0.1, acetone 0.2. Low soly in other organic solvents. Vapor pressure (20°): $<1 \times 10^{-5}$ Pa. LD_{50} in rats (mg/kg): >5000 orally, >2000 dermally (Wuerzer).

USE: Herbicide.

8067. Quinocide. [525-61-1] N^1-(6-Methoxy-8-quinolinyl)-1,4-pentanediamine; 8-(4-aminopentylamino)-6-methoxyquinoline; 8-[(4-amino-4-methylbutyl)amino]-6-methoxyquinoline; 6-methoxy-8-(4-aminopentylamino)quinoline; chinocide; khinocyde. $C_{15}H_{21}N_3O$; mol wt 259.35. C 69.47%, H 8.16%, N 16.20%, O 6.17%. Prepn: Braude, Stavrovskaya, *J. Gen. Chem. USSR* **26**, 999 (1956); modified method: *idem, Med. Prom. SSSR* **11**(7), 19 (1957), *C.A.* **52**, 11043 (1958); B. Balkrishen *et al., Chem. Ind. (London)* **1983**, 899.

bp$_1$ 183-186°. mp 46°.

Hydrochloride. $C_{15}H_{21}N_3O$·HCl. Crystals from abs alcohol, mp 224-224.5°.

Dihydrochloride. $C_{15}H_{21}N_3O$·2HCl. mp 227-227.5°.

Diphosphate. $C_{15}H_{27}N_3O_9P_2$. mp 174-176°.

THERAP CAT: Antimalarial.

8068. Quinoline. [91-22-5] Leucoline; chinoleine; 1-benzazine; benzo[*b*]pyridine. C_9H_7N; mol wt 129.16. C 83.69%, H

8-Quinolineboronic Acid

5.46%, N 10.84%. Occurs in small amounts in coal tar. Prepd by the Skraup synthesis by heating aniline with glycerol and nitrobenzene in presence of sulfuric acid: Clarke, Davis, *Org. Synth.* **coll. vol. I,** 478 (2nd ed., 1941) 478; alternate syntheses: Manske, *Chem. Rev.* **30,** 113 (1942); Bergstrom, *ibid.* **35,** 150 (1944). Process based on the interaction of aniline with acetaldehyde and a formaldehyde hemiacetal: Cislak, Wheeler, **US 3020281** (1962 to Reilly Tar & Chem.). Toxicity data: Smyth *et al., Arch. Ind. Hyg. Occup. Med.* **4,** 119 (1951).

Hygroscopic liquid. Absorbs as much as 22% water. Darkens on storage in ordinary, stoppered bottle. Penetrating odor, not as offensive as pyridine. Volatile with steam. d_4^{25} 1.0900; mp $-15°$; bp_{760} 237.7°; bp_{100} 163.2°; bp_{40} 136.7°; bp_{20} 119.8°; bp_{10} 103.8°; bp_5 89.6°; $bp_{1.0}$ 59.7°. n_D^{20} 1.62683. Absorption spectrum: Hantzsch, *Ber.* **44,** 1824 (1911). Weak base (neutral to phenolphthalein), forms water-soluble salts with strong acids: pK 9.5. Difficultly sol in cold water, more easily in hot water. Miscible with alcohol, ether, carbon disulfide. Dissolves sulfur, phosphorus, arsenic trioxide. *Protect from light and moisture.* LD_{50} orally in rats: 460 mg/kg (Smyth).

Bisulfate. $C_9H_9NO_4S$. White to grayish-white, crystalline powder. mp 163-165°. Freely sol in water; one gram dissolves in 50 ml cold, in 9 ml boiling abs alcohol. *Protect from light.*

Hydrochloride. $C_9H_7N.HCl$. White deliquesc crystals. mp 93-94°. Freely sol in water, alcohol, hot benzene, chloroform, sparingly in cold ether. *Keep well closed and protected from light.*

Salicylate. $C_{16}H_{13}NO_3$. Reddish-gray crystalline powder. Sol in 80 parts water; freely sol in alcohol, benzene, ether, glycerol, oils. *Protect from light.*

Tartrate. $C_{43}H_{45}N_3O_{24}$. White crystals, pungent odor, sharp taste. mp 125° (dec). Sol in 80 parts water, 150 parts alcohol. Insol in ether.

USE: Manuf dyes; prepn hydroxyquinoline sulfate, niacin. As preservative for anatomical specimens. Solvent for resins, terpenes.

THERAP CAT: Antimalarial.

8069. 8-Quinolineboronic Acid. [86-58-8] $C_9H_8BNO_2$; mol wt 172.98. C 62.49%, H 4.66%, B 6.25%, N 8.10%, O 18.50%. Prepd by reacting 8-bromoquinoline with butyllithium and tributyl borate: Letsinger, Dandegaonker, *J. Am. Chem. Soc.* **81,** 498 (1959).

Crystals from alc, mp >300°.

Butyl diester. $C_{17}H_{24}BNO_2$. bp_4 180°. n_D^{25} 1.4840.

Chloroethyl diester. $C_{13}H_{14}BCl_2NO_2$. Crystals from toluene, mp 193-194°.

8070. 8-Quinolinecarboxylic Acid. [86-59-9] $C_{10}H_7NO_2$; mol wt 173.17. C 69.36%, H 4.07%, N 8.09%, O 18.48%. Prepd by heating 2-aminobenzoic acid with 2-nitrobenzoic acid, glycerol and sulfuric acid: Schlosser, Skraup, *Monatsh. Chem.* **2,** 530 (1881); by oxidizing 8-quinolylaldehyde with chromic acid: Howitz, *Ber.* **35,** 1275 (1902).

Needles from water. mp 186-187.5°. Sublimes above mp. Slightly sol in cold water, appreciably sol in hot water and in alcohol. Freely sol in acids and alkalies.

USE: Detection of cadmium, copper, iron, lead, mercury, silver, thallium; quantitative determination of copper.

8071. Quinoline Yellow. [8004-92-0] C.I. Acid Yellow 3; D & C Yellow No. 10; Acid Yellow 3; Food Yellow 13; C.I. 47005. Synthetic dye. A mixture of the sodium salts of the mono- and disulfonic acids of quinoline yellow spirit soluble, *q.v.* Principal constituents: sodium salts of *2-(2,3-dihydro-1,3-dioxo-1H-indene-2-yl)-6-quinolinesulfonic acid* and *2-(2,3-dihydro-1,3-dioxo-1H-indene-2-yl)-8-quinolinesulfonic acid*. Prepn of sulfonic acids: M. C. Traub, *Ber.* **16,** 297 (1883); *Colour Index* vol. 4 (3rd ed., 1971) p 4435. HPLC determn: J. Chudy *et al., J. Chromatogr.* **154,** 306 (1978). Purification: N. A. Ambrosiano *et al.,* **US 4398916** (1983 to Sterling Drug). Stability: H. Delonca *et al., Pharm. Acta Helv.* **58,** 332 (1983). ^{13}C-NMR spectrum: M. Gelbcke *et al., Bull. Soc. Chim. Belg.* **91,** 237 (1982). TLC identification: J. A. Steele, *J. Assoc. Off. Anal. Chem.* **67,** 540 (1984). Composition and skin sensitivity: Y. Sata *et al., Contact Dermatitis* **10,** 30 (1984). LC determn of unsulfonated impurity: A. L. Goldberg, *J. Assoc. Off. Anal. Chem.* **68,** 477 (1985). Toxicity: F. C. Lu, A. Lavalle, *Can. Pharm. J.* **97,** 30 (1964).

Bright greenish yellow. Orange in conc H_2SO_4. Sol in water, slightly sol in ethanol. Practically insol in vegetable oils. LD_{50} in rats (g/kg): >2 orally (Lu, Lavalle).

USE: Textile dye for wool, nylon, silk. Paper dye. Barium salt in printing inks. Color for food, drugs, cosmetics.

8072. Quinoline Yellow Spirit Soluble. [8003-22-3] C.I. Solvent Yellow 33; quinoline yellow base; quinoline yellow A; D & C Yellow No. 11; C.I. 47000. Synthetic dye consisting principally of *quinophthalone (2-(2-quinolinyl)-1H-indene-1,3-(2H)-dione)*. Prepn: M. C. Traub, *Ber.* **16,** 297 (1883); E. Jacobsen, C. L. Reimer, *ibid.* 1082; *Colour Index* vol. 4 (3rd ed., 1971) p 4435. ^{13}C-NMR spectrum: M. Gelbcke *et al., Bull. Soc. Chim. Belg.* **91,** 237 (1982). Composition and skin sensitivity: Y. Sato *et al., Contact Dermatitis* **10,** 30 (1984); S. Kita *et al., ibid.* **11,** 210 (1984). Inhalation toxicity in animals: T. C. Marrs *et al., Hum. Toxicol.* **3,** 289 (1984).

Quinophthalone

Bright greenish yellow. Insol in water. Slightly sol in ethanol (yellow), linseed oil, mineral oil, oleic acid, paraffin wax, stearic acid, turpentine. Sol in acetone, chloroform, benzene, toluene. Yellow brown in conc H_2SO_4, yellow flocculent ppt in dilution.

USE: In spirit lacquers, polystyrenes, polycarbonates, polyamides, and acrylic resins. In colored smokes. Occasionally in hydrocarbon solvents. In externally applied drugs and cosmetics.

8073. Quinolinic Acid. [89-00-9] 2,3-Pyridinedicarboxylic acid. $C_7H_5NO_4$; mol wt 167.12. C 50.31%, H 3.02%, N 8.38%, O 38.29%. Metabolite of tryptophan, *q.v.* Prepn: S. Hoogewerff, W. A. van Dorp, *Ber.* **12,** 747 (1879); W. Koenigs, *ibid.* 983; O. Fischer, E. Renouf, *ibid.* **17,** 755 (1884); E. Sucharda, *ibid.* **58B,** 1727 (1925); V. Yu. Stiks, S. A. Bulgach, *ibid.* **65B,** 11 (1932); A. F. Lindenstruth, C. A. VanderWerf, *J. Am. Chem. Soc.* **71,** 3020 (1949). Metabolism studies: L. M. Henderson *et al., J. Biol. Chem.* **181,** 667, 677, 687, 731 (1949); H. P. Sarett, *ibid.* **193,** 627 (1951). Neuroexcitatory activity and possible role in neurodegenerative disorders: R. Schwarcz *et al., Science* **219,** 316 (1983).

Odorless crystals. mp 190° when rapidly heated, with decompn into CO_2 and nicotinic acid. Sol in 180 parts water, in alkalies, slightly in alcohol. Almost insol in ether or benzene.

8074. Quinone. [106-51-4] 2,5-Cyclohexadiene-1,4-dione; p-quinone; 1,4-benzoquinone; 1,4-cyclohexadienedione. $C_6H_4O_2$; mol wt 108.09. C 66.67%, H 3.73%, O 29.60%. Made by oxidation of aniline with sodium dichromate in presence of sulfuric acid. Laboratory prepn from hydroquinone: Vliet, *Org. Synth.* **2**, 85 (1922); also *Org. Synth.* **coll. vol. I** (2nd ed., 1941). *Cf.* Underwood, Walsh, *ibid.* **16**, 73 (1936). Toxicity study: Woodard *et al., Fed. Proc.* **8**, 348 (1949).

Yellow monoclinic prisms from water or petr ether. Penetrating odor resembling that of chlorine. Irritating vapors. d_4^{20} 1.318. mp 115.7°. Sublimes [sublimation velocities *in vacuo:* Kempf, *J. Prakt. Chem.* [2] **78**, 236 (1908)]. Volatile with steam. Absorption spectrum: Hantzsch, *Ber.* **49**, 522 (1916). Dipole moment: 0.67. Polemic over correct values: Paoloni, *J. Am. Chem. Soc.* **80**, 3879 (1958). Slightly sol in water; sol in alcohol, ether, hot petr ether, alkalies. LD_{50} orally in rats: 130 mg/kg (Woodard).

Caution: Potential symptoms of overexposure are eye and skin irritation, conjunctivitis; keratitis. *See NIOSH Pocket Guide to Chemical Hazards* (DHHS/NIOSH 97-140, 1997) p 272.

USE: Oxidizing agent; in photography; manuf dyes; manuf hydroquinone; tanning hides; making gelatin insol; strengthening animal fibers; as reagent.

8075. Quinovic Acid. [465-74-7] (3β)-3-Hydroxyurs-12-ene-27,28-dioic acid; quinovaic acid; chinovic acid; chinova acid. $C_{30}H_{46}O_5$; mol wt 486.68. C 74.04%, H 9.53%, O 16.44%. Isoln from cinchona bark as the glycoside quinovin: Hlasiwetz, *Ann.* **79**, 129 (1851); **111**, 182 (1859); Votocek, Rác, *Collect. Czech. Chem. Commun.* **1**, 234 (1929); Tschesche *et al., Ann.* **667**, 151 (1963); from *Zygophyllum coccineum* L., *Zygophyllaceae:* Soliman, *J. Chem. Soc.* **1939**, 1760; from bark of *Mitragyna inermis* Kuntze and leaves of *M. ciliata* Aubrev & Pellegr. and *M. rubrostipulacea* Havil., *Rubiaceae:* Badger *et al., ibid.* **1950**, 867. Structure: Brossi *et al., Helv. Chim. Acta* **34**, 244 (1951); Barton, de Mayo, *J. Chem. Soc.* **1953**, 3111. *Review:* J. Simonsen, W. C. J. Ross, *The Terpenes* vol. **5** (University Press, Cambridge, 1957) pp 75-113.

Prisms from dil pyridine, decomp 297°. Very bitter taste. $[\alpha]_D^{20}$ +99° (c = 2.48 in pyridine). Practically insol in water and other solvents except pyridine.

O-Acetylquinovic acid. $C_{32}H_{48}O_6$. Needles from dilute acetone, mp 282-284°.

Dimethyl ester. $C_{32}H_{50}O_5$. Needles from dil acetone, mp 175°. $[\alpha]_D^{19}$ +117.4° (c = 2.2 in $CHCl_3$). Sol in organic solvents.

8076. Quinovin. [53516-73-7] Quinova-bitter; chinovin. Isoln from cinchona bark (*cortex chinae*): Hlasiwetz, *Ann.* **111**, 182 (1859); Liebermann, Giesel, *Ber.* **16**, 926 (1883). A mixture of three glycosides, 60% A, 5% B and 30% C: Tschesche *et al., Ann.* **667**, 151 (1963).

Glycoside A. Quinovic acid β-D-quinovoside. $C_{36}H_{56}O_9$. Crystals from methanol + water, mp 237-238°. $[\alpha]_D^{21}$ +57 ± 2° (ethanol).

Glycoside B. Cincholic acid β-D-quinovoside. $C_{36}H_{56}O_9$. Crystals from methanol + water, mp 193-195°. $[\alpha]_D^{19}$ +78 ± 3° (c = 0.78 in ethanol).

Glycoside C. Quinovic acid β-D-glucoside. $C_{36}H_{56}O_{10}$. Crystals from methanol + water, mp 247-250°. $[\alpha]_D^{20}$ +62 ±2° (ethanol).

8077. Quinovose. [7658-08-4] 6-Deoxy-D-glucose; D-glucomethylose; D-isorhamnose; D-epirhamnose; isorhodeose; epifucose; chinovose. $C_6H_{12}O_5$; mol wt 164.16. C 43.90%, H 7.37%, O 48.73%. Isoln from cinchona bark: Freudenerg, *Ber.* **62**, 373 (1929). Identity with D-glucomethylose: Votocek, Rác, *Collect. Czech. Chem. Commun.* **1**, 239 (1929). Structure: Karrer, Boettcher, *Helv. Chim. Acta* **36**, 570 (1953). Synthesis from 6-*O*-p-tolylsulfonyl-D-glucose: Schmidt, "6-Deoxy-α-D-glucose" in *Methods in Carbohydrate Chemistry* vol. I, R. L. Whistler, M. L. Wolfrom, Eds. (Academic Press, New York, 1962) pp 198-201. Alternate facile synthesis: V. K. Srivastava, L. M. Lerner, *Carbohydr. Res.* **64**, 263 (1978).

Crystals from ethyl acetate, mp 146°. $[\alpha]_D^{20}$ +73° (5 min) → +30° (3 hr, final) (c = 8.3 in water). Sol in water, ethanol. Practically insol in ether, acetone.

8078. Quinoxaline. [91-19-0] 1,4-Benzodiazine; benzo[*a*]pyrazine; benzoparadiazine; phenpiazine. $C_8H_6N_2$; mol wt 130.15. C 73.83%, H 4.65%, N 21.52%. Prepd from *o*-phenylenediamine and glyoxal or glyoxal sodium bisulfite: Hinsberg, *Ber.* **17**, 320 (1884); *Ann.* **237**, 334 (1887); Jones, McLaughlin, *Org. Synth.* **30**, 86 (1950).

Crystals, mp 29-30°. Odor of quinoline when cool, odor of piperidine when hot. d_4^{48} (liq) 1.1334. $bp_{760.3}$ 229.5°. bp_{12} 108-111°. n_D^{48} 1.6231. Very freely sol in water, alc, ether, benzene.

Monohydrate. Crystals, mp 37°.

Sulfate. $C_8H_6N_2 \cdot H_2SO_4$. Leaflets, mp 186-187°. Freely sol in water. Less sol in alcohol.

8079. Quinoxyfen. [124495-18-7] 5,7-Dichloro-4-(4-fluorophenoxy)quinoline; DE-795; Fortress; Quintec. $C_{15}H_8Cl_2FNO$; mol wt 308.13. C 58.47%, H 2.62%, Cl 23.01%, F 6.17%, N 4.55%, O 5.19%. Quinoline fungicide for powdery mildew control in cereals, grapes and hops; inhibits formation of appressoria through which the fungus invades the plant. Prepn: W. R. Arnold *et al.*, **EP 326330** (1989 to Eli Lilly); *eidem,* **US 5145843** (1992 to DowElanco). Properties and field trials: C. Longhurst *et al., Brighton Crop Prot. Conf. - Pests Dis.* **1996**, 27. Resistance profile: D. W. Hollomon *et al., ibid.* 701. Metabolism and environmental fate: G. L. Reeves *et al., ibid.* 1169. Determn and fate in grapes, raisins and wine: P. Cabras *et al., J. Agric. Food Chem.* **48**, 6128 (2000).

Crystals from heptane, mp 105-106°. LD_{50} orally in rats: >5000 mg/kg; dermally in rabbits: >2000 mg/kg; by inhalation in rats: >3.38 mg/l (Longhurst).

USE: Agricultural fungicide.

8080. Quintozene. [82-68-8] Pentachloronitrobenzene; PCNB; terrachlor; PKhNB; Botrilex; Brassicol; Folosan; Pentagen;

Terraclor; Tilcarex. $C_6Cl_5NO_2$; mol wt 295.33. C 24.40%, Cl 60.02%, N 4.74%, O 10.83%. Prepd by treating pentachlorobenzene with fuming nitric acid: Jungfleisch, *Ann. Chim.* [4] **15**, 286 (1868); A. Roedig, K. Kiepert, *Ann.* **593**, 71 (1955). Persistence of residues in foods: P. B. Baker, B. Flaherty, *Analyst* **97**, 378 (1972); A. R. P. Paxton, D. Purser, *Pestic. Sci.* **13**, 401 (1982); in soil: J. Beck, K. E. Hansen, *ibid.* **5**, 41 (1974). Metabolism by sheep and goats: P. W. Aschbacher, V. J. Feil, *J. Agric. Food Chem.* **31**, 1150 (1983). Toxicity data: J. K. Finnegan *et al.*, *Arch. Int. Pharmacodyn. Ther.* **114**, 38 (1958). *Review: WHO Environmental Health Criteria* **41**, 1-38 (1984). Comparative review of the effects on soil organisms: E. R. Ingham, *Crop Prot.* **4**, 3-32 (1985).

Fine needles from alcohol, platelets from carbon disulfide. d_4^{25} 1.718. mp 144°. bp_{760} 328° (some dec). Practically insol in water, cold alcohol. Freely sol in carbon disulfide, benzene, chloroform. LD_{50} in male, female rats (g/kg): 1.71 ±0.20, 1.65 ±0.17 by gavage (Finnegan).

USE: Fungicide for seed and soil treatment.

8081. Quinuclidine. [100-76-5] 1-Azabicyclo[2.2.2]-octane; 1,4-ethylenepiperidine. $C_7H_{13}N$; mol wt 111.18. C 75.62%, H 11.79%, N 12.60%. Prepn: Löffler, Stietzel, *Ber.* **42**, 124 (1909); Meisenheimer *et al.*, *Ann.* **420**, 191 (1920); Clemo, Metcalfe, *J. Chem. Soc.* **1937**, 1989; Prelog, **US 2192840** (1940); Wawzonek *et al.*, *J. Am. Chem. Soc.* **73**, 2806 (1951); Leonard, Elkin, *J. Org. Chem.* **27**, 4635 (1962).

Prisms from petr ether. Sublimes. mp 156° (sealed tube). Very sol in water and the usual organic solvents.

Hydrochloride. $C_7H_{13}N.HCl$. Crystals from abs ethanol, mp 364-365°.

8082. 3-Quinuclidinol. [1619-34-7] 1-Azabicyclo[2.2.2]-octan-3-ol; 3-hydroxyquinuclidine. $C_7H_{13}NO$; mol wt 127.18. C 66.11%, H 10.30%, N 11.01%, O 12.58%. Prepn and resolution of *dl*-forms: Sternbach, Kaiser, *J. Am. Chem. Soc.* **74**, 2215 (1952); Sternbach, **US 2648667** (1953 to Hoffmann-La Roche); of free alcohol, acetate and/or benzoate esters: Grob *et al.*, *Helv. Chim. Acta* **40**, 2170 (1957); Mikhalina, Rubtsov, *Zh. Obshch. Khim.* **30**, 163 (1960), *C.A.* **54**, 22632h (1960). Structure activity of esters: M. D. Mashkovsky in *Proc. 1st Int. Pharmacol. Mtg. Stockholm, 1961* vol. **7** (Macmillan, New York, 1963) pp 359-366.

dl-**Form.** [3684-26-2] Crystals from benzene or acetone, mp 221-223° also reported as 225-227°. Sublimes at 120° and 20 mm Hg. Very sol in water.

dl-**Form hydrochloride.** [25333-43-1] Prisms from methanol + acetone, mp >300°.

dl-**Form acetate (ester).** Aceclidine; 3-acetoxyquinuclidine; 3-quinuclidinyl acetate. $C_9H_{15}NO_2$. Oily liq, $bp_{0.4}$ 73-74°, bp_{11} 113-115°. n_D^{25} 1.4675.

dl-**Form acetate hydrochloride.** [6109-70-2] Glaucostat; Glaucotat; Glaudin. $C_9H_{15}NO_2.HCl$; mol wt 205.68. Crystals, mp 166°.

dl-**Form benzilate (ester).** 3-Quinuclidinyl benzilate; BZ; QNB; Ro-2-3308. $C_{21}H_{23}NO_3$; mol wt 337.41. Prepn: Sternbach, Kaiser, *loc. cit.*, 2219. Crystals from acetone-ether, mp 164-165°.

dl-**Form benzoate (ester).** [66-93-3] 3-Benzoyloxyquinuclidine; 3-quinuclidinyl benzoate. $C_{14}H_{17}NO_2$. Oily liquid, $bp_{0.3}$ 148-150°.

dl-**Form benzoate hydrochloride.** [25333-48-6] Oksilidin; oxylidine. $C_{14}H_{17}NO_2.HCl$. Crystals, mp 238-240°.

l-**Form.** [25333-42-0] Prisms from acetone, mp 220-222°. $[\alpha]_D^{25}$ -2.0° (c = 6.5), -43.8° (c = 3 in 1N HCl).

USE: Benzilate (ester) has been used as an incapacitating agent in chemical warfare: *Health Aspects of Chemical and Biological Weapons* (WHO, Geneva, 1970) pp 49-51.

THERAP CAT: Hypotensive; acetate (ester) as cholinergic.

8083. Quinupramine. [31721-17-2] 5-(1-Azabicyclo-[2.2.2]oct-3-yl)-10,11-dihydro-5H-dibenz[b,f]azepine; 10,11-dihydro-5-(3-quinuclidinyl)-5H-dibenz[b,f]azepine; LM-208; Kinupril; Kevopril. $C_{21}H_{24}N_2$; mol wt 304.43. C 82.85%, H 7.95%, N 9.20%. Analog of imipramine, *q.v.* Prepn: C. Gueremy, P. C. Wirth, **DE 2030492** (1971 to Sogeras), *C.A.* **74**, 141581e (1971). Animal studies: W. Van Dorsser, A. Dresse, *Arch. Int. Pharmacodyn. Ther.* **208**, 373 (1974); *eidem, ibid.* **220**, 164 (1976). Clinical study: R. Volmat *et al.*, *Clin. Neurol. Psychiat.* **239**, 445 (1978).

Crystals, mp 150°.
THERAP CAT: Antidepressant.

8084. Quinupristin. [120138-50-3] 4-[4-(Dimethylamino)-N-methyl-L-phenylalanine]-5-[(2S,5R)-5-[[[(3S)-1-azabicyclo[2.2.-2]oct-3-yl]thio]methyl]-4-oxo-2-piperidinecarboxylic acid]virginiamycin S1; 5δ-[(3S)-3-quinuclidinyl]thiomethylpristinamycin IA; RP-57669. $C_{53}H_{67}N_9O_{10}S$; mol wt 1022.22. C 62.27%, H 6.61%, N 12.33%, O 15.65%, S 3.14%. Semisynthetic depsipeptide type I streptogramin, *q.v.* Marketed in combination with dalfopristin, *q.v.* Prepn: J.-C. Barriere *et al.*, **EP 248703**, *eidem*, **US 4798827** (1987, 1989 both to Rhone-Poulenc). *In vitro* activity: H. C. Neu *et al.*, *J. Antimicrob. Chemother.* **30**, Suppl. A, 83 (1992). HPLC determn in plasma: A. Le Liboux *et al.*, *J. Chromatogr. B* **708**, 161 (1998).

White crystals in combination with methanol, mp ~200°.
THERAP CAT: Antibacterial.

8085. Quisqualic Acid. [52809-07-1] (αS)-α-Amino-3,5-dioxo-1,2,4-oxadiazolidine-2-propanoic acid; L-quisqualic acid; β-(3,5-dioxo-1,2,4-oxadiazolidin-2-yl)-L-alanine. $C_5H_7N_3O_5$; mol wt 189.13. C 31.75%, H 3.73%, N 22.22%, O 42.30%. Excitatory amino acid (EAA) used to identify a specific subset of EAA receptors; consequently, the receptors are known as quisqualate receptors. *See also* NMDA, kainic acid. Isoln from the seeds of *Quisqualis chinesis* and anthelmintic activity: Y.-C. Tuan *et al., Yao Hsueh Hsueh Pao* **5,** 87 (1957), *C.A.* **56,** 14896b (1958); from *Q. indica:* S.-T. Fang, J.-H. Chu, *Hua Hsueh Hsueh Pao* **30,** 226 (1964), *C.A.* **61,** 7359f (1962); from *Q. fructus:* T. Takemoto *et al., Yakugaku Zasshi* **95,** 176 (1975), *C.A.* **82,** 152211a (1975). Enzymic synthesis: I. Murakoshi *et al., Chem. Pharm. Bull.* **22,** 473 (1974). Total synthesis: J. E. Baldwin *et al., Chem. Commun.* **1985,** 256. Crystal structure: J. L. Flippen, R. D. Gilardi, *Acta Crystallogr.* **B32,** 951 (1976). Identification as a neuroexcitant: H. Shinozaki, I. Shibuya, *Neuropharmacology* **13,** 665 (1974). Receptor binding studies: K. Koshiya, *Life Sci.* **37,** 1373 (1985); J. T. Greenamyre, *J. Pharmacol. Exp. Ther.* **233,** 254 (1985). Review of isolation of quisqualic acid and other EAAs: T. Takemoto, in *Kainic Acid as a Tool in Neurobiology,* R. G. McGeer *et al.,* Eds. (Raven Press, New York, 1978) pp 1-15.

Crystals from water-ethanol, mp 190-191°. $[\alpha]_D^{20}$ +17.0° (c = 2.0 in 6*M* HCl).

8086. Quizalofop-ethyl. [76578-14-8] 2-[4-[(6-Chloro-2-quinoxalinyl)oxy]phenoxy]propanoic acid ethyl ester; ethyl 2-[4-(6-chloro-2-quinoxalinyloxy)phenoxy]propionate; quinofop-ethyl; DPX-Y6202; NCI-96683; NC-302; Assure; Targa; Pilot. $C_{19}H_{17}$-ClN_2O_4; mol wt 372.80. C 61.21%, H 4.60%, Cl 9.51%, N 7.51%, O 17.17%. Post-emergence herbicide for control of grassy weeds in broad-leaved crops. Prepn and herbicidal activity: Y. Ura *et al.,* **DE 3004770** (1980 to Nissan), *C.A.* **94,** 103421h (1981). Prepn and structure-activity relationships: G. Sakata *et al., J. Pestic. Sci.* **10,** 61 (1985). Pharmacological effects in laboratory animals: K. Inokuchi *et al., Oyo Yakuri* **30,** 509 (1985), *C.A.* **104,** 30101s (1986). Site of action studies: T. Ikai *et al., Proc. Br. Crop Prot. Conf. - Weeds* **1985,** 163. Account of properties, toxicity, crop tolerance: G. Sakata *et al., Proc. 10th Conf. Int. Congr. Plant Prot.* **1,** 315 (1983).

White crystals, mp 92-93°. $bp_{0.2}$ 220°. Practically insol in water (0.3 × 10^{-6} g/ml at 20°). Soly in acetone, ethanol, benzene, xylene at 20° (g/ml): 0.11, 0.009, 0.29, 0.12. LD_{50} in male, female rats, male, female mice (mg/kg): 1670, 1480, 2350, 2360 orally; all 10,000 dermally. LC_{50} (96 hr) in rainbow trout: 10.7 mg/l (Sakata).

USE: Herbicide.

8087. Quorn®. Myco-protein. High protein, meat substitute derived from the biomass of the filamentous fungus, *Fusarium graminearum* (Schwabe). Description of production: J. Edelman *et al., Nutr. Abstr. Rev.* **53,** 471 (1983). See also: R. A. Marsh, **US 4555485** (1985 to Ranks Hovis McDougall). Nutritional profile: M. Sadler, *Nutr. Food Sci.* **112,** 9 (1988). Metabolic study in comparison with meat: W. H. Turnbull *et al., Am. J. Clin. Nutr.* **52,** 646 (1990). Effect on blood lipids: *eidem, ibid.* **55,** 415 (1992). *Review:* A. P. J. Trinci, *Mycol. Res.* **96,** 1-13 (1992).

Very mild, wheaty taste; slight aroma of mushrooms. Fibrous texture resembling that of meat.

USE: Meat substitute.

R

8088. R-11. [126-15-8] 1,5a,6,9,9a,9b-Hexahydro-4a(4*H*)-dibenzofurancarboxaldehyde; 2,3,4,5-bis(2-butenylene)tetrahydrofurfural; MGK-11; MGK Repellent 11. $C_{13}H_{16}O_2$; mol wt 204.26. C 76.44%, H 7.90%, O 15.67%. Prepd by heating furfuraldehyde with butadiene and water under pressure: Hillyer, Nicewander, **US 2683151** (1954 to Phillips Petroleum). Clinical efficacy vs sand flies: F. P. Fossati, M. Maroli, *Trans. R. Soc. Trop. Med. Hyg.* **80**, 771 (1986).

Liquid, bp 307°. d_4^{20} 1.10. mp −80°. n_D^{20} 1.5254. Practically insol in water.
Oxime. mp 97.2°.
Dinitrophenylhydrazone. mp 152.8°.
USE: Insect repellent.

8089. Rabeprazole. [117976-89-3] 2-[[[4-(3-Methoxypropoxy)-3-methyl-2-pyridinyl]methyl]sulfinyl]-1*H*-benzimidazole; pariprazole. $C_{18}H_{21}N_3O_3S$; mol wt 359.44. C 60.15%, H 5.89%, N 11.69%, O 13.35%, S 8.92%. Partially reversible gastric proton pump inhibitor. Prepn: S. Souda *et al.*, **EP 268956**; *idem*, **US 5045552** (1988, 1991 both to Eisai). Pharmacology: H. Goto *et al.*, *Arzneim.-Forsch.* **41**, 635 (1991). Mode of action: M. Morii, N. Takeguchi, *J. Biol. Chem.* **268**, 21553 (1993). HPLC determn in plasma: H. Nakai *et al.*, *J. Chromatogr. B* **660**, 211 (1994). Clinical pharmacokinetics: S. Yasuda *et al.*, *Int. J. Clin. Pharmacol. Ther.* **32**, 466 (1994). Review of clinical trials in acid peptic diseases: M. L. Cloud *et al.*, *Dig. Dis. Sci.* **43**, 993-1000 (1998); of pharmacology and clinical experience in gastro-esophageal reflux disease: B. Thjodleifsson, *Expert Opin. Pharmacother.* **5**, 137-149 (2004).

White crystals from CH_2Cl_2/ether, mp 99-100° (dec).
Sodium salt. [117976-90-6] E-3810; Aciphex; Pariet. $C_{18}H_{20}N_3NaO_3S$; mol wt 381.42. White crystals from ether, mp 140-141° (dec). Very sol in water, methanol; freely sol in ethanol, chloroform, ethyl acetate. Insol in ether, *n*-hexane.
THERAP CAT: Antiulcerative.

8090. Racecadotril. [81110-73-8] *N*-[2-[(Acetylthio)methyl]-1-oxo-3-phenylpropyl]glycine phenylmethyl ester; *N*-[(*R*,*S*)-3-acetylthio-2-benzylpropanoyl]glycine benzyl ester; acetorphan; Hidrasec; Tiorfan. $C_{21}H_{23}NO_4S$; mol wt 385.48. C 65.43%, H 6.01%, N 3.63%, O 16.60%, S 8.32%. Antisecretory enkephalinase inhibitor. Prepn: B. Roques *et al.*, **EP 38758** (1981); *idem*, **US 4513009** (1985 to Bioprojet). Pharmacology: J.-M. Lecomte *et al.*, *J. Pharmacol. Exp. Ther.* **237**, 937 (1986). Effect on intestinal transit: J. F. Bergmann *et al.*, *Aliment. Pharmacol. Ther.* **6**, 305 (1992). Clinical trial in acute diarrhea: P. Baumer *et al.*, *Gut* **33**, 753 (1992); in children: E. Salazar-Lindo *et al.*, *N. Engl. J. Med.* **343**, 463 (2000). Symposium on pharmacology and clinical experience: *Aliment. Pharmacol. Ther.* **13**, Suppl. 6, 1-32 (1999). Review of clinical development: J.-C. Schwartz, *Int. J. Antimicrob. Agents* **14**, 75-79 (2000); J. M. Lecomte, *ibid.* 81-87.

White crystals from ether mp 89°.
(S)-Form. [112573-73-6] Ecadotril; sinorphan; Bay-y-7432. $C_{21}H_{23}NO_4S$; mol wt 385.48. C 65.43%, H 6.01%, N 3.63%, O 16.60%, S 8.32%. Prepn: P. Duhamel *et al.*, **EP 318377**; *idem*, **US 5208255** (1989, 1993 both to Bioprojet); and pharmacology: B. Giros *et al.*, *J. Pharmacol. Exp. Ther.* **243**, 666 (1987). Clinical effect on plasma ANP levels in CHF: J. C. Kahn *et al.*, *Lancet* **335**, 118 (1990); on renal function: F. Schmitt *et al.*, *Am. J. Physiol.* **267**, F20 (1994). Clinical trial in heart failure: C. M. O'Connor *et al.*, *Am. Heart J.* **138**, 1140 (1999); J. G. F. Cleland, K. Swedberg, *Lancet* **351**, 1657 (1998). mp 71°. $[\alpha]_D^{25}$ −24.1° (c = 1.3 in methanol). LD_{50} i.v. in mice: >100 mg/kg (Duhamel, 1993).
THERAP CAT: Antidiarrheal.

8091. Racemethorphan. [510-53-2] (±)-3-Methoxy-17-methylmorphinan; *dl-cis*-1,3,4,9,10,10a-hexahydro-6-methoxy-11-methyl-2*H*-10,4a-iminoethanophenanthrene; *dl-cis*-1,2,3,9,10,10a-hexahydro-6-methoxy-11-methyl-4*H*-10,4a-iminoethanophenanthrene; deoxydihydrothebacodine; methorphan. $C_{18}H_{25}NO$; mol wt 271.40. C 79.66%, H 9.28%, N 5.16%, O 5.90%. Prepn: Schnider, Grüssner, **US 2676177** (1954 to Hoffmann-La Roche). Prepn of *d*-form: *eidem*, *ibid.*; Häfliger *et al.*, *Helv. Chim. Acta* **39**, 2053 (1956). Prepn of *l*-form hydrobromide: Corrodi *et al.*, *ibid.* **42**, 215 (1959). Crystal structure and absolute configuration of *d*-form hydrobromide: L. Gylbert, D. Carlstrom, *Acta Crystallogr. B*, 2833 (1977).

Hydrobromide. [6031-86-3] Ro-1-5470. $C_{18}H_{25}NO.HBr$; mol wt 352.31. Crystals, mp 124-126°.
d-Form hydrobromide. [125-69-9] Dextromethorphan hydrobromide; demorphan hydrobromide; Ro-1-5470/5; Benylin; Canfodion; Cosylan; Hihustan. HPLC-MS/MS determn of free base in urine: M. L. Constanzer *et al.*, *J. Chromatogr. B* **816**, 297 (2005). Occurs as the monohydrate, crystals, mp 122-124°. $[\alpha]_D^{20}$ +27.6° (c = 1.5 in water). Approx soly in water: 1.5% at 25°, 5% at 50°, 25% at 85°. Soly (w/w): 25% in 95% ethanol at room temp, 10% in glycerol. Sol in propylene glycol, chloroform. Practically insol in ether. pH of a 1% aq soln: 5.2-6.5. Long range stability of aq solns obtained by adjusting pH within 4-5.6. Reacts with alkalies forming the free base which is practically insol in water.
l-Form hydrobromide. [125-68-8] Levomethorphan hydrobromide; Ro-1-5470/6; Ro-1-7788. Occurs as the dihydrate, crystals, mp 124-126°. $[\alpha]_D^{20}$ −26.3°.
Note: Racemethorphan and levomethorphan are controlled substances (opiates): **21 CFR**, 1308.12.
THERAP CAT: Antitussive.

8092. Ractopamine. [97825-25-7] 4-Hydroxy-α-[[[3-(4-hydroxyphenyl)-1-methylpropyl]amino]methyl]benzenemethanol; 1-(4-hydroxyphenyl)-2-[1-methyl-3-(4-hydroxyphenyl)-propylamino]ethanol; *N*-[2-(4-hydroxyphenyl)-2-hydroxyethyl]-1-methyl-3-(4-hydroxyphenyl)propylamine. $C_{18}H_{23}NO_3$; mol wt 301.38. C 71.73%, H 7.69%, N 4.65%, O 15.93%. β-Adrenergic agonist; repartitioning agent. Prepn (stereochemistry unspecified): A. van Dijk, H. D. Moed, *Rec. Trav. Chim.* **92**, 1281 (1973). Prepn of *R,R*-isomer: J. Mills *et al.*, **EP 7205** (1980 to Lilly). Prepd (not claimed): D. B. Anderson *et al.*, **US 4690951** (1987 to Lilly).

Consult the Name Index before using this section.

LC determn in animal feeds: M. P. Turberg *et al., J. AOAC Int.* **77**, 840 (1994). Metabolism and tissue residue studies: J. E. Dalidowicz *et al., ACS Symp. Ser.* **503**, 234 (1992). Effect on growth, carcass characteristics and meat quality in swine: B. E. Uttaro *et al., J. Anim. Sci.* **71**, 2439 (1993). Effect on β-receptor affinity and density in pigs: M. E. Spurlock *et al., ibid.* **72**, 75 (1994).

Hydrochloride. [90274-24-1] EL-737; LY-031537; Optaflexx; Paylean. $C_{18}H_{23}NO_3 \cdot HCl$; mol wt 337.84. Mixture of 4 stereoisomers in approx equal proportions. Product containing 51% *RR,-SS*- and 49% *RS,SR*-diastereomers, mp 124-129°.

R,R-Form Hydrochloride. [74432-68-1] Butopamine hydrochloride. Crystals from ethanol + diethyl ether, mp 176-176.5° (dec). $[\alpha]_D$ −22.7°; $[\alpha]_{365}$ −71.2° (c = 3.7 mg/ml in methanol).

THERAP CAT (VET): Animal growth promotant.

8093. Radicinin. [10088-95-6] [2S-[2α,3β,7(E)]]-2,3-Dihydro-3-hydroxy-2-methyl-7-(1-propenyl)-4H,5H-pyrano[4,3-b]pyran-4,5-dione; stemphylone. $C_{12}H_{12}O_5$; mol wt 236.22. C 61.01%, H 5.12%, O 33.87%. A mold metabolite from the plant pathogen *Stemphylium radicinum*: Clark, Nord, *Arch. Biochem. Biophys.* **45**, 469 (1953); **59**, 269 (1955). Structure and identity with stemphylone: Grove, *J. Chem. Soc.* **1964**, 3234. Absolute configuration: M. Nukina, S. Marumo, *Tetrahedron Lett.* **1977**, 3271. Synthesis of dl-form: Kato *et al., Chem. Commun.* **1969**, 95.

Needles from ethanol, dec 238-240°. $[\alpha]_D^{27}$ −217.4° (c = 2.37 in pyridine); $[\alpha]_D^{27}$ −175.7° (c = 0.2 in ethanol); $[\alpha]_D^{27}$ −208° (c = 1.25 in chloroform). uv max: 343, 280, 270 nm (log ε 4.27, 3.62, 3.79). Soluble in alkali. Practically insol in dil acids, sodium bicarbonate, sodium carbonate.

Monoacetate. $C_{14}H_{14}O_6$. Crystals from methanol, mp 197°. $[\alpha]_D^{27}$ −267° (c = 0.69 in pyridine).

8094. Radium. [7440-14-4] Ra; at. no. 88; valence 2. Group IIA (2). Radioactive alkaline earth metal. Occurrence in earth's crust: approx 10^{-11}% by wt. No stable nuclides. Naturally occurring isotopes: 223, *actinium X* (T½ ll.435 days, α emitter, rel. at. mass 223.0185); 224, *thorium X* (T½ 3.66 days, α emitter, rel. at. mass 224.0202); 226 (longest-lived isotope, T½ 1599 years, α emitter, rel. at. mass 226.0254); 228, *mesothorium I* (T½ 5.75 years, β⁻ emitter, rel. at. mass 228.0311). Known radioactive isotopes: 205-222, 225, 227, 229-234. ^{226}Ra is a product of disintegration of uranium and is present in all ores contg uranium. Separated in the form of a salt by P. and M. S. Curie from the pitchblende of Joachimsthal, Bohemia: Curie *et al., Compt. Rend.* **127**, 1215 (1898). Isoln of the element by electrolysis of an aq soln of radium chloride: Curie, Debierne, *ibid.* **151**, 523 (1910). Production of ^{228}Ra by disintegration of thorium (^{232}Th) discovered in 1907 by O. Hahn in monazite residues from isolating thorium. Determn in environmental and monitoring samples: W. C. Lawrie *et al., Appl. Radiat. Isot.* **53**, 133 (2000). Clinical evaluation in brachytherapy of tongue: J. Horiuchi *et al., Int. J. Radiat. Oncol. Biol. Phys.* **8**, 82 (1982); M. Hoshina *et al., Br. J. Radiol.* **62**, 59 (1989); in intracavitary radiation of uterus: D. A. Jones, R. Stout, *Clin. Radiol.* **37**, 169 (1986). Review of radiotherapy in cervical carcinoma: P. R. Reddi *et al., Obstet. Gynecol.* **43**, 238-247 (1974); in rectal carcinoma: *Dis. Colon Rectum* **29**, 600-614 (1986), reprint of C. Gordon-Watson, *Br. J. Surg.* **17**, 649-669 (1930). Comprehensive reviews: K. W. Bagnall, *Chemistry of the Rare Radioelements* (New York, Academic Press, 1957); Goodenough, Stenger, "Magnesium, Calcium, Strontium, Barium, and Radium" in *Comprehensive Inorganic Chemistry* vol. **1**, J. C. Bailar, Jr. *et al.*, Eds.

(Pergamon Press, Oxford, 1973) pp 591-664. Review of toxicology and human exposure: *Toxicological Profile for Radium* (PB 91-180414, 1990) 138 pp; of discovery and medical use: J.-J. Mazeron, A. Gerbaulet, *Radiother. Oncol.* **49**, 205-216 (1998); of industrial use: D. I. Harvie, *Endeavour* **23**, 100-105 (1999).

Brilliant, white metal; body-centered cubic structure; blackens on exposure to air. mp 700°; bp 1737°; d 5.5. One gram of radium evolves about 1000 kcal per year. Undergoes spontaneous disintegration with formation of radon. One gram of radium produces about 0.0001 ml of radon per day at normal temp and pressure. Radium is produced and used in the form of its salts: the chloride, bromide, carbonate, sulfate. Its compds closely resemble those of barium; the element itself is more volatile than barium. Radium salts impart a carmine-red color to a flame.

Bromide. [10031-23-9] Br_2Ra. White or slightly brownish crystals. d 5.79. mp 728°. Sublimes at 900°. Sol in water. The salt of commerce is usually a mixture with barium bromide.

Chloride. [10025-66-8] Cl_2Ra. White or slightly brownish crystals. d 4.91. mp 1000°. Sol in water. The salt of commerce is usually a mixture with barium chloride.

Caution: Potential symptoms of overexposure to radioactive emissions are anemia, cataracts, fractured teeth and cancer, esp. bone cancer (*Toxicological Profile*).

USE: In physical research. In radiography of metals because the penetration of gamma rays is more pronounced than that of x-rays. As source of radon. No longer used to make luminous paints.

THERAP CAT: Antineoplastic (radiation source).

8095. Radon. [10043-92-2] Rn; at. no. 86. Obsolete synonyms: *niton*, symbol Nt, and **radium emanation** or **emanation**, symbol Em. Group VIIIA (18), also known as Group 0. A noble gas characterized by an electronic structure in which the outer *p* subshell is entirely filled. No stable nuclides; naturally occurring isotope (mass number): 222 (longest-lived known isotope, T½ 3.825 days, rel. at. mass 222.0176, α-emitter, member of decay chain of ^{238}U). Known artificial radioactive isotopes: 200-221, 223-226. Isotope ^{220}Rn (T½ 55.6 sec, α-emitter, rel. at. mass 220.0114, formed in decay chain of ^{232}Th), unofficial name *Thoron*, symbol Tn, was discovered by Owens and Rutherford in 1900. ^{222}Rn was discovered by Dorn in 1900 and isolated by Rutherford and Sody in 1902. Isotope ^{219}Rn (T½ 3.96 sec, α-emitter, formed in decay chain of ^{235}U), unofficial name *actinon*, symbol An, was discovered by Debièrne and Giesel in 1902. Concentration in air: 6×10^{-14} ppm by vol; in igneous rock of the earth's crust: 1.7 × 10^{-10} ppm by wt. Prepn of fluoride: Fields *et al., J. Am. Chem. Soc.* **84**, 4164 (1962); Stein, *Science* **168**, 362 (1970). Prepn of gas from radium salt: Jennings, Russ, *Radon: Its Technique and Use* (Murray, London, 1948) pp 79-95. Reviews of chemistry and compds: *Argon, Helium and the Rare Gases*, G. A. Cook, Ed. (Interscience, New York, 1961); Haissinsky, Adloff, *Radiochemical Survey of the Elements* (Elsevier, New York, 1965) pp 126-128; Cockett, Smith, "The Monatomic Gases" in *Comprehensive Inorganic Chemistry* vol. **1**, J. C. Bailar, Jr. *et al.*, Eds. (Pergamon Press, Oxford, 1973) pp 139-211; Bartlett, Sladky, *ibid.*, pp. 213-330; S.-C. Hwang, W. R. Weltner, Jr. in *Kirk-Othmer Encyclopedia of Chemical Technology* vol. **13** (John Wiley & Sons, 4th ed., 1995) pp 1-38; G. J. Schrobilgen, J. M. Whalen, *ibid.* pp 38-53; *Chemistry of the Elements*, N. N. Greenwood, A. Earnshaw, Eds. (Pergamon Press, New York, 1984) pp 1042-1059. Reviews of sources and health effects of indoor radon exposure: E. P. Radford, *Environ. Health Perspect.* **62**, 281-287 (1985); D. L. Henshaw, *Contemp. Phys.* **34**, 31-48 (1993).

Colorless, odorless, tasteless, inert, monatomic gas; will form compds with highly electronegative elemnts such as O, F, Cl. Soly of gas in water (20°) 230 cm^3/l water. Soluble in organic solvents. Strongly adsorbed on various surfaces. Heat capacity at 25° and 1 atm: 4.9860 cal/g-atom/K. Triple point temp 202 K, press 70 kPa. Critical temp 378 K, critical press 6280 kPa. Gas: d^0 (101.3 kPa) 9.73 kg/m³. Liquid: normal bp −62°, d (normal bp) 4400 kg/m³, heat of vaporization (normal bp) 18,100 J/mol. Heat of fusion (triple point) 3247 J/mol. Solid form exists as face-centered cubic crystals at normal pressure.

Caution: Toxicity due to ionizing radiation (α-emitter). Increased incidences of lung cancer have been reported due to occupational exposure to high doses of radon, especially in hard rock miners. Max permissible concn of ^{222}Rn in air: 10^{-8} μ-Curie/cc: *Natl. Bur. Stand. Handb.* **69,** 79 (1959). The U.S. EPA has established an action level of 4 pCi/l (0.02 working levels) for home indoor radon and radon decay product measurements. *See: Interim Protocols for Screening and Follow-up Radon and Radon Decay Product Measurements* (PB89-224265, EPA-520/1-86-014-1, 1987) 22 p. Radon and its isotopic forms, ^{222}Rn and ^{220}Rn, are listed as known human carcinogens: *Report on Carcinogens, Eleventh Edition* (PB2005-104914, 2004) p III-152

USE: To initiate and influence chemical reactions, as a surface label in the study of surface reactions; in the determination of radium or thorium; in the study of the behavior of filters; in combination with Be or other light materials as a source of neutrons.

THERAP CAT: Antineoplastic (radiation source).

8096. Raffinose. [512-69-6] β-D-Fructofuranosyl-*O*-α-D-galactopyranosyl-(1 → 6)-α-glucopyranoside; gossypose; melitose; melitriose. $C_{18}H_{32}O_{16}$; mol wt 504.44. C 42.86%, H 6.39%, O 50.75%. A trisaccharide built from 1 mol each of D-galactose, D-glucose, and D-fructose which are obtained from it by acid hydrolysis. Invertase splits it into melibiose and saccharose. Occurs in Australian manna (from *Eucalyptus* spp, *Myrtaceae); in* cottonseed meal. Prepn: C. S. Hudson, T. S. Harding, *J. Am. Chem. Soc.* **36,** 2110 (1914); E. P. Clark, *ibid.* **44,** 210 (1922); Harding, *Sugar* **25,** 82 (1923); Hungerford, Nees, *Ind. Eng. Chem.* **26,** 462 (1934). Configuration: Haworth *et al., J. Chem. Soc.* **1923,** 3125; Charlton *et al.;* Haworth *et al., ibid.* **1927,** 1527, 3146. Structure: Hassid, Ballou in W. Pigman, *The Carbohydrates* (Academic Press, New York, 1957) p 517. Synthesis: Suami *et al., Carbohydr. Res.* **26,** 234 (1973). Review: E. B. Rathbone, *Dev. Food Carbohydr.* **2,** 145-185 (1980).

Pentahydrate. Crystals in clusters from dil alc. Indifferent taste. d 1.465. mp 80°. Loses water of crystn upon slow heating to 100°. The anhydrous form dec 118-119°. $[α]_D^{20}$ +105.2° (c = 4). One gram dissolves in 7 ml water (soly table: Hungerford, Nees), in 10 ml methanol. Sol in pyridine, slightly sol in alc. Does not form an osazone and does not reduce Fehling's soln.

8097. Rafoxanide. [22662-39-1] *N*-[3-Chloro-4-(4-chlorophenoxy)phenyl]-2-hydroxy-3,5-diiodobenzamide; 3′-chloro-4′-(*p*-chlorophenoxy)-3,5-diiodosalicylanilide; MK-990; Flukanide; Ranide. $C_{19}H_{11}Cl_2I_2NO_3$; mol wt 626.01. C 36.45%, H 1.77%, Cl 11.33%, I 40.54%, N 2.24%, O 7.67%. Prepn: **NL 6815783; BE 724668** (both 1969 to Merck & Co.); Mrozik *et al., Experientia* **25,** 883 (1969). Trials in sheep and cattle: Snijders, Horak, Louw, *J. S. Afr. Vet. Med. Assoc.* **43,** 397 (1972); **44,** 251 (1973); **46,** 265 (1975); Horak, Snijders, *Vet. Rec.* **94,** 12 (1974).

Crystals, mp 168-170°. Moderately sol in acetone and acetonitrile. Practically insol in water.

THERAP CAT (VET): Fasciolicide; anthelmintic.

8098. Raloxifene. [84449-90-1] [6-Hydroxy-2-(4-hydroxyphenyl)benzo[*b*]thien-3-yl][4-[2-(1-piperidinyl)ethoxy]phenyl]-methanone; keoxifene; LY-139481. $C_{28}H_{27}NO_4S$; mol wt 473.58. C 71.01%, H 5.75%, N 2.96%, O 13.51%, S 6.77%. Nonsteroidal, selective estrogen receptor modulator (SERM). Prepn: C. D. Jones, **EP 62503;** *idem,* **US 4418068** (1982, 1983 both to Lilly);

idem et al., J. Med. Chem. **27,** 1057 (1984). Review of pharmacology and toxicology: J. Buelke-Sam *et al., Reprod. Toxicol.* **12,** 217-221 (1998); of clinical pharmacology and pharmacokinetics: D. Hochner-Celnikier, *Eur. J. Obstet. Gynecol. Reprod. Biol.* **85,** 23-29 (1999); of clinical efficacy in osteoporosis: D. Agnusdei, *ibid.* 43-46. Clinical effect on risk of breast cancer: S. R. Cummings *et al., J. Am. Med. Assoc.* **281,** 2189 (1999); on reduction of fracture risk: B. Ettinger *et al., ibid.* **282,** 637 (1999).

Crystals from acetone, mp 143-147°. uv max (ethanol): 290 nm (ε 34000).

Hydrochloride. [82640-04-8] LY-156758; Evista. $C_{28}H_{27}NO_4S.HCl$; mol wt 510.04. Crystals from methanol/water, mp 258°. uv max (ethanol): 286 nm (ε 32800).

THERAP CAT: Antiosteoporotic.

8099. Raltitrexed. [112887-68-0] *N*-[[5-[[(1,4-Dihydro-2-methyl-4-oxo-6-quinazolinyl)methyl]methylamino]-2-thienyl]carbonyl]-L-glutamic acid; *N*-(5-[*N*-(3,4-dihydro-2-methyl-4-oxoquinazolin-6-ylmethyl)-*N*-methylamino]-2-thenoyl)-L-glutamic acid; ICI-D-1694; ZD-1694; Tomudex. $C_{21}H_{22}N_4O_6S$; mol wt 458.49. C 55.01%, H 4.84%, N 12.22%, O 20.94%, S 6.99%. Folate-based inhibitor of thymidylate synthase; rapidly and extensively metabolized to its more potent polyglutamate derivatives. Prepn: L. R. Hughes, **EP 239362** (1987 to ICI; Natl. Res. Dev.); *idem,* **US 4992550** (1991 to ICI); P. R. Marsham *et al., J. Med. Chem.* **34,** 1594 (1991). Pharmacokinetics: D. I. Jodrell *et al., Cancer Chemother. Pharmacol.* **28,** 331 (1991). HPLC determn of metabolites in cultured cells: W. Gibson *et al., Biochem. Pharmacol.* **45,** 863 (1993). Review of clinical toxicology: S. J. Clarke *et al., Adv. Exp. Med. Biol.* **338,** 601-604 (1993); of mechanism of action: A. L. Jackman *et al., ibid.* **339,** 265-276. Historical development, pharmacology, and clinical evaluation: S. J. Clarke *et al., ibid.* 277-287; A. L. Jackman *et al., Eur. J. Cancer* **31A,** 1277-1282 (1995).

Pale yellow powder. Sol in water.
Monohydrate. $C_{21}H_{22}N_4O_6S.H_2O$. mp 180-184°.
THERAP CAT: Antineoplastic.

8100. Ramatroban. [116649-85-5] (3*R*)-3-[[(4-Fluorophenyl)sulfonyl]amino]-1,2,3,4-tetrahydro-9*H*-carbazole-9-propanoic acid; (+)-(3*R*)-3-(*p*-fluorobenzenesulfonamido)-1,2,3,4-tetrahydrocarbazole-9-propionic acid; (+)-3-(4-fluorophenylsulfonamido)-9-(2-carboxyethyl)-1,2,3,4-tetrahydrocarbazole; Bay u 3405; Baynas. $C_{21}H_{21}FN_2O_4S$; mol wt 416.47. C 60.56%, H 5.08%, F 4.56%, N 6.73%, O 15.37%, S 7.70%. Thromboxane A_2 receptor antagonist. Prepn: H. Böshagen *et al.,* **DE 3631824;** *eidem,* **US 4965258** (1988, 1990 both to Bayer); and absolute configuration: U. Rosentreter *et al., Arzneim.-Forsch.* **39,** 1519 (1989). Series of articles on pharmacology: *ibid.* 1522-1530. Clinical evaluation in asthma: H. Aizawa *et al., Chest* **109,** 338 (1996).

Crystals from ether, mp 134-135°. $[\alpha]_D$ +70.1° (c = 1.0 in methanol).

THERAP CAT: Antiasthmatic; antiallergic.

8101. Ramelteon. [196597-26-9] N-[2-[(8S)-1,6,7,8-Tetra-hydro-2H-indeno[5,4-b]furan-8-yl]ethyl]propanamide; TAK-375; Rozerem. $C_{16}H_{21}NO_2$; mol wt 259.34. C 74.10%, H 8.16%, N 5.40%, O 12.34%. Melatonin MT_1/MT_2 receptor agonist. Prepn: S. Ohkawa et al., **WO 9732871**; eidem **US 6034239** (1997, 2000 both to Takeda); O. Uchikawa et al., J. Med. Chem. **45**, 4222 (2002). Pharmacology: N. Yukuhiro et al., Brain Res. **1027**, 59 (2004). Receptor binding study: K. Kato et al., Neuropharmacology **48**, 301 (2005). Reviews of development and therapeutic potential: C. Cajochen, Curr. Opin. Invest. Drugs **6**, 114-121 (2005); N. N. Nguyen et al., Formulary **40**, 146-155 (2005).

Crystals from ethyl acetate, mp 113-115°. $[\alpha]_D^{20}$ −57.8° (c = 1.004 in chloroform).

THERAP CAT: Sedative, hypnotic.

8102. Ramifenazone. [3615-24-5] 1,2-Dihydro-1,5-di-methyl-4-[(1-methylethyl)amino]-2-phenyl-3H-pyrazol-3-one; 4-isopropylamino-2,3-dimethyl-1-phenyl-3-pyrazolin-5-one; 4-iso-propylaminoantipyrine; isopropylaminophenazone; isopyrin. $C_{14}H_{19}N_3O$; mol wt 245.32. C 68.54%, H 7.81%, N 17.13%, O 6.52%. Prepn: E. Skita, W. Stühmer, **DE 930328**; **DE 932677** (both 1955), C.A. **52**, 16372i, 20200h (1958). Acute toxicity: E. Tubaro et al., Arzneim.-Forsch. **20**, 1024 (1970). Clinical evaluation of combination with phenylbutazone, q.v., in migraine: W. Sacks, S. Afr. Med. J. **58**, 444 (1980).

Crystals from acetone + glacial acetic acid, mp 80°. LD_{50} in mice (mg/kg): 843 i.p.; 1070 orally (Tubaro).

Hydrochloride monohydrate. $C_{14}H_{19}N_3O\cdot HCl\cdot H_2O$.

Mixture with phenylbutazone. [76120-72-4] Tomanol.

THERAP CAT: Analgesic, antipyretic, anti-inflammatory.

8103. Ramipril. [87333-19-5] [2S,3aS,6aS]-1-[(2S)-2-[[(1S)-1-(Ethoxycarbonyl)-3-phenylpropyl]amino]-1-oxopropyl]-octahydrocyclopenta[b]pyrrole-2-carboxylic acid; N-(1S-carboeth-oxy-3-phenylpropyl)-S-alanyl-cis,endo-2-azabicyclo[3.3.0]octane-3S-carboxylic acid; (2S,3aS,6aS)-1-[(S)-N-[(S)-1-carboxy-3-phenyl-propyl]alanyl]octahydrocyclopenta[b]pyrrole-2-carboxylic acid 1-ethyl ester; HOE-498; Altace; Cardace; Delix; Pramace; Quark; Ramace; Triatec; Tritace; Unipril; Vesdil. $C_{23}H_{32}N_2O_5$; mol wt 416.51. C 66.32%, H 7.74%, N 6.73%, O 19.21%. Angiotensin converting enzyme (ACE) inhibitor; converted to active, diacid metabolite, *ramiprilat*. Prepn: V. Teetz et al., **EP 79022** (1983 to Hoechst A.G.), C.A. **100**, 52012h (1984); E. H. Gold et al., **US 4587258** (1986 to Schering Corp.); V. Teetz et al., Arzneim.-Forsch. **34**, 1399 (1984). Radioimmunoassay determn in human serum and plasma: H. G. Eckert et al., ibid. **35**, 1251 (1985). Toxicology: H. H. Donaubauer, D. Mayer, ibid. **38**, 14 (1988). Symposium on pharmacology and clinical efficacy: Am. J. Cardiol. **59**, 1D-177D (1987). Clinical trial in chronic nephropathy: P. Ruggenenti et al., Lancet **352**, 1252 (1998). Clinical prevention of cardiovascular events in high-risk patients: HOPE Study Investigators, N. Engl.

J. Med. **342**, 145 (2000). Clinical trial in prevention of stroke: J. Bosch et al., Br. Med. J. **324**, 1 (2002).

Felty needles from ether, mp 109°. $[\alpha]_D^{24}$ +33.2° (c = 1 in 0.1N ethanolic HCl). LD_{50} (14 day) in male, female mice, male, female rats (mg/kg): 1194, 1158, 687, 608 i.v.; 10933, 10048, >10000, >10000 orally (Donaubauer, Mayer).

THERAP CAT: Antihypertensive.

8104. Ramoplanin. [76168-82-6] A-16686; MDL-62198; Glycolipodepsipeptide antibiotic complex consisting of 6 related components (A_1, A_2, A_3, A'_1, A'_2, A'_3) of which A_2 is the most abundant. Isoln and inital characterization from Actinoplanes sp.: B. Cavalleri et al., **DE 3013246**; eidem, **US 4303646** (1980, 1981 both to Gruppo Lepetit); idem et al., J. Antibiot. **37**, 309 (1984). Bactericidal activity: R. Pallanza et al., ibid. 318. Structure elu-cidation: R. Ciabatti et al., ibid. **42**, 254 (1989); and sequence determn: J. K. Kettenring et al., ibid. 268. 3D structure: M. Kurz, W. Guba, Biochemistry **35**, 12570 (1996). Isoln and characteriza-tion of the A' factors: L. Gastaldo et al., J. Indus. Microbiol. **11**, 13 (1992). Determn in sera: M. T. Kenny et al., Diagn. Microbiol. Infect. Dis. **18**, 117 (1994). Clinical evaluation against vancomycin resistant enterococci (VRE): M. T. Wong et al., Clin. Infect. Dis. **33**, 1476 (2001). Review of discovery and chemistry: F. Parenti et al., Drugs Exp. Clin. Res. **16**, 451-455 (1990); of chemistry and mechanism of action: S. Walker et al., Chem. Rev. **105**, 449-475 (2005); of pharmacology and clinical potential: D. K. Farver et al., Ann. Pharmacother. **39**, 863-868 (2005).

Ramoplanin A_2

White powder, slightly hygroscopic. mp 210-230°. $[\alpha]_D^{20}$ +78.3° (c = 1.04 in H_2O). Sol in DMF and lower alcohols. Insol in ethyl ether, petroleum ether and benzene. LD_{50} in mice (mg/kg): 328 i.p., 122 i.v.; orally in rats: 2000 mg/kg (Pallanza).

Ramoplanin A_2. [81988-88-7] $C_{119}H_{154}ClN_{21}O_{40}$; mol wt 2554.07. C 55.96%, H 6.08%, Cl 1.39%, N 11.52%, O 25.06%. Total synthesis: W. Jiang et al., J. Am. Chem. Soc. **124**, 5288 (2002); eidem, ibid. **125**, 1877 (2003). White powder, mp 210-220°. $[\alpha]_D^{20}$ +73±4° (c = 0.49 in H_2O). uv max in methanol: 234, 268 nm ($E_{1cm}^{1\%}$ 206, 114).

THERAP CAT: Antibacterial.

8105. Ramosetron. [132036-88-5] (1-Methyl-1H-indol-3-yl)[(5R)-4,5,6,7-tetrahydro-1H-benzimidazol-5-yl]methanone; (R)-5-[(1-methylindol-3-yl)carbonyl]-4,5,6,7-tetrahydrobenzimidazole; Nor-YM-060. $C_{17}H_{17}N_3O$; mol wt 279.34. C 73.09%, H 6.13%,

N 15.04%, O 5.73%. Selective serotonin 5HT$_3$ receptor antagonist; structurally different from ondansetron, granisetron, q.q.v. Prepn: M. Ohta et al., **EP 381422**; eidem, **US 5344927** (1990, 1994 both to Yamanouchi). Pharmacology: K. Miyata et al., J. Pharmacol. Exp. Ther. **259**, 15 (1991). Effects on gastric emptying in rodents: K. Miyata et al., Jpn. J. Pharmacol. **69**, 205 (1995). Toxicity evaluation: H. Tabata et al., Arzneim.-Forsch. **45**, 760 (1995). HPLC determn in plasma and urine: H. Miura et al., Biomed. Chromatogr. **8**, 103 (1994). Clinical prevention of postoperative nausea and vomiting: Y. Fujii et al., Anesth. Analg. **90**, 472 (2000).

Foam. $[\alpha]_D^{20}$ − 16.5° (c 1.13 in methanol).

Hydrochloride. [132907-72-3] YM-060; Nasea. C$_{17}$H$_{17}$N$_3$·O.HCl; mol wt 315.80. Slightly yellowish-white, odorless crystalline powder. Easily sol in water (Tabata). Also as crystals from ethanol, mp 215-230°. $[\alpha]_D$ −42.9° (c 1.02 in methanol).

THERAP CAT: Antiemetic.

8106. Ranelic Acid. [135459-90-4] 5-[Bis(carboxymethyl)-amino]-2-carboxy-4-cyano-3-thiopheneacetic acid; 2-[N,N-di(carboxymethyl)amino]-3-cyano-4-carboxymethylthiophene-5-carboxylic acid. C$_{12}$H$_{10}$N$_2$O$_8$S; mol wt 342.28. C 42.11%, H 2.94%, N 8.18%, O 37.39%, S 9.37%. Prepn: M. Wierzbicki et al., **EP 415850**; eidem, **US 5128367** (1991, 1992 both to Adir & Co.).

Crystals from ethyl ether, contains 4% ether.

Strontium salt. [135459-87-9] Strontium ranelate; S-12911; Osseor; Protelos; Protos. C$_{12}$H$_6$N$_2$O$_8$SSr$_2$; mol wt 513.49. Bone metabolism modulator; inhibits bone resorption while maintaining bone formation. Effect on human chondrocytes in vitro: Y. Henrotin et al., J. Bone Miner. Res. **16**, 299 (2001). Effect on bone remodeling in monkeys: J. Buehler et al., Bone **29**, 176 (2001). Clinical trial in postmenopausal osteoporosis: P. J. Meunier et al., N. Engl. J. Med. **350**, 459 (2004).

THERAP CAT: Strontium salt as antiosteoporotic.

8107. Raney® Nickel. [7440-02-0] Raney nickel catalyst. Prepd by fusing 50 parts nickel with 50 parts aluminum: Raney, **US 1628190** (1927); **US 1915473** (1933); pulverizing the alloy and dissolving out most of the aluminum with NaOH soln: Covert, Adkins, J. Am. Chem. Soc. **54**, 4116 (1932); Ruggli, Preiswerk, Helv. Chim. Acta **22**, 494 (1939); Mozingo, Org. Synth. **21**, 15 (1941). Absorption studies: Kokes, Emmett, J. Am. Chem. Soc. **83**, 29 (1961). The residual aluminum, which amounts to several percent, appears to be necessary for proper catalytic activity. Review: J. S. Pizey, Synthetic Reagents vol. 2 (John Wiley, New York, 1974) pp 175-311.

Grayish-black powder or cubic crystals. Ignites on contact with air. Contains hydrogen and has been attributed the formula Ni$_2$H. Generally stored under alcohol, although ether, water, methylcyclohexane, and dioxane may be used. Raney nickel loses its hydrogen slowly on storage and becomes inactive. Properly prepd and stored it should remain active for 6 months.

USE: Catalyst for the hydrogenation of organic compds with gaseous hydrogen. Usually from 1 to 10% of the substance to be reduced is employed. Is active at room temp and 1 atm pressure, but is also used at high temps and high pressures, see H. B. Adkins, Reactions of Hydrogen (Madison, 1937).

8108. Ranibizumab. [347396-82-1] Anti-(human vascular endothelial growth factor) immunoglobulin G1 Fab fragment (hu-

man-mouse monoclonal rhuFAB V2 γ$_1$-chain) disulfide with human-mouse monoclonal rhuFAB V2 light chain; rhuFabV2; Lucentis. Recombinant humanized monoclonal antibody fragment directed against VEGF; approx 48 kDa. Exhibits antiangiogenic activity. Prepn: M. Baca et al., **WO 9845331**; eidem, **US 6884879** (1998, 2005 both to Genentech). Intraocular biodistribution study: J. Mordenti et al., Toxicol. Pathol. **27**, 536 (1999). In vivo efficacy vs choroid neovascularization: M. G. Krzystolik et al., Arch. Ophthalmol. **120**, 338 (2002); in combination with verteporfin: D Husain et al., ibid. **123**, 509 (2005). Pharmacokinetics: J. Gaudreault et al., Invest. Ophthalmol. Visual Sci. **46**, 726 (2005). Clinical evaluation: J. S. Heier et al., Ophthalmology **113**, 633 (2006).

THERAP CAT: Treatment of age-related macular degeneration.

8109. Ranimustine. [58994-96-0] Methyl 6-[[[(2-chloroethyl)nitrosoamino]carbonyl]amino]-6-deoxy-α-D-glucopyranoside; methyl N-carbamyl-N′-(2-chloroethyl)-N′-nitroso-6-amino-6-deoxy-α-D-glucopyranoside; 6-[3-(2-chloroethyl)-3-nitrosoureido]-6-deoxy-α-D-glucopyranoside; 3-(methyl-α-D-glucopyranos-6-yl)-1-(2-chloroethyl)-1-nitrosourea; ranomustine; MCNU; NSC-0270516; Cymerin; Thymerin. C$_{10}$H$_{18}$ClN$_3$O$_7$; mol wt 327.72. C 36.65%, H 5.54%, Cl 10.82%, N 12.82%, O 34.17%. Chloroethylnitrosourea derivative with antitumor activity. Similar to carmustine, chlorozotocin, lomustine, nimustine, q.q.v. Prepn: **NL 7507973**; G. Kimura, J. Sekine, **US 4057684**; **NL 7800920**; G. Kimura, **US 4156777** (1976, 1977, 1978, 1979, all to Tokyo Tanabe). Antitumor activity in rodents, comparison with other nitrosoureas: S. Sekido et al., Cancer Treat. Rep. **63**, 961 (1979); S. Fujimoto, M. Ogawa, Cancer Chemother. Pharmacol. **9**, 134 (1982); S. Fujimoto et al., Gann **75**, 937 (1984). Mechanism of action: R. Kanamaru et al., Curr. Chemother. Immunother. **2**, 1377 (1982). Effect of sugar alcohols on toxicity in mice: T. Tashiro et al., Cancer Chemother. Pharmacol. **8**, 183 (1982). Series of articles on metabolic fate in rats: Y. Esumi et al., Iyakuhin Kenkyu **16**, 381-428 (1985), C.A. **103**, 115620q, 115621r, 134369f (1985). Clinical study in hematological malignant diseases: T. Masaoka et al., Chemotherapy (Tokyo) **33**, 271 (1985).

Pale yellowish needles from anhydrous ethanol-ethyl ether (1:1), mp 111-112°. $[\alpha]_D^{20}$ +93.2° (c = 0.5 in methanol) (Kimura). Also reported as 101-103° (dec) from isopropanol. $[\alpha]_D^{25}$ +73.2° (c = 0.3 in methanol) (Kimura, Sekine). Solubility in water: 900 mg/ml at 25°. LD$_{50}$ in male rats (mg/kg): 42 i.p., 42 i.v., 50 orally (Kimura).

THERAP CAT: Antineoplastic.

8110. Ranitidine. [66357-35-5] N-[2-[[[5-[(Dimethylamino)methyl]-2-furanyl]methyl]thio]ethyl]-N′-methyl-2-nitro-1,1-ethenediamine. C$_{13}$H$_{22}$N$_4$O$_3$S; mol wt 314.40. C 49.66%, H 7.05%, N 17.82%, O 15.27%, S 10.20%. Histamine H$_2$-receptor antagonist which inhibits gastric acid secretion. Prepn: B. J. Price et al., **FR 2384765**; eidem, **US 4128658** (both 1978 to Allen & Hanburys). HPLC determn in plasma: P. F. Carey, L. E. Martin, J. Liq. Chromatogr. **1979**, 1291. Pharmacological studies: J. Bradshaw et al., Br. J. Pharmacol. **66**, 464 (1979); M. J. Daly et al., Gut **21**, 408 (1980). Efficacy in treatment of duodenal ulcers: A. Berstad et al., Scand. J. Gastroenterol. **15**, 637 (1980); R. P. Walt et al., Gut **22**, 49 (1981). Review of pharmacology and therapeutic use: R. N. Brogden et al., Drugs **24**, 267-303 (1982). Comprehensive description: M. Hohnjec et al., Anal. Profiles Drug Subs. **15**, 533-561 (1986).

Solid, mp 69-70°.

Hydrochloride. [66357-59-3] AH-19065; Azantac; Melfax; Noctone; Raniben; Ranidil; Raniplex; Sostril; Taural; Terposen; Trigger; Ulcex; Ultidine; Zantac; Zantic. $C_{13}H_{22}N_4O_3S.HCl$; mol wt 350.86. Off-white solid, mp 133-134°. Freely sol in acetic acid and water, sol in methanol, sparingly sol in ethanol. Practically insol in chloroform.

Bismuth citrate. [128345-62-0] Ranitidine bismutrex; GR-122311X; Pylorid; Tritec. $C_{13}H_{22}N_4O_3S.C_6H_5BiO_7$; mol wt 712.48. Pharmacology and activity vs *Helicobacter* sp: R. Stables *et al., Aliment. Pharmacol. Ther.* **7**, 237 (1993).

THERAP CAT: Antiulcerative.

8111. Ranolazine. [95635-55-5] *N*-(2,6-Dimethylphenyl)-4-[2-hydroxy-3-(2-methoxyphenoxy)propyl]-1-piperazineacetamide; (±)-4-[2-hydroxy-3-(*o*-methoxyphenoxy)propyl]-1-piperazineaceto-2′,6′-xylidide; (±)-1-[3-(2-methoxyphenoxy)-2-hydroxypropyl]-4-[*N*-(2,6-dimethylphenyl)carbamoylmethyl]piperazine; Ranexa. $C_{24}H_{33}N_3O_4$; mol wt 427.54. C 67.42%, H 7.78%, N 9.83%, O 14.97%. Anti-ischemic agent which modulates myocardial metabolism. Prepn: A. F. Kluge *et al., EP 126449; eidem, US 4567264* (1984, 1986 both to Syntex). HPLC resolution of enantiomers: E. Delée *et al., Chromatographia* **24**, 357 (1987). Clinical trial in angina: B. R. Chaitman *et al., J. Am. Coll. Cardiol.* **43**, 1375 (2004). Review of pharmacology and clinical development: J. G. McCormack *et al., Gen. Pharmacol.* **30**, 639-645 (1998); R. S. Schofield, J. A. Hill, *Expert Opin. Invest. Drugs* **11**, 117-123 (2002).

Dihydrochloride. [95635-56-6] RS-43285. $C_{24}H_{33}N_3O_4$.-2HCl; mol wt 500.46. White crystalline powder from methanol/-ether, mp 164-166°. Readily sol in water.

THERAP CAT: Antianginal.

8112. Ranpirnase. [133737-96-9] Ribonuclease (*Rana pipiens* reduced); P-30 protein; Onconase. Antitumor ribonuclease isolated from oocytes and early embryos of *Rana pipiens*. Single chain protein containing 104 amino acid residues; mol wt ~12 kDa. Description of cytotoxic activity: Z. Darzynkiewicz *et al., Cell Tissue Kinet.* **21**, 169 (1988). Amino acid sequence and identification as a ribonuclease: W. Ardelt *et al., J. Biol. Chem.* **266**, 245 (1991). Crystallization: S. C. Mosimann *et al., Proteins: Struct. Funct. Genet.* **14**, 392 (1992). Mechanism of action: Y. Wu *et al., J. Biol. Chem.* **268**, 10686 (1993). Prepn by recombinant technology: E. Notomista *et al., FEBS Lett.* **463**, 211 (1999). Clinical trial in malignant mesothelioma: S. M. Mikulski *et al., J. Clin. Oncol.* **20**, 274 (2002).

THERAP CAT: Antineoplastic.

8113. Rapacuronium Bromide. [156137-99-4] 1-[(2β,3α,-5α,16β,17β)-3-(Acetyloxy)-17-(1-oxopropoxy)-2-(1-piperidinyl)-androstan-16-yl]-1-(2-propenyl)piperidinium bromide; 1-allyl-2-(3α,17β-dihydroxy-2β-piperidino-5α-androstan-16β-yl)piperidinium bromide 3-acetate 17-propionate; Org-9487; Raplon. $C_{37}H_{61}$-N_2O_4.Br; mol wt 677.80. C 65.56%, H 9.07%, N 4.13%, O 9.44%, Br 11.79%. Aminosteroid, competitive neuromuscular blocker. Prepn: T. Sleigh *et al., CA 2094457; eidem, US 5418226* (both to Akzo). Clinical pharmacodynamics: P. M. C. Wright *et al., Anesthesiology* **90**, 16 (1999). Clinical trial in pediatric patients: R. F. Kaplan *et al., Anesth. Analg.* **89**, 1172 (1999). Review of pharmacology and use in endotracheal intubation: S. V. Onrust, R. H. Foster, *Drugs* **58**, 887-918 (1999).

Crystals from diethyl ether-acetone, mp 184°. $[\alpha]_D^{20}$ -12.7° (c = 1.01 in $CHCl_3$).

THERAP CAT: Neuromuscular blocking agent.

8114. Rapamycin. [53123-88-9] Sirolimus; RAPA; RPM; AY-22989; NSC-226080; Rapamune. $C_{51}H_{79}NO_{13}$; mol wt 914.17. C 67.01%, H 8.71%, N 1.53%, O 22.75%. Triene macrolide antibiotic isolated from *Streptomyces hygroscopicus*. Name derived from the native word for Easter Island, Rapa Nui. Isoln: S. N. Sehgal *et al., DE 2347682; eidem, US 3929992* (1974, 1975 both to Ayerst McKenna Harrison); purification and characterization: C. Vézina *et al., J. Antibiot.* **28**, 721 (1975); S. N. Sehgal *et al., ibid.* 727. Inhibition of immune response: R. R. Martel *et al., Can. J. Physiol. Pharmacol.* **55**, 48 (1977); of graft rejection in mice: C. P. Eng *et al., Transplant. Proc.* **23**, 868 (1991). Total synthesis: K. C. Nicolaou *et al., J. Am. Chem. Soc.* **115**, 4419 (1993); D. Romo *et al., ibid.* 7906. Series of articles on therapeutic monitoring and pharmacokinetics: *Clin. Ther.* **22**, Suppl. 2, B1-B132 (2000); on pharmacology and clinical experience in transplantation: *Transplant. Proc.* **35**, Suppl. 1, S1-S233 (2003). Clinical trial in prevention of coronary restenosis: D. R. Holmes, Jr. *et al., Circulation* **109**, 634 (2004).

Colorless crystalline solid from ether, mp 183-185°. uv max (95% ethanol): 267, 277, 288 nm ($E_{1cm}^{1\%}$ 417, 541, 416). $[\alpha]_D^{25}$ -58.2° (methanol). Sol in ether, chloroform, acetone, methanol and DMF; very sparingly sol in hexane and petr ether. Substantially insol in water. LD_{50} in mice (mg/kg): ≈600 i.p.; >2,500 orally (Vézina).

USE: Tool for immunochemistry.

THERAP CAT: Immunosuppressant; antirestenotic.

8115. Rapeseed Oil. Colza oil. Oil expressed from seeds of *Brassica campestris* L., *Cruciferae*. Pale yellow, rather viscid liq. d 0.913-0.917; n_D^{20} 1.4720-1.4752. Solidif -2° to -10°. Sapon no. 170-177. Iodine no. 97-105. Sol in chloroform, ether, CS_2.

USE: Lubricant; manuf rubber substitutes, margarine, soft soaps, blown oils; oiling woolens.

8116. Rasagiline. [136236-51-6] (1*R*)-2,3-Dihydro-*N*-2-propynl-1*H*-inden-1-amine; (*R*)-*N*-2-propynyl-1-indanamine; *N*-propargyl-1-(*R*)-aminoindan; AGN-1135. $C_{12}H_{13}N$; mol wt 171.24. C 84.17%, H 7.65%, N 8.18%. Irreversible MAO-B inhibitor. Prepn: M. B. H. Youdim *et al., EP* **436492**; *eidem.* US **5457133** (1991, 1995 both to Teva). Pharmacology: J. P. M. Finberg, M. B. H. Youdim, *Neuropharmacology* **43**, 1110 (2002); of metabolites: S. Glezer, J. P. M. Finberg, *Eur. J. Pharmacol.* **472**, 173 (2003). Mechanism of action: M. B. H. Youdim *et al., Biochem. Pharmacol.* **66**, 1635 (2003). Double-blind clinical trial as adjunctive therapy to levodopa: J. M. Rabey *et al., Clin. Neuropharmacol.* **23**, 324 (2000); multicenter trial in early Parkinson's disease: *Arch. Neurol.* **59**, 1937 (2002); in levodopa-treated Parkinson's patients: Parkinson Study Group, *ibid.* **62**, 241 (2005); O. Rascol *et al., Lancet* **365**, 947 (2005). Review of pharmacology: J. Chen, D. M. Swope, *J. Clin. Pharmacol.* **45**, 878-894 (2005); of clinical development: O. Rascol, *Expert Opin. Pharmacother.* **6**, 2061-2075 (2005); F. Stocchi, *Int. J. Clin. Pract.* **60**, 215-221 (2006).

Methanesulfonate. [161735-79-1] Rasagiline mesylate; TVP-1012; Agilect; Azilect. $C_{12}H_{13}N.CH_3SO_3H$; mol wt 267.34.

THERAP CAT: Antiparkinsonian.

8117. Rasburicase. [134774-45-1] Urate oxidase (*Aspergillus flavus* clone 9C/9A reduced); SR-29142; Elitek; Fasturtec. Recombinant form of fungal urate oxidase expressed in *Saccharomycese cerevisiae*; converts uric acid into the more soluble compound, allantoin, which is readily excreted by the kidneys. The natural enzyme is endogenous in most mammals but is absent in higher primates where uric acid is the end-product of purine metabolism. Prepn: D. Caput *et al., EP* **408461**; *eidem*, US **5382518** (1991, 1995 both to Sanofi); P. Leplatois *et al., Gene* **122**, 139 (1992). Comparison with natural enzyme: A. Bayol *et al., Biotechnol. Appl. Biochem.* **36**, 21 (2002). Radioimmunoassay in plasma: D. Dussossoy *et al., J. Pharm. Sci.* **85**, 955 (1996). Clinical pharmacokinetics in cancer patients: C.-H. Pui *et al., J. Clin. Oncol.* **19**, 697 (2001). Clinical comparison with allopurinol in pediatric hyperuricemia: S. C. Goldman *et al., Blood* **97**, 2998 (2001). *Review:* C.-H. Pui, *Expert Opin. Pharmacother.* **3**, 433-452 (2002); V. Oldfield, C. M. Perry, *Drugs* **66**, 529-545 (2006).

THERAP CAT: In treatment of malignancy associated hyperuricemia.

8118. Raspberry. Red raspberry. Deciduous, woody bush, *Rubus idaeus* L., *Rosaceae*, bearing edible fruit. The leaf has been used medicinally for diarrhea, nausea, vomiting and to prepare the uterus for childbirth. *Habit.* Europe, Asia, cultivated in Canada and U.S. *Constit.* Anthocyanins, ellagitannins, terpenoids, flavonoids, sugar, malic and citric acids. HPLC determn of antioxidants in fruit: J. Beekwilder *et al., J. Agric. Food Chem.* **53**, 3313 (2005). Clinical trial of raspberry leaf in pregnancy: M. Simpson *et al., J. Midwifery Women's Health* **46**, 51 (2001). Review of therapeutic constituents: A. V. Patel *et al., Curr. Med. Chem.* **11**, 1501-1512 (2004); of pharmacology and medicinal uses: J. Barnes *et al., Herbal Medicines* (Pharmaceutical Press, London, 2nd Ed., 2002) pp 397-398; J. Gruenwald *et al., PDR for Herbal Medicines* (Medical Economics, Montvale, 3rd Ed., 2004) pp 675-676.

USE: Fruit in jams, desserts, sauces, beverages. Pharmaceutic aid (flavor).

THERAP CAT: Astringent.

8119. Raubasine. [483-04-5] (19α)-16,17-Didehydro-19-methyloxayohimban-16-carboxylic acid methyl ester; δ-yohimbine; pytetrahydroserpentine; tetrahydroserpentine; ajmalicine; Circolene; Hydrosarpan; Isoarteril; Lamuran. $C_{21}H_{24}N_2O_3$; mol wt 352.43. C 71.57%, H 6.86%, N 7.95% O 13.62%. α₁-Adrenergic blocker isolated from bark of *Corynanthe johimbe* K. Schum., *Ru-*

biaceae: H. Heinemann, *Ber.* **67**, 15 (1934); from roots of *Rauwolfia serpentina* (L.) Benth., *Apocynaceae:* S. Siddiqui, R. H. Siddiqui, *J. Indian Chem. Soc.* **8**, 667 (1931); A. H. Popelak *et al., Naturwissenschaften* **40**, 625 (1953); A. Hofmann, *Helv. Chim. Acta* **37**, 849 (1954); M. W. Klohs *et al., J. Am. Chem. Soc.* **76**, 1332 (1954). Review of early literature: R. E. Woodson *et al., Rauwolfia: Botany, Pharmacognosy, Chemistry and Pharmacology* (Little, Brown and Co., Boston, 1957) 147 pp. Structure: Goutarel, Le Hir, *Bull. Soc. Chim. Fr.* **18**, 909 (1951). Stereochemistry: Wenkert *et al., J. Am. Chem. Soc.* **83**, 5037 (1961); Shamma, Richey, *ibid.* **85**, 2507 (1963). Total synthesis of *dl*-form: van Tamelen, Placeway, *ibid.* **83**, 2594 (1961); van Tamelen *et al., ibid.* **91**, 7359 (1969); J. Gutzwiller *et al., Helv. Chim. Acta* **64**, 1663 (1981); T. Kametani *et al., J. Chem. Soc. Perkin Trans. 1* **1981**, 3168. Biosynthesis: N. Nagakura *et al., ibid.* **1979**, 2308; M. Rueffer *et al., Chem. Commun.* **1979**, 1016. Pharmacokinetics: A. Marzo *et al., Farmaco Ed. Prat.* **36**, 173 (1981). Clinical evaluation of platelet anti-aggregant activity: J. Neuman *et al., Arzneim.-Forsch.* **36**, 1394 (1986). Evaluation of combination with almitrine, *q.v.*, in cerebral ischemia in rats: M. G. Borzeix, J. Cahn, *ibid.* **37**, 491 (1987).

Prisms from methanol, dec 257°. $[\alpha]_D^{20}$ −60° (c = 0.5 in chloroform); $[\alpha]_D^{20}$ −45° (c = 0.5 in pyridine); $[\alpha]_D^{20}$ −39° (c = 0.25 in methanol). uv max (methanol): 227, 292 nm (log ε 4.61, 3.79).

Hydrochloride. $C_{21}H_{24}N_2O_3.HCl$. Leaflets from ethanol, mp 290° (dec). $[\alpha]_D^{20}$ −17° (c = 0.5 in methanol). Sparingly sol in water or dil HCl.

Hydrobromide. $C_{21}H_{24}N_2O_3.HBr$. Diamond-shaped platelets from methanol, mp 295-296°.

THERAP CAT: Antihypertensive, anti-ischemic (cerebral and peripheral).

8120. Rauwolfia serpentina. Hiwolfia; Koglucoid; Raudixin; Rauserpol; Rauverid; Rauwoldin; Rauwolfemms; Serfolia; Serpina; Wolfina. Powdered, dried root of *Rauwolfia serpentina* (L.) Benth. *Apocynaceae*, a small shrub native to the Orient from India to Sumatra. Contains many indole alkaloids of which reserpine, rescinnamine and deserpidine are the primary constituents. Others include: reserpiline, yohimbine, ajmaline, serpentine, serpetinine. Review and bibliography: Monachino, *Econ. Bot.* **8**, 349-365 (1954). Clinical trial in hypertension: M. C. Srivastava *et al., Indian Pract.* **20**, 279 (1967); in combination with chlorothiazide: W. M. Smith, *Circ. Res.* **40**, Suppl I, I98 (1977). LC determn of reserpine-rescinnamine content: U. R. Cieri, *J. Assoc. Off. Anal. Chem.* **70**, 540 (1987).

Alseroxylon. [8001-95-4] Austrawolf; Egalin; Gendon; Rautensin; Rauwiloid; Ra-Valeas; Rivadescin. Alkaloidal extract of the dried root. Red, amorphous powder with characteristic odor. Contains 0.15-0.2% reserpine-rescinnamine alkaloids.

THERAP CAT: Antihypertensive.

8121. Ravuconazole. [182760-06-1] 4-[2-[(1*R*,2*R*)-2-(2,4-Difluorophenyl)-2-hydroxy-1-methyl-3-(1*H*-1,2,4-triazol-1-yl)propyl]-4-thiazolyl]benzonitrile; (2*R*,3*R*)-3-[4-(4-cyanophenyl)thiazol-2-yl]-2-(2,4-difluorophenyl)-1-(1*H*-1,2,4-triazol-1-yl)-2-butanol; BMS-207147; ER-30346. $C_{22}H_{17}F_2N_5OS$; mol wt 437.47. C 60.40%, H 3.92%, F 8.69%, N 16.01%, O 3.66%, S 7.33%. Ergosterol biosynthesis inhibitor. Prepn (stereochemistry unspecified): T. Naito *et al, EP* **667346**; *eidem,* US **5648372** (1995, 1997 both to Eisai); of optically acitve form: A. Tsuruoka *et al., Chem. Pharm. Bull.* **46**, 623 (1998). Chiral synthesis: Y. Kaku *et al., ibid.* 1125. *In vitro* comparative antifungal spectrum: J. C. Fung-Tomc *et al., Antimicrob. Agents Chemother.* **42**, 313 1998. Antifungal activity in candidosis: K. V. Clemons, D. A. Stevens, *ibid.* **45**, 3433 (2001);

in aspergillosis: W. R. Kirkpatrick *et al., J. Antimicrob. Chemother.* **49**, 353 (2002). Clinical evaluation in onychomycosis: A. K. Gupta *et al., J. Eur. Acad. Dermatol. Venereol.* **19**, 437 (2005). Review of development and therapeutic potential: S. Arikan, J. H. Rex, *Curr. Opin. Invest. Drugs* **3**, 555-561 (2002).

Colorless prisms from diisopropyl ether/*n*-hexane, mp 164-166°. $[\alpha]_D^{24}$ −29.1° (c = 1.03 in methanol).

THERAP CAT: Antifungal.

8122. Rayon. Regenerated cellulose. The Code of Federal Regulations defines rayon as a manufactured fiber composed of regenerated cellulose, as well as manufactured fibers composed of regenerated cellulose in which substituents have replaced not more than 15 percent of the hydrogens of the hydroxyl groups. Now produced almost exclusively by the viscose process. *Review:* J. Lundberg, A. Turbak in *Kirk-Othmer Encyclopedia of Chemical Technology* **Vol. 19** (Wiley-Interscience, New York, 3rd ed., 1982) pp 855-880.

Purified rayon. Avisco Rayon. A medicinal grade of rayon.

USE: Purified rayon as surgical aid.

8123. Razoxane. [21416-67-1] 4,4′-(1-Methyl-1,2-ethane-diyl)bis-2,6-piperazinedione; (±)-4,4′-propylenedi-2,6-piperazine-dione; (±)-(3,5,3′,5′-tetraoxo)-1,2-dipiperazinopropane; (±)-1,2-bis(3,5-dioxopiperazinyl)propane; ICI-59118; ICRF-159; NSC-129943. $C_{11}H_{16}N_4O_4$; mol wt 268.27. C 49.25%, H 6.01%, N 20.88%, O 23.86%. Cyclized analog of EDTA, *q.v.*; exhibits intracellular iron chelating activity. Plays role in preventing the formation of doxorubicin-iron complexes which generate radical oxygen species that are associated with cardiotoxicity. Prepn: A. M. Creighton *et al., Nature* **222**, 384 (1969); *idem,* **GB 1234935**; *idem,* **US 3941790** (1971, 1976 both to Natl. Res. Dev. Corp.). Mode of action: H. B. A. Sharpe *et al., Nature* **226**, 524 (1970). Metabolism: R. E. Bellet *et al., Eur. J. Cancer* **13**, 1293 (1977). Pharmacology: A. Atherton, *ibid.* **11**, 383 (1975). Clinical studies: M. T. Bakowski *et al., Int. J. Radiat. Oncol. Biol. Phys.* **4**, 115 (1978); H. W. Bruckner *et al., Cancer Treat. Rep.* **66**, 1713 (1982). Toxicity study: E. Hassenstein, K. Renner, *Strahlentherapie* **154**, 122 (1978). Clinical evaluation in renal cell cancer: J. P. Bray-brooke *et al., Clin. Cancer Res.* **6**, 4697 (2000). Review of antineoplastic activity and radiosensitization: M. T. Bakowski, *Cancer Treat. Rev.* **3**, 95-107 (1976); K. Hellmann, W. Rhomberg, *ibid.* **18**, 225-240 (1991).

Pale cream microcrystalline solid, mp 237-239°.

(+)-Form. [24584-09-6] Dexrazoxane; ADR-529; ICRF-187; NSC-169780; Zinecard. Clinical pharmacokinetics: R. H. Earhart *et al., Cancer Res.* **42**, 5255 (1982). HPLC determn in plasma and urine: R. C. Lewis *et al., Pharm. Res.* **9**, 101 (1992). Clinical study of protection vs doxorubicin-associated cardiomyopathy: J. L. Speyer *et al., J. Clin. Oncol.* **10**, 117 (1992); S. E. Lipshultz *et al., N. Engl. J. Med.* **351**, 145 (2004). Review of pharmacology and clinical studies: J. Koning *et al., Cancer Treat. Rev.* **18**, 1-19 (1991); of therapeutic role as a cardioprotectant: S. M. Swain, P.

Vici, *J. Cancer Res. Clin. Oncol.* **130**, 1-7 (2004). Crystals from aq methanol/ether, mp 193°. $[\alpha]_D$ +11.35° (c = 5 in DMF). Soly (mg/ml): 10-12 water, 35-43 0.1*N* HCl, 25-34 0.1*N* NaOH, 6.7-10 10% ethanol, 1 methanol, 7.1-10 H_2O/DMA (1:1), 9.7-14.5 0.1*M* citrate buffer (pH 4), 8.7-13 0.1*M* borate buffer (pH 9). pKa 2.1. Partition coefficient (octanol/water): 0.025. Degrades rapidly above pH 7.0.

(+)-Form hydrochloride. [149003-01-0] Cardioxane; Eucardion.

THERAP CAT: Racemate as antineoplastic. (+)-Form as cardioprotectant.

8124. Rebamipide. [90098-04-7] α-[(4-Chlorobenzoyl)-amino]-1,2-dihydro-2-oxo-4-quinolinepropanoic acid; (±)-α-(*p*-chlorobenzamido)-1,2-dihydro-2-oxo-4-quinolinepropionic acid; 2-(4-chlorobenzoylamino)-3-[2(1*H*)-quinolinon-4-yl]propionic acid; proamipide; OPC-12759; Mucosta. $C_{19}H_{15}ClN_2O_4$; mol wt 370.79. C 61.55%, H 4.08%, Cl 9.56%, N 7.56%, O 17.26%. Gastric cytoprotectant. Prepn: M. Uchida *et al.,* **DE 3324034**; *eidem,* **US 4578381**; (1984, 1986 both to Otsuka). Synthesis and pharmacology: M. Uchida *et al., Chem. Pharm. Bull.* **33**, 3775 (1985); of enantiomers: *eidem, ibid.* **35**, 853 (1987). Antiulcer activity in rats: K. Yamasaki *et al., Eur. J. Pharmacol.* **142**, 23 (1987); K. Yamasaki *et al., Jpn. J. Pharmacol.* **49**, 441 (1989). HPLC determn in plasma and urine: Y. Shioya, T. Shimizu, *J. Chromatogr.* **434**, 283 (1988).

White powder from DMF-water, mp 288-290° (dec) as hemihydrate.

(−)-Form. Colorless needles from DMF, mp 305-306° (dec). $[\alpha]_D^{20}$ −116.7° (c = 1.0 in DMF).

(+)-Form. Colorless needles from DMF, mp 305-306° (dec). $[\alpha]_D^{20}$ +116.9° (c = 1.0 in DMF).

THERAP CAT: Antiulcerative.

8125. Reboxetine. [98769-81-4] (2*R*)-rel-2-[(*R*)-(2-Ethoxy-phenoxy)phenylmethyl]morpholine; (±)-(2*R**)-2-[(α*R**)-α-(*o*-eth-oxyphenoxy)benzyl]morpholine. $C_{19}H_{23}NO_3$; mol wt 313.39. C 72.82%, H 7.40%, N 4.47%, O 15.32%. Selective noradrenaline reuptake inhibitor. Prepn: P. Melloni *et al.,* **DE 2901032**; *eidem,* **US 4229449** (1979, 1980 both to Farmitalia Carlo Erba); *eidem et al., Eur. J. Med. Chem. - Chim. Ther.* **19**, 235 (1984). Configuration: P. Melloni *et al., Tetrahedron* **41**, 1393 (1985). HPLC determn of enantiomers in plasma: E. Frigerio *et al., J. Chromatogr. A* **660**, 351 (1994). Metabolism: G. Cocchiara *et al., Eur. J. Drug Metab. Pharmacokinet.* **16**, 231 (1991). Stereoselective kinetics: M. S. Benedetti *et al., Chirality* **7**, 285 (1995). Clinical pharmacokinetics: C. Pellizzoni *et al., Biopharm. Drug Dispos.* **17**, 623 (1996). Clinical trial in depression and social phobia: S. A. Montgomery, *J. Psychopharmacol.* **11**, Suppl., S9 (1997); A. Dubini *et al., ibid.* S17.

mp 170-171°.

Methanesulfonate. [98769-82-5] Reboxetine mesylate; FCE-20124; Edronax; Prolift; Vestra. $C_{19}H_{23}NO_3 \cdot CH_3SO_3H$; mol wt 409.50. mp 145-146°.

THERAP CAT: Antidepressant.

8126. Red Fluorescent Protein. RFP. Tetrameric, 28kDa, fluorescent protein responsible for the red coloration of the *Discosoma* coral. Named following the pattern of two lower case letters indicating the species, FP for fluorescent protein, and the emission maximum wavelength in nm. Identification and cloning from *Discosoma* by homology to green fluorescent protein, *q.v.*: M. V. Matz *et al., Nat. Biotechnol.* **17,** 969 (1999); S. A. Lukyanov *et al.,* **WO 0034324** (2000 to Clontech). Structure and biochemical characterization: G. S. Baird *et al., Proc. Natl. Acad. Sci. USA* **97,** 11984 (2000). Chromophore structure: L. A. Gross *et al., ibid.* 11990; molecular spectroscopy and hydrodynamics: A. A. Heikal *et al., ibid.* 11996. Brief review in measurement of signal transduction: D. A. Zacharias *et al., Curr. Opin. Neurobiol.* **10,** 416-421 (2000).

drFP583. [251925-26-5] Fluorescent protein (Discosoma clone FP583); DsRed. Abs max (excitation aq. soln): 558 nm (ε 75000 $M^{-1}cm^{-1}$). Abs max (emission): 583 nm.

USE: Reagent for fluorescent imaging of cell signals.

8127. Reductic Acid. [80-72-8] 2,3-Dihydroxy-2-cyclopenten-1-one; 2-cyclopenten-2,3-diol-1-one. $C_5H_6O_3$; mol wt 114.10. C 52.63%, H 5.30%, O 42.07%. Antioxidant obtained from pectic substances: Reichstein, Oppenauer, *Helv. Chim. Acta* **16,** 988 (1933); **17,** 390 (1934); Goldstein, **US 2854484** (1958). Alternate syntheses: Hesse *et al., Ann.* **563,** 31 (1949); **592,** 137 (1955); **736,** 134 (1970). Crystal structure: D. Semmingsen, *Acta Chem. Scand. B* **31,** 81 (1977). Similar to vitamin C in structure but not activity.

Pale yellow crystals (has been obtained colorless) from ethyl acetate, dec 213-213.5° (also reported as 207.5° and 211°). Soluble in water, methanol, ethanol. Sparingly sol in ether, ethyl acetate, acetone. Insol in benzene.

5-Methylreductic acid. mp 71°. Stronger reducing agent than reductic acid.

USE: As antioxidant, like isoascorbic or ascorbic acid.

8128. Reinecke Salt. [13573-16-5] Ammonium diamminetetrakis(thiocyanato-*N*)chromate(1−); ammonium reineckate; ammonium tetrathiocyanodiammonochromate. $C_4H_{10}CrN_7S_4$; mol wt 336.43. C 14.28%, H 3.00%, Cr 15.46%, N 29.14%, S 38.12%. $NH_4[Cr(NH_3)_2(SCN)_4]$. Exists as monohydrate; made by fusing ammonium thiocyanate with ammonium dichromate. Prepn: Dakin, *Org. Synth.* **coll. vol. II,** 555 (1943).

Monohydrate. Dark red crystals or red cryst powder. Sparingly sol in cold water; sol in hot water, alcohol. Dec in aq soln with formation of a blue color and free HCN; dec occurs in about 2 weeks at room temp, rapidly above 65°. A similar decompn takes place in boiling alcohol.

Note: The K-salt is also known as Reinecke salt.

USE: Precipitant for primary and secondary amines, proline, hydroxyproline, and certain amino acids; also a reagent for mercury with which it gives a red color or precipitate.

8129. Relaxin. [9002-69-1] Cervilaxin; Releasin (formerly). Polypeptide hormone secreted by the corpora lutea of many mammalian species during pregnancy; also produced in several nonmammalians, including the shark. Facilitates the birth process by causing a softening and lengthening of the pubic symphysis and cervix; also inhibits contraction of the uterus and may play a role in timing of parturition. First discovered in estrogen-primed guinea pigs: F. L. Hisaw, *Proc. Soc. Exp. Biol. Med.* **23,** 661 (1926). Extraction from corpora lutea: Fevold *et al., J. Am. Chem. Soc.* **52,** 3340 (1930); Albert *et al., Endocrinology* **40,** 370 (1947); from pregnant rabbit serum: Abramowitz *et al., Anat. Rec.* **84,** 456 (1942); *cf.* Hall, Newton, *J. Physiol.* **106,** 18 (1947). Can be obtained commercially from pregnant sows' ovaries: Isoln procedure and purification by resin chromatography: Lehrman *et al., J. Am. Pharm. Assoc.* **44,** 206 (1955); R. L. Kroc, G. E. Phillips, **US 2852431**; G. E. Phillips, **US 2852432** (both 1958 to Warner-Lambert). Isoln from ovarian tissue using glacial acetic acid: Cohen,

US **2930737** (1960 to Princeton Laboratories). Alternate method: Keck, **US 3008878** (1961 to Thomae). Prepn from hog ovaries: Doczi, **US 3096246** (1963 to Warner-Lambert). Porcine relaxin has a mol wt of approx 6000 and consists of two peptide chains, A and B, of 22 and 31 residues respectively, linked covalently by one intra- and two inter-chain disulfide bonds. Purification, characterization of porcine relaxin: O. D. Sherwood, E. O'Byrne, *Arch. Biochem. Biophys.* **160,** 185 (1974). Structure of the A chain: C. Schwabe *et al., Biochem. Biophys. Res. Commun.* **70,** 397 (1976); of the B chain: *eidem, ibid.* **75,** 503 (1977). Relaxin is structurally homologous to insulin and related growth factors: R. A. Bradshaw, *Rev. Biochem.* **47,** 191 (1978); S. Bedarkar *et al., Nature* **270,** 449 (1977); N. Isaacs *et al., ibid.* **271,** 278 (1978). Complete amino acid sequence of porcine relaxin: R. James *et al., ibid.* **267,** 544 (1977); of rat: M. J. John *et al., Endocrinology* **108,** 726 (1981). Isoln, characterization of relaxin from the sand tiger shark (*Odontaspis taurus*): J. W. Reinig *et al., ibid.* **109,** 537 (1981); structure: L. K. Gowan *et al., FEBS Lett.* **129,** 80 (1981). Demonstration of synthesis of rat relaxin as a preprorelaxin molecule with a connecting peptide of 105 amino acid residues, using molecular cloning: P. Hudson *et al., Nature* **291,** 127 (1981). Structure of a genomic clone from which the amino acid sequence of biologically active human relaxin was predicted: *eidem, ibid.* **301,** 628 (1983). *Reviews:* C. Schwabe *et al., Recent Prog. Horm. Res.* **34,** 123-211 (1978); *Ann. N.Y. Acad. Sci.* **380,** entitled "Relaxin: Structure, Function, and Evolution", B. G. Steinetz *et al.,* Eds. (1982) pp 1-244.

Amorphous powder. Diffusion constant 12.6×10^{-7} cm²/sec. Sedimentation constant 1.6×10^{-13} sec. Isoelec pt around pH 7.0. uv max (water, pH 7.0): 277.5 nm ($E_{1cm}^{1\%}$ 7.20). Slightly sol in water and 95% alcohol. Sol in acid or alkaline solns. Insol in abs alcohol, ether, acetone, petr ether, benzene. Dec above pH 9. Neutral or acid solns which are free from oxidizing agents, are stable. Ampuled solns at pH 7.0 and 3.2 have been kept in refrigerator for one year without loss of activity.

THERAP CAT: Hormone (ovarian).

8130. Remacemide. [128298-28-2] 2-Amino-*N*-(1-methyl-1,2-diphenylethyl)acetamide. $C_{17}H_{20}N_2O$; mol wt 268.35. C 76.09%, H 7.51%, N 10.44%, O 5.96%. NMDA receptor antagonist. Prepn: R. C. Griffith, J. J. Napier, **EP 279937** (1988 to Pennwalt); *see also: eidem,* **US 5331007** (1994 to Fisons). Pharmacology, metabolism and pharmacokinetics: K. T. Muir, G. C. Palmer, *Epilepsy Res. Suppl.* **3,** 147 (1991). HPLC determn in plasma: J. W. Flynn, J. E. O'Brien, *J. Chromatogr.* **583,** 91 (1992). Mechanism of action study: S. Subramaniam *et al., J. Pharmacol. Exp. Ther.* **276,** 161 (1996). Neuroprotective properties: G. C. Palmer *et al., Ann. N.Y. Acad. Sci.* **765,** 236 (1995). Clinical evaluation in neuroprotection during cardiac surgery: J. E. Arrowsmith *et al., Stroke* **29,** 2357 (1998); in Parkinson's disease: Parkinson Study Group, *Neurology* **56,** 455 (2001). Review of mechanism of action and clinical applications: S. C. Schachter, D. Tarsy, *Expert Opin. Invest. Drugs* **9,** 871-883 (2000).

Hydrochloride. [111686-79-4] FPL-12924AA; PR-934-423A. $C_{17}H_{20}N_2O.HCl$; mol wt 304.81. Crystals from isopropanol + methanol, mp 253-254°. Soly (g/l): water 40; normal saline 22; dilute HCl 26; ethanol 24. LD_{50} (calculated as base) in rats (mg/kg): ~50 i.v., ~900 orally (Muir, Palmer).

THERAP CAT: Neuroprotective.

8131. Remifentanil. [132875-61-7] 4-(Methoxycarbonyl)-4-[(1-oxopropyl)phenylamino]-1-piperidinepropanoic acid methyl ester; 4-carboxy-4-(*N*-phenylpropionamido)-1-piperidinepropionic acid dimethyl ester; remifentanyl; GI-87084. $C_{20}H_{28}N_2O_5$; mol wt 376.45. C 63.81%, H 7.50%, N 7.44%, O 21.25%. Synthetic *mu*-opioid agonist. Prepn: P. L. Feldman *et al.,* **EP 383579**; *eidem,* **US 5019583** (1990, 1991 both to Glaxo); *eidem et al., J. Med. Chem.* **34,** 2202 (1991). Opioid receptor activity: M. K. James *et al., J.*

Pharmacol. Exp. Ther. **259,** 712 (1991). Pharmacology: W. E. Hoffman *et al., Anesthesiology* **79,** 107 (1993). Clinical pharmacokinetics: T. D. Egan *et al., ibid.* 881; C. L. Westmoreland *et al., ibid.* 893. HPLC determn in blood: K. Selinger *et al., J. Pharm. Biomed. Anal.* **12,** 243 (1994). Review of safety of bolus injection: S. P. Richardson, T. D. Egan, *Expert Opin. Drug Saf.* **4,** 643-651 (2005).

Hydrochloride. [132539-07-2] GI-87084B; Ultiva. $C_{20}H_{28}$-N_2O_5.HCl; mol wt 412.91.

Note: This is a controlled substance (opiate): **21 CFR,** 1308.12.

THERAP CAT: Analgesic (narcotic).

8132. Remoxipride. [80125-14-0] 3-Bromo-*N*-[[(2*S*)-1-ethyl-2-pyrrolidinyl]methyl]-2,6-dimethoxybenzamide; (−)-*N*-eth-yl-2-(3-bromo-2,6-dimethoxybenzamidomethyl)pyrrolidine. C_{16}-$H_{23}BrN_2O_3$; mol wt 371.27. C 51.76%, H 6.24%, Br 21.52%, N 7.55%, O 12.93%. Specific dopamine D_2-receptor antagonist. Prepn: G. L. Florvall, S. O. Ogren, **EP 4831;** *eidem,* **US 4232037** (1979, 1980 both to Astra); *eidem, J. Med. Chem.* **25,** 1280 (1982). Antidopaminergic activity: S. O. Ogren *et al., Eur. J. Pharmacol.* **102,** 459 (1984). Radiometric determn in urine: A. C. Veltkamp *et al., J. Chromatogr.* **384,** 357 (1987). Clinical pharmacology and pharmacokinetics: L. Farde *et al., Psychopharmacology* **95,** 157 (1988). Clinical evaluation in tardive dyskinesia: U. Andersson *et al., ibid.* **94,** 167 (1988); in schizophrenia: R. G. McCreadie *et al., Acta Psychiatr. Scand.* **78,** 49 (1988).

$[\alpha]_D^{20}$ −64° (c = 2 in ethanol).

Hydrochloride monohydrate. [117591-79-4]; [73220-03-8]. A-33547; FLA-731; Roxiam. $C_{16}H_{23}BrN_2O_3$.HCl.H_2O; mol wt 425.75. White to off-white crystalline solid. Loss of water at 105°; mp 173°. $[\alpha]_D^{20}$ −11° (c = 2 in water). pKa 8.9. uv max in water, ethanol, 0.1*N* HCl: 286, 287, 286 nm (ε 2280, 2260, 2280). Soly (mg/ml): water 300; ethanol 400; dichloromethane 80; acetone 20. LD_{50} i.p. in rats: 794 μmol/kg (Florvall, Ogren, 1982).

THERAP CAT: Antipsychotic.

8133. Renin. [9015-94-5] Highly specific aspartyl proteinase of mol wt about 40000 Da, produced and secreted by the kidney. Found also in amniotic fluid. Conc. of renin in the human kidney is about 20 times less than in hog kidney. Purification from hog kidneys: Haas *et al., Arch. Biochem. Biophys.* **42,** 368 (1953); from kidneys of various species: Haas *et al., ibid.* **48,** 256 (1954). Prepn of human renin: Haas *et al., ibid.* **110,** 534 (1965). Exists in α, β and γ configurations: Haas *et al., ibid.* **44,** 79 (1953). Purification on DEAE cellulose columns: Passananti, *Biochim. Biophys. Acta* **34,** 246 (1959); Maier, Morgan, *ibid.* **128,** 193 (1966). Has been observed to exist in high molecular weight inactive forms which upon acid treatment decrease in molecular size and increase in enzymic activity. *See* review of purification studies: E. Haber, E. E. Slater, *Circ. Res.* **40,** Suppl. I, I36 (1977). Renin is secreted by juxtaglomerular cells and acts on the plasma substrate, angiotensinogen, to split off the inactive decapeptide angiotensin I which is converted to the active pressor agent angiotensin II, *q.v.* Renin itself has no activity. Secretion of renin is stimulated by constriction of a renal artery, blood loss, low sodium levels, adrenal insufficiency. Increased levels of renin shown also in pregnancy. Cloning and sequence analysis of human renin cDNA: T. Imai *et*

al., Proc. Natl. Acad. Sci. USA **80,** 7405 (1983). Crystal structure of human recombinant renin: A. R. Sielecki *et al., Science* **243,** 1346 (1989). *Review:* W. S. Peart, "The Renin-Angiotensin System" in *Pharmacol. Rev.* **17,** 143 (1965); *idem, Proc. Roy. Soc. Ser. B* **173,** 317 (1969); Smeby, Bumpus, "Renin" in *Renal Hypertension,* I. Page, J. McCubbin, Eds. (Year Book Medical Publishers, Chicago, 1968) pp 14-61. Books: M. R. Lee, *Renin and Hypertension* (Williams & Wilkins, Baltimore, 1969); *Renin* **vol. 5,** S. Oparil *et al.,* Eds. (Eden Press, Quebec, 1980) 368 pp. Review of the renin-angiotensin system: J. C. Romero, F. G. Knox, *Hypertension* **11,** 724-738 (1988).

8134. Rennin. [9001-98-3] Chymosin; rennase; lab; abomasal enzyme; Lab Ferment (German). Mol wt about 31,000. The predominant milk-clotting enzyme from the true stomach or abomasum of the suckling calf: Tauber, Kleiner, *J. Biol. Chem.* **96,** 745 (1932). Secreted as an inactive precursor called *prorennin* and converted in the acid environment of the stomach to the active enzyme. Obtained by extracting dried strips of calf stomach with 5 to 10% NaCl soln contg boric acid for 5 days; improved process: Keil, **US 2339931** (1942). Structure consists of a single polypeptide chain with internal disulfide bridges. Amino acid composition: Schwander *et al., Helv. Chim. Acta* **35,** 553 (1952). Determn of *N*-terminal amino acid sequence: Foltmann, *Philos. Trans. R. Soc. London* **257B,** 147 (1970). Homologies in amino acid sequences of rennin and pepsin: Tang, Hartley, *Biochem. J.* **118,** 611 (1970). *Reviews:* Berridge, *Adv. Enzymol.* **15,** 423 (1954); Foltmann, *Milk Proteins* **2,** 217 (1971).

Yellowish powder, grains or scales. Peculiar, not unpleasant odor. Characteristic, slightly salty taste. Slightly hygroscopic. Can be purified enough to crystallize. The dry substance (sometimes diluted with NaCl or lactose) is stable, aq solns are not. Partially sol in water, dil alcohol. Insol at pH values near its isoelectric point of pH 4.5. pH of aq soln 5.8 (acceptable range 5.3-6.3). Strongly affected by ultraviolet (sunlight). Causes milk to coagulate, optimum temp 37-43°, optimum pH of milk 5.8. Not active below 15° nor above 55°. When a commercial prepn is labeled 1:10,000 it means that one gram will curdle 10 liters of milk at 35° within 40 minutes. Other strengths are 1:100,000 to 1:7,600,000.

USE: *Rennet* (a dried extract contg rennin) is used in the manuf of cheese and rennet casein, also sold retail for the making of junket or rennet custards.

THERAP CAT: Digestive enzyme.

8135. Renzapride. [112727-80-7] *rel*-4-Amino-*N*-(1*R*,4*S*,-5*R*)-1-azabicyclo[3.3.1]non-4-yl-5-chloro-2-methoxybenzamide; (±)-*endo*-4-amino-5-chloro-2-methoxy-*N*-(1-azabicyclo[3.3.1]-non-4-yl)benzamide; ATL-1251; BRL-24924. $C_{16}H_{22}ClN_3O_2$; mol wt 323.82. C 59.35%, H 6.85%, Cl 10.95%, N 12.98%, O 9.88%. Serotonin receptor 5-HT_4 agonist/5-HT_3 antagonist. Prepn: F. D. King, **EP 94742;** *idem,* **US 4612319** (1983, 1986 both to Beecham); *idem et al., J. Med. Chem.* **36,** 683 (1993). 5-HT_4 receptor selectivity as quaternary salt: G. S. Baxter *et al., Bioorg. Med. Chem. Lett.* **3,** 633 (1993). Clinical pharmacology: D. H. Staniforth, M. Pennick, *Eur. J. Clin. Pharmacol.* **38,** 161 (1990). Clinical evaluation in irritable bowel syndrome: M. Camilleri *et al., Clin. Gastroenterol. Hepatol.* **2,** 895 (2004). *Review:* P. Norman, *Curr. Opin. Cent. Peripher. Nerv. Syst. Invest. Drugs* **2,** 355-368 (2000).

mp >260°.

THERAP CAT: Gastroprokinetic. In treatment of irritable bowel syndrome.

8136. Repaglinide. [135062-02-1] 2-Ethoxy-4-[2-[[(1S)-3-methyl-1-[2-(1-piperidinyl)phenyl]butyl]amino]-2-oxoethyl]benzoic acid; (+)-2-ethoxy-α-[[(S)-α-isobutyl-o-piperidinobenzyl]carbamoyl]-p-toluic acid; (S)-(+)-2-ethoxy-4-[N-[1-(2-piperidinophenyl)-3-methyl-1-butyl]aminocarbonylmethyl]benzoic acid; AG-EE-623 ZW; Novonorm; Prandin. $C_{27}H_{36}N_2O_4$; mol wt 452.59. C 71.65%, H 8.02%, N 6.19%, O 14.14%. Non-sulfonylurea oral hypoglycemic agent. Prepn: W. Grell et al., **WO 9300337** (1993 to Thomae). HPLC determn of racemate in human plasma: A. Greischel et al., J. Chromatogr. **568**, 246 (1991). Clinical pharmacokinetics: F. J. Ampudia-Blasco et al., Diabetologia **37**, 703 (1994). Comparative clinical evaluation in NIDDM: B. H. R. Wolffenbuttel et al., Eur. J. Clin. Pharmacol. **45**, 113 (1993).

White, odorless, crystalline powder. Crystals from ethanol/water (2:1), mp 126-128°. Crystals from neutralized water, mp 130-131°. $[\alpha]_D^{20}$ +6.97° (c = 0.975 in methanol); $[\alpha]_D^{20}$ +7.45° (c = 1.06 in methanol). LD_{50} orally in rats: >1 g/kg (Grell).

THERAP CAT: Antidiabetic.

8137. Repinotan. [144980-29-0] 2-[4-[[[(2R)-3,4-Dihydro-2H-1-benzopyran-2-yl]methyl]amino]butyl]-1,2-benzisothiazol-3(2H)-one 1,1-dioxide; R-(−)-2-[4-[(chroman-2-ylmethyl)amino]-butyl]-1,1-dioxobenzo[d]isothiazolone; (−)-2-[N-[4-(1,1-dioxido-3-oxo-2,3-dihydrobenzisothiazol-2-yl)butyl]aminomethyl]chroman. $C_{21}H_{24}N_2O_4S$; mol wt 400.49. C 62.98%, H 6.04%, N 6.99%, O 15.98%, S 8.01%. Serotonin 5-HT$_{1A}$-receptor agonist. Prepn: B. Junge et al., **EP 352613**; eidem, **US 5137901** (1990, 1992 both to Bayer AG). Pharmacology and receptor binding study: J. De Vry et al., J. Pharmacol. Exp. Ther. **284**, 1082 (1998). Neuroprotective effect in vitro and in vivo: I. Semkova et al., Eur. J. Pharmacol. **359**, 251 (1998). Review: H. A. M. Mucke, Curr. Opin. Cent. Peripher. Nerv. Syst. Invest. Drugs **1**, 621-628 (1999).

Hydrochloride. [144980-77-8] Bay x 3702. $C_{21}H_{24}N_2O_4$-S.HCl; mol wt 436.95. mp 192-194°. $[\alpha]_D$ −42.2° (c = 1 in trichloromethane).

THERAP CAT: Neuroprotective.

8138. Repirinast. [73080-51-0] 5,6-Dihydro-7,8-dimethyl-4,5-dioxo-4H-pyrano[3,2-c]quinoline-2-carboxylic acid 3-methylbutyl ester; isopentyl 5,6-dihydro-7,8-dimethyl-4,5-dioxo-4H-pyrano[3,2-c]quinoline-2-carboxylate; MY-5116; Romet. $C_{20}H_{21}$-NO$_5$; mol wt 355.38. C 67.59%, H 5.96%, N 3.94%, O 22.51%. Prepn: **BE 876751**; Y. Morinaka, K. Takahashi, **US 4298610** (1979, 1981 both to Mitsubishi Yuka); Y. Morinaka et al., Eur. J. Med. Chem. - Chim. Ther. **16**, 251 (1981). General pharmacology in animals: K. Takahashi et al., Oyo Yakuri **32**, 233 (1986), C.A. **105**, 218691j (1986). Anti-allergic effects: S. Kono, K. Ohata, Arerugi **35**, 1105 (1986), C.A. **106**, 165870z (1987). Toxicity: M. Nagase et al., Iyakuhin Kenkyu **17**, 545 (1986), C.A. **106**, 108121r (1987).

Crystals from chloroform + n-hexane, mp 236-241°. LD_{50} in rats, mice (mg/kg): >5000 orally, >5000 s.c. both species (Nagase).

THERAP CAT: Antiallergic.

8139. Reproterol. [54063-54-6] 7-[3-[[2-(3,5-Dihydroxyphenyl)-2-hydroxyethyl]amino]propyl]-3,7-dihydro-1,3-dimethyl-1H-purine-2,6-dione; 7-[3-[(β,3,5-trihydroxyphenethyl)amino]-propyl]theophylline; D-1959. $C_{18}H_{23}N_5O_5$; mol wt 389.41. C 55.52%, H 5.95%, N 17.98%, O 20.54%. Theophylline deriv which has selective activity on β$_2$ receptors. Prepn: **FR M5969** (1968 to Degussa), C.A. **71**, 70644c (1969). See also **FR Addn. 0308** (1970 to Degussa), C.A. **78**, 72216h (1973). Synthesis: K. H. Klingler, Arzneim.-Forsch. **27**, 4 (1977). Toxicology: S. Habersang, ibid. 45. Series of articles on metabolism, pharmacology and clinical trials: ibid. 15-76. Other clinical studies: D. Nolte et al., Dtsch. Med. Wochenschr. **102**, 619 (1977); H. Budmiger et al., Schweiz. Med. Wochenschr. **108**, 1190 (1978).

Hydrochloride. [13055-82-8] W-2946M; Asmaterolo; Bronchodil; Bronchospasmin. $C_{18}H_{23}N_5O_5$.HCl; mol wt 425.87. Crystals, mp 249-250°. LD_{50} in mice (mg/kg): 148 i.v., >10,000 orally (Habersang).

THERAP CAT: Bronchodilator.

8140. Resacetophenone. [89-84-9] 1-(2,4-Dihydroxyphenyl)ethanone; 2',4'-dihydroxyacetophenone. $C_8H_8O_3$; mol wt 152.15. C 63.15%, H 5.30%, O 31.55%. Made by heating resorcinol, glacial acetic acid, and anhydr zinc chloride at 145-150°: Cooper, Org. Synth. **21**, 103 (1941); from resorcinol, acetic anhydride and boron trifluoride: Killelea, Lindwall, J. Am. Chem. Soc. **70**, 428 (1948).

Needles or leaflets, mp 145-147°. Gradually dec by water; sol in pyridine, in warm alcohol, in glacial acetic acid; practically insol in benzene, ether, chloroform.

USE: Reagent for iron as a 10% alcoholic soln. A red color is obtained with ferric ions in slightly acid soln: Cooper, Ind. Eng. Chem. Anal. Ed. **9**, 334 (1937).

8141. Resazurin. [550-82-3] 7-Hydroxy-3H-phenoxazin-3-one 10-oxide; "diazoresorcinol"; resazoin. $C_{12}H_7NO_4$; mol wt 229.19. C 62.89%, H 3.08%, N 6.11%, O 27.92%. Prepn from resorcinol: Rast et al., **DE 961829** (1957 to Bayer), C.A. **53**, 15098 (1959).

Dark red, small crystals with greenish luster. Insol in water, ether; sparingly sol in alcohol, glacial acetic acid; sol in dil alkali hydroxides.

USE: As indicator, using a soln of 0.1 g in 20 ml 0.1*N* NaOH, and water to make 500 ml. pH: 3.8 orange, 6.5 dark violet. In the detection of hyposulfite (sulfoxylate). In food research (reductase test).

8142. Rescinnamine. [24815-24-5] (3β,16β,17α,18β,20α)-11,17-Dimethoxy-18-[[1-oxo-3-(3,4,5-trimethoxyphenyl)-2-propenyl]oxy]-3,20-yohimban-16-carboxylic acid methyl ester; methyl 3,4,5-trimethoxycinnamic acid ester of methyl reserpate; methyl 3,4,5-trimethoxycinnamoyl reserpate; reserpinine; Cartric; Cinnaloid. $C_{35}H_{42}N_2O_9$; mol wt 634.72. C 66.23%, H 6.67%, N 4.41%, O 22.69%. Found in *Rauwolfia serpentina* Benth., *Apocynaceae:* Haack *et al., Naturwissenschaften* **41**, 214 (1954); Ordway, Guercio, **US 2876228** (1959 to Pfizer); Klohs *et al., US 2974144* (1961 to Riker); from *Rauwolfia* spp: Banes *et al., J. Am. Pharm. Assoc.* **47**, 625 (1958). Identity with reserpinine: Haack *et al., Naturwissenschaften* **42**, 47 (1955). Structure: Klohs *et al., J. Am. Chem. Soc.* **77**, 2241 (1955). LC-ED determn in urine: J. Wang, M. Bonakdar, *J. Chromatogr.* **382**, 343 (1986). LC determn in rauwolfia preparations: U. R. Cieri, *J. AOAC Int.* **81**, 373 (1998).

Fine needles from benzene, mp 238-239° (vac). $[\alpha]_D^{24}$ -97° (c = 1 in chloroform). uv max (methanol): 228, 302 nm (log ε 4.79, 4.48). Practically insol in water. Moderately sol in methanol, benzene, chloroform, other organic solvents.

THERAP CAT: Antihypertensive.

8143. Reserpic Acid. [83-60-3] (3β,16β,17α,18β,20α)-18-Hydroxy-11,17-dimethoxyyohimban-16-carboxylic acid; reserpinolic acid. $C_{22}H_{28}N_2O_5$; mol wt 400.47. C 65.98%, H 7.05%, N 7.00%, O 19.98%. Obtained by controlled alkaline hydrolysis of reserpine: Dorfman *et al., Helv. Chim. Acta* **37**, 59 (1954); Schlittler, **US 2824874** (1958).

Crystals from methanol, mp 241-243°.
Hydrochloride hemihydrate. $C_{22}H_{28}N_2O_5$.HCl.½H_2O. Crystals, mp 257-259°. $[\alpha]_D^{23}$ -81°.
Methyl ester. $C_{23}H_{30}N_2O_5$. Needles from methanol, mp 235-240°. $[\alpha]_D^{25}$ -106°.
Methyl ester hydrochloride. mp ~228°.

8144. Reserpiline. [131-02-2] (3β,19α,20α)-16,17-Didehydro-10,11-dimethoxy-19-methyloxayohimban-16-carboxylic acid

methyl ester. $C_{23}H_{28}N_2O_5$; mol wt 412.48. C 66.97%, H 6.84%, N 6.79%, O 19.39%. Isoln from *Rauwolfia serpentina* Benth., *Apocynaceae:* Klohs *et al., Chem. Ind. (London)* **1954**, 1264; from *R. canescens* L.: Stoll *et al., Helv. Chim. Acta* **38**, 270 (1955). Stereochemistry: Shamma, Richey, *J. Am. Chem. Soc.* **85**, 2507 (1963). Partial synthesis: S.-I. Sakai *et al., Heterocycles* **17**, 99 (1982).

Amorphous powder. $[\alpha]_D^{20}$ -38° (ethanol); -14° (c = 1.5 in pyridine); -12° (c = 1.7 in chloroform). uv max (ethanol): 229, 300-304 nm (log ε 4.57, 4.03). Freely sol in ethanol, acetone, chloroform, benzene.
Hydrochloride. $C_{23}H_{28}N_2O_5$.HCl. Crystals, mp 205-207°. $[\alpha]_D^{24}$ -40° (c = 0.44 in ethanol).
Reserpilic acid dimethylaminoethyl ester dihydrochloride. [3735-84-0] Paratensiol; Resporisan. $C_{26}H_{35}N_3O_5$.2HCl; mol wt 542.50.

THERAP CAT: Antihypertensive.

8145. Reserpine. [50-55-5] (3β,16β,17α,18β,20α)-11,17-Dimethoxy-18-[(3,4,5-trimethoxybenzoyl)oxy]yohimban-16-carboxylic acid methyl ester; 3,4,5-trimethoxybenzoyl methyl reserpate; Rivasin; Serpasil. $C_{33}H_{40}N_2O_9$; mol wt 608.68. C 65.12%, H 6.62%, N 4.60%, O 23.66%. Indole alkaloid found in *Rauwolfia* spp. Isoln from the roots of *Rauwolfia serpentina* L. Benth., *Apocynaceae:* J. M. Müller *et al., Experientia* **8**, 338 (1952); and structural studies: L. Dorfman *et al., Helv. Chim. Acta* **37**, 59 (1954); N. Neuss *et al., J. Am. Chem. Soc.* **76**, 2463 (1954). Stereochemistry: P. E. Aldrich *et al., ibid.* **81**, 2481 (1959); Y. Ban, O. Yonemitsu, *Tetrahedron* **20**, 2877 (1964). First total synthesis: R. B. Woodward *et al., J. Am. Chem. Soc.* **78**, 2023 (1956); *eidem, Tetrahedron* **2**, 1 (1958). Review of total syntheses: F.-E. Chen, J. Huang, *Chem. Rev.* **105**, 4671-4706 (2005). Comprehensive description: R. E. Schirmer, *Anal. Profiles Drug Subs.* **4**, 384-430 (1975). *Review:* A. Scriabine, Ed. in *Pharmacology of Antihypertensive Drugs* (Raven, New York, 1980) pp 119-125. Review of carcinogenicity studies: *IARC Monographs* **10**, 217-229 (1976); R. M. Diener *et al., Toxicol. Pathol.* **8**, 1-21 (1980).

Long prisms from dil acetone, dec 264-265° (dec 277-277.5° in evac tube). $[\alpha]_D^{23}$ -118° (CHCl₃); $[\alpha]_D^{26}$ -164° (c = 0.96 in pyridine); $[\alpha]_D^{26}$ -168° (c = 0.624 in DMF). uv max (CHCl₃): 216, 267, 295 nm (ε 61700, 17000, 10200). Weak base. pK 6.6. Very sparingly sol in water. Freely sol in chloroform (~1 g/6 ml), methylene chloride, glacial acetic acid. Sol in benzene, ethyl acetate. Slightly sol in acetone, methanol, alcohol (1 g/1800 ml), ether, and in aq solns of acetic and citric acids.
Hydrochloride hydrate. $C_{33}H_{40}N_2O_9$.HCl.H_2O. Crystals, dec 224°.
Caution: Reserpine is reasonably anticipated to be a human carcinogen: *Report on Carcinogens, Eleventh Edition* (PB2005-104914, 2004) p III-228.

THERAP CAT: Antihypertensive.

THERAP CAT (VET): Hypotensive, tranquilizer. Has been used to prevent aortic rupture in turkeys.

8146. Resibufogenin. [465-39-4] (3β,5β,15β)-14,15-Epoxy-3-hydroxy-5-bufa-20,22-dienolide; Respigon. $C_{24}H_{32}O_4$; mol wt 384.51. C 74.97%, H 8.39%, O 16.64%. Cytotoxic constituent of toad venom. Isoln: Meyer, *Helv. Chim. Acta* **35**, 2444 (1952); Linde, Meyer, *Pharm. Acta Helv.* **33**, 327 (1958). Structure: Thiessen, *Chem. Ind. (London)* **1958**, 440; Linde, Meyer, *Experientia* **14**, 238 (1958); *eidem, Helv. Chim. Acta* **42**, 807 (1959). Synthesis: Pettit *et al., J. Org. Chem.* **36**, 3736 (1971); Haede *et al., Ann.* **1973**, 5. Stereochemical study of cytotoxic properties: Y. Kamono *et al., J. Chem. Res. Synop.* **1977**, 78. Pharmacology: Leigh, Caldwell, *J. Pharm. Pharmacol.* **21**, 708 (1969).

Crystals from acetone + water, mp 113-140°/155-168°. $[\alpha]_D^{22}$ −7.1° (c = 1.259 in chloroform). Also obtained as an amorphous solid, $[\alpha]_D^{16}$ −5.4° (c = 2.030 in chloroform).

Hydrochloride. $C_{24}H_{33}ClO_4$. Crystals from acetone, dec 230-232°. $[\alpha]_D^{15}$ +15.1° (c = 0.5302 in chloroform). uv max (alc): 298 nm (log ε 3.74).

THERAP CAT: Cardiotonic.

8147. Resilin. Highly amorphous rubberlike protein found in insect cuticle. Isoln and characterization: Weis-Fogh, *J. Exp. Biol.* **37**, 889 (1960). The structure is a cross-linked random network of flexible protein chains, incorporating 15 of the more common amino acids and involving covalent bonds. Cross-links have been identified as di- and trityrosine. Biosynthesis: Coles, *J. Insect Physiol.* **12**, 679 (1966). Similar to elastin, *q.v.,* but does not form fibers; occurs as masses or typically as 2-5 μ layers. Elasticity approaches that of the ideal cross-linked rubber. Responsible for various springlike actions of winged insects. In flea: Rothschild, *Nature* **239**, 45 (1972). *Review:* Andersen, *Acta Physiol. Scand.* **66**, Suppl. 263 (1966); *idem,* "Resilin" in *Comprehensive Biochemistry* vol. **26C**, M. Florkin, E. H. Stotz, Eds. (Elsevier, New York, 1971) pp 633-657.

The colorless material is insol in water <140° and in all other solvents not rupturing peptide bonds. Swells in water and protein solvents; shrinks and becomes hard in absolute methanol, ethanol, dioxane, acetone. Shows no tendency to crystallize at all. Fluorescent in uv light.

8148. Resin Ipomea. [9000-34-4] Resin of Mexican scammony. Made by extracting the dried roots of *Ipomoea orizabensis* Ledenois, *Convolvulaceae* with alcohol and pptg with water.

Brown, translucent, brittle fragments or pale brown powder. Insol in water; sol in alc, chloroform, partially in ether.

THERAP CAT: Cathartic.

8149. Resin Jalap. [9000-35-5] Prepd by extracting the powdered root of *Exogonium purga* (Hayne) Lindl. (*E. jalapa* Baill., *Ipomoea purga* Hayne), *Convolvulaceae* with alcohol and pptg with water.

Yellow to brown, amorphous mass or powder. Insol in water, benzene, carbon disulfide, oils; freely sol in alc.

THERAP CAT: Cathartic.

8150. Resin Scammony. [9000-58-2] Made by extracting the tubers of *Convolvulus scammonia* L., *Convolvulaceae* with alcohol and pptg with water.

Brown, amorphous mass. Freely sol in alc; not less than 95% sol in ether and in caustic alkalies (with gentle heat).

THERAP CAT: Cathartic.

8151. Resiquimod. [144875-48-9] 4-Amino-2-(ethoxymethyl)-α,α-dimethyl-1H-imidazo[4,5-c]quinoline-1-ethanol; R-848; S-28463. $C_{17}H_{22}N_4O_2$; mol wt 314.38. C 64.95%, H 7.05%, N 17.82%, O 10.18%. Immune response modulator structurally similar to imiquimod, *q.v.* Induces cytokine secretion by monocytes and activates antibody secretion by B cells. Prepn: J. F. Gerster *et al.,* WO 9215582; *eidem,* US 5389640 (1992, 1995 both to 3M). Immunomodulating and antiviral activities: M. A. Tomai *et al., Antiviral Res.* **28**, 253 (1995). Mechanism of action study: G. A. Bishop *et al., Cell. Immunol.* **208**, 9 (2001). Clinical evaluation in genital herpes: S. L. Spruance *et al., J. Infect. Dis.* **184**, 196 (2001). Review of development: J. J. Wu *et al., Antiviral Res.* **64**, 79-83 (2004).

Colorless, crystalline solid, mp 190-193°.

THERAP CAT: Antiviral.

8152. Resistomycin. [20004-62-0] 3,5,7,10-Tetrahydroxy-1,1,9-trimethyl-2H-benzo[cd]pyrene-2,6(1H)-dione; X-340. $C_{22}H_{16}O_6$; mol wt 376.36. C 70.21%, H 4.29%, O 25.51%. Unusually stable antibiotic substance produced by *Streptomyces resistomycificus*: Brockmann, Schmidt-Kastner, *Naturwissenschaften* **38**, 479 (1951); *Ber.* **87**, 1460 (1954); Brockmann, DE 888918 (1953). Structure: Brockmann, *Angew. Chem.* **76**, 863 (1964). Revised structure: Bailey *et al., Chem. Commun.* **1968**, 374; Brockmann *et al., Ber.* **102**, 1224 (1969). Synthetic studies: J. F. Kingston, L. Weiler, *Can. J. Chem.* **55**, 785 (1977); K. James, R. A. Raphael, *Tetrahedron Lett.* **1979**, 3895. Total synthesis: B. A. Keay, R. Rodrigo, *J. Am. Chem. Soc.* **104**, 4725 (1982). Isoln from *Streptomyces griseoflavus* B71, ¹³C-NMR and biosynthesis: G. Höfle, H. Wolf, *Ann.* **1983**, 835.

Yellow needles from dioxane, dec 315°. Sublimes at 200-205° (10^{-4} mm) without activity loss. Stable to hot conc H_2SO_4 or hot N KOH. Weakly acid. Absorption max: 268, 290, 320, 337, 366, 457 nm (ε 24000, 23000, 14400, 13900, 11000, 15400). Slight soly in water; fair in ether, benzene, alcohol, acetone, acetic acid. Orange-red in sodium hydroxide and piperidine; red in pyridine. Fluoresces in alcohol, benzene, and acetone solns, also in sulfuric acid.

Note: The name Resistomycin is also used as a trademark for Kanamycin A sulfate.

8153. Resmethrin. [10453-86-8] 2,2-Dimethyl-3-(2-methyl-1-propenyl)cyclopropanecarboxylic acid [5-(phenylmethyl)-3-furanyl]methyl ester; 5-benzyl-3-furanmethanol-2,2-dimethyl-3-(2-methylpropenyl) cyclopropanecarboxylate; (5-benzyl-3-furyl)methyl chrysanthemate; (5-benzyl-3-furyl)methyl *cis, trans*-(±)-2,2-dimethyl-3-(2-methylpropenyl)cyclopropanecarboxylate; FMC-17370; SBP-1382; Chryson. $C_{22}H_{26}O_3$; mol wt 338.44. C 78.07%, H 7.74%, O 14.18%. Synthetic pyrethroid insecticide. Prepn: M. Elliott, GB 1168797; *idem,* US 3465007 (both 1969 to Natl. Res. Dev. Corp.); *idem et al., Nature* **213**, 493 (1967). GLC determn in corn, cornmeal, flour, wheat: R. A. Simonaitis, R. S. Cail, *J. AOAC* **58**, 1032 (1975); and infrared spec in nonaqueous

Consult the Name Index before using this section.

aerosols: M. W. Law *J. AOAC Int.* **59**, 745 (1976). LC determn in urine and water: B. L. Loper, K. A. Anderson, *ibid.* **86**, 1236 (2003). Photodecomposition: K. Ueda *et al., J. Agric. Food Chem.* **22**, 212 (1974). Environmental fate and ectoxicological effects in aquatic systems: G. M. Rand, *Ecotoxicology* **11**, 101 (2002). Efficacy against greenhouse pests: R. E. Webb *et al., J. Econ. Entomol.* **67**, 295 (1974); against *Anopheles quadrimaculatus*: C. A. Sandoski *et al. ibid,* **76**, 646 (1983). Review of toxicology and human exposure: *Toxicological Profile for Pyrethrins and Pyrethroids* (PB2004-100004, 2003) 332 pp.

Pred as a mixture of a 70-80% (±)-trans isomer and a 20-30% (±)-cis isomer. bp >180° (dec). d^{20} 0.96-0.97. Flash pt, closed cup: 264.2°F (129°C). Log P (octanol/water): 5.43. Vapor pressure: <10^{-5} mm Hg. Soly at 25° in water (μg/l): 35-40. Sol in organic solvents. LC$_{50}$ (96 hr) in rainbow trout, bluegill sunfish (μg/l): 3.14, 7.2 (Rand).

(+)-*trans*-Form see Bioresmethrin.
USE: Insecticide.

8154. Resorantel. [20788-07-2] *N*-(4-Bromophenyl)-2,6-dihydroxybenzamide; 4′-bromo-γ-resorcylanilide; 4′-bromo-2,6-dihydroxybenzanilide; 2,6-dihydroxybenzoic acid 4′-bromoanilide; resorcylam; HOE-296V; Terenol. C$_{13}$H$_{10}$BrNO$_3$; mol wt 308.13. C 50.67%, H 3.27%, Br 25.93%, N 4.55%, O 15.58%. Prepn: LeMaire *et al., J. Pharm. Sci.* **50**, 831 (1961); **GB 1124613**; H. Ruschig *et al., US 3449420* (1968, 1969 to Hoechst). Animal studies: Düwel; Behrens, Matschullat; Pfeiffer, *Dtsch. Tieraerztl. Wochenschr.* **77**, 97-107 (1970); Christ *et al., Berl. Muench. Tieraerztl. Wochenschr.* **83**, 61 (1970).

Colorless powder, mp 229-230°. Also reported as mp 183-186° (LeMaire). Stable at room temp for at least two years. Very resistant to acids and alkalies. Highly sensitive to iron compds which stain it deep red or violet. Very soluble in DMF; slightly sol in lower alcohols. Insol in water, hydrocarbons, vegetable oils.

THERAP CAT (VET): Anthelmintic (sheep and other ruminants).

8155. Resorcinol. [108-46-3] 1,3-Benzenediol; *m*-dihydroxybenzene; resorcin. C$_6$H$_6$O$_2$; mol wt 110.11. C 65.45%, H 5.49%, O 29.06%. Is at least 99.5% pure. Made by fusing *m*-benzenedisulfonic acid with excess NaOH. *Review:* J. Varagnat in *Kirk-Othmer Encyclopedia of Chemical Technology* vol. 13 (Wiley-Interscience, New York, 3rd ed., 1981) pp 39-69. Review of toxicology and risk assessment: B. S. Lynch *et al., Regul. Toxicol. Pharmacol.* **36**, 198-210 (2002).

White, needle-like crystals; sweetish taste. Becomes pink on exposure to light and air, or by contact with iron. d 1.272. mp 109-111°. bp 280°, but volatilizes at lower temp and is slightly volatile with steam. pH: 5.2. One gram dissolves in 0.9 ml water, 0.2 ml water at 80°, 0.9 ml alcohol; freely sol in ether, glycerol; slightly sol in chloroform. *Protect from light.*

Monoacetate. [102-29-4] Acetylresorcinol; Euresol. C$_8$H$_8$O$_3$; mol wt 152.15. Golden-yellow, thick, syrupy, oily liquid. bp

~283° with decompn. Insol in water. Miscible with alc, benzene, chloroform, acetone. Sol in solns of alkali hydroxides.

Caution: Potential symptoms of overexposure are irritation of eyes, skin, nose, throat, upper respiratory system; dermatitis; methemoglobinemia, cyanosis, convulsions; restlessness, bluish skin, increased heart rate, dyspnea; dizziness, drowsiness, hypothermia, hemoglobinuria; spleen, kidney, liver changes. *See NIOSH Pocket Guide to Chemical Hazards* (DHHS/NIOSH 97-140, 1997) p 272; *Patty's Industrial Hygiene and Toxicology* vol. 2B, G. D. Clayton, F. E. Clayton, Eds. (Wiley-Interscience, New York, 4th ed., 1994) pp 1586-1590.

USE: In tanning, photography; manuf of resins, resin adhesives, hexylresorcinol, *p*-aminosalicylic acid, explosives, dyes, tires, rubber products; in cosmetics; dyeing and printing textiles; as a reagent for zinc.

THERAP CAT: Keratolytic; antiseborrheic.

THERAP CAT (VET): Topical antipruritic and antiseptic. Has been used as an intestinal antiseptic.

8156. β-Resorcylaldehyde. [95-01-2] 2,4-Dihydroxybenzaldehyde; 2,4-dihydroxybenzenecarbonal. C$_7$H$_6$O$_3$; mol wt 138.12. C 60.87%, H 4.38%, O 34.75%. Prepd by saturating with HCl a soln of resorcinol and anhydr hydrocyanic acid in abs ether and boiling the precipitated resorcylaldimide-HCl with water: Gattermann, Köbner, *Ber.* **32**, 278 (1899); *DE 106508; Chem. Zentralbl.* **1900**, I, 742. By adding POCl$_3$ to a soln of resorcinol and formanilide in ether, then boiling with dil NaOH, acidifying with H$_2$SO$_4$ and extracting with ether: Dimrath, Zöppritz, *Ber.* **35**, 995 (1902); by passing HCl into a mixture of resorcinol, ether, anhydr zinc chloride and cyanogen bromide, then boiling the precipitate with water: Karrer, *Helv. Chim. Acta* **2**, 92 (1919).

Needles from water or ether + ligroin. mp 135-136°. bp$_{22}$ 226°. Freely sol in water, alcohol, ether, chloroform, glacial acetic acid. Difficultly sol in cold benzene. β-Resorcylaldehyde is easily dec by acids and alkalies. Prolonged exposure to moist air converts it to a brown, amorphous powder which is insol in ether.

8157. β-Resorcylic Acid. [89-86-1] 2,4-Dihydroxybenzoic acid; 2,4-dihydroxybenzenecarboxylic acid; BRA. C$_7$H$_6$O$_4$; mol wt 154.12. C 54.55%, H 3.92%, O 41.52%. Prepared from resorcinol and KHCO$_3$ in glycerol or water by heating and passing CO$_2$ through the mixture: Brunner, *Ann.* **351**, 320 (1907). *Cf.* Bistrzycki, Kostanecki, *Ber.* **18**, 1984 (1885); Nierenstein, Clibbens, *Org. Synth.* **coll. vol. II**, 557 (1943).

Hydrated crystals from water. Becomes anhydr at 100°, mp 213° (rapid heating). pK (25°) 3.30. Sol in hot water, alcohol, ether, olive oil. Boiling with water, acids or salt solns results in loss of CO$_2$.

USE: Intermediate for dyestuffs and drugs; spot test reagent for iron.

8158. Resveratrol. [501-36-0] 5-[(1E)-2-(4-hydroxyphenyl)ethenyl]-1,3-benzenediol; *trans*-resveratrol; (E)-5-(p-hydroxystyryl)resorcinol; 3,4′,5-stilbenetriol; 3,5,4′-trihydroxystilbene. C$_{14}$H$_{12}$O$_3$; mol wt 228.24. C 73.67%, H 5.30%, O 21.03%. Phytoalexin found in a variety of plants; active ingredient of Asian folk medicine "Kojo-Kon" which is the powdered root of the Japanese knotweed. Isoln from white hellebore and structure:

M. Takaoka, *J. Fac. Sci., Hokkaido Imp. Univ. Ser. 3* **3**, 1 (1940); *C.A.* **34**, 7887 (1940); from fescue grass: R. G. Powell *et al., Phytochemistry* **35**, 335 (1994). Isoln of monomers, oligomers, isomers and glucosides from wine: F. Mattivi *et al., J. Agric. Food Chem.* **43**, 1820 (1995). GC-MS determn: D. M. Goldberg *et al., J. Am. Enol. Viticult.* **46**, 159 (1995). Produced as stress metabolite in response to fungal infection or injury: G. H. Dai *et al., Physiol. Mol. Plant Pathol.* **46**, 177 (1995); P. Jeandet *et al., J. Phytopathol.* **143**, 135 (1995). Antiplatelet aggregating activity: A. A. E. Bertelli *et al., Int. J. Tissue React.* **17**, 1 (1995); and implications in coronary heart disease: C. R. Pace-Asciak *et al., Clin. Chim. Acta* **235**, 207 (1995).

Off-white powder from MeOH, mp 253-255°.

3-β-mono-D-glucoside. [27208-80-6] Polydatin; piceid. $C_{20}H_{22}O_8$. Isoln from fresh root of *Polygonum cuspidatum* Sieb. & Zucc., *Polygonaceae*, and structure: Nonomura *et al., Yakugaku Zasshi* **83**, 988 (1963).

(Z)-Form. [61434-67-1] *cis*-Resveratrol. GC-MS determn in wine: D. M. Goldberg *et al., J. Agric. Food Chem.* **43**, 1245 (1995).

8159. Retamine. [2122-29-4] Dodecahydro-7,14-methano-2*H*,6*H*-dipyrido[1,2-*a*:1′,2′-*e*][1,5]diazocin-1-ol. $C_{15}H_{26}N_2O$; mol wt 250.38. C 71.95%, H 10.47%, N 11.19%, O 6.39%. From bark and young branches of *Genista sphaerocarpa* Lam. (*Retama sphaerocarpa* (Lam.) Boiss.), *Leguminosae*. Isoln: Battandier, Malosse, *Compt. Rend.* **125**, 360, 450 (1897); Ribas *et al., An. Fis. Quim.* **42**, 516 (1946), *C.A.* **41**, 4894c (1947). Structure: Bohlmann *et al., Ber.* **98**, 659 (1965). Synthesis: Bohlmann *et al., ibid.* 653. Stereochemistry: Ribas *et al., Tetrahedron Lett.* **1965**, 3181.

Bitter crystals from alc, mp 165-166°. $[\alpha]_D^{20}$ +46.2° (c = 1.017 in abs ethanol). Practically insol in water; slightly sol in ether; sol in chloroform, alcohol, methanol; very sol in benzene.

Hydrochloride. mp 272-273°.

8160. Retene. [483-65-8] 1-Methyl-7-(1-methylethyl)phenanthrene. $C_{18}H_{18}$; mol wt 234.34. C 92.26%, H 7.74%. Occurs in pine tar, in fossilized pine, in high-boiling tar oils. Formed by Se or Pd dehydrogenation of abietic acid: Ruzicka, Waldmann, *Helv. Chim. Acta* **16**, 842 (1933). Synthesis starting with methyl β-(6-isopropyl-2-naphthoyl)propionate: Bardhan, Sengupta, *J. Chem. Soc.* **1932**, 2520, 2798; *cf.* Bogert, *Science* **77**, 289 (1933). Review and bibliography: Fieser, Fieser, *Natural Products Related to Phenanthrene* (New York, 3rd ed., 1949).

Plates, scales from alc, mp 99°. bp$_{10}$ 208°; bp$_{760}$ 390-394°. Absorption spectrum: Askew, *J. Chem. Soc.* **1935**, 509. Insol in water. Sol in hot alcohol, benzene, hot ether, carbon disulfide. Upon treatment with CrO_3 in acetic acid forms retenequinone, $C_{18}H_{16}O_2$, mp 197.5°.

8161. Reteplase. [133652-38-7] 173-L-serine-174-L-tyrosine-175-L-glutamine-173-527-plasminogen activator (human tissue-type); r-PA; BM-06022; Rapilysin; Retavase. Genetically engineered deletion variant of human tissue plasminogen activator (t-

PA), *q.v.* Single-chain, nonglycosylated form containing only the protease and kringle-2 domains of native, human t-PA. Expression in *E. coli* cells and chromatographic purifn: A. Stern *et al.,* **EP 382174**; *eidem,* **US 5223256** (1990, 1993 both to Boehringer, Mann.). Clinical pharmacokinetics: U. Martin *et al., Thromb. Haemostasis* **66**, 569 (1991). Review of pharmacology, toxicology and clinical evaluation: *idem et al., Cardiovasc. Drug Rev.* **11**, 299-311 (1993). Clinical comparison with alteplase in acute myocardial infarction: C. Bode *et al., Circulation* **94**, 891 (1996); E. J. Topol *et al., N. Engl. J. Med.* **337**, 1118 (1997); in pulmonary embolism: U. Tebbe *et al., Am. Heart J.* **138**, 39 (1999).

THERAP CAT: Thrombolytic.

8162. Reticulin. One of the connective tissue proteins occurring wherever connective tissue forms a boundary: Jacobson, *Nature and Structure of Collagen*, J. T. Randall, Ed. (Butterworths, London, 1953) pp 6-13, *C.A.* **48**, 10814e (1954). Found together with collagen and elastin. Particularly abundant in membranes of the glomeruli and tubules of the kidney and in supportive structure of the vasculature and lung alveoli. Isoln from kidney tissue slices: Kramer, Little, *ibid.* pp 33-43, *C.A.* **48**, 10815a (1954). Contains about 85% protein, the amino acid content of which is very similar to that of collagen. Also contains about 4.2% carbohydrate and approx 11% bound lipid which yields, on hydrolysis, 95% myristic acid and 5% palmitic acid: Windrum *et al., Br. J. Exp. Pathol.* **36**, 49 (1955). Lacks hydroxyproline; glycine content is that of normal proteins: Pras, Glynn, *ibid.* **54**, 449 (1973).

Stable in boiling water and in 1*N* HCl. Can be dispersed in distilled water but precipitated by physiological saline (0.15 mol/l).

8163. Reticuline. [485-19-8] 1,2,3,4-Tetrahydro-1-[(3-hydroxy-4-methoxyphenyl)methyl]-6-methoxy-2-methyl-7-isoquinolinol; 1,2,3,4-tetrahydro-6-methoxy-2-methyl-1-vanillyl-7-isoquinolinol; 2-methyl-7-hydroxy-6-methoxy-1-(3-hydroxy-4-methoxybenzyl)-1,2,3,4-tetrahydroisoquinoline; coclanoline. $C_{19}H_{23}NO_4$; mol wt 329.39. C 69.28%, H 7.04%, N 4.25%, O 19.43%. Precursor of many aporphine and morphine-type alkaloids. Isoln of *d*-form from *Anona reticulata* Linn., *Anonaceae*: Gopinath *et al., Ber.* **92**, 776 (1959); *dl*-form from opium: Brochmann-Hanssen, Furuya, *J. Pharm. Sci.* **53**, 575 (1964); *Planta Med.* **12**, 328 (1964). Structure: Brochmann-Hanssen, Nielson, *Tetrahedron Lett.* **1965**, 1271. Configuration: Battersby, Evans, *ibid.* 1275. Synthesis of amorphous *dl*-form: Gopinath *et al., Ber.* **92**, 1657 (1959); P. Kerekes *et al., Acta Chim. Acad. Sci. Hung.* **98**, 491 (1978). Synthesis of crystalline *dl*-form: Baxter *et al., J. Chem. Soc. C* **1965**, 3645; Chan, Maitland, *ibid.* **1966**, 753; K. C. Rice, A. Brossi, *J. Org. Chem.* **45**, 592 (1980); G. Dornyei *et al., Tetrahedron Lett.* **1982**, 2913. Asymmetric synthesis of (*S*)-reticuline: Konda *et al., Chem. Pharm. Bull.* **23**, 1063 (1975). Biosynthesis: D. S. Dewan *et al., J. Chem. Soc. Perkin Trans. 1* **1977**, 1662; A. Barrett *et al., ibid.* **1979**, 652.

dl-**Form.** Pink crystals, mp 146°. uv max: 284 nm (log ε 3.85). Sol in aqueous buffer of pH <7.5 or >11. Practically insol in water at pH 8-10.

(*S*)-**Form perchlorate.** $C_{19}H_{23}NO_4$·$HClO_4$. Colorless prisms from ethanol, mp 203-204°. $[\alpha]_D^{18}$ +88.3° (c = 0.21 in alc).

8164. Retinal. [116-31-4] Retinaldehyde; retinene$_1$; vitamin A aldehyde; axerophthal. $C_{20}H_{28}O$; mol wt 284.44. C 84.45%, H 9.92%, O 5.62%. Carotenoid component of the visual pigments. Of the 16 possible stereoisomers, 13 have been synthesized. The 11-*cis* isomer is the chromophore of the majority of naturally occurring opsins, *q.v.* Isoln from retinas: G. Wald, *J. Gen. Physiol.* **19**, 351 (1935); recognition as vitamin A aldehyde: R. A. Morton, *Nature* **153**, 69 (1944). Prepd by the oxidation of vitamin A: Ball *et al., Biochem. J.* **42**, 516 (1948); by the oxidation of β-carotene: Wendler *et al., J. Am. Chem. Soc.* **72**, 234 (1950); from β-ionone: Eiter, Truscheit, **US 3060229** (1962 to Bayer); Jacobs *et al., Rec. Trav. Chim.* **84**, 1113 (1965). Synthesis *in vitro* from vitamin A₁: G. Wald, R. Hubbard, *Proc. Natl. Acad. Sci. USA* **36**, 92 (1950). Synthesis of 11-*cis* isomer: J. M. Dieterle, C. D. Robeson, *Science* **120**, 219 (1954). X-ray crystallography of retinals: R. Gilardi *et al., Nature* **232**, 187 (1971); H. Matsumoto *et al., J. Am. Chem. Soc.* **102**, 4259 (1980). Exposure of opsin-bound retinal to light initiates the *cis-trans* isomerization and resultant dissociation of retinal from the apoprotein. This catalyzes an enzyme cascade which leads to visual excitation: R. Hubbard, A. Kropf, *Proc. Natl. Acad. Sci. USA* **44**, 130 (1958); B. Honig *et al., ibid.* **76**, 2503 (1979). Bioregulation of absorption maxima: B. Honig *et al., J. Am. Chem. Soc.* **101**, 7084 (1979). HPLC determn in biological material: T. Suzuki, M. Makino-Tasaka, *Anal. Biochem.* **129**, 111 (1983). Review of syntheses: V. Balogh-Nair, K. Nakanishi, *Methods Enzymol.* **88**, 496-506 (1982); R. Liu, A. Asata, *ibid.* 506-516. Role in vision: D. F. O'Brien, *Science* **218**, 961-966 (1982); P. S. Zurer, *Chem. Eng. News* **61**, 24-35 (Nov. 28, 1983). Book: *The Retinoids* **Vol. 1-2**, M. B. Sporn *et al.,* Eds. (Academic Press, New York, 1984).

11-*cis* Retinal

all-*trans* Retinal

***trans*-Isomer.** Orange colored crystals from petr ether, mp 61-64°. uv max (hexane): 368 nm (ε 48000). Sol in ethanol, chloroform, cyclohexane, petr ether, oils. Practically insol in water.

11-*cis*-Isomer. Orange prisms from petr ether, mp 63.5-64.4°. uv max (hexane): 365 nm (ε 26360).

8165. Retinoic Acid. [302-79-4] (*all-E*)-3,7-Dimethyl-9-(2,6,6-trimethyl-1-cyclohexen-1-yl)-2,4,6,8-nonatetraenoic acid; *all-trans*-retinoic acid; vitamin A acid; tretinoin; Aberel; Airol; Avita; Epi-Aberel; Eudyna; Kerlocal; Renova; Retin-A; Retinova; Vesanoid. C₂₀H₂₈O₂; mol wt 300.44. C 79.95%, H 9.39%, O 10.65%. Physiological metabolite of vitamin A, *q.v.* Effects gene expression via nuclear retinoic acid receptors (RAR); mediates cellular growth and differentiation. Prepn: D. A. van Dorp, J. R. Arens, *Rec. Trav. Chim.* **65**, 338 (1946); C. D. Robeson *et al., J. Am. Chem. Soc.* **77**, 4111 (1955). Single-step process: R. Marbet, **DE 2061507**; **US 3746730** (1971, 1973 both to Hoffmann-La Roche). Crystal structure: C. H. Stam, C. H. MacGillavry, *Acta Crystallogr.* **16**, 62 (1963). Toxicology: J. J. Kamm, *J. Am. Acad. Dermatol.* **6**, 652 (1982). Clinical evaluation in treatment of photoaged skin: J. S. Weiss *et al., J. Am. Med. Assoc.* **259**, 527 (1988); in promyelocytic leukemia: R. P. Warrell, Jr. *et al., Leukemia* **8**, 929 (1994). Review of pharmacology and therapeutic potential: G. D. Goss *et al., Crit. Rev. Clin. Lab. Sci.* **29**, 185-215 (1992). Book: *The Retinoids*, M. B. Sporn *et al.,* Eds. (Raven Press, New York, 2nd ed., 1994) 679 pp.

all-*trans* Retinoic Acid

Yellow to light orange crystalline powder with characteristic floral odor. Crystals from ethanol, mp 180-182°. uv max (methanol): 351 nm (ε 45000). Sol in DMSO; slightly sol in poly-

ethylene glycol 400, octanol, ethanol. Practically insol in water, mineral oil, glycerin. LD₅₀ (10 day) in mice, rats (mg/kg): 790, 790 i.p.; 2200, 2000 orally (Kamm).

9-*cis*-Form *see* Alitretinoin.

13-*cis*-Form *see* Isotretinoin.

α-Tocopheryl ester *see* Tocoretinate.

THERAP CAT: Antiacne; adjunct in treatment of photodamaged skin; antineoplastic (hormonal).

8166. Retronecine. [480-85-3] (1*R-trans*)-2,3,5,7a-Tetrahydro-1-hydroxy-1*H*-pyrrolizine-7-methanol. C₈H₁₃NO₂; mol wt 155.19. C 61.91%, H 8.44%, N 9.03%, O 20.62%. The most common base portion of pyrrolizidine alkaloids. *"Necine" bases* are *1-methylpyrrolizidines* of different stereochemical configurations and degrees of hydroxylation that occur in the form of esters in alkaloids of *Senecio, Crotalaria* and a number of genera of the *Boraginaceae*. Retronecine occurs in nature in the (+)-form. It is the necine base of monocrotaline, senecionine, seneciphylline, retrorsine, *q.q.v.,* and numerous other hepatotoxic pyrrolizidine alkaloids. Structure: R. Adams, E. F. Rogers, *J. Am. Chem. Soc.* **63**, 228 (1941). Total synthesis: T. A. Geissman, A. C. Waiss, *J. Org. Chem.* **27**, 139 (1962). Stereospecific synthesis: E. Vedejs, G. R. Martinez, *J. Am. Chem. Soc.* **102**, 7993 (1980); H. Niwa *et al., Tetrahedron Lett.* **27**, 4605 (1986). Total synthesis of (−)-form: J. Cooper *et al., Chem. Commun.* **1988**, 509. Toxicity data: P. N. Harris *et al., J. Pharmacol. Exp. Ther.* **75**, 78 (1942). Biosynthesis: D. J. Robins, J. R. Sweeney, *Chem. Commun.* **1979**, 120; G. Grue Sorensen, I. D. Spenser, *J. Am. Chem. Soc.* **103**, 3208 (1981). Comprehensive reviews on retronecine and other necine bases: F. L. Warren, *Fortschr. Chem. Org. Naturst.* **12**, 198-269 (1955); **24**, 329-406 (1966); D. J. Robins, *ibid.* **41**, 115-203 (1982); F. L. Warren in *Alkaloids* **Vol. XII**, R. H. F. Manske, Ed. (Academic Press, New York, 1970) pp 245-331.

Crystals from acetone, mp 119-120°. [α]²⁰_D +4.95° (c = 0.58 in alc). LD₅₀ i.v. in mice: 634.0 ±26.0 mg/kg (Harris).

(±)-Form. Crystals from acetone, mp 130-131°.

8167. Retrorsine. [480-54-6] 12,18-Dihydroxysenecionan-11,16-dione; β-longilobine. C₁₈H₂₅NO₆; mol wt 351.39. C 61.52%, H 7.17%, N 3.99%, O 27.32%. Hepatotoxic pyrrolizidine alkaloid; common constituent of *Senecio* species. Isoln from *Senecio retrorsus* DC, *Compositae:* R. H. F. Manske, *Can. J. Chem.* **5**, 651 (1931); G. Barger *et al., J. Chem. Soc.* **1935**, 11; from *Crotalaria usaramoensis* E. G. Baker, *Leguminosae:* C. C. J. Culvenor, L. W. Smith, *Aust. J. Chem.* **19**, 2127 (1966). Structure: S. M. H. Christie *et al., J. Chem. Soc.* **1949**, 1700; E. C. Leisegang, F. L. Warren, *ibid.* **1950**, 702. Identity with β-longilobine: F. L. Warren *et al., J. Am. Chem. Soc.* **72**, 1421 (1950). Review and evaluation of toxicity and carcinogenicity studies: *IARC Monographs* **10**, 303-312, 333-342 (1976). Comprehensive reviews of pyrrolizidine alkaloids: L. B. Bull *et al., The Pyrrolizidine Alkaloids* (North Holland, Amsterdam, 1968) 293 pp; F. L. Warren in *The Alkaloids* **vol. 12**, R. H. F. Manske, Ed. (Academic Press, New York, 1970) pp 245-331.

Crystals from ethyl acetate, mp 212° (Barger *et al.*); 216-216.5° (Bull *et al.*). [α]¹⁸_D −17.6° (c = 1.99 in ethanol). uv max (water):

217 nm (log ε 3.85). Readily sol in alcohol, chloroform; slightly sol in water, acetone, ethyl acetate; practically insol in ether.

N-Oxide. Isatidine; 12,18-dihydroxysenecionan-11,16-dione-4-oxide; retrorsine N-oxide. $C_{18}H_{25}NO_7$. Isolated from *Senecio* species. Review and evaluation of carcinogenicity and toxicity studies: *IARC Monographs* **10**, 269-273 (1976). Crystals from ethanol, mp 140.5-141.5° (Christie *et al.*).

8168. Revaprazan. [199463-33-7] 4-(3,4-Dihydro-1-methyl-2(1H)-isoquinolinyl)-N-(4-fluorophenyl)-5,6-dimethyl-2-pyrimidinamine; 5,6-dimethyl-2-(4-fluorophenylamino)-4-(1-methyl-1,2,3,4-tetrahydroisoquinolin-2-yl)pyrimidine. $C_{22}H_{23}FN_4$; mol wt 362.44. C 72.90%, H 6.40%, F 5.24%, N 15.46%. Gastric proton pump inhibitor. Prepn: J. W. Lee *et al.*, **WO 9605177**; *eidem*, **US 5750531** (1996, 1998 both to Yuhan). HPLC determn in plasma and urine: K. S. Han *et al., J. Chromatogr. B* **696**, 312 (1997). Clinical pharmacokinetics: K.-S. Yu *et al., J. Clin. Pharmacol.* **44**, 73 (2004).

Hydrochloride. [178307-42-1] YH-1885; Revanex. $C_{22}H_{23}$-FN_4.HCl; mol wt 398.90. mp 205-208°.

THERAP CAT: Antiulcerative.

8169. Reversine. [656820-32-5] N^6-Cyclohexyl-N^2-[4-(4-morpholinyl)phenyl]-1H-purine-2,6-diamine; 2-(4-morpholinoanilino)-6-cyclohexylaminopurine; 2-(4-morpholinoanilino)-N^6-cyclohexyladenine. $C_{21}H_{27}N_7O$; mol wt 393.49. C 64.10%, H 6.92%, N 24.92%, O 4.07%. Synthetic small molecule reported to induce murine myoblasts to dedifferentiate into multipotent progenitor cells. Discovery of induction of cell dedifferentiation: S. Chen *et al., J. Am. Chem. Soc.* **126**, 410 (2004). Prepn: S. Chen *et al.*, **WO 05047524**; *eidem*, **US 050176707** (both 2005 to Scripps); *see also* combinatorial synthesis method: S. Ding *et al., J. Am. Chem. Soc.* **124**, 1594 (2002). A_3 adenosine receptor antagonist activity: M. Perreira *et al., J. Med. Chem.* **48**, 4910 (2005).

Pale white solid.

8170. Reviparin Sodium. LU-47311; Clivarin(e). Low molecular weight heparin, prepared by controlled nitrous acid degradation of a standard heparin extracted from porcine intestinal mucosa. Mean molecular weight 3900 Da (range: 3500-4500 Da). Biochemical and pharmacological profile: W. Jeske *et al., Semin. Thromb. Hemostasis* **19**, Suppl 1, 229 (1993). Clinical pharmacokinetics: K. Andrassy *et al., Thromb. Res.* **73**, 95 (1994). Symposium on pharmacology and clinical efficacy in the prevention of thromboembolism and restenosis: *Blood Coagulation Fibrinolysis* **4**, S3-S60 (1993). Clinical trial in deep-vein thrombosis: H. K. Breddin *et al., N. Engl. J. Med.* **344**, 626 (2001).

THERAP CAT: Antithrombotic.

8171. Rhamnetin. [90-19-7] 2-(3,4-Dihydroxyphenyl)-3,5-dihydroxy-7-methoxy-4H-1-benzopyran-4-one; 3,3′,4′,5-tetrahydroxy-7-methoxyflavone; 7-methylquercetin; β-rhamnocitrin; cya-

nidenolon-7-methyl ether 1537. $C_{16}H_{12}O_7$; mol wt 316.26. C 60.76%, H 3.82%, O 35.41%. The aglucon of xanthorhamnin. From fruit of *Rhamnus cathartica* L., *Rhamnaceae:* Krassowski, *J. Russ. Phys. Chem. Soc.* **40**, 1510 (1909); from commercial xanthorhamnin: Nystrom *et al., J. Org. Chem.* **22**, 1272 (1957). Structure: Oesch, Perkin, *J. Chem. Soc.* **105**, 2354 (1914); Jurd, Horowitz, *J. Org. Chem.* **22**, 1618 (1957). Synthesis: Kuhn, Low, *Ber.* **77**, 211 (1944); Jurd, *J. Am. Chem. Soc.* **80**, 5531 (1958); **US 2892845** (1959 to USDA); Anand *et al., J. Sci. Ind. Res.* **21B**, 322 (1962), *C.A.* **57**, 13712f (1962); Kawano *et al., Chem. Pharm. Bull.* **15**, 711 (1967).

Yellow needles from acetone + methanol, mp 292-294°. uv max (ethanol): 371, 256 nm (log ε 4.41, 4.40). Sol in hot phenol. Slightly sol in hot water, hot alcohol, hot glacial acetic acid, hot acetone. Freely sol in dil alkalies with intense yellow color.

Tetraacetate. $C_{24}H_{20}O_{11}$. Needles from acetone + methanol, mp 189-190°.

USE: Has been used for dyeing wool and cotton.

8172. Rhamnose. [3615-41-6] 6-Deoxy-L-mannose; L-rhamnose; L-mannomethylose; isodulcit. $C_6H_{12}O_5$; mol wt 164.16. C 43.90%, H 7.37%, O 48.73%. Occurs free in poison sumac *(Rhus toxicodendron* L., *Anacardiaceae)*, combined in the form of glycosides of many plants. Preparation: Clark, *J. Biol. Chem.* **38**, 255 (1919). Structure and configuration: Fischer, Morrell, *Ber.* **27**, 384 (1894); Fischer, Zach, *ibid.* **45**, 3762 (1912); Hirst, Macbeth, *J. Chem. Soc.* **1926**, 23; Avery, Hirst, *ibid.* **1929**, 2466. Isoln from walls of gram-negative bacteria: Salton, *Biochim. Biophys. Acta* **45**, 364 (1960); from *Afraegle paniculata* Engl., *Rutaceae:* Torto, *J. Chem. Soc.* **1961**, 5234; from rabbit skin: Malawista, Davidson, *Nature* **192**, 871 (1961); from leaves of *Solanum chacoense* Bitter, *Solanaceae:* Kuhn, Löw, *Ber.* **94**, 1088 (1961).

α-Form. Always obtained by crystn from H_2O or EtOH. Monohydrate, holohedric rods from water, hemihedric monoclinic columns from alcohol. Loses water of crystn on heating and partially changes to the β-modification. Very sweet taste. mp 82-92°: Ghosh, *Proc. R. Soc. Edinburgh* **36**, 216 (1915/16). Sublimes at 105° and 2 mm Hg. d_4^{20} 1.4708. Shows mutarotation. $[\alpha]_D^{20} -7.7°$ → +8.9°: Hudson, Yanovsky, *J. Am. Chem. Soc.* **39**, 1032 (1917).

β-Form. Prepd by heating α-rhamnose monohydrate on a steam bath; crystallized from anhydr acetone + alcohol. Needles, mp 122-126° (rapid heating). $[\alpha]_D^{20} +31.5°$ (1 min, p = 10). After a short time the rotation adjusts to the same final value as α-rhamnose. The β-form is hygroscopic and changes into crystals of the α-modification upon exposure to moist air.

8173. Rhamnus cathartica. Buckthorn bark. Dried, ripe fruit of *Rhamnus cathartica* L., *Rhamnaceae. Habit.* Europe, Northern Africa to Middle Asia. *Constit.* Rhamnocathartin, rhamnotannic acid, rhamnin, rhamnetin.

THERAP CAT: Cathartic.

8174. Rhapontin. [155-58-8] (E)-3-Hydroxy-5-[2-(3-hydroxy-4-methoxyphenyl)ethenyl]phenyl β-D-glucopyranoside; 4′-methoxy-3,3′,5-stilbenetriol 3-glucoside; rhaponticin; ponticin. $C_{21}H_{24}O_9$; mol wt 420.41. C 59.99%, H 5.75%, O 34.25%. From root of *Rheum rhaponticum* L., *Polygonaceae:* Hesse, *J. Prakt. Chem.* **77**, 321 (1908); Schürhoff, Plettner, *Arch. Pharm.* **275**, 281 (1937). On hydrolysis yields rhapontigenin and glucose:

Kawamura, *J. Pharm. Soc. Jpn.* **58**, 405 (1938), *C.A.* **32**, 6655[4] (1938). Constitution of rhapontigenin: Takaoka, *Proc. Imp. Acad. Tokyo* **16**, 408 (1940), *C.A.* **35**, 1399[2] (1941).

Crystals, dec 236-237°. $[\alpha]_D^{32}$ −59.5° (acetone). Exhibits bright blue fluorescence. Sol in dil alcohol, hot acetone, hot water; slightly sol in ether, alc, acetone, cold water; practically insol in benzene, petr ether, chloroform.

8175. Rheadine. [2718-25-4] (8β)-8-methoxy-16-methyl-2,3:10,11-bis[methylenebis(oxy)]rheadan; rhoeadine. $C_{21}H_{21}NO_6$; mol wt 383.39. C 65.79%, H 5.52%, N 3.65%, O 25.04%. Isoln from the seed capsules of corn poppy *(Papaver rhoeas* L., *Papaveraceae):* Hesse, *Ann.* **140**, 145 (1866); *Arch. Pharm.* **228**, 7 (1890); Awe, *ibid.* **274**, 439 (1936); Awe, Winkler, *ibid.* **290**, 367 (1957); Nemecková, Santavy, *Collect. Czech. Chem. Commun.* **27**, 1210 (1962). Structure and stereochemistry: Santavy *et al., ibid.* **30**, 3479 (1965); **32**, 4452 (1967). Total synthesis: Klotzer *et al., Helv. Chim. Acta* **54**, 2057 (1971); **55**, 2228 (1972); Irie *et al., J. Chem. Soc. Perkin Trans. 1* **1972**, 2986.

Crystals from ethanol, mp 252-254°. $[\alpha]_D^{23}$ +235° (c = 1.01 in chloroform); $[\alpha]_D^{22}$ +174° (c = 0.69 in pyridine). uv max (ethanol): 239, 290 nm (ε 9150, 9180). Slightly sol in ethyl acetate, methylene chloride. Practically insol in water, alcohol, chloroform, ether, benzene.

8176. Rhein. [478-43-3] 9,10-Dihydro-4,5-dihydroxy-9,10-dioxo-2-anthracenecarboxylic acid; 1,8-dihydroxyanthraquinone-3-carboxylic acid; 4,5-dihydroxyanthraquinone-2-carboxylic acid; chrysazin-3-carboxylic acid; monorhein; rheic acid; cassic acid; parietic acid; rhubarb yellow. $C_{15}H_8O_6$; mol wt 284.22. C 63.39%, H 2.84%, O 33.78%. Found in the free state and as glucoside in *Rheum* spp, *Polygonaceae)* and in Senna leaves; also in several spp of *Cassia (Leguminosae).* Diacetate used as antirheumatic. Isoln from Chinese rhubarb: J. Schlossberger, O. Doepping, *Ann.* **50**, 196 (1844); O. Hesse, *ibid.* **309**, 32 (1899); F. Tutin, H. W. B. Clewer, *J. Chem. Soc.* **99**, 946 (1911); from aloeemodin, *q.v.:* O. A. Oesterle, *Arch. Pharm.* **241**, 604 (1903); from *Cassia alata* L.: H. Hauptmann, L. L. Nazario, *J. Am. Chem. Soc.* **72**, 1492 (1950); from *C. fistula:* V. K. Murty *et al., Tetrahedron* **23**, 515 (1967). Prepn from chrysophanic diacetate: Fischer *et al., J. Prakt. Chem.* [2] **83**, 208; **84**, 369 (1911). Structure: H. Nawa *et al., J. Org. Chem.* **26**, 979 (1961). Use in arthritis: C. A. Friedmann, *DE 2711493; idem, US 4244968* (1977, 1981 both to Proter). Spectrophotometric study: A. A. Habib, N. A. El-Sebakhy, *J. Nat. Prod.* **43**, 452 (1980). Determn by gas chromatography, mass spectroscopy: G. W. Van Eijk, H. J. Roeijmans, *J. Chromatogr.* **295**, 497 (1984); HPLC: A. J. J. Van den Berg, R. P. Labadie, *ibid.* **329**, 311 (1985). Pharmacological effects on colonic mucosa: R. Wanitschke, *Pharmacology* **20**, Suppl. 1, 21 (1980); K. Ewe, *ibid.* 27. Metabolism study: J. Lemli, L. Lemmons, *ibid.* 50. In electron transport: P. Egerer *et al., Z. Physiol. Chem.* **363**, 627 (1982). Inhibition of proteases: L. Raimondi *et al., Pharmacol. Res. Commun.* **14**, 103 (1982). Effect on prostaglandin biosynthesis: S. Franchi-Micheli *et al., J. Pharm. Pharmacol.* **35**, 262 (1983).

Yellow needles by sublimation, mp 321-322°, dec 330°. Absorption max (methanol): 229, 258, 435 nm (ε 36800, 20100, 11100). Practically insol in water. Sol in alkalies, pyridine; slightly sol in alc, benzene, chloroform, ether, petr ether. Forms a red potassium salt and a pink sodium salt. Red precips are also obtained with $Ca(OH)_2$ and $Ba(OH)_2$.

Diacetate *see* Diacerein.

8177. Rhenium. [7440-15-5] Re; at. wt 186.207; at. no. 75; valences 1-7; the heptavalent state is the most stable. Group VIIB(7). Two naturally occurring isotopes: 185 (37.07%); 187 (62.93%); the latter is radioactive, $T_{1/2} \sim 10^{11}$ years. Artificial, radioactive isotopes: 177-184; 186; 188-192. Occurs in gadolinite, molybdenite, columbite, rare earth minerals, and some sulfide ores. Average concn in earth's crust 1×10^{-9} (0.001 ppm). Discovered by Noddack *et al., Naturwissenschaften* **13**, 567, 571 (1925). Prepn of metallic rhenium by reduction of potassium perrhenate or ammonium perrhenate: Hurd, Brim, *Inorg. Synth.* **1**, 175 (1939). Prepn of high purity rhenium: Rosenbaum *et al., J. Electrochem. Soc.* **103**, 518 (1956). *Reviews:* Melaven in *Rare Metals Handbook,* C. A. Hampel, Ed. (Reinhold, New York, 1954) pp 347-364; Peacock in *Comprehensive Inorganic Chemistry* vol. 3, J. C. Bailar, Jr. *et al.,* Eds. (Pergamon Press, Oxford, 1973) pp 905-978; P. M. Treichel in *Kirk-Othmer Encyclopedia of Chemical Technology* vol. **20** (Wiley-Interscience, New York, 3rd ed., 1982) pp 249-258.

Hexagonal close-packed crystals, black to silver-gray. d 21.02. mp 3180°. bp 5900° (estimated). Specific heat 0-20° 0.03263 cal/g/°C. Specific electrical resistance: 0.21×10^{-4} ohm/cm at 20°. Brinell hardness: 250. Latent heat of vaporization 152 kcal/mol. Reacts with oxidizing acids, nitric and concd sulfuric; not with HCl.

USE: Electron tube and semiconductor applications, in alloys for electrical contacts, as catalyst; possibly in high temp thermocouples and to improve the workability of tungsten and molybdenum alloys; plating jewelry, medical instruments, high vac equipment, mirror backings.

8178. Rhenium Heptoxide. [1314-68-7] Dirhenium heptoxide. O_7Re_2; mol wt 484.41. O 23.12%, Re 76.88%. Re_2O_7. Prepd from rhenium metal or its lower oxides in a stream of air or oxygen at 400-425°: Noddack, Noddack, *Naturwissenschaften* **17**, 93 (1929); *Z. Anorg. Allg. Chem.* **181**, 1 (1929); **215**, 129 (1933); Briscoe *et al., Nature* **129**, 618 (1932); Melaven *et al., Inorg. Synth.* **3**, 188 (1950). Crystal structure: Krebs *et al., Chem. Commun.* **1968**, 263.

Canary-yellow, very deliquescent crystals. Begins to sublime at 250°. mp 300.3°; bp 360.3°: Smith *et al., J. Am. Chem. Soc.* **74**, 4964 (1952). Freely sol in water, alcohol, ether, ethyl acetate, dioxane, pyridine. Readily absorbs water forming perrhenic acid, $HReO_4$.

8179. Rhenium Hexafluoride. [10049-17-9] F_6Re; mol wt 300.20. F 37.97%, Re 62.03%. ReF_6. Prepd by direct fluorination of rhenium metal: Ruff, Kwasnik, *Z. Anorg. Allg. Chem.* **209**, 113 (1932); **219**, 65 (1934); Malm, Selig, *J. Inorg. Nucl. Chem.* **20**, 189 (1961). The product obtained by Ruff was probably a mixture of ReF_6 and ReF_7: *eidem, J. Am. Chem. Soc.* **82**, 1510 (1960).

Yellow, cubic crystals or liquid; colorless gas; extremely hygroscopic. Forms bluish vapors on contact with air, discolors to a dark purple liquid. mp 18.5°. bp 33.7°. Sol in nitric acid. Soly in anhyd HF: 1.75 moles/1000 g HF, Frlec, Hyman, *Inorg. Chem.* **6**, 1596 (1967). Does not attack dried Pyrex glass or silica. May be handled in copper up to 150°.

8180. Rhenium Trioxide. [1314-28-9] Rhenic anhydride. O_3Re; mol wt 234.21. O 20.49%, Re 79.50%. ReO_3. Prepd by reduction of Re_2O_7 with dioxane: Nechamkin, Hiskey, *Inorg. Synth.* **3**, 186 (1950); with CO: Melaven *et al., ibid.* 187.

Red cubic crystals; green luster by transmitted light; the color of the powder may appear blue (***rhenium blue***). At 400° disproportionates *in vacuo* to Re_2O_7 and ReO_2. bp 750°. d 6.9-7.4. Practically insol in water, alkalies, non-oxidizing acids; oxidized by HNO_3 to $HReO_4$.

8181. Rhizoxin. [90996-54-6] WF-1360; NSC-332598. $C_{35}H_{47}NO_9$; mol wt 625.75. C 67.18%, H 7.57%, N 2.24%, O 23.01%. Rice seedling blight pathogen; phytotoxin which inhibits tubulin polymerization. Isoln from *Rhizopus chinensis*: S. Iwasaki *et al., J. Antibiot.* **37**, 354 (1984). Absolute configuration: *eidem, ibid.* **39**, 424 (1986). Antitumor activity in comparison with vincristine, *q.v.*: T. Tsuruo *et al., Cancer Res.* **46**, 381 (1986). Mechanism of action: M. Takahashi *et al., Biochim. Biophys. Acta* **926**, 215 (1987); Y. Li *et al., Biochem. Biophys. Res. Commun.* **187**, 722 (1992). Angiogenesis inhibition: K. Aoki *et al., Eur. J. Pharmacol.* **459**, 131 (2003). Clinical pharmacology: A. W. Tolcher *et al., Ann. Oncol.* **11**, 333 (2000). Review of chemistry and biology: J. Hong, J. D. White, *Tetrahedron* **60**, 5653-5681 (2004).

Pale yellow powder, mp 131-135°. $[\alpha]_D^{24}$ +155.5° (c = 0.8 in methanol). uv max (methanol): 295, 308, 325 nm (ε 42300, 54000, 39000).

8182. Rhod-2. [132523-91-2] 9-[4-[Bis(carboxymethyl)-amino]-3-[2-[2-[bis(carboxymethyl)amino]-5-methylphenoxy]eth-oxy]phenyl]-3,6-bis(dimethylamino)xanthylium chloride. $C_{40}H_{43}$-ClN_4O_{11}; mol wt 791.24. C 60.72%, H 5.48%, Cl 4.48%, N 7.08%, O 22.24%. Rhodamine-based calcium specific fluorescent dye. Prepn: R. Y. Tsien, A. Minta, *EP 314480; eidem, US 5049673* (1989, 1991 both to Univ. California); A. Minta *et al, J. Biol. Chem.* **264**, 8171 (1989). Use in monitoring intramitochondrial Ca^{2+}: M. Hoth, R. S. Lewis in *Imaging Neurons*, R. Yuste *et al.*, Eds. (Cold Spring Harbor Laboratory Press, Cold Spring Harbor, NY, 2000) pp 1-14; in free/intracellular Ca^{2+} levels: M.-P. Muriel *et al., J. Comp. Neurol.* **426**, 297 (2000); G. A. MacGowan *et al., J. Biomed. Opt.* **6**, 23 (2001).

Dark purplish solid. K_D for Ca^{2+}: 1μM.
USE: Indicator for calcium measurement in biological systems.

8183. Rhodamine B. [81-88-9] 9-(2-carboxyphenyl)-3,6-bis(diethylamino)xanthylium chloride; *N*-[9-(2-Carboxyphenyl)-6-

(diethylamino)-3*H*-xanthen-3-ylidene]-*N*-ethylethanaminium chloride; tetraethylrhodamine; D & C Red No. 19; C.I. Basic Violet 10; C.I. 45170. $C_{28}H_{31}ClN_2O_3$; mol wt 479.01. C 70.21%, H 6.52%, Cl 7.40%, N 5.85%, O 10.02%. Prepn: *Colour Index* **vol. 4** (3rd ed., 1971) p 4420. Toxicity study: J. M. Webb *et al., Toxicol. Appl. Pharmacol.* **3**, 696 (1961).

Green crystals or reddish-violet powder. Very sol in water with a bluish-red color, dil solns being strongly fluorescent; very sol in alcohol; slightly sol in HCl, NaOH. LD_{50} i.v. in rats: 89.5 mg/kg (Webb).
USE: As a dye, especially for paper; as a reagent for antimony, bismuth, cobalt, niobium, gold, manganese, mercury, molybdenum, tantalum, thallium, tungsten; as biological stain. Provisionally listed for use in drugs and cosmetics.

8184. Rhodanine. [141-84-4] 2-Thioxo-4-thiazolidinone; 2-thio-4-ketothiazolidine; 4-oxo-2-thionothiazolidine; rhodanic acid. $C_3H_3NOS_2$; mol wt 133.19. C 27.05%, H 2.27%, N 10.52%, O 12.01%, S 48.15%. Prepd by the action of sodium chloroacetate on ammonium dithiocarbamate: Julian, Sturgis, *J. Am. Chem. Soc.* **57**, 1126 (1935); Redemann *et al., Org. Synth.* **coll. vol. III**, 763 (1955).

Pale yellow crystals (long blades) from glacial acetic acid or water. d 0.868. mp 168.5° (capillary); mp 170.5-171° (hot stage). May explode on rapid heating. pK (25°) 5.52. Freely sol in boiling water, in methanol, ethanol, DMF, ether, alkalies, ammonia, hot acetic acid.
USE: In the synthesis of phenylalanine.

8185. Rhodinol. [6812-78-8] (3*S*)-3,7-Dimethyl-7-octen-1-ol; α-citronellol. $C_{10}H_{20}O$; mol wt 156.27. C 76.86%, H 12.90%, O 10.24%. Name that has been used to describe a group of related chemicals as well as a single chemical. The term, at times, was applied to what was considered the most important alcohol in geranium oil, ***1-citronellol***. See: Barbier, Bouveault, *Ber.* **29**, 289 (1896). Prepn in pure form: Sutherland, *J. Am. Chem. Soc.* **73**, 2385 (1951). Synthesis from *cis*-pinane: Rienäcker, *Chimia* **27**, 97 (1973).

Oily liquid, odor of rose. d_4^{20} 0.8549. bp_{12} 114-115°. n_D^{20} 1.4556. $[\alpha]_D^{20}$ -2.88°. uv max: 186-189 nm (ε 9000). Very slightly sol in water, miscible with alcohol, ether.
USE: In perfumery. *See also* β-Citronellol.

8186. Rhodium. [7440-16-6] Rh; at. wt 102.90550; at. no. 45; valences 1-6; most common states 1, 3. Group VIII (9). One naturally occurring isotope: 103; artificial radioactive isotopes: 97-102; 104-110. Member of platinum group of metals. One of the rarest elements, constitutes about $1 \times 10^{-7}\%$ of the earth's crust; found in small quantities associated with all native platinum; in the minerals rhodite, sperrylite, iridosmine; in some nickel-copper ores. Discovered in 1803 by Wollaston, *Philos. Trans. R. Soc. London* **94**, 419 (1804). Prepn: Vauquelin, etc., cited by Mellor, *A Comprehensive Treatise on Inorganic and Theoretical Chemistry* **15**, 546 (1936). Practical methods of separation: Wichers, Gilchrist, *Trans. Am. Inst. Min. Metall. Eng.* **76**, 619 (1928). Reviews of prepn, properties and chemistry of rhodium and other platinum metals: Gilchrist, *Chem. Rev.* **32**, 277-372 (1943); Beamish *et al.*, in *Rare Metals Handbook*, C. A. Hampel, Ed. (Reinhold, New York, 1956) pp 291-328; W. P. Griffith, *The Chemistry of the Rarer Platinum Metals* (John Wiley, New York, 1967) pp 1-41, 313-430; Livingstone in *Comprehensive Inorganic Chemistry* **Vol. 3**, J. C. Bailar Jr. *et al.*, Eds. (Pergamon Press, Oxford, 1973) pp 1163-1189, 1233-1253.

Silvery-white, soft, ductile, malleable metal; face-centered cubic structure. mp 1966°: Roeser, Wensel, *Natl. Bur. Stand. J. Res.* **12**, 519 (1934); d^{20} 12.41. Electr resistivity (0°) 4.51 μ-ohms-cm. Brinell hardness: 100. Not attacked by acids even aqua regia when in compact form; the finely divided metal reacts with aqua regia. Absorbs oxygen when melted; at a red heat is slowly oxidized to the sesquioxide. Converted to the trihalide by chlorine or bromine at a red heat; not attacked by fluorine.

Caution: Potential symptom of overexposure to metal fumes and insoluble compds is respiratory sensitization. Potential symptoms of overexposure to soluble compds in exptl animals are eye irritation, CNS damage. *See NIOSH Pocket Guide to Chemical Hazards* (DHHS/NIOSH 97-140, 1997) p 272-275.

USE: As an alloy with platinum; as a corrosion-resistant electroplate for protecting silverware from tarnishing; for making high-reflectivity mirrors for cinema projectors, searchlights. Spongy or black rhodium is used as a catalyst in various organic hydrogenation and oxidation reactions.

8187. Rhodium Carbonyl Chloride. [14523-22-9] Tetracarbonyldi-μ-chlorodirhodium; dichlorotetracarbonyldirhodium; chlorodicarbonylrhodium(I) dimer. $C_4Cl_2O_4Rh_2$; mol wt 388.76. C 12.36%, Cl 18.24%, O 16.46%, Rh 52.94%. $[Rh(CO)_2Cl]_2$. Prepn: Hieber, Lagally, *Z. Anorg. Allg. Chem.* **251**, 96 (1943); McCleverty, Wilkinson, *Inorg. Synth.* **8**, 211 (1966); Colton *et al.*, *Aust. J. Chem.* **23**, 1351 (1970); Cramer, *Inorg. Synth.* **15**, 14 (1974). Structure: Dahl *et al.*, *J. Am. Chem. Soc.* **83**, 1761 (1961).

Orange-red crystalline solid or red crystalline sublimate. mp 124-125°. Sol in most organic solvents (except aliphatic hydrocarbons). Stable to dry air. Solutions in organic solvents decompose when exposed to air.

USE: Catalyst.

8188. Rhodium Chloride. [10049-07-7] Rhodium trichloride. Cl_3Rh; mol wt 209.26. Cl 50.83%, Rh 49.18%. $RhCl_3$. Similar to the chlorides of other platinum group metals, rhodium chloride readily forms double salts with alkali chlorides. The chloride is obtainable also as a water-sol hydrate with variable amounts of water. Prepn of trihydrate: Anderson, Basolo, *Inorg. Synth.* **7**, 214 (1963). Toxicity data: Landolt *et al.*, *Toxicol. Appl. Pharmacol.* **21**, 589 (1972).

Red powder. Insol in water. Sol in alkali hydroxide or cyanide solns. LD_{50} in rats (mg/kg): 198 i.v. (Landolt).

8189. Rhododendrin. [497-78-9] 3-(4-Hydroxyphenyl)-1-methylpropyl β-D-glucopyranoside; betuloside. $C_{16}H_{24}O_7$; mol wt 328.36. C 58.52%, H 7.37%, O 34.11%. From leaves of *Rhododendron* spp., *Ericaceae*: Archangelski, *Arch. Exp. Pathol. Pharmakol.* **46**, 313 (1901); Kawaguchi *et al.*, *J. Pharm. Soc. Jpn.* **62**, 4 (1942), *C.A.* **44**, 9634a (1950). Structure: Kim, *ibid.* 455, *C.A.* **45**, 4222h (1951). Identity with betuloside: Kim, *ibid.* 63, 103 (1943), *C.A.* **45**, 4222i (1951). Chemotaxonomic significance: Thieme, Winkler, *Pharmazie* **24**, 703 (1969).

Bitter crystals, mp 187°. Sol in hot water, alcohol; slightly sol in chloroform, ether.

Pentaacetate. Needles, mp 96-97°.

Methyl ether. Prisms from warm water, mp 102-103°. $[\alpha]_D^{21}$ −17.1° (96% alcohol).

USE: In systematic classification of *Rhododendron* species.

8190. Rhodomycins. Antibiotic substance produced by *Streptomyces purpurascens* nov. sp.: Brockmann, Bauer, *Naturwissenschaften* **37**, 492 (1950); Brockmann *et al., Ber.* **84**, 700 (1951); GB 708749 (1954 to Bayer). Separation of rhodomycin A and rhodomycin B: Brockmann, Patt, *Ber.* **88**, 1455 (1955). Isoln and structural elucidation of additional rhodomycins produced by *Streptomyces stammes:* Biedermann, Brauniger, *Pharmazie* **27**, 782 (1972); Brockmann *et al., Tetrahedron Lett.* **1973**, 3699. Total synthesis of racemic rhodomycinones (the aglycones of the rhodomycins): A. S. Kende, Y.-G. Tsay, *Chem. Commun.* **1977**, 140.

Rhodomycin A

Rhodomycin A. [23666-50-4] [7R-(7α,8β,10β)]-8-Ethyl-7,8,-9,10-tetrahydro-1,6,8,11-tetrahydroxy-7,10-bis[[2,3,6-trideoxy-3-(dimethylamino)-α-L-lyxo-hexopyranosyl]oxy]-5,12-naphthacenedione; β-rhodomycin II. $C_{36}H_{48}N_2O_{12}$; mol wt 700.77. Dec on mild acidic hydrolysis into 1 mole β-rhodomycinone and 2 moles rhodosamine: Brockmann, Spohler, *Naturwissenschaften* **48**, 716 (1961). Structure of β-rhodomycinone: Brockmann, Niemeyer, *ibid.* 570. Structure of rhodosamine: Brockmann, Spohler, *ibid.* **42**, 154 (1955). Total structure: Brockmann *et al., Tetrahedron Lett.* **1969**, 415.

Dihydrochloride. $C_{36}H_{48}N_2O_{12}$.2HCl. Red prisms from ethanol + isopropanol, mp 205°. Freely sol in water, lower alcohols; sparingly sol in benzene, chloroform; practically insol in ether, petr ether.

Perchlorate. $C_{36}H_{48}N_2O_{12}$.2HClO$_4$. Minute red needles, mp 188°. Freely sol in methanol, acetone; sparingly sol in water, butanol.

Rhodomycin B. [1404-52-0] [7R-(7α,8β,10β)]-8-Ethyl-7,8,9,-10-tetrahydro-1,6,7,8,11-pentahydroxy-10-[[2,3,6-trideoxy-3-(dimethylamino)-α-L-lyxo-hexopyranosyl]oxy]-5,12-naphthacenedione. $C_{28}H_{31}NO_9$; mol wt 525.55. Dec on mild acidic hydrolysis into 1 mole β-rhodomycinone and 1 mole rhodosamine: Brockmann, Spohler, *ibid.* **48**, 716 (1961).

Hydrochloride. Red prisms, mp 180°. Freely sol in lower alcohols; sparingly sol in water, acetone. Practically insol in chloroform, benzene.

8191. Rhodopin. [105-92-0] 1,2-Dihydro-1-hydroxy-ψ,ψ-carotene; 1,2-dihydro-1-hydroxylycopene. $C_{40}H_{58}O$; mol wt 554.89. C 86.58%, H 10.54%, O 2.88%. Pigment from *Rhodovibrio* and *Thiocystis* bacteria: Karrer, Solmssen, *Helv. Chim. Acta* **18**, 1306 (1935); **19**, 1019 (1936); Karrer *et al., ibid.* **21**, 1938 (1938); from *Rhodomicrobium vannielii:* Volk, Pennington, *J. Bacteriol.* **59**, 169 (1950); Ryvarden, Jensen, *Acta Chem. Scand.* **18**, 643 (1964). Structure: Jensen, *ibid.* **13**, 842, 2142 (1959). Synthesis: Bonnett *et al., ibid.* **18**, 1739 (1964); Surmatis *et al., J. Org. Chem.* **31**, 186 (1966). Synthesis of deuterated rhodopin: Johansen, Liaaen-Jensen, *Acta Chem. Scand.* **28B**, 301 (1974).

Aggregates of dark red crystals from carbon disulfide + petr ether, mp 171° (preliminary sintering). Absorption max (chloroform): 521, 486, 453 nm.

8192. Rhodopsin. [9009-81-8] Visual purple. Mol wt ~40,000. A photoreceptor protein found in the rods of the retina of the eye. Composed of 11-*cis* retinal, *q.v.*, bound as a protonated Schiff base to a lysine moiety in the apoprotein opsin, *q.v.* Prepn from retinal and opsin: G. Wald, P. K. Brown, *Proc. Natl. Acad. Sci. USA* **36**, 84 (1950); R. Hubbard, G. Wald, *ibid.* **37**, 69 (1951). Purification and amino acid compn of bovine rhodopsin: Shields *et al., Biochim. Biophys. Acta* **147**, 238 (1967). Synthesis of labelled rhodopsin and studies on the active site: Hirtenstein, Akhtar, *Biochem. J.* **119**, 359 (1970). Characterization in synthetic membranes: W. L. Hubbell, *Acc. Chem. Res.* **8**, 85 (1975). Amino acid sequence of bovine rhodopsin: P. A. Hargrave *et al., Biophys. Struct. Mech.* **9**, 235 (1983). Studies on transmembrane molecular structure: E. A. Dratz, P. A. Hargrave, *Trends Biochem. Sci.* **8**, 128 (1983); Crystal structure: K. Palczewski *et al., Science* **289**, 739 (2000). Isoln and sequence of gene encoding bovine rhodopsin: J. Nathans, D. S. Hogness, *Cell* **34**, 807 (1983); of gene encoding human rhodopsin: *eidem, Proc. Natl. Acad. Sci. USA* **81**, 4851 (1984). Exposure to light initiates the conversion of rhodopsin through a series of distinct intermediates to yield opsin + *trans*-retinal: R. Hubbard, A. Kropf, *ibid.* **44**, 130 (1958); R. Hubbard *et al., Nature* **183**, 142 (1959); B. Honig *et al., Proc. Natl. Acad. Sci. USA* **76**, 2503 (1979). Review of visual transduction and bioregulation of absorption maxima: K. Nakanishi, *Pure Appl. Chem.* **57**, 769-776 (1985). *Reviews:* T. G. Ebrey, B. Honig, *Q. Rev. Biophys.* **8**, 129-184 (1975); D. F. O'Brien, *Science* **218**, 961-966 (1982); A. Maeda, T. Yoshizawa, *Photochem. Photobiol.* **35**, 891-898 (1982); P. S. Zurer, *Chem. Eng. News* **61**, 24-35 (Nov. 28, 1983). *See also: Methods Enzymol.* **81** and **88**, Lester Packer, Ed. (Academic Press, New York, 1982).

8193. Rhodoquinone. [5591-74-2] 2-Amino-5-(3,7,11,15,-19,23,27,31,35,39-decamethyl-2,6,10,14,18,22,26,30,34,38-tetracontadecaenyl)-3-methoxy-6-methyl-2,5-cyclohexadiene-1,4-dione; rhodoquinone-10. $C_{58}H_{89}NO_3$; mol wt 848.33. C 82.12%, H 10.57%, N 1.65%, O 5.66%. Isoln from *Rhodospirillum rubrum*: Gloves, Threlfall, *Biochem. J.* **85**, 14P (1962). Structure and synthesis: Moore, Folkers, *J. Am. Chem. Soc.* **87**, 1409 (1965); **88**, 567 (1966); Daves *et al., ibid.* **90**, 5587 (1968).

Violet needles, mp 70-71°. uv max (cyclohexane): 280, 500 nm ($E_{1cm}^{1\%}$ 154, 14).

8194. Rhodoviolascin. [34255-08-8] 3,3',4,4'-Tetradehydro-1,1',2,2'-tetrahydroxy-1,1'-dimethoxy-ψ,ψ-carotene; 3,3',4,4'-tetradehydro-1,1',2,2'-tetrahydro-1,1'-dimethoxylycopene; spirilloxanthin. $C_{42}H_{60}O_2$; mol wt 596.92. C 84.51%, H 10.13%, O 5.36%. Carotenoid pigment isolated from *Rhodovibrio* and *Thioceptis* bacteria: Karrer, Solmssen, *Helv. Chim. Acta* **18**, 1306 (1935). Identity with spirilloxanthin: Zechmeister *et al., Arch. Biochem.* **5**, 243 (1944). Structure: Karrer, Koenig, *Helv. Chim. Acta* **23**, 460 (1940); Barber *et al., Proc. Chem. Soc. London* **1959**, 96. Synthesis: Surmatis, Ofner, *J. Org. Chem.* **28**, 2735 (1963); Surmatis, US 3160658 (1964 to Hoffmann-La Roche).

Dark red, spindle-shaped crystals from benzene, mp 218°. Absorption max (chloroform): 544, 507, 476 nm. Almost insol in petr ether, ligroin, methanol, somewhat more sol in hot benzene.

8195. Rhodoxanthin. [116-30-3] 4',5'-Didehydro-4,5-*retro*-β,β-carotene-3,3'-dione. $C_{40}H_{50}O_2$; mol wt 562.82. C 85.36%, H 8.95%, O 5.69%. Carotenoid pigment found widely distributed in nature, but in very small amounts only. One of very few carotenoids with retro configuration. Best isolated from the arils of *Taxus baccata* L., *Taxaceae*: Kuhn, Brockmann, *Ber.* **66**, 828 (1933). Occurs also in the feathers of birds such as *Phoenicircus nigricollis, Megaloprepia magnifica.* Isoln: Volker, *Z. Physiol. Chem.* **292**, 75 (1953). Structure: Kuhn, Brockmann, *loc. cit.;* Karrer, Solmssen, *Helv. Chim. Acta* **18**, 477 (1935). Synthesis: Mayer *et al., ibid.* **50**, 1606 (1967); Surmatis, Walser, US **3466331**; US 3624105 (1969, 1971 to Hoffmann-La Roche); Ellis *et al., Helv. Chim. Acta* **64**, 1092 (1981); E. Widmer *et al., ibid.* **65**, 944 (1982). *Review:* Liaaen-Jensen in *Aspects Terpenoid Chem. Biochem., Proc. Phytochem. Soc. Symp.*, 2nd, 1970, T. W. Goodwin, Ed. (Academic Press, London, 1971) p 223-254.

Rosettes of deep purple, lancet-shaped crystals from benzene: methanol (1:4). mp 219° (evacuated tube). Absorption max (chloroform): 546, 510, 482 nm. Freely sol in pyridine; sol in benzene, chloroform. Sparingly sol in ethanol and methanol. Practically insol in hexane, petr ether.

USE: Coloring material for food, beverages, pharmaceuticals and cosmetics.

8196. Rhubarb. Rhizome and roots of *Rheum officinale* Baill., *R. palmatum* L., or other *Rheum* spp, *Polygonaceae. Habit.* Central Asia; cultivated in Europe, Southern Siberia, North America. *Constit.* Chrysophanic acid, emodin, rhein, rheotannic acid, erythroretin, methylchrysophanic acid, rhabarberon, cinnamic and gallic acids, calcium oxalate. Comprehensive studies: Workman, Hiner, *J. Am. Pharm. Assoc.* **49**, 118 (1960). *Incompat.* Mineral acids, iron salts, lead acetate, zinc salts, lime water; infusions of catechu, cinchona, and nutgall; tartar emetic, tannic acid.

THERAP CAT: Cathartic.

THERAP CAT (VET): Has been used as a laxative.

8197. Rhynchophylline. [76-66-4] (7β,16E,20α)-16,17-Didehydro-17-methoxy-2-oxocorynoxan-16-carboxylic acid methyl ester; rhyncophylline; mitrinermine. $C_{22}H_{28}N_2O_4$; mol wt 384.47. C 68.73%, H 7.34%, N 7.29%, O 16.65%. From stems and roots of *Uncaria rynchophylla* Miq. [*Ourouparia rynchophylla* (Miq.)] Matsum, *Rubiaceae:* Kondo *et al., J. Pharm. Soc. Jpn.* **48**, 54 (1928); from *Mitragyna rotundifolia* (Roxb.), *Rubiaceae:* Barger *et al., J. Org. Chem.* **4**, 418 (1939). Structure: Seaton, Marion, *Can. J. Chem.* **35**, 1102 (1957); **38**, 1035 (1960). Stereochemistry: Nozoye, *Chem. Pharm. Bull.* **6**, 309 (1958); Ban, Oishi, *Tetrahedron Lett.* **1961**, 791; *eidem, Chem. Pharm. Bull.* **11**, 441, 446, 451 (1963). Partial synthesis: Finch, Taylor, *J. Am. Chem. Soc.* **84**, 1318, 3871 (1962). Total synthesis: Ban *et al., Tetrahedron Lett.* **1972**, 2113.

Crystals from methanol, mp 216°; *dl*-form reported as colorless pillars from ethyl acetate-ether, mp 197-199° (Ban *et al., loc. cit.*). $[\alpha]_D^{13}$ −14.7° (c = 2.5 in chloroform). pKa 6.4. uv max: 245, 280 nm (log ε 4.24, 3.15). Sol in chloroform; moderately sol in acetone, alcohol, benzene; sparingly sol in ether, ethyl acetate. Practically insol in petr ether.

8198. Ribavirin. [36791-04-5] 1-β-D-Ribofuranosyl-1*H*-1,2,4-triazole-3-carboxamide; RTCA; tribavirin; ICN-1229; Copegus; Rebetol; Viramid; Virazide; Virazole. $C_8H_{12}N_4O_5$; mol wt 244.20. C 39.35%, H 4.95%, N 22.94%, O 32.76%. Purine nucleoside analog; inhibits inosine monophosphate dehydrogenase (IMPDH). Prepn: J. T. Witkowski, R. Robins, **DE 2220246**; *eidem*, **US 3798209** (1972, 1974 both to ICN); J. T. Witkowski *et al.*, *J. Med. Chem.* **15**, 1150 (1972); *eidem, J. Carbohydr. Nucleosides Nucleotides* **5**, 363 (1978). Regioselective synthesis: Y. Ito *et al.*, *Tetrahedron Lett.* **1979**, 2521. NMR study: G. P. Kreishman *et al.*, *J. Am. Chem. Soc.* **94**, 5894 (1972). Crystal structure: P. Prusiner, M. Sundaralingam, *Nature New Biol.* **244**, 116 (1973). Teratogenicity study: D. M. Kochhar *et al.*, *Toxicol. Appl. Pharmacol.* **52**, 99 (1980). Review of antiviral activity: R. W. Sidwell *et al.*, *Pharmacol. Ther.* **6**, 123-146 (1979); of clinical experience: H. Fernandez *et al.*, *Eur. J. Epidemiol.* **2**, 1-14 (1986); of molecular modes of action: J. L. Patterson, R. Fernandez-Larsson, *Rev. Infect. Dis.* **12**, 1139-1146 (1990). Clinical trial in infants with respiratory syncytial viral infection: C. B. Hall *et al.*, *N. Engl. J. Med.* **308**, 1443 (1983); in combination with interferon alfa-2b in hepatitis C: O. Reichard *et al.*, *Lancet* **351**, 83 (1998).

White to off-white powder. Freely sol in water; slightly sol in anhydrous alcohol. Exists in two polymorphic forms: mp 166-168° (aq ethanol); mp 174-176° (ethanol) (Witkowski, 1972). Also reported as mp 180-182° (Ito). $[\alpha]_D^{25} -36.5°$ (c = 1 in water); $[\alpha]_D^{20} -38°$ (c = 1 in water). LD$_{50}$ i.p. in mice: 1.3 g/kg; orally in rats: 5.3 g/kg (Witkowski, 1972).

THERAP CAT: Antiviral.

8199. α-Ribazole. [132-13-8] 5,6-Dimethyl-1-α-D-ribofuranosyl-1*H*-benzimidazole. $C_{14}H_{18}N_2O_4$; mol wt 278.30. C 60.42%, H 6.52%, N 10.07%, O 23.00%. Nucleoside moiety of vitamin B$_{12}$, *q.v.* Isoln by acid hydrolysis of vitamin B$_{12}$: N. G. Brink *et al., J. Am. Chem. Soc.* **72**, 1866 (1950); N. G. Brink, K. Folkers, *ibid.* **74**, 2856 (1952). Syntheses of α- and β-anomers: F. W. Holly *et al., ibid.* 4521; R. S. Wright *et al., ibid.* **80**, 2004 (1958); J. D. Stevens *et al., J. Org. Chem.* **33**, 1806 (1968). Biosynthetic study: J. Hörig, P. Renz, *FEBS Lett.* **80**, 337 (1977). Spectroscopic characterization: K. L. Brown *et al., Inorg. Chem.* **23**, 1463 (1984).

Crystals from water, mp 198-199°. $[\alpha]_D^{23} +14°$ (c = 0.9 in pyridine).

8200. Riboflavin. [83-88-5] Vitamin B$_2$; lactoflavine; vitamin G; 7,8-dimethyl-10-(D-*ribo*-2,3,4,5-tetrahydroxypentyl)isoalloxazine; 7,8-dimethyl-10-ribitylisoalloxazine; Beflavin; Flavaxin. $C_{17}H_{20}N_4O_6$; mol wt 376.36. C 54.25%, H 5.36%, N 14.89%, O 25.51%. Nutritional factor found in milk, eggs, malted barley, liver, kidney, heart, leafy vegetables. Richest natural source is yeast. Minute amounts present in all plant and animal cells. Occurs in the free form only in the retina of the eye, in whey, and in urine. Bioactive forms occurring in tissues and cells are riboflavin monophosphate and flavine-adenine dinucleotide, *q.q.v.* Syntheses: Karrer *et al., Helv. Chim. Acta* **18**, 426, 522 (1935); Kuhn *et al., Naturwissenschaften* **23**, 260 (1935); Howe, **US 2807611** (1957 to Merck & Co.); F. Yoneda *et al., J. Chem. Soc. Perkin Trans. 1* **1978**,

348. May also be produced by fermentation: Malzahn *et al.*, **US 2876169** (1959 to Grain Processing Corp.). Toxicity studies: Kuhn, Boulanger, *Z. Physiol. Chem.* **241**, 233 (1936); K. Unna, J. G. Greslin, *J. Pharmacol. Exp. Ther.* **76**, 75 (1942). Early reviews: Rosenberg in *The Vitamins* (New York, 1945); Sebrell, Harris, *The Vitamins* vol. III (Academic Press, New York, 1954) pp 299-402; Vogel-Knobloch, *Chemie und Technik der Vitamine* vol. II, part 1 (Enke, Stuttgart, 1955). Review of metabolism: Rivlin, *N. Engl. J. Med.* **283**, 463 (1970). Review of extraction and assay methods: Pearson, *The Vitamins* vol. VII, P. György, W. N. Pearson, Eds. (Academic Press, New York, 2nd ed., 1967) pp 99-136. Comprehensive reviews: *ibid.* vol. V, pp 1-96 (1972); F. J. Al-Shammary *et al., Anal. Profiles Drug Subs.* **19**, 429-476 (1990).

Fine orange-yellow needles from 2*N* acetic acid, alcohol, water, or pyridine. Dec at 278-282° (darkens at about 240°). Three different crystal forms having different solubilities in water: Dale, **US 2603633**; **US 2797215**. $[\alpha]_D^{25} -112$ to $-122°$ (50 mg in 2 ml 0.1*N* alcoholic NaOH dil to 10 ml with water). Absorption max: 220-225, 266, 371, 444, 475 nm. One gram dissolves in from 3000 to about 15,000 ml of water, the variations in the soly being due to differences in the crystal structure. Soly in alcohol (27.5°): 0.0045 g/100 ml of abs ethanol. Slightly sol in cyclohexanol, amyl acetate, benzyl alcohol, phenol; very sol in dil alkalies (with decompn). Insol in ether, chloroform, acetone, benzene. pKa 10.2; pKb 1.7. pH of satd aq soln: ~6. Isoelectric pt: pH 6. Aq solns are yellow showing a green fluorescence with max at 565 nm. Sensitive to alkalies; stable to mineral acids in the dark. Visible or ultraviolet irradiation of alkaline solns causes the formation of lumiflavine, *q.v.*, whereas irradiation of acid or neutral solns gives rise to the production of lumichrome, *q.v.*, together with varying amounts of lumiflavine. LD$_{50}$ in rats (g/kg): >10 orally, 5.0 s.c., 0.56 i.p. (Unna, Greslin).

2',3',4',5'-Tetrabutyrate. [752-56-7] Bituvitan; Eyekas; Hibon; Lacflavin; Ribolact; Wakaflavin L; Viras. $C_{33}H_{44}N_4O_{10}$; mol wt 656.72.

THERAP CAT: Vitamin (enzyme cofactor).

THERAP CAT (VET): Vitamin (enzyme cofactor).

8201. Riboflavin Monophosphate. [146-17-8] Riboflavin 5'-(dihydrogen phosphate); flavin mononucleotide; FMN; vitamin B$_2$ phosphate. $C_{17}H_{21}N_4O_9P$; mol wt 456.34. C 44.74%, H 4.64%, N 12.28%, O 31.55%, P 6.79%. One of the bioactive forms of riboflavin, *q.v.* Prepd by phosphorylation of riboflavin with chlorophosphoric acid: L. A. Flexser, W. G. Farkas, **US 2610179** (1952 to Hoffmann-La Roche); with pyrophosphoric acid: Breivogel, Ridge, **US 2535385** (1950 to White Labs.); with metaphosphoric acid: Viscontini *et al., Helv. Chim. Acta* **35**, 457 (1952); **US 2740775** (1956 to Hoffmann-La Roche); with pyrocatechol cyclic phosphate: Ukita *et al.*, **US 3118876** (1964 to Takeda).

Monosodium salt. [130-40-5] Hyryl; Ribo. $C_{17}H_{20}N_4NaO_9$-P; mol wt 478.33. Occurs as the dihydrate. Yellow crystals. Soly in water at pH 6.9 = 112 mg/ml; at pH 5.6 = 68 mg/ml; at pH 3.8 = 43 mg/ml. *Protect from light.*

THERAP CAT: Vitamin (enzyme cofactor).

THERAP CAT (VET): Vitamin (enzyme cofactor).

8202. Ribonuclease. [9001-99-4] RNase. An enzyme that digests RNA. First isolated from beef pancreas in 1920. Crystallization from acid extracts of pancreas: Kunitz, *J. Gen. Physiol.* **24**, 15 (1940). Isoln: Kunitz, McDonald, *Biochem. Prep.* **3**, 9 (1953). Bovine pancreatic RNase A is a single-chain peptide of 124 amino acid residues. Primary structure: C. H. W. Hirs *et al., J. Biol.*

Chem. **235,** 633 (1960). Amino acid sequence: D. H. Spackman *et al., ibid.* 648. Pictorial representation of entire structure: Stein, Moore, *Sci. Am.* **204,** no. 2, 81-92 (Feb. 1961). Ribonuclease from plant leaves has slightly different characteristics: Markham, Strominger, *Biochem. J.* **64,** 46P (1956). Can be obtained as a by-product of microbial erythromycin production: **JP 63 26938** (1963 to Shionogi). Chemical synthesis of materials possessing partial RNase enzyme activity: Gutte, Merrifield, *J. Am. Chem. Soc.* **91,** 501 (1969); Denkewalter, Hirschmann *et al., ibid.* 502. Series of articles describing the total synthesis of a protein having the full enzymic activity of bovine pancreatic RNase: N. Fujii, H. Yajima, *J. Chem. Soc. Perkin Trans. 1* **1981,** 789-841. Specifically catalyzes the cleavage of the phosphodiester bond between the 3′ and 5′ positions of the ribose moieties in RNA with the formation of oligonucleotides terminating in 2′,3′-cyclic phosphate derivs: Roberts *et al., Proc. Natl. Acad. Sci. USA* **62,** 1151 (1969). *Reviews:* Anfinsen, White, *The Enzymes* vol. 5, P. D. Boyer *et al.,* Eds. (Academic Press, New York, 2nd ed., 1961) pp 95-122; Richards, Wyckoff, *ibid.* vol. 4 (3rd ed., 1971) pp 647-806.

Crystals. $[\alpha]_D^{25}$ (per mg N) $-0.47°$ (c = 5). uv max (0.1*M* KCl soln): 277.5 nm (ε 9700). Isoelec pt about pH 8.0. Freely sol in water. Aq solns of cryst ribonuclease are quite stable at temps below 25°. The region of maximum stability is between pH 2 and 4.5. Stable for years stored as refrigerated dry powder or in frozen soln. Aggregates on lyophilization and storage. Shows affinity for glass surfaces. The optimum temp for digestion of yeast ribonucleic acid is 65°. The optimum pH is 7.7. Inhibited by heavy metal ions; by magnesium ions at concns as low as 0.0005*M*. Competitively inhibited by DNA, the effect of denatured DNA being greater than that of the native nucleic acid. Ribonuclease is precipitated by trichloroacetic acid, and does not diffuse through collodion or cellophane.

8203. Ribonucleic Acid. RNA; yeast nucleic acid. Polynucleotide directly involved in protein synthesis; found in both the nucleus and the cytoplasm of cells. The four primary nucleosides are adenosine, guanosine, cytidine and uridine, *q.q.v.*; minor nucleosides are also found. The nucleosides are linked by phosphate diester bonds from the 3′-hydroxyl of one D-ribose to the 5′-hydroxyl of the next. The secondary structure of RNA is that of an incompletely organized single-stranded polynucleotide consisting of some areas with helical structure alternating with nonhelical lengths. *Compare* Deoxyribonucleic Acid (DNA). Structure: Brown, Todd in *The Nucleic Acids* vol. 1, E. Chargaff, J. N. Davidson, Eds. (Academic Press, New York, 1955) pp 409-439; Spirin, *Prog. Nucleic Acid Res.* **1,** 301-345 (1963); J. N. Davidson, *The Biochemistry of Nucleic Acids* (Academic Press, New York, 7th ed., 1972) pp 106-128. Review of NMR studies: B. R. Reid, *Annu. Rev. Biochem.* **50,** 969-996 (1981). Book: *The Ribonucleic Acids,* P. R. Stewart, D. S. Letham, Eds. (Springer-Verlag, New York, 2nd ed., 1977).

Ribosomal RNA. rRNA. Metabolically stable form; about 80% of the RNA found in cells; an important component of ribosomes, which play a central role in protein synthesis. Two rRNA species of high molecular weight have been isolated from ribosomes: mol wts approx 0.6×10^6 and 1.1×10^6 in bacterial cells; higher in eukaryotic cells. In addition, at least one rRNA species of low mol wt, 5S RNA, has been identified; approx 120 nucleotides. *Reviews:* Attardi, Amaldi, *Annu. Rev. Biochem.* **39,** 183-226; Möller, Garrett, "The Ribonucleic Acids of the Bacterial Ribosome" in *Protein Synthesis* vol. 1, E. H. McConkey, Ed. (Dekker, New York, 1971) pp 229-272; Craig, "Ribosomal RNA Synthesis in Eukaryotes and its Regulation" in *MTP Int. Rev. Sci.: Biochem., Ser. One* vol. 6, K. Burton, Ed. (University Park Press, Baltimore, 1974) pp 255-288.

Messenger RNA. mRNA; informational RNA. A short-lived form of high molecular weight; acts as template for protein synthesis in the cell; complementary to one strand of DNA. A linear relationship exists between the sequence of amino acids in a polypeptide and the sequence of nucleotides in the corresponding mRNA and DNA. The genetic code has been proposed to explain the necessary translation process. The four purine and pyrimidine bases are treated as letters which can be combined to form 3-letter words or *codons*; 4^3 or 64 codons can be formed. 61 have been found to code for specific amino acids; the remaining three are probably chain termination codons. Reviews of mRNA and the genetic code: Lipmann, "Messenger Ribonucleic Acid" in *Prog. Nucleic Acid*

Res. **1,** 135-161 (1963); Crick, "The Recent Excitement in the Coding Problem" *ibid.,* pp 163-217; Woese, "The Present Status of the Genetic Code" in *Prog. Nucleic Acid Res. Mol. Biol.* **7,** 107-172 (1967); Hadjiolov, "Ribonucleic Acids and Information Transfer in Animal Cells" *ibid.* 195-242; Jukes, Gatlin, "Recent Studies Concerning the Coding Mechanism" *ibid.* **11,** 303-350 (1971); J. N. Davidson, *The Biochemistry of the Nucleic Acids* (Academic Press, New York, 7th ed., 1972) pp 290-383; Mathews, "Mammalian Messenger RNA" in *Essays in Biochemistry* vol. 9, P. N. Campbell, F. Dickens, Eds. (Academic Press, New York, 1973) pp 59-102; Brawerman, *Annu. Rev. Biochem.* **43,** 621-642 (1974); Watts, Watts, "The Genetic Code" in *MTP Int. Rev. Sci.: Biochem., Ser. One* vol. **7,** H. R. V. Arnstein, Ed. (University Park Press, Baltimore, 1975) pp 255-294.

Transfer RNA. tRNA; soluble RNA; sRNA. Low mol wt: 23,000-27,000; approx 75-85 nucleotides. Each tRNA is specific for and binds with a particular amino acid; more than one may exist for each amino acid. Performs three functions during protein synthesis: binds with its specific amino acid; recognizes the corresponding codon on mRNA and places the amino acid in the correct position for attachment to the polypeptide chain being formed; binds the polypeptide to the ribosome. First determination of total structure of a transfer RNA (yeast alanine tRNA): Holley *et al., Science* **147,** 1462 (1965). Reviews of structure and function: Miura, "Specificity in the Structure of Transfer RNA" in *Prog. Nucleic Acid Res. Mol. Biol.* **6,** 39-82 (1967); Cramer, "Three-Dimensional Structure of tRNA", *ibid.* **11,** 391-421 (1971); *Nucleic Acid Sequence Analysis,* S. Mandeles (Columbia University Press, New York, 1972) pp 256-280; Nishimura, "Transfer RNA: Structure and Biosynthesis" in *MTP Int. Rev. Sci.: Biochem., Ser. One* vol. 6, K. Burton, Ed. (University Park Press, Baltimore, 1974) pp 289-322; A. Rich, V. L. Raj Bhandary, *Annu. Rev. Biochem.* **45,** 805-860 (1976); P. F. Agris, *The Modified Nucleosides of Transfer RNA* **II** (A. R. Liss, New York, 1983) 220 pp.

8204. D-Ribose. [50-69-1] $C_5H_{10}O_5$; mol wt 150.13. C 40.00%, H 6.71%, O 53.29%. Prepd by hydrolysis of yeast-nucleic acid: Levene, Jacobs, *Ber.* **42,** 1201, 3247 (1909); Levene, Clark, *J. Biol. Chem.* **46,** 19 (1921); Bredereck, *Ber.* **71,** 408 (1938); Bredereck *et al., ibid.* **73,** 956 (1940); Phelps, *US 2152662* (1939 to U.S. Gov't); by ion-exchange resin chromatography: Cohn, *Science* **109,** 377 (1949); *J. Am. Chem. Soc.* **71,** 2275 (1949); **72,** 1471 (1950). From glucose: Karrer, *Helv. Chim. Acta* **18,** 1435 (1935); Austin, Humoller, *J. Am. Chem. Soc.* **56,** 1152 (1934); Kuhn *et al., Ber.* **68,** 1765 (1935); from nucleosides: Laufer, Charney, *US 2379913; US 2379914* (both 1945 to Schwarz Labs.); from D-erythrose: Sowden, *J. Am. Chem. Soc.* **72,** 808 (1950); from L-glutamic acid: Koga *et al., Tetrahedron Lett.* **1971,** 263. Reduction of D-ribonic acid: van Ekenstein, Blanksma, *Chem. Zentralbl.* **1913, II,** 1562; Steiger, *Helv. Chim. Acta* **19,** 189 (1936). *Review:* Overend, Stacey, in *Nucleic Acids* vol. I, E. Chargaff, J. N. Davidson, Eds. (Academic Press, New York, 1955) pp 1-80.

Plates from abs alcohol, mp 87°. Shows complex mutarotation: Phelps *et al., J. Am. Chem. Soc.* **56,** 748 (1934). Final $[\alpha]_D^{24}$ $-25°$ (water). Sol in water, slightly sol in alc.

Phenylosazone. $C_{17}H_{20}N_4O_3$. Yellow needles from pyridine + water, mp 163-164°.

Methyl-D-riboside. Crystals from ethyl acetate, mp 83-84°. $[\alpha]_D^{20}$ $-113.6°$ (p = 3), Minsaas, *Ann.* **512,** 286 (1934).

8205. D-Ribose-5-phosphoric Acid. [4300-28-1] 5-(Dihydrogen phosphate)-D-ribose; D-ribofuranose-5-phosphoric acid; D-ribose-5-phosphate. $C_5H_{11}O_8P$; mol wt 230.11. C 26.10%, H 4.82%, O 55.62%, P 13.46%. From inosinic acid: Levene, Jacobs, *Ber.* **41,** 2703 (1908); **44,** 746 (1911); Levene, Mori, *J. Biol. Chem.* **81,** 215 (1929); Levene, Stiller, *ibid.* **104,** 299 (1934); LePage, Umbreit, *ibid.* **148,** 255 (1943); Marmur *et al., Arch. Biochem. Biophys.* **34,** 209 (1951). Purification: Groth *et al., J. Biol. Chem.* **199,** 389 (1952). Differentiation between ribose-5-phosphate and ribose-3-phosphate by means of the orcinol-pentose reaction: Albaum, Umbreit, *ibid.* **167,** 369 (1947).

Barium salt hemihendecahydrate. $C_5H_9BaO_8P.5\frac{1}{2}H_2O$. Hexagonal plates from water. Sparingly soluble in cold water. Reduces Fehling's soln.

8206. Ribostamycin. [25546-65-0] *O*-2,6-Diamino-2,6-dideoxy-α-D-glucopyranosyl-(1→4)-*O*-[β-D-ribofuranosyl-(1→5)]-2-deoxy-D-streptamine; SF-733 antibiotic. $C_{17}H_{34}N_4O_{10}$; mol wt 454.47. C 44.93%, H 7.54%, N 12.33%, O 35.20%. Aminocyclitol antibiotic belonging to the neomycin, *q.v.*, group of antibiotics. Produced by *Streptomyces ribosidificus* (formerly called *S. thermoflavus*). Taxonomy, isoln and toxicity data: T. Shomura *et al.*, *J. Antibiot.* **23**, 155 (1970). Prepn: *eidem*, **DE 1814735** corresp to **US 3661892**, **US 3799842** (1969, 1972, 1974 all to Meiji). Structure: E. Akita *et al.*, *J. Antibiot.* **23**, 173 (1970). Synthesis from neamine, *q.v.*: Ito *et al.*, *Antimicrob. Agents Chemother.* **1970**, 33; *eidem*, *Agric. Biol. Chem.* **34**, 980 (1970); V. Kumar, W. A. Remers, *J. Org. Chem.* **43**, 3327 (1978); **46**, 4298 (1981). Total synthesis: H. Fukami *et al.*, *Tetrahedron Lett.* **1976**, 545; *eidem*, *Agric. Biol. Chem.* **41**, 1689 (1977). *In vitro* antibacterial activity: E. Yourassowsky, M. P. Vander Linden, *Arzneim.-Forsch.* **26**, 184 (1976).

Colorless needles from methanol, mp 192-195°. Also reported as monohydrate from water-methanol-ethanol, mp 175-180° (dec). $[\alpha]_D^{23}$ +42°. pKa′ 7.70. Stable in neutral and alkaline solns; slightly unstable in acidic media. Sol in water; slightly sol in methanol. Practically insol in acetone, *n*-butanol, ethyl acetate, benzene, hexane, ether.

Sulfate. [53797-35-6] Ibistacin; Landamycine; Ribostamin; Ribomycine; Vistamycin. White or yellowish powder. $[\alpha]_D^{20}$ +39° (c = 1). LD$_{50}$ i.v. in mice: 225 mg/kg (Shomura).

THERAP CAT: Antibacterial.

8207. D-Ribulose. [488-84-6] D-*erythro*-2-Pentulose; D-adonose; D-*erythro*-2-ketopentose. $C_5H_{10}O_5$; mol wt 150.13. C 40.00%, H 6.71%, O 53.29%. Prepn from D-arabinose: Glatthaar, Reichstein, *Helv. Chim. Acta* **18**, 80 (1935); from 2-keto-D-gluconic acid: Hall *et al.*, *Biochem. J.* **60**, 271 (1955); from D-fructose: P. M. Collins *et al.*, *J. Chem. Soc. Perkin Trans. 1* **1980**, 277. Stereoselective synthesis: M. Yamaguchi, T. Mukaiyama, *Chem. Lett.* **1981**, 1005; K. Suzuki *et al.*, *ibid.* 1529.

Sweet syrup. $[\alpha]_D^{24}$ −15° (c = 0.5 in water).

Diphosphate. $C_5H_{12}O_{11}P_2$. Prepn from D-ribose-5-phosphate: Horecker *et al.*, *Biochem. Prep.* **6**, 83 (1958).

8208. Rice Bran Oil. Oil of rice bran; rice oil. Extracted from bran obtained in making white or polished rice (which is actually the endosperm of the seed of *Oryza sativa* L., *Gramineae*). Rice bran separated by milling of hulled rice consists of bran, aleurone layer and germ, and contains about 15% oil. The oil is usually obtained by solvent extraction, *see* J. R. Loeb, N. J. Morris:

Abstract Bibliography of the Chemistry, Processing, and Utilization of Rice Bran and Rice Bran Oil, U.S. Dept. of Agriculture, Ms. no **AIC**-328 (1952 and suppl.). Rice bran contains an unusually active lipase which raises the free fatty acid content on storage. A variety of methods to inhibit this rise can be found in the literature: Williams *et al.*, *J. Am. Oil Chem. Soc.* **42**, 151 (1965). The free fatty acid content of the oil should not exceed 4 to 5%, but may run as high as 70%. Acceptable rice bran oil contains 15-20% of satd and 80-85% unsatd fatty acids as glycerides: Myristic 0.4-1%, palmitic 12-18%, stearic 1-3%, C_{20}-C_{22} satd 1%, oleic 40-50%, linoleic 29-42%, linolenic trace to 1%, palmitoleic 0.2-0.4%. *See also* Sreenivasan, *J. Am. Oil Chem. Soc.* **45**, 263 (1968).

Golden yellow oil, difficult to bleach. Not affected by temporary heating to 160°. d_{25}^{25} 0.916-0.921. n_D^{25} 1.470-1.473; n_D^{40} 1.465-1.468. Titer (solidification pt) 24-28. Saponification value 181-189. Acid value 4-120 (see above comments on the lipase content of the bran). Iodine value 99-108. Thiocyanogen value 69-76. Hydroxyl value 5-14. Reichert-Meissl value <0.5. Polenské value <0.5. Hehner value 95.3. Unsaponifiable matter 3-5%. The high refractive index is ascribed to the presence of squalene. Also contains other antioxidants such as tocopherols. Miscible with hexane and other fat solvents.

USE: Soaps, hydrogenated shortenings. Edible oil, also suitable for cosmetics and pharmaceuticals when low in free fatty acids and all the lipase has been deactivated.

8209. Ricin. [9009-86-3] A toxic lectin and hemagglutinin isolated from castor bean, *Ricinus communis* L., *Euphorbiaceae*: Stillmark, *Arb. Pharmak. Inst. Dorpat* **1889**, 59; T. Osborne *et al.*, *Am. J. Physiol.* **14**, 259 (1905); H. L. Craig *et al.*, **US 3060165** (1962 to U.S. Dept. Army). Purification of toxic ricin protein: M. Ishiguro *et al.*, *J. Biochem.* **55**, 587 (1964). The hemagglutinating activity of ricin was initially believed to be the cause of its high toxicity, but later studies have shown that separate proteins are responsible for the toxicity and hemagglutination: S. Olsnes, A. Pihl, *Biochemistry* **12**, 3121 (1973). "Ricin", the original term for the mixed extract, is now used in various ways. Two ricin agglutinins (*RCL I*, *RCL II* (agglutinins), *RCL III* or *Ricin D* and *RCL IV* (toxins), *cf.* T. T. Lin, S. S. Li, *Eur. J. Biochem.* **105**, 453 (1980). All four lectins consist of two different polypeptide chains joined by a disulfide bond; the toxins are dimers of an A-chain (30,000 Da) and a B-chain (33,000 Da) and the agglutinins occur as a tetramer composed of two 30,000 and two 33,000 mol wt subunits. Ricin has been shown to have anti-tumor properties: J. Y. Lin *et al.*, *Nature* **227**, 92 (1970); P. E. Thorp *et al.*, *ibid.* **297**, 594 (1982). Synergistic effect with daunorubicin, cisplatin, and vincristine, *q.q.v.*, in systemic L 1210 leukemia: O. Fodstad, A. Pihl, *Cancer Res.* **42**, 2152 (1982). Conjugates of ricin and cell-binding antigens or antibodies, called immunotoxins, have been used in cancer therapy: E. S. Vitetta *et al.*, *Science* **219**, 644 (1983). Experimental study with ricin-A chain conjugate in AIDS: M. A. Till *et al.*, *Science* **242**, 1166 (1988). RIA determn in blood: A. Godal *et al.*, *J. Toxicol. Environ. Health* **8**, 409 (1981). *Reviews:* M. Funatsu, "The Structure and Toxic Function of Ricin" in *Proteins, Structure and Function* vol. 2, M. Funatsu *et al.*, Eds. (Kodansha, Tokyo, Wiley, New York, 1972) pp 103-139; G. A. Balint, *Toxicology* **2**, 77-122 (1974); C. Winder, *J. Toxicol. Toxin Rev.* **23**, 97-103 (2004). *See also* Abrin, Lectins.

Isoelectric pt 7.1. uv max: 280 nm (ε 85000). MLD i.p. in mice at 48 hrs: 0.001 μg ricin nitrogen/g body wt (Ishiguro).

Caution: Ricin is among the most toxic compounds known. Seeds of *R. communis*, if thoroughly masticated, can produce serious poisoning and death: J. M. Kingsbury, *Poisonous Plants of the United States and Canada* (Prentice-Hall, New Jersey, 1964) pp 194-197. Potential symptoms of overexposure by inhalation are weakness, fever, cough, pulmonary edema, respiratory distress, hypoxia; by ingestion are abdominal pain, GI hemorrhage, liver, spleen and kidney damage (Widner).

USE: As a tool in studies of cell-surface properties; exptly in cancer research.

8210. Ricinine. [524-40-3] 1,2-Dihydro-4-methoxy-1-methyl-2-oxo-3-pyridinecarbonitrile; 1,2-dihydro-4-methoxy-1-methyl-2-oxonicotinonitrile; ricidine. $C_8H_8N_2O_2$; mol wt 164.16. C 58.53%, H 4.91%, N 17.06%, O 19.49%. From seeds and leaves of the castor plant, *Ricinus communis* L., *Euphorbiaceae*. Extraction procedure: Böttcher, *Ber.* **51,** 673 (1918). Synthesis starting with polymerization of cyanoacetyl chloride: Schroeter *et al., Ber.* **65,** 432 (1932). Biosynthesis: Waller, Henderson, *J. Biol. Chem.* **236,** 1186 (1961); Essery *et al., Can. J. Chem.* **41,** 1142 (1963).

Prisms, needles from alc, mp 201.5°. Sublimes at 170-180° under 20 mm pressure. Sparingly sol in water, alc, chloroform, ether. Neutral to litmus. Does not form salts with acids.

Caution: Ingestion may cause nausea, vomiting, hemorrhagic gastroenteritis, hepatic and renal damage, convulsions, coma, hypotension, respiratory depression, death.

8211. Ricinoleic Acid. [141-22-0] (9*Z*,12*R*)-12-Hydroxy-9-octadecenoic acid; *d*-12-hydroxyoleic acid. $C_{18}H_{34}O_3$; mol wt 298.46. C 72.44%, H 11.48%, O 16.08%. $CH_3(CH_2)_5CH(OH)$-$CH_2CH=CH(CH_2)_7COOH$. Found primarily in oils from the seeds of *Ricinus* spp, *Euphorbiaceae*. Accounts for about 90% of the triglyceride fatty acids of castor oil, and up to about 40% of the glyceride fatty acids of ergot oil. Bibliography on its isoln: Ralston, *Fatty Acids* (New York, 1948) p 189. Also isolated from *Linum mucronatum* (flax), *Linaceae:* Kleiman, Spencer, *Lipids* **6,** 962 (1971). Structure: Goldsobel, *Ber.* **27,** 3121 (1894). Mechanism of biosynthesis: Morris, *Biochem. Biophys. Res. Commun.* **29,** 311 (1967).

Liquid. $d_4^{27.4}$ 0.940; mp 5.5°; bp_{10} 245°. $[\alpha]_D^{22}$ +6.67°; $[\alpha]_D^{26}$ +7.15° (c = 5 in acetone). n_D^{20} 1.4716. Neutralization value 187.98; iodine value 85.05. Sol in alcohol, acetone, ether, chloroform (*cf.* the solubilities of castor oil).

Acid sulfate. Ricinolsulfuric acid. $C_{18}H_{34}O_6S$. Obtained by the action of chlorosulfonic acid. Viscous brown liquid with weak blue fluorescence. Sol in water (about 10%), alcohol, ether, chloroform.

Sodium salt. [5323-95-5] Soricin; Colidosan. Sodium salts of the fatty acids from castor oil. White or slightly yellow, odorless or almost odorless powder. Sol in water or alcohol. The aq soln is alkaline.

USE: In textile finishing; sometimes added to Turkey red oil, dry-cleaning soaps.

THERAP CAT: Has been used in contraceptive jellies. The sodium salt has been used as sclerosing agent.

8212. Ridogrel. [110140-89-1] 5-[[(*E*)-[3-Pyridinyl[3-(tri-fluoromethyl)phenyl]methylene]amino]oxy]pentanoic acid; R-68070. $C_{18}H_{17}F_3N_2O_3$; mol wt 366.33. C 59.02%, H 4.68%, F 15.56%, N 7.65%, O 13.10%. Combined thromboxane A_2 synthase inhibitor and thromboxane A_2/prostaglandin endoperoxide receptor antagonist. Prepn: E. J. E. Freyne *et al., EP 221601; eidem,* **US 4963573** (1987, 1990 both to Janssen). Clinical pharmacology: B. Hoet *et al., Thromb. Haemostasis* **64,** 87 (1990); C. Weber *et al., ibid.* **68,** 214 (1992). Clinical study in peripheral arterial obstructive disease: J. De Cree *et al., Int. Angiol.* **12,** 59 (1993); as adjunct to thrombolysis in acute myocardial infarction: RAPT Investigators, *Circulation* **89,** 588 (1994).

Crystals from diisopropyl ether/hexane (2:1), mp 70.3°.
THERAP CAT: Antithrombotic.

8213. Rifabutin. [72559-06-9] 1′,4-Didehydro-1-deoxy-1,4-dihydro-5′-(2-methylpropyl)-1-oxorifamycin XIV; (9*S*,12*E*,-14*S*,15*R*,16*S*,17*R*,18*R*,19*R*,20*S*,21*S*,22*E*,24*Z*)-6,16,18,20-tetrahy-droxy-1′-isobutyl-14-methoxy-7,9,15,17,19,21,25-heptamethyl-spiro[9,4-(epoxypentadeca[1,11,13]trienimino)-2*H*-furo[2′,3′:7,-8]naphth[1,2-*d*]imidazole-2,4′-piperidine]-5,10,26-(3*H*,9*H*)-trione-

16-acetate; 4-deoxo-3,4-[2-spiro-(*N*-isobutyl-4-piperidyl)]-(1*H*)-imidazo-(2,5-dihydro)rifamycin S; 4-*N*-isobutylspiropiperidylrifamycin S; LM-427; Ansatipine; Mycobutin. $C_{46}H_{62}N_4O_{11}$; mol wt 847.00. C 65.23%, H 7.38%, N 6.61%, O 20.78%. Semisynthetic derivative of rifamycin S that inhibits nucleic acid synthesis. Prepn: L. Marsili *et al.,* **DE 2825445** (1979 to Farmitalia); *eidem,* **US 4219478** (1980 to Archifar Labs). *In vitro* and *in vivo* antibacterial activity: A. Sanfilippo *et al., J. Antibiot.* **33,** 1193 (1980); C. Della Bruna *et al., ibid.* **36,** 1502 (1983). Mechanism of action: D. Ungheri *et al., Drugs Exp. Clin. Res.* **10,** 681 (1984). Comparative *in vitro* antimycobacterial spectrum: J. M. Dickinson, D. A. Mitchison, *Tubercle* **68,** 177 (1987). *In vitro* inhibition of HIV-1 replication: R. Anand *et al., Antimicrob. Agents Chemother.* **32,** 684 (1988). Clinical pharmacokinetics: M. H. Skinner *et al., ibid.* **33,** 1237 (1989). Pharmacology and clinical efficacy in mycobacterial infections: R. J. O'Brien *et al., Rev. Infect. Dis.* **9,** 519 (1987).

Violet-red crystalline powder. Highly sol in chloroform, sol in methanol, slightly sol in ethanol, minimally sol in water. uv max (methanol): 493, 315, 274, 238 nm.
THERAP CAT: Antibacterial (tuberculostatic).

8214. Rifalazil. [129791-92-0] 1′,4-Didehydro-1-deoxy-1,4-dihydro-3′-hydroxy-5′-[4-(2-methylpropyl)-1-piperazinyl]-1-oxorifamycin VIII; (2*S*,16*Z*,18*E*,20*S*,21*S*,22*R*,23*R*,24*R*,25*S*,26*R*,-27*S*,28*E*)-5,12,21,23,25-pentahydroxy-10-(4-isobutyl-1-piperazinyl)-27-methoxy-2,4,16,20,22,24,26-heptamethyl-2,7-(epoxypentadeca[1,11,13]trienimino)-6*H*-benzofuro[4,5-*a*]phenoxazine-1(2*H*),6,15-trione 25-acetate; 3′-hydroxy-5′-(4-isobutyl-1-piperazinyl)benzoxazinorifamycin; KRM-1648. $C_{51}H_{64}N_4O_{13}$; mol wt 941.07. C 65.09%, H 6.85%, N 5.95%, O 22.10%. Semisynthetic derivative of rifamycin S, *q.v.* Prepn: T. Yamane *et al., EP 366914; eidem,* **US 4983602** (1990, 1991 both to Kanegafuchi); *eidem, Chem. Pharm. Bull.* **41,** 148 (1993). Antimycobacterial efficacy in comparison with rifampin, *q.v.:* T. Yamamoto *et al., Antimicrob. Agents Chemother.* **40,** 426 (1996). Pharmacokinetics: K. Hosoe *et al., ibid.* 2749. HPLC determn in biological fluids: *eidem, J. Chromatogr. B* **653,** 177 (1994). Review of pharmacology and clinical studies: D. M. Rothstein *et al., Expert Opin. Invest. Drugs* **12,** 255-271 (2003).

Crystals from chloroform-hexane, mp 195-200° (dec).
THERAP CAT: Antibacterial (tuberculostatic).

8215. Rifamide. [2750-76-7] 4-*O*-[2-(Diethylamino)-2-oxoethyl]-rifamycin; 2-[(1,2-dihydro-5,6,17,19,21-pentahydroxy-23-methoxy-2,4,12,16,18,20,22-heptamethyl-1,11-dioxo-2,7-(epoxypentadeca[1,11,13]trienimino)naphtho[2,1-*b*]furan-9-yl)oxy]-*N*,*N*-diethylacetamide 21-acetate; *N*,*N*-diethylrifomycin B amide; rifamycin B diethylamide; M-14; Rifocin M. $C_{43}H_{58}N_2O_{13}$; mol wt 810.93. C 63.69%, H 7.21%, N 3.45%, O 25.65%. Prepn: **BE 632770**; Sensi, Maggi, **US 3313804** (1963, 1967 both to Lepetit); Sensi *et al., J. Med. Chem.* **7**, 596 (1964). Physical and chemical properties: Maggi *et al., Farmaco Ed. Prat.* **20**, 147 (1965). Activity data: Pallanza *et al., Arzneim.-Forsch.* **15**, 800 (1965); Monnier, Bourse, *Pathol. Biol.* **16**, 901 (1968). Metabolic studies: Fürész *et al., Arzneim.-Forsch.* **15**, 802 (1965); Maffii, Shiatti, *Toxicol. Appl. Pharmacol.* **8**, 138 (1966). Toxicology: Dezulian *et al., ibid.* 126.

Yellow-orange ppt, crystallized from benzene + hexane. No definite mp, begins to soften at 140°, melts completely at 170° (dec). $[\alpha]_D^{20}$ −48.7° (c = 0.4 in methanol). Absorption max in phosphate buffer (pH 7.38): 222, 302, 421 nm (ε 42820, 20770, 16200). LD_{50} in mice, rats (mg/kg): 2450, >4000 orally; 640, 2500 s.c.; 320, 535 i.v. (Dezulian).
THERAP CAT: Antibacterial.

8216. Rifampin. [13292-46-1] 3-[[(4-Methyl-1-piperazinyl)imino]methyl]rifamycin; 5,6,9,17,19,21-hexahydroxy-23-methoxy-2,4,12,16,18,20,22-heptamethyl-8-[*N*-(4-methyl-1-piperazinyl)formimidoyl]-2,7-(epoxypentadeca[1,11,13]trienimino)-naphtho[2,1-*b*]furan-1,11(2*H*)-dione 21-acetate; rifampicin; rifaldazine; rifamycin AMP; R/AMP; Abrifam; Eremfat; Rifa; Rifadin(e); Rifaldin; Rifapiam; Rifaprodin; Rifoldin; Rimactan(e). $C_{43}H_{58}N_4O_{12}$; mol wt 822.94. C 62.76%, H 7.10%, N 6.81%, O 23.33%. Semisynthetic antibiotic obtained by reacting 3-formylrifamycin SV with 1-amino-4-methylpiperazine in tetrahydrofuran. Prepn and structure: Maggi *et al., Chemotherapia* **11**, 285 (1966); **NL 6509961**; Maggi, Sensi, **US 3342810** (1966, 1967 both to Lepetit). Chemical and biological properties: Fürész, *Antibiot. Chemother.* **16**, 316 (1970). Activity studies and clinical survey: Arioli *et al., Arzneim.-Forsch.* **17**, 523 (1967); Pallanza *et al., ibid.* 529; Bergamini, *ibid.* **20**, 1546 (1970); Dans *et al., Am. J. Med. Sci.* **259**, 120 (1970). Metabolism: Meyer-Brunot *et al., Int. Congr. Chemother. Proc., 5th, Vienna 1967* **1**(2), 763; Fürész *et al., Arzneim.-Forsch.* **17**, 534 (1967); Maggi *et al., ibid.* **19**, 651 (1969). Inhibition of protein synthesis in mammalian cells: W. C. Buss *et al., Science* **200**, 432 (1978). Comprehensive reviews: Binda *et al., Arzneim.-Forsch.* **21**, 1907-1978 (1971); Lester, *Annu. Rev. Microbiol.* **26**, 88-102 (1972). Comprehensive description: G. G. Gallo, P. Radaelli, *Anal. Profiles Drug Subs.* **5**, 467-513 (1976). Symposium on the use of rifampin in the treatment of nontuberculous infections: *Rev. Infect. Dis.* **5**, Suppl. 3, S399-S632 (1983).

Red to orange platelets from acetone, dec 183-188°. Absorption max (pH 7.38): 237, 255, 334, 475 nm (ε 33200, 32100, 27000, 15400). Rifampin is a "zwitterion" with pKa 1.7 related to the 4-hydroxy and pKa 7.9 related to the 3-piperazine nitrogen. Very stable in DMSO; rather stable in water. Freely sol in CH_3Cl,

DMSO; sol in ethyl acetate, methanol, tetrahydrofuran; slightly sol in water (pH <6), acetone, carbon tetrachloride. LD_{50} in mice, rats (mg/kg): 885, 1720 orally; 260, 330 i.v.; 640, 550 i.p. (Fürész).

THERAP CAT: Antibacterial (tuberculostatic).

8217. Rifamycins. Rifomycins. Group of antibiotics characterized by a natural ansa structure (chromophoric naphtho-hydroquinone group spanned by a long aliphatic bridge) not previously found in other known antibiotics. Isoln from the fermentation broths of *Streptomyces mediterranei*: P. Sensi *et al., Antibiot. Annu.* **1959-1960**, 262. Among rifamycins, rifamycin B, O, S, SV and X are the more studied members. Prepn of rifamycin B derivs: P. Sensi *et al.,* **US 3313804** (1967 to Lepetit). Structure: Prelog, *Pure Appl. Chem.* **7**, 551 (1963); *Chemotherapia* **7**, 133 (1963); Oppolzer *et al., Experientia* **20**, 336 (1964); Oppolzer, Prelog, *Helv. Chim. Acta* **56**, 2287 (1973). Total synthesis of rifamycin S: H. Nagaoka *et al., J. Am. Chem. Soc.* **102**, 7962 (1980); H. Iio *et al., ibid.* 7965; H. Nagaoka, Y. Kishi, *Tetrahedron* **37**, 3873 (1981); S. Hanessian *et al., J. Am. Chem. Soc.* **104**, 6164 (1982). Review of chemistry of ansamycin antibiotics: K. L. Rinehart *et al., Fortschr. Chem. Org. Naturst.* **33**, 231-307 (1976). General reviews: P. Sensi, *Research Progress in Organic-Biological & Medicinal Chemistry* vol. **1**, U. Gallo, L. Santamaria, Eds. (Società Editoriale Farmaceutica, Milan, Italy, 1964) pp 337-421; Wehrli, Staehelin, in *Antibiotics* vol. **3**, J. W. Corcoran, F. E. Hahn, Eds. (Springer-Verlag, New York, 1975) pp 252-268; C. Gurgo *et al.,* "Rifamycins" in *Handbook of Experimental Pharmacology* vol. **61**, G. V. R. Born *et al.,* Eds., entitled "Chemotherapy of Viral Infections", P. E. Came, L. A. Caliguiri, Eds. (Springer-Verlag, New York, 1982) pp 519-555.

	R	R'
Rifamycin B	—OCH_2COOH	—OH
Rifamycin O	—(1,3-dioxolan-4-on)-2-yl	=O
Rifamycin S	=O	=O
Rifamycin X	=N$\overset{+}{=}$N$^-$	=O

Rifamycin AMP *see* Rifampin.
Rifamycin B. [13929-35-6] 4-*O*-(Carboxymethyl)rifamycin; nancimycin. $C_{39}H_{49}NO_{14}$; mol wt 755.80. Yellow prismatic needles from benzene, mp 300° (dec 160-164°). $[\alpha]_D^{20}$ −11° (methanol). Absorption max (phosphate buffer soln pH 7.3): 223, 304, 425 nm ($E_{1cm}^{1\%}$ 555, 275, 220). Dibasic acid. Very stable. Solubili-

ties: water 0.027% (w/w), methanol 2.62%, ethanol 0.44%. LD_{50} in mice (mg/kg): 2040 i.v., >3000 i.p., s.c., and orally (Sensi, 1964).

Rifamycin O. [14487-05-9] 4-O-(Carboxymethyl)-1-deoxy-1,4-dihydro-4-hydroxy-1-oxorifamycin γ-lactone. $C_{39}H_{47}NO_{14}$; mol wt 753.79. Prepn: P. Sensi et al., Farmaco Ed. Sci. **15,** 228 (1960); Umezawa, **JP 66 15518** (1966), C.A. **66,** 1583v (1967). Pale yellow crystals from methanol, mp 300° (dec 160°). Also reported as mp 180-185° (Umezawa). $[\alpha]_D^{20}$ +71.5° (c = 1 in dioxane). uv max (methanol contg 5% acetate buffer soln pH 4.62): 226, 273, 370 nm ($E_{1cm}^{1\%}$ 365, 440, 60). Weak acid. Slowly sol in alkaline soln with red-violet color. Sol in acetone, tetrahydrofuran; slightly sol in methanol, ethanol, ethyl acetate. Practically insol in ether, petr ether, water, dilute acids.

Rifamycin S. [13553-79-2] 1,4-Dideoxy-1,4-dihydro-1,4-dioxorifamycin. $C_{37}H_{45}NO_{12}$; mol wt 695.75. Activation product found in solns of rifamycin B and rifamycin O: P. Sensi et al., Experientia **16,** 412 (1960). Yellow-orange crystals from methanol, dec 179-181°. $[\alpha]_D^{20}$ +476° (c = 0.1 in methanol). Absorption max (phosphate buffer soln pH 7.3): 317, 525 nm ($E_{1cm}^{1\%}$ 426, 62). LD_{50} in mice (mg/kg): 122 i.v.; 258 i.p.; 3000 orally (Sensi, 1964).

Rifamycin SV see separate entry.

Rifamycin X. $C_{37}H_{45}N_3O_{11}$; mol wt 707.77. Prepn: Greco et al., Farmaco Ed. Sci. **16,** 766 (1961). Yellow crystals, no definite mp, dec 135-140°. Unstable to light. $[\alpha]_D^{20}$ +491.8° (c = 0.981 in dioxane). Absorption max (acetate buffer soln): 286, 317, 402 nm ($E_{1cm}^{1\%}$ 400, 362, 195). Practically insol in water. Sol in methanol, ethanol, ethyl acetate, benzene.

Rifamycin AG. A condensation product of rifamycin O and aminoguanidine: P. Sensi et al., Antibiot. Chemother. **12,** 448 (1962).

8218. Rifamycin SV. [6998-60-3] 5,6,9,17,19,21-Hexahydroxy-23-methoxy-2,4,12,16,18,20,22-heptamethyl-2,7-(epoxypentadeca[1,11,13]trienimino)naphtho[2,1-b]furan-1,11(2H)-dione 21-acetate; rifomycin SV; rifamicine SV. $C_{37}H_{47}$-NO_{12}; mol wt 697.77. C 63.69%, H 6.79%, N 2.01%, O 27.52%. Semi-synthetic antibiotic derived from Rifamycin S. Prepn: Sensi et al., Experientia **16,** 412 (1960); Farmaco Ed. Sci. **16,** 165 (1961). Comprehensive review: Bergamini, Fowst, Arzneim.-Forsch. **15,** 951-1002 (1965). For general refs see Rifamycins.

Yellow-orange crystals, mp 300° (dec 140°). $[\alpha]_D^{20}$ −4° (methanol). uv max (phosphate buffer soln pH 7.3): 223, 314, 445 nm ($E_{1cm}^{1\%}$ 586, 322, 204). Acid reaction. Slightly sol in water, petr ether; sol in ether, bicarbonate soln; very sol in methanol, ethanol, acetone, ethyl acetate. A reducing substitute, such as ascorbic acid, should be added to aq solns of rifamycin SV to prevent its transformation to rifamycin S. LD_{50} in mice (mg/kg): 550 i.v.; 625 i.p.; 2120 orally (Bergamini, Fowst).

Sodium salt. [14897-39-3] Rifamastene; Rifocin. Orange-red crystals. Soly in water pH 7.2: ~5 g/100 ml.

THERAP CAT: Antibacterial.

THERAP CAT (VET): Antibacterial.

8219. Rifapentine. [61379-65-5] 3-[[(4-Cyclopentyl-1-piperazinyl)imino]methyl]rifamycin; MDL-473; DL-473; R-773; Priftin. $C_{47}H_{64}N_4O_{12}$; mol wt 877.03. C 64.37%, H 7.36%, N 6.39%, O 21.89%. Semi-synthetic rifamycin. Prepn: R. Cricchio, V. Arioli, **DE 2608218**; idem, **US 4002752** (1976, 1977 both to

Lepetit). Antibacterial activity: V. Arioli et al., J. Antibiot. **34,** 1026 (1981); H. C. Neu, Antimicrob. Agents Chemother. **24,** 457 (1983). Pharmacokinetics: A. Assandri et al., J. Antibiot. **37,** 1066 (1984). HPLC determn in plasma: E. Riva et al., J. Chromatogr. **553,** 35 (1991). Clinical trial in tuberculosis: Natl. Co-op Group Clin. Study Rifapentine, Chin. J. Antibiot. **17,** 313 (1992), B.A. **95,** 70840 (1993). Review of pharmacology and clinical efficacy: B. Jarvis, H. M. Lamb, Drugs **56,** 607-616 (1998).

Crystals from ethyl acetate, mp 179-180°. uv max: 475, 334 nm (ε 15200, 26700). LD_{50} in mice (mg/kg): >2000 orally; 750 i.p. (Cricchio). Also reported as LD_{50} in mice (mg/kg): 3300 orally; 710 i.p. (Aroli).

THERAP CAT: Antibacterial (tuberculostatic).

8220. Rifaximin. [80621-81-4] (2S,16Z,18E,20S,21S,22R,-23R,24R,25S,26R,27S,28E)-25-(Acetyloxy)-5,6,21,23-tetrahydroxy-27-methoxy-2,4,11,16,20,22,24,26-octamethyl-2,7-(epoxypentadeca[1,11,13]trienimino)benzofuro[4,5-e]pyrido[1,2-a]benzimidazole-1,15(2H)-dione; 4-deoxy-4'-methylpyrido[1',2'-1,2]imidazo[5,4-c]rifamycin SV; rifamycin L 105; rifaxidin; L-105; Fatroximin; Flonorm; Normix; Rifacol; Xifaxan. $C_{43}H_{51}N_3O_{11}$; mol wt 785.88. C 65.72%, H 6.54%, N 5.35%, O 22.39%. Non-absorbable semisynthetic rifamycin antibiotic. Prepn: **BE 888895**; E. Marchi, L. Montecchi, **US 4341785** (1981, 1982 both to Alfa); E. Marchi et al., J. Med. Chem. **28,** 960 (1985); and NMR study: M. Brufani et al., J. Antibiot. **37,** 1611 (1984). X-ray crystal structure: idem et al., ibid. 1623. In vitro and in vivo antibacterial activity: A. P. Venturini, E. Marchi, Chemioterapia **5,** 257 (1986). Toxicological study: G. Borelli, D. Bertoli, ibid. 263. Clinical trial in travelers' diarrhea: R. Steffen et al., Am. J. Gastroenterol. **98,** 1073 (2003). Review of activity, pharmacokinetics and clinical experience in gastrointestinal infections: J. C. Gillis, R. N. Brogden, Drugs **49,** 467-484 (1995); D. B. Huang, H. L. DuPont, J. Infection **50,** 97-106 (2005).

Red orange powder, mp 200-205° (dec). uv max: 232, 260, 292, 320, 370, 450 nm ($E_{1cm}^{1\%}$ 489, 339, 295, 216, 119, 159). Sol in alcohols, ethyl acetate, chloroform, toluene. Insol in water. LD_{50} orally in rats: >2000 mg/kg (Borelli, Bertoli).

THERAP CAT: Antibacterial.

THERAP CAT (VET): Antibacterial.

8221. Rilmazafone. [99593-25-6] 5-[[(Aminoacetyl)amino]methyl]-1-[4-chloro-2-(2-chlorobenzoyl)phenyl]-*N,N*-dimethyl-1*H*-1,2,4-triazole-3-carboxamide; 1-(2-*o*-chlorobenzoyl-4-chlorophenyl)-5-glycylaminomethyl-3-dimethylcarbamoyl-1*H*-1,2,4-triazole; 2′,5-dichloro-2-(3-dimethylcarbamoyl-5-glycylaminomethyl-1*H*-1,2,4-triazol-1-yl)benzophenone. $C_{21}H_{20}Cl_2N_6O_3$; mol wt 475.33. C 53.06%, H 4.24%, Cl 14.92%, N 17.68%, O 10.10%. Ring-opened triazolobenzodiazepine derivative. Prepn: K. Hirai, H. Sugimoto, **DE 2725164**; *eidem,* **US 4159374** (1977, 1979 both to Shionogi); and CNS activity: K. Hirai *et al., J. Heterocycl. Chem.* **19,** 1363 (1982). Receptor binding study of rilmazafone and its closed ring active metabolites: M. Fujimoto *et al., Biochem. Pharmacol.* **33,** 1645 (1984). Combined HPLC determn and enzyme immunoassay in plasma: G. Kominami *et al., J. Chromatogr.* **417,** 216 (1987). Series of articles on teratogenicity studies: *Oyo Yakuri* **30,** 749-833 (1985), *C.A.* **104,** 81885h-81887k; 102328w (1986).

Monohydrochloride dihydrate. 450191-S; Rhythmy. $C_{21}H_{20}$-$Cl_2N_6O_3 \cdot HCl \cdot 2H_2O$; mol wt 547.82. Solid from 95% ethanol, mp 107°. LD_{50} orally in mice: >1500 mg/kg (Hirai, 1979).
THERAP CAT: Sedative, hypnotic.

8222. Rilmenidine. [54187-04-1] *N*-(Dicyclopropylmethyl)-4,5-dihydro-2-oxazolamine; 2-[*N*-(dicyclopropylmethyl)amino]oxazoline; oxaminozoline; S-3341. $C_{10}H_{16}N_2O$; mol wt 180.25. C 66.63%, H 8.95%, N 15.54%, O 8.88%. α_2-Adrenoceptor agonist. Prepn: C. Malen *et al.,* **DE 2362754**; *eidem,* **US 4102890** (1974, 1978 both to Sci. Union et Cie. - Soc. Franc. Recher. Med.). Adrenoceptor binding study: P. Guicheney *et al., J. Pharmacol.* **12,** 255 (1981). Pharmacokinetics in hypertensive subjects: J. Velly *et al., ibid.* **13,** 413 (1982). Animal pharmacology: M. Laubie *et al., ibid.* **16,** 259 (1985); P. A. van Zwieten *et al., Arch. Int. Pharmacodyn.* **279,** 130 (1986). Hypotensive effect in humans: K. Weerasuriya *et al., Eur. J. Clin. Pharmacol.* **27,** 281 (1984). Mechanism of action study: R. E. Gomez *et al., Eur. J. Pharmacol.* **195,** 181 (1991). *Review:* T. J. Verbeuren *et al., Cardiovasc. Drug Rev.* **8,** 56-70 (1990).

Crystals from hexane, mp 106-107°.
Phosphate. S-3341-3; Hyperium. $C_{10}H_{16}N_2O \cdot H_3PO_4$; mol wt 278.24. pKa 9.3. Soly in H_2O: ~19% w/v; in methanol: ~7% w/v; in chloroform and ethanol: ~0.7% w/v. LD_{50} orally in mice, rats: 375, 295 mg/kg (Verbeuren).
Fumarate. $C_{14}H_{20}N_2O_5$. Crystals from ethanol, mp 170°.
THERAP CAT: Antihypertensive.

8223. Riluzole. [1744-22-5] 6-(Trifluoromethoxy)-2-benzothiazolamine; 2-amino-6-(trifluoromethoxy)benzothiazole; PK-26124; RP-54274; Rilutek. $C_8H_5F_3N_2OS$; mol wt 234.20. C 41.03%, H 2.15%, F 24.34%, N 11.96%, O 6.83%, S 13.69%. Modulates glutamatergic transmission. Prepn: L. M. Yagupol'skii, L. Z. Gandel'sman, *Zh. Obshch. Khim.* **33,** 2301 (1963), *C.A.* **60,** 692a (1964). Prepd but not claimed: J. Mizoule, **EP 50551**; *idem,* **US 4370338** (1982, 1983 both to Pharmindustrie). Pharmacology:

J. Mizoule *et al., Neuropharmacology* **24,** 767 (1985); F. Wahl *et al., Eur. J. Pharmacol.* **230,** 209 (1993). Mechanism of action studies: M.-W. Debono *et al., ibid.* **235,** 283; D. Martin *et al., ibid.* **250,** 473. Use in treatment of motor nerve diseases: E. Louvel, **EP 558861** (1993 to Rhône-Poulenc Rorer). Clinical study in amyotrophic lateral sclerosis: G. Bensimon *et al., N. Engl. J. Med.* **330,** 585 (1994). Review: J. Wokke, *Lancet* **348,** 795-799 (1996).

Crystals from ethanol/water (1:1), mp 119°. LD_{50} in mice (mg/kg): 46 i.p.; 67 orally (Mizoule).
THERAP CAT: Neuroprotective.

8224. Rimantadine. [13392-28-4] α-Methyltricyclo-[3.3.1.1^{3,7}]decane-1-methanamine; α-methyl-1-adamantanemethylamine; remantadin(e). $C_{12}H_{21}N$; mol wt 179.30. C 80.38%, H 11.81%, N 7.81%. Deriv of adamantane, *q.v.* Prepn: **NL 6408505**; W. W. Prichard, **US 3352912** (1965, 1967 both to du Pont). Antiviral activity: A. Tsunoda *et al., Antimicrob. Agents Chemother.* **1965,** 553. Effects on influenza in mice: J. W. McGahen *et al., Ann. N.Y. Acad. Sci.* **173,** 557 (1970). Mechanism of action study: A. Bukrinskaya *et al., Arch. Virol.* **66,** 275 (1980); *eidem, J. Gen. Virol.* **60,** 49 (1982). Pharmacokinetics in humans: R. J. Wills *et al., Antimicrob. Agents Chemother.* **31,** 826 (1987). Clinical trial in prophylaxis of influenza A infection: R. Dolin *et al., N. Engl. J. Med.* **307,** 580 (1982). Comparative toxicity of rimantadine and amantadine in healthy adults: F. G. Hayden *et al., Antimicrob. Agents Chemother.* **19,** 226 (1981). Controlled study of CNS effects: V. M. Millet *et al., ibid.* **21,** 1 (1982). Review of studies in the USSR on exptl and clinical pharmacology: D. M. Zlydnikov *et al., Rev. Infect. Dis.* **3,** 408-421 (1981).

Hydrochloride. [1501-84-4] EXP-126; Flumadine; Meradan(e); Roflual. $C_{12}H_{21}N \cdot HCl$; mol wt 215.76. White crystals, mp 373-375° (sealed tube).
THERAP CAT: Antiviral.

8225. Rimazolium Metilsulfate. [28610-84-6] 3-(Ethoxycarbonyl)-6,7,8,9-tetrahydro-1,6-dimethyl-4-oxo-4*H*-pyrido[1,2-*a*]pyrimidinium methyl sulfate; 3-carboxy-6,7,8,9-tetrahydro-1,6-dimethyl-4-oxo-4*H*-pyrido[1,2-*a*]pyrimidinium methyl sulfate, ethyl ester; 1,6-dimethyl-3-carbethoxy-4-oxo-6,7,8,9-tetrahydro-homopyrimidazole methyl sulfate; MZ-144; MZ-0780; Ro-11-780; Dolcuran; Probon; Probonal; Rimagina. $C_{14}H_{22}N_2O_7S$; mol wt 362.40. C 46.40%, H 6.12%, N 7.73%, O 30.90%, S 8.85%. Prepn: Z. Mészáros *et al.,* **HU Teljes 519** (1970 to Chinoin), *C.A.* **74,** 42374h (1971); *eidem, Arzneim.-Forsch.* **22,** 815 (1972). Anti-inflammatory and analgesic effects in animals: K. Gyires *et al., Drugs Exp. Clin. Res.* **11,** 493 (1985). Clinical analgesic effect: H. Graber, *Int. J. Clin. Pharmacol. Ther. Toxicol.* **6,** 354 (1972); M. Haataja *et al., Curr. Ther. Res.* **22,** 784 (1977). Series of articles on pharmacology, pharmacodynamics and toxicology: *Arzneim.-Forsch.* **21,** 717-738 (1971). Toxicity data: J. Knoll *et al., ibid.* **21,** 719.

White crystals, mp 165-166°. uv max: 336, 258 nm (ε 3630, 27500). Readily sol in water. LD_{50} in rats (mg/kg): 220 i.v.; 720 i.p.; 790 s.c.; 1600 orally (Knoll).

THERAP CAT: Analgesic.

8226. Rimexolone. [49697-38-3] (11β,16α,17β)-11-Hydroxy-16,17-dimethyl-17-(1-oxopropyl)androsta-1,4-dien-3-one; 11β-hydroxy-16α,17α-dimethyl-17-propionylandrosta-1,4-dien-3-one; 11β-hydroxy-16α,17α,21-trimethylpregna-1,4-diene-3,20-dione; trimexolone; Org-6216; Rimexel; Vexol. $C_{24}H_{34}O_3$; mol wt 370.52. C 77.80%, H 9.25%, O 12.95%. Prepn: NL 7300313; G. F. Woods *et al.*, US 3947478 (1973, 1976 both to Akzo); J. Cairns *et al., J. Chem. Soc. Perkin Trans. 1* 1981, 2306. Pharmacology: P. K. Fox *et al., Arzneim.-Forsch.* **30,** 55 (1980). Clinical trial in rheumatoid arthritis: E. van Vliet-Daskalopoulou *et al., Br. J. Rheumatol.* **26,** 450 (1987). Clinical pharmacokinetics: G. Gevers *et al., Clin. Rheumatol.* **13,** 103 (1994).

Crystals, mp 258-268°. [α]_D +100° (c = 0.92 in pyridine). uv max: 244 nm (ε 14600).

THERAP CAT: Anti-inflammatory (local).

8227. Rimiterol. [32953-89-2] 4-(Hydroxy-2-piperidinyl-methyl)-1,2-benzenediol; *erythro*-α-(3,4-dihydroxyphenyl)-2-piperidinemethanol; *erythro*-3,4-dihydroxyphenyl-2-piperidinylcarbinol. $C_{12}H_{17}NO_3$; mol wt 223.27. C 64.55%, H 7.67%, N 6.27%, O 21.50%. Prepn: G. H. Sankey, K. D. E. Whiting, DE 2024049; idem, US 3910934 (1970, 1975 to 3M); C. Kaiser, S. T. Ross, DE 2047937; idem, US 3705169 (1971, 1972 to SK & F); G. H. Sankey, K. D. E. Whiting, *J. Heterocycl. Chem.* **9,** 1049 (1972). Pharmacology: Carney *et al., Arch. Int. Pharmacodyn. Ther.* **194,** 334 (1971); Griffin, Turner, *J. Clin. Pharmacol.* **11,** 280 (1971); Bowman, Rodger, *Br. J. Pharmacol.* **45,** 574 (1972).

Crystals from ethyl acetate, mp 203-204°.

Hydrobromide. [31842-61-2] R-798; WG-253; Asmaten; Pulmadil. $C_{12}H_{17}NO_3$·HBr; mol wt 304.18. White powder, mp 220° (dec).

THERAP CAT: Bronchodilator.

8228. Rimocidin. [1393-12-0] $C_{39}H_{61}NO_{14}$; mol wt 767.90. C 61.00%, H 8.01%, N 1.82%, O 29.17%. Polyene antifungal antibiotic produced by *Streptomyces rimosus* along with oxytetracycline, *q.v.* Recovered from fermentation broth by extracting the mycelium with butanol. Isoln and antifungal activity: Davisson *et al., Antibiot. Chemother.* **1,** 289 (1951); Seneca *et al., ibid.* **2,** 435 (1952); Davisson *et al.,* US 2963401 (1960 to Pfizer). Partial structure: Cope *et al., J. Am. Chem. Soc.* **87,** 5452 (1965). Structure: L. Falkowski *et al., J. Antibiot.* **29,** 197 (1976); R. Pandey, K. L. Rinehart, *ibid.* **30,** 146 (1977).

Dec above 110°. [α]_D^{25} +116° (pyridine). uv max (80% methanol): 279, 291, 304, 318 nm. Slightly sol in water, acetone, lower alcohols. A cryst sodium salt was prepd by reaction with NaOH in methanol.

Sulfate heptahydrate. Large plates from dil methanol, dec 151°. [α]_D^{25} +75.2° (methanol). Sol in water. LD_{50} i.v. in mice: 20 mg/kg (Seneca).

8229. Rimonabant. [168273-06-1] 5-(4-Chlorophenyl)-1-(2,4-dichlorophenyl)-4-methyl-*N*-1-piperidinyl-1*H*-pyrazole-3-carboxamide; *N*-(piperidin-1-yl)-5-(4-chlorophenyl)-1-(2,4-dichlorophenyl)-4-methyl-1*H*-pyrazole-3-carboxamide; SR-141716; Acomplia. $C_{22}H_{21}Cl_3N_4O$; mol wt 463.79. C 56.97%, H 4.56%, Cl 22.93%, N 12.08%, O 3.45%. Brain cannabinoid receptor (CB$_1$) antagonist. Prepn: F. Barth *et al.*, EP 576357; idem., US 5624941 (1993, 1997 both to Sanofi); H. H. Seltzman *et al., J. Chem. Soc. Chem. Commun.* 1995, 1549; and pharmacology: A. K. Dutta *et al., Med. Chem. Res.* **5,** 54 (1994). Receptor antagonist activity: M. Rinaldi-Carmona *et al., FEBS Lett.* **350,** 240 (1994). Clinical trial in blockade of effects of smoked marijuana: M. A. Huestis *et al., Arch. Gen. Psychiatry* **58,** 322 (2001). Clinical trials in obesity: L. F. Van Gaal *et al., Lancet* **365,** 1389 (2005); J.-P. Després *et al., N. Engl. J. Med.* **353,** 2121 (2005). Review of therapeutic potential in obesity and drug addiction: M. A. M. Carai *et al., Life Sci.* **77,** 2339-2350 (2005).

Hydrochloride. [158681-13-1] SR-141716A. $C_{22}H_{21}Cl_3N_4$·O.HCl; mol wt 500.25. White crystals from ether + petr ether, mp 154-156° (Dutta); also reported as mp 157-159° (Seltzman).

THERAP CAT: Antiobesity agent.

8230. Rimsulfuron. [122931-48-0] *N*-[[(4,6-Dimethoxy-2-pyrimidinyl)amino]carbonyl]-3-(ethylsulfonyl)-2-pyridinesulfonamide; DPX-E9636; Matrix; Titus. $C_{14}H_{17}N_5O_7S_2$; mol wt 431.44. C 38.97%, H 3.97%, N 16.23%, O 25.96%, S 14.86%. Sulfonylurea herbicide; blocks branched-chain amino acid synthesis by inhibiting the plant enzyme, acetolactate synthase. Prepd (not claimed): P. H. Liang, US 4774337 (1988 to DuPont); and use in herbicidal mixtures: idem, EP 341011 (1989 to DuPont), C.A. **113,** 6360 (1990). Comprehensive description: H. L. Palm *et al., Brighton Crop Prot. Conf. - Weeds* 1989, 23-28. HPLC, TLC determn and environmental fate: G. E. Schneiders *et al., J. Agric. Food Chem.* **41,** 2402 (1993). Field trials in potatoes: C. V. Eberlein *et al., Weed Technol.* **8,** 428 (1994).

mp 176-178°. pKa 4.1. Vapor pressure at 25°: 1.1×10^{-8} Torr. Soly in water at 25° (ppm): 135 (pH 5); 7300 (pH 7); 5560 (pH 9). Partition coefficient (octanol/water): 0.034 (pH 7). LD_{50} orally in rats: >5000 mg/kg; dermally in rabbits: >2000 mg/kg (Palm).

USE: Herbicide.

8231. Rioprostil. [77287-05-9] (11α,13E)-1,11,16-Trihydroxy-16-methylprost-13-en-9-one; (2R,3R,4R)-4-hydroxy-2-(7-

hydroxyheptyl)-3-[(E)-(4RS)-(4-hydroxy-4-methyl-1-octenyl)]-cyclopentanone; 16-methyl-1,11α,16RS-trihydroxyprost-13E-en-9-one; Bay o 6893; ORF-15927; TR-4698; Rostil. $C_{21}H_{38}O_4$; mol wt 354.52. C 71.15%, H 10.80%, O 18.05%. Prostaglandin E_1 analog with cytoprotective and gastric antisecretory activity. Prepn: H. C. Kluender *et al.*, *US 4132738* (1979 to Miles). Pharmacology: D. A. Shriver *et al.*, *Arzneim.-Forsch.* **35**, 839 (1985). Effect on human gastric secretion: P. Demol *et al.*, *ibid.* 861; B. Vaona *et al.*, *Adv. Prostaglandin Thromboxane Leukotriene Res.* **17**, 328 (1987). Clinical evaluation in duodenal ulcer: H. G. Dammann *et al.*, *ibid.* 303.

$[\alpha]_D$ −58.6° (c = 1 in chloroform).

THERAP CAT: Antiulcerative.

8232. Risedronic Acid. [105462-24-6] [1-Hydroxy-2-(3-pyridinyl)ethylidene]bisphosphonic acid; 2-(3-pyridinyl)-1-hydroxyethane diphosphonic acid. $C_7H_{11}NO_7P_2$; mol wt 283.11. C 29.70%, H 3.92%, N 4.95%, O 39.56%, P 21.88%. Bisphosphonate antiresorptive agent. Prepn: J. J. Benedict, C. M. Perkins, **EP 186405**; *eidem*, **US 5583122** (1986, 1996 both to Procter & Gamble). Pharmacology: W. S. S. Jee *et al.*, *Bone* **14**, 493 (1993). Clinical trial in Paget's disease: E. S. Siris *et al.*, *J. Bone Miner. Res.* **13**, 1032 (1998); in postmenopausal bone loss: L. Mortensen *et al.*, *J. Clin. Endocrinol. Metab.* **83**, 396 (1998). Clinical effect on reduction of fracture risk: S. T. Harris *et al.*, *J. Am. Med. Assoc.* **282**, 1344 (1999). Review of pharmacology and clinical efficacy: K. L. Goa, J. A. Balfour, *Drugs Aging* **13**, 83-91 (1998).

Monosodium salt. [115436-72-1] Risedronate sodium; NE-58095; Actonel; Optinate. $C_7H_{10}NNaO_7P_2$; mol wt 305.09. Fine, white to off-white, odorless crystalline powder. Occurs as the hemi-pentahydrate. Sol in water. Essentially insol in common organic solvents.

THERAP CAT: Bone resorption inhibitor.

8233. Risperidone. [106266-06-2] 3-[2-[4-(6-Fluoro-1,2-benzisoxazol-3-yl)-1-piperidinyl]ethyl]-6,7,8,9-tetrahydro-2-methyl-4H-pyrido[1,2-a]pyrimidin-4-one; R-64766; Belivon; Risperdal. $C_{23}H_{27}FN_4O_2$; mol wt 410.48. C 67.30%, H 6.63%, F 4.63%, N 13.65%, O 7.80%. Combined serotonin (5-HT$_2$) and dopamine (D$_2$) receptor antagonist. Prepn: L. E. J. Kennis, J. Vandenberk, **EP 196132**; *eidem*, **US 4804663** (1986, 1989 both to Janssen). Pharmacology: P. A. J. Janssen *et al.*, *J. Pharmacol. Exp. Ther.* **244**, 685 (1988). Receptor binding studies: J. E. Leysen *et al.*, *ibid.* **247**, 661 (1988). HPLC determn in plasma: A. Avenoso *et al.*, *J. Chromatogr. B* **746**, 173 (2000). Clinical study in psychoses: Y. G. Gelders *et al.*, *Pharmacopsychiatry* **23**, 206 (1990); in autism: L. Scahill *et al.*, *N. Engl. J. Med.* **347**, 314 (2002). Brief review: M. G. Livingston, *Lancet* **343**, 457-460 (1994). Review of pharmacology and therapeutic potential: S. Grant, A. Fitton, *Drugs* **48**, 253-273 (1994); B. Green, *Curr. Med. Res. Opin.* **16**, 57-65 (2000); of clinical experience in schizophrenia: H.-J. Möller, *Expert Opin. Pharmacother.* **6**, 803-818 (2005),

Crystals from DMF + 2-propanol, mp 170.0°. LD$_{50}$ in male, female mice, rats, dogs (mg/kg): 29.7, 26.9, 34.3, 35.4, 14.1, 18.3 i.v.; 82.1, 63.1, 113, 56.6, 18.3, 18.3 orally (Janssen, 1988).

THERAP CAT: Antipsychotic.

8234. Ristocetin. [1404-55-3] Ristomycin; Spontin; Riston. Glycopeptide antibiotic complex produced by the actinomycete *Nocardia lurida*. Ristocetin A and the more active ristocetin B differ in the number of glucose, mannose, rhamnose and D-arabinose groups in their side chains. Isoln, crystallizn and chemical properties: J. E. Philip *et al.*, *Antibiot. Annu.* **1956-57**, p 699; *eidem*, **US 2990329** (1961 to Abbott). Total structure determn of ristocetin A: D. H. Williams *et al.*, *Chem. Commun.* **1979**, 906; J. R. Kalman, D. H. Williams, *J. Am. Chem. Soc.* **102**, 897 (1980). Identity of ristocetin A with ristomycin A: D. H. Williams *et al.*, *J. Chem. Soc. Perkin Trans. 1* **1979**, 787. ^{13}C-NMR studies: F. Sztaricskai *et al.*, *Tetrahedron Lett.* **21**, 2983 (1980); M. P. Williamson, D. H. Williams, *J. Chem. Soc. Perkin Trans. 1* **1981**, 1483. Revised configuration: C. M. Harris, T. M. Harris, *J. Am. Chem. Soc.* **104**, 363 (1982). Biosynthesis: S. J. Hammond *et al.*, *Chem. Commun.* **1983**, 116. Tool for investigation of platelet aggregation: Howard, Firkin, *Thromb. Diath. Haemorrh.* **26**, 362 (1971). *Review:* D. C. Jordan, *Antibiotics* vol. 1, D. Gottlieb, P. Shaw, Eds. (Springer-Verlag, New York, 1967) pp 84-89.

Ristocetin A

Crystalline sulfates. Sol in acidic aq solns; much less sol in the neutral pH range. Generally insol in organic solvents. Both components show good stability in aq acidic solns, but are readily inactivated above pH 7.0. Commercial prepns are mixtures of both with >90% ristocetin A.

Ristocetin A. [11021-66-2] Ristomycin A. $C_{95}H_{110}N_8O_{44}$; mol wt 2067.92. C 55.18%, H 5.36%, N 5.42%, O 34.04%. Cryst sulfate, $[\alpha]_D$ −120 to −133° (water).

Ristocetin B. [1405-59-0] Ristomycin B. $C_{84}H_{92}N_8O_{35}$. Cryst sulfate, $[\alpha]_D$ −144 to −149° (water).

USE: Peptide-based probe for platelet aggregation.

THERAP CAT: Antibacterial.

8235. Ritanserin. [87051-43-2] 6-[2-[4-[Bis(4-fluorophenyl)methylene]-1-piperidinyl]ethyl]-7-methyl-5H-thiazolo[3,2-a]-pyrimidin-5-one; R-55667; Tiserton. $C_{27}H_{25}F_2N_3OS$; mol wt 477.57. C 67.90%, H 5.28%, F 7.96%, N 8.80%, O 3.35%, S 6.71%. Selective serotonin (5-HT$_2$) receptor antagonist. Prepn: L. E. J. Kennis *et al.*, **EP 110435**; *eidem*, **US 4533665** (1984, 1985 both to Janssen). Pharmacological profile: F. Awouters *et al.*, *Drug Dev. Res.* **15**, 61 (1988). GC/MS determn in plasma and pharmacokinetics: P. Timmerman *et al*, *Biomed. Environ. Mass Spectrom.* **18**, 498 (1989). Clinical studies: G. Nappi *et al.*, *Headache* **30**, 439 (1990); G. Bersani *et al.*, *Acta Psychiatr. Scand.* **83**, 244 (1991); J. M. Monti *et al.*, *Sleep* **16**, 647 (1993).

Crystals from acetonitrile, mp 145.5°. LD$_{50}$ in male, female mice, rats, dogs (mg/kg): 28.2, 28.2, 20.0, 22.2, 24.1, 33.2 i.v.; 626, 993, 956, 515, ~1280, 640-1280 orally (Awouters).

L-Tartrate. [93076-39-2] $C_{27}H_{25}F_2N_3OS.C_4H_6O_6$. Solid from 2-propanol, mp 198.7°.

THERAP CAT: Anxiolytic; antidepressant.

8236. Ritipenem. [84845-57-8] (5R,6S)-3-[[(Aminocarbonyl)oxy]methyl]-6-[(1R)-1-hydroxyethyl]-7-oxo-4-thia-1-azabicyclo[3.2.0]hept-2-ene-2-carboxylic acid; (5R,6S,8R)-6α-hydroxyethyl-2-carbamoyloxymethyl-2-penem-3-carboxylic acid; (5R,6S)-6-[(1R)-1-hydroxyethyl]-3-(hydroxymethyl)-7-oxo-4-thia-1-azabicyclo[3.2.0]hept-2-ene-2-carboxylic acid, 3-carbamate. $C_{10}H_{12}N_2O_6S$; mol wt 288.28. C 41.66%, H 4.20%, N 9.72%, O 33.30%, S 11.12%. Prepn: M. Alpegiani *et al.,* **DE 3245270**; M. Foglio *et al.,* **US 4482565** (1983, 1984 both to Carlo Erba). Synthesis: G. Franceschi *et al., J. Antibiot.* **36**, 938 (1983). Total synthesis: W. Cabri *et al., Tetrahedron Lett.* **34**, 3491 (1993). Toxicity study: M. Brughera *et al., J. Antimicrob. Chemother.* **23**, Suppl. C, 129 (1989). Series of articles on synthesis, *in vitro* activity, metabolism: *ibid.,* 1-204 (1989). Clinical pharmacokinetics of acid and ester forms: S. R. Norrby *et al., ibid.* **25**, 371 (1990); A. M. Lovering *et al., ibid.* **29**, 179 (1992). HPLC determn in serum and urine: R. Mendez *et al., J. Chromatogr.* **579**, 115 (1992).

Sodium salt. [84845-58-9] FCE-22101. $C_{10}H_{11}N_2NaO_6S$; mol wt 310.26. $[\alpha]_D^{20}$ +140°. uv max (H$_2$O): 258, 306 nm (ε 4150, 6030). LD$_{50}$ in male, female mice, male, female rats (mg/kg): 3872, 4493, 2000, 2201 i.v. (Brughera).

Acetoxymethyl ester. [87238-52-6] Ritipenem acoxil; FCE-22891. $C_{13}H_{16}N_2O_8S$; mol wt 360.34. LD$_{50}$ in male, female mice, male, female rats (mg/kg): 4363, 6167, >5000, >5000 orally (Brughera).

THERAP CAT: Antibacterial.

8237. Ritodrine. [26652-09-5] (αS)-*rel*-4-Hydroxy-α-[(1R)-1-[[2-(4-hydroxyphenyl)ethyl]amino]ethyl]benzenemethanol; *erythro*-p-hydroxy-α-[1-[(p-hydroxyphenethyl)amino]ethyl]benzyl alcohol; N-[2-(p-hydroxyphenyl)ethyl]-N-[2-(p-hydroxyphenyl)-2-hydroxy-1-methylethyl]amine; 1-(4-hydroxyphenyl)-2-[2-(4-hydroxyphenyl)ethylamino]propanol; N-(p-hydroxyphenylethyl)-4-hydroxynorephedrine. $C_{17}H_{21}NO_3$; mol wt 287.35. C 71.06%, H 7.37%, N 4.87%, O 16.70%. β_2-Adrenergic agonist. Prepn: **BE 660244** (1965 to N.V. Philips); Claassen *et al.,* **US 3410944** (1968 to No. Am. Philips). Clinical investigations: Coutinho *et al., Am. J. Obstet. Gynecol.* **104**, 1053 (1969); Landesman *et al., ibid.* **110**, 111 (1971); Wesselius-De Casparis *et al., Br. Med. J.* **3**, 144 (1971). Clinical efficacy in treatment of preterm labor: J. F. Larsen *et al., Obstet. Gynecol.* **67**, 607 (1986).

Base. Resinous mass, mp 88-90°.

Hydrochloride. [23239-51-2] DU-21220; Miolene; Prempar; Pre-Par; Utemerin; Utopar; Yutopar. $C_{17}H_{21}NO_3.HCl$; mol wt 323.81. mp 193-195° (dec) from ethanol-ether. uv max: 267.5 nm (ε 3310).

THERAP CAT: Tocolytic.

8238. Ritonavir. [155213-67-5] (5S,8S,10S,11S)-10-Hydroxy-2-methyl-5-(1-methylethyl)-1-[2-(1-methylethyl)-4-thiazolyl]-3,6-dioxo-8,11-bis(phenylmethyl)-2,4,7,12-tetraazatridecan-13-oic acid 5-thiazolylmethyl ester; (2S,3S,5S)-5-[N-[N-[[N-methyl-N-[(2-isopropyl-4-thiazolyl)methyl]amino]carbonyl]valinyl]amino]-2-[N-[(5-thiazolyl)methoxycarbonyl]amino]-1,6-diphenyl-3-hydroxyhexane; A-84538; Abbott 84538; ABT-538; Norvir. $C_{37}H_{48}N_6O_5S_2$; mol wt 720.94. C 61.64%, H 6.71%, N 11.66%, O 11.10%, S 8.90%. Peptidomimetic HIV-1 protease inhibitor. Prepn: D. J. Kempf *et al.,* **WO 9414436**; *eidem,* **US 5541206** (1994, 1996 both to Abbott). Antiretroviral spectrum, pharmacokinetics: *idem et al., Proc. Natl. Acad. Sci. USA* **92**, 2484 (1995). Structural model for drug resistance: M. Markowitz *et al., J. Virol.* **69**, 701 (1995). HPLC determn in biological fluids: R. M. W. Hoetelmans *et al., J. Chromatogr. B* **705**, 119 (1998). Review of clinical experience: A. P. Lea, D. Faulds, *Drugs* **52**, 541-546 (1996). Clinical trial with nucleoside analogs in HIV-infected children: S. A. Nachman *et al., Med. Assoc.* **283**, 492 (2000). Clinical trial with lopinavir, *q.v.,* in HIV infection: S. Walmsley *et al., N. Engl. J. Med.* **346**, 2039 (2002).

THERAP CAT: Antiviral.

8239. Rituximab. [174722-31-7] Anti-(human CD20 antigen) immunoglobulin G1 (human-mouse monoclonal IDEC-C2B8 γ_1-chain) disulfide with human-mouse monoclonal IDEC-C2B8 κ-chain, dimer; IDEC-C2B8; Mabthera; Rituxan. Genetically engineered chimeric murine-human monoclonal antibody directed against the CD20 antigen found on normal and malignant B lymphocyte surfaces. Contains murine light and heavy-chain variable regions and γ_1 heavy-chain and κ light chain human constant regions. Composed of 2 heavy chains of 451 amino acids and 2 light chains of 213 amino acids; approx mol wt 145 kD. Prepn: D. R. Anderson *et al.,* **WO 9411026**; *eidem,* **US 5763137** (1994, 1998 both to IDEC); M. E. Reff *et al., Blood* **83**, 435 (1994). HPLC determn of product purity: K. G. Moorhouse *et al., J. Pharm. Biomed. Anal.* **16**, 593 (1997). Clinical pharmacokinetics: N. L. Berinstein *et al., Ann. Oncol.* **9**, 995 (1998). Clinical trial in lymphoma: P. McLaughlin *et al., J. Clin. Oncol.* **16**, 2825 (1998); in combination with CHOP chemotherapy: M. S. Czuczman *et al., ibid.* **17**, 268 (1999). Review of clinical studies: C. A. White, *Cancer Biother. Radiopharm.* **14**, 241-250 (1999); and pharmacology: S. V. Onrust *et al., Drugs* **58**, 79-88 (1999). Clinical evaluation in hematologic autoimmune diseases: F. Zaja *et al., Haematologica* **87**, 189 (2002).

THERAP CAT: Antineoplastic.

8240. Rivastigmine. [123441-03-2] Ethylmethylcarbamic acid 3-[(1S)-1-(dimethylamino)ethyl]phenyl ester; (S)-N-ethyl-3-[(1-dimethylamino)ethyl]-N-methylphenylcarbamate. $C_{14}H_{22}N_2O_2$; mol wt 250.34. C 67.17%, H 8.86%, N 11.19%, O 12.78%. Brain selective acetylcholinesterase inhibitor. Prepn: A. Enz, **DE 3805744**; *idem,* **US 5602176** (1988, 1997 both to Sandoz); and activity: R. Amstutz *et al., Helv. Chim. Acta* **73**, 739 (1990). Pharmacology: A. Enz *et al., Prog. Brain Res.* **98**, 431 (1993). Clinical trial in Alzheimer's disease: M. Rösler *et al., Br. Med. J.* **318**, 633 (1999).

$[\alpha]_D^{20}$ −32.1° (c = 5 in ethanol).

Hydrogen tartrate. [129101-54-8] ENA-713; SDZ-ENA-713; SDZ-212-713; Exelon. $C_{14}H_{22}N_2O_2 \cdot C_4H_6O_6$; mol wt 400.42. Crystals from ethanol, mp 123-125°. $[\alpha]_D^{20}$ +4.7° (c = 5 in ethanol).

THERAP CAT: Nootropic.

8241. Rizatriptan. [144034-80-0] N,N-Dimethyl-5-(1H-1,2,4-triazol-1-ylmethyl)-1H-indole-3-ethanamine; 3-[2-(dimethylamino)ethyl]-5-(1H-1,2,4-triazol-1-ylmethyl)indole; N,N-dimethyl-2-[5-(1,2,4-triazol-1-ylmethyl)-1H-indol-3yl]ethylamine. $C_{15}H_{19}$-N_5; mol wt 269.34. C 66.89%, H 7.11%, N 26.00%. Selective serotonin 5-HT$_{1D}$ receptor agonist; structurally derived from tryptamine. Prepn: R. Baker *et al.*, **EP 497512**; *eidem*, **US 5298520** (1992, 1994 both to Merck Sharp & Dohme); and binding characteristics: L. J. Street *et al.*, *J. Med. Chem.* **38**, 1799 (1995). Synthesis: C. Chen *et al.*, *Tetrahedron Lett.* **35**, 6981 (1994). Clinical pharmacokinetics: H. Cheng *et al.*, *Biopharm. Drug Dispos.* **17**, 17 (1996). LC-MS determn in plasma: D. A. McLoughlin *et al.*, *J. Chromatogr. A* **726**, 115 (1996). Comparative clinical trial in treatment of migraine: J. U. Adelman *et al.*, *Neurology* **57**, 1377 (2001). Review of pharmacology and therapeutic efficacy: K. Wellington, G. L. Plosker, *Drugs* **62**, 1539-1574 (2002).

mp 120-121°.

Benzoate. [145202-66-0] MK-0462; MK-462; Maxalt. C_{15}-$H_{19}N_5 \cdot C_6H_5COOH$; mol wt 391.47. mp 178-180°.

THERAP CAT: Antimigraine.

8242. Robenidine. [25875-51-8] Bis[(4-chlorophenyl)methylene]carbonimidic dihydrazide; 1,3-bis[(p-chlorobenzylidene)amino]guanidine. $C_{15}H_{13}Cl_2N_5$; mol wt 334.20. C 53.91%, H 3.92%, Cl 21.22%, N 20.96%. Prepn: Tomcufcik, **DE 1933112** (1970 to Am. Cyanamid), *C.A.* **72**, 90113c (1970). Activity studies: Kantor *et al.*, *Science* **168**, 373 (1970); Wong *et al.*, *Biochem. Biophys. Res. Commun.* **46**, 621 (1972). Metabolism: Zulalian *et al.*, 163rd Am. Chem. Soc. Meeting (Boston, April 1972) *Abstracts of Papers*, PEST 12, 13. Animal studies: Millard, *Res. Vet. Sci.* **11**, 394 (1970); Joyner, Norton, *ibid.* **13**, 279 (1972).

Hydrochloride. [25875-50-7] Robenzidene; Cycostat; Robenz. $C_{15}H_{13}Cl_2N_5 \cdot HCl$; mol wt 370.66. Crystals from ethanol, mp 289-290°.

THERAP CAT (VET): Coccidiostat.

8243. Robinin. [301-19-9] 3-[[6-O-(6-Deoxy-α-L-mannopyranosyl)-β-D-galactopyranosyl]oxy]-7-[(6-deoxy-α-L-mannopyranosyl)oxy]-5-hydroxy-2-(4-hydroxyphenyl)-4H-1-benzopyran-4-one; kaempferol 3-robinoside 7-rhamnoside. $C_{33}H_{40}O_{19}$; mol wt 740.66. C 53.51%, H 5.44%, O 41.04%. Dimorphic flavanoid isolated from the leaves and flowers of *Robinia pseudoacacia* L., *Leguminosae*: C. Zwenger, F. Dronke, *Ann.* **suppl. 1**, 257 (1861); C. Sando, *J. Biol. Chem.* **94**, 675 (1932). Structure: Zemplén, Bognár, *Ber.* **74B**, 1783 (1941). Total synthesis and structure: L. Farkas *et al.*, *Phytochemistry* **15**, 215 (1976).

β-Form. Yellow crystals, mp 250-254° (Farkas); also reported as straw-yellow needles from alc, mp 249-250° (Sando). uv max (ethanol): 352, 368 nm (log ε 4.14, 4.18), Jurd, Horowitz, *J. Org. Chem.* **22**, 1619 (1957). Sol in hot water, hot alc; practically insol in ether. On hydrolysis yields kaempferol, *q.v.*

α-Form. Obtained by crystallization from water and dehydrating, mp 195-197° (Sando). Also reported as hydrate, yellow needles from aq methanol, mp 196-199° (Farkas).

8244. Roccellic Acid. [29838-46-8] (2R,3S)-2-Dodecyl-3-methylbutanedioic acid; (2R,3S)-2-dodecyl-3-methylsuccinic acid; d-α-dodecyl-β-methylsuccinic acid; d-α-methyl-α'-dodecylsuccinic acid. $C_{17}H_{32}O_4$; mol wt 300.43. C 67.96%, H 10.74%, O 21.30%. Occurs in lichens. Isoln from *Lecanora sordida* (Pers.) Th. Fries, *Parmeliaceae*: Hesse, *J. Prakt. Chem.* **58**, 497 (1898); Kennedy *et al.*, *Sci. Proc. R. Dublin Soc.* **21**, 557 (1937); from *Roccella montagnei*, *Graphidaceae*: Subbaraya, Seshadri, *Proc. Indian Acad. Sci.* **12A**, 466 (1940); from *Crocynia membranacae* (Dicks.)Zahlbr., *Chrysotrichaceae*: Akermark *et al.*, *Acta Chem. Scand.* **13**, 1855 (1959). Structure: Kennedy *et al.*, *loc. cit.* Absolute configuration: Akermark, *Acta Chem. Scand.* **16**, 599 (1962).

Rectangular rods from acetone, mp 132-133°. $[\alpha]_D^{20}$ +18° (c = 1.84 in ethanol). Practically insol in water. Freely sol in alcohol, ether; sol in aq sodium bicarbonate solns. Forms a water-sol sodium salt.

8245. Rociverine. [53716-44-2] 1-Hydroxy[1,1'-bicyclohexyl]-2-carboxylic acid 2-(diethylamino)-1-methylethyl ester; 2-(diethylamino)-1-methylethyl cis-1-hydroxy[bicyclohexyl]-2-carboxylate; LG-30158; Rilaten. $C_{20}H_{37}NO_3$; mol wt 339.51. C 70.75%, H 10.98%, N 4.13%, O 14.14%. Spasmolytic agent with balanced neurotropic and myotropic properties. Prepn: L. Turbanti, **ZA 6705649** *C.A.* **70**, 47117d (1969) and **US 3700675** (1968, 1972 both to Guidotti). Antispasmodic activity *in vitro* and *in vivo*: G. Toson *et al.*, *Arzneim.-Forsch.* **28**, 1130 (1978). Effect in cystitis or bladder spasm: A. Manganelli, *Farmaco Ed. Prat.* **34**, 384 (1979). Clinical studies: M. Petrillo *et al.*, *Curr. Med. Res. Opin.* **7**, 73 (1980); R. Assisi, S. deStefano, *Acta Ther.* **6**, 353 (1980); F. Marsala, *Minerva Med.* **73**, 2179 (1982).

Oil, bp$_{0.1}$ 148-150°. n_D^{20} 1.4820. Sol in alc, ether, chloroform, benzene, dil mineral acids. Insol in water.

THERAP CAT: Antispasmodic.

8246. Rocuronium. [143558-00-3] 1-[(2β,3α,5α,16β,17β)-17-(Acetyloxy)-3-hydroxy-2-(4-morpholinyl)androstan-16-yl]-1-(2-propenyl)pyrrolidinium; 1-allyl-1-(3α,17β-dihydroxy-2β-morpholino-5α-androstan-16β-yl)pyrrolidinium 17-acetate. $[C_{32}H_{53}$-$N_2O_4]^+$. Aminosteroid, competitive neuromuscular blocker. Prepn: D. S. Savage *et al.*, **EP 287150**; T. Sleigh *et al.*, **US 4894369** (1988, 1990 both to Akzo). Pharmacology: A. W. Muir *et al.*, *Br. J. Anaesth.* **63**, 400 (1989); K. Khuenl-Brady *et al.*, *Anesthesiology* **72**, 669 (1990). Clinical pharmacodynamics: T. J. Quill *et al.*, *Anesth. Analg.* **72**, 203 (1991); and pharmacokinetics in the elderly: R. S. Matteo *et al., ibid.* **77**, 1193 (1993). Comparative clinical trial: T. Magorian *et al., Anesthesiology* **79**, 913 (1993). HPLC determn: U. W. Kleef *et al., J. Chromatogr.* **621**, 65 (1993). Review: T. C. Wicks, *J. Am. Assoc. Nurse Anesth.* **62**, 33-38 (1994).

Bromide. [119302-91-9] Org-9426; Esmeron; Zemuron. $C_{32}H_{53}BrN_2O_4$; mol wt 609.68. Crystals, mp 161-169°. $[\alpha]_D^{20}$ +18.7° (c = 1.03 in $CHCl_3$).
THERAP CAT: Neuromuscular blocking agent.

8247. Roentgenium. [54386-24-2] Element 111; ununnium. Rg, Uuu; at. no. 111. Group Ib (11). Transuranium element. No stable nuclides. Prepn and decay of isotope ^{272}111 ($T_{1/2}$ ~1.5 msec, α decay) by ^{209}Bi(^{64}Ni,n): S. Hofmann *et al., Z. Phys. A* **350**, 281 (1995). Synthesis and decay chains: *idem et al,, Eur. Phys. J. A* **14**, 147 (2002). Name and symbol approved: J. Corish, G. M. Rosenblatt, *Pure Appl. Chem.* **76**, 2101 (2004). Review of production and properties: *idem, Rep. Prog. Phys.* **61**, 639-689 (1998).

8248. Rofecoxib. [162011-90-7] 4-[4-(Methylsulfonyl)-phenyl]-3-phenyl-2(5*H*)-furanone; MK-0966; Vioxx. $C_{17}H_{14}O_4S$; mol wt 314.36. C 64.95%, H 4.49%, O 20.36%, S 10.20%. Selective cyclooxygenase-2 (COX-2) inhibitor. Prepn: Y. Ducharme *et al.,* **WO 9500501**; *idem,* **US 5474995** (both 1995 to Merck Frosst). HPLC determn in plasma: C. M. Chavez-Eng *et al., J. Chromatogr. B* **748**, 31 (2000). Enzyme inhibition and clinical evaluation in dental pain: E. W. Ehrich *et al., Clin. Pharmacol. Ther.* **65**, 336 (1999). Evaluation of risk of gastrointestinal effects in patients with osteoarthritis: M. J. Langman *et al., J. Am. Med. Assoc.* **282**, 1929 (1999); with rheumatoid arthritis: C. Bombardier *et al., N. Engl. J. Med.* **343**, 1520 (2000). Review of pharmacology and clinical experience: A. J. Matheson, D. P. Figgitt, *Drugs* **61**, 833-865 (2001).

White to off-white to light yellow powder. Sparingly sol in acetone; slightly sol in methanol, isopropyl acetate; very slightly sol in ethanol. Practically insol in octanol; insol in water.
THERAP CAT: Anti-inflammatory; analgesic.

8249. Roflumilast. [162401-32-3] 3-(Cyclopropylmethoxy)-*N*-(3,5-dichloro-4-pyridinyl)-4-(difluoromethoxy)benzamide; BY-217; Daxas. $C_{17}H_{14}Cl_2F_2N_2O_3$; mol wt 403.21. C 50.64%, H 3.50%, Cl 17.59%, F 9.42%, N 6.95%, O 11.90%. Selective phosphodiesterase 4 (PDE4) inhibitor. Prepn: D. Flockerzi *et al.,* **WO 9501338**; H. Amschler, **US 5712298** (1995, 1998 both to Byk-Gulden). Pharmacology: A. Hatzelmann, C. Schudt, *J. Pharmacol. Exp. Ther.* **297**, 267 (2001); D. S. Bundschuh *et al., ibid.* 280. Clinical evaluation in allergic rhinitis: B. M. W. Schmidt *et al., J. Allergy Clin. Immunol.* **108**, 530 (2001); in exercise-induced asthma: W. Timmer *et al., J. Clin. Pharmacol.* **42**, 297 (2002); in COPD: K. F. Rabe *et al., Lancet* **366**, 563 (2005). Comparative

review with cilomilast: M. A. Giembycz, *Monaldi Arch. Chest Dis.* **57**, 48-64 (2002).

Crystals from isopropanol, mp 158°.
THERAP CAT: Antiasthmatic; in treatment of chronic obstructive pulmonary disease.

8250. Rokitamycin. [74014-51-0] Leucomycin V 4B-butanoate 3B-propanoate; 3″-propionylleucomycin A5; 5-[*O*-(2,6-dideoxyhexopyranosyl)-(1 → 4)-3,6-dideoxy-3-dimethylamino-β-D-glucopyranosyloxy]-6-formylmethyl-3,9-dihydroxy-4-methoxy-8-methyl-10,12-hexadecadien-15-olide; rikamycin; M-19-Q; TMS-19Q; Ricamycin; Rokital. $C_{42}H_{69}NO_{15}$; mol wt 827.99. C 60.92%, H 8.40%, N 1.69%, O 28.98%. Macrolide antibiotic active against Mycoplasma and macrolide resistant strains of *Staphylococcus aureus* and *Streptococcus pyogenes*. Prepn: H. Sakakibara *et al.,* **DE 2918954** corresp to **US 4242504** (1979, 1980 both to Toyo Jozo); *eidem, J. Antibiot.* **34**, 1001 (1981). Series of articles on antibacterial activity, pharmacology, metabolism, toxicology: *Chemotherapy (Tokyo)* **32**, Suppl. 6, 1-627 (1984). Toxicity data: K. Matsumoto *et al., ibid.* 138.

mp 116°. $[\alpha]_D^{20}$ −71° (c = 1.0 in chloroform). uv max (ethanol): 232 nm (ε 28000).
THERAP CAT: Antibacterial.

8251. Rolipram. [61413-54-5] 4-[3-(Cyclopentyloxy)-4-methoxyphenyl]-2-pyrrolidinone; ZK-62711. $C_{16}H_{21}NO_3$; mol wt 275.34. C 69.79%, H 7.69%, N 5.09%, O 17.43%. Prototypical selective phosphodiesterase 4 (PDE4) inhibitor. Prepn: **BE 826923**; R. Schmiechen *et al.,* **US 4193926** (1975, 1980 both to Schering AG). Selective enzyme inhibition and enhancement of cAMP accumulation in rat brain tissue: U. Schwabe *et al., Mol. Pharmacol.* **12**, 900 (1976). Antidepressant mechanism of action study: H. Wachtel, *Neuropharmacology* **22**, 267 (1983). Receptor binding study: H. H. Schneider *et al., Eur. J. Pharmacol.* **127**, 105 (1986). Pharmacokinetics: W. Krause, G. Kühne, *Xenobiotica* **18**, 561 (1988). Clinical evaluation in severe depression: F. Eckmann *et al., Curr. Ther. Res.* **43**, 291 (1988). Pharmacology and efficacy in exptl autoimmune encephalomyelitis: N. Sommer *et al., Nat. Med.* **1**, 244 (1995).

Crystals from ethyl acetate, mp 132°.
USE: Pharmacological tool for characterization of phosphodiesterase isoenzymes.
THERAP CAT: Antidepressant.

8252. Rolitetracycline. [751-97-3] [4*S*-(4α,4aα,5aα,6β,12aα)]-4-(Dimethylamino)-1,4,4a,5,5a,6,11,12a-octahydro-3,6,10,-12,12a-pentahydroxy-6-methyl-1,11-dioxo-*N*-(1-pyrrolidinylmethyl)-2-naphthacenecarboxamide; *N*-(pyrrolidinomethyl)tetracycline; *N*-(1-pyrrolidinylmethyl)tetracycline; Reverin; Syntetrin; Tetraverin; Transcycline. $C_{27}H_{33}N_3O_8$; mol wt 527.57. C 61.47%, H 6.30%, N 7.96%, O 24.26%. Semi-synthetic antibiotic prepd from tetracycline: Siedel *et al.*, *Muench. Med. Wochenschr.* **100**, 661 (1958); Lindner *et al.*, **ZA 5703169**. Alternate procedure and structure: Gottstein *et al.*, *J. Am. Chem. Soc.* **81**, 1198 (1959); Cheney *et al.*, **US 3104240** (1963 to Bristol-Myers). Toxicity: E. I. Goldenthal, *Toxicol. Appl. Pharmacol.* **18**, 185 (1971).

Fine, pale yellow needles, dec 162-165°. Amphoteric. More sol than tetracycline and tetracycline hydrochloride. Soly in water at 25°: 1.25 g/ml. Freely sol in alc. Sol in dil acids and alkalies.

Nitrate sesquihydrate. [26657-13-6] Bristacin; Pyrrocycline-N. $C_{27}H_{33}N_3O_8.HNO_3.1\frac{1}{2}H_2O$; mol wt 599.59. LD₅₀ i.v. in rats: 91 mg/kg (Goldenthal).

Compd with chloramphenicol succinate. [4154-10-3] Cafrolicycline; gradocycline; levocycline; senociclin; Clorociclin; Crovicina; Metilcaf; Proterciclina; Reicaf; Tecaf; Tetrafenicol. $C_{27}H_{33}N_3O_8.C_{15}H_{16}Cl_2N_2O_8$; mol wt 950.77. Prepn: **BE 636234**; Scevola, **US 3218335** (1963, 1965 both to Lab. Pro-Ter). Bright yellow powder, dec 140-144°. Bitter taste. Very sol in water. Practically insol in ether, ligroin, hexane.

THERAP CAT: Antibacterial.

8253. Romurtide. [78113-36-7] N^2-[N^2-[N-(N-Acetylmuramoyl)-L-alanyl]-D-α-glutaminyl]-N^6-(1-oxooctadecyl)-L-lysine; N^2-(N-acetylmuramoyl-L-alanyl-D-isoglutaminyl)-N^6-stearoyl-L-lysine; MDP-Lys (L18); muroctasin; DJ-7041; Nopia. $C_{43}H_{78}N_6O_{13}$; mol wt 887.11. C 58.22%, H 8.86%, N 9.47%, O 23.45%. Derivative of muramyl dipeptide, *q.v.*, with immunostimulating activity. Prepn: T. Shiba *et al.*, **EP 21367**; *eidem*, **US 4317771** (1981, 1982 both to Daiichi Seiyaku). Immunopotentiating effect *in vitro*: Y. Osada *et al.*, *Infect. Immun.* **38**, 848 (1982); *in vivo*: K. Matsumoto *et al.*, *ibid.* **39**, 1029 (1983); M. Akasaki *et al.*, *Agents Actions* **22**, 144 (1987). Enzyme immunoassay in plasma: H. Masayasu *et al.*, *Chem. Pharm. Bull.* **33**, 5522 (1985). Supplement on pharmacology, toxicology and clinical studies: *Arzneim.-Forsch.* **38**, Suppl. 7A, 951-1074 (1988). Acute toxicity: Y. Ono *et al.*, *ibid.* 1022.

Odorless, tasteless white powder, mp 176-178°. $[\alpha]_D^{20}$ +24.9° (c = 1 in methanol). pKa 5.70. Soly at 20°: DMF 1 g/72 ml; methanol 1 g/190 ml; ethanol 1 g/330 ml. Practically insol in acetone, acetonitrile, chloroform, water. LD₅₀ in male, female mice, male, female rats, dogs (mg/kg): 436, 625, 761, 801, >200 s.c. (Ono).

THERAP CAT: Immunostimulant.

8254. Ronidazole. [7681-76-7] 1-Methyl-5-nitroimidazole-2-methanol carbamate (ester); carbamic acid (1-methyl-5-nitroimidazol-2-yl)methyl ester; 1-methyl-2-[(carbamoyloxy)methyl]-5-nitroimidazole; (1-methyl-5-nitroimidazol-2-yl)methyl carbamate; MCMN; Ridzol. $C_6H_8N_4O_4$; mol wt 200.15. C 36.01%, H 4.03%, N 27.99%, O 31.97%. Prepn and antiprotozoal activity: **NL 6609552**; **NL 6609553** (both 1967 to Merck & Co.), *C.A.* **67**,

54123u, 11487y (1967); Verdi; Kollonitsch, **US 3450710**; **US 3459764** (both 1969 to Merck & Co.).

Pale yellow crystals, mp 167-169°. Soly in water (at pH 6.5) ~2.9 mg/ml at room temp. More sol in acid solns. Unstable in alkaline solns. pKa 1.2. Freely sol in acetone. Sol in methanol, ethanol, chloroform and ethyl acetate.

THERAP CAT (VET): Antimicrobial.

8255. Ronifibrate. [42597-57-9] 3-Pyridinecarboxylic acid 3-[2-(4-chlorophenoxy)-2-methyl-1-oxopropoxy]propyl ester; 3-(nicotinoyloxy)propyl *p*-chlorophenoxyisobutyrate; 3-[α-(*p*-chlorophenoxy)isobutyryloxy]propyl nicotinate; I-612; Cloprane. $C_{19}H_{20}ClNO_5$; mol wt 377.82. C 60.40%, H 5.34%, Cl 9.38%, N 3.71%, O 21.17%. Diester of clofibric and nicotinic acids, *q.q.v.* Prepn: Y. Hirata *et al.*, **JP Kokai 73 40777** (1973 to Yamanouchi), *C.A.* **79**, 66180w (1973); H. Shindo *et al.*, **JP Kokai 74 30377** (1974 to Kowa Pharm.), *C.A.* **81**, 135984s (1974). Clinical trial in hyperdyslipidemia: A. Bucalossi *et al.*, *Clin. Ter.* **89**, 127 (1979). Efficacy and tolerability: G. Buzzelli *et al.*, *ibid.* 251.

LD₅₀ orally in mice: 4.08 g/kg (Bucalossi).

THERAP CAT: Antilipemic.

8256. Ronnel. [299-84-3] Phosphorothioic acid *O,O*-dimethyl *O*-(2,4,5-trichlorophenyl)ester; fenchlorphos; dimethyl trichlorophenyl thiophosphate; Trolene; Etrolene; Nankor; Korlan; Viozene. $C_8H_8Cl_3O_3PS$; mol wt 321.55. C 29.88%, H 2.51%, Cl 33.08%, O 14.93%, P 9.63%, S 9.97%. Cholinesterase inhibitor. Prepn: Schrader, **DE 814152** (1948 to Bayer); Moyle, **US 2599516** (1952 to Dow). Description of mfg process: *Can. Dept. Agr. Bull.* (3rd ed., Oct. 1957) p 136. Toxicity study: T. B. Gaines, *Toxicol. Appl. Pharmacol.* **14**, 515 (1969).

White powder, mp 41°. Vapor pressure at 25°: 8×10^{-4} mm Hg. Practically insol in water (0.004 g/100 ml at 25°). Freely sol in acetone, carbon tetrachloride, ether, methylene chloride, toluene, kerosene. LD₅₀ in male, female rats (mg/kg): 1250, 2630 orally (Gaines).

Caution: Potential symptoms of overexposure in exptl animals are cholinesterase inhibition; eye irritation; liver and kidney damage. *See NIOSH Pocket Guide to Chemical Hazards* (DHHS/NIOSH 97-140, 1997) p 274.

USE: Insecticide.

8257. Ropinirole. [91374-21-9] 4-[2-(Dipropylamino)ethyl]-1,3-dihydro-2*H*-indol-2-one; 4-[2-(di-*n*-propylamino)ethyl]-2(3*H*)-indolone; SKF-101468. $C_{16}H_{24}N_2O$; mol wt 260.37. C 73.81%, H 9.29%, N 10.76%, O 6.14%. Selective dopamine D₂-receptor agonist. Prepn: G. Gallagher, Jr., **US 4452808** (1984 to Smithkline Beckman); *idem et al.*, *J. Med. Chem.* **28**, 1533 (1985). HPLC determn in plasma: J. E. Swagzdis, B. A. Mico, *J. Pharm. Sci.* **75**, 90 (1986). Pharmacology and receptor binding study: R. J. Eden *et al.*, *Pharmacol. Biochem. Behav.* **38**, 147 (1991). Clinical pharmacology, pharmacokinetics: C. de Mey *et al.*, *Br. J. Clin. Pharmacol.* **32**, 483 (1991). Clinical trials in Parkinson's disease: O. Rascol *et al.*, *Mov. Disord.* **13**, 39 (1998); A. D. Korczyn *et al.*, *ibid.* 46; in restless legs syndrome: A. S. Walters *et al.*, *ibid.* **19**, 1414 (2004).

Hydrochloride. [91374-20-8] SKF-101468A; Requip. C_{16}-$H_{24}N_2O \cdot HCl$; mol wt 296.84. Crystals from acetonitrile, mp 241-243°.

THERAP CAT: Antiparkinsonian.

8258. Ropivacaine. [84057-95-4] $(2S)$-N-(2,6-dimethyl-phenyl)-1-propyl-2-piperidinecarboxamide; (S)-$(-)$-1-propyl-2′,6′-pipecoloxylidide; l-N-n-propylpipecolic acid-2,6-xylidide; LEA-103. $C_{17}H_{26}N_2O$; mol wt 274.40. C 74.41%, H 9.55%, N 10.21%, O 5.83%. Prepn: A. F. Thuresson, C. Bovin, **WO 8500599** (1985 to Apothekernes); H.-J. Federsel et al., Acta Chem. Scand. **B41**, 757 (1987). Physicochemical properties: G. R. Strichartz et al., Anesth. Analg. **71**, 158 (1990). HPLC determn in human plasma: Z. Yu et al., J. Chromatogr. B **654**, 221 (1994). In vitro metabolism: Y. Oda et al., Anesthesiology **82**, 214 (1995). Clinical pharmacokinetics: D. J. Kopacz et al., ibid. **81**, 1139 (1994). Toxicity study in sheep: A. C. Santos et al., ibid. **82**, 734 (1995). Clinical evaluation in relief of surgical pain: I. Cederholm et al., Reg. Anesth. **19**, 18 (1994); B. Johansson et al., Anesth. Analg. **78**, 210 (1994); labor pain: R. Stienstra et al., ibid. **80**, 285 (1995).

Crystals from toluene, mp 144-146°. $[\alpha]_D^{25}$ −82.0° (c = 2 in methanol). pKa 8.16. Distribution coefficient (1-octanol/aq buffer, pH 7.4): 115.0.

Hydrochloride. [98717-15-8] Naropin. $C_{17}H_{26}N_2O \cdot HCl$; mol wt 310.86. Crystals from isopropyl alcohol, mp 260-262°. $[\alpha]_D^{25}$ −6.6° (c = 2 in water).

Hydrochloride monohydrate. [132112-35-7] Crystals from acetone + water, mp 269.5-270.6°. $[\alpha]_D^{20}$ −7.28° (c = 2 in water).

THERAP CAT: Anesthetic (local).

8259. Roquinimex. [84088-42-6] 1,2-Dihydro-4-hydroxy-N,1-dimethyl-2-oxo-N-phenyl-3-quinolinecarboxamide; N-phenyl-N-methyl-1,2-dihydro-4-hydroxy-1-methyl-2-oxoquinoline-3-carboxamide; 1,2-dihydro-4-hydroxy-N,1-dimethyl-2-oxo-3-quino-linecarboxanilide; LS-2616; Linomide. $C_{18}H_{16}N_2O_3$; mol wt 308.33. C 70.12%, H 5.23%, N 9.09%, O 15.57%. Biological response modifier. Prepn: E. Eriksson et al., **EP 59698**; eidem, **US 4738971** (1982, 1988 both to AB Leo). Immunopharmacology: A. Tarkowski et al., Immunology **59**, 589 (1986). Mechanism of action study: E.-L. Larsson et al., Int. J. Immunopharmacol. **9**, 425 (1987). Clinical evaluation in cancer patients: J. C. S. Bergh et al., Cancer Invest. **15**, 204 (1997).

Crystals from pyridine, mp 200-204°.

THERAP CAT: Antineoplastic.

8260. Rosaprostol. [56695-65-9] 2-Hexyl-5-hydroxycyclo-pentaneheptanoic acid; 9-hydroxy-19,20-bisnorprostanoic acid; C-83; IBI-C83; Rosal. $C_{18}H_{34}O_3$; mol wt 298.46. C 72.44%, H 11.48%, O 16.08%. Prostaglandin analog. Prepn, hypolipemic,

platelet aggregation inhibitory activity: U. Valcavi, **DE 2535343**, eidem, **US 4073938** (1976, 1978 both to Ist. Biochim. Ital.). Alternate process: V. Marotta, G. Zabban, **EP 155392** (1985 to Ist. Biochim. Ital.). Gastric antisecretory, cytoprotective activity: U. Valcavi et al., Arzneim.-Forsch. **32**, 657 (1982). Effect on mucus and gastrin secretion in duodenal ulcer: D. Foschi et al., Prosta-glandins Leukotrienes Med. **15**, 147 (1984). Comparison with cimetidine, q.v.: eidem, Drugs Exp. Clin. Res. **10**, 427 (1984). Clinical evaluation in treatment of ulcers: G. P. Tincani et al., Minerva Med. **78**, 847 (1987).

Oil.

Sodium salt. [56695-66-0] $C_{18}H_{33}NaO_3$. White solid. LD_{50} orally in mice: ~3000 mg/kg (Valcavi, 1978); orally in rats: >5 g/kg (Valcavi, 1982).

THERAP CAT: Antiulcerative.

8261. Rosaramicin. [35834-26-5] 4′-Deoxycirramycin A_1; 3-ethyl-7-hydroxy-2,8,12,16-tetramethyl-5,13-dioxo-9-[[3,4,6-tri-deoxy-3-(dimethylamino)-β-D-$xylo$-hexopyranosyl]oxy]-4,17-di-oxabicyclo[14.1.0]heptadec-14-ene-10-acetaldehyde; antibiotic 67-694; juvenimicin A_3; rosamicin; M-4365A2; Sch-14947. $C_{31}H_{51}$-NO_9; mol wt 581.74. C 64.00%, H 8.84%, N 2.41%, O 24.75%. Macrolide antibiotic isolated from fermentations of Micromono-spora rosaria NRRL-3718. Isoln and properties: M. J. Weinstein et al., **ZA 7100402**; **FR 2081448** (1971, 1972 both to Sherico), C.A. **76**, 139065n (1972); **78**, 109310n (1973); G. H. Wagman et al., J. Antibiot. **25**, 641 (1972). Biological studies: J. A. Waitz et al., ibid. 647. Structure: H. Reimann, R. S. Jaret, Chem. Commun. **1972**, 1270. Crystal structure: A. K. Ganguly et al., Tetrahedron Lett. **21**, 4699 (1980). Biosynthesis: A. K. Ganguly et al., J. Antibiot. **29**, 976 (1976). Identity with juvenimicin A_3: T. Kishi et al., ibid. 1171. Isoln from M. capillata MCRL 0940 and identity with antibiotic M-4365A2: A. Kinumaki et al., ibid. **30**, 450 (1977). In vitro activity: S. Feltham et al., J. Antimicrob. Chemo-ther. **5**, 731 (1979). Use in experimental pneumococcal meningitis: C. M. Nolan et al., Antimicrob. Agents Chemother. **16**, 776 (1979).

Crystals from chloroform, mp 119-122°. $[\alpha]_D^{26}$ −35° (ethanol). uv max (methanol): 240 nm (ε 14600). Very sol in methanol, acetone, chloroform, benzene. Sparingly sol in ether. Slightly sol in water. LD_{50} in mice (mg/kg): 625 s.c.; 350 i.p.; 155 i.v. (Wagman).

THERAP CAT: Antibacterial.

8262. Rose Bengal. [632-68-8] 4,5,6,7-Tetrachloro-3′,6′-di-hydroxy-2′,4′,5′,7′-tetraiodospiro[isobenzofuran-1(3H),9′-[9H]xan-then]-3-one dipotassium salt; 4,5,6,7-tetrachloro-2′,4′,5′,7′-tetra-iodofluorescein dipotassium salt; C.I. Acid Red 94; Rose Bengale B; C.I. 45440. $C_{20}H_2Cl_4I_4K_2O_5$; mol wt 1049.85. C 22.88%, H 0.19%, Cl 13.51%, I 48.35%, K 7.45%, O 7.62%. Discovered by Gnehm 1882; tetraiodinate of 4,5,6,7-tetrachlorofluorescein (from resorcinol and tetrachlorophthalic anhydride) converted to potas-sium salt: Colour Index vol. 4 (3rd ed., 1971) 4428. Labeling with [131]I: Liebster, Andrysek, Nature **184**, 913 (1959). See also: H. J. Conn's Biological Stains, R. D. Lillie, Ed., (Williams & Wilkins, Baltimore, 9th ed., 1977) p 350. Diagnostic use in hepatic function: K. S. Nijran, D. C. Barber, Phys. Med. Biol. **31**, 563 (1986).

Bright bluish pink. Soluble in water (bluish red without fluorescence); brown soln in concd H_2SO_4, on dilution gives flesh pink ppt.

Disodium salt. [632-69-9] Rose Bengal Extra. $C_{20}H_2Cl_4I_4$-Na_2O_5.

131I-Labeled disodium salt. [50291-21-9] Sodium rose bengal I 131; rose bengal sodium I 131; Robenogatope I-131.

Note: C.I. Acid Red 94 and C.I. 45440 also used for disodium salt.

USE: As a dye, biological stain; in coloring straw, wood chips, and inks; for coloring edible products and cosmetics.

THERAP CAT: Diagnostic aid (corneal trauma indicator). Sodium Rose Bengal I 131 as diagnostic aid (hepatic function).

8263. Rose Hips. Hipberries. The fruits or berries from wild rose bushes, notably *Rosa canina* L., *R. gallica* L., *R. condita* Scop. and *R. rugosa* Thunb., *Rosaceae*. Rich in ascorbic acid: M. Szczyglowa *et al., Rocz. Panstw. Zakl. Hig.* **1**, 523-532 (1950), *C.A.* **46**, 1177d. Ascorbic acid content of hips of *R. canina* reported as 19-27 mg/g dry weight: Å. Gustafsson, J. Schröderheim, *Nature* **153**, 196 (1944); as 33.1 mg/g dry weight: I. Roubani *et al., J. Hortic. Sci.* **51**, 375 (1976). Comparison of methods for determn of ascorbic acid in hips: K. Gliniecki *et al., Pharm. Z.* **127**, 823 (1982).

8264. Rosemary. Low, branched perennial shrub, *Rosmarinus officinalis* L., *Labiatae*. *Habit.* Mediterranean basin; widely cultivated in gardens. Medicinal parts are the essential oil and the dried or fresh leaves and leafy stems. *Constit.* Volatile oil (1.0-2.5%); diterpenoids incl. carnosol, carnosic acid, rosmadial, rosmanol, epirosmarol, methyl carnosate; flavonoids incl. genkwanin, cirsimarin; rosmarinic acid. Extraction of volatile components: A. Basile *et al., J. Agric. Food Chem.* **46**, 5205 (1998); of antioxidants: E. Ibañez *et al., ibid.* **51**, 375 (2003). Botanical description and medicinal uses: J. Gruenwald *et al., PDR for Herbal Medicines* (Medical Economics, Montvale, 2nd Ed., 2000) pp 645-646. Review of pharmacology: J. Barnes *et al., Herbal Medicines* (Pharmaceutical Press, London, 2nd Ed., 2002) pp 403-407.

Volatile oil. [8000-25-7] Oil of rosemary. Obtained from the fresh flowering tops. *Constit.* α-Pinene (15-25%), 1,8-cineole (20-50%), camphor (10-25%), camphene, limonine, borneol, linalool. Colorless or pale yellow liquid; characteristic rosemary odor; camphoraceous taste. d_{25}^{25} 0.894-0.912. α_D^{25} -5 to $+10°$. n_D^{20} 1.464-1.476. Almost insol in water; sol in 10 vols 80% alcohol. *Keep well closed, cool and protected from light.*

USE: In hair conditioners, mouth rinses, fragrances; flavoring agent in foods.

THERAP CAT: Carminative; rubefacient; antimicrobial.

8265. Rosiglitazone. [122320-73-4] 5-[[4-[2-(Methyl-2-pyridinylamino)ethoxy]phenyl]methyl]-2,4-thiazolidinedione; 5-[4-[2-[N-methyl-N-(2-pyridinyl)amino]ethoxy]benzyl]-2,4-thiazolidinedione; BRL-49653. $C_{18}H_{19}N_3O_3S$; mol wt 357.43. C 60.49%, H 5.36%, N 11.76%, O 13.43%, S 8.97%. Insulin sensitizer; binds to peroxisome proliferator activated receptor gamma (PPAR-γ). Prepn: R. M. Hindley, **EP 306228**; *idem,* **US 5002953** (1989, 1991 both to Beecham); B. C. C. Cantello *et al., J. Med. Chem.* **37**, 3977 (1994). Pharmacology: N. D. Oakes *et al., Diabetes* **43**, 1203 (1994). Binding study: D. E. Mais *et al., Med. Chem. Res.* **7**, 325 (1997). Clinical pharmacokinetics and bioavailability: M. I. Freed *et al., Eur. J. Clin. Pharmacol.* **55**, 53 (1999). Review of pharmacology and clinical experience: J. A. Barman Balfour, G. L. Plosker, *Drugs* **57**, 921-930 (1999).

Colorless crystals from methanol, mp 153-155°.

Maleate. [155141-29-0] BRL-49653c; Avandia. $C_{18}H_{19}N_3$-$O_3S.C_4H_4O_4$; mol wt 473.50. White to off-white solid, mp 122-123°. pKa 6.1; 6.8. Readily sol in ethanol and in buffered aq soln with pH of 2.3; soly decreases with increasing pH in the physiological range.

THERAP CAT: Antidiabetic.

8266. Rosin. Colophony; yellow resin; abietic anhydride. Residue left after distilling off the volatile oil from the oleoresin obtained from *Pinus palustris* and other species of *Pinus, Pinaceae.* Offered as wood rosin (from Southern pine stumps), gum rosin (the exudate from incisions in the living tree, *P. palustris* and *P. caribaea*), and tall oil rosin, *see* Tall Oil. Rosin is chiefly produced in the U.S.A. *Constit.* About 90% resin acids and 10% neutral matter. Of the resin acids about 90% are isomeric with abietic acid ($C_{20}H_{30}O_2$); the other 10% is a mixture of dihydroabietic acid (C_{20}-$H_{32}O_2$) and dehydroabietic acid ($C_{20}H_{28}O_2$).

Pale yellow to amber, translucent fragments; brittle fracture at ordinary temp; slight turpentine odor and taste. Readily fusible when heated. d 1.07-1.09. Acid no. not less than 150. Insol in water. Freely sol in alc, benzene, ether, glacial acetic acid, oils, carbon disulfide; also sol in dil solns or fixed alkali hydroxides.

USE: Manuf varnishes, varnish and paint driers, printing inks, cements, soap, sealing wax, wood polishes, floor coverings, paper, plastics, fireworks, tree wax, sizes, rosin oil; for water-proofing cardboard, walls, etc. Pharmaceutic aid (stiffening agent).

8267. Rosin Oil. Rosinol. Obtained by dry distillation of rosin.

Yellow, viscid, fluorescent, oily liquid. bp >280°. Insol in water; sol in ether, oil turpentine and other oils. It dissolves phosphorus, sulfur, camphor, phenols, and many other organic compds.

USE: Manuf of carbon black for lithography and printing inks; in varnishes, retinol colors, lacquers, brewers' pitch, axle greases.

8268. Rosoxacin. [40034-42-2] 1-Ethyl-1,4-dihydro-4-oxo-7-(4-pyridinyl)-3-quinolinecarboxylic acid; acrosoxacin; Win-35213; Eracine; Eradacil; Eradacin; Winuron. $C_{17}H_{14}N_2O_3$; mol wt 294.30. C 69.38%, H 4.79%, N 9.52%, O 16.31%. Quinolone antibacterial. Prepn: G. Y. Lesher, P. M. Carabateas, **DE 2224090**; *eidem*, **US 3753993** (1972, 1973 both to Sterling). HPLC determn in plasma and urine: M. P. Kullberg *et al., J. Chromatogr.* **173**, 155 (1979). Pharmacological studies: S. Maigaard *et al., Urol. Res.* **8**, 113 (1980); *eidem, Invest. Urol.* **17**, 149 (1979). Clinical study in gonorrhea: B. M. Limson *et al., Curr. Ther. Res.* **26**, 842 (1979).

Yellow crystals from DMF, mp 290°. Stable in dry heat at 70°. Light sensitive. Solns and suspensions stable at pH 2.0-9.5.

THERAP CAT: Antibacterial.

8269. Rostaporfin. [284041-10-7] (*OC*-6-13)-Dichloro[*rel*-ethyl (18*R*,19*S*)-3,4,20,21-tetrahydro-4,9,14,19-tetraethyl-18,19-dihydro-3,8,13,18-tetramethyl-20-phorbinecarboxylato(2−)-$\kappa N^{23},\kappa N^{24},\kappa N^{25},\kappa N^{26}$]tin; SnET2; tin ethyl etiopurpurin dichloride; tin etiopurpurin dichloride; Photrex; Purlytin. $C_{37}H_{42}Cl_2N_4O_2Sn$; mol wt 764.37. C 58.14%, H 5.54%, Cl 9.28%, N 7.33%, O 4.19%, Sn 15.53%. Metalloporphin photosensitizer for photodynamic therapy. Prepn: A. R. Morgan *et al., SPIE* **847**, 172 (1987); *eidem, Cancer Res.* **48**, 194 (1988). Pharmacokinetics in dogs and rats: D. L. Frazier *et al., J. Vet. Pharmacol. Ther.* **15**, 275 (1992). Intracranial tissue uptake and specificity: L. Lilge, B. C. Wilson, *J. Clin. Laser Med. Surg.* **16**, 81 (1998). Photophysical properties: B. W. Pogue *et al.*, *Photochem. Photobiol.* **68**, 809 (1998). Clinical evaluation in cutaneous metastatic breast cancer: T. S. Mang *et al.*, *Cancer J. Sci. Am.* **4**, 378 (1998). Review of clinical development in wet age-related macular degeneration: D. W. C. Hunt, *IDrugs* **5**, 180-186 (2002).

Crystals from dichloromethane:methanol(10:1). Absorption max (dichloromethane): 659 nm (ε 30347). Absorption max: 656 nm (methanol); 661 (phosphate-buffered saline); (ε 42800; 15200).

THERAP CAT: In treatment of age-related macular degeneration.

8270. Rosuvastatin. [287714-41-4] (3R,5S,6E)-7-[4-(4-Fluorophenyl)-6-(1-methylethyl)-2-[methyl(methylsulfonyl)amino]-5-pyrimidinyl]-3,5-dihydroxy-6-heptenoic acid. $C_{22}H_{28}FN_3O_6S$; mol wt 481.54. HMG-CoA reductase inhibitor. Prepn: K. Hirai *et al.*, **EP 521471**; *eidem*, **US 5260440** (both 1993 to Shionogi); M. Watanabe *et al.*, *Bioorg. Med. Chem.* **5**, 437 (1997). Pharmacology: F. McTaggart *et al.*, *Am. J. Cardiol.* **87**, Suppl., 28B (2001). Comparative clinical trial with atorvastatin: M. Davidson *et al.*, *ibid.* **89**, 268 (2002); in metabolic syndrome: A. F. H. Stalenhoef *et al.*, *Eur. Heart J.* **26**, 2664 (2005); in African-American patients: K. C. Ferdinand *et al.*, *Am. J. Cardiol.* **97**, 229 (2006). Pharmacokinetics and pharmacogenetics in Asian and white ethnic groups: E. Lee *et al.*, *Clin. Pharmacol. Ther.* **78**, 330 (2005). Review of therapeutic potential: K. C. Ferdinand, *Expert Opin. Pharmacother.* **6**, 1897-1910 (2005).

Partition coefficient (octanol/water): 0.13 (pH 7.0).

Calcium salt. [147098-20-2] S-4522; ZD-4522; Crestor. $C_{44}CaH_{54}F_2N_6O_{12}S_2$; mol wt 1001.14. White powder from water as the monohydrate; begins to melt at 155° with no definitive mp. $[\alpha]_D^{24}$ +14.8° (c = 1.012 in 50% methanol). Sparingly sol in water, methanol; slightly sol in ethanol.

THERAP CAT: Antilipemic.

8271. Rotenone. [83-79-4] [2R-(2α,6aα,12aα)]-1,2,12,12a-Tetrahydro-8,9-dimethoxy-2-(1-methylethenyl)-[1]benzopyrano[3,4-*b*]furo[2,3-*h*][1]benzopyran-6(6a*H*)-one; Canex; Noxfire. $C_{23}H_{22}O_6$; mol wt 394.42. C 70.04%, H 5.62%, O 24.34%. Principal insecticidal constituent of derris root, cubé, etc. Powerful inhibitor of mitochondrial electron transport. Isoln from *Lonchocarpus nicou* (Aubl.) DC., *Leguminosae*: Geoffrey, *Ann. Inst. Colon. Marseille* **2**, 1 (1895). Review of structure: La Forge *et al.*, *Chem. Rev.* **12**, 181 (1933); Butenandt, McCartney, *Ann.* **494**, 17 (1932); King, *Annu. Rep. Prog. Chem.* **29**, 186 (1932). Absolute configuration: Büchi *et al.*, *J. Chem. Soc.* **1961**, 2843; Nakazaki, Arakawa, *Bull. Chem. Soc. Jpn.* **34**, 1246 (1961); Begley *et al.*, *Chem. Commun.* **1975**, 850. NMR spectrum: Crombie, Lown, *ibid.* **1962**, 775.

Total synthesis: Miyano *et al.*, *Agric. Biol. Chem.* **25**, 673 (1961); Miyano, *J. Am. Chem. Soc.* **87**, 3958 (1965). Alternate synthesis: Crombie *et al.*, *J. Chem. Soc. Perkin Trans. 1* **1973**, 1277, *eidem*, *Chem. Commun.* **1979**, 1142; I. Sasaki, K. Yamashita, *Agric. Biol. Chem.* **43**, 137 (1979). Synthesis of stereoisomers: Unai, Yamamoto, *ibid.* **37**, 897 (1973). Toxicology: Santi, Toth, *Farmaco Ed. Sci.* **20**, 270 (1965). Toxicity data: J.-I. Fukami *et al.*, *Science* **155**, 713 (1967). *Review:* H. Fukami, M. Nakajima in *Naturally Occurring Insecticides*, M. Jacobson, D. G. Crosby, Eds. (Dekker, New York, 1971) pp 71-97; S. B. Soloway, *Environ. Health Perspect.* **14**, 109-117 (1976); T. J. Haley, *J. Environ. Pathol. Toxicol.* **1**, 315-337 (1978).

Orthorhombic, six-sided plates from trichloroethylene, mp 165-166° (dimorphic form, mp 185-186°). $[\alpha]_D^{20}$ −228° (c = 2.22 in benzene). uv spectra: Büchi *et al.*, *loc. cit.* Practically insol in water. Sol in alcohol, acetone, carbon tetrachloride, chloroform, ether, and many other organic solvents. Dec upon exposure to light and air. Colorless solns in organic solvents oxidize upon exposure and become yellow, orange and then deep red and may deposit crystals of dehydrorotenone and rotenonone which are toxic to insects. LD_{50} i.p. in mice: 2.8 mg/kg (Fukami); in rats (mg/kg): 132 orally; 6 i.v. (Soloway).

Caution: Potential symptoms of overexposure are irritation of eyes, skin, respiratory system; numbness of mucous membranes; nausea, vomiting, abdominal pain; muscle tremors, incontinence, clonic convulsions, stupor. *See NIOSH Pocket Guide to Chemical Hazards* (DHHS/NIOSH 97-140, 1997) p 274. Inhalation may cause severe pulmonary irritation. *See Clinical Toxicology of Commercial Products*, R. E. Gosselin *et al.*, Eds. (Williams & Wilkins, Baltimore, 5th ed., 1984) Section III, pp 366-368.

USE: Pesticide.

THERAP CAT (VET): Ectoparasiticide.

8272. Rottlerin. [82-08-6] (*E*)-1-[6-[(3-Acetyl-2,4,6-trihydroxy-5-methylphenyl)methyl]-5,7-dihydroxy-2,2-dimethyl-2*H*-1-benzopyran-8-yl]-3-phenyl-2-propen-1-one; 5,7-dihydroxy-2,2-dimethyl-6-(2,4,6-trihydroxy-3-methyl-5-acetylbenzyl)-8-cinnamoyl-1,2-chromene; mallotoxin. $C_{30}H_{28}O_8$; mol wt 516.54. C 69.76%, H 5.46%, O 24.78%. Principal phenolic component of kamala, *q.v.*, an anthelmintic dye obtained from *Mallotus philippinensis* (Lam.) Muell. Arg. (also known as *Rottlera tinctoria* Roxb.), *Euphorbiaceae*. Isoln: H. Telle, *Arch. Pharm.* **244**, 446 (1906); S. Dutt, *J. Chem. Soc.* **127**, 2044 (1925); A. McGookin *et al.*, *ibid.* **1937**, 748. Structure: Brockmann, Maier, *Ann.* **535**, 149 (1938); A. McGookin *et al.*, *J. Chem. Soc.* **1939**, 1579. Synthesis of tetrahydrorottlerin: Backhouse *et al.*, *ibid.* **1948**, 113. Review of isoln and chemistry: M. Lounasmaa *et al.*, *Planta Med.* **28**, 16 (1975). Activity as protein kinase inhibitor: M. Gschwendt *et al.*, *Biochem. Biophys. Res. Commun.* **199**, 93 (1994). HPTLC determn in serum and pharmacokinetics: V. D. Mody *et al.*, *J. Pharm. Technol.* **10**, 71 (1994).

Light reddish-brown plates or needles with golden lustre from ethyl acetate, mp 212° (McGookin). Also reported as brownish-yellow plates from toluene, mp 206-207° (Dutt). Sol in ether, chloroform, benzene, ethyl acetate; sparingly sol in cold alc, acetic acid. Practically insol in water.

5,7-Dimethyl ether. $C_{32}H_{32}O_8$. Yellow crystals from ethyl acetate + acetone or chloroform + methanol, dec 245-246°. Sol in chloroform, pyridine, hot glacial acetic acid; slightly sol in cold methanol, ethyl acetate, acetone, benzene, ether.

Pentamethyl ether. $C_{35}H_{38}O_8$. Crystals from petr ether, methanol or 90% alcohol, mp 144°. Very sol in acetone, glacial acetic acid, benzene, ethyl acetate.

Pentaacetate. $C_{40}H_{38}O_{13}$. Leaflets from benzene + alcohol or acetone + alcohol, prisms from ethyl acetate, mp 212°.

Tetrahydrorottlerin. $C_{30}H_{32}O_8$. Yellow prisms from alcohol, mp 214°.

8273. Roxarsone. [121-19-7] 4-Hydroxy-3-nitrophenyl-arsonic acid; 4-hydroxy-3-nitrobenzenearsonic acid; 3-nitro-4-hydroxyphenylarsonic acid; 2-nitro-1-hydroxybenzene-4-arsonic acid; nitrophenolarsonic acid; NSC-2101; Ren-o-sal. $C_6H_6AsNO_6$; mol wt 263.04. C 27.40%, H 2.30%, As 28.48%, N 5.32%, O 36.49%. Prepd by treating sodium *p*-hydroxyphenylarsonate with a mixture of nitric and sulfuric acids at 0°: Benda, Bertheim, *Ber.* **44**, 3446 (1911); *DE 224953 C.A.* **5**, 156 (1911). Toxicity study: Kerr *et al.*, *Toxicol. Appl. Pharmacol.* **5**, 507 (1963). Review of toxicology and human exposure: *Toxicological Profile for Arsenic* (PB2000-108021, 2000) 468 pp.

Tufts of pale-yellow needles or rhombohedral plates from water. Puffs up and deflagrates on heating. Slightly sol in cold water; sol in ~30 parts boiling water; freely sol in methanol, ethanol, acetic acid, acetone, alkalies; sparingly sol in dil mineral acids. Insol in ether, ethyl acetate. Forms mono-, di-, and trisodium salts. LD_{50} in rats, chickens (mg/kg): 155, 110-123 orally; 66, 34 i.p. (Kerr).

USE: Formerly in manuf arsphenamines; as reagent for zirconium.

THERAP CAT (VET): Control of enteric infections. To improve growth and feed efficiency.

8274. Roxatidine Acetate. [78628-28-1] 2-(Acetyloxy)-*N*-[3-[3-(1-piperidinylmethyl)phenoxy]propyl]acetamide; aceroxatidine. $C_{19}H_{28}N_2O_4$; mol wt 348.44. C 65.49%, H 8.10%, N 8.04%, O 18.37%. Histamine H_2-receptor antagonist. Prepn and anti-ulcerative activity: K. Shibata *et al.*, **EP 24510**; *eidem*, **US 4293557** (both 1981 to Teikoku Hormone). Pharmacology in animals: M. Tarutani *et al.*, *Arzneim.-Forsch.* **35**, 703 (1985). Comparison with cimetidine of effect on gastric acid secretion and ulcer formation in animals: *eidem, ibid.* 844. Metabolism in humans: S. Honma *et al.*, *Oyo Yakuri* **30**, 555 (1985); *C.A.* **104**, 61453n (1985).

mp 59-60°. LD_{50} orally in male mice: 1000 mg/kg (Shibata).
Hydrochloride. [93793-83-0] Pifatidine; HOE-760; TZU-0460; Altat; Gastralgin; Neo H2; Roxit. $C_{19}H_{28}N_2O_4 \cdot HCl$; mol wt 384.90. mp 145-146°.
THERAP CAT: Antiulcerative.

8275. Roxindole. [112192-04-8] 3-[4-(3,6-Dihydro-4-phenyl-1(2*H*)-pyridinyl)butyl]-1*H*-indol-5-ol; 5-hydroxy-3-[4-(1,2,3,6-tetrahydro-4-phenyl-1-pyridyl)butyl]indole. $C_{23}H_{26}N_2O$; mol wt 346.47. C 79.73%, H 7.56%, N 8.09%, O 4.62%. Dopamine D_2-receptor agonist. Synthesis: H.-H. Hausberg *et al., Acta Pharm. Suec.* **1983**, Suppl 2, 213; H. Böttcher *et al., J. Med. Chem.* **35**, 4020 (1992). Pharmacology: C. A. Seyfried *et al., Eur. J.*

Pharmacol. **160**, 31 (1989). Clinical pharmacology: K. Wiedemann, M. Kellner, *Exp. Clin. Endocrinol.* **102**, 284 (1994). Clinical evaluation in schizophrenia: H. Wetzel *et al., Am. J. Psychiatry* **151**, 1499 (1994); in depression: G. Gründer *et al., Psychopharmacology* **111**, 123 (1993). Neuroendocrinology in schizophrenics: G. Gründer *et al., ibid.* **117**, 472 (1995).

Hydrochloride. [108050-82-4] EMD-38362. $C_{23}H_{26}N_2 \cdot$ O.HCl; mol wt 382.93. Monoclinic crystals, mp 274°.
Methanesulfonate. [119742-13-1] Roxindole mesylate; EMD-49980
THERAP CAT: Antidepressant.

8276. Roxithromycin. [80214-83-1] Erythromycin 9-[*O*-[(2-methoxyethoxy)methyl]oxime]; oxacyclotetradecane erythromycin deriv; 9-(2',5'-dioxahexyloxyimino)erythromycin; RU-28965; RU-965; Assoral; Claramid; Forilin; Overal; Rossitrol; Rotramin; Rulid; Surlid. $C_{41}H_{76}N_2O_{15}$; mol wt 837.05. C 58.83%, H 9.15%, N 3.35%, O 28.67%. Semisynthetic erythromycin derivative. Prepn: S. Gouin d'Ambrieres *et al.*, **FR 2473525**; *eidem*, **US 4349545** (1981, 1982 both to Roussel-UCLAF). *In vitro* antibacterial spectrum: R. N. Jones *et al., Antimicrob. Agents Chemother.* **24**, 209 (1983); Y. J. Drabu *et al., Drugs Exp. Clin. Res.* **13**, 201 (1987). Antiprotozoal activity in mice: B. J. Luft, *Eur. J. Clin. Microbiol.* **6**, 479 (1987); H. R. Chang, J.-C. R. Pechere, *Antimicrob. Agents Chemother.* **31**, 1147 (1987). Pharmacokinetics: R. Wise *et al., ibid.* 1051. Bioassay in biological fluids: A. L. Barry, R. R. Packer, *Eur. J. Clin. Microbiol.* **5**, 536 (1986). Clinical evaluations in respiratory tract infections: J. M. Lachat *et al., Schweiz. Med. Wochenschr.* **116**, 1739 (1986); C. Grassi *et al., Chemioterapia* **6**, 41 (1987). Series of articles on antimicrobial activity, pharmacokinetics and clinical efficacy: *J. Antimicrob. Chemother.* **20**, Suppl. B, 1-185 (1987).

$[\alpha]_D^{25} -77.5 \pm 2°$ (c = 0.45 in chloroform).
THERAP CAT: Antibacterial.

8277. Royal Jelly. Queen bee jelly; apilak; Weiselfuttersaft (German); Gelée royale (French). Secretion from the salivary glands of the worker honey bee which is essential for the development of queen bees. *See also* Queen Substance. Production from bee hives: Ritschel, *Oesterr. Drogisten-Ztg.* **12**, 4-7 (1958). Synthetic mixture fed to bee larvae maintains life, but does not produce queens. The presence of hormones affecting mammals has not been demonstrated: Hinglais, Gautherie, *Compt. Rend.* **242**, 2483 (1956). No practical utility in human nutrition because of the very large amounts required for any definite effect: Moreaux, *Bull. Soc. Sci. Nancy* **14**, 49-53 (1955), *C.A.* **50**, 13214f (1956). Review of composition and biological activity: A. D. Dayan, *J. Pharm. Pharmacol.* **12**, 377-383 (1960). Monographs: B. deBelvefer, *Royal Jelly* (Paris, Librairie Maloine, 1958) 270 pp; H. Rem-

bold, *Biologically Active Substances in Royal Jelly* in *Vitam. Horm.*
23, 359-382 (1965).

Royal Jelly Acid

Milky white, highly viscous secretion. Analysis of fresh specimen (% wt at pH 5): moisture 65-70, protein 15-20, carbohydrate 10-15, lipid 1.7-6, ash 0.7-2.0; elemental analysis: P up to 0.5, S up to 0.6; trace elements present: Na, K, Fe, Cu, Mg, Mn, Ca. Vitamins (μg/g): thiamine 2, riboflavine 10, pyridoxine 2, nicotinic acid 75, biotin 2, folic acid 0.3, inositol 100, pantothenic acid 250, ascorbic acid 3-5, vitamin D trace, vitamin E trace. When stored at room temp, changes to a lightly yellow gum, and after some weeks, to a brittle amber solid.

Royal jelly acid. *trans*-10-Hydroxy-Δ^2-decenoic acid. $C_{10}H_{18}O_3$; mol wt 186.25. Constitutes ~10% of the dried royal jelly. Isoln: Townsend, Lucas, *Biochem. J.* **34**, 1155 (1940); Butenandt, Rembold, *Z. Physiol. Chem.* **308**, 284 (1957). Synthesis: Fray *et al., Tetrahedron Lett.* **4**, 15 (1960); Smissman *et al., J. Org. Chem.* **29**, 3517 (1964); Bestmann *et al., Ann.* **699**, 33 (1966); J. Tsuji *et al., Bull. Chem. Soc. Jpn.* **50**, 2507 (1977); T. Fujisawa *et al., Chem. Lett.* **1982**, 219; R. Chiron, *J. Chem. Ecol.* **8**, 709 (1982). Leukemia prevention in mice: Townsend *et al., Nature* **183**, 1270 (1959). Prisms from ether + petr ether or methanol + water, mp 64-65°. uv max: 211 nm (ε 12000).

8278. Rubber. Caoutchouc; India rubber. Primarily obtained by coagulating the milk juice (latex) of several tropical trees, chiefly *Hevea brasiliensis* Muell.-Arg., *Euphorbiaceae. Habit.* Brazil, East Indies, Java, etc. Rubber also occurs in a number of plants, among which **guayule** (*Parthenium argentatum* Gray), a shrub which grows primarily in the northern Mexican desert, represents a potentially useful renewable source. Guayule produces rubber which is chemically identical to *Hevea* rubber in amounts ranging from 10-20% (dry basis) distributed in the roots and stems. *See* E. Campos-Lopez, *J. Polym. Sci. Polym. Lett. Ed.* **14**, 649 (1976); *J. Polym. Sci. Polym. Chem. Ed.* **14**, 1561 (1976); J. D. Johnson, C. W. Hinman, *Science* **208**, 460 (1980). Possible biosynthesis from acetate through mevalonic acid and isopentenyl pyrophosphate: Archer *et al., Nature* **184**, 268 (1959). Comprehensive review of chemistry: Ellis, *Chem. Ind. (London)* **1962**, 1447. Book: L. G. Polhamus, *Rubber* (Wiley, New York, 1962). *Review:* Jirgenson's, *Natural Organic Macromolecules* (Pergamon Press, New York, 1962) pp 115-124; D. R. St. Cyr in *Kirk-Othmer Encyclopedia of Chemical Technology* vol. 20 (Wiley-Interscience, New York, 3rd ed., 1982) pp 468-491. Natural rubber is defined as a *cis*-1,4-polyisoprene with a molecular weight varying from 100,000 to one million.

The best grades of raw rubber (pale crepe or smoked sheet) contain ~95% rubber hydrocarbon. The rest consists of proteins (2-3%), acetone-sol resins and fatty acids (2%), small amounts of sugar and a little mineral matter. Vulcanization, which consists of heating rubber with 1-3% of sulfur, introduces cross links between chains to produce a three-dimensional lattice of improved elasticity, strength, and temp sensitivity. Accelerators such as zinc dimethyldithiocarbamate greatly decrease the time or lower the temp required for vulcanization. Pure rubber is nearly colorless and transparent in thin layers; odorless and tasteless. It is very elastic and lighter than water. Dec at about 120°. Burns with smoky flame. Emits characteristic offensive odor while burning. Practically insol in water, alcohol, dil acids, or alkali; sol in abs ether, chloroform, most fixed and volatile oils, petr ether, carbon disulfide, oil of turpentine.

8279. Rubeanic Acid. [79-40-3] Ethanedithioamide; dithiooxamide. $C_2H_4N_2S_2$; mol wt 120.20. C 19.98%, H 3.35%,

N 23.31%, S 53.35%. $NH_2CSCSNH_2$. Review of rubeanic acid and derivs as chelating ligands and analytical reagents: Ray, Xavier, *J. Indian Chem. Soc.* **38**, 535 (1961).

Red crystals or cryst powder; dec ~200°. Slightly sol in water; sol in alcohols. Insol in ether.

USE: As a reagent for copper, cobalt, and nickel. As a stabilizer of ascorbic acid solns: Smoczkiewicz, Grochmalicka, *Nature* **192**, 16 (1961).

8280. Ruberythric Acid. [152-84-1] 1-Hydroxy-2-[(6-*O*-β-D-xylopyranosyl-β-D-glucopyranosyl)oxy]-9,10-anthracenedione; 1-hydroxy-2-anthraquinonyl 6-*O*-β-D-xylopyranosyl-β-D-glucopyranoside; β-2-alizarin primeveroside; ruberythrinic acid; rubian; rubianic acid. $C_{25}H_{26}O_{13}$; mol wt 534.47. C 56.18%, H 4.90%, O 38.92%. Isoln from root of *Rubia tinctorium* L., *Rubiaceae:* Hill, Richter, *Proc. R. Soc. London Ser. B* **121**, 547 (1937). Structure: Richter, *J. Chem. Soc.* **1936**, 1701. Synthesis: Zemplén, Bognár, *Ber.* **72B**, 913 (1939). Metabolism: Maehner, Dulce, *Z. Klin. Chem. Klin. Biochem.* **6**, 99 (1968).

Golden-yellow, silky, lustrous prisms or long needles. mp 259-261° (from water). Sol in hot water, alkalies; slightly sol in alc, ether. Practically insol in benzene.

8281. Rubiadin. [117-02-2] 1,3-Dihydroxy-2-methyl-9,10-anthracenedione; 1,3-dihydroxy-2-methylanthraquinone. $C_{15}H_{10}O_4$; mol wt 254.24. C 70.86%, H 3.96%, O 25.17%. From *Rubia tinctorum* L., *Coprosma* var., *Morinda citrifolia* Linn, *Rubiaceae:* Schunck, *Ann.* **87**, 344 (1853); Briggs, Nicholls, *J. Chem. Soc.* **1949**, 1241; Briggs *et al., ibid.* **1952**, 1718; Borvie, Cooke, *Aust. J. Chem.* **15**, 332 (1962). Structure: Marchlewski, *J. Chem. Soc.* **63**, 1137 (1893); Schunck, Marchlewski, *ibid.* **65**, 182 (1894); Jones, Robertson, *ibid.* **1930**, 1699. Synthesis: Joshi *et al., J. Sci. Ind. Res.* **14B**, 87 (1955); Hirase, *Chem. Pharm. Bull.* **8**, 417 (1960).

Yellow plates from glacial acetic acid, mp 302°; yellow slender plates from alc, mp 290°. Absorption max (ethanol): 246, 280, 415 nm (log ε 4.39, 4.52, 3.87). Sol in alc, ether. Practically insol in water, alkalies.

Diacetate. Yellow rods from acetic anhydride, mp 228°.
Dimethyl ether. Yellow needles from alc, mp 160.5°.

8282. Rubidium. [7440-17-7] Rb; at. wt 85.4678; at. no. 37; valence 1. Group IA (1). Alkali metal. Widely distributed in very small quantities in earth's crust: 0.0034% by wt. Naturally occurring isotopes: 85 (72.15%); 87 (27.85%); ^{87}Rb is radioactive, $T_{1/2}$ 4.88×10^{10} yr, β^- emitter. Artificial isotopes (mass nos.): 74-102. Found with other alkali metals in *rhodizite* (borate), *lepidolite* (aluminosilicate), *rubidium carnallite* (chloride); in sea water; in mineral springs and salt lakes. Discovered by Bunsen and Kirchhoff in 1861. Prepn: Hackspill, *Helv. Chim. Acta* **11**, 1003 (1928). *Review:* Whaley, "Sodium, Potassium, Rubidium, Cesium and Francium" in *Comprehensive Inorganic Chemistry* vol. I, J. C. Bailar Jr. *et al.*, Eds. (Pergamon Press, Oxford, 1973) pp 369-529; *Chemistry of the Elements* N. N. Greenwood, A. Earnshaw, Eds. (Pergamon Press, New York, 1984) pp 75-116; F. S. Wagner in *Kirk-Othmer Encyclopedia of Chemical Technology* vol. 21 (Wiley-Interscience, New York, 4th ed., 1997) pp 591-600.

Lustrous, silvery-white, soft metal; body-centered cubic structure; rapidly tarnishes on exposure to air. mp 39°. bp 688°. d^{20} 1.532. Specific heat 0.0802 cal/g deg. One of the most active metals. E° (aq) Rb/Rb$^+$ 2.924 V. Emits characteristic red-violet color (780.0 nm) in flame. Chemical properties closely resemble potassium. Reacts violently with water, ice, steam, lower alcohols, chlorinated hydrocarbons. Ignites spontaneously in oxygen; when molten readily takes fire in the air. Reacts vigorously with the halogens. Forms a series of solid solns with potassium, cesium, sodium. Combines vigorously with mercury. *Keep under benzene, petroleum, or other liq not containing oxygen.*

USE: In making rubidium salts; as a reagent in making zeolite catalysts; in photoelectric cells.

8283. Rubidium Bromide. [7789-39-1] BrRb; mol wt 165.37. Br 48.32%, Rb 51.68%. RbBr.

White, cryst powder; d 3.35; mp 682°; bp 1340°. Sol in about 1 part cold water, 0.5 part boiling water. The aq soln is neutral.

8284. Rubidium Chloride. [7791-11-9] Rubinorm. ClRb; mol wt 120.92. Cl 29.32%, Rb 70.68%. RbCl. Causes shock-induced aggression in rats: B. S. Eichelman, *Psychopharmacol. Bull.* **9**, 21 (1973). Biochemical, behavioral and metabolic studies in humans: R. R. Fieve *et al., Am. J. Psychiatry* **130**, 55 (1973). Clinical evaluations in depression: C. Paschalis *et al., J. R. Soc. Med.* **71**, 343 (1978); G. Placidi *et al., J. Clin. Psychopharmacol.* **8**, 184 (1988).

White, crystalline powder. d 2.76. mp 715°. bp 1390°. One gram dissolves in 1 ml cold, 0.7 ml boiling water, 90 ml methanol, 1650 ml alc. The aq soln is neutral.

USE: As catalyst; as gasoline octane number improver.

THERAP CAT: Antidepressant.

8285. Rubidium Hydroxide. [1310-82-3] HORb; mol wt 102.48. H 0.98%, O 15.61%, Rb 83.40%. RbOH. Book: L. S. Itkina, *Lithium, Rubidium and Cesium Hydroxide* (Nauka, Moscow, USSR, 1973) 136 pp. Toxicological study: G. T. Johnson *et al., Toxicol. Appl. Pharmacol.* **32**, 239 (1975).

Grayish-white, deliquesc mass. d 3.203. Melts at red heat. Sol in 0.6 part water; sol in alcohol. It is a stronger base than potassium hydroxide. *Keep well closed.*

USE: Catalyst in oxidative chlorination.

8286. Rubidium Iodide. [7790-29-6] IRb; mol wt 212.37. I 59.76%, Rb 40.24%. RbI.

White crystals or cryst powder; discolors on exposure to air and light; d 3.55; mp 642°; bp 1300°. Sol in 0.66 part water; sol in alcohol. The aq soln is neutral or slightly alkaline. *Keep well closed and protected from light.*

THERAP CAT: Iodine source.

8287. Rubijervine. [79-58-3] (3β,12α)-Solanid-5-ene-3,12-diol; Δ⁵-3β,12α-dihydroxysolanidene; rubigervine. C₂₇H₄₃NO₂; mol wt 413.64. C 78.40%, H 10.48%, N 3.39%, O 7.74%. From various species of *Veratrum, Liliaceae.* Isoln: Wright, Luff, *J. Chem. Soc.* **35**, 405 (1879); Salzberger, *Arch. Pharm.* **228**, 462 (1890); Jacobs, Craig, *J. Biol. Chem.* **148**, 41 (1943); Sato, Jacobs, *ibid.* **179**, 623 (1949); Pelletier, Locke, *J. Am. Chem. Soc.* **79**, 4531 (1957). Stereochemistry: Höhne *et al., Tetrahedron* **22**, 673 (1966). Comparative toxicity: O. Krayer *et al., J. Pharmacol. Exp. Ther.* **82**, 167 (1944).

Solvated needles from alc, mp 240-246°. $[\alpha]_D^{25}$ +19.0° (ethanol). Very sparingly sol in water. Sol in ethanol, methanol, benzene, chloroform. Slightly sol in ether, petr ether. Red color in concd H₂SO₄. Precipitated by digitonin. LD₅₀ i.v. in mice: 70 mg/kg (Krayer).

Hydrobromide. C₂₇H₄₃NO₂.HBr. Needles from methanol + acetone, dec 265-270°.

THERAP CAT: Antifungal.

8288. Rubitecan. [91421-42-0] (4S)-4-Ethyl-4-hydroxy-10-nitro-1H-pyrano[3′,4′:6,7]indolizino[1,2-b]quinoline-3,14(4H,-12H)-dione; 9-nitrocamptothecin; 9-nitro-(20S)-camptothecin; 9-NC; Orathecin. C₂₀H₁₅N₃O₆; mol wt 393.35. C 61.07%, H 3.84%, N 10.68%, O 24.40%. Semisynthetic camptothecin which inhibits DNA topoisomerase I. Prodrug of 9-aminocamptothecin, (9-AC), *q.v.* Prepn: **JP Kokai 59 51288** (1984 to Yakult Honsha), *C.A.* **101**, 91322 (1984); M. C. Wani *et al., J. Med. Chem.* **29**, 2358 (1986); and activity: S. Sawada *et al., Chem. Pharm. Bull.* **39**, 3183 (1991). Conversion to 9-AC by human cells: P. Pantazis *et al., Eur. J. Haematol.* **53**, 246 (1994); *eidem, ibid.* **55**, 211 (1995). Clinical trial in pancreatic cancer: J. S. Stehlin *et al., Int. J. Oncol.* **14**, 821 (1999). *Review:* C. F. Verschraegen, *Curr. Opin. Oncol. Endocr. Metab. Invest. Drugs* **1**, 184-190 (1999).

Yellow amorphous powder from CH₃OH-CHCl₃ (13:87), mp 182-186°. $[\alpha]_D^{23}$ +27° (c = 0.2 in CH₃OH-CHCl₃, 1:4).

THERAP CAT: Antineoplastic.

8289. Rubixanthin. [3763-55-1] (3R)-β,ψ-Caroten-3-ol. C₄₀H₅₆O; mol wt 552.87. C 86.90%, H 10.21%, O 2.89%. Carotenoid isomeric with cryptoxanthin. Isolated from hipberries (rose hips, *Rosa rubiginosa* L., *Rosaceae*): Kuhn, Grundmann, *Ber.* **67**, 339, 1133 (1934); from the flowers of *Tagetes patula* L., *Compositae.* Found also in other *Rosa* varieties. Structural studies: Brown, Weedon, *Chem. Commun.* **1968**, 382. Abs config: L. Bartlett *et al., J. Chem. Soc. C* **1969**, 2527. Biosynthesis studies: McDermott *et al., Biochem. J.* **134**, 1115 (1973). Has no vitamin A activity.

Deep red needles with metallic luster from benzene + methanol. Orange crystals from benzene + petr ether, mp 160°. Absorption max (chloroform): 509, 474, 439 nm. Sol in benzene, chloroform; slightly sol in petr ether, alcohol.

8290. Ruboxistaurin. [169939-94-0] (9S)-9-[(Dimethyl-amino)methyl]-6,7,10,11-tetrahydro-9H,18H-5,21:12,17-dimeth-enodibenzo[e,k]pyrrolo[3,4h][1,4,13]oxadiazacyclohexadecine-18,20(19H)-dione; (S)-3,4-[(N,N′-1,1′-((2″-ethoxy)-3‴(O)-4‴-(N,N-dimethylamino)butane)-bis-(3,3′-indolyl)]-1(H)-pyrrole-2,3-dione; LY-333531. C₂₈H₂₈N₄O₃; mol wt 468.55. C 71.77%, H 6.02%, N 11.96%, O 10.24%. Protein kinase Cβ (PKCβ) inhibitor; macrocyclic bisindolylmaleimide. Prepn: W. F. Heath, Jr. *et al.,* **EP 657458**; *eidem,* **US 5552396** (1995, 1996 both to Eli Lilly); M. R. Jirousek *et al., J. Med. Chem.* **39**, 2664 (1996); M. M. Faul *et al., J. Org. Chem.* **63**, 1961 (1998). Characterization of salt forms: G. L. Engel *et al., Int. J. Pharm.* **198**, 239 (2000). Enantioselective synthesis: B. M. Trost, W. Tang, *Org. Lett.* **3**, 3409 (2001). Antiangiogenic activity: R. P. Danis *et al., Invest. Ophthalmol. Visual Sci.* **39**, 171 (1998). Clinical trial in diabetic retinopathy: PKC-DRS Study Group, *Diabetes* **54**, 2188 (2005); in diabetic neuropathy: A. I. Vinik *et al., Clin. Ther.* **27**, 1164 (2005); in diabetic nephropathy: K. R. Tuttle *et al., Diabetes Care* **28**, 2686 (2005). Review of pharmacology and therapeutic potential: S. V. Joy *et al., Ann. Pharmacother.* **39**, 1693-1699 (2005); A. Vinik, *Expert Opin. Invest. Drugs* **14**, 1547-1559 (2005).

uv max (ethanol): 493, 382, 282, 232, 204 nm (ε 3944, 3796, 9946, 38382, 43887). Soly in water: <1 μg/ml.

Hydrochloride. [169939-93-9] $C_{28}H_{28}N_4O_3$·HCl; mol wt 505.01. Orange cake. $[\alpha]_D^{25}$ −28.7° (c = 1.0 in ethanol). Soly in water: 0.1 mg/ml.

Methanesulfonate monohydrate. [202260-21-7]; [192050-59-2] (anhydrous). Ruboxistaurin mesylate monohydrate; Arxxant. $C_{28}H_{28}N_4O_3$·CH_4O_3S·H_2O; mol wt 582.67. Thin red or red-orange plates from acetone/water. Dec 270°. Soly in water: 0.5 mg/ml.

THERAP CAT: In treatment of diabetic microvascular complications.

8291. Rubus. Blackberry bark. Dried bark of rhizome and roots of the section *Eubatus* Focke of the genus *Rubus* L. or *R. nigrobaccus* Bailey, *Rosaceae. Habit.* Eastern U.S. *Constit.* Tannin, gallic acid, villosin (a saponin).

THERAP CAT: Antidiarrheal.

8292. Rufigallol. [82-12-2] 1,2,3,5,6,7-Hexahydroxy-9,10-anthracenedione; 1,2,3,5,6,7-hexahydroxyanthraquinone; rufigallic acid; C.I. 58600. $C_{14}H_8O_8$; mol wt 304.21. C 55.27%, H 2.65%, O 42.07%. Prepd by the action of H_2SO_4 on gallic acid: Robiquet, *Ann.* **19**, 204 (1836); by dry distn of gallic acid: Kunz-Krause, Manicke, *Ber.* **53**, 190 (1920). *See also: Colour Index vol.* **4** (3rd ed., 1971) p 4520.

Red needles. Does not melt, but sublimes with partial decompn upon heating. Absorption spectrum: Treibs, Steinmetz, *Ann.* **506**, 171, 191 (1933). Practically insol in water. Freely sol in acetone; slightly sol in alcohol, ether, with yellow color. Sol in alkali hydroxide solns with violet color, but is soon dec by oxidation.

Hexamethyl ether. $C_{20}H_{20}O_8$. Yellow needles, mp 240°.

USE: For color reactions with Zr and Hf.

8293. Rufinamide. [106308-44-5] 1-[(2,6-Difluorophenyl)-methyl]-1H-1,2,3-triazole-4-carboxamide; 1-(2,6-difluorobenzyl)-1H-1,2,3-triazole-4-carboxamide; CGP-33101; Inovelon. $C_{10}H_8$-F_2N_4O; mol wt 238.19. C 50.42%, H 3.39%, F 15.95%, N 23.52%, O 6.72%. Antiepileptic triazole derivative which decreases firing by neurons at sodium channels. Prepn: R. Meier, **EP 199262**; *eidem*, **US 4789680** (1986, 1988 both to Ciba-Geigy). HPLC determn in human plasma: L. A. Brunner, M. L. Powell, *Biomed. Chromatogr.* **6**, 278 (1992). Clinical pharmacokinetics: W. K. Cheung *et al., Pharm. Res.* **12**, 1878 (1995); tolerability: J.-M. Cardot *et al., Biopharm. Drug Dispos.* **19**, 259 (1998). Clinical study in epilepsy: S. Palhagen *et al., Epilepsy Res.* **43**, 115 (2001). Review of clinical experience: K. K. Jain *et al., Exp. Opin. Invest. Drugs* **9**, 829-840 (2000).

Crystals from ethanol, mp 237-240°. Moderate soly in 0.1N HCl.

THERAP CAT: Anticonvulsant.

8294. Rufloxacin. [101363-10-4] 9-Fluoro-2,3-dihydro-10-(4-methyl-1-piperazinyl)-7-oxo-7H-pyrido[1,2,3-*de*]-1,4-benzo-thiazine-6-carboxylic acid; MF-934. $C_{17}H_{18}N_3O_3S$; mol wt 363.41. C 56.18%, H 4.99%, F 5.23%, N 11.56%, O 13.21%, S 8.82%. Fluorinated quinolone; structurally similar to ofloxacin, *q.v.* Prepn: G. Mascellani *et al.*, **AU 85 39142**; *eidem*, **US 4684647** (1985, 1987 both to Mediolanum); V. Cecchetti *et al., J. Med. Chem.* **30**, 465 (1987). *In vitro* activity: R. Wise *et al., Antimicrob. Agents Chemother.* **29**, 649 (1992). Mechanism of action and resistance: L. J. V. Piddock *et al., J. Antimicrob. Chemother.* **31**, 855 (1993). Pharmacokinetics and safety: J. C. Kisicki *et al., ibid.* **36**, 1296 (1992). HPLC determn in biological fluids: F. Lombardi *et al., J. Chromatogr.* **576**, 129 (1992). Clinical study in cystitis and urinary tract infections: R. Mattina *et al., Infection* **21**, 106 (1993); in bronchitis: W. Klietmann *et al., Antimicrob. Agents Chemother.* **37**, 2298 (1993).

Hydrochloride. [106017-08-7] ISF-09334; Qari; Monos; Tebraxin. $C_{17}H_{18}FN_3O_3S$·HCl; mol wt 399.87. Crystals from ethanol/water, mp 322-324° (Cecchetti). LD_{50} in rats, mice (mg/kg): 285, 224 i.v.; LD_{50} in rabbits, male, female rats (mg/kg): 660, 631, 501 orally (Cecchetti).

THERAP CAT: Antibacterial.

8295. Rugulovasines. $C_{16}H_{16}N_2O_2$; mol wt 268.31. C 71.62%, H 6.01%, N 10.44%, O 11.93%. Mixture of the interconvertible diastereomers, rugulovasine A (*cis*-form) and rugulovasine B (*trans*-form). Isolated as the hydrochlorides from surface cultures of *Penicillium concavo-rugulosum* Abe and other *penicillium* strains: Abe *et al., Agric. Biol. Chem.* **33**, 469 (1969); R. J. Cole *et al., Can. J. Microbiol.* **22**, 741 (1976). Prepn and separation of isomers: Abe, **DE 1919255** (1969 to Takeda), *C.A.* **72**, 30311f (1970). Structure: Yamatodani *et al., Agric. Biol. Chem.* **34**, 485 (1970). Abs config and mechanism of interconversion of the isomers: R. J. Cole *et al., Tetrahedron Lett.* **1976**, 3849. Total synthesis: J. Rebek, Y. K. Shue, *J. Am. Chem. Soc.* **102**, 5426 (1980). Hypotensive and cardiovascular activity studies of the hydrochloride isomers: Nagaoka *et al., Arzneim.-Forsch.* **22**, 137, 143 (1972).

Rugulovasine A   Rugulovasine B

Rugulovasine A. [26909-33-1] *cis*-(±)-3,4-Dihydro-4′-methyl-4-(methylamino)spiro[benz[*cd*]indole-5(1H),2′(5′H)-furan]-5′-one. Colorless prisms from benzene, chloroform, or acetonitrile, mp 138° (dec). $[\alpha]_{436}^{22}$ −3.0° (pyridine). uv max (ethanol): 224, 277, 288, 295 nm (log ε 4.37, 3.70, 3.78, 3.77). Sparingly sol in water, petr ether. Moderately sol in ether, chloroform, benzene, acetonitrile. Readily sol in ethyl acetate, acetone, methanol, ethanol, pyridine, and dil acids.

Hydrochloride. [28375-03-3] $C_{16}H_{16}N_2O_2$·HCl. Colorless prisms from water, mp 225° (dec).

Rugulovasine B. [26909-34-2] Difficult to crystallize from common solvents. Separated from benzene as colorless resinous oil. $[\alpha]_{436}^{22}$ +1.4° (pyridine). uv max (ethanol): 227, 278, 288, 295 nm (log ε 4.16, 3.68, 3.73, 3.72). Same solubilities as rugulovasine A.

Hydrochloride. [28510-15-8] $C_{16}H_{16}N_2O_2$.HCl. White prisms from water, mp 187° (dec).

8296. Rumex. Yellow dock; curled dock. Dried root of *Rumex crispus* L., or of *R. obtusifolius* L., *Polygonaceae. Habit.* Europe, North America. *Constit.* Chrysophanic acid, emodin, tannin, calcium oxalate, lapathin.

THERAP CAT: Cathartic, astringent.

8297. Rupatadine. [158876-82-5] 8-Chloro-6,11-dihydro-11-[1-[(5-methyl-3-pyridinyl)methyl]-4-piperidinylidene]-5H-benzo[5,6]cyclohepta[1,2-b]pyridine; UR-12592. $C_{26}H_{26}ClN_3$; mol wt 415.96. C 75.07%, H 6.30%, Cl 8.52%, N 10.10%. Dual antagonist of histamine H_1 and platelet-activating factor receptors. Prepn: E. Carceller *et al.*, **ES 2042421**; *eidem*, **US 5407941** (1993, 1995 both to Uriach); *eidem, J. Med. Chem.* **37**, 2697 (1994). Mechanism of action: M. Merlos *et al., J. Pharmacol. Exp. Ther.* **280**, 114 (1997). Clinical trial in seasonal allergic rhinitis: F. Saint-Martin *et al., J. Invest. Allergol. Clin. Immunol.* **14**, 34 (2004); and comparison with ebastine: E. M. Guadaño *et al., Allergy* **59**, 766 (2004). Review of pharmacology and clinical development: N. Y. Van Den Anker-Rakhmanina, *Curr. Opin. Anti-Inflam. Immunomod. Invest. Drugs* **2**, 127-132 (2000).

Creamy solid, mp 58-61°.

Fumarate. [182349-12-8] Rupafin. $C_{26}H_{26}ClN_3 \cdot C_4H_4O_4$; mol wt 532.03.

Trihydrochloride. [156611-76-6] $C_{26}H_{26}ClN_3$.3HCl; mol wt 525.34. Crystals from ethyl acetate + ether, mp 213-217°.

THERAP CAT: Antihistaminic.

8298. Rutecarpine. [84-26-4] 8,13-Dihydroindolo[2′,3′:3,-4]pyrido[2,1-b]quinazolin-5(7H)-one; rutaecarpine. $C_{18}H_{13}N_3O$; mol wt 287.32. C 75.24%, H 4.56%, N 14.62%, O 5.57%. From fruit of *Evodia rutaecarpa* Hook. & Thoms. and *Hortia arborea* Engl., *Rutaceae:* Asahina, Kashiwaki, *J. Pharm. Soc. Jpn.* **1915**, 1293; Pachter *et al., J. Am. Chem. Soc.* **82**, 5187 (1960). Structure: Y. Asahina, *J. Pharm. Soc. Jpn.* **1924**, 1. Synthesis: Y. Asahina *et al., J. Chem. Soc.* **1927**, 1708; T. Kametani *et al., J. Am. Chem. Soc.* **99**, 2306 (1977); *eidem, Chem. Pharm. Bull.* **26**, 1922 (1978); H. Möhrle *et al., Arch. Pharm.* **313**, 990 (1980); J. Bergman, S. Bergman, *Heterocycles* **16**, 347 (1981). Simple synthesis: J. Kökösi *et al., Tetrahedron Lett.* **22**, 4861 (1981). Synthesis under physiological conditions: Schöpf, *Angew. Chem.* **50**, 779, 797 (1937). Biosynthesis: M. Yamazaki *et al., Tetrahedron Lett.* **1966**, 3221; **1967**, 3317. Mass spec.: J. Tamas *et al., Acta Chim. Acad. Sci. Hung.* **89**, 85 (1976).

Needles from ethyl acetate, mp 259.5-260°. uv max (ethanol): 278, 290, 332, 345, 364 nm (log ε 3.83, 3.88, 4.49, 4.54, 4.44). Sol in alc, benzene, chloroform, ether. Practically insol in water.

8299. Ruthenium. [7440-18-8] Ru; at. wt 101.07; at. no. 44; valences 1-8; most common states 2, 3, 4. Group VIII (8). Naturally occurring isotopes: 96 (5.46%); 98 (1.87%); 99 (12.63%); 100 (12.53%); 101 (17.02%); 102 (31.6%); 104 (18.87%); artificial radioactive isotopes: 93-95; 97; 103; 105-108. Belongs to the platinum group of metals. Found in the minerals osmiridium, laurite, in platinum ores, in some copper-nickel ores. Discovered in 1828 by Osann; prepd in the pure state in 1845 by Klaus. Constitutes about 0.0004 ppm of the crust of the earth. Prepn from osmiridium: Fremy *et al.*, cited by Mellor, *A Comprehensive Treatise on Inorganic and Theoretical Chemistry* **15**, 499 (1936). Reviews of prepn, properties and chemistry of ruthenium and other platinum metals: Gilchrist, *Chem. Rev.* **32**, 277-372 (1943); W. P. Griffith, *The Chemistry of the Rarer Platinum Metals* (John Wiley, New York, 1967) pp 1-41, 126-226; Livingstone in *Comprehensive Inorganic Chemistry* vol. 3, J. C. Bailar, Jr. *et al.*, Eds. (Pergamon Press, Oxford, 1973) pp 1163-1209.

Lustrous, hard metal; hexagonal, close-packed structure. d_4^{20} 12.45. mp about 2450°; bp about 4150°. Sp heat (0°): 0.057 cal/g/°C. Does not react with acids, even aqua regia. Not oxidized by air in the cold; on heating combines readily with oxygen; the powdered metal forms the dioxide on igniting in air. Superficially attacked by concd alkaline hypochlorites. The powdered metal is attacked by chlorine above 200°; by bromine between 300-700°. Oxidized by fused alkali hydroxides. Forms alloys with platinum, palladium, cobalt, nickel, tungsten; forms definite compds with zinc and with tin.

USE: As substitute for platinum in jewelry; for pen nibs; as hardener in electrical contact alloys, electrical filaments; in ceramic colors; catalyst in synthesis of long chain hydrocarbons.

8300. Ruthenium Red. [1307-52-4] Ruthenium oxychloride ammoniated; C.I. 77800. $Cl_6H_{42}N_{14}O_2Ru_3$; mol wt 786.35. Cl 27.05%, H 5.38%, N 24.94%, O 4.07%, Ru 38.56%. [(NH$_3$)$_5$-Ru—O—Ru(NH$_3$)$_4$—O—Ru(NH$_3$)$_5$]Cl$_6$. Exists as tetrahydrate. Identification: A. Joly, *C.R. Hebd. Seances Acad. Sci.* **115**, 1299 (1893). Prepn and structure: Fletcher *et al., J. Chem. Soc.* **1961**, 2000. Mössbauer study: Clausen *et al., Inorg. Nucl. Chem. Lett.* **7**, 485 (1971). Alternate structure and composition: Sterling, *Am. J. Bot.* **57**, 172 (1970). Use as microscopic stain: L. Mangin, *C.R. Hebd. Seances Acad. Sci.* **116**, 653 (1893); in electron microscopy: R. Dierichs, *Histochemistry* **64**, 171 (1979). Differential staining: P. R. Blanquet, *ibid.* **47**, 175 (1976); M. G. Gutierrez-Gonzalvez *et al., J. Microsc.* **145**, 333 (1987). Series of articles on chemistry, mechanism of action, specific uses: *Anat. Rec.* **171**, 347-442 (1971). Conversion *in situ* to *ruthenium violet:* J. R. Luft, *ibid.* 347; M. G. Guiterrez-Gonzalvez *et al., loc. cit.*

Brownish-red powder. Sol in water, ammonia.

USE: In microscopy as a general stain.

8301. Ruthenium Tetroxide. [20427-56-9] Ruthenium-(VIII) oxide. O_4Ru; mol wt 165.07. O 38.77%, Ru 61.23%. RuO_4. Prepd by fusing Ru with $KMnO_4$ and KOH in a proportion of 1:2:20. Lab procedures: Ruff, Vidic, *Z. Anorg. Allg. Chem.* **136**, 49 (1924); Grube in *Handbook of Preparative Inorganic Chemistry* vol. 2, G. Brauer, Ed. (Academic Press, New York, 2nd ed., 1965) p 1599. Crystal structure: Tréhoux *et al., C.R. Seances Acad. Sci. Ser. C* **268**, 246 (1969). Review of use as oxidizing agent: P. N. Rylander, *Organic Syntheses with Noble Metal Catalysts* (Academic Press, New York, 1973) pp 134-144.

Golden-yellow monoclinic prisms. Very volatile, sublimes at room temp. *Handle in hood only. Vapors irritating to eyes and respiratory tract.* mp 25.4°. bp 40°. Sparingly sol in water, about 2.0% (w/v) at 20°. Freely sol in carbon tetrachloride, other chlorinated solvents. Also sol in bromine, liquid SO_2. Reacts explosively with alcohol and filter paper.

USE: Oxidizing agent similar to osmium tetroxide, but more difficult to handle. The solvents normally employed in OsO_4 oxidations (ether, benzene, pyridine) cannot be used because of their violent reaction with RuO_4. Only CCl_4 is recommended: Djerassi, Engle, *J. Am. Chem. Soc.* **75**, 3838 (1953).

8302. Ruthenium Trichloride. [10049-08-8] Cl_3Ru; mol wt 207.43. Cl 51.27%, Ru 48.72%. $RuCl_3$. Two forms, α and β, are known. Prepn: Fletcher *et al., Nature* **199**, 1089 (1963).

α-RuCl₃. Black lustrous crystals. Insol in alcohol, water.

β-RuCl₃. Dark-brown, fluffy, hexagonal crystals. Sol in alcohol.

8303. Rutherfordium. [53850-36-5] Element 104; kurchatovium; unnilquadium. Rf, Ku, Unq; at. no. 104. Group IVB(4). No stable nuclides. Initial production claimed by two groups. Prepn of isotope $^{260}104$ ($T_{1/2}$ ~300 msec; spontaneous fission) by ^{242}Pu ($^{22}Ne,4n$): G. N. Flerov et al., At. Energ. **17**, 310 (1964), C.A. **62**, 189d (1965); eidem, Phys. Lett. **13**, 73 (1964); I. Zvara et al., Radiokhimiya **11**, 161, 163 (1969). Prepn of two α-emitting isotopes, $^{257}104$ ($T_{1/2}$ 4.5 seconds) by ^{249}Cf ($^{12}C,4n$) and $^{259}104$ ($T_{1/2}$ 3 seconds) by ^{249}Cf ($^{13}C,3n$): A. Ghiorso et al., Phys. Rev. Lett. **22**, 1317 (1969). Ten isotopes reported; mass numbers 253-262. Longest-lived known isotope, $^{261}104$, α-emitter, $T_{1/2}$ 65 ±10 seconds, rel. at. mass 261.1089; produced by ^{248}Cm ($^{18}O,5n$): A. Ghiorso et al., Phys. Lett. B **32**, 95 (1970). Chemical properties of isotopes and revised $T_{1/2}$ 21 ±1 msec for $^{260}104$: L. P. Somerville et al., Phys. Rev. **C31**, 1801-1815 (1985). Solution chemistry: K. R. Czerwinski et al., Radiochim. Acta **64**, 23 (1994); eidem, ibid. 29. Reviews of history, prepn and properties: C. Keller, The Chemistry of the Transuranium Elements (Verlag Chemie, Weinheim, English Ed., 1971) pp 613-618; Silva, "Trans-Curium Elements" in MTP Int. Rev. Sci.: Inorg. Chem., Ser. One **vol. 8**, A. G. Maddock, Ed. (University Park Press, Baltimore, 1972) pp 71-105; R. J. Silva in The Chemistry of the Actinide Elements **vol. 2**, J. J. Katz et al., Eds. (Chapman and Hall, New York, 1986) pp 1103-1104; E. K. Hyde et al., Radiochim. Acta **42**, 57-102 (1987); Transfermium Working Group, Pure Appl. Chem. **65**, 1757-1814 (1993); M. Schädel, Inst. Phys. Conf. Ser. **132**, 413-422 (1993). Review of chemistry: D. C. Hoffman, Proc. Robert A. Welch Found. Conf. on Chem. Res., XXXIV, Fifty Years with Transuranium Elements (Houston, Texas, 1990) pp 255-276.

8304. Rutin. [153-18-4] 3-[[6-O-(6-Deoxy-α-L-mannopyranosyl)-β-D-glucopyranosyl]oxy]-2-(3,4-dihydroxyphenyl)-5,7-dihydroxy-4H-1-benzopyran-4-one; rutoside; quercetin-3-rutinoside; 3,3',4',5,7-pentahydroxyflavone-3-rutinoside; melin; phytomelin; eldrin; ilixathin; sophorin; globularicitrin; paliuroside; osyritrin; osyritin; myrticolorin; violaquercitrin; Birutan. $C_{27}H_{30}O_{16}$; mol wt 610.52. C 53.12%, H 4.95%, O 41.93%. Identity with ilixanthin: Schindler, Herb, Arch. Pharm. **288**, 372 (1955). Found in many plants, especially the buckwheat plant (Fagopyrum esculentum Moench., Polygonaceae) which contains about 3% (dry basis): Couch et al., Science **103**, 197 (1946). From tobacco (Nicotiana tabacum L., Solanaceae) Couch, Krewson, U.S. Dept. Agr., Eastern Regional Res. Lab. AIC-123 (1946). In forsythia [Forsythia suspensa (Thunb.) Vahl. var. fortunei (Lindl.) Rehd., Oleaceae], in hydrangea (Hydrangea paniculata Sieb., Saxifragaceae), in pansies (Viola sp., Violaceae). General extraction procedure: Beilstein XXXI, 376. From leaves of Eucalyptus macroryncha F. v. Muell., Myrtaceae: Attree, Perkin, J. Chem. Soc. **1927**, 234. Industrial production from Eucalyptus spp.: Humphreys, Econ. Bot. **18**, 195 (1964). Structure: Zemplén, Gerecs, Ber. **68B**, 1318 (1935). Synthesis: Shakhova et al., Zh. Obshch. Khim. **32**, 390 (1962), C.A. **58**, 1426e (1963). Rutin is hydrolyzed by rhamnodiastase from the seed of Rhamnus utilis Decne, Rhamnaceae (Chinese buckthorn); emulsin is not effective: Bridel, Charaux, Compt. Rend. **181**, 925 (1925). Toxicity data: Harrison et al., J. Am. Pharm. Assoc. **39**, 557 (1950). Book: J. Q. Griffith, Jr., Rutin and Related Flavonoids (Mack, Easton, Pa., 1955). Comprehensive description: T. I. Khalifa et al., Anal. Profiles Drug Subs. **12**, 623-681 (1983).

Pale yellow needles from water, gradual darkening on exposure to light. The crystals contain 3 H_2O and become anhydr after 12 hrs at 110° and 10 mm Hg. Anhydr rutin browns at 125°, becomes plastic at 195-197°, and dec 214-215° (with effervescence). $[\alpha]_D^{23}$ +13.82° (ethanol); $[\alpha]_D^{23}$ −39.43° (pyridine). Anhydr rutin is hygroscopic. One gram dissolves in about 8 liters water, about 200 ml boiling water, 7 ml boiling methanol. Sol in pyridine, formamide and alkaline solns; slightly sol in alcohol, acetone, ethyl acetate. Practically insol in chloroform, carbon bisulfide, ether, benzene, petr

solvents. Dil solns give green color with ferric chloride. Rutin is colored brown by tobacco enzyme under experimental conditions: Neuberg, Kobel, Naturwissenschaften **23**, 800 (1935). LD$_{50}$ i.v. in mice: 950 mg/kg (propylene glycol soln) (Harrison).

THERAP CAT: Capillary protectant.

8305. Rutinose. [90-74-4] 6-O-(6-Deoxy-α-L-mannopyranosyl)-D-glucose; 6-O-α-L-rhamnosyl-D-glucose. $C_{12}H_{22}O_{10}$; mol wt 326.30. C 44.17%, H 6.80%, O 49.03%. A disaccharide present in glycosides. Prepn from rutin by enzymatic hydrolysis using rhamnodiastase: Charaux, Compt. Rend. **178**, 1312 (1924); Bull. Soc. Chim. Biol. **6**, 634 (1924); Zemplén, Gerecs, Ber. **68B**, 1320 (1935). Synthesis: eidem, Ber. **67B**, 2049 (1934); **68B**, 1318 (1935). Structure: Gorin, Perlin, Can. J. Chem. **37**, 1930 (1959).

Very hygroscopic powder from alcohol and ether turning into a syrup on exposure to air. The freshly pptd material loses about 6% of its wt at 100°. The dried rutinose softens around 140°, dec 189-192°. $[\alpha]_D^{20}$ +3.2° → +0.8° (c = 4 in water). $[\alpha]_D^{20}$ −10° (95% alc). Very sol in water. Sol in alc. Hydrolysis with dil HCl yields 1 mol L-rhamnose and 1 mol D-glucose.

Heptaacetylrutinose. mp 169-170°. $[\alpha]_D^{20}$ −27.7° (chloroform).

8306. Ryania. [8047-13-0] A genus of tropical American shrubs and trees belonging to the Flacourtiaceae family. The wood of various species is insecticidal. Ground stem wood of Ryania speciosa Vahl., Flacourtiaceae is employed in the commercial insecticide formulations **Ryanex, Ryanicide** (formerly). See Folkers et al., US 2400295 (1946 to Merck & Co.); Pepper, Carruth, J. Econ. Entomol. **38**, 59 (1945); Heal, Agric. Chem. **4**, 37 (May, 1949). Insecticidal components such as ryanodine, q.v., are extractable by water, chloroform, or methanol. Toxicity data: Kuna, Heal, J. Pharmacol. Exp. Ther. **93**, 407 (1948).

LD$_{50}$ orally in rats, mice, rabbits, guinea pigs (mg/kg): 1200, 650, 650, 2500 (Kuna, Heal).

Caution: In exptl animals causes weakness, deep and slow respiration, vomiting, diarrhea, tremors, convulsions, coma; death may occur.

USE: Insecticide.

8307. Ryanodine. [15662-33-6] Ryanodol 3-(1H-pyrrole-2-carboxylate). $C_{25}H_{35}NO_9$; mol wt 493.55. C 60.84%, H 7.15%, N 2.84%, O 29.18%. Insecticidal principle isolated from Ryania speciosa Vahl., Flacourtiaceae: E. F. Rogers et al., J. Am. Chem. Soc. **70**, 3086 (1948); R. B. Kelly et al., Can. J. Chem. **29**, 905 (1951). Structure: D. R. Babin et al., Experientia **21**, 425 (1965); J. Santroch et al., ibid. **21**, 730 (1965); K. Wiesner et al., Tetrahedron Lett. **1967**, 221; K. Wiesner, Adv. Org. Chem. **8**, 295 (1972). Crystal structure: S. N. Srivastava, M. Przybylska, Can. J. Chem. **46**, 795 (1968). ¹H-NMR: A. L. Waterhouse et al., Chem. Commun. **1984**, 1265. Synthetic studies: P. Deslongchamps, Pure Appl. Chem. **49**, 1329 (1977). Effect on calcium ion uptake by cardiac sarcoplasmic reticulum vesicles: L. R. Jones et al., J. Pharmacol. Exp. Ther. **209**, 48 (1979); L. R. Jones, S. E. Cala, J. Biol. Chem. **256**, 11809 (1981).

Crystals, dec 219-220°. $[\alpha]_D^{25}$ +26° (methanol). uv max (alc): 268.5 nm (log ε 4.18). Sol in water, alcohol, acetone, ether, chloroform. Practically insol in benzene, petr ether.

USE: Insecticide.

S

8308. Sabadilla. [8051-02-3] Cevadilla; caustic barley. The dried ripe seeds of *Schoenocaulon officinale* (Schlecht. & Cham.) A. Gray (*Sabadilla officinarum* Brandt, *Asagraea officinalis* Lindl.), *Liliaceae*. *Habit*. The Andes of Mexico, Guatemala, Venezuela. *Constit.* About 3 to 6% total alkaloids of which cevadine (cryst veratrine) and veratridine (amorphous veratrine) are the most important; other alkaloids are sabadinine, sabadilline, and sabadine; also contains sabadillic and veratric acids; fatty oil, resin. Toxicity data: E. D. Swiss, R. O. Bauer, *Proc. Soc. Exp. Biol. Med.* **76**, 847 (1951).

LD$_{50}$ i.p. in mice: 7.5 mg/kg (Swiss, Bauer).

THERAP CAT: Pediculicide.

THERAP CAT (VET): Has been used as an insecticide.

8309. Sabcomeline. [159912-53-5] *R*-(*Z*)-α-(Methoxyimino)-1-azabicyclo[2.2.2]octane-3-acetonitrile; SB-202026. C$_{10}$H$_{15}$-N$_3$O; mol wt 193.25. C 62.15%, H 7.82%, N 21.74%, O 8.28%. Selective muscarinic M$_1$-receptor partial agonist. Prepn: B. S. Orlek *et al.*, **EP 392803**; *eidem*, **US 5278170**; (1990, 1994 both to Beecham); S. M. Bromidge *et al.*, *J. Med. Chem.* **40**, 4265 (1997). Pharmacology: J. M. Loudon *et al.*, *J. Pharmacol. Exp. Ther.* **283**, 1059 (1997). Cognition improvement in rats: H. Hodges *et al.*, *Behav. Brain Res.* **99**, 81 (1999).

White crystals from methanol-acetone, mp 154-156°. [α]$_D^{20}$ +14.4° (c = 0.424 in EtOH).

Hydrochloride. [159912-58-0] Memric. C$_{10}$H$_{15}$N$_3$O.HCl; mol wt 229.71. mp 218-219°. [α]$_D^{20}$ +25.3° (c = 1.00 in EtOH).

THERAP CAT: Nootropic.

8310. Sabeluzole. [104383-17-7] 4-(2-Benzothiazolylmethylamino)-α-[(4-fluorophenoxy)methyl]-1-piperidineethanol; *N*-methyl-*N*-[1-[3-(4-fluorophenoxy)-2-hydroxypropyl]piperidin-4-yl]benzothiazole-2-amine; R-58735. C$_{22}$H$_{26}$FN$_3$O$_2$S; mol wt 415.52. C 63.59%, H 6.31%, F 4.57%, N 10.11%, O 7.70%, S 7.72%. Prepn: R. A. Stokbroekx *et al.*, **EP 184257** (1986 to Janssen). Pharmacology: A. Wauquier *et al.*, *Drug Dev. Res.* **8**, 373 (1986). Comparative activity of racemate and enantiomers: L. Werbrouck *et al.*, *ibid.* **24**, 41 (1991). Clinical pharmacokinetics: P. P. DeDeyn *et al.*, *Eur. J. Clin. Pharmacol.* **43**, 661 (1992). Clinical evaluation of effects on memory functions: G. H. C. Clincke *et al.*, *Psychopharmacology* **94**, 52 (1988). Clinical studies in age-associated memory impairment: L. Tritsmans *et al.*, *Drug Dev. Res.* **20**, 473 (1990); G. Clincke *et al.*, *ibid.* **23**, 301 (1991); in memory functions of epileptics: A. P. Aldenkamp *et al.*, *Neuropsychobiology* **32**, 37 (1995).

mp 101.7°.

THERAP CAT: Nootropic.

8311. Saccharin. [81-07-2] 1,2-Benzisothiazol-3(2*H*)-one 1,1-dioxide; 2,3-dihydro-3-oxobenzisosulfonazole; 1,2-dihydro-2-ketobenzisosulfonazole; saccharin insoluble; benzosulfimide; *o*-sulfobenzimide; benzoic sulfimide; *o*-sulfobenzoic acid imide; Gluside; Glucid; Garantose; Saccharinol; Saccharinose; Saccharol; Saxin; Sykose; Hermesetas. C$_7$H$_5$NO$_3$S; mol wt 183.18. C 45.90%, H 2.75%, N 7.65%, O 26.20%, S 17.50%. Prepn from

o-sulfamoylbenzoic acid: Remsen, Fahlberg, *Ber.* **12**, 470 (1879). History and comparison with other sweetening agents: R. W. Moncrieff, *The Chemical Senses* (Wiley, New York, 1946). Mfg processes: O. Beyer, *Handbuch der Saccharinfabrikation* (Rascher, Zürich, 1923); *FIAT Report* **PB 901** (1945); *Chem. Eng. (N.Y.)* **61**, 128, 150 (July 1954). Maumee Chemical's process: *Chem. Eng. News* **41**, 76-78 (Dec. 9, 1963). Stability studies: DeGarmo *et al.*, *J. Am. Pharm. Assoc. Sci. Ed.* **41**, 17 (1952). Toxicity data: J. D. Taylor *et al.*, *Food Cosmet. Toxicol.* **6**, 313 (1968). Series of articles on toxicology and metabolism: *Food Chem. Toxicol.* **23**, 419-546 (1985). Review of toxicology and carcinogenicity studies of saccharin and its salts: *IARC Monographs* **22**, 111-170 (1980); D. L. Arnold, *Fundam. Appl. Toxicol.* **4**, 674-685 (1984). *Review:* R. Mazur, "Sweeteners" in *Kirk-Othmer Encyclopedia of Chemical Technology* **vol. 22** (John Wiley & Sons, New York, 3rd ed., 1983) pp 448-464.

Monoclinic crystals, mp 228.8-229.7°. Twinning on (001). Perfect 100 cleavage. Acicular crystals by vacuum sublimation. In dil aq soln it is 500 times as sweet as sugar; the sweet taste is still detectable in 1:100,000 dilution. Bitter, metallic aftertaste. d 0.828. Heat of combustion at constant volume: 4753.1 cal/g. uv max (0.1*N* NaOH): 267.3 nm (ε 1570). One gram dissolves in 290 ml water, 25 ml boiling water, 31 ml alcohol, 12 ml acetone, about 50 ml glycerol; freely sol in solns of alkali carbonates; slightly sol in chloroform, ether. pH of 0.35% aq soln 2.0. Hydrolysis products of saccharin are *o*-sulfamoylbenzoic acid (alkaline hydrolysis) and ammonium *o*-sulfobenzoic acid (acid hydrolysis).

Ammonium salt. Saccharin ammonium; Daramin; Sucline. C$_7$-H$_8$N$_2$O$_3$S; mol wt 200.22.

Sodium salt dihydrate. Soluble saccharin; saccharin sodium; Kristallose; Crystallose; Dagutan; Sucaryl; Sucromat. C$_7$H$_4$-NNaO$_3$S.2H$_2$O; mol wt 241.20. Crystalline powder; effloresces in dry air. In dil aq soln it is 300-500 times as sweet as sugar. One gram dissolves in 1.2 ml water, in about 50 ml alcohol. Aq solns are neutral or alkaline to litmus, but not alkaline to phenolphthalein. LD$_{50}$ in mice, rats (g/kg): 6.3, 7.1 i.p.; 17.5, 17.0 orally (Taylor). Anhydrous form, *Sucrédulcor.*

Note: Saccharin was formerly listed as reasonably anticipated to be a human carcinogen: *Eighth Report on Carcinogens* (PB99-128746, 1998) p III-905; delisted because the cancer data are not sufficient to meet the current criteria for this listing: *Ninth Report on Carcinogens* (PB2000-107509, 2000) p B-3.

USE: Non-nutritive sweetener; pharmaceutic aid (flavor). In formulations for electroplating-bath brighteners.

8312. L-Saccharopine. [997-68-2] *N*-(5-Amino-5-carboxypentyl)-L-glutamic acid; ε-*N*-(L-glutar-2-yl)-L-lysine. C$_{11}$H$_{20}$N$_2$-O$_6$; mol wt 276.29. C 47.82%, H 7.30%, N 10.14%, O 34.74%. A lysine precursor in the aminoadipic acid-lysine pathway in yeast: Darling, Larsen, *Acta Chem. Scand.* **15**, 743 (1961); Kjaer, Larsen, *ibid.* 750; Kuo *et al.*, *Biochem. Biophys. Res. Commun.* **8**, 227 (1962); Trupin, Broquist, *J. Biol. Chem.* **240**, 2524 (1965); Jones, Broquist, *ibid.* **241**, 3430 sqq. (1966). Isoln from mycelium of the yeast *Candida utilis:* Marimoto, Yamano, *Biochem. Z.* **340**, 155 (1964).

Hydrated crystals; loses water of crystn over P$_2$O$_5$ at 100°. Dec 240-248°, when anhydr. [α]$_D^{23}$ +33.6° (c = 1 in 0.5*N* HCl); [M]$_D$ +93°. pK$_2$ 2.6; pK$_3$ 4.1; pK$_4$ 9.2; pK$_5$ 10.3. Sparingly sol in water, ethanol. Readily sol in alkaline solns and in strong acids.

8313. Safflower Oil. The oil from the seed of *Carthamus tinctorius* L., *Compositae*. Milling and extraction procedures: Winter, *J. Am. Oil Chem. Soc.* **27**, 82 (1950). Purification and stabilization: Freedman, Shapiro, **US 2978381** (1961). Monograph: R. E. Woodward, G. M. Severson, *Industrial Survey of Safflower*, Chemurgy Dept. Report no. S-3 (Agricult. Expt. Sta., Lincoln, Nebraska, 1951). Fatty acids present as glycerides: palmitic 6.4%, stearic 3.1%, arachidic 0.2%, oleic 13.4%, linoleic 76.6-79.0%, linolenic 0.04-0.13%.

Edible drying oil, intermediate between soybean and linseed oil. d_{25}^{25} 0.9211-0.9215. Titer: 15-18°. n_D^{25} 1.472-1.475. n_D^{40} 1.4690-1.4692. Acid value 1.0-9.7. Saponif value 188-194. Iodine value 140-150. Thiocyanogen value 82.5-86.0. Reichert-Meissl value below 0.5. Hydroxyl value 2.9-6.0. Unsaponifiable below 1.5%. Thickens and becomes rancid on prolonged exposure to air. Sol in the usual oil and fat solvents.

USE: As linseed oil in paints. For salad oil blends, in hydrogenated state as shortening.

THERAP CAT: Dietary supplement in hypercholesteremia (and possible prophylaxis and treatment of atherosclerosis).

8314. Saffron. Crocus; Spanish saffron; French saffron. Stigmas of *Crocus sativus* L., *Iridaceae. Habit.* Western Asia, Southern Europe. *Constit.* About 1% volatile oil, picrocrocin—a bitter glucoside, crocin (polychroit), fixed oil, wax.

Flattish-tubular, almost thread-like stigmas ~1.25 inches (3 cm) long; orange-brown color; strong, peculiar, aromatic odor; bitterish, aromatic taste.

USE: Coloring and flavoring.

8315. Safinamide. [133865-89-1] (2*S*)-2-[[[4-[(3-Fluorophenyl)methoxy]phenyl]methyl]amino]propanamide; (*S*)-(+)-2-[[4-(3-fluorobenzoxy)benzyl]amino]propanamide; FCE-26743. $C_{17}H_{19}FN_2O_2$; mol wt 302.34. C 67.53%, H 6.33%, F 6.28%, N 9.27%, O 10.58%. Voltage-dependent sodium and calcium channel blocker; selective and reversible inhibitor of monoamine oxidase B (MAO-B). Prepn: P. Dostert *et al.,* **EP 400495**; *eidem,* **US 5236957** (1990, 1993 both to Farmitalia); and anticonvulsant activity: P. Pevarello *et al., J. Med. Chem.* **41**, 579 (1998). Mechanism of action study: P. Salvati *et al., J. Pharmacol. Exp. Ther.* **288**, 1151 (1999). Review of early clinical development: P. L. Chazot, *Curr. Opin. Invest. Drugs* **2**, 809-813 (2001). Clinical pharmacokinetics and pharmacodynamics: A. Marzo *et al., Pharmacol. Res.* **50**, 77 (2004). Clinical evaluation in Parkinson's disease: F. Stocchi *et al., Neurology* **63**, 746 (2004).

mp 208-212°.

Methanesulfonate. [202825-46-5] Safinamide mesylate; NW-1015; PNU-151774E. $C_{17}H_{19}FN_2O_2 \cdot CH_4O_3S$; mol wt 398.45. mp 210° (dec). $[\alpha]_D^{25}$ +12.9° (c = 1.1% in 98% acetic acid).

THERAP CAT: Antiparkinsonian; anticonvulsant.

8316. Safranal. [116-26-7] 2,6,6-Trimethyl-1,3-cyclohexadiene-1-carboxaldehyde; 2,2,6-trimethyl-4,6-cyclohexadien-1-aldehyde. $C_{10}H_{14}O$; mol wt 150.22. C 79.95%, H 9.39%, O 10.65%. Prepn from picrocrocin: Kuhn, Winterstein, *Ber.* **67**, 354 (1934). Synthesis: Kuhn, Wendt, *Ber.* **69**, 1549 (1936); Könst *et al., Tetrahedron Lett.* **1974**, 3175. Biogenetic synthesis: T. Kametani *et al., Chem. Pharm. Bull.* **29**, 105 (1981).

Liquid. d_4^{19} 0.9734. $bp_{1.0}$ 70° (bath temp). n_D^{19} 1.5281. Sol in methanol, ethanol, petr ether, glacial acetic acid.

8317. Safrole. [94-59-7] 5-(2-Propenyl)-1,3-benzodioxole; 4-allyl-1,2-methylenedioxybenzene; allylcatechol methylene ether; allyldioxybenzene methylene ether; *m*-allylpyrocatechin methylene ether. $C_{10}H_{10}O_2$; mol wt 162.19. C 74.05%, H 6.21%, O 19.73%. Constituent of several essential oils, notably of sassafras in which it is present to the extent of about 75%. Has been used as topical antiseptic; pediculicide. Metabolism studies: Oswald *et al., Biochim. Biophys. Acta* **230**, 237 (1971). Toxicity data: Hagan *et al., Toxicol. Appl. Pharmacol.* **7**, 18 (1965). Review of carcinogenic risk: *IARC Monographs* **10**, 231-241 (1976).

Colorless or slightly yellow liq; sassafras odor. d^{20} 1.096. mp ~11°. bp 232-234°. n_D^{20} 1.5383. Insol in water. Very sol in alcohol. Miscible with chloroform, ether. LD_{50} in rats, mice (mg/kg): 1950, 2350 orally (Hagan).

Caution: This substance is reasonably anticipated to be a human carcinogen: *Report on Carcinogens, Eleventh Edition* (PB2005-104914, 2004) p III-229.

USE: In perfumery; denaturing fats in soap manuf; also in manuf of heliotropin. Formerly as flavoring agent in foods, drugs and beverages.

8318. SAICAR. [3031-95-6] *N*-[[5-Amino-1-(5-*O*-phosphono-β-D-ribofuranosyl)-1*H*-imidazol-4-yl]carbonyl]-L-aspartic acid; *N*-[(5-amino-1-ribofuranosylimidazol-4-yl)carbonyl]aspartic acid 5′-phosphate; 5-amino-*N*-(1,2-dicarboxyethyl)-1-ribofuranosylimidazole-4-carboxamide 5′-phosphate; 5-amino-4-imidazole-*N*-succinocarboxamide ribonucleotide; 5-amino-4-imidazole-*N*-succinocarboxamide ribotide; *N*-[5-amino-1-(5′-phosphoribofuranosyl)-4-imidazolecarbonyl]aspartic acid; succino-AICAR. $C_{13}H_{19}N_4O_{12}P$; mol wt 454.28. C 34.37%, H 4.22%, N 12.33%, O 42.26%, P 6.82%. Important purine precursor. Synthesis by enzymic reaction according to the equation AIR + ATP + aspartic acid + $CO_2 \rightarrow$ SAICAR + ADP + orthophosphate: Lukens, Buchanan, *J. Biol. Chem.* **234**, 1791 (1959). Production by adenine-requiring mutants of *Bacillus subtilis*: Ohmura *et al.,* **US 3280007** (1966 to Takeda). Synthesis of SAICAR and derivatives: Burrows, Shaw, *J. Chem. Soc. C* **1967**, 1088; Burrows *et al., ibid.* **1968**, 40.

Dibarium salt. $C_{13}H_{15}Ba_2N_4O_{12}P$. uv max (pH 1): 269, 244 nm (ε 11850, 9580). If the Bratton-Marshall procedure [*J. Biol. Chem.* **128**, 537 (1939)] is modified by keeping the sample in ice during, and for 10 minutes after the addition of the reagents, SAICAR produces a purple chromophore having max absorption at 550 nm. The diazonium salt of SAICAR is very unstable and dec before it can couple under the usual test conditions.

8319. Sakuranetin. [2957-21-3] 2,3-Dihydro-5-hydroxy-2-(4-hydroxyphenyl)-7-methoxy-4*H*-1-benzopyran-4-one; 4′,5-dihydroxy-7-methoxyflavanone; naringin 7-methyl ether. $C_{16}H_{14}O_5$; mol wt 286.28. C 67.13%, H 4.93%, O 27.94%. Isoln by hydrolysis of 5-glucoside obtained from bark of *Prunus yedoensis* Matsum., *Rosaceae*: Asahina, *Arch. Pharm.* **246**, 259 (1908); from wood of various *Prunus* species: Hasegawa, Shirato, *J. Am. Chem. Soc.* **76**, 5559 (1954); **77**, 3557 (1955); Hasegawa, *ibid.* **79**, 1738 (1957). Structure: Asahina *et al., J. Pharm. Soc. Jpn.* No. **550**,

Consult the Name Index before using this section.

1007 (1927); Shinoda, Sato, *ibid.* **48**, 220 (1928). Synthesis: Zemplén *et al., Ber.* **75B**, 1432 (1942). Absolute configuration of (+)-isomer: Arakawa, Nakazaki, *Ann.* **636**, 111 (1960).

Needles, mp 152°. Also reported as dihydrate, mp 131-132° (Arakawa, Nakazaki, *loc. cit.*). (+)-Isomer, $[\alpha]_D^{16}$ +8.0° (c = 7.92 in acetone); $[\alpha]_D^{12}$ +8.4° (c = 6.28 in methanol). Sol in alcohol, ether, chloroform, benzene, ethyl acetate, pyridine; slightly sol in boiling water. Practically insol in cold water.

5-Glucoside. 4′,5-dihydroxy-7-methoxyflavanone 5-glucoside; sakuranin. $C_{22}H_{24}O_{10}$. Tetrahydrate, bitter needles from dil alcohol. Begins to lose water at 100°. mp 212-214°. $[\alpha]_D^{28}$ −106.6° (tetrahydrate in acetone); $[\alpha]_D^{28}$ −123.2° (anhydr compd in acetone); $[\alpha]_D^{16}$ −97.4° (c = 1.58 for anhydr compd in 75% acetone). Very sol in dil alcohol, pyridine; slightly sol in abs alcohol, hot water, ethyl acetate. Practically insol in ether, cold water.

8320. Salatrim. [64706-27-0] Family of low-calorie fats composed of mixtures of long-chain saturated fatty acids (predominantly stearic) and short-chain saturated fatty acids (acetic, propionic, and/or butyric) esterified to the glycerol backbone. Name is an acronym derived from *s*hort *a*nd *l*ong acyl*tri*glyceride *m*olecule. Prepd but not claimed: T. A. Pelloso *et al., WO* 9418290; *eidem, US* 5434278 (1994, 1995 both to Nabisco). Series of articles on prepn, characterization, HPLC determn, pharmacology, and clinical assessment: *J. Agric. Food Chem.* **42**, 432-604 (1994). GC/MS determn in foods: A. S. Huang *et al., ibid.* **43**, 1834 (1995).

Average caloric availability in humans: 4.9 kcal/g.

USE: Alternative fat used in foods.

8321. Salazosulfadimidine. [2315-08-4] 5-[[4-[[(4,6-Dimethyl-2-pyrimidinyl)amino]sulfonyl]phenyl]azo]-2-hydroxybenzoic acid; 5-[*p*-[(4,6-dimethyl-2-pyrimidinyl)sulfamoyl]phenylazo]salicylic acid; 4′-(4,6-dimethylpyrimidin-2-ylsulfamoyl)-4-hydroxyazobenzene-3-carboxylic acid; 5-[*p*-[(4,6-dimethyl-2-pyrimidinyl)aminosulfonyl]phenylazo]salicylic acid; salicylazosulfadimidine; salicylazosulfamethazine; Azudimidine. $C_{19}H_{17}N_5O_5S$; mol wt 427.43. C 53.39%, H 4.01%, N 16.38%, O 18.72%, S 7.50%. Prepn: Korkuczanski, *Przem. Chem.* **37**, 162 (1958), *C.A.* **52**, 13727 (1958); Malatesta, Lotti, *Ann. Chim. (Rome)* **50**, 114 (1960), *C.A.* **56**, 8613g (1962).

Brown crystals, mp 207°.

THERAP CAT: Antibacterial.

8322. Salen. [129409-01-4] (*E,E*-form); [94-93-9] (unspecified stereo). (*E,E*)-2,2′-[1,2-Ethanediylbis(nitrilomethylidyne)]bisphenol; *N,N*′-bis[(2-hydroxyphenyl)methylene]-1,2-ethanediamine; *N,N*′-ethylenebis(salicylideneimine); H$_2$sal$_2$en. $C_{16}H_{16}N_2O_2$; mol wt 268.31. C 71.62%, H 6.01%, N 10.44%, O 11.93%. Tetradentate Schiff base chelating ligand. Prepn: A. T. Mason, *Ber.* **20**, 267 (1887); and spectral analysis of Cu(II) complex: G. V. Panova *et al., J. Gen. Chem. USSR* **53**, 1452 (1983). Prepn of transition metal complexes: P. Pfeiffer *et al., Ann.* **505**, 84 (1933); and their physicochemical properties: A. Z. El-Sonbati *et al., Transition Met. Chem.* **17**, 66 (1992); M. M. Bhadbhade, D. Srinivas, *Inorg. Chem.* **32**, 6122 (1993). Mass spectra of transition metal complexes: S. M. Schildcrout *et al., ibid.* **34**, 4117 (1995). Thermodynamic properties of salen and its metal complexes: F. Lloret *et al., Inorg. Chim. Acta* **189**, 195 (1991). Use of Mn(III) complex as catalyst in

epoxidation of olefins: K. Srinivasan *et al., J. Am. Chem. Soc.* **108**, 2309 (1986); as specific DNA cleaving agent: D. J. Gravert, J. H. Griffin, *J. Org. Chem.* **58**, 820 (1993).

Crystals from alcohol, mp 125-126°. Insol in water.

USE: As stabilizing ligand for a variety of oxidation states of metal ions.

8323. Salep. Dried tubers of several species of *Orchis, Orchidaceae. Habit.* Europe, Asia Minor. *Constit.* Mucilage, starch.

USE: Nutrient, demulcent; as a vehicle for acrid remedies.

8324. Salicin. [138-52-3] 2-(Hydroxymethyl)phenyl-β-D-glucopyranoside; salicoside; salicyl alcohol glucoside; saligenin-β-D-glucopyranoside. $C_{13}H_{18}O_7$; mol wt 286.28. C 54.54%, H 6.34%, O 39.12%. Usually obtained by making hot water extracts from the ground bark of poplar *(Populus)* and willow *(Salix)*; also found in the leaves and female flowers of the willow. Isoln from root bark of *Viburnum prunifolium* L., *Caprifoliaceae:* Evans *et al., J. Am. Pharm. Assoc.* **34**, 207 (1945). Structure and synthesis: Irvine, Rose, *J. Chem. Soc.* **89**, 814 (1906); Kunz, *J. Am. Chem. Soc.* **48**, 262 (1926). Hydrolysis by acids: Moelwyn-Hughes, *Trans. Faraday Soc.* **25**, 503 (1929). Enzymatic hydrolysis: Pigman, *J. Res. Natl. Bur. Stand.* **27**, 6 (1941). Enzymatic hydrolysis in heavy water: Stacie, *Z. Phys. Chem.* **28B**, 236 (1935).

Orthorhombic crystals from water, mp 199-202°. $[\alpha]_D^{25}$ −62 to −67° (c = 3). $[\alpha]_D^{20}$ −45.6° (c = 0.6 in abs alc), Brauns, *J. Am. Chem. Soc.* **47**, 1292 (1925). One gram dissolves in 23 ml water, 3 ml boiling water, 90 ml alcohol, 30 ml alcohol at 60°. Soluble in alkalies, pyridine, glacial acetic acid. Practically insol in ether, chloroform. Aq solns are neutral to litmus and have a bitter taste.

USE: Standard substrate in evaluating enzyme prepns contg β-glucosidase: Weidenhagen, *Z. Ver. Zucker-Ind.* **79**, 591 (1929).

THERAP CAT: Analgesic.

THERAP CAT (VET): Has been used as a bitter stomachic, as an antirheumatic and as an analgesic.

8325. Salicyl Alcohol. [90-01-7] 2-Hydroxybenzenemethanol; saligenin; saligenol; *o*-hydroxybenzyl alcohol. $C_7H_8O_2$; mol wt 124.14. C 67.73%, H 6.50%, O 25.78%. Prepd by the action of emulsin on salicin; by heating phenol with methylene chloride and aq NaOH.

Plates or cryst powder. d 1.16. mp 86-87°; sublimes at 100°. Soluble in 15 parts water; very sol in alcohol, chloroform, ether, sol in benzene. Gives a red color with H_2SO_4.

THERAP CAT: Anesthetic (local).

8326. Salicylaldehyde. [90-02-8] 2-Hydroxybenzaldehyde; salicylic aldehyde. $C_7H_6O_2$; mol wt 122.12. C 68.85%, H 4.95%, O 26.20%. Made by heating sodium phenolate and chloroform with NaOH. Toxicity data: Binet, *Rev. Med. Suisse Romande* **15**, 561 (1895).

Clear, colorless, oily liq; bitter almond-like odor; burning taste. d_4^{20} 1.167; mp $-7°$; bp 196-197°; n_D^{20} 1.5735. Slightly sol in water; sol in alc, ether. Gives an orange color with H_2SO_4. MLD in rats (mg/kg): 900-1000 s.c. (Binet).

USE: In perfumery.

8327. Salicylaldoxime. [94-67-7] 2-Hydroxybenzaldehyde oxime; Saldox. $C_7H_7NO_2$; mol wt 137.14. C 61.31%, H 5.14%, N 10.21%, O 23.33%. $HOC_6H_4CH\!=\!NOH$.

Prisms, mp 57°. Slightly sol in cold water; more sol in hot water; freely sol in alcohol, ether, benzene, dil HCl. Insol in petr ether. On heating it dec into salicylaldehyde and hydroxylamine.

USE: As a reagent for copper and nickel.

8328. Salicylamide. [65-45-2] 2-Hydroxybenzamide; Salamid; Samid; Cidal; Salizell; Salymid; Urtosal. $C_7H_7NO_2$; mol wt 137.14. C 61.31%, H 5.14%, N 10.21%, O 23.33%. Prepn: A. Cahours, *Ann.* **48,** 60 (1843); D. S. Hoffenberg, C. R. Hauser, *J. Org. Chem.* **20,** 1496 (1955); J. B. Chattopadhyaya, A. V. Rama Rao, *Tetrahedron* **30,** 2899 (1974). Toxicity data: Hart, *J. Pharmacol. Exp. Ther.* **89,** 205 (1947). Clinical efficacy in headache: W. J. Murray, *J. Clin. Pharmacol. J. New Drugs* **7,** 150 (1967). Pharmacokinetics: A. G. de Boer *et al., Biopharm. Drug Dispos.* **4,** 321 (1983).

White or slightly pink, crystalline powder, somewhat bitter taste. Sensation of warmth on tongue. mp 140°. Soly in water at 30° = 0.2%, at 47° = 0.8%; in glycerol at 5° = 2.0%, at 39° = 5.0%, at 60° = 10.0%; in propylene glycol at 5° = 10.0%. Sol in hot water, alcohol, chloroform, ether. pH of satd aq soln at 28° about 5. Forms a water-soluble sodium salt at pH 9. LD_{50} orally in mice: 1.4 g/kg (Hart).

THERAP CAT: Analgesic.

8329. Salicylamide O-Acetic Acid. [25395-22-6] [2-(Aminocarbonyl)phenoxy]acetic acid; *o*-(carbamylphenoxy)acetic acid; α-(2-carbamoylphenoxy)acetic acid. $C_9H_9NO_4$; mol wt 195.17. C 55.39%, H 4.65%, N 7.18%, O 32.79%. Prepn: Merriman, *J. Chem. Soc.* **103,** 1838 (1913); Tzofin, *J. Gen. Chem. USSR* **3,** 17 (1933); Klosa, *Arch. Pharm.* **288,** 389 (1955); Izumi *et al.,* **JP 56 874** (1956 to Yoshitomi). Pharmacokinetics and efficacy: D. Loew *et al., Int. J. Clin. Pharmacol. Ther. Toxicol.* **30,** 509 (1992).

Crystals, mp 221°. Sol in aq alkali.

Sodium salt. [3785-32-8] Salizell (amp.). $C_9H_8NNaO_4$; mol wt 217.15. Crystals, mp 212-215°.

Diethylamine salt. Akistin. $C_{13}H_{22}N_2O_4$; mol wt 270.32.

THERAP CAT: Analgesic; anti-inflammatory; antipyretic.

8330. Salicylanilide. [87-17-2] 2-Hydroxy-*N*-phenylbenzamide; *N*-phenylsalicylamide; Salinidol. $C_{13}H_{11}NO_2$; mol wt 213.23. C 73.23%, H 5.20%, N 6.57%, O 15.01%. Usually made by the reaction of salicylic acid with aniline in the presence of PCl_3 at an elevated temp. Better yields are obtained by using an inert organic solvent such as toluene or carbon tetrachloride as a reaction diluent. Novel process using ion-exchange resins: Ma-

jewski, Skelly, **US 3221051** (1965). Alternate process: Majewski *et al.,* **US 3231611** (1966 to Dow).

Odorless leaflets. mp 135.8-136.2°. Slightly sol in water; freely sol in alcohol, ether, chloroform, benzene.

Caution: In concd form may cause irritation of skin, mucous membranes. *See also* Salicylic Acid.

USE: Anti-mildew, fungicide.

THERAP CAT: Antifungal (topical).

THERAP CAT (VET): Antifungal (topical).

8331. Salicylhydroxamic Acid. [89-73-6] *N*,2-Dihydroxybenzamide; 2-hydroxybenzhydroxamic acid. $C_7H_7NO_3$; mol wt 153.14. C 54.90%, H 4.61%, N 9.15%, O 31.34%. HOC_6H_4CO-$NHOH$ or $HOC_6H_4C(OH)\!=\!NOH$. Prepn: Jeanrenaud, *Ber.* **22,** 1272 (1889); Urbanski, *Nature* **166,** 267 (1950). Trypanocidal activity: F. Opperdoes *et al., Exp. Parasitol.* **40,** 198 (1976); A. B. Clarkson, F. H. Brohn, *Science* **194,** 204 (1976); A. J. Barnicoat *et al., Experientia* **37,** 1291 (1981).

Needles from acetic acid, mp 168° (slow heating), mp 176-178° (quick heating). Sublimes. pK (25°) 4.19.

Sodium salt. $C_7H_6NNaO_3$. Plates. Freely sol in water. pH of 0.1*N* soln 7.7.

USE: Complexing agent.

8332. Salicylic Acid. [69-72-7] 2-Hydroxybenzoic acid; Acnisal; Duofilm; Duoplant; Keralyt; Occlusal; Verrugon. C_7H_6-O_3; mol wt 138.12. C 60.87%, H 4.38%, O 34.75%. Occurs in the form of esters in several plants, notably in wintergreen leaves and the bark of sweet birch. Manuf by heating sodium phenolate with carbon dioxide under pressure: W. L. Faith *et al., Industrial Chemicals* (Wiley, New York, 3rd ed., 1965) pp 652-655. Review of prepns, properties, and uses of salicylic acid and derivatives: S. H. Erickson in *Kirk-Othmer Encyclopedia of Chemical Technology* **vol. 20** (John Wiley & Sons, New York, 3rd ed., 1982) pp 500-524. Toxicity data: K. Sota *et al., J. Pharm. Soc. Jpn.* **89,** 1392 (1969). HPLC determn in foods: B. H. Chen, S. C. Fu, *Chromatographia* **41,** 43 (1995). Clinical evaluation to treat warts: B. J. Bart *et al., J. Am. Acad. Dermatol.* **20,** 74 (1989); M. E. Bender *et al., Cutis* **47,** 199 (1991). Review of use in acne: E. Zander, S. Weisman, *Clin. Ther.* **14,** 247 (1992). Comprehensive description: M. A. Abounassif *et al., Anal. Profiles Drug Subs. Excip.* **23,** 421-470 (1994).

White crystals, fine needles, or fluffy white crystalline powder, mp 159°; sublimes at 76°. Gradually discolors in sunlight. d_4^{20} 1.443. bp_{20} 211°. pKa 2.98. *n* 1.565. Flash point (closed cup): 157°C. uv max (4 mg% in ethanol): 210, 234, 303 nm (ε 8343, 5466, 3591). Soly (Wt %): water 0.20 (20°), 2.21 (80°); carbon tetrachloride 0.262 (25°); benzene 0.775 (25°); propanol 27.36 (21°); abs ethanol 34.87 (21°); acetone 396 (23°). pH of satd aq soln 2.4. *Keep protected from light.* LD_{50} i.v. in mice: 500 mg/kg (Sota).

Sodium salt. [54-21-7] Sodium salicylate; Enterosalicyl; Enterosalil; Idocyl; Saliglutin. $C_7H_5NaO_3$; mol wt 160.10. Clinical trial in rheumatoid arthritis: S. J. Preston *et al., Br. J. Clin. Pharmacol.* **27,** 607 (1989). Toxicity data: E. I. Goldenthal, *Toxicol. Appl. Pharmacol.* **18,** 185 (1971). White crystalline powder, mp 440°. Soly (g/100 cc): water 125; methanol 17. *Protect from light.* LD_{50} i.p. in rats: 780 mg/kg (Goldenthal).

Caution: Ingestion of large amounts can cause vomiting, abdominal pain, increased respiration, acidosis, mental disturbances.

May cause skin rashes in sensitive individuals. *See: Clinical Toxicology of Commercial Products*, R. E. Gosselin *et al.*, Eds. (Williams & Wilkins, Baltimore, 5th ed., 1984) pp 368-375.

USE: In manuf aspirin, methyl salicylate, and other salicylates. Coupling agent for azo dyes. Has been used as food preservative.

THERAP CAT: Keratolytic. Sodium salt as anti-inflammatory, analgesic, antipyretic.

THERAP CAT (VET): Keratolytic.

8333. 4-Salicyloylmorpholine. [3202-84-4] 4-(2-Hydroxybenzoyl)morpholine; salicyl morpholide; L-1102; Tardisal. $C_{11}H_{13}NO_3$; mol wt 207.23. C 63.75%, H 6.32%, N 6.76%, O 23.16%. Prepn: Carron, **FR 1096209** (1955 to Robert & Carrière); Schweitzer, **US 2906728** (1959 to Dow).

Crystals, mp 175°. Soly (g/100 ml): water 0.41; alcohol 3.3; ether 0.22. pH of satd aq soln 6.2.

THERAP CAT: Choleretic.

8334. Salicylsulfuric Acid. [89-45-2] 2-(Sulfooxy)benzoic acid; salicylic acid, acid sulfate; salicylic acid sulfuric acid ester. $C_7H_6O_6S$; mol wt 218.18. C 38.53%, H 2.77%, O 44.00%, S 14.70%. Prepd by treating salicylic acid with chlorosulfonic acid in pyridine: Loeper *et al.*, *C.R. Seances Soc. Biol. Ses Fil.* **135**, 917 (1941); *Chim. Ind. (Paris)* **49**, 99 (1943).

Monosodium salt. [6155-64-2] Sodium salicylsulfate; Salcyl; Salcylix. Fine needles. Sol in water. Insol in organic solvents.

THERAP CAT: Analgesic, anti-inflammatory.

8335. Salinazid. [495-84-1] [(2-Hydroxyphenyl)methylene]hydrazide 4-pyridinecarboxylic acid; 1-isonicotinoyl-2-salicylidenehydrazine; isonicotinic acid salicylidenehydrazide; saliniazid; *N'-o*-hydroxybenzylidenepyridine-4-carboxyhydrazide; *o*-hydroxybenzal isonicotinylhydrazone; Nupa-Sal; Acozid. $C_{13}H_{11}N_3O_2$; mol wt 241.25. C 64.72%, H 4.60%, N 17.42%, O 13.26%. Prepd by the interaction of isoniazid and salicyl-aldehyde in water: Hart *et al.*, *Antibiot. Chemother.* **4**, 803 (1954); *cf.* Yale *et al.*, *J. Am. Chem. Soc.* **75**, 1933 (1953). Tuberculostatic activity and toxicity: Bavin *et al.*, *J. Pharm. Pharmacol.* **7**, 1032 (1955).

Crystals from ethanol, mp 232-233° (also given as 251°). Soly at 25° in 100 ml water: 0.005 g; in 100 ml abs ethanol: 0.18 g; in 100 ml propylene glycol: 0.212 g. Sol in dil aq acids and alkalies forming a yellow soln.

THERAP CAT: Antibacterial (tuberculostatic).

8336. Salinomycin. [53003-10-4] $C_{42}H_{70}O_{11}$; mol wt 751.00. C 67.17%, H 9.39%, O 23.43%. Polyether ionophoric antibiotic having a unique tricyclic spiroketal ring system and an unsaturated 6-membered ring in the molecule. Produced by a strain of *Streptomyces albus* (FERM-P No. 419 and ATCC 21838). Production: Y. Miyazaki *et al.*, **JP Kokai 72 25392** (1972 to Kaken Chem.), *C.A.* **78**, 41561 (1973). Structure: H. Kinashi *et al.*, *Tetrahedron Lett.* **1973**, 4955. Taxonomy, production, isolation and physicochemical and biological properties: Y. Miyazaki *et al.*, *J. Antibiot.* **27**, 814 (1974). Use as a coccidiostat: Y. Tanaka *et al.*, **DE 2253031**; *eidem*, **US 3857948** (1973, 1974 to Kaken Chem.). Anticoccidial efficacy: T. T. Migaki *et al.*, *Poult. Sci.*

58, 1192 (1979). Total synthesis: Y. Kishi *et al.*, *Front. Chem., Plenary Keynote Lect. IUPAC Congr., 28th* **1981**, K. J. Laidler, Ed. (Pergamon, Oxford, 1982) pp 287-304; R. C. D. Brown, P. J. Kocienski, *Synlett* **1994**, 415, 417. HPLC determn in animal feeds: M. R. LaPointe, H. Cohen, *J. Assoc. Off. Anal. Chem.* **71**, 480 (1988).

mp 112.5-113.5°. pKa' 6.4 (DMF). $[\alpha]_D^{25}$ $-63°$ (c = 1 in ethanol). uv max (ethanol-water, 2:1): 284 nm (ε 126). LD_{50} in mice (mg/kg): 18 i.p.; 50 orally (Miyazaki).

Sodium salt. [55721-31-8] Bio-Cox; Sacox; Salocin. $C_{42}H_{69}NaO_{11}$; mol wt 772.98. mp 140-142°. $[\alpha]_D^{25}$ $-37°$ (c = 1 in ethanol).

THERAP CAT (VET): Anticoccidial agent.

8337. Salmeterol. [89365-50-4] 4-Hydroxy-α^1-[[[6-(4-phenylbutoxy)hexyl]amino]methyl]-1,3-benzenedimethanol; ($\pm$)-4-hydroxy-α^1-[[[6-(4-phenylbutoxy)hexyl]amino]methyl]-*m*-xylene-α,α^1-diol; GR-33343X. $C_{25}H_{37}NO_4$; mol wt 415.57. C 72.25%, H 8.97%, N 3.37%, O 15.40%. β_2-Adrenergic agonist; structural analog of albuterol, *q.v.* Prepn: I. F. Skidmore *et al.*, **DE 3414752**; *eidem*, **US 4992474** (1984, 1991 both to Glaxo). Pharmacology: M. Johnson, *Lung* **168**, Suppl., 115 (1990). Preliminary evaluations in asthma: A. Ullman *et al.*, *Am. Rev. Respir. Dis.* **142**, 571 (1990); O. P. Twentyman *et al.*, *Lancet* **336**, 1338 (1990). Review of pharmacology and therapeutic use: R. N. Brogden, D. Faulds, *Drugs* **42**, 895-912 (1991).

mp 75.5-76.5°.

1-Hydroxy-2-naphthoate. [94749-08-3] Salmeterol xinafoate; GR-33343G; Arial; Salmetedur; Serevent. $C_{25}H_{37}NO_4 \cdot C_{11}H_8O_3$; mol wt 603.75. mp 137-138°. Freely sol in methanol; slightly sol in ethanol, chloroform, isopropanol; sparingly sol in water.

THERAP CAT: Bronchodilator.

8338. Salmine Sulfate. [53597-25-4] A protamine found in the sperm of salmon. Contains arginine, proline, serine, glycine, valine, leucine, alanine, threonine, isoleucine, lysine, histidine, aspartic and glutamic acids. Mol wt 6000 to 7000. N about 25%. Prepn and properties: Fisher, Scott, *J. Pharmacol. Exp. Ther.* **58**, 78 (1936); Felix, *Am. Sci.* **43**, 431 (1955); Callanan *et al.*, *J. Biol. Chem.* **229**, 279 (1957); Carroll *et al.*, *ibid.* **234**, 2314 (1959). Separation of components and amino acid sequence of major component: Ando, Watanabe, *Int. J. Protein Res.* **1**, 221 (1969). Toxicity study: Starbuck *et al.*, *Arch. Int. Pharmacodyn. Ther.* **165**, 374 (1967).

Salmine base is a powder sol in disodium phosphate buffer; the sulfate separates from water in the cold as a clear, immiscible liquid. LD_{50} i.v. in rats: 75 mg/kg (Starbuck).

8339. Salsalate. [552-94-3] 2-Hydroxybenzoic acid 2-carboxyphenyl ester; disalicylic acid; salicylic acid bimolecular ester; salicyloxysalicylic acid; salicylsalicylic acid; NSC-49171; Disalcid; Disalgesic; Mono-Gesic; Salflex. $C_{14}H_{10}O_5$; mol wt 258.23. C 65.12%, H 3.90%, O 30.98%. Nonacetylated aspirin analog. Prepn: **DE 211403** and **DE 214044** (1909, both to Boehringer, Mann.), *Frdl.* **9**, 928 and *C.A.* **4**, 368 (1910); W. Baker *et al.*, *J. Chem. Soc.* **1951**, 201. Metabolism: S. M. Dromgoole *et al.*, *J. Pharm. Sci.* **73**, 1657 (1984). Clinical evaluation in arthritis: T. C. McPherson, *Clin. Ther.* **6**, 388 (1984). Mechanism of action studies: C. A. Divincenzo, F. R. Venezio, *Curr. Ther. Res.* **42**, 720 (1987). HPLC determn in plasma and urine: L. I. Harrison *et al.*, *J. Pharm. Sci.* **69**, 1268 (1980). Review of chemistry, pharmacokinetics, safety and clinical efficacy: P. T. Singleton, *Clin. Ther.* **3**, 80-102 (1980).

Crystals from benzene. mp 148-149°. Practically insol in water but gradually hydrolyzed by it into 2 mols of salicylic acid. Sol in alc, ether; sparingly sol in benzene.

THERAP CAT: Analgesic, anti-inflammatory.

8340. Salsoline. [101467-40-7] (R)-1,2,3,4-Tetrahydro-7-methoxy-1-methyl-6-isoquinolinol; 6-hydroxy-7-methoxy-1-methyl-1,2,3,4-tetrahydroisoquinoline; (+)-salsoline. $C_{11}H_{15}NO_2$; mol wt 193.24. C 68.37%, H 7.82%, N 7.25%, O 16.56%. In *Salsola richteri* Karel., *Chenopodiaceae*. Extraction procedure: A. Orechoff, N. Proskurnina, *Ber.* **66**, 841 (1933); N. Proskurnina, A. Orekhoff, *Bull. Soc. Chim. Fr.* **1937**, 1265. Structure and synthesis: E. Späth *et al.*, *Ber.* **67**, 1214 (1934); O. Kovács, G. Fodor, *Ber.* **84**, 795 (1951). Abs config: A. R. Battersby, T. P. Edwards, *J. Chem. Soc.* **1960**, 1214. Biosynthetic studies: I. McFarlane, M. Slaytor, *Phytochemistry* **11**, 235 (1972). Synthesis of enantiomers: S. Teitel *et al.*, *J. Med. Chem.* **17**, 134 (1974). HPLC study: J. Strömbom, J. G. Bruhn, *J. Chromatogr.* **147**, 513 (1978).

Crystals from alc, mp 221°. $[\alpha]_D^{20}$ +34.5° (c = 1 in 0.1N HCl). Sol in chloroform, hot alc, dil NaOH. Slightly sol in water, benzene. Almost insol in ether, petr ether.

Hydrochloride. [51424-33-0] mp 174-175°. $[\alpha]_D$ +31.0° (methanol). uv max (isopropanol): 204, 227, 284, 286 nm (ε 39400, 5900, 3540, 3530). Sol in water, hot alcohol. Very sparingly sol in acetone, chloroform. LD_{50} in mice (mg/kg): 140 i.v.; >1000 orally (Teitel).

(−)-Form. [89-31-6] (S)-1,2,3,4-Tetrahydro-7-methoxy-1-methyl-6-isoquinolinol. mp 214-215°.

8341. Salutaridine. [1936-18-1] 5,6,8,14-Tetradehydro-4-hydroxy-3,6-dimethoxy-17-methylmorphinan-7-one; floripavine. $C_{19}H_{21}NO_4$; mol wt 327.37. C 69.71%, H 6.47%, N 4.28%, O 19.55%. Intermediate in morphine synthesis; naturally occurring in (+)-form. Isolated from various species of *Croton* and *Papaver*: Barton *et al.*, *J. Chem. Soc.* **1965**, 2423; Pfeifer, Kühn, *Pharmazie* **23**, 267 (1968). Structure and identity with floripavine: Mndzhoyan *et al.*, *C.A.* **68**, 114787w (1968). Synthesis: T. Kametani *et al.*, *J. Chem. Soc. C* **1969**, 2030; G. Horvath, S. Makleit, *Acta Chim. Acad. Sci. Hung.* **106**, 37 (1981); of racemate: T. Kametani *et al.*, *J. Chem. Soc. Perkin Trans. 1* **1972**, 1435; C. Szántay *et al.*, *J. Org. Chem.* **47**, 594 (1982); of racemate and (−)-form: W. Ludwig, H. J. Schafer, *Angew. Chem. Int. Ed.* **25**, 1025 (1986). *Review:* Stuart, *Chem. Rev.* **1971**, 47.

Rods from ethyl acetate, mp 197-198°. $[\alpha]_D^{12}$ +114° (c = 0.5 in methanol). uv max (methanol): 236, 279 nm (log ε 4.23, 3.76).

(−)-Form. Sinoacaline. $[\alpha]_D^{20}$ −98° (c = 0.55 g/100 ml CH_3-OH). uv max (methanol): 276, 240 nm (log ε 3.76, 4.24).

8342. Salverine. [6376-26-7] 2-[2-(Diethylamino)ethoxy]-N-phenylbenzamide; 2-[2-(diethylamino)ethoxy]benzanilide. C_{19}-

$H_{24}N_2O_2$; mol wt 312.41. C 73.05%, H 7.74%, N 8.97%, O 10.24%. Prepn: **AT 239779** (1965 to Montavit), *C.A.* **63**, 4211h (1965).

Hydrochloride. $C_{19}H_{24}N_2O_2$.HCl. Crystals, mp 173°.

THERAP CAT: Analgesic.

8343. Salvia. Sage. Dried leaves of *Salvia officinalis* L., *Labiatae*. *Habit.* Southern Europe; cultivated in U.S., England, France. *Constit.* 1-2.5% volatile oil; resin, tannin, bitter principles.

USE: Flavoring, condiment.

THERAP CAT: Antisecretory agent.

8344. Salvinorins. Divinorins. Family of neoclerodane diterpenes isolated from the hallucinogenic Mexican mint *Salvia divinorum*. Traditional medicine used by the Mazatec people of Oaxaca, Mexico. Isoln of Salvinorin A: A. Ortega *et al.*, *J. Chem. Soc. Perkin Trans. 1* **1982**, 2505; of A and B and biologic activity: L. J. Valdés, III *et al.*, *J. Org. Chem.* **49**, 4716 (1984); of C: L. J. Valdés, III *et al.*, *Org. Lett.* **3**, 3935 (2001). Stereochemistry: M. Koreeda *et al.*, *Chem. Lett.* **1990**, 2015. Pharmacologic effects: D. J. Siebert, *J. Ethnopharmacol.* **43**, 53 (1994). *Review:* L. J. Valdés III, *J. Psychoactive Drugs* **26**, 277-283 (1994).

Salvinorin A

Salvinorin A. [83729-01-5] (2S,4aR,6aR,7R,9S,10aS,10bR)-9-(Acetyloxy)-2-(3-furanyl)dodecahydro-6a,10b-dimethyl-4,10-dioxo-2H-naphtho[2,1-c]-pyran-7-carboxylic acid methyl ester; divinorin A. $C_{23}H_{28}O_8$; mol wt 432.46. One of the most potent natural hallucinogens known. First naturally occurring non-nitrogenous κ opioid receptor (KOR) agonist identified. HPLC quantification in *S. divinorum* extracts: J. W. Gruber *et al.*, *Phytochem. Anal.* **10**, 22 (1999). LC determn in biological fluids: M. S. Schmidt *et al.*, *J. Chromatogr. B* **818**, 221 (2005). KOR binding profile: B. L. Roth *et al.*, *Proc. Natl. Acad. Sci. USA* **99**, 11934 (2002). Brief review: D. J. Sheffler, B. L. Roth, *Trends Pharmacol. Sci.* **24**, 107-109 (2003). Colorless crystals from methanol, mp 238-240° (Ortega); also reported as mp 242-244° (Valdes, 1984). $[\alpha]_D^{22}$ −45.3° (c = 8.530 in $CHCl_3$). $[\alpha]_D^{25}$ −41° (c = 1 in $CHCl_3$).

USE: In traditional medicine, the leaves are used for divination and for treatment of anemia and excretory functions.

8345. Samaderins. Antitumor agents isolated from the bark and seed of *Samadera indica* Gaertn, *Simaroubaceae:* van der Marck, *Arch. Pharm.* **239**, 96 (1901). Separable into three components, samaderins A, B and C: Polonsky *et al.*, *Bull. Soc. Chim. Fr.* **1962**, 1715. According to Zylber *et al.*, *ibid.* **1963**, 1322, samaderin C is identical with *samaderoside A* isolated by Mitra, Gregg, *Naturwissenschaften* **14**, 327 (1962). Structure of B and C: Zylber, Polonsky, *Bull. Soc. Chim. Fr.* **1964**, 2016. Structure of A: M. C. Wani *et al.*, *Chem. Commun.* **1977**, 295. Crystal structure of A: K. D. Onan, A. T. McPhail, *J. Chem. Res. Synop.* **1978**, 14.

Samaderin A

Samaderin B ══O
Samaderin C ──OH

Samaderin A. $C_{18}H_{18}O_6$; mol wt 330.33. mp 253-255°. $[\alpha]_D^{25}$ −31.3° (c = 0.259 in pyridine). uv max (methanol): 288 nm (ε 13400).

Samaderin B. $C_{19}H_{22}O_7$; mol wt 362.37. Prisms from ethyl acetate, mp 235-240°.

Samaderin C. $C_{19}H_{24}O_7$; mol wt 364.39. Shiny plates from ethyl acetate+ alcohol, mp 265-268°. Sol in pyridine. Practically insol in ether. Very sparingly sol in other org solvents.

8346. Samandarine. [467-51-6] $1\alpha,4\alpha$-Epoxy-3-aza-A-homoandrostan-16β-ol. $C_{19}H_{31}NO_2$; mol wt 305.45. C 74.71%, H 10.23%, N 4.59%, O 10.48%. Constitutes together with samandarone approx 75% of the alkaloid content in the skin glands of the European fire and Alpine salamanders: *Salamandra maculosa* resp. *atra* Laur., *Salamandridae*. Isoln: Schöpf, Braun, *Ann.* **514,** 69 (1934). Structure and configuration: Wölfel *et al., Ber.* **94,** 2361 (1961).

Needles from abs methanol or 50% acetone, mp 187-188°. Solvated crystals from dil methanol. $[\alpha]_D^{17}$ +43.3° (acetone). Freely sol in most organic solvents. Practically insol in water and NaOH solns.

Hydrochloride. $C_{19}H_{31}NO_2$.HCl. Crystals from methanol, mp 312-313°; from water, mp 321-322° (monohydrate).

Samandarone. $C_{19}H_{29}NO_2$; mol wt 303.44. ketone corresponding to the secondary alcohol in samandarine. Synthesis: Hara, Oka, *J. Am. Chem. Soc.* **89,** 1041 (1967). Needles from methyl ethyl ketone, mp 191-192°; from 35% acetone, mp 189-191°. $[\alpha]_D^{21}$ −115.7° (acetone).

8347. Samarium. [7440-19-9] Sm; at. wt 150.36; at. no. 62; valences 2, 3. A lanthanide belonging to the cerium group of rare earth metals; named for the mineral "samarskite" from which it was isolated. Naturally occurring isotopes (mass numbers): 144 (3.1%); 147 (15.0%), radioactive, $T_{1/2}$ 1.06×10^{11} years, α-emitter; 148 (11.3%), radioactive, $T_{1/2}$ 7×10^{15} years, α-emitter; 149 (13.8%); 150 (7.4%); 152 (26.7%); 154 (22.7%). Known artificial radioactive isotopes: 133-143; 145; 146; 151; 153; 155-158. Abundance in earth's crust: 6.47-7.0 ppm. Commercially important sources are the rare earth minerals monazite and bastnaesite; also occurs in samarskite, cerite, orthite, ytterbite, and fluorspar. Isoln: L. de Boisbaudran, *Compt. Rend.* **88,** 322 (1879); **89,** 212 (1880). Sepn by crystn of the nitrates: Demarcay, *ibid.* **122,** 728 (1896); Feit, Przibylla, *Z. Anorg. Chem.* **43,** 203 (1905). Sepn of metal: Schumacher, Harris, *J. Am. Chem. Soc.* **48,** 3108 (1926); by reduction of salts: Marsh, *J. Chem. Soc.* **1942,** 398, 523; **1943,** 8; Daane *et al., J. Am. Chem. Soc.* **75,** 2272 (1953); Onstott, *ibid.* **75,** 5128 (1953); **77,** 812 (1955). Toxicity study: Haley, *J. Pharm. Sci.* **54,** 663 (1965). Reviews of prepn, properties and compds: Prandtl, *Z. Anorg. Allg. Chem.* **238,** 321-334 (1938); *The Rare Earths,* F. H. Spedding, A. H. Daane (Krieger, Huntington, N.Y., 1971, reprint of 1961 ed) 641 pp; Hulet, Bode, "Separation Chemistry of the Lanthanides and Transplutonium Actinides" in *MTP Int. Rev. Sci.: Inorg. Chem., Ser. One* **Vol. 7,** K. W. Bagnall, Ed. (University

Park Press, Baltimore, 1972) pp 1-45; Moeller, "The Lanthanides" in *Comprehensive Inorganic Chemistry* **Vol. 4,** J. C. Bailar Jr. *et al.,* Eds. (Pergamon Press, Oxford, 1973) pp 1-101; F. H. Spedding in *Kirk-Othmer Encyclopedia of Chemical Technology* **vol. 19,** (John Wiley & Sons, New York, 3rd ed., 1982) pp 833-854; *Chemistry of the Elements,* N. N. Greenwood, A. Earnshaw, Eds. (Pergamon Press, New York, 1984) pp 1423-1449. Brief review of properties: G. T. Seaborg, *Radiochim. Acta* **61,** 115-122 (1993).

Yellow metal; tarnishes on exposure to air. Hardest metal of the cerium group. Crystalline forms: rhombohedral α-form, d 7.536, transforms to β-form at 917°; body-centered cubic β-form exists at >917°. mp 1074°. bp 1794°. Heat of fusion: 8.623 kJ/mol. Heat of sublimation (25°): 206.7 kJ/mol. E°(aq) Sm^{3+}/Sm −2.41 V (calc).

Oxide. Sm_2O_3. Yellowish-white powder. d 8.347.

Hydroxide. $Sm(OH)_3$. Gelatinous precipitate.

Trichloride. $SmCl_3$. White-yellowish powder. d 4.465, mp 686°. Forms addition compds with ammonia. Forms a hexahydrate, $SmCl_3.6H_2O$, d 2.382, yellow crystalline plates. By reducing the anhydr trichloride at high temps with hydrogen, ammonia or aluminum powder, samarium dichloride is obtained. LD_{50} in mice (mg/kg): 585 i.p.; >2000 orally (Haley).

Dichloride. $SmCl_2$. Dark brown crystalline mass. d^{22} 3.687. Practically insol in alcohol. Dec by water.

Sulfate. $Sm_2(SO_4)_3$. Octahydrate, light yellow crystals, d^{18} 2.930. Sparingly sol in water.

USE: Oxide in control rods of some commercial nuclear power reactors. Alloys with cobalt to produce extremely stong permanent magnets.

8348. Samarium Cobalt. [12017-68-4] Cobalt compd with samarium (5:1); samarium pentacobalt. Co_5Sm; mol wt 445.03. Co 66.21%, Sm 33.79%. $SmCo_5$. Prepd by sintering or mechanical alloying to yield a single phase, highly efficient permanent magnetic material. Prepn: K. J. Strnat, A. E. Ray, *Z. Metallkunde* **61,** 461 (1970). Synthesis by mechanical alloying: J. Wecker *et al., J. Appl. Phys.* **69,** 6058 (1991). Prepn and magnetic properties of nanoparticles: E. M. Kirkpatrick *et al., IEEE Trans. Magnetics* **32,** 4502 (1996). Studies on use as a dental material: H. Tsutsui *et al., J. Dent. Res.* **58,** 1597 (1979). Biocompatibility study: L. Bondemark *et al., Am. J. Orthod. Dentofac. Orthop.* **105,** 568 (1994). Review of magnetic properties: R. A. McCurrie, *Cobalt* **1,** 23-24, 28 (1973); of properties, production and applications: H. J. Marik, K. Schlenk, *Powder Metallurgy Int.* **9,** 142-144 (1977). mp ~1325°. Curie temp: 724° (Strnat); also reported as 680° (Tsutsui). d 8.60.

Samarium Cobalt (Sm_2Co_{17}). [12052-78-7] Cobalt compd with samarium (17:2). $Co_{17}Sm_2$; mol wt 1302.58. Sm_2Co_{17}. Prepn and crystal structure: W. Ostertag, K. J. Strnat, *Acta Crystallogr.* **21,** 560 (1966); and magnetic properties: K. Strnat *et al., J. Appl. Phys.* **37,** 1252 (1966). ^{147}Sm and ^{149}Sm NMR study: H. Figiel *et al., J. Magn. Magnet. Mater.* **101,** 401 (1991). Orthodontic tooth movement study in animals: M. A. Darendeliler *et al., Am. J. Orthod. Dentofac. Orthop.* **107,** 578 (1995).

USE: In permanent magnetic materials including: computer disk drives, sensors, traveling wave tubes, actuators, satellite systems, motors; in dental applications.

8349. Samarium Iodide. [32248-43-4] Diiodosamarium; samarium diiodide; samarium(II) iodide. I_2Sm; mol wt 404.17. I 62.80%, Sm 37.20%. SmI_2. One-electron reducing agent. Prepn: C. Matignon, E. Cazes, *Ann. Chim. Phys.* **8,** 417 (1906); and use in organic synthesis: J. L. Namy *et al., Nouv. J. Chim.* **1,** 5 (1977); P. Girard *et al., J. Am. Chem. Soc.* **102,** 2693 (1980). Coordination chemistry and crystal structure of adducts with THF: W. J. Evans *et al., ibid.* **117,** 8999 (1995). Review of properties: S.-H. Wang, *Rev. Inorg. Chem.* **11,** 1-20 (1990); of uses in organic chemistry: G. A. Molander, C. R. Harris, *Chem. Rev.* **96,** 307-338 (1996); H. B. Kagan, *Tetrahedron* **59,** 10351-10372 (2003).

Black to light black solid, mp 526 ±3°. Deep blue-green soln in THF. Absorption max (THF): 565, 617 nm. Sol in ether, THF. Redox potential: E⁰ −1.55 v. *Unstable in the presence of oxygen or moisture; store under an inert atmosphere.*

USE: In organic synthesis and electron transfer reactions; in discharge lamps.

8350. Samarium ^{153}Sm Lexidronam. [154247-83-5] (*OC*-6-21)-[[[1,2-Ethanediylbis[(nitrilo-κN)bis(methylene)]]tetrakis[phosphonato-κO]](8−)]-samarate(5−)-^{153}Sm; samarium 153 ethylenediaminetetramethylenephosphonic acid; ^{153}Sm-EDTMP. $C_6H_{12}N_2O_{12}P_4{}^{153}$Sm. Tetraphosphonate chelating agent bound to a β-emitting radionuclide; targets areas of increased bone turnover. Prepn: J. Simon *et al.*, **EP 164843**; *eidem*, **US 4898724** (1985, 1990 both to Dow); W. F. Goeckeler *et al.*, *Nucl. Med. Biol.* **13**, 479 (1986). Biodistribution studies: *idem et al.*, *J. Nucl. Med.* **28**, 495 (1987). Pharmacokinetics and clinical evaluation of pain palliation in metastatic bone cancer: M. Farhanghi *et al.*, *ibid.* **33**, 1451 (1992). HPLC determn in urine: W. F. Goeckeler *et al.*, *Nucl. Med. Biol.* **20**, 657 (1993). Chromatographic determn of radiochemical purity: H. T. Gasiglia, H. Okada, *J. Radioanal. Nucl. Chem. Lett.* **199**, 295 (1995). Review of therapeutic potential: R. A. Holmes, *Semin. Nucl. Med.* **22**, 41-45 (1992). Clinical trial in palliation of bone pain in hormone-refractory prostate cancer: O. Sartor *et al.*, *Urology* **63**, 940 (2004).

Pentasodium salt. [160369-78-8] CYT-424; Quadramet. $C_6H_{12}N_2Na_5O_{12}P_4{}^{153}$Sm.

THERAP CAT: Antineoplastic.

8351. Sambucus. Elder; American elder; sweet elder. Flowers of *Sambucus canadensis* L., or of *S. nigra* L., *Caprifoliaceae*. *Habit.* U.S., east of Rocky Mts. *Constit.* Volatile oil, resin, fat, mucilage, tannin.

THERAP CAT: Diaphoretic, diuretic, cathartic.

8352. Sampatrilat. [129981-36-8] N^2-(Methylsulfonyl)-L-lysyl-1-[(2*S*)-3-amino-2-carboxypropyl]cyclopentanecarbonyl-L-tyrosine; UK-81252. $C_{26}H_{40}N_4O_9S$; mol wt 584.68. C 53.41%, H 6.90%, N 9.58%, O 24.63%, S 5.48%. Dual inhibitor of neutral endopeptidase (NEP) and angiotensin converting enzyme (ACE). Prepn: J. C. Danilewicz *et al.*, **EP 358398**; *idem*, **US 4975444** (both 1990 to Pfizer). Determn in plasma: R. F. Venn *et al.*, *J. Pharm. Biomed. Anal.* **16**, 875 (1998); and urine: *eidem*, *ibid.* 883. Clinical evaluations in hypertension: E. J. Wallis *et al.*, *Clin. Pharmacol. Ther.* **64**, 439 (1998); G. R. Norton *et al.*, *Am. J. Hypertens.* **12**, 563 (1999).

THERAP CAT: Antihypertensive.

8353. Sandalwood. White saunders; yellow saunders. Heartwood of *Santalum album* L., *Santalaceae*. *Habit.* India; cultivated in Timor and Sunda Islands. *Constit.* Volatile oil (3-5%), resin, tannin. Botanical description and medicinal uses: J. Gruenwald *et al.*, *PDR for Herbal Medicines* (Medical Economics, Montvale, 2nd Ed., 2000) pp 659-660.

Volatile oil. [8006-87-9] Oil of Santal; sandalwood oil. Obtained by steam distillation from the dried heartwood. *Constit.* Santalols, α-bergamotol, α-bergamotal. Fragrance monograph: *J. Food Cosmet. Toxicol.* **12**, 989 (1974). Pale yellow, somewhat viscid liquid; characteristic sandalwood odor and taste. d_{25}^{25} 0.965-0.980. n_D^{20} 1.500-1.510. Sol in most fixed oils, propylene glycol, mineral oil; in 5 vols 70% alcohol. Insol in glycerin. *Keep well closed, cool and protected from light.*

USE: Wood in boxes and carvings, as incense. Oil in perfumes and as fragrance in creams and lotions.

THERAP CAT: In treatment of urinary tract inflammations.

8354. Sandarac. Resin from *Callitris quadrivalvis* Vent., *Pinaceae*. *Habit.* Morocco. *Constit.* About 80% pimaric acid, about 10% callitrolic acid; sandaricinic acid.

Light yellow, brittle, elongated tears; translucent with vitreous fracture; crumbles to powder when masticated. Insol in water, benzene, petr ether. Sol in alcohol, ether, acetone, hot caustic alkalies; partially sol in chloroform, volatile oils, oil turpentine, carbon disulfide.

USE: Tooth cements, lacquers, varnishes; as an incense. Pharmaceutic aid (in ointments and plasters).

8355. Sanguinaria. Bloodroot; red puccoon; red root; puccoon root; tetterwort. Dried rhizome and roots of *Sanguinaria canadensis* L., *Papaveraceae*. *Habit.* North America. *Constit.* Sanguinarine, chelerythrine, protopine, homochelidonine, resin. An extract of *Sanguinaria canadensis* has been used in cough syrup; used experimentally as toothpaste base, in gingivitis and in periodontal disease: P. A. Ladanyi, **US 4145412** (1979 to Vipont Chem. Co.).

8356. Sanguinarine. [2447-54-3] 13-Methyl[1,3]benzodioxolo[5,6-*c*]-1,3-dioxolo[4,5-*i*]phenanthridinium; pseudochelerythrine; ψ-chelerythrine. $[C_{20}H_{14}NO_4]^+$. Principal alkaloid in sanguinaria extract. Isolated from the root of *Sanguinaria canadensis* L., and other *Papaveraceae*: Schmidt *et al.*, *Arch. Pharm.* **231**, 145 (1893). Widely distributed in poppy-fumaria species; constituent of argemone oil: S. A. E. Hakim *et al.*, *Nature* **189**, 198 (1961). Identity with pseudochelerythrine: Gadamer, Stichel, *ibid.* **262**, 488 (1924). Structure: Späth, Kuffner, *Ber.* **64**, 370, 2034 (1931); Beke, *Acta Chim. Acad. Sci. Hung.* **17**, 463 (1958). Biosynthesis: Leete, *J. Am. Chem. Soc.* **85**, 473 (1963). Synthesis: Dyke *et al.*, *Tetrahedron Lett.* **1968**, 3933; Sainsbury *et al.*, *J. Chem. Soc. C* **1970**, 1797; Onda *et al.*, *Chem. Pharm. Bull.* **17**, 404 (1969); **19**, 31 (1971); M. Hanaoka *et al.*, *Chem. Lett.* **22**, 739 (1986). Purification procedure: Stipanovic *et al.*, *J. Heterocycl. Chem.* **9**, 1453 (1972). Studies of effect of sanguinarine and argemone oil on intraocular pressure: S. A. E. Hakim, *Br. J. Ophthalmol.* **38**, 193 (1954); G. C. Dobbie, M. E. Langham, *ibid.* **45**, 61 (1961). Antiinflammatory activity in rats: J. Lenfeld *et al.*, *Planta Med.* **43**, 161 (1981). Clinical study of sanguinarine oral rinse as antiplaque agent: G. L. Southard *et al.*, *J. Am. Dent. Assoc.* **108**, 338 (1984). Acute toxicity study: P. J. Becci *et al.*, *J. Toxicol. Environ. Health* **20**, 199 (1987). *Review:* M. Shamma, *The Isoquinoline Alkaloids* (Academic Press, New York, 1972) pp 315-343. Symposium on chemistry, antimicrobial effects, clinical studies and toxicology: *J. Can. Dent. Assoc.* **56**, Suppl 7, 5-47 (1990).

Monohydrate. $C_{20}H_{13}NO_4 \cdot H_2O$. Crystals from water, mp 278-280° (Stipanovic). Soluble in alcohol, chloroform, acetone, ethyl acetate.

Chloride. Viadent. $C_{20}H_{14}ClNO_4$; mol wt 367.78. LD_{50} in male mice (mg/kg): 15.9 i.v.; in female mice (mg/kg): 102.0 s.c. (Lenfeld). LD_{50} in rats (mg/kg): 29 i.v.; 1658 orally (Becci).

Chloride dihydrate. $C_{20}H_{14}ClNO_4 \cdot 2H_2O$. Fine orange needles, mp 273-274° (dec). uv max (methanol): 234, 283, 325 nm (log ε 4.50, 4.52, 4.18).

USE: In mouthwash and toothpaste.

8357. α-Santalol. [115-71-9] 5-(2,3-Dimethyltricyclo[2.2.1.0^{2,6}]hept-3-yl)-2-methyl-2-penten-1-ol. $C_{15}H_{24}O$; mol wt 220.35. C 81.76%, H 10.98%, O 7.26%. A sesquiterpene alcohol which together with β-santalol comprises about 90% of commercial sandalwood oil: F. W. Semmler, K. Bode, *Ber.* **40**, 1124 (1907); E. Gruenther, *The Essential Oils* vol. **2** (Van Nostrand, New York, 1949) pp 266-269. Structure: F. W. Semmler, *Ber.* **43**, 1893 (1910). Separation of α- and β-santalols of high purity: A. E. Bradfield *et al.*, *J. Chem. Soc.* **1935**, 309. Synthesis of α-santalol and conversion to β-santalol: S. C. Bhattacharyya, *Sci. Cult.* **13**,

207 (1947), *C.A.* **43**, 5484gh (1949); *see also* V. M. Sathe *et al.*, *Indian J. Chem.* **4**, 393 (1966); S. Y. Kamat *et al.*, *Tetrahedron* **23**, 4487 (1967). Stereochemistry studies: G. Brieger, *Tetrahedron Lett.* **1963**, 2123. Natural α-santalol has a *cis*-(+)-configuration. Total synthesis: R. G. Lewis *et al.*, *ibid.* **1967**, 401. Stereospecific synthesis: E. J. Corey *et al.*, *J. Am. Chem. Soc.* **92**, 226, 6314 (1970); M. Julia, P. Ward, *Bull. Soc. Chim. Fr.* **1973**, 3065; M. Tamura, G. Suzukamo, *Tetrahedron Lett.* **22**, 577 (1981). Synthesis and separation of *cis*- and *trans*-isomers: K. Sato *et al.*, *Bull. Chem. Soc. Jpn.* **49**, 3351 (1976). *Review:* J. Simonsen, D. H. R. Barton, *The Terpenes* **vol. 3** (Univ. Press, Cambridge, 1961) pp 178-188; A. Bhati, *Flavour Ind.* **1**, 235-251 (1970).

Liquid. bp$_{14}$ 166-167°. d$_{25}^{25}$ 0.9770. n$_D^{25}$ 1.5017. α$_{5461}$ +10.3°. [α]$_D^{20}$ +17.20° (c = 0.8 in chloroform). Sol in alcohol; slightly sol in propylene glycol, glycerine. Practically insol in water.

USE: In perfumes, soaps and detergents.

8358. β-Santalol. [77-42-9] [1*S*-[1α,2α(*Z*),4α]]-2-Methyl-5-(2-methyl-3-methylenebicyclo[2.2.1]hept-2-yl)-2-penten-1-ol; 2-methyl-5-(2-methyl-3-methylene-2-norbornyl)-2-penten-1-ol. C$_{15}$H$_{24}$O; mol wt 220.35. C 81.76%, H 10.98%, O 7.26%. A sesquiterpene alcohol from sandalwood oil. Isoln and purification and additional refs: *see* α-santalol. Structure: L. Ruzicka, G. Thomann, *Helv. Chim. Acta* **18**, 355 (1935). Synthesis: S. C. Bhattacharyya, *Sci. Cult.* **13**, 209 (1957), *C.A.* **43**, 5385a (1949); H. C. Kretschmar, W. F. Erman, **US 3662008**, **US 3679756** (1972 to Procter & Gamble). Natural β-santalol has a *cis*-(−)-configuration. Total synthesis: *eidem, Tetrahedron Lett.* **1970**, 41. Synthesis of *dl*-form: P. A. Christenson, B. J. Willis, *J. Org. Chem.* **44**, 2012 (1979); M. Baumann, W. H. Hoffman, *Ann.* **1979**, 743; K. Sato *et al.*, *Chem. Lett.* **1981**, 1183.

Liquid. bp$_{17}$ 177-178°. d$_{25}^{25}$ 0.9717. n$_D^{25}$ 1.5100. α$_{5461}$ −87.1°. Sol in alcohol; practically insol in water.

dl-**Form.** bp$_{0.1}$ 101-103°.

USE: In perfumes, soaps and detergents.

8359. Santonica. Levant wormseed. Dried, unexpanded flower heads of *Artemisia maritima* L., sens. lat., *Compositae*. *Habit.* Iran, Turkestan. *Constit.* 2-4% santonin, 2-3% volatile oil; artemisin, resin.

THERAP CAT: Anthelmintic.

8360. Santonic Acid. [510-35-0] (α*S*,1*R*,3a*S*,4*R*,5*S*,7a*S*)-Octahydro-α,3a,5-trimethyl-6,8-dioxo-1,4-methano-1*H*-indene-1-acetic acid; hexahydro-α,3a,5-trimethyl-6,8-dioxo-1,4-methanoindan-1-acetic acid. C$_{15}$H$_{20}$O$_4$; mol wt 264.32. C 68.16%, H 7.63%, O 24.21%. Prepd from santonin by the action of hot concd aq bases, preferably potassium hydroxide: v. Oettingen, *Dissertation*, Göttingen, 1913; Woodward *et al.*, *J. Am. Chem. Soc.* **70**, 4216 (1948). Structure: Wedekind, Engel, *J. Prakt. Chem.* **139**, 115 (1934); Woodward *et al.*, *loc. cit.*; Woodward, Yates, *Chem. Ind. (London)* **1954**, 1391. Chemistry: Hortmann, Daniel, *J. Org. Chem.* **37**, 4446 (1972).

Crystals from water or alcohol, mp 170-172°; bp$_{15}$ 285°; [α]$_D^{20}$ −74.0° (chloroform). Soluble in 190 parts of water at 17°. Freely sol in alc, chloroform, ether, glacial acetic acid.

8361. α-Santonin. [481-06-1] [3*S*-(3α,3aα,5aβ,9bβ)]-3a,5,-5a,9b-Tetrahydro-3,5a,9-trimethylnaphtho[1,2-*b*]furan-2,8(3*H*,4*H*)-dione; 1,2,3,4,4a,7-hexahydro-1-hydroxy-α,4a,8-trimethyl-7-oxo-2-naphthaleneacetic acid γ-lactone; *l*-santonin. C$_{15}$H$_{18}$O$_3$; mol wt 246.30. C 73.15%, H 7.37%, O 19.49%. Anthelmintic isolated from the dried unexpanded flower heads of *Artemisia maritima* L., sens. lat., *Compositae* [Levant wormseed] and other species of *Artemisia* found principally in Russian and Chinese Turkestan and the Southern Ural region. Structure: Clemo *et al.*, *J. Chem. Soc.* **1930**, 1110; Ruzicka, Steiner, *Helv. Chim. Acta* **17**, 614 (1934). Stereochemistry: Corey, *J. Am. Chem. Soc.* **77**, 1044 (1955); Cocker, McMurry, *Tetrahedron* **8**, 181 (1960); Asher, Sim, *Proc. Chem. Soc. London* **1962**, 111, 335; Nakazaki, Arakawa, *Bull. Chem. Soc. Jpn.* **37**, 464 (1964); Pregosin *et al.*, *J. Chem. Soc. Perkin Trans. 1* **1972**, 299. Total synthesis: Abe *et al.*, *Proc. Jpn. Acad.* **30**, 116 (1954); *J. Am. Chem. Soc.* **78**, 1422 (1956); **US 2836604** (1958 to Takeda); J. A. Marshall, P. G. M. Wuts, *J. Org. Chem.* **43**, 1086 (1978). Mass spectral studies of the santonins and derivs: Woseda *et al.*, *Tetrahedron* **23**, 4623 (1967). *Review:* C. H. Heathcock in *The Total Synthesis of Natural Products* **vol. 2**, J. W. ApSimon, Ed. (Wiley, New York, 1973) pp 315-324.

(−)-**Form.** Tabular crystals, orthorhombic sphenoidal, mp 170-173°. Almost tasteless with bitter aftertaste. [α]$_D^{25}$ −170 to −175° (c = 2 in alc). Becomes yellow on exposure to light. Irritating to mucous membranes. d 1.187. One part dissolves in 5000 parts of cold water, in 250 parts of boiling water, in 280 parts of 50% alcohol at 17°, in 10 parts of boiling 50% alcohol, in 44 parts of cold 90% alcohol, in 3 parts of boiling 90% alcohol, in 125 parts of cold ether, in 72 parts of boiling ether, in 4.3 parts of cold chloroform.

(±)-**Form.** Colorless plates from methanol, mp 181°. uv max (ethanol): 241 nm (log ε 4.10).

(+)-**Form.** Colorless plates from methanol, mp 172°. [α]$_D^{20}$ +165.9° (c = 1.92 in ethanol).

4-Hydroxysantonin see Artemisin.

THERAP CAT: Anthelmintic (Nematodes).

THERAP CAT (VET): Has been used as an anthelmintic.

8362. Saperconazole. [110588-57-3] 4-[4-[4-[4-[[2-(2,4-Difluorophenyl)-2-(1*H*-1,2,4-triazol-1-ylmethyl)-1,3-dioxolan-4-yl]methoxy]phenyl]-1-piperazinyl]phenyl]-2,4-dihydro-2-(1-methylpropyl)-3*H*-1,2,4-triazol-3-one; (±)-1-*sec*-butyl-4-[*p*-[4-[*p*-[[(2*R**,4*S**)-2-(2,4-difluorophenyl)-2-(1*H*-1,2,4-triazol-1-ylmethyl)-1,3-dioxolan-4-yl]methoxy]phenyl]-1-piperazinyl]phenyl]-Δ^2-1,2,4-triazolin-5-one; R-66905. C$_{35}$H$_{38}$F$_2$N$_8$O$_4$; mol wt 672.72. C 62.49%, H 5.69%, F 5.65%, N 16.66%, O 9.51%. Orally active, fluorinated triazole antifungal. Prepn: J. Heeres *et al.*, **EP 283992**; *eidem*, **US 4916134** (1988, 1990 both to Janssen). *In vitro* antifungal activity: F. C. Odds, *J. Antimicrob. Chemother.* **24**, 533 (1989); D. W. Denning *et al.*, *Eur. J. Clin. Microbiol. Infect. Dis.* **9**, 693 (1990). *In vivo* efficacy vs *Aspergillus* species: J. Van Cutsem *et al.*, *Antimicrob. Agents Chemother.* **33**, 2063 (1989).

Crystals from acetonitrile, mp 189.5°. Poorly sol in water.

THERAP CAT: Antifungal.

8363. Saponaria. Soapwort; soaproot; fuller's herb; bruisewort; bouncing bet. *Saponaria officinalis* L., *Caryophyllaceae*; herbaceous perennial plant having sharp-pointed leaves and large pale pink flowers. Habit. Europe to Middle Asia; naturalized in U.S. *Constit.* Saponins, saponarin, saporins, *q.q.v.* Produces soapy lather when bruised and agitated with water. Root has been used in traditional medicine as antitussive or as a wash for skin irritations. Brief review: M. Wichtl, N. G. Bisset, *Herbal Drugs and Phytopharmaceuticals*, English Ed. (CRC Press, Boca Raton, 1994) pp 453-454.

8364. Saponarin. [20310-89-8] 6-β-D-Glucopyranosyl-7-(β-D-glucopyranosyloxy)-5-hydroxy-2-(4-hydroxyphenyl)-4H-1-benzopyran-4-one. $C_{27}H_{30}O_{15}$; mol wt 594.52. C 54.55%, H 5.09%, O 40.37%. From leaves of *Saponaria officinalis* L., *Caryophyllaceae:* Barger, *J. Chem. Soc.* **89**, 1210 (1906); from *Hibiscus syriacus* L., *Malvaceae:* Nakoaki, *J. Pharm. Soc. Jpn.* **64**, 304 (1944), *C.A.* **46**, 108d (1952); from *Lemna (Spirodela) oligorrhiza* Kurz., *Lemnaceae:* Jurd *et al., Arch. Biochem. Biophys.* **67**, 284 (1957). Structure: Seikel, Geissman, *ibid.* **71**, 17 (1957). Revised structure: Hörhammer *et al., Tetrahedron Lett.* **1965**, 1707. On acidic hydrolysis yields the aglycone, *saponaretin.*

Monohydrate. Pale yellow granules, mp 228°. $[\alpha]_D$ −7.9° (aq pyridine). uv max (ethanol): 335, 272 nm. Practically insol in cold water. Sparingly sol in hot water, alcohol; sol in alkalies with yellow color and in concd H_2SO_4 with blue fluorescence; sol in pyridine.

8365. Saponins. Sapogenin glycosides. A type of glycoside widely distributed in plants. Each saponin consists of a sapogenin which constitutes the aglucon moiety of the molecule, and a sugar. The sapogenin may be a steroid or a triterpene and the sugar moiety may be glucose, galactose, a pentose, or a methylpentose. Poisonous towards the lower forms of life and used for killing fish by the aborigines of South America. *Review and bibliography:* R. J. McIlroy, *The Plant Glycosides* (Edward Arnold & Co., London, 1951) Chapter IX; Y. Birk, I. Peri in *Toxic Const. Plant Foodst.,* I. E. Liener, Ed. (Academic Press, New York, 2nd ed., 1980) pp 161-182.

Bitter taste. All saponins foam strongly when shaken with water. They form oil-in-water emulsions and act as protective colloids.

Caution: Although practically non-toxic to man upon oral ingestion, they act as powerful hemolytics when injected into the blood stream, dissolving the red corpuscles even at extreme dilutions.

8366. Saporins. Single chain ribosome inactivating proteins (type 1 RIPs); found in the seeds, leaves and roots of the soapwort plant, *Saponaria officinalis* L., *Caryophyllaceae*. Used to produce targeted immunotoxins by conjugating with a specific monoclonal antibody or other cell receptor ligand. At least 7 isoforms have been identified. Saporin-6 is the most abundant and is often referred to as "saporin". Isoln from seeds: F. Stirpe *et al., Biochem. J.* **216**, 617 (1983). Purification and distribution in plant tissues: J. M. Ferreras *et al., Biochim. Biophys. Acta* **1216**, 31 (1993). Production by plant cell culture: A. Di Cola *et al., Plant Cell Rep.* **17**, 55 (1997). Review of use as neural lesioning tools: R. G. Wiley, *Trends Neurosci.* **15**, 285-290 (1992); in model for Alzheimer's disease: R. Schliebs *et al., Prog. Brain Res.* **109**, 253-264 (1996). Discussion of therapeutic potential in cancer: D. J. Flavell, *Curr. Top. Microbiol. Immunol.* **234**, 57-61 (1998).

Saporin-6. [166944-16-7] SO6. Isoform constituting 7% of the total seed protein. Composed of 259 amino acid residues; mol wt 29 kDa. Review of isoln, properties and production by recombinant technology: M. R. Soria *et al., Targeted Diagn. Ther.* **7**, 193-212 (1992). Crystal structure: C. Savino *et al., Acta Crystallogr.* **D54**, 636 (1998). pI >9.5. LD$_{50}$ i.p. in mice: 4 mg/kg (Stirpe).

USE: Biological research tool.

8367. Sapphire. [1317-82-4] The corundum modification of aluminum oxide, Al_2O_3. Mined in Montana, Siam, Burma, Ceylon. The highest priced variety of the native gem has the blue color of cornflowers. Easily prepd synthetically. Hydrothermal synthesis: Laudise, Ballman, *J. Am. Chem. Soc.* **80**, 2655 (1958).

USE: In jewelry, as phonograph needles, industrial abrasive, watch and instrument bearings.

8368. Sapropterin. [62989-33-7] (6*R*)-2-Amino-6-[(1*R*,2*S*)-1,2-dihydroxypropyl]-5,6,7,8-tetrahydro-4(1*H*)-pteridinone; (6*R*)-L-*erythro*-tetrahydrobiopterin; dapropterin; *R*-THBP; 6*R*-BH$_4$. $C_9H_{15}N_5O_3$; mol wt 241.25. C 44.81%, H 6.27%, N 29.03%, O 19.90%. Natural cofactor of the aromatic amino acid hydroxylases required for catecholamine and serotonin biosynthesis. Identification of cofactor activity: S. Kaufman, *Proc. Natl. Acad. Sci. USA* **50**, 1085 (1963). Prepn of (6*R*,*S*)-BH$_4$: B. Schircks *et al., Helv. Chim. Acta* **61**, 2731 (1978). Chromatographic separation of diastereoisomers: S. W. Bailey, J. E. Ayling, *J. Biol. Chem.* **253**, 1598 (1978). Absolute configuration of natural isomer: W. L. F. Armarego *et al., Aust. J. Chem.* **35**, 785 (1982). Stereospecific synthesis: S. Matsuura *et al., Heterocycles* **23**, 3115 (1985); H. Sakai, T. Kanai, *EP* 191335; *eidem, US* 4713454 (1986, 1987 both to Shiratori; Suntory). Bioavailability: G. Kapatos, S. Kaufman, *Science* **212**, 955 (1981). Effect on neurotransmitter monoamine biosynthesis: S. Miwa *et al., Arch. Biochem. Biophys.* **239**, 234 (1985). LC determn in biological samples: Y. Tani, T. Ishihara, *Life Sci.* **46**, 373 (1990). Therapeutic potential in hyperphenylalaninemia: S. Kaufman, *J. Nutr. Sci. Vitaminol,* Suppl., 601 (1992).

pK' 5.05. uv max (0.1 *N* HCl): 265 nm (ε 14000).

Dihydrochloride. [69056-38-8] SUN-0588; Biopten. C_9H_{15}-N_5O_3.2HCl; mol wt 314.17. Crystals from HCl, mp 245-246° (dec). $[\alpha]_D^{25}$ −6.81° (c = 0.665 in 0.1 *M* HCl). uv max (2 *M* HCl): 264 nm (ε 16770).

THERAP CAT: In treatment of hyperphenylalaninemia.

8369. Saquinavir. [127779-20-8] (2*S*)-*N*^{1}[(1*S*,2*R*)-3-[(3*S*,-4a*S*,8a*S*)-3-[[(1,1-Dimethylethyl)amino]carbonyl]octahydro-2(1*H*)-isoquinolinyl]-2-hydroxy-1-(phenylmethyl)propyl]-2-[(2-quinolinylcarbonyl)amino]butanediamide; (*S*)-*N*-[(α*S*)-α-[(1*R*)-2-[(3*S*,4a*S*,-8a*S*)-3-(*tert*-butylcarbamoyl)octahydro-2(1*H*)-isoquinolyl]-1-hydroxyethyl]phenethyl]-2-quinaldamido succinamide; *N*-*tert*-butyl-decahydro-2-[2[*R*)-hydroxy-4-phenyl-3(*S*)-[[*N*-(2-quinolylcarbonyl)-L-asparaginyl]amino]butyl](4a*S*,8a*S*)-isoquinoline-3(*S*)-carboxamide; Ro-31-8959. $C_{38}H_{50}N_6O_5$; mol wt 670.84. C 68.04%, H 7.51%, N 12.53%, O 11.92%. Selective HIV protease inhibitor. Prepn: J. A. Martin, S. Redshaw, *EP* 432695; *eidem, US* 5196438 (1991, 1993 both to Hoffmann-LaRoche); K. E. B. Parkes *et al., J. Org. Chem.* **59**, 3656 (1994). *In vitro* HIV proteinase inhibition: N. A. Roberts *et al., Science* **248**, 358 (1990). Antiviral properties: J. C. Craig *et al., Antiviral Res.* **16**, 295 (1991); S. Galpin *et al., Antiviral Chem. Chemother.* **5**, 43-45 (1994). Clinical evaluation of tolerability and activity: V. S. Kitchen *et al., Lancet* **345**, 952 (1995). Review of pharmacology and clinical experience: S. Kravcik, *Expert Opin. Pharmacother.* **2** 303-315 (2001).

White crystalline solid. $[\alpha]_D^{20}$ −55.9° (c = 0.5 in methanol). Soly (21°): 0.22 g/100 ml water.

Methanesulfonate salt. [149845-06-7] Saquinavir mesylate; Ro-31-8959/003; Fortovase; Invirase. $C_{38}H_{50}N_6O_5 \cdot CH_3SO_3H$; mol wt 766.95.

THERAP CAT: Antiviral.

8370. Sarafloxacin. [98105-99-8] 6-Fluoro-1-(4-fluorophenyl)-1,4-dihydro-4-oxo-7-(1-piperazinyl)-3-quinolinecarboxylic acid. $C_{20}H_{17}F_2N_3O_3$; mol wt 385.36. C 62.33%, H 4.45%, F 9.86%, N 10.90%, O 12.46%. Fluorinated quinolone antibacterial. Prepn: D. T. W. Chu, **EP 131839**; *idem*, **US 4730000** (1985, 1988 both to Abbott); D. T. W. Chu *et al.*, *J. Med. Chem.* **28**, 1558 (1985); H. Narita *et al.*, **JP Kokai 85 237069** (1985 to Toyama). Comparative *in vitro* antibacterial spectrum: A. Digranes, W. L. Dibb, *Chemotherapy* **34**, 298 (1988). *In vivo* antibacterial activity: P. B. Fernandes *et al.*, *Antimicrob. Agents Chemother.* **29**, 201 (1986). HPLC determn: J. F. Bauer *et al.*, *Pharm. Res.* **7**, 1177 (1990).

Monohydrochloride. [91296-87-6] Abbott 56620; A-56620. $C_{20}H_{17}F_2N_3O_3 \cdot HCl$; mol wt 421.83. mp as monohydrate >275°.

THERAP CAT (VET): Antibacterial.

8371. Sarafotoxins. SRTx. Family of vasoactive toxins isolated from the venom of the Israeli burrowing asp, *Atractaspis engaddensis*. Several isoforms exist, all are closely related in structure and biological activity to the mammalian endothelins, *q.v.*; both families show highly conserved sequences of 21 amino acids with 2 fixed disulfide bridges. Isoln: E. Kochva *et al.*, *Toxicon* **20**, 581 (1982). Purification of a-c: C. Takasaki *et al.*, *ibid.* **26**, 543 (1988); of d: A. Bdolah *et al.*, *FEBS Lett.* **256**, 1 (1989). Structure-activity studies: A. M. Doherty *et al.*, *J. Cardiovasc. Pharmacol.* **17**, Suppl 7, S59 (1991). Conformational stability: A. R. Atkins *et al.*, *Int. J. Pept. Protein Res.* **44**, 372 (1994). Review of structure and evolution: E. Kochva *et al.*, *Toxicon* **31**, 541-568 (1993); of biological activity: M. Sokolovsky in *Toxins and Signal Transduction*, Y. Gutman, P. Lazarovici, Eds. (Harwood Academic Publishers, Netherlands, 1997) pp 53-67.

C–S–C–K–D–M–T–D–K–E–C–L–N–F–C–H–Q–D–V–I–W

Sarafotoxin A

8372. Saralasin. [34273-10-4] 1-(*N*-Methylglycine)-5-L-valine-8-L-alanineangiotensin II; *N*-[1-[*N*-[*N*-[*N*-[*N*-[*N*²-(*N*-methylglycyl)-L-arginyl]-L-valyl]-L-tyrosyl]-L-valyl]-L-histidyl]-L-prolyl]-L-alanine; 1-sar-8-ala-angiotensin II. $C_{42}H_{65}N_{13}O_{10}$; mol wt 912.05. C 55.31%, H 7.18%, N 19.96%, O 17.54%. A specific antagonist of angiotensin II. Prepn: Sipos *et al.*, **DE 2127393** corresp to **US 3751404** (1972, 1973 to Norwich Pharmacal). Activity studies: Pals *et al.*, *Circ. Res.* **29**, 673 (1971); Pals, Fulton, *Arch. Int. Pharmacodyn. Ther.* **204**, 20 (1973); Solomon, Buckley, *J. Pharm. Sci.* **63**, 1109 (1974); Streeten *et al.*, *N. Engl. J. Med.* **292**, 657 (1975). Comprehensive review of the acetate: C. T. Huang *et al.*, in *Pharmacological and Biochemical Properties of Drug Substances* vol. 3, M. E. Goldberg, Ed. (Am. Pharm. Assoc., Washington, DC, 1981) pp 176-225.

Sar–Arg–Val–Tyr–Val–His–Pro–Ala

Hydrated acetate. [39698-78-7] Saralasin acetate; P-113; Sarenin. Described as $C_{42}H_{65}N_{13}O_{10} \cdot xC_2H_4O_2 \cdot xH_2O$. Fluffy white powder, mp 256°. Sol in water, 5% aq dextrose, 90-95% aq alcohol. LD_{50} i.v. in male mice: 1171 mg/kg (Huang).

THERAP CAT: Antihypertensive, diagnostic aid (renin-dependent hypertension).

8373. Sarcosine. [107-97-1] *N*-Methylglycine; *N*-methylaminoacetic acid; Sar; *N*-methylglycocoll; methylaminoethanoic acid. $C_3H_7NO_2$; mol wt 89.09. C 40.44%, H 7.92%, N 15.72%, O 35.92%. CH_3NHCH_2COOH. Has been found in starfish and sea urchins: A. Kossel, S. Edlbacher, *Z. Physiol. Chem.* **94**, 264 (1915); in rock lobsters: L. Novellie, H. M. Schwartz, *Nature* **173**, 450 (1954). Formation from caffeine by dec with barium hydroxide: Paulmann, *Arch. Pharm.* **232**, 601 (1894). Prepd on a large scale from formaldehyde, sodium cyanide, and methylamine: Eschweiler, *Ann.* **279**, 39 (1894); Baumann, *J. Biol. Chem.* **21**, 563 (1915); Caverly, **US 2720540** (1955 to du Pont); Leake, Brakebill, **US 3009954** (1961 to Allied Chem.). Synthesis: M. Ebata *et al.*, *Bull. Chem. Soc. Jpn.* **39**, 2535 (1966). Review of syntheses: T. Shirai, *Synthetic Production and Utilization of Amino Acids*, T. Kaneko *et al.*, Eds. (Wiley, New York, 1974) pp 184-186.

Orthorhombic, deliquescent crystals from dil methanol. Dec 212°. Sweetish taste. pK_1' 2.23; pK_2' 10.01. Sol in water: 5 ml of a satd aq soln contain 2.1412 g sarcosine. Slightly sol in alc.

Sodium salt. Usually sold as aq soln, pH 12.0.

Hydrochloride. $C_3H_7NO_2 \cdot HCl$. Needles from alcohol, dec 171°. Freely sol in water; slightly sol in alcohol, ether.

USE: Intermediate in the synthesis of antienzyme agents for toothpaste.

8374. Sarin. [107-44-8] Methylphosphonofluoridic acid 1-methylethyl ester; isopropoxymethylphosphoryl fluoride; isopropylmethylphosphonofluoridate; GB. $C_4H_{10}FO_2P$; mol wt 140.09. C 34.29%, H 7.19%, F 13.56%, O 22.84%, P 22.11%. Nerve gas; potent cholinesterase inhibitor similar in structure and activity to soman and tabun, *q.q.v.* Prepn: Holmstedt, *Acta Physiol. Scand.* **25**, suppl. 90, p 106 (1951); *Protar* **14**, 113 (1948); **16**, 131 (1950). Additional syntheses: Schrader, *B.I.O.S.* **714**, 41 (1947); B. C. Saunders, *Some Aspects of the Chemistry and Toxic Action of Organic Compounds Containing Phosphorus and Fluorine* (Cambridge, 1957) p 92 sqq; Bryant *et al.*, *J. Chem. Soc.* **1960**, 1553. Absolute configuration: Benschop *et al.*, *Rec. Trav. Chim.* **87**, 387 (1968). Toxicity study: B. Holmstedt, *Pharmacol. Rev.* **11**, 567 (1959). Epidemiological study of chronic effects: Y. Nishiwaki *et al.*, *Environ. Health Perspect.* **109**, 1169 (2001). Brief review: Schrader, *Die Entwicklung neuer insektizider Phosphorsäure-Ester* (Verlag Chemie, Weinheim, 1963) p 4; B. L. Harris in *Kirk-Othmer Encyclopedia of Chemical Technology* vol. 5 (Wiley-Interscience, New York, 4th ed., 1993) pp 795-816.

Liquid, d_4^{20} 1.10. mp −57°. bp_{760} 147°; bp_{16} 56°. Miscible with and hydrolyzed by water. Rapidly hydrolyzed by dil aq sodium hydroxide or sodium carbonate forming relatively non-toxic products. Water alone removes the fluorine atom producing the non-toxic acid $CH_3PO[OCH(CH_3)_2]OH$. LD_{50} i.p. in mice: 0.42 mg/kg (Holmstedt, 1959).

Caution: Potential symptoms of overexposure by inhalation are constriction of pupils of the eye, difficulty breathing followed by bronchial constriction, convulsions, and death. Also toxic due to absorption through skin and eyes. *See Chem. Eng. News* **31**, 4676 (1953).

USE: Chemical warfare agent.

8375. Sarizotan. [351862-32-3] *N*-[[(2*R*)-3,4-Dihydro-2*H*-1-benzopyran-2-yl]methyl]-5-(4-fluorophenyl)-3-pyridinemethanamine; (*R*)-(−)-2-[5-(4-fluorophenyl)-3-pyridylmethylaminomethyl]chromane; (*R*)-(−)-1-*N*-[5-(4-fluorophenyl)-3-pyridylmethyl]-*N*-2-chromanylmethylamine; EMD-77697. $C_{22}H_{21}FN_2O$; mol wt 348.41. C 75.84%, H 6.08%, F 5.45%, N 8.04%, O 4.59%. Dual serotonin 5-HT$_{1A}$ receptor agonist and dopamine D$_2$ receptor antagonist. Prepn: H. Böttcher *et al.*, **EP 707007**; *eidem*, **US 5767132** (1996, 1998 both to Merck Patent GmbH). PET receptor binding study: E. A. Rabiner *et al.*, *J. Psychopharmacol.* **16**, 195 (2002). Neurochemical profile: G. D. Bartoszyk *et al.*, *J. Neural Transm.* **111**, 113 (2004). Clinical evaluation in dyskinesia in Parkinson's disease: C. W. Olanow *et al.*, *Clin. Neuropharmacol.* **27**, 58 (2004); W. Bara-Jimenez *et al.*, *Mov. Disord.* **20**, 932 (2005).

Dihydrochloride. [177976-12-4] EMD-128130. $C_{22}H_{21}FN_2 \cdot 0.2HCl$; mol wt 421.34. mp 234-235°. $[\alpha]^{20}$ $-65°$ (c = 1 in methanol).

THERAP CAT: Antidyskinetic.

8376. Sarkomycin. [11031-48-4] Sarcomycin. Antibiotic and antitumor substance produced by *Streptomyces erythrochromogenes*, strain W-115-C, from soil found at Kamakura, Japan: Umezawa *et al.*, *J. Antibiot.* **6A**, 101, 147, 153 (1953); *eidem, Antibiot. Chemother.* **4**, 514 (1954). Structure of sarkomycin A, the active principle: Hooper *et al.*, *ibid.* **5**, 585 (1955). Characterization of sarkomycins A, A' and B: Maeda, Kondo, *J. Antibiot.* **11A**, 37 (1958). Sarkomycin reacts with H_2S to form sarkomycins S_1, S_2 and S_3: Tatsuoka *et al.*, *ibid.* **9B**, 107, 110 (1956). Structure of S_1 and S_2: *eidem, ibid.* **11B**, 275 (1958). Synthesis of *d-* and *l-*sarkomycin A: Toki, *ibid.* **10A**, 35, 226 (1957). Synthesis of *dl-*sarkomycin A: Toki, *Bull. Chem. Soc. Jpn.* **30**, 450 (1957); R. K. Boeckman, Jr. *et al.*, *J. Org. Chem.* **45**, 752 (1980); J. N. Marx, G. Minaskanian, *ibid.* **47**, 3306 (1982); B. A. Wexler *et al.*, *ibid.* 3333; A. P. Kozikowski, P. D. Stein, *J. Am. Chem. Soc.* **104**, 4023 (1982). Abs config of A: Sato *et al.*, *Chem. Pharm. Bull.* **11**, 829 (1963). Revised config of A: Hill *et al.*, *J. Org. Chem.* **32**, 2330 (1967). *Review:* S. A. Waksman, H. A. Lechevalier, *The Actinomycetes* **vol. III** (Williams & Wilkins, Baltimore, 1962) pp 362-364; Sung in *Antibiotics* **vol. I**, D. Gottlieb, P. Shaw, Eds. (Springer-Verlag, New York, 1967) pp 156-165.

Sarkomycin A

Oily liquid. $[\alpha]_D^{15}$ $-32.5°$ (c = 1 in methanol). uv max (water): 230 nm. Sol in water, methanol, ethanol, butanol, ethyl acetate. Sparingly sol in petr ether.

Sarkomycin A. [489-21-4] (*R*)-2-Methylene-3-oxocyclopentanecarboxylic acid. $C_7H_8O_3$; mol wt 140.14.

8377. Sarmentose. [13484-14-5] 2,6-Dideoxy-3-*O*-methyl-*xylo-*hexose. $C_7H_{14}O_4$; mol wt 162.18. C 51.84%, H 8.70%, O 39.46%. A methyl ether of a 2-desoxyhexomethylose, isomeric with cymarose. Obtained on hydrolysis of sarmentocymarin, a glycoside isolated from seeds of *Strophanthus sarmentosus* DC., *Apocynaceae* by the enzymic method: Jacobs, Heidelberger, *J. Biol. Chem.* **81**, 765 (1929); Jacobs, Bigelow, *ibid.* **96**, 355 (1932). Synthesis: H. Hauenstein, T. Reichstein, *Helv. Chim. Acta* **33**, 446 (1950).

Prisms, plates from ether + petr ether, mp 78-79°. Shows mutarotation. $[\alpha]_D^{20}$ +12° (20 min) → +15.8° (24 hrs c = 1.08): Elderfield, *Adv. Carbohydr. Chem.* **1**, 172 (1945).

8378. Sarpagine. [482-68-8] Sarpagan-10,17-diol; raupine. $C_{19}H_{22}N_2O_2$; mol wt 310.39. C 73.52%, H 7.14%, N 9.03%, O 10.31%. Isoln from *Rauwolfia serpentina* (L.) Benth., *Apocynaceae:* Stoll, Hofmann, *Helv. Chim. Acta* **36**, 1143 (1953). Structure: Stauffacher *et al.*, *ibid.* **40**, 508 (1957); Poisson *et al.*, *Bull. Soc. Chim. Fr.* **1957**, 610; Biemann, *J. Am. Chem. Soc.* **83**, 4801

(1961). Stereochemistry: Bartlett *et al.*, *ibid.* **84**, 622 (1962); Ohashi *et al.*, *Tetrahedron* **19**, 2241 (1963).

Needles from methanol or ethanol, long plates from acetone, dec >320°. $[\alpha]_D^{20}$ +54° (c = 0.5 in pyridine). uv max (ethanol): 230, 278 nm (log ε 4.30, 3.92). One gram dissolves in 60 ml boiling ethanol, 250 ml boiling methanol, 400 ml boiling acetone. Practically insol in chloroform.

Hydrochloride. $C_{19}H_{22}N_2O_2 \cdot HCl$. Needles from alcohol, dec >220°.

8379. Sarsaparilla. Dried root of *Smilax aristolochiaefolia* Mill. (*S. medica* Cham. & Schlecht.) (Mexican Sarsap.), or *S. regelii* Killip & Morton (*S. ornata* Hook f.) (Jamaica or Central American Sarsap.), *Liliaceae*. *Habit.* Honduras, Jamaica, Mexico (Vera Cruz), Brazil, Guatemala. *Constit.* Sarsaponin, smilacin (parillin), paroaparic acid, resin, volatile oil.

USE: As flavor in beverages. Pharmaceutic aid (flavor).

8380. Sarsasapogenin. [126-19-2] (3β,5β,25S)-Spirostan-3-ol; parigenin. $C_{27}H_{44}O_3$; mol wt 416.64. C 77.83%, H 10.64%, O 11.52%. Steroid sapogenin from *Smilax ornata* Hooker, fil., *Liliaceae* (Sarsaparilla): Power, Salway, *J. Chem. Soc.* **105**, 201 (1914); Jacobs, Simpson, *J. Biol. Chem.* **105**, 501 (1934); **109**, 573 (1935). Partial structure: Hirschmann *et al.*, *J. Chem. Soc.* **20**, 572 (1955). Stereochemistry: Taylor, *Chem. Ind. (London)* **1954**, 1066; Wall, Serota, *J. Am. Chem. Soc.* **76**, 2850 (1954); Callow, Massey-Beresford, *J. Chem. Soc.* **1957**, 4482; Rosen *et al.*, *J. Am. Chem. Soc.* **81**, 1687 (1959). *Reviews:* Turner, *The Steroidal Sapogenins* Pub. no. **361**, (Univ. Microfilms, Ann Arbor, Mich., 1941) 249 pp; Shabica, *Sarsasapogenin and Related Compounds, Univ. Microfilms* (Ann Arbor, Mich.), Pub. no. **549**, 89 pp (1943); L. F. Fieser, M. Fieser, *Steroids* (Reinhold, New York, 1959) p 810. *See also* Smilagenin.

Large prismatic needles from acetone, mp 199-199.5°. $[\alpha]_D^{25}$ $-75°$, $[\alpha]_{546}^{25}$ $-89°$ (c = 0.5 in $CHCl_3$). uv spectrum: Smith, Eddy, *Anal. Chem.* **31**, 1539 (1959). Sol in alcohol, acetone, benzene, chloroform. Is precipitated by digitonin.

Acetate. $C_{29}H_{46}O_4$. Flat needles from methanol, mp 144-145°. $[\alpha]_D^{25}$ $-70.2°$; $[\alpha]_{546}^{25}$ $-83.1°$ (c = 1.18 in $CHCl_3$).

USE: In the manuf of compds of the pregnane series.

8381. Sassafras. Saxifrax; ague tree; cinnamon wood; saloop. Deciduous tree, *Sassafras albidum* (Nutt.) Nees, *Lauraceae*; also known as *S. variifolium* (Salisb.) Kuntze, and *S. officinale* Nees & Eberm. Medicinal parts are the peeled and dried root bark, root wood, and essential oil of the root wood; traditionally used as carminative, diuretic, dermatologic and antirheumatic. *Habit.* North America. *Constit.* Volatile oil (5-9%), isoquinoline alkaloids (<0.1%), lignins such as sesamin, resin, sitosterol, starch, tannins, wax. Review of pharmacology: D. Hutson, M. J. Cupp in *Toxicology and Clinical Pharmacology of Herbal Products*, M. J.

Cupp, Ed. (Humana Press, Totowa, 2000) pp 245-252; of constituents and traditional uses: J. Barnes *et al., Herbal Medicines* (Pharmaceutical Press, London, 2nd Ed., 2002) pp 414-416.

Volatile oil. [8006-80-2] Oil of sassafras. Obtained from the root. *Constit.* 80-90% safrole, eugenol, α-pinene, α- and β-phellandrene, asarone, *d*-camphor, myristicin. Yellow to reddish-yellow liquid; characteristic odor and taste of sassafras. d_{25}^{25} 1.065-1.077. α_D^{25} +2 to +4°. n_D^{20} 1.5250-1.5350. Very slightly sol in water; sol in 2 vols 90% alcohol. *Keep well closed, cool and protected from light.*

Caution: Reported to be toxic and carcinogenic due to the content of safrole, *q.v.* Potential symptoms of overexposure include vomiting, stupor, spasm followed by paralysis (Barnes).

USE: Formerly as flavoring in beverages such as root beer. Oil as scent in perfumes and soaps.

8382. Sassy Bark. Saucy bark; Mancona bark; ordeal bark; red-water tree bark; casca bark; Saxon bark; doom bark; teli; bondou. Bark of *Erythrophleum guineense* G. Don, *Leguminosae.* *Habit.* Central and Western Africa. *Constit.* Erythrophleine, tannin, resin.

8383. Satigrel. [111753-73-2] 4-Cyano-5,5-bis(4-methoxyphenyl)-4-pentenoic acid; E-5510. $C_{20}H_{19}NO_4$; mol wt 337.37. C 71.20%, H 5.68%, N 4.15%, O 18.97%. Platelet aggregation inhibitor; inhibits phosphodiesterases and cyclooxygenase-1. Prepn: Y. Yamagishi *et al.,* **EP 238973;** *eidem,* **US 4978767** (1987, 1990 both to Eisai). Pharmacology: T. Fujimori *et al., Arzneim.-Forsch.* **37,** 1143 (1987); *eidem, Cardiovasc. Drug Rev.* **9,** 264 (1991). Selectivity for cyclooxygenase and phosphodiesterase isoforms: N. Nagakura *et al., Biol. Pharm. Bull.* **19,** 828 (1996). GC-MS determn in plasma: Y. Yamano *et al., J. Chromatogr.* **528,** 199 (1990). Clinical trial to prevent transient ischemic attacks: S. Maruyama *et al., Angiology* **46,** 999 (1995).

Crystals from ethyl acetate/hexane, mp 124-125°.
THERAP CAT: Antithrombotic.

8384. Satraplatin. [129580-63-8] (*OC*-6-43)-Bis(acetato-κ*O*)amminedichloro(cyclohexanamine)-platinum; bis-acetato-ammine-dichloro-cyclohexylamine-platinum(IV); BMS-182751; BMY-45594; JM-216. $C_{10}H_{22}Cl_2N_2O_4Pt$; mol wt 500.28. C 24.01%, H 4.43%, Cl 14.17%, N 5.60%, O 12.79%, Pt 38.99%. Orally active analog of cisplatin, *q.v.* Prepn: M. J. Abrams *et al.,* **EP 328274;** *eidem,* **US 5072011** (1989, 1991 both to Johnson Matthey). Clinical pharmacokinetics: S. Vouillamoz-Lorenz *et al., Anticancer Res.* **23,** 2757 (2003). Clinical evaluation in small-cell lung cancer: E. Fokkema *et al., J. Clin. Oncol.* **17,** 3822 (1999); in hormone-refractory prostate cancer: C. N. Sternberg *et al., Oncology* **68,** 2 (2005). Review of clinical development: L. R. Kelland, *Expert Opin. Invest. Drugs* **9,** 1373-1382 (2000).

Soly (mg/ml): water ~0.3; saline 0.4; 1-octanol 0.7. Partition coefficient (octanol/water): 0.1. LD_{50} in mice (mg/kg): 30 i.p.; 330 orally (Kelland).
THERAP CAT: Antineoplastic.

8385. Satumomab. [144058-40-2] Anti-(human tumor-associated glycoprotein 72) immunoglobulin G1 (mouse monoclo-

nal B72.3 γ1-chain) disulfide with mouse monoclonal B72.3 light chain, dimer; B72.3; CYT-099. Murine monoclonal antibody that targets a high molecular weight tumor-associated glycoprotein, *TAG-72*, expressed on the surface of certain human colon, breast and ovarian carcinoma cell lines. Prepn and characterization of MAb: D. Colcher *et al., Proc. Natl. Acad. Sci. USA* **78,** 3199 (1981); J. Schlom *et al.,* **US 4612282** (1986 to USA Secy. Dept. Health Human Services). Pharmacokinetics of ^{111}In labeled MAb: B. A. Brown *et al., Cancer Res.* **47,** 1149 (1987). Clinical studies of immunoscintigraphy in colorectal cancer: B. D. Collier *et al., Radiology* **185,** 179 (1992); in ovarian cancer: E. A. Surwit *et al., Gynecol. Oncol.* **48,** 285 (1993). Review of prepn and diagnostic use: R. T. Maguire *et al., Cancer* **72,** 3453-3462 (1993). Book: *Diagnosis of Colorectal and Ovarian Carcinoma,* R. T. Maguire, D. Van Nostrand, Eds. (Marcel Dekker, Inc., New York, 1992) 237 pp.

Indium ^{111}In satumomab pendetide. [138955-27-8] ^{111}In-CYT-103; monoclonal antibody B72.3-GYK-DTPA-In-111; B72.3-glycyl-tyrosyl-*N*-ε-diethylenetriaminepentaacetic acid-In-111; OncoScint.

THERAP CAT: ^{111}In-labeled form as diagnostic aid (radioactive tumor-targeting agent).

8386. Saunders, Red. Red sandalwood; ruby wood. Heartwood of *Pterocarpus santalinus* L. f., *Leguminosae. Habit.* East Indies. *Constit.* Santalin (santalinic acid), santal pterocarpin, tannin.

USE: For coloring tinctures and similar medicinal prepns; formerly used as a dye.

8387. Savin. Young shoots of *Juniperus sabina* L., *Cupressaceae;* used in traditional medicine as emmenagogue and antirheumatic. *Habit.* Europe, Northern Asia, Northern U.S. *Constit.* 3-5% volatile oil, tannin, savinin, podophyllotoxin. Isoln and structure of *savinin:* Hartwell *et al., J. Am. Chem. Soc.* **75,** 235 (1953); Schrecker, Hartwell, ibid. **76,** 4896 (1954). *Review:* J. Gruenwald *et al., PDR for Herbal Medicines* (Medical Economics, Montvale, 3rd Ed., 2004) pp 706-707.

Volatile oil. [8024-00-8] Oil of savin. *Constit.* Chiefly sabinyl acetate, sabinene; β-myrcene, terpin-4-ol, γ-terpinene, α-pinene, limonene. Colorless or pale yellow liquid. d_{15}^{15} 0.903-0.923. α_D +40 to +60°. n_D^{20} 1.470-1.478. Very slightly sol in water; very sol in alcohol. *Keep well closed, cool and protected from light.*

Caution: Potential symptoms of overexposure include queasiness, spasm, hematuria, central paralysis, unconsciousness. External application may cause skin irritation, blistering, necrosis (Gruenwald).

THERAP CAT: In treatment of warts.

8388. Saw Palmetto. Low shrubby palm, *Serenoa repens* (Bartr.) Small, *Palmae;* also known as *Sabal serrulata* Roem. et Schult. *Habit.* Southeastern U.S. Traditionally used in Native American medicine for genitourinary conditions. Medicinal formulations are prepared from the dried fruits. *Constit.* Phytosterols, fatty acids, polysaccharides, flavonoids. Description of botany, constituents and medicinal uses: E. Bombardelli, P. Morazzoni, *Fitoterapia* **68,** 99-113 (1997). Effect of climate on growth: H. L. Gholz *et al., Can. J. Forest Res.* **29,** 1248 (1999). Review of clinical trials in treatment of urinary tract symptoms in BPH: T. J. Wilt *et al., J. Am. Med. Assoc.* **280,** 1604-1609 (1998). *Review:* A. Meadows, M. J. Cupp in *Toxicology and Clinical Pharmacology of Herbal Products,* M. J. Cupp, Ed. (Humana Press, Totowa, NJ, 2000) pp 133-139.

Lipidosterolic extract. Capistan; Libeprosta; Permixon; Sereprostat. *n*-Hexane extract of entire fruit (pulp and seed). Constituents of extract: G. Jommi *et al., Gazz. Chim. Ital.* **118,** 823 (1988). Tissue distribution in rats: G. Chevalier *et al., Eur. J. Drug Metab. Pharmacokinet.* **22,** 73 (1997). Pharmacology: F. Van Coppenolle *et al., Prostate* **43,** 49 (2000). Review of clinical trials in BPH: P. Boyle *et al., Urology* **55,** 533-539 (2000).

THERAP CAT: In treatment of micturitional disorders due to benign prostatic hypertrophy.

8389. Saxitoxin. [35554-08-6] Mussel poison; clam poison; paralytic shellfish poison; gonyaulax toxin; STX. $[C_{10}H_{17}N_7O_4]^{2+}$. Powerful neurotoxin produced by the dinoflagellates *Go-*

nyaulax catenella, or *G. tamarensis,* the consumption of which causes the California sea mussel *Mytilus californianus,* the Alaskan butterclam *Saxidomus giganteus* and the scallop to become poisonous: Sommer *et al., Arch. Pathol.* **24,** 537, 560 (1937); Schantz *et al., Can. J. Chem.* **39,** 2117 (1961); Ghazarossian *et al., Biochem. Biophys. Res. Commun.* **59,** 1219 (1974). These poisonous shellfish have been connected to instances of toxic "red-tides" where the high concentrations of algae discoloring the water were of the *Gonyaulax* genus. Isoln and partial characterization: Schantz *et al., J. Am. Chem. Soc.* **79,** 5230 (1957); Mold *et al., ibid.* 5235. Purifn and biochemical data: Schantz *et al., Biochemistry* **5,** 1191 (1966); Schantz, *Ann. N.Y. Acad. Sci.* **90,** 843 (1960). pKa values: R. S. Rogers, H. Rapoport, *J. Am. Chem. Soc.* **102,** 7335 (1980). Toxicity: G. S. Wiberg, N. R. Stephenson, *Toxicol. Appl. Pharmacol.* **2,** 607 (1960). Structural studies: Schuett, Rapoport, *J. Am. Chem. Soc.* **84,** 2266 (1962); Wong *et al., ibid.* **93,** 4633, 7344 (1971). Revised structure: Schantz *et al., ibid.* **97,** 1238 (1975); Bordner *et al., ibid.* **97,** 6008 (1975). Pharmacology including study of sodium transport inhibition: Cheymol *et al., Arch. Int. Pharmacodyn. Ther.* **174,** 393 (1968); Evans, *Br. Med. Bull.* **25,** 263 (1969). Stereospecific total synthesis of *dl*-saxitoxin: H. Tanino *et al., J. Am. Chem. Soc.* **99,** 2818 (1977); Y. Kishi, *Heterocycles* **14,** 1477 (1980). *Reviews:* Kao, *Pharmacol. Rev.* **18,** 997 (1966); Kao, *Fed. Proc.* **31,** 1117 (1972); Narahashi, *ibid.* 1124, Evans, *Int. Rev. Neurobiol.* **15,** 83 (1972); Y. Shimizu in *Progress in the Chemistry of Natural Products* **vol. 45,** W. Herz *et al.,* Eds. (Springer-Verlag, New York, 1984) pp 239-246. *See also* Brevetoxins.

Dihydrochloride. White, hygroscopic solid. pKa in water: 8.24, 11.60. $[\alpha]_D^{25}$ +130°. Very sol in water, methanol; sparingly sol in ethanol, glacial acetic acid. Practically insol in lipid solvents. Stable in acid solns; decomposes rapidly in alkaline media. Boiling 3-4 hrs at pH 3 causes loss of activity. LD$_{50}$ in mice (μg/kg): 10 i.p.; 263 orally; 3.4 i.v. (Wiberg, Stephenson).

USE: As a tool in neurochemical research.

8390. SBR Rubber. Styrene-butadiene rubber; GR-S; Government Rubber Styrene. General-purpose synthetic rubbers that were originally produced in government owned plants as GR-S. They are copolymers obtained by the polymerization of butadiene and styrene in a ratio of approx 3:1. The chains contain a random sequence of the two monomers. Very similar in composition to *Buna S, Kraton, Solprene, Stereon.* Review: P. Schneider *et al.,* in Ullmann, *Encyklopädie der technischen Chemie,* 3 Aufl., Bd. IX (München-Berlin, 1957) p 331; M. Morton, *Introduction to Rubber Technology* (Reinhold, 1959) pp 56 and 256-284; R. G. Bauer in *Kirk-Othmer Encyclopedia of Chemical Technology* vol. 8 (Wiley-Interscience, New York, 3rd ed., 1979) pp 608-625.

USE: In tires, adhesives, chewing gum.

8391. Scammony Root. Root of *Convolvulus scammonia* L., *Convolvulaceae,* yielding not less than 8% resin. *Habit.* Eastern Mediterranean region, especially Syria. *Constit.* 8-13% resin; dihydroxycinnamic acid, β-methylesculetin, ipuranol, a reducing sugar, starch.

THERAP CAT: Cathartic.

8392. Scandium. [7440-20-2] Sc; at. wt 44.955912; at. no. 21; valence 3. Group IIIb (3). Rare earth metal. Naturally occurring isotope (mass number): 45; known artificial radioactive isotopes: 40-44, 46-51. Abundance in earth's crust: 5-25 ppm. Widely dispersed in nature. Occurs in the minerals thortveitite [(Sc,Y)$_2$Si$_2$O$_7$] and in other rare earth minerals such as davidite, ytterbite, orthite and cerrite; frequently associated with tin or zirconium. Predicted and called "ekaboron" by Mendeleev. Discovered by Nilson: *Ber.* **12,** 551, 554 (1879); **13,** 1430, 1439 (1880).

Sepn from wolframite: Lukens, *J. Am. Chem. Soc.* **35,** 1470 (1913); on basis of solubility: Fischer, Bock, *Z. Anorg. Chem.* **249,** 146 (1942). Toxicity of the chloride: Haley *et al., J. Pharm. Sci.* **51,** 1043 (1962). Review of isolns including ion-exchange techniques: F. H. Spedding *et al., J. Electrochem. Soc.* **105,** 683-686 (1958). Review of prepn, properties and compds: R. C. Vickery, *The Chemistry of Yttrium and Scandium* (Pergamon Press, New York, 1960) 123 pp; *idem,* "Scandium, Yttrium and Lanthanum" in *Comprehensive Inorganic Chemistry* **vol. 3,** J. C. Bailar, Jr. *et al.,* Eds. (Pergamon Press, Oxford, 1973) pp 329-353; T. Moeller, "The Lanthanides", *ibid.* **vol. 4,** pp 1-101; F. H. Spedding in *Kirk-Othmer Encyclopedia of Chemical Technology* **vol. 19** (John Wiley & Sons, New York, 3rd ed., 1982) pp 833-854; *Chemistry of the Elements,* N. N. Greenwood, A. Earnshaw, Eds. (Pergamon Press, New York, 1984) pp 1102-1110, 1423-1449.

Metal. Reported to be dimorphic. Crystalline forms: hexagonal close-packed α-form, d 2.9890; evidence of existence of face-centered cubic β-form, d 3.19, is inconclusive. mp 1541°. bp 2836°. Heat of fusion: 14.10 kJ/mol. Heat of sublimation (25°): 377.8 kJ/mol. E°(aq) Sc^{3+}/Sc −2.08 V (calc). Salts are hydrolyzed in aq soln.

Oxide. Scandia. O$_3$Sc$_2$. Fine white powder, d 3.864. Obtained by igniting the metal or its compds. Readily sol in hot or concd acids.

Hydroxide. Sc(OH)$_3$. White gelatinous precipitate forming a hard, horny mass on exposure to air; obtained by the action of alkalies on solns of the salts; dissolves readily in dil acids.

Chloride. ScCl$_3$. White deliquescent solid. Prepd by the action of a mixture of sulfur chloride and chlorine on the heated oxide; mp 960°; crystallizes with 6 mols of water. Sol in water. Practically insol in alc. LD$_{50}$ in mice: 755 mg/kg i.p.; 4 g/kg orally (Haley).

Sulfate. Sc$_2$(SO$_4$)$_3$. Pentahydrate, d 2.519. Most sol of the sulfates of the rare earths (54.6 g/100 ml at 25°). Converted to the dihydrate on heating above 100°.

Nitrate. Sc(NO$_3$)$_3$. Crystallizes as the tetrahydrate, prismatic deliquescent crystals, readily dissolves in water or alc.

8393. Scarlet Red. [85-83-6] 1-[[2-Methyl-4-[(2-methylphenyl)azo]phenyl]azo]-2-naphthalenol; C.I. Solvent Red 24; *o*-tolylazo-*o*-tolylazo-β-naphthol; 1-(4-*o*-tolylazo-*o*-tolylazo)-2-naphthol; C.I. 26105; Biebrich Scarlet Red; Sudan IV; Fat Ponceau R. C$_{24}$H$_{20}$N$_4$O; mol wt 380.44. C 75.77%, H 5.30%, N 14.73%, O 4.21%. Prepd by diazotizing *o*-aminoazotoluene and coupling with β-naphthol: *Colour Index* **vol. 4** (3rd ed., 1971) p 4227. Review of carcinogenicity studies: *IARC Monographs* **8,** 217 (1975).

Dark brown powder. Softens at 175°; mp 181-188°; dec completely at 260°. Practically insol in water. One gram dissolves in 15 ml chloroform. Sol in oils, fats, warm petrolatum, paraffin, phenol. Slightly sol in acetone, alcohol, benzene.

USE: Fat stain.

THERAP CAT: Has been used to promote wound healing.

THERAP CAT (VET): Has been used to stimulate healing of wounds.

8394. Schiff Bases. R-CH=N-C$_6$H$_5$. Condensation products of aldehydes and ketones with primary amines. The compounds are stable if there is at least one aryl group on the nitrogen or carbon. H. Schiff, *Ann. Suppl.* **3,** 343 (1864-1865). *Reviews:* N. V. Sidgewick, *Organic Chemistry of Nitrogen* (Clarendon Press, Oxford, 3rd ed., 1966) p 164-166; R. L. Reeves, *Chemistry of the Carbonyl Group,* S. Patai, Ed. (Wiley, New York, 1966) pp 608-614; J. Fastrez, *Ind. Chim. Belge* **34,** 835 (1969); A. Bruylants, E. Feymantis-de Medicis, *Chemistry of the Carbon-Nitrogen Double Bond,* S. Patai, Ed. (Wiley, New York, 1970) pp 465-502. Metal complexes: S. Yamada, *Coord. Chem. Rev.* **1,** 415 (1966); E. Sinn, C. M. Harris, *ibid.* **4,** 391 (1969); L. F. Lindsy, *Q. Rev. Chem. Soc.* **25,** 379 (1971).

8395. Schradan. [152-16-9] Octamethyldiphosphoramide; octamethyl pyrophosphoramide; bis[bisdimethylaminophosphonous] anhydride; bis-*N,N,N',N'*-tetramethylphosphorodiamidic anhydride; OMPA; Pestox III; Sytam. $C_8H_{24}N_4O_3P_2$; mol wt 286.25. C 33.57%, H 8.45%, N 19.57%, O 16.77%, P 21.64%. Synthesis: Schrader, *BIOS Final Report* No. 1808 (1948); Gardiner, Kilby, *J. Chem. Soc.* **1950**, 1769; *Biochem. J.* **51**, 79 (1952); Hartley *et al.*, *J. Sci. Food Agric.* **2**, 303, 310 (1951); **3**, 60 (1952); Toy, Costello, US **2717249** (1955 to Victor Chem.); Toy, Walsh, *Inorg. Synth.* **7**, 73 (1963). Has been found to inhibit peripheral cholinesterase without pronounced effects on the central nervous system: DuBois *et al.*, *J. Pharmacol. Exp. Ther.* **99**, 376 (1950). Toxicity study: T. B. Gaines, *Toxicol. Appl. Pharmacol.* **14**, 515 (1969).

Viscous liquid, d_4^{25} 1.09. $bp_{0.5}$ 120-125°. $bp_{2.0}$ 154°. mp 14-20°. n_D^{25} 1.462. Vapor pressure at 25°: 1×10^{-3} mm Hg. Misc with water. Sol in most organic solvents, including ketones, nitriles, esters, aromatic hydrocarbons and alcohols. Practically insol in higher aliphatic hydrocarbons. Hydrolyzed by acids. LD_{50} in male, female rats (mg/kg): 9.1, 42 orally; 15, 44 dermally (Gaines).

USE: Insecticide.

8396. Schwartz's Reagent. [37342-97-5] Chlorobis(η^5-2,4-cyclopentadien-1-yl)hydrozirconium; Cp$_2$Zr(H)Cl; (η^5-C$_5$H$_5$)$_2$-Zr(H)Cl. $C_{10}H_{11}ClZr$; mol wt 257.87. C 46.58%, H 4.30%, Cl 13.75%, Zr 35.38%. Hydrozirconation reagent for a range of unsaturated compounds. Prepn: P. C. Wailes, H. Weigold, *J. Organomet. Chem.* **24**, 405 (1970); with high yield: S. L. Buchwald *et al.*, *Tetrahedron Lett.* **28**, 3895 (1987); *in situ* prepn: B. H. Lipshutz *et al.*, *ibid.* **31**, 7257 (1990). Stereoselectivity: E. Cesarotti *et al.*, *Inorg. Chim. Acta* **64**, L207 (1982). Use as general reducing agent: J. Schwartz, J. A. Labinger, *Angew. Chem. Int. Ed.* **15**, 333 (1976); reduction of halides in presence of triethylborane, *q.v.*: K. Fujita *et al.*, *J. Am. Chem. Soc.* **123**, 3137 (2001); in silylation of alkenes: J. Terao *et al.*, *Tetrahedron* **60**, 1301 (2004). Review of applications in phosphorous chemistry: J.-P. Majoral *et al.*, *Ber.* **129**, 879-886 (1996); of mechanism and reduction of amides: J. M. White *et al.*, *Chem. Innovation* **30**, 23-28 (2000).

White solid turning pink in light.

USE: Functionalization of unsaturated systems via an organozirconium intermediate.

8397. Schweizer's Reagent. [17500-49-1] Tetraamminecopper dihydroxide. Approximately [Cu(NH$_3$)$_4$](OH)$_2$. Usually applied in the form of an ammoniacal soln which is easily obtained by dissolving Cu(OH)$_2$ in 20% ammonia water. The soln is an intense azure color. Evaporation yields long, blue needles: Schweizer, *J. Prakt. Chem.* **72**, 109, 344 (1857).

USE: Dissolves cellulose; used in rayon production.

8398. Schwesinger P$_4$ Base. [111324-04-0] (1,1-Dimethylethyl)tris[tris(dimethylamino)phosphoranylidene]phosphorimidic triamide; *t*-Bu-P$_4$. $C_{22}H_{63}N_{13}P_4$; mol wt 633.72. C 41.70%, H 10.02%, N 28.73%, P 19.55%. Sterically hindered polyiminophosphazene base. Prepn: R. Schwesinger, H. Schlemper, *Angew. Chem. Int. Ed.* **26**, 1167 (1987); and properties: R. Schwesinger *et al.*, *Ann.* **1996**, 1055. Use as promoter for ethylene oxide polymerization: B. Esswein *et al.*, *Macromol. Symp.* **107**, 331 (1996); for copolymer formation: S. Förster, E. Krämer, *Macromolecules* **32**, 2783 (1999).

Colorless crystalline solid, mp 207°. Sublimes at 0.001 torr. Hydrophilic and lipophilic; deliquesces in moist air and hexane vapors at room temp.

USE: Promoter for polymerizations; nonnucleophilic base.

8399. Scillaren. [11003-70-6] A mixture of glycosides, scillaren A and B in the proportions in which they occur in fresh squill, *Urginea (Scilla) maritima* (L.) Baker, *Liliaceae*, about 2 parts of A to 1 part of B. Isolation of scillaren and separation of A and B: Stoll *et al.*, *Helv. Chim. Acta* **16**, 703 (1933).

Scillaren A

Granular, very bitter powder. On drying in high vacuum at 78° for 15 hrs it loses not more than 6% of its wt. $[\alpha]_D^{20}$ −25 to −35° (0.5 g in 25 ml of 75% w/w alcohol). One gram dissolves in 3000 ml water, in 5 ml abs alcohol, in 5 ml methanol. Practically insol in ether and chloroform. Aq solns are neutral to litmus.

Scillaren A. [124-99-2] (3β)-3-[(6-Deoxy-4-*O*-β-D-glucopyranosyl-α-L-mannopyranosyl)oxy]-14-hydroxybufa-4,20,22-trienolide; glucoproscillaridin A; transvaalin. $C_{36}H_{52}O_{13}$; mol wt 692.79. C 62.41%, H 7.57%, O 30.02%. Characterization and structure: Stoll *et al.*, *Z. Physiol. Chem.* **222**, 24 (1933); *Helv. Chim. Acta* **17**, 641, 1334 (1934); **18**, 82, 120, 401, 644, 1247 (1935); **24**, 1380 (1941); Zoller, Tamm, *ibid.* **36**, 1744 (1953). Pharmacology: K. K. Chen, F. G. Henderson, *J. Pharmacol. Exp. Ther.* **111**, 365 (1954); G. Vogel, E. Kluge, *Arzneim.-Forsch.* **11**, 848 (1961). Very bitter taste. Two crystal modifications from methanol: prisms, mp 184-186°; leaflets, mp 208-211°. $[\alpha]_D^{23}$ −71.9° (c = 1.011 in methanol). Tendency to form solvated crystals. Six-sided plates, tablets contg 1 mol CH$_3$OH + 1 mol H$_2$O from dil methanol, mp 230-240°. Anhydr from 85% alcohol, solvent-free: mp 270°; $[\alpha]_D^{20}$ −72 to −78° (c = 1 to 3 in 75% alcohol), $[\alpha]_D^{20}$ −73.8°. Soluble in 350 parts alcohol, in 80 parts methanol, in 40 parts dil alcohol (4 vols ethanol + 1 vol water). Practically insol in chloroform, ether. Sparingly sol in water. LD_{50} i.v. in rats: 15.5 mg/kg (Vogel, Kluge).

Scillaren B. An undefined water-sol mixture of glucosides remaining after extraction of scillaren A. Amorphous, granular powder. Very bitter taste. Scillaren B dried in a high vacuum at 78°C for 15 hrs loses not more than 5% of its weight. Completely dried scillaren B contains approx 99.5% active glycosidal substance. $[\alpha]_D^{20}$ +35 to 41° (0.5 g in 25 ml of 75% w/w ethanol). Freely sol in water. Soluble in alcohol, methanol (about 1 in 5); very slightly sol in chloroform (about 1 in 10,000). Practically insol in ether. Aq solns are neutral to litmus.

THERAP CAT: Cardiotonic.

8400. Scillarenin. [465-22-5] (3β)-3,14-Dihydroxybufa-4,20,22-trienolide. $C_{24}H_{32}O_4$; mol wt 384.51. C 74.97%, H 8.39%, O 16.64%. Prepn by adaptive enzymic decompn of proscillaridin A: Stoll *et al., Helv. Chim. Acta* **34**, 2301 (1951); from *Urginea burkei* Baker, *Liliaceae:* Zoller, Tamm, *ibid.* **36**, 1744 (1953). Structure: Stoll *et al., ibid.* **35**, 1934 (1952). Toxicity study: Chen, Henderson, *J. Pharmacol. Exp. Ther.* **111**, 365 (1954).

Prisms from methanol, mp 232-238°. $[\alpha]_D^{20}$ −16.8° (c = 0.357 in methanol); $[\alpha]_D^{20}$ +17.9° (c = 0.39 in chloroform). uv max: 300 nm (log ε 3.72). Mean LD i.v. in cats: 0.1567 mg/kg (Chen, Henderson).

3-Acetate. $C_{26}H_{34}O_5$. Crystals from methanol, dec 240-243°. $[\alpha]_D^{20}$ −23.4° (c = 1.365 in chloroform).

THERAP CAT: Cardiotonic.

8401. Scilliroside. [507-60-8] (3β,6β)-6-(Acetyloxy)-3-(β-D-glucopyranosyloxy)-8,14-dihydroxybufa-4,20,22-trienolide. $C_{32}H_{44}O_{12}$; mol wt 620.68. C 61.92%, H 7.15%, O 30.93%. Glycoside from red squill, the red variety of *Urginea maritima* (L.) Baker, *Liliaceae:* Stoll, Renz, *Helv. Chim. Acta* **25**, 43 (1942); Wichtt, Fuchs, *Arch. Pharm.* **295**, 361 (1962). Structure: Stoll *et al., Helv. Chim. Acta* **26**, 648 (1943); von Wartburg, Renz, *ibid.* **42**, 1620 (1959). Toxicity data: F. Dybing *et al., Acta Pharmacol. Toxicol.* **8**, 391 (1952).

Long prisms from dilute methanol. The crystals are solvated and lose about 8% of their wt in high vacuum, but retain ½ mol H_2O. For the hemihydrate, indistinct mp 168-170°, dec 200°. $[\alpha]_D^{20}$ −59 to −60° (methanol). Absorption max (96% ethanol): 300 nm (log ε 3.73); (98% H_2SO_4): 295, 505 nm ($E_{1cm}^{1\%}$ 260, 315). Freely sol in the lower alcohols, in ethylene glycol, dioxane, glacial acetic acid. Slightly sol in water, acetone, chloroform, ethyl acetate. Practically insol in ether, petr ether. LD_{50} in mice (mg/kg): 0.471 s.c.; 0.440 orally (Dybing).

Tetraacetyl scilliroside. $C_{40}H_{52}O_{16}$. Rosettes of long needles from methanol, mp 199°. Sol in chloroform. The four additional acetyl groups are on the sugar.

8402. Scoparin. [301-16-6] 8-β-D-Glucopyranosyl-5,7-dihydroxy-2-(4-hydroxy-3-methoxyphenyl)-4H-1-benzopyran-4-one; 8-glycosyl-4',5,7-trihydroxy-3'-methoxyflavone; scoparoside. $C_{22}H_{22}O_{11}$; mol wt 462.40. C 57.14%, H 4.80%, O 38.06%. From

leaves and branches of *Spartium scoparium* L., *Leguminosae:* Stenhouse, *Ann.* **78**, 15 (1851); Mascré, Paris, *Compt. Rend.* **204**, 1270 (1937). Structural study: Hörhammer *et al., Naturwissenschaften* **49**, 393 (1962). Revised structure: Prox, *Tetrahedron* **24**, 3697 (1968).

Needles from 80% methanol, mp 253°. uv max (methanol): 345, 270 nm (log ε 4.27, 4.18). Practically insol in cold water, ether, chloroform, benzene. Sol in hot water, ethanol, methanol, acetic acid, ethyl acetate, acetone, pyridine.

Heptaacetate. $C_{36}H_{36}O_{18}$. Crystals, mp 240-241°.

8403. Scoparius. Broom; green broom; Scotch broom; Irish broom; hogweed; bannal. Dried tops of *Cytisus scoparius* (L.) Link, *Leguminosae*. The seeds and flowers are also used, though not officially. *Habit.* Western Asia, Southern and Western Europe; cultivated in U.S.A., particularly in Oklahoma. *Constit.* Sparteine, scoparin, genisteine, sarothamnine, volatile oil, tannin, fat, wax, sugar.

THERAP CAT: Diuretic, cathartic.

8404. Scoparone. [120-08-1] 6,7-Dimethoxy-2H-1-benzopyran-2-one; 6,7-dimethoxycoumarin; esculetin dimethyl ether. $C_{11}H_{10}O_4$; mol wt 206.19. C 64.08%, H 4.89%, O 31.04%. Isolation from *Zanthoxylum* and *Artemisia* spp: Araki, Miyashita, *J. Pharm. Soc. Jpn.* **48**, 437 (1928); Sera, Shibuye, *C.A.* **24**, 5742 (1930); Parihar, Dutt, *Proc. Indian Acad. Sci.* **25A**, 153 (1947); King *et al., J. Chem. Soc.* **1954**, 1392; Singh *et al., J. Sci. Ind. Res.* **15B**, 190 (1956); Ban'kovskaya, Ban'kovskaya, *C.A.* **55**, 17776c (1961). Structure and synthesis: Singh *et al., Chem. Ind. (London)* **1954**, 1294. Improved synthesis: R. S. Mali *et al., Indian J. Chem.* **21B**, 759 (1982).

Crystals, mp 145-146°. Absorption spectra: Cingolani, *Gazz. Chim. Ital.* **89**, 985, 999 (1959).

8405. Scopola. Dried rhizome of *Scopola carniolica* Jacq., *Solanaceae. Habit.* Germany (Bavaria), Hungary, Russia. *Constit.* Scopolamine (hyoscine), atropine, hyoscyamine; total about 0.7% alkaloids.

THERAP CAT: Anticholinergic.

8406. Scopolamine. [51-34-3] (αS)-α-(Hydroxymethyl)-benzeneacetic acid (1α,2β,4β,5α,7β)-9-methyl-3-oxa-9-azatricyclo[3.3.1.0²,⁴]non-7-yl ester; 6β,7β-epoxy-1αH,5αH-tropan-3α-ol (−)-tropate; 6β,7β-epoxy-3α-tropanyl S-(−)-tropate; 6,7-epoxytropine tropate; scopine tropate; tropic acid ester with scopine; hyoscine; l-hyoscine; Scopoderm TTS; Transcop; Transderm Scop. $C_{17}H_{21}NO_4$; mol wt 303.35. C 67.31%, H 6.98%, N 4.62%, O 21.10%. Anticholinergic, tropane alkaloid isolated from *Datura metel* L., *Scopola carniolica* Jacq. and other *Solanaceae*. Constituent of impure duboisine from *Duboisia myoporoides* R. Br., pure duboisine is l-hyoscyamine, q.v. Isoln: A. Ladenburg, *Ann.* **206**, 274 (1881); E. Schmidt, *Arch. Pharm.* **230**, 207 (1892). Identity with hyoscine: O. Hesse, *Ann.* **271**, 100 (1892); *idem, J. Prakt. Chem.* **66**, 194 (1902). Absorption spectra: J. J. Dobbie, J. J.

Fox, *J. Chem. Soc.* **103,** 1194 (1913). Resolution of isomers and review of early literature: H. King, *ibid.* **1919,** 476. Extraction procedure: F. Chemnitius, *J. Prakt. Chem.* **120,** 221 (1928). Structural studies: J. Gadamer, F. Hammer, *Arch. Pharm.* **259,** 122 (1921); K. Hess, O. Wahl, *Ber.* **55,** 1979 (1922); R. Willstätter, E. Berner, *ibid.* **56,** 1079 (1923); W. Steffens, *Arch. Pharm.* **262,** 205 (1924). Configuration: G. Fodor, *Nature* **170,** 278 (1952); J. Meinwald, *J. Chem. Soc.* **1953,** 712. Review of stereochemistry: G. Fodor, *Tetrahedron* **1,** 86 (1957). Absolute configuration of tropic acid moiety: G. Fodor, G. Csepreghy, *Tetrahedron Lett.* **1959,** 16; *eidem, J. Chem. Soc.* **1961,** 3222. Synthesis of DL-form: G. Fodor *et al., Chem. Ind. (London)* **1956,** 764; P. Dobo *et al., J. Chem. Soc.* **1959,** 3461. Clinical evaluation in motion sickness: J. J. Brand, P. Whittingham, *Lancet* **2,** 232 (1970); in peripheral vertigo: T. Rahko, P. Karma, *J. Laryngol. Otol.* **99,** 653 (1985). Acute toxicity of the hydrobromide: Stockhaus, Wick, *Arch. Int. Pharmacodyn. Ther.* **180,** 155 (1969). Review of CNS effects in humans: D. J. Safer, R. P. Allen, *Biol. Psychiatry* **3,** 347-355 (1971); of use in anesthesia: L. E. Shutt, J. B. Bowles, *Anaesthesia* **34,** 476-490 (1979); of pharmacology and clinical efficacy: S. P. Clissold, R. C. Heel, *Drugs* **29,** 189-207 (1985). Comprehensive description: F. J. Muhtadi, M. M. A. Hassan, *Anal. Profiles Drug Subs.* **19,** 477-551 (1990).

Viscous liquid. pKa 7.55-7.81. $[\alpha]_D^{20}$ $-28°$ (c = 2.7). Sol in 9.5 parts water at 15°. Forms a cryst monohydrate, mp 59°. Freely sol in hot water, in alcohol, ether, chloroform, acetone. Sparingly sol in benzene, petr ether. Easily hydrolyzed by acids or alkalies. Dec on standing.

Hydrobromide trihydrate. [114-49-8] Scopolammonium bromide. $C_{17}H_{21}NO_4 \cdot HBr \cdot 3H_2O$; mol wt 438.31. Orthorhombic sphenoidal crystals from water, slightly efflorescent in dry air. mp 195° (after drying at 105° for 3 hours). $[\alpha]_D^{25}$ -24 to $-26°$ (c = 5, calculated on anhydrous basis). uv max (methanol) 246, 252, 258, 264 nm ($A_{1cm}^{1\%}$ 3.5, 4.0, 4.5, 3.0). pH of 0.05M soln 5.85. One gram dissolves in 1.5 ml water, 20 ml alcohol. Slightly sol in chloroform. Practically insol in ether. LD_{50} in rats (mg/kg): 3800 s.c. (Stockhaus, Wick).

Hydrochloride. [55-16-3] $C_{17}H_{21}NO_4 \cdot HCl$. Crystals from acetone, mp 200°. Dihydrate, prisms from water, melts in water of crystn at 80°. Very sol in water and alcohol. pH of 0.05M soln 5.85.

Methyl bromide *see* Methscopolamine Bromide.

Methyl nitrate. [6106-46-3] Methscopolamine nitrate. $C_{17}H_{21}NO_4 \cdot CH_3NO_3$; mol wt 380.39. Crystals. Freely sol in water, dil alcohol; slightly sol in abs alcohol.

DL-Form. Atroscine. Dihydrate, chisel-shaped prisms from ethanol + water, mp 38-40°. Monohydrate, efflorescent crystals, mp 55-57°. Anhydrous, long prisms, mp 82-83°. Very slightly sol in water; sol in alc, chloroform, ether, oils.

THERAP CAT: In treatment of motion sickness; antiemetic; antispasmodic; mydriatic; preanesthetic medicant.

THERAP CAT (VET): Preanesthetic medicant.

8407. Scopolamine *N*-Oxide. [97-75-6] (αS)-α-(Hydroxymethyl)benzeneacetic acid $(1\alpha,2\beta,4\beta,5\alpha,7\beta)$-9-methyl-9-oxido-3-oxa-9-azatricyclo[3.3.1.0^{2,4}]non-7-yl ester *N*-oxide; 6β,7β-epoxy-1αH,5αH-tropan-3α-ol (−)-tropate 8-oxide; scopolamine aminoxide. $C_{17}H_{21}NO_5$; mol wt 319.35. C 63.94%, H 6.63%, N 4.39%, O 25.05%. Anticholinergic. Prepn: Polonovski, Polonovski, *Compt. Rend.* **180,** 1755 (1925). Absolute configuration: Huber *et al., Can. J. Chem.* **49,** 3258 (1971).

White powder, mp ~80°. $[\alpha]_D^{20}$ $-14°$ in water.

Hydrobromide. [6106-81-6] Genoscopolamine. $C_{17}H_{22}BrNO_5$; mol wt 400.26. Prisms from water, mp 135-138°. $[\alpha]_D^{25}$ $-25°$ (c = 2). Soly in water about 10 g/100 ml. Slightly sol in alcohol, acetone. pH of 3% aq soln about 3.2.

THERAP CAT: Antiparkinsonian.

8408. Scopoletin. [92-61-5] 7-Hydroxy-6-methoxy-2*H*-1-benzopyran-2-one; 7-hydroxy-6-methoxycoumarin; 6-methoxy-umbelliferone; β-methylesculetin; chrysatropic acid; gelseminic acid. $C_{10}H_8O_4$; mol wt 192.17. C 62.50%, H 4.20%, O 33.30%. The aglucone of scopolin. Occurs in root of *Scopolia japonica* Maxim., *Scopolia carniolica* Jacq., *Atropa belladonna* L., *Solanaceae, Convolvulus scammonia* L., *Convolvulaceae.* Isoln: Eykman, *Ber.* **17 III,** 442 (1884). Synthesis: Crosby, *J. Org. Chem.* **26,** 1215 (1961); Desai, Desai, *J. Indian Chem. Soc.* **40,** 456 (1963).

Needles or prisms from chloroform or acetic acid, mp 204°. uv max: 230, 254, 260, 298, 346 nm (log ε 4.11, 3.68, 3.63, 3.68, 4.07), Ballantyne *et al., Tetrahedron* **27,** 871 (1971). Slightly sol in water or cold alcohol; sol in hot alcohol or hot glacial acetic acid; moderately sol in chloroform. Practically insol in benzene. Its alcoholic soln has a blue fluorescence. Reduces Fehling's soln.

8409. Scopolin. [531-44-2] 7-(β-D-Glucopyranosyloxy)-6-methoxy-2*H*-1-benzopyran-2-one. $C_{16}H_{18}O_9$; mol wt 354.31. C 54.24%, H 5.12%, O 40.64%. Mono-β-glucopyranoside of scopoletin. From root of *Scopolia japonica* Maxim., *S. carniolica* Jacq., *Solanaceae* and *Nerium odorum* Sol., *Apocynaceae.* Isoln: Eykman, *Ber.* **17 III,** 442 (1884); Ritter *et al., Helv. Chim. Acta* **36,** 434 (1953). Synthesis: Merz, *Arch. Pharm.* **270,** 476 (1932). Possible identity with **murrayin:** Bose, Mookerjee, *J. Indian Chem. Soc.* **14,** 489 (1937). Chromatography, and spectrum of murrayin: Chakraborty, Bose, *ibid.* **33,** 905 (1956); Chakraborty, Chakrabarty, *Trans. Bose Res. Inst. (Calcutta)* **24** (1), 15 (1961), *C.A.* **55,** 24228c (1961). Needles. mp 218°. Soluble in water, alcohol. Practically insol in chloroform, ether.

Tetraacetate. $C_{24}H_{26}O_{13}$. Polymorphous crystals, prisms, mp 166° or flat plates, mp 184-185°.

8410. Scopoline. [487-27-4] Hexahydro-4-methyl-2,5-methano-2*H*-furo[3,2-*b*]pyrrol-6-ol; 3β,7β-epoxy-1βH,5βH-tropan-6α-ol; 3α,6α-epoxy-7β-hydroxytropane; Oscine. $C_8H_{13}NO_2$; mol wt 155.19. C 61.91%, H 8.44%, N 9.03%, O 20.62%. Decomposition product of scopolamine: Fodor, Kovács, *J. Chem. Soc.* **1953,** 2341. Prepn from teloidine: Zeile, Heusner, *Ber.* **90,** 2800, 2809 (1957); DE 1056617; DE 1062703 (1959 to Boehringer, Ing.). Structure: Fodor *et al., J. Chem. Soc.* **1955,** 3504. Stereochemistry: Fodor, *Tetrahedron* **1,** 86 (1957).

Crystals from petr ether, mp 107-109°. bp 248°. Sol in water, alcohol, acetone, ether.

Hydrochloride. $C_8H_{13}NO_2.HCl$. Crystals from ethanol, mp 255-257°.

Acetate. $C_{10}H_{15}NO_3$. Crystals from petr ether, mp 56-57°.

8411. Scotophobin. [33579-45-2] L-Seryl-L-aspartyl-L-asparaginyl-L-asparaginyl-L-glutaminyl-L-glutaminylglycyl-L-lysyl-L-seryl-L-alanyl-L-glutaminyl-L-glutaminylglycylglycyl-L-tyrosinamide. $C_{62}H_{97}N_{23}O_{26}$; mol wt 1580.57. C 47.11%, H 6.19%, N 20.38%, O 26.32%. Pentadecapeptide, isolated from the brains of rats with acquired fear of the dark, which induces dark avoidance in untrained mice. (From the Greek *skotos*, dark and *phobos*, fear.) Thought to be the first isolation, identification and synthesis of one of the "chemical code words" that control memory and learning. See Ungar *et al.*, *Nature* **238**, 198 (1972). Original training, testing and extraction procedures: Ungar *et al.*, *ibid.* **217**, 1259 (1968); *eidem*, *Proc. West. Pharmacol. Soc.* **13**, 149 (1970). Structural elucidation: Desiderio *et al.*, *Chem. Commun.* **1971**, 432. Synthesis of preliminary structures: Ali *et al.*, *Experientia* **27**, 1138 (1971); *eidem*, *Int. J. Pept. Protein Res.* **4**, 395 (1972). Solid phase synthesis of revised structure: Parr, Holzer, *Z. Physiol. Chem.* **352**, 1043 (1971); *eidem*, *Experientia* **28**, 884 (1972). Passive transfer of dark avoidance to mice: Malin, Guttman, *Science* **178**, 1219 (1972); to goldfish: Guttman *et al.*, *Nature New Biol.* **235**, 126 (1972); Bryant *et al.*, *Science* **177**, 635 (1972). Chemistry and critical analysis of published data on scotophobin: Stewart, *Nature* **238**, 202-210 (1972).

Ser–Asp–Asn–Asn–Gln–Gln–Gly–Lys–Ser–Ala–Gln–Gln–Gly–Gly–TyrNH₂

8412. Scutellarein. [529-53-3] 5,6,7-Trihydroxy-2-(4-hydroxyphenyl)-4*H*-1-benzopyran-4-one; 4′,5,6,7-tetrahydroxyflavone; 6-hydroxypelargidenon 1465. $C_{15}H_{10}O_6$; mol wt 286.24. C 62.94%, H 3.52%, O 33.54%. By hydrolysis of scutellarin: Molisck, Goldschmidt, *Monatsh. Chem.* **22**, 679 (1901); Marsh, *Biochem. J.* **59**, 58 (1955). From *Digitalis lanata* Ehrh., *Scrophulariaceae*: Rangaswami, Rao, *Proc. Indian Acad. Sci.* **54A**, 51 (1961), *C.A.* **56**, 10076f (1962). Structure: Wessely, Moser, *Monatsh. Chem.* **56**, 97 (1930). Synthesis: Sastri, Seshadri, *Proc. Indian Acad. Sci.* **23A**, 262 (1946), *C.A.* **41**, 449a (1947); Zemplén *et al.*, *Acta Chim. Acad. Sci. Hung.* **16**, 445 (1958); Jouanne, Mentzer, *C.R. Seances Acad. Sci. Ser. C* **263**, 1022 (1966).

Yellow leaflets from methanol, does not melt below 300°. uv max (ethanol): 286, 339 nm (ε 16600; 18300).

Tetraacetate. $C_{23}H_{18}O_{10}$. Prisms from ethyl acetate, mp 235-237°.

Glucuronide. $C_{21}H_{18}O_{12}$. From leaves of *Scutellaria altissima* Linn., *Labiatae*: Goldschmiedt, Zerner, *Monatsh. Chem.* **31**, 439 (1910); from *Centaurea scabiosa* L., *Compositae*: Charaux, Rabaté, *J. Pharm. Chim.* **9**, 155 (1940); from *Scutellaria* spp.: Marsh, *Biochem. J.* **59**, 58 (1955); *Nature* **183**, 1824 (1959). Synthesis: Farkas *et al.*, *Ber.* **107**, 3878 (1974). Needles from alc, darkens above 230°, does not melt below 300°. $[\alpha]_D^{18}$ −14° (water); $[\alpha]_D^{20}$ −139° (pyridine). uv max (ethanol): 285, 335 nm (ε 20000; 26100). Practically insol in water. Sol in alkali hydroxides, glacial acetic acid; slightly sol in organic solvents.

8413. Scutellaria. Skullcap; helmet flower. Dried overground portion of *Scutellaria lateriflora* L., *Labiatae*. *Habit.* North America. *Constit.* Scutellarin, volatile oil, tannin.

8414. Seaborgium. [54038-81-2] Element 106; unnilhexium. Sg, Unh; at. no. 106. Group VIB (6). No stable nuclides. Prepn of isotope 263106 (α-emitter; $T_{1/2}$ 0.9 ±0.2 sec; longest-lived known isotope; rel. at. mass 263.1186) by 249Cf (18O,4n): A. Ghiorso *et al.*, *Phys. Rev. Lett.* **33**, 1490 (1974). Four known

isotopes: 259-261, 263. Confirmation of discovery: K. E. Gregorich *et al.*, *ibid.* **72**, 1423 (1994). Review of history, prepn and properties: R. J. Silva in *The Chemistry of the Actinide Elements* vol. **2**, J. J. Katz *et al.*, Eds. (Chapman and Hall, New York, 1986) pp 1108-1110; P. Armbruster, *Proc. Int. Sch. Phys. "Enrico Fermi"* 222-240 (1986); G. N. Flerov, G. M. Ter-Akopian, *Prog. Particle Nucl. Phys.* **19**, 197-239 (1987); G. T. Seaborg, W. D. Loveland, *The Elements Beyond Uranium* (John Wiley & Sons, Inc., New York, 1990) p 54-56; Transfermium Working Group, *Pure Appl. Chem.* **65**, 1757-1814 (1993).

8415. Sebacic Acid. [111-20-6] Decanedioic acid; 1,8-octanedicarboxylic acid. $C_{10}H_{18}O_4$; mol wt 202.25. C 59.39%, H 8.97%, O 31.64%. $HOOC(CH_2)_8COOH$. Obtained on a large scale by heating castor oil or ricinoleic acid with sodium hydroxide. Convenient lab procedures: Topchiev, Pavlov, *C.A.* **47**, 8002h (1953); Dominguez *et al.*, *J. Chem. Educ.* **29**, 446 (1952). Also prepd by ozonization of undecylenic acid: Noorduyn, *Rec. Trav. Chim.* **38**, 326 (1919); Verkade *et al.*, *ibid.* 385. Toxicity study: P. M. Jenner *et al.*, *Food Cosmet. Toxicol.* **2**, 327 (1964). Review and bibliography: Jones, *Chimia* **5**, 169-173 (1951).

Monoclinic prismatic tablets, leaflets from acetone + petr ether (commercial product is a white, free-flowing powder having a mild fatty acid odor). d_4^{20} 1.207. mp 134.5°. bp_{100} 294.5°; bp_{50} 273°; bp_{15} 243.5°; bp_{10} 232°. Sp heat (solid) 0.48 cal/g; sp heat (liq) 0.53 cal/g. Sublimes slowly at 750 mm when heated to mp. n_D^{134} 1.422. $pK_1 = 4.59$; $pK_2 = 5.59$. Aq solns are neutral to methyl orange. Soly in water: 0.004% at 0°; 0.10% at 20°; 0.42% at 65°; 2.0% at 100°. Freely sol in alcohols, esters, ketones. Soly in ether: 0.1% at 17°. Sparingly sol in hydrocarbons and chlorinated hydrocarbons.

Ethyl ester. Ethyl sebacate; diethyl sebacate. $C_{14}H_{26}O_4$. Colorless to yellowish fluid. d_4^{20} 0.965. bp ~307° with some decompn. n_D^{20} 1.4369. Sol in about 700 parts cold, 50 parts boiling water; misc with alc, ether and other organic solvents. LD_{50} orally in rats: 14470 mg/kg (Jenner).

USE: Raw material in the manuf of synthetic resins of the alkyd or polyester type, non-migrating plasticizers, polyester rubbers, synthetic fibers of the polyamide type.

8416. Sebacil. [96-01-5] 1,2-Cyclodecanedione. $C_{10}H_{16}O_2$; mol wt 168.23. C 71.39%, H 9.59%, O 19.02%. Prepd by oxidation of sebacoin with chromium trioxide in acetic acid: Blomquist *et al.*, *J. Am. Chem. Soc.* **74**, 3640 (1952); *cf.* Prelog *et al.*, *Helv. Chim. Acta* **35**, 1610 (1952); Blomquist, Goldstein, *Org. Synth.* **coll. vol. IV**, 838 (1963).

Crystals, mp 40-41°. bp_{18} 120-125°; bp_{10} 104-105°.

8417. Sebacoin. [96-00-4] 2-Hydroxycyclodecanone; 1-cyclodecanol-2-one. $C_{10}H_{18}O_2$; mol wt 170.25. C 70.55%, H 10.66%, O 18.80%. Prepd by cyclization of methyl or ethyl sebacate with sodium metal: Hansley, US 2228268 (1941 to du Pont); Prelog *et al.*, *Helv. Chim. Acta* **35**, 1598 (1952); Allinger, *Org. Synth.* **coll. vol. IV**, 840 (1963).

Prisms from ether + petr ether, mp 42°. bp_6 113-114°; $bp_{0.1}$ 77°.

8418. Secalonic Acids. $C_{32}H_{30}O_{14}$; mol wt 638.57. C 60.19%, H 4.74%, O 35.08%. Toxic mold metabolites which are diastereoisomeric dimeric hydroxanthone derivatives manifest as yellow pigments. First isolation studies: Stoll *et al.*, *Helv. Chim. Acta* **35**, 2022 (1952). Seven isomers have been isolated: *secalonic acid A*, *secalonic acid B*, and *secalonic acid C* from ergot: Aberhart *et al.*, *Tetrahedron* **21**, 1417 (1965); Franck *et al.*, *Ber.* **99**,

3842, 3875 (1966); *secalonic acid D* from *Penicillium oxalicum:* Steyn, *Tetrahedron* **26**, 51 (1970); *secalonic acid E* from *Phoma terrestris:* Hansen, Howard *et al., Chem. Commun.* **1973**, 464; *secalonic acid F* from *Aspergillus aculeatus:* R. Andersen *et al., J. Org. Chem.* **42**, 352 (1977); *secalonic acid G* from *Pyrenochaeta terrestris:* I. Kurobane, C. E. Vining, *Tetrahedron Lett.* **1978**, 4633. Secalonic acid A is enantiomeric with D; secalonic acid B is enantiomeric with E. Chromatographic separation of the ergot pigments: Franck, *Angew. Chem. Int. Ed.* **8**, 251 (1969); structures: ApSimon *et al., J. Chem. Soc.* **1965**, 4144. Revised structures of secalonic acids A, B, C, D: Hooper *et al., Chem. Commun.* **1971**, 111; *eidem, J. Chem. Soc. C* **1971**, 3580. Crystal and molecular structure of secalonic acid A: C. C. Howard *et al., J. Chem. Soc. Perkin Trans. 1* **1976**, 1820. Identity of secalonic acid A with **entothein:** Yoshioka *et al., Chem. Pharm. Bull.* **16**, 2090 (1968). Biosynthesis of secalonic acid A: I. Kurobane *et al., Tetrahedron Lett.* **1978**, 1379. Review of secalonic acids and other ergochromes: Franck, Flasch in *Fortschr. Chem. Org. Naturst.* **30**, 151-206 (1973).

Secalonic acid A

Secalonic acid A. [35287-72-0] (3*R*,3'*R*,4*S*,4'*S*,4a*S*,4'a*S*)-2,2',-3,3',4,4',9,9'-Octahydro-1,1',4,4',8,8'-hexahydroxy-3,3'-dimethyl-9,9'-dioxo-[7,7'-bi-4a*H*-xanthene]-4a,4'a-dicarboxylic acid dimethyl ester; 6,6',7,7'-tetrahydro-1,1',5β,5'β,8,8'-hexahydroxy-6α,6'α-dimethyl-9,9'-dioxo-[2,2'-bixanthene]-10aβ,10'aβ(5*H*,5'*H*)-dicarboxylic acid dimethyl ester; ergochrome AA(2,2'). Fine lemon-yellow needles from dioxane + petr ether + chloroform, mp 246-248° (dec); also reported as mp 260° (Yoshioka *et al., loc. cit.*). [α]$_D$ −73° (CHCl$_3$). uv max (methanol): 247, 340 nm (ε 18140, 31200). pK$_{DMF}$ 8.7. Readily soluble in pyridine, dimethylformamide, dioxane; moderately sol in chloroform, methylene chloride, acetone. Gives a wine-red color reaction with 5% FeCl$_3$ in methanol.

8419. Secnidazole. [3366-95-8] α,2-Dimethyl-5-nitro-1*H*-imidazole-1-ethanol; 1-(2-hydroxypropyl)-2-methyl-5-nitroimidazole; 1-(2-methyl-5-nitroimidazol-1-yl)-2-propanol; PM-185184; RP-14539; Flagentyl. C$_7$H$_{11}$N$_3$O$_3$; mol wt 185.18. C 45.40%, H 5.99%, N 22.69%, O 25.92%. Analog of metronidazole, *q.v.* Prepn: **FR M3270** (1965 to Rhône-Poulenc), *C.A.* **63**, 11571d (1965); C. Cosar *et al., Arzneim.-Forsch.* **16**, 23 (1966). Antiamebic and trichomonacidal activities: F. Benazet, L. Guillaume, *Bull. Soc. Pathol. Exot. Ses Fil.* **69**, 309 (1976), *C.A.* **90**, 145922v (1979). Serum half-life: J. Symonds, *J. Antimicrob. Chemother.* **5**, 484 (1979). Therapeutic use: D. Videau *et al., Br. J. Vener. Dis.* **54**, 77 (1978).

Cryst from toluene, mp 76° (Cosar).
THERAP CAT: Antiamebic. Antiprotozoal (Trichomonas).

8420. Secobarbital Sodium. [309-43-3] 5-(1-Methylbutyl)-5-(2-propenyl)-2,4,6(1*H*,3*H*,5*H*)-pyrimidinetrione monosodium salt; sodium 5-allyl-5-(1-methylbutyl)barbiturate; 5-allyl-5-(1-methylbutyl)barbituric acid sodium salt; 5-allyl-5-(1-methylbutyl)-malonylurea sodium salt; meballymal sodium; quinalbarbitone sodium; Barbosec; Immenoctal; Pramil; Quinalspan; Sedutain; Seconal Sodium; Seotalnatrium. C$_{12}$H$_{17}$N$_2$NaO$_3$; mol wt 260.26. C

55.38%, H 6.58%, N 10.76%, Na 8.83%, O 18.44%. Prepn: **US 1954429** (1934). Comprehensive description: I. Comer, *Anal. Profiles Drug Subs.* **1**, 343-365 (1972). Toxicity data: E. W. Schafer, *Toxicol. Appl. Pharmacol.* **21**, 315 (1972).

White, hygroscopic powder. Bitter taste. Very sol in water. Sol in alc. Practically insol in ether. Aq solns are alkaline to litmus. The soly in elixirs is increased by the presence of methenamine. LD$_{50}$ orally in rats: 125 mg/kg (Schafer).
Free acid. C$_{12}$H$_{18}$N$_2$O$_3$. mp 100°.
Note: This is a controlled substance (depressant): **21 CFR**, 1308.12 and 1308.13.
THERAP CAT: Sedative; hypnotic.
THERAP CAT (VET): Short-acting hypnotic; sedative. Pre-anesthetic.

8421. Secretin. [1393-25-5] A strongly basic polypeptide gastrointestinal hormone, produced primarily in the duodenum and jejunum. Released in response to gastric acid delivered into the duodenal lumen; stimulates exocrine pancreatic secretion of water and bicarbonate and inhibits gastric acid secretion and emptying. Discovered by W. M. Bayliss and E. H. Starling, *Ergeb. Physiol.* **5**, 664 (1905). Isoln of porcine secretin: J. E. Jorpes, *Acta Chem. Scand.* **15**, 1790 (1961). Structure: J. E. Jorpes *et al., Biochem. Biophys. Res. Commun.* **9**, 275 (1962); V. Mutt *et al., Biochemistry* **4**, 2358 (1965). Synthesis: M. Bodanszky *et al., J. Am. Chem. Soc.* **89**, 685, 6753 (1967); M. A. Ondetti *et al., ibid.* **90**, 4711 (1968). Solid phase synthesis: B. Hemmasi, E. Bayer, *Int. J. Pept. Protein Res.* **9**, 63 (1977); D. H. Coy *et al., Peptides* **3**, 137 (1982). Isoln of bovine secretin and amino acid sequence (identical to porcine): M. Carlquist *et al., FEBS Lett.* **127**, 71 (1981); of human secretin: *idem et al., IRCS Med. Sci.* **13**, 217 (1985). Comparison of natural porcine secretin with synthetic porcine and human forms in pancreatic function testing: L. Somogyi *et al., Pancreas* **27**, 230 (2003). Review of radioimmunoassay methods: T. M. Chang, W. Y. Chey, *Dig. Dis. Sci.* **25**, 529-552 (1980). General reviews: W. H. Häcki, *Clin. Gastroenterol.* **9**, 609-632 (1980); W. Y. Chey, T.-M. Chang, *J. Gastroenterol.* **38**, 1025-1035 (2003).

$$\overset{1}{\text{His}}-\text{Ser}-\text{Asp}-\text{Gly}-\text{Thr}-\text{Phe}-\text{Thr}-\text{Ser}-\text{Glu}-\text{Leu}-\text{Ser}-\text{Arg}-\text{Leu}-\text{Arg}$$
$$\overset{27}{\text{Val}}-\text{Leu}-\text{Gly}-\text{Gln}-\text{Leu}-\text{Leu}-\text{Arg}-\text{Gln}-\text{Leu}-\text{Arg}-\text{Ala}-\text{Ser}-\text{Asp}$$

Porcine Secretin

Porcine secretin. [17034-35-4] Secretin (swine); secretin (pig). C$_{130}$H$_{220}$N$_{44}$O$_{41}$; mol wt 3055.41.
Porcine secretin acetate salt. [17034-34-3] RG-1068; Secreflo. Synthetic porcine secretin; amino acid sequence identical to natural form. Efficacy in pancreatic function testing: L. Somogyi *et al., Pancreas* **21**, 262 (2000); in diagnosis of Zollinger-Ellison syndrome: D. C. Metz *et al., Aliment. Pharmacol. Ther.* **15**, 669 (2001). Use in pancreatic duct cannulation: B. M. Devereaux *et al., Am. J. Gastroenterol.* **97**, 2279 (2002).
Human secretin. [108153-74-8] 15-L-Glutamic acid-16-glycine-secretin (pig). C$_{130}$H$_{220}$N$_{44}$O$_{40}$; mol wt 3039.41.
THERAP CAT: Diagnostic aid (pancreatic function).

8422. Securinine. [5610-40-2] Securinan-11-one. C$_{13}$H$_{15}$-NO$_2$; mol wt 217.26. C 71.87%, H 6.96%, N 6.45%, O 14.73%. From leaves and roots of *Securinega suffruticosa* Rehder, *Euphorbiaceae* found in the Ussuri region: Murav'eva, Ban'kovskii, *C.A.* **50**, 17335c (1956); *eidem, Dokl. Akad. Nauk SSSR* **110**, 998 (1956), *C.A.* **51**, 8121a (1957). Improved extraction process: Kogan *et al., GB 1169471* (1959 to All-Union Sci. Res. Inst. of Medicinal Plants), *C.A.* **72**, 47349x (1970) corresp to **US 3538103** (1970). Structure: Satoda *et al., Tetrahedron Lett.* **1962**, 1199; Mukherjee *et al., Na-*

turwissenschaften **50**, 155 (1963); Saito *et al., Tetrahedron* **19**, 2085 (1963). Stereochemistry: Nakano *et al., Chem. Ind. (London)* **1963**, 1034; Parello *et al., Bull. Soc. Chim. Fr.* **1963**, 898; Nakano *et al., J. Org. Chem.* **28**, 2619 (1963); Horii *et al., Tetrahedron* **19**, 2101 (1963); Imado *et al., Chem. Ind. (London)* **1964**, 1691. Synthesis of the racemate: Saito *et al., Chem. Pharm. Bull.* **14**, 313, 1059 (1966); Horii *et al., Tetrahedron* **23**, 1165 (1967). Toxicology study: S. L. Friess *et al., Toxicol. Appl. Pharmacol.* **3**, 347 (1961).

Yellow crystals from alcohol, mp 142-143°. $[\alpha]_D^{20}$ −1042° (c = 1 in alc). uv max (alc): 256, 330 nm (log ε 4.27, 3.30).

Hydrochloride. mp 230°. $[\alpha]_D^{20}$ −259.2° (alcohol).

Nitrate. mp 205°. $[\alpha]_D^{20}$ −312.12° (alcohol). LD$_{50}$ i.v. in mice: 3.5 ± 0.9 mg/kg (Friess).

8423. Seidlitz Mixture. [8014-63-9] Mixture of 3 parts Rochelle salt and 1 part sodium bicarbonate. Ten grams of the mixture are employed with 2.17 g tartaric acid for one Seidlitz powder.

THERAP CAT: Cathartic.

8424. Selamectin. [220119-17-5] (5Z)-25-Cyclohexyl-4′-O-de(2,6-dideoxy-3-O-methyl-α-L-*arabino*-hexopyranosyl)-5-demethoxy-25-de(1-methylpropyl)-22,23-dihydro-5-(hydroxyimino)-avermectin A$_{1a}$; 5-oxoimino-25-cyclohexyl avermectin B$_1$ monosaccharide; Revolution. C$_{43}$H$_{63}$NO$_{11}$; mol wt 769.96. C 67.08%, H 8.25%, N 1.82%, O 22.86%. Antiparasitic semisynthetic avermectin, *q.v.* Prepn: B. F. Bishop *et al.,* **WO 9415944**; *eidem,* **US 5981500** (1994, 1999 both to Pfizer).

Waterfast, no unpleasant odor.

THERAP CAT (VET): Anthelmintic; ectoparasiticide.

8425. Selectfluor®. [140681-55-6] 1-(Chloromethyl)-4-fluoro-1,4-diazoniabicyclo[2.2.2]octane bis[tetrafluoroborate(1−)]; F-TEDA-BF$_4$. C$_7$H$_{14}$B$_2$ClF$_9$N$_2$; mol wt 354.26. C 23.73%, H 3.98%, B 6.10%, Cl 10.01%, F 48.27%, N 7.91%. Electrophilic N—F fluorinating agent. Prepn: R. E. Banks, **US 5086178** (1992 to Air Prods. Chem.); *idem et al., J. Chem. Soc. Chem. Commun.* **1992**, 595; and applications as an electrophilic fluorinating agent: *idem et al., J. Chem. Soc. Perkin Trans. 1* **1996**, 2069. X-ray crystal structure: *idem et al., Acta Crystallogr.* **C49**, 492 (1993). Review of properties and applications in organic synthesis: R. E. Banks, *J. Fluorine Chem.* **87**, 1-17 (1998); of commercial development: J. J. Hart, R. G. Syvret, *ibid.* **100**, 157-161 (1999); of applications and mechanism of fluorination: P. T. Nyffeler *et al., Angew. Chem. Int. Ed.* **44**, 192-212 (2005).

White, free-flowing, non-hygroscopic crystalline solid, mp 225° (dec). Soly (g/l): water 176 (20°); acetonitrile 50. Slightly sol in lower alcohols, acetone. LD$_{50}$ in male rats: 640 mg/kg orally; >2 g/kg dermally (Banks, 1998).

Caution: Exothermic decompn can occur at temp >80° (Banks, 1996).

USE: Mild, versatile fluorinating reagent used in pharmaceutical and agricultural applications.

8426. Selectins. Family of calcium-dependent cell adhesion molecules (CAMs) that initiate leukocyte adhesion to activated platelets or vascular endothelium in reponse to tissue injury or infection. Involved in lymphocyte homing to lymph nodes and in the extravasation of neutrophils into inflamed tissues. Binds to specific carbohydrate ligands on the surface of target cells. Three types have been identified and are designated according to the cell type from which they were originally discovered: L-selectin, from lymphocytes; E-selectin, from endothelial cells; and P-selectin, from platelets. Structures consist of an amino terminal lectin domain, an epidermal growth factor type repeat, and a discreet number of short consensus repeats similar to those found in complement-regulatory proteins (CR domains). The term "selectin" was proposed to highlight the presence of the lectin domain and to emphasize their selective expression and function. *Reviews:* D. Vestweber, *Semin. Cell Biol.* **3**, 211-220 (1992); M. P. Bevilacqua, R. M. Nelson, *J. Clin. Invest.* **91**, 379-387 (1993); R. P. McEver, *Curr. Opin. Immunol.* **6**, 75-84 (1994). Review of role in inflammation: M. A. Jutila, *Adv. Pharmacol.* **25**, 235-262 (1994); as potential therapeutic targets: J. K. Welply *et al., Biochim. Biophys. Acta* **1197**, 215-226 (1994). Review of selectin ligands: A. Varki, *Proc. Natl. Acad. Sci. USA* **91**, 7390-7397 (1994).

L-Selectin. Lymphocyte adhesion molecule-1; LAM-1; leukocyte-endothelial cell adhesion molecule-1; LECAM-1; leu-8. Constitutively expressed on the surface of almost all leukocytes; rapidly shed upon cell activation. Binds to activated endothelial cells and to the high endothelial venule of lymph nodes. Human form contains 2 CR domains. Originally described as a lymphocyte homing receptor: W. M. Gallatin *et al., Nature* **304**, 30 (1983).

E-Selectin. Endothelial-leukocyte adhesion molecule-1; ELAM-1. Expressed by endothelial cells following stimulation by endotoxin or inflammatory cytokines such as IL-1 or TNF. Binds to neutrophils, monocytes, eosinophils, certain lymphocytes and some tumor cells. Human form contains 6 CR domains. Identification: M. P. Bevilacqua *et al., Proc. Natl. Acad. Sci. USA* **84**, 9238 (1987). Crystal structure of lectin domain: W. I. Weis, *Structure* **2**, 147 (1994).

P-Selectin. α-Granule membrane protein 140; GMP-140; platelet activation-dependent granule-external membrane protein; PADGEM. Synthesized constitutively by endothelial cells and platelets; stored in platelet α-granules or in Weibel-Palade bodies of endothelial cells. Rapidly mobilized to the cell surface following activation by histamine or thrombin. Binds to neutrophils, monocytes, and certain lymphocyte subsets. Human form contains 9 CR domains. Identification on activated platelets: S.-C. Hsu-Lin *et al., J. Biol. Chem.* **259**, 9121 (1984).

8427. Selectride®. Group of stereoselective trialkyl borohydride reducing agents. Reduction of cycloalkenones: J. M. Fortunato, B. Ganem, *J. Org. Chem.* **41**, 2194 (1976). Review of synthetic applications: S. Wittmann, B. Schönecker, *J. Prakt. Chem. Chem.-Ztg.* **338**, 759-762 (1996).

L-Selectride

L-Selectride. [38721-52-7] Lithium (T-4)-hydrotris(1-methylpropyl)borate(1−); lithium tri-*sec*-butylborohydride. C$_{12}$H$_{28}$BLi; mol wt 190.10. C 75.82%, H 14.85%, B 5.69%, Li 3.65%. Prepn and use in stereoselective reduction of cyclic ketones: H. C. Brown,

S. Krishnamurthy, *J. Am. Chem. Soc.* **94**, 7159 (1972). Synthetic use in reduction of cyclic anhydrides: M. A. Makhlouf, B. Rickborn, *J. Org. Chem.* **46**, 4810 (1981); in cleavage of carbamates and *O*-demethylation of alkaloids: A. Coop *et al.*, *ibid.* **63**, 4392 (1998).

K-Selectride. [54575-49-4] Potassium (*T*-4)-hydrotris(1-methylpropyl)borate(1−); potassium tri-*sec*-butylborohydride. $C_{12}H_{28}$-BK; mol wt 222.26. Prepn: C. A. Brown, *J. Am. Chem. Soc.* **95**, 4100 (1973); *idem, Inorg. Synth.* **17**, 26 (1977). Synthetic use in conjugate reduction and reductive alkylation of α,β-unsaturated cyclohexenones: B. Ganem, *J. Org. Chem.* **40**, 146 (1975); in reduction of diketo steroids: D. M. Tal *et al.*, *Tetrahedron* **40**, 851 (1984). Prepd as a viscous, clear, water-white to yellow soln in THF. *Reacts vigorously with water.*

Caution: Solutions in THF may cause skin irritation and chemical burns (C. A. Brown, 1977).

USE: Mild reducing agents in organic synthesis.

8428. Selegiline. [14611-51-9] (α*R*)-*N*,α-Dimethyl-*N*-2-propynylbenzeneethanamine; L-(−)-*N*,α-dimethyl-*N*-2-propynyl-phenethylamine; (−)-deprenil; L-deprenyl. $C_{13}H_{17}N$; mol wt 187.28. C 83.37%, H 9.15%, N 7.48%. Monoamine oxidase-B inhibitor related structurally to pargyline, *q.v.* Prepn of racemate: **FR M 2635** (1964 to Chinoin), *C.A.* **63**, 2927e (1965); of (−)-form: **NL 6605956** (1966 to Chinoin), *C.A.* **67**, 21611y (1967); J. S. Fowler, *J. Org. Chem.* **42**, 2637 (1977). *See also:* Z. Ecsery *et al.*, *US 4564706* (1986 to Chinoin). Effects of racemate on CNS: J. Knoll *et al.*, *Arch. Int. Pharmacodyn.* **155**, 154 (1965). Comparative pharmacology of isomers: K. Magyar *et al.*, *Acta Physiol. Acad. Sci. Hung.* **32**, 377 (1967). Preliminary study in Alzheimer's disease: L. S. Schneider *et al.*, *Am. J. Psychiatry* **150**, 321 (1993). Review of pharmacology: E. H. Heinonen, R. Lammintausta, *Acta Neurol. Scand.* **84**, Suppl 136, 44-59 (1991); of efficacy in Parkinson's disease: D. W. Robin, *Am. J. Med. Sci.* **302**, 392-395 (1991). Symposium: *Mov. Disord.* **8**, Suppl. 1, S1-S44 (1993). Review of veterinary use in canine cognitive dysfunction: W. W. Ruehl, B. L. Hart in *Psychopharmacology of Animal Behavior Disorders*, N. H. Dodman, L. Shuster, Eds. (Blackwell Sci., Malden, Mass., 1998) pp 283-304.

Oil, $bp_{0.8}$ 92-93°. n_D^{20} 1.5180. $[α]_D^{20}$ −11.2°.

Hydrochloride. [14611-52-0] Anipryl; Antiparkin; Amindan; Carbex; Déprényl; Egibren; Eldepryl; Jumex; Movergan; Otrasel; Plurimen; Seledat; Selegam; Selepark; Selgimed; Xilopar; Zelapar. $C_{13}H_{17}N\cdot HCl$; mol wt 223.74. Crystals, mp 141-142°. $[α]_D^{25}$ −10.8° (c = 6.48 in water). Freely sol in water, chloroform, methanol. LD_{50} in rats (mg/kg): 81 i.v., 280 s.c. (Magyar).

(±)-**Form.** [2323-36-6] Deprenyl; phenylisopropyl-*N*-methyl-propinylamine. Oil, bp_5 103-110°. n_D^{20} 1.5224.

(±)-**Form hydrochloride.** E-250. LD_{50} in rats (mg/kg): 63 i.v., 126 s.c., 385 orally (Knoll).

THERAP CAT: Antiparkinsonian.

THERAP CAT (VET): In treatment of canine cognitive dysfunction syndrome.

8429. Selenic Acid. [7783-08-6] H_2O_4Se; mol wt 144.97. H 1.39%, O 44.15%, Se 54.47%. H_2SeO_4. Prepd by treating lead selenate with hydrogen sulfide and concentrating the filtered soln by evaporation: Mitscherlich, *Pogg. Ann.* **9**, 623 (1827); **11**, 327 (1827); *Ann. Chim. Phys.* [2] **36**, 100 (1827); by treating calcium selenate with cadmium oxalate and hydrogen sulfide: von Hauer, *J. Prakt. Chem.* [1] **80**, 214, 317 (1860); by treating a soln of silver selenite with bromine and evaporating the filtered soln: Thomsen, *Ber.* **2**, 598 (1869); by oxidizing selenium oxide with 30% hydrogen peroxide and removing water: Gilbertson, King, *J. Am. Chem. Soc.* **58**, 180 (1936); *Inorg. Synth.* **3**, 137 (1950).

Hexagonal prisms; mp 58°; d_4^{15} 2.9508; bp 260°. Very sol in water; sol in sulfuric acid; insol in ammonia; dec in alcohol. Very deliquescent. Reduced by hydrobromic acid, hydriodic acid, hydrogen sulfide, hydroxylamine hydrochloride, phenylhydrazine, formic acid, oxalic acid, malonic acid, pyruvic acid, acetyl chloride, and several metals.

8430. Selenious Acid. [7783-00-8] Monohydrated selenium dioxide; selenous acid. H_2O_3Se; mol wt 128.97. H 1.56%, O 37.22%, Se 61.22%. H_2SeO_3. Prepd by dissolving selenium dioxide in hot water and cooling: Berzelius, *Acad. Handl. Stockholm* **39**, 13 (1818).

Deliquescent hexagonal prisms; d_4^{15} 3.004. Vapor press. (mm Hg): 2 at 15°; 4.5 at 35°; 7 at 40.3°. $K_1 = 0.0024$; $K_2 = 4.8 \times 10^{-9}$. Gives off water upon heating and selenium oxide sublimes. Oxidized to selenic acid by strong oxidizing agents such as ozone, hydrogen dioxide, chlorine. Reduced to selenium by most reducing agents including hydriodic acid, sulfurous acid, sodium hyposulfite, hydroxylamine salts, hydrazine salts, hypophosphorous acid, phosphorous acid. 90 parts dissolve in 100 parts water at 0°, 400 parts at 90°; very sol in alcohol; insol in ammonia.

USE: As a reagent for alkaloids; as oxidizing agent.

8431. Selenium. [7782-49-2] Se; at. wt 78.96; at. no. 34; valences 2, 4, 6. Group VIA (16). Six stable isotopes: 74 (0.87%); 76 (9.02%); 77 (7.58%); 78 (23.52%); 80 (49.82%); 82 (9.19%); artificial, radioactive isotopes: 70-73; 75; 79; 81; 83-85; 87. Discovered in 1817 by Berzelius. Constitutes about 0.09 ppm of the earth's crust. Occurs in nature usually in the sulfide ores of the heavy metals; found in small quantities in pyrite; in the minerals *clausthalite* (PbSe), *naumannite* [(Ag,Pb)Se], *tiemannite* (HgSe); in selenosulfur. Essential trace element in human and animal diets; constituent of selenoproteins. Prepn: Waitkins *et al.*, *Ind. Eng. Chem.* **34**, 899 (1942). Purification: Nielsen, Heritage, *J. Electrochem. Soc.* **106**, 39 (1959); Oberbacher, Schlier, *US 2930678* (1960 to Norddeutsche Raffinerie). Symposium on organic selenium and tellurium compds: Y. Okamoto, W. H. H. Gunther, Eds., *Ann. N.Y. Acad. Sci.* **192**, 1-225 (1972). Reviews of selenium and its compds: K. W. Bagnall, *The Chemistry of Selenium, Tellurium and Polonium* (Elsevier, New York, 1966) 200 pp; Bagnall in *Comprehensive Inorganic Chemistry* vol. **2**, J. C. Bailar, Jr. *et al.*, Eds. (Pergamon Press, Oxford, 1973) pp 935-1008; *Selenium*, R. A. Zingaro, W. C. Cooper, Eds. (Van Nostrand, Reinhold, New York, 1974) 835 pp; E. M. Elkin in *Kirk-Othmer Encyclopedia of Chemical Technology* vol. **20** (Wiley-Interscience, New York, 3rd ed., 1982) pp 575-601. Reviews of nutritional properties and toxicology: E. J. Underwood, *Trace Elements in Human and Animal Nutrition* (Academic Press, New York, 1971) pp 323-368; Frost, *Crit. Rev. Toxicol.* **1**, 467-514 (1972); Allaway, *Cornell Vet.* **63**, 151-170 (1973); Frost, Lish, *Annu. Rev. Pharmacol.* **15**, 259-284 (1975) of biochemistry: T. C. Stadtman, *Annu. Rev. Biochem.* **49**, 93-110 (1980); *idem, FASEB J.* **1**, 375-379 (1987). Review of role in human health: M. P. Rayman, *Lancet* **356**, 233-241 (2000); of toxicology and human exposure: *Toxicological Profile for Selenium* (PB2004-100005, 2003) 457 pp.

Exists in several allotropic forms: amorphous, cryst or red, and gray or metallic. Liq is a brownish red, boils at 685° forming dark red vapors. Sol in dil aq caustic alkali solns; in aq potassium cyanide soln, in potassium sulfite soln. Burns in air with a bright blue flame forming the dioxide and emitting a characteristic odor resembling rotten horseradish. Combines directly with hydrogen, with the halogens (excluding iodine). Oxidized to selenious acid by nitric acid, to selenic acid by sulfuric acid. Reduces hot aqueous solutions of silver and gold salts with formation of silver selenide and metallic gold, respectively. Reacts with many metals.

Amorphous forms. Vitreous, black selenium; dark red-brown to bluish-black solid; formed when molten Se is cooled rapidly. d 4.28. Softens at 50-60° and becomes elastic at 70°. Red, amorphous form; formed by reduction of selenious acid in water; by condensation of Se vapor on a cold surface. d 4.26. Review of structural studies: Richter, Breitling, *Z. Naturforsch.* **26B**, 1699-1708, 2074-2075 (1971). When freshly precipitated, reacts with water at 50° forming selenious acid and hydrogen. Sol in carbon disulfide, methylene iodide, benzene, or quinoline.

Crystalline or red. Two monoclinic forms; dark red, transparent crystals. α-Form prepd by slow evaporation of CS_2 soln of Se; β-form by rapid evaporation of soln. mp below 200°. d (α-form) 4.46. Structure of α-form: Cherin, Unger, *Acta Crystallogr.* **28B**, 513 (1972); *see also* Bagnall, *loc. cit.* Both forms are metastable and change into gray form on heating.

Gray or metallic. Lustrous gray to black hexagonal crystals. The most stable form. d_4^{20} 4.81. mp 217°. Mohs' hardness: 2.0. Latent heat of fusion 16.4 cal/g. Latent heat of vaporization 20.6

kcal/mol. Linear coefficient of thermal expansion per degree C = 37×10^{-6}. Specific heat (28°): 0.084 cal/g/°C. Surface tension (217°): 92.5 dynes/cm. Thermal conductivity (25°): 0.0007-0.00183 cal/(cm)(°C)(sec). Insol in water, alcohol; very slightly sol in carbon disulfide (2 mg/100 ml at ord temp). Sol in ether. Conducts electricity and rectifies alternating current; the conductivity increases up to a thousand times on exposure to light.

Caution: Potential symptoms of overexposure are irritation of eyes, skin, nose and throat; visual disturbance; headache; chills, fever; dyspnea, bronchitis; metallic taste, garlic breath, GI disturbance; dermatitis; skin and eye burns. *See NIOSH Pocket Guide to Chemical Hazards* (DHHS/NIOSH 97-140, 1997) p 276.

USE: As ingredient of toning baths in photography; as pigment in manuf ruby-, pink-, orange-, or red-colored glass; as metallic base in making electrodes for arc lights, electrical instruments and apparatus, as rectifier in radio and television sets; in selenium photocells, in semiconductor fusion mixtures, selenium cells, telephotographic apparatus; as vulcanizing agent in processing of rubber; as catalyst in determination of nitrogen by Kjeldahl method; for dehydrogenation of organic compds.

THERAP CAT (VET): Nutritional factor (interrelationship with vitamin E), chiefly to prevent muscle degenerative diseases.

8432. Selenium Chloride. [10025-68-0] Selenium monochloride. Cl_2Se_2; mol wt 228.83. Cl 30.99%, Se 69.01%. Se_2Cl_2. Prepd from the elements: Sacc *et al.*, cited in *Mellor's* vol. X, 894 (1930); by the action of PCl_5 on selenium, on the selenide of phosphorus or antimony, on SeO_2 or on $SeOCl_2$: Baudrimont, *Ann. Chim. Phys.* [4] **2**, 5 (1864); Michaelis, *Z. Chem.* [2] **6**, 460 (1870); by the action of HCl on a soln of selenium in fuming sulfuric acid: Divers, Shimose, *J. Chem. Soc.* **45**, 194, 198, 201 (1884); from Se, SeO_2 and HCl: Lenher, Kao, *J. Am. Chem. Soc.* **47**, 772 (1925); **48**, 1550 (1926).

Deep red, oily liquid. bp_{733} 127° (dec). d_4^{25} 2.7741. mp −85°. Sol in chloroform, benzene, carbon tetrachloride, carbon disulfide, fuming sulfuric acid; dec in water.

8433. Selenium Hexafluoride. [7783-79-1] F_6Se; mol wt 192.95. F 59.08%, Se 40.92%. SeF_6. Prepd by passing gaseous fluorine over finely divided selenium in a copper vessel: Klemm, Henkel, *Z. Anorg. Allg. Chem.* **207**, 74 (1932); Yost, Claussen, *J. Am. Chem. Soc.* **55**, 885 (1933); Yost, *Inorg. Synth.* **1**, 121 (1939). *Review:* Kemmitt, Sharp, *Adv. Fluorine Chem.* **4**, 235 (1965).

Gas. mp −50.8°; sublimes −63.8°. Vapor press. (mm Hg): 651.2 (−48.7°); 213.1 (−64.8°); 30.4 (−87.5°). Insol in water. Reacts with ammonia gas at 200° to give selenium, nitrogen, and hydrogen fluoride. Covalently satd, does not attack glass.

Caution: Potential symptoms of overexposure in exptl animals are pulmonary irritation and edema. *See NIOSH Pocket Guide to Chemical Hazards* (DHHS/NIOSH 97-140, 1997) p 276.

USE: Gaseous electric insulator.

8434. Selenium Oxide. [7446-08-4] Selenium dioxide; selenious anhydride. O_2Se; mol wt 110.96. O 28.84%, Se 71.16%. SeO_2. Prepd by burning selenium in oxygen: Berzelius, *Acad. Handl. Stockholm* **39**, 13 (1818); *Ann. Chim. Phys.* [2] **9**, 160, 225, 337 (1818); by burning selenium in oxygen and nitrogen dioxide: Lenher, *J. Am. Chem. Soc.* **20**, 559 (1898); by oxidizing selenium with nitric acid: A. P. Julien, *ibid.* **47**, 1799 (1925). Toxicology: E. A. Cerwenka, W. C. Cooper, *Arch. Environ. Health* **3**, 189 (1961). *Review:* Waitkins, Clark, *Chem. Rev.* **36**, 235-289 (1945).

Lustrous, tetragonal needles. Acidic taste; leaves a burning sensation. Its yellowish green vapor has a pungent, sour smell. mp 340°; d_4^{15} 3.954. Vapor pressure (mm Hg): 12.5 at 70°; 20.2 at 94°; 39.0 at 181°; 760.0 at 315°; 848.0 at 320°. n_D^{20} <1.76. Soly (parts/100 parts solvent) in water: 38.4 (14°); in methanol: 10.16 (11.8°); in 93% ethanol: 6.67 (14°); in acetone: 4.35 (15.3°); in acetic acid: 1.11 (13.9°). Sol in concd H_2SO_4. Stable to light and heat. Rapidly absorbs dry hydrogen fluoride, hydrogen chloride, hydrogen bromide, and hydrogen iodide to form the corresponding selenium oxyhalide. Reacts with ammonia to form nitrogen and selenium; in alcohol soln forms ammonium ethyl selenite, $HN_4(C_2H_5)SeO_3$. Yields nitrogen and black amorphous selenium with hydrazine; nitrogen and reddish-brown amorphous selenium with hydroxylamine hydrochloride. Forms selenic acid with nitric acid. Reduced by carbon and other organic substances.

Caution: Direct contact may cause intense local irritation of skin and eyes (Cerwenka, Cooper).

USE: In the manuf of other selenium compounds; as a reagent for alkaloids; as oxidizing agent: L. F. Fieser, M. Fieser, *Reagents for Organic Chemistry* vol. 1 (New York, Wiley, 1967) p 992.

8435. Selenium Oxychloride. [7791-23-3] Seleninyl chloride. Cl_2OSe; mol wt 165.87. Cl 42.75%, O 9.65%, Se 47.60%. $SeOCl_2$. Prepd by passing chlorine into SeO_2 suspended in carbon tetrachloride: Lenher, *J. Am. Chem. Soc.* **42**, 2498 (1920); Hönigschmid, Görnhardt, *Z. Naturforsch.* **1**, 661 (1946); by dehydration of dichloroselenious acid: Smith, Jackson, *Inorg. Synth.* **3**, 130 (1950); from $SOCl_2$ and SeO_2: Paetzold, Aurich, *Z. Anorg. Allg. Chem.* **315**, 72 (1962); from $AlCl_3$ and SeO_2: Drago, Whitten, *Inorg. Chem.* **5**, 677 (1966). Acute toxicity: C. G. Wilber, *Clin. Toxicol.* **17**, 171 (1980).

Nearly colorless or yellowish, corrosive liquid; fumes in the air. d_4^{16} 2.44. Solidif ~5°. bp 180°. n_D^{20} 1.651. Dec by water into HCl and selenious acid. Miscible with carbon tetrachloride, chloroform, carbon disulfide, benzene, toluene. It is an excellent solvent for many substances including metals. LD_{50} s.c. in rabbits: 7 mg/kg (Wilber).

Caution: Strong irritant, vesicant. *See Clinical Toxicology of Commercial Products*, R. E. Gosselin *et al.*, Eds. (Williams & Wilkins, Baltimore, 5th ed., 1984) Section II, p 129.

8436. Selenium Sulfides. Prepn from selenious acid and H_2S; product may be a mixture of the elements: *Gmelins, Selenium* (8th ed.) **10** (part B), 159-176 (1949). Prepn by fusion of the elements; solid solns of sulfur (S_8), selenium (Se_8) and selenium sulfides (S_nSe_{8-n}; n = 1-7) formed: Fergusson *et al.*, *J. Inorg. Nucl. Chem.* **24**, 157 (1962); Hawes, *Nature* **198**, 1267 (1963); Cooper, Culka, *J. Inorg. Nucl. Chem.* **27**, 755 (1965); **29**, 1217 (1967).

Se_4S_4. Red tabular crystals from benzene, d 3.20. mp 113° (dec). Sol in CS_2. Solubility in benzene (20°): 0.4 g/l.

Se_2S_6. Light-orange needles from benzene, d 2.44. mp 121.5°. Sol in CS_2. Solubility in benzene (20°): 12 g/l.

Selenium disulfide. [7488-56-4] Exsel; Selsun. SeS_2; mol wt 143.09. Prepn of shampoo: M. M. Baldwin, A. P. Young, Jr., US **2694669** (1954 to Abbott). Toxicity studies: L. M. Cummins, E. T. Kimura, *Toxicol. Appl. Pharmacol.* **20**, 89 (1971). Review of use as antidandruff agent: Matson, *J. Soc. Cosmet. Chem.* **7**, 459-466 (1956). Insol in water, in 0.01N HCl. LD_{50} orally in rats: 138 mg/kg (Cummins, Kimura).

Caution: Selenium sulfide (as SeS) is reasonably anticipated to be a human carcinogen: *Report on Carcinogens, Eleventh Edition* (PB2005-104914, 2004) p III-230. *See also Bioassay of Selenium Sulfide (Gavage) for Possible Carcinogenicity* (PB82-164955, 1980) 113p.

THERAP CAT: Disulfide as topical antiseborrheic.

THERAP CAT (VET): Topically in eczemas and dermatomycoses.

8437. Selenium Tetrabromide. [7789-65-3] Br_4Se; mol wt 398.58. Br 80.19%, Se 19.81%. $SeBr_4$. Prepd by adding excessive bromine to selenium: Schneider, *Pogg. Ann.* **128**, 327 (1866); **129**, 450, 634 (1866); by dissolving selenium dioxide in hydrobromic acid: Muthmann, Schäfer, *Ber.* **26**, 1008 (1893).

Red-brown, cryst powder. Unpleasant odor. Dec 70-80°. Dec in moist air and water. Sol in carbon disulfide, chloroform, ethyl bromide.

8438. Selenium Tetrachloride. [10026-03-6] Cl_4Se; mol wt 220.77. Cl 64.24%, Se 35.77%. $SeCl_4$. Prepd by the action of an excess of chlorine on selenium: Berzelius, cited in *Mellor's* vol X, 898 (1930); by the action of thionyl chloride or phosphorus trichloride on selenium oxychloride or by the action of phosphorus pentachloride on selenium oxide: Michaelis, *Z. Chem.* [2] **6**, 460 (1870); by the action of anhydr selenic acid on acetyl chloride at 0°: Lamb, *Am. Chem. J.* **30**, 209 (1903). Crystal structure: Shoemaker, Abrahams, *Acta Crystallogr.* **18**, 296 (1965).

White to pale yellow crystals. d 2.6. Sublimes when heated. Dec in water and moist air. Insol in liquid bromine. Dec by dry ammonia.

8439. Selenium Tetrafluoride. [13465-66-2] F_4Se; mol wt 154.95. F 49.04%, Se 50.96%. SeF_4. Fluorinating agent. Prepn from $SeCl_4$ and AgF: Prideaux, Cox, *J. Chem. Soc.* **1927**, 928;

1928, 1603; from Se and F_2: Aynsley *et al., ibid.* **1952,** 1231; J. Carre *et al., J. Fluorine Chem.* **14,** 139 (1979); from Se and AgF: Glemser *et al., Naturwissenschaften* **52,** 130 (1965); from Se_2Cl_2 and F_2: Goggin, *J. Inorg. Nucl. Chem.* **28,** 661 (1966); from Se and ClF: Pitts, Jache, US 3373000 (1968 to Olin Mathieson); from Se and ClF_3: Olah *et al., J. Am. Chem. Soc.* **96,** 925 (1974).

Colorless liquid; fumes in air. mp $-9.5°$. bp $106°$. d^{18} 2.75. Forms a white hygroscopic solid. Hydrolyzed violently by water. Attacks glass slowly when perfectly dry. Completely miscible with ether, ethanol, iodine pentafluoride, sulfuric acid; sol in chloroform, carbon tetrachloride.

USE: Fluorination of alcohols, carboxylic acids and carbonyl compds: Olah *et al., loc. cit.*

8440. Selenocysteine. [10236-58-5] 3-Selenyl-L-alanine; selenium cysteine. $C_3H_7NO_2Se$; mol wt 168.05. C 21.44%, H 4.20%, N 8.33%, O 19.04%, Se 46.99%. Naturally occurring amino acid found in the active site of certain prokaryotic and eukaryotic enzymes. Highly oxidizable making synthesis difficult. Easily prepared from its oxidized form **selenocystine.** Prepn of *dl*-selenocystine: A. Fredga, *Sven. Kem. Tidskr.* **48,** 160 (1936); E. P. Painter, *J. Chem. Soc.* **69,** 229 (1947); of *l*-form: H. Tanaka, K. Soda, *Methods Enzymol.* **143,** 240 (1987). Reduction of selenocystine and separation of L-selenocysteine: J. N. Burnell *et al., J. Inorg. Biochem.* **12,** 343 (1980). Chemical properties: R. E. Huber, R. S. Criddle, *Arch. Biochem. Biophys.* **122,** 164 (1967). Determn by HPLC/MS: H. E. Ganther *et al., Methods Enzymol.* **107,** 582 (1984); colorimetric determn: N. Esaki, K. Soda, *ibid.* **143,** 148 (1987). Identification of Se as a component in protein: S.-H. Oh *et al., Biochemistry* **13,** 1825 (1974). Characterization of selenocysteine as the Se containing amino acid moiety in various enzymes: J. E. Cone *et al., Proc. Natl. Acad. Sci. USA* **73,** 2659 (1976); J. B. Jones *et al., Arch. Biochem. Biophys.* **195,** 255 (1979); presence in the catalytic site of mammalian glutathione peroxidase: J. W. Forstrom *et al., Biochemistry* **17,** 2639 (1978); J. J. Zabrowski *et al., Biochem. Biophys. Res. Commun.* **84,** 248 (1978). Metabolism in animals: H. Tanaka *et al., Curr. Top. Cell. Regul.* **27,** 487 (1985). Identification of selenocysteine-specific tRNA: W. C. Hawkes *et al., Biochim. Biophys. Acta* **699,** 183 (1982); W. Leinfelder *et al., Nature* **331,** 723 (1988). *Review:* T. C. Stadtman, *FASEB J.* **1,** 375-379 (1987).

pK 5.2. Unstable to acid hydrolysis.

8441. Selenomethionine. [1464-42-2] 2-Amino-4-(methylseleno)butanoic acid; α-amino-γ-(methylseleno)butyric acid. $C_5H_{11}NO_2Se$; mol wt 196.11. C 30.62%, H 5.65%, N 7.14%, O 16.32%, Se 40.26%. $CH_3SeCH_2CH_2CH(NH_2)COOH$. Selenium analog of methionine. Prepn of DL-form: E. P. Painter, *J. Am. Chem. Soc.* **69,** 232 (1949); H. J. Klosterman, E. P. Painter, *ibid.* 2009; G. Zdansky, *Ark. Kemi* **19,** 559 (1962), *C.A.* **58,** 6919h (1963). Prepn of L-form: *idem, ibid.* **29,** 437 (1968); C. S. Pande *et al., J. Org. Chem.* **35,** 1440 (1970). Biosynthesis of radioactive (^{75}Se) form: M. Blau, *Biochim. Biophys. Acta* **49,** 389 (1961). Metabolism: M. Blau, J. F. Holland in *Radioactive Pharmaceuticals,* G. A. Andrews *et al.,* Eds. (USAEC Symposium Series #6, 1976) pp 409-421. Review of use in pancreatic scanning: J. E. Agnew *et al., Br. J. Radiol.* **49,** 979-995 (1976).

DL-Form. Transparent, hexagonal sheets or plates from methanol and water, metallic luster; mp $265°$ (dec). IR spectrum: Zdansky, *loc. cit.* (1962).

L-Form. Crystals from aqueous acetone; mp 266-268° (dec). $[\alpha]_D^{22}$ +21.6° (c = 0.5 in 2N HCl).

^{75}Se-Injection. [1187-56-0] Sethotope.

THERAP CAT: ^{75}Se as diagnostic aid (radioactive imaging agent).

8442. Sematilide. [101526-83-4] N-[2-(Diethylamino)ethyl]-4-[(methylsulfonyl)amino]benzamide; CK-1752. $C_{14}H_{23}N_3$-O_3S; mol wt 313.42. C 53.65%, H 7.40%, N 13.41%, O 15.31%, S 10.23%. Prepn: D. D. Davey *et al.,* US 4544654 (1985 to Schering AG); W. C. Lumma, Jr. *et al., J. Med. Chem.* **30,** 755

(1987). Pharmacology: S. S. Greenberg *et al., Drug Dev. Res.* **25,** 283 (1992). Pharmacokinetics and HPLC determn in plasma: S. Dancik *et al., J. Pharm. Sci.* **80,** 157 (1991). Clinical pharmacology: W. Wong *et al., Am. J. Cardiol.* **69,** 206 (1992). Electrophysiologic profile: P. T. Sager *et al., Circulation* **88,** 1072 (1993). *Review:* T. A. Argentieri, *Cardiovasc. Drug Rev.* **10,** 182-198 (1992).

Monohydrochloride. [101526-62-9] CK-1752A. $C_{14}H_{23}N_3$-$O_3S.HCl$; mol wt 349.88. Crystals from acetone/methanol. mp 141-142° (Lumma). Also reported as having two polymorphic crystalline forms, mp 137° and mp 142° (Argentieri). Apparent pKa_1 7.60; pKa_2 9.51. Distribution coefficient (octanol/pH 7.4 buffer): 0.104 at 10 mM. uv max (0.1N NaOH): 289 nm (ε 1.91×10^4). uv max (0.1N HCl): 254 nm (ε 1.78×10^4). LD_{50} i.p. in mice: 250-300 mg/kg (Lumma). LD_{50} in mice, rats, dogs (mg/kg): 96, 92, 143-175 i.v.; 1,800, 3,200, 500-1,000 orally (Argentieri).

THERAP CAT: Antiarrhythmic (class III).

8443. Semduramicin. [113378-31-7] (2R,3S,4S,5R,6S)-Tetrahydro-2,4-dihydroxy-6-[(1R)-1-[(2S,5R,7S,8R,9S)-9-hydroxy-2,8-dimethyl-2-[(2S,2'R,3'S,5R,5'R)-octahydro-2-methyl-5'-[(2S,-3S,5R,6S)-tetrahydro-6-hydroxy-3,5,6-trimethyl-2H-pyran-2-yl]-3'-[[(2S,5S,6R)-tetrahydro-5-methoxy-6-methyl-2H-pyran-2-yl]oxy][2,2'-bifuran]-5-yl]-1,6-dioxaspiro[4.5]dec-7-yl]ethyl]-5-methoxy-3-methyl-2H-pyran-2-acetic acid; UK-61689. $C_{45}H_{76}$-O_{16}; mol wt 873.08. C 61.91%, H 8.77%, O 29.32%. Semi-synthetic polyether ionophore antibiotic. Prepn: A. C. Goudie, N. D. A. Walshe, EP 255335; *eidem,* US 4804680 (1988, 1989 both to Pfizer). LC determn in poultry liver: J. F. Ericson *et al., J. AOAC Int.* **77,** 577 (1994). Metabolism and tissue residue studies in broiler chickens: M. J. Lynch *et al., ACS Symp. Ser.* **503,** 49-69 (1992). Anticoccidial effects in chickens: M. E. McKenzie *et al., Poult. Sci.* **72,** 2052 (1993); N. B. Logan *et al., ibid.,* 2058.

Sodium salt. [119068-77-8] UK-61689-2; Aviax. $C_{45}H_{75}$-NaO_{16}; mol wt 895.06. Crystals from isopropyl ether. mp 175-176°. $[\alpha]_D^{25}$ +19.3° (c = 0.5 in methanol).

THERAP CAT (VET): Coccidiostat.

8444. Semicarbazide Hydrochloride. [563-41-7] Hydrazinecarboxamide monohydrochloride; aminourea hydrochloride; carbamylhydrazine hydrochloride. CH_6ClN_3O; mol wt 111.53. C 10.77%, H 5.42%, Cl 31.79%, N 37.68%, O 14.35%. NH_2NH-$CONH_2.HCl$. Prepd by electrolytic reduction of nitrourea with cathodes of copper, nickel, lead, and mercury in hydrochloric acid solution: Ingersoll *et al., Org. Synth.* **5,** 93 (1925). Commercial prepn from hydrazine hydrate, iron carbonyl, and carbon monoxide: Sampson, US 2589289 (1952 to du Pont).

Prisms from dil alc, dec 175-185°. Freely sol in water with acid reaction. Dissociation consts of free base: Kb at $20°$ = 29 $\times$ 10^{-11}; Ka = 1.6×10^{-11}. Very slightly sol in hot alcohol, insol in anhydr ether. Ammonolysis with liq NH_3 gives a 95% yield of the free base; mp 96°: Audrieth, *J. Am. Chem. Soc.* **52,** 1250 (1930).

Acetone semicarbazone. $C_4H_9N_3O$. Needles from water, mp 192° (heated stage); mp 188° (open capillary tube).

USE: As a reagent for ketones and aldehydes with which it affords cryst compds having characteristic melting points.

8445. Semioxamazide. [515-96-8] Aminooxoacetic acid hydrazide; aminooxamide; oxamic acid hydrazide. $C_2H_5N_3O_2$; mol wt 103.08. C 23.30%, H 4.89%, N 40.76%, O 31.04%. H_2N-COCONHNH$_2$. Made from hydrazine sulfate, ethyl oxamate and KOH. *Ref:* Wilson, Pickering, *J. Chem. Soc.* **123**, 394 (1923); Leonard, Boyer, *J. Org. Chem.* **15**, 42 (1950).

Lustrous leaflets, mp ~220° with decompn. Soluble in 400 parts water; more sol in hot water; easily sol in acids and alkalies with formation of salts; insol in alcohol, ether.

USE: As a reagent for aldehydes and ketones.

8446. Semotiadil. [116476-13-2] (2R)-2-[2-[3-[[2-(1,3-Benzodioxol-5-yloxy)ethyl]methylamino]propoxy]-5-methoxyphenyl]-4-methyl-2H-1,4-benzothiazin-3(4H)-one; (+)-(R)-3,4-dihydro-2-[5-methoxy-2-[3-[N-methyl-[N-2-[3,4-(methylenedioxy)phenoxy]ethyl]amino]propoxy]phenyl]-4-methyl-3-oxo-2H-1,4-benzothiazine; sesamodil; DS-4823. $C_{29}H_{32}N_2O_6S$; mol wt 536.64. C 64.91%, H 6.01%, N 5.22%, O 17.89%, S 5.98%. Benzothiazine calcium antagonist. Prepn: J. Iwao *et al.,* **WO 8700838;** *eidem,* US **4786635** (1987, 1988 both to Santen). Synthesis: M. Fujita *et al., J. Med. Chem.* **33**, 1898 (1990). LC determn in plasma: K. Morishima *et al., J. Chromatogr.* **527**, 381 (1990). Molecular conformation and crystal structure: A. Ota *et al., Chem. Pharm. Bull.* **41**, 1681 (1993). Electrophysiology: N. Miyawaki *et al., J. Cardiovasc. Pharmacol.* **16**, 769 (1990); and antiarrhythmic effects: *eidem, Drug Dev. Res.* **22**, 293 (1991). Antihypertensive effects in rats: A. Kanda, H. Hashimoto, *Jpn. J. Pharmacol.* **63**, 121 (1993). Mechanism of action study: K. Murakami *et al., J. Cardiovasc. Pharmacol.* **25**, 262 (1995).

Fumarate. [116476-14-3] SD-3211. $C_{29}H_{32}N_2O_6S \cdot C_4H_4O_4$; mol wt 652.71. Crystals from EtOH, mp 134-135°. $[\alpha]_D^{25}$ +195° (in DMSO).

THERAP CAT: Antihypertensive; antianginal.

8447. Sempervirine. [6882-99-1] 2,3,4,13-Tetrahydro-1H-benz[g]indolo[2,3-a]quinolizin-6-ium; 3,4,5,6,14,15,20,21-octadehydroyohimbanium; sempervirene. $C_{19}H_{16}N_2$; mol wt 272.34. C 83.79%, H 5.92%, N 10.29%. Found in rhizome and roots of Carolina jessamine (yellow jessamine) *Gelsemium sempervirens* (L.) Ait. f., *Loganiaceae:* Stevenson, Sayre, *J. Am. Pharm. Assoc.* **4**, 60 (1915); **8**, 708 (1919); Hasenfratz, *Bull. Soc. Chim. Fr.* [4] **53**, 1084 (1933); Forsyth *et al., J. Chem. Soc.* **1945**, 579; Prelog, *Helv. Chim. Acta* **31**, 588 (1948). Believed to exist primarily as inner salt depicted below: Woodward, Witkop, *J. Am. Chem. Soc.* **71**, 379 (1949). Synthesis: Woodward, McLamore, *ibid.* 379; Swan, *J. Chem. Soc.* **1958**, 2039; Ban, Seo, *Tetrahedron* **16**, 11 (1961); Potts, Mattingly, *J. Org. Chem.* **33**, 3985 (1968).

Monohydrate. Yellow needles from chloroform, mp 228°. Brownish-yellow leaflets from dil ethanol, mp 258°. uv max (ethanol): 243, 249, 297, 345, 387 nm (log ε 4.58, 4.57, 4.20, 4.26, 4.24). Dipole moment: 8.5 (dioxane); 7.5 (benzene). Soluble in alcohol, chloroform, pyridine. Slightly sol in acetone. Practically insol in ether, benzene.

Methochloride. $C_{20}H_{19}ClN_2$. Minute yellow needles from ethanol, mp 330-332°. Soluble in water giving yellow solns with purple fluorescence. uv max: 241, 292, 330, 395 nm (log ε 4.56, 4.20, 4.28, 4.22).

8448. Senecialdehyde. [107-86-8] 3-Methyl-2-butenal; 3,3-dimethylacrolein; 3-methylcrotonaldehyde; senecioaldehyde; β,β-dimethylacrolein. C_5H_8O; mol wt 84.12. C 71.39%, H 9.59%, O 19.02%. $(CH_3)_2C=CHCHO$. Prepn from isoamyl alcohol: Fischer *et al., Ber.* **64**, 30 (1931); Fischer, Löwenberg, *Ann.* **494**, 272 (1932); *cf.* Burkhardt *et al.,* GB **512465** (1939); Montavon, Saucy, US **2902515** (1959 to Hoffmann-La Roche).

Liquid. Odor more pungent than that of isovaleraldehyde. Autooxidizes easily, but the pure substance can be stored under vacuum. d_4^{20} 0.8722; bp_{730} 133°; n_D^{20} 1.4526. Absorption spectrum: Forbes, Skilton, *J. Org. Chem.* **24**, 436 (1959).

Caution: Irritant to mucous membranes. Narcotic in high concentrations.

8449. Senecic Acid. [13588-16-4] (2R,3R,5Z)-5-Ethylidene-2-hydroxy-2,3-dimethylhexanedioic acid. $C_{10}H_{16}O_5$; mol wt 216.23. C 55.55%, H 7.46%, O 37.00%. One of the most widely studied *necic acids* which are constituent acids of the hepatotoxic pyrrolizidine alkaloids and are isolated from these alkaloids by hydrolysis or by hydrogenolysis. Necic acids are C_5- to C_{10}-acids; many are γ- or δ-hydroxy acids and have structures that may be dissected into isoprene units. Synthesis of senecic acid: C. C. J. Culvenor, T. A. Geissman, *J. Am. Chem. Soc.* **83**, 1647 (1961). uv spectra of senecic acid and its isomers: V. Simanek *et al., Collect. Czech. Chem. Commun.* **34**, 1832 (1969). Biosynthesis: D. H. G. Crout *et al., J. Chem. Soc. Perkin Trans. 1* **1972**, 671. Comprehensive reviews on necic acids: F. L. Warren, *Fortschr. Chem. Org. Naturst.* **12**, 198-269 (1955); **24**, 329-406 (1966); D. J. Robins *ibid.* **41**, 115-203 (1982); F. L. Warren in *Alkaloids* Vol. XII, R. H. F. Manske, Ed. (Academic Press, New York, 1970) pp 245-331.

Needles from benzene or ethyl acetate, mp 145-146°. Sublimes readily at ~125°.

8450. Senecio. Golden ragwort; squaw weed; life root. Dried plant of *Senecio aureus* L., *Compositae. Habit.* Canada and Eastern U.S. *Constit.* The alkaloids, senecifoline, senecine, etc., resins.

THERAP CAT: Emmenagogue.

8451. Senecionine. [130-01-8] 12-Hydroxysenecionan-11,16-dione; aureine. $C_{18}H_{25}NO_5$; mol wt 335.39. C 64.46%, H 7.51%, N 4.18%, O 23.85%. Hepatotoxic pyrrolizidine alkaloid from whole plant of *Senecio vulgaris* L., *Compositae* and several other *Senecio* spp. Isoln: Barger, Blackie, *J. Chem. Soc.* **1936**, 743. Structure: Adams, Govindachari, *J. Am. Chem. Soc.* **71**, 1953 (1949); Koekmoer, Warren, *J. Chem. Soc.* **1955**, 63. Conformation: Culvenor, *Tetrahedron Lett.* **1966**, 1091. Toxicity study: P. N. Harris *et al., J. Pharmacol. Exp. Ther.* **75**, 69 (1942). Review of toxicology of senecionine and other pyrrolizidine alkaloids: E. K. McLean, *Pharmacol. Rev.* **22**, 429-483 (1970). Comprehensive reviews of pyrrolizidine alkaloids: L. Bull *et al., The Pyrrolizidine Alkaloids* (North-Holland, Amsterdam, 1968) 293 pp; F. L. Warren in *The Alkaloids* vol. 12, R. H. F. Manske, Ed. (Academic Press, New York, 1970) pp 245-331; D. J. Robins, *Fortschr. Chem. Org. Naturst.* **41**, 115-203 (1982).

Bitter plates, mp 236°. $[\alpha]_D^{25}$ −55.1° (c = 0.034 in chloroform). Practically insol in water. Freely sol in chloroform; slightly sol in alcohol, ether. LD_{50} i.v. in mice: 64.12 ±2.24 mg/kg (Harris).

C_{15}-*trans* Isomer. Integerrimine; squalidine; [15(20)*E*]-12-hydroxysenecionan-11,16,dione. Isolated from several *Senecio* and *Crotalaria* spp.: L. Bull *et al., loc. cit.*; F. L. Warren, *loc. cit.* Identity of squalidine and integerrimine: A. G. Gonzalez, A. Calero, *Chem. Ind. (London)* **1958**, 126. mp 172-172.5°; $[\alpha]_D^{28}$ +4.3° (c = 0.8 in methanol).

8452. Seneciphylline. [480-81-9] 13,19-Didehydro-12-hydroxysenecionan-11,16-dione; jacodine; α-longilobine. $C_{18}H_{23}$-NO_5; mol wt 333.38. C 64.85%, H 6.95%, N 4.20%, O 24.00%. Hepatotoxic pyrrolizidine alkaloid, common constituent of *Senecio* species. Isoln from *Senecio platyphllus* DC. *Compositae:* A. Orechoff, W. Tiedebel, *Ber.* **68**, 650 (1935); from *S. jacobaea* L.: G. Barger, J. J. Blackie, *J. Chem. Soc.* **1937**, 584; from *Crotalaria juncea* L. *Leguminosae:* R. Adams, M. Gianturco, *J. Am. Chem. Soc.* **78**, 1919 (1956). Identity with α-longilobine: R. Adams, J. H. Looker, *ibid.* **73**, 134 (1951). Identity with jacodine: R. B. Bradbury, C. C. J. Culvenor, *Chem. Ind. (London)* **1954**, 1021. Structural study: R. Adams *et al., J. Am. Chem. Soc.* **74**, 700 (1952). Revised structure: S. Masume, *Chem. Ind. (London)* **1959**, 21. Review and evaluation of toxicity and carcinogenicity studies: *IARC Monographs* **10**, 319-325, 333-342 (1976). Comprehensive reviews of seneciphylline and other pyrrolizidine alkaloids: L. Bull *et al., The Pyrrolizidine Alkaloids* (North-Holland, Amsterdam, 1968) 293 pp; F. L. Warren in *The Alkaloids* vol. **12**, R. H. F. Manske, Ed. (Academic Press, New York, 1970) pp 245-331.

Small rhombic platelets from hot alcohol or acetone, mp 217-218°. $[\alpha]_D$ −128° (chloroform). Easily sol in chloroform, ethylene chloride; less sol in alc, acetone. Difficultly sol in ether, ligroin.

8453. Senega. Senega snakeroot; Seneca snakeroot; rattlesnake root. Dried root of *Polygala senega* L., *Polygalaceae. Habit.* North America. Used by native Americans as a treatment for snakebite. *Constit.* Triterpenoid saponins, 6-12%, with presenegenin as the main sapogenin; ~5% lipids; mono- and oligosaccharides; phenolic acid esters; traces of essential oil containing methyl salicylate which imparts a slight aromatic odor. Quantitative analysis of senega saponins: Kita *et al., Yakugaku Zasshi* **89**, 1111 (1969). Brief review: M. Wichtl, N. G. Bisset, *Herbal Drugs and Phytopharmaceuticals*, English Ed. (CRC Press, Boca Raton, 1994) pp 384-385.

THERAP CAT: Expectorant.

8454. Senna. Dried leaflets of *Cassia senna* L. (*C. acutifolia* Delile), (Alexandria senna), or of *C. angustifolia* Vahl (India or Tinnevelly senna), *Leguminosae. Habit.* Egypt and neighboring districts, Southern India (Tinnevelly). *Constit.* Sennosides A and B; glucosides of rhein and chrysophanic acid: Becker, *Planta Med.* **7**, 390 (1959); Fairbairne, *ibid.* **12**, 260 (1964). Prepn of senna powder: Friedmann, Ryan, **GB 832017** (1960 to Westminster Labs.); Corran, **GB 852343** (1960 to C. E. Fulford); Baetz, **DE 1158211** (1963 to Ludwig Heumann). *Incompat.* Mineral acids, carbonates, infusion cinchona, lime water, salts of heavy metals, tartar emetic.

THERAP CAT: Cathartic.

THERAP CAT (VET): Has been used as a purgative.

8455. Sennosides. Colonorm; Glysennid; Nytilax; Pursennid. $C_{42}H_{38}O_{20}$; mol wt 862.74. C 58.47%, H 4.44%, O

37.09%. Anthraquinone glucosides found in senna in equal amts and in the rhubarbs where sennoside A predominates. Isoln from Tinnevelly senna (*Cassia angustifolia* Vahl, *Leguminosae):* Stoll *et al., Helv. Chim. Acta* **32**, 1892 (1949); **GB 804232** (1958 to Byk-Gulden); Khorana, Sanghavi, *J. Pharm. Sci.* **53**, 110 (1964); Menssen *et al., US 3517269* (1970 to Nattermann & Cie). Isoln from the rhyzome of *Rheum palmatum* L.: Zwaving, *Planta Med.* **13**, 474 (1965). Isoln of sennoside A from rhubarb: Miyamoto *et al., Yakugaku Zasshi* **87**, 1040 (1967). Sennosides B, C, D, E, and F have also been isolated from rhubarb, *see* Oshio *et al., Chem. Pharm. Bull.* **22**, 823 (1974). Structure: Stoll *et al., Helv. Chim. Acta* **33**, 313 (1950). Sennoside A is built up from the dextrorotatory aglucon sennidin A and D-glucose. Sennoside B is built up from the intramolecularly compensated *meso*-sennidin B and D-glucose. *Review:* Stoll, Becker, *Fortschr. Chem. Org. Naturst.* **7**, 248 (1950). Transport and mechanism of action studies: Dobbs *et al., Farmaco Ed. Sci.* **30**, 147 (1975).

Sennoside A. [81-27-6] (*R**,*R**)-5,5'-Bis(β-D-glucopyranosyloxy)-9,9',10,10'-tetrahydro-4,4'-dihydroxy-10,10'-dioxo[9,9'-bianthracene]-2,2'-dicarboxylic acid. Rectangular yellow plates from dil acetone, dec 200-240°. $[\alpha]_D^{20}$ −164° (c = 0.1 in 60% acetone); $[\alpha]_D^{20}$ −147° (c = 0.1 in 70% acetone); $[\alpha]_D^{20}$ −24° (c = 0.2 in 70% dioxane). Insol in water, benzene, ether, chloroform. Sparingly sol in methanol, Carbitol, acetone, dioxane. The soly increases tremendously in water-miscible organic solvents contg an optimum of 30% w/w of water. Sol in aq solns of sodium bicarbonate. Sennoside A can be slowly isomerized to B in $NaHCO_3$ soln at 80°.

Sennoside B. [128-57-4] (9*R*,9'*S*)-5,5'-Bis(β-D-glucopyranosyloxy)-9,9',10,10'-tetrahydro-4,4'-dihydroxy-10,10'-dioxo[9,9'-bianthracene]-2,2'-dicarboxylic acid. Light yellow prisms from dil acetone; fine needles from water, dec 180-186°. $[\alpha]_D^{20}$ −100° (c = 0.2 in 70% acetone); $[\alpha]_D^{20}$ −67° (c = 0.4 in 70% dioxane). uv max (0.5% $NaHCO_3$): 270, 308, 355 nm. Has the same soly characteristics as sennoside A, but is more sol. Can be recrystallized from large amounts of hot water. *Keep protected from air and light.*

THERAP CAT: Cathartic.

8456. Seocalcitol. [134404-52-7] (1*R*,3*S*,5*Z*)-5-[(2*E*)-[(1*R*,3a*S*,7a*R*)-1-[(1*R*,2*E*,4*E*)-6-Ethyl-6-hydroxy-1-methyl-2,4-octadienyl]octahydro-7a-methyl-4*H*-inden-4-ylidene]ethylidene]-4-methylene-1,3-cyclohexanediol; (5*Z*,7*E*,22*E*,24*E*)-24a,26a,27a-trihomo-9,10-secocholesta-5,7,10(19),22,24-pentaene-1α,3β,25-triol; 1(*S*),3(*R*)-dihydroxy-20(*R*)-(5'-ethyl-5'-hydroxyhepta-1'(*E*),3'(*E*)-dien-1'-yl)-9,10-secopregna-5(*Z*),7(*E*),10(19)-triene; EB-1089. $C_{30}H_{46}O_3$; mol wt 454.68. C 79.25%, H 10.20%, O 10.56%. Antiproliferative vitamin D analog with reduced effects on calcium metabolism. Prepn: E. Binderup, M. J. Calverley, **WO 9100855**; **US 5190935** (1991, 1993 both to Leo Pharm.). LC-MS-MS determn in serum: A.-M. Kissmeyer *et al., J. Chromatogr. B* **740**, 117 (2000). Pharmacokinetics and metabolism: A.-M. Kissmeyer, J. T. Mortensen, *Xenobiotica* **30**, 815 (2000). Mechanism of action study: G. A. DeMasters *et al., J. Steroid Biochem. Mol. Biol.* **92**, 365 (2004). Clinical evaluation in pancreatic cancer: T. R. J. Evans *et al., Br. J. Cancer* **86**, 680 (2002); in hepatocellular carcinoma: K. Dalhoff *et al., Br. J. Cancer* **89**, 252 (2003). Review of pharmacology and clinical experience: C. M. Hansen *et al., Curr. Pharm. Des.* **6**, 803-828 (2000).

Needles from methyl formate-hexane, mp 123-125°. uv max: 232, 264 nm (ε 43745, 18060).

THERAP CAT: Antineoplastic.

8457. Sepia. Cuttle-fish bone. Calcareous substance found under the skin of the back of *Sepia officinalis* L., *Cephalopoda. Habit.* Mediterranean Sea, Atlantic and Pacific Oceans. *Constit.* Calcium carbonate and phosphate, gluten.

USE: As a polishing agent and in tooth powders.

8458. Sepiomelanin. The eumelanin isolated from ink sacs of the cuttlefish, *Sepia officinalis* L., *Cephalopoda.* Present in the raw ink as a suspension of small, dark granules in a colorless plasma. Structure is a macromolecule or probably a mixture of polyacid polymers in which the predominant chemical unit is of the indole type. Structure studies: Piattelli, Nicolaus, *Tetrahedron* **15**, 66 (1961); Piattelli *et al., ibid.* **19**, 2061 (1963). *Review:* R. A. Nicolaus, *Melanins* (Hermann, Paris, 1968) pp 68-91.

In the dry form, an amorphous, hygroscopic, black powder. Insol in all solvents.

USE: Pigment.

8459. Seratrodast. [112665-43-7] ζ-(2,4,5-Trimethyl-3,6-dioxo-1,4-cyclohexadien-1-yl)benzeneheptanoic acid; (±)-7-(3,5,6-trimethyl-1,4-benzoquinon-2-yl)-7-phenylheptanoic acid; AA-2414; Abbott 73001; Bronica. $C_{22}H_{26}O_4$; mol wt 354.44. C 74.55%, H 7.39%, O 18.06%. Thromboxane A_2-receptor antagonist. Prepn: S. Terao, Y. Maki, **EP 171251**; *eidem,* **US 5180742** (1986, 1993 both to Takeda); M. Shiraishi *et al., J. Med. Chem.* **32**, 2214 (1989). Effect on thromboxane A_2/prostaglandin endoperoxidase-receptor: Y. Imura *et al., Jpn. J. Pharmacol.* **52**, 35 (1990). Clinical effect in asthma: M. Fujimura *et al., J. Allergy Clin. Immunol.* **87**, 23 (1991). Clinical pharmacokinetics: Z. Hussein *et al., Clin. Pharmacol. Ther.* **55**, 441 (1994).

Crystals from ethanol, mp 128-129°.

THERAP CAT: Antiasthmatic.

8460. Serine. [56-45-1] L-Serine; Ser; S; 2-amino-3-hydroxypropionic acid; β-hydroxyalanine; (*S*)-2-amino-3-hydroxypropanoic acid; α-amino-β-hydroxypropionic acid. $C_3H_7NO_3$; mol wt 105.09. C 34.29%, H 6.71%, N 13.33%, O 45.67%. A non-essential amino acid for human development. A major intracellular source of one carbon units for *de novo* purine synthesis. Found in the active site of serine proteases such as trypsin. Isoln from the silk protein, sericine: E. Cramer, *Prakt. Chem.* **96**, 76 (1865). Structure and synthesis as DL-form: E. Fischer, H. Leuchs, *Ber.* **35**, 3787 (1902). Early chemistry and biochemistry: *Amino Acids and Proteins,* D. M. Greenberg, Ed. (Charles C. Thomas, Springfield, IL,

1951) 950 pp., *passim*; J. P. Greenstein, M. Winitz, *Chemistry of the Amino Acids* **vols 1-3** (John Wiley and Sons, Inc., New York, 1961) pp. 2202-2237, *passim.* Enzymatic determn in biological samples: R. D. Hurst *et al., Anal. Biochem.* **117**, 339 (1981). Synthetic reviews: K. Toi in *Synthetic Production and Utilization of Amino Acids,* T. Kaneko *et al.,* Eds. (Halsted, New York, 1974) pp 187-195; of DL-forms: L. Bassignani *et al., Ber.* **112**, 148-160 (1979). Review of role in enzyme active sites: B. S. Hartley, *Ann. N.Y. Acad. Sci.* **227**, 438-445 (1974); J. Lamotte-Brasseur *et al., Biotechnol. Genet. Eng. Rev.* **12**, 189-230 (1994). Review of metabolism: K. Snell, D. A. Fell, *Adv. Enzyme Regul.* **30**, 13-32 (1990).

Hexagonal plates or prisms. Sweetish taste, insipid aftertaste. Dec 228°. Sublimes at 150° in high vac (10^{-4} mm Hg). $[\alpha]_D^{20}$ −6.83° (c = 10.41); $[\alpha]_D^{25}$ +14.95° (c = 9.34 in 1*N* HCl). Absorption spectrum: *Z. Physiol. Chem.* **176**, 257 (1928). Sol in water. Insol in common neutral solvents.

DL-Form. [302-84-1] Monoclinic prismatic leaflets from water. d 1.537. Dec 246° (closed capillary, bath preheated to 225°). Sublimes at 150° in high vac (10^{-4} mm Hg). pK_1 2.21; pK_2 9.15. Soly in water (g/l) at 0° = 22.04; at 25° = 50.23; at 50° = 103; at 75° = 192; at 100° = 322. Insol in common neutral solvents.

D-Form. [312-84-5] Presence in rat brain: A. Hashimoto *et al., FEBS Lett.* **296**, 33 (1992). As synaptic modulator: M. J Schell *et al., Proc. Natl. Acad. Sci. USA* **92**, 3948 (1995).

8461. Sermorelin. [86168-78-7] Human growth hormone-releasing factor(1-29)amide; human pancreatic somatoliberin(1-29)amide; GRF(1-29)NH₂; hpGRF(1-29)NH₂; SM-8144; Geref; Groliberin. $C_{149}H_{246}N_{44}O_{42}S$; mol wt 3357.88. C 53.30%, H 7.38%, N 18.35%, O 20.01%, S 0.95%. Amidated fragment of human somatoliberin, *q.v.* Characterization of *in vitro* activity: J. Rivier *et al., Nature* **300**, 276 (1982). Prepn: N. Ling *et al., Biochem. Biophys. Res. Commun.* **123**, 854 (1984); J. E. F. Rivier *et al.,* **US 4703035** (1987 to Salk Inst. Biol. Stud.). Clinical pharmacology: M. Losa *et al., Klin. Wochenschr.* **62**, 1140 (1984). Clinical evaluation in growth hormone deficiency: M. B. Ranke *et al., Eur. J. Pediatr.* **145**, 485 (1986); R. Hümmelink *et al., Acta Paediatr. Scand.* **Suppl. 331**, 48 (1987). Field trial in pigs and dairy heifers: D. Petitclerc *et al., J. Anim. Sci.* **65**, 996 (1987).

¹Tyr-Ala-Asp-Ala-Ile-Phe-Thr-Asn-Ser-Tyr-Arg-Lys-Val-Leu-Gly

²⁹NH₂Arg-Ser-Met-Ile-Asp-Gln-Leu-Leu-Lys-Arg-Ala-Ser-Leu-Gln

$[\alpha]_D^{20}$ −63.1° (c = 1 in 30% acetic acid).

THERAP CAT: Growth hormone releasing factor.

8462. Serotonin. [50-67-9] 3-(2-Aminoethyl)-1*H*-indol-5-ol; 5-hydroxytryptamine; 3-(β-aminoethyl)-5-hydroxyindole; 5-hydroxy-3-(β-aminoethyl)indole; enteramine; thrombocytin; thrombotonin; 5-HT. $C_{10}H_{12}N_2O$; mol wt 176.22. C 68.16%, H 6.86%, N 15.90%, O 9.08%. Vasoactive amine found in tissues and fluids of vertebrates and invertebrates. Extraction of enteramine from rabbit tissue, pharmacology: V. Erspamer, *Arch. Exp. Pathol. Pharmakol.* **196**, 343 (1940). Isoln of 5-HT from beef serum: M. M. Rapport *et al., Science* **108**, 329 (1948); *eidem, J. Biol. Chem.* **176**, 1237, 1243 (1948); M. M. Rapport, *ibid.* **180**, 961 (1949). Identity with enteramine, the enterochromaffin cell hormone: V. Erspamer, B. Asero, *Nature* **169**, 800 (1952). Ultrastructural localization in enterochromaffin cells: R. D. Dey, J. Hoffpauir, *J. Histochem. Cytochem.* **32**, 661 (1984). Synthesis starting with 5-benzyloxyindole: M. E. Speeter *et al., J. Am. Chem. Soc.* **73**, 5514 (1951); K. E. Hamlin, **US 2715129** (1955 to Abbott). Alternate routes: R. Justoni, R, Pessina, **US 2947757** (1960 to Vismara). Pharmacology: G. Reid, M. Rand, *Nature* **169**, 801 (1952). Existence of multiple serotonin receptors: S. J. Peroutka, S. H. Snyder, *Mol. Pharmacol.* **16**, 687 (1979); G. Engel *et al., Arch. Pharmacol.* **324**, 116 (1983); W. Feniuk *et al., Eur. J. Pharmacol.* **96**, 71 (1983). Extraneural syn-

Consult the Name Index before using this section.

thesis in CNS: C. Maruki *et al., J. Neurochem.* **43,** 316 (1984). Effect on smooth muscle: W. Feniuk *et al., loc. cit.* Activity as neurotransmitter: S. G. Griffith *et al., Brain Res.* **247,** 388 (1982). Role in hemostasis: F. De Clerck *et al., Agents Actions* **15,** 627 (1984). Series of articles on role in hypertension, Raynaud's phenomenon and platelet activation: *J. Cardiovasc. Pharmacol.* **7,** Suppl. 7, 1-182 (1985). Review of role in migraine: E. T. MacKenzie *et al., Cephalalgia* **5,** 69-78 (1985). *Review:* V. Erspamer in E. Jucker, *Prog. Drug Res.* **3,** 151-367 (1961). Books: *Serotonin in Health and Disease* vols. I-V, W. B. Essman, Ed. (Spectrum, New York, 1978); *Adv. Exp. Med.* **133,** entitled "Serotonin: Current Aspects of Neurochemistry and Function," B. Haber, Ed. (1981) 824 pp; *Serotonin and the Cardiovascular System*, P. M. Vanhoutte, Ed. (Raven Press, New York, 1985) 280 pp. *See also* Bufotenine and Ketanserin.

Hydrochloride. $C_{10}H_{12}N_2O.HCl$. Hygroscopic crystals, sensitive to light, mp 167-168°. Water sol. Aq solns are stable at pH 2-6.4.

Complex with creatinine sulfate, monohydrate. Antemovis. $C_{14}H_{21}N_5O_6S.H_2O$; mol wt 405.43. Plates, 215° dec. uv max (water at pH 3.5): 275 nm (ε 15000). $pK_1' = 4.9$; $pK_2' = 9.8$. pH of 0.01 molar aq soln: 3.6. Sol in glacial acetic acid. Very sparingly sol in methanol, 95% ethanol. Insol in abs ethanol, acetone, pyridine, chloroform, ethyl acetate, ether, benzene.

8463. Serpentaria. Snakeroot; snakeweed; sangrel; birthwort. Dried rhizome and roots of *Aristolochia serpentaria* L. (Virginia snakeroot), and of *Aristolochia reticulata* Nutt. (Texas snakeroot), *Aristolochiaceae. Habit.* U.S. *Constit.* Aristolochic acid, volatile oil (~1%), resin, tannin.

THERAP CAT: Bitter tonic.

8464. Serpentine (Alkaloid). [18786-24-8] 3,4,5,6,16,17-Hexadehydro-16-(methoxycarbonyl)-19α-methyloxayohimbanium. $C_{21}H_{20}N_2O_3$; mol wt 348.40. C 72.40%, H 5.79%, N 8.04%, O 13.78%. From roots of *Rauwolfia serpentina* (L.) Benth., *Apocynaceae:* Schlittler, Schwarz, *Helv. Chim. Acta* **33,** 1463 (1950). Structure: Schlittler *et al., ibid.* **37,** 1912 (1954); Klohs *et al., J. Am. Chem. Soc.* **76,** 1332 (1954); Wenkert, Roychaudhuri, *ibid.* **80,** 1613 (1958). Stereoisomer of alstonine, *q.v.* Stereochemistry: Fritz, *Ann.* **655,** 148 (1962); Shamma, Richey, *J. Am. Chem. Soc.* **85,** 2507 (1963).

Solvated, yellow rods or leaflets from abs ethanol, mp 158° (air-dried), mp 175° (after drying at 120° in a high vacuum, but still not entirely solvent-free). Dec and turns red on drying at 150°. $[\alpha]_D^{25}$ +292° (c = 0.27 in methanol); $[\alpha]_D^{25}$ +267° (c = 0.21 in ethanol). uv max (ethanol): 252, 308, 370 nm (log ε 4.49, 4.30, 3.61). Freely sol in methanol. Sol in 10% acetic acid, in other organic solvents.

Nitrate. $C_{21}H_{20}N_2O_3.HNO_3$. Yellow crystals, mp 170-172°. Only slightly sol in water.

Hydrochloride monohydrate. $C_{21}H_{20}N_2O_3.HCl.H_2O$. Yellow crystals, mp 246-248°. $[\alpha]_D^{23}$ +178°. Sol in water.

Perchlorate. $C_{21}H_{20}N_2O_3.HClO_4$. Yellow crystals, mp 255-256°. $[\alpha]_D^{22}$ +185° (c = 0.5 in acetone). uv max (methanol): 252, 306-308, 365-370 nm (log ε 4.54, 4.35, 3.68).

8465. Sertaconazole. [99592-32-2] 1-[2-[(7-Chlorobenzo[*b*]thien-3-yl)methoxy]-2-(2,4-dichlorophenyl)ethyl]-1*H*-imidazole; (±)-1-[2,4-dichloro-β-[(7-chlorobenzo[*b*]thien-3-yl)meth-

oxy]phenethyl]imidazole; 7-chloro-3-[1-(2,4-dichlorophenyl)-2-(1*H*-imidazol-1-yl)ethoxy-methyl]benzo[*b*]thiophene; FI-7045. $C_{20}H_{15}Cl_3N_2OS$; mol wt 437.77. C 54.87%, H 3.45%, Cl 24.30%, N 6.40%, O 3.65%, S 7.32%. Prepn: R. Foguet *et al.,* **EP 151477;** *eidem,* **US 5135943** (1985, 1992 both to Ferrer). Synthesis, antifungal activity, pharmacology, toxicology and clinical evaluations: Arzneimittel-Forsch. **42,** 689-774 (1992). Physical props: C. Albet *et al., ibid.* 695. HPLC determn: *eidem, J. Pharm. Biomed. Anal.* **10,** 205 (1992).

mp 146-147°.

Nitrate. [99592-39-9] FI-7056; Dermofix; Zalain. $C_{20}H_{15}Cl_3-N_2OS.HNO_3$; mol wt 500.78. Odorless, white crystalline powder, mp 158-160°. Fairly sol in ethanol (1.7%); chloroform (1.5%); slightly sol in acetone (0.95%); very slightly sol in *n*-octanol (0.069%). Practically insol in water (<0.01%). pKb: 7.26. uv max (methanol): 302.3 ($A_{1cm}^{1\%}$ 79.8), 292.9 260.3 nm.

THERAP CAT: Antifungal.

8466. Sertindole. [106516-24-9] 1-[2-[4-[5-Chloro-1-(4-fluorophenyl)-1*H*-indol-3-yl]-1-piperidinyl]ethyl]-2-imidazolidinone; 5-chloro-1-(4-fluorophenyl)-3-[1-[2-(2-imidazolidinon-1-yl)-ethyl]-4-piperidyl]-1*H*-indole; Lu-23-174; Serdolect. $C_{24}H_{26}-ClFN_4O$; mol wt 440.94. C 65.37%, H 5.94%, Cl 8.04%, F 4.31%, N 12.71%, O 3.63%. Combined dopamine (D_2) and serotonin (5-HT$_2$) receptor antagonist. Prepn: J. K. Perregaard, **EP 200322;** *idem,* **US 4710500** (1986, 1987 both to Lundbeck); *idem et al., J. Med. Chem.* **35,** 1092 (1992). Neuropharmacology and receptor binding study: C. Sanchez *et al., Drug Dev. Res.* **22,** 239 (1991). Reviews of clinical efficacy and safety: J. M. Kane, *Int. Clin. Psychopharmacol.* **13,** Suppl. 3, S59-S64 (1997); A. S. Hale, *ibid.* S65-S70.

Crystals from acetone, mp 154-155°. Second crystal modification from 2-propanol + ethyl acetate, mp 166°.

THERAP CAT: Antipsychotic.

8467. Sertraline. [79617-96-2] (1*S*,4*S*)-4-(3,4-Dichlorophenyl)-1,2,3,4-tetrahydro-*N*-methyl-1-naphthalenamine. $C_{17}H_{17}-Cl_2N$; mol wt 306.23. C 66.68%, H 5.60%, Cl 23.15%, N 4.57%. Selective serotonin reuptake inhibitor (SSRI). Prepn: W. M. Welch *et al.,* **EP 30081;** *eidem,* **US 4536518** (1981, 1985 both to Pfizer); and stereospecific activity: W. M. Welch *et al., J. Med. Chem.* **27,** 1508 (1984). GC determn in plasma: H. G. Fouda *et al., J. Chromatogr.* **417,** 197 (1987). Comprehensive description: B. M. Johnson, P.-T. L. Chang, *Anal. Profiles Drug Subs. Excip.* **24,** 443-486 (1996). Review of pharmacology and clinical efficacy in depression and obsessive-compulsive disorder: D. Murdoch, D. McTavish, *Drugs* **44,** 604-624 (1992). Clinical trial in posttraumatic stress disorder: K. Brady *et al., J. Am. Med. Assoc.* **283,** 1837 (2000).

Hydrochloride. [79559-97-0] CP-51974-1; Lustral; Zoloft. $C_{17}H_{17}Cl_2N \cdot HCl$; mol wt 342.69. Crystals, mp 243-245°. $[\alpha]_D^{23}$ +37.9° (c = 2 in methanol). Soly room temp. (mg/ml): water 3.8; 0.1N HCl 0.51; 0.1N NaOH 0.002; ethanol 15.7; isopropyl alcohol 4.3; chloroform 110; acetone 1.1; N,N-dimethylformamide 88; dimethylsulfoxide 147; ethyl acetate 0.20; acetonitrile 0.85; methanolic 0.1N HCl 47; chloroform/methanol (1:1) 134. pKa (water): 9.48 ± 0.04. pKa (methanol:water, 40:60 v/v): 8.6. pKa (ethanol:water, 1:1 v/v): 8.5. d 1.37.

THERAP CAT: Antidepressant; antiobsessional.

8468. Serum Albumin. [9048-46-8] Most abundant of the plasma proteins (comprising ~60%). Structure characterized as a single, carbohydrate-free polypeptide chain consisting of 580-585 amino acid residues; stabilized by seventeen S-S bridges. Main biological functions include maintenance of osmotic pressure and the transport of sparingly soluble physiological and pharmacological substances, esp long-chain fatty acids and bilirubin. Trace amounts present in normal urine, excreted as the major protein constit in the condition of proteinuria. Review of determn in serum and plasma: P. G. Hill, *Ann. Clin. Biochem.* **22**, 565-578 (1985); of biosynthesis and biological function: M. A. Rothschild *et al.*, *Hepatology* **8**, 385-401 (1988); of structural studies: D. C. Carter, J. X. Ho, *Adv. Protein Chem.* **45**, 153-203 (1994).

Human serum albumin. HSA; Albuminar; Buminate; Pro-Bumin. Review of biochemistry and clinical experience: *Proceedings of the Workshop on Albumin*, J. T. Sgouris, A. René, Eds. (DHEW Publication No. (NIH) 76-925, 1975) 355 pp; of therapeutic use: G. E. Hastings, P. G. Wolf, *Arch. Fam. Med.* **1**, 281-287 (1992). Mol wt 65,000. Net charge per molecule (pH 7.4) −19. High solubility at neutrality: 30% solns prepd in water, 40% solns prepd in methanol or ethanol. Below pH 3, sol in 80-100% methanol, ethanol or acetone. Low viscosity. Stable, even at high temperatures.

^{131}I-labelled form. Iodinated (^{131}I) human serum albumin; ^{131}I HSA; Albumotope-^{131}I. Normal human serum albumin mildly iodinated with radioactive iodine (^{131}I) which has a half-life of 8 days, and emits beta and gamma rays. Contains not more than one atom of iodine per molecule of albumin. Physical and chemical properties essentially the same as those of albumin. Stable at 10° for at least 3 weeks. Supplied for injection in aq isotonic sodium chloride soln.

Sonicated human serum albumin. [150103-82-5] Albunex. Suspension of air filled albumin microspheres in a 5% (w/v) human albumin soln. Prepn: M. W. Keller *et al.*, *J. Am. Coll. Cardiol.* **12**, 1039 (1988); D. Cerny *et al.*, **EP 359246**; *eidem*, **US 4957656** (both 1990 to Molecular Biosystems). Pharmacology: M. W. Keller *et al.*, *J. Am. Soc. Echocardiogr.* **2**, 48 (1989). Diagnostic use in echocardiography: L. J. Crouse *et al.*, *J. Am. Coll. Cardiol.* **22**, 1494 (1993). Physical and biochemical properties: C. Christiansen *et al.*, *Biotechnol. Appl. Biochem.* **19**, 307 (1994). *Review:* N. Sponheim *et al.*, *IEEE Conf. Publ., Acoustic Sensing and Imaging* **369**, 103-108 (1993). pH 6.79-6.86. Osmolality 253-264 mmol/kg. Viscosity 1.44.

THERAP CAT: Plasma volume expander; treatment of hypoproteinemia. ^{131}I-labelled form as diagnostic aid (blood volume determination). Sonicated form as diagnostic aid (ultrasound contrast agent).

8469. Sesame Oil. Benne oil; teel oil; gingilli oil. From the seeds of cultivated varieties of *Sesamum indicum* L., *Pedaliaceae*. Constit. Olein, stearin, palmitin, myristin, linolein, sesamin, sesamolin. *Review:* Budowski, Markley, *Chem. Rev.* **48**, 125 (1951).

Pale yellow oil; almost odorless; bland taste. d 0.916-0.920. Solidif about −5°. $[\alpha]_D^{25}$ +1 to +9°. n_D^{40} 1.4650-1.4665. Sapon

no. 188-193. Iodine no. 103-122. Soluble in chloroform, ether, petr ether, carbon disulfide; slightly sol in alcohol. Insol in water.

USE: Manuf oleomargarine, cosmetics, iodized oil, etc. Pharmaceutic aid (solvent).

THERAP CAT (VET): Formerly as emollient, pediculicide.

8470. Sesamin. [607-80-7] 5,5′-(Tetrahydro-1H,3H-furo[3,4-c]furan-1,4-diyl)bis-1,3-benzodioxole; tetrahydro-1,4-bis[3,4-(methylenedioxy)phenyl]-1H,3H-furo[3,4-c]furan; 2,6-bis(3,4-methylenedioxyphenyl)-3,7-dioxabicyclo[3.3.0]octane. $C_{20}H_{18}O_6$; mol wt 354.35. C 67.79%, H 5.12%, O 27.09%. Isolated from the bark of various *Fagara* species; from sesame oil: Bertram *et al.*, *Biochem. Z.* **197**, 1 (1928); from fruit of *Piper lowong* Blume, *Piperaceae*: Peinemann, *Arch. Pharm.* **234**, 238 (1896). Structure: Cohen, *Rec. Trav. Chim.* **57**, 653 (1938). Synthesis of *dl*-form: Beroza, Schechter, *J. Am. Chem. Soc.* **78**, 1242 (1956); Freudenberg, *Naturwissenschaften* **43**, 16 (1956). Identity of *dl*-form with *fagarol*: Carnmalm, *Acta Chem. Scand.* **9**, 1111 (1955); identity of *d*-form with *pseudocubebin*: *idem, ibid.* **10**, 134 (1956). Stereochemistry of the *d*-isomer: Freudenberg, Sidhu, *Ber.* **94**, 851 (1961); Becker, Beroza, *Tetrahedron Lett.* **1962**, 157. *Review:* Budowski, *J. Am. Oil Chem. Soc.* **41**, 280 (1964).

(+)-Sesamin

d-Form. Needles from ethanol, mp 122-123°. $[\alpha]_D^{20}$ +64.5° (c = 1.75 in chloroform).

dl-Form. Crystals from ethanol, mp 125-126°. Freely sol in chloroform, benzene, acetic acid, acetone. Practically insol in water, alkaline solns and hydrochloric acid.

USE: Insecticide synergist.

8471. Sesamolin. [526-07-8] 5-[4-(1,3-Benzodioxol-5-yloxy)tetrahydro-1H,3H-furo[3,4-c]furan-1-yl]-1,3-benzodioxole; tetrahydro-1-[3,4-(methylenedioxy)phenoxy]-4-[3,4-(methylenedioxy)phenyl]-1H,3H-furo[3,4-c]furan. $C_{20}H_{18}O_7$; mol wt 370.35. C 64.86%, H 4.90%, O 30.24%. Constituent of sesame seeds, the seeds of *Sesamum indicum* L., *Pedaliaceae*. Isoln: Canzoneri, Perciabosco, *Gazz. Chim. Ital.* **33**, II, 253 (1907). Structure and synthesis: J. Boseken, W. D. Cohen, *Rec. Trav. Chim.* **55**, 815 (1936); E. Haslam, R. D. Haworth, *J. Chem. Soc.* **1955**, 827. Stereochemistry: E. Haslam, *ibid.* **1970**, 2332.

White plates from ethanol, mp 93-94°. $[\alpha]_D^{20}$ +212° (chloroform).
USE: Synergist for pyrethrum insecticides.

8472. Setastine. [64294-95-7] 1-[2-[1-(4-Chlorophenyl)-1-phenylethoxy]ethyl]hexahydro-1H-azepine; 1-[2-[(p-chloro-α-methyl-α-phenylbenzyl)oxy]ethyl]hexahydro-1H-azepine; 1-[2-(4-chloro-α-methyl-α-phenylbenzyloxy)ethyl]azepam; N-[2-(4-methyl-p-chlorobenzhydryloxy)ethyl]hexamethyleneimine; N-[2-[(4-chloro-α-methyl-α-phenylbenzyl)oxy]ethyl]hexamethylenimine. $C_{22}H_{28}ClNO$; mol wt 357.92. C 73.83%, H 7.89%, Cl 9.91%, N 3.91%, O 4.47%. Nonsedating-type histamine H_1-receptor antagonist; structurally similar to clemastine, *q.v.* Prepn: I. Beck *et al.*, **DE 2528194** (1976 to EGYT), *C.A.* **85**, 46439h (1976). *In vitro* antihistaminic activity: A. Németh, Z. Huszti, *Agents Actions* **23**,

194 (1988). Clinical pharmacology: Z. Vezekényi *et al.*, *Acta Med. Hung.* **44**, 55 (1987).

Hydrochloride. [59767-13-4] EGIS-2062; EGYT-2062; Loderix. $C_{22}H_{28}ClNO.HCl$; mol wt 394.38.

THERAP CAT: Antihistaminic.

8473. Sethoxydim. [74051-80-2] 2-[1-(Ethoxyimino)butyl]-5-[2-(ethylthio)propyl]-3-hydroxy-2-cyclohexen-1-one; BAS-9052; NP-55; Poast. $C_{17}H_{29}NO_3S$; mol wt 327.48. C 62.35%, H 8.93%, N 4.28%, O 14.66%, S 9.79%. Selective post-emergence herbicide. Prepn: JP Kokai 81 75408 (1981 to Nippon Soda), *C.A.* **95**, 110175e (1981). Activity: C. M. Knott, *Proc. Br. Crop Prot. Conf. - Weeds* **1980**, 39; G. H. Ingram *et al.*, *ibid.* 91.

USE: Herbicide.

8474. Sevelamer. [52757-95-6] 2-Propen-1-amine polymer with (chloromethyl)oxirane; allylamine polymer with 1-chloro-2,3-epoxypropane; allylamine-epichlorohydrin copolymer; poly(allylamin-co-*N,N'*-diallyl-1,3-diamino-2-hydroxypropane). Polymeric non-absorbed phosphate binder consisting of polyallylamine crosslinked with epichlorohydrin to form a hydrogel where 40% of the amines are protonated. Follows the general formula of $(C_3H_7N.C_3-H_5ClO)_n$. Binds dietary phosphate leading to increased fecal excretion, decreased absorption and decreased serum phosphorous levels. Prepd not claimed: S. R. Holmes-Farley *et al.*, **WO 9505184**; *eidem*, **US 5496545** (1995, 1996 both to GelTex). Mechanism of action: S. R. Holmes-Farley *et al.*, *J. Macromol. Sci. Pure Appl. Chem.* **A36**, 1085 (1999). Determn of phosphate binding capacity: J. R. Mazzeo *et al.*, *J. Pharm. Biomed. Anal.* **19**, 911 (1999). Clinical studies in end stage renal disease: E. A. Slatopolsky *et al.*, *Kidney Int.* **55**, 299 (1999).

Hydrochloride. [152751-57-0] PB-94; GT16-026A; Renagel. Insol in water. Hydrophilic.

THERAP CAT: Antihyperphosphatemic.

8475. Sevoflurane. [28523-86-6] 1,1,1,3,3,3-Hexafluoro-2-(fluoromethoxy)propane; fluoromethyl 2,2,2-trifluoro-1-(trifluoromethyl)ethyl ether; fluoromethyl 1,1,1,3,3,3-hexafluoro-2-propyl ether; Sevofrane; Sevorane. $C_4H_3F_7O$; mol wt 200.05. C 24.02%, H 1.51%, F 66.48%, O 8.00%. $(CF_3)_2CHOCH_2F$. Prepn: B. M. Regan, J. C. Longstreet, **DE 1954268**; *eidem*, **US 3689571** (1970, 1972 both to Baxter Labs.). Pharmacology and physicochemical properties: R. F. Wallin *et al.*, *Anesth. Analg.* **54**, 758 (1975). Clinical pharmacology and metabolism: D. A. Holaday, F. R. Smith, *Anesthesiology* **54**, 100 (1981). Toxicity study: D. P. Strum *et al.*, *Anesth. Analg.* **66**, 769 (1987). Minimum alveolar concentration (MAC) in man: T. Katoh, K. Ikeda, *Anesthesiology* **66**, 301 (1987). Preliminary clinical evaluation in pheochromocytoma: M. Doi, K. Ikeda, *ibid.* **70**, 360 (1989).

Volatile liquid; bp_{751} 58.1-58.2°; bp_{760} 58.5°. d_4^{23} 1.505. Vapor pressure (25°): 200 torr; (20°): 160 torr. Nonflammable in air at ambient temps; flammability limit in O_2: 11 vol. percent; in N_2O:

10 vol. percent. Partition coefficient at 37° (blood/gas): 0.60±0.07; (water/gas): 0.36±0.01; (corn oil/gas): 41.6±2.1.

THERAP CAT: Anesthetic (inhalation).

8476. Seyferth-Gilbert Reagent. [27491-70-9] (Diazomethyl)phosphonic acid dimethyl ester; dimethyl diazomethylphosphonate. $C_3H_7N_2O_3P$; mol wt 150.07. C 24.01%, H 4.70%, N 18.67%, O 31.98%, P 20.64%. Divalent carbon transfer reagent. Prepn: D. Seyferth, R. S. Marmor, *Tetrahedron Lett.* **11**, 2493 (1970); and applications in organophosphorus syntheses: D. Seyferth *et al.*, *J. Org. Chem.* **36**, 1379 (1971). Reactions with aldehydes and aryl ketones to form alkynes: J. C. Gilbert, U. Weerasooriya, *ibid.* **47**, 1837 (1982). Improved prepn: D. G. Brown *et al.*, *ibid.* **61**, 2540 (1996).

Distillable yellow liquid; $bp_{0.42}$ 59°. n_D^{25} 1.4585.

USE: Reagent for one-carbon homologation of aldehydes and ketones to alkynes.

8477. Shark Liver Oil. [68990-63-6] Robecote. Oil expressed from the livers of sharks and other *Elasmobranchii* species. *Constit:* Squalene, pristane, vitamins A and D, esters of fatty acids (esp. palmitic and oleic), glycerol ethers, triglycerides, cholesterol and fatty alcohols. Isoln: A. Ehrenreich, **GB 284657** (1927); C. E. Brown, S. A. Reed, **GB 1021542** (1966 to Marfleet Refining Co. Ltd.). Composition: N. A. Sörensen, J. Mehlum, *Acta Chem. Scand.* **2**, 140 (1948); E. Gelpi, J. Oro, *J. Am. Oil Chem. Soc.* **45**, 144 (1968); R. Lombardi *et al.*, *Ann. Pharm. Fr.* **29**, 429 (1971). Comparison with cod liver oil: A. O. Banjo, *J. Food Technol.* **14**, 107 (1979).

Clear, yellow oil. Phys props of liver oil from basking shark: n_D^{20} 1.4784; d^{20} 0.922; sapon no. 140-146; iodine no. 140-145 (Lombardi).

THERAP CAT: Topical protectant.

8478. Shellac. [9000-59-3] Lacca; lac. A resinous excretion of the insect *Laccifer (Tachardia) lacca* Kerr, order *Homoptera*, family *Coccidae*. Different resiniferous trees of India serve as host trees as the season progresses. The insects suck the juice of the tree and excrete "stick-lac" almost continuously. Whitest shellac is produced while the kusum tree (*Schleichera trijuga*) is the host. Most shellac is produced in the Central and in the United provinces of India and in the states of Bihar and Orissa. The major component of lac is a resin which upon mild hydrolysis gives a complex mixture of aliphatic and alicyclic hydroxy acids and their polyesters. The composition of the hydrolysate depends on the lac source and the time of collection. The major component of the aliphatic fraction is aleuritic acid, *q.v.*; the major component of the alicyclic fraction is shellolic acid, *q.v.*: Yates, Field, *Tetrahedron* **26**, 3135 (1970). Physical and chemical properties of shellac: Cockeran, Levine, *J. Soc. Cosmet. Chem.* **12**, 316 (1961). Trends in shellac chemistry: *eidem, Am. Ink Maker* **39** (7), 26 (1961); E. Hicks, *Shellac, Its Origin and Applications* (Chemical Publ. Co., New York, 1961). Review: J. Martin in *Kirk-Othmer Encyclopedia of Chemical Technology* **vol. 20** (Wiley-Interscience, New York, 3rd ed., 1982) pp 737-747.

Brittle, yellowish, transparent sheets or crushed pieces or powder. d 1.035-1.140. mp 115-120°. Sapon no. 185-210; iodine no. 10-18. Solubility in alcohol 85-95% w/w (very slowly sol); in ether 13-15%; in benzene 10-20%; in petr ether 2-6%. Sparingly sol in oil of turpentine. Insol in water; sol in aq solns of ethanolamines, of alkalies or borax with slightly purple color.

USE: Chiefly in lacquers and varnishes; also in manuf buttons, grinding wheels, sealing wax, cements, inks, phonograph records, paper; for stiffening hats; in electrical machines; coating confections and medicinal tablets; finishing leather.

8479. Shellolic Acid. [4448-95-7] [3R-(3α,3aβ,4α,7β,8α,-8aα)]-2,3,4,7,8,8a-Hexahydro-4-hydroxy-8-(hydroxymethyl)-8-methyl-1*H*-3a,7-methanoazulene-3,6-dicarboxylic acid; 10β,13-dihydroxycedr-8-ene-12,15-dioic acid. $C_{15}H_{20}O_6$; mol wt 296.32.

C 60.80%, H 6.80%, O 32.40%. Major component of the alicyclic fraction of shellac hydrolysate of which it usually constitutes 5-8%. Isoln: Harries, Nagel, *Ber.* **55**, 3833 (1922); Nagel, Mertens, *ibid.* **70**, 2173 (1937); Kirk *et al., J. Am. Chem. Soc.* **63**, 1243 (1941). Structure studies: Carruthers *et al., J. Chem. Soc.* **1961**, 5251; Cookson *et al., Tetrahedron* **18**, 547, 1321 (1962); Yates, Field, *ibid.* **26**, 3135 (1970). Stereochemistry: Yates *et al., ibid.* **26**, 3159 (1970).

Crystals, mp 204-207°.

Dimethyl ester. Crysts from ethyl acetate, mp 153-154.5°. uv max (ethanol): 231 nm (ε 6200).

8480. Shikimic Acid. [138-59-0] [3*R*-(3α,4α,5β)]-3,4,5-Trihydroxy-1-cyclohexene-1-carboxylic acid. $C_7H_{10}O_5$; mol wt 174.15. C 48.28%, H 5.79%, O 45.94%. Naturally occurring (−)-form is a major biosynthetic precursor of phenylalanine, tyrosine, and tryptophan and hence of the majority of plant alkaloids. It is also involved in the biosynthesis of lignin, *q.v.,* flavonoids and other important aromatic compounds. Isoln from the fruit of the oriental plant *Illicium religiosum* Sieb. et Zucc., *Magnoliaceae* (called in Japanese *shikimi-no-ki*): J. F. Eykman, *Rec. Trav. Chim.* **4**, 32 (1885); *idem, Ber.* **24**, 1278 (1891). Structural study: H. O. L. Fischer, G. Dangshat, *Helv. Chim. Acta* **17**, 1200 (1934). Configuration: *eidem, ibid.* **18**, 1206 (1935); **20**, 705 (1937). Conformation in soln: L. D. Hall, *J. Org. Chem.* **29**, 297 (1964). Enzymatic synthesis: P. R. Srinivasan *et al., J. Am. Chem. Soc.* **77**, 4943 (1955). Stereospecific synthesis: R. McCrindle *et al., J. Chem. Soc.* **1960**, 1560; E. E. Smissman *et al., J. Am. Chem. Soc.* **84**, 1040 (1962). Improved synthesis: J. L. Pawlak, G. A. Berchtold, *J. Org. Chem.* **52**, 1765 (1987). Synthesis of the (±)-form: R. Grewe, I. Hinrichs, *Ber.* **97**, 443 (1964); R. Grewe, S. Kersten, *Angew. Chem.* **77**, 859 (1965). Carcinogenicity study: I. A. Evans, M. A. Osman, *Nature* **250**, 348 (1974). *Reviews:* B. A. Bohm, *Chem. Rev.* **65**, 435-466 (1965); B. Ganem, *Tetrahedron* **34**, 3353-3383 (1978); J. B. Harborne, *Biosynthesis* **6**, 40-75 (1980). Books: E. Haslam, *The Shikimate Pathway* (Halsted Press, New York, 1974) 316 pp; *idem,* "Shikimic Acid Metabolites" in *Comprehensive Organic Chemistry* vol. 5 (Pergamon Press, Oxford, 1979) pp 1167-1205; U. Weiss, J. M. Edwards, *The Biosynthesis of Organic Compounds* (Wiley, New York, 1980) 728 pp.

Needles from methanol/ethyl acetate, mp 183-184.5°. Sublimes. [α]$_D$ −161° (c = 0.57 in methanol). [α]$_D^{18}$ −183.8° (c = 4.03 in water). uv max (alcohol): 213 nm (ε 8900). pK (14.1°) 5.19. Soly in water about 18 g/100 ml. Soly at 23° (g/100 m): 2.25 in abs alcohol: 0.015 in anhydr ether. Practically insol in chloroform, benzene, petr ether. LD$_5$ i.p. in mice: 1000 mg/kg (Evans, Osman).

(±)-**Form.** Needles from methanol/ethyl acetate, mp 191-192°. uv max (ethanol): 212 nm (ε 8200).

8481. Shionone. [10376-48-4] (1*R*,4a*S*,4b*S*,6a*S*,8*R*,10a*R*,-10b*S*,12a*S*)-Hexadecahydro-1,4b,6a,8,10a,12a-hexamethyl-8-(4-methyl-3-pentenyl)-2(1*H*)-chrysenone; *D:A*-friedo-18,19-secolup-19-en-3-one; 3β,5α,8,17aβ-tetramethyl-3-(4-methyl-3-pentenyl)-*D*-homoandrostan-17-one. $C_{30}H_{50}O$; mol wt 426.72. C 84.44%, H 11.81%, O 3.75%. From the fruit of *Aster tartaricus* L., *Compositae:* Nakaoki, *J. Pharm. Soc. Jpn.* **52**, 499 (1932); *C.A.* **26**, 4821[4] (1932); Takahashi *et al., ibid.* **79**, 1281 (1959); *C.A.* **54**, 4667g (1960). Structure: Y. Tanahashi *et al., Bull. Soc. Chim. Fr.* **1966**, 1670. Conformation: Y. Moriyama *et al., ibid.* **1968**, 2890.

Crystals from alc, mp 161-162°. [α]$_D^{26.5}$ −56.1° (c = 1.07 in chloroform). uv max (chloroform): 290 nm (log ε 1.47).

8482. Showdomycin. [16755-07-0] 3-β-D-Ribofuranosyl-1*H*-pyrrole-2,5-dione; 2-β-D-ribofuranosylmaleimide. $C_9H_{11}NO_6$; mol wt 229.19. C 47.16%, H 4.84%, N 6.11%, O 41.89%. Nucleoside antibiotic isolated from *Streptomyces showdoensis:* Nishimura *et al., J. Antibiot.* **17A**, 148 (1964); Nishimura, **FR M2751** corresp to **US 3316149** (1964, 1967, both to Shionogi). Structure: Nakagawa *et al., Tetrahedron Lett.* **1967**, 4105; Darnall *et al., Proc. Natl. Acad. Sci. USA* **57**, 548 (1967). Synthesis: Kalvoda *et al., Tetrahedron Lett.* **1970**, 2297; Trummlitz, Moffatt, *J. Org. Chem.* **38**, 1841 (1973); T. Sato *et al., Tetrahedron Lett.* **1978**, 1829; J. G. Buchanan *et al., J. Chem. Soc. Perkin Trans. 1* **1979**, 225; T. Inoue, I. Kuwajima, *Chem. Commun.* **1980**, 251; A. P. Kozikowski, A. Ames, *J. Am. Chem. Soc.* **103**, 3923 (1981); Y. Araki *et al., Tetrahedron Lett.* **29**, 351 (1988). Exhibits antitumor activity: Shinzo *et al., J. Antibiot.* **17A**, 234 (1964). *Review:* D. W. Visser, S. Roy-Burman in *Antibiotics* vol. 5(pt. 2), F. E. Hahn, Ed. (Springer-Verlag, New York, 1979) pp 363-371.

Leaflets from acetone + benzene, mp 153-154°. [α]$_D^{22.5}$ +49.9° (H$_2$O). uv max: 220-221 nm (E$_{1cm}^{1\%}$ 422). Sol in water, alcohol, acetone, dioxane; insol in ethyl ether, benzene, petr ether. More stable in acid media than in neutral or alkaline. LD$_{50}$ in mice (mg/kg): 25 i.p.; 18 s.c.; 110 i.v. (Nishimura).

8483. Shvo Catalyst. [104439-77-2] Tetracarbonyl-μ-hydro[(1,2,3,4,5-η)-1-hydroxylato-2,3,4,5-tetraphenyl-2,4-cyclopentadien-1-yl][(1,2,3,4,5-η)-1-hydroxy-2,3,4,5-tetraphenyl-2,4-cyclopentadien-1-yl]diruthenium; [(η^4-tetracyclone)(CO)$_2$Ru]$_2$. C_{62}H$_{42}$O$_6$Ru$_2$; mol wt 1085.13. C 68.62%, H 3.90%, O 8.85%, Ru 18.63%. Diruthenium catalyst especially for hydrogen-transfer reactions. Prepn: Y. Blum, Y. Shvo, *J. Organomet. Chem.* **282**, C7 (1985); Y. Shvo *et al., J. Am. Chem. Soc.* **108**, 7400 (1986). X-ray structure study: M. J. Mays *et al., Organometallics* **8**, 1162 (1989). Mechanism of hydrogen transfer: J. B. Johnson, J.-E. Bäckvall, *J. Org. Chem.* **68**, 7681 (2003). Catalytic disproportionation of aldehydes: N. Menashe, Y. Shvo, *Organometallics* **10**, 3885 (1991). Resolution of alcohols: B. A. Persson *et al., J. Am. Chem. Soc.* **121**, 1645 (1999); oxidation of alcohols: J. H. Choi *et al., Tetrahedron Lett.* **45**, 4607 (2004). Brief review: R. Prabhakaran, *Synlett* **2004**, 2048-2049.

Orange crystalline solid.

USE: Catalyst in organic syntheses for hydrogen transfers including disproportionation of aldehydes, reduction of ketones and aldehydes, oxidation and/or racemization of alcohols and amines.

8484. Sialic Acids. Nonulosaminic acids. Family of amino sugars contg 9 or more carbon atoms, *N*- and *O*-substituted derivatives of neuraminic acid, *q.v.* Widely distributed throughout the animal kingdom; appear to be regular components of all types of mucoproteins, mucopolysaccharides and certain mucolipids. Bovine and ovine submaxillary gland sialic acids are diacetyl derivs. Pig submaxillary mucin, and pig, horse, and ox erythrocytes contain sialic acids having an *N*-glycolyl group. *Reviews:* A. Gottschalk, *The Chemistry and Biology of Sialic Acids and Related Substances* (Cambridge U. Press, 1960); *idem, Rev. Pure Appl. Chem.* **12,** 46 (1962). Books: *Biological Roles of Sialic Acid,* A. Rosenberg, C.-L. Schengrund, Eds. (Plenum Press, New York, 1976) 393 pp; *Sialic Acids: Chemistry, Metabolism & Function,* R. Schauer, Ed. (Springer-Verlag, New York, 1983) 346 pp.

N-Acetylneuraminic acid

N-Acetylneuraminic acid. 5-(Acetylamino)-3,5-dideoxy-D-*glycero*-D-*galacto*-2-nonulosonic acid; NAN; NANA; lactaminic acid; O-sialic acid. $C_{11}H_{19}NO_9$; mol wt 309.27. The most important of the 5 sialic acids. Isoln: Klenk, Faillard, *Z. Physiol. Chem.* **298,** 230 (1954). Prepn from sheep submaxillary mucins: Blix, *Methods Carbohydr. Chem.* **1,** 246 (1962). Synthesis: Cornforth *et al., Biochem. J.* **68,** 57 (1958); R. Csuk *et al., Helv. Chim. Acta* **71,** 609 (1988). First synthesis from non-carbohydrate sources: M. P. DeNinno, S. J. Danishevsky, *J. Org. Chem.* **51** 2615 (1986). Configuration: Kuhn, Brossmer, *Angew. Chem. Int. Ed.* **1,** 218 (1962). Crystals from water/acetic acid (0.8:12) at 5°, mp 180-182° (dec). $[\alpha]_D^{20}$ -33.1° (c = 0.9 in water).

8485. Sibutramine. [106650-56-0] 1-(4-Chlorophenyl)-*N,N*-dimethyl-α-(2-methylpropyl)cyclobutanemethanamine; *N*-1-[1-(4-chlorophenyl)cyclobutyl]-3-methylbutyl-*N,N*-dimethylamine. $C_{17}H_{26}ClN$; mol wt 279.85. C 72.96%, H 9.36%, Cl 12.67%, N 5.01%. Serotonin and noradrenaline reuptake inhibitor (SNRI); decreases calorie intake and increases energy expenditure. Prepn: J. E. Jeffery *et al.,* **DE 3212682;** *idem,* **US 4929629** (1982, 1990 both to Boots). Clinical trial in obesity: C. Hanotin *et al., Int. J. Obes.* **22,** 32 (1998). Review of pharmacology and mechanism of action: D. J. Heal *et al., ibid.,* Suppl. 1, S18-S28.

Hydrochloride monohydrate. [125494-59-9] BTS-54524; Reductil; Meridia. $C_{17}H_{26}ClN.HCl.H_2O$; mol wt 334.32. Crystals from water, mp 193-195.5°. Partition coefficient (octanol/water): 30.9 (pH 5.0). Soly in water: 2.9 mg/ml at pH 5.2.

Note: This is a controlled substance (stimulant): **21 CFR,** 1308.14.

THERAP CAT: Antiobesity agent.

8486. Siccanin. [22733-60-4] (4a*S*,6a*S*,11b*R*,13a*S*,13b*S*)-1,2,3,4,4a,5,6,6a,11b,13b-Decahydro-4,4,6a,9-tetramethyl-13*H*-

benzo[*a*]furo[2,3,4-*mn*]xanthen-11-ol; Tackle. $C_{22}H_{30}O_3$; mol wt 342.47. C 77.16%, H 8.83%, O 14.02%. Antibiotic obtained from the cultured broth of *Helminthosporium siccans* Drechsler, a parasitic organism of rye grass (*Lolium multiflorum* Lam). Isoln: K. Ishibashi, **JP 62 3548** (1962 to Sankyo); *idem, J. Antibiot.* **15A,** 161 (1962). The *cis* formation of the decahydronaphthalene system may be the first example of the naturally occurring drimane skeleton. Structure: K. Hirai *et al., Tetrahedron Lett.* **1967,** 2177; K. Hirai *et al., Tetrahedron* **27,** 6057 (1971). Approach to synthesis: H. Oida *et al., Chem. Pharm. Bull.* **20,** 2634 (1972); T. Yoshida *et al., ibid.* 2642. Total synthesis of racemate: M. Kato *et al., J. Am. Chem. Soc.* **103,** 2434 (1981); *eidem, Tetrahedron* **43,** 711 (1987). CD spectral study: S. Nozoe *et al., Tetrahedron* **30,** 2773 (1974). *In vitro* activity studies: M. Arai *et al., Antimicrob. Agents Chemother.* **1969,** 247; M. G. Bellotti, L. Riviera, *Chemioterapia* **4,** 431 (1985); *in vivo* studies: S. Sugarwara, *Antimicrob. Agents Chemother.* **1969,** 253. Toxicology: Y. Suzuki *et al., Sankyo Kenkyusho Nempo* **21,** 120 (1969), *C.A.* **72,** 130939k (1970). Mode of action: K. Nose, A. Endo, *J. Bacteriol.* **105,** 176 (1971). Biosynthesis: K. Suzuki *et al., Bioorg. Chem.* **3,** 72 (1974). Clinical evaluation in surface mycosis: D. Crippa *et al., G. Ital. Dermatol. Venereol.* **120,** 57 (1985).

White to pale yellow odorless crystals, mp 139-140°. $[\alpha]_D^{20}$ -136° (c = 2 in chloroform), uv max (ethanol): 210, 285 nm (ε 45690, 1717). pK 10.9. Very sol in chloroform, dimethylformamide, benzene; freely sol in acetone, ether, ethyl acetate; sol in alcohol. Practically insol in water. LD_{50} in mice, rats (mg/kg): >6000, >1000 orally; >3000, >600 s.c. or i.p. (Suzuki).

THERAP CAT: Antifungal.

8487. Siduron. [1982-49-6] *N*-(2-Methylcyclohexyl)-*N'*-phenylurea; Tupersan. $C_{14}H_{20}N_2O$; mol wt 232.32. C 72.38%, H 8.68%, N 12.06%, O 6.89%. Prepn: Luckenbaugh, **BE 631289** (1963 to du Pont), *C.A.* **60,** 15775h (1964), corresp to **GB 1028818.** Prepn of *trans*-form: Hayman *et al., J. Pharm. Pharmacol.* **16,** 538 (1964).

Solid, mp 133-138°. Sol in water (18 ppm); sol to the extent of 10% or more in ethanol, dimethylacetamide, dimethylformamide, methylene chloride.

trans-**Form.** Crystals, mp 157-159°.

USE: Herbicide.

8488. Silane. [7803-62-5] Silicon tetrahydride; silicane; monosilane. H_4Si; mol wt 32.12. H 12.55%, Si 87.44%. SiH_4. Prepd from aluminum silicide and hydrochloric acid or by electrolysis of an aq soln of sodium, ammonium, manganese, or ferrous chloride using an aluminum-silicon alloy as the positive pole: Buff, Wöhler, *Ann.* **102,** 128 (1857); from magnesium silicide and HCl: Wöhler, *ibid.* **106,** 56 (1858); Stock, Somiesky, *Ber.* **49,** 111 (1916); from zinc silicide and acid: Deville, Caron, *Compt. Rend.* **45,** 163 (1857); from lithium silicide and acid: Moissan, *ibid.* **135,** 1284 (1902); from magnesium silicide and ammonium bromide or chloride in liquid ammonia: Johnson, Isenberg, *J. Am. Chem. Soc.* **57,** 1349 (1935); Clasen, **DE 926069** (1952); *Angew. Chem.* **70,** 179 (1958); from lithium aluminum hydride in ether and silicon tetrachloride: Finholt *et al., J. Am. Chem. Soc.* **69,** 2692 (1947); from silica gel, aluminum oxide and hydrogen: Jackson, **US 3068069** (1962 to du Pont); from silicon tetrachloride and sodium aluminum hydride: Mason, Kelly, **US 3043664** (1962 to Allied Chem.).

Purification: Jacob, Trenner, **US 3019087** (1962 to Merck & Co.); Shoemaker, Sumrell, **US 3041141** (1962 to Baker Chem.).

Gas, repulsive odor. d^{-185} (liq) 0.68. Solidifies at approx $-200°$. mp $-185°$; bp $-112°$. Stable at ordinary temps; completely dec ~$400°$ into silicon and hydrogen; dec by an electric discharge; ignites in an atm of chlorine; ignites in air by raising the temp. Slowly dec in water; practically insol in alc, ether, benzene, chloroform, silicochloroform and silicon tetrachloride. Dec in potassium hydroxide solns.

Caution: Potential symptoms of overexposure are irritation of eyes, skin, mucous membranes; nausea, headache. *See NIOSH Pocket Guide to Chemical Hazards* (DHHS/NIOSH 97-140, 1997) p 278.

USE: Source of hyperpure silicon for semiconductors.

8489. Sildenafil. [139755-83-2] 1-[[3-(4,7-Dihydro-1-methyl-7-oxo-3-propyl-1*H*-pyrazolo[4,3-*d*]pyrimidin-5-yl)-4-ethoxyphenyl]sulfonyl]-4-methylpiperazine; 5-[2-ethoxy-5-(4-methylpiperazinylsulfonyl)phenyl]-1-methyl-3-*n*-propyl-1,6-dihydro-7*H*-pyrazolo[4,3-*d*]pyrimidin-7-one; UK-92480. $C_{22}H_{30}N_6O_4S$; mol wt 474.58. C 55.68%, H 6.37%, N 17.71%, O 13.49%, S 6.76%. Orally active, selective type 5 cGMP phosphodiesterase inhibitor. Prepn: A. S. Bell *et al., EP 463756; eidem,* **US 5250534** (1992, 1993 both to Pfizer). Structure-activity study: N. K. Terrett *et al., Bioorg. Med. Chem. Lett.* **6,** 1819 (1996). Clinical trial in impotence: I. Goldstein *et al., N. Engl. J. Med.* **338,** 1397 (1998). Review of pharmacology: M. Boolell *et al., Int. J. Impot. Res.* **8,** 47-52 (1996); of clinical experience: D. G. Hatzichristou, *ibid.* **14,** Suppl. 1, S43-S52 (2002). Clinical evaluation in pulmonary hypertension: B. K. S. Sastry *et al., J. Am. Coll. Cardiol.* **43,** 1149 (2004).

Crystals, mp 187-189°.

Citrate. [171599-83-0] Revatio; Viagra. $C_{22}H_{30}N_6O_4S.C_6H_8O_7$; mol wt 666.70.

THERAP CAT: In treatment of male erectile dysfunction. Antihypertensive.

8490. Silicic Acid. [1343-98-2] Precipitated silica. Approx H_2SiO_3. Occurs in nature as *opal.* Monograph: E. A. Hauser, *Silicic Science* (Van Nostrand, Princeton, 1958). Short review of chemistry: S. A. Greenberg, *J. Chem. Educ.* **36,** 218-219 (1959).

White, amorphous powder. Insol in water or acids except hydrofluoric (*see under* Silicon Dioxide); sol in hot fixed alk hydroxide solns.

Silica gel. Pptd silicic acid in form of lustrous granules, esp prepd and adapted for absorption of various vapors.

8491. Silicon. [7440-21-3] Si; at. wt 28.0855; at. no. 14; valence 4, also 2. Group IVA (14). Three naturally occurring isotopes: 28 (92.18%); 29 (4.71%); 30 (3.12%); artificial isotopes: 25-27; 31; 32. Does not occur free in nature; found as silica (quartz, sand, sandstone) or as silicate (feldspar or orthoclase, kaolinite, anorthite, etc.). Constitutes about 27.6% of the earth's crust; second most abundant element on earth, oxygen being first. Prepd industrially by carbon reduction of silica in an electric arc furnace. Purification by zone refining (*see* ref. *under* Germanium). Very pure silicon is obtained by decompn of silicon tetraiodide: Litton, Anderson, *J. Electrochem. Soc.* **101,** 287 (1954); *Chem. Eng. News* **34,** 5007 (1956). From silicon tetrachloride: Lyon *et al., Trans. Electrochem. Soc.* **96,** 359 (1949); Klyuchnikov, *J. Appl. Chem. USSR* **29,** 139 (1956). By thermal decompn of a chlorosilane: Schering, **US 3041144** (1962 to Siemens-Schuckertwerke). Review of silicon and its compounds: Rochow, "Silicon" in *Comprehensive Inorganic Chemistry* **vol. 1,** J. C. Bailar, Jr. *et al.,* Eds. (Pergamon Press, Oxford, 1973) pp 1323-1467; W. Runyan in *Kirk-Othmer Encyclopedia of Chemical Technology* **vol. 20** (Wiley-Inter-

science, New York, 3rd ed., 1982) pp 826-845. The uses of silicon compounds in organic chemistry: E. W. Colvin, *Chem. Soc. Rev.* **7,** 15 (1978); I. Fleming, *ibid.* **10,** 83 (1981); L. A. Paquette, *Science* **217,** 793 (1982).

Black to gray, lustrous, needle-like crystals or octahedral platelets (cubic system). The amorphous form is a dark brown powder. Poor conductor of electricity. d_4^{25} 2.33. mp 1410°. Average heat capacity (16-100°): 0.1774 cal/g/°C. Lattice constant (25°): 5.41987 × 10^{-8} cm. Compressibility (V/V_0) at 25 × 10^3 kg/cm²: 0.978; at 100 × 10^3 kg/cm²: 0.940, *Gmelins, Silicon* (8th ed.) **15B** (1959) p 57. Dielectric const: 13. Covalent bond ionization energy at 0 K = 1.2 ev. Band gap: 1.106 ev. Impurity atom ionization energy: ~0.04 ev. Intrinsic resistivity at 300 K = 0.23 megohm. Electron mobility at 300 K: 1500 cm²/volt/sec. Hole mobility at 300 K: 500 cm²/volt/sec. Intrinsic charge density at 300 K: 1.5 × 10^{10}. Electron diffusion constant at 300 K: 38. Hole diffusion constant at 300 K: 13. Practically insol in water. Attacked by hydrofluoric or a mixture of hydrofluoric and nitric acids (depending upon cryst modifications). Soluble in molten alkali oxides. Burns in fluorine, chlorine.

Caution: Potential symptoms of overexposure are irritation of eyes, skin, upper respiratory system; cough. *See NIOSH Pocket Guide to Chemical Hazards* (DHHS/NIOSH 97-140, 1997) p 278.

USE: In making silanes and silicones, the Si—C bond being about as strong as a C—C bond. In the manuf of transistors, silicon diodes and similar semiconductors. For making alloys such as ferrosilicon, silicon bronze, silicon copper. As a reducing agent like aluminum in high temp reactions.

8492. Silicon Carbide. [409-21-2] CSi; mol wt 40.10. C 29.95%, Si 70.04%. SiC. Made by heating coke and sand (and salt as flux) in electric furnace.

Exceedingly hard, green to bluish-black, iridescent, sharp crystals; hardness = 9.5. d 3.23. Dielectric constant: 7.0. Electron mobility: >100 cm²/volt-sec. Hole mobility: >20 cm²/volt-sec. Band gap energy: 2.8 ev.

Caution: Potential symptoms of overexposure are irritation of eyes, skin, upper respiratory system; cough. *See NIOSH Pocket Guide to Chemical Hazards* (DHHS/NIOSH 97-140, 1997) p 278.

USE: Polishing glass, granite; smoothing bisque ware; in sharpening-stones; abrasive; manuf porcelain, "emery" paper and wheels, shoe soles, refractory brick, furnace linings; antiskid pavements; in semiconductor technology.

8493. Silicon Dioxide. [7631-86-9] Silica; silicic anhydride. O_2Si; mol wt 60.08. O 53.26%, Si 46.75%. SiO_2. Occurs in nature as *agate, amethyst, chalcedony, cristobalite, flint, quartz, sand, tridymite.* Reviews: *Kirk-Othmer Encyclopedia of Chemical Technology* **vol. 18** (Interscience, New York, 2nd ed., 1969) pp 46-111; Rochow in *Comprehensive Inorganic Chemistry* **vol. 1,** J. C. Bailar, Jr. *et al.,* Eds. (Pergamon Press, Oxford, 1973) pp 1388-1402. Toxicology: L. T. Fairhall, *Industrial Toxicology* (Hafner, New York, 1969) pp 105-107.

Transparent, tasteless crystals, or amorphous powder. d (amorphous) 2.2. d^0 (quartz) 2.65. Melts to a glass. Silica has the lowest coefficient of expansion by heat of any known substance. It is practically insol in water and acids, except hydrofluoric acid in which it readily dissolves forming the gas silicon tetrafluoride; it is also slowly attacked by heating with concd phosphoric acid. The crystallized forms of silica are scarcely attacked by alkalies, while the amorphous is sol, especially when finely divided. *See also* Infusorial Earth.

Caution: Potential symptom of overexposure to amorphous silica are eye irritation and pneumoconiosis. Potential symptoms of overexposure to crystalline silica as respirable dust are cough, dyspnea, wheezing; decreased pulmonary function, progressive respiratory symptoms (silicosis). *See NIOSH Pocket Guide to Chemical Hazards* (DHHS/NIOSH 97-140, 1997) p 276-279. Crystalline silica (respirable size), primarily quartz dusts occurring in industrial and occupational settings, is listed as a known human carcinogen: *Report on Carcinogens, Eleventh Edition* (PB2005-104914, 2004) p III-231.

USE: Manuf glass, water glass, refractories, abrasives, ceramics, enamels; decolorizing and purifying oils, petroleum products, etc.; in scouring and grinding-compounds, ferrosilicon, molds for castings; as anticaking and defoaming agent.

8494. Silicon Disulfide. [13759-10-9] S_2Si; mol wt 92.22. S 69.54%, Si 30.45%. SiS_2. Prepd from SiO_2 and Al_2S_3: Tiede, *Ber.* **59**, 1703 (1926); Zintl, Loosen, *Z. Phys. Chem.* **A174**, 301 (1935).

White, fibrous mass or needles. Yields H_2S on contact with moist air. d 2.02. mp 1090° (sublimes). Burns when held in flame. Sol with decompn in water, alcohol, alkaline solns. Insol in benzene.

8495. Silicones. Broad family of synthetic polymers containing a repeating silicon-oxygen backbone with organic side groups attached via carbon-silicon bonds. Classified into three major types: fluids, resins and elastomers. The name was coined by F. S. Kipping under the supposition that the compounds were analogous to ketones; now used to designate a variety of complex polymeric siloxanes which may be linear, branched or cross-linked. Structural unit is represented by the formula, $[R_nSiO_{(4-n/2)}]_m$, where $n = 1$-3 and $m > 1$. R groups are usually methyl, longer alkyl, fluoroalkyl, phenyl, vinyl, alkoxy or alkylamino. Silicones are characterized by thermal and oxidative stability, chemical inertness, resistance to weathering, good dielectric strength and low surface tension. Prepd commercially by the direct reaction of silicon with an organic halide, hydrolysis of the resulting organohalosilanes and condensation of the unstable diols. Review of chemistry, properties and uses: B. Hardman, A. Torkelson in *Encyclopedia of Polymer Science and Engineering* vol. **15** (Wiley-Interscience, New York, 1989) pp 204-308. Review of silicone surfactants: B. Grüning, G. Koerner, *Tenside Surfactants Deterg.* **26**, 312-317 (1989); and their uses in cosmetics and toiletries: C. Gould, *Spec. Chem.* **11**, 354-359 (1991). Clinical use of silicone elastomers in reconstructive surgery: M. B. Habal in *Advances in Biomedical Polymers*, C. G. Gebelein, Ed. (Plenum Press, New York, 1987) pp 17-29. Review of properties and commercial uses of silicone fluids: D. H. Demby *et al.* in *Synthetic Lubricants and High-Performance Functional Liquids*, R. L. Shubkin, Ed. (Marcel Dekker, New York, 1993) pp 183-203.

Polydimethylsiloxane *see* Dimethicone.

Polyether copolymers. Silicone polyethers; dimethicone copolyols; silicone glycol copolymers; silicone glycols. Branched siloxanes modified at the chain ends with a polyether, *e.g.* polyoxyethylene and/or polyoxypropylene. Trade marks for such products include: *Abil, Stilwet L.*

USE: As lubricants; wetting agents; defoamers; surfactants; hydraulic oils; dielectric oils; protective coatings; adhesives and caulking compounds; release agents; in paints, enamels, and varnishes; water repellents for textiles, paper, masonry, and concrete; damping fluids; electrical insulation; dental molds; medical implants; contact lenses; and in cosmetic and pharmaceutical formulations. A specialty product known as "bouncing putty" or "silly putty" has unusual rheological properties which allow it to be stretched, shattered, molded, or to rebound like rubber when dropped on hard surface.

8496. Silicon Monoxide. [10097-28-6] OSi; mol wt 44.08. O 36.30%, Si 63.71%. SiO. Prepd by high vacuum sublimation of a mixture of silicon and quartz: Schenk in *Handbook of Preparative Inorganic Chemistry* vol. **1**, G. Brauer, Ed. (Academic Press, New York, 2nd ed., 1963) pp 696-697. Existence below 1200° in doubt; may disproportionate to a mixture of Si and SiO_2: Benyon, *Vacuum* **20**, 293 (1970). *Review:* Rochow in *Comprehensive Inorganic Chemistry* vol. **1**, J. C. Bailar, Jr. *et al.*, Eds. (Pergamon Press, Oxford, 1973) pp 1353-1355.

Brownish-black scales by sublimation. Has been crystallized. Cubic system. About as hard as silicon. Nonconductor of electricity even at red heat. d 2.18.

8497. Silicon Nitride. [12033-89-5] Trisilicon tetranitride. N_4Si_3; mol wt 140.28. N 39.94%, Si 60.06%. Si_3N_4. Non-oxide ceramic material of high thermal stability. Manuf by direct nitridation of pure silicon. Prepn by pyrolysis of silicon diimide $(Si(NH_2)_2)$: O. Glemser, P. Naumann, *Z. Anorg. Allg. Chem.* **298**, 134 (1954); and characterization: K. S. Mazdiyasni, C. M. Cooke, *J. Am. Ceram. Soc.* **56**, 628 (1973); *eidem*, **US 3959446** (1976 to USA); by pyrolysis of silazanes: D. Seyferth *et al.*, *J. Am. Ceram. Soc.* **66**, C-13 (1983); *eidem*, **US 4397828** (1983 to M.I.T.). Brief review: D. L. Segal, *Chem. Ind. (London)* **1985**, 544.

Exists in two crystalline forms, α-Si_3N_4 and β-Si_3N_4. α-Form occurs when powdered Si_3N_4 is heated to 1200° >4 hr; increasing the temperature to >1450°C for 2 hr produces the β-form. White when pure but often brown or black powder. mp 2173°K (sublimes). d 3.2 kg/dm³. Coefficient of thermal expansion K^{-1}: 2.5 $\times 10^{-6}$.

USE: As high temp engineering material for use in gas turbines, diesel engines.

8498. Silicon Tetraacetate. [562-90-3] Acetic acid tetraanhydride with silicic acid. $C_8H_{12}O_8Si$; mol wt 264.26. C 36.36%, H 4.58%, O 48.44%, Si 10.63%. $Si(CH_3COO)_4$. Prepd from $SiCl_4 + (CH_3CO)_2O$: Balthis, *Inorg. Synth.* **4**, 45 (1953).

Extremely hygroscopic cryst mass. Hydrolyzed rapidly by moist air. mp 110°. Dec at 160-170° with evolution of acetic anhydride. $bp_{6.0}$ 148°. Violent reaction on contact with water. Forms SiO_2 and ethyl acetate on contact with alcohol. Moderately sol in acetone, benzene.

8499. Silicon Tetrabromide. [7789-66-4] Silicon bromide. Br_4Si; mol wt 347.70. Br 91.92%, Si 8.08%. $SiBr_4$. Prepd from the elements: Gattermann, *Ber.* **22**, 189 (1889).

Colorless, fuming liq; disagreeable odor; becomes yellow on exposure to air. d 2.8. Solidif $-12°$; mp 5°; bp 153°. Dec by water into silicic acid and HBr with great evolution of heat. Reacts violently with metallic potassium.

8500. Silicon Tetrachloride. [10026-04-7] Silicon chloride. Cl_4Si; mol wt 169.90. Cl 83.47%, Si 16.53%. $SiCl_4$. Prepd from the elements: Schenk in *Handbook of Preparative Inorganic Chemistry* vol. **1**, G. Brauer, Ed. (Academic Press, New York, 2nd ed., 1963) pp 682-683.

Colorless, clear, mobile, fuming liq; suffocating odor. d_4^0 1.52. mp $-70°$; bp 59°. Dec by water with much heat into silicic acid and HCl. Miscible with benzene, ether, chloroform, petr ether.

Caution: May be irritating to eyes, respiratory tract.

USE: Producing smoke screens in warfare. In the prepn of pure silicon.

8501. Silicon Tetrafluoride. [7783-61-1] Silicon fluoride. F_4Si; mol wt 104.08. F 73.01%, Si 26.98%. SiF_4. Commercial prepn from waste gases of phosphate fertilizer production: Molstad, **US 2833628** (1958 to W. R. Grace). Lab prepns: Booth, Swinehart, *J. Am. Chem. Soc.* **57**, 1337 (1935); Hoffman, Gutowski, *Inorg. Synth.* **4**, 145 (1953); Belf, *Chem. Ind. (London)* **1955**, 1296.

Colorless gas; very pungent odor similar to that of hydrogen chloride. Forms heavy clouds with moist air. Dec by water into silicic acid and HF. Sublimes $-95.7°$; mp $-90.2°$ (under pressure): d (liq; $-80°$) 1.590. Critical temp $-1.5°$; critical pressure 50 atm.

8502. Silicotungstic Acid. [12520-88-6] Tungstosilicic acid. $H_4O_{40}SiW_{12}$; mol wt 2878.17. H 0.14%, O 22.24%, Si 0.98%, W 76.65%. $H_4[SiO_4.(W_3O_9)_4]$. Prepn of hydrated compd: Grüttner, Jander in *Handbook of Preparative Inorganic Chemistry* vol. **2**, G. Brauer, Ed. (Academic Press, New York, 2nd ed., 1965) pp 1717-1718.

Hydrate. White to slightly yellow, deliquesc crystals. Very sol in water, alcohol. *Keep tightly closed.*

USE: Preparing heavy solns for separating minerals; as a mordant for basic aniline dyes; as a reagent for pptn and determination of alkaloids.

8503. Silodosin. [160970-54-7] 2,3-Dihydro-1-(3-hydroxypropyl)-5-[(2R)-2-[[2-[2-(2,2,2-trifluoroethoxy)phenoxy]ethyl]amino]propyl]-1H-indole-7-carboxamide; KMD-3213. $C_{25}H_{32}F_3N_3O_4$; mol wt 495.53. C 60.60%, H 6.51%, F 11.50%, N 8.48%, O 12.91%. α_{1a}-Adrenoceptor antagonist. Prepn: M. Kitazawa *et al.*, **EP 600675**; *eidem*, **US 5387603** (1994, 1995 both to Kissei). Adrenoceptor binding study: K. Shibata *et al.*, *Mol. Pharmacol.* **48**, 250 (1995); and tissue selectivity: S. Murata *et al.*, *J. Urol.* **164**, 578 (2000). Pharmacology: K. Akiyama *et al.*, *Pharmacology* **64**, 140 (2002). Series of articles on pharmacology, pharmacokinetcs and toxicology: *Yakugaku Zasshi* **126**, 187-263 (2006). Review of development and therapeutic potential: F. Kamali, *Curr. Opin. Cent. Peripher. Nerv. Syst. Invest. Drugs* **1**, 248-252 (1999).

$[\alpha]_D^{25}$ −14.0° (c = 1.01 in methanol).

THERAP CAT: In treatment of benign prostatic hypertophy.

8504. Silver. [7440-22-4] Ag; at. wt 107.8682; at. no. 47; valence 1, 2. Group IB (11). Occurrence in the earth's crust: 0.1 ppm; also present in seawater: 0.01 ppm. Natural isotopes: 107 (51.35%); 109 (48.65%); artificial isotopes (mass numbers): 100-106, 108, 110-117. One of the earliest known metals. Found native or associated with copper, gold and lead. Principle ores are *argentite*, *cerargyrite* or *horn silver* (mixture of halides), *proustite* (3Ag₂-S.As₂S₃), *pyrargyrite* (Ag₂S.Sb₂S₃). Extraction from ores: Percy *et al.*, cited by Mellor, *A Comprehensive Treatise on Inorganic and Theoretical Chemistry* **3**, 301 (1928); *Silver, Its Economics, Extraction, Use*, A. Butts, C. D. Coxe, Eds. (Van Nostrand, Princeton, 1967) 480 pp. *Reviews:* Thompson, "Silver" in *Comprehensive Inorganic Chemistry* **vol. 3**, J. C. Bailar, Jr. *et al.*, Eds. (Pergamon Press, Oxford, 1973) pp 79-128; G. H. Sistare and H. B. Lockhart in *Kirk-Othmer Encyclopedia of Chemical Technology* **vol. 21** (Wiley-Interscience, New York, 3rd ed., 1983) pp 1-32. Review of toxicology and human exposure: *Toxicological Profile for Silver* (PB91-180430, 1990) 157 pp.

White metal, face-centered cubic structure. More malleable and ductile than any other metal except gold; excellent conductor of heat and electricity. mp 960.5°. bp ~2000°. d^{15} 10.49. Not attacked by water or atmospheric oxygen; blackened by ozone, by hydrogen sulfide, by sulfur. Inert to most acids; readily reacts with dil nitric acid, hot concd sulfuric acid; superficially attacked by hydrochloric acid. Sol in fused alkali hydroxides in presence of air, in fused alkali peroxides, in alkali cyanides in presence of air or oxygen. Most silver salts are light-sensitive.

Caution: Potential symptoms of overexposure to dust are blue-gray eyes, nasal septum, throat and skin; irritation and ulceration of skin; GI disturbance. *See NIOSH Pocket Guide to Chemical Hazards* (DHHS/NIOSH 97-140, 1997) p 280. Blue-gray discoloration, known as argyria or argyrosis, results from chronic exposure to silver or silver salts. *See Patty's Industrial Hygiene and Toxicology* **vol. 2A**, G. D. Clayton, F. E. Clayton, Eds. (Wiley-Interscience, New York, 3rd ed., 1981) pp 1881-1894.

USE: For coinage, most frequently alloyed with copper or gold; for manuf tableware, mirrors, jewelry, ornaments; for electroplating; for making vessels and apparatus used in manuf medicinal chemicals, in processing foods and beverages, in handling organic acids; as catalyst in hydrogenation and oxidation processes; as ingredient of dental alloys. Has been used for purification of drinking water because of toxicity to bacteria and lower forms of life. Some salts used in photography.

8505. Silver Acetate. [563-63-3] $C_2H_3AgO_2$; mol wt 166.91. C 14.39%, H 1.81%, Ag 64.63%, O 19.17%. CH_3CO-OAg.

White to slightly grayish, lustrous needles or cryst powder. d 3.26. Sol in 100 parts of cold water, 35 parts of boiling water; freely sol in dil nitric acid. *Protect from light.*

USE: Oxidizing agent for use in liquid ammonia: Kline, Kershner, *Inorg. Chem.* **5**, 932 (1966).

8506. Silver Bromide. [7785-23-1] AgBr; mol wt 187.77. Ag 57.45%, Br 42.55%.

Yellowish, odorless powder; darkens on exposure to light. d 6.47; mp 432°. Soly in water (25°): 0.135 mg/l. Insol in alcohol, or most acids. Slightly sol in dil ammonia, but moderately sol in concd ammonia. One liter of 10% ammonia dissolves 3.3 g at 12°; sol in solns of alkali cyanides, sparingly sol in solns of thiocyanates or thiosulfates; sol in 220 parts saturated NaCl, in 35 parts saturated KBr solns; slightly sol in ammonium carbonate soln. *Protect from light.*

USE: In photography.

THERAP CAT: Topical anti-infective; astringent.

8507. Silver Carbonate. [534-16-7] Carbonic acid disilver(1+) salt. CAg_2O_3; mol wt 275.75. C 4.36%, Ag 78.24%, O 17.41%. Ag_2CO_3. Silver carbonate pptd on Celite, *q.v.*, is known as *Fétizon's reagent*. Thermal decompn studies: M. Centnerszwer, B. Bruzs, *J. Phys. Chem.* **29**, 733 (1925); P. Norby *et al.*, **41**, 3628 (2002). Prepn from silver nitrate and sol carbonate soln: Poyer *et al.*, *Inorg. Synth.* **5**, 19 (1957). Crystal structure: R. Masse *et al.*, *Acta Crystallogr.* **B35**, 1428 (1979). Mechanism of alcohol oxidation using silver carbonate pptd on celite: M. Fetizon, M. Golfier, *C.R. Acad. Sci. Ser. C* **267**, 900 (1968); M. Fetizon *et al.*, *Tetrahedron Lett.* **13**, 4445 (1972); F. J. Kakis *et al.*, *J. Org. Chem.* **39**, 523 (1974). Biological staining method: J. M. López-Cepero, *J. Histochem. Cytochem.* **52**, 211 (2004).

Light yellow powder when freshly pptd, but becomes darker on drying and on exposure to light. Dec at about 220° into Ag_2O and CO_2 and at higher temp into metal Ag. d 6.08. Sol in 30,000 parts cold water, 2000 parts boiling water; readily sol in dil nitric acid, ammonia, or alkali cyanides. *Protect from light.*

USE: Mild oxidizing agent for conversion of alcohols to aldehydes and ketones. Biological stain.

8508. Silver Chlorate. [7783-92-8] Argentous chlorate. $AgClO_3$; mol wt 191.32. Ag 56.38%, Cl 18.53%, O 25.09%. Prepd from $AgNO_3$ and $NaClO_3$: Nicholson, Holley, Jr., *Inorg. Synth.* **2**, 4 (1946).

White, tetragonal crystals. d_4^{20} 4.430. mp 230°, dec 270° forming silver chloride and oxygen. Solubility in water (g/100 ml): 10 (15°); 20 (27°); 50 (80°). Slightly sol in alc. Darkens upon exposure to light due to slow decompn. *Keep away from light, organic vapors and oxidizable substances.*

USE: In organic synthesis as an effective oxidizing agent for certain organic compds.

8509. Silver Chloride. [7783-90-6] AgCl; mol wt 143.32. Ag 75.26%, Cl 24.74%.

White powder; darkens on exposure to light. d 5.56; mp 455°; bp 1550°. Soly in water (25°): 1.93 mg/l; hydrochloric acid increases its soly. Sol in 250 parts of concd HCl, in 13 parts of 10% ammonia; more sol in stronger ammonia and also at higher temps. Sol in solns of alkali cyanides, thiosulfates, ammonium carbonates; appreciably sol in concd aq solns of ammonium chloride; mercuric nitrate, and silver nitrate. The freshly pptd chloride dissolves more readily than the dried precipitate. Insol in alcohol, or dil acids. *Protect from light.*

USE: In silver plating, in making antiseptic silver prepns.

8510. Silver Chromate(VI). [7784-01-2] Ag_2CrO_4; mol wt 331.73. Ag 65.03%, Cr 15.67%, O 19.29%.

Dark brownish-red, cryst powder. d^{25} 5.625. Soly in water (0°): 0.0014%. Sol in nitric acid and ammonia.

USE: Catalyst for formation of aldol from alcohol; formed at end point of Mohr titration of halides.

8511. Silver Citrate. [126-45-4] 2-Hydroxy-1,2,3-propanetricarboxylic acid silver salt; Itrol. $C_6H_5Ag_3O_7$; mol wt 512.70. C 14.06%, H 0.98%, Ag 63.12%, O 21.84%.

White, odorless, heavy, crystalline powder; darkens in light. Sol in 3500 parts water, more sol in boiling water; readily sol in dil HNO_3, ammonia. *Protect from light.*

USE: Anti-infective dusting powder.

8512. Silver Cyanide. [506-64-9] CAgN; mol wt 133.89. C 8.97%, Ag 80.56%, N 10.46%. AgCN.

White or grayish, odorless powder; stable in dry air; darkens on exposure to light; dec at 320°. *Poisonous!* d 3.95. Insol in water, alcohol, or dil acids; sol in alkali cyanides and in boiling concd nitric acid; converted by dil HCl into hydrocyanic acid and silver chloride; sparingly sol in concd ammonia. *Protect from light.*

USE: For silver plating; formerly used for extemporaneous prepn of dil hydrocyanic acid by treatment with HCl.

8513. Silver Difluoride. [7783-95-1] Argentic fluoride. AgF_2; mol wt 145.87. Ag 73.95%, F 26.05%. Prepd by the action of fluorine on silver: Ebert *et al.*, *J. Am. Chem. Soc.* **55**, 3056 (1933); by the interaction of fluorine and silver halides: Ruff, Giese, *Z. Anorg. Allg. Chem.* **219**, 143 (1934); v. Wartenberg, *ibid.* **242**, 406 (1939); Struve *et al.*, *Ind. Eng. Chem.* **39**, 353 (1947).

Laboratory procedure according to the equation $2AgCl + 2F_2 \rightarrow 2AgF_2 + Cl_2$: Priest, Swinehart, *Inorg. Synth.* **3,** 176 (1950); Kwasnik in *Handbook of Preparative Inorganic Chemistry* vol. 1, G. Brauer, Ed. (Academic Press, New York, 2nd ed., 1963) pp 241-242. Prepd from silver chloride and chlorine trifluoride: Rochow, Kukin, *J. Am. Chem. Soc.* **74,** 1615 (1952).

White when pure. Usually obtained as a gray-black or brownish, amorphous solid showing a yellow bloom. Sensitive to light. d 4.7. mp 690°. Very hygroscopic, is converted to a greasy black mass on exposure to atmospheric moisture. Violent reaction with water (instant hydrolytic cleavage). Powerful oxidizing agent giving off some ozone when treated with dil acids. Liberates iodine from iodides. May be stored in quartz or iron ampuls.

Caution: Symptoms due to fluoride. Highly toxic.

USE: In the fluorination of hydrocarbons.

8514. Silver Fluoride. [7775-41-9] Argentous fluoride; silver monofluoride. AgF; mol wt 126.87. Ag 85.02%, F 14.97%. Prepared according to the equation $Ag_2CO_3 + 2HF \rightarrow 2AgF + CO_2 + H_2O$; also prepd by reduction of AgF_2 with H_2: Ruff, *Die Chemie des Fluors* (Berlin, 1920) p 37; Eméléus in *J. H. Simons' Fluorine Chemistry* vol. I (Academic Press, New York, 1950) p 32; Kwasnik in *Handbook of Preparative Inorganic Chemistry* vol. 1, G. Brauer, Ed. (Academic Press, New York, 2nd ed., 1963) pp 240-241.

Flexible leaflets (cubic, NaCl lattice). Very hygroscopic. Darkens on exposure to light. d 5.852. mp 435°. bp ~1150°. Soly in water when freshly prepd: 182 g/100 ml at 15.5°. In moist air it gradually becomes insol because of basic fluoride formation. Aq solns are neutral and are solvents for silver oxide which renders them alkaline. Also sol in HF, NH_3, CH_3CN. Forms several hydrates. The dihydrate is stable to 39.5° and the tetrahydrate is stable from $-14°$ to $+18.7°$. In addition, an acid fluoride, AgF.3HF can be prepd by cooling a soln of AgF in HF. This loses HF at 0°, forming AgF.HF.

Caution: Prolonged absorption may cause mottling of teeth, skeletal changes.

USE: To convert organic Br and Cl compds to their fluoro analogs; as antiseptic.

THERAP CAT: Anti-infective.

8515. Silver Iodate. [7783-97-3] $AgIO_3$; mol wt 282.77. Ag 38.15%, I 44.88%, O 16.97%.

White, cryst powder. d 5.53. mp >200°. Sol in 1875 parts water at 25°, in about 1000 parts of 35% nitric acid, in 2.5 parts of 10% ammonia. *Protect from light.*

USE: As reagent for determining small quantities of chloride, e.g., in blood: Sendroy, *J. Biol. Chem.* **120,** 335-445 (1937).

8516. Silver Iodide. [7783-96-2] AgI; mol wt 234.77. Ag 45.95%, I 54.05%. Prepd according to the equation $AgNO_3 + KI \rightarrow AgI + KNO_3$: Kolkmeijer, van Hengel, *Z. Kristallogr.* **A88,** 317 (1934).

Light yellow, odorless powder; slowly darkened by light. Crystals are hexagonal or cubic. d 5.67; mp 552°. Practically insol in water (0.03 mg/l); in acid (except concd HI in which it dissolves readily on heating); in ammonium carbonate. Freely sol in solns of alkali cyanides or iodides; 35 mg dissolve in a liter of 10% ammonia; appreciably sol in concd solns of alkali bromides, chlorides, thiocyanates, thiosulfates, mercuric and silver nitrates. It is slowly attacked by boiling concd acids, but not affected by hot solns of alkali hydroxides.

USE: In cloud precipitation (rain-making).

THERAP CAT: Local anti-infective.

THERAP CAT (VET): In colloidal suspensions as local antiseptic for mucous membranes.

8517. Silver Lactate. [128-00-7] 2-Hydroxypropanoic acid silver salt. $C_3H_5AgO_3$; mol wt 196.94. C 18.30%, H 2.56%, Ag 54.77%, O 24.37%. $CH_3CH(OH)COOAg$.

Monohydrate. White or slightly gray, cryst powder readily affected by light. Sol in about 15 parts water; slightly sol in alcohol. *Protect from light.*

THERAP CAT: Topical anti-infective; astringent.

8518. Silver Nitrate. [7761-88-8] Nitric acid silver(1+) salt. $AgNO_3$; mol wt 169.87. Ag 63.50%, N 8.25%, O 28.26%. Prepn: T. W. Richards, G. S. Forbes, *J. Am. Chem. Soc.* **29,** 808 (1907).

Clinical prophylactic use in neonatal conjunctivitis: Credé, *Arch. Gynaekol.* **17,** 50 (1881). Raman and IR structural studies: Z. X. Shen, W. F. Sherman, *J. Mol. Struct.* **271,** 175 (1992). Clinical evaluation in molluscum contagiosum: K. Niizeki, K. Hashimoto, *Pediatr. Dermatol.* **16,** 395 (1999); of histological effects in epithelial cautery: J. Hanif *et al., Clin. Otolaryngol.* **28,** 368 (2003). Review of prophylactic use in neonatal gonococcal conjunctivitis: G. Schneider, *Can. Med. Assoc. J.* **131,** 193-196 (1984); of toxicology: S. D. M. Humphreys, P. A. Routledge, *Adverse Drug React. Toxicol. Rev.* **17,** 115-143 (1998); of chromatographic applications: C. M. Williams, L. N. Mander, *Tetrahedron* **57,** 425-447 (2001).

Colorless, rhombic crystals or white small crystals. d 4.352. Dimorphic; transition temp: 159.8°. mp 212°, forming a yellowish liq solidifying to a white, cryst mass on cooling. Dec at 440° into metallic silver, nitrogen and nitrogen oxides. Soly in water at 25° (g/100 g H_2O): 2.16×10^2. Soly (g/L): ethanol 20.8; methanol 35; benzene 2.2. Not photosensitive when pure; trace amts of organic material promote photoreduction.

Toughened silver nitrate. [8007-31-6] Nitric acid silver (1+) salt mixt with silver chloride (AgCl); lunar caustic; molded silver nitrate. Contains not less than 94.5% silver nitrate, remainder is silver chloride. White or grayish, hard rods or thin small cones. Darkens on exposure to light. *Protect from light.*

Caution: Potential symptoms of overexposure by direct contact are tissue corrosion and burns; absorption through mucous membranes or damaged areas of skin may be followed by systemic toxicity (Humphreys). *See also* Silver.

USE: In chromatography; photography; manuf of mirrors; other silver salts; silver plating; in sympathetic and indelible inks; dyeing hair; coloring porcelain; etching ivory; as a reagent in analytical chemistry.

THERAP CAT: Astringent, antiseptic, caustic.

THERAP CAT (VET): Astringent, antiseptic, caustic.

8519. Silver Nitrite. [7783-99-5] $AgNO_2$; mol wt 153.87. Ag 70.10%, N 9.10%, O 20.80%.

Pale yellow, odorless needles; non-hygroscopic; becomes gray in light. d 4.45. Dec at 140°. Sol in 300 parts water; more sol in boiling water; less sol in aqueous solns of silver nitrate; partly dec on prolonged boiling with water; insol in alcohol; dec by dil acids. *Protect from light.*

USE: For prepn of standard $NaNO_2$ soln for water analysis; prepn of aliphatic nitro-compds; as reagent for primary, secondary, and tertiary alcohols.

8520. Silver Oxalate. [533-51-7] Ethanedioic acid silver salt. $C_2Ag_2O_4$; mol wt 303.76. C 7.91%, Ag 71.02%, O 21.07%. AgOOCCOOAg.

White, cryst powder; at 140° dec violently. d 5.03. Sol in 24,000 parts water; sol in moderately concd nitric acid, in ammonia.

USE: Exptl photographic emulsion (low sensitivity).

8521. Silver Oxide. [20667-12-3] Argentous oxide. Ag_2O; mol wt 231.74. Ag 93.09%, O 6.90%. Prepd by making sol silver salt solns alkaline: Madsen, *Z. Anorg. Allg. Chem.* **79,** 197 (1913). Toxicity study: H. F. Smyth *et al., Am. Ind. Hyg. Assoc. J.* **30,** 470 (1969).

Brownish-black, heavy, odorless powder. d_4^{25} 7.22. Begins to dec at about 200° and at 250-300° decompn is rapid; it also breaks up into its constituents in sunlight. Reduced by hydogen, carbon monoxide and most metals. Moist silver oxide absorbs carbon dioxide. Sol in 40,000 parts water; freely sol in dil nitric acid, in ammonia; somewhat sol in NaOH solns. Practically insol in alcohol. *Protect from light.* LD_{50} orally in rats: 2.82 g/kg (Smyth).

USE: As catalyst; in the purification of drinking water; in the glass industry (polishing, coloring glass yellow).

THERAP CAT (VET): Has been used as germicide and parasiticide.

8522. Silver(II) Oxide. [1301-96-8] Argentic oxide; silver peroxide; silver suboxide; Divasil. AgO; mol wt 123.87. Ag 87.08%, O 12.92%. Is actually a silver(I)-silver(III) oxide: McMillan, *Chem. Rev.* **62,** 65 (1962). Prepd by the oxidation of silver nitrate with potassium peroxydisulfate in an alk medium: Hammer, Kleinberg, *Inorg. Synth.* **4,** 12 (1953). Prepn of single crystals: *Chem. Eng. News* **47,** 32 (Aug 11, 1969).

Charcoal-gray powder. *Avoid contact with skin, organic matter, strong ammonia and alkalies.* Malleable. Cubic or orthorhombic system when cryst. d_4^{25} 7.483. The dry solid is stable at 100° for 18 hrs, dec above 100° into silver and oxygen. Possesses semiconductor properties and is diamagnetic. *Strong oxidizing agent.* Ka 7.9 × 10⁻¹³. Practically insol in water: 27 mg/l at 25° (decompn). Sol in alkalies and NH₄OH (with decompn and evolution of N₂). In dil acids oxygen is evolved immediately, in concd acid intensely colored solns are formed (brown in nitric acid and olive green in sulfuric acid).

Caution: Highly irritating to skin, eyes, mucous membranes, respiratory tract.

USE: In the manuf of silver oxide-zinc alkali batteries.

8523. Silver Perchlorate. [7783-93-9] AgClO₄; mol wt 207.32. Ag 52.03%, Cl 17.10%, O 30.87%. Prepn from NOClO₄ + AgBr: Markowitz *et al., J. Inorg. Nucl. Chem.* **16,** 159 (1960).

Deliquescent crystals, dec 486°. d²⁵ 2.806. Freely sol in water: 557 g/100 ml; a satd aq soln contains 84.8% w/w at 25°: Smith, Ring, *J. Am. Chem. Soc.* **59,** 1889 (1937). Much less sol in 60% perchloric acid (5.63% w/w). Forms a monohydrate stable to 43°. Sol in many organic solvents, e.g., aniline, pyridine, benzene, toluene, nitromethane, glycerol, nitrobenzene, and chlorobenzene. Solvated crystals have been obtained contg 6 mols aniline, 4 mols pyridine, 1 mol benzene, 1 mol toluene. These compds explode readily when struck: Brinkley, *J. Am. Chem. Soc.* **62,** 3524 (1940).

Caution: Irritating to skin, mucous membranes.

USE: In the explosives industry.

8524. Silver Permanganate. [7783-98-4] Silver manganate (VII). AgMnO₄; mol wt 226.80. Ag 47.56%, Mn 24.22%, O 28.22%. Prepn: Büssem, Herrmann, *Z. Kristallogr.* **A74,** 459 (1930).

Violet, cryst powder; dec in light. d 4.49. Soly in water at room temps about 9 g/l. More sol in hot water; dec by alcohol. *Protect from light.*

USE: In gas masks.

8525. Silver Phosphate. [7784-09-0] Silver orthophosphate. Ag₃O₄P; mol wt 418.58. Ag 77.31%, O 15.29%, P 7.40%. Ag₃PO₄.

Yellow, odorless powder; darkens in light. d 6.37. mp 849°. Reduced by hydrogen. Soluble in 15,500 parts water, the soly in water is decreased by presence of silver nitrate; slightly sol in dil acetic acid; freely sol in dil nitric acid, in ammonia, ammonium carbonate, also in alkali cyanides and thiosulfates. *Protect from light.*

USE: In photography for collodion emulsions.

8526. Silver Picrate. [146-84-9] 2,4,6-Trinitrophenol silver salt; picric acid silver derivative; silver trinitrophenolate; Picragol; Picrotol. C₆H₂AgN₃O₇; mol wt 335.96. C 21.45%, H 0.60%, Ag 32.11%, N 12.51%, O 33.34%. (O₂N)₃C₆H₂OAg.

Monohydrate. Yellow crystals. Sol in about 50 parts water; sparingly sol in alc; slightly sol in acetone or glycerol. Insol in chloroform, ether.

THERAP CAT: Antiprotozoal (Trichomonas).

THERAP CAT (VET): Has been used in bovine granular vaginitis.

8527. Silver Protein. [9015-51-4] Argentoproteinum; protargin; silver proteinate; silver nucleate; silver nucleinate. Group of compounds characterized as colloidal combinations of silver and protein. Variably prepd from silver oxide, silver nitrate or other silver salts with gelatin, serum albumin, casein or peptone. Examples of prepns: **DE 105866** (1897 to Bayer); **GB 18478** (1897); H. P. Kaufmann, *Arzneimittel-Synthese* (Springer, 1953) p 588. Generally classified as mild or strong based on their germicidal and irritant properties. Differentiated by the amount of ionizable silver present: Van Deripe, Konnerth, *Am. J. Pharm.* **111,** 65 (1939). Use to stain nerve fibers: D. Bodian, *Anat. Rec.* **65,** 89 (1936). Neuronal selectivity and use in light and electron microscopy: I. S. Zagon, J. H. Haring, *Acta Anat.* **114,** 193 (1982); in Alzheimer's disease: C. Duyckaerts *et al., Acta Neuropathol.* **73,** 167 (1987).

Mild silver protein. Argentum vitellinum; Argyrol; Silvol. Brown, dark-brown, or almost black, odorless, lustrous scales or granules. Contains ~20% silver. Somewhat hygroscopic. Freely sol in water. Almost insol in alcohol, chloroform, ether. *Keep well closed and protected from light.*

Strong silver protein. Albumose silver; Protargol. Pale yellowish-orange to brownish-black, odorless powder. Contains ~8% silver, most of which is present in ionic form. Somewhat hygroscopic. Freely sol in water. Almost insol in alcohol, ether, chloroform. *Keep well closed and protected from light.*

USE: Neuronal-selective histological stain; general contrast medium for electron microscopy.

THERAP CAT: Antiseptic.

THERAP CAT (VET): Antiseptic.

8528. Silver Selenide. [1302-09-6] Ag₂Se; mol wt 294.70. Ag 73.21%, Se 26.79%. Occurs in nature as the mineral naumannite. Prepd by melting silver and selenium together and by passing hydrogen selenide into a soln of silver nitrate: Berzelius, cited by Mellor, *A Comprehensive Treatise on Inorganic and Theoretical Chemistry* **10,** 771 (1930); by combination of ions or elements in solns or melts: Kulifay, **US 3026175** (1962 to Monsanto).

Gray, hexagonal, microscopic needles. mp 880°. d¹⁵ 8.216. Two forms exist; transition temp at 133°. Forms metallic silver and selenium oxide when heated in oxygen; transformed by chlorine into silver and selenium chlorides; oxidized to silver selenite by fuming nitric acid. Sol in molten silver or bismuth without chemical change. Practically insol in water.

8529. Silver Sulfate. [10294-26-5] Ag₂O₄S; mol wt 311.80. Ag 69.19%, O 20.53%, S 10.28%. Ag₂SO₄. Prepd from silver nitrate and sulfuric acid: Richards, Jones, *Z. Anorg. Allg. Chem.* **55,** 72 (1907).

Crystals or cryst powder; slowly darkens on exposure to light. mp 657°; dec 1085°. d 5.45. Slowly sol in 125 parts water, 71 parts boiling water; sol in nitric acid, ammonia, concd sulfuric acid. Soly in AgNO₃ solns: Lietzke, Stoughton, *J. Inorg. Nucl. Chem.* **28,** 1877 (1966). *Protect from light.*

8530. Silver Sulfide. [21548-73-2] Argentous sulfide. Ag₂S; mol wt 247.80. Ag 87.06%, S 12.94%. Occurs in nature as the mineral *argentite.* Usually prepd from the elements: Hönigschmid, Sachtleben, *Z. Anorg. Allg. Chem.* **207,** 1931 (1931).

Grayish-black, heavy powder. The cryst structure is orthorhombic, changing to cubic when heated above 179°. d₄²⁰ 7.234. mp 845°. Insol in water. Sol in nitric acid, in solns of alkali cyanides.

USE: In ceramics.

8531. Silver Tetraiodomercurate(II). [7784-03-4] Mercuric silver iodide. Ag₂HgI₄; mol wt 923.94. Ag 23.35%, Hg 21.71%, I 54.94%.

Deep yellow thermochromic powder. Insol in water or dil acids; sol in solns of alkali iodides or cyanides.

USE: Thermal sensor to detect overheating in journal bearings, etc., becomes blood-red at 40-50° and yellow again on cooling.

8532. Silymarin. [65666-07-1] Apihepar; Laragon; Legalon; Pluropon; Silarine; Silepar; Silirex; Silliver; Silmar. Antihepatotoxic principle isolated from the seeds of the milk thistle, *Silybum marianum* (L.) Gaertn. (*Carduus marianus* L.). Comprised mainly of three isomers: *silidianin, silicristin* and the major component, *silybin* (formerly called silymarin). Characterized as a new class of substances, flavonolignans, almost certainly produced in the plant by a radical coupling of a flavonoid and coniferyl alcohol: Hänsel *et al., Dtsch. Apoth. Ztg.* **108,** 1988 (1968). Isoln and chemistry: Wagner *et al., Arzneim.-Forsch.* **18,** 688 (1968); **24,** 466 (1974). Structural work: Janiak, Hänsel, *Planta Med.* **8,** 71 (1960); Hänsel, Schöpflin, *Tetrahedron Lett.* **1967,** 3645; Pelter, Hänsel, *ibid.* **1968,** 2911. Pharmacology and toxicology: Hahn *et al., Arzneim.-Forsch.* **18,** 698 (1968); H. M. Rauen, H. Schriewer, *ibid.* **23,** 148-170 (1973); Halbach, Trost, *ibid.* **24,** 866 (1974).

Silybin. [22888-70-6] (2R,3R)-2-[(2R,3R)-2,3-Dihydro-3-(4-hydroxy-3-methoxyphenyl)-2-(hydroxymethyl)-1,4-benzodioxin-6-

yl]-2,3-dihydro-3,5,7-trihydroxy-4*H*-1-benzopyran-4-one; silibinin; silybum substance E$_6$; silymarin I. C$_{25}$H$_{22}$O$_{10}$; mol wt 482.44. Revised structure and synthetic studies: R. Hänsel *et al.*, *Chem. Commun.* **1972**, 195; *eidem*, *Ber.* **110**, 3664 (1977). Total synthesis: L. Merlini *et al.*, *Chem. Commun.* **1979**, 695; *eidem*, *J. Chem. Soc. Perkin Trans. 1* **1980**, 775. Anhydrous subst, mp 158°, dec 180°. [α]$_D^{20}$ +11° (c = 0.25 in acetone + alcohol). uv max (methanol): 288 nm (log ε 4.33). Sol in acetone, ethyl acetate, methanol, ethanol; sparingly sol in CHCl$_3$. Practically insol in water. Also occurs as the monohydrate, crystals from acetone + petr ether, mp 167°, dec 180°; from methanol + water, mp 180°.

THERAP CAT: Hepatoprotectant.

8533. Simazine. [122-34-9] 6-Chloro-*N,N'*-diethyl-1,3,5-triazine-2,4-diamine; 2-chloro-4,6-bis(ethylamino)-*s*-triazine; 2,4-bis(ethylamino)-6-chloro-s-triazine; G-27692; Gesatop; Princep; Simanex. C$_7$H$_{12}$ClN$_5$; mol wt 201.66. C 41.69%, H 6.00%, Cl 17.58%, N 34.73%. Selective pre-emergence herbicide. Prepn: Hofmann, *Ber.* **18**, 2776 (1885); Pearlman, Banks, *J. Am. Chem. Soc.* **70**, 3726 (1948); Thurston *et al.*, *ibid.* **73**, 2981 (1951). As herbicide: Gysin, Knüsli, *US 2891855* (1959 to Geigy). Toxicity studies: G. W. Bailey, J. L. White, *Residue Rev.* **10**, 97 (1965).

Crystals from ethanol or methyl Cellosolve, mp 226-227°. Practically insol in water. Slightly sol in dioxane, ethyl Cellosolve. LD$_{50}$ orally in rats: 5000 mg/kg (Bailey, White).

USE: Herbicide.

8534. Simeconazole. [149508-90-7] α-(4-Fluorophenyl)-α-[(trimethylsilyl)methyl]-1*H*-1,2,4-triazole-1-ethanol; 2-(4-fluorophenyl)-1-(1*H*-1,2,4-triazol-1-yl)-3-trimethylsilylpropan-2-ol; F-155; Mongarit; Sanlit. C$_{14}$H$_{20}$FN$_3$OSi; mol wt 293.41. C 57.31%, H 6.87%, F 6.48%, N 14.32%, O 5.45%, Si 9.57%. Broad spectrum triazole fungicide for use in food crops and turf; sterol demethylation inhibitor (DMI). Prepn: J. Tobitsuka *et al.*, **EP 537957**; *eidem*, *US 5306712* (1993, 1994 both to Sankyo); H. Itoh *et al.*, *Chem. Pharm. Bull.* **48**, 1148 (2000). Comprehensive description: M. Tsuda *et al.*, *Brighton Crop Prot. Conf. - Pests Dis.* **2000**, 557. Systemic activity in plants: M. Tsuda *et al.*, *Pest Manage. Sci.* **60**, 881 (2004); and comparison with other DMI fungicides: *eidem*, *ibid*, 875. Pharmacokinetics in rodents: K. Wakabayashi *et al.*, *J. Pestic. Sci.* **30**, 90 (2005).

Colorless crystals from diisopropyl ether, mp 118-119°. Log P (*n*-octanol/water): 3.2. Vapor pressure at 25°: 5.4 × 10^{-5} Pa. Soly in water (20°): 57.5 mg/l. LD$_{50}$ in male, female rats (mg/kg): 611, 682 orally (Tsuda).

USE: Agricultural fungicide.

8535. Simetride. [154-82-5] 1,4-Bis[(2-methoxy-4-propylphenoxy)acetyl]piperazine; AP2; Kyorin AP2. C$_{28}$H$_{38}$N$_2$O$_6$; mol wt 498.61. C 67.45%, H 7.68%, N 5.62%, O 19.25%. Prepn: FR M2936 (1964 to Kyorin Pharmaceutical Co., Ltd.); T. Irikura *et al.*, *US 3184463* (1965). Pharmacological studies: T. Irikura *et al.*, *Yakugaku Zasshi* **83**, 785 (1963), *C.A.* **60**, 1008b (1964). Analgesic activity: K. Nishino *et al.*, *Yakugaku Zasshi* **85**, 715 (1965), *C.A.* **63**, 16957b (1965).

Crystals, mp 128-130° (**FR M2936**); also reported as mp 138.5-139° (Irikura, 1963). Practically insoluble in water, ethanol. Sol in CHCl$_3$. LD$_{50}$ i.p. in mice: 15000 mg/kg (Irikura).

THERAP CAT: Analgesic.

8536. Simetryn. [1014-70-6] *N,N*-Diethyl-6-(methylthio)-1,3,5-triazine-2,4-diamine; 2,4-bis(ethylamino)-6-(methylthio)-*s*-triazine; 2,4-bis(ethylamino)-6-(methylthio)-1,3,5-triazine; 2-methylthio-4,6-bis(monoethylamino)-*s*-triazine; G-32911; Gy-bon. C$_8$H$_{15}$N$_5$S; mol wt 213.30. C 45.05%, H 7.09%, N 32.83%, S 15.03%. Prepn: Gysin, Knüsli, CH 337019 (1959 to Geigy), *C.A.* **57**, 14226c (1962). Crystal structure: A. J. Graham *et al.*, *Cryst. Struct. Commun.* **7**, 227 (1978). Toxicity study: E. F. Edson *et al.*, *World Rev. Pest Control* **1**, 36 (1965).

Crystals, mp 82-83°. LD$_{50}$ orally in rats: 1830 mg/kg (Edson).
USE: Herbicide.

8537. Simfibrate. [14929-11-4] 2-(4-Chlorophenoxy)-2-methylpropanoic acid 1,3-propanediyl ester; 2-(*p*-chlorophenoxy)-2-methylpropionic acid trimethylene ester; 1,3-propanediol bis[α-(*p*-chlorophenoxy)isobutyrate]; 1,3-propanediol bis[2-(4-chlorophenoxy)-2-methylpropionate]; sinfibrate; CLY-503; Cholesolvin; Liposolvin. C$_{23}$H$_{26}$Cl$_2$O$_6$; mol wt 469.35. C 58.86%, H 5.58%, Cl 15.11%, O 20.45%. Prepn: NL 6600044 corresp to Nakanishi *et al.*, **US 3494957** (1966, 1970 to Yoshitomi). Activity and toxicology studies: Nakanishi *et al.*, *J. Pharm. Soc. Jpn.* **90**, 267, 921, 926 (1970). Activity on postheparin lipoprotein lipase: L. Cavallini *et al.*, *Clin. Ter.* **92**, 25 (1980).

Crystals, mp 51-53°. bp$_{0.03}$ 197-200°, bp$_{0.15}$ 220-230°. LD$_{50}$ in mice, rats (g/kg): 3.3-3.5; 7.3-8.0 orally (Nakanishi, *J. Pharm. Soc. Japan*).

THERAP CAT: Antilipemic.

8538. Simplesse®. Protein-based fat substitute. Prepn from microparticulated, denatured dairy whey protein: N. S. Singer *et al.*, **EP 250623**; *eidem*, **US 4734287** (both 1988 to John LaBatt Ltd.). Brief description: D. D. Duxbury, *Food Process.* **49**, 21 (1988). Review: N. A. Bringe, D. R. Clark, *Front. Foods Food Ingredients* **1**, 51-68 (1993).

USE: Fat substitute for use in foods.

8539. Simvastatin. [79902-63-9] 2,2-Dimethylbutanoic acid (1*S*,3*R*,7*S*,8*S*,8a*R*)-1,2,3,7,8,8a-hexahydro-3,7-dimethyl-8-[2-[(2*R*,4*R*)-tetrahydro-4-hydroxy-6-oxo-2*H*-pyran-2-yl]ethyl]-1-naphthalenyl ester; 2,2-dimethylbutyric acid 8-ester with (4*R*,6*R*)-6-[2-[(1*S*,2*S*,6*R*,8*S*,8a*R*)-1,2,6,7,8,8a-hexahydro-8-hydroxy-2,6-dimethyl-1-naphthyl]ethyl]tetrahydro-4-hydroxy-2*H*-pyran-2-one; synvinolin; MK-733; Denan; Liponorm; Lodalès; Simovil; Sivacor; Sivastin; Zocor; Zocord. C$_{25}$H$_{38}$O$_5$; mol wt 418.57. C 71.74%, H 9.15%, O 19.11%. HMG-CoA reductase inhibitor; synthetic analog of lovastatin, *q.v.* Prepn: A. K. Willard *et al.*, **EP 33538**; W. F. Hoffman *et al.*, **US 4444784** (1981, 1984 both to Merck & Co.); W. F. Hoffman *et al.*, *J. Med. Chem.* **29**, 849 (1986). Comprehensive description: D. K. Ellison *et al.*, *Anal. Profiles Drug Subs. Excip.* **22**, 359-388 (1993). Effect on survival in

CHD: Scandinavian Simvastatin Survival Study Group, *Lancet* **344**, 1383 (1994). Clinical trial in primary hypercholesterolemia: L. Ose *et al., Clin. Cardiol.* **23**, 39 (2000); in mixed hyperlipidemia: E. Stein *et al., Am. J. Cardiol.* **86**, 406 (2000).

Crystals from *n*-butyl chloride + hexane, mp 135-138°. Soly (mg/ml): chloroform 610; DMSO 540; methanol 200; ethanol 160; *n*-hexane 0.15; $0.1M$ HCl 0.06; polyethylene glycol-400 70; propylene glycol 30; $0.1M$ NaOH 70; water 0.03. uv max (acetonitrile): 231, 238, 247 nm ($A_{1\ cm}^{1\%}$ 516, 604, 408). $[\alpha]_D^{25}$ +292° (c = 0.5% in acetonitrile).

THERAP CAT: Antilipemic.

8540. Sinalbin. [20196-67-2] Sinapine glucosinalbate. $C_{30}H_{42}N_2O_{15}S_2$; mol wt 734.79. C 49.04%, H 5.76%, N 3.81%, O 32.66%, S 8.73%. Mustard oil glucoside from white or yellow mustard *(Sinapis alba* L., *Cruciferae):* Gadamer, *Arch. Pharm.* **235**, 38, 83, 570 (1897); Viehoever, Nelson, *J. Assoc. Off. Agric. Chem.* **21**, 488 (1938); *Am. J. Pharm.* **110**, 411 (1938). Structure: Schulz, Gmelin, *Z. Naturforsch.* **7b**, 500 (1952); Ettlinger, Lundeen, *J. Am. Chem. Soc.* **78**, 4172 (1956).

Needles from 95% ethanol, mp 100-102°. (Also reported as 83-84° for the hydrated, 138-140° for the anhydr.) $[\alpha]_D^{20}$ −8.76° (c = 0.29). Soluble in hot alcohol, cold water.

8541. Sinapine. [18696-26-9] 2-[[3-(4-Hydroxy-3,5-dimethoxyphenyl)-1-oxo-2-propenyl]oxy]-*N,N,N*-trimethylethanaminium; sinapic acid choline ester. $[C_{16}H_{24}NO_5]^+$. From black mustard seeds, the seeds of *Brassica nigra* Koch, *Cruciferae*. Extraction procedure: Remsen, Coale, *Am. Chem. J.* **6**, 52 (1884). Synthesis: Späth, *Monatsh. Chem.* **41**, 271 (1920).

Chloride. $(C_{16}H_{24}NO_5)Cl$. Does not crystallize, very sol in water, alcohol.
Bromide trihydrate. $(C_{16}H_{24}NO_5)Br.3H_2O$. Needles, mp 92°; mp 107-115° when anhydr, very sol in water.
Iodide trihydrate. $(C_{16}H_{24}NO_5)I.3H_2O$. Crystals, becomes anhydr over H_2SO_4, mp 179° (anhydr). Sparingly sol in water.
Acid sulfate trihydrate. $(C_{16}H_{24}NO_5)HSO_4.3H_2O$. Tablets, dec 127°; dec 187° when anhydr. Freely sol in water, hot alcohol; very sparingly sol in ether.
Neutral sulfate pentahydrate. $(C_{16}H_{24}NO_5)_2SO_4.5H_2O$. Tablets from hot alcohol, mp 193° (anhydr). Not very stable; very sol in water, sparingly in alcohol.

8542. Sinapultide. [138531-07-4] KL4. $C_{126}H_{238}N_{26}O_{22}$; mol wt 2469.40. C 61.28%, H 9.71%, N 14.75%, O 14.25%. Synthetic pulmonary surfactant protein consisting of 21 amino acid residues in a repeating sequence of one lysine and four leucines.

Mimics *surfactant protein-B* (*SP-B*), a naturally occurring, hydrophobic protein found in human lung surfactant. Prepn: C. G. Cochrane, S. D. Revak, **WO 9222315**; *eidem*, **US 5407914** (1992, 1995 both to Scripps Res. Inst.). Surface behavior in phospholipid systems: J. Ma *et al., Biophys. J.* **74**, 1899 (1998).

Lys–Leu–Leu–Leu–Leu–Lys–Leu–Leu–Leu–Leu–Lys–Leu–Leu–Leu–Leu
Lys–Leu–Leu–Leu–Leu–Lys

Lucinactant. KL$_4$-surfactant; Surfaxin. Mixture of sinapultide with dipalmitoyl phosphatidylcholine and palmitoyl oleoylphosphatidyl glycerol (3:1) and palmitic acid. Effect on pulmonary function in animal models of meconium aspiration syndrome: C. G. Cochrane *et al., Pediatr. Res.* **44**, 705 (1998). Clinical evaluation in meconium aspiration syndrome: T. E. Wiswell *et al., Pediatrics* **109**, 1081 (2002). Clinical trial in premature infant respiratory distress syndrome: S. K. Sinha *et al., ibid.* **115**, 1030 (2005). Review of chemistry and clinical experience: S. M. Donn, *Expert Opin. Invest. Drugs* **14**, 329-334 (2005).

THERAP CAT: Pulmonary surfactant; in treatment of respiratory distress syndrome.

8543. Sincalide. [25126-32-3] 1-De(5-oxo-L-proline)-2-*de*-L-glutamine-5-L-methioninecaerulein; cholecystokinin *C*-terminal octapeptide; CCK *C*-terminal octapeptide; pancreozymin *C*-terminal octapeptide; SQ-19844; Kinevac. $C_{49}H_{62}N_{10}O_{16}S_3$; mol wt 1143.27. C 51.48%, H 5.47%, N 12.25%, O 22.39%, S 8.41%. The *C*-terminal octapeptide of cholecystokinin-pancreozymin (*see* cholecystokinin). Structurally similar to caerulein, *q.v.*, it evokes a variety of biological responses similar to CCK-PZ, including smooth-muscle contraction of the gall bladder and small intestine, relaxation of the choledochoduodenal junction, protein secretion by the pancreas and acid secretion by the stomach. It is more active than cholecystokinin on a weight or molar basis. Initial isoln: V. Mutt, J. E. Jorpes, *Eur. J. Biochem.* **6**, 156 (1968). Prepn: M. A. Ondetti *et al.*, **DE 1922185** corresp to **US 3723406** (1969, 1970, both to Squibb); *eidem, J. Am. Chem. Soc.* **92**, 195 (1970). Mechanical and metabolic effects: K. E. Andersson *et al., Acta Physiol. Scand.* **96**, 495 (1976). *In vitro* study: M. Deschodt-Lanckman *et al., Gastroenterology* **68**, 819 (1975). Use in clinical radiology: W. M. Thompson, J. R. Amberg, *Gastrointest. Radiol.* **3**, 191 (1978). Effect on food intake: M. A. Della-Fera, C. A. Baile, *Science* **206**, 471 (1979). Review of synthesis: L. Balaspiri, *Acta Physiol. Acad. Sci. Hung.* **47**, 299 (1976). Review of pharmacology: S. L. Engel *et al.*, in *Pharmacological and Biochemical Properties of Drug Substances* vol. 2, M. E. Goldberg, Ed. (Am. Pharm. Assoc., Washington, DC, 1979) pp 516-526.

SO$_3$H
Asp–Tyr–Met–Gly–Trp–Met–Asp–PheNH$_2$

Solid. $[\alpha]_D^{23}$ −18.4° (c = 0.7 in $1N$ NH$_3$). uv max (0.1N NaOH): 280, 288 nm (ε 4850, 4230).

THERAP CAT: Choleretic.

8544. Sinefungin. [58944-73-3] 6,9-Diamino-1-(6-amino-9*H*-purin-9-yl)-1,5,6,7,8,9-hexadeoxy-D-glycero-α-L-*talo*-decofuranuronic acid; Compd 57926; Antibiotic 32232RP; A-9145. $C_{15}H_{23}N_7O_5$; mol wt 381.39. C 47.24%, H 6.08%, N 25.71%, O 20.98%. Adenine-containing antibiotic produced by *Streptomyces griseoleus* NRRL 3739. Isoln: R. L. Hamill, M. M. Hoehn, **US 3758681** (1973 to Lilly); *eidem, J. Antibiot.* **26**, 463 (1973). Antifungal activity: R. S. Gordee, T. F. Butler, *ibid.* 466. Antiprotozoal activity: D. K. Dube *et al., Am. J. Trop. Med. Hyg.* **32**, 31 (1983); A. Ferrante *et al., Trans. R. Soc. Trop. Med. Hyg.* **78**, 837 (1984); P. Paolantonacci *et al., Antimicrob. Agents Chemother.* **28**, 528 (1985); E. Zweygarth *et al., Trop. Med. Parasitol.* **37**, 255 (1986); *in vivo* antileishmanial activity: J. L. Avila *et al., Am. J. Trop. Med. Hyg.* **43**, 139 (1990). Synthesis: M. Geze *et al., J. Am. Chem. Soc.* **105**, 7638 (1983); stereoselective synthesis: M. P. Maguire *et al., J. Org. Chem.* **55**, 948 (1990). Inhibition of methyltransferase: R. T. Borchardt *et al., Biochem. Biophys. Res. Commun.* **89**, 919 (1979).

White powder. Sol in water, very slightly sol in methanol and ethanol. Insol in organic solvents. Stable at room temp in aq soln from pH 1 to 11. pKa (66% DMF): 2.9, 3.9, 8.9, 10.2. uv max in neutral solns: 206 nm, 258 nm ($E_{1cm}^{1\%}$ 520, 325); in basic solns: 256 nm ($E_{1cm}^{1\%}$ 325). $[\alpha]_D^{25}$ $-2.61°$ (c = 5 in water). Also reported as $[\alpha]_D^{23}$ +12 ±2° (c = 0.227 in water). LD$_{50}$ s.c. in mice: 185 mg/kg (Hamill, Hoehn, *J. Antibiot.*)

8545. Sinigrin. [3952-98-5] 1-Thio-β-D-glucopyranose 1-[*N*-(sulfooxy)-3-butenimidate] monopotassium salt; sinigroside; myronate potassium; potassium myronate; allyl glucosinolate. $C_{10}H_{16}KNO_9S_2$; mol wt 397.46. C 30.22%, H 4.06%, K 9.84%, N 3.52%, O 36.23%, S 16.13%. A β-glucopyranoside isolated from black mustard seeds and from the horseradish root *Alliaria officinalis* Andrz., *Cruciferae*: A. Bussy, *J. Pharm. Chim.* **26**, 39 (1840); Gadamer, *Arch. Pharm.* **235**, 44 (1897); Stoll, Seebeck, *Helv. Chim. Acta* **31**, 1432 (1948). Structure: Ettlinger, Lundeen, *J. Am. Chem. Soc.* **78**, 4173 (1956); **79**, 1764 (1957). Hydrolysis: Ettlinger *et al.*, *Proc. Natl. Acad. Sci. USA* **47**, 1875 (1961). Crystal structure: Waser, Watson, *Nature* **198**, 1297 (1963). Synthesis: Benn, Ettlinger, *Chem. Commun.* **1965**, 445; A. Kjaer, *Acta Chem. Scand.* **22**, 3324 (1968).

Monohydrate. Crystals, mp 127-129°. When anhydr mp 179°. $[\alpha]_D^{18}$ $-16.4°$. Freely sol in water, hot alcohol; insol in benzene, chloroform, ether.

Tetraacetate. $C_{18}H_{24}KNO_{13}S_2$. Crystals, mp 193-195°. $[\alpha]_D^{26}$ $-16°$ (c = 0.14).

8546. Sinomenine. [115-53-7] (9α,13α,14α)-7,8-Didehydro-4-hydroxy-3,7-dimethoxy-17-methylmorphinan-6-one; cucoline; coculine; kukoline. $C_{19}H_{23}NO_4$; mol wt 329.39. C 69.28%, H 7.04%, N 4.25%, O 19.43%. An optical isomer of methoxythebainone, is the mirror image of those in morphine. From root of *Sinomenium acutum* (Thunb.) Rehd. & Wils. (*Cocculus diversifolius* DC.), *Menispermaceae*: Goto, *J. Chem. Soc. Jpn.* **44**, 795 (1923), *C.A.* **18**, 2710 (1924); Ohta, *Kitasato Arch. Exp. Med.* **6**, 259 (1925), *C.A.* **21**, 3233² (1927). Structure: Kondo, Ochiai, *Ann.* **470**, 224 (1929); Sasaki, *Yakugaku Zasshi* **80**, 270 (1960), *C.A.* **54**, 11702g (1960). Biogenesis: Cohen, *Chem. Ind. (London)* **1956**, 1391. Pharmacology: S. Fu *et al.*, *Yao Hsueh Hsueh Pao* **10**, 673 (1963), *C.A.* **60**, 8525h (1964). *Reviews:* Holmes in R. H. F. Manske, H. L. Holmes, *The Alkaloids* vol. **II** (Academic Press, New York, 1952) pp 219-260; K. W. Bentley, *The Chemistry of the Morphine Alkaloids* (Oxford, 1954).

Clusters of needles from benzene, mp 161°. After melting once, the mp is raised to 182°. $[\alpha]_D^{26}$ $-71°$ (c = 2.1 in alc). Sol in alc, acetone, chloroform, dil alkali; slightly sol in water, ether, benzene. LD$_{50}$ orally in mice: 580 mg/kg (Fu).

Hydrochloride dihydrate. $C_{19}H_{24}ClNO_4 \cdot 2H_2O$. Long prisms from water, dec 231° when anhydr. $[\alpha]_D^{17}$ $-82°$ (c = 4.4). Sol in about 1.5 parts water.

8547. Sipuleucel-T. APC-8015; Provenge. Autologous dendritic cell product loaded *ex vivo* with the recombinant fusion protein *PA2024* consisting of human granulocyte macrophage-colony stimulating factor (GM-CSF) linked to human prostatic acid phosphatase (PAP). Therapeutic vaccine designed to stimulate immunity against PAP expressed on prostate cancer cells. Prepn of target antigen: R. Laus *et al.*, **WO 9724438**; *eidem*, **US 5976546** (1997, 1999 both to Dendreon); of antigen presenting cells and pharmacology: E. J. Small *et al.*, *J. Clin. Oncol.* **18**, 3894 (2000). Clinical evaluation in androgen-independent prostate cancer: P. A. Burch *et al.*, *Prostate* **60**, 197 (2004); P. F. Schellhammer, R. M. Hershberg, *World J. Urol.* **23**, 47 (2005). Review of development and therapeutic potential: F. H. Valone *et al.*, *Cancer J.* **7**, Suppl. 2, S53-S61 (2001); B. I. Rini, *Curr. Opin. Mol. Ther.* **4**, 76-79 (2002).

THERAP CAT: Antineoplastic, immunomodulator.

8548. Sirius Red. [2610-10-8] 7,7'-(Carbonyldiimino)-bis[4-hydroxy-3-[[2-sulfo-4-[(4-sulfophenyl)azo]phenyl]azo]-2-naphthalenesulfonic acid] hexasodium salt; C.I. 35780; C.I. Direct Red 80; Sirius Red F3B. $C_{45}H_{26}N_{10}Na_6O_{21}S_6$; mol wt 1373.07. C 39.36%, H 1.91%, N 10.20%, Na 10.05%, O 24.47%, S 14.01%. Sulphonated tetrakisazo dye. Dye molecules bind parallel to helical native collagen. Water and light stability: J. J. Porter, *Text. Res. J.* **43**, 735 (1973). Spectral study: J. P. Hart, W. F. Smyth, *Spectrochim. Acta* **36A**, 279 (1980). Staining mechanisms: L. Feldskov Nielsen *et al.*, *Biotech. Histochem.* **73**, 71 (1998). Use as stain for collagen: F. Sweat *et al.*, *Arch. Pathol.* **78**, 69 (1964); D. A. Lee *et al.*, *J. Mater. Sci.: Mater. Med.* **9**, 47 (1998).

uv max (buffered): 220, 235, 290 nm (ε 1.2 × 10⁴, 1.3 × 10⁴, 1.2 × 10⁴). vis max (buffered): 420, 520, 545 nm (ε 0.8 × 10⁴, 2.5 × 10⁴, 2.6 × 10⁴). pK$_{1-6}$ < 2; pK$_{7,8}$ >13.

USE: Stain for connective tissue. Dye for cellulose fibers.

8549. Sisal. Henequem; yaxci; potosina. *Agave sisalana* Perrine, Amaryllidaceae; one of the plants native to the American desert. Process of treating juice and extracting steroidal material and waxes: Spray, **US 3019193** (1962). *Habit.* Principally the Mexican tableland. Abundant in the Mexican states Yucatan and Chiapas. *Constit.* Hemp, sapogenins such as hecogenin and tigogenin. *Review: Chem. Week* 41-48 (April 20, 1957).

Caution: The dust is irritating to respiratory tract.

USE: Manuf sisal ropes, steroid intermediates.

8550. Sisomicin. [32385-11-8] *O*-3-Deoxy-4-*C*-methyl-3-(methylamino)-β-L-arabinopyranosyl-(1 → 6)-*O*-[2,6-diamino-2,3,-4,6-tetradeoxy-α-D-*glycero*-hex-4-enopyranosyl-(1 → 4)]-2-deoxy-D-streptamine; (2*S-cis*)-4-*O*-[3-amino-6-(aminomethyl)-3,4-dihydro-2*H*-pyran-2-yl]-2-deoxy-6-*O*-[3-deoxy-4-*C*-methyl-3-(methylamino)-β-L-arabinopyranosyl]-D-streptamine; rickamicin; antibiotic 6640; Sch-13475. $C_{19}H_{37}N_5O_7$; mol wt 447.53. C 50.99%, H 8.33%, N 15.65%, O 25.03%. Gentamicin-like aminoglycoside antibiotic produced by *Micromonospora inyoesis* (NRRL 3292): M. J. Weinstein *et al.* **DE 1932309**; *eidem*, **US 3832286** (1970, 1974 both to Schering); *eidem, J. Antibiot.* **23**, 551 (1970). Isoln: G. H. Wagman *et al., ibid.* 555. Chemical and physical studies:

Cooper *et al., Chem. Commun.* **1971**, 285, 924; Kugelman *et al., J. Antibiot.* **26**, 394 (1973). Structure consists of 2-deoxystreptamine, *q.v.*, linked to two saccharide units, **garosamine** and **sisosamine**: Keiman *et al., J. Org. Chem.* **39**, 1451 (1974). Synthesis: D. H. Davies *et al., J. Med. Chem.* **21**, 189 (1978). Synthesis of sisosamine derivs: Cleophax *et al., Chem. Commun.* **1975**, 11. Has broad spectrum antibiotic activity: Waitz *et al., J. Antibiot.* **23**, 559 (1970). Biotransformation of sisomicin to gentamicin: B. K. Lee *et al., Antimicrob. Agents Chemother.* **12**, 335 (1977). Clinical studies: R. Lorber *et al., Clin. Ther.* **4**, 263 (1981); J. P. Sculier *et al., J. Antimicrob. Chemother.* **9**, 63 (1982). *Review:* P. Noone, *Drugs* **27**, 548-578 (1984).

Monohydrate. Needles from ethanol, mp 198-201°. $[\alpha]_D^{26}$ +189° (c = 0.3).

Penta-*N*-acetyl deriv. $C_{29}H_{47}N_5O_{12}$. Amorphous white powder from methanol-ethyl ether, mp 188-198° (dec). $[\alpha]_D^{26}$ +200° (c = 0.3).

Sulfate. [53179-09-2] Baymicin; Extramycin; Mensiso; Siseptin; Sisobiotic; Sisolline; Sisomin. $(C_{19}H_{37}N_5O_7)_2 \cdot 5H_2SO_4$; mol wt 1385.45. LD_{50} in mice (mg/kg): 34 i.v., 221 i.p., 288 s.c. (Weinstein).

THERAP CAT: Antibacterial.

8551. Sitafloxacin. [127254-12-0] 7-[(7S)-7-Amino-5-azaspiro[2.4]hept-5-yl]-8-chloro-6-fluoro-1-[(1R,2S)-2-fluorocyclopropyl]-1,4-dihydro-4-oxo-3-quinolinecarboxylic acid; DU-6859. $C_{19}H_{18}ClF_2N_3O_3$; mol wt 409.81. C 55.69%, H 4.43%, Cl 8.65%, F 9.27%, N 10.25%, O 11.71%. Fluorinated quinolone antibacterial. Prepn: I. Hayakawa, Y. Kimura, **EP 341493**; *idem*, **US 5587386** (1989, 1996 both to Daiichi); Y. Kimura *et al., J. Med. Chem.* **37**, 3344 (1994). Antibacterial spectrum: L. M. Deshpande, R. N. Jones, *Diagn. Microbiol. Infect. Dis.* **37**, 139 (2000). HPLC determn in serum and urine: H. Aoki *et al., J. Chromatogr. B* **660**, 365 (1994). Clinical pharmacokinetics: M. Nakashima *et al., Antimicrob. Agents Chemother.* **39**, 170 (1995). Clinical evaluation: N. Shetty, A. P. R. Wilson, *J. Antimicrob. Chemother.* **46**, 633 (2000).

Sesquihydrate. [163253-35-8] DU-6859a. Crystals from ethanol, water + ammonium hydroxide, mp 225° (dec). $[\alpha]_{589}$ −199.9° (c = 1 in 1 *N* NaOH). Soly in water: 131 μg/ml.

THERAP CAT: Antibacterial.

8552. Sitagliptin. [486460-32-6] 7-[(3R)-3-Amino-1-oxo-4-(2,4,5-trifluorophenyl)butyl]-5,6,7,8-tetrahydro-3-(trifluoromethyl)-1,2,4-triazolo[4,3-*a*]pyrazine; (2R)-4-oxo-4-[3-(trifluoromethyl)-5,6-dihydro[1,2,4]triazolo[4,3-*a*]pyrazin-7(8H)-yl]-1-(2,4,5-trifluorophenyl)butan-2-amine. $C_{16}H_{15}F_6N_5O$; mol wt 407.31. C 47.18%, H 3.71%, F 27.99%, N 17.19%, O 3.93%. Selective

inhibitor of dipeptidyl peptidase IV (DPP-IV). Prepn: S. D. Edmondson *et al.,* **WO 03004498**; *eidem*, **US 6699871** (2003, 2004 both to Merck & Co.); and enzyme inhibitory profile: D. Kim *et al., J. Med. Chem.* **48**, 141 (2005). Improved process: K. B. Hansen *et al., Org. Process Res. Dev.* **9**, 634 (2005). Clinical pharmacokinetics and pharmacodynamics: G. A. Herman *et al., Clin. Pharmacol. Ther.* **78**, 675 (2005). *Review:* C. F. Deacon, *Curr. Opin. Invest. Drugs* **6**, 419-426 (2005).

Viscous oil.

Monophosphate monohydrate. [654671-77-9]; [654671-78-0] (anhydrous). Sitagliptin phosphate; MK-0431; Januvia. $C_{16}H_{15}F_6N_5O \cdot H_3PO_4 \cdot H_2O$; mol wt 523.32. mp 215-217°. $[\alpha]_D$ −74.4° (c = 1.0 in water).

THERAP CAT: Antidiabetic.

8553. Sitamaquine. [57695-04-2] N,N-Diethyl-N'-(6-methoxy-4-methyl-8-quinolinyl)-1,6-hexanediamine; 8-(6'-diethylaminohexylamino)-6-methoxylepidine; 6-methoxy-8-(6-diethylaminohexylamine)-4-methylquinoline; kalazaquine; WR-6026. $C_{21}H_{33}N_3O$; mol wt 343.51. C 73.43%, H 9.68%, N 12.23%, O 4.66%. 8-Aminoquinolone; analog of the antimalarial agent primaquine, *q.v.* Prepn: K. N. Campbell *et al., J. Am. Chem. Soc.* **68**, 1556 (1946); *idem*, **US 2508937** (1950 to USA, as represented by the Secy. of War). Antileishmanial activity in hamsters: K. E. Kinnamon *et al., Am. J. Trop. Med. Hyg.* **27**, 751 (1978). HPLC determn in plasma: J. C. Anders *et al., J. Chromatogr.* **311**, 117 (1984). Clinical evaluation in AIDS-associated *Pneumocystis carinii* pneumonia: B. G. Petty *et al., J. Acquir. Immune Defic. Syndr.* **21**, 26 (1999); in visceral leishmaniasis: R. Dietze *et al., Am. J. Trop. Med. Hyg.* **65**, 685 (2001). *Ex vivo* use in prevention of transfusion-associated Chagas' disease: H. Moraes-Souza *et al., Rev. Soc. Bras. Med. Trop.* **35**, 563 (2002). Review of clinical development: C. Yeates, *Curr. Opin. Invest. Drugs* **3**, 1446-1452 (2002); H. Sangraula *et al., J. Assoc. Physicians India* **51**, 686-690 (2003).

bp$_{0.05}$ 190-200°.

Dihydrochloride. [5330-29-0] $C_{21}H_{33}N_3O \cdot 2HCl$; mol wt 416.43. Yellow crystals from propanol, mp 179-180°.

THERAP CAT: Antiprotozoal (Leishmania).

8554. Sitaxsentan. [184036-34-8] N-(4-Chloro-3-methyl-5-isoxazolyl)-2-[(6-methyl-1,3-benzodioxol-5-yl)acetyl]-3-thiophenesulfonamide; N-(4-chloro-3-methyl-5-isoxazolyl)-2-[3,4-(methylenedioxy)-6-methyl]phenylacetyl-3-thiophenesulfonamide; IPI-1040; TBC-11251. $C_{18}H_{15}ClN_2O_6S_2$; mol wt 454.90. C 47.53%, H 3.32%, Cl 7.79%, N 6.16%, O 21.10%, S 14.10%. Selective endothelin A (ET_A) receptor antagonist. Prepn: M. F. Chan *et al.,* **WO 9631492**; *eidem*, **US 5594021** (1996, 1997 both to Texas Biotech.); C. Wu *et al., J. Med. Chem.* **40**, 1690 (1997). Pharmacology: R. G. Tilton *et al., Pulm. Pharmacol. Ther.* **13**, 87 (2000). Clinical evaluation in heart failure: M. M. Givertz *et al., Circulation* **101**, 2922 (2000); in pulmonary arterial hypertension: D. Langleben *et al., Chest* **126**, 1377 (2004). Review of

Consult the Name Index before using this section.

development and therapeutic potential: E. M. Horn *et al., Expert Opin. Invest. Drugs* **13**, 1483-1492 (2004).

Yellow powder, mp 42-45°.

Sodium salt. [210421-74-2] Thelin. $C_{18}H_{14}ClNaN_2O_6S_2$; mol wt 476.89.

THERAP CAT: Antihypertensive. In treatment of chronic heart failure.

8555. α_1-Sitosterol. [474-40-8] (3β,4α,5α,24Z)-4-Methylstigmasta-7,24(28)-dien-3-ol; citrostadienol. $C_{30}H_{50}O$; mol wt 426.72. C 84.44%, H 11.81%, O 3.75%. Occurs in plants. Isoln from wheat germ oil: Anderson *et al., J. Am. Chem. Soc.* **48**, 2987 (1926); Wallis, Fernholz, *ibid.* **58**, 2446 (1936). Structure: Bernstein, Wallis, *ibid.* **61**, 2308 (1939); Mazur, Sondheimer, *ibid.* **80**, 6293, 6296 (1958). Identity with citrostadienol: Schreiber, Osske, *Experientia* **19**, 69 (1963); *eidem, Tetrahedron* **20**, 2575 (1964). Stereochemistry: C. Brooks *et al., Steroids* **20**, 487 (1972).

Needles from alcohol, mp 164-166°. $[\alpha]_D^{28}$ −1.7° (c = 2 in chloroform). Is pptd by digitonin.

8556. β-Sitosterol. [83-46-5] (3β)-Stigmast-5-en-3-ol; 22:23-dihydrostigmasterol; α-dihydrofucosterol; Δ^5-stigmasten-3β-ol; 24β-ethyl-Δ^5-cholesten-3β-ol; α-phytosterol; cinchol; cupreol; rhamnol; quebrachol; sitosterin; Harzol; Prostasal; Sito-Lande. $C_{29}H_{50}O$; mol wt 414.71. C 83.99%, H 12.15%, O 3.86%. Common sterol in plants. Isoln from wheat germ oil, corn oil: Anderson *et al., J. Am. Chem. Soc.* **48**, 2987 (1926); from rye germ oil: Gloyer, Schuette, *ibid.* **61**, 1901 (1939); from cottonseed oil: Wallis, Chakravorty, *J. Org. Chem.* **2**, 335 (1937); from tall oil: Sandqvist, Bengtsson, *Ber.* **64**, 2167 (1931). Also occurs in soy and calabar beans, in rice embryos: Tanaka, *J. Biochem.* **17**, 483 (1933); in cascara, cinchona bark and cinchona wax: Dirscherl, *Z. Physiol. Chem.* **235**, 1 (1935). Prepn from tall oil: G. I. Fujimoto, A. E. Jacobson, *J. Org. Chem.* **29**, 3377 (1964). Identity with 22:23-dihydrostigmasterol: W. Dirscherl, H. Nahm, *Ann.* **555**, 57 (1944). Identity with cinchol: *eidem, Ann.* **558**, 231 (1947). Structure: Bernstein, Wallis, *J. Org. Chem.* **2**, 341 (1937); Bergmann, Low, *ibid.* **12**, 67 (1947); Shoppee, *J. Chem. Soc.* **1948**, 1032. Stereospecific synthesis: W. Sucrow, M. Slopianka, *Ber.* **108**, 3721 (1975). Clinical efficacy in treatment of type II hyperlipoproteinemia: R. S. Lees, A. M. Lees, in *Lipoprotein Metabolism*, H. Greten, Ed. (Springer-Verlag, New York, 1976) pp 119-124; P. Oster *et al., ibid.* pp 125-130. Studies on inhibition of cholesterol absorption: S. M. Grundy, H. Y. I. Mok, *ibid.* pp 112-118; I. Ikeda, M. Sugano, *Biochim. Biophys. Acta* **732**, 651 (1983). Inhibition of induced carcinogenesis: N. D. Nigro *et al., J. Natl. Cancer Inst.* **69**, 103 (1982). Clinical trial in treatment of prostatic adenoma: H.-P. Szutrely, *Med. Klin.* **77**, 520 (1982). Book: *Monographs on Athe-*

roclerosis **Vol. 10**, T. B. Clarkson *et al.,* Eds. entitled "Sitosterol" by O. J. Pollak, D. Kritchevsky (Karger, Basel, 1981) 219 pp.

Plates from alcohol, mp 140°. $[\alpha]_D^{25}$ −37° (c = 2 in chloroform).

Acetate. $C_{31}H_{52}O_2$. mp 127-128°. $[\alpha]_D^{25}$ −41° (c = 2 in chloroform).

THERAP CAT: Antilipemic. Treatment of prostatic adenoma.

8557. γ-Sitosterol. [83-47-6] (3β,24S)-Stigmast-5-en-3-ol; clionasterol. $C_{29}H_{50}O$; mol wt 414.71. C 83.99%, H 12.15%, O 3.86%. Principal sterol of soybean oil: Bonstedt, *Z. Physiol. Chem.* **176**, 269 (1928). Isoln from corn oil: Anderson, Shriner, *J. Am. Chem. Soc.* **48**, 2976 (1926); from venom of Chinese toad, *Bufo gargarizans:* Rukstuhl, Meyer, *Helv. Chim. Acta* **40**, 1270 (1957). Differs from β-sitosterol in spatial configuration at C-24: Bergmann, Low, *J. Org. Chem.* **12**, 67 (1947). Structure: Pavanaram, *Helv. Chim. Acta* **46**, 1377 (1963). Stereospecific synthesis: W. Sucrow, M. Slopianka, *Ber.* **108**, 3721 (1975).

Monohydrate. Plates from alcohol. When dry, mp 147-148°. $[\alpha]_D^{20}$ −43° (c = 1.9 in chloroform). Table of mp's and $[\alpha]_D$'s: Dirscherl, *Z. Physiol. Chem.* **257**, 242 (1939).

Acetate. $C_{31}H_{52}O_2$. mp 143-144°. $[\alpha]_D^{20}$ −45.3° (c = 1.9 in chloroform).

8558. Sivelestat. [127373-66-4] N-[2-[[[4-(2,2-Dimethyl-1-oxopropoxy)phenyl]sulfonyl]amino]benzoyl]glycine; N-[o-(p-pivaloyloxybenzene)sulfonylaminobenzoyl]glycine; N-[2-[4-(2,2-dimethylpropionyloxy)phenylsulfonylamino]benzoyl]aminoacetic acid. $C_{20}H_{22}N_2O_7S$; mol wt 434.46. C 55.29%, H 5.10%, N 6.45%, O 25.78%, S 7.38%. Neutrophil elastase inhibitor. Prepn: K. Imaki *et al.*, **EP 347168**; *eidem,* **US 5017610** (1989, 1991 both to Ono); and structure-activity study: K. Imaki *et al., Bioorg. Med. Chem.* **4**, 2115 (1996). Pharmacology: K. Kawabata *et al., Biochem. Biophys. Res. Commun.* **177**, 814 (1991). HPLC determn in plasma and urine: T. Shintani *et al., J. Pharm. Biomed. Anal.* **12**, 397 (1994). Pharmacokinetics and metabolism in rats: F. Watanabe *et al., Biol. Pharm. Bull.* **20**, 392 (1997). Enzyme inhibition in *ex vivo* human pleural effusion: T. Sakuma *et al., Eur. J. Pharmacol.* **353**, 273 (1998). Acute toxicity: H. Yanagi *et al., J. Toxicol. Sci.* **23**, Suppl. 3, 409 (1998), *C.A.* **130**, 20355 (1998). Review: L. Pradella, *Curr. Opin. Anti-Inflam. Immunomod. Invest. Drugs* **1**, 485-501 (1999).

mp 218-220°.

Sodium salt tetrahydrate. [201677-61-4]; [150374-95-1] (anhydrous). EI-546; ONO-5046; Elaspol. $C_{20}H_{21}N_2NaO_7S.4H_2O$; mol wt 528.51. LD_{50} in rats (mg/kg): 450 i.v. (Yanagi).

THERAP CAT: In treatment of lung injury resulting from systemic inflammatory response syndrome.

8559. Sizofiran. [9050-67-3] Schizophyllan; SPG; Sonifilan. Immunostimulant polysaccharide produced by the fungus *Schizophyllum commune* Fries. Polymer of repeating tetrasaccharide units composed of three β-(1 → 3)-linked D-glucopyranose residues, to one of which is attached a single β-(1 → 6)-linked D-glucopyranosyl side chain. Forms triple-stranded helix of mol wt ~450,000 in neutral aqueous solution. Prepn by fermentation: S. Kikumoto *et al., JP 67 12000* (1967 to Taito), *C.A.* **67,** 107386r (1967). Synthesis of the 3 possible tetrasaccharide units: K. Takeo, S. Tei, *Carbohydr. Res.* **145,** 293 (1986). Host-mediated antitumor activity: N. Komatsu *et al., Gann* **60,** 137 (1969). Pharmacology, toxicology and antitumor activity in mice: T. Matsuo *et al., Arzneim.-Forsch.* **32,** 647 (1982). Macrophage stimulant activity *in vitro:* I. Sugawara *et al., Cancer Immunol. Immunother.* **16,** 137 (1984). Clinical trial in cervical cancer: K. Okamura *et al., Cancer* **58,** 865 (1986).

White, amorphous powder. Sol in water, forming highly viscous soln.

THERAP CAT: Antineoplastic.

8560. Skatole. [83-34-1] 3-Methyl-1*H*-indole. C_9H_9N; mol wt 131.17. C 82.41%, H 6.92%, N 10.68%. Constituent of feces, beetroot, nectandra wood, and coal tar. Obtained by fusing egg albumin with KOH. Toxicity data: Bin-Ichi, *Tohoku J. Exp. Med.* **25,** 407 (1935).

White to brownish scales; fecal odor; mp 95°; bp 265-266°. Sol in hot water, alc, benzene, chloroform, ether. With potassium ferrocyanide and sulfuric acid it gives a violet color. MLD in frogs (mg/kg): 1000 s.c. (Bin-Ichi).

8561. Skimmianine. [83-95-4] 4,7,8-Trimethoxyfuro[2,3-*b*]quinoline; β-fagarine; 7,8-dimethoxydictamnine. $C_{14}H_{13}NO_4$; mol wt 259.26. C 64.86%, H 5.05%, N 5.40%, O 24.68%. In *Skimmia japonica* Thunb., *Fagara* spp., *Glycosmis pentaphylla* Corr., *Ruta graveolens* L., Rutaceae: Honda, *Arch. Exp. Pathol. Pharmakol.* **52,** 83 (1904); Paris, Moyse-Mignon, *Ann. Pharm. Fr.* **5,** 410 (1947), *C.A.* **42,** 3909h (1948); Chatterjee, Majumdar, *J. Am. Chem. Soc.* **76,** 2459 (1954); Schneider, *Arzneim.-Forsch.* **14,** 435 (1964). Identity with β-fagarine: Deulofeu *et al., J. Am. Chem. Soc.* **64,** 2326 (1942). Structure: Asahina, Inubuse, *Ber.* **63,** 2052 (1930).

Pyramids, octahedral rods from alcohol. mp 178°. uv max (ethanol): 212, 251, 321, 331 nm (log ε 4.10, 4.91, 3.89, 3.91). Neutral to litmus. Sol in alcohol, chloroform; slightly in ether, amyl alcohol and carbon disulfide; practically insol in water and petr ether.

8562. Skimmin. [93-39-0] 7-(β-D-Glucopyranosyloxy)-2*H*-1-benzopyran-2-one; 7-(glucosyloxy)coumarin; 7-hydroxycoumarin-7-glucoside; umbelliferone glucoside. $C_{15}H_{16}O_8$; mol wt 324.28. C 55.56%, H 4.97%, O 39.47%. In bark and wood of *Skimmia japonica* Thunb., Rutaceae. Isoln, structure and synthesis: Späth, Neufeld, *Rec. Trav. Chim.* **57,** 535 (1938).

Crystals with one H_2O from water. After drying at 100° and 10 mm: mp 219-221° (evac tube). $[\alpha]_D^{18}$ −80° (c = 10 in pyridine). uv max (ethanol): 320 nm. Moderately sol in hot water, alcohol; practically insol in ether, chloroform.

8563. Slendid®. Natural food ingredient made from pectin extracted from citrus peels. Analysis of interaction with flavor compounds: J. P. Schirle-Keller *et al., J. Food Sci.* **59,** 813 (1994). Brief review: D. D. Duxbury, *Food Process.* **52,** 54-55 (1991).

Light cream to light tan, granular free-flowing powder. Tasteless and odorless. Completely sol in 25 parts of water at 60° with adequate agitation.

USE: Fat replacer in foods.

8564. SMEAH. [22722-98-1] Dihydrobis(2-methoxyethanolato-*O,O'*)aluminate(1−) sodium; sodium bis(2-methoxyethoxy)aluminum hydride; Red-Al; Vitride. $C_6H_{15}AlNaO_4$; mol wt 202.16. C 35.65%, H 7.98%, Al 13.35%, Na 11.37%, O 31.66%. $NaAlH_2(OCH_2CH_2OCH_3)_2$. Prepn: B. Casensky *et al., US 3507895* (1970). Properties: J. Vit, *Eastman Organic Chemical Bulletin* **42**(3), 1 (1970). Review of reductions by metal alkoxyaluminum hydrides: J. Málek, *Org. React.* **34,** 1-317 (1985); *idem, ibid.* **36,** 252-590 (1987).

Highly viscous liquid at room temp. Miscible in a great variety of inert solvents (e.g., aromatic hydrocarbons and ethers). Immiscible in paraffinic hydrocarbons. Thermally stable at 200°C; thermal decomposition starts at 205°C and is vigorous.

USE: Reducing agent.

8565. Smilagenin. [126-18-1] (25*R*)-Spirostan-3β-ol; isosarsasapogenin. $C_{27}H_{44}O_3$; mol wt 416.64. C 77.83%, H 10.64%, O 11.52%. Steroid sapogenin from *Smilax ornata* Hooker, Liliaceae (Sarsaparilla): Ashew *et al., J. Chem. Soc.* **1936,** 1399; from *Agave lecheguilla* Tou., Amaryllidaceae: Nord, *US 2897192* (1959). C_{25} isomer of sarsasapogenin: Scheer *et al., J. Am. Chem. Soc.* **77,** 1955 (1955). Obtained by acid isomerization of sarsasapogenin: Marker, Rohrmann, *ibid.* **61,** 846 (1939); Wall *et al., ibid.* **77,** 3086 (1955). For structure and stereochemistry *see* Sarsasapogenin.

Silky needles from acetone, mp 185°. $[\alpha]_D^{25}$ −69° (c = 0.5 in chloroform). Absorption spectrum: Smith, Eddy, *Anal. Chem.* **31,** 1539 (1959).

Acetate. $C_{29}H_{46}O_4$. Needles from methanol, mp 152°.

USE: In making compds of the pregnane series.

8566. Soap. Any salt of a fatty acid, usually made by saponification of a vegetable oil with caustic soda. Hard soap consists largely of sodium oleate (low titer) or of sodium palmitate or stearate (high titer); soft soap, of potassium and sodium salts of coconut and/or palm oil fatty acids. Rosin acid salts have detergent properties and are often incorporated in laundry soaps. Shaving soaps contain glycerol and gum to prevent rapid drying. Medicated soaps contain antiseptics such as phenols or mercury salts. Soaps also may be prepd from the fatty acid and an amine, *e.g.,* triethanolamine. Nonalkali-metal salts of the fatty acids are water insol and as such have certain uses.

Hard soap (olive-oil castile) is a white or yellowish white powder or bar, sol in water, alc. The aq soln is alkaline due to hydrolysis; the alc soln is only slightly alkaline. Transparent hard soap is obtained by adding additional glycerol during saponification. Floating soaps are made by adding air after saponification during the so-called "crutching" process. Soft soap (green soap) is a yellowish-white to brownish-yellow (or green) soft mass, more sol than hard soap.

USE: Hard soap—detergent; in soln as a vehicle for liniments; as ingredient of pills contg resinous drugs like aloe, etc. Soft soap—detergent; extern. as vehicle for active medicaments applied in ointment form or liniment. Insoluble soaps —fungicides (Cu), disinfectants (Pb, Cu, Hg), face powders and ointments (Zn), waxes and polishes (Al), greases (Al, Ca), and surface coatings (Ca).

THERAP CAT: Topical anti-infective. Antidote (mineral acid and heavy metal poisoning).

THERAP CAT (VET): Topically as detergent (cleansing agent) and mild antiseptic. In liniments as counterirritant. Has been used internally as laxative, antacid and as an antidote for mineral acids and heavy metals.

8567. Sobrerol. [498-71-5] 5-Hydroxy-$\alpha,\alpha,4$-trimethyl-3-cyclohexene-1-methanol; *p*-menth-6-ene-2,8-diol; 6,8-carvomenthenediol; 1-*p*-menthene-6,8-diol; pinol hydrate. $C_{10}H_{18}O_2$; mol wt 170.25. C 70.55%, H 10.66%, O 18.80%. An oxidation product of oil of turpentine formed by the autooxidation of α-pinene, *q.v.*, in the presence of water and especially in sunlight. First obtained by Margueron in 1797. Confused with terpin hydrate, *q.v.*, until fully characterized by Sobrero in 1851. The naturally occurring form is the *trans*-form. For a review of early structure and prepn work, *see* J. L. Simonsen, *The Terpenes* vol. II (University Press, Cambridge, 2nd ed., 1949) pp 137-138. Summary of general methods of prepn: Lombard, Heywang, *Bull. Soc. Chim. Fr.* **1954**, 1210. Prepn of *dl*-*trans*-form: Ward, *J. Am. Chem. Soc.* **60**, 325 (1938); Schenck *et al., Ann.* **584**, 177 (1953); Moore *et al., J. Am. Chem. Soc.* **78**, 1173 (1956); Brook, Wright, *J. Org. Chem.* **22**, 1314 (1957); of *l*-*trans*-form: Klein, US 2815378 (1958 to Glidden). Prepn of *cis*- and *trans*-forms and analysis of stereochemistry: Blumann, Wood, *J. Chem. Soc.* **1952**, 4420; H. Schmidt, *Ber.* **86**, 1437 (1953). Pharmacology and chemistry of *dl*-*trans*-form: GB 1176817; C. Corvi-Mora, US 3592908 (1970, 1971 to Camillo Corvi); V. Dalla Valle, *Boll. Chim. Farm.* **109**, 761 (1970). Clinical evaluation: C. F. Marchioni, G. Monzali, *Clin. Ter.* **60**, 135 (1972). Activity on mucociliary transport: P. Braga, *Clin. Trials J.* **18**, 30 (1981). Pharmacokinetics: P. C. Braga *et al., Eur. J. Clin. Pharmacol.* **24**, 209 (1983). Metabolism: P. Ventura *et al., Xenobiotica* **13**, 139 (1983); *eidem, ibid.* **15**, 317 (1985). GLC determn in human plasma: U. A. Shulka, *J. Chromatogr.* **308**, 189 (1984).

(−)-*trans* form

***dl*-*trans*-Form.** Lysmucol; Sobrepin. Crystals, mp 130-131.5°. bp 270-271°. Soly in water: 3.3 g/100 ml (15°). LD$_{50}$ in rats, mice (mg/kg): both 580 i.v. (Dalla Valle).
***d*-*trans*-Form.** mp 148-149°. $[\alpha]_D^{20}$ +150° (Schmidt).
***l*-*trans*-Form.** mp 148-149°. $[\alpha]_D^{20}$ −150° (Schmidt).
THERAP CAT: Mucolytic.

8568. Sobuzoxane. [98631-95-9] 1,2-Ethanediylbis[(2,6-dioxo-4,1-piperazinediyl)methylene]carbonic acid bis(2-methylpropyl) ester; 4,4'-ethylenebis[1-(hydroxymethyl)-2,6-piperazinedione] bis(isobutyl carbonate) (ester); 4,4'-(1,2-ethanediyl)bis(1-isobutoxycarbonyloxymethyl)-2,6-piperazinedione; 1,2-bis(4-isobutoxycarbonyloxymethyl-3,5-dioxopiperazin-1-yl)ethane; MST-16; Perazolin. $C_{22}H_{34}N_4O_{10}$; mol wt 514.53. C 51.35%, H 6.66%, N 10.89%, O 31.10%. Noncleavable complex-stabilizing DNA topoisomerase II inhibitor. Prepn: J.-C. Cai, M. Takase, EP 140327; *eidem,* US 4650799 (1985, 1987 both to Zenyaku Kogyo); *idem et al., Chem. Pharm. Bull.* **37**, 2976 (1989). Antitumor activity: T. Narita *et al., Cancer Chemother. Pharmacol.* **28**, 235 (1991). Clinical evaluation in non-Hodgkin's lymphoma: R. Ohno *et al., J. Natl. Cancer Inst.* **84**, 435 (1992); in adult T-cell leukemia-lymphoma: *idem et al., Cancer* **71**, 2217 (1993). Acute toxicity study: T. Tokiwa *et al., Iyakuhin Kenkyu* **22**, 435 (1991). *C.A.* **115**, 222916k (1991).

Crystals from ethylene glycol monomethylether, mp 128-130°. Also reported as crystals from ethanol, mp 132-133° (Cai, 1989). Practically insol in water. LD$_{50}$ in male, female mice, rats (mg/kg): 807, 960, 877, 567 i.p.; 400, 673, 3025, 2821 s.c.; >5 g/kg orally in all species (Tokiwa).
THERAP CAT: Antineoplastic.

8569. Soda Lime. [8006-28-8] Sodium hydroxide with lime. A mixture of calcium oxide with 5-20% sodium hydroxide and contg 6-18% water. It absorbs 25-35% its wt of CO_2.
White or gray-white granules. Rapidly deteriorates on exposure to air through absorption of carbon dioxide. *Keep tightly closed.*
Caution: Strongly corrosive and irritating to skin, mucous membranes, eyes. Ingestion can cause severe damage to G.I. tract, death.
USE: To absorb carbon dioxide in basal metabolism tests, in rebreathing anesthesia systems, in submarines, and in carbon determinations.

8570. Sodium. [7440-23-5] Natrium. Na; at. no. 11; at. wt 22.98976928; valence 1. Group IA (1). Alkali metal. Occurrence in earth's crust: 2.83% by wt; principal cation in hydrosphere. Naturally occurring isotope: 23 (100%); radioactive isotopes (mass number): 19-22; 24-35. Prepd by Davy in 1807 by electrolysis of fused sodium hydroxide. Found in form of its compds, halides, silicates, carbonates; does not occur free. Industrial prepns primarily in Downs cells, also in Castner cells: Batsford, *Chem. Metall. Eng.* **26**, 888, 932 (1932); Regelsberger, *Chemische Technologie der Leichtmetalle* Leipzig, 1926; Hardie, *Ind. Chem.* **30**, 161 (1954). *Reviews: ACS Monograph Series* no. 133, entitled "Sodium," M. Sittig, Ed. (Reinhold, New York, 1956); Whaley, "Sodium, Potassium, Rubidium, Cesium and Francium" in *Comprehensive Inorganic Chemistry* Vol. 1, J. C. Bailar, Jr. *et al.,* Eds. (Pergamon Press, Oxford, 1973) pp 369-529; *Chemistry of the Elements* N. N. Greenwood, A. Earnshaw, Eds. (Pergamon Press, New York, 1984) pp 75-116; C. H. Lemke, V. H. Markant in *Kirk-Othmer Encyclopedia of Chemical Technology* vol. 22 (Wiley-Interscience, New York, 4th ed., 1997) pp 327-354.
Light, silvery-white metal; body-centered cubic structure; lustrous when freshly cut; tarnishes on exposure to air, becoming dull and gray. Soft at ordinary temp, fairly hard at −20°. mp 97.82°; bp 881.4°; d^{20} 0.968. Heat capacity of solid: 0.292 cal/g deg; heat capacity of liquid at mp: 0.331 cal/g deg. Heat of fusion: 27.05 cal/g; thermal conductivity (cal/sec °C cm): 0.205 (97.82°) 0.170 (400°). E^0 (aqueous) Na/Na$^+$ 2.714 V. Violently decomposes water, forming sodium hydroxide and hydrogen which may ignite spontaneously. Decomposes alc. Reacts vigorously with oxygen, burning with a yellow flame. Emits characteristic yellow color (589.2 nm) in flame. Combines directly with the halogens, with phosphorus. Reduces most oxides to the elemental state, reduces metallic chlorides. Dissolves in liq ammonia to give a blue soln; when heated in ammonia gas yields sodamide. Dissolves in mercury, forming sodium amalgam. *Keep under liquids contg no oxygen, such as kerosene, naphtha.*
Caution: Direct contact with metal be may corrosive and cause skin and eye burns. *See: Fire Protection Guide to Hazardous Materials* (National Fire Protection Assoc., Quincy, MA, 12th ed., 1997) Section 49, p 117.
USE: Manuf of sodium compds, such as the cyanide, azide, peroxide, etc.; manuf of tetraethyllead; manuf of refractory metals; in org syntheses; for photoelectric cells; in sodium lamps; as catalyst for many polymerization reactions. Alloyed with potassium in heat transfer media.

8571. Sodium Acetate. [127-09-3] $C_2H_3NaO_2$; mol wt 82.03. C 29.28%, H 3.69%, Na 28.03%, O 39.01%. CH$_3$COONa. Crystal structure of the trihydrate: K.-T. Wei, D. L. Ward, *Acta Crystallogr.* **B33**, 522 (1977).
Hygroscopic powder. Very sol in water; moderately sol in alcohol.
Trihydrate. Transparent crystals or granules. Efflorescent in warm air. d 1.45. mp 58°; becomes anhyd at 120°; dec at higher temp. One gram dissolves in 0.8 ml water, 0.6 ml boiling water, 19 ml alcohol. pH of 0.1 molar aq soln at 25°: 8.9.
USE: Anhydrous form as auxiliary in acetylations. Trihydrate in photography; as reagent in anal. chemistry to eliminate effect of strong acids (buffer); for foot warmers and milk-bottle warmers.

Technical grades are used as a mordant in dyeing. As acidulant in food. Pharmaceutic aid (in dialysis solutions).

THERAP CAT (VET): Has been used in bovine ketosis.

8572. Sodium Acid Pyrophosphate. [7758-16-9] Disodium dihydrogen pyrophosphate. $H_2Na_2O_7P_2$; mol wt 221.94. H 0.91%, Na 20.72%, O 50.46%, P 27.91%. $Na_2H_2P_2O_7$. Prepn: Bell, *Inorg. Synth.* **3**, 98 (1950).

White, fused masses or powder. Dec at 220°. d (hexahydrate) 1.86. Sol in water, the soln having an acid reaction.

USE: Chiefly in baking powders.

8573. Sodium Alizarinesulfonate. [130-22-3] 9,10-Dihydro-3,4-dihydroxy-9,10-dioxo-2-anthracenesulfonic acid monosodium salt; alizarine S; alizarine carmine; C.I. Mordant Red 3; C.I. 58005. $C_{14}H_7NaO_7S$; mol wt 342.26. C 49.13%, H 2.06%, Na 6.72%, O 32.72%, S 9.37%. Prepn: *Colour Index* **vol. 4** (3rd ed., 1971) p 4514.

Monohydrate. Orange-yellow powder. Freely sol in water with yellow color; sol in alcohol.

USE: As acid-base indicator and in the determination of fluorine, usually used as a 1% aq soln. pH: 3.7 yellow, 5.2 purple; as a reagent for aluminum and stain in microscopy.

8574. Sodium Aluminate. [1302-42-7] Aluminum sodium oxide. $AlNaO_2$; mol wt 81.97. Al 32.92%, Na 28.05%, O 39.04%.

White granular mass. mp 1650°. Very sol in water. Insol in alcohol. The aq soln is strongly alkaline.

USE: Printing on fabrics; manuf lake colors; sizing paper; manuf milk-glass, soap; hardening building stones; water softener.

8575. Sodium Amalgam. [11110-52-4] An alloy of sodium and mercury. Readily prepd by adding sodium metal in small portions at a time to mercury. The combination takes place with evolution of much heat. The sodium contents of the amalgam can be varied, as desired, up to about 20% sodium, corresponding to approx Na_2Hg. The consistency and mp vary with the sodium content; the amalgam corresponding to $NaHg_2$, 5.4% Na, has the highest mp, +360°.

Sodium amalgams are dec by water similarly to sodium metal, but more slowly. *Keep tightly closed.*

8576. Sodium Amide. [7782-92-5] Sodamide. H_2NNa; mol wt 39.01. H 5.17%, N 35.91%, Na 58.93%. $NaNH_2$. Prepd from sodium metal and gaseous ammonia (or liq ammonia with ferric nitrate catalyst): Dennis, Browne, *Inorg. Synth.* **1**, 74 (1939); Greenlee, Henne, *ibid.* **2**, 128 (1946); Schenk in *Handbook of Preparative Inorganic Chemistry* **vol. 1**, G. Brauer, Ed. (Academic Press, New York, 2nd ed., 1963) pp 465-468. Alternate method: Bergstrom, *Org. Synth.* **coll. vol. III**, 778 (1955).

Crystals, mp 210°. The commercial product may be a white to olive-green solid with sea-shell fracture. Begins to volatilize at 400° and dec into its elements between 500 and 600°. Heat of formation of solid (18°; 1 atm): −32.26 kcal/mole. Heat of soln (21°): −31.06 kcal/mole. Soly in liq ammonia at 20° = about 0.1%. Reacts violently with water forming NaOH and NH_3. The reaction with alcohol is considerably slower. Should be stored in sealed containers which prevent all contact with air during storage: Bergstrom, Fernelius, *Chem. Rev.* **12**, 63, 75, 78 (1933). When exposed to the atmosphere, sodium amide rapidly absorbs H_2O and CO_2. When only limited absorption takes place, as in poorly sealed containers, products are formed which render the resulting mixture highly explosive. The formation of oxidation products is accompanied by the development of a yellow or brownish color. If such a change is noticed, the substance should be destroyed at once. This is conveniently accomplished by covering with much benzene, toluene, or kerosene and slowly adding dil ethanol with stirring.

Caution: Intensely irritating to skin, eyes, mucous membranes.

USE: Dehydrating agent. In the production of indigo and hydrazine. Intermediate in the prepn of sodium cyanide. In ammonolysis reactions, in Claisen condensations, alkylation of nitriles and ketones, synthesis of ethynyl compds, acetylenic carbinols. Fused $NaNH_2$ dissolves metallic Mg, Zn, Mo, W, quartz, glass, silicates and other substances.

8577. Sodium Amylosulfate. [9010-01-9] Sulfated potato amylopectin sodium salt; sodium amylopectin sulfate; SN-263; Depepsen. This product has substantially 1.6 sulfate groups per glucose unit and a mol wt of $2.0-8.0\times10^7$ and contains 15-16.5% of sulfur. Prepn: P. S. Camarata, S. Eich, **BE 645762** corresp to **US 3271388** (1964, 1966 to Searle).

THERAP CAT: Enzyme inhibitor.

8578. Sodium Arsanilate. [127-85-5] (4-Aminophenyl)-arsonic acid sodium salt; arsanilic acid sodium salt; sodium aminarsonate; sodium *p*-aminophenylarsonate; sodium anilarsonate; Arsamin; Atoxyl; Nuarsol; Protoxyl; Soamin; Sonate; Piglet Pro-Gen V; Trypoxyl. $C_6H_7AsNNaO_3$; mol wt 239.04. C 30.15%, H 2.95%, As 31.34%, N 5.86%, Na 9.62%, O 20.08%. Review of toxicology and human exposure: *Toxicological Profile for Arsenic* (PB2000-108021, 2000) 468 pp.

Tetrahydrate. White, odorless, cryst powder. *Poisonous!* Soluble in about 6 parts water, about 100 parts alcohol. The aq soln is moderately acid to litmus.

THERAP CAT: Formerly as antisyphilitic.

THERAP CAT (VET): Has been used as an anthelmintic in swine dysentery and other enteric conditions of pigs and poultry.

8579. Sodium Arsenate, Dibasic. [7778-43-0] Disodium arsenate. $AsHNa_2O_4$; mol wt 185.91. As 40.30%, H 0.54%, Na 24.73%, O 34.42%. Na_2HAsO_4. Toxicity study: Franke, Moxon, *J. Pharmacol. Exp. Ther.* **58**, 454 (1936). Review of toxicology and human exposure: *Toxicological Profile for Arsenic* (PB2000-108021, 2000) 468 pp.

Powder. Very sol in water; slightly sol in alcohol.

Heptahydrate. Odorless crystals; effloresces in warm air. *Poisonous*, but less so than the arsenite. Loses 5 H_2O (29%) at about 50°; becomes anhydr at 100°. At 150° or higher it is converted into pyroarsenate. d 1.87. mp 57° when rapidly heated. Sol in 1.3 parts water; sol in glycerol, slightly in alcohol. The aq soln is alkaline to litmus. LD_{75} i.p. in rats: 14-18 mg As/kg (Franke, Moxon).

USE: The technical grade, about 98% pure, is used in dyeing with Turkey-red oil and in printing fabrics; manuf of other arsenates.

THERAP CAT: Formerly as antimalarial; dermatologic.

THERAP CAT (VET): Has been used in parasitism (internally and externally), also for nonparasitic skin and blood diseases, in rheumatism, asthma and heaves, and as an alterative.

8580. Sodium Arsenite. [7784-46-5] Sodium meta-arsenite. $AsHNaO_2$; mol wt 130.92. As 57.23%, H 0.77%, Na 17.56%, O 24.44%. Product of commerce is 95-98% pure. Toxicity study: H. F. Smyth *et al.*, *Am. Ind. Hyg. Assoc. J.* **30**, 470 (1969). Review of toxicology and human exposure: *Toxicological Profile for Arsenic* (PB2000-108021, 2000) 468 pp.

White or grayish-white powder; somewhat hygroscopic. Absorbs CO_2 from air. *Very poisonous!* Freely sol in water, slightly in alcohol. *Keep well closed.* LD_{50} orally in rats: 0.041 g/kg (Smyth).

USE: Technical grade in manuf of arsenical soap for use on skins, for treating vines against certain scale diseases; as insecticide especially for termites.

THERAP CAT (VET): Topical acaricide.

8581. Sodium Azide. [26628-22-8] Smite. N_3Na; mol wt 65.01. N 64.64%, Na 35.36%. NaN_3. Cytochrome oxidase inhibitor. Prepd from $NaNH_2 + N_2O$: Dennis, Browne, *Z. Anorg. Allg.*

Chem. **40**, 95 (1904); Schenk in *Handbook of Preparative Inorganic Chemistry* **Vol. 1**, G. Brauer, Ed. (Academic Press, New York, 2nd ed., 1963) pp 474-475. Alternate procedures: *Inorg. Synth.* **1**, 79 (1939); **2**, 139 (1946). Large scale manuf processes: B. T. Fedoroff *et al.*, *Encyclopedia of Explosives and Related Items* **Vol. 1** (Picatinny Arsenal, Dover, N.J., 1960) pp A601-A619. *Review:* L. E. Audrieth, *Chem. Rev.* **15**, 169 (1934). Review of toxicology: K. A. Frederick, J. G. Babish, *Regul. Toxicol. Pharmacol.* **2**, 308-322 (1982); of human health effects: S. Chang, S.H. Lamm, *Int. J. Toxicol.* **22**, 175-186 (2003).

Colorless hexagonal crystals, d 1.846. On heating dec into sodium and nitrogen. Highly sol in water. Rapidly converted to hydrazoic acid, *q.v.* Soly in water: 40.16% at 10°, 41.7% at 17°. pK = 4.8, aq solns contains HN_3 which escapes readily at 37°. Slightly sol in alcohol. Insol in ether. Sol in liquid ammonia. LD_{50} in rats (mg/kg): 45 orally (Frederick, Babish).

Caution: Potential symptoms of overexposure are irritation of eyes, skin; nausea, vomiting, restlessness, diarrhea; headache, dizziness, weakness, blurred vision; dyspnea; hypotension, tachycardia, bradycardia, tachypnea; hypothermia; acidosis; convulsions; kidney changes. *See NIOSH Pocket Guide to Chemical Hazards* (DHHS/-NIOSH 97-140, 1997) p 280; *Clinical Toxicology of Commercial Products*, R. E. Gosselin *et al.*, Eds. (Williams & Wilkins, Baltimore, 5th ed., 1984), Section II, p 114; *Prudent Practices for Handling Hazardous Chemicals in Laboratories* (National Academy Press, Washington, D.C., 1981) pp 145-147.

USE: In organic syntheses; in the preparation of hydrazoic acid, lead azide, pure sodium. In the differential selection of bacteria; in automatic blood counters; as preservative for laboratory reagents. Propellant for inflating automotive safety bags. Agricultural nematocide; herbicide; in fruit rot control.

8582. Sodium Benzoate. [532-32-1] $C_7H_5NaO_2$; mol wt 144.10. C 58.34%, H 3.50%, Na 15.95%, O 22.21%. Toxicity: Smyth, Carpenter, *J. Ind. Hyg. Toxicol.* **30**, 63 (1948).

White, odorless granules or crystalline powder; sweetish, astringent taste. One gram dissolves in 1.8 ml water, 1.4 ml boiling water, about 75 ml alcohol, in 50 ml of a mixture of 47.5 ml alcohol and 3.7 ml water. The aq soln is slightly alkaline to litmus. pH about 8. *Incompat:* Acids, ferric salts. LD_{50} orally in rats: 4.07 g/kg (Smyth, Carpenter).

USE: Antimicrobial agent, flavoring agent and adjuvant in food; not to exceed a maximum level of 0.1% in food (**21 CFR**, 184.1733, 582.3733). Antifungal and bacteriostatic preservative in pharmaceuticals at concentrations of ~0.1%. Clinical reagent (bilirubin assay).

THERAP CAT: Diagnostic aid (hepatic function).

8583. Sodium Bicarbonate. [144-55-8] Sodium hydrogen carbonate; sodium acid carbonate; baking soda. $CHNaO_3$; mol wt 84.01. C 14.30%, H 1.20%, Na 27.37%, O 57.13%. $NaHCO_3$. The bicarbonate of commerce is about 99.8% pure. Prepd from sodium carbonate, water and carbon dioxide. Manuf: *Faith, Keyes & Clark's Industrial Chemicals*, F. A. Lowenheim, M. K. Moran, Eds. (Wiley-Interscience, New York, 4th ed., 1975) pp 702-705.

White cryst powder or granules. Begins to lose CO_2 at about 50° and at 100° it is converted into Na_2CO_3. Readily dec by weak acids. In aq soln it begins to break up into carbon dioxide and sodium carbonate at about 20° and completely on boiling. Sol in 10 parts water at 25°, in 12 parts water at about 18°. Insol in alcohol. Its aq soln prepd with cold water and without agitation is only slightly alkaline to litmus or phenolphthalein; on standing or rise in temp the alkalinity increases. pH of freshly prepd 0.1 molar aq soln at 25°: 8.3.

USE: Manuf many sodium salts; source of CO_2; ingredient of baking powder, effervescent salts and beverages; in fire extinguishers, cleaning compds.

THERAP CAT: Antacid; systemic alkalinizing agent.

THERAP CAT (VET): Systemic and urinary alkalinizing agent.

8584. Sodium Bifluoride. [1333-83-1] F_2HNa; mol wt 61.99. F 61.30%, H 1.63%, Na 37.09%. NaF.HF.

White, cryst powder. Sol in water. The aq soln corrodes glass.

USE: As a "sour" in laundering.

8585. Sodium Bismuthate(V). [12232-99-4] $BiNaO_3$; mol wt 279.97. Bi 74.64%, Na 8.21%, O 17.14%. $NaBiO_3$. The bismuthate of commerce contains about 85% $NaBiO_3$; the balance is chiefly water and Bi_2O_3.

Yellow to yellowish-brown, somewhat hygroscopic. Slowly dec on keeping; decompn accelerated by moisture and higher temp. Insol in cold, dec by hot water forming Bi_2O_3, NaOH, and liberating oxygen; dec by acids; with HCl chlorine is formed; with oxy-acids oxygen is liberated. LD_{50} orally in rats: 720 mg/kg, Hanzlik *et al., J. Pharmacol. Exp. Ther.* **62**, 372 (1938).

USE: For the determination of manganese in iron and steel, etc., the manganese being oxidized by it in hot HNO_3 or H_2SO_4 soln to permanganate.

8586. Sodium Bisulfate. [7681-38-1] Sodium acid sulfate; sodium hydrogen sulfate; sodium pyrosulfate. $NaHO_4S$; mol wt 120.06. H 0.84%, Na 19.15%, O 53.30%, S 26.71%. $NaHSO_4$.

Fused $NaHSO_4$, hygroscopic pieces. d 2.435. mp ~315°. Sol in 2 parts water, 1 part boiling water; dec by alcohol into sodium sulfate and free H_2SO_4. *Keep well closed.*

Monohydrate. Odorless crystals. When strongly heated it changes into pyrosulfate. Sol in about 0.8 part water; dec by alcohol into sodium sulfate and free H_2SO_4. The aq soln is strongly acid. pH of 0.1 molar soln: 1.4.

USE: Fusion of minerals to make them sol for analysis; for liberating CO_2 in carbonic acid baths. Technical grades are used for pickling metals, carbonizing wool, bleaching and swelling leather, manuf magnesia cements, etc.

8587. Sodium Bisulfide. [16721-80-5] Sodium sulfhydrate; sodium hydrosulfide; sodium hydrogen sulfide. HNaS; mol wt 56.06. H 1.80%, Na 41.01%, S 57.20%. NaSH. Prepd from sodium ethylate and hydrogen sulfide: Rule, *J. Chem. Soc.* **99**, 558 (1911); Teichert, Klemm, *Z. Anorg. Allg. Chem.* **243**, 86 (1939); Eibeck, *Inorg. Synth.* **7**, 128 (1963). The technical grade may be obtained by reacting sodium bisulfate with calcium sulfide in the cold or by saturating NaOH solns with H_2S.

Rhombohedric-cubic crystals. White to colorless. Odor of hydrogen sulfide. Very hygroscopic. Readily hydrolyzed in moist air to NaOH and Na_2S. d 1.79. Turns yellow upon heating in dry air, changing to orange at higher temps. mp 350° forming a black liquid. Sol in water, alcohol, ether. Gives a blue-green soln in dimethylformamide.

Dihydrate. Needles or flakes, mp 55°. Completely and rapidly sol in water, alcohol, ether. *Note:* The commercial product is usually the dihydrate. Can be shipped in lacquer-lined steel drums.

Trihydrate. Shiny rhombs, mp 22°.

USE: Dehairing hides; desulfurizing viscose rayon; in the manuf of sulfur-contg dyes and other thio compds such as thioamides, thiourea, thioglycolic acid, thio- and dithiobenzoic acids, sodium thiosulfate.

8588. Sodium Bisulfite. [7631-90-5] Sodium acid sulfite. $HNaO_3S$; mol wt 104.06. H 0.97%, Na 22.09%, O 46.13%, S 30.81%. $NaHSO_3$. The bisulfite of commerce consists chiefly of sodium metabisulfite, $Na_2S_2O_5$, and for all practical purposes possesses the same properties as the true bisulfite. Toxicity: Hoppe, Goble, *J. Pharmacol. Exp. Ther.* **101**, 101 (1951).

White, crystalline powder; SO_2 odor; disagreeable taste; on exposure to air it loses some SO_2 and is gradually oxidized to sulfate. d 1.48. Sol in 3.5 parts cold water, 2 parts boiling water, in about 70 parts alcohol. Its aq soln is acid. *Keep well closed and in a cool place.* LD_{50} i.v. in rats: 115 mg/kg (Hoppe, Goble).

Caution: Potential symptoms of overexposure are irritation of eyes, skin, mucous membranes. *See NIOSH Pocket Guide to Chemical Hazards* (DHHS/NIOSH 97-140, 1997) p 282.

USE: As disinfectant and bleach, particularly for wool; in dyeing for preparing hot and cold indigo vats; in paper-making in place of sodium hyposulfite to remove Cl from bleached fibers; as stripper (reducer) in laundering; to remove permanganate stains from skin and clothing; to render certain dyes sol; manuf sodium hydrosulfite;

coagulating rubber latex; as preservative for deteriorative liqs or solns used for technical purposes; as antiseptic in fermentation industries. As preservative and bleach in food. Pharmaceutic aid (antioxidant).

8589. Sodium Bitartrate. [526-94-3] Sodium acid tartrate. $C_4H_5NaO_6$; mol wt 172.07. C 27.92%, H 2.93%, Na 13.36%, O 55.79%. $NaHC_4H_4O_6$.
Monohydrate. White crystals. Sol in about 9 parts water, 2 parts boiling water. Almost insol in alcohol. The aq soln is acid.
USE: For detecting potassium; in nutrient media.

8590. Sodium Borate. [1330-43-4] Boron sodium oxide ($B_4Na_2O_7$); anhydrous borax; borax glass; fused borax; sodium biborate; sodium pyroborate; sodium tetraborate. $B_4Na_2O_7$; mol wt 201.22. B 21.49%, Na 22.85%, O 55.66%. $Na_2B_4O_7$. Toxicity: H. F. Smyth *et al., Am. Ind. Hyg. Assoc. J.* **30,** 470 (1969). Review of toxicology and human exposure: *Toxicological Profile for Boron* (PB93-110674, 1992) 110 pp.
Powder or glass-like plates becoming opaque on exposure to air. Slowly sol in water.
Decahydrate. [1303-96-4] Borax; Jaikin. Hard odorless crystals, granules or cryst powder; efflorescent in dry air, the crystal often being coated with white powder. d 1.73. Melts when rapidly heated at 75°; at 100° loses $5H_2O$; at 150° loses $9H_2O$; becomes anhydr at 320°. One gram dissolves in 16 ml water, 0.6 ml boiling water, about 1 ml glycerol. Insol in alcohol. The aq soln is alkaline to litmus and phenolphthalein. pH about 9.5. Borax dissolves many metallic oxides when fused with them. LD_{50} orally in rats: 5.66 g/kg (Smyth).
Caution: Potential symptoms of overexposure are irritation of eyes, skin, upper respiratory system; dermatitis; epistaxis; cough, dyspnea. *See NIOSH Pocket Guide to Chemical Hazards* (DHHS/NIOSH 97-140, 1997) p 30.
USE: Soldering metals; manuf glazes and enamels; tanning; in cleaning compds; artificially aging wood; as preservative, either alone or with other antiseptics against wood fungus; fireproofing fabrics and wood; curing and preserving skins; in cockroach control. Pharmaceutic aid (alkalizer).
THERAP CAT (VET): Has been used as antiseptic, detergent, astringent for mucous membranes.

8591. Sodium Borate Solution Compound. Dobell's soln. Made from 1.5 g sodium borate, 1.5 g sodium bicarbonate, 0.3 ml liquefied phenol, 3.5 ml glycerol and water to make 100 ml.
Yellowish, clear liquid.
THERAP CAT: Wash for mucous membranes.
THERAP CAT (VET): Has been used as a nonirritant wash for mucous membranes.

8592. Sodium Borohydride. [16940-66-2] Sodium tetrahydroborate. BH_4Na; mol wt 37.83. B 28.58%, H 10.66%, Na 60.77%. $NaBH_4$. Prepn: H. I. Schlesinger *et al., J. Am. Chem. Soc.* **75,** 205 (1953); H. C. Brown *et al., J. Am. Chem. Soc.* **79,** 5400 (1957). *Reviews*: R. M. Adams, A. R. Siedle, in *Boron, Metalloboron Compounds, and Boranes* (Interscience, New York, 1964) 765 pp; B. D. James, M. G. H. Walbridge, *Prog. Inorg. Chem.* **11,** 99-231 (1970).
Hygroscopic, cubic crystals forming a dihydrate, mp 36-37°. The anhydr material (d 1.074) is stable in dry air to 300°; dec slowly at 400° and rapidly at 500°. Supports combustion. Soly (g/100 g) in water at 25°: 55; at 60°: 88.5; liq ammonia at 25°: 104; ethylenediamine at 75°: 22; morpholine at 25°: 1.4; pyridine at 25°: 3.1; methanol at 20°: 16.4 (reacts); ethanol at 20°: 4.0 (reacts slowly); tetrahydrofurfuryl alcohol at 20°: 14.0 (reacts slowly); tetrahydrofuran at 20°: 0.1; diglyme at 25°: 5.5; dimethylformamide at 20°: 18.0.
USE: Reducing agent for aldehydes, ketones and Schiff bases in nonaqueous solvents. Also reduces acids, esters, acid chlorides, disulfides, nitriles, inorganic anions. Further used to generate diborane, as foaming agent, as scavenger for traces of aldehyde, ketones and peroxides in organic chemicals.

8593. Sodium Bromate. [7789-38-0] $BrNaO_3$; mol wt 150.89. Br 52.96%, Na 15.24%, O 31.81%. $NaBrO_3$. The article of commerce contains about 99% $NaBrO_3$.

Colorless, odorless crystals, white granules or cryst powder. d 3.34. mp 381° with dec and liberation of oxygen. Sol in 2.5 parts water, 1.1 parts boiling water. The aq soln is neutral. *Keep from contact with organic matter.*
Caution: See Potassium Bromate.
USE: As a mixture with sodium bromide for dissolving gold from its ores.

8594. Sodium Bromide. [7647-15-6] Sedoneural. BrNa; mol wt 102.89. Br 77.66%, Na 22.34%. NaBr. Prepd commercially by adding some excess bromine to a sodium hydroxide soln forming a mixture of bromide and bromate. The reaction products are evaporated to dryness and treated with carbon to reduce the bromate to bromide. Prepn: J. H. van der Meulen, **US 1775598** (1930). Toxicity study: Smith, Hambourger, *J. Pharmacol. Exp. Ther.* **55,** 200 (1935). Brief review of physical and chemical properties and pharmacology: T. O. Soine, C. O. Wilson, *Roger's Inorganic Pharmaceutical Chemistry* (Lea & Febiger, Philadelphia, 8th ed., 1967) pp 213-216.
White crystals, granules or powder; saline, feebly bitter taste. Absorbs moisture from air but is not deliquescent. d 3.21. mp 755°; volatilizes at somewhat higher temp. One gram dissolves in 1.1 ml water, about 16 ml alcohol, 6 ml methanol. The aq soln is practically neutral. pH 6.5-8.0. *Keep well closed.* From water of room temp, sodium bromide crystallizes with $2H_2O$ in the form of colorless crystals. *Incompat.* Acids, alkaloidal and heavy metal salts. LD_{50} orally in rats: 3.5 g/kg (Smith, Hambourger).
USE: In photography.
THERAP CAT: Sedative; hypnotic; anticonvulsant.
THERAP CAT (VET): Sedative. Has been used to control convulsions, chorea, hysteria.

8595. Sodium Cacodylate. [124-65-2] [(Dimethylarsino)oxy]sodium As-oxide; sodium dimethylarsonate; Arsecodile; Arsicodile; Arsycodile; Rad-e-cate; Silvisar. $C_2H_6AsNaO_2$; mol wt 159.98. C 15.02%, H 3.78%, As 46.83%, Na 14.37%, O 20.00%. An organic compd of arsenic yielding inorganic, trivalent arsenic in the body (is excreted partly unchanged, also yields dimethylarsine oxide. Prepd by the distillation of a mixture of arsenic trioxide and potassium acetate which yields Cadet's liquid, contg mostly dimethylarsine oxide. This is oxidized with mercuric oxide yielding crystals of cacodylic acid which is neutralized with Na_2CO_3 or NaOH: Cadet de Gassicourt, *Mem. savants étrangers* **3,** 633 (1760); Valeur, Gaillot, *Compt. Rend.* **185,** 956 (1927). Use in treatment of psoriasis: S. I. Dawes, H. C. Jackson, *J. Am. Med. Assoc.* **48,** 2020 (1903). Metabolism and excretion: A. Heffter, *Arch. Exp. Pathol. Pharmakol.* **46,** 230 (1901). Use as herbicide: M. A. Sprague, **US 3056663** (1962 to Ansul). Possible use in radiation dosimetry: H. S. Levinson, E. B. Garber, *Nature* **207,** 751 (1965). Review of toxicology and human exposure: *Toxicological Profile for Arsenic* (PB2000-108021, 2000) 468 pp.

$$H_3C-\underset{\underset{CH_3}{|}}{\overset{\overset{O}{\parallel}}{As}}-O^-\ Na^+$$

Trihydrate. Crystals, granules. Slight odor. Liquefies in its water of hydration at about 60°. Becomes anhyd at 120°. Burns with a bluish flame, emitting a garlic-like odor. One gram dissolves in 0.5 ml water, 2.5 ml alcohol. pH about 8-9. *Keep well closed.*
USE: Herbicide.
THERAP CAT (VET): Has been used in chronic eczema, anemia, as a tonic.

8596. Sodium Carbonate. [497-19-8] CNa_2O_3; mol wt 105.99. C 11.33%, Na 43.38%, O 45.29%. Na_2CO_3. Occurs in nature as the hydrate, *thermonatrite*, and the decahydrate, *natron* or *natrite*. Produced by the ammonia-soda or Solvay process, or from lake brines or sea water by electrolytic processes: *Faith, Keyes & Clark's Industrial Chemicals*, F. A. Lowenheim, M. K. Moran, Eds. (Wiley-Interscience, New York, 4th ed., 1975) pp 706-715. Toxicity: C. Norde *et al., Compt. Rend.* **257,** 791 (1963). *Reviews*: Bailey in *Mellor's* vol **II**, suppl II, *The Alkali Metals* (part 1), 1058-1205 (1961).
Anhydrous. Solvay soda. The technical grade (about 99% pure) is known as *soda ash*. Odorless, hygroscopic powder; alka-

line taste; d 2.53. mp 851° but begins to lose CO_2 even at 400°. On exposure to air it will gradually absorb one mol water, about 15%. Sol in glycerol; in 3.5 parts water at room temp, 2.2 parts water at 35°. Insol in alcohol. Dec by acids with effervescence. Combines with water with evolution of heat. Its aq soln is strongly alkaline. pH 11.6. *Keep well closed.* LD_{50} (30 day) i.p. in mice: 116.6 mg/kg (Norde).

Monohydrate. Odorless, small crystals or cryst powder; alkaline taste. Stable at ordinary temps and atmospheric conditions; dries out somewhat in warm, dry air or above 50°; becomes anhydr at 100°. d 2.25; also reported as 1.55. Sol in 3 parts water, 1.8 parts boiling water, 7 parts glycerol. Insol in alcohol.

Decahydrate. Nevite; Soda. The technical product is known as *sal soda* or *washing soda*. Transparent crystals; readily effloresces on exposure to air. d 1.46. mp 34°. Sol in 2 parts cold, 0.25 part boiling water, in glycerol. Insol in alcohol. The aq soln is strongly alkaline to litmus. *Keep well closed and in a cool place.*

Caution: Potential symptoms of overexposure to dusts or vapors of sodium carbonate are irritation of mucous membranes with subsequent coughing and shortness of breath. Chronic overexposure may lead to perforation of the nasal septum. Direct contact may cause skin irritation and redness, with concentrated solutions causing erythema. Chronic skin exposures may cause dermatitis and ulceration. *See Patty's Industrial Hygiene and Toxicology* vol. 2A, G. D. Clayton, F. E. Clayton, Eds. (Wiley-Interscience, New York, 4th ed., 1993) pp 769-771.

USE: In manuf of Na salts, glass, soap; for washing wool; textiles, etc.; in bleaching linen, cotton; general cleanser; in water-softening; in photography; as reagent in analytical chemistry. Pharmaceutic aid (alkalizer).

THERAP CAT (VET): Has been used as an emetic. In solution to cleanse skin, in eczema, to soften scabs of ringworm.

8597. Sodium Cellulose Phosphate. [9038-41-9] SCP; Calcibind; Calcisorb. Non-absorbable ion exchange resin with high affinity for calcium ions. Prepn: G. P. Touey, US 2759924 (1956 to Eastman Kodak). Use in treatment of hypercalcemia: C. Y. C. Pak *et al., J. Clin. Endocrinol. Metab.* **28,** 1828 (1968). Mechanism of action: C. Y. C. Pak, *J. Clin. Pharmacol.* **13,** 15 (1973). Clinical pharmacology: *idem, ibid.* **19,** 451 (1979). Use in treatment of calcium urolithiasis: U. Backman *et al., J. Urol.* **123,** 9 (1980); C. Y. C. Pak, *Invest. Urol.* **19,** 187 (1981).

Powder. Insol in water.

USE: As ion exchange resin.

THERAP CAT: Treatment of calcium urolithiasis.

8598. Sodium Chlorate. [7775-09-9] Atlacide; Defol; Dervan. $ClNaO_3$; mol wt 106.44. Cl 33.31%, Na 21.60%, O 45.09%. $NaClO_3$. The chlorate of commerce is about 99% pure. Produced from sodium chloride by electrolysis: *Faith, Keyes & Clark's Industrial Chemicals,* F. A. Lowenheim, M. K. Moran, Eds. (Wiley-Interscience, New York, 4th ed., 1975) pp 716-721. Toxicity: Ulrich, *J. Pharmacol. Exp. Ther.* **35,** 1 (1929).

Colorless, odorless crystals or white granules. d 2.5. mp 248°; at about 300° liberates oxygen; entirely dec at higher temp. Sol in about 1 ml cold, 0.5 ml boiling water, about 130 ml alcohol, about 50 ml boiling alcohol, 4 ml glycerol. Sodium chloride diminishes its soly in water. The aq soln is neutral. *Keep out of contact with organic matter or other oxidizable substances.* LD orally in rats: 12000 mg/kg (Ulrich).

USE: An oxidizer, like potassium chlorate, in manuf of dyes; explosives and matches; dyeing and printing fabrics; tanning and finishing leather. Herbicide. Pharmaceutical aid (oxidizing agent).

8599. Sodium Chloride. [7647-14-5] Salt; common salt. ClNa; mol wt 58.44. Cl 60.67%, Na 39.34%. NaCl. The article of commerce is also known as *table salt*, *rock salt* or *sea salt*. Occurs in nature as the mineral *halite*. Produced by mining (rock salt), by evaporation of brine from underground salt deposits and from sea water by solar evaporation: *Faith, Keyes & Clark's Industrial Chemicals,* F. A. Lowenheim, M. K. Moran, Eds. (Wiley-Interscience, New York, 4th ed., 1975) pp 722-730. Toxicity studies: E. M. Boyd, M. N. Shanas, *Arch. Int. Pharmacodyn.* **144,** 86 (1963). Comprehensive monograph: D. W. Kaufmann, *Sodium Chloride,* ACS Monograph Series no. 145 (Reinhold, New York, 1960) 743 pp.

Cubic, white crystals, granules, or powder; colorless and transparent or translucent when in large crystals. d 2.17. The salt of commerce usually contains some calcium and magnesium chlorides which absorb moisture and make it cake. mp 804° and begins to volatilize at a little above this temp. One gram dissolves in 2.8 ml water at 25°, in 2.6 ml boiling water, in 10 ml glycerol; very slightly sol in alcohol. Its soly in water is decreased by HCl. Almost insol in concd HCl. Its aq soln is neutral. pH: 6.7-7.3. d of satd aq soln at 25° is 1.202. A 23% aq soln of sodium chloride freezes at −20.5°C (5°F). LD_{50} orally in rats: 3.75 ±0.43 g/kg (Boyd, Shanas).

Note: Blusalt, a brand of sodium chloride contg trace amounts of cobalt, iodine, iron, copper, manganese, zinc is used in farm animals.

USE: Natural salt is the source of chlorine and of sodium as well as of all, or practically all, their compds, e.g., hydrochloric acid, chlorates, sodium carbonate, hydroxide, etc.; for preserving foods; manuf soap, to salt out dyes; in freezing mixtures; for dyeing and printing fabrics, glazing pottery, curing hides; metallurgy of tin and other metals.

THERAP CAT: Electrolyte replenisher; emetic; topical anti-inflammatory.

THERAP CAT (VET): Essential nutrient factor. May be given orally as emetic, stomachic, laxative or to stimulate thirst (prevention of calculi). Intravenously as isotonic solution to raise blood volume, to combat dehydration. Locally as wound irrigant, rectal douche.

8600. Sodium Chlorite. [7758-19-2] $ClNaO_2$; mol wt 90.44. Cl 39.20%, Na 25.42%, O 35.38%. $NaClO_2$. Prepd on a commercial scale by passing chlorine dioxide into a soln of sodium hydroxide contg carbonaceous matter and lime: Vincent, US 2092944; US 2092945 (both 1937 to Mathieson). Review of manuf and properties: Kesting, *Pulp Paper Mag. Can.* **53,** no. 8, 99-104 (1952); of toxicology and human exposure: *Toxicological Profile for Chlorine Dioxide and Chlorite* (PB2003-101465, 2002) 182 pp.

Slightly hygroscopic crystals or flakes, does not cake. Dec 180-200°. Powerful oxidizer, but will not explode on percussion unless in contact with oxidizable material. Soly in water (g/100 g soln): at 5°: 34; at 17°: 39; at 30°: 46; at 45°: 53; at 60°: 55.

Trihydrate. Triclinic leaflets, becomes anhydr at 38° or in desiccator over KOH at room temp.

USE: In the preparation of chlorine dioxide for immediate use; in water purification; as bleaching agent for textiles, paper pulp; disinfectant.

8601. Sodium Chromate(VI). [7775-11-3] Neutral sodium chromate. $CrNa_2O_4$; mol wt 161.97. Cr 32.10%, Na 28.39%, O 39.51%. Na_2CrO_4. Crystallizes as a tetra- or decahydrate. Manuf: *Faith, Keyes & Clark's Industrial Chemicals,* F. A. Lowenheim, M. K. Moran, Eds. (Wiley-Interscience, New York, 4th ed., 1975) pp 731-736. Diagnostic use of labeled compound in GI bleeding: A. Lussier *et al., Semin. Arthritis Rheum.* **17,** Suppl. 2, 40-45 (1988). Review of use as radiolabel for blood elements: *Diagnostic and Investigational Uses of Radiolabeled Blood Elements,* R. J. Davey, M. E. Wallace, Eds., (Am. Assoc. Blood Banks, Arlington, 1987) 118 pp.

Tetrahydrate. Yellow, somewhat deliquesc crystals. Sol in about 1 part water, insol in alcohol. The aq soln is alkaline. *Keep well closed.* The decahydrate is unstable with respect to water content. mp ~20°.

51Cr-Labeled compound. [10039-53-9] Sodium chromate-51Cr; sodium radio-chromate(51Cr); Chromitope Sodium; Rachromate-51. $^{51}CrNa_2O_4$. Prepd from radioactive chromium (^{51}Cr) which has a half-life of 27.7 days. The emission of gamma rays is applicable to biological tagging and tracing. Other properties identical to those of unlabeled sodium chromate.

Caution: Chromium hexavalent compounds are listed as known human carcinogens: *Report on Carcinogens, Eleventh Edition* (PB2005-104914, 2004) p III-63.

USE: Protection of iron against corrosion and rusting.

THERAP CAT: ^{51}Cr-labeled compound as diagnostic aid (blood volume determination; blood cell survival).

8602. Sodium Citrate. [68-04-2] 2-Hydroxy-1,2,3-propanetricarboxylic acid trisodium salt; trisodium citrate; Citrosodine; Cystemme; Urisal. $C_6H_5Na_3O_7$; mol wt 258.07. C 27.92%, H

1.95%, Na 26.73%, O 43.40%. Anticoagulant use in blood transfusion: R. Weil, *J. Am. Med. Assoc.* **64**, 425 (1915); *cf. ibid.* **250**, 1901 (1983). Toxicity study: C. M. Gruber, Jr., W. A. Halbeisen, *J. Pharmacol. Exp. Ther.* **94**, 65 (1948). Clinical evaluation of antacid efficacy: C. P. Gibbs *et al., Anesthesiology* **57**, 44 (1982); of effects on athletic performance: V. Oöpik *et al., Br. J. Sports Med.* **37**, 485 (2003).

$$Na^+ {}^-OOC \qquad COO^- Na^+$$
$$HO \qquad COO^- Na^+$$

LD$_{50}$ in rats, mice (mmol/kg): 6.0, 5.5 i.p. (Gruber, Halbeisen).

Dihydrate. [6132-04-3] White, odorless crystals, granules or powder; cool, saline taste. Stable in air; becomes anhydrous at 150°. Sol in 1.3 parts water, 0.6 part boiling water. Insol in alcohol. The aq soln is slightly alkaline to litmus. pH about 8.

USE: Anticoagulant for collection of blood. In photography; as sequestering agent to remove trace metals; as emulsifier, acidulant and sequestrant in foods.

THERAP CAT: Systemic alkalinizing agent.

8603. Sodium Cobaltinitrite. [13600-98-1] Trisodium hexakis(nitrato-*N*)cobaltate(3−); sodium hexanitrocobaltate(III). CoN$_6$Na$_3$O$_{12}$; mol wt 403.94. Co 14.59%, N 20.81%, Na 17.07%, O 47.53%. Na$_3$Co(NO$_2$)$_6$.

Yellow to brownish-yellow, cryst powder. Very sol in water, slightly in alc. Dec by mineral acids, but unaffected by dil acetic or similar organic acids. The aq soln dec gradually but if a few drops of acetic acid are added it may be kept for about 3 months.

USE: For the detection of potassium with which it forms a slightly sol compd.

8604. Sodium Cyanate. [917-61-3] Cyanic acid sodium salt. CNNaO; mol wt 65.01. C 18.48%, N 21.55%, Na 35.36%, O 24.61%. NaOCN. Prepn and properties: *Gmelins, Sodium* (8th ed.) **21**, 799-801 (1928) and supplement, part 4, 1382-1386 (1967). Used experimentally in treatment of sickle cell anemia. Effect of cyanate on sickling: May *et al., Lancet* **1**, 658 (1972); P. N. Gillette *et al., N. Engl. J. Med.* **290**, 654 (1974). Pharmacology and toxicology: Cerami *et al. J. Pharmacol. Exp. Ther.* **185**, 653 (1973). Clinical studies: Peterson *et al., ibid.* **189**, 577 (1974).

Colorless needles from alcohol. d$_4^{20}$ 1.893. mp 550°. Sol in water; decomposes to form Na$_2$CO$_3$ and urea. Soly in alc (0°): 0.22 g/100 g solvent. Insol in ether. LD$_{50}$ i.p. in mice: 260 mg/kg (Cerami).

8605. Sodium Cyanide. [143-33-9] Cyanogran. CNNa; mol wt 49.01. C 24.51%, N 28.58%, Na 46.91%. NaCN. This cyanide of commerce is 95-98% pure. Mixtures of sodium cyanide with sodium chloride or carbonate for special uses are also marketed. Toxicity study: Smyth *et al., Am. Ind. Hyg. Assoc. J.* **30**, 470 (1969). Review of toxicology and human exposure: *Toxicological Profile for Cyanide* (PB98-101207, 1997) 291 pp.

White granules or fused pieces. *Violent poison!* Odorless when perfectly dry; somewhat deliquesc in damp air and emits slight odor of HCN. mp 563°. Freely sol in water, slightly in alcohol. The aq soln is strongly alkaline and rapidly decomposes; the soln readily dissolves gold and silver in presence of air. *Keep well closed.* LD$_{50}$ orally in rats: 15 mg/kg (Smyth).

Caution: Potential symptoms of overexposure are irritation of eyes and skin; weakness, headache and confusion; nausea, vomiting; increased rate of respiration; slow gasping respiration; asphyxia; thyroid and blood changes. *See NIOSH Pocket Guide to Chemical Hazards* (DHHS/NIOSH 97-140, 1997) p 282.

USE: Extracting gold and silver from ores; electroplating baths; case hardening steel by liquid nitriding; manuf hydrocyanic acid and other cyanides.

8606. Sodium Cyanoborohydride. [25895-60-7] Sodium (cyano-*C*)trihydroborate(1−); sodium borocyanohydride; sodium cyanohydridoborate. CH$_3$BNNa; mol wt 62.84. C 19.11%, H 4.81%, B 17.20%, N 22.29%, Na 36.58%. NaBH$_3$CN. Reducing agent prepared from NaBH$_4$ and HCN: R. C. Wade *et al., Inorg. Chem.* **9**, 2146 (1970); R. C. Wade, **DE 2028569** corresp to **US 3667923** (1971, 1972 both to Ventron). Review of prepn, properties and use: C. F. Lane, *Synthesis* **1975**, 135-146.

White, hygroscopic powder, mp 240-242° (dec). d^{28} 1.199. Soly (g/100 g solvent) in water (29°): 212; in THF (28°): 37.2; in diglyme (25°): 17.6. Very sol in methanol; slightly sol in ethanol, isopropylamine; insol in ethyl ether, benzene, hexane. Stable in acid to pH 3; undergoes rapid hydrolysis in 12*N* HCl. Rate of hydrolysis 10^{-8} that of NaBH$_4$.

USE: Selective reducing agent for aldehydes, ketones, oximes, enamines; does not reduce amides, ethers, lactones, nitriles, nitro compds and epoxides. Also used for reductive amination of ketones and aldehydes, reductive alkylation of amines and hydrazines, reductive displacement of halides and tosylates, deoxygenation of aldehydes and ketones. *See* Lane, *loc. cit.*

8607. Sodium Diacetate. [126-96-5] Sodium acid acetate; Dykon. C$_4$H$_7$NaO$_4$; mol wt 142.09. C 33.81%, H 4.97%, Na 16.18%, O 45.04%. CH$_3$COONa.CH$_3$COOH. Described as a "bound" compd of sodium acetate and acetic acid.

White powder, dec above 150°. Sol in water, liberating 42.25% available acetic acid.

USE: Acetic acid in solid form; sequestrant; food preservative to inhibit molds and rope-forming bacteria in bread: Glabe, *Food Ind.* **14**, no. 2, 46 (1942).

8608. Sodium Dibunate. [14992-59-7] 2,6-Bis(1,1-dimethylethyl)-1-naphthalenesulfonic acid sodium salt; L-1633; 1633 Labaz; Becantal; Becantex; Dibunafon; Keuten; Linctussal. C$_{18}$H$_{23}$NaO$_3$S; mol wt 342.43. C 63.13%, H 6.77%, Na 6.71%, O 14.02%, S 9.36%. Although most sources refer to this compound as sodium 2,6-di-*tert*-butylnaphthalene sulfonate, it is a mixture of at least two isomers. Prepn and separation of isomers: Menard *et al., Can. J. Chem.* **39**, 729 (1961).

Slightly hygroscopic crystals, dec >300°. Slightly sol in cold water (0.5-1.0%); freely sol in hot water; sol in methanol, less sol in ethanol. Aq solns are stable to boiling.

THERAP CAT: Antitussive.

8609. Sodium Dichromate(VI). [10588-01-9] Sodium bichromate; bichromate of soda. Cr$_2$Na$_2$O$_7$; mol wt 261.97. Cr 39.70%, Na 17.55%, O 42.75%. Na$_2$Cr$_2$O$_7$. Usually prepd from Na$_2$CrO$_4$ and H$_2$SO$_4$. Description of industrial processes: Müller, Glissmann in *Ullmanns Encyklopädie der technischen Chemie* **vol. 5** (Munich, 3rd ed., 1954) p 575; *Faith, Keyes & Clark's Industrial Chemicals*, F. A. Lowenheim, M. K. Moran, Eds. (Wiley-Interscience, New York, 4th ed., 1975) pp 731-736.

Dihydrate. Reddish to bright orange, somewhat deliquescent crystals. Crystal system: monoclinic sphenoidal. Crystal habit: elongated prismatic. d$_4^{25}$ 2.348. Bulk density: 96 lbs/cu ft. Becomes anhydr on prolonged heating at ~100°. The anhydr salt mp 356.7° and starts to dec at ~400°. Heat of soln −28.2 cal/g. Very sol in water. A satd aq soln contains at 0°: 70.6% Na$_2$Cr$_2$O$_7$.·2H$_2$O; at 20°: 73.18%; at 40°: 77.09%; at 60°: 82.04%; at 80°: 88.39%; at 100°: 91.43%. A 20% soln freezes at −3.5°, a 30% soln at −6°, a 60% soln at −26°, a 69% soln at −48°. Specific heat of 20% soln at 25°: 0.85 cal/g/°C. Solns are acidic: pH of 1% soln: 4.0; pH of 10% soln: 3.5.

Caution: Potential symptoms of overexposure by ingestion are violent gasteroenteritis, peripheral vascular collapse, vertigo, muscle cramps, coma, hemorrhagic diathesis, fever, liver damage and acute renal failure. Direct contact may be highly corrosive to skin and mucous membranes. *See Clinical Toxicology of Commercial Products*, R. E. Gosselin *et al.*, Eds. (Williams & Wilkins, 5th ed., 1984) Section II, p 108. Chromium hexavalent compounds are listed as known human carcinogens: *Report on Carcinogens, Eleventh Edition* (PB2005-104914, 2004) p III-63.

USE: Oxidizing agent in manuf of dyes, many other synthetic organic chemicals, inks, etc.; in chrome-tanning of hides; in electric batteries; bleaching fats, oils, sponges, resins; refining petroleum; manuf chromic acid, other chromates and chrome pigments; in corrosion-inhibitors, corrosion-inhibiting paints; in many metal treatments; electroengraving of copper; mordant in dyeing; for hardening gelatin; for the defoliation of cotton plants and other plants and shrubs, La Lande, **US 2760854** (1956 to Pennsylvania Salt).

THERAP CAT: Anti-infective (topical).

8610. Sodium Dicyanoaurate(I). [15280-09-8] Gold sodium cyanide; sodium aurocyanide. C_2AuN_2Na; mol wt 271.99. C 8.83%, Au 72.42%, N 10.30%, Na 8.45%. $NaAu(CN)_2$.

White, cryst powder. Sol in water. *Poison!*

USE: Goldplating.

8611. Sodium Dithionate. [7631-94-9] Dithionic acid disodium salt. $Na_2O_6S_2$; mol wt 206.11. Na 22.31%, O 46.58%, S 31.11%. Prepd according to the equations $MnO_2 + 2SO_2 \rightarrow MnS_2O_6$ and $MnS_2O_6 + Na_2CO_3 \rightarrow MnCO_3 + Na_2S_2O_6$: de Baat, *Rec. Trav. Chim.* **45**, 237 (1926); Pfanstiel, *Inorg. Synth.* **2**, 170 (1946).

Dihydrate. Colorless, water-clear, orthorhombic crystals. Very stable in air. d 2.189. Loses all of its water of crystn at 110°. When heated to 267° it is dissociated into Na_2SO_4 and SO_2. Soly in water at 0°: 6.05% (w/w); at 20°: 13.39%; at 30°: 17.32%. Insol in alc.

8612. Sodium Dodecylbenzenesulfonate. [25155-30-0] Dodecylbenzenesulfonic acid sodium salt; dodecylbenzene sodium sulfonate; Conoco C-50; Conoco SD 40; Conoco C-60. $C_{18}H_{29}NaO_3S$; mol wt 348.48. C 62.04%, H 8.39%, Na 6.60%, O 13.77%, S 9.20%. $C_{12}H_{25}C_6H_4SO_3Na$. Manuf: *Chem. Eng.* **61**, no. 6, 372 (1954); Huber *et al., J. Am. Oil Chem. Soc.* **33**, 57 (1956); **GB 761095**; Seaton, **US 2782230** (1956, 1957 both to Monsanto); **GB 773423**; Gerhart, Karwacki, **US 2820056** (1957, 1958 both to Continental Oil). Toxicity study: Hopper *et al., J. Am. Pharm. Assoc. Sci. Ed.* **38**, 428 (1949).

LD_{50} in mice: 2 g/kg orally; 105 mg/kg i.v. (Hopper).

Caution: May cause skin irritation. If swallowed will cause vomiting.

USE: Anionic detergent.

8613. Sodium Ethoxide. [141-52-6] Sodium ethylate; caustic alcohol. C_2H_5NaO; mol wt 68.05. C 35.30%, H 7.41%, Na 33.78%, O 23.51%.

White or yellowish, hygroscopic powder. Dec on exposure to air and becomes darker on keeping. Dec by water into NaOH and alcohol. Sol without decompn in abs alc. *Keep tightly closed, protected from light and in a cool place.*

8614. Sodium Ethyl Sulfate. [546-74-7] Sodium sulfovinate. $C_2H_5NaO_4S$; mol wt 148.11. C 16.22%, H 3.40%, Na 15.52%, O 43.21%, S 21.65%. $NaC_2H_5SO_4$.

Monohydrate. White, very hygroscopic crystals. Sol in 0.7 part water, in alcohol. *Keep well closed.*

USE: In organic syntheses.

8615. Sodium Ferric Gluconate. [34089-81-1] D-Gluconic acid iron(3+) sodium salt. Bioavailable iron supplement containing a ferric hydroxide core stabilized and solubilized by simple carbohydrates. Prepn: W. Traube *et al., Ber.* **66B**, 1545 (1933). Intestinal absorption of clinical formulations: L. Samochowiec, *Clin. Ter.* **56**, 341 (1971).

Sodium ferric gluconate complex. Ferlixit; Ferrlecit; Ferrosprint; Sanifer. Aqueous iron formulation administered as an injectable, stable, macromolecular iron saccharate complex. Gluconate bridges the iron centers. Mol formula is approximately: $[NaFe_2O_3(C_6H_{11}O_7)(C_{12}H_{22}O_{11})_5]_n$. Apparent mol wt 289-440 kDa. Safety profile: G. Faich, J. Strobos, *Am. J. Kidney Dis.* **33**, 464 (1999). Clinical evaluation in hemodialysis patients: A. R. Nissenson *et al., ibid.* 471; and comparison with iron dextran: B. Michael *et al., Kidney Int.* **61**, 1830 (2002). Clinical pharmacokinetics: P. A. Seligman *et al., Pharmacotherapy* **24**, 574 (2004). Clinical evaluation in renal transplant patients: R. S. Gillespie, J. M. Symons, *Pediatr. Transplant.* **9**, 43 (2005). Review of therapeutic applications: S. Fishbane, J. Wagner, *Am. J. Kidney Dis.* **37**, 879-883 (2001). Deep red color indicative of ferric oxide linkages.

THERAP CAT: Hematinic.

8616. Sodium Ferrocyanide. [13601-19-9] Tetrasodium hexakis(cyano-*C*)ferrate(4−); sodium hexacyanoferrate(II); yellow prussiate of soda; sodium prussiate yellow. $C_6FeN_6Na_4$; mol wt 303.91. C 23.71%, Fe 18.38%, N 27.65%, Na 30.26%. $Na_4Fe(CN)_6$. Review of properties, chemistry and syntheses: *The Chemistry of Ferrocyanides,* American Cyanamid Co. (Beacon Press, New York, 1953) 112 pp.

Decahydrate. Pale yellow, monoclinic, slightly efflorescent crystals. Steady dehydration occurs >50°. Becomes anhyd at 81.5°. Dec 435°, forming sodium cyanide, iron, carbon, and nitrogen. Soly in water at 1°: 10.2% (calcd as the anhyd salt); at 17°: 14.7%; at 25°: 17.6%; at 53°: 28.1%; at 85°: 39%; at 96.6°: 39.7%. Practically insol in most organic solvents.

Caution: Do not mix with hot or concd acids and do not expose solns to sunlight for any length of time to avoid generation of hydrogen cyanide. Waste ferrocyanides in streams and lakes should not exceed 2 ppm because irradiated solns become toxic to fish, G. E. Burdick, M. Lipscheutz, *C.A.* **44**, 10939f (1950). *Toxicity:* Because of strong chemical bondage between the cyanide groups and the iron, ferrocyanides have a low order of toxicity.

USE: Addition of sodium ferrocyanide solns to slightly acidic solns of iron salts causes precipitation of insol Prussian blue (ferric ferrocyanide), $Fe_4[Fe(CN)_6]_3$. Alkaline solns yield sol Prussian blue, $NaFe[Fe(CN)_6]$. Sodium ferrocyanide forms gels with heavy metals in general. Used in ore flotation. In photography for bleaching, toning, and fixing. To prevent caking of rock salt and foods. Additive to pickling baths. Peptizing agent in rubber. Arc stabilizer in welding rod coatings. Emulsion polymerization catalyst.

8617. Sodium Fluoborate. [13755-29-8] Sodium tetrafluoroborate; sodium borofluoride. BF_4Na; mol wt 109.79. B 9.85%, F 69.22%, Na 20.94%. $NaBF_4$. Prepd according to the equation $2H_3BO_3 + 8HF + Na_2CO_3 \rightarrow 2NaBF_4 + 7H_2O + CO_2$: Balz, Wilke-Dörfurt, *Z. Anorg. Allg. Chem.* **159**, 197 (1927); Kwasnik in *Handbook of Preparative Inorganic Chemistry* vol. 1, G. Brauer, Ed. (Academic Press, New York, 2nd ed., 1963) p 222.

Orthorhombic, stout rectangular prisms, d^{20} 2.47. mp 384° (slight decompn). Does not etch glass when absolutely dry. Soly in water (g/100 ml): 108 (26°); 210 (100°). Sparingly sol in alcohol. Aq solns have a bitter taste and are acid to litmus.

USE: Fluorinating agent, *see* Lawton, Levy, *J. Am. Chem. Soc.* **77**, 6083 (1955).

8618. Sodium Fluoride. [7681-49-4] Chemifluor; Duraphat; Florocid; Fluoros; Flura-Drops; Karidium; Lemoflur; Luride-SF; Ossalin; Ossin; Osteo-F; Osteofluor; Slow-Fluoride; Villiaumite; Zymafluor. FNa; mol wt 41.99. F 45.25%, Na 54.75%. NaF. Prepd by fusing cryolite with NaOH or by adding equiv amounts of NaOH or Na_2CO_3 to 40% HF (precipitation is instantaneous and crystal size depends on pH, but too much HF yields sodium bifluoride, $NaHF_2$): Müller, *Chem. Ztg.* **52**, 5 (1928); Kwasnik in *Handbook of Preparative Inorganic Chemistry* vol. 1, G. Brauer, Ed. (Academic Press, New York, 2nd ed., 1963) pp 235-236. Technical grades are 90% and 95% NaF, light (37 cu in/lb) and dense (23 cu in/lb), and 98%. The impurities are mainly sodium and aluminum fluosilicates. Pharmacology: Caruso *et al., Handb. Exp. Pharmakol.* **XX** (Part 2), F. Smith, Ed. (Springer, Berlin, 1970) pp 144-165. Toxicity: H. F. Smyth *et al., Am. Ind. Hyg. Assoc. J.* **30**, 470 (1969). Carcinogenicity studies: J. R. Bucher *et al., Int. J. Cancer* **48**, 733 (1991). Review of toxicology: D. W. Banting, *J. Am. Dent. Assoc.* **122**, 86-91 (1991); and human exposure: *Toxicological Profile for Fluorides, Hydrogen Fluoride, and Fluorine* (PB2004-100002, 2003) 404 pp. Review of clinical efficacy in prevention of dental caries: L. G. Petersson, *Caries Res.* **27**, Suppl 1, 35-42 (1993); of clinical experience in osteoporosis: M. Kleerekoper, D. B. Mendlovic, *Endocr. Rev.* **14**, 312-323 (1993).

Cubic or tetragonal crystals (NaCl lattice). d 2.78. mp 993°. bp 1704°. *Poisonous!* Soly in water (g/100 ml): 4.0 (15°); 4.3 (25°); 5.0 (100°). Insol in alc. Aq solns have an alkaline reaction caused by partial hydrolysis. pH of freshly prepd satd soln 7.4. Aq solns etch glass, but the dry crystals or powder may be kept in glass bottles. Sodium fluoride sold as household insecticide must be tinted Nile Blue. LD_{50} orally in rats: 0.18 g/kg (Smyth).

Caution: Potential symptoms of overexposure by ingestion are salty or soapy taste; salivation, nausea, abdominal pain, vomiting, diarrhea; dehydration, thirst; sweating; stiff spine; muscle weakness, tremors; CNS depression; shock; arrhythmia. Direct contact may cause dermatitis; irritation of eyes, respiratory system. Potential symptoms of chronic ingestion are mottling of tooth enamel; osteosclerosis, calcification of ligaments of ribs, pelvis. *See NIOSH Pocket Guide to Chemical Hazards* (DHHS/NIOSH 97-140, 1997) p 282; *Clinical Toxicology of Commercial Products*, R. E. Gosselin *et al.*, Eds. (Williams & Wilkins, Baltimore, 5th ed., 1984) Section III, pp 185-193.

USE: As insecticide, particularly for roaches and ants; in other pesticide formulations; constituent of vitreous enamel and glass mixes; as a steel degassing agent; in electroplating; in fluxes; in heat-treating salt compositions; in the fluoridation of drinking water; for disinfecting fermentation apparatus in breweries and distilleries; preserving wood, pastes and mucilage; manuf of coated paper; frosting glass; in removal of HF from exhaust gases to reduce air pollution. Dental caries prophylactic.

THERAP CAT: In treatment of osteoporosis.

THERAP CAT (VET): Anthelmintic, pediculicide, acaricide.

8619. Sodium Folate. [6484-89-5] *N*-[4-[[(2-Amino-1,4-dihydro-4-oxo-6-pteridinyl)methyl]amino]benzoyl]-L-glutamic acid monosodium salt; folic acid sodium salt; sodium pteroylglutamate; sodium Folvite. $C_{19}H_{18}N_7NaO_6$; mol wt 463.38. C 49.25%, H 3.92%, N 21.16%, Na 4.96%, O 20.72%.

Sold only as sterile soln in ampuls. Clear, mobile liquid. Yellow to orange-yellow color. pH between 8.5 and 11.0. For spectrophotometric data *see* Folic Acid.

THERAP CAT: Water-soluble hematopoietic vitamin.

8620. Sodium Formaldehydesulfoxylate. [149-44-0] Hydroxymethanesulfinic acid sodium salt; formaldehyde sodium sulfoxylate; formaldehydesulfoxylic acid sodium salt; sodium hydroxymethanesulfinate; sodium methanalsulfoxylate; Aldanil; Rongalite; Rongalite C. CH_3NaO_3S; mol wt 118.09. C 10.17%, H 2.56%, Na 19.47%, O 40.65%, S 27.15%. $Na[HOCH_2SO_2]$. Prepn: Heyl, Greer, *Am. J. Pharm.* **94**, 80 (1922); Binns, US 2013125 (1935 to Virginia Smelting); Postnikov, Kunin, *J. Appl. Chem. USSR* **13**, 185 (1940). Structure of dihydrate: Truter, *J. Chem. Soc.* **1955**, 3064; **1962**, 3400. Of limited value in treatment of mercuric chloride poisoning: Modell *et al., J. Pharmacol. Exp. Ther.* **61**, 66 (1937).

Dihydrate. Crystals, mp 63-64°, dec at higher temp. Odorless when freshly prepd, but quickly develops a characteristic (garlic) odor. Freely sol in water; practically insol in abs alcohol, ether, benzene. Readily dec by dil acids. Aq soln is practically neutral. *Keep well closed in a cool place.* LD s.c. in mice, 4.0 g/kg: Rosenthal, *Public Health Rep.* **49**, 908 (1934).

USE: In vat color printing pastes: Borstelmann, Fordemwalt, US 2597281 (1952 to Am. Cyanamid). In polymerization of ethylenic compds: GB 816252; GB 852593 (1959 to Hercules Powder; 1960 to Air Reduction). In manuf of arsphenamines: Krumwiede, *J. Am. Pharm. Assoc.* **8**, 795 (1919); Heyl, Miller, *ibid.* **11**, 432 (1922).

THERAP CAT: Treatment of mercury poisoning.

8621. Sodium Formate. [141-53-7] $CHNaO_2$; mol wt 68.01. C 17.66%, H 1.48%, Na 33.80%, O 47.05%. HCOONa.

White, deliquesc granules or cryst powder; slight odor of formic acid. d 1.92. mp 253°; at higher temp dec into sodium oxalate and hydrogen, then into sodium carbonate. Sol in ~1.3 parts water; sol in glycerol, slightly in alcohol. The aq soln is neutral. pH ~7. Has buffering action. *Keep well closed.*

USE: In dyeing and printing fabrics; also in anal. chemistry as a precipitant for the "noble" metals. Solubilizes trivalent metal ions in soln by forming complex ions. Buffering action adjusts the pH of strong mineral acids to higher values.

THERAP CAT: Caustic, astringent.

8622. Sodium Glycerophosphate. [1334-74-3] 1,2,3-Propanetriol mono(dihydrogen phosphate) disodium salt. $C_3H_7Na_2$ O_6P; mol wt 216.04. C 16.68%, H 3.27%, Na 21.28%, O 44.43%, P 14.34%. Three isomers exist: The β-glycerophosphoric acid disodium salt ($(HOCH_2)_2CHOPO_3Na_2$) and D(+)- and L(−)-α-glycerophosphoric acid disodium salt ($HOCH_2CH(OH)CH_2OPO_3Na_2$). Prepn: H. King, F. L. Pyman, *Pharm. J.* **92**, 511 (1914). Exptl use in diagnosis of prostatic carcinoma: M. K. Schwartz *et al., Ann. N.Y. Acad. Sci.* **166**, 775 (1969). Chronic toxicity study of β-form: K. L. Raheja *et al., Toxicology* **8**, 115 (1977). Efficacy of β-form as cariostatic agent: T. H. Grenby, J. M. Bull. *Arch. Oral Biol.* **20**, 717 (1975). GC determn: Y. Handa *et al., J. Chromatogr.* **206**, 387 (1981).

β-Form hemiundecahydrate. White, odorless, scale-like crystals; dec >130°. Sol in ~1.5 parts water; more sol in hot water. (pH of aq soln: ~9.5). Insol in alcohol.

THERAP CAT: Tonic.

THERAP CAT (VET): Has been used as a tonic.

8623. Sodium Hexachloroplatinate(IV). [16923-58-3] Disodium hexachloroplatinate(2−); sodium platinichloride; sodium chloroplatinate. Cl_6Na_2Pt; mol wt 453.78. Cl 46.88%, Na 10.13%, Pt 42.99%. $Na_2[PtCl_6]$. Prepn: Grube in *Handbook of Preparative Inorganic Chemistry* vol. **2**, G. Brauer, Ed. (Academic Press, New York, 2nd ed., 1965) pp 1571-1572; Cox, Peters, *Inorg. Synth.* **13**, 173 (1971).

Yellow, hygroscopic crystals. Easily forms hexahydrate at 25° and relative humidity >50% (reconverted to anhydr salt by heat at 110° for one hour). uv max (1 formal HCl): 262 nm (ε 24500). Sol in water, alcohol.

USE: Catalyst.

8624. Sodium Hexafluorosilicate. [16893-85-9] Sodium fluosilicate; sodium silicofluoride; Salufer. F_6Na_2Si; mol wt 188.06. F 60.61%, Na 24.45%, Si 14.93%. Na_2SiF_6. Toxicity study: C. W. Muehlberger, *J. Pharmacol. Exp. Ther.* **39**, 246 (1930). Review of toxicology of fluoride compounds: G. L. Waldbott, *Acta Med. Scand. Suppl.* **400**, 1-44 (1963).

White, granular powder. d 2.68. Melts at red heat with decompn. Sol in 150 parts cold, 40 parts boiling water. Insol in alc. The soln in cold water is neutral. LD in rabbits (mg F/kg): 76 intragastric; in rats (mg F/kg): 42 s.c. (Muehlberger). LD in guinea pigs (mg/kg): 250 orally, 500 s.c. (Waldbott).

USE: In enamels for china and porcelain; manuf opal glass; as insecticide, rodenticide; mothproofing of woolens. Fluoridating agent for drinking water. Intermediate in prodn of synthetic cryolite.

THERAP CAT (VET): Pediculicide.

8625. Sodium Hydride. [7646-69-7] HNa; mol wt 24.00. H 4.20%, Na 95.79%. NaH. Prepd by passing hydrogen into molten sodium dispersed in oil or mixed with a catalyst such as anthracene above 250°: Hansley, Carlisle, *Chem. Eng. News* **23**, 1332 (1945). Laboratory procedure by hydrogenating sodium dispersions: Mattson, Whaley, *Inorg. Synth.* **5**, 10 (1957). Book: J. Plesek, S. Hermanek, *Sodium Hydride, Its Use in the Laboratory and in Technology* (Iliffe Books, London, 1968) 185 pp.

Silvery needles; the commercial product is a gray-white powder. d 1.396. Dec 425°. Reacts explosively with water, violently with lower alcohols, ignites spontaneously on standing in moist air. Sol in molten sodium hydroxide, insol in liq ammonia but forms sodamide at moderate temps.

USE: At low temps where reducing properties of sodium are undesirable as in the condensation of ketones and aldehydes with acid esters; in soln with molten sodium hydroxide for the reduction of oxide scale on metals; at high temps as a reducing agent and reduction catalyst.

8626. Sodium Hydrosulfite. [7775-14-6] Sodium sulfoxylate; sodium dithionite. $Na_2O_4S_2$; mol wt 174.11. Na 26.41%, O

36.76%, S 36.83%. $Na_2S_2O_4$. The hydrosulfite of commerce contains 85-90% $Na_2S_2O_4$.

White or grayish-white, cryst powder; slight characteristic odor. Oxidizes in air (more readily so in presence of moisture or when in soln) to bisulfite and bisulfate and acquires an acid reaction. Very sol in water, slightly in alcohol.

Note: The name sodium hydrosulfite is applied also to $NaHSO_2$, mol wt 88.06, sol in water, alcohol. Still more confusion results when "sodium hyposulfite" is applied to this compd ($Na_2S_2O_4$) *see* 1957 Subject Index to *Chem. Abstracts,* p 2218s *under* sodium dithionite.

USE: As reducing agent, particularly in dyeing with indigo and vat dyes; bleaching soaps, straw; removing dyes from dyed fabrics.

8627. Sodium Hydroxide. [1310-73-2] Caustic soda; soda lye; sodium hydrate. HNaO; mol wt 40.00. H 2.52%, Na 57.47%, O 40.00%. NaOH. By reacting calcium hydroxide with sodium carbonate; from sodium chloride by electrolysis; from sodium metal and water vapor at low temp. Description of industrial processes: *Faith, Keyes & Clark's Industrial Chemicals,* F. A. Lowenheim, M. K. Moran, Eds. (Wiley-Interscience, New York, 4th ed., 1975) pp 737-745. Toxicity: Fazekas, *Arch. Exp. Pathol. Pharmakol.* **184,** 587 (1937).

Fused solid with crystalline fracture. Rapidly absorbs carbon dioxide and water from the air. Very corrosive (caustic) to animal and vegetable tissue and to aluminum metal in the presence of moisture. Sold as lumps, sticks, pellets, chips, etc. When kept in tight containers, the usual grades contain 97-98% NaOH. mp 318°. d^{25} 2.13. One gram dissolves in 0.9 ml water, 0.3 ml boiling water, 7.2 ml abs alcohol, 4.2 ml methanol, also sol in glycerol. Generates considerable heat while dissolving, or when the soln is mixed with an acid. Volumetric NaOH solns used in the laboratory must be protected from air to avoid formation of carbonate. Concentrated NaOH solns dissolve practically no sodium carbonate. The pH of a 0.05% w/w soln ~12, of a 0.5% soln ~13, of a 5% soln ~14. Density, boiling and freezing pt data for (w/w) water solns. d_4^{15}: 5% 1.056, 10% 1.111, 20% 1.222, 30% 1.333, 40% 1.434, 50% 1.530. bp: 5% 102°, 10% 105°, 20% 110°, 30% 115°, 40% 125°, 50% 140°. fp: 5% −4°, 10% −10°, 20% −26°, 30% 1°, 40% 15°, 50% 12°. LD orally in rabbits: 500 mg/kg (10% soln) (Fazekas).

Caution: Potential symptoms of overexposure are irritation of eyes, skin and mucous membranes; pneumonitis; eye and skin burns; temporary loss of hair. *See NIOSH Pocket Guide to Chemical Hazards* (DHHS/NIOSH 97-1140, 1997) p 284.

USE: NaOH solutions are used to neutralize acids and make sodium salts, *e.g.,* in petroleum refining to remove sulfuric and organic acids; to treat cellulose in making viscose rayon and cellophane; in reclaiming rubber to dissolve out the fabric; in making plastics to dissolve casein. NaOH solns hydrolyze fats and form soaps; they precipitate alkaloids (bases) and most metals (as hydroxides) from water solns of their salts. Pharmaceutic aid (alkalizer).

THERAP CAT (VET): Caustic; dehorning of calves.

8628. Sodium Hypochlorite. [7681-52-9] ClNaO; mol wt 74.44. Cl 47.63%, Na 30.88%, O 21.49%. NaClO. Strong oxidizing and hydrolyzing agent; used in aqueous solutions of various strengths for its bactericidal properties. Prepn as the pentahydrate from NaOH and Cl_2 in the presence of water: Sanfourche, Gardent, *Bull. Soc. Chim.* [4] **35,** 1089 (1924); Schmeisser in *Handbook of Preparative Inorganic Chemistry* vol. 1, G. Brauer, Ed. (Academic Press, New York, 2nd ed., 1963) pp 309-310. Review of prepn and uses of *Dakin's solution,* a diluted antiseptic formulation: H. Plagge, *Pharm. Ztg.* **138,** No. 14, 26-31 (1993). Review of toxicology and use as household bleach: F. Racioppi *et al., Food Chem. Toxicol.* **32,** 845-861 (1994); of use in health care facilities: W. A. Rutala, D. J. Weber, *Clin. Microbiol. Rev.* **10,** 597-610 (1997). Review of use as endodontic irrigant: R. M. Clarkson, A. J. Moule, *Aust. Dent. J.* **43,** 250-256 (1998).

Prepd as the pentahydrate, crystals, mp 18°. Dec by CO_2 from air. Anhyd NaClO may be obtained by freeze-drying in a vacuum (over concd H_2SO_4). *Anhyd NaClO is very explosive.* Soly at 0°: 29.3 g/100 ml H_2O. Aqueous solutions for household bleach contain ~5.25%. Solutions for use as antiseptics contain ~0.5% sodium hypochlorite and are buffered or stabilized with various agents.

Caution: Potential symptoms of overexposure by ingestion are pain and inflammation of the mouth, pharynx, esophagus, stomach; vomiting; circulatory collapse, cold and clammy skin, cyanosis, shallow respirations; confusion, delirium, coma; edema of pharynx, larynx, glottis with stridor and obstruction; perforation of esophagus, stomach. Potential symptoms of overexposure by fume inhalation are severe respiratory tract irritation, pulmonary edema. Direct contact may cause vesicular eruptions on skin and eczematoid dermatitis. *See Clinical Toxicology of Commercial Products,* R. E. Gosselin *et al.,* Eds. (Williams & Wilkins, Baltimore, 5th ed., 1984) Section III, pp 202-205.

USE: Aq soln as bleach, disinfectant; chlorination of swimming pools; sanitation of drinking water.

THERAP CAT: Antiseptic, disinfectant.

8629. Sodium Hypophosphite. [7681-53-0] Phosphinic acid, sodium salt. H_2NaO_2P; mol wt 87.98. H 2.29%, Na 26.13%, O 36.37%, P 35.21%. NaH_2PO_2. Solubility data: Palit, *J. Am. Chem. Soc.* **69,** 3120 (1947).

Monohydrate. White, odorless, deliquesc granules; saline taste. When strongly heated, it dec with evolution of phosphine which ignites spontaneously in the air. *It explodes when triturated with chlorates or other oxidizing agents.* Sol in 1 part water, 0.15 part boiling water; freely sol in glycerol and in boiling alcohol; sol in cold alcohol, slightly in abs alcohol. Insol in ether. Soly of anhydr NaH_2PO_2 at 25° in ethylene glycol: 33.0 g/100 g; in propylene glycol: 9.7 g/100 g. The aq soln is neutral. *Keep well closed.*

USE: As reagent for arsenic and iodates; prepn of hypophosphites syrup.

8630. Sodium Iodate. [7681-55-2] $INaO_3$; mol wt 197.89. I 64.13%, Na 11.62%, O 24.25%. $NaIO_3$. The article of commerce contains about 99% $NaIO_3$. Acute toxicity study: S. H. Webster *et al., J. Pharmacol. Exp. Ther.* **120,** 171 (1957). Review of safety assessment: *J. Am. Coll. Toxicol.* **14,** 231-239 (1995).

White, cryst powder. d 4.28. Sol in acetone, acetic acid. Sol in ~11 parts water, 3 parts boiling water. Insol in alc. The aq soln is neutral. LD_{50} in female mice (mg/kg): 119 ±4 i.p., 108 ±4 i.v., 505 ±26 orally (Webster).

THERAP CAT: Antiseptic (mucous membranes).

8631. Sodium Iodide. [7681-82-5] Ioduril; Anayodin. INa; mol wt 149.89. I 84.67%, Na 15.34%. NaI. U.S.P. NaI is at least 99% pure.

White, odorless, deliquesc crystals or granules. Gradually absorbs up to about 5% (½ mol) moisture on exposure to air. Slowly becomes brown in the air due to liberation of iodine. Its aq soln is similarly affected. d 3.67. One gram dissolves in 0.5 ml water, ~2 ml alc, 1 ml glycerol; sol in acetone. It is made slightly alkaline to render it more stable. pH: 8-9.5. *Keep well closed and protected from light.* At ordinary room temp crystallizes from water with $2H_2O$ in the form of colorless, prismatic crystals. *Incompat.* As of potassium iodide. MLD i.v. in rats: 1.3 g/kg, Loeser, Konwiser, *J. Lab. Clin. Med.* **15,** 35 (1929).

THERAP CAT: Iodine supplement; expectorant.

THERAP CAT (VET): Actinobacillosis, actinomycosis. Expectorant. Has been used for ringworm, hyperplastic fibrous lesions, paraplegia from pachymeningitis of dogs.

8632. Sodium Iodide, Radioactive. [7790-26-3] Sodium radio-iodide (^{131}I); sodium iodide ^{131}I; Na^{131}I; Iodotope; Oriodide; Radiocaps-131; Theriodide-131. Prepd from radioactive iodine (^{131}I) which has a half-life of 8 days and emits beta and gamma rays. Other properties identical with those of ordinary sodium iodide. Dispensed as carrier-free sodium radioiodide in capsules for oral use or in aq soln for oral or parenteral administration.

THERAP CAT: Diagnostic aid (thyroid function); antineoplastic.

8633. Sodium Iodomethamate. [519-26-6] 1,4-Dihydro-3,5-diiodo-1-methyl-4-oxo-2,6-pyridinedicarboxylic acid disodium salt; 3,5-diiodo-1-methylchelidamic acid sodium salt; disodium *N*-methyl-3,5-diiodo-4-pyridone-2,6-dicarboxylate; iodoxyl; D-40; Neo-Iopax; Pyelectan; Uropac. $C_8H_3I_2NNa_2O_5$; mol wt 492.90. C 19.49%, H 0.61%, I 51.49%, N 2.84%, Na 9.33%, O 16.23%. Prepn: Chelidonic acid is converted to chelidamic acid by the action of NH_3, chelidamic acid is iodinated with iodine in a boiling aq alkaline soln, the iodinated product is methylated at the nitrogen with dimethyl sulfate in hot alkaline soln, *cf.* Dohrn, Diedrich, *Ann.* **494**, 284 (1932); **DE 545916**; **DE 545266**; **DE 556142**; **US 1919417** (1933).

Crystals, dec around 200° with effervescence. Freely sol in water (1:1). Practically insol in chloroform, ether, acetone, petr ether.

THERAP CAT: Diagnostic aid (radiopaque medium).

8634. Sodium Isopropyl Xanthate. [140-93-2] Isopropyl-xanthic acid sodium salt; Good-Rite Nix. $C_4H_7NaOS_2$; mol wt 158.22. C 30.36%, H 4.46%, Na 14.53%, O 10.11%, S 40.53%. $(CH_3)_2CHOCSSNa$.

Deliquescent, white to yellowish powder or lumps, dec 150°. Slightly unpleasant odor. Soly in water: 30% at 4°; 46% at 24°; 54% at 35°.

Caution: Irritating to skin, eyes, mucous membranes, respiratory tract.

USE: Control of annual weeds in bean and pea fields.

8635. Sodium Lactate. [72-17-3] Lacolin. $C_3H_5NaO_3$; mol wt 112.06. C 32.15%, H 4.50%, Na 20.52%, O 42.83%. Commercially available as a mixture with water containing 70-80% sodium lactate. *Ref:* Shaw, **US 2856326** (1958 to Nat. Dairy Prod. Corp.).

Colorless or almost colorless, thick, odorless liquid. Miscible with water, alcohol. The soln is neutral.

USE: Instead of glycerol in calico printing; as a plasticizer for casein; as a corrosion inhibitor in alc antifreeze mixture.

THERAP CAT: Electrolyte replenisher; systemic and urinary alka-linizing agent.

THERAP CAT (VET): Has been used in bovine ketosis.

8636. Sodium Lauryl Sulfate. [151-21-3] Sulfuric acid monododecyl ester sodium salt; sodium dodecyl sulfate; SDS; Irium. $C_{12}H_{25}NaO_4S$; mol wt 288.38. C 49.98%, H 8.74%, Na 7.97%, O 22.19%, S 11.12%. $CH_3(CH_2)_{10}CH_2OSO_3Na$. Anionic detergent prepd by sulfation of lauryl alcohol, followed by neutral-ization with sodium carbonate: A. Lottermoser, F. Stoll, *Kolloid-Z.* **63**, 50 (1933). Surfactant properties: J. Powney, C. C. Addison, *Trans. Faraday Soc.* **33**, 1244 (1937); E. E. Dreger *et al., Ind. Eng. Chem.* **36**, 610 (1944). Use in electrophoretic sepn and mol wt estimation of proteins: A. L. Shapiro *et al., Biochem. Biophys. Res. Commun.* **28**, 815 (1967); K. Weber, M. Osborn, *J. Biol. Chem.* **244**, 4406 (1969); of glycopolypeptides: B. S. Leach *et al., Biochemistry* **19**, 5734 (1980). Toxicity study: A. I. T. Walker *et al., Food Cosmet. Toxicol.* **5**, 763 (1967). Review of toxicology: Ch. Glox-huber, *Arch. Toxicol.* **32**, 245-270 (1974).

White or cream-colored crystals, flakes, or powder. Faint odor of fatty substances. Smooth feel. Neutral reaction. One gram dis-solves in 10 ml water, giving an opalescent soln. Lowers the surface tension of aq solns. Emulsifies fats. LD_{50} orally in rats: 1288 mg/kg (Walker).

USE: Wetting agent, detergent, esp in the textile industry. Elec-trophoretic separation of proteins and lipids. Ingredient of tooth-pastes.

8637. Sodium-Lead Alloy. [12740-44-2] Lead-sodium al-loy; sodium-lead; Drynap; Dri-Na. Usually contains a minimum of 9.5% active sodium. For tetraethyllead manufacture the sodium-lead alloy is produced in large quantities by making a melt of 90 parts of lead with 10.5 parts of sodium (w/w). The reaction is strongly exothermic and starts at 225°. Prepn of the alloy on a laboratory scale: Soroos, *Ind. Eng. Chem. Anal. Ed.* **11**, 657 (1939).

Obtained in brittle lumps which can be stored in an air-tight container. It reacts only slowly with air or water, yet dries ether as completely as sodium wire. Residues of ether or other liquids still containing some active alloy can be destroyed safely by the addition of water, as the reaction never reaches the violence ob-served with pure sodium metal. The alloy may be ground to a very

fine powder under the surface of a non-polar solvent such as kero-sine or ether.

Caution: Finely ground powder, if not protected by a suitable liquid, may react with excess moisture from the air sufficiently to catch fire.

USE: In manuf of tetraethyllead by reaction of alloy with ethyl chloride; for drying ether and for reductions: Tabei *et al., Bull. Chem. Soc. Jpn.* **40**, 1538 (1967); as a sodium substitute in many chemical reactions where the presence of lead is not objectionable.

8638. Sodium Metabisulfite. [7681-57-4] Sodium pyrosul-fite. $Na_2O_5S_2$; mol wt 190.11. Na 24.19%, O 42.08%, S 33.73%. $Na_2S_2O_5$. Crystallizes from cold water with $7H_2O$.

White crystals or powder; odor of SO_2. Freely sol in water, glycerol; slightly sol in alcohol. The aq soln is acid.

Caution: Potential symptoms of overexposure are irritation of eyes, skin and mucous membranes. *See NIOSH Pocket Guide to Chemical Hazards* (DHHS/NIOSH 97-140, 1997) p 284.

USE: Pharmaceutic aid (antioxidant).

8639. Sodium Metaborate. [7775-19-1] $BNaO_2$; mol wt 65.80. B 16.43%, Na 34.94%, O 48.63%. $NaBO_2$. Obtained by fusing equivalent mol wts of borax and sodium carbonate.

White pieces or powder. mp 966°. Sol in water, the soln being strongly alkaline.

8640. Sodium Metaperiodate. [7790-28-5] Sodium period-ate. $INaO_4$; mol wt 213.89. I 59.33%, Na 10.75%, O 29.92%. $NaIO_4$. Synthesis starting with sodium iodide: *Inorg. Synth.* **2**, 212 (1946) and **1**, 170 (1939).

White, tetragonal crystals, d_4^{16} 3.865. Dec ~300°. Sol in cold water, sulfuric, nitric, acetic acids.

Trihydrate. White, efflorescent, trigonal crystals, d_4^{18} 3.219. Dec 175°. One gram dissolves in 8 ml water at 20°.

8641. Sodium Metaphosphate. $(NaPO_3)_n$ where "n" may be 2 or more. Prepd by dehydration of sodium phosphates (e.g. $Na_2H_2P_2O_7$, NaH_2PO_4, Na_2HPO_4). Several different forms are known. *Reviews:* J. R. Van Waser, *Phosphorus and Its Compounds* **vol. 1** (Interscience, New York, 1958) pp 601-800; Pantony in *Mellor's* **vol. II** supplement II, *The Alkali Metals* (Part 1), 1316-1349 (1961); Thilo in *Adv. Inorg. Chem. Radiochem.* **4**, 1-75 (1962). *See also* Sodium Hexametaphosphate; Sodium Trimetaphosphate; Maddrell's Salt.

8642. Sodium Metasilicate. [6834-92-0] Na_2O_3Si; mol wt 122.06. Na 37.67%, O 39.32%, Si 23.01%. Na_2SiO_3. Usually prepared from sand (SiO_2) and soda ash (Na_2CO_3) by fusion: Schwarz, *Z. Anorg. Allg. Chem.* **126**, 62 (1923); *Faith, Keyes & Clark's Industrial Chemicals*, F. A. Lowenheim, M. K. Moran, Eds. (Wiley-Interscience, New York, 4th ed., 1975) pp 755-761. *Review: Gmelins, Sodium* (8th ed. supplement) **21**, pp 1474-1478 (1967).

Usually obtained as a glass; also orthorhombic crystals. d 2.614. mp 1089°. n_D^{25} (glass) 1.520. Specific heat (20°): 0.217. Heat of formation: -371.2 kcal/mol. Heat of soln (cryst) -7.45 kcal/-mol. Heat of fusion: 10.3 kcal/mol. Sol in cold water, hydrolyzed by hot water. Insol in alcohol, acids, salt solns.

Nonahydrate. Efflorescent, orthorhombic bipyramidal platelets, mp 48° in water of crystn. Heat of hydration: -24.15 kcal/mol.

8643. Sodium Methoxide. [124-41-4] Sodium methylate. CH_3NaO; mol wt 54.02. C 22.23%, H 5.60%, Na 42.56%, O 29.62%. CH_3ONa. Prepn: Burness, *Org. Synth.* **39**, 51 (1959).

White, free-flowing powder. Sensitive to air and moisture. Dec by water. Sol in methanol, ethanol. Also exists in solvated form, $CH_3ONa.2CH_3OH$, white powder. Apparent density of solvent-free material ~4.6 lb/gal.

USE: In organic syntheses.

8644. Sodium Methylsulfinylmethylide. [15590-23-5] Sodium sulfinylbismethane ion(1−); dimsyl sodium; methylsulfinyl sodium; sodium dimethylsulfoxylate; sodium DMSO. C_2H_5NaOS; mol wt 100.12. C 23.99%, H 5.03%, Na 22.96%, O 15.98%, S 32.03%. Conjugate base of dimethyl sulfoxide, *q.v.*; nucleophilic reagent in organic chemistry. Prepn: E. J. Corey, M. Chaykovsky, *J. Am. Chem. Soc.* **87**, 1345 (1965); of stable solns: K. Sjöberg, *Tetrahedron Lett.* **7**, 6383 (1966). Reactivity: T. J. Broxton *et al., Aust. J. Chem.* **19**, 521 (1966). Synthetic applications: A. J. Birch *et al., ibid.* **24**, 2179 (1971); T. G. Warner, A. A. Benson, *J. Lipid Res.* **18**, 548 (1977); L. Petrus *et al., Carbohydr. Res.* **268**, 319 (1995). Brief review: M. Mondal, *Synlett* **2005**, 2697-2698.

Highly sol in DMSO. *DMSO solns are sensitive to heat and air; dec above 85°.*

USE: Nucleophile in organic synthesis.

8645. Sodium Molybdate(VI). [7631-95-0] (*T*-4)-Disodium molybdate (MoO_4^{2-}); sodium molybdenum oxide. $MoNa_2O_4$; mol wt 205.92. Mo 46.59%, Na 22.33%, O 31.08%. Na_2MoO_4.

Dihydrate. [10102-40-6] Molyhibit 100. $MoNa_2O_4 \cdot 2H_2O$; mol wt 241.95. Cryst powder. Loses its water of crystn at 100°. Sol in 1.7 parts cold water, ~0.9 part boiling water. pH of 5% aq soln at 25° = 9.0-10.0. Has been reported to be less toxic than the other corresponding compds of group 6B in the periodic table: Fairhall *et al., Public Health Bull.* no. 293 (1945).

USE: Manuf of inorganic and organic pigments, corrosion inhibitor, bath additive for metals finishing, reagent for alkaloids, micronutrient for plants and animals.

8646. Sodium β-Naphthoquinone-4-sulfonate. [521-24-4] 3,4-Dihydro-3,4-dioxo-1-naphthalenesulfonic acid sodium salt; sodium 1,2-naphthoquinone-4-sulfonate; 1,2-naphthoquinone-4-sulfonic acid sodium salt; β-naphthoquinone-4-sulfonic acid sodium salt. $C_{10}H_5NaO_5S$; mol wt 260.20. C 46.16%, H 1.94%, Na 8.84%, O 30.74%, S 12.32%. Prepn: Folin, *J. Biol. Chem.* **51**, 377 (1922).

Yellow crystals from dil alc. Readily sol in water; slightly sol in 95% alcohol; moderately sol in acetone; practically insol in ether, chloroform, carbon disulfide, benzene, petr ether. Aq solns fade slowly on exposure to light but may be stabilized by HCl.

USE: Colorimetric determn of amino acids and amines.

8647. Sodium Nitrate. [7631-99-4] Chile saltpeter; cubic niter; soda niter. $NNaO_3$; mol wt 84.99. N 16.48%, Na 27.05%, O 56.48%. $NaNO_3$. The purified grade contains at least 99% $NaNO_3$. Occurs as a mineral in Chile. Toxicity data: Dollahite, Rowe, *Southwest. Vet.* **27**, 246 (1974).

Colorless, transparent crystals, white granules or powder; deliquesc in moist air. d 2.26. mp 308°. One gram dissolves in 1.1 ml water, 0.6 ml boiling water, 125 ml alcohol, 52 ml boiling alcohol, 3470 ml abs alcohol, 300 ml abs methanol. When dissolved in water the temp of the soln is lowered. The aq soln is neutral. *Keep well closed.* LD_{50} orally in rabbits: 1.955 g anion/kg (Dollahite, Rowe).

USE: Manuf of nitric acid and as catalyst in the manuf of sulfuric acid. Manuf sodium nitrite, glass, enamels for pottery; in matches; for improving burning properties of tobacco; pickling meats; as color fixative in meats. Clinical reagent (parasites). The technical grade is used as fertilizer.

8648. Sodium Nitrite. [7632-00-0] Nitrous acid sodium salt; erinitrit. $NNaO_2$; mol wt 69.00. N 20.30%, Na 33.32%, O 46.38%. Contains 96-98% $NaNO_2$. Thermodynamic properties: Plekhotkun, *Zh. Prikl. Khim.* **40**, 1843 (1967), *C.A.* **68**, 33797x (1968). Toxicity studies: Faccini *et al., Ind. Aliment. (Pinerolo, Italy)* **8**, 77 (1969), *C.A.* **71**, 100583b (1969); H. F. Smyth *et al., Am. Ind. Hyg. Assoc. J.* **30**, 470 (1969). Review of chemistry of $NaNO_2$ in a biological system as related to meat curing: Bard, Townsend, *Science of Meat & Meat Products*, J. F. Price, B. S. Schweigert, Eds. (W. H. Freeman, 2nd ed. 1971) pp 452-470.

White or slightly yellow, hygroscopic granules, rods, or powder. Very slowly oxidizes to nitrate in air. d 2.17. mp 271°; dec above

320°. Sol in 1.5 parts cold water, 0.6 part boiling water, slightly in alc. Dec even by weak acids with evolution of brown fumes of N_2O_3. The aq soln is alkaline. pH ~9. *Keep well closed.* LD_{50} orally in rats: 180 mg/kg (Smyth). *Incompat:* Acetanilide, antipyrine, chlorates, hypophosphites, iodides, mercury salts, permanganate, sulfites, tannic acid, vegetable astringent decoctions, infusions or tinctures.

Caution: Consult latest Government regulation to determine max amounts allowable in food.

USE: Manuf diazo dyes, nitroso compds, and in many other processes of manuf of organic chemicals; dyeing and printing textile fabrics; bleaching flax, silk, and linen; photography. In meat curing, coloring and preserving; in processing smoked chub. Also as reagent in anal. chemistry.

THERAP CAT: Vasodilator; antidote (cyanide poisoning).

THERAP CAT (VET): In cyanide poisoning. Has been used as a vasodilator, as a circulatory (blood pressure) depressant and to relieve smooth muscle spasm.

8649. Sodium Nitroprusside. [14402-89-2] Pentakis(cyano-*C*)nitrosylferrate(2−) disodium; sodium nitrosylpentacyanoferrate(III); sodium nitroferricyanide; sodium nitroprusside; Nipruss. $C_5FeN_6Na_2O$; mol wt 261.92. C 22.93%, Fe 21.32%, N 32.09%, Na 17.55%, O 6.11%. $Na_2[Fe(CN)_5NO]$. Prepn: L. Playfair, *Proc. Roy. Soc. London* **5**, 846 (1849). Pharmacology: Fernandez *et al., Arch. Inst. Farmacol. Exp. Madrid* **23**, 1-51 (1971). *Review:* I. H. Tuzel, *J. Clin. Pharmacol.* **14**, 494-503 (1974). Review of pharmacology, toxicology and therapeutic uses: J. H. Tinker, J. D. Michenfelder, *Anesthesiology* **45**, 340 (1976). Comprehensive description: R. Rucki, *Anal. Profiles Drug Subs.* **6**, 487-513 (1977); A. Bult *et al., ibid.* **15**, 781-792 (1986). Clinical trial in critically ill patients with heart failure: U. N. Khot *et al., N. Engl. J. Med.* **348**, 1756 (2003).

Dihydrate. [13755-38-9] Nipride; Nitropress. Ruby-red, practically odorless, transparent crystals. Sol in ~2.3 parts water, slightly in alcohol. Slowly dec in aq soln.

USE: Reagent for the detection of many organic compds, e.g., acetone, aldehydes, also of alkali sulfides, zinc, SO_2.

THERAP CAT: Antihypertensive.

8650. Sodium Oxalate. [62-76-0] Ethanedioic acid disodium salt. $C_2Na_2O_4$; mol wt 134.00. C 17.93%, Na 34.31%, O 47.76%. $Na_2C_2O_4$.

White, odorless, cryst powder. Sol in 27 parts water, 16 parts boiling water; insol in alcohol. The aq soln is practically neutral.

Caution: Potential symptoms of overexposure by ingestion are burning pain in throat, esophagus, stomach; vomiting; weak, irregular pulse; hypotension, cardiovascular collapse; headache, muscle cramps, tetany, convulsions, stupor, coma; kidney damage. See *Clinical Toxicology of Commercial Products*, R. E. Gosselin *et al.,* Eds. (Williams & Wilkins, Baltimore, 5th ed., 1984) Section III, pp 326-328.

USE: Finishing textiles, tanning and finishing leather; for standardizing potassium permanganate soln.

8651. Sodium Oxide. [1313-59-3] Sodium monoxide. Na_2O; mol wt 61.98. Na 74.18%, O 25.81%.

White, amorphous pieces or powder. d 2.27. Melts at a dull red heat and begins to dec >400° into sodium peroxide and metal. It is very reactive and combines violently with water, forming sodium hydroxide. *Handle with tongs and not with bare hands, and keep tightly closed.*

USE: As a dehydrating agent; in certain chemical reactions as a polymerizing or condensing agent.

8652. Sodium Perborate. [7632-04-4] Dexol. $BNaO_3$; mol wt 81.80. B 13.22%, Na 28.10%, O 58.68%. $NaBO_3$. Contains, when reasonably fresh, ~95% of the perborate corresp to 9.9% available oxygen. Prepn from sodium metaborate and hydrogen peroxide: Leblon, Lambert, **US 3109706** (1963 to Solvay & Cie).

Tetrahydrate. White, odorless, cryst powder; saline taste. Stable when kept cool and dry, but is dec with liberation of oxygen in warm or moist air. Dec >60°. Sol in ~40 parts water, the soln being alkaline and dec with the liberation of H_2O_2, and then of oxygen. In the presence of acids, H_2O_2 is formed. *Keep well closed and in a cool place.*

Caution: Prevent swallowing of soln.

USE: Bleaching straw and other fibers, ivory, sponges, bristles, waxes, textiles; in laundering, dentifrices, soaps.

THERAP CAT: Antiseptic (topical).

THERAP CAT (VET): Mouthwash.

8653. Sodium Perchlorate. [7601-89-0] Irenat. ClNaO$_4$; mol wt 122.44. Cl 28.96%, Na 18.78%, O 52.27%. NaClO$_4$.

Monohydrate. White, deliquesc crystals. Dec ~130°. d 2.02. Very sol in water. *Keep well closed.*

USE: In the explosives industry.

THERAP CAT: Thyroid inhibitor.

8654. Sodium Permanganate. [10101-50-5] MnNaO$_4$; mol wt 141.93. Mn 38.71%, Na 16.20%, O 45.09%. NaMnO$_4$.

Trihydrate. Reddish-black, very hygroscopic granules. Very sol in water; dec by alcohol.

8655. Sodium Peroxide. [1313-60-6] Sodium dioxide; sodium superoxide; Solozone. Na$_2$O$_2$; mol wt 77.98. Na 58.96%, O 41.03%. The product of commerce contains 90-95% Na$_2$O$_2$. Prepd by heating sodium metal to 300° in aluminum vessels with a current of air from which carbon dioxide has been removed. Prepn of the octahydrate: Penneman, *Inorg. Synth.* **3,** 1 (1950).

Yellowish-white, granular powder. Absorbs water and CO$_2$ from the air. Freely sol in water, forming sodium hydroxide and hydrogen peroxide, the latter quickly dec into oxygen and water. With dil acids H$_2$O$_2$ is formed which remains stable. In contact with organic matter or readily oxidizable substances ignition and explosion may take place. *Keep tightly closed and protected from contact with organic or oxidizable substances.*

Caution: Irritant and corrosive. *See* Sodium Hydroxide.

USE: Bleaching animal and vegetable fibers, feathers, bones, ivory, wood, wax, sponges, coral; rendering air charged with CO$_2$ respirable as in torpedo boats, submarines, diving bells, etc.; purifying air in sick rooms; dyeing and printing textiles; chemical analysis. General oxidizing agent.

8656. Sodium Persulfate. [7775-27-1] Sodium peroxydisulfate. Na$_2$O$_8$S$_2$; mol wt 238.10. Na 19.31%, O 53.76%, S 26.93%. Na$_2$S$_2$O$_8$. Toxicity data: DaVal, *Arch. Ital. Sci. Farmacol.* **2,** 445 (1933).

White, cryst powder. Gradually dec; decompn is promoted by moisture and higher temp. Initial soly in water at 20°: 549 g/l; dec by alcohol and silver ions. MLD in rabbits (mg/kg): 178 i.v. (DaVal).

Caution: Highly irritating to skin, mucous membranes.

USE: Bleaching and oxidizing agent; promoter for emulsion polymerization reactions.

8657. Sodium Pertechnetate ^{99m}Tc. [23288-60-0] Pertscan; Ultra-Technekow. NaO$_4$^{99m}Tc. Na^{99m}TcO$_4$. Prepn: Keller, Kanellakopulos, *Radiochim. Acta* **1,** No. 2, 107 (1963), *C.A.* **59,** 1256a (1963); Kanellakopulos, **AEC Accession** No. **31424,** Rept. No. **KFK-197,** 73 pp (1964), *C.A.* **62,** 7350d (1965). Clinical application for labelling red blood cells: D. Ducassou *et al., Br. J. Radiol.* **49,** 344 (1976). Diagnostic use in Meckel's diverticulum: D. R. Cooney *et al., J. Pediatr. Surg.* **17,** 611 (1982); in thyroid neoplasm: M. Vorne, K. Jarve, *Eur. J. Nucl. Med.* **13,** 362 (1987). Review of diagnostic use in brain scanning: J. G. McAfee *et al., J. Nucl. Med.* **5,** 811-827 (1964); in thyroid function: M. S. Sucupira *et al., Int. J. Nucl. Med. Biol.* **10,** 29-33 (1983).

THERAP CAT: Diagnostic aid (radioactive imaging agent).

8658. Sodium Phenolsulfonate. [1300-51-2] Hydroxybenzenesulfonic acid sodium salt; sodium sulfocarbolate. C$_6$H$_5$NaO$_4$S; mol wt 196.16. C 36.74%, H 2.57%, Na 11.72%, O 32.63%, S 16.35%. HOC$_6$H$_4$SO$_3$Na.

Dihydrate. White, odorless crystals; slightly bitter taste; somewhat efflorescent in dry air. One gram dissolves in 4.2 ml water, 0.8 ml boiling water, 140 ml alcohol, 13.5 ml boiling alcohol, 5 ml glycerol. The aq soln is neutral.

THERAP CAT: Intestinal antiseptic.

THERAP CAT (VET): Has been used as an intestinal antiseptic, in dusting powders for ulcers, slowly granulating wounds and in dilute solution in the eye.

8659. Sodium Phosphate, Dibasic. [7558-79-4] Dibasic sodium phosphate; disodium hydrogen phosphate; disodium orthophosphate; disodium phosphate; DSP; phosphate of soda; secondary sodium phosphate. HNa$_2$O$_4$P; mol wt 141.96. H 0.71%, Na 32.39%, O 45.08%, P 21.82%. Na$_2$HPO$_4$. Industrial production: *Faith, Keyes & Clark's Industrial Chemicals* (John Wiley, New York, 4th ed., 1975) pp 746-754. Toxicity of heptahydrate: H. F. Smyth *et al., Am. Ind. Hyg. Assoc. J.* **30,** 470 (1969).

Anhydr, *exsiccated sodium phosphate.* Hygroscopic powder. On exposure to air will absorb from 2 to 7 mols H$_2$O, depending on the humidity and temp. Sol in ~8 parts water, much more sol in hot water. Soly per 100 gal water increases from ~14 lbs at slightly >0° to over 900 lbs at 95°. Insol in alc. pH of 1% aq soln at 25°: 9.1. *Keep well closed.*

Dihydrate. Sorensen's phosphate; Sorensen's sodium phosphate.

Heptahydrate. Crystals or granular powder. Stable in the air. d ~1.7. Sol in 4 parts water, more sol in boiling water; practically insol in alcohol. The aq soln is alkaline, pH ~9.5. LD$_{50}$ orally in rats: 12.93 g/kg (Smyth).

Dodecahydrate. Translucent crystals or granules; readily loses 5 mols of water on exposure to air at ordinary temp. mp 34-35° (when it contains the full 12 mols of H$_2$O). d ~1.5. Sol in 3 parts water; practically insol in alcohol. Aq soln is alkaline, pH ~9.5. *Keep well closed and in a cool place. Incompat:* Alkaloids, antipyrine, chloral hydrate, lead acetate, pyrogallol, resorcinol.

Caution: Anhydr form may cause mild irritation to skin, mucous membranes; intern. causes purging.

USE: As sequestrant, emulsifier and buffer in foods. As mordant in dyeing; for weighting silk; in tanning; in manuf of enamels, ceramics, detergents, boiler compds; as fireproofing agent; in soldering and brazing instead of borax; as reagent and buffer in analytical chemistry.

THERAP CAT: Cathartic.

THERAP CAT (VET): Laxative.

8660. Sodium Phosphate, Monobasic. [7558-80-7] Sodium biphosphate; sodium dihydrogen phosphate; acid sodium phosphate; monosodium orthophosphate; primary sodium phosphate. H$_2$NaO$_4$P; mol wt 119.98. H 1.68%, Na 19.16%, O 53.34%, P 25.82%. NaH$_2$PO$_4$. It is about 99% pure.

Monohydrate. White, odorless, slightly deliquesc crystals or granules. At 100° loses all its water; when ignited it converts into metaphosphate. Freely sol in water; practically insol in alcohol. The aq soln is acid. pH of 0.1 molar aq soln at 25°: 4.5.

Dihydrate. Orthorhombic bisphenoidal colorless crystals, mp 60°. d 1.915. At room temp crystallizes with 2H$_2$O. Directions for max yield: Beans, Kiehl, *J. Am. Chem. Soc.* **49,** 1878 (1927).

USE: In baking powders; in boiler water treatment; as dry acidulant and sequestrant for foods: Tidridge, Pals, **US 3030213** (1962 to FMC).

THERAP CAT: Urinary acidifier.

THERAP CAT (VET): Urinary acidifier.

8661. Sodium Phosphate, Radioactive. [8027-28-9] Sodium phosphate ^{32}P; radioactive sodium phosphate; sodium radiophosphate (^{32}P); Phosphotope.

Aq soln of mixed radioactive phosphates with a pH range of 5.0-6.0. Contains radioactive monobasic sodium phosphate (NaH$_2$^{32}PO$_4$) and radioactive dibasic sodium phosphate (Na$_2$H^{32}PO$_4$). ^{32}P is a pure beta emitter with a half-life of 14.3 days.

THERAP CAT: Antineoplastic; antipolycythemic; diagnostic aid (neoplasm).

8662. Sodium Phosphate, Tribasic. [7601-54-9] Trisodium orthophosphate; trisodium phosphate; TSP; Oakite. Na$_3$O$_4$P; mol wt 163.94. Na 42.07%, O 39.04%, P 18.89%. Na$_3$PO$_4$. Crystallizes with 8 and 12 mols of H$_2$O.

Dodecahydrate. Colorless or white crystals. When rapidly heated melts at ~75°. Does not lose the last mol of water even on moderate ignition. d 1.6. Sol in 3.5 parts water, 1 part boiling water; insol in alcohol. The aq soln is strongly alkaline. pH of 0.1% soln: 11.5; of 0.5% soln: 11.7; of 1.0% soln: 11.9. Technical crystals are sometimes made with excess alkali to prevent caking and give more alkaline solutions. LD$_{50}$ orally in rats: 7.40 g/kg, H. F. Smyth *et al., Am. Ind. Hyg. Assoc. J.* **30,** 470 (1969).

Consult the Name Index before using this section.

USE: In photographic developers; clarifying sugar; removing boiler scale, softening water; manuf paper; laundering; tanning leather; in detergent mixture.

8663. Sodium Phosphite. [13708-85-5] HNa_2O_3P; mol wt 125.96. H 0.80%, Na 36.50%, O 38.11%, P 24.59%. Na_2HPO_3.

Pentahydrate. White, hygroscopic cryst powder. Heat of formation (25°): −684.2 kcal/mole. Freely sol in water. *Keep well closed.*

8664. Sodium Phosphomolybdate. [1313-30-0] Sodium molybdophosphate. $Mo_{12}Na_3O_{40}P$; mol wt 1891.20. Mo 60.88%, Na 3.65%, O 33.84%, P 1.64%. $Na_3PO_4 \cdot 12MoO_3$.

White crystals. Freely sol in water.

USE: As reagent in chemical analysis.

8665. Sodium Phosphotungstate. [51312-42-6] Sodium tungstophosphate. Approx $2Na_2O \cdot P_2O_5 \cdot 12WO_3 \cdot 18H_2O$.

White, granular powder. Sol in water.

USE: As reagent for alkaloids, uric acid, potassium.

8666. Sodium Polyanetholesulfonate. [52993-95-0] Polyanetholesulfonic acid sodium salt; anetholesulfonic acid sodium salt polymer. A polymer of anetholesulfonic acid. Originally developed as an anticoagulant, it was soon found that it possesses anti-complement action and lowers the bactericidal action of blood. *Ref:* Demole, Reinert, *Arch. Exp. Pathol. Pharmakol.* **158**, 211 (1930); Friedmann, *Klin. Wochenschr.* **14**, 215 (1935); Stuart, *J. Clin. Pathol.* **1**, 311 (1948).

Light brown powder. Insol in alcohol. Swells in water and slowly goes in soln with neutral reaction. Aq solns are stable to heat, dil alkalies and dil acids.

USE: To inhibit blood coagulation *in vitro,* and as diagnostic reagent to encourage the growth of pathogens in blood. To stabilize colloidal solns such as milk and gelatin.

8667. Sodium Polymetaphosphate. [50813-16-6] Graham's salt; "sodium hexametaphosphate"; glassy sodium metaphosphate; Hy-Phos. $(NaPO_3)_x$. A mixture of polymeric metaphosphates; not a hexamer. Prepd by rapidly chilling molten sodium metaphosphate: Bell, *Inorg. Synth.* **3**, 103 (1950). *Reviews: see* Sodium Metaphosphate.

Clear, hygroscopic glass. mp 628°. Sol in water, but dissolves slowly. Depolymerizes in aqueous soln to form sodium trimetaphosphate and sodium orthophosphates.

Sodium hexametaphosphate detergents. Calgon; Giltex; Quadrafos; Hagan phosphate; Micromet. Mixtures contg Graham's salt as the principal agent. Supplied in the form of a powder, flakes, and as small, broken, glass-like particles. Sol in water (pH adjusted to 8-8.6). Insol in organic solvents. Possess dispersing and deflocculating properties, coagulate albumins, and inhibit the crystn of slightly sol compds such as calcium carbonate and calcium sulfate.

USE: Water softeners and detergents. For leather tanning, dyeing, laundry work, textile processing; for the "threshold treatment" of softening industrial water supplies.

8668. Sodium Polystyrene Sulfonate. [9003-59-2] Resonium A; Kayexalate. A cation exchange resin charged with sodium.

Marketed as a powder, insol in water; also as an emulsion with methyl cellulose.

THERAP CAT: Ion-exchange resin (potassium).

8669. Sodium Propionate. [137-40-6] Propionic acid sodium salt; Impedex. $C_3H_5NaO_2$; mol wt 96.06. C 37.51%, H 5.25%, Na 23.93%, O 33.31%. CH_3CH_2COONa.

Transparent crystals, granules. Deliquescent in moist air. Neutral or slightly alkaline reaction to litmus. One gram dissolves in ~1 ml water, in ~0.65 ml boiling water, in ~24 ml alcohol at 25°. Most active at acid pH: Wolford, Andersen, *Food Ind.* **17**, 622 (1945); Olsen, Macy, *J. Dairy Sci.* **29**, 173 (1946).

USE: Fungicide, mold preventative.

THERAP CAT: Antifungal (topical).

THERAP CAT (VET): In ketosis of ruminants (glucose precursor). Antifungal agent. Has been used in dermatoses, wound infections, conjunctivitis.

8670. Sodium Rhodizonate. [523-21-7] 5,6-Dihydroxy-5-cyclohexene-1,2,3,4-tetrone disodium salt; [(3,4,5,6-tetraoxo-1-cyclohexen-1,2-ylene)dioxy]disodium. $C_6Na_2O_6$; mol wt 214.04. C 33.67%, Na 21.48%, O 44.85%.

Violet crystals. Sol in water with an orange-yellow color; slightly sol in soda soln; insol in alc. Solns are unstable even in the refrigerator, and must be prepd fresh every other day.

USE: As a reagent for barium and strontium.

8671. Sodium Selenate. [13410-01-0] Na_2O_4Se; mol wt 188.94. Na 24.34%, O 33.87%, Se 41.79%. Na_2SeO_4. Acute toxicity study: C. Nofre *et al., C.R. Hebd. Seances Acad. Sci.* **257**, 791 (1963). Review: *NTP Technical Report on Toxicity Studies of Sodium Selenate and Sodium Selenite* (NIH 94-3387, 1994) 121 pp.

Decahydrate. [10102-23-5] White crystals; very sol in water. LD_{50} i.p. in mice: 18.45 mg/kg (Nofre).

USE: Insecticide in some horticultural applications.

THERAP CAT (VET): Dietary growth promoter for poultry and livestock.

8672. Sodium Selenide. [1313-85-5] Na_2Se; mol wt 124.94. Na 36.80%, Se 63.20%. Prepd by adding selenium to a soln of sodium in liquid ammonia: Hugot, *Compt. Rend.* **129**, 299 (1899); *Ann. Chim. Phys.* [7] **21**, 34 (1900); Feher in *Handbook of Preparative Inorganic Chemistry* vol. **1**, G. Brauer, Ed. (Academic Press, New York, 2nd ed., 1963) p 421.

Amorphous crystals. d^{10} 2.625. mp >875°. Turns red on exposure to air and deliquesces. Dec in water. Insol in ammonia.

Hemienneahydrate. Fine needles. Turns red on exposure to air and deliquesces.

Decahydrate. Needles. Turns red and then brown on exposure to air.

Hexadecahydrate. Prisms. mp 40°. Dec in air to sodium carbonate, selenium and a small amount of sodium selenide.

8673. Sodium Selenite. [10102-18-8] Selenious acid disodium salt; Selenase. Na_2O_3Se; mol wt 172.94. Na 26.59%, O 27.75%, Se 45.66%. Na_2SeO_3. Prepd by evaporating an aqueous solution of sodium hydroxide and selenious acid between 60° and 100°: Krak, *J. Am. Ceram. Soc.* **12**, 530 (1929); by heating a mixture of sodium chloride and selenium oxide: Cameron, Macallan, *Proc. Roy. Soc.* **46**, 13 (1890). Metabolism: M. Sandholm, *Acta Pharmacol. Toxicol.* **33**, 6 (1973); H. W. Symonds *et al., Br. J. Nutr.* **45**, 117 (1981). Mutagenicity study: M. Nodo *et al., Mutat. Res.* **66**, 175 (1979). Toxicity study: Cummins, Kimura, *Toxicol. Appl. Pharmacol.* **20**, 89 (1971). Clinical effect of selenium supplementation on immune cell function: M. Roy *et al., Biol. Trace Elem. Res.* **46**, 115 (1994); L. Kiremidjian-Schumacher *et al., ibid.* 183. Clinical evaluation as immunostimulant in head and neck cancer: *eidem, ibid.* **73**, 97 (2000); in treatment of radiation-associated secondary lymphedema: O. Micke *et al., Int. J. Radiat. Oncol. Biol. Phys.* **56**, 40 (2003).

Tetragonal prisms. Stable in air. Freely sol in water. Insol in alcohol. LD_{50} orally in rats: 7 mg/kg (Cummins, Kimura).

USE: Removing green color from glass during its manuf; alkaloidal reagent.

THERAP CAT: Selenium supplement.

THERAP CAT (VET): Selenium supplement for livestock.

8674. Sodium Sesquicarbonate. [533-96-0] Urao; trona. $C_2HNa_3O_6$; mol wt 190.00. C 12.64%, H 0.53%, Na 36.30%, O

50.52%. $Na_2CO_3.NaHCO_3$. Found in nature as the dihydrate, e.g., Owens Lake, Searles Lake (U.S.A.); Lake Magadi (Kenya). Produced on a large scale from sodium carbonate and a slight excess of sodium bicarbonate: Schenk in *Winnacker-Weingaertner, Chemische Technologie* vol. **I** (München, 1950) p 427.

Dihydrate. Monoclinic needles, d 2.112. Crystals are stable in air. Soly in water (g/100 ml) at 0°: 13; at 100°: 42. Aq solns are mildly alkaline. pH of 0.1*M* soln = 10.1.

Caution: Irritating to skin, mucous membranes.

USE: Chiefly in laundering in conjunction with soap.

8675. Sodium Silicate. [1344-09-8] Water glass; soluble glass. Manuf: *Faith, Keyes & Clark's Industrial Chemicals*, F. A. Lowenheim, M. K. Moran, Eds. (Wiley-Interscience, New York, 4th ed., 1975) pp 755-761.

The compositions of the commonly available sodium silicates in dry form are: Na_2SiO_3, $Na_6Si_2O_7$, and $Na_2Si_3O_7$, with variable amounts of water, the first-named containing approx $5H_2O$. They are in the form of colorless to white or grayish-white, crystal-like pieces or lumps. These silicates are very slightly sol or almost insol in cold water. They are best brought into soln by heating with water under pressure. They are less readily sol in large amounts of water than in small amounts of water, and the anhydr dissolve with more difficulty than the hydrated silicates; also, the silicates containing more sodium dissolve more readily. The aq solns are strongly alkaline. The dry sodium silicates are used relatively little. *See also* Sodium Metasilicate.

Caution: Irritating and caustic to skin, mucous membranes. If swallowed causes vomiting and diarrhea.

USE: Lining Bessemer converters, acid concentrators. Manuf grindstones, abrasive wheels (as binder only).

8676. Sodium Silicate Solution. [1344-09-8] Sodium silicate solns of varying composition with respect to the ratio between sodium and silica, as well as of various densities, are available. One of the most commonly used sodium silicate solns, also known as "egg preserver", contains ~40% $Na_2Si_3O_7$. Solns of sodium silicate are strongly alkaline and are readily dec by acids with separation of silicic acid. The greater the ratio of Na_2O to SiO_2 (the greater the alkalinity) the more tacky is the soln.

USE: For preserving eggs; fireproofing fabrics; as a detergent in soaps; as adhesive; waterproofing walls; in cements; in cold-water paints; manuf of abrasive wheels; weighting silk, etc.

8677. Sodium Stannate(IV). [12058-66-1] Sodium tin oxide. Na_2O_3Sn; mol wt 212.69. Na 21.62%, O 22.57%, Sn 55.81%. Na_2SnO_3.

Trihydrate. White or colorless crystals; gradually dec in the air; dec by weak acids. Sol in ~1.7 parts water; insol in alcohol. The aq soln is alkaline. *Keep well closed.*

USE: As mordant in dyeing and printing calico; for fireproofing of curtains, etc.

8678. Sodium Stearate. [822-16-2] Stearic acid sodium salt. Approx $C_{18}H_{35}NaO_2$. Usually contains sodium palmitate.

White powder; soapy feel; slight, tallow-like odor. Slowly soluble in cold water or cold alcohol; freely sol in the hot solvents. The aq soln is strongly alkaline, due to hydrolysis; the alcohol soln is practically neutral.

USE: Pharmaceutic aid (emulsifying and stiffening agent). In glycerol suppositories; also in toothpaste; as waterproofing agent.

8679. Sodium Succinate. [150-90-3] Succinic acid sodium salt; disodium succinate. $C_4H_4Na_2O_4$; mol wt 162.05. C 29.65%, H 2.49%, Na 28.37%, O 39.49%. Crystal structure of hexahydrate: I. Fonseca *et al., Acta Crystallogr.* **C42**, 1123 (1986). Acute toxicity and clinical experience: M. Zuckerbrod, I. Graef, *Ann. Intern. Med.* **32**, 905 (1950).

LD_{50} i.v. in mice: 4.5 g/kg (Zuckerbrod, Graef).

Hexahydrate. [6106-21-4] $C_4H_4Na_2O_4.6H_2O$; mol wt 270.14. Granules or crystalline powder. Loses all its water at 120°. Sol in ~5 parts water. Insol in alcohol. The aq soln is neutral or slightly alkaline.

USE: Acidulant and flavoring agent in foods. As protective coating for fruits and vegetables.

8680. Sodium Sulfate. [7757-82-6] Na_2O_4S; mol wt 142.04. Na 32.37%, O 45.06%, S 22.57%. Na_2SO_4. Occurs in nature as the minerals *mirabilite, thenardite*. Industrial production: *Faith, Keyes & Clark's Industrial Chemicals*, F. A. Lowenheim, M. K. Moran, Eds. (Wiley-Interscience, New York, 4th ed., 1975) p 762-768.

Anhydrous form, *salt cake* (technical grade). Powder or orthorhombic bipyramidal crystals, mp ~800°. d 2.7. Sol in ~3.6 parts water. Max soly at 33°: 1 in 2. Above this temp the soly gradually decreases and at 100° requires 2.4 parts water. Insol in alcohol.

Decahydrate. Glauber's salt. $Na_2O_4S.10H_2O$. Odorless, efflorescent crystals or granules, mp 32.4°. d 1.46. Loses all its water at 100°. Sol in 1.5 parts water at 25°, in 3.3 parts water at 15°. Soly in water decreased by NaCl. Sol in glycerol; insol in alcohol. The aq soln is neutral. pH 6-7.5. *Keep well closed in a cool place.*

USE: For standardizing dyes; in freezing mixtures; in dyeing and printing textiles. The *anhydrous* form for drying organic liquids; in Kjeldahl nitrogen determination; in manuf of glass, ultramarine, paper pulp.

THERAP CAT: Cathartic.

THERAP CAT (VET): Purgative.

8681. Sodium Sulfide. [1313-82-2] Sodium monosulfide; sodium sulfuret. Na_2S; mol wt 78.04. Na 58.92%, S 41.09%. Best prepd from the elements in liq ammonia, also obtained by dehydration of the nonahydrate: Courtois, *Compt. Rend.* **207**, 1220 (1938); Klemm *et al., Z. Anorg. Allg. Chem.* **241**, 281 (1939); Feher in *Handbook of Preparative Inorganic Chemistry* vol **1**, G. Brauer, Ed. (Academic Press, New York, 2nd ed., 1963) pp 358-360. Review: C. Drum in *Kirk-Othmer Encyclopedia of Chemical Technology* vol. **21** (Wiley-Interscience, New York, 3rd ed., 1983) pp 256-262.

Cubic crystals or granules. Extremely hygroscopic. Discolors upon exposure to air. d_4^{14} 1.856. mp 1180° *(in vacuo)*; also reported as mp 920°. Soly in water (g/100 g H_2O): 8.1 (−9.0°); 12.4 (0°); 18.6 (20°); 29.0 (40°); 35.7 (48°); 39.0 (50°). Slightly sol in alcohol. Insol in ether. Aq solns are strongly alkaline.

Pentahydrate. Flat, shiny, four-sided, prismatic crystals. Loses 3 mols water at 100°. mp 120° (with loss of all water of crystn). Freely sol in water. Also sol in alcohol. Aq solns are strongly alkaline. Insol in ether. Dec by acids with evolution of H_2S.

Nonahydrate. Tetragonal, deliquescent crystals. Odor of hydrogen sulfide. Discolors upon exposure to light and air (first yellow, then brownish-black). d_4^{16} 1.427. mp ~50°. One gram dissolves in 0.5 ml water, also reported as 18 g dissolve in 100 ml water at 25°. Slightly sol in alcohol, insol in ether. Dec by acids, even by carbonic acid. Aqueous solns are very alkaline and upon standing in contact with air are slowly converted according to the equation: $2Na_2S + 2O_2 + H_2O \rightarrow Na_2S_2O_3 + 2NaOH$. Exposure of the crystals to air produces hydrogen sulfide according to the equation $Na_2S + H_2O + CO_2 \rightarrow Na_2CO_3 + H_2S$. *Keep well closed and in a cool place. Do not handle with bare hands.*

USE: In dehairing hides and wool pulling; desulfurizing viscose rayon; in the manuf of rubber, sulfur dyes; in ore flotation, metal refining, engraving, cotton printing, as chemical intermediate, as laboratory reagent; in paper-pulping process.

8682. Sodium Sulfite. [7757-83-7] Na_2O_3S; mol wt 126.04. Na 36.48%, O 38.08%, S 25.44%. Na_2SO_3.

Small crystals or powder. It is fairly stable and does not oxidize as readily as the hydrated sulfite. Sol in 3.2 parts water; sol in glycerol; almost insol in alcohol. pH about 9. *Keep well closed.* LD_{50} i.v. in mice: 175 mg/kg, Hoppe, Goble, *J. Pharmacol. Exp. Ther.* **101**, 101 (1951).

Heptahydrate. Efflorescent crystals. Unstable, oxidizing in the air to sulfate. Sol in 1.6 parts water, about 30 parts glycerol; sparingly sol in alc. The aq soln is alkaline and dissolves sulfur. pH ~9. *Keep well closed in a cool place. Note:* The commercial heptahydrate (about 90% pure, the remainder consisting chiefly of the sulfate) has been largely replaced by the commercial anhydr salt (about 96-99% pure) which is more stable.

USE: Chiefly in photographic developers and instead of "hypo" for fixing prints; bleaching wool, straw, silk; generating SO_2; as reducer in manuf dyes; silvering glass; removing traces of Cl in bleached textiles and paper; preserving meat, egg yolks, etc.

8683. Sodium β-Sulfopropionitrile. [513-15-5] 2-Cyanoethanesulfonic acid sodium salt; sodium 2-cyanoethanesulfonate.

$C_3H_4NNaO_3S$; mol wt 157.12. C 22.93%, H 2.57%, N 8.91%, Na 14.63%, O 30.55%, S 20.41%. $NaO_3SCH_2CH_2CN$.

Crystals, mp 243-244°. Sol in water, hot methanol, glacial acetic acid. Insol in most other organic solvents.

USE: In organic synthesis for introducing the sulfonic acid group into a variety of molecules, especially surface active agents.

8684. Sodium Tartrate. [868-18-8] $C_4H_4Na_2O_6$; mol wt 194.05. C 24.76%, H 2.08%, Na 23.69%, O 49.47%. $Na_2C_4H_4O_6$.

Dihydrate. White crystals or granules. Loses its water at about 120°. d 1.82. Sol in about 3 parts cold water, 1.5 parts boiling water; insol in alcohol. The aq soln is slightly alkaline to litmus, pH 7 to 9.

USE: Dihydrate as standard for standardizing Karl Fischer reagent (determination of water).

THERAP CAT: Cathartic.

8685. Sodium Tellurate(IV). [10102-20-2] Sodium tellurite. Na_2O_3Te; mol wt 221.58. Na 20.75%, O 21.66%, Te 57.59%. Na_2TeO_3. Review of toxicology: B. Venugopal, T. P. Luckey, *Environ. Qual. Safety* Suppl. 1, 4-73 (1975).

White powder. Soluble in water. LD_{50} in rats (mg/kg): 56.78 i.p., 55.85 i.v.; in rabbits (mg/kg): 104 orally (Venugopal, Luckey).

8686. Sodium Tellurate(VI). [10101-83-4] Na_2O_4Te; mol wt 237.58. Na 19.35%, O 26.94%, Te 53.71%. Na_2TeO_4. Toxicity data: Franke, *J. Pharmacol. Exp. Ther.* **58,** 454 (1936).

White powder. Sol in 130 parts cold water, 50 parts boiling water. MLD in rats (mg/kg): 37.2-55.8 i.p. (Franke).

8687. Sodium Tetrachloroaluminate. [7784-16-9] Aluminum sodium chloride; sodium chloroaluminate. $AlCl_4Na$; mol wt 191.78. Al 14.07%, Cl 73.95%, Na 11.99%. $AlCl_3.NaCl$. Prepn: *Gmelins, Aluminum* (8th ed.) **35B,** p 376 (1934); Good, Batha, US 2867499 (1959 to Olin Mathieson).

Yellowish powder. Sol in water.

USE: Catalyst for organic reactions.

8688. Sodium Tetrachloroaurate(III). [15189-51-2] Gold sodium chloride; sodium chloroaurate(III). $AuCl_4Na$; mol wt 361.77. Au 54.45%, Cl 39.20%, Na 6.35%. Prepd by evapn of a soln of $HAuCl_4$ and NaCl.

Dihydrate. Orange-yellow, rhombic, bipyramidal crystals. Stable to 100°. Dec before all H_2O of hydration lost. Freely sol in water; sol in alcohol, ether.

USE: For paper-toning in photography, in electroplating baths.

8689. Sodium Tetradecyl Sulfate. [139-88-8] 7-Ethyl-2-methyl-4-undecanol hydrogen sulfate sodium salt; sodium 2-methyl-7-ethyl-4-hendecanol sulfate sodium salt; sodium 7-ethyl-2-methylundecyl-4-sulfate; Sotradecol; Tergitol 4; Trombavar; Trombovar. $C_{14}H_{29}NaSO_4$; mol wt 316.43. C 53.14%, H 9.24%, Na 7.27%, S 10.13%, O 20.22%.

White, waxy solid. Sol in water, alcohol, ether. The pH of a 5% soln is from 6.5 to 9.0. Surface tension (dynes/cm) of aq soln at 25°: 56.5 dynes/cm (0.05% w/w); 52 (0.10%); 47 (0.20%); 40 (0.50%); 35 (1.0%). LD_{50} orally in rats: 4.95 g/kg, H. F. Smyth, C. P. Carpenter, *J. Ind. Hyg. Toxicol.* **30,** 63 (1948).

USE: Wetting agent.

THERAP CAT: Sclerosing agent.

8690. Sodium Tetraphenylborate. [143-66-8] Tetraphenylboron sodium; Kalignost. $C_{24}H_{20}BNa$; mol wt 342.22. C 84.23%, H 5.89%, B 3.16%, Na 6.72%. $Na[B(C_6H_5)_4]$. Prepn: Wittig, Raff, *Ann.* **573,** 195 (1950); US 2853525 (1958); Heyl, **GB** 705719 (1954); Kozlova, Pal'm, *Zh. Obshch. Khim.* **31,** 2922 (1961); Holtzapfel, Richter, *ibid.* **32,** 1358 (1962).

Snow-white crystals from chloroform. Freely sol in water, acetone. Less sol in ether, chloroform. Practically insol in petr ether.

Aq solns should be adjusted to a pH of about 5 and can be stored at room temp or lower. Such solns have been stored at 45° for 5 days without deterioration. The solv in polar solvents increases as the temp decreases.

USE: As reagent for determination of potassium, ammonium, rubidium and cesium ions: Barnard, Buechl, *Chemist-Analyst* **48,** 44, 49 (1959); Montequi, Serrano, *An. R. Acad. Farm.* **26,** 107 (1960).

8691. Sodium Thiocarbonate. [534-18-9] Sodium sulfocarbonate. CNa_2S_3; mol wt 154.19. C 7.79%, Na 29.82%, S 62.39%. Na_2CS_3.

USE: Usually supplied as a 40°Bé soln for destroying insects injurious to plants, especially vines.

8692. Sodium Thioglycolate. [367-51-1] Mercaptoacetic acid sodium salt; sodium mercaptoacetate. $C_2H_3NaO_2S$; mol wt 114.10. C 21.05%, H 2.65%, Na 20.15%, O 28.04%, S 28.10%. $HSCH_2COONa$.

Hygroscopic crystals. Slight characteristic odor. Discolors on exposure to air or iron. Freely sol in water; slightly sol in alc. LD_{50} i.p. in rats: 148 mg/kg, Freeman, Rosenthal, *Fed. Proc.* **11,** 347 (1952).

USE: In cold-waving of hair; as depilatory; in bacteriology for the prepn of thioglycolate media; as analytical reagent, *see* Thioglycolic Acid.

8693. Sodium Thiophosphate. [10101-88-9] Sodium phosphorothioate; sodium monothiophosphate. Na_3O_3PS; mol wt 180.01. Na 38.31%, O 26.66%, P 17.21%, S 17.81%. Na_3PO_3S. Conveniently prepd from $NaPO_3 + Na_2S$: Zintl, Bertram, *Z. Anorg. Allg. Chem.* **245,** 16 (1940); from $PSCl_3 + NaOH$: Tridot, Tudo, *Bull. Soc. Chim. Fr.* **1960,** 1231. Several alternate routes, e.g. from P_2S_5 and NaOH, *see* Klement in *Handbook of Preparative Inorganic Chemistry* vol. 1, G. Brauer, Ed. (Academic Press, New York, 2nd ed., 1963) pp 569-570.

Dodecahydrate. Thin, six-sided leaflets from water. Effloresces in dry air. mp 60°. Freely sol in warm water. Aq solns are strongly alkaline.

8694. Sodium Thiosulfate. [7772-98-7] Sodium hyposulfite; "hypo"; antichlor; Sodothiol; Sulfothiorine; Ametox. $Na_2O_3S_2$; mol wt 158.11. Na 29.08%, O 30.36%, S 40.56%. $Na_2S_2O_3$. Review of mfg processes: *Faith, Keyes & Clark's Industrial Chemicals,* F. A. Lowenheim, M. K. Moran, Eds. (Wiley-Interscience, New York, 4th ed., 1975) pp 769-773. Crystal structure of the pentahydrate: A. A. Uraz, N. Armagan, *Acta Crystallogr.* **B33,** 1396 (1977). Toxicity of the pentahydrate: C. Voegtlin *et al., J. Pharmacol. Exp. Ther.* **25,** 297 (1925).

Powder. Sol in water; practically insol in alcohol.

Pentahydrate. Odorless crystals or granules, mp 48° when rapidly heated. Effloresces in warm dry air; slightly deliquesces in moist air. d 1.69. Loses all its water at 100°; dec at higher temp. Sol in water; insol in alcohol. Slowly dec in aq soln at ordinary temp, more rapidly when heated. The aq soln is practically neutral, pH 6.5-8.0. It dissolves silver halides and many other salts of silver. *Incompat:* Iodine, acids; lead, mercury, and silver salts. LD i.v. in rats: >2.5 g/kg (Voegtlin).

USE: To remove chlorine from solns according to the eq: $Na_2S_2O_3 + 4Cl_2 + 5H_2O \rightarrow 2NaHSO_4 + 8HCl$ and $Na_2S_2O_3 + 2HCl \rightarrow 2NaCl + H_2O + S + SO_2$. As "antichlor" in bleaching of paper pulp; as fixer in photography; for extraction of silver from ores; as mordant in dyeing and printing textiles; reducer in chrome dyeing; manuf leather; bleaching bone, straw, ivory; also as reagent in analytical chemistry.

THERAP CAT: Antidote (cyanide).

THERAP CAT (VET): Antidote (cyanide). Has been used as a "general detoxifier", in bloat, and externally in ringworm, mange.

8695. Sodium Triacetoxyborohydride. [56553-60-7] Sodium (*T*-4)-tris(acetato-κO)hydroborate(1−). $C_6H_{10}BNaO_6$; mol wt 211.94. C 34.00%, H 4.76%, B 5.10%, Na 10.85%, O 45.29%. Mild borohydride reagent. Prepn and use in reduction of aldehydes: G. W. Gribble, D. C. Ferguson, *J. Chem. Soc. Chem. Commun.* **1975,** 535. Reductive amination of aldehydes and ketones: A. F. Abdel-Magid *et al., J. Org. Chem.* **61,** 3849 (1996); L.-X. Yang, K. G. Hofer, *Tetrahedron Lett.* **37,** 6081 (1996); of amino acid esters: J.

M. Ramanjulu, M. M. Joullié, *Synth. Commun.* **26**, 1379 (1996). Reductive alkylation of amines: Y. Han, M. Chorev, *J. Org. Chem.* **64**, 1972 (1999). Reduction of conjugated aldehydes: J. Singh *et al., Synth. Commun.* **30**, 1515 (2000). Stereoselective reduction of ketones: Y.-T. Liu *et al., Tetrahedron Lett.* **45**, 6097 (2004).

USE: Selective reducing agent in organic synthesis.

8696. Sodium Trimetaphosphate. [7785-84-4] Metaphosphoric acid trisodium salt. $Na_3O_9P_3$; mol wt 305.89. Na 22.55%, O 47.07%, P 30.38%. $(NaPO_3)_3$. Prepd by tempering sodium hexametaphosphate at about 500° for 8-12 hrs; by heating Na_2HPO_4 and NH_4NO_3 to 320° or by heating NaH_2PO_4 at 530°: Fleitmann, Henneberg, *Ann.* **65**, 304 (1848); v. Knoore, *Z. Anorg. Allg. Chem.* **24**, 381 (1900); Karbe, Jander, *Kolloid-Beih.* **54**, 35 (1942); Bell, *Inorg. Synth.* **3**, 103 (1950); Lee, Bond, *J. Appl. Chem.* **18**, 345 (1968). Crystal structure of hexahydrate: Caglioti *et al., Atti Acad. Italia Rend.* **3** [7], 761 (1942), *C.A.* **40**, 6927[b] (1946); of anhydrate: Ondik, *Acta Crystallogr.* **18**, 226 (1965). Use in detergent processing: Shen, *J. Am. Oil Chem. Soc.* **45**, 510 (1968). Toxicity study: Behrens, Seelkopf, *Arch. Exp. Pathol. Pharmakol.* **169**, 238 (1932). *Reviews: see* Sodium Metaphosphate.

Hexahydrate. Efflorescent, triclinic-rhombohedral prisms. d 1.786. mp 53°. Loses water on storage at 20°, becomes definitely anhyd at 100°. d (anhydr) 2.49. One gram dissolves in 4.5 ml water. Insol in alc. LD orally in mice: >100 mg/kg (Behrens, Seelkopf).

USE: In detergent processing.

8697. Sodium Tripolyphosphate. [7758-29-4] Triphosphoric acid pentasodium salt; sodium triphosphate; tripolyphosphate; STPP; poly; pentasodium triphosphate. $Na_5O_{10}P_3$; mol wt 367.86. Na 31.25%, O 43.49%, P 25.26%. $Na_5P_3O_{10}$. Prepd by molecular dehydration of mono- and disodium phosphates: Audrieth, Bell, *Inorg. Synth.* **3**, 85 (1950). Toxicity study: H. F. Smyth *et al., Am. Ind. Hyg. Assoc. J.* **30**, 470 (1969).

Slightly hygroscopic granules. Soly in water (g/100 ml) at 25°: 20; at 100°: 86.5. pH of 1% soln at 25° = 9.7-9.8. Its properties are between those of tetrasodium pyrophosphate and sodium metaphosphate. Stability: With prolonged heating of STPP solns, it tends to revert to the orthophosphate. More stable than the higher (i.e., meta-) phosphates, but less stable than tetrasodium pyrophosphate. LD_{50} orally in rats: 6.50 g/kg (Smyth).

Caution: Moderately irritating to skin, mucous membranes. Ingestion can cause violent purging.

USE: In water softening (calcium and magnesium hardness is sequestered from soln without precipitation); peptizing agent, emulsifier and dispersing agent, ingredient of cleansers in drilling fluids to control mud viscosity in oil fields; as preservative, sequestrant and texturizer in foods.

8698. Sodium Tungstate(VI). [13472-45-2] $(T-4)$-Disodium tungstate (WO_4^{2-}). Na_2O_4W; mol wt 293.82. Na 15.65%, O 21.78%, W 62.57%. Na_2WO_4. Crystals have a spinel structure isomorphous with sodium molybdate(VI), *q.v.* Mfr: N. T. Gordon, A. F. Spring, *Ind. Eng. Chem.* **16**, 555 (1924). Properties of sodium tungstate derivatives: E. F. Smith, *J. Am. Chem. Soc.* **44**, 2027 (1922). Crystal structure: I. Lindqvist, *Acta Chem. Scand.* **4**, 1066 (1950). Polymerization study: M. L. Freedman, *J. Am. Chem. Soc.* **80**, 2072 (1958). Thermochemistry study: R. L. Graham, L. G. Hepler, *ibid.* 3538. HPLC and CZE analysis: K. Hettiarachchi *et al., J. Pharm. Biomed. Anal.* **13**, 515 (1995). Pharmacokinetics in rats: S. Le Lamer-Déchamps *et al., Int. J. Pharm.* **248**, 131 (2002). Antidiabetic effects in rats: A. Barberà *et al., Diabetologia* **44**, 507 (2001). Review of toxicity: B. Venugopal, T. D. Luckey, *Environ. Qual. Safety,* Suppl. 1, 4-73 (1975); of toxicology and human expo-

sure: *Toxicological Profile for Tungsten* (PB2006-100007, 2005) 203 pp.

Dihydrate. [10213-10-2] Colorless crystals or white, cryst powder. mp 665°. Effloresces in dry air. Loses its water at 100°. Sol in about 1.1 parts water. Insol in alcohol. The aq soln is slightly alkaline, pH 8-9. LD_{50} (mg tungstate/kg) in rabbits: 105 i.m.; in rats: 240 s.c. (Venugopal, Luckey).

USE: Fireproofing and waterproofing fabrics; preparing complex compds such as phosphotungstate and silicotungstate; as a protective colloid in biological development methods; precipitant for alkaloids; catalyst in oxidation reactions; corrosion inhibitor for steel.

8699. Sodium Uranate(VI). [13721-34-1] Sodium diuranate; uranium oxide yellow; uranium yellow. $Na_2O_7U_2$; mol wt 634.03. Na 7.25%, O 17.66%, U 75.08%. $Na_2U_2O_7$.

Monohydrate. Yellow powder. Insol in water; sol in acids.

USE: Manuf yellowish-green fluorescent glass; painting on porcelain and enameling.

8700. Sodium Vanadate(V). [13718-26-8] Sodium metavanadate. NaO_3V; mol wt 121.93. Na 18.85%, O 39.37%, V 41.78%. $NaVO_3$.

Tetrahydrate. Yellowish-white, cryst powder. Sol in hot water. LD_{75} i.p. in rats: 4-5 mg V/kg, Franke, Moxon, *J. Pharmacol. Exp. Ther.* **58**, 454 (1936).

USE: In photography and manuf of inks.

8701. Sofalcone. [64506-49-6] [5-[(3-Methyl-2-butenyl)-oxy]-2-[3-[4-[(3-methyl-2-butenyl)oxy]phenyl]-1-oxo-2-propenyl]-phenoxy]acetic acid; 2′-carboxymethoxy-4,4′-bis(3-methyl-2-butenyloxy)chalcone; Su-88; Solon. $C_{27}H_{30}O_6$; mol wt 450.52. C 71.98%, H 6.71%, O 21.31%. Substituted chalcone with anti-ulcer activity. Prepn: K. Kyogoku *et al., DE 2705603; eidem, US 4085135* (1977, 1978 both to Taisho); *eidem, Chem. Pharm. Bull.* **27**, 2943 (1979). Effects on exptl ulcer models: R. Saziki *et al., Oyo Yakuri* **18**, 579 (1979), *C.A.* **92**, 174433h (1980). Absorption, distribution, excretion: T. Nozu *et al., ibid.* 815, *C.A.* **92**, 191017t (1980). Reproduction studies: T. Yamada *et al., ibid.* **19**, 543 (1980), *C.A.* **93**, 230875j (1980). Toxicity study: Y. Tarumoto *et al., Yakuri to Chiryo* **10**, 61 (1982), *C.A.* **96**, 193205j (1982). Effect on gastric blood flow: Y. Matsuo *et al., Arzneim.-Forsch.* **33**, 242 (1983). Gastric cytoprotective effect in rats: T. Suwa *et al., Jpn. J. Pharmacol.* **35**, 47 (1984); S. Kishimoto *et al., Arzneim.-Forsch.* **31**, 944 (1987).

Light yellow needles from ethanol, mp 143-144°. LD_{50} in mice, rats: >10 g/kg orally (Tarumoto).

THERAP CAT: Antiulcerative.

8702. Solan. [2307-68-8] *N*-(3-Chloro-4-methylphenyl)-2-methylpentanamide; 3′-chloro-2-methyl-*p*-valerotoluidide; Niagara 4512. $C_{13}H_{18}ClNO$; mol wt 239.74. C 65.13%, H 7.57%, Cl 14.79%, N 5.84%, O 6.67%. Prepn: Dorschner *et al., GB 869169; US 3020142* (1961, 1962 both to FMC). Toxicity study: G. W. Bailey, J. L. White, *Residue Rev.* **10**, 97 (1965).

Crystals, mp 79-80°. Sol in pine oil, diisobutylketone, isophorone, xylene. Practically insol in water. LD_{50} orally in rats: 10000 mg/kg (Bailey, White).

USE: Herbicide.

8703. Solanesol. [13190-97-1] (2*E*,6*E*,10*E*,14*E*,18*E*,22*E*,-26*E*,30*E*,)-3,7,11,15,19,23,27,31,35-Nonamethyl-2,6,10,14,18,22,-26,30,34-hexatriacontanonaen-1-ol; nonaisoprenol. $C_{45}H_{74}O$; mol wt 631.07. C 85.65%, H 11.82%, O 2.54%. High molecular weight isoprenoid alcohol isolated from tobacco leaf. Associated with the particulate fraction of tobacco smoke. Isoln: R. L. Rowland *et al., J. Am. Chem. Soc.* **78**, 4680 (1956). Synthesis: R. Rüegg *et al., Helv. Chim. Acta* **43**, 1745 (1960). Stereoselective synthesis: K. Sato *et al., J. Chem. Soc. Perkin Trans. 1* **1981**, 761. Structural analysis: N. J. Jensen, T. Sumpter, *Beitr. Tabakforsch. Int.* **16**, 85 (1995). Determn in tobacco smoke: M. W. Ogden, K. C. Maiolo, *LC-GC* **10**, 459 (1992); in tobacco extracts: K. Z. Liu *et al., Anal. Lett.* **31**, 1947 (1998).

White waxy solid, mp 41.5-42.5°. Sol in organic solvents. Insol in water.

USE: Tracer for environmental exposure to tobacco smoke.

8704. Solanidine. [80-78-4] (3β)-Solanid-5-en-3-ol; solatubine. $C_{27}H_{43}NO$; mol wt 397.64. C 81.55%, H 10.90%, N 3.52%, O 4.02%. From *Solanum* spp., *Solanaceae*. Potato sprouts contain about 0.008%. Obtained by hydrolysis of solanine. Extraction procedure: Soltys, Wallenfels, *Ber.* **69**, 811 (1936). Review on structure: Reichstein, Reich, *Annu. Rev. Biochem.* **15**, 155 (1946). Stereochemistry: Rosen, Rosen, *Chem. Ind. (London)* **1954**, 1581. Revised stereochemistry: Höhne *et al., Tetrahedron* **22**, 673 (1966). Synthesis: Schreiber, Roensch, *Ber.* **97**, 2362 (1964); *Tetrahedron* **21**, 645 (1965); Kessar *et al., ibid.* **27**, 2153 (1971).

Long needles from chloroform-methanol, mp 218-219°. Sublimes near mp with slight decompn. $[\alpha]_D^{21}$ −29° (c = 0.5 in chloroform). Freely sol in benzene, chloroform; slightly in alcohol, methanol; almost insol in ether, water.

Hydrochloride. $C_{27}H_{43}NO.HCl$. Prisms from 80% alcohol, dec 345°.

Methyliodide. $C_{27}H_{43}NO.CH_3I$. Crystals from 50% alcohol, dec 286°.

Acetylsolanidine. $C_{29}H_{45}NO_2$. Crystals from alc, mp 208°.

8705. Solanine. [20562-02-1] (α-form); [51938-42-2] (unspecified stereo). Solatunine. $C_{45}H_{73}NO_{15}$; mol wt 868.06. C 62.26%, H 8.48%, N 1.61%, O 27.65%. From *Solanum* species, especially from *S. tuberosum* L. (potato), *S. nigrum* L. (woody nightshade), and *Lycopersicon esculentum* Mill., *Solanaceae* (tomato). Fresh potato sprouts contain about 0.04%. Extraction procedure: Soltys, Wallenfels, *Ber.* **69**, 811 (1936). Separated by chromatography into six components: α-, β-, γ-solanine and α-, β-, γ-chaconine. Main constituent α-solanine: Kuhn, Löw, *Angew. Chem.* **66**, 639 (1954); Kuhn *et al., Ber.* **88**, 1492 (1955); Paseshnichenko, Guseva, *Biokhimiya* **21**, 585 (1956); *eidem, ibid.* **22**, 843 (1957). Pharmacology: Nishie *et al., Toxicol. Appl. Pharmacol.* **19**, 81 (1971). Toxicity study: B. C. Patil *et al., Food Cosmet. Toxicol.* **10**, 395 (1972); and teratogenicity study: S. Chaube, C. A. Swinyard, *Toxicol. Appl. Pharmacol.* **36**, 227 (1976).

Slender needles from 85% alc, browns and sinters about 190°, dec about 285°. $[\alpha]_D^{20}$ −60° (pyridine). pK (15°) 6.65. Readily sol in hot alc. Practically insol in water (25 mg/l at pH 6.0), ether, chloroform. LD_{50} i.p. in mice: 32.3 mg/kg (Patil). LD_{50} i.p. in rats: 67.0 mg/kg (Chaube, Swinyard).

Hydrochloride. [40816-40-8] $C_{45}H_{73}NO_{15}.HCl$. Usually amorphous and gummy, but has been crystallized, dec about 212°. Sol in water.

USE: Has been used as an agricultural insecticide.

8706. Solanocapsine. [639-86-1] (3β,5α,16α,22α,23β,25β)-3-Amino-16,23-epoxy-16,28-secosolanidan-23-ol; solanocapsin; 3β-amino-22,26-imino-16β,23-oxido-5α,22α,23β,25α-cholestan-23-ol; 3β-amino-22,26-imino-16β,23-oxido-5α,22R,23S,25R-cholestan-23-ol. $C_{27}H_{46}N_2O_2$; mol wt 430.67. C 75.30%, H 10.77%, N 6.50%, O 7.43%. From *Solanum pseudocapsicum* L., *S. capsicastrum* Link, *S. hendersonii* hort., *Solanaceae*. Isolation: Barger, Fraenkel-Conrat, *J. Chem. Soc.* **1936**, 1537; K. Schreiber, H. Ripperger, *Z. Naturforsch.* **17B**, 217 (1962). Structure: *eidem, Experientia* **16**, 536 (1960). Revised structure and synthesis: *eidem, Ann.* **723**, 159 (1969). Stereochemistry: *eidem, Tetrahedron Letters* no. 27, 9 (1960); *Ann.* **655**, 114 (1962). Synthesis: Ripperger *et al., Tetrahedron Lett.* **1970**, 5251; *eidem, Tetrahedron* **28**, 1629 (1972).

Monohydrate, needles from methanol, mp 213-215°. $[\alpha]_D^{20}$ +26.3° (c = 1.80 in methanol); $[\alpha]_D^{20}$ +24.9° (c = 2.13 in methanol).

N'-Acetylsolanocapsine. $C_{29}H_{48}N_2O_3$. Needles from ethanol, mp 233-234°. $[\alpha]_D^{23}$ −33.7° (c = 1.59 in pyridine).

N,N'-Diacetylsolanocapsine. $C_{31}H_{50}N_2O_4$. Crystals from chloroform + acetone, mp 281-283°. $[\alpha]_D^{22}$ −38.6° (c = 1.31 in pyridine).

N,N,N'-Trimethylsolanocapsine. $C_{30}H_{52}N_2O_2$. Needles from abs methanol, mp 222-224°. $[\alpha]_D^{22}$ +53.2° (c = 1.09 in pyridine).

N-Benzylidenesolanocapsine. $C_{34}H_{50}N_2O_2$. Needles from pyridine + abs methanol, mp 249-251°. $[\alpha]_D^{18}$ +31.4° (c = 0.78 in pyridine).

8707. Solanone. [1937-54-8] (5S,6E)-8-Methyl-5-(1-methylethyl)-6,8-nonadien-2-one; L-(+)-2-methyl-5-isopropyl-1,3-nonadien-8-one. $C_{13}H_{22}O$; mol wt 194.31. C 80.36%, H 11.41%, O 8.23%. Stereochemically unique terpene. Isoln from tobacco, structure and synthesis: Johnson, Nicholson *J. Org. Chem.* **30**, 2918 (1965). Stereoselective synthesis: A. Kohda, T. Sato, *Chem. Commun.* **1981**, 951.

Liquid. bp$_1$ 60°. n_D^{20} 1.4755. d_4^{20} 0.870. $[\alpha]_D^{23}$ +13.6° (neat). uv max (ethanal and hexane): 230 nm (log ε 4.07).

8708. Solanum. Bull nettle; radical weed; sand-brier; horse nettle. Air-dried ripe fruit of *Solanum carolinense* L., *Solanaceae*. *Habit.* South America, Florida and other sections of U.S.A. *Constit.* Solanine, solanidine.

THERAP CAT: Sedative, anticonvulsant.

8709. Solasodine. [126-17-0] (3β,22α,25R)-Spirosol-5-en-3-ol; solasod-5-en-3β-ol; Δ⁵-20β$_F$,22α$_F$,25α$_F$,27-azaspirosten-3β-ol; solancarpidine; solanidine-S; purapuridine. C$_{27}$H$_{43}$NO$_2$; mol wt 413.64. C 78.40%, H 10.48%, N 3.39%, O 7.74%. Steroidal alkaloid isolated from various *Solanum* species. By hydrolysis of solasonine: Rochelmeyer, *Arch. Pharm.* **277**, 329 (1939). *See also* ref *under* Solasonine and Solanidine. Structure: Briggs *et al.*, *J. Chem. Soc.* **1950**, 3013. Synthesis: Uhle, *J. Org. Chem.* **27**, 656 (1962); Schreiber, Rönsch, *Tetrahedron* **20**, 1939 (1964); Kessar *et al., ibid.* **27**, 2869 (1971). Comprehensive description: G. Indrayanto *et al., Anal. Profiles Drug Subs. Excip.* **24**, 487-522 (1996).

Hexagonal plates from methanol or by sublimation in high vacuum, mp 200-202°. $[\alpha]_D^{25}$ −98° (c = 0.14 in methanol); $[\alpha]_D$ −113° (CHCl$_3$). Alkaline reaction to litmus in alcoholic soln. pKb 6.30. uv max (methanol): 206 nm. Freely sol in benzene, pyridine and chloroform. Practically insol in ether. Soly at 30° (mg/ml): methanol 9.5; 95% ethanol 5.0; acetone 3.5; *n*-hexane <1.0; water <1.0.

USE: Starting material for steroidal drugs.

8710. Solasonine. [19121-58-5] (3β,22α,25R)-Spirosol-5-en-3-yl O-6-deoxy-α-L-mannopyranosyl-(1 → 2)-O-[β-D-glucopyranosyl-(1 → 3)]-β-D-galactopyranoside; solanine-S; purapurine. C$_{45}$H$_{73}$NO$_{16}$; mol wt 884.06. C 61.14%, H 8.32%, N 1.58%, O 28.96%. From *Solanum aviculare* Forst F., *S. sodomeum* L., *S. xanthocarpum* Schrad & Wendl., *Solanaceae*: Bell, Briggs, *J. Chem. Soc.* **1942**, 1; Briggs *et al., ibid.* **1942**, 3; Kuhn, Löw, *Ber.* **88**, 289 (1955). Isoln from other *S.* spp: Briggs, Cambie, *J. Chem. Soc.* **1958**, 1422; Briggs *et al., ibid.* **1961**, 4645. Paper chromatography: Szendey, *Arch. Pharm.* **290**, 563 (1957). Structure: Briggs *et al., J. Chem. Soc.* **1963**, 2848. Enzymic decompn: Guseva, Pasechnichenko, *Biokhimiya* **24**, 563 (1959).

Needles from methanol, sinters 296°, mp 301-303°. $[\alpha]_D^{23}$ −88° (c = 1.01 in pyridine); $[\alpha]_D^{22}$ −74.5° (c = 0.51 in methanol). Sol in hot alc, hot dioxane; slightly sol in hot water, dil acetic acid. Practically insol in chloroform, ether.

8711. Solasulfone. [133-65-3] 1,1′-[Sulfonylbis(4,1-phenyleneimino)]bis[3-phenyl-1,3-propanedisulfonic acid] tetrasodium salt; di(γ-phenylpropylamino)-4,4′-diphenylsulfone α,α′,γ,γ′-sodium tetrasulfonate; tetrasodium 4,4′-bis(γ-phenylpropylamino)diphenylsulfone α,γ,α′,γ′-tetrasulfonate; phenopryldiasulfone sodium; sol-

apsone; RP-3668; Cimedone; Sulphetrone. C$_{30}$H$_{28}$N$_2$Na$_4$O$_{14}$S$_5$; mol wt 892.83. C 40.36%, H 3.16%, N 3.14%, Na 10.30%, O 25.09%, S 17.96%. Prepared by reacting 4,4′-diaminodiphenyl sulfone with more than 2 mols cinnamic aldehyde in the cold and treating the resulting 4,4′-dicinnamylideneaminodiphenyl sulfone with NaHSO$_3$ soln: Gray, Henry, **GB 491265** (1938 to Wellcome Foundation); Buttle *et al., Biochem. J.* **32**, 1101 (1938). Improved process: Henry, Gray, **GB 562216** (1944 to Wellcome Foundation). Properties and estimation: Brownlee *et al., Br. J. Pharmacol.* **3**, 15 (1948).

Crystals contg 5-7% H$_2$O from alc. Becomes anhyd at 110° *in vacuo*. Exceedingly sol in cold water, giving a neutral soln. 20% and 40% (w/v) aq solns are stable when neutral or slightly alkaline and may be autoclaved. Practically insol in cold alc. Solns are incompatible with acids. Absorption spectrum of dye obtained by diazotization and coupling to *N*-(1-naphthyl)ethylenediamine hydrochloride: Brownlee, *loc. cit.*

THERAP CAT: Antibacterial (leprostatic).

8712. Solifenacin. [242478-37-1] (1S)-3,4-Dihydro-1-phenyl-2(1H)-isoquinolinecarboxylic acid (3R)-1-azabicyclo-[2.2.2]oct-3-yl ester; (1S,3′R)-3′quinuclidinyl-1-phenyl-1,2,3,4-tetrahydro-2-isoquinolinecarboxylate. C$_{23}$H$_{26}$N$_2$O$_2$; mol wt 362.46. C 76.21%, H 7.23%, N 7.73%, O 8.83%. Muscarinic M$_3$ receptor antagonist. Prepn: M. Takeuchi *et al.*, **WO 9620194**; *eidem*, **US 6017927** (1996, 2000 both to Yamanouchi). Receptor binding studies: K. Ikeda *et al., Arch. Pharmacol.* **366**, 97 (2002); selectivity profile: A. Ohtake *et al., Eur. J. Pharmacol.* **492**, 243 (2004). Clinical study in overactive bladder: C. R. Chapple *et al., Br. J. Urol.* **93**, 303 (2004); F. Habb *et al., Eur. Urol.* **47**, 376 (2005). Clinical comparison with tolterodine: C. R. Chapple *et al., ibid.* **48**, 464 (2005). Review of efficacy and tolerability studies: S. Brunton, L. Kuritzky, *Curr. Med. Res. Opin.* **21**, 71-80 (2005); of clinical development: C. K. Payne, *Drugs* **66**, 175-190 (2006).

Yellow oil.

Succinate. [242478-38-2] YM-905; Vesicare. C$_{23}$H$_{26}$N$_2$O$_2$.-C$_4$H$_6$O$_4$; mol wt 480.55. White to slightly yellowish crystals, mp ~145°. Freely sol in acetic acid, water, methanol, dimethylsulfoxide.

THERAP CAT: In treatment of urinary incontinence.

8713. Soman. [96-64-0] Methylphosphonofluoridic acid 1,2,2-trimethylpropyl ester; pinacoloxymethylphosphoryl fluoride; pinacolyl methylphosphonofluoridate; GD. C$_7$H$_{16}$FO$_2$P; mol wt 182.17. C 46.15%, H 8.85%, F 10.43%, O 17.57%, P 17.00%. Nerve gas; potent cholinesterase inhibitor similar in structure and activity to sarin and tabun, *q.q.v.* Prepn: Holmstedt, *Acta Physiol. Scand.* **25**, suppl. 90, p 106 (1951); *Protar* **16**, 131 (1950); G. Schrader, *Die Entwicklung neuer Insektizide auf Grundlage organischer Fluor- und Phosphor-Verbindungen* [Monographie Nr. 62 zu Angewandte Chemie und Chemie-Ingenieur-Technik (Verlag Chemie 1951)]; B. C. Saunders, *Some Aspects of the Chemistry and Toxic Action of Organic Compounds Containing Phosphorus and Fluorine* (Cambridge, 1957) p 94. Toxicity study: Loomis,

Salafsky, *Toxicol. Appl. Pharmacol.* **5**, 685 (1963). Brief description: B. L. Harris in *Kirk-Othmer Encyclopedia of Chemical Technology* vol. 5 (Wiley-Interscience, New York, 4th ed., 1993) pp 795-816.

$$(H_3C)_3C \quad CH_3 \quad O$$

LD$_{50}$ in mice (mg/100 g): 0.062 i.p.; 0.78 dermally (Loomis, Salafsky).

Caution: Potential symptoms of overexposure by inhalation are constriction of pupils of the eye, difficulty breathing followed by bronchial constriction, convulsions, death. Also toxic due to absorption through skin and eyes. *See Chem. Eng. News* **31**, 4676 (1953).

USE: Chemical warfare agent.

8714. Somatoliberin. [83930-13-6] Growth hormone-releasing factor; GH-RF; GH-RH; GRF; growth hormone-releasing hormone; hGRF; hpGRF; somatocrinin. Stimulatory growth-hormone releasing factor of the hypothalamus that mediates, together with somatostatin, *q.v.*, the neuroregulation of somatotropin secretion. The concept of hypothalamic regulation of growth hormone release was postulated on the basis of physiological and biochemical evidence, *cf.* A. V. Schally *et al., Recent Prog. Horm. Res.* **24**, 497 (1968); J. B. Martin in *Frontiers in Neuroendocrinology*, L. Martini, W. F. Ganong, Eds. (Raven Press, New York, 1976) pp 129-168. Demonstration of the existence of a GH-RH: R. Deuben, J. Meites, *Endocrinology* **74**, 408 (1964); A. V. Schally *et al., ibid.* **82**, 271 (1968); E. Dickermann *et al., Neuroendocrinology* **4**, 75 (1969). Isoln of a decapeptide originally believed to be GRF: A. V. Schally *et al., Endocrinology* **84**, 1493 (1969). Review of early literature: *eidem, Science* **179**, 341 (1973). Isoln and characterization of hpGRF, a fully bioactive, 44 amino acid peptide from human pancreatic tumor: R. Guillemin *et al., Science* **218**, 585 (1982); J. Rivier *et al., Nature* **300**, 276 (1982). Cloning and sequence analysis of cDNA for hpGRF precursor: U. Gubler *et al., Proc. Natl. Acad. Sci. USA* **80**, 4311 (1983). Expression-cloning of cDNA for hpGRF: K. E. Mayo *et al., Nature* **306**, 86 (1983). Isoln, primary structure and synthesis of native human hypothalamic GRF (hGRF), identity with hpGRF and comparison with GRF from other species: N. Ling *et al., Proc. Natl. Acad. Sci. USA* **81**, 4302 (1984). Immunohistochemical detection of GRF in brain: B. Bloch *et al., ibid.* **301**, 607 (1983). Potent interaction of glucocorticoids with GRF *in vivo:* W. B. Wehrenberg *et al., Science* **221**, 556 (1983). Series of articles on clinical pharmacology: *Horm. Res.* **22**, 32-57 (1985). Clinical evaluation in treatment of hypopituitary dwarfism: M. O. Thorner *et al., N. Engl. J. Med.* **312**, 4 (1985). *Reviews:* R. Guillemin *et al., Recent Prog. Horm. Res.* **40**, 233-299 (1984); W. B. Wehrenberg *et al., Annu. Rev. Pharmacol. Toxicol.* **25**, 463-483 (1985).

Porcine GRF is destroyed by trypsin, chymotrypsin, pepsin. Biological activity remains after incubation at pH 8.5 for 4 hours at 37°, but is destroyed after similar incubation at pH 2.

8715. Somatostatin. [38916-34-6] Growth hormone-release inhibiting factor; GH-RIF; SRIF; SRIF-14. $C_{76}H_{104}N_{18}O_{19}S_2$; mol wt 1637.88. C 55.73%, H 6.40%, N 15.39%, O 18.56%, S 3.92%. Widely occurring cyclic tetradecapeptide that mediates, together with somatoliberin, *q.v.*, the neuroregulation of somatotropin secretion. Inhibits release of growth hormone, insulin and glucagon. Also a potent inhibitor in a number of systems, including central and peripheral neural, gastrointestinal, and vascular smooth muscle. Isoln from ovine hypothalamic extracts: P. Brazeau *et al., Science* **179**, 77 (1973). Structure: Burgus *et al., Proc. Natl. Acad. Sci. USA* **70**, 684 (1973); Ling *et al., Biochem. Biophys. Res. Commun.* **50**, 127 (1973). Synthesis: Rivier *et al., C.R. Seances Acad. Sci. Ser. D* **276**, 2737 (1973); Sarantakis, McKinley, *Biochem. Biophys. Res. Commun.* **54**, 234 (1973); Yamashiro, Li, *ibid.* 882; Coy *et al., ibid.* 1267; A. M. Felix *et al., Int. J. Pept. Protein Res.* **15**, 342 (1980); B. Hartrodt *et al., Pharmazie* **37**, 403 (1982). Synthesis and bacterial expression of somatostatin gene: K. Itakura *et al., Science* **198**, 1056 (1977); K. Itakura, A. D. Riggs, *BE 871782*; K. Itakura, US

4356270; A. D. Riggs, US 4366246 (1979, 1982, 1982 all to Genentech). Isoln of a 28-amino acid somatostatin, termed *SRIF-28*, from porcine gastrointestinal tract: L. Pradayrol *et al., Biochem. Biophys. Res. Commun.* **85**, 701 (1978). Primary structure: *eidem, FEBS Lett.* **109**, 55 (1980). Synthesis: E. Wunsch, *Z. Naturforsch.* **35B**, 911 (1980). Isoln of a 25-amino acid somatostatin, *SRIF-25*, and structure: P. Brazeau *et al., C.R. Seances Acad. Sci. Ser. D* **290**, 1369 (1980). Both of these peptides consist of an *N*-terminal extension of SRIF-14. They are more potent than SRIF-14 in inhibition of insulin release but less potent in inhibition of glucagon release: L. Mandarino *et al., Nature* **291**, 76 (1981). Synthetic linear SRIF-14 exhibits the same bioactivity as the natural cyclic form: P. Brazeau *et al., Endocrinology* **94**, 184 (1974). Activity studies in humans: T. M. Siler *et al., J. Clin. Endocrinol. Metab.* **37**, 632 (1973). Inhibitory effects on the secretion of thyrotropin: Vale *et al., Fed. Proc.* **32**, 211 (1973); of insulin: K. G. Alberti *et al., Lancet* **2**, 1299 (1973); Koeker *et al., Science* **184**, 482 (1974). Role in diabetes: Maugh, *ibid.* **188**, 920 (1975). Clinical trial in controlling acute variceal hemorrhage: S. A. Jenkins *et al., Br. Med. J.* **290**, 275 (1985). Review of distribution, secretion, physiology of gastrointestinal somatostatin: C. H. S. McIntosh, *Life Sci.* **37**, 2043-2058 (1985). Symposium of biosynthesis, bioactivity, and clinical applications: *Adv. Exp. Med. Biol.* **188**, 1-524 (1985). *Reviews:* Vale *et al., Recent Prog. Horm. Res.* **31**, 365-397 (1975); Guillemin, Gerich, *Annu. Rev. Med.* **27**, 379-388 (1976); R. L. Moss, *Annu. Rev. Physiol.* **41**, 617 (1979); A. Arimura, J. B. Fishback, *Neuroendocrinology* **33**, 246-256 (1981); several authors in *Gut Hormones*, S. R. Bloom, J. M. Polack, Eds. (Churchill, New York, 2nd ed., 1981) 605 pp; S. M. McCann, *Annu. Rev. Pharmacol. Toxicol.* **22**, 491-515 (1982); N. Bethge *et al., J. Clin. Chem. Clin. Biochem.* **20**, 603-613 (1982). Book: *Somatostatin* Vol. 2, M. T. McQuillan, Ed. (Eden Press, Quebec, 1980) 238 pp.

Ala–Gly–Cys–Lys–Asn–Phe–Phe–Trp

Cys–Ser–Thr–Phe–Thr–Lys

Acetate. SRIF-A; Aminopan; Modustatina; Somatofalk; Stilamin.

THERAP CAT: Treatment of severe, acute hemorrhage of gastroduodenal ulcers. Treatment of erosive or hemorrhagic gastritis. Experimental antidiabetic. Growth hormone inhibitor.

8716. Somatotropin. [9002-72-6] Adenohypophyseal growth hormone; GH; hypophyseal growth hormone; anterior pituitary growth hormone; growth hormone; phyone; pituitary growth hormone; somatotropic hormone; STH. Species-specific anabolic protein that promotes somatic growth, stimulates protein synthesis, and regulates carbohydrate and lipid metabolism. Increases serum levels of somatomedins, *q.v.* Secreted by the anterior pituitary under the regulation of the hypothalamic hormones, somatoliberin and somatostatin, *q.q.v.* Growth hormones from various species differ in amino acid sequence, antigenicity, isoelectric point, and in the range of animals in which they can produce biological responses. Isoln from bovine anterior pituitary substance: C. H. Li *et al., J. Biol. Chem.* **159**, 353 (1945); A. E. Wilhelmi *et al., ibid.* **176**, 735 (1948); C. H. Li, US 3118815 (1964 to Upjohn). Isoln from human pituitaries: Lewis, Brink, US 2974088 (1961 to Merck & Co.); Reisfeld *et al., Endocrinology* **71**, 559 (1962). Amino acid sequence of human growth hormone (HGH): C. H. Li *et al., J. Am. Chem. Soc.* **88**, 2050 (1966); *eidem, Arch. Biochem. Biophys.* **133**, 70 (1969). Total synthesis: C. H. Li, D. Yamashiro, *J. Am. Chem. Soc.* **92**, 7608 (1970). Revised sequence of HGH: H. D. Niall, *Nature New Biol.* **230**, 90 (1971). Review of structural studies and comparison with the lactogenic hormones: H. D. Niall *et al., Recent Prog. Horm. Res.* **29**, 387-416 (1973). Review of protein chemistry: C. H. Li, *Mol. Cell. Biochem.* **46**, 31-41 (1982). Cloning and expression of cDNA for HGH in *E. coli:* D. V. Goeddel *et al., Nature* **281**, 544 (1979); D. V. Goeddel, H. L. Heyneker, *BE 884012; eidem, US 4342832* (1980, 1982 both to Genentech); in mammalian cells: G. N. Pavakis *et al., Proc. Natl. Acad. Sci. USA* **78**, 7398 (1981). Purification and bioactivity of recombinant HGH: K. C. Olson *et al., Nature* **293**, 408 (1981). Clinical comparison of natural and recombinant HGH: R. L. Hintz *et al., Lancet* **1**, 1276 (1982). Use of recombinant bovine GH to increase milk production in cows: D. E. Bauman *et al., J. Dairy Sci.* **68**, 1352 (1985).

Discussion of use of recombinant GH in applied animal agriculture: J. L. Burton, B. W. McBride, *J. Agric. Ethics* **2**, 129-159 (1989). Review of GH gene studies: D. D. Moore *et al., Recent Prog. Horm. Res.* **38**, 197-225 (1982). Review of bioregulation of HGH secretion: D. G. Johnston *et al., J. R. Soc. Med.* **78**, 319-327 (1985); of mechanism of action on target cells: O. G. P. Isaksson *et al., Annu. Rev. Physiol.* **47**, 483-499 (1985). Symposium on pharmacology and clinical efficacy: *Horm. Res.* **33**, Suppl. 4, 1-107 (1990). Books: *Growth and Growth Hormone*, A. Pecile, E. Muller, Eds. (Excerpta Medica, Amsterdam, 1972); *Human Growth Hormone and Gonadotrophins in Health and Disease*, P. Franchimont, H. Burger, Eds. (Elsevier, New York, 1975) 494 pp; *Growth Hormone and Other Biologically Active Peptides*, A. Pecile, E. Muller, Eds. (Elsevier, New York, 1980); *Evaluation of Growth Hormone Secretion*, Z. Laron, O. Butenandt, Eds. (S. Karger, New York, 1983); *Use of Somatotropin in Livestock Production*, K. Sejrsen *et al.*, Eds. (Elsevier, New York, 1989).

Human growth hormone. [12629-01-5] HGH; somatropin; CB-311; Crescormon; Genotropin; Grorm; Humatrope; Nanormon; Norditropin; Nutropin; Nutropinaq; Saizen; Umatrope; Zomacton. $C_{990}H_{1529}N_{263}O_{299}S_7$; mol wt 22123.77. A single polypeptide chain of 191 amino acids having a molecular weight of 22,124. Isoelectric point 4.9. $[\alpha]^{25} -38.7°$ (0.1M acetic acid).

Methionyl human growth hormone. [82030-87-3] Somatrem; met-HGH; Protropin; Somatonorm. $C_{995}H_{1537}N_{263}O_{301}S_8$; mol wt 22255.95. Produced in bacteria from recombinant DNA. Contains the complete amino acid sequence of the natural hormone plus an additional *N*-terminal methionine.

Bovine somatotropin. One of the four naturally occurring molecular variants is known as *somavubove*, $C_{976}H_{1533}N_{265}O_{286}S_8$. Several variants have been produced by recombinant DNA technology: *somagrebove*, $C_{987}H_{1550}N_{268}O_{291}S_9$, *CL-291894*, *Quest*; *sometribove*, $C_{978}H_{1537}N_{265}O_{286}S_9$; *somidobove*, $C_{1020}H_{1596}N_{274}$-$O_{302}S_9$, *EL-349, LY-177837, Optiflex*.

Porcine somatotropin. Somacton. Several variants have been produced by recombinant DNA technology: *somalapor*, C_{977}-$H_{1527}N_{265}O_{287}S_7$; *somenopor*, $C_{938}H_{1469}N_{255}O_{275}S_7$; *sometripor*, $C_{979}H_{1527}N_{265}O_{287}S_8$; *somfasepor*, $C_{938}H_{1465}N_{257}O_{278}S_6$, *Grolean, Leanstar*.

THERAP CAT: Growth stimulant.

THERAP CAT (VET): Growth stimulant. Bovine somatotropin as galactopoietic.

8717. Songorine. [509-24-0] (1α,15β)-21-Ethyl-1,15-dihydroxy-4-methyl-16-methylene-7,20-cycloveatchan-12-one; napellonine; zongorine. $C_{22}H_{31}NO_3$; mol wt 357.49. C 73.91%, H 8.74%, N 3.92%, O 13.43%. From *Aconitum songoricum* Popov, *Ranunculaceae:* Yunusov, *J. Gen. Chem. USSR* **18**, 515 (1948); Kuzovkov, *ibid.* **23**, 504 (1953); **25**, 2006 (1955). Identity with napellonine: Kuzovkov, *Zh. Obshch. Khim.* **28**, 2283 (1958); **29**, 1728 (1959). Structure: Sugasawa, *Chem. Pharm. Bull.* **9**, 889, 897 (1961). Absolute configuration: Okamoto *et al., ibid.* **13**, 1270 (1965). Synthesis of the aromatic intermediate: Wiesner *et al., Can. J. Chem.* **51**, 3978 (1973). Pharmacology: Sadritdinov, *Farmakol. Alk.* No. 312 (1965), *C.A.* **66**, 93772d (1967). Mass spectra data: Yunusov *et al., Khim. Prir. Soedin.* **6**, 101 (1970), *C.A.* **73**, 131178u (1970). Pharmacology and toxicity data: N. G. Bisset, *J. Ethnopharmacol.* **4**, 247-336 (1981).

Crystals, mp 201-202°. $[\alpha]_D^{20} -135.4°$. uv max: 290 nm (log ε 2.6). LD$_{50}$ in mice (mg/kg): 1575 orally, 630 s.c., 485 i.p., 142.5 i.v.; in rats (mg/kg): 407.5 i.p. (Bisset).

Hydrochloride. Crystals, mp 257-258°. $[\alpha]_D^{20} -114°$ (c = 2 in water).

8718. Sophorabioside. [2945-88-2] 3-[4-[[2-*O*-(6-Deoxy-α-L-mannopyranosyl)-β-D-glucopyranosyl]oxy]phenyl]-5,7-dihydroxy-4*H*-1-benzopyran-4-one; genistein-4'-glucosidorhamnoside. $C_{27}H_{30}O_{14}$; mol wt 578.52. C 56.05%, H 5.23%, O 38.72%. From fruits of *Sophora japonica* L., *Leguminosae*. Isoln and structure: Zemplén, Bognár, *Ber.* **75B**, 482 (1942). The biose is not identical with rutinose.

The anhydr substance mp 248° (slight decompn). $[\alpha]_D^{19} -73°$ (0.27 g in 10 ml pyridine). Freely sol in pyridine; sol in hot alcohol, hot acetone; slightly sol in boiling water. The alcoholic soln gives a purple color with ferric chloride.

Trihydrate. Needles from dil alcohol, mp 156-160°. The water of crystn can be removed by drying at 100° over P_2O_5 *in vacuo* for 12 hours.

8719. Sophorose. [534-46-3] 2-*O*-β-D-Glucopyranosyl-α-D-glucose. $C_{12}H_{22}O_{11}$; mol wt 342.30. C 42.11%, H 6.48%, O 51.41%. From pods of *Sophora japonica* L., *Leguminosae:* Rebaté, *Bull. Soc. Chim. Fr.* **7**, 565 (1940); Clancy, *J. Chem. Soc.* **1960**, 4213; Clancy in *Methods in Carbohydrate Chemistry* vol. I, R. L. Whistler, M. L. Wolfrom, Eds. (Academic Press, New York, 1962) pp 345-349. Structure and synthesis: Coxon, Fletcher, *J. Org. Chem.* **26**, 2892 (1961); Koeppen, *Carbohydr. Res.* **7**, 410 (1968). Crystal structure: J. Ohanessian *et al., Acta Crystallogr.* **B34**, 3666 (1978).

Monohydrate. Needles from 80% aq methanol, mp 196-198°. $[\alpha]_D^{18} +19°$ (c = 1.2 in water).

Octa-*O*-acetyl-β-sophorose. $C_{28}H_{38}O_{19}$. Needles from ethanol, mp 193-194°. $[\alpha]_D^{18} -3.2°$ (c = 2.5 in chloroform).

8720. Sorafenib. [284461-73-0] 4-[4-[[[[4-Chloro-3-(trifluoromethyl)phenyl]amino]carbonyl]amino]phenoxy]-*N*-methyl-2-pyridinecarboxamide; *N*-4-(Chloro-3-(trifluoromethyl)phenyl)-*N'*-(4-(2-(*N*-methylcarbamoyl)-4-pyridyloxy)phenyl)urea; Bay-43-9006. $C_{21}H_{16}ClF_3N_4O_3$; mol wt 464.82. C 54.26%, H 3.47%, Cl 7.63%, F 12.26%, N 12.05%, O 10.33%. Multiple kinase inhibitor targeting both RAF kinase and receptor tyrosine kinases that promote angiogensis. Prepn: B. Riedl *et al., WO 0041698* (2000 to Bayer); *eidem, US 03139605* (2003); D. Bankston *et al., Org. Process Res. Dev.* **6**, 777 (2002). Structure-activity study: U. R. Khire *et al., Bioorg. Med. Chem. Lett.* **14**, 783 (2004). Characterization of kinase inhibition: S. M. Wilhelm *et al., Cancer Res.* **64**, 7099 (2004). Mechanism of action study: D. J. Panka *et al., Cancer Res.* **66**, 1611 (2006). LC determn in serum: S. Afify *et al., J. Chromatogr. B* **809**, 99 (2004). Clinical pharmacokinetics: H. Richly *et al., Int. J. Clin. Pharmacol. Ther.* **41**, 620 (2003). Analysis of clinical safety and efficacy: D. Strumberg *et al., Eur. J. Cancer* **42**, 548 (2006). Clinical evaluation and brief review: H. DeGrendele, *Clin. Colorectal Cancer* **3**, 16-18 (2003). Review of clinical development: B. I. Rini, *Expert Opin. Pharmacother.* **7**, 453-461 (2006).

White solid, mp 205.6°.

Tosylate. [475207-59-1] Nexavar. $C_{21}H_{16}ClF_3N_4O_3 \cdot C_7H_8$-$O_3S$; mol wt 637.03.

THERAP CAT: Antineoplastic.

8721. Sorbic Acid. [110-44-1] $(2E,4E)$-2,4-Hexadienoic acid; 2-propenylacrylic acid. $C_6H_8O_2$; mol wt 112.13. C 64.27%, H 7.19%, O 28.54%. $CH_3CH=CHCH=CHCOOH$. May be obtained from berries of the mountain ash, *Sorbus aucuparia* L., *Rosaceae* where it occurs as the lactone, called parasorbic acid: Hofmann, *Ann.* **110**, 129 (1859). Synthesis by condensing crotonaldehyde and malonic acid in pyridine soln: Doebner, *Ber.* **33**, 2140 (1900); Allen, Van Allan, *Org. Synth.* **coll. vol. III**, 783 (1955); by condensing crotonaldehyde and ketene in the presence of boron trifluoride: Hagemeyer, Jr., *Ind. Eng. Chem.* **41**, 768 (1949). Prepn from 1,1,3,5-tetraalkoxyhexane: Parker, MacLean, US **2921090** (1960 to Celanese). Additional syntheses: Fernholz, Mundlos, DE **1049852**; US **3021365** (1959, 1962 both to Hoechst). Prepn of sodium salt: Horn, Fernholz, DE **1045390** (1958 to Hoechst); of calcium salt: C. M. Gooding, US **3139736** (1964 to Corn Products Co.). Purification: Fernholz, DE **1044803** (1958 to Hoechst). The *trans,trans*-isomer is usually obtained and is the commercial product. Toxicity study: Smyth, Carpenter, *J. Ind. Hyg. Toxicol.* **30**, 63 (1948).

Needles from water, mp 134.5°. Should be stored at temps below 40°. bp 228° (dec). Vapor pressure at 20° <0.01 mm, at 143° 50 mm. Flash pt 260°F (127°C). pK (25°) = 4.76. Soly in water at 30° 0.25%, at 100° 3.8%, in propylene glycol at 20° 5.5%, in abs ethanol or methanol 12.90%, in 20% ethanol 0.29%, in glacial acetic acid 11.5%, in acetone 9.2%, in benzene 2.3%, in carbon tetrachloride 1.3%, in cyclohexane 0.28%, in dioxane 11.0%, in glycerol 0.31%, in isopropanol 8.4%, in isopropyl ether 2.7%, in methyl acetate 6.1%, in toluene 1.9%. LD_{50} orally in rats: 7.36 g/kg (Smyth, Carpenter).

USE: Mold and yeast inhibitor. Fungistatic agent for foods, especially cheeses. To improve the characteristics of drying oils. In alkyd type coatings to improve gloss. To improve milling characteristics of cold rubber. *See also* Potassium Sorbate.

8722. Sorbic Alcohol. [111-28-4] 2,4-Hexadien-1-ol; 1-hydroxy-2,4-hexadiene; hexadenol; Hexene-Ol; Hexakose. $C_6H_{10}O$; mol wt 98.14. C 73.43%, H 10.27%, O 16.30%. CH_3-$CH=CHCH=CHCH_2OH$. Prepd from sorbic aldehyde by means of aluminum isopropylate in isopropanol: Reichstein *et al., Helv. Chim. Acta* **15**, 264 (1932).

Long needles. Agreeable odor of new mown grass. mp 30.5-31.5°. bp_{12} ~80°. Volatile with steam. Insol in water. Sol in alcohol, ether, oils. Not stable to air; must be sealed in evacuated ampuls for storage.

Diphenylurethan. $C_{19}H_{19}NO_2$. Crystals from petr ether, mp 78-79°.

3,5-Dinitrobenzoate. Yellowish needles from petr ether, mp 85°.

8723. Sorbinil. [68367-52-2] (4′S)-6-Fluoro-2,3-dihydro-spiro[4H-1-benzopyran-4,4′-imidazolidine]-2′,5′-dione; (+)-(4S)-6-fluorospiro[chroman-4,4′-imidazolidine]-2′,5′-dione; CP-45634. $C_{11}H_9FN_2O_3$; mol wt 236.20. C 55.93%, H 3.84%, F 8.04%, N 11.86%, O 20.32%. Spirohydantoin aldose reductase inhibitor. Prepn of racemate and resolution of isomers: R. Sarges, DE **2821966**; *idem*, US **4130714** (both 1978 to Pfizer). Synthesis: R. Sarges *et al., J. Org. Chem.* **47**, 4081 (1982); N. L. Dirlam *et al., J. Org. Chem.* **52**, 3587 (1987). Absolute configuration: R. Sarges *et al., J. Med. Chem.* **28**, 1716 (1985). Effect on polyol accumulation in diabetic rats: M. J. Peterson *et al., Metabolism* **28**, Suppl. 1, 456 (1979). Pharmacokinetics in humans: G. Foulds *et al., Clin. Pharmacol. Ther.* **30**, 693 (1981). HPLC determn in human lens and plasma: P. Lloyd, M. J. C. Crabbe, *J. Chromatogr.* **343**, 402 (1985). Preliminary clinical trials in diabetic neuropathy: R. J. Young *et al.,*

Diabetes **32**, 938 (1983); J. Jaspan *et al., Lancet* **2**, 758 (1983). Symposium on pharmacology and clinical efficacy: *Metabolism* **35**, Suppl 1, 1-121 (1986).

Crystals from ethanol, mp 241-243°. $[\alpha]_D^{25}$ +54.0° (c = 1 in methanol).

8724. Sorbitan Esters. Sorbitan fatty acid esters; SFAE. Nonionic surface active agents; partial esters of the common fatty acids (lauric, palmitic, stearic, and oleic) and hexitol anhydrides derived from sorbitol. Commercial products may be mixtures of fatty acid esters of 1,4- and 1,5 anhydrosorbitol and 1,4,3,6-dianhydrosorbitol, but generally conform to the structure depicted below. Prepn: K. R. Brown, US **2322820** (1943 to Atlas Powder Co.). Improved process: G. J. Stockburger, US **4297290** (1981 to ICI). Comprehensive description: P. Becher, "Polyol Surfactants" in *Nonionic Surfactants*, M. J. Schick, Ed. (Dekker, New York, 1967) pp 247-299. Description of prepn and uses: L. R. Chislett, J. Walford, *Int. Flavours Food Addit.* **7**, 61 (1976). GLC determn of sorbitan monolaurate in plasma: S. H. Giovanetto, *Anal. Lett.* **16**, 867 (1983). Analysis by HPLC: N. Garti *et al., J. Am. Oil Chem. Soc.* **60**, 1151 (1983). Series of toxicity studies: *Food Cosmet. Toxicol.* **16**, 519-542 (1978). Review: Cosmetic, Toiletry and Fragrance Assoc., *J. Am. Coll. Toxicol.* **4**, 65-121 (1985).

Sorbitan Laurate	R = OOC($C_{11}H_{23}$)
Sorbitan Stearate	R = OOC($C_{17}H_{35}$)
Sorbitan Oleate	R = OOC($C_{17}H_{33}$)

Polyoxyethylene derivatives *see* Polysorbates.

Sorbitan Laurate. [1338-39-2] Sorbitan monolaurate; Alkamuls SML; Arlacel 20; Emsorb 2515; Glycomul L; Span 20. C_{18}-$H_{34}O_6$; mol wt 346.46. Yellow liquid. Acid value: <8. Saponification value: 150-165. Hydroxyl value: 330-360. Sol in mineral oil, cottonseed oil, methanol, ethanol, isopropyl alc, ethylene glycol. Insol in water, propylene glycol.

Sorbitan Stearate. [1338-41-6] Sorbitan monostearate; Alkamuls SMS; Arlacel 60; Glycomul S; Span 60. $C_{24}H_{46}O_6$; mol wt 430.62. White to tan waxy solid, mp 49-65°. Acid value: 5-11. Saponification value: 140-157. Hydroxyl value: 230-260. Sol in alcohols, carbon tetrachloride, toluene. Insol in water, acetone, mineral spirits.

Sorbitan Oleate. [1338-43-8] Sorbitan monooleate; Alkamuls SMO; Arlacel 80; Capmul O; Emsorb 2500; Glycomul O; Span 80. $C_{24}H_{44}O_6$; mol wt 428.60. Yellow to amber colored oily liquid. Acid number: 5-8. Saponification value: 140-160. Hydroxyl value: 193-215. Sol in ethanol, isopropyl alc, mineral oil, vegetable oil. Insol in water, propylene glycol.

USE: use: As emulsifiers, stabilizers, and thickeners in foods, cosmetics, and medicinal products. In the textile industry as fiber lubricants and softeners. Pharmaceutic aid (surfactant).

8725. Sorbitol. [50-70-4] D-Glucitol; D-sorbitol; L-gulitol; sorbit; Resulax; Sorbilax; Sorbo; Sorbostyl; Sorbilande. $C_6H_{14}O_6$; mol wt 182.17. C 39.56%, H 7.75%, O 52.70%. First found in the ripe berries of the mountain ash *Pyrus aucuparia* Ehrh. (L.) (*Sorbus aucuparia* L.), *Rosaceae*. Occurs also in many other berries (except grapes) and in cherries, plums, pears, apples, seaweed and algae. Has been detected in blackstrap molasses. Isoln from berries: Embden, Griesbach, *Z. Physiol. Chem.* **91**, 268 (1914). Prepd industrially from glucose by high pressure hydrogenation or by electrolytic reduction: Boye, *Chem. Ztg.* **82**, 657 (1958); Fedor *et al.*, *Ind. Eng. Chem.* **52**, 282 (1960); from dextrose by catalytic hydrogenation: *Faith, Keyes & Clark's Industrial Chemicals*, F. A. Lowenheim, M. K. Moran, Eds. (Wiley-Interscience, New York, 4th ed., 1975) pp 774-778. Review of uses: Kempf, *Staerke* **6**, 269-274 and 303-306 (1954); **9**, 234-237 (1955).

CH$_2$OH
HC—OH
HO—CH
HC—OH
HC—OH
CH$_2$OH

Needles with ½ or 1H$_2$O. Sweet taste, ~60% as sweet as sugar (w/w). In the healthy human organism 1.0 g of sorbitol yields 3.994 calories which is comparable to 3.940 calories from 1.0 g of cane sugar. Seventy percent of orally ingested sorbitol is converted to CO$_2$ without appearing as glucose in the blood: Adcock, Gray, *Biochem. J.* **65**, 554 (1957). The hydrated crystals melt somewhat below 100°. When completely anhydr mp 110-112°. $[\alpha]_D^{20}$ −2.0° (H$_2$O). In the presence of molybdate the rotation is reversed and increased to +56°. Freely sol in water (up to 83%). High % sorbitol solns are much more viscous than corresp glycerol solns. Quite sol in hot alcohol, sparingly sol in cold alcohol. Also sol in methanol, isopropanol, butanol, cyclohexanol, phenol, acetone, acetic acid, DMF, pyridine, acetamide solns. Practically insol in most other organic solvents. Not attacked in the cold when mixed with dil acids, alkalies or mild oxidizing substances. pKa (17.5°): 13.6. pH about 7.0. A commercial 70% aq soln may have the following characteristics: d_{20}^{20} 1.2879; n_D^{25} 1.45831; $[\alpha]_D^{20}$ −2.10°; bp$_{760}$ 105°; pH between 6 and 7; viscosity (25°): 110 cP. d_4^{20} for various % solns: 5% 1.014; 10% 1.038; 25% 1.099; 50% 1.198; 60% 1.249; 70% 1.299; 83% 1.391. Viscosity in cP at 20°: 5% soln 1.230; 10% 1.429; 25% 2.689; 50% 11.09; 60% 35.73; 70% 185; 83% >10,000.

USE: In manuf of sorbose, ascorbic acid, propylene glycol, synthetic plasticizers and resins; as humectant (moisture conditioner) on printing rolls, in leather, tobacco. In writing inks to insure a smooth flow and to prevent crusting on the point of the pen. In antifreeze mixtures with glycerol or glycols. In candy manuf to increase shelf life by retarding the solidification of sugar; as humectant and softener in shredded coconut and peanut butter; as texturizer in foods; as sequestrant in soft drinks and wines. Used to reduce the undesirable aftertaste of saccharin in foodstuffs; as sugar substitute for diabetics. Pharmaceutic aid (flavor; tablet excipient); to increase absorption of vitamins and other nutrients in pharmaceutical preparations: *Chem. Eng. News* **36**, 59 (Feb. 24, 1958).

THERAP CAT: Laxative.

THERAP CAT (VET): In ruminant ketosis, osmotic diuretic, laxative.

8726. Sorbose. [87-79-6] L-Sorbose; sorbin; sorbinose. C$_6$H$_{12}$O$_6$; mol wt 180.16. C 40.00%, H 6.71%, O 53.28%. From sorbitol by fermentation with *Acetobacter suboxydans*: Perlman, *J. Chem. Educ.* **36**, 60 (1959); Lockwood, *Methods Carbohydr. Chem.* **1**, 151 (Academic Press, New York, 1962).

CH$_2$OH
C=O
HO—CH
HC—OH
HO—CH
CH$_2$OH

Orthorhombic, bisphenoidal crystals. About as sweet as sucrose. d^{15} 1.65. mp 165°. $[\alpha]_D^{30}$ −42.7° (c = 5). pKa (17.5°): 11.55. Freely sol in water; almost insol in alcohol. Reduces Fehling's soln.

USE: In the manuf of vitamin C (accounts for nearly 1000 tons of ascorbic acid produced every year). For conversion of L-sorbose to

2-keto-L-gulonic acid *see* Reichstein, Grüssner, *Helv. Chim. Acta* **17**, 311 (1934).

8727. Sorivudine. [77181-69-2] 1-β-D-Arabinofuranosyl-5-[(1E)-2-bromoethenyl]-2,4(1H,3H)-pyrimidinedione; 1-β-D-arabinofuranosyl-(E)-5-(2-bromovinyl)uracil; 5-bromovinyl-araU; brovavir; BV-araU; BVAU; YN-72; SQ-32756; Usevir. C$_{11}$H$_{13}$BrN$_2$O$_6$; mol wt 349.13. C 37.84%, H 3.75%, Br 22.89%, N 8.02%, O 27.50%. Orally active antiviral agent; inhibits viral DNA synthesis. Prepn: H. Machida, S. Sakata, **EP 31128**; *eidem*, **US 4386076** (1981, 1983 both to Yamassa Shoyu); S. Sakata *et al.*, *Nucleic Acids Symp. Ser.* **8**, s39 (1980); R. Busson *et al.*, *ibid.* **9**, 49 (1981). Antiviral activity and toxicity: H. Machida, S. Sakata, *Antiviral Res.* **4**, 135 (1984). Mechanism of action studies: T. Yokota *et al.*, *Mol. Pharmacol.* **36**, 312 (1989); H. Machida, *Adv. Exp. Med. Biol.* **278**, 255 (1990). Clinical trial in herpes zoster infection: M. Niimura, *ibid.* 267.

mp 182° (Sakata, 1980); also reported as white crystals from ethanol, mp 195-200° (dec) (Machida, Sakata, 1983). $[\alpha]_D^{25}$ +0.5° (1N NaOH). LD$_{50}$ in mice (mg/kg): ~3300 i.p.; >5000 s.c.; >10000 orally (Machida, Sakata, 1984).

THERAP CAT: Antiviral.

8728. Sotalol. [3930-20-9] N-[4-[1-Hydroxy-2-[(1-methylethyl)amino]ethyl]phenyl]methanesulfonamide; 4'-[1-hydroxy-2-(isopropylamino)ethyl]methanesulfonanilide. C$_{12}$H$_{20}$N$_2$O$_3$S; mol wt 272.36. C 52.92%, H 7.40%, N 10.29%, O 17.62%, S 11.77%. β-Adrenergic blocker. Prepn: Uloth *et al.*, *J. Med. Chem.* **9**, 88 (1966). Pharmacology and toxicology: Larsen, Lish, *Nature* **203**, 1283 (1964); Lish *et al.*, *J. Pharmacol. Exp. Ther.* **149**, 161 (1965); Stanton *et al.*, *ibid.* 175; Kvam *et al.*, *ibid.* 183. Activity of the d- and l-forms: Somani, Watson, *ibid.* **164**, 317 (1968); Somani, Bachand, *Eur. J. Pharmacol.* **7**, 239 (1969). HPLC determn in body fluids: W. P. Gluth *et al.*, *Arzneim.-Forsch.* **38**, 408 (1988). Review of pharmacology and therapeutic use: B. N. Singh *et al.*, *Drugs* **34**, 311-349 (1987); S. H. Hohnloser, R. L. Woosley, *N. Engl. J. Med.* **331**, 31-38 (1994). Comprehensive description: R. T. Foster, R. A. Carr, *Anal. Profiles Drug Subs. Excip.* **21**, 501-533 (1992).

Crystals. uv max (chloroform): 242.2, 275.2 nm. pK$_1$ 8.2, pK$_2$ 9.8.

Hydrochloride. [959-24-0] MJ-1999; Beta-Cardone; Betapace; Darob; Sotacor; Sotalex. C$_{12}$H$_{20}$N$_2$O$_3$S.HCl; mol wt 308.82. White crystalline solid, mp 206.5-207° (dec), also reported as mp 218-219° (Singh). Freely sol in water; slightly sol in chloroform. Partition coefficient (water/n-octanol): 0.24; (octan-1-ol/pH 7.4 phosphate buffer) at 37°: 0.09. LD$_{50}$ in male mice, rats (mg/kg): 2600, 3450 orally; 670, 680 i.p.; LD$_{50}$ orally in rabbits: 1000 mg/kg; LD$_{50}$ i.p. in dogs: 330 mg/kg (Lish).

THERAP CAT: Antianginal; antiarrhythmic (class II + III); antihypertensive.

8729. Soterenol. [13642-52-9] N-[2-Hydroxy-5-[1-hydroxy-2-[(1-methylethyl)amino]ethyl]phenyl]methanesulfonamide; 2'-hydroxy-5'-[1-hydroxy-2-(isopropylamino)ethyl]methanesulfonanilide; MJ-1992. C$_{12}$H$_{20}$N$_2$O$_4$S; mol wt 288.36. C 49.98%, H

6.99%, N 9.71%, O 22.19%, S 11.12%. β-Adrenergic agonist. Prepn: Larsen *et al.*, *J. Med. Chem.* **10**, 462 (1967). Pharmacological study: K. W. Dungan *et al.*, *J. Pharmacol. Exp. Ther.* **164**, 290 (1968).

Monohydrochloride. [14816-67-2] $C_{12}H_{20}N_2O_4S$·HCl. Crystals from methanol-isopropyl ether, mp 195.5-196.5° (dec). LD_{50} (7 day) in mice (mg/kg): 41 i.v.; 315 i.p.; 660 orally (Dungan).

THERAP CAT: Bronchodilator.

8730. Soybean. Soya bean; soja bean; Lincoln bean; Manchurian bean; Chinese pea. Seed of *Glycine max* (L.) Merrill [*G. soja* Sieb. & Zucc., *G. hispida* (Moench) Maxim., *Soja hispida* Moench], *Leguminosae. Habit.* Eastern Asia, especially Manchuria. Cultivated in the midwestern U.S.A., Brazil, some European countries, such as Italy and Yugoslavia. *Constit.* Proteins 40%, carbohydrates 17%, oil 18%, ash 4.6%. The ash content equals K 1.67%, Na 0.34%, Ca 0.28%, Mg 0.22%, Cl 0.024%, I 0.000054%, Fe 0.0097%, Cu 0.0012%, Mn 0.0028%, Zn 0.0022%, P 0.66%, S 0.41%, Al 0.0007%. The chief proteins are glycinin, a globulin, phaseolin, another globulin, and 2 albumins: legumelin and soy legumelin. The carbohydrates are sucrose, raffinose, stachyose, and pentosans. Phosphorus compds (about 3%) are phospholipids, nucleic acid phosphates, phytin, and inorganic phosphates. The phospholipids contain lecithin, cephalin, and inositol. The vitamin content is moderate: Vitamin A 110 i.u./100g; thiamine 1.14 mg/100 g; riboflavin 0.31 mg/100 g; niacin 2.1 mg/100 g; ascorbic acid: trace. Food energy: 350 cal/100 g. Amino acid analysis of the protein fraction: Glutamic acid 18.4%, leucine 8.1%, arginine 7.5%, lysine 6.7%, valine 5.4%, isoleucine 5.3%, phenylalanine 5.2%, threonine 3.9%, histidine 2.3%, tryptophan 1.6%, methionine 1.4%. Ten kg of soybeans yield 15 g of the isoflavone glycoside genistin, the mother liquor contains daidzin. Soybeans contain a small amount of enzymes such as lipoxidase, urease, uricase, protease, antienzymes such as antitrypsin, and a growth-inhibiting factor. Bitter principles and saponins are also found. *Reviews:* K. S. Markley, *Soybeans and Soybean Products,* 2 vols. (Interscience, New York, 1951); Cowan in *Kirk-Othmer Encyclopedia of Chemical Technology* vol. **18** (Interscience, New York, 2nd ed., 1969) pp 599-614.

Whitish or yellowish-green to brownish-black, ovoid beans, about 8 mm long, 7 mm wide, and 6 mm thick. Most varieties have a wt of 20 g/100 seeds.

USE: In the production of soybean oil. As food and feedstuff. Debittered soybean flour contains practically no starch and is widely used in dietetic foods. Soybean meal obtained after expressing the oil is a preferred source of protein for feedstuffs. Other products are soybean lecithin, genistin, monosodium glutamate, soybean milk, soy sauce; *tofu,* a soybean curd; *miso,* a fermented mixture with barley or rice; *natto,* which is soybean cheese. Soybean proteins are used also in the adhesive and plastics industries.

THERAP CAT: Nutrient.

8731. Soybean Oil. Obtained from soybeans by solvent extraction using petroleum hydrocarbons or, to a lesser extent, by expression using continuous screw press operations. *Constit.* Triglycerides of oleic acid 26%, of linoleic acid 49%, of linolenic acid 11%, of saturated acids 14%. Free fatty acids are usually less than 1%. Phospholipids (lecithin) 1.5-4%. Another 0.8% consists of stigmasterol, sitosterols, and tocopherols. The phospholipids and sterols are removed by refining with alkali. Reviews and bibliographies: K. S. Markley, *Soybeans and Soybean Products,* 2 vols. (Interscience, New York, 1951); E. W. Eckey, *Vegetable Fats and Oils* (Reinhold, New York, 1954); W. J. Wolf in *Kirk-Othmer Encyclopedia of Chemical Technology* vol. **21** (Wiley-Interscience, New York, 3rd ed., 1983) pp 417-442.

Pale yellow to brownish-yellow oil. Slight characteristic odor and taste. The flavor of crude soybean oil has been described as paint-like and grass-like, and is somewhat distasteful to the palate of occidentals. d_{25}^{25} 0.916-0.922. Flash pt 540°F (282°C). Ignition

temp 833°F (445°C). n_D^{25} 1.471-1.475. Titer 22-27. Solidifies at −10 to −16°. Viscosity (cP): 172.9 (0°); 99.7 (10°); 50.09 (25°); 28.86 (40°). Acid value 0.3-3.0. Saponification value 189-195. Iodine value 127-138. Thiocyanogen value 77-85. Diene no. 0.7. Hydroxyl value 4-8. Reichert-Meissl value 0.2-0.7. Polenske value 0.2-1.0. Miscible with abs alcohol, ether, petr ether, chloroform, carbon disulfide.

USE: Directly as food in the Orient, also in blends with olive oil. In the manuf of margarine, shortenings, candy, soap. In drying oil industries (paints, varnishes, linoleum, printing ink). The foots or residue from refining has been used to obtain soybean fatty acids which can be used in the manuf of alkyd resins.

8732. Soy Sauce. Soy sauce is a hydrolysis product of soybeans. A combination of mold fermentation and acid hydrolysis is used. The molds employed are *Aspergillus flavus, A. niger,* and *A. oryzae.* Soy sauce consists of a mixture of amino acids, peptides, polypeptides, peptones, simple proteins, purines, carbohydrates, and lesser organic compds suspended in an 18% sodium chloride soln. Adenine, arginine, choline, lysine, betaine, and glutamic acid have been isolated. In the manuf of soy sauce, during the fermentation process, 60-70% of the vitamins present in soybeans are destroyed. Review and bibliography: K. S. Markley, *Soybeans and Soybean Products,* 2 vols. (Interscience, N.Y., 1951).

8733. Spandex. Lycra; Vyrene. An elastic, segmented polyurethane fiber obtained by the interaction of a diisocyanate with a glycol. The term "segmented" indicates that it is made from a block copolymer in which reasonably long flexible chains are joined to shorter stiff chains through the urethane linkages. *Ref: Mod. Text. Mag.* **40**, 38 (Dec. 1959); Hicks Jr., *Am. Dyest. Rep.* **52**, no. 1, 33 (1963). Book: Moncrieff, *Man-Made Fibres* (Heywood, London, 4th ed., 1963) pp 396-403. *See:* **US 2692873** (1954 to du Pont) and **US 2751363** (1956 to U.S. Rubber). Compare also Smith, **US 3061574**; Frazer, Shivers **US 3071557** (1962, 1963 to du Pont). Historical review of industrial production with extensive patents list: L. Rose, *Rep. Prog. Appl. Chem.* **51**, 609-612 (1966). Monograph: M. McDonald, *Spandex Manufacture* (Noyes, Park Ridge, N.J., 1970) 190 pp.

All linkages are hydrolytically stable to acids, alkalies.

Caution: Can cause allergic contact dermatitis if any diisocyanate is present as impurity.

USE: Snap-back fiber, stronger and lighter than rubber. Used mainly for elastic garments such as belts, girdles, corsets, brassieres, garters, surgical stockings and sock tops. Can be used bare, giving lighter fabrics and eliminating the costly covering process needed for rubber.

8734. Sparassol. [520-43-4] 2-Hydroxy-4-methoxy-6-methylbenzoic acid methyl ester; 4-methoxy-2,6-cresotic acid methyl ester; everninic acid methyl ester; orsellinic acid methyl ester 4-methyl ether. $C_{10}H_{12}O_4$; mol wt 196.20. C 61.22%, H 6.16%, O 32.62%. Antibiotic substance produced by the fungus *Sparassis ramosa:* Falck, *Ber.* **56**, 2555 (1923). Also obtained in methanol extracts of the lichen *Evernia prunasti:* Stenhouse, *Ann.* **68**, 55 (1848); Späth, Jeschki, *Ber.* **57**, 471 (1924). Structure: Fischer, Hoesch, *Ann.* **391**, 347 (1912); Wedekind, Fleischer, *Ber.* **56**, 2556 (1923). Synthesis: G. Nicollier *et al., Helv. Chim. Acta* **61**, 2899 (1978).

Prisms from water, mp 67-68°. Slightly sol in hot water; freely sol in acetone, ether, chloroform; moderately sol in methanol, ethanol, petr ether. Alkaline hydrolysis yields free everninic acid, mp 170°.

8735. Sparfloxacin. [110871-86-8] *rel*-5-Amino-1-cyclopropyl-7-[(3*R*,5*S*)-3,5-dimethyl-1-piperazinyl]-6,8-difluoro-1,4-dihydro-4-oxo-3-quinolinecarboxylic acid; AT-4140; CI-978; PD-131501; Spara; Zagam. $C_{19}H_{22}F_2N_4O_3$; mol wt 392.40. C 58.16%, H 5.65%, F 9.68%, N 14.28%, O 12.23%. Fluorinated quinolone antibacterial. Prepn: J. Matsumoto *et al.,* **EP 221463**; *eidem,* **US 4795751** (1987, 1989 both to Dainippon). Synthesis and structure-activity relationship: T. Miyamoto *et al., J. Med. Chem.* **33**, 1645 (1990). Antibacterial activity: S. Nakamura *et al., Antimicrob. Agents Chemother.* **33**, 1167 (1989). Comparative *in vitro* antimicrobial spectrum: T. Kojima *et al., ibid.* 1980. Pharmacokinetics: S. Nakamura *et al., ibid.* **34**, 89 (1990). Subacute toxicity studies: M. Yasuba *et al., Chemotherapy* **39**, Suppl. 4, 180 (1991), *C.A.* **115**, 247561d (1991); M. Iida *et al., ibid.* 195, *C.A.* **115**, 247562e (1991).

Crystals from chloroform + ethanol, mp 266-269° (dec). pKa$_1$ 6.25, pKa$_2$ 9.30.

THERAP CAT: Antibacterial.

8736. Sparsomycin. [1404-64-4] (2*E*)-*N*-[(1*S*)-1-(Hydroxymethyl)-2-[(*R*)-[(methylthio)methyl]sulfinyl]ethyl]-3-(1,2,3,4-tetrahydro-6-methyl-2,4-dioxo-5-pyrimidinyl)-2-propenamide; (*E*)-(1*S*)-1,2,3,4-tetrahydro-*N*-[1-(hydroxymethyl)-2-[[(methylthio)methyl]sulfinyl]ethyl]-6-methyl-2,4-dioxo-5-pyrimidine-acrylamide; (+)-sparsomycin; NSC-59729; U-19183. $C_{13}H_{19}N_3O_5S_2$; mol wt 361.44. C 43.20%, H 5.30%, N 11.63%, O 22.13%, S 17.74%. Protein synthesis inhibitor with antibiotic and antitumor activity. Isoln from fermentation broth of *Streptomyces sparsogenes* var *sparsogenes*: S. P. Owen *et al., Antimicrob. Agents Chemother.* **1962**, 772; **GB 974541** (1964 to Upjohn); from *S. cuspidosporus*: E. Higashide *et al., Takeda Kenkyusho Nempo* **25**, 1 (1966), *C.A.* **66**, 54238q (1967). Characterization and purification: A. D. Argoudelis, R. R. Herr, *Antimicrob. Agents Chemother.* **1962**, 780. Structural elucidation: P. F. Wiley, F. A. MacKellar, *J. Org. Chem.* **41**, 1858 (1976). Total synthesis: H. C. J. Ottenheijm *et al., ibid.* **46**, 3273 (1981); R. M. J. Liskamp *et al., ibid.* 5408. HPLC determn in plasma and urine: B. Winograd *et al., J. Chromatogr.* **275**, 145 (1983). Pharmacokinetics and toxicology: Z. Zylicz *et al., Cancer Chemother. Pharmacol.* **20**, 115 (1987). Ribosomal binding studies: E. Lazaro *et al., Antimicrob. Agents Chemother.* **35**, 10 (1991). Biosynthetic studies: R. J. Parry *et al., J. Am. Chem. Soc.* **114**, 5946 (1992). Review of chemistry and biological activity: H. C. J. Ottenheijm *et al., Prog. Med. Chem.* **23**, 220-268 (1986).

Crystals, mp 208-209° (dec). $[\alpha]_D^{25}$ +69° (c = 0.5 in water). pKa' 8.67 in water, 9.05 in 40% ethanol. uv max: 302 nm (water or 0.1*N* aq sulfuric acid), 328 nm (0.1*N* aq potassium hydroxide). Slightly sol in water and lower alcohols. Insol in less polar organic solvents. LD$_{50}$ in dogs, rats, mice (mg/kg): 0.5-1.0, 2.25, 4.32 i.v. (Ottenheijm, 1986). LD$_{50}$ i.p. in mice: 2.4 mg/kg (Owen).

USE: Research tool for studying protein biosynthesis.

8737. Sparteine. [90-39-1] [7*S*-(7α,7aα,14α,14aβ)]-Dodecahydro-7,14-methano-2*H*,6*H*-dipyrido[1,2-*a*:1',2'-*e*][1,5]diazocine; *l*-sparteine; lupinidine. $C_{15}H_{26}N_2$; mol wt 234.38. C 76.87%, H 11.18%, N 11.95%. In yellow and black lupin beans, *Lupinus luteus* L. and *L. niger* Hort.; also in *Cytisus scoparius* (L.) Link. and *Anagyris foetida* L., *Leguminosae.* Extraction procedure: Karrer *et al., Helv. Chim. Acta* **11**, 1062 (1928). Structure: Clemo *et al., J. Chem. Soc.* **1931**, 429; Ing, *ibid.* **1933**, 504; Schirm, Besendorf, *Arch. Pharm.* **280**, 64 (1942); Galinovsky, Stern, *Ber.*

77B, 132 (1944); Clemo *et al., J. Chem. Soc.* **1949**, 663. Biosynthesis: Anet *et al., Nature* **165**, 35 (1950); Schöpf *et al., Angew. Chem.* **65**, 161 (1953); **69**, 69 (1957); van Tamelen, Foltz, *J. Am. Chem. Soc.* **82**, 2400 (1960). Absolute configuration: Okuda *et al., Chem. Ind. (London)* **1961**, 1116. Conformation: Bohlmann *et al., Tetrahedron Lett.* **1965**, 2705; Wiewiorowski *et al., Can. J. Chem.* **45**, 1447 (1967). Synthesis of racemate: Bohlmann *et al., Ber.* **106**, 3026 (1973); N. Takatsu *et al., Chem. Pharm. Bull.* **35** 4990 (1987). Chemistry: Binnig, *Arzneim.-Forsch.* **24**, 752 (1974). Studies of cardiovascular effects: Raschak, *ibid.* 753.

Viscous, oily liquid. bp$_8$ 173°. Volatile with steam. $[\alpha]_D^{21}$ −16.4° (c = 10 in abs alc). n_D^{20} 1.5312. d$_4^{20}$ 1.020. pK$_1$ at 20°: 2.24; pK$_2$: 9.46; pH of 0.01 molar soln 11.6. One gram dissolves in 325 ml water. Freely sol in alcohol, chloroform or ether.

Sulfate pentahydrate. [6160-12-9] Depasan; Tocosamine. $C_{15}H_{26}N_2.H_2SO_4.5H_2O$; mol wt 422.54. Columnar crystals, loses water of crystn at 100° turning brown, dec 136°. pH of 0.05 molar soln 3.3. One gram dissolves in 1.1 ml water, 3 ml alcohol. Practically insol in chloroform and ether.

l-α-**Isosparteine.** [446-95-7] Genisteine (alkaloid). 14aα-stereoisomer. Isoln from *Cytisus scoparius* (L.) Link, (*Spartium scoparium* L.), *Leguminosae:* Valeur, *Compt. Rend.* **167**, 23, 163 (1918); from *Lupinus caudatus* Kellog, *Leguminosae:* Marion *et al., Can. J. Chem.* **29**, 22 (1951). Identity as stereoisomer: Marion, Leonard, *ibid.* 297. Structure: Leonard *et al., J. Am. Chem. Soc.* **77**, 1552 (1955). Absolute configuration: Okuda, Tsuda, *Chem. Ind. (London)* **1961**, 1115. Monohydrate, needles from boiling acetone, mp 108-110°. $[\alpha]_D^{22}$ −51.6° (c = 0.7 in abs. ethanol).

THERAP CAT: In treatment of cardiac insufficiency.

8738. Spearmint. Green mint; curled mint. Hardy perennial herb, *Mentha spicata* L., *Labiatae.* Medicinal portions include the dried leaves and tops and essential oil. *Habit.* Mediterrean region; cultivated in U.S. and Europe. *Constit.* Volatile oil (0.8-2.5%), flavonoids incl. thymonin. Botanical description and medicinal uses: J. Gruenwald *et al., PDR for Herbal Medicines* (Medical Economics, Montvale, 2nd Ed., 2000) pp 709-710. Extraction of volatile constituents and effect of drying method: M. C. Diaz-Maroto *et al., J. Agric. Food Chem.* **51**, 1265 (2003).

Volatile oil. [8008-79-5] Oil of spearmint. Obtained by steam distillation of flowering tops. *Constit.* Primarily carvone (~50%), (−)-limonene, 1,8-cineole. Colorless, yellow or greenish-yellow liq; characteristic spearmint odor and taste. d$_{25}^{25}$ 0.917-0.934. α_D^{20} −48 to −59°. n_D^{20} 1.484-1.491. Very slightly sol in water; sol in equal vol 80% alcohol. *Keep well closed, cool and protected from light.*

Spirit of spearmint. An alcoholic soln contg per liter 100 ml oil of spearmint and the alcohol-soluble principles from 10 g coarsely powdered spearmint leaves previously macerated with water.

USE: As flavor in foods, dental products, chewing gum, pharmaceuticals.

THERAP CAT: Carminative.

8739. Spectinomycin. [1695-77-8] [2*R*-(2α,4aβ,5aβ,6β,-7β,8β,9α,9aα,10aβ)]-Decahydro-4a,7,9-trihydroxy-2-methyl-6,8-bis(methylamino)-4*H*-pyrano[2,3-*b*][1,4]benzodioxin-4-one; actinospectacin; espectinomicina; CHX-3101; M-141. $C_{14}H_{24}N_2O_7$; mol wt 332.35. C 50.59%, H 7.28%, N 8.43%, O 33.70%. Antibiotic isolated from fermentation broth of *Streptomyces spectabilis:* D. J. Mason *et al., Antibiot. Chemother.* **11**, 118 (1961); M. E. Bergy *et al., ibid.* 661; M. E. Bergy, C. De Boer, **US 3234092** (1966 to Upjohn). Purification and crystallization: H. K. Jahnke, **US 3206360**; V. J. Peters, **US 3272706** (1965, 1966 both to Upjohn). Isoln and characterization: A. C. Sinclair, A. F. Winfield, *Antimicrob. Agents Chemother.* **1961**, 503. Structure: H. Hoeksema *et al., J. Am. Chem. Soc.* **84**, 3212 (1962); P. F. Wiley *et al., ibid.* **85**, 2652 (1963). Solubility data: J. R. Marsh, P. J. Weiss, *J. Assoc. Off. Anal. Chem.* **50**, 457 (1967). Stereochemistry and abs config:

T. G. Cochran *et al., Chem. Commun.* **1972,** 494. Biosynthesis: L. A. Mitscher *et al., ibid.* **1971,** 1541; H. Otsuka *et al., J. Am. Chem. Soc.* **102,** 6817 (1980). Enantioselective synthesis: D. R. White *et al., Tetrahedron Lett.* **1979,** 2737; S. Hanessian, R. Roy, *Can. J. Chem.* **63,** 163 (1985). Mechanism of action study: M. F. Brink *et al., Nucleic Acids Res.* **22,** 325 (1994). HPLC determn in animal plasma: N. Haagsma *et al., J. Chromatogr.* **615,** 289 (1993). Clinical pharmacokinetics: J. G. Wagner *et al., Int. Z. Klin. Pharmakol. Ther. Toxikol.* **1,** 261 (1968). Clinical evaluation in gonorrhea: Y. H. Kouri *et al., Genitourin. Med.* **65,** 342 (1989); in chancroid: M. Guzmán *et al., Sex. Transm. Dis.* **19,** 291 (1992). Co-treatment with lincomycin, *q.v.,* for footrot in sheep: C. M. Venning *et al., Aust. Vet. J.* **67,** 258 (1990). *Reviews:* W. M. McCormack, M. Finland, *Ann. Intern. Med.* **84,** 712-716 (1976); W. J. Holloway, *Med. Clin. North Am.* **66,** 169-173 (1982).

Amorphous powder. $[\alpha]_D^{25}$ $-20°$ (water). pKa'$_1$ 6.95, pKa'$_2$ 8.70. Sol in water, methanol, ethanol. Insol in acetone, hydrocarbon solvents.

Dihydrochloride pentahydrate. [22189-32-8] Spectam; Stanilo; Trobicin. $C_{14}H_{24}N_2O_7.2HCl.5H_2O$; mol wt 495.35. Exists as a ketone hydrate and not in the carbonyl form (Cochran *et al.*). Colorless needles from aq acetone, mp 205-207° (dec). $[\alpha]_D$ +14.8° (c = 0.42 in water). Soly in water, methanol, propylene glycol, formamide, DMSO, 0.1N NaOH, 0.1N HCl: >20 mg/ml. Soly (mg/ml): chloroform 0.042; acetone 0.015; diethyl ether 0.010.

Sulfate tetrahydrate. [64058-48-6] $C_{14}H_{24}N_2O_7.H_2SO_4$.-$4H_2O$. White crystals from aq acetone, mp ~185° (dec). $[\alpha]_D^{25}$ +17.0° (c = 1 in water). pKa'$_1$ 7.00, pKa'$_2$ 8.75. Soly in water, DMSO: 225, 5-10 (mg/ml). Practically insol in pyridine, chloroform, ethanol, ethyl acetate, cyclohexane, benzene, acetone, DMF, dioxane, acetonitrile.

THERAP CAT: Antibacterial.

THERAP CAT (VET): Antibacterial.

8740. Spectrin. Tektin A. Major protein component of the membrane cytoskeleton of mammalian and avian erythroid cells. Responsible for maintaining the normal shape, strength and stability of the erythrocyte. A ubiquitous family of proteins, spectrin analogs have also been isolated from a variety of non-erythroid cells. Given the name spectrin because of its original isolation from hemoglobin-free red cell membranes known as erythrocyte "ghosts": V. T. Marchesi, E. Steers, *Science* **159,** 203 (1968). Comparison with actin, *q.v.:* E. Steers, V. Marchesi, *J. Gen. Physiol.* **54,** 65 S (1969). Isoln from human red cells and species comparison: T. W. Tillack *et al., Biochim. Biophys. Acta* **200,** 125 (1970). Spectrin is a heterodimer composed of 2 high mol wt polypeptide subunits referred to as band 1 or α-spectrin (mol wt ~240 kDa) and band 2 or β-spectrin (mol wt ~220 kDa). Structural studies: M. Clarke, *Biochem. Biophys. Res. Commun.* **45,** 1063 (1971); T. L. Steck, *J. Cell Biol.* **62,** 1 (1974); J. M. Anderson, *J. Biol. Chem.* **254,** 939 (1979); D. W. Speicher *et al., ibid.* **257,** 9093 (1982). The β-subunit of spectrin is bound to the red cell membrane by proteins known as *ankyrin:* V. Bennett, P. J. Stenbuck, *ibid.* **254,** 2533 (1979); or *syndeins:* J. Yu, S. R. Goodman, *Proc. Natl. Acad. Sci. USA* **76,** 2340 (1979). The spectrin heterodimers aggregate on the membrane surface and, together with actin and other proteins, form a filamentous network that covers the surface of the cytoplasmic membrane: S. E. Lux, *Nature* **281,** 426 (1979); *idem, Semin. Hematol.* **16,** 21 (1979). Identification of spectrin analogs from nonerythroid cells: S. R. Goodman *et al., Proc. Natl. Acad. Sci. USA* **78,** 7580 (1981). Isoln of *fodrin,* also known as brain or neural cell spectrin: J. Levine, M. Willard, *J. Cell Biol.* **90,** 631 (1981); V. Bennett *et al., Nature* **299,** 126 (1982). Isoln of *TW 260/240,* a spectrin analog from chicken intestinal epithelial cells: J. R. Glenney *et al., Cell* **28,** 843 (1982). Comparison of erythroid and nonerythroid spectrins: J. R. Glenney *et al., Proc. Natl. Acad. Sci. USA*

79, 4002 (1982); J. R. Glenney, P. Glenney, *Eur. J. Biochem.* **144,** 529 (1984). Review of erythrocyte spectrin: S. R. Goodman, K. Shiffer, *Am. J. Physiol.* **244,** C121-C141 (1983); of neural cell spectrin: S. R. Goodman, I. S. Zagon, *ibid.* **250,** C347-C360 (1986). Comprehensive review: S. R. Goodman *et al., Crit. Rev. Biochem.* **23,** 171-234 (1988).

8741. Spermaceti. Cetaceum; Spermwax. A waxy substance from the head of the sperm whale. *Constit.* Chiefly cetyl palmitate; free cetyl alcohol present in appreciable amounts; esters of lauric, stearic, and myristic acids; esters of higher alcohols also present.

White, somewhat translucent, slightly unctuous masses with crystalline fracture and pearly luster; almost odorless and tasteless but becomes yellow and rancid on long exposure to air. d 0.938-0.944; mp 42-50°; n_D^{80} ~1.4330. Sapon no. 120-136. Iodine no. 3-4.4. Insol in water or cold alcohol. Sol in chloroform, ether, carbon disulfide, oils, boiling alcohol; slightly sol in petr ether.

USE: As a base for ointments, cerates, etc., and as emulsion with egg yolk or expressed almond oil. In manuf of candles, soaps, cosmetics, laundry wax; finishing and lustering linens. Emollient.

8742. Spermidine. [124-20-9] *N*-(3-Aminopropyl)-1,4-butanediamine; *N*-(γ-aminopropyl)tetramethylenediamine. $C_7H_{19}N_3$; mol wt 145.25. C 57.88%, H 13.18%, N 28.93%. $NH_2(CH_2)_4$-$NH(CH_2)_3NH_2$. Biogenic polyamine formed from putrescine; a precursor of spermine, *q.q.v.* First detected in human sperm, but occurs widely in nature. Essential for both normal and neoplastic tissue growth. Synthesis: H. W. Dudley *et al., Biochem. J.* **20,** 1082 (1926); **21,** 97 (1927); J. V. Braun, W. Pinkernelle, *Ber.* **70,** 1234 (1937); M. Danzig, H. P. Schultz, *J. Am. Chem. Soc.* **74,** 1836 (1952). For reviews of the early literature, *see* M. Guggenheim, *Die biogenen Amine* (S. Karger, Basel, 4th ed., 1951) 619 pp; H. Tabor *et al., Annu. Rev. Biochem.* **30,** 579-604 (1961). Role in cell growth processes: C. W. Tabor, H. Tabor, *ibid.* **45,** 285 (1976); J. Janne *et al., Biochim. Biophys. Acta* **473,** 241 (1978); C. W. Porter, R. J. Bergeron, *Science* **219,** 1083 (1983). Formation and interconversion of spermidine and putrescine in mammalian cells: A. E. Pegg *et al., Adv. Enzyme Regul.* **19,** 427 (1980). Effect on polypeptide chain elongation *in vitro:* A. K. Abraham, A. Pihl, *Eur. J. Biochem.* **106,** 257 (1980). Regulation of tRNA methyltransferase activity: M. Mach *et al., Biochem. J.* **202,** 153 (1982). HPLC study: C. E. Prussak, D. H. Russell, *J. Chromatogr.* **229,** 47 (1982). Interaction with actin, *q.v.:* C. Oriol-Audit, *Biochem. Biophys. Res. Commun.* **105,** 1096 (1982). Studies on use as a biochemical tool in cancer research: A. Thyss *et al., Eur. J. Cancer Clin. Oncol.* **18,** 611 (1982); V. Quemener *et al., J. Nat. Prod.* **45,** 608 (1982); C. W. Porter *et al., Cancer Res.* **42,** 4072 (1982). Toxicity study: P. R. Langford *et al., J. Antibiot.* **35,** 1387 (1982). *Reviews:* T. C. Theoharides, *Life Sci.* **27,** 703-713 (1980); O. Heby, *Differentiation* **19,** 1-20 (1981); L. Stevens, *Med. Biol.* **59,** 308-313 (1981). Book: *Polyamines in Biology and Medicine,* D. R. Morris, L. J. Marton, Eds. (Dekker, New York, 1981) 512 pp.

Liq, bp$_{14}$ 128-130°. Sol in water, ethanol, ether.

Trihydrochloride. $C_7H_{22}Cl_3N_3$. Cryst from ethanolic HCl (65:2). mp 256-258°.

USE: As a tool in biochemical research.

8743. Spermine. [71-44-3] *N,N'*-Bis(3-aminopropyl)-1,4-butanediamine; *N,N'*-bis(3-aminopropyl)tetramethylenediamine; gerontine; musculamine. $C_{10}H_{26}N_4$; mol wt 202.34. C 59.36%, H 12.95%, N 27.69%. $H_2N(CH_2)_3NH(CH_2)_4NH$-$(CH_2)_3NH_2$. Biogenic polyamine formed from spermidine, *q.v.,* and occurring in almost all tissues. Essential for both normal and neoplastic tissue growth. First observed in human semen and described as the cryst phosphate salt by A. von Leeuwenhoek, *Philos. Trans. R. Soc. London* **12,** 1040 (1678). For a description of the history, occurrence, formation, and early prepns of spermine, *see Beilstein* **vol. IV,** Suppl. 1, 704; M. Guggenheim, *Die biogenen Amine* (S. Karger, Basel, 4th ed., 1951) 619 pp; H. Tabor *et al., Annu. Rev. Biochem.* **30,** 579-604 (1961). Prepn of spermine and its tetrahydrochloride: Israel *et al., J. Med. Chem.* **7,** 710 (1964). Role in cell growth processes: C. W. Tabor, H. Tabor, *Annu. Rev. Biochem.* **45,** 285 (1976); J. Janne *et al., Biochim. Biophys. Acta* **473,** 241 (1978). Modulation of calcium-dependent immune processes: T. C. Theoharides, *Life Sci.* **27,** 703 (1980). Biosynthesis in fungi:

L. Stevens, *Med. Biol.* **59**, 308 (1981). HPLC study: C. E. Prussak, D. H. Russell, *J. Chromatog.* **229**, 47 (1982). Use as a biochemical marker for malignant tumors: Y. Horn *et al.*, *Cancer Res.* **42**, 3248 (1982). Metabolic study: A. E. Pegg *et al.*, *Biochemistry* **21**, 5082 (1982). Review of role in cell proliferation and differentiation: O. Heby, *Differentiation* **19**, 1-20 (1981). Book: *Polyamines in Biology and Medicine* D. R. Morris, L. J. Marton, Eds. (Dekker, New York, 1981) 512 pp.

Needles, mp 55-60°. Liq, bp$_{0.5}$ 141-142°. Strong base, absorbs carbon dioxide from air. *Keep well closed.* Sol in water, lower alcohols, chloroform. Practically insol in ether, benzene, petr ether.

Diphosphate hexahydrate. Spermine phosphate. $C_{10}H_{32}N_4 \cdot O_8P_2 \cdot 6H_2O$. Cryst from water, mp 230-234° (dec). Soly in water: 0.037% at 20°; 1% at 100°. Insol in alc, ether and other organic solvents. Sol in dilute acids and alkali. Known as **Charcot-Neumann crystals**, also found in spleen, blood, bone marrow in leukemia and secretions in asthma.

Tetrahydrochloride. $C_{10}H_{30}Cl_4N_4$. Cryst from ethanol, mp 312-314.5°.

USE: As a tool in biochemical research.

8744. Sperm Oil. From sperm whale. *Constit.* Esters of fatty acids; small quantities of spermaceti.

Yellow, thin liquid; slight fishy odor if not of good quality. d 0.875-0.884. Sapon no. 123-147. Iodine no. 80-84. Insoluble in water, cold alcohol, or petr ether; sol in chloroform, ether.

USE: As lubricant, in lamps, hardening steel, manuf soap.

8745. Sphingofungins. Family of six antifungal agents, sphingofungins A-F, isolated from *Aspergillus fumigatus* of which sphingofungin C is the most abundant. Specific inhibitors of serine palmitoyltransferase. Isoln and charaterization of sphingofungins A-D: F. VanMiddlesworth *et al.*, *J. Antibiot.* **45**, 861 (1992); of sphingofungins E-F: W. S. Horn *et al.*, *ibid.* 1692. Stereochemistry of A-D: F. VanMiddlesworth *et al.*, *Tetrahedron Lett.* **33**, 297 (1992). Mechanism of action: M. M. Zweerink *et al.*, *J. Biol. Chem.* **267**, 25032 (1992). Synthesis of D: K. Mori, K. Otaka, *Tetrahedron Lett.* **35**, 9207 (1994); and stereochemistry of E: B. Wang *et al.*, *Synlett* **2001**, S1 904.

Sphingofungin C

Sphingofungin C. [121025-46-5] 5-(Acetyloxy)-2-amino-3,4,14-trihydroxy-6-eicosenoic acid. $C_{22}H_{41}NO_7$; mol wt 431.56. Cream colored solid.

8746. Sphingomyelins. Rowamyelin. Sphingosine phosphatides occurring in the myelin sheaths of nerves. Prepn of beef heart sphingomyelin: Rapport, Lerner, *J. Biol. Chem.* **232**, 63 (1958). Isoln from human and rat brain: Hausheer *et al.*, *Helv. Chim. Acta* **46**, 601 (1963). Structure: Fujino, *J. Biochem. (Tokyo)* **39**, 45 (1952); Rouser *et al.*, *J. Am. Chem. Soc.* **75**, 310 (1953); Marinetti *et al.*, *ibid.* 313. Structure of honey bee (*Apis mellifera*) sphingomyelin: Karlander *et al.*, *Biochim. Biophys. Acta* **270**, 117 (1972). Synthesis of dihydrosphingomyelins: Shapiro *et al.*, *J. Am. Chem. Soc.* **80**, 2339 (1958). Synthesis of sphingomyelins: Shapiro *et al.*, *ibid.* **81**, 3743, 4360 (1959). Configuration: Shapiro, Flowers, *ibid.* **84**, 1047 (1962). Monograph: S. R. Korey, *The Biology of Myelin* (Hoeber-Harper, New York, 1959).

R = different fatty acids such as stearic, palmitic, lignoceric, nervonic acids.

Slightly hygroscopic powder. Occurs as a hydrate. Sol in hot abs alcohol, acetic acid, chloroform; slightly sol in pyridine. Practically insol in ether, acetone, water.

8747. Sphingosine. [123-78-4] (2*S*,3*R*,4*E*)-2-Amino-4-octadecene-1,3-diol; (*E*)-D-*erythro*-4-octadecene-1,3-diol; 1,3-dihydroxy-2-amino-4-octadecene; 4-sphingenine. $C_{18}H_{37}NO_2$; mol wt 299.49. C 72.19%, H 12.45%, N 4.68%, O 10.68%. Important membrane component; long-chain amino-dialcohol; moiety of certain phosphatides, such as sphingomyelins, cerebrosides, and gangliosides. Natural sphingosine is D-(+)-*erythro*-1,3-dihydroxy-2-amino-4-*trans*-octadecene. Does not exist in the free state in animals, plants or microorganisms. First obtained by hydrolysis of cerebrosides from brains: J. L. W. Thudichum, *Die Konstitution des Gehirns des Menschen und der Tiere* (Tübingen, 1901). Separation procedures: Carter *et al.*, *J. Biol. Chem.* **170**, 269 (1947); Wittenberg, *ibid.* **216**, 379 (1955); Tipton, *Biochem. Prep.* **9**, 127 (1962). Stereospecific synthesis of DL-*erythro-trans*-form and isomers: C. A. Grob, F. Gadient, *Helv. Chim. Acta* **40**, 1145 (1957). Stereoselective synthesis: H. Newman, *J. Am. Chem. Soc.* **95**, 4098 (1973); B. Bernet, A. Vasella, *Tetrahedron Lett.* **24**, 5491 (1983). Comprehensive review: C. A. Grob, *Record Chem. Progr. (Kresge-Hooker Sci. Lib.)* **18**, 55-66 (1957); D. Shapiro, *Chemistry of Sphingolipids* (Hermann, Paris, 1969) 111 pp. Bibliography: *Rodd's Chemistry of Carbon Compounds* **Vol. I**, part E, S. Coffey, Ed. (Elsevier, New York, 2nd ed., 1976) pp 394-397.

DL-Sphingosine. Waxy crystals from ether + pentane, mp 67°.

DL-Triacetylsphingosine. $C_{24}H_{43}NO_5$. Crystals from pentane + ether, mp 91-92°.

Triacetyl derivative of natural sphingosine. $C_{24}H_{43}NO_5$. Crystals, mp 101-102°. $[\alpha]_D^{25}$ −11.7° (chloroform).

8748. Spigelia. Pinkroot; Indian pink; Carolina pink; Maryland pink; wormgrass. Dried rhizome and roots of *Spigelia marilandica* L., *Loganiaceae*. *Habit.* North America (New Jersey to Florida and west to Wisconsin). *Constit.* Spigeline, resin, tannin, bitter principle, volatile oil.

THERAP CAT: Anthelmintic.

8749. α-Spinasterol. [481-18-5] (3*β*,5*α*,22*E*)-Stigmasta-7,22-dien-3-ol; α-spinasterin; bessisterol; hitodesterol. $C_{29}H_{48}O$; mol wt 412.69. C 84.40% H 11.72%, O 3.88%. Stereoisomeric with chondrillasterol, *q.v.* Extracted from spinach leaves: Hart, Heyl, *J. Biol. Chem.* **95**, 311 (1932); from *Citrullus colocynthis* Schrad., *Cucurbitaceae*: Hamilton, Kermack, *J. Chem. Soc.* **1952**, 5051. Structure: Fieser *et al.*, *J. Am. Chem. Soc.* **71**, 2226 (1949). Prepn: Kircher, Rosenstein, *J. Org. Chem.* **38**, 2259 (1973); M. Anastasia *et al.*, *J. Chem. Soc. Perkin Trans. 1* **1981**, 2561.

Crystals from alcohol + light petr, mp 168-169°. $[\alpha]_D^{25}$ −3.6° (c = 2.8 in chloroform).

Benzoate. $C_{36}H_{52}O_2$. Plates from ethyl acetate, mp 200°. $[\alpha]_D^{25}$ +1.8° (c = 1.7 in chloroform).

8750. Spinosyns. [131929-60-7] Class of fermentation derived 12 membered macrocyclic lactones in a unique tetracyclic ring. At least 20 spinosyns have been isolated from *Saccharopoly-*

spora spinosa; variations in the two sugars account for most of the structural and insecticidal activity differences. Isolation and biological activity: L. D. Boeck *et al.*, **EP 375316** (1990 to Lilly); *eidem*, **US 5496931** (1996 to DowElanco); and structure determn: H. A. Kirst *et al.*, *Tetrahedron Lett.* **32**, 4839 (1991). Soil degradation: K. A. Hale, D. E. Portwood, *J. Environ. Sci. Health* **B31**, 477 (1996). HPLC determn in vegetables: L.-T. Yeh *et al.*, *J. Agric. Food Chem.* **45**, 1746 (1997); in soil and water: S. D. West, *ibid.* 3107. Uptake and metabolism in larvae: T. C. Sparks *et al.*, *Proc. Beltwide Cotton Conf.* **2**, 1259 (1997). Mode of action study: V. L. Salgado *et al.*, *Pestic. Biochem. Physiol.* **60**, 103 (1998). Review of physical and biological properties: C. V. De-Amicis *et al.*, *ACS Symp. Ser.* **658**, 144-154 (1997). *Review:* G. D. Crouse, T. C. Sparks, *Rev. Toxicol.* **2**, 133-146 (1998).

Spinosyn A   R = H
Spinosyn D   R = CH₃

Spinosyn A. (2*R*,3a*S*,5a*R*,5b*S*,9*S*,13*S*,14*R*,16a*S*,16b*R*)-2-[(6-Deoxy-2,3,4-tri-*O*-methyl-α-L-mannopyranosyl)oxy]-13-[[(2*R*,5*S*,6*R*)-5-(dimethylamino)tetrahydro-6-methyl-2*H*-pyran-2-yl]oxy]-9-ethyl-2,3,3a,5a,5b,6,9,10,11,12,13,14,16a,16b-tetradecahydro-14-methyl-1*H*-*as*-indaceno[3,2-*d*]oxacyclododecin-7,15-dione; lepicidin A; A-83543A; LY-232105. $C_{41}H_{65}NO_{10}$; mol wt 731.96. Total synthesis: L. A. Paquette *et al.*, *J. Am. Chem. Soc.* **120**, 2553 (1998). White, odorless crystalline solid, mp 118°. pKa 8.1. uv max (methanol): 243 nm (ε 11000). $[\alpha]_D^{27}$ −262.7° (methanol). Vapor pressure: 2.4×10^{-10}. Soly in water (ppm): 290 (pH 5), 235 (pH 7), 16 (pH 9), distilled 20. Soly (w/v%): methanol 19, acetone 17, dichloromethane >50, hexane 0.45%. LD_{50} in rats (mg/kg): 3783-5000 orally (Crouse).

Spinosyn D. [131929-63-0] A-83543D. $C_{42}H_{67}NO_{10}$; mol wt 745.98. Odorless, white crystalline solid. mp 169°. pKa 7.8. uv max (methanol): 243 nm (ε 11000). $[\alpha]_D^{27}$ −297.5° (methanol). Vapor pressure: 2.0×10^{-10}. Soly in water (ppm): 28 (pH 5), 0.329 (pH 7), 0.04 (pH 9), distilled 1.3. Soly (w/v%): methanol 0.25, acetone 1.0, dichloromethane 45, hexane 0.07%.

Spinosad. [168316-95-8] XDE-105; DE-105; Conserve; Justice; Naturalyte; SpinTor; Success; Tracer. Mixture of spinosyns A and D. Effect on beneficial insects: D. Murray, R. Lloyd, *Australian Cottongrower* **18**, 62 (1997). Light grey to white crystals (tech). LD_{50} in rats, mallard ducks, quail (mg/kg): >3600, >2000, >2000 orally (Crouse).

USE: Insecticide.

8751. Spiperone. [749-02-0] 8-[4-(4-Fluorophenyl)-4-oxobutyl]-1-phenyl-1,3,8-triazaspiro[4.5]decan-4-one; 8-[3-(*p*-fluorobenzoyl)propyl]-1-phenyl-1,3,8-triazaspiro[4.5]decan-4-one; 4-phenyl-8-[3-(4-fluorobenzoyl)propyl]-1-oxo-2,4,8-triazaspiro[4.5]decane; Spiropitan. $C_{23}H_{26}FN_3O_2$; mol wt 395.47. C 69.85%, H 6.63%, F 4.80%, N 10.63%, O 8.09%. Prepn: Janssen, **US 3155669**; **US 3155670** and **US 3161644** (all 1964 to Janssen).

Crystals, mp 190-193.6°.
THERAP CAT: Antipsychotic.

8752. Spiramycin. [8025-81-8] RP-5337; Selectomycin; Rovamicina; Rovamycin. Antibiotic substance classified in the erythromycin-carbomycin group and produced by *Streptomyces ambofaciens* from soil of northern France: Cosar *et al.*, *C.R. Seances Soc. Biol. Ses Fil.* **234**, 1498 (1952); Pinnert-Sindico *et al.*, *Antibiot. Annu.* **1954-1955**, 724; Ninet, Verrier, **US 2943023** (1960 to Rhône-Poulenc), *see also* **US 3000785** (1961 to Rhône-Poulenc). Antibacterial activity and toxicity: H. Sous *et al.*, *Arzneim.-Forsch.* **8**, 386 (1958). Separation into 3 components named spiramycin I, II and III: Preud'homme, Charpentier, **US 2978380** and **US 3011947** (1961 to Rhône-Poulenc). Structure: Kuehne, Benson, *J. Am. Chem. Soc.* **87**, 4660 (1965). Revised structure: Omura *et al.*, *ibid.* **91**, 3401 (1969); Mitscher *et al.*, *J. Antibiot.* **26**, 55 (1973). Revised configuration at C-9: Freiberg *et al.*, *J. Org. Chem.* **39**, 2474 (1974). Symposium on pharmacology, antibacterial spectrum, and clinical efficacy: *J. Antimicrob. Chemother.* **22**, Suppl. B, 1-213 (1988).

Spiramycin I   R = H
Spiramycin II   R = COCH₃
Spiramycin III   R = COCH₂CH₃

Amorphous base, slightly sol in water. $[\alpha]_D^{20}$ −80° (methanol). uv max (ethanol): 231 nm. Sol in most organic solvents. Active on gram-positive bacteria and rickettsiae. Cross resistance between microorganisms resistant to erythromycin and carbomycin. LD_{50} in rats (mg/kg): 9400 orally; 1000 s.c.; 170 i.v. (Sous).

Embonate. Spira 200.

Hexanedioate. Spiramycin adipate; Stomamycin; Suanovil.

Spiramycin I. [24916-50-5] Foromacidin A. $C_{43}H_{74}N_2O_{14}$; mol wt 843.05. Crystals, mp 134-137°. $[\alpha]_D^{20}$ −96°.

Spiramycin I triacetate. Crystals, mp 140-142°. $[\alpha]_D^{20}$ −92.5°.

Spiramycin II. [24916-51-6] Foromacidin B. $C_{45}H_{76}N_2O_{15}$; mol wt 885.09. Crystals, mp 130-133°. $[\alpha]_D^{20}$ −86°.

Spiramycin II diacetate. Crystals from cyclohexane, mp 156-160°. $[\alpha]_D^{20}$ −98.4°.

Spiramycin III. [24916-52-7] Foromacidin C. $C_{46}H_{78}N_2O_{15}$; mol wt 899.12. Crystals, mp 128-131°. $[\alpha]_D^{20}$ −83°.

Spiramycin III diacetate. Crystals from cyclohexane, mp 140-142°. $[\alpha]_D^{20}$ −90.4°.

THERAP CAT: Antibacterial.
THERAP CAT (VET): Antibacterial; growth promotant.

8753. Spirapril. [83647-97-6] (8*S*)-7-[(2*S*)-2-[[(1*S*)-1-(Ethoxycarbonyl)-3-phenylpropyl]amino]-1-oxopropyl]-1,4-dithia-7-azaspiro[4.4]nonane-8-carboxylic acid; (8*S*)-7-[(*S*)-*N*-[(*S*)-1-carboxy-3-phenylpropyl]alanyl]-1,4-dithia-7-azaspiro[4.4]nonane-8-carboxylic acid 1-ethyl ester. $C_{22}H_{30}N_2O_5S_2$; mol wt 466.61. C 56.63%, H 6.48%, N 6.00%, O 17.14%, S 13.74%. Angiotensin-converting enzyme (ACE) inhibitor. Prepn: E. H. Gold *et al.*, **US 4470972** (1984 to Schering); E. M. Smith *et al.*, *J. Med. Chem.* **32**, 1600 (1989). Pharmacology: E. J. Sybertz *et al.*, *Arch. Int. Pharmacodyn. Ther.* **286**, 216 (1987); T. Baum *et al.*, *ibid.* 230. Radioimmunoassay in plasma: M. Hossein-Nia *et al.*, *Ther. Drug Monit.* **14**, 234 (1992). Pharmacokinetics and evaluation in CHF: S. A. J. van den Broek *et al.*, *J. Cardiovasc. Pharmacol.* **18**, 614 (1991). Clinical evaluation in essential hypertension: G. P. Reams *et al.*, *J. Clin. Pharmacol.* **33**, 348 (1993). *Review:* P. Jerie, H.-J. Kremer, *Cor Vasa* **34**, 82-87 (1992).

Consult the Name Index before using this section.

Hemihydrate. White foam. $[\alpha]_D^{26}$ −29.5° (c = 0.2 in ethanol).
Hydrochloride. [94841-17-5] Sch-33844; TI-211-950; Renormax; Renpress; Sandopril. $C_{22}H_{30}N_2O_5S_2$.HCl; mol wt 503.07. White solid, mp 192-194° (dec). $[\alpha]_D^{26}$ −11.2° (c = 0.4 in ethanol).
Diacid. [83602-05-5] Spiraprilat; spiraprilic acid; Sch-33861. $C_{20}H_{26}N_2O_5S_2$; mol wt 438.56. Hemihydrate, mp 163-165°. $[\alpha]_D^{26}$ +4.1° (c = 0.4 in ethanol).
THERAP CAT: Antihypertensive.

8754. Spirit of Ammonia, Aromatic. [8013-59-0] Spirit of hartshorn, aromatic. A soln contg 34 g ammonium carbonate, 90 ml 10% ammonia water, 10 ml lemon oil, 1 ml oil of lavender, 1 ml oil of myristica, 700 ml alcohol and a sufficient quantity of water to make 1 liter. Absolute alc by vol, ~66%.
Almost colorless to slightly yellow liquid with an aromatic, pungent odor and the taste of ammonia. d 0.90. Forms an opalescent mixture with water; miscible with alcohol.
THERAP CAT: Reflex respiratory stimulant.
THERAP CAT (VET): By inhalation: respiratory and circulatory stimulant. Internally: expectorant, diaphoretic, antacid, carminative. Externally: counterirritant, and in diluted form to relieve the irritation of insect stings and bites.

8755. Spirit of Ether. [8013-43-2] Hoffmann's drops. A mixture of alcohol and ether. Made by mixing 325 ml ether U.S.P. with sufficient U.S.P. alcohol (~690 ml) to make 1000 ml. Absolute alc by vol, ~66%.
Colorless, volatile liquid. d 0.785.
THERAP CAT: Carminative.

8756. Spirit of Ether Compound. [8013-44-3] Hoffmann's anodyne. A mixture of 325 ml ether U.S.P., 25 ml ethereal oil and sufficient alcohol (~665 ml) to make 1000 ml. Absolute alc by vol, ~64%.
Colorless, clear liquid. d ~0.785.
THERAP CAT: Carminative.
THERAP CAT (VET): Has been used as a stomachic, carminative, in colic.

8757. Spirodiclofen. [148477-71-8] 2,2-Dimethylbutanoic acid 3-(2,4-dichlorophenyl)-2-oxo-1-oxaspiro[4,5]dec-3-en-4-yl ester; BAJ2740; Envidor. $C_{21}H_{24}Cl_2O_4$; mol wt 411.32. C 61.32%, H 5.88%, Cl 17.24%, O 15.56%. Tetronic acid acaricide for use in fruit, grapevines and nuts. Prepn: R. Fischer et al., **DE 4216814**; *eidem*, **US 5262383** (both 1993 to Bayer). Comprehensive description of properties and activity: U. Wachendorff et al., *BCPC Conf. - Pests Dis.* **2000**, 53. Greenhouse trials vs spider mites: R. Nauen et al., *ibid.* 453.

White powder, mp 101-108°. Log P (n-octanol/water): 5.8 (pH 4 at 20°). Vapor pressure (20°): 3×10^{-7} Pa. Soly in water (pH 4): 50 µg/l at 20°. LD_{50} in rats (mg/kg): >2500 orally; >2000 dermally (24 hr). LC_{50} (4 hr) in rats (mg/m³): >5000 by inhalation; LC_{50} (96 hr) in fish: >68 mg/l (Wachendorff).
USE: Acaricide.

8758. Spirogermanium. [41992-23-8] 8,8-Diethyl-N,N-dimethyl-2-aza-8-germaspiro[4.5]decane-2-propanamine; 2-[3-(dimethylamino)propyl]-8,8-diethyl-2-aza-8-germaspiro[4.5]decane. $C_{17}H_{36}GeN_2$; mol wt 341.12. C 59.86%, H 10.64%, Ge 21.29%, N 8.21%. Cytostatic germanium deriv. Prepn: L. M. Rice, **DE 2243550**; *idem*, **US 3825546** (1973, 1974 both to Geschickter Fund for Med. Res.); L. M. Rice et al., *J. Heterocycl. Chem.* **11**, 1041 (1974). Toxicology study: M. C. Henry et al., *Preclinical Toxicologic Evaluation* (PB-264117, 1977) 213 pp. Metabolism study: D. Garteiz et al., *Drug Metab. Dispos.* **19**, 44 (1991). Clinical evaluation: P. S. Schein et al., *Cancer Treat. Rep.* **64**, 1051 (1980); C. Tropie et al., *ibid.* **65**, 119 (1981). Toxicity study: M. C. Henry et al., *ibid.* **64**, 1207 (1980).

Oil, bp$_{0.03}$ 106-109°.
Dihydrochloride. [41992-22-7] NSC-192965; Spiro-32. $C_{17}H_{36}GeN_2$.2HCl; mol wt 414.04. Crystals, mp 287-288°. LD_{50} in rats (mg/kg): 75 i.p.; in mice (mg/kg): 150 i.p., 324 orally (Rice et al.). LD_{50} in male, female mice (mg/kg): 44.5, 41.5 i.v.; 142.9, 119 i.m. (Henry, 1980).
THERAP CAT: Antineoplastic.

8759. Spiromesifen. [283594-90-1] 3,3-Dimethyl butanoic acid 2-oxo-3-(2,4,6-trimethylphenyl)-1-oxaspiro[4.4]non-3-en-4-yl ester; 3-(2,4,6-trimethylphenyl)-4-neopentylcarbonyloxy-5,5-tetramethylene-Δ^3-dihydrofuran-2-one; BSN-2060; Oberon. $C_{23}H_{30}O_4$; mol wt 370.48. C 74.56%, H 8.16%, O 17.27%. Tetronic acid acaricide and whitefly insecticide for use in cotton, vegetables and ornamentals. Prepn: R. Fischer et al., **EP 528156**; *eidem*, **US 5262383** (both 1993 to Bayer); *see also*: U. Wachendorff-Neumann, **US 6436988** (2002 to Bayer). Review of properties and activity: R. Nauen et al., *BCPC Conf. - Pests Dis.* **2002**, 39-44. Series of articles on discovery, properties, ecological profile, and field trials: *Pflanzenschutz-Nachr. Bayer* **58**, 307-502 (2005).

White solid, mp 98°. d²⁰ 1.13. Log P (n-octanol/water): 4.55 (pH 2 and 7.5). Vapor pressure (20°): 7×10^{-6} Pa. Soly in water: 0.13 mg/ml. LD_{50} in rats (mg/kg): >2500 orally; >2000 dermally (24 hr); LC_{50} (4 hr) in rats (mg/m³): >4873 by inhalation (Nauen).
USE: Insecticide.

8760. Spironolactone. [52-01-7] (7α,17α)-7-(Acetylthio)-17-hydroxy-3-oxopregn-4-ene-21-carboxylic acid γ-lactone; 17-hydroxy-7α-mercapto-3-oxo-17α-pregn-4-ene-21-carboxylic acid γ-lactone, acetate; 3-(3-oxo-7α-acetylthio-17β-hydroxy-4-androsten-17α-yl)propionic acid γ-lactone; SC-9420; Aldactone; Aquareduct; Practon; Osyrol; Sincomen; Spirobeta; Spiroctan; Spirolone; Spironone; Verospiron; Xenalon. $C_{24}H_{32}O_4S$; mol wt 416.57. C 69.20%, H 7.74%, O 15.36%, S 7.70%. Aldosterone antagonist. Prepn: Cella, Tweit, *J. Org. Chem.* **24**, 1109 (1959); **US 3013012** (1961 to Searle); Tweit et al., *J. Org. Chem.* **27**, 3325 (1962). Activity and metabolic studies: Gerhards, Engelhardt, *Arzneim.-Forsch.* **13**, 972 (1963). Crystal and molecular structure: Dideberg, Dupont, *Acta Crystallogr.* **B28**, 3014 (1972). Comprehensive description: J. L. Sutter, E. P. K. Lau, *Anal. Profiles Drug Subs.* **4**, 431-451 (1975). Review of carcinogenetic risk: *IARC Monographs* **24**, 259-273 (1980). Review of antiandrogen effects and clinical use in hirsutism: R. R. Tremblay, *Clin. Endocrinol. Metab.* **15**, 363-371 (1986); of clinical efficacy in hypertension: A. N. Brest, *Clin. Ther.* **8**, 568-585 (1986). Review of pharmacology: H. A. Skluth, J. G. Gums, *DICP Ann. Pharmacother.* **24**, 52-59

(1990). Clinical trial in congestive heart failure: B. Pitt *et al.*, *N. Engl. J. Med.* **341**, 709 (1999).

Crystals from methanol, mp 134-135° (resolidifies and dec 201-202°). [α]$_D^{20}$ −33.5° (chloroform). uv max: 238 nm (ε 20200). Practically insol in water. Sol in alcohol; freely sol in benzene, chloroform. LD$_{50}$ in rats, mice, rabbits (mg/kg): 790, 360, 870 i.p. (IARC, 1980).

THERAP CAT: Diuretic.

THERAP CAT (VET): Diuretic.

8761. Spiroxamine. [118134-30-8] 8-(1,1-Dimethylethyl)-*N*-ethyl-*N*-propyl-1,4-dioxaspiro[4.5]decane-2-methanamine; KWG-4168; Impulse. C$_{18}$H$_{35}$NO$_2$; mol wt 297.48. C 72.67%, H 11.86%, N 4.71%, O 10.76%. Spiroketalamine fungicide for use on cereal crops; inhibits ergosterol synthesis. Prepn: W. Kraemer *et al.*, **DE 3735555**; *eidem*, **US 4851405** (1988, 1989 both to Bayer). Mode of action and field trials: S. Dutzmann *et al.*, *Brighton Crop Prot. Conf. - Pests Dis.* **1996**, 47. Series of articles on chemistry, activity, determn and ecobiology: *Pflanzenschutz-Nachr.* **50**, 5-98 (1997).

Colorless liquid, mixture of stereoisomers. bp 120° at 0.067 hPa. n$_D^{20}$ 1.4662. Log P (*n*-octanol/water): <3. pKa: 6.9. Soly in acetone, acetonitrile, dichlormethane, *n*-hexane, 2-propanol, toluene, water (pH 3): all >200 g/l at 20°. LD$_{50}$ in rats (mg/kg): ~595 orally; >1600 dermally. LC$_{50}$ in rats (mg/m³): ~2772 by inhalation; LC$_{50}$ (96 hr) in rainbow trout: 18.5 mg/l (Dutzmann).

USE: Agricultural fungicide.

8762. Splendipherin. [149152-95-4] Caerin 2.3. First reported aquatic sex pheromone from frogs or toads; specific for the magnificent tree frog, *Litoria splendida*. 25 L-amino acid peptide produced by males to attract females. Isoln from skin secretions of *Litoria caerula* as one of the hypotensive caerin peptides: D. J. M. Stone *et al.*, *J. Chem. Res. Synop.* **1993**, 138; from *L. splendida* and identification of pheromonal activity: P. A. Wabnitz *et al.*, *Nature* **401**, 444 (1999). Seasonal distribution and specificity of effect: *eidem, Eur. J. Biochem.* **267**, 269 (2000).

1
Gly–Leu–Val–Ser–Ser–Ile–Gly–Lys–Ala–Leu–Gly
25 |
                                                  Gly
Ala–Pro–Gln–Gly–Lys–Ser–Lys–Val–Val–Asp–Ala–Leu–ˈLeu

8763. Splenin. [1416-60-0] Thymopoietin III; SP. Polypeptide hormone of the spleen which induces differentiation and maturation of both T- and B-cell precursors. Originally detected by its cross reactivity with thymopoietin, *q.v.*, in radioimmunoassay. Human splenin (hSP) contains 48 amino acids; bovine splenin (bSP) contains 49. *Splenopentin*, a pentapeptide corresponding to residues 32-36, exhibits full bioactivity. The amino acid sequence of splenin is highly homologous with that of thymopoietin; the differences in bioactivity are attributed to a single amino acid substitution at position 34. Unlike the thymic hormone, splenin exhibits no neuromuscular effects. Isoln from bovine spleen and complete amino acid sequence: T. Audhya *et al.*, *Biochemistry* **20**, 6195 (1981). Synthesis: T. Abiko *et al.*, *Chem. Pharm. Bull.* **34**, 2133 (1986). Isoln and sequence of human splenin: T. Audhya *et al.*, *Proc. Natl. Acad. Sci. USA* **84**, 3545 (1987). Biological activities of

bSP and comparison with thymopoietin: T. Audhya *et al.*, *ibid.* **81**, 2847 (1984). Effect on antibody production *in vivo*: W. Diezel *et al.*, *Biomed. Biochim. Acta* **45**, 1349 (1986). Effect of hSP on B-cell number *in vitro*: T. Abiko, H. Sekino, *Chem. Pharm. Bull.* **37**, 391 (1989).

Arg–Lys–Ala–Val–Tyr

Human Splenopentin

Note: The term, splenin, formerly referred to a crude mixture of bioactive substances extracted from mammalian spleen: G. Ungar, *Endocrinology* **37**, 329 (1945).

8764. Sporidesmins. Toxic fungal mixture from *Pithomyces chartarum* Ellis (*Sporidesmium bakeri* Sydow), composed of sporidesmins A-H and J, as causative agent of "facial eczema" in sheep. First isoln of A (major metabolite): R. L. M. Synge, E. P. White, *Chem. Ind. (London)* **1959**, 1546. Isoln of A and B: J. W. Ronaldson *et al.*, *J. Chem. Soc. C* **1963**, 3172. Structure of A: J. Fridrichsons, A. M. Mathieson, *Tetrahedron Lett.* **1962**, 1265. Abs config of A: A. F. Beecham *et al.*, *ibid.* **1966**, 3131. Isoln and structure of D and F: W. D. Jamieson *et al.*, *J. Chem. Soc. C* **1969**, 1564; of E: R. Rahman *et al.*, *ibid.* 1665; of G: E. Francis *et al.*, *J. Chem. Soc. Perkin Trans. 1* **1972**, 470; of H and J: R. Rahman *et al.*, *ibid.* **1978**, 1476. Total synthesis of A: Y. Kishi *et al.*, *J. Am. Chem. Soc.* **95**, 6493 (1973).

Sporidesmin A

Sporidesmin A. [1456-55-9] (3α,5aα,10bα,11β,11aα)-9-Chloro-2,3,5a,6,10b,11-hexahydro-10b,11-dihydroxy-7,8-dimethoxy-2,3,6-trimethyl-3,11a-epidithio-11a*H*-pyrazino[1′,2′:1,5]pyrrolo[2,-3-*b*]indole-1,4-dione; sporidesmin. C$_{18}$H$_{20}$ClN$_3$O$_6$S$_2$; mol wt 473.95. Colorless needles with a faint green sheen, from aq methanol, mp 179° (dependent on rate of heating). [α]$_D^{20}$ −45° (c = 0.98 in methanol). uv max: 219, 253, 305 nm (E$_{1cm}^{1\%}$ 700, 220, 40). Very slightly sol in water, light petroleum, CCl$_4$. Readily sol in most organic solvents.

8765. Sporidesmolides. Cyclodepsipeptides containing both D and L amino acids, isolated from the pasture fungus *Sporidesmium bakeri* Syd. (*Pithomyces chartarum* (Berk. & Curt.) Ellis): D. W. Russell, *Biochim. Biophys. Acta* **45**, 411 (1960); W. S. Bertaud *et al.*, *J. Gen. Microbiol.* **32**, 385 (1963); E. Bishop, D. W. Russell, *Biochem. J.* **92**, 19P (1964).

cyclo–Hiv–Val–MeLeu–Hiv–D-Val–D-Leu

Sporidesmolide I

Hiv = α-hydroxyisovaline

Sporidesmolide I. [2900-38-1] C$_{33}$H$_{58}$N$_4$O$_8$; mol wt 638.84. Structure: D. W. Russell, *J. Chem. Soc.* **1962**, 753. Synthesis: M. M. Shemyakin *et al.*, *Tetrahedron* **19**, 995 (1963). Biosynthetic study: D. W. Russell, *Biochim. Biophys. Acta* **261**, 469 (1972). MS determn: B. C. Das *et al.*, *J. Antibiot.* **32**, 569 (1979). Needles from 70% acetic acid, mp 261-263°. [α]$_D^{17}$ −217° (c = 1.5 in chloroform). Practically insol in water; very sol in chloroform; sparingly sol in other common organic solvents.

Sporidesmolide II. [3200-75-7] 2-D-Alloisoleucine sporidesmolide I. C$_{34}$H$_{60}$N$_4$O$_8$; mol wt 652.86. Structure and synthesis: M. M. Shemyakin *et al.*, *Tetrahedron Lett.* **1963**, 1927. Crystals, mp 228-230°. [α]$_D^{20}$ −195° (c = 0.6 in chloroform).

Sporidesmolide III. [1803-67-4] 6-L-Leucine sporidesmolide I. C$_{32}$H$_{56}$N$_4$O$_8$; mol wt 624.81. Synthesis: Y. A. Ovchinnikov *et al.*, *ibid.* **1965**, 1111. Crystals, mp 277-278°. [α]$_D$ −80° (c = 1.6 in acetic acid).

Sporidesmolide IV. [10252-34-3] 4-(4-Methyl-L-2-hydroxy-pentanoic acid) sporidesmolide I. $C_{34}H_{60}N_4O_8$; mol wt 652.86. Structure and synthesis: A. A. Kiryushkin *et al., ibid.* **1965**, 143; E. Bishop, D. W. Russell, *J. Chem. Soc. C* **1967**, 634. Crystals, mp 227-228°. $[\alpha]_D$ −195° (c = 1 in chloroform). Practically insol in water, sol in chloroform, moderately sol in common organic solvents.

8766. Squalamine. [148717-90-2] (3β,5α,7α)-3-[[3-((4-Aminobutyl)amino)propyl]amino]-cholestane-7,24-diol 24-hydrogen sulfate; 3β-(N-[3-aminopropyl]-1,4-butanediamine)-7α,24ζ-dihydroxy-5α-cholestane 24-sulfate; 3β-N-1-[N-[3-(4-aminobutyl)]-1,3-diaminopropane]-7α,24ζ-dihydroxy-5α-cholestane 24-sulfate. $C_{34}H_{67}N_3O_5S$; mol wt 629.98. C 64.82%, H 10.72%, N 6.67%, O 12.70%, S 5.09%. Broad-spectrum aminosterol antibiotic present in shark tissues; novel indication for steroid as vertebrate host-defense agent. Isoln from the stomach of the spiny dogfish shark, *Squalus acanthias*: M. Zasloff *et al.,* US 5192756 (1993 to Children's Hospital of Penn.). Structural determn and antimicrobial activity: K. S. Moore *et al., Proc. Natl. Acad. Sci. USA* **90**, 1354 (1993). NMR spectral studies: S. L. Wehrli *et al., Steroids* **58**, 370 (1993). Synthesis of trihydrochloride: R. M. Moriarty *et al.,* WO 9419366 (1994 to Magainin Pharm.).

Sol in water.

8767. Squalane. [111-01-3] 2,6,10,15,19,23-Hexamethyltetracosane; perhydrosqualene; dodecahydrosqualene; spinacane; Cosbiol; Robane; Wax-O-Sol. $C_{30}H_{62}$; mol wt 422.81. C 85.22%, H 14.78%. [$(CH_3)_2CHCH_2CH_2CH_2CH(CH_3)CH_2CH_2$-$CH_2CH(CH_3)CH_2CH_2$—]$_2$. Prepn by complete hydrogenation of squalene, *q.v.*: Chapman, *J. Chem. Soc.* **123**, 770 (1923); Heilbron *et al., ibid.* **1926**, 3135. Commercial grades are obtained by direct hydrogenation of shark liver oil and may contain some batyl alcohol: Tsujimoto, *Chem. Umschau Fette* **34**, 256 (1927), *C.A.* **21**, 4081 (1927). Synthesis: J. W. Scott, D. Valentine, *Org. Prep. Proced. Int.* **12**, 7 (1980); T. Mandai *et al., Tetrahedron Lett.* **22**, 763 (1981). Oil. Stable to air and oxygen. d_4^{15} 0.8115. mp ~−38°. bp_{760} ~350°; bp_{10} 263°; bp_5 248°. Flash pt 425°F (218°C). n_D^{15} 1.4530. Specific heat at 20° ~0.62. Viscosity (Engler) at 20° ~6.08. Readily sol in ether, gasoline, petr ether, benzene, chloroform, oils. Slightly sol in methanol, ethanol, acetone, glacial acetic acid. Concd H_2SO_4 at 70° is discolored, but the squalane remains unchanged.

USE: Lubricant, transformer oil. Ingredient of watch and chronometer oils. Perfume fixative. In pharmacy and cosmetics as skin lubricant, ingredient of suppositories, carrier of lipid-soluble drugs.

THERAP CAT (VET): Cerumenolytic.

8768. Squalene. [111-02-4] (all-E)-2,6,10,15,19,23-Hexamethyl-2,6,10,14,18,22-tetracosahexaene; Spinacene; Supraene. $C_{30}H_{50}$; mol wt 410.72. C 87.73%, H 12.27%. All trans isoprenoid contg six isoprene units. Found in large quantities in shark liver oil. Occurs in smaller amounts (0.1 to 0.7%) in olive oil, wheat germ oil, rice bran oil, and yeast. Intermediate in biosynthesis of cholesterol. Isoln: Heilbron *et al., J. Chem. Soc.* **1926**, 1630. Structure: *eidem, ibid.* **1929**, 873; Heilbron, Thompson, *ibid.* 883; Karrer *et al., Helv. Chim. Acta* **13**, 1084 (1930); Karrer, Helfenstein, *ibid.* **14**, 78 (1931); Karrer *et al., ibid.* 435. Crystal structure: J. Ernst *et al., Angew. Chem. Int. Ed.* **15**, 778 (1976). Synthesis: Trippett, *Chem. Ind. (London)* **1956**, 80; Dicker, Whiting, *J. Chem. Soc.* **1958**, 1994; Cornforth *et al., ibid.* **1959**, 2539; Johnson *et al., J. Am. Chem. Soc.* **92**, 741 (1970); Hirai *et al., Tetrahedron Lett.* **1971**, 4359; P. A. Grieco, Y. Masaki, *J. Org. Chem.* **39**, 2135 (1974). Synthesis of squalene and *trans-cis-trans-trans* isomer: Biellmann, Ducep, *Tetrahedron* **27**, 5861 (1971).

Oil. Faint, agreeable odor. Absorbs oxygen and becomes viscous like linseed oil. d_4^{20} 0.8584; bp_{25} 285°; bp_2 240°; $bp_{0.15}$ 203°. Crystals from ether/methanol, mp −5°. n_D^{20} 1.4965. Viscosity at 25°: 12 cP. Iodine no. 360-380. Practically insol in water. Freely sol in ether, petr ether, CCl_4, acetone, other fat solvents; sparingly sol in alc, glacial acetic acid.

USE: Bactericide; intermediate in manuf of pharmaceuticals, organic coloring materials, rubber chemicals, aromatics and surface active agents.

8769. Squaric Acid. [2892-51-5] 3,4-Dihydroxy-3-cyclobutene-1,2-dione; 1,2-dihydroxycyclobutenedione; diketocyclobutenediol. $C_4H_2O_4$; mol wt 114.06. C 42.12%, H 1.77%, O 56.11%. Dibasic acid; two-dimensional molecular antiferroelectric material. Prepn: S. Cohen *et al., J. Am. Chem. Soc.* **81**, 3480 (1959); J. D. Park *et al., ibid.* **84**, 2919 (1962). Aqueous dissociation study: L. M. Schwartz, L. O. Howard, *J. Phys. Chem.* **74**, 4374 (1970). Structure determn studies: D. Semmingsen, *Acta Chem. Scand.* **27**, 3961 (1973); Y. Wang *et al., J. Chem. Soc. Perkin Trans. 2* **1974**, 35. Review of syntheses and reactivity: G. Maahs, P. Hegenberg, *Angew. Chem. Int. Ed.* **5**, 888-893 (1966); of coordination chemistry: L. A. Hall, D. J. Williams, *Adv. Inorg. Chem.* **52**, 249-291 (2001).

Crystals from water, dec 293°. d 1.90. uv max (H_2O): 269.5 nm (ε 37000). Soly: 7% boiling water; 2% room temp water. Insol in acetone, ether. pK_1 0.6 (25°). pK_2 3.480 ±0.023 (25°).

Dibutylester. [2892-62-8] 3,4-Dibutoxy-3-cyclobutene-1,2-dione; dibutyl squarate. $C_{12}H_{18}O_4$; mol wt 226.27. Prepn: G. Maahs, *Ann.* **686**, 55 (1965). Clinical evaluation in alopecia: G. Micali *et al., Int. J. Dermatol.* **35**, 52 (1996); in treatment of warts: *idem et al., Pediatr. Dermatol.* **17**, 315 (2000). $bp_{0.5}$ 138-139°. n_D^{20} 1.4943.

USE: Squaric acid and its derivatives are used in synthesis of pharmaceutical intermediates, squarylium dyes, and photoconducting squaraines.

THERAP CAT: Dibutylester as contact sensitizer for treatment of alopecia and warts.

8770. Squill. Sea onion; Bulbus Scillae; Meerzwiebel. The fleshy inner bulb scales of the white variety of *Urginea maritima* (L.) Baker (*Scilla maritima* L.), *Liliaceae.* Habit. Lands of the Mediterranean seacoast. *Constit.* Glucoscillaren A (scillarenin + rhamnose + glucose + glucose); scillaren A (scillarenin + rhamnose + glucose); proscillaridin A (scillarenin + rhamnose); scillaridin A; scilliglaucoside; scillipheoside; glucoscillipheoside; scillicyanoside; scillicoeloside; scilliazuroside; scillicryptoside. *Review:* G. Baumgarten, W. Förster, *Die Herzwirksamen Glykoside* (Thieme, Leipzig, 1963) pp 70-75 *et passim.*

USE: Rodenticide.

THERAP CAT: Diuretic, emetic, expectorant, cardiotonic.

THERAP CAT (VET): Has been used as expectorant, emetic.

8771. Stachydrine. [471-87-4] (2S)-2-Carboxy-1,1-dimethylpyrrolidinium inner salt; methyl hygrate betaine; hygric acid methylbetaine. $C_7H_{13}NO_2$; mol wt 143.18. C 58.72%, H 9.15%, N 9.78%, O 22.35%. Occurs widely in nature, especially in alfalfa, chrysanthemum, citrus and stachys species. May be prepd by methylation of proline. Isoln: Planta, Schulze, *Ber.* **26**, 939 (1893); Jahns, *ibid.* **29**, 2065 (1896); Yoshimura, *Z. Physiol. Chem.* **88**, 334 (1913); Vickery, *J. Biol. Chem.* **61**, 117 (1924). Structure: Schulze, Trier, *Z. Physiol. Chem.* **67**, 59 (1910). Synthesis: Karrer, Widmer, *Helv. Chim. Acta* **8**, 364 (1925). Biosynthesis: Robertson, Marion, *Can. J. Chem.* **38**, 396 (1960). *Review:* Marion in *The Alkaloids* vol. 1, R. H. F. Manske, H. L. Holmes, Eds. (Academic Press, New York, 1950) pp 101-103.

H₃C   CH₃
[structure: pyrrolidine ring with N bearing two methyl groups and a COO⁻ group]

Monohydrate. Deliquescent crystals, sweetish taste, mp 235° when anhydr. Isomerizes at the mp to methyl hygrate. Sol in water, alcohol, dil acids. Practically insol in ether, chloroform.

Hydrochloride. $C_7H_{13}NO_2.HCl$. Large prisms from abs alcohol, dec 235°, very sol in water, sol in 13 parts alcohol.

Acid oxalate. $C_7H_{13}NO_2.C_2H_2O_4$. Needles, mp 106°. Practically insol in abs alcohol.

Aurichloride. $C_7H_{13}NO_2.HAuCl_4$. Yellow leaflets, mp 225° (rapid heating). Practically insol in cold water. Quite sol in hot water.

Platinichloride tetrahydrate. $(C_7H_{13}NO_2)_2.H_2PtCl_6.4H_2O$. Orange crystals, dec 210-220° (rapid heating), very sol in water and dil alc. Also obtained with 2 mols H_2O of crystn.

8772. Stallimycin. [636-47-5] N-[5-[[(3-Amino-3-imino-propyl)amino]carbonyl]-1-methyl-1H-pyrrol-3-yl]-4-[[[4-(formyl-amino)-1-methyl-1H-pyrrol-2-yl]carbonyl]amino]-1-methyl-1H-pyrrole-2-carboxamide; β-[1-methyl-4-[1-methyl-4-(1-methyl-4-formylaminopyrrole-2-carboxamido)pyrrole-2-carboxamido]-pyrrole-2-carboxamido]propionamidine; distamycin A; F.I. 6426. $C_{22}H_{27}N_9O_4$; mol wt 481.51. C 54.88%, H 5.65%, N 26.18%, O 13.29%. Antibiotic substance with antiviral and oncolytic properties, obtained from *Streptomyces distallicus:* Arcamone *et al.,* **DE 1039198** (1958 to Farmaceutici Italia), *C.A.* **55,** 2012f (1961). Structure and synthesis: Arcamone *et al., Nature* **203,** 1064 (1964); *eidem, Gazz. Chim. Ital.* **97,** 1097, 1110 (1964). Total synthesis: M. Bialer *et al., Tetrahedron* **1978,** 2389; L. Grehn, U. Ragnarsson, *J. Org. Chem.* **46,** 3492 (1981). Toxicity and antitumor activity: A. DiMarco *et al., Cancer Chemother. Rep.* **18,** 15 (1962). *Review:* Hahn in *Antibiotics* vol. 3, J. W. Corcoran, F. E. Hahn, Eds. (Springer-Verlag, New York, 1975) pp 79-100.

[structure diagram of stallimycin]

mp 154-156°.

Hydrochloride. [6576-51-8] Herperal. $C_{22}H_{27}N_9O_4.HCl$; mol wt 517.97. Crystals from dil HCl, mp 184-187° (Arcamone, 1967). Also reported as 189-193° from ethanol-ethyl acetate (Bialer). uv max (96% ethanol): 237, 303 nm (ε 30000, 37000). LD_{50} in mice (mg/kg): 75 i.v.; 500 i.p. (DiMarco).

THERAP CAT: Antiviral.

8773. Stannic Bromide. [7789-67-5] Tin tetrabromide. Br_4Sn; mol wt 438.33. Br 72.92%, Sn 27.08%. $SnBr_4$.
White, cryst mass; fumes strongly on exposure to air. d 3.34; mp 31°; bp 202°. Very sol in water with evolution of heat; also sol in alcohol. *Keep tightly closed.*
USE: In metallurgical separation of minerals.

8774. Stannic Chloride. [7646-78-8] Tin tetrachloride; fuming spirit of Libavius. Cl_4Sn; mol wt 260.52. Cl 54.43%, Sn 45.57%. $SnCl_4$. Improperly called *"tin bichloride".*
Fuming, caustic liquid. d 2.26; mp −33°; bp 114°. Sol in water and evolution of much heat; sol in alcohol, carbon tetrachloride, benzene, toluene, acetone, kerosene, gasoline. *Keep tightly closed.*
Pentahydrate. White or slightly yellow crystals or fused small lumps; slight HCl odor. Very sol in H_2O; sol in alc.
Caution: May be highly irritating to eyes, mucous membranes.
USE: As mordant; reviving colors; stabilizer for colors and perfumes in soap; in dyeing of fabrics, weighting silk, tinning vessels; dehydrating agent in organic syntheses; in ceramics to produce abrasion-resistant or light-reflecting coatings.

8775. Stannic Chromate(VI). [38455-77-5] Cr_2O_8Sn; mol wt 350.70. Cr 29.65%, O 36.50%, Sn 33.85%. $Sn(CrO_4)_2$.
Brownish-yellow, cryst powder; dec when heated. Sol in water.
USE: Decorating porcelain and china in rose and violet colors.

8776. Stannic Fluoride. [7783-62-2] Tin tetrafluoride. F_4Sn; mol wt 194.70. F 39.03%, Sn 60.97%. SnF_4. Lewis acid. Prepd from $SnCl_4$ and HF: Ruff, Plato, *Ber.* **37,** 673 (1904); or from stannous fluoride and chlorine or bromine: Forbes, Anderson, *J. Am. Chem. Soc.* **67,** 1911 (1945); from stannous oxide or sulfide and fluorine: Haendler *et al., J. Am. Chem. Soc.* **76,** 2179 (1954). *Review:* Kemmitt, Sharp, *Adv. Fluorine Chem.* **4,** 185-186 (1965).
Snow-white, tetragonal crystals. Very hygroscopic. d_4^{19} 4.78. Sublimes at 705°. Hydrolyzes readily, but is more resistant to water than stannic chloride. Forms complexes with donor molecules.
USE: Friedel-Crafts catalyst.

8777. Stannic Iodide. [7790-47-8] Tin tetraiodide. I_4Sn; mol wt 626.33. I 81.05%, Sn 18.95%. SnI_4. Toxicity data: Kolmer, *J. Pharmacol. Exp. Ther.* **43,** 515 (1931).
Yellow to reddish crystals. d 4.46. mp ~143°; sublimes at about 180°. bp 340°. Dec by water; sol in alcohol, benzene, chloroform, ether, carbon disulfide. MLD in rats (mg/kg): 200 i.v. (Kolmer).

8778. Stannic Oxide. [18282-10-5] White tin oxide; tin dioxide; stannic anhydride; flowers of tin. O_2Sn; mol wt 150.71. O 21.23%, Sn 78.77%. SnO_2. Occurs in nature as the mineral *cassiterite.* The commercial grade is also known as *polishing powder,* *putty powder,* or *tin ash.* Review of toxicology and human exposure: *Toxicological Profile for Tin* (PB2006-100006, 2005) 426 pp.
White or slightly gray powder. d 6.95. Insol in water, alcohol, or cold acids. Slowly sol in hot concd potassium or sodium hydroxide soln.
Caution: Potential symptoms of overexposure are stannosis (benign pneumoconiosis); dyspnea, decreased pulmonary function. *See NIOSH Pocket Guide to Chemical Hazards* (DHHS/NIOSH 97-140, 1997) p 308.
USE: Polishing glass and metals; manuf milk-colored, ruby and alabaster glass, enamels, pottery, putty; mordant in printing and dyeing fabrics; in fingernail polishes.

8779. Stannic Selenide. [20770-09-6] Tin diselenide. Se_2Sn; mol wt 276.63. Se 57.09%, Sn 42.91%. $SnSe_2$. Prepd by passing the vapor of selenium over heated tin: Little, *On Selenium and Some of the Metallic Selenides,* Göttingen (Thesis, 1859); by treating a soln of stannic chloride with hydrogen selenide: Berzelius, cited in *Mellor's* vol. X, 785 (1930); by treating a soln of an alkali selenostannate or sulfoselenostannate with hydrochloric acid: Ditte, *Compt. Rend.* **95,** 641 (1882).
Red-brown crystals. d 5.133 (Little); d 4.85 [Schneider, *Pogg. Ann.* **127,** 624 (1866)]. mp 650°. Soluble in alkali, concd sulfuric acid, aqua regia, aq ammonia. Insol in water, dilute acids. Dec in nitric acid. Forms potassium selenostannate with potassium selenide; sodium selenostannate with sodium selenide.

8780. Stannic Sulfide. [1315-01-1] Tin disulfide; mosaic gold; tin bronze. S_2Sn; mol wt 182.84. S 35.07%, Sn 64.93%. SnS_2.
Golden leaflets with metallic luster; fatty feel to the touch. d 4.5. Insol in water or dil acids. Sol in aqua regia, in solns of alkali hydroxides or sulfides.
Note: The term "mosaic gold" is also used to designate an alloy consisting of 65.3% copper and 34.7% zinc.
USE: Gilding and bronzing metals; gypsum, wood and paper, usually by suspending in lacquer or varnish.

8781. Stannous Acetate. [638-39-1] $C_4H_6O_4Sn$; mol wt 236.80. C 20.29%, H 2.55%, O 27.03%, Sn 50.13%. $Sn(C_2H_3O_2)_2$. Prepd by refluxing granulated tin with 98% acetic acid: Colonna, *Gazz. Chim. Ital.* **35 II,** 224 (1905); by refluxing SnO with 50% (v/v) acetic acid under nitrogen: Donaldson *et al., J. Chem. Soc.* **1964,** 5942.
White, orthorhombic crystals; dec by water. mp 182.5-183°. d 2.31. Sol in dil HCl. *Keep well closed.*
USE: Reducing agent.

8782. Stannous Bromide. [10031-24-0] Tin dibromide. Br_2Sn; mol wt 278.52. Br 57.38%, Sn 42.62%. $SnBr_2$.
Yellowish powder; oxidizes in air. d 5.12; mp 215°; bp 623°. Sol in little water, gradually dec by much water; sol in alcohol, ether, acetone. *Keep tightly closed and protected from light.*

8783. Stannous Chloride. [7772-99-8] Tin dichloride; tin protochloride; Stannochlor. Cl_2Sn; mol wt 189.62. Cl 37.39%, Sn 62.60%. $SnCl_2$. Prepn: Stephen, *J. Chem. Soc.* **1930**, 2786; Williams, *Org. Synth.* **coll. vol. III**, 627 (1955). Metabolism and toxicity studies: M. Marciniak, *Acta Physiol. Pol.* **32**, 193 (1981); P. P. Singh, A. Y. Junnarkar, *Indian J. Pharmacol.* **23**, 153 (1991). Review of toxicology and human exposure: *Toxicological Profile for Tin* (PB2006-100006, 2005) 426 pp.

Orthorhombic cryst mass or flakes; fatty appearance. bp 247°; d 3.95. Sol in water, ethanol, acetone, ether, methyl acetate, methyl ethyl ketone, isobutyl alcohol. Practically insol in mineral spirits, petr naphtha, xylene. LD_{50} in mice, rats (mg/kg): 1710.0, 2000.0 orally; 271.0, 316.0 i.p.; 34.8, 43.0 i.v. (Singh, Junnarkar).

Dihydrate. [10025-69-1] $Cl_2Sn.2H_2O$. Crystals; absorbs oxygen from air and forms insol oxychloride. d 2.71. mp 37-38° when rapidly heated; dec on strong heating. Sol in less than its own wt of water; with much water it forms an insol basic salt; very sol in dil or in concd hydrochloric acid; also sol in alcohol, ethyl acetate, glacial acetic acid, sodium hydroxide soln. *Keep tightly closed, in a cool place.*

USE: Powerful reducing agent, particularly in manuf of dyes and ^{99m}Tc radiopharmaceuticals; in tinning by galvanic methods; in liquor finishing of wire; in sensitizing of glass and plastics before metallizing; as soldering flux; as mordant in dyeing with cochineal; in manufacture of tin chemicals, color pigments, pharmaceuticals, sensitized paper, lubricating oil additives; as tanning agent; in removing ink stains; in yeast revivers; as reagent in analytical chemistry; as catalyst in organic reactions.

8784. Stannous Fluoride. [7783-47-3] Tin difluoride; Fluoristan. F_2Sn; mol wt 156.71. F 24.25%, Sn 75.75%. SnF_2. Prepd by evaporating a soln of stannous oxide in hydrofluoric acid in the absence of oxygen: Gay-Lussac, Thénard, *Mém. Phys. Chim.* **2**, 317 (1809); Nebergall *et al., J. Am. Chem. Soc.* **74**, 1604 (1952); from tin and hydrogen fluoride: Muetterties, *Inorg. Chem.* **1**, 342 (1962). *Review:* Kemmitt, Sharp, *Adv. Fluorine Chem.* **4**, 186 (1965). Review of toxicology and human exposure: *Toxicological Profile for Tin* (PB2006-100006, 2005) 426 pp.

Monoclinic, lamellar plates. mp 213°. d^{25} 4.57. Sol in water (about 30%). Forms an oxyfluoride, $SnOF_2$, on exposure to air.

USE: Dental caries prophylactic.

8785. Stannous Iodide. [10294-70-9] Tin diiodide. I_2Sn; mol wt 372.52. I 68.13%, Sn 31.87%. SnI_2. Preparation and crystal structure: Moser, Trevena, *Chem. Commun.* **1969**, 25.

Red, cryst powder or needles. d 5.28; mp 320°; bp 720° with decompn. Slightly sol in and dec by water; sol in solns of alkali chlorides or iodides, in benzene, chloroform, carbon disulfide. *Keep tightly closed.*

8786. Stannous Oxalate. [814-94-8] C_2O_4Sn; mol wt 206.73. C 11.62%, O 30.96%, Sn 57.42%. SnC_2O_4.

White, heavy powder. d 3.56. Insol in water. Sol in dil hydrochloric acid.

USE: Dyeing and printing textiles.

8787. Stannous Oxide. [21651-19-4] Tin monoxide; tin protoxide. OSn; mol wt 134.71. O 11.88%, Sn 88.12%. SnO. Prepn of high purity SnO: Kwestroo, Vromans, *J. Inorg. Nucl. Chem.* **29**, 2187 (1967). Prepn of metastable, red, orthorhombic form: Donaldson *et al., J. Chem. Soc.* **1961**, 839.

Brownish-black powder; burns to SnO_2 on heating in air. d 6.45. Insol in water or alcohol. Sol in acids, in concd sodium or potassium hydroxide solns.

Caution: Potential symptoms of overexposure are stannosis (benign pneumoconiosis); dyspnea, decreased pulmonary function. *See NIOSH Pocket Guide to Chemical Hazards* (DHHS/NIOSH 97-140, 1997) p 308.

USE: Reducing agent; prepn of stannous salts.

8788. Stannous Pyrophosphate. [15578-26-4] Diphosphoric acid tin(2+) salt (1:2); ditin diphosphate; ditin pyrophosphate. $O_7P_2Sn_2$; mol wt 411.36. O 27.23%, P 15.06%, Sn 57.72%. $Sn_2P_2O_7$. Prepd by thermal dehydration of stannous hydrogen phosphate: Jablczynski, Wieckowski, *Z. Anorg. Allg. Chem.* **152**, 207 (1926); from $Na_2H_2P_2O_7$ and $SnCl_2$: Klement, Haselbeck, *Ber.* **96**, 1022 (1958); from pyrophosphoric acid and stannous chloride:

Nelson, **US 3401012** (1968 to Monsanto). Clinical application for labelling red blood cells: D. Ducasson *et al., Br. J. Radiol.* **49**, 344 (1976). Chemical characterization of complexes: J. Kroesbergen *et al., Nucl. Med. Biol.* **15**, 209 (1988). Diagnostic application in bone scanning: N. S. Anderton *et al., Am. J. Roentgenol. Radium Ther. Nucl. Med.* **124**, 625 (1975); in myocardial infarction: D. E. Jansen *et al., Circulation* **75**, 611 (1987).

Amorphous powder. $d^{16.4}$ 4.009. Insol in water. Sol in concd acid, excess alkali.

^{99m}Technetium complex. ^{99m}Tc-PPi; ^{99m}Tc-PYP; TechneScan PYP.

USE: Ingredient in caries-preventing toothpaste: Norris, Schweizer, **US 2946725** (1960 to Proctor & Gamble).

THERAP CAT: ^{99m}Tc complex as diagnostic aid (radioactive imaging agent).

8789. Stannous Selenide. [1315-06-6] Tin monoselenide. SeSn; mol wt 197.67. Se 39.95%, Sn 60.05%. SnSe. Prepd by direct fusing of the elements: Ditte, *Compt. Rend.* **95**, 641 (1882); **96**, 1792 (1883); **97**, 44 (1883); Berzelius cited in *Mellor's* **vol. X**, 784 (1930); by adding powdered selenium to molten, anhydr stannous chloride: Schneider, *Pogg. Ann.* **127**, 624 (1866).

Steel-gray prisms. d^0 6.18; mp 861°. Insol in water. Sol in aqua regia and alkali sulfides and selenides.

8790. Stannous Sulfate. [7488-55-3] O_4SSn; mol wt 214.77. O 29.80%, S 14.93%, Sn 55.27%. $SnSO_4$. Prepn: Donaldson, Moser, *J. Chem. Soc.* **1960**, 4000.

Snow-white, orthorhombic crystals; dec at 378° to SnO_2 and SO_2. Sol in water, the soln soon decomposing with pptn of a basic sulfate; sol in dil H_2SO_4. *Keep well closed.*

USE: In tin plating; prepn of stannous salts.

8791. Stannous Sulfide. [1314-95-0] Tin monosulfide; tin protosulfide. SSn; mol wt 150.78. S 21.27%, Sn 78.73%. SnS. Dark-gray crystals or black, amorphous powder. d 5.08. Insol in water or alkali hydroxide or alkali sulfide soln. Sol in concd HCl, hot concd H_2SO_4.

USE: Polymerization catalyst.

8792. Stannous Tartrate. [815-85-0] $C_4H_4O_6Sn$; mol wt 266.78. C 18.01%, H 1.51%, O 35.98%, Sn 44.50%. $SnC_4H_4O_6$. White powder. Sol in water, dil HCl. *Keep well closed.*

USE: Dyeing and printing textiles.

8793. Stanolone. [521-18-6] $(5\alpha,17\beta)$-17-Hydroxyandrostan-3-one; 17β-hydroxy-3-androstanone; 3-oxo-17β-hydroxyandrostane; androstan-17β-ol-3-one; 4-dihydrotestosterone; androstanolone; Anabolex; Andractim; Androlone. $C_{19}H_{30}O_2$; mol wt 290.44. C 78.57%, H 10.41%, O 11.02%. Prepd by hydrogenation of testosterone: Butenandt *et al., Ber.* **68**, 2097 (1935); from dehydroepiandrosterone: Ruzicka, Kagi, *Helv. Chim. Acta* **20**, 1557 (1937); Ruzicka *et al., ibid.* **24**, 1151 (1941); from 3,17-androstandione: Oliveto, Hershburg, **US 2927921** (1960 to Schering).

Crystals from ethyl acetate + hexane. Sublimes$_{0.01}$ 135°. mp 181°. $[\alpha]_D^{20}$ +32.4° (alcohol). Infrared absorption data: *J. Am. Chem. Soc.* **75**, 903 (1953). Sol in acetone, ether, alcohol, ethyl acetate. Practically insol in water.

Note: This is a controlled substance (anabolic steroid): **21 CFR**, 1308.13, as defined in 1300.01.

THERAP CAT: Androgen.

8794. Stanozolol. [10418-03-8] (2'H form); [302-96-5] (1'H form). $(5\alpha,17\beta)$-17-Methyl-2'H-androst-2-eno[3,2-c]pyrazol-17-ol; 1,2,3,3a,3b,4,5,5a,6,8,10,10a,10b,11,12,12a-hexadecahydro-1,-10a,12a-trimethylcyclopenta[7,8]phenanthro[2,3-c]pyrazol-1-ol; 17β-hydroxy-17α-methylandrostano[3,2-c]pyrazole; androstanazole; stanazol; NSC-43193; Win-14833; Stromba; Strombaject; Winstrol. $C_{21}H_{32}N_2O$; mol wt 328.49. C 76.78%, H 9.82%, N 8.53%, O 4.87%. Prepn: Clinton *et al., J. Am. Chem. Soc.* **81**, 1513 (1959); **83**, 1478 (1961); Manson, US 3030358 (1962 to Sterling Drug).

Crystals from alc, mp 229.8-242.0°. $[\alpha]_D$ +35.7° (chloroform); $[\alpha]_D$ +48.6° (methanol). uv max: 223 nm (ε 4740).

Note: This is a controlled substance (anabolic steroid): **21 CFR**, 1308.13, as defined in 1300.01.

THERAP CAT: Androgen.

THERAP CAT (VET): Anabolic steroid.

8795. Staphisagria. Stavesacre. Ripe seed of *Delphinium staphisagria* L., Ranunculaceae. *Habit.* Mediterranean basin; cultivated in France, Italy. *Constit.* Delphinine, delphinoidine, delphisine, staphisagrine, staphisagroine, malic acid, fixed oil.

THERAP CAT: Parasiticide (external).

8796. Staphylokinase. [9040-61-3] Fibrin-specific plasminogen activator lacking enzymatic activity; produced by certain strains of *Staphylococcus aureus*. Consists of 136 amino acids in a single polypeptide chain without disulfide bridges; several molecular forms have been purified, mol wt 16,500-18,000. Forms a stoichiometric complex with the proenzyme plasminogen, *q.v.*, that becomes biologically active after the conversion of plasminogen to the proteolytic enzyme plasmin, *q.v.* Profibrinolytic properties: C. H. Lack, *Nature* **161**, 559 (1948); E. B. Gerheim, *et al., Proc. Soc. Exp. Biol. Med.* **68**, 246 (1948). Cloning and expression in *Escherichia coli*: T. Sako *et al., Mol. Gen. Genet.* **190**, 271 (1983); in *Bacillus subtilis*: D. Behnke, D. Gerlach, *ibid.* **210**, 528 (1987). High yield production and purification of recombinant form: B. Schlott *et al., Biotechnology* **12**, 185 (1994). Series of articles on isoln, characterization, structure, biochemistry and pharmacology of natural (*STAN*) and recombinant (*STAR*) forms: *Fibrinolysis* **6**, 203-242 (1992). Determn in plasma by bioimmunoassay: H. R. Lijnen *et al., Thromb. Haemostasis* **70**, 491 (1993); by ELISA: A. Mike *et al., Biol. Pharm. Bull.* **17**, 564 (1994). Clinical evaluation in peripheral arterial occlusion: S. Vanderschueren *et al., Circulation* **92**, 2050 (1995). Comparative clinical trial vs alteplase, *q.v.: idem et al., ibid.* 2044. Series of articles on recombinant variants with altered immunoreactivity: D. Collen *et al., ibid.* **94**, 197-216 (1996); **95**, 455-472 (1997). Reviews: D. Collen, H. R. Lijnen, *Blood* **84**, 680-686 (1994); H. R. Lijnen, D. Collen, *Fibrinolysis* **10**, 119-126 (1996).

THERAP CAT: Thrombolytic.

8797. Star Anise. Chinese anise. Fruit of *Illicium verum* Hook. f., Magnoliaceae. *Habit.* Southeastern Asia and subtropical countries; commercial supply chiefly from China. *Constit.* About 5% volatile and fixed oils; anisic acid, tannin, resin, pectin. *Note:* Japanese star anise is *Illicium anisatum* L. (*I. religiosum* Sieb. & Zucc.; *I. japonicum* Sieb.) and contains a toxic lactone called anisatin. Chinese star anise does not contain this toxic principle. Shikimic acid has been found in both.

USE: Manufacture of liqueurs and the volatile oil. The fruit as source of oil of anise.

THERAP CAT: Hemostatic.

8798. Starch. Amylum. $(C_6H_{10}O_5)_n$. Carbohydrate polymer stored by plants; analogous to storage of fats by animals. Occurs as discrete granules in the mature grain of corn, *Zea mays* Linné, *Gramineae* or of wheat, *Triticum aestivum* Linné, *Gramineae* or tubers of potato, *Solanum tuberosum* Linné, *Solanaceae* or rice, *Oryza sativa* Linné, *Gramineae*. Starches are mixtures of two polymers: *amylose,* a linear (1 → 4)-α-D-glucan and *amylopectin,* a branched D-glucan with mostly α-D-(1 → 4) and approx 4% α-D-(1 → 6) linkages. The starch in corn contains approx 27% amylose

and 73% amylopectin, with these two polymers so associated in the crystal lattice that they are practically insol in cold water or alcohol. *Refs:* J. N. BeMiller, "Starch Amylose" in *Industrial Gums*, R. L. Whistler, Ed. (Academic Press, New York, 2nd ed., 1973) pp 545-566; E. L. Powell, "Starch Amylopectin", *ibid.*, pp 567-576.

Although hydrolysis will not take place in cold water, and starch is comparatively resistant to naturally occurring enzymes, the reaction may be brought about by the use of acids or enzymes (α-amylase, β-amylase, amyloglucosidase). The hydrolysis reaction follows a different path depending on whether acids or enzymes are used. While acid hydrolysis produces a mixture of saccharides, the enzymes give more specific products. β-Amylase, for example, breaks off mostly maltose units, and amyloglucosidase yields mainly D-glucose. Chemistry and technology: R. L. Whistler, E. F. Paschall, Eds., *Starch: Chemistry and Technology* 2 vols. (Academic Press, New York, 1965); J. A. Radley, Ed., *Starch and Its Derivatives* (Chapman & Hall, London, 4th ed., 1968). Comprehensive description: A. W. Newman *et al., Anal. Profiles Drug Subs. Excip.* **24**, 523-577 (1996).

Caution: Potential symptoms of overexposure are irritation of eyes, skin, mucous membranes; cough, chest pains; dermatitis; rhinorrhea. *See NIOSH Pocket Guide to Chemical Hazards* (DHHS/NIOSH 97-140, 1997) p 284.

USE: Starching and sizing fabrics, etc.; paste; as indicator in iodometric analyses. In the food industry. Pharmaceutic aid (tablet disintegrant, filler, binder); dusting powder. Dietetic grades of corn starch are marketed as *Maizena; Mondamin.*

THERAP CAT: Antidote (iodine poisoning).

THERAP CAT (VET): Internally: demulcent, mild astringent, in diarrhea, as an antidote for iodine poisoning. Externally: absorbent, emollient, in dusting powders and in ointments.

8799. Starch, Soluble. [9005-84-9] Amylodextrin; amylogen. Prepd by treating potato or corn starch with dilute hydrochloric acid.

White, odorless, tasteless powder. Readily soluble in hot water; forms transparent mobile liquid.

USE: For determination of diastatic power of malt, etc.; as indicator in iodometric analyses.

8800. Statine. [49642-07-1] (3S,4S)-4-Amino-3-hydroxy-6-methylheptanoic acid; AHMHA. $C_8H_{17}NO_3$; mol wt 175.23. C 54.83%, H 9.78%, N 7.99%, O 27.39%. Amino acid present in pepstatin, *q.v.* Synthesis: H. Morishima *et al., J. Antibiot.* **26**, 115 (1973). Abs config and stereospecific synthesis of all four isomers: M. Kinoshita *et al., ibid.* 249. Crystal structure: H. Nakamura *et al., ibid.* 255. Biosynthesis: H. Morishima *et al., ibid.* **27**, 267 (1974). Alternate syntheses: M. Kinoshita *et al., Bull. Chem. Soc. Jpn.* **48**, 570 (1975); W.-S. Liu, G. I. Glover, *J. Org. Chem.* **43**, 754 (1978); D. H. Rich *et al., ibid.* 3624; K. E. Rittle *et al., ibid.* **47**, 3016 (1982). Distribution in rats: D. A. Grant *et al., Biochem. Pharmacol.* **31**, 2302 (1982).

mp 201-203° (dec). $[\alpha]_D^{15}$ −20° (c = 0.64 in water).

8801. Statolon. [11006-77-2] An antiviral substance which appears to be a macromolecular polyanionic polysaccharide composed of galacturonic acid, galactose, galactosamine, glucose, arabinose, xylose, and rhamnose. Prophylactically active against a wide range of viruses, including those causing canine distemper, lymphomatosis in fowl, shipping fever in cattle, transmissible gastroenteritis in swine, and coryza and other upper respiratory illnesses, as well as against ECHO viruses, enteroviruses in monkeys, MM neurotropic virus, Semliki Forest virus, and NEF 1 poliomyelitis virus. Antitumor activity demonstrated in experimental leukemia and sarcoma. Produced by submerged culture fermentation, using *Penicillium stoloniferum* var. ATCC 14586: Stark *et al.*, US 3108047 (1963 to Lilly).

THERAP CAT: Antiviral.

8802. Staurosporine. [62996-74-1] (9S,10R,11R,13R)- 2,-3,10,11,12,13-Hexahydro-10-methoxy-9-methyl-11-(methylamino)-9,13-epoxy-1H,9H-diindolo[1,2,3-gh:3',2',1'-lm]pyrrolo[3,4-j]-[1,7]benzodiazonin-1-one; AM-2282; CGP-39360. $C_{28}H_{26}N_4O_3$; mol wt 466.53. C 72.09%, H 5.62%, N 12.01%, O 10.29%. Protein kinase C inhibitor; alkaloid isolated from *Streptomyces staurosporeus*. Isoln: S. Omura *et al., J. Antibiot.* **30**, 275 (1977). Crystal and molecular structure: A. Furusaki *et al., J. Chem. Soc. Chem. Commun.* **1978**, 800; *eidem, Bull. Chem. Soc. Jpn.* **55**, 3681 (1982). Corrected stereochemistry: N. Funato *et al., Tetrahedron Lett.* **35**, 1251 (1994). Total synthesis: J. T. Link *et al., J. Am. Chem. Soc.* **117**, 552 (1995); *idem et al., ibid.* **118**, 2825 (1996). Biosynthetic studies: D. Meksuriyen, G. A. Cordell, *J. Nat. Prod.* **51**, 884, 893 (1988); S.-W. Yang *et al., ibid.* **62** 1551 (1999). HPLC determn in blood and pharmacokinetics in rats: L. R. Gurley *et al., J. Chromatogr. B* **712**, 211 (1998). Inhibition of protein kinase C: T. Tamaoki *et al., Biochem. Biophys. Res. Commun.* **135**, 397 (1986); of other protein kinases: U. T. Rüegg, G. M. Burgess, *Trends Pharmacol. Sci.* **10**, 218 (1989). Induction of apoptosis: E. Falcieri *et al., Biochem. Biophys. Res. Commun.* **193**, 19 (1993); R. Bertrand *et al., Exp. Cell Res.* **211**, 314 (1994); of tyrosine phosphorylation: D. Rasouly, P. Lazarovici, *Eur. J. Pharmacol.* **269**, 255 (1994).

Pale yellow needles from chloroform-methanol as the methanol solvate, mp 270° (dec) (Omura). Also reported as yellow crystals from methanol, mp 288-291° (Meksuriyen, Cordell). $[\alpha]_D^{25}$ +35.0° (c = 1 in methanol); $[\alpha]_D^{22}$ +56.1° (c = 0.14 in methanol). uv max (methanol): 241.0, 266.0, 292.5, 321.5, 335.0, 355.0, 372.5 nm (log ε 4.25, 4.26, 4.53, 3.88, 3.96, 3.81, 3.85). Sol in DMSO, DMF. Slightly sol in chloroform, methanol.

Hydrochloride. $C_{28}H_{26}N_4O_3 \cdot HCl$; mol wt 502.99. LD_{50} in mice (mg/kg): 6.6 i.p. (Omura).

USE: Pharmacological tool to study signal transduction pathways, tyrosine phosphorylation and to induce apoptosis.

8803. Stavudine. [3056-17-5] 2',3'-Didehydro-3'-deoxythymidine; 1-(2,3-dideoxy-β-*glycero*-pent-2-enofuranosyl))thymine; 3'-deoxy-2'-thymidinene; D4T; BMY-27857; Zerit. $C_{10}H_{12}N_2O_4$; mol wt 224.21. C 53.57%, H 5.39%, N 12.49%, O 28.54%. Analog of thymidine, *q.v.*; reverse transcriptase inhibitor. Prepn: J. P. Horwitz *et al., J. Org. Chem.* **31**, 205 (1966); J. W. Beach *et al., ibid.* **57**, 3887 (1992). Large scale production: J. E. Starrett *et al.*, EP 334368; *eidem*, US 5130421 (1989, 1992 both to Bristol-Myers). *In vitro* activity against HIV and toxicology: M. M. Mansuri *et al., Antimicrob. Agents Chemother.* **34**, 637 (1990). Mechanism of action study: H.-T. Ho, M. J. M. Hitchcock, *ibid.* **33**, 844 (1989). Disposition and metabolism: E. M. Cretton *et al., ibid.* **37**, 1816 (1993). Clinical pharmacokinetics: M. N. Dudley *et al., J. Infect. Dis.* **166**, 480 (1992). HPLC determn in plasma and urine: J. S. Janiszewski *et al., J. Chromatogr.* **577**, 151 (1992). Clinical evaluation in AIDS and ARC: M. J. Browne *et al., J. Infect. Dis.* **167**, 21 (1993).

Colorless, granular solid from ethanol/benzene, mp 165-166° (Horwitz). Also reported as crystals from ethanol-ether, mp 174° (Beach). uv max (water): 266 nm (ε 10149). $[\alpha]_D^{25}$ −39.4° (c = 0.701 in water); $[\alpha]_D^{20}$ −46.1° (c = 0.7 in water).

THERAP CAT: Antiviral.

8804. Stearic Acid. [57-11-4] Octadecanoic acid; Emersol 132. $C_{18}H_{36}O_2$; mol wt 284.48. C 76.00%, H 12.76%, O 11.25%. $CH_3(CH_2)_{16}COOH$. Occurs as a glyceride in tallow and other animal fats and oils, as well as in some vegetable oils; also prepd synthetically by hydrogenation of cottonseed and other vegetable oils.

White leaflets. d^{70} 0.847; mp 69-70°; bp 383°; n_D^{80} 1.4299. Slowly volatilizes at 90-100°. Very slightly sol in water. One gram dissolves in 21 ml alcohol, 5 ml benzene, 2 ml chloroform, 26 ml acetone, 6 ml carbon tetrachloride, 3.4 ml carbon disulfide; also sol in amyl acetate, toluene. LD_{50} i.v. in mice, rats: 23±0.7, 21.5±1.8 mg/kg, L. Örö, A. Wretlind, *Acta Pharmacol. Toxicol.* **18**, 141 (1961). U.S.P. stearic acid consists chiefly of a mixture of stearic and palmitic acids. It is in the form of white or slightly yellow, crystal masses, or a white to slightly yellow powder; slight tallow-like odor. Does not congeal below 54°.

Ethyl ester. Ethyl stearate. $C_{20}H_{40}O_2$. White, cryst solid; odorless or practically so. mp 33-35°. bp 224°. Ethyl stearate of commerce solidifies at 20-24°; bp_4 180°. Insol in water; sol in alcohol or ether.

Methyl ester. Methyl stearate. $C_{19}H_{38}O_2$. White crystals. mp 38-39°. bp_{15} 215°. Insol in water; sol in alcohol, ether.

USE: For suppositories, coating enteric pills, ointments, and for coating bitter remedies. Manuf stearates of aluminum, zinc, and other metals, stearin soap for opodeldoc, candles, phonograph records, insulators, modeling compds; impregnating plaster of Paris; in vanishing creams and other cosmetics.

8805. Stearyl Alcohol. [112-92-5] 1-Octadecanol; stenol. $C_{18}H_{38}O$; mol wt 270.49. C 79.93%, H 14.16%, O 5.91%. CH_3-$(CH_2)_{16}CH_2OH$. The official substance is a mixture of solid alcohols consisting chiefly of stearyl alcohol. Preparation from ethyl stearate: Brown, Rao, *J. Am. Chem. Soc.* **78**, 2582 (1956); Hesse, Schrödel, *Ann.* **607**, 24 (1954). Prepn of technical grade from sperm whale oil: Maiorov *et al., Zh. Prikl. Khim.* **37**, 1344 (1964).

Unctuous white flakes or granules, mp 56-60° (the pure substance, mp 59.4-59.8°, bp_{15} 210°). Sol in alcohol, ether, benzene, acetone.

USE: Substitute for cetyl alc in pharmaceutical dispensing, in cosmetic creams, for emulsions, textile oils and finishes, as antifoam agent, lubricant, and chemical raw material.

8806. Stellar®. [151031-37-7] Starch based fat replacer produced by controlled acid hydrolysis of corn starch. Shears to create a firm, deformable creme consisting of loosely aggregated submicron-sized starch particles. Consists of branched amylodextrins; average mol wt <20000. Prepn: D. W. Harris, K. D. Stanly, EP 529891 (1992 to Staley Manuf.). Functional properties in relationship to structure: D. W. Harris, G. A. Day, *Starch/Staerke* **45**, 221 (1993). Brief description: *Prepared Foods* **161**, 77 (1992).

Bland taste, slick fat-like mouthfeel. Hydrophilic. pH of 10% slurry, 3.0-5.0. Caloric value: 16 kJ/g. Exhibits thixotropic rheological behavior similar to hydrogenated vegetable shortening.

USE: Fat substitute for reduced calorie foods.

8807. Stem Cell Factor. Steel factor; mast cell growth factor; kit ligand; SCF. Hematopoietic growth factor that interacts with other cytokines to stimulate primitive, undifferentiated blast cells and is particularly active in mast cell and erythroid lineages. The full length, membrane bound protein consists of 248 amino acids that is cleaved to produce a soluble form consisting of 165 residues. The soluble form exists as a glycosylated homodimer; mol wt ~45 kDa. Identification: D. E. Williams *et al., Cell* **63**, 167 (1990); K. M. Zsebo *et al., ibid.* 195. Review of discovery and bioactivity: D. E. Williams, S. D. Lyman, *Prog. Growth Factor Res.* **3**, 235-242 (1991). Crystal structure of human soluble dimer: Z. Zhang *et al., Proc. Natl. Acad. Sci. USA* **97**, 7732 (2000). Review of biology and clinical potential: I. K. McNiece, R. A. Briddell, *J. Leukocyte Biol.* **57**, 14-22 (1995); J. Glaspy *et al., Cancer Chemother. Pharmacol.* **38**, Suppl., S53-S57 (1996). Review of role in hematopoietic system: L. K. Ashman, *Int. J. Biochem. Cell Biol.*

31, 1037-1051 (1999); and therapeutic potential: S. Nakagawa, T. Kitoh, *Curr. Opin. Hematol.* **7**, 133-142 (2000).

Ancestim. [163545-26-4] *N*-L-Methionyl-1-165-hematopoietic cell growth factor KL (human clone V19.8:hSCF162) dimer; rhSCF; Stemgen. Produced in *E. coli* by recombinant DNA technology. Prepn: K. M. Zsebo *et al.,* **EP 423980** (1991 to Amgen). Clinical trial in combination with filgrastim for hematopoietic reconstitution in chemotherapy patients: E. J. Shpall *et al., Blood* **9**, 2491 (1999).

THERAP CAT: Hematopoietic.

8808. Stenbolone. [5197-58-0] (5α,17β)-17-Hydroxy-2-methylandrost-1-en-3-one; 2-methyl-5α-androst-1-en-17β-ol-3-one; 2-methyl-17β-hydroxy-5α-androst-1-en-3-one; stenobolone (rescinded USAN). $C_{20}H_{30}O_2$; mol wt 302.45. C 79.42%, H 10.00%, O 10.58%. Preparation of free alcohol and acetate: R. Mauli *et al., J. Am. Chem. Soc.* **82**, 5494 (1960); Kaspar *et al.,* **DE 1096356** (1961 to Schering AG), *C.A.* **55**, 27440b (1961); R. E. Counsell *et al., J. Org. Chem.* **27**, 248 (1962); **GB 925849** (1963 to Syntex).

Crystals from acetone + hexane, mp 155-158°. [α]$_D$ +52° (chloroform) (Mauli). [α]$_D^{26}$ +47° (chloroform) (Counsell). uv max (95% ethanol): 241 nm (log ε 3.99).

Acetate. [1242-56-4] $C_{22}H_{32}O_3$; mol wt 344.49. Crystals from acetone + hexane, mp 146-149°. [α]$_D$ +32° (chloroform) (Mauli). [α]$_D^{26}$ +60° (chloroform) (Counsell). uv max (95% ethanol): 241 nm (log ε 4.03).

Note: This is a controlled substance (anabolic steroid): **21 CFR**, 1308.13, as defined in 1300.01.

8809. Stepronin. [72324-18-6] *N*-[1-Oxo-2-[(2-thienylcarbonyl)thio]propyl]glycine; 2-(α-thenoylthio)propionylglycine; *N*-(2-mercaptopropionyl)glycine 2-thiophenecarboxylate (ester); TTPG; prostenoglycine; Tiase. $C_{10}H_{11}NO_4S_2$; mol wt 273.33. C 43.94%, H 4.06%, N 5.12%, O 23.41%, S 23.46%. Prepn, properties and toxicology: F. Bolasco, **BE 875186**; *eidem,* **US 4242354** (1979, 1980 to Mediolanum Farmaceutici). Clinical trials in bronchitis: M. Lingetti *et al., Int. J. Clin. Pharmacol. Res.* **1**, 273 (1981); F. Dotta *et al., Clin. Ter.* **105**, 307 (1983); G. C. Morandini *et al., Curr. Ther. Res.* **35**, 783 (1984). Effect on human lung mucus: M. C. Morale *et al., Int. J. Tissue React.* **5**, 231 (1983).

Colorless crystals from acetonitrile, mp 168-170°. uv max: 292 nm. LD$_{50}$ in mice (mg/kg): >2500 orally, >1250 i.v.; in rats (mg/kg): >2500 orally, 1801 i.m. (Bolasco).

Lysine salt. [113790-28-6] Masor; Mucodil.

Sodium salt. [78126-10-0] Broncoplus; Tioten. $C_{10}H_{10}NNaO_4S_2$; mol wt 295.31.

THERAP CAT: Mucolytic.

8810. Stevioside. [57817-89-7] (4α)-13-[(2-*O*-β-D-Glucopyranosyl-β-D-glucopyranosyl)oxy]kaur-16-en-18-oic acid β-D-glucopyranosyl ester; steviosin. $C_{38}H_{60}O_{18}$; mol wt 804.87. C 56.71%, H 7.51%, O 35.78%. Isolated from leaves of *Stevia rebaudiana* (Bert.) Hemsl. (*Eupatorium rebaudianum* Bert.), *Compositae*, also called *yerba dulce*. *Habit.* Paraguay. Isoln and structure: Wood *et al., J. Org. Chem.* **20**, 875 (1955). Review of botany: Samaniego, *Rev. Farm. (Buenos Aires)* **88**, 199 (1946). Review of chemistry and use as sweetening agent: Bell, *Chem. Ind. (London)* **1954**, 897; Fletcher, Jr., *Chemurg. Dig.* **14**, 7, 18 (July-Aug. 1955); *Chem. Eng. News* **34**, 124 (1956). Total synthesis: *eidem, Tetrahedron* **36**, 2641 (1980). Synthesis and sensory evaluation of analogs: G. E. Dubois *et al., J. Med. Chem.* **24**, 1269 (1981).

Hygroscopic crystals, mp 198°. [α]$_D^{25}$ −39.3° (c = 5.7 in H$_2$O). 300 times as sweet as cane sugar. One gram dissolves in 800 ml water. Sol in dioxane. Slightly sol in alc.

Steviol. [471-80-7] (4α)-13-Hydroxykaur-16-en-18-oic acid; hydroxydehydrostevic acid. Aglucon of stevioside, the sweet glucoside abundant in leaves and stems of *Stevia rebaudiana* Bert. Absolute configuration: Mosettig *et al., ibid.* **85**, 2305 (1963). Biosynthesis: Ruddat *et al., Arch. Biochem. Biophys.* **110**, 496 (1965). Total synthesis of *dl*-form: Mori *et al., Tetrahedron Lett.* **1970**, 2411; Cook, Knox, *ibid.* 4091; *eidem, Tetrahedron* **28**, 3217 (1972). Needles from methanol or ethanol + water, mp 215°. [α]$_D$ −94.7°.

USE: Has been proposed as non-nutritive sweetening agent.

8811. Stibine. [7803-52-3] Antimony hydride. H$_3$Sb; mol wt 124.78. H 2.42%, Sb 97.58%. SbH$_3$. Conveniently prepd by dissolving zinc-antimony or magnesium-antimony alloy in dil HCl: Hurd, *Chemistry of the Hydrides* (Wiley, New York, 1952) p 132. Detailed directions (including prepn of the alloy from powdered Sb and Mg): Schenk in *Handbook of Preparative Inorganic Chemistry* **vol. 1**, G. Brauer, Ed. (Academic Press, New York, 2nd ed., 1963) pp 606-608. Review of preparative methods: Jolly, Norman, "Hydrides of Groups IV and V" in *Preparative Inorganic Reactions* **vol. 4**, W. L. Jolly, Ed. (Interscience, New York, 1968) pp 1-58.

Colorless gas. *Intensely poisonous.* Disagreeable odor. mp −88°. bp −18.4°. d 2.204 g/ml at bp. Heat of formation +34.68 kcal/mole: Gunn, Green, *J. Phys. Chem.* **65**, 779 (1961). Thermally less stable than arsine. Dec slowly on standing at room temp. Quickly destroyed at 200°. The decomposition products are hydrogen and metallic antimony, generally deposited in the form of a mirror. The gas is slightly sol in water. Freely sol in alcohol, carbon disulfide, other organic solvents. Lethal concn in air for mice: about 100 ppm.

Caution: Potential symptoms of overexposure are headache, weakness; nausea; abdominal pain; lumbar pain, hemoglobinuria, hematuria and hemolytic anemia; jaundice; pulmonary irritation. *See NIOSH Pocket Guide to Chemical Hazards* (DHHS/NIOSH 97-140, 1997) p 284.

USE: Has been used as fumigating agent.

8812. Stibocaptate. [27279-76-1] 2,2′-[(1,2-Dicarboxy-1,2-ethanediyl)bis(thio)]bis-1,3,2-dithiastibolane-4,5-dicarboxylic acid hexasodium salt; 2,3-dimercaptosuccinic acid cyclic ester with antimonic acid, diester with 2,3-dimercaptosuccinic acid hexasodium salt; 2,3-dimercaptosuccinic acid cyclic thioantimonate (III) *S,S*-diester with 2,3-dimercaptosuccinate hexasodium salt; sodium antimony-2,3-*meso*-dimercaptosuccinate; "antimony dimercaptosuccinate"; TWSb; Ro-4-1544/6; SB-58; Astiban. $C_{12}H_6Na_6O_{12}S_6Sb_2$; mol wt 916.02. C 15.73%, H 0.66%, Na 15.06%, O 20.96%, S 21.00%, Sb 26.58%. Prepn: Friedheim, **US 2880222** (1959). Prepn and antischistosomal activity: J.-K. Hsu, M.-K. Ch'en, *K'o Hsueh T'ung Pao* **1966**, 978, *C.A.* **65**, 17580e (1966). Toxicity data: Ercoli, *Proc. Soc. Exp. Biol. Med.* **129**, 284 (1968).

White or slightly yellowish-green powder. Hygroscopic, unstable when moistened. Sol in water. LD_{50} s.c. in mice: 500 mg Sb/kg (Ercoli).

Note: Stibocaptate described as the tripotassium salt: Friedheim *et al., Am. J. Trop. Med. Hyg.* **3**, 714 (1954).

THERAP CAT: Anthelmintic (Schistosoma).

8813. Stibophen. [15489-16-4] (*T*-4)-Bis[4,5-dihydroxy-1,3-benzenedisulfonato(4−)-*O⁴,O⁵*]-antimonate(5−) pentasodium heptahydrate; sodium antimony bis(pyrocatechol-2,4-disulfonate) heptahydrate; antimony pyrocatechol sodium disulfonate heptahydrate; Sdt-91; Fuadin; Fouadin; Fantorin; Neoantimosan; Repodral. $C_{12}H_4Na_5O_{16}S_4Sb.7H_2O$; mol wt 895.23. C 16.10%, H 2.03%, Na 12.84%, O 41.11%, S 14.33%, Sb 13.60%. Prepn of potassium salt: GB 213285 (1923 to Heyden). Prepn from sodium pyrocatechol-3,5-disulfonate and antimony trioxide in alkaline soln: H. Schmidt, DE 448800 (1924 to I. G. Farbenind.), *Frdl.* **16**, 2546 (1931); *idem,* US 1549154 (1925); *idem, Z. Angew. Chem.* **43**, 963 (1930); *idem,* US 1873668 (1932 to Winthrop). Toxicity: H. Eagle *et al., J. Pharmacol. Exp. Ther.* **89**, 196 (1947). Clinical trial in schistosomiasis: J. Azar *et al., Am. J. Trop. Med.* **29**, 595 (1949); in leishmaniasis: H. S. Girgla *et al., Br. J. Dermatol.* **97**, 307 (1977). UV spectrophotometric analysis: A. Besada *et al., Anal. Lett.* **21**, 447 (1988).

Fine crystals. Almost insol in abs alcohol, ether, chloroform, acetone, petr ether. Readily sol in cold water. Unless the colorless neutral water soln is acidified it acquires a yellowish tint and finally reaches lemon-yellow color. LD_{50} i.v. in rabbits: ~90 mg/kg (Eagle).

Potassium salt. Antimosan; Heyden 611.

THERAP CAT: Anthelmintic (Schistosoma).

THERAP CAT (VET): Has been used in schistosomiasis.

8814. Stigmastanol. [83-45-4] (3β,5α)-Stigmastan-3-ol; dihydro-β-sitosterol; β-sitostanol; 24α-ethylcholestanol; fucostanol. $C_{29}H_{52}O$; mol wt 416.72. C 83.58%, H 12.58%, O 3.84%. Occurs along with β-sitosterol and stigmasterol. Formation from β-sitosterol: Bernstein, Wallis, *J. Org. Chem.* **2**, 341 (1937); from β-sitostenone: Marker, Wittle, *J. Am. Chem. Soc.* **59**, 2704 (1937). Antihypercholesteremic activity in rabbits: I. Ikeda *et al., J. Nutr. Sci. Vitaminol.* **27**, 243 (1981).

Monohydrate. Crystals, mp 138-139°. When dry mp 144-145°. $[\alpha]_D^{20}$ +25° (c = 1.1 in chloroform).

Acetate. $C_{31}H_{54}O_2$. mp 137-138°. $[\alpha]_D^{20}$ +14° (c = 1.8 in chloroform).

8815. Stigmasterol. [83-48-7] (3β,22E)-Stigmasta-5,22-dien-3-ol; 3β-hydroxy-24-ethyl-Δ⁵,²²-cholestadiene. $C_{29}H_{48}O$; mol wt 412.69. C 84.40%, H 11.72%, O 3.88%. Usually isolated

from the phytosterol mixture from soy or calabar beans, *cf.* Thornton *et al., J. Am. Chem. Soc.* **62**, 2006 (1940); Byerrum, Ball, *Biochem. Prep.* **7**, 86 (1959). Structure: Fernholz, *Ann.* **507**, 128 (1933); **508**, 215 (1933); Fernholz, Chakravorty, *Ber.* **67**, 2021 (1934). Identity with *guinea-pig-anti-stiffness factor*: H. Rosenkrantz *et al., Proc. Soc. Exp. Biol. Med.* **76**, 408 (1951). Synthesis: W. Sucrow, M. Slopianka, *Ber.* **108**, 3721 (1975). HPLC separation from plant oils: H. Colin *et al., Anal. Chem.* **51**, 1661 (1979).

Monohydrate. Crystals from alcohol. When dry, mp 170°. $[\alpha]_D^{22}$ −51° (c = 2 in chloroform). Insol in water. Sol in the usual organic solvents.

Acetate. $C_{31}H_{50}O_2$. mp 144°. $[\alpha]_D^{20}$ −55.6° (c = 2 in chloroform).

p-Nitrobenzoate. $C_{36}H_{51}NO_4$. mp 203°. $[\alpha]_D^{17}$ −13° (c = 2 in alcohol).

8816. Stilbamidine. [122-06-5] 4,4′-(1,2-Ethenediyl)-bisbenzenecarboximidamide; 4,4′-stilbenedicarboxamidine; 4,4′-di-amidinostilbene. $C_{16}H_{16}N_4$; mol wt 264.33. C 72.70%, H 6.10%, N 21.20%. Prepn: A. J. Ewins, J. N. Ashley, GB 510097 (1939 to May & Baker); J. N. Ashley *et al., J. Chem. Soc.* **1942**, 103; of isethionate: G. Newbery, A. P. T. Easson, US 2394003 (1946 to May & Baker). Trypanocidal activity: E. M. Lourie, W. Yorke, *Ann. Trop. Med. Parasitol.* **33**, 289 (1939). Preliminary pharmacology: R. Wien, *ibid.* **37**, 1 (1943). Mechanism of action studies: M. J. Pine, *Biochem. Pharmacol.* **17**, 75 (1968); G. Weissmann *et al., ibid.* **19**, 1251 (1970). Crystal structure: C. Courseille *et al., C.R. Seances Acad. Sci. Ser. C* **272**, 1115 (1971). DNA binding study: N. Gresh, B. Pullman, *Mol. Pharmacol.* **25**, 452 (1984). Early review of pharmacology, mode of action and clinical applications: E. B. Schoenbach, E. M. Greenspan, *Medicine* **27**, 327-377 (1948).

Dihydrochloride. $C_{16}H_{18}Cl_2N_4$. Needles from water. LD_{50} in mice (mg/g): 0.031 i.v.; 0.18 s.c. (Wien).

Isethionate. [140-59-0] M & B 744. $C_{20}H_{28}N_4O_8S_2$; mol wt 516.59. Crystals, discolored by light, dec 290°. uv max: 330 nm ($E_{1cm}^{1\%}$ 750). Soly in water: approx 1 g in 2.5 to 3.0 ml H_2O; in methanol: 1.5 g/100 ml. pH of 0.5% aq soln 5.5-6.5.

THERAP CAT: Antiprotozoal (Leishmania, Trypanosoma).

8817. Stilbene. [588-59-0] 1,1′-(1,2-Ethenediyl)bis[benzene]; α,β-diphenylethylene; bibenzal; bibenzylidene. $C_{14}H_{12}$; mol wt 180.25. C 93.29%, H 6.71%. *trans*-Form prepd by Clemmensen reduction of benzoin: Shriner, Berger, *Org. Synth.* **coll. vol. III**, 786 (1955); *cis*-form by copper-chromite decarboxylation of α-phenylcinnamic acid: Buckles, Wheeler, *ibid.* **coll. vol. IV**, 857 (1963). Synthesis of *cis*- and *trans*-forms by the Wittig reaction and by decarboxylation of phenylcinnamic acids: Wheeler, Batlle de Pabon, *J. Org. Chem.* **30**, 1473 (1965).

trans-Form   *cis*-Form

trans-Form. [103-30-0] Crystals from 95% ethanol, mp 124°. bp_{760} 306-307°. uv max (95% ethanol): 296, 305 nm (ε 28100;

26700). Volatile with steam. Practically insol in water. Sol in 90 parts cold alc, 13 parts boiling alc, freely in benzene, ether.

cis-**Form.** [645-49-8] Liquid, solidifies at $-5°$. bp_{10} 135°; $bp_{1.0}$ 96°. n_D^{25} 1.6188. uv max (95% ethanol): 278 nm (ε 10200). Completely sol in cold abs alcohol.

8818. Stillingia. Queen's root; yaw root; silver leaf. Dried roots of *Stillingia sylvatica* L., *Euphorbiaceae*. *Habit.* Southeastern U.S. *Constit.* Acrid resin (sylvacrol), fixed and volatile oils, a glucoside.

THERAP CAT: Emetic, cathartic.

8819. Storax. [8023-62-9] Styrax; sweet oriental gum. Balsam obtained from the trunk of *Liquidambar orientalis* Mill., known as Levant Storax, or of *L. styraciflua* L., known as American Storax (family *Hamamelidaceae*). *Habit.* Levant storax is native to Asia Minor. American storax is produced chiefly in Honduras; found along the Atlantic coast from Connecticut to Central America. *Constit.* 33-50% α- and β-storesin and its cinnamic ester; 5-10% styracin; 10% phenylpropyl cinnamate; small amounts of ethyl cinnamate; benzyl cinnamate; 5-15% free cinnamic acid; styrene; 0.4% levorotatory oil; $C_{10}H_{16}O$, and traces of vanillin.

Semiliquid, grayish, sticky, opaque mass (Levant storax) or a semisolid, sometimes solid mass softened by warming (American storax). Storax is transparent in thin layers, has characteristic taste and odor, and is denser than water. Insol in water. Almost completely sol in 1 part warm alcohol, ether, acetone, carbon disulfide. Ingredient of Compound Benzoin Tincture, *see* Benzoin.

USE: In fumigating pastilles and powders; in perfumery; as imbedding material in microscopy.

THERAP CAT: Topical protectant. Expectorant.

THERAP CAT (VET): As a component of Compound Benzoin Tincture. Has been used as a parasiticide.

8820. Stramonium. Thorn apple; Jamestown weed; Jimpson weed; Jimson weed; stinkweed; devil's apple; apple of Peru. Dried leaves and flowering tops of *Datura stramonium* L., Solanaceae or its varieties. Used in traditional medicine in treatment of asthma. *Habit.* Europe, Asia, America. *Constit.* Leaves: 0.25-0.45% alkaloids consisting of atropine, hyoscyamine, and scopolamine; proteins, albumin. Seed: the same alkaloids but in lesser amounts; fixed oil, malic acid proteins. Comprehensive monograph: A. F. Blakeslee, *The Genus Datura* (Ronald Press, New York, 1959) 289 pp. *Review:* V. E. Tyler *et al.* in *Pharmacognosy*, 9th Ed., (Lea & Febiger, Philadelphia, 1988) pp 197-199.

8821. Strepogenin. [11000-03-6] A name for the biologically active principle capable of stimulating growth of certain microorganisms, and originally found present in products of natural origin, such as liver extract, flour, yeast, and tomato juice. Its peptide nature was indicated by its presence in hydrolyzates of purified proteins. To compare the activities of various protein hydrolyzates, a strepogenin unit was introduced and defined as: 1 mg of a standard liver extract (Wilson's liver fraction L) has the strepogenin activity of one unit (using *Lactobacillus casei* as test organism). The different structures of strepogenin-active peptides subsequently obtained from natural sources or by synthesis, indicate that strepogenin is not a distinct, chemically defined, biologically active peptide, but rather represents a biological phenomenon of a multitude of peptides. From the large number of strepogenin-active peptides known, no conclusion can be drawn with regard to structure-function relationships; these peptides have been suspected to be nothing more than easily accessible amino acids, particularly since they (peptides) are not essential for the growth of the microorganisms. Early isolation from liver extract and from tryptic digests of pure proteins: Sprince, Woolley, *J. Exp. Med.* **80**, 213 (1944); *eidem, J. Am. Chem. Soc.* **67**, 1734 (1945). *Review:* E. Schröder, K. Lübke, *The Peptides* vol. II (Academic Press, New York, 1966) pp 267-270.

8822. Streptidine. [85-17-6] *N,N'*-Bis(aminoiminomethyl)-streptamine; *N,N'*-diamidinostreptamine; *N,N''''*-(2,4,5,6-tetrahydroxy-1,3-cyclohexanediyl)bisguanidine; 1,3-diguanido-2,4,5,6-cyclohexanetetrol. $C_8H_{18}N_6O_4$; mol wt 262.27. C 36.64%, H 6.92%, N 32.04%, O 24.40%. The aglycone component of the streptomycin molecule joined with streptobiosamine through a glycosidic linkage. Obtained from streptomycin by acid hydrolysis:

Peck *et al., J. Am. Chem. Soc.* **68**, 29 (1946); Fried *et al., J. Biol. Chem.* **162**, 391 (1946). Structure: Carter *et al., Science* **103**, 53, 540 (1946). Synthesis: Wolfrom *et al., J. Am. Chem. Soc.* **72**, 1724 (1950). Absolute configuration: Dyer, Todd, *ibid.* **85**, 3896 (1963); Tatsuoka, Horii, *J. Antibiot.* **17A**, 88 (1964). Biosynthesis studies: Bruton *et al., J. Biol. Chem.* **242**, 813 (1967).

Optically inactive, diacidic base.

Dipicrate dihydrate. $C_{20}H_{24}N_{12}O_{18}\cdot2H_2O$. Yellow needles from water, dec 283-284° (becomes anhydrous *in vacuo* at 56°, dec 284-285°).

Sulfate. $C_8H_{18}N_6O_4\cdot H_2SO_4$. Crystals from dilute sulfuric acid + acetone, not melted at 300°. Forms solvated crystals from methanol.

Dihydrochloride. $C_8H_{18}N_6O_4\cdot2HCl$. Hygroscopic, amorphous powder, dec 170-210°. Forms solvated crystals from methanol.

8823. Streptodornase. [37340-82-2] Streptococcal deoxyribonuclease. DNAase produced by various strains of β-hemolytic streptococci. Identification in culture medium: W. S. Tillett *et al., Proc. Soc. Exp. Biol. Med.* **68**, 184 (1948); M. McCarty, *J. Exp. Med.* **88**, 181 (1948). Purification: J. H. Mowat *et al.*, US 2753291 (1956 to Am. Cyanamid). Clinical use with streptokinase in wound debridement: J. Poulsen *et al., Acta Chir. Scand.* **149**, 245 (1983).

Mixture with streptokinase. [8048-16-6] Ernodasa; Varidase.

THERAP CAT: Debriding agent.

8824. Streptogramins. Family of related antibiotic complexes produced by variety of soil organisms of the genus *Streptomyces*. Consists of two types of antibacterial components: a polyunsaturated macrolactone (Group A, Type II) and a cyclic hexadepsipeptide (Group B, Type I). Both groups inhibit bacterial growth by preventing the translation of mRNA by binding to the bacterial ribosome and act synergistically. Isoln of complex from *Streptomyces graminofaciens*: J. Charney *et al., Antibiot. Chemother.* **3**, 1283 (1953). Each strain specific complex and its respective components were named to reflect the producing strain, however structural studies showed considerable overlap *see* Pristinamycin, Virginiamycin, *q.q.v.* Nomenclature: P. Crooy, R. De Neys, *J. Antibiot.* **25**, 371 (1972). Mechanism of action: B. T. Porse, R. A. Garrett, *J. Mol. Biol.* **286**, 375 (1999). Review of isolations, identification and activity: D. Vazquez, *Antibiotics* vol. 1, D. Gottlieb, P. D. Shaw, Eds. (Springer-Verlag, New York, 1967) pp 387-403; vol. 3, J. W. Corcoran, F. E. Hahn, Eds. (1975) pp 521-534. *Review:* J.-C. Pechère, *Drugs* **51**, Suppl. 1, 13-19 (1996); of chemistry and biological activity: J. C. Barrière *et al., Curr. Pharm. Des.* **4**, 155-180 (1998).

Streptogramin A *see* Virginiamycin M1.
Streptogramin B *see* Pristinamycin IA.

8825. Streptokinase. [9002-01-1] Streptococcal fibrinolysin; plasminokinase; Kabikinase; Streptase. Single-chain protein produced by β-hemolytic streptococci; mol wt ~47 kDa. Activates plasminogen to produce plasmin which dissolves fibrin. Discovery: W. S. Tillet, R. L. Garner, *J. Exp. Med.* **58**, 485 (1933). Isoln from streptococcal culture filtrates: L. R. Christensen, *J. Gen. Physiol.* **28**, 363 (1945). Purification: M. Siegel *et al.*, US 3042586 (1962 to Merck & Co.); P. K. Siiteri, R. D. Mills, US 3226304 (1965 to Am. Cyanamid); and characterization: E. C. De Renzo *et al., J. Biol. Chem.* **242**, 533 (1967). Review of isoln, assay and properties: F. B. Taylor, R. H. Tomar, *Methods Enzymol.* **19**, 807-821 (1970); F. Castellino, Jr. *et al., ibid.* **45B**, 244-257 (1976); of mechanism of action: K. N. N. Reddy in *Fibrinolysis*, D. L. Kline, K. N. N. Reddy, Eds. (CRC, Boca Raton, 1980) pp 71-94. Clinical trials in acute myocardial infarction: J. L. Anderson *et al., N. Engl. J. Med.* **308**, 1312 (1983); ISIS-2 Collaborative Group, *Lancet* **2**, 349 (1988). Clinical comparison with alteplase (tPA): GISSI-2 and Int. Study

Group, *Eur. Heart J.* **13**, 1692 (1992). Pharmacokinetics: D. S. Grierson, T. D. Bjornsson, *Clin. Pharmacol. Ther.* **41**, 304 (1987). Review of clinical efficacy in deep venous thrombosis: L. Q. Rogers, C. L. Lutcher, *Am. J. Med.* **88**, 389-395 (1990); in myocardial infarction: K. L. Goa *et al., Drugs* **39**, 693-719 (1990); P. E. Battershill *et al., Drugs Aging* **4**, 63-86 (1994).

THERAP CAT: Thrombolytic.

8826. Streptomycin. [57-92-1] *O*-2-Deoxy-2-(methylamino)-α-L-glucopyranosyl-(1 → 2)-*O*-5-deoxy-3-*C*-formyl-α-L-lyxofuranosyl-(1 → 4)-*N,N'*-bis(aminoiminomethyl)-D-streptamine; streptomycin A. $C_{21}H_{39}N_7O_{12}$; mol wt 581.57. C 43.37%, H 6.76%, N 16.86%, O 33.01%. Antibiotic substance produced by the soil Actinomycete *Streptomyces griseus* (Krainsky) Waksman et Henrici (Fam. *Actinomycetaceae*). Isolation: Schatz *et al., Proc. Soc. Exp. Biol. Med.* **55**, 66 (1944). Production by aerobic fermentation and purification: Tishler in *Streptomycin*, Selman A. Waksman, Ed. (Williams & Wilkins, Baltimore, 1949) pp 32-54. Isoln and purification by ion exchange: Bartels *et al., Chem. Eng. Prog.* **54** (8), 49-51 (Aug. 1958); Bartels *et al., US 2868779* (1959 to Olin Mathieson). Structure: Brink, Folkers, *J. Am. Chem. Soc.* **69**, 1234 (1947); Wolfrom *et al., ibid.* **76**, 3675 (1950). Total synthesis: Umezawa *et al., J. Antibiot.* **27**, 997 (1974). Mechanism of action: B. J. Wallace *et al.,* in *Antibiotics* vol. 5(pt. 1), F. E. Hahn, Ed. (Springer-Verlag, New York, 1979) pp 272-303. *Review:* Lemieux, Wolfrom, "The Chemistry of Streptomycin" in W. W. Pigman, M. L. Wolfrom, *Adv. Carbohydr. Chem.* **3**, 337-384 (1948). Comprehensive description: J. Mossa *et al., Anal. Profiles Drug Subs.* **16**, 507-609 (1986).

Streptomycin is usually available as the trihydrochloride, trihydrochloride-calcium chloride double salt, phosphate, or sesquisulfate, which occur as granules or powder. Odorless or nearly so, with a slightly bitter taste. Most salts are hygroscopic and deliquesce on exposure to air, but are not affected by air or light. The salts are very sol in water; but almost insol in alc, chloroform, ether. Solns are levorotatory.

Trihydrochloride. Streptomycin hydrochloride. $C_{21}H_{39}N_7$- O_{12}.3HCl. $[\alpha]_D^{25}$ −84°. Solubilities as determined by Weiss *et al., Antibiot. Chemother.* **7**, 374 (1957) in mg/ml at about 28°: water >20; methanol >20; ethanol 0.90; isopropanol 0.12; isoamyl alcohol 0.117; petr ether 0.02; carbon tetrachloride 0.042; ether 0.01.

Trihydrochloride-calcium chloride double salt. Streptomycin hydrochloride-calcium chloride complex. $(C_{21}H_{39}N_7O_{12}.3HCl)_2$- $CaCl_2$Prepn from the trihydrochloride: Peck, *US 2446102* (1948 to Merck & Co.). Very hygroscopic, dec about 200°. $[\alpha]_D^{25}$ −76°.

Pantothenate. Streptothenat. Prepn: **GB 771338** (1957 to Grünenthal). The commercial prepn may contain the sulfate.

Sesquisulfate. [3810-74-0] Streptomycin sulfate; AgriStrep; Streptobrettin; Vetstrep. $(C_{21}H_{39}N_7O_{12})_2$.3$H_2SO_4$; mol wt 1457.38. White to light gray or pale buff powder with faint amine-like odor. Solubilities as determined by Weiss *et al., loc. cit.,* in mg/ml at about 28°: water >20; methanol 0.85; ethanol 0.30; isopropanol 0.01; petr ether 0.015; carbon tetrachloride 0.035; ether 0.035.

THERAP CAT: Antibacterial (tuberculostatic).

THERAP CAT (VET): Antibacterial.

8827. Streptonigrin. [3930-19-6] 5-Amino-6-(7-amino-5,8-dihydro-6-methoxy-5,8-dioxo-2-quinolyl)-4-(2-hydroxy-3,4-dimethoxyphenyl)-3-methyl-2-pyridinecarboxylic acid; 5-amino-6-(7-amino-5,8-dihydro-6-methoxy-5,8-dioxo-2-quinolyl)-4-(2-hydroxy-3,4-dimethoxyphenyl)-3-methylpicolinic acid; bruneomycin; NSC-45383. $C_{25}H_{22}N_4O_8$; mol wt 506.46. C 59.29%, H 4.38%, N 11.06%, O 25.27%. Antitumor antibiotic produced by *Streptomyces flocculus*: Rao, Cullen, *Antibiot. Annu.* **1959-1960**, 950. Structure: Rao *et al., J. Am. Chem. Soc.* **85**, 2532 (1963). Crystal and molecular structure: Y. Y. H. Chiu, W. N. Lipscomb, *ibid.* **97**, 2525 (1975). Identity with bruneomycin: Brazhnikova *et al., Antibiotiki* **13**, 99 (1968), *C.A.* **68**, 89890q (1968). Synthetic studies: Kametani *et al., C.A.* **76**, 14272w (1972); **79**, 31817g (1973). Total synthesis: F. Z. Basha *et al., J. Am. Chem. Soc.* **102**, 3962 (1980); A. S. Kende *et al., ibid.* **103**, 1271 (1981); S. M. Weinreb *et al., ibid.* **104**, 536 (1982). Biosynthesis: S. J. Gould, D. E. Cane, *ibid.* 343. *Reviews:* N. S. Mizuno in *Antibiotics* vol. 5, pt. 2, F. E. Hahn, Ed. (Springer-Verlag, New York, 1979) pp 372-384; S. J. Gould, S. M. Weinreb, *Fortschr. Chem. Org. Naturst.* **41**, 77-111 (1982). Review of genotoxicity: A. D. Bolzán, M. S. Bianchi, *Mutat. Res.* **488**, 25-37 (2001).

Coffee-brown to almost black rectangular plates from acetone or dioxane, dec 275°; brown needles, mp 262-263° (Brazhnikova). uv max (methanol): 248, 375-380 nm (ε 38400, 17400). Weak acid. pKa 6.2-6.4 (1:1 aq dioxane). Sol in dioxane, pyridine, dimethylformamide, aq sodium bicarbonate with decompn; slightly sol in water, lower alcohols, ethyl acetate, chloroform.

Caution: Potential symptoms of overexposure include severe and prolonged bone marrow depression (Bolzán, Bianchi).

8828. L-Streptose. [13008-73-6] 5-Deoxy-3-*C*-formyl-L-lyxose; 3-*C*-formyl-5-deoxy-L-lyxofuranose. $C_6H_{10}O_5$; mol wt 162.14. C 44.45%, H 6.22%, O 49.34%. A sugar which is part of the streptomycin molecule: Kuehl *et al., J. Am. Chem. Soc.* **68**, 2096 (1946). Structure: *eidem, ibid.* **68**, 2679 (1946). Configuration: Wolfrom, DeWalt, *ibid.* **70**, 3148 (1948); Kuehl *et al., ibid.* **71**, 1445 (1949). Biosynthesis: Hough, Jones, *Nature* **167**, 180 (1951). Synthesis of α- and β-L-streptose: Dyer *et al., J. Am. Chem. Soc.* **87**, 654 (1965); Paulsen *et al., Ber.* **105**, 1978 (1972).

Colorless, strongly hygroscopic glass. $[\alpha]_D^{20}$ −18° (c = 0.65).

8829. Streptothricins. Racemomycins; yazumycins. A mixture of antibiotics, originally thought to be a single substance, differing only in the number of repeating residues in the peptide side chain. Streptothricins F, E, D, C, B, A, and X are known and have 1 to 7 β-lysine residues resp.: Khokhlov, Shutova, *J. Antibiot.* **25**, 501 (1972). Separation of isomers: Khokhlov, Reshetov, *J. Chromatogr.* **14**, 495 (1964). Identity with racemomycins: H. Taniyama *et al., Chem. Pharm. Bull.* **19**, 1627 (1971). Identity with yazumycins: *eidem, J. Antibiot.* **24**, 390 (1971). Activity studies: Germanova, Goncharskaya, *Antibiotiki* **14**, 48, 137 (1969), *C.A.* **70**, 66547, 85906t (1969). Biosynthetic studies: Voronina *et al., ibid.* 1063, *C.A.* **72**, 77387a (1970); Y. Sawada *et al., Chem. Pharm. Bull.* **26**, 885 (1978). Partial syntheses: M. Kinoshita, Y. Suzuki, *Bull.*

Chem. Soc. Jpn. **50**, 2375 (1977); S. Kusumoto *et al., Chem. Lett.* **1981**, 1317. Prepn of semi-synthetic racemomycins: Y. Sawada, H. Taniyama, *Chem. Pharm. Bull.* **25**, 1302 (1977). *Streptolin* was formerly used for the streptothricin components where n equals 2 or 3.

Streptothricin F. Racemomycin A; streptothricin VI; yazumycin A. $C_{19}H_{34}N_8O_8$; mol wt 502.52. n = 1. Originally known as streptothricin. Produced by variants of *Actinomyces lavendulae.* Isoln: Waksman, Woodruff, *Proc. Soc. Exp. Biol. Med.* **49**, 207 (1942). Purification: Peck *et al., J. Am. Chem. Soc.* **68**, 772 (1946); Kocholaty, Junowicz-Kocholaty, *Arch. Biochem.* **15**, 55 (1947). Identity with streptothricin VI: Hutchinson *et al., Arch. Biochem.* **22**, 16 (1949); Swart; *J. Am. Chem. Soc.* **71**, 2942 (1949). Prepn: Carter *et al., J. Am. Chem. Soc.* **76**, 566 (1954). Structure: van Tamelen *et al., ibid.* **83**, 4295 (1961); Johnson, Westley, *J. Chem. Soc.* **1962**, 1642. Revised structure: S. Kusumoto *et al., J. Antibiot.* **35**, 925 (1982). Biosynthesis: S. J. Gould *et al., J. Am. Chem. Soc.* **103**, 2871 (1981). Total synthesis: S. Kusumoto *et al., Tetrahedron Lett.* **23**, 2961 (1982). Amorphous, white powder. Thermostable. Water sol; slightly sol in most organic solvents. Stable between pH 1 and 8.5. LD_{50} i.v. in mice: 300 mg/kg (Taniyama).

Hydrochloride. White powder. $[\alpha]_D^{25}$ −51.3° (c = 1.4). Sol in water and dil mineral acids. Practically insol in ether, petr ether, chloroform.

8830. Streptovaricin. [1404-74-6] Streptovarycin. A complex of ansamycin antibiotics consisting of streptovaricins A, B, C, D, E, F, G, J and K of which streptovaricin C is the major component. Isolation from *Streptomyces spectabilis:* Siminoff *et al., Am. Rev. Tuberc. Pulm. Dis.* **75**, 576 (1957); Whitfield *et al., ibid.* 584; and resolution of components: Dietz *et al.,* **US 3116202** (1963 to Upjohn). Characterization of complex: Rinehart *et al., Chem. Commun.* **1974**, 861. Preliminary structural studies: Rinehart *et al., J. Am. Chem. Soc.* **88**, 3149, 3150 (1966); **90**, 6241 (1968); Rinehart *et al., ibid.* **93**, 6273 (1971). Revised structure of streptovaricin C: Sasaki *et al., J. Antibiot.* **25** 68 (1972); Rinehart, Antosz, *ibid.* 71. Activity studies: Quintrell, McAuslan, *J. Virol.* **6**, 485 (1970); Tan, McAuslan, *Biochem. Biophys. Res. Commun.* **42**, 230 (1971); Carter *et al., Nature New Biol.* **232**, 212, 214 (1971). Biosynthetic study: P. V. Deshmukh *et al., J. Am. Chem. Soc.* **98**, 870 (1976). ^{13}C-NMR studies: K. B. Kakinuma *et al., J. Org. Chem.* **41**, 1358 (1976). Synthesis of a key intermediate for the total synthesis of streptovaricin A: P. A. McCarthy, *Tetrahedron Lett.* **23**, 4199 (1982). Synthesis of the naphthalene core of streptovaricin D: B. M. Trost, W. H. Pearson, *ibid.* **24**, 269 (1983). Review of the chemistry of streptovaricins: K. L. Rinehart *et al., Fortschr. Chem. Org. Naturst.* **33**, 231-307 (1976).

Streptovaricin C

The complex yields yellow crystals from ethyl acetate + hexane. Neutral or weakly acidic substance which hydrolyzes on treatment with dil alkali. Stable at room temp for 3-4 days at pH 2.0-6.0. Gradually loses its antibiotic activity while standing at room temp for 2-4 days at pH 7.8.

Streptovaricin A. [23344-16-3] $C_{42}H_{53}NO_{16}$; mol wt 827.87. mp 194-196°. $[\alpha]_D$ in chloroform +61°. uv max (95% ethanol): 245, 260, 320, 430 nm ($E_{1cm}^{1\%}$ 418.9, 352.1, 139.8, 136.2).

Streptovaricin B. [11031-82-6] $C_{42}H_{53}NO_{15}$; mol wt 811.87. mp 185-187°. $[\alpha]_D$ in chloroform +576° (Dietz, +454°). uv max (95% ethanol): 245, 266, 320, 432 nm ($E_{1cm}^{1\%}$ 408.3, 338.5, 140.1, 109.7).

Streptovaricin C. [23344-17-4] $C_{40}H_{51}NO_{14}$; mol wt 769.83. mp 189-191° (Dietz, 168-171°). $[\alpha]_D$ in chloroform +602° (Dietz, +317°). uv max (95% ethanol): 245.5, 260, 320, 430 nm ($E_{1cm}^{1\%}$ 443.5, 389.7, 153.1, 121.9). Solubility data: March, Weiss, *J. Assoc. Off. Anal. Chem.* **50**, 457 (1967).

Streptovaricin D. [32164-26-4] $C_{40}H_{51}NO_{13}$; mol wt 753.83. mp 167-170° (Dietz, 115-118°). $[\alpha]_D$ in chloroform +436° (Dietz, +102°). uv max (95% ethanol): 246, 264, 320, 433 nm ($E_{1cm}^{1\%}$ 431.4, 370.3, 147.7, 105.3).

Streptovaricin E. [35413-63-9] $C_{40}H_{49}NO_{14}$; mol wt 767.82. mp 102-105°. $[\alpha]_D^{24}$ in chloroform +164°, also reported as +613°. uv max (95% ethanol): 245, 273, 320, 437 nm ($E_{1cm}^{1\%}$ 382.2, 346.9, 190.4, 91.9).

Streptovaricin F. [35512-37-9] $C_{39}H_{47}NO_{14}$; mol wt 753.79.

Streptovaricin G. [11031-85-9] $C_{40}H_{51}NO_{15}$; mol wt 785.83. mp 190-192°. $[\alpha]_D$ in chloroform +473°.

Streptovaricin J. [52275-61-3] $C_{42}H_{53}NO_{15}$; mol wt 811.87. mp 177-180°. $[\alpha]_D$ +326° (c = 0.25 in ethanol); +436° (c = 0.094 in chloroform).

8831. Streptovirudin. [56833-74-0] Nucleoside antibiotic complex produced by *Streptomyces griseoflavus* subsp. *thuringiensis,* strain JA 10124, that has inhibitory activity vs gram-positive bacteria, mycobacteria, and several RNA and DNA viruses. Isoln: K. Eckardt *et al., Z. Allg. Mikrobiol.* **13**, 625 (1973); *eidem, J. Antibiot.* **28**, 274 (1975). Taxonomy, fermentation, production: H. Thrum *et al., ibid.* 514. Streptovirudin is related chemically to tunicamycin, *q.v.,* and contains at least 10 components, of which 8 have been isolated in pure form. The complex is divided into 2 series of compounds: series I (streptovirudins A_1 through D_1) contains dihydrouracil and series II (streptovirudins A_2 through D_2) contains uracil. Differentiation of streptovirudin and tunicamycin by gel chromatography, HPLC, and hydrolysis: K. Eckardt *et al., ibid.* **33**, 908 (1980). Structures of streptovirudins and identity of components B_{2a} and C_2 with tunicamycin components: *eidem, ibid.* **34**, 1631 (1981); W. Ihn *et al., Tetrahedron* **38**, 1781 (1982). Biological activities of isolated streptovirudin and tunicamycin components, identity of streptovirudin C_2 with tunicamycin A: R. W. Keenan *et al., Biochemistry* **20**, 2968 (1981). Chemical and biological properties of streptovirudins: A. D. Elbein *et al., ibid.* 4210. Viral inhibition study: M. S. Kang *et al., Biochem. Biophys. Res. Commun.* **99**, 422 (1981).

Streptovirudin A_1

White amorphous solid. uv max (methanol): 212 nm. Sol in methanol, pyridine. Slightly sol in water, ethanol. Insol in chloroform, acetone, benzene, ethyl acetate. Stable up to 5 hours at 90°. No loss of activity was observed after standing at 37° for 4 weeks. LD_{50} in mice (mg/kg) of the antibiotic complex from culture filtrate: 250 orally; 15 s.c.; 15-17.5 i.p.; 17.5 i.v.; of the complex from mycelium: 150 orally; 5-10 s.c.; 3.5-7.5 i.p. (Thrum).

8832. Streptozocin. [18883-66-4] 2-Deoxy-2-[[(methyl-nitrosoamino)carbonyl]amino]-D-glucopyranose; 2-deoxy-2-(3-methyl-3-nitrosoureido)-D-glucopyranose; streptozotocin; NSC-85998; U-9889; Zanosar. $C_8H_{15}N_3O_7$; mol wt 265.22. C 36.23%, H 5.70%, N 15.84%, O 42.23%. Isoln from *Streptomyces achromogenes* fermentation broth: Herr *et al., Antibiot. Annu.* **1959-1960**, 236; Bergy *et al.,* FR 1434920 (1966 to Upjohn), *C.A.* **65**, 17661h (1966). Structure and synthesis: Herr *et al., J. Am. Chem. Soc.* **89**, 4808 (1967); Hardegger *et al., Helv. Chim. Acta* **52**, 2555 (1969); Hessler, Jahnke, *J. Org. Chem.* **35**, 245 (1970); P. F. Wiley *et al., ibid.* **44**, 9 (1979). Diabetogenic effect: Rakieten *et al., Cancer Chemother. Rep.* **29**, 91 (May 1963). Comparison of streptozotocin- and alloxan-induced diabetes: C. Rerup, F. Tarding, *Eur. J. Clin. Pharmacol.* **7**, 89 (1969). Antileukemic activity: Bhuyan *et al., Cancer Chemother. Rep. Part 1* **56**, 709 (1972). Biosynthetic study: S. Singaram *et al., J. Antibiot.* **32**, 379 (1979). Review and evaluation of studies of carcinogenicity in laboratory animals: *IARC Monographs* **4**, 221-227 (1974). Toxicity data: M. Iwasaki *et al., J. Med. Chem.* **19**, 918 (1976). *Review:* B. Rudas, *Arzneim.-Forsch.* **22**, 830-861 (1972); P. F. Wiley, *Anticancer Agents Based on Natural Product Models,* J. M. Cassidy, J. D. Douros, Eds. (Academic Press, New York, 1980) pp 167-200. Book: *Streptozotocin: Fundamentals and Therapy,* M. K. Agarwal, Ed. (Elsevier/North Holland Biomedical Press, New York, 1981) 309 pp.

Pointed platelets or prisms, from 95% ethanol, mp 115° (dec). Sol in H_2O, lower alcohols and ketones. uv max (ethanol): 228 nm (ε 6360). A mixture of α and β anomers; aq solns rapidly undergo mutarotation to an equilibrium value of $[\alpha]_D^{25}$ +39°. LD_{50} in female mice (mg/kg): 360 i.p.; 275 i.v.; in male dogs (mg/kg): 50 i.v. (Iwasaki).

Tetraacetate. $C_8H_{11}N_3O_7(COCH_3)_4$. Crystals, mp 111-114° (dec). $[\alpha]_D^{25}$ +41° (c = 0.78 in 95% ethanol).

Caution: Streptozocin is reasonably anticipated to be a human carcinogen: *Report on Carcinogens, Eleventh Edition* (PB2005-104914, 2004) p III-234.

USE: Production of experimental diabetes in laboratory animals.

THERAP CAT: Antineoplastic.

8833. Strigol. [11017-56-4] (3E,3aR,5S,8bS)-3-[[[(2R)-2,5-Dihydro-4-methyl-5-oxo-2-furanyl]oxy]methylene]-3,3a,4,5,6,7,8,-8b-octahydro-5-hydroxy-8,8-dimethyl-2H-indeno[1,2-b]furan-2-one. $C_{19}H_{22}O_6$; mol wt 346.37. C 65.88%, H 6.40%, O 27.71%. Potent seed germination stimulant for the root parasite, witchweed, *Striga lutea* Lour. isolated from root exudates of cotton, *Gossypium hirsutum* L.: C. E. Cook *et al., Science* **154**, 1189 (1966). Structure: *eidem, J. Am. Chem. Soc.* **94**, 6198 (1972). Crystal structure: P. Coggan *et al., J. Chem. Soc. Perkin Trans. 2* **1973**, 465. Synthesis: J. B. Heather *et al., J. Am. Chem. Soc.* **98**, 3661 (1976); of (±)-form: G. A. MacAlpine *et al., Chem. Commun.* **1974**, 834; *eidem, J. Chem. Soc. Perkin Trans. 1* **1976**, 410. Synthesis of analogs: A. W. Johnson *et al., ibid.* **1981**, 1734. Witchweed seed germination stimulating activity: A. L. Hsiao *et al., Weed Sci.* **29**, 101 (1981); A. B. Pepperman *et al., ibid.* **30**, 561 (1982).

White needles from benzene-hexane, mp 200-202° (dec). $[\alpha]_D^{25}$ +293° (c = 0.15 in $CHCl_3$). uv max: 234 nm (ε 17700). Sol in acetone, methylene chloride. Moderately sol in benzene; insol in hexane.

8834. Strobilurins. Class of antifungal antibiotics found in wood-rotting mushrooms. Strobilurins A-H have been isolated. Strobilurin A is the parent compound for a new class of agricultural antifungals which inhibit mitochondrial respiration at the cytochrome bc_1 complex. *See* synthetic analogs: azoxystrobin, kresoxim methyl. Identification of activity in *Oudemansiella mucida*: V. Musilek *et al., Folia Microbiol.* **14**, 377 (1969). Isoln of A and B from *Strobilurus tenacellus*: T. Anke *et al., J. Antibiot.* **30**, 806 (1977); of F, G, H from *Bolinea lutea* Sacc.: A. Fredenhagen *et al., ibid.* **43**, 655 (1990). Identity with mucidin and mechanism of action: G. Von Jagow *et al., Biochemistry* **25**, 775 (1986). Revised stereostructure and synthesis of A: T. Anke *et al., Ann.* **1984**, 1616. Stereosynthesis: K. Beautement, J. M. Clough, *Tetrahedron Lett.* **28**, 475 (1987). Brief review: T. Anke, *Can. J. Bot.* **73** Suppl. 1, S940-S945 (1995).

Strobilurin A

Strobilurin A. [52110-55-1] (E,Z,E)-2-(Methoxymethylene)-3-methyl-6-phenyl-3,5-hexadienoic acid methyl ester; mucidin. $C_{16}H_{18}O_3$; mol wt 258.31. Colorless, homogeneous oil. uv max (ethanol): 230, 237, 294 nm (ε 16900, 15330, 21850). Sol in methanol, ethanol. acetone, ethyl acetate, $CHCl_3$, CCl_4; very poorly sol in water.

8835. Strontium. [7440-24-6] Sr; at. wt 87.62; at. no. 38; valence 2. Group IIA (2). Alkaline earth metal. Naturally occurring, stable isotopes: 88 (82.58%); 86 (9.86%); 87 (7.00%); 84 (0.56%). Known radioactive isotopes: 76-83, 85, 89, 90 (longest lived isotope, $T_{1/2}$ 28.78 yr, β^- decay), 91-102. Occurs in the minerals, *celestine* ($SrSO_4$) and *strontianite* ($SrCO_3$); found in small quantities associated with calcium or barium minerals. Abundance in earth's crust 384 ppm. First prepared in 1807 by Davy. Commercial production by thermal reduction of strontium oxide with aluminum. Prepn: Glascock, *J. Am. Chem. Soc.* **32**, 1222 (1910); Matignon, *Compt. Rend.* **177**, 1116 (1923); *J. Chem. Soc.* **126**[ii], 44 (1924); Guntz *et al.,* cited in *Gmelins, Strontium* (8th ed.) **29**, 35 (1931). *Reviews:* Goodenough, Stenger, "Magnesium, Calcium, Strontium, Barium and Radium" in *Comprehensive Inorganic Chemistry* vol. 1, J. C. Bailar, Jr. *et al.,* Eds. (Pergamon Press, Oxford, 1973) pp 591-774; *Chemistry of the Elements* N. N. Greenwood, A. Earnshaw, Eds. (Pergamon Press, New York, 1984) pp 117-154; S. G. Hibbins in *Kirk-Othmer Encyclopedia of Chemical Technology* vol. 22 (Wiley-Interscience, New York, 4th ed., 1997) pp 947-955. Review of clinical use of ^{89}Sr in pain palliation for metastatic bone cancer: G. B. Altman, C. A. Lee, *Oncol. Nurs. Forum* **32**, 523-527 (1996). Review of toxicology and human exposure: *Toxicological Profile for Strontium* (PB2004-104400, 2004) 445 pp.

Silvery-white metal; face-centered cubic structure; rapidly becomes yellow on exposure to air and assumes an oxide film. The finely divided metal ignites spontaneously in air. d 2.6; mp 757 ±1°; bp 1366°. E^0 (aq) Sr^{2+}/Sr −2.89 V. Undergoes reactions characteristic of alkaline earth metals. Strong reducing agent. *Keep under liquid containing no oxygen.* The heated metal combines with hydrogen to form **strontium hydride** and with nitrogen to form **strontium nitride**. Metal and its salts emit characteristic brilliant red color in flame.

Note: The problems of internal radiation hazards from radio-strontium are discussed by A. Engström *et al., Bone and Radio-strontium* (Wiley, New York, 1958).

USE: In fireworks, in red signal flares; on tracer bullets. Eutectic modifier in Al-Ag casting alloys to improve strength and ductility. Innoculant in ductile iron casting to control graphite formation.

THERAP CAT: [89]Sr as antineoplastic (radiation source).

8836. Strontium Acetate. [543-94-2] $C_4H_6O_4Sr$; mol wt 205.71. C 23.35%, H 2.94%, O 31.11%, Sr 42.59%. $Sr(C_2H_3-O_2)_2$. Toxicity: V. V. Cole *et al.*, *J. Pharmacol. Exp. Ther.* **71**, 1 (1941).

Hemihydrate. White crystalline powder. Loses its water at 150°; on ignition is converted into $SrCO_3$. Sol in 2.5 parts water; slightly sol in alcohol. The aq soln is practically neutral to litmus. LD i.v. in rats: 1.16 mmol/kg (Cole).

8837. Strontium Bromide. [10476-81-0] Br_2Sr; mol wt 247.43. Br 64.59%, Sr 35.41%. $SrBr_2$. Acute toxicity: K. W. Cochran *et al.*, *Arch. Ind. Hyg. Occup. Med.* **1**, 637 (1950).

Hexahydrate. Colorless, deliquesc crystals or white granules; bitter saline taste. mp 88° when rapidly heated; mp 643° when anhydr. Loses all its water at 180°. Sol in 0.35 part water; sol in alcohol. Insol in ether. The aq soln is neutral. *Incompat:* Soluble sulfates. LD_{50} i.p. in rats: 1000 mg/kg (Cochran).

THERAP CAT: Has been used as anticonvulsant.

THERAP CAT (VET): Has been used as sedative, anticonvulsant.

8838. Strontium Carbonate. [1633-05-2] CO_3Sr; mol wt 147.63. C 8.14%, O 32.51%, Sr 59.35%. $SrCO_3$. Occurs in nature as the mineral *strontianite*.

White, odorless, tasteless powder. d 3.5. Dec at 1100° into SrO and CO_2. Sol in 100,000 parts water, in about 1000 parts of water saturated with CO_2; sol in dil acids.

USE: In pyrotechnics; manuf iridescent glass; refining sugar.

8839. Strontium Chlorate. [7791-10-8] Cl_2O_6Sr; mol wt 254.52. Cl 27.86%, O 37.72%, Sr 34.43%. $Sr(ClO_3)_2$.

Colorless or white crystals. d 3.15. mp 120° with decomposition and evolution of O_2. Sol in 0.6 part water, slightly in alcohol. *Handle with caution like potassium chlorate.*

USE: In pyrotechnics to produce red fire.

8840. Strontium Chloride. [10476-85-4] Cl_2Sr; mol wt 158.53. Cl 44.73%, Sr 55.27%. $SrCl_2$. Acute toxicity: I. B. Syed, F. Hosain, *Toxicol. Appl. Pharmacol.* **22**, 150 (1972).

⁸⁹Sr-Labeled form. [38270-90-5] Metastron. Clinical studies in pain palliation for metastatic bone cancer: R. G. Robinson *et al.*, *RadioGraphics* **9**, 271 (1989); K. M. Kälkner *et al.*, *Anticancer Res.* **20**, 1109 (2000). $T_{1/2}$ 50.52 days, β^- emitter.

Hexahydrate. [10025-70-4] Colorless, odorless crystals or white granules. Effloresces in air; deliquesces in moist air. At 100° loses $5H_2O$; at 150° all its H_2O; d 1.96; mp 61° when rapidly heated; the anhydr salt melts at 868°. Soluble in 0.8 part water, 0.5 part boiling water; sol in alcohol. The aq soln is neutral. *Keep well closed.* LD_{50} i.v. in mice: 147.6 mg/kg (Syed, Hosain).

USE: Manuf strontium salts; in pyrotechnics; pharmaceutic aid (dental desensitizer).

THERAP CAT: Antineoplastic (radiation source).

8841. Strontium Chromate(VI). [7789-06-2] CrO_4Sr; mol wt 203.61. Cr 25.54%, O 31.43%, Sr 43.03%. $SrCrO_4$.

Yellow powder. d 3.89. Soluble in 840 parts cold water, about 5 parts boiling water; freely sol in dil hydrochloric, nitric or acetic acids.

Caution: Chromium hexavalent compounds are listed as known human carcinogens: *Report on Carcinogens, Eleventh Edition* (PB2005-104914, 2004) p III-63.

USE: Corrosion inhibitor in pigments; in electrochemical processes to control sulfate concn of solns.

8842. Strontium Fluoride. [7783-48-4] F_2Sr; mol wt 125.62. F 30.25%, Sr 69.75%. SrF_2. Prepd by dissolving $SrCO_3$ in an excess of 40% HF and evaporating to dryness: Berzelius, *Pogg. Ann.* **1**, 20 (1824); final drying should be done at 150° *in vacuo.*

White powder or cubic crystals. d 4.24. mp ~1400°. bp 2460°. Stable in air up to 1000°. Above this temp it is oxidized to strontium oxide. Heat of evaporation 78.2. Trouton const 28.6. Soly in water (18°) 11.7 mg/100 ml. More sol in dil acids. Dec by strong acids. May be stored in glass bottles.

8843. Strontium Hydroxide. [18480-07-4] Strontium hydrate. H_2O_2Sr; mol wt 121.63. H 1.66%, O 26.31%, Sr 72.04%. $Sr(OH)_2$.

Octahydrate. Colorless, deliquesc crystals or white powder; absorbs CO_2 from air forming carbonate. Loses part of its water at about 100°. Sol in 50 parts water, 2.1 parts boiling water. The soln is very alkaline. pH about 13.5. *Keep tightly closed.*

USE: Refining beet sugar; separating crystallizable sugar from molasses.

8844. Strontium Iodide. [10476-86-5] I_2Sr; mol wt 341.43. I 74.34%, Sr 25.66%. SrI_2. The article of commerce is hydrated. Toxicity data: K. W. Cochran *et al.*, *Arch. Ind. Hyg. Occup. Med.* **1**, 637 (1950).

Hexahydrate. Colorless to yellowish, deliquesc, fused masses or granules with bitterish saline taste; becomes yellow on exposure to air and light due to liberation of iodine. Melts when rapidly heated, at about 120°. mp 402° (anhydrous). d 4.42. Sol in 0.2 part water; sol in alcohol. The aq soln is practically neutral. *Keep well closed and protected from light.* LD_{50} i.p. in rats: 800 mg/kg (Cochran).

THERAP CAT: Iodine source.

THERAP CAT (VET): Has been used in iodide therapy.

8845. Strontium Nitrate. [10042-76-9] N_2O_6Sr; mol wt 211.63. N 13.24%, O 45.36%, Sr 41.40%. $Sr(NO_3)_2$.

White granules or powder. d 2.99. mp 570°. Sol in 1.5 parts water; slightly sol in alcohol or acetone. The aq soln is neutral. At low temps strontium nitrate crystallizes with $4H_2O$ (25.4%). LD_{50} i.p. in rats: 540 mg/kg, Cochran *et al.*, *Arch. Ind. Hyg.* **1**, 637 (1950).

USE: In pyrotechnics (red fire), signal lights, marine signals, railroad flares, matches.

8846. Strontium Oxide. [1314-11-0] Strontia; strontium monoxide. OSr; mol wt 103.62. O 15.44%, Sr 84.56%. SrO.

White to grayish-white, porous, caustic mass. d 4.7. mp 2430°. When treated with water, forms the hydroxide with evolution of much heat. *Keep tightly closed.*

USE: Manuf of strontium salts.

8847. Strontium Peroxide. [1314-18-7] O_2Sr; mol wt 119.62. O 26.75%, Sr 73.25%. SrO_2. The peroxide of commerce contains about 85% SrO_2.

White, odorless, tasteless powder; gradually dec on exposure to air. Almost insol in water, but is gradually dec by it with evolution of oxygen; forms hydrogen peroxide with dil acids. *Keep well closed.*

THERAP CAT: Antiseptic.

8848. Strontium Sulfate. [7759-02-6] O_4SSr; mol wt 183.68. O 34.84%, S 17.46%, Sr 47.70%. $SrSO_4$. Occurs in nature as the mineral *celestine* or *celestite*.

White, odorless, crystalline powder. d 3.96. One gram dissolves in ~8800 ml water, 800 ml 2% HCl, 700 ml 3% HNO_3; appreciably sol in alkali chloride solns.

USE: In ceramics, pyrotechnics.

8849. Strontium Sulfide. [1314-96-1] SSr; mol wt 119.69. S 26.79%, Sr 73.21%. SrS. The article of commerce contains 65-75% SrS. Strontium sulfide made by reduction of the sulfate is not luminous; the luminous sulfide is prepared by heating strontium hydroxide with sulfur.

Gray powder; has the odor of H_2S in moist air. d 3.70. Slightly sol in water; sol in acids with decompn. *Keep dry.*

USE: In luminous paints; as a depilatory.

8850. Strontium Titanate. [12060-59-2] Strontium titanium oxide ($SrTiO_3$). O_3SrTi; mol wt 183.49. O 26.16%, Sr 47.75%, Ti 26.09%. $SrTiO_3$. Dielectric and photoelectric material. Occurs in nature as the mineral *tausonite*. Optical properties: H. A. Weakliem *et al.*, *RCA Rev.* **36**, 149 (1975). Electrical conductivity: U. Balachandran, N. G. Eror, *J. Solid State Chem.* **39**, 351 (1981). Dielectric properties of glass-ceramics: S. L. Swartz, A. S. Bhalla, *Ferroelectrics* **87**, 141 (1988). Review of growth and properties of single crystals: K. Nassau, A. E. Miller, *J. Cryst. Growth* **91**, 373-381 (1988). Prepn by sol-gel method: J. Moreno *et al.*, *J. Mater. Chem.* **5**, 509 (1995); by solution-precipitation method: V. Kumar, *J. Am. Ceram. Soc.* **82**, 2580 (1999). Prepn of thin films by ECR plasma sputtering: S. Miyake *et al.*, *Surface Coatings Technol.* **169-170**, 27 (2003); by spray pyrolysis: G. Brankovic *et al.*, *J.*

Eur. Ceram. Soc. **24**, 989 (2004). Piezoelectric response at cryogenic temperatures: D. E. Grupp, A. M. Goldman, *Science* **276**, 392 (1997). IR characterization of thin films: B. G. Almeida *et al., Appl. Surface Sci.* **238**, 395 (2004). Room-temperature ferroelectricity: J. H. Haeni *et al., Nature* **430**, 758 (2004).

d 5.12. n_D 2.409. Hardness 5½ on Moh's scale. Specific heat: ~10 J s⁻¹ K⁻¹ m⁻¹. Thermal conductivity: ~52 mW cm⁻¹ K⁻¹.

USE: In electronics and electrochemical insulation; in photocatalysis; sputtering target for thin film capacitors; substrate for epitaxial growth of high temperature superconductor thin films. Diamond simulant gemstone.

8851. Strophanthidin. [66-28-4] (3β,5β)-3,5,14-Trihydroxy-19-oxocard-20(22)-enolide; apocynamarin; convallatoxigenin; corchorin; cymarigenin; cynotoxin; corchorgenin; corchsularin. C₂₃H₃₂O₆; mol wt 404.50. C 68.29%, H 7.97%, O 23.73%. By acid or enzymic hydrolysis of glycosides present in several species of *Strophanthus, Apocynaceae.* Isoln: Jacobs, Heidelberger, *J. Biol. Chem.* **54**, 253 (1922). Structure: Kon, *Chem. Ind. (London)* **53**, 593, 956 (1934); Jacobs, Elderfield, *Science* **80**, 533 (1934). Identity with corchorin, corchorgenin and corchsularin: Sen *et al., Helv. Chim. Acta* **40**, 588 (1957). Synthesis from pregnenolone acetate, *q.v.:* E. Yoshii *et al., J. Org. Chem.* **43**, 3946 (1978). Toxicity study: Graebner, Geisel, *Arzneim.-Forsch.* **22**, 1854 (1972). *Reviews:* Elderfield, *Chem. Rev.* **17**, 187 (1935); Tschesche, *Ergeb. Physiol.* **38**, 31 (1936); Stoll, *The Cardiac Glycosides* (Pharmaceutical Press, London, 1937); Strain in *Organic Chemistry* **vol. II**, Gilman, Ed. (New York, 2nd ed., 1943); Fieser, Fieser, *Steroids* (Reinhold, New York, 1959) pp 729-730, 736-750.

Orthorhombic tablets from 5 parts methanol and 10 parts water. *Very poisonous!* Contains ½ mol H₂O which is given up at 110° over P₂O₅ at 20 mm Hg. mp 171-175° with effervescence. Occasionally a few isolated crystals are found which melt at ~230°. [α]D²⁵ +43.1° (c = 2.8 in methanol). Sol in alcohol, acetone, chloroform, benzene, and glacial acetic acid. Practically insol in water, ether, petr ether. Color reaction with H₂SO₄ and Ac₂O like cholesterol. LD₁₀₀ i.v. in cats: 0.337 mg/kg (Graebner, Geisel).

3-Benzoylstrophanthidin. C₃₀H₃₆O₇. mp 230°. [α]D²⁶ +47.8° (c = 1.07 in acetone).

3-(p-Bromobenzoyl)strophanthidin. C₃₀H₃₅BrO₇. mp 222-224°. [α]D²⁰ +42.0° (c = 1.094 in acetone).

Dihydrostrophanthidin. C₂₃H₃₄O₆. mp 100-103°, resolidifies and again melts at 190-195°. [α]D²³ +34.9° (methanol).

16-Hydroxystrophanthidin. Strophadogenin. C₂₃H₃₂O₇. Long prisms from ethanol, dec 238-241°. [α]D²⁵ +52.9° (c = 1.24 in 96% alc). uv max: 219 nm (log ε 4.3).

8852. Strophanthin. [11005-63-3] K-Strophanthin; K-strophanthoside; Kombetin. A glycoside or a mixture of glycosides obtained from *Strophanthus kombé* Oliv., *Apocynaceae.* Properly speaking K-strophanthoside contains α-glucose 19%, β-glucose 19%, cymarose 15%, strophanthidin 47%. K-Strophanthin-β (Strophosid) contains β-glucose, cymarose, and strophanthidin: Geissberger, *Schweiz. Med. Wochenschr.* **91**, 241 (1961). Pharmacology and acute toxicity: H. Mehnert, *Arch. Pharmacol.* **184**, 181 (1937).

White or yellowish powder contg as much as 10% water, which it does not lose entirely without decompn. *Very poisonous!* Stable in air, but affected by light. Soluble in water and in dil alcohol; less sol in abs alcohol. Nearly insol in chloroform, ether, benzene. Aq solns are neutral to litmus. When bioassayed, strophanthin shall possess a potency per mg equivalent to 0.5 mg of U.S.P. Ouabain

Reference Standard. A deviation of 20% is permitted. MLD in cats, rats (mg/kg): 0.11, 9.4 i.v. (Mehnert).

G-strophanthin *see* Ouabain.

THERAP CAT: Cardiotonic.

THERAP CAT (VET): Has been used as a cardiotonic.

8853. Strophanthus. Dried ripe seeds of *Strophanthus kombé* Oliv., or of *S. hispidus* DC., *Apocynaceae,* deprived of the awns. *Habit.* East and Central Africa. *Constit.* 2-5% Strophanthin, kombic acid, choline, trigonelline, ~30% oil. *Poisonous!*

USE: As arrow poison by African natives.

THERAP CAT: Cardiotonic.

THERAP CAT (VET): Has been used as a cardiotonic.

8854. Struvite. [15490-91-2] Magnesium ammonium phosphate hexahydrate; guanite. H₆MgNO₅P.6H₂O; mol wt 263.42. H 6.89%, Mg 9.23%, N 5.32%, O 66.81%, P 11.76%. (NH₄)-MgPO₄.6H₂O. Phosphate mineral named in honor of H. C. G. von Sturve, a Russian naturalist, in 1845 by Ulex, a Swedish geologist. A component of urinary calculi and bat guano also found as a contaminant in canned foods, in waste management systems. Production by urease-splitting bacteria: H. Robinson, *Proc. Cambridge Philos. Soc.* **6**, 360 (1889); J. Beavon, N. G. Heatley, *J. Gen. Microbiol.* **31**, 167 (1962); M. T. Gonzalez-Munoz *et al., Chemosphere* **26**, 1881 (1993). Identification in tinned seafood: M. T. Gilles, Seafood Processing in *Food Processing Review* **22**, (Noyes Data Corp., Park Ridge, NJ, 1971) pp 31-58; in homecanned beef: J. G. Sebranek *et al., J. Muscle Foods* **4**, 81 (1993). Precipitation in sludge digesters: C. Maqueda *et al., Water Res.* **28**, 411 (1994). Crystal growth: R. J. C. McLean *et al., Urol. Res.* **18**, 39 (1990). Thermodynamics of formation: J. R. Buchanan *et al., Trans. ASAE* **37**, 617 (1994). Chemical control in waste systems: J. R. Buchanan *et al., ibid.* 1301. Review of struvite urolithiasis: formation, detection and dissolution: C.A. Osborne *et al., Adv. Vet. Sci. Compar. Med.* **29**, 1-101 (1985). Review of struvite calculi: M. J. Gleeson, D. P. Griffith, *Br. J. Urol.* **71**, 503-511 (1993).

Glass like crystals.

8855. Strychnine. [57-24-9] Strychnidin-10-one. C₂₁H₂₂-N₂O₂; mol wt 334.41. C 75.42%, H 6.63%, N 8.38%, O 9.57%. Occurs most abundantly in seeds of *Strychnos nux-vomica* L., *Loganiaceae* and beans of *S. ignatii*, Berg. One of the first alkaloids isolated in pure form. Isoln: Pelletier, Caventou, *Ann. Chim. Phys.* **8**, 323 (1818); *ibid.* **10**, 142 (1819). Extraction procedure: C. Srinivasulu *et al., Res. Ind.* **23**, 224 (1978). Structure elucidation: L. H. Briggs *et al., J. Chem. Soc.* **1946**, 903; H. T. Openshaw, R. Robinson, *Nature* **157**, 438 (1946); R. B. Woodward *et al., J. Am. Chem. Soc.* **69**, 2250 (1947). Total synthesis: R. B. Woodward *et al., ibid.* **76**, 4749 (1954); *eidem, Tetrahedron* **19**, 247 (1963). Abs config: A. F. Peerdeman, *Acta Crystallogr.* **9**, 824 (1956); K. Nagarajan *et al., Helv. Chim. Acta* **46**, 1212 (1963). Stereoselective total synthesis: S. D. Knight *et al., J. Am. Chem. Soc.* **115**, 9293 (1993). ¹H- and ¹³C-NMR analysis: E. Wenkert *et al., J. Org. Chem.* **43**, 1099 (1978). Pharmacology and pharmacokinetics: S. Weiss, R. A. Hatcher, *J. Pharmacol. Exp. Ther.* **19**, 419 (1921). Acute toxicity: I. Setnikar, M. J. Magistretti, *Arzneim.-Forsch.* **14**, 996 (1964). HPLC determn in urine and tissues: T. Egloff *et al., J. Clin. Chem. Clin. Biochem.* **20**, 203 (1982); GC/EI-MS determn in whole blood: M. Barroso *et al., J. Chromatogr. B* **816**, 29 (2005). *Review:* J. B. Hendrickson in *The Alkaloids* **vol. VI**, R. H. F. Manske, Ed. (Academic Press, New York, 1960) pp 179-195; G. F. Smith, *ibid.* **vol. VIII** (1965) pp 591-671. Comprehensive description: F. J. Muhtadi, M. S. Hifnawy, *Anal. Profiles Drug Subs.* **15**, 563-646 (1986). Brief review of synthesis: U. Beifuss, *Angew. Chem. Int. Ed.* **33**, 1144-1149 (1994).

Brilliant, colorless cubes from chloroform-ether, mp 275-285°. d¹⁸ 1.359. [α]D¹⁸ −104.3° (c = 0.254 in alc); [α]D²⁵ −139° (c = 0.4 in chloroform). pKa (25°) 8.26: A. J. Everett *et al., J. Chem. Soc.* **1957**, 1120. uv max (95% ethanol): 255, 280, 290 nm ($E_{1\,cm}^{1\%}$ 377, 130, 101): A. I. Biggs, *J. Pharm. Pharmacol.* **13**, 547 (1952). One gram dissolves in 182 ml ethanol, 6.5 ml chloroform, 150 ml benzene, 250 ml methanol, 83 ml pyridine; very slightly sol in ether, water. LD$_{50}$ i.v. (slow infusion) in rats: 0.96 mg/kg (Setnikar, Magistretti).

Hydrochloride dihydrate. [6101-04-8] $C_{21}H_{22}N_2O_2$.HCl.2H$_2$O; mol wt 406.90. Efflorescent, trimetric prisms. One gram dissolves in ~35 ml cold water, ~80 ml alc. Insol in ether. pH of 0.01M soln 5.4.

Nitrate. [66-32-0] $C_{21}H_{22}N_2O_2$.HNO$_3$; mol wt 397.42. Colorless, odorless needles or white, cryst powder. At 25°, one gram dissolves in 42 ml water, 120 ml alcohol, 156 ml chloroform. Insol in ether. pH ~5.7. *Protect from light.*

Sulfate. [60-41-3] $(C_{21}H_{22}N_2O_2)_2$.H$_2$SO$_4$; mol wt 766.90. Usually crystallizes as pentahydrate. Properties of pentahydrate: colorless, odorless, very bright crystals, or white, cryst powder. Effloresces in dry air; loses all its water of crystn at 100°. mp when anhydr ~200° with decompn. At 25°, one gram dissolves in 31 ml water, 65 ml alcohol, 325 ml chloroform. Insol in ether. pH 5.5 in 1:100 soln. *Protect from light.* LD$_{50}$ orally in rats: 5 mg/kg, E. W. Schafer, *Toxicol. Appl. Pharmacol.* **21**, 315 (1972).

Caution: Extremely poisonous, *see:* G. D. Osweiler, *Curr. Vet. Ther.* **6**, 115 (1977). Potential symptoms of overexposure to strychnine are stiff neck and facial muscles; restlessness, apprehension and increased acuity of perception; increased reflex excitability; cyanosis; tetanic convulsions with opisthotonos. *See NIOSH Pocket Guide to Chemical Hazards* (DHHS/NIOSH 97-140, 1997) p 286.

USE: Chiefly in poison baits for rodents.

THERAP CAT (VET): Has been used as a tonic and central stimulant.

8856. Strychnine N^6-Oxide. [7248-28-4] Strychnidin-10-one 19-oxide; Genostrychnine. $C_{21}H_{22}N_2O_3$; mol wt 350.41. C 71.98%, H 6.33%, N 7.99%, O 13.70%. Prepn: Pictet, Mattison, *Ber.* **38**, 2782 (1905); Bailey, Robinson, *J. Chem. Soc.* **1948**, 703; Zellner, **US 2758113** (1956 to Donau-Pharmazie).

Monoclinic prisms from water, dec 207°. pK 5.17. Freely sol in alc, glacial acetic acid, chloroform; fairly sol in water; sparingly sol in benzene. Practically insol in ether, petr ether.

Hydriodide. Light yellow plates from hot water, dec 253°.
Nitrate. Small transparent prisms from water, dec 250°.

8857. Stryker's Reagent. [33636-93-0] Octahedrohexa-μ^3-hydrohexakis(triphenylphosphine)hexacopper; hexa-μ-hydrohexakis(triphenylphosphine) hexacopper; triphenylphosphine copper(I) hydride hexamer. $C_{108}H_{96}Cu_6P_6$; mol wt 1961.04. C 66.15%, H 4.93%, Cu 19.44%, P 9.48%. [(C$_6$H$_5$)$_3$PCuH]$_6$. Copper(I) hydride cluster; mild hydride donor in organic synthesis. Prepn and crystal characterization: S. A. Bezman *et al., J. Am. Chem. Soc.* **93**, 2063 (1971); M. R. Churchill *et al., Inorg. Chem.* **11**, 1818 (1972). Improved prepns: D. M. Brestensky *et al., Tetrahedron Lett.* **29**, 3749 (1988); P. Chiu *et al., ibid.* **44**, 455 (2003). Use in reduction of α,β-unsaturated carbonyl compds: W. S. Mahoney *et al., J. Am. Chem. Soc.* **110**, 291 (1988); W. S. Mahoney, J. M. Stryker, *ibid.* **111**, 8818 (1989); in hydrosilylation of aldehydes and ketones: B. H. Lipshutz *et al., J. Organomet. Chem.* **624**, 367 (2001). Brief review: A. de Fátima, *Synlett* **2005**, 1805-1806 (2005).

Isolated as H$_6$Cu$_6$(PPh$_3$)$_6$.DMF. Bright red crystals, mp 111° (dec). d 1.367. Sol in benzene; slightly sol in DMF. Insol in acetonitrile, water. Dec in alcohols, ethers, chlorinated hydrocarbons. *Air sensitive in soln. Store under nitrogen.*

USE: Stoichiometric reducing agent or catalyst in reduction reactions.

8858. Stylopine. [7461-02-1] 6,7,12b,13-Tetrahydro-4*H*-bis[1,3]benzodioxolo[5,6-*a*:4′,5′-*g*]quinolizine; 2,3:9,10-bis(methylenedioxy)-13a-berbine; tetrahydrocoptisine. $C_{19}H_{17}NO_4$; mol wt 323.34. C 70.58%, H 5.30%, N 4.33%, O 19.79%. From root of *Stylophorum diphyllum* (Michx.) Nutt, *Corydalis cava* Schwg. and *Chelidonium majus* L., *Papaveraceae:* Schlotterbeck, Watkins, *Ber.* **35**, 7 (1902); Späth, Julian, *Ber.* **64**, 1131 (1931); Manske, *Can. J. Res.* **B20**, 53 (1942); Slavik, *Collect. Czech. Chem. Commun.* **20**, 198 (1955); Bandelin, Malesh, *J. Am. Pharm. Assoc.* **45**, 702 (1956); Slavik, *Collect. Czech. Chem. Commun.* **26**, 2933 (1961).

dl-**Form.** Crystals from chloroform + methanol, mp 222-224°.
Hydrochloride. $C_{19}H_{18}ClNO_4$. Needles from methanol + HCl, mp 266-269°.
l-**Form.** Needles from chloroform + ethanol, mp 203°. $[\alpha]_D^{25}$ −300° (c = 0.53 in chloroform). Practically insol in water; sol in alc, glacial acetic acid; slightly sol in dil acids.
d-**Form.** Crystals from alcohol, mp 203-204°. $[\alpha]_D^{25}$ +310° (c = 0.88 in chloroform). Sol in chloroform; slightly sol in ether, ethanol, methanol.

8859. Styphnic Acid. [82-71-3] 2,4,6-Trinitro-1,3-benzenediol; 2,4,6-trinitroresorcinol; 2,4-dihydroxy-1,3,5-trinitrobenzene. $C_6H_3N_3O_8$; mol wt 245.10. C 29.40%, H 1.23%, N 17.14%, O 52.22%. May be prepd from natural sources, such as Pernambuco wood extract or quebracho extract by the action of nitric acid: Einbeck, Jablonski, *Ber.* **54**, 1086 (1921). Prepd industrially by first sulfonating, then nitrating resorcinol: Merz, Zetter, *Ber.* **12**, 681, 2037 (1879); Datta, Varma, *J. Am. Chem. Soc.* **41**, 2043 (1919). Prepd by nitrating 2,4-dinitroresorcinol: Kametani, Ogasawara, *Chem. Pharm. Bull.* **15**, 893 (1967).

Hexagonal yellow crystals from dil alc. Astringent, but not bitter taste. Solvated crystals from acetic acid. Sublimes in high vacuum. Becomes almost colorless upon vacuum sublimation, but turns deep yellow on contact with air. When dry, mp 175.5°; also reported as mp 179-180°. One gram dissolves in 156 ml water at 14°, in 88 ml water at 62°. Freely sol in alcohol, ether. Acid to litmus. Dibasic acid. Deflagrates on rapid heating.

USE: Has been used in the manuf of explosives.

8860. Styrene. [100-42-5] Ethenylbenzene; styrol; styrolene; cinnamene; cinnamol; phenylethylene; vinylbenzene. C_8H_8; mol wt 104.15. C 92.26%, H 7.74%. $C_6H_5CH{=}CH_2$. Isolated from storax by Bonastre in 1831. Manuf from benzene and ethylene: *Faith, Keyes & Clark's Industrial Chemicals*, F. A. Lowenheim, M. K. Moran, Eds. (Wiley-Interscience, New York, 4th ed., 1975) pp 779-785. Synthesis starting with 1-phenylethanol and leading to polystyrene: Wilen *et al., J. Chem. Educ.* **38**, 304 (1961). When heated to 200° it is converted into the polymer, polystyrene, which is a clear plastic having excellent insulating properties even at ultra-high radio frequencies. Toxicity data: H. J. Meyer, R. Kretzschmar, *Arzneim.-Forsch.* **19**, 617 (1969). Monograph: W. C. Teach, G. C. Kiessling, *Polystyrene* (Reinhold, New York, 1960). Reviews of styrene monomer and polymers: Boyer *et al.*, "Styrene Polymers" in *Encyclopedia of Polymer Science and Technology* **vol. 13** (Interscience, New York, 1970) pp 128-447; Coulter *et al.*, "Styrene and Related Monomers" in *Vinyl and Diene*

Monomers (part 2), E. C. Leonard, Ed. (Wiley-Interscience, New York, 1971) pp 479-576. Review of neurotoxicity: R. Pahwa, J. Kalra, *Vet. Hum. Toxicol.* **35**, 516-520 (1993); of toxicology and carcinogenic risk: *IARC Sci. Publ.* **127**, 1-412 (1993); of toxicology and human exposure: *Toxicological Profile for Styrene* (PB93-110849, 1992) 164 p.

Colorless to yellowish, very refractive, oily liq; penetrating odor. On exposure to light and air it slowly undergoes polymerization and oxidation with formation of peroxides, etc. d^{20} 0.9059. mp $-30.6°$. bp 145-146°. n_D^{20} 1.5463. Flash pt, closed cup: 87°F (31°C). Sparingly sol in water; sol in alcohol, ether, methanol, acetone, carbon disulfide. LD_{50} in mice (mg/kg): 660 ± 44.3 i.p.; 90 ± 5.2 i.v. (Meyer, Kretzschmar).

Polystyrene. Dylene; Trycite. Physical properties of unmodified polystyrene: d_4^{20} 1.04-1.065; n_D^{25} 1.60; water-clear solid plastic, begins to soften at ~85°. Dielectric constant at 100 megacycles: 2.4-2.65.

Caution: Potential symptoms of overexposure are irritation of eyes, nose, respiratory system; headache, fatigue, dizziness, confusion, malaise, drowsiness, weakness and unsteady gait; narcosis; defatting dermatitis; liver injury, reproductive effects. *See NIOSH Pocket Guide to Chemical Hazards* (DHHS/NIOSH 97-140, 1997) p 286.

USE: Manuf plastics; synthetic rubber; resins; insulator.

8861. Styrene Glycol. [93-56-1] 1-Phenyl-1,2-ethanediol; phenylglycol; phenylethyleneglycol; α,β-dihydroxyethylbenzene. $C_8H_{10}O_2$; mol wt 138.16. C 69.55%, H 7.30%, O 23.16%. Prepd by reduction of phenylglyoxylic acid with $LiAlH_4$: Nystrom, Brown, *J. Am. Chem. Soc.* **69**, 2548 (1947); by reduction of styrene peroxide: Russel, *J. Am. Chem. Soc.* **75**, 5011 (1953). Prepn of optically active styrene glycol: Wilhelm, Bright, *Helv. Chim. Acta* **37**, 221 (1954).

Needles from ligroin, mp 67-68°. bp_{755} 272-274°. Freely sol in water, alcohol, benzene, ether, chloroform, acetic acid; slightly sol in ligroin.

USE: Esters as plasticizers.

8862. Suberic Acid. [505-48-6] Octanedioic acid; 1,6-hexanedicarboxylic acid. $C_8H_{14}O_4$; mol wt 174.19. C 55.16%, H 8.10%, O 36.74%. $COOH(CH_2)_6COOH$. Made by heating castor oil or ricinoleic acid with nitric acid: Dominguez, Lopez, *Ciencia (Mexico City)* **20**, 73 (1959), *C.A.* **54**, 18990f (1960). Prepn from diethyl malonate + ω-bromocapronitrile: Cason *et al., J. Org. Chem.* **14**, 37 (1949); by oxidation of oleic acid with nitric acid: Cavanaugh, Weir, US 2560156 (1951 to du Pont).

Crystals, mp 140-144°. bp_{100} 279°. Sublimes at 300° without decompn. One gram dissolves in 625 ml water, 172 ml ether; sol in alcohol; almost insol in chloroform.

USE: In the plastics industry.

8863. Substance P. [11035-08-8] SP. $C_{63}H_{98}N_{18}O_{13}S$; mol wt 1347.63. C 56.15%, H 7.33%, N 18.71%, O 15.43%, S 2.38%. An undecapeptide belonging to a group of proteins named tachykinins characterized by contractile action on extravascular smooth muscle. Discovered by von Euler and Gaddum, *J. Physiol.* **72**, 74 (1931). Present in the brain of all vertebrates including man, in spinal ganglia, and in the intestines, esp the duodenum and jejunum. Isoln from cattle brain: Zuber, Jaques, *Angew. Chem. Int. Ed.* **1**, 160 (1962); from horse intestine: Studer *et al., Helv. Chim. Acta* **56**, 860 (1973). Purification from bovine hypothalami and amino acid composition: N. N. Chang, S. E. Leeman, *J. Biol. Chem.* **245**, 4784 (1970). Amino acid sequence and solid-phase synthesis: Chang *et al., Nature New Biol.* **232**, 86 (1971); Tregear *et al., ibid.* 87; G. H. Fisher *et al., J. Med. Chem.* **17**, 843 (1974). Additional syntheses: Yajima, Kitigawa, *Chem. Pharm. Bull.* **21**, 682 (1973); Bayer, Mutter, *Ber.* **107**, 1344 (1974); K. Neubert *et al., Pharmazie* **36**, 10 (1981); A. Fournier *et al., J. Med. Chem.* **25**, 64 (1981). Substance P acts as a vasodilator, a depressant, stimulates

salivation and produces increased capillary permeability. It is also capable of producing both analgesia and hyperalgesia in animals, depending on dose and pain responsiveness of the animal, *see* R. C. A. Frederickson *et al., Science* **199**, 1359 (1978); P. Oehme *et al., ibid.* **208**, 305 (1980); role in sensory transmission and pain perception: T. M. Jessell, *Adv. Biochem. Psychopharmacol.* **28**, 189 (1981). Mechanism of action studies: Stern *et al., Arch. Pharmacol.* **281**, 233 (1974); B. G. Livett *et al., Nature* **278**, 256 (1979). *Reviews:* Haefeli, Huelimann, *Experientia* **18**, 297 (1962); Lembeck, Zetler in *International Encyclopedia of Pharmacology and Therapeutics* sect. 72, vol. 1, J. M. Walker, Ed. (Pergamon Press, New York, 1971) pp 29-71; J. L. Barker, *Physiol. Rev.* **56**, 435 (1976); D. R. Brown, R. J. Miller, *Annu. Rep. Med. Chem.* **17**, 271-280 (1982). Books: U.S. Von Euler, B. Pernow, Eds., *Substance P* (Raven Press, New York, 1977) 360 pp; *Substance P* vol. 2, P. Skrabanek, D. Powell, Eds. (Eden Press, Quebec, 1980) 175 pp; *Substance P in The Nervous System: Ciba Foundation Symposium* **91**, R. Porter, M. O'Connor, Eds. (Pitman, London, 1982) 350 pp.

Arg–Pro–Lys–Pro–Gln–Gln–Phe–Phe–Gly–Leu–MetNH₂

Behaves during isoln as a basic polypeptide (R_f value = 0.5 in the thin layer chromatogram: silica gel *n*-butanol/pyridine/AcOH/H_2O = 30:20:6:24). Upon high voltage electrophoresis (pH 1.9; acetic acid/formic acid/H_2O = 15:3:100) it migrates approx as far as glutamic acid or serine, and at pH 9.5 (0.25M triethylammonium carbonate buffer) it behaves in a manner similar to arginine. Biological activity is destroyed by pepsin and chymotrypsin. Aqueous solns of highly purified material lose biological activity in a few minutes. This loss is prevented by storage at low pH, under nitrogen, or with various antioxidants. Addition of Tween 80, gelatin, human plasma albumin, or bovine γ-globulin increases stability of aq SP solns. Crude SP solns are stable though rapidly destroyed above pH 8.

8864. Subtilin. [1393-38-0] Polypeptide antibiotic structurally similar to nisin, *q.v.*, but contains no methionine. Produced by *Bacillus subtilis* (NRRL no. B-543): E. F. Jansen, D. J. Hirshmann, *Arch. Biochem.* **4**, 297 (1944); Lewis *et al., ibid.* **14**, 415 (1947); Dimick *et al., ibid.* **15**, 1 (1947). Isoln by partition chromatography on silica gel: Alderton, Snell, *J. Am. Chem. Soc.* **81**, 701 (1959). Early structural studies: Stracher, Craig, *ibid.* 696. Structure is a heterodetic pentacyclic peptide consisting of 32 amino acid residues and containing unusual amino acids such as lanthionine, β-methyllanthionine, D-alanine, dehydroalanine and dehydrobutyrine: E. Gross *et al., Z. Physiol. Chem.* **354**, 799 (1973). Biosynthetic studies: C. Nishio *et al., Biochem. Biophys. Res. Commun.* **116**, 751 (1983); S. Banerjee, J. N. Hansen, *J. Biol. Chem.* **263**, 9508 (1988).

Amorphous powder. $[\alpha]_D^{23}$ -29 to $-35°$ (c = 1 in 1% acetic acid). Diffuses quickly through cellophane. Readily sol in dilute acids; sparingly sol (less than 5 mg/ml) in water at pH 6-9. Sol in methanol, 80% alc. Soly in butanol satd with water: about 5 mg/ml. Easily salted out of soln by NaCl.

USE: Food preservative.

8865. Succimer. [304-55-2] (2R,3S)-*rel*-2,3-Dimercaptobutanedioic acid; *meso*-2,3-dimercaptosuccinic acid; DMS; DMSA; Ro-1-7977; Chemet. $C_4H_6O_4S_2$; mol wt 182.22. C 26.37%, H 3.32%, O 35.12%, S 35.19%. $HOOCCH(SH)CH(SH)COOH$. A water soluble chelating agent. Prepn: L. N. Owen, M. U. S. Sultanbawa, *J. Chem. Soc.* **1949**, 3109. Pharmacology, toxicity and activity in heavy metal poisoning in animals: E. Friedheim, C. Corvi, *J. Pharm. Pharmacol.* **27**, 624 (1975); J. H. Graziano *et al., J. Pharmacol. Exp. Ther.* **207**, 1051 (1978). GC determn in urine: J. J. Knudsen, E. L. McGown, *J. Chromatogr.* **424**, 231 (1988). Clinical evaluations in heavy metal poisoning: E. Friedheim *et al., Lancet* **2**, 1234 (1978); L. Fournier *et al., Med. Toxicol.* **3**, 499 (1988). Diagnostic use of complex with technetium in urinary tract imaging: I. G. Verber *et al., Arch. Dis. Child.* **63**, 1320 (1988); in tumor imaging: H. Ohta *et al., Nucl. Med. Commun.* **9**, 105 (1988). *Review:* H. V. Aposhian, "Biological Chelation: 2,3-Dimercaptopropanesulfonic Acid and Meso-Dimercaptosuccinic Acid" in *Adv. Enzyme Regul.* **20**, G. Weber, Ed. (Pergamon Press, Oxford, 1982) pp 301-319. Review of pharmacology and clinical use in heavy metal poisoning: *idem, Annu. Rev. Pharmacol.*

Toxicol. **23,** 193-215 (1983); J. H. Graziano, *Med. Toxicol.* **1,** 155-162 (1986).

White crystals from aqueous methanol, mp 192-194°. LD_{50} i.p. in mice: >3000 mg/kg (Friedheim, Corvi).

USE: Chelating agent.

THERAP CAT: Antidote (heavy metal poisoning). ^{99m}Tc complex as diagnostic aid (radioactive imaging agent).

8866. Succinamide. [110-14-5] Butanediamide. $C_4H_8N_2$-O_2; mol wt 116.12. C 41.37%, H 6.94%, N 24.12%, O 27.56%. $H_2NOCCH_2CH_2CONH_2$. Made by the action of ammonia water on the dimethyl or diethyl ester of succinic acid.

Needles. mp 260° with decompn; also stated as 242°. Sol in 220 parts cold, 9 parts boiling water; insol in alc, ether.

8867. Succinanil. [83-25-0] 1-Phenyl-2,5-pyrrolidinedione; *N*-phenylsuccinimide; *N*-phenylbutanimide. $C_{10}H_9NO_2$; mol wt 175.18. C 68.56%, H 5.18%, N 8.00%, O 18.27%. Prepd by treating succinanilic acid with acetyl chloride: Ruggli, *Ann.* **412,** 4 (1916); Warren, Briggs, *Ber.* **64,** 29 (1931); L. F. Fieser, *Experiments in Organic Chemistry* (Boston, 1955) p 106.

Monoclinic prisms from water or alcohol, mp 154.5°. d_4^{20} 1.356. bp_{760} ~400°. Sol in ether, boiling alcohol. Slightly sol in boiling water.

8868. Succinanilic Acid. [102-14-7] 4-Oxo-4-(phenylamino)butanoic acid; succinic acid monoanilide; *N*-phenylsuccinamic acid; *N*-phenylbutanedioic acid monoamide. $C_{10}H_{11}NO_3$; mol wt 193.20. C 62.17%, H 5.74%, N 7.25%, O 24.84%. Prepd by boiling succinic anhydride with aniline in benzene: Menschutkin, *Ann.* **162,** 176 (1872); Warren, Briggs, *Ber.* **64,** 29 (1931); L. F. Fieser, *Experiments in Organic Chemistry* (Boston, 3rd ed., 1955) p 105.

Needles from benzene, mp 150°. pK (25°) 4.69. Soluble in alcohol, ether, boiling water (some dec).

8869. Succinic Acid. [110-15-6] Butanedioic acid; amber acid; ethylenesuccinic acid; Bernsteinsäure (German); Asuccin. $C_4H_6O_4$; mol wt 118.09. C 40.68%, H 5.12%, O 54.19%. $HOOCCH_2CH_2COOH$. Observed by Agricola in 1546, in the distillate from amber. Occurs in fossils, fungi, lichens, etc. Prepn from acetic acid: Coffman *et al., J. Am. Chem. Soc.* **80,** 2864 (1958). Manuf: Crosby, Braunwarth, US 2862028 (1958 to Pure Oil); Chafetz, Patterson, US 2978473 (1961 to Texaco). Toxicity study: H. F. Smyth *et al., Arch. Ind. Hyg. Occup. Med.* **4,** 119 (1951).

Odorless, monoclinic prisms; very acid taste; d 1.56; mp 185-187°; bp 235° with partial conversion into the anhydride. One gram dissolves in 13 ml cold water, 1 ml boiling water, 18.5 ml alcohol, 6.3 ml methanol, 36 ml acetone, 20 ml glycerol, 113 ml ether. Practically insol in benzene, carbon disulfide, carbon tetrachloride, petr ether. pH of 0.1 molar aq soln 2.7.

Potassium salt trihydrate. Potassium succinate. $C_4H_4K_2$-O_4.3H_2O. Hygroscopic crystalline powder. d 1.564. Freely sol in water; the aq soln is practically neutral. *Keep tightly closed.*

Diethyl ester. Ethyl succinate. $C_8H_{14}O_4$. Colorless, clear liq; faint, pleasant odor. d_2^{20} 1.040. bp 217-218°. mp $-21°$. n_D^{20} 1.4201. Insol in water. Miscible with alcohol, ether. LD_{50} orally in rats: 8.53 g/kg (Smyth).

Dimethyl ester. Methyl succinate. $C_6H_{10}O_4$. Colorless liquid. d_4^{18} 1.1202. mp 19.5°. bp_{760} 195.3°; bp_{25} 103.5°. Sol in 120 parts water, 35 parts alcohol.

USE: Manuf lacquers, dyes, esters for perfumes, succinates; in photography.

8870. Succinic Anhydride. [108-30-5] Dihydro-2,5-furandione; succinic acid anhydride; succinyl oxide; 2,5-diketotetrahydrofuran; butanedioic anhydride; Bernsteinsäureanhydrid (German). $C_4H_4O_3$; mol wt 100.07. C 48.01%, H 4.03%, O 47.96%. Usually prepd by warming succinic acid with acetic anhydride, acetyl chloride, or phosphorus oxychloride: Shriner, Struck, *Org. Synth.* **12,** 66 (1932); L. F. Fieser, *Experiments in Organic Chemistry* (Boston, 3rd ed., 1955) p 105.

Orthorhombic prisms from abs alc. d 1.503 (also given as 1.104 and 1.234). Rate of sublimation: Kempf, *J. Prakt. Chem.* [2] **78,** 257 (1908). mp 119.6°; bp_{760} 261°; bp_{400} 237°; bp_{200} 212°; bp_{100} 189°; bp_{60} 174°; bp_{40} 163°; bp_{20} 145°; bp_{10} 128°. Sublimes at 115° and 5 mm pressure, at 92° and 1.0 mm pressure. Soluble in chloroform, carbon tetrachloride, alcohol; very slightly sol in ether and water.

8871. Succinimide. [123-56-8] 2,5-Pyrrolidinedione; butanimide; 2,5-diketopyrrole; 3,4-dihydropyrrole-2,5-dione; dihydro-3-pyrroline-2,5-dione; 2,5-dioxopyrrolidine; Orotric. C_4H_5-NO_2; mol wt 99.09. C 48.48%, H 5.09%, N 14.14%, O 32.29%. Prepd by rapid distillation of ammonium succinate: Clarke, Behr, *Org. Synth.* **coll. vol. II** (1943) p 562; Fehling, *Ann.* **49,** 198 (1844); Bunge, *Ann. Suppl.* **7,** 118 (1870); Menschutkin, *Ann.* **162,** 166 (1872). Prepn by heating succinic acid with ammonia: Fehling, *loc. cit.*; Franchimont, Friedmann, *Rec. Trav. Chim.* **25,** 79 (1906); with urea: Ma, Sah, *C.A.* **28,** 6108 (1934); *see also* Tafel, Stern, *Ber.* **33,** 2232 (1900); Koller, *Ber.* **37,** 1598 (1904). Prevention of oxalic lithiasis in rats: J. M. Melon *et al., Therapie* **26,** 991 (1971).

Orthorhombic bipyramidal crystals from acetone or alc. mp 125-127°. d 1.41. bp 287-289° (slight decompn). pKa 9.5. One gram dissolves in 3 ml water, 0.7 ml boiling water, 24 ml alc, 5 ml alc at 60°. Insol in ether, chloroform. LD_{50} orally in rats: 14 g/kg (Melon).

THERAP CAT: Antiurolithic.

8872. Succinonitrile. [110-61-2] Butanedinitrile; ethylene dicyanide; succinic acid dinitrile; *sym*-dicyanoethane; ethylene cyanide; Dinile; Suxil. $C_4H_4N_2$; mol wt 80.09. C 59.99%, H 5.03%, N 34.98%. $NCCH_2CH_2CN$. Prepd from ethylene bromide and KCN in alcohol: Fauconnier, *Bull. Soc. Chim. Fr.* **50,** 214 (1888).

Waxy isometric crystals. d_4^{45} 1.023. mp 57.15°. d_4^{60} (liq) 0.9868. n_D^{60} (liq) 1.41734. May be heated to 200° for 72 hrs without decompn. bp_{760} 265-267°; bp_{60} 185°; bp_{20} 158-160°. Sol in acetone, chloroform, dioxane. Slightly sol in water, ethanol, benzene, ether, carbon disulfide.

Caution: Potential symptoms of overexposure are irritation of eyes, skin, respiratory system; headache, dizziness, weakness, giddiness, confusion, convulsions; blurred vision; dyspnea; abdominal pain, nausea, vomiting. *See NIOSH Pocket Guide to Chemical Hazards* (DHHS/NIOSH 97-140, 1997) p 288.

8873. Succinyl Chloride. [543-20-4] Butanedioyl chloride; succinyl dichloride. $C_4H_4Cl_2O_2$; mol wt 154.98. C 31.00%, H 2.60%, Cl 45.75%, O 20.65%. $ClOCCH_2CH_2COCl$.

Fuming, highly refractive liq; d_4^{15} 1.395; n_D^{15} 1.473; mp 17°; also stated as 20°; bp 192-193°. Solidif at 0° to cryst leaflets.

8874. Succinylcholine Bromide. [55-94-7] 2,2'-[(1,4-Dioxo-1,4-butanediyl)bis(oxy)]bis[*N,N,N*-trimethylethanaminium] dibromide; bis[2-dimethylaminoethyl]succinate bis[methobromide]; 3,8-dioxadecane-4,7-dione-1,10-bis[trimethylammonium bromide]; suxamethonium bromide; IS-370; compd 48/268; LT-1; M & B 2207; Brevidil M. $C_{14}H_{30}Br_2N_2O_4$; mol wt 450.21. C 37.35%, H 6.72%, Br 35.50%, N 6.22%, O 14.22%. Prepd by reacting β-bromoethyl succinate with trimethylamine: Glick, *J. Biol. Chem.* **137**, 357 (1941); Fusco *et al., Gazz. Chim. Ital.* **79**, 129, 837 (1949); Walker, *J. Chem. Soc.* **1950**, 193. Alternate prepns: Phillips, *J. Am. Chem. Soc.* **71**, 3264 (1949); Tammelin, *Acta Chem. Scand.* **7**, 185 (1953).

Slightly hygroscopic crystals, mp 225°. Freely sol in water or normal saline, giving solns which are very slightly acidic. Aq solns undergo progressive hydrolysis with corresponding loss of activity and increase in acidity. *Prepare solns just before using.* The rate of this decompn increases with temp and autoclaving or prolonged exposure to warmth should be avoided.

THERAP CAT: Neuromuscular blocking agent.

8875. Succinylcholine Chloride. [71-27-2] 2,2'-[(1,4-Di-oxo-1,4-butanediyl)bis(oxy)]bis[*N,N,N*-trimethylethanaminium] dichloride; bis[2-dimethylaminoethyl]succinate bis[methochloride]; 2-dimethylaminoethyl succinate dimethochloride; diacetylcholine dichloride; suxamethonium chloride; choline succinate dichloride; succinic acid bis[β-dimethylaminoethyl] ester dimethochloride; choline chloride succinate (2:1); listenon; Anectine; Lysthenon; Midarine; Quelicin; Scoline; Sucostrin. $C_{14}H_{30}Cl_2N_2O_4$; mol wt 361.31. C 46.54%, H 8.37%, Cl 19.62%, N 7.75%, O 17.71%. Prepn: R. Fusco *et al., Gazz. Chim. Ital.* **79**, 129 (1949); Tammelin, *Acta Chem. Scand.* **7**, 185 (1953); O. Schmid, *AT 171411* (1952 to OSSW), *C.A.* **47**, 4902f (1953); C. H. Wang *et al., Org. Prep. Proced. Int.* **11**, 93 (1979). Crystal structure: B. Jensen, *Acta Chem. Scand. B* **30**, 1002 (1976). Toxicity data: P. Anttila, P. Ertama, *Med. Biol.* **56**, 152 (1978). Comprehensive description: P. R. B. Foss, S. A. Benezra, *Anal. Profiles Drug Subs.* **10**, 691-704 (1981).

Exists as a dihydrate at room temp, crystals, mp 156-163°. Anhydr form mp ~190°. Slightly bitter taste. Freely sol in water (about 1 g/1 ml water). Soly in 95% ethanol: 0.42 g/100 ml. Sparingly sol in benzene, chloroform. Practically insol in ether. The pH of a 2-5% aq soln may vary from 4.5 to 3.0. Solns without stabilizers (e.g., 0.1% methyl *p*-hydroxybenzoate) must be kept refrigerated, they are incompatible with alkaline agents, such as thiopental sodium. LD_{50} i.v. in mice: 0.45 mg/kg (Anttila, Ertama).

THERAP CAT: Neuromuscular blocking agent.
THERAP CAT (VET): Muscle relaxant (skeletal).

8876. Succinylcholine Iodide. [541-19-5] *O,O*-Succinyl-dicholine iodide; diacetylcholine iodide; diacetylcholine diiodide; suxamethonium iodide; bis(β-dimethylaminoethyl)succinate bis(methyl iodide); Celocurine. $C_{14}H_{30}I_2N_2O_4$; mol wt 544.21. C 30.90%, H 5.56%, I 46.64%, N 5.15%, O 11.76%. Prepd by reacting β-bromoethyl succinate with trimethylamine: Glick, *J. Biol. Chem.* **137**, 357 (1941); Fusco *et al., Gazz. Chim. Ital.* **79**, 129, 837 (1949); Walker, *J. Chem. Soc.* **1950**, 193. Succinic acid chloride may be coupled with choline chloride directly or with dimethylaminoethanol, followed by quaternization with methyl iodide: Tammelin, *Acta Chem. Scand.* **7**, 185 (1953). A third method is to start with the diethyl ester of succinic acid, then bring about the exchange reaction with dimethylaminoethanol, and quaternize with methyl iodide: Phillips, *J. Am. Chem. Soc.* **71**, 3264 (1949).

Slightly hygroscopic crystals, mp 243-245°. Freely sol in water or normal saline, giving solns which are very slightly acidic. Most stable at pH 4-5. Aq solns undergo progressive hydrolysis with corresp loss of activity and increase in acidity. *Prepare solns just before using.* Incompatible with solns of alkaline salts.

THERAP CAT: Neuromuscular blocking agent.
THERAP CAT (VET): Muscle relaxant (skeletal).

8877. Succinylsulfathiazole. [116-43-8] 4-Oxo-4-[[4-[(2-thiazolylamino)sulfonyl]phenyl]amino]butanoic acid; 4'-(2-thiazol-ylsulfamoyl)succinanilic acid; *p*-2-thiazolylsulfamylsuccinanilic acid; 2-(*N*⁴-succinylsulfanilamido)thiazole; Sulfasuxidine. $C_{13}H_{13}N_3O_5S_2$; mol wt 355.39. C 43.93%, H 3.69%, N 11.82%, O 22.51%, S 18.04%. Prepd by refluxing sulfathiazole with a slight excess of succinic anhydride in alcohol: Moore, Miller, *J. Am. Chem. Soc.* **64**, 1572 (1942); *US 2324013*; *US 2324014* (both 1943); by refluxing *p*-succinimidobenzenesulfonyl chloride with 2-aminothiazole in benzene: *GB 578004* (1946). Toxicology: A. D. Welch *et al., J. Pharmacol. Exp. Ther.* **75**, 231 (1942).

Monohydrate. Crystals with unclear mp. Has been reported as mp 184-186°; also reported as mp 192-195°. Emits pungent fumes on heating to mp. One gram dissolves in about 4800 ml water. Soluble in solns of alkali hydroxides and in solns of sodium bicarbonate with the evolution of carbon dioxide; sparingly sol in alcohol and in acetone. Insol in chloroform and ether. LD_{50} i.p. in mice: ~5.7 g/kg (Welch).

THERAP CAT: Antibacterial.
THERAP CAT (VET): Antibacterial, esp in enteric infections.

8878. Succisulfone. [5934-14-5] 4-[[4-[(4-Aminophenyl)-sulfonyl]phenyl]amino]-4-oxobutanoic acid; 4'-sulfanilyl-succinanilic acid; 4-amino-4'-(β-carboxypropylamino)phenyl-sulfonylbenzene; 4-amino-4'-β-carboxypropylaminodiphenyl-sulfone; 4-(β-carboxypropionylamino)-4'-aminodiphenyl sulfone; 4-succinylamido-4'-aminodiphenylsulfone; F-1500; Fourneau 1500; Exosulfonyl. $C_{16}H_{16}N_2O_5S$; mol wt 348.37. C 55.16%, H 4.63%, N 8.04%, O 22.96%, S 9.20%. Prepn: Fourneau, Tré-fouel, **FR 866619** (1941 to Rhône-Poulenc); Kharasch, Reinmuth, **US 2268754** (1942 to Lilly); Bauer, *J. Am. Chem. Soc.* **70**, 2254 (1948); Rohls, Behnish, **DE 895600** (1953 to Bayer); Liberman, **FR 1020713** (1953 to Chimie et Atomistique).

Crystals, mp 157°. Soluble in ammonia.
2,2'-Iminodiethanol salt. [547-36-4] $C_{20}H_{27}N_3O_7S$. Prepn: **FR 992112** (1951 to Theraplix).

THERAP CAT: Antibacterial (leprostatic).

8879. Sucralfate. [54182-58-0] Hexadeca-μ-hydroxytetra-cosahydroxy[μ₈-[1,3,4,6-tetra-*O*-sulfo-β-D-fructofuranosyl-α-D-glucopyranoside tetrakis(hydrogen sulfato)(8−)]]hexadecaalumi-num; β-D-fructofuranosyl-α-D-glucopyranoside octakis(hydrogen sulfate) aluminum complex; sucrose octakis(hydrogen sulfate) aluminum complex; Antepsin; Carafate; Citogel; Hexagastron; Keal; Succosa; Sucralfin; Sucrate; Sugast; Sulcrate; Ulcar; Ulcerlmin; Ulcogant. $C_{12}H_{54}Al_{16}O_{75}S_8$; mol wt 2086.74. C 6.91%, H 2.61%, Al 20.69%, O 57.50%, S 12.29%. A basic aluminum sucrose sulfate complex which inhibits peptic hydrolysis and stomach acidity. Prepn: M. Nametaka *et al., Yakugaku Zasshi* **87**, 889 (1967), *C.A.* **68**, 20831d (1968); **FR 1500571**; N. Yoshihiro *et al.*, **US 3432489** (1967, 1969 both to Chugai). Structure and properties: R. Nagashima, N. Yoshida, *Arzneim.-Forsch.* **29**, 1668 (1979). *In* *vitro* and *in vivo* study of antipeptic and antiulcer activity: L. E. Borella, *et al., ibid.* 793. Series of articles on mode of action: *ibid.* **30**, 73-88 (1980). Pharmacokinetics, metabolism and selective binding studies: K. Steiner *et al., ibid.* **32**, 512 (1982). Clinical studies: J. F. Mayberry *et al., Br. J. Clin. Pract.* **32**, 291 (1978). Symposium on clinical studies: *J. Clin. Gastroenterol.* **3**, Suppl. 2, 103-184 (1981); *Scand. J. Gastroenterol.* **18**, Suppl. 83, 1-82 (1983). Review of pharmacology and clinical studies: R. N. Brogden *et al., Drugs* **27**, 194 (1984). Series of articles on clinical efficacy in peptic ulcer disease and gastritis: *Am. J. Med.* **79**, Suppl. 2C, 1-64 (1985).

R = SO₃[Al₂(OH)₅]

White amorphous powder. Sol in dil HCL and NaOH solns. Practically insol in water, ethanol, CHCl₃. pKa = 0.43 to 1.19. Dissolution of aluminum occurs at pH <3; of sucrose sulfate at pH >4.

THERAP CAT: Antiulcerative.

8880. Sucralose. [56038-13-2] 1,6-Dichloro-1,6-dideoxy-β-D-fructofuranosyl-4-chloro-4-deoxy-α-D-galactopyranoside; 4,1′,6′-trichloro-4,1′,6′-trideoxy-*galacto*-sucrose; 1′,4,6′-trichloro-galactosucrose; TGS; Splenda. $C_{12}H_{19}Cl_3O_8$; mol wt 397.63. C 36.25%, H 4.82%, Cl 26.75%, O 32.19%. Chlorinated sucrose derivative with enhanced sweetness. Prepn: P. H. Fairclough *et al., Carbohydr. Res.* **40**, 285 (1975). Prepn of crystalline anhydrous and pentahydrate: M. R. Jenner, D. Waite, *EP 30804* (1981 to Tate & Lyle; Talres Dev.); *eidem, US 4343934* (1982 to Talres Dev.). Use as non-nutritive sweetener: *BE 850180*; L. Hough *et al., US 4435440* (1977, 1984 both to Tate & Lyle). *In vitro* activity vs cariogenic bacteria: J. Verran, D. B. Drucker, *Arch. Oral Biol.* **27**, 693 (1982). Structure-sweetness relationship: M. Mathlouthi *et al., Carbohydr. Res.* **152**, 47 (1986). *Review:* L. Hough, R. Khan, *Trends Biochem. Sci.* **3**, 61-63 (1978).

Syrup, [α]_D +68.2° (c = 1.1 in ethanol). Anhydrous crystalline form: orthorhombic, needle-like crystals, mp 130°. Intensely sweet taste.

Pentahydrate. mp 36.5°.

8881. Sucrose. [57-50-1] β-D-Fructofuranosyl-α-D-glucopyranoside; α-D-glucopyranosyl-β-D-fructofuranoside; sugar; saccharose; cane sugar; beet sugar. $C_{12}H_{22}O_{11}$; mol wt 342.30. C 42.11%, H 6.48%, O 51.41%. Obtained from sugar cane (*Saccharum officinarum* L., *Gramineae*) and sugar beet (*Beta valgaris* L., *Chenopodiaceae*). Sugar cane contains from 15-20% and sugar beet from 10-17% sucrose. Structure: Avery *et al., J. Chem. Soc.* **1927**, 2308; Beevers, Cochrane, *Proc. Roy. Soc.* **190A**, 257 (1947). Synthesis: Pictet, Vogel, *Helv. Chim. Acta* **11**, 436 (1928); Lemieux, Huber, *J. Am. Chem. Soc.* **78**, 4117 (1956). Ref. with extensive bibliography: Bates, *Polarimetry, Saccharimetry, and the Sugars, National Bureau of Standards Circular* C440, Washington, 1942; W. Pigman, *The Carbohydrates* (Academic Press, New York, 1957) pp 501-506. *Reviews:* M. R. Jenner, *Dev. Food Carbohydr.* **2**, 91-143 (1980); R. Khan, *Pure Appl. Chem.* **56**, 833 (1984).

Monoclinic sphenoidal crystals, cryst masses, blocks, or powder. Sweet taste. Stable in air. Finely divided sugar is hygroscopic and absorbs up to 1% moisture which is given up on heating to 90°. d_4^{25} 1.587. Dec 160-186°. Chars and emits characteristic odor of caramel. [α]_D^{20} not less than +65.9° (c = 26); usual value [α]_D^{25} +66.47 to +66.49°. One gram dissolves in 0.5 ml water; in slightly more than 0.2 ml boiling water, in 170 ml alcohol; in about 100 ml methanol. Moderately sol in glycerol, pyridine. pKa 12.62. d_4^{20} of water solns (g/100 g): 2% 1.0060; 6% 1.0219; 10% 1.0381; 20% 1.0810; 30% 1.1270; 40% 1.1764; 50% 1.2296; 60% 1.2865; 70% 1.3471; 76% 1.3854. n_D^{20} of 10% soln 1.34783. Sucrose does not reduce Fehling's soln, form an osazone, or show mutarotation. It is hydrolyzed to glucose and fructose by dil acids and by invertase, a yeast enzyme. Upon hydrolysis the optical rotation falls and is negative when the hydrolysis is complete. The mixture of glucose and fructose is known as "invert sugar." Sucrose is fermentable, but resists bacterial decompn when in high concentrations.

Caution: Potential symptoms of overexposure are irritation of eyes, skin, upper respiratory system; cough. *See NIOSH Pocket Guide to Chemical Hazards* (DHHS/NIOSH 97-140, 1997) p 288.

USE: Sweetening agent and food. Starting material in the fermentative production of ethanol, butanol, glycerol, citric and levulinic acids. Used in pharmaceuticals as a flavor, as a preservative, as an antioxidant (in the form of invert sugar), as a demulcent, as substitute for glycerol, as granulation agent and excipient for tablets, as coating for tablets. In the plastics and cellulose industry, in rigid polyurethane foams, manuf of ink and of transparent soaps.

8882. Sucrose Octaacetate. [126-14-7] $C_{28}H_{38}O_{19}$; mol wt 678.59. C 49.56%, H 5.64%, O 44.80%. Prepn from sucrose: Linstead *et al., J. Am. Chem. Soc.* **62**, 3260 (1940). Synthesis: Lemieux, Huber, *ibid.* **78**, 4117 (1956).

Hygroscopic, intensely bitter needles from alcohol, mp 89°; dec above 285°; bp₁ 260°. [α]_D^{25.4} +58.5° (c = 2.56 in abs alcohol). n_D 1.4660. Sol in 1100 parts water, 1.1 parts acetal, 0.7 part glacial acetic acid, 0.3 part acetone, 11 parts alcohol, 0.6 part benzene, 22 parts carbon tetrachloride, about 0.5 part methyl acetate, 7 parts paraldehyde, about 0.5 part toluene.

USE: Adhesive; impregnating and insulating papers; in lacquers and plastics; as a denaturant for alcohol.

8883. Sucrose Polyester. Olestra; SPE; Olean. Non-absorbable, non-digestible lipid; noncaloric substitute for fat in foods. Mixture of hexa-, hepta- and octa-fatty acid esters of sucrose. Analysis by gel permeation chromatography: C. G. Birch, F. E. Crowe, *J. Am. Oil Chem. Soc.* **53**, 581 (1976). Effect on absorption of dietary cholesterol in rats: F. H. Mattson *et al., J. Nutr.* **106**, 747 (1976); L. Aust *et al., Ann. Nutr. Metab.* **25**, 255 (1981). Effects as a dietary agent for lowering plasma cholesterol in man: R. W. Fallat *et al., Am. J. Clin. Nutr.* **29**, 1024 (1976); C. J. Glueck *et al., ibid.* **32**, 1636 (1979). Effects on cholesterol metabolism in man: J. R. Crouse, S. M. Grundy, *Metab. Clin. Exp.* **28**, 994 (1979); R. J. Jandacek *et al., Am. J. Clin. Nutr.* **33**, 251 (1980). Caloric dilution study in obese patients: C. J. Glueck *et al., ibid.* **35**, 1352 (1982). Review of properties and clinical safety studies: K. D. Lawson *et al., Drug Metab. Rev.* **29**, 651-703 (1997); of clinical effects on GI functions: J. W. Freston *et al., Regul. Toxicol. Pharmacol.* **26**, 210-218 (1997).

Smoke point 480°F. Flash point 550°F. Fire point 625°F.

USE: Dietary fat replacement in savory snack foods.

8884. Sudan III. [85-86-9] 1-[[4-(Phenylazo)phenyl]azo]-2-naphthalenol; 1-(*p*-phenylazophenylazo)-2-naphthol; tetrazobenzene-β-naphthol; D & C Red No. 17; C.I. Solvent Red 23; C.I. 26100; Sudan Red BK; Tony Red. $C_{22}H_{16}N_4O$; mol wt 352.39. C 74.98%, H 4.58%, N 15.90%, O 4.54%. Weakly acidic azo dye; originally introduced as a fat stain in 1896. Prepn: R. Nietzki, *Ber.* **13**, 1838 (1880); *Colour Index* vol. 4 (3rd ed., 1971) p 4227. Description: *H. J. Conn's Biological Stains*, R. D. Lillie, Ed. (Williams & Wilkins, Baltimore, 9th ed., 1977) pp 168-169, 576. HPLC determn in cosmetics: J. W. Wegener *et al., Chromatographia* **24**, 865 (1987); LC/electrospray-MS determn as environmental contaminant: H.-Y. Lin, R. D. Voyksner, *Anal. Chem.* **65**, 451 (1993). Use as biological stain: W. Frisch-Niggemeyer, *J. Virol. Methods* **5**, 135 (1982); A. Kishida *et al., J. Controlled Release* **13**, 83 (1990). Structure effects on dye adsorption: H. L. Needles *et al., Colourage Annu.* **1995**, 115.

Brown leaves with green metallic shine, mp ~195°. Insol in water or lye. Slightly sol in hot glacial acetic acid. Sol in chloroform; moderately sol ether, acetone, petr ether, fixed and volatile oils, hot glycerol. Sol in alcohol 0.15%.

USE: Dye. Biological stain.

8885. Sudan Black B. [4197-25-5] 2,3-Dihydro-2,2-dimethyl-6-[[4-(phenylazo)-1-naphthalenyl]azo]-1*H*-perimidine; C.I. Solvent Black 3; C.I. 26150; SBB; SSB; SBB-II; SSB-II. $C_{29}H_{24}N_6$; mol wt 456.54. C 76.29%, H 5.30%, N 18.41%. Lipid dye comprised of two major blue components SBB-I, SBB-II and at least 12 secondary components. SBB-II is defined by the chemical name and CAS registry number cited. Introduced: L. Lison, *C.R. Seances Soc. Biol. Ses Fil.* **115**, 202 (1934). TLC purification and histochemistry: A. G. W. Lansink, *Histochemie* **16**, 68 (1968); and solvent effects: W. M. Frederiks *et al.*, *Acta Histochem. Suppl.* **24**, 259 (1981). Structure elucidation: U. Pfüller *et al.*, *Histochemistry* **54**, 237 (1977). Staining technique: D. A. Nelson, F. R. Davey, "Sudan Black B Staining" in *Hematology*, W. J. Williams *et al.*, Eds. (McGraw-Hill Publishing Co., New York, 1990) pp 1747-1748. Use as lipid stain: H. N. Subramaniam, K. A. Chaubal, *J. Biochem. Biophys. Methods* **21**, 9 (1990).

Sudan Black B II

Basic compound completely decomposed at 180-186°.
Sudan Black B I. SBB-I; SSB-I; 2,3-dihydro-2,2-dimethyl-4[(4-phenylazo-1-naphthalenyl)-azo]-1*H*-perimidine. Neutral compound, mp 180-186° (dec). Sublimates 140-160° at 10^{-3} torr without decompositon.

USE: Biological stain for lipids.

8886. Suet, Prepared. Mutton suet. The internal fat of abdomen of sheep purified by melting and straining.

White, solid fat with slight odor and taste; bland if fresh, but rancid after long exposure to air. mp 45-50°; n_D^{60} 1.449-1.451. Sapon no. 192-195. Iodine no. 33-46. Insol in water or cold alcohol; one gram dissolves in 45 ml boiling alcohol, about 60 ml ether.

USE: Preparing ointments.

8887. Sufentanil. [56030-54-7] *N*-[4-(Methoxymethyl)-1-[2-(2-thienyl)ethyl]-4-piperidinyl]-*N*-phenylpropanamide; *N*-[4-(methoxymethyl)-1-[2-(2-thienyl)ethyl]-4-piperidyl]propionanilide; sufentanyl; R-30730. $C_{22}H_{30}N_2O_2S$; mol wt 386.55. C 68.36%, H 7.82%, N 7.25%, O 8.28%, S 8.30%. Potent deriv of fentanyl, *q.v.* Prepn: P. A. J. Janssen, G. H. P. Van Daele, **DE 2610228**; *eidem*, **US 3998834** (both 1976 to Janssen); G. H. P. Van Daele *et al.*, *Arzneim.-Forsch.* **26**, 1521 (1976). *In vitro* binding properties to *mu*-opiate receptor: J. E. Leysen, W. Gommeren, *Arch. Int. Pharmacodyn. Ther.* **260**, 287 (1982); J. E. Leyson *et al.*, *Eur. J. Pharmacol.* **87**, 209 (1983). Analgesic activity and safety assessment: W. F. M. Van Bever *et al.*, *Arzneim.-Forsch.* **26**, 1548 (1976); C. J. E. Niemegeers *et al.*, *ibid.* 1551. GC determn in biological fluids: R. Woestenborghs *et al.*, *J. Chromatogr.* **224**, 122 (1981); T. J. Gillespie *et al.*, *J. Anal. Toxicol.* **5**, 133 (1981). Radioimmunoassay: M. Michaels *et al.*, *J. Pharm. Pharmacol.* **35**, 86 (1983). Comparison to fentanyl for coronary artery surgery: S. de Lange *et al.*, *Anes-*

thesiology **56**, 112 (1982). EEG effects in man: J. G. Bovill *et al.*, *Br. J. Anaesth.* **54**, 45 (1982). Review of pharmacokinetics: L. E. Mather, *Clin. Pharmacokinet.* **8**, 422-426 (1983).

Crystals from petr ether, mp 96.6°. LD_{50} i.v. in mice: 18.7 mg/kg (Van Bever).
Citrate. [60561-17-3] R-33800; Sufenta. $C_{22}H_{30}N_2O_2S.C_6H_8O_7$; mol wt 578.67.
Note: This is a controlled substance (opiate): **21 CFR, 1308.12.**

THERAP CAT: Analgesic (narcotic).

8888. Suint. Portion of the sheep's fleece which is sol in cold water after the wax has been removed. Complex mixture of metallic ions, organic acids, peptides, weak bases, neutral substances, and inorganic cations. The following acids have been identified: acetic, propionic, butyric, valeric, oxalic, succinic, and glutaric. Paper chromatography indicates the presence of adipic and pimelic acids: Deane, Truter, *Biochim. Biophys. Acta* **18**, 435 (1955); *J. Chem. Soc.* **1959**, 2746. Determination of ion content: Mohsin, Shah, *Pak. J. Sci. Ind. Res.* **12**, 286 (1970), *C.A.* **73**, 4778q (1970).

8889. Sulbactam. [68373-14-8] (2*S*,5*R*)-3,3-Dimethyl-7-oxo-4-thia-1-azabicyclo[3.2.0]heptane-2-carboxylic acid 4,4-dioxide; penicillanic acid sulfone; penicillanic acid 1,1-dioxide; CP-45899. $C_8H_{11}NO_5S$; mol wt 233.24. C 41.20%, H 4.75%, N 6.01%, O 34.30%, S 13.75%. Semi-synthetic β-lactamase inhibitor. Prepn and use with β-lactam antibiotics: **BE 867859**; W. E. Barth, **US 4234579** (1978, 1980 both to Pfizer); R. A. Volkmann *et al.*, *J. Org. Chem.* **47**, 3344 (1982). β-Lactamase activity and antibacterial spectrum *in vitro*: A. R. English *et al.*, *Antimicrob. Agents Chemother.* **14**, 414 (1978); R. N. Jones *et al.*, *Diagn. Microbiol. Infect. Dis.* **3**, 489 (1985). HPLC determn in human plasma and urine: J. Haginaka *et al.*, *J. Chromatogr.* **341**, 115 (1985). Pharmacokinetics in humans: G. Foulds *et al.*, *Antimicrob. Agents Chemother.* **23**, 692 (1983). Clinical study of synergistic effect with ampicillin: S. Mehtar *et al.*, *J. Antimicrob. Chemother.* **17**, 389 (1986); B. V. Stromberg *et al.*, *Surg. Gynecol. Obstet.* **162**, 575 (1986). Review of activity and therapeutic use of sulbactam with ampicillin: D. M. Campoli-Richards, R. N. Brogden, *Drugs* **33**, 577-609 (1987).

White, crystalline solid, mp 148-151° (Barth); also reported as mp 154-155.5° (dec) (Barth); also reported as mp 170° (dec) (Volkmann). $[\alpha]_D^{20}$ +251° (c = 0.01 in pH 5.0 buffer). Sol in water.
Sodium salt. [69388-84-7] CP-45899-2; Betamaze. $C_8H_{10}NNaO_5S$; mol wt 255.22.
Mixture of sodium salt with ampicillin sodium. [117060-71-6] Loricin; Unacim; Unasyn (inj.).
Mixture of sodium salt with cefoperazone sodium. Sulperazone.
Compd with ampicillin see Sultamicillin.

THERAP CAT: In combination with β-lactam antibiotics as antibacterial.

8890. Sulbenicillin. [41744-40-5] (2*S*,5*R*,6*R*)-3,3-Dimethyl-7-oxo-6-[[(2*R*)-phenylsulfoacetyl]amino]-4-thia-1-azabicyclo[3.2.0]heptane-2-carboxylic acid; α-sulfobenzylpenicillin; sulfocillin. $C_{16}H_{18}N_2O_7S_2$; mol wt 414.45. C 46.37%, H 4.38%, N 6.76%, O 27.02%, S 15.47%. Semi-synthetic antibiotic related to penicillin. Prepn: S. Morimoto *et al.*, **DE 1948943** corresp to **US 3660379** (1970, 1972 both to Takeda); *eidem, J. Med. Chem.* **15,** 1105, 1108 (1972). *In vitro* activity studies: Tsuchiya *et al., J. Antibiot.* **24,** 607 (1971); *in vivo:* Yamazaki, Tsuchiya, *ibid.* 620. Metabolism: Tsuchiya *et al., ibid.* **25,** 336 (1972). Toxicity: Y. Murata *et al., Takeda Kenkyushoho* **30,** 262 (1971), *C.A.* **76,** 147x (1972). Pharmacokinetics: A. Montanari *et al., Clin. Ter.* **89,** 163 (1979); *eidem, Int. J. Clin. Pharmacol. Ther. Toxicol.* **18,** 225 (1980).

Disodium salt. Kedacillina; Sulpelin; Lilacillin. $C_{16}H_{16}N_2$-$Na_2O_7S_2$; mol wt 458.42. Prepd as a 3:1 mixture of D($-$) and L($+$) isomers. Yellowish-white powder, mp 195-198° (dec). $[\alpha]_D^{22}$ +169-173°. uv max: 257, 262, 268 nm. Very sol in water; sol in methanol. Almost insol in *n*-propanol, acetone, chloroform, benzene, ethyl acetate. LD_{50} in male, female mice, male, female rats (mg/kg): 7900, 8000, 6000, 6200 i.v.; 9600, 10000, 7200, 7500 i.p.; 11500, 13500, 11000, 11800 s.c.; 11000, 10500, 8300, 8600 i.m.; all >15000 orally (Murata).

THERAP CAT: Antibacterial.

8891. Sulbenox. [58095-31-1] (4,5,6,7-Tetrahydro-7-oxo-benzo[*b*]thien-4-yl)urea; CL-206576; Vigazoo. $C_9H_{10}N_2O_2S$; mol wt 210.25. C 51.41%, H 4.79%, N 13.32%, O 15.22%, S 15.25%. Prepn: **NL 7610270** (1977 to Am. Cyanamid), *C.A.* **88,** 22607x (1978). Activity: G. Asato, R. D. Wilbur, *Experientia* **35,** 1458 (1979).

Crystals, mp 245-246°. LD_{50} orally in rats: >5000 mg/kg (Asato, Wilbur).

THERAP CAT (VET): Growth stimulant.

8892. Sulbentine. [350-12-9] Tetrahydro-3,5-bis(phenylmethyl)-2*H*-1,3,5-thiadiazine-2-thione; 3,5-dibenzyltetrahydro-2*H*-1,3,5-thiadiazine-2-thione; 2-thioxo-3,5-dibenzyltetrahydro-1,3,5-thiadiazine; dibenzthione; Fungiplex; Refungine. $C_{17}H_{18}N_2S_2$; mol wt 314.47. C 64.93%, H 5.77%, N 8.91%, S 20.39%. Prepn: Rieche *et al., Arch. Pharm.* **293,** 957 (1960); **DD 20634** (1961), *C.A.* **56,** 487e (1962).

Crystals from acetone or methanol, mp 101-102°.

THERAP CAT: Antifungal.

8893. Sulconazole. [61318-90-9] 1-[2-[[(4-Chlorophenyl)-methyl]thio]-2-(2,4-dichlorophenyl)ethyl]-1*H*-imidazole; ($\pm$)-1-[2,4-dichloro-β-[(*p*-chlorobenzyl)thio]phenethyl]imidazole. C_{18}-$H_{15}Cl_3N_2S$; mol wt 397.75. C 54.35%, H 3.80%, Cl 26.74%, N 7.04%, S 8.06%. Prepn: K. A. M. Walker, **DE 2541833**; *idem*, **US 4055652** (1976, 1977 both to Syntex). HPLC determn in plasma: M. Fass *et al., J. Pharm. Sci.* **70,** 1338 (1981). Mechanism of action study: W. H. Beggs, *Biochem. Arch.* **10,** 117 (1994). Clinical trial in tinea pedis: W. A. Akers *et al., J. Am. Acad. Dermatol.* **21,** 686 (1989). Review of pharmacology and clinical efficacy: P. Benfield, S. P. Clissold, *Drugs* **35,** 143-153 (1988).

Nitrate. [61318-91-0] RS-44872; Exelderm; Myk; Sulcosyn. $C_{18}H_{15}Cl_3N_2S.HNO_3$; mol wt 460.76. Colorless crystals from acetone, mp 130.5-132°.

THERAP CAT: Antifungal.

8894. Sulcotrione. [99105-77-8] 2-[2-Chloro-4-(methylsulfonyl)benzoyl]-1,3-cyclohexanedione; ICIA-0051; SC-0051; Mikado. $C_{14}H_{13}ClO_5S$; mol wt 328.77. C 51.15%, H 3.99%, Cl 10.78%, O 24.33%, S 9.75%. Triketone bleaching herbicide for use in maize. Inhibits 4-hydroxyphenylpyruvate dioxygenase, an enzyme involved in the biosynthesis of plastoquinones. Prepn: W. J. Michaely, G. W. Kraatz, **EP 137963**; *eidem*, **US 4780127** (1983, 1988 both to Stauffer Chem.). Field trials in corn: J. S. Wilson, C. L. Foy, *Weed Technol.* **4,** 731 (1990). Soil adsorption: *eidem, ibid.* **6,** 583 (1992). Mode of action study: J. Secor, *Plant Physiol.* **106,** 1429 (1994). Comprehensive description: J. M. Beraud *et al., Brighton Crop Prot. Conf. - Weeds* **1991,** 51-56.

Light tan solid, mp 139°. Vapor pressure (25°): 4×10^{-8} mm Hg. Soly in water (25°): 165 mg/l. Sol in acetone, chlorobenzene.

USE: Herbicide.

8895. Sulesomab. [167747-19-5] Anti-(human NCA-90 granulocyte cell antigen) immunoglobulin G1 Fab' fragment (mouse monoclonal IMMU-MN3 γ_1-chain) disulfide with mouse monoclonal IMMU-MN3 light chain. Murine antigranulocyte monoclonal Fab' antibody fragment directed against nonspecific crossreactive antigen-90 (NCA-90), a surface glycoprotein on granulocytes, and cross reactive with carcinoembryonic antigen (CEA). ^{99m}Technetium radiolabeled immunoconjugate designed for imaging activated granulocytes. Prepn and characterization as an anti-CEA antibody: H. J. Hansen *et al., Cancer* **71,** 3478 (1993). Prepn of radiolabeled form: *idem et al.*, **US 5328679** (1994 to Immunomedics). Pharmacology and immunoscintigraphy: W. Becker *et al., Semin. Nucl. Med.* **24,** 142 (1994). Clinical study in detection of osteomyelitis: S. J. Harwood *et al., Clin. Infect. Dis.* **28,** 1200 (1999); of appendicitis: B. Baron *et al., Surgery* **125,** 288 (1999).

^{99m}**Tc-Labeled form.** [157856-25-2] ImmuRAID-MN3-Tc-99m; LeukoScan.

THERAP CAT: ^{99m}Tc-labeled form as diagnostic aid (radioactive imaging agent).

8896. Sulfabenz. [127-77-5] 4-Amino-*N*-phenylbenzenesulfonamide; sulfanilanilide; *p*-aminobenzenesulfonanilide; *p*-aminophenylsulfonamidobenzene; N^1-phenylsulfanilamide. $C_{12}H_{12}$-N_2O_2S; mol wt 248.30. C 58.05%, H 4.87%, N 11.28%, O 12.89%, S 12.91%. Prepn: Gelmo, *J. Prakt. Chem.* **77,** 369 (1908); Mastryukova *et al., Tetrahedron* **19,** 357 (1963).

Needles from dil alc, mp 200°. Practically insol in water; readily sol in warm alcohol, acetone. pKa: 10.94 (in 50% aq alc); 11.59 (in 80% aq alc).

THERAP CAT (VET): Antibacterial; coccidiostat (for poultry).

8897. Sulfabenzamide. [127-71-9] *N*-[(4-Aminophenyl)-sulfonyl]benzamide; *N*-sulfanilylbenzamide; *N*[1]-benzoylsulfanil-amide; *N*-(*p*-aminobenzenesulfonyl)benzamide; Sulfabenzide. $C_{13}H_{12}N_2O_3S$; mol wt 276.31. C 56.51%, H 4.38%, N 10.14%, O 17.37%, S 11.60%. Prepn: Crossley *et al.*, *J. Am. Chem. Soc.* **61**, 2950 (1939); Dvornikoff, US 2240496 (1941 to Monsanto); GB 541958 (1942 to Schering AG); Siebenmann, Schnitzer, *J. Am. Chem. Soc.* **65**, 2126 (1943).

Long, hexagonal prisms from 60% alcohol, mp 181.2-182.3°. pKa (25°): 4.57. Substantially insol in water. One gram dissolves in 3225 ml of water at 30°, in 33 ml of 95% ethanol, in 9 ml of acetone. Soly in 1*N* NaOH or KOH: ~16 g/100 ml; pH just above 7.0. Aq solns of the water-soluble sodium salt have the same pH.

THERAP CAT: Antibacterial.

THERAP CAT (VET): Antimicrobial.

8898. Sulfabromomethazine. [116-45-0] 4-Amino-*N*-(5-bromo-4,6-dimethyl-2-pyrimidinyl)benzenesulfonamide; *N*[1]-(5-bromo-4,6-dimethyl-2-pyrimidinyl)sulfanilamide; 4-amino-4,6-di-methyl-2-sulfanilamidopyrimidine; 2-sulfanilamido-5-bromo-4,6-dimethyl pyrimidine; 5-bromosulfamethazine; SN-3517. $C_{12}H_{13}BrN_4O_2S$; mol wt 357.23. C 40.35%, H 3.67%, Br 22.37%, N 15.68%, O 8.96%, S 8.98%. Prepn: English *et al.*, *J. Am. Chem. Soc.* **68**, 453 (1946). Pharmacology: C. M. Stowe *et al.*, *Am. J. Vet. Res.* **29**, 345 (1958).

Crystals, dec 250-252°. uv max (methanol): 238, 272 nm (A 428, 635); min: 250 nm (A 290). Sol in alkaline solns.

Sodium salt monohydrate. Sulfabrom. $C_{12}H_{12}BrN_4NaO_2$-S.H_2O; mol wt 397.22. Cream-colored powder. Sol in water.

THERAP CAT (VET): Antibacterial.

8899. Sulfacetamide. [144-80-9] *N*-[(4-Aminophenyl)sul-fonyl]acetamide; *N*-sulfanilylacetamide; *N*[1]-acetylsulfanilamide; *p*-aminobenzenesulfonoacetamide. $C_8H_{10}N_2O_3S$; mol wt 214.24. C 44.85%, H 4.70%, N 13.08%, O 22.40%, S 14.97%. Incorrectly called *sulfacetimide*. Prepn: M. L. Crossley *et al.*, *J. Am. Chem. Soc.* **61**, 2950 (1939); M. Dohrn, P. Diedrich, *Muench. Med. Wochenschr.* **85**, 2017 (1938); *eidem*, US 2411495 (1946 to Schering). Toxicity: R. S. Fisher, H. B. Haag, *J. Urol.* **47**, 183 (1942). Antimicrobial activity: R. D. Houlsby *et al.*, *J. Pharm. Sci.* **72**, 1401 (1983). GC determn in animal tissues: A. E. Mooser, H. Koch, *J. AOAC Int.* **76**, 976 (1993). Clinical trial in conjunctivitis: J. A. Lohr *et al.*, *Pediatr. Infect. Dis. J.* **7**, 626 (1988); in acne: D. L. Breneman, M. C. Ariano, *Int. J. Dermatol.* **32**, 365 (1993). Comprehensive description: I. Ahmad *et al.*, *Anal. Profiles Drug Subs. Excip.* **23**, 471-509 (1994).

White or yellowish white prisms, mp 182-184°. Acidic, slightly saline taste. uv max (water, 0.1*M* HCl, 0.1*M* HCl, 0.1*M* NaOH): 258, 217, 270, 256 (a_m 17700, 18900, 8900, 17300). Soluble in 150 parts water at 20°, in 15 parts alcohol, in 7 parts acetone. Sol in mineral acids and soln of alkali hydroxides and carbonates.

Slightly sol in ether; very slightly sol in chloroform. An aq soln is acid to litmus. LD_{50} orally in dogs: 8000 mg/kg (Fisher).

Sodium salt. [127-56-0]; [6209-17-2] (monohydrate). Soluble sulfacetamide; Ak-Sulf; Albucid; Antébor; Beocid-Puroptal; Bleph-10; Cetamide; Prontamid; Sebizon; Sodium Sulamyd; Sulf-10; Sulten-10. $C_8H_9N_2NaO_3S$; mol wt 236.22. Minute prisms from dil alcohol, mp 257°. Occurs as the monohydrate; white, odorless, crystalline powder with slightly bitter taste. uv max (pH 7.0 phosphate buffer, 0.1*M* HCl, aq. acid, 0.1*M* NaOH, aq alkali): 255, 271, 271, 256, 256 ($A_{1cm}^{1\%}$ 660-720, 207, 260, 626, 750). Sol in 1.5 parts water. Slightly sol in 96% ethanol; sparingly sol in acetone. Practically insol in ether and chloroform. pKa_1 (amino group): 1.8; pKa_2 (sulfonamide group at 25°): 5.4.

THERAP CAT: Antibacterial.

THERAP CAT (VET): Antibacterial.

8900. Sulfachlorpyridazine. [80-32-0] 4-Amino-*N*-(6-chloro-3-pyridazinyl)benzenesulfonamide; *N*[1]-(6-chloro-3-pyridazinyl)sulfanilamide; 3-chloro-6-sulfanilamidopyridazine; 3-sulfanilamido-6-chloropyridazine; 3-(*p*-aminophenylsulfonamido)-6-chloropyridazine; Ciba 10370; Ba-10370; Cosumix; Sonilyn. $C_{10}H_9ClN_4O_2S$; mol wt 284.72. C 42.18%, H 3.19%, Cl 12.45%, N 19.68%, O 11.24%, S 11.26%. Prepn: Lester, English, US 2790798 (1957 to Am. Cyanamid). Comparative antibacterial spectrum: G. E. Burrows *et al.*, *J. Vet. Diagn. Invest.* **5**, 541 (1993). Pharmacokinetics and therapeutic potential in horses: E. van Duijkeren *et al.*, *Vet. Rec.* **137**, 483 (1995). ELISA determn in food of animal origin: C. A. Spinks *et al.*, *Food Addit. Contam.* **18**, 11 (2001).

Sodium salt. [23282-55-5] Vetisulid. $C_{10}H_8ClN_4NaO_2S$; mol wt 306.70.

THERAP CAT: Antibacterial.

THERAP CAT (VET): Antibacterial agent. In enteric infections.

8901. Sulfachrysoidine. [485-41-6] 3,5-Diamino-2-[[4-(aminosulfonyl)phenyl]azo]benzoic acid; 3,5-diamino-2-[*p*-(sulfamoylphenyl)azo]benzoic acid; carboxysulfamidochrysoidine; Azo Compd No. 4; Rubiazol. $C_{13}H_{13}N_5O_4S$; mol wt 335.34. C 46.56%, H 3.91%, N 20.88%, O 19.08%, S 9.56%. Prepn: Gley, Girard, *C.R. Seances Soc. Biol. Ses Fil.* **125**, 1027 (1937).

Deep red crystals. mp above 300°.

THERAP CAT: Antibacterial.

8902. Sulfacytine. [17784-12-2] 4-Amino-*N*-(1-ethyl-1,2-dihydro-2-oxo-4-pyrimidinyl)benzenesulfonamide; *N*'-(1-ethyl-1,2-dihydro-2-oxo-4-pyrimidinyl)sulfanilamide; 1-ethyl-*N*-sulfanilylcytosine; *N*-sulfanilyl-1-ethylcytosine; CL-636; Renoquid. $C_{12}H_{14}N_4O_3S$; mol wt 294.33. C 48.97%, H 4.79%, N 19.04%, O 16.31%, S 10.89%. Prepn: NL 6610815 corresp to Doub, Krolls, US 3375247 (1967, 1968 to Parke, Davis). Prepn and activity: Doub *et al.*, *J. Med. Chem.* **13**, 242 (1970).

Crystals from butyl alcohol, methanol, mp 166.5-168°, (monohydrate, mp 104°). uv max (methanol): 263, 297 nm ($E_{1cm}^{1\%}$ 584,

762). Equilibrium soly in pH 5 buffer at 37°: approx 175 mg/100 ml. Soly increases with increasing pH. pK' 6.9.

THERAP CAT: Antibacterial.

8903. Sulfadiazine. [68-35-9] 4-Amino-*N*-2-pyrimidinyl-benzenesulfonamide; 2-sulfanilamidopyrimidine; *N¹*-2-pyrimidin-ylsulfanilamide; *N¹*-2-pyrimidylsulfanilamide; 2-sulfanilylamino-pyrimidine; sulfapyrimidine; Adiazine. $C_{10}H_{10}N_4O_2S$; mol wt 250.28. C 47.99%, H 4.03%, N 22.39%, O 12.79%, S 12.81%. Prepd by condensing 2-aminopyrimidine with acetylsulfanilyl chloride followed by hydrolysis of the acetyl group with NaOH: Roblin *et al., J. Am. Chem. Soc.* **62**, 2002 (1940); Barber, **GB 557055** (1943); Sprague, **US 2407966** (1946 to Sharp & Dohme); Winnek, Roblin, **US 2410793** (1946 to Am. Cyanamid). Toxicological, chemotherapeutic and pharmacokinetic studies: Böhni *et al., Chemotherapy* **14**, 195-226 (1969). *In vitro* activity of silver salt: Carr *et al., Antimicrob. Agents Chemother.* **4**, 585 (1973). Use of silver salt in burns: C. L. Fox, *Arch. Surg.* **96**, 184 (1968). Comprehensive description: H. Stober, W. DeWitte, *Anal. Profiles Drug Subs.* **11**, 523-551 (1982).

White or slightly yellow powder. mp 252-256°. Sparingly sol in water at 37°: 13 mg/100 ml at pH 5.5; 200 mg/100 ml at pH 7.5. Sparingly sol in alcohol, acetone. One gram dissolves in about 620 ml of human serum at 37°. Freely sol in dil mineral acids and in solns of potassium and sodium hydroxides and in ammonia water.

Mixture with trimethoprim (usually 5:1). Co-trimazine; Nordine; Scorprin; Tribrissen; Triglobe; Vesuprim.

Sodium salt. Sulfadiazine sodium; soluble sulfadiazine. $C_{10}H_9N_4NaO_2S$. White powder. On prolonged exposure to humid air, it absorbs carbon dioxide with the liberation of sulfadiazine and becomes incompletely sol in water. One gram dissolves in about 2 ml of water. Slightly sol in alc. Solns are alkaline to phenol-phthalein (pH 9-11).

Silver salt. [22199-08-2] Flamazine; Flammazine; Silvadene.

THERAP CAT: Antibacterial.

THERAP CAT (VET): Antibacterial.

8904. Sulfadicramide. [115-68-4] *N*-[(4-Aminophenyl)sul-fonyl]-3-methyl-2-butenamide; 3-methyl-*N*-sulfanilylcrotonamide; *N¹*-senecioylsulfanilamide; *N*-sulfanilylseneciamide; *N¹*-dimethyl-acroylsulfanilamide; *N*-sulfanilyl-β,β-dimethylacrylamide; Irgamide. $C_{11}H_{14}N_2O_3S$; mol wt 254.31. C 51.95%, H 5.55%, N 11.02%, O 18.87%, S 12.61%. Prepd from β,β-dimethylacrylamide by treatment with sodamide and *p*-nitrobenzenesulfonyl chloride; the resulting 4-nitro-*N*-(β,β-dimethylacrylyl)benzenesulfonamide is reduced with Fe and dil AcOH: Martin, Häfliger, **US 2417005** (1947), *cf.* **US 2383874** (1945).

Crystals from alc. mp 184-185°. Slightly sol in water, ether. Freely sol in alcohol, acetone. For the prepn of solns the water-soluble sodium salt is marketed. A 20% aq soln of the sodium salt has a pH of 8.3.

THERAP CAT: Antibacterial.

8905. Sulfadimethoxine. [122-11-2] 4-Amino-*N*-(2,6-di-methoxy-4-pyrimidinyl)benzenesulfonamide; *N¹*-(2,6-dimethoxy-4-pyrimidinyl)sulfanilamide; 2,6-dimethoxy-4-sulfanilamidopyri-midine; 2,4-dimethoxy-6-sulfanilamido-1,3-diazine; 6-sulfanilami-do-2,4-dimethoxypyrimidine; 2,6-dimethoxy-4-(*p*-aminobenzene-sulfonamido)pyrimidine; Albon; Sulforal; Ultrasulfon. $C_{12}H_{14}N_4O_4S$; mol wt 310.33. C 46.44%, H 4.55%, N 18.05%, O 20.62%, S 10.33%. Prepn: Bretschneider, Klötzer, **US 2703800** (1955 to Oesterr. Stickstoffwerke); *eidem, Monatsh. Chem.* **87**, 136 (1956);

Langley, **GB 866843** (1961 to I.C.I.); Bretschneider *et al., Monatsh. Chem.* **92**, 128 (1961); **US 3127398** (1964 to Hoffmann-La Roche); Shepherd *et al., J. Org. Chem.* **26**, 2764 (1961). Toxicity data: Seki *et al., Arzneim.-Forsch.* **15**, 1441 (1965). Toxicological, chemotherapeutic and pharmacokinetic studies: Böhni *et al., Chemotherapy* **14**, 195-226 (1969); *see also* Aviado *et al., ibid.* 37.

Crystals from dil alc, mp 201-203°. Sol in dil HCl and in aq solns of sodium carbonate. Soly in water at 37° (mg/100 ml): 4.6 at pH 4.10; 29.5 at pH 6.7; 58.0 at pH 7.06; 5170 at pH 8.71. LD_{50} orally in mice: >10 g/kg (Seki).

Sodium salt. [1037-50-9] Di-Methox. $C_{12}H_{13}N_4NaO_4S$; mol wt 332.31. Crystals from methanol + ether. Freely sol in water. pH of 5% solution: 8.1; of 10% soln: 8.6.

THERAP CAT (VET): Antibacterial.

8906. Sulfadoxine. [2447-57-6] 4-Amino-*N*-(5,6-dimeth-oxy-4-pyrimidinyl)benzenesulfonamide; *N'*-(5,6-dimethoxy-4-pyrimidinyl)sulfanilamide; 6-(4-aminobenzenesulfonamido)-4,5-dimethoxypyrimidine; 4-sulfanilamido-5,6-dimethoxypyrimidine; sulforthomidine; sulphormethoxine; Ro-4-4393; Fanasil. $C_{12}H_{14}N_4O_4S$; mol wt 310.33. C 46.44%, H 4.55%, N 18.05%, O 20.62%, S 10.33%. Dihydropteroate synthetase inhibitor. Prepn: **BE 618639**; H. Bretschneider *et al.*, **US 3132139** (1962, 1964 both to Hoffmann-La Roche). Toxicological, chemotherapeutic and phar-macokinetic studies: E. Böhni *et al., Chemotherapy* **14**, 195-226 (1969). Comprehensive description: V. K. Kapoor, *Anal. Profiles Drug Subs.* **17**, 571-605 (1988). Enzyme inhibition *in vitro*: Y. Zhang, S. R. Meshnick, *Antimicrob. Agents Chemother.* **35**, 267 (1991). Determn in plasma using supercritical fluid chromatogra-phy: S. I. Bhoir *et al., J. Chromatogr. B* **757**, 39 (2001). Clinical trial of combination with pyrimethamine, *q.v.*, for malaria: C. V. Plowe *et al., Br. Med. J.* **328**, 545 (2004).

Crystals from 50% aq alc, mp 190-194°. Practically insol in ether. Very slightly sol in water, slightly sol in alcohol, methanol. Sol in dilute mineral acids, solutions of alkali hydroxides and car-bonates. LD_{50} in mice (microcrystals, mg/kg): 5200 orally, 2900 s.c., 2900 i.p. (Böhni).

Mixture with trimethoprim. [39295-60-8] Animar; Bimo-trim; Borgal.

THERAP CAT: Antibacterial; antimalarial.

THERAP CAT (VET): Antibacterial.

8907. Sulfaethidole. [94-19-9] 4-Amino-*N*-(5-ethyl-1,3,4-thiadiazol-2-yl)benzenesulfonamide; *N¹*-(5-ethyl-1,3,4-thiadiazol-2-yl)sulfanilamide; 5-ethyl-2-sulfanilamido-1,3,4-thiadiazole; 2-(*p*-aminobenzenesulfonamido)-5-ethylthiadiazole; sulfaethylthia-diazole; VK-55; Sul-Spantab. $C_{10}H_{12}N_4O_2S_2$; mol wt 284.36. C 42.24%, H 4.25%, N 19.70%, O 11.25%, S 22.55%. The commercial prepn (Schering AG) is described in P.B. reports, no. 245, p 5, and no. 1361, p 73. Prepn: Wojahn, Wuckel, *Arch. Pharm.* **284**, 53 (1951).

Crystals, mp 185.5-186.0°. One gram dissolves in 4000 ml water, in 40 g methanol, in 30 g ethanol, in 10 g acetone, in 1350 g ether, in 2800 g chloroform, in 20,000 g benzene. Faintly acid to litmus.

Sodium salt. pH of 20% soln: 7.5.

THERAP CAT: Antibacterial.

THERAP CAT (VET): Antimicrobial.

8908. Sulfaguanidine. [57-67-0] 4-Amino-*N*-(aminoimino-methyl)benzenesulfonamide; 4-amino-*N*-(diaminomethylene)ben-zenesulfonamide; N^1-amidinosulfanilamide; N^1-guanylsulfanil-amide; *p*-aminobenzenesulfonylguanidine; sulfanilylguanidine; RP-2275; Diacta; Ganidan; Guanicil; Resulfon; Shigatox. C_7H_{10}-N_4O_2S; mol wt 214.24. C 39.24%, H 4.70%, N 26.15%, O 14.94%, S 14.97%. Prepd by condensing acetylsulfanilyl chloride with guanidine nitrate in the presence of much NaOH in water-acetone: Winnek, **US 2218490** (1940); **US 2229784** (1941); **US 2233569** (1941); or by fusing N^4-acetylsulfanilamide and dicyanodiamide: Haworth, Rose, **GB 551524** (1943). Additional syntheses: *ACS Monograph Series* no. **106**, entitled "Sulfonamides and Allied Compounds," E. H. Northey, Ed. (Reinhold, New York, 1948). Revised structure: G. R. Sullivan, J. D. Roberts, *J. Org. Chem.* **42**, 1095 (1977). Review of pharmacology: E. K. Marshall, Jr. *et al., Bull. Johns Hopkins Hosp.* **67**, 163-188 (1940); E. Pick, *J. Mt. Sinai Hosp.* **10**, 343-354 (1943).

Monohydrate. Needles. When anhydr, mp 190-193°. One gram dissolves in about 1000 ml water at 25° and in about 10 ml at 100°. Sparingly sol in alcohol or acetone. Freely sol in dil mineral acids. Insol in NaOH solns at room temp.

THERAP CAT: Antibacterial.

THERAP CAT (VET): Antimicrobial. In enteric infections.

8909. Sulfaguanole. [27031-08-9] 4-Amino-*N*-[[(4,5-di-methyl-2-oxazolyl)amino]iminomethyl]benzenesulfonamide; N^1-[(4,5-dimethyl-2-oxazolyl)amidino]sulfanilamide; 1-(4,5-dimethyl-oxazol-2-yl)-3-sulfanilylguanidine; 1-(*p*-aminophenylsulfonyl)-3-(4,5-dimethyl-2-oxazolyl)guanidine; sulfadimethyloxazolylguani-dine; Enterocura. $C_{12}H_{15}N_5O_3S$; mol wt 309.34. C 46.59%, H 4.89%, N 22.64%, O 15.52%, S 10.37%. Prepn: Loop *et al.*, **GB 1185139** *C.A.* **73**, 3909w (1970); *eidem,* **US 3562258** (1970, 1971 both to Nordmark-Werke); Loop, Kohlmann, *Arzneim.-Forsch.* **23**, 171 (1973). Toxicology: J. Kuhne *et al., ibid.* 178. Series of articles on pharmacology: *ibid.* 172-192.

Almost colorless crystals from 9:1 acetone-water, mp 233-236°; from water-methanol, mp 228-230°. pKa 7.76. Practically insol in water. Sol in dil NaOH solns. No deaths in mice or rats for oral doses of 5 g/kg (Kuhne).

THERAP CAT: Antibacterial.

8910. Sulfalene. [152-47-6] 4-Amino-*N*-(3-methoxypyra-zinyl)benzenesulfonamide; N^1-(3-methoxy-2-pyrazinyl)sulfanil-amide; 2-(*p*-aminobenzenesulfonamido)-3-methoxypyrazine; 3-methoxy-2-sulfanilamidopyrazine; 2-sulfanil-amido-3-methoxypyrazine; sulfamethopyrazine; sulfapyrazine-methoxyine; Farmitalia 204/122; Dalysep; Kelfizina; Kelfizine W; Longum; Policydal; Vetkelfizina. $C_{11}H_{12}N_4O_3S$; mol wt 280.30. C 47.13%, H 4.32%, N 19.99%, O 17.12%, S 11.44%. Prepn: B. Camerino, G. Palamidessi, *Gazz. Chim. Ital.* **90**, 1815 (1960); **GB 928151**; **US 3098069** (both 1963 to Farmitalia). *Review:* Gaspar-ini, *Veterinaria (Milan)* **20**, 302 (1971). Also used in combination with trimethoprim, *q.v.* Toxicology: V. De Pascale *et al., Boll.*

Chim. Farm. **116**, 155 (1977). Pharmacodynamics: D. S. Reeves *et al., J. Antimicrob. Chemother.* **6**, 647 (1980). Clinical assessment: H. Harazim *et al., J. Int. Med. Res.* **11**, 197 (1983); M. L. Colombo *et al., Pharmatherapeutica* **3**, 556 (1984). Review of clinical efficacy: F. Celotti *et al., J. Int. Med. Res.* **14**, 236-241 (1986).

Crystals from alcohol, mp 176°. LD_{50} in mice (g/kg): 2.164 orally; 1.41 i.v. (**US 3098069**).

Mixture with trimethoprim. [50933-06-7] Kelfiprim. LD_{50} in mice, rats (mg/kg): 3500; 3550 orally (De Pascale).

THERAP CAT: Antibacterial.

THERAP CAT (VET): Antibacterial.

8911. Sulfallate. [95-06-7] Diethylcarbamodithioic acid 2-chloro-2-propenyl ester; diethyldithiocarbamic acid 2-chloroallyl ester; 2-chloroallyl diethyldithiocarbamate; CDEC; CP-4742; Ve-gadex. $C_8H_{14}ClNS_2$; mol wt 223.79. C 42.94%, H 6.31%, Cl 15.84%, N 6.26%, S 28.66%. Selective pre-planting or pre-emer-gence herbicide. Prepn: Harman, D'Amico, *J. Am. Chem. Soc.* **75**, 4081 (1953); **GB 769222** (1957 to Monsanto). Toxicity data: G. W. Bailey, J. L. White, *Residue Rev.* **10**, 97 (1965). Review of carcinogenic risk: *IARC Monographs* **30**, 283-291 (1983).

Amber liquid, bp_1 128-130°. n_D^{25} 1.5822. d^{25} 1.088. Soly in water at 25°: 100 ppm. Sol in most organic solvents. LD_{50} orally in rats: 850 mg/kg (Bailey, White).

Caution: Prolonged contact with skin and eyes may cause mod-erate irritation. *See Clinical Toxicology of Commercial Products,* R. E. Gosselin *et al.,* Eds. (Williams & Wilkins, Baltimore, 5th ed., 1984) Section II, p 313. This substance is reasonably anticipated to be a human carcinogen: *Report on Carcinogens, Eleventh Edition* (PB2005-104914, 2004) p III-238.

USE: Herbicide.

8912. Sulfaloxic Acid. [14376-16-0] 2-[[[4-[[[[(Hydroxy-methyl)amino]carbonyl]amino]sulfonyl]phenyl]amino]carbonyl]-benzoic acid; 4'-(carbamoylsulfamoyl)phthalanilic acid hydroxy-methyl derivative; 4'-(carbamoylsulfamoyl)-*N*-(hydroxymethyl)-phthalanilic acid; formophthaloylsulfanilyl urea; 2-[4-(hydroxy-methylureidosulfonyl)phenylcarbamoyl]benzoic acid; sulphaloxic acid. $C_{16}H_{15}N_3O_7S$; mol wt 393.37. C 48.85%, H 3.84%, N 10.68%, O 28.47%, S 8.15%. Prepn: Wiedemann, Strassburger, **DE 960190** (1957 to von Heyden), *C.A.* **53**, 6547i (1959).

Crystals, mp 160-165°. Soluble in dil bases.

Calcium salt. [59672-20-7] Enteromide; Intestin-Euvernil. $C_{32}H_{28}CaN_6O_{14}S_2$; mol wt 824.80.

THERAP CAT: Antibacterial.

8913. Sulfamerazine. [127-79-7] 4-Amino-*N*-(4-methyl-2-pyrimidinyl)benzenesulfonamide; N^1-(4-methyl-2-pyrimidyl)sulfa-nilamide; N^1-(4-methyl-2-pyrimidinyl)sulfanilamide; 2-sulfanil-amido-4-methylpyrimidine; sulfamethyldiazine; RP-2632; Mesulfa; Percoccide. $C_{11}H_{12}N_4O_2S$; mol wt 264.30. C 49.99%, H 4.58%, N 21.20%, O 12.11%, S 12.13%. Prepd by condensing 2-amino-4-

methylpyrimidine with acetylsulfanilyl chloride followed by hydrolysis of the acetyl group: Roblin et al., J. Am. Chem. Soc. **62**, 2002 (1940); Sprague et al., ibid. **63**, 3028 (1941); Sprague, **US 2407966** (1946 to Sharp & Dohme). For prepn of 2-amino-4-methylpyrimidine see Benary, Ber. **63**, 2601 (1930); Backer, Grevenstuk, Rec. Trav. Chim. **61**, 291 (1942); cf. E. H. Northey, Sulfonamides (Reinhold, New York, 1948). Antimicrobial activity: Gill et al., Indian J. Vet. Sci. **32**, 240 (1962); Vaichulis, Vedros, Chemotherapia **11**, 315 (1966). Toxicity studies: Simunek et al., Vet. Med. (Prague) **13**, 619 (1968). Kinetics of sulfamerazine decompn: Zajac, Diss. Pharm. Pharmacol. **22**, 455 (1970). Comprehensive description: R. D. G. Woolfenden, Anal. Profiles Drug Subs. **6**, 515-577 (1977).

Crystals, mp 234-238°. uv max (water): 243, 257 nm ($E_{1cm}^{1\%}$ 875, 822); (0.1M HCl): 243, 307 nm ($E_{1cm}^{1\%}$ 625, 200); (ethanol): 271 nm ($E_{1cm}^{1\%}$ 835). Slowly darkens on exposure to light. Soly in water at 37°: 35 mg/100 ml at pH 5.5; 170 mg/100 ml at pH 7.5. Readily sol in dil mineral acids and in solns of potassium, ammonium and sodium hydroxides. Sparingly sol in acetone, slightly sol in alcohol, very slightly sol in ether, chloroform.

Monosodium salt. [127-58-2] Soluble sulfamerazine; Solumédine. $C_{11}H_{11}N_4NaO_2S$; mol wt 286.29. Crystals. Bitter, caustic taste. Hygroscopic. On prolonged exposure to humid air, it absorbs CO_2 with the liberation of sulfamerazine and becomes incompletely sol in water. Its solns are alkaline to phenolphthalein (pH 10 or more). One gram dissolves in 3.6 ml water. Slightly sol in alc. Insol in ether, chloroform.

THERAP CAT: Antibacterial.

THERAP CAT (VET): Antibacterial.

8914. Sulfameter. [651-06-9] 4-Amino-N-(5-methoxy-2-pyrimidinyl)benzenesulfonamide; N^1-(5-methoxy-2-pyrimidinyl)-sulfanilamide; sulfa-5-methoxypyrimidine; 2-sulfanilamido-5-methoxypyrimidine; 2-(p-aminobenzenesulfonamido)-5-methoxypyrimidine; 5-methoxysulfadiazine; sulfamethoxydiazine; sulfametin (rescinded USAN); sulfametorine; methoxypyrimal; AHR-857; I-2586; Bayrena; Durenat; Kinecid; Kiron; Kirocid; Sulla; Ultrax. $C_{11}H_{12}N_4O_3S$; mol wt 280.30. C 47.13%, H 4.32%, N 19.99%, O 17.12%, S 11.44%. Prepn: **DE 1101428**; P. Diedrich, **US 3214335** (1961, 1965 both to Schering AG); Horstmann et al., Arzneim.-Forsch. **11**, 682 (1961); Budesinky et al., Experientia **17**, 129 (1961); **CS 98818**; **BE 633513** (1963 to SPOFA); Collect. Czech. Chem. Commun. **29**, 2980 (1964). Toxicity study: G. Hecht et al., Arzneim.-Forsch. **11**, 695 (1961). Toxicology, chemotherapeutics and pharmacokinetics: Böhne et al., Chemotherapy **14**, 195-226 (1969).

Minute, bitter crystals, mp 214-216°. uv max: 230, 271 nm ($E_{1cm}^{1\%}$ 562, 726). Very sparingly sol in water, alcohol, ether. Sol in dil acids, alkalies.

Sodium salt. Water soluble. pK about 6.8. pH of 1% aq soln: about 8.9. LD_{50} in mice, rats (g/kg): 1.1 ±0.2, 1.2 i.v.; 1.5, 1.1 i.p.; 3.0, 1.0 orally (Hecht).

THERAP CAT: Antibacterial.

8915. Sulfamethazine. [57-68-1] 4-Amino-N-(4,6-dimethyl-2-pyrimidinyl)benzenesulfonamide; N^1-(4,6-dimethyl-2-pyrimidinyl)sulfanilamide; N^1-(4,6-dimethyl-2-pyrimidyl)sulfanilamide; 4,6-dimethyl-2-sulfanilamidopyrimidine; sulfamezathine; sulfadimerazine; sulfadimidine; sulfamidine; sulfadimethylpyrimidine; Diazil; Sulfadine; S-Dimidine; Dimidin-R; Neazina; Sulmet. $C_{12}H_{14}N_4O_2S$; mol wt 278.33. C 51.78%, H 5.07%, N 20.13%, O 11.50%,

S 11.52%. Prepn: Caldwell et al., J. Am. Chem. Soc. **63**, 2188 (1941); Roblin et al., ibid. **64**, 567 (1942); Weisner, Katscher, **GB 546158** (1942 to Ward, Blenkinsop); Sprague, **US 2407966** (1946 to Sharp & Dohme). Alternate prepn: Haworth, Rose, **GB 552887** (1943 to I.C.I.); Garzia, **US 3119818** (1964 to Ist. Chemioterap. Ital.). Anticoccidiosis activity: Zarin, Feodorova, C.A. **66**, 114, 435p-436q (1967). Metabolic studies: Turco et al., Clin. Pharmacol. Ther. **7**, 603 (1966); Parker et al., Hum. Hered. **19**, 402 (1969). Solubility studies: Shkadova et al., Farm. Zh. (Kiev) **24**, 39 (1969). Acute toxicity: B. Bobranski et al., Arch. Immunol. Ther. Exp. **16**, 804 (1968). Comprehensive description: C. Papostephanou, M. Frantz, Anal. Profiles Drug Subs. **7**, 401-422 (1978).

Crystals from dioxane-water, mp 176° (also reported as mp 178-179°; mp 198-199°; mp 205-207°). uv max (water, pH 6.6): 241 nm ($E_{1cm}^{1\%}$ 670); (0.01N NaOH): 243, 257 nm ($E_{1cm}^{1\%}$ 765, 776); (0.01N HCl): 241, 297 nm ($E_{1cm}^{1\%}$ 561, 266). Soly in water at 29°: 150 mg/100 ml; at 37°: 192 mg/100 ml at pH 7.0. pK_1 7.4±0.2, pK_2 2.65±0.2. The soly increases rapidly with an increase in pH. LD_{50} i.p. in mice: 1.06 g/kg (Bobranski).

Sodium salt. [1981-58-4] Intradine; Sulfoxine 33; Vesadin. $C_{12}H_{13}N_4NaO_2S$; mol wt 300.31.

THERAP CAT: Antibacterial.

THERAP CAT (VET): Antibacterial.

8916. Sulfamethizole. [144-82-1] 4-Amino-N-(5-methyl-1,3,4-thiadiazol-2-yl)benzenesulfonamide; N^1-(5-methyl-1,3,4-thiadiazol-2-yl)sulfanilamide; 2-sulfanilamido-5-methyl-1,3,4-thiadiazole; 5-methyl-2-sulfanilamido-1,3,4-thiadiazole; 2-(p-aminobenzenesulfonamido)-5-methylthiadiazole; sulfamethylthiadiazole; Lucosil; Rufol; Urolucosil. $C_9H_{10}N_4O_2S_2$; mol wt 270.33. C 39.99%, H 3.73%, N 20.73%, O 11.84%, S 23.72%. Prepn: Hübner, **US 2447702** (1948 to Lundbeck).

Crystals from water, mp 208°. pKa 5.45. One gram dissolves in 4000 ml water at pH 6.5, in 5 ml water at pH 7.5, in 40 g methanol, in 30 g ethanol, in 10 g acetone, in 1370 g ether, in 2800 g chloroform. Practically insol in benzene.

THERAP CAT: Antibacterial.

THERAP CAT (VET): Antibacterial.

8917. Sulfamethomidine. [3772-76-7] 4-Amino-N-(6-methoxy-2-methyl-4-pyrimidinyl)benzenesulfonamide; N^1-(6-methoxy-2-methyl-4-pyrimidinyl)sulfanilamide; 2-methyl-4-methoxy-6-sulfanilamidopyrimidine; 4-sulfanilamido-2-methyl-6-methoxypyrimidine; 2-methyl-4-methoxy-6-sulfanilamido-1,3-diazine; 4-(p-aminobenzenesulfonyl)amino-2-methyl-6-methoxypyrimidine; Duroprocin; Methofadin; Télémid. $C_{12}H_{14}N_4O_3S$; mol wt 294.33. C 48.97%, H 4.79%, N 19.04%, O 16.31%, S 10.89%. Prepn: Loop, Lührs, Ann. **580**, 225 (1953); Loop, **DE 926131** (1955 to Nordmark).

Crystals, mp 146°. Also obtained as the monohydrate.

THERAP CAT: Antibacterial.

8918.   **Sulfamethoxazole.** [723-46-6] 4-Amino-N-(5-methyl-3-isoxazolyl)benzenesulfonamide; N^1-(5-methyl-3-isoxazolyl)sulfanilamide; 5-methyl-3-sulfanilamidoisoxazole; 3-sulfanilamido-5-methylisoxazole; 3-(p-aminophenylsulfonamido)-5-methylisoxazole; sulfisomezole; sulfamethylisoxazole; sulfamethoxizole; Gantanol; Sinomin. $C_{10}H_{11}N_3O_3S$; mol wt 253.28. C 47.42%, H 4.38%, N 16.59%, O 18.95%, S 12.66%. Prepn starting with ethyl 5-methylisoxazole-3-carbamate: Kano et al., **US 2888455** (1959 to Shionogi); Annu. Rep. Shionogi Res. Lab. **7,** 1 (1957), C.A. **51,** 17889 (1957). Toxicity data: Yamamoto et al., Chemotherapy (Tokyo) **21,** 187 (1973), C.A. **79,** 73738n (1973). Clinical trial of mixture with trimethoprim in Pneumocystis carinii pneumonia: J. M. Wharton et al., Ann. Intern. Med. **105,** 37 (1986). Comprehensive description: B. C. Rudy, B. Z. Senkowski, Anal. Profiles Drug Subs. **2,** 467-486 (1973). Review of antibacterial activity and clinical efficacy of mixture with trimethoprim: G. P. Wormser et al., Drugs **24,** 459-518 (1982). Symposium on clinical intravenous therapy: Rev. Infect. Dis. **9,** Suppl. 2, S152-S229 (1987).

Bitter crystals from dil ethanol, mp 167°. LD_{50} orally in mice: 3662 mg/kg (Yamamoto).

Mixture with trimethoprim. [8064-90-2] Co-trimoxazole; Abacin; Apo-Sulfatrim; Bactramin; Bactrim; Baktar; Chemotrim; Drylin; Eusaprim; Fectrim; Gantaprim; Gantrim; Imexim; Kepinol; Laratrim; Linaris; Microtrim; Nopil; Oraprim; Septra; Septrin; Sigaprim; Sulfotrim; Sulprim; Sumetrolim; Supracombin; Suprim; Teleprim; Thiocuran; Trigonyl; Trimesulf; Uroplus. LD_{50} orally in mice: 5513 mg/kg (Yamamoto).

N^4-**Acetylsulfamethoxazole.** [21312-10-7] Crystals from alcohol, mp 209-210°.

THERAP CAT: Antibacterial; antipneumocystic.

THERAP CAT (VET): Antibacterial.

8919.   **Sulfamethoxypyridazine.** [80-35-3] 4-Amino-N-(6-methoxy-3-pyridazinyl)benzenesulfonamide; N^1-(6-methoxy-3-pyridazinyl)sulfanilamide; 6-methoxy-3-sulfanilamidopyridazine; 3-(p-aminobenzenesulfamido)-6-methoxypyridazine; CL-13494; RP-7522; Lederkyn; Midicel; Midikel. $C_{11}H_{12}N_4O_3S$; mol wt 280.30. C 47.13%, H 4.32%, N 19.99%, O 17.12%, S 11.44%. Prepn: Clark, **US 2712012** (1955 to Am. Cyanamid). Toxicity: Seki et al., Arzneim.-Forsch. **15,** 1441 (1965). Toxicological, chemotherapeutic and pharmacokinetic studies: Böhni et al., Chemotherapy **14,** 195-226 (1969).

Bitter crystals from water, mp 182-183°. pKa 6.7. Soly in water at 37° (mg/100 ml): 110 at pH 5; 120 at pH 6; 147 at pH 6.5. Slightly sol in methanol, ethanol (about 1:200); more sol in acetone (1:50), in dimethylformamide (1 g/ml). Freely sol in aq solns of alkali hydroxides. LD_{50} orally in mice: 1750 mg/kg, (Seki).

Sodium salt. [2577-32-4] Davosin; Sulfoxine LA. $C_{11}H_{11}N_4$-NaO_3S; mol wt 302.28.

THERAP CAT: Antibacterial.

THERAP CAT (VET): Antibacterial.

8920.   **Sulfametrole.** [32909-92-5] 4-Amino-N-(4-methoxy-1,2,5-thiadiazol-3-yl)benzenesulfonamide; N^1-(4-methoxy-1,2,5-thiadiazol-3-yl)sulfanilamide; 3-methoxy-4-(4'-aminobenzenesulfonamido)-1,2,5-thiadiazole. $C_9H_{10}N_4O_3S_2$; mol wt 286.33. C 37.75%, H 3.52%, N 19.57%, O 16.76%, S 22.40%. Anti-infective sulfanilamide, related structurally to sulfadiazine, q.v. Prepn: **BE**

629551 corresp to K. Menzl, **US 3247193** (1963, 1966 both to OSSW). Improved prepn: idem, **US 4151164** (1979 to Chemie Linz). Bacteriological study (of mixture with trimethoprim): G. Nabert-Bock, H. Grims, Arzneim.-Forsch. **27,** 1109 (1977). Tolerance, therapeutic effect, pharmacokinetics: S. Breyer et al., Wien. Med. Wochenschr. **130,** 448 (1980). Renal excretion mechanism, pharmacokinetics: T. B. Vree et al., Eur. J. Clin. Pharmacol. **20,** 283 (1981). Pharmacokinetics of sulfametrole and its metabolite in man: Y. A. Hester et al., J. Antimicrob. Chemother. **8,** 133 (1981). Crystal and molecular structures: C. H. Koo et al., Bull. Korean Chem. Soc. **3,** 9 (1982), C.A. **96,** 208771 (1982). Single-dose therapy of chancroid with trimethoprim-sulfametrole: F. A. Plummer et al., N. Engl. J. Med. **309,** 67 (1983).

Cryst from dilute acetic acid, mp 149-150°.

Mixture with trimethoprim. [63749-94-0] Lidaprim; Maderan.

THERAP CAT: Antibacterial.

8921.   **Sulfamic Acid.** [5329-14-6] Amidosulfonic acid. H_3NO_3S; mol wt 97.09. H 3.11%, N 14.43%, O 49.44%, S 33.03%. H_2NSO_3H. Obtained from chlorosulfonic acid and ammonia, or by heating urea with H_2SO_4. Purification: Sisler et al., Inorg. Synth. **2,** 178 (1946). Toxicity data: Ambrose, J. Ind. Hyg. Toxicol. **25,** 26 (1943). Reviews: Audrieth et al., Chem. Rev. **26,** 49 (1940); Burton, Nickless, "Amido- and Imido-Sulfonic Acids" in Inorganic Sulphur Chemistry, G. Nickless, Ed. (Elsevier, New York, 1968) pp 607-627, 661-667; E. B. Bell in Kirk-Othmer Encyclopedia of Chemical Technology **vol. 21** (Wiley-Interscience, New York, 3rd ed., 1983) pp 949-960. Brief review of synthetic applications: B. Wang, Synlett **2005,** 1342-1343.

Orthorhombic crystals. d 2.15. mp ~205° (dec). Stable when dry but in soln slowly hydrolyzes forming ammonium bisulfate. Sol in 6.5 parts water at 0°, in about 2 parts water at 80°. Sulfuric acid decreases soly in water. Sparingly sol in alcohol, methanol; slightly sol in acetone. Insol in ether. Freely sol in nitrogenous bases, e.g., liq ammonia, also in nitrogen contg organic solvents, e.g., pyridine, formamide, dimethylformamide. Immiscible with toluene, THF. A strong acid; pH of a 1% soln at 25° 1.18. Can be titrated with bases by means of indicators showing color change between pH 4.5 to 9. MLD orally in rats: 1.6 g/kg (Ambrose).

Caution: Moderately irritating to skin, mucous membranes.

USE: As standard in alkalimetry; in acid cleaning; in nitrite removal; in chlorine stabilization for use in swimming pools, cooling towers, paper mills. Solid-acid catalyst in organic synthesis. The acid or its ammonium salt has been recommended for flameproofing fabrics and wood. Metal salts are used in electroplating. Ammonium sulfamate, q.v., is also widely used as a weed killer.

8922.   **Sulfamide.** [7803-58-9] Sulfuryl amide. $H_4N_2O_2S$; mol wt 96.11. H 4.19%, N 29.15%, O 33.29%, S 33.36%. H_2-NSO_2NH_2. Prepd from sulfuryl chloride and gaseous ammonia: Traube, Ber. **25,** 2427 (1892); **26,** 610 (1893); Hantzsch, Holl, Ber. **34,** 3430 (1902); Schenk in Handbook of Preparative Inorganic Chemistry **vol. 1,** G. Brauer, Ed. (Academic Press, New York, 2nd ed., 1963) pp 482-483.

Orthorhombic, tasteless plates from abs alcohol, mp 93°; dec 250°. Dipole moment: 3.9. Freely sol in water, hot alcohol, acetone. Sparingly sol in cold alc. Solid and solns are stable.

Note: Not to be confused with ammonium sulfamate or with sulfanilamide.

USE: Similar to urea in many of its reactions, but is more acidic, and can act as a dibasic acid.

8923.   **Sulfamidochrysoidine.** [103-12-8] 4-[(2,4-Diaminophenyl)azo]benzenesulfonamide; 2,4-diaminoazobenzene-4'-sulfonamide; 4'-sulfamyl-2,4-diaminoazobenzene. $C_{12}H_{13}N_5O_2S$; mol wt 291.33. C 49.47%, H 4.50%, N 24.04%, O 10.98%, S 11.01%. Prototype compd leading to the development of sulfonamide antibacterials. Prepn: F. Mietzsch, J. Klarer, **DE 607537**

(1935 to I. G. Farbenind.); *eidem,* **US 2085037** (1937 to Winthrop). Antibacterial activity *in vivo:* G. Domagk, *Dtsch. Med. Wochenschr.* **61,** 573 (1935); (for English translation *see Rev. Infect. Dis.* **8,** 163 (1986)). Identification of sulfanilamide as active metabolite: J. Tréfouel *et al., C.R. Seances Soc. Biol. Ses Fil.* **120,** 756 (1935); L. Colebrook *et al., Lancet* **2,** 1323 (1936). Polymorphic forms in commercial prepns: L. Kofler, A. Kofler, *Monatsh. Chem.* **81,** 321 (1950). Use to visualize carbonic anhydrase during isoelectric focusing in polyacrylamide gels: W. Siffert *et al., J. Biochem. Biophys. Methods* 8, 331 (1983). Historical review: M. H. Bickel, *Gesnerus* **45,** 67-86 (1988).

Hydrochloride. [33445-35-1] Prontosil; Prontosil flavum; Prontosil rubrum; Rubiazol I; Septosan; Streptozon. $C_{12}H_{13}N_5O_2 \cdot$ S.HCl; mol wt 327.79. Orange-red crystals, mp 248-250°. One gram dissolves in 400 ml water; much more sol in hot water. Sol in alcohol, acetone, fats, oils.

USE: Specific stain for carbonic anhydrase in polyacrylamide gels.

THERAP CAT: Antibacterial.

8924. Sulfamoxole. [729-99-7] 4-Amino-*N*-(4,5-dimethyl-2-oxazolyl)benzenesulfonamide; N^1-(4,5-dimethyl-2-oxazolyl)-sulfanilamide; 2-(*p*-aminobenzenesulfonamido)-4,5-dimethyl-oxazole; 4,5-dimethyl-2-sulfanilamidooxazole; *p*-aminobenzene-sulfonyl-2-amino-4,5-dimethyloxazole; sulfadimethyloxazole; Justamil; Sulfmidil; Sulfuno; Tardamide. $C_{11}H_{13}N_3O_3S$; mol wt 267.30. C 49.43%, H 4.90%, N 15.72%, O 17.96%, S 12.00%. Prepn: Loop *et al., US 2809966* (1957 to Nordmark-Werke). Series of articles on antimicrobial activity, pharmacology and clinical efficacy of mixture with trimethoprim: *Arzneim.-Forsch.* **26,** 595-684 (1976). Toxicity data: F. Lagler *et al., ibid.* 634.

Crystals, mp 193-194°. Soly in mg/100 ml at 20°: water 85; 0.01*N* HCl 163; 0.01*N* NaOH 196; methanol 2315; chloroform 240. uv max (4.91 µg/ml methanol): 210, 250, 270 nm (ε 740, 546, 857). LD$_{50}$ in mice, rats (g/kg): >10.0, >12.5 orally; 1.80, ~2.50 i.p. (Lagler).

Mixture with trimethoprim. [57197-43-0] Co-trifamole; CN-3123; Co-Fram; Dibactil; Nevin; Supristol. LD$_{50}$ in mice, rats (g/kg): >12.0, 14.0 orally; 1.87, 2.00 i.p. (Lagler).

THERAP CAT: Antibacterial.

8925. Sulfanilamide. [63-74-1] 4-Aminobenzenesulfonamide; *p*-anilinesulfonamide; *p*-sulfamidoaniline; 1162-F; Prontosil album; Prontylin; Streptocide. $C_6H_8N_2O_2S$; mol wt 172.20. C 41.85%, H 4.68%, N 16.27%, O 18.58%, S 18.62%. Active metabolite of the antibacterial dye, sulfamidochrysoidine, *q.v.* Prepn: P. Gelmo, *J. Prakt. Chem.* **77,** 369 (1908); A. Galat, *Ind. Eng. Chem.* **36,** 192 (1944); Hurdis, Yang, *J. Chem. Educ.* **46,** 697 (1969). Large-scale process: F. Mietzsch, J. Klarer, **US 2132178;** *eidem et al., US 2276664* (1938, 1942 both to Winthrop). Antibacterial activity: J. Tréfouel *et al., C.R. Seances Soc. Biol. Ses Fil.* **120,** 756 (1935); and clinical efficacy: L. Colebrook, A. W. Purdie, *Lancet* **233,** 1291 (1937). Toxicity study: E. K. Marshall, Jr. *et al., J. Am. Med. Assoc.* **110,** 252 (1938). Historical review: M. H. Bickel, *Gesnerus* **45,** 67-86 (1988).

Crystals from boiling water, mp 164.5-166.5°. Neutral to litmus. pH (0.5% aq soln): 5.8-6.1. uv max: 255, 312 nm. One gram dissolves in about 37 ml alcohol; in about 5 ml acetone; in about 2 ml boiling water. Sol in glycerol, HCl, solns of K and Na hydroxides. Practically insol in chloroform, ether, benzene. LD$_{50}$ orally in mice: 3.8 g/kg (Marshall).

N^4-**Acetylsulfanilamide.** [121-61-9] *N*-[4-(Aminosulfonyl)-phenyl]acetamide. $C_8H_{10}N_2O_3S$; mol wt 214.24. Major metabolite of sulfanilamide: E. K. Marshall, Jr. *et al., Science* **85,** 202 (1937). Needles from water, mp 219°.

THERAP CAT: Antibacterial.

THERAP CAT (VET): Antibacterial.

8926. Sulfanilic Acid. [121-57-3] 4-Aminobenzenesulfonic acid; *p*-anilinesulfonic acid. $C_6H_7NO_3S$; mol wt 173.19. C 41.61%, H 4.07%, N 8.09%, O 27.71%, S 18.51%. Readily prepd from aniline and sulfuric acid: I. G. Farben, *FIAT* Final Rept. **1313** (I), 255 (1948); Fierz-David, Blangey, *Fundamental Processes of Dye Chemistry* (Interscience, New York, 1949) pp 126-128; A. I. Vogel, *Practical Organic Chemistry* (Longmans, London, 3rd ed., 1959) p 586; R. Q. Brewster *et al., Unitized Experiments in Organic Chemistry* (Van Nostrand, Princeton, 2nd ed., 1964) pp 162-163. Improved procedure: Jacobs *et al., Ind. Eng. Chem.* **35,** 321-323 (1943).

Monohydrate. [6101-32-2] Orthorhombic plates from water (very slow crystn can yield the dihydrate), becomes anhydr at around 100°. Dec without melting at ~288° (also reported as >360°). pK$_2$ (25°): 3.23. Slowly sol in water: ~1% at 20°, 1.45% at 30°, 1.94% at 40° (w/w anhydr). Almost insol in ethanol, benzene, ether. Slightly sol in hot methanol.

Sodium salt dihydrate. [6106-22-5] $C_6H_6NNaO_3S.2H_2O$. Orthorhombic bipyramidal plates. Freely sol in water, sol in hot methanol.

Zinc salt tetrahydrate. [31884-76-1] Zinc sulfanilate tetrahydrate; Nizin. $C_{12}H_{12}N_2O_6S_2Zn.4H_2O$; mol wt 481.83.

Amide *see* Sulfanilamide.

USE: Manuf various dyes and organic chemicals; as reagent in anal. chemistry (Ehrlich's reagent, detn of nitrites).

THERAP CAT: Antibacterial.

8927. 2-*p*-Sulfanilylanilinoethanol. [80-02-4] 2-[[4-[(4-Aminophenyl)sulfonyl]phenyl]amino]ethanol; 4-amino-4'-(β-hydroxyethylamino)diphenyl sulfone; *p*-aminophenyl *p*-(2-hydroxy-ethylamino)phenyl sulfone; Smith's sulfone. $C_{14}H_{16}N_2O_3S$; mol wt 292.35. C 57.52%, H 5.52%, N 9.58%, O 16.42%, S 10.97%. Preparation: Jackson, *J. Am. Chem. Soc.* **70,** 680 (1948); Weijlard, Swanezy, *ibid.* **71,** 4134 (1949); Jackson, *ibid.* **72,** 395 (1950); Anand *et al., J. Sci. Ind. Res.* **13B,** 260 (1954); Onishi, Fukagawa, **JP 56 2975** (1956 to Yoshitomi Drug).

Exists in diamorphic forms, crystals, mp 130.5-131.5° and crystals, mp 144°. The lower melting crystals' soly in water: 74 mg/100 ml at 37°. The higher melting form is readily sol in acetone; sol in ethanol, dioxane, cold 1% HCl; fairly sol in hot water; slightly sol in cold water.

THERAP CAT: Antibacterial (Mycobacterium).

8928. *p*-Sulfanilylbenzylamine. [4393-19-5] 4-[(4-Aminophenyl)sulfonyl]benzenemethanamine; *p*-sulfanilidobenzylamine; 4-aminomethyl-4'-aminodiphenyl sulfone; *p*-aminophenyl-*p*-aminomethylphenyl sulfone; Alphamide. $C_{13}H_{14}N_2O_2S$; mol wt

262.33. C 59.52%, H 5.38%, N 10.68%, O 12.20%, S 12.22%. Prepn: Dewing, *J. Chem. Soc.* **1946**, 466; Wenner, *J. Org. Chem.* **22**, 1508 (1957).

Needles from water, mp 159°.
Monohydrochloride monohydrate. $C_{13}H_{14}N_2O_2S.HCl.H_2O$. Crystals, mp 195°. Very sol in water.
Dihydrochloride. $C_{13}H_{14}N_2O_2S.2HCl$. mp 285°.
THERAP CAT: Antibacterial.

8929. Sulfanilyl Fluoride. [98-62-4] *p*-Aminobenzenesulfonyl fluoride. $C_6H_6FNO_2S$; mol wt 175.18. C 41.14%, H 3.45%, F 10.85%, N 8.00%, O 18.27%, S 18.30%. Prepd by heating potassium fluoride with 4-acetamidobenzenesulfonyl chloride: Parker, Hofmann, **US 2576037** (1951 to Am. Cyanamid).

Crystals, mp 68-69°.
USE: In the prepn of dyes which pick up light readily.

8930. N^4-Sulfanilylsulfanilamide. [547-52-4] 4′-Sulfamoylsulfanilanilide; 4-aminobenzenesulfono-*p*-sulfamoylanilide; 4-(4′-aminobenzenesulfonamido)benzenesulfonamide; DB-32; Diseptal C; Uliron C; Disulon; Neosanamid II; Albasil C; Disulfan. $C_{12}H_{13}N_3O_4S_2$; mol wt 327.38. C 44.02%, H 4.00%, N 12.84%, O 19.55%, S 19.59%. Prepn: **FR 817034** (to I. G. Farben.), *C.A.* **32**, 1714i (1938); Sakai, Yamamoto, *J. Pharm. Soc. Jpn.* **58**, 683 (1938); Golovchinskaya, *J. Appl. Chem. USSR* **18**, 647 (1945); Sasa, *J. Soc. Org. Syn. Chem. Jpn.* **12**, 211 (1954), *C.A.* **51**, 2780h (1957); Grigorovskii, Dykhanov, *J. Appl. Chem. USSR* **30**, 1284 (1957).

Needles from water, mp 133-134°. Absorption max: Maschka *et al., Monatsh. Chem.* **84**, 1071 (1953). Slightly sol in cold water; considerably more sol in hot water. Sol in methanol, ethanol, ether, dil NH_3, dil HCl; practically insol in petr ether, chloroform.
Note: The name Disulon is also used for disulfanilamide, H_2-$NC_6H_4SO_2NHSO_2C_6H_4NH_2$, esp. in the French literature.
THERAP CAT: Antibacterial (topical).

8931. Sulfanilylurea. [547-44-4] 4-Amino-*N*-(aminocarbonyl)benzenesulfonamide; *N*-sulfanilylcarbamide; sulfacarbamide; sulfaurea; Euvernil; Uractyl; Uramid; Urenil; Urosulfan. C_7-$H_9N_3O_3S$; mol wt 215.23. C 39.06%, H 4.21%, N 19.52%, O 22.30%, S 14.90%. Prepd by treating N^4-acetylsulfanilamide with potassium cyanate or with carbamyl chloride or with urea (or with nitrourea and sodium carbonate) in 80% alcohol. The *p*-AcNHC$_6$-$H_4SO_2NHCONH_2$ is saponified by slight warming with dil KOH and then acidified: Martin *et al.*, **US 2411661** (1946 to Geigy). By boiling sulfanilamide with urea and sodium carbonate in 75% alcohol: Haack, *Alien Prop. Custodian, Serial* **369**, 118 (1943). By warming calcium acetylsulfanilylcyanamide with dil HCl: Winnek *et al., J. Am. Chem. Soc.* **64**, 1684 (1942); improved procedure: Leitch *et al., Can. J. Res.* **23B**, 139 (1945).

Crystals from water. mp 146-148° (slight dec). Solubility in water at 37°: 811 mg/100 ml. Soluble in alkalies. Forms a very soluble sodium salt.
Monohydrate. mp 125-127°.
THERAP CAT: Antibacterial.

8932. *N*-Sulfanilyl-3,4-xylamide. [120-34-3] *N*-[(-4-Aminophenyl)sulfonyl]-3,4-dimethylbenzamide; N^1-(3,4-dimethylbenzoyl)sulfanilamide; Geigy 867; Irgafen. $C_{15}H_{16}N_2O_3S$; mol wt 304.36. C 59.19%, H 5.30%, N 9.20%, O 15.77%, S 10.54%. Prepd from *p*-nitrobenzenesulfonamide and 3,4-dimethylbenzoyl chloride; the resulting *p*-nitro-*N*-(3,4-dimethylbenzoyl)benzenesulfonamide is reduced with Fe and dil AcOH: Martin *et al.*, **US 2383874** (1945).

Needles from alcohol, mp 222-223°. Sparingly sol in water. Marketed as the water-soluble sodium salt for making solns; a 5% aq soln having a pH of 8.2.
THERAP CAT: Antibacterial.

8933. Sulfanitran. [122-16-7] *N*-[4-[[(4-Nitrophenyl)amino]sulfonyl]phenyl]acetamide; 4′-[(*p*-nitrophenyl)sulfamoyl]acetanilide; N^4-acetyl-N^1-(*p*-nitrophenyl)sulfanilamide; 4-acetaminobenzenesulfon-4′-nitroanilide; *N*-(*p*-acetylaminobenzene sulfonyl)-*p*-nitroaniline; APNPS. $C_{14}H_{13}N_3O_5S$; mol wt 335.34. C 50.14%, H 3.91%, N 12.53%, O 23.86%, S 9.56%. Prepn: Webster, Powers, *J. Am. Chem. Soc.* **60**, 1553 (1938); Kaufmann, Bückmann, *Arch. Pharm.* **279**, 194 (1941); Shepherd, *J. Org. Chem.* **12**, 275 (1947).

Crystals from dil alcohol, mp 239-240° (Kaufmann); mp 264° (Shepherd). Freely sol in acetone; sol in hot ethanol, methanol; sparingly sol in water, ether.
Note: Ingredient of **Unistat**, **Novastat W**.
THERAP CAT (VET): Antibacterial; coccidiostat (poultry).

8934. Sulfaperine. [599-88-2] 4-Amino-*N*-(5-methyl-2-pyrimidinyl)benzenesulfonamide; N^1-(5-methyl-2-pyrimidinyl)-sulfanilamide; 5-methyl-2-sulfanilamidopyrimidine; 2-sulfanilamido-5-methylpyrimidine; isosulfamerazine; 5-methylsulfadiazine; Pallidin; Retardon; Rexulfa; Sintosulfa; Sulfatreis. $C_{11}H_{12}N_4O_2$-S; mol wt 264.30. C 49.99%, H 4.58%, N 21.20%, O 12.11%, S 12.13%. Prepd by condensing 2-amino-5-methylpyrimidine with acetylsulfanilyl chloride followed by hydrolysis of the acetyl group with NaOH: Sprague, **US 2407966** (1946 to Sharp & Dohme).

Minute, cream-colored crystals, mp 262-263°. Very sparingly sol in water, ethanol; ~40 mg/100 ml H_2O at pH 5.5. Sol in aq solns of acids and alkalies. Forms a water-sol sodium salt.

THERAP CAT: Antibacterial.

8935. Sulfaphenazole. [526-08-9] 4-Amino-*N*-(1-phenyl-1*H*-pyrazol-5-yl)benzenesulfonamide; *N'*-(1-phenylpyrazol-5-yl)-sulfanilamide; 1-phenyl-5-sulfanilamidopyrazole; 3-(*p*-aminobenzenesulfonamido)-2-phenylpyrazole. $C_{15}H_{14}N_4O_2S$; mol wt 314.36. C 57.31%, H 4.49%, N 17.82%, O 10.18%, S 10.20%. Synthesis: Schmidt, Druey, *Helv. Chim. Acta* **41**, 309 (1958); Druey, Schmidt, US 2858309 (1958 to Ciba). Toxicity study: Seki *et al., Arzneim.-Forsch.* **15**, 1441 (1965).

Crystals from alcohol, mp 179-183°. Very sparingly sol in water: 0.15 g/100 ml H_2O at pH 7.0 and 25°. More sol in methanol, ethanol, glacial acetic acid. LD_{50} orally in mice: 5800 mg/kg (Seki).

Sodium salt monohydrate. $C_{15}H_{13}N_4NaO_2S.H_2O$. White powder. Sol in water. A 10% soln (w/w) has a pH of ~9.

THERAP CAT: Antibacterial.

THERAP CAT (VET): Antibacterial.

8936. Sulfaproxyline. [116-42-7] *p*-Isopropoxy-*N*-sulfanil-ylbenzamide; *N*[1]-(*p*-isopropoxybenzoyl)sulfanilamide; *N*[1]-(4-iso-propoxybenzoyl)-*p*-aminobenzenesulfonamide; sulphaproxyline. $C_{16}H_{18}N_2O_4S$; mol wt 334.39. C 57.47%, H 5.43%, N 8.38%, O 19.14%, S 9.59%. Prepn: Gysin, US 2503820 (1950 to Geigy).

Crystals, mp 172-173°.

THERAP CAT: Antibacterial.

8937. Sulfapyrazine. [116-44-9] 4-Amino-*N*-(pyrazinyl)-benzenesulfonamide; *N*[1]-2-pyrazinylsulfanilamide; 2-sulfanilami-dopyrazine. $C_{10}H_{10}N_4O_2S$; mol wt 250.28. C 47.99%, H 4.03%, N 22.39%, O 12.79%, S 12.81%. Prepd by reacting acetyl-sulfanilyl chloride with 2-aminopyrazine in pyridine, followed by hydrolysis and neutralization: Ellingson, US 2420703 (1947). Biological properties: Ghione *et al., Chemotherapia* **6**, 344 (1962).

Crystals, dec 250-254°. Very slightly sol in alc; slightly sol in acetone. Sol in aq solns of sodium, potassium, and barium hydrox-ides, in ammonia water, and in dil and concd mineral acid solns. Practically insol in water (5 mg/100 ml at 25°, and 5.2 mg/100 ml at 37°).

Sodium salt monohydrate. $C_{10}H_9N_4NaO_2S.H_2O$. Bitter pow-der. Freely soluble in water (1 g/3.33 ml at 25°). Alkaline to litmus. pH of 10% aq soln 9.1. Very sol in acetone, slightly sol in alc. Insol in ether, chloroform. Aq solns of sulfapyrazine sodi-um may absorb carbon dioxide which causes precipitation of sulfa-pyrazine.

THERAP CAT: Antibacterial.

THERAP CAT (VET): Antibacterial.

8938. Sulfapyridine. [144-83-2] 4-Amino-*N*-2-pyridinyl-benzenesulfonamide; dagenan; *N*[1]-2-pyridylsulfanilamide; 2-sulfa-nilamidopyridine; 2-(*p*-aminobenzenesulfonamido)pyridine; M & B 693. $C_{11}H_{11}N_3O_2S$; mol wt 249.29. C 53.00%, H 4.45%, N 16.86%, O 12.84%, S 12.86%. Prepn: A. J. Ewins, M. A. Phillips, GB 512145 (1939); *eidem*, US 2275354 (1942); R. Winterbottom, *J. Am. Chem. Soc.* **62**, 160 (1940). Metabolism: R. Wien, J. Hamp-ton, *J. Pharmacol. Exp. Ther.* **84**, 211 (1945). Toxicology: R. Wien *et al., ibid.* 203. GC-MS determn in edible animal tissues: A. E. Mooser, H. Koch, *J. AOAC Int.* **76**, 976 (1993). Efficacy and proposed mechanism of action in dermatological disease: O. J. Stone, *Med. Hypotheses* **31**, 99 (1990). Clinical evaluation in oc-ular cicatricial pemphigoid: M. J. Elder *et al., Br. J. Ophthalmol.* **80**, 549 (1996).

Crystals from alc, mp 190-191°. One gram dissolves in ~3500 ml water, 440 ml alcohol, 65 ml acetone. Freely sol in dil mineral acids and in aq solns of KOH and NaOH. More sol in warm sugar solns than in water alone. The aq soln is neutral. LD_{50} orally in mice: 7.5 mg/g (Wien).

Sodium salt monohydrate. [127-57-1] Soluble sulfapyridine. $C_{11}H_{10}N_3NaO_2S.H_2O$; mol wt 289.29. On prolonged exposure to humid air it absorbs CO_2, liberates sulfapyridine, becomes incom-pletely sol in water. One gram dissolves in ~1.5 ml water, 10 ml alcohol. pH of 5% aq soln: 11.4. LD_{50} orally in mice: 2.7 mg/g (Wien).

THERAP CAT: In treatment of dermatitis herpetiformis; antibac-terial.

THERAP CAT (VET): Antibacterial.

8939. Sulfaquinoxaline. [59-40-5] 4-Amino-*N*-2-quinoxa-linylbenzenesulfonamide; *N*[1]-(2-quinoxalinyl)sulfanilamide; 2-sul-fanilamidoquinoxaline; *N*[1]-(2-quinoxalyl)sulfanilamide; sulfabenz-pyrazine; Compd 3-120; S.Q.; Sulquin. $C_{14}H_{12}N_4O_2S$; mol wt 300.34. C 55.99%, H 4.03%, N 18.65%, O 10.65%, S 10.68%. Prepd by treating 2-aminoquinoxaline with acetylsulfanilyl chloride in the presence of pyridine and hydrolyzing the resulting acetyl deriv: Weijlard *et al., J. Am. Chem. Soc.* **66**, 1957 (1944); Weijlard, Tishler, US 2404199 (1946 to Merck & Co.). Anticoccidial spec-trum: G. F. Mathis *et al., Poult. Sci.* **63**, 1149 (1984). Evaluation of antibacterial and anticoccidial efficacy of mixture with trimetho-prim: G. White, R. B. Williams, *Vet. Rec.* **113**, 608 (1983); D. W. T. Piercy *et al., ibid.* **114**, 60 (1984). Drug residue study in poultry muscle and liver: M. Patthy, *J. Chromatogr.* **275**, 115 (1983). HPLC determn in rabbit plasma and urine: J. G. Eppel, J. J. Thiessen, *J. Pharm. Sci.* **73**, 1635 (1984).

Minute crystals, mp 247-248°. uv max (pH 6.6 in H_2O): 252, 360 nm ($E_{1cm}^{1\%}$ 1110, 275). Solubility in water at pH 7: 0.75 mg/100 ml; in 95% alcohol: 73 mg/100 ml; in acetone: 430 mg/100 ml. Sol in aq Na_2CO_3 and NaOH solns.

Sodium salt. Aviochina. $C_{14}H_{11}N_4NaO_2S$; mol wt 322.32. Very sol in water; pH of 1% soln ~10. The amorphous salt is deliquescent and absorbs CO_2 which liberates the practically insol sulfaquinoxaline.

THERAP CAT (VET): Coccidiostat.

8940. Sulfarside. [1134-98-1] [2-Amino-4-(aminosulfo-nyl)phenyl]arsinous acid; 4-sulfamoyl-*o*-arsanilic acid; 2-amino-4-aminosulfonylphenylarsinic acid; RP-4482; Bemarside. C_6H_9-AsN_2O_5S; mol wt 296.13. C 24.34%, H 3.06%, As 25.30%, N 9.46%, O 27.01%, S 10.83%. Prepn: Trefouel, US 2616913 (1953 to Rhône-Poulenc).

THERAP CAT: Sodium salt as antiamebic.

8941. Sulfarsphenamine. [618-82-6] [1,2-Diarsenediyl-bis[(6-hydroxy-3,1-phenylene)imino]]bismethanesulfonic acid disodium salt; disodium 3,3′-diamino-4,4′-dihydroxyarsenobenzene N-dimethylenesulfonate; sulfarsenobenzene; Karsulphan; Myosalvarsan; Myarsenol; Metarsenobillon; Thiosarmine. $C_{14}H_{14}As_2N_2$-$Na_2O_8S_2$; mol wt 598.22. C 28.11%, H 2.36%, As 25.05%, N 4.68%, Na 7.69%, O 21.40%, S 10.72%. Prepn: C. Voegtlin, J. M. Johnson, *J. Am. Chem. Soc.* **44**, 2573 (1922); W. J. C. Dyke, H. King, *J. Chem. Soc.* **1935**, 1745.

Yellow, odorless, or almost odorless powder. Very sol in water, slightly in alcohol. The aq soln is usually slightly acid. *Keep in evacuated or in inert gas-filled ampuls.*

THERAP CAT: Formerly as antisyphilitic.

THERAP CAT (VET): Has been used as antibacterial.

8942. Sulfasalazine. [599-79-1] 2-Hydroxy-5-[[4-[(2-pyridinylamino)sulfonyl]phenyl]azo]benzoic acid; 5-[p-(2-pyridylsulfamoyl)phenylazo]salicylic acid; salazosulfapyridine; 5-[4-(2-pyridylsulfamoyl)phenylazo]-2-hydroxybenzoic acid; 4-(pyridyl-2-amidosulfonyl)-3′-carboxy-4′-hydroxyazobenzene; salicylazosulfapyridine; sulphasalazine; Azulfidine; Colo-Pleon; Salazopyrin. C_{18}-$H_{14}N_4O_5S$; mol wt 398.39. C 54.27%, H 3.54%, N 14.06%, O 20.08%, S 8.05%. Conjugate of 5-aminosalicylic acid and sulfapyridine, q.q.v. Prepn and bactericidal effect: E. E. A. Askelof *et al., US 2396145* (1946 to Pharmacia); Doraswamy, Guha, *J. Indian Chem. Soc.* **23**, 278 (1946). Physicochemical properties: B. Nygard *et al., Acta Pharm. Suec.* **3**, 313-342 (1966). Metabolism studies: H. Schroder, D. E. S. Campbell, *Clin. Pharmacol. Ther.* **13**, 539 (1972); M. A. Peppercorn, P. Goldman, *J. Pharmacol. Exp. Ther.* **181**, 555 (1972). HPLC determn in biological fluids: R. A. Hogezand *et al., J. Chromatogr.* **305**, 470 (1984). Clinical trial in rheumatoid arthritis: D. E. Bax, R. S. Amos, *Ann. Rheum. Dis.* **44**, 194 (1985). Review of clinical pharmacokinetics: U. Klotz, *Clin. Pharmacokinet.* **10**, 285-302 (1985); of pharmacology and clinical use in inflammatory bowel disease: M. A. Peppercorn, *Ann. Intern. Med.* **3**, 377 (1984); G. Watkinson, *Drugs* **32**, Suppl. 1, 1-11 (1986). Comprehensive description: J. P. McDonnell, *Anal. Profiles Drug Subs.* **5**, 515-532 (1976).

Minute, brownish-yellow crystals, dec 240-245°. uv max: 237 ($E_{1cm}^{1\%}$ ~658) and 359 nm. Slightly sol in alc. Practically insol in water, benzene, chloroform, ether.

THERAP CAT: Anti-inflammatory (gastrointestinal).

THERAP CAT (VET): Has been used in granulomatous colitis.

8943. Sulfathiazole. [72-14-0] 4-Amino-N-2-thiazolylbenzenesulfonamide; N^1-2-thiazolylsulfanilamide; 2-sulfanilamidothiazole; 2-(sulfanilylamino)thiazole; 2-(p-aminobenzenesulfonamido)thiazole; norsulfazole; RP-2090; M & B 760; Thiazamide; Cibazol; Enterobiocine; Duatok; Sulfamul; Sulfavitina; Sulzol. C_9-$H_9N_3O_2S_2$; mol wt 255.32. C 42.34%, H 3.55%, N 16.46%, O

12.53%, S 25.12%. Prepn: R. J. Fosbinder, L. A. Walter, *J. Am. Chem. Soc.* **61**, 2032 (1939); W. A. Lott, F. H. Bergeim, *ibid.* 3593; G. Newbery, P. Viaud, **GB 517272**; G. Newbery, **US 2362087** (1940, 1944 both to May & Baker). Antibacterial activity *in vivo*: O. W. Barlow, E. Homburger, *Proc. Soc. Exp. Biol. Med.* **42**, 792 (1939). Toxicology: H. B. van Dyke *et al., ibid.* 410; P. H. Long *et al., ibid.* **43**, 328 (1940). Review of early literature: *ACS Monograph Series* **no. 106,** entitled "Sulfonamides and Allied Compounds," E. H. Northey, Ed. (Reinhold, New York, 1948) 660 pp. HPLC determn in milk: V. K. Agarwal, *J. Liq. Chromatogr.* **16**, 3793 (1993). Oral bioavailability in ruminants: K. Weijkamp *et al., Vet. Q.* **16**, 33 (1994). Comprehensive description: V. K. Kapoor, *Anal. Profiles Drug Subs. Excip.* **22**, 389-430 (1993).

mp 202-202.5°. pKa 7.2. Soly at 26° (mg/100 ml): water 60 (pH 6.03); alcohol 525. Sol in acetone, dil mineral acids, KOH and NaOH solns, ammonia water. Very slightly sol in water; sparingly sol in ethanol. Practically insol in chloroform, ether.

Sodium salt sesquihydrate. Soluble sulfathiazole. $C_9H_8N_3$-$NaO_2S_2.1\frac{1}{2}H_2O$. Crystals or white powder or granules. Also occurs as the monohydrate and pentahydrate. One gram dissolves in ~2.5 ml water, in ~15 ml alc. pH of 1% aq soln 9.35; of 10% soln 10.2. LD_{50} s.c. in mice: 1.45 g/kg (van Dyke); also reported as 1.95 g/kg (Long).

Polymer with formaldehyde. [12041-72-4] Formosulfathiazole; formaldehyde-sulfathiazole; Forbina. $(C_9H_9N_3O_2S_2.CH_2$-$O)_x$. Contains ~11% formaldehyde. Prepn: J. Druey, A. Becker, *Helv. Chim. Acta* **31**, 2184 (1948). Intrauterine use in cows: D. P. Dobson, D. E. Noakes, *Vet. Rec.* **127**, 128 (1990). Amorphous powder. Practically insol in water.

THERAP CAT: Antibacterial.

THERAP CAT (VET): Antibacterial.

8944. Sulfathiourea. [515-49-1] 4-Amino-N-(aminothioxomethyl)benzenesulfonamide; 1-sulfanilyl-2-thiourea; sulfathiocarbamide; RP-2255; Badional; Fontamide. $C_7H_9N_3O_2S_2$; mol wt 231.30. C 36.35%, H 3.92%, N 18.17%, O 13.83%, S 27.73%. Prepd by reacting acetylsulfanilylcyanamide with hydrogen sulfide. Has also been prepd directly from sulfanilyl cyanamide and ammonium sulfide: Leitch *et al., Can. J. Res.* **23B**, 139 (1945); alternate method: Földi *et al., US 2332906* (1943).

Crystals, dec 171.5-172°. Soly in water at 37°: 1.1 g/100 ml.

Sodium salt. [6101-34-4] $C_7H_8N_3NaO_2S$. Dec 245-245.5°. Very sol in water. pH of 1% aq soln: 7.

Water sol form. Solufontamide. Marketed as a slightly viscous soln contg 33% of 1-sulfanilyl-2-thiourea. d_4^{15} 1.16. pH 6.8-7.2.

THERAP CAT: Antibacterial.

8945. Sulfazamet. [852-19-7] 4-Amino-N-(3-methyl-1-phenyl-1H-pyrazol-5-yl)benzenesulfonamide; N^1-(3-methyl-1-phenylpyrazol-5-yl)sulfanilamide; 5-(p-aminobenzenesulfonamido)-3-methyl-1-phenylpyrazole; 3-(p-aminobenzenesulfonamido)-2-phenyl-5-methylpyrazole; 3-methyl-1-phenyl-5-(sulfanilamido)pyrazole; sulfamethylphenazole; sulfapyrazole; Vesulong. $C_{16}H_{16}N_4O_2S$; mol wt 328.39. C 58.52%, H 4.91%, N 17.06%, O 9.74%, S 9.76%. Prepn: Crippa, Guarneri, *Gazz. Chim. Ital.* **85**, 199 (1955); **GB 848627** (1960 to Ciba); Seydel, Krueger-Theimer, *Arzneim.-Forsch.* **14**, 1294 (1964). Amino-imino tautomerism: *eidem, ibid.*

Consult the Name Index before using this section.

Crystals from alc, mp 195° (Seydel, Krueger-Theimer); mp 181-182° (**GB 848627**). pKa' 5.69.

THERAP CAT (VET): Antibacterial.

8946. Sulfazecin. [77912-79-9] D-γ-Glutamyl-*N*-[(3*R*)-3-methoxy-2-oxo-1-sulfo-3-azetidinyl]-D-alaninamide; 3-γ-D-glutamyl-D-alanylamino-3-methoxyazetidin-2-one-1-sulfonic acid; (3*R*)-3-(γ-D-glutamyl-D-alanylamino)-3-methoxy-2-oxoazetidine-1-sulfonic acid; antibiotic G-6302. $C_{12}H_{20}N_4O_9S$; mol wt 396.37. C 36.36%, H 5.09%, N 14.13%, O 36.33%, S 8.09%. Novel monocyclic β-lactam (monobactam) antibiotic, produced by *Pseudomonas acidophila* and *P. mesoacidophila*. Isoln, description of physico-chemical and bacteriostatic properties: A. Imada *et al.*, **DE 2855949** corresp to **US 4229436** (1979, 1980 both to Takeda); *eidem, Nature* **289**, 590 (1981); M. Asai *et al., J. Antibiot.* **34**, 621 (1981). X-ray crystallographic structure determn: K. Kamiya *et al., Acta Crystallogr.* **B37**, 1626 (1981). Prepn of fluorinated sulfazecin analogs: K.Yoshioka *et al., J. Org. Chem.* **49**, 1427 (1984); P. F. Bevilacqua *et al., ibid.* 1430.

Crystallizes from methanol/water as the alcoholate-hemihydrate; colorless needles, mp 168-170°. $[\alpha]_D^{25}$ +82° (c = 1.0 in water). pKa: 3.4 (COO^-); 9.2 (NH_3^+). Sol in water, DMF, DMSO. Slightly sol in methanol, THF. Practically insol in ethanol, acetone, ethyl acetate, chloroform and other organic solvents. Relatively stable in neutral and weakly acidic solns; unstable in alkaline and strongly acidic solns.

Sodium salt monohydrate. $C_{12}H_{19}N_4NaO_9S.H_2O$. Colorless powder, browns at 170°, no sharp mp. $[\alpha]_D^{20}$ +85° (c = 0.37 in water).

8947. Sulfentrazone. [122836-35-5] *N*-[2,4-Dichloro-5-[4-(difluoromethyl)-4,5-dihydro-3-methyl-5-oxo-1*H*-1,2,4-triazol-1-yl]phenyl]methanesulfonamide; 2′,4′-dichloro-5′-(4-difluoromethyl-4,5-dihydro-3-methyl-5-oxo-1*H*-1,2,4-triazol-1-yl)methanesulfonanilide; F-6285; FMC-97285; Authority. $C_{11}H_{10}Cl_2F_2N_4O_3S$; mol wt 387.19. C 34.12%, H 2.60%, Cl 18.31%, F 9.81%, N 14.47%, O 12.40%, S 8.28%. Aryltriazolinone herbicide; inhibits protoporphyrinogen oxidase in the chlorophyll biosynthetic pathway. Prepn: G. Theodoridis, **US 4818275** (1989 to FMC); and structure-activity study: *idem et al., ACS Symp. Ser.* **504**, 134 (1992). Metabolism and distribution in animals: L. Y. Leung *et al., J. Agric. Food Chem.* **39**, 1509 (1991). Properties and field trials in soybeans: W. A. Van Saun *et al., Brighton Crop Prot. Conf. -Weeds* 1991, 77. Field trial in peanuts: W. C. Johnson, III, B. G. Mullinix, Jr., *Peanut Sci.* **21**, 65 (1994).

Tan solid, mp 75-78°. pKa 6.56. vapor pressure (25°): 1 × 10^{-9} mm Hg. Soly in water at 25° (mg/g): 0.11 (pH 6.0); 0.78 (pH 7.0); 16 (pH 7.5). LD$_{50}$ orally in rats: 2855 mg/kg; dermally in

rabbits: >2000 mg/kg; LC$_{50}$ (96 hr) in bluegill sunfish, rainbow trout (ppm): 92.8, >130 (Van Saun).

USE: Herbicide.

8948. Sulfinalol. [66264-77-5] 4-Hydroxy-α-[[[3-(4-methoxyphenyl)-1-methylpropyl]amino]methyl]-3-(methylsulfinyl)-benzenemethanol; 4-hydroxy-α-[[[3-(*p*-methoxyphenyl)-1-methylpropyl]amino]methyl]-3-(methylsulfinyl)benzyl alcohol. $C_{20}H_{27}NO_4S$; mol wt 377.50. C 63.63%, H 7.21%, N 3.71%, O 16.95%, S 8.49%. β-Adrenergic blocker. Prepn: R. E. Philion, **DE 2728641** (1978 to Sterling), *C.A.* **90**, 137468 (1979). Pharmacological activity profile: P. H. Hernández *et al., Fed. Proc.* **38**, 738 (1979). Chromatographic determn in human plasma and urine: G. B. Park *et al., Anal. Chem.* **53**, 604 (1981). Metabolism, disposition in animals: D. P. Benziger *et al., Drug Metab. Dispos.* **9**, 493 (1981).

Hydrochloride. [63251-39-8] Win-40808-7; Perifadil. C_{20}-$H_{27}NO_4S.HCl$; mol wt 413.96. Crystals, mp 172-175°.

THERAP CAT: Antihypertensive.

8949. Sulfinpyrazone. [57-96-5] 1,2-Diphenyl-4-[2-(phenylsulfinyl)ethyl]-3,5-pyrazolidinedione; 1,2-diphenyl-3,5-dioxo-4-(2-phenylsulfinylethyl)pyrazolidine; 4-(phenylsulfoxyethyl)-1,2-diphenyl-3,5-pyrazolidinedione; 4-(2-benzenesulfinylethyl)-1,2-diphenylpyrazolidine-3,5-dione; sulfoxyphenylpyrazolidine; G-28315; Anturan; Anturane; Anturano; Enturen. $C_{23}H_{20}N_2O_3S$; mol wt 404.48. C 68.30%, H 4.98%, N 6.93%, O 11.87%, S 7.93%. Prepn: F. Häfliger, **US 2700671** (1955 to Geigy AG); R. Pfister, F. Häfliger, *Helv. Chim. Acta* **44**, 232 (1961). Uricosuric effect: J. J. Burns *et al., J. Pharmacol. Exp. Ther.* **119**, 418 (1957). Clinical trial in prevention of sudden cardiac death: Anturane Reinfarction Trial Research Group, *N. Engl. J. Med.* **298**, 289 (1978); **302**, 250 (1980); as antithrombotic: R. D. Sautter *et al., J. Am. Med. Assoc.* **250**, 2649 (1983); D. T. Domoto *et al., Thromb. Res.* **62**, 737 (1991). *Review:* E. H. Margulies, A. M. White, in *Pharmacological and Biochemical Properties of Drug Substances* vol. 2, M. E. Goldberg, Ed. (Am. Pharm. Assoc., Washington, DC, 1979) pp 255-278; E. H. Margulies *et al., Drugs* **20**, 179-197 (1980).

Crystals from chloroform + heptane, mp 136-137°. Stable to light and air. uv max (1.0*N* NaOH): 255 nm. Sol in ethyl acetate, chloroform. Slightly sol in water, alcohol, ether, mineral oils, fats.

d-Form. Crystals from ethanol, mp 130-133°. $[\alpha]_D^{22}$ +67.1° (c = 2.04 in ethanol); $[\alpha]_D$ +109.3° (c = 0.5 in CHCl$_3$).

l-Form. Crystals, mp 130-133°. $[\alpha]_D^{23}$ −64.2° (c = 2.14 in ethanol); $[\alpha]_D^{26}$ −104.5° (c = 0.5 in CHCl$_3$).

THERAP CAT: Uricosuric; antithrombotic.

8950. Sulfiram. [95-05-6] Tetraethylthiodicarbonic diamide; bis(diethylthiocarbamoyl)sulfide; tetraethylthiuram monosulfide; monosulfiram; TTMS; Kutkasin; Tetmosol. $C_{10}H_{20}N_2S_3$; mol wt 264.47. C 45.41%, H 7.62%, N 10.59%, S 36.37%. Prepn: Davies, Sexton, *Biochem. J.* **40**, 331 (1946); Ritter, **US 2524081** (1950 to Sharples Chem.); Sahasrabudhey, Radhakrishnan, *J. Indian Chem. Soc.* **31**, 853 (1954); Zbirovsky, Ettel, *Chem. Listy* **51**, 2094 (1957); **52**, 95 (1958).

Crystals from benzene + petr ether, mp 30-32°.
USE: As vulcanization agent.
THERAP CAT: Ectoparasiticide.
THERAP CAT (VET): Ectoparasiticide.

8951. Sulfisomidine. [515-64-0] 4-Amino-N-(2,6-dimethyl-4-pyrimidinyl)benzenesulfonamide; N^1-(2,6-dimethyl-4-pyrimidinyl)sulfanilamide; 2,6-dimethyl-4-sulfanilamidopyrimidine; 6-sulfanilamido-2,4-dimethylpyrimidine; 6-(sulfanilamido)-2,4-dimethyl-1,3-diazine; 6-(p-aminophenylsulfonamido)-2,4-dimethylpyrimidine; 6-(p-aminobenzenesulfonyl)amino-2,4-dimethylpyrimidine; sulfadimetine; sulfaisodimidine; sulphasomidine; Elkosin; Elcosine; Elkosil; Domian; Aristamid. $C_{12}H_{14}N_4O_2S$; mol wt 278.33. C 51.78%, H 5.07%, N 20.13%, O 11.50%, S 11.52%. Prepn: **FR 886009** (1943 to Nordmark); Gysin, **US 2351333** (1944 to Geigy); Hartmann et al., **US 2386852**; **US 2429184** (1945, 1947, both to Ciba); Matsukawa et al., J. Pharm. Soc. Jpn. **70**, 283 (1950); Loop, Lührs, Ann. **580**, 225 (1953).

Needles from ethanol, mp 243°. Soly in water at 15°: 0.12 g/100 ml, at 30°: 0.30 g/100 ml. More sol in hot water (about 1:60). Aq solns are neutral to litmus. Soly in urine at 37°: 360 mg/100 ml at pH 5.5 to 1100 mg/100 ml at pH 7.5. Slightly sol in alcohol, acetone. Practically insol in benzene, ether, chloroform. Freely sol in dil HCl and NaOH. Compared with sulfanilamide it is but slightly acetylated in the body. *Do not confuse with sulfamethazine.*
THERAP CAT: Antibacterial.
THERAP CAT (VET): Antimicrobial.

8952. Sulfisoxazole. [127-69-5] 4-Amino-N-(3,4-dimethyl-5-isoxazolyl)benzenesulfonamide; N^1-(3,4-dimethyl-5-isoxazolyl)sulfanilamide; 3,4-dimethyl-5-sulfanilamidoisoxazole; 5-(4-aminophenylsulfonamido)-3,4-dimethylisoxazole; 5-(4-aminobenzenesulfonamido)-3,4-dimethylisooxazole; sulfafurazole; sulphafurazole. $C_{11}H_{13}N_3O_3S$; mol wt 267.30. C 49.43%, H 4.90%, N 15.72%, O 17.96%, S 12.00%. Prepn: H. M. Wuest, M. Hoffer, **US 2430094** (1947 to Hoffmann-La Roche). Toxicity study: Seki et al., Arzneim.-Forsch. **15**, 1441 (1965). Comprehensive description: B. C. Rudy, B. Z. Senkowski, Anal. Profiles Drug Subs. **2**, 487-506 (1973). HPLC determn in biological fluids: D. Jung, S. Oie, Clin. Chem. **26**, 51 (1980). Clinical trial in otitis media: P. A. M. Bernard et al., Pediatrics **88**, 215 (1991).

White to slightly yellowish crystalline powder. Bitter taste. mp 194°. pKa 5. Soly in water (25°): 0.13 mg/ml. Sol in alcohol. LD_{50} orally in mice: 6800 mg/kg (Seki).
Diethanolamine salt. [4299-60-9] Sulfisoxazole diolamine. $C_{11}H_{13}N_3O_3S.C_4H_{11}NO_2$; mol wt 372.44. White to off-white, odorless, crystalline powder. Sol in alcohol; freely sol in water. A 4% soln is about isotonic with tears.
Acetyl sulfisoxazole. [80-74-0] N-[(4-Aminophenyl)sulfonyl]-N-(3,4-dimethyl-5-isoxazolyl)acetamide; N^1-monoacetyl sulfisoxazole; Gantrisin. $C_{13}H_{15}N_3O_4S$; mol wt 309.34. Prepn: M. Hoffer, **US 2721200** (1955 to Hoffmann-La Roche). Should not be confused with N^4-acetyl sulfisoxazole which is a metabolite.

Tasteless crystals, mp 193-194°. Soly (mg/ml): 0.07 in water; 4.93 in methanol; 5.7 in 95% ethanol; 0.94 in ether; 29.0 in chloroform.
THERAP CAT: Antibacterial.
THERAP CAT (VET): Antibacterial.

8953. Sulfoacetic Acid. [123-43-3] Sulfoethanoic acid. $C_2H_4O_5S$; mol wt 140.12. C 17.14%, H 2.88%, O 57.09%, S 22.88%. HO_3SCH_2COOH.
Monohydrate. Hygroscopic crystals. mp 84-86° when anhydr. bp 245° with decompn. Sol in water, alcohol; insol in ether, chloroform. *Keep well closed.* LD_{50} orally in rats: 3.16 g/kg, Smyth et al., J. Ind. Hyg. Toxicol. **31**, 60 (1949).

8954. Sulfobromophthalein Sodium. [71-67-0] 3,3'-(4,5,6,7-Tetrabromo-3-oxo-1(3H)-isobenzofuranylidene)bis[6-hydroxybenzenesulfonic acid] disodium salt; disodium phenoltetrabromophthalein sulfonate; bromosulfophthalein; BSP; Bromsulphalein; Bromthalein. $C_{20}H_8Br_4Na_2O_{10}S_2$; mol wt 838.00. C 28.67%, H 0.96%, Br 38.14%, Na 5.49%, O 19.09%, S 7.65%. Prepd by the condensation of phenol and tetrabromophthalic acid or its anhydride, followed by sulfonation and conversion to the disodium salt. Pharmacology and use as liver function test: S. M. Rosenthal, E. C. White, J. Pharmacol. **24**, 265 (1924); W. Häcki et al., J. Lab. Clin. Med. **88**, 1019 (1976).

Hygroscopic crystals. Bitter taste. Sol in water. Insol in alcohol, acetone. Alkaline solns have an intense bluish-purple color.
THERAP CAT: Diagnostic aid (hepatic function).
THERAP CAT (VET): Diagnostic aid (hepatic function).

8955. Sulfolane. [126-33-0] Tetrahydrothiophene 1,1-dioxide; tetrahydrothiophene 1-dioxide; thiophan sulfone. $C_4H_8O_2S$; mol wt 120.17. C 39.98%, H 6.71%, O 26.63%, S 26.68%. Prepn by catalytic hydrogenation of sulfolene oxides: Mahan, Fauske, **US 2578565** (1951 to Phillips Petroleum); from butadiene and sulfur dioxide: Staaterman et al., Chem. Eng. Prog. **43**, 148 (1947); Evans, Morris, **US 2360859** (1944 to Shell). Toxicity study: H. F. Smyth et al., Am. Ind. Hyg. Assoc. J. **30**, 470 (1962).

Liquid, d_4^{30} 1.2606. mp 27.4-27.8°. bp_{760} 285°. n_D^{30} 1.481. Viscosity at 30° = 10.34 cP. Flash pt, open cup: 350°F (176°C). At 30°, miscible with water, acetone, toluene; partially misc with octanes, olefins and naphthenes. LD_{50} orally in rats: 1.54 ml/kg (Smyth).
USE: Selective solvent for liquid-vapor extractions.

8956. 3-Sulfolene. [77-79-2] 2,5-Dihydrothiophene 1,1-dioxide; 1-thia-3-cyclopentene 1,1-dioxide; butadiene sulfone. $C_4H_6O_2S$; mol wt 118.15. C 40.66%, H 5.12%, O 27.08%, S 27.14%. Preparation: Staudinger, Rizenthaler, Ber. **68**, 455 (1935); de Roy van Zuydewijn, Rec. Trav. Chim. **56**, 1047 (1937); Hooker et al., **US 2395050** (1946 to Dow); Morris, Finch, **US 2420834** (1947 to Shell).

Crystals, mp 64-65.5°. Sol in water, organic solvents.

8957. Sulfometuron-methyl. [74222-97-2] 2-[[[[(4,6-Dimethyl-2-pyrimidinyl)amino]carbonyl]amino]sulfonyl]benzoic acid methyl ester; N-[(4,6-dimethylpyrimidin-2-yl)aminocarbonyl]-2-methoxycarbonylbenzenesulfonamide; 2-[3-(4,6-dimethylpyrimidin-2-yl)ureidosulfonyl]benzoic acid methyl ester; Aa-5648; DPX-5648; Oust. $C_{15}H_{16}N_4O_5S$; mol wt 364.38. C 49.44%, H 4.43%, N 15.38%, O 21.95%, S 8.80%. Nonselective pre- and post-emergence sulfonylurea herbicide for noncropland use; inhibits branched chain amino acid biosynthesis. Prepn: G. Levitt, **EP 7687**; idem, **US 4394506** (1980, 1983 both to Du Pont); idem, Pestic. Chem.: Hum. Welfare Environ., Proc. 5th Int. Congr. Pestic. **1**, 243 (1983). Herbicidal activity and toxicity: R. H. Harding et al., Proc. West. Soc. Weed Sci. **34**, 120 (1981). Mechanism of action: T. B. Ray, Proc. Br. Crop Prot. Conf. - Weeds 1985, 131. HPLC determn in soil and water: E. W. Zahnow, J. Agric. Food Chem. **33**, 479 (1985). Degradation and bioaccumulation studies: J. Harvey et al., ibid. 590; J. J. Anderson, J. J. Dulka, ibid. 596. Field trials: R. L. Atkins et al., Proc. South. Weed Sci. Soc. **36**, 300 (1983); in afforested areas: A. Nir, Z. Arenstein, Proc. Br. Crop Prot. Conf. - Weeds **1987**, 787.

White solid, mp 198-202°. Soly in water at 25° (ppm): 10 at pH 5, 300 at pH 7. pKa 5.7. LD_{50} in male, female rats (mg/kg): >5000, >5000 orally (Harding).

USE: Herbicide.

8958. Sulfonethylmethane. [76-20-0] 2,2-Bis(ethylsulfonyl)butane; diethylsulfonmethylethylmethane; methylsulfonal; Trional. $C_8H_{18}O_4S_2$; mol wt 242.36. C 39.65%, H 7.49%, O 26.41%, S 26.46%. Prepd by condensing ethylmercaptan with methyl ethyl ketone and oxidizing the resulting mercaptol with $KMnO_4$: Fromm, Ann. **253**, 135 (1889); cf. Baumann, Ber. **18**, 883 (1885); Arch. Pharm. **226**, 511 (1888); Bayer, Pharm. Z. **34**, 98 (1889); **DE 46333**; Moragas, Uthoff, Chim. Ind. (Paris) **17**, 284 (1927); Ramberg, Samén, C.A. **28**, 6103 (1934); Suter, Organic Chemistry of Sulfur (New York, 1944) pp 735, 742.

Lustrous leaflets, scales from water. Bitter taste. mp 74-76°. Upon further heating dec with evolution of SO_2. One gram dissolves in 200 ml cold, about 30 ml boiling water, in 8 ml alc. Sol in ether. A satd aq soln is neutral to litmus.

Note: This is a controlled substance (depressant): **21 CFR, 1308.13.**

THERAP CAT: Sedative, hypnotic.

THERAP CAT (VET): Has been used as a hypnotic.

8959. Sulfoniazide. [3691-81-4] 4-Pyridinecarboxylic acid [(3-sulfophenyl)methylene]hydrazide; isonicotinic acid m-sulfobenzylidene hydrazide; isonicotinyl hydrazonotoluene-m-sulfonic acid; G-605. $C_{13}H_{11}N_3O_4S$; mol wt 305.31. C 51.14%, H 3.63%, N 13.76%, O 20.96%, S 10.50%. Prepn: Girard, **US 2727041** (1955 to Lab. Français Chimiother.); Sugimoto, **JP 57 1117** (1957 to Tanake), C.A. **52**, 4696e (1958).

Needles, dec 250-253°. Slightly sol in water.

Sodium salt trihydrate. Sulfon-Niazone. $C_{13}H_{10}N_3NaO_4S$.-$3H_2O$; mol wt 381.34. Crysts from water. Soly in water (18°): 1 g/33 cc.

THERAP CAT: Antibacterial (tuberculostatic).

8960. Sulfonmethane. [115-24-2] 2,2-Bis(ethylsulfonyl)propane; diethylsulfondimethylmethane; propane-diethyl sulfone; sulfonal. $C_7H_{16}O_4S_2$; mol wt 228.33. C 36.82%, H 7.06%, O 28.03%, S 28.09%. Prepd by condensing ethyl mercaptan with acetone, then oxidizing with $KMnO_4$: Fromm, Ann. **253**, 140 (1889); cf. Baumann, Ber. **18**, 883 (1885); Arch. Pharm. **226**, 511 (1888); Bayer, Pharm. Z. **34**, 98 (1889); **DE 46333**; Moragas, Uthoff, Chim. Ind. (Paris) **17**, 284 (1927); Ramberg, Samén, C.A. **28**, 6103 (1934); Suter, Organic Chemistry of Sulfur (New York, 1944) pp 735, 742. Soly data: Falck, J. Pharm. Chim. [7] **21**, 279 (1920).

Crystals, almost tasteless, mp 124-126°. bp 300°. One gram dissolves in 365 ml water, 16 ml boiling water, 60 ml alcohol, 3 ml boiling alcohol, 64 ml ether, 11 ml chloroform. Soluble in benzene. Insol in glycerol.

Note: This is a controlled substance (depressant): **21 CFR, 1308.13.**

THERAP CAT: Hypnotic.

THERAP CAT (VET): Has been used as a hypnotic.

8961. Sulfonyldiacetic Acid. [123-45-5] Sulfonediacetic acid; dimethylenesulfone-α,α'-dicarboxylic acid. $C_4H_6O_6S$; mol wt 182.15. C 26.38%, H 3.32%, O 52.70%, S 17.60%. $HOOCCH_2SO_2CH_2COOH$. Prepd by oxidation of thiodiglycolic acid: Lovén, Ber. **17**, 2818 (1884).

Tabular crystals, mp 182°. Freely sol in water. Sol in alc. Slightly sol in ether.

USE: Detection of barium, lead, mercury and silver.

8962. Sulforaphane. [142825-10-3]; [4478-93-7] (unspecified stereo). (R)-1-Isothiocyanato-4-(methylsulfinyl)butane; 4-methylsulfinylbutyl isothiocyanate. $C_6H_{11}NOS_2$; mol wt 177.29. C 40.65%, H 6.25%, N 7.90%, O 9.02%, S 36.17%. Potent, selective inducer of phase II detoxification enzymes with anticarcinogenic properties. Occurs naturally in broccoli. Prepn: H. Schmid, P. Karrer, Helv. Chim. Acta **31**, 1497 (1948). Absolute configuration: K. Mislow et al., J. Am. Chem. Soc. **87**, 665 (1965). Isoln from SAGA broccoli and enzyme inducing activities: Y. Zhang et al., Proc. Natl. Acad. Sci. USA **89**, 2399 (1992). Asymmetric synthesis: J. K. Whitesell, M.-S. Wong, J. Org. Chem. **59**, 597 (1994). In vivo antitumor activity: Y. Zhang et al., Proc. Natl. Acad. Sci. USA **91**, 3147 (1994). Mechanism of action study: M. C. Myzak et al., Cancer Res. **64**, 5767 (2004). Review of antioxidant activitiy: J. W. Fahey, P. Talalay, Food Chem. Toxicol. **37**, 973-979 (1999).

$[\alpha]_D^{22}$ −79.3 ±1° (c = 1.223 in chloroform). $[\alpha]_D^{25}$ −78.6° (c = 1.19 in chloroform). uv max (water): 238 nm (ε 910 $M^{-1}cm^{-1}$); upon addition of 0.1M NaOH uv max: 226 nm (ε 15300 $M^{-1}cm^{-1}$).

8963. Sulforidazine. [14759-06-9] 10-[2-(1-Methyl-2-piperidinyl)ethyl]-2-(methylsulfonyl)-10H-phenothiazine; 3-(methylsulfonyl)-10-[2-(1-methyl-2-piperidyl)ethyl]phenothiazine; thioridazine-2-sulfone; TPN-12; Imagotan; Inofal. $C_{21}H_{26}N_2O_2S_2$; mol wt 402.57. C 62.65%, H 6.51%, N 6.96%, O 7.95%, S 15.93%. Dopamine receptor blocker; metabolite of thioridazine and mesoridazine, q.q.v. Prepn: Renz et al., **FR 1363683** and **FR 1459476** (1964, 1966, both to Sandoz). Pharmacology: Maruyama et al., C.A. **68**, 20799z (1968). Effects on dopaminergic function in comparison with mesoridazine and thioridazine: D. M. Niedzwiecki *et al., J. Pharmacol. Exp. Ther.* **228,** 636 (1984); C. D. Kilts *et al., ibid.* **231,** 334 (1984). Clinical evaluation as antipsychotic: R. Axelsson, *Curr. Ther. Res.* **21,** 587 (1977). HPLC determn in plasma: D. A. Ganes, K. K. Midha, *J. Chromatogr.* **423,** 227 (1987).

Crystals from acetone, mp 121-123°.
THERAP CAT: Antipsychotic.

8964. Sulfosalicylic Acid. [97-05-2] 2-Hydroxy-5-sulfobenzoic acid; 3-carboxy-4-hydroxybenzenesulfonic acid; 5-sulfosalicylic acid; 2-hydroxybenzoic-5-sulfonic acid; salicylsulfonic acid. $C_7H_6O_6S$; mol wt 218.18. C 38.53%, H 2.77%, O 44.00%, S 14.70%. Prepn: Pusca *et al., Rev. Chim. (Bucharest)* **13,** no. 1, 49-50 (1962), *C.A.* **57,** 14994b (1962).

Dihydrate. White crystals or cryst powder. Colored pink by traces of iron. mp ~120° when anhydr; at higher temp dec into phenol and salicylic acid. Very sol in water or alcohol; sol in ether. Generally sol in polar solvents. *Keep well closed and protected from light.*
Caution: Irritating to skin, mucous membranes.
USE: Clinical reagent for albumin in urine; colorimetric reagent for ferric ion with which it gives a violet color. It is a trifunctional aromatic compound, undergoing reactions typical of phenols, carboxylic and sulfonic acid groups. Suggested industrial uses: metal chelating agent, intermediate in the manuf of surface-active agents, organic catalysts and grease additives.

8965. Sulfosulfuron. [141776-32-1] *N*-[[(4,6-Dimethoxy-2-pyrimidinyl)amino]carbonyl]-2-(ethylsulfonyl)imidazo[1,2-*a*]-pyridine-3-sulfonamide; 1-(2-ethylsulfonylimidazol[1,2-*a*]pyridin-3-ylsulfonyl)-3-(4,6-dimethoxypyrimidin-2-yl)urea; MON-37500; Maverick; Monitor; Sundance. $C_{16}H_{18}N_6O_7S_2$; mol wt 470.48. C 40.85%, H 3.86%, N 17.86%, O 23.80%, S 13.63%. Sulfonylurea herbicide to control grassy weeds in wheat. Prepn: Y. Ishida *et al.,* **EP 477808** (1992 to Takeda). Description of physical properties, toxicity and activity: S. K. Parrish *et al., Brighton Crop Prot. Conf. - Weeds* **1995,** 57. Soil degradation: *idem et al., ibid.* 667. Field trial in winter wheat: R. E. Blackshaw, W. M. Hamman, *Weed Technol.* **12,** 421 (1998). Absorption and translocation in grass species: B. L. S. Olson *et al., Weed Sci.* **47,** 37 (1999).

White, odorless crystals, mp 201.1-201.7°. Soly in water (ppm): 18 (pH 5); 1627 (pH 7); 482 (pH 9). Vapor pressure: $<10^{-6}$ Pa. Log P (octanol/water): <10. LD_{50} in rats (mg/kg): >5000 orally; >5000 dermally; LC_{50} (96 hr) in rainbow trout, carp (mg/l): >95, >91 (Parrish).
USE: Herbicide.

8966. Sulfotep. [3689-24-5] Thiodiphosphoric acid tetraethyl ester; thiopyrophosphoric acid tetraethyl ester; sulfotepp; thiotepp; dithio; dithione; dithiophos; TEDP; ASP-47; Bayer E 393; ENT-16273; Bladafum. $C_8H_{20}O_5P_2S_2$; mol wt 322.32. C 29.81%, H 6.25%, O 24.82%, P 19.22%, S 19.90%. Prepn: A. D. F. Toy, *J. Am. Chem. Soc.* **73,** 4670 (1951); G. Schrader, R. Mühlmann, **DE 848812** (1952 to Bayer), *C.A.* **47,** 5426a (1953); R. Appel, H. Einig, *Z. Anorg. Allg. Chem.* **414,** 236 (1975). Activity: F. F. Smith *et al., J. Econ. Entomol.* **43,** 627 (1950). Toxicity data: B. Holmstedt, *Pharmacol. Rev.* **11,** 567 (1959).

Pale yellow liquid, bp_2 136-139°. *Poisonous!* Vapor press. at 20°: 1.7×10^{-4} mm Hg. d_4^{25} 1.196. n_D^{25} 1.4753. Soly in water: 25 mg/l. Miscible with most organic solvents. Corrosive to iron. LD_{50} s.c. in mice: 8 mg/kg (Holmstedt).
Caution: Potential symptoms of overexposure are eye pain, blurred vision, lacrimation and rhinorrhea; headache; cyanosis; anorexia, nausea, vomiting and diarrhea; local sweating, weakness, twitching, paralysis, Cheyne-Stokes respiration, convulsions, low blood pressure and cardiac irregularities; skin and eye irritation. *See NIOSH Pocket Guide to Chemical Hazards* (DHHS/NIOSH 97-140, 1997) p 294.
USE: Insecticide; miticide.

8967. Sulfoxide. [120-62-7] 5-[2-(Octylsulfinyl)propyl]-1,3-benzodioxole; 1,2-(methylenedioxy)-4-[2-(octylsulfinyl)propyl]benzene; *n*-octylsulfoxide of isosafrole; 1-methyl-2-(3,4-methylenedioxyphenyl)ethyl octyl sulfoxide; Sulfox-Cide. $C_{18}H_{28}O_3S$; mol wt 324.48. C 66.63%, H 8.70%, O 14.79%, S 9.88%. Prepn: M. E. Synerholm *et al., Contrib. Boyce Thompson Inst.* **15,** 35 (1947); M. E. Synerholm, **US 2486579** (1949 to Boyce Thompson Inst. for Plant Res.). Synergistic use with pyrethrum, allethrin, rotenone, ryania, etc.: *idem,* **US 2486445** (1949 to Boyce Thompson Inst. for Plant Res.). Acute toxicity: T. B. Gaines, R. E. Linder, *Fundam. Appl. Toxicol.* **7,** 299 (1986).

Pale yellow, sweet-smelling, viscous oil. Practically insol in water. Sol in most organic solvents except petr ether. LD_{50} in adult male, female rats (mg/kg): 3957, 3477 orally (Gaines, Linder).
USE: Insecticide.

8968. Sulfoxone Sodium. [144-75-2] Disodium[sulfonyl-bis(*p*-phenylenimino)]dimethanesulfinate; 4,4'-diaminodiphenyl-sulfone disodium formaldehyde sulfoxylate; disodium formaldehydesulfoxylate-diaminodiphenylsulfone; aldesulfone sodium; Diazon; Novotrone; Diasone. $C_{14}H_{14}N_2Na_2O_6S_3$; mol wt 448.45. C 37.50%, H 3.15%, N 6.25%, Na 10.25%, O 21.41%, S 21.45%. Prepn: H. Bauer, *J. Am. Chem. Soc.* **61,** 617 (1939); S. M. Rosenthal, H. Bauer, **US 2234981** (1941); G. W. Raiziss *et al., J. Am. Pharm. Assoc.* **33,** 43 (1944); **US 2256575** (1941). Therapeutic use in dermatitis herpetiformis: T. Cornbleet, *Arch. Dermatol. Syphilol.* **64,** 684 (1951); S. I. Katz, *Arch. Dermatol.* **118,** 809 (1982); in leprosy: J. H. Peters *et al., Lepr. Rev.* **46,** 171 (1975). Comprehensive description: V. K. Kapoor, *Anal. Profiles Drug Subs.* **19,** 553-573 (1990).

Dihydrate. Needles or amorphous powder. After drying at 100-110° it dec 263-265°. Easily sol in water. Slightly sol in alcohol. Practically insol in the usual organic solvents. Must be stored in vacuum-sealed ampuls. The addition of 10% sodium bicarbonate helps to prevent oxidative changes.

THERAP CAT: Antibacterial (leprostatic).

8969. Sulfur. [7704-34-9] Brimstone; sulphur. S; at. wt 32.066; at. no. 16; valences 2, 4, 6. Group VIA (16). Four naturally occurring isotopes: 32 (95.0%); 33 (0.76%); 34 (4.22%); 36 (0.014%); artificial, radioactive isotopes: 29-31; 35; 37; 38. Has been known from very early times. Occurs both in the free state and in combination, mainly as sulfides and sulfates; constitutes 0.05% of the crust of the earth. Industrial prepn by Frasch process: *Faith, Keyes & Clark's Industrial Chemicals*, F. A. Lowenheim, M. K. Moran, Eds. (Wiley-Interscience, New York, 4th ed., 1975) pp 786-794. Exists in several allotropic modifications; at S.T.P. only the orthorhombic, cyclooctasulfur (S_α) is thermodynamically stable: Meyer, *Chem. Rev.* **64**, 429 (1964). Prepn of cyclohexasulfur: Bartlett *et al., J. Am. Chem. Soc.* **83**, 10 (1961); of cycloheptaand cyclodecasulfur: Schmidt *et al., Angew. Chem. Int. Ed.* **7**, 632 (1968); of cyclononasulfur: Schmidt, Wilhelm, *Chem. Commun.* **1970**, 1111; of cyclododecasulfur: *eidem, Angew. Chem. Int. Ed.* **5**, 964 (1966). Review of structures of elemental sulfur: Meyer in *Adv. Inorg. Chem. Radiochem.* **18**, 287-317 (1976). Reviews of sulfur and its compds: W. N. Tuller, *The Sulphur Data Book* (McGraw-Hill, New York, 1954); B. Meyer, *Elemental Sulfur* (Interscience-Wiley, 1965); *Inorganic Sulphur Chemistry*, G. Nickless, Ed. (Elsevier, New York, 1968); Schmidt, Siebert in *Comprehensive Inorganic Chemistry* vol. **2**, J. C. Bailar, Jr. *et al.*, Eds. (Pergamon, Oxford, 1973) pp 795-933. *See also* Sulfur, Pharmaceutical.

Sulfur is insol in water. Sparingly sol in ether; sol in carbon disulfide (one gram/2 ml); sol in benzene (about 2.4% at 30°, much more at higher temps.), in toluene. Liquid ammonia (anhydr) dissolves 38.5% S at −78°; acetone dissolves 2.65% at 25°; methylene iodide dissolves 9.1% at 10°; chloroform dissolves about 1.5% at 18°. For other solvents *see* Tuller, *op. cit.* Ignites in air above 261°, in oxygen below 260°, burning to the dioxide; combines readily with hydrogen; combines in the cold with fluorine, chlorine, and bromine; combines with carbon at high temperatures; reacts with silicon, phosphorus, arsenic, antimony and bismuth at their melting points; combines with nearly all metals; with lithium, sodium, potassium, copper, mercury and silver in the cold on contact with the solid; with magnesium, zinc and cadmium very slightly in the cold, more readily on heating; with other metals at high temperatures. Does not react with iodine, nitrogen, tellurium, gold, platinum and iridium.

α-Sulfur. Orthorhombic cyclooctasulfur. Amber-colored crystals; the stable form at ordinary temperature. d 2.06; when heated to 94.5° becomes opaque owing to the formation of monoclinic sulfur.

β-Sulfur. Monoclinic cyclooctasulfur. Opaque, light-yellow, brittle, needle-like crystals; stable between 94.5-120°. Passes slowly into the rhombic form on standing. d 1.96; mp 115.21°: West, *J. Am. Chem. Soc.* **81**, 29 (1959). bp ~444.6°.

γ-Sulfur. Mother-of-pearl sulfur. A second monoclinic form, mp 106.8°.

Polymeric sulfur. Crystex. Amorphous form; mol wt approx 200,000. Metastable, gradually reverts to the α-form. Insol in solvents used for orthorhombic form. *Reviews:* Meyer, *loc. cit.* (1964); A. V. Tobolsky, W. J. MacKnight, *Polymeric Sulfur and Related Polymers* (Interscience, New York, 1965) pp 87-97.

Caution: May cause irritation of skin, mucous membranes.

USE: In mfg sulfuric acid, carbon disulfide, sulfites, insecticides, plastics, enamels, metal-glass cements; in vulcanizing rubber; in syntheses of dyes; in making gunpowder; matches; for bleaching wood pulp, straw, wool, silk, felt, linen.

8970. Sulfur Chloride. [10025-67-9] Disulfur dichloride; sulfur monochloride; sulfur subchloride. Cl_2S_2; mol wt 135.04. Cl 52.51%, S 47.49%. S_2Cl_2. Prepared by passing chlorine into molten sulfur, can be purified by fractional distillation: Fehér in *Handbook of Preparative Inorganic Chemistry* vol. **1**, G. Brauer, Ed. (Academic Press, New York, 2nd ed., 1963) pp 371-372. Hydrolysis: H. L. Olin, *J. Am. Chem. Soc.* **48**, 167 (1926).

Non-flammable, light amber to yellowish red, fuming, oily liquid. Penetrating odor. $d_{15.5}^{15.5}$ 1.6885. n_D^{20} 1.670. mp −77°. bp$_{760}$ 138°; bp$_{100}$ 72.0°; bp$_{10}$ 19.1°. Dielectric constant 4.9 at 22°. Dipole moment 1.60. Sol in alcohol, benzene, ether, carbon disulfide, carbon tetrachloride, oils. Readily dissolves sulfur (up to 67% at room temp). Dec by water yielding sulfur, hydrogen chloride, sulfur dioxide, hydrogen sulfide, sulfite, thiosulfate. In acid solns pentathionic and other polythionic acids are formed. *Keep tightly closed and out of contact with water.*

Caution: Potential symptoms of overexposure are irritation of eyes, skin and mucous membranes; lacrimation; coughing; eye and skin burns; pulmonary edema. *See NIOSH Pocket Guide to Chemical Hazards* (DHHS/NIOSH 97-140, 1997) p 290.

USE: Intermediate and chlorinating agent in the manuf of organic chemicals, sulfur dyes, insecticides, synthetic rubbers; in cold vulcanization of rubber; as polymerization catalyst for vegetable oils; for hardening soft woods.

8971. Sulfur Dioxide. [7446-09-5] Sulfurous anhydride; sulfurous oxide. O_2S; mol wt 64.06. O 49.95%, S 50.05%. SO_2. Liquid SO_2 used as solvent: Waddington, *Non-aqueous Solvent Systems*, T. C. Waddington, Ed. (Academic Press, New York, 1965) pp 253-284. Review of toxicology and human exposure: *Toxicological Profile for Sulfur Dioxide* (PB99-122020, 1998) 223 pp. Brief review of synthetic applications: F. Fonquerne, *Synlett* **2005**, 1340-1341.

Colorless, nonflammable gas; strong suffocating odor. Condenses at −10° and ordinary pressure to a colorless liquid. d (liq) 1.5. mp −72°. bp −10°. Mixed with oxygen and passed over red-hot Pt, it is converted into SO_3. With water forms sulfurous acid (H_2SO_3). Bleaches vegetable colors. Soly: in water 17.7% at 0°, 11.9% at 15°, 8.5% at 25°, 6.4% at 35°; in alcohol 25%; in methanol 32%; also sol in chloroform or ether.

Caution: Potential symptoms of overexposure are irritation of eyes, nose and throat, rhinorrhea; choking, coughing; reflex bronchoconstriction; direct contact with liquid may cause frostbite. *See NIOSH Pocket Guide to Chemical Hazards* (DHHS/NIOSH 97-140, 1997) p 288.

USE: Preserving fruits, vegetables, etc.; disinfectant in breweries and food factories; bleaching textile fibers, straw, wicker ware, gelatin, glue, beet sugars. Solvent and reagent in organic synthesis.

8972. Sulfuretin. [120-05-8] (Z)-2-[(3,4-Dihydroxyphenyl)methylene]-6-hydroxy-3(2H)-benzofuranone; 2-(3,4-dihydroxybenzylidene)-6-hydroxy-3(2H)-benzofuranone; 3',4',6-trihydroxyaurone; 3',4',6-trihydroxybenzalcoumaranone. $C_{15}H_{10}O_5$; mol wt 270.24. C 66.67%, H 3.73%, O 29.60%. Flavonoid pigment responsible for the yellow color of certain species of *Compositae*. Isoln from *Cosmos sulphureus* Cav., *Compositae*: Shimokoriyama, Hattori, *J. Am. Chem. Soc.* **75**, 1900 (1953); from *Dahlia variabilis* Desf., *Compositae*: Nordström, Swain, *Arch. Biochem. Biophys.* **60**, 329 (1956). Prepn by condensation of 6-hydroxy-3-coumaranone and protocatechuic alcohol: Nordström, Swain, *ibid.* Prepn and structure studies: Geissman, Jurd, *J. Am. Chem. Soc.* **76**, 4475 (1954); Farkas *et al., Ber.* **92**, 2847 (1959). Structure: Shimokoriyama, Geissman, *J. Org. Chem.* **25**, 1956 (1960).

Orange crystals from dil alc, mp 280-285° (Shimokoriyama), mp 315° (dec) (Nordström), mp 302-304° (Farkas). uv max: 398 nm.

Triacetate. $C_{21}H_{16}O_8$. Pale yellow needles from methanol, mp 191-194° (Shimokoriyama), mp 167-168° (Nordström).

8973. Sulfur Hexafluoride. [2551-62-4] F_6S; mol wt 146.06. F 78.04%, S 21.95%. SF_6. Prepd by direct fluorination of sulfur or sulfur dioxide: Moissan, Lebeau, *Compt. Rend.* **130**, 865, 984 (1900); *eidem, Ann. Chim. Phys.* [7] **26**, 147 (1902); Schumb, *Inorg. Synth.* **3**, 119 (1950); Kwasnik in *Handbook of Preparative Inorganic Chemistry* Vol. **1**, G. Brauer, Ed. (Academic Press, New York, 2nd ed., 1963) pp 169-170. Reviews: Cady, "Fluorine-Containing Compounds of Sulfur" in *Adv. Inorg. Chem. Radiochem.* **2**, 105-157 (1960); Kemmitt, Sharp, *Adv. Fluorine Chem.* **4**, 218-219 (1965).

Colorless, odorless gas. One of the heaviest known gases; density approx 5 times that of air. mp −50.8°. Sublimes at −63.8°. Crit temp 45.6°. d (liq; −50.8°) 1.88. Sparingly sol in water, somewhat more in alcohol. At 25° and 1 atm 0.297 ml SF_6 dissolves in 1.0 ml of transformer oil. Thermodynamically unstable but kinetically stable gas. This stability explained by symmetrical, octahedral structure of the molecule. Inert to nucleophilic attack. Does not attack glass. No fluorine exchange with HF. Stable to silent electrical discharge. Unchanged at 500°.

Caution: Potential symptoms of overexposure are asphyxia; increased breathing rate and pulse rate; slight muscle incoordination, emotional upset; fatigue, nausea, vomiting, convulsions. See *NIOSH Pocket Guide to Chemical Hazards* (DHHS/NIOSH 97-140, 1997) p 288.

USE: In electrical circuit interrupters. In electronic ultra-high frequency piping.

8974. Sulfuric Acid. [7664-93-9] Oil of vitriol. H_2O_4S; mol wt 98.08. H 2.06%, O 65.25%, S 32.69%. H_2SO_4. Prepd by the Contact Process according to the reactions $2SO_2 + O_2 \rightarrow 2SO_3$, and $SO_3 + H_2O \rightarrow H_2SO_4$; by the Chamber Process according to the reactions $2NO + O_2 \rightarrow 2NO_2$, and $NO_2 + SO_2 + H_2O \rightarrow H_2SO_4 + NO$. Sulfuric acid of commerce contains 93-98% H_2SO_4; the remainder is water. Monograph: W. W. Duecker, J. R. West, *The Manufacture of Sulfuric Acid* (Reinhold, New York, 1959) 515 pp. Review of manuf: Pearce, "Sulphuric Acid: Physico-Chemical Aspects of Manufacture" in *Inorganic Sulphur Chemistry*, G. Nickless, Ed. (Elsevier, New York, 1968) pp 535-561; *Faith, Keyes & Clark's Industrial Chemicals*, F. A. Lowenheim, M. K. Moran, Eds. (Wiley-Interscience, New York, 4th ed., 1975) pp 795-806. Toxicity data: H. F. Smyth *et al., Am. Ind. Hyg. Assoc. J.* **30**, 470 (1969). Review of toxicology and human exposure: *Toxicological Profile for Sulfur Trioxide and Sulfuric Acid* (PB99-122038, 1998) 224 pp.

Clear, colorless, odorless, oily liquid. *Very corrosive!* Has a very great affinity for water, abstracting it from the air and also from many organic substances; hence it chars sugar, wood, etc. d ~1.84. bp ~290°; dec 340° into sulfur trioxide and water. mp 10° (anhydrous acid). 98% H_2SO_4 freezes at +3°; 93% at −32°; 78% at −38°; 74% at −44°; 65% at −64°. Misc with water and alcohol with the generation of much heat and with contraction in vol. When diluting, the acid should be added to the diluent. *Keep tightly closed. Handle with caution. Avoid contact with skin.* LD$_{50}$ orally in rats: 2.14 g/kg (Smyth).

Sulfuric acid, fuming. [8014-95-7] H_2SO_4 with free SO_3, designated in commerce as *oleum*. Available grades contain up to about 80% free SO_3. Colorless or slightly colored, viscous liquid, emitting choking fumes of sulfur trioxide. *Extremely corrosive. Handle with great care. Avoid contact with skin. Keep tightly closed in glass-stoppered bottles.*

Caution: Potential symptoms of overexposure are eye, skin, nose and throat irritation; pulmonary edema, bronchitis; emphysema; conjunctivitis; stomatis; dental erosion; tracheobronchitis; skin and eye burns; dermatitis. See *NIOSH Pocket Guide to Chemical Hazards* (DHHS/NIOSH 97-140, 1997) p 290. See also *Clinical Toxicology of Commercial Products*, R. E. Gosselin *et al.,* Eds. (Williams & Wilkins, Baltimore, 5th ed., 1984) section III, pp 8-12. Occupational exposure to strong inorganic acid mists containing sulfuric acid is listed as a known human carcinogen: *Report on Carcinogens, Eleventh Edition* (PB2005-104914, 2004) p III-234.

USE: In manuf of fertilizers, explosives, dyestuffs, other acids, parchment paper, glue, purification of petroleum, pickling of metal.

THERAP CAT: Dil acid formerly in treatment of gastric hypoacidity. Concd acid formerly as a topical caustic.

8975. Sulfur Iodide. [1312-15-8] Iodosulfane. Approx SI. Obtained by fusing together 4 parts iodine with 1 part sulfur. It probably contains free iodine as well as free sulfur.

Grayish-black masses of metallic luster and iodine odor. Insol in water; sol in carbon disulfide, alcohol, ether, in about 50 parts glycerol. KI soln dissolves a portion of the iodine leaving free sulfur. *Keep well closed.*

THERAP CAT: Dermatologic.

THERAP CAT (VET): Has been used in chronic eczema, ringworm, mange.

8976. Sulfurous Acid. [7782-99-2] Sulfur dioxide soln. A soln of ~6% sulfur dioxide in water.

Colorless, clear, acid liquid; suffocating odor of sulfur dioxide. d ~1.03. Gradually oxidizes in the air to sulfuric acid. *Keep in nearly full, tightly closed containers, in a cool place.*

USE: Dental bleach.

THERAP CAT: Antiseptic.

8977. Sulfur, Pharmaceutical. [7704-34-9] Two forms of sulfur of 99.5% purity or better are recognized in pharmacy: *sublimed sulfur*, also known as *flowers of sulfur*, and *precipitated sulfur*, also known as *milk of sulfur*, made by boiling sublimed sulfur with lime and pptg with hydrochloric acid. Other sulfur preparations include: *washed sulfur*, made by treating sublimed sulfur with ammonia and washing with water to dissolve impurities, particularly arsenic; *sulfurated lime*, the active component of *Vleminckx's lotion*, made by boiling sublimed sulfur with lime, resulting in formation of calcium pentasulfide and calcium thiosulfate; and *sulfurated potash* ($K_2(S_x)$), also known as *liver of sulfur*, made by heating sublimed sulfur with potassium carbonate. Review of dermatological applications: C. W. McMurtry, *J. Cutan. Dis.* **1913**, 322-328, 399-408; of chemistry, biologic effects and clinical use: A. N. Lin *et al., J. Am. Acad. Dermatol.* **18**, 553-558 (1988).

Sublimed sulfur forms a fine, yellow crystalline powder. Insol in water, alcohol. Precipitated sulfur forms a very fine, pale yellow, amorphous or microcryst powder. Practically insol in water. Very slightly sol in alcohol. Soly in ether at 23°: 0.97%; in acetone at 25°: 2.084%; in carbon disulfide at 20°: 29.5%; in olive oil at 15°: 2.3%. Sulfurated potash forms irregular, liver-brown pieces; dec in air. Sol in water.

THERAP CAT: Keratolytic; scabicide.

THERAP CAT (VET): Antiseptic and parasiticidal; in lotions, ointments and dips.

8978. Sulfur Tetrafluoride. [7783-60-0] F_4S; mol wt 108.06. F 70.33%, S 29.67%. SF_4. First prepd from cobalt trifluoride and elemental sulfur: Fischer, Jaenckner, *Angew. Chem.* **42**, 810 (1929); Kwasnik in *Handbook of Preparative Inorganic Chemistry* vol. **1**, G. Brauer, Ed. (Academic Press, New York, 2nd ed., 1963) pp 168-169. Best prepared from SCl_2 and NaF suspended in acetonitrile; also from sulfur, chlorine and sodium fluoride: Tullock *et al., J. Am. Chem. Soc.* **82**, 539 (1960); Arth, Fried, US **3046094** (1962 to Merck & Co.); Fawcett, Tullock, *Inorg. Synth.* **7**, 119 (1963). Reviews of prepn and chemistry: Smith, *Angew. Chem. Int. Ed.* **1**, 467-475 (1962); Kemmitt, Sharp, *Adv. Fluorine Chem.* **4**, 220-222 (1965); Martin, *Ann. N.Y. Acad. Sci.* **145**, 161-168 (1967).

Colorless gas. Thermostable to 600°. mp −121.0°. bp −38°. d (liq; −78°) 1.95. d (solid; −183°) 2.349. Freely sol in benzene. Violent reaction with water. Hydrofluoric acid released on exposure to moisture. Dec by concd H_2SO_4. Attacks glass but not quartz or mercury.

Caution: Potential symptoms of overexposure are irritation of eyes, mucous membranes; direct contact with liquid may cause frostbite; eye and skin burns from released hydrofluoric acid. See *NIOSH Pocket Guide to Chemical Hazards* (DHHS/NIOSH 97-140, 1997) p 290.

USE: Selective fluorinating agent.

8979. Sulfur Trioxide. [7446-11-9] Sulfuric anhydride. O_3S; mol wt 80.06. O 59.95%, S 40.05%. SO_3. Prepd by the contact process, *i.e.*, by the action of oxygen on sulfur dioxide in the presence of catalysts such as platinized asbestos, platinized magnesium sulfate, ferric oxide, or vanadium compds. Extensive review and bibliography: Fairlie, *Sulfuric Acid Manufacture*, A.C.S. Monograph Series no. **69** (New York, 1936). Exists in 3 modifications. May be prepd in the laboratory by heating fuming sulfuric acid and collecting the sublimate in a cooled receiver. If the vapor is condensed above 27°, the γ-form is obtained as a liquid. If the vapor is condensed below 27° and in the presence of a trace of moisture, a mixture of all 3 forms is obtained. The 3 forms can be separated by fractional distillation. The α-form is the stable modification, the β- and γ-forms are metastable. Review of toxicology and human exposure: *Toxicological Profile for Sulfur Trioxide and Sulfuric Acid* (PB99-122038, 1998) 224 pp.

Melted SO_3 exists in the γ-form and on solidifying tends to the α-form. The difference in vapor pressures explains the so-called "alpha explosion" of sulfur trioxide. Heating of high-melting SO_3 in glass vessels should be avoided to prevent possible shattering of the container. Absolutely dry SO_3 is not corrosive to metals and shows no acid reaction. On exposure to air, it absorbs moisture rapidly, emitting dense white fumes. Combines with water with explosive violence (heat of dilution 504 cals/g) forming sulfuric acid. Due to this avidity for water, SO_3 chars many organic substances. On contact with wood shavings the heat produced by dehydration is sufficient to cause fire.

α-Form. Asbestos-like needles, mp 62.3°. Vapor pressure at 25° = 73 mm.

β-Form. Asbestos-like neeedles, mp 32.5°. Vapor pressure at 25° = 344 mm.

γ-Form. Ice-like mass, mp 16.8° or liquid, d 1.9224. bp_{760} 44.8°. Vapor pressure at 25° = 433 mm.

Caution: Potential symptoms of overexposure by inhalation are tooth erosion and respiratory tract irritation; by ingestion are mouth and throat burns, gastric erosion; direct contact may cause irritation or chemical burns of skin, eyes, respiratory and gastrointestinal tracts. *See* PB99-122038.

USE: Intermediate in sulfuric acid manuf; in sulfonations for formation of addition compds with amines; in the manuf of explosives.

8980. Sulfuryl Chloride. [7791-25-5] Cl_2O_2S; mol wt 134.97. Cl 52.53%, O 23.71%, S 23.76%. SO_2Cl_2. Prepd by passing a mixture of dry sulfur dioxide and chlorine through activated charcoal (other catalysts, such as camphor, can be used): Danneel, *Angew. Chem.* **39**, 1553 (1926); Durrans, *J. Soc. Chem. Ind.* **45**, 347 (1926); Meyer, *Angew. Chem.* **44**, 41 (1931); Danneel, Hesse, *Z. Anorg. Allg. Chem.* **212**, 214 (1933); Allen, Maxson, *Inorg. Synth.* **1**, 114 (1939).

Colorless, mobile liquid, very pungent odor. *Even the vapors are corrosive to human skin and mucous membranes.* Turns yellow upon prolonged standing because of slight dissociation into SO_2 and Cl_2. d_4^{20} 1.6674. d_4^0 1.7045. mp −54.1° (also given as −46°). bp 69.3°. n_D^{20} 1.4437. Dipole moment 1.86. Trouton constant 20.7. Slowly dec by water, forming H_2SO_4 and HCl. With ice-cold water it forms a hydrate, $SO_2Cl_2 \cdot 15H_2O$, resembling camphor in appearance. Violent reaction on contact with alkalies. Miscible with benzene, toluene, ether, glacial acetic acid, other organic solvents.

USE: Chlorinating and sulfonating or chlorosulfonating agent in organic syntheses, e.g., in the manufacture of chlorophenol and chlorothymol. Has been used in war gas formulations.

8981. Sulfuryl Fluoride. [2699-79-8] Profume; Vikane. F_2O_2S; mol wt 102.06. F 37.23%, O 31.35%, S 31.42%. SO_2F_2. Prepn: H. Moissan, P. Lebeau, *C.R. Hebd. Seances Acad. Sci.* **132**, 374 (1901); M. Trautz, K. Ehrmann, *J. Prakt. Chem.* [2] **142**, 79 (1935). Insecticidal properties and use as fumigant: E. E. Kenaga, US 2875127 (1959 to Dow). Review of prepn and properties: W. Kwasnik in *Handbook of Preparative Inorganic Chemistry* **vol. 1,** G. Brauer, Ed. (Academic Press, New York, 2nd ed., 1963) pp 173-174; R. D. W. Kemmitt, D. W. A. Sharp, *Adv. Fluorine Chem.* **4**, 225-227 (1965). Ion chromatographic determn in air: S. A. Bouyoucos *et al., Am. Ind. Hyg. Assoc. J.* **44**, 57 (1983). Efficacy vs termite species during structural fumigation: N.-Y. Su, R. H. Scheffrahn, *J. Econ. Entomol.* **79**, 903 (1986). Comparison with methyl bromide, *q.v.*, of residue potential in packaged foods: R. H. Scheffrahn *et al., Bull. Environ. Contam. Toxicol.* **48**, 821 (1992).

Odorless, colorless gas. Not very reactive. Stable to 400°. mp −135.82°. bp −55.38°. Vapor pressure (20°): 15.2 atm. Vapor density (20°): 4.3 g/l. Specific gravity (20°): 1.35. Soly at 16.5° (ml gaseous F_2SO_2/100 ml solvent): 4-5 (water); 24-27 (alcohol); 210-220 (toluene); 136-138 (CCl_4). Not hydrolyzed by water. Hydrolyzed by NaOH solns. May be stored in compressed form in steel cylinders or in a gasometer over H_2SO_4.

Caution: Potential symptoms of overexposure are conjunctivitis, rhinitis and pharyngitis; paresthesia; direct contact with liquid may cause frostbite. *See NIOSH Pocket Guide to Chemical Hazards* (DHHS/NIOSH 97-140, 1997) p 292.

USE: Fumigant insecticide; termiticide.

8982. Sulindac. [38194-50-2] (1*Z*)-5-Fluoro-2-methyl-1-[[4-(methylsulfinyl)phenyl]methylene]-1*H*-indene-3-acetic acid; *cis*-5-fluoro-2-methyl-1-[*p*-(methylsulfinyl)benzylidene]indene-3-acetic acid; MK-231; Aflodac; Algocetil; Arthrocine; Artribid; Citireuma; Clinoril; Clisundac; Reumofil; Reumyl; Sudac; Sulinol; Sulreuma. $C_{20}H_{17}FO_3S$; mol wt 356.41. C 67.40%, H 4.81%, F 5.33%, O 13.47%, S 9.00%. Non-steroidal anti-inflammatory drug. Prepn: T.-Y. Shen *et al.*, DE 2039426; *eidem*, US 3654349 (1971, 1972 both to Merck & Co.). Stereospecific synthesis: R. F. Shuman *et al., J. Org. Chem.* **42**, 1914 (1977); enantioselective synthesis: A. R. Maguire *et al., Synlett* **2001**, 41. ^{13}C-NMR study: A. W. Douglas, *Can. J. Chem.* **56**, 2129 (1978). Metabolism and disposition: H. B. Hucker *et al., Drug Metab. Dispos.* **1**, 721 (1973). HPLC determn in biological fluids: D. G. Musson *et al., J. Pharm. Sci.* **73**, 1270 (1984). Book: *Current Concepts on Anti-inflammatory Drugs*, K. Miehlke, Ed. (Biomedical Information Corp., New York, 1980) 240 pp. Review of pharmacology and efficacy in rheumatic disease: R. N. Brogden *et al., Drugs* **16**, 97-114 (1978); in treatment of colorectal polyps: F. Tonelli *et al., Dig. Dis.* **12**, 259-264 (1994). Review of clinical pharmacokinetics: N. M. Davies, M. S. Watson, *Clin. Pharmacokinet.* **32**, 437-459 (1997).

Yellow odorless crystals from ethyl acetate, mp 182-185° (dec). uv max (methanolic 0.1*N* HCl): 327, 285, 256, 226 nm ($E_{1cm}^{1\%}$ 375, 420, 410, 540). pKa (25°) 4.7. Sparingly sol in methanol, U.S.P. alcohol; slightly sol in ethyl acetate. Practically insol in water at pH <4.5. Soly increases with rising pH to ~3.0 mg/ml at pH 7. Stable in aq acid and base. Solid stable for at least three days in air at 100°.

THERAP CAT: Anti-inflammatory.

8983. Sulisobenzone. [4065-45-6] 5-Benzoyl-4-hydroxy-2-methoxybenzenesulfonic acid; 3-benzoyl-4-hydroxy-6-methoxy-benzenesulfonic acid; 2-benzoyl-5-methoxy-1-phenol-4-sulfonic acid; 2-hydroxy-4-methoxybenzophenone-5-sulfonic acid; benzophenone-4; NSC-60584; Spectra-Sorb UV 284; Sungard; Uval; Uvinul MS-40. $C_{14}H_{12}O_6S$; mol wt 308.31. C 54.54%, H 3.92%, O 31.14%, S 10.40%. Prepn: A. J. Cofrancesco, GB 1136525 (1968 to GAF). Activity: J. M. Knox *et al., J. Invest. Dermatol.* **34**, 51 (1960).

Light-tan powder, mp 145°. 1 g dissolves in 2 ml methanol, 3.3 ml alc, 4 ml water, 100 ml ethyl acetate.

USE: Ultraviolet absorber for leather and textile fibers; in cosmetics and shampoos.

THERAP CAT: Ultraviolet screen.

8984. Sulmarin. [29334-07-4] 4-Methyl-6,7-bis(sulfooxy)-2H-1-benzopyran-2-one; 6,7-dihydroxy-4-methylcoumarin disulfate; 4-methylesculetin bis(hydrogen sulfate); 4-methyl-6,7-dihydroxycoumarindisulfate; 4-methylesculetindisulfonic acid; 4-methylesculetin-6,7-disulfuric ester; MG-143; Idro P$_2$. $C_{10}H_8O_{10}S_2$; mol wt 352.29. C 34.09%, H 2.29%, O 45.42%, S 18.20%. Prepn: Cavallini, Mazzucchi, *Farm. Sci. Tec.* **3**, 297 (1948), *C.A.* **42**, 8900d (1948). Description: Maggiorelli, *G. Med. Mil.* **101**, 365 (1951), *C.A.* **47**, 6412d (1951); Banchetti, *Farmaco Ed. Sci.* **10**, 970 (1955). Polarographic method for determn: A. M. Contri, *Farmaco Ed. Prat.* **25**, 231 (1970).

Disodium salt trihydrate. $C_{10}H_6Na_2O_{10}S_2 \cdot 3H_2O$. Crystals from 60% alc, dec 252-253°. uv max (pH 11.85): 304 nm.

THERAP CAT: Hemostatic.

8985. Sulmazole. [73384-60-8] 2-[2-Methoxy-4-(methylsulfinyl)phenyl]-1H-imidazo[4,5-b]pyridine; AR-L 115BS; Vardax. $C_{14}H_{13}N_3O_2S$; mol wt 287.34. C 58.52%, H 4.56%, N 14.62%, O 11.14%, S 11.16%. Prepn: **NL 7401254**; E. Kutler *et al.*, **US 3985891** (1974, 1976 both to Thomae). Toxicity study: W. Diederen, R. Kadatz, *Arzneim.-Forsch.* **31**, 141 (1981). Series of articles on pharmacology, pharmacokinetics, metabolism, clinical studies: *ibid.* 129-278. Brief review of pharmacology: H. Koch, *Pharm. Int.* **3**, 5 (1982).

Solid, mp 203-205°. LD$_{50}$ in albino mice (mg/kg): 560 orally; 163 i.v. (Diederen, Kadatz).

THERAP CAT: Cardiotonic.

8986. Sulodexide. [57821-29-1] Glucuronylglucosamineglicane sulfate; KRX-101; Provenal; Ravenol; Vessel. Orally active heparinoid prepared from porcine intestinal mucosa. Mixture of 80% electrophoretically fast moving heparin and 20% dermatan sulfate; average mol wt <8000. Preparative method: P. Bianchini, **DE 2426586**; *idem*, **US 3936351** (1975, 1976 both to Opocrin). Review of pharmacology: F. A. Ofosu, *Semin. Thromb. Hemostasis* **24**, 127-138 (1998); J. Harenberg, *Med. Res. Rev.* **18**, 1-20 (1998). Effect on albuminuria in diabetic patients: J. Skrha *et al.*, *Diabetes Res. Clin. Pract.* **38**, 25 (1997). Clinical trial in venous leg ulcers: S. Coccheri *et al.*, *Thromb. Haemostasis* **87**, 947 (2002); in deep venous thrombosis: B. M. Errichi *et al.*, *Angiology* **55**, 243 (2004); in diabetic nephropathy: A. Achour *et al.*, *J. Nephrol.* **18**, 568 (2005).

THERAP CAT: Antithrombotic; in treatment of chronic leg ulcers and diabetic nephropathy.

8987. Sulphan Blue. [129-17-9] N-[4-[[4-(Diethylamino)phenyl](2,4-disulfophenyl)methylene]-2,5-cyclohexadien-1-ylidene]-N-ethylethanaminium inner salt, sodium salt; C.I. Acid Blue 1; [4-[α-[p-(diethylamino)phenyl]-2,4-disulfobenzylidene]-2,5-cyclohexadien-1-ylidene]diethylammonium hydroxide inner salt sodium salt; anhydro-4,4'-bis(diethylamino)triphenylmethanol-2'',4''-disulfonic acid monosodium salt; C.I. Food Blue 3; C.I. 42045; Disulphine Blue. $C_{27}H_{31}N_2NaO_6S_2$; mol wt 566.66. C 57.23%, H 5.51%, N 4.94%, Na 4.06%, O 16.94%, S 11.32%. Prepn from 4-formylbenzene-1,3-disulfonic acid and diethylaniline: *Colour Index* **vol. 4** (3rd ed., 1971) p 4382.

Violet powder. One gram dissolves in 20 ml water at 20°. Dilute aq solns are blue and turn yellow upon the addition of concd hydrochloric acid. In the absence of strong acid or caustic the blue color is stable over a wide pH range. Partly sol in alcohol.

2,5-Disulfophenyl isomer. [68238-36-8] Isosulfan blue; Lymphazurin.

USE: Coloring medicinal products; in dyeing and printing wool, silk.

THERAP CAT: Isosulfan blue as diagnostic aid (lymphangiography).

8988. Sulphenone. [80-00-2] 1-Chloro-4-(phenylsulfonyl)benzene; p-chlorophenyl phenyl sulfone; 4-chlorodiphenyl sulfone; sulfenone; R-242. $C_{12}H_9ClO_2S$; mol wt 252.72. C 57.03%, H 3.59%, Cl 14.03%, O 12.66%, S 12.69%. May also contain 20% related diaryl sulfones. Prepn: Bender, Pitt, **US 2593001** (1952 to Stauffer Chem.). Toxicology: L. W. Hazleton *et al.*, *J. Agric. Food Chem.* **3**, 836 (1955).

Dimorphic crystals, mp 94°. Slight aromatic odor. Tasteless. Soly at 20° (g/100 ml): acetone 74.4; dioxane 65.6; isopropanol 21; hexane 0.4; benzene 44.4; toluene 29.4; xylene 18.2; carbon tetrachloride 4.9. Practically insol in water. Slightly sol in petr oils. Stable to oxidizing and reducing agents, acids and alkalies found in spray formulations. LD$_{50}$ orally in mice: 2.7 g/kg (Hazleton).

USE: Acaricide.

8989. Sulpiride. [15676-16-1] 5-(Aminosulfonyl)-N-[(1-ethyl-2-pyrrolidinyl)methyl]-2-methoxybenzamide; N-[(1-ethyl-2-pyrrolidinyl)methyl]-5-sulfamoyl-o-anisamide; N-[(1-ethyl-2-pyrrolidinyl)methyl]-2-methoxy-5-sulfamoylbenzamide; Abilit; Aiglonyl; Coolspan; Dobren; Dogmatil; Dogmatyl; Dolmatil; Guastil; Meresa; Miradol; Mirbanil; Misulvan; Neogama; Omperan; Pyrikappl; Sernevin; Splotin; Sulpitil; Sulpor; Sursumid; Synédil; Trilan. $C_{15}H_{23}N_3O_4S$; mol wt 341.43. C 52.77%, H 6.79%, N 12.31%, O 18.74%, S 9.39%. Dopamine D$_2$ and D$_3$-receptor antagonist. Prepn: C. S. Miller *et al.*, **US 3342826** (1964 to Soc. d'Etudes Sci. Ind. de l'Ile-de-France); of *l*-form: F. Mauri, **DE 2903891** (1979 to Ravizza), *C.A.* **91**, 211259h (1979). Crystal structure: L. Y. Y. Ma *et al.*, *Acta Crystallogr.* **B38**, 2861 (1982). Mechanism of action: P. Jenner *et al.*, *J. Pharm. Pharmacol.* **32**, 39 (1980). Structure-activity study: P. Dostert *et al.*, *Eur. J. Med. Chem. - Chim. Ther.* **17**, 437 (1982). Physical properties: D. Pitrè, E. Valoti, *Arch. Pharmacol.* **320**, 859 (1987). Comprehensive description: D. Pitrè *et al.*, *Anal. Profiles Drug Subs.* **17**, 607-641 (1988). Review of clinical efficacy in psychiatry: A. J. Wagstaff *et al.*, *CNS Drugs* **2**, 313-333 (1994); of levosulpiride in gastroenterology: M. Guslandi, *Curr. Ther. Res.* **53**, 484-501 (1993).

White, odorless crystalline powder, mp 178-180°. Sparingly sol in methanol. Practically insol in water, ether, chloroform, benzene. pKa_1 9.00, pKa_2 10.19. $[\alpha]_D^{25}$ −66.8° (c = 0.5 in DMF). LD_{50} in mice (mg/kg): 170 i.p.; 2250 orally (Dostert).

l-**Form.** [23672-07-3] Levosulpiride; $S(-)$-sulpiride; Levobren; Levopraid. Monomorphic crystalline solid, mp 185-187°.

THERAP CAT: Antipsychotic; antidepressant; antiemetic.

8990. Sulprofos. [35400-43-2] *O*-Ethyl *O*-[4-(methylthio)-phenyl]phosphorodithioic acid *S*-propyl ester; *O*-ethyl *O*-[4-(methylmercapto)phenyl]-*S*-*n*-propylphosphorothionothioate; *O*-ethyl *O*-[4-(methylthio)phenyl] *S*-propylphosphorodithioate; BAY NTN 9306; Bolstar; Helothion. $C_{12}H_{19}O_2PS_3$; mol wt 322.45. C 44.70%, H 5.94%, O 9.92%, P 9.61%, S 29.83%. Prepn: S. Kishino *et al.*, **DE 2111414**; *eidem*, **US 3947529** (1971, 1976 both to Bayer). Metabolism: D. L. Bull, G. W. Ivie, *J. Agric. Food Chem.* **24**, 143 (1976); G. W. Ivie *et al.*, *ibid.* 147; D. L. Bull *et al.*, *ibid.* 601. Photodegradation: G. W. Ivie, D. L. Bull, *ibid.* 1053.

Tan liquid, phosphorus odor, $bp_{0.1}$ 155-158°. d_{20}^{20} 1.20, n_D^{20} 1.5859. Low soly in water, sol in organic solvents. LD_{50} orally in rats: 227 mg/kg (Bull, Ivie).

Caution: Potential symptoms of overexposure are nausea, vomiting, abdominal cramps, diarrhea, salivation; headache, giddiness, vertigo, weakness; rhinorrhea, chest tightness; blurred vision, miosis; cardiac irregularities; muscle fasciculations; dyspnea. *See NIOSH Pocket Guide to Chemical Hazards* (DHHS/NIOSH 97-140, 1997) p 292.

USE: Insecticide.

8991. Sulprostone. [60325-46-4] (5*Z*)-7-[(1*R*,2*R*,3*R*)-3-Hydroxy-2-[(1*E*,3*R*)-3-hydroxy-4-phenoxy-1-butenyl]-5-oxocyclopentyl]-*N*-(methylsulfonyl)-5-heptenamide; CP-34089; SHB-286; ZK-57671; Nalador. $C_{23}H_{31}NO_7S$; mol wt 465.56. C 59.34%, H 6.71%, N 3.01%, O 24.06%, S 6.89%. Analog of prostaglandin E_2, *q.v.*, with uterine stimulant activity. Prepn: J. Bindra, M. R. Johnson, **DE 2355540** (1974 to Pfizer), *C.A.* **81**, 49330u (1974); *eidem*, **US 4024179** (1977 to Pfizer). Antifertility effects: H. Hess *et al.*, *Experientia* **33**, 1076 (1977). Influence on platelet function: R. C. Briel, T. H. Lippert, *Adv. Prostaglandin Thromboxane Res.* **6**, 351 (1980). Biological action and half-life: *eidem*, *Prostaglandins Med.* **6**, 1 (1981). Induction of abortion: K. Schmidt-Gollwitzer, *Int. J. Fertil.* **26**, 86 (1981).

Colorless oil.

THERAP CAT: Abortifacient.

8992. Sultamicillin. [76497-13-7] (2*S*,5*R*,6*R*)-6-[[(2*R*)-Aminophenylacetyl]amino]-3,3-dimethyl-7-oxo-4-thia-1-azabicyclo[3.2.0]heptane-2-carboxylic acid [[[(2*S*,5*R*)-3,3-dimethyl-4,4-dioxido-7-oxo-4-thia-1-azabicyclo[3.2.0]hept-2-yl]carbonyl]oxy]methyl ester; 1,1-dioxopenicillanoyloxymethyl 6-(D-α-amino-α-phenylacetamido)penicillanate; 6′-(2-amino-2-phenylacetamido)penicillanoyloxymethyl penicillanate 1,1-dioxide; CP-49952; VD-1827. $C_{25}H_{30}N_4O_9S_2$; mol wt 594.66. C 50.49%, H 5.08%, N 9.42%, O 24.21%, S 10.78%. Orally absorbed double ester of sulbactam and ampicillin, *q.q.v.* Prepn: E. C. Bigham, **DE 3018590**; *eidem*, **US 4244951** (1980, 1981 both to Pfizer); and pharmacology: B. Baltzer *et al.*, *J. Antibiot.* **33**, 1183 (1980). HPLC determn and pharmacokinetics: H. J. Rogers *et al.*, *J. Antimicrob. Chemother.* **11**, 435 (1983). Clinical trial in pediatric otitis

media: K. H. Chan *et al.*, *Pediatr. Infect. Dis. J.* **12**, 24 (1993). Review of antibacterial activity, pharmacokinetics and therapeutic efficacy: H. A. Friedel *et al.*, *Drugs* **37**, 491-522 (1989).

mp 190°.
Tosylate. [83105-70-8] Bacimex; Unacid PD oral; Unacim; Unasyn. $C_{25}H_{30}N_4O_9S_2 \cdot C_7H_8O_3S$; mol wt 766.86.
THERAP CAT: Antibacterial.

8993. Sulthiame. [61-56-3] 4-(Tetrahydro-2*H*-1,2-thiazin-2-yl)benzenesulfonamide *S*,*S*-dioxide; *N*-(4′-sulfamylphenyl)-1,4-butanesultam; tetrahydro-2-(*p*-sulfamoylphenyl)-1,2-thiazine 1,1-dioxide; 2-(*p*-aminosulfonylphenyl)tetrahydro-1,2-thiazine dioxide; 1-(*p*-amidosulfonylphenyl)-2-thiapiperidine 2,2-dioxide; *N*-(*p*-aminosulfonylphenyl)-1,4-butanesultam; Elisal; Ospolot; Trolone. $C_{10}H_{14}N_2O_4S_2$; mol wt 290.36. C 41.36%, H 4.86%, N 9.65%, O 22.04%, S 22.09%. Prepn of this type of compd: Helferich, Behnisch, **US 2916489** (1959 to Schenley).

Crystalline powder, mp 180-182°. Practically insol in cold water. Partly sol in boiling water; slightly sol in alcohol, acids; readily sol in alkalies.
THERAP CAT: Anticonvulsant.

8994. Sultopride. [53583-79-2] *N*-[(1-Ethyl-2-pyrrolidinyl)methyl]-5-(ethylsulfonyl)-2-methoxybenzamide; *N*-[(1-ethyl-2-pyrrolidinyl)methyl]-5-(ethylsulfonyl)-*o*-anisamide. $C_{17}H_{26}N_2O_4S$; mol wt 354.46. C 57.60%, H 7.39%, N 7.90%, O 18.05%, S 9.05%. Dopamine D_2-receptor antagonist. Prepn: C. S. Miller *et al.*, **FR M 5916**; *see also*: G. Bulteau *et al.*, **US 3975434** (1966, 1976 both to Soc. Etudes Sci. Ind. l'Ile-de-France). Pharmacology: C. Lavelle, J. Margarit, *J. Pharmacol.* **5**, Suppl. 2, 58 (1974); B. Bruguerolle *et al.*, *ibid.* **12**, 27 (1981). Clinical trial in psychosis: D. Morel, *Sem. Hop.* **59**, 2337 (1983). GC determn in serum: A. Kamizono *et al.*, *J. Chromatogr.* **567**, 113 (1991). Pharmacokinetics of enantiomers: *idem et al.*, *Biol. Pharm. Bull.* **16**, 1121 (1993).

Hydrochloride. [23694-17-9] LIN-1418; Barnetil; Barnotil. $C_{17}H_{26}N_2O_4S \cdot HCl$; mol wt 390.93. Crystals from methyl ethyl ketone, mp 181-182° (Miller); also reported as crystals from ethanol, mp 190° (Bulteau).
THERAP CAT: Antipsychotic.

8995. Sultosilic Acid. [57775-26-5] 2-Hydroxy-5-[[(4-methylphenyl)sulfonyl]oxy]benzenesulfonic acid; 2-hydroxy-5-tosyloxybenzenesulfonic acid; 2,5-dihydroxybenzenesulfonic acid 5-*p*-toluenesulfonate. $C_{13}H_{12}O_7S_2$; mol wt 344.36. C 45.34%, H 3.51%, O 32.52%, S 18.62%. Prepn: **NL 7305916** (1973 to Lab. del Esteve); J. Esteve *et al.*, *Eur. J. Med. Chem.* **11**, 43 (1976); of piperazine salt: A. Esteve-Subirana, **US 3954767** (1976). Toxicology: L. Rodriguez *et al.*, *Arch. Farmacol. Toxicol.* **5**, 281 (1979).

Metabolism: S. G. Wood *et al., Xenobiotica* **12**, 165 (1982). Clinical evaluation: H. Vinazzer, J. C. Farine, *Atherosclerosis* **49**, 109 (1983). HPLC determn and pharmacokinetics: R. Roser *et al., Eur. J. Drug Metab. Pharmacokinet.* **11**, 1 (1986).

Piperazine salt. [57775-27-6] Diethylenediamine sultosylate; piperazine sultosylate; A-585; Mimedran. $C_{13}H_{12}O_7S_2.C_4H_{10}N_2$; mol wt 430.50. Crystals from ethanol, mp 174°. LD_{50} i.p. in beagles, male rats, female rats: 605, 833.6, 1272 mg/kg; orally in rats: >11 g/kg (Rodriguez).

THERAP CAT: Antilipemic.

8996. Sumach. Name used for several plants of the *Rhus* species. Leaves of *Rhus glabra* L. and *Rhus typhina* L., *Anacardiaceae* are known commercially as **North American Sumach.** They contain fisetin, dihydrofisetin, 27% tannin and gallic acid esters. Constituents of the *Rhus typhina* fruit: J. Tischer, *Pharmazie* **15**, 83 (1960).

USE: North American sumach as black dye; as scenting agent for tobacco.

8997. Sumatriptan. [103628-46-2] 3-[2-(Dimethylamino)ethyl]-*N*-methyl-1*H*-indole-5-methanesulfonamide; GR-43175. $C_{14}H_{21}N_3O_2S$; mol wt 295.40. C 56.92%, H 7.17%, N 14.22%, O 10.83%, S 10.85%. Serotonin $5HT_1$-receptor agonist. Prepn: M. D. Dowle, I. H. Coates, **DE 3320521**; *eidem,* **US 4816470**; A. W. Oxford, **GB 2162522** (1983, 1989, 1986 all to Glaxo). Receptor binding studies: P. P. A. Humphrey *et al., Br. J. Pharmacol.* **94**, 1123 (1988); P. Schoeffter, D. Hoyer, *Arch. Pharmacol.* **340**, 135 (1989). LC-MS determn in plasma: J. Oxford, M. S. Lant, *J. Chromatogr.* **496**, 137 (1989). Clinical evaluations in migraine: A. Doenicke *et al., Lancet* **1**, 1309 (1988); Subcutaneous Sumatriptan International Study Group, *N. Engl. J. Med.* **325**, 316 (1991); in acute cluster headache: Sumatriptan Cluster Headache Study Group, *ibid.* 322. Review of pharmacology and clinical experience: S. J. Peroutka, *Headache* **30** (Suppl. 2), 554-560 (1990).

mp 169-171°.
Succinate. [103628-48-4] GR-43175C; Imigran; Imitrex; Imiject. $C_{14}H_{21}N_3O_2S.C_4H_6O_4$; mol wt 413.49. mp 165-166°.

THERAP CAT: Antimigraine.

8998. Sumbul. Musk root. Dried rhizome and roots of *Ferula sumbul* (Kauffm.) Hook. f. (*Euryangium sumbul* Kauffm.), or of other closely related species of *Ferula* having a musk-like odor (*Umbelliferae*). Habit. Central Asia, East Indies. Constit. Angelic (sumbulic) acid, valeric acid, methylcrotonic acid, resin, 0.2-0.4% volatile oil.

THERAP CAT: Sedative.

8999. Sunflower Seed Oil. The oil obtained by milling the seeds of *Helianthus annuus* L., *Compositae.* Classified as a semi-drying oil. Alternately classified as an oleic-linoleic acid oil. Produced on a large scale in U.S.S.R., the Baltic region, India, Egypt, Canada, Argentina. Composition: palmitic acid 6.4%, stearic acid 1.3%, arachidic acid 4.0%, behenic acid 0.8%, oleic acid 21.3%, linoleic acid 66.2% (the glycerides in sunflower oil consist mainly of mixed triglycerides, each contg one or two linoleic acid radicals), linolenic acid <0.1%. Vitamin E (mixed tocopherols) 75 mg/100 g. This approaches the tocopherol content of wheat germ oil which is 103 mg/100 g. *Reviews:* E. W. Eckey, *Vegetable Fats and Oils* (Reinhold, New York, 1954) pp 772-777; L. H. Bailey,

Standard Cyclopedia of Horticulture **vol. II** (Macmillan, New York, 1953) pp 1445-1449.

Pale yellow oil. Bland, agreeable taste. d_{15}^{15} 0.922-0.926. d_{25}^{25} 0.915-0.919. mp −18°. Titer: 16-20°. Acid value: 0.6. Saponif value: 188-194. Iodine value: 125-136. Thiocyanogen value: 78. Hydroxyl value: 14-16. Reichert-Meissl value below 0.5. Polenske value below 0.5. Unsaponifiable below 1.5%. n_D^{25} 1.472-1.474. n_D^{40} 1.466-1.468. Slightly sol in alc. Miscible with benzene, chloroform, carbon tetrachloride. Forms a "skin" after exposure to air for 2-3 weeks.

USE: Food and salad oil, in candy manuf, in oleomargarine. Like wheat germ oil in dietary supplements. Industrially in oil-modified alkyd resins and soap manuf.

9000. Sunitinib. [557795-19-4] *N*-[2-(Diethylamino)ethyl]-5-[(Z)-(5-fluoro-1,2-dihydro-2-oxo-3*H*-indol-3-ylidene)methyl]-2,4-dimethyl-1*H*-pyrrole-3-carboxamide; 5-[5-fluoro-2-oxo-1,2-di-hydroindol-(3*Z*)-ylidenemethyl]-2,4-dimethyl-1*H*-pyrrole-3-car-boxylic acid (2-diethylaminoethyl)amide. $C_{22}H_{27}FN_4O_2$; mol wt 398.47. C 66.31%, H 6.83%, F 4.77%, N 14.06%, O 8.03%. Tyrosine kinase inhibitor targeting VEGF-R2, PDGF-Rβ, KIT and FLT3. Prepn: P. C. Tang *et al.,* **WO 0160814** (2001 to Sugen); *eidem,* **US 6573293** (2003 to Sugen; Pharmacia & Upjohn); and kinase inhibition activity: L. Sun *et al., J. Med. Chem.* **46**, 1116 (2003). Pharmacology: D. B. Mendel *et al., Clin. Cancer Res.* **9**, 327 (2003). Clinical pharmacokinetics and evaluation in acute myeloid leukemia: A.-M. O'Farrell *et al., ibid.* 5465. LC-MS-MS determn in biological samples: S. Baratté *et al., J. Chromatogr. A* **1024**, 87 (2004). Formulation development: A. Sistla *et al., Drug Dev. Ind. Pharm.* **30** 19 (2004). Review of development and therapeutic potential: K. M. Sakamoto, *Curr. Opin. Invest. Drugs* **5**, 1329-1339 (2004).

Orange solid. pKa 8.5. Log P (octanol/water): 3.1. Soly at 22° (μg/ml): 2582 in 20mM KCl/HCl buffer (pH 2); 364 in 20 mM phosphate buffer (pH 6).
Maleate. [341031-54-7] SU-11248; Sutent. $C_{22}H_{27}FN_4O_2.$-$C_4H_6O_5$; mol wt 532.56.

THERAP CAT: Antineoplastic.

9001. Sunset Yellow FCF. [2783-94-0] 6-Hydroxy-5-[(4-sulfophenyl)azo]-2-naphthalenesulfonic acid disodium salt; 1-*p*-sul-fophenylazo-2-naphthol-6-sulfonic acid disodium salt; FD & C Yellow No. 6; C.I. Food Yellow 3; C.I. 15985. $C_{16}H_{10}N_2Na_2O_7S_2$; mol wt 452.37. C 42.48%, H 2.23%, N 6.19%, Na 10.16%, O 24.76%, S 14.18%. Prepn: P. Griess, *Ber.* **11**, 2191 (1878). Metabolism: J. L. Radomski, T. J. Mellinger, *J. Pharmacol. Exp. Ther.* **136**, 259 (1962). Toxicology: I. F. Gaunt *et al., Food Cosmet. Toxicol.* **5**, 747 (1967); **7**, 9 (1969); **12**, 1 (1974). *Review: IARC Monographs* **8**, 257-266 (1967). *See also: Colour Index* **vol. 4** (3rd ed., 1971) p 4087.

Orange-red crystals. Absorption max (0.02 *N* CH_3COONH_4): 480 nm. Sol in water; slightly sol in ethanol. Reddish-orange soln in conc H_2SO_4, changing to yellow on dilution. LD_{50} in rats, mice (g/kg): >10, >6 orally (Gaunt, 1967).

USE: Provisionally listed for use in food, drugs and cosmetics.

9002. Superoxide Dismutase. [9054-89-1] SOD. Family of naturally occurring metalloenzymes that act as free oxygen radical scavengers and protect against the deleterious effects of biologically generated superoxide oxygen radicals ($O_2^{\cdot-}$) by dismutation to hydrogen peroxide (H_2O_2) + molecular oxygen (O_2). Three metallotypes have been described; distinguished by the metal found at the active site: cupro-zinc containing (Cu/Zn SOD), manganese containing (Mn SOD), and iron containing (Fe SOD). Widely distributed, present in almost all aerobic organisms and some anaerobes. Isoln and purification of Cu/Zn SOD from bovine erythrocytes and identity with *erythrocuprein (hemocuprein)*: J. M. McCord, I. Fridovich, *J. Biol. Chem.* **244,** 6049 (1969); of Mn SOD from *E. coli:* B. B. Keele *et al., ibid.* **245,** 6176 (1970); of Fe SOD from *E. coli:* F. J. Yost, Jr., I. Fridovich, *ibid.* **248,** 4905 (1973). Enzyme immunoassay for determn of human Cu/Zn SOD: N. Kurobe *et al., Clin. Chim. Acta* **187,** 11 (1990); of human Mn SOD: *idem et al., ibid.* **192,** 171 (1990). Review of biological activity and therapeutic use: A. Petkau, *Cancer Treat. Rev.* **13,** 17-44 (1986); of protective effect vs radiation injury: *eidem, Br. J. Cancer* **55,** Suppl. 8, 87-95 (1987); of structure and function: J. V. Bannister *et al., Crit. Rev. Biochem.* **22,** 111-180 (1987); of chemical and biological characteristics: B. A. Omar *et al., Adv. Pharmacol.* **23,** 109-161 (1992). Books: *Superoxide and Superoxide Dismutases,* A. M. Michelson *et al.,* Eds. (Academic Press, New York, 1977) 568 p.; *Superoxide Dismutase* vols. I, II, III, L. W. Oberley, Ed. (CRC Press, Inc., Boca Raton, 1982, 1982, 1985).

Orgotein. Artrolasi; Ormetein (rescinded); Ontosein; Oxinorm; Palosein; Peroxinorm. Water-soluble Cu/Zn SOD produced from beef liver. Mol wt ~33,000 with a compact conformation maintained by about 4 gram atoms of chelated divalent metal. Isoln: W. Huber, **ZA 6902983**; *idem,* **US 3579495** (1969, 1971 both to Diagnostic Data). Purification: *idem,* **DE 2101866**; *idem,* **US 3624251** (both 1971 to Diagnostic Data). Toxicology: S. Carson *et al., Toxicol. Appl. Pharmacol.* **26,** 184 (1973). Clinical pharmacokinetics: G. Jadot *et al., Clin. Pharmacokinet.* **28,** 17 (1995). Clinical studies in osteoarthritis: K. Lund-Olesen, K. B. Menander-Huber, *Arzneim.-Forsch.* **33,** 1199 (1983); in Peyronie's disease: G. Primus, *Int. Urol. Nephrol.* **25,** 169 (1993). Clinical use of liposomal form vs radiation-induced fibrosis: S. Delanian *et al., Radiother. Oncol.* **32,** 12 (1994). Therapeutic use in animals: D. E. Breshears *et al., Mod. Vet. Pract.* **55,** 85 (1974); S. Ahlengard *et al., Equine Vet. J.* **10,** 122 (1978); J. R. Coffman *et al., J. Am. Vet. Med. Assoc.* **174** 261 (1979). Review of clinical trials: L. Flohé, *Mol. Cell. Biochem.* **84,** 123-131 (1988). LD_{50} in mice (mg/kg): >5800 s.c., >60 i.p., >4000 i.v.; in rats (mg/kg): >400 s.c., >284 i.p. (Jadot).

Pegorgotein. [155773-57-2] PEG-SOD; Win-22118; Dismutec. Orgotein polyethylene glycol conjugate; mol wt 71-105 kDa. Prepn and anti-inflammatory activity: P. S. Pyatak *et al., Res. Commun. Chem. Pathol. Pharmacol.* **29,** 113 (1980). Pharmacokinetics: E. Boccu *et al., Pharmacol. Res. Commun.* **14,** 113 (1982). Toxicology: A. T. Viau *et al., J. Free Radicals Biol. Med.* **2,** 283 (1986). Clinical trials in head injury: J. P. Muizelaar, *Adv. Exp. Med. Biol.* **366,** 389 (1994).

Recombinant human form. RhSOD. Pharmacokinetics: C. Tsao *et al., Clin. Pharmacol. Ther.* **50,** 713 (1991). Clinical study in renal transplantation: W. Land *et al., Transplantation* **57,** 211 (1994). Review of cloning and expression: D. Tuoati, *Free Radical Biol. Med.* **5,** 393-402 (1988).

USE: Research probe for O_2^- in biological and chemical reactions.

THERAP CAT: Anti-inflammatory; radioprotective agent.

THERAP CAT (VET): Anti-inflammatory; antirheumatic.

9003. Suplatast Tosylate. [94055-76-2] [3-[[4-(3-Ethoxy-2-hydroxypropoxy)phenyl]amino]-3-oxopropyl]dimethylsulfonium salt with 4-methylbenzenesulfonic acid; (±)-[2-[[*p*-(3-ethoxy-2-hydroxypropoxy)phenyl]carbamoyl]ethyl]dimethylsulfonium *p*-toluenesulfonate; IPD-1151T; IPD. $C_{16}H_{26}NO_4S \cdot C_7H_7O_3S$; mol wt 499.64. C 55.29%, H 6.66%, N 2.80%, O 22.42%, S 12.84%. Selective inhibitor of the IgE antibody response; inhibits interleukin-4 gene expression and mast cell differentiation. Prepn: A. Koda *et al.,* **DE 3408708**; *eidem,* **US 4556737** (1984, 1985 both to Taiho). Suppression of IL-4 production and the IgE response: Y. Yanagihara *et al., Jpn. J. Pharmacol.* **61,** 23, 31 (1993). Effect on mast cell differentiation: S. Konno *et al., Eur. J. Pharmacol.* **259,**

15 (1994). Series of articles on toxicology: *J. Toxicol. Sci.* **17,** Suppl. 2, 1-205, (1992); *C.A.* **117,** 103839-103846; 103995 (1992). Acute toxicity: K. Yamishita *et al., ibid.* 1. Clinical evaluation in asthma: J. Tamaoki *et al., Lancet* **356,** 273 (2000).

Crystals, mp 70-73°. LD_{50} in male, female mice, male, female rats (mg/kg): 81, 96, 96, 93 i.v.; in mice, rats (g/kg): >12.5, >10 orally (Yamashita).

THERAP CAT: Antiallergic; antiasthmatic.

9004. Suprasterol II. [562-71-0] (2α,7α,8R,19α,22E)-7,19:8,19-Dicyclo-9,10-secoergosta-5(10),22-dien-2-ol. $C_{28}H_{44}O$; mol wt 396.65. C 84.78%, H 11.18%, O 4.03%. Ultraviolet irradiation product of vitamin D_2. Isoln: Windaus *et al., Ann.* **483,** 17 (1930). Structure and stereochemistry: Dauben, Baumann, *Tetrahedron Lett.* **1961,** 565. Crystal structure: C. P. Saunderson *et al., ibid.* 573. Improved isoln and spectral data: T. Kobayashi *et al., J. Nutr. Sci. Vitaminol.* **23,** 291 (1977).

Rough prisms from acetone or methanol, mp 110°. $bp_{0.005}$ 190°. $[\alpha]_D^{19}$ +62.9° (methanol); $[\alpha]_D^{22}$ +47.8° (methanol). Sol in all organic solvents.

9005. Suprofen. [40828-46-4] α-Methyl-4-(2-thienylcarbonyl)benzeneacetic acid; *p*-(2-thenoyl)hydratropic acid; sutoprofen; R-25061; Masterfen; Srendam; Sulprotin; Supranol; Suprocil; Suprol; Topalgic. $C_{14}H_{12}O_3S$; mol wt 260.31. C 64.60%, H 4.65%, O 18.44%, S 12.32%. Prostaglandin biosynthesis inhibitor. Prepn: P. A. Janssen *et al.,* **DE 2353357**; *eidem,* **US 4035376** (1974, 1977 both to Janssen); P. G. H. Van Daele *et al., Arzneim.-Forsch.* **25,** 1495 (1975). Pharmacology: C. J. E. Niemegeers *et al., ibid.,* 1537. HPLC determn in plasma and urine: H. Muller *et al., ibid.* **32,** 257 (1982). Series of articles on pharmacology, toxicology and clinical trials: *ibid.* **25,** 1501-1542 (1975); *ibid.* **33,** 1322-1338 (1983); on pharmacology, efficacy and safety: *Pharmacology* **27,** Suppl. 1, 1-96 (1983); on pharmacokinetics and clinical efficacy: *Arzneim.-Forsch.* **35,** 738-759 (1985); *ibid.* **36,** 941-971 (1986).

White to slightly yellow microcryst powder, mp 124.3°. pKa 3.91. uv max (0.01*N* HCl-90% 2-propanol): 266, 292 nm (ε 15700, 15600). Freely sol in methanol, ethanol, chloroform, acetone, polyethylene glycol, 1.0*N* NaOH. Sol in ether. Slightly sol in 0.1*N* NaOH. Practically insol in *n*-hexane. Very slightly sol in water. LD_{50} (7 days post-drug) in mice, rats, guinea pigs, dogs (mg/kg): 590, 353, 280, 160 orally (Niemegeers).

THERAP CAT: Anti-inflammatory; analgesic.

9006. Suramin Sodium. [129-46-4] 8,8'-[Carbonylbis[imino-3,1-phenylenecarbonylimino(4-methyl-3,1-phenylene)carbonylimino]]bis-1,3,5-naphthalenetrisulfonic acid hexasodium salt; hexasodium *sym*-bis(*m*-aminobenzoyl-*m*-amino-*p*-methylbenzoyl-1-naphthylamino-4,6,8-trisulfonate) carbamide; Bayer 205; Fourneau 309; Antrypol; Germanin; Moranyl; Naganol; Naphuride. $C_{51}H_{34}$-$N_6Na_6O_{23}S_6$; mol wt 1429.17. C 42.86%, H 2.40%, N 5.88%, Na 9.65%, O 25.75%, S 13.46%. Discovered in 1917 by O. Dressel and R. Kothe: J. Dressel, *J. Chem. Educ.* **38**, 620 (1961). Prepn: E. Fourneau *et al., Compt. Rend.* **178**, 675 (1924); J. Trefouel, E. Fourneau, **GB 224849** (1923); B. Heymann, *Angew. Chem.* **37**, 585 (1924). Pharmacology, toxicology and clinical antiparasitic activity: F. Hawking, *Adv. Pharmacol. Chemother.* **15**, 289-322 (1978). Inhibition of reverse transcriptase *in vitro*: E. De Clercq, *Cancer Lett.* **8**, 9 (1979); vs HIV: H. Mitsuya *et al., Science* **226**, 172 (1984). HPLC determn in plasma: R. W. Klecker, J. M. Collins, *J. Liq. Chromatogr.* **8**, 1685 (1985). Pharmacokinetics: J. M. Collins *et al., J. Clin. Pharmacol.* **26**, 22 (1986). Pharmacology and virustatic effect in AIDS: S. Broder *et al., Lancet* **2**, 627 (1985); A. M. Levine *et al., Ann. Intern. Med.* **105**, 32 (1986). Clinical trial in onchocerciasis: H. Schultz-Key *et al., Trop. Med. Parasitol.* **36**, 244 (1985); in prostate cancer: C. Myers *et al., J. Clin. Oncol.* **10**, 881 (1992). *Review:* Olenick in *Antibiotics* vol. 3, J. W. Corcoran, F. E. Hahn, Eds. (Springer-Verlag, New York, 1975) pp 699-703; R. La Rocca *et al., Cancer Cells* **2**, 106-115 (1990).

White or slightly pink or cream-colored powder. Slightly saline taste. Hygroscopic. Freely sol in water, in physiological saline; sparingly sol in 95% alcohol. Insol in benzene, ether, petr ether, chloroform. Aq solns are neutral to litmus. LD_{50} in mice (mg/kg): ~620 i.v. (Hawking).

THERAP CAT: Anthelmintic (Nematodes); antiprotozoal (Trypanosoma).

THERAP CAT (VET): Antiprotozoal (Trypanosoma).

9007. Surinamine. [537-49-5] *N*-Methyl-L-tyrosine; andirine; angeline; geoffroyine; ratanhine. $C_{10}H_{13}NO_3$; mol wt 195.22. C 61.52%, H 6.71%, N 7.17%, O 24.59%. Isoln from bark of *Andira retusa* Kunth. (*Geoffroya retusa* Lam.), *Leguminosae:* Hiller-Bombein, *Arch. Pharm.* **230**, 513 (1892). Prepn of inactive compd: Kanevskaya, *J. Prakt. Chem.* **124**, 48 (1929). Prepn of L-form: Kanao, *J. Pharm. Soc. Jpn.* **66**, 4 (1946); Huguenin, Boissonnas, *Helv. Chim. Acta* **44**, 213 (1961). Prepn of D-form: Izumiya, Nagamatsu, *Bull. Chem. Soc. Jpn.* **25**, 265 (1952).

Crystals, mp 292-295°. $[\alpha]_D^{21}$ +19.6° (c = 3.8 in 10% HCl). Almost insol in water. Slightly sol in alcohol; sol in dil acids.

D-Form. Crystals, mp 273-274°. $[\alpha]_D^{15}$ −18.9° (c = 1.74 in 3*N* HCl).

DL-Form. Crystals from water.

9008. Survivin. Mammalian apoptosis inhibitor; member of the IAP (inhibitor of apoptosis protein) family. Selectively overexpressed in common human cancers and correlates with unfavorable prognosis. Also present in embryonic cells but not detectable in normal differentiated tissues. Cytoplasmic, 142 residue protein; mol wt 16.5 kDa. Expressed during mitosis in a cell cycle-dependent manner and localized to the mitotic spindle. Identification in human cancers: G. Ambrosini *et al., Nat. Med.* **3**, 917 (1997).

Developmentally regulated expression in fetal tissue: C. Adida *et al., Am. J. Pathol.* **152**, 43 (1998). Mechanism of action study: F. Li *et al., Nature* **396**, 580 (1998). Crystal structure of murine: S. W. Muchmore *et al., Mol. Cell* **6**, 173 (2000); of human: L. Chantalat *et al., ibid.* 183; M. A. Verdecia *et al., Nat. Struct. Biol.* **7**, 602 (2000). Determn in urine and clinical use in diagnosis of bladder cancer: S. D. Smith *et al., J. Am. Med. Assoc.* **285**, 324 (2001).

9009. Suxibuzone. [27470-51-5] Butanedioic acid mono-[(4-butyl-3,5-dioxo-1,2-diphenyl-4-pyrazolidinyl)methyl] ester; succinic acid monoester with 4-butyl-4-(hydroxymethyl)-1,2-diphenyl-3,5-pyrazolidinedione; 4-butyl-4-(hydroxymethyl)-1,2-diphenyl-3,5-pyrazolidinedione hydrogen succinate (ester); 1,2-diphenyl-4-*n*-butyl-4-hydroxymethyl-3,5-dioxopyrazolidine hemisuccinate; 4-hydroxymethylbutazolidine hemisuccinate; AE-17; Calibène; Danilon; Flogos; Solurol. $C_{24}H_{26}N_2O_6$; mol wt 438.47. C 65.74%, H 5.98%, N 6.39%, O 21.89%. Prodrug of phenylbutazone, *q.v.* Prepd (not claimed) and use as anti-inflammatory: A. Esteve, **DE 1936747**; *idem,* **US 3752894** (1970, 1973 both to Lab. Esteve). Pharmacology: A. Esteve *et al., Quim. Ind. (Madrid)* **17**, 107 (1971). HPLC determn in plasma and urine: T. Marunaka *et al., J. Pharm. Sci.* **69**, 1258 (1980). Metabolism in humans: Y. Yasuda *et al., ibid.* **71**, 565 (1982). Comparative clinical study with phenylbutazone in rheumatoid arthritis: Y. Mizushima *et al., Int. J. Tissue React.* **5**, 35 (1983).

White, bitter crystalline powder from alcohol, mp 126-127°. Sol in most organic solvents. Insol in water. LD_{50} orally in mice: 5.683 micromol/kg (Esteve, 1973).

THERAP CAT: Anti-inflammatory.

THERAP CAT (VET): Analgesic, antipyretic, anti-inflammatory.

9010. Swertiamarin. [17388-39-5] [4a*R*-(4aα,5β,6α)]-5-Ethenyl-6-(β-D-glucopyranosyloxy)-4,4a,5,6-tetrahydro-4a-hydroxy-1*H*,3*H*-pyrano[3,4-*c*]pyran-1-one; 4,4a,5,6-tetrahydro-4aα-hydroxy-1-oxo-5β-vinyl-1*H*,3*H*-pyrano[3,4-*c*]pyran-6-yl β-D-glucopyranoside. $C_{16}H_{22}O_{10}$; mol wt 374.34. C 51.34%, H 5.92%, O 42.74%. Bitter principle of *Swertia japonica* (Maxim.) Makino, *Gentianaceae.* Yields erythrocentaurin on hydrolysis with emulsin. Isoln: Kubota, Tomita, *Chem. Ind. (London)* **1958**, 229; Inouye *et al., Chem. Pharm. Bull.* **18**, 1856 (1970). Occurrence in gentianaceous plants: Inouye, Nakamura, *J. Pharm. Sci. Japan* **91**, 755 (1971), *C.A.* **75**, 95431b (1971). Structure: Kubota, Tomita, *Tetrahedron Lett.* **1961**, 176; *Bull. Chem. Soc. Jpn.* **34**, 1345 (1961); Koch *et al., Bull. Soc. Chim. Fr.* **1964**, 405. Stereochemistry: Inouye *et al., Tetrahedron Lett.* **1968**, 4429. Biosynthesis studies: Inouye *et al., Chem. Pharm. Bull.* **18**, 2043 (1970).

Plates from ethanol + chloroform + ether, mp 113-114°. $[\alpha]_D^{20}$ −127° (c = 1 in 96% ethanol). uv max (methanol): 238 nm (log ε 3.93).

Tetraacetate. $C_{24}H_{30}O_{14}$. Prisms, mp 190-191°. $[\alpha]_D$ −100.3° (CHCl₃). uv max: 206, 234 nm (log ε 3.20, 4.00).

9011. Sydnones. [50927-09-8] A term originally applied to the compd obtained by action of acetic anhydride on *N*-nitrosophenylglycine: Eade, Earl, *J. Chem. Soc.* **1946**, 591; Earl, *Chem.*

Ind. (London) **1953,** 746. Sydnones are 5-membered heterocyclic mesoionic compounds that are best represented by polar resonance structures: W. Baker, W. D. Ollis, *Q. Rev. Chem. Soc.* **11,** 15 (1957); Y. Noel, *Bull. Soc. Chim. Fr.* **1964,** 173. Photochromic properties: S. Nespurek, M. Sorm, *Collect. Czech. Chem. Commun.* **42,** 811 (1977). ^{14}N-NMR study: L. Stefaniak, *Tetrahedron* **33,** 2571 (1977). ^{15}N-NMR study: L. Stefaniak *et al., Org. Magn. Reson.* **13,** 274 (1980). Regioselectivity study: A. Padwa *et al., J. Org. Chem.* **47,** 786 (1982). Review of chemistry: F. H. C. Stewart, *Chem. Rev.* **64,** 129-147 (1964).

9012. Synephrine. [94-07-5] 4-Hydroxy-α-[(methylamino)methyl]benzenemethanol; *p*-hydroxy-α-[(methylamino)methyl]benzyl alcohol; 1-(4-hydroxyphenyl)-2-methylaminoethanol; *p*-methylaminoethanolphenol; β-methylamino-α-(4-hydroxyphenyl)-ethyl alcohol; methylaminomethyl 4-hydroxyphenyl carbinol; Analeptin; Ethaphene; Oxedrine; Parasympatol; Simpalon; Synephrin; Synthenate. $C_9H_{13}NO_2$; mol wt 167.21. C 64.65%, H 7.84%, N 8.38%, O 19.14%. Prepd by hydrogenating ω-methylamino-4-hydroxyacetophenone in water in the presence of Pt or Pd: **DE 566578** (1931 to Boehringer, Ing.), *Frdl.* **18,** 3025.

Crystals, mp 184-185°. Stable to air and light.

Hydrochloride. [5985-28-4] $C_9H_{13}NO_2$.HCl. Crystals, mp 151-152°. Freely sol in water.

Tartrate. [16589-24-5] Corvasymton; Simpadren; Sympathol. $2C_9H_{13}NO_2.C_4H_6O_6$; mol wt 484.50. Crystals, mp 188-190° (some dec). Freely sol in water; sol in alcohol.

Tartaric acid monoester. [6414-49-9] *p*-Methylaminoethanolphenol tartrate; Neupentedrin; Pentedrin. $C_{13}H_{17}NO_7$; mol wt 299.28.

THERAP CAT: Adrenergic; vasopressor.

9013. Synhexyl. [117-51-1] 3-Hexyl-7,8,9,10-tetrahydro-6,6,9-trimethyl-6*H*-dibenzo[*b,d*]pyran-1-ol; 1-hydroxy-3-hexyl-6,6,9-trimethyl-7,8,9,10-tetrahydro-6*H*-dibenzo[*b,d*]pyran; parahexyl; pyrahexyl. $C_{22}H_{32}O_2$; mol wt 328.49. C 80.44%, H 9.82%, O 9.74%. Psychotomimetic synthetic analog of the tetrahydrocannabinols, *q.v.* Prepn: Adams *et al., J. Am. Chem. Soc.* **63,** 1971 (1941); Adams, **US 2419935** (1947); Hughes *et al.,* **US 3576887** (1971 to Am. Home Products). Comparison of physiological effects with those of tetrahydrocannabinol: Hollister *et al., Clin. Pharmacol. Ther.* **9,** 783 (1968). Physical constants: Farmilo *et al., Bull. Narc.* **6,** 7 (1954). Toxicity data: Loewe, *J. Pharmacol. Exp. Ther.* **88,** 154 (1946).

Liquid, $bp_{1.0}$ 190-192°; n_D^{20} 1.5504. uv and ir spectra: *Bull. Narc.* **6,** 27 (1954); **7,** 42 (1955). LD_{50} in mice, dogs, rabbits (mg/kg): 170, 223, 143 i.v. (Loewe).

Note: This is a controlled substance (hallucinogen): **21 CFR,** 1308.11.

9014. Synsorbs. [83382-98-3] Synthetic mimics of toxin receptor binding sites consisting of a trisaccharide covalently coupled via an 8-methoxycarbonyloctyl linker to **Chromosorb® P,** a commercially available SiO_2-based column matrix. Preparative methods for trisaccharides and linkers: R. U. Lemieux *et al., J. Am. Chem. Soc.* **97,** 4076 (1975); D. D. Cox *et al., Carbohydr. Res.* **63,** 139 (1978); P. J. Garegg, S. Oscarson, *ibid.* **136,** 207 (1985).

Synsorb Pk. [192230-81-2] Synthetic analog of the *E. coli* shigatoxin (verotoxin) receptor. Trisaccharide component is αGal(1 → 4)βGal(1 → 4)βGlc. Characterization of specificity: G. D. Armstrong *et al., J. Infect. Dis.* **164,** 1160 (1991). Binding affinity: T. Takeda *et al., Microbiol. Immunol.* **43,** 331 (1999). Clinical pharmacokinetics: G. D. Armstrong *et al. J. Infect. Dis.* **171,** 1042 (1995). Review of clinical experience: *idem et al.,* in *Escherichia coli O157:H7 and Other Shiga Toxin-Producing E. coli Strains,* J. B. Kaper, A. D. O'Brien, Eds. (American Society for Microbiology, Washington D.C., 1998) pp 374-384.

Synsorb CD. Synsorb 90. Synthetic analog of the *Clostridium difficile* toxin A receptor. Trisaccharide component is αGal(1 → 3)βGal(1 → 4)βGlc. Characterization of specificity: L. D. Heerze *et al., J. Infect. Dis.* **169,** 1291 (1994); I. Castagliuolo *et al., Gastroenterology* **111,** 433 (1996).

THERAP CAT: Synsorb Pk in the treatment of verotoxigenic *E. coli* gastroenteritis; Synsorb CD in the treatment of *Clostridium difficile* associated disease.

9015. Syringaldehyde. [134-96-3] 4-Hydroxy-3,5-dimethoxybenzaldehyde; syringic aldehyde; 3,5-dimethoxy-4-hydroxybenzene carbonal; gallaldehyde 3,5-dimethyl ether. $C_9H_{10}O_4$; mol wt 182.17. C 59.34%, H 5.53%, O 35.13%. Widely distributed in plants. Hydrolysis product of the naturally occurring glycosyringic aldehyde: Körner, *Gazz. Chim. Ital.* **18,** 215 (1888). Prepn from heat-treated beechwood and lignin: Kratzl, Silbernagel, *C.A.* **50,** 6040 (1956). Synthesis from pyrogallol 1,3-dimethyl ether: Pearl, *J. Am. Chem. Soc.* **70,** 1746 (1948), *cf.* Graebe, Martz, *Ber.* **36,** 1032 (1903); Allen, Leubner, *Org. Synth.* **31,** 92 (1951); **coll. vol. IV,** 866 (1963).

Very pale yellow needles from petr ether, mp 113°. bp_{14} 192-193°. uv max (dioxane): 305 nm. Very sparingly sol in water, petr ether. Sol in alcohol, ether, chloroform, hot benzene, glacial acetic acid. Forms yellow sodium and potassium salts.

9016. Syringin. [118-34-3] (*E*)-4-(3-Hydroxy-1-propenyl)-2,6-dimethoxyphenyl-β-D-glucopyranoside; 4-(3-hydroxypropen-yl)-2,6-dimethoxyphenyl-D-glucoside; syringoside; ligustrin; lilacin; methoxyconiferine. $C_{17}H_{24}O_9$; mol wt 372.37. C 54.83%, H 6.50%, O 38.67%. First isolated by Meillet in 1841 from bark of *Syringa vulgaris* L. (lilac): *Ann.* **40,** 319 (1841). Prepn: Pauly, Strassberger, *Ber.* **62,** 2277 (1929); Freudenberg, Schraube, *Ber.* **86,** 16 (1955). Isoln from lilac bark: Freudenberg *et al., Ber.* **84,** 472 (1951); from various plants: Plouvier, *Compt. Rend.* **254,** 4196 (1962); from cambial sap of spruce: Freudenberg, Harkin, *Phytochemistry* **2,** 189 (1963).

Monohydrate. Crystals from water, mp 192°. $[\alpha]_D^{20}$ −8.2° (c = 2.43 in chloroform), −17.25° (water). Slightly sol in cold water; sol in hot water, alc. Practically insol in ether.

9017.   Syrosingopine. [84-36-6] 18-[[4-[(Ethoxycarbonyl)-oxy]-3,5-dimethoxybenzoyl]oxy]-11,17-dimethoxyyohimban-16-carboxylic acid methyl ester; methyl carbethoxysyringoyl reserpate; carbethoxysyringoyl methyl reserpate; methyl *O*-(*O'*-carbethoxy-syringoyl)reserpate; syringopine; Su-3118; Isotense; Londomin; Raunova; Seniramin; Siringina. $C_{35}H_{42}N_2O_{11}$; mol wt 666.71. C 63.05%, H 6.35%, N 4.20%, O 26.40%. Prepn: Lucas *et al.*, *J. Am. Chem. Soc.* **81**, 1928 (1959); US 2813871 (1957 to Ciba).

Crystals from acetone, mp 175-179°.
THERAP CAT: Antihypertensive.

9018.   Systemin. [137181-56-7] L-Alanyl-L-valyl-L-gluta-minyl-L-seryl-L-lysyl-L-prolyl-L-prolyl-L-seryl-L-lysyl-L-argininyl-L-α-aspartyl-L-prolyl-L-prolyl-L-lysyl-L-methionyl-L-glutaminyl-L-threonyl-L-aspartic acid. First known polypeptide signal in plants. Systemically induces plant defenses in response to wounding of leaves by insects or pathogens. Proline-rich palindromic structure. Identification of activity: C. A. Ryan, *Plant Physiol.* **54**, 328 (1974). Isolation from tomato leaves and characterization: G. Pearce *et al.*, *Science* **253**, 895 (1991). Purification by capillary electrophoresis: P. Mucha *et al.*, *J. Chromatogr. A* **734**, 410 (1996). Proton NMR assignments: D. J. Russell *et al.*, *J. Protein Chem.* **11**, 265 (1992). Structure-activity: T. Meindl *et al.*, *Plant Cell* **10**, 1561 (1998). Tertiary structure and mechanism of action: T. Specht *et al.*, *Plants Proteins Eur. Crops* **1998**, 41. *Review:* C. A. Ryan, G. Pearce, *Annu. Rev. Cell Dev. Biol.* **14**, 1-17 (1998).

Ala–Val–Gln–Ser–Lys–Pro–Pro–Ser–Lys–Arg–Asp–Pro–Pro–Lys–Met–Gln–Thr–Asp

Insol in lipid solvents.
USE: Wound hormone in plants.

T

9019. 2,4,5-T. [93-76-5] (2,4,5-Trichlorophenoxy)acetic acid; Esteron 245; Trioxone. $C_8H_5Cl_3O_3$; mol wt 255.48. C 37.61%, H 1.97%, Cl 41.63%, O 18.79%. Post-emergence herbicide. Prepd from 2,4,5-trichlorophenol: Pokorny, *J. Am. Chem. Soc.* **63**, 1768 (1941); from benzenehexachloride: Galat, *ibid.* **74**, 3890 (1952). Activity: C. L. Hamner, T. B. Tukey, *Science* **100**, 154 (1944). Contains trace levels of TCDD, *q.v.*, as a contaminant: J. Smith, *Science* **203**, 1090 (1979); *Chem. Eng. News* **59**, 6 (Jan. 5, 1981). Toxicity: V. A. Rowe, T. A. Hymas, *Am. J. Vet. Res.* **15**, 622 (1954). *See also* 2,4-D.

Crystals from benzene, mp 153°. d_{20}^{20} 1.80. Soly in water at 30°: 238 mg/kg. Sol in alcohol. Forms water-soluble sodium and alkanolamine salts. Commercial products are usually in the form of amines or esters, often in mixture with 2,4-D. LD_{50} orally in mice, rats: 389, 500 mg/kg (Rowe, Hymas).

Caution: Potential symptoms of overexposure in exptl animals are ataxia; skin irritation, acne-like rash; liver damage. *See NIOSH Pocket Guide to Chemical Hazards* (DHHS/NIOSH 97-140, 1997) p 292.

Note: In March 1985 the E.P.A. terminated all registrations for the use of this herbicide on rice fields, orchards, sugarcane, rangeland and other noncrop sites. This follows the 1970 action of the Department of Agriculture halting the use of the pesticide on all food crops except rice: *Chem. Eng. News* **63**, 6 (Mar. 25, 1985).

USE: Formerly as herbicide.

9020. Tabernanthine. [83-94-3] 13-Methoxyibogamine. $C_{20}H_{26}N_2O$; mol wt 310.43. C 77.38%, H 8.44%, N 9.02%, O 5.15%. Indole alkaloid isolated from root of *Tabernanthe iboga* Baill., *Apocynaceae*: Delourme-Houdé, *Ann. Pharm. Fr.* **4**, 30 (1946); Dickel *et al.*, *J. Am. Chem. Soc.* **80**, 123 (1958). Also in *Tabernaemontana* and *Stemmadenia* spp.; usually found in ibogaine mother liquors: Walls *et al.*, *Tetrahedron* **2**, 173 (1958). Isoln from genus *Conopharingia*, *Apocynaceae*: Renner, Prins, US 3008954 (1961) to Geigy. Structure: Bartlett *et al.*, *J. Am. Chem. Soc.* **80**, 126 (1958). Mass spectrum: Biemann, Friedmann-Spiteller, *ibid.* **83**, 4805 (1961). Derivs: Taylor, US 2877229 (1959 to Ciba). Interaction with benzodiazepine receptors: J.-H. Trouvin *et al.*, *Eur. J. Pharmacol.* **140**, 303 (1987).

Needles or shiny leaflets from ethanol, mp 213.5-215°. Sublimes at 160° (0.005 mm pressure). $[\alpha]_D^{20}$ −40° (acetone). pKa 6.04 in 80% methylcellosolve. uv max (ethanol): 228, 271, 299 nm (log ε 4.53, 3.64, 3.77). Sol in alcohol, benzene, ether, chloroform. Practically insol in water.

Hydrochloride. $C_{20}H_{26}N_2O.HCl$. Crystals from water, dec 275-277°. $[\alpha]_D^{25}$ −66° (methanol, Dickel, *loc. cit.*); mp 210°, $[\alpha]_D^{20}$ −76.5° (methanol, Delourme-Houdé). Sol in water. More sol in chloroform than ibogaine hydrochloride.

9021. Tabun. [77-81-6] Dimethylphosphoramidocyanidic acid, ethyl ester; ethyl *N*-dimethylphosphoramidocyanidate; dimethylamidoethoxyphosphoryl cyanide; GA. $C_5H_{11}N_2O_2P$; mol wt 162.13. C 37.04%, H 6.84%, N 17.28%, O 19.74%, P 19.10%. Nerve gas; potent cholinesterase inhibitor similar in structure and activity to sarin and soman, *q.q.v.* Prepd from dimethylamidophosphoryl dichloride and sodium cyanide in the presence of ethanol:

Holmstedt, *Acta Physiol. Scand.* **25**, Suppl. 90, 26 (1951). Synthesis of dimethylamidophosphoryl dichloride: Michaelis, *Ann.* **326**, 129 (1903). Alternate synthetic route: B. C. Saunders, *Some Aspects of the Chemistry and Toxic Action of Organic Compounds Containing Phosphorus and Fluorine* (Cambridge, 1957) p 91. Toxicity study: B. Holmstedt, *Pharmacol. Rev.* **11**, 567 (1959). Brief review: Schrader, *Die Entwicklung neuer insektizider Phosphorsäure-Ester* (Verlag Chemie, Weinheim, 1963) p 3; B. L. Harris in *Kirk-Othmer Encyclopedia of Chemical Technology* vol. **5** (Wiley-Interscience, New York, 4th ed., 1993) pp 795-816.

Liquid. Fruity odor reminiscent of bitter almonds. d 1.077. mp −50°. bp760 240°; bp10 120°; bp9 100-108°. n_D^{20} 1.4250. IR absorption: *Acta Chem. Scand.* **5**, 1179 (1951). Readily sol in organic solvents. Miscible with water, but quickly hydrolyzed. Destroyed by bleaching powder (chlorinated lime), but gives rise to cyanogen chloride. *Extremely poisonous!* LD_{50} i.p. in mice: 0.6 mg/kg (Holmstedt).

Caution: Potential symptoms of overexposure by inhalation are constriction of pupils of the eye, difficulty breathing followed by bronchial constriction, convulsions, death. Also toxic due to absorption through skin and eyes. *See Chem. Eng. News* **31**, 4676 (1953).

USE: Chemical warfare agent.

9022. Tacalcitol. [57333-96-7] (1α,3β,5Z,7E,24R)-9,10-Secocholesta-5,7,10(19)-triene-1,3,24-triol; 1α,24(R)-dihydroxycholecalciferol; 1α,24R-dihydroxyvitamin D_3; TV-02; Bonealfa; Curatoderm. $C_{27}H_{44}O_3$; mol wt 416.64. C 77.83%, H 10.64%, O 11.52%. Bioactive, synthetic vitamin D_3 analog; exhibits antiproliferative effect on keratinocytes. Prepn: T. Takeshita *et al.*, **DE 2526981**; *eidem*, **US 4022891** (1976, 1977 both to Teijin); M. Morisaki *et al.*, *J. Chem. Soc. Perkin Trans. 1* **1975**, 1421; K. Ochi *et al.*, *ibid.* **1979**, 165. Pharmacology: T. Matsunaga *et al.*, *J. Dermatol.* **17**, 135 (1990). Clinical evaluation in psoriasis: M. J. P. Gerritsen *et al.*, *Br. J. Dermatol.* **131**, 57 (1994). *Review:* M. Nishimura *et al.*, *Eur. J. Dermatol.* **3**, 255-261 (1993).

White solid. uv max (ethanol): 265 nm.
THERAP CAT: Antipsoriatic.

9023. Tachysterol. [115-61-7] (3β,6E,22E)-9,10-Secoergosta-5(10),6,8,22-tetraen-3-ol. $C_{28}H_{44}O$; mol wt 396.65. C 84.78%, H 11.18%, O 4.03%. From ergosterol or lumisterol by ultraviolet irradiation: Windaus *et al.*, *Ann.* **492**, 226 (1932); *Ann.* **499**, 188 (1932); Dimroth, *Ber.* **70**, 1631 (1937). From calciferol by adsorption on acid clay: Thibaudet, *Compt. Rend.* **220**, 751 (1945). From precalciferol: Velluz, Goffinet, US 2847426 (1958 to UCLAF). Structure: Grundmann, *Z. Physiol. Chem.* **252**, 151 (1938); Thibaudet, *loc. cit.* Stereochemistry of the tachysterol system: Inhoffen, *Ber.* **88**, 1424 (1955); Verloop, *Rec. Trav. Chim.* **76**, 689 (1957); Delaroff *et al.*, *Bull. Soc. Chim. Fr.* **1963**, 1739.

Oil. $[\alpha]_D^{18}$ −70° (24.6 mg in 2 ml petr ether); $[\alpha]_{546}^{18}$ −86.3° (petr ether). uv max: 280 nm. Not pptd by digitonin. Insol in water. Sol in organic solvents, but not in methanol. Very easily oxidized by air.

4-Methyl-3,5-dinitrobenzoate. $C_{36}H_{48}N_2O_6$. Pale yellow crystals, mp 155°.

Dihydro derivative see Dihydrotachysterol.

9024. Tacrine. [321-64-2] 1,2,3,4-Tetrahydro-9-acridinamine; 9-amino-1,2,3,4-tetrahydroacridine; 5-amino-1,2,3,4-tetrahydroacridine; 1,2,3,4-tetrahydro-5-aminoacridine. $C_{13}H_{14}N_2$; mol wt 198.26. C 78.75%, H 7.12%, N 14.13%. Centrally active anticholinesterase; cognition enhancer. Prepn: Braun et al., Ber. **64**, 227 (1931); Albert, Gledhill, J. Soc. Chem. Ind. **64**, 169T (1945); Petrow, J. Chem. Soc. **1947**, 634; J. A. Moore, L. D. Kornreich, Tetrahedron Lett. **4**, 1277 (1963). Pharmacology and toxicity: S. Gershon, F. H. Shaw, J. Pharm. Pharmacol. **10**, 638 (1958). Enzyme inhibiting activity: P. N. Kaul, ibid. **14**, 243 (1962). Neuropharmacology: B. Drukarch et al., Life Sci. **42**, 1011 (1988). Spectrofluorimetric determn in serum: I. Aparico et al., Analyst **123**, 1575 (1998). Clinical trial in severe Alzheimer's disease: W. K. Summers et al., N. Engl. J. Med. **315**, 1241 (1986). See also: ibid. **316**, 1603-1606. Clinical evaluation of reduced mortality in dementia: B. R. Ott, K. L. Lapane, J. Am. Geriatr. Soc. **50**, 35 (2002). Review of pharmacology and clinical uses: W. K. Summers et al., Clin. Toxicol. **16**, 269-281 (1980); of cholinesterase inhibition in Alzheimer's disease: N. Qizilbash et al., J. Am. Med. Assoc. **280**, 1777-1782 (1998).

Octahedra from very dil alc, mp 183-184°.

Hydrochloride. [1684-40-8] Cognex; THA. $C_{13}H_{14}N_2 \cdot HCl$; mol wt 234.72. Yellow needles from concd hydrochloric acid, mp 283-284°. Bitter taste. Sol in water. pH of 1.5% soln: 4.5-6. uv max (acetate buffer, pH 1-7): 242 nm. Emission max: 362 nm.

THERAP CAT: Nootropic. Antidote to curare. Respiratory stimulant.

9025. Tacrolimus. [104987-11-3] (3S,4R,5S,8R,9E,12S,-14S,15R,16S,18R,19R,26aS)-5,6,8,11,12,13,14,15,16,17,18,19,24,-25,26,26a-Hexadecahydro-5,19-dihydroxy-3-[(1E)-2-[(1R,3R,4R)-4-hydroxy-3-methoxycyclohexyl]-1-methylethenyl]-14,16-dimethoxy-4,10,12,18-tetramethyl-8-(2-propenyl)-15,19-epoxy-3H-pyrido[2,1-c][1,4]oxaazacyclotricosine-1,7,20,21(4H,23H)-tetrone; 17-allyl-1,14-dihydroxy-12-[2-(4-hydroxy-3-methoxycyclohexyl)-1-methylvinyl]-23,25-dimethoxy-13,19,21,27-tetramethyl-11,28-dioxa-4-azatricyclo[22.3.1.0^{4,9}]octacos-18-ene-2,3,10,16-tetraone. $C_{44}H_{69}NO_{12}$; mol wt 804.02. C 65.73%, H 8.65%, N 1.74%, O 23.88%. Macrolide isolated from Streptomyces tsukubaensis no. 9993: M. Okuhara et al., EP 184162 (1986 to Fujisawa); and

characterization: T. Kino et al., J. Antibiot. **40**, 1249 (1987). Structure determn: H. Tanaka et al., J. Am. Chem. Soc. **109**, 5031 (1987). Total synthesis of (−)-form: T. K. Jones et al., J. Am. Chem. Soc. **111**, 1157 (1989). In vitro immunosuppressant activity in comparison with cyclosporin, q.v.: T. Kino et al., J. Antibiot. **40**, 1256 (1987). Toxicology: K. Ohara et al., Transplant. Proc. **22**, 83 (1990). Symposium on pharmacology and clinical trials: ibid. **23**, 2709-3376 (1991). Review of mechanism of action: G. Wiederrecht et al., Ann. N.Y. Acad. Sci. **696**, 9-19 (1993); of clinical trials in comparison with cyclosporin in renal transplantation: G. A. Knoll, R. C. Bell, Br. Med. J. **318**, 1104-1107 (1999). Review of use in dermatoses: A. K. Gupta et al., J. Eur. Acad. Dermatol. Venereol. **16**, 100-114 (2002).

Monohydrate. [109581-93-3] FK-506; FR-900506; Prograf; Protopic. $C_{44}H_{69}NO_{12} \cdot H_2O$. Colorless prisms from acetonitrile, mp 127-129°. $[\alpha]_D^{23}$ −84.4° (c = 1.02 in chloroform). Sol in methanol, ethanol, acetone, ethyl acetate, chloroform, diethyl ether; sparingly sol in hexane, petroleum ether. Insol in water. LD_{50} i.p. in mice: >200 mg/kg (Kino). LD_{50} in male, female rats (mg/kg): 57.0, 23.6 i.v.; 134, 194 orally (Ohara).

THERAP CAT: Immunosuppressant.

9026. Tacryl®. Acrylic fiber of a specific multichain type. The structure could be described as a spider molecule with up to six long straight linear legs which can orient independently and build up a fibrous structure. The molecular structure is built up by a controlled cross-linking process, so that Tacryl is like wool as it has a specific chain molecular interlinking which contributes to its mechanical and elastic properties. Synthesis of multichain polymers: Schaefgen, Flory, J. Am. Chem. Soc. **70**, 2709 (1948). Tacryl has a higher shear modulus and a higher strength than linear acrylics with the same degrees of orientation. It undergoes very slow hydrolysis under hot acid aq conditions, and is very resistant to dry and wet heat (neutral conditions): Sundén, Tappi **41**, 173A (1958).

9027. Tadalafil. [171596-29-5] (6R,12aR)-6-(1,3-Benzodioxol-5-yl)-2,3,6,7,12,12a-hexahydro-2-methylpyrazino[1′,2′:1,-6]pyrido[3,4-b]indole-1,4-dione; (6R,12aR)-2,3,6,7,12,12a-hexahydro-2-methyl-6-[3,4-(methylenedioxy)phenyl]pyrazino[1′,2′:1,-6]pyrido[3,4-b]indole-1,4-dione; GF-196960; IC-351; Cialis. C_{22}-$H_{19}N_3O_4$; mol wt 389.40. C 67.86%, H 4.92%, N 10.79%, O 16.43%. Selective type 5 cGMP phosphodiesterase (PDE-5) inhibitor. Prepn: A. C. Daugan, WO 9519978 (1995 to Glaxo); eidem, US 5859006 (1999 to ICOS); and PDE-5 inhibition: idem et al., J. Med. Chem. **46**, 4525, 4533 (2003). HPLC determn in plasma: C.-L. Cheng, C.-H. Chou, J. Chromatogr. B **822**, 278 (2005). Clinical pharmacokinetics: S. T. Forgue et al., Br. J. Clin. Pharmacol. **61**, 280 (2005). Clinical trial in erectile dysfunction: G. B. Brock et al., J. Urol. **168**, 1332 (2002); in comparison with sildenafil: I. Eardley et al., BJU Int. **96**, 1323 (2005). Review of pharmacology and clinical experience: H. Porst, Int. J. Impotence Res. **14**, Suppl.

1, S57-S64 (2002); in comparison with other phosphodiesterase inhibitors: S. A. Doggrell, *Expert Opin. Pharmacother.* **6**, 75-84 (2005).

White crystals from 2-propanol, mp 302-303°. $[\alpha]_D^{20}$ +71.0° (c = 1.00 in CHCl$_3$). Very slightly sol in ethanol. Practically insol in water.

THERAP CAT: In treatment of male erectile dysfunction.

9028. TAED. [10543-57-4] *N,N'*-1,2-ethanediylbis[*N*-acetylacetamide]; *N,N,N',N'*-tetraacetylethylenediamine; TAED 4303. C$_{10}$H$_{16}$N$_2$O$_4$; mol wt 228.25. C 52.62%, H 7.07%, N 12.27%, O 28.04%. Bleach activator for peroxide-based detergents. Prepn: A. P. N. Franchimont, J. V. Dubsky, *Rec. Trav. Chim.* **30**, 184 (1911); R. P. Mariella, K. H. Brown, *J. Org. Chem.* **36**, 735 (1971). Chemical degradation studies: D. M. Davies, M. E. Deary, *J. Chem. Soc. Perkin Trans. 2* **1991**, 1549; N. Brand et al., *Chemosphere* **34**, 2637 (1997). Determn by iodometric titration in household detergents: L. Baini et al., *Riv. Ital. Sostanze Grasse* **69**, 615 (1992). Biocidal efficacy: V. B. Cloud, I. M. George, *Household Pers. Prod. Ind.* **34**, 82 (1997). Enhancement of whiteness of cellulosic blends: A. J. Mathews, S. J. Scarborough, *Proc. Beltwide Cotton Conf.* **1998**, 732; of wool/cotton blends: P. A. Duffield et al., *ibid.*, 816; of paper pulp: C. Leduc et al., *Appita J.* **51**, 306 (1998).

Solid, mp 149-150°. Sol in water up to 10^{-3} mol/l. uv max (water): 213 nm (ε 18000 mol^{-1}cm^{-1}).

USE: Peroxide bleach activator for household detergents, paper pulp.

9029. Tafenoquine. [106635-80-7] *N*^{4}-[2,6-Dimethoxy-4-methyl-5-[3-(trifluoromethyl)phenoxy]-8-quinolinyl]-1,4-pentanediamine; 8-[(4-amino-1-methylbutyl)amino]-2,6-dimethoxy-4-methyl-5-[3-(trifluoromethyl)phenoxy]quinoline; WR-238605. C$_{24}$H$_{28}$F$_3$N$_3$O$_3$; mol wt 463.49. C 62.19%, H 6.09%, F 12.30%, N 9.07%, O 10.36%. Analog of primaquine, *q.v.* Prepn: P. Blumbergs, M. P. LaMontagne, **US 4617394** (1986 to U.S. Sec. Army); M. P. LaMontagne et al., *J. Med. Chem.* **32**, 1728 (1989). HPLC determn in blood and plasma: D. A. Kocisko et al., *Ther. Drug Monit.* **22**, 184 (2000). Metabolism: O. R. Idowu et al., *Drug Metab. Dispos.* **23**, 1 (1995). Clinical pharmacokinetics: M. D. Edstein et al., *Br. J. Pharmacol.* **52**, 663 (2001). Clinical evaluation in prevention of malaria relapse: D. S. Walsh et al., *J. Infect. Dis.* **180**, 1282 (1999); in malaria prophylaxis: B. Lell et al., *Lancet* **355**, 2041 (2000); B. R. Hale et al., *Clin. Infect. Dis.* **36**, 541 (2003).

Succinate. [106635-81-8] Etaquine. C$_{24}$H$_{28}$F$_3$N$_3$O$_3$.C$_4$H$_6$O$_4$. Crystals from acetonitrile, mp 146-149°. LD$_{50}$ in male, female rats (mg/kg): 102, 71 i.p.; 429, 416 orally (LaMontagne).

THERAP CAT: Antimalarial.

9030. D-Tagatose. [87-81-0] D-*lyxo*-Hexulose; Naturlose. C$_6$H$_{12}$O$_6$; mol wt 180.16. C 40.00%, H 6.71%, O 53.28%. Uncommon, but naturally occurring ketohexose. Isoln from *Sterculia setigera* gum: E. L. Hirst et al., *J. Chem. Soc.* **1949**, 3145. Prepn from D-galactose: C. A. L. De Bruyn, W. A. Van Ekenstein, *Rec. Trav. Chim.* **16**, 262 (1897); T. Reichstein, W. Bosshard, *Helv. Chim. Acta* **17**, 753 (1934); by biochemical oxidation of D-talitol: E. L. Totton, H. A. Lardy, *J. Am. Chem. Soc.* **71**, 3076 (1949); from lactose in heated milk: S. Adachi, *Nature* **181**, 840 (1958). Synthesis: M. L. Wolfrom, R. B. Bennett, *J. Org. Chem.* **30**, 1284 (1965); A. A. H. Al-Jobore et al., *Carbohydr. Res.* **16**, 474 (1971). Crystal structure: S. Takagi, R. D. Rosenstein, *ibid.* **11**, 156 (1969). Manuf process from whey: J. R. Beadle et al., **US 5002612** (1991 to Biospherics). Stability and sweetening properties in toothpaste: Y. Lu, *Int. J. Cosmet. Sci.* **23**, 175 (2001). Review of use as bulk sugar substitute: G. V. Levin et al., *Am. J. Clin. Nutr.* **62**, Suppl., 1161S-1168S (1995). Series of articles on toxicology and gastrointestinal tolerance: *Regul. Toxicol. Pharmacol.* **29**, S1-S93 (1999).

Crystals from aq ethanol, mp 131-133°. $[\alpha]_D^{25}$ −5° (c = 1 in water). Sucrose-like taste, approx 92% as sweet as sucrose.

L-Tagatose. [17598-82-2] Prepn: C. Glatthaar, T. Reichstein, *Helv. Chim. Acta* **20**, 1537 (1937). Stereoselective synthesis: T. Mukaiyama et al., *Chem. Lett.* **1982**, 1169. Crystals, mp 134-135°. $[\alpha]_D^{16}$ +1° (c = 2 in water).

USE: Non-nutritive sweetener. Sweetening agent for pharmaceuticals and personal aid products.

9031. Taka-Diastase. [9001-19-8] α-Amylase (*Aspergillus oryzae*); Koji; Aspergillus diastase; Sanzyme. A purified multienzyme produced by the microorganism *Aspergillus oryzae* (Ahl.) Cohn, *Aspergillaceae*, grown on sterilized wheat bran or on rice hulls. Represents more than 30 different enzymatic functions. It is not only amylolytic but digests proteins and fats also.

Whitish-yellow, very hygroscopic powder. Converts 450 times its wt of starch into maltose. *Keep tightly closed.*

USE: Preparing the Japanese national drink "sake"; in converting maizes into sugar in manuf of whiskey.

THERAP CAT: Amylolytic.

9032. Talampanel. [161832-65-1] (8*R*)-7-Acetyl-5-(4-aminophenyl)-8,9-dihydro-8-methyl-7*H*-1,3-dioxolo[4,5-*h*][2,3]-benzodiazepine; *R*-(−)-1-(4-aminophenyl)-3-acetyl-4-methyl-7,8-methylenedioxy-3,4-dihydro-5*H*-2,3-benzodiazepine; LY-300164. C$_{19}$H$_{19}$N$_3$O$_3$; mol wt 337.37. C 67.64%, H 5.68%, N 12.46%, O 14.23%. Noncompetitive AMPA receptor antagonist. Prepn: F. Andrasi et al., **EP 492485**; *eidem*, **US 5536832** (1992, 1996 both to Gyogyszerkutato Intezet KFT). Enantioselective synthesis: I. Ling et al., *J. Chem. Soc. Perkin Trans. 1* **1995**, 1423. HPLC determn in plasma: J. A. Eckstein, S. P. Swanson, *J. Chromatogr. B* **668**, 153 (1995). Stereoselective electropharmacology and neuroprotective effects: D. Lodge et al., *Neuropharmacology* **35**, 1681 (1996). Review of manufacturing process: B. A. Anderson et al. in *Process*

Chemistry in the Pharmaceutical Industry, K. G. Gadamasetti, Ed. (Marcel Dekker, New York, 1999) pp 263-282. Review of clinical development: C. Q. Meng, *Curr. Opin. Cent. Peripher. Nerv. Syst. Invest. Drugs* **1**, 637-643 (1999).

Crystals, mp 169-172°. $[\alpha]_D$ −321.34° (c = 1 in methanol).

THERAP CAT: Anticonvulsant.

9033. Talampicillin. [47747-56-8] (2*S*,5*R*,6*R*)-6-[[(2*R*)-Aminophenylacetyl]amino]-3,3-dimethyl-7-oxo-4-thia-1-azabicyclo[3.2.0]heptane-2-carboxylic acid 1,3-dihydro-3-oxo-1-isobenzofuranyl ester; (2*S*,5*R*,6*R*)-6-[(*R*)-2-amino-2-phenylacetamido]-3,3-dimethyl-7-oxo-4-thia-1-azabicyclo[3.2.0]heptane-2-carboxylic acid ester with 3-hydroxyphthalide; 6-[D(−)-α-aminophenylacetamido]penicillanic acid phthalide ester; ampicillin 1-oxo-1,3-dihydroisobenzofuran-3-yl ester; phthalidyl D-α-aminobenzylpenicillanate. $C_{24}H_{23}N_3O_6S$; mol wt 481.52. C 59.86%, H 4.81%, N 8.73%, O 19.94%, S 6.66%. Semi-synthetic antibiotic related to penicillin. Prepn: H. Ferres, M. P. Clayton, **DE 2228012**; *eidem*, **US 3860579** (1972, 1975 both to Beecham). *See also:* M. Murakami *et al.*, **US 3951954** (1976 to Yamanouchi). Pharmacology: Clayton *et al.*, *Antimicrob. Agents Chemother.* **5**, 670 (1974). HPLC determn in urine and comparison of pharmacokinetics with other aminopenicillins: T. Uno *et al.*, *Chem. Pharm. Bull.* **29**, 1957 (1981). Clinical comparison with ampicillin, *q.v.:* H. N. Williams *et al.*, *Br. J. Clin. Pract.* **35**, 147 (1981).

Hydrochloride. [39878-70-1] BRL-8988; Talat; Talpen; Yamacillin. $C_{24}H_{23}N_3O_6S$.HCl; mol wt 517.98. White powder, mp 154-157° (dec).

THERAP CAT: Antibacterial.

9034. Talaporfin. [110230-98-3] *N*-[[(7*S*,8*S*)-3-Carboxy-7-(2-carboxyethyl)-13-ethenyl-18-ethyl-7,8-dihydro-2,8,12,17-tetramethyl-21*H*,23*H*-porphin-5-yl]acetyl]-L-aspartic acid; (2*S*,3*S*)-18-carboxy-20-[*N*-(*S*)-1,2-dicarboxyethyl]carbamoylmethyl-13-ethyl-3,7,12,17-tetramethyl-8-vinylchlorin-2-propanoic acid; mono-L-aspartyl chlorin e₆; NPe6. $C_{38}H_{41}N_5O_9$; mol wt 711.76. C 64.12%, H 5.81%, N 9.84%, O 20.23%. Semisynthetic derivative of chlorin e₆, *q.v.* Photosensitizer activated at 664 nm by laser or light-emitting diode-based light infusion device. Causes irreversible tumor blood vessel closure. Prepn: J. C. Bommer, B. F. Burnham, **EP 168831**; *eidem*, **US 4675338** (1986, 1987 both to Nippon Petrochemicals). Photophysical properties: J. D. Spikes, J. C. Bommer, *J. Photochem. Photobiol. B* **17**, 135 (1993); L. Li *et al.*, *ibid.* **67**, 51 (2002). Chemical and NMR structural studies: S. Gomi *et al.*, *Heterocycles* **48**, 2231 (1998). Safety assessment in treatment of refractory solid tumors: R. A. Lustig *et al.*, *Cancer* **98**, 1767 (2003). Clinical evaluation in lung cancer: H. Kato *et al.*, *Lung Cancer* **42**, 103 (2003).

Dark blue-green powder. Sol in water. Absorption max (phosphate buffer, pH 7.4): 400, 654 nm (ε 180000, 40000). Absorption

max (*p*-dioxane): 401.7, 663.5 nm (E_{mM} 111, 38). Hygroscopic and light sensitive. *Store under vacuum; protect from light.*

Tetrasodium salt. [220201-34-3] Talaporfin sodium; LS-11; ME-2906; Laserphyrin. $C_{38}H_{37}N_5Na_4O_9$; mol wt 799.69.

THERAP CAT: Antineoplastic (photosensitizer).

9035. Talastine. [16188-61-7] 2-[2-(Dimethylamino)ethyl]-4-(phenylmethyl)-1(2*H*)-phthalazinone; 4-benzyl-2-[2-(dimethylamino)ethyl]-1(2*H*)-phthalazinone. $C_{19}H_{21}N_3O$; mol wt 307.39. C 74.24%, H 6.89%, N 13.67%, O 5.20%. Prepn: Engelbrecht *et al.*, **DE 1046625**; *eidem*, **US 3017411** (1958, 1962, both to VEB Deutsches Hydrierwerk Rodleben). Pharmacology: D. Lenke, *Arzneim.-Forsch.* **7**, 678 (1957).

Liquid, bp₀.₃ 215-222°.

Hydrochloride. [16188-76-4] HL-2186; Ahanon. $C_{19}H_{21}N_3$-O.HCl; mol wt 343.85. Crystals, mp 178°. LD₅₀ i.p. in mice: 116 mg/kg (Lenke).

THERAP CAT: Antihistaminic.

9036. Talbutal. [115-44-6] 5-(1-Methylpropyl)-5-(2-propenyl)-2,4,6(1*H*,3*H*,5*H*)-pyrimidinetrione; 5-allyl-5-*sec*-butylbarbituric acid; 5-allyl-5-(1-methylpropyl)barbituric acid; Lotusate. $C_{11}H_{16}N_2O_3$; mol wt 224.26. C 58.91%, H 7.19%, N 12.49%, O 21.40%. Prepn: Volwiler, *J. Am. Chem. Soc.* **47**, 2236 (1925). Acute toxicity: E. W. Schafer, *Toxicol. Appl. Pharmacol.* **21**, 315 (1972).

Crystals from water or dil alcohol, mp 108-110°. Slightly bitter taste. Practically insol in water and petr ether. Sol in alcohol, chloroform, ether, acetone, glacial acetic acid, also in solns of fixed alkali hydroxides. A satd aq soln is acid to litmus. LD₅₀ orally in rats: 57.5 mg/kg (Schafer).

Note: This is a controlled substance (depressant): **21 CFR,** 1308.13.

THERAP CAT: Sedative, hypnotic.

9037. Talc. [14807-96-6] Talcum; French chalk. The lumps are also known as *soapstone* or *steatite*. Finely powdered native hydrous magnesium silicate. Comprehensive description: A. W. Newman *et al.*, *Anal. Profiles Drug Subs. Excip.* **23**, 511-542 (1994).

White to grayish-white, very fine odorless, crystalline powder; unctuous, and adheres readily to the skin. Insol in water, cold acids or in alkalies. Sol in hot concentrated phosphoric acid.

Caution: Potential symptoms of overexposure to talc containing no asbestos and less than 1% quartz are fibriotic pneumoconiosis; irritation of eyes. Potential symptoms of overexposure to soapstone containing less than 1% quartz are pneumoconiosis; cough, dyspnea; digital clubbing; cyanosis; basal crackles, cor pulmonale. *See NIOSH Pocket Guide to Chemical Hazards* (DHHS/NIOSH 97-140, 1997) p 292, 280.

USE: Dusting powder, either alone or with starch or boric acid, for medicinal and toilet prepns; excipient and filler for pills, tablets and for dusting tablet molds; clarifying liquids by filtration. As pigment in paints, varnishes, rubber; filler for paper, rubber, soap; in fireproof and cold-water paints for wood, metal and stone; lubricating molds and machinery; glove and shoe powder; electric and heat insulator.

9038. Talinolol. [57460-41-0] *N*-Cyclohexyl-*N'*-[4-[3-[(1,1-dimethylethyl)amino]-2-hydroxypropoxy]phenyl]urea; 1-(4-cyclohexylureidophenoxy)-2-hydroxy-3-*tert*-butylaminopropane; (±)-1-[*p*-[3-(*tert*-butylamino)-2-hydroxypropoxy]phenyl]-3-cyclohexylurea; 02-115; Cordanum. $C_{20}H_{33}N_3O_3$; mol wt 363.49. C 66.09%, H 9.15%, N 11.56%, O 13.20%. Selective β_1-adrenergic blocker structurally related to practolol, *q.v.* Prepn: R. Eckardt *et al.*, *DE 2153024* (1972 to Arzneimittelwerke VEB), *C.A.* **77**, 61639b (1972); *idem et al.*, *Pharmazie* **30**, 633 (1975). Series of articles on pharmacology, toxicology: *ibid.* 638-683. Acute toxicity: K. Femmer *et al.*, *ibid.* 642. Clinical pharmacokinetics and bioavailability: B. Trausch *et al.*, *Biopharm. Drug Dispos.* **16**, 403 (1995). Review of clinical experience: I. Assmann, *Curr. Med. Res. Opin.* **13**, 325-342 (1995).

Cryst from isopropanol, mp 142-144°. LD_{50} in rats, mice (mg/kg): 1180, 593 orally; 54.3, 74.7 i.p.; 29.7, 25.0 i.v. (Femmer).

THERAP CAT: Antihypertensive; antiarrhythmic.

9039. Talipexole. [101626-70-4] 5,6,7,8-Tetrahydro-6-(2-propenyl)-4*H*-thiazolo[4,5-*d*]azepin-2-amine; 6-allyl-5,6,7,8-tetrahydro-4*H*-thiazolo[4,5-*d*]azepine. $C_{10}H_{15}N_3S$; mol wt 209.31. C 57.38%, H 7.22%, N 20.08%, S 15.32%. α_2-Adrenoceptor and dopamine D_2-receptor agonist. Prepn: G. Griss *et al.*, *DE 2040510* (1972 to Thomae); *eidem*, *US 3804849* (1974 to Boehringer, Ing.). Dopaminergic effects: P. A. Johansen *et al.*, *Life Sci.* **43**, 515 (1988); S. K. Kulkarni, K. Chopra, *Methods Find. Exp. Clin. Pharmacol.* **12**, 99 (1990). Clinical evaluation in Parkinson's disease: Y. Mizuno *et al.*, *Drug Invest.* **5**, 186 (1993).

Dihydrochloride. [36085-73-1] B-HT-920; Domin. $C_{10}H_{15}N_3S.2HCl$; mol wt 282.23. mp 245° (dec).

THERAP CAT: Antiparkinsonian.

9040. Tall Oil. Liquid rosin; Acintol C; tallol; talleol. "Tall" is Swedish for "pine". A by-product of the wood pulp industry. Usually recovered from pine wood "black liquor" of the sulfate or kraft paper process. Contains rosin acids, oleic and linoleic acids. Long chain alcohols and small amounts of sterols, especially phytosterol, have also been found. Comprehensive collection of 1660 abstracts: J. Weiner, *Tall Oil* (The Institute of Paper Chemistry, Appleton, Wisconsin, 3rd ed., 1959) 450 pp; J. Weiner, J. Byrne, 1st supplement (1965).

Dark brown liquid. Acrid odor similar to that of burnt rosin. d 0.95 to 1.0. $n_D^{20} \sim 1.5$. Acid no. 170-180. Sapon no. 172-185. Iodine no. 120-188. Fatty acids 50-60%. Rosin acids 34-40%. Unsaponifiable matter 5-10%.

USE: Mfg soap pastes, flotation agents, greases, paint, alkyd resins, linoleum, soaps, fungicides, asphalt emulsions, rubber formulations, cutting oils, sulfonated oils. Review of possible uses: Cannon, *Chem. Eng.* **61**, 142 (June 1954).

9041. Tallow. In North America designates the fat from the fatty tissue of bovine cattle and sheep only. It may be offered separately as beef tallow and as sheep or mutton tallow. The term horse tallow is generally no longer admitted. *Oleo stock* is the highest grade of beef tallow. Contains (as glycerides): Oleic acid (37-43%), palmitic (24-32%), stearic (20-25%), myristic (3-6%), linoleic (2-3%). Minor constituents are cholesterol, arachidonic, elaidic, and vaccenic acids. Perhaps the most observed characteristic of tallow is its titer (solidif pt) which ranges from 40° to 46°.

9042. Tallow Alcohol. A name for commercial mixtures of *n*-octadecanol and *n*-hexadecanol.

Fatty crystalline mass, mp 46-47°.

USE: Defoaming agent, emollient, intermediate for surface active agents.

9043. Tallysomycin. [67995-68-0] Talisomycin; BU-2231; Antitumor antibiotic complex and third generation analog of bleomycins, *q.v.*, produced by *Streptoalloteichus hindustanus* E 465-94. Prodn, isoln, properties of the major components, tallysomycins A and B: H. Kawaguchi *et al.*, *BE 845513*; *eidem*, *US 4051237* (both 1977 to Bristol-Myers); *eidem*, *J. Antibiot.* **30**, 779 (1977). Structure of A and B, based on originally proposed bleomycin structure: M. Konishi *et al.*, *ibid.* 789; *cf.* bleomycin for revised structure. Antitumor activity: H. Imanishi *et al.*, *ibid.* **31**, 667 (1978). Radioimmunoassay: A. Broughton *et al.*, *Cancer Treat. Rep.* **63**, 1829 (1979). Pharmacokinetics: J. E. Strong *et al.*, *ibid.* 1821. ^{13}C-NMR spectra of tallysomycin and its zinc complex: F. T. Greenaway *et al.*, *Org. Magn. Reson.* **13**, 270 (1980). Biosynthetic derivs: T. Miyaki *et al.*, *J. Antibiot.* **34**, 658, 665 (1981). Relative pulmonary toxicity: A. Broughton *et al.*, *Cancer Treat. Rep.* **64**, 659 (1980). *Review:* S. T. Crooke *et al.*, *Recent Results Cancer Res.* **76**, 83-90 (1981).

Tallysomycin A   R =

Tallysomycin B   R =

Tallysomycin A. [65057-90-1] N^1-[4-Amino-6-[[3-[(4-aminobutyl)amino]propyl]amino]-6-oxohexyl]-13-[(4-amino-4,6-dideoxy-α-L-talopyranosyl)oxy]-19-demethyl-12-hydroxybleomycinamide; BU-2231A. $C_{68}H_{110}N_{22}O_{27}S_2$; mol wt 1731.86. The term "talisomycin" has also been used to refer to tallysomycin A. White amorphous solid. No definite mp; gradually dec >210°. Sol in water, methanol, DMF; slightly sol in ethanol. Practically insol in other organic solvents. $[\alpha]_D^{23}$ −21° (c = 0.5 in water). uv max (water): 290 nm ($E_{1cm}^{1\%}$ 67). LD$_{50}$ s.c. in mice: 28 mg/kg (**US 4051237**).

Tallysomycin B. [65057-91-2] N^1-[3-[(4-Aminobutyl)amino]-propyl]-13-[(4-amino-4,6-dideoxy-α-L-talopyranosyl)oxy]-19-demethyl-12-hydroxybleomycinamide; talisomycin B; BU-2231B. $C_{62}H_{98}N_{20}O_{26}S_2$; mol wt 1603.69. Mp, soly similar to tallysomycin A. $[\alpha]_D^{23}$ −19° (c = 0.5 in water). uv max (water): 289.5 ($E_{1cm}^{1\%}$ 77). LD$_{50}$ s.c. in mice: >50 mg/kg (**US 4051237**).

9044. Talniflumate. [66898-62-2] 2-[[3-(Trifluoromethyl)phenyl]amino]-3-pyridinecarboxylic acid 1,3-dihydro-3-oxo-1-isobenzofuranyl ester; phthalidyl 2-(3-trifluoromethylanilino)nicotinate; phthalidyl 2-(α,α,α-trifluoro-m-toluidino)nicotinate; BA-7602-06; Somalgen. $C_{21}H_{13}F_3N_2O_4$; mol wt 414.33. C 60.88%, H 3.16%, F 13.76%, N 6.76%, O 15.45%. Prodrug of niflumic acid, *q.v.* Prepn: **BE 858864** (1978 to Bago), *C.A.* **89**, 109104 (1978); S. Bago, **US 4168313** (1979). Synthesis and pharmacologic study: M. Los *et al.*, *Farmaco Ed. Sci.* **36**, 372 (1981). HPLC determn in plasma: D.-J. Jang *et al.*, *Biomed. Chromatogr.* **19**, 32 (2005). Review of clinical development as a mucoregulator: D. Knight, *Curr. Opin. Invest. Drugs* **5**, 557-562 (2004).

White or pale yellow crystalline powder, mp 165-166°. uv max (chloroform): 287, 357 nm (ε 25600, 7800). LD$_{50}$ orally in rats: 12000 mg/kg (Los).

THERAP CAT: Anti-inflammatory; analgesic.

9045. Taltirelin. [103300-74-9] N-[[(4S)-Hexahydro-1-methyl-2,6-dioxo-4-primidinyl]carbonyl]-L-histidyl-L-prolinamide; (S)-N-(1-methyl-4,5-dihydroorotyl)-L-histidyl-L-prolinamide. $C_{17}H_{23}N_7O_5$; mol wt 405.41. C 50.36%, H 5.72%, N 24.18%, O 19.73%. Analog of thyrotropin releasing hormone TRH, *q.v.*, with pronounced CNS activity. Prepn: H. Sugano *et al.*, **EP 168042**; *eidem*, **US 4665056** (1986, 1987 both to Tanabe Seiyaku); M. Suzuki *et al.*, *J. Med. Chem.* **33**, 2130 (1990). Radioimmunoassay determn in plasma and urine: S. Morikawa *et al.*, *J. Pharm. Biomed. Anal.* **16**, 1267 (1998). CNS pharmacology: M. Yamamura *et al.*, *Jpn. J. Pharmacol.* **53**, 451 (1990). Effect on motor neuron survival: Y. Iwasaki *et al.*, *Neurol. Res.* **19**, 613 (1997). Review of pharmacology, toxicology, and clinical trials: K. Kinoshita *et al.*, *CNS Drug Rev.* **4**, 25-41 (1998).

Crystals from water as the hemiheptahydrate, mp 72-75°. $[\alpha]_D^{25}$ −13.6° (c = 1 in water).

Tetrahydrate. [201677-75-0] TA-0910; Ceredist. $C_{17}H_{21}N_7O_5 \cdot 4H_2O$; mol wt 475.45. White, odorless crystals, bp 72-75°. Sol in water, acetic acid, ethanol. Slightly sol in methanol, acetonitrile. $[\alpha]_D^{23}$ −13.6°. LD$_{50}$ in mice, rats (mg/kg): >5000, >5000 orally; in mice, male, female rats (mg/kg): >2000, 799, 946 i.v. (Kinoshita).

THERAP CAT: In treatment of spinocerebellar degeneration.

9046. Tamarind. Partially dried ripe fruit of *Tamarindus indica* L., *Leguminosae*, preserved in sugar or syrup. *Habit.* East Indies, India, Africa; naturalized in West Indies. *Constit.* The pulp contains about 10% tartaric acid, also some citric and malic acids; 25-40% invert sugar, pectin. *Review:* Rao, Srivastava, in *Indus-*

trial Gums, R. L. Whistler, Ed. (Academic Press, New York, 2nd ed., 1973) pp 369-411.

USE: The pulp as souring agent in Indian curries. The seed kernel powder with water as sizing agent.

9047. Tamibarotene. [94497-51-5] 4-[[(5,6,7,8-Tetrahydro-5,5,8,8-tetramethyl-2-naphthalenyl)amino]carbonyl]benzoic acid; p-(5,6,7,8-Tetrahydro-5,5,8,8-tetramethyl-2-naphthylcarbamoyl)benzoic acid; AM-80; Tamibaro. $C_{22}H_{25}NO_3$; mol wt 351.44. C 75.19%, H 7.17%, N 3.99%, O 13.66%. Synthetic retinoic acid receptor-α/β-selective retinoid. Prepn: K. Shudo, **EP 170105** (1986 to Sumitomo; Yoshitomi); *idem*, **US 4703110** (1987); H. Kagechika *et al.*, *J. Med. Chem.* **31**, 2182 (1988). HPLC determn in plasma: M. Itoh, G. Kominami, *J. Immunoassay Immunochem.* **22**, 213 (2001). Receptor binding studies in human leukemia cells: Y. Hashimoto *et al.*, *Jpn. J. Cancer Res.* **79**, 473 (1988). Series of articles on pharmacokinetics and reproductive and developmental toxicity: K. Mizojiri *et al.*, *Arzneim.-Forsch.* **47**, 59, 195, 201, 259, 270 (1997). Inhibition of myeloma cell-induced angiogeneis: T. Sanda *et al.*, *Leukemia* **19**, 901 (2005). Clinical evaluation in acute promyelocytic leukemia: K. Shinjo *et al.*, *Int. J. Hematol.* **72**, 470 (2000).

Colorless prisms from ethyl acetate-n-hexane, mp 231-232°.

THERAP CAT: Antineoplastic.

9048. Tamoxifen. [10540-29-1] (Z)-2-[4-(1,2-Diphenyl-1-butenyl)phenoxy]-N,N-dimethylethanamine; 1-p-β-dimethylaminoethoxyphenyl-*trans*-1,2-diphenylbut-1-ene. $C_{26}H_{29}NO$; mol wt 371.51. C 84.06%, H 7.87%, N 3.77%, O 4.31%. Nonsteroidal estrogen antagonist. Prepn: **BE 637389** (1964 to ICI). Identification and separation of isomers: G. R. Bedford, D. N. Richardson, *Nature* **212**, 733 (1966); **BE 678807**; M. J. K. Harper *et al.*, **US 4536516** (1966, 1985 both to ICI). Stereospecific synthesis: R. B. Miller, M. I. Al-Hassan, *J. Org. Chem.* **50**, 2121 (1985). Review of chemistry and pharmacology: B. J. A. Furr, V. C. Jordan, *Pharmacol. Ther.* **25**, 127-205 (1984). Reviews of clinical experience in treatment and prevention of breast cancer: I. A. Jaiyesimi *et al.*, *J. Clin. Oncol.* **13**, 513-529 (1995); C. K. Osborne, *N. Engl. J. Med.* **339**, 1609-1618 (1998).

Crystals from petr ether, mp 96-98°.

Citrate. [54965-24-1] ICI-46474; Kessar; Nolvadex; Tamofène; Zemide; Zitazonium. $C_{26}H_{29}NO \cdot C_6H_8O_7$; mol wt 563.64. Fine, white, odorless crystalline powder, mp 140-142°. Slightly sol in water; sol in ethanol, methanol, acetone. Hygroscopic at high relative humidities. Sensitive to uv light. LD$_{50}$ in mice, rats (mg/kg): 200, 600 i.p.; 62.5, 62.5 i.v.; 3000-6000, 1200-2500 orally (Furr, Jordan).

(*E*)-**Form.** [13002-65-8] mp 72-74° from methanol.

(*E*)-**Form citrate.** ICI-47699. mp 126-128°.

Caution: Tamoxifen is listed as a known human carcinogen: *Report on Carcinogens, Eleventh Edition* (PB2005-104914, 2004) p III-239.

THERAP CAT: Antineoplastic (hormonal).

9049. Tamsulosin. [106133-20-4] 5-[(2R)-2-[[2-(2-Ethoxy-phenoxy)ethyl]amino]propyl]-2-methoxybenzenesulfonamide; am-sulosin. $C_{20}H_{28}N_2O_5S$; mol wt 408.51. C 58.80%, H 6.91%, N 6.86%, O 19.58%, S 7.85%. Specific α_1-adrenoceptor antagonist. Prepn: K. Imai *et al.*, **EP 34432**; *eidem*, **US 4703063** (1981, 1987 both to Yamanouchi). Comparative pharmacology of enantiomers and racemate: K. Honda *et al.*, *Arch. Pharmacol.* **336**, 295 (1987). HPLC determn in plasma: Y. Soeishi *et al.*, *J. Chromatogr.* **533**, 291 (1990). Clinical trials in benign prostatic hypertrophy: K. Kawabe *et al.*, *J. Urol.* **144**, 908 (1990); P. Abrams *et al.*, *Br. J. Urol.* **76**, 325 (1995). Review of pharmacology and clinical experience in uro-logical disorders: M. C. Michel, J. J. de la Rosette, *Expert Opin. Pharmacother.* **5**, 151-160 (2004).

Hydrochloride. [106463-17-6] LY-253351; YM-12617-1; YM-617; Flomax; Flomaxtra; Harnal; Omnic; Pradif. $C_{20}H_{28}N_2$-$O_5S.HCl$; mol wt 444.97. mp 228-230°. $[\alpha]_D^{24}$ −4.0° (c = 0.35 in methanol).

THERAP CAT: In treatment of benign prostatic hypertrophy.

9050. Tanacetin. [1401-54-3] [3aS-(3aα,5aβ,6β,9aα,9bβ)]-Decahydro-6,9a-dihydroxy-5a-methyl-3,9-bis(methylene)naphtho-[1,2-b]furan-2(3H)-one; 1β,5α-dihydroxy-6β,7αH-selina-4(15),11-(13)-dien-6,12-olide. $C_{15}H_{20}O_4$; mol wt 264.32. C 68.16%, H 7.63%, O 24.21%. Isoln from seed, herb, and flowers of *Tanacetum vulgare* L., *Compositae*: Homolle, *J. Pharm. Chim.* **7**, 57 (1845); Jaretzky, Kühne, *Arch. Pharm.* **271**, 353 (1933); Suchy, *Collect. Czech. Chem. Commun.* **27**, 1058 (1962). Structure and absolute config: Samek *et al.*, *ibid.* **38**, 1971 (1973).

Crystals, mp 205°. $[\alpha]_D^{22}$ +179.5° (c = 2.3 in ethanol).

9051. Tandospirone. [87760-53-0] (3aα,4β,7β,7aα)-Hexa-hydro-2-[4-[4-(2-pyrimidinyl)-1-piperazinyl]butyl]-4,7-methano-1H-isoindole-1,3(2H)-dione; (1R*,2S*,3R*,4S*)-N-[4-[4-(2-pyri-midinyl)-1-piperazinyl]butyl]-2,3-bicyclo[2.2.1]heptanedicarbox-imide. $C_{21}H_{29}N_5O_2$; mol wt 383.49. C 65.77%, H 7.62%, N 18.26%, O 8.34%. Serotonin (5-HT$_{1A}$) receptor agonist. Prepn: K. Ishizumi *et al.*, **EP 82402**; *eidem*, **US 4507303** (1983, 1985 both to Sumitomo); *idem et al.*, *Chem. Pharm. Bull.* **39**, 2288 (1991). Behavioral pharmacology: C. A. Sannerud *et al.*, *Drug Alcohol Depend.* **32**, 195 (1993). Clinical efficacy in treatment of bulimia: H. Tamai *et al.*, *Int. J. Obes.* **14**, 289 (1990). Clinical evaluation of potential adverse effects: M. Suzuki *et al.*, *Jpn. J. Psychopharma-col.* **13**, 213 (1993); of abuse liability: S. M. Evans *et al.*, *J. Pharmacol. Exp. Ther.* **271**, 683 (1994). Review of pharmacology: P. A. Seymour *et al.*, *Prog. Clin. Biol. Res.* **361**, 453-460 (1990).

Crystals from toluene/*n*-hexane, mp 112-113.5°.

Citrate. [112457-95-1] SM-3997; Sediel. $C_{21}H_{29}N_5O_2.C_6$-H_8O_7; mol wt 575.61. mp 169.5-170°.

Hydrochloride. $C_{21}H_{29}N_5O_2.HCl$. Crystals from isopropanol, mp 227-229°.

THERAP CAT: Anxiolytic; antidepressant.

9052. Tannic Acid. Tannin; gallotannin; gallotannic acid. Incorrectly *"digallic acid"*. Tannic acid of commerce usually con-tains about 10% H_2O. Occurs in the bark and fruit of many plants, notably in the bark of the oak species, in sumac and myrobalan. It is produced from Turkish or Chinese nutgall, the former contg 50-60%, the latter about 70%. The chemistry of the tannins is most complex and non-uniform. Tannins may be divided into 2 groups: (*a*) derivatives of flavanols, so-called condensed tannins and (*b*) hydrolyzable tannins (the more important group) which are esters of a sugar, usually glucose, with one or more trihydroxybenzene-carboxylic acids. The structure given here is that of a tannin named *corilagin*: Schmidt *et al.*, *Ann.* **587**, 67 (1954). The empirical formula of corilagin is $C_{27}H_{22}O_{18}$. For the commercial tannic acid, whose specifications follow, the empirical formula is usually given as $C_{76}H_{52}O_{46}$. Toxicity study: Robinson, Graessle, *J. Pharmacol. Exp. Ther.* **77**, 63 (1943). Comprehensive reviews: M. Nierenstein, *The Natural Organic Tannins* (London, 1934); O. Th. Schmidt, "Gallotannine" in *Fortschr. Chem. Org. Naturst.* **13**, 70-136 (1956); *Symposium on the Chemistry of Vegetable Tannins* (Soc. Leather Trades Chemists, Croydon 1956).

Corilagin

Yellowish-white to light brown, amorphous, bulky powder or flakes, or spongy masses; faint characteristic odor; astringent taste. Gradually darkens on exposure to air and light; at 210-215° dec mostly into pyrogallol and CO_2. Gives insol ppts with albumin, starch, gelatin, most alkaloidal and metallic salts; produces a bluish-black color or precip with ferric salts. One gram dissolves in 0.35 ml water, 1 ml warm glycerol; very sol in alc, acetone. Practically insol in benzene, chloroform, ether, petr ether, carbon disulfide, carbon tetrachloride. *Keep well closed and protected from light.* LD_{100} orally in mice: 6.0 g/kg (Robinson, Graessle).

USE: Mordant in dyeing; manuf ink; sizing paper and silk; printing fabrics; with gelatin and albumin for manuf of imitation horn and tortoise shell; tanning; clarifying beer or wine; in photo-graphy; as coagulant in rubber manuf; manuf gallic acid and pyro-gallol; as reagent in analytical chemistry.

THERAP CAT: Astringent.

THERAP CAT (VET): Astringent, hemostatic, in solutions for burns. Has been used internally as an astringent and as a heavy metal antidote.

9053. Tantalum. [7440-25-7] Ta; at. wt 180.94788; at. no. 73; valence 5, also 4, 3, 2. Group VB (5). Two naturally occurring isotopes: 181 (99.9877%); 180 (0.0123%), $T_{1/2} > 10^{12}$ years; arti-ficial radioactive isotopes: 172-179; 182-186. Occurs almost in-variably with niobium; less abundant than niobium. Found in the minerals *columbite* [(Fe,Mn)(Nb,Ta)$_2O_6$], *tantalite* [(Fe,Mn)(Ta, Nb)$_2O_6$] and *microlite* [(Na,Ca)$_2$Ta$_2O_6$(O,OH,F)]. Discovered by Ekeberg in 1802; first obtained pure by Bolton: *Z. Elektrochem.* **11**, 45 (1905). Prepn: Schoeller, Powell, *J. Chem. Soc.* **119**, 1927 (1921). Reviews of tantalum and its compounds: G. L. Miller, *Tantalum and Niobium* (Academic Press, New York, 1959) 767 pp; Brown, "The Chemistry of Niobium and Tantalum" in *Comprehen-*

sive Inorganic Chemistry vol. 3, J. C. Bailar, Jr. *et al.*, Eds. (Pergamon Press, Oxford, 1973) pp 553-622.

Gray, very hard, malleable, ductile metal; can readily be drawn in fine wires. mp 2996°. bp 5429°. d 16.69. Spec heat (0°): 0.036 cal/g/°C. Electrical resistivity (18°): 12.4 μohm-cm. Insol in water. Very resistant to chemical attack; not attacked by acids other than hydrofluoric; not attacked by aq alkalies; slowly attacked by fused alkalies. Reacts with fluorine, chlorine, and oxygen only on heating. At high temps absorbs several hundred times its volume of hydrogen; combines with nitrogen, with carbon.

Caution: Potential symptoms of overexposure to metal and oxide dust are irritation of eyes and skin. *See NIOSH Pocket Guide to Chemical Hazards* (DHHS/NIOSH 97-140, 1997) p 294.

USE: In pen points; analytical weights; apparatus and instruments for chemical, surgical, and dental use instead of platinum, in tantalum capacitors (a type of electrolytic condenser, trademarked "Tantalytic").

9054. Tantalum Pentachloride. [7721-01-9] Tantalum chloride (TaCl₅). Cl_5Ta; mol wt 358.21. Cl 49.49%, Ta 50.51%. $TaCl_5$. Prepn: Rolsten, *J. Am. Chem. Soc.* **80**, 2952 (1958). Review of tantalum halides: Fairbrother in *Halogen Chemistry* vol. 3, V. Gutmann, Ed. (Academic Press, New York, 1967) pp 123-178. Acute toxicity: K. W. Cochran *et al.*, *Arch. Ind. Hyg. Occup. Med.* **1**, 637 (1950).

White or light yellow, cryst powder; monoclinic; dec in moist air. d 3.68; mp 216.5-220°. Begins to volatilize at 144°, bp 239.3°. Dec by water; sol in abs alcohol. LD_{50} in rats (mg/kg): 75 i.p.; 1900 orally (Cochran).

9055. Tantalum Pentafluoride. [7783-71-3] F_5Ta; mol wt 275.94. F 34.42%, Ta 65.58%. TaF_5. Prepd from tantalum pentachloride by the halide exchange method according to the equation $TaCl_5 + 5HF \rightarrow TaF_5 + 5HCl$: Ruff, Zedner, *Ber.* **42**, 492 (1909); Ruff, Schiller, *Z. Anorg. Allg. Chem.* **72**, 329 (1911); Kwasnik in *Handbook of Preparative Inorganic Chemistry* vol. 1, G. Brauer, Ed. (Academic Press, New York, 2nd ed, 1963) pp 255-256. Prepn from the elements: Fairbrother, Frith, *J. Chem. Soc.* **1951**, 3051. Review of transition metal pentafluorides: Peacock, *Adv. Fluorine Chem.* **7**, 113-145 (1973).

Deliquescent, strongly refractive prisms. d^{20} 4.74. mp 96.8°. Also reported as 95.1°: Fairbrother, Frith, *loc. cit.* bp 229.5°. Sol in water and ether with formation of oxyfluoro complexes. Also sol in concd nitric acid, more sol in fuming nitric acid. Sparingly sol in hot carbon disulfide and hot carbon tetrachloride. Etches glass slowly.

USE: Friedel-Crafts catalyst.

9056. Tantalum Pentoxide. [1314-61-0] Tantalum oxide (Ta₂O₅); tantalic acid anhydride. O_5Ta_2; mol wt 441.89. O 18.10%, Ta 81.90%. Ta_2O_5. Acute toxicity: K. W. Cochran *et al.*, *Arch. Ind. Hyg. Occup. Med.* **1**, 637 (1950).

White, microcrystalline, infusible powder. Insol in water, alcohol, mineral acids. Sol in HF. Dec by fusing with $KHSO_4$ or KOH, forming potassium tantalate with the latter. LD_{50} orally in rats: 8000 mg/kg (Cochran).

9057. Taprostene. [108945-35-3] 3-[(Z)-[(3aR,4R,5R,6aS)-4-[(1E,3S)-3-Cyclohexyl-3-hydroxy-1-propenyl]hexahydro-5-hydroxy-2H-cyclopenta[b]furan-2-ylidene]methyl]benzoic acid; α-[(2Z,3aR,4R,5R,6aS)-4-[(1E,3S)-3-cyclohexyl-3-hydroxypropenyl]-hexahydro-5-hydroxy-2H-cyclopenta[b]furan-2-ylidene]-*m*-toluic acid; [(5Z,13E,9α,11α,15S)-2,3,4-trinor-1,5-inter-*m*-phenylene-6,9-epoxy-11,15-dihydroxy-15-cyclohexyl-16,17,18,19,20-pentanor]-prosta-5,13-dienoic acid. $C_{24}H_{30}O_5$; mol wt 398.49. C 72.34%, H 7.59%, O 20.08%. Prostacyclin analog; platelet aggregation inhibitor. Prepn: U. Seipp *et al.*, *EP 45842*; *eidem*, *US 4372971* (1982, 1983 both to Grünenthal); L. Flohé *et al.*, *Arzneim.-Forsch.* **33**, 1240 (1983). As adjuvant to thrombolytic therapy in acute myocardial infarction: F. W. Bär *et al.*, *Eur. Heart J.* **14**, 1118 (1993). Review of pharmacology and clinical experience: J. Schneider *et al.*, *Cardiovasc. Drug Rev.* **11**, 479-500 (1993).

Sodium salt. [87440-45-7] CG-4203; Rheocyclan. $C_{24}H_{29}NaO_5$; mol wt 420.47. $[\alpha]_D^{22}$ +249° (c = 0.68 in methanol). LD_{50} in mice, rats (mg/kg): 164, 20 i.v. (Schneider).

THERAP CAT: Antithrombotic.

9058. TAPS. [29915-38-6] 3-[[2-Hydroxy-1,1-bis(hydroxymethyl)ethyl]amino]-1-propanesulfonic acid; *N*-tris[(hydroxymethyl)methyl]-3-aminopropanesulfonic acid. $C_7H_{17}NO_6S$; mol wt 243.28. C 34.56%, H 7.04%, N 5.76%, O 39.46%, S 13.18%. Zwitterionic *N*-substituted sulfonic acid in the style of the "Good" buffers; active in the pH range 6-8.5. Prepn: I. Zeid, I. Ismail, *Ann.* **1974**, 667. Dissociation: A. M. El-Nady, H. A. Azab, *Acta Chim. Hung.* **130**, 665 (1993). Use as eluent: R. H. P. Reid, *J. Chromatogr. A* **684**, 221 (1994). Effect of buffer concentration on pH-activity relationship: C. G. Bevans, A. L. Harris, *J. Biol. Chem.* **274**, 3711 (1999).

Crystals, mp 194°. pKa: 8.55; pKa (37°): 8.1; pKa_2 (25°): 8.28.

TAPSO. [68399-81-5] 2-Hydroxy-3-[[2-hydroxy-1,1-bis(hydroxymethyl)ethyl]amino]-1-propanesulfonic acid. $C_7H_{17}NO_7S$; mol wt 259.28. Hydroxy analog of TAPS. Prepn: W. J. Ferguson *et al.*, *Anal. Biochem.* **104**, 300 (1980). Crystal structure: J. Wouters, D. Stalke, *Acta Crystallogr.* **C52**, 1684 (1996). Thermodynamics of dissociation: R. N. Roy *et al.*, *J. Chem. Eng. Data* **42**, 446 (1997). Triclinic colorless crystals, mp 226-228° (dec). pKa (20°): 7.7. ΔpKa/°C: −0.018. Soly in water (0°): 1M.

USE: Biological buffer.

9059. Taraxacum. Dandelion; lion's tooth. Dried rhizome and roots of *Taraxacum palustre* (Lyons) Lam. & DC. (*T. officinale* Weber, *Leontodon taraxacum* L.), *Compositae*. *Habit.* Europe; naturalized in North America. *Constit.* Taraxerol, choline, levulin, inulin, pectin.

9060. Taraxasterol. [1059-14-9] (3β,18α,19α)-Urs-20(30)-en-3-ol; taraxast-20(30)-en-3β-ol; α-tarucerol; taraxasterin. $C_{30}H_{50}O$; mol wt 426.72. C 84.44%, H 11.81%, O 3.75%. A monohydroxy triterpene. Isoln from *Taraxacum officinale*, Wiggers, *Compositae:* Power, Browning, *J. Chem. Soc.* **101**, 2411 (1912). Structure and configuration: Ames *et al.*, *ibid.* **1954**, 1905. Identity with anthesterin: Power, Browning *ibid.* **105**, 1829 (1914); with α-lactucerol: Zellner, *Monatsh. Chem.* **47**, 681 (1926).

Needles from alcohol, mp 221-222°. $[\alpha]_D$ +96.3° (CHCl$_3$). Very sol in alcohol, ether, petr ether; slightly sol in chloroform, benzene, carbon disulfide, acetone.

Acetate. Lactucerin; lactucon. C$_{32}$H$_{52}$O$_2$. Hexagonal plates. mp 251-252° (from ethyl acetate + alcohol). $[\alpha]_D$ +100.5°.

9061. Taraxein. [9010-30-4] A protein complex isolated from the blood serum of schizophrenics; thought to be an antibrain antibody. Method of isolation: R. G. Heath *et al.*, *Am. J. Psychiatry* **114**, 14 (1957). Studies of relationship to schizophrenia: *idem et al.*, *Arch. Gen. Psychiatry* **16**, 1, 10, 24 (1967); J. R. Bergen *et al.*, *Biol. Psychiatry* **15**, 369 (1980). Review: R. G. Heath in *Nutrients and Brain Function*, W. B. Essman, Ed. (Karger, Basel, 1987) pp 186-192.

9062. Taraxerol. [127-22-0] (3β)-D-Friedoolean-14-en-3-ol; isoolean-14-en-3β-ol; skimmiol; alnulin; tiliadin. C$_{30}$H$_{50}$O; mol wt 426.72. C 84.44%, H 11.81%, O 3.75%. Found in *Tilia cordata* Mill., *Tiliaceae:* Bräutigam, *Arch. Pharm.* **238**, 555 (1900); in *Alnus glutinosa* (L.) Gaertn., *Betulaceae:* Zellner, Weiss, *Sitzungsber. Akad. Wiss. Wien* **132**, 258 (1923); in *Taraxacum officinale* Weber, *Compositae:* Burrows, Simpson, *J. Chem. Soc.* **1938**, 2042; in *Litsea dealbata* Nees, *Lauraceae:* Dunstan *et al.*, *Aust. J. Chem.* **6**, 321 (1953); from *Befaria racemosa* (Vent.), *Ericaceae:* Euda *et al.*, *J. Org. Chem.* **26**, 271 (1961). Structure: Beaton *et al.*, *J. Chem. Soc.* **1955**, 2131. Partial synthesis from β-amyrin: *eidem*, *Chem. Ind. (London)* **1955**, 35.

Plates from chloroform + methanol, needles from benzene, mp 282-285°. uv max (ethanol): 210, 215, 220, 223 nm (ε 3900, 2400, 700, 250). Sol in benzene, chloroform, ether, ethyl acetate, acetic anhydride, acetic acid, phenol, pyridine, xylene; less sol in alcohol.

Acetate. C$_{32}$H$_{52}$O$_2$. Plates from chloroform + methanol, mp 303-305°. $[\alpha]_D$ +10.5° (c = 1.8 in chloroform).

Benzoate. C$_{37}$H$_{54}$O$_2$. Needles from benzene or chloroform + alc, mp 292-293°. $[\alpha]_D^{23}$ +35.7° (c = 0.7 in chloroform).

9063. Taribavirin. [119567-79-2] 1-β-D-Ribofuranosyl-1H-1,2,4-triazole-3-carboximidamide; 1-β-D-ribofuranosyl-1,2,4-triazole-3-carboxamidine; ribamidine. C$_8$H$_{13}$N$_5$O$_4$; mol wt 243.22. C 39.51%, H 5.39%, N 28.79%, O 26.31%. Liver-targeting antiviral nucleoside analog; 3-carboxamidine prodrug of ribavirin, *q.v.* Prepn of hydrochloride: J. T. Witkowski *et al.*, *DE* **2220246**; *eidem*, *US* **3798209** (1972, 1974 both to ICN); *idem et al.*, *ibid.* **32**, 1447 (1989); B. Gabrielsen *et al.*, *ibid.* **35**, 3231 (1992). In vitro and in vivo efficacy vs *Phlebovirus*: R. W. Sidwell *et al.*, *Antiviral Res.* **10**, 193 (1988); vs influenza: *idem et al.*, *ibid.* **68**, 10 (2005). LC/MS/MS determn in plasma: Y. Liu *et al.*, *J. Chromatogr. B* **832**, 17 (2006). Liver-targeting properties and safety profile in animals: C. Lin *et al.*, *Antivir. Chem. Chemother.* **14**, 145 (2003). Mechanism of action study: J. Z. Wu *et al.*, *Antimicrob. Agents Chemother.* **48**, 4006 (2004). Clinical pharmacokinetics in hepatitis C patients: S. Aora *et al.*, *J. Clin. Pharmacol.* **45**, 275 (2005).

Hydrochloride. [40372-00-7] Viramidine. C$_8$H$_{13}$N$_5$O$_4$.HCl; mol wt 279.68. Crystals from acetonitrile + ethanol, mp 177-179° (dec).

THERAP CAT: Antiviral.

9064. Tariquidar. [206873-63-4] N-[2-[[[4-[2-(3,4-Dihydro-6,7-dimethoxy-2(1H)-isoquinolinyl)ethyl]phenyl]amino]carbonyl]-4,5-dimethoxyphenyl]-3-quinolinecarboxamide; XR-9576. C$_{38}$H$_{38}$N$_4$O$_6$; mol wt 646.73. C 70.57%, H 5.92%, N 8.66%, O 14.84%. Multidrug resistance modulator; selective inhibitor of P-glycoprotein (P-gp), *q.v.* Prepn: H. Ryder *et al.*, **WO 9817648**; *eidem*, **US 6218393** (1998, 2001 both to Xenova); M. Roe *et al.*, *Bioorg. Med. Chem. Lett.* **9**, 595 (1999). Molecular interaction with P-gp: C. Martin *et al.*, *Br. J. Pharmacol.* **128**, 403 (1999). Effect on multidrug resistant cell lines: P. Mistry *et al.*, *Cancer Res.* **61**, 749 (2001). Clinical pharmacology: A. Stewart *et al.*, *Clin. Cancer Res.* **6**, 4186 (2000). Effect on accumulation of ^{99m}Tc-sestamibi, *q.v.*, in patients with metastatic cancers: M. Agrawal *et al.*, *Clin. Cancer Res.* **9**, 650 (2003).

THERAP CAT: Antineoplastic adjunct (chemosensitizer).

9065. Tar Oil. Volatile oil distilled from wood tar. *Principal constit.* Phenolic substances and hydrocarbons.

Almost colorless liquid when fresh, but soon becomes dark brownish-red. d 0.860-0.900. Insol in water; sol in alcohol, ether.

9066. Tar Oil, Rectified. Pine tar oil. The volatile oil from pine tar rectified by steam distillation. Chief active constituents are phenolic substances.

Dark reddish-brown, thin liquid; strong empyreumatic odor and taste. d$_{25}^{25}$ 0.960-0.990. Insol in water; miscible with alcohol.

THERAP CAT: Antiseptic (topical); dermatologic.

THERAP CAT (VET): Antiseptic, antipruritic. For chronic skin conditions and in hoof dressings. Has been used internally as an expectorant.

9067. Tarragon. Estragon. The dried leaves and flowering tops of the perennial herb, *Artemisia dracunculus* L., *Compositae*. *Habit.* Siberia, Caspian Sea region; cultivated in Western Europe. Yields up to 0.8% oil of tarragon. *Constit.* p-Allylanisole (estragole; methyl chavicol); ocimene; myrcene; phellandrene(?); p-methoxycinnamaldehyde.

USE: The herb for culinary purposes, the oil as flavoring agent in liqueurs, soups, sauces and salad dressings. In perfumery to improve the note of chypre type perfumes.

9068. D-Tartaric Acid. [147-71-7] (2S,3S)-2,3-Dihydroxybutanedioic acid; unusual tartaric acid; unnatural tartaric acid; l-tartaric acid; (−)-tartaric acid; levotartaric acid; D-threo-2,3-dihydroxysuccinic acid. C$_4$H$_6$O$_6$; mol wt 150.09. C 32.01%, H 4.03%, O 63.96%. Levorotatory tartaric acid having a dextro configuration. Although termed "unnatural," its occurrence in nature has been demonstrated. Obtained in small amounts from racemic tartaric acid through biochemical cleavage using *Penicillium notatum*, *Aspergillus griseus*, *A. niger* or other microorganisms: Pasteur, *Compt. Rend.* **51**, 298 (1860). Alternate route using salt formation with d-methylamphetamine: Walton, *J. Soc. Chem. Ind.* **64**, 219 (1945). Monograph: K. Freudenberg, *Stereochemie* I, (1933), reprinted by J. W. Edwards (Ann Arbor, 1945). Crystallographic data: A. N. Winchell, *The Optical Properties of Organic Compounds* (Academic Press, New York, 2nd ed., 1954) p 47.

Monoclinic sphenoidal prisms. d_4^{20} 1.7598. mp 168-170°. $[\alpha]_D^{20}$ −12.0° (c = 20 in H$_2$O). pKa$_1$ 2.93; pKa$_2$ 4.23. One gram dissolves in 0.75 ml water at room temp, in 0.5 ml boiling water, 1.7 ml methanol, 3 ml ethanol, 0.5 ml propanol, 250 ml ether. Also sol in glycerol. Insol in chloroform. Maximum soly in water at 20°: 139 g/100 ml.

9069.   DL-Tartaric Acid. [133-37-9] 2,3-Dihydroxybutanedioic acid; racemic tartaric acid; racemic acid; *dl*-tartaric acid; resolvable tartaric acid; uvic acid; paratartaric acid; *dl*-Weinsäure (German); Vogesensäure (German); Traubensäure (German). C$_4$H$_6$O$_6$; mol wt 150.09. C 32.01%, H 4.03%, O 63.96%. Probably never a natural product, although sometimes found in small amounts during wine-making. Prepn from L-tartaric acid by boiling with aq NaOH (*meso*-tartaric acid is obtained as a byproduct): Holleman, *Org. Synth.* **6**, 82 (1926); **coll. vol. I** (2nd ed., 1941) p 497. Synthesis by oxidation of fumaric acid: Milas, Terry, *J. Am. Chem. Soc.* **47**, 1412 (1925); Milas, Sussman, *ibid.* **58**, 1302 (1936); **US 2000213** (1935 to Standard Brands). From maleic acid: Church, Blumberg, *Ind. Eng. Chem.* **43**, 1780 (1951).

Anhyd acid, triclinic pinacoidal crystals from abs alc, from water above 73°, or by drying the monohydrate at 100°. mp 206°. pKa$_1$ 2.96; pKa$_2$ 4.24. Less soluble in water than L-tartaric acid. pH of 0.1M aq soln: 2.0. Soly in alcohol (g/100 g): 2.006 at 0°; 3.153 at 15°; 5.01 at 25°; 6.299 at 40°. Soly in ether about 1%.
Monohydrate. Triclinic pinacoidal crystals from water. d_4^{20} 1.697. One hundred parts (w/w) of water dissolve 14.00 parts at 10°; 20.60 at 20°; 29.10 at 30°; 43.32 at 40°; 99.88 at 70°; 184.91 at 100°.

9070.   L-Tartaric Acid. [87-69-4] (2R,3R)-2,3-Dihydroxybutanedioic acid; ordinary tartaric acid; natural tartaric acid; *d*-tartaric acid; (+)-tartaric acid; dextrotartaric acid; L-2,3-dihydroxybutanedioic acid; *d-α,β*-dihydroxysuccinic acid; Weinsäure (German); Weinsteinsäure (German). C$_4$H$_6$O$_6$; mol wt 150.09. C 32.01%, H 4.03%, O 63.96%. Dextrorotatory tartaric acid having a levo configuration. Widely distributed in nature, classified as a fruit acid. Occurs in many fruits, free and combined with potassium, calcium or magnesium. Observed in antiquity as the acid potassium salt found deposited as a fine crystalline crust during fermentation of grape juice or tamarind juice and termed *faecula* (little yeast) by the Romans. The derivation from *Tartarus* is of medieval, alchemical origin. In modern processes the acid potassium tartrate obtained during wine-making is first converted to calcium tartrate which is then hydrolyzed to tartaric acid and calcium sulfate: Metzner, *Chem. Eng. Prog.* **43**, 160 (1947); several modifications, e.g., **IT 490221** (1954 to Procedimenti Chimici), *C.A.* **50**, 11607c (1956). Extraction from tamarind pulp in about 10% yield: **IN 52167** (1955), *C.A.* **50**, 5249g (1956). Synthesis by hydroxylation of maleic acid: Church, Blumberg, *Ind. Eng. Chem.* **43**, 1780 (1951). Practically all of the L-tartaric acid sold today is a byproduct of the wine industry. Monograph: U. Roux, *La Grande Industrie des Acides Organiques* (Dounod, Paris, 1939). Example of a modern process: Dabul, **US 3114770** (1963 to Orandi & Massera).

Monoclinic sphenoidal prisms, mp 168-170°. Stable to air and light. Strong acid taste. Refreshing when in dil aq soln. d_4^{20} 1.7598. Odor of burnt sugar when heated to mp. $[\alpha]_D^{20}$ +12.0° (c

= 20 in H$_2$O). Strong organic acid. At 25° pKa$_1$ 2.98; pKa$_2$ 4.34. pH of 0.1N soln: 2.2. Heat of combustion: −275.1 kcal/mol. Specific heat: 0.288 cal/g/°C at 21 to 51°; 0.296 at 0 to 99.6°. Dielectric constant 36.0 for 1200 cm waves. Freely sol in water. d_4^{15} of aq solns (w/w at 15°): 1% 1.0045; 10% 1.0469; 20% 1.0969; 30% 1.1505; 40% 1.2078; 50% 1.2696. Max soly in water in g/100 ml at various temps: 0° = 115; 10° = 126; 20° = 139; 30° = 156; 40° = 176; 50° = 195; 60° = 217; 70° = 244; 80° = 273; 90° = 307; 100° = 343. One gram dissolves in 0.75 ml water at room temp, in 0.5 ml boiling water, 1.7 ml methanol, 3 ml ethanol, 10.5 ml propanol, 250 ml ether. Also sol in glycerol. Insol in chloroform.
Caution: Can cause local irritation. *See Patty's Industrial Hygiene and Toxicology* vol. 2C, G. D. Clayton, F. E. Clayton, Eds. (Wiley-Interscience, New York, 3rd ed., 1982) p 4937, 4943-4945.
USE: In the soft drink industry, confectionery products, bakery products, gelatin desserts, as an acidulant. In photography, tanning, ceramics, manuf tartrates. The common commercial esters are the diethyl and dibutyl derivs used for lacquers and in textile printing. Pharmaceutic aid (buffering agent).

9071.   meso-Tartaric Acid. [147-73-9] (2R,3S)-*rel*-2,3-Dihydroxybutanedioic acid; mesotartaric acid; internally compensated tartaric acid; unresolvable tartaric acid; Antiweinsäure (German). C$_4$H$_6$O$_6$; mol wt 150.09. C 32.01%, H 4.03%, O 63.96%. Prepd by boiling L-tartaric acid with alkali; as byproduct of racemization: Winther, *Z. Phys. Chem.* **56**, 507 (1906); Holleman, *Org. Synth.* **coll. vol. I** (2nd ed., 1941) p 497; Milas, **US 2414385** (1947). Microbial prepn: Martin, Foster, *J. Bacteriol.* **70**, 405 (1955); Foster, **US 2947665** (1960). Explanation of optical inactivity: Noller, *Science* **102**, 508 (1945); C. R. Noller, *Chemistry of Organic Compounds* (Philadelphia, 2nd ed., 1957) p 339.

(2R,3S)-rel-form

Monohydrate. Rectangular plates, d_4^{20} 1.666 (also reported as 1.737). mp 140° (also reported as 159-160°). pKa$_1$ 3.11; pKa$_2$ 4.80. Maximum soly in water at 20°: 125 g/100 ml.

9072.   Tartrazine. [1934-21-0] 4,5-Dihydro-5-oxo-1-(4-sulfophenyl)-4-[(4-sulfophenyl)azo]-1H-pyrazole-3-carboxylic acid trisodium salt; C.I. Acid Yellow 23; 3-carboxy-5-hydroxy-1-*p*-sulfophenyl-4-*p*-sulfophenylazopyrazole trisodium salt; 5-hydroxy-1-(*p*-sulfophenyl)-4-[(*p*-sulfophenyl)azo]pyrazole-3-carboxylic acid trisodium salt; hydrazine yellow; C.I. 19140; FD & C Yellow No. 5; C.I. Food Yellow 4. C$_{16}$H$_9$N$_4$Na$_3$O$_9$S$_2$; mol wt 534.36. C 35.96%, H 1.70%, N 10.48%, Na 12.91%, O 26.95%, S 12.00%. Prepn: **US 2457823** (1949 to Ilford); Freeman *et al., J. Assoc. Off. Agric. Chem.* **33**, 937 (1950). *See also: Colour Index* **vol. 4** (3rd ed., 1971) p 4132.

Bright orange-yellow powder. Freely sol in water. The aq soln is not changed by HCl but becomes redder with sodium hydroxide.
USE: As a dye for wool and silks; as colorant in food, drugs and cosmetics. In biochemistry as an adsorption-elution indicator for chloride estimations.

9073.   Tartronic Acid. [80-69-3] Hydroxypropanedioic acid; hydroxymalonic acid. C$_3$H$_4$O$_5$; mol wt 120.06. C 30.01%, H 3.36%, O 66.63%. HOCH(COOH)$_2$. Prepd by ozonization of malonic acid in aq soln: Dobinson, *Chem. Ind. (London)* **1959**, 853.
Colorless, odorless crystals. Crystallizes from water with ½ and 1H$_2$O. Becomes anhyd at 60°. Sublimes 110-120°. mp 158-160°

with decompn (CO_2 evolved). pK_1 2.42; pK_2 4.54, *see* Grandjean, *Bull. Soc. R. Sci. Liege* **38**, 288 (1969), *C.A.* **72**, 42684t (1970). Very sol in water, alcohol; the anhydrous acid is sol in ether.

9074. Taurine. [107-35-7] 2-Aminoethanesulfonic acid. $C_2H_7NO_3S$; mol wt 125.15. C 19.19%, H 5.64%, N 11.19%, O 38.35%, S 25.62%. $NH_2CH_2CH_2SO_3H$. Conditionally essential nutrient, important during mammalian development, especially for cells of the cerebellum and retina. Conjugates bile acids, present in most milk (but only minimally in that of dairy cows); occurs also in lungs and flesh extract of oxen, in shark blood, in mussels, in oysters. Isoln from ox bile: Hammarsten, *Z. Physiol. Chem.* **32**, 456 (1901); from the large muscle of abalone *(Haliotis)*: Schmidt, Watson, *J. Biol. Chem.* **33**, 499 (1918). Synthesis starting with 2-bromoethanesulfonate: C. S. Marvel, C. F. Bailey, *Org. Synth.* **coll. vol. II**, 563 (1943). Synthesis by sodium sulfite sulfonation of ethylene chloride followed by ammonolysis with anhydr NH_3 or with aq NH_3 and ammonium carbonate: Schick, Degering, *Ind. Eng. Chem.* **39**, 906 (1947). Importance to retinal function in cats: A. R. Rabin *et al., Invest. Ophthalmol.* **12**, 694 (1973); K. C. Ha *et al., Science* **188**, 949 (1975); E. L. Berson *et al., Invest. Ophthalmol.* **15**, 52 (1976); K. C. Hayes, *Can. Vet. J.* **23**, 2 (1982). Comparison of taurine depletion in humans and other mammals: K. C. Hayes, J. A. Sturman, *Adv. Exp. Med. Biol.* **139**, 79 (1982). Presence in human milk: G. E. Gaull, *J. Pediatr. Gastroenterol. Nutr.* **2**, Suppl. 1, 266 (1983); *idem, Acta Paediatr. Scand. Suppl.* **296**, 38 (1982). Concn in plasma and urine of breast-fed and formula-fed infants: A.-L. Järvenpää *et al., Pediatrics* **70**, 221 (1982). Association of retinal dysfunction with low plasma taurine levels in adults: H. S. Geggel *et al., N. Engl. J. Med.* **312**, 142 (1985). Books: *Taurine*, R. Huxtable, A. Barbeau, Eds. (Raven Press, New York, 1975) 480 pp; *Taurine: Nutritional Value and Mechanisms of Action*, J. B. Lombardini *et al.*, Eds. (Plenum Press, New York, 1992) 456 pp.

Large monoclinic prismatic rods, dec about 300°. pK_1' 1.5; pK_2' 8.74. Sol in 15.5 parts of water at 12°. 100 parts of 95% alc dissolve 0.004 parts at 17°. Insol in abs alc.

Note: Some infant formulas are being reformulated to increase the concn of taurine to that found in human milk, *Chem. Eng. News* **62**, 22 (July 30, 1984).

9075. Taurocholic Acid. [81-24-3] 2-[[(3α,5β,7α,12α)-3,7,12-Trihydroxy-24-oxocholan-24-yl]amino]ethanesulfonic acid; *N*-choloyltaurine; cholaic acid; cholyltaurine. $C_{26}H_{45}NO_7S$; mol wt 515.70. C 60.55%, H 8.80%, N 2.72%, O 21.72%, S 6.22%. The product of conjugation of cholic acid with taurine. Its sodium salt is the chief ingredient of the bile of carnivorous animals. Prepn from dog bile: Hammarsten in Abderhalden, *Handbuch der Biol. Arbeitsmethoden*, Abt. **I**, Teil 6, p 219 (1925). Separation from bile acids: Ahrens, Craig, *J. Biol. Chem.* **195**, 763 (1952). Enzymic synthesis: Siperstein, Murray, *Science* **123**, 377 (1956). Prepn of the sodium salt: Cortese, *J. Am. Chem. Soc.* **59**, 2532 (1937); Norman, *Ark. Kemi* **8**, 331 (1955); of the barium salt: Kazuno, Yanazaki, *Z. Physiol. Chem.* **224** 160 (1934). Binding of taurocholic acid to serum proteins: Burke *et al., Clin. Chim. Acta* **32**, 207 (1971). Toxicity data: Klaassen, *Toxicol. Appl. Pharmacol.* **24**, 37 (1973).

Clusters of slender, four-sided prisms from alcohol + ether, stable to air. (Commercial prepns are usually amorphous, very hygroscopic, and of yellow color.) Dec about 125°. $[\alpha]_D^{18}$ +38.8° (c = 2 in alcohol). pK 1.4. Freely sol in water, sol in alcohol. Almost insol in ether, ethyl acetate. Is hydrolyzed to cholic acid and taurine by acids and alkalies. LD_{50} in newborn rats: 380 mg/kg (Klaassen).

Sodium salt. Sodium taurocholate. $C_{26}H_{44}NNaO_7S$. Crystals with 1.5 and 2 mols H_2O. Sweet taste with bitter aftertaste. Dec about 230°. $[\alpha]_D^{20}$ +24° (c = 3). Very freely sol in water or alcohol. Solvent action on cholesterol: Rosin, *Z. Physiol. Chem.* **124**, 282 (1923).

Barium salt. Barium taurocholate. $C_{52}H_{88}BaN_2O_{14}S_2$. Crystals with 5 mols H_2O, dec 225-227°. $[\alpha]_D^{20}$ +25.6°. Converted to taurocholic acid by treatment with sulfuric acid.

USE: Sodium salt is a lipase accelerator. *See also* Ox Bile Extract.

THERAP CAT: Choleretic.

9076. Taurolidine. [19388-87-5] 4,4'-Methylenebis(tetrahydro-1,2,4-thiadiazine) 1,1,1',1'-tetraoxide; 4,4'-methylenebis-(perhydro-1,2,4-thiadiazine 1,1-dioxide); bis(1,1-dioxoperhydro-1,2,4-thiadiazin-4-yl)methane; Drainasept; Taurolin; Tauroflex. $C_7H_{16}N_4O_4S_2$; mol wt 284.36. C 29.57%, H 5.67%, N 19.70%, O 22.51%, S 22.55%. Broad spectrum, synthetic formaldehyde carrier formed by the condensation of two molecules of taurine and three molecules of formaldehyde. Prepn: **FR 1458701**; R. W. Pfirrmann, **US 3423408** (1966, 1969 both to Ed. Geistlich Söhne). Antibacterial activity in mice: M. K. Browne *et al., J. Appl. Bacteriol.* **41**, 363 (1976). Anti-endotoxin activity in lab animals: R. W. Pfirrmann, G. B. Leslie, *ibid.* **46**, 97 (1979). Mechanism of action: E. Myers *et al., ibid.* **48**, 89 (1980). HPLC determn of metabolites in plasma: A. D. Woolfson *et al., Int. J. Pharm.* **49**, 135 (1989). Pharmacokinetics: C. Steinbach-Lebbin *et al., Arzneim.-Forsch.* **32**, 1542 (1982). Metabolism in humans: B. I. Knight *et al., Br. J. Clin. Pharmacol.* **12**, 695 (1981). Clinical trials in peritonitis: M. K. Browne *et al., Surg. Gynecol. Obstet.* **146**, 721 (1978); G. Wesch *et al., Fortschr. Med.* **101**, 545 (1983); in wound sepsis: A. K. Halsall *et al., Pharmatherapeutica* **2**, 673 (1981); in pleural infection: A. A. Conlan *et al., S. Afr. Med. J.* **64**, 653 (1983).

White crystals, mp 154-158°. Sol in water.
THERAP CAT: Antibacterial.

9077. Taxicins. Acyl-free polyols from which the taxines are prepared by partial esterfication: Baxter *et al., J. Chem. Soc.* **1962**, 2964. Structure of taxicin-I and -II: Eyre *et al, Proc. Chem. Soc. London* **1963**, 271. Structure and stereochemical studies of taxicin-I and -II: Dukes *et al., Tetrahedron Lett.* **1965**, 4765; *J. Chem. Soc. C* **1967**, 448; Eyre *et al., ibid.* 452. Structure of *O*-cinnamoyl-taxicin-II triacetate (taxinine): Kurono *et al., Tetrahedron Lett.* **1963**, 2153; Nakanishi, Kurono, *ibid.* **1963**, 2161; Ueda *et al., ibid.* **1963**, 2167; Uyeo *et al., J. Pharm. Soc. Jpn.* **84**, 762 (1964). Stereochemistry of taxinine: Kurono *et al., Tetrahedron Lett.* **1965**, 1917; Shiro *et al., Chem. Commun.* **1966**, 97.

	R	R'	R"
Taxicin-I	OH	H	H
O-cinnamoyltaxicin-I	OH	H	COCH=CHC₆H₅
O-cinnamoyltaxicin-I triacetate	OH	COCH₃	COCH=CHC₆H₅
Taxicin-II	H	H	H
O-cinnamoyltaxicin-II triacetate	H	COCH₃	COCH=CHC₆H₅

Taxicin-I. [5308-89-4] [3*S*-(3α,4aα,5α,6α,11β,12α,12aβ)]-1,3,-4,4a,5,6,7,11,12,12a-Decahydro-3,5,6,11,12-pentahydroxy-9,12a,-13,13-tetramethyl-4-methylene-6,10-methanobenzocyclodecen-8(2*H*)-one. $C_{20}H_{30}O_6$; mol wt 366.45.

O-**Cinnamoyltaxicin-I.** [11034-45-0] $C_{29}H_{36}O_7$. mp 233-234°. $[\alpha]_D^{21}$ +285° (chloroform). uv max (alc): 282 nm (ε 28200).

O-**Cinnamoyltaxicin-I triacetate.** [13452-36-3] $C_{35}H_{42}O_{10}$. Prisms from alc. mp 237-239°. $[\alpha]_D^{18}$ +218° (chloroform).

Taxicin-II. [5308-90-7] $C_{20}H_{30}O_5$; mol wt 350.45.

O-Cinnamoyltaxicin-II triacetate. [3835-52-7] Taxinine. $C_{35}H_{42}O_9$. Prisms from alc, mp 265-267°. $[\alpha]_D^{18}$ +137° (chloroform). uv max: 217, 223, 278 nm (ε 20500; 16000; 28600).

9078. Taxine. [12607-93-1] A mixture of alkaloids from needles and berries of the yew tree, *Taxus baccata* L., *Taxaceae:* Lucas, *Arch. Pharm.* **85**, 145 (1856); Winterstein, Iatrides, *Z. Physiol. Chem.* **117**, 240 (1921); Winterstein, Guyer, *ibid.* **128**, 175 (1923); Callow *et al., J. Chem. Soc.* **1931**, 2138. Structural studies of *taxine-I*: Baxter *et al., ibid.* **1962**, 2964e; of *taxine-II*: Dukes *et al., ibid.* **1967**, 448; Eyre *et al., ibid.* 452. Sepn of cryst *taxine A* and amorph *taxine B* from the amorph mixture: E. Graf, H. Bertholdt, *Pharm. Zentralhalle* **96**, 385 (1957). Structure of taxine A: E. Graf *et al., Ann.* **1982**, 376. *Review:* B. Lythgoe, *The Alkaloids* **vol. X**, R. H. F. Manske, Ed. (Academic Press, New York, 1968) pp 597-626. Toxicity data: Y. Tekol, *Vet. Hum. Toxicol.* **33**, 337 (1991).

Taxine A

Granular amorphous powder, mp 121-124°. $[\alpha]_D^{17}$ +95.7° (c = 4.59 in ethanol). Sol in ether, chloroform, alcohol. Practically insol in water, petr ether. LD_{50} (as the sulfate salt) in mice (mg/kg): 19.72 orally, 21.88 i.p.; in rats (mg/kg): 20.18 s.c. (Tekol).

Taxine A. [1361-49-5] $(\alpha R,\beta S)$-β-(Dimethylamino)-α-hydroxy benzenepropanoic acid $(1S,2R,3E,5S,7S,8S,10R,13S)$-2,13-bis(acetyloxy)-7,10-dihydroxy-8,12,15,15-tetramethyl-9-oxotricyclo[9.3.1.1^{4,8}]hexadeca-3,11-dien-5-yl ester. $C_{35}H_{47}NO_{10}$; mol wt 641.75. mp 204-206°. $[\alpha]_D$ −140° (CHCl$_3$).

Caution: Taxine is undoubtedly responsible for the poisonous properties of the yew. Fatalities among domestic animals due to yew poisoning are not uncommon. Human fatal symptoms are those of gastrointestinal irritation, cardiac and respiratory failure.

9079. Taxodione. [19026-31-4] (4bS-*trans*)-4b,5,6,7,8,8a-Hexahydro-4-hydroxy-4b,8,8-trimethyl-2-(1-methylethyl)-3,9-phenanthrenedione; 11-hydroxy-13-isopropylpodocarpa-7,9(11),-13-triene-6,12-dione. $C_{20}H_{26}O_3$; mol wt 314.42. C 76.40%, H 8.33%, O 15.27%. Diterpenoid quinone methide with tumor-inhibitory properties. Isoln of naturally occurring (+)-form from *Taxodium distichum* Rich, *Taxodiaceae:* S. M. Kupchan *et al., J. Am. Chem. Soc.* **90**, 5923 (1968). Structure: *eidem, J. Org. Chem.* **34**, 3912 (1969). Total synthesis of the racemate: K. Mori, M. Matsui, *Tetrahedron* **26**, 3467 (1970); T. Matsumoto *et al., Bull. Chem. Soc. Jpn.* **44**, 2766 (1971); **50**, 1575 (1977); D. L. Snitman *et al., Tetrahedron Lett.* **1979**, 2477; R. V. Stevens, G. S. Bisacchi, *J. Org. Chem.* **47**, 2396 (1982). Total synthesis of the (+)-form: T. Matsumoto *et al., Bull. Chem. Soc. Jpn.* **50**, 266 (1977); R. H. Burnell *et al., Can. J. Chem.* **65**, 775 (1987). Antitumor activity studies: Hanson *et al., Science* **168**, 378 (1970).

Golden plates from methanol, mp 115-116°. $[\alpha]_D^{28}$ +56° (c = 1 in CHCl$_3$). uv max (methanol): 320, 332, 400 nm (ε 25000, 26000, 2000).

9080. Tazanolast. [82989-25-1] Oxo[[3-(1*H*-tetrazol-5-yl)-phenyl]amino]acetic acid butyl ester; butyl 3′-(1*H*-tetrazol-5-yl)-oxanilate; TO-188; WP-833; Tazalest; Tazanol. $C_{13}H_{15}N_5O_3$; mol wt 289.29. C 53.97%, H 5.23%, N 24.21%, O 16.59%. Mast-cell degranulation inhibitor. Prepn: **JP Kokai 82 11975** (1982 to Wakamoto), *C.A.* **96**, 217856a (1982). Immunopharmacology: M. Agata *et al., Jpn. J. Pharmacol.* **32**, 689 (1982). Series of articles on pharmacology and mechanism of action: *Arzneim.-Forsch.* **38**, 70-92 (1988).

THERAP CAT: Antiallergic.

9081. Tazarotene. [118292-40-3] 6-[(3,4-Dihydro-4,4-dimethyl-2*H*-1-benzothiopyran-6-yl)ethynyl]-3-pyridinecarboxylic acid ethyl ester; ethyl 6-[2-(4,4-dimethylthiochroman-6-yl)ethynyl]nicotinate; AGN-190168; Avage; Tazorac; Zorac. $C_{21}H_{21}NO_2S$; mol wt 351.46. C 71.76%, H 6.02%, N 3.99%, O 9.10%, S 9.12%. Acetylenic retinoid prodrug converted to the active metabolite, *tazarotenic acid*, with selective affinity for retinoic acid receptors RARβ and RARγ. Prepn: R. A. S. Chandraratna, **EP 284288**; *idem*, **US 5089509** (1988, 1992 both to Allergan). Clinical evaluation in psoriasis: T. Esgleyes-Ribot *et al., J. Am. Acad. Dermatol.* **30**, 581 (1994). Clinical trial in treatment of photodamage: S. Kang *et al., ibid.* **52**, 268 (2005). Review of pharmacokinetics and metabolism: D. D.-S. Tang-Liu *et al., Clin. Pharmacokinet.* **37**, 273-287 (1999); of mechanism of action and treatment strategies: A. Roeder *et al., Skin Pharmacol. Physiol.* **17**, 111-118 (2004).

White solid.
THERAP CAT: Antiacne; antipsoriatic. In treatment of photodamaged skin.

9082. Tazettine. [507-79-9] Sekisanine; sekisanoline; ungernine. $C_{18}H_{21}NO_5$; mol wt 331.36. C 65.24%, H 6.39%, N 4.23%, O 24.14%. From *Narcissus tazetta* L., *Lycoris radiata* Herb., *Ungernia sewerzowi* (Rgl.) Fedtsch., and other *Amaryllidaceae:* Späth, Kahovec, *Ber.* **67**, 1501 (1934). Structure and stereochemistry: Ikeda *et al., J. Chem. Soc.* **1956**, 4749. Abs config: Highet, Highet, *Tetrahedron Lett.* **1966**, 4099. Synthesis: Hendrickson *et al., J. Am. Chem. Soc.* **92**, 5538 (1970); Tsuda *et al., Tetrahedron Lett.* **1972**, 3153. Biosynthesis: Fales, Wildman, *J. Am. Chem. Soc.* **86**, 294 (1964). Identity with sekisanine and sekisanoline: Ikeda *et al., loc. cit.* Stereospecific total synthesis: Hendrickson *et al., J. Am. Chem. Soc.* **96**, 7781 (1974); S. Danishefsky *et al., ibid.* **102**, 2838 (1980); **104**, 7591 (1982).

Crystals, mp 210-211° (evac tube); racemate reported as mp 237-238° (Tsuda) and mp 175-176° (Danishefsky). $[\alpha]_D^{25}$ +150.3° (82 mg in 2 ml chloroform). Sol in methanol, ethanol, choroform. Sparingly sol in ether.

Hydrochloride. Crystals, mp 206°, water soluble.

Methiodide. Crystals, dec 220° (evacuated tube).

9083. Tazobactam. [89786-04-9] (2S,3S,5R)-3-Methyl-7-oxo-3-(1H-1,2,3-triazol-1-ylmethyl)-4-thia-1-azabicyclo[3.2.0]heptane-2-carboxylic acid 4,4-dioxide; 2β-[(1,2,3-triazol-1-yl)methyl]-2α-methylpenam-3α-carboxylic acid 1,1-dioxide; YTR-830H; CL-298741. $C_{10}H_{12}N_4O_5S$; mol wt 300.29. C 40.00%, H 4.03%, N 18.66%, O 26.64%, S 10.68%. β-Lactamase inhibitor. Prepn: R. G. Micetich *et al.*, *EP 97446*; *eidem*, *US 4562073* (1984, 1985 both to Taiho); R. G. Micetich *et al.*, *J. Med. Chem.* **30**, 1469 (1987). Degradation in solution: T. Marunaka *et al.*, *Chem. Pharm. Bull.* **36**, 4478 (1988); in solid state: E. Matsushima *et al.*, *ibid.* 4593. β-Lactamase inhibiting activity in comparison with clavulanic acid and sulbactam, *q.q.v.*, vs aerobes: M. R. Jacobs *et al.*, *Antimicrob. Agents Chemother.* **29**, 980 (1986); vs anaerobes: P. C. Appelbaum *et al.*, *ibid.* **30**, 789. HPLC determn in biological materials: T. Marunaka *et al.*, *J. Chromatogr.* **431**, 87 (1988). Clinical trial in combination with piperacillin, *q.v.*: I. M. Gould *et al.*, *Drugs Exp. Clin. Res.* **17**, 187 (1991).

Sodium salt. [89785-84-2] YTR-830; CL-307579. $C_{10}H_{11}$-N_4NaO_5S; mol wt 322.27. Amorphous solid, mp >170° (dec).

Combination of sodium salt with piperacillin sodium. Tazocilline; Tazocin; Zosyn.

THERAP CAT: In combination with β-lactam antibiotics as antibacterial.

9084. TCDD. [1746-01-6] 2,3,7,8-Tetrachlorodibenzo[b,e]-[1,4]dioxin; 2,3,7,8-tetrachlorodibenzo-p-dioxin; 2,3,6,7-tetrachlorodibenzodioxin; dioxin; TCDBD. $C_{12}H_4Cl_4O_2$; mol wt 321.97. C 44.76%, H 1.25%, Cl 44.05%, O 9.94%. Highly toxic contaminant; produced as a by-product during the manuf of chlorinated phenols (2,4,5-trichlorophenol, *q.v.*) and phenoxyherbicides (2,4-D and 2,4,5-T, *q.q.v.*), chlorine bleaching of paper pulp and combustion of chlorine-containing waste. Prepn: W. Sandermann, *Ber.* **90**, 690 (1957); M. Tomita *et al.*, *Yakugaku Zasshi* **79**, 186 (1959), *C.A.* **53**, 13152d (1959). Crystal structure: F. P. Boer *et al.*, *Acta Crystallogr.* **28B**, 1023 (1972). Environmental degradation: D. G. Crosby, A. S. Wong, *Science* **195**, 1337 (1976). Comprehensive review of formation, chemistry, and toxic and environmental effects: *Adv. Chem. Ser.* **120**, entitled "Chlorodioxins: Origin and Fate," E. H. Blair, Ed. (ACS, Washington DC, 1973) 141 pp. Toxicity and metabolism: B. A. Schwetz *et al.*, *ibid.* 55-69; A. Poland, A. Kende, *Fed. Proc.* **35**, 2404 (1976). Special issue: *Chem. Eng. News* **61** (June 6, 1983). Review of toxicology and human exposure: *Toxicological Profile for 2,3,7,8-Tetradichlorodibenzo-p-dioxin* (PB89-214522, 1989) 135 pp; of epidemiological data: L. Tollefson, *Regul. Toxicol. Pharmacol.* **13**, 150-169 (1991); of receptor binding and mechanism of toxicity: J. P. Whitlock, Jr., *Annu. Rev. Pharmacol. Toxicol.* **30**, 251-277 (1990); of carcinogenicity: J. Huff *et al.*, *ibid.* **34**, 343-372 (1994). Review of GC high resolution mass spectrometric analysis: J.-F. Focant *et al.*, *J. Chromatogr. A* **1067**, 265-275 (2005).

Needles, mp 295° (Tomita); crystals from anisole, mp 320-325° (Sandermann). LD_{50} in male, female rats (mg/kg): 0.022, 0.045 orally (Schwetz).

Note: An industrial accident during the manufacture of 2,4,5-trichlorophenol in Seveso, Italy on July 10, 1976 caused the release of an estimated two to ten pounds of TCDD into the environment. Concentrations as high as 51.3 ppm TCDD were found in some samples: R. Rawls, D. A. O'Sullivan, *Chem. Eng. News* **54**, 27

(Aug. 23, 1976); A. Hay, *Nature* **262**, 636 (1976). TCDD, as a contaminant created in the manufacture of *Agent Orange*, a widely used defoliant in Vietnam during the 1960's, has also been implicated as the causative agent of various symptoms described by veterans exposed to the defoliant, *see* C. Holden, *Science* **205**, 770 (1979).

Caution: Potential symptoms of overexposure to TCDD are eye irritation; allergic dermatitis, chloracne; porphyria; GI disturbances; possible reproductive and teratogenic effects. *See NIOSH Pocket Guide to Chemical Hazards* (DHHS/NIOSH 97-140, 1997) p 298. Toxic effects in animals include the wasting syndrome, gastric ulcers, immunotoxicity, hepatotoxicity, hepatoporphyria, vascular lesions, chloracne, teratogenicity, fetotoxicity, impaired reproductive performance, endometriosis and delayed death. *See* Poland, Kende, *loc. cit.*; C. D. Carter *et al.*, *Science* **188**, 738 (1975). This substance is listed as a known human carcinogen: *Report on Carcinogens, Eleventh Edition* (PB2005-104914, 2004) p III-241.

9085. TCEP. [5961-85-3] 3,3′,3″-Phosphinidynetrispropanoic acid; tris(2-carboxyethyl)phosphine. $C_9H_{15}O_6P$; mol wt 250.19. C 43.21%, H 6.04%, O 38.37%, P 12.38%. Disulfide reducing agent. Prepn: M. M. Rauhut *et al.*, *J. Am. Chem. Soc.* **81**, 1103 (1959); and mechanism: J. A. Burns *et al.*, *J. Org. Chem.* **56**, 2648 (1991). Use as a reducing agent in measurement of redox activity: M. Neuburger *et al.*, *Eur. J. Biochem.* **267**, 2882 (2000); in determn of aminothiols: J. Krijt *et al.*, *Clin. Chem.* **47**, 1821 (2001); in protein sequencing: T.-Y. Yen *et al.*, *J. Mass Spectrom.* **37**, 15 (2002); B. P. English *et al.*, *J. Am. Chem. Soc.* **124**, 4995 (2002).

Hydrochloride. [51805-45-9] Odorless, air-stable, white crystalline solid. mp 176°. uv max: 192, 218 nm (ε 150, 180 L mol^{-1} cm^{-1}). Water soluble. pKa 7.66. When pH of dilute solutions is less than pKa, air oxidation occurs slowly.

USE: Biochemical tool for selective reduction of disulfide bridges at low pH; reductant for redox assays.

9086. TCMTB. [21564-17-0] Thiocyanic acid (2-benzothiazolylthio)methyl ester; 2-(thiocyanomethylthio)benzothiazole; Bulab 6009; Busan 72; Busan 1118. $C_9H_6N_2S_3$; mol wt 238.35. C 45.35%, H 2.54%, N 11.75%, S 40.36%. Antimicrobial agent used as a substitute for chlorophenols in industrial applications. Prepn: A. G. M. Willems *et al.*, *Rec. Trav. Chim.* **90**, 97 (1971). Antimicrobial spectrum and field study: W. G. Guthrie, R. Elsmore, *Spec. Chem.* **10**, 345 (1990). Environmental fate: T. Reemtsma *et al.*, *Environ. Sci. Technol.* **29**, 478 (1995). HPLC determn in wastewater: J. S. Warner *et al.*, *Determination of MBTS and TCMTB in Industrial and Municipal Wastewaters* (PB85-189025, 1985) 45 p; in seawater: K. Martínez *et al.*, *J. Chromatogr. A* **879**, 27 (2000). Use as wood preservative: K. Tsunoda, *Wood Res.* **77**, 28 (1990); as biocide vs zebra mussels: I. D. Martin *et al.*, *Arch. Environ. Contam. Toxicol.* **24**, 381 (1993); as fungicide on leather: L. Muthusubramanian *et al.*, *J. Soc. Leather Technol. Chem.* **82**, 22 (1998). Toxicity studies: R. E. Rush *et al.*, *Acute Toxic. Data* **1**, 206, 207 (1992).

Oil with pungent odor. d^{25} 1.05 (c = 0.30). Flash point (open cup): 66°C. Insol in water. Sol in most organic solvents. LD_{50} in male, female rats (mg/kg): 752, 679 orally (Rush).

USE: Wood preservative, marine biocide, fungicide.

9087. TDCPP. [13674-87-8] 1,3-Dichloro-2-propanol phosphate (3:1); phosphoric acid tris(1,3-dichloro-2-propyl)ester; tris(1,3-dichloroisopropyl)phosphate; tris[2-chloro-1-(chloromethyl)ethyl]phosphate; Fyrol FR-2. $C_9H_{15}Cl_6O_4P$; mol wt 430.90. C 25.09%, H 3.51%, Cl 49.37%, O 14.85%, P 7.19%. Flame retardant formerly used in children's sleepwear; once considered as a potential replacement for Tris-BP, *q.v.* Prepn: W. J. Jones *et al.*, *J. Chem. Soc.* **1946**, 824. Use in flameproofing: R. J. Polacek,

US 3041293 (1962 to Celanese). Thermal studies: K. Paciorek *et al., Am. Ind. Hyg. Assoc. J.* **39**, 633 (1978); N. Inagaki *et al., J. Appl. Polym. Sci.* **21**, 217 (1977); **24**, 1 (1979). Mutagenicity studies: M. D. Gold *et al., Science* **200**, 785 (1978); A. Nakamura *et al., Mutat. Res.* **66**, 373 (1979); D. Brusick *et al., J. Environ. Pathol. Toxicol.* **3**, 207 (1979). Toxicity study: J. K. Piotrowski *et al., Bromatol. Chem. Toksykol.* **9**, 141 (1976), *C.A.* **85**, 104825u (1976).

Viscous liquid, bp$_5$ 236-237°. n_D^{20} 1.5022. Soly in water ~100 ppm. LD$_{50}$ orally in rats: 1.85 g/kg (Piotrowski).

USE: Flame retardant.

9088. Tea. Evergreen shrub or tree, *Camellia sinensis* (L.) O. Kuntze, *Theaceae*, also known as *Thea sinensis*. Tender leaves and buds used commercially to produce the beverage; tea extracts are also used in traditional medicine, esp for their antineoplastic, stimulant, and diuretic properties. *Habit.* Discovered in China 4-6000 yrs ago, also indigenous to India, Japan, Sri Lanka, and other tropical and subtropical countries. Approx. 2.5 million tons of dried leaves are used in tea production each yr. Leaves are quickly steamed to prevent enzymatic oxidation in production of *green tea*, partially oxidized to a green/brown color in *oolong tea*, and rolled, sifted and oxidized to a copper color in *black tea*. *Constit.* Caffeine, theobromine, theophylline, amino acids, proteins, flavonoids, lignin, organic acids, chlorophyll, polysaccharides, polyphenols. Beneficial health effects have been linked to the polyphenols known as catechins, esp epigallocatechin gallate (EGCG), *q.v.* Determn of catechins: J. J. Dalluge, B. C. Nelson, *J. Chromatogr. A* **881**, 411 (2000). Review of tea manufacture: M. A. Bokuchava, N. I. Skobeleva, *Crit. Rev. Food Sci. Nutr.* **12**, 303-370 (1980); and plant history, tea chemistry and consumption: H. N. Graham in *The Methylxanthine Beverages and Foods: Chemistry, Consumption, and Health Effects*, G. A. Spiller, Ed. (Alan R. Liss, New York, 1984) pp 29-74; of chromatographic determn: A. Finger *et al., J. Chromatogr.* **624**, 293-315 (1992); of potential therapeutic antioxidant properties: L. A. Mitscher *et al., Med. Res. Rev.* **17**, 327-365 (1997); of botany and horticulture: L. Manivel, *Hort. Rev.* **22**, 267-295 (1998); of potential therapeutic dermatologic applications: A. F. Alexis *et al., Int. J. Dermatol.* **38**, 735-743 (1999); of anti-cariogenic properties: J. M. T. Hamilton-Miller, *J. Med. Microbiol.* **50**, 299-302 (2001); of inhibition of carcinogenesis: C. S. Yang *et al., Annu. Rev. Pharmacol. Toxicol.* **42**, 25-54 (2002).

Astringent, bitter taste. Black tea is faintly aromatic; green tea is practically odorless.

USE: Stimulant beverage; flavoring in food products; ingredient in skincare products and shampoos.

9089. Tea Tree Oil. [68647-73-4] Melaleuca oil; tea tree (melaleuca alternafolia) oil. Native Australian medicinal oil obtained from the leaves and terminal branchlets of the tea tree, *Melaleuca alternifolia* Myrtaceae. A complex mixture of hydrocarbons and terpenes of ~100 components; the two standardized components for commercial use are 1,6-cineole (max of 15%) and the 1-terpinen-4-ol (min of 30%). Description: A. R. Penfold, *J. Proc. R. Soc. N.S.W.* **59**, 306 (1925). Analysis and composition: J. J. Brophy *et al., J. Agric. Food Chem.* **37**, 1330 (1989). Toxicity study: D. Villar *et al., Vet. Hum. Toxicol.* **36**, 139 (1994). Antimicrobial activity: C. F. Carson, T. V. Riley, *J. Appl. Bacteriol.* **78**, 264 (1995); and mode of action: S. D. Cox *et al., ibid.* **88**, 170 (2000). Antifungal activity: K. A. Hammer *et al., Antimicrob. Agents Chemother.* **44**, 467 (2000). Clinical evaluation in oral candidiasis in AIDS patients: A. Jandourek *et al., AIDS* **12**, 1033 (1998). Review of early work: A. R. Penfold, F. R. Morrison, "Tea Tree Oils" in *The Essential Oils* **4**, E. Guenther, Ed. (Van Nostrand Co., New York, 1950) pp 526-548. Review: J. A. Staton, *Proc. 3rd. Sci. Conf. Asian Soc. Cosmet. Sci. Taipei*, 18-24 (1997). Review of clinical trials: E. Ernst, A. Huntley, *Forsch. Komplemen-*

tärmed. **7**, 17-20 (2000); of antimicrobial properties and clinical potential: L. Halcón, K. Milkus, *Am. J. Infect. Control* **32**, 402-408 (2004).

Colorless to pale-yellow, clear, mobile liquid with fresh terpene type odor with nutmeg associations and possibly with citrus or floral undertones. n_D^{20} 1.4760-1.4810. [α]$_D$ +6°48' to +9°48'. d$_{15}^{15}$ 0.8950-0.9050. Soly in 80% alcohol (w/w): 0.6 to 0.8 volumes. LD$_{50}$ orally in rats: 1.9-2.6 ml/kg; dermally in rabbits: 5.0 g/kg (Halcón).

USE: Flavoring and antiseptic agent in personal hygiene items such as toothpaste; as a cosmeceutical.

9090. Tebanicline. [198283-73-7] 5-[(2R)-2-Azetidinylmethoxy]-2-chloropyridine; ABT-594. C$_9$H$_{11}$ClN$_2$O; mol wt 198.65. C 54.42%, H 5.58%, Cl 17.85%, N 14.10%, O 8.05%. Non-opioid 3-pyridyl ether analgesic acting acting via a neuronal nicotinic acetylcholine receptor mediated mechanism. Prepn: M. W. Holladay *et al., WO 9640682*; M. A. Abreo *et al., US 5948793* (1996, 1999 both to Abbott); as hydrochloride: M. W. Holladay *et al., J. Med. Chem.* **41**, 407 (1998). Asymmetric synthesis: J. K. Lynch *et al., Tetrahedron: Asymmetry* **9**, 2791 (1998). Analgesic activity and receptor affinity: A. W. Bannon *et al., Science* **279**, 77 (1998). Pharmacology *in vitro:* D. L. Donnelly-Roberts *et al., J. Pharmacol. Exp. Ther.* **285**, 777 (1998); *in vivo:* A. W. Bannon *et al., ibid.* 787. Efficacy in neuropathic pain models: *idem et al., Brain Res.* **801**, 158 (1998).

Hydrochloride. [203564-54-9] mp 116-117°. [α]$_D^{23}$ +8.6° (c = 0.52 in methanol).

Tosylate. [198283-74-8] C$_9$H$_{11}$ClN$_2$O.C$_7$H$_8$O$_3$S; mol wt 370.85.

USE: Analgesic agent in pain models.

9091. Tebbe Reagent. [67719-69-1] μ-Methylene-μ-chlorobis(η⁵-2,4-cyclopentadien-1-yl)(dimethylaluminum)titanium; (μ-chloro)(μ-methylene)bis(cyclopentadienyl)(dimethylaluminum)titanium. C$_{13}$H$_{18}$AlClTi; mol wt 284.58. C 54.87%, H 6.38%, Al 9.48%, Cl 12.46%, Ti 16.82%. Titanium-aluminum complex used in the Tebbe Olefination. Prepn: F. N. Tebbe *et al., J. Am. Chem. Soc.* **100**, 3611 (1978). Improved prepn: L. F. Cannizzo, R. H. Grubbs, *J. Org. Chem.* **50**, 2386 (1985). Ab initio structural model: M. M. Francl, W. J. Hehre, *Organometallics* **2**, 457 (1983). Carbonyl methylenation applications compared with Wittig reactions: S. H. Pine *et al., J. Org. Chem.* **50**, 1212 (1985); *idem et al., Synthesis* **1991**, 165. Review of methylenation chemistry: *Org. Synth. Highlights*, J. Mulzer *et al.,* Eds. (VCH, Weinheim, 1991) pp 192-196.

Reddish-orange crystals. Sol in toluene, benzene. *Sensitive to air and water.*

USE: Reagent for the methylenation of carbonyl groups.

9092. Tebuconazole. [107534-96-3] α-[2-(4-Chlorophenyl)ethyl]-α-(1,1-dimethylethyl)-1H-1,2,4-triazole-1-ethanol; (RS)-1-(4-chlorophenyl)-4,4-dimethyl-3-(1H-1,2,4-triazol-1-ylmethyl)-pentan-3-ol; ethyltrianol; fenetrazole; terbuconazole; terbutrazole; BAY HWG 1608; HWG-1608; Corail; Elite; Folicur; Horizon; Lynx; Raxil. C$_{16}$H$_{22}$ClN$_3$O; mol wt 307.82. C 62.43%, H 7.20%, Cl 11.52%, N 13.65%, O 5.20%. Ergosterol biosynthesis inhibitor. Prepn: G. Holmwood *et al., EP 40345; eidem, US 4723984* (1981, 1988 both to Bayer). Synthesis of enantiomers: J. Kaulen, *Angew. Chem. Int. Ed.* **28**, 462 (1989). Photodegradation: H. Wamhoff *et al., Z. Naturforsch.* **49b**, 280 (1994). GC determn in plant material, soil and water: W. Maasfeld, *Pflanzenschutz-Nachr. Bayer (Engl. Ed.)* **40**, 29 (1987). Review of chemistry and biochemistry: D. Berg *et al., ibid. 111*-132. Series of articles on field trials: *ibid.* **42**, 91-222 (1989); *BCPC Monograph* **57**, 97-108 (1994).

Colorless crystals, mp 104.7°. Vapor pressure (20°) <10^{-5} mbar. Soly (g/l at 20°): water 0.032, dichloromethane >200, *n*-hexane 2-5, 2-propanol, 100-200, toluene 50-100.

USE: Fungicide.

9093. Tebufenozide. [112410-23-8] 3,5-Dimethylbenzoic acid 1-(1,1-dimethylethyl)-2-(4-ethylbenzoyl)hydrazide; *N-tert*-butyl-*N'*-(4-ethylbenzoyl)-3,5-dimethylbenzoylhydrazide; RH-5992; Confirm; Mimic. $C_{22}H_{28}N_2O_2$; mol wt 352.47. C 74.97%, H 8.01%, N 7.95%, O 9.08%. Synthetic nonsteroidal ecdysone agonist causing premature molting; novel insect growth regulator specific to lepidopteran species. Prepn: A. C. Hsu, H. E. Aller, **AU 64289**; *idem*, **US 4985461** (1986, 1991 both to Rohm & Haas). Properties and field evaluation: J. J. Heller *et al., Brighton Crop Prot. Conf. - Pests Dis.* **1992**, 59. Determn by LC in environmental samples: K. M. S. Sundaram *et al., J. AOAC Int.* **76**, 668 (1993); by GC and LC in formulations: *idem, et al., J. Chromatogr. A* **687**, 323 (1994). Soil adsorption: *idem, J. Environ. Sci. Health* **B29**, 415 (1994). Insecticidal activity: G. Smagghe, D. Degheele, *Pestic. Sci.* **42**, 85 (1994). Mechanism of action: A. Retnakaran *et al., Insect Biochem. Mol. Biol.* **25**, 109 (1995). Aquatic toxicology: D. P. Kreutzweiser *et al., Ecotoxicol. Environ. Saf.* **28**, 14 (1994). Review of biological activity and use: H. Oberlander *et al., Arch. Insect Biochem. Physiol.* **28**, 209-223 (1995).

mp 191°. Also reported as mp 186-188° (Sundaram, 1081). Vapor pressure (25°): 3×10^{-8} mm Hg. Also reported as vapor pressure (25°): 1.7×10^{-6} mm Hg (Sundaram, 415). Soly (25°): 0.83 μg/ml water. Partition coefficient (octanol/water): 32000. LD_{50} orally in rats, mice: >5000 mg/kg; dermally in rats: >5000 mg/kg; LD_{50} in honey bees (96 hr, contact): >234 μg/bee; LC_{50} in mallard duck (8-day dietary): >5000 mg/kg; LC_{50} in rainbow trout (96 hr): 5.7 mg/l (Heller).

USE: Insecticide.

9094. Tebufenpyrad. [119168-77-3] 4-Chloro-*N*-[[4-(1,1-dimethylethyl)phenyl]methyl]-3-ethyl-1-methyl-1*H*-pyrazole-5-carboxamide; *N*-(4-*t*-butylbenzyl)-4-chloro-3-ethyl-1-methylpyrazole-5-carboxamide; MK-239; Pyranica. $C_{18}H_{24}ClN_3O$; mol wt 333.86. C 64.76%, H 7.25%, Cl 10.62%, N 12.59%, O 4.79%. Used to control plant-feeding mites on cotton, citrus, fruits, vegetables, and ornamentals; inhibits electron transport during mitochondrial respiration. Prepn: I. Okada *et al.*, **EP 289879**; *idem*, **US 4950668** (1988, 1990 both to Mitsubishi Kasei). GC/MS determn in water, soil, and urine samples: A. Navalón *et al., Chromatographia* **54**, 377 (2001). Field trial vs mites in apple orchards: W. G. Thwaite *et al., Exp. Appl. Acarol.* **20**, 177 (1996); in honey bee colonies: M. A. Ali *et al., J. Econ. Entomol.* **96**, 259 (2003). Mite toxicity study: Y.-J. Kim *et al., ibid.* **92**, 187 (1999). *Review*: K. Inoue, T. Fukuchi, *Agrochem. Jpn.* **64**, 12-14 (1994).

Off-white solid, slight aromatic odor, mp 61-62°. Vapor pressure (25°): 1.0×10^{-5} Pa. LD_{50} in male, female rats (mg/kg): 595, 997 orally; >2000, >2000 dermally. LC_{50} in male rats (mg/m³): 2660 by inhalation (Inoue, Fukuchi).

USE: Acaricide.

9095. Tebuthiuron. [34014-18-1] *N*-[5-(1,1-Dimethylethyl)-1,3,4-thiadiazol-2-yl]-*N,N'*-dimethylurea; 1-(5-*tert*-butyl-1,3,4-thiadiazol-2-yl)-1,3-dimethylurea; EL-103; Graslan; Perflan; Spike. $C_9H_{16}N_4OS$; mol wt 228.31. C 47.35%, H 7.06%, N 24.54%, O 7.01%, S 14.04%. Broad spectrum pre- and post-emergent herbicide. Prepn: **GB 1266172** (1972 to Air Prod. Chem.); E. V. P. Tao, **BE 799575**; *idem*, **US 3803164** (1973, 1974 both to Lilly); *idem, Synth. Commun.* **4**, 249 (1974). Herbicidal activity: A. T. Perkins *et al., Proc. South. Weed Sci. Soc.* **30**, 326 (1977). Toxicity study: G. C. Todd *et al., Food Cosmet. Toxicol.* **12**, 461 (1974). Metabolism in animals: D. M. Morton, D. G. Hoffman, *J. Toxicol. Environ. Health* **1**, 757 (1976). Determn by HPLC: J. H. Kennedy, *J. Chromatogr. Sci.* **15**, 79 (1977); by GC: A. Loh *et al., J. Agric. Food Chem.* **26**, 410 (1978). Field trial against woody shrubs: C. H. Herbel *et al., J. Range Manage.* **38**, 391 (1985).

mp 160-163°. Moderately sol in water (2500 ppm); sol in methanol (170,000 ppm) (company literature). LD_{50} in mice, rats, rabbits (mg/kg): 579, 644, 286 orally (Todd).

USE: Herbicide.

9096. Tecadenoson. [204512-90-3] *N*-[(3*R*)-Tetrahydro-3-furanyl]adenosine; CVT-510. $C_{14}H_{19}N_5O_5$; mol wt 337.33. C 49.85%, H 5.68%, N 20.76%, O 23.71%. Selective adenosine A_1-receptor agonist. Prepn: R. T. Lum *et al.*, **WO 9808855**; *idem*, **US 5789416** (both 1998 to CV Therapeutics). Clinical effect on AV nodal conduction: B. B. Lerman *et al., J. Cardiovasc. Pharmacol. Ther.* **6**, 237 (2001). Clinical evaluation in paroxysmal supraventricular tachycardia: E. N. Prystowsky *et al., J. Am. Coll. Cardiol.* **42**, 1098 (2003); K. A. Ellenbogen *et al., Circulation* **111**, 3202 (2005). Review of pharmacology and clinical experience: A. Zaza, *Curr. Opin. Invest. Drugs* **3**, 96-100 (2002); J. W. Cheung, B. B. Lerman, *Cardiovasc. Drug Rev.* **21**, 277-292 (2003).

THERAP CAT: Antiarrhythmic.

9097. Technetium. [7440-26-8] Tc; at. no. 43. Usual valences 4 and 7; 3 less common. Group VIIB (7). Radioactive element; no stable nuclides. Discovery claimed by Noddack, Tacke, and Berg who called it "masurium"; the existence of masurium has never been confirmed by isoln of the element. First artificially produced element. Named from the Greek word for "artificial"; separated from a molybdenum plate that had been bombarded for a few months with a strong beam of deuterons in the Berkeley cyclotron: Perrier, Segré, *Nature* **140**, 193 (1937); *eidem, J. Chem. Phys.* **5**, 712 (1937); Cacciapuoti, Segré, *Phys. Rev.* **52**, 1252 (1937). Most commonly available isotope (mass number): 99 ($T_{1/2}$ 2.12×10^5 years, rel. at. mass 98.9063). Other long-lived isotopes: 97 ($T_{1/2}$ 2.6×10^6 years, rel. at. mass 96.9064); 98 ($T_{1/2}$ 4.2×10^6 years, longest-lived isotope, rel. at. mass 97.9072). Known artificial isotopes: 92-107. Prepn of metal: Cobble *et al., J. Am. Chem. Soc.* **74**, 1852 (1952). Comprehensive reviews: Boyd, *J. Chem. Educ.* **36**, 3-14 (1959); Schwochau, *Angew. Chem.*

76, 9-19 (1964); Kotegov *et al.*, in *Adv. Inorg. Chem. Radiochem.* **11,** 1-90 (1968); Peacock in *Comprehensive Inorganic Chemistry* **vol. 3,** J. C. Bailar Jr. *et al.*, Eds. (Pergamon Press, Oxford, 1973) pp 877-903. Pharmacokinetics and organ distribution of radiopharmaceuticals: O. P. D. Noronha, K. S. Venkateswarlu, *Eur. J. Nucl. Med.* **6,** 121 (1980).

Close-packed hexagonal structure; isomorphous with rhodium, ruthenium, and osmium. The element obtained by hydrogen reduction of ammonium pertechnate is a silver-gray spongy mass which tarnishes slowly in moist air. mp 2250 $\pm 50°$. In its chemical behavior resembles rhenium. The element is precipitated by hydrogen sulfide from hydrochloric acid (diluted up to 5N); for higher acid concns the precipitation is not complete. Is oxidized by hydrogen peroxide in alkaline soln into sol anions: Perrier, Segré, *Atti R. Accad. Lincei* [6] **27,** 579 (1938); Segré, *Nature* **143,** 460 (1939). Reacts with dil or concd nitric acid, in aqua regia, in concd sulfuric acid; not with HCl. Burns in fluorine to form penta- and hexafluorides. Combines with sulfur at high temp to form disulfide; with carbon to form TcC.

USE: Minute quantities of TcO_4^- ion exert remarkable inhibition of the corrosion of soft iron in neutral aq soln: Cartledge, *J. Am. Chem. Soc.* **77,** 2658 (1955).

THERAP CAT: ^{99m}Tc as diagnostic aid (radioactive imaging agent).

9098. Technetium ^{99m}Tc Apcitide. [178959-14-3] ^{99m}Tc-P246; AcuTect. Radiolabeled synthetic peptide that preferentially binds to glycoprotein GP IIb/IIIa receptors on the surface of activated platelets. Monomer designed as a scintigraphic imaging agent for detection and localization of acute deep vein thrombosis (DVT). Prepn: R. T. Dean, J. Lister-James, **WO 9325244;** *eidem,* **US 5508020** (1993, 1996 both to Diatech); D. A. Pearson *et al., J. Med. Chem.* **39,** 1372 (1996). Pharmacology and immunoscintigraphy: J. Lister-James *et al., J. Nucl. Med.* **37,** 755 (1996). Clinical study in DVT: R. Taillefer *et al., ibid.* **41,** 1214 (2000).

Dimer. [153507-46-1] Bibapcitide; P-280. $C_{112}H_{162}N_{36}O_{43}$-$S_{10}$; mol wt 3021.35. C 44.52%, H 5.40%, N 16.69%, O 22.77%, S 10.61%. Synthetic peptide consisting of 26 amino acids; exhibits the same GP IIb/IIIa binding activity as the monomer. Splits to form monomer upon reaction with sodium pertechnetate ^{99m}Tc, *q.v.*

THERAP CAT: Diagnostic aid (radioactive imaging agent).

9099. Technetium ^{99m}Tc Bicisate. [121281-41-2] (SP-5-35)-[[Diethyl-N,N'-1,2-ethanediylbis[L-cysteinato]](3$-$)-N,N',S,S']oxotechnetium-^{99m}Tc; [N,N'-ethylenedi-L-cysteinato(3$-$)]oxo-[^{99m}Tc]technetium(V) diethyl ester; technetium ^{99m}Tc ethyl cysteinate dimer; ^{99m}Tc-L,L-ECD; RP-217; Neurolite. $C_{12}H_{21}N_2O_5$-S_2 ^{99m}Tc. Neutral, lipophilic complex which rapidly crosses bloodbrain barrier. Prepn: P. L. Bergstein *et al.,* **EP 279417** (1988 to DuPont); *eidem,* **US 5279811** (1994 to DuPont Merck). Pharmacology: R. C. Walovitch *et al., J. Nucl. Med.* **30,** 1892 (1989). Clinical pharmacokinetics: S. Vallabhajosula *et al., ibid.* 599. Metabolism in humans: R. C. Walovitch *et al., Neuropharmacology* **30,** 283 (1991). TLC determn of radiochemical purity: J. M. Green *et al., J. Nucl. Med. Technol.* **22,** 21 (1994). Series of articles on clinical pharmacology and diagnostic use in SPECT brain imaging: *J. Cereb. Blood Flow Metab.* **14,** Suppl. 1, S1-S120 (1994).

THERAP CAT: Diagnostic aid (radioactive imaging agent).

9100. Technetium ^{99m}Tc Fanolesomab. [225239-31-6] Anti-(human CD15 (antigen))(mouse monoclonal RB5 μ-chain)immunoglobulin M disulfide with mouse monoclonal RB5 light chain pentamer technetium-^{99m}Tc salt; ^{99m}Tc-anti-SSEA-1; LeuTech; NeutroSpec. Murine monoclonal antibody directed against stage-specific embryonic antigen-1 (SSEA-1); binds to cluster designation 15 (CD15) antigen expressed on human neutrophils. Antigranulocyte antibody designed for *in vivo* functional imaging and diagnosis of infection. Prepn of antibody: D. Solter, B. B. Knowles, *Proc. Natl. Acad. Sci. USA* **75,** 5565 (1978); of labeled form: M. L. Thakur *et al., J. Nucl. Med.* **29,** 1817 (1988). *See also* for diagnostic

use: *idem,* **US 4917878** (1990 to Thomas Jefferson Univ.). *In vivo* labeling and imaging of neutrophils: *idem et al., J. Nucl. Med.* **37,** 1789 (1996). Clinical biodistribution and radiation dosimetry study: P. D. Mozley *et al., ibid.* **40,** 625 (1999). Clinical evaluation as imaging agent for osteomyelitis: C. J. Palestro *et al., J. Foot Ankle Surg.* **42,** 2 (2003); for appendicitis: E. B. Rypins *et al., Ann. Surg.* **235,** 232 (2002). Review of development and clinical use: C. Love, C. J. Palestro, *IDrugs* **6,** 1079-1085 (2003).

THERAP CAT: Diagnostic aid (radioactive imaging agent).

9101. Technetium ^{99m}Tc Mertiatide. [125224-05-7]; [104348-91-6]. (SP-5-25)-[N-[N-[N-(Mercaptoacetyl)glycyl]glycyl]glycinato(5$-$)-N,N',N'',S]oxotechnetate(2$-$)-^{99m}Tc disodium; ^{99m}Tc-MAG$_3$; ^{99m}Tc mercaptoacetyltriglycine; TechneScan MAG3. $C_8H_8N_3Na_2O_6S$ ^{99m}Tc. Nonisomeric mercaptide compound complexed with technetium; radioactive renal function imaging agent. Prepn and biodistribution: A. R. Fritzberg *et al., J. Nucl. Med.* **27,** 111 (1986); *idem et al.,* **EP 284071** (1988 to Neorx). Stability and HPLC determn of radiochemical purity: A. M. Millar *et al., Nucl. Med. Commun.* **11,** 405 (1990). Clinical pharmacokinetics: B. Bubeck *et al., J. Nucl. Med.* **31,** 1285 (1990). Diagnostic use in captopril renography: I. E. Datseris *et al., ibid.* **35,** 251 (1994); in renal transplant evaluation: J. P. O'Malley *et al., Clin. Nucl. Med.* **18,** 22 (1993). Review of synthesis and diagnostic use: D. Eshima, A. Taylor, Jr., *Semin. Nucl. Med.* **22,** 61-73 (1992).

THERAP CAT: Diagnostic aid (radioactive imaging agent).

9102. Technetium ^{99m}Tc Sestamibi. [109581-73-9] (OC-6-11)-Hexakis(1-isocyano-2-methoxy-2-methylpropane)technetium-(1+)-^{99m}Tc; hexakis(2-methoxy-2-methylpropyl isocyanide)[^{99m}Tc] technetium(1+); ^{99m}Tc hexakis(2-methoxyisobutylisonitrile); ^{99m}Tc-HEXAMIBI; ^{99m}Tc-MIBI; ^{99m}Tc-RP-30A; Cardiolite. C_{36}-$H_{66}N_6O_6$ ^{99m}Tc. Lipophilic, cationic isonitrile compound complexed with technetium; radioactive myocardial perfusion imaging agent. Prepn: P. L. Bergstein, N. Subramanyam, **EP 233368** (1987 to Du Pont); P. Angelberger, E. Zbiral, *Oesterr. Forschungszent. Seibersdorf* **4411,** I (1987). Preparative TLC purification: A. Proulx *et al., Appl. Radiat. Isot.* **40,** 95 (1989). Biodistribution and comparative clinical evaluation as myocardial perfusion imaging agent: F. J. Th. Wackers *et al., J. Nucl. Med.* **30,** 301 (1989). Clinical evaluation as parathyroid imaging agent: A. J. Coakley *et al., Nucl. Med. Commun.* **10,** 791 (1989). Symposium on pharmacology and clinical studies: *Am. J. Cardiol.* **66,** 1E-96E (1990). Review of cardiac imaging: J. A. Leppo *et al., J. Nucl. Med.* **32,** 2012-2022 (1991).

THERAP CAT: Diagnostic aid (radioactive imaging agent).

9103. Technetium ^{99m}Tc Teboroxime. [104716-22-5] (TPS-7-1-232′4′54)-[Bis[(1,2-cyclohexanedione dioximato)(1$-$)-

O] [(1,2-cyclohexanedione dioximato)(2−)-*O*]methylborato(2−)-*N*,*N* ′,*N* ″,*N* ‴,*N* ⁗,*N* ⁗′]chlorotechnetium-99mTc; CDO-MeB; SQ-30217; Cardiotec. $C_{19}H_{29}BClN_6O_6$99mTc. Neutral, lipophilic technetium complex classified as a boronic acid adduct of technetium dioxime (BATO); radioactive myocardial perfusion imaging agent. Prepn: A. D. Nunn *et al., EP 199260; eidem, US 4705849* (1986, 1987 both to Squibb); and structural characterization: E. N. Treher *et al., Inorg. Chem.* **28**, 3411 (1989). Pharmacokinetics: R. E. Stewart *et al., J. Nucl. Med.* **31**, 1183 (1990). Reviews of physiologic properties and pharmacology: D. J. Meerdink, J. A. Leppo, *Am. J. Cardiol.* **66**, 9E-15E (1990); of clinical pharmacokinetics and comparative studies of myocardial imaging: L. L. Johnson, D. W. Seldin, *ibid.* 63E-67E; of diagnostic use in coronary artery disease: J. A. Leppo *et al., J. Nucl. Med.* **32**, 2012-2022 (1991).

THERAP CAT: Diagnostic aid (radioactive imaging agent).

9104. Teclothiazide. [4267-05-4] 6-Chloro-3,4-dihydro-3-trichloromethyl-2*H*-1,2,4-benzothiadiazine-7-sulfonamide 1,1-dioxide; 6-chloro-3,4-dihydro-7-sulfamoyl-3-trichloromethyl-2*H*-1,2,4-benzothiadiazine 1,1-dioxide; 3-trichloromethylhydrochlorothiazide; tetrachlormethiazide. $C_8H_7Cl_4N_3O_4S_2$; mol wt 415.10. C 23.15%, H 1.70%, Cl 34.16%, N 10.12%, O 15.42%, S 15.45%. Prepn: Close *et al., J. Am. Chem. Soc.* **82**, 1132 (1960); Novello *et al., J. Org. Chem.* **25**, 970 (1960). Pharmacology and toxicology: M. Auclair *et al., Therapie* **18**, 131, 137 (1963).

Crystals, mp 300-303° (Close); mp 287° (Novello).
Potassium salt. [5306-80-9] PS-207; K-33; Depleil. C_8H_6-$Cl_4KN_3O_4S_2$; mol wt 453.19. LD_{50} i.p. in mice: 4.75 g/kg (Auclair).
THERAP CAT: Diuretic.

9105. Teclozan. [5560-78-1] *N*,*N* ′-[1,4-Phenylenebis(methylene)]-bis[2,2-dichloro-*N*-(2-ethoxyethyl)acetamide]; *N*,*N* ′-bis-(ethoxyethyl)-*N*,*N* ′-bis(dichloroacetyl)-1,4-xylylenediamine; *N*,*N* ′-bis(dichloroacetyl)-*N*,*N* ′-bis(2-ethoxyethyl)-1,4-bis(aminomethyl)benzene; teclosan; teclosine; teclozine; NSC-107433; Win-13146; Win-AM-13146; Falmonox. $C_{20}H_{28}Cl_4N_2O_4$; mol wt 502.26. C 47.83%, H 5.62%, Cl 28.23%, N 5.58%, O 12.74%. Prepn: Surrey, Mayer, *J. Med. Pharm. Chem.* **3**, 409 (1961). Amebicidal activity and toxicity: Berberian *et al., Am. J. Trop. Med. Hyg.* **10**, 503 (1961).

Crystals, mp 137.6-143.9°. LD_{50} orally in mice: >8000 mg/kg (Berberian).
THERAP CAT: Antiamebic.

9106. Tecomanine. [6878-83-7] [4*R*-(4α,7β,7aβ)]-1,2,3,4,-7,7a-Hexahydro-2,4,7-trimethyl-6*H*-2-pyridin-6-one; tecomine.

$C_{11}H_{17}NO$; mol wt 179.26. C 73.70%, H 9.56%, N 7.81%, O 8.93%. Principal alkaloid isolated from *Tecoma stans* (L.) H.B.K. *(Bignonia stans* L.), Bignoniaceae: Y. Hammouda, M. M. Motawi, *Egypt. Pharm. Bull.* **41**, 73 (1959), *C.A.* **54**, 21646c (1960). Structure: G. Jones *et al., Tetrahedron Lett.* **1963**, 397. Stereochemistry, abs config and crystal structure: G. Jones *et al., Chem. Commun.* **1971**, 994; G. Ferguson, W. C. Marsh, *J. Chem. Soc. Perkin Trans. 2* **1975**, 1124. Hypoglycemic activity of salts: Y. Hammouda *et al., J. Pharm. Pharmacol.* **16**, 833 (1964); Y. Hammouda, M. S. Amer, *J. Pharm. Sci.* **55**, 1452 (1966). Stereoselective total synthesis of (±)-form: T. Imanishi *et al., Tetrahedron Lett.* **22**, 667 (1981). Facile synthesis of (+)-form: T. Kametani *et al., Heterocycles* **26**, 1491 (1987).

Liquid. bp$_{0.1}$ 125°. $[\alpha]_D^{24}$ −175° (c = 1.17 in CHCl$_3$). uv max (alc): 226 nm (log ε 4.10).
Methiodide. $C_{12}H_{20}INO$. Crystals, dec 240-242°.
Methoperchlorate. $C_{12}H_{20}ClNO_5$. Crystals from methanol, mp 242°.

9107. Tectorigenin. [548-77-6] 5,7-Dihydroxy-3-(4-hydroxyphenyl)-6-methoxy-4*H*-1-benzopyran-4-one; 4′,5,7-trihydroxy-6-methoxyisoflavone. $C_{16}H_{12}O_6$; mol wt 300.26. C 64.00%, H 4.03%, O 31.97%. Phytoalexin aglycon isolated from rhizomes of *Iris tectorum* Maxim., Iridaceae, the extract of which is used as a traditional Chinese medicine. Isoln of the glycoside and aglycon: S. Shibata, *J. Pharm. Soc. Jpn.* **37**, 380 (1927), *C.A.* **21**, 3050⁸ (1927); from *Iris germanica* Linnaeus: A. Kawase *et al., Agric. Biol. Chem.* **37**, 145 (1973). Structure: Asahina *et al., J. Pharm. Soc. Jpn.* **48**, 1087 (1928), *C.A.* **23**, 2718¹ (1929); Shriner *et al., J. Am. Chem. Soc.* **61**, 2322 (1939). Synthesis: Farkas, Várady, *Ber.* **93**, 1269 (1960); W. Baker *et al., J. Chem. Soc. C* **1970**, 1219. Inhibition of cyclooxygenase-2 induction: K. Ohuchi *et al., Recent Adv. Nat. Prod. Res., Proc. 3rd Int. Symp. 1999*, 12-24. Antioxidant effects: K.-T. Lee *et al., Arch. Pharmacal Res.* **23**, 461 (2000).

Pale yellow needles from ethanol, mp 225-226°. uv max (ethanol): 267-269, 338 nm (log ε 4.41, 3.40).
Tectoridin. [611-40-5] Tectorigenin-7-glucoside; shekanin. $C_{22}H_{22}O_{11}$; mol wt 462.40. Identity with shekanin and structure: Mannich *et al., Arch. Pharm.* **275**, 317 (1937). Synthesis: Várady, *Acta Chim. Acad. Sci. Hung.* **48**, 181 (1966). Colorless needles from ethanol, mp 256-258°. uv max (ethanol): 267-269, 336 nm (log ε 4.62, 3.65). $[\alpha]_D^{20}$ −29.4° (pyridine). Sol in pyridine, alcohol, water. Practically insol in organic solvents.

9108. Tedisamil. [90961-53-8] 3′,7′-Bis(cyclopropylmethyl)spiro[cyclopentane-1,9′-[3,7]diazabicyclo[3.3.1]nonane]. C_{19}-$H_{32}N_2$; mol wt 288.47. C 79.11%, H 11.18%, N 9.71%. Potassium channel blocking bradycardic agent. Prepn: U. Schön *et al., DE 3234697; eidem, US 4550112* (1984, 1985 both to Kali-Chemie); and pharmacology: *idem et al., J. Med. Chem.* **41**, 318 (1998). Suppression of the outward transient K⁺ current in rat myocytes: I. D. Dukes, M. Morad, *Am. J. Physiol.* **275**, H1746 (1989). Toxicity in rats: E. Hayes *et al., Pharmacol. Toxicol.* **73**, 257 (1993). Comparative clinical study in coronary artery disease: V. Mitrovic, *et al., Clin. Cardiol.* **21**, 492 (1998). Clinical study in stable angina: K. M. Fox *et al., Heart* **83**, 167 (2000). Review of pharmacology and clinical development: B. Freestone, G. Y. H. Lip, *Expert Opin. Invest. Drugs* **13**, 151-160 (2004).

Solid, mp 44°. d 1.48 g/cm³. bp$_{1.33hPa}$ 156°. Vapor pressure (20°): 8 × 10⁻⁶ mPa. Soly in water: 2 × 10⁻² mg/l; in acetone, dichloromethane, hexane and toluene: >500 g/l. LD$_{50}$ technical grade in rats (mg/kg): 35 orally; 200-1000 dermally (Marrs, Gordon).

USE: Insecticide.

9112. Tegafur. [17902-23-7] 5-Fluoro-1-(tetrahydro-2-furanyl)-2,4(1*H*,3*H*)-pyrimidinedione; 5-fluoro-1-(tetrahydro-2-furyl)uracil; *N*$_1$-(2′-furanidyl)-5-fluorouracil; FT-207; MJF-12264; NSC-148958; Citofur; Coparogin; Exonal; Fental; Franrose; Ftorafur; Fulaid; Fulfeel; Furafluor; Furofutran; Futraful; Lamar; Lifril; Neberk; Nitobanil; Riol; Sinoflurol; Sunfural; Tefsiel C. C$_8$H$_9$FN$_2$-O$_3$; mol wt 200.17. C 48.00%, H 4.53%, F 9.49%, N 13.99%, O 23.98%. Prepn: S. A. Hillers *et al., Dokl. Akad. Nauk SSSR* **176,** 332 (1967), *C.A.* **68,** 29664j (1968); *eidem,* **GB 1168391** (1969), *C.A.* **72,** 43715r (1970) and **FR 1574684** (1969), *C.A.* **73,** 77281g (1970). Alternate synthesis: T. Kametani *et al., J. Heterocycl. Chem.* **14,** 473 (1977). Synthesis, antitumor activity, toxicity study: M. Yasumoto *et al., J. Med. Chem.* **21,** 738 (1978). Crystal structure: Y. Nakai, *Chem. Pharm. Bull.* **30,** 2629 (1982). Pharmacokinetics, metabolism in man: J. L. Au *et al., Cancer Treat. Rep.* **63,** 343 (1979). Evaluation of efficacy and toxicity: C. R. Smart *et al., Cancer* **36,** 103 (1975). Evaluation in colorectal cancer: T. Buroker *et al., Cancer* **44,** 48 (1979). *In vivo* and *in vitro* studies on Walker carcinoma in rats: J. Mattern *et al., Arzneim.-Forsch.* **30,** 981 (1980).

Dihydrochloride. [132523-84-3] KC-8857. C$_{19}$H$_{32}$N$_2$.2HCl; mol wt 361.39. White crystals, mp 195-197°. bp 230° (0.1 Torr). Sol in water.

THERAP CAT: Antiarrhythmic (class III); antianginal.

9109. Teflubenzuron. [83121-18-0] *N*-[[(3,5-Dichloro-2,4-difluorophenyl)amino]carbonyl]-2,6-difluorobenzamide; 1-(3,5-dichloro-2,4-difluorophenyl)-3-(2,6-difluorobenzoyl)urea; CME-134; Nomolt. C$_{14}$H$_6$Cl$_2$F$_4$N$_2$O$_2$; mol wt 381.11. C 44.12%, H 1.59%, Cl 18.61%, F 19.94%, N 7.35%, O 8.40%. Insect growth regulator; inhibits chitin biosynthesis and moulting. Prepn: H.-M. Becher *et al.,* **EP 52833**; *eidem,* **US 4457943** (1982, 1984 both to Celamerck). Physical properties and bioactivity: *eidem et al., Proc. 10th Int. Congr. Plant Prot.* **1,** 408 (1983). Field trials in soybeans: D. A. Herbert, J. D. Harper, *J. Econ. Entomol.* **78,** 333 (1985). Efficacy vs fire ants (*Solenopsis invicta* Buren): D. F. Williams *et al., Fla. Entomol.* **80,** 84 (1997).

mp 221-224°. Vapor pressure (20°): 8 × 10⁻¹² mbar. Soly at 20-23° (g/100 ml): hexane 0.005; toluene 0.085; ethanol 0.14; acetone 1.0; DMSO 6.6. Soly in water (20-23°): 20 ppb. LD$_{50}$ orally in rats: >5000 mg/kg (Becher).

USE: USE: Insecticide.

9110. Teflurane. [124-72-1] 2-Bromo-1,1,1,2-tetrafluoroethane; 1,1,1,2-tetrafluoro-2-bromoethane; Abbott 16900; DA-708; Terflurane. C$_2$HBrF$_4$; mol wt 180.93. C 13.28%, H 0.56%, Br 44.16%, F 42.00%. FBrCHCF$_3$. Prepn: Larsen, **US 2971990** (1961 to Dow). Pharmacology: Black *et al., Br. J. Anaesth.* **41,** 288 (1969).

Gas, bp 8°. Nonexplosive; nonflammable.

THERAP CAT: Anesthetic (inhalation).

9111. Tefluthrin. [79538-32-2] (1*R*,3*R*)-*rel*-3-[(1*Z*)-2-Chloro-3,3,3-trifluoro-1-propenyl]-2,2-dimethylcyclopropanecarboxylic acid (2,3,5,6-tetrafluoro-4-methylphenyl)methyl ester; (±)-*cis*-4-methyltetrafluorobenzyl 3-(2-chloro-3,3,3-trifluoro-prop-1-en-1-yl)-2,2-dimethylcyclopropane carboxylate; 2,3,5,6-tetrafluoro-4-methylbenzyl-(Z)-(1*RS*,3*RS*)-3-(2-chloro-3,3,3-trifluoro-1-propenyl)-2,2-dimethylcyclopropanecarboxylate; JF-6064; PP-993; R-151993; Force; Forza; Komet. C$_{17}$H$_{14}$ClF$_7$O$_2$; mol wt 418.73. C 48.76%, H 3.37%, Cl 8.47%, F 31.76%, O 7.64%. Synthetic pyrethroid insecticide. Prepn: N. Punja, **EP 31199**; *idem,* **US 4405640** (1981, 1983 both to ICI). Evaluation as seed treatment: G. J. Marrs, R. F. S. Gordon, *Br. Crop Prot. Counc. Monogr.* **39,** 17 (1988); for sugar beet: D. Cooke *et al., Br. Sugar Beet Rev.* **59,** 30 (1991). Effects on non-target organisms: J. M. Coulson *et al., Brighton Crop Prot. Conf. - Pests Dis.* **1990,** 975; A. M. Dewar *et al., ibid.* 987. Review of properties and insecticidal activity: M. Konradt, C. Hemmen, *Gesunde Pflanz.* **44,** 64-68 (1992); of toxicology and human exposure: *Toxicological Profile for Pyrethrins and Pyrethroids* (PB2004-100004, 2003) 332 pp.

Z-(1S)-form

Crystals from ethanol, mp 164-165°. uv max: 270 nm [ε 8460 (pH 2); ε 8050 (pH 7); ε 6700 (pH 12)]. Easily sol in hot water, alcohol, DMF. Practically insol in ether. LD$_{50}$ in mice (mg/kg): 900 orally (3 days) (Yasumoto); 750 i.p. (**FR 1574684**), also reported as 1150 i.p. (Smart).

THERAP CAT: Antineoplastic.

9113. Tegaserod. [145158-71-0] 2-[(5-Methoxy-1*H*-indol-3-yl)methylene]-*N*-pentylhydrazinecarboximidamide. C$_{16}$H$_{23}$N$_5$-O; mol wt 301.39. C 63.76%, H 7.69%, N 23.24%, O 5.31%. Selective serotonin 5HT$_4$-receptor partial agonist. Prepn: R. K. A. Giger, H. Mattes, **EP 505322**; *eidem,* **US 5510353** (1992, 1996 both to Sandoz); K.-H. Buchheit *et al., J. Med. Chem.* **38,** 2331 (1995). Clinical pharmacology: S. Appel *et al., Clin. Pharmacol. Ther.* **62,** 546 (1997); and pharmacokinetics: *idem et al., J. Clin. Pharmacol.* **37,** 229 (1997). Clinical trial in irritable bowel syndrome: S. A. Müller-Lissner *et al., Aliment. Pharmacol. Ther.* **15,** 1655 (2001); in female patients: J. Novick *et al., ibid.* **16,** 1877 (2002). Review of clinical efficacy: B. W. Jones *et al., J. Clin. Pharm. Ther.* **27,** 343-352 (2002); of mechanism of action, efficacy and safety: M. Corsetti, J. Tack, *Expert Opin. Pharmacother.* **3,** 1211-1218 (2002).

mp 155°.

Maleate. [189188-57-6] SDZ-HTF-919; Zelmac; Zelnorm. C$_{16}$H$_{23}$N$_5$O.C$_4$H$_4$O$_4$; mol wt 417.46.

THERAP CAT: Gastroprokinetic; in treatment of irritable bowel syndrome.

9114. Teichoic Acids. Major components of walls and membranes of a number of bacteria, accounting for 20 to 60% of the dry weight of cell walls. Teichoic acids vary considerably in structure but are all rich in phosphodiester linkages. Depending on their location, they can be divided into two classes: membrane and cell-wall teichoic acids. *Reviews:* Baddiley, *Endeavour* **23**, 33 (1964); *idem, Proc. Roy. Soc. London* **170B**, 331 (1968); *idem, Acc. Chem. Res.* **3**, 98 (1970); M. Duckworth in *Surface Carbohydrates of the Procaryotic Cell,* I. W. Sutherland, Ed. (Academic Press, London, 1977) pp 177-208.

Membrane teichoic acids. Contain polyglycerol phosphate chains linking positions 1 and 3 on adjacent glycerol units through the phosphodiesters, with glycosyl substituents and alanine residues on some or all of the 2 positions. Structural studies: Kelemen, Baddiley, *Biochem. J.* **80**, 246 (1961). Biosynthetic studies: Burger, Glaser, *J. Biol. Chem.* **239**, 3168, 3187 (1964); **241**, 494 (1966). Synthesis of a membrane teichoic acid fragment of *Staphylococcus aureus:* J. Oltvoort *et al., Rec. Trav. Chim.* **101**, 87 (1982).

Wall teichoic acids. Have greater structural diversity and include also polyribitol phosphate chains linking positions 1 and 5 on adjacent ribitol residues. Polymers may contain 6 to 20 repeating units. Structural studies: Armstrong *et al., Biochem. J.* **76**, 610 (1960); Baddiley, *ibid.* **85**, 49 (1962). Biosynthetic studies: Glaser, *J. Biol. Chem.* **239**, 3178 (1964). Molecular arrangement in cell wall of *Staphylococcus lactis:* Archibald *et al., Nature New Biol.* **241**, 29 (1973).

9115. Teicoplanin. [61036-64-4] Teicoplanin A₂; teichomycin A₂; MDL-507; Targocid; Targosid. Glycopeptide antibiotic complex produced by *Actinoplanes teichomyceticus* nov. sp.; structurally related to vancomycin, *q.v.* Comprised of 5 major components differentiated by a specific fatty acid moiety. Inhibits peptidoglycan synthesis in the cell wall of gram-positive bacteria. Isoln: **BE 839259**; C. Coronelli *et al.,* **US 4239751** (1976, 1980 both to Lepetit); F. Parenti *et al., J. Antibiot.* **31**, 276 (1978); M. R. Bardone *et al., ibid.* 170. Separation of components: A. Borghi *et al.,* **DE 3320342**; *eidem,* **US 4542018** (1983, 1985 both to Lepetit); *eidem, J. Antibiot.* **37**, 615 (1984). Structural studies: C. Coronelli *et al., ibid.* 621; J. C. J. Barna *et al., J. Am. Chem. Soc.* **106**, 4895 (1984). Comparative *in vitro* activity: M. H. Cynamon, P. A. Granato, *Antimicrob. Agents Chemother.* **21**, 504 (1982); H. C. Neu, P. Labthavikul, *idem,* **24**, 425 (1983). Human pharmacokinetics: L. Verbist *et al., ibid.* **26**, 881 (1984); P. L. Carver *et al., ibid.* **33**, 82 (1989). Mechanism of action: S. Somma *et al., ibid.* **26**, 917 (1984). Synergism with rifampin, *q.v.:* C. Watanakunakorn, *J. Antimicrob. Chemother.* **19**, 439 (1987). HPLC determn in human serum: J. Levy *et al., ibid.* **533**. Clinical trial in gram-positive bacterial infections: Y. Glupczynski *et al., Antimicrob. Agents Chemother.* **29**, 52 (1986). Brief review: A. H. Williams, R. N. Grüneberg, *J. Antimicrob. Chemother.* **14**, 441 (1984). Symposium on chemistry, pharmacology, activity, and clinical trials: *J. Hosp. Infect.* **7**, Suppl. A, 47-112 (1986).

Teicoplanin A₂-1	(Z)-4-decenoic acid
A₂-2	8-methylnonanoic acid
A₂-3	n-decanoic acid
A₂-4	8-methyldecanoic acid
A₂-5	9-methyldecanoic acid

Amorphous powder, mp 260° (dec). uv max in 0.1*N* HCl: 278 ($E_{1cm}^{1\%}$ 53); in 0.1*N* NaOH: 297 ($E_{1cm}^{1\%}$ 74). Sol in aq soln at pH 7.0; partially sol in methanol, ethanol. Insol in dil mineral acids, in nonpolar organic solvents.

Teicoplanin A₂-1. [91032-34-7] $C_{88}H_{95}Cl_2N_9O_{33}$; mol wt 1877.64. White amorphous powder, darkens at 220°, dec 255°.

Teicoplanin A₂-2. [91032-26-7] $C_{88}H_{97}Cl_2N_9O_{33}$; mol wt 1879.66. White amorphous powder, darkens at 210°, dec 250°.

Teicoplanin A₂-3. [91032-36-9] $C_{88}H_{97}Cl_2N_9O_{33}$; mol wt 1879.66. White amorphous powder, darkens at 210°, dec 250°.

Teicoplanin A₂-4. [91032-37-0] $C_{89}H_{99}Cl_2N_9O_{33}$; mol wt 1893.68. White amorphous powder, darkens at 210°, dec 250°.

Teicoplanin A₂-5. [91032-38-1] $C_{89}H_{99}Cl_2N_9O_{33}$; mol wt 1893.68. White amorphous powder, darkens at 210°, dec 250°.

THERAP CAT: Antibacterial.

9116. Telavancin. [372151-71-8] $N^{3''}$-[2-(Decylamino)ethyl]-29-[[(phosphonomethyl)amino]methyl]vancomycin. $C_{80}H_{106}$-$Cl_2N_{11}O_{27}P$; mol wt 1755.63. C 54.73%, H 6.09%, Cl 4.04%, N 8.78%, O 24.61%, P 1.76%. Broad spectrum, semi-synthetic glycopeptide antibiotic; inhibits bacterial cell wall formation and disrupts cell membrane integrity. Prepn: M. R. Leadbetter, M. S. Linsell, **WO 0198328**; *eidem,* **US 6635618** (2001, 2003 both to Advanced Medicine). Chemistry and antibacterial properties: *idem et al., J. Antibiot.* **57**, 326 (2004). Comparative *in vitro* antimicrobial activity: A. King *et al., J. Antimicrob. Chemother.* **53**, 797 (2004). Mechanism of action study: D. L. Higgins *et al., Antimicrob. Agents Chemother.* **49**, 1127 (2005). Clinical pharmacology: J. P. Shaw *et al., Antimicrob. Agents Chemother.* **49**, 195 (2005). Clinical trial in complicated skin and soft-tissue infections: M. E. Stryjewski *et al., Clin. Infect. Dis.* **40**, 1601 (2005). Review of discovery: J. K. Judice, J. L. Pace, *Bioorg. Med. Chem. Lett.* **13**, 4165-4168 (2003); of clinical development: J. L. Pace, J. K. Judice, *Curr. Opin. Invest. Drugs* **6**, 216-225 (2005).

Hydrochloride. [560130-42-9] TD-6424; Arbelic. $C_{80}H_{106}$-$Cl_2N_{11}O_{27}P$.HCl; mol wt 1792.10.

THERAP CAT: Antibacterial.

9117. Telbivudine. [3424-98-4] 1-(2-Deoxy-β-L-*erythro*-pentofuranosyl)-5-methyl-2,4(1*H*,3*H*)-pyrimidinedione; 1,2'-deoxy-β-L-ribofuranosylthymine; 2'-deoxy-L-thymidine; LdT; L-thymidine. $C_{10}H_{14}N_2O_5$; mol wt 242.23. C 49.58%, H 5.83%, N 11.56%, O 33.03%. Nucleoside analog; specific inhibitor of hepatitis B virus (HBV) replication. Prepn: J. Smejkal, F. Sorm, *Collect. Czech. Chem. Commun.* **29**, 2809 (1964); A. Holy, *ibid.* **37**, 4072 (1972). Anti-HBV activity: M. L. Bryant *et al., Nucleosides Nucleotides Nucleic Acids* **20**, 597 (2001). *In vitro* pharmacology: B. Hernandez-Santiago *et al., Antimicrob. Agents Chemother.* **46**, 1728 (2002). Clinical evaluation in hepatitis B: C.-L. Lai *et al., Hepatology* **40**, 719 (2004). Review of mechanism of action and pharmacology: D. N. Standring *et al., Antiviral Chem. Chemother.* **12**, Suppl. 1, 119-129 (2001); of clinical development: S.-H. B. Han, *Expert Opin. Invest. Drugs* **14**, 511-519 (2005). *See also* Thymidine.

Crystals from ethanol, mp 186°(Smejkal, Sorm). $[\alpha]_D^{20} -20.3°$ (c = 0.192 in water). Also reported as mp 189° (Holy). uv max (pH 2): 267 nm (ε 9800).

THERAP CAT: Antiviral.

9118. Teleocidins. [78474-55-2] Indole alkaloid tumor promoters isolated from the mycelia of *Streptomyces*. Consists of *teleocidin A* (two isomers) and, the major component, *teleocidin B* (four isomers). The mixture is known as telocidin; the name is derived from its toxicity to fish (Teleostei). Isoln: M. Takashima, H. Sakai, *Bull. Agric. Chem. Soc. Jpn.* **24**, 647 (1960). Resolution into A and B and their isomers: H. Fujiki, T. Sugimura, *Cancer Surv.* **2**, 539 (1983). Structure: S. Sakai *et al., Chem. Pharm. Bull.* **32**, 354 (1984). Abs config: Y. Endo *et al., ibid.* 358. Structure determn of B isomers: Y. Hitotsuyanagi *et al., ibid.* 4233. Structure-activity study: T. Kawai *et al., J. Med. Chem.* **35**, 2248 (1992). Tumor promotion: H. Fujiki *et al., Biochem. Biophys. Res. Commun.* **90**, 976 (1979); *eidem, Carcinogenesis* **3**, 895 (1982). *Review:* H. Fujiki, T. Sugimura, *Adv. Cancer Res.* **49**, 233-264 (1987).

Teleocidin B₄

White-crystal like powder, dec >61°. Easily sol in methanol, ethanol, ether, acetone, ethyl-acetate, benzene, chloroform, carbon tetrachloride; slightly sol in petroleum-ether, petroleum-benzine, ligroin. Almost insol in water, %5 HCl and 5% NaOH solution. LD_{50} orally in mice: 2 mg/kg (Takashima).

Teleocidin B₄. [11032-05-6] (4S,7S,10R,13R)-13-Ethenyl-1,3,-4,5,7,8,10,11,12,13-decahydro-4-(hydroxymethyl)-8,10,13-trimethyl-7,10-bis(1-methylethyl)-6H-benzo[g][1,4]diazonino[7,6,5-cd]indol-6-one; olivoretin D. $C_{28}H_{41}N_3O_2$; mol wt 451.64.

Dihydroteleocidin B. Structure: H. Harada *et al., Bull. Chem. Soc. Jpn.* **39**, 1773 (1966). Tumor promoting activity: H. Fujiki *et al., Proc. Natl. Acad. Sci. USA* **78**, 3872 (1981).

USE: use: Tumor promoting agent.

9119. Telithromycin. [191114-48-4] 3-De[(2,6-dideoxy-3-C-methyl-3-O-methyl-α-L-ribohexopyranosyl)oxy]-11,12-dideoxy-6-O-methyl-3-oxo-12,11-[oxycarbonyl[[4-[4-(3-pyridinyl)-1H-imidazol-1-yl]butyl]imino]]erythromycin; HMR-3647; RU-66647; Ketek. $C_{43}H_{65}N_5O_{10}$; mol wt 812.00. C 63.60%, H 8.07%, N 8.62%, O 19.70%. Semisynthetic macrolide antibiotic of the ketolide class, a group of erythromycin derivatives in which the L-cladinose residue has been replaced by a 3-keto group. Prepn: C. Agouridas *et al.,* EP 680967; *eidem,* US 5635485 (1995, 1997 both to Roussel Uclaf); A. Denis *et al., Bioorg. Med. Chem. Lett.* **9**, 3075 (1999). *In vitro* activity vs anaerobic bacteria: L. M. Ednie *et al., Antimicrob. Agents Chemother.* **41**, 2019 (1997); vs gram-positive bacteria: K. Malathum *et al., ibid.* **43**, 930 (1999). Time-kill kinetics: F. J. Boswell *et al., J. Antimicrob. Chemother.* **41**, 149 (1998). HPLC analysis: B. Lingerfelt, W. S. Champney, *J. Pharm. Biomed. Anal.* **20**, 459 (1999). Review of pharmacology and clinical trials: G.

Ackermann, A. C. Rodloff, *J. Antimicrob. Chemother.* **51**, 497-511 (2003).

Crystals from ether, mp 187-188°.

THERAP CAT: Antibacterial.

9120. Telluric(VI) Acid. [7803-68-1] Orthotelluric acid. H_6O_6Te; mol wt 229.64. H 2.63%, O 41.80%, Te 55.57%. $Te(OH)_6$. Most stable form. Prepd by oxidizing tellurium or its dioxide with chromic acid or potassium permanganate in nitric acid: Staudenmaier, *Z. Anorg. Chem.* **10**, 189 (1895); Mathers *et al., Inorg. Synth.* **3**, 145 (1950); from tellurium by oxidation with chloric acid: Meyer, Franke, *Z. Anorg. Allg. Chem.* **193**, 191 (1930); Meyer, Holowatyj, *Ber.* **81**, 119 (1948); Fehér in *Handbook of Preparative Inorganic Chemistry* vol. 1, G. Brauer, Ed. (Academic Press, New York, 2nd ed., 1963) pp 451-453°. Forms *poly-metatelluric acid* $(H_2TeO_4)_n$ when heated in air at 100-200°; *n* approx 11. Concd soln of polymerized form called *allotelluric acid*; formed when orthotelluric acid is heated in a sealed tube and dissolves in its water of constitution. *Review:* Datton, Cooper, *Chem. Rev.* **66**, 657-675 (1966).

White solid; dimorphic: monoclinic, d 3.068; cubic, d 3.163: Avinens, Petit, *C.R. Seances Acad. Sci. Ser. C* **266**, 981 (1968). Crystallizes as tetrahydrate at temp below 10°. Very weak acid: $K_1 = 2 \times 10^{-8}$; $K_2 = 1 \times 10^{-11}$. Soly in water about 33% at 30°: Mylius, *Ber.* **34**, 2208 (1901). Strong tendency to polymerize (like stannic acid) as the mol wt increases the soly becomes less and less and aq solns become truly colloidal. Sparingly sol in concd nitric acid. Soly in dil nitric acid: *Inorg. Syn. (loc. cit.)*.

9121. Tellurium. [13494-80-9] Aurum paradoxum; metallum problematicum. Te; at. wt 127.60; at. no. 52; valence 2, 4, 6. Group VIA (16). Diatomic (Te_2) in the vapor state. Eight stable isotopes: 120 (0.089%); 122 (2.46%); 123 (0.87%); 124 (4.61%); 125 (6.99%); 126 (18.71%); 128 (31.79%); 130 (34.48%); artificial radioactive isotopes: 114-119; 121; 127; 129; 131-134. Present in the earth's crust to the extent of 0.002 ppm. Discovered by von Reichenstein in 1782; named by Klaproth in 1798. Occurs as tellurides in combination with metals in the minerals tetradymite, altaite, coloradolite; found as the dioxide, tellurite; found also native, associated with silver and gold. Prepn: Kracek, *J. Am. Chem. Soc.* **63**, 1989 (1941); Fehér in *Handbook of Preparative Inorganic Chemistry* vol. 1, G. Brauer, Ed. (Academic Press, New York, 2nd ed., 1963) pp 437-438. Prepn of spectrally pure Te for semiconductor devices: Weidel, *Z. Naturforsch.* **9a**, 697 (1954). Symposium on organic selenium and tellurium compds: Y. Okamoto, W. H. H. Gunther, Eds., *Ann. N.Y. Acad. Sci.* **192**, 1-225 (1972). *Reviews:* Stone, Caron in *Rare Metals Handbook*, C. A. Hampel, Ed. (Reinhold, New York, 1954) pp 405-415; Bagnall in *Comprehensive Inorganic Chemistry* vol. 2, J. C. Bailar, Jr. *et al.,* Eds. (Pergamon Press, Oxford, 1973) pp 935-1008; E. M. Elkin in *Kirk-Othmer Encyclopedia of Chemical Technology* vol. 22 (Wiley-Interscience, New York, 3rd ed., 1983) pp 658-679.

Grayish-white, lustrous, brittle, crystalline solid, hexagonal, rhombohedral structure, or dark-gray to brown, amorphous powder with metal characteristics. d (cryst) 6.11-6.27. mp 449.8°. bp 989.9°. Electrical resistivity (19.6°): 200,000 μ-ohms-cm. Latent heat of fusion: 4.27 kcal/mole. Linear coefficient of thermal expansion: 16.8×10^{-6}/°C. Modulus of elasticity: 6,000,000 psi. Specific heat (solid): 0.047 cal/g/°C. Magnetic susceptibility (18°): -0.31×10^{-6} cgs. Hardness (Mohs): 2.3. Thermal conductivity: 0.014 at 20°. Burns in air with a greenish-blue flame, forming the dioxide. Insol in water, in benzene, in carbon disulfide. Not attacked by hydrochloric acid; reacts with nitric acid; with concd or fuming sulfuric acids, forming a red soln; in presence of air dissolves in potassium hydroxide with formation of a deep-red soln. Combines with the halogens; does not react with sulfur or selenium.

Caution: Potential symptoms of overexposure are garlic odor on breath and sweat; dry mouth, metal taste; somnolence; anorexia, nausea and no sweating; dermatitis. *See NIOSH Pocket Guide to Chemical Hazards* (DHHS/NIOSH 97-140, 1997) p 294.

USE: As coloring agent in chinaware, porcelains, enamels, glass; reagent in producing black finish on silverware; in manuf special alloys of marked electrical resistance; in semiconductor research.

9122. Tellurium Dichloride. [10025-71-5] Tellurous chloride. Cl_2Te; mol wt 198.51. Cl 35.72%, Te 64.28%. $TeCl_2$. Prepn from CCl_2F_2 and Te: Aynsley, *J. Chem. Soc.* **1953**, 3016.

Black, amorphous solid; black liquid; purple vapor. mp 208°. bp 328°. Disproportionates in ether, dioxane, dibutyl ether. Insol in CCl_4.

9123. Tellurium Dioxide. [7446-07-3] Tellurium oxide (TeO_2). O_2Te; mol wt 159.60. O 20.05%, Te 79.95%. TeO_2. Prepd by oxidation of Te by HNO_3: Norris, *J. Am. Chem. Soc.* **28**, 1675 (1906); Marshall, *Inorg. Synth.* **3**, 143 (1950); Fehér in *Handbook of Preparative Inorganic Chemistry* vol. 1, G. Brauer, Ed. (Academic Press, New York, 2nd ed., 1963) pp 447-449. The orthorhombic form occurs in nature as the mineral *tellurite*. Review: Dutton, Cooper, *Chem. Rev.* **66**, 657-675 (1966).

White crystals, dimorphic: tetragonal, d 5.75; orthorhombic, d 6.04. Turns yellow on heating, mp 733°, forming a deep yellow liquid. Soly in water about 1:150,000. Sol in sodium hydroxide solns and in hydrochloric acid. Practically insol in ammonia water.

9124. Tellurium Hexafluoride. [7783-80-4] F_6Te; mol wt 241.59. F 47.18%, Te 52.82%. TeF_6. Prepd by direct fluorination of tellurium metal: Prideaux, *J. Chem. Soc.* **89**, 322 (1906); Klemm, Henkel, *Z. Anorg. Allg. Chem.* **207**, 74 (1932); Yost, Claussen, *J. Am. Chem. Soc.* **55**, 885 (1933); Yost, *Inorg. Synth.* **1**, 121 (1939).

Colorless gas. Repulsive odor. mp −37.6°. Sublimes at −38.9°. Critical temperature 83°. d (solid; −191°) 4.006; d (liq; −10°) 2.499. Not as inert chemically as SeF_6 and SF_6 because the covalence maximum of tellurium is higher than 6. Slowly absorbed by water with hydrolysis to telluric acid, H_6TeO_6; more quickly hydrolyzed by aq KOH. Does not attack glass when pure. Corrodes mercury.

Caution: Potential symptoms of overexposure are headache; dyspnea; garlic odor on breath. *See NIOSH Pocket Guide to Chemical Hazards* (DHHS/NIOSH 97-140, 1997) p 294.

9125. Tellurium Tetrabromide. [10031-27-3] Telluric bromide. Br_4Te; mol wt 447.22. Br 71.47%, Te 28.53%. $TeBr_4$. Prepd from the elements: Fehér in *Handbook of Preparative Inorganic Chemistry* vol. 1, G. Brauer, Ed. (Academic Press, New York, 2nd ed., 1963) pp 445-446.

Orange crystals when cold, red when hot. d 4.3. mp ~380°. bp 414-420°, dec into dibromide and bromine; can be sublimed without dec at 300° in vacuum. Soluble in a little water, but hydrolyzed by much water. Sol in HBr, ether, glacial acetic acid. *Keep well closed.*

9126. Tellurium Tetrachloride. [10026-07-0] Telluric chloride. Cl_4Te; mol wt 269.41. Cl 52.64%, Te 47.36%. $TeCl_4$. Prepd from the elements: Suttle, Smith, *Inorg. Synth.* **3**, 140 (1950).

White, very hygroscopic, cryst solid. d 3.01. mp 225°. Melts to a yellow liquid, becoming dark red at higher temp. bp 380° without decompn. Dec by water into TeO_2 and HCl. Sol in abs alcohol and toluene. *Keep tightly closed.*

9127. Tellurium Tetraiodide. [7790-48-9] I_4Te; mol wt 635.22. I 79.91%, Te 20.09%. TeI_4. Prepd from $Te(OH)_6$ and

HI, Gutbier, Flury, *Z. Anorg. Allg. Chem.* **32**,108 (1902); Damiens, *Ann. Chim.* [9] **19**, 44 (1923); Fehér in *Handbook of Preparative Inorganic Chemistry* vol. 1, G. Brauer, Ed. (Academic Press, New York, 2nd ed., 1963) p 447.

Gunmetal-gray crystals. Stable in moist air. d_4^{15} 5.05. mp 280°. Gives off I_2 when heated. Hydrolyzed slowly by cold, quickly by hot water, forming TeO_2 and HI. Sol in HI; somewhat sol in acetone.

9128. Tellurous Acid. [10049-23-7] Telluric(IV) acid. H_2O_3Te; mol wt 177.61. H 1.14%, O 27.02%, Te 71.84%. H_2TeO_3.

White crystals or cryst powder. d 3.0. Slightly sol in water; sol in dil acids or alkalies. Its potassium salt is reduced by many microorganisms, producing dark-colored solns.

9129. Telmisartan. [144701-48-4] 4'-[[(1,4'-Dimethyl-2'-propyl[2,6'-bi-1*H*-benzimidazol]-1'-yl)methyl][1,1'-biphenyl]-2-carboxylicacid;4'-[[4-methyl-6-(1-methyl-2-benzimidazolyl)-2-propyl-1-benzimidazolyl]methyl]-2-biphenylcarboxylic acid; BIBR 277; Kinzalmono; Micardis; Pritor. $C_{33}H_{30}N_4O_2$; mol wt 514.62. C 77.02%, H 5.88%, N 10.89%, O 6.22%. Angiotensin II receptor antagonist. Prepn: N. Hauel *et al.*, **EP 502314** (1992 to Thomae), *C.A.* **117**, 251352 (1992); U. J. Ries *et al.*, *J. Med. Chem.* **36**, 4040 (1993). Pharmacology: W. Wienen *et al.*, *Br. J. Pharmacol.* **110**, 245 (1993). Binding study: W. Wienen, M. Entzeroth, *J. Hypertens.* **12**, 119 (1994). Clinical pharmacology, pharmacokinetics: J. M. Neutel, D. H. G. Smith, *Adv. Ther.* **15**, 206 (1998). Clinical trial in hypertension: D. H. G. Smith *et al.*, *ibid.* 229. Review of pharmacology and clinical efficacy: K. J. McClellan, A. Markham, *Drugs* **56**, 1039-1044 (1998).

White solid, mp 261-263°. Practically insol in water (pH 3-9). Sparingly sol in strong acid (except insol in hydrochloric acid); sol in strong base.

THERAP CAT: Antihypertensive.

9130. Telomerase. Telomere terminal transferase. RNA-containing enzyme found in unicellular organisms and germline cells. Also produced by tumor cells and by immortalized cell lines; not expressed in normal somatic cells. Specialized reverse transcriptase that adds short, tandemly repeated segments of DNA onto the ends of eukaryotic chromosomes (telomeres) using its RNA component as a template. Replenishes the small amount of telomeric DNA that is normally lost during replication. In the absence of telomerase, this incremental loss of DNA continues with each cell division until the chromosome can no longer replicate and ultimately results in cell death. Activation of telomerase is associated with the unlimited proliferation of tumor cells. Discovery in the ciliate, *Tetrahymena thermophila:* C. W. Greider, E. H. Blackburn, *Cell* **43**, 405 (1985). Overview and potential physiological significance: C. W. Greider, *BioEssays* **12**, 363-369 (1990). Proposed role in cell immortalization: C. M. Counter *et al.*, *EMBO J.* **11**, 1921 (1992). Detection in human ovarian carcinoma cells: *idem et al., Proc. Natl. Acad. Sci. USA* **91**, 2900 (1994). Structural studies: A. Bhattacharyya, E. H. Blackburn, *EMBO J.* **13**, 5721 (1994); M. McCormick-Graham, D. P. Romero, *Nucleic Acids Res.* **23**, 1091 (1995). Clinical implications in cancer diagnosis and therapy: N. W. Kim, *Eur. J. Cancer* **33**, 781 (1997). Effect on life-span of normal human cells *in vitro:* A. G. Bodnar *et al., Science* **279**, 349 (1998).

9131. Telomycin. [19246-24-3] $C_{59}H_{77}N_{13}O_{19}$; mol wt 1272.32. C 55.70%, H 6.10%, N 14.31%, O 23.89%. Polypeptide antibiotic produced by *Streptomyces* spp. from Florida soil: Misiek *et al., Antibiot. Annu.* **1957-1958**, 852. Structure: Sheehan *et al., J. Am. Chem. Soc.* **85**, 2867 (1963); **90**, 462 (1968). NMR spectrum and conformation: Kumar, Urry, *Biochemistry* **12**, 3811, 4392 (1973). Antibacterial spectrum: A. Gourevitch *et al., Antibiot. Annu.* **1957-1958**, 856. Pharmacology: D. E. Tisch *et al., ibid.* 863.

Asp–Ser–Thr–*a*-Thr–Ala–Gly–*t*-3-Hyp–*e*-3-Hyl

c-3-Hyp–Δ-Trp–β-MeTrp

a-Thr =	*allo*-threonine
t-3-Hyp =	*trans*-3-hydroxyproline
c-3-Hyp =	*cis*-3-hydroxyproline
Δ-Trp =	α,β-didehydrotryptophan
e-3-Hyl =	*erythro*-3-hydroxyleucine

Amorphous, gray solid. $[\alpha]_D^{28}$ −133° (c = 1 in 2:1 methanol-water). uv max (ethanol:water, 2:1): 222.5, 277, 290, 339 nm (ε 63732; 13746; 11890; 22058). Minimum soly in water at pH 3.0 to 3.3 = 4 mg/ml. Maximum soly is above pH 8.5 = >150 mg/ml. Soly in 10% sodium chloride soln less than 1 mg/ml. Moderately sol in methanol, ethanol. Very slightly sol in acetone, ethyl acetate. Insol in ether, chloroform, hydrocarbons. Aq solns are stable to heat. LD_{50} in mice (mg/kg): >1000 orally, i.v., i.p., i.m. (Tisch).

9132. Temafloxacin. [108319-06-8] 1-(2,4-Difluorophenyl)-6-fluoro-1,4-dihydro-7-(3-methyl-1-piperazinyl)-4-oxo-3-quinolinecarboxylic acid; T-1258; A-63004; Teflox; Temac; Omniflox. $C_{21}H_{18}F_3N_3O_3$; mol wt 417.38. C 60.43%, H 4.35%, F 13.66%, N 10.07%, O 11.50%. Trifluorinated quinolone antibacterial. Prepn: D. T. W. Chu, **EP 131839**; *idem*, **US 4730000** (1985, 1988 to Abbott). Antibacterial activities: D. J. Hardy *et al., Antimicrob. Agents Chemother.* **31**, 1768 (1987); K. V. I. Rolston *et al., Eur. J. Clin. Microbiol. Infect. Dis.* **7**, 684 (1988); in comparison with other fluoroquinolones: A. L. Barry, R. N. Jones, *J. Antimicrob. Chemother.* **23**, 527 (1989).

Hydrochloride. [105784-61-0] A-62254. $C_{21}H_{18}F_3N_3O_3$·HCl; mol wt 453.84.

9133. Temazepam. [846-50-4] 7-Chloro-1,3-dihydro-3-hydroxy-1-methyl-5-phenyl-2*H*-1,4-benzodiazepin-2-one; 3-hydroxydiazepam; *N*-methyloxazepam; oxydiazepam; ER-115; K-3917; Ro-5-5345; Wy-3917; Euhypnos; Euipnos; Gelthix; Levanxene; Levanxol; Normison; Perdorm; Planum; Remestan; Restoril. $C_{16}H_{13}$-ClN_2O_2; mol wt 300.74. C 63.90%, H 4.36%, Cl 11.79%, N 9.31%, O 10.64%. Pharmacologically active metabolite of diazepam, *q.v.* Prepn: S. C. Bell, S. J. Childress, *J. Org. Chem.* **27**, 1691 (1962); S. C. Bell, **US 3197467** (1965 to Am. Home. Prod.). *See also:* E. Reeder *et al.*, **US 3340253** and **US 3374225** (1967, 1968, both to Hoffmann-La Roche). Metabolism: H. J. Schwandt *et al., Xenobiotica* **4**, 733 (1974); S. H. Curry *et al., Br. J. Pharmacol.* **57**, 427P (1976). Pharmacology: L. O. Randall *et al., Arch. Int. Pharmacodyn.* **185**, 135 (1970); S. Garattini *et al.,* "Metabolic Studies on Benzodiazepines in Various Animal Species" in *Benzodiazepines,* S. Garattini, Ed. (Raven Press, New York, 1973) pp 73-97. Pharmacology and toxicity study: L. O. Randall *et al., Curr. Ther. Res.* **7**, 590 (1965). Clinical study: P. Sarteschi *et al., Arzneim.-Forsch.* **22**, 93 (1972). Review of pharmacology and therapeutic efficacy: R. C. Heel *et al., Drugs* **21**, 321-340 (1981).

Crystals from cyclohexane, mp 119-121°.
Note: This is a controlled substance (depressant): **21 CFR**, 1308.14.
THERAP CAT: Sedative, hypnotic.

9134. TEMED. [110-18-9] *N,N,N',N'*-Tetramethyl-1,2-ethanediamine; TMEDA. $C_6H_{16}N_2$; mol wt 116.20. C 62.02%, H 13.88%, N 24.11%. Prepn: M. Freund, H. Michaels, *Ber.* **30**, 1374 (1897); W. Hanhart, C. K. Ingold, *J. Chem. Soc.* **1927**, 997. Base strength: L. Spialter, R. W. Moshier, *J. Am. Chem. Soc.* **79**, 5955 (1957). Effect on kinetics of gel polymerization: Y. Pegon, C. Quincy, *J. Chromatogr.* **100**, 11 (1974). Use as initiator in electrophoresis: B. J. Bassam, S. Bentley, *BioTechniques* **19**, 568 (1995); as chelator in biological redox systems: H. C. Chang, J. A. Bumpus, *Proc. Natl. Sci. Counc. ROC(B)* **25**, 26 (2001); as solvent in RPLC: L. Palego *et al., Prog. Neuro-Psychopharmacol. Biol. Psychiatry* **25**, 519 (2001); in capillary isoelectric focusing: D. Mohan, C. S. Lee, *J. Chromatogr. A* **979**, 271 (2002).

Basic liquid. fp −55.1°. bp$_{724}$ 119.4-119.5°. n_D^{18} 1.4196. pKa$_1$ 5.85; pKa$_2$ 8.97.
USE: Polymerization accelerator in gel electrophoresis, solvent and oxidizing reagent.

9135. Temephos. [3383-96-8] *O,O'*-(Thiodi-4,1-phenylene)phosphorothioic acid *O,O,O',O'*-tetramethyl ester; *O,O'*-(thiodi-4,1-phenylene)bis(*O,O'*-dimethylphosphorothioate); *O,O,O',O'*-tetramethyl *O,O'*-thiodi-*p*-phenylene phosphorothioate; phosphorothioic acid *O,O*-dimethyl ester *O,O*-diester with 4,4'-thiodiphenol; ENT-27165; AC-52160; Abate; Biothion. $C_{16}H_{20}O_6P_2S_3$; mol wt 466.47. C 41.20%, H 4.32%, O 20.58%, P 13.28%, S 20.62%. Prepn: J. B. Lovell, R. W. Baer, **BE 648531** *C.A.* **63**, 11433e (1965); *eidem,* **US 3317636** (1964, 1967 both to Am. Cyanamid). Metabolism: R. C. Blinn, *J. Agric. Food Chem.* **17**, 118 (1969). Toxicity study: T. B. Gaines, *Toxicol. Appl. Pharmacol.* **14**, 515 (1969).

Crystalline solid, mp 30.0-30.5°. Optimum stability at pH 5-7. Sol in acetonitrile, carbon tetrachloride, ether, dichloroethane, toluene. Almost insol in water, hexane. LD_{50} in male, female rats (mg/kg): 8600, 13000 orally (Gaines).
Caution: Potential symptoms of overexposure are eye irritation, blurred vision; dizziness, confusion; dyspnea; salivation; abdominal cramps, nausea, diarrhea, vomiting. *See NIOSH Pocket Guide to Chemical Hazards* (DHHS/NIOSH 97-140, 1997) p 296.
USE: Insecticide.

9136. Temocapril. [111902-57-9] (2*S*,6*R*)-6-[[(1*S*)-1-(Ethoxycarbonyl)-3-phenylpropyl]amino]tetrahydro-5-oxo-2-(2-thienyl)-1,4-thiazepine-4(5*H*)-acetic acid; (+)-(2*S*,6*R*)-6-[[(1*S*)-1-carboxy-3-phenylpropyl]amino]tetrahydro-5-oxo-2-(2-thienyl)-1,4-thiazepine-4(5*H*)-acetic acid, 6-ethyl ester. $C_{23}H_{28}N_2O_5S_2$; mol wt 476.61. C 57.96%, H 5.92%, N 5.88%, O 16.78%, S 13.46%. Angiotensin-converting enzyme (ACE) inhibitor. Hydrolyzed *in* *vivo* to the active diacid metabolite. Prepn: H. Yanagisawa *et al.*, **EP 161801**; *idem*, **US 4699905** (1985, 1987 both to Sankyo); *idem et al.*, *J. Med. Chem.* **30**, 1984 (1987). Pharmacology: K. Oizumi *et al.*, *Jpn. J. Pharmacol.* **48**, 349 (1988). GC/MS determn in human plasma and urine: H. Shioya *et al.*, *J. Chromatogr.* **496**, 129 (1989). Clinical evaluation: M. Arita *et al.*, *Clin. Exp. Pharmacol. Physiol.* **21**, 195 (1994); and pharmacokinetics: S. Tokunaga *et al.*, *Drug Invest.* **7**, 161 (1994). *Review:* H. Koike *et al.*, *Annu. Rep. Sankyo Res. Lab.* **44**, 1-81 (1992).

Cryst powder, mp 168°. $[\alpha]^{23}$ +40° (c = 1.1 in DMF).

Hydrochloride. [110221-44-8] CS-622; Acecol. Solid from ethanol/ethyl acetate, mp 187° (dec). $[\alpha]_D^{25}$ +47.7° (c = 1 in DMF). LD_{50} in mice, rats, dogs (mg/kg): >5000, >5000, >800 orally (Koike).

Diacid. [110221-53-9] Temocaprilat; RS-5139. $C_{21}H_{24}N_2O_5$-S_2; mol wt 448.56. Solid from ethanol, mp 246° (dec). $[\alpha]_D^{25}$ +63.4° (c = 1 in DMF).

THERAP CAT: Antihypertensive.

9137. Temocillin. [66148-78-5] (2S,5R,6S)-6-[(Carboxy-3-thienylacetyl)amino]-6-methoxy-3,3-dimethyl-7-oxo-4-thia-1-azabicyclo[3.2.0]heptane-2-carboxylic acid; (6S)-6-[2-carboxy-2-(3-thienyl)acetamido]-6-methoxypenicillanic acid. $C_{16}H_{18}N_2O_7S_2$; mol wt 414.45. C 46.37%, H 4.38%, N 6.76%, O 27.02%, S 15.47%. Semi-synthetic injectable penicillin deriv with high activity vs a large number of gram-negative bacteria, but with little activity vs gram-positive organisms. Prepn: J. P. Clayton, P. H. Bentley, **DE 2600866** (1976 to Beecham), *C.A.* **86**, 55420t (1977); P. H. Bentley *et al.*, *J. Chem. Soc. Perkin Trans. 1* **1979**, 2455. *In vitro* antibacterial activity and β-lactamase susceptibility: I. Phillips *et al.*, *J. Antimicrob. Chemother.* **10**, 271 (1982). Comparison to other penicillins vs *H. influenzae* and intestinal gram-negative rods: H. Y. Chen, J. D. Williams, *ibid.* 279. Pharmacokinetics and tissue penetration in healthy volunteers: R. M. Brown *et al.*, *ibid.* 295. *In vivo* and *in vitro* comparison to ampicillin: R. Yogev *et al.*, *Antimicrob. Agents Chemother.* **23**, 182 (1983). Series of articles on microbiology, pharmacology and clinical studies: *Drugs* **29**, Suppl. 5, 1-243 (1985).

Disodium salt. [61545-06-0] BRL-17421; Temopen. $C_{16}H_{16}$-$N_2Na_2O_7S_2$; mol wt 458.42. Amorphous solid.

THERAP CAT: Antibacterial.

9138. Temoporfin. [122341-38-2] 3,3′,3″,3‴-(2,3-Dihydro-21H,23H-porphine-5,10,15,20-tetrayl)tetrakisphenol; 2,3-dihydro-5,10,15,20-tetra(m-hydroxyphenyl)porphyrin; 5,10,15,20-tetra(m-hydroxyphenyl)chlorin; m-THPC; dihydro meta-HK7; EF-9; Foscan. $C_{44}H_{32}N_4O_4$; mol wt 680.75. C 77.63%, H 4.74%, N 8.23%, O 9.40%. Second generation systemic photosensitizing agent. Prepn: R. Bonnett, M. C. Berenbaum, **EP 337601**; *idem*, **US 4992257** (1989, 1991 both to Efamol Holdings); R. Bonnett *et al.*, *Biochem. J.* **261**, 277 (1989). NMR study: *idem et al.*, *J. Chem. Soc. Perkin Trans. 2* **1994**, 1839. Toxicology study: R. B. Veenhuizen *et al.*, *Int. J. Cancer* **59**, 830 (1994). HPLC determn in plasma and tissue: M. Barberi-Heyob *et al.*, *J. Chromatogr. B* **688**, 331 (1997). Clinical pharmacokinetics: T. Glanzmann *et al.*, *Photochem. Photobiol.* **67**, 596 (1998). Clinical evaluation in photodynamic therapy of malignancies: J.-F. Savary *et al.*, *Arch. Otolaryngol. Head Neck Surg.* **123**, 162 (1997).

Purple solid from methanol/water. Absorption max (methanol): 284, 306, 415, 516, 543, 591, 650 nm (ε 16900, 15600, 146000, 11000, 7300, 4400, 22400 l/mol-cm). Sol in polar solvents.

THERAP CAT: Antineoplastic (photosensitizer).

9139. Temozolomide. [85622-93-1] 3,4-Dihydro-3-methyl-4-oxoimidazo[5,1-d]-1,2,3,5-tetrazine-8-carboxamide; 8-carbamoyl-3-methylimidazo[5,1-d]-1,2,3,5-tetrazin-4(3H)-one; methazolastone; M & B 39831; CCRG-81045; NSC-362856; Temodal; Temodar. $C_6H_6N_6O_2$; mol wt 194.15. C 37.12%, H 3.11%, N 43.29%, O 16.48%. Imidazotetrazine alkylating agent. Prepn: E. Lunt *et al.*, **DE 3231255** (1983 to May & Baker); *eidem*, **US 5260921** (1993 to Cancer Res. Campaign Technol.); M. F. G. Stevens *et al.*, *J. Med. Chem.* **27**, 196 (1984). Crystal structure and structure-activity study: P. R. Lowe *et al.*, *ibid.* **35**, 3377 (1992). Synthesis: Y. Wang *et al.*, *J. Org. Chem.* **62**, 7288 (1997). HPLC determn in plasma and urine: F. Shen *et al.*, *J. Chromatogr. B* **667**, 291 (1995). Review of pharmacology and clinical efficacy in melanoma and brain tumor: E. S. Newlands *et al.*, *Cancer Treat. Rev.* **23**, 35-61 (1997); S. J. Danson, M. R. Middleton, *Expert Rev. Anticancer Ther.* **1**, 13-19 (2001).

Crystals from dichloromethane, mp 212° (dec). uv max (95% ethanol): 327 nm.

THERAP CAT: Antineoplastic.

9140. TEMPO. [2564-83-2] 2,2,6,6-Tetramethyl-1-piperidinyloxy; 2,2,6,6-tetramethylpentamethylene nitroxide. C_9H_{18}-NO; mol wt 156.25. C 69.18%, H 11.61%, N 8.96%, O 10.24%. Stable nitroxide free radical used as reversible capping agent in "living" free radical polymerizations and as catalyst for selective oxidation of alcohols. Prepn: E. G. Ruzantsev *et al.*, *Bull. Acad. Sci. USSR Div. Chem. Sci.* **1962**, 2152. Crystal structure: Z. Ciunik, *J. Mol. Struct.* **412**, 27 (1997). Thermal stability: M. V. Ciriano *et al.*, *J. Am. Chem. Soc.* **121**, 6375 (1999). Effect of acids on reaction rates: M. V. Baldovi *et al.*, *Macromolecules* **29**, 5497 (1996). Use in oxidation of alcohols: M. Zhao *et al.*, *J. Org. Chem.* **64**, 2564 (1999); in production of aminyl radicals: W. Huang *et al.*, *J. Am. Chem. Soc.* **121**, 3939 (1999); in polymerization: L. I. Gabaston *et al.*, *Polymer* **40**, 4505 (1999).

Monoclinic dark red crystals, mp 36-40°. Flash pt: 67°C (Acros Organics Data Sheet).

USE: In organic chemistry as a radical trap, a catalyst and in polymerization mediation.

9141. TEMPOL. [2226-96-2] 4-Hydroxy-2,2,6,6-tetramethyl-1-piperidinyloxy; 4-hydroxy-TEMPO; 4-hydroxy-2,2,6,6-tetramethyl piperidine *N*-oxide; 4-hydroxy-2,2,6,6-tetramethylpiperidinooxy. $C_9H_{18}NO_2$; mol wt 172.24. C 62.76%, H 10.53%, N 8.13%, O 18.58%. Stable nitroxyl radical; water-soluble analogue of TEMPO, *q.v.* Functions as a membrane-permeable radical scavenger. Prepn: E. G. Rozantsev, *Bull. Acad. Sci. USSR Div. Chem. Sci.* **12**, 2085 (1964). Energy transfer studies: N. N. Quan, A. V. Guzzo, *J. Phys. Chem.* **85**, 140 (1981). IR conformation study: W. A. Bueno, L. Degrève, *J. Mol. Struct.* **74**, 291 (1981). Solid state NMR spectra: C. J. Groombridge, M. J. Perkins, *J. Chem. Soc. Chem. Commun.* **1991**, 1164. LC/MS/MS determn: I. D. Podmore, *J. Chem. Res. Synop.* **2002**, 574. Use as a phase transfer catalyst: X.-Y. Wang *et al., Synth. Commun.* **29**, 157 (1999). Review of effects in animal models for shock, ischemia-reperfusion injury, and inflammation: C. Thiemermann, *Crit. Care Med.* **31**, S76-S84 (2003).

Crystals from ether + hexane, mp 71.5°. uv max (hexane): 240, 450-500 ($\varepsilon \sim 1800, \sim 5$). uv max (ethanol): 242, 435-455 ($\varepsilon \sim 3800, \sim 10$). Sol in water.
USE: Spin label for EPR studies; phase transfer dehydration catalyst; antioxidant; inhibitor of olefin free radical polymerization.

9142. Temsirolimus. [162635-04-3] Rapamycin 42-[3-Hydroxy-2-(hydroxymethyl)-2-methylpropanoate]; rapamycin 42-ester with 2,2-bis(hydroxymethyl)propionic acid; CCI-779. $C_{56}H_{87}NO_{16}$; mol wt 1030.29. C 65.28%, H 8.51%, N 1.36%, O 24.85%. Ester analog of rapamycin, *q.v.*; selectively inhibits mammalian target of rapamycin (mTOR). Prepn: J. S. Skotnicki *et al., US 5362718* (1994 to Am. Home Prod.). Lipase-catalyzed synthesis from rapamycin: J. Gu *et al., Org. Lett.* **7**, 3945 (2005). Clinical pharmacology: E. Raymond *et al., J. Clin. Oncol.* **22**, 2336 (2004). Clinical study in advanced refractory renal cell carcinoma: M. B. Atkins *et al., ibid.* 909. Clinical evaluation in glioblastoma multiforme: E. Galanis *et al., J. Clin. Oncol.* **23**, 5294 (2005); in breast cancer: S. Chan *et al., ibid.* 5314; in mantle cell lymphoma: T. E. Witzig *et al., ibid.* 5347.

White solid. Sol in water. Lipophilic.
THERAP CAT: Antineoplastic.

9143. Tenecteplase. [191588-94-0] 103-L-Asparagine-117-L-glutamine-296-L-alanine-297-L-alanine-298-L-alanine-299-L-ala-

nineplasminogen activator (human tissue-type); TNK-tPA; Metalyse. Genetically engineered variant of human tissue plasminogen activator (t-PA), *q.v.*; expressed in Chinese hamster ovary cells. mol wt ~65 kDa. Constructed by oligonucleotide-directed mutagenesis at 3 specific sites. Prepn: W. F. Bennett *et al., WO 9324635* (1993 to Genentech); B. A. Keyt *et al., Proc. Natl. Acad. Sci. USA* **91**, 3670 (1994). Pharmacology: C. R. Benedict *et al., Circulation* **92**, 3032 (1995). Clinical pharmacokinetics: N. B. Modi *et al., Thromb. Haemostasis* **79**, 134 (1998). Clinical trial in acute myocardial infarction: ASSENT-2 Investigators, *Lancet* **354**, 716 (1999).
THERAP CAT: Thrombolytic.

9144. Tenidap. [120210-48-2] (*Z*)-5-Chloro-2,3-dihydro-3-(hydroxy-2-thienylmethylene)-2-oxo-1*H*-indole-1-carboxamide; 5-chloro-2,3-dihydro-2-oxo-3-(2-thienylcarbonyl)-1*H*-indole-1-carboxamide; 5-chloro-3-(2-thenoyl)-2-oxindole-1-carboxamide; CP-66248. $C_{14}H_9ClN_2O_3S$; mol wt 320.75. C 52.42%, H 2.83%, Cl 11.05%, N 8.73%, O 14.96%, S 10.00%. Inhibitor of 5-lipoxygenase and interleukin-1 (IL-1) activity. Prepn: S. B. Kadin, *EP 156603; idem, US 4556672* (both 1985 to Pfizer). Effect on 5-lipoxygenase activity *in vitro:* K. Fogh *et al., Arch. Dermatol. Res.* **280**, 430 (1988). Effect on IL-1 activity in patients with rheumatoid arthritis: B. McDonald *et al., Arthritis Rheum.* **31**, Suppl., S52 (1988). Clinical evaluation: P. Katz *et al., ibid.* S52.

Fluffy, yellow crystals from acetic acid, mp 230° (dec).
Sodium salt. [119784-94-0] CP-66248-2. $C_{14}H_8ClN_2NaO_3S$; mol wt 342.73. Crystals from methanol-isopropanol, mp 237-238°.
THERAP CAT: Anti-inflammatory.

9145. Teniposide. [29767-20-2] (5*R*,5a*R*,8a*R*,9*S*)-5,8,8a,9-Tetrahydro-5-(4-hydroxy-3,5-dimethoxyphenyl)-9-[[4,6-*O*-[(*R*)-2-thienylmethylene]-β-D-glucopyranosyl]oxy]furo[3′,4′:6,7]naphtho[2,3-*d*]-1,3-dioxol-6(5a*H*)-one; 4′-demethylepipodophyllotoxin 9-(4,6-*O*-2-thenylidene-β-D-glucopyranoside); 4′-demethylepipodophyllotoxin-β-D-thenylidine glucoside; ETP; NSC-122819; VM-26; Vehem-Sandoz; Vumon. $C_{32}H_{32}O_{13}S$; mol wt 656.65. C 58.53%, H 4.91%, O 31.67%, S 4.88%. Semi-synthetic derivative of podophyllotoxin, *q.v.* Prepn: A. Von Wartburg, *ZA 6607585*; C. Keeler-Juslen *et al., US 3524844* (1968, 1970 both to Sandoz). Mechanism of action: H. Stähelin, *Eur. J. Cancer* **6**, 303 (1970). Pharmacology: M. Hacker, D. Roberts, *Cancer Res.* **37**, 3287 (1977); S. M. Sieber *et al., Teratology* **18**, 31 (1978); T. J. Vietti *et al., Cancer Treat. Rep.* **62**, 1313 (1978). Metabolism: L. Allen, *Drug Metab. Rev.* **8**, 119 (1978); *Cancer Res.* **38**, 2549 (1978). Clinical studies: N. M. Gadel-Mawla *et al., Cancer Treat. Rep.* **62**, 993 (1978); R. E. Bellet *et al., ibid.* 445. Studies on delayed toxicity in mice after i.p. injections: M. Hacker, D. Roberts, *Cancer Res.* **35**, 1756 (1975); H. Stählin, *Eur. J. Cancer* **12**, 925 (1976). Review of pharmacology, pharmacokinetics and assay methods: P. I. Clark, M. L. Slevin, *Clin. Pharmacokinet.* **12**, 223-252 (1987). Comprehensive description: J. J. Kettenes-van den Bosch *et al., Anal. Profiles Drug Subs.* **19**, 575-600 (1990).

Crystals from abs ethanol, mp 242-246°. $[\alpha]_D^{20}$ $-107°$ (9:1 chloroform/methanol). uv max (methanol): 283 nm ($E_{1cm}^{1\%}$ 64.1). pKa 10.13.

THERAP CAT: Antineoplastic.

9146. Tenofovir. [147127-20-6] [[(1R)-2-(6-Amino-9H-purin-9-yl)-1-methylethoxy]methyl]phosphonic acid; (R)-9-(2-phosphonomethoxypropyl)adenine; (R)-PMPA; GS-1278. $C_9H_{14}N_5O_4$-P; mol wt 287.21. C 37.64%, H 4.91%, N 24.38%, O 22.28%, P 10.78%. Acyclic phosphonate nucleotide analog; reverse transcriptase inhibitor. Prepn: I. Rosenberg et al., Collect. Czech. Chem. Commun. **53**, 2753 (1988); A. Holy et al., ibid. **60**, 1390 (1995); L. M. Schultze et al., Tetrahedron Lett. **39**, 1853 (1998). Prepn of ester prodrug: M. N. Arimilli et al., Antiviral Chem. Chemother. **8**, 557 (1997); idem et al., WO 9804569; eidem, US 5922695 (1998, 1999 both to Gilead Sci.). Antiretroviral activity in vitro: J. Balzarini et al., Biochem. Biophys. Res. Commun. **219**, 337 (1996). Metabolism and pharmacokinetics of prodrugs: J.-P. Shaw et al., Pharm. Res. **14**, 1824 (1997). Clinical trial in HIV-infected patients: J. E. Gallant et al., J. Am. Med. Assoc. **292**, 191 (2004).

Crystals from boiling water + ethanol, mp 279°. $[\alpha]_D$ +21° (c = 1 in 0.1M HCl).

Bis(isopropyloxycarbonyloxymethyl) ester. [201341-05-1] 5-[[(1R)-2-(6-Amino-9H-purin-9-yl)-1-methylethoxy]methyl]-2,4,6,-8-tetraoxa-5-phosphanononanedioic acid bis(1-methylethyl) ester 5-oxide; tenofovir disoproxil; (R)-bis(POC)PMPA. $C_{19}H_{30}N_5O_{10}P$; mol wt 519.44. Log P (1-octanol/aqueous phosphate buffer, pH 6.5): 1.3.

Disoproxil fumarate. [202138-50-9] Tenofovir DF; GS-4331-05; Viread. $C_{19}H_{30}N_5O_{10}P \cdot C_4H_4O_4$; mol wt 635.51. White, fine, powder-like crystals.

THERAP CAT: Antiviral.

9147. Tenonitrozole. [3810-35-3] N-(5-Nitro-2-thiazolyl)-2-thiophenecarboxamide; 2-(α-thenoylamino)-5-nitrothiazole; thenitrazole; TC-109; Atrican; Moniflagon. $C_8H_5N_3O_3S_2$; mol wt 255.27. C 37.64%, H 1.97%, N 16.46%, O 18.80%, S 25.12%. Prepd from 2-thenoyl chloride and 2-amino-5-nitrothiazole: FR M715 (1961 to Chantereau), C.A. **59**, 7533g (1963).

Crystals from dioxane or DMF, mp 255-256°.

THERAP CAT: Antiprotozoal (Trichomonas); antifungal.

9148. Tenoxicam. [59804-37-4] 4-Hydroxy-2-methyl-N-2-pyridinyl-2H-thieno[2,3-e]-1,2-thiazine-3-carboxamide 1,1-dioxide; Ro-12-0068; Alganex; Dolmen; Liman; Mobiflex; Rexalgan; Tilatil; Tilcotil. $C_{13}H_{11}N_3O_4S_2$; mol wt 337.37. C 46.28%, H 3.29%, N 12.46%, O 18.97%, S 19.01%. Nonsteroidal anti-inflammatory agent. Prepn: O. Hromatka et al., DE 2537070 (1976 to Hoffmann-La Roche), C.A. **85**, 63077 (1976). Pharmacology: Y. Tanaka et al., Nippon Yakurigaku Zasshi **77**, 531 (1981), C.A. **95**, 35473 (1981). HPLC determn in plasma: M. E. Pickup et al., J. Chromatogr. **225**, 493 (1981). Comparative study vs aspirin in normal volunteers: H. A. Bird et al., Curr. Med. Res. Opin. **8**, 9 (1982). Preliminary review of pharmacology, therapeutic efficacy and mechanism of action: J. P. Gonzalez, P. A. Todd, Drugs **34**, 289-310 (1987). Comprehensive description: A. M. Al-Obaid, M. S. Mian, Anal. Profiles Drug Subs. Excip. **22**, 431-459 (1993).

Crystals from xylene, mp 209-213° (dec). Soly (mg/ml): water 0.045; ethanol <1; methanol <1; acetone 2; dichloromethane 10; chloroform 8; DMSO 63. uv max (ethanol): 205, 265, 360 nm (ε 16422.12, 10127.42, 12544.21). pKa₁ 5.3, pKa₂ 1.1. Partition coefficient (octanol/water): 0.3 (pH 7.4); 3.5 (pH 1.2).

THERAP CAT: Anti-inflammatory; analgesic.

9149. Tenuazonic Acid. [610-88-8] (5S)-3-Acetyl-1,5-dihydro-4-hydroxy-5-[(1S)-1-methylpropyl]-2H-pyrrol-2-one; L-3-acetyl-5-sec-butyl-4-hydroxy-3-pyrrolin-2-one; L-3-acetyl-5-sec-butyltetramic acid. $C_{10}H_{15}NO_3$; mol wt 197.23. C 60.90%, H 7.67%, N 7.10%, O 24.34%. Mycotoxin produced by Alternaria alternata and other fungal species; contaminant found in wheat and other grains, sunflower seeds, tomatoes and other fruits. Isoln from culture filtrates of Alternaria tenuis Auct.: T. Rosett et al., Biochem. J. **67**, 390 (1957). Structure: C. E. Stickings, Biochem. J. **72**, 332 (1959). Biosynthesis: C. E. Stickings, R. J. Townsend, ibid. **78**, 412 (1961). Chemical synthesis: R. N. Lacey, J. Chem. Soc. **1954**, 850; S. A. Harris et al., J. Med. Chem. **8**, 478 (1965); R. Schobert et al., Org. Biomol. Chem. **2**, 3524 (2004). Tumor inhibitory properties: E. A. Kaczka et al., Biochem. Biophys. Res. Commun. **14**, 54 (1964); C. O. Gitterman et al., Cancer Res. **24**, 440 (1964). Toxicity of isolates from agricultural samples: R. A. Meronuck et al., Appl. Microbiol. **23**, 613 (1972). Review of analytical methods and occurrence in foods: P. M. Scott, J. AOAC Int. **84**, 1809-1817 (2001).

Pale brown, viscous, gummy substance, $[\alpha]_D^{20}$ $-128°$ (c = 1.0 in methanol); $-132 \pm 2°$ (c = 0.5 in CHCl₃). bp₀.₀₃₅ 117°. Readily sol in organic solvents incl petr ether; sparingly sol in water. On long standing, changes into the crystalline iso-form.

Sodium salt. [1013-59-8] Sodium L-tenuazonate. $C_{10}H_{14}$-NNaO₃. $[\alpha]_{546}$ $-96.7°$ (c = 2.0 in methanol). uv max (pH 7): 280, 241 nm ($E_{1 cm}^{1\%}$ 573, 400).

9150. Tephrosin. [76-80-2] (7aR-cis)-13,13a-Dihydro-7a-hydroxy-9,10-dimethoxy-3,3-dimethyl-3H-bis[1]benzopyrano[3,4-b:6',5'-e]pyran-7(7aH)-one; hydroxydeguelin; toxicarol. $C_{23}H_{22}$-O₇; mol wt 410.42. C 67.31%, H 5.40%, O 27.29%. Occurs in leaves of Tephrosia vogelii Hook. f., Leguminosae, in derris root, cubé root: Hanriot, Compt. Rend. **144**, 150 (1907); Clark, J. Am. Chem. Soc. **53**, 729 (1931). Structure: Butenandt, Hilgetag, Ann. **495**, 172 (1932).

Prisms. mp 198° (218-220°). Practically insol in water. Sol in chloroform, ether, acetone; sparingly sol in methanol.

9151. Tepoxalin. [103475-41-8] 5-(4-Chlorophenyl)-N-hydroxy-1-(4-methoxyphenyl)-N-methyl-1H-pyrazole-3-propanamide; 3-[5-(4-chlorophenyl)-1-(4-methoxyphenyl)-3-pyrazolyl]-*N*-hydroxy-*N*-methylpropanamide; ORF-20485; RWJ-20485; Zubrin. $C_{20}H_{20}ClN_3O_3$; mol wt 385.84. C 62.26%, H 5.22%, Cl 9.19%, N 10.89%, O 12.44%. Dual inhibitor of cyclooxygenase and 5-lipoxygenase. Prepn: M. P. Wachter, M. P. Ferro, **EP 248594**; *eidem*, **US 4826868** (1987, 1989, both to Ortho); W. V. Murray, S. K. Hadden, *J. Org. Chem.* **57**, 6662 (1992). LC/MS characterization of impurities and degradation products: D. J. Burinsky *et al., J. Pharm. Sci.* **85**, 159 (1996). Mechanism of action: S. S. C. Tam *et al., J. Biol. Chem.* **270**, 13948 (1995). Toxicity study in rats, dogs: E. V. Knight *et al., Fundam. Appl. Toxicol.* **33**, 38 (1996). Pharmacological profile in animal models: D. C. Argentieri *et al., J. Pharmacol. Exp. Ther.* **271**, 1399 (1994); in man: M. Depré *et al., Int. J. Clin. Pharmacol. Res.* **16**, 1 (1996). Bioavailability in dogs: L. M. Homer *et al., J. Vet. Pharmacol. Ther.* **28**, 287 (2005).

Crystals from ethyl acetate + hexane, mp 124-126°.
THERAP CAT (VET): Anti-inflammatory.

9152. Tepraloxydim. [149979-41-9] 2-[1-[[[(2*E*)-3-Chloro-2-propenyl]oxy]imino]propyl]-3-hydroxy-5-(tetrahydro-2*H*-pyran-4-yl)-2-cyclohexen-1-one; 2-[1-[(2*E*)-3-chloroallyloxyimino]-propyl]-3-hydroxy-5-perhydropyran-4-ylcyclohex-2-en-1-one; caloxydim; BAS-620H; Aramo; Equinox. $C_{17}H_{24}ClNO_4$; mol wt 341.83. C 59.73%, H 7.08%, Cl 10.37%, N 4.10%, O 18.72%. Graminicide for use in broad-leaf crops. Inhibits acetyl CoA carboxylase which catalyzes the first step in fatty acid formation. General prepn: R. Becker *et al., EP 071707; eidem US 4422864* (both 1983 to BASF). Comprehensive description: E. Kibler *et al., Brighton Crop Prot. Conf. - Weeds* **1999**, 59-64. Efficacy vs blackgrass: R. E. Ruske, S. R. Moss, *ibid.* 191. HPLC-UV determn in drinking water: P. Sandin-España *et al., Chromatographia* **55**, 681 (2002). Mechanism of action study: A. Takahashi *et al., Weed Biol. Manage.* **2**, 84 (2002).

Beige solid, slight characteristic odor. mp 71.5°. Vapor pressure (20°): 1.1×10^{-5} Pa. Soly in water: 0.14 mg/l. LD_{50} in rats (mg/kg): > 2200 orally; >2000 dermally; LC_{50} in rats (mg/l): 5.1 by inhalation. LC_{50} (96 hr) in trout: > 100 mg/l (Kibler).
USE: Herbicide.

9153. Teprenone. [6809-52-5] 6,10,14,18-Tetramethyl-5,-9,13,17-nonadecatetraen-2-one; geranylgeranylacetone; GGA; E-0671; E36U31; Selbex. $C_{23}H_{38}O$; mol wt 330.55. C 83.57%, H 11.59%, O 4.84%. Acyclic polyisoprenoid 2:3 mixture of (5*Z*,9*E*,-13*E*) and all *trans* (5*E*,9*E*,13*E*) isomers. Prepn from geranylgeranyl bromide: L. Ruzicka, L. Castro, *Helv. Chim. Acta* **28**, 590 (1945); from substituted acetylenes: K. Sato *et al., J. Org. Chem.* **35**, 565 (1970). Anti-ulcer and toxicity studies: M. Murakami *et al., Arzneim.-Forsch.* **31**, 799 (1981). *In vivo* effects on aspirin induced gastric ulcer: *eidem, Jpn. J. Pharmacol.* **32**, 299 (1982); on stress induced gastric ulcer: *eidem, ibid.* **33**, 549 (1983). Mechanism of action studies: Y. Nishizawa *et al., Biochem. Biophys. Res. Commun.* **103**, 706 (1981); K. Oketani *et al., Jpn. J. Pharmacol.* **33**, 593 (1983). Metabolism in rats: Y. Nishizawa *et al., Xenobiotica* **17**, 575 (1987). Determn in serum by GC-MS: M. Tanaka *et al., J.*

Chromatogr. **231**, 301 (1982); by HPLC: T. Seki *et al., ibid.* **424**, 410 (1988).

all *trans*-form

Yellow oil, $bp_{0.01}$ 155-160°. $d_4^{20.5}$ 0.9081. n_D^{20} 1.4947.
THERAP CAT: Antiulcerative.

9154. Terazosin. [63590-64-7] 1-(4-Amino-6,7-dimethoxy-2-quinazolinyl)-4-[(tetrahydro-2-furanyl)carbonyl]piperazine; 2-[(4-tetrahydro-2-furoyl)-1-piperazinyl]-4-amino-6,7-dimethoxyquinazoline. $C_{19}H_{25}N_5O_4$; mol wt 387.43. C 58.90%, H 6.50%, N 18.08%, O 16.52%. α_1-Adrenergic blocker related to prazosin, *q.v.* Prepn: M. Winn *et al., DE 2646186; eidem, US 4026894* (both 1977 to Abbott); of the hydrochloride dihydrate: R. Roteman, **DE 2831112**; *idem, US 4251532* (1979, 1981 both to Abbott). HPLC determn in biological fluids: S. E. Patterson, *J. Chromatogr.* **311**, 206 (1984). Toxicity in rats: F. L. Fort *et al., Drug Chem. Toxicol.* **7**, 435 (1984). Clinical study in essential hypertension: P. A. Abraham *et al., Pharmacotherapy* **5**, 285 (1985); in treatment of benign prostatic hyperplasia: H. Lepor *et al., J. Urol.* **148**, 1467 (1992). Symposium on pharmacology, pharmacokinetics, and clinical efficacy in hypertension: *Am. J. Med.* **80**, Suppl. 5B, 1-105 (1986). Comprehensive description: Z. L. Chang, J. F. Bauer, *Anal. Profiles Drug Subs.* **20**, 693-727 (1991). Review of pharmacology and therapeutic efficacy: R. Achari, A. Laddu, *J. Clin. Pharmacol.* **32**, 520-523 (1992).

Fine, white, odorless crystals, mp 272.6-274°. Soly at 25°C (mg/ml): methanol 33.7; water 29.7; 95% ethanol 4.1; 0.1*N* HCl 3.8; chloroform 1.2; acetone 0.01. Practically insol in hexane. uv max (0.005% in water): 212, 245, 330 nm (a 65.7, 127.5, 24.0). pKa (0.1*N* NaOH): 7.1.
Hydrochloride. $C_{19}H_{25}N_5O_4$·HCl. Hygroscopic crystals from isopropyl alc, mp 278-279°. Soly in water: 761.2 mg/ml. LD_{50} in mice (mg/kg): 259.3 i.v. (Winn).
Hydrochloride dihydrate. [70024-40-7] Abbott 45975; Heitrin; Hytrin; Hytrinex; Itrin; Urodie; Vasocard; Vasomet; Vicard. $C_{19}H_{25}N_5O_4$·HCl.$2H_2O$; mol wt 459.92. mp 271-274°. Soly in water: 24.2 mg/ml. LD_{50} in male, female rats (mg/kg): 277, 293 i.v. (Fort).
THERAP CAT: Antihypertensive. In treatment of benign prostatic hyperplasia.

9155. Terbacil. [5902-51-2] 5-Chloro-3-(1,1-dimethylethyl)-6-methyl-2,4(1*H*,3*H*)-pyrimidinedione; 3-*tert*-butyl-5-chloro-6-methyluracil; Du Pont Herbicide 732; Sinbar. $C_9H_{13}ClN_2O_2$; mol wt 216.66. C 49.89%, H 6.05%, Cl 16.36%, N 12.93%, O 14.77%. Prepn: Loux, **US 3235357** (1966 to du Pont). Herbicidal activity and physical properties: G. D. Hill, Jr. *et al., 2nd Symp. New Herbic.* **1965**, 313, *C.A.* **66**, 18234b (1967). Metabolism and mode of action: Herholdt, *Diss. Abstr. Int. B* **30**, 1978 (1969).

Crystals, mp 175-177°. Soly in water at 25°: 710 ppm. Sol in DMF, dimethylacetamide, cyclohexanone; moderately sol in methyl

isobutyl ketone, butyl acetate, xylene. Approx. LD orally in rats: >5000 mg/kg (Hill).
USE: Herbicide.

9156. Terbinafine. [91161-71-6] *N*-[(2*E*)-6,6-Dimethyl-2-hepten-4-ynyl]-*N*-methyl-1-naphthalenemethanamine; *trans-N*-methyl-*N*-(1-naphthylmethyl)-6,6-dimethylhept-2-en-4-ynyl-1-amine. $C_{21}H_{25}N$; mol wt 291.43. C 86.55%, H 8.65%, N 4.81%. Orally active, antimycotic allylamine related to naftifine, *q.v.* Specific inhibitor of squalene epoxidase, a key enzyme in fungal ergosterol biosynthesis. Prepn: A. Stütz, **EP 24587**; *idem*, **US 4755534** (1981, 1988 both to Sandoz); A. Stütz, G. Petranyi, *J. Med. Chem.* **27**, 1539 (1984). Mode of action: G. Petranyi *et al.*, *Science* **224**, 1239 (1984); N. S. Ryder, *Antimicrob. Agents Chemother.* **27**, 252 (1985). *In vitro* antifungal activity: S. Shadomy *et al.*, *Sabouraudia* **23**, 125 (1985). Toxicity data: U. Ganzinger *et al.*, *Proc. 13th Int. Congr. Chemother.* **6**, 116/52 (1983). Symposium on pharmacology and clinical trials: *J. Am. Acad. Dermatol.* **23**, Suppl., 775-812 (1990). Clinical trial as systemic treatment of toenail onychomycosis: E. G. V. Evans *et al.*, *Br. Med. J.* **318**, 1031 (1999).

Hydrochloride. [78628-80-5] SF-86-327; Lamisil. $C_{21}H_{25}$-N.HCl; mol wt 327.89. Crystals from 2-propanol + diethyl ether, mp 195-198° (change in crystal structure begins ~150°). Freely sol in methanol, methylene chloride; sol in ethanol; slightly sol in water. LD_{50} in mice, rats (mg/kg): 4000, 4000 orally; 393, 213 i.v. (Ganzinger).
THERAP CAT: Antifungal.

9157. Terbium. [7440-27-9] Tb; at. wt 158.92535; at. no. 65; valences 3, 4. A lanthanide; belongs to the yttrium group of rare earth metals. Naturally occurring isotope (mass number): 159; known artificial radioactive isotopes: 144-158; 160-164. Abundance in earth's crust: 0.91-1.2 ppm; occurs in small quantities in monazite, cerite, gadolinite and other rare earth minerals. Discovered by Mosander, *Skand. Naturför. Förh.* **3**, 387 (1842); *Philos. Mag.* [3] **23**, 241 (1843). Sepn by fractional crystn and precipitation: Urbain, *Compt. Rend.* **139**, 736 (1904); **141**, 521 (1905); James, Bissel, *J. Am. Chem. Soc.* **36**, 2060 (1914); by ion exchange: Spedding *et al.*, *ibid.* **76**, 2557 (1954). Prepn of metal by electrodeposition: *idem*, *J. Electrochem. Soc.* **100**, 442 (1953). Absorption spectrum: Urbain, *loc. cit.* Toxicity study: Haley, *J. Pharm. Sci.* **54**, 663 (1965). Reviews of prepn, properties and compds: *The Rare Earths*, F. H. Spedding, A. H. Daane, Eds. (Krieger, Huntington, N.Y., 1971, reprint of 1961 ed.) 641 pp; Hulet, Bode, "Separation Chemistry of the Lanthanides and Transplutonium Actinides" in *MTP Int. Rev. Sci.: Inorg. Chem., Ser. One* vol. 7, K. W. Bagnall, Ed. (University Park Press, Baltimore, 1972) pp 1-45; Moeller, "The Lanthanides" in *Comprehensive Inorganic Chemistry* vol. 4, J. C. Bailar, Jr. *et al.*, Eds. (Pergamon Press, Oxford, 1973) pp 1-101; F. H. Spedding in *Kirk-Othmer Encyclopedia of Chemical Technology* vol. **19** (John Wiley & Sons, New York, 3rd ed., 1982) pp 833-854; *Chemistry of the Elements*, N. N. Greenwood, A. Earnshaw, Eds. (Pergamon Press, New York, 1984) pp 1423-1449. Brief review of properties: G. T. Seaborg, *Radiochim. Acta* **61**, 115-122 (1993).

Silver-gray metal, easily oxidized in air. Hexagonal close-packed crystals at room temp; d 8.27 (Spedding, Daane, *loc. cit.* p. 183). mp 1356°. bp 3230°; also reported as bp 2480° (Moeller).

Oxide. Terbia. O_3Tb_2. A white solid.

Oxide. Non-stoichiometric, approx composition, Tb_4O_7, for this formula Tb^{3+} and Tb^{4+} present in equal amounts. Dark brown or black solid; obtained by igniting the oxalate or the sulfate. Dissolves in hot concd acids with formation of salts; loses oxygen on heating; forms the oxide when heated in hydrogen.

Nitrate. $Tb(NO_3)_3$. Occurs as the hexahydrate, monoclinic crystals, mp 89.3°. *See* Urbain, cited by Mellor, *A Comprehensive Treatise on Inorganic and Theoretical Chemistry* **5**, 695 (1929). LD_{50} in rats (mg/kg): 260 i.p.; >5000 orally (Haley).

Chloride hexahydrate. $TbCl_3.6H_2O$. Prismatic deliquesc crystals. Very sol in water; forms supersaturated solns. Dehydrated on heating in hydrogen chloride at 180-200°. The anhydr chloride, crystals, d^0 4.35; mp 588°; dissolves in water without hydrolysis. LD_{50} in mice (mg/kg): 550 i.p.; 5100 orally (Haley).

9158. Terbufos. [13071-79-9] Phosphorodithioic acid *S*-[[(1,1-dimethylethyl)thio]methyl] *O,O*-diethyl ester; phosphorodithioic acid *S*-[(*tert*-butylthio)methyl] *O,O*-diethyl ester; AC-92100; Counter. $C_9H_{21}O_2PS_3$; mol wt 288.43. C 37.48%, H 7.34%, O 11.09%, P 10.74%, S 33.35%. Organophosphate insecticide. Prepn: Ikeda *et al.*; Takahashi *et al.*, **JP 66 16799**; **JP 67 1743**; **JP 67 4455** (all to Hokko), *C.A.* **66**, 18510p, 85467p, **67**, 11205e (all 1967). As insecticidal soil treatment: F. M. Gordon, **DE 2258528** (1973 to Am. Cyanamid), *C.A.* **79**, 62601m (1973). Toxicity to birds: E. F. Hill, M. B. Camardese, *Ecotoxicol. Environ. Saf.* **8**, 551 (1984).

Technical product (85 to 88% purity): clear, colorless to pale yellow liq, d^{24} 1.105. $bp_{0.01}$ 69°. mp −29.2°. Flash pt 88°C (tag open cup). Sol in acetone, alcs, aromatic and chlorinated hydrocarbons. Soly in water: 10-15 ppm. LD_{50} orally in quail: 15 mg/kg (Hill, Camardese).
Caution: Cholinesterase inhibitor.
USE: Soil insecticide.

9159. Terbutaline. [23031-25-6] 5-[2-[(1,1-Dimethylethyl)amino]-1-hydroxyethyl]-1,3-benzenediol; α-[(*tert*-butylamino)methyl]-3,5-dihydroxybenzyl alcohol; 1-(3,5-dihydroxyphenyl)-2-(*tert*-butylamino)ethanol. $C_{12}H_{19}NO_3$; mol wt 225.28. C 63.98%, H 8.50%, N 6.22%, O 21.31%. β-Adrenergic agonist. Prepn: K. Wetterlin, L. A. Svensson, **BE 704932**; *idem*, **US 3937838** (1968, 1976 both to Draco). Pharmacology: Bergman *et al.*, *Experientia* **25**, 899 (1969). Resolution of isomers and activity studies: K. Wetterlin, *J. Med. Chem.* **15**, 1182 (1972). Clinical study in treatment of preterm labor: S. N. Caritis *et al.*, *Am. J. Obstet. Gynecol.* **150**, 7 (1984). *Review:* J. J. McPhillips in *Pharmacological and Biochemical Properties of Drug Substances* vol. 1, M. E. Goldberg, Ed. (Am. Pharm. Assoc., Washington, DC, 1977) pp 311-328. Review of clinical toxicology: J. D. Truwit, *Crit. Care Clin.* **7**, 639-657 (1991). Comprehensive description: S. Ahuja, J. Ashman, *Anal. Profiles Drug Subs.* **19**, 601-625 (1990).

Crystals from abs ether, mp 119-122°.
Sulfate. [23031-32-5] Brethaire; Brethine; Bricanyl; Butaliret; Monovent; Terbasmin; Terbul. $(C_{12}H_{19}NO_3)_2.H_2SO_4$; mol wt 548.65. mp 246-248°. uv max (0.1*N* HCl): 276 nm ($A_{1cm}^{1\%}$ 67.6). pKa_1 8.8, pKa_2 10.1, pKa_3 11.2. Soly at 25° (mg/ml): water >20; 0.1*N* HCl >20; 0.1*N* NaOH >20; ethanol 1.2; 10% ethanol >20; methanol 2.7.
THERAP CAT: Bronchodilator; tocolytic.

9160. Terconazole. [67915-31-5] *rel*-1-[4-[[(2*R*,4*S*)-2-(2,4-Dichlorophenyl)-2-(1*H*-1,2,4-triazol-1-ylmethyl)-1,3-dioxolan-4-yl]methoxy]phenyl]-4-(1-methylethyl)piperazine; triaconazole; R-42470; Fungistat; Gyno-Terazol; Terazol; Tercospor. $C_{26}H_{31}Cl_2$-N_5O_3; mol wt 532.46. C 58.65%, H 5.87%, Cl 13.32%, N 13.15%, O 9.01%. Topical triazole antifungal. Prepn: J. Heeres *et al.*, **DE 2804096**; *idem*, **US 4144346**; **US 4223036** (1978, 1979, 1980 all to Janssen); *idem*, *J. Med. Chem.* **26**, 611 (1983). Pharmacology: J. Van Cutsem *et al.*, *Chemotherapy* **29**, 322 (1983). Clinical comparison with clotrimazole in vaginal candidiasis: A. Kjaeldgaard, *Pharmacotherapeutica* **4**, 525 (1986).

Crystals from isopropyl ether, mp 126.3°.

THERAP CAT: Antifungal.

9161. Terebic Acid. [79-91-4] Tetrahydro-2,2-dimethyl-5-oxo-3-furancarboxylic acid; tetrahydro-2,2-dimethyl-5-oxo-3-furoic acid; terebinic acid; (1-hydroxy-1-methylethyl)succinic acid γ-lactone. $C_7H_{10}O_4$; mol wt 158.15. C 53.16%, H 6.37%, O 40.47%. Prepared from fumaric or maleic acid: Schenck, Steinmetz, *Tetrahedron Letters* no. 21, 1 (1960); Lipp *et al., Ann.* **644,** 37 (1961). Prepn of optical isomers: Fredga, *C.A.* **42,** 123g (1948); Delépine, Badoche, *Compt. Rend.* **235,** 1069 (1952).

Crystals, mp 174-175°, but begins to volatilize at 100°. d 0.815. Slightly sol in cold water, freely in boiling water or warm alcohol.

(+)-Form. $[\alpha]_D^{25}$ +13.2° (c = 0.03 in acetone).

(−)-Form. mp 201-205° (dec). $[\alpha]_D^{25}$ −13.2° (c = 0.03 in acetone).

9162. Terephthalic Acid. [100-21-0] 1,4-Benzenedicarboxylic acid; *p*-phthalic acid; Tephthol. $C_8H_6O_4$; mol wt 166.13. C 57.84%, H 3.64%, O 38.52%. Prepd by oxidation of *p*-methylacetophenone: Koelsch, *Org. Synth.* **coll. vol. III,** 791 (1955). Manuf processes: US 3014961 (1959 to VEB Chemie Werke Buna); Sherwood, *Chem. Ind. (London)* **1960,** 1096. *Review: Faith, Keyes & Clark's Industrial Chemicals*, F. A. Lowenheim, M. K. Moran, Eds. (Wiley-Interscience, New York, 4th ed., 1975) pp 807-813; A. G. Bemis *et al.,* "Phthalic Acids" in *Kirk-Othmer Encyclopedia of Chemical Technology* **vol. 17** (Wiley-Interscience, New York, 3rd ed., 1982) pp 732-777.

Crystals. Sublimes at 402°. Practically insol in water, chloroform, ether, acetic acid; slightly sol in cold alcohol, more in hot alcohol; sol in alkalies.

Dimethyl ester. Dimethyl terephthalate; DMT. $C_{10}H_{10}O_4$. White crystals, mp 140.6°. bp 288°.

Caution: Mild irritant.

USE: Forms polyesters with glycols which are made into plastic films and sheets; in analytical chemistry.

9163. Terfenadine. [50679-08-8] α-[4-(1,1-Dimethylethyl)phenyl]-4-(hydroxydiphenylmethyl)-1-piperidinebutanol; 1-(*p*-*tert*-butylphenyl)-4-[4′-(α-hydroxydiphenylmethyl)-1′-piperidyl]-butanol; α-(*p*-*tert*-butylphenyl)-4-(α-hydroxy-α-phenylbenzyl)-1-piperidinebutanol; MDL-9918; Allerplus; Cyater; Seldane; Teldane; Teldanex; Terfex; Ternadin; Triludan. $C_{32}H_{41}NO_2$; mol wt 471.67. C 81.49%, H 8.76%, N 2.97%, O 6.78%. Nonsedating-type histamine H_1-receptor antagonist. Prepn: A. A. Carr, C. R. Kinsolving, DE 2303306; *eidem,* US 3878217 (1973, 1975 both to Richardson-Merrell); A. A. Carr, D. R. Meyer, *Arzneim.-Forsch.* **32,** 1157 (1982). Series of articles on chemistry, pharmacology, toxicology and clinical studies: *ibid.* **32,** 1153-1218 (1982). Metabolism in human liver: M. Jurima-Romet *et al., Drug Metab. Dispos.* **22,** 849

(1994). Comprehensive description: A. A. Badwan *et al., Anal. Profiles Drug Subs.* **19,** 627-662 (1990). *Review:* H. C. Masheter, *Clin. Rev. Allergy* **11,** 5-34 (1993).

Crystals from acetone, mp 146.5-148.5°; may exist in three polymorphic forms, mp 149-152°, 146-148°, 142-144°. Soly at 30° (g/100ml): water 0.001; ethanol 3.780; methanol 3.750; hexane 0.034; 0.1*M* HCl 0.012; 0.1*M* citric acid 0.110; 0.1*M* tartaric acid 0.045. uv max (methanol): 260 nm (A 660.4); (ethanol): 260 nm (A 671.4); (dichloromethane): 260 nm (A 762.2). LD_{50} orally in mice: >2000 mg/kg (Carr, Meyer).

THERAP CAT: Antihistaminic.

9164. Terguride. [37686-84-3] *N,N*-Diethyl-*N′*-[(8α)-6-methylergolin-8-yl]urea; *N*-(D-6-methyl-8-isoergolin-1-yl)-*N′,N′*-diethylurea; 6-methyl-8α-(diethylcarbamoylamino)ergoline; 9,10α-dihydrolisuride; 9,10-transdihydrolisuride; TDHL. $C_{20}H_{28}N_4O$; mol wt 340.46. C 70.56%, H 8.29%, N 16.46%, O 4.70%. Ergot derivative; dihydrogenated analog of lisuride, *q.v.* Exhibits dopamine agonist and antagonist activity. Prepn: V. Zikán *et al., Collect. Czech. Chem. Commun.* **37,** 2600 (1972); *eidem,* DE 2238540; *eidem,* US 3953454 (1973, 1976 both to Spofa). Physical properties: A. Cerny *et al., Collect. Czech. Chem. Commun.* **52,** 1331 (1987). Pharmacology in animals and humans: H. Wachtel, R. Dorow, *Life Sci.* **32,** 421 (1983). Receptor binding studies in rat brain: W. Kehr *et al., Acta Pharm. Suec.* **1983,** Suppl. 2, 98; M. W. Valchár *et al., Eur. J. Pharmacol.* **136,** 97 (1987). Evaluation in animal models of Parkinson's disease: W. C. Koller, G. Herbster, *Neurology* **37,** 723 (1987); T. Brücke *et al., Eur. J. Pharmacol.* **148,** 445 (1988). Radioreceptor assay in biological fluids: R. Lapka *et al., J. Pharmacol. Methods* **11,** 263 (1984). Pharmacokinetics in humans: W. Krause *et al., Eur. J. Clin. Pharmacol.* **27,** 335 (1984). Clinical evaluation in Huntington's disease: S. Bassi *et al., Neurology* **36,** 984 (1986); in Parkinson's disease: T. Brücke *et al., Adv. Neurol.* **45,** 573 (1986); I. Suchy *et al., ibid.* 577; in hyperprolactinemia and acromegaly: D. Dallabonzana *et al., J. Clin. Endocrinol. Metab.* **63,** 1002 (1986).

Crystals from ethanol, mp 203-204° (dec). $[\alpha]_D^{20}$ +30° (c = 1 in pyridine). Also reported as crystals from ethanol, mp 205-207° (dec) (Cerny). $[\alpha]_D^{20}$ +29.0° (c = 0.2 in pyridine). uv max: 292, 281, 224 nm (log ε 3.72, 3.81, 4.42). Practically insol in water.

Hydrogen maleate. [37686-85-4] SH-406; VUFB-6638; ZK-31224; Dironyl; Mysalfon. $C_{20}H_{28}N_4O·C_4H_4O_4$; mol wt 456.53. Crystals from ethanol, mp 190-191°.

Hydrogen maleate hydrate. Crystals from ethanol, mp 150-153°. $[\alpha]_D^{20}$ −15.0° (c = 0.1 in H_2O). Soly in water: 1.26 mg/ml.

THERAP CAT: Antiparkinsonian; antihyperprolactinemic.

9165. Teriflunomide. [163451-81-8]; [108605-62-5] (unspecified stereo). (2*Z*)-2-Cyano-3-hydroxy-*N*-[4-(trifluoromethyl)phenyl]-2-butenamide; A-771726. $C_{12}H_9F_3N_2O_2$; mol wt 270.21. C

53.34%, H 3.36%, F 21.09%, N 10.37%, O 11.84%. Disease modifying antirheumatic drug (DMARD); active metabolite of leflunomide, *q.v.* Prepn: R. R. Bartlett, F.-J. Kämmerer, **WO 9117748**; *eidem*, **US 5494911** (1991, 1996 both to Hoechst). Identification as active metabolite: J. W. Patterson *et al.*, *J. Med. Chem.* **35**, 507 (1992). Phamacokinetics: J. Lucien *et al.*, *Ther. Drug Monit.* **17**, 454 (1995). Inhibits dihydroorotate dehydrogenase: J. P. Davis *et al.*, *Biochemistry* **35**, 1270 (1996). Configurational study: G. Bertolini *et al.*, *J. Med. Chem.* **40**, 2011 (1997); and crystal structure: C. Papageorgiou *et al.*, *Bioorg. Chem.* **25**, 233 (1997). HPLC determn in plasma: V. Chan *et al.*, *J. Chromatogr. B* **803**, 331 (2004).

THERAP CAT: Immunomodulator; in treatment of multiple sclerosis.

9166. Teriparatide Acetate. [99294-94-7] hPTH 1-34 acetate; MN-10T; Parathar; Forteo. $C_{181}H_{292}N_{55}O_{51}S_2 \cdot yC_2H_4O_2 \cdot xH_2O$. Synthetic, biologically active polypeptide consisting of the 1-34 amino-terminal fragment of human parathyroid hormone (hPTH), *q.v.* Amino acid sequence: H. B. Brewer *et al.*, *Proc. Natl. Acad. Sci. USA* **69**, 3585 (1972). Prepn: R. H. Andreatta *et al.*, *Helv. Chim. Acta* **56**, 470 (1973). Revised structure: H. D. Niall *et al.*, *Proc. Natl. Acad. Sci. USA* **71**, 384 (1974). Prepn: R. L. Colescott, **DE 2649727**; *idem*, **DE 2649848**; G. W. Tregear, **US 4086196** (1977, 1977, 1978 all to Armour Pharm.). Solid phase synthesis and biological activity: G. W. Tregear *et al.*, *Z. Physiol. Chem.* **355**, 415 (1974). Solution synthesis and biological activity: M. Takai *et al.*, *Pept. Chem.* **17**, 187 (1980). Clinical pharmacology: R. M. Neer *et al.*, *J. Clin. Endocrinol. Metab.* **38**, 420 (1977). RIA determn in plasma: J. M. Zanelli *et al.*, *J. Immunoassay* **1**, 289 (1980). Clinical pharmacokinetics: G. N. Kent *et al.*, *Clin. Sci.* **68**, 171 (1985). Clinical evaluation in osteoporosis: J. Reeve *et al.*, *Br. Med. J.* **280**, 1340 (1980); D. M. Slovik *et al.*, *J. Clin. Invest.* **68**, 1261 (1981). Diagnostic use: T. Igarashi *et al.*, *Pharmatherapeutica* **3**, 79 (1982); L. E. Mallette *et al.*, *J. Clin. Endocrinol. Metab.* **67**, 964 (1988). Review of diagnostic use in modified Ellsworth-Howard test: L. E. Mallette, *Ann. Intern. Med.* **109**, 800-804 (1988); of pharmacology and clinical efficacy: H. Dobnig, *Expert Opin. Pharmacother.* **5**, 1153-1162 (2004).

THERAP CAT: Treatment of osteoporosis. Diagnostic aid (hypocalcemia).

9167. Terlipressin. [14636-12-5] *N*-[*N*-(*N*-Glycylglycyl)-glycyl]-8-L-lysinevasopressin; N^α-glycylglycylglycylvasopressin; 1-triglycyl-8-lysinevasopressin; Glypressin. $C_{52}H_{74}N_{16}O_{15}S_2$; mol wt 1227.37. C 50.89%, H 6.08%, N 18.26%, O 19.55%, S 5.22%. Analog of lypressin, *q.v.* Prepn: E. Kasafirek *et al.*, *Collect. Czech. Chem. Commun.* **31**, 4581 (1966); Z. Procházka *et al.*, *ibid.* **43**, 1285 (1978). Pharmacological studies: J. Kynčl *et al.*, *Eur. J. Pharmacol.* **28**, 294 (1974); P. O. B. Sjöquist *et al.*, *Acta Pharmacol. Toxicol.* **40**, 369 (1977). Use in treatment of uterine bleeding: V. Pavlin *et al.*, *Br. J. Obstet. Gynaecol.* **85**, 801 (1978). Hemostatic effects in cirrhosis patients: C. V. Prowse *et al.*, *Eur. J. Clin. Invest.* **10**, 49 (1980). Conversion to lysine vasopressin in man: M. L. Forsling *et al.*, *J. Endocrinol.* **85**, 237 (1980). Uterine effects in first trimester of pregnancy: T. Laudanski, M. Aakerlund, *Contraception* **22**, 199 (1980). Single-dose effects on renal potassium excretion in humans: H. Nadvornikova, O. Schueck, *Int. J. Clin. Pharmacol. Ther. Toxicol.* **20**, 155 (1982).

Gly–Gly–Gly–Cys–Tyr–Phe–Gln–Asn–Cys–Pro–Lys–GlyNH₂

Diacetate pentahydrate. Glycylpressin. $C_{56}H_{82}N_{16}O_{19}S_2 \cdot 5H_2O$; mol wt 1437.55. $[\alpha]_D^{25}$ −82° (c = 0.2 in 1*M* acetic acid).

THERAP CAT: Vasopressor (treatment of uterine and esophogeal bleeding).

9168. Terofenamate. [29098-15-5] 2-[(2,6-Dichloro-3-methylphenyl)amino]benzoic acid ethoxymethyl ester; *N*-(2,6-di-

chloro-*m*-tolyl)anthranilic acid ethoxymethyl ester; etoclofene; Etofen. $C_{17}H_{17}Cl_2NO_3$; mol wt 354.23. C 57.64%, H 4.84%, Cl 20.02%, N 3.95%, O 13.55%. Anti-inflammatory deriv of anthranilic acid, *q.v.* Prepn: **GB 1199386**; E. Manghisi, **US 3642864** (1970, 1972 both to Lusofarmaco); A. Salembeni *et al.*, *Farmaco Ed. Sci.* **30**, 276 (1975). Biological properties: G. B. Fregnan *et al.*, *ibid.* **353**. Absorption, distribution, excretion: *eidem*, *Boll. Chim. Farm.* **114**, 85 (1975). Pharmacological and toxicity studies: T. Chieli *et al.*, *ibid.* **115**, 41 (1976).

Crystals from ethanol, mp 73-74°. LD₅₀ in mice, rats (mg/kg): 918, 307 orally; 300, 274 i.p. (Chieli).

THERAP CAT: Anti-inflammatory; analgesic.

9169. Terpin. [80-53-5] 4-Hydroxy-α,α,4-trimethylcyclohexanemethanol; *p*-menthane-1,8-diol; dipenteneglycol. $C_{10}H_{20}O_2$; mol wt 172.26. C 69.72%, H 11.70%, O 18.58%. Both *cis*- and *trans*-modifications are known. The *cis*-compd is obtained most readily in the hydrated form, *cis*-terpin hydrate. Prepn of *cis*-form from oil of turpentine: Hempel, *Ann.* **180**, 71 (1876); Wallach, *Ann.* **230**, 225 (1885); Schmitt, *Manuf. Chem.* **26**, 350 (1955). From *d*-limonene: Sword, *J. Chem. Soc.* **127**, 1632 (1925). Prepn of *trans*-form from 1,8-cineole, α-terpineol or *cis*-terpin hydrate: Matsuura *et al.*, *Bull. Chem. Soc. Jpn.* **31**, 990 (1958); Lombard, Ambroise, *Bull. Soc. Chim. Fr.* **1961**, 230. Structure of *cis*- and *trans*-forms: Baeyer, *Ber.* **26**, 2861 (1893); Wagner, *ibid.* **27**, 1636 (1894).

cis-form

cis-Form hydrate. [2451-01-6] Terpin hydrate; terpinol. Rhombic pyramids from water, mp 116-117°; sublimes at ~100° when heated slowly; slight characteristic odor and slightly bitter taste; efflorescent in dry air. Anhydr *cis*-form: mp 104-105°; bp 258°; rapidly re-forms hydrate on exposure to air. One gram dissolves in 34 ml boiling water, 13 ml alcohol, 3 ml boiling alcohol, 135 ml chloroform, 140 ml ether, ~1 ml boiling glacial acetic acid. At 20°, one gram dissolves in 13 ml methanol, 13 ml ethyl acetate, 250 ml water, 77 ml benzene, 290 ml carbon tetrachloride, 250 ml carbon disulfide. Practically insol in petr ether.

trans-Form. [565-50-4] Monoclinic prisms, mp 158-159°. One gram dissolves at 20° in 11 ml methanol, 20 ml ethyl acetate, 100 ml water, 250 ml benzene, 250 ml carbon tetrachloride, 500 ml carbon disulfide.

THERAP CAT: *cis*-Form hydrate as expectorant.

THERAP CAT (VET): Expectorant.

9170. Terpinene. $C_{10}H_{16}$; mol wt 136.23. C 88.16%, H 11.84%. Mixture of three isomeric hydrocarbons: α-terpinene and γ-terpinene which occur naturally and β-terpinene which has been prepd synthetically. Isoln of α-terpinene from cardamom and marjoram oils: Weber, *Ann.* **238**, 101 (1887); Beltz, *Ber.* **32**, 996 (1899). Isoln of α-terpinene from oils of *Mosla japonica, M. grosserrata* and *Cupressus macrocarpa:* Richter, Wolff, *Ber.* **60**, 477 (1927); Briggs, Sutherland, *J. Org. Chem.* **7**, 397 (1942). Prepn of β-terpinene from sabinene: Wallach, *Ann.* **357**, 64 (1907); **362**, 285 (1908). Structure: Wallach, *ibid.* **362**, 293 (1908). *Review:* J. L. Simonsen, *The Terpenes* **vol. I** (University Press, Cambridge, 2nd ed., 1947) pp 172-193.

α   β   γ

α-Terpinene. Oil, pleasant odor of lemons. bp 173.5-174.8°; bp$_{13.5}$ 65.4-66°, d$_4^{19.6}$ 0.8375. n$_D^{20}$ 1.4784. Practically insol in water. Miscible with alcohol, ether.

β-Terpinene. Oil, bp 173-174°. d^{22} 0.838. n$_D^{22}$ 1.4754.

γ-Terpinene. Oil, bp 183°. d$_4^{15}$ 0.853. n$_D^{15.6}$ 1.4754.

Dihydrochloride. C$_{10}$H$_{18}$Cl$_2$. Crystals, mp 51-52°.

9171. α-Terpineol. [98-55-5] α,α,4-Trimethyl-3-cyclohexene-1-methanol; p-menth-1-en-8-ol. C$_{10}$H$_{18}$O; mol wt 154.25. C 77.87%, H 11.76%, O 10.37%. Terpineol exists as three isomers, α-, β-, and γ-terpineol: J. L. Simonsen, *The Terpenes* vol. I (University Press, Cambridge, 2nd ed., 1947) pp 256-274. Isoln of d-α-terpineol from petitgrain oil: Walbaum, Hüthig, *J. Prakt. Chem.* **67**, 322 (1903). Isoln of l-α-terpineol from long leaf pine oil: Teeple, *J. Am. Chem. Soc.* **30**, 412 (1908). Isoln of dl-α-terpineol from cajeput oil: Voiry, *Compt. Rend.* **106**, 1540 (1888). Synthesis of d-α-terpineol: Cologne, Crabalona, *Bull. Soc. Chim. Fr.* **1960**, 102. Synthesis of l-α-terpineol: *eidem, ibid.* **1959**, 1505. Stereochemistry: Henbest, McElkinney, *J. Chem. Soc.* **1959**, 1834. *Review:* Wagner, *Manuf. Chem.* **22**, 98, 153 (1951).

d-Form. Liquid. bp$_{4.5}$ 81-82°; bp$_{731}$ 206-207°. d$_4^{20}$ 0.9338. n$_D^{20}$ 1.4818. [α]$_D^{20}$ +92.45°. Solidifies at 31°.

Phenylurethan. C$_{17}$H$_{23}$NO$_2$. Crystals from petr ether, mp 111°. [α]$_D^{20}$ +30.50° (benzene).

l-Form. Liquid. bp$_5$ 80-81.5°. d$_4^{20}$ 0.935. n$_D^{20}$ 1.4820. [α]$_D^{20}$ -100° (c = 20 in alc). Solidifies at 36.4°.

Dinitrobenzoate. C$_{17}$H$_{20}$N$_2$O$_6$. Crystals from alcohol, mp 101.5°. [α]$_D^{20}$ -31° (c = 9.5 in carbon tetrachloride).

dl-Form. Liquid. bp$_3$ 85°; bp$_{752}$ 218.8-219.4°, d^{15} 0.9386. n$_D^{20}$ 1.4831.

Phenylurethan. C$_{17}$H$_{23}$NO$_2$. Crystals, mp 113°.

USE: Perfumes; denaturing fats for soap manufacture.

THERAP CAT: Antiseptic.

9172. Terreic Acid. [121-40-4] (1R)-3-Hydroxy-4-methyl-7-oxabicyclo[4.1.0]hept-3-ene-2,5-dione; 2-hydroxy-3-methyl-1,4-benzoquinone 5,6-epoxide; 5,6-epoxy-3-hydroxy-p-toluquinone. C$_7$H$_6$O$_4$; mol wt 154.12. C 54.55%, H 3.92%, O 41.52%. Antibiotic metabolite produced by the mold *Aspergillus terreus;* naturally occurring as the (−)-form: Wilkins, Harris, *Br. J. Exp. Pathol.* **23**, 166 (1942); Abraham, Florey, in H. W. Florey *et al., Antibiotics* vol. I (Oxford Univ. Press, New York, 1949) p 337; Kaplan *et al., Antibiot. Chemother.* **4**, 746 (1954). Structure: Sheehan *et al., J. Am. Chem. Soc.* **80**, 5536 (1958). Synthesis of the racemate: Rashid, Read, *J. Chem. Soc. C* **1967**, 1323. Alternate synthesis and resolution of isomers: Sheehan, Lo, *J. Med. Chem.* **17**, 371 (1974). Improved synthesis: A. Enhsen *et al., J. Org. Chem.* **55**, 1177 (1990).

Pale yellow plates from benzene or hexane. Easily sublimed *in vacuo.* mp 127-127.5°. Rotation varies considerably with the solvent: [α]$_D^{22}$ -16.6° (chloroform); [α]$_D^{22}$ -28.6° (methanol-benzene 1:1); [α]$_D^{22}$ +74.3° (pH 7 phosphate buffer). uv max (ethanol): 214, 316 nm (log ε 4.03, 3.88). Enol-type acid, pKa 4.5. Slightly sol in water. Soluble in ether, lower alcohols, acetone, hot cyclohexane. Moderately stable to mineral acid, but dec rapidly in alkaline soln.

9173. Tertatolol. [34784-64-0] 1-[(3,4-Dihydro-2H-1-benzothiopyran-8-yl)oxy]-3-[(1,1-dimethylethyl)amino]-2-propanol; (±)-1-tert-butylamino-3-(1-thiachroman-8-yloxy)-2-propanol; dl-8-[2-hydroxy-3-[(tert-butylamino)propyl]oxy]thiochromane. C$_{16}$H$_{25}$NO$_2$S; mol wt 295.44. C 65.05%, H 8.53%, N 4.74%, O 10.83%, S 10.85%. Nonselective β-adrenergic blocker. Prepn: C. Malen, M. Laubie, DE 2115201; *eidem,* US 3960891 (1971, 1976 both to Sci. Union et Cie). Pharmacology in animals: M. Laubie *et al., Arch. Int. Pharmacodyn. Ther.* **201**, 323, 334 (1973); B. R. Walker *et al., J. Cardiovasc. Pharmacol.* **7**, 1193 (1985). Synergistic effect with indapamide, *q.v.:* E. Marmo *et al., Drugs Exp. Clin. Res.* **11**, 709 (1985). GC-MS determn in plasma and urine: S. Staveris *et al., J. Chromatogr.* **339**, 97 (1985). Pharmacology in humans and mechanism of action study: A. De Blasi *et al., Clin. Pharmacol. Ther.* **39**, 245 (1986). Preliminary evaluation in hypertension: J. P. Degaute *et al., Am. J. Hypertens.* **1**, 263S (1988).

Crystals from hexane, mp 70-72°.

Hydrochloride. [33580-30-2] S-2395; SE-2395; Artex; Artexal; Prenalex. C$_{16}$H$_{25}$NO$_2$S.HCl; mol wt 331.90. Crystals from acetonitrile, mp 180-183°. pKa 9.8. LD$_{50}$ in rats, mice (mg/kg): 40, 37 i.v.; 90, 120 i.p. (Laubie).

THERAP CAT: Antihypertensive.

9174. α-Terthienyl. [1081-34-1] 2,2':5'2''-Terthiophene; 5-(2-thienyl)-2,2'-bithiophene. C$_{12}$H$_8$S$_3$; mol wt 248.39. C 58.03%, H 3.25%, S 38.73%. Biocidal constituent of various species of marigolds. Isoln from *Tagetes erecta* L., *Compositae:* L. Zechmeister, J. W. Sease, *J. Am. Chem. Soc.* **69**, 273 (1947). Isoln and distribution in *Tageteae:* K. R. Downum, G. H. N. Towers, *J. Nat. Prod.* **46**, 98 (1983). Synthesis: W. Steinkopf *et al., Ann.* **546**, 180 (1941); H. J. Kooreman, H. Wynberg, *Rec. Trav. Chim.* **86**, 37 (1967); J.-P. Beny *et al., J. Org. Chem.* **47**, 2201 (1982). Biological activity as nematocide: J. H. Uhlenbroek, J. D. Bijloo, *Rec. Trav. Chim.* **77**, 1004 (1958); J. D. Bijloo *et al.,* DE 1075891; *eidem,* US 3050442 (1960, 1962, both to North American Philips); J. Bakker *et al., J. Biol. Chem.* **254**, 1841 (1979); as herbicide: J. Harvey, Jr., US 3086854 (1963 to Du Pont); G. Campbell *et al., J. Chem. Ecol.* **8**, 961 (1982); as antimicrobial: J. R. Kagan *et al., Bull. Photochem. Photobiol.* **31**, 465 (1980); T. Arnason *et al., ibid.* **33**, 821 (1981); F. DiCosmo *et al., Pestic. Sci.* **13**, 589 (1982).

Yellow-orange plates from methanol, mp 93-94°. uv max (methanol): 254, 350 nm (ε 7100, 21300). Sol in carbon bisulfide, ether, benzene, acetone, petr ether; slightly sol in methanol, ethanol. Insol in water.

9175. Tertiapin. [58694-52-3] TPN. Neurotoxic 21 residue peptide isolated from the venom of the European honey bee, *Apis mellifera.* Characterized by 2 disulfide linkages and the complete absence of negatively charged residues, it selectively inhibits G-protein inwardly rectifying potassium channels (GIRK) by binding to the external vestibule of the channel. Isoln: J. Gauldie *et al., Eur. J. Biochem.* **61**, 369 (1976); B. E. C. Banks *et al., Bull. Instit. Pasteur* **74**, 137 (1976). Primary structure: Y. A. Ovchinnikov *et al., Soviet J. Bioorg. Chem.* **6**, 187 (1980); 3D-structure: X. Xu, J.

W. Nelson, *Proteins Struct. Funct. Genet.* **17**, 124 (1993). Inhibition of GIRK-channels: W. Jin, Z. Lu, *Biochemistry* **37**, 13291 (1998); of muscarinic inwardly rectifying potassium channels ($I_{K(ACh)}$): M.-D. Drici *et al., Br. J. Pharmacol.* **131**, 569 (2000); D. E. Benavides-Haro *et al., Arch. Pharm.* **368**, 309 (2003).

Ala-Lys-Cys-Asn-Cys-Asn-Arg-Ile-Ile-Ile-Phe-His-Met-Cys-Trp-Lys-Lys-Cys-Gly-Lys-LysNH₂

Tertiapin Q. [252198-49-5] TPN_Q. Non-air-oxidizable derivative of TPN in which Met-13 is replaced with Gln. Synthesis: W. Jin, Z. Lu, *Biochemistry* **38**, 14286 (1999). Mechanism of inhibition: W. Jin *et al., ibid.* 14294. Proton titration of TPN_Q binding: Y. Ramu *et al., ibid.* **40**, 3601 (2001).
USE: Biochemical probe for potassium channels.

9176. TES. [7365-44-8] 2-[[2-Hydroxy-1,1-bis(hydroxymethyl)ethyl]amino]ethanesulfonic acid; *N*-[2-hydroxy-1,1-bis(hydroxymethyl)ethyl]taurine; *N*-tris(hydroxymethyl)methyl-2-aminoethanesulfonic acid. $C_6H_{15}NO_6S$; mol wt 229.25. C 31.43%, H 6.60%, N 6.11%, O 41.87%, S 13.99%. One of the zwitterionic amino acids known as "Good" buffers; active in the pH range 6.5 to 8.0. Prepn: N. E. Good *et al., Biochemistry* **5**, 467 (1966). Thermodynamic constants: C. A. Vega, R. G. Bates, *Anal. Chem.* **48**, 1293 (1976). Effect of temperature and solvent systems on pK_2: H. A. Azab *et al., Monatsh. Chem.* **125**, 233 (1994). Use as buffer: F. C. Molinia *et al., Reprod. Nutr. Dev.* **34**, 491 (1994); K. Isobe, H. Nishise, *J. Biotechnol.* **75**, 265 (1999).

Crystals from alcohol/water, mp 226-228°, dec 231°. pKa of 0.1M soln: (0°) 7.92; (20°) 7.5; (37°) 7.14. Δ pKa/°C −0.020.
USE: Biological buffer.

9177. Tesaglitazar. [251565-85-2] (αS)-α-Ethoxy-4-[2-[4-[(methylsulfonyl)oxy]phenyl]ethoxy]benzenepropanoic acid; (*S*)-2-ethoxy-3-[4-[2-(4-methanesulfonyloxyphenyl)ethoxy]phenyl]-propanoic acid; AZ-242; Galida. $C_{20}H_{24}O_7S$; mol wt 408.47. C 58.81%, H 5.92%, O 27.42%, S 7.85%. Dual-acting peroxisome proliferator-activated receptor (PPAR) α and γ agonist. Prepn: K. Andersson, **WO 9962872** (1999 to Astra); *idem*, **US 6258850** (2001 to AstraZeneca). Crystal structure in complex with the PPARα and PPARγ ligand binding domains: P. Cronet *et al., Structure* **9**, 699 (2001). Solid-phase extraction LC/MS/MS determn in plasma: H. Svennberg *et al., J. Chromatogr. B* **787**, 231 (2003). Mechanism of action study: B. D. Hegarty *et al., Endocrinology* **145**, 3158 (2004). Clinical pharmacokinetics: H. Ericsson *et al., Drug Metab. Dispos.* **32**, 923 (2004). Clinical effects on lipid and glucose metabolism in hypertriglyceridaemia and abdominal obesity: B. Fagerberg *et al., Diabetologia* **48**, 1716 (2005). Review of clinical development: N. Kamber, T. M. E. Davis, *IDrugs* **8**, 927-935 (2005).

THERAP CAT: Antidiabetic.

9178. Tesmilifene. [98774-23-3] *N,N*-Diethyl-2-[4-(phenylmethyl)phenoxy]ethanamine; DPPE. $C_{19}H_{25}NO$; mol wt 283.41. C 80.52%, H 8.89%, N 4.94%, O 5.65%. Intracellular histamine antagonist with chemopotentiating and cytoprotective activity. Structurally similar to tamoxifen, *q.v.*, although binds anti-estrogen binding site (AEBS) with no affinity for the estrogen receptor. Prepn: L. J. Brandes, M. W. Hermonat, *Biochem. Biophys. Res. Commun.* **123**, 724 (1984); and use as antineoplastic: *eidem*, **US 4803227** (1989 to Univ. Manitoba); and study of binding affinity: M. Poirot *et al., Bioorg. Med. Chem.* **8**, 2007 (2000). Spectral analysis of interaction with P450 isozymes: L. J. Brandes *et al., Cancer Chemother. Pharmacol.* **45**, 298 (2000). Clinical evaluation in combination with cyclophosphamide in prostate can-

cer: L. J. Brandes *et al., J. Clin. Oncol.* **13**, 1398 (1995); in combination with doxorubicin in breast cancer: L. Reyno *et al., J. Clin. Oncol.* **22**, 269 (2004).

Hydrochloride. [92981-78-7] BMS-217380-01; BMY-33419. $C_{19}H_{25}NO.HCl$; mol wt 319.87. White crystals from isopropanol + acetone (3:1), mp 156-158°. pKa 10.9.
THERAP CAT: Antineoplastic adjunct (chemosensitizer).

9179. Testolactone. [968-93-4] (4a*S*,4b*R*,10a*R*,10b*S*,12a*S*)-3,4,4a,5,6,10a,10b,11,12,12a-Decahydro-10a,12a-dimethyl-2*H*-phenanthro[2,1-b]pyran-2,8(4b*H*)-dione; D-homo-17a-oxaandrosta-1,4-diene-3,17-dione; 13-hydroxy-3-oxo-13,17-secoandrosta-1,4-dien-17-oic acid δ-lactone; 1,2,3,4,4a,4b,7,9,10,10a-decahydro-2-hydroxy-2,4b-dimethyl-7-oxo-1-phenanthrenepropionic acid δ-lactone; delta-1-testololactone; 1-dehydrotestololactone; 17α-oxo-*D*-homo-1,4-androstadiene-3,17-dione; Δ¹-testolactone; NSC-23759; SQ-9538; Fludestrin; Teslac. $C_{19}H_{24}O_3$; mol wt 300.39. C 75.97%, H 8.05%, O 15.98%. Obtained by microbial transformation of progesterone, Reichstein's substance S, or testosterone: Fried *et al., J. Am. Chem. Soc.* **75**, 5764 (1953); *eidem*, **US 2744120** (1956 to Olin Mathieson); Brannon *et al., J. Org. Chem.* **30**, 760 (1965). Comprehensive description: K. Florey, *Anal. Profiles Drug Subs.* **5**, 533-553 (1976).

Crystals from acetone, mp 218-219°. $[\alpha]_D^{23}$ −45.6° (c = 1.24 in chloroform). uv max (ethanol): 242 nm (ε 15800).
Note: This is a controlled substance (anabolic steroid): **21 CFR,** 1308.13, as defined in 1300.01.
THERAP CAT: Antineoplastic.

9180. Testosterone. [58-22-0] (17β)-17-Hydroxyandrost-4-en-3-one; Δ⁴-androsten-17β-ol-3-one; *trans*-testosterone; Andro; Androderm; Andropatch; Mertestate; Oreton; Testoderm; Testogel; Testolin; Testro AQ; Virosterone. $C_{19}H_{28}O_2$; mol wt 288.42. C 79.12%, H 9.79%, O 11.09%. Principal hormone of the testes, produced by the interstitial cells. Major circulating androgen; converted by 5α-reductase in androgen-dependent target tissues to **5α-dihydrotestosterone** which is required for normal male sexual differentiation. Also converted by aromatization to estradiol, *q.v.* Isoln from bull testes: David *et al., Z. Physiol. Chem.* **233**, 281 (1935). Prepn from cholesterol and confirmation of structure: A. Butenandt, G. Hanisch, *Ber.* **68**, 1859 (1935); *eidem, Z. Physiol. Chem.* **237**, 89 (1935); from dehydroandrosterone: L. Ruzicka, A. Wettstein, *Helv. Chim. Acta* **18**, 1264 (1935); from mixed esters: L. Ruzicka *et al., ibid.* 1478. Crystal structure: P. J. Roberts *et al., J. Chem. Soc. Perkin Trans. 2* **1973**, 1978. Historical review: J. M. Hoberman, C. E. Yesalis, *Sci. Am.* **272**, 76-81 (Feb. 1995). Review of role in aging males: F. E. Kaiser, J. E. Morley, *Neurobiol. Aging* **15**, 559-563 (1994); of clinical relevance in females: R. S. Rittmaster, *Am. J. Med.* **98**, Suppl. 1A, 17S-21S (1995).

Needles from dil acetone, mp 155°. $[\alpha]_D^{24}$ +109° (c = 4 in alc). uv max: 238 nm. Insol in water. Sol in alcohol, ether, and other organic solvents.
Acetate. [1045-69-8] $C_{21}H_{30}O_3$. mp 140-141°.

17β-Cyclopentanepropionate. [58-20-8] Testosterone cypionate; depAndro; Depotest; Depo-Testosterone; Depovirin; Pertestis; Virilon. $C_{27}H_{40}O_3$; mol wt 412.60. Pharmacology: A. C. Ott *et al., J. Clin. Endocrinol. Metab.* **12**, 15 (1952). Crystals, mp 101-102°. $[\alpha]_D^{25}$ +87° (CHCl₃). Sol in oils.

Enanthate. [315-37-7] Andro LA; Androtardyl; Delatestryl; Everone; Primoteston; Testinon; Testo-Enant. $C_{26}H_{40}O_3$; mol wt 400.59. Prepn: Junkmann *et al.*, **US 2840508** (1958 to Schering AG). Comprehensive description: K. Florey, *Anal. Profiles Drug Subs.* **4**, 452-465 (1975). Crystals, mp 36-37.5°.

Propionate. [57-85-2] Anertan; Enarmon; Neo-Hombreol (amp.); Orchisterone; Synandrol; Testex; Testoviron; Virormone. $C_{22}H_{32}O_3$; mol wt 344.49. Prepn: K. Miescher *et al.*, **US 2109400** (1938 to Soc. Chem. Ind. Basel). Stout prisms from alcohol + water, mp 118-122°. $[\alpha]_D^{25}$ +83 to +90° (100 mg in 10 ml dioxane). Insol in water. Freely sol in alcohol, ether, pyridine, in other organic solvents. Sol in vegetable oils.

Undecanoate. [5949-44-0] Testosterone 17β-undecylate; Andriol; Pantestone; Restandol. $C_{30}H_{48}O_3$; mol wt 456.70.

Note: This is a controlled substance (anabolic steroid): **21 CFR**, 1308.13, as defined in 1300.01.

THERAP CAT: Androgen.

THERAP CAT (VET): Androgen.

9181. Tetraamminecopper Sulfate. [14283-05-7] Cuprammonium sulfate; ammonium cupric sulfate; cupric sulfate, ammoniated; Eau Celeste. $CuH_{12}N_4O_4S$; mol wt 227.73. Cu 27.90%, H 5.31%, N 24.60%, O 28.10%, S 14.08%. $[Cu(NH_3)_4]SO_4$. Prepd by dissolving copper sulfate in ammonia water and pptg with alcohol: Mazzi, *Acta Crystallogr.* **8**, 137 (1955). Crystal structure of monohydrate: Morosin, *ibid.* **25B**, 19 (1969).

Monohydrate. Large, dark blue crystals. d_4^{20} 1.81. Ammonia odor, dec in air. Loses H_2O and $2NH_3$ on heating to 120°, remaining $2NH_3$ at 160°. Soly in water at 21.5°: 18.5 g/100 ml. Practically insol in the lower alcohols.

USE: In textile printing, especially in calico finishing. As fungicide.

9182. Tetrabenazine. [58-46-8] 1,3,4,6,7,11b-Hexahydro-9,10-dimethoxy-3-(2-methylpropyl)-2H-benzo[a]quinolizin-2-one; 2-oxo-3-isobutyl-9,10-dimethoxy-1,2,3,4,6,7-hexahydro-11bH-benzo[a]quinolizine; Ro-1-9569. $C_{19}H_{27}NO_3$; mol wt 317.42. C 71.89%, H 8.57%, N 4.41%, O 15.12%. Dopamine depleting agent. Prepn: Brossi *et al.*, *Helv. Chim. Acta* **41**, 119 (1958); **US 2830993** (1958 to Hoffmann-La Roche); Osbond, *J. Chem. Soc.* **1961**, 4711. Pharmacology: Leusen *et al.*, *Arch. Int. Pharmacodyn.* **119**, 225 (1959). Metabolism: Schwartz *et al.*, *Biochem. Pharmacol.* **15**, 645 (1966). Clinical trials in hyperkinetic movement disorders: J. Janovic, *Ann. Neurol.* **11**, 41 (1982); J. Janovic, J. Orman, *Neurology* **38**, 391 (1988).

Prisms from methanol, mp 125-126°.

Oxime. Crystals from dil alcohol, mp 158°.

Hydrochloride. [2105-47-7] $C_{19}H_{27}NO_3 \cdot HCl$. Crystals, mp 208-210°. Soluble in hot water. Practically insol in acetone. uv max (alcohol): 230, 284 nm (ε 7780, 3820).

Methanesulfonate. [804-53-5] Nitoman. $C_{19}H_{27}NO_3 \cdot CH_3SO_3H$; mol wt 413.53. Bitter crystals, sensitive to light, mp 126-130°. Sparingly sol in water, sol in alcohol. Practically insol in ether.

THERAP CAT: Antidyskinetic; antipsychotic.

9183. Tetraborane(10). [18283-93-7] Tetraboron decahydride; borobutane. B_4H_{10}; mol wt 53.32. B 81.10%, H 18.90%. Prepd by the reaction of magnesium boride with hydrochloric or phosphoric acid: Stock, Kuss, *Ber.* **56B**, 789 (1923); from dihydropentaborane: Burg, Schlesinger, *J. Am. Chem. Soc.* **55**, 4009 (1933); from diborane: Stock, Mathing, *Ber.* **69B**, 1456 (1936);

Klein *et al., J. Am. Chem. Soc.* **80**, 4149 (1958). *Review:* Greenwood in *Comprehensive Inorganic Chemistry* **vol. 1**, J. C. Bailar, Jr. *et al.*, Eds. (Pergamon Press, Oxford, 1973) pp 785-791.

Gas; disagreeable odor; mp −120°; bp 18°. Vapor pressure 580 mm Hg at 6°; 388 mm at 0°. Dec at room temp in a few hours. Dec rapidly at 100°. Ignites spontaneously in air or oxygen. Hydrolyzes in water to boric acid and hydrogen. Reacts with ammonia to form a tetraammoniate.

9184. 3,4,5,6-Tetrabromo-o-cresol. [576-55-6] $C_7H_4Br_4$-O; mol wt 423.72. C 19.84%, H 0.95%, Br 75.43%, O 3.78%. Prepd by bromination of o-cresol or its methyl or ethyl ether: Zincke, Hedenström, *Ann.* **350**, 269 (1906); Bonneaud, *Bull. Soc. Chim. Fr.* **7**, 776 (1910); Treacy, **US 2319960** (1943 to Merck & Co.).

White to buff, cryst powder, mp 205-208° with dec. Practically insol in water. Sol in alcohol, ether, alkali hydroxides.

Acetate. $C_9H_6Br_4O_2$. Needles from dil alcohol, mp 154°. Slightly sol in alcohol and glacial acetic acid.

Caution: Irritating to skin, mucous membranes.

USE: Fungicide.

9185. sym-Tetrabromoethane. [79-27-6] 1,1,2,2-Tetrabromoethane; acetylene tetrabromide; Muthmann's liquid. $C_2H_2Br_4$; mol wt 345.65. C 6.95%, H 0.58%, Br 92.47%. $Br_2CHCHBr_2$. Manuf by bromination of acetylene: **GB 889649** (1962 to Associated Ethyl Co.). Toxicity studies: Gray, *Arch. Ind. Hyg. Occup. Med.* **2**, 407 (1950); D. L. Wolff, *Acta Biol. Med. Ger.* **41**, 945 (1982).

Yellowish, heavy, very refractive liquid; odor of camphor and iodoform. d 2.964; bp_{54} 151°; mp 0°; n_D^{20} 1.638. Insol in water. Miscible with alc, chloroform, ether, aniline, glacial acetic acid. LD_{50} i.p. in mice: 443.3 mg/kg (Wolff).

Caution: Potential symptoms of overexposure are irritation of eyes and nose; anorexia, nausea; severe headaches; abdominal pain; jaundice; monocytosis; CNS depression. *See NIOSH Pocket Guide to Chemical Hazards* (DHHS/NIOSH 97-140, 1997) p 6.

USE: In microscopy, as solvent, separating minerals by density.

9186. 3′,3″,5′,5″-Tetrabromophenolphthalein. [76-62-0] 3,3-Bis(3,5-dibromo-4-hydroxyphenyl)-1(3H)-isobenzofuranone. $C_{20}H_{10}Br_4O_4$; mol wt 633.91. C 37.89%, H 1.59%, Br 50.42%, O 10.10%. Prepd by direct bromination of phenolphthalein: Blicke *et al., J. Am. Chem. Soc.* **54**, 1465 (1932). Diagnostic use: E. A. Graham, W. H. Cole, *J. Am. Med. Assoc.* **250**, 2975 (1984), reprint of *J. Am. Med. Assoc.* **82**, 613 (1924).

Crystals from alcohol, glacial acetic acid, or ether, mp 295-297° (dec). Practically insol in water. Slightly sol in alc, glacial acetic acid; sol in ether, in alkali with a violet color.

Disodium salt. [860-07-1] Tetrabromophenolphthalein sodium; Brom-Tetragnost; Cholegnostyl; Tetrabrom. $C_{20}H_8Br_4Na_2O_4$; mol wt 677.87. Blue crystals, dec on exposure to air becoming partially insol. Freely sol in water; slightly sol in alcohol. Insol in ether. pH of aq soln is 9-10. *Keep well closed and protected from light.*

THERAP CAT: Disodium salt as diagnostic aid (radiopaque medium).

9187. Tetrabutylammonium Fluoride. [429-41-4] *N,N,N*-Tributyl-1-butanaminium fluoride; TBAF. $C_{16}H_{36}FN$; mol wt 261.46. C 73.50%, H 13.88%, F 7.27%, N 5.36%. Catalytic reagent which is both a potent base and a source of nucleophilic fluoride. Prepn as hydrated form: D. L. Fowler *et al., J. Am. Chem. Soc.* **62**, 1140 (1940). Instability of anhydrous form: R. K. Sharma, J. L. Fry, *J. Org. Chem.* **48**, 2112 (1983). Use as fluoride source: D. P. Cox *et al., ibid.* **49**, 3216 (1984); T. Kobayashi *et al., ibid.* **67**, 3156 (2002). Synthesis and/or use as catalyst in cyclization reactions: J. Pless, *ibid.* **39**, 2644 (1974); A. R. Gangloff *et al., Tetrahedron Lett.* **42**, 1441 (2001); in addition reactions: P. Molina *et al., Synlett* **2003**, 714. Deprotecting agent: M. Namikoshi *et al., J. Org. Chem.* **56**, 5464 (1991); J. J. Parlow *et al., Bioorg. Med. Chem. Lett.* **8**, 2391 (1998). Brief review in cleavage of silyl protecting groups: M. B. Kumar, *Synlett* **2002**, 2125-2126.

Colorless oil which crystallizes on exposure to humidity.

USE: Reagent in organic syntheses in addition, condensation, base-catalyzed cyclization reactions, fluorination and desulfonylation reactions and as a deprotecting agent. Typically dried prior to use.

9188. Tetracaine Hydrochloride. [136-47-0] 4-(Butylamino)benzoic acid 2-(dimethylamino)ethyl ester monohydrochloride; *p*-butylaminobenzoyl-2-dimethylaminoethanol hydrochloride; 2-dimethylaminoethyl 4-*n*-butylaminobenzoate hydrochloride; dicain; amethocaine hydrochloride; Anethaine; Decicain; Pantocaine; Pontocaine Hydrochloride; Tonexol. $C_{15}H_{25}ClN_2O_2$; mol wt 300.82. C 59.89%, H 8.38%, Cl 11.79%, N 9.31%, O 10.64%. Prepn: US **1889645** (1932); GB **815144** (1959 to Abbott). Prepn of pharmaceutical dosage forms: Shupe, US **3272700** (1966 to Sterling Drug). Mechanism of action studies: Y.-W. Leung *et al., J. Infect. Dis.* **136**, 679 (1977). Toxicity study: Dawes, *Br. J. Pharmacol. Chemother.* **1**, 90 (1946). Acute toxicity: B. A. Bopp *et al., J. Pharm. Sci.* **67**, 882 (1978). Comprehensive description: M. Riaz, *Anal. Profiles Drug Subs.* **18**, 379-411 (1989).

Faintly bitter crystals producing transient numbness of the tongue. mp 147-150°. pKa 8.39. uv max (water): 225, 310 nm (ε 14108, 26352); (0.1*N* H_2SO_4): 229, 281, 312 nm ($\varepsilon_{1cm}^{1\%}$ 509, 55, 76); (methanol): 226, 310 nm (ε 7586, 29512); (chloroform): 308 nm (ε 27542). Sol at 20° in 7.5 parts water, 40 parts alcohol; 30 parts chloroform. Practically insol in ether, benzene, acetone. The aq soln is neutral to litmus. Aq solns are stable and may be sterilized by brief boiling. LD_{50} i.p. in mice: 70 mg/kg (Dawes); also reported as LD_{50} in female mice (mg/kg): 13 i.v.; 35 s.c. (Bopp).

THERAP CAT: Anesthetic (local).

THERAP CAT (VET): Anesthetic (topical).

9189. Tetrachloroethane. [79-34-5] 1,1,2,2-Tetrachloroethane; *sym*-tetrachloroethane; acetylene tetrachloride; Cellon; Bonoform. $C_2H_2Cl_4$; mol wt 167.85. C 14.31%, H 1.20%, Cl 84.49%. $Cl_2CHCHCl_2$. Manuf by catalytic addition of chlorine to acetylene: Peters, Neumann, *Angew. Chem.* **45**, 261 (1932); by chlorination of ethylene: Pye, US **2752402** (1956 to Dow); by catalytic chlorination of ethane: Joseph, US **2752401** (1956 to Dow); by chlorination of 1,2-dichloroethane: Conrad, US **2725412** (1955 to Ethyl Corp.); Fox, US **2846484** (1958 to Monsanto). Toxicity study: H. F. Smyth *et al., Am. Ind. Hyg. Assoc. J.* **30**, 470 (1969). Review of toxicology and human exposure: *Toxicological Profile for 1,1,2,2-Tetrachloroethane* (PB97-121099, 1996) 186 pp.

Nonflammable, heavy, mobile liquid. Sweetish, suffocating, chloroform-like odor. d_4^{25} 1.58658. mp −44°. bp_{760} 146.5°. n_D^{20} 1.49419. Very sparingly sol in water. At 25° one gram dissolves in 350 ml H_2O. Misc with methanol, ethanol, benzene, ether, petr ether, carbon tetrachloride, chloroform, carbon disulfide, dimethylformamide, oils. Has the highest solvent power of the chlorinated hydrocarbons. LD_{50} orally in rats: 0.20 ml/kg (Smyth).

Caution: Potential symptoms of overexposure are nausea, vomiting and abdominal pain; finger tremors; jaundice, hepatitis, tender liver; dermatitis; monocytosis; kidney damage. Potential occupational carcinogen. *See NIOSH Pocket Guide to Chemical Hazards* (DHHS/NIOSH 97-140, 1997) p 300.

USE: Nonflammable solvent for fats, oils, waxes, resins, cellulose acetate, rubber, copal, phosphorus, sulfur. As solvent in certain types of Friedel-Crafts reactions or phthalic anhydride condensations. In the manuf of paint, varnish, and rust removers. In soil sterilization and weed killer and insecticide formulations. In the determination of theobromine in cacao. As immersion fluid in crystallography. In the biological laboratory to produce pathological changes in gastrointestinal tract, liver, and kidneys. Intermediate in the manuf of trichloroethylene and other chlorinated hydrocarbons having two carbon atoms.

9190. Tetrachloroethylene. [127-18-4] Tetrachloroethene; perchloroethylene; ethylene tetrachloride; tetrachlorethylene; Nema; Tetracap; Tetropil; Perclene; Ankilostin; Didakene. C_2Cl_4; mol wt 165.83. C 14.49%, Cl 85.52%. $Cl_2C=CCl_2$. Prepd by Faraday in 1821. Manuf by catalytic oxidation of 1,1,2,2-tetrachloroethane: Ellsworth, Vancamp, US **2951103** (1960 to Columbia-Southern Chem.); Feathers, Rogerson, US **3040109** (1962 to Pittsburgh Plate Glass); by catalytic chlorination of acetylene: Thermet, Parvi, US **2938931** (1960 to Société d'électrochimie, d'électrométallurgie et des aciéries électriques d'Ugine). Review of mfg processes: *Faith, Keyes & Clark's Industrial Chemicals*, F. A. Lowenheim, M. K. Moran, Eds. (Wiley-Interscience, New York, 4th ed., 1975) pp 604-611. Physical properties: Mumford, Phillips, *J. Chem. Soc.* **1950**, 75. Toxicity data: Dybing, *Acta Pharmacol. Toxicol.* **2**, 223 (1946); Lazarew, *Arch. Exp. Pathol. Pharmakol.* **141**, 19 (1929). Review of toxicology and human exposure: *Toxicological Profile for Tetrachloroethylene* (PB98-101181, 1997) 318 pp.

Colorless, nonflammable liq; ethereal odor; d_4^{15} 1.6311; d_4^{20} 1.6230. bp 121°. mp ~−22°. n_D^{20} 1.5055. Sol in about 10,000 vol water; misc with alcohol, ether, chloroform, benzene. LD_{50} orally in mice: 8.85 g/kg (Dybing). LC for mice in air: 5925 ppm (Lazarew).

Caution: Potential symptoms of overexposure are irritation of eyes, nose and throat; nausea; flushing of face and neck; vertigo, dizziness, incoordination; headache, somnolence; skin erythema; liver damage. *See NIOSH Pocket Guide to Chemical Hazards* (DHHS/NIOSH 97-140, 1997) p 300. This substance is reasonably anticipated to be a human carcinogen: *Report on Carcinogens, Eleventh Edition* (PB2005-104914, 2004) p III-243

USE: Dry cleaning; textile processing; degreasing metals; solvent; chemical intermediate in production of fluorocarbons. Insulating fluid and cooling gas in electrical transformers.

THERAP CAT: Anthelmintic (Nematodes, Trematodes).

THERAP CAT (VET): Anthelmintic.

9191. 3,3′,4′,5-Tetrachlorosalicylanilide. [1154-59-2] 3,5-Dichloro-*N*-(3,4-dichlorophenyl)-2-hydroxybenzamide; Irgasan BS200. $C_{13}H_7Cl_4NO_2$; mol wt 351.01. C 44.48%, H 2.01%, Cl 40.40%, N 3.99%, O 9.12%. Prepn of polyhalosalicylanilides: Bindler, Model, US **2703332** (1955 to Geigy). Bacteriostat in the manuf of thermoplastic articles: Teller, US **3005720** (1961 to Weco Products).

Crystals, mp 161°. Fluoresces under ultraviolet light. Practically insol in water. Sol in alkaline aq solns and in solns of wetting agents. Sol in many organic solvents.

USE: Bacteriostat in formulations of surgical soaps, laundry soaps, rinses, polishes, shampoos, deodorants. Also as preservative in textile finishes, certain petroleum products, cellulose esters, cutting oils, coolants.

9192. Tetrachlorvinphos. [22248-79-9] Phosphoric acid (Z)-2-chloro-1-(2,4,5-trichlorophenyl)ethenyl dimethyl ester; 2,4,5-trichloro-α-(chloromethylene)benzyl phosphate ester; 2-chloro-1-(2,4,5-trichlorophenyl)vinyl dimethyl phosphate; stirofos; ENT-25841; SD-8447; Gardona; Rabon; Rabond. $C_{10}H_9Cl_4O_4P$; mol wt 365.96. C 32.82%, H 2.48%, Cl 38.75%, O 17.49%, P 8.46%. Organophosphate insecticide; cholinesterase inhibitor. Prepn: D. D. Phillips, L. F. Ward, Jr., **US 3102842**; D. E. Ramey, **US 3553297** (1963, 1971 both to Shell). Properties: Whetstone *et al., J. Agric. Food Chem.* **14,** 352 (1966). Soil persistence: N. P. Agnihotri *et al., Indian J. Agric. Chem.* **14,** 27 (1981). Metabolism: M. H. Akhtar, T. S. Foster, *J. Agric. Food Chem.* **28,** 698 (1980); *eidem, ibid.* **29,** 766 (1981). Determn of residues in foods: V. Leoni *et al., J. AOAC Int.* **75,** 511 (1992). Toxicology studies: T. B. Gaines, *Toxicol. Appl. Pharmacol.* **14,** 515 (1969); A. I. T. Walker *et al., Pestic. Sci.* **3,** 517 (1972). Review of agricultural use: A. G. Jennings, *Int. Pest Control* **12,** 28-33 (1970); of carcinogenic risk: *IARC Monographs* **30,** 197-206 (1983).

mp 97-98°. Vapor pressure at 20° = 4.2 × 10^{-8}. Soly in water: 11 ppm; in xylene: <15%; 40-50% in chloroform at room temp. LD_{50} in male, female rats (mg/kg): 1100, 1125 orally (Gaines).

USE: Insecticide.

THERAP CAT (VET): Insecticide.

9193. Tetraconazole. [112281-77-3] 1-[2-(2,4-Dichlorophenyl)-3-(1,1,2,2-tetrafluoroethoxy)propyl]-1H-1,2,4-triazole; (RS)-2-(2,4-dichlorophenyl)-3-(1H-1,2,4-triazol-1-yl)propyl 1,1,2,2-tetrafluoroethyl ether; M-14360; Domark; Eminent; Lospel. C_{13}-$H_{11}Cl_2F_4N_3O$; mol wt 372.15. C 41.96%, H 2.98%, Cl 19.05%, F 20.42%, N 11.29%, O 4.30%. Systemic triazole antifungal; inhibitor of sterol biosynthesis. Prepn: **JP Kokai 87 169773**; R. Colle *et al.,* **US 5081141** (1987, 1992 both to Montedison). Chemical and biological properties: C. Garavaglia *et al., Brighton Crop Prot. Conf. - Pests Dis.* **1988,** 49. Chemoenzymatic stereospecific synthesis and biological activity of racemate and enantiomers: D. Bianchi *et al., J. Agric. Food Chem.* **39,** 197 (1991); stereoselective inhibition of ergosterol biosynthesis: F. Gozzo *et al., Pestic. Biochem. Physiol.* **53,** 10 (1995). ELISA of commercial prepns: F. Forlani *et al., J. Agric. Food Chem.* **40,** 328 (1992). Field trial on wheat: D. Pancaldi, I. Alberti, *Informat. Fitopatolog.* **44,** 48 (1994).

Viscous colorless oil. Vapor pressure (20°): 1.2× 10^{-5} mmHg. Log P (octan-1-ol/water): 3.1 (pH 7). Stable in dil. aq. soln at pH 5-9. Stable in sunlight. Soly (20°) mg/l: water 150. Readily sol in dichloromethane, acetone and methanol. LD_{50} orally in rats: 1150 mg/kg (Garavaglia).

USE: Agricultural fungicide.

9194. Tetracosamethylhendecasiloxane. [107-53-9] Tetracosamethylundecasiloxane. $C_{24}H_{72}O_{10}Si_{11}$; mol wt 829.76. C 34.74%, H 8.75%, O 19.28%, Si 37.23%. Prepd by reaction of

hexamethyldisiloxane with octamethylcyclotetrasiloxane and sulfuric acid: Patnode, Wilcock, *J. Am. Chem. Soc.* **68,** 362 (1946); by cohydrolysis of ethoxytrimethylsilane and diethoxydimethylsilane: Hyde, **US 2457677** (1948 to Corning Glass).

Liquid; $bp_{4.7}$ 201°; $bp_{0.5}$ 152°; d_4^{25} 0.9247; n_D^{20} 1.3994. Stable. Inert to most chemical reagents and rubber. Maintains about the same viscosity over a wide temperature range. Sol in benzene and the lighter hydrocarbons; slightly sol in alcohol and the heavy hydrocarbons.

USE: As a basis for silicone oils or fluids designed to withstand extremes of temperature; as a foam suppressant in petroleum lubricating oil.

9195. Tetracyanoethylene. [670-54-2] Ethenetetracarbonitrile; 1,1,2,2-tetracyanoethene; $\Delta^{2,2'}$-bimalononitrile; TCNE. C_6-N_4; mol wt 128.09. C 56.26%, N 43.74%. Prepd by debromination of dibromomalononitrile with copper powder in boiling benzene: Cairns *et al., J. Am. Chem. Soc.* **80,** 2775 (1958).

Crystals, mp 200°. Begins to sublime at 120°.

USE: In the synthesis of spiro compds, in modified Diels-Alder reactions, as aromatizing agent: Longone, Smith, *Tetrahedron Lett.* **1962,** 205.

9196. Tetracycline. [60-54-8] [4S-(4α,4aα,5aα,6β,12aα)]-4-(Dimethylamino)-1,4,4a,5,5a,6-11,12a-octahydro-3,6,10,12,12a-pentahydroxy-6-methyl-1,11-dioxo-2-naphthacenecarboxamide; deschlorobiomycin; tsiklomitsin; Liquamycin. $C_{22}H_{24}N_2O_8$; mol wt 444.43. C 59.45%, H 5.44%, N 6.30%, O 28.80%. Antibiotic substance produced by *Streptomyces spp.* Prepn: J. H. Boothe *et al., J. Am. Chem. Soc.* **75,** 4621 (1953); L. H. Conover *et al., ibid.* 4622; Conover, **US 2699054** (1955). Production by *Streptomyces viridifaciens:* Gourevitch, Lein, Heinemann *et al.,* **US 2712517;** **US 2886595** (1955, 1959 both to Bristol Labs.); by *S. aureofaciens:* Miller, Arishima, Sekizwa, **US 3005023; US 3019173** (1961, 1962 both to Am. Cyanamid). Purification: Kaplan, Granatek, **US 3301899** (1967 to Bristol-Myers). Total synthesis of tetracyclines: J. H. Boothe *et al., J. Am. Chem. Soc.* **81,** 1006 (1959); L. H. Conover *et al., ibid.* **84,** 3222 (1962). Graphic outline of Woodward synthesis: *Chem. Eng. News* **40,** 36 (Oct. 8, 1962). Abs config: V. N. Dobrynin *et al., Tetrahedron Lett.* **1962,** 901. Solubility studies: Weiss *et al., Antibiot. Chemother.* **7,** 374 (1957). Toxicity: E. I. Goldenthal, *Toxicol. Appl. Pharmacol.* **18,** 185 (1971). Review: "Tetracycline" in *The Technology of the Tetracyclines* vol. I, R. C. Evans, Ed. (Quadrangle Press, New York, 1968) pp 209-426. Mechanism of action: A. Kaji, M. Ryoji in *Antibiotics* vol. 5 (pt. 1), F. E. Hahn, Ed. (Springer-Verlag, New York, 1979) pp 304-328. Review of biosynthesis: C. R. Hutchinson in *Antibiotics* vol. 4, J. W. Corcoran, Ed. (Springer-Verlag, New York, 1981) pp 1-12. Review of anticollagenase activity of tetracyclines: L. M. Golub *et al., Crit. Rev. Oral Biol. Med.* **2,** 297-322 (1991).

Trihydrate, crystals. Swells at 165°. Dec 170-175°. Becomes anhydr by drying *in vacuo* at 60° for 8 hrs. $[\alpha]_D^{25}$ −257.9° (0.1N HCl); $[\alpha]_D^{25}$ −239° (methanol). uv max (0.1N HCl): 220, 268, 355 nm (ε 13000, 18040, 13320). pKa (50% aq DMF): 8.3, 10.2. Stable in neutral and in alkaline soln. Soly at about 28°: 1.7

mg/ml water; >20 mg/ml methanol. LD$_{50}$ in rats, mice (mg/kg): 807, 808 orally (Goldenthal).

Hydrochloride. [64-75-5] Achromycin; Ambramicina; Diocyclin; Helvecyclin; Hexacycline; Hostacyclin; Imex; Panmycin; Robitet; Steclin; Sumycin; Supramycin; Sustamycin; Tefilin; Tetracyn; Tetralution; Tetsol; Topicycline. C$_{22}$H$_{24}$N$_2$O$_8$·HCl; mol wt 480.90. Crystals from butanol + HCl, dec 214°. [α]$_D^{25}$ −257.9° (c = 0.5 in 0.1*N* HCl). Freely sol in water, sol in methanol, ethanol. Insol in ether, hydrocarbons. pH (2% aq soln): 2.1-2.3. LD$_{50}$ orally in rats: 6443 mg/kg (Goldenthal).

Phosphate complex. [1336-20-5] Tetrex. Prepn: Seiger, Weidenheimer, **US 3053892** (1962 to Am. Cyanamid). Yellow, odorless powder. Sparingly sol in water; slightly sol in ethanol.

THERAP CAT: Antiamebic; antibacterial; antirickettsial.

THERAP CAT (VET): Antibacterial.

9197. Tetradecamethylhexasiloxane. [107-52-8] C$_{14}$H$_{42}$O$_5$Si$_6$; mol wt 458.99. C 36.63%, H 9.22%, O 17.43%, Si 36.71%. Prepd by hydrolysis of dimethyldichlorosilane and trimethylchlorosilane: Patnode, Wilcock, *J. Am. Chem. Soc.* **68,** 358 (1946); by reaction of hexamethyldisiloxane with octamethylcyclotetrasiloxane and sulfuric acid: *eidem, ibid.* 362; Patnode, **US 2469888** (1949 to General Electric); by cohydrolysis of ethoxytrimethylsilane and diethoxydimethylsilane: Hunter *et al., J. Am. Chem. Soc.* **68,** 2284 (1946); Hyde, **US 2457677** (1948 to Corning Glass).

$$(H_3C)_3Si\left[O-\underset{\underset{CH_3}{|}}{\overset{\overset{CH_3}{|}}{Si}}-O\right]_2 Si(CH_3)_3$$

Liquid; bp$_{20}$ 142°; d$_4^{20}$ 0.8910; n$_D^{20}$ 1.3948; flash pt 118.33°C. Freezes below −100°. Stable. Inert to most chemical reagents and rubber. Maintains about the same viscosity over a wide temp range. Sol in benzene and the lighter hydrocarbons; slightly sol in alcohol and the heavy hydrocarbons.

USE: As a basis for silicone oils or fluids designed to withstand extremes of temp; as a foam suppressant in petroleum lubricating oil.

9198. Tetradifon. [116-29-0] 1,2,4-Trichloro-5-[(4-chlorophenyl)sulfonyl]benzene; *p*-chlorophenyl 2,4,5-trichlorophenyl sulfone; 2,4,5,4'-tetrachlorodiphenyl sulfone; tedion; Tedion-V18. C$_{12}$H$_6$Cl$_4$O$_2$S; mol wt 356.05. C 40.48%, H 1.70%, Cl 39.83%, O 8.99%, S 9.01%. Prepn: Meltzer, Huisman, **US 2812281** (1957 to Phillips); and soly data: Huisman *et al., Rec. Trav. Chim.* **77,** 103 (1958). Toxicity study: Ben-dyke *et al., World Rev. Pest Control* **9,** 119 (1970).

Crystals from benzene; mp 146.5-147.5°. Stable to concd and dil alkalies, mineral acids, high temp, and uv light. LD$_{50}$ orally in rats: 556 mg/kg (Ben-dyke).

USE: Acaricide. Ovicide on deciduous fruits, citrus, cotton and other crops.

9199. Tetraethylammonium Bromide. [71-91-0] *N,N,N*-Triethylethanaminium bromide; TEAB; TMD-10; Etylon; Etambro; Sympatektoman; Tetranium. C$_8$H$_{20}$BrN; mol wt 210.16. C 45.72%, H 9.59%, Br 38.02%, N 6.66%. (C$_2$H$_5$)$_4$NBr. Ganglion blocking agent. Prepd from triethylamine and ethyl bromide: Hofmann, *Ann.* **78,** 263 (1851). Review of the pharmacology of the tetraethylammonium ion: Moe, Freyburger, *Pharmacol. Rev.* **2,** 61-95 (1950).

Deliquesc crystals. Freely sol in water, alc, chloroform, acetone. Slightly sol in benzene. pH of a 10% aq soln 6.5. The pH is not changed by heating for 28 hrs at 95°.

9200. Tetraethylammonium Chloride. [56-34-8] *N,N,N*-Triethylethanaminium chloride; etamon chloride; TEA chloride. C$_8$H$_{20}$ClN; mol wt 165.70. C 57.99%, H 12.17%, Cl 21.40%, N

8.45%. N(C$_2$H$_5$)$_4$Cl. Potassium-selective ion channel blocker. Prepn: H. Schiff, U. Monsacchi, *Z. Phys. Chem.* **24,** 513 (1897). Synthetic applications: G. Coppens *et al., J. Org. Chem.* **27,** 3299 (1962); S. Gervat *et al., Tetrahedron Lett.* **34,** 2115 (1993). Hydrogen bonding structural studies: K. M. Harmon, J. M. Gabriele, *Inorg. Chem.* **20,** 4013 (1981); idem *et al., J. Mol. Struct.* **216,** 53 (1990). Toxicity studies: J. F. Keith, Jr. *et al., Circulation* **6,** 902 (1952). Mechanistic study of selective potassium channel binding: W. Jarolimek *et al., Mol. Pharmacol.* **49,** 165 (1996).

Deliquescent crystals. d$_4^{21}$ 1.0801. Freely sol in water, alcohol, chloroform, acetone; slightly sol in benzene. pH of 10% aq soln 6.48. LD$_{50}$ i.v. in dogs: 55.7-72.4 mg/kg (Keith, Jr.).

Tetrahydrate. [6024-76-6] Monoclinic prismatic crystals. mp 37.5°. d 1.084.

USE: Dehydrogenation catalyst; phase transfer catalyst in polymerization reactions. Electrolyte in membrane transport studies.

9201. Tetraethylammonium Hydroxide. [77-98-5] C$_8$H$_{21}$NO; mol wt 147.26. C 65.25%, H 14.37%, N 9.51%, O 10.86%. (C$_2$H$_5$)$_4$NOH. Made from the corresp halide by treating with silver oxide or with a soln of potassium hydroxide in methanol.

Marketed as an aq soln. A 10% soln has a d$_4^{20}$ ~1.01. The free base is known only in soln or as hydrates. Dec on boiling. It is a very strong base readily absorbing CO$_2$ from the air. The aq soln is colorless, odorless, bitter, caustic, strongly alkaline, and imparts a soapy feel to the skin. *Keep well closed.*

Tetrahydrate. mp 49-50°.

Hexahydrate. mp 55°.

9202. Tetraethyllead. [78-00-2] Tetraethylplumbane; lead tetraethyl; TEL. C$_8$H$_{20}$Pb; mol wt 323.44. C 29.71%, H 6.23%, Pb 64.06%. Pb(C$_2$H$_5$)$_4$. Prepd by the action of PbCl$_2$ on zinc ethyl or on a Grignard reagent; by heating C$_2$H$_5$Cl and sodium-lead alloy in an autoclave. Production from lead, ethylene, and hydrogen using triethylaluminum as intermediate was first described by K. Ziegler at the 14th International Congress of Pure and Applied Chemistry (July 1955): *Chem. Eng. News* **33,** 3486 (1955). Alternate synthesis using nonhalide compds: Pearson *et al.* in *Adv. Chem. Ser.* **23,** entitled "Metal-Organic Compounds," M. Sittig, Ed. (ACS, Washington DC, 1959) pp 299-305. *See also* Milde, Beatty, *ibid.,* 306-318. Toxicity study: Schroeder *et al., Experientia* **28,** 923 (1972). Review of toxicology and human exposure: *Toxicological Profile for Lead* (PB99-166704, 1999) 640 pp.

Colorless liq; burns with an orange-colored flame with green margin. *Extremely poisonous!* d^{20} 1.653. bp ~200° also stated as 227.7° with decompn. n$_D^{20}$ 1.5198. Practically insol in water. Sol in benzene, petr ether, gasoline, slightly in alcohol. LD$_{50}$ orally in rats: 12.3 mg/kg (Schroeder).

Caution: Potential symptoms of overexposure are insomnia, lassitude and anxiety; tremor, hyper-reflexia and spasticity; bradycardia, hypotension, hypothermia, pallor, nausea, anorexia and weight loss; confusion, disorientation, hallucinations, psychosis, mania, convulsions and coma; eye irritation. *See NIOSH Pocket Guide to Chemical Hazards* (DHHS/NIOSH 97-140, 1997) p 302. *See also Patty's Industrial Hygiene and Toxicology* vol. 2A, G. D. Clayton, R. E. Clayton, Eds. (Wiley-Interscience, New York, 3rd ed., 1981) pp 1687-1728; *Clinical Toxicology of Commercial Products,* R. E. Gosselin *et al.,* Eds. (Williams & Wilkins, Baltimore, 5th ed., 1984) Section II, p 139, Section III, pp 226-239.

USE: As a gasoline additive to prevent "knocking" in motors.

9203. *N,N,N',N'*-Tetraethylphthalamide. [83-81-8] *N,N,N',N'*-Tetraethyl-1,2-benzenedicarboxamide; orthophthalic acid didiethylamide; *o*-phthalic acid bis[diethylamide]; tetraethylbis-(phthalamide); Analetil; Neo-Cardiamine; Neospiran; Unispiran. C$_{16}$H$_{24}$N$_2$O$_2$; mol wt 276.37. C 69.53%, H 8.75%, N 10.14%, O 11.58%. Prepd by treating phthalyl chloride with diethylamine: **FR 785428; GB 443396; US 2057145** (1936 to Chem. Fabrik Grünau); by heating sodium phthalate with diethylamine phosphate: **FR 866229** (1941 to Corbière).

Crystals, mp 39°. bp 175-180°. Soluble in water, physiol saline.
THERAP CAT: Analeptic.

9204.   Tetraethyl Pyrophosphate. [107-49-3] Diphosphoric acid tetraethyl ester; pyrophosphoric acid tetraethyl ester; bis-*O,O*-diethylphosphoric anhydride; TEPP; Bladan; Nifos T; Kilmite 40; Vapotone; Tetron; Killax; Mortopal. $C_8H_{20}O_7P_2$; mol wt 290.19. C 33.11%, H 6.95%, O 38.59%, P 21.35%. Cholinesterase inhibitor. Prepd commercially by controlled hydrolysis of *O,O*-diethylphosphoric acid chloride: Kosolapoff, **US 2479939** (1947 to Monsanto); Toy, *J. Am. Chem. Soc.* **70**, 3882 (1948). Chemical history and comparison of various syntheses: G. Schrader, *Die Entwicklung neuer insektizider Phosphorsäure-Ester* (Verlag Chemie, Weinheim, 3rd ed., 1963) pp 68-79. Toxicity study: T. B. Gaines, *Toxicol. Appl. Pharmacol.* **14**, 515 (1969).

Mobile liquid. Agreeable odor. Hygroscopic. d_4^{20} 1.185. Thermal decompn range 170-213° with copious formn of ethylene. $bp_{0.05}$ 82°; $bp_{1.0}$ 124°; $bp_{2.3}$ 138°. Vapor pressure at 30° = 4.7 × 10^{-4} mm Hg. n_D^{20} 1.4196. Misc with water, but slowly hydrolyzed by it (half life at 25° about 7 hrs in a 50 v/v mixt.). Also misc with acetone, methanol, ethanol, benzene, chloroform, carbon tetrachloride, glycerol, ethylene glycol, propylene glycol, toluene, xylene. Not misc with petr ether, kerosene, other petr oils. LD$_{50}$ orally in male rats: 1.1 mg/kg (Gaines).
Caution: Potential symptoms of overexposure are eye pain, blurred vision, lacrimation, rhinorrhea, headache, tight chest and cyanosis; anorexia, nausea, vomiting and diarrhea; weakness, twitching, paralysis, Cheyne-Stokes respiration and convulsions; low blood pressure, cardiac irregularities; sweating. *See NIOSH Pocket Guide to Chemical Hazards* (DHHS/NIOSH 97-140, 1997) p 296.
USE: Insecticide.

9205.   Tetrafluoroethylene. [116-14-3] Tetrafluoroethene; perfluoroethene; TFE. C_2F_4; mol wt 100.02. C 24.02%, F 75.98%. $CF_2{=}CF_2$. Monomer of the plastic, polytetrafluoroethylene, *q.v.* Prepn: O. Ruff, O. Bretschneider, *Z. Anorg. Allg. Chem.* **210**, 173 (1933). Structural study: T. T. Broun, R. L. Livingston, *J. Am. Chem. Soc.* **74**, 6084 (1952). Physical properties: M. M. Renfrew, E. E. Lewis, *Ind. Eng. Chem.* **38**, 870 (1946). Addition reactions: D. D. Coffman *et al., J. Org. Chem.* **14**, 747 (1949). Thermodynamics and kinetics of mfr by pyrolysis of chlorodifluoromethane: P. B. Chinoy, P. D. Sunavala, *Ind. Eng. Chem. Res.* **26**, 1340 (1987). Review of mfr: Y. Venkateswarlu, P. S. Murti, *Chem. Process. Eng.* **4**, 25-36 (1970); of chemistry: M. Saijwani, Dinkar, *Labdev J. Sci. Tech.* **9-A**, 1-12 (1971); of toxicology: G. L. Kennedy, Jr., *Crit. Rev. Toxicol.* **21**, 149-170 (1990).
Colorless, odorless gas, bp_{760} −76.3°. mp −142.5°. d 1.519. Critical temp: 33.3°. Critical press.: 572 lb/sq in. Critical d 0.58. Insol in water. LC$_{50}$ (4 hr) in rats, mice, hamsters, guinea pigs (ppm): 37500-45000, 35000, 28500, 28000 (Kennedy). *Highly flammable when exposed to heat or flame. Reacts violently with oxygen.*
Caution: This substance is reasonably anticipated to be a human carcinogen: *Report on Carcinogens, Eleventh Edition* (PB2005-104914, 2004) p III-245.
USE: In mfr of polymers and synthesis of fluorinated refrigerants, dielectric media and solvents. In vinyl polymerization, cyclo-alkylation and addition reactions.

9206.   2,2,3,3-Tetrafluoro-1-propanol. [76-37-9] C_3-Fluoroalcohol. $C_3H_4F_4O$; mol wt 132.06. C 27.28%, H 3.05%, F 57.54%, O 12.12%. $HCF_2CF_2CH_2OH$. Prepn: Bestian, Rehn, **DE 1007771** (1957 to Hoechst).
Liquid. d_4^{20} 1.4853. mp −15°. bp_{760} 109-110°. n_D^{20} 1.3197. Surface tension at 20° = 27.6 dyn/cm.
p-Nitrobenzoate. mp 47°.
USE: To introduce fluoroalkyl groups into an organic molecule. Proposed intermediate for plastics, surface active agents, lubricants, elastomers.

9207.   Tetraglycine Hydroperiodide. [7097-60-1] Globaline. $C_{16}H_{42}I_7N_8O_{16}$; mol wt 1490.88. C 12.89%, H 2.84%, I 59.58%, N 7.52%, O 17.17%. 2[(NH$_2$CH$_2$COOH)$_4$HI].2½I$_2$. Prepn: Frost, Eddy, *J. Am. Chem. Soc.* **74**, 1346 (1952); Morris *et al., Ind. Eng. Chem.* **45**, 1013 (1953).
Flat needles with brassy-bronze metallic luster in reflected light, dec 162-167°. Soly in water at 25° = 380 g/l.
USE: Decontamination of drinking water in emergencies. Used in amounts sufficient to yield 8 ppm of active iodine. A tablet contg 20 mg plus 96 mg Na$_2$H$_2$PO$_7$ plus 4 mg talc will decontaminate one quart of water. Such tablets after 7 days' storage at 60° retained 60% of their original active iodine. Less stable than aluminum hexaurea sulfate triiodide.

9208.   Tetraglyme. [143-24-8] 2,5,8,11,14-Pentaoxapentadecane; tetraethylene glycol dimethyl ether; dimethoxytetraethylene glycol. $C_{10}H_{22}O_5$; mol wt 222.28. C 54.03%, H 9.98%, O 35.99%. $CH_3O(CH_2CH_2O)_4CH_3$. Prepd from ethylene glycol methyl ether and 2,2'-dichlorodiethyl ether: Zellhoefer, **US 2111234** (1935); *Ind. Eng. Chem.* **29**, 550 (1937). Purification: Vogel, *J. Chem. Soc.* **1948**, 618. Toxicity study: H. F. Smyth *et al., J. Ind. Hyg. Toxicol.* **23**, 259 (1941).
Liquid. d_4^{20} 1.0087; d_4^{86} 0.9514. mp −27°. bp_{760} 275.3°; bp_2 118°. n_D^{20} 1.4325. Sol in water. Misc with hydrocarbon solvents. LD$_{50}$ orally in rats: 5.14 g/kg (Smyth).
USE: Solvent.

9209.   Tetrahydrocannabinols. Psychoactive constituents of cannabis, *q.v.* (*Cannabis sativa* L. *Cannabinaceae*). The (−)-*trans*-Δ^9 isomer (Δ^9-THC) is the principal active constituent; the (−)-*trans*-Δ^8 isomer (Δ^8-THC), although physiologically active, is present to a lesser extent. Δ^9 analogs with shorter alkyl side chains have also been identified. Isoln from cannabis resin: H. J. Wollner *et al., J. Am. Chem. Soc.* **64**, 26 (1942). Isoln and structure of Δ^9-THC: Y. Gaoni, R. Mechoulam, *ibid.* **86**, 1646 (1964). Isoln of Δ^8-THC: R. L. Hively *et al., ibid.* **88**, 1832 (1966). Abs config of (−)-*trans*-Δ^9 isomer: R. Mechoulam, Y. Gaoni, *Tetrahedron Lett.* **1967**, 1109. Stereospecific synthesis of Δ^8- and Δ^9-THC: R. Mechoulam *et al., J. Am. Chem. Soc.* **89**, 4552 (1967); of Δ^9-THC: R. K. Razden *et al., ibid.* **96**, 5860 (1974); *eidem, Experientia* **31**, 16 (1975). IR, NMR, MS data: T. Petrzilka, C. Sikemeier, *Helv. Chim. Acta* **50**, 1416, 2111 (1967). Toxicity studies: H. Rosenkranz *et al., Toxicol. Appl. Pharmacol.* **28**, 18 (1974); H. Yoshimura *et al., J. Med. Chem.* **21**, 1079 (1978). Clinical experience with Δ^9-THC in chemotherapy induced nausea and vomiting: D. S. Poster *et al., J. Am. Med. Assoc.* **245**, 2047 (1981); as appetite stimulant in AIDS-associated anorexia: J. E. Beal *et al., J. Pain Symptom Manage.* **14**, 7 (1997). Chromatographic determn in cannabis products: L. Vollner *et al., Regul. Toxicol. Pharmacol.* **6**, 348-358 (1986). GC/MS determn in hair: M. J. Baptista *et al., Forensic Sci. Int.* **128**, 66 (2002). Review of pharmacology: W. L. Dewey, *Pharmacol. Rev.* **38**, 151-178 (1986); of pharmacokinetics and metabolism: F. Grotenhermen, *Clin. Pharmacokinet.* **42**, 327-360 (2003).

Δ^9-THC

(−)-*trans*-Δ^9-**Form.** [1972-08-3] (6a*R*,10a*R*)-6a,7,8,10a-Tetrahydro-6,6,9-trimethyl-3-pentyl-6*H*-dibenzo[*b,d*]pyran-1-ol; (−)-Δ^1-3,4-*trans*-tetrahydrocannabinol; Δ^9-THC; Δ^1-THC; dronabinol; QCD-84924; Marinol. $C_{21}H_{30}O_2$; mol wt 314.46. C 80.21%, H 9.62%, O 10.18%. Light yellow resinous oil; hardens upon refrigeration. $bp_{0.02}$ 200°. $[α]_D$ −150.5° (c = 0.53 in CHCl$_3$). pKa 10.6. uv max (ethanol): 283, 276 nm (log ε 3.21, 3.20). Essentially insol in water. LD$_{50}$ (sesame oil emulsion) in male rats (mg/kg): 800 orally; 35.5 i.v.; 672 i.p. (Rosenkranz).

(−)-*trans*-Δ^8-**Form.** [5957-75-5] (−)-Δ^6-3,4-*trans*-tetrahydrocannabinol; Δ^8-THC; Δ^6-THC. $bp_{0.001}$ 200°. $[α]_D^{18}$ −264° (c = 0.11 in ethanol). uv max (ethanol): 282, 275 nm (log ε 3.22,

3.22); shoulder at 230 nm (log ε 4.07). LD_{50} i.v. in mice: 27.5 mg/kg (Yoshimura).

Note: This is a controlled substance (hallucinogen): **21 CFR,** 1308.11.

THERAP CAT: Antiemetic; appetite stimulant.

9210. Tetrahydrocortisone. [53-05-4] $(3\alpha,5\beta)$-3,17,21-Tri-hydroxypregnane-11,20-dione; $3\alpha,17\alpha,21$-pregnanetriol-11,20-di-one; 11,20-pregnanedione-3α,17α,21-triol; THE. $C_{21}H_{32}O_5$; mol wt 364.48. C 69.20%, H 8.85%, O 21.95%. A normal mammalian metabolite of cortisone: Schneider, *J. Biol. Chem.* **183**, 365 (1950). Prepn by microbial reduction using a *Streptomyces* sp.: Barke-meyer *et al., Appl. Microbiol.* **8**, 237 (1960). Prepn of the triacetate: **GB 737291** (1955 to Merck & Co.). Prepn of the 21-acetate: Julian *et al.,* **US 2752339** (1956 to Glidden).

Crystals from ethyl acetate, mp 190°. $[\alpha]_D^{25}$ +85.5° (abs ethanol).
21-Acetate. $C_{23}H_{34}O_6$. Crystals from acetone, mp 227°.
Triacetate. $C_{27}H_{38}O_8$. Crystals from methanol, mp 150-152°; solvated crystals from ethyl acetate, mp 112-118°.

9211. Tetrahydrofuran. [109-99-9] Diethylene oxide; tetramethylene oxide. C_4H_8O; mol wt 72.11. C 66.62%, H 11.18%, O 22.19%. Prepn from 1,4-butanediol: Schmoyer, Case, *Nature* **187**, 592 (1960). Manuf by catalytic hydrogenation of maleic anhydride: Gilbert, Howk, **US 2772293** (1956 to du Pont); of furan: Banford, Manes, **US 2846449** (1958 to du Pont); Manly, **US 3021342** (1962 to Quaker Oats). Stabilization to prevent excessive peroxide formation on storage with 0.05-1.0% *p*-cresol, 0.05-0.1% hydroquinone, or less than 0.01-0.1% 4,4'-thiobis(6-*tert*-butyl-*m*-cresol): Bordner, Hinegardner, **US 2489260**; **US 2525410**; Campbell, **US 3029257** (1949, 1950, 1962 all to du Pont). Review of toxicology and biological effects: D. E. Moody, *Drug Chem. Toxicol.* **14**, 319-342 (1991).

Liquid. Ether-like odor. mp −108.5°. d_4^{20} 0.8892. bp$_{760}$ 66°; bp$_{176}$ 25°. Flash pt 1°F. n_D^{20} 1.4070. Dipole moment: 1.70. uv cut-off for spectro grade: 220 nm. Miscible with water, alcohols, ketones, esters, ethers, and hydrocarbons. *Caution:* Distil only in presence of a reducing agent, such as ferrous sulfate; peroxide explosions have occurred: *Angew. Chem.* **68**, 182 (1956).
Caution: Potential symptoms of overexposure are irritation of eyes and upper respiratory system; nausea, dizziness and headache; CNS depression. *See NIOSH Pocket Guide to Chemical Hazards* (DHHS/NIOSH 97-140, 1997) p 302.
USE: Solvent for high polymers, esp polyvinyl chloride. As reaction medium for Grignard and metal hydride reactions. In the synthesis of butyrolactone, succinic acid, 1,4-butanediol diacetate. Solvent in histological techniques. May be used under Federal Food, Drug & Cosmetic Act for fabrication of articles for packaging, transporting, or storing of foods if residual amount does not exceed 1.5% of the film: *Fed. Regist.* **27**, 3919 (Apr. 25, 1962).

9212. 2,5-Tetrahydrofurandimethanol. [104-80-3] THF glycol; 2,5-bis(hydroxymethyl)tetrahydrofuran. $C_6H_{12}O_3$; mol wt 132.16. C 54.53%, H 9.15%, O 36.32%. Prepd from diallyl by oxidation with perbenzoic acid in chloroform, boiling with dil sul-furic acid and hydrolyzing the reaction product with KOH soln: Böeseken, *Rec. Trav. Chim.* **45**, 838 (1926); by Raney nickel reduc-tion of 5-hydroxymethylfurfural or of dimethyl furan-2,5-dicarbox-ylate: Cope, Baxter, *J. Am. Chem. Soc.* **77**, 393 (1955). The usual form obtained is the *cis* form, described here.

Hygroscopic liquid. Faint odor. *Avoid contact with eyes.* d_4^0 1.1719; d_4^{25} 1.1542; d_4^{50} 1.1359. mp below −50°. bp$_{760}$ 265°; bp$_{96}$ 200°; bp$_{11}$ 155°; bp$_{0.25}$ 105°. n_D^{25} 1.4766. Viscosity (cP): 1926 at 0°; 225 at 25°; 51.9 at 50°. Coefficient of expansion: 0.00063 per °C at 25°. Specific heat 0.5 cal/g/°C. Heat of vaporization 115 cal/g. Miscible with water, methanol, ethanol, acetone, benzene, methyl acetate, methyl ethyl ketone, chloroform. Moderately sol in ether, toluene. Almost insol in heptane, methylcyclohexane.
Caution: Highly irritating to eyes, skin, mucous membranes.
USE: Solvent, softener, humectant. In the synthesis of plasticiz-ers, resins, surfactants, agricultural chemicals.

9213. Tetrahydrofurfuryl Alcohol. [97-99-4] Tetrahydro-2-furanmethanol; tetrahydro-2-furancarbinol; tetrahydro-2-furyl-methanol; THFA. $C_5H_{10}O_2$; mol wt 102.13. C 58.80%, H 9.87%, O 31.33%. Prepn by catalytic hydrogenation of furfuryl alcohol: Lukes, Nelson, *J. Org. Chem.* **21**, 1096 (1956). Manuf by catalytic hydrogenation of furfural or furfuryl alcohol: Dunlop, Schegulla, **US 2838523** (1958 to Quaker Oats). Occurs in two isomeric forms: D-isomer (levorotatory), L-isomer (dextrorota-tory). Abs config: Gagnaire, Butt, *Bull. Soc. Chim. Fr.* **1961**, 312; Hartman, Barker, *J. Org. Chem.* **29**, 873 (1964). *Review:* A. P. Dunlop, F. N. Peters, *The Furans* (Reinhold, New York, 1953).

Liquid. Hygroscopic. d_{20}^{20} 1.0543; d_{24}^{24} 1.0511; d_{31}^{31} 1.0450. Melts below −80°. bp$_{760}$ 178°. n_D^{20} 1.4520; n_D^{25} 1.4499. Flash pt, open cup: 183°F (84°C). Flammability in air: Upper limit 9.7% by vol, lower limit 1.5% by vol. Heat capacity at 30-37°: 0.432 cal/g/°C. Heat of combustion at constant vol: 708.6 cal/g mole. Viscosity at 20°: 6.24 cP. Surface tension at 25°: 37 dyn/cm. Octane no. 82.5. Evaporation rate: 7 (*n*-butyl acetate = 100). Kauributanol value 71.5. Dilution ratio (lacquer ingredi-ents): 4.5. Dielectric constant at 23°: 13.6. Miscible with water, alcohol, ether, acetone, chloroform, benzene.
L-Isomer. Prepn *see* Hartman, Barker, *loc. cit.* $[\alpha]_D^{24}$ +14.9° (c = 5.0 in nitromethane).
Caution: Moderately irritating to skin, mucous membranes.
USE: Solvent for fats, waxes, resins. In organic synthesis: Undergoes the reactions of a primary alcohol, while the ring exhibits characteristics of a saturated cyclic ether.

9214. Tetrahydrogestrinone. [618903-56-3] (17α)-13-Eth-yl-17-hydroxy-18,19-dinorpregna-4,9,11-trien-3-one; 18a-homo-pregna-4,9,11-trien-17β-ol-3-one; THG. $C_{21}H_{28}O_2$; mol wt 312.45. C 80.72%, H 9.03%, O 10.24%. Androgen and progestin; hydrogenation product of gestrinone, *q.v.* Discovery, synthesis, LC/MS/MS and GC/MS determn in urine: D. H. Catlin *et al., Rapid Commun. Mass Spectrom.* **18**, 1245 (2004). Hormonal prop-erties: A. K. Death *et al., J. Clin. Endocrinol. Metab.* **89**, 2498 (2004). *In vitro* metabolism study: J.-F. Lévesque *et al., Anal. Chem.* **77**, 3164 (2005).

Absorption max: 345 nm.
Note: This is a controlled substance (anabolic steroid): **21 CFR,** 1308.13, as defined in 1300.01.

9215. Tetrahydropalmatine. [10097-84-4] 5,8,13,13a-Tetrahydro-2,3,9,10-tetramethoxy-6*H*-dibenzo[*a,g*]quinolizine; 2,-3,9,10-tetramethoxyberbine; 2,3,9,10-tetramethoxydibenzo[*a,g*]-quinolizidine; hyndarin. $C_{21}H_{25}NO_4$; mol wt 355.43. C 70.96%,

H 7.09%, N 3.94%, O 18.01%. Synthesis of *dl*-form: Haworth *et al., J. Chem. Soc.* **1927**, 548; Bradsher, Dutta, *J. Org. Chem.* **26**, 2231 (1961); T. Kametani, M. Ihara, *J. Chem. Soc. C* **1967**, 530; G. D. Pandey, K. P. Tiwari, *Indian J. Chem.* **18B**, 545 (1979); Z. Kiparissides *et al., Can. J. Chem.* **58**, 2770 (1980); N. S. Narasimhan *et al., Tetrahedron Lett.* **22**, 2797 (1981). Biosynthesis: D. S. Bhakuni *et al., Tetrahedron* **36**, 2491 (1980). *See also* Palmatine. Both optically active forms are found in plants.

l-**Form.** Caseanine; gindarine; rotundine. Crystals from dil methanol, mp 147°. $[\alpha]_D^{20}$ −291° (c = 0.8 in 95% alcohol). Also a hydrate, mp 115° (effervescence).

Hydrochloride. $C_{21}H_{25}NO_4 \cdot HCl$. Crystals.

d-**Form.** Crystals from methanol, mp 141-142° (evac tube). $[\alpha]_D^{14}$ +292° (c = 0.8 in 95% alcohol).

Hydrochloride. Crystals, mp 266°.

dl-**Form.** Crystals from methanol upon addition of water. mp 148-149°.

Hydrochloride. Needles from methanol, mp 215-216°.

9216. Tetrahydropapaveroline. [4747-99-3] 1-[(3,4-Dihydroxyphenyl)methyl]-1,2,3,4-tetrahydro-6,7-isoquinolinediol; 1-(3,4-dihydroxybenzyl)-1,2,3,4-tetrahydro-6,7-isoquinolinediol; 6,7-dihydroxy-1-(3,4-dihydroxybenzyl)-1,2,3,4-tetrahydroisoquinoline; norlaudanosoline; THP. $C_{16}H_{17}NO_4$; mol wt 287.31. C 66.89%, H 5.96%, N 4.88%, O 22.27%. Alkaloid deriv of dopamine and a biosynthetic precursor of morphine, *q.v.* Prepn of the racemic hydrochloride: F. L. Pyman, *J. Chem. Soc.* **95**, 1610 (1909); of the (+)- and (−)-form hydrochlorides: S. Teitel *et al., J. Med. Chem.* **15**, 845 (1972). Chromatographic study: K. D. McMurtrey *et al., J. Liq. Chromatogr.* **3**, 663 (1980). Possible role of THP in the biochemical mediation of alcohol addiction: V. E. Davis, M. J. Walsh, *Science* **167**, 1005 (1970); G. Cohen, M. Collins, *ibid.* 1749; R. D. Meyers, C. L. Melchior, *ibid.* **196**, 554 (1977); M. Sandler *et al., Prog. Clin. Biol. Res.* **90**, 215 (1982). Biosynthetic study: D. K. Choudhary, B. L. Kaul, *Indian Drugs* **19**, 229 (1982). *In vivo* and *in vitro* effects on rat pituitary function: D. R. Britton *et al., Biochem. Pharmacol.* **31**, 1205 (1982). Effect on dopaminergic neurons: I. S. Hoffman, L. X. Cubeddu, *J. Pharmacol. Exp. Ther.* **220**, 16 (1982). Comparison to opioid effects in brain regions: G. R. Siggins *et al., Prog. Clin. Biol. Res.* **90**, 275 (1982).

(±)-Form hydrochloride. $C_{16}H_{18}ClNO_4$. Colorless microscopic prisms, mp 291-293° (dec). Practically insol in water, alc.

(−)-Form hydrochloride. Cryst from 6*N* HCl, mp 285-286°. $[\alpha]_D^{25}$ −32.4° (c = 1 in water). uv max (ethanol): 230, 286 nm (ε 11100, 6700).

(+)-Form hydrochloride. Cryst, mp 285-286°. $[\alpha]_D^{25}$ +32.1° (c = 1 in water).

USE: As a research tool in neurological biochemistry.

9217. Tetrahydropyran. [142-68-7] Pentamethylene oxide. $C_5H_{10}O$; mol wt 86.13. C 69.72%, H 11.70%, O 18.58%. Prepd by hydrogenation of dihydropyran (from furfural): Paul, *Bull. Soc. Chim. Fr.* [4] **53**, 1489 (1933); Andrus, Johnson, *Org. Synth.* **23**, 90 (1943); Cass, *Ind. Eng. Chem.* **40**, 219 (1948).

Mobile, flammable liquid. Pungent, sweetish odor. d_4^{20} 0.8814. mp −49.2°. bp 88°. n_D^{20} 1.4211. Dipole moment 1.87. Flash pt −4.0°F. Azeotrope with water, bp 71°, contains 8.5% H_2O. Sol in water [relative solubilities: Bennett, Philip, *J. Chem. Soc.* **1928**, (1939)]. Miscible with alcohol, ether, many other organic solvents. Forms peroxides on exposure to air. All technical tetrahydropyran is stabilized against peroxide formation.

9218. Tetrahydrothiophene. [110-01-0] Tetramethylene sulfide; thiacyclopentane; THT; THTP. C_4H_8S; mol wt 88.17. C 54.49%, H 9.15%, S 36.37%. Prepn: J. v. Braun, A. Trümpler, *Ber.* **43**, 545 (1910); J. K. Lawson *et al., Org. Synth.* **coll. vol. IV**, 892 (1963). Method for odorizing liquified natural gas: D. K. Mulliner, *Proc., Opec. Sect., Am. Gas Assoc.* **D**, 27 (1974). GC/MS determn in water: G. Carlucci *et al., J. Chromatogr.* **287**, 425 (1984). On-site GC determn in natural gas: R. C. M. de Nijs *et al., J. High Resolut. Chromatogr.* **16**, 379 (1993).

Colorless liquid, bp 119-121°. n_D^{25} 1.5000-1.5014. LD_{50} by inhalation in mice: 26.7 mg/l (Carlucci).

USE: Natural gas odorant.

9219. Tetrahydrozoline. [84-22-0] 4,5-Dihydro-2-(1,2,3,4-tetrahydro-1-naphthalenyl)-1*H*-imidazole; 2-(1,2,3,4-tetrahydro-1-naphthyl)-2-imidazoline; tetryzoline. $C_{13}H_{16}N_2$; mol wt 200.28. C 77.96%, H 8.05%, N 13.99%. Prepn from ethylenediamine, ethylenediamine hydrochloride, and methyl 1,2,3,4-tetrahydro-1-naphthoate: Synerholm *et al.*, **US 2731471** (1956 to Sahyun Labs.). Use as potentiator for veterinary depressants: Gardocki *et al.*, **US 2842478** (1958 to Pfizer).

Hydrochloride. [522-48-5] Rhinopront; Tyzine; Visine; Yxin. $C_{13}H_{16}N_2 \cdot HCl$; mol wt 236.74. Crystals from alcohol, dec 256-257°. uv max: 264.5, 271.5 nm ($A_{1cm}^{1\%}$ 17.5, 15.5). Freely sol in water, alcohol. Very slightly sol in chloroform. Practically insol in ether. pH of a 1% aq soln 5.0 to 6.5.

THERAP CAT: Adrenergic (vasoconstrictor); nasal decongestant.

9220. Tetraiodoethylene. [513-92-8] Tetraiodoethene; diiodoform; ethylene periodide; ethylene tetraiodide. C_2I_4; mol wt 531.64. C 4.52%, I 95.48%. $I_2C=CI_2$. Prepd by the action of iodine on diiodoacetylene obtained from calcium carbide and iodine. Crystal and molecular structure: B. C. Haywood, R. Shirley, *Acta Crystallogr.* **B33**, 1765 (1977).

Light yellow, heavy, small, practically odorless crystals; characteristic odor. On exposure to light turns brown. d 2.98. mp 187°. Insol in water; sol in benzene, chloroform, toluene, CS_2, slightly in ether. *Protect from light.*

9221. Tetralin®. [119-64-2] 1,2,3,4-Tetrahydronaphthalene; Tetranap. $C_{10}H_{12}$; mol wt 132.20. C 90.85%, H 9.15%. Prepd by catalytic hydrogenation of purified naphthalene. Toxicity study: Smyth *et al., Arch. Ind. Hyg. Occup. Med.* **4**, 119 (1951). *See* references under Decalin.

Liquid. Odor resembling that of a mixture of benzene and menthol. d_4^{20} 0.9702; d_4^{25} 0.9662. Volatile with steam; mp −31.0°;

bp_{760} 207.2°; bp_{400} 181.8°; bp_{200} 157.2°; bp_{100} 135.3°; bp_{60} 121.3°; bp_{40} 110.4°; bp_{20} 93.8°; bp_{10} 79.0°; bp_5 65.3°; $bp_{1.0}$ 38.0°. n_D^{20} 1.54135; n_D^{25} 1.53919. Flash pt, open cup 171°F (77°C), closed cup 180°F (82°C). Insol in water; miscible with ethanol, butanol, acetone, benzene, ether, chloroform, petr ether, Decalin; soluble in methanol: 50.6% w/w. Prolonged, intimate contact with air may cause the formn of tetralin peroxide which may cause explosion of tetralin distn residues. Peroxide formn is prevented by the addn of an antioxidant, such as hydroquinone. LD_{50} orally in rats: 2.86 g/kg (Smyth).

Caution: Irritating to skin, eyes, mucous membranes, and, in high concns, narcotic. In exptl animals has produced cataracts: E. Browning, *Toxicity and Metabolism of Industrial Solvents* (Elsevier, New York, 1965) pp 119-124.

USE: Degreasing agent. Solvent for naphthalene, fats, resins, oils, waxes, used instead of turpentine in lacquers, shoe polishes, floor waxes.

9222. Tetralol. [530-91-6] 1,2,3,4-Tetrahydro-2-naphthalenol; *ac*-tetrahydro-β-naphthol; *ac*-β-tetralol. $C_{10}H_{12}O$; mol wt 148.20. C 81.04%, H 8.16%, O 10.80%. Prepd by hydrogenation of 2-naphthol in the presence of a palladium catalyst: Foreman, Stork, **US 2526859** (1950 to Lakeside Labs.); by reduction of 2-naphthol with sodium: Hueckel *et al., Ann.* **645,** 162 (1961). Toxicity study: Draize *et al., J. Pharmacol. Exp. Ther.* **93,** 26 (1948).

Liquid, bp_{12} 140°; mp 15.5°. Crystallizes on prolonged storage at −50° and then at −15°. LD_{50} orally in rats: 1.0 ml/kg (Draize).

p-**Tosylate.** $C_{10}H_{11}O_3S.C_6H_4CH_3$. Crystals from petr ether + benzene, mp 86°.

Methyl ether. $C_{10}H_{11}OCH_3$. bp_{11} 114.5°, d_4^{20} 1.0239, n_D^{20} 1.5326.

9223. Tetramethrin. [7696-12-0] 2,2-Dimethyl-3-(2-methyl-1-propenyl)cyclopropanecarboxylic acid (1,3,4,5,6,7-hexahydro-1,3-dioxo-2*H*-isoindol-2-yl)methyl ester; 2,2-dimethyl-3-(2-methylpropenyl)cyclopropanecarboxylic acid ester with *N*-(hydroxymethyl)-1-cyclohexene-1,2-dicarboximide; *N*-(3,4,5,6-tetrahydrophthalimide)methyl-*cis,trans*-chrysanthemate; *N*-(chrysanthemoxymethyl)-1-cyclohexene-1,2-dicarboximide; phthalthrin; FMC-9260; SP-1103; Neo-Pynamin. $C_{19}H_{25}NO_4$; mol wt 331.41. C 68.86%, H 7.60%, N 4.23%, O 19.31%. Synthetic pyrethroid insecticide. Prepn of racemic mixture: T. Kato *et al.,* **JP 65 8535**; *eidem,* **US 3268398** (1965, 1966 both to Sumitomo). Activity: *eidem, Agric. Biol. Chem.* **28,** 914 (1965). Comparative activity of isomers: Y. Okuno *et al.,* **DE 2348930**; *eidem,* **US 3934023** (1973, 1976 both to Sumitomo). Metabolism: J. Miyamoto *et al., Agric. Biol. Chem.* **32,** 628 (1968). Photodecompn: Y.-L. Chen, J. E. Casida, *J. Agric. Food Chem.* **17,** 208 (1969). Toxicity study: T. Kato *et al., Agric. Biol. Chem.* **28,** 914 (1965). Review of toxicology and human exposure: *Toxicological Profile for Pyrethrins and Pyrethroids* (PB2004-100004, 2003) 332 pp.

(1R-trans)-form

The commercial product is a mixture of isomers. White crystalline solid, mp 65-80°. d_{20}^{20} 1.108; $n_D^{21.5}$ 1.5175. LD_{50} orally in mice: 1000 mg/kg (Kato).

USE: Insecticide.

9224. Tetramethylammonium Hydroxide. [75-59-2] *N,N,N*-Trimethylmethanaminium hydroxide. $C_4H_{13}NO$; mol wt 91.15. C 52.71%, H 14.38%, N 15.37%, O 17.55%. $(CH_3)_4NOH$. Usually marketed in 10% aq soln. Strong ammonia-like odor. d_4^{25} ~1.00. The free base is known only in soln or as a solid pentahydrate, forming colorless, deliquesc needles, mp 63°. On

distillation, it dec to trimethylamine and CH_3OH. It is a very strong base, readily absorbing CO_2 from the air. *Keep well closed.*

9225. Tetramethylammonium Iodide. [75-58-1] C_4H_{12}-IN; mol wt 201.05. C 23.90%, H 6.02%, I 63.12%, N 6.97%. $(CH_3)_4NI$.

Pale yellow crystals. Begins to dec at about 230°. d 1.84. Sparingly sol in water, freely in abs alcohol; insol in chloroform, ether.

USE: Emergency disinfection of drinking water. Required dosage: 8 ppm of iodine.

9226. Tetramethyldiaminobutane. [111-51-3] *N,N,N',N'*-Tetramethyl-1,4-butanediamine; *N,N,N',N'*-tetramethylputrescine. $C_8H_{20}N_2$; mol wt 144.26. C 66.61%, H 13.97%, N 19.42%. $(CH_3)_2N(CH_2)_4N(CH_3)_2$. From root and herb of *Hyoscyamus reticulatus* L. and *H. muticus* L., *Solanaceae:* Willstätter, Heuber, *Ber.* **40,** 3869 (1907); Konowalowa, Magidson, *Arch. Pharm.* **266,** 449 (1928). Synthesis: Lunsford *et al., J. Org. Chem.* **22,** 1225 (1957); Solov'ev, Skoldinov, *Zh. Obshch. Khim.* **33,** 1821 (1963), *C.A.* **59,** 7360f (1963).

White crystals; penetrating odor and sharp, scratching taste. bp 169°; bp_{28} 78-80°; bp_7 43°. n_D^{20} 1.4280. d^{20} 0.7861. Volatile with steam. Sol in water, alc, ether.

Dihydrochloride. $C_8H_{20}N_2.2HCl$. Crystals from alc, mp 273°.

Dipicrate. $C_8H_{20}N_2.2C_6H_3N_3O_7$. Needles from hot water, mp 203-205°.

9227. Tetramethylenedisulfotetramine. [80-12-6] 2,6-Dithia-1,3,5,7-tetraazatricyclo[3.3.1.1^{3,7}]decane 2,2,6,6-tetraoxide; 2,6-dithia-1,3,5,7-tetraazaadamantane 2,2,6,6-tetraoxide. $C_4H_8N_4$-O_4S_2; mol wt 240.26. C 20.00%, H 3.36%, N 23.32%, O 26.64%, S 26.69%. Prepd from sulfamide, $H_2NSO_2NH_2$ and formaldehyde in 60% H_2SO_4: Hecht, Henecka, *Angew. Chem.* **61,** 365 (1949). Toxicity: Hagen, *Dtsch. Med. Wochenschr.* **75,** 183 (1950).

Cubic crystals from acetone, dec 255-260°. *Violent convulsive poison!* Stable to acids and alkalies in dilutions up to 0.1*N*. Dec upon prolonged boiling of aq solns. Soly in water about 0.25 mg/ml. Slightly sol in acetone. Insol in methanol, ethanol. LD in mice (mg/kg): 0.20 orally or s.c. (Hagen).

9228. Tetramethyl-*p*-phenylenediamine. [100-22-1] *N,N,-N',N'*-Tetramethyl-1,4-benzenediamine; Wurster's reagent; Wurster's blue. $C_{10}H_{16}N_2$; mol wt 164.25. C 73.12%, H 9.82%, N 17.06%. Prepn: Meyer, *Ber.* **36,** 2979 (1903); Cox, Smith, *J. Org. Chem.* **29,** 488 (1964).

Crystals from petr ether, mp 51-52°. bp 260°. Slightly sol in cold water; more sol in hot water; freely sol in alc, chloroform, ether, petr ether.

USE: In the form of the hydrochloride as a reagent in analytical chemistry.

9229. Tetramethylsilane. [75-76-3] TMS; silicon tetramethyl. $C_4H_{12}Si$; mol wt 88.22. C 54.46%, H 13.71%, Si 31.84%. $(CH_3)_4Si$. Two crystalline forms exist, α and β; β form is more stable. Prepn and properties: E. Krause, A. von Grosse in *Die Chemie der metall-organischen Verbindungen,* (Gebrüder Borntraeger, Berlin, 1937) pp 258-262; J. G. Aston *et al., J. Am. Chem. Soc.* **63,** 2343 (1941); S. Tannenbaum *et al., ibid.* **75,** 3753 (1953). Dielectric properties: A. P. Altshuller, L. Rosenblum, *ibid.* **77,** 272 (1955). Temperature dependence of magnetic susceptibility, ^1H, and ^{13}C chemical shifts: F. G. Morin *et al., J. Magn. Reson.* **48,** 138 (1982). Thermodynamic properties: W. V. Steele, *J. Chem. Thermodynam.* **15,** 595 (1983). Use in chemical vapor deposition of films of silicon carbide, *q.v.*: N. Herlin *et al.*, *J. Phys. Chem.* **96,** 7063 (1992); A. Grill, V. Patel, *J. Appl. Phys.* **85,** 3314 (1999). Definition of ^1H resonance of TMS as the NMR primary standard: R. K. Harris *et al.*, *Pure Appl. Chem.* **73,** 1795 (2001).

Liquid, mp $-102.12°$ (α-form), $-99.04°$ (β-form). bp 26.6°. d 0.636 at bp. d_4^0 0.6688. d_4^{20} 0.6464. n_D^{20} 1.3588. Heat of vaporization at normal bp: 5785.1 ± 16.0 cal/mole. Dielectric constant at 20°: 1.921.

USE: NMR reference standard. In semiconductor applications (chemical vapor deposition).

9230. Tetramethylurea. [632-22-4] TMU; Temur. C_5H_{12}-N_2O; mol wt 116.16. C 51.70%, H 10.41%, N 24.12%, O 13.77%. $[(CH_3)_2N]_2CO$. Prepn: Lawson, Croom, *J. Org. Chem.* **28,** 232 (1963). Review of prepn, manuf, properties and use as solvent and as reagent: Lüttringhaus, Dirksen, *Angew. Chem. Int. Ed.* **3,** 260 (1964).

Liquid with faint, pleasant odor, bp 176.5°, bp_{74} 174.5°, bp_{12} 63-64°. mp $-1.2°$. Flash pt ~75°C. d_4^{25} 0.9687. n_D^{25} 1.4493. Dipole moment: 3.47 D in benzene. pKb 2. uv max: 217.5 nm (ε 1940). Miscible with water and with all common organic solvents including petr ether. LD_{50} i.v. in rats: 1.1 g/kg (Lüttringhaus, Dirksen).

USE: As solvent and reagent.

9231. Tetrandrine. [518-34-3] (1β)-6,6',7,12-Tetramethoxy-2,2'-dimethylberbaman. $C_{38}H_{42}N_2O_6$; mol wt 622.75. C 73.29%, H 6.80%, N 4.50%, O 15.41%. From root of *Stephania tetrandra* S. Moore, *Menispermaceae*. Isoln: Kondo, Yano, *Ann.* **497,** 90 (1932). Structure: Fujita, Murai, *J. Pharm. Soc. Jpn.* **71,** 1039 (1951). Synthesis: Kataoka, *C.A.* **51,** 16501i (1957). Total synthesis: Inubushi *et al.*, *Tetrahedron Lett.* **1968,** 3399; *eidem, J. Chem. Soc. C* **1969,** 1547. Present in the Chinese drug han-fang-chi.

Needles. mp 217-218°. $[\alpha]_D^{26}$ +252.4° (chloroform). Practically insol in water, petr ether; sol in ether and some other organic solvents.

l-**Form.** [1263-79-2] Phaenthine. mp 210°. $[\alpha]_D^{20}$ $-278°$ (chloroform).

THERAP CAT: Analgesic; antipyretic.

9232. Tetranectin. [109489-77-2] Tetrameric protein isolated from human plasma. Enhances plasminogen activation catalyzed by tissue plasminogen activator, *q.v.* Composed of four identical, non-covalently bound, polypeptide chains each containing 181 amino acids, with mol wt 20,100 daltons. Isoln from human serum: I. Duhl Clemmensen, C. Kluft, **EP 206400** (1986 to Ned. Cent. Org. Toegepast-Natuurwetenschappelijk Onderzoek). Purification, characterization and plasminogen binding activity: I. Clemmensen *et al.*, *Eur. J. Biochem.* **156,** 327 (1986). Primary structure: J. Fuhlendorff *et al.*, *Biochemistry* **26,** 6757 (1987). Enzyme-linked immunoassay in human plasma: B. A. Jensen *et al.*, *J. Lab. Clin. Med.* **110,** 612 (1987). Distribution in human endocrine tissue: L. Christensen *et al.*, *Histochemistry* **87,** 195 (1987). Possible role in cancer metastasis: B. A. Jensen, I. Clemmensen, *Cancer* **62,** 869 (1988).

Isoelectric point 5.8. $E_{280nm}^{1\%}$ 12.5.

9233. Tetranitromethane. [509-14-8] CN_4O_8; mol wt 196.03. C 6.13%, N 28.58%, O 65.29%. $C(NO_2)_4$. Prepd by nitration of acetic anhydride with anhydrous nitric acid: Liang, *Org. Synth.* **coll. vol. III,** p 803 (1955).

Pale yellow liquid. d_4^{25} 1.6229; d_4^{25} 1.638 (tech). mp 13.8°. bp_{760} 126°; $bp_{25.8}$ 40°; $bp_{14.9}$ 30°; $bp_{8.4}$ 20°; $bp_{5.7}$ 13.8°; $bp_{1.9}$ 0°. n_D^{20} 1.4384; n_D^{25} 1.4358. Viscosity at 20° = 1.76 cP. Energy of decompn: Tschinkel, *Ind. Eng. Chem.* **48,** 732 (1956). Insol in water. Freely sol in alcohol, ether, alcoholic KOH. Attacks iron, copper, brass, zinc, rubber. Highly explosive in the presence of impurities.

Caution: Potential symptoms of overexposure are irritation of eyes, skin, nose and throat; dizziness; headache; chest pain, dyspnea; methemoglobinuria, cyanosis; skin burns. *See NIOSH Pocket Guide to Chemical Hazards* (DHHS/NIOSH 97-140, 1997) p 304. *See also Patty's Industrial Hygiene and Toxicology* vol. **2A,** G. D. Clayton, F. E. Clayton, Eds. (John Wiley & Sons, New York, 4th ed., 1994) 614-617. This substance is reasonably anticipated to be a human carcinogen: *Report on Carcinogens, Eleventh Edition* (PB2005-104914, 2004) p III-246.

USE: Oxidizer in rocket propellants. As explosive in admixture with toluene. To increase cetane number of diesel fuels. Reagent for detecting the presence of double bonds in organic compds and for mild nitrations. Has been proposed as irritant war gas.

9234. Tetrantoin. [52094-70-9] 3',4'-Dihydrospiro[imidazolidine-4,2'(1'H)-naphthalene]-2,5-dione; 7,8-benzo-1,3-diazaspiro[4.5]decane-2,4-dione; S-2-676; Spirodon. $C_{12}H_{12}N_2O_2$; mol wt 216.24. C 66.65%, H 5.59%, N 12.95%, O 14.80%. Prepn: Novelli, *An. Farm. Bioquim.* **21,** 81 (1954), *C.A.* **50,** 4922 (1956); Faust *et al.*, *J. Am. Pharm. Assoc.* **46,** 118 (1957); Jules *et al.*, **US 2716648** (1955 to Cutter Labs.).

Crystals from ethanol or glacial acetic acid, mp 267-268°.

THERAP CAT: Anticonvulsant.

9235. Tetraphenylarsonium Bromide. [507-27-7] $C_{24}H_{20}$-AsBr; mol wt 463.24. C 62.23%, H 4.35%, As 16.17%, Br 17.25%. $(C_6H_5)_4AsBr$.

Dihydrate. Crystals. *Poisonous!* Loses all its water over sulfuric acid or at 100°. mp 281-284°. Sol in ~60 parts water; sol in alcohol or methanol, sparingly in acetone.

9236. Tetraphenylarsonium Chloride. [507-28-8] C_{24}-$H_{20}AsCl$; mol wt 418.79. C 68.83%, H 4.81%, As 17.89%, Cl 8.47%. $(C_6H_5)_4AsCl$. Willard, Smith, *Ind. Eng. Chem. Anal. Ed.* **11,** 186 (1939).

Dihydrate. Crystals. *Poisonous!* Loses all its water at 100°. mp 258-260°. Freely sol in water; sol in alcohol or methanol, sparingly in acetone.

USE: As a reagent for Cd, Hg, Zn, perchlorate, periodate, and other ions.

9237. Tetraphenylphosphonium. [18198-39-5] TPP^+. $[C_{24}H_{20}P]^+$. Membrane-permeable, lipophilic cation. Prepd as bromide: J. Dodonov, H. Medox, *Ber.* **61B,** 907 (1928); D. B. Denney, F. J. Gross, *J. Org. Chem.* **32,** 3710 (1967). As analytical reagent for identification of metals and their salts: H. H. Willard, L. R. Perkins, *Anal. Chem.* **25,** 1634 (1953); R. Neeb, *Z. Anal. Chem.* **154,** 17 (1957). Enhanced metal -TPP^+ complex determn by extraction-visible spectrophotometry: M. Siroki, L. Maric, *ibid.* **276,** 371 (1975). Solvent interactions: J. F. Coetzee, W. R. Sharpe, *J. Phys. Chem.* **75,** 3141 (1971). Use in determn of membrane potential in liposomes: K. Nakazato *et al.*, *Biochim. Biophys. Acta* **946,** 143 (1988); in hepatocytes: S. Saito *et al.*, *ibid.* **1111,** 221 (1992). NMR determn of TPP^+ driven potential: C. M. Franzin, P. M. Macdonald, *Biochemistry* **35,** 851 (1996).

USE: As analytical reagent for metals and their salts. As a probe for measuring membrane potential.

9238. Tetraphosphorus Trisulfide. [1314-85-8] Phosphorus sesquisulfide; trisulfurated phosphorus. P_4S_3; mol wt 220.09.

P 56.29%, S 43.71%. Prepn by fusing red phosphorus with sulfur: Stock, *Ber.* **43**, 150 (1910); also from white phosphorus and sulfur in a high-boiling solvent such as α-chloronaphthalene: Frary, **DE 309618** (1918); *Chem. Zentralbl.* **1919**, II, 55.

Yellowish-green, long, rhombic needles from benzene. Stable to air. d_4^{20} 2.03. mp 172.5°. bp 407.5°. Insol in cold water. Dec by hot water, yielding H_2S. Soly in carbon disulfide (20°): about 60% (w/w). Sol in benzene, similar hydrocarbons, phosphorus trichloride.

USE: In match tips.

9239. Tetrasilane. [7783-29-1] Tetrasilicon decahydride; silicobutane; tetrasilicane; tetrasilicobutane. $H_{10}Si_4$; mol wt 122.42. H 8.23%, Si 91.77%. Si_4H_{10}. Prepn by the action of hydrochloric acid on magnesium silicide: Stock, Somiesky, *Ber.* **49**, 111 (1916); **54B**, 524 (1921); **56B**, 247 (1923); Stock *et al., Ber.* **56**, 1695 (1923); Emeleus, Maddock, *J. Chem. Soc.* **1946**, 1131.

Liquid. mp ~ −90°; bp 109°; vapor pressure 7.8 mm Hg at 0° (Stock *et al., loc. cit.*). mp −84.3°; bp (calc) 107.4°; vapor pressure 9.1 mm Hg at 0° (Emeleus, Maddock, *loc. cit.*). d^0 0.825. Dec at room temp; explodes in air. Reacts vigorously with CCl_4 and $CHCl_3$. Dec in water.

9240. Tetrasodium Pyrophosphate. [7722-88-5] TSPP; pyro; sodium pyrophosphate. $Na_4O_7P_2$; mol wt 265.90. Na 34.58%, O 42.12%, P 23.30%. $Na_4P_2O_7$. Available alkalinity as Na_2O 4.4%, total alkalinity 22.7%. Produced by molecular dehydration of dibasic sodium phosphate at 500°: Bell, *Inorg. Synth.* **3**, 98 (1950).

Crystals, d 2.534. mp 988°. Soly in water (g/100 ml) at 0°: 2.61; at 25°: 6.70; at 100°: 42.2. pH of a 1% soln = 10.2. Hydrolyzes to orthophosphate in aq soln, but the rate of hydrolysis is much slower than for the more acid pyrophosphate. No noticeable hydrolysis within 60 hrs at 70°: Bell, *Ind. Eng. Chem.* **39**, 136 (1947).

Decahydrate. Crystals, d 1.82. mp 79.5°. Slight efflorescence in dry air. Soly in water (g/100 ml) at 0°: 3.16; at 20°: 6.23; at 25°: 8.14; at 60°: 21.83; at 80°: 30.04. pH of 1% soln at 25° = 10.2. Insol in alc.

Caution: Potential symptoms of overexposure are irritation of eyes, skin, nose, throat; dermatitis. *See NIOSH Pocket Guide to Chemical Hazards* (DHHS/NIOSH 97-140, 1997) p 304.

USE: In cleansing compds, oil-well drilling, water treatment, cheese emulsification, as general sequestering agent, to remove rust stains, as ingredient of one-fluid ink eradicators, in electrodeposition of metals.

9241. Tetrasulfur Tetranitride. [28950-34-7] Schwefelstickstoff. N_4S_4; mol wt 184.29. N 30.40%, S 69.60%. S_4N_4. Prepd by the interaction of disulfur dichloride and ammonia: Becke-Goehring, *Inorg. Synth.* **6**, 124 (1960).

Orange-red, monoclinic needles from benzene, mp 178°. Additional purification by sublimation in high vacuum, (bath temp 100°), mp 180°. bp$_{760}$ ~185°. Further heating results in deflagration and explosion. Practically insol in cold water, hydrolyzed by boiling water. Slightly sol in benzene, abs ethanol, carbon disulfide. *Handle with caution:* May dec explosively on striking or at temps much above 100°.

9242. Tetrathiafulvalene. [31366-25-3] 2-(1,3-Dithiol-2-ylidene)-1,3-dithiole; Δ 2,2'-bi-1,3-dithiole; bis-1,3-dithiole; 1,4,5,8-tetrathiafulvalene; TTF. $C_6H_4S_4$; mol wt 204.36. C 35.26%, H 1.97%, S 62.76%. Of interest in solid state chemistry as a conductor, catalyst or sensor due to its unusual electronic and magnetic properties. Primarily used as the parent compound for supramolecular assemblies. Prepn: F. Wudl *et al., Chem. Commun.* **1970**, 1453. In combination with TCNQ (*tetracyano-p-quinodimethane*) to form first "organic metal": J. Ferraris *et al., J. Am. Chem. Soc.* **95**, 948 (1973); electronic structure: R. Gleiter *et al., J. Electron. Spectrosc. Relat. Phenom.* **2**, 207 (1973). Use as a catalyst in radical reactions: R. J. Fletcher *et al., J. Chem. Soc. Perkin Trans. 1* **1995**, 623; J. A. Murphy, S. J. Roome, *ibid.* 1349. TTF-mediated biosensors for glucose: T. Yu *et al., J. Appl. Polym. Sci.* **58**, 973 (1995); for NADH: X. Zhang *et al., Anal. Commun.* **33**, 111 (1996); for gln and glu: A. Mulchandani, A. S. Bassi, *Biosens. Bioelectron.* **11**, 271 (1996). *Review:* T. Jorgensen *et al., Chem. Soc. Rev.* **23**, 41-51 (1994). Review of electrical properties and structural data of unsymmetric TTF cmpds: J. M. Fabre *et al., Synth. Met.* **35**, 57-64

(1990); of role in superconductors: M. R. Bryce, *J. Mater. Chem.* **5**, 1481-1496 (1995).

Orange solid in its neutral state; loses electrons to form purple cation radical and subsequent yellow dication. Also reported as yellow solid, mp 118.5-119°. Sublimes 100°, 0.3 mm. uv max (CH_2Cl_2): 290, 310 nm (ε 4 × 10^4, 4 × 10^4). Insol in water. Readily photo-oxidized in air to violet water-soluble radical cation. The cation is a deep purple crystalline solid, mp 155-165° (dec). uv max (H_2O): 250 nm (ε 4.7 × 10^4); absorption max (H_2O): 340, 405, 435, 575 nm (ε 4.4 × 10^4; 3.6 × 10^4; 5.6 × 10^4; 1.6 × 10^4). A counter ion is necessary to prevent further oxidation to the dication. Ethanolic solutions of the cation are stable for prolonged periods of time (>48hr).

USE: Molecular sensors; radical catalyst.

9243. Tetrazepam. [10379-14-3] 7-Chloro-5-(1-cyclohexen-1-yl)-1,3-dihydro-1-methyl-2*H*-1,4-benzodiazepin-2-one; 7-chloro-5-(1-cyclohexenyl)-1-methyl-2-oxo-2,3-dihydro-1*H*-[1,4]-benzo[*f*]diazepine; CB-4261; Musaril; Muskelat; Myolastan. C_{16}-$H_{17}ClN_2O$; mol wt 288.77. C 66.55%, H 5.93%, Cl 12.28%, N 9.70%, O 5.54%. Prepn: Schmitt, **NL 6600095** and **US 3426014**; **US 3551412** (1966, 1969, 1970 to Clin-Byla); Schmitt *et al., Chim. Ther.* **2**, 254 (1967). Spectroscopic and chromatographic studies: Lafargue *et al., Ann. Pharm. Fr.* **28**, 343, 477 (1970). GC-MS determn in urine: H. Maurer, K. Pfleger, *J. Chromatogr.* **422**, 85 (1987). Pharmacokinetics: H. Bun *et al., Arzneim.-Forsch.* **37**, 199 (1987). Pharmacology and benzodiazepine receptor study: P. E. Keane *et al., J. Pharmacol. Exp. Ther.* **245**, 692, 699 (1988). Clinical evaluation in post-stroke spasticity: I. Milanov, *Acta Neurol. Belg.* **92**, 5 (1992).

Yellow-brown crystals from ethyl acetate, mp 144°. uv max (ethanol): 227 nm (ε 28500). LD_{50} in mice (mg/kg): 415 i.p.; 2000 orally (Schmitt).

Note: This is a controlled substance (depressant): **21 CFR**, 1308.14.

THERAP CAT: Muscle relaxant (skeletal).

9244. Tetrazolium Blue. [1871-22-3] 3,3'-(3,3'-Dimethoxy[1,1'-biphenyl]-4,4'-diyl)bis[2,5-diphenyl-2*H*-tetrazolium] dichloride; 3,3'-dianisolebis[4,4'-(3,5-diphenyl)tetrazolium chloride]; blue tetrazolium; dimethoxy neotetrazolium; ditetrazolium chloride; BT. $C_{40}H_{32}Cl_2N_8O_2$; mol wt 727.64. C 66.03%, H 4.43%, Cl 9.74%, N 15.40%, O 4.40%. Prepn: A. M. Rutenburg *et al., Cancer Res.* **10**, 113 (1950); L. J. Pannone, J. B. Rust, **US 2713581** (1955 to Montclair Res. Corp. and Ellis-Foster Co.).

Lemon-yellow crystals, dec 242-245°. Freely sol in methanol, ethanol, chloroform. Slightly sol in water. Insol in ethyl acetate, acetone, ether. Reduction potential about −0.08 volt. Yields a dark blue diformazan pigment in the presence of a reducing agent.

USE: For research in seed germination, as stain for bacteria and molds, in histochemical studies, to demonstrate oxidation-reduction enzymes in normal and cancerous tissues. *See also* Triphenyltetrazolium Chloride.

9245. Tetrin. Polyene antifungal antibiotic produced by Streptomyces *Illinois* #155-2: Pote, *Diss. Abstr.* **19**, 2778 (1959); Gottlieb, Pote, *Phytopathology* **50**, 817 (1960). Isoln of the two tetraenes, tetrin A and B: Rinehart *et al., Ann.* **668**, 77 (1963); German, *Diss. Abstr.* **25**, 97 (1964). Structure of tetrin A: Pandey *et al., J. Am. Chem. Soc.* **93**, 3738 (1971); of tetrin B: Rinehart *et al., ibid.* 3747. Revised structure: R. C. Pandey, K. L. Rinehart, *J. Antibiot.* **29**, 1035 (1976). Mode of action of tetrin A: van Etten, Gottlieb, *J. Gen. Microbiol.* **46**, 377 (1967).

Tetrin A   R = H
Tetrin B   R = OH

Tetrin A. $C_{34}H_{51}NO_{13}$; mol wt 681.77. Fine, colorless needles from methanol or aqueous *n*-butanol, mp >350° (dec). $[\alpha]_D^{21}$ +8.3° (c = 0.72 in pyridine). $[\alpha]_D^{28}$ +27.5° (c = 1.0 in pyridine). uv max: 214, 278, 290, 303, 318 nm ($E_{1cm}^{0.1\%}$ 19.4, 44.2, 81.2, 115.0, 110.9). Monobasic, pKa' 8.30 in 60% ethanol. Sol in pyridine, dil alkalies, dil mineral acids; moderately sol in lower alcohols; practically insol in acetone, ether, water.

Tetrin B. $C_{34}H_{51}NO_{14}$; mol wt 697.77. Brown, amorphous powder, mp >360° (darkens at 160-165°, blackens at 250-295°). $[\alpha]_D^{24}$ +43.5° (c = 0.14 in methanol); $[\alpha]_D^{28}$ +45° (c = 0.3 in pyridine). uv max: 214, 278, 290, 303, 318 nm ($E_{1cm}^{0.1\%}$ 18.6, 51.4, 80.1, 112.8, 108.9). Readily sol in ethanol + water, dioxane + water; fairly sol in water, lower alcohols, dioxane, pyridine, dimethyl sulfoxide; slightly sol in acetone. Practically insol in ethyl acetate, chloroform, ether, ethylene dichloride.

9246. Tetrodotoxin. [4368-28-9] Octahydro-12-(hydroxymethyl)-2-imino-5,9:7,10a-dimethano-10a*H*-[1,3]dioxocino[6,5-*d*]pyrimidine-4,7,10,11,12-pentol; maculotoxin; spheroidine; tarichatoxin; tetrodontoxin; fugu poison; TTX. $C_{11}H_{17}N_3O_8$; mol wt 319.27. C 41.38%, H 5.37%, N 13.16%, O 40.09%. Toxin from the ovaries and liver of many species of *Tetraodontidae*, esp the globe fish *(Spheroides rubripes):* Yokoo, *J. Chem. Soc. Jpn.* **71**, 590 (1950), *C.A.* **45**, 6759c (1951). Identity with tarichatoxin: Buchwald *et al., Science* **143**, 474 (1963); with maculotoxin: D. D. Sheumack *et al., ibid.* **199**, 188 (1978). Structure studies: Goto *et al., Tetrahedron Lett.* **1963**, 2105, 2115; **1964**, 779, 1831. Structure: Woodward, *Pure Appl. Chem.* **9**, 49 (1964); Tsuda *et al., Chem. Pharm. Bull.* **12**, 1357 (1964); Goto *et al., Tetrahedron* **21**, 2059 (1965). Synthetic studies: Kishi *et al., Tetrahedron Lett.* **1970**, 5127, 5129. Total synthesis: Kishi *et al., J. Am. Chem. Soc.* **94**, 9219 (1972). Pharmacology: Evans, *Br. Med. Bull.* **25**, 263 (1969); Kao, *Fed. Proc.* **31**, 1117 (1972). Mechanism of action: Narahashi, *ibid.* 1124. Toxicity study: C. Y. Kao, F. A. Fuhrman, *J. Pharmacol. Exp. Ther.* **140**, 31 (1963). *Review:* Scheuer, *Fortschr. Chem. Org. Naturst.* **22**, 265 (1964); Mosher *et al., Science* **144**, 1100 (1964); Kao, *Pharmacol. Rev.* **18**, 997 (1966); Evans, *Int. Rev. Neurobiol.* **15**, 83 (1972); of total syntheses: U. Koert, *Angew. Chem. Int. Ed.* **43**, 5572-5576 (2004).

Darkens above 220° without dec. $[\alpha]_D^{25}$ −8.64° (c = 8.55 in dil acetic acid). pKa: 8.76 (water); 9.4 (50% alc). Sol in dil acetic acid; slightly sol in water, dry alc, ether. Practically insol in other organic solvents. Toxin destroyed in strong acids and in alkaline solns. LD_{50} i.p. in mice: 10 µg/kg (Kao, Fuhrman).

9247. Tetrofosmin. [127502-06-1] 6,9-Bis(2-ethoxyethyl)-3,12-dioxa-6,9-diphosphatetradecane; ethylenebis[bis(2-ethoxyethyl)phosphine]; P53. $C_{18}H_{40}O_4P_2$; mol wt 382.46. C 56.53%, H 10.54%, O 16.73%, P 16.20%. Prepn: J. D. Kelly *et al.,* **EP 337654**; *eidem,* **US 5045302** (1989, 1991 both to Amersham). Pharmacology and determn of radiochemical purity: *idem et al., J. Nucl. Med.* **34**, 222 (1993). Clinical biodistribution: B. Higley *et al., ibid.* 30. Clinical trial as a myocardial perfusion imaging agent: B. L. Zaret *et al., Circulation* **91**, 313 (1995).

^{99m}Tc-Complex. [127455-27-0] ^{99m}Tc tetrofosmin; $[^{99m}$Tc-(tetrofosmin)$_2$O$_2]^+$; PPN1011; Myoview. $C_{36}H_{80}O_{10}P_4{}^{99m}$Tc.
THERAP CAT: ^{99m}Tc-Complex as diagnostic aid (radioactive imaging agent).

9248. Tetronasin. [75139-06-9] 4-Hydroxy-3-[(2*S*)-2-[(1*S*,2*S*,6*R*)-2-[(1*E*)-3-hydroxy-2-[(2*R*,3*R*,6*S*)-tetrahydro-3-methyl-6-[(1*E*,3*S*)-3-[(2*R*,3*S*,5*R*)-tetrahydro-5-[(1*S*)-1-methoxyethyl]-3-methyl-2-furanyl]-1-butenyl]-2*H*-pyran-2-yl]-1-propenyl]-6-methylcyclohexyl]-1-oxopropyl]-2(5*H*)-furanone; antibiotic M139603; ICI-139603; M-139603. $C_{35}H_{54}O_8$; mol wt 602.80. C 69.74%, H 9.03%, O 21.23%. Polyether antibiotic produced by *Streptomyces longisporoflavus* NCIB 11426. Possesses a biosynthetically rare acid grouping in the form of an acyl tetronic acid moiety. Isoln and use in ruminants: D. H. Davies, G. L. Norris, **GB 2027013**; *eidem,* **US 4279894** (1980, 1981 both to ICI). Physical data and crystal structure: D. H. Davies *et al., Chem. Commun.* **1981**, 1073. Solution conformation and cation-binding properties: J. Grandjean, P. Laszlo, *Tetrahedron Lett.* **24**, 3319 (1983). Synthetic studies: A. M. Doherty, S. V. Ley, *ibid.* **27**, 105 (1986). Biosynthetic studies: J. M. Bulsing *et al., Chem. Commun.* **1984**, 1301; D. M. Doddrell *et al., ibid.* 1302; A. K. Demetriadou *et al., ibid.* **1985**, 408. Antimicrobial activity: C. J. Newbold *et al., Appl. Environ. Microbiol.* **54**, 544 (1988). Effect on gain efficiency in cattle: S. J. Bartle *et al., J. Anim. Sci.* **66**, 1502 (1988).

Sodium salt. $C_{35}H_{53}NaO_8$. mp 176-178°. $[\alpha]_D^{23}$ −82° (c = 0.2 in methanol). uv max (ethanol): 234, 270 nm (ε 13000, 11000). pKa 1.8 ±0.3 (methanol/H$_2$O 1:9). Sol in most organic solvents. Insol in water.
THERAP CAT (VET): Ruminant performance enhancer.

9249. Tetroquinone. [319-89-1] 2,3,5,6-Tetrahydroxy-2,5-cyclohexadiene-1,4-dione; tetrahydroxy-*p*-benzoquinone; tetrahydroxyquinone; THQ; HPEK-1; NSC-112931. $C_6H_4O_6$; mol wt 172.09. C 41.88%, H 2.34%, O 55.78%. Prepn from glyoxal: A. J. Fatiadi, W. F. Sager, *Org. Synth.* **coll. vol. V**, 1011 (1973). Clinical evaluation for ophthalmic fibrosis: R. Ching, *Eye Ear Nose Throat Mon.* **50**, 101, 144 (1971).
Dark, odorless, tasteless crystals with blue-black metallic luster in reflected light. mp 280°. Sol (1:200) in cold water; sol (1:100) in

hot water or in alcohol; slightly sol in ether. It acts like a strong dibasic acid.

Disodium salt. $Na_2C_6H_2O_6$. Almost black crystals with a green metallic luster, sparingly sol in water.

USE: Disodium salt is used as an indicator in the volumetric determination of sulfate by means of barium chloride solution.

9250. Tetroxoprim. [53808-87-0] 5-[[3,5-Dimethoxy-4-(2-methoxyethoxy)phenyl]methyl]-2,4-pyrimidinediamine; 2,4-diamino-5-[3,5-dimethoxy-4-(2-methoxyethoxy)benzyl]pyrimidine; HE-781. $C_{16}H_{22}N_4O_4$; mol wt 334.37. C 57.47%, H 6.63%, N 16.76%, O 19.14%. Analog of trimethoprim, q.v. Prepn: W. Liebenow, J. Prikryl, **FR 2221147**; *eidem*, **US 3992379** (1974, 1976 both to Heumann). Series of articles on tetroxoprim and other antibacterial folate inhibitors: *J. Antimicrob. Chemother.* **5,** Suppl. B, 1-239 (1979); on synthesis of radioactive tetroxoprim, tissue distribution, kinetics, HPLC determn: *Arzneim.-Forsch.* **30,** 307-319 (1980). Effect on bacterial growth kinetics: J. K. Seydel, E. Wempe, *Chemotherapy* **26,** 361 (1980). *In vitro* activity of the tetroxoprim-sulfadiazine combination: H. Hahn, A. Kirov, *Arzneim.-Forsch.* **30,** 1047 (1980).

Crystals from water, mp 153-156° (Liebenow, Prikryl); also reported as mp 160.1° (*eidem, J. Antimicrob. Chemother.* **5,** Suppl B, 15 (1979)). Soly at 30° (mg/ml): water 2.65; chloroform 69; *n*-octanol 1.61. pKb 8.25. LD_{50} orally in rats: 1357 mg/kg (Liebenow, Prikryl).

Mixture with sulfadiazine. [73173-12-3] Co-tetroxazine; Biroxin; Sterinor; Tibirox; Troximin.

THERAP CAT: Antibacterial.

9251. Texanol Isobutyrate. [6846-50-0] 2-Methylpropanoic acid 2,2-dimethyl-1-(1-methylethyl)-1,3-propanediyl ester; 2,2,4-trimethyl-1,3-pentanediol diisobutyrate; TXIB; $C_{16}H_{30}O_4$; mol wt 286.41. C 67.10%, H 10.56%, O 22.34%. Plasticizer for PVC and other resins. Prepn: U. Schwenk, A. Becker, *Ann.* **756,** 162 (1972). GC determn in PVC plastisol formulations: W. P. Hayes *et al., J. Chromatogr.* **139,** 395 (1977). Toxicology: B. D. Astill *et al., Toxicol. Appl. Pharmacol.* **22,** 387 (1972). Technical data sheet: "Eastman TXIB Plasticizer" (Eastman Chemical Co., publication L-151K, April 1998) 18 pp.

Colorless liquid, slightly fruity odor. bp_{760} 281.5°. fp −70°. Flash pt, closed cup: 262°F (128°C). d_{20}^{20} 0.942-0.948. n_D^{25} 1.4300. Soly in water (20°): 0.42 g/l. Viscosity (25°): 9 cP.

USE: In mfr of vinyl flooring, toys and other vinyl products.

9252. Tezosentan. [180384-57-0] *N*-[6-(2-Hydroxyethoxy)-5-(2-methoxyphenoxy)-2-[2-(1*H*-tetrazol-5-yl)-4-pyridinyl]-4-pyrimidinyl]-5-(1-methylethyl)-2-pyridinesulfonamide; 5-isopropylpyridine-2-sulfonic acid 6-(2-hydroxyethoxy)-5-(2-methoxyphenoxy)-2-(2-1*H*-tetrazol-5-ylpyridin-4-yl)pyrimidin-4-ylamide. $C_{27}H_{27}N_9O_6S$; mol wt 605.62. C 53.55%, H 4.49%, N 20.82%, O 15.85%, S 5.29%. Dual endothelin (ET_A/ET_B) receptor antagonist. Prepn: V. Breu *et al.,* **WO 9619459**; *eidem,* **US 6004965** (1996, 1999 both to Hoffmann-La Roche). Pharmacology and receptor binding: M. Clozel *et al., J. Pharmacol. Exp. Ther.* **290,** 840 (1999). Clinical pharmacokinetics: J. Dingemanse *et al., Br. J. Clin. Pharmacol.* **53,** 355 (2002). Clinical evaluation in advanced heart failure: C. Schalcher *et al., Am. Heart J.* **142,** 340 (2001). LC-MS determn in plasma: P. L. M. van Giersbergen *et al., J. Chromatogr. B* **792,** 369 (2003).

White solid from acetonitrile, mp 198-200°.

Sodium salt. [180384-58-1] Ro-61-0612; Veletri. $C_{27}H_{25}N_9$-Na_2O_6S; mol wt 649.59. White powder from sodium methylate. pKa_1 4.4; pKa_2 4.1. Sol in water.

THERAP CAT: In treatment of congestive heart failure.

9253. TFM. [88-30-2] 4-Nitro-3-(trifluoromethyl)phenol; α,α,α-trifluoro-4-nitro-*m*-cresol; 3-trifluoromethyl-4-nitrophenol; HOE-2770; Lamprecid. $C_7H_4F_3NO_3$; mol wt 207.11. C 40.59%, H 1.95%, F 27.52%, N 6.76%, O 23.18%. A substance toxic to the parasitic sea lamprey, *Petromyzon marinus,* which preys upon commercial fish species of the Great Lakes: Scherer *et al.,* **DE 1068505** *C.A.* **55,** 9774d (1961) corresp to **US 3157571** (1959, 1964, both to Hoechst). Toxicological studies in fish, and bibliography: Kawatski, McDonald, *Comp. Gen. Pharmacol.* **5,** 67 (1974). Physical properties: Smith, *J. Chem. Eng. Data* **6,** 607 (1961). *Review:* Schnick, *Investigations in Fish Control,* no. 44 (Sport Fisheries and Wildlife Bureau) 31 pp.

mp 76°. pK 6.07. uv max (acid): 280 nm (ε 1930); in 1% NaOH: 300, 395 nm (ε 4650, 13,130); in 95% ethanol: 290 nm (ε 14,700).

USE: Lamprey killer.

9254. Thalicarpine. [5373-42-2] (6a*S*)-9-[4,5-Dimethoxy-2-[[(1*S*)-1,2,3,4-tetrahydro-6,7-dimethoxy-2-methyl-1-isoquinolinyl]methyl]phenoxy]-5,6,6a,7-tetrahydro-1,2,10-trimethoxy-6-methyl-4*H*-dibenzo[de,g]quinoline. $C_{41}H_{48}N_2O_8$; mol wt 696.83. C 70.67%, H 6.94%, N 4.02%, O 18.37%. Tumor-inhibitory alkaloid from *Thalictrum dasycarpum* Fisch. & Lall., *Ranunculaceae:* Kupchan *et al., J. Pharm. Sci.* **52,** 985 (1963). Structure: Kupchan, Yokoyama, *J. Am. Chem. Soc.* **86,** 2177 (1964); Tomita *et al., Tetrahedron Lett.* **1965,** 4309. Total synthesis: Kupchan, Liepa, *Chem. Commun.* **1971,** 599; Kupchan *et al., J. Am. Chem. Soc.* **95,** 2995 (1973). Pharmacology: Herman, Chadwick, *Toxicol. Appl. Pharmacol.* **26,** 137 (1973); S. M. Sieber *et al., Cancer Treat. Rep.* **60,** 1127 (1976). Antimicrobial and hypotensive activity: W. N. Wu *et al., Lloydia* **40,** 508 (1977). Biosynthesis: D. S. Bhakuni, S. Jain, *Tetrahedron* **38,** 729 (1982).

Needles from ethyl acetate, mp 160-161°. $[\alpha]_D^{25}$ +133° (c = 0.83 in methanol); $[\alpha]_D^{25}$ +89° (c = 0.88 in chloroform). uv max (methanol): 282, 302 nm (ε 17,000, 13,000).

9255. Thalidomide. [50-35-1] 2-(2,6-Dioxo-3-piperidinyl)-1*H*-isoindole-1,3(2*H*)-dione; *N*-(2,6-dioxo-3-piperidyl)phthalimide; α-phthalimidoglutarimide; 3-phthalimidoglutarimide; 2,6-dioxo-3-phthalimidopiperidine; *N*-phthalylglutamic acid imide; *N*-phthaloylglutamimide; K-17; Contergan; Neurosedyn; Softenon; Thalomid. $C_{13}H_{10}N_2O_4$; mol wt 258.23. C 60.47%, H 3.90%, N 10.85%, O 24.78%. Selective inhibitor of tumor necrosis factor α (TNF-α). Formerly used as sedative, hypnotic. Prepn: **GB 768821** (1957 to Chemie Grünenthal). Teratogenicity studies: I. D. Fratta *et al., Toxicol. Appl. Pharmacol.* **7,** 268 (1965). Review of proposed mechanisms of embryopathy: T. D. Stephens, *Teratology* **38,** 229-239 (1988). HPLC determn in plasma: A. Delon *et al., J. Liq. Chromatogr.* **18,** 297 (1995). Stereospecific determn and pharmacokinetics of enantiomers: T. Eriksson *et al., Chirality* **7,** 44 (1995). Clinical trial in HIV wasting syndrome: G. Reyes-Terán *et al., AIDS* **10,** 1501 (1996); in aphthous ulcers related to HIV infection: J. M. Jacobson *et al., N. Engl. J. Med.* **336,** 1487 (1997). Review of chemistry, pharmacokinetics and clinical safety: V. Günzler, *Drug Saf.* **7,** 116-134 (1992); of effect on TNF-α and clinical use in leprosy and tuberculosis: J. D. Klausner *et al., Clin. Immunol. Immunopathol.* **81,** 219-223 (1996); of pharmacology, history and potential clinical uses: D. Stirling *et al., J. Am. Pharm. Assoc.* **NS37,** 307-313 (1997); of use in multiple myeloma: S. V. Rajkumar, *Expert Rev. Anticancer Ther.***1,** 20-28 (2001); of pharmacology and toxicology: C. Meierhofer, C. J. Wiedermann, *Curr. Opin. Drug Disc. Devel.* **6,** 92-99 (2003); of clinical experience: S. J. Matthews, C. McCoy, *Clin. Ther.* **25,** 342-395 (2003).

Needles, mp 269-271°. uv max (neutral soln): 220, 300 nm. Soly in water: ~2×10^{-4} mol/L; 45-60 mg/L. Sparingly sol in water, methanol, ethanol, acetone, ethyl acetate, butyl acetate, glacial acetic acid. Very sol in dioxane, DMF, pyridine. Practically insol in ether, chloroform, benzene.

THERAP CAT: Immunomodulator.

9256. Thallium. [7440-28-0] Tl; at. wt 204.3833; at. no. 81; valence 1, 3. Group IIIA(13). Naturally occurring isotopes: 203 (29.50%), 205 (70.50%); artificial, radioactive isotopes: 191-202; 204; 206-210. Occurs in crookesite, $(Cu,Tl,Ag)_2Se$, found in Sweden; in lorandite, $TlAsS_2$, found in Greece; in hutchinsonite, (Tl,-Cu,Ag)$_2$S.PbS.2As$_2$S$_3$, found in Switzerland. Occurrence in the earth's crust: 0.7 ppm. Discovered by Crookes in 1861. Prepn: Sanderson, *Can. Mining J.* **65,** 624 (1944). Use in organic syntheses: McKillop *et al., Tetrahedron Lett.* **1970,** 5281; Taylor *et al., ibid.* 5285. *Review:* Wade, Banister in *Comprehensive Inorganic Chemistry* vol. 1, J. C. Bailar, Jr. *et al.,* Eds. (Pergamon Press, Oxford, 1973) pp 997-1000, 1119-1172. Review of toxicity: E. Browning, *Toxicity of Industrial Metals* (Appleton-Century-Crofts, New York, 2nd ed., 1969) pp 317-322; of toxicology and human exposure: *Toxicological Profile for Thallium* (PB93-110856, 1992) 114 pp.

Bluish-white, very soft, inelastic, easily fusible, heavy metal; leaves a streak on paper. Oxidizes superficially in air forming a coating of Tl_2O. Forms alloys with other metals and readily amalgamates with mercury. d 11.85. Begins to volatilize at 174°. mp 303.5°. bp 1457°. Specific heat at 20° 0.031 cal/g/°C. Latent heat of fusion 5.04 cal/g. Brinell hardness: 2. May be distilled in a stream of hydrogen. Insol in water; reacts with nitric or sulfuric acid; difficultly soluble with hydrochloric acid.

Caution: Potential symptoms of overexposure are nausea, diarrhea, abdominal pain and vomiting; ptosis, strabismus; peripheral neuritis, tremor; retrosternal tightness, chest pain and pulmonary edema; seizure, chorea and psychosis; liver and kidney damage; alopecia; paresthesia of legs. *See NIOSH Pocket Guide to Chemical Hazards* (DHHS/NIOSH 97-140, 1997) p 304. *See also Patty's Industrial Hygiene and Toxicology* vol. **2A,** G. D. Clayton, F. E. Clayton, Eds. (Wiley-Interscience, New York, 3rd ed., 1981) 1914-1931.

USE: In semi-conductor industry; alloyed with mercury for switches and closures which operate at subzero temps. In manuf of highly refractive optical glass. Has been used in admixture with 97-98% of inert substances as poison for rats and other rodents.

9257. Thallium Acetate. [563-68-8] Thallous acetate. C_2-H_3O_2Tl; mol wt 263.43. C 9.12%, H 1.15%, O 12.15%, Tl 77.59%. Toxicity study: W. L. Downs *et al., Am. Ind. Hyg. Assoc. J.* **21,** 399 (1960). Brief review: *Dangerous Prop. Ind. Mater. Rep.* **7,** 92-94 (1987).

White, deliquesc crystals, mp 131°. Specific gravity 3.68. *Poisonous!* Sol in water, alcohol. *Keep well closed.* LD_{50} in female rats (mg Tl/kg): 23 i.p., 32 orally (Downs).

USE: Rodenticide, insecticide; fireworks dye; in optical glass; depilatory.

9258. Thallium Bromide. [7789-40-4] Thallous bromide. BrTl; mol wt 284.29. Br 28.11%, Tl 71.89%. TlBr.

Pale yellow, cryst powder. *Poisonous!* d 7.5. mp ~460°. Sol in 2360 parts water.

9259. Thallium Carbonate. [6533-73-9] Thallous carbonate. CO_3Tl_2; mol wt 468.78. C 2.56%, O 10.24%, Tl 87.20%. Tl_2CO_3.

White crystals. *Poisonous!* d 7.1. mp 272°. Soluble in 24 parts water, 3.7 parts boiling water; insol in alc.

USE: Manuf imitation diamonds.

9260. Thallium Chloride. [7791-12-0] Thallous chloride. ClTl; mol wt 239.84. Cl 14.78%, Tl 85.22%. TlCl.

White, cryst powder. *Poisonous!* d 7.0. mp 430°. Sol in 260 parts cold water, 70 parts boiling water. Insol in alcohol. HCl decreases its soly in water.

USE: As catalyst in chlorinations.

9261. Thallium Cyanide. [13453-34-4] Thallous cyanide. CNTl; mol wt 230.40. C 5.21%, N 6.08%, Tl 88.71%. TlCN. Prepn: *Gmelins, Thallium* (8th ed.) **38,** 390 (1940); E. C. Taylor *et al., J. Org. Chem.* **43,** 2280 (1978).

White, hexagonal platelets. d 6.523. Soly in water: 16.8 g/100 ml. Sol in alcohol, acid. Aqueous soln is alkaline.

USE: In organic synthesis.

9262. Thallium Fluoride. [7789-27-7] Thallous fluoride. FTl; mol wt 223.38. F 8.50%, Tl 91.50%. TlF. Prepared from Tl_2CO_3 and HF: Ketelaar, *Z. Kristallogr.* **92,** 30 (1935); Hayek, *Z. Anorg. Allg. Chem.* **225,** 47 (1935); Barrow *et al., Trans. Faraday Soc.* **51,** 1650 (1955); from Tl and HF: Keneshea, Cubicciotti, *J. Phys. Chem.* **69,** 3910 (1965); Tranquard, *Bull. Soc. Chim. Fr.* **1967,** 2578.

Hard, shiny, crystals which deliquesce when breathed upon, but which resolidify immediately in dry air. Not hygroscopic in the usual sense. Orthorhombic (deformed NaCl lattice). d_4^{25} 8.36. mp 322°. Begins to sublime at 300°. Very freely sol in water. Concd solns show strong alkalinity.

USE: In the prepn of fluoro esters.

9263. Thallium Hydroxide. [12026-06-1] Thallous hydroxide. HOTl; mol wt 221.39. H 0.46%, O 7.23%, Tl 92.32%. TlOH.

Yellow needles. *Poisonous!* Very sol in water; the soln is strongly alkaline and turns turmeric paper brown.

9264. Thallium Iodide. [7790-30-9] Thallous iodide. ITl; mol wt 331.29. I 38.31%, Tl 61.69%. TlI.

Yellow, cryst powder. *Poisonous!* d 7.1; mp 440°; bp 824°. Almost insol in water. Insol in alcohol. Sol in KI soln.

9265. Thallium Mononitrate. [10102-45-1] Nitric acid thallium(1+) salt; thallium(I) nitrate; thallous nitrate. NO_3Tl; mol wt 266.39. N 5.26%, O 18.02%, Tl 76.72%. TlNO₃. Toxicity study: M. W. Williams *et al., Toxicol. Appl. Pharmacol.* **63,** 461 (1982).

White crystals. *Poisonous!* d 5.55. mp 206°; dec at 450°. Sol in 10 parts cold water, 0.3 part boiling water. Insol in alcohol. LD_{50} i.p. in mice: 0.14 mmol/kg (Williams).

USE: As a reagent in analytical chemistry, esp for the determination of iodine in presence of Br and Cl; also with $KClO_3$, HgCl and resin for green fire for signalling at sea.

9266. Thallium Oxide. [1314-12-1] Thallous oxide. OTl_2; mol wt 424.77. O 3.77%, Tl 96.23%. Tl_2O.

Black powder. *Poisonous!* mp about 300°. Sol in water, forming the hydroxide; also sol in alcohol. On exposure to air it gradually oxidizes to thallic oxide and becomes insol.

USE: In manuf of glass of a high coefficient of refraction for optical purposes (thallium flint glass) and for artificial gems.

9267. Thallium Selenide. [15572-25-5] Thallous selenide. $SeTl_2$; mol wt 487.73. Se 16.19%, Tl 83.81%. Tl_2Se. Prepared by the action of hydrogen selenide on a soln of thallous carbonate: Kuhlmann, *Bull. Soc. Chim.* [2] **1,** 330 (1864).

Dark gray plates with a metallic luster. mp 340° (Kuhlmann); mp 338° [Palabon, *Compt. Rend.* **145,** 118 (1907); **173,** 142 (1921)]. Insol in water and acids.

9268. Thallium Sesquioxide. [1314-32-5] Thallic oxide; thallium peroxide. O_3Tl_2; mol wt 456.76. O 10.51%, Tl 89.49%. Tl_2O_3.

Brown powder. d 9.65. mp 717°. Insol in water. Dec by HCl with evolution of chlorine and by H_2SO_4 with evolution of oxygen.

9269. Thallium Sulfate. [7446-18-6] Thallous sulfate; Eccothal. O_4STl_2; mol wt 504.83. O 12.68%, S 6.35%, Tl 80.97%. Tl_2SO_4.

White, rhomboid prisms. *Poisonous!* d 6.77; mp 632°. Soly in 100 ml water at 0°: 2.70 g; at 20°: 4.87 g; at 100°: 18.45 g. LD_{50} orally in rats: 25 mg/kg, E. W. Schafer, *Toxicol. Appl. Pharmacol.* **21,** 315 (1972).

Caution: Potential symptoms of overexposure are nausea, diarrhea, abdominal pain, vomiting, ptosis, strabismus; peripheral neuritis, tremor; retrosternal tightness, chest pain, pulmonary edema; seizures, chorea, psychosis; liver, kidney damage; alopecia; leg paresthesia. *See NIOSH Pocket Guide to Chemical Hazards* (DHHS/NIOSH 97-140, 1997) p 304; *Clinical Toxicology of Commercial Products,* R. E. Gosselin *et al.,* Eds. (Williams & Wilkins, Baltimore, 5th ed., 1984) section III, pp 379-383. *See also* Thallium.

USE: As rat poison, as ant bait and as a reagent in analytical chemistry.

9270. Thallium Sulfide. [1314-97-2] Thallous sulfide. STl_2; mol wt 440.83. S 7.27%, Tl 92.73%. Tl_2S.

Bluish-black, cryst powder. d 8.39. mp 448.5°. Almost insol in water, alkali hydoxides, sulfides or cyanides. Sol in mineral acids.

9271. Thallium Trinitrate. [13746-98-0] Nitric acid thallium (3+) salt; thallium(III) nitrate. TlN_3O_9; mol wt 390.40. Tl 52.35%, N 10.76%, O 36.88%. $Tl(NO_3)_3$. Oxidizing reagent. Prepn and use for olefin rearrangement: A. McKillop *et al., Tetrahedron Lett.* **1970,** 5275. Review of early uses: *idem,* E. C. Taylor, *Endeavour* **35,** 88-93 (1976). Phenolic oxidation for isodityrosine functionality: K. Nakamura *et al., Tetrahedron Lett.* **42,** 6311 (2001); promotion of ring contractions for indans: H. M. C. Ferraz *et al., Tetrahedron* **57,** 1709 (2001). *Review: idem et al., Synthesis* **1999,** 2001-2023; T. O. Vieira, *Synlett* **2002,** 1017-1018.

Colorless crystals. Readily sol in methanol, dilute mineral acids and mixed sovent systems such as aqueous glyme.

USE: In organic syntheses for a wide variety of oxidations including rearrangement of ketones, olefins, electrophilic cyclization

transformations, phenolic oxidative couplings and hydrolysis of dithianes.

9272. Thapsigargin. [67526-95-8] Octanoic acid [3S-[3α,-3aβ,4α,6β,6aβ,7β,8α(Z),9bα]]-6-(acetyloxy)-2,3,3a,4,5,6,6a,7,8,9b-decahydro-3,3a-dihydroxy-3,6,9-trimethyl-8-[(2-methyl-1-oxo-2-butenyl)oxy]-2-oxo-4-(1-oxobutoxy)azuleno[4,5-*b*]furan-7-yl ester; thapsigargine; Tg. $C_{34}H_{50}O_{12}$; mol wt 650.75. C 62.75%, H 7.74%, O 29.50%. Sesquiterpene lactone which inhibits intracellular Ca^{2+} transport ATPases. Isolated from the root of *Thapsia garganica* L., *Apiaceae,* traditionally used as a counter-irritant: U. Rasmussen *et al., Acta Pharm. Suec.* **15,** 133 (1978). Structure elucidation: S. B. Christensen *et al., Tetrahedron Lett.* **21,** 3829 (1980); stereochemistry from x-ray analysis: *idem et al., J. Org. Chem.* **47,** 649 (1982). Absolute configuration: S. B. Christensen, E. Norup, *Tetrahedron Lett.* **26,** 107 (1985). Inhibition of ATPases: J. Lytton *et al., J. Biol. Chem.* **266,** 17067 (1991). Effect on gene expression: K. D. Rodland *et al., Mol. Endocrinol.* **11,** 281 (1997). Review of mechanism of action: G. Inesi, Y. Sagara, *Arch. Biochem. Biophys.* **298,** 313-317 (1992). Review of use as molecular probe: O. Thastrup *et al., Agents Actions* **27,** 17-23 (1989); T. B. Rogers *et al., Biosci. Rep.* **15,** 341-349 (1995).

Colorless amorphous powder.

USE: Reagent for defining and manipulating intracellular calcium pools.

9273. Thaumatin. [53850-34-3] Talin. Sweet-tasting basic protein extracted from the fruit of the tropical plant, *Thaumatococcus danielli* Benth., *Marantaceae,* found in Western Africa from Sierra Leone to Zaire, in Sudan and Uganda. Composed of five different forms, thaumatins I, II, III, b and c; thaumatins I and II predominate. All are nearly 100,000 times sweeter than sucrose and have molecular weights of about 22,000. Isoln and characterization: H. van der Wel, K. Loeve, *Eur. J. Biochem.* **31,** 221 (1972). Extraction process: J. Higgenbotham, US **4011206** (1976 to Tate and Lyle Ltd.). Electrophysical study of effects on taste receptors: Brouwer *et al., Acta Physiol. Scand.* **89,** 550 (1973). Spectrometric investigation: O. Korver *et al., Eur. J. Biochem.* **35,** 554 (1973). Studies on the primary structure of thaumatin I: R. B. Iyengar *et al., ibid.* **96,** 193 (1979). Thaumatins I and II consist of almost identical sequences of 207 amino acids. Thaumatin I crystallizes in two different forms: H. van der Wel *et al., FEBS Lett.* **56,** 316 (1975). The crystal structure shows two distinct regions with the amino acids either in sheets or in complex loops. Crystal structure: A. M. de Vos *et al., Proc. Natl. Acad. Sci. USA* **82,** 1406 (1985). Cloning and expression in *E. coli* of the structural gene of thaumatin II: L. Edens *et al., Gene* **18,** 1 (1982); C. T. Verrips, EP **54330;** EP **54331** (both 1982 to Unilever). Cloning of the natural gene: A. M. Ledeboer *et al., Gene* **30,** 23 (1984). *Reviews:* R. Cagan, *Science* **181,** 32 (1973); H. van der Wel, *Chem. Ind. (London)* **1983,** 19.

Intensely sweet taste, licorice aftertaste. Strongly cationic, isoelectric pt greater than or equal to 11.7. uv max: 278 nm (pH 5.6); 283, 290 nm (pH 13.0). About 750-1600 times sweeter than sucrose on a wt basis; 30,000-100,000 times on a molar basis. Threshold values are near 10^{-4}%. The proteins lose sweetness on heating, on splitting of disulfide bridges and also at pH < 2.5 which points to the importance of the tertiary structure for the sweetness.

USE: Potential low-calorie sweetener.

9274. Theaflavine. [4670-05-7] 1,8-Bis[(2R,3R)-3,4-dihydro-3,5,7-trihydroxy-2*H*-1-benzopyran-2-yl]-3,4,6-trihydroxy-5*H*-benzocyclohepten-5-one. $C_{29}H_{24}O_{12}$; mol wt 564.49. C 61.70%,

H 4.29%, O 34.01%. From black tea extracts: Roberts, Myers, *J. Sci. Food Agric.* **10**, 176 (1959). Structure: Takino *et al., Tetrahedron Lett.* **1965**, 4019. Configuration: Brown *et al., ibid.* **1966**, 1193.

Crystals from water, dec 237-240°. Absorption max (ethanol): 216, 271, 384, 470 nm (ε 35500, 19500, 8700, 3600).

Nonaacetate. $C_{47}H_{42}O_{21}$. Crystals, mp 167-168°. uv max (alc): 211, 250, 314, 353 nm (ε 25100, 13200, 7100, 4700).

9275. Thearubigins. [12698-96-3] Weakly acidic class of orange-brown phenolic pigments produced during the fermentation step of tea manufacture. Accounts for as much as 20% of dry weight of black tea; in combination with theaflavine, *q.v.*, determines the color, brightness and body of a tea infusion. Isolation: E. A. H. Roberts *et al., J. Sci. Food Agric.* **8**, 72 (1957); E. A. H. Roberts, *ibid.* **9**, 212 (1958). Effects on tea characteristics: R. F. Smith, *ibid.* **19**, 530 (1968); M. Hazarika *et al., ibid.* **35**, 1208 (1984). Structure studies: A. G. Brown *et al., Phytochemistry* **8**, 2333 (1969); J. E. Berkowitz *et al., ibid.* **10**, 2271 (1971); D. J. Cattell, H. E. Nursten, *ibid.* **15**, 1967 (1976). HPLC analysis: B. L. Wedzicha, T. J. Donovan, *J. Chromatogr.* **478**, 217 (1989); R. G. Bailey *et al., ibid.* **542**, 115 (1991).

9276. Thebaine. [115-37-7] (5α)-6,7,8,14-Tetradehydro-4,5-epoxy-3,6-dimethoxy-17-methylmorphinan; paramorphine. $C_{19}H_{21}NO_3$; mol wt 311.37. C 73.29%, H 6.80%, N 4.50%, O 15.42%. From opium, which contains from 0.3-1.5% depending on its origin. Discussion of structure and bibliography: Small, Lutz, "Chemistry of the Opium Alkaloids" in *U.S. Public Health Reports* **Suppl. No. 103** (Washington, 1932); Small, Browning, *J. Org. Chem.* **3**, 618 (1938); Cherbuliez, Araqui, *Helv. Chim. Acta* **26**, 2251 (1943); Ghosh, Robinson, *J. Chem. Soc.* **1944**, 506; K. W. Bentley, *The Chemistry of the Morphine Alkaloids* (Oxford, 1954) p 184 sqq. Config: Kalvoda *et al., Helv. Chim. Acta* **38**, 1847 (1955). Syntheses: Rapoport *et al., J. Am. Chem. Soc.* **89**, 1942 (1967); Schwartz, Mami, *ibid.* **97**, 1239 (1975); Barber, Rapoport, *J. Med. Chem.* **18**, 1074 (1975). Absorption spectrum: Csokán, *Z. Anal. Chem.* **124**, 344 (1942). Toxicity data: Eddy, *J. Pharmacol. Exp. Ther.* **66**, 182 (1939).

Orthorhombic, rectangular plates by sublimation at 170-180° under atmospheric pressure and a 1 mm distance. mp 193° (rapid heating). $[\alpha]_D^{15}$ −219° (p = 2 in alc); $[\alpha]_D^{23}$ −230° (p = 5 in chloroform). pK at 15° = 6.05. pH of satd water soln 7.6. One gram dissolves in 1460 ml water at 15° [Kolthoff, *Biochem. Z.* **162**, 336 (1925)], in about 15 ml hot alcohol or 13 ml chloroform, about 200 ml ether, 25 ml benzene, 12 ml pyridine; not very sol in petr ether.

Hydrochloride monohydrate. $C_{19}H_{21}NO_3 \cdot HCl \cdot H_2O$. Orthorhombic prisms from alcohol, $[\alpha]_D^{23}$ −164° (p = 2). Sol in about 12 parts water, in alcohol; pH of 0.05 molar soln 4.95. LD_{50} s.c. in rabbits: 14 mg/kg (Eddy).

Oxalate hexahydrate. $2C_{19}H_{21}NO_3 \cdot C_2H_2O_4 \cdot 6H_2O$. Prisms, sol in about 10 parts water, in alcohol. Almost insol in ether.

Binoxalate monohydrate. $C_{19}H_{21}NO_3 \cdot C_2H_2O_4 \cdot H_2O$. Prisms, sol in 45 parts water.

Bitartrate monohydrate. $C_{19}H_{21}NO_3 \cdot C_4H_6O_6 \cdot H_2O$. Prisms, sol in 130 parts water, quite sol in hot water, hot alcohol.

Salicylate. $C_{19}H_{21}NO_3 \cdot C_7H_6O_3$. Crystals, sol in 750 parts water.

Note: This is a controlled substance (opiate): **21 CFR**, 1308.12.

9277. Thebainone. [467-98-1] 7,8-Didehydro-4-hydroxy-3-methoxy-17-methylmorphinan-6-one; thebainone-A. $C_{18}H_{21}$-NO_3; mol wt 299.36. C 72.22%, H 7.07%, N 4.68%, O 16.03%. Prepn from thebaine, codeinone or β-ethylthiocodide: Morris, Small, *J. Am. Chem. Soc.* **56**, 2159 (1934). Earlier references and discussion of structure: Small, Lutz, "Chemistry of the Opium Alkaloids" in *U.S. Public Health Reports* **Suppl. No. 103** (Washington, 1932). About anomalies in nomenclature and difference from metathebainone *see* Henry, *Plant Alkaloids* (London, 1939) p 249. Description of all thebainones: K. W. Bentley, *The Chemistry of the Morphine Alkaloids* (Oxford, 1954) p 219.

Crystals from ethyl acetate, mp 146°. $[\alpha]_D^{28}$ −47° (c = 1.16 in 95% alc). One gram dissolves in 250 ml water, about 120 ml boiling water. Sol in chloroform, benzene, acetone; sparingly sol in ether, alcohol, methanol.

Sesquihydrate. Crystals from water, mp 90°.

Methanolate. Crystals from methanol, mp 118°.

Hydrochloride. $C_{18}H_{21}NO_3 \cdot HCl$. Crystals from alcohol, mp 256° (turns red at mp). $[\alpha]_D^{30}$ −25° (c = 1.63).

Hydriodide. $C_{18}H_{21}NO_3 \cdot HI$. Crystals, mp 165°, solidifies and remelts 260°.

Methiodide. mp 251°.

9278. Thenaldine. [86-12-4] 1-Methyl-*N*-phenyl-*N*-(2-thienylmethyl)-4-piperidinamine; 1-methyl-4-*N*-2-thenylanilinopiperidine; 1-methyl-4-amino-*N*-phenyl-*N*-(2-thenyl)piperidine; thenophenopiperidine; 1-methyl-4-[phenyl-(2-thenyl)amino]piperidine; thenalidine; Sandostene. $C_{17}H_{22}N_2S$; mol wt 286.43. C 71.29%, H 7.74%, N 9.78%, S 11.19%. Prepn: Stoll, Bourquin, **US 2717251** and **US 2757175** (1955 and 1956 to Sandoz).

bp$_{0.02}$ 158-160°, mp 95-97°.

Tartrate. Crystals, mp 170-172°.

THERAP CAT: Tartrate as antihistaminic; antipruritic.

9279. 3-Thenoic Acid. [88-13-1] 3-Thiophenecarboxylic acid; β-thiophenic acid. $C_5H_4O_2S$; mol wt 128.15. C 46.86%, H 3.15%, O 24.97%, S 25.02%. Prepd by the oxidation of 3-thenaldehyde with silver oxide: Campaigne, LeSuer, *Org. Synth.* **33**, 94 (1953).

Crystals from water, mp 137-138°. Soly in water at 25°: 0.43 g/100 g. pKa 6.23. Volatile with steam.

9280. Thenyldiamine. [91-79-2] *N*,*N*-Dimethyl-*N*'-2-pyridinyl-*N*'-(3-thienylmethyl)-1,2-ethanediamine; 2-[(2-dimethylaminoethyl)-3-thenylamino]pyridine; *N*,*N*-dimethyl-*N*'-(α-pyridyl)-*N*'-(3-methylthienyl)ethylenediamine; *N*-(α-pyridyl)-*N*-(β-thenyl)-*N*',*N*'-dimethylethylenediamine; *N*-(2-dimethylaminoethyl)-*N*-2-pyridyl-3-thenylamine; dethylandiamine; Win-2848; Thenfadil. $C_{14}H_{19}N_3S$; mol wt 261.39. C 64.33%, H 7.33%, N 16.08%, S 12.27%. Prepn: Campaigne, LeSuer, *J. Am. Chem. Soc.* **71**, 333 (1949). Toxicity study: Hoppe, Lands, *J. Pharmacol. Exp. Ther.* **97**, 371 (1949).

Free base, liquid. bp$_{1.0}$ 169-172°. n_D^{20} 1.5915.
Hydrochloride. $C_{14}H_{19}N_3S.HCl$. Crystals from methanol, mp 169.5-170°. Bitter taste. Sol in water up to 20%. Slightly sol in alc. pH of 1% aq soln 6.5. LD$_{50}$ orally in rats: 525 mg/kg (Hoppe, Lands).

THERAP CAT: Hydrochloride as antihistaminic.

9281. Theobroma Oil. Cacao butter; cocoa butter. From roasted seeds of *Theobroma cacao* L., *Sterculiaceae. Constit.* Chiefly glycerides of stearic, palmitic, oleic, arachidic, and linoleic acids.
Yellowish-white solid; brittle below 25°; chocolate odor and taste; d$_{25}^{100}$ 0.858-0.864; mp 30-35°; n_D^{40} 1.4537-1.4578. Sapon. no. 188-195. Iodine no. 35-40. Insoluble in water. Slightly sol in alcohol; sol in boiling abs alc; very sol in chloroform, ether, benzene, petr ether.
USE: Lubricant in massage; base for suppositories and ointments. Manuf chocolate, toilet soaps, creams, etc.

9282. Theobromine. [83-67-0] 3,7-Dihydro-3,7-dimethyl-1*H*-purine-2,6-dione; 3,7-dimethylxanthine. $C_7H_8N_4O_2$; mol wt 180.16. C 46.67%, H 4.48%, N 31.10%, O 17.76%. The principal alkaloid of the cacao bean which contains 1.5-3% of the base. Also present in cola nuts and in tea. Usually extracted from the hull of cacao beans which contains 0.7-1.2%. Extraction process: Schwyzer, *Die Fabrikation pharmazeutischer und chemisch-technischer Produkte* (Berlin, 1931). Synthesis starting with 3-methyluric acid: Fischer, Ach, *Ber.* **31**, 1980 (1898); *cf.* Gebner, Krebs, *J. Gen. Chem. USSR* **16**, 179-186 (1946). Comparison with theophylline, *q.v.*, of metabolism in humans: D. J. Birkett *et al., Drug Metab. Dispos.* **13**, 725 (1985). Pharmacokinetics: A. Lelo *et al., Br. J. Clin. Pharmacol.* **22**, 177 (1986). Bronchodilator effect in asthma: F. E. R. Simons *et al., J. Allergy Clin. Immunol.* **76**, 703 (1985).

Monoclinic needles (lamellar twinning on 001) from water, mp 357°. Sublimes 290-295°. Kb at 18°: 1.3×10^{-14}; Ka 0.9×10^{-10}. Absorption spectrum: Hartley, *J. Chem. Soc.* **87**, 1803, 1810 (1905). One gram dissolves in about 2000 ml water, 150 ml boiling water, 2220 ml 95% alcohol; sol in the fixed alkali hydroxides, concd acids, in about 22 parts of 20% aq tribasic sodium phosphate soln; moderately sol in ammonia. Almost insol in benzene, ether, chloroform, carbon tetrachloride. Forms salts which are dec by water, and compds with bases which are more stable.
Calcium salicylate. [8065-51-8] Theocalcin; Calcium Diuretin. Double salt or mixture of calcium theobromine and calcium

salicylate. Contains no less than 44% theobromine. White, amorphous powder. Slightly saline taste. Partly sol in water. Aq solns are alkaline to phenolphthalein.
Sodium acetate. [8002-88-8] Thesodate. Equimolar mixture of sodium theobromine and sodium acetate, containing 1H$_2$O. Theobromine 59.6%, anhyd sodium acetate 27.1%. White, odorless or almost odorless, hygroscopic powder. Absorbs CO$_2$ from the air becoming incompletely sol. Very sol in water, sparingly sol in cold alcohol; the solns are strongly alkaline. pH about 10. *Keep tightly closed.*
Sodium salicylate. [8048-31-5] Diuretin. Equimolar mixture of sodium theobromine and sodium salicylate, containing 1H$_2$O. Theobromine 47.3%, sodium salicylate 42.1%. White, odorless or almost odorless, hygroscopic powder. Absorbs CO$_2$ from the air and becomes incompletely soluble. Soluble in 1 part water; slightly sol in alcohol; the solns are strongly alkaline. pH about 10.

THERAP CAT: Diuretic, bronchodilator, cardiotonic.
THERAP CAT (VET): Diuretic, myocardial stimulant, vasodilator.

9283. 1-Theobromineacetic Acid. [5614-56-2] 2,3,6,7-Tetrahydro-3,7-dimethyl-2,6-dioxo-1*H*-purine-1-acetic acid; 3,6-dihydro-3,7-dimethyl-2,6-dioxo-1(2*H*)-purineacetic acid; 3,6-dihydro-2,6-diketo-3,7-dimethyl-1(2)-purineacetic acid. $C_9H_{10}N_4O_4$; mol wt 238.20. C 45.38%, H 4.23%, N 23.52%, O 26.87%. Prepd from sodium theobromine + chloroacetic acid: E. Merck *et al.,* **DE** 352980 *C.A.* **17**, 1307[1] (1923).

Crystals, mp 260°.
Sodium salt. [32245-40-2] Sodium theobromine acetate; Técarine. $C_9H_9N_4NaO_4$; mol wt 260.18. Crystalline powder, freely sol in water, forming a neutral soln.

THERAP CAT: Bronchodilator.

9284. Theofibrate. [54504-70-0] 2-(4-Chlorophenoxy)-2-methylpropanoic acid 2-(1,2,3,6-tetrahydro-1,3-dimethyl-2,6-dioxo-7*H*-purin-7-yl)ethyl ester; 2-(*p*-chlorophenoxy)-2-methylpropionic acid ester with 7-(2-hydroxyethyl)theophylline; 1-(theophyllin-7-yl)ethyl 2-(*p*-chlorophenoxy)isobutyrate; etofylline clofibrate; ML-1024; Duolip. $C_{19}H_{21}ClN_4O_5$; mol wt 420.85. C 54.22%, H 5.03%, Cl 8.42%, N 13.31%, O 19.01%. Deriv of clofibric acid, *q.v.*, with antilipemic, antithrombotic, and platelet-aggregation inhibitory activity: Prepn: G. Metz, M. Specker, **DE 2308826**; *eidem*, **US 3984413** (1974, 1976 both to Merckle); *eidem, Arzneim.-Forsch.* **25**, 1686 (1975). Hypolipemic activity: G. Metz *et al., ibid.* **27**, 1173 (1977). Series of articles on chemistry, biopharmaceutic evaluation, pharmacology, toxicology, clinical studies: *ibid.* **30**, 2013-2074 (1980).

Colorless crystals from ethanol, mp 133-135°. Practically insol in water at pH 2-7.4 and in cold alcohols. Sol in acetone, chloroform, hot alcohols. LD$_{50}$ in mice, rats, dogs (g/kg): 11.7, 17.0, >10.0 orally (Metz *et al.*).

THERAP CAT: Antilipemic.

9285. Theophylline. [58-55-9] 3,7-Dihydro-1,3-dimethyl-1*H*-purine-2,6-dione; 1,3-dimethylxanthine; Aerobin; Aerolate; Bronchoretard; Diffumal; Duraphyllin; Elixophyllin; Etheophyl; Euphylline; Euphylong; Lasma; Nuelin; PulmiDur; Pulmo-Timelets; Respbid; Slo-Phyllin; Solosin; Teosona; Theobid; Theochron;

Theolair; Theon; Theograd; Theostat; Unifyl; Uniphyl; Uniphyllin; Xanthium. $C_7H_8N_4O_2$; mol wt 180.16. C 46.67%, H 4.48%, N 31.10%, O 17.76%. Xanthine derivative with diuretic, cardiac stimulant and smooth muscle relaxant activities; isomeric with theobromine, q.v. Small amounts occur in tea. Synthesis starting with dimethylurea and ethyl cyanoacetate: Traube, *Ber.* **33**, 3035 (1900); Grinberg, *J. Appl. Chem. USSR* **13**, 1461 (1940); Gebner, Krebs, *J. Gen. Chem. USSR* **16**, 179 (1946). Bioavailability: K. Svedmyr *et al., Allergy* **37**, 111 (1982). Comprehensive description: J. L. Cohen, *Anal. Profiles Drug Subs.* **4**, 466-493 (1975). Symposium on clinical experience in asthma and allergy: *Am. J. Med.* **79**(6A), 1-78 (1985); on pharmacology, bioavailability, pharmacokinetics and efficacy in obstructive pulmonary disease: *J. Allergy Clin. Immunol.* **78**(4 Part 2), 669-824 (1986). Review of clinical toxicology: J. D. Truwit, *Crit. Care Clin.* **7**, 639-657 (1991).

Monohydrate, thin monoclinic tablets from water, mp 270-274°. Bitter taste. pKa (25°): 8.77; pKb: 13.5, 11.5. One gram dissolves in 120 ml water, 80 ml alcohol, about 110 ml chloroform. Sol in hot water, in alkali hydroxides, ammonia, dil HCl or HNO_3; sparingly sol in ether. uv max (0.1*N* NaOH): 274 nm.

Ethanolamine. [573-41-1] $C_9H_{15}N_5O_3$; mol wt 241.25. White, crystalline, nonhygroscopic powder contg 75% anhydr theophylline and 25% ethanolamine. Sol in water.

Isopropanolamine. [5600-19-1] $C_{10}H_{17}N_5O_3$; mol wt 255.27. Prepn: Greenbaum, *Am. J. Pharm.* **109**, 550 (1937). Prisms from alcohol. Very sol in water. pH of aq solns 9.20.

Lysine salt. Paidomal.

Sodium acetate. [8002-89-9] Equimolar mixture of theophylline sodium and sodium acetate, containing $1H_2O$. White, odorless, crystalline powder; bitter taste. Sol in about 25 parts water. Insol in alcohol, chloroform or ether.

Sodium glycinate. [8000-10-0] Afonilum. Prepn: Krantz *et al., J. Am. Pharm. Assoc.* **36**, 248 (1947). Equimolar mixture of theophylline sodium and glycine. Darkens at 180°. Soly in water 18% w/v. Saturated soln has a pH of 8.7-9.1, d^{20} 1.05, and is stable to carbon dioxide.

THERAP CAT: Bronchodilator.

THERAP CAT (VET): Bronchodilator.

9286. Thermolysin. [9073-78-3] Bacillus thermoproteolyticus neutral proteinase; EC 3.4.24.27. Proteolytic enzyme of mol wt 37,500 that hydrolyzes protein bonds on the *N*-terminal side of hydrophobic amino acid residues. Contains a zinc atom essential for activity and four Ca^{2+} ions essential for thermal and conformational stability. Isoln from *Bacillus thermoproteolyticus*: S. Endo, *J. Ferment. Technol.* **40**, 346 (1962). Properties and amino acid composition: Y. Ohta *et al., J. Biol. Chem.* **241**, 5919 (1966). Site of enzymatic hydrolysis: Y. Ohta, Y. Ogura, *J. Biochem.* **58**, 607 (1965). Substrate specificity studies: H. Matsubara *et al., Biochem. Biophys. Res. Commun.* **21**, 242 (1965); **24**, 427 (1966); K. Morihara, H. Tsuzuki, *Biochim. Biophys. Acta* **118**, 215 (1966). Stability studies: Y. Ohta, *J. Biol. Chem.* **242**, 509 (1967). Inhibition studies: H. Matsubara *et al., Biochem. Biophys. Res. Commun.* **34**, 719 (1969); J. Murphy *et al., Arch. Biochem. Biophys.* **202**, 405 (1980). Purification: H. Matsubara, *Methods Enzymol.* **19**, 642 (1970). Structure studies: K. Titani *et al., Nature* **238**, 35 (1972); B. W. Matthews *et al., ibid.* **37**, 41; P. M. Colman *et al., J. Mol. Biol.* **70**, 701 (1972). Function of the metal ions: J. Feder *et al., Biochemistry* **10**, 4552 (1971); G. Voordouw, R. S. Roche, *ibid.* **14**, 4667 (1975); R. S. Roche, G. Voordouw, *Crit. Rev. Biochem.* **5**, 1 (1978). Effect of the histidyl residue on the mechanism of action: S. Blumberg *et al., Isr. J. Chem.* **12**, 643 (1974); M. K. Pangburn, K. A. Walsch, *Biochemistry* **14**, 4050 (1975). *Review:* Experientia **26**, Suppl., 31-59 (1976).

Crystals. uv max: 280 nm (ε 66,300). Optimum pH 7.0-8.5; stable at pH 6.0-9.0. The refrigerated lyophilized enzyme is stable

for months; frozen enzyme soln can be kept for weeks without significant loss of activity. Not deactivated at 65°, but loses half of its activity upon heating at 80° for 1 hr.

USE: In studies of protein sequences.

9287. Thermorubin. [11006-83-0] Antibiotic substances isolated from *Thermoactinomyces antibioticus*: Craveri *et al., Clin. Med.* **71**, 511 (1964); *eidem,* DE 1180891; *eidem,* US 3300379 (1964, 1967 both to Lepetit). Structure of thermorubin A, the major component: Moppett *et al., J. Am. Chem. Soc.* **94**, 3269 (1972); revised structure: F. Johnson *et al., ibid.* **102**, 5580 (1980). Inhibition of bacterial protein synthesis: G. Pirali *et al., Biochim. Biophys. Acta* **366**, 310 (1974). Studies on mechanism of action: F. Lin, A. Wishnia, *Biochemistry* **21**, 477, 484 (1982).

Thermorubin A

Orange-red rosettes and needles from chloroform, darkens 190°, chars 300° without melting. $[\alpha]_D^{25}$ −14° (c = 0.4 in dioxane). Absorption max [dioxane-cyclohexane (1:1)]: 300, 328, 414, 430 nm ($E_{1cm}^{1\%}$ 1041, 1066, 313, 332). Sol in dioxane, pyridine, tetrahydrofuran, DMF, DMSO, concd alkalies, concd H_2SO_4, glacial acetic acid; slightly sol in methanol, ethanol, butanol, ethyl acetate, acetone, chloroform, benzene, cyclohexane. Practically insol in water, ether, petr ether, hexane. LD_{50} i.p. in mice: 300 mg/kg (Craveri, 1967).

Diacetate. Crystals from ethyl acetate. Absorption max [0.1*N* HCl-dioxane (1:1)]: 337, 436, 462 nm ($E_{1cm}^{1\%}$ 1500, 113, 162).

Thermorubin A. $C_{32}H_{24}O_{12}$; mol wt 600.53. Dihydrate, orange-red rosettes from ethyl acetate. Absorption max (ethanol): 250, 300, 328, 435 nm (ε 33700, 54640, 49980, 16300). pKa values: 4.7, 7.0, 9.0. Easily tautomerizes in soln. Thermally labile, decomposes rapidly in soln at temps >60°.

9288. Thevetin A. [37933-66-7] (3β,5β)-3-[(O-β-D-Glucopyranosyl-(1 → 6)-O-D-glucopyranosyl-(1 → 4)-6-deoxy-3-O-methyl-α-L-glucopyranosyl)oxy]-14-hydroxy-19-oxocard-20(22)-enolide. $C_{42}H_{64}O_{19}$; mol wt 872.95. C 57.79%, H 7.39%, O 34.82%. Glycoside isolated from *Thevetia neriifolia* Juss., *Apocynaceae:* Bloch *et al., Helv. Chim. Acta* **43**, 652 (1960). Separation from thevetin B: Delalande, Baisse, US 3030355; US 3043829 (1962). Structure: K. Tori *et al., Tetrahedron Lett.* **1977**, 717.

Crystals from water. mp 208-210°. $[\alpha]_D^{24}$ −72.0 ±1.5° (c = 1.48 in methanol).

Acetyl deriv. $C_{58}H_{80}O_{27}$. Crystals from methanol + ether, mp 143-149°. $[\alpha]_D^{26}$ −54.2 ±1° (c = 1.86 in chloroform).

9289. Thiabendazole. [148-79-8] 2-(4-Thiazolyl)-1*H*-benzimidazole; 4-(2-benzimidazolyl)thiazole; MK-360; Equizole; Mertect; Mintezol; Tecto. $C_{10}H_7N_3S$; mol wt 201.25. C

59.68%, H 3.51%, N 20.88%, S 15.93%. Prepd by the reaction of 4-thiazolecarboxamide with *o*-phenylenediamine in polyphosphoric acid: H. D. Brown *et al.*, *J. Am. Chem. Soc.* **83**, 1764 (1961); L. H. Sarett, H. D. Brown, US 3017415 (1962 to Merck & Co.). Synthesis of labeled thiabendazole: D. J. Tocco *et al.*, *J. Med. Chem.* **7**, 399 (1964). Alternate route of synthesis: V. J. Grenda *et al.*, *J. Org. Chem.* **30**, 259 (1965). Anthelmintic props: H. D. Brown *et al.*, *loc. cit.*; K. C. Kates *et al.*, *J. Parasitol.* **57**, 356 (1971). Fungicidal props: H. J. Robinson *et al.*, *J. Invest. Dermatol.* **42**, 479 (1966). Systemic props in plants: D. C. Erwin *et al.*, *Phytopathology* **58**, 860 (1968). Toxicity: H. J. Robinson *et al.*, *Toxicol. Appl. Pharmacol.* **7**, 53 (1965). Residue analysis: IUPAC Appl. Chem. Div., *Pure Appl. Chem.* **52**, 2567 (1980). Comprehensive description: V. K. Kapoor, *Anal. Profiles Drug Subs.* **16**, 611-639 (1986).

Colorless crystals, mp 304-305°. uv max (methanol): 298 nm (ε 23330). Fluorescence max in acid soln: 370 nm (310 nm excitation). Max soly in water at pH 2.2: 3.84%. Soluble in DMF, DMSO. Slightly soluble in alcohols, esters, chlorinated hydrocarbons. LD_{50} in mice, rats, rabbits (g/kg): 3.6, 3.1, >3.8 orally (Robinson).

Hypophosphite. [28558-32-9] Arbotect. Amber liquid. d^{25} 1.103.

USE: Fungicide for spoilage control of citrus fruit; for treatment and prevention of Dutch elm disease in trees; for control of fungal diseases of seed potatoes.

THERAP CAT: Anthelmintic (Nematodes).

THERAP CAT (VET): Anthelmintic, fungicide.

9290. Thiacetazone. [104-06-3] *N*-[4-[[(Aminothioxomethyl)hydrazono]methyl]phenyl]acetamide; 2-[[4-(acetylamino)-phenyl]methylene]hydrazinecarbothioamide; 4′-formylacetanilide thiosemicarbazone; *p*-acetamidobenzaldehyde thiosemicarbazone; *p*-acetylaminobenzaldehyde thiosemicarbazone; *p*-acetaminobenzylidenethiosemicarbazone; amithiozone; thibone; thioacetazone; Tb I-698; Conteben; Livazone; Myrizone; Neustab; Panrone; Seroden; Tebethion; Thiocarbazil; Thioparamizone; Tibione; Tiobicina. $C_{10}H_{12}N_4OS$; mol wt 236.29. C 50.83%, H 5.12%, N 23.71%, O 6.77%, S 13.57%. Prepn: G. Domagk *et al.*, *Naturwissenschaften* **33**, 315 (1946); Behnisch *et al.*, *Angew. Chem.* **60A**, 113 (1948); Chabrier, Cattelain, *Bull. Soc. Chim. Fr.* **1950M**, 52; Das, Mukherjee, *J. Am. Chem. Soc.* **75**, 1241 (1953). Toxicity data: Bavin *et al.*, *J. Pharm. Pharmacol.* **2**, 764 (1950). HPLC determn in body fluids: P. J. Jenner, *J. Chromatogr.* **276**, 463 (1983). Review of clinical experience: H. C. Hinshaw, W. McDermott, *Am. Rev. Tuberc.* **61**, 145-157 (1950); of clinical safety and efficacy: P. Nunn *et al.*, *Trans. R. Soc. Trop. Med. Hyg.* **87**, 578 (1993).

Minute, pale yellow crystals from abs alc. Bitter taste. Darkens on exposure to light. Dec 225-230°. uv max (ethanol): 328 nm, extinction 0.580. Sol in hot alc; very sparingly sol in cold alc. Insol in water, acetone, benzene, carbon tetrachloride, chloroform, carbon disulfide, petr ether. Practically insol in the other common organic solvents except glycols. Soly in propylene glycol ~1%. LD_{50} s.c. in mice: 1-2 g/kg (Bavin).

THERAP CAT: Antibacterial (tuberculostatic).

9291. Thiacloprid. [111988-49-9] [3-[(6-Chloro-3-pyridinyl)methyl]-2-thiazolidinylidene]cyanamide; 1-(2-chloro-5-pyridylmethyl)-2-cyanoiminothiazolidine; Calypso. $C_{10}H_9ClN_4S$; mol wt 252.72. C 47.53%, H 3.59%, Cl 14.03%, N 22.17%, S 12.69%. Chloronicotinyl insecticide for use in fruits and vegetables. Prepn: K. Shiokawa *et al.*, EP 235725; *eidem*, US 4849432 (1987, 1989 both to Nihon Tokushu Noyaku Seizo KK). LC-MS

determn in fruits and vegetables: D. Zywitz *et al.*, *Deutsche Lebens.-Rundschau* **99**, 188 (2003). Review of properties and bioactivity: A. Elbert *et al.*, *Brighton Crop Prot. Conf. - Pests Dis.* **2000**, 21-26.

Z-form

Crystals from ether, mp 128-129°. Remaining data is for *Z*-form: yellowish powder. Vapor pressure (20°): 3×10^{-10} Pa. Soly in water (20°): 185 mg/l. Log P (octanol/water): 1.26. LD_{50} in male, female rats (mg/kg): 836, 444 orally; >2000, >2000 dermally. LC_{50} (4 hr) in male, female rats (mg/m³): >2535, 1223. LC_{50} (96 hr) in rainbow trout (mg/l): 30.5 (Elbert).

USE: Insecticide.

9292. Thialbarbital. [467-36-7] 5-(2-Cyclohexen-1-yl)dihydro-5-(2-propenyl)-2-thioxo-4,6(1*H*,5*H*)-pyrimidinedione; 5-allyl-5-(2-cyclohexen-1-yl)-2-thiobarbituric acid; 5-(2-cyclohexen-1-yl)-5-allyl-2-thiobarbituric acid; thialbarbitone; Kemithal. $C_{13}H_{16}N_2O_2S$; mol wt 264.34. C 59.07%, H 6.10%, N 10.60%, O 12.11%, S 12.13%. Prepn: Volwiler, Tabern, US 2153730 (1939 to Abbott).

Crystals, mp 148-150°.

Sodium salt. $C_{13}H_{15}N_2NaO_2S$. Pale yellow crystals from methanol, mp 130-132°. Very sol in water, alc. Practically insol in benzene, ether. pH of 2.5% soln in water: 10.5.

Note: This is a controlled substance (depressant): **21 CFR**, 1308.13.

THERAP CAT: Anesthetic (intravenous).

THERAP CAT (VET): Anesthetic.

9293. Thiambutene. [86-14-6] *N,N*-Diethyl-1-methyl-3,3-di-2-thienylallylamine; 3-diethylamino-1,1-di(2′-thienyl)but-1-ene; diethylthiambutene; 191C49; NIH-4185. $C_{16}H_{21}NS_2$; mol wt 291.47. C 65.93%, H 7.26%, N 4.81%, S 22.00%. Prepn: Adamson, *J. Chem. Soc.* **1950**, 885; US 2561899 (1951 to Burroughs Wellcome). Toxicity data: J. S. McKenzie, N. R. Beechey, *Arch. Int. Pharmacodyn. Ther.* **135**, 376 (1962). Use: Hayes, *Vet. Rec.* **83**, 528 (1968). Evaluation as analgesic and preanesthetic agent: W. D. Harbison *et al.*, *Aust. Vet. J.* **50**, 543 (1974). HPLC determn: I. Jane *et al.*, *J. Chromatogr.* **323**, 191 (1985).

$bp_{0.03}$ 122-128°. LD_{50} i.p. in mice: 90 mg/kg (McKenzie, Beechey).

Hydrochloride. Themalon. $C_{16}H_{21}NS_2 \cdot HCl$; mol wt 327.94. Crystals, mp 152-153°.

Note: This is a controlled substance (opiate): **21 CFR**, 1308.11.

THERAP CAT (VET): Analgesic (narcotic).

9294. Thiamethoxam. [153719-23-4] 3-[(2-Chloro-5-thiazolyl)methyl]tetrahydro-5-methyl-*N*-nitro-4*H*-1,3,5-oxadiazin-4-imine; CGA-293343; Actara; Adage; Cruiser. $C_8H_{10}ClN_5O_3S$; mol wt 291.71. C 32.94%, H 3.46%, Cl 12.15%, N 24.01%, O

16.45%, S 10.99%. Broad-spectrum chloronicotinyl insecticide. Prepn: P. Maienfisch, L. Gsell, **CA 2100924** (1994 to Ciba-Geigy); *eidem*, **US 5852012** (1998 to Novartis); T. Göbel *et al., Pestic. Sci.* **55,** 343 (1999). Effect on feeding behavior of aphids: P. Harrewijn *et al., Brighton Crop Prot. Conf. - Pests Dis.* **1998,** 813. LC-MS determn in fruits and vegetables: D. Zywitz *et al., Deutsche Lebens.-Rundschau* **99,** 188 (2003). Review of physical properties and field trials: R. Senn *et al., ibid.* 27-36; of biological activity, metabolism, and physical properties: D. S. Lawson *et al., Proc. Beltwide Cotton Conf.* **2,** 1106-1109 (1999).

Crystalline powder, mp 139.1°. Soly in water at 25°: 4100 mg/l. Vapor pressure at 25°: 6.6×10^{-9} Pa. Log P (octanol/water) at 25°: −0.13. LD$_{50}$ in rats (mg/kg): 1563 orally, >2000 dermally; LD$_{50}$ in bobwhite quail, mallard duck (mg/kg): 1552, 576 orally. LC$_{50}$ (96hr) in rainbow trout, bluegill (mg/l): >100, >114 (Senn).

USE: Insecticide.

9295. Thiamine. [59-43-8] 3-[(4-Amino-2-methyl-5-pyrimidinyl)methyl]-5-(2-hydroxyethyl)-4-methylthiazolium chloride; vitamin B$_1$; aneurin; thiamine monochloride; thiaminium chloride. C$_{12}$H$_{17}$ClN$_4$OS; mol wt 300.81. C 47.91%, H 5.70%, Cl 11.79%, N 18.63%, O 5.32%, S 10.66%. Essential nutrient required for carbohydrate metabolism; also involved in nerve function. Biosynthesized by microorganisms and plants. Dietary sources include whole grains, meat products, vegetables, milk, legumes and fruit. Also present in rice husks and yeast. Converted *in vivo* to thiamine diphosphate, a coenzyme in the decarboxylation of α-keto acids. Chronic deficiency may lead to neurological impairment, beriberi, Wernicke-Korsakoff syndrome. Isoln from rice bran: B. C. P. Jansen, W. F. Donath, *Chem. Weekbl.* **23,** 201 (1926). Structure: R. R. Williams, *J. Am. Chem. Soc.* **58,** 1063 (1936); R. R. Williams, J. K. Cline, *ibid.* 1504; R. R. Williams *et al., ibid.* **59,** 526 (1937). Review of syntheses: Knobloch in H. Vogel, *Chemie und Technik der Vitamine* vol. **II** (Stuttgart, 1953) pp 1-128. Toxicity data: D. Winter *et al., Int. Z. Vitaminforsch.* **37,** 82 (1967). HPLC determn in foods, pharmaceuticals, body tissues: T. Kawaski, *Methods Enzymol.* **122,** 15 (1986); in plasma and pharmacokinetics: H. Mascher, C. Kikuta, *J. Pharm. Sci.* **82,** 56 (1993). Review of bioavailability, absorption, and role in nutrition: F. L. Iber *et al., Am. J. Clin. Nutr.* **36,** 1067-1082 (1982). *Reviews:* "Thiamin: Twenty Years of Progress", *Ann. N.Y. Acad. Sci.* **378,** H. Z. Sable, C. J. Grubier, Eds. (1982) 470 pp; "Thiamin, Vitamin B$_1$, Aneurin" in *Vitamins,* W. Friedrich, Ed. (de Gruyter, Berlin, 1988) pp 339-401.

Hydrochloride. [67-03-8] Thiamine chloride hydrochloride; thiamine dichloride; Benerva; Betabion; Betalin S; Betaxin; Bewon; Metabolin; Vitaneurin. C$_{12}$H$_{17}$ClN$_4$OS.HCl; mol wt 337.27. Comprehensive description: K. A. M. Al-Rashood *et al., Anal. Profiles Drug Subs.* **18,** 413-458 (1989). Monoclinic plates in rosette-like clusters. Slight thiazole odor. Bitter taste. dec 248°. One gram dissolves in ~1 ml water, 18 ml glycerol, 100 ml 95% alcohol, 315 ml abs alcohol; more sol in methanol. Sol in propylene glycol. Practically insol in ether, benzene, hexane, chloroform. pH of a 1% w/v soln in water 3.13; pH of a 0.1% w/v soln in water 3.58. On exposure to air of average humidity, the vitamin absorbs an amount of water corresponding to nearly one mol, forming a hydrate. LD$_{50}$ in mice (mg/kg): 89.2 i.v.; 8224 orally (Winter).

Mononitrate. [532-43-4] C$_{12}$H$_{17}$N$_5$O$_4$S. Prepn: R. J. Turner, G. J. Schmitt, **US 2844579** (1958 to Am. Cyanamid). Crystals, mp 196-200° (dec). Practically nonhygroscopic. pKa 4.8. Soly in water (g/100 ml): 2.7 (25°); ~30 (100°). pH of 2% aq soln 6.5 to 7.1. More stable than the hydrochloride; suitable for enrichment of flours and feeds, multivitamin prepns.

THERAP CAT: Vitamin (enzyme cofactor).

THERAP CAT (VET): Vitamin (enzyme cofactor).

9296. Thiamine Diphosphate. [154-87-0] 3-[(4-Amino-2-methyl-5-pyrimidinyl)methyl]-4-methyl-5-(4,6,6-trihydroxy-3,5-dioxa-4,6-diphosphahex-1-yl)thiazolium chloride P,P'-dioxide; thiamine trihydrogen pyrophosphate (ester); cocarboxylase; thiamine pyrophosphate; thiamine diphosphate ester chloride; TDP; TPP; Berolase; Bivitasi; Cocalose; Cocarvit; Nutrase; Pyrolase. C$_{12}$H$_{19}$ClN$_4$O$_7$P$_2$S; mol wt 460.77. C 31.28%, H 4.16%, Cl 7.69%, N 12.16%, O 24.31%, P 13.44%, S 6.96%. Coenzyme required for the decarboxylation of α-keto acids. Most abundant form of thiamine in animal tissues. Identification as cofactor and enzymatic synthesis: K. Lohmann, P. Schuster, *Biochem. Z.* **294,** 183 (1937). Chemical synthesis: Weijlard, Tauber, *J. Am. Chem. Soc.* **60,** 2263 (1938); Weil-Malherbe, *Biochem. J.* **34,** 980 (1940); Weijlard, *J. Am. Chem. Soc.* **63,** 1160 (1941); Karrer, Viscontini, *Helv. Chim. Acta* **29,** 711 (1946). LC determn in blood: J. W. I. Brunnekreeft *et al., J. Chromatogr.* **491,** 89 (1989). Role in pathogenesis of Wernicke-Korsakoff Syndrome: R. F. Butterworth *et al., Alcohol. Clin. Exp. Res.* **17,** 1084 (1993). Review of enzyme activity: J. Ullrich *et al., Vitam. Horm.* **28,** 365 (1970); of mechanism of action: R. Kluger, *Chem. Rev.* **87,** 863-876 (1987); M. Louloudi, N. Hadjiliadis, *Coord. Chem. Rev.* **135,** 429-468 (1994).

Monohydrate. Crystals from alc contg some HCl, dec 240-244°. mp 238-240° from abs ethanol. uv max: 242 nm. Soluble in water. pH of 0.3% soln 2.23. The dry substance is very stable.

Free ester tetrahydrate. C$_{12}$H$_{18}$N$_4$O$_7$P$_2$S.4H$_2$O. Prepn: Wenz *et al.,* **US 2991284** (1961 to E. Merck). Dec 220-225°.

Thiamine monophosphate. [532-40-1] 3-[(4-Amino-2-methyl-5-pyrimidinyl)methyl]-4-methyl-5-[2-(phosphonooxy)ethyl]thiazolium chloride; thiamine monophosphate chloride. C$_{12}$H$_{18}$ClN$_4$O$_4$PS; mol wt 380.79. Prepd by sulfuric acid hydrolysis of thiamine diphosphate: Lohmann, Schuster, *loc. cit.* Monohydrate; prisms from dil acetone or water, mp ~200°. Freely sol in water.

THERAP CAT: Vitamin (enzyme cofactor).

9297. Thiamine Disulfide. [67-16-3] N,N'-[Dithiobis[2-(2-hydroxyethyl)-1-methyl-2,1-ethenediyl]]bis[N-[(4-amino-2-methyl-5-pyrimidinyl)methyl]formamide]; aneurin disulfide; vitamin B$_1$ disulfide; Aktivin; Neolamin. C$_{24}$H$_{34}$N$_8$O$_4$S$_2$; mol wt 562.71. C 51.23%, H 6.09%, N 19.91%, O 11.37%, S 11.40%. Isoln: Zima, Williams, *Ber.* **73,** 941 (1940). Prepn: Warnat, **US 2458453** (1949 to Hoffmann-La Roche); Matsukawa, Hirano, *J. Pharm. Soc. Jpn.* **73,** 379 (1953); Hirano, Iwatsu, *ibid.* **73,** 1115 (1953); Kawasaki, *ibid.* **76,** 706 (1956). Bioavailability: N. Aoyagi *et al., Chem. Pharm. Bull.* **34,** 281 (1986).

(Z,Z)-isomer

When anhydr, mp 177° with intense yellow coloration. Very sparingly sol in benzene, acetone, ether, ethanol; freely sol if the crystals contain solvated acetone or water. Soly in water at 37° (mg/ml): 37.7 (pH 1.2); 3.0 (pH 3); 1.33 (pH 5); 0.568 (pH 7.2).

Hydrochloride. [18642-10-9] Crystals from methanol + water, dec 231°.

Phosphate. [992-46-1] Thiamine monophosphate disulfide; Biotinin; Vitamogen. $C_{24}H_{36}N_8O_{10}P_2S_2$; mol wt 722.67.

O,O-Diisobutyrate. [3286-46-2] O-Isobutyrylthiamine disulfide; bisibutiamine; sulbutiamine; Arcalion; Neodaian; Vitaberin. $C_{32}H_{46}N_8O_6S_2$; mol wt 702.89.

THERAP CAT: Vitamin (enzyme cofactor).

9298. Thiamine Triphosphate. [3475-65-8] 3-[(4-Amino-2-methyl-5-pyrimidinyl)methyl]-4-methyl-5-(4,6,8,8-tetrahydroxy-3,5,7-trioxa-4,6,8-triphosphaoct-1-yl)thiazolium inner salt P,P',P''-trioxide; thiamine triphosphoric acid ester; TTP. $C_{12}H_{19}N_4O_{10}P_3$-S; mol wt 504.29. C 28.58%, H 3.80%, N 11.11%, O 31.73%, P 18.43%, S 6.36%. One of the bioactive forms of thiamine; concentrated in neurons and in excitable tissues such as skeletal muscle. Believed to have a noncofactor role in nerve function. Prepn: L. Velluz et al., Bull. Soc. Chim. Fr. **15**, 871 (1948); Roux et al., Bull. Soc. Chim. Biol. **30**, 592 (1948); M. Viscontini et al., Helv. Chim. Acta **32**, 1478 (1949). Relation to thiamine diphosphate: L. Velluz et al., J. Biol. Chem. **180**, 1137 (1949). Identification in rat liver: A. Rossi-Fanelli et al., Science **116**, 711 (1952). Biosynthesis by baker's yeast: K.-H. Kiessling, Nature **172**, 1187 (1953). Enzymatic synthesis: J. R. Cooper, K. Nishino, Methods Enzymol. **122**, 24 (1986). Chromatographic determn in brain extracts: J. R. Cooper, T. Matsuda, ibid. 20. Review of metabolism, tissue distribution and potential neurophysiological role: J. R. Cooper, J. H. Pincus, Neurochem. Res. **4**, 223-239 (1979); L. Bettendorff, Metab. Brain Dis. **9**, 183-209 (1994).

Hemihydrate. Very hygroscopic, rhomb-shaped microcrystals from water-alcohol-acetone, dec 228-232°. Freely sol in water. Insol in the usual organic solvents.

9299. Thiamiprine. [5581-52-2] 6-[(1-Methyl-4-nitro-1H-imidazol-5-yl)thio]-1H-purin-2-amine; 2-amino-6-[(1-methyl-4-nitroimidazol-5-yl)thio]purine; 2-amino-6-(1'-methyl-4'-nitro-5'-imidazolyl)mercaptopurine; Guaneran. $C_9H_8N_8O_2S$; mol wt 292.28. C 36.98%, H 2.76%, N 38.34%, O 10.95%, S 10.97%. Prepd from thioguanine and 1-methyl-4-nitro-5-chloroimidazole: Hitchings, Elion, US 3056785 (1962 to Burroughs Wellcome).

Crystals, dec slowly >200°. uv max: 320 nm at pH 1; 315 nm at pH 11.

THERAP CAT: Antineoplastic.

9300. Thiamorpholine. [123-90-0] Thiomorpholine; tetrahydro-1,4-thiazine; 1,4-thiazan; parathiazan. C_4H_9NS; mol wt 103.19. C 46.56%, H 8.79%, N 13.57%, S 31.07%. Prepd by heating β,β'-dichlorodiethyl sulfide with alcoholic ammonia under pressure: Davies, J. Chem. Soc. **117**, 298, 306 (1920).

Mobile liquid. Strong odor resembling that of piperidine. Absorbs CO_2 from air. bp_{758} 169°; bp_{743} 166-167°. Volatile with steam. Miscible with water and many organic liquids.

Hydrochloride. $C_4H_9NS.HCl$. Hygroscopic needles from alcohol + ether, dec 163°. Freely sol in water.

Picrolonate. $C_4H_9NS.C_{10}H_8N_4O_5$. Deep orange prisms from alcohol, dec 242° (darkens at 210°).

9301. Thiamphenicol. [15318-45-3] 2,2-Dichloro-N-[(1R,-2R)-2-hydroxy-1-(hydroxymethyl)-2-[4-(methylsulfonyl)phenyl]-ethyl]acetamide; D-d-threo-2-dichloroacetamido-1-(4-methylsulfonyl)phenyl-1,3-propanediol; dextrosulphenidol; Win-5063-2; 8053CB; Hyrazin; Igralin; Neomyson; Rigelon; Thiamcol; Thionicol; Thiophenicol; Urfamycine; Urophenil. $C_{12}H_{15}Cl_2NO_5S$; mol wt 356.22. C 40.46%, H 4.24%, Cl 19.91%, N 3.93%, O 22.46%, S 9.00%. Synthesis: Cutler et al., J. Am. Chem. Soc. **74**, 5475 (1952); Suter et al., ibid. **75**, 4330 (1953); Suter, US 2759927; US 2759970; US 2759971; US 2759972; US 2759976 (all 1956 to Sterling Drugs); GB 770277 (1957 to Parke, Davis).

Crystals, mp 164.3-166.3°. $[\alpha]_D^{25}$ +12.9° (ethanol). uv max (95% ethanol): 224, 266, 274 nm (ε 13,700, 800, 700). Appreciably sol in water. Soluble in alcohol.

DL-Form. [847-25-6] Raceophenidol; racephenicol; Dexawin; Thiocymetin.

THERAP CAT: Antibacterial.

THERAP CAT (VET): D-Form as antimicrobial; DL-form in control of fowl cholera.

9302. Thiamylal. [77-27-0] Dihydro-5-(1-methylbutyl)-5-(2-propenyl)-2-thioxo-4,6(1H,5H)-pyrimidinedione; 5-allyl-5-(1-methylbutyl)-2-thiobarbituric acid; thioseconal. $C_{12}H_{18}N_2O_2S$; mol wt 254.35. C 56.67%, H 7.13%, N 11.01%, O 12.58%, S 12.61%. Prepn: GB 613704 (1948 to Lilly); Abe et al., J. Pharm. Soc. Jpn. **75**, 891 (1955); Izumi, Nakanishi, JP 56 8785 (1956 to Yoshitomi); Donnison, US 2876225 (1959 to Abbott).

Crystals from dil ethanol, mp 132-133°.

Sodium salt. [337-47-3] Surital. $C_{12}H_{17}N_2NaO_2S$; mol wt 276.33.

Note: This is a controlled substance (depressant): **21 CFR**, 1308.13.

THERAP CAT: Anesthetic (intravenous).

THERAP CAT (VET): Anesthetic (intravenous).

9303. Thianaphthene. [95-15-8] Benzo[b]thiophene; benzothiofuran. C_8H_6S; mol wt 134.20. C 71.60%, H 4.51%, S 23.89%. Occurs in lignite tar. Catalytic synthesis from styrene and hydrogen sulfide: Moore, Greensfelder, J. Am. Chem. Soc. **69**, 2008 (1947); from ethyl benzene and hydrogen sulfide: Hansch, Hawthorne, ibid. **70**, 2495 (1948).

Leaflets. Odor similar to that of naphthalene. mp 32°; bp_{760} 221°; bp_{20} 103-105°. Volatile with steam. Sol in the usual organic solvents.

USE: Manuf of pharmaceuticals, thioindigo.

9304. Thiarubrines. $C_{13}H_8S_2$; mol wt 228.33. C 68.38%, H 3.53%, S 28.09%. Class of dark red bioactive dithiacyclohexadiene polyacetylenes found in various *Asteraceae*; A and B forms are most common. Used medicinally in Africa: J. M. Watt, M. G. Breyer-Brandwijk, *The Medicinal and Poisonous Plants of Southern and Eastern Africa* (E. & S. Livingstone Ltd., Edinburgh, 2nd edition, 1962) pp 202-205; leaves are consumed by chimpanzees possibly as a pharmaceutic: E. Rodriguez *et al., Experientia* **41**, 419 (1985). Isoln: F. Bohlmann, K.-M. Kleine, *Ber.* **98**, 3081 (1965); and separation by HPLC: R. A. Norton *et al., Phytochemistry* **24**, 356 (1985); from *Ambrosia chamissonis:* S. Ellis *et al., ibid.* **33**, 224 (1993). NMR spectra and biosynthetic study of A: M. L. Gomez-Barrios *et al., ibid.* **31**, 2703 (1992). Synthesis of A: M. Koreeda, W. Yang, *J. Am. Chem. Soc.* **116**, 10793, (1994); of B: E. Block *et al., ibid.* 9403. Antibiotic properties of A: G. H. N. Towers *et al., Planta Med.* **51**, 225 (1985); photo-enhancement of activity: G. P. Constabel, G. H. N Towers, *ibid.* **55**, 35 (1989). Antiviral properties of A: J. B. Hudson *et al., ibid.* **52**, 51 (1986); photo-enhancement of activity against HIV: J. B. Hudson *et al., Photochem. Photobiol.* **57**, 675 (1993).

Thiarubrine A

Thiarubrin(e) A. [63543-09-9] 3-(5-Hexene-1,3-diynyl)-6-(1-propynyl)-1,2-dithiin. Red liquid. λmax (EtOH): 490 nm. uv max (EtOH): 345, 233 nm.

Thiarubrin(e) B. [71539-72-5] 3-(3-Buten-1-ynyl)-6-(1,3-pentadiynyl)-1,2-dithiin. λMax (EtOH): 490 nm. uv max (EtOH): 345, 243 nm.

9305. Thiazesim. [5845-26-1] 5-[2-(Dimethylamino)ethyl]-2,3-dihydro-2-phenyl-1,5-benzothiazepin-4(5H)-one; thiazenone; tiazesim. $C_{19}H_{22}N_2OS$; mol wt 326.46. C 69.90%, H 6.79%, N 8.58%, O 4.90%, S 9.82%. Prepn of the hydrochloride: Krapcho *et al., J. Med. Chem.* **6**(5), 544 (1963); Krapcho, US **3075967** (1963 to Olin Mathieson). Metabolism: J. Dreyfuss *et al., J. Pharm. Sci.* **57**, 1497, 1505 (1968).

Hydrochloride. [3122-01-8] SQ-10496; Altinil. $C_{19}H_{22}N_2$-OS.HCl; mol wt 362.92. Crystals from acetonitrile, mp 222-224°.
THERAP CAT: Antidepressant.

9306. Thiazinamium Methylsulfate. [58-34-4] *N,N,N,α*-Tetramethyl-10H-phenothiazine-10-ethanaminium methyl sulfate; trimethyl(1-methyl-2-phenothiazin-10-ylethyl)ammonium methyl sulfate; trimethyl[1-methyl-2-(10-phenothiazinyl)ethyl]ammonium methyl sulfate; *N*-[β-(10-phenothiazinyl)propyl]trimethylammonium methyl sulfate; RP-3554; Multergan; Padisal. $C_{19}H_{26}N_2O_4$-S_2; mol wt 410.55. C 55.58%, H 6.38%, N 6.82%, O 15.59%, S 15.62%. Prepd by treating promethazine with dimethyl sulfate: **GB 641452** (1950 to Rhône-Poulenc). Crystal structure: P. Marsau, Y. Cam, *Acta Crystallogr.* **B29**, 980 (1973). Determn in body fluids: J. H. G. Jonkman *et al., J. Pharm. Pharmacol.* **27**, 849 (1975). Bioavailability: *idem et al., Clin. Pharmacol. Ther.* **21**, 457 (1977). Pharmacokinetics: *idem et al., Arzneim.-Forsch.* **23**, 223 (1983); *idem et al., Int. J. Clin. Pharmacol. Ther. Toxicol.* **21**, 454 (1983).

Crystals, mp 206-210° (some dec). Discolors on exposure to light. Soly in water (25°): ~10%. Freely sol in abs ethanol; sparingly sol in acetone. Practically insol in ether, benzene.
THERAP CAT: Antihistaminic.

9307. Thiazole. [288-47-1] C_3H_3NS; mol wt 85.13. C 42.33%, H 3.55%, N 16.45%, S 37.67%. First described as the pyridine of the thiophene series: A. Hantzsch, J. Weber, *Ber.* **20**, 3118 (1887); A. Hantzsch, *Ann.* **249**, 1 (1888). Book: *The Chemistry of Heterocyclic Compounds* **vol. 34**, A. Weissberger, E. C. Taylor, Eds. (New York, Wiley, 1979).

Colorless or pale yellow liquid. Characteristic foul odor; d^{17} ~1.20; bp 115-118°. Slightly sol in water; sol in many organic solvents. Forms compds with auric, mercuric, and platinic chlorides.

9308. Thiazole Orange. 1-Methyl-4-[(3-methyl-2(3H)-benzothiazolylidene)methyl] quinolinium; TO. $[C_{19}H_{17}N_2S]^+$. Asymmetric cyanine dye; fluoresces when intercalated with DNA or RNA. Prepn of tosylate and use in reticulocyte analysis: L. G. Lee *et al., Cytometry* **7**, 508 (1986). Interactions with DNA: J. Nygren *et al., Biopolymers* **46**, 39 (1998). Use in detection of reticulated platelets: T. Fujii *et al., Thromb. Res.* **97**, 431 (2000); L. Joutsi-Korhonen *et al., Eur. J. Haematol.* **65**, 66 (2000); in fluorescent intercalator displacement assays: D. L. Boger, W. C. Tse, *Bioorg. Med. Chem.* **9**, 2511 (2001).

Dimer. [143413-84-7] 1,1'-[1,3-Propanediylbis[(dimethylimino)-3,1-propanediyl]]bis[4-(3-methyl-2(3H)-benzothiazolylidene)methyl] quinolinium tetraiodide; TOTO. $C_{49}H_{58}I_4N_6S_2$; mol wt 1302.77. Synthesis and characterization: H. S. Rye *et al., Nucleic Acids Res.* **20**, 2803 (1992). ^{1}H NMR soln structure of complex with DNA: H. P. Spielmann *et al., Biochemistry* **34**, 8542 (1995). Interactions with DNA: J. Bunkenborg *et al., Bioconjugate Chem.* **11**, 861 (2000). Absorption max (4 mM TAE, pH 8.2): 481 nm. $ε_{507}$ 131.7×10³ in methanol.
Iodide. [24147-36-2] $C_{19}H_{17}IN_2S$; mol wt 432.32. Absorption max (4 mM TAE, pH 8.2): 501 nm. $ε_{502}$ 77.0×10³ in methanol.
Methyl Sulfate. [172668-52-9] $C_{19}H_{17}N_2S.CH_3O_4S$; mol wt 416.51. Prepn: T. G. Deligeorgiev *et al., Dyes Pigments* **29**, 315 (1995). Crystals from acetone, mp 225-227°. Absorption max (methanol): 500 nm (ε 80700).
Tosylate. [107091-89-4] $C_{19}H_{17}N_2S.C_7H_7O_3S$; mol wt 476.61. Sol in methanol. Absorption max (methanol): 512 nm.
Note: The term "thiazole orange" is used to describe various salt forms in the chemical literature.
USE: Stains DNA or RNA in flow cytometry reticulocyte analysis, in agarose gels, in capillary electrophoresis.

9309. Thiazolsulfone. [473-30-3] 5-[(4-Aminophenyl)sulfonyl]-2-thiazolamine; 2-amino-5-sulfanilylthiazole; 4-aminophenyl-2'-aminothiazolyl-5'-sulfone; thiazosulfone; thiazolesulfone;

Promizole. $C_9H_9N_3O_2S_2$; mol wt 255.32. C 42.34%, H 3.55%, N 16.46%, O 12.53%, S 25.12%. Prepd from the reaction products of *p*-nitrobenzenesulfonyl chloride and 2 mols of 2-aminothiazole: Bambas, *J. Am. Chem. Soc.* **67**, 671 (1945); Bambas, **US 2389126** (1945 to Parke, Davis).

Fine needles from alc, mp 219-221° (some decompn). Sol in water at pH 6.5 to the extent of 30-40 mg per 100 ml at 28-30°. Freely sol in acetone, dioxane, 70% alc, dil acids. Moderately sol in abs alcohol, ethyl acetate and ether. It is a very weak acid, dissolves in 10% alkali (decompn) and forms an alkali metal salt at pH 10.

THERAP CAT: Antibacterial.

9310. Thiazol Yellow G. [1829-00-1] 2,2'-(1-Triazene-1,3-diyldi-4,1-phenylene)bis[6-methyl-7-benzothiazolesulfonic acid] disodium salt; C.I. Direct Yellow 9; 2,2'-[(diazoamino)di-*p*-phenylene]bis[6-methyl-7-benzothiazolesulfonic acid] disodium salt; C.I. 19540; Chlorazol Yellow 2G; Clayton yellow; Diazamine Golden Yellow T; Titan yellow. $C_{28}H_{19}N_5Na_2O_6S_4$; mol wt 695.72. C 48.34%, H 2.75%, N 10.07%, Na 6.61%, O 13.80%, S 18.44%. Prepn from 2-(*p*-aminophenyl)-6-methyl-7-benzothiazolesulfonic acid ("dehydrothio-*p*-toluidinesulfonic acid"): *Beilstein* **vol. 27**, 2nd suppl, 509; F. J. Welcher, *Organic Analytical Reagents* **vol. 4** (Van Nostrand, New York, 1948) p 391; H. King *et al.*, *Analyst* **92**, 695 (1967). *See also: Colour Index* **vol. 2** (3rd ed., 1971) p 2010; *H. J. Conn's Biological Stains*, R. D. Lillie, Ed. (Williams & Wilkins, Baltimore, 9th ed., 1977) p 371.

Yellowish-brown powder. Sol in water, or alc (yellow solns), NaOH (reddish-yellow soln), H_2SO_4 (brownish-yellow soln). *Protect from light.*

USE: Dyeing cotton, viscose rayon, natural silk; as biological stain; as an analytical reagent, most often for the determination of Mg; as pH indicator, yellow 11.0 to red 13.0; as fluorescent dye for microscopy.

9311. Thiazopyr. [117718-60-2] 2-(Difluoromethyl)-5-(4,-5-dihydro-2-thiazolyl)-4-(2-methylpropyl)-6-(trifluoromethyl)-3-pyridinecarboxylic acid methyl ester; RH-123652; MON-13200; Mandate; Visor. $C_{16}H_{17}F_5N_2O_2S$; mol wt 396.38. C 48.48%, H 4.32%, F 23.96%, N 7.07%, O 8.07%, S 8.09%. Pre-emergent herbicide for use in crops. Prepn: Y.-L. L. Sing, L. F. Lee, **EP 278944**; *eidem*, **US 4988384** (1988, 1991 both to Monsanto). GC determn in soil and plant samples: R. A. Pérez *et al.*, *J. Chromatogr. A* **778**, 193 (1997). Metabolism in plants: P. C. C. Feng *et al.*, *Pestic. Sci.* **45**, 203 (1995). Field trials in perennial crops: H. L. Warner, J. A. Holmdal, *Brighton Crop Prot. Conf. - Weeds* **1995**, 942.

Pale orange crystals from hexanes, mp 79-81°.
USE: Herbicide.

9312. Thibenzazoline. [6028-35-9] 1,3-Dihydro-1,3-bis-(hydroxymethyl)-2*H*-benzimidazole-2-thione; 1,3-bis(hydroxymethyl)-2-benzimidazolinethione; 2-mercaptobenzimidazole-1,3-dimethylol; Thyreocordon. $C_9H_{10}N_2O_2S$; mol wt 210.25. C

51.41%, H 4.79%, N 13.32%, O 15.22%, S 15.25%. Prepn: Monti, Venturi, *Gazz. Chim. Ital.* **76**, 365 (1946).

Very bitter. mp 160-162°. Soluble dil in alkalies.
THERAP CAT: Antihyperthyroid.

9313. Thidiazuron. [51707-55-2] *N*-Phenyl-*N'*-1,2,3-thiadiazol-5-ylurea; 5-(*N*-phenylcarbamoylamino)-1,2,3-thiadiazole; thiadiazuron; TDZ; Dropp; Ginstar. $C_9H_8N_4OS$; mol wt 220.25. C 49.08%, H 3.66%, N 25.44%, O 7.26%, S 14.56%. Non-purine containing urea derivative with cytokinin activity. Prepn: H. Schulz, F. Arndt, **DE 2214632**; *eidem*, **US 3883547** (1973, 1975 both to Schering AG). Field trial in cotton: A. R. Hopkins, R. F. Moore, *J. Econ. Entomol.* **73**, 768 (1980). Effect of temperature and adjuvants on activity in cotton: C. E. Snipes, G. D. Wills, *Weed Sci.* **42**, 13 (1994). Review of effect on shoot formation and axillary shoot proliferation: C.-Y. Lu, *In Vitro Cell. Dev. Biol.* **29P**, 92-96 (1993); on woody plant tissue culture: C. A. Huetteman, J. E. Preece, *Plant Cell Tissue Organ Cult.* **33**, 105-119 (1993).

Crystals from isopropanol, mp 217° (dec). Very sol in DMSO, DMF, acetone, cyclohexanone, isophorone. Slightly sol in aliphatic and aromatic hydrocarbons and water.
USE: Cotton defoliant; plant growth regulator in tissue culture.

9314. Thienamycin. [59995-64-1] (5*R*,6*S*)-3-[(2-Amino-ethyl)thio]-6-[(1*R*)-1-hydroxyethyl]-7-oxo-1-azabicyclo[3.2.0]-hept-2-ene-2-carboxylic acid. $C_{11}H_{16}N_2O_4S$; mol wt 272.32. C 48.52%, H 5.92%, N 10.29%, O 23.50%, S 11.77%. The first member of a family of des-thia-carbapenem nucleus antibiotics having a thioethylamine side-chain on the enamine portion of the fused 5-membered ring. Produced by *Streptomyces cattleya:* J. S. Kahan *et al.*, **US 3950357** (1976 to Merck & Co.). Discovery, isoln, taxonomy, physical properties: *eidem, J. Antibiot.* **32**, 1 (1979). Structure, absolute configuration: G. Albers-Schönberg *et al., J. Am. Chem. Soc.* **100**, 6491 (1978). Synthesis of the (±)-form: D. B. R. Johnston *et al., ibid.* 313; F. A. Bouffard *et al., J. Org. Chem.* **45**, 1130 (1980); S. M. Schmitt *et al., ibid.* 1135, 1142; D. G. Melillo *et al., Tetrahedron Lett.* **21**, 2783 (1980); *eidem, ibid.* **22**, 913 (1981); M. Shiozaki, T. Hiraoka, *Tetrahedron* **38**, 3457 (1982). Alternate prepn of key intermediate: J. D. Buynak *et al., Chem. Commun.* **1986**, 941. Stereocontrolled synthesis of the naturally occurring (+)-form: T. Salzmann *et al., J. Am. Chem. Soc.* **102**, 6161 (1980); S. Karady *et al., ibid.* **103**, 6765 (1981). Alternate synthetic routes: S. T. Hodgson *et al., Tetrahedron* **41**, 5871 (1985); T. Iimori, M. Shibasaki, *Tetrahedron Lett.* **26**, 1523 (1985); T. Chiba, T. Nakai, *ibid.* 4647; D. J. Hart, D. C. Ha, *ibid.* 5493; T. Kametani *et al., J. Org. Chem.* **50**, 2327 (1985); H. Maruyama, T. Hiraoka, *ibid.* **51**, 399 (1986); D. G. Melillo *et al., ibid.* 1498. Continuous production in immobilized cell systems: E. J. Arcuri *et al., Biotechnol. Bioeng.* **28**, 842 (1986). Biosynthesis: J. M. Williamson *et al., J. Biol. Chem.* **260**, 4637 (1985). *In vitro* antibacterial activity: F. P. Tally *et al., Antimicrob. Agents Chemother.* **14**, 436 (1978); S. S. Weaver *et al., ibid.* **15**, 518 (1979). Evaluation of *in vitro* and *in vivo* activities: H. Kropp *et al., Antimicrob. Agents Chemother.* **17**, 993 (1980). Comparative study vs gram-positive and gram-negative aerobic and anaerobic species and β-lactamase stability: H. C. Neu, P. Labthavikul, *ibid.* **21**, 180 (1982). *N*-Acyl derivatives as anti-inflammatory agents: J. B. Doherty *et al.*, **US 4465687** (1984 to Merck & Co.). Pharmacokinetics, bacteriological efficacy: P. Patamasucon, G. H. McCracken, *Antimicrob. Agents Chemother.* **21**, 390 (1982). Review of early syntheses of the carbapenems: T. Kametani, *Heterocycles* **17**, 463-506 (1982).

White hygroscopic solid. $[\alpha]_D^{27}$ +82.7° (c = 1.0 in water). uv max (water, pH 4-8): 296.5 nm (ε 7900); (pH 2): 309 nm; (pH 12): 300.5 nm. Freely sol in water, sparingly sol in methanol. In dilute soln, stability is optimal between pH 6-7, declining with unusual rapidity above that range. Susceptible to inactivation by dilute solns of hydroxylamine and cysteine.

N-Formimidoylthienamycin monohydrate *see* Imipenem.

9315. Thiethylperazine. [1420-55-9] 2-(Ethylthio)-10-[3-(4-methyl-1-piperazinyl)propyl]phenothiazine; 3-ethylmercapto-10-(1'-methylpiperazinyl-4'-propyl)phenothiazine. $C_{22}H_{29}N_3S_2$; mol wt 399.62. C 66.12%, H 7.31%, N 10.52%, S 16.05%. Prepn: Bourquin *et al., Helv. Chim. Acta* **41,** 1072 (1958).

Crystals from acetone, mp 62-64°. bp$_{0.01}$ 227°.
Dimaleate. [1179-69-7] GS-95; NSC-130044; Torecan; Toresten. $C_{22}H_{29}N_3S_2 \cdot 2C_4H_4O_4$; mol wt 631.76. Crystals from methanol, dec 188-190°.
Dihydrochloride. $C_{22}H_{29}N_3S_2 \cdot 2HCl$. Crystals from ethanol, mp 214-216°.
Dimalate. [52239-63-1] $C_{22}H_{29}N_3S_2 \cdot 2C_4H_6O_5$. Crystals from ethanol, mp 139°.
THERAP CAT: Antiemetic.

9316. Thifensulfuron-methyl. [79277-27-3] 3-[[[[(4-Methoxy-6-methyl-1,3,5-triazin-2-yl)amino]carbonyl]amino]sulfonyl]-2-thiophenecarboxylic acid methyl ester; methyl 3-(3-(4-methoxy-6-methyl-1,3,5-triazin-2-yl)ureidosulfonyl)thiophene-2-carboxylate; thiameturon-methyl; DPX-M6316; Pinnacle; Harmony. $C_{12}H_{13}N_5O_6S_2$; mol wt 387.39. C 37.20%, H 3.38%, N 18.08%, O 24.78%, S 16.55%. Sulfonylurea herbicide for postemergence broadleaf weed control in food crops. Prepn: G. Levitt, **EP 30142;** *idem,* **US 4481029** (1981, 1984 both to DuPont). Degradation in soil: H. M. Brown *et al., J. Agric. Food Chem.* **45,** 955 (1997). HPLC determn in cotton seed: J. J. Stry *et al., J. AOAC Int.* **83,** 651 (2000). Metabolism in soybeans: H. M. Brown *et al., Pestic. Biochem. Physiol.* **37,** 303 (1990). Review of physical properties, mode of action and field trials: S. D. Sionis *et al., Proc. Br. Crop Prot. Conf. - Weeds* **1985,** 49-54.

White solid, mp 186°. pKa at 25°: 4.0. Soly in water at 25° (mg/l): 24 (pH 4); 260 (pH 5); 2400 (pH 6). Vapor pressure at 25°: 2.7×10^{-6} mmHg. Partition coefficient (octanol/water): 0.027.
USE: Herbicide.

9317. Thimerosal. [54-64-8] Ethyl[2-mercaptobenzoato-(2−)-O,S]mercurate(1−) sodium; [(o-carboxyphenyl)thio]ethylmercury sodium salt; sodium ethylmercurithiosalicylate; thiomersalate; mercurothiolate; Merthiolate; Merzonin; Vitaseptol. $C_9H_9HgNaO_2S$; mol wt 404.81. C 26.70%, H 2.24%, Hg 49.55%, Na 5.68%, O 7.90%, S 7.92%. Prepd by reacting ethylmercuric chlo-

ride (or ethylmercuric hydroxide) with thiosalicylic acid: Kharasch, **US 1672615** (1928); Trikojus, *Nature* **158,** 472 (1946); Swirska *et al., Przem. Chem.* **39,** 371 (1960), *C.A.* **55,** 3507a (1961). Toxicity: Mason *et al., Clin. Toxicol.* **4,** 185 (1971). Review of health effects from vaccine exposure: M. Bigham, R. Copes, *Drug Saf.* **28,** 89-101 (2005).

Cream-colored, crystalline powder. Stable in air, but not in sunlight. One gram dissolves in about 1 ml water, in about 8 ml alcohol. Practically insol in ether and benzene. Stabilization of solns with EDTA: Davisson, **US 2864844** (1958 to Lilly). pH of 1% aq soln: 6.7. LD$_{50}$ s.c. in rats: 98 mg/kg (Mason).
USE: Pharmaceutic aid (preservative).
THERAP CAT: Anti-infective.
THERAP CAT (VET): Antibacterial, antifungal (topical).

9318. Thioacetaldehyde. [2765-04-0] 2,4,6-Trimethyl-*s*-trithiane; trithioacetaldehyde. $C_6H_{12}S_3$; mol wt 180.35. C 39.96%, H 6.71%, S 53.34%. Occurs in α- and β-forms. Prepn: Baumann, Fromm, *Ber.* **22,** 2600 (1889); Fromm, Engler, *Ber.* **58,** 1916 (1925). Molecular structure: Hassel, Viervoll, *Acta Chem. Scand.* **1,** 164 (1947). Stereochemistry: Schönberg, Barakat, *J. Chem. Soc.* **1947,** 693.

α-**Form.** Monoclinic plates, mp 101°.
β-**Form.** Needles from acetone, mp 126°.

9319. Thioacetamide. [62-55-5] Ethanethioamide. C_2H_5NS; mol wt 75.13. C 31.97%, H 6.71%, N 18.64%, S 42.68%. CH_3CSNH_2. Prepd by heating ammonium acetate and aluminum sulfide: Kindler, Finndorf, *Ber.* **54,** 1080 (1921); from acetonitrile + H_2S: Kindler, *Ann.* **431,** 203 (1923); from acetamide + K_3PS_4: Schultz, Ranke, *Arch. Pharm.* **294,** 82 (1961). Toxicity data: Ambrose *et al., J. Ind. Hyg. Toxicol.* **31,** 158 (1949). Review of uses: H. F. Walton, *Thioacetamide as Analytical Reagent,* Arapahoe Chemicals, Inc., Boulder, Colorado.
Crystals from benzene, mp 113-114°. Slight odor of mercaptans. uv max (water): 210, 261, 318 nm (log ε 3.66, 4.08, 1.8). Soly in water at 25° 16.3 g/100 ml; in ethanol 26.4 g/100 g. Sparingly sol in ether. MLD orally in rats: 200 mg/kg (Ambrose).
Caution: This substance is reasonably anticipated to be a human carcinogen: *Report on Carcinogens, Eleventh Edition* (PB2005-104914, 2004) p III-247.
USE: Substitute for H_2S in laboratory qualitative analyses.

9320. Thioacetic Acid. [507-09-5] Ethanethioic acid; thiolacetic acid; thiacetic acid. C_2H_4OS; mol wt 76.12. C 31.56%, H 5.30%, O 21.02%, S 42.12%. CH_3COSH. Prepn by distilling glacial acetic acid with phosphorus pentasulfide: Kekulé, *Ann.* **90,** 309 (1854); from acetic anhydride and hydrogen sulfide: Ellingboe, *Org. Synth.* **31,** 105 (1951).
Yellow, fuming liquid; pungent odor. d$_4^{10}$ 1.075; bp 93°. Not solidified at −17°. Sol in water, particularly hot; very sol in alcohol.

9321. Thiobarbital. [77-32-7] 5,5-Diethyldihydro-2-thioxo-4,6(1H,5H)-pyrimidinedione; 5,5-diethyl-2-thiobarbituric acid; Ibition. $C_8H_{12}N_2O_2S$; mol wt 200.26. C 47.98%, H 6.04%, N 13.99%, O 15.98%, S 16.01%. Prepn: Fischer, Dilthey, *Ann.* **335,** 350 (1904); Carrington, *J. Chem. Soc.* **1944,** 124. Metabolism in man: Bush *et al., J. Pharmacol. Exp. Ther.* **134,** 110 (1961).

Pale yellow needles from water, mp 180°. Sol in about 88 parts hot water, in ethanol, chloroform, ether, acetone, ammonia, alkalies. Sparingly sol in toluene. Practically insol in benzene.

THERAP CAT: Antihyperthyroid.

9322. Thiobenzyl Alcohol. [100-53-8] Benzenemethanethiol; benzyl mercaptan; α-toluenethiol. C_7H_8S; mol wt 124.20. C 67.69%, H 6.49%, S 25.82%. $C_6H_5CH_2SH$.

Colorless liquid; odor of leek; d^{20} 1.058; bp 194-195°. Oxidizes in air to dibenzyl disulfide.

Caution: Can cause mild irritation to mucous membranes.

9323. Thiobutabarbital. [2095-57-0] 5-Ethyldihydro-5-(1-methylpropyl)-2-thioxo-4,6(1H,5H)-pyrimidinedione; 5-*sec*-butyl-5-ethyl-2-thiobarbituric acid; 5-ethyl-5-(1-methylpropyl)-2-thiobarbituric acid; thibutabarbital. $C_{10}H_{16}N_2O_2S$; mol wt 228.31. C 52.61%, H 7.06%, N 12.27%, O 14.02%, S 14.04%. Prepn: Volwiler, Tabern, US 2153729; US 2153731 (both 1939 to Abbott).

Crystals, mp 163-165°.

Sodium salt. [947-08-0] Inactin; Brevinarcon. $C_{10}H_{15}N_2$-NaO_2S; mol wt 250.29. Crystalline, slightly hygroscopic solid. Readily sol in water.

Note: This is a controlled substance (depressant): **21 CFR, 1308.13.**

THERAP CAT: Anesthetic (intravenous).

9324. Thiocolchicine. [2730-71-4] *N*-[(7S)-5,6,7,9-Tetrahydro-1,2,3-trimethoxy-10-(methylthio)-9-oxobenzo[*a*]heptalen-7-yl]acetamide. $C_{22}H_{25}NO_5S$; mol wt 415.50. C 63.59%, H 6.06%, N 3.37%, O 19.25%, S 7.72%. Prepn: Velluz, Muller, *Bull. Soc. Chim. Fr.* **1954,** 755; Muller, Velluz, US 2820029 (1958 to UCLAF). Prepn of 2-glucoside analog: Velluz, Muller, *Bull. Soc. Chim. Fr.* **1955,** 194; Muller, Velluz, *loc. cit.*

Yellow cubic crystals from ethyl acetate, mp 192-194°. $[\alpha]_D^{20}$ −221°. Sol in ethanol, acetone, chloroform. Practically insol in water, ether.

2-Glucoside analog. [602-41-5] Thiocolchicoside; 2-demethoxy-2-glucosidoxythiocolchicine; Coltramyl; Coltrax; Miorel; Musco-Ril. $C_{27}H_{33}NO_{10}S$; mol wt 563.62. Crystals from ethanol + 1N NaOH, dec 220°. $[\alpha]_D$ −609° (water), −240° (ethanol).

THERAP CAT: Thiocolchicoside as muscle relaxant (skeletal).

9325. Thiocresol. [26445-03-4] Methylbenzenethiol; methylthiophenol; tolylmercaptan; toluenethiol. C_7H_8S; mol wt 124.20. C 67.69%, H 6.49%, S 25.82%. $CH_3C_6H_4SH$. Prepn of *m*-isomer: D. S. Tarbell, D. K. Fukushima, *Org. Synth.* **Coll. Vol. 3,** 809 (1955).

All three isomers boil at ~195°. Insol in water. Sol in alcohol or ether.

o-**Thiocresol.** [137-06-4] Colorless to pale yellow liquid, mp 15°; volatile with steam. Flash point, closed cup: 147°F (64°C).

m-**Thiocresol.** [108-40-7] Liquid, mp below −20°. bp$_{25}$ 90-93°. d_4^{20} 1.044. n_D^{25} 1.568-1.571. Flash point, closed cup: 163°F (73°C).

p-**Thiocresol.** [106-45-6] Leaflets, mp 43-44°. Flash point, closed cup: 154°F (68°C).

Caution: May be irritating to skin, eyes, and respiratory tract.

9326. Thioctic Acid. [62-46-8] 1,2-Dithiolane-3-pentanoic acid; 1,2-dithiolane-3-valeric acid; 6,8-thioctic acid; α-lipoic acid; 5-(1,2-dithiolan-3-yl)valeric acid; 5-[3-(1,2-dithiolanyl)]pentanoic acid; δ-[3-(1,2-dithiacyclopentyl)]pentanoic acid; protogen A; acetate replacing factor; pyruvate oxidation factor; Biletan; Thioctacid; Thioctan; Tioctan. $C_8H_{14}O_2S_2$; mol wt 206.33. C 46.57%, H 6.84%, O 15.51%, S 31.08%. Growth factor for many bacteria and protozoa; prosthetic group, coenzyme, or substrate in plants, microorganisms, and animal tissues. Isoln of naturally occurring *d*-form: L. J. Reed *et al., Science* **114,** 93 (1951); *eidem, J. Am. Chem. Soc.* **75,** 1267 (1953); Patterson *et al., ibid.* **76,** 1823 (1954). Syntheses of *dl*-form: Bullock *et al., ibid.* **74,** 1868, 3455 (1952); Hornberger *et al., ibid.* 2382; Reed, US 2980716 and US 3049549 (1961, 1962 to Res. Corp.); Lewis, Raphael, *J. Chem. Soc.* **1962,** 4263; Ose *et al.,* US 3223712 (1965 to Yamanouchi); J. Tsuji *et al., J. Org. Chem.* **43,** 3606 (1978). Biosynthesis via linoleic acid: J. P. Carreau *Methods Enzymol.* **62,** 152-158 (1974). Enantioselective synthesis of *d*-form: P. C. Bulmanpage *et al., Chem. Commun.* **1986,** 1408. Clinical study in treatment of Wilson's disease: S. F. Gomes da Costa, *Arzneim.-Forsch.* **20,** 1210 (1970). Use in treatment of mushroom poisoning: R. Plotzker *et al., Am. J. Med. Sci.* **283,** 79 (1982); J. P. Hanrahan, M. A. Gordon, *J. Am. Med. Assoc.* **251,** 1057 (1984). *Reviews:* Wagner, Folkers, *Vitamins and Coenzymes* (Interscience, New York, 1964) pp 244-263; Schmidt *et al., Angew. Chem. Int. Ed.* **4,** 846 (1965); Schmidt *et al., Adv. Enzymol. Relat. Areas Mol. Biol.* **32,** 423 (1969).

d-Form

Sodium salt. [2319-84-8] $C_8H_{13}NaO_2S_2$. White powder, sol in water. pH of aq solns about 7.4.

d-**Form.** [1200-22-2] Crystals by vacuum sublimation (at 85-90° and 25 microns). mp 46-48° (microblock). $[\alpha]_D^{23}$ +104° (c = 0.88 in benzene). uv max (methanol): 333 nm (ε 150). pKa 5.4. Practically insol in water. Sol in fat solvents.

dl-**Form.** [1077-28-7] Yellow needles from cyclohexane, mp 60-61°. bp 160-165°. uv spectrum: Calvin, *Fed. Proc.* **13,** 703 (1954). Practically insol in water. Sol in fat solvents. Forms a water-soluble sodium salt.

l-**Form.** [1077-27-6] Crystals from cyclohexane, mp 45-47.5° (microblock). $[\alpha]_D^{23}$ −113° (c = 1.88 in benzene). uv max (methanol): 330 nm (ε 140).

Ethylenediamine. Tioctidasi.

THERAP CAT: Treatment of liver disease; antidote to poisonous mushrooms (*Amanita* species).

9327. Thiocyanate Sodium. [540-72-7] Sodium sulfocyanate; sodium rhodanide; sodium thiocyanate. CNNaS; mol wt 81.07. C 14.82%, N 17.28%, Na 28.36%, S 39.55%. NaSCN. Contains at least 98% NaSCN. Toxicity study: Anderson, Chen, *J. Am. Pharm. Assoc.* **29,** 152 (1940).

Colorless or white, deliquesc crystals. mp about 300°. Sol in about 0.6 part water; freely sol in alcohol, acetone. When dissolved in water the temp is considerably lowered. The solns are neutral. *Keep well closed.* LD$_{50}$ orally in rats: 764 mg/kg; i.v. in mice: 484 mg/kg (Anderson, Chen).

USE: Manuf other thiocyanates, especially organic.

9328. Thiocyanic Acid. [463-56-9] Hydrogen thiocyanate; Rhodanwasserstoffsäure (German). CHNS; mol wt 59.09. C 20.33%, H 1.71%, N 23.70%, S 54.26%. HSCN. Thiocyanic acid is believed to be a tautomeric mixture of HSCN and HNCS (*isothiocyanic acid*): Beard, Dailey, *J. Chem. Phys.* **18**, 1437 (1950). Conveniently prepd in the laboratory from KNCS + KHSO$_4$: Birckenbach, Bucher, *Ber.* **73**, 1153 (1940). Dil aq solns may be prepd from ammonium thiocyanate by the action of ion exchange resins: Klement, *Z. Anorg. Allg. Chem.* **260**, 268 (1949). Toxicology of organic thiocyanates: Y. Yokoi, *Jpn. J. Pharmacol.* **3**, 99 (1954), *C.A.* **48**, 13965f (1954).

Colorless gas or white solid depending upon degree of polymerization. Freely sol in water. Very strong acid. A 5% aq soln may be kept refrigerated for several weeks. Also sol in some organic solvents.

Ethyl ester. Ethyl thiocyanate; ethyl sulfocyanate. C$_3$H$_5$NS. Liquid. d$_4^{23}$ 1.007. bp 146°. n$_D^{15}$ 1.4684. Insol in water. Misc with alcohol, ether. MLD in mice (mg/kg): 52 orally; 39.1 s.c.; 18.3 i.p.; 6 i.v. (Yokoi).

9329. Thiodicarb. [59669-26-0] *N,N'*-[Thiobis[(methylimino)carbonyloxy]]bisethanimidothioic acid dimethyl ester; bis-[*O*-(1-methylthioethylimino)-*N*-methylcarbamic acid]-*N,N'*-sulfide; *N,N'*-bis[1-methylthioacetaldehyde *O*-(*N*-methylcarbamoyl)oxime]sulfide; *O*-[[*N*-[*N'*-(1-methylthioethylideneiminooxycarbonyl)-*N'*-methylaminosulfenyl]-*N*-methylcarbamoyl]]-*S*-methylacetohydroximate; dicarbosulf; bismethomyl thioether; UC-51762; CGA-45156; Larvin. C$_{10}$H$_{18}$N$_4$O$_4$S$_3$; mol wt 354.47. C 33.88%, H 5.12%, N 15.81%, O 18.05%, S 27.14%. Prepn: **NL 7508197** (1976 to Ciba-Geigy); T. D. J. D'Silva, **DE 2654331**; *eidem*, **US 4382957** (1977, 1983 both to Union Carbide). Activity: A. A. Sousa *et al.*, *J. Econ. Entomol.* **70**, 803 (1977). Field trials: E. P. Pieters, D. L. Pitts, *J. Ga. Entomol. Soc.* **15**, 207 (1980); J. R. Bradley, Jr., A. M. Agnello, *J. Econ. Entomol.* **81**, 706 (1988).

Crystals, mp 173-174°. LD$_{50}$ in rats (mg/kg): 160 orally, >1600 dermally (Sousa).

USE: Insecticide.

9330. 2,2'-Thiodiethanol. [111-48-8] 2,2'-Thiobisethanol; thiodiglycol; thiodiethylene glycol; bis(hydroxyethyl)sulfide. C$_4$H$_{10}$O$_2$S; mol wt 122.19. C 39.32%, H 8.25%, O 26.19%, S 26.24%. Prepd from ethylene oxide and hydrogen sulfide: Chichibabin, Bestuzher, *Compt. Rend.* **200**, 242 (1935); Nenitzescu, Scarlatescu, *Ber.* **68**, 587 (1935); Headlee, cited in G. O. Curme, F. Johnston, *Glycols* (Reinhold, New York, 1952) p 103.

Liquid. d$_4^{20}$ 1.1824. mp −16°. bp$_{14}$ 168°. n$_D^{20}$ 1.519. Flash pt, open cup: 320°F (160°C). Misc with water, alc. Slightly sol in ether.

9331. Thiodiglycolic Acid. [123-93-3] 2,2'-Thiobis[acetic acid]; dimethylsulfide-α,α'-dicarboxylic acid; mercaptodiacetic acid. C$_4$H$_6$O$_4$S; mol wt 150.15. C 32.00%, H 4.03%, O 42.62%, S 21.36%. Prepn from sodium chloroacetate and hydrogen sulfide: Loven, *Ber.* **27**, 3059 (1894).

Crystals from water. mp 129°. Sol in water, alcohol.

USE: Detection of copper, lead, mercury, silver: Dubsky *et al.*, *C.A.* **34**, 6185 (1940).

9332. 3,3'-Thiodipropionic Acid. [111-17-1] 3,3'-Thiobis-[propanoic acid]; β,β-thiodipropionic acid; thiodihydracrylic acid; diethyl sulfide 2,2'-dicarboxylic acid. C$_6$H$_{10}$O$_4$S; mol wt 178.21. C 40.44%, H 5.66%, O 35.91%, S 17.99%. Prepn: **GB 571628** (1945 to Am. Cyanamid); Gresham, Shaver, **US 2449992** (1948 to B. F. Goodrich).

Nacreous leaflets from hot water, mp 134°. pK (25°) 4.11. One gram dissolves in 26.9 ml water at 26°. Freely sol in hot water, alcohol, acetone.

USE: Antioxidant for soap products and polymers of ethylene. In plasticizers and lubricants. Proposed for edible fats, oils, other foods.

9333. Thioformamide. [115-08-2] Methanethioamide. CH$_3$NS; mol wt 61.11. C 19.65%, H 4.95%, N 22.92%, S 52.47%. HCSNH$_2$. Prepd by the action of phosphorus pentasulfide on formamide: Willstätter, Wirth, *Ber.* **42**, 1911 (1909). Synthesis: Erlenmeyer, Menzi, *Helv. Chim. Acta* **31**, 2071 (1948); Schmitz, **US 2682558** (1954 to du Pont); R. Tull, L. M. Weinstock, *Angew. Chem. Int. Ed.* **8**, 278 (1969). Spectroscopic studies: R. Sugisaki *et al., J. Mol. Spectrosc.* **49**, 241 (1974); R. H. Judge *et al., Can. J. Chem.* **65**, 2100 (1987). Use in synthesis of thiazoles: T. J. Cousineau, J. A. Secrist III, *J. Org. Chem.* **44**, 4351 (1979); H. Fukatsu *et al., Heterocycles* **29**, 1517 (1989).

Prisms from ethyl acetate or from ether + petr ether, mp 26-27°. uv max (CH$_3$OH): 263 nm (ε 12500). Turns yellow and dec to a dark-colored mass. May be stored as soln in abs ether, preferably over P$_2$O$_5$. Sol in water (with considerable cooling). Freely sol in tetrahydrofuran, alcohol, ether, acetone, ethyl acetate; sparingly sol in cold chloroform, benzene, petr ether, carbon disulfide. The decompn products are hydrogen cyanide, hydrogen sulfide, ammonia, and some solid, amorphous, sulfur-contg compounds.

Monohydrate. Yellow oil.

USE: In the synthesis of the thiazole containing compds.

9334. 5-Thio-D-glucose. [20408-97-3] 5-Thio-α-D-glucopyranose; α-D-glucothiopyranose. C$_6$H$_{12}$O$_5$S; mol wt 196.22. C 36.73%, H 6.16%, O 40.77%, S 16.34%. The nearest analog of normal D-glucose available to date. Thought to interfere with cellular transport systems utilizing D-glucose due to this structural similarity. The first chemical other than a hormone or alkylating agent which can interfere reversibly with spermatogenesis and which also has been effective against malignant cultured cells. Prepn: M. S. Feather, R. L. Whistler, *Tetrahedron Lett.* **1962**, 667; Rowell, Whistler, *J. Org. Chem.* **31**, 1514 (1966); U. G. Nayak, R. L. Whistler, *ibid.* **34**, 97 (1969); Abd El-Rahman, Whistler, *Org. Prep. Proced. Int.* **5**, 245 (1973); H. Driguez, B. Henrissat, *Tetrahedron Lett.* **22**, 5061 (1981). Pharmacology: D. J. Hoffman, R. L. Whistler, *Biochemistry* **7**, 4479 (1968); R. L. Whistler, W. C. Lake, *Biochem. J.* **130**, 919 (1972). Radioprotective effect on tissue *in vivo:* V. L. Schuman *et al., Int. J. Radiat. Oncol. Biol. Phys.* **8**, 589 (1982). Brief review: *Science* **186**, 431 (1974).

Crystals from methanol, mp 135-136°. [α]$_D^{20}$ +188° (c = 1.56 in water). LD$_{50}$ i.p. in mice: 5.5 g/kg (Schuman).

USE: Tool for examination of D-glucose biochemistry.

9335. Thioglycerol. [96-27-5] 3-Mercapto-1,2-propanediol; α-monothioglycerol; thioglycerin. C$_3$H$_8$O$_2$S; mol wt 108.16. C 33.31%, H 7.46%, O 29.58%, S 29.65%. Prepn: L. Carius, *Ann.* **124**, 221 (1862); B. Sjöberg, *Ber.* **75**, 13 (1942). Use in fast atom bombardment MS: C. Dass, *J. Mass Spectrom.* **31**, 77 (1996); as antioxidant in cell culture media: M. Brielmeier *et al., Nucleic Acids Res.* **26**, 2082 (1998).

Yellowish, very viscous, hygroscopic liquid; slight sulfidic odor. bp$_1$ 100-101°. d 1.246. n$_D^{20}$ 1.527. Flash point, closed cup: 235°F (113°C). Slightly sol in water; miscible with alcohol. Insol in ether.

USE: Antioxidant preservative; reagent in analytical chemistry, cell culture research. Matrix substrate in fast atom bombardment mass spectrometry.

9336. Thioglycolic Acid. [68-11-1] Mercaptoacetic acid; thioglycollic acid. $C_2H_4O_2S$; mol wt 92.12. C 26.08%, H 4.38%, O 34.74%, S 34.81%. $HSCH_2COOH$. Prepd by the action of sodium sulfhydrate on sodium chloroacetate; by electrolysis of dithioglycollic acid (from sodium sulfide and sodium chloroacetate). Toxicity study: Deichmann, Mergard, *J. Ind. Hyg. Toxicol.* **30,** 373 (1948).

Liquid, strong, unpleasant odor. Readily oxidized by air. d 1.325. mp $-16.5°$. bp$_{29}$ 123°. bp$_{15}$ 108°. bp$_5$ 96°. K_1 at 25° $= 2.1 \times 10^{-4}$; $K_2 = 2.1 \times 10^{-11}$. Miscible with water, alcohol, ether, chloroform, benzene, and many other organic solvents. LD$_{50}$ orally in rats: 0.15 ml/kg (Deichmann, Mergard).

Caution: Potential symptoms of overexposure are irritation of eyes, skin, nose, throat; lacrimation, corneal damage; skin burns, blisters. *See NIOSH Pocket Guide to Chemical Hazards* (DHHS/-NIOSH 97-140, 1997) p 306.

USE: Sensitive reagent for iron, molybdenum, silver, tin. With ferric iron a blue color appears, and when an alkali hydroxide is added to a soln contg ferrous salts and thioglycolic acid, a yellow precipitate forms. Used in the manuf of thioglycolates. The ammonium and sodium salts are commonly used for cold waving and the calcium salt is a depilatory. The sodium salt also is used in bacteriology in the prepn of thioglycolate media.

9337. Thioguanine. [154-42-7] 2-Amino-1,7-dihydro-6*H*-purine-6-thione; 2-aminopurine-6-thiol; Lanvis; Tabloid. $C_5H_5N_5$-S; mol wt 167.19. C 35.92%, H 3.01%, N 41.89%, S 19.18%. Prepn: Elion, Hitchings, *J. Am. Chem. Soc.* **77,** 1676 (1955); Hitchings, Elion, **US 2697709; US 2800473; US 2884667;** Hitchings *et al.,* **US 3019224; US 3132144** (1954, 1957, 1959, 1962, and 1964, all to Burroughs Welcome).

Needles from water, mp >360°.
THERAP CAT: Antineoplastic.

9338. Thioguanosine. [85-31-4] 2-Amino-6-mercapto-9-β-D-ribofuranosylpurine. $C_{10}H_{13}N_5O_4S$; mol wt 299.31. C 40.13%, H 4.38%, N 23.40%, O 21.38%, S 10.71%. Prepn: Fox *et al., J. Am. Chem. Soc.* **80,** 1669 (1948).

Hemihydrate. Tiny tapered prisms from water, dec 224-227°. $[\alpha]_D^{22} -64°$ (c = 1.3 in 0.1*N* NaOH). uv max (pH 4-6): 257, 342 nm (ε 8820, 24800). pKa 8.33.

USE: In cancer research, *cf.* 6-Mercaptopurine and Nebularine.

9339. Thiokol®. Polysulfide rubber; thiorubber. Polysulfide polymers prepd from dihaloalkanes and sodium polysulfide. Reviews of prepn, chemistry and applications: Berenbaum in *High Polymers,* H. Mark *et al.,* Eds., **vol. 13** entitled *Polyethers* **part 3,** N. G. Gaylord, Ed. (Interscience, New York, 1962) pp 43-114; Panek, *ibid.* pp 115-224; Berenbaum in *Encyclopedia of Polymer Science and Technology* **vol. 11** (Interscience, New York, 1969) pp 425-447.

Thiokol A

Thiokol A. Ethanite; Perduren. The first commercial polysulfide polymer, prepd from ethylene dichloride and sodium polysulfide. Sulfur content 84%; d about 1.6. Mixes with natural rubber. Cured polymer retains unpleasant odor; irritating fumes evolve during manuf. Stable to the usual organic solvents and dil mineral acids. Unstable to alkalies and oxidizing substances. Of low tensile strength and abrasion resistance. Not recommended where tropic or arctic climates prevail.

Thiokol FA. Prepd from ethylene dichloride, dichlorodiethyl formal and sodium polysulfide. Sulfur content 47%; d 1.34. No odor. Excellent solvent resistant characteristics but not as good as Thiokol A. Low temperature flexibility to −50°F.

USE: In rubber and resin manuf. As lining for flexible oil pipes and self-sealing gasoline tanks.

9340. Thiolactic Acid. [79-42-5] 2-Mercaptopropanoic acid; 2-mercaptopropionic acid; 2-thiolpropionic acid; α-mercaptopropanoic acid. $C_3H_6O_2S$; mol wt 106.14. C 33.95%, H 5.70%, O 30.15%, S 30.21%. $CH_3CH(SH)COOH$. First prepd from α-chloropropionic acid and potassium hydrosulfide: Schacht, *Ann.* **129,** 3 (1864); prepn from α-chloropropionic acid and sodium thiosulfate: Martin, **US 2413361** (1946 to Martin Labs). From sodium sulfide, sulfur and α-bromopropionic acid: Dumesnil, **US 2985557** (1961 to Frank E. Jonas). *Review:* Reid, *Organic Chemistry of Bivalent Sulfur* **vol. I** (Chemical Publ. Co., New York, 1958) p 449.

Oil, disagreeable odor. Solidif on cooling, crystals mp about 10°. d$_4^{15}$ 1.220. bp$_{16}$ 117°. n_D^{16} 1.4823. Miscible with water, alcohol, ether, acetone.

Copper salt. $C_3H_5CuO_2S$. Yellow precipitate. Practically insol in water and in dil HNO$_3$.

Barium salt. $Ba(C_3H_5O_2S)_2$. Rubbery compd, very sol in water. Practically insol in alcohol.

Mercury salt. $Hg(C_3H_5O_2S)_2$. Small shiny platelets, sparingly sol in water, very sol in alcohol.

Sodium salt pentahydrate. $C_3H_5NaO_2S.5H_2O$. Crystals. Dec about 250°. Sol in water, methanol, ethanol. Less sol in propanol.

Calcium salt decahydrate. $Ca(C_3H_5O_2S)_2.10H_2O$. Crystals. Dec 270°. Sol in water, methanol, ethanol. Less sol in propanol.

Platinum salt. $Pt(C_3H_5O_2S)_2$. Greenish-yellow precipitate. Practically insol in water and dil acids. Sol in sodium hydroxide and sodium carbonate.

Silver salt. $C_3H_5AgO_2S$. Yellow precipitate. Practically insol in water and dil HNO$_3$.

USE: In depilatory and hair waving prepns.

9341. 2-Thiolhistidine. [13552-61-9] α-Amino-2,3-dihydro-2-thioxo-1*H*-imidazole-4-propanoic acid; 2-mercaptohistidine; α-amino-2-mercapto-4-imidazolepropionic acid. $C_6H_9N_3O_2S$; mol wt 187.22. C 38.49%, H 4.85%, N 22.44%, O 17.09%, S 17.13%. Prepn from histidine: Ashley, Harington, *J. Chem. Soc.* **1930,** 2586; from aspartic acid: Harington, Overhoff, *Biochem. J.* **27,** 338 (1933). Alternate procedures: Hegedüs, *Helv. Chim. Acta* **38,** 22 (1955); Marei, Raphael, *J. Chem. Soc.* **1958,** 2624. *Review:* J. P. Greenstein, M. Winitz, *Chemistry of the Amino Acids* **vol. 3** (John Wiley, New York, 1961) pp 2671-2675.

L-Form. Plates from water, darkens at 290°, not melted at 310°. $[\alpha]_D^{20} -10°$ (c = 2 in *N* HCl). pK$_1^1$ 1.84; pK$_2^1$ 8.47; pK$_3^1$ 11.4. Readily sol in hot water, sparingly sol in water at room temp. Tends to form supersaturated solns. Practically insol in alcohol, other organic solvents.

Dihydrochloride. $C_6H_9N_3O_2.2HCl$. Large prisms, dec 197-199°. Freely sol in water, sparingly sol in alcohol.

9342. Thiolutin. [87-11-6] 6-(Acetamido)-4-methyl-1,2-dithiolo[4,3-*b*]pyrrol-5(4*H*)-one; *N*-(4,5-dihydro-4-methyl-5-oxo-1,2-dithiolo[4,3-*b*]pyrrol-6-yl)acetamide; 3-acetamido-5-methylpyrrolin-4-one[4,3-*d*]-1,2-dithiole; acetopyrrothine. $C_8H_8N_2O_2S_2$; mol wt 228.29. C 42.09%, H 3.53%, N 12.27%, O 14.02%, S 28.09%. Antibiotic isolated from several strains of *Streptomyces albus*: F. W. Tanner, Jr. *et al.,* 118th Am. Chem. Soc. Meet. (Chicago, Sept.

1950), *Abstracts of Papers,* p 18A; F. W. Tanner, Jr. *et al.,* **US 2689854** (1954 to Pfizer). Characterization, similarity to aureothricin, *q.v.:* W. D. Celmer *et al., J. Am. Chem. Soc.* **74**, 6304 (1952). Structure: W. D. Celmer, I. A. Solomons, *ibid.* **77**, 2861 (1955). Total synthesis: U. Schmidt, F. Geiger, *Ann.* **664**, 168 (1963); K. Hagio, N. Yoneda, *Bull. Chem. Soc. Jpn.* **47**, 1484 (1974). Bactericidal, protozoicidal, fungicidal properties: H. Seneca *et al., Antibiot. Chemother.* **2**, 357 (1952). Mode of action: A. Jimenez *et al., Antimicrob. Agents Chemother.* **3**, 729 (1973). Inhibition of microbiological growth in beer: J. B. Bockelmann, F. B. Strandskov, **US 2798811** (1957 to Schaefer Brewing Co.). Activity against soil borne pathogens: P. R. Deb, B. K. Dutta, *Curr. Sci.* **53**, 659 (1984). As allergy inhibitor: P. Stahl *et al.,* **DE 3434562** (1986 to Boehringer, Mannheim), *C.A.* **105**, 54609k (1986).

Brilliant yellow needles from *n*-butanol, dec 273-276°. Sublimes 200°/0.1 mm. uv max (methanol): 250, 311, 388 nm (ε 6300, 5700, 11,000) (Celmer, Solomons). Sparingly sol in water (210 mg/l); more sol in methanol, ethanol, chloroform, acetone (1% solns in acetone have been prepd), glacial acetic acid, methyl isobutyl ketone. Less sol in ether, benzene, hexane. Stable in acid and neutral solns, decomp in alkaline soln. Effective vs gram-positive and gram-negative bacteria, fungi and ameboid parasites. LD_{50} in mice (mg/kg): 25 s.c.; 25 orally (Seneca).

9343. Thiomalic Acid. [70-49-5] Mercaptobutanedioic acid; mercaptosuccinic acid. $C_4H_6O_4S$; mol wt 150.15. C 32.00%, H 4.03%, O 42.62%, S 21.36%.

White crystals; sulfidic odor. mp 149-150°. Soly in water at 40° about 50 g/100 ml; in ethanol at 25° about 50 g/100 ml. Also sol in acetone. Moderately sol in ether. Practically insol in benzene. The aq soln gives a transitory blue color with ferric chloride.

9344. Thionalide. [93-42-5] 2-Mercapto-*N*-2-naphthalenylacetamide; thioglycollic-β-aminonaphthalide. $C_{12}H_{11}NOS$; mol wt 217.29. C 66.33%, H 5.10%, N 6.45%, O 7.36%, S 14.76%.

White to ivory-colored needles. mp 111-112°. Insol in water. Freely sol in most organic solvents.
USE: As a reagent for copper, mercury, silver, thallium, and bismuth.

9345. Thionaphthene-2-carboxylic Acid. [6314-28-9] Benzo[*b*]thiophene-2-carboxylic acid; 2-benzothiophenecarboxylic acid; TNCA; BL-5583. $C_9H_6O_2S$; mol wt 178.21. C 60.66%, H 3.39%, O 17.96%, S 17.99%. Prepn: R. Weissgerber, O. Kruber, *Ber.* **53**, 1551 (1920); *eidem,* **DE 341837** (1921), *Frdl.* **13**, 279 (1921); D. A. Shirley, M. D. Cameron, *J. Am. Chem. Soc.* **72**, 2788 (1950); T. Higa, A. J. Krubsack, *J. Org. Chem.* **41**, 3399 (1976). Use as anti-osteoporotic agent: C. M. Samour, J. A. Vida, **US 4101668** (1978 to Bristol-Myers). Effect on total skeletal calcium in mice: J. C. Robin *et al., J. Med.* **11**, 15 (1980). Mechanism of action study: J. C. Robin *et al., Calcif. Tissue Int.* **36**, 194 (1984). Hypocalcemic effect: A. J. Johannesson *et al., Endocrinology* **117**, 1508 (1985).

Prisms from alcohol or needles from water, mp 236° (Weissgerber). Also reported as crystals from benzene-ethyl acetate, mp 236-238° (Higa).

9346. Thionine. [135-59-1] 3,7-Diaminophenothiazin-5-ium chloride; Lauth's violet; C.I. 52000. $C_{12}H_{10}ClN_3S$; mol wt 263.75. C 54.65%, H 3.82%, Cl 13.44%, N 15.93%, S 12.16%. Prepn from *p*-phenylenediamine: Lauth, *Compt. Rend.* **82**, 1441 (1876); *Bull. Soc. Chim. Fr.* [2] **26**, 422 (1876); Bernthsen, **DE 25150** (1883 to BASF), *Frdl.* **1**, 253; Loiseleur, *Ann. Inst. Pasteur* **86**, 262 (1954); Loiseleur, Petit, *Compt. Rend.* **250**, 2573 (1960); Balestic, Magat, *C.A.* **55**, 23542g (1961). *See also: Colour Index* vol. **4** (3rd ed., 1971) p 4469.

Blackish-green glistening needles. Absorption max (water): 602.5 nm. Difficultly sol in cold, easily sol in hot water, giving first a blue, then a violet soln. The soln becomes somewhat bluer when HCl is added. Brownish-red precipitate with NaOH. Yellowish-green soln with concd H_2SO_4 which upon dilution turns blue, then violet on further dilution.
USE: For general nuclear staining; for counting bacteria in milk; as antioxidant for linseed oil. Has been used as catalyst in condensation of 1,3-butadienyl ethyl ether with maleic anhydride.

9347. Thionyl Bromide. [507-16-4] Br_2OS; mol wt 207.87. Br 76.88%, O 7.70%, S 15.43%. $SOBr_2$. Prepd from thionyl chloride and hydrogen bromide: Besson, *Compt. Rend.* **122**, 320 (1896); **123**, 884 (1896); Hibbert, Pullman, *Inorg. Synth.* **1**, 113 (1939).
Orange-yellow liquid. d_4^{20} 2.688. mp $-52°$. bp_{773} 138°; bp_{20} 48°. Somewhat less stable than thionyl chloride. Dec slowly on standing in glass-stoppered bottles. Hydrolyzed by water. Miscible with benzene, chloroform, carbon tetrachloride.
Caution: Highly irritating to skin, eyes, mucous membranes, respiratory tract.

9348. Thionyl Chloride. [7719-09-7] Sulfurous oxychloride. Cl_2OS; mol wt 118.97. Cl 59.60%, O 13.45%, S 26.95%. $SOCl_2$. Prepn by the oxidation of sulfur with sulfur trioxide: Michaelis, *Ann.* **274**, 173 (1893); Edwards, **US 2362057** (1944 to Hooker Electrochemical); Fehér in *Handbook of Preparative Inorganic Chemistry* vol. 1, G. Brauer, Ed. (Academic Press, New York, 2nd ed., 1963) pp 382-383; Macaluso, "Sulfur Compounds" in *Kirk-Othmer Encyclopedia of Chemical Technology* vol. **19** (Interscience, New York, 2nd ed., 1969) pp 398-401. Purification by distilling from quinoline and boiled linseed oil: Martin, Fieser, *Org. Synth.* **coll. vol. II**, 570 (1943). Alternate methods of purification: Cottle, *J. Am. Chem. Soc.* **68**, 1380 (1946); Kunkel; Rosenberg, Flaxman, **US 3155457**; **US 3156529** (both 1964 to Hooker Chem.); Friedman, Wetter, *J. Chem. Soc. A* **1967**, 36.
Colorless to pale yellow or reddish, fuming, refractive liquid. *Suffocating odor.* d_4^0 1.676; d_4^{10} 1.655; d_4^{20} 1.638. mp $-104.5°$. bp_{760} 76°; $bp_{96.6}$ 20°. n_D^{20} 1.517. Dec when heated above 140° forming Cl_2, SO_2, and S_2Cl_2. Hydrolyzed by water forming SO_2 and HCl. Miscible with benzene, chloroform, carbon tetrachloride.
Caution: Potential symptoms of overexposure are irritation of eyes, skin, mucous membranes; eye, skin burns. *See NIOSH Pocket Guide to Chemical Hazards* (DHHS/NIOSH 97-140, 1997) p 306.
USE: For making acyl chlorides, to replace OH or SH groups with chlorine atoms; reacts with Grignard reagents to form the corresp sulfoxides. Review of use in organic synthesis: J. S. Pizey, *Synthetic Reagents* vol. 1 (John Wiley, New York, 1974) pp 321-357.

9349. Thionyl Fluoride. [7783-42-8] Thionyl difluoride. F_2OS; mol wt 86.06. F 44.15%, O 18.59%, S 37.26%. SOF_2. Usually prepd by the action of antimony trifluoride on thionyl chloride in the presence of antimony pentafluoride: Booth, Mericola, *J. Am. Chem. Soc.* **62**, 640 (1940); Smith, Muetterties, *Inorg. Synth.* **6**, 162 (1960). May also be prepared by the action of other fluorides on thionyl chloride: Kemmitt, Sharp, *Adv. Fluorine Chem.* **4**, 228-229 (1965).

Colorless gas. Suffocating odor. Does not attack glass. Stored in compressed form in steel cylinders. mp −129.5°. bp −43.8°. Crit temp +88°. d (liq; −100°) 1.780. d (solid; −183°) 2.095. Trouton constant 22.6. Very slowly hydrolyzed by cold water. Sol in ether, benzene.

Caution: Highly irritating to eyes, respiratory tract.

9350. Thiopental Sodium. [71-73-8] 5-Ethyldihydro-5-(1-methylbutyl)-2-thioxo-4,6(1*H*,5*H*)-pyrimidinedione monosodium salt; 5-ethyl-5-(1-methylbutyl)-2-thiobarbituric acid sodium salt; thiomebumal sodium; penthiobarbital sodium; thiopentone sodium; thionembutal; Intraval Sodium; Nesdonal Sodium; Pentothal Sodium; Trapanal. $C_{11}H_{17}N_2NaO_2S$; mol wt 264.32. C 49.98%, H 6.48%, N 10.60%, Na 8.70%, O 12.11%, S 12.13%. Prepn: **US 2153729** (1939); **US 2876225** (1959). Prepn of nonhygroscopic crystals: Hartop, **US 3109001** (1963 to Abbott). Acute toxicity: Christensen, Lee, *Toxicol. Appl. Pharmacol.* **26**, 495 (1973). Comprehensive description: M. J. McLeish, *Anal. Profiles Drug Subs. Excip.* **21**, 535-572 (1992).

Yellowish-white, hygroscopic powder. Alliaceous, garlic-like odor. Sol in water, alcohol. Insol in ether, benzene, petr ether. Aq solns are alkaline to litmus. Solns dec on standing; on boiling precipitation occurs. LD_{50} in mice (mg/kg): 149 i.p.; 78 i.v. (Christensen, Lee).

Note: This is a controlled substance (depressant): **21 CFR,** 1308.13.

THERAP CAT: Anesthetic (intravenous).

THERAP CAT (VET): Short-acting anesthetic.

9351. Thiopeptin. [12609-84-6] Thiofeed. Sulfur containing peptide antibiotic complex produced by *Streptomyces tateyamensis* no. 7906: Miyairi *et al.*, **DE 1929355** (1969 to Fujisawa), *C.A.* **72**, 88921w (1970). Consists of the a and b series of thiopeptins A₁, A₂, A₃, A₄, and B (major component). Structurally similar to thiostrepton, *q.v.* Biological and chemical studies: Miyairi *et al.*, *Antimicrob. Agents Chemother.* **1**, 192 (1972). Characterization of thiopeptins B: Miyairi *et al.*, *J. Antibiot.* **23**, 113 (1970); structural studies: Muramatsu *et al.*, *ibid.* **25**, 537 (1972); **30**, 383 (1977). Total structures of components: O. D. Hensens, G. Albers-Schönberg, *Tetrahedron Lett.* **1978**, 3649.

Thiopeptins B. Faint yellow crystals, mp 219-222° (dec). $[\alpha]_D^{23}$ −80° (c = 1 in chloroform). uv spectrum (methanol): shoulders at 230-250, 295, 305 nm. Sol in dioxane, DMSO, DMF, pyridine, chloroform. Insol in ether, benzene, *n*-hexane, petr ether, water. Fairly sol in methanol, acetone, ethyl acetate.

THERAP CAT (VET): Antibiotic feed additive.

9352. Thiophanate. [23564-06-9] [1,2-Phenylenebis-(iminocarbonothioyl)]biscarbamic acid diethyl ester; 4,4'-*o*-phenylenebis[3-thioallophanic acid]diethyl ester; 1,2-bis(3-ethoxycarbonyl-2-thioureido)benzene; Cercobin; Topsin; Nemafax. $C_{14}H_{18}N_4O_4S_2$; mol wt 370.45. C 45.39%, H 4.90%, N 15.12%, O 17.28%, S 17.31%. Prepn: T. Noguchi *et al.*, **DE 1806123**; *eidem*, **US 4020095** (1969, 1977 both to Nippon Soda Co.). Photodegradation: H. Buchenauer *et al.*, *Pestic. Sci.* **5**, 343 (1973). Activity vs nematode infection in ruminants: Eichler, *Br. Vet. J.* **129**, 533 (1973). Toxicology in animals: *idem, ibid.* **130**, 570 (1974).

Colorless plates from acetone, dec 194°. LD_{50} orally in mice and rats: >15 g/kg (Eichler).

O,O-**Dimethyl analog.** [23564-05-8] Thiophanate-methyl; Cercobin-M; Topsin-M. $C_{12}H_{14}N_4O_4S_2$; mol wt 342.39. Prepn: T. Noguchi *et al., loc. cit.* Persistence in soil: J. R. Fleeker *et al., J. Agric. Food Chem.* **22**, 592 (1974). Pharmacology, toxicity: Y. Hashimoto *et al., Toxicol. Appl. Pharmacol.* **23**, 606, 616 (1972). Colorless prisms, mp 181.5-182.5°. Sol in acetone, methanol, chloroform, acetonitrile; slightly sol in other organics. Practically insol in water. LD_{50} in rats, mice, guinea pigs, rabbits (g/kg): 3.40, 6.64, 3.64, 2.27 orally (Hashimoto).

USE: Systemic fungicide.

THERAP CAT (VET): Anthelmintic (Nematodes).

9353. Thiophene. [110-02-1] Thiofuran; thiofurfuran; thiole; thiotetrole; divinylene sulfide. C_4H_4S; mol wt 84.14. C 57.10%, H 4.79%, S 38.11%. Found in coal tar, in coal gas, and in technical benzene: V. Meyer, *Ber.* **16**, 1471 (1883); **17**, 2642 (1884). Made available in commercial quantities by a process utilizing the dehydrogenation of butane with sulfur as the dehydrogenating agent, followed by cyclization with sulfur to form the thiophene ring: Rasmussen, Ray, *Chem. Inds.* **60**, 593, 620 (1947). Laboratory prepn by heating sodium succinate with phosphorus trisulfide: R. Phillips, *Org. Synth.* **coll. vol. II**, 578 (1943). Also prepd by passing ethylene or acetylene into boiling sulfur; or by passing acetylene and hydrogen sulfide over hot bauxite or nickel hydroxide: **US 1421743** *C.A.* **16**, 3093 (1922). *Review:* B. Buchholz in *Kirk-Othmer Encyclopedia of Chemical Technology* **vol. 22** (Wiley-Interscience, New York, 3rd ed., 1983) pp 965-973.

Liquid. Slight aromatic odor resembling that of benzene. d_4^0 1.0873; d_4^{25} 1.0573; d_4^{50} 1.0285. mp −38.3°. bp_{760} 84.4°; bp_{400} 64.7°; bp_{200} 46.5°; bp_{100} 30.5°; bp_{60} 20.1°; bp_{40} 12.5°; bp_{20} 0.0°; bp_{10} −10.9°; bp_5 −20.8°; n_D^{25} 1.52684. Absorption spectrum: Purvis, *J. Chem. Soc.* **97**, 1653, 1656 (1910). Insol in water; miscible with most organic solvents. May be heated to 850° without decompn.

USE: Solvent similar to benzene, but suitable for lower and higher temps; manuf of resins from thiophene-phenol mixtures and formaldehyde; manuf of dyes and pharmaceuticals.

9354. 2-Thiophenecarboxylic Acid. [527-72-0] 2-Thenoic acid. $C_5H_4O_2S$; mol wt 128.15. C 46.86%, H 3.15%, O 24.97%, S 25.02%. Prepn: Voerman, *Rec. Trav. Chim.* **26**, 293 (1907); Sy, de Malleray, *Bull. Soc. Chim. Fr.* **1963**, 1276; Gross *et al.*, *Ber.* **96**, 1382 (1963).

Needles from water, mp 128.5°. Very sol in ether, alc, hot water; moderately sol in CHCl₃; slightly sol in petr ether.

Sodium salt. Sodium 2-thiophenecarboxylate; sodium 2-thenoate; Trophires. $C_5H_3NaO_2S$; mol wt 150.13.

USE: Sodium salt as lubricating-grease thickener, Morway, Kolfenbach, **US 2576031** (1951 to Standard Oil).

9355. Thiophenol. [108-98-5] Benzenethiol; phenylmercaptan. C_6H_6S; mol wt 110.18. C 65.41%, H 5.49%, S 29.10%. C_6H_5SH. Prepd by the reduction of benzenesulfonyl chloride with zinc dust in sulfuric acid: Adams, Marvel, *Org. Synth.* **1**, 71 (1921).

Liquid. Repulsive, penetrating, garlic-like odor, esp when impure. d_4^{25} 1.0728; bp_{760} 168.3°; bp_{100} 103.6°; bp_{50} 86.2°; bp_{20} 69.7°; $bp_{1.0}$ 18.6°; n_D^{25} 1.58603. Heat of fusion 24.90 cal/g; spec heat at 25°: 0.3829; entropy at 25°: 52.6. Insol in water. Very sol in alc; miscible with ether, benzene, CS_2. Feebly acidic. Oxidizes in air, esp when dissolved in alcoholic ammonia, forming diphenyl disulfide, $C_6H_5SSC_6H_5$. The hydrogen of the SH group is easily replaced by metals.

Caution: Potential symptoms of overexposure are irritation of eyes, skin and respiratory system; dermatitis; cyanosis; coughing, wheezing, dyspnea, pulmonary edema, pneumonitis; headache, dizziness, CNS depression; nausea, vomiting; kidney, liver and spleen damage. *See NIOSH Pocket Guide to Chemical Hazards* (DHHS/NIOSH 97-140, 1997) p 26.

9356. Thiopropazate. [84-06-0] 4-[3-(2-Chlorophenothia-zin-10-yl)propyl]-1-piperazineethanol acetate; 2-chloro-10-[3-[1-(2-acetoxyethyl)-4-piperazinyl]propyl]phenothiazine; 10-[3-[1-(2-acetoxyethyl)-4-piperazinyl]propyl]-2-chlorophenothiazine; N-(β-acetoxyethyl)-N'-[γ-(2'-chloro-10'-phenothiazinyl)propyl]pipera-zine; 1-(2-acetoxyethyl)-4-[3-(2-chloro-10-phenothiazinyl)propyl]-piperazine. $C_{23}H_{28}ClN_3O_2S$; mol wt 446.01. C 61.94%, H 6.33%, Cl 7.95%, N 9.42%, O 7.17%, S 7.19%. Prepd from 2-chloro-10-(γ-chloropropyl)phenothiazine and piperazine in buta-none followed by treatment with β-bromoethyl acetate in toluene: Cusic, **US 2766235** (1956); Anderson et al., Arzneim.-Forsch. **12**, 937 (1962).

Free base, $bp_{0.1}$ 214-218°. Sol in ether.
Dihydrochloride. [146-28-1] Dartal; Dartalan. $C_{23}H_{28}ClN_3$-$O_2S.2HCl$; mol wt 518.93. Crystals from 95% ethanol, dec 223-229°. Freely sol in water; much less sol in alc, chloroform; almost insol in ether.
Dimaleate. [104999-18-0] $C_{23}H_{28}ClN_3O_2S.2C_4H_4O_4$. Crys-tals from methanol + ethanol, mp 167-169°.
THERAP CAT: Antipsychotic.

9357. Thioproperazine. [316-81-4] N,N-Dimethyl-10-[3-(4-methyl-1-piperazinyl)propyl]phenothiazine-2-sulfonamide; 3-di-methylsulfamoyl-10-[3-(4-methylpiperazino)propyl]phenothiazine; 2-dimethylsulfamoyl-10-[3'-(4''-piperazino)propyl]phenothiazine; thioperazine; RP-7843; SKF-5883. $C_{22}H_{30}N_4O_2S_2$; mol wt 446.63. C 59.16%, H 6.77%, N 12.54%, O 7.16%, S 14.36%. Prepn: **GB 814512** (1959 to Rhône-Poulenc).

Crystals, mp 140°.
Fumarate. $C_{22}H_{30}N_4O_2S_2.C_4H_4O_4$. Crystals, mp 182°.
Dimethanesulfonate. [2347-80-0] Thioproperazine mesylate; Majeptil; Vontil. $C_{22}H_{30}N_4O_2S_2.2CH_3SO_3H$; mol wt 638.84.
THERAP CAT: Antipsychotic; antiemetic.

9358. Thioredoxin. [52500-60-4] Ubiquitous, small, hydro-gen carrier protein that participates in a wide variety of biochemical reactions, e.g., ribonucleotide reduction, methionine sulfoxide, sul-fate and disulfide reduction, phosphate transfer reactions. Thio-redoxin is oxidized from a dithiol to a disulfide during ribonucleo-tide reduction, and regenerated by reduced triphosphopyridine nu-cleotide (TPNH) and the flavoprotein thioredoxin reductase: Lau-rent et al., J. Biol. Chem. **239**, 3436 (1964). Prepn from Escherichia coli: Williams et al., ibid. **242**, 5226 (1967). Complete amino acid sequence: A. Holmgren, Eur. J. Biochem. **6**, 475 (1968). Purifica-tion and characterization: A. Holmgren et al., J. Biol. Chem. **256**, 3118 (1981). Prepn of bacteriophage T4-induced thioredoxin: Berglund, Sjoberg, ibid. **245**, 6030 (1970). Amino acid sequence: Sjoberg, Holmgren, ibid. **247**, 8063 (1972). The T4 thioredoxin shows no structural homology with thioredoxin from E. coli. Pu-rification, characterization and amino acid sequence of thioredoxin from Corynebacterium nephridii: M. Meng, H. P. C. Hogenkamp, ibid. **256**, 9174 (1981).

9359. Thioridazine. [50-52-2] 10-[2-(1-Methyl-2-piperidi-nyl)ethyl]-2-(methylthio)-10H-phenothiazine; 2-methylmercapto-10-[2-(N-methyl-2-piperidyl)ethyl]phenothiazine; 3-methylmercap-

to-N-[2'-(N'-methyl-2-piperidyl)ethyl]phenothiazine. $C_{21}H_{26}N_2$-S_2; mol wt 370.57. C 68.06%, H 7.07%, N 7.56%, S 17.31%. Dopamine receptor blocker; parent compound of sulforidazine and mesoridazine, q.q.v. Prepn: Bourquin et al., Helv. Chim. Acta **41**, 1072 (1958). Toxicity: E. I. Goldenthal, Toxicol. Appl. Pharma-col. **18**, 185 (1971). Effect on dopaminergic function: D. M. Niedzwiecki et al., J. Pharmacol. Exp. Ther. **228**, 636 (1984); C. D. Kilts et al., ibid. **231**, 334 (1984). GLC determn in plasma: E. C. Dinovo et al., J. Pharm. Sci. **65**, 667 (1976). HPLC sepn of isomers: R. Whelpton et al., J. Chromatogr. **426**, 223 (1988). Clinical evaluation: R. Axelsson et al., Curr. Ther. Res. **21**, 587 (1977). Comprehensive description: E. M. Abdel-Moety, K. A. Al-Rashood, Anal. Profiles Drug Subs. **18**, 459-525 (1989).

Crystals from acetone, mp 72-74°. $bp_{0.02}$ 230°. uv max (95% ethanol): 263, 314 nm (ε 38172, 4595); (0.1N HCl): 230, 263 nm (ε 20939, 45954); (0.1 N NaOH): 313 nm (ε 5226). pKa 9.5. Sol in alcohol (1 in 6), chloroform (1 in 0.81), ether (1 in 3); freely sol in dehydrated alcohol. Insol in water. LD_{50} orally in rats: 995 ±39 mg/kg (Goldenthal).
Hydrochloride. [130-61-0] TP-21; Aldazine; Mellaril; Meller-etten; Melleril; Mallorol; Novoridazine; Orsanil; Ridazin; Stalleril. $C_{21}H_{26}N_2S_2.HCl$; mol wt 407.04. Crystals from acetone, mp 158-160°. uv max (water): 262, 310 nm (ε 41842, 3215); (95% etha-nol): 264, 310 nm (ε 41598, 3256); (0.1N HCl): 264, 305 nm (ε 42371, 5495); (0.1N NaOH): 263 nm (ε 18392). Sol in water (1 in 9); freely sol in ethanol (1 in 10), methanol, chloroform (1 in 5). Insol in ether.
THERAP CAT: Antipsychotic.

9360. Thiosalicylic Acid. [147-93-3] 2-Mercaptobenzoic acid; o-sulfhydrylbenzoic acid. $C_7H_6O_2S$; mol wt 154.19. C 54.53%, H 3.92%, O 20.75%, S 20.80%. Prepd by heating o-halogenated benzoic acids with an alkaline hydrosulfide in the presence of copper: **DE 189200** (1906); by reduction of dithio-salicylic acid: Claasz, Ber. **45**, 2427 (1912); **DE 205450**; C. F. H. Allen, D. D. MacKay, Org. Synth. coll. vol. II, 580 (1943).

Sulfur-yellow flakes, plates, needles from glacial acetic acid or alcohol. Softens at 158°. mp 164-165°. Sublimes. Slightly sol in hot water; freely in glacial acetic acid, alc. Exposure to air yields dithiosalicylic acid, which is produced also when an alcoholic soln of thiosalicylic acid comes in contact with FeCl$_3$ (resulting in a transitory blue color).
Sodium salt. Jecto-Sal; Thiocyl. $C_7H_5NaO_2S$; mol wt 176.17. Crystals, sol in water.
USE: Manuf thioindigo dyes, reagent for determn of iron.

9361. Thiosemicarbazide. [79-19-6] Hydrazinecarbothio-amide. CH_5N_3S; mol wt 91.14. C 13.18%, H 5.53%, N 46.11%, S 35.18%. $NH_2CSNHNH_2$.
White, cryst powder. mp 182-184°. Sol in water or alc. LD_{50} orally in adult Norway rats: 13 mg/kg, Dieke, Proc. Soc. Exp. Biol. Med. **70**, 688 (1949).
USE: As a reagent for detection of metals.

9362. Thiosinamine. [109-57-9] (2-Propenyl)thiourea; al-lyl thiourea; allylthiocarbamide; Aminosin; Rhodalline. $C_4H_8N_2S$; mol wt 116.18. C 41.35%, H 6.94%, N 24.11%, S 27.60%. $CH_2=CHCH_2NHCSNH_2$. Made by warming a mixture of equal parts of allyl mustard oil and abs alcohol with an equal amount of 30% ammonia. Growth regulating activity: Karanov, Vasilev, *Izv. Inst. Fiziol. Rast. Bulg. Akad. Nauk* **16**, 167 (1970), *C.A.* **73**, 119454y (1970). Mechanism of action studies as an egg suppressive agent in schistosomiasis, A. B. Machado *et al., J. Parasitol.* **56**, 392 (1970). *In vivo* and *in vitro* effects: I. Popiel, D. A. Erasmus, *Trans. R. Soc. Trop. Med. Hyg.* **75**, 287 (1981). Toxicity study: S. H. Dieke *et al., J. Pharmacol. Exp. Ther.* **90**, 260 (1947).

White crystals; bitter taste; slight garlic odor; d 1.22; mp 78°. Sol in about 30 parts water; sol in alcohol, slightly sol in ether. Insol in benzene. LD$_{50}$ orally in rats: 200 mg/kg (Dieke).

THERAP CAT (VET): Has been used to minimize scar tissue.

9363. 1-Thiosorbitol. [24531-57-5] 1-Thio-D-glucitol. C$_6$-H$_{14}$O$_5$S; mol wt 198.24. C 36.35%, H 7.12%, O 40.35%, S 16.17%. CH$_2$OH(CHOH)$_4$CH$_2$SH. Prepd by heating an aq soln of glucose with a catalyst, sulfur, and hydrogen at 150° and 1500 psi for 3 hrs: Farlow *et al., J. Am. Chem. Soc.* **70**, 1392 (1948).

Crystals from abs alcohol, mp 92-93°. Nonhygroscopic. [α]$_D^{27}$ −1.9° (c = 2). Readily sol in water, pyridine, ethylene glycol, formamide; practically insol in benzene, petr ether, carbon tetrachloride; carbon disulfide. Solubilities at 20° in g/100 ml solvent: 1.7 in abs alcohol; 1.2 in dioxane; 0.016 in ethyl ether; 0.016 in trichloroethylene; 0.010 in acetone. Strong reducing agent.

USE: Suggested as a polymer stabilizer; anticorrosion agent for pickling baths; in plating baths.

9364. Thiostrepton. [1393-48-2] Bryamycin; Thiactin. C$_{72}$H$_{85}$N$_{19}$O$_{18}$S$_5$; mol wt 1664.89. C 51.94%, H 5.15%, N 15.98%, O 17.30%, S 9.63%. Polypeptide antibiotic contg sulfur. Produced by *Streptomyces azureus* isolated from New Mexican soil: Pagano *et al., Antibiot. Annu.* **1955-56**, 554; Vandeputte, Dutcher, *ibid.* 560; **GB 795570** (1958); Donovick *et al.;* Platt, **US 2982689**; **US 2982698** (1961 all to Olin Mathieson). Structure studies: Bodanszky *et al., J. Am. Chem. Soc.* **84**, 2003 (1962); **86**, 2478 (1964); Anderson *et al., Nature* **225**, 233 (1970). Total structure determn: K. Tori *et al., Tetrahedron Lett.* **1976**, 185; *eidem, J. Antibiot.* **32**, 1072 (1979). ^{13}C-NMR study: *eidem, ibid.* **34**, 124 (1981). Total synthesis: K. C. Nicolaou *et al., Angew. Chem. Int. Ed.* **43**, 5087, 5092 (2004). Mode of action as an inhibitor of protein synthesis: Cannon, Burns, *FEBS Lett.* **18**, 1 (1971); Cundliffe, *Biochem. Biophys. Res. Commun.* **44**, 912 (1971). Identity with thiactin: Bodanszky *et al., J. Antibiot.* **16A**, 76 (1963). Comprehensive description: K. Florey, *Anal. Profiles Drug Subs.* **7**, 423-444 (1978). *Review:* Pestka, Bodley, in *Antibiotics* vol. 3, J. W. Corcoran, F. E. Hahn, Eds. (Springer-Verlag, New York, 1975) pp 551-573; E. Cundliffe, *ibid.* **vol. 5** (pt. 1), F. E. Hahn, Ed. (1979) pp 329-343.

Crystals from chloroform + methanol, dec 246-256°. [α]$_D^{23}$ −98.5° (glacial acetic acid); −61° (dioxane); −20° (pyridine). Sol in chloroform, dioxane, pyridine, glacial acetic acid, DMF.

Practically insol in water, the lower alcohols, nonpolar organic solvents, dil aq acid or base. Dissolved by methanolic acid or base with decompn. Stable in the presence of gastric and intestinal juices and urine. No uv maxima but shows characteristic shoulders at 225, 250, 280 nm (E$_{1cm}^{1\%}$ 520, 380, 255).

Hemisuccinate. Prepn: Bodanszky, Fried, **US 3181995** (1965 to Olin Mathieson). mp 200-220°, forms a water-soluble potassium salt.

THERAP CAT: Antibacterial.

THERAP CAT (VET): Antibacterial.

9365. Thiothixene. [5591-45-7] *N,N*-Dimethyl-9-[3-(4-methyl-1-piperazinyl)propylidene]thioxanthene-2-sulfonamide; *cis*-9-[3-(4-methyl-1-piperazinyl)propylidene]-2-(dimethylsulfonamido)thioxanthene; tiotixene; Navane; Orbinamon. C$_{23}$H$_{29}$N$_3$O$_2$S$_2$; mol wt 443.63. C 62.27%, H 6.59%, N 9.47%, O 7.21%, S 14.46%. Prepn of *cis/trans*-isomer mixture and sepn of isomers: Bloom, Muren, **BE 647066** corresp to **US 3310553** (1964, 1967 both to Pfizer); Muren, Bloom, *J. Med. Chem.* **13**, 17 (1970). Only *cis*-isomer exhibits therapeutic activity. Structure studies: J. P. Schaefer, *Chem. Commun.* **1967**, 743. Pharmacological studies: A. Weissman, *Psychopharmacologia* **12**, 142 (1968). HPLC determn in serum: C. Dilger *et al., Arzneim.-Forsch.* **38**, 1522 (1988). Book: T. A. Ban, *Psychopharmacology of Thiothixene* (Raven Press, New York, 1978) 485 pp. Comprehensive description: D. K. Wyatt, L. T. Grady, *Anal. Profiles Drug Subs.* **18**, 527-565 (1989).

cis-form

cis-Isomer. Crystals, mp 147.5-149°. uv max (methanol): 228, 260, 310 nm (log ε 4.6, 4.3, 3.9). Has greater pharmacologic activity than *trans*-isomer. LD$_{50}$ in mice, rats (mg/kg): 100, 55 i.p. (Weissman).

trans-Isomer. mp 123-124.5°. uv max (methanol): 229, 252, 301 nm (log ε 4.5, 4.2, 3.9). LD$_{50}$ i.p. in mice: 235 mg/kg (Weissman).

cis-trans-Isomer mixture. Crystals, mp 114-118°.

Dimaleate. mp 158-160.5°.

Dioxalate. mp 229°.

THERAP CAT: Antipsychotic.

9366. 2-Thiouracil. [141-90-2] 2,3-Dihydro-2-thioxo-4-(1*H*)-pyrimidinone; 2-mercapto-4-hydroxypyrimidine; 4-hydroxy-2(1*H*)-pyrimidinethione; 2-mercapto-4(1*H*)-pyrimidinone; 6-hydroxy-2-mercaptopyrimidine; 2-mercapto-4-pyrimidone; Deracil. C$_4$H$_4$N$_2$OS; mol wt 128.15. C 37.49%, H 3.15%, N 21.86%, O 12.48%, S 25.02%. Occurs in seeds of *Brassica, Cruciferae:* Purves, *Br. J. Exp. Pathol.* **22**, 241 (1941). Prepd by condensing ethyl formylacetate with thiourea: Wheeler, Liddle, *Am. Chem. J.* **40**, 550 (1908). Antithyroid activity results from its interference with the iodination of thyroxine precursors: *see* Maloof, Soodak, *Pharmacol. Rev.* **15**, 72-79 (1963). Inhibition of nucleic acid metabolism: Cardeilhac, *Proc. Soc. Exp. Biol. Med.* **125**, 692 (1967). Toxicology: K. K. Carroll, R. L. Noble, *J. Pharmacol. Exp. Ther.* **97**, 478 (1949).

Minute, bitter crystals, no definite mp. Very slightly soluble in water (1:2000); practically insol in alcohol, ether, acids. Readily sol in alkaline solns. LD_{100} i.p. in rats: 1500 mg/kg (Carroll, Noble).

THERAP CAT: Treatment of hyperthyroidism; angina pectoris; congestive heart failure.

THERAP CAT (VET): Thyroid depressant. In hyperthyroidism and to promote fattening.

9367. Thiourea. [62-56-6] Thiocarbamide. CH_4N_2S; mol wt 76.12. C 15.78%, H 5.30%, N 36.80%, S 42.12%. H_2NCSNH_2. Made by fusing ammonium thiocyanate: Powers and Powers, Mitchell, US 2552584; US 2560596 (both 1951 to Koppers); by treating cyanamide with hydrogen sulfide: Robin, Jr., US 2173067 (1940 to Am. Cyanamid); Lewis, US 2393917 (1946 to Monsanto); Van de Kamp, US 2357149 (1944 to Merck & Co.). Toxicity data: Dieke et al., J. Pharmacol. Exp. Ther. **90**, 262 (1947).

Crystals, mp 176-178°. d 1.405. Soluble in 11 parts water, in alcohol; sparingly sol in ether. Neutral reaction. Forms addition compds with metallic salts. LD_{50} orally in wild Norway rats: 1830 mg/kg (Dieke).

Caution: Chronic administration in rats has resulted in hepatic tumors, bone marrow depression and goiters: Clinical Toxicology of Commercial Products, R. E. Gosselin et al., Eds. (Williams & Wilkins, Baltimore, 5th ed., 1984) Section II, p 350. This substance is reasonably anticipated to be a human carcinogen: Report on Carcinogens, Eleventh Edition (PB2005-104914, 2004) p III-250.

USE: In animal glue liquifiers and silver tarnish removers. Photographic fixing agent and to remove stains from negatives; manuf resins; vulcanization accelerator; a reagent for bismuth, selenite ions.

9368. Thioxanthene. [261-31-4] Thiaxanthene; dibenzothiopyran; dibenzopenthiophene; diphenylenemethane sulfide. $C_{13}H_{10}S$; mol wt 198.28. C 78.75%, H 5.08%, S 16.17%. Conveniently obtained from thioxanthone in 74% yield by reduction with lithium aluminum hydride: Mustafa, Hilmy, J. Chem. Soc. **1952**, 1345.

Needles or rods from alcohol + chloroform. Sublimes easily. mp 128°. bp_{730} 340°. Dipole moment: 1.44 D. Freely sol in chloroform. Moderately sol in alcohol, ether.

9369. Thioxanthone. [492-22-8] Thioxanthen-9-one; thiaxanthone; 9-oxothioxanthone. $C_{13}H_8OS$; mol wt 212.27. C 73.56%, H 3.80%, O 7.54%, S 15.11%. Prepd by the interaction of diphenyl sulfide and phosgene with aluminum chloride as catalyst: Szmant et al., J. Org. Chem. **18**, 745 (1953).

Yellow needles from chloroform, mp 211°. bp_{715} 273°. Freely sol in benzene, chloroform, carbon disulfide, hot glacial acetic acid. Slightly sol in alc. Practically insol in water, alkaline solns. Sol in concd sulfuric acid, giving a yellow soln with strong green fluorescence in visible light.

9370. Thiphenamil. [82-99-5] α-Phenylbenzeneethanethioic acid S-[2-(diethylamino)ethyl]ester; diphenylthioacetic acid S-(2-diethylaminoethyl) ester; diphenylthiolacetic acid 2-diethylaminoethyl ester; S-[2-(diethylamino)ethyl]diphenylthioacetate; β-diethylaminoethyl diphenylthioacetate. $C_{20}H_{25}NOS$; mol wt 327.48. C 73.35%, H 7.69%, N 4.28%, O 4.89%, S 9.79%. Smooth muscle relaxant. Prepn: Richardson, US 2390555 (1945 to Wm. P. Poythress); Clinton, US 2510773 (1950 to Sterling Drug); Richardson, J. Pharm. Sci. **55**, 1316 (1966). Mechanism of action study: Y. Kimoto et al., J. Urol. **144**, 1497 (1990). Clinical evaluation in detrusor incontinence: C. E. Constantinou, Urol. Int. **48**, 42 (1992).

Hydrochloride. [548-68-5] Trocinate. $C_{20}H_{25}NOS.HCl$; mol wt 363.94. Rosettes of tiny needles from benzene + petr ether, large prisms from abs ethanol + ethyl acetate, mp 129-130°. Sol in water. Aq solns are about neutral to litmus.

THERAP CAT: Antispasmodic.

9371. Thiram. [137-26-8] Tetramethylthioperoxydicarbonic diamide; bis(dimethylthiocarbamoyl) disulfide; bis(dimethylthiocarbamyl) disulfide; tetramethylthiuram disulfide; TMTD; ENT-987; SQ-1489; NSC-1771; Thiurad; Thylate; Fernasan; Nomersan; Rezifilm; Pomarsol; Tersan; Tuads; Arasan. $C_6H_{12}N_2S_4$; mol wt 240.43. C 29.97%, H 5.03%, N 11.65%, S 53.35%. Prepn: v. Braun, Stechele, Ber. **35**, 820 (1902); **36**, 2280 (1903); Romani, C.A. **16**, 854 (1922); Cummings, Simmons, Ind. Eng. Chem. **20**, 1173 (1928). Acute toxicity: Gaines, Toxicol. Appl. Pharmacol. **14**, 515 (1969). Review of carcinogenic risk: IARC Monographs **12**, 225 (1976).

Crystals from chloroform + alcohol, mp 155-156° (commercial grades, mp 146°). d 1.29. Insol in water, dil caustic, gasoline. Soly in alcohol and in ether less than 0.2%; soly in acetone 1.2%; in benzene 2.5%. Sol in chloroform, acetone. LD_{50} orally in rats: 640 mg/kg (Gaines).

Caution: Potential symptoms of overexposure are irritation of eyes, skin, mucous membranes; dermatitis; Antabuse-like effects. See NIOSH Pocket Guide to Chemical Hazards (DHHS/NIOSH 97-140, 1997) p 306. A potent skin sensitizer. Toxicity greater in presence of fats, oils, fat solvents. See Clinical Toxicology of Commercial Products, R. E. Gosselin et al., Eds. (Williams & Wilkins, Baltimore, 5th ed., 1984) section III, pp 383-386.

USE: Rubber accelerator; vulcanizer; seed disinfectant; fungicide; bacteriostat in soap; animal repellent.

THERAP CAT: Antiseptic.

9372. Thomas Phosphate. [1306-01-0] Thomas flour; calcium phosphate, tetrabasic. $Ca_3(PO_4)_2.CaO$ also represented by $4CaO.P_2O_5$. A byproduct of the Thomas steel process used in Europe: Iron ore of the "Minette" type from Alsace and the Rhineland contains about 2% phosphates which are combined with calcium and separated during the refining process.

USE: Agricultural fertilizer.

9373. Thonzylamine Hydrochloride. [63-56-9] N-[(4-Methoxyphenyl)methyl]-N′,N′-dimethyl-N-2-pyrimidinyl-1,2-ethanediamine monohydrochloride; 2-[(2-dimethylaminoethyl)(p-methoxybenzyl)amino]pyrimidine hydrochloride; N,N-dimethyl-N′-(p-methoxybenzyl)-N′-(2-pyrimidyl)ethylenediamine hydrochloride; Anahist; Tonamil. $C_{16}H_{23}ClN_4O$; mol wt 322.83. C 59.53%, H 7.18%, Cl 10.98%, N 17.35%, O 4.96%. Histamine H_1-receptor antagonist. Prepd by treating the sodium salt of 2-(p-methoxybenzyl)aminopyrimidine with N,N-dimethyl-2-chloroethylamine: Friedman, Tolstoouhov, US 2465865 (1949). Toxicity study: Reinhard, Seudi, Proc. Soc. Exp. Biol. Med. **66**, 512 (1947). Spectroscopic determn in nasal drops: S. M. Sabry et al., J. Pharm. Biomed. Anal. **22**, 257 (2000).

Consult the Name Index before using this section.

Crystals, mp 173-176° (free base, oily liq, $bp_{2.2}$ 185-187°). Freely sol in water; sol in alcohol, chloroform. Practically insol in ether. pH 5.1-5.7 (2% aq solution). LD_{50} orally in guinea pigs: 493 mg (base)/kg (Reinhard, Seudi).

THERAP CAT: Antihistaminic.

9374. Thorium. [7440-29-1] Th; at. wt 232.03806 (characteristic terrestrial isotopic composition); at. no. 90; valence 4. No stable nuclides. Naturally occurring isotopes (mass numbers): 232 (~100%, $T_{1/2}$ 1.40 × 10^{10} years, longest-lived known isotope, α-decay, rel. at. mass 232.0380); 228 (natural decay product of ^{232}Th); 227, 231 (natural decay products of ^{235}U); 230 ($T_{1/2}$ 7.54×10^4 years, rel. at. mass 230.0331), 234 (natural decay products of ^{238}U); other isotopes: 213-226, 229, 233, 235, 236. ^{232}Th found in nature undergoes natural decay by the emission of α-, β-, and γ-rays, eventually forming ^{208}Pb. Occurs in the minerals thorite, thorianite, orangite, yttrocrasite; in monazite sand (principal ore of commercial significance); present in the earth's crust 8-15 ppm. Isoln from thorite ($ThSiO_4$): J. J. Berzelius, *K. Sven. Ventenskapsakad. Handl.* **9**, 1 (1829); *Pogg. Ann.* **16**, 385 (1829). Prepn of metal: *idem, Ann. Phys.* **16**, 385 (1829); Marden, *Trans. Electrochem. Soc.* **66**, 39 (1934). Monographs: F. L. Cuthbert, *Thorium Production Technology* (Addison-Wesley, Reading, Mass., 1958); L. Grainger, *Uranium and Thorium* (Pitman, London, 1958). *Reviews: Mellor's* vol. **7**, 174-253 (1930); "The Actinides," in *Comprehensive Inorganic Chemistry* vol. **5**, J. C. Bailar, Jr., *et al.*, Eds. (Pergamon Press, Oxford, 1973) pp 1-715; L. I. Katzin in *Kirk-Othmer Encyclopedia of Chemical Technology* vol. **22** (Wiley-Interscience, New York, 3rd ed., 1983) pp 989-1002; L. I. Katzin, D. C. Sonnenberger in *The Chemistry of the Actinide Elements* vol. **1**, J. J. Katz *et al.*, Eds. (Chapman and Hall, New York, 1986) pp 41-101. Review of prepn and purification: J. C Spirlet *et al., Adv. Inorg. Chem.* **31**, 1-40 (1987). Review of toxicology and health effects: *Toxicological Profile for Thorium* (PB91-180448, 1990) 174 pp; *Patty's Industrial Hygiene and Toxicology* vol. **2C,** G. D. Clayton, F. E. Clayton, Eds. (Wiley-Interscience, New York, 4th ed., 1994) pp 2249-2258.

Grayish-white, lustrous, radioactive metal; somewhat ductile and malleable. Two alloptropic phases: face-centered cubic α-form, d^{25} 11.724, transforms to β-form at 1360°; body-centered cubic β-form transforms to liquid at mp 1750° (Katzin, Sonnenberger). Also reported as mp 1690° (Cuthbert). bp ~3800°. Heat of fusion <19.2 kJ/mol. Heat of vaporization ~586 kJ/mol. Heat capacity (25°) 27.32 J/mol.K. Darkens on prolonged exposure to air. Finely divided metal is pyrophoric in air. HCl attacks metal vigorously, leaving up to 25% as an undissolved residue. Nitric acid passivates metal. Dilute HF and H_2SO_4 and concentrated H_3PO_4 and $HClO_4$ attack thorium slowly, with evolution of H. Metal not attacked by alkali hydroxides.

USE: As fuel in nuclear reactors, as source of fissionable ^{233}U. In manuf incandescent gas-light mantles, welding electrodes, ceramics. As hardener in Mg alloys; for filament coatings in incandescent lamps and vacuum tubes; as chemical catalyst.

9375. Thorium Chloride. [10026-08-1] Thorium tetrachloride. Cl_4Th; mol wt 373.85. Cl 37.93%, Th 62.07%. $ThCl_4$. It may contain from 7 to 9 mols H_2O. Prepn of the octahydrate: Kremer, *J. Am. Chem. Soc.* **64**, 1009 (1942).

White, odorless crystals; d 4.59; mp 770°. bp 921°. Sol in water, alcohol. Sol in ethylenediamine.

9376. Thorium Nitrate. [13823-29-5] $N_4O_{12}Th$; mol wt 480.06. N 11.67%, O 39.99%, Th 48.34%. $Th(NO_3)_4$. Commercial form obtained as tetrahydrate; also crystallizes with 6 and 12 mols H_2O. Obtained from monazite: Pearce *et al., Inorg. Synth.* **II,** 38 (1946).

Tetrahydrate. White, slightly deliquesc crystals. Very sol in water, alcohol, the soln having an acid reaction. *Keep well closed.*

USE: Thorium nitrate with 1% cerium nitrate constitutes the usual impregnating liq for incandescent mantles. As a reagent for determination of fluorine.

9377. Thorium Oxide. [1314-20-1] Thorium dioxide; thoria. O_2Th; mol wt 264.04. O 12.12%, Th 87.88%. ThO_2. *Review:* Keller in *Comprehensive Inorganic Chemistry* vol. **5**, J. C. Bailar, Jr. *et al.*, Eds. (Pergamon Press, Oxford, 1973) pp 221-223.

White, heavy, infusible, cryst powder; when heated is incandescent. d 10.0. mp 3390°. Insol in water or alkalies. Sol in acids with difficulty.

Suspension contg 20-25% ThO_2. Thorotrast. Reviews of tumor induction by Thorotrast: Looney, *Am. J. Roentgenol. Radium Ther. Nucl. Med.* **83**, 163-185; Smoron, Battifora, *Cancer* **30**, 1252-1259 (1972).

Caution: Thorium oxide is listed as a known human carcinogen: *Report on Carcinogens, Eleventh Edition* (PB2005-104914, 2004) p III-154.

THERAP CAT: Has been used as diagnostic aid (radiopaque medium).

9378. Thorium Tetracyanoplatinate(II). [14481-33-5] Thorium(4+) tetrakis(cyano-*C*)platinate(2−) (1:2); platinous thorium cyanide; thorium platinocyanide. $C_8N_8Pt_2Th$; mol wt 830.35. C 11.57%, N 13.49%, Pt 46.99%, Th 27.94%. $Th[Pt(CN)_4]_2$.

Hexadecahydrate. Yellow crystals. Sparingly sol in water.

USE: For fluorescent screens, *see* Barium Platinous Cyanide.

9379. Thozalinone. [655-05-0] 2-(Dimethylamino)-5-phenyl-4(5*H*)-oxazolone; 2-(dimethylamino)-5-phenyl-2-oxazolin-4-one; 5-phenyl-2-(dimethylamino)-2-oxazolin-4-one; tozalinone; Stimsen. $C_{11}H_{12}N_2O_2$; mol wt 204.23. C 64.69%, H 5.92%, N 13.72%, O 15.67%. Prepn: Hardy, Jr. *et al.*, US 3037990 (1962 to Am. Cyanamid). Pharmacological studies: B. M. Bernstein, C. N. Latimer, *Psychopharmacologia* **12**, 338 (1968); U. H. Lindberg, J. Pedersen, *Acta Pharm. Suec.* **5**, 15 (1968). In treatment of Parkinsonism: W. D. Gray, C. E. Edward, US 3665075 (1972 to Am. Cyanamid).

Crystals from water, mp 133-136°.

THERAP CAT: Antidepressant.

9380. Threonine. [72-19-5] L-Threonine; Thr; T; (2*S*,3*R*)-2-amino-3-hydroxybutyric acid; α-amino-β-hydroxybutyric acid. $C_4H_9NO_3$; mol wt 119.12. C 40.33%, H 7.62%, N 11.76%, O 40.29%. An essential amino acid for human development; last of the common amino acids to be discovered. Identified in oat protein: S. B. Schryver, H. W. Buston, *Proc. Roy. Soc. London* **99B,** 476 (1925/6); isolated from blood fibrin: W. C. Rose, *J. Biol. Chem.* **109**, 77 (1935). Structure: C. E. Meyer, W. C. Rose, *ibid.* **115**, 721 (1936). Early chemistry and biochemistry: *Amino Acids and Proteins*, D. M. Greenberg, Ed. (Charles C. Thomas, Springfield, IL, 1951) 950 pp., *passim*; J. P. Greenstein, M. Winitz, *Chemistry of the Amino Acids* vols **1-3** (John Wiley and Sons, Inc., New York, 1961) pp. 2238-2258, *passim*. GC/MS metabolism study: O. Ballevre *et al., Anal. Biochem.* **193**, 212 (1991). Clinical evaluation in amyotrophic lateral sclerosis: J. B. Roufs, *Med. Hypotheses* **34**, 20 (1991); O. Blin *et al., J. Neurol.* **239**, 79 (1992). Review of microbial production: Daoust, *Dev. Ind. Microbiol.* **7**, 41 (1966); R. Bhattacharyya *et al., Hind. Antibiot. Bull.* **30**, 54-65 (1988). Review of biosynthesis: G. N. Cohen in *Amino Acids, Biotechnol. Ser.* **3**, 147-171 (1983); of regulation of biosynthesis: G. Galili, *Plant Cell* **7**, 899-906 (1995).

Crystals, dec 255-257°. $[\alpha]_D^{26}$ −28.3° (c = 1.09). pK_1' 2.63; pK_2' 10.43. Freely sol in water. Insol in common neutral solvents.

DL-Form hemihydrate. Orthorhombic crystals, dec 229-230°.

9381. D-Threose. [95-43-2] (2*S*,3*R*)-2,3,4-Trihydroxybutanal. $C_4H_8O_4$; mol wt 120.10. C 40.00%, H 6.71%, O 53.29%. From calcium D-xylonate by oxidation with H_2O_2: Ruff, *Ber.* **34**, 1370 (1901). Improved procedure using strontium D-xylonate and ferric acetate catalyst: Hockett, *J. Am. Chem. Soc.* **57**, 2260, 2265 (1935). From tetraacetyl-D-xylononitrile: Maquenne, *Compt. Rend.* **130**, 1403 (1900); *Ann. Chim.* [7] **24**, 404 (1901); Bonner, Roth, *J. Am. Chem. Soc.* **81**, 5454 (1959); from monobenzylidene-D-arabitol: Steiger, Reichstein, *Helv. Chim. Acta* **19**, 1016 (1939); from 1,1-diethylsulfonyl-D-*threo*-3,4,5-trihydroxypent-1-ene: Hough, Taylor, *J. Chem. Soc.* **1955**, 1212; from D-galactose: Perlin, Brice, *Can. J. Chem.* **34**, 541 (1956). Synthesis of DL-threose: Lake, Glattfeld, *J. Am. Chem. Soc.* **66**, 1091 (1944); Schmid, Grob, *Helv. Chim. Acta* **32**, 77 (1949); Sonogashira, Nakagawa, *Bull. Chem. Soc. Jpn.* **45**, 2616 (1972).

Syrup. Shows mutarotation. Final $[\alpha]_D^{20}$ −12.3° (20 min, c = 4). Very sol in water; slightly in alcohol. Practically insol in ether, petr ether.

Phenylosazone. $C_{16}H_{18}N_4O_2$. Dec 164-165°. Identical with D-erythrose phenylosazone.

Triacetate. $C_{10}H_{14}O_7$. Prisms from abs ethanol, mp 117-118°. $[\alpha]_D^{25}$ +34.4° (c = 2 in chloroform). Soluble in hot water, chloroform, acetone, ethyl acetate; sparingly sol in abs alcohol, methanol, ether.

9382. L-Threose. [95-44-3] (2R,3S)-2,3,4-Trihydroxybutanal. $C_4H_8O_4$; mol wt 120.10. C 40.00%, H 6.71%, O 53.29%. By degradation of L-xylose through the oxime and tetraacetyl-L-xylononitrile to L-threose diacetamide: Hockett *et al., J. Am. Chem. Soc.* **60**, 278 (1938); from D-glucitol: Hutson, Weigel, *J. Chem. Soc.* **1961**, 1546.

Shows mutarotation; final $[\alpha]_D^{20}$ +13.2° (c = 4.5). Sol in water.
Phenylosazone. $C_{16}H_{18}N_4O_2$. Dec 162°.

9383. Thrombin. [9002-04-4] Blood-coagulation factor IIa; factor IIa; fibrinogenase; EC 3.4.21.5. Multifunctional serine protease generated at the site of vascular injury from prothrombin, *q.v.* Key enzyme in the coagulation cascade; converts fibrinogen into fibrin and activates factor XIII, *q.v.*, which cross-links and stabilizes the fibrin polymer. Enhances inflammation and tissue repair via receptor-mediated cellular responses; activates platelets and endothelial cells and stimulates proliferation of fibroblasts and smooth muscle cells. The mature enzyme is glycosylated and consists of two polypeptide chains, designated A and B, covalently linked by a disulfide bridge. Exists in several forms, the largest and most active being the 39 kDa α-thrombin. The human α-thrombin A chain contains 36 amino acids; the B chain contains 259 residues. Purification by conversion from bovine prothrombin: W. H. Seegers *et al., J. Biol. Chem.* **126**, 91 (1938); W. H. Seegers, D. A. McGinty *ibid.* **146**, 511 (1942); H. P. Smith, US 2398077 (1946 to Parke, Davis). Sequence of bovine A chain: S. Magnussen, *Biochem. J.* **110**, 25P (1968). Primary structure of human α-thrombin: R. J. Butkowski *et al., J. Biol. Chem.* **252**, 4942 (1977). Review of structure: M. T. Stubbs, W. Bode, *Thromb. Res.* **69**, 1-58 (1993). Review of cloning, structure and function of thrombin receptors: S. R. Coughlin *et al., Cold Spring Harbor Symp. Quant. Biol.* **57**, 149-154 (1992); C. Tapparelli *et al., Trends Pharmacol. Sci.* **14**, 426-428 (1993). Review of role in hemostasis: J. W. Fenton *et al., Hematol. Oncol. Clin. North Am.* **7**, 1107-1119 (1993); in cell adhesion and proliferation: R. Bar-Shavit *et al., Am. J. Resp. Cell Mol.* **6**, 123-130 (1992); in inflammation and healing and effects in RA: R. Morris *et al., Ann. Rheum. Dis.* **53**, 72-79 (1994).

Topical thrombin. Thrombinar; Thrombogen; Thrombostat. A standardized prepn of bovine thrombin. Review of clinical experience: R. T. Tidrick *et al., Surgery* **14**, 191-196 (1943); in combination with fibrin: M. Brennan, *Blood Rev.* **5**, 240-244 (1991). White powder. Sol in water, isotonic saline.

THERAP CAT: Hemostatic (local).

9384. Thrombomodulin. Thrombin-binding protein present on the surface of vascular endothelial cells that modulates the pro-vs anti-coagulant activities of thrombin, *q.v.* Alters the macromolecular specificity of thrombin, decreasing its ability to catalyze clot formation and converting it to a potent activator of protein C, *q.v.* Also expressed by platelets, synovial cells, and certain tumor cells. Identification: C. T. Esmon, W. G. Owen, *Proc. Natl. Acad. Sci. USA* **78**, 2249 (1981). Isoln from rabbit lung: N. L. Esmon *et al., J. Biol. Chem.* **257**, 859 (1982); from human placenta: H. H. Salem *et al., ibid.* **259** 12246 (1984). Human thrombomodulin is a single-chain glycoprotein containing 559 amino acids; mol wt ~75 kDa. A soluble, truncated form has been isolated from human plasma and urine: H. Ishii, P. W. Majerus, *J. Clin. Invest.* **76**, 2178 (1985). Review: N. L. Esmon, *Prog. Hemostasis Thromb.* **9**, 29-55 (1989); of structure and function: W. A. Dittman, P. W. Majerus, *Blood* **75**, 329-336 (1990); of tissue distribution and expression by tumor cells: L. M. Fink *et al., Int. J. Dev. Biol.* **37**, 221-226 (1993).

9385. Thromboplastin. [9035-58-9] Blood-coagulation factor III; Factor III; cytozyme; thrombokinase; thrombokinin; tissue factor; tissue thromboplastin; zymoplastic substance; thrombo-stop; Tachostyptan. An integral membrane glycoprotein which, in the presence of Ca^{2+} ions, initiates coagulation by augmenting the proteolytic attack of factor VII on factors IX and X, *q.q.v.*: Nemerson, *Biochemistry* **5**, 601 (1966). Prepn from cattle brains: Hess, *J. Am. Med. Assoc.* **66**, 558 (1916). From rabbit brains or lung tissue: Singher, Swart, US 2842480 (1958 to Ortho); *see also* US 2847347 and US 2847350 (1958 to Ortho). Purification of bovine tissue factor: R. Bach *et al., J. Biol. Chem.* **256**, 8324 (1981). The tissue thromboplastin activity seems to be brought about by a lipoprotein comprising a combination of phospholipids: phosphatidyl ethanolamine (PE), phosphatidyl serine (PS), and phosphatidyl choline (PC): R. B. Hunter, *et al., Fibrinogen and Fibrin Turnover of Clotting Factors* (Schattauer, Stuttgart, 1963) pp 429-454. Removal of phospholipids from tissue factor results in loss of coagulant activity as well as solubilizing the protein component. Purification and characterization of the protein component: Nemerson, Pitlick, *Biochemistry* **9**, 5100 (1970); of tissue factor apoprotein: F. A. Pitlick, Y. Nemerson, *Methods Enzymol.* **45B**, 37-48 (1976). Located on the plasma membrane of endothelial cells readily available for complexing with clotting factors: Zeldis *et al., Science* **175**, 766 (1972). Synthesis by cultured cells: Zacharski, McIntyre, *J. Med.* **4**, 118 (1973). Possibly a vitamin K dependent clotting factor: L. R. Zacharski *et al., Ann. N.Y. Acad. Sci.* **370**, 311 (1981). Use as clinical reagent: F. D. Ziegler *et al., Ann. Clin. Lab. Sci.* **11**, 202 (1981); A. L. Suchman, P. F. Griner, *Ann. Intern. Med.* **104**, 810 (1986).

THERAP CAT: Hemostatic.

9386. Thrombopoietin. Thrombocytopoiesis-stimulating factor; TSF; TPO; c-Mpl ligand; megakaryocyte potentiating factor. Glycopeptide hormone which is the major physiological regulator of platelet production. Promotes the maturation of megakaryocytes and increases platelet size and number. Produced in the kidney; detectable in plasma and urine of thrombocytopenic animals and humans. Identification of humoral factor that increases platelet levels: E. Kelemen *et al., Acta Haematol.* **20**, 350 (1958). Partial purification from rabbit plasma: B. L. Evatt *et al., J. Lab. Clin. Med.* **83**, 364 (1974); from human plasma: A. Vannucchi *et al., Leukemia* **2**, 236 (1988). Production by cultured human embryonic kidney cells: T. P. McDonald *et al., J. Lab. Clin. Med.* **85**, 59 (1975). Purification: *idem et al., Exp. Hematol.* **17**, 865 (1989). Review of biological activity and properties: *idem, Am. J. Pediatr. Hematol. Oncol.* **14**, 8-21 (1992). Recombinant TPO acts both as a proliferative and a maturation factor for megakaryocytes. Cloning and characterization of human TPO: F. J. de Sauvage *et al., Nature* **369**, 533 (1994); of murine: S. Lok *et al., ibid.* 565; K. Kaushansky *et al., ibid.* 568; F. Wendling *et al., ibid.* 571.

9387. Thrombospondin. Glycoprotein G; thrombin-sensitive protein; TSP. A major glycoprotein constituent of human platelet α-granules that is released in response to platelet activation by α-thrombin, and plays an important role in mediating platelet aggregation. Discovery and initial isoln and properties: N. L. Baenziger *et al., Proc. Natl. Acad. Sci. USA* **68**, 240 (1971); *eidem, J. Biol. Chem.* **247**, 2723 (1972). Thrombospondin was initially thought to be a single polypeptide of mol wt about 190,000, but has been shown to be a disulfide-linked trimer of mol wt 450,000: I. Hagen, *Biochim. Biophys. Acta* **392**, 242 (1975); D. R. Phillips, P. P. Agin, *J. Biol. Chem.* **252**, 2121 (1977); J. W. Lawler *et al.*, *Thromb. Haemostasis* **37**, 355 (1977); *eidem*, *J. Biol. Chem.* **253**, 8609 (1978); S. S. Margossian *et al.*, *ibid.* **256**, 7495 (1981). Synthesis and secretion by cells in culture: G. J. Raugi *et al.*, *J. Cell Biol.* **95**, 351 (1982). Quantitative analysis: J. N. George *et al.*, *J. Lab. Clin. Med.* **92**, 430 (1978). The binding of secreted thrombospondin to platelet membranes is dependent on Ca^{2+}: D. R. Phillips *et al.*, *J. Biol. Chem.* **255**, 11629 (1980). Evidence for calcium-sensitive structure: J. Lawler *et al.*, *ibid.* **257**, 12257 (1982). Radioimmuno-assay: S. D. Saglio, H. S. Slayter, *Blood* **59**, 162 (1982). Identity of thrombospondin with the endogenous lectin secreted by activated platelets: E. A. Jaffee *et al.*, *Nature* **295**, 246 (1982). *See also* Fibrinogen.

Partial specific volume: 0.714 ml/g. Intrinsic viscosity: 40 ml/g in buffered saline at pH 7.6, 20°.

9388. Thromboxanes. Compounds derived from prostaglandin endoperoxides that cause platelet aggregation, contraction of arteries and other biological effects. Found in platelets, leucocytes, lung tissue, spleen, kidney, and umbilical artery. They are important mediators of the actions of polyunsaturated fatty acids transformed by cyclooxygenase. Discovery and structure of thromboxane B_2 (originally referred to as PHD): M. Hamberg, B. Samuelsson, *Proc. Natl. Acad. Sci. USA* **71**, 3400 (1974). Discovery and structure of thromboxane A_2 and identity with the unstable component of RCS (rabbit aorta contracting substance) *see* P. J. Piper, J. R. Vane, *Nature* **223**, 29 (1969); M. Hamberg *et al.*, *Proc. Natl. Acad. Sci. USA* **72**, 2994 (1975). Biosynthesis and biological properties: P. Needleman *et al.*, *Science* **193**, 163 (1976). Physiological review: J. R. Vane *et al.*, *Int. Rev. Exp. Pathol.* **23**, 161-207 (1982). *Reviews:* B. Samuelsson in *Organic Chemistry*, A. T. Blomquist, H. H. Wasserman, Eds. vol. **36**, entitled "Prostaglandin Research", P. Crabbe, Ed. (Academic Press, New York, 1977) pp 17-46; E. Granström *et al.*, *Adv. Prostaglandin Thromboxane Leukotriene Res.* **10**, 15-58 (1982); L. J. Roberts *et al.*, *ibid.* 211-225. Books: *Advances in Prostaglandin and Thromboxane Research* vols. **1-8**, B. Samuelsson, R. Paoletti, Eds. (Raven Press, New York, 1976-1980); *New Synthetic Routes to Prostaglandins and Thromboxanes* S. M. Roberts, F. Scheinmann, Eds. (Academic Press, New York, 1982).

Thromboxane A₂

Thromboxane B₂

Thromboxane A₂. [57576-52-0] (5Z,9α,11α,13E,15S)-9,11-Epoxy-15-hydroxythromboxa-5,13-dien-1-oic acid; [1S-[1α,3α(1E,-3R*)4β(Z),5α]]-7-[3-(3-hydroxy-1-octenyl)-2,6-dioxabicyclo[3.1.1]hept-4-yl]-5-heptenoic acid; TXA₂. $C_{20}H_{32}O_5$; mol wt 352.47. Highly unstable, biologically active bicyclic oxitane-oxane compound derived from the endoperoxide **PGG₂** and rapidly converted to thromboxane B₂ by addition of water. Formed by incubation of arachidonic acid or PGG₂ with washed platelets. It induces irreversible platelet aggregation and causes contraction of the isolated rabbit aorta and release of serotonin and ADP from platelets in platelet-rich plasma. Synthesis of stable analogs: E. J. Corey *et al.*, *Tetrahedron Lett.* **1980**, 137; K. M. Massey, G. M. Bundy, *ibid.* 445; S. Ohuchida *et al.*, *J. Am. Chem. Soc.* **103**, 4597 (1981); V. N. Kale, D. L. J. Clive, *J. Org. Chem.* **49**, 1554 (1984). Synthesis of biologically active unstable analogs: S. S. Bhagwat *et al.*, *Tetrahedron Lett.* **1985**, 1955. Total synthesis and structure of thromboxane A2: *eidem*, *Nature* **315**, 511 (1985). Formation and effects

in human platelets: J. Svensson *et al.*, *Acta Physiol. Scand.* **98**, 285 (1970). Biological half-life: 32 ±2 sec at 37°.

Thromboxane B₂. [54397-85-2] (5Z,9α,13E,15S)-9,11,15-tri-hydroxythromboxa-5,13-dien-1-oic acid; [2R-[2α(1E,3S*),3β(Z),-4β,6α]]-7-[tetrahydro-4,6-dihydroxy-2-(3-hydroxy-1-octenyl)-2H-pyran-3-yl]-5-heptenoic acid; TXB₂; PHD. $C_{20}H_{34}O_6$; mol wt 370.48. A stable metabolite of thromboxane A₂ in platelets, initially considered biologically inactive. It is released during anaphylaxis in isolated guinea pig lungs and has been isolated from guinea pig brain homogenates and carrageenin-induced granuloma. TXB₂ has also been reported as possessing chemotactic properties. Total synthesis: N. A. Nelson, R. W. Jackson, *Tetrahedron Lett.* **1976**, 3275; R. C. Kelly *et al.*, *ibid.* 3279; from a prostaglandin $F_{2α}$ derivative: W. P. Schneider, R. A. Morge, *ibid.* 3283; stereospecific synthesis from D-glucose: S. Hanessian, P. Lavallee, *Can. J. Chem.* **55**, 562 (1977); E. J. Corey *et al.*, *Tetrahedron Lett.* **1977**, 1625; S. Hanessian, P. Lavallee, *Can. J. Chem.* **59**, 870 (1981). Metabolism: L. J. Roberts *et al.*, *J. Biol. Chem.* **252**, 7415 (1966). Biological properties: J. R. Boot *et al.*, *J. Physiol.* **257**, 47P (1976); L. S. Wolfe *et al.*, *Biochem. Biophys. Res. Commun.* **70**, 907 (1976); W.-C. Chang *et al.*, *Prostaglandins* **13**, 3 (1977). Plates from ethyl acetate/ether/petr ether, mp 95-96°. $[\alpha]_D^{25}$ +57.4° (c = 0.26 in ethyl acetate).

9389. Thuja. Arbor vitae; white cedar; tree of life. Coniferous, pyramidal evergreen tree, *Thuja occidentalis* L., *Cupressaceae*, used as an ornamental plant and in traditional medicine to treat respiratory infection, warts, scurvy and rheumatism. *Habit.* North America, Europe. Medicinal portions include the dried, leafy young branches and the oil extracted from the leaves and branch tips. *Constit.* Volatile oil (1.4-4%); *p*-coumaric acid; umbelliferone; flavonoids incl. quercetin, mearusitrin; tannic acid (~1.3%); polysaccharides and proteins (~4%). Botanical description and medicinal uses: J. Gruenwald *et al.*, *PDR for Herbal Medicines* (Medical Economics, Montvale, 2nd Ed., 2000) pp 759-760. Review of pharmacology and clinical experience: B. Naser *et al.*, *Evid. Based Complement. Alternat. Med.* **2**, 69-78 (2005). Books:

Volatile oil. [8007-20-3] Oil of thuja; cedar leaf oil; oil of white cedar. *Constit.* α-thujone (69%), β-thujone (7-10%), fenchone (10-15%). Fragrance monograph: *Food Cosmet. Toxicol.* **12**, 843-844 (1974). Colorless to yellow liquid. d_{25}^{25} 0.906-0.916. n_D^{20} 1.4560-1.4590. Sol in most fixed oils, mineral oil, propylene glycol; 1 ml dissolves in 3 ml 70% alcohol. Practically insol in glycerin.

Caution: Symptoms of overexposure may include queasiness, vomiting, painful diarrhea, mucous membrane hemorrhaging, death (Gruenwald).

USE: As fragrance in soaps, detergents, perfumes.

THERAP CAT: Immunostimulant.

9390. β-Thujaplicin. [499-44-5] 2-Hydroxy-4-(1-methylethyl)-2,4,6-cycloheptatrien-1-one; hinokitiol; 4-isopropyltropolone. $C_{10}H_{12}O_2$; mol wt 164.20. C 73.15%, H 7.37%, O 19.49%. Tropolone derivative found in the heartwood of cupressaceous plants including western red cedar, eastern white cedar, and hiba; β-thujaplicin antimicrobial activity contributes to the decay-resistance of these trees. Isoln from western red cedar, *Thuja plicata* D. Don: H. Erdtman, J. Gripenberg, *Nature* **161**, 719 (1948); and characterization: A. B. Anderson, J. Gripenberg, *Acta Chem. Scand.* **2**, 644 (1948). Synthesis: W. von E. Doering, L. H. Knox, *J. Am. Chem. Soc.* **75**, 297 (1953). Biosynthesis in *Cupressus lusitanica*: J. Zhao, K. Sakai, *J. Exp. Bot.* **54**, 647 (2003). HPLC determn in cosmetics: M. Endo *et al.*, *J. Chromatogr.* **455**, 430 (1988). CZE determn in aqueous solns: L. Dyrskov *et al.*, *J. Agric. Food Chem.* **52**, 1452 (2004). Antibacterial activity in atopic dermatitis: Y. Arima *et al.*, *J. Antimicrob. Chemother.* **51**, 113 (2003).

mp 52-52.5° (Erdtman); also reported as mp 50-51° (Doering).

uv max (isooctane): 236, 322, 353 nm (log ε 4.37, 3.72, 3.66).

USE: Antibacterial additive in foods, cosmetics, eye drops and toothpaste.

9391. Thujic Acid. [499-89-8] 5,5-Dimethyl-1,3,6-cyclo-heptatriene-1-carboxylic acid; 4,4-dimethylcyclohepta-2,5,7-triene-carboxylic acid; dehydroperillic acid. $C_{10}H_{12}O_2$; mol wt 164.20. C 73.15%, H 7.37%, O 19.49%. Antibiotic substance from heart-wood of *Thuja plicata* D. Don, *Cupressaceae* (Western red cedar). Isoln: Anderson, Sherrard, *J. Am. Chem. Soc.* **55**, 3813 (1933); Erdtman, Gripenberg, *Acta Chem. Scand.* **2**, 625 (1948). Structure: Gripenberg, *ibid.* **3**, 1137 (1949); **5**, 995 (1951); **10**, 487 (1956); Davis, Tulinsky, *Tetrahedron Lett.* **1962**, 839.

Crystals from petr ether, mp 88-89°. uv max: 220, 280 nm (log ε 4.3, 3.7); min: 240 nm (log ε 3.0).
Methyl ester. $C_{11}H_{14}O_2$. Crystals, mp 34.5-35° or liq with pleasant odor, bp$_{14}$ 112-113°. d$_4^{22}$ 1.0225. n$_D^{22}$ 1.5130.
Hexahydrothujic acid. $C_{10}H_{18}O_2$. Liq, bp$_{14}$ 150-152°. n$_D^{20}$ 1.4671.

9392. Thujone. 4-Methyl-1-(1-methylethyl)bicyclo[3.1.0]-hexan-3-one; 3-thujanone. $C_{10}H_{16}O$; mol wt 152.23. C 78.90%, H 10.59%, O 10.51%. A constituent of many essential oils; present in thuja, etc. Equilibrium mixture contains 33% α-thujone and 67% β-thujone: Eastman, Winn, *J. Am. Chem. Soc.* **82**, 5908 (1960). α- and β-Thujones differ only in the stereochemistry of the 4-methyl group. Conformation: Hach *et al.*, *Tetrahedron Lett.* **1970**, 3175. Chemistry: J. P. Kutney *et al.*, *Bioorg. Chem.* **7**, 289 (1978); *eidem, Can. J. Chem.* **57**, 3145 (1979); **58**, 2641 (1980). Toxicity study: K. C. Rice, R. S. Wilson, *J. Med. Chem.* **19**, 1054 (1976). *Review:* J. L. Simonsen, *The Terpenes* vol. II (University Press, Cambridge, 1949) pp 32-52.

α-Thujone   β-Thujone

Colorless or almost colorless liquid. uv max (isooctane): 300 nm (ε 23). Practically insol in water. Sol in alc and many other organic solvents. LD$_{50}$ s.c. in mice: 134.2 mg/kg (Rice, Wilson).
α-Thujone. [546-80-5] (1S,4R,5R)-(−)-3-Thujanone. bp$_{17}$ 83.8-84.1°. d$_4^{25}$ 0.9109. n$_D^{15}$ 1.4490. [α]$_D^{20}$ −19.2°. LD$_{50}$ s.c. in mice: 87.5 mg/kg (Rice, Wilson).
β-Thujone. [471-15-8] *d*-Isothujone; (1S,4S,5R)-(+)-3-thuja-none. bp$_{17}$ 85.7-86.2°. d$_4^{25}$ 0.9135. n$_D^{25}$ 1.4500. [α]$_D^{15}$ +72.5°. LD$_{50}$ s.c. in mice: 442.2 mg/kg (Rice, Wilson).
Caution: Ingestion may cause convulsions.

9393. Thujopsene. [470-40-6] 1,1a,4,4a,5,6,7,8-Octahy-dro-2,4a,8,8-tetramethylcyclopropa[d]naphthalene; widdrene. $C_{15}H_{24}$; mol wt 204.35. C 88.16%, H 11.84%. From wood oil of the Japanese Hiba tree, *Thujopsis dolobrata* Sieb, and Zucc., *Cupressaceae:* Yano, *J. Soc. Chem. Ind. Jpn.* **16**, 443 (1913); Uchida, *ibid.* **31**, 501 (1928). Identity with widdrene: Erdtman, Thomas, *Acta Chem. Scand.* **12**, 267 (1958). Structure: Norin, *ibid.* **15**, 1676 (1961). Stereochemistry: Sisido *et al., J. Org. Chem.* **26**, 1964 (1961); Norin *Acta Chem. Scand.* **17**, 738 (1963). Synthesis: Dauben, Ashcraft, *J. Am. Chem. Soc.* **85**, 3673 (1963); Büchi, White, *ibid.* **86**, 2884 (1964).

Liquid. bp$_{10}$ 120°. [α]$_D$ −110° (c = 2 in chloroform). n$_D^{25}$ 1.5031. d^{24} 0.932. uv max (alc): 212 nm (ε 4680).

9394. Thulium. [7440-30-4] Tm; at. wt 168.93421; at. no. 69; valences 2, 3. A rare earth metal of the yttrium group; member of the lanthanide series. Naturally occurring isotope (mass number): 169; known artificial radioactive isotopes: 147; 148; 150-168; 170-176. Estimated abundance in earth's crust: 0.2-0.5 ppm. Found in small quantities in euxenite, ytterspar, sipylite, gadolinite, and other rare earth minerals. Discovered in crude erbium oxide: Cleve, *Compt. Rend.* **89**, 478, 521, 708 (1879). Obtained in a state of high purity by fractional crystn of its bromide: James, *J. Am. Chem. Soc.* **32**, 517 (1910); **33**, 1332 (1911). Sepn from other rare earths by ion exchange: Spedding *et al., ibid.* **76**, 2557 (1954). Toxicity study: Haley, *J. Pharm. Sci.* **54**, 663 (1965). Review of prepn, properties and compds: *The Rare Earths,* F. H. Spedding, A. H. Daane, Eds. (Krieger, Huntington, N.Y., 1971, reprint of 1961 ed.) 641 pp; Hulet, Bode, "Separation Chemistry of the Lanthanides and Transplutonium Actinides" in *MTP Int. Rev. Sci.: Inorg. Chem., Ser. One* vol. 7, K. W. Bagnall, Ed. (University Park Press, Baltimore, 1972) pp 1-45; Moeller, "The Lanthanides" in *Comprehensive Inorganic Chemistry* vol. 4, J. C. Bailar, Jr. *et al.,* Eds. (Pergamon Press, Oxford, 1973) pp 1-101; F. H. Spedding in *Kirk-Othmer Encyclopedia of Chemical Technology* vol. 19 (John Wiley & Sons, New York, 3rd ed., 1982) pp 833-854; *Chemistry of the Elements,* N. N. Greenwood, A. Earnshaw, Eds. (Pergamon Press, New York, 1984) pp 1423-1449. Brief review of properties: G. T. Seaborg, *Radiochim. Acta* **61**, 115-122 (1993).

Silvery-white, easily worked metal. Hexagonal close-packed crystals, d 9.3208. mp 1545°. bp 1725°; also reported as bp 1950° (Spedding, 1982). Heat of fusion: 16.84 kJ/mol. Heat of sublimation (25°): 232.2 kJ/mol. Solns of thulium salts show a characteristic absorption spectrum: Exner, Haschek, cited in *Mellor's* vol. V, 698 (1929).
Oxide. Thulia. O$_3$Tm$_2$. Dense powder of greenish-white color. Prepd by igniting the oxalate; dissolves slowly in strong acids; exhibits a reddish glow on gentle heating.
Hydroxide. Tm(OH)$_3$. White precipitate.
Chloride heptahydrate. TmCl$_3$.7H$_2$O. Deliquesc crystals. Sol in water, in alcohol. LD$_{50}$ in mice: 485 mg/kg i.p.; 6.25 g/kg orally (Haley).
Sulfate octahydrate. Tm$_2$(SO$_4$)$_3$.8H$_2$O. Obtained by ppting an aq soln of thulium chloride and sulfuric acid with alc.
Oxalate hexahydrate. Tm$_2$(C$_2$O$_4$)$_3$.6H$_2$O. Greenish-white precipitate. Sol in aq alkali oxalates with formation of double oxalates.

9395. Thurfyl Nicotinate. [70-19-9] Nicotinic acid tetrahy-drofurfuryl ester; tetrahydrofurfuryl nicotinate; nicotafuryl; Trafuril. $C_{11}H_{13}NO_3$; mol wt 207.23. C 63.75%, H 6.32%, N 6.76%, O 23.16%. Prepn: Hartmann, Merz, *US 2485152* (1949 to Ciba). Brief review: A. A. Fisher, *Cutis* **51**, 225-227 (1993).

Oil, bp$_{0.25}$ 114-116°. Sol in water, oil.
THERAP CAT: Rubefacient.

9396. Thyme. Dried leaves and flowering tops of *Thymus vulgaris* L., *Labiatae. Habit.* Southern Europe; cultivated in gardens. *Constit.* Volatile oil; tannin, gum.
USE: As a seasoning in foods.

9397. Thymidine. [50-89-5] 1-(2-Deoxy-β-D-ribofurano-syl)-5-methyluracil; thymine-2-desoxyriboside. $C_{10}H_{14}N_2O_5$;

mol wt 242.23. C 49.58%, H 5.83%, N 11.56%, O 33.03%. Constituent of deoxyribonucleic acid, *q.v.* Isoln from thymonucleic acid: Levene, London, *J. Biol. Chem.* **83**, 793 (1929). Structure: Levene, Tipson, *ibid.* **109**, 623 (1935). Conformation: Lemieux, *Can. J. Chem.* **39**, 116 (1961); Tollin *et al.*, *Nature* **217**, 1148 (1968). Prepn of thymidine-3'-phosphate and of thymidine-5'-phosphate: Tener, *J. Am. Chem. Soc.* **83**, 165 (1961). *Review: Basic Principles in Nucleic Acid Chemistry* vol. 1, P. O. P. Ts'o, Ed. (Academic Press, New York, 1974) *passim.*

Rosettes of needles from ethyl acetate. mp 185°. Yields a sublimate of thymine when heated. $[\alpha]_D^{25}$ +30.6° (c = 1.029). uv max (pH 7.2): 206.5, 267 nm ($\varepsilon \times 10^{+3}$ 9.8, 9.7). Absorption spectra: D. Voet *et al.*, *Biopolymers* **1**, 193 (1963). Sol in water, methanol, hot alcohol, hot acetone, hot ethyl acetate, pyridine, glacial acetic acid; sparingly sol in hot chloroform.

Monotrityl thymidine. $C_{29}H_{28}N_2O_5$. Prepd by the action of triphenylmethyl chloride on thymidine in pyridine. mp 125°. $[\alpha]_D^{24}$ +11.4° (c = 1.01 in acetone).

9398. Thymine. [65-71-4] 5-Methyl-2,4(1*H*,3*H*)-pyrimidinedione; 5-methyluracil; 2,4-dihydroxy-5-methylpyrimidine. $C_5H_6N_2O_2$; mol wt 126.11. C 47.62%, H 4.80%, N 22.21%, O 25.37%. A pyrimidine derivative; constituent of nucleic acids. Originally isolated from thymus nucleic acid: Levene, *Z. Physiol. Chem.* **39**, 4 (1903). Prepn by heating 2-ethylmercapto-4-hydroxy-5-methylpyrimidine: Wheeler, Merriam, *Am. Chem. J.* **29**, 478 (1903); **43**, 29 (1910). From methylcyanacetylurea by catalytic reduction: Bergmann, Johnson, *J. Am. Chem. Soc.* **55**, 1733 (1933). From β-methylmalic acid: Scherp, *J. Am. Chem. Soc.* **68**, 912 (1946). Crystal structure of monohydrate: Gerdil, *Acta Crystallogr.* **14**, 333 (1961). *Review:* Ts'o, "Bases, Nucleosides and Nucleotides" in *Basic Principles in Nucleic Acid Chemistry* vol. **1**, P. O. P. Ts'o, Ed. (Academic Press, New York, 1974) pp 453-584.

Dendritic or star-shaped plates from water, sometimes short needles. Sublimes in platelets. Dec 335-337° (Kofler stage). Weak acid, pK at 25° = 9.94. uv max (pH 7.0): 205, 264.5 nm ($\varepsilon \times 10^3$ 9.5, 7.9). Absorption spectra: D. Voet *et al.*, *Biopolymers* **1**, 193 (1963). Sol in hot water; slightly sol in cold water (4 g/l at 25°). Somewhat sol in alc; sparingly sol in ether; readily sol in alkalies with formation of salts. Oxidation yields urea, ethanal, pyruvic acid, formic acid. Hydrazine reacts with thymine forming urea and 4-methylpyrazolone. Thymine forms a silver salt which is sol in excess ammonia. Its mercuric and lead salts are insol.

Thymine-2-desoxyriboside see Thymidine.

USE: In biochemical research.

9399. Thymol. [89-83-8] 5-Methyl-2-(1-methylethyl)phenol; 5-methyl-2-isopropyl-1-phenol; 1-methyl-3-hydroxy-4-isopropylbenzene; 3-*p*-cymenol; 3-hydroxy-*p*-cymene; thyme camphor; *m*-thymol. $C_{10}H_{14}O$; mol wt 150.22. C 79.95%, H 9.39%, O 10.65%. Isolated by Neumann in 1719. Obtained from the essential oil of *Thymus vulgaris* L. and *Monarda punctata* L., *Labiatae:* Arppe, *Ann.* **58**, 41 (1846); Meyer, *Pharm. Ztg.* **81**, 192, 205 (1936). Also occurs in other volatile oils. Produced synthetically from *p*-cymene, piperitone, or *m*-cresol: Austerweil, **GB 221227** (1923); Jennen, Verdroncken, *Compt. Rend.* **245**, 183 (1957); Bottoms, **US**

2840616 (1958 to Natl. Cylinder Gas). Bactericidal activity: J. M. Schaffer, F. W. Tilley, *J. Bacteriol.* **14**, 259 (1927). Mold elimination on surfaces: O. W. Richards, K. J. Hawley, *J. Chem. Educ.* **16**, 6 (1939). In vitro antifungal activity: H. B. Myers, *J. Am. Med. Assoc.* **89**, 1834 (1927). Effectiveness as antifungal preservative: M. Dersarkissian, M. Goodberry: *Stud. Conserv.* **25**, 28 (1980). Use as clinical preservative: T. Z. Liu, *Clin. Chem.* **25**, 336 (1979); T. Z. Liu *et al.*, *ibid.* **27**, 1144 (1981). Toxicity: P. M. Jenner *et al.*, *Food Cosmet. Toxicol.* **2**, 327 (1964).

Crystals, mp 51.5°. bp ~233°. Appreciably volatile at 100°; volatilizes in water vapors. Characteristic odor; pungent, somewhat caustic taste. d_4^{25} 0.9699. n_D^{20} 1.5227; n_D^{25} 1.5204. One gram dissolves in ~1000 ml water, 1 ml alcohol, 0.7 ml chloroform, 1.5 ml ether, 1.7 ml olive oil at 25°. Sol in glacial acetic acid, oils, fixed alkali hydroxides. LD_{50} orally in rats: 980 mg/kg (Jenner). *Incompat:* Acetanilide, antipyrine, camphor, monobromated camphor, chloral hydrate, menthol, quinine sulfate, salol, urethane, spirit nitrous ether; in triturations because of liquefaction.

Acetate. [528-79-0] Acetylthymol; thymyl acetate. $C_{12}H_{16}$-O_2. Yellowish, oily liq; thymol odor. d^0 1.009. bp 243.5-245.5°. Practically insol in water. Miscible with alcohol, benzene chloroform, ether.

Caution: Mild irritant.

Carbonate. [552-93-2] $C_{21}H_{26}O_3$. White crystals; thymol odor; volatilizes with steam. mp 49°. Insol in water, acids, alkalies. Sol in hot alcohol, chloroform, ether, carbon tetrachloride.

USE: For destroying mold; preserving documents, art objects and urine. Stabilizer (antioxidant) for trichloroethylene, halothane.

THERAP CAT: Antiseptic (topical); anthelmintic (Nematodes).

THERAP CAT (VET): Has been used as anthelmintic, and as an antiseptic, external and internal.

9400. Thymol Blue. [76-61-9] 4,4'-(3*H*-2,1-Benzoxathiol-3-ylidene)bis[5-methyl-2-(1-methylethyl)phenol] *S*,*S*-dioxide; α-hydroxy-α,α-bis(5-hydroxycarvacryl)-*o*-toluenesulfonic acid γ-sultone; thymolsulfonephthalein. $C_{27}H_{30}O_5S$; mol wt 466.59. C 69.50%, H 6.48%, O 17.15%, S 6.87%.

Brownish-green, cryst powder; characteristic odor. Insol in water. Sol in alcohol, dil alkali solns.

USE: As as acid-base indicator; pH: red 1.2 to yellow 2.8; also yellow 8.0 to blue 9.6.

9401. Thymolphthalein. [125-20-2] 3,3-Bis[4-hydroxy-2-methyl-5-(1-methylethyl)phenyl]-1(3*H*)-isobenzofuranone; 5',5"-diisopropyl-2',2"-dimethylphenolphthalein. $C_{28}H_{30}O_4$; mol wt 430.54. C 78.11%, H 7.02%, O 14.86%. Obtained by heating phthalic anhydride with thymol at 110° in the presence of stannic chloride.

Needles, mp ~253°. Insol in water; sol in alcohol, acetone; also sol in dil alkalies with a blue color, in H_2SO_4 with a carmine-red color.

USE: As pH indicator: colorless 9.3 to blue 10.5. Also as reagent for blood after decolorizing the alkaline soln by boiling with zinc dust.

9402. Thymomodulin. [90803-92-2] Leucotrofina. Cell-free thymic hormone preparation extracted from calf thymus by acid hydrolysis. Composed of a mixture of biologically active acidic peptides of mol wt <10,000. Modulates the maturation of T-cells. Prepn of crude extract from calf thymus: B. Brunetti, E. Pini, US 3657417 (1972 to Ellem). Electrophoretic characterization: C. Secchi et al., Riv. Eur. Sci. Med. Farmacol. 4, 499 (1982), C.A. 101, 21878m (1984). Biological activity and comparison with other thymic hormones: J. J. Twomey, N. M. Kouttab, Cell. Immunol. 72, 186 (1982). Purification and pharmacodynamics: eidem, Drugs Exp. Clin. Res. 10, 921 (1984). Antileukopenic activity in myelodepressed cancer patients: Z. Uray et al., Agressologie 21, 215 (1980); C. Gallo Curcio et al., Int. J. Immunother. 2, 189 (1986). Use in prophylaxis of infantile asthma: R. Genova, A. Guerra, Pediatr. Med. Chir. 5, 395 (1983). Preliminary study in AIDS: G. Valesini et al., Eur. J. Cancer Clin. Oncol. 22, 531 (1986).

THERAP CAT: Immunoregulator.

9403. Thymopentin. [69558-55-0] N-(N-(N-(N-(N^2-L-Arginyl-L-lysyl)-L-α-aspartyl)-L-valyl)-L-tyrosine; thymopoietin pentapeptide; TP-5; ORF-15244; Immunox; Sintomodulina; Timunox. C_{30}-$H_{49}N_9O_9$; mol wt 679.76. C 53.01%, H 7.27%, N 18.54%, O 21.18%. Thymic hormone analog corresponding to residues 32-36 of thymopoietin, q.v., which exhibits the full biological activity of the natural hormone. Synthesis: G. Goldstein et al., Science 204, 1309 (1979); eidem, US 4190646 (1980 to Sloan-Kettering). Bioavailability: T. Audhya, G. Goldstein, Int. J. Pept. Protein Res. 22, 187 (1983). Pharmacology: K. Bolla et al., Int. J. Clin. Pharmacol. Res. 4, 431 (1984). Comparison of biological activity with thymopoietin and splenin: T. Audhya et al., Proc. Natl. Acad. Sci. USA 81, 2847 (1984). Clinical study in treatment of primary immunodeficiencies: F. Aiuti et al., Lancet 1, 551 (1983); in AIDS: N. Clumeck et al., Int. J. Clin. Pharmacol. Res. 4, 459 (1984); in rheumatoid arthritis: M. G. Malaise et al., Lancet 1, 832 (1985). Review: E. A. Boyse, Surv. Immunol. Res. 4, 6-10 (1985).

Arg–Lys–Asp–Val–Tyr

THERAP CAT: Immunoregulator.

9404. Thymopoietin. Thymin (formerly); TP. A polypeptide thymic hormone which selectively induces T-cell maturation from prothymocytes and inhibits B-cell differentiation. mol wt ~5500 daltons. First detected as a factor causing impaired neuromuscular transmission in myasthenia gravis, a neuromuscular disease associated with thymic abnormalities: G. Goldstein, S. Wittingham, Lancet 2, 315 (1966); G. Goldstein, ibid. 2, 119 (1968). Isoln from bovine thymus as two closely homologous forms, thymopoietins I and II: idem, Nature 247, 11 (1974); idem, Ann. N.Y. Acad. Sci. 249, 177 (1975); idem, US 4077949 (1978 to Sloan-Kettering). Bovine TPs contain 49 amino acids; I differs from II only in residues 1, 2, and 43. The active site corresponds to residues 32-36. Human TP contains 48 amino acids. Human and bovine forms are highly homologous and are identical at the active site. Proposed sequence of bTP-II: D. H. Schlesinger, G. Goldstein, Cell 5, 361 (1975). Revised sequence of II, sequence of I, isoln and sequence of splenin, q.v., a thymopoietin-like peptide found in spleen: T. Audhya et al., Biochemistry 20, 6195 (1981). Isoln and sequence of human thymopoietin: T. Audhya et al., Proc. Natl. Acad. Sci. USA 84, 3545 (1987). First synthesis of a bioactive fragment: D. H. Schlesinger, Cell 5, 367 (1975). Identification of active site and synthesis of thymopentin, q.v., the pentapeptide corresponding to the active site: G. Goldstein et al., Science 204, 1309 (1979). Total synthesis of originally proposed amino acid sequence of II: M. Fujino et al., Chem. Pharm. Bull. 25, 1486 (1977); of revised sequence: T. Abiko, H. Sekino, ibid. 35, 2016 (1987). Effect on T-cell differentiation: R. S. Basch, G. Goldstein, Proc. Natl. Acad. Sci. USA 71, 1474 (1974); M. P. Scheid et al., Ann. N.Y. Acad. Sci. 249, 531 (1975). Comparison of bioactivities of thymopoietin and splenin: T. Audhya et al., Proc. Natl. Acad. Sci. USA 81, 2847 (1984). Review of thymopoietin and other thymic hormones: J. F. Bach, J. Immunopharmacol. 1, 277-310 (1979); of thymopoietin and immunoregulation: G. Goldstein, C. Lau in Polypeptide Hormones, R. F. Beers, E. G. Bassett, Eds. (Raven Press, New York, 1980) pp 459-467; E. A. Boyse, Surv. Immunol. Res. 4, 6-10 (1985).

9405. Thymosins. Family of thymic peptide hormones that regulate immune and endocrine events. Extraction from calf thymus and partial purification: A. L. Goldstein et al., Proc. Natl. Acad. Sci. USA 56, 1010 (1966). Purification and characterization of thymosins and isoln of one of the active components, **thymosin fraction 5**: eidem, ibid. 69, 1800 (1972). Improved isoln and properties: J. A. Hooper et al., Ann. N.Y. Acad. Sci. 249, 125 (1975). Thymosin fraction 5 is a mixture of polypeptides ranging in mol wt from ~1000 to 15,000; it has a very low content of non-protein material; it is heat stable up to 80°. It is an immunopotentiating agent that can act in place of the thymus gland in immuno-deprived or thymus-deprived patients to restore some immune functions. Nomenclature of the polypeptide fragments of fraction 5 is based on isoelectric points: α-region below 5.0, β-region 5.0-7.0, and γ-region above 7.0. **Thymosin α1** is an acidic (pI 4.2), 28 amino acid polypeptide (mol wt 3108) found in the highly acidic region of fraction 5. It is a biologically active proteolytic fragment of pro-thymosin α1. Isoln and preliminary structural determination of thymosin α1: A. L. Goldstein et al., Proc. Natl. Acad. Sci. USA 74, 725 (1977). Isoln, characterization, biological activities, and amino acid sequence analysis of α1 and **polypeptide β1**, a 74 amino acid peptide identical with ubiquitin, q.v.: T. L. K. Low et al., J. Biol. Chem. 254, 981 (1979); T. L. K. Low, A. L. Goldstein, ibid. 987. Synthesis of α1 by solution methods: S. S. Wang et al., J. Am. Chem. Soc. 101, 253 (1979). **Thymosin β4** is a biologically active, G-actin sequestering peptide consisting of 43 amino acids; mol wt 4.9 kDa; pI 5.1. Amino acid sequence of β4: T. L. K. Low et al., Proc. Natl. Acad. Sci. USA 78, 1162 (1981). Automated solid phase synthesis of β4: S. S. Wang et al., Int. J. Pept. Protein Res. 18, 413 (1981). Role of β4 in wound healing: K. M. Malinda et al., J. Invest. Dermatol. 113, 364 (1999). Series of articles on prepn, purification and characterization of thymic hormones and peptides: Methods Enzymol. 116, 213-291 (1985). Review of immune and endocrine modulation: P. H. Naylor, A. L. Goldstein, Adv. Pigment Cell Res. 256, 489-502 (1988); of immunological activities and therapeutic uses of thymic hormones and factors: S. Ben-Efraim et al., Crit. Rev. Immunol. 19, 261-284 (1999); of β-thymosins: V. T. Nachmias, Curr. Opin. Cell Biol. 5, 56-62 (1993); T. Huff et al., Int. J. Biochem. Cell Biol. 33, 205-220 (2001).

AcSer-Asp-Ala-Ala-Val-Asp-Thr-Ser-Ser-Glu-Ile-Thr-Thr
|
Lys
|
Asp
|
HO-Asn-Glu-Ala-Glu-Glu-Val-Val-Glu-Lys-Lys-Glu-Lys-Leu

Human Thymosin α1

Thymalfasin. [62304-98-7] Human thymosin α1; bovine thymosin α1; Zadaxin; Timosina. Synthetic peptide; mol wt 3108. Synthesis: S. S. Wang et al., Int. J. Pept. Protein Res. 15, 1 (1980). Clinical trial in influenza vaccine enhancement: S. Gravenstein et al., J. Am. Geriatr. Soc. 37, 1 (1989). Clinical pharmacokinetics: K. L. Rost et al., Int. J. Clin. Pharmacol. Ther. 37, 51 (1999). Review of use in combined chemo-immunotherapy in treatment of cancer: E. Garaci et al., Int. J. Immunopharmacol. 22, 1067-1076 (2000); of clinical efficacy in hepatitis: P. H. Naylor, Expert Opin. Invest. Drugs 8, 281-287 (1999); A. Billich, Curr. Opin. Invest. Drugs 3, 698-707 (2002). pI 3.8.

THERAP CAT: Thymalfasin as immunomodulator.

9406. Thymostatin. Calf thymic extract which markedly inhibits in vitro and in vivo the incorporation of labelled nucleosides into the DNA and RNA of lymphocytes. Also inhibited incorporation of labelled nucleosides in vitro into other cell types both lymphoid and non-lymphoid, but did not affect incorporation in vitro of labelled amino acids into cellular protein. A carbohydrate containing peptide with a particle size <2000. Prepn and properties: Goldstein et al., Proc. Natl. Acad. Sci. USA 57, 821 (1967).

Relatively heat stable; insol in chloroform but sol in chloroform-methanol (2:1).

9407. Thymostimulin. [117149-90-3] TP-1. Biological response modifier; partially purified extract of calf thymus composed of a mixture of bovine thymic peptides. Extraction and purification: G. Bergesi, R. Falchetti, *Folia Allergol. Immunol. Clin.* **24**, 204 (1977). Pharmacology and biological properties: R. Falchetti *et al., Drugs Exp. Clin. Res.* **3**, 39 (1977). Clinical studies in combination with antimicrobial therapy: P. Periti *et al., J. Chemother.* **5**, 37 (1993); as an adjunct to cancer chemotherapy: M. Federico *et al., Am. J. Clin. Oncol.* **18**, 8 (1995); with zidovudine vs HIV infection: G. Barbaro *et al. Curr. Ther. Res.* **56**, 369 (1995). Review of pharmacology and therapeutic use: K. L. Dechant, H. M. Bryson, *Clin. Immunother.* **1**, 378-398 (1994).

THERAP CAT: Immunomodulator.

9408. o-Thymotic Acid. [548-51-6] 2-Hydroxy-6-methyl-3-(1-methylethyl)benzoic acid; 3-hydroxy-2-*p*-cymenecarboxylic acid; *o*-thymotinic acid; 6-methyl-3-isopropylsalicylic acid. $C_{11}H_{14}O_3$; mol wt 194.23. C 68.02%, H 7.27%, O 24.71%. Prepn from thymol: Kolbe, Lautemann, *Ann.* **115**, 205 (1861); Spallino, Provenzal, *Gazz. Chim. Ital.* **39** (II), 326 (1909); Royer *et al., Bull. Soc. Chim. Fr.* **1955**, 1421.

Monoclinic prismatic needles from water, mp 127°. Volatile with steam. One gram dissolves in 10 liters of water at 20°. Sol in alc, ether, chloroform, benzene, petr ether.

Sodium salt. $C_{11}H_{13}NaO_3$. White cryst mass, freely sol in water.

Amide. $C_{11}H_{15}NO_2$. Needles from alc, mp 137°, dec 205°. Sol in org solvents and in aq solns of sodium carbonate.

Acetonyl ester. $C_{14}H_{18}O_4$. Needles from alcohol, mp 75°. Sol in alcohol.

USE: As salicylic acid and salicylates.

9409. Thymyl N-Isoamylcarbamate. [578-20-1] Isoamylcarbamic acid thymyl ester; isopropyl-*m*-cresyl ester of isoamylcarbamic acid; Egressin. $C_{16}H_{25}NO_2$; mol wt 263.38. C 72.96%, H 9.57%, N 5.32% O 12.15%. Prepd by interaction of isoamylamine and thymyl chloroformate: Zima, v. Werder, US 2524185 (1949 to E. Merck).

Needles from petr ether, mp 57°. Practically insol in water (<1:50,000). Upon alkaline saponification, it is split into isoamylamine and thymol (along with CO_2).

THERAP CAT: Anthelmintic (Nematodes).

9410. Thyroid. Tiroidina; Thyradin; Thyrocrine. Thyroid gland of domesticated animals that are used as food by man, freed from connective tissue and fat, dried and powdered. Contains not less than 0.17% and not over 0.23% iodine in thyroid combination. 1 part ≃ 5 parts fresh gland. Chemistry and physiology: Rawson *et al., The Hormones* **vol. III** (Academic Press, New York, 1955) pp 433-519.

Yellowish powder; slight meat-like odor; saline taste.

THERAP CAT: Thyroid hormone.

THERAP CAT (VET): In myxedema. Has been used in obesity, renal insufficiency, chronic skin conditions and to increase spermatogenesis, libido, lactation.

9411. Thyroidin. Iodothyrin. A dried extract of thyroid diluted with milk sugar or other suitable diluent, equal in potency to official thyroid.

THERAP CAT: Thyroid hormone.

9412. Thyropropic Acid. [51-26-3] 4-(4-Hydroxy-3-iodo-phenoxy)-3,5-diiodohydrocinnamic acid; 3,3′,5-triiodothyropropionic acid; β-[4-(3′-iodo-4′-hydroxyphenoxy)-3,5-diiodophenyl]propionic acid; Birodan. $C_{15}H_{11}I_3O_4$; mol wt 635.96. C 28.33%, H 1.74%, I 59.86%, O 10.06%. Thyroid hormone analog. Prepd by iodination of 3,5-diiodothyropropionic acid: Tomita, Lardy, *J. Biol. Chem.* **219**, 595 (1956).

Crystals from abs ethanol, mp 200°.

THERAP CAT: Antilipemic.

9413. Thyroprotein. [9005-97-4] Thyroactive protein; Protamone-D. Iodinated casein. Use in feed supplements: Kohler, *The Use of Thyroactive Protein in Dairy Cattle Feeding,* The Texas Nutrition Conference Oct. **1953**, Abstracts of papers, pp 5-7. Prepn: Reineke *et al., J. Biol. Chem.* **143**, 285 (1942); **147**, 115 (1943); Turner, Reineke, US 2329445, US 2379842, US 2385117, US 2478065 (1944, 1945, 1945, 1949 to Am. Dairies & Quaker Oats); Whitmoyer, Moore, US 2382193 (1945 to Whitmoyer Labs.); West, Van Bruggen, US 2642426, US 2709671 (1953, 1955 to Feed Prods).

USE: Feed supplement, *Fed. Regist.* **45**, 41360 (1980).

9414. Thyrotropin. [9002-71-5] TSH; thyroid-stimulating hormone; thyrotropic hormone. Glycoprotein hormone secreted by the anterior pituitary under the regulation of TRH, *q.v.* Stimulates the uptake of iodine, synthesis of thyroglobulin and release of thyroxine, *q.v.*, by the thyroid. Structure is a heterodimer of α- and β- subunits; analogous with chorionic gonadotropin, luteinizing hormone, and follicle-stimulating hormone, *q.q.v.* Reviews of early literature: W. T. Salter, *Hormones* **2**, 301-349 (1950); M. Sonnenberg, *Vitam. Horm.* **16**, 205-261 (1958). Purification from bovine pituitaries: T.-H. Liao *et al., J. Biol. Chem.* **244**, 6458 (1969). Amino acid sequence of bovine TSH: B. Shome *et al., ibid.* **246**, 833 (1971); T.-H. Liao, J. G. Pierce, *ibid.* 850; of human α and β subunits: J. G. Pierce *et al., Recent Prog. Horm. Res.* **27**, 165 (1971). Use in diagnosis of thyroid function: C. W. H. Havard, M. Boss, *Br. Med. J.* **3**, 678 (1974). Review of structure and bioactivity: J. A. Magner, *Endocr. Rev.* **11**, 354-385 (1990); and therapeutic potential: M. Grossmann *et al., ibid.* **18**, 476-501 (1997).

Biological activity is destroyed by heating and by proteolysis with pepsin, trypsin, and chymotrypsin. Also inactivated by oxidizing agents, such as potassium permanganate and elemental iodine.

Thyrotropin alfa. [194100-83-9] Thyrotropin (human β-subunit) complex with chorionic gonadotropin (human α-subunit); Thyrogen. Recombinant human TSH produced in Chinese hamster ovary cells. Prepn and pharmacology: E. S. Cole *et al., Biotechnology* **11**, 1014 (1993). *See also:* C. A. Kelton *et al.,* US 5240832 (1993 to Genzyme). Use in diagnosis of differentiated thyroid carcinoma (DTC): P. W. Ladenson *et al., N. Engl. J. Med.* **337**, 888 (1997). Clinical evaluation as adjunct to radioablative treatment of DTC: M. Luster *et al., J. Clin. Endocrinol. Metab.* **85**, 3640 (2000). Review of clinical studies: R. J. Robbins, A. K. Robbins, *ibid.* **88**, 1933-1938 (2003).

THERAP CAT: Diagnostic aid (thyroid tumor imaging).

THERAP CAT (VET): Diagnostic aid (thyroid function).

9415. Thyroxine. [51-48-9] *O*-(4-Hydroxy-3,5-diiodophenyl)-3,5-diiodo-L-tyrosine; (−)-3-[4-(4-hydroxy-3,5-diiodophenoxy)-3,5-diiodophenyl]alanine; 3,5,3′,5′-tetraiodo-L-thyronine; levothyroxine; T_4. $C_{15}H_{11}I_4NO_4$; mol wt 776.87. C 23.19%, H 1.43%, I 65.34%, N 1.80%, O 8.24%. One of the thyroid hormones involved in the maintenance of metabolic homeostasis. Synthesized and stored as amino acid residues of *thyroglobulin*, the major protein component of the thyroid follicular colloid. Synthesis and secretion are regulated by the pituitary hormone, TSH, *q.v.* Circulates in the serum bound to specific proteins, primarily *thyroxine-binding globulin*, *transthyretin*, and albumin. Deiodinated in peripheral tissues to the active metabolite, liothyronine, *q.v.* The D-form has very little activity as a thyroid hormone, but has been used to treat hyperlipidemia. Isoln from thyroid: E. C. Kendall, *J. Am.*

Med. Assoc. **64,** 2042 (1915); *idem, J. Biol. Chem.* **39,** 125 (1919). Structure: C. R. Harington, *Biochem. J.* **20,** 293, 300 (1926). Synthesis: C. R. Harington, G. Barger, *ibid.* **21,** 169 (1927); of naturally occurring L-form: J. R. Chalmers *et al., J. Chem. Soc.* **1949,** 3424; of isomers and racemate: L. G. Ginger, P. Z. Anthony, US 2889363; US 2889364 (both 1959 to Baxter Labs.). Direct determn in serum by RIA: J. C. Nelson, R. T. Tomel, *Clin. Chem.* **34,** 1737 (1988). Comprehensive description of levothyroxine sodium: A. Post, R. J. Warren, *Anal. Profiles Drug Subs.* **5,** 225-281 (1976). Review of pharmacology: E. Sypniewski, *Ann. Thorac. Surg.* **56,** S2-S8 (1993); of therapeutic use: A. D. Toft, *N. Engl. J. Med.* **331,** 174-180 (1994). Review of thyroid physiology: D. A. Fisher, *Clin. Chem.* **42,** 135-139 (1996); R. R. Cavalieri, *Thyroid* **7,** 177-181 (1997).

Crystals, dec 235-236°. $[\alpha]_{546}^{25}$ −3.2° (0.66 g in 6.07 g of 0.5*N* NaOH and 13.03 g alc); $[\alpha]_D^{20}$ −4.4° (3% in 0.13*N* NaOH in 70% EtOH).

Sodium salt. [55-03-8] Levothyroxine sodium; Eferox; Eltroxin; Euthyrox; Levaxin; Levothroid; Levothyrox; Levoxyl; Oroxine; Soloxine; Synthroid; Thyro-Tabs. $C_{15}H_{10}I_4NNaO_4$; mol wt 798.85. Occurs as the hydrate. Triclinic crystals or cream-colored powder. Odorless, tasteless, somewhat hygroscopic. d_4^{20} 2.381. $[\alpha]_D^{20}$ −4.4° (c = 3 in 70% ethanol). Soly in water (25°): about 15 mg/100 ml. Sol in mineral acids and in solns of alkali hydroxides and carbonates. More sol in alcohol. Very slightly sol in chloroform, ether. pH of a satd water soln: 8.35 to 9.35.

DL-Thyroxine. [300-30-1] Needle-like crystals. Dec 231-233°. Insol in water, in alcohol, and in the other usual organic solvents, but in the presence of mineral acids or alkalies it dissolves in alcohol; sol in solns of the alkali hydroxides and in hot solns of the alkali carbonates.

D-Thyroxine. [51-49-0] Dextrothyroxine. Crystals, dec 237°. $[\alpha]_{546}^{21}$ +2.97° (0.74 g in 6 g of 0.5*N* NaOH and 14 g of alcohol).

D-Thyroxine sodium salt. [137-53-1] Dextrothyroxine sodium; Choloxin; Debetrol; Dethyrona; Dextroid; Dynothel; Eulipos.

THERAP CAT: Thyroid hormone. Dextrothyroxine as antilipemic.

THERAP CAT (VET): Thyroid hormone.

9416. Tiadenol. [6964-20-1] 2,2′-[1,10-Decanediylbis(thio)]bisethanol; 2,2′-(decamethylenedithio)diethanol; 1,10-bis(2-hydroxyethylthio)decane; LL-1558; Delipid; Eulip; Fonlipol; Tiaden; Tiaterol. $C_{14}H_{30}O_2S_2$; mol wt 294.52. C 57.09%, H 10.27%, O 10.86%, S 21.77%. $HOCH_2CH_2S(CH_2)_{10}SCH_2CH_2OH$. Prepn: Williams, Cossar, US 3021215 (1962 to Eastman Kodak); Lafon, DE 2038836 (1971 to Orsymonde), *C.A.* **75,** 35528d (1971). Series of articles on pharmacology, metabolism, and toxicology: *Therapie* **27,** 395-444 (1972).

Crystals, mp 69.5°. uv max (ethanol): 212 nm. Soluble in ethanol, chloroform. Practically insol in water.

THERAP CAT: Antilipemic.

9417. Tiagabine. [115103-54-3] (3*R*)-1-[4,4-Bis(3-methyl-2-thienyl)-3-butenyl]-3-piperidinecarboxylic acid; (−)-(*R*)-1-[4,4-bis(3-methyl-2-thienyl)-3-butenyl]nipecotic acid; TGB; NO-328; NO-05-0328; NNC-05-0328; A-70569. $C_{20}H_{25}NO_2S_2$; mol wt 375.55. C 63.96%, H 6.71%, N 3.73%, O 8.52%, S 17.08%. GABA uptake inhibitor. Prepn: F. C. Groenvald, C. Braestrup, WO 8700171 (1987 to Novo); F. C. Gronvald, C. Braestrup, US 5010090 (1991 to Novo Nordisk); K. E. Andersen *et al., J. Med. Chem.* **36,** 1716 (1993). Pharmacology: C. L. Faingold *et al., Exp. Neurol.* **126,** 225 (1994). HPLC determn in human plasma: L. E. Gustavson, S. Chu, *J. Chromatogr.* **574,** 313 (1992). Clinical evaluation as add-on therapy: J. Bauer *et al., J. Epilepsy* **8,** 83 (1995). Review of pharmacology: W. J. Giardina, *ibid.* **7,** 161-166 (1994); and chemistry: H. Mengel, *Epilepsia* **35,** Suppl. 5, S81-S84 (1994). Review of clinical experience: J. P. Leach, M. J. Brodie, *Lancet* **351,** 203 (1998).

Hydrochloride. [145821-59-6] Gabitril. $C_{20}H_{25}NO_2S_2$·HCl; mol wt 412.01. White to off-white, odorless crystalline powder. mp 192° (dec) (Mengel). $[\alpha]_D^{20}$ −11°. pKa$_1$ 3.3; pKa$_2$ 9.4. Partition coefficient (octanol/water): 39.3 (pH 7.4). Soly in water: 3%. Practically insol in hexane.

THERAP CAT: Anticonvulsant.

9418. Tiamenidine. [31428-61-2] *N*-(2-Chloro-4-methyl-3-thienyl)-4,5-dihydro-1*H*-imidazol-2-amine; 2-[(2-chloro-4-methyl-3-thienyl)amino]-2-imidazoline; 2-chloro-4-methyl-3-(2′-imidazolin-2′-ylamino)thiophene; thiamenidine. $C_8H_{10}ClN_3S$; mol wt 215.70. C 44.55%, H 4.67%, Cl 16.44%, N 19.48%, S 14.87%. A thiophene analog of clonidine, *q.v.* Prepn: R. Rippel *et al., DE 1941761; idem, US 3758476 (1971, 1973, both to Hoechst). Structural studies: J. M. Leger, *C.R. Seances Acad. Sci. Ser. C* **289,** 93 (1979); A. Carpy *et al., Mol. Pharmacol.* **21,** 400 (1981). GC mass spectrum determn in human plasma: T. A. Bryce, J. L. Burrows, *Biomed. Mass Spectrom.* **6,** 27 (1979). Pharmacology: E. Lindner, J. Kaiser, *Arch. Int. Pharmacodyn. Ther.* **211,** 305 (1974). Activity as α-adrenoceptor agonist: A. G. Roach *et al., J. Pharmacol. Exp. Ther.* **227,** 421 (1983).

Crystals from isopropanol + petr ether, mp 152°.

Hydrochloride. [51274-83-0] HOE-440; Sundralen. $C_8H_{10}ClN_3S$·HCl; mol wt 252.16. Crystals from isopropanol + petr ether, mp 228-229°. LD$_{50}$ in rats, mice (mg/kg): 40, 45 i.v.; in mice: 170 s.c., 400 orally (Lindner, Kaiser).

THERAP CAT: Antihypertensive.

9419. Tiamulin. [55297-95-5] (3a*S*,4*R*,5*S*,6*S*,8*R*,9*R*,9a*R*,-10*R*)-[[2-(Diethylamino)ethyl]thio]acetic acid 6-ethenyldecahydro-5-hydroxy-4,6,9,10-tetramethyl-1-oxo-3a,9-propano-3a*H*-cyclopentacycloocten-8-yl ester; 14-desoxy-14-[(2-diethylaminoethyl)-mercaptoacetoxy]mutilin; thiamutilin; SQ-14055. $C_{28}H_{47}NO_4S$; mol wt 493.74. C 68.11%, H 9.59%, N 2.84%, O 12.96%, S 6.49%. Derivative of pleuromutilin, *q.v.* Prepn: H. Egger, DE 2248237 corresp to US 3919290 (1973, 1975 both to Sandoz); H. Egger, H. Reinshagen, *J. Antibiot.* **29,** 915 (1976). Biosynthesis: F. Knauseder, E. Brandl, *ibid.* 125. *In vitro* activity: H. Werner *et al., ibid.* **31,** 756 (1978). Metabolism: J. Dreyfuss *et al., ibid.* **32,** 496 (1979). Effect vs *Mycoplasma*: C. O. Baughn *et al., Avian Dis.* **22,** 620 (1978); R. F. Goodwin, *Vet. Rec.* **104,** 194 (1979). Mechanism of action: G. Högenauer in *Antibiotics* vol. 5(pt. 1), F. E. Hahn, Ed. (Springer-Verlag, New York, 1979) pp 344-360. Treatment of swine dysentery: M. D. Anderson, *Vet. Med. Small Anim. Clin.* **78,** 98 (1983).

Fumarate. [55297-96-6] 81723 hfu; SQ-22947; Denagard; Dynamutilin; Tiamutin. $C_{32}H_{51}NO_8S$; mol wt 609.81. Crystals from acetone, mp 147-148° (after stirring in ethyl acetate and drying at 60° and 80° overnight).

THERAP CAT (VET): Antibacterial.

9420. Tianeptine. [66981-73-5] 7-[(3-Chloro-6,11-dihydro-6-methyldibenzo[c,f][1,2]thiazepin-11-yl)amino]heptanoic acid S,S-dioxide. $C_{21}H_{25}ClN_2O_4S$; mol wt 436.95. C 57.72%, H 5.77%, Cl 8.11%, N 6.41%, O 14.65%, S 7.34%. Tricyclic compound with psychostimulant, anti-ulcer and anti-emetic properties. Prepn: C. Malen et al., **DE 2011806** corresp to **US 3758528** (1970, 1973 both to Sci. Union et Cie-Soc. Franc. Rech. Med.). Neuropharmacology study: C. Malen, J. Poignant, *Experientia* **28**, 811 (1972).

Sodium salt. [30123-17-2] S-1574; Stablon. $C_{21}H_{24}ClN_2$-NaO_4S; mol wt 458.93. Solid, mp 180°.

THERAP CAT: Antidepressant.

9421. Tiapride. [51012-32-9] N-[2-(Diethylamino)ethyl]-2-methoxy-5-(methylsulfonyl)benzamide; N-[2-(diethylamino)ethyl]-5-(methylsulfonyl)-o-anisamide; thiapride; FLC-1374. $C_{15}H_{24}$-N_2O_4S; mol wt 328.43. C 54.86%, H 7.37%, N 8.53%, O 19.49%, S 9.76%. Dopamine receptor antagonist structurally related to sulpiride, *q.v.* Prepn: G. Bulteau et al., **DE 2327192**; **GB 1394563** (1973, 1975 both to Soc. d'Etudes Sci. Ind. de L'Ile-de-France). Crystal structure: C. Houttemane et al., *Acta Crystallogr.* **C39**, 585 (1983). Dopamine receptor binding studies: T. Arima et al., *Jpn. J. Pharmacol.* **41**, 419 (1986). Pharmacokinetics: E. Rey et al., *Int. J. Clin. Pharmacol. Ther. Toxicol.* **20**, 62 (1982). Clinical evaluation in neuroleptic-induced dyskinesia: W. Greil et al., *Neuropsychobiology* **14**, 17 (1985); in alcohol withdrawal syndrome: R. Agricola et al., *J. Int. Med. Res.* **10**, 160 (1982); G. K. Shaw et al., *Br. J. Psychiatry* **150**, 164 (1987).

Crystals, mp 123-125°.
Hydrochloride. [51012-33-0] Gramalil; Italprid; Luxoben; Sereprile; Tiapridal; Tiapridex. $C_{15}H_{24}N_2O_4S$.HCl; mol wt 364.89.

THERAP CAT: Antidyskinetic.

9422. Tiaprofenic Acid. [33005-95-7] 5-Benzoyl-α-methyl-2-thiopheneacetic acid; α-methyl-5-benzoyl-2-thienylacetic acid; FC-3001; RU-15060; Suralgan; Surgam. $C_{14}H_{12}O_3S$; mol wt 260.31. C 64.60%, H 4.65%, O 18.44%, S 12.32%. Non-steroidal anti-inflammatory. Prepn: F. Clémence, O. Le Martret, **DE 2055264** and **FR 2112111** (1971 and 1972 to Roussel-UCLAF), *C.A.* **75**, 63597u (1971) and **78**, 97473c (1973); F. Clémence et al., *Eur. J. Med. Chem. - Chim. Ther.* **9**, 390 (1974). Pharmacology: eidem, ibid.; H. Fujimura et al., *Oyo Yakuri* **9**, 715 (1975), *C.A.* **83**, 188321w (1975). Review of pharmacology and efficacy in rheumatic diseases and pain control: E. M. Sorkin, R. N. Brogden, *Drugs* **29**, 208-235 (1985).

mp 96° (isopropyl ether).
THERAP CAT: Anti-inflammatory.

9423. Tiaprost. [71116-82-0] 7-[3,5-Dihydroxy-2-[3-hydroxy-4-(3-thienyloxy)-1-butenyl]cyclopentyl]-5-heptenoic acid; (15-R,S)-16-(3-thienyloxy)-ω-tetranor-PGF$_{2\alpha}$. $C_{20}H_{28}O_6S$; mol wt 396.50. C 60.58%, H 7.12%, O 24.21%, S 8.09%. Analog of prostaglandin F$_{2\alpha}$, *q.v.* Prepn: W. Bartmann et al., **DE 2524955** corresp to **US 4258053** (1977, 1981 both to Hoechst); eidem, *Prostaglandins* **17**, 301 (1979). Efficacy in bovine endometritis: W. Bentele et al., *Tieraerztl. Umsch.* **35**, 676, 678, 683 (1980). Pharmacological effects: W. v. Rechenberg et al., *Blue Book for the Vet. Profession* (Hoechst AG) **30**, 417 (1981). Administration in cattle: R. Humble, ibid. 425.

Tromethamine salt. Tiaprost trometamol; Iliren. $C_{24}H_{39}NO_9$-S; mol wt 517.63.

THERAP CAT (VET): Luteolytic.

9424. Tiaramide. [32527-55-2] 4-[(5-Chloro-2-oxo-3(2H)-benzothiazolyl)acetyl]-1-piperazineethanol; 5-chloro-3-[4-(2-hydroxyethyl)-1-piperazinyl]carbonylmethyl-2-benzothiazolinone; tialamide. $C_{15}H_{18}ClN_3O_3S$; mol wt 355.84. C 50.63%, H 5.10%, Cl 9.96%, N 11.81%, O 13.49%, S 9.01%. Prepn: Umio et al., **JP 71 15302** *C.A.* **75**, 36127j (1971); eidem, **JP 71 18752** *C.A.* **75**, 63824r (1971); Umio, **US 3661921** (1971, 1971, 1972 all to Fujisawa). Pharmacology: Takashima et al., *Arzneim.-Forsch.* **22**, 711 (1972); Tsurumi et al., ibid. 716, 724. Metabolism: Noda et al., ibid. 732. Toxicity studies: Watanabe et al., ibid. **23**, 504 (1973). Mode of antiasthmatic action: G. C. Folco et al., *Pharmacol. Res. Commun.* **11**, 703 (1979).

pKa 6.2.
Hydrochloride. [35941-71-0] NTA-194; FK-1160; Solantal. $C_{15}H_{18}ClN_3O_3S$.HCl; mol wt 392.30. White, odorless, bitter tasting crystalline powder, mp 159-161°. pH (10% aqueous soln): 3.4-3.7. Very soluble in water; slightly sol in organic solvents. LD$_{50}$ in male mice, rats (mg/kg): 178, 203 i.v.; 298, 540 i.p.; 564, 3600 orally (Watanabe).

THERAP CAT: Antiasthmatic; anti-inflammatory.

9425. Tiazofurin. [60084-10-8] 2β-D-Ribofuranosyl-4-thiazolecarboxamide; riboxamide; TCAR; CI-909; NSC-286193; Tiazole. $C_9H_{12}N_2O_5S$; mol wt 260.27. C 41.53%, H 4.65%, N 10.76%, O 30.74%, S 12.32%. Nucleoside analog that inhibits inosine monophosphate dehydrogenase (IMPDH). Prepn: M. Fuertes et al., *J. Org. Chem.* **41**, 4074 (1976); and antiviral activity: P. C. Srivastava et al., *J. Med. Chem.* **20**, 256 (1977). Structure-activity study: G. Gebeyehu et al., ibid. **28**, 99 (1985). HPLC determn in plasma: R. W. Klecker, Jr., J. M. Collins, *J. Chromatogr.* **307**, 361 (1984). Clinical pharmacokinetics: D. Raghavan et al., *Cancer Chemother. Pharmacol.* **16**, 160 (1986). Clinical evaluation in leukemia: G. Tricot et al, *Int. J. Cell Cloning* **8**, 161 (1990). Series of articles on pharmacology and clinical experience: *Anticancer Res.* **16**, 3307-3354 (1996).

Crystals from ethanol-ethyl acetate, mp 145-146°. $[\alpha]_D^{25}$ -9° (c = 0.5 in ethanol). uv max in ethanol: 215, 237 nm (ε 9450, 7625).

THERAP CAT: Antineoplastic.

9426. Tibezonium Iodide. [54663-47-7] *N,N*-Diethyl-*N*-methyl-2-[[4-[4-(phenylthio)phenyl]-3*H*-1,5-benzodiazepin-2-yl]-thio]ethanaminium iodide; diethylmethyl[2-[[4-[*p*-(phenylthio)-phenyl]-3*H*-1,5-benzodiazepin-2-yl]thio]ethyl]ammonium iodide; 2-[β-(*N*-diethylamino)ethylthio]-4-(*p*-phenylthio)phenyl-3*H*-1,5-benzodiazepine methiodide; thiabenzazonium iodide; Rec-15-0691; Antoral. $C_{28}H_{32}IN_3S_2$; mol wt 601.61. C 55.90%, H 5.36%, I 21.09%, N 6.98%, S 10.66%. 1,5-Benzodiazepine deriv with bactericidal activity. Prepn: D. Nardi *et al.*, **CH 555347** (1974 to Recordati), *C.A.* **82**, 43480 (1975). Synthesis, physical characteristics, antibacterial activity: *eidem, Experientia* **31**, 440 (1975); *eidem, Farmaco Ed. Sci.* **30**, 248 (1975). Structure activity study: C. Greico *et al., ibid.* **32**, 909 (1977). Antimicrobial activity: M. Veronese *et al., Chemotherapy* **23**, 90 (1977). Toxicity study: D. Nardi *et al., Experientia* **31**, 440 (1975).

Crystals from isopropanol, mp 162°. LD_{50} in mice, rats (mg/kg): 9000, >10000 orally; 42, 35 i.p. (Nardi).

THERAP CAT: Antibacterial.

9427. Tibolone. [5630-53-5] (7α,17α)-17-Hydroxy-7-methyl-19-norpregn-5(10)-en-20-yn-3-one; 7α-methyl-17α-ethynyl-17β-hydroxy-19-norandrost-5(10)-en-3-one; 7α-methyl-17α-ethynyl-17β-hydroxyestr-5(10)-en-3-one; Org-OD-14; Livial. $C_{21}H_{28}O_2$; mol wt 312.45. C 80.72%, H 9.03%, O 10.24%. Synthetic steroid with weak estrogenic, androgenic and progestogenic activity. Prepn: **NL 6406797**; H. P. de Jongh, N. P. van Vliet, **US 3340279** (1965, 1967 both to Organon). Improved process: M. S. de Winter, E. A. Harryvan, **US 3475465** (1969 to Organon). Endocrinological profile: J. de Visser *et al., Arzneim.-Forsch.* **34**, 1010 (1984). Series of articles on pharmacology and clinical efficacy in post-menopausal women: *Maturitas* Suppl 1, 1-72 (1987). Clinical effect in osteoporosis: P. Geusens *et al., ibid.* **13**, 155 (1991).

Crystals, mp 165-169°.

THERAP CAT: In treatment of menopausal syndrome.

9428. Ticarcillin. [34787-01-4] (2*S*,5*R*,6*R*)-6-[[(2*R*)-Carboxy-3-thienylacetyl]amino]-3,3-dimethyl-7-oxo-4-thia-1-azabicyclo[3.2.0]heptane-2-carboxylic acid; *N*-(2-carboxy-3,3-dimethyl-7-oxo-4-thia-1-azabicyclo[3.2.0]hept-6-yl)-3-thiophenemalonamic acid; 6-[D(−)-α-carboxy-3-thienylacetamido]penicillanic acid; α-carboxy-3-thienylmethylpenicillin. $C_{15}H_{16}N_2O_6S_2$; mol wt 384.43. C 46.86%, H 4.20%, N 7.29%, O 24.97%, S 16.68%. Broad spectrum semi-synthetic antibiotic related to penicillin. Prepn: **BE 646991**; E. G. Brain, J. H. Nayler, **US 3282926** (1964, 1966 to Beecham Group Ltd.). *In vitro* studies: H. C. Neu, E. B. Winshell, *Antimicrob. Agents Chemother.* **1970**, 385; R. Sutherland *et al., ibid.* 390; N. J. Legakis, J. Papavassiliou, *J. Antibiot.* **28**, 912 (1975). *In vivo* studies: P. Acred *et al., Antimicrob. Agents Chemother.* **1970**, 396. Absorption and excretion: R. Sutherland, P. J. Wise, *ibid.* 402. Clinical pharmacology: V. Rodriguez *et al., Antimicrob. Agents Chemother.* **4**, 31 (1973); R. D.

Libke *et al., Clin. Pharmacol. Ther.* **17**, 441 (1975). Review of pharmacology and therapeutic efficacy: R. N. Brogden *et al., Drugs* **20**, 325-352 (1980).

Disodium salt. [4697-14-7] BRL-2288; Monapen; Ticar; Ticarpen; Ticillin. $C_{15}H_{14}N_2Na_2O_6S_2$; mol wt 428.39. Creamy-white hygroscopic non-crystalline powder. Readily sol in water (>100 g/100 ml water) giving a clear soln with pH between 6.0 and 8.0. Aq solns are relatively stable; acid solns relatively unstable (Sutherland).

THERAP CAT: Antibacterial.

THERAP CAT (VET): Antibacterial.

9429. Ticlopidine. [55142-85-3] 5-[(2-Chlorophenyl)methyl]-4,5,6,7-tetrahydrothieno[3,2-*c*]pyridine; 5-(*o*-chlorobenzyl)-4,-5,6,7-tetrahydrothieno[3,2-*c*]pyridine. $C_{14}H_{14}ClNS$; mol wt 263.79. C 63.74%, H 5.35%, Cl 13.44%, N 5.31%, S 12.16%. Platelet aggregation inhibitor. Prepn: **DE 2404308**; A. R. J. Castaigne, **US 4051141** (1974, 1977 both to Cent. Etudes Ind. Pharm.); E. Braye, **US 4127580** (1978 to Parcor). Metabolism: P. Godard *et al., Eur. J. Drug Metab. Pharmacokinet.* **3**, 67 (1978); *eidem, ibid.* **4**, 133 (1979); A. Tuong *et al., ibid.* **6**, 91 (1981). Mode of action: G. Leblondel, P. Allain, *Biochem. Pharmacol.* **27**, 2099 (1978); J. R. O'Brien *et al., Thromb. Res.* **13**, 245 (1978); J. J. Bruno, *ibid.* **1983**, Suppl. 4, 59. Pharmacology: A. Akashi *et al., Arzneim.-Forsch.* **30**, 409, 415 (1980). Clinical studies: J. J. Thebault *et al., J. Int. Med. Res.* **5**, 405 (1977); C. Lecrubier *et al., Therapie* **32**, 189 (1977); T. Katsumura *et al., Angiology* **33**, 357 (1982). Review of pharmacodynamics, pharmacokinetics and therapeutic use: E. Saltiel, A. Ward, *Drugs* **34**, 222-262 (1987). Comprehensive description: F. J. Al-Shammary, N. A. A. Mian, *Anal. Profiles Drug Subs. Excip.* **21**, 573-609 (1992).

Hydrochloride. [53885-35-1] 4-C-32; 53-32 C; Anagregal; Caudaline; Panaldine; Ticlid; Ticlodix; Ticlodone; Ticlosin; Tiklid. $C_{14}H_{14}ClNS.HCl$; mol wt 300.25. uv max (water): 214, 268, 295 nm ($A_{1cm}^{1\%}$ 303.8, 13.14, 2). pKa 7.64. Almost sol in water; sol in 95% alcohol, methanol, chloroform. Insol in ether. LD_{50} in mice (mg/kg/24 hrs): 55 i.v.; >300 orally (Castaigne).

THERAP CAT: Antithrombotic.

9430. Ticrynafen. [40180-04-9] [2,3-Dichloro-4-(2-thienylcarbonyl)phenoxy]acetic acid; [2,3-dichloro-4-(2-thenoyl)phenoxy]acetic acid; [2,3-dichloro-4-(2-thiophenecarbonyl)phenoxy]-acetic acid; tienilic acid; thienylic acid; ANP-3624; CE-3624; SKF-62698; Diflurex; Selacryn. $C_{13}H_8Cl_2O_4S$; mol wt 331.17. C 47.15%, H 2.43%, Cl 21.41%, O 19.32%, S 9.68%. A heterocyclic derivative of phenoxyacetic acid. Prepn: J. Godfroid, J. Thuillier, **DE 2048372**; **US 3758506** (1971, 1973 both to C.E.R.-P.H.A.) and **FR 2115042** (1972 to C.E.R.P.H.A.). Synthesis and pharmacology: G. Thuillier *et al., Eur. J. Med. Chem.* **9**, 625 (1974). Pharmacokinetics in healthy volunteers: A. L. Kerremans *et al., Eur. J. Clin. Pharmacol.* **22**, 515 (1982). Comparative study in hypertensive patients: B. T. Emmerson *et al., ibid.* 203. Hepatotoxicity study: J. W. Manier *et al., Am. J. Gastroenterol.* **77**, 401 (1982).

Crystals from 50% ethanol, mp 148-149°; also reported as mp 157°. LD$_{50}$ in mice (mg/kg): 225 i.v., 1275 orally (**US 3758506**).

THERAP CAT: Diuretic; uricosuric; antihypertensive.

9431. Tiemonium Iodide. [144-12-7] 4-[3-Hydroxy-3-phenyl-3-(2-thienyl)propyl]-4-methylmorpholinium iodide; *N*-methyl-*N*-[3-hydroxy-3-phenyl-3-(α-thienyl)propyl]morpholinium iodide; Visceralgina. C$_{18}$H$_{24}$INO$_2$S; mol wt 445.36. C 48.54%, H 5.43%, I 28.49%, N 3.15%, O 7.18%, S 7.20%. Anticholinergic. Prepn: **GB 953386** (1964 to C.E.R.M.).

Solid, mp 189-191°.
THERAP CAT: Antispasmodic.

9432. Tigecycline. [220620-09-7] (4*S*,4a*S*,5a*R*,12a*S*)-4,7-Bis(dimethylamino)-9-[[[(1,1-dimethylethyl)amino]acetyl]amino]-1,4,4a,5,5a,6,11,12a-octahydro-3,10,12,12a-tetrahydroxy-1,11-dioxo-2-naphthacenecarboxamide; 9-*t*-butylglycylamido-minocycline; TBG-MINO; GAR-936; Tygacil. C$_{29}$H$_{39}$N$_5$O$_8$; mol wt 585.65. C 59.47%, H 6.71%, N 11.96%, O 21.86%. Broad spectrum glycylcycline antibiotic; semisynthetic tetracycline analogue. Prepn: J. J. Hlavka *et al.*, **EP 536515**; *eidem*, **US 5494903** (1993, 1996 both to Am. Cyanamid); P.-E. Sum, P. Petersen, *Bioorg. Med. Chem. Lett.* **9**, 1459 (1999). *In vivo* pharmacodynamics: M. L. van Ogtrop *et al.*, *Antimicrob. Agents Chemother.* **44**, 943 (2000). *In vitro* activity vs clinical bacterial isolates: A. C. Gales, R. N. Jones, *Diagn. Microbiol. Infect. Dis.* **36**, 19 (2000); D. Milatovic *et al.*, *Antimicrob. Agents Chemother.* **47**, 400 (2003). Mode of action study: G. Bauer *et al.*, *J. Antimicrob. Chemother.* **53**, 592 (2004). Clinical pharmacology: A. K. Meagher *et al.*, *Diagn. Microbiol. Infect. Dis.* **52**, 165 (2005). Clinical evaluation in complicated skin and skin-structure infections: R. G. Postier *et al.*, *Clin. Ther.* **26**, 704 (2004); E. J. Ellis-Grosse *et al.*, *Clin. Infect. Dis.* **41**, S341 (2005); in complicated intra-abdominal infections: T. Babinchak *et al.*, *ibid.* S354. Review of chemistry, pharmacology and clinical development: E. Rubinstein, D. Vaughan, *Drugs* **65**, 1317-1336 (2005); R. A. Squires, R. G. Postier, *Expert Opin. Invest. Drugs* **15**, 155-162 (2006).

Orange powder or cake.
THERAP CAT: Antibacterial.

9433. Tiglic Acid. [80-59-1] (2*E*)-2-Methyl-2-butenoic acid; (*E*)-2-methylcrotonic acid; *trans*-2,3-dimethylacrylic acid. C$_5$H$_8$O$_2$; mol wt 100.12. C 59.98%, H 8.05%, O 31.96%. The stable isomer of angelic acid. Found as glyceride in croton oil, as butyl ester in the oil of the Roman camomile, *Anthemis nobilis* L., *Compositae*, and as geranyl tiglate in oil of geranium. Is formed during the charcoaling of maple wood. Formation by the intestinal roundworm, *Ascaris lumbricoides*: Bueding, *J. Biol. Chem.* **202**, 505 (1953). Has been found in crude sodium penicillin: Cram, Tishler, *J. Am. Chem. Soc.* **70**, 4238 (1948). Sepn by partition chromatography: Bueding, *loc. cit.* Synthesis from 2-hydroxy-2-methylbutyronitrile: Crawford, *J. Soc. Chem. Ind. London* **64**, 231 (1945). Review and bibliography: Buckles *et al.*, *Chem. Rev.* **55**, 659-677 (1955).

Triclinic plates, rods from water. Spicy odor. *Vesicant.* d 0.972. mp 63.5-64°. bp$_{760}$ 198.5°; bp$_{11.5}$ 95.0-96°. Volatile with steam. n_D^{81} 1.4342. pK (25°) 5.02. uv max (H$_2$O): 216-217 nm (ε 10700). Molar heat of combustion 635.1 kcal. Sparingly sol in cold water; freely sol in hot water. Sol in alcohol, ether.

Calcium salt trihydrate. Ca(C$_5$H$_7$O$_2$)$_2$.3H$_2$O. Leaflets. Much less sol in water than calcium angelate: 100 parts of aq soln satd at 17° contains 6.05 parts of anhydr calcium tiglate.

Amide. C$_5$H$_9$NO. Crystals, mp 75-76°.

Methyl ester. C$_6$H$_{10}$O$_2$. Liquid; d$_4^{20}$ 0.9498; bp$_{766}$ 139.6°; n_D^{20} 1.4370.

Ethyl ester. C$_7$H$_{12}$O$_2$. Liquid; d$_4^{19.5}$ 0.9247; bp$_{752}$ 156°; bp$_{11}$ 55.5°. n_D^{20} 1.4350. Heat of formn at constant vol: 953.2 kcal, at constant pressure: 954.4 kcal.

Geranyl ester. C$_{15}$H$_{24}$O$_2$. Liquid; pleasant odor; d$_{15}^{15}$ 0.9279; bp$_7$ 149-151°.

USE: The esters in perfumes and flavoring agents. The free acid as a breaker of emulsions.

9434. Tigloidine. [495-83-0] 2-Methyl-2-butenoic acid [1α,3α(*E*),5α]- 8-methyl-8-azabicyclo[3.2.1]oct-3-yl ester; (*E*)-1α*H*,5α*H*-tropan-3β-ol 2-methylcrotonate; tiglylpseudotropeine; 3β-tigloyloxytropane; tiglic acid ester with pseudotropine. C$_{13}$H$_{21}$-NO$_2$; mol wt 223.31. C 69.92%, H 9.48%, N 6.27%, O 14.33%. Isoln from *Duboisia myoporoides* R. Br., *Solanaceae* and prepn from tropine and tigloyl chloride: Barger *et al.*, *J. Chem. Soc.* **1937**, 1820; isoln from *Datura innoxia* Miller, *Solanaceae*: Evans, Wellendorf, *ibid.* **1959**, 1406. Pharmacology: Sanghvi *et al.*, *Eur. J. Pharmacol.* **4**, 246 (1968).

Hydrobromide. Tiglyssin. C$_{13}$H$_{21}$NO$_2$.HBr; mol wt 304.22. mp 234-235°. Soluble in chloroform.
THERAP CAT: Antispasmodic.

9435. Tigogenin. [77-60-1] (3β,5α,25*R*)-Spirostan-3-ol. C$_{27}$H$_{44}$O$_3$; mol wt 416.64. C 77.83%, H 10.64%, O 11.52%. The aglycon of tigonin; C-5 epimer of smilagenin, *q.v.* Obtained from leaves of *Digitalis lanata* Ehrh., *Scrophulariaceae*: Windhaus, *Z. Physiol. Chem.* **150**, 205 (1925); Jacobs, Fleck, *J. Biol. Chem.* **88**, 545 (1930). From the sisal plant *Agave sisalana* L., *Amaryllidaceae*: Rubin, **US 2991282** (1961); **US 3303187** (1967). Structure: Marker, Rohrmann, *J. Am. Chem. Soc.* **62**, 898 (1940); and synthesis: Mazur, Sondheimer, *ibid.* **81**, 3161 (1959); Caglioti, Magi, *Tetrahedron* **19**, 1127 (1963). In synthesis of steroids: T. Ohta *et al.*, *Org. Process Res. Dev.* **1**, 420 (1997); L. Amiranshvili *et al.*, *Bull. Georgian Acad. Sci.* **161**, 252 (2000).

Crystals from dil methanol, mp 203°. [α]$_D^{20}$ −62°. More sol in acetone, in ether, and esp in petr ether than gitogenin. Pptd by digitonin.

Tigonin. [1329-83-5] C$_{56}$H$_{92}$O$_{27}$; mol wt 1197.31. Isoln from *Digitalis* sp: Tschesche, *Ber.* **69**, 1665 (1936); Liang, Noller, *J. Am. Chem. Soc.* **57**, 525 (1935). Built from 2 glucose, 2 galactose, 1 xylose, and 1 tigogenin unit. Hygroscopic, amorphous flakes from 95% alc. After drying at 118° over P$_2$O$_5$ *in vacuo* sinters at 220°.

mp ~260° *(in vacuo)*. Sol in water. Not pptd by ether from water (difference from digitonin); amorphous ppt with amyl alcohol.

9436. Tiliacorine. [27073-72-9] (1α,1'α)-6',7-Didemethoxy-6',7-epoxyrodiasine. $C_{36}H_{36}N_2O_5$; mol wt 576.68. C 74.98%, H 6.29%, N 4.86%, O 13.87%. From bark of *Tiliarcora acuminata* Miers, and *T. racemosa* Colebr., *Menispermaceae*. Isoln: Van Itallie, Steenhauer, *Pharm. Weekbl.* **59**, 1381 (1922). Structure: Anjaneyulu *et al., Chem. Ind. (London)* **1959**, 1119; Rao, Row, *J. Org. Chem.* **25**, 981 (1960). Revised structure: Anjaneyula *et al., J. Sci. Ind. Res.* **21B**, 602 (1962); *eidem, Tetrahedron* **25**, 3091 (1969); M. Shamma, J. E. Foy, *J. Org. Chem.* **41**, 1293 (1976). Abs config and biosynthesis: D. S. Bhakuni *et al., Chem. Commun.* **1978**, 226.

Bitter crystals, mp 271-272°. [α]$_D$ +105.3°. uv max: 295, 265 nm (log ε 3.91, 3.48). Sol in alcohol, benzene, chloroform, ether.

9437. Tilidine. [20380-58-9] (1R,2S)-rel-2-(Dimethylamino)-1-phenyl-3-cyclohexene-1-carboxylic acid ethyl ester; ethyl 2-(dimethylamino)-1-phenyl-3-cyclohexene-1-carboxylate; 3-*trans*-dimethylamino-4-phenyl-4-*trans*-carbethoxy-Δ¹-cyclohexene. $C_{17}H_{23}NO_2$; mol wt 273.37. C 74.69%, H 8.48%, N 5.12%, O 11.71%. Prepn: **ZA 6606476**; **GB 1120186**; G. Satzinger, **US 3557127** (1967, 1968, 1971, all to Warner-Lambert). Synthesis of 6-C¹⁴ hydrochloride: K.-O. Vollmer, F. W. Koss, *Arzneim.-Forsch.* **20**, 990 (1970). Pharmacology and toxicity data: M. Hermann *et al., ibid.* 977, 983. Metabolism: K.-O. Vollmer, H. Achenbach, *ibid.* **24**, 1237 (1974). HPLC determn in pharmaceutics: D. Zivanov-Stakic *et al., Farmaco* **44**, 759 (1989). Clinical trial in comparison with nefopam, *q.v.*: J. Abeloos *et al., Acta Anaesthesiol. Belg.* **34**, 283 (1983); in combination with naloxone, *q.v.*: H. Van Cauwenberge *et al., Int. J. Clin. Pharmacol. Res.* **12**, 1 (1992).

bp$_{0.01}$ 95.5-96°.
Hydrochloride hemihydrate. Gö-1261C; W-5759A; Lucayan; Valoron. $C_{17}H_{23}NO_2 \cdot HCl \cdot \frac{1}{2}H_2O$; mol wt 318.84. Crystals, mp 125°. Easily sol in water. LD$_{50}$ (7 day) in mice, rats (mg/kg): 437.0, 417.7 i.g.; 490.0, 400.0 s.c.; 52.0, 74.1 i.v. (Herrmann).
Hydrochloride. [27107-79-5] Crystals from ethyl acetate-methyl ethyl ketone, mp 159°.
cis-(±)-**Form.** [112244-09-4] bp$_{0.01}$ 97.5-98°.
cis-(±)-**Hydrochloride.** $C_{17}H_{23}NO_2 \cdot HCl \cdot 1\frac{1}{2}H_2O$. Crystals from ethyl acetate-methyl ethyl ketone, mp 84°.
Note: This is a controlled substance (opiate): **21 CFR**, 1308.11.
THERAP CAT: Analgesic (narcotic).

9438. Tilisolol. [85136-71-6] 4-[3-[(1,1-Dimethylethyl)-amino]-2-hydroxypropoxy]-2-methyl-1(2H)-isoquinolinone; 4-[3-(*tert*-butylamino)-2-hydroxypropoxy]-N-methylisocarbostyril. $C_{17}H_{24}N_2O_3$; mol wt 304.38. C 67.08%, H 7.95%, N 9.20%, O 15.77%. β-Adrenergic blocker. Prepn: H. Fukushima, Y. Suzuki, **DE 2631080**; *eidem,* **US 4129565** (1977, 1978 both to Nisshin). Antiarrhythmic activity: K. Hashimoto *et al., J. Pharmacol. Exp.*

Ther. **223**, 801 (1982); and pharmacological profile: Y. Nakagawa *et al., Arzneim.-Forsch.* **34**, 194 (1984). Receptor binding study: T. Nagatomo *et al., Jpn. J. Pharmacol.* **34**, 249 (1984). Vasodilating activity in humans: T. Imaizumi *et al., Arzneim.-Forsch.* **38**, 1342 (1988). HPLC determn in plasma: K. Yonezawa *et al., J. Chromatogr.* **339**, 219 (1985). Toxicity data: S. Kawase *et al., Oyo Yakuri* **34**, 499 (1987), *C.A.* **108**, 161293m (1988).

Hydrochloride. [62774-96-3] N-696; Selecal. $C_{17}H_{24}N_2O_3 \cdot$ HCl; mol wt 340.85. White crystals from ethyl acetate, mp 203-205°. LD$_{50}$ in male, female mice and rats (mg/kg): 1393, 1290, 145, 188 orally; 1219, 1245, 176, 169 s.c.; 578, 557, 39.5, 29.2 i.p.; 74.3, 104.7, 75.8, 38.1 i.v. (Kawase).
THERAP CAT: Antiarrhythmic; antihypertensive.

9439. Tilmicosin. [108050-54-0] 4ᴬ-O-De(2,6-dideoxy-3-C-methyl-α-L-*ribo*-hexopyranosyl)-20-deoxo-20-(3,5-dimethyl-1-piperidinyl)tylosin; 20-deoxo-20-(3,5-dimethylpiperidin-1-yl)desmycosin; EL-870; LY-177370; Micotil; Pulmotil. $C_{46}H_{80}N_2O_{13}$; mol wt 869.13. C 63.57%, H 9.28%, N 3.22%, O 23.93%. Macrolide antibiotic; structurally related to tylosin, *q.v.* Prepd as 85:15 mixture of *cis/trans* isomers: M. Debono, H. A. Kirst, **EP 103465**; *eidem,* **US 4820695** (1984, 1989 both to Lilly); M. Debono *et al., J. Antibiot.* **42**, 1253 (1989). *In vitro* antibacterial activity: E. E. Ose, *ibid.* **40**, 190 (1987). Metabolism and tissue residue studies in cattle: A. L. Donoho *et al., ACS Symp. Ser.* **503**, 158-167 (1992). Trial in treatment of calf pneumonia: E. E. Ose, L. V. Tonkinson, *Vet. Rec.* **123**, 367 (1988). Prophylactic efficacy in bovine respiratory tract disease: D. W. Morck *et al., J. Am. Vet. Med. Assoc.* **202**, 273 (1993).

cis-form

uv max: 283 nm (ε 22643). pKa' (66% DMF): 7.4, 8.5. [α]$_D^{23}$ +12.75° (c = 0.010004 in CHCl$_3$, 5 cm).
THERAP CAT (VET): Antibacterial.

9440. Tilorone. [27591-97-5] 2,7-Bis[2-(diethylamino)ethoxy]-9H-fluoren-9-one; bis-DEAE-fluorenone. $C_{25}H_{34}N_2O_3$; mol wt 410.55. C 73.14%, H 8.35%, N 6.82%, O 11.69%. The first recognized synthetic, small mol wt compound that is an orally active interferon inducer: Krueger, Mayer, *Science* **169**, 1213 sqq. (1970). Prepn: Fleming *et al.,* **DE 1964761** corresp to **US 3592819** (1970, 1971 to Richardson Merrell); E. R. Andrews *et al., J. Med. Chem.* **17**, 882 (1974); H. M. Burke, M. M. Joullie, *ibid.* **21**, 1084 (1978). Mechanism of action: De Clercq, Merigan, *J. Infect. Dis.* **123**, 190 (1971). Toxicity studies: Kaufman *et al., Proc. Soc. Exp. Biol. Med.* **137**, 357 (1971). Review: P. Chandra *et al.,* "Tilorone Hydrochloride" in *Antibiotics* vol. 5(pt. 2), F. E. Hahn, Ed. (Springer-Verlag, New York, 1979) pp 385-413.

Dihydrochloride. [27591-69-1] $C_{25}H_{34}N_2O_3 \cdot 2HCl$. Crystals from butanone-methanol, mp 235-237°. uv max (water): 269 nm ($E_{1cm}^{1\%}$ 1600). LD_{50} in mice, rats (single dose): 959, 852 mg/kg orally; 145, 244 mg/kg i.p. (Krueger, Mayer).

9441. Tiludronic Acid. [89987-06-4] [[(4-Chlorophenyl)-thio]methylene]bisphosphonic acid; ACPMD; Cl-TMBP; ME-3737. $C_7H_9ClO_6P_2S$; mol wt 318.61. C 26.39%, H 2.85%, Cl 11.13%, O 30.13%, P 19.44%, S 10.06%. Bisphosphonate antiresorptive agent. Prepn: J. C. Breliere et al., **EP 100718**; eidem, **US 4876248** (1984, 1989 both to Sanofi). HPLC determn in plasma and urine: J.-P. Fels et al., J. Chromatogr. **430**, 73 (1988). Determn of dissociation constants: M. Bonnery et al., Bull. Soc. Chim. Fr. **1988**, 49. Symposium on pharmacology and clinical experience: Bone **17**, Suppl., 471S-519S (1995). Clinical trial in Paget's disease: W. D. Fraser et al., Postgrad. Med. J. **73**, 496 (1997).

pK_1 10.85; pK_2 6.90; pK_3 2.95; pK_4 1.30.
Disodium salt. [149845-07-8]; [155453-10-4] (hemihydrate). Tiludronate disodium; SR-41319B; Skelid. $C_7H_7ClNa_2O_6P_2S$; mol wt 362.57. Occurs as the hemihydrate.
Di-tert-butylamine salt. mp 253° (dec).
THERAP CAT: Bone resorption inhibitor.

9442. Timepidium Bromide. [35035-05-3] 3-(Di-2-thienylmethylene)-5-methoxy-1,1-dimethylpiperidinium bromide; SA-504; Mepidium; Sesden. $C_{17}H_{22}BrNOS_2$; mol wt 400.40. C 50.99%, H 5.54%, Br 19.96%, N 3.50%, O 4.00%, S 16.02%. Anticholinergic. Prepn: M. Kawazu et al., **DE 2128808** corresp to **US 3764607** (1971, 1973 both to Tanabe). Pharmacological properties: H. Tamaki et al., Jpn. J. Pharmacol. **22**, 685 (1972), C.A. **78**, 52812 (1973). Metabolism: J. Sugihara, N. Taga, Radioisotopes **26**, 238 (1977). Absorption, distribution, excretion: M. Yoshikawa, Oyo Yakuri **14**, 179 (1977), C.A. **88**, 163772 (1978). Teratological study: Y. Fujisawa et al., ibid. **7**, 1293 (1973), C.A. **81**, 99413 (1974). Chronic toxicity study: K. Doi et al., ibid. **13**, 851 (1977), C.A. **88**, 32014 (1978).

Colorless cryst from acetone/ether, mp 198-200°.
THERAP CAT: Antispasmodic.

9443. Timiperone. [57648-21-2] 4-[4-(2,3-Dihydro-2-thioxo-1H-benzimidazol-1-yl)-1-piperidinyl]-1-(4-fluorophenyl)-1-butanone; 1-[1-[3-(4-fluorobenzoyl)propyl]-4-piperidyl]-2-mercaptobenzimidazole; 4-fluoro-4-[4-(2-thioxo-1-benzimidazolinyl)piperidino]butyrophenone; 1-[1-[3-(4-fluorobenzoyl)propyl]-4-piperidyl]-2,3-dihydrobenzimidazole-2-thione; DD-3480; Tolopelon. $C_{22}H_{24}FN_3OS$; mol wt 397.51. C 66.47%, H 6.09%, F 4.78%, N 10.57%, O 4.02%, S 8.07%. Butyrophenone derivative with neuroleptic activity. Prepn: M. Sato et al., **JP Kokai 75 84578**; K. Ueno et al., **US 3963727** (1975, 1976 both to Daiichi); M. Sato et al., J. Med. Chem. **21**, 1116 (1978). Improved synthesis: M. Sato, M. Arimoto, Chem. Pharm. Bull. **30**, 719 (1982). Pharmacology: T. Yamasaki et al., Jpn. J. Pharmacol. **27** (Suppl.), 124P (1977); eidem, Arzneim.-Forsch. **31**, 701, 707 (1981); T. Shibuya et al., Int. J. Clin. Pharmacol. Ther. Toxicol. **20**, 251 (1982). Pharmacokinetics and metabolism: H. Tachizawa et al., Drug Metab. Dispos. **9**, 442 (1981); K. Sudo et al., Xenobiotica **11**, 685 (1981). Multicenter

controlled clinical trials in schizophrenia: R. Takahashi et al., J. Int. Med. Res. **10**, 257 (1982); T. Kariya et al., ibid. **11**, 66 (1983).

Crystals from acetone, mp 201-203°. uv max (ethanol): 226.5, 246, 309 nm. Slightly sol in water. LD_{50} in male rats, mice (mg/kg): 232, 478 orally (Yamasaki).
THERAP CAT: Antipsychotic.

9444. Timolol. [26839-75-8] (2S)-1-[(1,1-Dimethylethyl)-amino]-3-[[4-(4-morpholinyl)-1,2,5-thiadiazol-3-yl]oxy]-2-propanol; S-(−)-3-(3-tert-butylamino-2-hydroxypropoxy)-4-morpholino-1,2,5-thiadiazole; (−)-3-morpholino-4-(3-tert-butylamino-2-hydroxypropoxy)-1,2,5-thiadiazole. $C_{13}H_{24}N_4O_3S$; mol wt 316.42. C 49.35%, H 7.65%, N 17.71%, O 15.17%, S 10.13%. β-Adrenergic blocker. Prepn: B. K. Wasson, **DE 1925956**; idem, **US 3655663** (1969, 1972 both to Frosst). Manufacturing process: L. M. Weinstock et al., **DE 1925955**; eidem, **US 3657237** (1970, 1972 both to Frosst). Synthesis and activity data: Wasson et al., J. Med. Chem. **15**, 651 (1972). Pharmacology: Franciosa et al., Clin. Pharmacol. Ther. **13**, 138 (1972); Ulrych et al., ibid. 232. Review of efficacy in glaucoma: R. C. Heel et al., Drugs **17**, 38-55 (1979). Clinical evaluation in hypertension: B. A. Rofman et al., Hypertension **2**, 643 (1980). Multicenter study of effect in myocardial infarction: N. Engl. J. Med. **304**, 801 (1981); of efficacy in limiting infarct size: M. Sederholm et al., ibid. **310**, 9 (1984). Comprehensive description: D. J. Mazzo, A. E. Loper, Anal. Profiles Drug Subs. **16**, 641-692 (1987).

Hemihydrate. White, odorless, crystalline powder. Slightly sol in water; freely sol in ethanol.
Hydrogen maleate salt. [26921-17-5] MK-950; Aquanil; Betim; Betimol; Blocadren; Proflax; Temserin; Tenopt; Timacar; Timacor; Timoptic; Timoptol. $C_{13}H_{24}N_4O_3S \cdot C_4H_4O_4$; mol wt 432.49. White crystals from ethanol, mp 201.5-202.5°. $[\alpha]_{405}^{24}$ −12.0° (c = 5 in 1N HCl), $[\alpha]_D^{25}$ −4.2°. uv max (0.1N HCl): 294 nm ($A_{1cm}^{1\%}$ 200). Sol in water, ethanol, methanol; sparingly sol in chloroform; very slightly sol in cyclohexane. Practically insol in isooctane, ether. Stable in soln up to pH 12.
(±)-Free base. Crystalline solid from isopropyl ether, mp 71.5-72.5°.
THERAP CAT: Antihypertensive; antiarrhythmic (class II); antianginal; antiglaucoma agent.

9445. Timonacic. [444-27-9] 4-Thiazolidinecarboxylic acid; ATC; norgamen; thioproline; NSC-25855; Detoxepa; Hepalidine; Heparegen; Tiazolidin. $C_4H_7NO_2S$; mol wt 133.17. C 36.08%, H 5.30%, N 10.52%, O 24.03%, S 24.08%. Prepd from DL- or L-cysteine and formaldehyde. Prepn of l-form: Ratner, Clarke, J. Am. Chem. Soc. **59**, 200 (1937); of dl- and l-forms: Werner et al., Helv. Chim. Acta **30**, 432 (1947); **FR M3184** (1965 to Sogespar S.A.), C.A. **63**, 12980h (1965). Proton magnetic resonance and conformation: Martin, Mathur, J. Am. Chem. Soc. **87**, 1065 (1965). Series of articles on pharmacology and toxicology: Gazz. Med. Ital. **131**, 251-286 (1972). Toxicity data: Bertrand, Piton, ibid. 265. Induces reverse transformation of tumor cells to normal. Clinical evaluation in cancer: A. Brugarolas, M. Gosalvez, Lancet **1**, 68 (1980).

dl-**Form.** Crystals, mp 195°. LD$_{50}$ orally in mice: 400 mg/kg (Bertrand, Piton).

l-**Form.** Crystals from water, dec 196-197°. Readily sol in hot water, acid, alkali; sparingly sol in cold water. Practically insol in alcohol.

THERAP CAT: Hepatoprotectant.

9446. Tin. [7440-31-5] Sn; at. wt 118.710; at. no. 50; valence 2, 4. Group IVA (14). Naturally occurring isotopes: 112 (0.95%); 114 (0.65%); 115 (0.34%); 116 (14.24%); 117 (7.57%); 118 (24.01%); 119 (8.59%); 120 (32.97%); 122 (4.71%); 124 (5.98%); artificial, radioactive isotopes: 108-111; 113; 121; 123; 125-132. Found in cassiterite, stannite, and tealite. Occurrence in earth's crust: 6×10^{-4}%. The metal of commerce is about 99.8% pure. Prepn of high purity tin: Baralis, Marone, *Met. Ital.* **59**, 494 (1967), *C.A.* **67**, 119613a (1967). Physical properties: Kirshenbaum, Cahill, *J. Inorg. Nucl. Chem.* **25**, 232 (1963). *Monograph:* C. L. Mantell, *Tin: Its Mining, Production, Technology and Applications* (Reinhold, New York, 1949). *Reviews:* Abel in *Comprehensive Inorganic Chemistry* **vol. 2**, J. C. Bailar, Jr. *et al.,* Eds. (Pergamon Press, Oxford, 1973) pp 43-104; W. Germain *et al.,* in *Kirk-Othmer Encyclopedia of Chemical Technology* **vol. 23** (Wiley-Interscience, New York, 3rd ed., 1983) pp 18-42. Review of toxicology and human exposure: *Toxicological Profile for Tin* (PB-2006-100006, 2005) 426 pp.

Silver-white, lustrous, soft, very malleable and ductile metal; only slightly tenacious; easily powdered. When being bent, emits the crackling "tin cry". Brittle at 200°. At $-40°$ crumbles to gray amorphous powder ("gray tin"), slowly changing back above 20° to white tin. Available in the form of bars, foil, powder, shot, etc. Stable in air, but when in powder form it oxidizes, esp in presence of moisture. d 7.31. mp 231.9°. bp 2507° (2780 K). Specific heat (25°) 0.053 cal/g/°C. Brinell hardness 2.9. Insol in water. Reacts slowly with cold dil HCl or dil HNO$_3$, hot dil H$_2$SO$_4$; readily with concd HCl, aqua regia; very slowly attacked by acetic acid; slowly attacked by cold, more readily by hot caustic alkali; concd HNO$_3$ converts it into insol metastannic acid.

Caution: Potential symptoms of overexposure to metallic tin are irritation of eyes, skin, respiratory system. Potential symptoms of overexposure to organic tin compounds are irritation of eyes, skin, respiratory system; headache, vertigo; psychoneurologic disturbances; sore throat, cough; abdominal pain, vomiting; urine retention; paresis, focal anesthesia; skin burns; pruritis. *See NIOSH Pocket Guide to Chemical Hazards* (DHHS/NIOSH 97-140, 1997) p 308. *See also Patty's Industrial Hygiene and Toxicology* **vol. 2A**, G. D. Clayton, F. E. Clayton, Eds. (Wiley-Interscience, New York, 3rd ed., 1981) pp 1940-1968.

USE: Chiefly for tin-plating and manuf of food, beverage and aerosol containers, soldering alloys, babbitt and type metals, manuf tin salts, collapsible tubes, coating for copper wire. Principle component in pewter. Alloys as dental materials (silver-tin-mercury), nuclear reactor components (tin-zirconium), aircraft components (tin-titanium), bronze (copper-tin), brass.

9447. Tinidazole. [19387-91-8] 1-[2-(Ethylsulfonyl)ethyl]-2-methyl-5-nitro-1*H*-imidazole; ethyl[2-(2-methyl-5-nitro-1-imidazolyl)ethyl]sulfone; CP-12574; Fasigin; Simplotan; Tindamax; Tricolam; Trimonase. C$_8$H$_{13}$N$_3$O$_4$S; mol wt 247.27. C 38.86%, H 5.30%, N 16.99%, O 25.88%, S 12.97%. Prepn: K. Butler, US 3376311 (1968 to Pfizer); M. W. Miller *et al., J. Med. Chem.* **13**, 849 (1970). Series of articles on prepn, antiprotozoal activity and pharmacokinetics: *Antimicrob. Agents Chemother.* **1969**, 257-270. Review of antiprotozoal activity: P. R. Sawyer *et al., Drugs* **11**, 423-440 (1976); of antibacterial activity, pharmacology and therapeutic efficacy vs anaerobes: A. A. Carmine *et al., ibid.* **24**, 85-117 (1982). Symposium on clinical experience in anaerobic infection: *J. Antimicrob. Chemother.* **10**, Suppl. A, 1-184 (1982). Clinical trial in *Helicobacter pylori* positive gastritis: G. Oderda *et al., Gut* **33**, 1328 (1992).

Colorless crystals from benzene, mp 127-128°. LD$_{50}$ in mice (mg/kg): >3600 orally; >2000 i.p. (Miller).

THERAP CAT: Antiprotozoal (Trichomonas, Giardia); antiamebic; antibacterial.

9448. Tinoridine. [24237-54-5] 2-Amino-4,5,6,7-tetrahydro-6-(phenylmethyl)thieno[2,3-*c*]pyridine-3-carboxylic acid ethyl ester; 2-amino-6-benzyl-4,5,6,7-tetrahydrothieno[2,3-*c*]pyridine-3-carboxylic acid ethyl ester; 2-amino-3-ethoxycarbonyl-6-benzyl-4,-5,6,7-tetrahydrothieno[2,3-*c*]pyridine; ethyl 2-amino-6-benzyl-4,5,-6,7-tetrahydrothieno[2,3-*c*]pyridine-3-carboxylate; Y-3642. C$_{17}$-H$_{20}$N$_2$O$_2$S; mol wt 316.42. C 64.53%, H 6.37%, N 8.85%, O 10.11%, S 10.13%. Prepn: M. Nakanishi *et al.,* **DE 1812404**; *eidem,* **US 3563997** (1969, 1971 both to Yoshitomi). Pharmacological studies: M. Nakanishi *et al., J. Pharm. Soc. Jpn.* **90**, 272-334 (1970), *C.A.* **73**, 54504t-54510s (1970); *eidem, Arzneim.-Forsch.* **20**, 998, 1004 (1970); *Yakuri to Chiryo* **2**, 1028 (1974). Protective effect vs carbon tetrachloride hepatotoxicity: H. Yasuda *et al., Toxicol. Appl. Pharmacol.* **52**, 407 (1980).

Slightly sol in H$_2$O, mp 112-113°. LD$_{50}$ in mice, rats (mg/kg): 5400, >10200 orally; 1600, 1250 i.p. (Nakanishi, 1970).

Hydrochloride. [25913-34-2] Dimaten; Nonflamin. C$_{17}$H$_{20}$-N$_2$O$_2$S.HCl; mol wt 352.88. Yellowish white to yellow powder, mp 234-235° (dec). Practically odorless with a bitter taste. Slightly sol in methanol; very slightly sol in water, ether, acetone, benzene. LD$_{50}$ orally in mice: 1601 mg/kg (Nakanishi).

THERAP CAT: Analgesic; antipyretic; anti-inflammatory.

9449. Tin Phosphides. Several stoichiometries reported: *Mellor's* **vol. VIII**, 847-849 (1931). Crystal structure of Sn$_4$P$_3$ and discussion of other phases: Olofsson, *Acta Chem. Scand.* **21**, 1659 (1967); **24**, 1153 (1970).

USE: Tin phosphide with a phosphorus content >10% used in manuf of phosphor bronze.

9450. Tinzaparin. Innohep; Logiparin. Low molecular weight heparin prepared by enzymatic depolymerization of porcine mucosal heparin with heparinase from *Flavobacterium heparinum.* Approx mol wt 4900 Da. Manufacturing process: J. I. Nielsen, P. B. Ostergaard, **EP 244236**; J. I. Nielsen, **US 5106734** (1987, 1992 both to Novo). Pharmacokinetics: P. C. Pedersen *et al., Thromb. Res.* **61**, 477 (1991). Multicenter clinical trial: A. Liezorovicz *et al., Br. J. Surg.* **78**, 412 (1991).

THERAP CAT: Antithrombotic.

9451. Tioclomarol. [22619-35-8] 3-[3-(4-Chlorophenyl)-1-(5-chloro-2-thienyl)-3-hydroxypropyl]-4-hydroxy-2*H*-1-benzo-pyran-2-one; 3-[5-chloro-α-(*p*-chloro-β-hydroxyphenethyl)-2-thenyl]-4-hydroxycoumarin; Apegmone. C$_{22}$H$_{16}$Cl$_2$O$_4$S; mol wt 447.33. C 59.07%, H 3.61%, Cl 15.85%, O 14.31%, S 7.17%. Slow-acting anticoagulant, related structurally to warfarin, *q.v.* Prepn: E. Boschetti *et al.,* **ZA 6707267** corresp to **US 3574234** (1968, 1971 both to Lipha). Synthesis and anticoagulant activity: *eidem, Chim. Ther.* **7**, 20 (1972).

     Consult the Name Index before using this section.

White cryst from methanol, mp 104°.

THERAP CAT: Anticoagulant.

9452. Tioconazole. [65899-73-2] 1-[2-[(2-Chloro-3-thien-yl)methoxy]-2-(2,4-dichlorophenyl)ethyl]-1*H*-imidazole; 1-[2,4-di-chloro-β-[(2-chloro-3-thenyl)oxy]phenethyl]imidazole; UK-20349; Fungibacid; Gyno-Trosyd; Trosyd; Trosyl; Vagistat; Zoniden. C_{16}-$H_{13}Cl_3N_2OS$; mol wt 387.71. C 49.57%, H 3.38%, Cl 27.43%, N 7.23%, O 4.13%, S 8.27%. Antimycotic imidazole derivative. Prepn: G. E. Gymer, **BE 841309**; *idem*, **US 4062966** (1976, 1977 both to Pfizer). Antifungal spectrum: S. Jevons, *Antimicrob. Agents Chemother.* **15**, 597 (1979); F. C. Odds, *J. Antimicrob. Chemother.* **6**, 749 (1980). Pharmacology: M. S. Marriott *et al.*, *Dermatologica* **166**, Suppl. 1, 1 (1983). Clinical trial in dermato-mycosis: Y. M. Clayton *et al.*, *Clin. Exp. Dermatol.* **7**, 543 (1982). Series of articles on pharmacology and clinical efficacy in gyneco-logical use: *Gynak. Rundsch.* **23**, Suppl. 1, 1-60 (1983).

Hydrochloride. $C_{16}H_{13}Cl_3N_2OS.HCl$. Crystals, mp 168-170°.

THERAP CAT: Antifungal (topical).

9453. Tiopronin. [1953-02-2] *N*-(2-Mercapto-1-oxopro-pyl)glycine; *N*-(2-mercaptopropionyl)glycine; α-mercaptopropio-nylglycine; Acadione; Capen; Epatiol; Mucolysin; Thiola; Thiosol. $C_5H_9NO_3S$; mol wt 163.19. C 36.80%, H 5.56%, N 8.58%, O 29.41%, S 19.65%. Prepn: Mita *et al.*, **US 3246025** (1966 to Santen). Antidotal effects in mice: H. Fujimura *et al.*, *Nippon Yakurigaku Zasshi* **60**, 278 (1964); *C.A.* **62**, 972h (1965). Anti-inflammatory pharmacology in animals: F. Capasso, *Agents Ac-tions* **11**, 741 (1981). Clinical trial in chronic hepatitis: F. Ichida *et al.*, *J. Int. Med. Res.* **10**, 325 (1982). Clinical comparison with D-penicillamine in rheumatoid arthritis: B. Amor *et al.*, *Arthritis Rheum.* **25**, 698 (1982); G. Pasero *et al.*, *ibid.* 923.

Crystals from ethyl acetate, mp 95-97°. LD$_{50}$ i.v. in mice: 2.1 g/kg (Fujimura).

THERAP CAT: Antidote (heavy metal poisoning); hepatoprotect-ant; mucolytic.

9454. Tiotropium Bromide. [136310-93-5] (1α,2β,4β,5α,-7β)-7-[(Hydroxydi-2-thienylacetyl)oxy]-9,9-dimethyl-3-oxa-9-azo-niatricyclo[3.3.1.0^{2,4}]nonane bromide; 6β,7β-epoxy-3β-hydroxy-8-methyl-1αH,5αH-tropanium bromide, di-2-thienylglycolate; Ba-679 BR; Ba-679; Spiriva. $C_{19}H_{22}BrNO_4S_2$; mol wt 472.42. C 48.31%, H 4.69%, Br 16.91%, N 2.96%, O 13.55%, S 13.57%. Muscarinic receptor antagonist. Prepn: R. Banholzer *et al.*, **EP 418716**; *ei-dem*, **US 5610163** (1991, 1997 both to Boehringer Ingelheim). Pharmacology: T. Takahashi *et al.*, *Am. J. Respir. Crit. Care Med.* **150**, 1640 (1994). Binding study: E.-B. Haddad *et al.*, *Mol. Pharmacol.* **45**, 899 (1994). Comparative clinical trial with salmeterol, *q.v.*, in chronic obstructive pulmonary disease (COPD): J. F. Donohue *et al.*, *Chest* **122**, 47 (2002).

mp 218-220°.

THERAP CAT: Bronchodilator.

9455. Tioxidazole. [61570-90-9] (6-Propoxy-2-benzothia-zolyl)carbamic acid methyl ester; methyl 6-propoxy-2-benzothia-zolylcarbamate; Sch-21480; Tiox. $C_{12}H_{14}N_2O_3S$; mol wt 266.32. C 54.12%, H 5.30%, N 10.52%, O 18.02%, S 12.04%. Structurally related to benzimidazole anthelmintics. Prepn and anthelmintic activity: M. M. Nafissi-Varchei, **BE 840945**; **US 4006242** (1976, 1977 both to Schering). Physical data, activity against round-worms: E. Panitz *et al.*, *Experientia* **34**, 733 (1978). Anthelmintic effect against gastrointestinal parasites in naturally infected horses: J. H. Drudge *et al.*, *Am. J. Vet. Res.* **41**, 1383 (1980); E. T. Lyons *et al.*, *ibid.* **42**, 1048 (1981).

White odorless solid, mp 178-180°. Insoluble in water. Slightly sol in organic solvents.

THERAP CAT (VET): Anthelmintic for horses.

9456. Tioxolone. [4991-65-5] 6-Hydroxy-1,3-benzoxa-thiol-2-one; 6-hydroxy-2-oxo-1,3-benzoxathiole; thioxolone; Ca-myna; Stepin. $C_7H_4O_3S$; mol wt 168.17. C 49.99%, H 2.40%, O 28.54%, S 19.07%. Prepd from resorcinol and ammonium thio-cyanate in presence of copper sulfate: Werner, **US 2332418** (1943 to Winthrop); Urushibara, Koga, *Bull. Chem. Soc. Jpn.* **29**, 419 (1956); Berg, Fiedler, **US 2886488** (1959 to Thomae). Formerly believed to be the 4-hydroxy isomer: Fiedler, *Ber.* **95**, 1771 (1962).

Crystals from water, mp 160°. Practically insol in water. Sol in ethanol, isopropanol, propylene glycol, ether, benzene, toluene. Hydrolyzed by alkali.

Combination with hydrocortisone. [8064-73-1] Psoil.

THERAP CAT: Antiseborrheic; antiacne.

9457. Tipepidine. [5169-78-8] 3-(Di-2-thienylmethylene)-1-methylpiperidine; 1-methyl-3-piperidylidenedi(2-thienyl)meth-ane; tipepidine; AT-327; CR-662. $C_{15}H_{17}NS_2$; mol wt 275.43. C 65.41%, H 6.22%, N 5.09%, S 23.28%. Prepn: Okumura *et al.*, *Tanabe Seiyaku Kenkyu Nempo* **3**, 30 (1958), *C.A.* **53**, 10214 (1959); Ponomarev, Martem'yanova, **SU 176903** (1965), *C.A.* **64**, 12648b (1966). Synthesis: *eidem*, *Khim. Geterosikl. Soedin.* **1967**, 174, *C.A.* **67**, 73501g (1967). Prepn of hibenzate: M. Yamamoto, H. Yoshikawa, **JP 62 17988** *C.A.* **59**, 11446a (1963); **GB 924544** (1962, 1963 both to Tanabe Seiyaku). Pharmacology and clinical efficacy: Higaki *et al.*, *Tanabe Seiyaku Kenkyu Nempo* **4**, 35 (1959), *C.A.* **54**, 3725h (1960); Kase *et al.*, *Chem. Pharm. Bull.* **7**, 372 (1959). Metabolism: Watanabe *et al.*, *Yakugaku Zasshi* **89**, 29 (1969); Sasaki *et al.*, *ibid.* 345.

Yellow crystals from petr ether, mp 64-65°. bp$_{4.5}$ 178-184°. LD$_{50}$ in mice (mg/kg): 294 i.p.; 308 i.m.; 867 orally (Higaki).

Citrate monohydrate. Bithiodine. $C_{15}H_{17}NS_2.C_6H_8O_7.H_2O$. Yellow crystals, mp 138-139°. Sol in water, ethanol, propylene glycol.

Hibenzate. [31139-87-4] Asverin; Sotal. $C_{29}H_{27}NO_4S_2$; mol wt 517.66. Crystals from acetone, mp 187-190°. Sparingly sol in water.

THERAP CAT: Antitussive.

9458. Tipifarnib. [192185-72-1]; [192185-68-5] (unspecified stereo). 6-[(R)-Amino(4-chlorophenyl)(1-methyl-1H-imidazol-5-yl)methyl]-4-(3-chlorophenyl)-1-methyl-2(1H)-quinolinone; R-115777; Zarnestra. $C_{27}H_{22}Cl_2N_4O$; mol wt 489.40. C 66.26%, H 4.53%, Cl 14.49%, N 11.45%, O 3.27%. Farnesyl transferase inhibitor. Prepn: M. G. Venet *et al.,* **WO 9721701**; *eidem,* **US 6037350** (1997, 2000 both to Janssen). Review of syntheses: P. R. Angibaud *et al., Eur. J. Org. Chem.* **2004,** 479-486. Inhibition of farnesyl protein transferase and antitumor effects *in vivo:* D. W. End *et al., Cancer Res.* **61,** 131 (2001). Clinical pharmacology and pharmacokinetics: J. Zujewski *et al., J. Clin. Oncol.* **18,** 927 (2000). Accelerator mass spec determn in biological samples: R. C. Garner *et al., Drug Metab. Dispos.* **30,** 823 (2002). Clinical evaluation in hematologic malignancies: J. Cortes *et al., Blood* **101,** 1692 (2003). Review of clinical experience: P. Norman, *Curr. Opin. Invest. Drugs* **3,** 313-319 (2002).

Crystals from 2-propanol, mp 234°. $[\alpha]_D^{20}$ +22.86° (c = 0.98 in methanol).

THERAP CAT: Antineoplastic.

9459. Tipranavir. [174484-41-4] N-[3-[(1R)-1-[(6R)-5,6-Dihydro-4-hydroxy-2-oxo-6-(2-phenylethyl)-6-propyl-2H-pyran-3-yl]propyl]phenyl]-5-(trifluoromethyl)-2-pyridinesulfonamide; 5-trifluoromethyl-N-[3(R)-[1-[5,6-dihydro-4-hydroxy-2-oxo-6(R)-(2-phenethyl)-6(R)-n-propyl-2H-pyran-3-yl]propyl]phenyl]-2-pyridinesulfonamide; PNU-140690; Aptivus. $C_{31}H_{33}F_3N_2O_5S$; mol wt 602.66. C 61.78%, H 5.52%, F 9.46%, N 4.65%, O 13.27%, S 5.32%. Nonpeptidic HIV protease inhibitor (NPPI). Prepn: K. R. Romines *et al.,* **WO 9530670** (1995 to Upjohn); *eidem,* **US 5852195** (1998 to Pharmacia & Upjohn); S. R. Turner *et al., J. Med. Chem.* **41,** 3467 (1998); K. S. Fors *et al., J. Org. Chem.* **63,** 7348 (1998). Antiviral activity: S. M. Poppe *et al., Antimicrob. Agents Chemother.* **41,** 1058 (1997); vs multidrug resistant clinical isolates: B. A. Larder *et al., AIDS* **14,** 1943 (2000). HPLC determn in plasma: E. Dailly *et al., J. Chromatogr. B* **832,** 317 (2006). Clinical pharmacokinetics in combination with ritonavir: T. R. MacGregor *et al., HIV Clin. Trials* **5,** 371 (2004). Clinical evaluation in HIV infection: S. McCallister *et al., J. Acquir. Immune Defic. Syndr.* **35,** 376 (2004). Review of pharmacologic interactions with other HIV medications: M. Boffito *et al., J. Clin. Pharmacol.* **46,** 130-139 (2006); of clinical development: B. Best, R. Haubrich, *Expert Opin. Invest. Drugs* **15,** 59-70 (2006).

White solid from ethyl acetate + heptane, mp 86-89°. $[\alpha]_D$ +20° (ethanol). Freely sol in dehydrated alcohol, propylene glycol. Insol in aq. buffer, pH 7.5.

THERAP CAT: Antiviral.

9460. Tiquizium Bromide. [71731-58-3] (5R,9aR)-rel-3-(Di-2-thienylmethylene)octahydro-5-methyl-2H-quinolizinium bromide; 3-(di-2-thienylmethylene)-5-methyl-trans-quinolizidinium bromide; HSR-902; HS-902; Thiaton. $C_{19}H_{24}BrNS_2$; mol wt 410.43. C 55.60%, H 5.89%, Br 19.47%, N 3.41%, S 15.63%. Quaternary ammonium salt with anticholinergic activity. Prepn: H. Kato *et al.,* **BE 866988** (1978 to Hokuriku), *C.A.* **90,** 151996p

(1979); H. Kato, E. Koshinaka, **US 4205074** (1980 to Hokuriku). Synthesis and anticholinergic activity: E. Koshinaka *et al., Chem. Pharm. Bull.* **27,** 1454 (1979). Pharmacological comparison with other antispasmodics: S. Kubo *et al., Jpn. J. Pharmacol.* **30,** 103P (1980). Pharmacology: M. Yamazaki *et al., Oyo Yakuri* **23,** 417, 423 (1981), *C.A.* **97,** 66016u, 66017v (1982). HPLC determn in biological fluids: T. Yamada *et al., Yakugaku Zasshi* **103,** 1319 (1983), *C.A.* **100,** 131957y (1984).

Needles from methanol-acetone, mp 278-281° (dec).

THERAP CAT: Antispasmodic.

9461. Tirapazamine. [27314-97-2] 1,2,4-Benzotriazin-3-amine 1,4-dioxide; 3-amino-1,2,4-benzotriazine 1,4-dioxide; NSC-130181; SR-4233; Win-59075; Tirazone. $C_7H_6N_4O_2$; mol wt 178.15. C 47.19%, H 3.39%, N 31.45%, O 17.96%. Bioreductive anticancer agent; selectively toxic to cells under hypoxic conditions. Prepn: R. F. Robbins, K. Schofield, *J. Chem. Soc.* **1957,** 3186; J. C. Mason, G. Tennant, *J. Chem. Soc. B* **1970,** 911. *See also:* K. Ley *et al.,* **DE 2204574**; *eidem,* **US 3868371** (1973, 1975 both to Bayer). HPLC determn in plasma: H. Robin, Jr. *et al., Cancer Chemother. Pharmacol.* **36,** 266 (1995). Review of pharmacology and mechanism of action studies: J. M. Brown, *Br. J. Cancer* **67,** 1163-1170 (1993). Clinical evaluation in combination with cisplatin: C. A. Johnson *et al., J. Clin. Oncol.* **15,** 773 (1997).

Orange needles from methanol, mp 229-230° (dec) (Robbins, Scholfield). Also reported as reddish-golden crystals from water + acetic acid, mp 220° (dec) (Ley). uv max: 272, 474 nm (log ε 4.24, 3.52).

THERAP CAT: Antineoplastic.

9462. Tiratricol. [51-24-1] [4-(4-Hydroxy-3-iodophenoxy)-3,5-diiodophenyl]acetic acid; 3,3′,5-triiodo-4-(4-hydroxyphenoxy)phenylacetic acid; 3,5-diiodo-4-(3-iodo-4-hydroxyphenoxy)phenylacetic acid; 3,3′,5-triiodothyroacetic acid; Triac; Triacana. $C_{14}H_9I_3O_4$; mol wt 621.93. C 27.04%, H 1.46%, I 61.21%, O 10.29%. Thyroid hormone analog. Prepd by iodination of 4-(4′-hydroxyphenoxy)-3,5-diiodophenylacetic acid: Wilkinson, *Biochem. J.* **63,** 601 (1956); Hems, **GB 803149** (1958 to Glaxo); Wilkinson, **GB 805761** (1958 to Nat. Res. Dev. Corp.); Meltzer *et al., J. Org. Chem.* **26,** 1418 (1961). Clinical evaluation in thyroidectomy: S. I. Sherman, P. W. Ladenson, *J. Clin. Endocrinol. Metab.* **75,** 901 (1992).

Needles from methanol+ water, mp 65°, resolidifies 110°, mp 180-183°.

THERAP CAT: Antihypothyroid.

9463. Tirilazad. [110101-66-1] (16α)-21-[4-(2,6-Di-1-pyrrolidinyl-4-pyrimidinyl)-1-piperazinyl]-16-methylpregna-1,4,-9(11)-triene-3,20-dione. $C_{38}H_{52}N_6O_2$; mol wt 624.86. C 73.04%, H 8.39%, N 13.45%, O 5.12%. Member of a novel class of non-

Consult the Name Index before using this section.

glucocorticoid, 21-aminosteroid antioxidants known as *lazaroids* which inhibit lipid peroxidation and have cytoprotectant activity. Prepn: J. M. McCall *et al.,* **WO 8701706**; *eidem,* **US 5175281** (1987, 1992 both to Upjohn). Inhibition of iron-dependent lipid peroxidation *in vitro:* J. M. Braughler *et al., J. Biol. Chem.* **262,** 10438 (1987). HPLC determn in plasma: J. W. Cox, R. H. Pullen, *J. Chromatogr.* **424,** 293 (1988). Clinical pharmacokinetics: J. C. Fleishaker *et al., J. Clin. Pharmacol.* **33,** 175, 182 (1993). Veterinary evaluation in endotoxemia of neonatal calves: M. L. Rose, S. D. Semrad, *Am. J. Vet. Res.* **53,** 2305 (1992). *Review:* E. D. Hall, *Ann. Neurol.* **32,** S137-S142 (1992). Review of efficacy and mechanism of action in experimental models of subarachnoid hemorrhage: *idem, Eur. J. Anaesthesiol.* **13,** 279-289 (1996); of clinical trials in acute ischemic stroke: Tirilazad International Steering Committee, *Stroke* **32,** 2257-2265 (2000).

Methanesulfonate monohydrate. [111793-42-1] Tirilazad mesylate; U-74006F; Freedox. $C_{38}H_{52}N_6O_5 \cdot CH_3SO_3H \cdot H_2O$; mol wt 738.98. mp 181-185° (dec). uv max: 234, 285 nm (ε 52000, 17000). Log P (octanol/water): 8.

9464. Tirofiban. [144494-65-5] *N*-(Butylsulfonyl)-*O*-[4-(4-piperidinyl)butyl]-L-tyrosine; *N*-(butylsulfonyl)-4-[4-(4-piperidyl)-butoxy]-L-phenylalanine; 2-*S*-(*n*-butylsulfonylamino)-3-[4-(piperidin-4-yl)butyloxyphenyl]propionic acid. $C_{22}H_{36}N_2O_5S$; mol wt 440.60. C 59.97%, H 8.24%, N 6.36%, O 18.16%, S 7.28%. Specific nonpeptide platelet fibrinogen receptor (GPIIb/IIIa) antagonist. Prepn: M. S. Egbertson *et al.,* **EP 478363**; M. E. Duggan *et al.,* **US 5292756** (1992, 1994 both to Merck & Co.); J. Y. L. Chung *et al., Tetrahedron* **49,** 5767 (1993). Physicochemical properties: J. A. McCauley *et al., J. Phys. D: Appl. Phys.* **26,** B85 (1993). Pharmacology: J. J. Lynch *et al., J. Pharmacol. Exp. Ther.* **272,** 20 (1995). Clinical pharmacokinetics and pharmacodynamics: J. S. Barrett *et al., Clin. Pharmacol. Ther.* **56,** 377 (1994). Clinical trials in angina: P. Théroux *et al., N. Engl. J. Med.* **338,** 1488 (1998); H. D. White *et al., ibid.* 1498. Clinical comparison with abciximab, *q.v.,* in coronary revascularization: D. J. Moliterno *et al., Lancet* **360,** 355 (2002).

White solid, mp 223-225°.
Hydrochloride monohydrate. [150915-40-5]; [142373-60-2] (hydrochloride). MK-383; Aggrastat. $C_{22}H_{36}N_2O_5S \cdot HCl \cdot H_2O$; mol wt 495.07. Solid, mp 131-132°. $[\alpha]_D^{25}$ −14.4° (c = 0.92 in methanol).

THERAP CAT: Antithrombotic; in treatment of unstable angina.

9465. Tiron. [149-45-1] 4,5-Dihydroxy-1,3-benzenedisulfonic acid disodium salt; 1,2-dihydroxybenzene-3,5-disulfonic acid disodium salt; disodium-1,2-dihydroxybenzene-3,5-disulfonate; sodium catechol disulfonate; sodium pyrocatechol-2,4-disulfonate; disodium pyrocatechol-3,5-disulfonate. $C_6H_4Na_2O_8S_2$; mol wt 314.20. C 22.94%, H 1.28%, Na 14.63%, O 40.74%, S 20.41%. Chelating agent. Prepn: Fukayama *et al.,* **JP 52 4327** (1952 to Sanwa Pure Chem.), *C.A.* **48,** 5215c (1954). Use in HPLC determn of iron, titanium, osmium and aluminum: E. Wang, A. Liu, *Microchem. J.* **43,** 191 (1991); in spectrophotometric determn of titanium: S. Honshi *et al., Anal. Sci.* **13,** 863 (1997).

Crystals, nonhygroscopic. Very freely sol in water. Produces water-sol, colored compds with metal salts. With ferric chloride the resulting complex yields a deep blue soln at pH below 5. Titanium salts give an orange color, copper salts produce a green-yellow, and hexavalent molybdenum a canary-yellow color.

USE: In determination of trace metals.

9466. Tiropramide. [55837-29-1] α-(Benzoylamino)-4-[2-(diethylamino)ethoxy]-*N,N*-dipropylbenzenepropanamide; DL-α-benzamido-*p*-[2-(diethylamino)ethoxy]-*N,N*-dipropylhydrocinnamide; *O*-(2-diethylaminoethyl)-*N*-benzoyl-DL-tyrosyl-di-*n*-propylamide; CR-605. $C_{28}H_{41}N_3O_3$; mol wt 467.64. C 71.91%, H 8.84%, N 8.99%, O 10.26%. Smooth muscle relaxant; deriv of tyrosine. Prepn: F. Makovec *et al.,* **DE 2503992**; *eidem,* **US 4004008** (1975, 1977 both to Rotta). Activity on gastrointestinal motility: P. Senin *et al., Gastrointestinal Motility in Health and Disease,* H. L. Duthie, Ed. (University Park Press, Baltimore, 1978) pp 417-427. Mechanism of action: R. R. Vidal y Plana *et al., J. Pharm. Pharmacol.* **33,** 19 (1981).

Cryst from petr ether, mp 65-67°. LD$_{50}$ in rats: 33.9 mg/kg i.v. (Makovec).
Hydrochloride. [53567-47-8] Alfospas; Maiorad. $C_{28}H_{41}N_3$-$O_3 \cdot HCl$; mol wt 504.10.

THERAP CAT: Antispasmodic.

9467. Tissue Factor Pathway Inhibitor. TFPI; lipoprotein-associated coagulation inhibitor; LACI. Endogenous inhibitor of the tissue factor mediated pathway of blood coagulation. Glycoprotein containing 276 amino acid residues; mol wt ~42 kDa. Structure consists of an acidic amino terminal region followed by three tandem Kunitz-type protease inhibitory domains and a basic carboxy terminal region. Forms a quaternary inhibitory complex with tissue factor, factor VIIa and factor Xa to block the formation of thrombin from prothrombin. Isoln of factor produced by hepatoma cells: G. J. Broze, Jr., J. P. Miletich, *Proc. Natl. Acad. Sci. USA* **84,** 1886 (1987); from human plasma: W. F. Novotny *et al., J. Biol. Chem.* **264,** 18832 (1989). Review of structure and physiology: G. J. Broze, Jr., *Annu. Rev. Med.* **46,** 103-112 (1995); of pharmacology and therapeutic potential: A. K. Lindahl, *Cardiovasc. Res.* **33,** 286-291 (1997); B. Kaiser *et al., Emerg. Drugs* **5,** 73-87 (2000).

Tifacogin. [148883-56-1] *N*-L-Alanyl-blood coagulation factor LACI (human clone λP9 protein moiety reduced); SC-59735. Recombinant human form; differs from the native protein by an additional alanine residue at the amino terminus and is not glycosylated. Prepn by expression in *E. coli:* G. J. Broze, Jr. *et al.,* **EP 318451**; *eidem,* **US 4966852** (1989, 1990 both to Monsanto Co.; Washington Univ.); M. E. Gustafson *et al., Protein Expression Purif.* **5,** 233 (1994). Production in *Saccharomyces cerevisiae:* M. A. Innis, A. A. Creasey, **WO 9604377**; *eidem,* **US 6103500** (1996, 2000 both to Chiron). Clinical pharmacokinetics: M. J. B. Kemme *et al., Clin. Pharmacol. Ther.* **67,** 504 (2000). Clinical evaluation in sepsis: E. Abraham, *Crit. Care Med.* **28,** Suppl., S31 (2000). *Review:* N. Sne *et al., IDrugs* **5,** 91-97 (2002).

THERAP CAT: Antithrombotic.

9468. Tissue Plasminogen Activator. Fibrinokinase; extrinsic plasminogen activator; t-PA; TPA. Serine protease catalyzing the enzymatic conversion of plasminogen to plasmin, *q.q.v.* Component of the mammalian fibrinolytic system; major physiological function is to provide plasmin that will dissolve fibrin clots. Shows high affinity and specificity for fibrin-bound plasminogen and weak affinity for circulating plasminogen. Plasminogen activation and fibrinolysis are therefore localized to the clot site, with limited systemic enzymatic activity. t-PA exists as 2 bioactive structural variants and can be isolated in either form depending on method of purification. Synthesized in vascular endothelial cells and released into circulation as the native single chain form, 527 amino acids, mol wt ~70,000. Converted to the two chain form by cleavage of Arg275-Ile276 bond to form two polypeptides connected by a disulfide bond. Discovery of *in vitro* plasminogen-activating ability in tissue fragments: T. Astrup, P. M. Permin, *Nature* **159**, 681 (1947); H. J. Tagnon, M. L. Petermann, *Proc. Soc. Exp. Biol. Med.* **70**, 359 (1949). Review of early literature: T. Astrup, *Fed. Proc.* **25**, 42-51 (1966). Purifn from human tissue: D. C. Rijken *et al., Biochim. Biophys. Acta* **580**, 140 (1979). Identification and purifn of 2 forms: P. Wallen *et al., Biochim. Biophys. Acta* **719**, 318 (1982); and comparison of biological activity: D. C. Rijken *et al., J. Biol. Chem.* **257**, 2920 (1982). Review of role in fibrinolytic system: D. Collen, *Thromb. Haemostasis* **43**, 77-89 (1980); of pharmacology and clinical efficacy: S. D. Rogers *et al., Pharmacotherapy* **7**, 111-121 (1987); D. Collen *et al., Drugs* **38**, 346-388 (1989); of production by cell cultures: J. B. Griffiths, A. Electricwala, *Adv. Biochem. Eng. Biotechnol.* **34**, 147-166 (1987).

Practically insol in solns of low ionic strength at neutral pH. Sol in 1.6*M* KSCN at neutral pH; 0.3*M* K-acetate at pH 4.2.

Alteplase. [105857-23-6] rt-PA; Actilyse; Actiplas; Activase. Recombinant form of human t-PA; purified glycoprotein of 527 amino acids with a sequence identical to the naturally occurring form. Cloning and expression of cDNA: D. Pennica *et al., Nature* **301**, 214 (1983). Review of pharmacokinetics: P. Tanswell *et al., Arzneim.-Forsch.* **41**, 1310-1319 (1991). Comparative clinical trial in myocardial infarction: C. P. Cannon *et al., J. Am. Coll. Cardiol.* **24**, 1602 (1994); in acute ischemic stroke: The Natl. Inst. Neurological Disorders and Stroke rt-PA Stroke Study Group, *N. Engl. J. Med.* **333**, 1581 (1995).

Duteplase. [120608-46-0] 245-L-Methionine-plasminogen activator (human tissue-type 2-chain form protein moiety); Solclot. Two-chain form of recombinant human t-PA. Clinical pharmacokinetics: R. W. Koster *et al., Clin. Pharmacol. Ther.* **50**, 267 (1991). Clinical efficacy in myocardial infarction: Z. G. Turi *et al., Am. J. Cardiol.* **71**, 1009 (1993).

THERAP CAT: Thrombolytic.

9469. Titanic(IV) Acid. [20338-08-3] Orthotitanic acid; titanic hydroxide. $Ti(OH)_4 \cdot xH_2O$. The H_2O content depends upon the method and time of drying.

White, amorphous powder. Insol in water; when freshly pptd it is sol in dil HCl or H_2SO_4 and in boiling caustic alkali solns; after drying it is almost insol.

9470. Titanium. [7440-32-6] Ti; at. wt 47.867; at. no. 22; valence 2, 3, 4 (mostly tetravalent). Group IVB (4). Five naturally occurring isotopes (mass numbers): 48 (73.94%); 46 (7.93%); 47 (7.28%); 49 (5.51%); 50 (5.34%). Artificial isotopes: 43-45; 51. Ninth most abundant element in earth's crust; 0.63% by wt. Occurs as the oxide in the minerals rutile, ilmenite, perovskite, anatase, or octahedrite and brookite; other minerals include **sphene** or **titanite** ($CaTiSiO_5$) and **benitoite** ($BaTiSi_3O_9$). Discovered by Gregor in 1789; investigated and named by Klaproth in 1795; isolated by Berzelius in 1825. Prepn: de Boer, *Ind. Eng. Chem.* **19**, 1256 (1927); Fast, *Z. Anorg. Chem.* **241**, 42 (1939); Ehrlich in *Handbook of Preparative Inorganic Chemistry* vol. 2, G. Brauer, Ed. (Academic Press, New York, 2nd ed., 1965) pp 1161-1172. *Reviews: Gmelins, Titanium* (8th ed.) **41** (1951); Everhart, *Titanium and Titanium Alloys* (Reinhold, New York, 1954); Brophy *et al., Titanium Bibliography* 1900-1951 + suppl (Washington, 1954); McQuillan & McQuillan, *Titanium* (Butterworth's, London, 1956); Barksdale, *Titanium, Its Occurrence, Chemistry and Technology* (Ronald Press, New York, 2nd ed, 1966); Clark, "Titanium" in *Comprehensive Inorganic Chemistry* vol. 3, J. C. Bailar, Jr. *et al.,* Eds. (Pergamon Press, Oxford, 1973) pp 355-417.

Dark gray, lustrous metal. Dimorphic; α-form: hexagonal structure below 882.5°; β-form: body-centered cubic crystals above 882.5°. Brittle when cold; malleable when hot. Ductile only when free of oxygen; traces of oxygen or nitrogen increase strength. mp 1677°. bp 3277°. Calculated d (α- form): 4.506 (25°); (β-form): 4.400 (900°). Specific heat (25°): 5.98 cal/g-atom/°C. Decomposes steam at 700-800°. Combines with oxygen at a red heat. Can burn in an atm of oxygen under certain conditions: *Chem. Eng. News* **36**, 36 (Aug. 4, 1958). Attacked by acids only on heating; oxidized by nitric acid to the dioxide. Reacts with fluorine at 150°, with chlorine at 300°, with bromine at 360°, with iodine above 360°. Combines with nitrogen at 800°. Forms alloys with aluminum, chromium, cobalt, copper, iron, lead, nickel, tin.

USE: As alloy with copper and iron in titanium bronze; as addition to steel to impart great tensile strength; to aluminum to impart resistance to attack by salt solns and by organic acids; to remove traces of oxygen and nitrogen from incandescent lamps. Surgical aid (fracture fixation).

9471. Titanium Dichloride. [10049-06-6] Cl_2Ti; mol wt 118.77. Cl 59.70%, Ti 40.30%. $TiCl_2$. Prepn: Clifton, McWood, *J. Phys. Chem.* **60**, 311 (1956); Ehrlich *et al., Z. Anorg. Allg. Chem.* **292**, 139 (1957).

Black crystals. mp 1035°. d 3.13. Burns like tinder when heated in air; dec by water. Sol in alcohol. Practically insol in chloroform, ether, carbon disulfide. *Keep dry and well closed.*

9472. Titanium Dioxide. [13463-67-7] Titanium oxide (TiO_2); unitane; C.I. Pigment White 6; C.I. 77891. O_2Ti; mol wt 79.87. O 40.06%, Ti 59.93%. TiO_2. Found in nature as the minerals **rutile** (tetragonal), **anatase** or **octahedrite** (tetragonal), **brookite** (orthorhombic), **ilmenite** ($FeTiO_3$), and **perovskite** ($CaTiO_3$). May be prepd by direct combination of titanium and oxygen; by treatment of titanium salts in aq soln; by the reaction of volatile, inorganic titanium compds with oxygen; by oxidation or hydrolysis of organic compds of titanium. Industrial prepn from ilmenite or rutile: *Faith, Keyes & Clark's Industrial Chemicals,* F. A. Lowenheim, M. K. Moran, Eds. (Wiley-Interscience, New York, 4th ed., 1975) pp 814-821. Prepn of synthetic rutile: Merker, **US 2760874** (1956 to National Lead). Prepn of spectroscopically pure material by dissolving titanium in an ammoniacal soln of 90% H_2O_2: Czanderna *et al., J. Am. Chem. Soc.* **79**, 5407 (1957). Comprehensive description: H. G. Brittain *et al., Anal. Profiles Drug Subs. Excip.* **21**, 659-691 (1992).

White powder. mp 1855°. d (rutile): 4.23; (anatase): 3.90; (brookite): 4.13. Insol in water, HCl, HNO_3, or dil H_2SO_4. Sol in hot concd H_2SO_4, in HF. The reactivity depends on a previous heat treatment; prolonged heating produces a less sol material. Also made sol by fusion with potassium bisulfate or with alkali hydroxides or carbonates to form alkali titanates. Possesses perhaps the greatest hiding power of all inorganic white pigments. *Titania* is a name applied to large TiO_2 crystals (translucent water-white or with yellowish cast) suitable for use in jewelry. These crystals have a refractive index (2.7) higher than diamonds (2.4), but lack the hardness of diamonds. When substantially pure, a massive single crystal (boule) of rutile has the properties of a precious gem with a very light straw color and with reflectance, refraction and brilliance measuring greater than those of a diamond.

Note: The rutile structure is common among metal fluorides and oxides of the type MF_2 and MO_2.

Caution: Potential symptom of overexposure is lung fibrosis. Potential occupational carcinogen. *See NIOSH Pocket Guide to Chemical Hazards* (DHHS/NIOSH 97-140, 1997) p 310.

USE: Airfloated ilmenite is used for titanium pigment manuf. Rutile sand is suitable for welding-rod-coating materials, as ceramic colorant, as source of titanium metal. As color in the food industry. Anatase titanium dioxide is used for welding-rod-coatings, acid resistant vitreous enamels, in specification paints, exterior white house paints, acetate rayon, white interior air-dry and baked enamels and lacquers, inks and plastics, for paper filling and coating, in water paints, tanners' leather finishes, shoe whiteners, and ceramics. High opacity and tinting values are claimed for rutile-like pigments.

THERAP CAT: Protectant (topical); ultraviolet sunscreen.

9473. Titanium Hydride. [7704-98-5] H_2Ti; mol wt 49.88. H 4.04%, Ti 95.96%. TiH_2. Prepd by the reduction of titanium oxide with calcium hydride in the presence of hydrogen above 600°: Alexander, US 2427338 (1947).

Gray-black metallic powder. Stable in air. Dissociation appreciable at 450°.

USE: Additive in powder metallurgy; getter for oxygen and nitrogen in electronic tubes; wetting agent for ceramic to metal seals; source of pure hydrogen.

9474. Titanium Nitride. [25583-20-4] NTi; mol wt 61.87. N 22.64%, Ti 77.37%. TiN. Refractory transition metal nitride with high chemical and thermal stability, good wear resistance, and high electrical conductivity. Prepn by plasma-enhanced chemical vapor deposition: N. J. Ianno et al., J. Electrochem. Soc. **136**, 276 (1989). Hydrazide sol-gel synthesis: I. Kim, P. N. Kumta, J. Mater. Chem. **13**, 2028 (2003). Low temp induced synthesis: X. Feng et al., Inorg. Chem. **43**, 3558 (2004). Prepn and catalytic properties: S. Kaskel et al., J. Mol. Catal. A **208**, 291 (2004). Physical-mechanical properties of TiN nanostructures: R. A. Andrievski, Nano-Struct. Mater. **9**, 607 (1997). Bioactivity of TiN-coated hip prostheses: S. Piscanec et al., Acta Mater. **52**, 1237 (2004). Review of chemistry, properties and prepn methods: L. E. Toth, Transition Metal Carbides and Nitrides (Academic Press, New York, 1971) 279 pp; of structure and properties of TiN coatings: J.-E. Sundgren, Thin Solid Films **128**, 21-44 (1985); S. Chatterjee et al., J. Mater. Sci. **27**, 1989-2006 (1992).

Golden-yellow solid, mp 2950°. d 5.39. Microhardness: 2000 kg/mm².

USE: As protective coating for cutting tools; in diffusion barriers for microelectronic devices; as crucibles in metal smelting; as a gold-colored surface for jewelry. In high-performance ceramic materials. As a coating for orthopedic and dental implants.

9475. Titanium Oxysulfate. [13825-74-6] Oxo[sulfato-(2−)-κO,κO']titanium; titanyl sulfate; titanium sulfate. O₅STi; mol wt 159.93. O 50.02%, S 20.05%, Ti 29.93%. TiO(SO₄). Prepn: E. Hayek, A. Engelbrecht, Monatsh. Chem. **80**, 640 (1949). Crystal structure: B. M. Gatehouse et al., Acta Crystallogr. **B49**, 428 (1993). Catalytic hydrolysis of chlorofluorocarbon: X. Deng et al., J. Catalysis **204**, 200 (2001). Prepn of titanium dioxide, q.v.,via thermal hydrolysis: A. V. Tolchev et al., Russ. J. Appl. Chem. **74**, 1631 (2001); L. G. Gerasimova et al., ibid. **75**, 875 (2002). Sol-gel synthesis of nanosized *anatase*, a mineral form of titanium dioxide: S. Sivakumar et al., Mater. Lett. **57**, 330 (2002). Brief review as whitening agent in tanning: S. Bangaruswamy et al., J. Soc. Leather Technol. Chem. **68**, 13-14 (1984).

Clear, colorless elongated prisms.

Note: The name titanium sulfate is used for both this compound and titanium(IV) sulfate (Ti(SO₄)).

USE: In tanning; in production of pigment grade and of anatase-structured titanium dioxide.

9476. Titanium Sesquisulfate. [10343-61-0] Titanous sulfate. O₁₂S₃Ti₂; mol wt 383.92. O 50.01%, S 25.06%, Ti 24.94%. Ti₂(SO₄)₃. (Crystallizes also as a hydrate with 8H₂O).

Green, cryst powder. Insol in water, alc, concd H₂SO₄. Sol in dil HCl or dil H₂SO₄, giving violet-colored solns.

USE: Same as titanium trichloride.

9477. Titanium Tetrabromide. [7789-68-6] Br₄Ti; mol wt 367.48. Br 86.98%, Ti 13.03%. TiBr₄. Prepn: Olsen, Ryan, J. Am. Chem. Soc. **54**, 2215 (1932).

Amber-yellow or orange, very hygroscopic crystals. mp 28.25°. bp 233.45°. d²⁰ 3.25. Also reported as 2.6: Duppa, Proc. Roy. Soc. London **8**, 42 (1857). Dec by water; sol in abs ether, abs alcohol. Keep tightly closed.

9478. Titanium Tetrachloride. [7550-45-0] Cl₄Ti; mol wt 189.68. Cl 74.76%, Ti 25.24%. TiCl₄. Purification: Baxter et al., J. Am. Chem. Soc. **45**, 1228 (1923); **48**, 3117 (1926). Survey of preparative methods: Ehrlich in Handbook of Preparative Inorganic Chemistry **Vol. 2**, G. Brauer, Ed. (Academic Press, New York, 2nd ed., 1965) pp 195-199. Review of toxicology and human exposure: Toxicological Profile for Titanium Tetrachloride (PB98-101082, 1997) 145 pp.

Colorless liquid; penetrating acid odor. Absorbs moisture from the air and evolves dense white fumes. Reacts with water to produce titanium dioxide and hydrochloric acid. d 1.726. mp −24.1°.

bp 136.4°. Vapor pressure (20°): 10.0 mm; (22°) 9.6 mm. Sol in cold water, alcohol; dec by hot water. Corrosive. Keep tightly closed.

Caution: Potential symptoms of overexposure by inhalation are coughing, tightness in chest, chemical bronchitis or pneumonia, congestion of mucous membranes of upper resp tract. Direct contact may cause irritation or burns of eyes, skin, mucous membranes and lungs (PB98-101082).

USE: Manuf titanium compounds, iridescent glass and artificial pearls. Formerly used with potassium bitartrate as a mordant in textile industry, and with dyewoods in dyeing leather; also as smoke-producing screen with ammonia.

9479. Titanium Tetrafluoride. [7783-63-3] F₄Ti; mol wt 123.86. F 61.35%, Ti 38.65%. TiF₄. Prepd by the reaction of hydrogen fluoride with titanium tetrachloride: Ruff, Ipsen, Ber. **36**, 1777 (1903); Ruff, Plato, ibid. **37**, 673 (1904); by the action of fluorine on the metal or the dioxide: Haendler et al., J. Am. Chem. Soc. **76**, 2177 (1954).

Powdery white mass. d₄²⁰ 2.798. Sublimes at 284°. mp >400°. Hisses on contact with water. Very hygroscopic; the dihydrate may be crystallized from aqueous soln (also obtained from solns of TiO₂ in HF). Aq solns hydrolyze slowly, and the existence of an oxy-fluoride, TiOF₂, has been established. Also sol in alcohol and pyridine from which the compds TiF₄.2EtOH and TiF₄.C₅H₅N have been isolated. Insol in ether. Dry ammonia is absorbed at room temp to form TiF₄.4NH₃, but at 120° TiF₄.2NH₃ is the stable phase. This is sol in water and is sufficiently stable to sublime. TiF₄ is also sol in phosphorus oxychloride, but at 30° a reaction occurs and POF₃ is evolved. See also Eméleus in Fluorine Chemistry vol. I, J. H. Simons, Ed. (Academic Press, New York, 1950) p 47.

9480. Titanium Tetraisopropoxide. [546-68-9] Isopropyl titanate(IV); Titanium Isopropylate. C₁₂H₂₈O₄Ti; mol wt 284.22. C 50.71%, H 9.93%, O 22.52%, Ti 16.84%. Ti[OCH(CH₃)₂]₄. Mild Lewis acid catalyst. Prepn: F. Bischoff, H. Adkins, J. Am. Chem. Soc. **46**, 256 (1924). Vibrational spectra: P. D. Moran et al., Inorg. Chem. **37**, 2741 (1998). Kinetic behavior in asymmetric epoxidation: S. S. Woodard et al., J. Am. Chem. Soc. **113**, 106 (1991). Kinetics in prepn of titanium dioxide, q.v., thin films: V. Gourinchas-Courtecuisse et al., High Press. Chem. Eng. **1996**, 133; G. A. Battiston et al., Metalurgija **8**, 183 (2002); of sol-gel process: A. Soloviev et al., J. Mater. Sci. **38**, 3315 (2003). Use as complexing agent in sol-gel process: B. Wang et al., Polym. Commun. **32**, 400 (1991); H. Arce et al., Rev. Soc. Quim. Mex. **47**, 73 (2003). Review as reagent in stereoselective synthesis: R. Mahrwald, J. Prakt. Chem. **341**, 191-194 (1999); as catalyst: F. Lake, C. Moberg, Russ. J. Org. Chem. **39**, 436-452 (2003). Brief review in a variety of organic syntheses: O. López, Synlett **2003**, 2261-2262.

Flammable, moisture-sensitive liquid. mp 18-20°. bp₇₄₀ 230°. Sol in a wide range of solvents including ethers, organohalides, alcohols and benzenes.

USE: Catalyst especially for asymmetric induction in organic syntheses; in preparation of nanosized TiO₂. Complexing agent in sol-gel process.

9481. Titanium Trichloride. [7705-07-9] Titanous chloride. Cl₃Ti; mol wt 154.23. Cl 68.96%, Ti 31.04%. TiCl₃. Prepn by reduction of the tetrachloride: Ingraham et al., Inorg. Synth. **6**, 52 (1960); Sherfey, ibid. 57.

Dark red-violet, unstable, deliquesc crystals; dec on heating above 500°. The dry powder is pyrophoric in air. Very reactive and readily dissociated by moisture in air. Sol in water, exothermic process; sol in alcohol. Practically insol in ether. Keep tightly closed.

USE: A powerful reducing agent. Reduces nitrate to ammonia; when boiled with aq SO₂, sulfur is separated; hence is used as an aq soln for estimation of nitro groups, ferric ions, per-salts, etc. Removes stains, etc. (stripper) in laundering.

9482. Titanocene Dichloride. [1271-19-8] Dichlorobis(η⁵-2,4-cyclopentadien-1-yl)titanium; dichlorodi-π-cyclopentadienyltitanium; biscyclopentadienyltitanium(IV) dichloride. C₁₀H₁₀Cl₂Ti; mol wt 248.96. C 48.24%, H 4.05%, Cl 28.48%, Ti 19.23%. Cp₂-TiCl₂. Prepn: Wilkinson, Birmingham, J. Am. Chem. Soc. **76**,

4281 (1954). Structure: Clearfield *et al., Can. J. Chem.* **53,** 1622 (1975).

Bright red acicular crystals from toluene. mp 289 ± 2°. d 1.60. Moderately sol in toluene, chloroform, alcohol, other hydroxylic solvents; sparingly sol in water, petr ether, benzene, ether, carbon disulfide, carbon tetrachloride.

USE: Catalyst; with aluminum alkyls as Ziegler-Natta polymerization catalyst.

9483. Titin. Connectin. Giant, elastic protein found in vertebrate skeletal and cardiac muscles; comprises ~10% of the myofibrillar mass. One of the largest polypeptides known; mol wt: ~3 × 10⁶ Da. Structure consists of repeats of 2 motifs, each with approximately 100 amino acid residues, organized into a super-repeating pattern. Enriched in proline (8-9 mole %) which contributes to its flexibility. Integral component of the cytoskeletal lattice of muscle cells (*see also* Nebulin). Thought to act as a "molecular ruler" that regulates the assembly of myosin and other thick filament proteins; connects the ends of the thick filament with the Z-line. Also responsible for the generation of resting tension in stretched muscle fibers. Identification in rabbit muscle: K. Maruyama *et al., Nature* **262,** 58 (1976). Characterization and localization in myofibrils: K. Wang *et al., Proc. Natl. Acad. Sci. USA* **76,** 3698 (1979). Purification methods: K. Wang, *Methods Enzymol.* **85B,** 264 (1982). Distribution and organization in the cytoskeletal matrix of striated muscle: *idem, Adv. Exp. Med. Biol.* **170,** 285-305 (1984). Quantitative determn in muscle fibers by gel electrophoresis: H. L. M. Granzier, K. Wang, *Electrophoresis* **14,** 56 (1993). *Reviews:* J. Trinick, *Trends Biochem. Sci.* **19,** 405-409 (1994); K. Maruyama, *Biophys. Chem.* **50,** 73-85 (1994).

9484. Tixocortol. [61951-99-3] (11β)-11,17-Dihydroxy-21-mercaptopregn-4-ene-3,20-dione; 11β,17α-dihydroxy-21-thio-3,20-dioxo-4-pregnene. $C_{21}H_{30}O_4S$; mol wt 378.53. C 66.63%, H 7.99%, O 16.91%, S 8.47%. Synthesis and biological activity: S. S. Simons *et al., J. Steroid Biochem.* **13,** 311 (1980). Use in fluorescent chemoaffinity labeling: *idem, Biochemistry* **18,** 4915 (1979). Prepn of the 21-pivalate: D. R. Torossian *et al.,* **DE 2357778;** *idem,* **US 4014909** (1974, 1977 both to Jouveinal). Series of articles on pharmacology, *in vitro* and *in vivo* activity of the pivalate: *Arzneim.-Forsch.* **31,** 453-469 (1981).

Fine white solid, dec 220-221°. uv max (95% ethanol): 241 nm (ε 1.65×10⁴).

21-Pivalate. [55560-96-8] (11β)-21-[(2,2-Dimethyl-1-oxopropyl)thio]-11,17-dihydroxypregn-4-ene-3,20-dione; JO-1016; Pivalone; Rectovalone; Tiovalon. $C_{26}H_{38}O_5S$; mol wt 462.64. Crystals from ethanol, mp 195-200°. [α]$_D^{20}$ +145° (c = 1 in dioxane). uv max (methanol): 229 nm (log ε 4.259).

USE: Free thiol in chemoaffinity labeling.

THERAP CAT: Anti-inflammatory.

9485. Tizanidine. [51322-75-9] 5-Chloro-*N*-(4,5-dihydro-1*H*-imidazol-2-yl)-2,1,3-benzothiadiazol-4-amine; 5-chloro-4-(2-imidazolin-2-ylamino)-2,1,3-benzothiadiazole. $C_9H_8ClN_5S$; mol wt 253.71. C 42.61%, H 3.18%, Cl 13.97%, N 27.60%, S 12.64%. α₂-Adrenergic agonist; centrally active myotonolytic. Prepn and antitremor activity: P. Neumann, **NL 7306228;** *idem,* **US 3843668** (1973, 1974 both to Wander-Sandoz). Pharmacology:

A. C. Sayers *et al., Arzneim.-Forsch.* **30,** 793 (1980); and mechanism of action studies: L. Turski *et al., Brain Res.* **379,** 367 (1986); H. Ono *et al., Gen. Pharmacol.* **17,** 137 (1986). Pharmacokinetics: V. Heazlewood *et al., Eur. J. Clin. Pharmacol.* **25,** 65 (1983). Clinical evaluation in spasticity of multiple sclerosis: P. M. Newman *et al., ibid.* **23,** 31 (1982); M. C. Hoogstraten *et al., Acta Neurol. Scand.* **77,** 224 (1988).

Crystals from methanol, mp 221-223°. LD₅₀ orally in mice: 235 mg/kg (Sayers).

Hydrochloride. [64461-82-1] AB-021; DS-103-282; Sirdalud; Ternelin; Zanaflex. $C_9H_8ClN_5S$.HCl; mol wt 290.17.

THERAP CAT: Muscle relaxant (skeletal).

9486. TMD. [60761-10-6] Decahydro-1,1,4a-trimethyl-2-naphthalenol; 1,1,10-trimethyl-*trans*-2-decalol; 4,4,10β-trimethyl-*trans*-decal-3β-ol. $C_{13}H_{24}O$; mol wt 196.33. C 79.53%, H 12.32%, O 8.15%. Prepn: B. Gaspert *et al., J. Chem. Soc.* **1958,** 624; C. Djerassi, D. Marshall, *J. Am. Chem. Soc.* **80,** 3986 (1958); T. G. Halsall *et al., J. Chem. Soc.* **1959,** 2798; S. L. Mukherjee, P. C. Dutta, *ibid.* **1960,** 67. Inhibitor of cholesterol biosynthesis: J. A. Nelson *et al., J. Am. Chem. Soc.* **100,** 4900 (1978); T.-Y. Chang *et al., J. Biol. Chem.* **254,** 11258 (1979).

Crystals, mp 60-65° (subl). Sol in alcohol; slightly sol in water.

d-Form. Crystals, mp 87-88° (subl). [α]$_D^{26}$ +15.9° (CHCl₃).

l-Form. Crystals, mp 87-88° (subl). [α]$_D^{26}$ −16.9° (CHCl₃).

9487. TNAZ. [97645-24-4] 1,3,3-Trinitroazetidine. $C_3H_4N_4O_6$; mol wt 192.09. C 18.76%, H 2.10%, N 29.17%, O 49.97%. Melt-castable nitramine explosive. Synthesis and crystal structure: T. G. Archibald *et al., J. Org. Chem.* **55,** 2920 (1990). Alternate synthesis: A. R. Katritzky *et al., J. Heterocycl. Chem.* **31,** 271 (1994); T. Axenrod *et al., J. Org. Chem.* **60,** 1959 (1995). Decomposition studies: P. Politzer, J. M. Seminario, *Chem. Phys. Lett.* **207,** 27 (1993). Thermolysis: J. C. Oxley *et al., J. Phys. Chem.* **98,** 7004 (1994). *Review:* S. Borman, *Chem. Eng. News* **72,** 18-22 (Jan. 17, 1994).

Explosive. White crystals from CCl₄, mp 100-101°. d 1.84 g/cm³.

USE: Munitions.

9488. TOAC. [15871-57-5] 4-Amino-4-carboxy-2,2,6,6-tetramethyl-1-piperidinyloxy; 2,2,6,6-tetramethylpiperidine-*N*-oxyl-4-amino-4-carboxylic acid. $C_{10}H_{19}N_2O_3$; mol wt 215.27. C 55.79%, H 8.90%, N 13.01%, O 22.30%. Conformationally-constrained, nitroxide, achiral, Cα-tetrasubstituted α-amino acid used as a spin-label for protein structure determination. Prepn: A. Rassat, P. Rey, **FR 1501917** (1967 to Commissariat à l'Energie Atomique); *eidem, Bull. Soc. Chim. Fr.* **1967,** 815. Use as probe for structure conformation studies: T. A. Pertinhez *et al., Biopolymers* **42,** 821 (1997); T. T. T. Bui *et al., J. Chem. Soc. Perkin Trans.* **2000,** 1043; of interchain interactions: A. Polese *et al., J. Am. Chem. Soc.* **121,** 11071 (1999).

Consult the Name Index before using this section.

Pale yellow crystals from water-ethanol (20%/80%), mp 228-230° (dec). uv max (water): 239, 416 nm (ε 1480, 8.4).

USE: EPR probe.

9489. Tobacco Mosaic Virus. TMV. Most thoroughly investigated and best known virus. A ribonucleoprotein contg 95% protein and 5% ribonucleic acid. Molecular weight is 39.0×10^6. TMV is a rod-shaped particle, ~3000 Å long, consisting of 2130 polypeptide chains arranged in some regular order to form a tubular molecule containing a core of RNA. The polypeptide chains consist of 158 amino acid residues each; their mol wt is 17,533. The RNA is responsible for the infectivity of the virus. The protein functions to protect the RNA and determine the macroscopic properties of the virus such as morphology and serological specificity. Isoln from diseased tobacco plants: Stanley, *Science* **81**, 644 (1935). Prepn and characterization of essentially uniform TMV particles: Boedtker, Simmons, *J. Am. Chem. Soc.* **80**, 2550 (1958); Knight, *Biochem. Prep.* **9**, 132 (1962). Sequential arrangement of the 158 amino acid residues of the protein subunit: Tsugita *et al.*, *Proc. Natl. Acad. Sci. USA* **46**, 1463 (1960). Synthesis of TMV-RNA by cell free extracts from infected tobacco leaves: Kim, Wildman, *Biochem. Biophys. Res. Commun.* **8**, 394 (1962); Cochran, *Chem. Eng. News* **40**, 64 (Sept. 17, 1962). Reviews: Anderer, *Adv. Protein Chem.* **18**, 1 (1963); Caspar, *ibid.* 37; Klug, Caspar, *Adv. Virus Res.* **7**, 233-277 (1960); Lauffer, Stevens, *ibid.* **13**, 1 (1968); Reddi, *ibid.* **17**, 51 (1972); L. Hirth, K. E. Richards, *ibid.* **26**, 145-199 (1981).

USE: Popular tool for studying the correlation between chemical structure and biological function.

9490. Tobramycin. [32986-56-4] *O*-3-Amino-3-deoxy-α-D-glucopyranosyl-(1 → 6)-*O*-[2,6-diamino-2,3,6-trideoxy-α-D-*ribo*-hexopyranosyl-(1 → 4)]-2-deoxy-D-streptamine; 4-[2,6-diamino-2,-3,6-trideoxy-α-D-glycopyranosyl)-6-[3-amino-3-deoxy-α-D-glyco-pyranosyl]-2-deoxystreptamine; nebramycin factor 6; NF 6; Tobracin; Tobralex; Tobramaxin; Tobrex. $C_{18}H_{37}N_5O_9$; mol wt 467.51. C 46.24%, H 7.98%, N 14.98%, O 30.80%. Aminoglycoside antibiotic; component of the **nebramycin** complex produced by *Streptomyces tenebrarius*. *See also* apramycin. Series of articles on isolation, separation and evaluation of the nebramycin complex: *Antimicrob. Agents Chemother.* **1967**, 314-348. Elucidation of structure: K. F. Koch, J. A. Rhoades, *Antimicrob. Agents Chemother.* **1970**, 309. Synthesis: Y. Takagi *et al.*, *Bull. Chem. Soc. Jpn.* **49**, 3649 (1976); M. Tanabe *et al.*, *Tetrahedron Lett.* **1977**, 3607. Toxicology: J. S. Welles *et al.*, *Toxicol. Appl. Pharmacol.* **22**, 332 (1972). Comprehensive description: A. K. Dash, *Anal. Profiles Drug Subs. Excip.* **24**, 579-613 (1996). Clinical trial in cystic fibrosis patients: B. W. Ramsey *et al.*, *N. Engl. J. Med.* **340**, 23 (1999). Review of clinical experience: H. Lode, *Curr. Ther. Res.* **59**, 420-453 (1998).

Basic substance. Freely sol in water (1 in 1.5 parts). Very slightly sol in ethanol (1 in 2000 parts). Practically insol in chloroform, ether. $[\alpha]_D^{20}$ +129° (c = 1 in water). LD_{50} in mice, rats (mg/kg): 441, 969 s.c. (Welles).

Sulfate. [79645-27-5] Gernebcin; Nebcin; Nebicina; Obracin; Tobra; Tobradistin.

THERAP CAT: Antibacterial.

9491. Tocainide. [41708-72-9] 2-Amino-*N*-(2,6-dimethyl-phenyl)propanamide; 2-aminopropiono-2′,6′-xylidide. $C_{11}H_{16}N_2$-

O; mol wt 192.26. C 68.72%, H 8.39%, N 14.57%, O 8.32%. Antiarrhythmic agent related to lidocaine, *q.v.* Prepn: R. N. Boys *et al.*, **DE 2235745** (1973 to Astra), *C.A.* **78**, 140411 (1973); and resolution of isomers: E. W. Byrnes *et al.*, *J. Med. Chem.* **22**, 1171 (1979). *In vitro* effects on muscle contractions: R. Dengler, R. Rüdel, *Arzneim.-Forsch.* **29**, 270 (1979). Inhibition of leucocyte locomotion in dogs: G. J. Stewart *et al.*, *Lab. Invest.* **42**, 302 (1980). Biotransformation in humans: A. T. Elvin *et al.*, *J. Pharm. Sci.* **69**, 47 (1980). Kinetics: C. Groffner, *Clin. Pharmacol. Ther.* **27**, 64 (1980). Use in refractory ventricular arrhythmias: D. M. Roden *et al.*, *Am. Heart J.* **100**, 15 (1980). HPLC resolution of enantiomers: K. M. McErlane, G. K. Pillai, *J. Chromatogr.* **274**, 129 (1983); determn in plasma: A. J. Sedman, J. Gal, *ibid.* **306**, 155 (1984). Pharmacokinetics of enantiomers: A. H. Thomson *et al.*, *Br. J. Pharmacol.* **21**, 149 (1986). *In vitro* and *in vivo* pharmacodynamics of enantiomers: A. J. Block *et al.*, *J. Cardiovasc. Pharmacol.* **11**, 216 (1988). Review of pharmacology and therapeutic efficacy: B. Holmes *et al.*, *Drugs* **26**, 93-123 (1983); D. M. Roden, R. L. Woosley, *N. Engl. J. Med.* **315**, 41-45 (1986).

(±)-Form hydrochloride. [71395-14-7] W-36095; Taquidil; Tonocard; Xylotocan. $C_{11}H_{16}N_2O$·HCl; mol wt 228.72. Crystals from ethanol/ether, mp 246-247°.

R-(−)-Form hydrochloride. [53984-74-0] Crystals from ethanol-diethyl ether, mp 265-266°. $[\alpha]_D$ −42.16° (c = 2.63 in methanol).

S-(+)-Form hydrochloride. [53984-76-2] Crystals from ethanol-diethyl ether, mp 264.5°. $[\alpha]_D$ +42.35° (c = 2.63 in methanol).

THERAP CAT: Antiarrhythmic (class IB).

9492. Tocamphyl. [5634-42-8] 1,2,2-Trimethyl-1,3-cyclo-pentanedicarboxylic acid 1-[1-(4-methylphenyl)ethyl] ester, compd with 2,2′-iminobis[ethanol] (1:1); camphoric acid 1-(*p*,α-dimethyl-benzyl) ester, compd with 2,2′-imidodiethanol (1:1); *p*,α-dimethyl-benzyl camphorate diethanolamine salt; *p*-toluoylmethylcarbinol-mono-*d*-camphoric acid ester diethanolamine salt; methyl *p*-tolyl-carbinol camphorate diethanolamine salt; *p*-tolylmethylcarbinol camphoric acid ester diethanolamine salt; diethanolamine *p*-tolyl-methylcarbinol camphorate; diethanolamine *d*-methyltoluylcarbinol camphorate; Biliphorine; Hepatoxane; Syncuma. $C_{23}H_{37}NO_6$; mol wt 423.54. C 65.22%, H 8.81%, N 3.31%, O 22.67%. Prepn: **CH 211203** (1940 to Chemiewerk Homburg); *Chem. Zentralbl.* **1941**, I, 2972.

Crystals, sol in water.

THERAP CAT: Choleretic.

9493. Tocilizumab. [375823-41-9] Anti-(human interleukin 6 receptor) immunoglobulin G1 (human-mouse monoclonal MRA heavy chain) disulfide with human-mouse monoclonal MRA κ-chain, dimer; atlizumab; MRA; rhPM-1; R-1569; Actemra. Recombinant humanized monoclonal antibody directed against human interleukin 6 receptor (IL-6R); designed to inhibit biological activities of IL-6. Prepn: M. Tsuchiya *et al.*, **WO 9219759**; *eidem*, **US 5795965** (1992, 1998 both to Chugai); K. Sato *et al.*, *Cancer Res.* **53**, 851 (1993). Pharmacology: H. Shinkura *et al.*, *Anticancer Res.* **18**, 1217 (1998). Clinical pharmacokinetics: N. Nishimoto *et al.*, *J. Rheumatol.* **30**, 1426 (2003). Clinical study in rheumatoid arthritis: *idem et al.*, *Arthritis Rheum.* **50**, 1761 (2004); in Crohn's disease: H. Ito *et al.*, *Gastroenterology* **126**, 989 (2004). Review of preclinical and clinical pharmacology: N. Nishimoto *et al.*, *Ann. Rheum. Dis.* **59**, Suppl. 1, i21-i27 (2000); and therapeutic potential: C. Ding, G. Jones, *Curr. Opin. Mol. Ther.* **5**, 64-69 (2003); of mechanism of action: H. Ito, *Expert Opin. Ther. Targets* **8**, 287-294 (2004).

THERAP CAT: Anti-inflammatory.

9494. Tocol. [119-98-2] 3,4-Dihydro-2-methyl-2-(4,8,12-trimethyltridecyl)-2*H*-1-benzopyran-6-ol; 2-methyl-2-(4,8,12-trimethyltridecyl)-6-chromanol; 2-methyl-2-phytyl-6-chromanol; 6-hydroxy-2-methyl-2-phytylchroman; 2-methyl-2-phytyl-6-hydroxychroman. $C_{26}H_{44}O_2$; mol wt 388.63. C 80.35%, H 11.41%, O 8.23%. Synthesis by the condensation of hydroquinone and phytol in the presence of anhydr formic acid: Pendse, Karrer, *Helv. Chim. Acta* **40**, 1837 (1957). Antioxidant activity of tocol and its methyl derivs: Olcott, van der Veen, *Lipids* **3**, 331 (1968).

Colorless, viscous oil. $bp_{0.001}$ 165-175°.

Acetate. $C_{28}H_{46}O_3$. Viscous oil. $bp_{0.001}$ 180-185°.

USE: Antioxidant.

9495. α-Tocopherol. [59-02-9] (2*R*)-3,4-Dihydro-2,5,7,8-tetramethyl-2-[(4*R*,8*R*)-4,8,12-trimethyltridecyl]-2*H*-1-benzopyran-6-ol; (+)-2,5,7,8-tetramethyl-2-(4′,8′,12′-trimethyltridecyl)-6-chromanol; *R,R,R*-α-tocopherol; *d*-α-tocopherol; 5,7,8-trimethyltocol; Optovit; Tocovital. $C_{29}H_{50}O_2$; mol wt 430.71. C 80.87%, H 11.70%, O 7.43%. Most bioactive of the naturally occurring forms of vitamin E, *q.v.* Richest sources are green vegetables, grains, and oils, particularly palm, safflower and sunflower oils. Isoln from wheat germ: H. M. Evans *et al., J. Biol. Chem.* **113**, 319 (1936). Structure: E. Fernholz, *J. Am. Chem. Soc.* **59**, 1154 (1937); **60**, 700 (1938). Synthesis of *dl*-form: P. Karrer *et al., Helv. Chim. Acta* **21**, 520, 820 (1938); F. Bergel *et al., J. Chem. Soc.* **1938**, 1382. Distillation from vegetable oils and prepn of esters: J. G. Baxter *et al., J. Am. Chem. Soc.* 918 (1943). Prepn of crystalline natural form: C. D. Robeson, *ibid.* 1660 (1942); of crystalline acetate: *idem, ibid.* **64**, 1487 (1942). Abs config of natural α-tocopherol: H. Mayer *et al., Helv. Chim. Acta* **46**, 963 (1963). Stereoselective synthesis: K.-K. Chan *et al., J. Org. Chem.* **43**, 3435 (1978). Total synthesis of all 8 stereoisomers: N. Cohen *et al., Helv. Chim. Acta* **64**, 1158 (1981). Clinical trial in Alzheimer's disease: M. Sano *et al., N. Engl. J. Med.* **336**, 1216 (1997); to improve immune function in healthy elderly: S. N. Meydani *et al., J. Am. Med. Assoc.* **277**, 1380 (1997). Review of bioavailability from vitamin E supplements: M. G. Traber, *BioFactors* **10**, 115-120 (1999). Review of clinical trials in heart disease: W. A. Pryor, *Free Radical Biol. Med.* **28**, 141-164 (2000).

Transparent needles, mp 2.5-3.5°. $[\alpha]_{546.1}^{25}$ −3.0° (benzene); $[\alpha]_{546.1}^{25}$ +0.32° (ethanol).

Acetate. [58-95-7] Spondyvit. $C_{31}H_{52}O_3$; mol wt 472.74. Light yellow oil. Crystallized at −30° as needle-like crystals, mp 26.5-27.5°. $[\alpha]_D^{25}$ +0.25° (c = 10 in chloroform); $[\alpha]_D^{25}$ +3.2° (in ethanol).

Succinate. [4345-03-3] *d*-α-Tocopheryl acid succinate; Tocovite. Needles from petr ether, mp 76-77°. uv max (ethanol): 286 nm ($E_{1cm}^{1\%}$ 38.5). Practically insol in water.

***dl*-α-Tocopherol.** [10191-41-0] *all-rac*-α-Tocopherol. Equimolar mixture of all four racemates. Slightly viscous, pale yellow oil. d_4^{25} 0.950; $bp_{0.1}$ 200-220°; n_D^{25} 1.5045. uv max: 294 nm ($E_{1cm}^{1\%}$ 71). Practically insol in water. Freely sol in oils, fats, acetone, alcohol, chloroform, ether, other fat solvents. Stable to heat and alkalies in the absence of oxygen. Not affected by acids up to 100°. Slowly oxidized by atm oxygen, rapidly by ferric and silver salts. Gradually darkens on exposure to light.

***dl*-α-Tocopherol acetate.** [52225-20-4] *dl*-α-Tocopheryl acetate; Detulin; Ephynal; Eusovit; Evion. Comprehensive description: B. C. Rudy, B. Z. Senkowski, *Anal. Profiles Drug Subs.* **3**, 111-126 (1974). Pale yellow, viscous liquid. mp −27.5°. $d_4^{21.3}$ 0.9533. $bp_{0.01}$ 184°; $bp_{0.025}$ 194°; $bp_{0.3}$ 224°. n_D^{20} 1.4950-1.4972. uv max (cyclohexane): 285.5 nm. Practically insol in water. Freely sol in acetone, chloroform, ether. Less readily sol in alc.

USE: As an antioxidant in vegetable oils and shortening.

THERAP CAT: Vitamin E supplement.

THERAP CAT (VET): Vitamin E supplement.

9496. β-Tocopherol. [16698-35-4]; [148-03-8] (*dl*-form). (2*R*)-3,4-Dihydro-2,5,8-trimethyl-2-[(4*R*,8*R*)-4,8,12-trimethyltridecyl]-2*H*-1-benzopyran-6-ol; (+)-2,5,8-trimethyl-2-(4,8,12-trimethyltridecyl)-6-chromanol; 5,8-dimethyltocol; cumotocopherol; neotocopherol; *p*-xylotocopherol. $C_{28}H_{48}O_2$; mol wt 416.68. C 80.71%, H 11.61%, O 7.68%. One of the naturally occurring forms of vitamin E, *q.v.* Is biologically less active than α-tocopherol. May be separated by fractional crystn: Emerson *et al., Science* **83**, 421 (1936); *J. Biol. Chem.* **113**, 319 (1936); Baxter *et al., J. Am. Chem. Soc.* **65**, 918 (1943).

Pale yellow, viscous oil. $bp_{0.1}$ 200-210°. $[\alpha]_{546.1}^{25}$ +2.9° (c = 7.15 in ethanol). uv max: 297 nm ($E_{1cm}^{1\%}$ 87.6). Insol in water. Freely sol in oils, fats, acetone, alcohol, chloroform, ether, other fat solvents. Very stable to heat and alkalies. Slowly oxidized by atmospheric oxygen, rapidly by ferric and silver salts. Gradually darkens on exposure to light.

9497. γ-Tocopherol. [54-28-4]; [7616-22-0] (*dl*-form). (2*R*)-3,4-Dihydro-2,7,8-trimethyl-2-[(4*R*,8*R*)-4,8,12-trimethyltridecyl]-2*H*-1-benzopyran-6-ol; (+)-2,7,8-trimethyl-2-(4,8,12-trimethyltridecyl)-6-chromanol; (*R,R,R*)-γ-tocopherol; 7,8-dimethyltocol; *o*-xylotocopherol. $C_{28}H_{48}O_2$; mol wt 416.68. C 80.71%, H 11.61%, O 7.68%. One of the naturally occurring forms of vitamin E, *q.v.* Most abundant tocopherol in soybean and corn oils. Isoln by fractional crystn: Emerson *et al., Science* **83**, 421 (1936); *J. Biol. Chem.* **113**, 319 (1936); J. G. Baxter *et al., J. Am. Chem. Soc.* **65**, 918 (1943). Prepn of crystalline natural form: C. D. Robeson, *J. Am. Chem. Soc.* **65**, 1660 (1943). Comparison of bioactivity with α-tocopherol, *q.v.*: J. G. Bieri, R. P. Evarts, *J. Nutr.* **104**, 850 (1974). Protective effects vs reactive nitrogen oxide species: R. V. Cooney *et al., Proc. Natl. Acad. Sci. USA* **90**, 1771 (1993); S. Christen *et al., ibid.* **94**, 3217 (1997). HPLC determn in serum: A. Sobczak *et al., J. Chromatogr. B* **730**, 265 (1999). Review of bioavailability, metabolism, and activity: Q. Jiang *et al., Am. J. Clin. Nutr.* **74**, 714-722 (2001).

Pale yellow, viscous oil. Has been crystallized as transparent needles, mp −3 to −2°. $bp_{0.1}$ 200-210°. $[\alpha]_{546.1}^{25}$ −2.4° (c = 8.59 in benzene); $[\alpha]_{546.1}^{25}$ +2.2° (c = 9.32 in ethanol). uv max: 298 nm ($E_{1cm}^{1\%}$ 92.8). Insol in water. Freely sol in oils, fats, acetone, alcohol, chloroform, ether, other fat solvents. Very stable to heat and alkalies. Slowly oxidized by atmospheric oxygen, rapidly by ferric and silver salts. Gradually darkens on exposure to light.

9498. δ-Tocopherol. [119-13-1] (2*R*)-3,4-Dihydro-2,8-dimethyl-2-[(4*R*,8*R*)-4,8,12-trimethyltridecyl]-2*H*-1-benzopyran-6-ol; 8-methyltocol. $C_{27}H_{46}O_2$; mol wt 402.65. C 80.54%, H 11.52%, O 7.95%. One of the naturally occurring forms of vitamin E, *q.v.* Isoln from soybean oil: Stern *et al., J. Am. Chem. Soc.* **69**, 869 (1947). Synthesis: Green *et al., J. Chem. Soc.* **1959**, 3374; GB **900085** (1961 to Hoffmann-La Roche).

Pale yellow, viscous oil. $[\alpha]_{546}^{25}$ +3.4° (c = 15.5 in alc); $[\alpha]_{546}^{25}$ +1.1° (c = 10.9 in benzene). uv max: 298 nm ($E_{1cm}^{1\%}$ 91.2).

9499. Tocoretinate. [40516-48-1] Retinoic acid *rel*-(2*R*)-3,4-dihydro-2,5,7,8-tetramethyl-2-[(4*R*,8*R*)-4,8,12-trimethyltridecyl]-2*H*-1-benzopyran-6-yl ester; (±)-(2*R**)-2,5,7,8-tetramethyl-2-[(4*R**,8*R**)-4,8,12-trimethyltridecyl]-6-chromanyl retinoate; tretinoin tocoferil; DL-α-tocopheryl retinoate; L-300; N-021; Olcenon. $C_{49}H_{76}O_3$; mol wt 713.13. C 82.53%, H 10.74%, O 6.73%. Wound healing agent that stimulates proliferation of normal skin fibroblasts. Prepn: H. Fukawa, K. Tanaka, **JP Kokai 73 00469**; *eidem*, **US 3878202** (1973, 1975 both to Nisshin Flour Milling Co.). Pharmacology: K. Sakyo *et al.*, *Oyo Yakuri* **43**, 111 (1992), *C.A.* **116**, 228223z (1992). Pharmacokinetics: T. Nakazawa *et al.*, *ibid.* 205, *C.A.* **117**, 19823 (1993). Mechanism of action study: N. Kawamura *et al.*, *Dig. Dis. Sci.* **39**, 2191 (1994). Clinical evaluation in skin ulcers: T. Doi, *Skin Res.* **36**, 384 (1994); K. Nakagawa *et al.*, *ibid.* 209. Acute toxicity study: Y. Harada *et al.*, *Oyo Yakuri* **43**, 227 (1992), *C.A.* **117**, 20721 (1992).

Light yellow oil. uv max (ethanol): 365 nm ($E_{1cm}^{1\%}$ 642). LD_{50} in mice (mg/kg): >1000 i.v.; >2000 orally (Fukawa, 1975).

THERAP CAT: Vulnerary.

9500. α-Tocotrienol. [58864-81-6]; [1721-51-3] (unspecified stereo). (2*R*)-3,4-Dihydro-2,5,7,8-tetramethyl-2-[(3*E*,7*E*)-4,8,12-trimethyl-3,7,11-tridecatrienyl]-2*H*-1-benzopyran-6-ol; 2,5,7,8-tetramethyl-2-(4,8,12-trimethyl-3,7,11-tridecatrienyl)-6-chromanol; ζ_1-tocopherol. $C_{29}H_{44}O_2$; mol wt 424.66. C 82.02%, H 10.44%, O 7.54%. One of the naturally occurring forms of vitamin E, *q.v.* Isoln from wheat bran: Green *et al.*, *J. Sci. Food Agric.* **6**, 274 (1955); Green *et al.*, *Chem. Ind. (London)* **1960**, 73. Structure: Green *et al.*, *J. Chem. Soc.* **1959**, 3362. Attempt at synthesis: McHale *et al.*, *ibid.* **1963**, 784. *Review:* M. Kofler *et al.*, "Physicochemical Properties and Assay of the Tocopherols" in R. S. Harris, I. G. Wood, *Vitam. Horm.* **20**, 407-439 (1962). Synthesis of all-*trans*-form: Schudel *et al.*, *Helv. Chim. Acta* **46**, 2517 (1963).

uv max (ethanol): 292.5 nm ($E_{1cm}^{1\%}$ 91).

9501. β-Tocotrienol. [490-23-3] (2*R*)-3,4-Dihydro-2,5,8-trimethyl-2-[(3*E*,7*E*)-4,8,12-trimethyl-3,7,11-tridecatrienyl]-2*H*-1-benzopyran-6-ol; 2,5,8-trimethyl-2-(4,8,12-trimethyltrideca-3,7,11-trienyl)chroman-6-ol; 5-methyltocol; ε-tocopherol. $C_{28}H_{42}O_2$; mol wt 410.63. C 81.90%, H 10.31%, O 7.79%. One of the naturally occurring forms of vitamin E, *q.v.* Isoln from wheat germ oil and from bran: Eggitt, Ward, *J. Sci. Food Agric.* **4**, 569 (1953); Eggitt, Norris, *ibid.* **6**, 689 (1955); **7**, 496 (1956). Structure: Green *et al.*, *J. Chem. Soc.* **1959**, 3362; *Chem. Ind. (London)* **1960**, 73; McHale *et al.*, *J. Chem. Soc.* **1963**, 784. Synthesis: Schudel *et al.*, *Helv. Chim. Acta* **46**, 2517 (1963).

Pale yellow oil. uv max (ethanol): 296 nm ($E_{1cm}^{1\%}$ 87).

9502. Todralazine. [14679-73-3] 2-(1-Phthalazinyl)hydrazinecarboxylic acid ethyl ester; 3-(1-phthalazinyl)carbazic acid ethyl ester; N^1-carbethoxy-N^2-phthalazinehydrazine; carboethoxyphthalazinohydrazine; ecarazine. $C_{11}H_{12}N_4O_2$; mol wt 232.24. C 56.89%, H 5.21%, N 24.12%, O 13.78%. Prepn: S. Biniecki *et al.*, *Bull. Acad. Pol. Sci. Ser. Sci.* **6**, 227 (1958), *C.A.* **52**, 18424g (1958); *eidem*, **BE 647722**; *eidem*, **US 3591588** (1964, 1971 both to Polfa). Spectrofluorometric determn in plasma: A. Ishii, T. Deguchi, *Chem. Pharm. Bull.* **26**, 2241 (1978). Pharmacological study: M. Filczewski, E. Boguka, *Pol. J. Pharmacol. Pharm.* **31**, 127 (1979), *C.A.* **91**, 204508 (1979). Absorption, distribution, excretion in rats and humans: A. Ishii *et al.*, *Oyo Yakuri* **18**, 61 (1979), *C.A.* **92**, 104012 (1980). Clinical study: W. Reiterer, H. Czitober, *Arzneim.-Forsch.* **27**, 2163 (1977). Toxicity study: F. Parravincini *et al.*, *Farmaco Ed. Sci.* **34**, 299 (1979).

Hydrochloride. [3778-76-5] CEPH; BT-621; Apiracohl; Aperdor; Apride; Atapren; Binazin; Illcut; Propat. $C_{11}H_{12}N_4O_2$·HCl; mol wt 268.70. LD_{50} i.p. in mice: 500 mg/kg (Parravincini).

THERAP CAT: Antihypertensive.

9503. Tofisopam. [22345-47-7] 1-(3,4-Dimethoxyphenyl)-5-ethyl-7,8-dimethoxy-4-methyl-5*H*-2,3-benzodiazepine; EGYT-341; Grandaxin; Seriel. $C_{22}H_{26}N_2O_4$; mol wt 382.45. C 69.09%, H 6.85%, N 7.32%, O 16.73%. The first 5*H*-2,3-benzodiazepine. Prepn: J. Korosi *et al.*, **HU 155572** (1969 to Pharm. Res. Inst.), *C.A.* **70**, 115026a (1969); **GB 1202579** corresp to **US 3736315** (1970, 1973 both to EGYT); J. Korosi, T. Lang, *Ber.* **107**, 3883 (1974). Synthesis and conformation: *eidem*, *Ther. Hung.* **23**, 132 (1975). FT ^{13}C NMR study: A. Neszmelyi *et al.*, *Ber.* **107**, 3894 (1974). Pharmacology: L. Petocz, I. Kosoczky, *Ther. Hung.* **23**, 134 (1975). Human pharmacokinetics: S. Ronai *et al.*, *ibid.* 139. Comparative efficacy: H. L. Goldberg, R. J. Finnerty, *Am. J. Psychiatry* **136**, 196 (1979).

Colorless to light cream cryst powder from isopropyl alcohol, mp 156-157°. uv max (methanol): 310, 272, 239 nm (ε 16100, 11200, 26300).

THERAP CAT: Anxiolytic.

9504. Tolan. [501-65-5] 1,1'-(1,2-Ethynediyl)bisbenzene; diphenylacetylene; diphenylethyne. $C_{14}H_{10}$; mol wt 178.23. C 94.34%, H 5.66%. $C_6H_5C \equiv CC_6H_5$. Prepd by the oxidation of benzil dihydrazone with mercuric oxide: Schlenk, Bergmann, *Ann.* **463**, 76 (1928); by dehydrohalogenation of stilbene dibromide: Söderbäck, *Ann.* **443**, 161 (1925); Smith, Hoehn, *J. Am. Chem.*

Soc. **63,** 1180 (1941); Smith, Falkof, *Org. Synth.* **coll. vol. III,** 350 (1955). Improved procedure: L. F. Fieser, *Experiments in Organic Chemistry* (Boston, 3rd ed., 1955) p 181.

Monoclinic, pseudo-rhombic rods or large spears from 95% ethanol. mp 60-61° (also reported as 62.5°). bp_{760} 300°; bp_{19} 170°. Dipole moment 0.3. Specific heat at 20°: 0.297. uv max: 216, 221, 269, 272, 279, 288, 297 nm (ε 20600, 20300, 23450, 25200, 33000, 23250, 29400). Insol in water. Freely sol in ether, hot alcohol.

9505. Tolazamide. [1156-19-0] N-[[(Hexahydro-1*H*-azepin-1-yl)amino]carbonyl]-4-methylbenzenesulfonamide; 1-(hexahydro-1*H*-azepin-1-yl)-3-(*p*-tolylsulfonyl)urea; N-(*p*-toluenesulfonyl)-N'-hexamethyleniminourea; tolazolamide; U-17835; Tolanase. $C_{14}H_{21}N_3O_3S$; mol wt 311.40. C 54.00%, H 6.80%, N 13.49%, O 15.41%, S 10.30%. Prepn: J. B. Wright, **GB 887886** (1962 to Upjohn); J. B. Wright, R. E. Willette, *J. Med. Pharm. Chem.* **5,** 815 (1962). Pharmacology: W. E. Dulin *et al., Proc. Soc. Exp. Biol. Med.* **107,** 245 (1961). Mode of action study: Marshall *et al., Metab. Clin. Exp.* **19,** 1046 (1970). Clinical experience and review of early literature: Balodimos, Marble, *Curr. Ther. Res.* **13,** 6-12 (1971). Clinical bioavailability and pharmacokinetics: P. G. Welling *et al., J. Pharm. Sci.* **71,** 1259 (1982). Structural studies: C. H. Koo *et al., Arch. Pharmacal Res.* **11,** 74 (1988). HPLC determn in serum: B. J. Starkey *et al., J. Liq. Chromatogr.* **12,** 1889 (1989). Comprehensive description: J. K. Lee *et al., Anal. Profiles Drug Subs. Excip.* **22,** 489-516 (1993).

Crystals, mp 170-173°. Very slightly sol in water; slightly sol in alcohol; sol in acetone; freely sol in chloroform. pKa (25°): 3.6, pKa (37.5°): 5.68. LD_{50} in rats, mice (mg/kg): >5000 orally, 2239 i.p. (Dulin).

THERAP CAT: Antidiabetic.

9506. Tolazoline. [59-98-3] 4,5-Dihydro-2-(phenylmethyl)-1*H*-imidazole; 2-benzyl-2-imidazoline; 2-benzyl-2-iminazoline; benzazoline; 2-benzyl-4,5-imidazoline; phenylmethylimidazoline. $C_{10}H_{12}N_2$; mol wt 160.22. C 74.96%, H 7.55%, N 17.48%. α-Adrenergic blocker. Prepn: Sonn, **US 2161938** (1939 to Ciba). HPLC determn in serum: L. M. L. Todesco *et al., Ther. Drug Monit.* **9,** 78 (1987). Review of pharmacology and clinical use: R. M. Ward, *Clin. Perinatol.* **11,** 703-713 (1984).

Hydrochloride. [59-97-2] Lambral; Priscol; Priscoline; Vaso-Dilatan. $C_{10}H_{12}N_2$·HCl; mol wt 196.68. Bitter crystals, mp 174°. Freely sol in water, alcohol; sol in chloroform; very slightly sol in ether, ethyl acetate. pH of 2.5% soln 4.9-5.3.

THERAP CAT: Vasodilator (peripheral).

9507. Tolbutamide. [64-77-7] N-[(Butylamino)carbonyl]-4-methylbenzenesulfonamide; 1-butyl-3-(*p*-tolylsulfonyl)urea; tolylsulfonylbutylurea; 3-(*p*-tolyl-4-sulfonyl)-1-butylurea; N-*n*-butyl-N'-tosylurea; N'-4-methylbenzenesulfonyl-N''-butylurea; N-(sulfonyl-*p*-methylbenzene)-N'-*n*-butylurea; D-860; U-2043; Artosin; Diaben; Dolipol; Mobenol; Orabet; Orinase; Oterben; Pramidex; Rastinon. $C_{12}H_{18}N_2O_3S$; mol wt 270.35. C 53.31%, H 6.71%, N 10.36%, O 17.75%, S 11.86%. Description: Ehrhart, *Naturwissenschaften* **43,** 93 (1956). Prepn: **GB 808071**; Aumüller, Herr, **DE 1066575** (both 1959 to Hoechst); Ruschig *et al.,* **US 2968158** (1961 to Upjohn). Comprehensive description: W. F. Beyer, E. H. Jensen, *Anal. Profiles Drug Subs.* **3,** 513-543 (1974).

Crystals, mp 128.5-129.5°.
Sodium salt. [473-41-6] $C_{12}H_{17}N_2NaO_3S$. mp 130-133°. Tetrahydrate, mp 41-43°.

THERAP CAT: Antidiabetic.
THERAP CAT (VET): Hypoglycemic agent.

9508. Tolcapone. [134308-13-7] (3,4-Dihydroxy-5-nitrophenyl)(4-methylphenyl)methanone; 3,4-dihydroxy-4'-methyl-5-nitrobenzophenone; Ro-40-7592; Tasmar. $C_{14}H_{11}NO_5$; mol wt 273.24. C 61.54%, H 4.06%, N 5.13%, O 29.28%. Orally active inhibitor of central and peripheral catechol-O-methyltransferase (COMT). Prepn: K. Bernauer *et al.,* **EP 237929**; *eidem,* **US 5236952** (1987, 1993 both to Hoffmann-La Roche). Pharmacology: G. Zürcher *et al., Adv. Neurol.* **53,** 497 (1990). HPLC determn in plasma: U. Timm, R. Erdin, *J. Chromatogr.* **593,** 63 (1992). Clinical pharmacokinetics: J. Dingemanse *et al., Clin. Pharmacol. Ther.* **57,** 508 (1995). Clinical evaluation as adjunct to levodopa: P. Limousin *et al., Clin. Neuropharmacol.* **18,** 258 (1995). Review of pharmacology and clinical experience: G. M. Keating, K. A. Lyseng-Williamson, *CNS Drugs* **19,** 165-184 (2005); of safety and efficacy: N. Borges, *Expert Opin. Drug Saf.* **4,** 69-73 (2005).

Crystals from methylene chloride, mp 146-148°.
THERAP CAT: Antiparkinsonian.

9509. Tolciclate. [50838-36-3] Methyl(3-methylphenyl)-carbamothioic acid O-(1,2,3,4-tetrahydro-1,4-methanonaphthalen-6-yl) ester; O-(1,4-methano-1,2,3,4-tetrahydro-6-naphthyl)-N-methyl-N-(*m*-tolyl)thiocarbamate; KC-9147; Fungifos; Kilmicen; Tolmicen. $C_{20}H_{21}NOS$; mol wt 323.45. C 74.27%, H 6.54%, N 4.33%, O 4.95%, S 9.91%. Topical antimycotic agent with high liposolubility. Prepn: P. Melloni *et al.,* **DE 2313845** corresp to **US 3855263** (1973, 1974 both to Carlo Erba). *In vitro* and *in vivo* study: I. deCarneri *et al., Arzneim.-Forsch.* **26,** 769 (1976). Antimycotic studies: A. Bianchi *et al., Antimicrob. Agents Chemother.* **12,** 429 (1977). Clinical studies in dermatomycosis: L. C. Cucé *et al., J. Int. Med. Res.* **8,** 144 (1980); C. Intini *et al., Pharmatherapeutica* **2,** 439 (1980).

White cryst powder from isopropanol, mp 92-94°. Practically insol in water. Soly (mg/ml): 14.9 in *n*-hexane; 23.9 in *n*-octanol. LD_{50} in mice, rats, dogs (mg/kg): 4000, 6000, 5000 orally (deCarneri).

THERAP CAT: Antifungal.

9510. Tolclofos-methyl. [57018-04-9] O-(2,6-Dichloro-4-methylphenyl)phosphorothioic acid O,O-dimethyl ester; O-(2,6-dichloro-*p*-tolyl) O,O-dimethyl phosphorothioate; tolclophos-methyl; S-3349; Rizolex. $C_9H_{11}Cl_2O_3PS$; mol wt 301.13. C 35.90%, H 3.68%, Cl 23.55%, O 15.94%, P 10.29%, S 10.65%. Organophosphorus fungicide; inhibits phospholipid biosynthesis. Prepn: T. Kato *et al.,* **DE 2501040**; **GB 1467561** (1975, 1977 both to Sumitomo). Properties and biological activity: S. Ohtsuki, A. Fujinami, *Jpn. Pestic. Inf.* **41,** 21 (1982). Synthesis: M. Sasaki *et al., J.*

Pestic. Sci. **9,** 737 (1984). Mode of action: S. Nakamura, T. Kato, *ibid.* 725; P. Leroux *et al., Pestic. Sci.* **36,** 255 (1992). GC determn in soil, lettuce: M. Gennari *et al., J. AOAC Int.* **80,** 1298 (1997). Control of bottom rot on lettuce: J. R. Coley-Smith *et al., Plant Pathol.* **40,** 359 (1991).

White crystals from methanol, mp 79-79.5°. Vapor pressure at 20°: 4.27×10^{-4} mm Hg. Soly at 23°: water 0.3-0.4 ppm. Easily sol in xylene, acetone, cyclohexanone, chloroform. LD_{50} in male, female rats, male, female mice (mg/kg): ~5000, ~5000, 3500, 3600 orally; all >5000 dermally; ~5000, 4900, 1070, 1260 i.p.; all >5000 s.c. (Ohtsuki, Fujinami).
USE: Agricultural fungicide.

9511. Tolcyclamide. [664-95-9] *N*-[(Cyclohexylamino)carbonyl]-4-methylbenzenesulfonamide; 1-cyclohexyl-3-*p*-tolylsulfonylurea; tolhexamide; glycyclamide; cyclamide; K-386; Diaboral. $C_{14}H_{20}N_2O_3S$; mol wt 296.39. C 56.73%, H 6.80%, N 9.45%, O 16.19%, S 10.82%. Prepn: Logemann, Artini, *Ber.* **90,** 2527 (1957).

Crystals from trichloroethylene, mp 174-176°.
THERAP CAT: Antidiabetic.

9512. Toldimfos Sodium. [575-75-7] (4-Dimethylamino-*o*-tolyl)phosphonous acid sodium salt; sodium (4-dimethylamino-*o*-tolyl)phosphonate; *p*-dimethylamino-*o*-toluenephosphonous acid sodium salt; Foston; Tonofosfan. $C_9H_{13}NNaO_2P$; mol wt 221.17. C 48.87%, H 5.92%, N 6.33%, Na 10.39%, O 14.47%, P 14.00%. Prepd from *N,N*-dimethyl-*m*-toluidine and phosphorus trichloride: Benda, Schmidt, **DE 397813** (1924 to Cassella), *Frdl.* **14,** 1409.

Trihydrate. [5787-63-3] Scales, needles, or prisms from alc. Freely sol in cold water, hot alcohol.
THERAP CAT (VET): Phosphorus source.

9513. Tolfenamic Acid. [13710-19-5] 2-[(3-Chloro-2-methylphenyl)amino]benzoic acid; *N*-(3-chloro-*o*-tolyl)anthranilic acid; *N*-(2-methyl-3-chlorophenyl)anthranilic acid; GEA-6414; Clotam; Tolfedine; Tolfine. $C_{14}H_{12}ClNO_2$; mol wt 261.70. C 64.25%, H 4.62%, Cl 13.55%, N 5.35%, O 12.23%. Deriv of anthranilic acid, related structurally to mefenamic and flufenamic acids, *q.q.v.* Prepn: **NL 6600251** (1966 to Gea A/S), *C.A.* **66,** 2377 (1967); R. A. Scherrer, F. W. Short, **US 3313848** (1967 to Parke, Davis). Inhibition of prostaglandin biosynthesis: I. B. Linden *et al., Scand. J. Rheumatol.* **5,** 129 (1976). HPLC determn: F. Nielsen-Kudsk, *Acta Pharmacol. Toxicol.* **47,** 267 (1980). Metabolism: T. Kuninaka *et al., Yakugaku Zasshi* **101,** 232 (1981), *C.A.* **95,** 168 (1981). Human pharmacokinetics: P. Pentikaeinen *et al., Eur. J. Clin. Pharmacol.* **19,** 359 (1981). Pharmacological studies: S. Yamashita *et al., Toho Igakkai Zasshi* **28,** 76-105 (1981), *C.A.* **95,** 16183, 180846 (1981). Clinical study: V. Rejholec *et al., Scand. J. Rheumatol.* **Suppl. 33,** 50 (1980); **Suppl. 36,** 1 (1980).

Crystals from abs ethanol, mp 207-207.5°.
THERAP CAT: Anti-inflammatory; analgesic.
THERAP CAT (VET): Anti-inflammatory.

9514. *o*-Tolidine. [119-93-7] 3,3'-Dimethyl-[1,1'-biphenyl]-4,4'-diamine; 3,3'-dimethylbenzidine; 4,4'-diamino-3,3'-dimethylbiphenyl. $C_{14}H_{16}N_2$; mol wt 212.29. C 79.21%, H 7.60%, N 13.20%. Made by alkaline reduction of *o*-nitrotoluene with zinc, and subsequent rearrangement of the *o*-hydrazotoluene formed, by boiling with HCl: Van Loon, *Chem. Weekbl.* **5,** 689 (1907). *See also* Schultz *et al., Ann.* **352,** 111 (1907). Crystal and molecular structure: Chawdhury *et al., Acta Crystallogr.* **B24,** 1222 (1968). Metabolism: Dieteren, *Arch. Environ. Health* **12,** 30 (1966). Carcinogenic activity: Pliss, Zebenzhinskii, *J. Natl. Cancer Inst.* **45,** 283 (1970).

White to reddish crystals or cryst powder. mp 129-131°. Slightly sol in water; sol in alcohol, ether, dil acids. *Keep well closed and protected from light.*
Sulfate. $C_{14}H_{16}N_2 \cdot H_2SO_4$. White to gray mass. Slightly sol in water, alcohol; sol in dil acids.
Caution: Potential symptoms of overexposure to *o*-tolidine are irritation of eyes and nose. *See NIOSH Pocket Guide to Chemical Hazards* (DHHS/NIOSH 97-140, 1997) p 310. *o*-Tolidine is reasonably anticipated to be a human carcinogen: *Report on Carcinogens, Eleventh Edition* (PB2005-104914, 2004) p III-104.
USE: Manuf dyes; also as very sensitive reagent for gold (1:10 million detectable), and for free chlorine in water.

9515. Tolindate. [27877-51-6] Methyl (3-methylphenyl)-carbamothioic acid *O*-(2,3-dihydro-1*H*-inden-5-yl) ester; *m,N*-dimethylthiocarbanilic acid *O*-5-indanyl ester; *O*-(5-indanyl) *m,N*-dimethylthiocarbanilate; Dalnate. $C_{18}H_{19}NOS$; mol wt 297.41. C 72.69%, H 6.44%, N 4.71%, O 5.38%, S 10.78%. Prepared by treating 5-indanyl thionochloroformate with *N*-methyl-*m*-toluidine: Elpern, Youlus, **US 3509200** (1970 to USV).

Crystals, mp 94-95°.
THERAP CAT: Antifungal.

9516. Toliprolol. [2933-94-0] 1-[(1-Methylethyl)amino]-3-(3-methylphenoxy)-2-propanol; 1-(isopropylamino)-3-(*m*-tolyloxy)-2-propanol; 1-(3-methylphenoxy)-3-(isopropylamino)-2-propanol; 1-(3-methylphenoxy)-2-hydroxy-3-isopropylaminopropane; MHIP. $C_{13}H_{21}NO_2$; mol wt 223.31. C 69.92%, H 9.48%, N 6.27%, O 14.33%. β-Adrenergic blocker. Prepn: **NL 6409883**; H. Koppe *et al.,* **US 3459782** (1965, 1969 both to Boehringer, Ing.); **NL 6410522**; R. Howe, **US 3432545** (1965, 1969 both to I.C.I.). The (−)-isomer is the more potent adrenergic β-receptor antagonist. Resolution of isomers: Howe, Rao, *J. Med. Chem.* **11,** 1118 (1968). Structure-activity studies: Crowther *et al., ibid.* **12,** 638 (1969); Somani, Laddu, *Eur. J. Pharmacol.* **14,** 209 (1971). Metabolism: Stock, Westermann, *Biochem. Pharmacol.* **14,** 227 (1965). Review of pharmacology and clinical data: Marmo *et al., Clin. Ter.* **62,** 11-51, 117-163 (1972).

Crystals from ethyl acetate-petr ether, mp 75-76°. Also reported as mp 79°.

Hydrochloride. [306-11-6] ICI-45763; Ko-592; Doberol; Sinorytmal. $C_{13}H_{22}NO_2 \cdot HCl$; mol wt 260.78. Crystals from ethanol-ether, mp 120-121°. uv max (water): 270 nm ($E_{1cm}^{1\%}$ 49.8).

THERAP CAT: Antianginal, antihypertensive.

9517. Tollens Reagent. A solution prepd from equal amounts of 10% silver nitrate and 10% sodium hydroxide solutions to which enough dilute ammonia solution has been added to dissolve the precipitated silver oxide. Tollens reagent oxidizes aldehydes to the corresponding acids; during the reaction the silver, bound in form of a complex, is reduced to metallic silver and forms a characteristic silver mirror. *Refs:* B. Tollens, *Ber.* **15**, 1635 (1882); W. Ponndorf, *ibid.* **64B**, 1913 (1937); S. Siggia, E. Segel, *Anal. Chem.* **25**, 640 (1953); J. M. Kolthoff, P. J. Elving, *Treatise on Analytical Chemistry* vol. 13 (New York, 1966) p 183.

Caution: Tollens reagent should always be prepared freshly; old, opaque or "dried out" solutions are explosive, H. Waldmann, *Chimia* **13**, 297 (1959).

USE: Reagent in characterization of sugars, aldehydes, hydrazides. As oxidizing agent.

9518. Tolmetin. [26171-23-3] 1-Methyl-5-(4-methylbenzoyl)-1*H*-pyrrole-2-acetic acid; 1-methyl-5-*p*-toluoylpyrrole-2-acetic acid; 5-(*p*-toluoyl)-1-methylpyrrole-2-acetic acid; McN-2559. $C_{15}H_{15}NO_3$; mol wt 257.28. C 70.03%, H 5.88%, N 5.44%, O 18.66%. Prepn: Carson, **FR 1574570** (1969 to McNeil Labs.), *C.A.* **72**, 100498y (1969). Pharmacology: Carson *et al., J. Med. Chem.* **14**, 646 (1971); S. Wong *et al., J. Pharmacol. Exp. Ther.* **185**, 127 (1973). *Review:* S. Wong in *Pharmacological and Biochemical Properties of Drug Substances* vol. 1, M. E. Goldberg, Ed. (Am. Pharm. Assoc., Washington, DC, 1977) pp 233-255. Review of pharmacology and therapeutic efficacy: R. N. Brogden *et al., Drugs* **15**, 429-450 (1978).

Crystals from acetonitrile, mp 155-157° (dec).

Sodium salt dihydrate. [64490-92-2] McN-2559-21-98; Reutol; Tolectin; Tolmene. $C_{15}H_{14}NNaO_3 \cdot 2H_2O$; mol wt 315.30.

THERAP CAT: Anti-inflammatory.

9519. Tolnaftate. [2398-96-1] Methyl(3-methylphenyl)-carbamothioic acid *O*-2-naphthalenyl ester; *m,N*-dimethylthiocarbanilic acid *O*-2-naphthyl ester; *O*-2-naphthyl *m,N*-dimethylthiocarbanilate; 2-naphthyl *N*-methyl-*N*-(3-tolyl)thionocarbamate; Sch-10144; Aftate; Chinofungin; Fungistop; Hi-Alarzin; Sporiline; Timoped; Tinactin; Tinaderm; Tonoftal. $C_{19}H_{17}NOS$; mol wt 307.41. C 74.23%, H 5.57%, N 4.56%, O 5.20%, S 10.43%. Prepn: **FR 1337797**; Miyazaki *et al.*, **US 3334126** (1963, 1967 to Japan Soda); Noguchi *et al., J. Pharm. Soc. Jpn.* **88**, 335 (1968). Pharmacology and toxicology: Noguchi *et al., Antimicrob. Agents Chemother.* **1962**, 259; Hashimoto *et al., Toxicol. Appl. Pharmacol.* **8**, 380 (1966); Noguchi *et al., ibid.* 368. Clinical comparison with undecylenic acid: J. F. Fuerst *et al., Cutis* **25**, 544 (1980); F. Battistini *et al., Int. J. Dermatol.* **22**, 388 (1983). Mode of action study: M. P. Gupta *et al., J. Vet. Med. Mycol.* **29**, 45 (1991). LC determn in pharmaceuticals: A. K. Dash, *J. Pharm. Biomed. Anal.* **11**, 847 (1993). Comprehensive description: *idem, Anal. Profiles Drug Subs. Excip.* **23**, 543-570 (1994).

Crystals from alcohol, mp 110.5-111.5°. Practically insol in water. Sparingly sol in methanol, ethanol. Sol in chloroform (1:1.5), acetone (1:7), CCl_4 (1:9). uv max (methanol): 258, 222 nm. LD_{50} in mice, rats (g/kg): >10, >6 orally; >6, >4 s.c. (Hashimoto).

THERAP CAT: Antifungal.

THERAP CAT (VET): Antifungal.

9520. Tolonium Chloride. [92-31-9] 3-Amino-7-(dimethylamino)-2-methylphenothiazin-5-ium chloride; 3-amino-7-dimethylamino-2-methylphenazathionium chloride; toluidine blue O; dimethyltoluthionine chloride; C.I. Basic Blue 17; C.I. 52040; Blutene; Klot; Tolazul. $C_{15}H_{16}ClN_3S$; mol wt 305.83. C 58.91%, H 5.27%, Cl 11.59%, N 13.74%, S 10.48%. Prepd from dimethyl-*p*-phenylenediamine, sodium thiosulfate, and *o*-toluidine: Dändliker, Bernthsen, **US 416055** (1888 to BASF). Prepn of hemostatic compositions contg tolonium chloride: D. A. Hoff, **US 2809913** (1957 to Warren-Teed). Prepn of clear, colorless, stable, isotonic solns of purified leucotoluidine blue O by reducing toluidine blue O with sodium hydrosulfite at pH 2.5-3.5: B. March, E. E. Moore, **US 2571593** (1951 to Abbott). Clinical studies in bleeding disorders: J. Allen *et al., Surg. Gynecol. Obstet.* **89**, 692 (1949). Clinical use for parathyroid identification during thyroidectomy: R. M. Yeager, E. T. Krementz, *Ann. Surg.* **169**, 829 (1969). Acute and chronic toxicity study: T. J. Haley, F. Stolarsky, *Stanford Med. Bull.* **9**, 96 (1951). Review of therapeutic and diagnostic use: A. Mashberg, *J. Am. Dent. Assoc.* **106**, 319-323 (1983). *See also Colour Index* vol. 4 (3rd ed., 1971) p 4471; *H. J. Conn's Biological Stains*, R. D. Lillie, Ed. (Williams & Wilkins, Baltimore, 9th ed., 1977) p 428.

Dark green powder. Sol in water (3.82 g/100 ml), giving a blue to violet soln; sol in alc (0.57 g/100 ml), giving a blue soln. Absorption max (water): 640.4 nm. LD_{50} in mice, rats, rabbits (mg/kg): 27.56, 28.93, 13.44 i.v. (Haley, Storlarsky).

USE: Direct dyeing, printing of wool, silk. Biological stain.

THERAP CAT: Hemostatic. Diagnostic aid (oral carcinoma).

9521. Toloxatone. [29218-27-7] 5-(Hydroxymethyl)-3-(3-methylphenyl)-2-oxazolidinone; 5-(hydroxymethyl)-3-*m*-tolyl-2-oxazolidinone; MD-69276; Humoryl; Perenum. $C_{11}H_{13}NO_3$; mol wt 207.23. C 63.75%, H 6.32%, N 6.76%, O 23.16%. Reversible monoamine oxidase type A inhibitor. Prepn: C. Fauran *et al.*, **DE 2012120**; *eidem*, **US 3655687** (1970, 1972 both to Delalande); *eidem, Chim. Ther.* **8**, 324 (1973). Pharmacology: G. Raynaud *et al., ibid.* 328. Psychopharmacological profile: J.-P. Kan *et al., Eur. J. Med. Chem.* **12**, 13 (1977); H. Giono-Barber *et al., Arzneim.-Forsch.* **27**, 1188 (1977). Pharmacokinetics: M. S. Benedetti *et al., ibid.* **32**, 276 (1982). Metabolism: A. Malnoe, M. S. Benedetti, *Xenobiotica* **9**, 281 (1979). GLC determn in plasma: S. Vajta *et al., J. Chromatogr.* **274**, 139 (1983). Clinical evaluation in panic disorder: G. Perna *et al., J. Clin. Psychopharmacol.* **14**, 414 (1994).

Crystals from isopropyl alcohol, mp 76°. LD_{50} orally in mice (mg/kg): 1850 (Fauran); also reported as 1500 (Raynaud).

THERAP CAT: Antidepressant.

9522. Tolperisone. [728-88-1] 2-Methyl-1-(4-methylphenyl)-3-(1-piperidinyl)-1-propanone; 2,4'-dimethyl-3-piperidinopropiophenone; 1-piperidino-2-methyl-3-(*p*-tolyl)-3-propanone; 2-methyl-3-piperidino-1-*p*-tolylpropan-1-one; mydetone. $C_{16}H_{23}NO$; mol wt 245.36. C 78.32%, H 9.45%, N 5.71%, O 6.52%. Prepn: Nádor *et al.*, **HU 144997** (1956); Yokoyama *et al.*, **JP 65**

Consult the Name Index before using this section.

20390 (1965 to Eisai). Pharmacology and toxicity: J. Porszasz *et al., Acta Physiol. Acad. Sci. Hung.* **18,** 149 (1960); *eidem, Arzneim.-Forsch.* **11,** 257 (1961).

Hydrochloride. [3644-61-9] N-553; Abbsa; Atmosgen; Arantoick; Besnoline; Isocalm; Kineorl; Menopatol; Metosomin; Minacalm; Muscalm; Mydocalm; Naismeritin; Tolisartine. $C_{16}H_{23}NO$.-HCl; mol wt 281.82. Crystals from methyl ethyl ketone, mp 176-177°. LD_{50} s.c. in mice: 620 mg/kg (Porszasz, 1961).
THERAP CAT: Muscle relaxant (skeletal).

9523. Tolpropamine. [5632-44-0] N,N,4-Trimethyl-γ-phenylbenzenepropanamine; N,N-dimethyl-3-phenyl-3-p-tolylpropylamine; 3-dimethylamino-1-phenyl-1-p-tolylpropane. $C_{18}H_{23}N$; mol wt 253.38. C 85.32%, H 9.15%, N 5.53%. Prepn: Bockmühl, Stein, **DE 925468** (1955 to Hoechst); Klosa, *J. Prakt. Chem.* **34,** 312 (1966). Pharmacology: Sendrail, Gleizes, *Therapie* **15,** 119 (1960).

Hydrochloride. Pragman Gelee. $C_{18}H_{23}N$.HCl; mol wt 289.84. mp 182-184°.
THERAP CAT: Topical antihistaminic, antipruritic.

9524. Tolrestat. [82964-04-3] N-[[6-Methoxy-5-(trifluoromethyl)-1-naphthalenyl]thioxomethyl]-N-methylglycine; tolrestatin; AY-27773; Alredase; Lorestat. $C_{16}H_{14}F_3NO_3S$; mol wt 357.35. C 53.78%, H 3.95%, F 15.95%, N 3.92%, O 13.43%, S 8.97%. Orally active aldose reductase inhibitor. Prepn and pharmacology: K. Sestanj *et al.,* **EP 59596** (1982 to Ayerst); *eidem, J. Med. Chem.* **27,** 255 (1984). Prevention of cataracts in galactosemic rats: N. Simard-Duquesne *et al., Proc. Soc. Exp. Biol. Med.* **178,** 599 (1985). Kinetics and metabolism in man: D. R. Hicks *et al., Clin. Pharmacol. Ther.* **36,** 493 (1984). Ultraviolet and HPLC determn in serum: D. R. Hicks, M. Kraml, *Ther. Drug Monit.* **6,** 328 (1984). Effect on erythrocyte sorbitol levels in diabetic patients: P. Raskin *et al., Clin. Pharmacol. Ther.* **38,** 625 (1985).

mp 164-165°.
Methyl ester. $C_{17}H_{16}F_3NO_3S$. mp 109-110°.
THERAP CAT: Treatment of diabetic neuropathy.

9525. Tolterodine. [124937-51-5] 2-[(1R)-3-[Bis(1-methylethyl)amino]-1-phenylpropyl]-4-methylphenol; (+)-(R)-2-[α-[2-(diisopropylamino)ethyl]benzyl]-p-cresol; (+)-N,N-diisopropyl-3-(2-hydroxy-5-methylphenyl)-3-phenylpropylamine; Kabi 2234. $C_{22}H_{31}NO$; mol wt 325.49. C 81.18%, H 9.60%, N 4.30%, O 4.92%. Muscarinic receptor antagonist. Prepn: N. A. Jönsson *et al.,* **EP 325571** (1989 to KabiVitrum); *eidem,* **US 5382600** (1995 to Pharmacia). Asymmetric total synthesis: C. Hedberg, P. G. Andersson, *Adv. Synth. Catal.* **347,** 662 (2005). Pharmacology: L. Nilvebrant *et al., Life Sci.* **60,** 1129 (1997). Receptor binding study: *idem et*

al., Eur. J. Pharmacol. **327,** 195 (1997). GC-MS determn in biological fluids: L. Palmér *et al., J. Pharm. Biomed. Anal.* **16,** 155 (1997). Clinical pharmacokinetics: N. Brynne *et al., Int. J. Clin. Pharmacol. Ther.* **35,** 287 (1997). Review of clinical trials: R. A. Appell, *Urology* **50,** Suppl. 6A, 90-96 (1997); of use in overactive bladder: E. S. Rovner, *Expert Opin. Pharmacother.* **6,** 653-666 (2005).

$[α]_D^{25}$ +72° (c = 1.0 in CH_2Cl_2).
Tartrate. [124937-52-6] PNU-200583E; Detrol; Detrusitol. $C_{22}H_{31}NO.C_4H_6O_6$; mol wt 475.57. Crystals from ethanol. $[α]_{546}^{25}$ +36.0°. pKa 9.87. Soly in water: 12 mg/ml. Sol in methanol; slightly sol in ethanol. Practically insol in toluene. Partition coefficient (n-octanol/water): 1.83 (pH 7.3). LD_{50} i.v. in male mice: 10-20 mg/kg (Jönsson).
THERAP CAT: In treatment of urinary incontinence.

9526. Toltrazuril. [69004-03-1] 1-Methyl-3-[3-methyl-4-[4-[(trifluoromethyl)thio]phenoxy]phenyl]-1,3,5-triazine-2,4,6(1H,-3H,5H)-trione; 1-methyl-3-[4-[p-[(trifluoromethyl)thio]phenoxy]-m-tolyl]-s-triazine-2,4,6(1H,3H,5H)-trione; Bay Vi 9142; Baycox. $C_{18}H_{14}F_3N_3O_4S$; mol wt 425.38. C 50.82%, H 3.32%, F 13.40%, N 9.88%, O 15.04%, S 7.54%. Triazinetrione anticoccidial. General prepn: **BE 826900**; J. H. Reisdorff *et al.,* **US 3966725** (1975, 1976 both to Bayer). Prepn and use as animal growth promotant: **BE 866389**; A. Haberkorn *et al.,* **US 4219552** (1978, 1980 both to Bayer). Series of articles on efficacy vs coccidia in chickens: E. Kutzer *et al., Wien. Tieraerztl. Monatssch.* **72,** 321-340 (1985). Field trial in sheep: B. Gjerde, O. Helle, *Acta Vet. Scand.* **27,** 124 (1986); in chickens: H. D. Chapman, *J. Comp. Pathol.* **97,** 21 (1987).

mp 194°.
THERAP CAT (VET): Coccidiostat.

9527. *o*-Tolualdehyde. [529-20-4] 2-Methylbenzaldehyde; o-toluylaldehyde. C_8H_8O; mol wt 120.15. C 79.97%, H 6.71%, O 13.32%. Prepd by reacting nitropropane with o-xylyl bromide in the presence of sodium ethanoate: Hass, Bender, *Org. Synth.* **30,** 99 (1950).

Liquid. d_4^{19} 1.0386. bp_{760} 200-202°; bp_{15} 94-96°; bp_6 68-72°. n_D^{25} 1.5430; n_D^{19} 1.549; $n_α^{19}$ 1.5423; $n_β^{19}$ 1.5650; $n_γ^{19}$ 1.5798.

9528. *o*-Toluamide. [527-85-5] 2-Methylbenzamide. C_8H_9NO; mol wt 135.16. C 71.09%, H 6.71%, N 10.36%, O 11.84%. Prepd by reacting o-tolunitrile, hydrogen peroxide, 95% alcohol, and sodium hydroxide at 40-50°: Noller, *Org. Synth.* **coll. vol. II,** 586 (1943). Also prepared by reacting the nitrile with boron fluoride in dil acetic acid: Hauser, Hoffenberg, *J. Org. Chem.* **20,** 1448 (1955).

Crystals from water, mp 144-145°. Very sol in alcohol, hot water, concd HCl, less sol in ether. Sparingly sol in benzene. Practically insol in cold water. *Explosive. Keep away from open flame.*

9529. Toluene. [108-88-3] Methylbenzene; toluol; phenylmethane; Methacide. C_7H_8; mol wt 92.14. C 91.25%, H 8.75%. Obtained mainly from tar oil. Review of mfg processes: *Faith, Keyes & Clark's Industrial Chemicals*, F. A. Lowenheim, M. K. Moran, Eds. (Wiley-Interscience, New York, 4th ed., 1975) pp 822-830. Solubility: F. P. Schwarz, *Anal. Chem.* **52**, 10 (1980). Myelotoxic potential: L. Greenburg *et al., J. Am. Med. Assoc.* **118**, 573 (1942). Comparison with benzene of effects on hematopoiesis and bone marrow metabolism: H. W. Gerarde, *AMA Arch. Ind. Health* **13**, 468 (1956). Acute toxicity: H. F. Smyth *et al., Am. Ind. Hyg. Assoc. J.* **30**, 470 (1969). Evaluation of chronic occupational exposure: H. Tahti *et al., Int. Arch. Occup. Environ. Health* **48**, 61 (1981). *Review:* M. C. Hoff in *Kirk-Othmer Encyclopedia of Chemical Technology* vol. 23 (Wiley-Interscience, New York, 3rd ed., 1983) pp 246-273. Review of reproductive toxicity: J. M. Donald *et al., Environ. Health Perspect.* **94**, 237-244 (1991); of toxicology and human exposure: *Toxicological Profile for Toluene* (PB2000-108028, 2000) 357 pp.

Flammable, refractive liq; benzene-like odor. d_4^{20} 0.866. mp $-95°$. bp 110.6°. n_D^{20} 1.4967. Flash pt, closed cup: 40°F (4.4°C). Soly in water at 23.5°C (w/w): 0.067%. Very slightly sol in water; misc with alc, chloroform, ether, acetone, glacial acetic acid, carbon disulfide. LD_{50} orally in rats: 7.53 g/kg (Smyth).

Caution: Readily absorbed by inhalation, ingestion and somewhat by skin contact. Direct contact may cause severe dermatitis due to drying and defatting action. May present lung aspiration hazard if ingested. Potential symptoms of acute overexposure by inhalation may include local irritation; CNS excitation and depression. Low concentrations may result in transitory mild upper respiratory tract irritation, mild eye irritation, lacrimation, metallic taste, slight nausea, hilarity, lassitude, drowsiness and impaired balance. High concentrations may cause paresthesia, vision disturbances, dizziness, nausea, headache, narcosis and collapse; death from respiratory failure or sudden ventricular fibrillation. Chronic overexposure by inhalation has been associated with hepatotoxicity and nephrotoxicity. Syndromes following chronic inhalation involve severe muscle weakness, cardiac arrhythmias, gastrointestinal and neuropsychiatric complaints. *See Patty's Industrial Hygiene and Toxicology* vol. 2B, G. D. Clayton, F. E. Clayton, Eds. (Wiley-Interscience, New York, 4th ed., 1994) pp 1326-1332; *Clinical Toxicology of Commercial Products*, R. E. Gosselin *et al.*, Eds. (Williams & Wilkins, Baltimore, 5th ed., 1984) Section II, p 153, Section III, p 397-404.

USE: In manuf benzoic acid, benzaldehyde, explosives, dyes, and many other organic compds; as a solvent for paints, lacquers, gums, resins; thinner for inks, perfumes, dyes; in the extraction of various principles from plants; as gasoline additive.

9530. Toluene 2,4-Diisocyanate. [584-84-9] 2,4-Diisocyanato-1-methylbenzene; 2,4-diisocyanatotoluene; 2,4-tolylene diisocyanate; TDI; Nacconate 100. $C_9H_6N_2O_2$; mol wt 174.16. C 62.07%, H 3.47%, N 16.08%, O 18.37%. Usually prepd from toluene-2,4-diamine and phosgene. *Review:* Astle, *Industrial Organic Nitrogen Compounds* (New York, 1961) pp 284-313; *Faith, Keyes & Clark's Industrial Chemicals*, F. A. Lowenheim, M. K. Moran, Eds. (Wiley-Interscience, New York, 4th ed., 1975) pp 831-835.

Liquid at room temperature. Sharp, pungent odor. mp 19.5-21.5°. d_4^{20} liq 1.2244. bp_{760} 251°; bp_{11} 126°. Darkens on exposure to sunlight. Reacts with water with evolution of carbon dioxide. Flash pt, open cup: 132°C (270°F). Misc with alcohol (decompn), diglycol monomethyl ether, ether, acetone, carbon tetrachloride, benzene, chlorobenzene, kerosene, olive oil. Concd alkaline compds such as NaOH or *tert*-amines may cause run-away polymerization.

Caution: Potential symptoms of overexposure are irritation of eyes, skin, nose and throat; choking, paroxysmal cough; chest pain, retrosternal soreness; nausea, vomiting and abdominal pain; bronchitis, bronchospasm, pulmonary edema; dyspnea, asthma; conjunctivitis, lacrimation; dermatitis, skin sensitization. *See NIOSH Pocket Guide to Chemical Hazards* (DHHS/NIOSH 97-140, 1997) p 312. *See also Clinical Toxicology of Commercial Products*, R. E. Gosselin *et al.*, Eds. (Williams & Wilkins, Baltimore, 5th ed., 1984) Section II, p 414. This substance is reasonably anticipated to be a human carcinogen: *Report on Carcinogens, Eleventh Edition* (PB2005-104914, 2004) p III-256.

USE: In the manuf of polyurethane foams and other elastomers.

9531. Toluene-3,4-dithiol. [496-74-2] 1,2-Dimercapto-4-methylbenzene; "dithiol". $C_7H_8S_2$; mol wt 156.27. C 53.80%, H 5.16%, S 41.04%. Prepd from toluene-3,4-disulfonyl chloride with tin and hydrochloric acid: Mills, Clark, *J. Chem. Soc.* **1936**, 178.

Crystals, mp 31°. bp_{84} 185-187°. Sol in benzene, in aq alkali hydroxide solns.

USE: For the detection of bismuth, molybdenum, rhenium, tin, tungsten, *see* Bickford *et al., J. Am. Pharm. Assoc. Sci. Ed.* **37**, 255 (1948).

9532. *p*-Toluenesulfinic Acid. [536-57-2] $C_7H_8O_2S$; mol wt 156.20. C 53.83%, H 5.16%, O 20.49%, S 20.53%. Prepd by reduction of *p*-toluenesulfonyl chloride with zinc dust: Whitmore, Hamilton, *Org. Synth.* **2**, 89 (1922). Because the sulfinic acid is difficult to dry without partial conversion to the sulfonic acid, the sodium salt, $CH_3C_6H_4SO_2Na.2H_2O$, is usually prepd. The free sulfinic acid is then obtained as needed by dissolving the sodium salt in cold water and carefully acidifying the soln with the exact amt of HCl needed.

Long, rhombic plates or needles from water. mp 85°. Freely sol in alc, ether; sparingly sol in water, hot benzene.

9533. *p*-Toluenesulfonic Acid. [104-15-4] 4-Methylbenzenesulfonic acid; tosic acid. $C_7H_8O_3S$; mol wt 172.20. C 48.82%, H 4.68%, O 27.87%, S 18.62%. $CH_3C_6H_4SO_3H$. Prepd by sulfonation of toluene with 96-100% H_2SO_4; when carried out at 75° the compn of the reaction product is 75% *para*-, 19% *ortho*- and 6% *meta*-toluenesulfonic acid. Convenient lab prepn: L. F. Fieser, *Experiments in Organic Chemistry* (Boston, 3rd ed., 1955) p 144. The separation of toluene from petroleum fractions can be accomplished by sulfonation with H_2SO_4 at 60°.

Monoclinic leaflets or prisms. Also reported as crystallizing with $1H_2O$ or $4H_2O$. When anhydrous, mp 106-107°. Metastable form, mp 38°. bp_{20} 140°. $bp_{0.1}$ 185-187°. Freely sol in water, about 67 g/100 ml. Sol in alc and ether.

Sodium salt. $C_7H_7NaO_3S$. Orthorhombic plates, very sol in water.

Caution: Highly irritating to skin, mucous membranes.

USE: In dye chemistry; in manuf of oral antidiabetic drugs.

9534. p-Toluenesulfonyl Chloride. [98-59-9] Tosyl chloride. $C_7H_7ClO_2S$; mol wt 190.65. C 44.10%, H 3.70%, Cl 18.60%, O 16.78%, S 16.82%. $CH_3C_6H_4SO_2Cl$. Made by treating toluene with chlorosulfonic acid.

Crystals, mp 69-71°. bp_{15} 146°. Insol in water; freely sol in alcohol, benzene, ether.

9535. Toluic Acid. Methylbenzoic acid. $C_8H_8O_2$; mol wt 136.15. C 70.57%, H 5.92%, O 23.50%. Prepn of *m*- and *o*-forms by oxidation of corresponding xylene: Toland, **US 2903480** (1959 to California Res. Corp.); Hay *et al., J. Org. Chem.* **25**, 616 (1960). Prepn of *p*-form by reaction of *p*-tolyldiazonium tetrafluoroborate with nickel carbonyl and acetic acid: Clark, Cookson, *J. Chem. Soc.* **1962**, 686; by oxidation of *p*-xylene: Taves, **US 3030413** (1962 to Hercules Powder). Manuf of *p*-form from toluene: Braunworth, **US 3046305** (1962 to Pure Oil).

m-Toluic acid. Prisms from water, mp 111-113°, bp 263°. Sublimes. Sol in 1170 parts water at 15°, 60 parts boiling water; very sol in alcohol, ether.

o-Toluic acid. Crystals, mp 107-108°; bp 258-260°; volatile with steam. Slightly sol in cold water; sol in 35 parts boiling water; very sol in alcohol.

p-Toluic acid. Crystals, mp 180-181°; bp 274-275°. Sparingly sol in hot water; very sol in alcohol, ether, methanol.

9536. Toluidine. C_7H_9N; mol wt 107.15. C 78.46%, H 8.47%, N 13.07%. Prepn: J. S. Muspratt, A. W. Hofmann, *Ann.* **54**, 1 (1845); of each isomer: F. Beilstein, A. Kuhlberg, *ibid.* **156**, 66 (1870); P. Kovacic, J. L. Foote, *J. Am. Chem. Soc.* **83**, 743 (1961); P. Kovacic *et al., ibid.* **84**, 759 (1962). Toxicity data: H. F. Smyth, *Am. Ind. Hyg. Assoc. J.* **23**, 95 (1962). GC determn in urine: K. El-Bayoumy *et al., Cancer Res.* **46**, 6064 (1986).

m-Toluidine. [108-44-1] 3-Methylbenzamine; 3-aminotoluene; 3-methylaniline. Liquid, mp ~ −50°. bp 203-204°. d_{25}^{25} 0.990. n_D^{22} 1.5711. Slightly sol in water; sol in alcohol, ether, dil acids.

o-Toluidine. [95-53-4] 2-Methylbenzamine; 2-aminotoluene; 2-methylaniline. Light yellow liquid becoming reddish brown on exposure to air and light. bp 200-202°. d_{20}^{20} 1.008. n_D^{20} 1.5688. Flash pt, closed cup: 185°F (85°C). Slightly sol in water; sol in alcohol, ether, dil acids. Keep well closed and protected from light. LD_{50} orally in rats: 0.94 g/kg (Smyth).

p-Toluidine. [106-49-0] 4-Methylbenzamine; 4-aminotoluene; 4-methylaniline. Lustrous plates or leaflets, mp 44-45°. bp 200-201°. d_4^{20} 1.046. n_D^{59} 1.5532. Flash pt, closed cup: 188°F (86°C). Sol in about 135 parts water; freely sol in alcohol, ether, acetone, methanol, carbon disulfide, oils, dil acids.

Caution: Potential symptoms of overexposure to *o*-toluidine are eye irritation; anoxia; headache, cyanosis; weakness, dizziness, drowsiness; microhematuria; eye burns; dermatitis. Potential symptoms of overexposure to *m*- or *p*- toluidine are eye, skin irritation; hematuria, methemoglobinemia; cyanosis, nausea, vomiting, low blood pressure, convulsions; anemia, weakness. *p*-Toluidine is a potential occupational carcinogen. *See NIOSH Pocket Guide to Chemical Hazards* (DHHS/NIOSH 97-140, 1997) p 312. *o*-Tolui-

dine and its hydrochloride are reasonably anticipated to be human carcinogens: *Report on Carcinogens, Eleventh Edition* (PB2005-104914, 2004) p III-258.

USE: Manufacture of various dyes and other organic chemicals. *o*-Isomer also in printing textiles blue black; making colors fast to acids. *p*-Isomer also as a reagent for lignin, nitrite, phloroglucinol.

9537. o-Tolunitrile. [529-19-1] 2-Methylbenzonitrile; 2-methylbenzenecarbonitrile; *o*-cyanotoluene; *o*-methylbenzonitrile. C_8H_7N; mol wt 117.15. C 82.02%, H 6.02%, N 11.96%. $CH_3C_6H_4CN$. Prepd from *o*-toluidine by diazotization in HCl soln and treatment of the diazonium chloride with potassium cuprocyanide: Herb, *Ann.* **258**, 9 (1890); Clarke, Read, *Org. Synth.* **coll. vol. I** (2nd ed., 1941) p 514.

Liquid; d_4^{20} 0.9955; d_4^{45} 0.9737; d_7^{75} 0.9481; mp −13°; bp_{760} 205.2°; bp_{100} 135°; bp_{40} 110°; bp_{20} 93°; bp_{10} 77.9°; bp_5 64°; $bp_{1.0}$ 36.7°; n_D^{23} 1.52720. Absorption spectrum: Baly, Ewbank, *J. Chem. Soc.* **87**, 1357 (1905); Purvis, *ibid.* **107**, 503 (1915). Insol in water. Miscible with alc, ether.

9538. p-Tolunitrile. [104-85-8] Prepd from *p*-toluidine in the manner described for *o*-tolunitrile.

Needles from alc. d_4^{30} 0.9785; d_4^{45} 0.9640; d_4^{60} 0.9512; d_7^{75} 0.9390; mp 29.5°; bp_{760} 217.6°; bp_{100} 145.2°; bp_{60} 130°; bp_{40} 109.5°; bp_{20} 101.7°; bp_{10} 85.8°; bp_5 71.3°; $bp_{1.0}$ 42.5°. Absorption spectrum: Baly, Ewbank, *J. Chem. Soc.* **87**, 1357 (1905); Purvis, *ibid.* **107**, 503 (1915). Insol in water. Very sol in alcohol, ether.

9539. 2-(p-Toluyl)benzoic Acid. [85-55-2] *p*-Toluyl-*o*-benzoic acid; 4′-methylbenzophenone-2-carboxylic acid. $C_{15}H_{12}O_3$; mol wt 240.25. C 74.99%, H 5.03%, O 19.98%. Prepd from phthalic anhydride and toluene in the presence of aluminum chloride: Friedel, Crafts, *Ann. Chim. Phys.* [6] **14**, 447 (1888); Fieser, *Org. Synth.* **4**, 73 (1925).

Monohydrate. Triclinic pinacoidal crystals from alcohol. Sweet taste. Becomes anhyd at 100°, then melts at 146°. Slightly sol in boiling water; freely sol in alcohol, benzene, ether, acetone, boiling toluene.

Methyl ester. $C_{16}H_{14}O_3$. Plates from methanol, mp 53°. Soluble in alcohol, benzene.

9540. Tolvaptan. [150683-30-0] N-[4-[(7-Chloro-2,3,4,5-tetrahydro-5-hydroxy-1*H*-1-benzazepin-1-yl)carbonyl]-3-methylphenyl]-2-methylbenzamide; 7-chloro-5-hydroxy-1-[2-methyl-4-(2-methylbenzoylamino)benzoyl]-2,3,4,5-tetrahydro-1*H*-1-benzazepine; OPC-41061. $C_{26}H_{25}ClN_2O_3$; mol wt 448.94. C 69.56%, H 5.61%, Cl 7.90%, N 6.24%, O 10.69%. Nonpeptide arginine vasopressin V_2 receptor antagonist. Prepn: H. Ogawa *et al.,* **WO 9105549**; *eidem,* **US 5258510** (1991, 1993 both to Otsuka); K. Kondo *et al., Bioorg. Med. Chem.* **7**, 1743 (1999). Pharmacology: Y. Yamamura *et al., J. Pharmacol. Exp. Ther.* **287**, 860 (1998). Clinical trial in heart failure: M. Gheorghiade *et al., J. Am. Med. Assoc.* **291**, 1963 (2004).

Colorless prisms, mp 225.9°.

THERAP CAT: In treatment of congestive heart failure.

9541. Tolycaine. [3686-58-6] 2-(2-Diethylaminoacetam-ido)-*m*-toluic acid methyl ester; 2-methyl-6-carbomethoxy-*N*-diethylaminoacetanilide; methyl 2-diethylaminoacetamido-*m*-toluate; 3-methyl-2-diethylaminoacetylaminobenzoic acid methyl ester. $C_{15}H_{22}N_2O_3$; mol wt 278.35. C 64.72%, H 7.97%, N 10.06%, O 17.24%. Prepn: Hiltmann *et al.*, **DE 1018070** (1957 to Bayer); **US 2921077** (1960 to Schenley).

Oil, bp$_5$ 190-192°.
Hydrochloride. [7210-92-6] Baycain. $C_{15}H_{22}N_2O_3$.HCl; mol wt 314.81. Crystals, mp 139-140.5°.
    THERAP CAT: Anesthetic (local).

9542. Tolylhydrazine. $C_7H_{10}N_2$; mol wt 122.17. C 68.82%, H 8.25%, N 22.93%. Prepd by stannous chloride reduction of the diazonium salt of the corresponding toluidine: Hunsberger *et al.*, *J. Org. Chem.* **21,** 394 (1956).

_m_-Tolylhydrazine. Oily liquid. bp$_{760}$ 243°, bp$_{16}$ 132-134°. d$_{15}^{15}$ 1.061-1.062, d$_4^{20}$ 1.057-1.058. Insol in water; sol in alc, chloroform, ether.
    Nitrate. $C_7H_{10}N_2$.HNO$_3$. Needles, mp 145-147°.
    _o_-Tolylhydrazine. Needles, mp 56-59°. Sparingly sol in water; sol in alcohol, chloroform, ether, slightly in cold petr ether.
    Nitrate. Leaflets, mp 98-100°. Very sol in water, alcohol; insol in ether.
    _p_-Tolylhydrazine. Rhombic bipyramids, mp 61° or 65-66°. bp 240-244° with slight decompn. Sparingly sol in water; sol in alcohol, benzene, ether.
    Nitrate. Leaflets, mp 152-153°.
    USE: *o*-Tolylhydrazine as reagent for galactose.

9543. _p_-Tolylsulfonylmethylnitrosamide. [80-11-5] *N*,4-Dimethyl-*N*-nitrosobenzenesulfonamide; *N*-methyl-*N*-nitroso-*p*-toluenesulfonamide; Diazald. $C_8H_{10}N_2O_3S$; mol wt 214.24. C 44.85%, H 4.70%, N 13.08%, O 22.40%, S 14.97%. Prepd by the action of nitrous acid on *p*-tolylsulfonylmethylamide: **DE 224388** (1910 to Bayer); *Frdl.* **10,** 1216; *Chem. Zentralbl.* **1910, II,** 609; Takizawa, *J. Pharm. Soc. Jpn.* **70,** 490 (1950); de Boer, Backer, *Rec. Trav. Chim.* **73,** 229 (1954); *Org. Synth.* **34,** 96 (1954).

Yellow crystals from benzene + petr ether, mp 62°. Stable in an ordinary brown bottle for several years. A white coating (formed of *p*-tolylsulfonylmethylamide) does no harm. Insol in water. Sol in ether, petr ether, benzene, chloroform, carbon tetrachloride. Yields diazomethane on treatment with alkali.
    USE: In the laboratory prepn of diazomethane. Directions for use: de Boer, Backer, *Rec. Trav. Chim.* **73,** 232 (1954).

9544. Tomatidine. [77-59-8] (3β,5α,22β,25S)-Spirosolan-3-ol; 5α-tomatidan-3β-ol; 5α,20β$_F$,22α$_F$,25β$_F$,27-azaspirostan-3β-ol. $C_{27}H_{45}NO_2$; mol wt 415.65. C 78.02%, H 10.91%, N 3.37%, O 7.70%. By hydrolysis of tomatine: Kuhn *et al.*, *Ber.* **83,** 448 (1950). Isoln from the roots of Rutgers tomato plant

[*Lycopersicon esculentum* Mill., cultivar. "Rutgers"]: Brink, Folkers, *J. Am. Chem. Soc.* **73,** 4018 (1951); Fontaine *et al.*, *ibid.* 878; Sato *et al.*, *ibid.* 880; Kuhn, Low, **US 2770618** (1956 to Amer. Home Prod.). Structure: Sato *et al.*, *J. Org. Chem.* **25,** 783 (1960); Schreiber, Adams, *Experientia* **17,** 13 (1961). Synthesis: Uhle, Moore, *J. Am. Chem. Soc.* **76,** 6412 (1954); Uhle, *ibid.* **83,** 1460 (1961); Kessar *et al.*, *Tetrahedron* **27,** 2869 (1971).

Plates from ethyl acetate, mp 202-206°. $[\alpha]_D^{25}$ +8° (chloroform).
Hydrochloride. $C_{27}H_{45}NO_2$.HCl. Crystals from abs ethanol, mp 265-270°. $[\alpha]_D^{25}$ −5° (methanol).

9545. Tomatine. [17406-45-0] (3β,5α,22β,25S)-Spirosolan-3-yl O-β-D-glucopyranosyl-(1 → 2)-O-[β-D-xylopyranosyl-(1 → 3)]-O-β-D-glucopyranosyl-(1 → 4)-β-D-galactopyranoside; lycopersicin. $C_{50}H_{83}NO_{21}$; mol wt 1034.19. C 58.07%, H 8.09%, N 1.35%, O 32.49%. Occurs in the extract of leaves of wild tomato plants: Fontaine *et al.*, *Arch. Biochem.* **18,** 467 (1948); Kuhn, Low, *Ber.* **81,** 552 (1948); Kuhn *et al.*, *ibid.* **83,** 448 (1950); Bognar, Makleit, *Pharmazie* **11,** 376 (1956). Yields on partial hydrolysis, besides α-tomatine, the main constituent, β_1-, β_2-, γ- and δ-tomatine: Kuhn *et al.*, *Ber.* **90,** 203 (1957). α-Tomatine consists of one mol tomatidine linked to a tetrasaccharide composed of 2 mols D-glucose, 1 mol D-xylose and 1 mol D-galactose: Kuhn *et al.*, *Angew. Chem.* **68,** 212 (1956). Proposed as an alternate precipitant to digitonin: Schultz, Sander, *Z. Physiol. Chem.* **308,** 122 (1957). Structure: Reichstein, *ibid.* **74,** 887 (1962). Toxicity study: Wilson *et al.*, *Toxicol. Appl. Pharmacol.* **3,** 39 (1961).

Needles from methanol, mp 263-268°. $[\alpha]_D^{20}$ −18° (c = 0.55 in pyridine). Sol in ethanol, methanol, dioxane, propylene glycol. Practically insol in water, ether, petr ether. Stable to strong alkali but hydrolyzed by acids to produce cryst tomatidine and a soln rich in reducing sugars. Has been found to inhibit the growth of various fungi and bacteria. LD orally in rats: 900-1000 mg/kg (Wilson).
    USE: Precipitating agent for steroids.

9546. Tonin. [53414-68-9] β-Angiotensin I converting enzyme (formerly). A converting enzyme that differs from renin, *q.v.*, in its ability to form angiotensin II directly from angiotensinogen by cleaving the Phe-His bond; it can also convert angiotensin I to angiotensin II. Its presence was discovered in rat submaxillary glands: R. Boucher *et al.*, *Hypertension 72,* J. Genest, E. Koiw, Eds. (Springer-Verlag, New York, 1972) p 512; *eidem, Circ. Res.* **Suppl. I,** 203 (1974). Purification and characterization: S. Demassieux *et al.*, *Can. J. Biochem.* **54,** 788 (1976). Crystal data: K. Hayakawa *et al.*, *J. Mol. Biol.* **123,** 107 (1978). Radioimmunoassay: J. Gutkowska *et al.*, *Can. J. Biochem.* **56,** 769 (1978).

Purification by affinity chromatography: M. Ikeda *et al., Hypertension* **3**, 81 (1981); by gel permeation and HPLC: C. Lazure *et al., Anal. Biochem.* **125**, 406 (1982). Isoln using chromatofocusing: E. S. P. Cheng, B. J. Morris, *ibid.* **126**, 295 (1982). *N*-Terminal amino acid sequence of rat tonin: N. G. Seidah *et al., Can. J. Biochem.* **56**, 920 (1978). Substrate specificity studies: *eidem, Proc. Am. Peptide Symp. 6th*, E. Gross, J. Meienhofer, Eds. (Pierce Chem. Co., Rockford, Ill., 1979) p 921; M. Chretien *et al., FEBS Lett.* **113**, 173 (1980). Formation of angiotensin II by tonin from partially purified human angiotensinogen: C. Grise *et al., Can. J. Biochem.* **59**, 250 (1981). Pressor effect in anephric animals: E. L. Schiffrin *et al., Can. J. Physiol. Pharmacol.* **59**, 864 (1981). Sequence homologies between tonin and other peptides: C. Lazure *et al., Nature* **292**, 383 (1981). Immunohistochemical study: T. B. Oerstavik *et al., J. Histochem. Cytochem.* **30**, 1123 (1982). Role as renin activator: J. Gutkowska *et al., Can. J. Biochem.* **60**, 843 (1982). Role in exptl hypertension: R. Garcia *et al., Hypertension, Int. Symp., 3rd*, H. Villarreal, Ed. (Wiley, New York, 1981) p 79. *Reviews:* R. Boucher *et al., Circ. Res.* **Suppl. II**, 26-29 (1977); R. Boucher, J. Genest, *Endocrine Functions of the Brain*, M. Motta, Ed. (Raven Press, New York, 1980) pp 373-384; J. Genest, *Heterogeneity of Renin and Renin Substrate*, M. P. Sambhi, Ed. (Elsevier, New York, 1981) pp 11-24.

Mol wt determn is 31,400 by gel filtration and 28,700 by sedimentation equilibrium. Activity is not affected by pepstatin. Can be incubated at 20° for 150 min, between pH 3.4-8 without significant loss of enzymatic activity; loses 15% of its original activity at pH 2.8. After 5 min of incubation at 100°, 60-65% activity remains.

9547. Topiramate. [97240-79-4] 2,3:4,5-Bis-*O*-(1-methylethylidene)-β-D-fructopyranose sulfamate; 2,3:4,5-di-*O*-isopropylidene-β-D-fructopyranose sulfamate; McN-4853; RWJ-17021-000; Topamax. $C_{12}H_{21}NO_8S$; mol wt 339.36. C 42.47%, H 6.24%, N 4.13%, O 37.72%, S 9.45%. Sulfamate substituted monosaccharide; structurally distinct antiepileptic agent. Prepn: B. E. Maryanoff, J. F. Gardocki, US 4513006 (1985 to McNeil); and anticonvulsant activity: B. E. Maryanoff *et al., J. Med. Chem.* **30**, 880 (1987). GC determn in plasma: M. L. Holland *et al., J. Chromatogr.* **433**, 276 (1988). Comparative pharmacokinetics: M. Bialer, *Clin. Pharmacokinet.* **24**, 441 (1993). Series of articles on pharmacology and clinical experience in epilepsy: *Epilepsia* **38**, Suppl. 1, 1-62 (1997). Review of clinical trials in migraine prevention: G. Bussone *et al., Int. J. Clin. Pract.* **59**, 961-968 (2005); of pharmacology and clinical experience: S. D. Silberstein *et al., Clin. Ther.* **27**, 154-165 (2005).

Crystals from ethyl acetate + hexane, mp 125-126°. $[\alpha]_D^{23}$ −34.0° (c = 0.4 in methanol).
THERAP CAT: Anticonvulsant; antimigraine.

9548. Topotecan. [123948-87-8] (4*S*)-10-[(Dimethylamino)methyl]-4-ethyl-4,9-dihydroxy-1*H*-pyrano[3',4':6,7]indolizino-[1,2-*b*]quinoline-3,14(4*H*,12*H*)-dione; 9-[(dimethylamino)methyl]-10-hydroxy-(20*S*)-camptothecin; hycamptamine; SKF-104864. $C_{23}H_{23}N_3O_5$; mol wt 421.45. C 65.55%, H 5.50%, N 9.97%, O 18.98%. DNA topoisomerase I inhibitor; semisynthetic analog of camptothecin, *q.v.* Prepn: J. C. Boehm *et al., EP 321122; eidem, US 5004758* (1989, 1991 both to SmithKline Beecham); W. D. Kingsbury *et al., J. Med. Chem.* **34**, 98 (1991). HPLC determn in plasma: J. H. Beijnen *et al., J. Pharm. Biomed. Anal.* **8**, 789 (1990). Clinical pharmacology: E. K. Rowinsky *et al., J. Clin. Oncol.* **10**, 647 (1992); and pharmacokinetics: L. J. C. van Warmerdam *et al., Cancer Chemother. Pharmacol.* **38**, 254 (1996). Clinical evaluation in ovarian cancer: A. P. Kudelka *et al., J. Clin. Oncol.* **14**, 1552 (1996); in small cell lung cancer: J. H. Schiller *et al., ibid.* 2345. Review of clinical toxicity: K. Seiter, *Expert Opin. Drug Safety* **4**, 45-53 (2005).

Hydrochloride. [119413-54-6] NSC-609669; SKF-104864A; Hycamtin. $C_{23}H_{23}N_3O_5 \cdot HCl$; mol wt 457.91. Light yellow to greenish powder, mp 213-218° (dec). Soluble in water up to 1 mg/ml.
THERAP CAT: Antineoplastic.

9549. Torcetrapib. [262352-17-0] (2*R*,4*S*)-4-[[[3,5-Bis(trifluoromethyl)phenyl]methyl](methoxycarbonyl)amino]-2-ethyl-3,4-dihydro-6-(trifluoromethyl)-1(2*H*)-quinolinecarboxylic acid ethyl ester; (2*R*,4*S*)-4-[(3,5-bis-trifluoromethylbenzyl)methoxycarbonylamino]-2-ethyl-6-trifluoromethyl-3,4-dihydro-2*H*-quinoline-1-carboxylic acid ethyl ester; CP-529414. $C_{26}H_{25}F_9N_2O_4$; mol wt 600.47. C 52.01%, H 4.20%, F 28.48%, N 4.67%, O 10.66%. Cholesteryl ester transfer protein (CETP) inhibitor. Prepn: M. P. DeNinno *et al., WO 0017164; eidem, US 6197786* (2000, 2001 both to Pfizer); of crystalline forms: D. J. M. Allen *et al., WO 0140190* (2001 to Pfizer). Mechanism of action study: R. W. Clark *et al., J. Lipid Res.* **47**, 537 (2006). Clinical evaluation of effects on HDL cholesterol levels: R. W. Clark *et al., Arterioscler. Thromb. Vasc. Biol.* **24**, 490 (2004); M. E. Brousseau *et al., N. Engl. J. Med.* **350**, 1505 (2004). Review of clinical development in combination with atorvastatin: J. R. Burnett, *Curr. Opin. Invest. Drugs* **6**, 944-950 (2005).

Anhydrous, non-hygroscopic crystals, mp 89-90°. d 1.406.
Ethanolate. [343798-00-5] $C_{26}H_{25}F_9N_2O_4 \cdot C_2H_6O$; mol wt 646.54. White crystalline powder, mp 54-58°. $[\alpha]_D$ −93.3° (c = 1.08 in methanol). d 1.402. Non-hygroscopic. Higher aqueous soly than anhydrous form.
THERAP CAT: Antilipemic; antiatherosclerotic.

9550. Toremifene. [89778-26-7] 2-[4-[(1*Z*)-4-Chloro-1,2-diphenyl-1-butenyl]phenoxy]-*N*,*N*-dimethylethanamine; (*Z*)-4-chloro-1,2-diphenyl-1-[4-[2-(*N*,*N*-dimethylamino)ethoxy]phenyl]-1-butene. $C_{26}H_{28}ClNO$; mol wt 405.96. C 76.92%, H 6.95%, Cl 8.73%, N 3.45%, O 3.94%. Nonsteroidal antiestrogen structurally similar to tamoxifen, *q.v.* Prepn: R. J. Toivola *et al., EP 95875; eidem, US 4696949* (1983, 1987 both to Farmos). Pharmacology: S. Kallio *et al., Cancer Chemother. Pharmacol.* **17**, 103 (1986). Antitumor effects *in vitro* and *in vivo*: L. Kangas *et al., ibid.* 109. HPLC determn in plasma: W. M. Holleran *et al., Anal. Lett.* **20**, 871 (1987). Clinical evaluation in high-grade prostatic intraepithelial neoplasia: M. S. Steiner, C. R. Pound, *Clin. Prostate Cancer* **2**, 24 (2003). Review of pharmacology and clinical efficacy in advanced breast cancer: L. R. Wiseman, K. L. Goa, *Drugs* **54**, 141-160 (1997); in postmenopausal breast cancer: J. U. Mäenpää, S.-L. Ala-Fossi, *Drugs Aging* **11**, 261-270 (1997).

mp 108-110°.

Citrate. [89778-27-8] FC-1157a; Acapodene; Fareston. C_{26}-$H_{28}ClNO.C_6H_8O_7$; mol wt 598.08. mp 160-162°.

THERAP CAT: Antineoplastic.

9551. Toril Oil. From the fruit of *Torilis anthriscus* (L.) Gmel., *Umbelliferae*. A Japanese folk remedy for ascaris. It is relatively non-toxic for higher animals and very toxic for Lumbricus, leech and ascaris.

9552. Torsemide. [56211-40-6] *N*-[[(1-Methylethyl)amino]carbonyl]-4-[(3-methylphenyl)amino]-3-pyridinesulfonamide; 1-isopropyl-3-[(4-*m*-toluidino-3-pyridyl)sulfonyl]urea; 3-isopropyl-carbamylsulfonamido-4-(3'-methylphenyl)aminopyridine; torasemide; AC-4464; BM-02015; JDL-464; Demadex; Toradiur; Torem; Unat. $C_{16}H_{20}N_4O_3S$; mol wt 348.42. C 55.16%, H 5.79%, N 16.08%, O 13.78%, S 9.20%. Sulfonylurea loop diuretic. Prepn: J. E. DeLarge *et al.*, **DE 2516025**; *idem*, **US 4018929** (1975, 1977 both to A. Christiaens, S.A.); J. DeLarge, C. L. Lapiere, *Ann. Pharm. Fr.* **36**, 369 (1978). Pharmacokinetics in humans: M. Lesne *et al.*, *Int. J. Clin. Pharmacol. Ther. Toxicol.* **20**, 382 (1982). Preliminary evaluation in acute heart failure: R. Stroobandt *et al.*, *Arch. Int. Pharmacodyn.* **260**, 151 (1982). Clinical pharmacology: D. C. Brater *et al.*, *Clin. Pharmacol. Ther.* **42**, 187 (1987). Series of articles on pharmacology, mode of action and renal effects in animals: *Arzneim.-Forsch.* **35**, 1520-1541 (1985); on pharmacology, pharmacokinetics and clinical studies: *Eur. J. Clin. Pharmacol.* **31**, Suppl., 1-55 (1986); *Arzneim.-Forsch.* **38**, 143-214 (1988). Clinical comparison with furosemide, *q.v.*, in congestive heart failure: J. Cosin *et al.*, *Eur. J. Heart Fail.* **4**, 507 (2002).

mp 163-164°. pKa 6.44.

THERAP CAT: Diuretic.

9553. Torularhodin. [514-92-1] 3',4'-Didehydro-β,ψ-caroten-16'-oic acid. $C_{40}H_{52}O_2$; mol wt 564.84. C 85.06%, H 9.28%, O 5.67%. Carotenoid pigment found in *Torula rubra* and *Rhodotorula mucilaginosa* yeasts. Isoln: Karrer, Rutschmann, *Helv. Chim. Acta* **26**, 2109 (1943). Structure and synthesis: Isler *et al.*, *ibid.* **42**, 864 (1959).

Fine dark purple needles from methanol + ether or toluene, mp 210-212° (vac, some decompn). Absorption max in CS_2: 582, 541, 502 nm; in methanol: 529, 493, 460 nm. Freely sol in carbon disulfide, chloroform, pyridine; less sol in ether, benzene, hot ethanol; sparingly sol in methanol. Practically insol in petr ether.

Methyl ester. $C_{41}H_{54}O_2$. Dark red needles from benzene + methanol, mp 172-173°.

9554. Tositumomab. [208921-02-2] Anti-(human CD20 antigen) immunoglobulin G2a (mouse monoclonal clone B1R1 $γ_{2a}$-chain) disulfide with mouse monoclonal clone B1R1 $λ_x$-chain, dimer; anti-B1 antibody. Murine monoclonal antibody targeted against CD-20 antigen located on mature B lymphocytes but not on normal stem cells or progenitor cells. [131]Iodine radioimmunoconjugate designed for tumor-targeted treatment of non-Hodgkin's lymphoma (NHL). Prepn: M. S. Kaminski *et al.*, **US 5595721** (1997 to Coulter); and clinical evaluation: *idem et al.*, *N. Engl. J. Med.* **329**, 459 (1993). Clinical study of radioimmunotherapy in NHL: *eidem*, *Blood* **96**, 1259 (2000). Review of mechanism of action and clinical application: A. K. Gopal, O. W. Press, *J. Lab. Clin. Med.* **134**, 445 (1999); of use in follicular lymphoma: A. J. Davies, *Expert Opin. Biol. Ther.* **5**, 577-588 (2005).

[131]I-Labeled form. [192391-48-3] SB-393229; Bexxar.

THERAP CAT: Antineoplastic.

9555. Tosufloxacin. [100490-36-6] 7-(3-Amino-1-pyrrolidinyl)-1-(2,4-difluorophenyl)-6-fluoro-1,4-dihydro-4-oxo-1,8-naphthyridine-3-carboxylic acid; A-61827. $C_{19}H_{15}F_3N_4O_3$; mol wt 404.34. C 56.44%, H 3.74%, F 14.10%, N 13.86%, O 11.87%. Trifluorinated quinolone antibacterial. Prepn: H. Narita *et al.*, **DE 3514076** (1985 to Toyama), *C.A.* **104**, 129888r (1986); D. T. W. Chu, **EP 153580**; *idem*, **US 4616019** (1985, 1986 both to Abbott); and activity: *idem et al.*, *J. Med. Chem.* **29**, 2363 (1986); H. Narita *et al.*, *Yakugaku Zasshi* **106**, 802 (1986), *C.A.* **106**, 196291v (1987). *In vitro* activity studies of the base: P. B. Fernandes *et al.*, *Antimicrob. Agents Chemother.* **32**, 27 (1988); and *in vivo* animal studies of the toluenesulfonate: M. Takahata *et al.*, *J. Antimicrob. Chemother.* **22**, 143 (1988). Series of articles on antibacterial activity and clinical evaluation: *Chemotherapy (Tokyo)* **36**, Suppl. 9, 1-1538 (1988).

Hydrochloride. [104051-69-6] A-60969. $C_{19}H_{15}F_3N_4O_3$.HCl; mol wt 440.80. Crystals from conc HCl-ethanol (1:3), mp 247-250° (dec).

Toluenesulfonate. [115964-29-9] Tosufloxacin tosylate; A-64730; T-3262; Ozex; Tosuxacin. $C_{19}H_{15}F_3N_4O_3.C_7H_8O_3S$; mol wt 576.54. Prepd as the monohydrate, mp 258-260°.

THERAP CAT: Antibacterial.

9556. Tosylmethyl Isocyanide. [36635-61-7] 1-[(Isocyanomethyl)sulfonyl]-4-methylbenzene; (4-methylphenylsulfonyl)-methyl isocyanide; *p*-toluenesulfonylmethyl isocyanide; TosMIC. $C_9H_9NO_2S$; mol wt 195.24. C 55.37%, H 4.65%, N 7.17%, O 16.39%, S 16.42%. Isonitrile reagent with reversed polarity; serves as a carbonyl anion equivalent in organic synthesis. Prepn: U. Schöllkopf *et al.*, *Ann.* **766**, 130 (1972); A. M. van Leusen *et al.*, *Tetrahedron Lett.* **13**, 2367 (1972); B. E. Hoogenboom *et al.*, *Org. Synth.* **57**, 102 (1977). Review of applications in organic synthesis: C. Lamberth, *J. Prakt. Chem. Chem.-Ztg.* **340**, 483-485 (1998); V. K. Tandon, S. Rai, *Sulfur Rep.* **24**, 307-385 (2003).

Crystals from methanol, mp 116-117° (dec).

USE: Versatile synthon in organic chemistry, esp in the synthesis of heterocyclic compds.

9557. Toxaphene. [8001-35-2] Chlorinated camphene; camphechlor; polychlorocamphene; Hercules 3956; Alltox; Geniphene; Motox; Phenacide; Phenatox; Strobane-T; Toxakil. A very complex, but reproducible mixture of at least 177 C_{10} polychloro derivs, having an approx overall empirical formula of $C_{10}H_{10}Cl_8$. Produced by the chlorination of camphene to 67-69% chlorine by weight and made up of compds of $C_{10}H_8Cl_{10}$, $C_{10}H_{18-n}Cl_n$ (mostly polychlorobornanes) and $C_{10}H_{16-n}Cl_n$ (polychlorobornenes and/or polychlorotricyclenes) with n = 6 to 9. Prepn: Buntin, US 2565471 (1951 to Hercules Powder). Isoln of components in crystalline form: Casida et al., Science 183, 520 (1974); eidem, J. Agric. Food Chem. 22, 939 (1974). Acute toxicity data: T. B. Gaines, Toxicol. Appl. Pharmacol. 14, 515 (1969). Mutagenicity studies: N. K. Hooper et al., Science 205, 591 (1979). Livestock toxicity and tissue residues: L. Penumarthy et al., Vet. Toxicol. 18, 60 (1976). Reviews: Liebmann et al., Arch. Pflanzenschutz 7, 131-150 (1971); F. Korte et al., Pure Appl. Chem. 51, 1583-1601 (1979); M. A. Saleh, Rev. Environ. Contam. Toxicol. 118, 1-85 (1990). Review of toxicology and human exposure: Toxicological Profile for Toxaphene (PB97-121057, 1996) 252 pp.

Yellow waxy solid, mp 65-90°. Pleasant piney odor. Vapor pressure at 20°: 3×10^{-7} mm Hg. d^{25} 1.630. Log P (octanol/water): 6.44. Dehydrochlorinates in the presence of alkali, prolonged exposure to sunlight, and at temps about 155°. Soly in water: 3 mg/l. Freely sol in aromatic hydrocarbons. Corrosive to iron. LD_{50} in male, female rats (mg/kg): 90, 80 orally; 1075, 780 dermally (Gaines).

Caution: Potential symptoms of overexposure are nausea, confusion, agitation, tremors, convulsions and unconsciousness; dry, red skin. See NIOSH Pocket Guide to Chemical Hazards (DHHS/NIOSH 97-140, 1997) p 58. See also Clinical Toxicology of Commercial Products, R. E. Gosselin et al., Eds. (Williams & Wilkins, Baltimore, 5th ed., 1984) Section III, pp 386-387. This substance is reasonably anticipated to be a human carcinogen: Report on Carcinogens, Eleventh Edition (PB2005-104914, 2004) p III-259

USE: Insecticide. Not recommended for use in dairy barns or on milking animals (Penumarthy).

9558. Toxiferine I. [6888-23-9] C-Toxiferine I. [$C_{40}H_{46}$-N_4O_2]$^{2+}$. Naturally occurring neuromuscular blocker. From calabash curare: Schmid, Karrer, Helv. Chim. Acta 30, 1162 (1947); from Strychnos toxifera Schomb., Loganiaceae: Wieland et al., Ann. 547, 156 (1941); King, J. Chem. Soc. 1949, 3263. Identity with **toxiferine V** and **toxiferine XI**: Battersby et al., ibid. 1960, 1848. Structure: Arnold et al., Helv. Chim. Acta 44, 620 (1961). Synthesis: Berlage et al., ibid. 42, 394 (1959); Grdinic et al., J. Am. Chem. Soc. 86, 3357 (1964). Pharmacokinetics: P. G. Waser, J. Reller, Agents Actions 2, 170 (1972). ^{13}C-NMR study: E. Wenkert et al., J. Org. Chem. 43, 1099 (1978).

Dichloride. $C_{40}H_{46}Cl_2N_4O_2$. Crystals. [α]$_D^{22}$ −546° (c = 0.30). uv max (ethanol): 292 nm (log ε 4.62). Sol in water.
C-Toxiferine II. [7257-29-6] C-Calebassine; C-strychnotoxine. [$C_{40}H_{48}N_4O_2$]$^{2+}$. From calabash-curare: Karrer, Schmidt, Helv. Chim. Acta 29, 1853 (1946); Zürcher et al., J. Am. Chem. Soc. 80, 1500 (1958). Identity as C-toxiferine II and C-strychnotoxine: Wieland, Merz, Ber. 85, 731 (1952). Structure: Hesse et al., Helv. Chim. Acta 44, 2211 (1961); Fehlmann et al., ibid. 48, 303 (1965).

9559. Toxoflavin. [84-82-2] 1,6-Dimethylpyrimido[5,4-e]-1,2,4-triazine-5,7(1H,6H)-dione; 1,6-dimethyl-5,7-dioxo-1,5,6,7-tetrahydropyrimido[5,4-e]-as-triazine; xanthothricin. $C_7H_7N_5O_2$; mol wt 193.16. C 43.53%, H 3.65%, N 36.26%, O 16.57%. Highly

toxic antibiotic from cultures of Pseudomonas cocovenenans which also produces bongkrekic acid, q.v. Isoln: van Veen, Mertens, Rec. Trav. Chim. 53, 257, 398 (1934); R. A. Machlowitz et al., Antibiot. Chemother. 4, 259 (1954). Structure: Van Damm et al., Rec. Trav. Chim. 79, 255 (1960). Synthesis: Daves et al., J. Am. Chem. Soc. 83, 3904 (1961); 84, 1724 (1962); Yoneda et al., Tetrahedron Lett. 1971, 851. Mode of action: Latuasan, Berends, Biochim. Biophys. Acta 52, 502 (1961). Biosynthesis: Levenberg, Linton, J. Biol. Chem. 241, 846 (1966). Production by Burkholderia glumae and pathogenicity to rice seedlings: K. Yoneyama et al., Ann. Phytopathol. Soc. Jpn. 64, 91 (1998).

Bright yellow platelets from propanol, dec 172-173°. uv max: 257.5, 394 nm (ε 16400, 2500). Acts as a pH indicator with a sharp loss of color at pH 10.5, but is destroyed by alkali. Sol in water, chloroform, ethyl acetate, ethanol. LD_{50} in mice (mg/kg): 1.7 i.v.; 8.4 orally (Machlowitz).

9560. Toxohormone. [9014-44-2] Name given in 1948 by Nakahara and Fukuoka to a factor produced by living cancer cells and released into the circulation to produce decreases in liver catalase activity, tryptophan pyrrolase activity, liver ferritin and plasma iron. See Nakahara, Fukuoka, Jpn. J. Cancer Res. 40, 45 (1949). This tumor-specific concept has been questioned: Greenfield, Meister, J. Natl. Cancer Inst. 11, 997 (1951); Olivares et al., Science 157, 327 (1967); Kampschmidt, Upchurch, Proc. Soc. Exp. Med. Biol. 127, 632 (1968). Described as a polypeptide of low mol wt having 30-40 amino acid residues of which 12-13 are different, and with a high content of glycine, glutamic acid, aspartic acid, alanine and leucine. Amino acid and lipid composition of a highly purified toxohormone prepd from human malignant tissue: Yunoki, Griffin, Cancer Res. 21, 537 (1961); from cell-free fluid of ascites sarcoma 180: H. Masuno et al., ibid. 41, 284 (1981). Reviews: W. Nakahara, F. Fukuoka, Chemistry of Cancer Toxin Toxohormone (C. C. Thomas, Springfield, Illinois, 1961) 75 pp; Nakahara, Methods Cancer Res. 2, 203-237 (1967); Olivares, Kampschmidt in Oncology, Proc. Int. Cancer Congr., 10th, Houston 1970 3, 158-170 (1971); S. Fujii, Gann Monogr. Cancer Res. 24, 215-222 (1979).

Thermostable, non-heat-coagulable, water-sol and alcohol precipitable.

9561. Toxopyrimidine. [73-67-6] 4-Amino-2-methyl-5-pyrimidinemethanol; 6-amino-5-hydroxymethyl-2-methylpyrimidine; 4-amino-5-hydroxymethyl-2-methylpyrimidine; pyramin; pyramine. $C_6H_9N_3O$; mol wt 139.16. C 51.79%, H 6.52%, N 30.20%, O 11.50%. A metabolite of thiamine. Prepd from 4-amino-5-aminomethyl-2-methylpyrimidine dihydrochloride or ethyl 4-amino-2-methyl-5-pyrimidinecarboxylate: Dornow, Petsch, Ber. 86, 1404 (1953); DiBella, Hennessy, J. Org. Chem. 26, 2017 (1961).

Needles from water, mp 193-198°; crystals from methanol + ether, mp 198-200°. Sublimes at 0.01 mm between 155-170°.

9562. Toyocamycin. [606-58-6] 4-Amino-7-β-D-ribofuranosyl-7H-pyrrolo[2,3-d]pyrimidine-5-carbonitrile; 4-amino-5-cyano-7-(D-ribofuranosyl)-7H-pyrrolo[2,3-d]pyrimidine; uramycin B; vengicide; antibiotic 1037; E-212. $C_{12}H_{13}N_5O_4$; mol wt 291.26. C 49.48%, H 4.50%, N 24.05%, O 21.97%. Antibiotic substance extracted from the culture filtrate and mycelium of Streptomyces toyocaensis. Isoln: Nishimura et al., J. Antibiot. 9A, 60 (1956). Structure: Ohkuma, ibid. 14A, 343 (1961). Synthesis of aglycone: Taylor, Hendess, *J. Am. Chem. Soc.* **86**, 951 (1964). Total synthesis: Tolman *et al., ibid.* **90**, 524 (1968); **91**, 2102 (1969). Biosynthesis: Uematsu, Suhadolnik, *Biochemistry* **9**, 1260 (1970); *eidem, J. Biol. Chem.* **245**, 4365 (1970). Crystal and molecular structure: P. Prusiner, M. Sundaralingam, *Acta Crystallogr.* **B34**, 517 (1978).

Fine needles from methanol or acetone, mp 243°. Recrystallization from water yields the hydrate, $C_{12}H_{13}N_5O_4.H_2O$, mp 239-243°. $[\alpha]_D^{16}$ −45.7° (c = 1.05 in 0.1*N* HCl). uv max (H_2O): 230, 277 nm ($E_{1cm}^{1\%}$ 400, 548). Soluble in acetic acid, acidic solns. Moderately sol in methanol, ethanol, acetone, dioxane, butanol, water, ether. Practically insol in chloroform, ethyl acetate, petr ether. LD_{100} s.c. in mice: 10-20 mg/kg (Nishimura).

9563. TPMPA. [182485-36-5] Methyl (1,2,3,6-tetrahydro-4-pyridinyl)phosphinic acid; (1,2,5,6-tetrahydropyridine-4-yl)methylphosphinic acid. $C_6H_{12}NO_2P$; mol wt 161.14. C 44.72%, H 7.51%, N 8.69%, O 19.86%, P 19.22%. Selective antagonist for $GABA_c$ receptors. Prepn: Y. Murata *et al., Bioorg. Med. Chem. Lett.* **6**, 2073 (1996); R. Miledi *et al.,* **US 5627169** (1997 to Univ. California). Design and *in vitro* pharmacology: D. Ragozzino *et al., Mol. Pharmacol.* **50**, 1024 (1996). Specificity vs human receptors and alternate synthesis: M. Chebib *et al., Eur. J. Pharmacol.* **357**, 227 (1998). Use as antagonist: A. Rozzo *et al., Neuroscience* **90**, 1085 (1999).

Off-white solid from ethanol, mp 252-254°. Soly in water 16 mg/ml. Insol in DMSO.
USE: Neurochemical tool.

9564. Tralkoxydim. [87820-88-0] 2-[1-(Ethoxyimino)propyl]-3-hydroxy-5-(2,4,6-trimethylphenyl)-2-cyclohexen-1-one; 2-[1-(ethoxyimino)propyl]-3-hydroxy-5-mesitylcyclohex-2-en-1-one; PP-604; Achieve; Grasp. $C_{20}H_{27}NO_3$; mol wt 329.43. C 72.92%, H 8.26%, N 4.25%, O 14.57%. Cereal selective post-emergent herbicide. Prepn: R. B. Warner *et al.,* **EP 80301**; *eidem,* **US 4717418** (1983, 1988 both to ICI). Physical properties and herbicidal activity: R. B. Warner *et al., Proc. Br. Crop Prot. Conf. - Weeds* **1987**, 19. Field trials on grass weeds: J. Rola, *ibid.* 363; P. B. Sutton *et al., ibid.* 389. Mechanism of action study: J. Secor, C. Cseke, *Plant Physiol.* **86**, 10 (1988).

White crystalline solid, mp 106°. Vapor pressure at 20°: 4×10^{-10} kPa. Soly at 20° (mg/l): water 6 at pH 6.5, 5 at pH 5.0; at 24° (g/l): hexane 18; toluene 213; dichloromethane >500; methanol 25; acetone 89; ethyl acetate 110. LD_{50} orally in male and female rats, male and female mice, male rabbit (mg/kg): 1324, 934, 1231, 1100, 519; dermally in male and female rats: >2000, >2000 mg/kg (Warner 1987).
USE: Post-emergent herbicide.

9565. Tralomethrin. [66841-25-6] 2,2-Dimethyl-3-(1,2,2,-2-tetrabromoethyl)cyclopropanecarboxylic acid cyano(3-phenoxyphenyl)methyl ester; (*S*)-α-cyano-3-phenoxybenzyl (1*R*)-*cis*-2,2-dimethyl-3-[(*RS*)-1,2,2,2-tetrabromoethyl]cyclopropanecarboxylate; RU-25474; OMS-3048; Saga; Scout; Tracker; Tralate; Tralox. $C_{22}H_{19}Br_4NO_3$; mol wt 665.01. C 39.73%, H 2.88%, Br 48.06%, N 2.11%, O 7.22%. Synthetic pyrethroid consisting of two active diastereomers whose absolute configurations differ at the monobrominated carbon atom. Prepn: **BE 873201**; J. Martel *et al.,* **US 4279835** (1979, 1981 both to Roussel-Uclaf). Insecticidal activity: M. Benoit *et al., Pestic. Biochem. Physiol.* **26**, 284 (1986). Mechanism of action study: M. Roche *et al., ibid.* **24**, 306 (1985). HPLC determn in water, sediment and fish tissue: J. Mao *et al., J. Agric. Food Chem.* **41**, 596 (1993). Field trials: D. D. Amalraj *et al., Indian J. Malariol.* **28**, 141 (1991); W. R. Halliday *et al., J. Agric. Entomol.* **9**, 145 (1992). Review of toxicology and human exposure: *Toxicological Profile for Pyrethrins and Pyrethroids* (PB2004-100004, 2003) 332 pp.

USE: Insecticide.

9566. Tramadol. [27203-92-5] (1*R*,2*R*)-*rel*-2-[(Dimethylamino)methyl]-1-(3-methoxyphenyl)cyclohexanol; E-265; CG-315E; U-26225A. $C_{16}H_{25}NO_2$; mol wt 263.38. C 72.96%, H 9.57%, N 5.32%, O 12.15%. Prepn: **GB 997399**; K. Flick, E. Frankus, **US 3652589** (1965, 1972 both to Grünenthal); K. Flick *et al., Arzneim.-Forsch.* **28**, 107 (1978). Series of articles on pharmacology and clinical studies: *ibid.* 114-219. Toxicology: F. Lagler *et al., ibid.* 164. Mechanism of action study: R. B. Raffa *et al., J. Pharmacol. Exp. Ther.* **267**, 331 (1993). HPLC determn in urine: B. Elsing, G. Blaschke, *J. Chromatogr.* **612**, 223 (1993). HPLC determn in plasma and pharmacokinetics: A. Küçük *et al., J. Chromatogr. B* **816**, 203 (2005). Symposium on pharmacology and clinical experience: *Drugs* **47**, Suppl. 1, 1-46 (1994).

Hydrochloride. [22204-88-2] Amadol; Contramal; Crispin; Tradonal; Tramal; Ultram; Zamadol; Zydol. $C_{16}H_{25}NO_2.HCl$; mol wt 299.84. White crystals, mp 180-181°. Sol in water. LD_{50} in mice, rats (mg/kg): 350, 228 orally; 200, 286 s.c. (Lagler).
THERAP CAT: Analgesic.

9567. Tramazoline. [1082-57-1] 4,5-Dihydro-*N*-(5,6,7,8-tetrahydro-1-naphthalenyl)-1*H*-imidazol-2-amine; 2-[(5,6,7,8-tetrahydro-1-naphthyl)amino]-2-imidazoline. $C_{13}H_{17}N_3$; mol wt 215.29. C 72.53%, H 7.96%, N 19.52%. α-Adrenergic agonist. Prepn: Berg, **DE 1191381**; **DE 1195323** (both 1965 to Thomae), *C.A.* **63**, 8373c; 13274d (1965). Pharmacology and toxicity data: R. Engelhorn, H. Klupp, *Arzneim.-Forsch.* **12**, 971 (1962). Activity studies: Sachsenröder *et al., ibid.* **22**, 392 (1972).

Crystals from isopropanol, mp 142-143°.
Hydrochloride monohydrate. [3715-90-0] KB-227; Biciron; Ellatun; Rhinaspray; Rhinogutt; Rhinospray; Rinogutt; Towk. C_{13}-

$H_{17}N_3 \cdot HCl \cdot H_2O$; mol wt 269.77. Crystals from alc + ether or acetone + ether, mp 172-174°. Sol in water. LD_{50} orally in mice: 195 mg/kg (Engelhorn, Klupp).

THERAP CAT: Decongestant.

9568. Trandolapril. [87679-37-6] (2S,3aR,7aS)-1-[(2S)-2-[[(1S)-1-(Ethoxycarbonyl)-3-phenylpropyl]amino]-1-oxopropyl]-octahydro-1H-indole-2-carboxylic acid; (3aR,7aS)-1-[N-[1(S)-(ethoxycarbonyl)-3-phenylpropyl]-(S)-alanyl]octahydroindole-2(S)-carboxylic acid; (2S,3aS,7aS)-1-[(S)-N-[(S)-1-carboxy-3-phenylpropyl]alanyl]hexahydro-2-indolinecarboxylic acid 1-ethyl ester; RU-44570; Mavik; Odrik; Gopten. $C_{24}H_{34}N_2O_5$; mol wt 430.54. C 66.95%, H 7.96%, N 6.51%, O 18.58%. Angiotensin converting enzyme (ACE) inhibitor. Prepn: H. Urbach et al., EP 84164; eidem, US 4933361 (1983, 1990 both to Hoechst). Enzyme inhibition and pharmacology: N. L. Brown et al., Eur. J. Pharmacol. 148, 79 (1988). Clinical pharmacology: F. De Ponti et al., Eur. J. Clin. Pharmacol. 40, 149 (1991). Clinical trial in prevention of death after myocardial infarction: L. Kober et al., N. Engl. J. Med. 333, 1670 (1995). Series of articles on pharmacology and clinical trials: Am. J. Hypertens. 8, 63S-74S (1995). Clinical trial in diabetic neuropathy: R. A Malik et al., Lancet 352, 1978 (1998).

Colorless, crystalline solid, mp 125°. Sol in chloroform, dichloromethane, methanol.

Diacid. [87679-71-8] Trandolaprilat; RU-44403. $C_{22}H_{30}N_2O_5$; mol wt 402.48.

THERAP CAT: Antihypertensive.

9569. Tranexamic Acid. [1197-18-8] trans-4-(Aminomethyl)cyclohexanecarboxylic acid; AMCHA; RP-18429; Anvitoff; Cyklokapron; Exacyl; Spiramin; Spotof; Tranex; Transamin; Ugurol. $C_8H_{15}NO_2$; mol wt 157.21. C 61.12%, H 9.62%, N 8.91%, O 20.35%. Antifibrinolytic agent; blocks lysine binding sites of plasminogen. Prepn: A. Einhorn, C. Ladisch, Ann. 310, 194 (1900); M. Levine, R. Sedlecky, J. Org. Chem. 24, 115 (1959); NL 6503605; T. Naito et al., US 3499925 (1965, 1970 to both Daiichi Seiyaku and Mitsubishi Chem.). Pharmacology: Andersson et al., Scand. J. Haematol. 2, 230 (1965). Resoln of isomers and antiplasmin activity: M. Shimizu et al., Chem. Pharm. Bull. 16, 357 (1968); T. Naito et al., ibid., 728. Toxicity data: B. Melander et al., Acta Pharmacol. Toxicol. 22, 340 (1965). Clinical study in treatment of acute upper gastrointestinal tract bleeding: D. Barer et al., N. Engl. J. Med. 308, 1571 (1983); in menorrhagia: J. Bonnar, B. L. Sheppard, Br. Med. J. 313, 579 (1996). Review of pharmacology and therapeutic use: C. J. Dunn, K. L. Goa, Drugs 57, 1005-1032 (1999).

mp 386-392° (dec). Soly in water: about 1 g/6 ml. Very slightly sol in alcohol, ether. Practically insol in most other organic solvents. Chemically stable; not hygroscopic. LD_{50} in mice, rats (mg/kg): 1500, 1200 i.v. (Melander).

cis-form. [1197-17-7] mp 236-238° (dec).

THERAP CAT: Hemostatic.

9570. Tranilast. [53902-12-8] 2-[[3-(3,4-Dimethoxyphenyl)-1-oxo-2-propenyl]amino]benzoic acid; N-(3',4'-dimethoxycinnamoyl)anthranilic acid; N-5'; Rizaben. $C_{18}H_{17}NO_5$; mol wt 327.33. C 66.05%, H 5.23%, N 4.28%, O 24.44%. Orally active anti-allergic agent. Prepn: K. Harita et al., DE 2402398; idem, US 3940422 (1974, 1976 both to Kissei). Pharmacological properties:

H. Azuma et al., Br. J. Pharmacol. 58, 483 (1976). Mechanism of action study: Y. Iijima et al., Biochem. Biophys. Res. Commun. 93, 912 (1980). Clinical study in pediatric bronchial asthma: H. Shioda, Allergy 34, 213 (1979). Toxicity studies: M. Nakazawa et al., Oyo Yakuri 12, 385, 407 (1976), C.A. 88, 115327-8 (1978). Series of articles on teratogenicity tests: Iyakuhin Kenkyu 9, 148-193 (1978), C.A. 88, 130930f, 146300m-303q (1978).

Crystals from chloroform, mp 211-213°. LD_{50} in male, female mice, male, female rats (mg/kg): 780, 680, 1600, 1100 orally; 410, 385, 405, 395 i.p.; 2630, 2820, 3630, 3060 s.c. (Nakazawa, p 385).

THERAP CAT: Antiallergic.

9571. Transferrins. A group of homologous non-heme, iron-binding glycoproteins of approx mol wts of 76,000-81,000. They are widely distributed in a variety of physiological fluids and cells, esp in the sera of most vertebrates, in egg whites and in mammalian milk, tears and leukocytes. They are involved in iron transport to developing red cells for hemoglobin synthesis. Each protein molecule specifically binds with two Fe^{3+} ions to form salmon-pink complexes; bicarbonate or carbonate ions are involved in the formation of these colored complexes. Reviews of isoln, properties and biological functions: Feeney, Komatsu, Struct. Bonding 1, 149-206 (1966); Aisen, "The Transferrins" in Inorganic Biochemistry vol. 1, G. L. Eichhorn, Ed. (Elsevier, New York, 1973) pp 280-305; Bezkorovainy, Zschocke, Arzneim.-Forsch. 24, 476-485, 726-737 (1974); P. Aisen, A. Leibman, Bioinorg. Chem. II, K. N. Raymond, Ed. (A.C.S., Washington, 1977) pp 104-126; P. Aisen, I. Listowsky, Annu. Rev. Biochem. 49, 357-393 (1980). Review of transferrin receptors: R. Newman et al., Trends Biochem. Sci. 7, 397-399 (1982).

Serum transferrin. β_1-Metal-combining protein; siderophilin. Commonly called transferrin. Structure of carbohydrate moiety: Jamieson et al., J. Biol. Chem. 246, 3686 (1971). Composed of two homologous domains, each containing a binding site for metal ions. The sites are similar, but not identical, in their metal-binding properties. X-ray studies: L. J. DeLucas et al., J. Mol. Biol. 123, 285 (1978). Resolution of the two sites by Eu(III) excitation spectroscopy: P. B. O'Hara, R. Bersohn, Biochemistry 21, 5269 (1982). N-Terminal amino acid sequence of human serum transferrin: M.-H. Metz-Boutigue et al., Biochim. Biophys. Acta 670, 243 (1981). Absorption max of human serum Fe^{3+}-transferrin: about 465 nm ($E_{1cm}^{1\%}$ 0.57); uv max: 280 nm ($E_{1cm}^{1\%}$ 14.3).

Conalbumin. Ovotransferrin; Diarconal. Isolated from egg white; distinguished from ovalbumin by its lower thermal coagulation point: Osborne, Campbell, J. Am. Chem. Soc. 22, 422 (1900). Sepn from other egg-white proteins: Longworth et al., ibid. 62, 2580 (1940). Primary structure of hen ovotransferrin: J. Williams et al., Eur. J. Biochem. 122, 297 (1982). Purification, characterization and function of the iron-binding fragments: W.-M. Keung et al., J. Biol. Chem. 257, 1177, 1184 (1982). Antibacterial activity: P. Valenti et al., Antimicrob. Agents Chemother. 21, 840 (1982). Absorption max of Fe^{3+}-complex: 470 nm ($E_{1cm}^{1\%}$ 0.62).

Lactoferrin. Lactotransferrin. Important component of the human milk bacteriostatic system; also found in human and bovine tear proteins. Isoln from human whey by a single chromatographic step: L. Bläckberg, O. Hernell, FEBS Lett. 109, 180 (1980). Sequential purification of lactoferrin, lysozyme, and secretory IgA from human milk: M. Boesman-Finkelstein, R. A. Finkelstein, ibid. 144, 1 (1982). Partial C-terminal amino acid sequence of human lactoferrin: M.-H. Metz-Boutigue et al., ibid. 142, 107 (1982).

9572. Transforming Growth Factor-β. TGF-β. Family of multifunctional cytokines that regulate cellular differentiation, motility and growth. Also regulate the synthesis and deposition of the extracellular matrix. Involved in various physiological processes including embryogenesis, immunoregulation, bone remodeling and wound healing. Secreted by virtually all cell types as a biologically inactive (latent) form which is stored at the cell surface and in the extracellular matrix. The mature, active cytokine is a homodimer; mol wt 25 kDa. At least 5 isoforms have been identified. The three mammalian isoforms (TGF-β_1, β_2, and β_3) exhibit 70-80% sequence homology, bind to the same receptors and exert similar biological effects. TGF-β_1 is the most abundant. Biological effects are mediated by binding to membrane receptors that exist on virtually all cells. Released from degranulating platelets at the site of a wound, TGF-β initiates angiogenesis and collagen synthesis. Acts as a chemoattractant and activator of macrophages and fibroblasts. Dysregulation is implicated in the pathogenesis of fibrotic diseases. Inhibits the growth of most epithelial and lymphoid cells. Escape from this normal control mechanism is implicated in carcinogenic transformation. Initial description: J. E. DeLarco, G. J. Todaro, *Proc. Natl. Acad. Sci. USA* **75**, 4001 (1978). Crystal structure of TGF-β_2: S. Daopin *et al., Science* **257**, 369 (1992). Review of physiological actions: A. B. Roberts, M. B. Sporn, *Growth Factors* **8**, 1-9 (1993); of latent forms, binding proteins and receptors: K. Miyazono *et al., ibid.,* 11-22. Proposed mechanisms for tumor cell transformation: M. J. Newman, *Cancer Metastasis Rev.* **12**, 239-254 (1993). Role in embryogenesis: N. L. McCartney-Francis, S. M. Wahl, *J. Leukocyte Biol.* **55**, 401-409 (1994); in tissue fibrosis: W. A. Border, N. A. Noble, *N. Engl. J. Med.* **331**, 1286-1292 (1994); in kidney disease: K. Sharma, F. N. Ziyadeh, *Am. J. Physiol.* **266**, F829-F842 (1994). Review of potential clinical applications in oncology: J. Kekow, G. J. Wiedemann, *Int. J. Oncol.* **7**, 177-182 (1995).

9573. Tranylcypromine. [155-09-9] (1*R*,2*S*)-*rel*-2-Phenyl-cyclopropanamine; SKF-385. $C_9H_{11}N$; mol wt 133.19. C 81.16%, H 8.32%, N 10.52%. Monoamine oxidase inhibitor. Prepn: Burger, Yost, *J. Am. Chem. Soc.* **70**, 2198 (1948); R. E. Tedeschi, US 2997422 (1961 to SK & F).

Liquid, bp$_{1.5-1.6}$ 79-80°.
Hydrochloride. $C_9H_{11}N$.HCl. Crystals from ethyl acetate + ether, mp 164-166°.
Sulfate. [13492-01-8] Parnate; Tylciprine. $(C_9H_{11}N)_2 \cdot H_2$-SO_4; mol wt 364.46. Crystals, sol in water; very slightly sol in alcohol, ether. Practically insol in chloroform.
THERAP CAT: Antidepressant.

9574. Trapidil. [15421-84-8] *N,N*-Diethyl-5-methyl-[1,2,-4]triazolo[1,5-*a*]pyrimidin-7-amine; 7-diethylamino-5-methyl-*s*-triazolo[1,5-*a*]pyrimidine; trapymin; AR-12008; Avantrin; Rocornal. $C_{10}H_{15}N_5$; mol wt 205.26. C 58.51%, H 7.37%, N 34.12%. First triazolopyrimidine registered as a drug. Prepn: E. Tenor *et al.,* **DD 55956** (1967), *C.A.* **67**, 90830f (1967); E. Tenor, R. Ludwig, *Pharmazie* **26**, 534 (1971). Physical and chemical properties: S. Pfeifer *et al., ibid.* 539. Pharmacology and toxicology: H. Fuller *et al., ibid.* 554. Metabolic studies: S. Pfeifer *et al., ibid.* 549; *ibid.* **27**, 752 (1972); I. Bornschein *et al., ibid.* **33**, 51 (1978). Mechanism of action: K. Satoh *et al., Arzneim.-Forsch.* **30**, 1264 (1980). Antiarrhythmic activities in rabbits: M. Sakanashi *et al., ibid.* **33**, 215 (1983). Clinical hemodynamic effects: M. Di Donato *et al., ibid.* **35**, 1295 (1985). GC determn in biological fluids: A. Marzo *et al., ibid.* **37**, 947 (1987).

White to yellowish, odorless and bitter crystalline powder, mp 98-99.4° (Pfeifer); 102-104° from heptane (Tenor). Eutectic temp of mixture with azobenzene: 48°. Very sol in water, 1*N* sulfuric acid, 10% ammonium hydroxide; easily sol in methanol, isopropanol, *n*-butanol, chloroform and benzene; sol in ether. Practically insol in hexane, heptane. pK$_s$ = 2.79. uv max (methanol): 222, 270, 307 nm (log ε 4.28, 3.83, 4.28). Very stable except under extremely alk

conditions. LD$_{50}$ in mice, rats (mg/kg): 115, 76 i.v.; 380, 235 orally; 155, 100 i.p.; 132, 100 s.c. (Fuller).
Hydrochloride. $C_{10}H_{15}N_5$.HCl. mp 212°.
THERAP CAT: Vasodilator (coronary).

9575. Trastuzumab. [180288-69-1] Anti-(human p185*neu* receptor) immunoglobulin G1 (human-mouse monoclonal rhuMab HER2 γ_1-chain) disulfide with human-mouse monoclonal rhuMab HER2 light chain, dimer; rhuMab HER2; Herceptin. Humanized monoclonal antibody directed against the protein product of the HER2/*neu* oncogene which is homologous to the human epidermal growth factor receptor and is overexpressed by certain tumor cells. Constructed by inserting the antigen binding regions of murine monoclonal antibody 4D5 into the framework of a consensus human immunoglobulin G$_1$. Prepn: R. M. Hudziak *et al.,* **WO 8906692**; *eidem,* US 5677171 (1989, 1997 both to Genentech); P. Carter *et al., Proc. Natl. Acad. Sci. USA* **89**, 4285 (1992). Analysis by capillary electrophoresis: G. Hunt *et al., J. Chromatogr. A* **744**, 295 (1996). Clinical evaluation in combination with cisplatin in breast cancer: M. D. Pegram *et al., J. Clin. Oncol.* **16**, 2659 (1998). Review of clinical efficacy: G. N. Hortobagyi, *Semin. Oncol.* **28**, Suppl. 18, 43-47 (2001); of clinical safety and tolerability in breast cancer: S. Rueckert *et al., Expert Opin. Biol. Ther.* **5**, 853-866 (2005).
THERAP CAT: Antineoplastic.

9576. Traumatic Acid. [6402-36-4] 2-Dodecenedioic acid; 1-decene-1,10-dicarboxylic acid. $C_{12}H_{20}O_4$; mol wt 228.28. C 63.14%, H 8.83%, O 28.03%. A wound hormone of plants. Isoln from pods of green beans: English *et al., Proc. Natl. Acad. Sci. USA* **25**, 323 (1939). The naturally occurring traumatic acid is the *trans*-form. Synthesis of the *trans*-form: *eidem, J. Am. Chem. Soc.* **61**, 3434 (1939); US 2339259 (1944); US 2391824 (1945); Truscheit, Eiter, *Ann.* **658**, 86 (1962); Dolezal, *Collect. Czech. Chem. Commun.* **35**, 1932 (1970); Schreurs *et al., Recl. Trav. Chim. Pays-Bas Belg.* **90**, 1331 (1971); Prakasa Rao, Nayak, *Synthesis* **1975**, 608; J. H. Babler, R. K. Moy, *Synth. Commun.* **9**, 669 (1979). Synthesis of the *cis*-form: Lauer, Gensler, *J. Am. Chem. Soc.* **67**, 1171 (1945).

trans-**Form.** Crystals from alc, acetone, or 1,2-dimethoxy-ethane, mp 166-167°. bp$_{0.001}$ 150-160°. Very sparingly sol in water; sol in alc, ether, benzene, chloroform.
cis-**Form.** Crystals from ethyl acetate and petr ether, mp 67-68°.

9577. Travoprost. [157283-68-6] (5*Z*)-7-[(1*R*,2*R*,3*R*,5*S*)-3,5-Dihydroxy-2-[(1*E*,3*R*)-3-hydroxy-4-[3-(trifluoromethyl)phenoxy]-1-butenyl]cyclopentyl]-5-heptenoic acid 1-methylethyl ester; (+)-16-[3-(trifluoromethyl)phenoxy]-17,18,19,20-tetranorprostaglandin F$_{2\alpha}$ isopropyl ester; (+)-9α,11α,15-trihydroxy-16-(3-trifluoromethylphenoxy)-17,18,19,20-tetranor-5-*cis*-13-*trans*-prostadienoic acid isopropyl ester; AL-6221; Travatan. $C_{26}H_{35}F_3O_6$; mol wt 500.55. C 62.39%, H 7.05%, F 11.39%, O 19.18%. Selective FP prostaglandin receptor agonist. Isopropyl ester of (+)-fluprostenol, *q.v.* General prepn (not claimed): J. W. Stjernschantz, **EP 364417** (1989 to Pharmacia). Large scale synthesis: L. T. Boulton *et al., Org. Process Res. Dev.* **6**, 138 (2002). Pharmacology: M. R. Hellberg *et al., J. Ocul. Pharmacol. Ther.* **17**, 421 (2001). LC/MS/MS determn in plasma: B. A. McCue *et al., J. Pharm. Biomed. Anal.* **28**, 199 (2002). Ocular hypotensive effects in dogs: A. B. Carvalho *et al., Vet. Ophthalmol.* **9**, 121 (2006). Clinical trial in glaucoma or ocular hypertension: R. L. Fellman *et al., Ophthalmology* **109**, 998 (2002); in combination with timolol: J. S. Schuman *et al., Am. J. Ophthalmol.* **140**, 242-250 (2005).

Colorless oil. $[\alpha]_D^{20}$ +14.6° (c = 1.0 in methylene chloride). Very sol in acetonitrile, methanol, octanol, chloroform. Practically insol in water.

THERAP CAT: Antiglaucoma.

THERAP CAT (VET): Antiglaucoma.

9578. Traxanox. [58712-69-9] 9-Chloro-7-(1H-tetrazol-5-yl)-5H-[1]benzopyrano[2,3-b]pyridin-5-one; 9-chloro-7-(5-1H-tetrazolyl)-5-oxo-5H-[1]benzopyrano[2,3-b]pyridine. $C_{13}H_6ClN_5O_2$; mol wt 299.67. C 52.10%, H 2.02%, Cl 11.83%, N 23.37%, O 10.68%. Antiallergic agent which selectively inhibits release of allergic mediators from mast cells. Prepn: T. Oe, M. Tsuruda, **DE 2521980**; eidem, **US 4085111** (1975, 1978 both to Yoshitomi). Antianaphylactic activity in animals: K. Goto et al., Jpn. J. Pharmacol. **30**, 537 (1980). Mechanism of action study: K. Goto et al., Int. Arch. Allergy Appl. Immunol. **68**, 332 (1982). Clinical pharmacology and pharmacokinetics: A. Ebihara et al., Arzneim.-Forsch. **37**, 1388 (1987). Metabolism in humans: M. Tateno et al., Yakuri to Chiryo **16**, 3251 (1988), C.A. **110**, 18040n (1989).

mp >300°.

Sodium salt pentahydrate. Y-12141; Clearnal. $C_{13}H_5ClN_5NaO_2 \cdot 5H_2O$; mol wt 411.73.

THERAP CAT: Antiallergic; antiasthmatic.

9579. Trazodone. [19794-93-5] 2-[3-[4-(3-Chlorophenyl)-1-piperazinyl]propyl]-1,2,4-triazolo[4,3-a]pyridin-3(2H)-one. $C_{19}H_{22}ClN_5O$; mol wt 371.86. C 61.37%, H 5.96%, Cl 9.53%, N 18.83%, O 4.30%. Prepn: Palazzo, Silvestrini, **US 3381009** (1968 to Angelini Francesco). Pharmacology: Catanese, Lisciani, Boll. Chim. Farm. **109**, 369 (1970); B. Silvestrini, E. Quadri, Eur. J. Pharmacol. **12**, 231 (1970). Analytical data: Baiocchi et al., Arzneim.-Forsch. **23**, 400 (1973). Crystal structure: J. P. Fillers, S. W. Hawkinson, Acta Crystallogr. **B35**, 498 (1979). Review of pharmacological properties and therapeutic use: R. N. Brogden et al., Drugs **21**, 401-429 (1981); B. Silvestrini et al., in Pharmacological and Biochemical Properties of Drug Substances vol. 3, M. E. Goldberg, Ed. (Am. Pharm. Assoc., Washington, DC, 1981) pp 94-119. Comprehensive description: D. Gorecki, R. Verbeeck, Anal. Profiles Drug Subs. **16**, 693-729 (1986). Symposium on clinical efficacy: Psychopharmacology **95**, Suppl., 1-56 (1988).

Crystals, mp 86-87°. Also reported as mp 96° (Baiocchi). pKa (50% ethanol): 6.14.

Hydrochloride. [25332-39-2] AF-1161; Bimaran; Desyrel; Molipaxin; Pragmazone; Thombran; Tombran; Trazolan; Trittico. $C_{19}H_{22}ClN_5O \cdot HCl$; mol wt 408.32. White, odorless plates from ethanol, mp 223°. Soluble in chloroform; sparingly sol in water, ethanol, methanol. Practically insol in common organic solvents. uv max (water): 211, 246, 274, 312 nm (ε 50100, 11730, 3840, 3840). LD_{50} i.v. in mice: 96 mg/kg (Silvestrini, Quadri).

THERAP CAT: Antidepressant.

9580. Trehalose. [99-20-7] α-D-Glucopyranosyl-α-D-glucopyranoside; mushroom sugar; mycose; α,α-trehalose. $C_{12}H_{22}O_{11}$; mol wt 342.30. C 42.11%, H 6.48%, O 51.41%. Non-reducing disaccharide found in fungi, bacteria, yeasts, and insects; 45% as sweet as sucrose. Provides the energy source for flight in many insects. Incorporated into mycobacterial structural glycolipids such as cord factors, q.v. Isoln from the ergot of rye: H. A. L. Wiggers, Ann. **1** 129 (1832). Prepn and review of early history: T. S. Harding, Sugar **25**, 476-478 (1923). Isoln from yeast: E. M. Koch, F. C. Koch, Science **61**, 570 (1925); L. C. Stewart et al., J. Am. Chem. Soc. **72**, 2059 (1950). Synthesis: Lemieux, Bauer, Can. J. Chem. **32**, 340 (1954). Crystal structure: G. A. Jeffrey, R. Nanni, Carbohydr. Res. **137**, 21 (1985). Review of metabolism: A. D. Elbein, Adv. Carbohydr. Chem. Biochem. **30**, 227-256 (1974). In vitro evaluation in cryopreservation of human oocytes: A. Eroglu et al., Fertil. Steril. **77**, 152 (2002). Use in freeze-drying human platelets: W. F. Wolkers et al., Cryobiology **42**, 79 (2001); eidem, Cell Preservation Technol. **1**, 175 (2003). Review of properties, toxicity and safety studies: A. B. Richards et al., Food Chem. Toxicol. **40**, 871-898 (2002); of stabilizing functions and applications: T. Higashiyama, Pure Appl. Chem. **74**, 1263-1269 (2002).

Dihydrate. [6138-23-4] Orthorhombic, bisphenoidal crystals from dil alcohol. Sweet taste. mp 96.5-97.5°. The water of crystn escapes around 130°. Anhydrous trehalose melts at 203°. $[\alpha]_D^{20}$ +178° (c = 7 of the dihydrate). Sol in water, hot alcohol. Insol in ether. Does not reduce Fehling's soln. Is fermented by yeast. Is not split by α-glucosidase. Acid hydrolysis gives 2 mols D-glucose.

USE: Stabilizes cells during freezing, freeze-drying and air-drying. Sweetener and stabilizer in foods; cryoprotectant for freeze-dried foods. Additive in cosmetics and personal care products.

9581. Tremetone. [4976-25-4] 1-[2,3-Dihydro-2-(1-methylethenyl)-5-benzofuranyl]ethanone; 2,3-dihydro-2-isopropenyl-5-benzofuranyl methyl ketone; 2-isopropenyl-2,3-dihydro-5-acetylbenzofuran. $C_{13}H_{14}O_2$; mol wt 202.25. C 77.20%, H 6.98%, O 15.82%. Principal ketone suspected of being the active toxin of Eupatorium urticaefolium Reichard, Compositae (white snakeroot). Isoln and structure: Bonner, DeGraw, Tetrahedron **18**, 1295 (1962). Synthesis of dihydrotremetone: DeGraw, Bonner, ibid. 1311. Synthesis of racemic tremetone: DeGraw et al., ibid. **19**, 19 (1963); Bohlmann, Buehmann, Ber. **105**, 863 (1972). Abs config: Bonner et al., Tetrahedron **20**, 1419 (1964). Review: Christensen, Econ. Bot. **19**, 293-300 (1965).

Liquid. $[\alpha]_D^{28}$ −59.6° (c = 5.52 in absolute ethanol). n_D^{25} 1.5658. d_4^{28} 1.080. uv max (ethanol): 227, 280, 285 nm (ε 11,950, 12,600, 12,300).

Dihydrotremetone. (R)-1-[2,3-Dihydro-2-(1-methylethyl)-5-benzofuranyl]ethanone. $C_{13}H_{16}O_2$. Liquid. bp 216-221°. $[\alpha]_D^{25}$ −47.0° (c = 1.78 in abs ethanol). uv max (ethanol): 231, 279 nm (ε 39,500; 18,800).

9582. Tremorine. [51-73-0] 1,1'-(2-Butyne-1,4-diyl)bispyrrolidine; 1,1'-(2-butynylene)dipyrrolidine; 1,4-dipyrrolidino-2-butyne. $C_{12}H_{20}N_2$; mol wt 192.30. C 74.95%, H 10.48%, N 14.57%. Prepn from pyrrolidine + 1,4-dichloro-2-butyne: Maier, **DE 896810** (1953 to BASF); Reppe et al., Ann. **596**, 79 (1955); Biel, DiPierro, J. Am. Chem. Soc. **80**, 4609 (1958). Review of chemical and biological studies: Karlen, Acta Pharm. Suec. **1970**, 169-200; see also Kolla, Obvintseva, Farmakol. Toksikol. **36**, 736-745 (1973).

Liquid. $bp_{2.5}$ 116-116.5°; $bp_{0.1}$ 93-95°.

Methiodide. $C_{12}H_{20}N_2 \cdot 2CH_3I$. Crystals, mp 239-240°.

USE: To produce exptl parkinsonism: Everett et al., Science **124**, 79 (1956).

9583. Trenbolone. [10161-33-8] (17β)-17-Hydroxyestra-4,9,11-trien-3-one; 4,9,11-estratrien-17β-ol-3-one; 17β-hydroxy-19-norandrosta-4,9,11-trien-3-one; 19-norandrosta-4,9,11-trien-17β-ol-3-one; trienbolone; trienolone. $C_{18}H_{22}O_2$; mol wt 270.37. C 79.96%, H 8.20%, O 11.84%. Prepn of base: Velluz et al., C.R. Hebd. Seances Acad. Sci. **257,** 569 (1963); Heller et al., Steroids **10,** 211 (1967). Base and 17-acetate: **FR M1958** and **GB 1035683** (1963 and 1966 to Roussel-UCLAF), C.A. **60,** 3039h (1964); **65,** 17027c (1966). 17-Cyclohexylmethylcarbonate: Nedelec, Costerousse, **FR M5979** (1968 to Roussel-UCLAF), C.A. **71,** 50356g (1969). Pharmacology of the acetate: Krüskemper et al., Arzneim.-Forsch. **17,** 449 (1967). Animal studies: Beranger, Malterre, C.R. Seances Soc. Biol. Ses Fil. **162,** 1157 (1968); Best, Vet. Rec. **91,** 624 (1972). Environmental degradation study: B. Schiffer et al., Environ. Health Perspect. **109,** 1145 (2001).

Crystals, mp 186°. $[\alpha]_D^{20}$ +19° (c = 0.45 in ethanol). Also reported as mp 183-186° from acetone-water. uv max: 239, 340.5 nm (ε 5260, 28000) (Heller).

Acetate. [10161-34-9] (17β)-17-Acetyloxyestra-4,9,11-trien-3-one; 17β-acetoxy-3-oxoestra-4,9,11-triene; 17β-acetoxyestra-4,9,11-trien-3-one; Finaplix; Parabolan. $C_{20}H_{24}O_3$; mol wt 312.40. Crystals, mp 96-97°. $[\alpha]_D^{20}$ +36.8° (c = 0.37 in methanol).

Cyclohexylmethylcarbonate. [23454-33-3] (17β)-17-[(cyclohexylmethoxy)carbonyl]oxyestra-4,9,11-trien-3-one; trenbolone hexahydrobenzylcarbonate. $C_{26}H_{34}O_4$; mol wt 410.55. Crystals from cyclohexane-petr ether, mp 90-95°. $[\alpha]_D^{20}$ +41.6° (c = 0.5 in ethanol).

Note: This is a controlled substance (anabolic steroid): **21 CFR,** 1308.13, as defined in 1300.01.

THERAP CAT (VET): Anabolic.

9584. Trengestone. [5192-84-7] (9β,10α)-6-Chloropregna-1,4,6-triene-3,20-dione; 6-chloro-1,6-didehydroretroprogesterone; 6-chloro-1,6-bisdehydroretroprogesterone; Ro-4-8347; Retroid. $C_{21}H_{25}ClO_2$; mol wt 344.88. C 73.13%, H 7.31%, Cl 10.28%, O 9.28%. A member of a class of hormonally active steroids termed "retrosteroids", which are characterized by a (9β, 10α)-configuration in contrast to the usual (9α,10β)-configuration of steroids. Prepn: Threadgold, **BE 652597** corresp to Reerink et al., **US 3422122** (1965, 1969 to Phillips). Activity studies: Sadovsky et al., Gynecol. Invest. **1,** 319 (1970); Kalra et al., J. Endocrinol. **51,** 675 (1971). Metabolism: Breuer et al., Acta Endocrinol. **74,** 127 (1973); Dixon et al., Steroids **22,** 35 (1973).

Crystals from acetone, mp 208-209° (dec). uv max: 229, 253, 302 nm (ε 11500, 10520, 10650).

THERAP CAT: Progestogen.

9585. Trepibutone. [41826-92-0] 2,4,5-Triethoxy-γ-oxobenzenebutanoic acid; 3-(2,4,5-triethoxybenzoyl)propionic acid; AA-149; Supacal. $C_{16}H_{22}O_6$; mol wt 310.34. C 61.92%, H 7.15%, O 30.93%. Prepn: T. Murata et al., **DE 2244324** corresp to **US 3943169** (1973, 1976 both to Takeda). Properties and stabilities: M. Mitani et al., Takeda Kenkyushoho **36,** 206 (1977), C.A. **88,** 126284f (1978). Pharmacokinetics: eidem, ibid. 215, C.A. **88,**

115067m (1978). Biotransformation: T. Kobayashi et al., Xenobiotica **8,** 535 (1978). Metabolism studies: S. Tanayama et al., ibid. 365, 377. Spasmolytic action in dogs: H. Satoh et al., Eur. J. Pharmacol. **48,** 309 (1978). Mechanism of choleretic action: eidem, ibid. 125. Toxicity studies: S. Sato et al., Takeda Kenkyushoho **36,** 263 (1977), C.A. **88,** 11535x (1978).

Colorless needles from aq ethanol or plates from aq acetone, mp 150-151°. Stable to heat, humidity, indoor diffused sunlight. Aq solns heated to 100° for 10 hr showed no degradation.

THERAP CAT: Choleretic; antispasmodic.

9586. Treprostinil. [81846-19-7] [[(1R,2R,3aS,9aS)-2,3,-3a,4,9,9a-Hexahydro-2-hydroxy-1-[(3S)-3-hydroxyoctyl]-1H-benz-[f]inden-5-yl]oxy]acetic acid; 9-deoxy-2',9α-methano-3-oxa-4,5,6-trinor-3,7-(1',3'-interphenylene)-13,14-dihydroprostaglandin F$_1$. $C_{23}H_{34}O_5$; mol wt 390.51. C 70.74%, H 8.78%, O 20.49%. Synthetic analog of prostacyclin, q.v. Prepn: P. A. Aristoff et al., **GB 2070596**; idem, **US 4306075** (both 1981 to Upjohn). Pharmacology: R. P. Steffen, M. de la Mata, Prostaglandins Leukotrienes Essen. Fatty Acids **43,** 277 (1991). Pharmacokinetics: M. J. McNulty et al., ibid. 159; of intravenous and subcutaneous administration: K. Laliberte et al., J. Cardiovasc. Pharmacol. **44,** 209 (2004). RIA determn in plasma: J. W. A. Findlay et al., ibid. 167. Clinical study in pulmonary arterial hypertension: G. Simonneau et al., Am. J. Respir. Crit. Care Med. **165,** 800 (2002); by s. c. infusion: R. J. Oudiz et al., Chest **126,** 420 (2004); by continuous i.v.: V. F. Tapson et al., ibid. **129,** 683 (2006).

Crystals from ethyl acetate in hexane, mp 121-123°.

Sodium salt. [289480-64-4] 15AU81; BW15AU; U-62840; UT-15; Remodulin. $C_{23}H_{33}NaO_5$; mol wt 412.49.

THERAP CAT: Antihypertensive.

9587. Tretoquinol. [21650-42-0] 1,2,3,4-Tetrahydro-1-[(3,4,5-trimethoxyphenyl)methyl]-6,7-isoquinolinediol; 1-(3',4',5'-trimethoxybenzyl)-6,7-dihydroxy-1,2,3,4-tetrahydroisoquinoline; trimethoquinol. $C_{19}H_{23}NO_5$; mol wt 345.39. C 66.07%, H 6.71%, N 4.06%, O 23.16%. Synthesis of dl-form: Yamato et al., Tetrahedron Suppl. **8,** 129 (1966). Pharmacology: Fogelman, Grundy, Br. J. Pharmacol. **38,** 416 (1970). Metabolic studies: Meshi et al., Biochem. Pharmacol. **19,** 2937 (1970); Satoh et al., Chem. Pharm. Bull. **19,** 667 (1971).

dl-Form hydrochloride. [18559-63-2] Pale yellow crystals from methanol + ether, decomp 224.5-226°.

l-Form hydrochloride. [18559-59-6] AQ-110; Inolin; Vems. $C_{19}H_{23}NO_5$·HCl; mol wt 381.85. Pale yellow crystals, freely sol in water; sol in alcohol.

THERAP CAT: Bronchodilator.

9588. TRH. [24305-27-9] 5-Oxo-L-prolyl-L-histidyl-L-prolinamide; thyrotropin-releasing factor; thyrotropin releasing hormone; TRF; protirelin; lopremone (rescinded USAN); TSH-releasing factor; pyroglutamylhistidylprolinamide; thyroliberin; Antepan; Stimu-TSH; Thypinone; Thyrefact. $C_{16}H_{22}N_6O_4$; mol wt 362.38. C 53.03%, H 6.12%, N 23.19%, O 17.66%. A hypothalamic neurohormone which stimulates the release and synthesis of TSH, *q.v.*, from the anterior pituitary via the hypophyseal portal system; the first of the hypothalamic regulatory hormones to be isolated, characterized, and synthesized. Isoln from bovine hypothalami: Schreiber *et al., Experientia* **18**, 338 (1962); Schally *et al., Endocrinology* **78**, 726 (1966). Purification from ovine hypothalami: Guillemin *et al., C.R. Seances Acad. Sci. Ser. D* **262**, 2278 (1966). Isoln from porcine hypothalami and properties: Schally *et al., Biochem. Biophys. Res. Commun.* **25**, 165 (1966); Schally *et al., J. Biol. Chem.* **244**, 4077 (1969). Structural studies: Folkers *et al., Biochem. Biophys. Res. Commun.* **37**, 123 (1969); Burgus *et al., C.R. Seances Acad. Sci. Ser. D* **269**, 226 (1969). Identity of isolated TRH with synthetic tripeptide: Burgus *et al., ibid.* 1870; Bowers *et al., Endocrinology* **86**, 573, 1143 (1970). Solubility: Burgus *et al., Experientia* **23**, 417 (1967). Synthesis: Flouret, *J. Med. Chem.* **13**, 843 (1970); Chang *et al., ibid.* **14**, 481 (1971); E. Gross *et al., Angew. Chem. Int. Ed.* **12**, 664 (1972); P. G. Pietta *et al., J. Org. Chem.* **39**, 44 (1974). Review of synthetic methods: Rivier, *Methods Enzymol.* **37**, 408 (1975). TRH is also believed to induce the secretion of the pituitary lactogenic hormone, prolactin, *q.v.*: Tasjian *et al., Biochem. Biophys. Res. Commun.* **43**, 516 (1971); Bowers *et al., ibid.* **51**, 512 (1973). It has been shown to block and reverse leukotriene-induced hypotension in the unanesthetized guinea pig: W. E. Lux *et al., Nature* **302**, 822 (1983). Clinical studies: Hershman, *N. Engl. J. Med.* **290**, 886 (1974). Reviews of TRH and other hypothalamic releasing hormones: Schally *et al., Recent Prog. Horm. Res.* **24**, 497 (1968); Burgus, Guillemin, *Annu. Rev. Biochem.* **39**, 499 (1970); *Polypeptide Hormones,* R. F. Beers, E. G. Bassett, Eds. (Raven Press, New York, 1980) pp 165-278.

5-oxo-Pro–His–ProNH₂

Purified TRH is partially sol in chloroform, highly sol in absolute methanol. Completely insol in pyridine. Inactivated by diazotized sulfanilic acid (Pauly reagent) and by plasma, serum, or whole blood *in vitro*. Resists inactivation by proteolytic enzymes.
Tartrate. [54974-54-8] Irtonin; Xantium. $C_{16}H_{22}N_6O_4 \cdot xC_4H_6O_6$
THERAP CAT: Prohormone.

9589. Triacetin. [102-76-1] 1,2,3-Propanetriol triacetate; glyceryl triacetate; triacetyl glycerine; Enzactin; Fungacetin. $C_9H_{14}O_6$; mol wt 218.20. C 49.54%, H 6.47%, O 43.99%. $C_3H_5(OCOCH_3)_3$. Prepd by acetylation of glycerol: Dunbar, Bolstad, *J. Org. Chem.* **21**, 1041 (1956); by reaction of oxygen with a liquid phase mixture of allyl acetate and acetic acid using a bromide as catalyst: Keith, **US 2911437** (1959 to Sinclair Refining). As an antifungal: **GB 845029** (1960 to Wisc. Alumni Res. Found.). Acute toxicity: A. Wretlind, *Acta Physiol. Scand.* **40**, 338 (1957).
Colorless, somewhat oily liquid having a slight, fatty odor and a bitter taste. d_4^{25} 1.1562, d_4^{20} 1.1596, d_{20}^{20} 1.163. mp $-78°$. bp 258-260°, bp_{40} 172°. n_D^{20} 1.4307. Sol in 14 parts water. Miscible with alcohol, ether, chloroform. Slightly sol in carbon disulfide. LD_{50} i.v. in mice: 1600 ±81 mg/kg (Wretlind).
USE: As fixative in perfumery; solvent in manuf celluloid, photographic films. Technical triacetin (a mixture of mono-, di-, and small quantities of triacetin) as a solvent for basic dyes, particularly indulines, and tannin in dyeing.
THERAP CAT: Antifungal (topical).

9590. Triacetone Triperoxide. [17088-37-8] 3,3,6,6,9,9-Hexamethyl-1,2,4,5,7,8-hexoxonane; 3,3,6,6,9,9-hexamethyl-1,4,7-cyclononatriperoxane; TATP; trimeric acetone peroxide. $C_9H_{18}O_6$; mol wt 222.24. C 48.64%, H 8.16%, O 43.19%. Explosive solid; decomposes via an entropically favorable mechanism to form 4 gas phase molecules. Prepn: R. Wolffenstein, *Ber.* **28**, 2265 (1895); A. Baeyer, V. Villiger, *ibid.* **33**, 858 (1900); F. Acree, Jr., H. L. Haller, *J. Am. Chem. Soc.* **65**, 1652 (1943). Crystal structure determn: P. Groth, *Acta Chem. Scand.* **23**, 1311 (1969). Spectroscopic characterization and detection by ion mobility spectrometry: G. A. But-

tigieg *et al., Forensic Sci. Int.* **135**, 53 (2003). Decompn study: F. Dubnikova *et al., J. Am. Chem. Soc.* **127**, 1146 (2005).

Crystals from methyl alcohol, mp 98°. d 1.22. *Explosive! Sensitive to mechanical stress and open flame. Highly volatile.*
USE: In explosives.

9591. 1-Triacontanol. [593-50-0] Melissyl alcohol; myricyl alcohol; 1-hydroxytriacontane. $C_{30}H_{62}O$; mol wt 438.81. C 82.11%, H 14.24%, O 3.65%. $CH_3(CH_2)_{28}CH_2OH$. Present in plant cuticle waxes and in beeswax as the palmitate. Prepn: Robinson, *J. Chem. Soc.* **1934**, 1545; K. Maruyama *et al., J. Org. Chem.* **45**, 737 (1980). Use as a plant growth regulator: S. K. Ries *et al., Science* **195**, 1339 (1977); S. K. Ries, **BE 854587** corresp to **US 4150970** (1977, 1979 to Michigan State Univ.). Use of colloidally dispersed triacontanol in plant growth enhancement studies: R. G. Laughlin *et al., Science* **219**, 1219 (1983).
Crystals. d_{95} 0.777. mp 87°. Practically insol in water; freely sol in benzene, ether; very slightly sol in cold, more sol in hot alcohol.
USE: Plant growth regulator.

9592. Triadimefon. [43121-43-3] 1-(4-Chlorophenoxy)-3,3-dimethyl-1-(1*H*-1,2,4-triazol-1-yl)-2-butanone; BAY MEB 6447; Bayleton. $C_{14}H_{16}ClN_3O_2$; mol wt 293.75. C 57.24%, H 5.49%, Cl 12.07%, N 14.30%, O 10.89%. Systemic fungicide active against mildews and rusts of grains, fruits, vegetables and ornamentals. Prepn and activity: W. Meiser *et al., DE 2201063* corresp to **US 3912752** (1973, 1975 to Bayer). Fungal metabolism: M. Gasztonyi, *Pestic. Sci.* **12**, 433 (1981). *Reviews:* F. Michel, P. Pourcharesse, *Def. Veg.* **31**, 97-109 (1977); T. J. Martin, D. B. Morris, *Pflanzenschutz-Nachr.* **32**, 31-79 (1979).

Crystals, mp 82°. Soly in water at 20°: 260 mg/l. Moderately sol in most organic solvents except aliphatics. LD_{50} in male, female rats (mg/kg): 568, 363 orally (Michel, Pourcharesse).
USE: Systemic agricultural fungicide.

9593. Triadimenol. [55219-65-3] β-(4-Chlorophenoxy)-α-(1,1-dimethylethyl)-1*H*-1,2,4-triazole-1-ethanol; 1-(4-chlorophenoxy)-3,3-dimethyl-1-(1*H*-1,2,4-triazol-1-yl)butan-2-ol; BAY KWG 0519; Bayfidan; Baytan; Spinnaker; Summit. $C_{14}H_{18}ClN_3O_2$; mol wt 295.76. C 56.85%, H 6.13%, Cl 11.99%, N 14.21%, O 10.82%. Agricultural fungicide systemically active against powdery mildews and rusts of grains. Commercial product is mixture of 2 diastereoisomers. Prepn: **BE 814831**; W. Kramer *et al.,* **US 3952002** (1974, 1976 both to Bayer AG). Comprehensive description: P. E. Frohberger, *Pflanzenschutz-Nachr.* **31**, 11 (1978). Field trials in cereal diseases: J. Trägner-Born, T. van den Boom, *ibid.* 25. Inhibits fungal ergosterol biosynthesis: H. Buchenauer, *Pestic. Sci.* **9**, 507 (1978). Active fungal metabolite of triadimefon, *q.v.*: M. Gasztonyi, *ibid.* **12**, 433 (1981). GC separation of enantiomers: T. Clark, A. H. B. Deas, *J. Chromatogr.* **329**, 181 (1985).

Crystals, mp 112-117°. Slight, non-specific odor. Soly in water at 20°: 0.012 g/100 g. Soluble in alcohol, ketones. LD_{50} in male, female rats (mg/kg): 1161, 1105 orally; >5000 dermally, 24-hr; LD_{50} in quail: >10000 mg/kg (Frohberger).

USE: Systemic agricultural fungicide; cereal seed protectant.

9594. Triallate. [2303-17-5] Bis(1-methylethyl)carbamothioic acid S-(2,3,3-trichloro-2-propenyl) ester; diisopropyl-thiocarbamic acid S-(2,3,3-trichloroallyl) ester; 2,3,3-trichloro-2-propene-1-thiol diisopropylcarbamate; S-2,3,3-trichloroallyl diisopropylthiocarbamate; S-(2,3,3-trichloro-2-propenyl) bis(1-methylethyl)carbamothioate; CP-23426; Avadex BW; Far-Go. $C_{10}H_{16}$-Cl_3NOS; mol wt 304.66. C 39.42%, H 5.29%, Cl 34.91%, N 4.60%, O 5.25%, S 10.52%. Selective herbicide for control of wild oats in wheat. Prepn: M. W. Harman, J. J. D'Amico, **US 3330821** (1967 to Monsanto). Herbicidal activity: R. Grover et al., *Weed Res.* **19**, 363 (1979). Mutagenic evaluation *in vitro* (Ames Test): F. De Lorenzo et al., *Cancer Res.* **38**, 13 (1978); G. R. Douglas et al., *Mutat. Res.* **85**, 45 (1981). Soil persistence: A. E. Smith, B. J. Hayden, *Bull. Environ. Contam. Toxicol.* **29**, 240 (1982). Field studies for pre-emergent use: T. G. Reeves, C. L. Touhey, *Aust. J. Exp. Agric. Anim. Husb.* **12**, 55 (1972); E. M. Randall, R. H. Jarvis, *Exp. Husb.* **38**, 32 (1982); post-emergent use: R. P. Garnett, *Aspects Appl. Biol.* **13**, 73 (1980). Determn in soils by GC: A. E. Smith, *J. Chromatogr.* **97**, 103 (1974); by HPLC: A. Pena Heras, F. Sanchez-Rasero, *ibid.* **358**, 302 (1986). Review of genotoxicity: C. E. Healy et al., *Int. J. Toxicol.* **22**, 233-251 (2003).

USE: Herbicide.

9595. Triamcinolone. [124-94-7] (11β, 16α)-9-Fluoro-11,-16,17,21-tetrahydroxypregna-1,4-diene-3,20-dione; Δ^1-9α-fluoro-16α-hydroxyhydrocortisone; 9α-fluoro-16α-hydroxyprednisolone; Δ^1-16α-hydroxy-9α-fluorohydrocortisone; 16α-hydroxy-9α-fluoroprednisolone; CL-19823; Aristocort; Kenacort; Ledercort (tabl.); Omcilon; Tricortale; Volon. $C_{21}H_{27}FO_6$; mol wt 394.43. C 63.95%, H 6.90%, F 4.82%, O 24.34%. Prepn: Bernstein et al., *J. Am. Chem. Soc.* **78**, 5693 (1956); **81**, 1689 (1959); Thoma et al., *ibid.* **79**, 4818 (1957); Bernstein et al., Allen et al., **US 2789118; US 3021347** (1957, 1962, both to Am. Cyanamid). Comprehensive description: K. Florey, *Anal. Profiles Drug Subs.* **1**, 367-396, 423-442 (1972); D. H. Sieh, *ibid.* **11**, 593-614, 651-661 (1982).

Crystals, mp 269-271°. mp also reported as 260-262.5°. $[\alpha]_D^{25}$ +75° (acetone). uv max: 238 nm (ε 15800).

16,21-Diacetate. [67-78-7] (11β,16α)-16,21-Bis(acetyloxy)-9-fluoro-11,17-dihydroxypregna-1,4-diene-3,20-dione; 16α,21-diacetoxy-9α-fluoro-11β,17α-dihydroxy-1,4-pregnadiene-3,20-dione; Cenocort; CINO-40; Tracilon. $C_{25}H_{31}FO_8$; mol wt 478.51. Solvated crystals, mp 186-188° (with effervescence, mp 235° after drying). $[\alpha]_D^{25}$ +22° (chloroform). uv max: 239 nm (ε 15200).

THERAP CAT: Glucocorticoid.

THERAP CAT (VET): Glucocorticoid.

9596. Triamcinolone Acetonide. [76-25-5] (11β,16α)-9-Fluoro-11,21-dihydroxy-16,17-[1-methylethylidenebis(oxy)]pregna-1,4-diene-3,20-dione; 9α-fluoro-11β,16α,17,21-tetrahydroxy-pregna-1,4-diene-3,20-dione cyclic 16,17-acetal with acetone; 9α-fluoro-16α-hydroxyprednisolone acetonide; triamcinolone 16α,17-acetonide; 9α-fluoro-11β,21-dihydroxy-16α,17α-isopropylidene-

dioxy-1,4-pregnadiene-3,20-dione; 9α-fluoro-16α,17-isopropylidenedioxyprednisolone; Adcortyl; Azmacort; Delphicort; Extracort; Ftorocort; Kenacort-A; Kenalog; Ledercort Cream; Nasacort; Respicort; Rineton; Solodelf; Tramacin; Triam; Tricinolon; Vetalog; Volon A; Volonimat. $C_{24}H_{31}FO_6$; mol wt 434.50. C 66.34%, H 7.19%, F 4.37%, O 22.09%. Prepd by stirring a suspension of triamcinolone in acetone in the presence of a trace of perchloric acid: Fried et al., *J. Am. Chem. Soc.* **80**, 2338 (1958); Bernstein et al., *ibid.* **81**, 1689 (1959); Bernstein, Allen, **US 2990401** (1961 to Am. Cyanamid). Alternate synthesis using 2,3-dibromo-5,6-dicyanoquinone: Hydorn, **US 3035050** (1962 to Olin Mathieson). Clinical trial in chronic asthma: I. L. Bernstein et al., *Chest* **81**, 20 (1982). Comprehensive description: K. Florey, *Anal. Profiles Drug Subs.* **1**, 397-421 (1972); D. H. Sieh, *ibid.* **11**, 615-649 (1982).

Crystals, mp 292-294°. $[\alpha]_D^{23}$ +109° (c = 0.75 in chloroform). uv max (abs alc.): 238 nm (ε 14600). Sparingly sol in methanol, acetone, ethyl acetate.

21-Acetate. Crystals, mp 268-270°. $[\alpha]_D^{23}$ +92° (c = 0.59 in chloroform).

21-Disodium phosphate. [1997-15-5] Aristosol. $C_{24}H_{30}$-FNa_2O_9P; mol wt 558.44.

21-Hemisuccinate. Solutedarol. $C_{28}H_{35}FO_9$; mol wt 534.57.

THERAP CAT: Glucocorticoid; antiasthmatic (inhalant); antiallergic (nasal).

THERAP CAT (VET): Glucocorticoid.

9597. Triamcinolone Benetonide. [31002-79-6] (11β,-16α)-21-[3-(Benzoylamino)-2-methyl-1-oxopropoxy]-9-fluoro-11-hydroxy-16,17-[(1-methylethylidene)bis(oxy)]pregna-1,4-diene-3,20-dione; 9-fluoro-11β,16α,17,21-tetrahydroxypregna-1,4-diene-3,20-dione cyclic 16,17-acetal with acetone 21-ester with N-benzoyl-2-methyl-β-alanine; 9α-fluoro-16α-hydroxyprednisolone 16α,17α-acetonide 21-(β-benzoylamino)isobutyrate; triamcinolone acetonide β-benzoylaminoisobutyrate; TBI; Tibicorten. $C_{35}H_{42}$-FNO_8; mol wt 623.71. C 67.40%, H 6.79%, F 3.05%, N 2.25%, O 20.52%. Prepn: C. Cavazza et al., **DE 2047218**; *eidem*, **US 3749712** (1971, 1973 both to Sigma-Tau). Pharmacology: E. T. Ordonez, *Arzneim.-Forsch.* **21**, 248 (1971). Percutaneous absorption by rats and rabbits: W. H. Down et al., *Toxicol. Lett.* **1**, 95 (1977). Clinical study: D. J. Tazelaar, *J. Int. Med. Res.* **5**, 338 (1977). HPLC analysis: S. Muck et al., *Boll. Chim. Farm.* **120**, 240 (1981). For structure *see* Triamcinolone Acetonide.

Crystalline powder, mp 203-207°. $[\alpha]_D^{20}$ +96 ±3° (c = 1 in ethanol). Sol in methanol, acetone, ethanol, dioxane, pyridine, DMF, chloroform. Insol in water.

THERAP CAT: Glucocorticoid; anti-inflammatory (topical).

9598. Triamcinolone Hexacetonide. [5611-51-8] (11β,16α)-21-(3,3-dimethyl-1-oxobutoxy)-9-fluoro-11-hydroxy-16,17-[(1-methylethylidene)bis(oxy)]pregna-1,4-diene-3,20-dione; 9-fluoro-11β,16α,17,21-tetrahydroxypregna-1,4-diene-3,20-dione cyclic 16,17-acetal with acetone, 21-(3,3-dimethylbutyrate); 21-tert-butylacetate-9α-fluoro-11β-hydroxy-16α,17α-(isopropylidenedioxy)pregna-1,4-diene-3,20-dione; 21-(3,3-dimethylbutyryloxy)-9α-fluoro-11β-hydroxy-16α,17α-(isopropylidenedioxy)pregna-1,4-diene-3,20-dione; triamcinolone acetonide tert-butyl acetate; TATBA; CL-34433; Aristospan; Hexatrione; Lederlon; Lederspan. $C_{30}H_{41}FO_7$; mol wt 532.64. C 67.65%, H 7.76%, F 3.57%, O 21.03%. The hexacetonide ester of the potent glucocorticoid, triamcinolone, *q.v.* Prepn of syringeable suspension: Nash, Naeger, **US 3457348** (1969 to Am. Cyanamid). Anti-inflammatory activity in rabbits: I. M. Hunneyball, *Agents Actions* **11**, 490 (1981). Early clinical studies: Bilka, *Minn. Med.* **50**, 483 (1967); Layman, Peterson, *ibid.* 669. Clinical studies of intra-articular therapy in arthritis: R. C. Allen et al., *Arthritis Rheum.* **29**, 997 (1986); M.

Talke, *Fortschr. Med.* **104,** 742 (1986). Toxicity study: Tonelli, *Steroids* **8,** 857 (1966). Comprehensive description: V. Zbinovsky, G. P. Chrekian, *Anal. Profiles Drug Subs.* **6,** 579-595 (1977). For structure *see* Triamcinolone Acetonide.

Fine, white, needle-like crystals, mp 295-296° (dec), also reported as mp 271-272° (dec). uv max (ethanol): 238 nm (ε 15500). $[\alpha]_D^{25}$ +90±2° (c = 1.13% in chloroform). Soly in g/100 ml at 25°: chloroform and dimethylacetamide >5; ethyl acetate 0.77, methanol 0.59, diethyl carbonate 0.50, glycerin 0.42, propylene glycol 0.13; absolute alcohol 0.03; water 0.0004.

THERAP CAT: Anti-inflammatory.

9599. Triamterene. [396-01-0] 6-Phenyl-2,4,7-pteridine-triamine; 2,4,7-triamino-6-phenylpteridine; 6-phenyl-2,4,7-triaminopteridine; ademin(e); pterofen; pterophene; NSC-77625; SKF-8542; Dyren; Dyrenium; Dytac; Jatropur; Teriam; Triteren; Urocaudal. $C_{12}H_{11}N_7$; mol wt 253.26. C 56.91%, H 4.38%, N 38.71%. Prepn: Spickett, Timmis, *J. Chem. Soc.* **1954,** 2887; Pachter, *J. Org. Chem.* **28,** 1191 (1963); Weinstock, Wiebelhaus, US **3081230** (1963 to SK & F); Osdene *et al., J. Med. Chem.* **10,** 431 (1967). *Review: Ther. Triamteren Wien. Symp.* **1966,** K. Fellinger, Ed. (Georg Thieme, Vienna, 1967). Comprehensive description: V. K. Kapoor, *Anal. Profiles Drug Subs. Excip.* **23,** 571-605 (1994).

Yellow plates from butanol, mp 316° (Spickett, Timmis); also reported as crystals from DMF, mp 327° (Osdene *et al.*). pKa 6.2. Practically insol in ether. Sol in formic acid. Slight sol in water (1 in 1000), ethanol (1 in 3000), chloroform (1 in 4000). uv max (4.5% formic acid): 356 nm (ε 21000).

THERAP CAT: Diuretic.

9600. Triasulfuron. [82097-50-5] 2-(2-Chloroethoxy)-*N*-[[(4-methoxy-6-methyl-1,3,5-triazin-2-yl)amino]carbonyl]benzene-sulfonamide; 1-[2-(2-chloroethoxy)phenylsulfonyl]-3-(4-methoxy-6-methyl-1,3,5-triazin-2-yl)urea; CGA-131036; Amber; Logran. $C_{14}H_{16}ClN_5O_5S$; mol wt 401.83. C 41.85%, H 4.01%, Cl 8.82%, N 17.43%, O 19.91%, S 7.98%. Sulfonylurea herbicide for broadleaf weeds. Prepn: W. Meyer, W. Föry, **EP 44808**; *eidem,* **US 4514212** (1982, 1985 both to Ciba-Geigy). Comprehensive description: J. Amrein, H. R. Gerber, *Proc. Br. Crop Prot. Conf. - Weeds* **1985,** 55-62. Uptake and metabolism in wheat: A. M. Meyer, F. Müller, *Brighton Crop Prot. Conf. - Weeds* **1989,** 441. Behavior in soil: F. K. Oppong, G. R. Sagar, *Weed Res.* **32,** 157, 167 (1992). Immunoassay in soil: J. A. Schlaeppi *et al., J. Agric. Food Chem.* **42,** 1914 (1994).

White crystals, mp 186°. Vapor pressure (20°): 7.5×10^{-13} mm Hg. Soly in water (20°): 1.5 g/l (pH 7). LD_{50} in rats (mg/kg): >5000 orally; >2000 dermally; LC_{50} (4 hr) in rats: >5185 mg/m³ by inhalation (Amrein, Gerber).

USE: Herbicide.

9601. Triazamate. [112143-82-5] [[1-[(Dimethylamino)-carbonyl]-3-(1,1-dimethylethyl)-1*H*-1,2,4-triazol-5-yl]thio]acetic acid ethyl ester; ethyl (3-*tert*-butyl-1-dimethylcarbamoyl-1*H*-1,2,4-triazol-5-ylthio)acetate; 1-dimethylcarbamoyl-3-*tert*-butyl-5-carbo-ethoxymethylthio-1,2,4-triazole; RH-7988; WL-145158; Aphistar; Aztec. $C_{13}H_{22}N_4O_3S$; mol wt 314.40. C 49.66%, H 7.05%, N 17.82%, O 15.27%, S 10.20%. Cholinesterase inhibitor. Prepn: R. M. Jacobson *et al.,* **EP 213718**; R. M. Jacobson, M. Thirugnanam, US **4742072** (1987, 1988 both to Rohm and Haas). Properties

and biological activity: A. Murray *et al., Brighton Crop Prot. Conf. - Pests Dis.* **1988,** 73. Field studies on sugar beets: A. M. Dewar *et al., ibid.* **1994,** 407. HPLC determn in crops: R. Weitzel, U. Zimmermann, *ibid.* **1996,** 983. Review of metabolism and aphicidal spectrum: R. M. Jacobson, M. Thriugnanam, *ACS Symp. Ser.* **443,** 322-339 (1991).

Light tan solid, mp 60°. Vapor pressure 4.8×10^{-6} torr. Soly of technical grade in water <1%; sol in methylene chloride, ethyl acetate. LD_{50} (14 d) in mice, rats (mg/kg): 61, 50-200 orally; in rats (mg/kg): >5000 dermally (Murray). LC_{50} (48 h) in daphnia: 0.048 mg/l; (96 h) in bluegill, trout: 1.0, 0.43 mg/l (Murray).

USE: Pesticide.

9602. s-Triazine. [290-87-9] 1,3,5-Triazine. $C_3H_3N_3$; mol wt 81.08. C 44.44%, H 3.73%, N 51.83%. Originally prepd in 1895 and incorrectly identified as "dimeric hydrocyanic acid," C_2-H_2N_2. Prepn: C. Grundmann, A. Kreutzberger, *J. Am. Chem. Soc.* **76,** 632, 5646 (1954). Reactivity and use in synthesis of heterocycles: *eidem, ibid.* **77,** 44, 6559 (1955). IR and Raman spectroscopy: J. Goubeau *et al., J. Phys. Chem.* **58,** 1078 (1954). X-ray crystal structure: P. J. Wheatley, *Acta Crystallogr.* **8,** 224 (1955). Determn of enthalpy of combustion and sublimation: K. Byström, *J. Chem. Thermodynam.* **14,** 865 (1982). Molecular structure: C. A. Morrison *et al., J. Phys. Chem. A* **101,** 10029 (1997). Review of applications in organic chemistry: T. Güthner, *Chim. Oggi* **17,** 12-14 (1999); G. Giacomelli *et al., Curr. Org. Chem.* **8,** 1497-1519 (2004).

Rhombohedral crystals, mp 86°. bp_{760} 114°. *Extremely volatile. Hydrolyzes to formamide upon contact with water. Store in a tightly sealed container.*

USE: Reagent in oxidation reactions, in synthesis of heterocycles. Triazine derivatives are used as herbicides, pharmaceuticals, complexation agents, peptidomimetic building blocks, and dyes.

9603. Triaziquone. [68-76-8] 2,3,5-Tris(1-aziridinyl)-2,5-cyclohexadiene-1,4-dione; 2,3,5-tris(1-aziridinyl)-*p*-benzoquinone; 2,3,5-tris(aziridino)-1,4-benzoquinone; 2,3,5-tris(ethyleneimino)-benzoquinone; trenimon; Bayer 3231. $C_{12}H_{13}N_3O_2$; mol wt 231.25. C 62.33%, H 5.67%, N 18.17%, O 13.84%. Polyfunctional alkylating agent. Prepn: Gauss, Domagk, US **2976279** (1961 to Schenley). Review of biochemical, physiological and genetic effects: G. Obe, B. Beek, *Mutat. Res.* **65,** 21-70 (1979); of structure and chemical reactivity: P. Rademacher, G. Obe, *ibid.* **340,** 37-49 (1995).

Purple acicular crystals from ethyl acetate, mp 162.5-163°. Sparingly sol in cold water; sol in acetone, benzene, chloroform, ethyl acetate, methanol and warm acetic acid.

USE: Alkylating reagent in mutation research.

9604. Triazolam. [28911-01-5] 8-Chloro-6-(2-chlorophenyl)-1-methyl-4*H*-[1,2,4]triazolo[4,3-*a*][1,4]benzodiazepine; 8-chloro-6-(*o*-chlorophenyl)-1-methyl-4*H*-*s*-triazolo[4,3-*a*][1,4]benzodiazepine; clorazolam; U-33030; Halcion; Songar. $C_{17}H_{12}Cl_2N_4$; mol wt 343.21. C 59.49%, H 3.52%, Cl 20.66%, N 16.32%. Prepn:

J. B. Hester, **DE 2012190**; *idem,* **US 3701782** (1970, 1972 both to Upjohn); J. B. Hester *et al., J. Med. Chem.* **14**, 1078 (1971). Pharmacology: T. Furukawa *et al., Igaku Kenkyu* **45**, 285 (1975), *C.A.* **84**, 130354p. Metabolism: F. S. Eberts, *Drug Metab. Dispos.* **5**, 547 (1977). HPLC determn in urine: T. Inoue, S. Suzuki, *J. Chromatogr.* **422**, 197 (1987). Clinical studies: K. K. Okawa, G. S. Allens, *J. Int. Med. Res.* **6**, 343 (1978); A. J. Bowen, *ibid.* 337; A. J. Puech *et al., Therapie* **33**, 287 (1978). Toxicity: *Pharm. Weekbl.* **113**, 725 (1978). Review of pharmacology and therapeutic efficacy: G. E. Pakes *et al., Drugs* **22**, 81-110 (1981).

Tan crystals from 2-propanol, mp 233-235°. Sol in alcohol. Poorly sol in water. LD_{50} in mice, rats (mg/kg): >100, >5000 orally *(Pharm. Weekblad.).*

Note: This is a controlled substance (depressant): **21 CFR,** 1308.14.

THERAP CAT: Sedative, hypnotic.

9605. 1*H*-1,2,4-Triazole. [288-88-0] Pyrrodiazole. $C_2H_3N_3$; mol wt 69.07. C 34.78%, H 4.38%, N 60.84%. Prepn starting with thiosemicarbazide and formic acid: Ainsworth, *Org. Synth.* **40**, 99 (1960).

Needles from ethanol + benzene, mp 120-121°. bp_{760} 260° (de-compn). Appreciably sol in water, alcohol.

Hydrochloride. $C_2H_3N_3 \cdot HCl$. Platelets, dec 169°.

9606. Triazophos. [24017-47-8] Phosphorothioic acid *O,O*-diethyl *O*-(1-phenyl-1*H*-1,2,4-triazol-3-yl)ester; 1-phenyl-3-(*O,O*-diethylthionophosphoryl)-1,2,4-triazole; HOE-2960; Hostathion. $C_{12}H_{16}N_3O_3PS$; mol wt 313.31. C 46.00%, H 5.15%, N 13.41%, O 15.32%, P 9.89%, S 10.23%. Cholinesterase inhibitor. Prepn: O. Scherer, H Mildenberger, **ZA 6803471**; *idem,* **US 3686200** (1968, 1972 both to Hoechst). Properties and analytical methods: W. G. Thier *et al. Anal. Methods Pestic. Plant Growth Regul.* **10**, 127 (1978). Degradation studies: K.-D. Bock *et al., Environ. Quality Safety, Suppl. 3 (Pesticides)* 833 (1975). GC determn: H.-J. Stan, D. Mrowetz, *J. Chromatogr.* **279**, 173 (1983). Soil adsorption studies: G. S. Rao *et al., Indian J. Agric. Sci.* **61**, 674 (1991). Field studies as insecticide and acaricide: S. J. B. Hay, *Proc. 6th Brit. Crop Prot. Council - Insect. Fungic.* 597 (1972). Nematicidal activity: A. Sirohi, Siyanand, *Indian J. Nematol.* **22**, 134 (1992).

Light brown oil, mp 0-5°. Vapor pressure 2.9×10^{-6} mbar (303 K). d 1.247. Soly at 296 K: 39 ppm in water. Soly at 298 K (g/100 ml): *n*-hexane 0.7, toluene 30, ethyl acetate 30, acetone 30, ethanol 30. LD_{50} in rats (mg/kg): 82 orally, 1100 dermally (Thier). LD_{50} in rats (mg/kg): 107 i.p.; in rabbits (mg/kg): 280 dermally (Hay).

USE: Pesticide.

9607. Triazoxide. [72459-58-6] 7-Chloro-3-(1*H*-imidazol-1-yl)-1,2,4-benzotriazine 1-oxide; 3-(imidazol-1-yl)-7-chloro-benzo-1,2,4-triazine-1-oxide; BAY SAS 9244. $C_{10}H_6ClN_5O$; mol

wt 247.64. C 48.50%, H 2.44%, Cl 14.32%, N 28.28%, O 6.46%. Prepn: K. Sasse *et al.,* **DE 2802488**; *idem,* **US 4239760** (1979, 1980 both to Bayer). GC determn in water: R. Brennecke, K. Vogeler, *Pflanzenschutz-Nachr.* **37**, 46 (1984). HPLC determn of adsorption coeff on soil: W. Kördel *et al., Sci. Total Environ.* **162**, 119 (1995). Physicochemical properties, toxicology, and fungicidal activity: S. Dutzmann, *Br. Crop Prot. Counc. Monogr.* **57**, 85 (1994). Field trials in combination with tebuconazole, *q.v.:* A. Wainwright *et al., ibid.* 103.

Light yellow crystals, mp 182° (Dutzmann); also reported as mp 172° (Sasse). Vapor pressure at 25°: 5.2×10^{-12} Pa. Soly at 20° (g/l): water 0.03; *n*-hexane <1; dichloromethane 50-100; 2-propa-nol 2-5; toluene 20-50. LD_{50} in rats (mg/kg): >5000 dermally; 100-200 orally. LC_{50} (4hr) in rats (mg/l): 0.8-3.2 by inhalation (Dutzmann).

USE: Fungicide.

9608. Tribenoside. [10310-32-4] Ethyl 3,5,6-tris-*O*-(phen-ylmethyl)-D-glucofuranoside; Ba-21401; Alven; Flebosan; Glyve-nol; Hemocuron; Venex. $C_{29}H_{34}O_6$; mol wt 478.58. C 72.78%, H 7.16%, O 20.06%. Prepn: Druey, Huber, **US 3157634** (1964 to Ciba). Pharmacology: Lecomte, *C.R. Seances Soc. Biol. Ses Fil.* **163**, 1469 (1969); Helfer, Jaques, *Pharmacology* **5**, 23 (1971). Increase in capillary resistance in patients with rheumatoid arthritis: W. C. Dick *et al., Ann. Rheum. Dis.* **28**, 187 (1969). GLC determn in plasma: A. Sioufi, F. Pommier, *J. Pharm. Sci.* **69**, 167 (1980). Excretion as hippuric acid: *idem, Eur. J. Drug Metab. Pharma-cokinet.* **7**, 223 (1982). Review of pharmacology: R. Jaques, *ibid.* **15**, 445-460 (1977).

$bp_{1.2}$ 270-280°. $[\alpha]_D^{26}$ +8° (chloroform).

THERAP CAT: Sclerosing agent.

9609. Tribromoacetic Acid. [75-96-7] $C_2HBr_3O_2$; mol wt 296.74. C 8.10%, H 0.34%, Br 80.78%, O 10.78%. CBr_3COOH. Prepn: Müller, **US 2057964** (1936 to Winthrop Chem.); A. M. Kovalevskaya, S. A. Shkylar, *Zh. Org. Khim.* **1**, 1540 (1965). Study of far IR spectrum: G. Statz, E. Lippert, *Ber. Bunsen-Ges. Phys. Chem.* **71**, 673 (1967).

Monoclinic prisms, mp 129-135°. bp 245° (dec). Sol in water, alcohol, ether; slightly sol in petr ether. Dec in boiling water to bromoform.

USE: Catalyst for polymerization; as brominating agent: W. J. Szczepek, *Pol. J. Chem.* **55**, 709 (1981).

9610. 2,4,6-Tribromoaniline. [147-82-0] Aniline tribro-mide. $C_6H_4Br_3N$; mol wt 329.81. C 21.85%, H 1.22%, Br 72.68%, N 4.25%. Prepd by controlled bromination of aniline: Suthers *et al., J. Org. Chem.* **27**, 447 (1962).

Needles; d 2.35; mp 120-122°; bp 300°. Insol in water. Sol in hot alc, chloroform, ether; slightly sol in cold alcohol.

9611. Tribromo-*tert*-butyl Alcohol. [76-08-4] 1,1,1-Tribromo-2-methyl-2-propanol; acetone-bromoform; brometone. $C_4H_7Br_3O$; mol wt 310.81. C 15.46%, H 2.27%, Br 77.12%, O 5.15%. $(CH_3)_2C(OH)CBr_3$. Prepd from acetone and bromoform in the presence of sodium or potassium hydroxide: Aldrich, *J. Am. Chem. Soc.* **33**, 386 (1911); Viehe *et al., Ber.* **96**, 426 (1963).

Crystals from dil alcohol, mp 167-176° (Aldrich), from ether, mp 169° (Viehe). Camphor-like odor and taste. Volatilizes in air. Slightly sol in water; sol in alcohol, ether.

USE: As modifier in polymerization of vinyl chloride, Seymour, **US 2716112** (1955 to U.S. Rubber).

9612. 2,4,6-Tribromo-*m*-cresol. [4619-74-3] 2,4,6-Tribromo-3-methylphenol; 2,4,6-tribromo-3-hydroxytoluene; Micatex. $C_7H_5Br_3O$; mol wt 344.83. C 24.38%, H 1.46%, Br 69.52%, O 4.64%. Prepn by bromination of *m*-cresol: Biilmann, Rimbert, *Bull. Soc. Chim. Fr.* [4] **33**, 1473 (1923).

Crystals from 50% aq alcohol, mp 84°.
THERAP CAT: Antifungal (topical).

9613. 2,4,6-Tribromophenol. [118-79-6] Bromol. $C_6H_3Br_3O$; mol wt 330.80. C 21.78%, H 0.91%, Br 72.46%, O 4.84%. Prepd by controlled bromination of phenol: Konecny, *J. Am. Chem. Soc.* **76**, 4993 (1954). Toxicity study: E. F. Stohlman, *Public Health Rep.* **66**, 1303 (1951).

Long crystals; d 2.55; mp 94-96°; bp 244°. Sublimable. Sol in 14,000 parts water at 15°; sol in alcohol, chloroform, ether, glycerol oils. LD_{50} orally in rats: <2000 mg/kg (Stohlman).

9614. 1,2,3-Tribromopropane. [96-11-7] *sym*-Tribromopropane; glycerol tribromohydrin; tribromohydrin; allyl tribromide. $C_3H_5Br_3$; mol wt 280.78. C 12.83%, H 1.79%, Br 85.37%. $BrCH_2CHBrCH_2Br$. Prepd by the addn of bromine to allyl bromide in carbon tetrachloride: Perkin, Simonsen, *J. Chem. Soc.* **87**, 859 (1905); Johnson, McEwen, *Org. Synth.* **5**, 99 (1925). By gentle heating of propylene bromide with bromine in the presence of iron wire: Kronstein, *Ber.* **54**, 7 (1921); Tapley, Giesy, *J. Am. Pharm. Assoc.* **15**, 173 (1926); by reaction of bromotrichloromethane with allyl bromide initiated by γ-rays: Heiba, Anderson, *J. Am. Chem. Soc.* **79**, 4940 (1957).

Liquid; d^{23} 2.436; mp 16.5°; bp_{760} 220°; bp_{200} 170°; bp_{100} 148°; bp_{60} 134°; bp_{40} 123°; bp_{20} 106°; bp_{10} 90°; bp_5 76°; $bp_{1.0}$ 47.5°; n_D^{18} 1.58436. Insol in water; sol in alcohol, ether, chloroform.

USE: As a nematocide: Youngson, Goring, **US 3003914** (1959 to Dow).

9615. Tribromosilane. [7789-57-3] Tribromomonosilane; silicobromoform. Br_3HSi; mol wt 268.81. Br 89.18%, H 0.37%, Si 10.45%. $SiHBr_3$. Prepd by passing hydrogen bromide over heated silicon or a silicide such as copper silicide: Schumb, Young, *Inorg. Synth.* **1**, 38 (1939); Schenk in *Handbook of Preparative Inorganic Chemistry* **vol. 1**, G. Brauer, Ed. (Academic Press, New York, 2nd ed., 1963) pp 692-694.

Mobile liquid. Spontaneously flammable when the contact surface with air is large. d_4^{17} 2.7. mp −73.5°. bp_{760} 111.8°. The vapor pressure at 0° is given as 8.8 mm Hg. Dipole moment 0.79. Hydrolyzed by water with the formation of silicoformic anhydride, $H_2Si_2O_3$ and HBr. Sol in chlorinated hydrocarbons.

9616. Tribromsalan. [87-10-5] 3,5-Dibromo-*N*-(4-bromophenyl)-2-hydroxybenzamide; 3,4′,5-tribromosalicylanilide; TBS; Temasept IV. $C_{13}H_8Br_3NO_2$; mol wt 449.92. C 34.70%, H 1.79%, Br 53.28%, N 3.11%, O 7.11%. Prepn: **GB 840366** (1960 to Unilever); Lemaire *et al., J. Pharm. Sci.* **50**, 831 (1961); Lamberti, **US 2967885**; Schramm, Lemaire, **US 3064048**; Schramm, **US 3057920** (1961, 1962, 1962 all to Lever Bros.); Majewski, **US 3254121** (1966 to Dow).

Crystals, mp 227-228°. Practically insol in water. Sol in hot acetone; very sol in DMF.
USE: Bacteriostat in detergents.

9617. Tribufos. [78-48-8] Phosphorotrithioic acid *S,S,S*-tributyl ester; *S,S,S*-tributyl phosphorotrithioate; B-1776; Def. $C_{12}H_{27}OPS_3$; mol wt 314.51. C 45.83%, H 8.65%, O 5.09%, P 9.85%, S 30.59%. Organophosphate defoliant used in preparation of cotton for harvesting. Preparative method: K. H. Rattenbury, J. R. Costello, **US 2943107** (1960 to Chemagro). Prepn: D. Voigt *et al., C.R. Hebd. Seances Acad. Sci* **260**, 2210 (1965). Comprehensive description: D. MacDougall, *Anal. Methods Pestic. Plant Growth Regul. Food Addit.* **4**, 89-93 (1964). Oxidative chemistry and toxicology: J. H. Hur *et al., J. Agric. Food Chem.* **40**, 1703 (1992). GC determn in water and fish tissue: C. Habig *et al., J. AOAC Int.* **70**, 103 (1987). Acute toxicity: T. B. Gaines, *Toxicol. Appl. Pharmacol.* **14**, 515 (1969). Human exposure studies: W. Kilgore *et al., Residue Rev.* **91**, 71 (1984). Soil dissipation study: T. L. Potter *et al., J. Agric. Food Chem.* **50**, 3795 (2002).

Colorless to pale yellow liquid, mp <−25°. $bp_{0.3}$ 150°. bp_4 166.5°. d_4^{20} 1.0552. n_D^{20} 1.534. Sol in aliphatic, aromatic, and chlorinated hydrocarbon solvents; alcohols. LD_{50} in male, female rats (mg/kg): 233, 150 orally; 360, 168 dermally (Gaines).
USE: Defoliant.

9618. Tributylamine. [102-82-9] *N,N*-Dibutyl-1-butanamine. $C_{12}H_{27}N$; mol wt 185.35. C 77.76%, H 14.68%, N 7.56%. $(CH_3CH_2CH_2CH_2)_3N$. Prepd by vapor phase alkylation of ammonia with butanol: Lemon, Myerly, **US 3022349** (1962 to Union Carbide Corp.).

Hygroscopic liquid; characteristic odor. d_{20}^{20} 0.7782; bp 216-217°. Sparingly sol in water; very sol in alcohol, ether. *Keep well closed.*
Caution: Causes CNS stimulation, skin irritation, sensitization.

9619. Tributyl Phosphate. [126-73-8] Phosphoric acid tributyl ester. $C_{12}H_{27}O_4P$; mol wt 266.31. C 54.12%, H 10.22%, O 24.03%, P 11.63%. $(C_4H_9)_3PO_4$. Prepd by reaction of $POCl_3$ with butyl alcohol: Pianfetti, Janey, **US 3020303** (1962 to FMC). Toxicity study: Smyth, Carpenter, *J. Ind. Hyg. Toxicol.* **26**, 269 (1944).

Colorless, odorless liq; d_{25}^{25} 0.976; bp 289° with decompn; bp_{27} 177-178°; mp below −80°. Flash pt 146°C. n_D^{25} 1.4215. One ml dissolves in about 165 ml water; miscible with usual organic solvents. LD_{50} orally in rats: 3.0 g/kg (Smyth, Carpenter).
Caution: Potential symptoms of overexposure are irritation of eyes, respiratory system and skin; headache; nausea. See *NIOSH Pocket Guide to Chemical Hazards* (DHHS/NIOSH 97-140, 1997) p 314.
USE: Plasticizer for cellulose esters, lacquers, plastics, and vinyl resins.

9620. Tributyrin. [60-01-5] Butanoic acid 1,2,3-propane-triyl ester; glyceryl tributyrate. $C_{15}H_{26}O_6$; mol wt 302.36. C 59.58%, H 8.67%, O 31.75%. $(C_3H_7COO)_3C_3H_5$. Prepd by esterification of glycerol with excess butyric acid: Weatherby *et al., J. Am. Chem. Soc.* **47**, 2249 (1925).

Oily liq; bitter taste; d_4^{20} 1.032; mp $-75°$; bp_{760} 305-310°. bp_{15} about 190°; n_D^{20} 1.4358. Insol in water. Very sol in alc, ether.

9621. Tricaine. [886-86-2] 3-Aminobenzoic acid ethyl ester methanesulfonate; tricaine methanesulfonate; ethyl *m*-aminobenzoate methanesulfonate; MS-222; Finquel. $C_{10}H_{15}NO_5S$; mol wt 261.29. C 45.97%, H 5.79%, N 5.36%, O 30.62%, S 12.27%. Prepn: **DE 454698**; O. Billeter *et al.,* **US 1678317** (both 1928 to Sandoz). Pharmacology in fish: D. W. Jolly *et al., Vet. Rec.* **91**, 424 (1972). Blood concentrations during anesthetization and recovery: A. H. Houston, R. J. Woods, *J. Fish Res. Board Can.* **29**, 1344 (1972). pH effects on anesthetic potency: E. A. Ohr, *Comp. Biochem. Physiol.* **54C**, 13 (1976). Toxicity study: J. M. McKim *et al., Environ. Toxicol. Chem.* **6**, 295 (1987). Use as anesthetic in fish: P. K. Bourne, *Aquaculture* **36**, 313 (1984); on fish larvae: K. C. Massee *et al., ibid.* **134**, 351 (1995); in amphibians: J. Letcher, *Zoo Biol.* **11**, 243 (1992).

Fine white needles from alcohol + ethyl acetate, mp 149-150°. Soly in water to 11%; it forms clear colorless acid solns. In ocean water solns are almost neutral. LC_{50} (96hr) in rainbow trout: 50.50 mg/l (McKim).

THERAP CAT (VET): Anesthetic for fish.

9622. Tricarballylic Acid. [99-14-9] 1,2,3-Propanetricarboxylic acid; β-carboxyglutaric acid. $C_6H_8O_6$; mol wt 176.12. C 40.92%, H 4.58%, O 54.51%. Natural product produced by rumen bacteria; structural component of fumonisin mycotoxins. Prepn from aconitic acid by reduction with sodium amalgam: Fittig, *Ann.* **314**, 15 (1901); by hydrolysis of ethyl propane-1,1,2,-3-tetracarboxylate: Clarke, Murray, *Org. Synth.* **coll. vol. I** (2nd ed., 1941) p 523. Absorption spectrum: Bielecki, Henri, *Ber.* **46**, 2596 (1913). Crystal structure: J. C. Barnes, J. D. Paton, *Acta Crystallogr.* **C44**, 758 (1988). Production by rumen microorganisms: J. B. Russell, N. Forsberg, *Br. J. Nutr.* **56**, 153 (1986). Review of chemistry: A. S. H. Elgazwy, *Curr. Org. Chem.* **8**, 1405-1423 (2004).

Large, orthorhombic prisms from water or ether, mp 166°. pK_1 (30°): 3.49; pK_2: 4.58; pK_3: 5.83. At 18° 50 g dissolve in 100 ml water and 0.9 g dissolve in 100 ml ether. Quite sol in alc.

Trimethyl ester. [6138-26-7] $C_9H_{14}O_6$. d_4^{20} 1.1822; bp_{13} 150°; n_D^{20} 1.4398.

9623. Trichlorfon. [52-68-6] (2,2,2-Trichloro-1-hydroxyethyl)phosphonic acid dimethyl ester; *O,O*-dimethyl-1-hydroxy-2,2,2-trichloroethylphosphonate; *O,O*-dimethyl 2,2,2-trichloro-1-hydroxyethylphosphonate; chlorofos; metrifonate; trichlorphene; Bayer L 1359; Bilarcil; Cekufon; Combot; Danex; Dipterex; Dylox; Neguvon; ProMem; Proxol; Tugon. $C_4H_8Cl_3O_4P$; mol wt 257.44. C 18.66%, H 3.13%, Cl 41.31%, O 24.86%, P 12.03%. Slow release cholinesterase inhibitor; transformed nonenzymatically to the active compd, dichlorvos, *q.v.* Prepn: W. Lorenz, **US 2701225** (1955 to Bayer); W. F. Barthel *et al., J. Am. Chem. Soc.* **76**, 4186 (1954); W. Lorenz *et al., ibid.* **77**, 2554 (1955). Insecticidal activity: R. L. Metcalf *et al., J. Econ. Entomol.* **52**, 44 (1959). Toxicity study: T. B. Gaines, *Toxicol. Appl. Pharmacol.* **14**, 515 (1969). Transformation and mode of action: E. Reiner *et al., Biochem. Pharmacol.* **24**, 717 (1975); I. Nordgren *et al., Arch. Toxicol.* **41**, 31 (1978). HPLC determn in plasma: L. K. Unni *et al., J. Chromatogr.* **573**, 99 (1992). Clinical pharmacokinetics: L. C. Pettigrew *et*

al., J. Clin. Pharmacol. **38**, 236 (1998). Clinical trial in Alzheimer's disease: R. E. Becker *et al., Alzheimer Dis. Assoc. Disord.* **10**, 124 (1996). Evaluation of carcinogenic risk: *IARC Monographs* **30**, 207-231 (1983). Review of clinical experience in schistosomiasis: H. Feldmeier, E. Doehring, *Acta Trop.* **44**, 357 (1987); in Alzheimer's disease: B. R. Williams, *Am. J. Health-Syst. Pharm.* **56**, 427 (1999).

White crystals, mp 83-84°. d_4^{20} 1.73. n_D^{20} 1.3439. Vapor pressure at 20°: 7.8×10^{-6} mm Hg. Soly in water (25°): 15.4 g/100 ml. Sol in benzene, ethanol. Poorly sol in CCl_4, diethyl ether. Insol in petroleum oils. Dec by alkali. LD_{50} in male, female rats (mg/kg): 630, 560 orally (Gaines).

Butanoic acid ester. [126-22-7] 2,2,2-Trichloro-1-(dimethoxyphosphinoyl)ethyl butyrate; butonate; T-113. $C_8H_{14}Cl_3O_5P$; mol wt 327.53. Prepn: Arthur, Casida, *J. Agric. Food Chem.* **6**, 360 (1958). Liquid. $bp_{0.5}$ 129°.

USE: Insecticide.

THERAP CAT: Anthelmintic (schistosoma).

THERAP CAT (VET): Anthelmintic (Nematodes); ectoparasiticide.

9624. Trichlormethiazide. [133-67-5] 6-Chloro-3-(dichloromethyl)-3,4-dihydro-$2H$-1,2,4-benzothiadiazine-7-sulfonamide 1,1-dioxide; 6-chloro-3-dichloromethyl-7-sulfamyl-3,4-dihydro-1,2,4-benzothiadiazine 1,1-dioxide; 3-dichloromethyl-6-chloro-7-sulfamyl-3,4-dihydro-1,2,4-benzothiadiazine 1,1-dioxide; 3-dichloromethylhydrochlorothiazide; hydrotrichlorothiazide; hydrochloromethiazide; Achletin; Anatran; Anistadin; Aponorin; Carvacron; Diurese; Esmarin; Fluitran; Flutra; Intromene; Kubacron; Metahydrin; Naqua; Salurin; Tachionin; Tolcasone; Triflumen. $C_8H_8Cl_3$-$N_3O_4S_2$; mol wt 380.66. C 25.24%, H 2.12%, Cl 27.94%, N 11.04%, O 16.81%, S 16.85%. Prepn: deStevens *et al., Experientia* **16**, 113 (1960); Sherlock *et al., ibid.* 184. Toxicity: E. I. Goldenthal, *Toxicol. Appl. Pharmacol.* **18**, 185 (1971).

Crystals from methanol + acetone + water, dec 266-273°, also reported as 248-250°. Soly (mg/ml) at 25°: water 0.8; ethanol 21; methanol 60. LD_{50} orally in rats: >20000 mg/kg (Goldenthal).

THERAP CAT: Diuretic; antihypertensive.

THERAP CAT (VET): Diuretic.

9625. Trichlormethine. [555-77-1] 2-Chloro-*N,N*-bis(2-chloroethyl)ethanamine; 2,2′,2″-trichlorotriethylamine; tris(β-chloroethyl)amine; trimustine; HN-3. $C_6H_{12}Cl_3N$; mol wt 204.53. C 35.23%, H 5.91%, Cl 52.00%, N 6.85%. $N(CH_2CH_2Cl)_3$. Nitrogen mustard formerly used as a chemical warfare agent. Prepd by the action of thionyl chloride on triethanolamine: Ward, *J. Am. Chem. Soc.* **57**, 914 (1935); **US 2072348** (1937 to Hercules Powder). Improved procedure: Wilson, Tishler, *J. Am. Chem. Soc.* **73**, 3635 (1951); Witten in *Kirk-Othmer Encyclopedia of Chemical Technology* **vol. 7** (Interscience, New York, 1951) p 130. Clinical use in treatment of Hodgkin's disease and leukemias: L. S. Goodman *et al., J. Am. Med. Assoc.* **132**, 126 (1946). Evaluation of carcinogenic risk: *IARC Monographs* **50**, 143 (1990). GC determn in air: J. R. Stuff *et al., J. Chromatogr. A* **849**, 529 (1999).

Mobile liquid. Faint odor of fish + soap. *Vesicant, necrotizing irritant. Never use without appropriate gas mask.* Volatility at 25° = 0.120 mg/l. d_4^{25} 1.2347, mp $-4°$. bp_{15} 144°. n_D^{25} 1.4925. Very slightly sol in water. Miscible with dimethylformamide, carbon disulfide, carbon tetrachloride, many other organic solvents and oils. The undiluted liq dec on standing and forms polymeric quaternary ammonium salts which are insol in the free base.

Hydrochloride. [817-09-4] Trillekamin. $C_6H_{12}Cl_3N.HCl$; mol wt 240.99. Crystals, mp 130-131°. Freely sol in water, sol in alcohol.

THERAP CAT: Antineoplastic.

9626. Trichloroacetaldehyde. [75-87-6] Chloral; anhydr chloral. C_2HCl_3O; mol wt 147.39. C 16.30%, H 0.68%, Cl 72.16%, O 10.86%. Cl_3CCHO. Prepn by chlorinating alcohol, treating with H_2SO_4 and then distilling: Liebig, *Ann.* **1**, 189 (1832); Personne, *J. Pharm. Chim.* [4] **10**, 350 (1869); **11**, 205 (1870); Brochet, *Bull. Soc. Chim. Fr.* [3] **17**, 228 (1897); *Ann. Chim.* [7] **10**, 332 (1897); Trillat, *Bull. Soc. Chim. Fr.* [3] **17**, 230 (1897); Besson, **DE 133021** (1902); *Chem. Zentralbl.* **1902, II**, 553; Ohse, **DE 734723** (1943), *C.A.* **38**, 3671 (1944). Prepn by chlorination of a mixture of alcohol and acetaldehyde: Société d'Electrochimie, **FR 612396**; *Chim. Ind. (Paris)* **21**, 567 (1929). Prepn from chloral hydrate by azeotropic distn: Mahoney, Pierson, **US 2584036** (1952 to Merck & Co.). From hypochlorous acid and trichloroethylene: Stevens *et al.*, **US 2759978** (1956 to Columbia-Southern). In the laboratory anhyd chloral may be quickly obtained by shaking pharmaceutical grade chloral hydrate with concd H_2SO_4, separating the two layers, and distilling: *cf.* Gattermann, Wieland, *Praxis des Organischen Chemikers* (de Gruyter, Berlin, 40th ed., 1961) p 334. *See also* Chloral Hydrate.

Oily liquid. Pungent, irritating odor; d_4^{20} 1.510; d_4^{25} 1.5050. mp $-57.5°$. bp_{760} 97.8°. n_D^{20} 1.45572; $n_{He}^{21.4}$ 1.45412. Freely sol in water forming chloral hydrate. Sol in alcohol forming chloral alcoholate; sol in ether. Polymerizes under the influence of light and in presence of sulfuric acid forming a white solid trimer called **metachloral**.

USE: Manuf chloral hydrate, DDT.

9627. Trichloroacetic Acid. [76-03-9] TCA. $C_2HCl_3O_2$; mol wt 163.39. C 14.70%, H 0.62%, Cl 65.10%, O 19.58%. CCl_3-COOH. Prepd by oxidation of chloral hydrate with nitric acid: Parkes, Hollingshead, *Chem. Ind. (London)* **1954**, 222. Manuf by chlorination of acetic acid: Eaker, **US 2832803** (1958 to Monsanto). Toxicity study: G. W. Bailey, J. L. White, *Residue Rev.* **10**, 97 (1965).

Very deliquesc crystals; slight characteristic odor. d_4^{61} 1.629; mp 57-58°; bp 196-197°. Sol in 0.1 part water; very sol in alcohol, ether; dec by heating with caustic alkalies into chloroform and alkali carbonate. Its aq soln is very acid. pH of 0.1 molar aq soln 1.2. *Keep tightly closed in a cool place.* Storage of trichloroacetic acid solns in water of less than 30% strength is not recommended. Decompn products are chloroform, hydrochloric acid, carbon dioxide and carbon monoxide. LD_{50} orally in rats: 5000 mg/kg (Bailey, White).

Ethyl ester. [515-84-4] Ethyl trichloroacetate. $C_4H_5Cl_3O_2$. Clear liq; odor resembling menthol. d_4^{20} 1.383. bp 168°. n_D^{20} 1.4507. Insol in water. Misc with alcohol, ether.

Sodium salt. [650-51-1] Sodium trichloroacetate; Konesta; Varitox. $C_2Cl_3NaO_2$; mol wt 185.37. Yellow deliquesc powder, mp >300°. Soly in water at 25°: 1.2 kg/l. Sol in ethanol.

Caution: Potential symptoms of overexposure are irritation of eyes, skin, nose, throat, respiratory system; cough, dyspnea, delayed pulmonary edema; eye and skin burns; dermatitis; salivation, vomiting, diarrhea. *See NIOSH Pocket Guide to Chemical Hazards* (DHHS/NIOSH 97-140, 1997) p 314.

USE: As a decalcifier and fixative in microscopy; also as a precipitant of protein. As herbicide.

THERAP CAT: Caustic.

THERAP CAT (VET): Caustic, vesicant.

9628. Trichloroacetonitrile. [545-06-2] Trichloromethylnitrile; Tritox. C_2Cl_3N; mol wt 144.39. C 16.64%, Cl 73.66%, N 9.70%. CCl_3CN. Prepd from ethyl trichloroacetate and aq ammonia, and physical and thermodynamic properties: Davies, Jenkin, *J. Chem. Soc.* **1954**, 2374; by action of phosphorus pentoxide on trichloroacetamide: Carpenter, *J. Org. Chem.* **27**, 2085 (1962). Manuf by reaction of methylnitrile, HCl and chlorine gas: Käbisch, **US 2745868** (1956 to Degussa). Toxicity study: H. F. Smyth *et al.*, *Am. Ind. Hyg. Assoc. J.* **23**, 95 (1962).

Liquid, bp_{760} 85.7°; d_4^{25} 1.4403, d_4^{35} 1.4223; $n_D^{20.0}$ 1.4409, $n_D^{27.0}$ 1.4375. LD_{50} orally in rats: 0.25 g/kg (Smyth).

Caution: A strong irritant to eyes, skin.

USE: Insecticide.

9629. 2,4,6-Trichloroanisole. [87-40-1] Tyrene. $C_7H_5Cl_3$-O; mol wt 211.47. C 39.76%, H 2.38%, Cl 50.30%, O 7.57%. Prepd by reaction of 2,4,6-trichlorophenol with dimethyl sulfate: Kohn, Heller, *Monatsh. Chem.* **46**, 91 (1925).

Monoclinic needles from alc, mp 60°, $bp_{738.2}$ 240°, bp_{28} 132°. Faint odor similar to that of acetophenone. Sublimes slowly at room temp. Volatile with steam. Practically insol in water. Sol in methanol, dioxane, benzene, cyclohexanone.

USE: Formerly as a dye assistant for polyester fibers.

9630. 1,2,3-Trichlorobenzene. [87-61-6] *vic*-Trichlorobenzene. $C_6H_3Cl_3$; mol wt 181.45. C 39.72%, H 1.67%, Cl 58.62%. Prepared from 3,4,5-trichloroaniline by diazotization: Cohen, Hartley, *J. Chem. Soc.* **87**, 1365 (1905); Holleman, *Rec. Trav. Chim.* **37**, 196 (1918); from 2,3,4-trichloroaniline by diazotization: Dadien *et al.*, *Monatsh. Chem.* **61**, 431 (1932); from 2,3,4-trichloroaniline by treatment with ethyl nitrite: Beilstein, Kurbatow, *Ann.* **192**, 234 (1878).

Platelets from alc, d 1.69. mp 52.6°. bp 221°. n_D^{19} 1.5776. Flash pt 113°C (235.4°F). Volatile with steam. Insol in water. Sparingly sol in alc. Freely sol in benzene, carbon disulfide.

Caution: Irritating to eyes, mucous membranes.

USE: A commercial grade (mixture of isomeric trichlorobenzenes) is used to combat termites.

9631. 1,2,4-Trichlorobenzene. [120-82-1] *unsym*-Trichlorobenzene. $C_6H_3Cl_3$; mol wt 181.45. C 39.72%, H 1.67%, Cl 58.62%. Prepd from 2,4-dichloroaniline or 2,5-dichloroaniline or 3,4-dichloroaniline by diazotization and treatment with Cu_2Cl_2: Beilstein, Kurbatow, *Ann.* **192**, 230 (1878); van der Lande, *Rec. Trav. Chim.* **51**, 104, 110 (1932); from 1,3-diaminobenzene by tetrazotization and treatment with Cu_2Cl_2: Cohn, Fischer, *Monatsh. Chem.* **21**, 278 (1900).

Liquid; mp 17°; d_{25}^{25} 1.4634; bp 213°; n_D^{25} 1.5524. Flash pt 110°C (230°F). Volatile with steam. Insol in water. Sparingly sol in alc.
Miscible with ether, benzene, petr ether, carbon disulfide.

Caution: Potential symptoms of overexposure are irritation of eyes, skin, mucous membranes. *See NIOSH Pocket Guide to Chemical Hazards* (DHHS/NIOSH 97-140, 1997) p 314.

9632. 1,3,5-Trichlorobenzene. [108-70-3] *sym*-Trichlorobenzene. $C_6H_3Cl_3$; mol wt 181.45. C 39.72%, H 1.67%, Cl 58.62%. Prepd from 2,4,6-trichloroaniline by diazotization and treatment with alcohol: Jackson, Lamar, *Am. Chem. J.* **18**, 667 (1896); Backer, van der Baan, *Rec. Trav. Chim.* **56**, 1177 (1937).

Crystals; mp 63.4°; bp 208.4°. n_D^{19} 1.5662. Flash pt 107°C (224.6°F). Volatile with steam. Insol in water. Sparingly sol in alc. Freely sol in ether, benzene, petr ether, carbon disulfide, glacial acetic acid.

9633. α,α,β-Trichloro-n-butyraldehyde. [76-36-8] 2,2,3-Trichlorobutanal; butylchloral; anhydr butylchloral; butyrchloral; crotonchloral. $C_4H_5Cl_3O$; mol wt 175.44. C 27.38%, H 2.87%, Cl 60.62%, O 9.12%. $CH_3CHClCCl_2CHO$. Prepd by the action of chlorine on acetaldehyde: Krämer, Pinner, *Ber.* **3**, 883 (1870); Pinner, *Ann.* **179**, 24 (1875); on paraldehyde: *idem;* on crotonaldehyde after saturation with gaseous HCl: High, **US 2280290** (1942); Brown, Plump, **US 2351000** (1944). From crotonaldehyde and chlorine: Ropp *et al., Org. Synth.* **coll. vol. IV**, 130 (1963).

Oily liquid. Pungent, disagreeable odor; d_4^{20} 1.3956; bp_{760} 164.5-165.5°; bp_{25} 57-60°. n_D^{20} 1.47554. Freely sol in water forming butylchloral hydrate; sol in alcohol forming an alcoholate; sol in ether. Polymerizes.

9634. 2,4,6-Trichloro-m-cresol. [551-76-8] 2,4,6-Trichloro-3-methylphenol; 2,4,6-trichloro-3-hydroxytoluene. $C_7H_5Cl_3O$; mol wt 211.47. C 39.76%, H 2.38%, Cl 50.30%, O 7.57%. Prepd by chlorination of *m*-cresol, chlorination of thymol in the presence of iron, or by action of concd sulfuric acid on 2,4,4-trichloro-3-methyl-6-isopropyl-$\Delta^{2,5}$-cyclohexadienone: Crowther, McCombie, *J. Chem. Soc.* **103**, 536 (1913).

Needles or plates from water or petr ether. mp 45-47°; bp 265°, bp_{14} 142-144°. Volatile with steam. Slightly sol in water, benzene, petr ether, glacial acetic acid. Freely sol in methanol, alc, chloroform, xylene, ether and in alkali solns.

9635. 4,5,6-Trichloro-o-cresol. [551-78-0] 2,3,4-Trichloro-6-methylphenol; 3,4,5-trichloro-2-hydroxytoluene; 1-methyl-2-hydroxy-3,4,5-trichlorobenzene. Prepd by chlorination of 1-methyl-2-hydroxy-4-chlorobenzene: Kohn, Syreia, *J. Am. Chem. Soc.* **70**, 3950 (1948).

Needles from petr ether, mp 77°. Slightly soluble in water; freely sol in the customary organic solvents and in caustic alkali solns.

9636. 1,1,1-Trichloroethane. [71-55-6] Methylchloroform; Chlorothene. $C_2H_3Cl_3$; mol wt 133.40. C 18.01%, H 2.27%, Cl 79.73%. CH_3CCl_3. Prepd by the action of chlorine on 1,1-dichloroethane: Sutton, *Proc. Roy. Soc.* **A133**, 673 (1931); by the catalytic addition of HCl to 1,1-dichloroethylene: **DE 523436** (1931); **US 2209000** (Nutting, Huscher, 1940). Review of mfg processes: *Faith, Keyes & Clark's Industrial Chemicals*, F. A. Lowenheim, M. K. Moran, Eds. (Wiley-Interscience, New York, 4th ed., 1975) pp 836-843; of toxicology and human exposure: *Toxicological Profile for 1,1,1-Trichloroethane* (PB95-264396, 1995) 307 pp.

Liquid; sweet sharp odor. Nonflammable. mp −32.5°. d_4^{20} 1.3376. bp_{760} 74.1°. n_D^{20} 1.43838. Insol in water. Absorbs some water. Sol in acetone, benzene, carbon tetrachloride, methanol, ether.

Caution: Potential symptoms of overexposure are irritation of eyes and skin; headache, lassitude, CNS depression, poor equilibrium; dermatitis; cardiac arrhythmias; liver damage. *See NIOSH Pocket Guide to Chemical Hazards* (DHHS/NIOSH 97-140, 1997) p 202.

USE: Solvent for adhesives, in cold type metal cleaning, in cleaning plastic molds.

9637. 1,1,2-Trichloroethane. [79-00-5] Vinyl trichloride. $C_2H_3Cl_3$; mol wt 133.40. C 18.01%, H 2.27%, Cl 79.73%. CH_2-ClCHCl$_2$. Prepd by catalytic chlorination of ethane or ethylene: Joseph, **US 2752401** and Pye, **US 2752402** (both 1956 to Dow); Reynolds, **US 2783286** (1957 to Olin Mathieson). Toxicity data: H. F. Smyth *et al., Am. Ind. Hyg. Assoc. J.* **30**, 470 (1969). Review of toxicology and human exposure: *Toxicological Profile for 1,1,2-Trichloroethane* (PB90-196411, 1989) 120 pp.

Nonflammable liquid; pleasant odor; d_4^{20} 1.4416. mp −35°. bp 113-114°. n_D^{20} 1.4711. Insol in water. Misc with alcohol, ether, and many other organic liquids. LD_{50} orally in rats: 0.58 ml/kg (Smyth).

Caution: Potential symptoms of overexposure are irritation of nose and eyes; CNS depression; liver and kidney damage; dermatitis. Potential occupational carcinogen. *See NIOSH Pocket Guide to Chemical Hazards* (DHHS/NIOSH 97-140, 1997) p 314.

USE: Solvent for fats, waxes, natural resins, alkaloids.

9638. 2,2,2-Trichloroethanol. [115-20-8] Trichloroethyl alcohol. $C_2H_3Cl_3O$; mol wt 149.40. C 16.08%, H 2.02%, Cl 71.19%, O 10.71%. CCl_3CH_2OH. Prepd by reduction of the corresponding ester, acid chloride, or acid with lithium aluminum hydride: Sroog *et al., J. Am. Chem. Soc.* **71**, 1710 (1949). Manufacture by reduction of chloral hydrate with an amine borane: Chamberlain, Schechter, **US 2898379** (1959 to Callery Chem.). Pharmacology: H. Molitor, H. Robinson, *Curr. Res. Anesth. Analg.* **17**, 258 (1938).

Hygroscopic liquid, ethereal odor. At low temps it crystallizes in rhombic tablets. mp at 18°; bp 151-153°; d_{20}^{20} 1.55. Sol in about 12 parts water; miscible with alcohol or ether. pH of aq soln is 5-6, but on prolonged contact with water some free acid is formed. *Keep well closed and protected from light.*

THERAP CAT: Sedative; hypnotic.

9639. Trichloroethylene. [79-01-6] Trichloroethene; ethinyl trichloride; Tri-Clene; Trilene; Trichloren; Algylen; Trimar; Triline; Trethylene; Westrosol; Chlorylen; Gemalgene; Germalgene. C_2HCl_3; mol wt 131.39. C 18.28%, H 0.77%, Cl 80.95%. Cl_2C=CHCl. Prepn from *sym*-tetrachloroethane by elimination of HCl (by boiling with lime): **DE 171900**; by passing tetrachloroethane vapor over $CaCl_2$ catalyst at 300°: **DE 263457**; without catalyst at 450-470°: **GB 575530** (1946 to du Pont). Physical properties: E. W. McGovern, *Ind. Eng. Chem.* **35**, 1230 (1943); S. A. Mumford, J. W. C. Phillips, *J. Chem. Soc.* **1950**, 75. Review of mfg processes: S. A. Miller, *Chem. Process Eng.* **47**, 268 (1966); *Faith, Keyes & Clark's Industrial Chemicals*, F. A. Lowenheim, M. K. Moran, Eds. (Wiley-Interscience, New York, 4th ed., 1975) pp 844-848. Toxicity data: H. S. Smyth *et al., Am. Ind. Hyg. Assoc. J.* **30**, 470 (1969). Review of carcinogenic risk: *IARC Monographs* **20**, 545-572 (1979); B. L. Van Duuren, *Environ. Res.* **49**, 333 (1989). Review of use as anesthetic: J. V. Farman, *Br. J. Anaesth.* **53**, Suppl. 3, 3S-9S (1981). Review of metabolism, toxicity and carcinogenicity: J. V. Bruckner *et al., Crit. Rev. Toxicol.* **20**, 31-50 (1989); of toxicology and human exposure: *Toxicological Profile for Trichloroethylene* (PB98-101165, 1997) 335 pp. Series of articles on toxicology and risk assessment: *Environ. Health Perspect.* **108**, Suppl. 2, 159-366 (2000).

Nonflammable, mobile liquid. Characteristic odor resembling that of chloroform. *Use with adequate ventilation.* d_4^0 1.4904; d_4^{15} 1.4695; d_4^{20} 1.4642; d_4^{25} 1.4559. Vapor density: 4.53 (air = 1.00). mp −84.8°. bp_{760} 86.9°; bp_{400} 67.0°; bp_{200} 48.0°; bp_{100} 31.4°; bp_{60} 20.0°; bp_{20} −1.0°; bp_{10} −12.4°; bp_5 −22.8°; $bp_{1.0}$ −43.8°; n_D^{17} 1.47914; n_D^{20} 1.4775; n_D^{25} 1.45560. Soly in water (25°): 0.11 g/100 g. Misc with ether, alcohol, chloroform. Dissolves most fixed and volatile oils. Slowly dec (with formn of HCl) by light in the presence of moisture. Preserve in sealed, light-resistant containers; avoid prolonged exposure to excessive heat. Medicinal trichloroethylene may contain thymol as a preservative; industrial grades may contain stabilizers such as triethylamine. LD_{50} orally in rats: 4.92 ml/kg; LC (4 hrs) in rats: 8000 ppm (Smyth).

Caution: Potential symptoms of overexposure are headache, vertigo; visual disturbance, fatigue, giddiness, tremors, somnolence, nausea and vomiting; irritation of eyes, skin; dermatitis; cardiac arrhythmias, paresthesia; liver injury. *See NIOSH Pocket Guide to Chemical Hazards* (DHHS/NIOSH 97-140, 1997) p 316. *See also Patty's Industrial Hygiene and Toxicology* vol. **2B**, G. D. Clayton, F. E. Clayton, Eds. (Wiley-Interscience, 3rd ed., 1982) pp 3553-3560; *Clinical Toxicology of Commercial Products*, R. E. Gosselin *et al.*, Eds. (Williams & Wilkins, Baltimore, 5th ed., 1984) Section II, pp 165-166. This substance is reasonably anticipated to be a human carcinogen: *Report on Carcinogens, Eleventh Edition* (PB2005-104914, 2004) p III-261.

USE: Solvent for fats, waxes, resins, oils, rubber, paints, and varnishes. Solvent for cellulose esters and ethers. Used for solvent extraction in many industries. In degreasing, in dry cleaning. In the manuf of organic chemicals, pharmaceuticals, such as chloroacetic acid.

THERAP CAT: Anesthetic (inhalation).

THERAP CAT (VET): Anesthetic (inhalation).

9640. Trichlorofluoromethane. [75-69-4] Trichloromonofluoromethane; fluorotrichloromethane; fluorocarbon 11; FC 11; Arcton 11; Freon 11; Frigen 11. CCl_3F; mol wt 137.37. C 8.74%, Cl 77.43%, F 13.83%. Prepn: Henne, *Org. React.* **2**, 64 (1944). Manuf: *Faith, Keyes & Clark's Industrial Chemicals*, F. A. Lowenheim, M. K. Moran, Eds. (Wiley-Interscience, New York, 4th ed., 1975) pp 325-330.

Liquid at temps below 23.7°. Faint ethereal odor. Nonflammable. $d_4^{17.2}$ 1.494; d_{gas}^{25} 5.04 (air = 1). mp −111°. bp_{760} 23.7°; bp_{400} 6.8°; bp_{200} −9.1°; bp_{100} −23.0°; bp_{60} −32.3°; bp_{40} −39.0°; bp_{20} −49.7°; bp_{10} −59.0°; bp_5 −67.6°; $bp_{1.0}$ −84.3°. Crit temp 198°; crit press. 43.2 atm (635 lb/sq inch, abs). $n_D^{18.5}$ 1.3865. Dipole moment 0.45. Practically insol in water. Sol in alcohol, ether, other, organic solvents.

Caution: Potential symptoms of overexposure are incoordination, tremors; dermatitis; cardiac arrhythmias, cardiac arrest; asphyxia; direct contact with liquid may cause frostbite. *See NIOSH Pocket Guide to Chemical Hazards* (DHHS/NIOSH 97-140, 1997) p 146. *See also Patty's Industrial Hygiene and Toxicology* **vol. 2B,** G. D. Clayton, F. E. Clayton, Eds. (Wiley-Interscience, New York, 3rd ed., 1981) p 3073-3091. *Note:* Consult latest Government regulations on use as aerosol propellant.

USE: In refrigeration machinery requiring a refrigerant effective at negative pressures. As aerosol propellant.

9641. Trichloroisocyanuric Acid. [87-90-1] 1,3,5-Trichloro-1,3,5-triazine-2,4,6-(1*H*,3*H*,5*H*)-trione; trichloroiminocyanuric acid; TCCA; ACL-85; Chloreal; Symclosene. $C_3Cl_3N_3O_3$; mol wt 232.41. C 15.50%, Cl 45.76%, N 18.08%, O 20.65%. Industrially significant bleaching agent and biocide. Prepn: F. D. Chattaway, J. M. Wadmore, *J. Chem. Soc.* **81**, 191 (1902); Hands, Whitt, *J. Soc. Chem. Ind.* **67**, 66 (1948). Structure determn: R. C. Petterson *et al., J. Org. Chem.* **25**, 1595 (1960). Review of synthetic applications as a chlorinating agent or oxidant: U. Tilstam, H. Weinmann, *Org. Process Res. Dev.* **6**, 384-393 (2002); J. C. Barros, *Synlett* **2005**, 2115-2116.

Needles from ethylene chloride, mp 246-247° (dec). May be stored in the dry state for at least a year. Releases hypochlorous acid on contact with water. pH of aq solns about 4.4. Soly in water at 25° about 0.2%. Sol in chlorinated and highly polar solvents.

Caution: Moderately irritating to eyes, skin, mucous membranes.

USE: Chlorinating agent, disinfectant, industrial deodorant. In household cleansers. In removing oil and protein in stainless steel. In nonshrink treatment for wool. Oxidant and chlorinating reagent in organic synthesis.

THERAP CAT: Anti-infective (topical).

9642. 3,4,6-Trichloro-2-nitrophenol. [82-62-2] 2-Nitro-3,4,6-trichlorophenol; 2,4,5-trichloro-6-nitrophenol; Dowlap. $C_6H_2Cl_3NO_3$; mol wt 242.44. C 29.72%, H 0.83%, Cl 43.87%, N 5.78%, O 19.80%. Prepd by dissolving 2,4,5-trichlorophenol in glacial acetic acid and treating with concd nitric acid: Kohn, Fink, *Monatsh. Chem.* **58**, 73 (1931); Harrison *et al., J. Chem. Soc.* **1943**, 235.

Pale yellow crystals from petr ether, mp 92-93°.

USE: To combat the sea lamprey, an eel-like fish which attacks trout, especially in the Great Lakes region.

9643. 2,4,5-Trichlorophenol. [95-95-4] Collunosol; Dowicide 2. $C_6H_3Cl_3O$; mol wt 197.45. C 36.50%, H 1.53%, Cl 53.87%, O 8.10%. Prepd by treating 1,2,4,5-tetrachlorobenzene with methanolic NaOH in autoclave at 160° for several hrs: Harrison *et al., J. Chem. Soc.* **1943**, 235; Agfa, *DE 411052* (1925); *Chem. Zentralbl.* **1925, I,** 2411. Toxicity data: Deichmann, *Fed. Proc.* **2,** 76 (1943). Review of toxicology and human exposure: *Toxicological Profile for Chlorophenols* (PB99-166639, 1999) 260 pp.

Needles from alcohol or ligroin. Strong phenolic odor. mp 67°. Sublimes. bp_{746} 248°. bp_{760} 253°. Weak monobasic acid. pK (25°) 7.37. Soly (g/100 g of solvent at 25°): acetone 615; benzene 163; carbon tetrachloride 51; ether 525; denatured alcohol formula 30, 525; methanol 615; liquid petrolatum (at 50°) 56; soybean oil 79; toluene 122; water <0.2. LD_{50} orally in rats: 0.82 g/kg (Deichmann).

Sodium salt sesquihydrate. Dowicide B. Prepn: US 1991329 (1935 to Dow). Flakes. Solubility (g/100 g solvent at 25°): acetone 163; denatured alcohol formula 30, 186; ethylene glycol 33; methanol 241; water 113. pH of satd aq soln 11.0-13.0.

USE: Fungicide, bactericide, biocide; intermediate in production of herbicides.

9644. 2,4,6-Trichlorophenol. [88-06-2] Dowicide 2S; Omal. $C_6H_3Cl_3O$; mol wt 197.45. C 36.50%, H 1.53%, Cl 53.87%, O 8.10%. Prepd by direct chlorination of phenol: Tiessens, *Rec. Trav. Chim.* **50**, 115 (1931); Chulkov *et al., Org. Chem. Ind. USSR* **3**, 97 (1937); *Chem. Zentralbl.* **1938, I,** 1419; *C.A.* **31**, 4967 (1937). Prepn of sodium salt monohydrate: Hunter, Seyfried, *J. Am. Chem. Soc.* **43**, 154 (1921). Review of toxicology and human exposure: *Toxicological Profile for Chlorophenols* (PB99-166639, 1999) 260 pp.

Crystals from ligroin. Strong phenolic odor. Volatile with steam, but not from alkaline soln. d 1.4901. mp 69°. bp_{760} 246°. Soly (g/100 g of solvent): Acetone 525; benzene 113; carbon tetrachloride 37; diacetone alcohol 335; ether 354; denatured alcohol formula 30, 400; methanol 525; pine oil 163; Stoddard solvent 16; toluene 100; turpentine 37; water <0.1.

Sodium salt monohydrate. Flaky crystals. Freely sol in water, alcohol, ether, acetone. pH of satd aq soln 11.0-13.0.

Caution: 2,4,6-Trichlorophenol is reasonably anticipated to be a human carcinogen: *Report on Carcinogens, Eleventh Edition* (PB2005-104914, 2004) p III-263.

USE: Fungicide, bactericide, wood preservative, biocide; intermediate in production of higher chlorinated phenols.

9645. 1,1,1-Trichloro-2-propanol. [76-00-6] 1,1,1-Trichloroisopropyl alcohol; trichloroisopropanol; Isopral. $C_3H_5Cl_3O$; mol wt 163.43. C 22.05%, H 3.08%, Cl 65.08%, O 9.79%. CCl_3-CH(OH)CH$_3$. Prepd by reaction of chloral and methylmagnesium bromide: Kharasch *et al., J. Am. Chem. Soc.* **63**, 2305 (1941). Toxicity study: Burtner, Lehmann, *J. Pharmacol. Exp. Ther.* **63**, 183 (1938).

Monoclinic crystals; camphor-like odor; pungent taste; mp 50°; bp 161-162°. Sublimes at ordinary temp. Sol in about 35 parts water; freely sol in alcohol or ether. *Keep well closed in a cool place.* LD_{50} orally in rats: 1 g/kg (Burtner, Lehmann).

9646. Trichlorosilane. [10025-78-2] Trichloromonosilane; silicochloroform. Cl_3HSi; mol wt 135.45. Cl 78.52%, H 0.74%, Si 20.73%. $SiHCl_3$. Prepd from Si and HCl or from SiH_4 and HCl in presence of $AlCl_3$: Gattermann, *Ber.* **22**, 190 (1889); Ruff, Albert, *Ber.* **38**, 2226 (1905); Stock, Zeidler, *Ber.* **56**, 986 (1923); Schenk in *Handbook of Preparative Inorganic Chemistry* **vol. 1**, G. Brauer, Ed. (Academic Press, New York, 2nd ed., 1963) pp 691-692. Toxicity study: H. F. Smyth *et al., J. Ind. Hyg. Toxicol.* **31**, 60 (1949).

Volatile, mobile liquid. Fumes in air. Supports combustion. d_4^0 1.3830; d_4^{20} 1.3417; d_4^{25} 1.3313. mp $-126.5°$. bp_{760} 31.8°, also reported as 36.5°. Viscosity in cP: 0.397 at 0°; 0.332 at 20°; 0.316 at 25°. n_D^{20} 1.4020; n_D^{25} 1.3983. Dec by water. Sol in benzene, carbon disulfide, chloroform, carbon tetrachloride. Dipole moment 0.97. LD_{50} orally in rats: 1.03 g/kg (Smyth).

USE: In organic synthesis.

9647. Trichodermin. [4682-50-2] 12,13-Epoxytrichothec-9-en-4-ol acetate; WG-696. $C_{17}H_{24}O_4$; mol wt 292.37. C 69.84%, H 8.27%, O 21.89%. Antifungal metabolite from *Trichoderma viride* ND8: **NL 302527** (1964 to Loevens); *C.A.* **62**, 1050f (1965); also isolated from *Myrothecium roridum*. Structure: Godtfredsen, Vangedal, *Proc. Chem. Soc. London* **1964**, 188; Gutzwiller *et al., Helv. Chim. Acta* **47**, 2234 (1964); Godtfredsen, Vangedal, *Acta Chem. Scand.* **19**, 1088 (1965); Abrahamsson, Nilsson, *ibid.* **20**, 1044 (1966). Total synthesis: Colvin *et al., Chem. Commun.* **1971**, 858; *eidem, J. Chem. Soc. Perkin Trans. 1* **1973**, 1989. Activity studies: Yamamoto *et al., Takeda Kenkyusho Nempo* **28**, 69 (1969), *C.A.* **72**, 76058g (1970). Inhibition of protein synthesis: F. Hernandez, M. Cannon, *J. Antibiot.* **35**, 875 (1982).

Crystals from pentane at $-70°$. mp 46°, 58-60° (Colvin). $bp_{0.05}$ 110-112°. $[\alpha]_D^{20}$ $-11°$ (c = 1 in chloroform). uv max (ethanol): 205 nm (ε 2400). Sparingly soluble in water; soluble in all common organic solvents. LD_{50} in mice (mg/kg): 500-1000 s.c.; >1000 orally (**NL 302527**).

Trichodermol. [2198-93-8] Roridan C. $C_{15}H_{22}O_3$; mol wt 250.33. Crystals, mp 124-125°. *See also* verrucarins.

9648. Trichosanthin. [60318-52-7] GLQ223. Active component of the traditional Chinese medicine, Tian Hua Fen (Radix Trichosanthis), known since 300 A.D. and used in gynecological disorders and abortion. Basic polypeptide of 234 amino acids, M_r 26,000 Da, isolated from the roots of *Trichosanthes kirilowii* Maxim, *Cucurbitaceae*. Purification, characterization, and amino acid sequence: W. Yu *et al., Pure Appl. Chem.* **58**, 789 (1986); J. M. Maraganore *et al., J. Biol. Chem.* **262**, 11628 (1987). Conformation: S. Kubota *et al., Biochim. Biophys. Acta* **871**, 101 (1986); and homology with ricin, *q.v.: eidem, Int. J. Pept. Protein Res.* **30**, 646 (1987). Inhibition of protein synthesis: H. W. Yeung *et al., ibid.* **31**, 265 (1988). Inhibition of HIV replication: M. S. McGrath *et al., Proc. Natl. Acad. Sci. USA* **86**, 2844 (1989). Abortifacient activity in animals: M. C. Chang *et al., Contraception* **19**, 175 (1979); S. K. Saksena *et al., ibid.* **20**, 367 (1979); I. F. Lau *et al., ibid.* **21**, 77 (1980). Clinical trial as abortifacient: K. F. Cheng, *Obstet. Gynecol.* **59**, 494 (1982).

Crystals. pI 9.4.

THERAP CAT: Abortifacient.

9649. Trichostatin(s). Antibiotic A-300; A-300-I. Antifungal antibiotic isolated from metabolites of *Streptomyces hygroscopicus*. It is composed of trichostatins A (major), B, the ferric chelate of trichostatin A, and C, the first glycosyl hydroxamate from a natural source. Isoln of A and B: N. Tsuji *et al., JP Kokai 74 14691, C.A.* **81**, 48547h (1974). Structural elucidation of A and B: *eidem, J. Antibiot.* **29**, 1 (1976). Isoln and structure of C: N. Tsuji, M. Kobayashi, *ibid.* **31**, 939 (1978).

Trichostatin A

Trichostatin A. [58880-19-6] [R-(E,E)]-7-[4-(Dimethylamino)phenyl]-N-hydroxy-4,6-dimethyl-7-oxo-2,4-heptadienamide. $C_{17}H_{22}N_2O_3$; mol wt 302.37. Crystals from ethyl acetate, mp 150-151°. $[\alpha]_D^{20.5}$ +62.8° ±1.1° (c = 1.007 in ethanol). uv max (ethanol): 252, 265, 341 nm ($E_{1cm}^{1\%}$ 531, 582, 648). Sol in lower alcohols, sparingly sol in chloroform, ethyl acetate, acetone, benzene.

Trichostatin B. [58895-00-4] Tris[7-[4-(dimethylamino)phenyl]-N-hydroxy-4,6-dimethyl-7-oxo-2,4-heptadienamidato-O^NO^1]iron. $C_{51}H_{63}FeN_6O_9$; mol wt 959.93. Trihydrate, dark reddish purple prisms from methanol, mp 192° (dec). uv max (ethanol): 253, 277, 341, 450 nm ($E_{1cm}^{1\%}$ 624, 651, 918, 50).

Trichostatin C. [68676-88-0] 7-[4-(Dimethylamino)phenyl]-N-(β-D-glucopyranosyloxy)-4,6-dimethyl-7-oxo-2,4-heptadienamide. $C_{23}H_{32}N_2O_8$; mol wt 464.51. Colorless prisms from methanol, mp 171-173°. $[\alpha]_D^{24}$ +50.5 ±0.9° (c = 0.987 in methanol). uv max (methanol): 268, 344 nm (ε 14600; 14300).

9650. Trichothecin. [6379-69-7] [4β(Z)]-12,13-Epoxy-4-[(1-oxo-2-butenyl)oxy]trichothec-9-en-8-one; 12,13-epoxy-4-hydroxytrichothec-9-en-8-one crotonate. $C_{19}H_{24}O_5$; mol wt 332.39. C 68.66%, H 7.28%, O 24.07%. Mycotoxin with antibiotic activity. Produced by *Trichothecium roseum*: Freeman, Morrison, *Nature* **162**, 30 (1948). Activity: G. G. Freeman, *J. Gen. Microbiol.* **12**, 213 (1955). Structure: Godtfredsen, Vangedal, *Proc. Chem. Soc. London* **1964**, 188; Gutzwiller *et al., Helv. Chim. Acta* **47**, 2234 (1964). Biogenesis: Jones, Lowe, *J. Chem. Soc.* **1960**, 3959. Biosynthetic studies: Achilladelis *et al., J. Chem. Soc. Perkin Trans. 1* **1972**, 1425; Machida, Nozoe, *Tetrahedron Lett.* **1972**, 1969; *eidem, Tetrahedron* **28**, 5113 (1972).

Slender needles from petrol ether, mp 118°. $[\alpha]_D^{18}$ +44° (c = 1 in $CHCl_3$). uv max (hexane): 217 nm (ε 18000); (methanol): 215 nm (ε 19000). Slightly sol in water (400 mg/l at 25°). Freely sol in most organic solvents. Aq solns are stable at pH 1-10 for at least 48 hrs at 20°. At pH 12 the antifungal activity is destroyed rapidly. Aq solns at pH 7 can be maintained at 100° for at least one hour without loss of activity. LD_{50} i.v. in mice: ~300 mg/kg (Freeman).

9651. Tricine. [5704-04-1] N-[2-Hydroxy-1,1-bis(hydroxymethyl)ethyl]glycine; N-[tris(hydroxymethyl)methyl]glycine. $C_6H_{13}NO_5$; mol wt 179.17. C 40.22%, H 7.31%, N 7.82%, O 44.65%. One of the zwitterionic amino acids known as "Good" buffers; active in the pH range 6-8.5. Prepn: N. E. Good, *Arch. Biochem. Biophys.* **96**, 653 (1962); and characterization: N. E. Good *et al., Biochemistry* **5**, 467 (1966). Temperature effects on pK: R. N. Roy *et al., J. Am. Chem. Soc.* **95**, 8231 (1973); M. L. Soni, R. C. Kapoor, *Int. J. Quantum Chem.* **20**, 385 (1981); and on pH: R. N. Roy *et al., Cryobiology* **22**, 589 (1985). Scavenger of hydroxyl radicals: M. Hicks, J. M. Gebicki, *FEBS Lett.* **199**, 92 (1986); B. Halliwell *et al., Anal. Biochem.* **165**, 215 (1987). Use as buffer: R. S. Gardner, *J. Cell Biol.* **42**, 320 (1969); R. S. Spendlove *et al., Proc. Soc. Exp. Biol. Med.* **137**, 258 (1971); H. Schaegger, G. Von Jagow, *Anal. Biochem.* **166**, 368 (1987).

Crystals from alcohol/water, mp 187°. pKa$_1$ ~2.3; pKa$_2$ (0.1M): 0°, 8.6; 20°, 8.15; 37°, 7.8. pKa$_2$ (20°): 8.15 (0.2M); 8.15 (0.01M). ΔpKa/°C −0.021. Saturated aqueous soln is 0.8M at 0°.

USE: Biological buffer.

9652. Triclabendazole. [68786-66-3] 5-Chloro-6-(2,3-di-chlorophenoxy)-2-methylthio-1H-benzimidazole; CGA-89317; Fasinex. C$_{14}$H$_9$Cl$_3$N$_2$OS; mol wt 359.66. C 46.75%, H 2.52%, Cl 29.57%, N 7.79%, O 4.45%, S 8.92%. Benzimidazole derivative effective against liver fluke. Prepn: J.-J. Gallay *et al., BE 865870* corresp to *US 4197307* (1978, 1980 both to Ciba-Geigy). Efficacy against immature and mature *Fasciola hepatica* in sheep, goats: K. Wolff *et al., Vet. Parasitol.* **13**, 145 (1983); in sheep: J. C. Boray *et al., Vet. Rec.* **113**, 315 (1983). Effective also against *F. gigantica* in sheep: N. Güralp, R. Tinar, *J. Helminthol.* **58**, 113 (1984). Brief review: J. Eckert *et al., Biol. Muench. Tieraerztl. Wochenschr.* **97**, 349 (1984).

Crystals, mp 175-176°.

THERAP CAT (VET): Anthelmintic (fasciola).

9653. Triclobisonium Chloride. [79-90-3] N,N,N',N'-Tetramethyl-N,N'-bis[1-methyl-3-(2,2,6-trimethylcyclohexyl)pro-pyl]-1,6-hexanediaminium dichloride; hexamethylenebis[dimeth-yl[1-methyl-3-(2,2,6-trimethylcyclohexyl)propyl]ammonium chloride]; N,N'-bis[1-methyl-3-(2,2,6-trimethylcyclohexyl)propyl]-N,N'-dimethyl-1,6-hexanediamine bis(methochloride); Ro-5-0810/1; Triburon. C$_{36}$H$_{74}$Cl$_2$N$_2$; mol wt 605.89. C 71.36%, H 12.31%, Cl 11.70%, N 4.62%. Obtained as the hemihydrate. Prepn: Goldberg, Teitel, *US 3064052* (1962 to Hoffmann-La Roche). Clinical application: Edelson *et al., Antibiot. Annu.* **1958-1959**, 110; Robinson, Harmon, *ibid.* 113. Comprehensive description: B. C. Rudy, B. Z. Senkowski, *Anal. Profiles Drug Subs.* **2**, 507-521 (1973).

White cryst powder, mp 243-253° (dec). Sol in water, chloroform, alcohol.

THERAP CAT: Antiseptic.

9654. Triclocarban. [101-20-2] N-(4-Chlorophenyl)-N'-(3,4-dichlorophenyl)urea; 3,4,4'-trichlorocarbanilide; 1-(3',4'-di-chlorophenyl)-3-(4'-chlorophenyl)urea; TCC; Cutisan; Nobacter; Solubacter. C$_{13}$H$_9$Cl$_3$N$_2$O; mol wt 315.58. C 49.48%, H 2.87%, Cl 33.70%, N 8.88%, O 5.07%. Prepn from 3,4-dichloroaniline and 4-chlorophenyl isocyanate: Beaver *et al., J. Am. Chem. Soc.* **79**, 1236 (1957); Beaver, Stoffel, *US 2818390* (1957 to Monsanto); *GB 769273* (1957).

Fine white plates, mp 255.2-256°.

USE: Bacteriostat and antiseptic in soaps and other cleansing compositions.

THERAP CAT: Antiseptic, disinfectant.

9655. Triclofos. [306-52-5] 2,2,2-Trichloroethanol dihydrogen phosphate; trichloroethyl phosphate. C$_2$H$_4$Cl$_3$O$_4$P; mol wt 229.38. C 10.47%, H 1.76%, Cl 46.37%, O 27.90%, P 13.50%. Prepn: Hems *et al., Br. Med. J.* **1**, 1834 (1962).

Monosodium salt. [7246-20-0] Sch-10159. C$_2$H$_3$Cl$_3$NaO$_4$P; mol wt 251.37. Sol in water. LD$_{50}$ orally in mice: 1.4 g/kg (Hems).

THERAP CAT: Sedative, hypnotic.

9656. Triclopyr. [55335-06-3] [(3,5,6-Trichloro-2-pyridin-yl)oxy]acetic acid; Dowco 233. C$_7$H$_4$Cl$_3$NO$_3$; mol wt 256.47. C 32.78%, H 1.57%, Cl 41.47%, N 5.46%, O 18.71%. Selective post-emergence herbicide. Prepn: L. D. Markley, *US 3862952* (1975 to Dow). Activity: B. C. Byrd *et al., Proc. South. Weed Sci. Soc.* **28**, 251 (1975). Acute toxicity: E. E. Kenaga, *Down Earth* **35**, 25 (1979).

Fluffy solid, mp 148-150°. Vapor pressure at 25°: 1.26 × 10^{-6} mm Hg. pKa 2.68. Subject to photolysis. Soly in water at 25°: 440 mg/l. Soly at 25° (g/kg): acetone 989; 1-octanol 307. LD$_{50}$ orally in rats: 713 mg/kg (Kenaga).

Butoxyethyl Ester. [64700-56-7] Garlon; Pathfinder; Remedy; Turflon. C$_{13}$H$_{16}$Cl$_3$NO$_4$; mol wt 356.63.

Triethylamine Salt. [57213-69-1] Grandstand. C$_7$H$_4$Cl$_3$-NO$_3$.C$_6$H$_{15}$N; mol wt 357.66.

USE: Herbicide.

9657. Triclosan. [3380-34-5] 5-Chloro-2-(2,4-dichloro-phenoxy)phenol; 2,4,4'-trichloro-2'-hydroxydiphenyl ether; CH-3635; Aquasept; Gamophen; Irgasan DP 300; Sapoderm; Ster-Zac. C$_{12}$H$_7$Cl$_3$O$_2$; mol wt 289.54. C 49.78%, H 2.44%, Cl 36.73%, O 11.05%. Prepn: *NL 6401526* corresp to E. Model, J. Bindler, *US 3506720* (1964, 1970 to Geigy). Physical and bacteriostatic properties: C. A. Savage, *Drug Cosmet. Ind.* **109**(3), 36, 161 (1971). Metabolism: J. G. Black *et al., Toxicology* **3**, 33 (1975). Toxicology: F. L. Lyman, T. Furia, *Ind. Med. Surg.* **38**(2), 64 (1969), *C.A.* **71**, 89601h (1969). Use as disinfectant and textile preservative: E. Model, J. Bindler, *US 3629477* (1971 to Geigy).

White to off-white crystalline powder, slight, faintly aromatic odor. mp 54-57.3°. Vapor pressure (20°C) 4 × 10^{-6} mm Hg. pKa 7.9. Insol in water. Readily sol in alkaline solns and many organic solvents.

USE: Bacteriostat and preservative for cosmetic and detergent prepns.

THERAP CAT: Antiseptic, disinfectant.

THERAP CAT (VET): Antiseptic.

9658. Tricromyl. [85-90-5] 3-Methyl-4H-1-benzopyran-4-one; 3-methylchromone; 3-methyl-γ-benzopyrone; Cromonalgina. C$_{10}$H$_8$O$_2$; mol wt 160.17. C 74.99%, H 5.03%, O 19.98%. Based on an ancient Egyptian drug now termed *bezr el khelda*. Prepn from *o*-hydroxypropiophenone: Clerc-Bory *et al., Bull. Soc. Chim. Fr.* **1955**, 1083; Mentzer, Meunier, *FR 980785* (1951 to Lab. Franc. Chimiother.); Mentzer, *US 2769015* (1956 one-half to Laroche-Navarron).

Crystals from ethanol, mp 68°. uv max (alc): 304 nm.

THERAP CAT: Antispasmodic; vasodilator (coronary).

9659. Tridecylbenzene. [123-02-4] 1-Phenyltridecane; Detergent Alkylate #5; Tridane. $C_{19}H_{32}$; mol wt 260.46. C 87.62%, H 12.38%. $C_6H_5(CH_2)_{12}CH_3$. Prepn: Ziegler *et al.*, *Ann.* **511**, 13 (1934). Manufacture: Williamson, Bieneman, **US 3207800** (1965 to Continental Oil).

Liquid, bp 346°, bp_{10} 188-189.5°. mp 10°. d_4^{20} 0.8550, d_4^{25} 1.8515. n_D^{20} 1.4821, n_D^{25} 1.4800. Forms stable foams in the presence of fat.

USE: In manuf of detergents and surface-active agents. Can be sulfonated.

9660. Tridemorph. [24602-86-6] 2,6-Dimethyl-4-tridecylmorpholine; *N*-tridecyl-2,6-dimethylmorpholine; 2,6-dimethyl-4-tridecyltetrahydro-1,4-oxazine. $C_{19}H_{39}NO$; mol wt 297.52. C 76.70%, H 13.21%, N 4.71%, O 5.38%. Prepn: W. Sanne *et al.*, **BE 614214**; *eidem*, **US 3468885** (1962, 1969 both to BASF); K.-H. König *et al.*, *Angew. Chem. Int. Ed.* **4**, 336 (1965). Structure determn of two diastereomers: D. Kost, E. Gurfinkel, *J. Chromatogr.* **108**, 207 (1975). Fungicidal activity: J. Kradel *et al.*, *Proc. 5th Brit. Insectic. Fungic. Conf.*, 16 (1969); *in vitro* activity comparison of tridemorph and commercial formulation Calixin: A. Kerkenaar, A. A. Sijpesteijn, *Pestic. Biochem. Physiol.* **12**, 124 (1979). Uptake and distribution in barley: E.-H. Pommer *et al.*, *Proc. 5th Brit. Insectic. Fungic. Conf.*, 347 (1969); R. H. Waring, M. S. Wolfe, *Pestic. Sci.* **6**, 169 (1975). Behavior in soil: S. Otto, N. Drescher, *Proc. 7th Brit. Insectic. Fungic. Conf.*, 257 (1973). Metabolic fate in rats: D. R. Hawkins *et al.*, *Pestic. Sci.* **5**, 535 (1974); of Calixin: R. H. Waring, *Xenobiotica* **4**, 717 (1974). Mode of action: A. Kerkenaar *et al.*, *Pestic. Biochem. Physiol.* **12**, 195 (1979). Comparison of toxicity of tridemorph and Calixin: J. Merkle *et al.*, *Teratology* **29**, 259 (1984). Field trials: P. Lakshmanan, S. Mohan, *Pesticides* **22**, 27 (1988).

Oil, $bp_{0.7}$ 130-133°; $bp_{1.3}$ 139-142°. n_D^{25} 1.4568.

Commercial product. Calixin. Reaction mixture of C_{11}-C_{14} 4-alkyl-2,6-dimethylmorpholine homologs containing 60-70% of tridemorph.

USE: Systemic agricultural fungicide.

9661. Tridihexethyl Iodide. [125-99-5] γ-Cyclohexyl-*N*,-*N*,*N*-triethyl-γ-hydroxybenzenepropanaminium iodide; (3-cyclohexyl-3-hydroxy-3-phenylpropyl)triethylammonium iodide; 3-diethylamino-1-cyclohexyl-1-phenyl-1-propanol ethiodide; 3-diethylamino-1-phenyl-1-cyclohexyl-1-propanol ethiodide; α-(2-diethylaminoethyl)-α-phenylcyclohexanemethanol ethiodide; propethonum iodide; tridihexethide; 921 C; Claviton. $C_{21}H_{36}INO$; mol wt 445.42. C 56.63%, H 8.15%, I 28.49%, N 3.14%, O 3.59%. Anticholinergic. Prepn: Lobby, **US 2913494** (1959 to Am. Cyanamid).

Bitter crystals, mp 179-184°. Solubility in water at 25°: 1.1 g/100 ml. Freely sol in alc, chloroform. Very slightly sol in ether. pH of a 1% aq soln 5.5-7.

Note: The name **Pathilon** previously used for the iodide is now used for **tridihexethyl chloride**.

THERAP CAT: Antispasmodic.

9662. Tridiphane. [58138-08-2] 2-(3,5-Dichlorophenyl)-2-(2,2,2-trichloroethyl)oxirane; Dowco 356. $C_{10}H_7Cl_5O$; mol wt 320.43. C 37.48%, H 2.20%, Cl 55.32%, O 4.99%. Prepn: L. D. Markley, E. J. Norton, **DE 2519073**; *eidem*, **US 4211549** (1975, 1980 both to Dow). Herbicidal activity: J. A. Jagschitz, *Proc. Annu. Meet. Northeast. Weed Sci. Soc.* **39**, 274 (1985); D. B. Vitolo *et al.*, *ibid.* **40**, 272 (1986). Field trial in combination with atrazine, *q.v.*: P. J. Dryden, M. J. Watson, *Proc. 38th N. Z. Weed Pest Control Conf.* **1985**, 191. Mechanism of action: G. L. Lamoureux, D. G. Rusness, *Pestic. Biochem. Physiol.* **26**, 323 (1986). Metabolism in mouse: J. Magdalou, B. D. Hammock, *Toxicol. Appl. Pharmacol.* **91**, 439 (1987). Toxicological studies: T. R. Hanley *et al.*, *Fundam. Appl. Toxicol.* **8**, 179 (1987); J. A. John-Greene *et al.*, *Toxicology* **43**, 325 (1987).

Yellow oil, n_D^{25} 1.5720. LD_{50} for technical grade (89-91% pure) in male, female mice, male, female rats (mg/kg): ~1200, ~740, 1700-2300, 1500-1900 orally (Hanley).

USE: Herbicide.

9663. Trientine. [112-24-3] *N*,*N'*-Bis(2-aminoethyl)-1,2-ethanediamine; triethylenetetramine; 1,8-diamino-3,6-diazaoctane; 3,6-diazaoctane-1,8-diamine; 1,4,7,10-tetraazadecane; trien; TETA; TECZA. $C_6H_{18}N_4$; mol wt 146.23. C 49.28%, H 12.41%, N 38.31%. $(NH_2CH_2CH_2NHCH_2—)_2$. Prepn: A. W. von Hoffmann, *Ber.* **23**, 3711 (1890); J. van Alphen, *Rec. Trav. Chim.* **55**, 412 (1936); G. D. Jones *et al.*, *J. Org. Chem.* **9**, 125 (1944); of the dihydrochloride: H. B. Dixon *et al.*, *Lancet* **1**, 853 (1972). Effects on the metabolism of copper in rats: F. W. Sunderman *et al.*, *Toxicol. Appl. Pharmacol.* **38**, 177 (1976); H. Harders *et al.*, *Arzneim.-Forsch.* **30**, 254 (1980). Use of the dihydrochloride in the treatment of Wilson's disease: J. M. Walshe, *Prog. Clin. Biol. Res.* **34**, 271 (1979); R. H. Haslam *et al.*, *Dev. Pharmacol. Ther.* **1**, 318 (1980); J. M. Walshe, *Lancet* **1**, 643 (1982). Review of chemistry, physical properties and industrial uses: R. D. Spitz, "Diamines and Higher Amines, Aliphatic" in *Kirk-Othmer Encyclopedia of Chemical Technology* **vol. 7** (Wiley-Interscience, New York, 3rd ed., 1979) pp 580-602. *Review:* J. M. Walshe, *Orphan Drugs*, F. E. Karch, Ed. (Marcel Dekker, New York, 1982) pp 57-71.

Oily liquid, mp 12°. bp 266-267°. n_D^{20} 1.4971; d^{15} 0.9817. Flash pt 290°F (143°C). pH 14. Sol in water, alc. *Corrosive!* LD_{50} orally in rats: 2.5 g/kg (Spitz).

Dihydrochloride. [38260-01-4] Syprine. $C_6H_{18}N_4.2HCl$; mol wt 219.16. Hygroscopic crystals, mp 115-118°.

USE: As thermosetting resin; epoxy curing agent; lubricating oil additive; analytical reagent for Cu, Ni.

THERAP CAT: Chelating agent (copper); Wilson's disease treatment.

9664. Trietazine. [1912-26-1] 6-Chloro-*N*,*N*,*N'*-triethyl-1,3,5-triazine-2,4-diamine; 2-chloro-4-diethylamino-6-ethylamino-*s*-triazine; 2-ethylamino-4-diethylamino-6-chloro-*s*-triazine; G-27901; NC-1667; Aventox. $C_9H_{16}ClN_5$; mol wt 229.71. C 47.06%, H 7.02%, Cl 15.43%, N 30.49%. Prepn: Pearlman, Banks, *J. Am. Chem. Soc.* **70**, 3726 (1948). Toxicity study: G. W. Bailey, J. L. White, *Residue Rev.* **10**, 97 (1965).

Crystals from propanol, mp 100-102°. Soly at 25°: 20 ppm in water; 17% in acetone; 20% in benzene; >50% in chloroform; 10% in dioxane; 3% in ethanol. LD$_{50}$ orally in rats: 1750 mg/kg (Bailey, White).

USE: Herbicide.

9665. Triethanolamine. [102-71-6] 2,2′,2″-Nitrilotriseth-anol; trihydroxytriethylamine; tris(hydroxyethyl)amine; triethylol-amine; trolamine. C$_6$H$_{15}$NO$_3$; mol wt 149.19. C 48.30%, H 10.13%, N 9.39%, O 32.17%. N(CH$_2$CH$_2$OH)$_3$. Produced along with mono- and diethanolamine by ammonolysis of ethylene oxide. See the refs under Ethanolamine. Monograph: E. J. Fischer, Tri-äthanolamin und andere Alkanolamine (Heidelberg, 4th ed., 1954).

Very hygroscopic, viscous liq. Slight ammoniacal odor. Turns brown on exposure to air and light. d$_4^{20}$ 1.1242; d$_4^{60}$ 1.0985. One gallon weighs 9.37 lbs. mp 21.57°. bp$_{760}$ 335.4°. See: McDonald et al., J. Chem. Eng. Data **4**, 311 (1959). Viscosity (cP): 590.5 (25°); 65.7 (60°). Strong base. pK (25°) 9.50. pH of 0.1N aq soln 10.5. n$_D^{20}$ 1.4852. Flash pt 365°F. Miscible with water, methanol, acetone. Soly at 25° in benzene, 4.2%; in ether, 1.6%; in carbon tetrachloride, 0.4%; in n-heptane, <0.1%.

Hydrochloride. [637-39-8] C$_6$H$_{15}$NO$_3$.HCl; mol wt 185.65. Crystals from ethanol, mp 177°.

Salicylate. [2174-16-5] Trolamine salicylate; Mobisyl; Myo-flex. C$_6$H$_{15}$NO$_3$.C$_7$H$_6$O$_3$; mol wt 287.31.

USE: Intermediate in the manuf of surface active agents, textile specialties, waxes, polishes, herbicides, petroleum demulsifiers, toilet goods, cement additives, cutting oils. In making emulsions with mineral and vegetable oils, paraffin and waxes. Solvent for casein, shellac, dyes; manuf synthetic resins; increasing the penetration of organic liquids into wood and paper. In the production of lubricants for the textile industry. Pharmaceutic aid (alkalizer).

THERAP CAT: Analgesic.

9666. Triethylamine. [121-44-8] N,N-Diethylethanamine. C$_6$H$_{15}$N; mol wt 101.19. C 71.22%, H 14.94%, N 13.84%. (C$_2$-H$_5$)$_3$N. Prepd by reaction of N,N-diethylacetamide with lithium aluminum hydride: Uffer, Schlittler, Helv. Chim. Acta **31**, 1397 (1948). Manuf by vapor phase alkylation of ammonia with ethanol: Lemon, Myerly, US 3022349 (1962 to Union Carbide). Toxicity study: H. F. Smyth et al., Arch. Ind. Hyg. Occup. Med. **4**, 119 (1951).

Liquid; strong ammoniacal odor; d$_4^{25}$ 0.7255; mp −115°; bp 89-90°; n$_D^{20}$ 1.4003. Flash pt, closed cup: 20°F (−6°C). Slightly sol in water above 18.7°; misc with alcohol, ether, also with water below 18.7°. Keep well closed. LD$_{50}$ orally in rats: 0.46 g/kg (Smyth).

Hydrochloride. C$_6$H$_{15}$N.HCl. Crystals from alcohol, mp 253-254°, sublimes at 245°; d 1.069. Sol in 0.7 parts water; sol in alcohol, chloroform; very slightly sol in benzene. Practically insol in ether.

Caution: Potential symptoms of overexposure to triethylamine are irritation of eyes, respiratory system and skin. See NIOSH Pocket Guide to Chemical Hazards (DHHS/NIOSH 97-140, 1997) p 318.

USE: In the prepn of quaternary ammonium compds.

9667. Triethylammonium Formate. [585-29-5] C$_7$H$_{17}$-NO$_2$; mol wt 147.22. C 57.11%, H 11.64%, N 9.51%, O 21.74%. (C$_2$H$_5$)$_3$N.HOOCH. Prepd by neutralizing 50% formic acid with triethylamine and evaporating the resulting soln on a steambath for twelve hours at 20 mm: Alexander, Wildman, J. Am. Chem. Soc. **70**, 1187 (1948).

Light brown syrup. Very sol in water. Sol in alc.

USE: In syntheses employing the Leuckart reaction.

9668. Triethylborane. [97-94-9] Triethylboron. C$_6$H$_{15}$B; mol wt 97.99. C 73.54%, H 15.43%, B 11.03%. Primarily as an initiator in radical reactions. Prepn: A. Stock, F. Zeidler, Ber. **78**, 531 (1921); E. C. Ashby, J. Am. Chem. Soc. **81**, 4791 (1959). Use as protecting group: C. Lutz et al., Tetrahedron **54**, 10317 (1998); as transfer reagent in polymerizations: V. Beraud et al., Macromol. Rapid Commun. **21**, 901 (2000); as stereoselective intiator for hydrometalation: K. Takami et al., J. Org. Chem. **68**, 6627 (2003). Review of radical reactivity in generation of carbon-centered radicals: C. Ollivier, P. Renaud, Chem. Rev. **101**, 3415-3434 (2001). Brief review of application in radical initiation and in non-radical processes: G. O'Mahony, Synlett **2004**, 572-573.

Colorless liquid. Spontaneously flammable! Burns in air with green flame.

USE: Reagent in organic syntheses blocking agent and radical initiator.

9669. Triethylenediamine. [280-57-9] 1,4-Diazabicyclo-[2.2.2]octane; Dabco. C$_6$H$_{12}$N$_2$; mol wt 112.17. C 64.25%, H 10.78%, N 24.97%. Prepn: Krause et al., GB 871754 (1958 to Houdry Process).

Crystals, extremely hygroscopic. Sublimes readily at room temp. mp 158°. bp 174°. pKa$_1$ 3.0; pKa$_2$ 8.7. Soly (g/100 g at 25°) in water: 45; acetone: 13; benzene: 51; ethanol: 77; methyl ethyl ketone: 26.1.

USE: Catalyst in making urethane foams.

9670. Triethylene Glycol. [112-27-6] 2,2′-[1,2-Ethanediyl-bis(oxy)]bisethanol; 2,2′-ethylenedioxybis(ethanol). C$_6$H$_{14}$O$_4$; mol wt 150.17. C 47.99%, H 9.40%, O 42.62%. Prepd from ethylene oxide and ethylene glycol in the presence of sulfuric acid: Matignon et al., Bull. Soc. Chim. [5] **1**, 1308 (1934). Manuf by forming ether-ester of HOCH$_2$COOH with glycol and then hydrogenating: Gresham, US 2654786 (1953 to du Pont). Toxicity data: Stenger et al., Arzneim.-Forsch. **18**, 1536 (1968).

Colorless, hygroscopic, practically odorless liquid. d$_4^{15}$ 1.1274; bp 285°; bp$_{14}$ 165°. mp −7.2°. Viscosity at 20°: 47.8 cP; n$_D^{15}$ 1.4578. Misc with water, alcohol, benzene, toluene; sparingly sol in ether. Practically insol in petr ether. LD$_{50}$ in mice, rats (g/kg): 21, 15-22 orally; 7.3-9.5, 11.7 i.v. (Stenger).

USE: In various plastics to increase pliability; in air disinfection.

9671. Triethylenemelamine. [51-18-3] 2,4,6-Tris(1-aziri-dinyl)-1,3,5-triazine; 2,4,6-tris(ethylenimino)-s-triazine; 2,4,6-tri-ethylenimino-1,3,5-triazine; triethanomelamine; tretamine; triame-lin; TEM; NSC-9706; Persistol. C$_9$H$_{12}$N$_6$; mol wt 204.23. C 52.93%, H 5.92%, N 41.15%. Prepd from ethylenimine and cyanuric chloride: Bestian, Ann. **566**, 210 (1950); Wystrach, Kaiser, US 2520619 (1950 to Am. Cyanamid); Kaiser, Schaefer, US 2653934 (1953); Wystrach et al., J. Am. Chem. Soc. **77**, 5915 (1955). Toxicology: F. S. Philips, J. B. Thiersch, J. Pharmacol. Exp. Ther. **100**, 398 (1950). Review of carcinogenic risk: IARC Monographs **9**, 95-105 (1975); of comparative mutagenicity: C. Ramel, Environ. Sci. Res. **24**, 943-976 (1981).

Minute crystals from chloroform, dec 139°. Soly (w/w) at 26°: in water 40%, chloroform 28.1%, methylene chloride 19.7%, methanol 12.5%, acetone 10.6%, dioxane 9.6%, ethanol 7.7%, benzene 5.6%, dimethyl Cellosolve 4.8%, methyl ethyl ketone 4.7%, ethyl acetate 4.5%, carbon tetrachloride 3.6%. Stable at reduced temps; ampuled aq solns stored at 4° are stable for about 3 months. At room temp, aq solns polymerize. LD_{50} in mice, rats (mg/kg): 2.8, 1.0 i.p.; 15, 13 orally (Philips).

USE: Manuf of resinous products, textile finishing agents. Insect sterilant. Research tool used as positive control for mutagenicity assays.

THERAP CAT: Antineoplastic.

9672. Triethylenephosphoramide. [545-55-1] 1,1',1"-Phosphinylidynetrisaziridine; tris(1-aziridinyl)phosphine oxide; phosphoric acid triethyleneimide; aphoxide; APO; TEPA. C_6H_{12}-N_3OP; mol wt 173.15. C 41.62%, H 6.99%, N 24.27%, O 9.24%, P 17.89%. Prepn: Bestian, *Ann.* **566**, 231 (1950). Toxicity study: Gaines, *Toxicol. Appl. Pharmacol.* **14**, 515 (1969).

Crystals, mp 41°. bp$_{23}$ 90-91°. Extremely sol in water. Very sol in alcohol, ether, acetone. LD_{50} orally in male rats: 37 mg/kg (Gaines).

USE: Insect chemosterilant; in dyeing, creaseproofing and flameproofing textiles; stabilizer for polymers; in photographic emulsion hardening.

THERAP CAT: Antineoplastic.

9673. Triethylenethiophosphoramide. [52-24-4] 1,1',1"-Phosphinothioylidynetrisaziridine; tris(1-aziridinyl)phosphine sulfide; thiotepa; Tespamin; Tifosyl. $C_6H_{12}N_3PS$; mol wt 189.22. C 38.08%, H 6.39%, N 22.21%, P 16.37%, S 16.95%. Preparation: Kuh, Seeger, US 2670347 (1954 to Am. Cyanamid); Saijo, Endo, **JP 55 218** (1955 to Semimoto Chem.). Toxicity data: Scherf *et al., Arzneim.-Forsch.* **20**, 1467 (1970). Review of carcinogenicity studies: *IARC Monographs* **9**, 85-94 (1975).

Crystals from pentane or ether, mp 51.5°. Soly in water at 25°: 19 g/100 ml. Freely sol in alc; sol in benzene, ether, chloroform. LD_{50} i.v. in rats: 15 mg/kg (Scherf).

Caution: This substance is listed as a known human carcinogen: *Report on Carcinogens, Eleventh Edition* (PB2005-104914, 2004) p III-249.

USE: Insect sterilant.

THERAP CAT: Antineoplastic.

9674. Triethyl Phosphate. [78-40-0] Ethyl phosphate. C_6-$H_{15}O_4P$; mol wt 182.15. C 39.56%, H 8.30%, O 35.13%, P 17.00%. $(C_2H_5)_3PO_4$. Prepd from tetraethyl hypophosphate with ethanol in the presence of aluminum ethoxide: Mukaiyama *et al., J. Org. Chem.* **27**, 1815 (1962). Manuf by treating triethyl phosphite with diethyl hydrogen phosphate: McCall, Coover, US 2960529 (1960 to Kodak).

Liquid; d^{19} 1.0725; bp 215-216°; bp$_{10}$ 90-95°; n_D^{17} 1.4067. Sol in water with some decompn; sol in alcohol, ether.

USE: As ethylating agent; formation of polyesters which are used as insecticides.

9675. Triethyl Phosphine. [554-70-1] $C_6H_{15}P$; mol wt 118.16. C 60.99%, H 12.80%, P 26.21%. $(C_2H_5)_3P$. Prepd from ethyllithium and phosphorus trichloride: Screttas, Isbell, *J. Org. Chem.* **27**, 2573 (1962). Manuf from white phosphorus, ethylene and hydrogen at elevated pressures: Oppegard, US 2687437 (1954 to du Pont).

Colorless liquid; odor of hyacinths; d_4^{15} 0.800; bp$_{744}$ 127-128°. Practically insol in water. Miscible with alcohol, ether.

USE: In organic syntheses.

9676. Triflic Acid. [1493-13-6] Trifluoromethanesulfonic acid; TFMSA. CHF_3O_3S; mol wt 150.08. C 8.00%, H 0.67%, F 37.98%, O 31.98%, S 21.37%. F_3CSO_2OH. One of the strongest acids known. Prepn: R. N. Haszeldine, J. M. Kidd, *J. Chem. Soc.*

1954, 4228. Acid-base equilibria study: Y. Y. Fialkov, V. I. Ligus, *J. Gen. Chem. USSR* **42**, 256 (1972). Deprotecting agent in peptide chemistry: H. Yajima *et al., J. Chem. Soc. Chem. Commun.* **1974**, 107. Hammett acidity function: S. Saito *et al., Chem. Pharm. Bull.* **39**, 2718 (1991). Electrochemical determn of ionic form: F. Favier, J. L. Pascal, *Analyst* **116**, 479 (1991). Ion chromatographic determn of triflic and trifluoroacetic acids: N. Simonzadeh, *J. Chromatogr.* **634**, 125 (1993). *Reviews:* R. D. Howells, J. D. McCown, *Chem. Rev.* **77**, 69-92 (1977); P. J. Stang, M. R. White, *Aldrichim. Acta* **16**, 15-22 (1983).

Clear, colorless, hygroscopic liquid, bp$_{760}$ 162°; bp$_{57.5}$ 91°; bp$_{37.5}$ 81°; bp$_1$ 42°. d^{25} 1.6980. n_D^{25} 1.325. Miscible with water; sol in alcohols, ketones, ethers, esters and many other polar organic solvents. Viscosity at 25°: 2.87 cP. Electrical conductivity at 25°: 2 $\times 10^{-4}$ Ω^{-1} cm^{-1}. Thermally stable; nonoxidizing.

Caution: Direct contact may cause skin burns (Haszeldine).

USE: As a catalyst in Friedel-Crafts type acylation, alkylation and polymerization reactions; as a solvent for ESR; as a nonaqueous strong acid titrant; with trifluoroacetic acid, *q.v.*, in solid-phase peptide synthesis.

9677. Trifloxystrobin. [141517-21-7] (αE)-α-(Methoxyimino)-2-[[[(E)-[1-[3-(trifluoromethyl)phenyl]ethylidene]amino]-oxy]methyl]benzeneacetic acid methyl ester; (E,E)-methoxyimino-[2-[1-(3-trifluoromethylphenyl)ethylideneaminooxymethyl]-phenyl]acetic acid methyl ester; CGA-279202; Flint; Compass; Gem; Twist. $C_{20}H_{19}F_3N_2O_4$; mol wt 408.37. C 58.82%, H 4.69%, F 13.96%, N 6.86%, O 15.67%. Strobilurin fungicide. Prepn: J. M. Clough *et al., EP 472300; eidem,* US 5238956 (1992, 1993 both to ICI). Field trial in fruit trees: M. Reuveni *et al., Crop Prot.* **19**, 335 (2000). Review of physical properties, biological properties and field trials: P. Margot *et al., Brighton Crop Prot. Conf. - Pests Dis.* **1998**, 375-382.

Odorless white powder, mp 72.9°. bp~312°; decompn starting at 285°. Soly in water at 25°: 610 μg/l. Vapor pressure at 25°: 3.4 $\times 10^{-6}$ Pa. Log P at 25° (*n*-octanol/water): 4.5. LD_{50} in rats (mg/kg): >5000 orally; >2000 dermally. LC_{50} by inhalation in rats (mg/m^3): >4646. LC_{50} in bobwhite quail (mg/kg): >2000. LC_{50} in rainbow trout (mg/l): 0.015 (Margot).

USE: Agricultural fungicide.

9678. Triflumuron. [64628-44-0] 2-Chloro-*N*-[[[4-(trifluoromethoxy)phenyl]amino]carbonyl]benzamide; *N*-(2-chlorobenzoyl)-*N'*-[4-(trifluoromethoxy)phenyl]urea; trifluron; SIR-8514; BAY SIR 8514; Alsystin; Baycidal; Starycide. $C_{15}H_{10}ClF_3N_2O_3$; mol wt 358.70. C 50.23%, H 2.81%, Cl 9.88%, F 15.89%, N 7.81%, O 13.38%. Arthropod insecticide which inhibits chitin biosynthesis: Prepn: W. Sirrenberg *et al., DE 2601780* corresp to US 4139636 (1977, 1979 both to Bayer AG); BE 867046 corresp to R. H. Rigterink, US 4170657 (1978, 1979 both to Dow Chemical). Insecticidal activity: C. H. Schaefer *et al., J. Econ. Entomol.* **71**, 427 (1978); S. C. Chang, *ibid.* **72**, 479 (1979). Stability under field conditions: C. H. Schaefer, E. F. Dupras, *J. Agric. Food Chem.* **27**, 1031 (1979). Comprehensive description: G. Zoebelein *et al., Z. Angew. Entomol.* **89**, 289-297 (1980).

Crystals, mp 198° (Sirrenberg). Also reported as mp 188-190° (Rigterink). Slightly toxic to fish. Safe to bees. LD_{50} in rats, mice (mg/kg): >5000, >5000 i.p., s.c., orally (Zoebelein).

USE: Insecticide (larvicide).

9679. Trifluomeprazine. [2622-37-9] *N,N,β*-Trimethyl-2-(trifluoromethyl)-10*H*-phenothiazine-10-propanamine; 10-[3-(dimethylamino)-2-methylpropyl]-2-(trifluoromethyl)phenothiazine; RP-7746. $C_{19}H_{21}F_3N_2S$; mol wt 366.44. C 62.28%, H 5.78%, F 15.55%, N 7.64%, S 8.75%. Prepn: **GB 813861** corresp to G. E. Ullyot, **US 2921069** (1959, 1962 both to SK&F). Metabolism study: T. L. Flanagan *et al., J. Pharm. Sci.* **51**, 996 (1962). Chromatographic studies: M. W. Anders, G. J. Mannering, *J. Chromatogr.* **7**, 258 (1962); R. J. Warren *et al., J. Pharm. Sci.* **55**, 144 (1966); B. B. Wheals, *J. Chromatogr.* **187**, 65 (1980). Pharmacological studies: R. C. Kelsey, G. J. Frishmuth, *Arch. Int. Pharmacodyn. Ther.* **173**, 44 (1968); E. W. Baur, *J. Pharmacol. Exp. Ther.* **177**, 219 (1971).

uv max (95% ethanol): 308, 258 nm (log ε 3.60, 4.55).
Maleate. Nortran. $C_{19}H_{21}F_3N_2S.C_4H_4O_4$; mol wt 482.52.
THERAP CAT (VET): Tranquilizer.

9680. Trifluoperazine. [117-89-5] 10-[3-(4-Methyl-1-piperazinyl)propyl]-2-(trifluoromethyl)-10*H*-phenothiazine; 2-trifluoromethyl-10-[3′-(1-methyl-4-piperazinyl)propyl]phenothiazine. $C_{21}H_{24}F_3N_3S$; mol wt 407.50. C 61.90%, H 5.94%, F 13.99%, N 10.31%, S 7.87%. Prepn: Craig *et al., J. Org. Chem.* **22**, 709 (1957); **GB 813861**; G. E. Ullyot, **US 2921069** (1959 and 1960 to SK & F). Metabolism: T. L. Flanagan *et al., J. Pharm. Sci.* **51**, 996 (1962); C. L. Huang, K. G. Bhansali, *ibid.* **57**, 1511 (1968). Toxicity: P. J. Fowler *et al., Arzneim.-Forsch.* **27**, 866 (1977). Comprehensive description: A. Post *et al., Anal. Profiles Drug Subs.* **9**, 543-581 (1980).

bp$_{0.6}$ 202-210°. uv max (ethanol): 258, 307.5 nm (log ε 4.50, 3.50). LD$_{50}$ orally in rats, mice: 542.7, 424.0 mg/ml (Fowler).
Dihydrochloride. [440-17-5] Triftazin; triphthasine; Eskazinyl; Eskazine; Jatroneural; Modalina; Stelazine; Terfluzine. $C_{21}H_{24}F_3N_3S.2HCl$; mol wt 480.42. Cream colored fine powder from abs alc, mp 242-243°. Hygroscopic. Freely sol in water. Insol in dil base, ether, benzene. pK$_1$ 3.9, pK$_2$ 8.1. pH of 5% aq soln 2.2.
THERAP CAT: Antipsychotic.

9681. Trifluoroacetic Acid. [76-05-1] Perfluoroacetic acid. $C_2HF_3O_2$; mol wt 114.02. C 21.07%, H 0.88%, F 49.99%, O 28.06%. CF$_3$COOH. Prepn: F. Swarts, *Bull. Sci. Acad. R. Belg.* **8**, 343 (1922); by oxidation of fluorine olefins: A. L. Henne, **US 2371757** (1945 to du Pont); A. L. Henne *et al., J. Am. Chem. Soc.* **67**, 918 (1945). Improved prepn: A. L. Henne, P. Trott, *ibid.* **69**, 1820 (1947). Photochemical prepn: R. N. Hazeldine, F. Nyman, *J. Chem. Soc.* **1959**, 387; *eidem, ibid.* 420. Toxicity and metabolism: M. M. Airaksinen, T. Tammisto, *Ann. Med. Exp. Biol. Fenn.* **46**, 242 (1968). *Review:* J. B. Milne in *Chem. Non-Aqueous Solvents* vol. **5B**, J. J. Lagowski, Ed. (Academic Press, New York, 1978) pp 1-52.
Liquid, sharp biting odor. bp 72.4°. mp −15.4°. d^{20} 1.5351. Miscible with ether, acetone, ethanol, benzene, CCl$_4$, hexane. Strong, non-oxidizing acid. pka 0.3. LD$_{50}$ i.v. in mice: 1200 mg/kg (Airaksinen, Tammisto).
USE: In organic synthesis; dissolves protein when mixed with liquid SO$_2$.

9682. Trifluoroethanol. [75-89-8] 2,2,2-Trifluoroethanol; TFE; 2,2,2-trifluoroethyl alcohol. $C_2H_3F_3O$; mol wt 100.04. C

24.01%, H 3.02%, F 56.97%, O 15.99%. CF$_3$CH$_2$OH. Weakly acidic alcohol. Prepn: F. Swarts, *Bull. Soc. Chim. Belg.* **43**, 471 (1934). Structural study: L. A. Curtiss *et al., J. Am. Chem. Soc.* **100**, 79 (1978). Interaction with peptides and proteins: R. Rajan, P. Balaram, *Int. J. Pept. Protein Res.* **48**, 328 (1996). Review of production and applications: S. Arai, *Spec. Chem.* **18**, 294-297 (1998); of effects on peptide and protein structures: M. Buck, *Q. Rev. Biophys.* **31**, 297-355 (1998).
Transparent, colorless liquid; bp 74.05°; mp −43.5°. d^0 1.4106. d^{22} 1.3739. n_D^{22} 1.2907. pK 12.4. Dielectric constant: 26.67. Dipole moment: 2.52 D. Miscible with water, alcohols, ethers, ketones, chloroform.
USE: In synthesis of medical anaesthetics, pharmaceuticals, and agrochemicals; in polymerizations. Protein denaturant; stabilizes peptide structures. Cleaning solvent; eluent in HPLC separations; working fluid in Rankine heat cycle systems. Environmentally friendly alternative to CFCs.

9683. Trifluoromethyltrimethylsilane. [81290-20-2] Trimethyl(trifluoromethyl)silane; Ruppert's reagent; TMS-CF$_3$. $C_4H_9F_3Si$; mol wt 142.19. C 33.79%, H 6.38%, F 40.08%, Si 19.75%. (CH$_3$)$_3$SiCF$_3$. Reagent used for fluoride ion catalyzed trifluoromethylation of organic substrates. Prepn: I. Ruppert *et al., Tetrahedron Lett.* **25**, 2195 (1984); and use in trifluoromethylation of aldehydes and ketones: G. K. S. Prakash *et al., J. Am. Chem. Soc.* **111**, 393 (1989). Review of chemistry: G. K. S. Prakash, A. K. Yudin, *Chem. Rev.* **97**, 757-786 (1997); R. P. Singh, J. M. Shreeve, *Tetrahedron* **56**, 7613-7632 (2000).
Colorless, volatile liquid, bp 45° (Ruppert); also reported as bp 54-55° (Prakash, Yudin).
USE: Nucleophilic trifluoromethylating reagent.

9684. Trifluperidol. [749-13-3] 1-(4-Fluorophenyl)-4-[4-hydroxy-4-[3-(trifluoromethyl)phenyl]-1-piperidinyl]-1-butanone; 4′-fluoro-4-[4-hydroxy-4-(α,α,α-trifluoro-*m*-tolyl)piperidino]butyrophenone; *p*-fluoro-4-[4′-hydroxy-4′-(3″-trifluoromethyl)phenyl]-piperidinobutyrophenone; 1-(3′-*p*-fluorobenzoylpropyl)-4-hydroxy-4-(3″-trifluoromethylphenyl)piperidine; ω-[4-hydroxy-4-(*m*-trifluoromethylphenyl)piperidino]-*p*-fluorobutyrophenone; flumoperone. $C_{22}H_{22}F_4NO_2$; mol wt 409.42. C 64.54%, H 5.66%, F 18.56%, N 3.42%, O 7.82%. Prepn: P. A. J. Janssen, **GB 895309**; *idem*, **US 3438991** (1962, 1969 both to Janssen). Pharmacology: *idem, Arzneim.-Forsch.* **11**, 932 (1961).

Hydrochloride. [2062-77-3] R-2498; Psicoperidol; Psychoperidol; Triperidol. $C_{22}H_{23}F_4NO_2.HCl$; mol wt 445.88. Crystals from acetone, mp 200.5-201.3°. Sol in water. LD$_{50}$ in rats (mg/kg): 14 i.v.; 70 s.c. (Janssen, 1961).
THERAP CAT: Antipsychotic.

9685. Triflupromazine. [146-54-3] *N,N*-Dimethyl-2-(trifluoromethyl)-10*H*-phenothiazine-10-propanamine; 10-[3-(dimethylamino)propyl]-2-trifluoromethylphenothiazine; 2-trifluoromethyl-10-(γ-dimethylaminopropyl)phenothiazine; fluopromazine. $C_{18}H_{19}F_3N_2S$; mol wt 352.42. C 61.35%, H 5.43%, F 16.17%, N 7.95%, S 9.10%. Prepn: Yale *et al., J. Am. Chem. Soc.* **79**, 4375 (1957); **GB 813861** (1959 to SK & F). Comprehensive description of the hydrochloride: K. Florey, *Anal. Profiles Drug Subs.* **2**, 523-550 (1973).

Liquid, bp$_{0.7}$ 176°; bp$_{0.4}$ 162-164°. n_D^{23} 1.5780.

Hydrochloride. [1098-60-8] Psyquil; Vesprin. C$_{18}$H$_{19}$F$_3$N$_2$-S.HCl; mol wt 388.88. Crystals from xylene, dec 173-174°. uv max: 255, 305 nm (E$_{1cm}^{1\%}$ 700, 90). Sol in water, ethanol, acetone. pH of 2% aq soln 4.1, if the pH is raised to 6.4, pptn of the free base results.

THERAP CAT: Antipsychotic.

THERAP CAT (VET): Tranquilizer.

9686. Trifluralin. [1582-09-8] 2,6-Dinitro-*N,N*-dipropyl-4-(trifluoromethyl)benzenamine; *α,α,α*-trifluoro-2,6-dinitro-*N,N*-di-propyl-*p*-toluidine; 2,6-dinitro-*N,N*-dipropyl-*α,α,α*-trifluoro-*p*-tolui-dine; 2,6-dinitro-*N,N*-dipropyl-4-trifluoromethylaniline; *N,N*-dipro-pyl-2,6-dinitro-4-trifluoromethylaniline; L-36352; Lilly 36352; Tre-flan; Tri-4; Triflurex. C$_{13}$H$_{16}$F$_3$N$_3$O$_4$; mol wt 335.28. C 46.57%, H 4.81%, F 17.00%, N 12.53%, O 19.09%. Pre-emergence herbi-cide used for grass control in crops. Prepn: **GB 917253** *C.A.* **59**, 9889b (1963); Soper, **US 3403180** (1963; 1968, both to Lilly). Photodecomposition: E. Leitis, D. G. Crosby, *J. Agric. Food Chem.* **22**, 842 (1974). Soil degradation: T. Golab *et al., ibid.* **27**, 163 (1979). Toxicity data: Goldenthal, *Toxicol. Appl. Phar-macol.* **18**, 185 (1971). Carcinogenicity study: J. F. Robens, *Vet. Hum. Toxicol.* **22**, 328 (1980). Review of toxicology: E. Ebert *et al., Food Chem. Toxicol.* **30**, 1031-1044 (1992).

Yellow crystals, mp 46-47°. bp$_{4.2}$ 139-140°. Slightly sol in water (0.0024 g/100 ml); freely sol in acetone, Stoddard solvent, xylene. LD$_{50}$ orally in rats: 500 mg/kg (Goldenthal).

USE: Herbicide.

9687. Trifluridine. [70-00-0] *α,α,α*-Trifluorothymidine; 2′-deoxy-5-(trifluoromethyl)uridine; 5-(trifluoromethyl)-2′-deoxyuri-dine; F3TDR; NSC-75520; TFT Thilo; Virophta; Viroptic. C$_{10}$-H$_{11}$F$_3$N$_2$O$_5$; mol wt 296.20. C 40.55%, H 3.74%, F 19.24%, N 9.46%, O 27.01%. Prepn: C. Heidelberger *et al., J. Am. Chem. Soc.* **84**, 3597 (1962); *eidem, J. Med. Chem.* **7**, 1 (1964); C. Hei-delberger, **US 3201387** (1965 to U.S. Dept. HEW). Crystal struc-ture: A. H. Tench, *Diss. Abstr. Int. B* **33**, 3587 (1973). NMR study: R. J. Cushley *et al., J. Am. Chem. Soc.* **90**, 709 (1968). Metabolism: D. L. Dexter *et al., Cancer Res.* **32**, 247 (1972); W. J. O'Brien, H. F. Edelhauser, *Invest. Ophthalmol. Visual Sci.* **16**, 1093 (1977). Phar-macodynamics: B. L. Wigdahl, J. R. Parkhurst, *Antimicrob. Agents Chemother.* **14**, 470 (1978); G. J. Smith *et al., Biochem. Biophys. Res. Commun.* **83**, 1538 (1978). Teratogenicity study: M. Itoi *et al., Arch. Ophthalmol.* **93**, 46 (1975). Cytotoxicity and mutagenic-ity study: E. Huberman, C. Heidelberger, *Mutat. Res.* **14**, 130 (1972). Clinical studies: H. E. Kaufman, *Invest. Ophthalmol. Visual Sci.* **17**, 941 (1978); R. A. Hyndiuk *et al., Arch. Ophthalmol.* **96**, 1839 (1978). Review of mechanism of antiviral activity: C. Heidelberger, *Ann. N.Y. Acad. Sci.* **255**, 317 (1975). Review of pharmacology and therapeutic use: A. A. Carmine *et al., Drugs* **23**, 329-353 (1982).

Cryst from ethyl acetate, mp 186-189°. uv max (0.1*N* HCl): 260 nm (ε 9960); (0.1*N* NaOH): 260 nm (ε 6590).

THERAP CAT: Antiviral (ophthalmic).

9688. Triflusal. [322-79-2] 2-(Acetyloxy)-4-(trifluorometh-yl)benzoic acid; *α,α,α*-trifluoro-2,4-cresotic acid acetate; acetyl-4-trifluoromethylsalicylic acid; UR-1501; Disgren. C$_{10}$H$_7$F$_3$O$_4$; mol wt 248.16. C 48.40%, H 2.84%, F 22.97%, O 25.79%. Analog of aspirin, *q.v.*; inhibits platelet aggregation. Prepn of free acid: M. Hauptschein, **US 3019253** (1962 to Pennsalt). Inhibition of platelet aggregation in man and rat: J. Garcia-Rafanell, J. Morell, *Therapie* **32**, 337 (1977). Effect on blood coagulation: M. Rutllant *et al., Curr. Ther. Res.* **22**, 510 (1977). Pharmacokinetics: V. Rimbau *et al., Arch. Farmacol. Toxicol.* **7**, 11 (1981). Clinical studies: R. M. Masso *et al., Curr. Ther. Res.* **25**, 791 (1979); E. Sala-Planell *et al., Angiologia* **33**, 71 (1981).

White cryst solid from petr ether/ether, mp 120-122° (upon slow heating); 110-112° (upon quick heating). Misc with ethanol. Prac-tically insol in water.

THERAP CAT: Antithrombotic.

9689. Triflusulfuron-methyl. [126535-15-7] 2-[[[[[4-(Di-methylamino)-6-(2,2,2-trifluoroethoxy)-1,3,5-triazin-2-yl]amino]-carbonyl]amino]sulfonyl]-3-methyl benzoic acid methyl ester; DPX-66037; Debut; Safari; Upbeet. C$_{17}$H$_{19}$F$_3$N$_6$O$_6$S; mol wt 492.43. C 41.46%, H 3.89%, F 11.57%, N 17.07%, O 19.49%, S 6.51%. Sulfonylurea herbicide for use in beets; acetolactate syn-thase inhibitor. Prepn: M. P. Moon, **WO 8909214**; *idem,* **US 5090993** (1989, 1992 both to DuPont). Comprehensive description: K. A. Peeples *et al., Brighton Crop Prot. Conf. - Weeds* **1991**, 25-30. Selectivity in sugar beets: V. A. Wittenbach *et al., Pestic. Biochem. Physiol.* **49**, 72 (1994).

White solid, mp 160-163°. Log P (octanol/water pH 7) at 25°: 9.2. pKa 4.4. Soly in water at 25° (ppm): 1 (pH 3); 3 (pH 5); 110 (pH 7); 11000 (pH 9). LD$_{50}$ orally in rats: >5000 mg/kg; dermally in rabbits: >2000 mg/kg (Peeples).

USE: Herbicide.

9690. Trifolium. Meadow clover; red clover; purple clover; cow clover. Perennial herb, *Trifolium pratense* L., *Leguminosae.* Important in agriculture as a forage legume; usually as a companion crop for cereal grains or pasture grass. Used in traditional medicine for coughs and bronchitis and as a dermatological agent. Medicinal formulations are prepared from the dried and fresh flowerheads (inflorescence). *Habit.* Europe, Asia, Northern Africa; naturalized in U.S. *Constit.* Diphenolic isoflavones, primarily biochanin A, formononetin, genistein, daidzein, *q.q.v.*; coumarin derivatives; vol-atile oil containing furfural, methyl salicylate; tannin, resins, poly-saccharides. Description of botany and uses in agriculture: N. L. Taylor, K. H. Quesenberry, *Red Clover Science* (Kluwer, Dordrecht, 1996) 226 pp. HPLC-ES-MS determn of flavonoids in botanical extracts: X. He *et al., J. Chromatogr. A* **755**, 127 (1996). Review of medicinal uses: J. Barnes *et al., Herbal Medicines* (Pharmaceut-ical Press, London, 2nd ed., 2002) pp 399-400.

Ethanolic extract. Menoflavin; Promensil; Rimostil. Estro-genic activity: E. Dornstauder *et al., J. Steroid Biochem. Mol. Biol.* **78**, 67 (2001). Clinical effect on lipid and bone metabolism: P. B. Clifton-Bligh *et al., Menopause* **8**, 259 (2001); on menopausal symptoms: P. H. M. van der Weijer, R. Barentsen, *Maturitas* **42**, 187 (2002).

THERAP CAT: In treatment of menopausal symptoms.

9691. Triforine. [26644-46-2] *N,N'*-[1,4-Piperazinediyl-bis(2,2,2-trichloroethylidene)]bisformamide; 1,4-di(2,2,2-trichloro-1-formamidoethyl)piperazine; 1,4-bis(1-formamido-2,2,2-trichloroethyl)piperazine; Cela W-524; CME-74770; Basforin; Funginex; Saprol. $C_{10}H_{14}Cl_6N_4O_2$; mol wt 434.96. C 27.61%, H 3.24%, Cl 48.91%, N 12.88%, O 7.36%. Prepn: W. Ost *et al.*, **DE 1901421** corresp to **US 3595916** (1969, 1971, both to Boehringer, Ing.).

White crystals, mp 155°. Vapor pressure at 25° = 2×10^{-7} mm Hg. Soly in water at 20°: 27-29 ppm. Sol in CMF, DMSO, *N*-methylpyrrolidone; moderately sol in tetrahydrofuran. Insol in acetone, benzene, carbon tetrachloride, chloroform, methylene chloride, petroleum ether. Dec to chloral and piperazine salts by conc H_2SO_4 and HCl; slowly dec to chloroform and piperazine by conc alk. Half life in the soil ~3 weeks. Low toxicity to fish and bees.

USE: Fungicide.

9692. Triglyme. [112-49-2] 2,5,8,11-Tetraoxadodecane; triethylene glycol dimethyl ether. $C_8H_{18}O_4$; mol wt 178.23. C 53.91%, H 10.18%, O 35.91%. $CH_3O(CH_2)_2O(CH_2)_2O(CH_2)_2$-$OCH_3$. Prepd by high pressure hydrogenation of 1,1,2,2-tetrakis(2-methoxyethoxy)ethane: McNamee, MacDowell, **US 2425042** (1947 to Carbide & Carbon Chem.).

Liquid. d_4^{20} 0.990. Flash pt 111°C. mp $-45°$. bp_{760} 216°; bp_{10} 103.5°; $bp_{0.9}$ 20°. n_D^{20} 1.4233. Miscible with water, hydrocarbon solvents.

USE: Solvent.

9693. Trigonellamide Chloride. [1005-24-9] 3-(Aminocarbonyl)-1-methylpyridinium chloride; N^1-methylnicotinamide chloride; 1-methylpyridine-3-carboxylic acid amide chloride; nicotinamide chloromethylate; nicotinamide methyl chloride. $C_7H_9ClN_2$-O; mol wt 172.61. C 48.71%, H 5.26%, Cl 20.54%, N 16.23%, O 9.27%. One of the principal excretion products of the metabolism of nicotinic acid in man, dog, and rat. Coenzyme action: Warburg, Christian, *Biochem. Z.* **287**, 291 (1936). Synthesis by refluxing nicotinamide with methyl iodide in methanol, then shaking the nicotinamide methiodide with AgCl: Karrer *et al.*, *Helv. Chim. Acta* **19**, 826 (1936); and isolation from urine: Huff, Perizweig, *J. Biol. Chem.* **150**, 395 (1943). Differentiation from NAD: Carpenter, Kodicek, *Biochem. J.* **46**, 421 (1950). *In vitro* metabolism: G. S. Johnson, *Eur. J. Biochem.* **112**, 635 (1980); H. Hoshino *et al.*, *Biochim. Biophys. Acta* **801**, 250 (1984). HPLC determn in urine: M. A. Kutnink *et al.*, *J. Liq. Chromatogr.* **7**, 969 (1984).

Crystals from methanol. Dec 240°. Moderately sol in water. More sol in alcohol, butanol, isobutanol. Insol in amyl alcohol, octyl alcohol, benzene, chlorobenzene, chloroform. Destroyed upon boiling the aq soln, more rapidly in the presence of alkali. At room temp it is destroyed in alkaline soln. Reacts with ketones in aq alkaline soln to produce a greenish-blue fluorescence; on acidification the fluorescence changes to blue, and is intensified by heating.

9694. Trigonelline. [535-83-1] 3-Carboxy-1-methylpyridinium inner salt; nicotinic acid *N*-methylbetaine; coffearine; caf-

fearine; gynesine; trigenolline. $C_7H_7NO_2$; mol wt 137.14. C 61.31%, H 5.14%, N 10.21%, O 23.33%. In seeds of *Trigonella foenumgraecum* L., *Leguminosae*, in coffee beans, in seeds of *Strophanthus* spp, *Apocynaceae* and of *Cannabis sativa* L., *Moraceae*, in seeds of many other plants; also in sea urchin, *Arabacia pustulosa*, and in jellyfish, *Velella spirans*. Excreted in urine after taking nicotinic acid: Ackermann, *Z. Biol.* **59**, 17 (1912). Isoln from normal urine: Linnewah, Renwein, *Z. Physiol. Chem.* **207**, 48 (1932); **209**, 110 (1932). Syntheses: Turnau, *Monatsh. Chem.* **26**, 551 (1905); Sarett *et al., J. Biol. Chem.* **135**, 483 (1940); Green, Tong, *J. Am. Chem. Soc.* **78**, 4896 (1956); Kosower, Patton, *J. Org. Chem.* **26**, 1318 (1961). Toxicity study: Brazda, Coulson, *Proc. Soc. Exp. Biol. Med.* **62**, 19 (1946).

Monohydrate. Crystals from ethanol, mp 230-233°. Salty taste. Very sol in water; sol in alcohol. Practically insol in ether, chloroform. LD_{50} s.c. in rats: 5.0 g/kg (Brazda, Coulson).

Hydrochloride. $C_7H_7NO_2$·HCl. Crystals from 90% alcohol, mp 258-259°. Very sol in water; slightly in alcohol. Practically insol in ether, benzene.

9695. Trihexyphenidyl Hydrochloride. [52-49-3] α-Cyclohexyl-α-phenyl-1-piperidinepropanol hydrochloride; 3-(1-piperidyl)-1-cyclohexyl-1-phenyl-1-propanol hydrochloride; 1-phenyl-1-cyclohexyl-3-piperidyl-1-propanol hydrochloride; benzhexol chloride; Aparkane; Artane; Broflex; Cyclodol; Pacitane; Paralest; Pargitan; Parkinane; Parkopan; Peragit; Pipanol; Sedrena; Tremin; Triphedinon; Triphenidyl; Tsiklodol. $C_{20}H_{32}ClNO$; mol wt 337.93. C 71.08%, H 9.54%, Cl 10.49%, N 4.14%, O 4.73%. Anticholinergic. Synthesis: Denton *et al., J. Am. Chem. Soc.* **71**, 2053 (1949); Adamson, Wilkinson, **US 2682543** (1954 to Burroughs Wellcome); Denton, **US 2716121** (1955 to Am. Cyanamid). Resolution into isomers: Adamson, Duffin, **GB 750156** (1956 to Wellcome Found.).

Crystals, dec 258.5°. Free base, mp 114.3-115.0°. Soly (g/100 ml): water at 25°, 1.0; alcohol 6; chloroform 5. More sol in methanol; very slightly sol in ether, benzene. pH of a 1% aq soln 5.5-6.0.

l-**Form.** Crystals from isopropyl alc, mp 264°. $[\alpha]_D^{20}$ $-30°$ (c = 0.4 in chloroform). Free base, mp 112-113°. $[\alpha]_D^{20}$ $-25°$ (c = 0.4 in ethanol).

THERAP CAT: Antiparkinsonian.

9696. Trillium. Beth root; Indian balm; ground lily; birthroot. Dried rhizome of *Trillium erectum* L. and other spp of *Trillium, Liliaceae. Habit.* Canada, south to Tennessee and Missouri; also Japan. *Constit.* Trilline, fixed oil, tannin.

THERAP CAT: Formerly in metrorrhagia, menorrhagia, various types of hemorrhage; astringent in diarrhea.

9697. Trilobine. [6138-73-4] (1'α)-6',7-Epoxy-6,12'-dimethoxy-2'-methyloxyacanthan. $C_{35}H_{34}N_2O_5$; mol wt 562.65. C 74.71%, H 6.09%, N 4.98%, O 14.22%. From root of *Cocculus trilobus* DC. and *C. sarmentosus* Diels, *Menispermaceae:* Tomita *et al., J. Pharm. Soc. Jpn.* **48**, 83 (1928); **50**, 127 (1930); **62**, 468, 481 (1942). Structure: Kondo, Tomita, *Ann.* **497**, 104 (1932); Inubushi, Nomura, *Tetrahedron Lett.* **1962**, 1133. Total synthesis of trilobine and isotrilobine: Y. Inubushi *et al., Chem. Pharm. Bull.* **25**, 1636 (1977).

Trilobine   R = H
Isotrilobine   R = CH₃

Crystals from benzene, mp 237°. $[\alpha]_D$ +307° (chloroform). Practically insol in water. Sparingly sol in alcohol, acetone, ether. Sol in chloroform.

Isotrilobine. [26195-62-0] Homotrilobine; *N*-methyltrilobine. $C_{36}H_{36}N_2O_5$. Crystals from acetone, mp 215°. $[\alpha]_D$ +317° (chloroform).

9698. Trilostane. [13647-35-3] ($4\alpha,5\alpha,17\beta$)-4,5-Epoxy-3,17-dihydroxyandrost-2-ene-2-carbonitrile; 4,5-epoxy-17-hydroxy-3-oxoandrostane-2-carbonitrile; 2α-cyano-$4\alpha,5\alpha$-epoxyandrostan-17β-ol-3-one; Win-24540; Desopan; Modrastane; Modrenal. $C_{20}H_{27}NO_3$; mol wt 329.43. C 72.92%, H 8.26%, N 4.25%, O 14.57%. Prepn: R. O. Clinton, A. J. Manson, US 3296255 (1967 to Sterling); H. C. Neumann *et al., J. Med. Chem.* **13**, 948 (1970). Inhibition of steroid biosynthesis: G. O. Potts *et al., Steroids* **32**, 257 (1978). Disposition in animals: J. F. Baker *et al., Arch. Int. Pharmacodyn. Ther.* **243**, 4 (1980). Metabolism in rats: Y. Mori *et al., Chem. Pharm. Bull.* **29**, 2646 (1981); in humans: D. T. Robinson *et al., J. Steroid Biochem.* **21**, 601 (1984). HPLC determn in plasma: P. Powles *et al., J. Chromatogr.* **311**, 434 (1984); and of major metabolite, *17-ketotrilostane*: R. R. Brown *et al., ibid.* **339**, 440 (1985). Clinical study in Cushing's syndrome: P. Komanicky *et al., J. Clin. Endocrinol. Metab.* **47**, 1042 (1978). Clinical trials in breast cancer: C. G. Beardwell *et al., Cancer Chemother. Pharmacol.* **10**, 158 (1983); C. J. Williams *et al., Cancer Treat. Rep.* **71**, 1197 (1987).

Tan crystals from pyridine/dioxane, mp 257.8-270° (dec). $[\alpha]_D^{25}$ +137.4° (c = 1 in pyridine). uv max (ethanol): 252 nm (ε 8300).

THERAP CAT: Adrenocortical suppressant; in treatment of breast cancer.

9699. Trimebutine. [39133-31-8] 3,4,5-Trimethoxybenzoic acid 2-(dimethylamino)-2-phenylbutyl ester. $C_{22}H_{29}NO_5$; mol wt 387.47. C 68.20%, H 7.54%, N 3.61%, O 20.65%. Opioid receptor agonist. Prepn by esterification: C. P. J. Roux, D. R. Torossian, FR 1344455 (1963 to Jouveinal), *C.A.* **60**, 15777g (1964); *see also*: D. R. Torossian, G. G. Aubard, GB 1342547 (1974 to Jouveinal). HPLC determn in plasma: M. Lavit *et al., Arzneim.-Forsch.* **50**, 640 (2000). Review of pharmacology and clinical experience: M. Delvaux, D. Wingate, *J. Int. Med. Res.* **25**, 225-246 (1997).

Crystals from ethanol, mp 78-80°C. Soluble in methylene chloride.

Maleate. [34140-59-5] TM-906; Cerekinon; Debridat; Digerent; Modulon; Polibutin; Spabucol; Transacalm. $C_{22}H_{29}NO_5\cdot C_4H_4O_4$; mol wt 503.54. Crystals from water, mp 105-106°.

THERAP CAT: Antispasmodic.

9700. Trimecaine. [616-68-2] 2-Diethylamino-2′,4′,6′-trimethylacetanilide; *N-sym*-trimethylphenyldiethylaminoacetamide; 2-diethylaminoacetyl-2′,4′,6′-trimethylanilide; S-203; Mesocaine; Mesidicaine; Mesokain. $C_{15}H_{24}N_2O$; mol wt 248.36. C 72.54%, H 9.74%, N 11.28%, O 6.44%. Prepn: Löfgren, Lundqvist, US 2441498 (1948 to Astra); A. Borovansky *et al., J. Am. Pharm. Assoc.* **48**, 402 (1959).

Crystals, mp 44°. bp₆ 187°; bp₀.₆ 154-155°. LD₅₀ s.c. in mice: 295 mg/kg (Borovansky).

Hydrochloride. $C_{15}H_{24}N_2O\cdot HCl$. Crystals from acetone, mp 140°.

THERAP CAT: Anesthetic.

9701. Trimedlure. [12002-53-8] 4(or 5)-Chloro-2-methylcyclohexanecarboxylic acid, 1,1-dimethylethyl ester; *tert*-butyl 4(or 5)-chloro-2-methylcyclohexanecarboxylate. $C_{12}H_{21}ClO_2$; mol wt 232.75. C 61.92%, H 9.09%, Cl 15.23%, O 13.75%. Synthetic sex pheromone developed as attractant for the Mediterranean fruit fly, or medfly, *Ceratitis capitata* (Weidemann). Prepn and physical props: M. Beroza *et al., J. Agric. Food Chem.* **9**, 361 (1961). Commercial product consists mainly of the four isomers having the methyl and ester substituents on the ring in a *trans* configuration. Separation and identification of isomers: T. P. McGovern, M. Beroza, *J. Org. Chem.* **31**, 1472 (1966). Extension of activity by fixatives: *eidem, J. Econ. Entomol.* **60**, 379 (1967). Controlled release: S. Nakagawa *et al., ibid.* **72**, 625 (1979). Repellent effect of high concns: *eidem, ibid.* **64**, 762 (1971). Rate of loss from wicks: J. R. King, P. J. Landolt, *ibid.* **77**, 221 (1984). Acute toxicity studies: M. Beroza *et al., Toxicol. Appl. Pharmacol.* **31**, 421 (1975).

trans-form

Oil, bp 107-113°. n_D^{20} 1.460. LD₅₀ in rats (mg/kg): 4556 ±1136 orally; in rabbits (mg/kg): >2025 dermally; LC₅₀ (24 hr) in rainbow trout, bluegill sunfish (ppm): 11.5, 14.7 (Beroza).

USE: As attractant in medfly traps.

9702. Trimellitic Acid. [528-44-9] 1,2,4-Benzenetricarboxylic acid; 1,2,4-tricarboxybenzene. $C_9H_6O_6$; mol wt 210.14. C 51.44%, H 2.88%, O 45.68%. Obtained by oxidation of coal with nitric acid: Grosskinsky, *Glueckauf* **88**, 376 (1952), *C.A.* **46**, 7731 (1952); by oxidation of β-indancarboxylic acid with nitric acid: Braun *et al., Ber.* **53**, 1160 (1920). Manuf by oxidation of pseudocumene: Backlund, US 3009953 (1961 to Union Oil of Calif.).

Crystals from acetic acid or dilute alcohol. mp 218-220° (also reported 229-234° dec). Solubilities at 25° in g/100 g solvent: carbon tetrachloride 0.004; ligroin 0.03; mixed xylenes 0.006; dimethylformamide 31.3; ethyl acetate 1.7; acetone 7.9; water 2.1; ethanol 25.3. Practically insol in chloroform, benzene, carbon disulfide.

USE: Intermediate in the prepn of resins, plasticizers, dyes, inks, adhesives.

9703. Trimellitic Anhydride. [552-30-7] 1,3-Dihydro-1,3-dioxo-5-isobenzofurancarboxylic acid; trimellitic acid 1,2-anhydride; anhydrotrimellitic acid; 1,3-dioxo-5-phthalancarboxylic acid. $C_9H_4O_5$; mol wt 192.13. C 56.26%, H 2.10%, O 41.64%. Prepd by subliming trimellitic acid above its mp: Alder, Dortmann, *Ber.* **85**, 556 (1952); by heating crude trimellitic acid with V_2O_5: McKinnis, US 2998431 (1959 to Union Oil of Calif.).

Crystals, mp 161-163.5°. bp_{14} 240-245°. Solubilities at 25° in g/100 g solvent: carbon tetrachloride 0.002; ligroin 0.06; mixed xylenes 0.4; dimethylformamide 15.5; acetone 49.6; ethyl acetate 21.6.

Caution: Potential symptoms of overexposure are irritation of eyes, skin, nose, respiratory system; pulmonary edema, respiratory sensitization; rhinitis, asthma, cough, wheezing, dyspnea, malaise, fever, muscle aches, sneezing. *See NIOSH Pocket Guide to Chemical Hazards* (DHHS/NIOSH 97-140, 1997) p 318.

USE: In the preparation of resins, adhesives, polymers, dyes, printing inks.

9704. Trimeprazine. [84-96-8] *N,N,β*-Trimethyl-10*H*-phenothiazine-10-propanamine; 10-[3-(dimethylamino)-2-methylpropyl]phenothiazine; 10-(2-methyl-3-dimethylaminopropyl)-phenothiazine; alimemazine; methylpromazine; Bayer 1219; RP-6549. $C_{18}H_{22}N_2S$; mol wt 298.45. C 72.44%, H 7.43%, N 9.39%, S 10.74%. Prepn: Jacob, Robert, US 2837518 (1958 to Rhône-Poulenc). Metabolism studies: Robinson, *J. Pharm. Pharmacol.* **18**, 19 (1966).

Crystals, mp 68°. $bp_{0.3}$ 150-175°.

Tartrate. [4330-99-8] Panectyl; Repeltin; Temaril; Theralene; Vallergan. $(C_{18}H_{22}N_2S)_2 \cdot C_4H_6O_6$; mol wt 746.98. Crystals. Sol in water; slightly sol in alcohol.

THERAP CAT: Antipruritic.

THERAP CAT (VET): Antipruritic.

9705. Trimetazidine. [5011-34-7] 1-[(2,3,4-Trimethoxyphenyl)methyl]piperazine. $C_{14}H_{22}N_2O_3$; mol wt 266.34. C 63.13%, H 8.33%, N 10.52%, O 18.02%. Coronary vasodilator. Prepn: Regnier, Canevari, FR 1302958 (1962 to Sci. Union et Cie, Soc. Franç. Rech. Med.); FR M805; J. Servier, US 3262852 (1961, 1966 to Biofarma). Pharmacology: Fujita, *Jpn. J. Pharmacol.* **17**, 19 (1967); Nagata *et al., ibid.* **19**, 628 (1969); **21**, 337 (1971). GC-MS determn in biological fluids: L. Fay *et al., J. Chromatogr.* **490**, 198 (1989). Review of pharmacology, toxicology and clinical studies: C. Harpey *et al., Cardiovasc. Drug Rev.* **6**, 292-312 (1989).

bp_2 200-205°.

Dihydrochloride. [13171-25-0] Kyurinett; Vastarel F; Yoshimilon. $C_{14}H_{22}N_2O_3 \cdot 2HCl$; mol wt 339.26. Crystals, mp 225-228°. LD_{50} in male, female mice, rats (mg/kg): 91, 107, 124, 124 i.v.; 264, 245, 327, 288 i.p.; 528, 608, 1147, 987 orally (Harpey).

THERAP CAT: Antianginal.

9706. Trimethadione. [127-48-0] 3,5,5-Trimethyl-2,4-oxazolidinedione; 3,5,5-trimethyl-2,4-dioxooxazolidine; troxidone; Absentol; Epidione; Petidon; Ptimal; Tridione. $C_6H_9NO_3$; mol wt 143.14. C 50.35%, H 6.34%, N 9.79%, O 33.53%. Synthesis: Spielman, *J. Am. Chem. Soc.* **66**, 1244 (1944); US 2575692 (1951 to Abbott); Davies, Hook, US 2559011 (1951 to Brit. Schering). Metabolism to dimethadione, *q.v.:* T. C. Butler, *J. Pharmacol. Exp. Ther.* **108**, 11 (1953); T. C. Butler, W. J. Waddell, *ibid.* **110**, 241 (1954). Anticonvulsant activity: H. Ferngren, *Acta Pharmacol. Toxicol.* **26**, 177 (1968); H. H. Frey, *ibid.* **27**, 295 (1969). Pharmacodynamics and metabolism in rats: D. O. Thueson *et al., Epilepsia* **15**, 563 (1974). Evaluation in teratogenesis: J. German *et al., Teratology* **3**, 349 (1970); A. B. Rifkind, *Toxicol. Appl. Pharmacol.* **30**, 452 (1974). GC determn in serum: E. Tanaka, S. Misawa, *J. Chromatogr.* **413**, 376 (1987); LC determn in serum: M. Okamoto *et al., Chromatographia* **23**, 325 (1987). Use in treatment of petit mal epilepsy: S. Livingston *et al., J. Am. Med. Assoc.* **194**, 227 (1965). Use in dissolution of pancreatic stones in humans and dogs: A. Noda *et al., Lancet* **2**, 351 (1984); *eidem, Gastroenterology* **93**, 1002 (1987).

Granules, crystals, mp 46-46.5°. bp_5 78-80°. Slight camphor-like odor. Burning, faintly bitter taste. Soly in water about 5%; increased by the addition of urethan. Freely sol in alcohol, benzene, chloroform, ether. Practically insol in petr ether. The pH of a 5% soln is ~6.0.

THERAP CAT: Anticonvulsant.

THERAP CAT (VET): Anticonvulsant.

9707. Trimethaphan Camsylate. [68-91-7] Decahydro-2-oxo-1,3-bis(phenylmethyl)thieno[1′,2′:1,2]thieno[3,4-*d*]imidazol-5-ium salt with (1*S*)-7,7-dimethyl-2-oxobicyclo[2.2.1]heptane-1-methanesulfonic acid (1:1); trimetaphan camphorsulfonate; methioplegium; trimethaphan camphorsulfonate; trimethaphen camphorsulfonate; 4,6-dibenzyl-5-oxo-1-thia-4,6-diazatricyclo[6.3.0.-0³·⁷]undecanium (+)-β-camphorsulfonate; *d*-3,4-(1′,3′-dibenzyl-2′-ketoimidazolido)-1,2-trimethylenethiophanium *d*-camphorsulfonate; Nu-2222; Arfonad. $C_{32}H_{40}N_2O_5S_2$; mol wt 596.80. C 64.40%, H 6.76%, N 4.69%, O 13.40%, S 10.75%. Available from the Roche synthesis of biotin: Randall *et al., J. Pharmacol. Exp. Ther.* **97**, 48 (1949); Scurr, Wyman, *Lancet* **1**, 338 (1954). May be prepd by treating (+)-3,4-(1,3-dibenzylureylene)tetrahydro-2-oxothiophene with 3-ethoxypropylmagnesium bromide, followed by reduction, ring closure, and conversion into the (+)-β-camphorsulfonate. Comprehensive description: K. W. Blessel *et al., Anal. Profiles Drug Subs.* **3**, 545-564 (1974).

Bitter crystals, dec ~245°. $[\alpha]_D^{20}$ +22.0° (c = 4 in water). One gram dissolves in less than 5 ml water and in less than 2 ml alcohol. Slightly sol in acetone, ether; pH of a 1% aq soln is 5.0-6.0.

THERAP CAT: Antihypertensive.

9708. Trimethobenzamide. [138-56-7] *N*-[(2-Dimethylaminoethyl)benzyl]-3,4,5-trimethoxybenzamide; 4-(2-dimethylaminoethoxy)-*N*-(3,4,5-trimethoxybenzoyl)benzylamine. $C_{21}H_{28}$-N_2O_5; mol wt 388.46. C 64.93%, H 7.27%, N 7.21%, O 20.59%. Prepn: M. W. Goldberg, S. Teitel, **US 2879293** (1959 to Hoffmann-La Roche). Pharmacology: K. W. Blessel *et al.*, *Anal. Profiles Drug Subs.* **2**, 551-570 (1973).

Hydrochloride. [554-92-7] Ro-2-9578; Anaus; Tigan; Xametina. $C_{21}H_{28}N_2O_5$.HCl; mol wt 424.92. Crystals, mp 187.5-190°. Freely sol in water (approx soly at 25° >50%). A 5% aq soln is stable to autoclaving at 120° for 20 min at pH 3-7.

THERAP CAT: Antiemetic.

9709. Trimethoprim. [738-70-5] 5-[(3,4,5-Trimethoxyphenyl)methyl]-2,4-pyrimidinediamine; 2,4-diamino-5-(3,4,5-trimethoxybenzyl)pyrimidine; Instalac; Monotrim; Proloprim; Syraprim; Tiempe; Trimanyl; Trimogal; Trimopan; Trimpex; Uretrim; Wellcoprim. $C_{14}H_{18}N_4O_3$; mol wt 290.32. C 57.92%, H 6.25%, N 19.30%, O 16.53%. Prepn from guanidine and β-ethoxy-3,4,5-trimethoxybenzylbenzalnitrile: Stenbuck, Hood, **US 3049544** (1962 to Burroughs Wellcome); Hoffer, **US 3341541** (1967 to Hoffmann-La Roche). Improved synthesis: B. Roth *et al.*, *J. Med. Chem.* **23**, 379, 535 (1980). Toxicity data: Yamamoto *et al.*, *Chemotherapy (Tokyo)* **21**, 187 (1973). *Review:* Burchall in *Antibiotics* vol. 3, J. W. Corcoran, F. E. Hahn, Eds. (Springer-Verlag, New York, 1975) pp 304-320. Comprehensive description: G. J. Manius, *Anal. Profiles Drug Subs.* **7**, 445-475 (1978). Review of antibacterial activity, pharmacokinetics and therapeutic use: R. N. Brogden *et al.*, *Drugs* **23**, 405-430 (1982).

White to cream, bitter crystalline powder, mp 199-203°. Soly in g/100 ml at 25°: DMAC 13.86; benzyl alcohol 7.29; propylene glycol 2.57; chloroform 1.82; methanol 1.21; water 0.04; ether 0.003; benzene 0.002. pKa 6.6. LD_{50} orally in mice: 7000 mg/kg (Yamamoto).

Note: See Sulfamethoxazole, Sulfadiazine, Sulfametrole, Sulfamoxole, and Sulfalene for lists of trade names of mixtures with Trimethoprim.

THERAP CAT: Antibacterial.

THERAP CAT (VET): Antibacterial.

9710. Trimethylamine. [75-50-3] *N,N*-Dimethylmethanamine. C_3H_9N; mol wt 59.11. C 60.96%, H 15.35%, N 23.70%. $(CH_3)_3N$. Together with other amines it is a degradation product of nitrogenous plant and animal substances. Formed during the distillation of sugar beet residues which contain betaine. Widely distributed as conjugated form in animal tissue and especially in fish. Converted to the free tertiary amine during putrefaction. Detected in menstrual blood, and in urine which was stored at room temp. Prepn from paraformaldehyde and ammonium chloride: Adams, Brown, *Org. Synth.* **1**, 75 (1921); **coll. vol. I**, 2nd ed., p 528; by the action of formaldehyde and formic acid on ammonia: Sommelet, Ferrand, *Bull. Soc. Chim.* [4] **35**, 446 (1924). Physical properties: J. G. Aston *et al.*, *J. Am. Chem. Soc.* **66**, 1171 (1944). Review as indicator of spoilage in stored fish: J. Oehlenschläger, *Dev. Food Sci.* **37**, 571-586 (1997).

Gas. Pungent, fishy, ammoniacal odor, saline taste. Liquefiable by pressure at ordinary temp or by condensation. mp −117.08°. bp_{760} 2.87°; bp_{747} 3.2-3.8°. d_4^0 0.6709. Strong base. pK$_b$ (25°): 4.13. Readily absorbed by water, alcohol with which it is miscible;

also sol in ether, benzene, toluene, xylene, ethylbenzene, chloroform.

Hydrochloride. [593-81-7] Trimethylammonium chloride. C_3H_9N.HCl. Prepn: *Org. Synth.* **coll. vol. I**, 2nd ed., p 531. Monoclinic deliquesc crystals from alc. Odor less intense than that of base. Dec 277-278°. Sinters and sublimes at 200°. Sol in water, alcohol; moderately sol in chloroform. Insol in ether. *Keep well closed.*

Caution: Potential symptoms of overexposure to trimethylamine are irritation of eyes, skin, nose, throat, respiratory system; cough, dyspnea, delayed pulmonary edema; blurred vision, corneal necrosis; skin burns; direct contact with liquid may cause frostbite. *See NIOSH Pocket Guide to Chemical Hazards* (DHHS/NIOSH 97-140, 1997) p 318.

USE: In the manuf of quaternary ammonium compds; as insect attractant; as warning agent for natural gas.

9711. Trimethylamine *N*-Oxide. [1184-78-7] *N,N*-Dimethylmethanamine *N*-oxide; TMAO. C_3H_9NO; mol wt 75.11. C 47.97%, H 12.08%, N 18.65%, O 21.30%. Naturally occurring osmolyte found in marine organisms; counteracts protein-destabilizing factors such as urea, temperature, salt, and hydrostatic pressure. The enzymatic reduction to trimethylamine, *q.v.*, is used as an indication of spoilage in stored fish. Prepn of the dihydrate: W. R. Dunstan, E. Goulding, *J. Chem. Soc.* **75**, 792 (1899); of the anhydrous compd: J. A. Soderquist, C. L. Anderson, *Tetrahedron Lett.* **27**, 3961 (1986). Determn in natural waters and biological media: A. D. Hatton, S. W. Gibb, *Anal. Chem.* **71**, 4886 (1999). Review of use as reagent in organometallic chemisty: T.-Y. Luh, *Coord. Chem. Rev.* **60**, 255-276 (1984); in organic synthesis: H.-J. Knölker, *J. Prakt. Chem.* **338**, 190-192 (1996). Review of distribution in marine animals of various habitats: R. H. Kelly, P. H. Yancey, *Biol. Bull.* **196**, 18-25 (1999); of biosynthesis, distribution and biological role: B. A. Seibel, P. J. Walsh, *J. Exp. Biol.* **205**, 297-306 (2002); P. H. Yancey *et al.*, *Comp. Biochem. Physiol. A* **133**, 667-676 (2002).

Free-flowing large colorless crystals, mp 225-227°. Very hygroscopic.

Dihydrate. [62637-93-8] $C_3H_9NO.2H_2O$; mol wt 111.14. Radiating needles, mp 96°. Sol in water, methanol. Insol in ether.

Caution: May be irritating to eyes, skin, respiratory system.

USE: Oxidizing reagent in organic synthesis.

9712. Trimethyl Borate. [121-43-7] Boric acid trimethyl ester; methyl borate. $C_3H_9BO_3$; mol wt 103.91. C 34.68%, H 8.73%, B 10.40%, O 46.19%. $B(OCH_3)_3$. Prepn from pyridineboron trichloride complex: Gerrard, Lappert, *Chem. Ind. (London)* **1952**, 53; from methanol and boric oxide, borax or boric acid: Schlesinger, *J. Am. Chem. Soc.* **75**, 213 (1953); from methyl orthosilicates and boron halide: Wiberg, Krüerke, *Z. Naturforsch.* **8b**, 608 (1953); from boric acid and methanol: Steinberg, Hunter, *Ind. Eng. Chem.* **49**, 174 (1957). Several mfg processes: **US 2689259**; **US 2884439**; **US 2937195** (to Callery Chem.); **US 2880227** and **US 2884440** (to Olin Mathieson); **US 2855427** (to Am. Potash & Chem.); **US 2739979** (to USAEC). Acute toxicity: H. F. Smyth *et al.*, *Am. Ind. Hyg. Assoc. J.* **23**, 95 (1962).

Liquid, d 0.915. bp 67-68°. Flash pt 29°C (84.2°F). Miscible with tetrahydrofuran, ether, isopropylamine, hexane, methanol, Nujol and other organic liquids. Stable in the absence of moisture, but hydrolyzes in the presence of water to methanol and boric acid. Forms an azeotrope with methanol: 70% $B(OCH_3)_3$ +30% methanol, d 0.87; bp 52-54°; flash pt 34°C (93.2°F). LD_{50} orally in rats: 6.14 ml/kg (Smyth).

USE: As solvent for waxes, resins, oils; catalyst in the manuf of ketones; analysis of paint and varnish ingredients; as neutron detector gas in the presence of a scintillation counter; as a promoter of diborane reactions.

9713. Trimethylene Bromide. [109-64-8] 1,3-Dibromopropane; α,γ-dibromopropane; ω,ω′-dibromopropane; trimethylene dibromide. $C_3H_6Br_2$; mol wt 201.89. C 17.85%, H 3.00%, Br 79.16%. $BrCH_2CH_2CH_2Br$. Prepd by the action of hydrobromic acid on trimethylene glycol in the presence of sulfuric acid: Kamm, Marvel, *Org. Synth.* **coll. vol. I**, p 30 (1941); *cf.* Derick, Hess, *J. Am. Chem. Soc.* **40**, 545 (1918); Norris, Mulliken, *ibid.* **42**, 2096 (1920): Kamm, Newcomb, *ibid.* **43**, 2229 (1921). From trimethylene glycol and PBr_3: Bogert, Slocum, *ibid.* **46**, 765 (1924).

Colorless liquid; d_4^{25} 1.9712; bp_{760} 167° (mp −36°); n_D^{15} 1.5249. Slightly sol in water (1.68 g/l at 30°); sol in alc, ether. Upon prolonged heating trimethylene bromide dec and part of it is converted to propylene bromide (1,2-dibromopropane). Boiling with water yields trimethylene glycol.

9714. Trimethylene Glycol. [504-63-2] 1,3-Propanediol. $C_3H_8O_2$; mol wt 76.09. C 47.35%, H 10.60%, O 42.05%. $HOCH_2CH_2CH_2OH$. Prepd by reduction of ethyl glycidate with lithium aluminum hydride: Walborsky, Colombini, *J. Org. Chem.* **27**, 2387 (1962).

Colorless to pale yellow, very viscid, sweet liquid. d_4^{20} 1.0597; bp 210-212°; n_D^{20} 1.4398. Miscible with water, alc.

9715. Trimethylene Oxide. [503-30-0] Oxetane; 1,3-epoxypropane. C_3H_6O; mol wt 58.08. C 62.04%, H 10.41%, O 27.55%. Prepd by dropwise addition of 3-chloropropyl acetate to hot potassium hydroxide soln: Noller, *Org. Synth.* **29**, 92 (1949); modified procedure: Searles, *J. Am. Chem. Soc.* **73**, 124 (1951).

Oil, agreeable aromatic odor. d_0^0 0.8975; d_4^{25} 0.8930. bp_{750} 48°; bp_{736} 45-46°. n_D^{25} 1.3895; n_D^{23} 1.3905. Reacts with Grignard reagents and organolithium compds to give, after hydrolysis, 3-substituted propanols.

9716. Trimethyl Isopropyl Butanamide. [51115-67-4] N,2,3-Trimethyl-2-(1-methylethyl)butanamide; 2-isopropyl-N,2,3-dimethylbutanamide; WS23. $C_{10}H_{21}NO$; mol wt 171.28. C 70.12%, H 12.36%, N 8.18%, O 9.34%. Prepn: D. G. Rowsell *et al.*, **DE 2317538**; *eidem*, **US 4296255** (1973, 1981 both to Wilkinson Sword). Structure-activity study: H. R. Watson *et al.*, *J. Soc. Cosmet. Chem.* **29**, 185 (1978). Brief review: M. A. Parrish, *Manuf. Chem.* **58**, 31-32 (February, 1987).

Colorless solid, mp 58-61° (Rowsell); also reported as white, crystalline solid, melting range 63° (Parrish). $bp_{0.35mm}$ 83-85°.

USE: Physiological coolant in foods, beverages, tobacco products, toiletries, cosmetics and pharmaceuticals.

9717. Trimethyl Orthovalerate. [13820-09-2] 1,1,1-Trimethoxypentane; methyl orthovalerate. $C_8H_{18}O_3$; mol wt 162.23. C 59.23%, H 11.18%, O 29.59%. Prepn: S. M. McElvain *et al.*, *J. Am. Chem. Soc.* **68**, 1922 (1946); J. W. Scheeren *et al.*, *Synthesis* **1978**, 283.

Liquid. d_4^{27} 0.9413. bp_{760} 164-166°; bp_{14} 60°. n_D^{24} 1.4090. n_D^{20} 1.4105.

9718. 2,4,6-Trimethylpyridine. [108-75-8] γ-Collidine; *sym*-collidine; 2,4,6-collidine; α,γ,α'-collidine. $C_8H_{11}N$; mol wt 121.18. C 79.29%, H 9.15%, N 11.56%. Found in small amts in coal tar, in shale oil. Produced commercially from coal tar to some extent; also produced by the Hantzsch pyridine synthesis: Hantzsch, *Ann.* **215**, 1 (1882); Mosher in *Heterocyclic Compounds* **vol. 1**, R. C. Elderfield, Ed., (John Wiley, New York, 1950) pp 462-

472; from acetone and ammonia: Mosher in *Kirk-Othmer Encyclopedia of Chemical Technology* **vol. 11** (New York, 1953) p 287, *cf.* Dürkopf, *Ber.* **21**, 2713 (1888); from paraldehyde, acetone, ammonium acetate, and ammonia water: **DE 349267**; *Frdl.* **14**, 539; from 3,5-dimethyl-2-cyclohexen-1-one, ammonium acetate, and ammonia water: Frank, Meikle, *J. Am. Chem. Soc.* **72**, 4184 (1950).

Liquid. Aromatic odor. $d_4^{16.4}$ 0.9191; $d_4^{22.1}$ 0.9166 (commercial grade: $d_{15.5}^{15.5}$ 0.920-0.935, approx 7.74 lbs/gal). mp −46°. bp_{762} 170.5°; bp_{760} 171°; bp_{31} 65°; $bp_{2.7}$ 10°. n_D^{25} 1.4959; $n_D^{22.1}$ 1.49770. pKa (25°): 6.69. Flash pt 136°F. Dielectric constant at 22° = 6.6 (λ = 70 cm). More sol in cold water than in hot water: 20.8 g/100 ml at 6°; 3.5 g/100 ml at 20°; 1.8 g/100 ml at 100°. Miscible with ether. Sol in methanol, ethanol, chloroform, benzene, toluene, dil acids.

9719. Trimethylsilyl Triflate. [27607-77-8] Trifluoromethanesulfonic acid trimethylsilyl ester; trimethylsilyltrifluoromethane sulfonate. $C_4H_9F_3O_3SSi$; mol wt 222.26. C 21.62%, H 4.08%, F 25.64%, O 21.60%, S 14.43%, Si 12.64%. $CF_3SO_2OSi(CH_3)_3$. Prepn: M. Schmeisser *et al.*, *Ber.* **103**, 868 (1970); H. W. Roesky, H. H. Giere, *Z. Naturforsch.* **25B**, 773 (1970); D. Haebich, F. Effenberger, *Synthesis* **1978**, 755; T. Morita *et al.*, *ibid.* **1981**, 745. As catalytic reagent: H. Vorbrueggen, K. Krolikiewicz, *Angew. Chem. Int. Ed.* **14**, 421 (1975); as silylating agent: G. A. Olah *et al.*, *J. Org. Chem.* **46**, 5212 (1981).

Liquid, bp_{760} 140°, bp_{10} 36.5°. n_D^{20} 1.3630. Fumes in air; sensitive to atm moisture.

USE: Catalyst and silylating agent for organic syntheses.

9720. Trimetozine. [635-41-6] 4-(3,4,5-Trimethoxybenzoyl)morpholine; N-(3,4,5-trimethoxybenzoyl)tetrahydro-1,4-oxazine; V-7; Opalène; Trioxazine. $C_{14}H_{19}NO_5$; mol wt 281.30. C 59.78%, H 6.81%, N 4.98%, O 28.44%. Prepd from morpholine and 3,4,5-trimethoxybenzoyl chloride: **GB 872350** (1961 to Egyesült Gyogyszer és Tápszergyár); Pettit *et al.*, *J. Med. Pharm. Chem.* **5**, 800 (1962).

Crystals, mp 120-122°. Slightly sol in water, alcohol.

THERAP CAT: Anxiolytic.

9721. Trimetrexate. [52128-35-5] 5-Methyl-6-[[(3,4,5-trimethoxyphenyl)amino]methyl]-2,4-quinazolinediamine; 2,4-diamino-5-methyl-6-[(3,4,5-trimethoxyanilino)methyl]quinazoline; TMQ; NSC-249008; JB-11; CI-898. $C_{19}H_{23}N_5O_3$; mol wt 369.42. C 61.77%, H 6.28%, N 18.96%, O 12.99%. Lipophilic dihydrofolate reductase inhibitor structurally related to methotrexate, *q.v.*, with antimicrobial and antitumor activity. Prepn: E. F. Elslager, L. M. Werbel, **GB 1345502** (1974 to Parke, Davis); E. F. Elslager *et al.*, *J. Med. Chem.* **26**, 1753 (1983); of water soluble salts: N. L. Colbry, **EP 51415**; *idem*, **US 4376858** (1982, 1983 both to Warner-Lambert). *In vitro* antifolate activity and *in vivo* antitumor effect: J. R. Bertino *et al.*, *Biochem. Pharmacol.* **28**, 1983 (1979). Pharmacology: E. C. Weir *et al.*, *Cancer Res.* **42**, 1696 (1982); R. C. Jackson *et al.*, *Adv. Enzyme Regul.* **22**, 187 (1984). GC-MS determn in human plasma: P. L. Stetson, W. D. Ensminger, *J. Chromatogr.* **383**, 69 (1986). Clinical evaluation with leucovorin vs *Pneumocystis carinii* in patients with AIDS: C. J. Allegra *et al.*, *N. Engl. J. Med.* **317**, 978 (1987). Review of pharmacology and clinical efficacy: J. T. Lin, J. R. Bertino, *J. Clin. Oncol.* **5**, 2032-2040 (1987); P. J. O'Dwyer *et al.*, *NCI Monogr.* **5**, 105-109 (1987).

Monoacetate monohydrate. [117381-09-6] $C_{19}H_{23}N_5O_3.C_2$-$H_4O_2.H_2O$. Crystals from aqueous acetic acid, mp 215-217°. Poorly sol in water. LD_{50} i.p. in mice: 175 mg/kg (Jackson).

D-Glucuronate. [82952-64-5] NSC-352122; Neutrexin. C_{19}-$H_{23}N_5O_3.C_6H_{10}O_7$; mol wt 563.56. Tan colored solid. Soly in water: >50 mg/ml.

THERAP CAT: Antineoplastic; antipneumocystis.

9722.   Trimipramine. [739-71-9] 10,11-Dihydro-N,N,β-trimethyl-$5H$-dibenz[b,f]azepine-5-propanamine; 5-[3-(dimethylamino)-2-methylpropyl]-10,11-dihydro-$5H$-dibenz[b,f]azepine; 5-(3-dimethylamino-2-methylpropyl)iminodibenzyl; trimeprimine; trimeproprimine; RP-7162; Sapilent. $C_{20}H_{26}N_2$; mol wt 294.43. C 81.59%, H 8.90%, N 9.51%. Prepn: Jacob, Messer, *Compt. Rend.* **252**, 2117 (1961). Toxicity studies: Okamoto, *C.A.* **72**, 77299y (1970). Chemistry: Bever, Bredenstein, *Dtsch. Apoth. Ztg.* **113**, 1562 (1973). Comprehensive description of the maleate: A. A. Al-Badr, *Anal. Profiles Drug Subs.* **12**, 683-712 (1983).

Crystals, mp 45°.

Maleate. [521-78-8] Stangyl (tabl); Surmontil (tabl). $C_{20}H_{26}$-$N_2.C_4H_4O_4$; mol wt 410.51. Crystals, mp 142°. Sol in chloroform; slightly sol in water, ethanol. Practically insol in ether.

Methanesulfonate. Stangyl (amp); Surmontil (amp).

THERAP CAT: Antidepressant.

9723.   Trimoprostil. [69900-72-7] (5Z,11α,13E,15R)-15-Hydroxy-11,16,16-trimethyl-9-oxoprosta-5,13-dien-1-oic acid; (Z)-7-[(1R,2R,3R)-2-[(E)-(3R)-3-hydroxy-4,4-dimethyl-1-octenyl]-3-methyl-5-oxocyclopentyl]-5-heptenoic acid; *nat*-11R,16,16-trimethyl-15R-hydroxy-9-oxoprosta-*cis*-5-*trans*-13-dienoic acid; 11R,16,16-trimethyl-(11-desoxyprostaglandin E_2); 11-deoxy-11α,16,16-trimethyl-PGE$_2$; TM-PGE$_2$; Ro-21-6937; Ulstar. C_{23}-$H_{38}O_4$; mol wt 378.55. C 72.97%, H 10.12%, O 16.91%. Synthetic prostaglandin E_2 analog with antisecretory activity. Prepn: G. W. Holland *et al.*, **DE 2437622**; *eidem*, **US 4052446**; **US 4190587** (1975, 1977, 1980 all to Hoffmann-La Roche). Pharmacology: D. E. Wilson, S. L. Winter, *Prostaglandins* **16**, 127 (1978); S. P. Lee *et al.*, *Eur. J. Clin. Invest.* **17**, 1 (1987). Effect on bicarbonate secretion: M. Feldman, *J. Clin. Invest.* **72**, 295 (1983); on inhibition of gastric acid secretion: R. J. Wills *et al.*, *Clin. Pharmacol. Ther.* **37**, 113 (1985). Metabolism: S. J. Kolis *et al.*, *Drug Metab. Dispos.* **14**, 465 (1986). Clinical pharmacokinetics: R. J. Wills *et al.*, *J. Clin. Pharmacol.* **26**, 48 (1986). Clinical evaluation: H. G. Dammann *et al.*, *Arzneim.-Forsch.* **36**, 500 (1986). Multicenter clinical comparison with cimetidine, *q.v.*: K. D. Bardhan *et al.*, *Scand. J. Gastroenterol.* **23**, 134 (1988); with aldioxa, *q.v.*: A. Ishimori *et al.*, *Acta Ther.* **15**, 27 (1989). Toxicity study: M. Shimizu *et al.*, *Shin'yaku to Rinsho* **35**, 2199 (1986), *C.A.* **106**, 150180e (1987).

Colorless oil. $[\alpha]_D$ −51.54° (c = 1 in $CHCl_3$). LD_{50} in mice, rats (mg/kg): 41, 23 orally; 70, 21 i.p.; 68, 29 s.c. (Shimizu).

THERAP CAT: Antiulcerative.

9724.   Trimyristin. [555-45-3] Myristin; glyceryl trimyristate. $C_{45}H_{86}O_6$; mol wt 723.16. C 74.74%, H 11.99%, O 13.27%. Occurs in many vegetable fats and oils, notably in coconut oil and nutmeg butter.

White to yellowish-gray solid; d_4^{60} 0.885; mp 56-57°; n_D^{60} 1.4429. Insol in H_2O; sol in alc, benzene, chloroform, ether.

9725.   Trinexapac-ethyl. [95266-40-3] 4-(Cyclopropyl-hydroxymethylene)-3,5-dioxocyclohexanecarboxylic acid ethyl ester; cimectacarb; CGA-163935; Palisade. $C_{13}H_{16}O_5$; mol wt 252.26. C 61.90%, H 6.39%, O 31.71%. Gibberellin biosynthesis inhibitor. Prepn: H.-G. Brunner, **EP 126713**; *idem*, **US 4693745** (1984, 1987 both to Ciba-Geigy). Comprehensive description: E. Kerber *et al.*, *Brighton Crop Prot. Conf. - Weeds* **1989**, 83-88. Field trials in cereals and oilseed rape: J. Amrein *et al.*, *ibid.* 89; in turfgrass: D. B. Vitolo *et al.*, *Proc. Plant Growth Regul. Soc. Am.* **18**, 136 (1991). Mechanism of action: R. Adams *et al.*, *Curr. Plant Sci. Biotechnol. Agric.* **13**, 818 (1992).

mp 36°. n_D^{30} 1.5350. pKa 4.7. Vapor pressure (20°): 1.6 × 10^{-3} Pa. Soly in water at 20° (g/l): 27 (pH 7); 5 (pH 5). Soly at 20° (g/ml): methanol >1; acetonitrile >1; cyclohexanone >1; isopropanol 0.9; n-octanol 0.18; hexane 0.035. Log P (n-octanol/water) pH 3: 2.1; pH 7: −0.4. LD_{50} in rats (mg/kg): 4460 orally; >4000 dermally (Kerber).

USE: Plant growth regulator.

9726.   sym-Trinitrobenzene. [99-35-4] 1,3,5-Trinitrobenzene; benzite. $C_6H_3N_3O_6$; mol wt 213.10. C 33.82%, H 1.42%, N 19.72%, O 45.05%. Prepared by decarboxylation of trinitrobenzoic acid, obtained by oxidation of TNT: Clarke, Hartman, *Org. Synth.* **2**, 93 (1922); by the action of alkali on 2,4,6-trinitrobenzaldehyde: Secareanu, *Bull. Soc. Chim.* **51**, 591 (1932). Use as explosive, less sensitive to impact than TNT but more powerful and brisant: Robertson, *J. Chem. Soc.* **119**, 8 (1921); van Duin, *Rec. Trav. Chim.* **39**, 687 (1920). Review of toxicology and human exposure: *Toxicological Profile for 1,3-Dinitrobenzene and 1,3,5-Trinitrobenzene* (PB95-264289, 1995) 168 p.

Orthorhombic bipyramidal plates from glacial acetic acid. mp 122.5°. bp 315°. d_4^{20} 1.76; d_4^{152} 1.4775. Log P (octanol:water) 1.18. Dimorphic, the other (rare) form melts at 61°. Can be sublimed by careful heating, explodes when heated rapidly. Absorption spectrum: Hatzsch, Picton, *Ber.* **42**, 2121 (1909). Soly (g/100 g solvent): water 0.035; benzene 6.2; methanol 4.9; alcohol 1.9; ether 1.5; carbon disulfide 0.25; petr ether 0.05. Freely sol in dil Na_2SO_3 soln. LD_{50} orally in rats: 275 mg/kg (*Toxicological Profile*).

USE: Explosive. Vulcanizing agent for natural rubber. Indicator for pH 12.0-14.0.

9727.   2,4,6-Trinitrobenzoic Acid. [129-66-8] *sym*-Trinitrobenzoic acid. $C_7H_3N_3O_8$; mol wt 257.11. C 32.70%, H 1.18%, N 16.34%, O 49.78%. Prepd by chromic acid oxidation of 2,4,6-trinitrotoluene: Clarke, Hartman, *Org. Synth.* **2**, 95 (1922); Kastens, Kaplan, *Ind. Eng. Chem.* **42**, 402 (1950).

O2N—⟨COOH, NO2, NO2⟩

Orthorhombic crystals from water, mp 228.7°. Sublimes with decompn forming CO_2 and trinitrobenzene. Soly at 25°: 2.05% (w/w) in water, 26.6% in alcohol, 14.7% in ether. Also sol in acetone, methanol; slightly sol in benzene.

9728. 2,4,7-Trinitrofluorenone. [129-79-3] 2,4,7-Trinitro-9H-fluoren-9-one; TNF. $C_{13}H_5N_3O_7$; mol wt 315.19. C 49.54%, H 1.60%, N 13.33%, O 35.53%. Prepn by nitration of fluorenone: Schmidt, Bauer, *Ber.* **38**, 3758 (1905); Orchin *et al., J. Am. Chem. Soc.* **69**, 1225 (1947); by nitration of 2,5-dinitrofluorenone: Ray, Francis, *J. Org. Chem.* **8**, 58 (1943). Structure: Bell, *J. Chem. Soc.* **1928**, 1990. Crystal structure: D. L. Dorset *et al., Acta Crystallogr.* **B28**, 3122 (1972); H. L. Ammon, *ibid.* **B29**, 2314 (1973). Carcinogenicity study: C. Huggins, N. C. Yang, *Science* **137**, 257 (1962). Evaluation of employee exposure to TNF in workplace using HPLC: M. J. Seymour, *J. Chromatogr.* **236**, 530 (1982); R. E. McCullen, A. N. Sanghvi, *ASTM Spec. Tech. Publ.* **786**, 26 (1982).

O2N—⟨fluorenone structure⟩—NO2, NO2

Yellow needles from acetic acid, mp 175.2-176°.
USE: In photocopiers; forms charge-transfer complexes with aromatic hydrocarbons and amines.

9729. Trinitromethane. [517-25-9] Nitroform. CHN_3O_6; mol wt 151.04. C 7.95%, H 0.67%, N 27.82%, O 63.56%. $CH(NO_2)_3$. Prepn from tetranitromethane and $K_4[Fe(CN)_6]$ in aq soln: Chattaway, Harrison, *J. Chem. Soc.* **109**, 171 (1916); by nitration of acetylene with nitric acid: Hager, *Ind. Eng. Chem.* **41**, 2168 (1949).

Crystals, mp 15° (the unstable *aci*-form, mp 50°). d_4^5 (liq) 1.469. Heat of combustion 746 cal/g. Dipole moment 2.61 (benzene). Dec above 25°. Explodes when heated rapidly. Sol in water, giving an intensely yellow soln, although the dry crystals are pure white.

Potassium salt. $CK(NO_2)_3$. Moderately stable crystals. Soly in water at 0°: 16.7 g/100 ml; at 60°: 193.8 g/100 ml. Soly in ethanol: 5.29 g/l.
Caution: Slightly irritating to eyes, mucous membranes.
USE: In the manuf of explosives and propellants.

9730. 2,4,6-Trinitrotoluene. [118-96-7] TNT; *α*-trinitrotoluol; *sym*-trinitrotoluene; 1-methyl-2,4,6-trinitrobenzene; trotyl; tolit; trilit. $C_7H_5N_3O_6$; mol wt 227.13. C 37.02%, H 2.22%, N 18.50%, O 42.26%. Prepn by nitration of toluene with mixed acid ($HNO_3 + H_2SO_4$) in three steps or by continuous flow according to the Schmid-Meissner and Biazi processes: Swift, Tittensor, *J. Soc. Chem. Ind.* **59**, 92 (1940); Johnston in *McGraw-Hill Encyclopedia of Science and Technology* **9**, 104 (1960). Physical constants and applications: Lothrop, Handrick, *Chem. Rev.* **44**, 419-445 (1949); *ACS Monograph Series* **no. 139**, entitled "The Science of High Explosives," M. A. Cook, Ed. (Reinhold, New York, 1958). Review of toxicology and human exposure: *Toxicological Profile for 2,4,6-Trinitrotoluene* (PB95-264297, 1995) 208 pp.

O2N—⟨CH3 toluene structure⟩—NO2, NO2

Monoclinic rhombohedra from alcohol. The commercial crystals (needles) are yellow. mp 80.1°. d_4^{20} 1.654. Burns at 295° when not confined. Can be distilled under reduced pressure. Vapors are toxic. Dipole moment 1.37. Very sparingly sol in water: About 0.01% at 25°, one gram dissolves in 700 ml of boiling water. Sol in acetone, benzene. Less sol than 2,4,6-trinitrophenol in alcohol, ether, carbon disulfide. Reacts vigorously with reducing agents.
Caution: Potential symptoms of overexposure are irritation of skin, mucous membranes; liver damage, jaundice; cyanosis; sneezing; coughing, sore throat; peripheral neuropathy, muscle pain; kidney damage; cataract; sensitization dermatitis; leukocytosis; anemia; cardiac irregularities. *See NIOSH Pocket Guide to Chemical Hazards* (DHHS/NIOSH 97-140, 1997) p 322.
USE: High explosive in military munitions. Must be detonated by a high velocity initiator such as nitramine or by efficient concussion.

9731. Trinitrotriazidobenzene. [29306-57-8] 1,3,5-Triazido-2,4,6-trinitrobenzene; TNTA. $C_6N_{12}O_6$; mol wt 336.14. C 21.44%, N 50.00%, O 28.56%. Nontoxic, metal-free, high energy density material. Explodes to produce gaseous nitrogen and carbon dioxide. Prepn: I. O. Turek, *Chim. Ind. (Paris)* **26**, 785 (1931). Use as a fixative in immunofluorescence microscopy: E. McBeath, K. Fujiwara, *J. Cell Biol.* **99**, 2061 (1984). Thermal decompn studies: A. D. Yoffe, *Proc. R. Soc. London Ser. A* **208**, 188 (1951); D. Adam *et al., Heteroatom Chem.* **10**, 548 (1999). Synthesis, crystal structure, and detonation properties: *idem et al., Propellants Explosives Pyrotechnics* **27**, 7 (2002).

O2N—⟨N3, triazide structure, N3⟩—NO2, N3, NO2

Bright yellow plates from acetic acid, mp 128-130° (dec). d 1.84.
Explosive!
Caution: Sensitive to electrostatic discharge, friction and impact; rapid heating above 168° causes explosion (Adam, 2002).
USE: Initiator or solid rocket propellant in military explosives.

9732. Triolein. [122-32-7] 9-Octadecenoic acid 1,2,3-propanetriyl ester; olein; glyceryl trioleate. $C_{57}H_{104}O_6$; mol wt 885.43. C 77.32%, H 11.84%, O 10.84%. One of the chief constituents of nondrying oils and fats. From Palestine olive oil: Hilditch, Madison, *J. Soc. Chem. Ind.* **60**, 258 (1941); from cacao butter: Meara, *J. Chem. Soc.* **1949**, 2154. Prepn by esterification of oleic acid: Wheeler *et al., J. Biol. Chem.* **132**, 687 (1940); Swicklik *et al., J. Am. Oil Chem. Soc.* **32**, 69 (1955). Synthesis: Serebrennikova *et al., Dokl. Akad. Nauk SSSR* **140**, 1083 (1961).

$$CH_2OC(CH_2)_7CH=CH(CH_2)_7CH_3$$
$$CHOC(CH_2)_7CH=CH(CH_2)_7CH_3$$
$$CH_2OC(CH_2)_7CH=CH(CH_2)_7CH_3$$

Colorless to yellowish, oily liquid; tasteless, odorless. d_4^{15} 0.915. mp −5 to −4°. bp_{15} 235-240°. n_D^{20} 1.4676; n_D^{60} 1.4561. Practically insol in water; sol in chloroform, ether, carbon tetrachloride; slightly sol in alcohol.

9733. Triostins. A *"quinoxaline antibiotic complex"* similar to echinomycin, q.v. Powerful, selective inhibitor of nucleic acid synthesis *in vitro*. Isoln of triostin C from *Streptomyces* S-2-210 resembling *S. aureus*: J. Shoji, K. Katagiri, *J. Antibiot.* **14A**, 335 (1961). Isoln of triostins A and B: H. Otsuka, J. Shoji, *ibid.* **19A**, 128 (1966). Structure of C: *eidem, Tetrahedron* **21**, 2931 (1965); of minor components: *eidem, ibid.* **23**, 1535 (1967); of A: H. Otsuka *et al., J. Antibiot.* **29**, 107 (1976). Biosynthesis: T. Yoshida, K. Katagiri, *Biochemistry* **8**, 2645 (1969). Synthesis of A: P. K. Chakravarty, R. K. Olsen, *Tetrahedron Lett.* **1978**, 1613; M. Shin *et al., Pept. Chem.* **18**, 207 (1980). Conformation of A in soln: J.

R. Kalman *et al., J. Chem. Soc. Perkin Trans. 1* **1979**, 1313. Review of chemistry and biochemistry: M. J. Waring in *Antibiotics* **vol. 5**(pt. 2), F. E. Hahn, Ed. (Springer-Verlag, New York, 1979) pp 173-194.

Triostin A   R = CH₃
Triostin C   R = CH(CH₃)₂

Needles from chloroform + methanol.

Triostin A. $C_{50}H_{62}N_{12}O_{12}S_2$; mol wt 1087.23. mp 245-248° (dec). $[\alpha]_D^{25}$ −157° (c = 0.97 in chloroform). uv max (methanol): 243, 320 nm (log ε 4.75, 4.11).

Triostin C. $C_{54}H_{70}N_{12}O_{12}S_2$; mol wt 1143.34. mp >260° (dec). $[\alpha]_D^{24}$ −143.9° (c = 1.2 in chloroform). uv max (methanol): 243, 320 nm (log ε 4.87, 4.13).

9734. *s*-Trioxane. [110-88-3] 1,3,5-Trioxane; 1,3,5-trioxacyclohexane; metaformaldehyde; trioxymethylene. $C_3H_6O_3$; mol wt 90.08. C 40.00%, H 6.71%, O 53.28%. *Review:* Walker, Carlisle, *Chem. Eng. News* **21**, 1250 (1943).

Stable, cyclic trimer of formaldehyde possessing characteristic chloroform-like odor. Crystalline solid, mp 64°, bp₇₅₉ 114.5° without dec. Sublimes readily. Easily sol in water (17.2 g/100 ml at 18°, 21.1 g/100 ml at 25°), alcohols, ketones, ether, acetone, chlorinated and aromatic hydrocarbons, and other organic solvents. Only slightly sol in pentane, petroleum ether, and lower paraffins. d_4^{65} 1.17. Flash pt 45°C. On distillation with water, forms an azeotrope boiling at 91.4° containing approx 70% trioxane by wt. Slowly depolymerized by strong acids in aq soln, but inert to alkalies. In non-aqueous systems, readily converted to monomeric formaldehyde by small concentrations of strong acids at a rate determined by the acid concentration.

9735. Trioxsalen. [3902-71-4] 2,5,9-Trimethyl-7*H*-furo[3,-2-*g*][1]benzopyran-7-one; 6-hydroxy-β,2,7-trimethyl-5-benzofuranacrylic acid δ-lactone; 4,5′,8-trimethylpsoralen; NSC-71047; Trisoralen. $C_{14}H_{12}O_3$; mol wt 228.24. C 73.67%, H 5.30%, O 21.03%. Synthetic trimethyl psoralen deriv. Prepn: K. D. Kaufman, *J. Org. Chem.* **26**, 117 (1961); US 3201421 (1965). Protective effect vs UV-B erythema: P. G. Agache, L. Coupez, *Arch. Dermatol. Res.* **268**, 85 (1980). Clinical study: N. Vaatainen *et al., Clin. Exp. Dermatol.* **6**, 133 (1981). Comprehensive description: M. M. A. Hassan, M. A. Loutfy, *Anal. Profiles Drug Subs.* **10**, 705-727 (1981). *See also* Psoralen, Methoxsalen.

Prisms from chloroform, mp 234.5-235°. uv max (methanol): 250, 295, 335 nm (log ε 4.35, 3.99, 3.80). Sol in methylene chloride. Slightly sol in alc, chloroform. Practically insol in water.

THERAP CAT: Pigmentation agent (photosensitizer).

9736. Tripalmitin. [555-44-2] Hexadecanoic acid 1,2,3-propanetriyl ester; palmitin; glyceryl tripalmitate. $C_{51}H_{98}O_6$; mol wt 807.32. C 75.87%, H 12.24%, O 11.89%. $(C_{15}H_{31}COO)_3C_3$-H_5. Occurs in fats. Prepd from glycerol and palmitic acid in the presence of Twitchell reagent: Ozaki, *Biochem. Z.* **177**, 159 (1926); or in the presence of trifluoroacetic anhydride: Bourne *et al., J. Chem. Soc.* **1949**, 2976.

Needles from ether, mp 66° (occurs also in lower-melting, unstable forms). bp 310-320°; d_4^{70} 0.8730; d_4^{80} 0.8663. n_D^{80} 1.43807. Saponification value 208.5. Insol in water. Practically insol in alcohol (0.0043 parts/100 parts of abs alcohol at 21°). Freely sol in ether, benzene, chloroform.

9737. Tripamide. [73803-48-2] (3aα,4α,7α,7aα)-3-(Aminosulfonyl)-4-chloro-*N*-(octahydro-4,7-methano-2*H*-isoindol-2-yl)-benzamide; 4-chloro-*N*-(*endo*-hexahydro-4,7-methanoisoindol-2-yl)-3-sulfamoylbenzamide; toripamide; ADR-033; E-614; Normonal. $C_{16}H_{20}ClN_3O_3S$; mol wt 369.87. C 51.96%, H 5.45%, Cl 9.59%, N 11.36%, O 12.98%, S 8.67%. Sulfonamide with diuretic and peripheral vasodilator activity. Prepn: H. Hamano *et al.*, **JP 73 5585** (1973 to Eisai), *C.A.* **78**, 136070r (1973). Synthesis of ¹⁴C-tripamide: T. Nakamura *et al., J. Labelled Compd. Radiopharm.* **14**, 191 (1978). Pharmacological study: T. Satoh *et al., Oyo Yakuri* **21**, 607 (1981), *C.A.* **96**, 28414u (1982). Metabolism: T. Horie *et al., Xenobiotica* **11**, 197, 693 (1981).

Colorless needles.

THERAP CAT: Antihypertensive; diuretic.

9738. Tripelennamine. [91-81-6] *N,N*-Dimethyl-*N*′-(phenylmethyl)-*N*′-2-pyridinyl-1,2-ethanediamine; 2-[benzyl(2-dimethylaminoethyl)amino]pyridine; *N*-benzyl-*N*′,*N*′-dimethyl-*N*-(2-pyridyl)ethylenediamine; *N,N*-dimethyl-*N*′-benzyl-*N*′-(α-pyridyl)-ethylenediamine; β-dimethylaminoethyl-2-pyridylbenzylamine; β-dimethylaminoethyl-2-pyridylaminotoluene. $C_{16}H_{21}N_3$; mol wt 255.36. C 75.26%, H 8.29%, N 16.46%. Prepn: C. P. Huttrer *et al., J. Am. Chem. Soc.* **68**, 1999 (1946); C. Djerassi *et al.*, US 2406594 (1946 to Ciba); R. J. Horclois, US 2502151 (1950 to Rhône-Poulenc). Crystal structure: M. Parvez, *Acta Crystallogr.* **C43**, 1408 (1987). Toxicity studies: D. P. Waller *et al., Clin. Toxicol.* **16**, 17 (1980). Comprehensive description: H. G. Piskorik, *Anal. Profiles Drug Subs.* **14**, 108-133 (1985).

Yellow oil. Amine odor. bp₀.₁ 138-142°, bp₁.₇ 185-190°, bp₂₀ 193-205°. n_D^{25} 1.5759-1.5765. Miscible with water.

Hydrochloride. [154-69-8] Dehistin; Azaron; Pyribenzamine; PBZ; Vetibenzamina. $C_{16}H_{21}N_3$·HCl; mol wt 291.82. Crystals from ethyl acetate + methanol, mp 192-193°. Bitter taste, produces temporary numbness of the tongue. uv max (water): 244, 305 (ε 14470, 4780). One gram dissolves in 0.77 ml water, in 6 ml alcohol, in 6 ml chloroform, in about 350 ml acetone. Practically insol in benzene, ether, ethyl acetate. About neutral to litmus. pH of aq soln contg 25 mg/ml: 6.71; 50 mg/ml: 6.67; 100 mg/ml: 5.56. LD_{50} in mice (mg/kg): 47 i.p. (Walker).

Citrate. [6138-56-3] $C_{16}H_{21}N_3 \cdot C_6H_8O_7$. Crystals, mp 106-110°. Less bitter than the hydrochloride. Freely sol in water, alcohol. Very slightly sol in ether. Practically insol in benzene, chloroform. 1% aq soln has a pH of 4.25.

THERAP CAT: Antihistaminic.

THERAP CAT (VET): Antihistaminic.

9739. Triphenylcarbinol. [76-84-6] Triphenylmethanol; tritanol. $C_{19}H_{16}O$; mol wt 260.33. C 87.66%, H 6.19%, O 6.15%. $(C_6H_5)_3COH$. Prepd by the action of phenylmagnesium bromide on benzophenone: Acree, *Ber.* **37**, 2755 (1904); Peters *et al., J. Am. Chem. Soc.* **47**, 452 (1925); Dubsky, Jacot-Guillarmod, *Helv. Chim. Acta* **53**, 1965 (1970); by the action of potassium permanganate on triphenylfluoro- or triphenylchloromethane: Blicke, *J. Am. Chem. Soc.* **46**, 1518 (1924). Convenient lab prepn from methyl benzoate and phenylmagnesium bromide: L. F. Fieser, *Experiments in Organic Chemistry* (Boston, 3rd ed., 1955) p 77.

Trigonal crystals from benzene; d_4^0 1.199; mp 164.2°. Distills between 360 and 380° without decompn. Absorption spectrum in alc: Orndorff *et al., J. Am. Chem. Soc.* **49**, 1543 (1927). Insol in water, petr ether. Easily sol in alc, ether, benzene. Sol in concd H_2SO_4 with an intensely yellow color, in glacial acetic acid without color.

9740. Triphenylene. [217-59-4] 9,10-Benzphenanthrene; 1,2,3,4-dibenznaphthalene; isochrysene. $C_{18}H_{12}$; mol wt 228.29. C 94.70%, H 5.30%. Occurs in coal tar: Kaffer, *Ber.* **68**, 1812 (1935). Synthesis from cyclohexanone: Mannich, *Ber.* **40**, 163 (1907); Nenitzescu, Curcaneanu, *Ber.* **70**, 346 (1937); from 9-phenanthrylmagnesium bromide and succinic anhydride: Bergmann, *J. Am. Chem. Soc.* **59**, 1441 (1937); from 1,2,3,4-tetrahydrophenanthrene: Bachmann, Struve, *J. Org. Chem.* **4**, 472 (1937); by reaction of 3 mols *o*-bromoiodobenzene in the presence of lithium: Heaney, Millar, *Org. Synth.* **40**, 105 (1960).

Long needles from alc or chloroform. Sublimes; d 1.302; mp 199°; bp 425°. Absorption spectrum: Clar, Lombardi, *Ber.* **65**, 1414 (1932). Solns have blue fluorescence. Does not react with maleic anhydride.

9741. Triphenylmethane. [519-73-3] 1,1′,1″-Methylidenetris[benzene]; Tritan. $C_{19}H_{16}$; mol wt 244.33. C 93.40%, H 6.60%. $(C_6H_5)_3CH$. Prepd by ether reduction of triphenylchloromethane obtained by reaction of carbon tetrachloride and benzene in the presence of aluminum chloride: Norris, *Org. Synth.* **4**, 81 (1925); from diphenylchloromethane and phenylmagnesium bromide: Sayles, Kharasch, *J. Org. Chem.* **26**, 4210 (1961).

Orthorhombic pyramidal, solvated crystals containing one mol benzene, mp 78.2°, dries on exposure to air. When dry, mp 93.4° (stable form; there are 2 metastable forms). d_4^{100} 1.0134; bp_{760} 360°; bp_{200} 239.7°; bp_{100} 228°; bp_{60} 221°; bp_{40} 215.5°; bp_{20} 206.8°; bp_{10} 197°; bp_5 188°; $bp_{1.0}$ 170°. n_D^{100} 1.59546. Absorption spectrum: Orndorff, *J. Am. Chem. Soc.* **49**, 1543 (1927); Anderson, *ibid.* **50**, 209 (1928); **51**, 1890 (1929). Very sol in ether, hot alcohol, chloroform. Sol in petr ether, benzene, CS_2. Slightly sol in glacial acetic acid. Soly (parts/100 parts satd soln (w/w) at 30°) 48.6 in chloroform; 12.5 in hexane; 53 in CS_2; 7.24 parts in benzene (19°).

9742. Triphenyl Phosphate. [115-86-6] $C_{18}H_{15}O_4P$; mol wt 326.28. C 66.26%, H 4.63%, O 19.61%, P 9.49%. $(C_6H_5O)_3$-PO. Prepd from P_2O_5 and phenol: Prahl, US 2805240 (1957); by reaction of triethyl phosphite with chloramine-T: Cadogan, Moulden, *J. Chem. Soc.* **1961**, 3079. Toxicology: Sutton *et al., Arch. Environ. Health* **1**, 33 (1960).

Nonflammable needles; mp 49-50°; bp_{11} 245°. Insol in water. Sol in benzene, chloroform, ether, acetone, moderately sol in alcohol.

Caution: Potential symptoms of overexposure are minor changes in blood enzymes. *See* NIOSH Pocket Guide to Chemical Hazards (DHHS/NIOSH 97-140, 1997) p 322.

USE: Noncombustible substitute for camphor in celluloid; rendering acetylcellulose, nitrocellulose, airplane "dope", etc., stable and fireproof; impregnating roofing paper; plasticizer in lacquers and varnishes.

9743. Triphenylphosphine. [603-35-0] $C_{18}H_{15}P$; mol wt 262.29. C 82.43%, H 5.76%, P 11.81%. $(C_6H_5)_3P$. Prepd from phenylmagnesium bromide and phosphorus trichloride: Pfeiffer, Pietsch, *Ber.* **37**, 4621 (1904); Sauvage, *Compt. Rend.* **139**, 675 (1904); Dodonon, Medox, *Ber.* **61**, 910 (1928); Denney *et al., J. Am. Chem. Soc.* **83**, 1729 (1961).

Odorless monoclinic platelets or prisms from ether, mp 80.5°. bp >360° (in inert gas). d_4^{25} 1.194; d_4^{80}(liq) 1.075. For more physical constants *see* Forward *et al., J. Chem. Soc.* **1949**, 5121. Is triboluminescent. Freely sol in ether; sol in benzene, chloroform, glacial acetic acid; less sol in alcohol; practically insol in water.

USE: In organic synthesis; polymerization initiator.

9744. Triphenyltetrazolium Chloride. [298-96-4] 2,3,5-Triphenyl-2H-tetrazolium chloride; red tetrazolium; TPTZ; TTC; RT; VitaStain. $C_{19}H_{15}ClN_4$; mol wt 334.80. C 68.16%, H 4.52%, Cl 10.59%, N 16.73%. Prepn: H. v. Pechmann, P. Runge, *Ber.* **27**, 2920 (1894); Atkinson *et al., Science* **111**, 385 (1950); R. Kuhn, D. Jerchel, *Ber.* **74**, 945 (1941); R. Price, *J. Chem. Soc. A* **1971**, 3379. Review of prepn and use of tetrazolium salts as indicators in biochemical and biological oxidation-reduction processes: W. Ried, *Angew. Chem.* **14**, 391 (1952).

Solvated nearly colorless needles from alcohol or chloroform, dry at 105°. Turns yellow on exposure to light. Dec 243°. Sol in water, alcohol, acetone. Insol in ether. Oxidizes aldoses and ketoses, as well as other α-ketols, and is thereby reduced to a water-insoluble, deep red pigment, a triphenylformazan.

USE: In analytical chemistry as a sensitive reagent for reducing sugars, and to distinguish between α-ketols and simple aldehydes. For staining plant and animal tissue. Germination indicator in testing the ability of seeds to germinate: G. Lakon, *Ber. Dtsch. Bot. Ges.* **60**, 299, 434 (1942). In histochemical studies. In determination of antibiotics; of dehydrogenases.

9745. Triphenyltin Hydroxide. [76-87-9] Hydroxytriphenylstannane; hydroxytriphenyltin; fentin hydroxide; fenolovo; Du-Ter. $C_{18}H_{16}OSn$; mol wt 367.03. C 58.90%, H 4.39%, O 4.36%, Sn 32.34%. $(C_6H_5)_3SnOH$. Prepn by alkaline hydrolysis of $(C_6H_5)_3SnCl$: Kushlefsky *et al., Inorg. Chem.* **2**, 187 (1963); of $(C_6H_5)_3SnI$: Poller, *J. Inorg. Nucl. Chem.* **24**, 593 (1963). GC determn in vegetable crops: H. H. Van den Broek *et al., Analyst* **113**, 1237 (1988). Review of analytical methods: A. Van Rossum *et al., Anal. Methods Pestic. Plant Growth Regul.* **11**, 227-246 (1980). *Reviews:* Ingham, *Chem. Rev.* **60**, 459-539 (1960); R. Bock, *Residue Rev.* **79**, 1-270 (1981). Review of toxicology and human exposure: *Toxicological Profile for Tin* (PB2006-100006, 2005) 426 pp.

Crystals. mp 122-123.5°. Thermally dec to $(C_6H_5)_4$Sn, $(C_6H_5)_2$SnO and H_2O. Slightly sol in alcohol, toluene. Practically insol in water.

Acetate. Triphenyltin acetate; acetoxytriphenyltin; fentin acetate; Brestan. $C_{20}H_{18}O_2Sn$; mol wt 409.07. Prepn from acetic acid and $(C_6H_5)_3SnOH$: van der Kirk, Luijten, *J. Appl. Chem.* **6**, 49 (1956); and $(C_6H_5)_3SnH$: Weber, Becker, *J. Org. Chem.* **27**, 1258 (1962). Small needles, mp 122-124°. Sol in ether, slightly sol in alcohol, benzene.

USE: Antifeeding compounds for insect pest control; non-systemic fungicide.

9746. Triprolidine. [486-12-4] 2-[(1E)-1-(4-Methylphenyl)-3-(1-pyrrolidinyl)-1-propenyl]pyridine; *trans*-2-[3-(1-pyrrolidinyl)-1-*p*-tolylpropenyl]pyridine; *trans*-1-(2-pyridyl)-3-pyrrolidino-1-*p*-tolylprop-1-ene; *trans*-1-(4-methylphenyl)-1-(2-pyridyl)-3-pyrrolidinoprop-1-ene. C$_{19}$H$_{22}$N$_2$; mol wt 278.39. C 81.97%, H 7.97%, N 10.06%. Histamine H$_1$-receptor antagonist. Prepn: Adamson, US 2712020; US 2712023 (both 1955 to Burroughs Wellcome); Adamson et al., J. Chem. Soc. **1958,** 312. Structure-activity studies: Ison, Casy, J. Pharm. Pharmacol. **23,** 848 (1971). Crystal and molecular structure: James, Williams, Can. J. Chem. **52,** 1880 (1974). Pharmacokinetics and antihistaminic effects in humans: K. J. Simons et al., J. Allergy Clin. Immunol. **77,** 326 (1986). Comprehensive description: S. A. Benezra, C.-H. Yang, Anal. Profiles Drug Subs. **8,** 509-528 (1979).

Crystals from light petr, mp 59-61°. uv max (ethanol): 236, 285 nm (ε 15300, 6800).

Hydrochloride monohydrate. [6138-79-0] 295C51; Actidil; Actidilon; Pro-Actidil; Pro-Entra; Venen. C$_{19}$H$_{22}$N$_2$.HCl.H$_2$O; mol wt 332.87. Crystals from water, mp 116-118°. uv max (ethanol): 235, 283 nm (ε 15000, 7400). Moderately sol in water, ethanol, methanol.

Oxalate. C$_{19}$H$_{22}$N$_2$.C$_2$H$_2$O$_4$. Crystals from methanol, dec 173-174°. uv max (ethanol): 233, 283 nm (ε 16200, 8200).

THERAP CAT: Antihistaminic.

9747. Triptolide. [38748-32-2] (3bS,4aS,5aS,6R,6aR,7aS,-7bS,8aS,8bS)-3b,4,4a,6,6a,7a,7b,8b,9,10-Decahydro-6-hydroxy-8b-methyl-6a-(1-methylethyl)trisoxireno[4b,5:6,7:8a,9]phenanthro[1,-2-c]furan-1(3H)-one; PG490. C$_{20}$H$_{24}$O$_6$; mol wt 360.40. C 66.65%, H 6.71%, O 26.64%. Diterpenoid triepoxide with immunosuppressant and antitumor properties; isolated from the Chinese medicinal herb, *Tripterygium wilfordii* Hook. f., Celastraceae. Isoln and structure determn: S. M. Kupchan et al., J. Am. Chem. Soc. **94,** 7194 (1972). Synthesis of racemate: R. S. Buckanin et al., ibid. **102,** 1200 (1980); of naturally occurring (−)-form: D. Yang et al., ibid. **121,** 5579 (1999). HPLC and SPE determn in *Tripterygium* root extracts: A. M. Brinker, I. Raskin, J. Chromatogr. A **1070,** 65 (2005). Animal studies of male antifertility effects: A. P. S. Hikim et al., J. Androl. **21,** 431 (2000); P. N. Huynh et al., ibid. 689. Mechanistic studies of apoptotic and antitumor activities: W.-T. Chang et al., J. Biol. Chem. **276,** 2221 (2001); T. M. Kiviharju et al., Clin. Cancer Res. **8,** 2666 (2002); S. J. Leuenroth, C. M. Crews, Chem. Biol. **12,** 1259 (2005). Review of anti-inflammatory and immunosuppressive properties: B. J. Chen, Leuk. Lymphoma **42,** 253-265 (2001).

mp 226-227°. [α]$_D^{25}$ −154° (c = 0.369 in CH$_2$Cl$_2$). uv max (ethanol): 218 nm (ε 14000). Sol in DMSO, ethanol. LD$_{50}$ i.p. in mice: 1.93 mg/kg (Chen).

14-Succinyl triptolide sodium salt. [195883-09-1] PG490-88. C$_{24}$H$_{27}$NaO$_9$; mol wt 482.46. Semi-synthetic water soluble prodrug. Prepn: Y. M. Qi, J. H. Musser, US 5663335 (1997 to Pharmagenesis). Animal model studies of prevention of graft-vs-

host disease: B. J. Chen et al., Transplantation **70,** 1442 (2000); of antitumor effects: J. M. Fidler et al., Mol. Cancer Ther. **2,** 855 (2003); of allograft survival in organ transplantation: F. Pan et al., Transplant. Proc. **37,** 134 (2005).

9748. Triptorelin. [57773-63-4] 6-D-Tryptophanluteinizing hormone-releasing factor (pig); 6-D-tryptophan-LH-RH; D-trp^6-LHRH; D-Trp^{6}LRH; D-trp^6-gonadorelin; détryptoréline; AY-25650; Wy-42462; Wy-42422. C$_{64}$H$_{82}$N$_{18}$O$_{13}$; mol wt 1311.45. C 58.61%, H 6.30%, N 19.22%, O 15.86%. Synthetic peptide agonist analog of LH-RH, q.v. Prepn: A. V. Schally, D. H. Coy, DE 2625843; eidem, US 4010125 (1976, 1977); D. H. Coy et al., J. Med. Chem. **19,** 423 (1976). Comparison with LH-RH of in vitro activity: D. H. Coy et al., Biochem. Biophys. Res. Commun. **67,** 576 (1975). Pharmacokinetics and metabolism in humans: J. L. Barron et al., J. Clin. Endocrinol. Metab. **54,** 1169 (1982). HPLC analysis: D. C. Serti et al., J. Liq. Chromatogr. **4,** 1135 (1981). RIA in human serum: M. Mason-Garcia et al., Proc. Natl. Acad. Sci. USA **82,** 1547 (1985). Clinical trial for in vitro fertilization: A. Hazout et al., Fertil. Steril. **59,** 596 (1993). Clinical trial in prostate cancer: C. F. Heyns et al., BJU Int. **92,** 226 (2003); in severe endometriosis: A. Y. K. Wong, L. Tang, Fertil. Steril. **81,** 1522 (2004).

5-oxoPro–His–Trp–Ser–Tyr–D-Trp–Leu–Arg–Pro–GlyNH$_2$

Fluffy, white solid. [α]$_D^{23}$ −58.8° (c = 0.33 in acetic acid).

Acetate. [140194-24-7] Gonapeptil. C$_{64}$H$_{82}$N$_{18}$O$_{13}$.C$_2$H$_4$-O$_2$; mol wt 1371.50.

Pamoate. [124508-66-3] Decapeptyl; Trelstar. C$_{64}$H$_{82}$N$_{18}$-O$_{13}$.C$_{23}$H$_{16}$O$_6$; mol wt 1699.82.

THERAP CAT: Antineoplastic (hormonal); in treatment of endometriosis and infertility.

9749. Triptycene. [477-75-8] 9,10-Dihydro-9,10-*o*-benzenoanthracene. C$_{20}$H$_{14}$; mol wt 254.33. C 94.45%, H 5.55%. Synthesis by three different methods: Bartlett et al., J. Am. Chem. Soc. **64,** 2649 (1942); Wittig, Org. Synth. **39,** 75 (1959); Friedman, Logullo, J. Am. Chem. Soc. **85,** 1549 (1963).

Crystals from cyclohexane or methylcyclohexane, mp 253-254°.

9750. 2,4,6-Tripyridyl-*s*-triazine. [3682-35-7] 2,4,6-Tri-2-pyridyl-*s*-triazine; 2,4,6-tripyridyl-1,3,5-triazine; tripyridyltriazine; TPTZ. C$_{18}$H$_{12}$N$_6$; mol wt 312.33. C 69.22%, H 3.87%, N 26.91%. Synthesis: Case, Kroft, J. Am. Chem. Soc. **81,** 905 (1959). Preparation: Schaefer, US 3294798 (1966 to Am. Cyanamid). Thermal stability data: Johns et al., J. Chem. Eng. Data **7,** 227 (1962). Review: "2,4,6-Tripyridyl-*s*-triazine" in Diehl et al., The Iron Reagents (The G. Frederick Smith Chem. Co., Columbus, Ohio, 1965) pp 41-56.

Crystals, mp 210-220° (Schaefer); trihydrate from aqueous ethanol, mp 244-245° (Case, Kroft). Reacts with ferrous ions to yield intense violet color over pH range 3.4-5.8. Absorption max Fe(TPTZ)$_2^{2+}$ (water): 593 nm (ε 22600), Collins et al., Anal. Chem. **31,** 1862 (1959).

USE: Reagent for the spectrophotometric determn of iron.

9751. Tris-BP. [126-72-7] 2,3-Dibromo-1-propanol phosphate(3:1); phosphoric acid tris(2,3-dibromopropyl) ester; tris(2,3-dibromopropyl) phosphate; Apex 462-5; Flammex AP; Flammex T

23P; Firemaster LV-T 23P; Firemaster T 23P; T 23P; Fyrol HB 32. $C_9H_{15}Br_6O_4P$; mol wt 697.61. C 15.50%, H 2.17%, Br 68.72%, O 9.17%, P 4.44%. Prepn: G. E. Walter, I. Hornstein, **US 2574515** (1951 to Glenn. L. Martin Co.); D. E. Overbeek, R. C. Nametz, **US 3046297** (1962 to Michigan Chem. Co.); R. W. Rimmer, **US 3223755** (1965 to duPont). Use in flameproofing: W. D. Paist, N. Van Gorder, **US 2662834** (1953 to Celanese). Mutagenicity studies: M. J. Prival *et al.*, *Science* **195**, 76 (1977); A. Nakamura *et al.*, *Mutat. Res.* **66**, 373 (1979). Carcinogenicity studies: B. L. Van Duuren *et al.*, *Cancer Res.* **38**, 3236 (1978); G. Reznik *et al.*, *J. Natl. Cancer Inst.* **63**, 205 (1979). Review of toxicology: F. A. Daniher, *Proc. Symp. Text. Flammability* **4**, 126-143 (1976). *Review:* A. Blum, B. N. Ames, *Science* **195**, 17 (1977).

Viscous liquid. LD_{50} orally in rats: >5.0 g/kg (Daniher).

Caution: This substance is reasonably anticipated to be a human carcinogen: *Report on Carcinogens, Eleventh Edition* (PB2005-104914, 2004) p III-84.

USE: Flame retardant. Formerly used in children's sleepwear.

9752. Tris(ethylenediamine)cadmium Dihydroxide. [14874-24-9] Tris(ethylenediamine)cadmium hydroxide; tri(en)-cadmium hydroxide; Cadoxen. $C_6H_{26}CdN_6O_2$; mol wt 326.72. C 22.06%, H 8.02%, Cd 34.41%, N 25.72%, O 9.79%. $[Cd(H_2-NCH_2CH_2NH_2)_3](OH)_2$. Prepared by shaking a given amount of cadmium oxide in 10 times its wt of 30% aq ethylenediamine soln for 15 minutes and centrifuging; the supernatant liquor is the product: Jayme, Neuschäfer, *Naturwissenschaften* **44**, 62 (1957). The soln contains about 4.5% Cd (w/w) and dissolves about 3% (w/w) cellulose, giving a clear, highly viscous soln.

USE: Solvent for cellulose: Jayme, **DE 1079318** (1960 to E. Merck), *C.A.* **55**, 18107d (1961); solvent for sulfite pulps.

9753. Tris(hydroxymethyl)nitromethane. [126-11-4] 2-(Hydroxymethyl)-2-nitro-1,3-propanediol; 2-nitro-2-(hydroxymethyl)-1,3-propanediol; trimethylolnitromethane. $C_4H_9NO_5$; mol wt 151.12. C 31.79%, H 6.00%, N 9.27%, O 52.94%. Prepn from trioxymethylene and nitromethane: Boileau, *Mem. Poudres* **35**, Annexe 7-76 (1953).

Crystals from ethyl acetate + benzene, mp 214° (pure); mp 180° (usual laboratory product); mp 175-176° (tech). Soly in water at 20°: 220 g/100 ml. Freely sol in alcohols. Sparingly sol in benzene, other hydrocarbons. pH of 0.1M aq soln 4.5.

Caution: Irritating to skin, mucous membranes.

USE: Bactericide for inanimate objects. To inhibit bacterial growth in circulating industrial water systems, cutting oils, nonprotein glues and sizings.

9754. Trisilane. [7783-26-8] Trisilicopropane; trisilicon octahydride; silicopropane; trisilicane. H_8Si_3; mol wt 92.32. H 8.73%, Si 91.27%. Si_3H_8. Obtained by separation of mixed silanes prepared from magnesium silicide and hydrochloric acid: Stock, Somiesky, *Ber.* **49**, 111 (1916); **54B**, 524 (1921); **56B**, 247 (1923); Culbertson, **US 2551571** (1951 to Union Carbide); prepared by conversion of silane to higher silanes in an ozonizer type of electric discharge: Spanier, MacDiarmid, *Inorg. Chem.* **1**, 432 (1962).

Liquid. mp −117.4°; bp 52.9°; d^0 0.743; vapor pressure 95.5 mm Hg at 0°. Much less stable than silane or disilane. Detonates in air. Dec in water. Reacts vigorously with CCl_4 and $CHCl_3$.

9755. Tris(pentafluorophenyl)boron. [1109-15-5] Tris-(pentafluorophenyl)borane. $C_{18}BF_{15}$; mol wt 511.98. C 42.23%,

B 2.11%, F 55.66%. Lewis acid catalyst. Prepn and characterization: A. G. Massey, A. J. Park, *J. Organomet. Chem.* **2**, 245 (1964); and NMR study of adducts: *eidem, ibid.* **5**, 218 (1966). Catalytic role in olefin polymerization: X. Yang *et al., J. Am. Chem. Soc.* **116**, 10015 (1994). Lewis acid properties: H. Jacobsen *et al., Organometallics* **18**, 1724 (1999). Prepn and properties of $B(C_6F_5)_3$ radical anion: R. J. Kwaan *et al., ibid.* **20**, 3818 (2001). Review of chemistry and uses: W. E. Piers, T. Chivers, *Chem. Soc. Rev.* **26**, 345-354 (1997).

White solid, mp 126-128°. Sol in many organic solvents. Monomeric in benzene at 30°. Hygroscopic. Thermally stable.

USE: Catalyst in organic transformations; cocatalyst with group IV metallocene alkyls in olefin polymerization.

9756. Tristearin. [555-43-1] Octadecanoic acid 1,2,3-propanetriyl ester; stearin; glyceryl tristearate. $C_{57}H_{110}O_6$; mol wt 891.48. C 76.79%, H 12.44%, O 10.77%. Present in many animal and vegetable fats, especially the hard ones like cacao butter and tallow. Prepd from stearic acid and glycerol in the presence of Al_2O_3: Ingram, **GB 663566** (1951 to I.C.I.); by catalytic hydrogenation of many oils: *Bailey's Industrial Oil and Fat Products* (Wiley, New York, 3rd ed.) pp 881-882.

White powder; d_4^{80} 0.862; mp ~55°; on further heating solidifies and melts again at 72°. n_D^{80} 1.4385. Insol in water. Sol in benzene, chloroform, hot alcohol; almost insol in cold alcohol, ether, petr ether.

USE: In textile sizes. Formerly in making candles.

9757. Tris(trimethylsilyl)silane. [1873-77-4] 1,1,1,3,3,3-Hexamethyl-2-(trimethylsilyl)trisilane. $C_9H_{28}Si_4$; mol wt 248.66. C 43.47%, H 11.35%, Si 45.18%. $((CH_3)_3Si)_3SiH$. Radical based mediator. Prepn: H. Gilman *et al., Chem. Ind. (London)* **1965**, 848; H. Bürger, W. Kilian, *J. Organomet. Chem.* **18**, 299 (1969). Si-H bond dissociation energies: J. M. Kanabus-Kaminska *et al., J. Am. Chem. Soc.* **109**, 5268 (1987). Identification as reducing agent: C. Chatgilialoglu *et al., J. Org. Chem.* **53**, 3641 (1988). Use as a reducing agent: M. Ballestri *et al., ibid.* **56**, 678 (1991); D. H. R. Barton *et al., Tetrahedron Lett.* **33**, 6629 (1992); in carbonylation: I. Ryu *et al., Synlett* **1993**, 143.

Liquid, bp_{8mm} 80-83°.

USE: Reducing and hydrosilyating agent.

9758. Tristriphenylphosphine Rhodium Carbonyl Hydride. [17185-29-4] Carbonylhydrotris(triphenylphosphine)rhodium; hydridocarbonyltris(triphenylphosphine)rhodium(I). $C_{55}H_{46}OP_3Rh$; mol wt 918.78. C 71.90%, H 5.05%, O 1.74%, P 10.11%, Rh 11.20%. $HRh(CO)[P(C_6H_5)_3]_3$. Prepn: Bath, Vaska, *J. Am. Chem. Soc.* **85**, 3500 (1963); Levison, Robinson, *J. Chem. Soc. A* **1970**, 2947; Ahmad *et al., J. Chem. Soc. Dalton Trans.* **1972**, 843; Ahmad *et al., Inorg. Synth.* **15**, 45 (1974). Structure: LaPlaca, Ibers, *J. Am. Chem. Soc.* **85**, 3501 (1963); *eidem, Acta Crystallogr.* **18**, 511 (1965). Chemistry: Evans *et al., J. Chem. Soc. A* **1968**, 2660; O'Connor, Wilkinson, *ibid.* 2665.

Yellow microcrystals, d 1.33. mp 120-122° in air; 172-174° under nitrogen. Moderately sol in benzene, chloroform, dichloromethane; sparingly sol in cyclohexane; insol in light petroleum. Dissociates extensively in organic solvents.

USE: Catalyst.

9759. Trithiocarbonic Acid. [594-08-1] Carbonotrithioic acid; dihydrogen thiocarbonate. CH_2S_3; mol wt 110.22. C

10.90%, H 1.83%, S 87.28%. Prepared by the treatment of $BaCS_3$ with ice-cold 10% HCl: v. Halban *et al.*, *Z. Elektrochem.* **29**, 445 (1923); Mills, Robinson, *J. Chem. Soc.* **1928**, 2326; Gattow, Krebs, *Angew. Chem.* **74**, 29 (1962).

Highly refractive red oil. mp $-26.9°$. bp 57.8°. d_4^{20} 1.483; d_4^{25} 1.476. n_D^{20} 1.8225. Dec by water, alcohol. Addition of sulfur produces tetrathiocarbonic acid CH_2S_4.

9760. Trithiozine. [35619-65-9] 4-[Thioxo(3,4,5-trimethoxyphenyl)methyl]morpholine; 4-(3,4,5-trimethoxythiobenzoyl)-morpholine; sulmetozine (rescinded INN); tritiozine; ISF-2001; Tresanil. $C_{14}H_{19}NO_4S$; mol wt 297.37. C 56.55%, H 6.44%, N 4.71%, O 21.52%, S 10.78%. Non-anticholinergic gastric secretion inhibitor. Prepn: G. Pifferi, **DE 2102246**; *idem*, **US 3862138** (1972, 1975 both to ISF). Synthesis and pharmacology: G. Pifferi *et al.*, *Chim. Ther.* **8**, 462 (1973). HPLC determn in plasma and urine: T. Crolla *et al.*, *J. Chromatogr.* **222**, 257 (1981). Clinical studies: M. Elakovic *et al.*, *J. Int. Med. Res.* **8**, 347 (1980); U. Marini *et al.*, *Clin. Ter.* **92**, 399 (1980). Evaluation of gastric acid suppression: K. Gibinski, *Curr. Med. Res. Opin.* **7**, 516 (1981).

Pale yellow solid from ethanol, mp 141-143°. LD_{50} i.p. in mice: 2000 mg/kg (Pifferi, 1973).

THERAP CAT: Antisecretory (gastric).

9761. Triticum. Agropyrum; couch grass; dog grass; graminis; quick grass. Dried rhizome and roots of *Agropyron repens* L., Beauv., *Gramineae*, gathered in spring. *Habit.* Europe, Northern Asia; naturalized in the U.S. *Constit.* Triticin, glucose, mannite, inosite.

9762. Tritium. [10028-17-8] Triterium. T or ^3_1H. at. wt 3.016. Exists in the diatomic state, T_2; mol wt 6.032. Naturally occurring radioactive isotope of hydrogen, *q.v.*, ($T_{1/2}$ 12.32 yr, low energy β^- emitter). Under normal conditions the total atmospheric content of molecular T_2 gas is only 11 g. First prepd by the bombardment of deuterophosphoric acid with fast deuterons: M. L. E. Oliphant *et al.*, *Proc. Roy. Soc.* **A144**, 692 (1934); T. W. Bonner, *Phys. Rev.* **53**, 711 (1938). Produced commercially from ^6Li by slow neutron bombardment: $^6_3Li + ^1_0n \rightarrow ^3_1H + ^4_2He$. Prepn by neutron irradiation of lithium fluoride: Jenks *et al.*, **US 3079317** (1963). *Reviews:* E. A. Evans, *Tritium and Its Compounds* (Butterworth, London, 1966) 441 pp; Mackay, Dove, "Deuterium and Tritium" in *Comprehensive Inorganic Chemistry* **vol. 1**, J. C. Bailar Jr. *et al.*, Eds. (Pergamon Press, Oxford, 1973) pp 77-116; *Chemistry of the Elements* N. N. Greenwood, A. Earnshaw, Eds. (Pergamon Press, New York, 1984) pp 38-74; J. J. Katz in *Kirk-Othmer Encyclopedia of Chemical Technology* **vol. 8** (Wiley-Interscience, New York, 4th ed., 1993) pp 17-30.

Gas, having properties similar to hydrogen. mp $-254.54°$ (20.62 K) at 162 mm (triple point). bp $-248.12°$ (25.04 K). Crit temp $-232.56°$. Crit press. 18.317 atm. Molar density of liquid: 45.35 moles/l (20.62 K).

USE: In fusion-based thermonuclear weapons (hydrogen bombs). Energy is released by deuteron bombardment according to the reaction: $^3_1H + ^2_1H \rightarrow ^4_2He + ^1_0n + 18$ meV. Widely used as a radioactive tracer in chemical, biochemical, biological and hydrological research.

9763. Tritolyl Phosphate. [1330-78-5] Phosphoric acid tris(methylphenyl) ester; tricresyl phosphate; TCP; PX-917; Celluflex 179; Kronitex TCP; Lindol. $C_{21}H_{21}O_4P$; mol wt 368.36. C 68.47%, H 5.75%, O 17.37%, P 8.41%. A mixture of isomeric tritolyl phosphates, usually excluding the very toxic *ortho*-isomer as much as possible. Prepd from cresol and phosphoric oxychloride, phosphoric acid or pentachloride: Prahl, **US 2805240** (1957); Bondy, Gumb, **GB 890642** (1962 to Coalite and Chem. Prod.); *Faith, Keyes & Clark's Industrial Chemicals*, F. A. Lowenheim,

M. K. Moran, Eds. (Wiley-Interscience, New York, 4th ed., 1975) pp 849-853.

Oily, flame resistant liquid. d_{25}^{25} 1.16; bp_{10} ~265°. Pour point $-28°$. n_D^{25} 1.55. Insol in water (<0.002% at 85°). Sp heat 0.38. Misc with all the common organic solvents and thinners, linseed oil, china wood oil, castor oil.

USE: As plasticizer in vinyl plastics manuf, as flame-retardant, solvent for nitrocellulose, in cellulosic molding compositions, as additive to extreme pressure lubricants, as a nonflammable fluid in hydraulic systems, as lead scavenger in gasoline: Yust, Bame, **US 2889212** (1959 to Shell); to sterilize certain surgical instruments.

9764. Tri-*o*-tolyl Phosphate. [78-30-8] Phosphoric acid tris(2-methylphenyl) ester; tri-*o*-cresyl phosphate. $C_{21}H_{21}O_4P$; mol wt 368.36. C 68.47%, H 5.75%, O 17.37%, P 8.41%.

Colorless or pale yellow liquid. *Poisonous!* mp 25.6°. bp ~410° with slight decompn. Flash pt 225°C. d 1.1955. n 1.5575. Sparingly sol in water, slightly sol in alcohol, sol in ether.

Caution: Potential symptoms of overexposure are GI disturbance; peripheral neuropathy; cramps in calves, paresthesia in feet or hands; weak feet, wrist drop and paralysis. *See NIOSH Pocket Guide to Chemical Hazards* (DHHS/NIOSH 97-140, 1997) p 322. Ingestion may cause acute nausea, vomiting, diarrhea. Following a latent period, polyneuritis progressing to paralysis of extremities has been seen in severe poisoning. *See Clinical Toxicology of Commercial Products*, R. E. Gosselin *et al.*, Eds. (Williams & Wilkins, Baltimore, 5th ed., 1984) Section III, pp 388-393; *Patty's Industrial Hygiene and Toxicology* **vol. 2D**, G. D. Clayton, F. E. Clayton, Eds. (John Wiley & Sons, New York, 4th ed., 1994) pp 3063-3085.

USE: As plasticizer in lacquers and varnishes.

9765. Tritoqualine. [14504-73-5] 7-Amino-4,5,6-triethoxy-3-(5,6,7,8-tetrahydro-4-methoxy-6-methyl-1,3-dioxolo[4,5-g]isoquinolin-5-yl)-1(3H)-isobenzofuranone; 7-amino-4,5,6-triethoxy-3-(5,6,7,8-tetrahydro-4-methoxy-6-methyl-1,3-dioxolo[4,5-g]isoquinolin-5-yl)phthalide; tritocaline; L-554; Hypostamine; Inhibostamin; Livalfa. $C_{26}H_{32}N_2O_8$; mol wt 500.54. C 62.39%, H 6.44%, N 5.60%, O 25.57%. Prepn: **FR 1295309** (1962 to Lab. de Recherches Biol. Laborec). Activity: Hahn *et al.*, *Arzneim.-Forsch.* **20**, 1490 (1970).

Crystals, mp 183°.

THERAP CAT: Antihistaminic.

9766. Triuret. [556-99-0] Diimidotricarbonic diamide; 1,3-dicarbamylurea; carbonyldiurea. $C_3H_6N_4O_3$; mol wt 146.10. C 24.66%, H 4.14%, N 38.35%, O 32.85%. $H_2NCONHCONHCONH_2$. Prepared by the action of phosgene on urea: Schiff, *Ann.* **291**, 374 (1896); Blair, *J. Am. Chem. Soc.* **48**, 101 (1926); Haworth, Mann, *J. Chem. Soc.* **1943**, 603; Werner, Gray, *Sci. Proc. R. Dublin Soc.* **24**, 111 (1946).

Crystals from ammonia water, dec 233°. Freely sol in liq ammonia. Forms a mono- and dipotassium salt, *see* Blair, *loc. cit.*

9767. Troclosene Potassium. [2244-21-5] 1,3-Dichloro-1,3,5-triazine-2,4,6(1H,3H,5H)-trione potassium salt; 3,5-dichloro-tetrahydro-2,4,6-trioxo-s-triazin-1(2H)-yl potassium; potassium troclosene; potassium dichloroisocyanurate; ACL-59. $C_3Cl_2KN_3O_3$; mol wt 236.05. C 15.26%, Cl 30.04%, K 16.56%, N 17.80%, O 20.33%. Structure studies and prepn: Petterson *et al.*, *J. Org. Chem.* **25**, 1595 (1960). Prepn from trisodium isocyanurate and gaseous Cl: Symes *et al.*, **US 3035056**; **US 3035057** (both 1962 to Monsanto).

USE: Useful source of available Cl in solid bleach and detergent formulations.

THERAP CAT: Anti-infective (topical).

9768. Trofosfamide. [22089-22-1] N,N,3-Tris(2-chloroethyl)tetrahydro-2H-1,3,2-oxazaphosphorin-2-amine 2-oxide; 2-[bis(2-chloroethyl)amino]-3-(2-chloroethyl)tetrahydro-2H-1,3,2-oxaphosphorine 2-oxide; N,N,N'-tris(2-chloroethyl)-N',O-propylene phosphoric acid ester diamide; trilophosphamide; trophosphamide; NSC-109723; Z-4828; Ixoten. $C_9H_{18}Cl_3N_2O_2P$; mol wt 323.58. C 33.41%, H 5.61%, Cl 32.87%, N 8.66%, O 9.89%, P 9.57%. The 3-(2-chloroethyl) deriv of cyclophosphamide, *q.v.* Prepn: **GB 1188159**, *C.A.* **73**, 44892d (1970); Arnold *et al.*, **DE 2107936**, *C.A.* **77**, 152238m (1972) (1970, 1972 both to Asta-Werke); K. Pankiewicz *et al.*, *J. Am. Chem. Soc.* **101**, 7712 (1979). Pharmacology: N. Brock, *Int. Congr. Chemother., Proc. 5th*, K. H. Spitzy, H. Haschek, Eds. (Verlag Wiener Med. Akad., Vienna, 1967) **II**(1), pp 155-161; J. Potel, N. Brock, *Arzneim.-Forsch.* **21**, 1250 (1971); N. Brock, J. Potel, *ibid.* **24**, 1149 (1974); Harrison, Fuquay, *Proc. Soc. Exp. Biol. Med.* **139**, 957 (1972). Crystal and molecular structure: A. Perales, S. Garcia-Blanco, *Acta Crystallogr.* **33B**, 1939 (1977).

Crystals from ether, mp 50-51°. $[\alpha]_D^{25} -28.6°$ (c = 2 in CH_3OH). LD_{50} i.p. in mice: 212 mg/kg (Brock, Potel).

THERAP CAT: Antineoplastic.

9769. Troglitazone. [97322-87-7] 5-[[4-[(3,4-Dihydro-6-hydroxy-2,5,7,8-tetramethyl-2H-1-benzopyran-2-yl)methoxy]phenyl]methyl]-2,4-thiazolidinedione; (±)-5-[4-[(6-hydroxy-2,5,7,8-tetramethylchroman-2-yl)methoxy]benzyl]-2,4-thiazolidinedione; romglizone; CS-045; CI-991; Noscal; Prelay; Rezulin. $C_{24}H_{27}NO_5S$; mol wt 441.54. C 65.28%, H 6.16%, N 3.17%, O 18.12%, S 7.26%. Oral hypoglycemic agent which improves insulin sensitivity and decreases hepatic glucose production. Prepn: **JP Kokai 85 51189**; T. Yoshioka *et al.*, **US 4572912** (1985, 1986 both to Sankyo); T. Yoshioka *et al.*, *J. Med. Chem.* **32**, 421 (1989). Mechanism of action studies: T. P. Ciaraldi *et al.*, *Metabolism* **39**, 1056 (1990); M. Kellerer *et al.*, *Diabetes* **43**, 447 (1994). Clinical evaluation: T. Kuzuya *et al.*, *Diabetes Res. Clin. Pract.* **11**, 147 (1991). Clinical metabolic effects: S. L. Suter *et al.*, *Diabetes Care* **15**, 193 (1992).

Crystals from benzene-acetone, mp 184-186°.

THERAP CAT: Antidiabetic.

9770. Troleandomycin. [2751-09-9] Oleandomycin triacetate ester; triacetyloleandomycin; NSC-108166; Cyclamycin; Wytrion; Evramycin; TAO; Triocetin. $C_{41}H_{67}NO_{15}$; mol wt 813.97. C 60.50%, H 8.30%, N 1.72%, O 29.48%. Semi-synthetic macrolide antibiotic. Prepd from oleandomycin: Celmer *et al.*, *Antibiot. Annu.* **1957-1958**, p 476; **GB 877730** (1958 to Pfizer); M. Khristov, N. Petkov, *Farmatsiya (Sofia)* **27**, 1 (1977), *C.A.* **90**, 23458c (1979). *Review:* S. Ross, *Antimicrobial Therapy*, B. M. Kagan, Ed. (Saunders, Philadelphia, 1970) pp 134-144.

$$R = \text{—}\overset{\displaystyle O}{\overset{\|}{C}}\text{—}CH_3$$

Crystals from isopropanol. Practically tasteless. Dec 176°. $[\alpha]_D^{25} -23°$ (methanol). pKa 6.6. Soly in water <0.1 g/100 ml.

THERAP CAT: Antibacterial.

9771. Tromantadine. [53783-83-8] 2-[2-(Dimethylamino)ethoxy]-N-tricyclo[3.3.1.1^{3,7}]dec-1-ylacetamide; N-1-adamantyl-N-[2-(dimethylamino)ethoxy]acetamide; 1-(dimethylaminoethoxyacetamido)adamantane. $C_{16}H_{28}N_2O_2$; mol wt 280.41. C 68.53%, H 10.06%, N 9.99%, O 11.41%. Prepn: Scherm, Peteri, **DE 1941218** (1971 to Merz), *C.A.* **74**, 99516k (1971); May, Peteri, *Arzneim.-Forsch.* **23**, 718 (1973). Chemistry and toxicology: Peteri, Sterner, *ibid.* 577.

Hydrochloride. [41544-24-5] D-41; Viru-Merz; Viruserol. $C_{16}H_{28}N_2O_2 \cdot HCl$; mol wt 316.87. Crystals, mp 157-158°. LD_{50} orally in rats: 630 mg/kg; i.v. in mice: 71.0 mg/kg (Peteri, Sterner).

THERAP CAT: Antiviral.

9772. Tromethamine. [77-86-1] 2-Amino-2-hydroxymethyl-1,3-propanediol; trimethylol aminomethane; tris(hydroxymethyl)aminomethane; trisamine; tris buffer; trometamol; tromethane; TRIS; THAM; Trizma. $C_4H_{11}NO_3$; mol wt 121.14. C 39.66%, H 9.15%, N 11.56%, O 39.62%. May be prepd by reduction or catalytic hydrogenation of the corresp nitro compd. Prepn of similar compds: Hass, Vanderbilt, **US 2174242** (1940); Johnson, Degering, *J. Org. Chem.* **8**, 7 (1943); Boileau, *Mem. Poudres* **35**, Annexe 7-76 (1953). Prepn by electrolytic reduction: McMillan,

US 2485982 (1949 to Comm. Solvents Corp.). Titrimetric standard: Whitehead, *J. Chem. Educ.* **36**, 297 (1959). Monograph: *Ann. N.Y. Acad. Sci.* **92**, Art. 2, pp 333-812 (June 17, 1961). Crystal structure: R. Rudman *et al.*, *Science* **200**, 531 (1978). GC determn in plasma: H. Hulshoff, H. B. Kostenbauder, *J. Chromatogr.* **145**, 155 (1978). Pharmacokinetics in rabbits: H. Brasch, H. Iven, *Arch. Int. Pharmacodyn.* **254**, 4 (1981). Use as a biological buffer: R. A. Durst, B. R. Staples, *Clin. Chem.* **18** 206 (1972); S. P. Fling, D. S. Gregerson, *Anal. Biochem.* **155**, 83 (1986); T. Higa, D. M. Desiderio, *ibid.* **173**, 463 (1988). Interaction with hydroxyl radicals: M. Hicks, J. M. Gebicki, *FEBS Lett.* **199**, 92 (1986). Review of clinical experience in treatment of acidemia: G. G. Nahas *et al.*, *Drugs* **55**, 191-224 (1998).

Crystalline mass, mp 171-172°. bp_{10} 219-220°. Weak, monoacidic base: pKb (25°): 5.91. pKa (20°): 8.3. pKa (37°): 7.82. pH of 0.1 molar aq soln 10.4. Aq solns do not absorb CO_2 from the air. Soly at 25° (mg/ml) in water: 550; ethylene glycol: 79.1; methanol: 26; anhydr ethanol: 14.6; 95% ethanol: 22.0; DMF: 14; acetone: 2.0; ethyl acetate: 0.5; olive oil: 0.4; cyclohexane: 0.1; chloroform: 0.05; carbon tetrachloride: <0.05.

USE: In the synthesis of surface-active agents, vulcanization accelerators, pharmaceuticals. As emulsifying agent for cosmetic creams and lotions, mineral oil and paraffin wax emulsions, leather dressings, textile specialties, polishes, cleaning compds, so-called soluble oils. Absorbent for acidic gases. Biological buffer.

THERAP CAT: Alkalinizing agent.

9773. Tropacine. [6878-98-4] α-Phenylbenzeneacetic acid (3-*endo*)-8-methyl-8-azabicyclo[3.2.1]oct-3-yl ester; 1αH,5αH-tropan-3α-ol diphenylacetate; diphenylacetic acid 3α-tropanyl ester; 3α-tropanyl diphenylacetate; tropine diphenylacetate. $C_{22}H_{25}NO_2$; mol wt 335.44. C 78.77%, H 7.51%, N 4.18%, O 9.54%. Anticholinergic. Prepd from tropine and diphenylacetyl chloride: **CH 202181** (1939 to Ciba), *C.A.* **33**, 8922[8] (1939); Friess *et al.*, *Toxicol. Appl. Pharmacol.* **2**, 574 (1960).

Hydrochloride. Crystals from chloroform + ether, mp 217-218°.

THERAP CAT: Antiparkinsonian

9774. Tropacocaine. [537-26-8] *exo*-8-Methyl-8-azabicyclo[3.2.1]octan-3-ol benzoate (ester); 1αH,5αH-tropan-3β-ol benzoate; benzoylpseudotropeine; benzoyl-ψ-tropeine; pseudotropine benzoate; ψ-tropine benzoate; tropacaine. $C_{15}H_{19}NO_2$; mol wt 245.32. C 73.44%, H 7.81%, N 5.71%, O 13.04%. From Javanese coca leaves. Prepared by heating pseudotropine with water and benzoic anhydride: Wilstätter, *Ber.* **29**, 943 (1896). Stereochemistry: Beyerman *et al.*, *Rec. Trav. Chim.* **75**, 1445 (1956).

Plates, tablets, mp 49°. Distills *in vacuo* without dec. pK (15°) 4.72. pH of 0.06*M* soln 8.4. Freely sol in alc, ether, chloroform,

benzene, petr ether, dil acids; slightly sol in water. MLD i.v. in rats: 15-20 mg/kg, Hirschfelder, *Physiol. Rev.* **12**, 262 (1932).

Hydrochloride. $C_{15}H_{19}NO_2$·HCl. Strongly refractive prisms from alcohol, dec 283°. Sol in water, slightly in abs alc, practically insol in ether. Aq solns are stable to boiling water for ~20 minutes. pH of 0.1*M* soln 5.8.

9775. Tropaeolin O. [547-57-9] 4-[(2,4-Dihydroxyphenyl)-azo]benzenesulfonic acid monosodium salt; C.I. Acid Orange 6; sodium *p*-(2,4-dihydroxyphenylazo)benzenesulfonate; sodium azoresorcinolsulfanilate; C.I. Food Yellow 8; C.I. 14270; Resorcinol Yellow; Yellow T; Tropeolin O; Tropaeolin R; Chrysoine; Gold Yellow. $C_{12}H_9N_2NaO_4S$; mol wt 316.27. C 45.57%, H 2.87%, N 8.86%, Na 7.27%, O 25.29%, S 10.14%. Prepd from resorcinol and a *p*-sulfobenzenediazonium salt, followed by reaction with an inorganic sodium salt: Sisley, *Bull. Soc. Chim. Fr.* [3] **25**, 869 (1901). *See also: Colour Index* vol. 4 (3rd ed., 1971) p 4064. Brief review: *H. J. Conn's Biological Stains*, R. D. Lillie, Ed. (Williams & Wilkins, Baltimore, 9th ed., 1977) p 106.

Brown powder. Sol in water with reddish-yellow color; sol in alcohol.

USE: As indicator. pH: yellow 11, orange-brown 12.7. Occasionally used as plasma stain.

9776. Tropaeolin OO. [554-73-4] 4-[[4-(Phenylamino)-phenyl]azo]benzenesulfonic acid monosodium salt; C.I. Acid Orange 5; *p*-[(*p*-anilinophenyl)azo]benzenesulfonic acid sodium salt; sodium *p*-[(*p*-anilinophenyl)azo]benzenesulfonate; Diphenylamine Orange; Orange GS; Orange N; Orange IV; Fast Yellow; Acid Yellow D; C.I. 13080. $C_{18}H_{14}N_3NaO_3S$; mol wt 375.38. C 57.59%, H 3.76%, N 11.19%, Na 6.12%, O 12.79%, S 8.54%. Prepd from diphenylamine and *p*-sulfobenzenediazonium chloride, followed by reaction with NaOH: Witt, *Ber.* **12**, 258 (1879); *Colour Index* vol. 4 (3rd ed., 1971) p 4045.

Orange-yellow scales or yellow powder. Sol in water.
USE: As indicator. pH: red 1.4 to yellow 2.6.

9777. Tropane. [529-17-9] 8-Methyl-8-azabicyclo[3.2.1]-octane; 1αH,5αH-tropane; 2,3-dihydro-8-methylnortropidine. C_8-$H_{15}N$; mol wt 125.21. C 76.74%, H 12.07%, N 11.19%. Structure and synthesis: Ladenburg, *Ber.* **16**, 1408 (1883); Merling, *Ber.* **25**, 3124 (1892); Willstätter, Iglauer, *Ber.* **30**, 721 (1897); **33**, 1170 (1900); *eidem, Ann.* **317**, 315, 350 (1901); Robinson, *J. Chem. Soc.* **111**, 762, 876 (1917); Hess, *Ber.* **51**, 1007 (1918); Schöpf, *Angew. Chem.* **50**, 779, 797 (1937); Ruggli, Maeder, *Helv. Chim. Acta* **27**, 436 (1944); Keagle, Hartung, *J. Am. Chem. Soc.* **68**, 1608 (1946).

Liquid; bp 163-169°; d_{15}^{15} 0.9259. Sparingly sol in water, the soly decreasing with an increase in temp. Tropane and water will mix provided the volume of tropane is in excess.

9778. Tropesin. [65189-78-8] 1-(4-Chlorobenzoyl)-5-methoxy-2-methyl-1*H*-indole-3-acetic acid 2-carboxy-2-phenylethyl ester; *d,l*-2-phenyl-3-[1-(4-chlorobenzoyl)-5-methoxy-2-methyl-indole-3-acetoxy]propionic acid; 1-*p*-chlorobenzoyl-5-methoxy-2-methyl-3-indolylacetic acid 2-phenyl-2-carboxyethyl ester; Repanidal. $C_{28}H_{24}ClNO_6$; mol wt 505.95. C 66.47%, H 4.78%, Cl 7.01%, N 2.77%, O 18.97%. Tropic acid ester of indomethacin, *q.v.* Prepn: L. Fisnerova *et al.*, **DE 2727629**; *eidem*, **US 4136194** (1978, 1979 both to Spofa). Clinical pharmacokinetics: I. Janku *et al.*, *Drugs Exp. Clin. Res.* **IX**, 407 (1983). Review of pharmacology and clinical experience: J. Grimová *et al.*, *Drugs Today* **27**, 391-400 (1991).

Crystals from nitromethane, mp 130-132°. Also reported as mp 127-129°; 128-130°. LD$_{50}$ in female mice, rats (mg/kg): 190, 140 orally (Fisnerova, 1979).

THERAP CAT: Anti-inflammatory; analgesic.

9779. Tropic Acid. [529-64-6] α-(Hydroxymethyl)benzene-acetic acid; 2-phenylhydracrylic acid; α-phenyl-β-hydroxypropionic acid; tropaic acid; tropeic acid. C$_9$H$_{10}$O$_3$; mol wt 166.17. C 65.05%, H 6.07%, O 28.88%. Degradation product of tropane alkaloids, esp atropine: Lossen, *Ann.* **133**, 351, 370 (1865). Resolution of isomers: McKenzie, Wood, *J. Chem. Soc.* **115**, 828 (1919). Absolute config of isomers: Fodor, Csepreghy, *ibid.* **1961**, 3222; Watson, Youngson, *J. Chem. Soc. Perkin Trans. 1* **1972**, 1597. Prepn: Sletzinger, Paulsen, **US 2390278** (1945 to Merck & Co.); Blicke, **US 2716650** (1955 to U. of Michigan); **DE 923426** (1955 to Sterling Drug). Biosynthetic studies: Louden, Leete, *J. Am. Chem. Soc.* **84**, 1510, 4507 (1962).

(±)-**Form.** Needles or plates from water or benzene, mp 118°. K at 25° = 7.5×10^{-5}. Absorption spectrum: Dobbie, Fox, *J. Chem. Soc.* **103**, 1194 (1913). 1 gram dissolves in 50 ml water; freely sol in boiling water; sol in alcohol, ether, slightly in benzene; practically insol in petr ether.

(+)-**Form.** mp 107°. [α]$_D^{20}$ +72° (c = 0.5 in water).
(−)-**Form.** mp 126-128°. [α]$_D^{20}$ −72° (c = 0.5 in water).

9780. Tropicamide. [1508-75-4] *N*-Ethyl-α-(hydroxymethyl)-*N*-(4-pyridinylmethyl)benzeneacetamide; *N*-ethyl-2-phenyl-*N*-(4-pyridylmethyl)hydracrylamide; *N*-ethyl-*N*-(γ-picolyl)tropamide; Mydriacyl; Mydriaticum. C$_{17}$H$_{20}$N$_2$O$_2$; mol wt 284.35. C 71.81%, H 7.09%, N 9.85%, O 11.25%. Ophthalmic anticholinergic. Prepn: Rey-Bellet, Spiegelberg, **US 2726245** (1955 to Hoffmann-La Roche). Comprehensive description: K. W. Blessel *et al.*, *Anal. Profiles Drug Subs.* **3**, 565-580 (1974).

Crystals, mp 96-97°. uv max (0.025 mg/ml in 0.1*N* HCl): 254 nm (ε 5.1×10^3).

THERAP CAT: Mydriatic.
THERAP CAT (VET): Mydriatic.

9781. Tropine. [120-29-6] *endo*-8-Methyl-8-azabicyclo-[3.2.1]octan-3-ol; 1αH,5αH-tropan-3α-ol; 2,3-dihydro-3α-hydroxy-8-methylnortropidine; 2,3-dihydro-3α-hydroxytropidine. C$_8$H$_{15}$-NO; mol wt 141.21. C 68.04%, H 10.71%, N 9.92%, O 11.33%. Prepd by reaction of tropidine and HBr, followed by hydrolysis and separation of isomers, tropine and pseudotropine: Ladenburg, *Ber.* **35**, 1159 (1902); by hydrogenation of tropinone in the presence of

Raney nickel: Van de Kamp, Sletzinger, **US 2366760** (1945 to Merck & Co.); Stoll *et al.*, **US 2746976** (1956 to Sandoz). Yield of tropine and pseudotropine under varying conditions of reduction: Beckett *et al.*, *Tetrahedron* **6**, 319 (1959). Separation of tropine and pseudotropine by gold salt formation: Ladenburg, *loc. cit.*; by fractional distillation under reduced pressure: Friess *et al.*, *Toxicol. Appl. Pharmacol.* **2**, 574 (1960). Stereochemistry: Beyerman *et al.*, *Rec. Trav. Chim.* **75**, 1445 (1956).

Hygroscopic plates from ether, mp 63°. bp 233°. pK at 15° = 3.80. pH of 0.05 molar soln 11.5. Freely sol in water and alcohol; sol in ether and chloroform.

Note: Esters of tropine are known as *tropeines*.

9782. Tropine Benzylate. [3736-36-5] *endo*-α-Hydroxy-α-phenylbenzeneacetic acid 8-methyl-8-azabicyclo[3.2.1]oct-3-yl ester; 1αH,5αH-tropan-3α-ol benzilate; benzilic acid 3α-tropanyl ester; glykin; BAT; BTE; BETE. C$_{22}$H$_{25}$NO$_3$; mol wt 351.44. C 75.19%, H 7.17%, N 3.99%, O 13.66%. Prepn: Hromatka *et al.*, *Monatsh. Chem.* **83**, 1321 (1952).

Prisms from ether or benzene, mp 152-153°.
Hydrochloride. C$_{22}$H$_{25}$NO$_3$.HCl. mp 239-240°.

9783. Tropisetron. [89565-68-4] 1*H*-Indole-3-carboxylic acid (3-*endo*)-8-methyl-8-azabicyclo[3.2.1]oct-3-yl ester; 3α-tropanyl-1*H*-indole-3-carboxylic acid ester; 1αH,5αH-tropan-3α-yl indole-3-carboxylate; ICS-205-930. C$_{17}$H$_{20}$N$_2$O$_2$; mol wt 284.35. C 71.81%, H 7.09%, N 9.85%, O 11.25%. Specific serotonin (5-HT$_3$) receptor antagonist. Prepn: P. Donatsch *et al.*, **DE 3322574** (1983 to Sandoz); *idem et al.*, **US 4789673** (1988). Pharmacology: B. P. Richardson *et al.*, *Nature* **316**, 126 (1985); F. M. Williams *et al.*, *J. Cardiovasc. Pharmacol.* **7**, 550 (1985). Receptor binding studies: C. Waeber *et al.*, *Neuroscience* **31**, 393 (1989). Clinical pharmacokinetics: V. Fischer *et al.*, *Drug Metab. Dispos.* **20**, 603 (1992). Series of articles on antiemetic efficacy in chemotherapy and radiotherapy: *Drugs* **43**, Suppl. 3, 6-39 (1992). Review of pharmacology: C. Seynaeve *et al.*, *Anti-Cancer Drugs* **2**, 343-355 (1991); and toxicology: K. Kutz, *Ann. Oncol.* **4**, Suppl. 3, S15-S18 (1993).

mp 201-202° (from methylene chloride/ethyl acetate).
Monohydrochloride. [105826-92-4] Navoban; Novaban. C$_{17}$H$_{20}$N$_2$O$_2$.HCl; mol wt 320.81. mp 283-285° (dec).

THERAP CAT: Antiemetic.

9784. Tropomyosins. Fibrous proteins involved in the regulation of muscle relaxation. They are present in all forms of striated and smooth muscles and probably in nonmuscle cells as well. Native tropomyosin consisting of two proteins, tropomyosin and *troponin*, is the Ca^{2+}-sensitive regulatory protein that controls the interaction between actin and myosin necessary for the production of force in muscle. In all skeletal tissues, there are two forms of tropomyosin chains, designated α and β. Their ratio depends on the muscle source. Troponin consists of three subunits, troponin T (the tropomyosin binding subunit), troponin I (the actomyosin ATPase inhibitory subunit) and troponin C (the Ca^{2+}-binding subunit). All three subunits, in addition to tropomyosin, are responsible for the native tropomyosin activity. Isoln of tropomyosin from skeletal muscle and cardiac muscle: K. Bailey, *Nature* **157**, 368 (1946); *idem, Biochem. J.* **43**, 271 (1948). Structure studies: R. S. Hodges, L. B. Smillie, *Biochem. Biophys. Res. Commun.* **41**, 987 (1970). Amino acid sequence studies: J. Sodek *et al., Proc. Natl. Acad. Sci. USA* **69**, 3800 (1972). X-ray crystal structure of troponin C: M. Sundaralingam *et al., Science* **227**, 945 (1985). *Reviews:* C. E. Bodwell, K. Laki, in *Contractile Proteins and Muscle*, K. Laki, Ed. (Dekker, New York, 1971); W. F. Harrington in *The Proteins* vol. 4, H. Neurath, R. L. Hill, Eds. (Academic Press, New York, 1979) pp 317-327. Comprehensive review of isolation, preparation, identification and role in the contractile process: "Structural and Contractile Proteins" in *Methods Enzymol.* **85**, Part B, 1-774 (1982).

9785. Tropylium Bromide. [5376-03-4] Cycloheptatrienylium bromide; cycloheptatrienocarbonium bromide. C_7H_7Br; mol wt 171.03. C 49.16%, H 4.13%, Br 46.72%. Prepd by bromination of 1,3,5-cycloheptatriene in carbon tetrachloride, followed by removal of the CCl_4 and heating the residue *in vacuo* for several days: von Doering, Knox, *J. Am. Chem. Soc.* **79**, 352 (1957); King, Stone, *Inorg. Synth.* **7**, 99 (1963).

Yellow prisms from ethanol, mp 203°. Freely sol in water. Practically insol in ether.

9786. Trospium Chloride. [10405-02-4] $(1\alpha,3\beta,5\alpha)$-3-[(Hydroxydiphenylacetyl)oxy]spiro[8-azoniabicyclo[3.2.1]octane-8,1'-pyrrolidinium] chloride; 3α-hydroxyspiro[1αH,5αH-nortropane-8,1'-pyrrolidinium] chloride benzilate; azoniaspiro(3α-benziloyloxynortropane-8,1'-pyrrolidine) chloride; azoniaspiro(3α-diphenylglycoloyloxynortropan-8,1'-pyrrolidine) chloride; 3α-benziloyloxyspiro(nortropane-8,1'-pyrrolidinium) chloride; Regurin; Relaspium; Sanctura; Spasmex; Spasmolyt. $C_{25}H_{30}ClNO_3$; mol wt 427.96. C 70.16%, H 7.07%, Cl 8.28%, N 3.27%, O 11.22%. Tropine derivative with anticholinergic activity. Prepn: **NL 6402155**; R. Pfleger *et al., US 3480626* (1964, 1969 both to Pfleger); H. Bertholdt *et al., Arzneim.-Forsch.* **17**, 719 (1967). Pharmacology and toxicology in animals: H. Antweiler *et al., ibid.* **16**, 1581 (1966). Inhibition of gastric motility and acid secretion in humans: G. Lux, P. Frühmorgen, *Fortschr. Med.* **96**, 2113 (1978). Fluorimetric determn in plasma and urine: G. Schladitz-Keil *et al., J. Chromatogr.* **345**, 99 (1985). Bioavailability: *eidem, Arzneim.-Forsch.* **36**, 984 (1986). Clinical trial in bladder hyper-reflexia: H. Madersbacher *et al., Br. J. Urol.* **75**, 452 (1995). Review in overactive bladder: N. R. Zinner, *Expert Opin. Pharmacother.* **6**, 1409-1420 (2005).

Crystals from ethanol-ether, mp 255-257° (dec). Soly in water: ~1 g/2 ml. LD_{50} in mice (mg/kg): 12.3 i.v. (Antweiler).

THERAP CAT: Antispasmodic; in treatment of urinary incontinence.

9787. Trovafloxacin. [147059-72-1] $(1\alpha,5\alpha,6\alpha)$-7-(6-Amino-3-azabicyclo[3.1.0]hex-3-yl)-1-(2,4-difluorophenyl)-6-fluoro-1,4-dihydro-4-oxo-1,8-naphthyridine-3-carboxylic acid; CP-99219. $C_{20}H_{15}F_3N_4O_3$; mol wt 416.35. C 57.70%, H 3.63%, F 13.69%, N 13.46%, O 11.53%. Fluorinated quinolone antibacterial. Prepn: K. E. Brighty, **US 5164402** (1992 to Pfizer). Voltammetric determn in urine and serum: J. L. Vílchez *et al., J. Pharm. Biomed. Anal.* **31**, 465 (2003). Antibacterial spectrum *in vitro*: H. C. Neu, N.-X. Chin, *Antimicrob. Agents Chemother.* **38**, 2615 (1994). Clinical pharmacokinetics: R. Teng *et al., J. Antimicrob. Chemother.* **36**, 385 (1995). Evaluation in gonorrhea: E. W. Hook *et al., Antimicrob. Agents Chemother.* **40**, 1720 (1996). Mechanism of hepatotoxicity: M. J. Liguori *et al., Hepatology* **41**, 177 (2005).

Hydrochloride. [146961-34-4] $C_{20}H_{15}F_3N_4O_3 \cdot HCl$. Pale yellow crystals from acetonitrile/methanol, mp 246°.

Methanesulfonate. [147059-75-4] Trovafloxacin mesylate; CP-99219-27; Trovan. $C_{20}H_{15}F_3N_4O_3 \cdot CH_3SO_3H$; mol wt 512.46.

THERAP CAT: Antibacterial.

9788. Troxacitabine. [145918-75-8] 4-Amino-1-[(2S,4S)-2-(hydroxymethyl)-1,3-dioxolan-4-yl]-2(1H)-pyrimidinone; $(-)$-2'-deoxy-3'-oxacytidine; β-L-$(-)$ dioxolane cytidine; $(-)$-(2S,4S)-1-[2-(hydroxymethyl)-1,3-dioxolan-4-yl]cytosine; L-OddC; $(-)$-BCH-204; BCH-4556; Troxatyl. $C_8H_{11}N_3O_4$; mol wt 213.19. C 45.07%, H 5.20%, N 19.71%, O 30.02%. Synthetic nucleoside analog with stereochemically unnatural β-L configuration. Prepn: Y.-C. Cheng *et al., WO 9218517* (1992 to Yale Univ. and Univ. Georgia Res. Found.); B. R. Belleau *et al., Tetrahedron Lett.* **33**, 6949 (1992); H. O. Kim *et al., J. Med. Chem.* **36**, 519 (1993). Resolution of enantiomers: M. P. DiMarco *et al., J. Chromatogr.* **645**, 107 (1993). Structure activity study: T. S. Mansour *et al., Nucleosid. Nucleotid.* **14**, 627 (1995). Clinical pharmacokinetics: J. S. deBono *et al. J. Clin. Oncol.* **20**, 96 (2001). Population pharmacokinetics: C. K. K. Lee *et al., Clin. Cancer Res.* **12**, 2158 (2006). Clinical evaluation in refractory leukemia: F. J. Giles *et al., ibid.* **20**, 656 (2002); in imatinib-resistant chronic myelogenous leukemia: *idem et al., Leukem. Res.* **27**, 1091 (2003); in pancreatic cancer: R. Lapointe *et al., Ann. Oncol.* **16**, 289 (2005). Review of pharmacology and clinical development: *idem, Expert Rev. Anticancer Ther.* **2**, 261-266 (2002); G. Ecker, Curr. Opin. Invest. Drugs **3**, 1533-1538 (2002).

mp 176-177°. $[\alpha]_D^{25}$ $-38.33°$ (c = 0.43 in MeOH). uv max (water): 270.0 (pH 7), 278.0 (pH 2), 269.0 (pH 11) (ε 7770, 11970, 8380).

THERAP CAT: Antineoplastic.

9789. Troxerutin. [7085-55-4] 2-[3,4-Bis(2-hydroxyeth-oxy)phenyl]-3-[[6-*O*-(6-deoxy-α-L-mannopyranosyl)-β-D-gluco-pyranosyl]oxy]-5-hydroxy-7-(2-hydroxyethoxy)-4*H*-1-benzopyran-4-one; 7,3′,4′-tris[*O*-(2-hydroxyethyl)]rutin; trioxyethylrutin; tri(hy-droxyethyl)rutoside; Posorutin; Ruven; Vastribil; Veinamitol; Ven-iten. $C_{33}H_{42}O_{19}$; mol wt 742.68. C 53.37%, H 5.70%, O 40.93%. The principal component of a mixture, the *O*-(β-hydroxyethyl)-rutosides, which also contains mono-, di-, tetra- and other trihy-droxyethyl derivs of rutin, *q.v.* The mixture is prepd by the hy-droxyethylation of the phenolic groups of rutin with glycochlorohy-drin in alk medium: J. Favre, **CH 349614** (1957); *see also* **GB 833174** (1960 to Zyma), *C.A.* **54,** 21135i (1960). Isolation and identification of major components of the mixture: P. Courbat *et al., Helv. Chim. Acta* **49,** 1203, 1420 (1966). Prepn of troxerutin: P. J. Courbat, **US 3420815** (1969 to Zyma). Metabolism in man: A. M. Hackett *et al., Arzneim.-Forsch.* **26,** 925 (1976).

Yellow powder, mp 181°. Sol in water, glycerol, propylene glycol. Practically insol in cold ethanol, methanol (forms alcohol-ate), ether, benzene, chloroform.

O-(β-Hydroxyethyl)rutinosides (mixture). [55965-63-4] HR; Paroven; Relvene; Varemoid; Venoruton. Yellow powder, mp 156°. Sol in water, methanol, glycerol, propylene glycol. Practically insol in cold ethanol (forms alcoholate), ether, benzene, chloroform.

THERAP CAT: Treatment of venous disorders.

9790. Troxipide. [99777-81-8] 3,4,5-Trimethoxy-*N*-3-piperidinylbenzamide; 3-(3,4,5-trimethoxybenzamido)piperidine; KU-54; Aplace. $C_{15}H_{22}N_2O_4$; mol wt 294.35. C 61.21%, H 7.53%, N 9.52%, O 21.74%. Prepn: **BE 736840**; T. Irikura *et al.,* **US 3647805** (1969, 1972 both to Kyorin). Anti-ulcer activity: T. Irikura, K. Kasuga, *J. Med. Chem.* **14,** 357 (1971). Pharmaco-kinetics in man: T. Irikura *et al., Iyakuhin Kenkyu* **12,** 971 (1981), *C.A.* **96,** 79377s (1982). Effect on gastric mucosa in rats: Y. Abe *et al., Nippon Yakurigaku Zasshi* **83,** 317 (1984), *C.A.* **101,** 456g (1984); on glucosamine synthetase: Y. Abe *et al., Oyo Yakuri* **27,** 521 (1984), *C.A.* **101,** 17001c (1984). Metabolism in rats: K. Tagaki *et al., ibid.* 1151, *C.A.* **101,** 103555t (1984); K. Tagaki, K. Endo, *ibid.* 1167, *C.A.* **101,** 103556u (1984). Toxicity: T. Irikura *et al., Kiso to Rinsho* **12,** 3422 (1978).

Needles from acetonitrile, mp 179-181.5°. Sol in ethanol. LD_{50} in male, female rats, male, female mice (mg/kg): 500, 2100, 2200, 2000 orally; >4150, >4150, 1600, 1550 s.c.; 340, 340, 300, 305 i.p. (Irikura, 1978).

Hydrochloride hemihydrate. $C_{15}H_{22}N_2O_4 \cdot HCl \cdot \frac{1}{2}H_2O$. Needles from acetonitrile, mp 206-209°. Sol in ethanol.

THERAP CAT: Antiulcerative.

9791. Truxillic Acid. [4462-95-7] 2,4-Diphenyl-1,3-cyclo-butanedicarboxylic acid. $C_{18}H_{16}O_4$; mol wt 296.32. C 72.96%, H 5.44%, O 21.60%. Cinnamic acid polymers obtained from the minor alkaloids of cocaine: Liebermann, *Ber.* **21,** 2342 (1888). Five stereoisomers have been obtained: α-, γ-, ε-, *peri*- and *epi*-isomers. Stereochemical configurations: Stoermer, Bacher, *Ber.* **57B,** 15-23 (1924).

	a	b	c	d	e	f
α-Isomer	COOH	H	H	C_6H_5	H	COOH
γ-Isomer	COOH	H	H	C_6H_5	COOH	H
ε-Isomer	H	COOH	C_6H_5	H	H	COOH
peri-Isomer	COOH	H	C_6H_5	H	COOH	H
epi-Isomer	COOH	H	C_6H_5	H	H	COOH

α-Isomer. γ-Isatropaic acid; cocaic acid. Prepd by irradiation of cinnamic acid in water: White, Dunathan, *J. Am. Chem. Soc.* **78,** 6055 (1956). Crystals from acetic acid, mp 284-285°. Sparingly sol in boiling water, in ether, benzene, carbon disulfide; sol in hot glacial acetic acid, hot alc; sparingly sol in acetone.

γ-Isomer. ε-Isatropaic acid. γ-Truxillic anhydride, obtained by heating α-truxillic acid with acetic anhydride and sodium acetate, was heated with alkali and the free acid pptd with HCl: Lieber-mann, *Ber.* **22,** 124 (1889). Needles from dil alc, mp 228°. Very slightly sol in hot water; sol in ether.

ε-Isomer. β-Cocaic acid. Prepd by fusion of α-truxillic acid with KOH: Hesse, *Ann.* **271,** 180 (1892). Needles from ether, mp 192°. Freely sol in glacial acetic acid, abs alcohol, chloroform; less sol in benzene. Practically insol in ligroin.

peri-Isomer. η-Truxillic acid. Prepn: γ-Truxillic anhydride heated at low pressure forms the *peri*-anhydride, converted to the acid by warming with alcoholic KOH: Stoermer, Bacher, *loc. cit.* Crystals from benzene + ligroin, mp 266° (effervescence). Soluble in alcohol. Practically insol in ether, benzene.

epi-Isomer. Prepd by boiling *peri*-truxillic acid with excess 10% NaOH: Stoermer, Bacher, *loc. cit.* Crystals from dil alc, mp 285-287°. By melting or heating with acetic anhydride in a tube, ε-isomer forms. Practically insol in ether, benzene.

9792. Trypan Blue. [72-57-1] 3,3′-[(3,3′-Dimethyl[1,1′-bi-phenyl]-4,4′-diyl)bis(azo)]bis[5-amino-4-hydroxy-2,7-naphthalene-disulfonic acid] tetrasodium salt; C.I. Direct Blue 14; C.I. 23850; 3,3′-[(3,3′-dimethyl-4,4′-biphenylene)bis(azo)]bis(5-amino-4-hy-droxy-2,7-naphthalenedisulfonic acid) tetrasodium salt; tetrasodium 3,3′-[(3,3′-dimethyl-4,4′-biphenylene)bis(azo)]bis(5-amino-4-hy-droxy-2,7-naphthalenedisulfonate); sodium ditolyl-diazobis-8-ami-no-1-naphthol-3,6-disulfonate; Benzamine Blue; Diamine Blue; Benzo Blue; Congo Blue; Dianil Blue; Naphthylamine Blue; Niag-ara Blue. $C_{34}H_{24}N_6Na_4O_{14}S_4$; mol wt 960.81. C 42.50%, H 2.52%, N 8.75%, Na 9.57%, O 23.31%, S 13.35%. Prepd by coupling diazotized *o*-tolidine with 5-amino-4-hydroxy-2,7-naph-thalenedisulfonic acid in sodium carbonate soln: Lewers, Lowy, *Ind. Eng. Chem.* **17,** 1289-1290 (1925); *Colour Index* vol. 4 (3rd ed., 1971) p 4198. Toxicity study: Anderson *et al., Proc. Soc. Exp. Biol. Med.* **31,** 825 (1934). Review of teratogenicity studies: R. L. Cahen, *Clin. Pharmacol. Ther.* **5,** 480 (1964).

Bluish-gray powder. Sol in water forming a deep blue soln with violet tinge. Almost insol in alcohol. LD_{100} i.v. in rats: 300 mg/kg (Anderson).

USE: Biological stain.

9793. Trypan Red. [574-64-1] 4,4′-[(3-Sulfo[1,1′-biphen-yl]-4,4′-diyl)bis(azo)]bis[3-amino-2,7-naphthalenedisulfonic acid] pentasodium salt; 4,4′-[(3-sulfo-4,4′-biphenylene)bis(azo)]bis(3-amino-2,7-naphthalenedisulfonic acid) pentasodium salt; pentaso-dium 4,4′-[(3-sulfo-4,4′-biphenylene)bis(azo)]bis(3-amino-2,7-naphthalenedisulfonate); C.I. 22850. $C_{32}H_{19}N_6Na_5O_{15}S_5$; mol wt 1002.80. C 38.33%, H 1.91%, N 8.38%, Na 11.46%, O 23.93%, S 15.99%. Prepd by coupling diazotized 4,4'-diaminobiphenyl-3-sulfonic acid with sodium 2-amino-3,6-naphthalenedisulfonate: Krauss, *J. Am. Chem. Soc.* **36**, 961 (1914); *Colour Index* **vol. 4** (3rd ed., 1971) p 4181.

Reddish-brown powder. Sol in water. Practically insol in alcohol.

USE: Biological stain.

THERAP CAT: Antiprotozoal (Trypanosoma).

THERAP CAT (VET): Has been used as a trypanocide.

9794. Tryparsamide. [554-72-3] [4-[(2-Amino-2-oxoethyl)amino]phenyl]arsonic acid monosodium salt; *N*-(carbamoylmethyl)arsanilic acid monosodium salt; monosodium *N*-phenylglycinamide-*p*-arsonate; Glyphenarsine; Tryparsone; Tryponarsyl; Trypothane. $C_8H_{10}AsN_2NaO_4$; mol wt 296.09. C 32.45%, H 3.40%, As 25.30%, N 9.46%, Na 7.76%, O 21.61%. Prepd by heating a soln of arsanilic acid in aq NaOH, Na_2CO_3 and chloroacetamide: Jacobs, Heidelberger, *J. Am. Chem. Soc.* **41**, 1590 (1919); *Org. Synth.* **8**, 100 (1928). US 1280119; US 1280124; US 1280126 (1918); US 2465308 (1949).

Hemihydrate. Platelets, slowly affected by light, stable to air. One gram dissolves in about 2 ml water. Slightly sol in alcohol. Insol in ether, chloroform. pH of 1:20 aq soln 6.5. *Keep tryparsamide in tight containers, preferably at a temp not above 20° and protected from light.*

THERAP CAT: Antiprotozoal (Trypanosoma).

9795. Trypsin. [9002-07-7] Parenzymol; Trypure. Mol wt 24,000. Proteolytic enzyme formed in the small intestine by the action of a peptidase, enterokinase, on the pancreatic cell product, trypsinogen. Acts on lysyl and arginyl bonds of peptide chains and hydrolyzes even esters and amides. *Reviews:* Desnuelle, "Trypsin" in *The Enzymes* **vol. 4**, P. D. Boyer *et al.,* Eds. (Academic Press, New York, 2nd ed., 1960) pp 119-132; Keil, *ibid.* **vol. 3** (3rd ed., 1971) pp 250-275; Inagami, "Trypsin" in *Proteins, Structure and Function* **vol. 1**, M. Funatsu *et al.,* Eds. (Kodansha, Tokyo, Wiley, New York, 1972) pp 1-83.

Yellow to grayish-yellow powder or crystals. Stable indefinitely in dry form at room temp. Sol in water. Practically insol in alcohol or glycerol. Readily sol in Sorensen's sodium phosphate buffer soln. Acts optimally at pH values between 7 and 9. Solns lose 75% of their potency within 3 hrs at room temp. Prepn of stabilized trypsin compositions contg partially hydrolyzed gelatin: Sullivan, Martin, US 2930736 (1960 to National Drug).

THERAP CAT: Enzyme (proteolytic).

THERAP CAT (VET): Enzyme (proteolytic).

9796. Tryptamine. [61-54-1] 1*H*-Indole-3-ethanamine; 3-(2-aminoethyl)indole; 2-(3-indolyl)ethylamine. $C_{10}H_{12}N_2$; mol wt 160.22. C 74.96%, H 7.55%, N 17.48%. Occurs in plants. Synthesis starting from nitroethylene and indole: Noland, Hartman, *J. Am. Chem. Soc.* **76**, 3227 (1954). Alternate routes: Thesing, Schulde, *Ber.* **85**, 324 (1952); Jackson, Smith, *J. Chem. Soc.* **1965**, 3498; Tacconi, *Farmaco Ed. Sci.* **20**, 902 (1965); S. Takano *et al., Heterocycles* **6**, 1167 (1977); I. Fleming, M. Woolias, *J. Chem. Soc. Perkin Trans. 1* **1979**, 829. X-ray structure determn: Wakahara *et al., Tetrahedron Lett.* **1970**, 4999. *Review* of tryptamine syntheses:

J. E. Saxton in R. H. F. Manske, *The Alkaloids* **vol. VIII** (1965) pp 8-10.

Needles from petr ether, mp 118°. uv max (ethanol): 222, 282, 290 nm (log ε 4.56, 3.78, 3.71). Sol in ethanol, acetone. Practically insol in water, ether, benzene, chloroform.

Hydrochloride. $C_{10}H_{12}N_2$.HCl. Needles from ethanol + ethyl acetate, mp 248°. uv max (95% ethanol): 221, 275, 281, 290 nm (log ε 4.52, 3.73, 3.75, 3.69).

9797. Tryptophan. [73-22-3] L-Tryptophan; Trp; W; (*S*)-α-amino-1*H*-indole-3-propanoic acid; *l*-α-aminoindole-3-propionic acid; *l*-α-amino-3-indolepropionic acid; 2-amino-3-indolylpropanoic acid; *l*-β-3-indolylalanine; Ardeytropin; Kalma; Optimax; Pacitron; Sedanoct; Trofan; Tryptan. $C_{11}H_{12}N_2O_2$; mol wt 204.23. C 64.69%, H 5.92%, N 13.72%, O 15.67%. An essential amino acid for human development; precursor of serotonin, *q.v.* Isoln from casein: F. G. Hopkins, S. W. Cole, *J. Physiol.* **27**, 418 (1902). Structure: A. Ellinger, *Ber.* **39**, 2515 (1906); A. Ellinger, A. C. Flamand, *Ber.* **40**, 3029 (1907). Early chemistry and biochemistry: *Amino Acids and Proteins*, D. M. Greenberg, Ed. (Charles C. Thomas, Springfield, IL, 1951) 950 pp., *passim*; J. P. Greenstein, M. Winitz, *Chemistry of the Amino Acids* **vols 1-3** (John Wiley and Sons, Inc., New York, 1961) pp. 2316-2347, *passim*. Intrinsic fluorescent/phosphorescent moiety in proteins; used in characterizing structure and conformational changes: E. A. Burstein *et al., Photochem. Photobiol.* **18**, 263 (1973); C. Pokalsky *et al., J. Biol. Chem.* **270**, 3809 (1995); review of phosphorescence: S. Papp, J. M. Vanderkooi, *Photochem. Photobiol.* **49**, 775-784 (1989). Review of microbial production: T. K. Maiti, S. P. Chatterjee, *Hind. Antibiot. Bull.* **33**, 26-61 (1991). Review of biosynthesis: I. P. Crawford, G. V. Stauffer, *Annu. Rev. Biochem.* **49**, 163-195 (1980); of nutrition and metabolism: J. C. Peters. *Adv. Exp. Med. Biol.* **294**, 345-358 (1991). Review of use in depression: S. N. Young, *J. Psychiatr. Neurosci.* **16**, 241-246 (1991); in neuropsychiatric disorders: R. Sandyk, *Int. J. Neurosci.* **67**, 127-144 (1992). Review as toxic agent in eosinophilia-myalgia syndrome (EMS): D. S. Milburn, C. W. Myers, *DICP Ann. Pharmacother.* **25**, 1259 (1991); L. D. Kaufman, R. M. Philen, *Drug Saf.* **8**, 89-98 (1993).

Leaflets or plates from dil alc, dec 289° (rapid heating). $[\alpha]_D^{23}$ −31.5° (c = 1); $[\alpha]_D^{20}$ +2.4° (0.5*N* HCl); $[\alpha]_D^{20}$ +0.15° (c = 2.43 in 0.5*N* NaOH). pK_1 2.38; pK_2 9.39. Soly in water (g/l): 8.23 at 0°; 10.57 at 20°; 11.36 at 25°; 17.66 at 50°; 27.95 at 75°; 49.87 at 100°. Sol in hot alcohol, in alkali hydroxides. Insol in chloroform.

Hydrochloride. $C_{11}H_{12}N_2O_2$.HCl. Needles from methanol, dec 251°.

USE: Probe for studying protein structure and dynamics.

THERAP CAT: In treatment of depression, schizophrenia and other neuropsychiatric disorders.

9798. Tryptophol. [526-55-6] 3-Indoleethanol; 3-ω-hydroxyethylindole; 2-(3-indolyl)ethyl alcohol; 2-indolyl(3)-ethanol; β-indolylethyl alcohol; 3-β-hydroxyethylindole. $C_{10}H_{11}NO$; mol wt 161.20. C 74.51%, H 6.88%, N 8.69%, O 9.93%. Prepd by treatment of indolemagnesium bromide with ethylene oxide: Oddo, Cambieri, *Gazz. Chim. Ital.* **60**, 19 (1939); Snyder, Pilgrim, *J. Am. Chem. Soc.* **70**, 1962 (1948); by Bouveault-Blanc reduction of 3-indoleacetic ester: Jackson, *J. Biol. Chem.* **88**, 659 (1930); by treatment of indolemagnesium iodide with ethylene chlorohydrin: Majima, Hoshino, *Ber.* **58**, 2042 (1925); from gramine: Snyder, Pilgrim, *J. Am. Chem. Soc.* **70**, 3770 (1948). By lithium aluminum hydride reduction of methyl 3-indoleglycolate: Speeter, Anthony, **US 3076814** (1963 to Upjohn).

Platelets from ether + petr ether, mp 59°. $bp_{2.0}$ 174°. Slightly sol in water. Sol in methanol, ethanol, ether, acetone, chloroform, ethyl acetate, glacial acetic acid. Moderately sol in benzene, amyl alcohol, hot carbon disulfide. Sparingly sol in petr ether.

9799. TSQ. [109628-27-5] *N*-(6-Methoxy-8-quinolinyl)-4-methylbenzenesulfonamide; 6-methoxy-8-(*p*-toluenesulfonyl)aminoquinoline. $C_{17}H_{16}N_2O_3S$; mol wt 328.39. C 62.18%, H 4.91%, N 8.53%, O 14.62%, S 9.76%. Fluorescent membrane permeant probe selective for Zn^{2+} in the presence of Ca^{2+} and Mg^{2+}. Prepn: G. B. Bachman *et al., J. Org. Chem.* **15**, 1278 (1950). Atomic absoportion determn of Zn^{2+} to picomole levels in biological systems: J. G. Reyes *et al., Biol. Res.* **27**, 49 (1994). Structure/mechanism analysis: M. S. Nasir *et al., J. Biol. Inorg. Chem.* **4**, 775 (1999). Visualization of reactive zinc in the brain: C. J. Frederickson *et al., J. Neurosci. Methods* **20**, 91 (1987); in extracellular areas of CNS: A. A. Larson *et al., Pain* **86**, 177 (2000); in apoptosis: G. R. Sauer *et al., J. Cell Biochem.* **88**, 954 (2003).

White crystalline solid from ethanol, mp 133-134°.
USE: Determn of extracellular and intracellular Zn^{2+} levels in biological systems.

9800. Tsuduranine. [517-97-5] (6a*R*)-5,6,6a,7-Tetrahydro-1,2-dimethoxy-4*H*-dibenzo[*de,g*]quinolin-10-ol; 1,2-dimethoxy-6aβ-noraporphin-10-ol; tuduranine. $C_{18}H_{19}NO_3$; mol wt 297.35. C 72.71%, H 6.44%, N 4.71%, O 16.14%. In sinomenine mother liquors. Isoln: Gotô, *Ann.* **521**, 175 (1935). Structure: Gotô, Shishido, *Ann.* **539**, 262 (1939). Synthesis of *dl*-form: Narayanaswami *et al., Indian J. Chem.* **7**, 945 (1969).

Difficult to crystallize. Minute needles from slowly evaporating ether, mp about 125° (softens at 105°), or 204° depending on cryst form. $[\alpha]_D^{20}$ −127.5° (c = 0.855 in ethanol). Freely sol in the usual organic solvents.
Hydrochloride. Shiny scales from water, dec 286°. $[\alpha]_D^{15}$ −148° (c = 0.88 in water + methanol). Sparingly sol in water.

9801. T-2 Toxin. [21259-20-1] (3α,4β,8α)-12,13-Epoxytrichothec-9-ene-3,4,8,15-tetrol 4,15-diacetate 8-(3-methylbutanoate); 3α-hydroxy-4β,15-diacetoxy-8α-(3-methylbutyryloxy)-12,-13-epoxy-Δ⁹-tricothecene; 8α-(3-methylbutyryloxy)-4β,15-diacetoxyscirp-9-en-3α-ol; fusariotoxin T-2; insariotoxin; mycotoxin T-2; NSC-138780. $C_{24}H_{34}O_9$; mol wt 466.52. C 61.79%, H 7.35%, O 30.87%. *Tricothecene mycotoxin* isolated from *Fusarium tricinctum:* J. R. Bamburg *et al., Tetrahedron* **24**, 3329 (1968). Physicochemical data: A. E. Pohland *et al., Pure Appl. Chem.* **54**, 2119 (1982). Synthesis: M. C. Wani *et al., J. Org. Chem.* **52**, 3468 (1987). Biosynthetic study: F. Van Middlesworth *et al., J. Org. Chem.* **55**, 1237 (1990). Toxicology studies: W. F. O. Mar-

asas *et al., Toxicol. Appl. Pharmacol.* **15**, 471 (1969); H. B. Schiefer, D. S. Hancock, *ibid.* **76**, 464 (1984); D. A. Creasia *et al., Fundam. Appl. Toxicol.* **14**, 54 (1990). Implicated as a chemical warfare agent in Southeast Asia with nivalenol, *q.v.:* N. Wade, *Science* **214**, 34 (1981); R. T. Rosen, J. D. Rosen, *Biomed. Mass Spectrom.* **9**, 443 (1982). *Review: Developments in Food Science* **vol. 4**, Y. Ueno, Ed., entitled "Trichothecenes: Chemical, Biological and Toxicological Aspects" (Kodansha Ltd. and Elsevier, New York, 1983) 310 pp. Review of pharmacokinetics and metabolism: B. Yagen, M. Bialer, *Drug Metab. Rev.* **25**, 281-323 (1993).

Crystals, mp 151-152°. $[\alpha]_D^{26}$ +15° (c = 2.58 in ethanol). Freely sol in ethyl alcohol, ethyl acetate, chloroform, DMSO and other organic solvents; slightly sol in petroleum ether; very slightly sol in water. LD_{50} orally in female rats: 4.0 mg/kg (Marasas). LD_{50} (mg/kg) in mice: 5.2 i.p., 4.2 i.v.; in rats: 7.0 intragastric, 0.9-1.3 i.p., 0.9 i.v., 2.0 s.c.; in guinea pigs: 3.0-4.0 orally, 5.3 intragastric, 1.0 i.m., 1.0-2.0 i.v., 1.0-2.0 s.c.; in pigs: 5.0 orally, 3.0 i.v. (Yagen, Bailer).
Caution: May be highly irritating to skin and mucous membranes. Direct contact may cause extensive inflammation and tissue necrosis (Marasas). Topical exposure has lead to systemic toxicity and death in experimental animals (Schiefer, Hancock).

9802. Tuaminoheptane. [123-82-0] 2-Heptanamine; 1-methylhexylamine; 2-aminoheptane; Tuamine. $C_7H_{17}N$; mol wt 115.22. C 72.97%, H 14.87%, N 12.16%. $CH_3(CH_2)_4CH(CH_3)$-NH_2. α-Adrenergic agonist; topical vasoconstrictor. Prepd by heating 2-bromoheptane on steam bath with alcoholic ammonia in pressure tube: Clarke, *J. Am. Chem. Soc.* **21**, 1027 (1899); by hydrogenation of methyl amyl ketone and ammonia in the presence of Raney nickel: Norton *et al., J. Org. Chem.* **19**, 1054 (1954).
Volatile liq; d_4^{25} 0.7600-0.7660; bp_{760} 142-144°; n_D^{25} 1.4150-1.4200. Slightly soluble in water. pH of 1% aq soln 11.45. Freely sol in alcohol, ether, petr ether, chloroform, benzene.
Hydrochloride. $C_7H_{17}N.HCl$. Needles, mp 133°. Soluble in water. pH about 5.4.
Sulfate. [6411-75-2] Heptedrine. $2C_7H_{17}N.H_2SO_4$; mol wt 328.51. Crystals, readily sol in water. The pH of a 1% soln is about 5.4.
THERAP CAT: Nasal decongestant.

9803. Tuberactinomycin. [11075-36-8] Polypeptide antibiotic mixture produced by *Streptomyces griseoverticillatus* var *tuberacticus:* Nagata *et al., J. Antibiot.* **21**, 681 (1968); *eidem*, **US 3639580** (1972). Composed of tuberactinomycins A, B, N, and O. Structures: Yoshioka *et al., Tetrahedron Lett.* **1971**, 2043; Wakamiya *et al., Bull. Chem. Soc. Jpn.* **46**, 949 (1973); Wakamiya, Shiba, *J. Antibiot.* **27**, 900 (1974); *eidem*, **28**, 292 (1975). Total synthesis of tuberactinomycin O: T. Teshima *et al., Tetrahedron Lett.* **1976**, 2343; *eidem, J. Antibiot.* **30**, 1073 (1977). Chemical studies on tuberactinomycin: T. Wakamiya *et al., Heterocycles* **15**, 999 (1981).

Tuberactinomycins

	A	B	N	O
R_1	OH	OH	H	H
R_2	OH	OH	H	H

Hydrochloride. White solid, mp 244-264° (dec). $[\alpha]_D^{25}$ $-31.5°$ (c = 1 in water). uv maxima in water: 268 nm ($E_{1cm}^{1\%}$ 330); in 1N HCl: 268.5 nm ($E_{1cm}^{1\%}$ 313); in 0.1N NaOH: 285 nm ($E_{1cm}^{1\%}$ 206.5). Sol in water; weakly sol in methanol. Practically insol in ethanol, pyridine, ether, chloroform, dioxane; insol in acetone, benzene. pKa_1 7.2; pKa_2 10.3.

Tuberactinomycin A. [33103-21-8] 1-[(3R,4R)-4-Hydroxy-L-3,6-diaminohexanoic acid]viomycin. $C_{25}H_{43}N_{13}O_{11}$; mol wt 701.69.

Tuberactinomycin B *see* Viomycin.

Tuberactinomycin N *see* Enviomycin.

Tuberactinomycin O. [33137-73-4] (R)-6-[L-2-(2-Amino-1,-4,5,6-tetrahydro-4-pyrimidinyl)glycine]viomycin. $C_{25}H_{43}N_{13}O_9$; mol wt 669.69.

THERAP CAT: Antibacterial (tuberculostatic).

9804. Tubercidin. [69-33-0] 7-β-D-Ribofuranosyl-7H-pyrrolo[2,3-d]pyrimidin-4-amine; 4-amino-7-β-D-ribofuranosyl-7H-pyrrolo[2,3-d]pyrimidine; 7-deazaadenosine; sparsamycin A; U-10071. $C_{11}H_{14}N_4O_4$; mol wt 266.25. C 49.62%, H 5.30%, N 21.04%, O 24.04%. Antibiotic substance produced in the culture broth of *Streptomyces tubericidus*. Isoln: Anzai *et al., J. Antibiot.* **10A**, 201 (1957). Structure: Susuki, Marumo, *ibid.* **14A**, 34 (1961). Total synthesis: Tolman *et al., J. Am. Chem. Soc.* **91**, 2102 (1969). Crystal structure: Stroud, *Acta Crystallogr.* **29B**, 690 (1973); Abola, Sundaralingham, *ibid.* 697.

Needles from water, dec 247-248°. $[\alpha]_D^{17}$ $-67°$ (50% acetic acid). uv max (0.01N NaOH): 270 nm (ε 12,100). Sol in acidic and alkaline soln. One gram dissolves in 330 ml water, 200 ml methanol, 2000 ml ethanol. Practically insol in acetone, ethyl acetate, chloroform, benzene, petr ether. LD_{50} i.v. in mice: 45 mg/kg (Anzai).

9805. Tuberculin. A filtrate from triturated *Mycobacteria tuberculosis*. **Old Tuberculin** is the culture filtrate prepd by boiling and then filtering the *M. tuberculosis* culture. Purified protein derivative is a more refined tuberculin prepd by precipitating the culture filtrate with ammonium sulfate. Purification and dermal reactivity: F. B. Seibert, J. T. Glenn, *Am. Rev. Tuberc.* **44**, 9 (1941). Review of tuberculin skin test: G. W. Comstock *et al., Am. Rev. Respir. Dis.* **124**, 356 (1981).

Purified Protein Derivative. [92129-86-7] PPD; Aplisol; Tubersol.

THERAP CAT: Diagnostic aid (tuberculosis).

9806. Tuberin. [53643-53-1] N-[2-(4-Methoxyphenyl)ethenyl]formamide; N-trans-(p-methoxystyryl)formamide; N-formyl trans-p-methoxystyrylamine. $C_{10}H_{11}NO_2$; mol wt 177.20. C 67.78%, H 6.26%, N 7.90%, O 18.06%. Antitubercular antibiotic isolated from the broth filtrate of *Streptomyces amakusaensis*: Ohkuma *et al., J. Antibiot.* **15A**, 115 (1962); Sumiki *et al.,* **JP 64 7399** (1964 to Inst. Phys. & Chem. Res.), *C.A.* **62**, 8355g (1965). Structure and synthesis: Anzai *et al., J. Antibiot.* **15A**, 110, 117, 123 (1962). Alternate synthesis: I. J. Massey, I. T. Harrison, *Chem. Ind. (London)* **1977**, 920. Biosynthetic studies: K. M. Cable *et al., J. Chem. Soc. Perkin Trans. 1* **1987**, 1593.

Prisms from benzene, mp 132-133°. Stable in weakly acidic or weakly alkaline solns. uv max (methanol): 219, 285 nm ($E_{1cm}^{1\%}$ 870, 1710). Sol in the lower alcohols, ethyl acetate, acetone; moderately sol in carbon tetrachloride, chloroform; sparingly sol in water, benzene. Practically insol in petr ether.

Dihydrotuberin. $C_{10}H_{13}NO_2$. Liquid. n_D^{19} 1.5349.

9807. Tubocurarine Chloride. [57-94-3] 7',12'-Dihydroxy-6,6'-dimethoxy-2,2',2'-trimethyltubocuraranium chloride hydrochloride; dextrotubocurarine chloride; Jexin; Tubarine. $C_{37}H_{42}$-$Cl_2N_2O_6$; mol wt 681.65. C 65.19%, H 6.21%, Cl 10.40%, N 4.11%, O 14.08%. Arrow tip poison of South American Indians. Induces neuromuscular block through interactions with acetylcholine receptor. Identification as active principle from museum specimen: H. King, *J. Chem. Soc.* **1935**, 1381. Isoln from *Chondodendron tomentosum R. & P. Menispermaceae:* J. D. Dutcher, *J. Am. Chem. Soc.* **68**, 419 (1946). Purification and structure determn: idem, *ibid.* **74**, 2221 (1952). Revised structure: A. J. Everett *et al., Chem. Commun.* **1970**, 1020. Conformational analysis: B. S. Zhorov, N. B. Brovtsyna, *J. Membr. Biol.* **135**, 19 (1993); by NMR: Y. Fraenkel *et al., Biochemistry* **33**, 644 (1994). Binding characterization: N. Shaker *et al., J. Pharmacol. Exp. Ther.* **220**, 172 (1982); M. E. O'Leary *et al., Am. J. Physiol.* **266**, C648 (1994). Clinical pharmacokinetics and dynamics: D. M. Fisher, *Anesthesiology* **57**, 203 (1982). Toxicity data: H. Rosen *et al., Proc. Soc. Exp. Biol. Med.* **120**, 511 (1965). Clinical trial in prevention of muscle fasciculations: S. C. Harvey *et al., Anesth. Analg.* **87**, 719 (1998). Review of clinial use: G. S. Perotti, *J. Am. Assoc. Nurse Anesth.* **45**, 182-186 (1977). Comprehensive description: C. Papastephanou, *Anal. Profiles Drug Subs.* **7**, 477-500 (1978).

Hexagonal and pentagonal microplatelets from water; can exist in the form of various hydrates. The anhydrous material (dec 274-275°) takes up water in moist atm until it reaches the pentahydrate stage, dec ~270°. uv max (H₂O): 280 nm ($E_{1cm}^{1\%}$ 118). $[\alpha]_D^{20-25}$ +215° (c = 0.25-0.3 g/100 ml). Soly (25°): ~50 mg/ml water; but supersatd solns are formed readily. Presence of 1.0N HCl diminishes soly by about one-third. Rather sol in ethanol and methanol. Insol in pyridine, chloroform, benzene, acetone, ether. pK: 7.4. LD_{50} in mice, rats (mg/kg): 33.2, 27.8 orally in DMSO; 59.5, 36.9 orally in water (Rosen).

l-Form. Isoln of *l*-form from *Ch. tomentosum:* H. King, *Nature* **158**, 515 (1946); idem, *J. Chem. Soc.* **1947**, 936. Needles from water as pentahydrate, mp 268° (effervescence). $[\alpha]_D^{20}$ $-258°$ (c = 0.38) for the anhydr salt.

THERAP CAT: Neuromuscular blocking agent.

THERAP CAT (VET): Neuromuscular blocking agent.

9808. Tubulin. Colchicine-binding protein. The subunit protein of *microtubules*, which are large protein assemblies that play an important role in eukaryotic cell form determination and dynamics. Microtubules have the general structure of long hollow cylinders within which 13 protofilaments of tubulin are arranged in a parallel manner to the cylinder axis. The axial arrangement of the protofilaments with respect to each other results in the appearance of a helical structure, and the *in vitro* microtubule assembly process generally follows the laws of helical protein polymerization, cf. *Thermodynamics of the Polymerization of Proteins,* F. Oosawa, S. Asakura, Eds. (Academic Press, New York, 1975). Tubulin is an asymmetric dimer consisting of two nearly identical molecules, *α-tubulin* and *β-tubulin*, each having mol wts of about 55,000. The two molecules can be separated due to differences in electrophoretic mobilities. Isoln from mammalian brain using colchicine binding: R. C. Weisenberg *et al., Biochemistry* **7**, 4466 (1968). Discovery of conditions for microtubule assembly *in vitro*: R. C. Weisenberg, *Science* **177**, 1104 (1972); G. G. Borisy, J. B. Olmstead, *ibid.* 1196.

Prepn of large quantities of brain tubulin through successive assembly-disassembly cycles: M. L. Shelanski *et al., Proc. Natl. Acad. Sci. USA* **70**, 765 (1973). Purification of tubulin from rat pancreas: J. F. Launay *et al., Biochem. Biophys. Res. Commun.* **111**, 253 (1983). Structure of two human α-tubulin genes: C. Wilde *et al., Proc. Natl. Acad. Sci. USA* **79**, 96 (1982). Structure and arrangement of protofilaments in microtubules and tubulin sheets: B. F. McEwen, *Diss. Abstr. B* **43**, 942 (1982). Series of articles on prepn, isoln, and purification of tubulin from various sources: *Methods Enzymol.* **85**, Pt. B, 376-417 (1982). *Reviews:* J. A. Snyder, J. R. McIntosh, *Annu. Rev. Biochem.* **45**, 699-720 (1976); S. N. Timasheff, L. M. Grisham, *ibid.* **49**, 565-591 (1980); M. F. Carlier, *Mol. Cell. Biochem.* **47**, 97-113 (1982).

Purified calf brain tubulin retains many of its *in vivo* biochemical characteristics, such as the ability to self-assemble into microtubules and the response of the assembly reaction to inhibitory effects of cold temperature, Ca^{2+}, and anti-microtubule agents, *e.g.* vinblastine and colchicine, *q.q.v.* uv max (PG buffer): 278 nm (ε 1.33 ml $mg^{-1} cm^{-1}$).

9809. Tuftsin. [9063-57-4] L-Threonyl-L-lysyl-L-prolyl-L-arginine; N^2-[1-(N^2-L-threonyl-L-lysyl)-L-prolyl]-L-arginine. $C_{21}H_{40}N_8O_6$; mol wt 500.59. C 50.39%, H 8.05%, N 22.38%, O 19.18%. A naturally occurring tetrapeptide having a variety of immunopotentiating properties, especially stimulation and enhancement of phagocytosis. It also exhibits antitumor and antibacterial activity and has been shown to possess chemotactic, migration-enhancing, and mitogenic properties for leukocytes. Discovered during research on the physiological role of cytophilic gammaglobulin: V. A. Najjar, K. Nishioka, *Nature* **228**, 672 (1970). Produced in the spleen; present in mammalian blood in the gamma globulin fraction as part of the larger molecule *leucokinin*. Isoln and characterization: K. Nishioka *et al., Biochim. Biophys. Acta* **310**, 217 (1973); V. A. Najjar, US 3778426 (1973 to Research Corp.). Solid phase synthesis: K. Nishioka *et al., Biochem. Biophys. Res. Commun.* **47**, 172 (1972); *eidem, Biochim. Biophys. Acta* **310**, 230 (1973). Synthesis by fragment condensation: J. Vicar *et al., Collect. Czech. Chem. Commun.* **41**, 3467 (1976); by liquid phase method: S. Nozaki *et al., Bull. Chem. Soc. Jpn.* **50**, 422 (1977). ^{13}C-NMR and circular dichroism studies: I. Z. Siemion *et al., Eur. J. Biochem.* **112**, 339 (1980). Conformational studies have provided conflicting evidence on the structure, *cf.* M. Blumenstein *et al., Biochemistry* **18**, 4247 (1979). Specific receptors on macrophages, monocytes, and granulocytes are thought to mediate the biological activity of tuftsin: A. Constantopoulos, V. A. Najjar, *J. Biol. Chem.* **248**, 3819 (1973); R. M. G. Nair *et al., Immunochemistry* **15**, 901 (1978); Z. Bar-Shavit *et al., Biochem. Biophys. Res. Commun.* **94**, 1445 (1980). Its physiological significance has been shown in patients in whom tuftsin deficiency has resulted in a human syndrome with increased incidence of severe infections: *Macrophages and Lymphocytes, Part A,* M. R. Escobar, H. Friedman, Eds. (Plenum Press, New York, 1980) pp 131-147; *Lymphokine Reports,* E. Pick, Ed. (Academic Press, New York, 1980) pp 157-159; V. A. Najjar, *Med. Biol.* **59**, 134 (1981). General biological properties: V. A. Najjar, *Mol. Cell. Biochem.* **41**, 1 (1981). Antitumor activity: K. Nishioka *et al., ibid.* 13. Bactericidal activity: J. Martinez, F. Winternitz, *ibid.* 123. Analogs: F. Z. Siemion, *ibid.* 99. *Reviews:* V. A. Najjar, *Exp. Cell Biol.* **46**, 114-126 (1978); *eidem, Adv. Exp. Med. Biol.* **121A**, 131-147 (1980); K. Nishioka *et al., Life Sci.* **28**, 1081-1090 (1981); V. A. Najjar, *Mol. Cell. Biochem.* **41**, 73-98 (1981). Conference proceedings: *Ann. N.Y. Acad. Sci.* **419**, entitled "Antineoplastic, Immunogenic and Other Effects of the Tetrapeptide Tuftsin: a Natural Macrophage Activator", V. A. Najjar, M. Fridkin, Eds. (1983) pp 1-273.

Thr–Lys–Pro–Arg

9810. Tulathromycin. Draxxin. $C_{41}H_{79}N_3O_{12}$; mol wt 806.08. C 61.09%, H 9.88%, N 5.21%, O 23.82%. Triamilide antibiotic for treatment of bovine and porcine respiratory disease. Exists as an equilibrium mixture of two isomeric forms, tulathromycin A (90%) and B (10%). HPLC determn in livestock plasma and lung homogenates: D. Gáler *et al., J. Agric. Food Chem.* **52**, 2179 (2004). Pharmacokinetics in cattle: M. A. Nowakowski *et al., Vet. Ther.* **5**, 60 (2004); in swine: H. A. Benchaoui *et al., J. Vet. Pharmacol. Ther.* **27**, 203 (2004).

Tulathromycin A

Tulathromycin A. [217500-96-4] (2R,3S,4R,5R,8R,10R,11R,-12S,13S,14R)-13-[[2,6-Dideoxy-3-C-methyl-3-O-methyl-4-C-[(propylamino)methyl]-α-L-*ribo*-hexopyranosyl]oxy]-2-ethyl-3,4,10-trihydroxy-3,5,8,10,12,14-hexamethyl-11-[[3,4,6-trideoxy-3-(dimethylamino)-β-D-*xylo*-hexopyanosyl]oxy]-1-oxa-6-azacyclopentadecan-15-one; CP-472295. Prepn: B. S. Bronk *et al.,* **WO 9856802**; *eidem,* **US 6420536** (1998, 2002 both to Pfizer); and crystal structure: M. A. Letavic *et al., Bioorg. Med. Chem. Lett.* **12**, 2771 (2002).

Tulathromycin B. [280755-12-6] (2R,3R,6R,8R,9R,10S,11S,-12R)-11-[[2,6-Dideoxy-3-C-methyl-3-O-methyl-4-C-[(propyl-amino)methyl]-α-L-*ribo*-hexopyranosyl]oxy]-2-[(1R,2R)-1,2-dihy-droxy-1-methylbutyl]-8-hydroxy-3,6,8,10,12-pentamethyl-9-[[3,4,6-trideoxy-3-(dimethylamino)-β-D-*xylo*-hexopyanosyl]oxy]-1-oxa-4-azacyclotridecan-13-one; CP-547272. Prepn: R. J. Rafka *et al.,* **WO 0031097**; *eidem,* **US 6329345** (2000, 2001 both to Pfizer).

THERAP CAT (VET): Antibacterial.

9811. Tulobuterol. [41570-61-0] 2-Chloro-α-[[(1,1-di-methylethyl)amino]methyl]benzenemethanol; α-[(*tert*-butylamino)-methyl]-o-chlorobenzyl alcohol. $C_{12}H_{18}ClNO$; mol wt 227.73. C 63.29%, H 7.97%, Cl 15.57%, N 6.15%, O 7.03%. A β-adrenergic receptor agonist, related structurally to terbutaline, *q.v.* Prepn: H. Kato, S. Kurata, DE 2244737 (1973 to Hokuriku), *C.A.* **78**, 147538a (1973). Pharmacology: S. Kubo *et al., Arzneim.-Forsch.* **25**, 1028 (1975); *eidem, ibid.* **27**, 1433 (1977); I. Uesaka *et al., ibid.* 1439. Metabolism: T. Fujiihashi *et al., Oyo Yakuri* **18**, 347 (1979), *C.A.* **92**, 121781 (1980); K. Matsumura *et al., Yakugaku Zasshi* **101**, 198 (1981), *C.A.* **94**, 167404 (1981). Determn of tulobuterol and its metabolites in human urine: *eidem, J. Chromatogr.* **222**, 53 (1981). Toxicological studies: S. Kubo *et al., Oyo Yakuri* **13**, 197, 317 (1977), *C.A.* **88**, 83591-2 (1978).

Crystals, mp 89-91°. LD_{50} in male mice, rats, rabbits (mg/kg): 305, 850, 563 orally; 170, 417, 164 s.c. (Kubo, 1975).
Hydrochloride. [56776-01-3] C-78; Atenos; Berachin; Brelomax; Bremax; Hokunalin; Respacal. $C_{12}H_{18}ClNO.HCl$; mol wt 264.19. White crystalline powder, mp 161-163°.
THERAP CAT: Bronchodilator.

9812. Tumor Necrosis Factor. TNF. Cytokine produced by activated macrophages as part of the cellular immune response. Originally characterized by its selective hemorrhagic necrosis of tumor cells. Identification in the sera of endotoxin treated mice previously sensitized with bacillus Calmette-Guerin (BCG): E. A. Carswell *et al., Proc. Natl. Acad. Sci. USA* **72**, 3666 (1975). Partial purification: S. Green *et al., ibid.* **73**, 381 (1976). Preliminary characterization of murine TNF: T. Haranaka, N. Satomi, *Jpn. J. Exp. Med.* **51**, 191 (1981); F. C. Kull, P. Cuatrecasas, *J. Immunol.* **126**, 1279 (1981); of rabbit TNF: M. R. Ruff, G. E. Gifford, *ibid.* **125**, 1671 (1980); N. Matthews *et al., Br. J. Cancer* **42**, 416 (1980). Identification of macrophages as cellular source of TNF: D. N. Männel *et al., Infect. Immun.* **30**, 523 (1980); N. Santomi *et al., Jpn. J. Exp. Med.* **51**, 317 (1981). Differentiation from interferon: N.

Bloksma *et al., Cancer Immunol. Immunother.* **14,** 41 (1982). Cytotoxic effect on the malaria parasite *Plasmodium falciparum:* C. G. Haidaris *et al., Infect. Immun.* **42,** 385 (1983); A. O. Wozencraft *et al., ibid.* **43,** 664 (1984). Activity against transplanted human and murine tumors in mice: T. Haranaka *et al., Int. J. Cancer* **34,** 263 (1984). Human TNF is a trimer of 3 identical subunits with 157 amino acid residues and mol wt 17,350 Da. Cloning and expression of cDNA for human TNF in *E. coli:* D. Pennica *et al., Nature* **312,** 724 (1984); T. Shirai *et al., ibid.* **313,** 803 (1985); A. M. Wang *et al., Science* **228,** 149 (1985). Identity with **cachectin:** B. Buetler, A. Cerami, *Nature* **320,** 584 (1986). Structure: E. Y. Jones *et al., ibid.* **338,** 225 (1989). Preliminary evaluation with interferon-γ in metastatic melanoma: S. Retsas *et al., Br. Med. J.* **298,** 1290 (1989). *Reviews:* M. R. Ruff, G. E. Gifford, *Lymphokines* **2,** 235 (1981); L. J. Old, *Sci. Am.* **258**(5), 59-60, 70-75 (1988).

Note: Lymphotoxin, a TNF-like factor produced by lymphocytes has been referred to as *TNF-β.*

9813. Tung Oil. China wood oil. A drying oil from seeds of *Aleurites cordata* Steud., *Euphorbiaceae,* indigenous to China and Japan, but now grown also in Florida. Chief fatty acid component is eleostearic acid. Unlike linseed and soybean oils, it need not be refined.

Pale yellow liquid; characteristic disagreeable odor. On long keeping, or on heating for a short time at 300°, polymerizes to a stiff jelly. d 0.936-0.943. Iodine no. 163-171. Sapon no. 190-197. Sol in chloroform, ether, carbon disulfide, oils; the polymerized product is practically insol in the usual organic solvents.

USE: Manuf quick-drying wood varnishes, linoleum, and floor cloth; in India rubber substitutes, insulating masses; for waterproofing paper and other tissues.

9814. Tungsten. [7440-33-7] Wolfram. W; at. wt 183.84; at. no. 74; valences 6, 5, 4, 3, 2. Group VIB(6). Naturally occurring isotopes: 180 (0.135%); 182 (26.4%); 183 (14.4%); 184 (30.6%); 186 (28.4%); artificial radioactive isotopes: 173-179; 181; 185; 187-189. Discovered by C. W. Scheele in 1781, isolated in 1783 by J. J. and F. de Elhuyar. One of the rarer metals, comprises about 1.5 ppm of the earth's crust. Chief ores are *wolframite* [(Fe,Mn)WO₄] and scheelite (CaWO₄). Found chiefly in China, Malaya, Mexico, Alaska, South America and Portugal. Scheelite ores mined in the U.S. carry from 0.4-1.0% WO₃. Description of isoln processes: K. C. Li, C. Y. Wang, *Tungsten,* A.C.S. Monograph Series no. **94** (Reinhold, New York, 3rd ed., 1955) pp 113-269; G. D. Rieck, *Tungsten and Its Compounds* (Pergamon Press, New York, 1967) 154 pp. *Reviews:* Parish, *Adv. Inorg. Chem. Radiochem.* **9,** 315-354 (1966); Rollinson, "Chromium, Molybdenum and Tungsten" in *Comprehensive Inorganic Chemistry* **vol. 3,** J. C. Bailar, Jr. *et al.,* Eds. (Pergamon Press, Oxford, 1973) pp 623-624, 742-769. Review of toxicology and human exposure: *Toxicological Profile for Tungsten* (PB2006-100007, 2005) 203 pp.

Steel-gray to tin-white metal; body centered cubic structure. d_4^{20} 18.7-19.3; depends on extent of working. Hardness 6.5-7.5. mp 3410°. bp₇₆₀ 5900°. Spec heat (20°): 0.032 cal/g/°C. Heat of fusion 44 cal/g. Heat of vaporization 1150 cal/g. Electrical resistivity (20°): 5.5 μohm-cm. Stable in dry air at ordinary temps, forms the trioxide at red heat. Not attacked by water, but oxidized to the dioxide by steam. Very stable to acids, attacked only superficially by concd nitric acid or aqua regia. Powdered tungsten can be pyrophoric under the right conditions. Slowly sol in fused potassium hydroxide or sodium carbonate in presence of air; sol in a fused mixture of NaOH and nitrate. Attacked by fluorine at room temp; by chlorine at 250-300° giving the hexachloride in absence of air, and the trioxide and oxychloride in the presence of air.

Caution: Potential symptoms of overexposure to tungsten are irritation of eyes, skin, respiratory system; diffuse pulmonary fibrosis; loss of appetite, nausea, cough; blood changes. Potential symptoms of overexposure to tungsten carbide (cemented) are irritation of eyes, skin, respiratory system; possible skin sensitization to cobalt, nickel; diffuse pulmonary fibrosis; loss of appetite, nausea, cough; blood changes. *See NIOSH Pocket Guide to Chemical Hazards* (DHHS/NIOSH 97-140, 1997) p 324.

USE: To increase hardness, toughness, elasticity and tensile strength of steel; manuf alloys; manuf filaments for incandescent lamps and in electron tubes; in contact points for automotive, tele-

graph, radio and television apparatus; in phonograph needles. *Tungsten carbides* (W₂C, WC) used in rock drills, metal-cutting tools, wire-drawing dies. WC used as catalyst instead of platinum: Bennett *et al., Science* **184,** 563 (1974).

9815. Tungsten Carbide. [12070-12-1] CW; mol wt 195.85. C 6.13%, W 93.87%. WC. Stable, wear-resistant material with hardness close to diamond. Prepn: S. Hilpert, M. Ornstein, *Ber.* **46,** 1669 (1913); M. R. Andrews, *J. Phys. Chem.* **27,** 270 (1923); A. E. Newkirk, I. Aliferis, *J. Am. Chem. Soc.* **79,** 4629 (1957). Heat of combustion: L. D. McGraw *et al., ibid.* **69,** 329 (1947). Development of WC dental burs: J. Osborne *et al., Br. Dent. J.* **90,** 229 (1951). Review of industrial-scale production and applications: A. S. Hester *et al., Ind. Eng. Chem.* **52,** 94-100 (1960). Structural and electronic properties: A. Y. Liu *et al., Phys. Rev. B* **38,** 9483 (1988). Catalytic properties: E. Iglesia *et al., Catal. Today* **15,** 307 (1992). Physical properties and calculated electronic structure: H. W. Hugosson, H. Engqvist, *Int. J. Refractory Metals Hard Mater.* **21,** 55 (2003). FTIR characterization of thin films and bulk samples: P. Hoffmann *et al., Mater. Charact.* **50,** 255 (2003). Combustion synthesis: G. Jiang *et al., Ceram. Int.* **30,** 185, 191 (2004). Review of toxicology and human exposure: *Toxicological Profile for Tungsten* (PB2006-100007, 2005) 203 pp.

mp 2600-2850°. Hardness: 16-22 GPa. Youngs modulus: 696 GN m⁻². Fracture toughness: 28 MPa m^{1/2}. Compressive strength (20°): 5 GPa. Heat of combustion ($\Delta H_{298.16}$): −285.80 ±0.07 kcal/mol.

USE: In drill tips, mining, metal cutting tools, dental burs, surgical instruments, wear-resistant coatings. In mfr of cemented carbide. Substitute for noble metals in catalysis.

9816. Tungsten Hexafluoride. [7783-82-6] F₆W; mol wt 297.83. F 38.27%, W 61.73%. WF₆. Prepd by direct fluorination of powdered tungsten. Can be purified by distillation, preferably under pressure: Ruff, Ascher, *Z. Anorg. Allg. Chem.* **196,** 413 (1931); Henkel, Klemm, *ibid.* **222,** 68 (1935); Marchi, *Inorg. Synth.* **3,** 181 (1950); from ClF and tungsten: Pitts, Jache, *Inorg. Chem.* **7,** 1661 (1968). Review of toxicology and human exposure: *Toxicological Profile for Tungsten* (PB2006-100007, 2005) 203 pp.

Colorless gas or pale yellow liquid. Orthorhombic, deliquescent crystals when solid. d_{liq}^{15} 3.441. mp 2.3°. bp 17.5°. Soly in anhydr HF: 3.14 moles/1000 g HF, Frlec, Hyman, *Inorg. Chem.* **6,** 1596 (1967). May be stored in glass pressure ampuls.

USE: In the electronics industry as a source of tungsten metal that connects the aluminum layers within semiconductor devices.

9817. Tungsten Trioxide. [1314-35-8] Tungsten oxide (WO₃); tungstic anhydride. O₃W; mol wt 231.84. O 20.70%, W 79.30%. WO₃. Prepn from sodium tungstate: Hein, Herzog, in *Handbook of Preparative Inorganic Chemistry* **vol. 2,** G. Brauer, Ed. (Academic Press, New York, 2nd ed., 1965) pp 1423-1424. Review of toxicology and human exposure: *Toxicological Profile for Tungsten* (PB2006-100007, 2005) 203 pp.

Canary yellow, heavy powder; dark orange when heated, regaining the original color on cooling. Insol in water. Sol in caustic alkalies; very slightly sol in acids.

USE: Manuf tungstates which are used for x-ray screens and for fireproofing fabrics.

9818. Tungstic(VI) Acid. [7783-03-1] H₂O₄W; mol wt 249.85. H 0.81%, O 25.61%, W 73.58%. H₂WO₄. Prepn: Morley, *J. Chem. Soc.* **1930,** 1990.

Yellow or greenish-yellow powder. Insol in water and acid except hydrofluoric acid. Slowly sol in solns of caustic alkalies. When freshly pptd from a soluble tungstate it contains 1 mol H₂O, and is appreciably sol in water.

9819. Tunicamycin. [11089-65-9] A family of nucleoside antibiotics produced by *Streptomyces lysosuperificus.* Isoln, characterization: A. Takatsuki *et al., J. Antibiot.* **24,** 215 (1971). Biological properties: A. Takatsuki, G. Tamura, *ibid.* 224. Effect on microorganisms: A. Takatsuki *et al., ibid.* **25,** 75 (1972). Tunicamycin is produced as a mixture of at least 10 homologous antibiotics, the main components being tunicamycins V, VII, II and X, also referred to respectively as A, B, C, D. They contain uracil, *N*-acetylglycosamine, an 11-carbon aminodialdose called *tunicamine,* and a fatty acid linked to the amino group of tunicamine. The homologs differ in their fatty acid components, which vary in degree of saturation and chain length and branching. Structural elucidation: A. Takatsuki *et al., Agric. Biol. Chem.* **41,** 2307 (1977); T. Ito *et al., ibid.* **44,** 695 (1980). HPLC sepn of components: W. C. Mahoney, D. Duskin, *J. Biol. Chem.* **254,** 6572 (1979). Approaches to synthesis: Y. Fukuda *et al., Bull. Chem. Soc. Jpn.* **55,** 880 (1982). Tunicamycin has been shown to interfere with glycoprotein synthesis in yeast and mammalian systems: A. Takatsuki *et al., Agric. Biol. Chem.* **39,** 2089 (1975); S. Kuo, J. O. Lampen, *Arch. Biochem. Biophys.* **172,** 574 (1976). Effect on epidermal glycoprotein and glycosaminoglycan synthesis *in vitro*: I. A. King, A. Tabiowo, *Biochem. J.* **198,** 331 (1981). Enhancement of antiviral and anticellular activity of interferon, *q.v.*: R. K. Maheshwari *et al., Science* **219,** 1339 (1983). *Review:* A. D. Elbein, *Trends Biochem. Sci.* **6,** 219-221 (1981). Book: *Tunicamycin*, G. Tamura, Ed. (Japan Sci. Soc., Tokyo, 1982) 220 pp. *See also* Streptovirudin.

Tunicamycins II, V, VII, X
(n = 8, 9, 10, 11)

White cryst powder, mp 234-235° (dec). $[\alpha]_D^{20}$ +52° (c = 0.5 in pyridine). uv max (methanol): 205, 260 nm ($E_{1cm}^{1\%}$ 230, 110). Sol in alk water, pyridine, hot methanol. Slightly sol in ethanol, butanol. Practically insol in acetone, ethyl acetate, chloroform, benzene, acidic water. When dissolved in water at 100° and held for 30 min, stable at neutral and alk pH; unstable at acidic pH.

USE: As a tool in studying glycoproteins in a wide variety of biological systems.

9820. Tunichrome B-1. [97689-87-7] (αE)-3,5-Dihydroxy-L-tyrosyl-α,β-didehydro-3,5-dihydroxy-N-[(1Z)-2-(3,4,5-trihydroxyphenyl)ethenyl]tyrosinamide; TB-1. $C_{26}H_{25}N_3O_{11}$; mol wt 555.49. C 56.22%, H 4.54%, N 7.56%, O 31.68%. Major component of a group of polyphenolic yellow blood pigments isolated from the sea squirt (tunicate) *Ascidia nigra* (Linnaeus). The *tunichromes* are strong biological reducing agents involved in the selective accumulation of vanadium by *A. nigra*. Isoln of crude tunichrome mixture from the blood cells of *A. nigra*, action in converting vanadium(V) to vanadium(III): I. G. Macara *et al., Biochem. J.* **181,** 457 (1979). Isoln of tunichrome B-1 by HPLC under anaerobic conditions, characterization and structure determn by mass spec, nmr: R. C. Bruening *et al., J. Am. Chem. Soc.* **107,** 5298 (1985). Brief account of the role of tunichromes in studies into the biochemical nature of vanadium and other trace metals: R. J. Seltzer, *Chem. Eng. News* **63,** 67 (Sept. 16, 1985). *Review:* R. C. Bruening *et al., J. Nat. Prod.* **49,** 193 (1986).

Yellow solid, sol in methanol. uv max (methanol): 210, 340 nm (ε 68000, 19600).

9821. Turanose. [547-25-1] 3-*O*-α-D-Glucopyranosyl-D-fructose; 3-(α-D-glucosido)-D-fructose. $C_{12}H_{22}O_{11}$; mol wt 342.30. C 42.11%, H 6.48%, O 51.41%. Prepd from melezitose: Tanret, *Compt. Rend.* **142,** 1424 (1906); Bridel, Aagard, *Bull. Soc. Chim. Biol.* **9,** 884 (1927); Hudson, Pacsu, *J. Am. Chem. Soc.* **52,** 2522 (1930); Pacsu in *Methods in Carbohydrate Chemistry* vol. I (Academic Press, New York, 1962) p 353. Structure: Isbell, Pigman, *J. Res. Natl. Bur. Stand.* **20,** 787 (1938); Isbell, *ibid.* **26,** 35 (1941); Hudson, *J. Org. Chem.* **9,** 117, 470 (1944); Hassid, Ballou in *The Carbohydrates*, W. Pigman, Ed. (Academic Press, New York, 1957) p 508. Crystal structure: A. Neuman *et al., Acta Crystallogr.* **B34,** 242 (1978).

Nonhygroscopic prisms from water + alc. Very sweet taste. Dec 157°. Shows mutarotation. $[\alpha]_D^{20}$ +27.3° → +75.8° (c = 4 in water). Freely sol in water, methanol. One gram dissolves in 19 ml of 95% alc. Acid hydrolysis yields 1 mol D-glucose and 1 mol D-fructose. Reducing power about ½ of D-glucose.

9822. Toluylene Blue. [97-26-7] *N*-[4-[(2,4-Diamino-5-methylphenyl)imino]-2,5-cyclohexadien-1-ylidene]-*N*-methyl-methanaminium chloride; [4-(4,6-diamino-*m*-tolyl)imino-2,5-cyclohexadien-1-ylidene]dimethylammonium chloride; C.I. 49410. $C_{15}H_{19}ClN_4$; mol wt 290.79. C 61.96%, H 6.59%, Cl 12.19%, N 19.27%. Prepd by condensation of *p*-nitrosodimethylaniline with 2,4-diaminotoluylene: Witt, *Ber.* **12,** 933 (1879); **DE 15272;** *Frdl.* **1,** 274. Also formed by irradiating a mixture of dimethyl-*p*-phenylenediamine and *m*-toluylenediamine: Loiseleur, *Compt. Rend.* **237,** 461 (1953). *See also Colour Index* vol. 4 (3rd ed., 1971) p 4443.

Monohydrate. Prismatic, copper-brown, shiny crystals. Gives blue soln with cold water, alc, acetic acid.

USE: Biological stain.

9823. Turkey-Red Oil. Sulfated castor oil; red oil. Prepd by treating castor oil with 15-30% H_2SO_4 at 25-30° for several hrs, followed by washing and neutralizing with NaOH soln. The product is an anion-active wetting agent. The commercial mfg process actually esterifies the 12-hydroxyl group in ricinoleic acid (the main constit of castor oil) thus producing a true sulfate ester, and not a sulfonate.

USE: In finishing cotton and linen; to obtain bright, clear colors in dyeing fabrics.

9824. Turmeric. Curcuma longa; tumeric; saffron Indian. From rhizome of *Curcuma longa* Linn. (*C. domestica* Valeton), *Zingiberaceae. Habit.* India, China, East Indies. *Constit.* Yellow coloring matter (curcumin), *p,p*-dihydroxydicinnamoylmethane, *p*-hydroxycinnamoylferuloylmethane, *p,α*-dimethylbenzyl alcohol, 1-methyl-4-acetyl-1-cyclohexene, turmerone, α-phellandrene, sabinene, zingiberene, cineol, borneol, caprylic acid. Isoln of curcumin from turmeric: Janaki, Bose, *J. Indian Chem. Soc.* **44,** 985 (1967).

Turmeric has an aromatic pepper-like but somewhat bitter taste and gives curry dishes their characteristic yellowish color.

USE: Condiment (as curry powder), color for ointments.

9825.   *ar*-Turmerone. [532-65-0] (6*S*)-2-Methyl-6-(4-methylphenyl)-2-hepten-4-one; 2-methyl-6-*p*-tolyl-2-hepten-4-one. $C_{15}H_{20}O$; mol wt 216.32. C 83.28%, H 9.32%, O 7.40%. Isoln of naturally occurring (+)-form from Curcuma oil *(Curcuma longa* Linn., *Zingiberaceae):* H. Rupe *et al., Helv. Chim. Acta* **17,** 372 (1934). Structure: H. Rupe, A. Gassmann, *ibid.* **19,** 569 (1936). Abs config: V. K. Honwad, A. S. Rao, *Tetrahedron* **20,** 2921 (1964). Total synthesis: A. I. Meyers, R. K. Smith, *Tetrahedron Lett.* **1979,** 2749; T. Sato *et al., ibid.* **1980,** 3377.

Oil. bp_{10} 159-160°. $[\alpha]_D^{20}$ +82.21° (Rupe, Gassman); also reported as $[\alpha]_D^{22}$ +59.9° (c = 4.5 in hexane) (Sato). d_4^{20} 0.9634.

(±)-form. [38142-58-4] Synthesis: J. Colonge, J. Chambion, *C.R. Hebd. Seances Acad. Sci.* **222,** 557 (1946); T.-L. Ho, *Synth. Commun.* **11,** 579 (1981). n_D^{21} 1.5218.

9826.   Turpentine. [9005-90-7] Gum thus; pine resin. Oleoresin from *Pinus palustris* Mill. and from other species of *Pinus, Pinaceae.* "Turpentine" also is used to designate the volatile oil. Review of production and properties: J. J. W. Coppen, G. A. Hone, *Gum Naval Stores: Turpentine and Rosin from Pine Resin* (FAO, Rome, 1995) 71 pp; of production and uses: S. K. Srivastava, M. C. Nigam, *Curr. Res. Med. Aromat. Plants* **3,** 49-70 (1981); T. Plocek, *Perfum. Flavor.* **23,** 1-6 (1998).

Yellowish, opaque, sticky masses; characteristic odor and taste. Insol in water. Sol in alc, chloroform, ether, glacial acetic acid.

Volatile oil. [8006-64-2] Oil of turpentine; spirit of turpentine; turpentine oil. Distilled from the oleoresin yielding only terpene oils. *Constit.* α- and β-pinenes, limonene, 3-carene. May be rectified to remove unpleasant odor and taste by treatment with NaOH and distillation. A mixture of 3 parts oil with 1 part sulfurated linseed oil is known as **Haarlem oil.** Colorless liq; characteristic odor and taste, both becoming more pronounced and less agreeable on aging or exposure to air. d_{25}^{25} 0.854-0.868. Greater part distills between 154-170°. n_D^{20} 1.4680-1.4780. Rotation is variable. Insol in water; sol in 5 vols alcohol; miscible with benzene, chloroform, ether, carbon disulfide, petr ether and oils. *Flammable!*

Caution: Absorbed through skin, lungs, intestine. Potential symptoms of overexposure are irritation of eyes, skin, nose, throat; headache, vertigo, convulsions; skin sensitization; hematuria, albuminuria; kidney damage; abdominal pain, nausea, vomiting, diarrhea; cough, choking, dyspnea, cyanosis; excitement, ataxia, confusion, stupor. Aspiration of liquid may cause chemical pneumonia. *See NIOSH Pocket Guide to Chemical Hazards* (DHHS/ NIOSH 97-140, 1997) p 324; *Clinical Toxicology of Commercial Products,* R. E. Gosselin *et al.,* Eds. (Williams & Wilkins, Baltimore, 5th ed., 1984) section III, pp 393-395.

USE: Solvent and thinner for paints, varnishes, polishes. In manufacture of aroma chemicals such as camphor, myrcene, linalool; source of pine oil.

9827.   Tutin. [2571-22-4] (1a*S*,1b*S*,2'*R*,5*R*,6*S*,6a*R*,7a*R*,- 8*S*)-Hexahydro-1b,6-dihydroxy-6a-methyl-8-(1-methylethenyl)- spiro[2,5-methano-7*H*-oxireno[3,4]cyclopent[1,2-*d*]oxepin-7,2'-oxiran]-3(2*H*)-one. $C_{15}H_{18}O_6$; mol wt 294.30. C 61.22%, H 6.16%, O 32.62%. Poisonous constituent of *Coriaria ruscifolia* L. or *C. japonica* A. Gray, (tutu) *Coriariaceae.* Naturally occurring form is (+)-tutin. Isoln: Easterfield, Aston, *J. Chem. Soc.* **79,** 125 (1901). Structure: Johns, Markham, *ibid.* **1961,** 3006; Craven, *Nature* **197,** 1193 (1963); Mackay, Mathieson, *Tetrahedron Lett.* **1963,** 1399. Absolute configuration: Okuda, Yoshida, *ibid.* **1965,** 2137. Biosynthesis: A. Corbella *et al., Chem. Commun.* **1969,** 634. NMR analysis: J. W. Blunt *et al., Aust. J. Chem.* **32,** 1339 (1979). Stereospecific synthesis: K. Watamatsu *et al., Tetrahedron* **42,** 5551 (1986). Determn in toxic honey: J. L. Love *et al., N.Z. J. Technol.* **2,** 179 (1986). Effect on central nervous system: D. R. Curtis *et al., Brain Res.* **63,** 419 (1973); A. Nistri *et al., Lancet* **1,** 996 (1974). Toxicity data: C. H. Jarboe *et al., J. Med. Chem.* **11,** 729 (1968).

White, odorless crystals. mp 209-212°; also reported as mp 204-205° (Wakamatsu). $[\alpha]_D^{20}$ +9.25° (alc); $[\alpha]_D^{17}$ +13.9° (c = 0.75, methanol). Sol in water, alcohol, ether. LD_{50} i.p. in female mice: 3.0 mg/kg (Jarboe).

Diacetate. $C_{19}H_{22}O_8$. Crystals from ethanol-water, mp 197-201°.

Caution: Poisoning from ingestion of *C. ruscifolia* has been reported and is due to presence of tutin. Symptoms include giddiness, stupor, coma, delirium, convulsions.

9828.   Twistane. [253-14-5] Tricyclo[4.4.0.0$^{3.8}$]decane. $C_{10}H_{16}$; mol wt 136.23. C 88.16%, H 11.84%. Synthesis: Whitlock, *J. Am. Chem. Soc.* **84,** 3412 (1962); Gautier, Deslongchamps, *Can. J. Chem.* **45,** 297 (1967); Whitlock, Siefken, *J. Am. Chem. Soc.* **90,** 4929 (1968). Absolute configuration: Keiichi *et al., Tetrahedron Lett.* **1968,** 5467.

Crystals, mp 163-164.8°.

9829.   Tybamate. [4268-36-4] Butylcarbamic acid 2-[[(aminocarbonyl)oxy]methyl]-2-methylpentyl ester; carbamate of 2-(hydroxymethyl)-2-methylpentyl ester of butylcarbamic acid; *N*-butyl-2-methyl-2-propyl-1,3-propanediol dicarbamate; 2-methyl-2-propyltrimethylene butylcarbamate carbamate; Nospan; Solacen; Tybatran. $C_{13}H_{26}N_2O_4$; mol wt 274.36. C 56.91%, H 9.55%, N 10.21%, O 23.33%. Prepd from 2-methyl-2-propyl-3-hydroxypropyl carbamate + butyl isocyanate: Berger, Ludwig, *US 2937119* (1960 to Carter Prod.). Comprehensive description: P. Reisberg *et al., Anal. Profiles Drug Subs.* **4,** 494-515 (1975).

Crystals from 1,1,2-trichloroethane + hexane (1:2), mp 49-51°, $bp_{0.06}$ 150-152°.

THERAP CAT: Anxiolytic.

9830.   Tylocrebrine. [6879-02-3] 9,11,12,13,13a,14-Hexahydro-2,3,5,6-tetramethoxydibenzo[*f*,*h*]pyrrolo[1,2-*b*]isoquinoline; 2,3,5,6-tetramethoxyphenanthro[9,10:6',7']indolizidine. $C_{24}H_{27}-NO_4$; mol wt 393.48. C 73.26%, H 6.92%, N 3.56%, O 16.26%. Phenanthroindolizidine alkaloid; isomeric with tylophorine, *q.v.* Isoln of *l*-isomer from *Tylophora crebriflora* S. T. Blake, *Asclepiadaceae:* E. Gellert *et al., J. Chem. Soc.* **1962,** 1008; K. V. Rao *et al., J. Pharm. Sci.* **59,** 1501 (1970). Antileukemic activity: E. Gellert, R. Rudzats, *J. Med. Chem.* **7,** 361 (1964). *d*-Isomer isolated from *Ficus septica, Moraceae.* Synthesis of the *dl*-form and structure: E. Gellert *et al., loc. cit.;* B. Chauncy, E. Gellert, *Aust. J. Chem.* **23,** 2503 (1970). Inhibits protein synthesis: G. R. Donaldson *et al., Biochem. Biophys. Res. Commun.* **31,** 104 (1968); E. Battaner, D. Vasquez, *Biochim. Biophys. Acta* **254,** 316 (1971). Mode of action studies: M. T. Huang, A. P. Grollman, *Mol. Pharmacol.* **8,** 538 (1972). *Review:* R. S. Gupta, *Antibiotics* **6,** 47 (1983).

dl-Form. Needles from chloroform + methanol, mp 219-221°.

l-Form. Crystals from methanol, dec 218-220°. uv max: 263, 342, 360 nm (log ε 4.81, 3.25, 3.09). $[\alpha]_D^{24}$ −45° (c = 0.74 in chloroform). pKa (50% aq ethanol): 6.7.

d-Form. Crystals from methanol, mp 220-222°. $[\alpha]_D^{22}$ +20.5°.

9831. Tylophorine. [482-20-2] (13a*S*)-9,11,12,13,13a,14-Hexahydro-2,3,6,7-tetramethoxydibenzo[*f,h*]pyrrolo[1,2-*b*]isoquinoline; 2,3,6,7-tetramethoxyphenanthro[9,10:6′,7′]indolizidine. $C_{24}H_{27}NO_4$; mol wt 393.48. C 73.26%, H 6.92%, N 3.56%, O 16.26%. Major alkaloid from *Tylophora asthmatica* Wight *et* Arn., *Asclepiadaceae*. Also found in other *Asclepiadaceae, Moraceae, Urticaceae* and *Lauraceae*. Naturally occurring form originally isolated and reported to be levorotatory; later corrected to dextrorotatory. Isoln: A. N. Ratnagiriswaran, K. Venkatachalam, *Indian J. Med. Res.* **22**, 433 (1935); R. N. Chopra *et al., Arch. Pharm.* **275**, 236 (1937); T. R. Govindachari *et al., J. Chem. Soc.* **1954**, 2801. Structure: *eidem, Tetrahedron* **9**, 53 (1960). Absolute configuration: *eidem, J. Chem. Soc. Perkin Trans. I* **1974**, 1161. Synthesis of the *dl*-form: *eidem, Chem. Ind. (London)* **1960**, 664; N. A. Khatri *et al., J. Am. Chem. Soc.* **103**, 6387 (1981). Synthesis and verification of dextrorotation of naturally occurring form: T. F. Buckley 3rd, H. Rapoport, *J. Org. Chem.* **48**, 4222 (1983); J. E. Nordlander, F. G. Njoroge, *ibid.* **52**, 1627 (1987). Stereoselective synthesis of *l*-form: M. Ihara *et al., Tetrahedron Lett.* **29**, 4135 (1988). Biosynthesis: Mulchandani *et al., Phytochemistry* **8**, 1931 (1969); *ibid.* **10**, 1047 (1971); D. S. Bhakuni, V. K. Mangla, *Tetrahedron* **37**, 401 (1981). Pharmacology: C. Gopalakrishnan *et al., Indian J. Med. Res.* **69**, 513 (1979); **71**, 940 (1980).

Crystals, dec 282-284°. $[\alpha]_D^{23}$ +15° (c = 0.7 in chloroform); $[\alpha]_D^{21}$ +73° (c = 0.7 in chloroform). uv max in ethanol: 257, 286, 339, 356 nm (log ε 4.7, 4.42, 3.28, 3.19). Unstable in solutions, decomposition with yellowing sets in promptly accompanied by decreasing rotatory strength.

l-Form. Colorless crystals, dec 286-287°. $[\alpha]_D^{27}$ −11.6° (c = 1.07 in chloroform). uv max 255, 290, 340, 352 nm (log ε 4.74, 4.49, 3.30, 2.93). Sol in chloroform; slightly sol in abs alc, ether, cold benzene. Practically insol in water.

dl-Form. Crystals from chloroform + ethanol, mp 292°.

9832. Tylosin. [1401-69-0] Tylan. $C_{46}H_{77}NO_{17}$; mol wt 916.10. C 60.31%, H 8.47%, N 1.53%, O 29.69%. Macrolide antibiotic isolated from a strain of *Streptomyces fradiae* found in soil from Thailand: Hamill *et al., Antibiot. Chemother.* **11**, 328 (1961); *eidem, US 3178341* (1965 to Lilly). Prodn in batch and chemostat cultures: P. P. Gray, S. Bhuwapathanapun, *Biotechnol. Bioeng.* **22**, 1785 (1980). Partial structure: Morin, Gorman, *Tetrahedron Lett.* **1964**, 2339. Structure: Morin *et al., ibid.* **1970**, 4737; Achenbach *et al., Ber.* **108**, 2481 (1975). Configurational study: S. Omura *et al., Tetrahedron Lett.* **1977**, 1045. Abs config: *eidem, J.*

Antibiot. **33**, 915 (1980); N. D. Jones *et al., ibid.* **35**, 420 (1982). Synthesis of *tylonolide*, the aglycone: S. Masamune *et al., J. Am. Chem. Soc.* **98**, 7874 (1976); K. Tatsuta *et al., Tetrahedron Lett.* **22**, 3997 (1981). Relationship of ribosomal binding and antibacterial properties: J. W. Corcoran *et al., J. Antibiot.* **30**, 1012 (1977). Biosynthesis studies: E. T. Seno *et al., Antimicrob. Agents Chemother.* **11**, 455 (1977); S. Omura *et al., J. Antibiot.* **31**, 254 (1978).

Crystals from water, mp 128-132°. $[\alpha]_D^{25}$ −46° (c = 2 in methanol). uv max: 282 nm ($E_{1cm}^{1\%}$ 245). Soly in water at 25°: 5 mg/ml. Sol in lower alcohols, esters and ketones, in chlorinated hydrocarbons, benzene, ether. Solns are stable at pH 4-9; at pH <4 another active compd, *desmycosin* is formed.

Hydrochloride. $C_{46}H_{77}NO_{17} \cdot HCl$. Crystals from ethanol + ether, mp 141-145°.

THERAP CAT (VET): Antibacterial.

9833. Tyloxapol. [25301-02-4] 4-(1,1,3,3-Tetramethylbutyl)phenol polymer with formaldehyde and oxirane; oxyethylated tertiary octylphenol formaldehyde polymer; *p*-isooctylpolyoxyethylenephenol formaldehyde polymer; tyloxypal; Alevaire; Superinone; Triton A-20; Triton WR-1339. Nonionic detergent with surface-tension-reducing properties. Prepn: Bock, Rainey, *US 2454541* (1948 to Rohm & Haas); J. W. Cornforth *et al., Nature* **168**, 150 (1951). Use to induce exptl hyperlipidemia: A. Kellner *et al., J. Exp. Med.* **93**, 373 (1951); P. E. Schurr *et al., Lipids* **7**, 68 (1972). Use as ophthalmic excipient: D. E. Guttman *et al., J. Pharm. Sci.* **50**, 305 (1961). Phase behavior of mixtures with water: K. Westesen, *Int. J. Pharm.* **102**, 91 (1994); K. Westesen, M. H. J. Koch, *ibid.* **103**, 225 (1994). Tissue distribution and excretion: R. L. DeAngelis *et al., Xenobiotica* **25**, 521 (1995).

R = (CH$_2$CH$_2$O)$_x$H

x = 8 - 10

m < 6

d^{20} 1.0963. Cloud point: 92-97°. Slowly but freely misc with water. Sol in benzene, toluene, chloroform, carbon tetrachloride, carbon disulfide, acetic acid. Alkaline pH. Oxidized by metals.

Combination with colfosceril palmitate and hexadecanol see Exosurf®.

USE: Pharmaceutic aid (dispersing agent; excipient). To induce exptl hyperlipidemia in animal models.

THERAP CAT: Mucolytic.

9834. Tymazoline. [24243-97-8] 4,5-Dihydro-2-[[5-methyl-2-(1-methylethyl)phenoxy]methyl]-1*H*-imidazole; 2-[(thymyloxy)methyl]-2-imidazoline; 2-(thymyloxymethyl)glyoxalidine; 2-[(*p*-mentha-1,3,5-trien-2-yloxy)methyl]-2-imidazoline. $C_{14}H_{20}N_2O$; mol wt 232.32. C 72.38%, H 8.68%, N 12.06%, O 6.89%. Prepd from an alkyl thymyloxyacetimidate and ethylenediamine: Sonn, *US 2149473* (1939 to Ciba); Djerassi, Scholz, *J. Am. Chem.*

Soc. **69,** 1688 (1947). Pharmacology: Pham-Huu-Chanh et al., *Therapie* **24,** 797 (1969).

Hydrochloride. Pernazene. $C_{14}H_{20}N_2O \cdot HCl$; mol wt 268.78. Crystals, mp 215-217° (Sonn); from water or methyl ethyl ketone + ethanol, mp 223.5-225° (Djerassi, Scholz).

THERAP CAT: Nasal decongestant.

9835. Tyramine. [51-67-2] 4-(2-Aminoethyl)phenol; 4-hydroxyphenethylamine; tyrosamine; 2-*p*-hydroxyphenylethylamine; *p*-β-aminoethylphenol; α-(4-hydroxyphenyl)-β-aminoethane. $C_8H_{11}NO$; mol wt 137.18. C 70.04%, H 8.08%, N 10.21%, O 11.66%. Decarboxylation product of tyrosine. Found in mistletoes, putrefied animal tissue, ripe cheese, ergot. Synthesis: Barger, *J. Chem. Soc.* **95,** 1127 (1909); Waser, *Helv. Chim. Acta* **8,** 766 (1925); Buck, *J. Am. Chem. Soc.* **55,** 3389 (1933). Crystal and molecular structure: A. Podder et al., *Acta Crystallogr.* **B35,** 649 (1979).

Crystals from benzene or alcohol, mp 164-165°. bp_{25} 205-207°; bp_2 166°. Alkaline reaction. One gram dissolves in 95 ml water at 15°; in 10 ml boiling alcohol. Sparingly sol in benzene, xylene.

Hydrochloride. [60-19-5] Mydrial. $C_8H_{11}NO \cdot HCl$; mol wt 173.64. Crystals from alcohol + ether, mp 269°. Sol in water with neutral reaction.

THERAP CAT: Adrenergic.

9836. Tyrocidine. [8011-61-8] Peptide antibiotic mixture produced by *Bacillus brevis:* major constituent of tyrothricin, *q.v.* Isoln: Hotchkiss et al., *J. Biol. Chem.* **141,** 155, 163 (1941); Moses, **US 3265572** (1966 to Penick). Separated into the three components, tyrocidines A, B, and C. Review of chemistry and biosynthesis: E. Katz, A. L. Demain, *Bacteriol. Rev.* **41,** 449-474 (1977). Regulatory role in bacterial sporogenesis: H. Ristow et al., *Nature* **280,** 165 (1979); *eidem, Eur. J. Biochem.* **129,** 395 (1982); W. Pschorn et al., *ibid.* 403. Structure-activity relationship: W. Danders et al., *Antimicrob. Agents Chemother.* **22,** 785 (1982).

Tyrocidine A

Hydrochloride mixture. Brevicidin; Rapicidin. Rods or needles from methanol, dec 240°. $[\alpha]_D^{20} -101°$ (c = 1.2 in 95% alc). Soluble in 95% alc, acetic acid, pyridine; slightly sol in water, acetone, abs alcohol. Practically insol in ether, chloroform, hydrocarbons.

Tyrocidine A. [1481-70-5] $C_{66}H_{87}N_{13}O_{13}$; mol wt 1270.48. Separation from the tyrocidine mixture: Battersby, Craig, *J. Am. Chem. Soc.* **74,** 4019, 4023 (1952). Structure: Paladine, Craig, *ibid.* **76,** 688 (1954). Synthesis: Ohno et al., *Bull. Chem. Soc. Jpn.* **39,** 1738 (1966); K. Okamoto et al., *ibid.* **50,** 231 (1977).

Tyrocidine A hydrochloride. Crystals from methanol + water, mp 240-242°. $[\alpha]_D^{25} -111°$ (c = 1.37 in 50% alc). Freely sol in aq methanol or alc; slightly sol in methanol, ethanol. Practically insol in chloroform, acetone, ether.

Tyrocidine B. [865-28-1] $C_{68}H_{88}N_{14}O_{13}$; mol wt 1309.51. Purification and amino acid sequence determination: King, Craig, *J. Am. Chem. Soc.* **77,** 6624, 6627 (1955). Synthesis: Kuromizu, Izumiya, *Experientia* **26,** 587 (1970). Possesses the same structure as tyrocidine A except that L-tryptophan replaces the L-phenylalanine. Crystals from methanol + isopropyl ether.

Tyrocidine B hydrochloride pentahydrate. Crystals, mp 236-237°. $[\alpha]_D -93.0°$ (c = 0.5 in methanol).

Tyrocidine C. [3252-29-7] $C_{70}H_{89}N_{15}O_{13}$; mol wt 1348.55. Separation from the tyrocidine mixture: Ruttenberg et al., *Biochemistry* **4,** 11 (1965). Possesses same structure as tyrocidine B except that D-tryptophan replaces D-phenylalanine attached to L-asparagine. Synthesis: Kuromizu, Izumiya, *Tetrahedron Lett.* **1970,** 1471.

THERAP CAT: Antibacterial.

9837. Tyropanoate Sodium. [7246-21-1] α-Ethyl-2,4,6-triiodo-3-[(1-oxobutyl)amino]benzenepropanoic acid monosodium salt; 3-butyramido-α-ethyl-2,4,6-triiodohydrocinnamic acid sodium salt; α-ethyl-β-(2,4,6-triiodo-3-butyramidophenyl)propionic acid sodium salt; sodium tyropanoate; Win-8851-2; Bilopaque; Lumopaque; Tyropaque. $C_{15}H_{17}I_3NNaO_3$; mol wt 663.00. C 27.17%, H 2.58%, I 57.42%, N 2.11%, Na 3.47%, O 7.24%. Prepn: S. Archer, J. O. Hoppe, **US 2895988** (1959 to Sterling Drug); and pharmacology: J. O. Hoppe et al., *J. Med. Chem.* **13,** 997 (1970). Clinical trials: S. Y. Han, D. M. Witten, *Radiology* **112,** 529 (1974); R. F. Thoeni, A. A. Moss, *ibid.* **144,** 271 (1982).

Colorless solid from ethyl ether, mp 208-210°. Soluble in water. LD_{50} i.v. in mice: 720 mg/kg (Hoppe).

Free acid. $C_{15}H_{18}I_3NO_3$. Crystals from ethyl oxyacetate, mp 182-184°.

THERAP CAT: Diagnostic aid (radiopaque medium—cholecystographic).

9838. Tyrosinase. [9002-10-2] A copper-containing enzyme widely distributed in plants, animals, and man. Catalyzes the hydroxylation of tyrosine in the liver and in melanin-forming cells to 3,4-dihydroxyphenylalanine (dopa). Causes the cut surface of many fruits and plants to darken. The enzyme, as isolated from the common edible mushroom or potato, is characterized by its ability to catalyze aerobic oxidation of both monohydric and *o*-dihydric phenols. These activities are commonly referred to as **cresolase** (**monophenolase, monophenoloxidase**) and **catecholase** (**o-dihydric phenolase**) activities. Since monophenolase activity is frequently lost during purification of the enzyme, the name **polyphenolase** (**polyphenoloxidase**) is preferred by some workers for prepns which have mainly *o*-dihydric phenolase activity. *Ref:* C. R. Dawson, W. B. Tarpley "Copper Oxidases" in J. B. Sumner, K. Myrbäck, *The Enzymes* vol. II, (Academic Press, New York, 1951) pp 456-483. Prepn from potato peels: Kubowitz, *Biochem. Z.* **299,** 32 (1938). Extraction from mushrooms: Cohen, Lerner, **US 2956929** (1960 to Gillette). Separation of α-, β-, γ-, and δ-tyrosinases of mushroom tyrosinase: Bouchilloux et al., *J. Biol. Chem.* **238,** 1699 (1963). Isoln and properties of crystalline tyrosinase from *Neurospora:* Fling et al., *ibid.,* p 2045. Isoln and properties of β-tyrosinase: Kumagai et al., *J. Biol. Chem.* **245,** 1767 (1970).

THERAP CAT: Antihypertensive.

9839. Tyrosine. [60-18-4] L-Tyrosine; Tyr; Y; β-(*p*-hydroxyphenyl)alanine; α-amino-*p*-hydroxyhydrocinnamic acid; (*S*)-α-amino-4-hydroxybenzenepropanoic acid. $C_9H_{11}NO_3$; mol wt 181.19. C 59.66%, H 6.12%, N 7.73%, O 26.49%. Non-essential amino acid for human development; precursor for the synthesis of thyroid hormones and select neurotransmitters, such as dopamine and norepinephrine. May be considered essential by the brain. Name derived from the Greek "tyros" for "cheese" from which it was first identified and isolated: J. Liebig, *Ann.* **57,** 127 (1846); *idem, ibid.* **62,** 257 (1847). Early chemistry and biochemistry: *Amino Acids and Proteins,* D. M. Greenberg, Ed. (Charles C. Thomas, Springfield, IL, 1951) 950 pp., *passim;* J. P. Greenstein, M. Winitz, *Chemistry of the Amino Acids* vol 1-3 (John Wiley and Sons, Inc., New York, 1961) pp. 2348-2367, *passim.* Synthesis of labeled form: Y. Watanabe et al., *Acta Radiol.* **376** (Suppl.), 110 (1991). Intrinsic fluorophore in proteins; used in characterizing structure and conformational changes: V. Giancotti et al., *Biochim. Biophys.*

Acta **624**, 60 (1980); S. T. Ferreira *et al., Biophys. J.* **66,** 1185 (1994); B. Kierdaszuk *et al., Photochem. Photobiol.* **61,** 319 (1995). Review of determn in blood: E. Robins, *Methods Biochem. Anal.* **17,** 287-309 (1969). Review of neurotransmitter synthesis: C. J. Gibson, *Retina* **2,** 332-340 (1982). Review of toxicity: C. Laberge *et al., Adv. Exp. Med. Biol.* **206,** 209-221 (1986). Review of post-translational phosphorylation: S. Atherton-Fessler *et al., Semin. Cell Biol.* **4,** 433-442 (1993); sulfation: C. Niehrs *et al., Chem. Biol. Interact.* **92,** 257-271 (1994).

Fine silky needles, dec 342-344° (closed capillary, bath preheated to 280°, rapid heating). d 1.456. pK_1 2.20; pK_2 9.11; pK_3 10.07. $[\alpha]_D^{22}$ -10.6° (c = 4 in HCl); $[\alpha]_D^{18}$ -13.2° (c = 4 in 3N NaOH). Soly in water (g/100 g): 0.02 at 0°; 0.045 at 25°; 0.105 at 50°; 0.244 at 75°; 0.565 at 100°. Insol in common neutral solvents, such as abs alcohol, ether, acetone, except water. Sol in alkaline solns.

DL-Form. Synthetic product. Stout needles. Dec 316°. Soly in water (g/100 g): 0.0147 at 0°; 0.351 at 25°; 0.0836 at 50°.

D-Form. Crystals. Dec 310-314°. $[\alpha]_D^{25}$ +10.3° (c = 4 in HCl). Soly in water (g/100 g): 0.196 at 0°; 0.1052 at 50°.

USE: Probe for studying protein structure and dynamics.

9840. *m*-Tyrosine. [587-33-7] 3-Hydroxy-L-phenylalanine; α-amino-3-hydroxyhydrocinnamic acid; metatyrosine. $C_9H_{11}NO_3$; mol wt 181.19. C 59.66%, H 6.12%, N 7.73%, O 26.49%. A possible precursor of catecholamines: Sourkes *et al., Nature* **189,** 577 (1961). An intermediate in an alternate pathway for the biosynthesis of catecholamines, where with the existing hydroxylating enzymes *m*-hydroxylation of phenylalanine to *m*-tyrosine occurs before *p*-hydroxylation (forming dopa) and is followed by subsequent decarboxylation to dopamine. Formation *in vitro* of dopa from L-*m*-tyrosine: Tong *et al., Biochem. Biophys. Res. Commun.* **43,** 819 (1971); *in vivo:* Hollunger, Persson, *Acta Pharmacol. Toxicol.* **34,** 391 (1974). Biosynthesis and metabolism studies: D'Iorio *et al., Adv. Neurol.* **5,** 265 (1974). Has also been isolated from a plant source, *Euphorbia myrsinites* L. *Euphorbiaceae:* Mothes *et al., Z. Naturforsch.* **19b,** 1161 (1964). *m*-Tyrosine has the ability to cross the blood-brain barrier and is decarboxylated to

m-tyramine which stimulates dopamine receptors, presumably accounting for the demonstrated pharmacological effects of *m*-tyrosine. Pharmacological studies: Carlsson, Lindqvist, *Eur. J. Pharmacol.* **2,** 187 (1967); Rubenson, *J. Pharm. Pharmacol.* **23,** 228, 412 (1971); Sandler *et al., Nature* **229,** 414 (1971); Ungerstedt *et al., Eur. J. Pharmacol.* **21,** 230 (1973). Crystal and molecular structure: Byrkjedal *et al., Acta Chem. Scand.* **28B,** 750 (1974).

mp 267-270° (dec). $[\alpha]_D^{22}$ -14.5° (70% ethanol); $[\alpha]_D^{22}$ +8.9° (70% ethanol, 2N HCl).

9841. Tyrothricin. [1404-88-2] "Dubos crude crystals"; Hydrotricine; Dermotricine; Tyri 10; Tyrosur. Polypeptide antibiotic mixture extracted from cultures of soil bacilli belonging to the *Tyrothrix* group of bacteria. Usually obtained by extracting acidified cultures of *Bacillus brevis* with alc and precipitating with NaCl soln. Surface, submerged, and aerated cultures are used. Tyrothricin contains from 10 to 20% gramicidin and from 40 to 60% tyrocidine. Solubility data: Weiss *et al., Antibiot. Chemother.* **7,** 374 (1957). Function in the sporulation process: Sarkar, Paulus, *Nature New Biol.* **239,** 228 (1972). Toxicity data: H. Sous *et al., Arzneim.-Forsch.* **7,** 98 (1957).

Gray to brown powder, decomp 215-220°. Has 2-3% absorbed or combined moisture. Stable to light, air and temps up to 50°. Practically insol in water. Sol in alcohol (about 28 mg/ml), in methanol and in propylene glycol. One part of a 2% alcoholic soln contg 10% formaldehyde soln U.S.P. dissolves in 49 parts of water without cloudiness. Tyrothricin should not be dissolved in ether or acetone as only the gramicidin component is soluble. Soly in mg/ml at about 28°: water 2.1; isopropanol 5.6; benzene 0.30; isooctane 0.042; carbon tetrachloride 0.455; ethyl acetate 2.65; acetone 6.8; ether 3.25; dioxane 11.1; chloroform 1.6. Aqueous suspensions may be attacked by microorganisms. Solutions and emulsions should not be sterilized by heat. Incompatible with alkalies and strong acids. Tyrothricin gives a positive biuret and Hopkins-Cole test. LD_{50} in mice (mg/kg): >1500 s.c.; 100 i.p.; >3000 orally (Sous).

THERAP CAT: Topical antibacterial.

THERAP CAT (VET): Topical antibacterial.

U

9842. Ubenimex. [58970-76-6] N-[(2S,3R)-3-Amino-2-hydroxy-1-oxo-4-phenylbutyl]-L-leucine; NK-421; Bestatin. $C_{16}H_{24}$-N_2O_4; mol wt 308.37. C 62.32%, H 7.84%, N 9.08%, O 20.75%. Dipeptide antitumor antibiotic produced by *Streptomyces olivoreticuli* with immunostimulant activity; inhibits leucine aminopeptidase and aminopeptidases B and N. Prepn from fermentation broth: H. Umezawa *et al., DE 2528984; eidem,* **US 4052449** (1976, 1977 both to Microbiochem. Res. Found., Japan); *eidem, J. Antibiot.* **29,** 97 (1976). Structure: H. Suda *et al., ibid.* 100. Synthesis of stereoisomers and structure-activity study: R. Nishizawa *et al., J. Med. Chem.* **20,** 510 (1977). Stereocontrolled synthesis: S. Kobayashi *et al., Tetrahedron Lett.* **25,** 5079 (1984). Crystal structure: J. S. Ricci, Jr. *et al., J. Org. Chem.* **47,** 3063 (1982). Cell surface binding studies: H. Umezawa *et al., J. Antibiot.* **29,** 857 (1976); W. E. Müller *et al., Int. J. Immunopharmacol.* **4,** 393 (1982). Acute toxicity: T. Sakakibara *et al., Jpn. J. Antibiot.* **36,** 2971 (1983). Review of pharmacology: G. Mathé, *Biomed. Pharmacother.* **45,** 49-54 (1991); of clinical studies: K. Ota, *ibid.* 55-60. Clinical trial in squamous-cell lung carcinoma: Y. Ichinose *et al., J. Natl. Cancer Inst.* **95,** 605 (2003).

Colorless needles, mp 233-236°. $[\alpha]_D^{20}$ $-15.5°$ (c = 1.0 in 1N HCl). pKa 8.1, 3.1. uv max: 241.5, 248, 253, 258, 264.5, 268 nm ($E_{1cm}^{1\%}$ 3.8, 4.0, 5.0, 6.0, 4.6, 2.7). Sol in acetic acid, DMSO, methanol. Less sol in water. Insol in ethyl acetate, benzene, hexane, chloroform. LD_{50} in male, female mice, male, female rats (g/kg): 1.3, 1.9, 1.9, 2.1 s.c.; 0.19, 0.19, 0.90, 0.78 i.p.; >4.0, >4.0, >2.0, >2.0 orally (Sakakibara).

THERAP CAT: Immunomodulator; antineoplastic.

9843. Ubiquinones. Coenzymes Q; mitoquinones; SA; Q-275. A group of lipid-soluble benzoquinones involved in electron transport in mitochondria, *i.e.*, in the oxidation of succinate or reduced nicotine adenine dinucleotide (NADH) via the cytochrome system. Occurs in the majority of aerobic organisms, from bacteria to higher plants and animals. Ubiquinone structures, analogous to the menaquinones, *q.v.*, are based on the 2,3-dimethoxy-5-methylbenzoquinone nucleus with a variable terpenoid side chain contg one to twelve mono-unsaturated *trans*-isoprenoid units with 10 units being the most common in animals. According to the existing dual system of nomenclature the compds can be described as: coenzyme Q_n in which n = 1-12, or ubiquinone(x) in which x designates the total number of carbon atoms in the side chain and can be any multiple of 5. Differences in properties are due to the difference in length of the side chain. Naturally occurring members are the coenzymes Q_6-Q_{10}. The entire series has been prepd synthetically. Recent syntheses of ubiquinone 50: S. Terao *et al., J. Org. Chem.* **44,** 868 (1979); Y. Naruta, *ibid.* **45,** 4097 (1980); K. Sato *et al., Chem. Commun.* **1982,** 153. *Reviews: Ciba Foundation Symposium on Quinones in Electron Transport,* Wolstenholme, O'Connor, Eds. (Churchill, London, 1961) 453 pp; Wagner, Folkers, *Vitamins and Coenzymes* (Interscience, New York, 1964) pp 435-468; Crane in *Progr. Chem. Fats Lipids* vol. 7(2), Holman, Ed. (Pergamon Press, 1964) pp 267-289; *Methods Enzymol.* **18C,** 135-237 (1971); R. A. Morton in *The Vitamins* vol. V, W. H. Sebrell, R. S. Harris, Eds. (Academic Press, New York, 2nd ed., 1972) pp 355-391. Series of books: *Biomedical and Clinical Aspects of Coenzyme Q* vols. **1-3,** K. Folkers, Y. Yamamura, Eds. (Elsevier, New York, 1977, 1980, 1981).

Ubiquinone 50. [303-98-0] Coenzyme Q_{10}; CoQ_{10}; coenzyme Q-199; ubidecarenone; ubiquinone 10; NSC-140865; Adelir; Cao-

met; Decafar; Decorenone; Dymion; Heartcin; Inokiten; Iuvacor; Mitocor; Neuquinon; Taidecanone; Ubicardio; Ubicor; Ubidenone; Ubifactor; Ubimaior; Ubisan; Ubiten-50; Ubivis; Udekinon. C_{59}-$H_{90}O_4$; mol wt 863.34. Clinical evaluation in early Parkinson disease: C. W. Shults *et al., Arch. Neurol.* **59,** 1541 (2002).

Ubichromenol 50. [2382-48-1] Cyclic isomer of ubiquinone 50.

Ubiquinone 50

THERAP CAT: Cardiotonic; coenzyme Q_{10} as antiparkinsonian.

9844. Ubiquitin. ATP-dependent proteolytic factor; APF-1; Ub; ubiquitous immunopoietic polypeptide; UBIP. Ubiquitous polypeptide, mol wt 8500 daltons, so named due to its presence in all eukaryotes including plants; widely distributed in the organism. Highly conserved sequence of 76 amino acids is identical in a wide variety of sources including humans, fish, and insects. Participates in diverse cellular functions, such as protein synthesis, chromatin structure, and heat shock, by conjugation to other proteins through its carboxyl terminus. Isoln: G. Goldstein *et al., Proc. Natl. Acad. Sci. USA* **72,** 11 (1975); as APF-1 and recognition of role as marker in protein degradation: A. Ciechanover *et al., Biochem. Biophys. Res. Commun.* **81,** 1100 (1978); A. Ciechanover *et al., Proc. Natl. Acad. Sci. USA* **77,** 1365 (1980); A. Hershko *et al., ibid.* 1783. Amino acid sequence: D. H. Schlesinger *et al., Biochemistry* **14,** 2214 (1975). Identity of APF-1 with ubiquitin and revised amino acid sequence: A. Ciechanover *et al., J. Biol. Chem.* **255,** 7525 (1980); K. D. Wilkinson *et al., ibid.* 7529; K. D. Wilkinson, T. K. Audhya, *ibid.* **256,** 9235 (1981). Structural studies: W. J. Cook *et al., J. Mol. Biol.* **130,** 353 (1979); S. Vijay-Kumar *et al., J. Biol. Chem.* **262,** 6396 (1987); P. L. Weber *et al., Biochemistry* **26,** 7282 (1987). Role of chromatin structure: D. C. Watson *et al., Nature* **276,** 196 (1978); R. D. Mueller *et al., J. Biol. Chem.* **260,** 5147 (1985); in receptor structure: M. Siegelman *et al., Science* **231,** 823 (1986). Identity as heat shock protein: U. Bond, M. J. Schlesinger, *Mol. Cell. Biol.* **5,** 949 (1985). Role as marker for protein degradation in polymeric form: A. Hershko, H. Heller, *Biochem. Biophys. Res. Commun.* **128,** 1079 (1985); V. Chau *et al., Science* **243,** 1576 (1989). Enzymic determn: I. A. Rose, J. V. B. Warms, *Proc. Natl. Acad. Sci. USA* **84,** 1477 (1987). Brief review of functions and mechanisms: D. Finley, A. Varshavsky, *Trends Biochem. Sci.* **10,** 343 (1985). Review of protein degradation: M. Rechsteiner, *Annu. Rev. Cell Biol.* **3,** 1-30 (1987); A. Hershko, *J. Biol. Chem.* **263,** 15327-15240 (1988). *Review:* K. D. Wilkinson, *Anti-Cancer Drug Des.* **2,** 211-229 (1987). Book: *Ubiquitin,* M. Rechsteiner, Ed. (Plenum Press, New York, 1988).

9845. Uliginosins. Antibiotics isolated from *Hypericum uliginosum* HBK, a woody herb found in Mexico and Central America. Isoln: Taylor, Brooker, *Lloydia* **32,** 217 (1969). Structure: Parker, Johnson, *J. Am. Chem. Soc.* **90,** 4716 (1968); Parker *et al., ibid.* 4723. Synthesis of uliginosin A and dihydrouliginosin B: Meikle, Stevens, *Chem. Commun.* **1972,** 123; *eidem, J. Chem. Soc. Perkin Trans. 1* **1978,** 1303. Synthesis of uliginosin B: *eidem, Tetrahedron Lett.* **1972,** 4787; *eidem, J. Chem. Soc. Perkin Trans. 1* **1979,** 2563.

Uliginosin A. [19809-78-0] 3,5-Dihydroxy-4,4-dimethyl-2-(2-methyl-1-oxopropyl)-6-[[2,4,6-trihydroxy-3-(3-methyl-2-butenyl)-5-(2-methyl-1-oxopropyl)phenyl]methyl]-2,5-cyclohexadien-1-one. $C_{28}H_{36}O_8$; mol wt 500.58. Pale yellow crystals, mp 160.5-161.5° from acetonitrile-chloroform (4:1). uv max (cyclohexane): 229, 293 nm (ε 31500, 25000).

Uliginosin A

Uliginosin B

Uliginosin B. [19809-79-1] 2-[[5,7-Dihydroxy-2,2-dimethyl-8-(2-methyl-1-oxopropyl)-2H-1-benzopyran-6-yl]methyl]-3,5-dihydroxy-4,4-dimethyl-6-(2-methyl-1-oxopropyl)-2,5-cyclohexadien-1-one. $C_{28}H_{34}O_8$; mol wt 498.56. Pale yellow crystals, mp 139.5-142.0° from nitromethane. uv max (cyclohexane): 230, 270 nm (ε 34000, 37000).

9846. Ultramarine. [1317-97-1] C.I. Pigment Blue 29; C.I. 77007. A blue pigment occurring naturally as the mineral lapis lazuli. Made by igniting a mixture of kaolin, Na_2CO_3 (or Na_2SO_4), S and carbon. The resulting aluminosulfosilicates resemble zeolites structurally and have the approx formula $Na_7Al_6Si_6O_{24}S_3$. *See: Colour Index* **vol. 4** (3rd ed., 1971) p 4653.

Blue lumps or powder. Insol in water; readily dec by acids, even carbonic acid, with liberation of H_2S.

USE: As a pigment in calico printing, wall paper, mottled soap; bluing in laundry use; for coloring tiles, cements, rubber, but is now largely replaced by coal tar dyes; as a color in food.

9847. Umbelliferone. [93-35-6] 7-Hydroxy-2H-1-benzo-pyran-2-one; 7-hydroxycoumarin; hydrangin; skimmetin. $C_9H_6O_3$; mol wt 162.14. C 66.67%, H 3.73%, O 29.60%. The aglucon of skimmin. Present in many plants. Obtained by distillation of resins from umbelliferae: Zwenger, *Ann.* **115**, 1, 15 (1860). Prepn: Bert, *Compt. Rend.* **214**, 230 (1942); Austerweil, *ibid.* **248**, 1810 (1959); Dressler, Reabe, US 3503996 (1970 to Koppers). Main product of metabolism of coumarin in man: Schilling *et al., Nature* **221**, 664 (1969). Metabolism studies of umbelliferone: Indahl, Scheline, *Xenobiotica* **1**, 13 (1971). Use in brain intracellular pH measurements: T. M. Sundt, R.E. Anderson, *Brain Res.* **186**, 355 (1980); *eidem, J. Neurophysiol.* **44**, 60 (1980). Use in fluorescent immunoassays: S. G. Thompson, J. F. Burd, *Antimicrob. Agents Chemother.* **18**, 264 (1980); T. M. Li *et al., Anal. Biochem.* **118**, 102 (1981).

Needles from water, mp 225-228°. Develops odor of coumarin on heating. Sublimes. Absorption spectrum: Sen, Bagchi, *J. Org. Chem.* **24**, 316 (1959). One gram dissolves in ~100 ml boiling water; freely sol in alcohol, chloroform, acetic acid; sol in dil alkalies; sparingly sol in ether. Solns show blue fluorescence.

USE: In sunscreen lotions and creams; as intracellular and pH sensitive fluorescent indicator and blood-brain barrier probe.

9848. Undecylenic Acid. [112-38-9] 10-Undecenoic acid; 10-hendecenoic acid; 9-undecylenic acid; Fungoid Solution; Myco-

décyl Solution. $C_{11}H_{20}O_2$; mol wt 184.28. C 71.69%, H 10.94%, O 17.36%. $CH_2=CH(CH_2)_8CO_2H$. Prepn from castor oil: Krafft, *Ber.* **10**, 2035 (1877); Perkins, Cruz, *J. Am. Chem. Soc.* **49**, 1073 (1927); G. Das *et al., J. Am. Oil Chem. Soc.* **66**, 938 (1989). Toxicology: G. W. Newell *et al., J. Invest. Dermatol.* **13**, 145 (1949). Clinical trials: A. L. Shapiro, S. Rothman, *Arch. Dermatol. Syphilol.* **52**, 166 (1945), republ. in *Arch. Dermatol.* **119**, 345 (1983); J. H. Chretien *et al., Int. J. Dermatol.* **19**, 51 (1980). Historical review: J. W. Landau, *Arch. Dermatol.* **119**, 351-353 (1983).

Liquid or crystals. Odor suggestive of perspiration. d_4^{24} (vac) 0.9072; d_{25}^{25} 0.9102; d_{45}^{45} 0.8993; $d_4^{79.9}$ (vac) 0.8653. mp 24.5°; bp$_{760}$ 275° (dec); bp$_{182}$ 232-235°; bp$_{130}$ 230-235°; bp$_{100}$ 213.5°; bp$_{90}$ 198-200°; bp$_{15}$ 168.3°; bp$_{1.0}$ 131°. n_D^{25} 1.4486. Neutralization value 304.5; iodine value 137.8. Insol in water. Sol in alcohol, chloroform, ether. LD_{50} in mice (g/kg): 8.15 orally; 0.960 i.p. (Newell).

Zinc salt. [557-08-4] Zinc undecylenate. $C_{22}H_{38}O_4Zn$. Amorphous white powder, mp 115-116°. Resembles zinc stearate in appearance and physical properties. Can be prepd by dissolving zinc oxide in dil undecylenic acid and concentrating the solution.

Mixture with zinc salt. Cruex; Desenex; Fungex; Turexan Crème.

Methyl ester. $C_{12}H_{22}O_2$. Liq; d_4^{15} 0.889; bp$_{760}$ 248°; bp$_{10}$ 124°; mp −27.5°; n_D^{20} 1.43928; n_D^{25} 1.43727. Sol in alcohol, chloroform, ether, petr ether, oils.

THERAP CAT: Antifungal (topical).

THERAP CAT (VET): Antifungal (topical).

9849. Unoprostone. [120373-36-6] (5Z)-7-[(1R,2R,3R,5S)-3,5-Dihydroxy-2-(3-oxodecyl)cyclopentyl]-5-heptenoic acid; 13,14-dihydro-15-keto-20-ethyl-$PGF_{2\alpha}$. $C_{22}H_{38}O_5$; mol wt 382.53. C 69.08%, H 10.01%, O 20.91%. Prepn: R. Ueno *et al., EP 289349; eidem,* US 5221763 (1988, 1993 both to Ueno). Pharmacological characterization: Y. Goh, J. Kishino, *Jpn. J. Ophthalmol.* **38**, 236 (1994). Mechanism of action study: M. Sakurai *et al., ibid.* **37**, 252 (1993). Comparative clinical trial in glaucoma and ocular hypertension: J.-P. Nordmann *et al., Am. J. Ophthalmol.* **133**, 1 (2002).

Isopropyl ester. [120373-24-2] UF-021; Rescula. $C_{25}H_{44}O_5$; mol wt 424.61.

THERAP CAT: Antiglaucoma; in treatment of ocular hypertension.

9850. Uracil. [66-22-8] 2,4(1H,3H)-Pyrimidinedione; 2,4-dioxopyrimidine; 2,4-pyrimidinediol; 4-hydroxy-2(1H)-pyrimidinone; 2-hydroxy-4(1H)-pyrimidinone; 2-hydroxy-4(3H)-pyrimidinone. $C_4H_4N_2O_2$; mol wt 112.09. C 42.86%, H 3.60%, N 24.99%, O 28.55%. Obtained by hydrolysis of nucleic acids, *cf.* Levene, Bass, *Nucleic Acids* (New York, 1931). Alternate routes of formation: Johnson, *J. Am. Chem. Soc.* **63**, 263 (1941); Fox, Harada, *Science* **133**, 1923 (1961); Takemoto, Yamamoto, *Synthesis* **1971**, 154. Several desmotropic forms. Crystal structure: Stewart, *Acta Crystallogr.* **23**, 1102 (1967). Review: Ts'o "Bases, Nucleosides and Nucleotides" in *Basic Principles in Nucleic Acid Chemistry* **vol. 1**, P. O. P Ts'o, Ed. (Academic Press, New York, 1974) pp 453-584.

Needles from water, mp 335° with effervescence. uv max (pH 7.0): 202.5, 259.5 nm ($\varepsilon \times 10^{-3}$ 9.2, 8.2). Freely sol in hot water;

sparingly in cold water (100 parts of water at 25° dissolves 0.358 part of uracil). Almost insol in alc, ether; sol in ammonia water and in other alkalies. pK = 9.45.

USE: In biochemical research.

9851. Uracil Mustard. [66-75-1] 5-[Bis(2-chloroethyl)-amino]-2,4-(1H,3H)-pyrimidinedione; 5-[bis(2-chloroethyl)amino]-uracil; 2,6-dihydroxy-5-bis[2-chloroethyl]aminopyramidine; 5-[di(β-chloroethyl)amino]uracil; uramustine; demethyldopan; desmethyldopan; NSC-34462; U-8344. $C_8H_{11}Cl_2N_3O_2$; mol wt 252.10. C 38.11%, H 4.40%, Cl 28.13%, N 16.67%, O 12.69%. Synthesis from 5-aminouracil: Lyttle, Petering, *J. Am. Chem. Soc.* **80**, 6459 (1958); Lyttle, US 2969364 (1961 to Upjohn). Teratology study: S. Chaube, M. L. Murphy, "The Teratogenic Effects of the Recent Drugs Active in Cancer Chemotherapy" in *Adv. Teratol.* **3**, D. H. M. Woollam, Ed. (Academic Press, New York, 1968) pp 181-237.

Crystals from methanol + water, dec 206°. Sparingly sol in water. uv max (0.01N H_2SO_4 in 95% ethanol): 257 nm (ε 5675). LD_{50} i.p. in rats: ~1.25-2.5 mg/kg (Chaube, Murphy).

THERAP CAT: Antineoplastic.

9852. Uramil. [118-78-5] 5-Amino-2,4,6(1H,3H,5H)-pyrimidinetrione; 5-aminobarbituric acid; dialuramide; 5-amino-2,4,6-pyrimidinetriol. $C_4H_5N_3O_3$; mol wt 143.10. C 33.57%, H 3.52%, N 29.36%, O 33.54%. Prepd by boiling alloxantin with ammonium chloride: Wöhler, Liebig, *Ann.* **26**, 241 (1838); by reduction of 5-nitrobarbituric acid with tin and HCl: Hartman, Sheppard, *Org. Synth.* **coll. vol. II**, 617 (1943); from barbituric acid, sodium nitrite and sodium hydrosulfite: Koppel, Robins, *J. Am. Chem. Soc.* **80**, 2751 (1958).

Crystals. Discolors in the air. Does not melt below 400°. Insol in cold water, in ether, chloroform; sparingly sol in hot water; sol in solns of alkali hydroxides, in ammonia and in sulfuric acid. Forms a slightly sol lead salt.

9853. Uranediol. [516-51-8] (3β,5α,17α,17aβ)-17-Methyl-D-homoandrostane-3,17a-diol. $C_{21}H_{36}O_2$; mol wt 320.51. C 78.69%, H 11.32%, O 9.98%. From pregnant mares' urine: Marker *et al., J. Am. Chem. Soc.* **60**, 210, 1061, 1561, 2719 (1938); Klyne, *Biochem. J.* **43**, 611 (1948); Brooks *et al., ibid.* **51**, 694 (1952). Structure: Klyne, *Nature* **166**, 559 (1950). Formation by acid hydrolysis of 5α-pregnane-3β,20β-diol: Hirschmann, Williams, *J. Biol. Chem.* **238**, 2305 (1963). Configuration: Hirschmann *et al., J. Org. Chem.* **31**, 375 (1966).

Needles from aq ethanol, mp 216-219°. Sublimes at 180° and 0.06-0.1 mm. $[\alpha]_D^{15}$ +3.7° (c = 1.8 in chloroform).

Diacetate. $C_{25}H_{40}O_4$. Plates from aq methanol, mp 159.5-160.5°. Sublimes at 190° and 0.1 mm. $[\alpha]_D^{20}$ −30.4° (c = 1.4 in chloroform); $[\alpha]_D^{22}$ −29.6° (ethanol).

Dibenzoate. $C_{35}H_{44}O_4$. Leaflets from chloroform + methanol, mp 209-210°. $[\alpha]_D^{29}$ +18.6° (c = 1.05 in chloroform). uv max: 230, 272 nm (log ε 4.43, 3.26).

9854. Uranium. [7440-61-1] U; at. wt 238.0289 (characteristic naturally occurring isotopic mixture); at. no. 92; valence 6, 5, 4, 3. No stable nuclides; three naturally occurring isotopes (mass numbers): 238, $T_{1/2}$ 4.47 × 10^9 years, rel. at. mass 238.0508 (99.275%); 235, $T_{1/2}$ 7.04 × 10^8 years, rel. at. mass 235.0439 (0.718%); 234, $T_{1/2}$ 2.46 × 10^5 years, rel. at. mass 234.0409 (0.005%); twelve artificial isotopes: 226-233; 236; 237; 239; 240. Occurrence in the earth's crust 2.1 ppm. Mined as uranium ore; main ores of commercial interest are carnotite, pitchblende, tobernite and autunite. Commercially important mines located in Elliot Lake−Blind River area in Canada, Rand gold fields in South Africa, Colorado and Utah in U.S., in Australia and France. Discovery from pitchblende: M. H. Klaproth, *Chem. Ann.* **II**, 387 (1789). Prepn of metal: E. Péligot, *C.R. Hebd. Seances Acad. Sci.* **12**, 735 (1841); *idem, Ann. Chim. Phys.* **5**, 5 (1842). Flowsheet and details of prepn of pure uranium metal: *Chem. Eng.* **62**, no. 10, 113 (1955); Spedding *et al.*, US 2852364 (1958 to U.S.A. E.C.). *Reviews: Mellor's* vol. XII, 1-138 (1932); C. D. Harrington, A. R. Ruehle, *Uranium Production Technology* (Van Nostrand, Princeton, 1959); E. H. P. Cordfunke, *The Chemistry of Uranium* (Elsevier, New York, 1969) 250 pp; several authors in *Handb. Exp. Pharmakol.* **36**, 3-306 (1973); "The Actinides," in *Comprehensive Inorganic Chemistry* vol. 5, J. C. Bailar, Jr., *et al.*, Eds. (Pergamon Press, Oxford, 1973) *passim;* F. Weigel in *Kirk-Othmer Encyclopedia of Chemical Technology* vol. 23 (Wiley-Interscience, New York, 3rd ed., 1983) pp 502-547; *idem* in *The Chemistry of the Actinide Elements* vol. 1, J. J. Katz *et al.*, Eds. (Chapman and Hall, New York, 1986) pp 169-442; J. C. Spirlet *et al., Adv. Inorg. Chem.* **31**, 1-40 (1987). Review of toxicology and health effects: *Toxicological Profile for Uranium* (PB99-163362, 1999) 462 pp.

Silver-white, lustrous, radioactive metal; malleable and ductile. Tarnishes rapidly in air, forming a layer of dark-colored oxide. Three allotropic modifications: orthorhombic α-form, d 19.07, transforms to β-form at 667.8° ±1.3°; tetragonal, β-form, d 18.11, transforms to γ-form at 774.9° ±1.6°; body-centered cubic γ-form, d 18.06, transforms to liquid at mp. mp 1132.8 ±0.8°. Heat of vaporization 446.7 kJ/mol; heat of fusion 19.7 kJ/mol; heat of sublimation 487.9 kJ/mol. Finely divided U metal and some U compounds may ignite spontaneously in air or oxygen. Rapidly soluble in aqueous HCl. Non-oxidizing acids, such as sulfuric, phosphoric and hydrofluoric, react only very slowly with U; nitric acid dissolves massive U at a moderate rate. Dissolution of finely divided U in nitric acid may approach explosive violence. Uranium metal is inert to alkalies.

Caution: Uranium is a chemical hazard as well as a radiological hazard. Potential symptoms of overexposure to U metal or insoluble U compds are dermatitis; kidney damage; blood changes. Potential symptoms of overexposure to soluble U compds are lacrimation, conjunctivitis; shortness of breath, cough, chest rales; nausea, vomiting, skin burns; red blood cells and casts in urine; albuminuria; high blood urea nitrogen. Radiation hazard is caused by the direct emission of α-particle radiation and by α-particles emitted from radon gas and its particulate daughters formed during the natural decay of U. U and U compds are potential occupational carcinogens. See *NIOSH Pocket Guide to Chemical Hazards* (DHHS/NIOSH 97-140, 1997) p 326; *Patty's Industrial Hygiene and Toxicology* vol. 2C, G. D. Clayton, F. E. Clayton, Eds. (Wiley-Interscience, New York, 4th ed., 1994) pp 2297-2317.

USE: ^{235}U in nuclear power reactors and nuclear weapons. Uranium depleted of ^{235}U to manuf armor-piercing ammunition, in inertial guidance devices and gyro compasses, as a counterweight for missile reentry vehicles, as radiation shielding material, and x-ray targets.

9855. Uranium Dioxide. [1344-57-6] Uranous oxide; black uranium oxide. O_2U; mol wt 270.03. O 11.85%. U 88.15%. UO_2. Occurs in nature as the minerals **uraninite** or **pitchblende**. Review of uranium oxides: Keller in *Comprehensive Inorganic Chemistry* vol. 5, J. C. Bailar, Jr. *et al.*, Eds. (Pergamon Press, Oxford, 1973) pp 224-233.

Brown to black powder, or cubic crystals. d 10.97. mp 2865°. When obtained by heating the urano-uranic oxide or the oxalate in hydrogen, it is brown or copper-red in color and is pyrophoric. Insol in water, dil acids; sol in concd acids.

USE: Nuclear fuel.

9856. Uranium Hexafluoride. [7783-81-5] F_6U; mol wt 352.02. F 32.38%, U 67.62%. UF_6. Prepd by the action of fluorine on uranium metal or carbide; on uranium pentachloride; on uranium tetrafluoride; on triuranium octaoxide in the presence of carbon. It appears that all uranium compds when heated with fluorine to a sufficiently high temp give UF_6: National Nuclear Energy Series VIII-5, J. J. Katz, E. Rabinowitch, *The Chemistry of Uranium*, part I (New York, 1951) pp 396-449.

Volatile, white monoclinic cryst solid. $d_4^{20.7}$ 5.09. d^{70} (liq) 3.595. mp 64.8°. Sublimes at 56.5°. Critical temp 230.2°, crit pressure 45.5 atm: Oliver *et al.*, *J. Am. Chem. Soc.* **75**, 2827 (1953). Reacts vigorously with water, forming mainly UO_2F_2 and HF. Sol in liq chlorine and bromine. Dissolves in nitrobenzene to give a dark red soln fuming in air. Sol in carbon tetrachloride, chloroform, and *sym*-tetrachloroethane, $Cl_2CHCHCl_2$, which forms the most stable soln, extensive reaction occurring only after several days at room temp. Sol in fluorocarbons (C_6F_{12} or C_7F_{16}) without reaction. Best handled in copper apparatus.

9857. Uranium Tetrachloride. [10026-10-5] Cl_4U; mol wt 379.84. Cl 37.33%, U 62.67%. UCl_4. Prepd from uranium(VI) oxide and hexachloropropene: Hermann, Suttle, *Inorg. Synth.* **5**, 143 (1957).

Dark green octahedral crystals (tetragonal symmetry). Oxidizes in air and dec on contact with water. Should be stored in sealed ampuls. d_4^{25} 4.725. mp 590°, bp_{760} 791°. Heat of formation (solid) 250.9 kcal/mol at 0°. Freely sol in water (dec). Also sol in polar organic solvents. Insol in nonpolar solvents such as hydrocarbons and ethyl ether.

9858. Uranium Tetrafluoride. [10049-14-6] F_4U; mol wt 314.02. F 24.20%, U 75.80%. UF_4. Prepd from uranyl oxide and dichlorodifluoromethane: Booth *et al.*, *J. Am. Chem. Soc.* **68**, 1969 (1946); also prepd by the action of hydrogen fluoride on uranium dioxide or by addition of hydrofluoric acid to a U(IV) soln: Eméléus in *Fluorine Chemistry* vol. I, J. H. Simons, Ed. (Academic Press, New York, 1950) p 59.

Monoclinic green crystals, mp >1100°. Changes to U_3O_8 when heated in air. Insol in water. Sol in concd acids and alkalies with decompn.

Hemipentahydrate. Orthorhombic green crystals, insol in water.

9859. Uranium Trichloride. [10025-93-1] Cl_3U; mol wt 344.39. Cl 30.88%, U 69.12%. UCl_3. Prepd by hydrogen reduction of uranium(IV) chloride: Suttle, *Inorg. Synth.* **5**, 145 (1957).

Dark purple crystals. Less hygroscopic than uranium(IV) chloride. d 5.51. mp 842°. Heat of formation at 25° 212.0 kcal/mol. Freely sol in water, giving a purple soln, which evolves hydrogen and turns green because of oxidation to uranium(IV). Less sol in polar organic solvents than uranium(IV) chloride and insol in nonpolar solvents.

9860. Uranium Trioxide. [1344-58-7] Uranic oxide; red uranium oxide. O_3U; mol wt 286.03. O 16.78%, U 83.22%. UO_3. Review of uranium oxides: Keller in *Comprehensive Inorganic Chemistry* vol. 5, J. C. Bailar, Jr. *et al.*, Eds. (Pergamon Press, New York, 1973) pp 224-233.

Red or brownish-yellow powder. d 7.29. Insol in water; sol in acids.

9861. Uranyl Acetate. [541-09-3] $C_4H_6O_6U$; mol wt 388.12. C 12.38%, H 1.56%, O 24.73%, U 61.33%. $UO_2(C_2H_3-O_2)_2$.

Dihydrate. Yellow, cryst powder; slight acetic odor. d 2.89. Sol in 10 parts of water, usually incompletely, due to the presence of basic salt. Freely sol in water acidulated with acetic acid, slightly in alcohol.

USE: As a reagent for pptn of sodium; in dry copying inks, and as activator in bacterial oxidation processes.

9862. Uranyl Chloride. [7791-26-6] Uranium dioxydichloride. Cl_2O_2U; mol wt 340.93. Cl 20.80%, O 9.39%, U 69.82%. UO_2Cl_2. Prepd by the reaction of O_2 with uranium(IV) chloride at 300-350°: Leary, Suttle, *Inorg. Synth.* **5**, 148 (1957).

Bright yellow crystals. Orthorhombic system. Very hygroscopic. Appreciably volatile above 775°. Dec *in vacuo* above 450° yielding chlorine and UO_2 plus U_3O_8. Very freely sol in water. Forms cryst hydrates. Sol in polar organic solvents such as acetone and alcohol, but insol in less polar solvents such as benzene. Aq solns are unstable.

9863. Uranyl Nitrate. [36478-76-9] N_2O_8U; mol wt 394.04. N 7.11%, O 32.48%, U 60.41%. $UO_2(NO_3)_2$.

Hexahydrate. Yellow crystals; greenish luster by reflected light. When shaken, rubbed, or crushed, the crystals show remarkable triboluminescence with occasional detonations. d 2.807; mp 60°. Sol in ~1.5 parts of water, freely in alcohol, ether. The aq soln is acid. Solns of uranium nitrate in ether should not be allowed to stand in sunlight as explosion may occur.

USE: As intensifier in photography; manuf uranium glaze, decorating porcelain; also as reagent in analytical chemistry.

9864. Uranyl Sulfate. [1314-64-3] O_6SU; mol wt 366.09. O 26.22%, S 8.76%, U 65.02%. UO_2SO_4.

Trihydrate. Lemon-yellow, cryst mass. d 3.28. Sol in ~5 parts water, 25 parts alcohol.

9865. Urapidil. [34661-75-1] 6-[[3-[4-(2-Methoxyphenyl)-1-piperazinyl]propyl]amino]-1,3-dimethyl-2,4(1H,3H)-pyrimidine-dione; 6-[[3-[4-(o-methoxyphenyl)-1-piperazinyl]propyl]amino]-1,3-dimethyluracil; B-66256; Ebrantil; Eupressyl; Uraprene. C_{20}-$H_{29}N_5O_3$; mol wt 387.48. C 61.99%, H 7.54%, N 18.07%, O 12.39%. α_1-Adrenergic antagonist; deriv of uracil, *q.v.* Prepn: W. Pruesse *et al.*, **DE 1942405**; *eidem*, **US 3957786** (1971, 1976 both to Byk Gulden); K. Klemm *et al.*, *Arzneim.-Forsch.* **27**, 1895 (1977). Series of articles on pharmacology, pharmacokinetics, metabolism: *ibid.* 1898-1932. Toxicity data: J. Koenig *et al.*, *ibid.* 1919. Mode of action: M. Eltze, *Eur. J. Pharmacol.* **59**, 1 (1979); H. R. Kaplan, R. D. Smith, *Fed. Proc.* **40**, 2268 (1981). Hemodynamic responses in man: G. G. Belz *et al.*, *Clin. Pharmacol. Ther.* **37**, 48 (1985). Clinical trials: A. Barankay *et al.*, *Arzneim.-Forsch.* **31**, 849 (1981); H. Liebau *et al.*, *J. Hypertens.* **4**, Suppl. 6, S141 (1986). Series of articles on clinical efficacy in hypertension: *Drugs* **35**, Suppl. 6, 147-192 (1988).

Crystals from water, mp 156-158°. uv max (methanol): 237, 268 nm (ε 1.10×10^4, 2.67×10^4). pKa 7.10. LD_{50} in male mice, rats (mg/kg): 750, 550 orally; 260, 145 i.v. (Koenig).

THERAP CAT: Antihypertensive.

9866. Urazole. [3232-84-6] 1,2,4-Triazolidine-3,5-dione; bicarbamimide; 1H-1,2,4-triazole-3,5(2H,4H)-dione; hydrazodicarbonimide; 3,5-diketotriazolidine. $C_2H_3N_3O_2$; mol wt 101.06. C 23.77%, H 2.99%, N 41.58%, O 31.66%. Prepd by heating biuret with hydrazine hydrate at 108°: Stolle, Krauch, *J. Prakt. Chem.* [2] **88**, 313 (1913). From methyl or ethyl allophanate: Gordon, Audrieth, *Inorg. Synth.* **5**, 52 (1957).

Leaflets from water, dec 249-250°. Weak acid, Ka: 1.6×10^{-6}. pH of satd aqueous soln at 25° = 3.15. Soly in water (g/100 ml): 2.83 (0°); 23.7 (65°). Sparingly sol in alc, practically insol in ether. Sol in concd HCl from which it crystallizes without change. Forms ammonium and sodium salts.

9867. Urea. [57-13-6] Carbamide; carbonyldiamide; Aquacare; Aquadrate; Basodexan; Hyanit; Keratinamin; Nutraplus; Onychomal; Pastaron; Ureaphil; Urepearl. CH_4N_2O; mol wt 60.06. C 20.00%, H 6.71%, N 46.64%, O 26.64%. H_2NCONH_2. Physiological regulator of nitrogen excretion in mammals; synthesized in the liver as an end-product of protein catabolism and excreted in urine. Also occurs normally in skin. First organic compd to be synthesized from inorganic reagents: Wöhler, *Ann. Phys.* **12**, 253 (1828). Review of mechanism of ammonium cyanate-urea conversion: J. Shorter, *Chem. Soc. Rev.* **7**, 1-14 (1978). Prepn from ammonia, carbon monoxide and sulfur in methanol: Applegath, US 2857430 (1958 to Monsanto); Franz, Applegath, *J. Org. Chem.* **26**, 3304, 3306, 3309 (1961). Review of commercial processes: *Faith, Keyes & Clark's Industrial Chemicals,* F. A. Lowenheim, M. K. Moran, Eds. (Wiley-Interscience, New York, 4th ed., 1975) pp 854-861; of uses and manufacture: I. Mavrovic, A. R. Shirley, Jr. in *Kirk-Othmer Encyclopedia of Chemical Technology* vol. 23 (Wiley-Interscience, New York, 3rd ed., 1983) pp 548-575. Review of physiological synthesis: A. J. Meijer in *Nitrogen Metabolism and Excretion,* P. J. Walsh, P. Wright, Eds. (CRC Press, Boca Raton, 1995) pp 193-204; of analytical methods: A. J. Taylor, P. Vadgama, *Ann. Clin. Biochem.* **29**, 245-264 (1992). Clinical use as emollient: G. Swanbeck, *Acta Derm. Venereol. Suppl.* **177**, 7 (1992). Diagnostic use in *Helicobacter pylori* infection: A. K. Hamlet *et al., Scand. J. Gastroenterol.* **30**, 1058 (1995).

Tetragonal prisms. Develops odor of NH_3. Cooling, saline taste. mp 132.7°. On further heating it decomposes to biuret, NH_3, and cyanuric acid. d_4^{18} 1.32; d_4^{18} of water solns (w/w): 10% 1.027; 20% 1.054; 50% 1.145. pH of a 10% water soln: 7.2. One gram dissolves in 1 ml water, 10 ml 95% alc, 1 ml boiling 95% alc, 20 ml abs alc, 6 ml methanol, 2 ml glycerol. Almost insol in chloroform, ether. Sol in concd HCl. Water solns hydrolyze slowly to ammonium carbonate with eventual decomp to ammonia and carbon dioxide.

Hydrochloride. [506-89-8] $CH_4N_2O \cdot HCl$. White to faintly yellow, deliquesc crystals. Dec at 145°. Sol in water.

USE: Nitrogen-release fertilizer. Starting material for resins and plastics. Condensed with malonic ester to form barbituric acid. Used in the manuf of paper.

THERAP CAT: Emollient; diuretic.

THERAP CAT (VET): Nutritional factor (partial source of dietary nitrogen in ruminants); debriding agent; diuretic.

9868. Ureaform. [9011-05-6] Uramite. Condensation product of urea and formaldehyde in the approx ratio of 1.2-1.5 to 1. Consists of a mixture of methylene-urea polymers of varying length. Total nitrogen content at least 35%. Prepn: E. T. Darden, US 2766283 (1956 to Du Pont). Long-term trial in turf grass: D. V. Waddington *et al., Soil Sci. Soc. Am. J.* **40**, 593 (1976). Availability and mineralization in soil: P. Sasson, *Soil Sci.* **128**, 285 (1979). *Review:* A. Alexander, H.-U. Helm, *Z. Pflanzenernaehr. Bodenkd.* **153**, 249-255 (1990).

n = 1-10

Yellow, granular material of small particle size. Cold water sol fraction is composed primarily of methylenediurea and dimethylenetriurea.

USE: Slow-release nitrogen fertilizer for turf grass.

9869. Urea Nitrate. [124-47-0] Acidogen nitrate. $CH_5N_3O_4$; mol wt 123.07. C 9.76%, H 4.09%, N 34.14%, O 52.00%. $CO(NH_2)_2 \cdot HNO_3$. Prepn: DE 285259 (1914 to Osterr. Ver. Chem. Metallurg. Prod.), *Frdl.* **12**, 97; and physicochemical props: T. R.

Narayanan Kutty, A. R. Vasudeva Murthy, *Indian J. Technol.* **10**, 305 (1972). Crystal structure: S. Harkema, D. Feil, *Acta Crystallogr.* B25, 589 (1969). Use to solubilize mineral phosphates in soils: D. N. Pathak, *Fert. Technol.* **15**, 154 (1978). Use for nitration of aromatic amines: T. P. Sura *et al., Synth. Commun.* **18**, 2161 (1988).

White, odorless leaflets. mp 152° with decompn. Flammable, may explode if exposed to heat, flame or shock. Soly (g/100g) at 0°: water 9.30, alcohol 1.35; at 65.3°: water 39.84, alcohol 8.84. The aq soln is acid.

USE: As sensitizer for explosives; fertilizer; organic reagent.

9870. Urease. [9002-13-5] Urea amidohydrolase. Nickel-dependent metalloenzyme which hydrolyzes urea to ammonium carbonate. First enzyme crystallized; mol wt approx 489,000 Da. Isolation from jack bean, *Canavalia ensiformis* and crystallization: J. B. Sumner, *J. Biol. Chem.* **69**, 435 (1926). Early structure-activity studies: G. Gorin *et al., Biochemistry* **1**, 911 (1962); C. J. Bailey, D. Boulter, *Biochem. J.* **113**, 669 (1969). Identification as nickel containing: N. E. Dixon *et al., J. Am. Chem. Soc.* **97**, 4131 (1975). Crystal structure: E. Jabri *et al., Science* **268**, 998 (1995). *Review:* J. E. Varner, "Urease" in *The Enzymes* vol. 4, P. D. Boyer *et al.,* Eds. (Academic Press, New York, 2nd ed., 1960) pp 247-256; F. J. Reithel, *ibid.* vol. 4 (3rd ed., 1971) pp 1-21.

Colorless, octahedral crystals. Soluble in water, in dil alkali and dil ammonia. uv max: 278.5 nm. Isoelectric point pH 5.0-5.1; also reported as pH 4.8 (Reithel).

USE: Clinical reagent in determination of urea in body fluid.

9871. Urea Stibamine. [1340-35-8] Carbostibamide. Pentavalent antimonial. Therapeutic efficacy in kala-azar: U. N. Brahmachari, *Indian J. Med. Res.* **10**, 492 (1922). Prepn and proposed structure as $NH_2CONHC_6H_4SbO(OH)ONH_4$: U. N. Brahmachari, J. Das, *ibid.* **12**, 423 (1924). Shown to be a mixture of products with *sym*-diphenylcarbamido-4,4'-distibonic acid as the active principal: W. H. Gray *et al., Proc. Roy. Soc.* B108, 54 (1931). Description of development: R. C. Guha *et al., Nature* **151**, 108 (1943); W. Peters, *Indian J. Med. Res.* **73** Suppl., 1 (1981). Improved prepn, characterization and activity: S. B. Mahato *et al., Biochem. Med. Metab. Biol.* **38**, 47 (1987).

Sol in water. Partially sol in alc, ether.

THERAP CAT: Antiprotozoal (Leishmania).

9872. Uredepa. [302-49-8] [Bis(1-aziridinyl)phosphinyl]-carbamic acid ethyl ester; ethyl [bis(1-aziridinyl)phosphinyl]carbamate; ethyl *N*-[bis(ethyleneimido)phosphoro]carbamate; bis(ethylenimido)phosphorylurethane; urethimine; AB-100; NSC-37095; Avinar. $C_7H_{14}N_3O_3P$; mol wt 219.18. C 38.36%, H 6.44%, N 19.17%, O 21.90%, P 14.13%. Outline of prepn: Bardos *et al., Nature* **183**, 399 (1959); Bardos, Papanastassiou, US 3201313 (1965 to Armour Pharm.).

Crystals from benzene + cyclohexane, mp 88-90°. Readily sol in water but dec in aq soln.

USE: Has been used experimentally as an insect chemosterilant.

THERAP CAT: Antineoplastic.

9873. Urena. Cadillo; caesarweed. A bast fiber from the plant *Urena lobata* Dill. ex L., *Malvaceae,* a common, perennial grass growing in tropical and subtropical areas. *Habit.* Brazil, India, Madagascar, and Africa. Harvested when in full bloom (pink flowers). The fiber is creamy white, lustrous, soft and flexible, comparable to jute. *Ref:* E. E. Stout, *Introduction to Textiles* (John Wiley, New York, 1960) pp 56-57; A. S. Roy, *Indian Textile J.* **81**, 73 (1981). Evaluation for use in pulp and paper: R. K. Dubey *et al., IPPTA* **18**, 52 (1981).

USE: In cordage and course textiles.

9874. Urethan. [51-79-6] Carbamic acid ethyl ester; ethyl carbamate; urethane; ethyl urethan. $C_3H_7NO_2$; mol wt 89.09. C

40.44%, H 7.92%, N 15.72%, O 35.92%. $NH_2COOC_2H_5$. Naturally occurring contaminant in fermented foods, particularly wine, stone-fruit brandies, and bread. Prepd by heating urea with alcohol under pressure; by warming urea nitrate with alcohol and sodium nitrite. Toxicity data: K. J. Franklin, *J. Pharmacol. Exp. Ther.* **42**, 1 (1931). Review of carcinogenic action and metabolism: S. S. Mirvish in *Adv. Cancer Res.* **11**, 1-42 (1968); of mutagenicity, metabolism and interactions with DNA: R. E. Sotomayor, T. F. X. Collins, *Toxicol. Ind. Health* **6**, 71-108 (1990); of physiological effects in animals: K. J. Field, C. M. Lang, *Lab. Animals* **22**, 255-262 (1988). Review of analysis, occurrence and formation in foodstuffs: R. Battaglia *et al., Food Addit. Contam.* **7**, 477-496 (1990); B. Zimmerli, J. Schlatter, *Mutat. Res.* **259**, 325-350 (1991).

Crystals, mp 48-50°. Cooling saline taste, d 1.1. bp 182-184°. Sublimes readily at 103° and 54 mm pressure. One gram dissolves in 0.5 ml water, 0.8 ml alcohol, 0.9 ml chloroform, 1.5 ml ether, 2.5 ml glycerol, 32 ml olive oil. The aq soln is neutral. MLD i.p. in mice: 2.1-2.2 g/kg (Franklin).

Caution: This substance is reasonably anticipated to be a human carcinogen: *Report on Carcinogens, Eleventh Edition* (PB2005-104914, 2004) p III-270.

USE: Intermediate in organic synthesis. In the prepn and modification of amino resins. As solvent, solubilizer and cosolvent for various organic materials. Animal anesthetic in laboratory procedures.

9875. Uric Acid. [69-93-2] 7,9-Dihydro-1*H*-purine-2,6,-8(3*H*)-trione; 8-hydroxyxanthine; purine-2,6,8-triol; purine-2,6,-8(1*H*,3*H*,9*H*)-trione; 2,6,8-trioxypurine. $C_5H_4N_4O_3$; mol wt 168.11. C 35.72%, H 2.40%, N 33.33%, O 28.55%. Discovered by Scheele and independently by Bergman in 1776. It forms the chief end-product of the nitrogenous metabolism of birds and scaly reptiles and is found in their excrement; present in the urine of all carnivorous animals. Prepn from urea: Bills *et al., J. Org. Chem.* **27**, 4633 (1962). Role in biological processes: Bishop, Talbott, *Pharmacol. Rev.* **5**, 231 (1953).

White, odorless, tasteless crystals; dec by heat without melting and with evolution of HCN. d 1.89. One gram dissolves in about 15,000 parts cold water, about 2000 parts boiling water; sol in glycerol, in solns of alkali hydroxides, their carbonates, sodium acetate and sodium phosphate. Insol in alcohol, ether. Gives murexide reaction.

9876. Uricase. [9002-12-4] Urate oxidase; uric oxidase; urico-oxidase; uriKoxidase. An enzyme responsible for the oxidative scission of the purine skeleton, and therefore of key importance to the catabolism of nitrogenous compds in general in organisms that do not eliminate intact uric acid or some other purine. All mammals except the primates (including man) are uricolytic organisms. Porcine liver or bovine kidney is the starting material for various purified prepns of uricase. Isoln from porcine liver: Holmberg, *Biochem. J.* **33**, 1901 (1939); Miller *et al., J. Biol. Chem.* **216**, 625 (1955); Robbins, Grant, US 2878161 (1959 to Armour). *Review:* Mahler, "Uricase" in *The Enzymes* vol. **8**, P. D. Boyer *et al.,* Eds. (Academic Press, New York, 1963) pp 285-296.

Pale, brownish-green crystals or shiny, transparent, striated plates. Practically insol in water. Slightly sol in buffered alkali solns. Solns at pH 7.5-10.5 are relatively stable. Shows unusually high absorption in the region of 330-350 nm (for highly purified uricase: $A_{276}^{1\%} = 11.3$, $A_{330}^{1\%} = 2.0$, both in 1% Na_2CO_3; $A_{280}/A_{330} = 5.6$). Isoelec. pt. pH 6.3. Copper content of the enzyme (specific activity 120-125) equals ~0.56 mg/g of enzyme protein. There appears to be a satisfactory correlation between copper content and activity of the purified enzyme. The enzyme is sensitive to cyanide ion; the presence of $10^{-4}M$ KCN inhibits its activity.

USE: In the determination of serum and urine uric acid.

9877. Uridine. [58-96-8] 1-β-D-Ribofuranosyluracil; uracil riboside. $C_9H_{12}N_2O_6$; mol wt 244.20. C 44.27%, H 4.95%, N 11.47%, O 39.31%. Nucleoside; widely distributed in nature. Prepd by hydrolysis of yeast nucleic acid with weak alkali, *cf.* Levene, Bass, *Nucleic Acids* (New York, 1931). Improved isolns: Harris, Thomas, *J. Chem. Soc.* **1948**, 1936; Elmore, *ibid.* **1950**, 2084; Lorine, Ploeser, *J. Biol. Chem.* **178**, 439 (1949). Crystal structure: Green *et al., Chem. Commun.* **1971**, 53. *Review: Basic Principles in Nucleic Acid Chemistry* vol. 1, P. O. P. Ts'o, Ed. (Academic Press, New York, 1974) *passim.*

Needles from dil alc, mp 165°. $[\alpha]_D^{20}$ +4° (c = 2). uv max (pH 7.3): 261, 205 nm (ε × 10^{-3} 10.1, 9.8), Voet *et al., Biopolymers* **1**, 193 (1963). Sol in water. Upon prolonged refluxing with HCl, furfurol is formed.

9878. Uridine 5'-Diphosphate. [58-98-0] Uridine 5'-(trihydrogen diphosphate); UDP; uridine 5'-pyrophosphate; uridine-5-pyrophosphoric acid. $C_9H_{14}N_2O_{12}P_2$; mol wt 404.16. C 26.75%, H 3.49%, N 6.93%, O 47.50%, P 15.33%. Can be isolated from calf's liver, thymus, and yeast. The commercial product is derived from yeast. Pentose nucleic acids (isolated from yeast) are digested with rattlesnake venom (freed of 5'-monoesterase) and the nucleotides are separated by chromatography: Cohn, Volkin, *Arch. Biochem. Biophys.* **35**, 465 (1952); *J. Biol. Chem.* **203**, 319 (1953). For alternate procedures *see* the refs under Uridine Diphosphate Glucose. Syntheses: Chambers, *J. Am. Chem. Soc.* **81**, 3032 (1959); Moffatt, Khorana, *ibid.* **83**, 649 (1961).

Lithium salt monohydrate. $C_9H_{12}N_2O_{12}P_2Li_2.H_2O$. Crystals, sol in water.

Sodium salt trihydrate. $C_9H_{12}N_2O_{12}P_2Na_2.3H_3O$. Crystals. pKa'_1 6.5; pKa'_2 9.4. uv max (pH 7): 262 nm; (pH 11): 261 nm. Freely sol in water.

9879. Uridine Diphosphate Glucose. [133-89-1] Uridine 5'-(trihydrogen diphosphate) P'-α-D-glucopyranosyl ester; UDPG; UDP-Glucose; uridine 5'-pyrophosphate glucose ester; uridine-5'-diphosphoglucose; co-waldenase; co-galactoisomerase. $C_{15}H_{24}$-$N_2O_{17}P_2$; mol wt 566.30. C 31.81%, H 4.27%, N 4.95%, O 48.03%, P 10.94%. The coenzyme of the galactowaldenase system which catalyzes the conversion of galactose-1-phosphate into glucose-1-phosphate. Isoln from baker's yeast: Caputto *et al., J. Biol. Chem.* **184**, 333 (1950). Also present in animal tissue. Synthesis: Michelson, Todd, *J. Chem. Soc.* **1956**, 3459; Moffatt, Khorana, *J. Am. Chem. Soc.* **80**, 3756 (1958). *Reviews:* Leloir, Cardini in *The Enzymes* vol. **2A**, P. D. Boyer *et al.,* Eds. (Academic Press, New York, 2nd ed., 1960) pp 39-61; A. M. Michelson, *The Chemistry of Nucleosides and Nucleotides* (Academic Press, New York, 1963) pp 153-250; D. W. Hutchison, *Nucleotides and Coenzymes* (John Wiley, New York, 1964) pp 36-82.

Isolated as the barium or calcium salt, white powder, sol in water.
Sodium salt dihydrate. $C_{15}H_{23}N_2O_{17}P_2Na.2H_2O$. White powder. uv max (pH 2.0): 262 nm. Freely sol in water.

9880. Uridine 5'-Triphosphate. [63-39-8] Uridine 5'-(tetrahydrogen triphosphate); UTP. $C_9H_{15}N_2O_{15}P_3$; mol wt 484.14. C 22.33%, H 3.12%, N 5.79%, O 49.57%, P 19.19%. Pyrimidine analog of ATP. Activates chloride channels in epithelial cells; increases ciliary beat frequency and induces degranulation of goblet cells in airway epithelia. Also effects inflammatory cell function and vascular reactivity. Isoln from rabbit muscle: Lipton *et al., J. Am. Chem. Soc.* **75**, 5450 (1953). Synthesis: Kenner *et al., J. Chem. Soc.* **1954**, 2288; Hall, Khorana, *J. Am. Chem. Soc.* **76**, 5056 (1954). Review of bioactivity mediated by nucleotide receptors: S. E. O'Connor, *Life Sci.* **50**, 1657-1664 (1992). Clinical effect on chloride secretion in cystic fibrosis: M. R. Knowles *et al., Am. J. Respir. Crit. Care Med.* **151**, S65 (1995); on mucociliary clearance in combination with amiloride, *q.v.:* W. D. Bennett *et al., ibid.* **153**, 1796 (1996).

Trisodium salt dihydrate. Uteplex. $C_9H_{12}N_2Na_3O_{15}P_3.2H_2O$; mol wt 586.12. White powder, sol in water, very sparingly sol in alcohol. pKa_1 6.6; pKa_2 9.5. uv max (pH 7): 262 nm (a_M 10,000); (pH 11): 261 nm (a_M 8100).
THERAP CAT: In treatment of cystic fibrosis.

9881. 5'-Uridylic Acid. [58-97-9] Uridine 5'-phosphoric acid; uridine 5'-monophosphate; UMP. $C_9H_{13}N_2O_9P$; mol wt 324.18. C 33.34%, H 4.04%, N 8.64%, O 44.42%, P 9.55%. Nucleotide; widely distributed in nature. Synthesis by phosphorylation of 2',3'-O-benzylidene uridine with diphenyl phosphorochloridate: Brown *et al., J. Chem. Soc.* **1950**, 408; Smith, *Biochem. Prep.* **8**, 130 (1961). Monograph on the synthesis of nucleotides: G. R. Pettit, *Synthetic Nucleotides* vol. 1 (Van Nostrand Reinhold, New York, 1972) 252 pp. Crystal structure of hydrated barium salt: Shefter, Trueblood, *Acta Crystallogr.* **18**, 1067 (1965). *Reviews: see* Uridine.

Free acid: pKa_1' 6.4, pKa_2' 9.5. uv max (pH 7.0): 262 nm (a_M 10,000).

Disodium salt dihydrate. $C_9H_{11}N_2Na_2O_9P.2H_2O$. White powder, characteristic meaty taste. uv max (0.1M HCl): 262 nm (ε 10,000). Soly in water at 20°: about 41 g/100 ml H_2O.

9882. Urinastatin. [80449-31-6] Bikunin trypsin inhibitor; mingin; urinary trypsin inhibitor; UTI; ulinastatin; Miraclid. Acid-stable glycoprotein (pI 2.8), mol wt ~67,000 by gel filtration. Consists of a single polypeptide chain of 147 amino acid residues containing two Kunitz-type protease inhibitor domains, and two carbohydrate side chains. Normally present in serum and urine. Isoln from human urine: N. R. Shulman, *J. Biol. Chem.* **213**, 655 (1955); and purification: G. J. Proksch, J. I. Routh, *J. Lab. Clin. Med.* **79**, 491 (1972). Characterization: M. Balduyck *et al., Eur. J. Biochem.* **158**, 417 (1986). Protease inhibition: H. Sumi, N. Toki, *Proc. Soc. Exp. Biol. Med.* **167** 530 (1981). Determn by enzyme immunoassay: N. Nishino *et al., Haemostasis* **19**, 112 (1989). Biodistribution and clinical kinetics: B.-M. Jönsson-Berling, K. Ohlsson, *Scand. J. Clin. Lab. Invest.* **51**, 549 (1991). Protective effect in exptl pancreatitis: T. Hirano, T. Manabe, *Arch. Surg.* **128**, 1322 (1993). Clinical evaluation vs ischemic myocardial injury: S. Shimai *et al., Jpn. Circ. J.* **53**, 1144 (1989); vs postoperative hyperamylasemia: D. Korenaga *et al., Eur. Surg. Res.* **23**, 214 (1991). Receptor binding studies: H. Kobayashi *et al., J. Biol. Chem.* **269**, 20642 (1994). Review of early literature: H. J. Faarvang, *Scand. J. Clin. Lab. Invest.* **17**, Suppl. 83, 11-77 (1965). Review of characterization as subunit of inter-α-trypsin inhibitor (inter-α-inhibitor): W. Gebhard, K. Hochstrasser in *Proteinase Inhibitors*, A. J. Barrett, G. Salvesen, Eds. (Elsevier, Amsterdam, 1986) pp 389-401; W. Gebhard *et al., Biol. Chem. Hoppe-Seyler* **371**, Suppl., 13-22 (1990).

THERAP CAT: Protease inhibitor.

9883. Urobilins. Bile pigments which occur in feces; and in urine. More specifically described as dipyrrylmethene compds joined at the two α-pyrrolyl positions by methylene bridges to either pyrrolenone or pyrrolidone rings. Reviews of occurrence, proposed structures, stereoisomerism, and interrelationships of *i-urobilin*, *d-urobilin*, *stercobilin*, *urobilin IXα*, and *d-urobilin IXα*: A. H. Jackson *et al., Nature* **209**, 581 (1966); C. H. Gray, D. C. Nicholson, *Medicine* **46**, 83 (1967); W. Rüdiger, *Fortschr. Chem. Org. Naturst.* **29**, 60-139 (1971). Structure of stercobilin and *d-urobilin*: C. H. Gray, D. C. Nicholson, *J. Chem. Soc.* **1958**, 3085. Revised structure of *d-urobilin*: S. D. Killilea, P. O'Carra, *Biochem. J.* **129**, 1179 (1972). Stereochemistry: W. J. Cole *et al., J. Chem. Soc.* **1965**, 4085. Spectral study: W. J. Cole *et al., J. Chem. Soc. C* **1966**, 1321. Synthesis of optically active stercobilin: H. Plieninger, J. Ruppert, *Ann.* **736**, 43 (1970); of optically active urobilins: H. Plieninger *et al., ibid.,* 62. Abs config of stercobilin: H. Brockmann, Jr. *et al., Proc. Natl. Acad. Sci. USA* **68**, 2141 (1971).

(−)-Stercobilin

USE: Spot-test reagent for detection of copper, mercury, zinc: F. J. Welcher, *Organic Analytical Reagents* vol. **IV** (Van Nostrand, New York, 1949).

9884. Urochloralic Acid. [97-25-6] 2,2,2-Trichloroethyl β-D-glucopyranosiduronic acid; 2,2,2-trichloroethyl β-D-glucosiduronic acid; β,β,β-trichloroethyl-D-glucuronide. $C_8H_{11}Cl_3O_7$; mol wt 325.53. C 29.52%, H 3.41%, Cl 32.67%, O 34.40%. Isolated from urine of man and dog after ingestion of chloral hydrate: von Mering, Musculus, *Ber.* **8**, 663 (1875); from urine of calves fed trichloroethylene: Seto, Schultze, *J. Am. Chem. Soc.* **78**, 1616 (1956).

Needles, mp 142°. $[\alpha]_D^{27}$ −50.0° (c = 0.7). Freely soluble in water, alcohol. One gram dissolves in 234 ml of anhydr ether at 20°.

9885. Urocortin. [176591-49-4] (human); [171543-83-2] (rat). Mammalian neuropeptide related to corticotropin releasing factor (CRF), *q.v.* Composed of 40 amino acid residues. Evokes secretion of ACTH; binds to CRF receptors and to CRF binding protein. Identification in rat brain: J. Vaughan *et al., Nature* **378**, 287 (1995). Cloning and characterization of human urocortin: C. J. Donaldson *et al., Endocrinology* **137**, 2167 (1996). Interaction with CRF binding protein: D. P. Behan *et al., Brain Res.* **725**, 263 (1996). Appetite suppressing effects: M. Spina *et al., Science* **273**, 1561 (1996).

9886. Urodilatin. [115966-23-9] Renal natriuretic peptide. Natriuretic hormone produced by the kidney and secreted into the urine; regulates sodium and water reabsorption in the medullary collecting duct. Derived from the same prohormone as atrial natriuretic peptide, *q.v.*, with similar pharmacological effects. Isoln from human urine: P. Schulz-Knappe *et al., Klin. Wochenschr.* **66**, 752 (1988). RIA determn in biological samples: C. Drummer *et al., Pflügers Arch.* **423**, 372 (1993). Role in body fluid regulation: C. Drummer, *Semin. Nephrol.* **21**, 239 (2001). Review of pharmacology and clinical implications: W.-G. Forssmann *et al., Cardiovasc. Res.* **51**, 450-462 (2001). Comparison of biological actions of natriuretic peptides in experimental heart failure: H. H. Chen *et al., Am. J. Physiol. Regul. Integr. Comp. Physiol.* **288**, 1093 (2005).

Thr–Ala–Pro–Arg–Ser–Leu–Arg–Arg–Ser–Ser–Cys–Phe–Gly–Gly–Arg–Met–Asp–Arg

32
Tyr–Arg–Phe–Ser–Asn–Cys–Gly–Leu–Gly–Ser–Gln–Ala–Gly
Ile

human Urodilatin

Ularitide. [118812-69-4] Human urodilatin; ANP 95-126; CDD 95-126. $C_{145}H_{234}N_{52}O_{44}S_3$; mol wt 3505.93. Nonglycosylated peptide of 32 amino acid residues. Solid phase synthesis: W.-G. Forssmann *et al., WO 8806596; eidem, US 5449751* (1988, 1995 both to Bissendorf Peptide).

9887. Urokinase. [9039-53-6] Win-22005; Abbokinase; Actosolv; Breokinase; Persolv; Purochin; Ukidan; Uronase; Win-Kinase. Serine protease which activates plasminogen to plasmin; present in mammalian blood and urine. Produced as prourokinase, *q.v.*, and converted to active form by plasmin or kallikrein, *q.q.v.* Description of fibrinolytic activity: J. R. B. Williams, *Br. J. Exp. Pathol.* **32**, 530 (1951). Isolation from human urine and activity: T. Astrup, I. Sterndorff, *Proc. Soc. Exp. Biol. Med.* **81**, 675 (1952); G. W. Sobel *et al., Am. J. Physiol.* **171**, 768 (1952). Species specificity and distribution in mammals: S. R. Mohler *et al., Am. J. Physiol.* **192**, 186 (1958). Isoln from human male urine: H. O. Singher, L. Zuckerman, *US 2961382* and *US 2989440* (1960, 1961 to Ortho); N. O. Kjeldgaard, J. Ploug, *US 2983647* (1961 to Lövens Kemiske Fabrik); J. Doczi, *US 3081236* (1963 to Warner-Lambert). Prepn of crystalline form: A. Lesuk *et al., Science* **147**, 880 (1965). Two variants of bioactive urokinase, high molecular weight (HMW-UK, ~50 KDa) and low molecular weight (LMW-UK, ~30 KDa) have been identified: W. F. White *et al., Biochemistry* **5**, 2160 (1966). Both are disulfide-linked dimers consisting of a heavy chain (B) and a light chain (A). HMW-UK is converted to LMW-UK by proteolytic cleavage of the A-chain to form the A_1-chain. Series of articles on plasminogen activation, fibrinolysis and clinical efficacy: *Proc. Serono Symp., Thrombosis and Urokinase* **9**, 1-257 (1977). *Review:* F. Duckert, *Handb. Exp. Pharmacol.* **46**, 209-237 (1978). Structural characterization: M. Nobuhara *et al., J. Biochem.* **90**, 225 (1981). Structure and amino acid sequences: W. A. Günzler *et al., Z. Physiol. Chem.* **363**, 133 (1982); G. J. Steffens *et al., ibid.* 1043;

W. A. Günzler *et al., ibid.* 1155. Expression of gene coding for human urokinase in *E. coli:* B. Ratzkin *et al., Proc. Natl. Acad. Sci. USA* **78**, 3313 (1981). Clinical evaluation in pulmonary embolism: P. Petitpretz *et al., Circulation* **70**, 861 (1984). Clinical trial following myocardial infarction: H. Kambara *et al., Jpn. Circ. J.* **51**, 1072 (1987). Clinical applications of urokinase-treated tubing: T. Ohshiro *et al., Methods Enzymol.* **137**, 529 (1988). Literature review of thrombolytic therapy: J. A. Kaufman, M. A. Bettmann, *Semin. Intervent. Radiol.* **9**, 159-165 (1992).

THERAP CAT: Thrombolytic.

9888. Urothion. [19295-31-9] 2-Amino-7-(1,2-dihydroxyethyl)-6-(methylthio)thieno[3,2-g]pteridin-4(3H)-one. $C_{11}H_{11}N_5-O_3S_2$; mol wt 325.37. C 40.61%, H 3.41%, N 21.52%, O 14.75%, S 19.71%. Constituent of normal human urine: Koschara, *Z. Physiol. Chem.* **277**, 284 (1943). Structure: Tschesche *et al., Ber.* **88**, 1251 (1955). Revised structure: Goto *et al., Tetrahedron Lett.* **1967**, 4507; *eidem, J. Biochem. (Tokyo)* **65**, 611 (1969). Synthesis: Sakurai, Goto, *Tetrahedron Lett.* **1968**, 2941; *eidem, J. Biochem. (Tokyo)* **65**, 755 (1969).

Orange-colored clusters of crystals, not melted at 360°. Shows mutarotation: $[\alpha]_D^{20}$ −20° (after 15 hrs in 0.05N NaOH). Soly in water at pH 6.6 about 1:10,000. More sol in alkaline soln. Also sol in acids. Practically insol in the usual organic solvents.

9889. Ursodiol. [128-13-2] (3α,5β,7β)-3,7-Dihydroxycholan-24-oic acid; 17β-(1-methyl-3-carboxypropyl)etiocholane-3α,7β-diol; 3α,7β-dioxycholanic acid; ursodeoxycholic acid; Actigall; Arsacol; Cholit-Ursan; Delursan; Desol; Destolit; Deursil; Litursol; Lyeton; Peptarom; Solutrat; Urdes; Ursacol; Urso; Ursochol; Ursofalk; Ursolvan. $C_{24}H_{40}O_4$; mol wt 392.57. C 73.43%, H 10.27%, O 16.30%. Epimeric with chenodiol, *q.v.*, with respect to the hydroxyl group at C_7. Found in bear bile (combined with taurine). Isoln: Shoda, *J. Biochem. (Tokyo)* **7**, 505 (1927). Structure: Kaziro, *Z. Physiol. Chem.* **185**, 511 (1929); **197**, 206 (1931); Iwasaki, *ibid.* **244**, 181 (1936). Toxicity data: M. Ardenne, P. G. Reitnauer, *Arzneim.-Forsch.* **20**, 323 (1970). Effect on cholesterol and bile acid metabolism: G. S. Tint *et al., Gastroenterology* **91**, 1007 (1986). Clinical trial in primary biliary cirrhosis: R. E. Poupon *et al., N. Engl. J. Med.* **324**, 1548 (1991). Review of pharmacology, toxicology, efficacy: A. Ward *et al., Drugs* **27**, 95-131 (1984). Brief review of clinical effects and comparison with chenodiol: H. Fromm, *Gastroenterology* **87**, 229-233 (1984).

Bitter plates from alc. mp 203°. $[\alpha]_D^{20}$ +57° (c = 2 in abs ethanol). Freely sol in ethanol, glacial acetic acid; slightly sol in chloroform, sparingly sol in ether. Practically insol in water. LD_{50} in mice (g/kg): 0.1 i.v. (Ardenne, Reitnauer); in rats, mice (mg/kg): 2000, 6000 s.c.; 1000, 1200 i.p., 310, 260 i.v. (Ward).

Diformate. $C_{26}H_{40}O_6$. Crystals, mp 170°.

Diacetate. $C_{28}H_{44}O_6$. Crystals, mp 98-102°.

THERAP CAT: Anticholelithogenic.

9890. Ursolic Acid. [77-52-1] (3β)-3-Hydroxyurs-12-en-28-oic acid; urson; prunol; micromerol; malol. $C_{30}H_{48}O_3$; mol wt 456.70. C 78.90%, H 10.59%, O 10.51%. In leaves and berries of *Arctostaphylos uva-ursi* (L.) Spreng (bearberry), of *Vaccinium* macrocarpon Ait. (cranberry), *Rhododendron hymenanthes* Makino, *Ericaceae*. In the protective wax-like coating of apples, pears, prunes, and other fruits. Isoln from apple peelings: Sando, *J. Biol. Chem.* **56**, 457 (1923). Structure: Ruzicka *et al., Helv. Chim. Acta* **28**, 199 (1945); Zurcher *et al., ibid.* **37**, 2145 (1954). Conversion from α-amyrin: Boar *et al., J. Chem. Soc. C* **1970**, 678. Chemistry: Mezzetti *et al., Planta Med.* **20**, 244 (1971).

Large, lustrous prisms from abs alcohol, fine hair-like needles from dil alcohol, mp 285-288°. $[\alpha]_D^{21}$ +67.5° (c = 1 in *N* alc KOH). Soly at 15°: One part dissolves in 88 parts methanol, 178 alcohol (35 boiling alcohol), 140 ether, 388 chloroform, 1675 carbon disulfide. Moderately sol in acetone. Sol in hot glacial acetic acid and in 2% alcoholic NaOH. Insol in water and petr ether.

Acetate. $C_{32}H_{50}O_4$. mp 289-290°. $[\alpha]_D$ +62.3° (c = 1.15 in chloroform).

Methyl ester. $C_{31}H_{50}O_3$. mp 171°. $[\alpha]_D^{20}$ +58° (c = 1.2 in pyridine).

Methyl ester acetate. $C_{33}H_{52}O_4$. mp 246-247°.

USE: As emulsifying agent in pharmaceuticals, foods.

9891. Urushiol. Main constituent of the irritant oil of poison ivy, *Toxicodendron radicans* (L.) Kuntze, poison oak, *T. diversilobum*, the Asiatic lacquer tree, *T. verniciferum* D.C. and other plants of the genus *Toxicodendron, Anacardiaceae*. Yoshida, *J. Chem. Soc.* **43**, 472 (1883); Hill *et al., J. Am. Chem. Soc.* **56**, 2736 (1934). Mixture of 4 catechols, 3 of which have unsaturated side chains, one of which is 3-(8-pentadecenyl)catechol; the fourth is 3-*n*-pentadecylcatechol. Component identification: Majima *et al., Ber.* **55**, 172 (1922); Corbett, Billets, *J. Pharm. Sci.* **64**, 1715 (1975). Urushiol from *T. verniciferum* is a mixture of I-IV and urushiol from *T. radicans* is a mixture of I, II, III, and V: Symes, Dawson, *J. Am. Chem. Soc.* **76**, 2959 (1954); Sunthankar, Dawson, *ibid.* **76**, 5070 (1954). Separation of components: Markiewitz, Dawson, *J. Org. Chem.* **30**, 1610 (1965). Structural characterization of urushiol from *T. diversilobum*: Corbett, Billets, *loc. cit.* Separation of urushiol congeners: C. Y. Ma *et al., J. Chromatogr.* **200**, 163 (1980). Isoln of pure urushiol from poison ivy or oak extracts and separation of congeners by reversed phase chromatography: M. A. El Sohly *et al., J. Nat. Prod.* **45**, 532 (1982). Allergenic properties of congeners: E. S. Watson *et al., J. Pharm. Sci.* **70**, 785 (1981). Review of extraction and compositional analysis: J. H. P. Tyman, *Chem. Soc. Rev.* **8**, 499 (1979).

| I | R = $(CH_2)_7CH_3$ |
| II | R = $CH=CH(CH_2)_5CH_3$ |

Pale yellow liq; $d_4^{21.5}$ 0.9687; bp 200-210°. Soluble in alcohol, ether, benzene. Moderately sol in petr ether.

Caution: An extremely active allergen causing skin reactions similar to poison ivy.

THERAP CAT: Antiallergic (hyposensitization therapy).

9892. Uscharidin. [24321-47-9] [2α(2S,3R,6R),3β,5α]-14-Hydroxy-19-oxo-2,3-[(tetrahydro-3-hydroxy-6-methyl-4-oxo-2*H*-pyran-3,2-diyl)bis(oxy)]card-20(22)-enolide. $C_{29}H_{38}O_9$; mol wt

530.61. C 65.64%, H 7.22%, O 27.14%. African arrow poison and cardiac glycoside produced by *Calotropis procera* R. Br., *Asclepiadaceae*: Hesse *et al., Ann.* **566**, 130 (1950). Prepn by hydrolysis of uscharin with 2*N* H_2SO_4 in methanol: Hesse *et al., Ann.* **537**, 67 (1938); by treatment of voruscharin with mercuric chloride: Hesse, Ludwig, *Ann.* **632**, 158 (1960). Structure: Crout *et al., J. Chem. Soc.* **1964**, 2187. Revised structure: Brüschweiler *et al., Helv. Chim. Acta* **52**, 2276 (1969). Stereochemistry: H. T. A. Cheung, T. R. Watson, *J. Chem. Soc. Perkin Trans. 1* **1980**, 2162.

Rhombic plates, decomp 290°. $[\alpha]_D^{20}$ +38° (c = 0.9 in methanol).

9893. Usnic Acid. [125-46-2] 2,6-Diacetyl-7,9-dihydroxy-8,9b-dimethyl-1,3(2*H*,9b*H*)-dibenzofurandione; usninic acid; usnein. $C_{18}H_{16}O_7$; mol wt 344.32. C 62.79%, H 4.68%, O 32.53%. Antibacterial substance found in lichens. Isoln from varieties of *Usnea barbata* (L.) Wigg., *Usneaceae*: Rochleder, Heldt, *Ann.* **48**, 11 (1843); Widman, *Ann.* **310**, 230 (1900); **324**, 139 (1902). Isoln from *Ramalina reticulata*: Marshak, *Public Health Rep.* **62**, 3 (1947); Stark *et al., J. Am. Chem. Soc.* **72**, 1819 (1950). Occurs in nature in both the *d*- and *l*-forms as well as a racemic mixture. Structure: Curd, Robertson, *J. Chem. Soc.* **1937**, 894; Schöpf, Ross, *Ann.* **546**, (1941); Barton, Brunn, *J. Chem. Soc.* **1953**, 603. Resolution of (±)-usnic acid: Dean *et al., ibid.* 1250. Synthesis: Barton *et al., ibid.* **1956**, 530. Biosynthesis *in vitro*: Penttila, Fales, *Chem. Commun.* **1966**, 656. Absolute configuration of (+)-form: S. Huneck *et al., Tetrahedron Lett.* **22**, 351 (1981). Toxicity study: *Antibiotics* **I**, D. Gottlieb, P. Shaw, Eds. (Springer Verlag, New York, 1967) p 611.

Yellow orthorhombic prisms from acetone, mp 204°. $[\alpha]_D^{16}$ +509.4° (c = 0.697 in chloroform). Monobasic acid. Soly at 25° (g/100 ml): water <0.01; acetone 0.77; ethyl acetate 0.88; ethanol 0.02; methyl Cellosolve 0.22; ethyl Cellosolve 0.32; furfural 7.32; furfuryl alcohol 1.21. LD_{50} i.v. in mice: 25 mg/kg (Gottlieb, Shaw).

Sodium salt dihydrate. $C_{18}H_{15}NaO_7.2H_2O$. Pale yellow, silky needles. Slightly sol in water.

9894. Ustilagic Acid. [8002-36-6] Ustizeain B. $C_{37}H_{62-66}O_{17}$; mol wt about 780. A mixture of partially acylated derivatives of a di-D-glucosyldihydroxyhexadecanoic acid. Antibiotic substance produced by the corn smut fungus *Ustilago zeae*: Haskins, *Can. J. Res.* **28C**, 213 (1950); Lemieux *et al., Can. J. Chem.* **29**, 409, 415 (1951); Reed, Holder, *Can. J. Med. Sci.* **31**, 505 (1953); Haskins, US 2698843 (1955 to National Research Council, Canada). Biosynthesis: Boothroyd *et al., Can. J. Biochem. Physiol.* **33**, 289 (1955). Production by submerged culture: Lemieux, CA 600121 (1960 to National Research Council, Canada).

Long crystals from ether, mp 146-147°. $[\alpha]_D^{23}$ +7° (pyridine). Freely sol in methanol, pyridine, 2,3-butanediol, 1,2-propanediol. Sparingly sol in ethanol, butanol, acetone. Insol in water, glycerol, ethyl acetate, ether, benzene, petr ether. Shows *in vitro* activity against *Cryptococcus neoformans, Candida albicans,* and some saprophytic fungi. Practically ineffective in rabbits and mice suffering from fungus diseases.

9895. Utrophin. Dystrophin-related protein; DRP; DMDL protein. Autosomal homolog of dystrophin, *q.v.,* the protein affected by mutation in Duchenne muscular dystrophy (DMD). Cytoplasmic protein; mol wt 395 kDa. Localized in the neuromuscular junctions of normal adult muscle. Widely distributed in a variety of other tissues including brain, stomach, kidney, spleen, liver, and lung. The name is derived from its ubiquitous pattern of expression. Like dystrophin, utrophin binds to actin and to a transmembrane glycoprotein complex, known as dystrophin-associated proteins (DAPs), to link the cytoskeleton with the extracellular matrix. Thought to partially compensate for the lack of dystrophin in DMD patients. Identification in mouse skeletal muscle: D. R. Love *et al., Nature* **339,** 55 (1989). Primary structure: J. M. Tinsley *et al., ibid.* **360,** 591 (1992). Association with DAPs: K. Matsumura *et al., ibid.* 588; J. M. Tinsley *et al., Proc. Natl. Acad. Sci. USA* **91,** 8307 (1994). Analysis of actin-binding: S. J. Winder *et al., J. Cell Sci.* **108,** 63 (1995). Expression in DMD patients: Y. Mizuno *et al., J. Neurol. Sci.* **119,** 43 (1993). Review and comparison with dystrophin: J. M. Tinsley *et al., Curr. Opin. Genet. Dev.* **3,** 484-490 (1993); D. R. Love *et al., Neuromuscul. Disord.* **3,** 5-21 (1993); J. M. Tinsley, K. E. Davies, *ibid.* 537-539.

9896. Uva Ursi. Bearberry. Dried leaves of *Arctostaphylos uva-ursi* (L.), Spreng., *Ericaceae,* a small evergreen shrub. *Habit.* Temperate regions of Europe, North America, Asia. *Constit.* Hydroquinone derivatives, primarily arbutin, *q.v.,* and methylarbutin; tannins of the gallic and ellagic acid types; flavonoids (quercetin, myricetin); piceoside; monotropein; ursolic, gallic and quinic acids; volatile oil. Discussion of active components: D. Frohne, *Planta Med.* **18,** 1 (1970). Bioavailability: D. H. Paper *et al., Pharm. Pharmacol. Lett.* **3,** 63 (1993). Brief review of use in phytomedicine: A. Y. Leung, S. Foster, *Encyclopedia of Common Natural Ingredients* (John Wiley & Sons, New York, 2nd ed., 1996) pp 505-506.

Leaf extract. Arctuvan; Uvalysat.

THERAP CAT: Antiseptic (urinary).

9897. Uzarin. [20231-81-6] (3β,5α)-3-[(2-*O*-β-D-Glucopyranosyl-β-D-glucopyranosyl)oxy]-14-hydroxycard-20(22)-eno-

lide. $C_{35}H_{54}O_{14}$; mol wt 698.79. C 60.16%, H 7.79%, O 32.05%. Isoln from the dried root of a *Gomphocarpus* sp, *Asclepiadaceae:* Windaus, Haack, *Ber.* **63,** 1377 (1930); Tschesche, Brathge, *ibid.* **85,** 1042 (1952); Schmid *et al., Helv. Chim. Acta* **42,** 72 (1959). Yields uzarigenin by enzymic cleavage. Structure: Tschesche, Bohle, *Ber.* **68,** 2252 (1935). Structure of uzarigenin: Rangaswami, Reichstein, *Helv. Chim. Acta* **32,** 939 (1949); Russel *et al., ibid.* **44,** 1320 (1961). Unlike all other known cardiac glycosides, has the A/B-*trans* configuration: L. F. Fieser, M. Fieser, *Steroids* (Reinhold, New York, 1959) pp 762-763. *Review:* Heusser, *Fortschr. Chem. Org. Naturst.* **7,** 101 (1950).

Uzarigenin

Prisms from pyridine + water, mp 266-270°; stout needles from methanol + ether, mp 206-208°. $[\alpha]_D^{20}$ −27° (c = 1.075 in pyridine); $[\alpha]_D^{19}$ −1.4° (c = 0.85 in methanol). uv max: 217 nm (log ε 4.23). Sol in pyridine, hot methyl Cellosolve; sparingly sol in water. Practically insol in ether, chloroform, acetone.

Uzarigenin. [466-09-1] (3β,5α)-3,14-Dihydroxycard-20(22)-enolide; odorigenin. $C_{23}H_{34}O_4$; mol wt 374.51. Synthesis: Stache *et al., Ann.* **726,** 136 (1969); Kamano *et al., J. Org. Chem.* **39,** 2319 (1974); *eidem, J. Chem. Soc. Perkin Trans. 1* **1975,** 1972. Crystals from methanol, mp 240-256°. $[\alpha]_D^{20}$ +10.5° (c = 1.056 in alc).

3-*O*-Acetyluzarigenin. $C_{25}H_{36}O_5$. Hexagonal plates from methanol, mp 262-266°. $[\alpha]_D^{22}$ +4.6° (c = 1.09 in chloroform).

THERAP CAT: Antidiarrheal.

V

9898. Vaccenic Acid. [693-72-1] (11*E*)-11-Octadecenoic acid; *trans*-Δ^{11}-octadecenoic acid. $C_{18}H_{34}O_2$; mol wt 282.46. C 76.54%, H 12.13%, O 11.33%. $CH_3(CH_2)_5CH=CH(CH_2)_9$-COOH. Found in butterfat and in other animal fats. Growth-promoting factor for rats. Isoln: Bertram, *Biochem. Z.* **197**, 433 (1928). Synthesis: Böeseken, Hoagland, *Rec. Trav. Chim.* **46**, 632 (1927); Ahmad *et al., J. Am. Chem. Soc.* **70**, 3391 (1948). Configuration and ir spectrum: Rao, Daubert, *ibid.* 1102.

Platelets from acetone, mp 43-44°; n_D^{60} 1.4439; n_D^{70} 1.4402. Neutralization equivalent 282.5; iodine no. 89.9.

Methyl ester. $C_{19}H_{36}O_2$. bp_3 172-173°.

9899. Valacyclovir. [124832-26-4] L-Valine 2-[(2-amino-1,6-dihydro-6-oxo-9*H*-purin-9-yl)methoxy]ethyl ester; L-valine ester with 9-[(2-hydroxyethoxy)methyl]guanine; valaciclovir; Val-ACV. $C_{13}H_{20}N_6O_4$; mol wt 324.34. C 48.14%, H 6.22%, N 25.91%, O 19.73%. L-Valine ester prodrug of acyclovir, *q.v.* Prepn: T. A. Krenitsky *et al.*, **EP 308065**; L. M. Beauchamp, **US 4957924** (1989, 1990 both to Wellcome). Evaluation as prodrug: L. M. Beauchamp *et al., Antiviral Chem. Chemother.* **3**, 157 (1992). Clinical pharmacokinetics: S. Weller *et al., Clin. Pharmacol. Ther.* **54**, 595 (1993). Review of pharmacology and clinical efficacy in herpes virus infections: C. M. Perry, D. Faulds, *Drugs* **52**, 754-772 (1996). Clinical trial to prevent cytomegalovirus disease in renal transplantation: D. Lowance *et al., N. Engl. J. Med.* **340**, 1462 (1999); to prevent transmission of genital herpes: L. Corey *et al., ibid.* **350**, 11 (2004).

Hydrochloride. [124832-27-5] 256U; BW-256U87; BW-256; Valtrex. Crystalline solid, occurs as hydrate. uv max (water): 252.8 nm (ε 8530). Soly in water: 174 mg/ml.

THERAP CAT: Antiviral.

9900. Valdecoxib. [181695-72-7] 4-(5-Methyl-3-phenyl-4-isoxazolyl)benzenesulfonamide; SC-65872; Bextra. $C_{16}H_{14}N_2O_3$-S; mol wt 314.36. C 61.13%, H 4.49%, N 8.91%, O 15.27%, S 10.20%. Selective cyclooxygenase-2 (COX-2) inhibitor. Active metabolite of parecoxib, *q.v.* Prepn: J. J. Talley *et al.,* **WO 9625405** (1996 to Searle); *eidem,* **US 5633272** (1997); and activity: *eidem, J. Med. Chem.* **43**, 775 (2000). Chromatographic determn of purity: D. A. Roston *et al., J. Pharm. Biomed. Anal.* **26**, 339 (2001). Gastrointestinal tolerability study: G. M. Eisen *et al., Aliment. Pharmacol. Ther.* **21**, 591 (2005). Clinical trial in hip arthroplasty: F. Camu *et al., Am. J. Ther.* **9**, 43 (2002). Clinical comparison with oxycodone/acetaminophen in dental pain: S. E. Daniels *et al., J. Am. Dent. Assoc.* **133**, 611 (2002). Clinical trial in migraine: D. Kudrow *et al., Headache* **45**, 1151 (2005). Review of clinical experience: M. Goldman, S. Schutzer, *Formulary* **37**, 68-77 (2002); of clinical efficacy and safety: G. P. Joshi, *Expert Rev. Neurother.* **5**, 11-24 (2005).

Crystals, mp 155-157°. Soly at 25°(μg/ml): water 10 (pH 7.0). Sol in methanol, ethanol; freely sol in organic solvents and alkaline (pH = 12) aqueous solns.

THERAP CAT: Anti-inflammatory; analgesic.

9901. Valdetamide. [512-48-1] 2,2-Diethyl-4-penten-amide; diethylallylacetamide; Novonal. $C_9H_{17}NO$; mol wt 155.24. C 69.63%, H 11.04%, N 9.02%, O 10.31%. Description: Bockmühl, Schaumann, *Dtsch. Med. Wochenschr.* **54**, 270 (1928). Pharmacokinetics and metabolism: H. Uehleke, M. Brinkschulte-Freitas, *Arch. Pharmacol.* **302**, 11 (1978). TLC determn in urine: E. Klug, P. Toffel, *Arzneim.-Forsch.* **29**, 1651 (1979).

White powder, mp 75-76°. Sol in 120 parts water; freely sol in alcohol, ether.

THERAP CAT: Sedative, hypnotic.

9902. *n*-Valeraldehyde. [110-62-3] Pentanal; valeral; valeric aldehyde. $C_5H_{10}O$; mol wt 86.13. C 69.72%, H 11.70%, O 18.58%. $CH_3(CH_2)_3CHO$. Prepn: Lieben, Rossi, *Ann.* **159**, 70 (1871); Olsen, **US 2548171** (1951 to GAF); Sisti *et al., J. Org. Chem.* **27**, 279 (1962). Toxicity study: H. F. Smyth *et al., Am. Ind. Hyg. Assoc. J.* **30**, 470 (1969).

Liquid, bp 102-103°. d_4^{20} 0.8095. n_D^{20} 1.3944. Very slightly sol in water; miscible with many organic solvents. LD_{50} orally in rats: 5.66 ml/kg (Smyth).

Caution: Potential symptoms of overexposure are irritation of eyes, skin, nose, throat. *See NIOSH Pocket Guide to Chemical Hazards* (DHHS/NIOSH 97-140, 1997) p 326.

USE: In flavoring compds, resin chemistry, rubber accelerators.

9903. Valerian. Perennial herb, *Valeriana officinalis* L., *Valerianaceae*. Medicinal portions are the dried rhizomes and roots; traditionally used to treat insomnia and anxiety. *Habit.* Europe, Northern Asia; naturalized in eastern U.S. Numerous other species exist throughout the world which are also used medicinally. *Constit.* Volatile oil (0.5-2%); iridoids (valepotriates) such as valtrate, didrovaltrate, isovaltrate; alkaloids incl. valerianine and chatinine; tannin, resin. Review of pharmacology: P. J. Houghton, *J. Ethnopharmacol.* **22**, 121-142 (1988); of constituents and medicinal uses: J. Barnes *et al., Herbal Medicines* (Pharmaceutical Press, London, 2nd Ed., 2002) pp 468-476; J. Gruenwald *et al., PDR for Herbal Medicines* (Medical Economics, Montvale, 3rd Ed., 2004) pp 852-856.

Volatile oil. [8008-88-6] Oil of valerian. *Constit.* Monoterpenes, incl. α- and β-pinene, camphene, borneol, eugenol; sesquiterpenes incl. β-bisabolene, caryophyllene, valeratone. Yellowish-green to brownish liquid. d_{15}^{15} 0.93-0.96. α_D −8 to −13°. Sapon no. 100-150. Acid no. 20-50. Slightly sol in water; very sol in alcohol, chloroform, ether. *Keep well closed, cool and protected from light.*

THERAP CAT: Sedative.

9904. *n*-Valeric Acid. [109-52-4] Pentanoic acid; valerianic acid; propylacetic acid. $C_5H_{10}O_2$; mol wt 102.13. C 58.80%, H 9.87%, O 31.33%. Obtained by decompn of *n*-propylmalonic acid: Fürth, *Monatsh. Chem.* **9**, 308 (1888); from *n*-butyl chloride: Gilman, Kirby, *Org. Synth.* **coll. vol. I**, 363 (2nd ed., 1941). Industrial synthesis by oxidation of amyl alcohol or by fermentation processes. Toxicity study: L. Orö, A. Wretlind, *Acta Pharmacol. Toxicol.* **18**, 141 (1961).

Colorless liquid; unpleasant odor; d_4^{20} 0.939; mp −34.5°; bp 186-187°; bp_{23} 96°; n_D^{20} 1.4086. Sol in 30 parts water; freely sol in alcohol, ether. LD_{50} i.v. in mice: 1290 ±53 mg/kg (Orö, Wretlind).

Ethyl ester. [539-82-2] Ethyl *n*-valerate. $C_7H_{14}O_2$. Liquid. d_4^{20} 0.877. bp 145-146°. n_D^{20} 1.3732. Insol in water. Misc with alcohol, ether.

USE: Intermediate in perfumery.

9905. Valeronitrile. [110-59-8] Pentanenitrile; 1-butyl cyanide; 1-cyanobutane. C_5H_9N; mol wt 83.13. C 72.24%, H 10.91%, N 16.85%. $CH_3(CH_2)_3CN$. Prepn: A. Lieben, A. Rossi, *Ann.* **158**, 137 (1871); W. Kantlehner *et al., ibid.* **1980**, 389; H. G. Thomas, H. D. Greyn, *Synthesis* **1990**, 129. Acute toxicity and metabolism: H. Tanii, K. Hashimoto, *Arch. Toxicol.* **55**, 47 (1984). Comparative toxicity of aliphatic nitriles: M. A. Wallig *et al., Food Chem. Toxicol.* **26**, 149 (1988).

bp$_{15}$ 45-47°. bp$_{739.3}$ 140.4°. bp 141°. d^0 0.8164. n_D^{20} 1.3962. Log P (*n*-octanol/water): 0.94. LD$_{50}$ orally in male mice: 2.297 mmol/kg (Tanii).

USE: Solvent.

9906. Valethamate Bromide. [90-22-2] *N,N*-Diethyl-*N*-methyl-2-[(3-methyl-1-oxo-2-phenylpentyl)oxy]ethanaminium bromide; 3-methyl-2-phenylvaleric acid diethyl(3-hydroxyethyl)methylammonium bromide ester; 2-phenyl-3-methylvaleric acid β-(diethylamino)ethyl ester bromomethylate; 3-methyl-2-phenylvaleric acid 2-diethylaminoethyl ester methyl bromide; 2-diethylaminoethyl 2-phenyl-3-methylvalerate methyl bromide; diethyl(2-hydroxyethyl)methylammonium 3-methyl-2-phenylvalerate bromide; Resitan; Epidosin. $C_{19}H_{32}BrNO_2$; mol wt 386.37. C 59.06%, H 8.35%, Br 20.68%, N 3.63%, O 8.28%. Anticholinergic. Prepn: Stühmer, Funke, **DE 969245**; **DE 971136**; **DE 1112989** (all 1958 to Kali-Chemie); Martin, Habicht, **DE 1091124**; **US 2987517** (1960, 1961 both to Cilag-Chemie).

Crystals from ethanol + ether or acetone, mp 100-101°. Freely sol in water, very sol in alcohol. Practically insol in ether. Aq solns are stable to storage; 0.6% ampuled solns showed no loss after one year at room temp.

THERAP CAT: Antispasmodic.

9907. Valganciclovir. [175865-60-8] L-Valine 2-[(2-amino-1,6-dihydro-6-oxo-9*H*-purin-9-yl)methoxy]-3-hydroxypropyl ester; 2-[(2-amino-1,6-dihydro-6-oxo-9*H*-purin-9-yl)methoxy]-3-hydroxypropanyl-L-valinate. $C_{14}H_{22}N_6O_5$; mol wt 354.36. C 47.45%, H 6.26%, N 23.72%, O 22.58%. Valine ester prodrug of ganciclovir, *q.v.* Prepn: J. J. Nestor *et al., EP 694547; eidem, US 6083953* (1996, 2000 both to Hoffmann-La Roche). HPLC determn in plasma: R. Chan *et al., J. Pharm. Biomed. Anal.* **21**, 647 (1999). Clinical pharmacokinetics in HIV- and CMV-positive patients: F. Brown *et al., Clin. Pharmacokinet.* **37**, 167 (1999); in liver transplant patients: M. D. Pescovitz *et al., Antimicrob. Agents Chemother.* **44**, 2811 (2000). Clinical trial in cytomegalovirus retinitis: D. F. Martin *et al., N. Engl. J. Med.* **346**, 1119 (2002).

Hydrochloride. [175865-59-5] Ro-107-9070/194; RS-79070-194; Cymeval; Valcyte. $C_{14}H_{22}N_6O_5 \cdot HCl$; mol wt 390.82. Crystals from water + isopropanol, undergoes phase change at 142°; dec 175°.

THERAP CAT: Antiviral.

9908. Validamycins. Antibiotic complex produced by *Streptomyces hygroscopicus* var *limoneus*. Consists of validamycins A (major component), B, C, D, E, and F. Isoln, characterization, and biological properties of validamycins A and B: Iwasa *et al., J.*

Antibiot. **24**, 107, 119 (1971). Isoln and characterization of validamycins C, D, E, F: Horii *et al., ibid.* **25**, 48 (1972). Manuf: Horii *et al., JP 72 39697* (1972 to Takeda), *C.A.* **78**, 122657a (1973). Structure of validamycin A: Horii, Kameda, *Chem. Commun.* **1972**, 747; revised structure: T. Suami *et al., J. Antibiot.* **33**, 98 (1980). Bioassay methods: Iwasa *et al., ibid.* **24**, 114 (1971). Total synthesis of (±)-validoxylamines A and B, constituents of validamycins: S. Ogawa *et al., J. Org. Chem.* **49**, 2594 (1984). Total synthesis of validamycin B: S. Ogawa, Y. Miyamoto, *Chem. Commun.* **1987**, 1843; of validamycin A: *eidem, Chem. Lett.* **1988**, 889.

Validamycin A

Validamycin A. [37248-47-8] [1*S*-(1α,4α,5β,6α)]-1,5,6-Trideoxy-4-*O*-β-D-glucopyranosyl-5-(hydroxymethyl)-1-[[4,5,6-trihydroxy-3-(hydroxymethyl)-2-cyclohexen-1-yl]amino]-D-*chiro*-inositol; Validacin; Valimon. $C_{20}H_{35}NO_{13}$; mol wt 497.49. Colorless hydrophilic powder. Does not show sharp mp; softens at 100°, dec at 135°. $[\alpha]_D^{24}$ +110° (c = 1 in water or pyridine), +92° (c = 1 in DMF). pKa 6.0. Sol in water, methanol, DMF, DMSO; sparingly sol in ethanol, acetone. Insol in ethyl acetate, diethyl ether.

Hydrochloride. $C_{20}H_{35}NO_{13} \cdot HCl$. Crystalline powder, mp 95° (dec). $[\alpha]_D^{22}$ +49° (c = 1 in water). Sol in water, alcohols. Insol in acetone, diethyl ether.

USE: Fungicide.

9909. Valine. [72-18-4] L-Valine; Val; V; 2-aminoisovaleric acid; 2-amino-3-methylbutyric acid; α-aminoisovaleric acid; (*S*)-2-amino-3-methylbutanoic acid. $C_5H_{11}NO_2$; mol wt 117.15. C 51.26%, H 9.46%, N 11.96%, O 27.31%. An essential amino acid for human development. Identified from organ extracts in 1856 by von Group-Besanez; isolated from proteins in 1879 by Schützenberger who proposed that it was aminovaleric acid. Structure confirmation: E. Fischer, *Ber.* **39**, 2320 (1906). Early chemistry and biochemistry: *Amino Acids and Proteins*, D. M. Greenberg, Ed. (Charles C. Thomas, Springfield, IL, 1951) 950 pp., *passim*; J. P. Greenstein, M. Winitz, *Chemistry of the Amino Acids* vols **1-3** (John Wiley and Sons, Inc., New York, 1961) pp. 2368-2380, *passim*. Conformation study: R. H. Yun, J. Hermans, *Protein Eng.* **4**, 761 (1991). Nutritional assessment study: V. R. Young *et al., J. Nutr.* **102**, 1159 (1972); in parenteral nutrition: P. Reiderer *et al., Nutr. Metab.* **24**, 209 (1980); in hemodialysis patients: G. A. Young *et al., Kidney Int.* **21**, 492 (1982). Brief review of metabolism: P. Kamoun, *Trends Biochem. Sci.* **17**, 175-176 (1992).

Leaflets from water + alcohol, mp 315° (closed capillary). d 1.230. Sublimes. [M]$_D$ +33.1° (5*N* HCl); +72.6° (glacial acetic acid); $[\alpha]_D^{23}$ +22.9° (c = 0.8 in 20% HCl). pK$_1$ 2.32; pK$_2$ 9.62. Soly in water at 0°: 83.4 g/l; at 25°: 88.5 g/l; at 50°: 96.2 g/l; at 65°: 102.4 g/l. Insol in common neutral solvents.

DL-Form. Sublimes without melting at ordinary speed of heating. Dec 298° (closed capillary, very rapid heating). One part dissolves in 11.7 parts of water at 15°, in 14.1 parts of water at 25°. Insol in common neutral solvents.

9910. Valinomycin. [2001-95-8] $C_{54}H_{90}N_6O_{18}$; mol wt 1111.32. C 58.36%, H 8.16%, N 7.56%, O 25.91%. Cyclododecadepsipeptide ionophore antibiotic produced by *Streptomyces fulvissimus* and related to the enniatins, *q.v.* Composed of 3 moles each of L-valine, D-α-hydroxyisovaleric acid, D-valine, and L-lactic acid linked alternately to form a 36-membered ring: Brockmann *et al., Ber.* **88**, 57 (1955); *Ann.* **603**, 216 (1957). Structural studies: Shemyakin *et al., Tetrahedron Lett.* **1963**, 351; *Tetrahedron* **19**, 995 (1963). Proposed structure: Brockmann *et al., Naturwissenschaften* **50**, 689 (1963). Structure and synthesis: Shemyakin *et al., Tetrahedron Lett.* **1963**, 1921. Solid phase synthesis: Gisin *et al., J. Am. Chem. Soc.* **91**, 2691 (1969); Losse, Klengel, *Tetrahedron* **27**, 1423 (1971). Biosynthesis: Smirnova *et al., C.A.* **73**, 97347m (1970); Ristow *et al., FEBS Lett.* **42**, 127 (1974). Conformation: Ivanov *et al., Biochem. Biophys. Res. Commun.* **34**, 803 (1969); Onishi, Urry, *ibid.* **36**, 194 (1969); Duax *et al., Science* **176**, 911 (1972). *Review:* Y. A. Ovchinnokov, V. T. Ivanov, "The Cyclic Peptides: Structure, Conformation, and Function", in *The Proteins* vol. **V**, H. Neurath, R. L. Hill, Eds. (Academic Press, New York, 3rd ed., 1982) pp 563-573.

Shiny rectangular platelets from dibutyl ether, mp 190° (hot stage). $[\alpha]_D^{20}$ +31.0° (c = 1.6 in benzene). Neutral reaction. Practically insol in water. Freely sol in petr ether, ether, benzene, chloroform, glacial acetic, butyl acetate, acetone. Active *in vitro* against *Mycobacterium tuberculosis*.

USE: Insecticide, nematocide, Patterson, Wright, US 3520973 (1970 to Am. Cyanamid).

9911. Valnemulin. [101312-92-9] [[2-[[(2R)-2-Amino-3-methyl-1-oxobutyl]amino]-1,1-dimethylethyl]thio]acetic acid (3aS,4R,5S,6S,8R,9R,9aR,10R)-6-ethenyldecahydro-5-hydroxy-4,6,9,10-tetramethyl-1-oxo-3a,9-propano-3aH-cyclopentacyclooocten-8-yl ester; 14-*O*-[1-(D-2-amino-3-methylbutyrylamino)-2-methylpropan-2-ylthioacetyl]mutilin. $C_{31}H_{52}N_2O_5S$; mol wt 564.82. C 65.92%, H 9.28%, N 4.96%, O 14.16%, S 5.68%. Semisynthetic antibiotic; derivative of pleuromutilin, *q.v.* Prepn: H. Berner, H. Vyplel, EP 153277; *eidem*, US 4675330 (1985, 1987 both to Sandoz). Comparative *in vitro* activity vs porcine bacterial pathogens: I. A. Aitken *et al., Vet. Rec.* **144**, 128 (1999). Mechanism of action study: S. M. Poulsen *et al., Mol. Microbiol.* **41**, 1091 (2001). Pharmacokinetics in pigs: S. Horkovics-Kovats, F. Schatz, *J. Pharm. Med.* **6**, 149 (1996). Efficacy vs *Mycoplasma gallisepticum* in chickens: F. T. W. Jordan *et al., Avian Dis.* **42**, 738 (1998); vs *Mycoplasma bovis* in calves: L. Stipkovits *et al., Res. Vet. Sci.* **78**, 207 (2005).

Hydrochloride. [133868-46-9] Econor. $C_{31}H_{52}N_2O_5S$.HCl; mol wt 601.28.

THERAP CAT (VET): Antibacterial.

9912. Valnoctamide. [4171-13-5] 2-Ethyl-3-methylpentanamide; 2-ethyl-3-methylvaleramide; α-ethyl-β-methylvaleramide; valmethamide; McN-X-181; Axiquel; Nirvanil. $C_8H_{17}NO$; mol wt 143.23. C 67.08%, H 11.96%, N 9.78%, O 11.17%. Isomer of valpromide, *q.v.* Prepn: Freifelder *et al., J. Org. Chem.* **26**, 203 (1961). GLC determn in plasma: M. Bialer, B. Hoch, *J. Chromatogr.* **337**, 408 (1985). Clinical pharmacokinetics: M. Bialer *et al., Eur. J. Clin. Pharmacol.* **38**, 289 (1990).

Crystals, mp 113.5-114°. Sol in water.
THERAP CAT: Anxiolytic.

9913. Valproic Acid. [99-66-1] 2-Propylpentanoic acid; 2-propylvaleric acid; di-*n*-propylacetic acid; Convulex; Depakene. $C_8H_{16}O_2$; mol wt 144.21. C 66.63%, H 11.18%, O 22.19%. Antiepileptic; increases levels of γ-aminobutyric acid (GABA) in the brain. Prepn: B. S. Burton, *Am. Chem. J.* **3**, 385 (1882); E. Oberreit, *Ber.* **29**, 1998 (1896); M. Tiffeneau, Y. Deux, *Compte Rend.* **212**, 105 (1941). Anticonvulsant activity: H. Meunier *et al., Therapie* **18**, 435 (1963). Toxicity data: Jenner *et al., Food Cosmet. Toxicol.* **2**, 327 (1964). Comprehensive description: Z. L. Chang, *Anal. Profiles Drug Subs.* **8**, 529-556 (1979). Review of teratogenicity studies: H. Nau *et al., Pharmacol. Toxicol.* **69**, 310-321 (1991); R. Alsdorf, D. F. Wyszynski, *Expert Opin. Drug Safety* **4**, 345-353 (2005). Review of pharmacology and clinical experience in epilepsy: E. M. Rimmer, A. Richens, *Pharmacotherapy* **5**, 171-184 (1985); in psychiatric disease: D. R. P. Guay, *ibid.* **15**, 631-647 (1995); in migraine prophylaxis: C. E. Shelton, J. F. Connelly, *Ann. Pharmacother.* **30**, 865-866 (1996). Review of pharmacodynamics and mechanisms of action: W. Löscher, *Prog. Neurobiol.* **58**, 31-59 (1999).

Colorless liquid with characteristic odor. bp 219.5°. $n_D^{24.5}$ 1.425. d_4^0 0.9215. pKa 4.6. Very sol in organic solvents. Soly in water: 1.3 mg/ml. LD$_{50}$ orally in rats: 670 mg/kg (Jenner).

Sodium salt (1:1). [1069-66-5] Sodium valproate; Depacon; Depakin; Dépakine; Epilim; Ergenyl; Leptilan; Orfiril. C_8H_{15}-NaO_2; mol wt 166.19. White, odorless, crystalline, deliquescent powder. pKa 4.8. Hygroscopic. One gram is sol in 0.4 ml water; 1.5 ml ethanol; 5 ml methanol. Practically insol in common organic solvents. LD$_{50}$ orally in mice: 1700 mg/kg (Meunier).

Sodium salt (2:1). [76584-70-8] Sodium hydrogen bis(2-propylpentanoate); divalproex sodium; valproate semisodium; Abbott 50711; Depakote; Valcote. $C_{16}H_{31}NaO_4$; mol wt 310.40.

Magnesium salt. Depamag. $C_{16}H_{30}MgO_4$; mol wt 310.71.

THERAP CAT: Anticonvulsant; antimanic; antimigraine.

9914. Valpromide. [2430-27-5] 2-Propylpentanamide; 2-propylvaleramide; 2-propylpentamide; dipropylacetamide; Depamide. $C_8H_{17}NO$; mol wt 143.23. C 67.08%, H 11.96%, N 9.78%, O 11.17%. Prodrug of valproic acid, *q.v.* Prepn: E. Fischer, A. Dilthey, *Ber.* **35**, 844 (1902); M. Tiffeneau, Y. Deux, *Compt. Rend.* **212**, 105 (1941). GC determn in plasma: M. Pokrajac *et al., Pharm. Acta Helv.* **67**, 237 (1992). Review of pharmacology and clinical activity: M. Bialer, *Clin. Pharmacokinet.* **20**, 114-122 (1991).

White, odorless and bitter crystalline powder, mp 125-126°. Practically insol in water.

THERAP CAT: Anticonvulsant.

9915. Valrubicin. [56124-62-0] Pentanoic acid 2-[(2S,4S)-1,2,3,4,6,11-hexahydro-2,5,12-trihydroxy-7-methoxy-6,11-dioxo-4-[[2,3,6-trideoxy-3-[(trifluoroacetyl)amino]-α-L-lyxo-hexopyranosyl]oxy]-2-naphthacenyl]-2-oxoethyl ester; N-trifluoroacetyladriamycin-14-valerate; AD-32; NSC-246131; Valstar. $C_{34}H_{36}F_3NO_{13}$; mol wt 723.64. C 56.43%, H 5.01%, F 7.88%, N 1.94%, O 28.74%. Semisynthetic doxorubicin, q.v., analog. Prepn: M. Israel et al., Cancer Res. **35**, 1365 (1975); M. Israel, E. J. Modest, US 4035566 (1977 to S. Farber Cancer Inst.). TLC determn in biological samples: B. Barbieri et al., J. Chromatogr. **163**, 195 (1979). Clinical pharmacokinetics: R. E. Greenberg et al., Urology **49**, 471 (1997). Clinical trial in refractory bladder cancer: G. Steinberg et al., J. Urol. **163**, 761 (2000). Review of pharmacology and clinical development: C. Doehn, Curr. Opin. Oncol. Endocr. Metab. Invest. Drugs **1**, 407-415 (1999); S. V. Onrust, H. M. Lamb, Drugs Aging **15**, 69-75 (1999).

Orange or orange-red powder, mp 135-136°. Highly lipophilic. Sol in methylene chloride, ethanol, methanol, acetone. Practically insol in water.

THERAP CAT: Antineoplastic

9916. Valsartan. [137862-53-4] N-(1-Oxopentyl)-N-[[2'-(1H-tetrazol-5-yl)[1,1'-biphenyl]-4-yl]methyl]-L-valine; N-[p-(o-1H-tetrazol-5-ylphenyl)benzyl]-N-valeryl-L-valine; (S)-N-(1-carboxy-2-methylprop-1-yl)-N-pentanoyl-N-[2'-(1H-tetrazol-5-yl)-biphenyl-4-ylmethyl]amine; CGP-48933; Diovan; Tareg. $C_{24}H_{29}N_5O_3$; mol wt 435.52. C 66.19%, H 6.71%, N 16.08%, O 11.02%. Nonpeptide angiotensin II AT$_1$-receptor antagonist. Prepn: P. Bühlmayer et al., EP 443983; eidem, US 5399578 (1991, 1995 both to Ciba Geigy); idem et al., Bioorg. Med. Chem. Lett. **4**, 29 (1994). Pharmacological profile: L. Criscione et al., Br. J. Pharmacol. **110**, 761 (1993). HPLC determn in human plasma: A. Sioufi et al., J. Liq. Chromatogr. **17**, 2179 (1994). Clinical pharmacology: P. Müller et al., Eur. J. Clin. Pharmacol. **47**, 231 (1994). Clinical comparison with captopril, q.v., in high risk patients following myocardial infarction: M. A. Pfeffer et al., N. Engl. J. Med. **349**, 1893 (2003). Review of pharmacology and clinical experience in heart failure: R. Latini et al., Expert Opin. Pharmacother. **5**, 181-193 (2004).

Crystals from diisopropyl ether, mp 116-117°. Partition coefficient (n-octanol/aq phosphate buffer): 0.033. Sol in water at 25°.

THERAP CAT: Antihypertensive.

9917. Valspodar. [121584-18-7] 6-[(2S,4R,6E)-4-Methyl-2-(methylamino)-3-oxo-6-octenoic acid]cyclosporin D; [3'-desoxy-3'-oxo-MeBmt]^1-[Val]^2-cyclosporin; [3'-keto-Bmt1]-[Val2]-cyclo-

sporin; PSC-833; SDZ-PSC-833; Amdray. $C_{63}H_{111}N_{11}O_{12}$; mol wt 1214.62. C 62.30%, H 9.21%, N 12.68%, O 15.81%. Non-immunosuppressive cyclosporin analog that reverses multidrug resistance (MDR) by inhibiting cellular drug efflux mediated by P-glycoprotein, q.v. Prepn: P. Bollinger et al., EP 296122; eidem, US 5525590 (1988, 1996 both to Sandoz). Pharmacology: D. Boesch et al., Exp. Cell Res. **196**, 26 (1991). Clinical pharmacokinetics: R. M. Lush et al., J. Clin. Pharmacol. **37**, 123 (1997). HPLC determn in blood: M. G. Scott et al., Clin. Chem. **43**, 509 (1997). Clinical evaluation in multiple myeloma: P. Sonneveld et al., Leukemia **10**, 1741 (1996); in acute myelogenous leukemia: R. Advani et al., Blood **93**, 787 (1999). Review of pharmacology and clinical efficacy: F. Loor, Expert Opin. Invest. Drugs **8**, 807-835 (1999).

Insol in water. Sol in ethanol, DMSO. $[\alpha]_D^{20}$ −255.1° (c = 0.5 in CHCl$_3$).

THERAP CAT: Antineoplastic adjunct (chemosensitizer).

9918. Vanadium. [7440-62-2] V; at. wt 50.9415; at. no. 23; valencies 2, 3, 4, 5. Group VB(5). Two naturally occurring isotopes: ^{51}V (99.75%); ^{50}V (0.25%); the latter is radioactive: T$_{1/2}$ 6 × 10^{15} years. Artificial isotopes: 46-49; 52-54. Abundance in earth's crust: 0.01% by wt. Widespread in nature; over 65 minerals known including **patronite** (polysulfide), **vanadinite** (9PbO.3V$_2$O$_5$.PbCl$_2$), **roscoelite** [2K$_2$O.2Al$_2$O$_3$.(Mg,Fe)O.3V$_2$O$_5$.10SiO$_2$.4 H$_2$O] and **carnotite** (K$_2$O.2U$_2$O$_3$.V$_2$O$_5$.3H$_2$O). [Carnotite is also an important source of uranium]. Discovered by Selström in 1830; prepd by Roscoe in 1869. Prepn: Prandtl, Manz, Z. Anorg. Allg. Chem. **79**, 209 (1912); Marden, Rich, J. Ind. Eng. Chem. **19**, 786 (1927); McKechnie, Seybolt, J. Electrochem. Soc. **97**, 311 (1950); Gregory, Lilliendahl, ibid. **98**, 395 (1951); Handbook of Preparative Inorganic Chemistry vol. 2, G. Brauer, Ed. (Academic Press, New York, 2nd ed., 1965) pp 1252-1255. Review: Clark, "Vanadium" in Comprehensive Inorganic Chemistry vol. 3, J. C. Bailar, Jr. et al., Eds. (Pergamon Press, Oxford, 1973) pp 491-551. Review of toxicology and human exposure: Toxicological Profile for Vanadium and Compounds (PB93-110880, 1992) 130 pp.

Light gray or white lustrous powder, fused hard lumps or body-centered cubic crystals; not tarnished in air and not appreciably affected by moisture at ordinary temp. mp 1917°. d$^{18.7}$ 6.11. Sp heat (20-100°) 0.12 cal/g/°C. Electrical resistivity 24.8 microhms/cm. Insol in water. Not attacked by hot or cold hydrochloric acid, by cold sulfuric acid. Reacts with hot sulfuric acid, hydrofluoric acid, nitric acid, aqua regia. Not attacked by bromine water, or by aq alkalies. The metal precipitates gold, silver and platinum from their salts; reduces mercuric salts to mercurous, ferric salts to ferrous.

Caution: Potential symptoms of overexposure to dust or fumes are irritation of eyes, skin, throat; green tongue, metallic taste, eczema; cough; fine rales, wheezing, bronchitis; dyspnea. See NIOSH Pocket Guide to Chemical Hazards (DHHS/NIOSH 97-140, 1997) p 328.

USE: Alloying agent in manuf of rust-resistant vanadium steel.

9919. Vanadium Carbonyl. [20644-87-5] Vanadium hexacarbonyl. C_6O_6V; mol wt 219.00. C 32.91%, O 43.83%, V 23.26%. V(CO)$_6$. Prepn: Natta et al., C.A. **54**, 16252 (1960); Ercoli et al., J. Am. Chem. Soc. **82**, 2966 (1960); Hileman in Prep. Inorg. React. **1**, 107 (1964).

Blue-green pyrophoric crystals. Sensitive to air. Should be stored under nitrogen. Dec 60-70° in a nitrogen-filled tube.

9920. Vanadium Pentafluoride. [7783-72-4] F$_5$V; mol wt 145.93. F 65.09%, V 34.91%. VF$_5$. Prepd from vanadium tetrafluoride by thermal disproportionation at 650° in N$_2$ current according to the eq $2VF_4 \rightarrow VF_5 + VF_3$: Ruff, Lickfett, *Ber.* **44**, 2548 (1911); Kwasnik in *Handbook of Preparative Inorganic Chemistry* **vol. 1**, G. Brauer, Ed. (Academic Press, New York, 2nd ed., 1963) p 253; from the elements: Trevorrow *et al., J. Am. Chem. Soc.* **79**, 5167 (1957); Clark, Emeleus, *J. Chem. Soc.* **1957**, 2119. Review of transition metal pentafluorides: Peacock, *Adv. Fluorine Chem.* **7**, 113-145 (1973).

Liquid. mp 19.5°; bp 47.9°. $d_4^{19.5}$ 2.502. Heat of vaporization 10.60 kcal/mole. Appreciable vapor pressure at room temp. Hydrolyzed by water, dil alkali. Soly in anhydrous HF: 3.3 moles/l. Freely sol in alcohol, chloroform, acetone, ligroin. Insol in carbon disulfide. Dec toluene and ether. Etches glass slowly at room temp; more rapidly in presence of moisture with formation of yellow color. May be stored in sealed vessels made from iron, nickel, copper, platinum.

9921. Vanadium Pentoxide. [1314-62-1] Vanadium oxide (V_2O_5); vanadic anhydride. O_5V_2; mol wt 181.88. O 43.98%, V 56.02%. V_2O_5. Prepd by heating ammonium metavanadate, NH_4-VO_3.

Yellow to rust-brown orthorhombic crystals; d 3.35; mp 690°. Loses oxygen reversibly in the region 700-1125°. One gram dissolves in ~125 ml water; sol in concd acids, forming red to yellow solns; sol in alkalies, forming vanadates; insol in alcohol. Its acid solutions are reduced by SO_2, Zn + HCl, and by evaporation with HCl.

Caution: Reported to be a respiratory irritant and to cause skin pallor, greenish-black tongue, chest pain, cough, dyspnea, palpitation, lung changes. When ingested, causes G.I. disturbances. May also cause a papular skin rash: Zenz *et al., Arch. Environ. Health* **5**, 542 (1962); E. Browning, *Toxicity of Industrial Metals* (Appleton-Century-Crofts, New York, 2nd ed., 1969) pp 340-347.

USE: As catalyst in the oxidation of SO_2 to SO_3, alcohol to acetaldehyde, etc.; for the manuf of yellow glass; inhibiting ultraviolet light transmission in glass; depolarizer; as developer in photography; in form of ammonium vanadate as mordant in dyeing and printing fabrics and in manuf of aniline black.

9922. Vanadium Trifluoride. [10049-12-4] F_3V; mol wt 107.94. F 52.80%, V 47.19%. VF_3. Prepd from VCl_3 and HF: Ruff, Lickfett, *Ber.* **44**, 2539 (1911); from VCl_2 and HF: Emeleus, Gutmann, *J. Chem. Soc.* **1949**, 2979; by thermal decompn in an inert atm of $(NH_4)_3VF_6$: Sturm, Sheridan, *Inorg. Synth.* **7**, 87 (1963).

Greenish-yellow powder. d 3.363. mp approx 1406°. Sublimes at bright red heat. Almost insol in water, alcohol, acetone, ethyl acetate, acetic anhydride, glacial acetic acid, toluene, carbon tetrachloride, chloroform, carbon disulfide. Black color with NaOH soln. Aq solns have strong reducing properties.

Trihydrate. Dark green rhombohedral crystals, obtained by crystallizing vanadium trioxide dissolved in hydrofluoric acid, or by electrolytic reduction of a soln of vanadium pentoxide in aq HF. Loses one molecule of water at 100°. Dissolves in water to some extent, forming autocomplexes.

9923. Vanadium Trioxide. [1314-34-7] Vanadium sesquioxide; vanadic oxide. O_3V_2; mol wt 149.88. O 32.02%, V 67.98%. V_2O_3. Prepd by reduction of V_2O_5 with hydrogen or carbon monoxide.

Black powder. On exposure to air it is gradually converted into indigo-blue crystals of V_2O_4. d 4.87; mp 1940°. Insol in water; difficultly sol in acids.

USE: Catalyst, e.g., when making ethanol from ethylene.

9924. Vanadium Trisulfide. [1315-03-3] Vanadium sesquisulfide. S_3V_2; mol wt 198.08. S 48.56%, V 51.44%. V_2S_3.

Greenish-black powder; d 4.7. Dec when heated. Insol in water, cold HCl, dil H_2SO_4; sol in hot HCl, hot dil H_2SO_4, HNO_3.

9925. Vanadyl Dichloride. [10213-09-9] Vanadium oxydichloride. Cl_2OV; mol wt 137.85. Cl 51.44%, O 11.61%, V 36.95%. $VOCl_2$. Usually contains some water. Prepd according to the eq $V_2O_5 + 3VCl_3 + VOCl_3 \rightarrow 6VOCl_2$: Funk, Weiss, *Z. Anorg. Allg. Chem.* **295**, 327 (1958); Oppermann, *ibid.* **351**, 113 (1967).

Green, very deliquesc tabular crystals. d 2.88. Disproportionates at 384° to VOCl and $VOCl_3$. Slowly dec by water. Sol in abs alcohol, glacial acetic acid. *Keep tightly closed.*

USE: Has been used as mordant in printing fabrics.

9926. Vanadyl Sulfate. [27774-13-6] Vanadium oxysulfate. O_5SV; mol wt 163.00. O 49.08%, S 19.67%, V 31.25%. $VOSO_4$.

Dihydrate. Blue, cryst powder. Sol in water.

USE: Dihydrate as mordant in dyeing and printing textiles; manuf colored glass; for blue and green glazes on pottery.

9927. Vanadyl Trichloride. [7727-18-6] (*T*-4)-Trichloro-oxovanadium; vanadium(V) trichloride oxide; vanadium oxytrichloride. Cl_3OV; mol wt 173.30. Cl 61.37%, O 9.23%, V 29.39%. $VOCl_3$. Prepn by the action of dry Cl_2 on V_2O_3 or V_2O_5: Brown, Griffitts, *Inorg. Synth.* **1**, 106 (1939); **4**, 80 (1953); Oppermann, *Z. Anorg. Allg. Chem.* **351**, 113 (1967). Toxicity data: Smyth *et al., Am. Ind. Hyg. Assoc. J.* **30**, 470 (1969).

Yellow liquid, emitting red fumes on exposure to moist air. d 1.84. bp 126-127°. mp −77°. Dec in presence of moisture into vanadic acid and HCl. When a small quantity of water is added, it becomes thick and almost blood-red because of formation of vanadic acid. *Keep tightly closed.* LD_{50} orally in rats: 0.14 g/kg (Smyth).

9928. Vanaspati. Manuf by hydrogenation of vegetable oils, peanut, cottonseed and sesame in the presence of activated-Ni catalyst: Gupta, *Indian Chem. Eng.* **3**, 163 (1961), *C.A.* **56**, 15895h (1962).

Product mp 33-37°; max free fatty acid (as oleic) 0.25%.

USE: Hydrogenated shortening. Used in the Orient.

9929. Vancomycin. [1404-90-6] $C_{66}H_{75}Cl_2N_9O_{24}$; mol wt 1449.25. C 54.70%, H 5.22%, Cl 4.89%, N 8.70%, O 26.50%. Amphoteric glycopeptide antibiotic produced by *Streptomyces orientalis* discovered in soil from Borneo. Inhibits bacterial cell wall synthesis by binding to peptidoglycan. Isoln: M. H. McCormick *et al., Antibiot. Annu.* **1955-56**, 606; *eidem,* **US 3067099** (1962 to Lilly). Pharmacology and toxicology: R. C. Anderson *et al., Antibiot. Annu.* **1956-57**, 75. Purif: H. M. Higgins *et al., ibid.* **1957-58**, 906. Structure studies: F. J. Marshall, *J. Med. Chem.* **8**, 18 (1965); W. D. Weringa *et al., J. Chem. Soc. Perkin Trans. 1* **1972**, 443; K. A. Smith *et al., ibid.* **1974**, 2369. Total structure determination by x-ray analysis: G. M. Sheldrick *et al., Nature* **271**, 223 (1978). Revised configuration: M. P. Williamson, D. H. Williams, *J. Am. Chem. Soc.* **103**, 6580 (1981). Further revision of structure: C. M. Harris *et al., ibid.* **105**, 6915 (1983). Total synthesis: K. C. Nicolaou *et al., Angew. Chem. Int. Ed.* **38**, 240 (1999). Review of mechanism of action studies: H. P. Perkins, M. Nieto, *Ann. N.Y. Acad. Sci.* **235**, 348-363 (1974). Series of articles on antimicrobial activity, pharmacokinetics and clinical usage: *J. Antimicrob. Chemother.* **14**, Suppl. D, 1-109 (1984). HPLC determn in serum: L. Li *et al., Ther. Drug Monit.* **17**, 366 (1995). Review of clinical experience: B. A. Cunha, *Med. Clin. North Am.* **79**, 817-831 (1995).

Monohydrochloride. [1404-93-9] Lyphocin; Vanco; Vancocin. $C_{66}H_{75}Cl_2N_9O_{24}\cdot HCl$; mol wt 1485.71. White solid; uv max (H_2O): 282 nm (E_{1cm}^1 40). Soly in water: >100 mg/ml. Moderately sol in dil methanol. Insol in the higher alcohols, acetone, ether. LD_{50} in mice (mg/kg): 489 i.v.; 1734 i.p.; 5000 s.c.; 5000 orally (Anderson).

THERAP CAT: Antibacterial.

9930. Vanilla. Cured, full-grown, unripe fruit of *Vanilla planifolia* Andr., *Orchidaceae. Habit.* Mexico, West Indies, Reunion, Mauritius, Seychelles. *Constit.* 2-2.75% vanillin, ~4% resin; vanillic acid, ~10% sugar.

USE: In manuf of confectionery and in various bakery products; perfumery; flavor for beverages; pharmaceutic aid (flavor).

9931. Vanillic Acid. [121-34-6] 4-Hydroxy-3-methoxybenzoic acid. $C_8H_8O_4$; mol wt 168.15. C 57.14%, H 4.80%, O 38.06%. Obtained from vanillin by oxidation with silver oxide or by controlled caustic fusion: Pearl, *Org. Synth.* **30**, 101 (1950).

White, odorless needles. mp 210°. Sublimes undecomposed. Sol in 860 parts water; very sol in alc; sol in ether. Not colored by $FeCl_3$. Its salts are freely sol in water.

9932. Vanillin. [121-33-5] 4-Hydroxy-3-methoxybenzaldehyde; methylprotocatechuic aldehyde; vanillic aldehyde; Rhonavil Extra Pure. $C_8H_8O_3$; mol wt 152.15. C 63.15%, H 5.30%, O 31.55%. Occurs naturally in a wide variety of foods and plants such as orchids; major commercial source of natural vanillin is from vanilla bean extract. Synthetically produced in-bulk from lignin-based byproducts of paper processes or from guaiacol. Known prior to literature identification, first reported in the literature by Bucholtz in 1816 but not isolated until 1858. Isoln from vanilla beans: M. Gobley, *Jahresber. Fortschr. Chem. Verw. Theile Anderer Wiss.* **1858**, 534. LC determn: S. Kahan, D. A. Krueger, *J. AOAC Int.* **80**, 564 (1997). Acute toxicity: P. M. Jenner *et al., Food Cosmet. Toxicol.* **2**, 327 (1964). Brief review of toxicology: D. L. J. Opdyke, *ibid.* **15**, 633-638 (1977). Review of NMR studies: G. J. Martin, *Ind. Chem. Libr.* **8**, 506-527 (1996). Review of synthetic prepn: M. B. Hocking, *J. Chem. Educ.* **74**, 1055-1059 (1997). Reviews: G. S. Clark, *Perfum. Flavor.* **15**, 45-54 (1990); L. J. Esposito *et al.* in *Kirk-Othmer Encyclopedia of Chemical Technology* **vol. 24** (Wiley-Interscience, New York, 4th ed., 1997) pp 812-825.

White or off-white nonhygroscopic crystalline powder. Pleasant aromatic vanilla odor and taste. Affected by light. d 1.056; bulk density ~0.6. mp 81-83°. $bp_{101.3\ kPa}$ 285°; $bp_{10\ mm\ Hg}$ 154°. Solubility in water >2%; in ethanol is 1:2 vanillin:ethanol. Freely sol in chloroform, ether, in solns of fixed alkali hydroxides; sol in glycerin and hot water. Solns are acid to litmus. LD_{50} orally in rats, guinea pigs: 1580, 1400 mg/kg (Jenner).

USE: Pharmaceutic aid (flavor). As a flavoring agent in confectionery, beverages, foods and animal feeds. Fragance and flavor in cosmetics. Reagent for synthesis.

9933. Vanilmandelic Acid. [55-10-7] α,4-Dihydroxy-3-methoxybenzeneacetic acid; 3-methoxy-4-hydroxymandelic acid; 4-hydroxy-3-methoxymandelic acid; VMA. $C_9H_{10}O_5$; mol wt 198.17. C 54.55%, H 5.09%, O 40.37%. Catecholamine metabolite. Urine levels elevated in various pathologies. Misnamed *vanillinemandelic acid* and *vanillylmandelic acid*. Prepn from vanillin cyanohydrin: Gardner, Hibbert, *J. Am. Chem. Soc.* **66**, 608 (1944). Improved procedure: Shaw *et al., J. Org. Chem.* **23**, 30 (1958); E. F. Recondo, H. Rinderknecht, *ibid.* **25**, 2248 (1960); I. Goodman *et al., Biochem. Prep.* **13**, 75 (1971). Resolution: Armstrong *et al., Biochim. Biophys. Acta* **25**, 422 (1957). Determination in urine: T. C. Stewart, J. A. Freeman, *Vanilmandelic Acid & Catecholamine Determinations* (Am. Soc. Clin. Pathol., Chicago, 1976) pp 1-81.

DL-Form. Scales from ether + benzene, dec 131-133°; also reported as mp 134-135° (Goodman). uv max (0.1*N* HCl): 230, 279 nm (ε 6320, 2810); (0.1*N* NaOH): 247, 285, 345 nm (ε 6860, 3960, 630). Readily resinifies on heating or on prolonged exposure to air. Freely sol in water, acetone. Mod sol in ether, acetonitrile. Sparingly sol in benzene. Mass spectral data: T. R. Sharp, *Org. Mass Spectrom.* **15**, 381 (1980).

L-Form. Crystals, dec 152°. $[\alpha]_D^{22}$ +128° (c = 0.7).
D-Form. Crystals, dec 152°. $[\alpha]_D^{23}$ −131°.

9934. Vapreotide. [103222-11-3] D-Phenylalanyl-L-cysteinyl-L-tyrosyl-D-tryptophyl-L-lysyl-L-valyl-L-cysteinyl-L-tryptophanamide cyclic (2 → 7)-disulfide; BMY-41606; RC-160; Octastatin. $C_{57}H_{70}N_{12}O_9S_2$; mol wt 1131.37. C 60.51%, H 6.24%, N 14.86%, O 12.73%, S 5.67%. Octapeptide somatostatin analog. Prepn: A. V. Schally, R. Z. Cai, **EP 203031** (1986 to Tulane); *eidem*, **US 4650787** (1987). Inhibition of growth hormone, insulin and glucagon release: T. Karashima *et al., Life Sci.* **41**, 1011 (1987); on pancreatic secretion: S. J. Konturek *et al., Proc. Soc. Exp. Biol. Med.* **187**, 241 (1988). RIA determn in serum: M. Mason-Garcia *et al., Proc. Natl. Acad. Sci. USA* **85**, 5688 (1988). Clinical pharmacology: M. A. Ritz *et al., Br. J. Clin. Pharmacol.* **47**, 195 (1999). Clinical trial for variceal bleeding in cirrhosis: P. Calès *et al., N. Engl. J. Med.* **344**, 23 (2001).

D-Phe–Cys–Tyr–D-Trp–Lys–Val–Cys–Trp–NH₂

THERAP CAT: Hemostatic.

9935. Vardenafil. [224785-90-4] 1-[[3-(1,4-Dihydro-5-methyl-4-oxo-7-propylimidazo[5,1-*f*][1,2,4]triazin-2-yl)-4-ethoxyphenyl]sulfonyl]-4-ethyl-piperazine. $C_{23}H_{32}N_6O_4S$; mol wt 488.60. C 56.54%, H 6.60%, N 17.20%, O 13.10%, S 6.56%. Orally active, selective phosphodiesterase type 5 (PDE5) inhibitor. Prepn: U. Niewöhner *et al.*, **WO 9924433**; *eidem*, **US 6362178** (1999, 2002 both to Bayer AG). Effect on cGMP in human corpus cavernosum muscle cells: N. N. Kim *et al., Life Sci.* **69**, 2249 (2001). Pharmacology: E. Bischoff *et al., J. Urol.* **165**, 1316 (2001). Clinical trial in impotence: H. Porst *et al., Int. J. Impotence Res.* **13**, 192 (2001); in erectile dysfunction: C. Stief *et al., Int. J. Clin. Pract.* **58**, 230 (2004); F. Giuliano *et al., BJU Int.* **95**, 110 (2005). Review of clinical experience in erectile dysfunction: S. Markou *et al., Int. J. Impotence Res.* **16**, 470-478 (2004); M. Kendirci *et al., Expert Opin. Pharmacother.* **5**, 923-932 (2004).

Hydrochloride trihydrate. [330808-88-3]; [224785-91-5] (anhydrous). Bay-38-9456; Levitra; Nuviva. $C_{23}H_{32}N_6O_4S$·HCl.-3H_2O; mol wt 579.11. Nearly colorless solid, mp 218°. Soly in water: 0.11 mg/ml.

THERAP CAT: In treatment of male erectile dysfunction.

9936. Varenicline. [249296-44-4] 7,8,9,10-Tetrahydro-6,10-methano-6*H*-pyrazino[2,3-*h*][3]benzazepine; 5,8,14-triaza-tetracyclo[10.3.1.0^{2,11}.0^{4,9}]hexadeca-2(11)-3,5,7,9-pentaene; CP-526555. $C_{13}H_{13}N_3$; mol wt 211.26. C 73.91%, H 6.20%, N 19.89%. Nicotinic $\alpha 4\beta 2$ acetylcholine receptor partial agonist. Prepn: P. R. P. Brooks, J. W. Coe, **WO 0162736** (2001 to Pfizer). Synthesis, receptor binding studies, and *in vivo* dopaminergic activity: J. W. Coe *et al., J. Med. Chem.* **48**, 3474 (2005). Metabolism: R. S. Obach *et al., Drug Metab. Dispos.* **34**, 121 (2006).

Tartrate. [375815-87-5] Champix. $C_{13}H_{13}N_3.C_4H_6O_6$; mol wt 361.35.

THERAP CAT: Aid in smoking cessation.

9937. Vasicine. [6159-55-3] 1,2,3,9-Tetrahydropyrrolo[2,1-b]quinazolin-3-ol; peganine. $C_{11}H_{12}N_2O$; mol wt 188.23. C 70.19%, H 6.43%, N 14.88%, O 8.50%. Isoln from *Adhatoda vasica* Nees, *Acanthaceae:* Hooper, *Pharm. J.* **18**, 841 (1888); Sen, Ghose, *J. Indian Chem. Soc.* **1**, 315 (1924); Mehta *et al., J. Org. Chem.* **28**, 445 (1963). Isoln from *Peganum harmala* L., *Zygophyllaceae:* Späth, Nikawitz, *Ber.* **67**, 45 (1934); Späth, Kuffner, *ibid.* **67**, 868 (1934). Structure and synthesis: Späth *et al., ibid.* **68**, 699 (1935); Späth, Platzer, *ibid.* **69**, 255 (1936). Synthesis of *dl*-vasicine: Southwick, Casanova, *J. Am. Chem. Soc.* **80**, 1168 (1958). *Reviews:* Späth, *Monatsh. Chem.* **72**, 115 (1938); H. T. Openshaw, "The Quinazoline Alkaloids" in *The Alkaloids* vol. III, R. H. F. Manske, H. L. Holmes, Eds. (Academic Press, New York, 1953) pp 101-118; Ray, *J. Indian Chem. Soc.* **35**, 697 (1958).

dl-**Form.** Needles from alc. mp 210°. Sublimes in high vacuum. Sol in acetone, alcohol, chloroform; slightly sol in water, ether, benzene.

l-**Form.** Needles from alc, mp 212°. $[\alpha]_D^{14}$ −254° (c = 2.4 in CHCl$_3$); $[\alpha]_D^{14}$ −62° (c = 2.4 in alc). In dil HCl this alkaloid is dextrorotatory.

Hydrochloride dihydrate. Needles, mp 208° (dry).

Hydriodide dihydrate. Needles, mp 195° (dry).

Methiodide. Needles from methanol, mp 187°.

Acetylvasicine. $C_{11}H_{11}N_2OCOCH_3$. Crystals, mp 123°, bp$_{0.01}$ 230-240°.

9938. Vasopressin. [9034-50-8] Antidiuretic hormone; beta-hypophamine; β-hypophamine; Pitressin; Pressyn. The water-soluble pressor principle prepd by synthesis or obtained from the posterior lobe of the pituitary of healthy domestic animals used for food by man: *U.S.P.* **XVIII**, 770. Separation from oxytocin: Kamm *et al., J. Am. Chem. Soc.* **50**, 573 (1928). Purification: Turner *et al., J. Biol. Chem.* **191**, 21 (1951). Two vasopressins, differing only in the amino acid at position 8, have been isolated: arginine vasopressin, from human, beef, chicken, horse and sheep pituitaries, and lysine vasopressin (lypressin, *q.v.*), from porcine pituitaries. *Review:* E. Schröder, K. Lübke, *The Peptides* vol. II (Academic Press, New York, 1966) pp 336-350; C. R. W. Edwards, "Vasopressin" in *Hormones in Blood* vol. 2, C. H. Gray, V. H. T. James, Eds. (Academic Press, London, 3rd ed., 1979) pp 423-450. Book: *Antidiuretic Hormone* vol. 4, M. L. Forsling, Ed. (Eden Press, Quebec, 1980) 165 pp.

Cys–Tyr–Phe–Gln–Asn–Cys–Pro–Arg–GlyNH$_2$

Arginine Vasopressin

Arginine vasopressin. Argipressin; rinder-vasopressin. C_{46}-$H_{65}N_{15}O_{12}S_2$; mol wt 1084.23. Structure: du Vigneaud *et al., J. Am. Chem. Soc.* **75**, 4880 (1953). Synthesis: du Vigneaud *et al., ibid.* **80**, 3355 (1958); Bodanszky *et al., ibid.* **86**, 4452 (1964); Meienhofer *et al., ibid.* **92**, 7199 (1970); Jones *et al., J. Org. Chem.* **38**, 2865 (1973). Fever suppressing activity: K. E. Cooper *et al., J. Physiol. (London)* **295**, 33 (1979). Effect on female sexual behavior in rats: P. Södersten *et al., Nature* **301**, 608 (1983).

Ornithine vasopressin *see* Ornipressin.

THERAP CAT: Antidiuretic and vasopressor hormone; hemostatic.

THERAP CAT (VET): Antidiuretic hormone; in deficiency conditions.

9939. Vatalanib. [212141-54-3] *N*-(4-Chlorophenyl)-4-(4-pyridinylmethyl)-1-phthalazinamine; 1-(4-chloroanilino)-4-(4-pyridylmethyl)phthalazine; CGP-79787. $C_{20}H_{15}ClN_4$; mol wt 346.81. C 69.26%, H 4.36%, Cl 10.22%, N 16.15%. Vascular endothelial growth factor (VEGF) receptor tyrosine kinase inhibitor; vascular endothelial angiogenesis inhibitor. Prepn: G. Bold *et al.,* **WO 9835958**; *eidem,* **US 6258812** (1998, 2001 both to Novartis); *eidem, J. Med. Chem.* **43**, 2310 (2000). Enzyme inhibition study and pharmacology: J. M. Wood *et al., Cancer Res.* **60**, 2178 (2000). Antiangiogenic activity: J. Drevs *et al., ibid.* **62**, 4015 (2002). Clinical pharmacokinetics: B. Morgan *et al., J. Clin. Oncol.* **21**, 3955 (2003). Review of mechanism of action: P. Furet, P. W. Manley *ACS Symp. Ser.* **796**, 282-298 (2001); and therapeutic potential: A. L. Thomas *et al., Semin. Oncol.* **30**, Suppl. 6, 32-38 (2003).

Crystals from water + diethyl ether, mp 209-212°.

Succinate. [212142-18-2] CGP-79787D; PTK-787; ZK-222584. $C_{20}H_{15}ClN_4.C_4H_6O_4$; mol wt 464.90. Crystals from ethanol, mp 195°.

THERAP CAT: Antineoplastic.

9940. Veatchine. [76-53-9] $C_{22}H_{33}NO_2$; mol wt 343.50. C 76.92%, H 9.68%, N 4.08%, O 9.32%. From bark of *Garrya veatchii* Kellogg, *Garryaceae,* where it occurs together with garryine and other alkaloids: Oneto, *J. Am. Pharm. Assoc.* **35**, 204 (1946); Wiesner *et al., Can. J. Chem.* **30**, 608 (1952). Structure: Wiesner *et al., J. Am. Chem. Soc.* **76**, 6068 (1954); Pelletier, *ibid.* **82**, 2398 (1960). Stereochemistry: Vorbrüggen, Djerassi, *Tetrahedron Lett.* **1961**, 119; *J. Am. Chem. Soc.* **84**, 2990 (1962). Coexistence of epimers found in crystal and molecular structure: S. W. Pelletier *et al., ibid.* **100**, 7976 (1978). ^{13}C-NMR study of epimers: N. V. Mody, S. W. Pelletier, *Tetrahedron* **34**, 2421 (1978). Racemic syntheses and resolution: Nagata *et al., ibid.* **86**, 929 (1964), **89**, 1499 (1967); Guthrie *et al., Collect. Czech. Chem. Commun.* **31**, 602 (1966). Total synthesis of optically active form: Wiesner *et al., Experientia* **26**, 471 (1970).

Crystals from dil acetone, mp 119-120°. Bitter taste. pH 11.5. $[\alpha]_D^{27.5}$ −69.01° (c = 1.06 in ethanol). Readily sol in water, ethanol.

Hydrochloride. $C_{22}H_{33}NO_2.HCl$. Crystals from abs ethanol + ether, dec 267-271°. Sol in water.

9941. Vecuronium Bromide. [50700-72-6] 1-[(2β,3α,5α,-16β,17β)-3,17-Bis(acetyloxy)-2-(1-piperidinyl)androstan-16-yl]-1-methylpiperidinium bromide; NC-45; Org-NC-45; Musculax; Norcuron. $C_{34}H_{57}BrN_2O_4$; mol wt 637.73. C 64.03%, H 9.01%, Br 12.53%, N 4.39%, O 10.04%. Aminosteroid, competitive neuromuscular blocker. Prepn: W. R. Buckett *et al., J. Med. Chem.* **16**,

1116 (1973); I. C. Carlyle *et al.*, **EP 8824** (1980 to Akzo), *C.A.* **93**, 155850 (1980). Series of articles on pharmacology, pharmacokinetics, pharmacodynamics, clinical studies: *Br. J. Anaesth.* **52**, Suppl. 1, 1S-72S (1980). Clinical pharmacology: M. R. Fahey *et al.*, *Anesthesiology* **55**, 6 (1981). Comparison with pancuronium bromide, *q.v.*: S. L. Son *et al.*, *ibid.* 12.

Crystals, mp 227-229°. LD$_{50}$ in mice: 0.061 mg/kg i.v. (Buckett).

THERAP CAT: Neuromuscular blocking agent.

THERAP CAT (VET): Neuromuscular blocking agent.

9942. Vedaprofen. [71109-09-6] 4-Cyclohexyl-α-methyl-1-naphthaleneacetic acid; 2-(4-cyclohexyl-1-naphthyl)-propionic acid; CERM-10202; PM-150; Quadrisol. C$_{19}$H$_{22}$O$_2$; mol wt 282.38. C 80.81%, H 7.85%, O 11.33%. Propionic acid type non-steroidal anti-inflammatory drug (NSAID). Prepn: J. J. Godfroid, E. Steiner, **BE 870553**; *eidem*, **US 4218473** (1979, 1980 both to CERM). Summary of field trials in dogs: J. G. H. Bergman, P. van Laar, *Vet. Q.* **18**, S20 (1996). Pharmacodynamics and pharmacokinetics in horses: P. Lees *et al.*, *J. Vet. Pharmacol. Ther.* **22**, 96 (1999).

Crystals from ethyl alcohol/water, mp 150°. LD$_{50}$ orally in rat: 400 mg/kg (Godfroid).

THERAP CAT (VET): Anti-inflammatory.

9943. Vedejs Reagent. [23319-63-3] (*PB*-7-34-1222′2′)-(Hexamethylphosphoric triamide-κ*O*)oxodiperoxy(pyridine)molybdenum; oxodiperoxymolybdenum(pyridine)(hexamethylphosphoric triamide); MoOPH. C$_{11}$H$_{23}$MoN$_4$O$_6$P; mol wt 434.24. C 30.43%, H 5.34%, Mo 22.09%, N 12.90%, O 22.11%, P 7.13%. Oxidizing agent. Prepn and structural characterization: H. Mimoun *et al.*, *Bull. Soc. Chim. Fr.* **1969**, 1481. Prepn and synthetic use in hydroxylation of enolates: E. Vedejs, *J. Am. Chem. Soc.* **96**, 5944 (1974); *idem et al.*, *J. Org. Chem.* **43**, 188 (1978); E. Vedejs, S. Larsen, *Org. Synth.* **64**, 127 (1986). Improved prepn: A. R. Daniewski, W. Wojciechowska, *Synth. Commun.* **16**, 535 (1986). Synthetic applications: K. Krohn *et al.*, *Ber.* **123**, 1729 (1990); K. Makino *et al.*, *Tetrahedron* **58**, 9737 (2002). Brief review: D. B. Weibel, *Synlett* **2000**, 1076.

Yellow crystalline powder, mp 103-105° (evolution of gas). *Protect from light and moisture; keep refrigerated.*

USE: Reagent for the hydroxylation of enolates.

9944. Vellosimine. [6874-98-2] Sarpagan-17-al; velosimine. C$_{19}$H$_{20}$N$_2$O; mol wt 292.37. C 78.05%, H 6.89%, N 9.58%, O 5.47%. From bark of *Geissosperum vellosii* Allem., *Apocynaceae*: Rapoport *et al.*, *J. Am. Chem. Soc.* **80**, 1601 (1958). Structure: Rapoport, Moore, *J. Org. Chem.* **27**, 2981 (1962); Ohashi *et al.*, *Tetrahedron* **19**, 2241 (1963).

Crystals from methanol, mp 305-306°. Can be sublimed at 180-100° (0.01 mm). [α]$_D^{26}$ +48°. uv max (ethanol): 280, 289 nm (ε 8000, 6430).

9945. Venice Turpentine. Larch turpentine. Oleoresin from *Larix decidua* Mill. (*L. europaea* Lam. & DC.), *Pinaceae. Habit.* Middle and Southern Europe. *Constit.* Volatile oil, resin. Use in light microscopy: D. A. Johansen, *Plant Microtechnique* (McGraw Hill, New York, 1940) pp 115-116.

Yellow, sometimes greenish, limpid, tenacious, thick liquid; pleasant, aromatic odor; hot, pungent, somewhat bitter taste. Becomes hard and brittle on prolonged exposure to air. Insol in water; sol in glacial acetic acid, amyl alcohol, acetone, caustic alkalies; slowly but freely sol in alc.

USE: As clearing agent and mounting medium for light microscopy.

9946. Venlafaxine. [93413-69-5] 1-[2-(Dimethylamino)-1-(4-methoxyphenyl)ethyl]cyclohexanol; (±)-1-[α-[(dimethylamino)-methyl]-*p*-methoxybenzyl]cyclohexanol; *N*,*N*-dimethyl-2-(1-hydroxycyclohexyl)-2-(4-methoxyphenyl)ethylamine; venlafaxine. C$_{17}$H$_{27}$NO$_2$; mol wt 277.40. C 73.61%, H 9.81%, N 5.05%, O 11.54%. Serotonin noradrenaline reuptake inhibitor (SNRI). Prepn: G. E. M. Husbands *et al.*, **EP 112669**; **US 4535186** (1984, 1985 both to Am. Home Prods.); and resolution of isomers: J. P. Yardley *et al.*, *J. Med. Chem.* **33**, 2899 (1990). Receptor binding studies: E. A. Muth *et al.*, *Biochem. Pharmacol.* **35**, 4493 (1986). HPLC determn in biological fluids: D. R. Hicks *et al.*, *Ther. Drug Monit.* **16**, 100 (1994). Clinical pharmacokinetics: K. J. Klamerus *et al.*, *J. Clin. Pharmacol.* **32**, 716 (1992). Clinical trial in major depression: E. Schweizer *et al.*, *J. Clin. Psychopharmacol.* **11**, 233 (1991). Review of pharmacology and clinical efficacy in depression: S. A. Montgomery, *J. Clin. Psychiatry* **54**, 119-126 (1993). Clinical trial in generalized anxiety disorder: A. J. Gelenberg *et al.*, *J. Am. Med. Assoc.* **283**, 3082 (2000).

Hydrochloride. [99300-78-4] Wy-45030; Effexor. C$_{17}$H$_{27}$NO$_2$.HCl; mol wt 313.86. White to off-white crystalline solid from methanol/ethyl acetate, mp 215-217°. Soly (mg/ml): 572 water. Partition coefficient (octanol/water): 0.43.

(+)-**Form.** Crystals from ethyl acetate, mp 102-104°. [α]$_D^{25}$ +27.6° (c = 1.07 in 95% ethanol).

(+)-**Form hydrochloride.** Wy-45655. Crystals from methanol/ether, mp 240-240.5°. [α]$_D^{25}$ −4.7° (c = 0.945 in ethanol).

(−)-**Form.** Crystals from ethyl acetate, mp 102-104°. [α]$_D^{25}$ −27.1° (c = 1.04 in 95% ethanol).

(−)-Form hydrochloride. Wy-45651. Crystals from methanol/ether, mp 240-240.5°. $[\alpha]_D^{25}$ +4.6° (c = 1.0 in ethanol).

THERAP CAT: Antidepressant.

9947. Venturicidins. Antifungal antibiotics isolated from *Streptomyces aureofaciens* strains. Preliminary isolation work: Rhodes *et al., Nature* **192**, 952 (1962). Isoln of venturicidins A and B and activity studies: Brufani *et al., Helv. Chim. Acta* **51**, 1293 (1968); *see also* Langcake *et al., Biochem. Soc. Trans.* **2**, 202 (1974). Final structures: Brufani *et al., Experientia* **27**, 604 (1971); *eidem, Helv. Chim. Acta* **55**, 2329 (1972).

Venturicidin A   R = NH₂CO
Venturicidin B   R = H

Venturicidin A. [33538-71-5] Venturicidin B 3′-carbamate. $C_{41}H_{67}NO_{11}$; mol wt 749.97. Needles from chloroform-petr ether, mp 145-147°. Also reported as mp 140-142°. $[\alpha]_D$ +119° (c = 0.5 in chloroform). uv max (alcohol): 206, 247 (shoulder), ~300 nm (shoulder) (log ε 3.80, 2.23, 2.08).

Venturicidin B. [33538-72-6] (3-Decarbamoyloxy)-3-hydroxyventuricidin A. $C_{40}H_{66}O_{10}$; mol wt 706.95. Amorphous white powder from chloroform-ether, mp 168-170°. Also reported as mp 145-149° (ethyl acetate-petr ether). $[\alpha]_D$ +100° (c = 0.847 in chloroform).

9948. Veralipride. [66644-81-3] 5-(Aminosulfonyl)-2,3-dimethoxy-*N*-[[1-(2-propenyl)-2-pyrrolidinyl]methyl]benzamide; *N*-[(1-allyl-2-pyrrolidinyl)methyl]-5-sulfamoyl-*o*-veratramide; LIR-1660; Agréal; Agradil; Veralipril. $C_{17}H_{25}N_3O_5S$; mol wt 383.46. C 53.25%, H 6.57%, N 10.96%, O 20.86%, S 8.36%. Prepn: **NL 7707982** (1978 to Soc. d'Etudes Sci. Ind. de l'Ile-de-France), *C.A.* **89**, 30768 (1978). Pharmacological studies: P. Bouyard *et al., Sem. Hop.* **56**, 1475 (1980); J. C. Czyba, *ibid.* 1483. Clinical studies: R. Renaud, J. Macler, *ibid.* **57**, 353 (1981); S. Angeli, P. Fougère, *ibid.* **58**, 111 (1982).

THERAP CAT: Treatment of menopausal disorders.

9949. Veralkamine. [17155-31-6] (3β,16β,17α,22α)-17-Methyl-18-nor-16,28-secosolanida-5,12-diene-3,16-diol; 17-methyl-20α-((2S,5S)-5-methyl-2-piperidyl)-18-nor-17α-pregna-5,12-diene-3β,16β-diol; (22S:25S)-12,26-epimino-17β-methyl-18-norcholesta-5,12-diene-3β,16β-diol; (17S:12S:25S)-22,26-epimino-18(13 → 17)-*abeo*-cholesta-5,12-diene-3β,16β-diol; veralcamine. $C_{27}H_{43}NO_2$; mol wt 413.64. C 78.40%, H 10.48%, N 3.39%, O 7.74%. Steroidal alkaloid isolated from *Veratrum album* sp. *lobelianium* (Bernh.) Suessenguth, *Liliaceae:* Tomko *et al., Pharm. Zentralhalle* **99**, 373 (1960), *C.A.* **55**, 2013e. Structure studies: Tomko *et al., Collect. Czech. Chem. Commun.* **27**, 1404 (1962). Complete structure: Tomko *et al., Tetrahedron Lett.* **1967**, 3907; *eidem, Tetrahedron* **24**, 4865 (1968); Hoehne *et al., ibid.* 4875.

Crystals from ethanol, mp 119-123° and 165-169°; $[\alpha]_D^{24}$ −84.1 ±3° (c = 0.533 in CHCl₃).

***N,O,O*-Triacetate.** mp 152-154°. $[\alpha]_D^{27}$ −8.0° (CHCl₃).

***N*-Monoacetate.** mp 191-193°. $[\alpha]_D^{23}$ −79.1° (CHCl₃).

9950. Verapamil. [52-53-9] α-[3-[[2-(3,4-Dimethoxyphenyl)ethyl]methylamino]propyl]-3,4-dimethoxy-α-(1-methylethyl)-benzeneacetonitrile; 5-[(3,4-dimethoxyphenethyl)methylamino]-2-(3,4-dimethoxyphenyl)-2-isopropylvaleronitrile; α-isopropyl-α-[(*N*-methyl-*N*-homoveratryl)-γ-aminopropyl]-3,4-dimethoxyphenyl-acetonitrile; iproveratril; D-365. $C_{27}H_{38}N_2O_4$; mol wt 454.60. C 71.33%, H 8.43%, N 6.16%, O 14.08%. Prototype calcium antagonist; vasodilating activity resides primarily in the (*S*)-isomer. Both isomers inhibit the p-glycoprotein efflux pump in multidrug resistant tumor cells. Prepn: **BE 615861**; Dengel, **US 3261859** (1962, 1966 both to Knoll). Pharmacology: H. Haas, G. Härtfelder, *Arzneim.-Forsch.* **12**, 549 (1962). Physical and chemical data: W. Appel, *ibid.* 562. Synthesis and absolute configuration of enantiomers: H. Ramuz, *Helv. Chim. Acta* **58**, 2050 (1975). Stereospecific synthesis: L. J. Theodore, W. L. Nelson, *J. Org. Chem.* **52**, 1309 (1987). HPLC determn of enantiomers and metabolites in plasma: G. Stagni, W. R. Gillespie, *J. Chromatogr. B* **667**, 349 (1995). Comprehensive description: Z. L. Chang, *Anal. Profiles Drug Subs.* **17**, 643-674 (1988). Review of pharmacology and therapeutic use in arrhythmias: B. N. Singh *et al., Drugs* **25**, 125-153 (1983); in hypertension: D. McTavish, E. M. Sorkin, *ibid.* **38**, 19-76 (1989). Clinical trial of dexverapamil as adjunct to cancer chemotherapy: G. Kornek *et al., Cancer* **76**, 1356 (1995); R. J. Motzer *et al., J. Clin. Oncol.* **13**, 1958 (1995).

Viscous, pale yellow oil, bp₀.₀₁ 243-246°. n_D^{25} 1.5448. Practically insol in water. Sparingly sol in hexane; sol in benzene, ether. Freely sol in the lower alcohols, acetone, ethyl acetate, chloroform.

Hydrochloride. [152-11-4] Berkatens; Calan; Cardibeltin; Covera-HS; Dignover; Falicard; Flamon; Geangin; Isoptin; Quasar; Securon; Tarka; Univer; Veracim; Veramex; Veraptin; Verelan; Vertab; Zolvera. $C_{27}H_{38}N_2O_4$·HCl; mol wt 491.06. Crystals, dec 138.5-140.5° (corr). pH of 0.1% aq soln: 5.25. uv max: 232, 278 nm. Soly (mg/ml): water 83, ethanol (200 proof) 26, propylene glycol 93, ethanol (190 proof) >100, methanol >100, 2-propanol 4.6, ethyl acetate 1.0, DMF >100, methylene chloride >100, hexane 0.001. pKa 8.6. LD₅₀ in mice, rats (mg/kg): 7.6, 16 i.v.; 68, 107 s.c.; 68, 67 i.p.; 163, 114 orally (Haas, Härtfelder).

(*R*)-Form hydrochloride. [38176-02-2]; [38321-02-7]. Dexverapamil hydrochloride. Crystals, mp 131-133°. $[\alpha]_D^{25}$ +8.9° (c = 5.01 in ethanol).

THERAP CAT: Antihypertensive; antianginal; antiarrhythmic (class IV).

9951. Veratraldehyde. [120-14-9] 3,4-Dimethoxybenzaldehyde; 3,4-dimethoxybenzenecarbonal; veratric aldehyde; protocatechualdehyde dimethyl ether. $C_9H_{10}O_3$; mol wt 166.17. C 65.05%, H 6.07%, O 28.88%. Prepd by methylation of vanillin: Kostanecki, Tambor, *Ber.* **39**, 4022 (1906); Buck, *Org. Synth.* **13**, 102 (1933); Alt, **US 3007968** (1957 to Monsanto); by oxidation of veratryl alcohol with chromium(VI) oxide-pyridine complex: Holum, *J. Org. Chem.* **26**, 4814 (1961).

Needles from ether, petr ether, toluene, or carbon tetrachloride. Odor of vanilla beans; mp 42-43°; bp$_{760}$ 281°; bp$_{53}$ 201°; bp$_{10}$ 155°. Slightly sol in hot water; freely sol in alcohol and ether. Solns are oxidized to veratic acid under the influence of light.

9952. Veratramine. [60-70-8] (3β,23β)-14,15,16,17-Tetradehydroveratraman-3,23-diol. C$_{27}$H$_{39}$NO$_2$; mol wt 409.60. C 79.17%, H 9.60%, N 3.42%, O 7.81%. Secondary base from *Veratrum grandiflorum* (Maxim.) Loes. f., and from *V. viride* Ait., *Liliaceae*. Isoln and structure: Saito, *Bull. Chem. Soc. Jpn.* **15,** 22 (1940); Jacobs, Craig, *J. Biol. Chem.* **160,** 555 (1945); Jacobs, Sato, *ibid.* **181,** 55 (1949); **191,** 71 (1951); Tamm, Wintersteiner, *J. Am. Chem. Soc.* **74,** 3842 (1952); Wintersteiner, *Festschrift Arthur Stoll* (Birkhäuser-Verlag, Basel) pp 166-176. Total synthesis: Masamune *et al., J. Am. Chem. Soc.* **89,** 4521 (1967); Johnson *et al., ibid.* 4523; Masamune *et al., Tetrahedron* **27,** 3369 (1971); Kutney *et al., Can. J. Chem.* **53,** 1796 (1975). Stereochemistry: Sicher, Tichy, *Tetrahedron Lett.* **1959**(12), 6 (1959); Kataoka, *Chem. Ind. (London)* **1961,** 512; Bailey *et al., Tetrahedron Lett.* **1963,** 555. Revised stereochemistry: Scott *et al., ibid.* **1967,** 2381; Kupchan, Suffness, *J. Am. Chem. Soc.* **90,** 2730 (1968); Sprague *et al., Tetrahedron* **27,** 4857 (1971). *See also:* Veratrum Viride.

Crystals, mp 206-207°. Slightly sol in water. Sol in methanol, alcohol. Precipitated by digitonin. [α]$_D^{25}$ −71.8° (c = 1.21); [α]$_D^{25}$ −70° (c = 1.56 in methanol). uv max: 268 nm.

Dihydroveratramine. Crystals, mp 192.5-194°. [α]$_D^{25}$ +26° (c = 1.26 in acetic acid).

9953. Veratric Acid. [93-07-2] 3,4-Dimethylbenzoic acid; dimethylprotocatechuic acid. C$_9$H$_{10}$O$_4$; mol wt 182.17. C 59.34%, H 5.53%, O 35.13%. Isolated from seed of *Schoenocaulon officinale* (Schlecht. & Cham.) A. Gray (*Sabadilla officinarum* Brandt). Prepn: Arthur, Ng, *J. Chem. Soc.* **1959,** 3094.

Monohydrate. Odorless crystals. At 100° becomes anhydr; mp 180-181° when anhydr. Sublimes in rhombic crystals. Sol in 2150 parts cold, 165 parts boiling water; very sol in alcohol or ether. Its barium salt is but slightly sol in water.

9954. Veratridine. [71-62-5] (3β,4α,16β)-4,9-Epoxycevane-3,4,12,14,16,17,20-heptol 3-(3,4-dimethoxybenzoate); 3-veratroylveracevine. C$_{36}$H$_{51}$NO$_{11}$; mol wt 673.79. C 64.17%, H 7.63%, N 2.08%, O 26.12%. From seed of *Schoenocaulon officinale* (Schlecht. & Cham.) A. Gray and also from the rhizome of *Veratrum album* L. *Liliaceae*. Can be isolated from commercial veratrine as the sparingly sol nitrate: Blount, *J. Chem. Soc.* **1935,** 122; Vejdelek *et al., Chem. Listy* **50,** 603 (1956); *Collect. Czech. Chem. Commun.* **22,** 98 (1957). Purification and properties: L. C. McKinney *et al., Anal. Biochem.* **153,** 33 (1986). Toxicity studies: O. Krayer *et al., J. Pharmacol. Exp. Ther.* **82,** 167 (1944); K. Tanaka,

ibid. **113,** 89 (1955); Swiss, Bauer, *Proc. Soc. Exp. Biol. Med.* **76,** 847 (1951). Review of chemistry and structure of veratridine and other *Veratrum* alkaloids: Kupchan, By, in *The Alkaloids* vol. 10, R. H. F. Manske, Ed. (Academic Press, New York, 1968) pp 193-285.

Yellowish-white, amorphous powder. Tenaciously retains water. mp 180° (after drying at 130°). [α]$_D^{20}$ +8.0° (ethanol). pKa 9.54 ±0.02. Insol in water. Slightly sol in ether. LD$_{50}$ in mice (mg/kg): 1.35 i.p. (Swiss, Bauer); 0.42 i.v. (Krayer); 6.3 s.c. (Tanaka).

Nitrate. Amorphous powder, sparingly sol in water.

Sulfate. Slender needles, very hygroscopic.

Perchlorate. Long thin needles from water, mp 259-260° (after drying at 120° *in vacuo*).

9955. Veratrine (Mixture). This veratrine is a mixture of the alkaloids cevadine, veratridine, cevadilline, sabadine, cevine from seeds of *Schoenocaulon officinale* (Schlecht & Cham.) A. Gray, *Liliaceae*.

White or grayish-white powder. mp 145-155°. One gram dissolves in about 1800 ml water, 1000 ml boiling water, 2.8 ml alcohol, 0.7 ml chloroform, 4.2 ml ether, 80 ml olive oil; freely sol in dil acids, benzene, amyl alcohol, slightly in glycerol; insol in petr ether.

Caution: Poisonous! Exceedingly irritating to mucous membranes; causing violent sneezing when inhaled.

THERAP CAT: Topical counterirritant.

THERAP CAT (VET): Has been used as emetic, ruminatoric.

9956. Veratrole. [91-16-7] 1,2-Dimethoxybenzene; *o*-dimethoxybenzene; pyrocatechol dimethyl ether. C$_8$H$_{10}$O$_2$; mol wt 138.16. C 69.55%, H 7.30%, O 23.16%. Prepd by methylation of pyrocatechol: Ullmann, *Ann.* **327,** 104 (1903); Drahowzal, Klamann, *Monatsh. Chem.* **82,** 588 (1951). Toxicity study: P. M. Jenner *et al., Food Cosmet. Toxicol.* **2,** 327 (1964).

Crystals or liquid; d$_{25}^{25}$ 1.084; mp 22-23°; bp 206-207°. Slightly sol in water; sol in alcohol, ether, fatty oils. LD$_{50}$ in rats, mice (mg/kg): 1360, 2020 orally (Jenner).

9957. Veratrum viride. American hellebore; green hellebore; American veratrum; Indian poke. Dried rhizome and roots of *Veratrum viride* Ait., *Liliaceae*. Habit. North America. Constit. The alkaloids jervine, pseudojervine, rubijervine, cevadine, germitrine, germidine, veratralbine, veratroidine. *See* Seiferle *et al., J. Econ. Entomol.* **35,** 35 (1942); Fried *et al., J. Am. Chem. Soc.* **72,** 4621 (1950). *Review:* Kupchan, *J. Pharm. Sci.* **50,** 273-287 (1961).

Mixture of the alkaloids of *Veratrum viride*. Alkavervir; Veriloid.

THERAP CAT: Antihypertensive.

THERAP CAT (VET): Has been used as antihypertensive and to improve digestion.

9958. Verbascose. [546-62-3] β-D-Fructofuranosyl *O*-α-D-galactopyranosyl-(1 → 6)-*O*-α-D-galactopyranosyl(1 → 6)-*O*-α-D-galactopyranosyl-(1 → 6)-α-D-glucopyranoside; *O*-α-D-galactopyrano-syl-(1→6)-[*O*-α-D-galactopyranosyl-(1→6)-]$_2$-*O*-α-D-glucopyrano-syl-(1 → 2)-β-D-fructofuranoside. $C_{30}H_{52}O_{26}$; mol wt 828.72. C 43.48%, H 6.32%, O 50.20%. Oligosaccharide isolated from roots of mullein *Verbascum thapsus* L., *Scrophulariaceae:* Bourquelot, Bridel, *Compt. Rend.* **151**, 760 (1910); from birch wood, *Betula verrucosa* Ehrh., *Betulaceae:* Lindberg, Selleby, *Acta Chem. Scand.* **12**, 1512 (1958). Structure: Wickström *et al., Bull. Soc. Chim. Fr.* **1956**, 827. *Review:* D. French "The Raffinose Family of Oligosaccharides" in *Adv. Carbohydr. Chem.* **9**, 180-181 (1954).

Needles, mp 219-220°, mp 253°. $[\alpha]_D^{20}$ +170° (water); $[\alpha]_D^{25}$ +146° (c = 2.1 in water).

9959. Verbenalin. [548-37-8] [1*S*-(1α,4aα,7α,7aα)]-1-(β-D-Glucopyranosyloxy)-1,4a,5,6,7,7a-hexahydro-7-methyl-5-oxo-cyclopenta[c]pyran-4-carboxylic acid methyl ester; cornin. C_{17}-$H_{24}O_{10}$; mol wt 388.37. C 52.57%, H 6.23%, O 41.20%. A glyco-side isolated from *Verbena officinalis* L., *Verbenaceae, Cornus florida* L., *Cornaceae. Refs:* Bourdier, *J. Pharm. Chim.* **27**(6), 49, 101 (1908); Holste, *Arch. Exp. Pathol. Pharmakol.* **101**, 46 (1924); Miller, *J. Am. Pharm. Assoc.* **17**, 744 (1928). Identity with cornin: Reichert, *Arch. Pharm.* **273**, 357 (1935). Structure: Büchi, Man-ning, *Tetrahedron Lett.* **1960**, 5 (1960); *eidem, Tetrahedron* **18**, 1049 (1962). Synthesis of *verbenalol*, the aglycone: P. Callant *et al., ibid.* **37**, 2085 (1981).

Bitter needles, mp 182-183°. $[\alpha]_D^{25}$ −173° (water). uv max: 238, 290 nm (ε 9600, 105) in ethanol. Freely sol in water, slightly in alcohol, ethyl acetate, acetone. Practically insol in chloroform, ether.

9960. *d*-Verbenone. [18309-32-5] (1*R*)-4,6,6-Trimethylbi-cyclo[3.1.1]hept-3-en-2-one; (1*R*,5*R*)-(+)-2-pinen-4-one. $C_{10}H_{14}$-O; mol wt 150.22. C 79.95%, H 9.39%, O 10.65%. A constituent of Spanish verbena oil (from *Verbena triphylla* L., *Verbenaceae*): Kerschbaum, *Ber.* **33**, 885 (1900). Prepn from α-pinene: Bain, Gary, *US* **2911442** (1959 to Glidden). Structure: Blumann, Zeit-schel, *Ber.* **46**, 1178 (1913); Weinhaus, Schumm, *Ann.* **439**, 20 (1924). Absolute configuration: Hurst, Whitham, *J. Chem. Soc.* **1960**, 2864. *Review:* J. L. Simonsen, *The Terpenes* **vol. II** (University Press, Cambridge, 2nd ed., 1949) p 232-239.

Oil. Characteristic odor. mp 6.5°. bp$_{12}$ 102-105°; bp$_{760}$ 227-228°. d^{20} 0.9780. n_D^{18} 1.4957. $[\alpha]_D^{18}$ +249.62°. uv max (ethanol): 253 nm (ε 6730). Practically insol in water. Miscible in all pro-portions with the usual organic solvents.

9961. Vermiculite. [1318-00-9] Hydrated magnesium-alu-minum-iron silicate. Typical analysis of Montana vermiculite ore: SiO_2 38.64%, MgO 22.68%, Al_2O_3 14.94%, Fe_2O_3 9.29%, K_2O 7.84%, CaO 1.23%, Cr_2O_3 0.29%, Mn_3O_4 0.11%, Cl 0.28%. Monoclinic crystals, pseudo-hexagonal characteristics. Soft, re-silient, glabrous feel. Dissolves in hot concd H_2SO_4. Has base

exchange capacities. Sold as the ore or in "expanded" form. The expanded grades can absorb large quantities of liquids and remain free flowing. The ore is not sol in weak acids or bases, but expanded grades may be attacked. Vermiculites should be classed as mont-morillonoids: Rustum Roy, *Chem. Eng. News* **32**, 4842 (1954).

Note: A food grade vermiculite is known as *Verxite.*

USE: As catalyst; loose fill insulation, filler and packing material.

9962. Vernolepin. [18542-37-5] [3a*R*-(3aα,4α,5aα,9aα,-9bβ)]-5a-Ethenyloctahydro-4-hydroxy-3,9-bis(methylene)-2*H*-furo[2,3-*f*][2]benzopyran-2,8(3*H*)-dione. $C_{15}H_{16}O_5$; mol wt 276.28. C 65.21%, H 5.84%, O 28.96%. The first recognized naturally occurring elemanolide dilactone; a sesquiterpene lactone with tumor inhibiting properties. Isoln from *Vernonia hymenolepsis* A. Rich, *Compositae* and structure: S. M. Kupchan *et al., J. Am. Chem. Soc.* **90**, 3596 (1968); structural elucidation: *eidem, J. Org. Chem.* **34**, 3903 (1969). Biological properties: S. M. Kupchan *et al., J. Med. Chem.* **14**, 1147 (1971). Approach to stereosynthesis of (+)-form: H. Iio *et al., Tetrahedron* **35**, 941 (1979); K. Kondo *et al. Tetrahedron Lett.* **34**, 4219 (1993). Total synthesis of (±)-form: P. A. Grieco *et al., J. Am. Chem. Soc.* **98**, 1612 (1976); F. Zutterman *et al., Tetrahedron* **35**, 2389 (1979).

Crystals from chloroform-petr ether, mp 181-182°. $[\alpha]_D^{28}$ +72° (c = 1.04 in acetone). uv max (methanol): 208 nm (ε 20300).

(±)-**Form.** [59598-29-7] Crystals from chloroform, mp 210-211°.

9963. Vernolic Acid. 11-(3-Pentyloxiranyl)-9-undecenoic acid; 12,13-epoxyoleic acid; *cis*-12,13-epoxyoctadec-*cis*-9-enoic acid; octadec-*cis*-12,13-epoxy-*cis*-9-enoic acid. $C_{18}H_{32}O_3$; mol wt 296.44. C 72.93%, H 10.88%, O 16.19%. Naturally occurring as the (+) and (−) forms. Principal seed-oil acid from *Vernonia anthelmintica* Willd. (*Serratula anthelmintica* Roxb., *Conyza an-thelmintica* Linn.) *Compositae.* Isoln and structure: Gunstone, *J. Chem. Soc.* **1954**, 1611; from *Plectranthus spp.:* C. M. J. Daulata-bad, A. M. Mirajkur, *J. Chem. Technol. Biotechnol.* **45**, 143 (1989). Synthesis and absorption spectrum: Osbond, *ibid.* **1961**, 5270; *idem*, **GB 909354** (1962 to Roche). Enantiospecific synthesis of (−)-form: C. A. Moustakis *et al., Tetrahedron Lett.* **27**, 303 (1986).

(−)-**Form.** [32381-42-3] [2*R*-[2α(*Z*),3α]]-11-(3-Pentyl-oxiranyl)-9-undecenoic acid; (12*R*,13*S*)-(−)-12,13-epoxyoleic acid. Crystals from acetone at −25°, mp 30-31°. Liq at room temp. $[\alpha]_D$ −8°.

(+)-**Form.** [503-07-1] [2*S*-[2α(*Z*),3α]]-11-(3-Pentyloxiranyl)-9-undecenoic acid; (12*S*,13*R*)-(+)-12,13-epoxyoleic acid.

9964. Verrucarins. Macrocyclic tricothecane derivs which are secondary metabolites of the soil fungi *Myrothecium verrucaria* (Albertini et Schweinitz) Ditmar ex Fries; they are characterized by antibiotic, antifungal, and cytostatic activity. Verrucarins are triest-ers of the sesquiterpene alcohol *verrucarol* and closely related to the *roridins*, which are diesters of the same alcohol. Isoln of verrucar-ins A (major), B, C, D, E, F, G: E. Haerri *et al., Helv. Chim. Acta* **45**, 840 (1962). Isoln of A: Symth, Kraskin, *US* **3087859** (1963 to Rohm & Haas); Vittimberga, *J. Org. Chem.* **28**, 1786 (1963). Identity with muconomycin A: Vittimberga, Vittimberga, *ibid.* **30**, 746 (1965). Structure of A: J. Gutzwiller, C. Tamm, *Helv. Chim. Acta* **48**, 157 (1965). Stereochemistry: W. Zürcher *et al., ibid.* 840; A. T. McPhail, G. T. Sim, *J. Chem. Soc. C* **1966**, 1394. Synthesis of A: W. C. Still, H. Ohmizu, *J. Org. Chem.* **46**, 5242

(1981). Isoln of B: W. Loeffler *et al.*, **BE 627002** (1963 to Sandoz), *C.A.* **60**, 10485b (1964). Structure of B: J. Gutzwiller, C. Tamm, *Helv. Chim. Acta* **48**, 177 (1965). Toxicological studies of A and B: Guarino *et al., Biotechnol. Bioeng.* **10**, 457 (1968); of A: Mortimer *et al., Res. Vet. Sci.* **12**, 508 (1971). Biosynthetic studies of A and B: B. Müller, C. Tamm, *Helv. Chim. Acta* **58**, 483 (1975); G. A. Cordell, *Chem. Rev.* **76**, 425 (1976). Isoln of J (muconomycin B): Vittimberga, Vittimberga, *loc. cit.;* of H and J: B. Boehner *et al., Helv. Chim. Acta* **48**, 1079 (1965). Structure of J: E. Fetz *et al., ibid.* 1669. Partial synthesis of tetrahydroverrucarin J and revised structure of J: W. Breitenstein, C. Tamm, *ibid.* **61**, 1975 (1978). Isoln and structure of K: *eidem, ibid.* **60**, 1522 (1977). Isoln of L: B. B. Jarvis *et al., J. Antibiot.* **34**, 121 (1981). Total synthesis of verrucarol: R. H. Schlessinger, R. A. Nugent, *J. Am. Chem. Soc.* **104**, 1116 (1982). Toxicity study: E. M. Rüsch, H. Stählin, *Arzneim.-Forsch.* **15**, 893 (1965). Comprehensive review of the verrucarins and roridins: C. Tamm, *Fortschr. Chem. Org. Naturst.* **31**, 64-117 (1974). For a description of the stereochemistry of the roridins *see* B. R. Jarvis *et al., J. Nat. Prod.* **45**, 440 (1982).

Verrucarin A

Verrucarin A. [3148-09-2] Muconomycin A. $C_{27}H_{34}O_9$; mol wt 502.55. Colorless rectangular plates from ether/acetone, mp >360° (dec). $[\alpha]_D^{23}$ +206° (c = 1.012 in chloroform); uv max (ethanol): 260 nm (log ε 4.25). LD_{50} in mice, rats, rabbits (mg/kg): 1.5, 0.87, 0.54 i.v. (Rüsch, Stählin).

Verrucarin B. [2290-11-1] (2′S,3′R)-2′-Deoxy-2′,3′-epoxyverrucarin A. $C_{27}H_{32}O_9$; mol wt 500.54. Colorless needles from acetone/ether, decomp >330°. $[\alpha]_D^{23}$ +147° (c = 1.066 in benzene). $[\alpha]_D^{22}$ +101 ±1.5° (c = 1.416 in dioxane). uv max (methanol): 258.5 nm (log ε 4.37).

Verrucarin J. [4643-58-7] (2′E)-2′,3′-Didehydro-2′-deoxyverrucarin A; muconomycin B. $C_{27}H_{32}O_8$; mol wt 484.54. Crystals from ether, dec >235°. $[\alpha]_D^{19}$ +54° (benzene). $[\alpha]_D^{22}$ +20 ± 2° (c = 1.011 in chloroform). uv max: 261, 220.5 nm (ε 22000, 21600).

Verrucarin K. [63739-93-5] 12,13-Deepoxy-12,13-didehydroverrucarin A. $C_{27}H_{34}O_8$; mol wt 486.55. Crystals from methylene chloride/ether, dec >320°. $[\alpha]_D^{23}$ +218 ±2° (c = 0.58 in chloroform). uv max (ethanol): 259 nm (log ε 4.19).

Caution: Verrucarins are extremely toxic; can cause severe local irritation and inflammation of the skin.

9965. Versalide®. [88-29-9] 1-(3-Ethyl-5,6,7,8-tetrahydro-5,5,8,8-tetramethyl-2-naphthalenyl)ethanone; 3′-ethyl-5′,6′,7′,8′-tetrahydro-5′,5′,8′,8′-tetramethyl-2′-acetonaphthone. $C_{18}H_{26}O$; mol wt 258.40. C 83.67%, H 10.14%, O 6.19%. Prepn: Davidson, Lusskin, **US 3045047** (1962 to Trubek Lab.). GC determn in fragrances: H. H. Wisneski *et al., J. Assoc. Off. Anal. Chem.* **65**, 598 (1982). Toxicity: K. R. Butterworth, P. L. Mason, *Food Cosmet. Toxicol.* **19**, 753 (1981).

Crystals, mp 46.5°. bp_2 130°. Soluble in alc.
USE: As musk for perfumes, cosmetics, soaps.

9966. Versenol®. [139-89-9] N-[2-[Bis(carboxymethyl)amino]ethyl]-N-(2-hydroxyethyl)glycine trisodium salt; N-(carboxymethyl)-N′-(2-hydroxyethyl)-N,N′-ethylenediglycine trisodium salt; N-hydroxyethylethylenediaminetriacetic acid trisodium salt; trisodium N-hydroxyethylethylenediaminetriacetate; HEDTA. $C_{10}H_{15}N_2Na_3O_7$; mol wt 344.20. C 34.89%, H 4.39%, N 8.14%, Na 20.04%, O 32.54%. Prepn: Young, **US 2811550** (1957 to Refined Prod.); Kroll, Dexter, **US 2845457** (1958 to Geigy).

USE: As chelating agent for trivalent iron from pH 7 to pH 10. Forms strong 1:1 ferric chelates. The iron chelates formed will then chelate other heavy metal or alkaline earth ions.

9967. Verteporfin. [129497-78-5] (4R,4aS)-rel-18-Ethenyl-4,4a-dihydro-3,4-bis(methoxycarbonyl)-4a,8,14,19-tetramethyl-23H,25H-benzo[b]porphine-9,13-dipropanoic acid monomethyl ester; BPD-MA; CL-318952; Visudyne. $C_{41}H_{42}N_4O_8$; mol wt 718.79. C 68.51%, H 5.89%, N 7.79%, O 17.81%. Benzoporphyrin photosensitizer. Preparative method: A. M. Richter *et al., J. Natl. Cancer Inst.* **79**, 1327 (1987). Photosensitizing efficiency: A. M. Richter *et al., Biochem. Pharmacol.* **43**, 2349 (1992). Spectral characterization: R. Gillies *et al., J. Photochem. Photobiol. B* **33**, 87 (1996). Tissue uptake parameters: R. K. Chowdhary *et al., Biopharm. Drug Dispos.* **19**, 395 (1998). Clinical trial in macular degeneration: TAP Study Group, *Arch. Ophthalmol.* **117**, 1329 (1999). Review of pharmacology and clinical experience: K. J. Mellish, S. B. Brown, *Expert Opin. Pharmacother.* **2**, 351-361 (2001); S. J. Bakri, P. K. Kaiser, *ibid.* **5**, 195-203 (2004).

Isomer A   R = H   R¹= CH_3
Isomer B   R = CH_3 R¹= H

Virtually insol in water. Absorption max: ~690 nm.
Note: The marketed form is a mixture of the two possible methyl esters.
THERAP CAT: In treatment of age-related macular degeneration.

9968. Verticillins. Three antibiotics, verticillins A, B and C, produced by a species of *Verticillium* (strain TM-759), an imperfect fungus isolated from a basidiocarp of *Coltricia cinnamomea (Polystictus cinnamomeus)*. Isoln, IR, NMR spectra of verticillin A: Katagiri *et al., J. Antibiot.* **23**, 420 (1970); *see also* Chepenko *et al., C.A.* **78**, 156654n (1973). Structure: Minato *et al., Chem. Commun.* **1971**, 44. Structure of verticillins A, B and C and absolute configuration of verticillins A and B: *eidem, J. Chem. Soc. Perkin Trans. 1* **1973**, 1819. Synthetic studies: Häusler, Schmidt, *Ber.* **107**, 2804 (1974); Schmidt *et al., ibid.* 2816.

Verticillin A

Verticillin A. [32164-16-2] $C_{30}H_{28}N_6O_6S_4$; mol wt 696.84. Pale yellow plates from chloroform, $C_{30}H_{28}N_6O_6S_4.CHCl_3$, mp 199-213° (dec); pale yellow needles from pyridine, $C_{30}H_{28}N_6O_6S_4.2/3C_5H_5N$, mp 202-217° (dec); pale yellow amorphous powder from tetrahydrofuran, mp 203-214° (dec). $[\alpha]_D$ +703.7° (c = 0.422 in dioxane). uv max (dioxane): 306 nm (ε 5960). LD_{50} i.p. in mice: 7.6 mg/kg (Katagiri).

Verticillin B. [52212-86-9] $C_{30}H_{28}N_6O_7S_4$; mol wt 712.84. The mono-3-hydroxymethyl analog of verticillin A. Pale yellow prisms from chloroform, mp 230-233° (dec). $[\alpha]_D^{21}$ +704.7° (c = 0.493 in dioxane). uv max (dioxane): 306 nm (ε 5600).

Verticillin C. $C_{30}H_{28}N_6O_7S_5$; mol wt 744.90. Differs from verticillin B by having a trisulfide rather than disulfide bridge in one of the two dioxopiperazine rings. Pale yellow amorphous powder from methanol-water, mp 230-235° (dec). $[\alpha]_D^{21}$ +765.0° (c = 0.506 in dioxane). uv max (dioxane): 303 nm (ε 5500).

9969. **Verticine.** [23496-41-5] $(3\beta,5\alpha,6\alpha)$-Cevane-3,6,20-triol; peimine. $C_{27}H_{45}NO_3$; mol wt 431.65. C 75.13%, H 10.51%, N 3.24%, O 11.12%. A member of the hexacyclic *Ce-veratrum* group of alkaloids. Isoln from *Fritillaria verticillata* Willd. var. *Thunbergii* Baker, *Liliaceae:* Fukuda: *Sci. Rep. Res. Inst. Tohoku Univ. Ser. A* **18**, 323 (1929); Morimoto, Kimata, *Chem. Pharm. Bull.* **8**, 302 (1960). Also isolated from *F. roylei* Hook: Chou, Chen, *Chin. J. Physiol.* **6**, 265 (1932), *C.A.* **26**, 5703 (1932). Structure: Ito *et al., ibid.* **11**, 1337 (1963). Abs config: S. Ito *et al., Tetrahedron Lett.* **1968**, 5373. Total synthesis: J. P. Kutney *et al., J. Am. Chem. Soc,* **99**, 964 (1977).

Needles from ethanol, mp 223-224°. $[\alpha]_D^{16}$ −19.4° (ethanol); $[\alpha]_D^{17}$ −20° (CHCl₃). pK'a 9.5. uv max (ethanol + HCl): 215 nm (ε 10).

Hydrochloride. $C_{27}H_{45}NO_3.HCl$. Prisms from water, dec 291-294°. $[\alpha]_D^{18}$ −18.5°.

Perchlorate. $C_{27}H_{45}NO_3.HClO_4$. Prisms from water, dec 273°. $[\alpha]_D^{23}$ −15° (c = 0.05).

Methiodide. $C_{27}H_{45}NO_3.CH_3I$. Crystals from butanol + ether, dec 205-210°. $[\alpha]_D^{18}$ −14.0° (water). Sol in water, methanol, ethanol; practically insol in chloroform, benzene, acetone.

3-Glucoside. Peiminoside. $C_{33}H_{55}NO_8$. Pale brown powder. Sol in water, methanol, alc; sparingly sol in benzene.

9970. **Vesnarinone.** [81840-15-5] 1-(3,4-Dimethoxybenzo-yl)-4-(1,2,3,4-tetrahydro-2-oxo-6-quinolinyl)piperazine; 3,4-dihy-dro-6-[4-(3,4-dimethoxybenzoyl)-1-piperazinyl]-2(1*H*)-quinoli-none; 6-[4-(3,4-dimethoxybenzoyl)-1-piperazinyl]-3,4-dihydro-carbostyril; 1-(1,2,3,4-tetrahydro-2-oxo-6-quinolyl)-4-veratroyl-piperazine; piteranometozine; OPC-8212; Arkin. $C_{22}H_{25}N_3O_4$; mol wt 395.45. C 66.82%, H 6.37%, N 10.63%, O 16.18%. Positive inotropic agent. Prepn: Y. H. Yang *et al.,* **BE 890942**; M. Tominaga *et al.,* **US 4415572** (1982, 1983 both to Otsuka); M. Tominaga *et al., Chem. Pharm. Bull.* **32**, 2100 (1984). Physico-chemical properties: T. Shimizu *et al., Arzneim.-Forsch.* **34**, 334 (1984). Series of articles on mechanism of action and pharmacol-ogy: *ibid.* 342-402. Effects on canine arrhythmias: K. Hashi-moto, H. Mitsuhashi, *Br. J. Pharmacol.* **88**, 915 (1986). Metabo-lism: G. Miyamoto *et al., Xenobiotica* **18**, 1143 (1988). Clinical pharmacokinetics: A. Ohnishi, T. Ishizaki, *J. Clin. Pharmacol.* **28**, 719 (1988). HPLC determn in plasma and urine: G. Miyamoto *et al., J. Chromatogr.* **338**, 450 (1985). Clinical evaluations in con-gestive heart failure: H. Asanoi *et al., J. Am. Coll. Cardiol.* **9**, 865 (1987); A. M. Feldman *et al., Am. Heart J.* **116**, 771 (1988).

Colorless granules from ethanol-chloroform, mp 238.1-239.5° (Tominaga); also reported as odorless, tasteless, pale yellow crys-talline powder, mp 238.1-239.8° (Shimizu). uv max (methanol, ethanol, chloroform): 271 nm (ε = 2.51 × 10⁴, 2.52 × 10⁴, 2.30 × 10⁴, c = 10 μg/ml). % solubility (25°): glacial acetic acid 18.68; chloroform 14.19; benzyl alcohol 5.913; N-methyl-2-pyrrolidone 3.407; DMSO 2.509; 60% sulfolane 1.229; DMF 1.179; dioxane 0.1653; methanol 0.1151; acetone 0.06389; ethanol 0.04005; water 0.002086. pKa 2.86.

THERAP CAT: Cardiotonic.

9971. **Vetivones.** $C_{15}H_{22}O$; mol wt 218.33. C 82.52%, H 10.16%, O 7.33%. Ketonic components of vetiver oil; from roots of *Vetiveria zizanioides (Andropogon muricatus* Retz., *Gramineae).* Two isomers, the α-form having the stronger odor. Isoln and struc-ture: Pfau, Plattner, *Helv. Chim. Acta* **22**, 640 (1939); Naves, Perrottet, *ibid.* **24**, 3 (1941).

α-Vetivone β-Vetivone

α-Vetivone. [15764-04-2] (4*R-cis*)-4,4a,5,6,7,8-Hexahydro-4,4a-dimethyl-6-(1-methylethylidene)-2(3*H*)-naphthalenone; 4*βH*,-5α-eremophila-1(10),7(11)-dien-2-one; isonootkatone. Structure: Endo, DeMayo, *Chem. Commun.* **1967**, 89; Marshall, Andersen, *Tetrahedron Lett.* **1967**, 1611. Total syntheses of the racemate: Marshall *et al., Chem. Commun.* **1967**, 753; Marshall, Warne, *J. Org. Chem.* **36**, 178 (1971); Vandergen *et al., Rec. Trav. Chim.* **90**, 1034, 1045 (1971); Dastur, *J. Am. Chem. Soc.* **96**, 2605 (1974). Crystals from pentane, strong agreeable odor. mp 51.5° (Naves, Perrottet); mp of racemate 30-35° (Marshall, Andersen). n_D^{20} 1.5384. $[\alpha]_D^{20}$ +248° (chloroform). d_4^{20} 1.003 (liquid, supercooled). uv max (ethanol): 233 nm (ε 13200).

β-Vetivone. [18444-79-6] (5*R-cis*)-6,10-Dimethyl-2-(1-meth-ylethylidene)spiro[4.5]dec-6-en-8-one; 2-isopropylidene-6,10-di-methylspiro[4.5]dec-6-en-8-one. Structure: Marshall *et al., J. Am. Chem. Soc.* **89**, 2748, 2750 (1967). Syntheses of racemate: Marshall, Johnson, *Chem. Commun.* **1968**, 391; *eidem, J. Org.*

Chem. **35**, 192 (1970); K. Uneyama *et al.*, *Chem. Lett.* **1977**, 493; S. Torii *et al.*, *Bull. Chem. Soc. Jpn.* **51**, 3590 (1978); E. Wenkert *et al.*, *J. Am. Chem. Soc.* **100**, 1267 (1978). Stereospecific synthesis of (−)-β-vetivone: Deighton *et al.*, *Chem. Commun.* **1975**, 662; M. Asaoka *et al.*, *Chem. Lett.* **1988**, 1225. Crystals from pentane, mp 44-46°. d_4^{20} 1.000 (liquid, supercooled). d_4^{45} 0.9804. $[\alpha]_D^{20}$ −38.9° (c = 10 in alcohol). n_D^{20} 1.5309 (liquid, supercooled), n_D^{45} 1.5216.

USE: Of potential interest in the perfume industry.

9972. Vetrabutine. [3735-45-3] α-(3,4-Dimethoxyphenyl)-*N*,*N*-dimethylbenzenebutanamine; *N*,*N*-dimethyl-α-(3-phenylpropyl)veratrylamine; 1-(3,4-dimethoxyphenyl)-1-dimethylamino-4-phenylbutane; 3,4-dimethoxy-*N*,*N*-dimethyl-α-(3-phenylpropyl)benzylamine; dimophebumine. $C_{20}H_{27}NO_2$; mol wt 313.43. C 76.64%, H 8.68%, N 4.47%, O 10.21%. Prepn: **GB 802723** (1958 to Thomae).

bp$_{0.1}$ 166-168°.

Hydrochloride. [5974-09-4] SP-281; Monzal; Monzaldon. $C_{20}H_{27}NO_2$.HCl; mol wt 349.89. Solid, mp 146-148°.

THERAP CAT (VET): Uterine relaxant.

9973. Viburnum opulus. Cramp bark; high bush cranberry; cranberry tree; water elder; squaw bush; snowball bush. Dried bark of *Viburnum opulus* L., var. *americanum* Ait., *Caprifoliaceae*. *Habit.* Europe, Asia, northern North America, south to Pennsylvania. *Constit.* Viburnin, bitter resin, tannin, sugar; citric, malic, oxalic, and valeric acids.

THERAP CAT: Antispasmodic (uterine).

9974. Viburnum prunifolium. Black hawk; sweet viburnum; sheep berry; stag bush; sloe-leaved viburnum. Dried root bark of *Viburnum prunifolium* L., *Caprifoliaceae*. *Habit.* U.S. *Constit.* Viburnin, bitter resin, tannin; citric, malic, oxalic, and valeric acids.

THERAP CAT: Antispasmodic (uterine).

9975. Vicine. [152-93-2] 2,6-Diamino-5-(β-D-glucopyranosyloxy)-4(1*H*)-pyrimidinone; 2,4-diamino-6-oxypyrimidine-5-(β-D-glucopyranoside); divicine 5-glucoside; vicioside; divicine-β-glucoside. $C_{10}H_{16}N_4O_7$; mol wt 304.26. C 39.48%, H 5.30%, N 18.41%, O 36.81%. Isoln from vetch seeds (*Vicia sativa* L., *Leguminosae*): Ritthausen, *Ber.* **9**, 301 (1876); Levene, *J. Biol. Chem.* **18**, 306 (1914); Levene, Senior, *ibid.* **25**, 611 (1916); Herissey, Cheymol, *Bull. Soc. Chim. Biol.* **13**, 29 (1931); Gmelin, Hasenmaier, *Arzneim.-Forsch.* **7**, 755 (1957). Structure: Bendich, *Trans. N.Y. Acad. Sci.* **15**, 58 (1952); Bendich, Clements, *Biochim. Biophys. Acta* **12**, 462 (1953).

Needles from water, dec 243-244°. $[\alpha]_D^{26}$ −11.7° (c = 3.9 in 0.2*N* NaOH). uv max (0.1*N* HCl): 274 nm (ε 16400); (0.1*N* NaOH): 269, 248, 235, 230 nm (ε 9520, 4360, 5180, 5090). One gram dissolves in about 100 ml water; slightly sol in alcohol; readily sol in dil acids and alkalies.

Note: Another *vicin*, a rhamnosidoglucoside from vetch flowers, is described by Karrer, Widmer, *Helv. Chim. Acta* **10**, 67 (1927). It has the formula: $C_{21}H_{21}O_{12}$.2H$_2$O.

9976. Vidarabine. [5536-17-4] 9-β-D-Arabinofuranosyl-9*H*-purine-6-amine monohydrate; 9-β-D-arabinofuranosyladenine

monohydrate; arabinosyladenine; adenine arabinoside; spongoadenosine; ara-A; CI-673; Arasena-A; Vira-A. $C_{10}H_{13}N_5O_4$.H$_2$O; mol wt 285.26. C 42.10%, H 5.30%, N 24.55%, O 28.04%. Purine nucleoside first synthesized as a potential anticancer agent: Lee *et al.*, *J. Am. Chem. Soc.* **82**, 2648 (1960); Reist *et al.*, *J. Org. Chem.* **27**, 3274 (1962); Glaudemans, Fletcher, *ibid.* **28**, 3004 (1963); Reist *et al.*, *ibid.* **29**, 3725 (1964). Fermentation process using a strain of *Streptomyces antibioticus:* **GB 1159290**; J. D. Howells, A. Ryder, **US 3616208** (1969, 1971 both to Parke, Davis). Crystal and molecular structure: Bunick, Voet, *Acta Crystallogr.* **30B**, 1641 (1974). Series of articles on antiviral activity: *Antimicrob. Agents Chemother.* **1968**, 136-179. Toxicity study: S. M. Kurtz *et al.*, *ibid.* 180. HPLC determn in plasma and urine: W. P. McCann *et al.*, *ibid.* **28**, 265 (1985). Clinical trial in immunocompromised patients: R. J. Whitley *et al.*, *J. Infect. Dis.* **165**, 450 (1992). Book: *Adenine Arabinoside: An Antiviral Agent*, D. Paven-Langston *et al.*, Eds. (Raven Press, New York, 1975) xviii + 425 pp. Review of pharmacology and clinical experience: R. A. Buchanan, F. Hess, *Pharmacol. Ther.* **8**, 143-171 (1980). Comprehensive description: W. Hong *et al.*, *Anal. Profiles Drug Subs.* **15**, 647-672 (1986).

Crystals from water, mp 257.0-257.5° (0.4 H$_2$O). $[\alpha]_D^{27}$ −5° (c = 0.25). uv max (pH 1): 257.5 nm (ε 12700); pH 7: 259 nm (ε 13400); pH 13: 259 nm (ε 14000). LD$_{50}$ in mice (mg/kg): 4677 i.p.; >7950 orally (Kurtz).

THERAP CAT: Antiviral.

9977. Viehe's Salt. [33842-02-3] *N*-(Dichloromethylene)-*N*-methylmethanaminium chloride; *N*-(dichloromethylene)-*N*,*N*-dimethyliminium chloride; *N*,*N*-dimethylphosgeniminium chloride; phosgeniminium chloride. $C_3H_6Cl_3N$; mol wt 162.45. C 22.18%, H 3.72%, Cl 65.47%, N 8.62%. Electrophilic chlorinating reagent. Prepn: H. G. Viehe, Z. Janousek, *Angew. Chem.* **83**, 614 (1971); and chemistry: *eidem*, *Angew. Chem. Int. Ed.* **12**, 806 (1973). ^{35}Cl NMR study: G. Jugie *et al.*, *J. Chem. Soc. Perkin Trans. 2* **1975**, 925. Review of chemistry: Z. Janousek, H. G. Viehe, *J. Prakt. Chem. Chem.-Ztg.* **336**, 561-562 (1994); of applications in synthesis of heterocyclic compounds: J. M. Quintela *et al.*, *Recent Res. Dev. Org. Chem.* **2**, 409-418 (1998).

Colorless, hygroscopic solid, fp ~180°.

USE: Chlorinating agent; introduces amide chloride groups into activated substrates. Building block in organic synthesis.

9978. Vigabatrin. [60643-86-9] 4-Amino-5-hexenoic acid; γ-vinyl-γ-aminobutyric acid; gamma-vinyl GABA; γ-vinyl GABA; GVG; MDL-71754; RMI-71754; Sabril. $C_6H_{11}NO_2$; mol wt 129.16. C 55.79%, H 8.58%, N 10.84%, O 24.77%. Irreversible inhibitor of γ-aminobutyric acid transaminase, the enzyme responsible for the degradation of the neurotransmitter γ-aminobutyric acid (GABA). Prepn: B. W. Metcalf, M. Jung, **US 3960927** (1976 to Richardson-Merrell); and *in vitro* enzyme inactivation: B. Lippert *et al.*, *Eur. J. Biochem.* **74**, 441 (1977). Mechanism of action study: P. J. Schechter *et al.*, *Eur. J. Pharmacol.* **45**, 319 (1977). Anticonvulsant activity and toxicity studies: W. Löscher, *Neuropharmacology* **21**, 803 (1982). HPLC determn in plasma and urine: J. A. Smithers *et al.*, *J. Chromatogr.* **341**, 232 (1985). The S(+)-enantiomer is the pharmacologically active form. Pharmacokinetics of enantiomers in humans: K. D. Haegele, P. J. Schechter, *Clin. Pharmacol. Ther.* **40**, 581 (1986). Clinical studies in treatment resistant epilepsy: C. A. Tassinari *et al.*, *Arch. Neurol.* **44**, 907 (1987); T. R. Browne *et al.*, *Neurology* **37**, 184 (1987). Series of articles on clinical use in adult and childhood epilepsy: *J. Child Neurol.* **6**, Suppl. 2, S3-S69 (1991). Reviews of early literature and mechanism of action: M. J. Iadarola, K. Gale, *Mol. Cell. Biochem.* **39**, 305-330 (1981); of pharmacology and toxicology: E. J. Hammond, B. J. Wilder, *Clin. Neuropharmacol.* **8**, 1-12 (1985). *Review:* S. M. Grant, R. C. Heel, *Drugs* **41**, 889-926 (1991).

Crystals from acetone/water, mp 209°. Freely sol in water. LD_{50} i.p. in mice: >2500 mg/kg (Löscher).

THERAP CAT: Anticonvulsant.

9979. Vildagliptin. [274901-16-5] (2*S*)-1-[[(3-Hydroxy-tricyclo[3.3.1.13,7]dec-1-yl)amino]acetyl]-2-pyrrolidinecarbonitrile; 1-[[(3-hydroxy-1-adamantyl) amino]acetyl]-2-cyano-(*S*)-pyrrolidine; LAF-237; NVP-LAF237; Galvus. $C_{17}H_{25}N_3O_2$; mol wt 303.40. C 67.30%, H 8.31%, N 13.85%, O 10.55%. Dipeptidyl peptidase-IV (DPP-IV) inhibitor. Prepn: E. Villhauer, **WO 0034241**; *idem*, **US 6166063** (both 2000 to Novartis); and pharmacology: *idem et al.*, *J. Med. Chem.* **46**, 2774 (2003). Clinical evaluation in type 2 diabetes: B. Ahrén *et al.*, *J. Clin. Endocrinol. Metab.* **89**, 2078 (2004); in combination with metformin: *idem et al.*, *Diabetes Care* **27**, 2874 (2004). Review of development and therapeutic potential: D. Barlocco, *Curr. Opin. Invest. Drugs* **5**, 1094-1100 (2004).

White solid from ethyl acetate, mp 138-140°; from 2-propanol, mp 148-150°. [α] −78.3° (c = 9.73 in methanol).

THERAP CAT: Antidiabetic.

9980. Viloxazine. [46817-91-8] 2-[(2-Ethoxyphenoxy)-methyl]morpholine; 2-(2-ethoxyphenoxymethyl)tetrahydro-1,4-oxazine; ICI-58834. $C_{13}H_{19}NO_3$; mol wt 237.29. C 65.80%, H 8.07%, N 5.90%, O 20.23%. Prepn: K. B. Mallion *et al.*, **GB 1138405**; *idem*, **US 3714161** (1969, 1973 both to I.C.I.). Manufacturing process: S. A. Lee, **GB 1260886**; *idem*, **US 3712890** (1972, 1973 both to I.C.I.). Pharmacology: Mallion *et al.*, *Nature* **238**, 157 (1972); Bereen, *Lancet* **1**, 379 (1973). Toxicity: R. D. Brosnan *et al.*, *J. Int. Med. Res.* **4**, 83 (1976). Clinical evaluation in narcolepsy: C. Guilleminault *et al.*, *Sleep* **9**, 275 (1986). Review of pharmacology and therapeutic efficacy: R. M. Pinder *et al.*, *Drugs* **13**, 401 (1977).

Hydrochloride. [35604-67-2] Vivalan; Vicilan; Vivarint. $C_{13}H_{19}NO_3 \cdot HCl$; mol wt 273.76. mp 185-186°. LD_{50} in mice (mg/kg): 1000 orally, 60 i.v. (Brosnan).

THERAP CAT: Antidepressant.

9981. Viminol. [21363-18-8] α-[[Bis(1-methylpropyl)amino]methyl]-1-[(2-chlorophenyl)methyl]-1*H*-pyrrole-2-methanol; 1-(*o*-chlorobenzyl)-α-[(di-*sec*-butylamino)methyl]pyrrole-2-methanol; 1-[α-(*N*-*o*-chlorobenzyl)pyrryl]-2-di-*sec*-butylaminoethanol; diviminol; Z-424. $C_{21}H_{31}ClN_2O$; mol wt 362.94. C 69.49%, H 8.61%, Cl 9.77%, N 7.72%, O 4.41%. Prepn: U. M. Teotino, D. Della Bella, **ZA 6702732**, *eidem*, **US 3539589** (1970 to Whitefin Holding). Synthesis and metabolic fate of ^{14}C-viminol: Cameron *et al.*, *Arzneim.-Forsch.* **23**, 708 (1973). Viminol possesses 3 asymmetric carbon atoms and thus is composed of 6 stereoisomers. Role

of stereoisomers in determining specific pharmacological effects: D. Della Bella *et al.*, *Nature New Biol.* **241**, 282 (1973). Additional pharmacology data: M. Babbini *et al.*, *Eur. J. Pharmacol.* **23**, 137 (1973). *Review:* D. Della Bella, *Boll. Chim. Farm.* **111**, 5-19 (1972).

$bp_{0.1 mm}$ 160-165°.

p-**Hydroxybenzoate.** [23784-10-3] Dividol. $C_{21}H_{31}ClN_2$-$O.C_7H_6O_3$; mol wt 501.06. mp 128-130° (dec). LD_{50} i.p. in rats: 205.9 mg/kg (Babbini).

THERAP CAT: Analgesic.

9982. Vinblastine. [865-21-4] Vincaleukoblastine; VLB. $C_{46}H_{58}N_4O_9$; mol wt 810.97. C 68.13%, H 7.21%, N 6.91%, O 17.76%. Antitumor alkaloid isolated from periwinkle, *Vinca rosea* Linn., *Apocynaceae*; inhibits microtubule assembly. Identification: R. L. Noble *et al.*, *Ann. N.Y. Acad. Sci.* **76**, 882-894 (1958). Isolation and characterization: M. Gorman *et al.*, *J. Am. Chem. Soc.* **81**, 4745, 4754 (1959); C. T. Beer *et al.*, **US 3097137** (1963 to CPD Ltd.). Structure: N. Neuss *et al.*, *J. Am. Chem. Soc.* **86**, 1440 (1964). ^{13}C-NMR spectral analysis: E. Wenkert *et al.*, *Helv. Chim. Acta* **58**, 1560 (1975). Synthesis from catharanthine and vindoline, *q.q.v.*: P. Mangeney *et al.*, *J. Am. Chem. Soc.* **101**, 2243 (1979); J. P. Kutney *et al.*, *Heterocycles* **27**, 1845 (1988). Enantioselective synthesis: M. E. Kuehne *et al.*, *J. Org. Chem.* **56**, 513 (1991). Toxicology: C. Lu, M. Meistrich, *Cancer Res.* **39**, 3575 (1979). Clinical trial in combination with bleomycin, methotrexate, *q.q.v.* in Hodgkin's disease: P. G. Gobbi *et al.*, *J. Clin. Oncol.* **14**, 527 (1996). Review of pharmacology, toxicology and pharmacokinetics: W. P. Brade, *Beitr. Onkol.* **6**, 95-123 (1981). Comprehensive description: F. J. Muhtadi, A. F. A. Afify, *Anal. Profiles Drug Subs. Excip.* **21**, 611-658 (1992).

Solvated needles from methanol, mp 211-216°. $[\alpha]_D^{23}$ −32° (c = 0.88 in methanol). uv max (ethanol): 214, 259 nm (log ε 4.74, 4.22). pKa_1 5.4; pKa_2 7.4. Practically insol in water, petr ether. Sol in alcohols, acetone, ethyl acetate, $CHCl_3$.

Sulfate. [143-67-9] 29060-LE; Exal; Velban; Velbe. $C_{46}H_{58}$-$N_4O_9 \cdot H_2SO_4$; mol wt 909.05. Crystallizes as hydrate, mp 284-285°. $[\alpha]_D^{26}$ −28° (c = 1.01 in methanol). uv max (methanol): 212, 262, 284, 292 nm (log ε 4.75, 4.28, 4.22, 4.18). Very slightly sol in ethanol. Practically insol in ether. One part is sol in 10 parts of water, 50 parts of chloroform. LD_{50} i.v. in mice: 9.5 mg/kg (Lu, Meistrich).

THERAP CAT: Antineoplastic.

9983. Vincamine. [1617-90-9] (3α,14β,16α)-14,15-Dihydro-14-hydroxyeburnamenine-14-carboxylic acid methyl ester; 13a-ethyl-2,3,5,6,12,13,13a,13b-octahydro-12-hydroxy-1*H*-indolo[3,2,1-*de*]pyrido[3,2,1-*ij*][1,5]naphthyridine-12-carboxylic acid methyl ester; Angiopac; Arteriovinca; Cetal; Oxygeron; Pervincamine; Vincafor; Vincagil; Vincimax; Vraap. $C_{21}H_{26}N_2O_3$; mol wt 354.44. C 71.16%, H 7.39%, N 7.90%, O 13.54%. Major indole alkaloid of *Vinca minor* L., *Apocynaceae* occurring naturally in the *d*-form: E. Schlittler, A. Furlenmeier, *Helv. Chim. Acta* **36**, 2017 (1953); Pailer, Belohlav, *Monatsh. Chem.* **85**, 1055 (1954); King *et al., J. Chem. Soc.* **1955**, 4206; J. Trojanek *et al., Collect. Czech. Chem. Commun.* **26**, 867 (1961). Isoln from *Tabernaemontana rigida* Miers, *Apocynaceae:* M. P. Cava *et al., J. Org. Chem.* **33**, 1055 (1968). Structure: J. Trojanek *et al., Tetrahedron Lett.* **1961**, 702; J. Mokry *et al., ibid.* **1962**, 433; O. Clauder, *ibid.* 1147; Plat *et al., Bull. Soc. Chim. Fr.* **1962**, 1082. Abs config: J. Trojanek *et al., Chem. Ind. (London)* **1965**, 1261; Blaha *et al., Collect. Czech. Chem. Commun.* **33**, 3833 (1968). X-ray determn of molecular structure: H. P. Weber, T. J. Petcher, *J. Chem. Soc. Perkin Trans. 2* **1973**, 2001. Total synthesis: C. Szantay *et al., Tetrahedron Lett.* **1973**, 191; *eidem, Tetrahedron* **33**, 1803 (1977); P. Pfäffli *et al., Helv. Chim. Acta* **58**, 1131 (1975); W. Oppolzer *et al., ibid.* **60**, 1801 (1977); of *dl*-form: M. E. Kuehne, *J. Am. Chem. Soc.* **86**, 2946 (1964); J. L. Herrmann *et al., ibid.* **96**, 3702 (1974); K. H. Gibson, J. E. Saxton, *Tetrahedron* **33**, 833 (1977); K. Irie, Y. Ban, *Heterocycles* **18**, 255 (1982); T. R. Govindachari, S. Rajeswari, *Indian J. Chem.* **22B**, 531 (1983). Synthesis of stereoisomers: J. Warnant *et al.,* **DE 2115718**; *eidem,* **US 3770724** (1971, 1973 both to Roussel-UCLAF); G. Rossey, A. Wick, *J. Org. Chem.* **47**, 4725 (1982). HPLC determn: A. Amato *et al., J. Chromatogr.* **270**, 387 (1983). Toxicity data: L. Szporny, K. Szász, *Arch. Exp. Pathol. Pharmakol.* **236**, 296 (1959). Hypotensive activity in dogs and man: Z. Szabo, Z. Nagy, *Arzneim.-Forsch.* **10**, 811 (1960). Clinical pharmacology: C. C. Lim *et al., Br. J. Clin. Pharmacol.* **9**, 100 (1980). Clinical pharmacokinetics: H. Millart, D. Lamiable *et al., Int. J. Clin. Pharmacol. Ther. Toxicol.* **21**, 581 (1983). Brief review: P. Cook, I. James, *N. Engl. J. Med.* **305**, 1562 (1981).

Yellow crystals from acetone or methanol, mp 232-233°. $[\alpha]_D^{23}$ +41° (in pyridine). uv max: 225, 278 nm (log ε 4.14, 3.61). LD_{50} in mice (mg/kg): 75 i.v.; >1000 s.c. (Szporny, Szász); 1000 orally (Szabo, Nagy).

Hydrochloride. [10592-03-7] Esberidin. $C_{21}H_{26}N_2O_3$·HCl; mol wt 390.90.

(±)-Form. Crystals from methanol, mp 228-229° (Gibson, Saxton).

Note: Other alkaloids found in the "vincamine fraction" of *Vinca minor* L. are: **vincine, vincaminine** and **vincinine**: Holubek *et al., Tetrahedron Lett.* **1963**, 897.

THERAP CAT: Vasodilator.

9984. Vinclozolin. [50471-44-8] 3-(3,5-Dichlorophenyl)-5-ethenyl-5-methyl-2,4-oxazolidinedione; 3-(3,5-dichlorophenyl)-5-methyl-5-vinyloxazolidine-2,4-dione; BAS-352F; Ronilan; Vorlan. $C_{12}H_9Cl_2NO_3$; mol wt 286.11. C 50.38%, H 3.17%, Cl 24.78%, N 4.90%, O 16.78%. Prepn: D. Mangold *et al.,* **DE 2207576** (1973 to BASF), *C.A.* **79**, 137120q (1973). Activity: C. Hess, F. Locher, *Proc. Brit. Insectic. Fungic. Conf.* **2**, 693 (1975). Comparative mechanism of action: A. C. Pappas, D. J. Fisher, *Pestic. Sci.* **10**, 239 (1979).

Crystalline solid, mp 108°. Soly in water at 20°: 1 g/l. Soly in (g/kg): acetone 435; benzene 146; chloroform 319; ethyl acetate

253. Slowly hydrolyzed in alkaline soln. LD_{50} orally in rats: 10 g/kg (Hess, Locher).

Caution: Causes eye and skin irritation; potential skin sensitizer (Mallinckrodt Technical Data Sheet).

USE: Agricultural fungicide.

9985. Vinconate. [70704-03-9] 3-Ethyl-2,3,3a,4-tetrahydro-1*H*-indolo[3,2,1-*de*][1,5]naphthyridine-6-carboxylic acid methyl ester; chanodesethylapovincamine. $C_{18}H_{20}N_2O_2$; mol wt 296.36. C 72.95%, H 6.80%, N 9.45%, O 10.80%. Synthetic hexahydrocanthane alkaloid; vincamine analog. Prepn: **BE 870887**; J. A. A. Hannart, **US 4200638** (1979, 1980 both to Omnium Chim.). Pharmacology: K. Ninomiya *et al., Iyakuhin Kenkyu* **23**, 620 (1992), *C.A.* **118**, 32823 (1992). Pharmacokinetics: M. Kinbara, Y. Satou, *ibid.* 275, *C.A.* **117**, 123938 (1992). Nootropic activity: H. Kinoshita *et al., Res. Commun. Chem. Pathol. Pharmacol.* **84**, 175 (1994). Clinical pharmacology: B. Saletu *et al., Arch. Gerontol. Geriatr.* **3**, 127 (1984). Acute toxicity study: N. Nishimura *et al., Yakuri to Chiryo* **20**, Suppl. 8, S1995 (1992), *C.A.* **118**, 52241 (1992).

mp 120-121°.

Monohydrochloride. [119600-43-0] OC-340; OM-853. $C_{18}H_{20}N_2O_2$·HCl; mol wt 332.82. mp 194-195°. LD_{50} in male, female mice, rats (mg/kg): 947, 699, 2582, 2348 orally; 127, 131, 112, 117 i.v.; 4073, 3446, >6000, >6000 s.c. (Nishimura).

THERAP CAT: Nootropic.

9986. Vincristine. [57-22-7] 22-Oxovincaleukoblastine; leurocristine; VCR; LCR. $C_{46}H_{56}N_4O_{10}$; mol wt 824.96. C 66.97%, H 6.84%, N 6.79%, O 19.39%. Antitumor alkaloid isolated from *Vinca rosea* Linn. (*Catharanthus roseus* G. Don), *Apocynaceae:* Svoboda, *Lloydia* **24**, 173 (1961). Structure: Neuss *et al., J. Am. Chem. Soc.* **86**, 1440 (1964); Moncrief, Lipscomb, *ibid.* **87**, 4963 (1965). Pharmacology: R. H. Adamson *et al., Arch. Int. Pharmacodyn. Ther.* **157**, 299 (1965); S. M. Sieber *et al., Cancer Treat. Rep.* **60**, 127 (1976). Prepn and pharmacology of [³H]vincristine: Owellen, Donigian, *J. Med. Chem.* **15**, 894 (1972). Symposium on vincristine: *Cancer Chemother. Rep.* **52**, 453-535 (1968). Biosynthesis from catharanthine and vindoline, *q.q.v.:* A. Rahman *et al., Tetrahedron Lett.* **1976**, 2351; P. Mangeney *et al., J. Am. Chem. Soc.* **101**, 2243 (1979). Comprehensive description of the sulfate: J. H. Burns, *Anal. Profiles Drug Subs.* **1**, 463-480 (1972); F. J. Muhtadi, A. F. A. Afify, *Anal. Profiles Drug Subs. Excip.* **22**, 517-533 (1993).

Blades from methanol, mp 218-220°. $[\alpha]_D^{25}$ +17°; $[\alpha]_D^{25}$ +26.2° (ethylene chloride). pKa: 5.0, 7.4 in 33% DMF. uv max (ethanol): 220, 255, 296 nm (log a_m 4.65, 4.21, 4.18). LD_{50} i.p. in mice: 5.2 mg/kg (Adamson).

Sulfate. [2068-78-2] Kyocristine; Oncovin; Vincrex. $C_{46}H_{56}$-$N_4O_{10}.H_2SO_4$; mol wt 923.04. Crystals from ethanol. mp 273-281°. One part sol in 2 parts water, in 30 parts chloroform. Slightly sol in ethanol. Practically insol in ether. $[\alpha]_D^{26}$ +8.5° (c = 0.8). uv max (methanol): 218, 252, 285, 293 nm (log ε 4.72, 4.24, 4.18, 4.23).

THERAP CAT: Antineoplastic.

9987. Vindesine. [53643-48-4] 3-(Aminocarbonyl)-O^4-deacetyl-3-de(methoxycarbonyl)vincaleukoblastine; desacetylvinblastine amide; VDS; Compound 112531; NSC-245467. $C_{43}H_{55}$-N_5O_7; mol wt 753.93. C 68.50%, H 7.35%, N 9.29%, O 14.85%. Synthetic deriv of the dimeric *Catharanthus* alkaloid vinblastine, *q.v.* Prepn: G. J. Cullinan, K. Gerzon, **DE 2415980** (1974 to Lilly), *C.A.* **82**, 72191r (1975); *see also* C. J. Burnett *et al., J. Med. Chem.* **21**, 88 (1978). ^{13}C-NMR spectroscopy: D. E. Dorman, J. W. Paschal, *Org. Magn. Reson.* **8**, 413 (1976). Antitumor activity in rodents: M. J. Sweeney *et al., Cancer Res.* **38**, 2886 (1978). Pharmacokinetics: R. J. Owellen *et al., ibid.* **37**, 2603 (1977). Use in acute lymphocytic leukemia of childhood: W. Krivit *et al., Cancer Chemother. Pharmacol.* **2**, 267 (1979). Brief review of preclinical and early clinical data: R. W. Dyke *et al., ibid.* 229. Toxicology: G. C. Todd *et al., Toxicol. Environ. Health* **1**, 843 (1976); R. J. Owellen *et al., Biochem. Pharmacol.* **26**, 1213 (1977).

Crystals from ethanol-methanol, mp 230-232°. $[\alpha]_D^{25}$ +39.4° (c = 1.0 in methanol). uv max (methanol): 214, 266, 288, 296 nm (ε 53400, 17450, 13950, 12500). pKa' (DMF 66%) 5.39, 7.36; (H_2O) 6.04, 7.67.

Sulfate salt. [59917-39-4] LY-099094; Eldisine; Fildesin. C_{43}-$H_{55}N_5O_7.H_2SO_4$; mol wt 852.00. Amorphous solid from ethanol-isopropyl alcohol, mp >250° (solvated form). LD_{50} in mice, rats (mg/kg): 6.3 ± 0.6, 2.0 ± 0.2 i.v. (Todd); in mice: 8.8 ± 2.5 i.p. (Owellen, *Biochem. Pharmacol.*).

THERAP CAT: Antineoplastic.

9988. Vindoline. [2182-14-1] (2β,3β,4β,5α,12β,19α)-4-(Acetyloxy)-6,7-didehydro-3-hydroxy-16-methoxy-1-methyl-aspidospermidine-3-carboxylic acid methyl ester. $C_{25}H_{32}N_2O_6$; mol wt 456.53. C 65.77%, H 7.07%, N 6.14%, O 21.03%. Major alkaloid from the leaves of *Vinca rosea* Linn. (*Catharanthus roseus* G. Don.), *Apocynaceae;* occurs naturally as the (−)-form: Gorman *et al., J. Am. Pharm. Assoc.* **48**, 256 (1959); Svoboda *et al., ibid.* 659; Moza, Trojánek, *Collect. Czech. Chem. Commun.* **28**, 1419 (1963). Structure: Gorman *et al., J. Am. Chem. Soc.* **84**, 1058 (1962); Neuss, *Bull. Soc. Chim. Fr.* **1963**, 1509. Stereochemistry: Moncrief, Lipscomb, *J. Am. Chem. Soc.* **87**, 4963 (1965). Review of chemistry: Neuss *et al., Adv. Chemother.* **1**, 133 (1964). Total synthesis of (±)-vindoline: Ando *et al., J. Am. Chem. Soc.* **97**, 6880 (1975); Y. Ban *et al., Tetrahedron Lett.* **1978**, 151; J. P. Kutney *et al., J. Am. Chem. Soc.* **100**, 4220 (1978). Lacks physiological activity alone but is contained as the pentacyclic moiety in the antineoplastic agents vinblastine and vincristine, *q.q.v.*

Vindoline   R = OCH₃
Demethoxyvindoline   R = H

Needles from acetone + petr ether, mp 164-165°; prisms, mp 174-175°; $[\alpha]_D^{20}$ −18° (chloroform); pKa 5.5 in 66% DMF (Moza, Trojánek). Also reported as crystals, mp 154-155°; $[\alpha]_D^{27}$ +42° (chloroform) (Gorman). uv max (ethanol): 212, 250, 304 nm (log ε 4.49, 3.74, 3.57).

Hydrochloride. $C_{25}H_{32}N_2O_6.HCl$. Crystals from acetone, mp 161-164°.

Demethoxyvindoline. [5231-60-7] Vindorosine; vindolidine. $C_{24}H_{30}N_2O_5$; mol wt 426.51. Structure: Moza, Trojánek, *Collect. Czech. Chem. Commun.* **28**, 1427 (1963). Needles from benzene + petr ether, mp 167°. $[\alpha]_D^{16}$ −31° (chloroform). uv max (methanol): 250, 302 nm (log ε 3.98, 3.52).

9989. Vinflunine. [162652-95-1] (2β,3β,4β,5α,12R,19α)-4-(Acetyloxy)-6,7-didehydro-15-[(2R,4R,6S,8S)-4-(1,1-difluoroethyl)-1,3,4,5,6,7,8,9-octahydro-8-(methoxycarbonyl)-2,6-methano-2H-azecino[4,3-b]indol-8-yl]-3-hydroxy-16-methoxy-1-methylaspidospermidine-3-carboxylic acid methyl ester; 4'-deoxy-20',20'-difluoro-8'-norvincaleukoblastine; 20',20'-difluoro-3',4'-dihydrovinorelbine. $C_{45}H_{54}F_2N_4O_8$; mol wt 816.93. C 66.16%, H 6.66%, F 4.65%, N 6.86%, O 15.67%. Semisynthetic *Vinca* alkaloid with microtubule destabilizing and antiangiogenic activity; derivative of vinorelbine, *q.v.* Prepn: J.-C. Jacquesy *et al.,* **FR 2707988**; *eidem,* **US 5620985** (1995, 1997 both to Pierre Fabre); J. Fahy *et al., J. Am. Chem. Soc.* **119**, 8576 (1997). NMR study of tubulin binding: C. Fabre *et al., Biochem. Pharmacol.* **64**, 733 (2002). Clinical pharmacokinetics and evaluation in solid tumors: J. Bennouna *et al., Ann. Oncol.* **14**, 630 (2003). Clinical evaluation in bladder cancer: S. Culine *et al., Br. J. Cancer* **2006**, 1. Review of clinical development and mechanism of action: A. Kruczynski, B. T. Hill, *Crit. Rev. Oncol. Hematol.* **40**, 159-173 (2001); J. Bennouna *et al. Expert Opin. Invest. Drugs* **14**, 1259-1267 (2005).

Ditartrate. [194468-36-5] Javlor. $C_{45}H_{54}F_2N_4O_8.2C_4H_6O_6$; mol wt 1117.10.

THERAP CAT: Antineoplastic.

9990. Vinorelbine. [71486-22-1] (2β,3β,4β,5α,12R,19α)-4-(Acetyloxy)-6,7-didehydro-15-[(2R,6R,8S)-4-ethyl-1,3,6,7,8,9-hexahydro-8-(methoxycarbonyl)-2,6-methano-2H-azecino[4,3-b]indol-8-yl]-3-hydroxy-16-methoxy-1-methylaspidospermidine-3-carboxylic acid methyl ester; 3',4'-didehydro-4'-deoxy-C'-norvincaleukoblastine; nor-5'-anhydrovinblastine; NVB; KW-2307. $C_{45}H_{54}N_4$-

O_8; mol wt 778.93. C 69.39%, H 6.99%, N 7.19%, O 16.43%. Semi-synthetic *Vinca* alkaloid; structurally related to vinblastine, *q.v.* Prepn: **JP Kokai 80 31096**; N. Langlois *et al., US 4307100* (1980, 1981 both to Agence Nat. Valorisation Recherche); P. Mangeney *et al., Tetrahedron* **35**, 2175 (1979). Pharmacology: G. Mathé, P. Reizenstein, *Cancer Lett.* **27**, 285 (1985). HPLC determn in biological fluids: F. Jehl *et al., J. Chromatogr.* **525**, 225 (1990). Veterinary trial in dogs with spontaneous neoplasia: V. J. Poirier *et al., J. Vet. Intern. Med.* **18**, 536 (2004). Symposium: *Semin. Oncol.* **16**, Suppl. 4, 1-45 (1989). Review of early clinical development: M. Marty *et al., Nouv. Rev. Fr. Hematol.* **31**, 77-84 (1989); of clinical pharmacokinetics: D. Leveque, F. Jehl, *Clin. Pharmacokinet.* **31**, 184-197 (1996); of use in advanced non-small cell lung cancer: M. P. Curran, G. L. Plosker, *Drugs Aging* **19**, 695-721 (2002).

Residue. $[\alpha]_D^{20}$ +52.4° (c = 0.3 in $CHCl_3$). uv max (ethanol): 215, 268, 282, 293, 310 nm (ε 3700, 11000, 9500, 7600, 4400). Partition coefficient (octanol/buffer pH 7.2): 16. LD_{50} in mice (mg/m^2): 72 i.v.; 78 orally (Mathé, Reizenstein).

Ditartrate. [125317-39-7] Eunades; Navelbine. $C_{45}H_{54}N_4$-$O_8.2C_4H_6O_6$; mol wt 1079.11. Yellow-white amorphous powder. Sol in water and ethanol.

THERAP CAT: Antineoplastic.

THERAP CAT (VET): Antineoplastic.

9991. Vinpocetine. [42971-09-5] ($3\alpha,16\alpha$)-Eburnamenine-14-carboxylic acid ethyl ester; $3\alpha,16\alpha$-apovincaminic acid ethyl ester; ethyl apovincamin-22-oate; RGH-4405; Cavinton. $C_{22}H_{26}$-N_2O_2; mol wt 350.45. C 75.40%, H 7.48%, N 7.99%, O 9.13%. Deriv of vincamine, *q.v.*, with vasodilating activity. Prepn: C. Lörincz *et al., DE 2253750; eidem, US 4035370* (1973, 1977 both to Gedeon Richter); *eidem, Arzneim.-Forsch.* **26**, 1907 (1976). Series of articles on pharmacology, biochemistry, metabolism, pharmacokinetics, clinical studies: *ibid.* 1908-1989. Toxicity studies: E. Pálosi, L. Szporny, *ibid.* 1926; E. Cholnoky, L. I. Dömök, *ibid.* 1939. HPLC studies: G. Szepesi, M. Gazdag, *J. Chromatogr.* **205**, 57, 341 (1981). Evaluation of effectiveness as antimotion drug: E. I. Matsnev, D. Bodo, *Aviat. Space Environ. Med.* **55**, 281 (1984). One-pot synthesis from vincamine: Y. Kuge *et al., Synth. Commun.* **24**, 759 (1994).

Crystals from benzene, mp 147-153° (dec). $[\alpha]_D^{20}$ +114° (c = 1 in pyridine). uv max (96% ethanol): 229, 275, 315 nm (log ε 4.45, 4.08, 3.85). LD_{50} in mice, rats (mg/kg): 534, 503 orally; 240, 133.8 i.p.; 58.7, 42.6 i.v. (Pálosi, Szporny), also reported as 161.2 mg/kg i.p. in mice (Cholnoky, Dömök).

THERAP CAT: Vasodilator (cerebral).

9992. Vinyl Acetate. [108-05-4] Acetic acid ethenyl ester; acetic acid vinyl ester. $C_4H_6O_2$; mol wt 86.09. C 55.81%, H 7.02%, O 37.17%. $CH_3COOCH=CH_2$. Prepn: Schnizer, *US 2859241* (1958 to Celanese); Sharp, Steitz, *US 2860159* (1958 to Pan Am. Petroleum); Foster, Tobler, *J. Am. Chem. Soc.* **83**, 851 (1961). Toxicity data: Smyth, Carpenter, *J. Ind. Hyg. Toxicol.* **30**, 63 (1948). Study of chronic human exposure: Deese, Joyner, *Am. Ind. Hyg. Assoc. J.* **30**, 449 (1969). *Reviews:* Leonard "Vinyl Acetate" in *Vinyl and Diene Monomers* (part 1), E. C. Leonard, Ed. (Wiley-Interscience, New York, 1970) pp 263-328; *Faith, Keyes & Clark's Industrial Chemicals*, F. A. Lowenheim, M. K. Moran, Eds (Wiley-Interscience, New York, 4th ed., 1975) pp 862-867; W. Daniels, "Poly(Vinyl Acetate)" in *Kirk-Othmer Encyclopedia of Chemical Technology* vol. 23 (Wiley-Interscience, New York, 3rd ed., 1983) pp 817-847. Review of toxicology and human exposure: *Toxicological Profile for Vinyl Acetate* (PB93-110898, 1992) 166 pp.

Liquid; sweet, fruity odor. Polymerizes in light to a colorless, transparent mass. bp 72.7°. mp −100°; also reported as mp −93° (Daniels). d_4^{20} 0.932. *Flammable.* Flash pt, closed cup: 18°F (−8°C). Soly in water (20°): 1 g/50 ml. Misc with alc, ether. Sol in acetone, benzene, chloroform. LD_{50} orally in rats: 2.92 g/kg (Smyth, Carpenter).

Caution: Potential symptoms of overexposure are irritation of eyes, skin, nose, throat; hoarseness, cough; loss of smell; eye burns, skin blisters. *See NIOSH Pocket Guide to Chemical Hazards* (DHHS/NIOSH 97-140, 1997) p 328.

USE: In polymerized form for plastic masses, films and lacquers; in plastic film for food packaging. As modifier for food starch.

9993. Vinylbital. [2430-49-1] 5-Ethenyl-5-(1-methylbutyl)-2,4,6(1H,3H,5H)-pyrimidinetrione; 5-(1-methylbutyl)-5-vinylbarbituric acid; 5-vinyl-5-(1-methylbutyl)barbituric acid; butyvinal; Speda; Optanox. $C_{11}H_{16}N_2O_3$; mol wt 224.26. C 58.91%, H 7.19%, N 12.49%, O 21.40%. Prepn: Seefelder, *Festschr. Carl Wurster* 1960, 71, *C.A.* **56**, 9928d (1962). Mechanism of action study: U. J. Jovanovic, *Arzneim.-Forsch.* **17**, 1369 (1967). Pharmacokinetics: D. D. Breimer, A. G. de Boer, *ibid.* **26**, 448 (1976). GC-MS screening method in urine: H. H. Maurer, *J. Chromatogr.* **530**, 307 (1990).

Crystals, mp 90-91.5°.

Note: This is a controlled substance (depressant): **21 CFR,** 1308.13.

THERAP CAT: Sedative, hypnotic.

9994. Vinyl Chloride. [75-01-4] Chloroethylene. C_2H_3Cl; mol wt 62.50. C 38.43%, H 4.84%, Cl 56.72%. $CH_2=CHCl$. Prepd from ethylene dichloride and alcoholic potassium: Regnault, *Ann.* **14**, 22 (1835); by halogenation of ethylene: Miller, Jenks, *US 2896000* (1959 to National Distillers and Chemical Corp.). Review of mfg processes: *Faith, Keyes & Clark's Industrial Chemicals*, F. A. Lowenheim, M. K. Moran, Eds. (Wiley-Interscience, New York, 4th ed., 1975) pp 868-873. Acute toxicity study: L. Prodan *et al., Ann. N.Y. Acad. Sci.* **246**, 154 (1975). Series of articles on toxicology and "vinyl chloride disease": *ibid.* 1-337. *Review:* in *Kirk-Othmer Encyclopedia of Chemical Technology* vol. 12 (John Wiley & Sons, 3rd ed., 1983) pp 865-885. Review of carcinogenic risk: *IARC Monographs* **19**, 377-437 (1979); of toxicology and human exposure: *Toxicological Profile for Vinyl Chloride* (PB98-101132, 1997) 277 pp.

Colorless gas; mild, sweet odor. Liquefies in a freezing mixture. Polymerizes in light or in presence of catalyst. mp −153.8°. bp −13.37°. d_4^{20} 0.9106. n_D^{20} 1.3700. Vapor pressure at 20°: 2530 mm Hg. *Flammable.* Flash pt, closed cup: −78°C (−112°F). Sol in alc, ether, carbon tetrachloride, benzene. Slightly sol in water. LD_{50} in mice, rats, guinea pigs, rabbits (mg/l): 293.75, 390, 595, 295 by inhalation (Prodan).

Caution: Potential symptoms of overexposure are weakness; abdominal pain, GI bleeding; hepatomegaly; pallor or cyanosis of extremities; direct contact with liquid may cause frostbite. *See NIOSH Pocket Guide to Chemical Hazards* (DHHS/NIOSH 97-140, 1997) p 330. *See also Patty's Industrial Hygiene and Toxicology* vol. **2E**, G. D. Clayton, F. E. Clayton, Eds. (John Wiley & Sons, Inc., New York, 4th ed., 1994) pp 4169-4177. This substance is listed as a known human carcinogen: *Report on Carcinogens, Eleventh Edition* (PB2005-104914, 2004) p III-272.

USE: In the plastics industry to manuf polyvinyl chloride; in organic syntheses. Has been used as refrigerant, spray can propellant.

9995. Vinyl Ether. [109-93-3] 1,1'-Oxybisethene; divinyl ether; divinyl oxide; ethenyloxyethene; Vinethene; Vinesthene. C_4-H_6O; mol wt 70.09. C 68.54%, H 8.63%, O 22.83%. $CH_2 = CHOCH = CH_2$. Prepn: Major, Ruigh, US 2021872 (1935 to Merck & Co.); Mittag, Smidt, US 2832807 (1958 to Consortium für electrochem. Ind. GmbH). Toxicity data: Molitar, *J. Pharmacol. Exp. Ther.* **57**, 274 (1936).

Very volatile, flammable liq; characteristic odor. Dec on exposure to light or to acid fumes, forming acetaldehyde, and polymerizes to a solid glass-like mass. d_{20}^{20} 0.774; d_4^{20} 0.773. bp 28.4°. n_D^{20} 1.3989. Crit temp 183° (calc). Critical press. ~30 atm. Specific heat ~0.53 cal/g. Explosives limits (% by vol in air), lower: 1.7, upper: 27.0. Autoignition temp 360° (680°F). 0.53 g dissolves in 100 g water at 37°. Oil-water soly coefficient at 37°: 41. Miscible with alcohol, ether, oils and other organic solvents. Pharmaceutical product contains not less than 96.0% and not more than 97.0% vinyl ether, the remainder consisting of dehydrated alcohol. *Keep protected from light and acid fumes, in a cool place, and away from an open flame.* LC$_{50}$ (3 hr in air) in mice, rats (mg/l): 146.8, 386.5 (Molitor).

THERAP CAT: Anesthetic (inhalation).

9996. Vinylidene Chloride. [75-35-4] 1,1-Dichloroethene; 1,1-dichloroethylene; *asym*-dichloroethylene. $C_2H_2Cl_2$; mol wt 96.94. C 24.78%, H 2.08%, Cl 73.14%. $CH_2 = CCl_2$. Prepn from ethylene chloride: Reilly, US 2140548 (1938 to Dow); by dehydrochlorination of 1,1,2-trichloroethane: Conrad, Gould, US 2989570 (1961 to Ethyl Corp.). Review of production, properties and uses: D. S. Gibbs *et al.* in *Kirk-Othmer Encyclopedia of Chemical Technology* vol. **23** (Wiley-Interscience, New York, 3rd ed., 1982) pp 764-798; of toxicology and human exposure: *Toxicological Profile for 1,1-Dichloroethene* (PB 95-100152, 1994) 200 pp.

Liquid. Mild, sweet odor resembling that of chloroform. d_4^{20} 1.2129. mp −122.5°. bp$_{760}$ 31.7°. n_D^{20} 1.4249. Practically insol in water. Sol in organic solvents. At temps >0° and especially in the presence of oxygen or other suitable catalysts polymerizes to a plastic. Several inhibitors to preserve the monomer have been invented. Uncontrolled polymerization may lead to explosive reaction products with oxygen or ozone: Reinhardt, *Chem. Eng. News* **25**, 2136 (1947).

Caution: Potential symptoms of overexposure are irritation of eyes, skin, throat; dizziness, headache, nausea; dyspnea; liver and kidney dysfunction; pneumonitis. Potential occupational carcinogen. *See NIOSH Pocket Guide to Chemical Hazards* (DHHS/-NIOSH 97-140, 1997) p 332; *Patty's Industrial Hygiene and Toxicology* vol. **2E**, G. D. Clayton, F. E. Clayton, Eds. (John Wiley & Sons, Inc., New York, 4th ed., 1994) pp 4181-4189.

USE: Intermediate in the production of "vinylidene polymer plastics" such as **Saran**.

9997. Violacein. [548-54-9] (*E*)-3-[1,2-Dihydro-5-(5-hydroxy-1*H*-indol-3-yl)-2-oxo-3*H*-pyrrol-3-ylidene]-1,3-dihydro-2*H*-indol-2-one; 3-[2-(5-hydroxyindol-3-yl)-5-oxo-2-pyrrolin-4-ylidene]-2-indolinone; 3-[2-(5-hydroxyindol-3-yl)-5-oxo-4-pyrrolin-4-ylidene]oxindole; 5-(5-hydroxy-3-indolyl)-3-(3-oxindolylidene)-2-oxopyrroline. $C_{20}H_{13}N_3O_3$; mol wt 343.34. C 69.96%, H 3.82%, N 12.24%, O 13.98%. Pigment isolated from *Chromobacterium violaceum* (*Bacillus violaceus*): Tobie, *J. Bacteriol.* **29**, 223 (1935); Strong, *Science* **100**, 287 (1944); Ballantine *et al.*, *J. Chem. Soc.* **1958**, 755. Structure and synthesis: Ballantine *et al.*, *ibid.* **1960**, 2292. *Review:* DeMoss in *Antibiotics* vol. 2, D. Gottlieb, P. D. Shaw, Eds. (Springer, New York, 1967).

Purplish-black needles, prisms. Practically insol in water; slightly sol in alcohol; moderately sol in dioxane.

9998. Violaxanthin. [126-29-4] 5,6:5',6'-Diepoxy-5,5',6,6'-tetrahydro-β,β-carotene-3,3'-diol; zeaxanthin diepoxide. $C_{40}H_{56}$-O_4; mol wt 600.87. C 79.96%, H 9.39%, O 10.65%. Widely distributed carotenoid pigment. Formed in plants from zeaxanthin. Isoln from yellow pansies (*Viola tricolor*): Kuhn, Winterstein, *Ber.* **64**, 326 (1931). Structure: Karrer *et al.*, *Helv. Chim. Acta* **14**, 1044 (1931); **16**, 977 (1933); **19**, 1024 (1936); **27**, 1684 (1944). Partial synthesis: Karrer, Jucker, *ibid.* **28**, 300 (1945). Abs config: Bartlett *et al.*, *J. Chem. Soc. C* **1969**, 2527. Isoln from *Viola tricolor* and configuration of the 15-*cis*-isomer: P. Molnar, J. Szabolcs, *Phytochemistry* **19**, 623 (1980).

Orange prisms from methanol, reddish-brown acicular crystals from CS_2. mp 200°. $[\alpha]_{Cd}^{20}$ +35° (c = 0.08 in chloroform). Absorption max (in alc): 471.5, 442.5, 417.5 nm. Sol in alcohol, methanol, carbon disulfide. ether; almost insol in petr ether.

15-*cis*-Isomer. Irregular yellow plates from benzene/petrol, mp 109°. uv max (benzene): 479, 448, 423, 337 nm (log ε 4.91, 4.98, 4.83, 4.77). Friction causes crystals to form orange prisms.

9999. Viologen. A term coined by Michaelis to designate the chlorides of certain quaternary bases derived from γ,γ'-dipyridyl. Presently used as dichlorides, dibromides and diiodides. Prepn: Michaelis, *Biochem. Z.* **250**, 564 (1932); Michaelis, Hill, *J. Am. Chem. Soc.* **55**, 1481 (1933); *J. Gen. Physiol.* **16**, 859-873 (1933). Viologens are useful as oxidation-reduction indicators when their potential range is very negative. In contrast to other redox indicators, the color is exhibited by the reduced form, whereas usually the oxidized form is the colored one and secondly, the redox potential of these substances is independent of pH. Review of electrochemistry: C. L. Bird, A. T. Kuhn, *Chem. Soc. Rev.* **10**, 49-82 (1981).

Ethyl viologen. 1,1'-Diethyl-4,4'-bipyridinium; *N,N*'-diethyl-γ,γ'-dipyridylium. Normal potential at 30°: −0.449 volts.

Benzyl viologen. 1,1'-Bis(phenylmethyl)-4,4'-bipyridinium; *N,N*'-dibenzyl-γ,γ'-dipyridylium. Normal potential at 30°: −0.359 volts.

Betaine viologen. *N,N*'-Dibetaine-γ,γ'-dipyridylium. Normal potential at 30°: −0.444 volts.

Dimethyl analog see Paraquat.

USE: As biological oxidation-reduction indicators.

10000. Violuric Acid. [87-39-8] 2,4,5,6(1*H*,3*H*)-Pyrimidine-tetrone 5-oxime; alloxan 5-oxime; 5-isonitrosobarbituric acid; 5-(hydroxyimino)barbituric acid. $C_4H_3N_3O_4$; mol wt 157.08. C 30.58%, H 1.93%, N 26.75%, O 40.74%. Known to exist as a mixture of keto-enol tautomers. Prepd from alloxan and hydroxylamine: Cresole, *Ber.* **16**, 1133 (1883); Guinchard, *Ber.* **32**, 1723 (1899).

Orthorhombic crystals, dec 240-241°. pK 4.7. Sparingly sol in water to a violet-colored soln; sol in alcohol. With $FeCl_3$ produces blue color.

USE: Analytical reagent for chromatographic separation of cations. Forms chelates: Leermakers, Hoffman, *J. Am. Chem. Soc.* **80**, 5663 (1958).

10001. Viomycin. [32988-50-4] Celiomycin; florimycin; tuberactinomycin B. $C_{25}H_{43}N_{13}O_{10}$; mol wt 685.69. C 43.79%, H 6.32%, N 26.56%, O 23.33%. Polypeptide antibiotic produced by various *Streptomyces* species including *S. puniceus, S. floridae, S. vinaceus.* Isoln: A. C. Finlay *et al., Am. Rev. Tuberc.* **63**, 1 (1951); Bartz *et al., ibid.* 4. Production: Marsh *et al.,* US 2633445 (1953 to Ciba); Freaney, US 2828245 (1958 to C.S.C.). Purification and chemical characterization: T. Kitagawa *et al., Chem. Pharm. Bull.* **20**, 2176 (1972). Proposed structure: Yoshioka *et al., Tetrahedron Lett.* **1971**, 2043. Alternate structure: B. W. Bycroft *et al., ibid.* **1968**, 5901; *eidem, Experientia* **27**, 501 (1971); *eidem, J. Chem. Soc. Perkin Trans. 1* **1972**, 820, 827. Confirmed structure: Noda *et al., J. Antibiot.* **25**, 427 (1972); T. Kitagawa *et al., Chem. Pharm. Bull.* **20**, 2215 (1972). X-ray crystallography: B. W. Bycroft, *Chem. Commun.* **1972**, 660. Biosynthesis: J. H. Carter II *et al., Biochemistry* **13**, 1221, 1227 (1974). Toxicological study: H. Keller *et al., Arzneim.-Forsch.* **6**, 61 (1956). Enzyme immunoassay for determn in body fluids: T. Kitagawa *et al., Chem. Pharm. Bull.* **30**, 2487 (1982).

Sulfate. [37883-00-4] Viocin. Hygroscopic plates, mp 266° (dec). $[\alpha]_D^{18}$ $-29.5°$ (c = 1 in H_2O). uv max (water or 0.1N HCl; 0.1N NaOH): 268 nm (log ε 4.4); 285 nm (log ε 4.2). LD_{50} in mice (mg/kg): 240 i.v. (Finlay); 1750 s.c. (Keller). Sol in water. Relatively insol in most organic solvents. Solns adjusted to pH 5-6 are quite stable. Soly data: Weiss *et al., Antibiot. Chemother.* **7**, 374 (1957).

Pantothenate sulfate. [1401-79-2] $C_{25}H_{43}N_{13}O_{10}.C_9H_{17}$-$NO_5.H_2SO_4$; mol wt 1003.00. Prepn: H. Keller, H. Mückter, DE 1011800 (1957 to Grünenthal), *C.A.* **53**, 13519c (1959). Crystals, mp 242° (dec).

Hydrochloride. Hygroscopic plates, mp 270° (dec). $[\alpha]_D^{18}$ $-16.6°$ (c = 1 in H_2O). uv max (water; 0.1N HCl; 0.1N NaOH): 268 nm (log ε 4.5); 268 nm (log ε 4.4); 285 nm (log ε 4.3).

THERAP CAT: Antibacterial (tuberculostatic).

10002. VIP. [37221-79-7] Vasoactive intestinal polypeptide; vasoactive intestinal peptide. Neuroactive polypeptide gastrointestinal hormone, related to glucagon and secretin, *q.q.v.* It exhibits a wide variety of biological activities, including relaxation of systemic and vascular smooth muscle and stimulation of the exocrine pancreas, of secretion of insulin and of cyclic-AMP formation in the small intestine. Initially isolated from porcine upper intestinal wall: S. I. Said, V. Mutt, *Science* **169**, 1217 (1970); *eidem, Eur. J. Biochem.* **28**, 199 (1972). Porcine VIP is a 28-residue peptide having an N-terminal seryl sequence: M. Bodanszky *et al., Proc. Natl. Acad. Sci. USA* **70**, 382 (1973); V. Mutt, S. I. Said, *Eur. J. Biochem.* **42**, 581 (1974). Synthesis: M. Bodanszky *et al., J. Am. Chem. Soc.* **96**, 4973 (1974); *see also* S. I. Said *et al.,* US 3862927 (1975). Solid-phase synthesis: D. H. Coy, J. Gardner, *Int. J. Pept. Protein Res.* **15**, 73 (1980); R. Colombo, *Experientia* **38**, 773 (1982). Isoln of chicken VIP: A. Nilsson, *FEBS Lett.* **47**, 284 (1974). Amino acid sequence: *idem, ibid.* **60**, 322 (1975). Synthesis of C-terminal fragment: M. Bodanszky *et al., Bioorg. Chem.* **5**, 339 (1976).

Solid-phase synthesis: R. Colombo, *Int. J. Pept. Protein Res.* **19**, 71 (1982). Multiple immunoreactive forms of VIP have also been found in human colonic mucosa: R. Dimaline, G. J. Dockray, *Gastroenterology* **75**, 387 (1978). The presence of a common form of VIP in brain and gastrointestinal tract has been demonstrated by radioimmunoassay and radioreceptor assay: J. Besson *et al., Acta Endocrinol.* **87**, 799 (1978). Although the precise effect of VIP on neuronal function is not completely known, it is believed to play an important role in neurotransmission, *cf.* M. G. Bryant *et al., Lancet* **1**, 991 (1976); Y. Matsuzaki *et al., Science* **210**, 1252 (1980). Review of possible functions as a neural peptide: S. I. Said *et al., Adv. Biochem. Psychopharmacol.* **22**, 75-82 (1980). Book: *Vasoactive Intestinal Peptide,* S. I. Said, Ed. (Raven Press, New York, 1982) 528 pp.

His–Ser–Asp–Ala–Val–Phe–Thr–Asp–Asn–Tyr–Thr–Arg–Leu–Arg

Asn–Leu–Ile–Ser–Asn–Leu–Tyr–Lys–Lys–Val–Ala–Met–Gln–Lys

Porcine VIP

10003. Viquidil. [84-55-9] (3*R-cis*)-3-(3-Ethenyl-4-piperidinyl)-1-(6-methoxy-4-quinolinyl)-1-propanone; quinicine; 1-(6-methoxy-4-quinolyl)-3-(3-vinyl-4-piperidyl)-1-propanone; chinicine; mequiverine; quinotoxine; quinotoxol; LM-192. $C_{20}H_{24}N_2$-O_2; mol wt 324.42. C 74.04%, H 7.46%, N 8.63%, O 9.86%. An isomer of quinine; occurs naturally as the *d*-form. Present in small quantities in cinchona barks; formed by heating quinine with glycerol at 180°: Howard, *J. Chem. Soc.* **24**, 61 (1871); **25**, 101 (1872); Miller, Rohde, *Ber.* **33**, 3214 (1900); Howard, Chick, *Pharm. J.* **99**, 143 (1917). Conversion to quinine: Rabe, Kindler, *Ber.* **51**, 466 (1918). Partial synthesis: Prostenik, Prelog, *Helv. Chim. Acta* **26**, 1965 (1943). Total synthesis: Woodward, Doering, *J. Am. Chem. Soc.* **66**, 849 (1944); **67**, 860 (1945); US 2500444 (1950 to Polaroid); Grethe *et al., Helv. Chim. Acta* **56**, 1485 (1973). Review of synthesis, chemistry and pharmacology: Quevauviller *et al., Ann. Pharm. Fr.* **24**, 39 (1966). Series of articles on pharmacology and metabolism: *Arzneim.-Forsch.* **22**, 1334-1346 (1972).

Yellow viscous oil, $[\alpha]_D$ +43°. Slightly sol in water; freely sol in alcohol, chloroform, ether.

Hydrochloride. [52211-63-9] Desclidium; Permiran. $C_{20}H_{24}$-$N_2O_2.HCl$; mol wt 360.88. Yellow, odorless and bitter tasting powder, mp 184 ±4°. uv max (chloroform): 246, 355 nm. Sol in alc; sparingly sol in water. Practically insol in acetone.

THERAP CAT: Vasodilator (cerebral).

10004. Virginiamycin. [11006-76-1] Staphylomycin; virgimycin; SKF-7988; Eskalin; Stafac; Staphylomycine. One of the streptogramins, *q.v.*, produced by a *Streptomyces virginiae*: P. De Somer, P. Van Dijck, *Antibiot. Chemother.* **5**, 632 (1955). Two principal components S_1 and M_1. Separation of factors M and S: H. Vanderhaeghe *et al., ibid.* **7**, 606 (1957); of the complex into six components: Gosselinckx, Parmentier, *Chromatogr. Symp., 2nd* **1962**, 1817. Nomenclature and identification with other streptogramins: P. Crooy, R. De Neys, *J. Antibiot.* **25**, 371 (1972). HPLC determn in animal feeds: F. Gossele *et al., Analyst* **116**, 1373 (1991). Quantitative determn of components from fermentation broth: B. V. Tyaglov *et al., J. Planar Chromatogr. Mod. TLC* **8**, 374 (1995). Mode of action: B. T. Porse, R. A. Garrett, *J. Mol. Biol.* **286**, 375 (1999). *Review:* A. M. Biot, *Drugs Pharm. Sci.* **22**, 695-720 (1984). Review of use in feed: W. Witte *et al., Acta Vet. Scand. Suppl.* **93**, 37-45 (2000).

Virginiamycin S₁

Virginiamycin M₁

Amorphous, reddish-yellow powder, mp 115-120°. Sol in methanol, ethanol, chloroform. Poorly sol in water. Practically insol in hexane and petroleum ether.

Virginiamycin S₁. [23152-29-6] Staphylomycin S. $C_{43}H_{49}$-N_7O_{10}; mol wt 823.89. C 62.69%, H 5.99%, N 11.90%, O 19.42%. Hexacyclicdepsipeptide antibiotic. Structure: H. Vanderhaeghe, G. Parmentier, *J. Am. Chem. Soc.* **82**, 4414 (1960). Crystals from methanol, mp 240-242°. $[\alpha]_D^{20}$ −28° (c = 1 in ethanol). uv max (ethanol): 305 nm (log ε 3.85).

Virginiamycin M₁. [21411-53-0] Mikamycin A; ostreogrycin A; pristinamycin II$_A$; staphylomycin M₁; streptogramin A; vernamycin A. $C_{28}H_{35}N_3O_7$; mol wt 525.59. C 63.99%, H 6.71%, N 7.99%, O 21.31%. Macrolactone antibiotic, *see also* Pristinamycin. Structure: G. R. Delpierre *et al., Tetrahedron Lett.* **1966**, 369; *eidem, J. Chem. Soc. C* **1966**, 1653; D. G. I. Kingston *et al., ibid.* 1669. Biosynthesis: *idem et al., Rev. Latinoam. Quim.* **20**, 128 (1989). Molecular dynamics: E. Surcouf *et al., Stud. Phys. Theor. Chem.* **71**, 719 (1990). Colorless laths from ethyl acetate, mp 203-205°. $[\alpha]_D^{20}$ −218° (c = 0.34 in ethanol). uv max (ethanol): 228 nm (log ε 4.51).

THERAP CAT: Antibacterial.

THERAP CAT (VET): Antibacterial; growth promotant.

10005. Viridicatin. [129-24-8] 3-Hydroxy-4-phenyl-2(1*H*)-quinolinone; 3-hydroxy-4-phenylcarbostyril; 2,3-dihydroxy-4-phenylquinoline. $C_{15}H_{11}NO_2$; mol wt 237.25. C 75.94%, H 4.67%, N 5.90%, O 13.49%. Antibiotic substance from the mycelium of *Penicillium viridicatum* Westling, the chief mold on stored corn: Cunningham, Freeman, *Biochem. J.* **53**, 328 (1953); from various strains of *P. cyclopium* Westling: Bracken *et al., ibid.* **57**, 587 (1954); from *P. puberulum* Bainier, Austin, Meyers, *J. Chem. Soc.* **1964**, 1197. Biosynthesis: Luckner, *Tetrahedron Lett.* **1962**, 1035; Luckner, Mothes, *Arch. Pharm.* **296**, 18 (1963); Framm *et al., Eur. J. Biochem.* **37**, 78 (1973). Synthesis: Eistert, Selzer, *Z. Naturforsch.* **17b**, 202 (1962). Mass spectra: Luckner *et al., Tetrahedron* **25**, 2575 (1969). Antibacterial activity and inhibitory effect on plant growth: Taniguchi, Satomura, *Agric. Biol. Chem.* **34**, 506 (1970).

Lustrous needles from methanol or ethanol, mp 268°. Sublimes unchanged in high vacuum at 160-170°. Very weak acid. uv and ir curves: Cunningham, Freeman, *loc. cit.* Practically insol in water,

aq $NaHCO_3$. Sparingly sol in cold organic solvents, cold concd HCl, dil mineral acids; sol in cold, aq 2*N* KOH, glacial acetic acid.

Sodium salt. $C_{15}H_{10}NNaO_2$. Prismatic needles from aq NaOH, dec 260-265°. Sol in water.

Monoacetylviridicatin. $C_{17}H_{13}NO_3$. Crystals from aq ethanol, mp 200-201°. Dec slowly on standing.

O,O-**Dimethylviridicatin.** $C_{17}H_{15}NO_2$. Plates from ethanol, mp 86-87°.

O,N-**Dimethylviridicatin.** $C_{17}H_{15}NO_2$. Plates from ethanol, mp 197-198°.

10006. Viridin. [3306-52-3] 1β-Hydroxy-2β-methoxy-18-norandrosta-5,8,11,13-tetraeno[6,5,4-*bc*]furan-3,7,17-trione. C_{20}-$H_{16}O_6$; mol wt 352.34. C 68.18%, H 4.58%, O 27.25%. Antibiotic substance from *Gliocladium virens*: Grove *et al., J. Chem. Soc.* **1965**, 3803. Previously reported isolation from *Trichoderma viride*: Brian, McGowan, *Nature* **156**, 144 (1945); Brian *et al., Ann. Appl. Biol.* **33**, 190 (1946). Epimerizes to β-viridin where methoxyl group is equatorial. Separation of the two isomers: Vischer *et al., Nature* **165**, 528 (1950). Structure: Grove *et al., Chem. Commun.* **1965**, 343. Configuration: *eidem, J. Chem. Soc. C* **1966**, 743; Neidle, Hursthouse, *J. Chem. Soc. Perkin Trans.* 2 **1972**, 760. Biosynthesis: Blight *et al., Chem. Commun.* **1968**, 1117; Grove, *J. Chem. Soc. C* **1969**, 549.

Prisms from benzene, mp 245° (dec). $[\alpha]_D^{19}$ −224°. uv max: 242, 300 nm (log ε 4.49, 4.22). Needles from acetone, mp 222-224° (dec). Prisms from glacial acetic acid, mp 200-205° (dec). Sol in water, chloroform; sparingly sol in carbon disulfide, carbon tetrachloride. Practically insol in ether, camphor. Aq solns lose activity rapidly unless acidified to pH 3.

β-Isomer. Prisms from benzene, mp 240-245° (dec). $[\alpha]_D^{16}$ −23°. uv max: 243, 300 nm (log ε 4.45, 4.25).

THERAP CAT: Antifungal.

10007. Virulizin®. [216586-46-8] Virulizin-2γ. Biological response modifier extracted from bovine bile. Prepn: R. Rang, **WO 9507089** (1995 to Imutec); *idem, US 6551623* (2003 to Lorus). *In vivo* antitumor activity: N. Feng *et al., Cancer Chemother. Pharmacol.* **51**, 247 (2003). Clinical evaluation in pancreatic cancer: E. Warner *et al., Clin. Invest. Med.* **17**, 37 (1994). Mechanism of action studies: M. Y. Cao *et al., Cancer Immunol. Immunother.* **54**, 229 (2005); H. Li *et al., ibid.* 1115. Review of pharmacology and therapeutic potential: E. S. Ferdinandi *et al., Expert Opin. Invest. Drugs* **8**, 1721-1735 (1999).

Aqueous soln containing 5% (w/v) solid material comprised of a mixture of inorganic salts (95-99% dry wt) and organic compds of mol wts <3000 Da (1-5% dry wt).

THERAP CAT: Immunomodulator.

10008. Viscose. A viscous orange-red aq soln of sodium cellulose xanthogenate obtained by dissolving wood pulp cellulose in sodium hydroxide soln and treating with carbon disulfide. Manuf: Bachlott, **US 2855321** (1958 to du Pont); Von Kohorn, **US 2985647** (1961).

USE: Intermediate in the manuf of rayon and cellophane.

10009. Viscosin. [27127-62-4] $C_{54}H_{95}N_9O_{16}$; mol wt 1126.38. C 57.58%, H 8.50%, N 11.19%, O 22.73%. Antibiotic substance produced by *Pseudomonas viscosa.* Isoln: Kochi *et al., Bact. Proc.* **1951,** 29; Groupé *et al., Proc. Soc. Exp. Biol. Med.* **78,** 354 (1951); Ohno *et al., J. Agric. Chem. Soc. Jpn.* **27,** 665 (1953); *C.A.* **49,** 3012 (1955); Toki, Ohno, *C.A.* **53,** 243b (1959). Synthesis studies: Fukuda, Bani, *C.A.* **56,** 10265i (1962). Structure: Toki, Ohno, *loc. cit.* Revised structure: Hiramoto *et al., Tetrahedron Lett.* **1970,** 1087; *eidem, Chem. Pharm. Bull.* **19,** 1308, 1315 (1971). Shows antitubercular activity.

D-CH₃(CH₂)₆CHCH₂C—Leu—D-Glu—D-*allo*-Thr—D-Val—Leu—D-Ser
            | ||
           OH   O   └ Ile—D-Ser—Leu ┘

Powder, dec 270-273°. $[\alpha]_D^{29}$ −168.3° (ethanol). Stable to heat. Practically insol in water. Sol in methanol, ethanol, ether, acetone, alkaline phosphate buffer solns.

10010. Visnadine. [477-32-7] (2*R*)-2-Methylbutanoic acid (9*R*,10*R*)-10-(acetyloxy)-9,10-dihydro-8,8-dimethyl-2-oxo-2*H*,8*H*-benzo[1,2-*b*:3,4-*b′*]dipyran-9-yl ester; 2-methylbutyric acid 9-ester with 9,10-dihydro-9,10-dihydroxy-8,8-dimethyl-2*H*,8*H*-benzo[1,2-*b*:3,4-*b′*]dipyran-2-one acetate; 8,8-dimethyl-2-oxo-9,10-dihydro-2*H*,8*H*-benzo[1,2-*b*:3,4-*b′*]dipyran-9,10-diyl-10-acetate-9-(α-methylbutyrate); 3,4,5-trihydroxy-2,2-dimethyl-6-chromanacrylic acid δ-lactone 4-acetate 3-(2-methylbutyrate); 4′-acetoxy-3′-(α-methylbutyryloxy)-2′,2′-dimethyldihydropyrano(7,8:6′,5′)coumarin; 3-(α-methylbutyryloxy)-4-acetoxy-3,4-dihydroseseline; Cardine; Carduben; Vibeline; Visnamine. $C_{21}H_{24}O_7$; mol wt 388.41. C 64.94%, H 6.23%, O 28.83%. Isoln from seeds of *Ammi visnaga* L., *Umbelliferae* (Bishop's weed): Smith *et al., Science* **115,** 520 (1952); *eidem, J. Am. Chem. Soc.* **79,** 3534 (1957); Smith, Haber; Smith, Hosansky, **US 2816118**; **US 2980699** (1957, 1961 both to Penick); Le Men, **US 2995574** (1961 to Lab. Roger Bellon); Baddar *et al., J. Chem. Soc.* **1963,** 4522. Synthesis of (±)-form: Shanbhag *et al., Tetrahedron* **21,** 3591 (1965). Pharmacology and toxicology: Nkondi *et al., Therapie* **21,** 1267 (1966); Erbring *et al., Arzneim.-Forsch.* **17,** 283 (1967); Eyraud, Aurousseau, *ibid.* **23,** 201 (1973).

Needles from light petr, or ether + hexane, mp 85-88°. $[\alpha]_D^{20}$ +9.2° (alc), $[\alpha]_D^{30}$ +42.5° (c = 2 in dioxane). Slightly sol in water; quite sol in ethanol, methanol. Very sol in chloroform, acetone, ether, benzene, DMF. LD₅₀ in mice (mg/kg): 2240 orally; >370 s.c. (Erbring).

(±)-**Form.** Crystals from petr ether, mp 150-152° (Shanbhag).

THERAP CAT: Vasodilator (coronary).

10011. Visnagin. [82-57-5] 4-Methoxy-7-methyl-5*H*-furo-[3,2-*g*][1]benzopyran-5-one; 5-methoxy-2-methylfuranochromone. $C_{13}H_{10}O_4$; mol wt 230.22. C 67.82%, H 4.38%, O 27.80%. Spasmolytic constituent of *Ammi visnaga* Lam., *Umbelliferae.* One of the active principles in the Egyptian traditional medicine known as "khella" that is used as a diuretic and vasodilator. *See also:* visnadine, khellin. Isoln and structure: Späth, Gruber, *Ber.* **74,** 1492 (1941). Synthesis: Aneja *et al., Tetrahedron* **3,** 230 (1958); Badawi, Fayez, *Tetrahedron Lett.* **1967,** 1029. HPLC de-

termn in *A. visnaga* fruit: M. M. El-Domiaty, *J. Pharm. Sci.* **81,** 475 (1992).

Thread-like needles from water. mp 142-145°. Very slightly sol in water; sparingly sol in alc; freely sol in chloroform.

10012. Vital Red. [574-65-2] 3-Amino-4-[[4′-[(2-amino-6-sulfo-1-naphthalenyl)azo]-3,3′-dimethyl[1,1′-biphenyl]-4-yl]azo]-2,7-naphthalenedisulfonic acid trisodium salt; C.I. Direct Red 34; C.I. 23570; brilliant vital red; Brilliant Congo R; Vital Red Evans; ditolyldiazo-3,6-disulfo-β-naphthylamine-β-naphthylamine-6-sulfonic acid sodium salt. $C_{34}H_{25}N_6Na_3O_9S_3$; mol wt 826.76. C 49.39%, H 3.05%, N 10.17%, Na 8.34%, O 17.42%, S 11.64%. Prepd by diazotization of *o*-tolidine and coupling the resulting tetrazotolidine first with 2-naphthylamine-3,6-disulfonic acid (amino R salt) and next with 2-naphthylamine-6-sulfonic acid (Brönner acid): Palkin, Evans, *J. Am. Chem. Soc.* **47,** 429 (1925); **DE 41095;** *Frdl.* **1,** 476; *Colour Index* **vol. 4** (3rd ed., 1971) p 4191.

Cherry-red crystals from water. Absorption max: 500 nm (aq soln). Sol in water giving a brownish-red soln. Gives blue solution with concd HCl. Slightly sol in alc.

USE: For blood volume determinations.

10013. Vitamin A. [68-26-8] Retinol; all-*trans*-retinol; (*all-E*)-3,7-dimethyl-9-(2,6,6-trimethyl-1-cyclohexen-1-yl)-2,4,6,8-nonatetraen-1-ol; anti-infective vitamin; antixerophthalmic vitamin; axerophthol; lard-factor; oleovitamin A; ophthalamin (obsolete); vitamin A₁; vitamin A alcohol; Aquasol A; Avibon; Avitol; Vogan. $C_{20}H_{30}O$; mol wt 286.45. C 83.86%, H 10.56%, O 5.59%. Fat soluble, essential micronutrient. Occurs preformed only in animals; metabolized from carotenoids, such as β-carotene, *q.v.,* in the intestinal mucosa. Dietary sources include liver, milk, butter, cheese, eggs and fish liver oils or as carotenoids from fruits and vegetables. Stored primarily in the liver in esterified form; transported in the blood by *retinol binding protein* (RBP). Oxidized to retinal, *q.v.,* a key component of the visual system, and to retinoic acid, *q.v.,* which effects gene expression via specific nuclear receptors. Identification as essential nutrient in butter and egg: E. V. McCollum, M. Davis, *J. Biol. Chem.* **15,** 167 (1913). Isoln from fish oil: P. Karrer *et al., Helv. Chim. Acta* **14,** 1036 (1931). Structure: *eidem, ibid.* 1431; I. M. Heilbron *et al., Biochem. J.* **26,** 1194 (1932). Synthesis: O. Isler *et al., Helv. Chim. Acta* **30,** 1911 (1947); N. L. Wendler *et al., J. Am. Chem. Soc.* **72,** 234 (1950); T. Mukaiyama, A. Ishida, *Chem. Lett.* **1975,** 1201. Stereospecific synthesis: P. S. Manchand *et al., Helv. Chim. Acta* **59,** 567 (1976); G. Cardillo *et al., J. Chem. Soc. Perkin Trans. I* **1979,** 1729. Toxicology: J. J. Kamm, *J. Am. Acad. Dermatol.* **6,** 652 (1982). Review: W. Friedrich in *Vitamins* (Walter de Gruyter, New York, 1988) pp 63-140. Book: *The Retinoids,* M. B. Sporn *et al.,* Eds. (Raven Press, New York, 1994) 679pp. Review of role in vision: R. K. Crouch *et al., Photochem. Photobiol.* **64,** 613-621 (1996); of physiological functions and dietary requirements in humans: H. Gerster, *Int. J. Vitam. Nutr. Res.* **67,** 71-90 (1997); of metabolism and transport: E. H. Harrison, *Annu. Rev. Nutr.* **18,** 259-276 (1998).

Solvated crystals from polar solvents, such as methanol or ethyl formate. mp 62-64°. Distills at 120-125° at 5×10^{-3} mm pressure. n_D^{22} 1.6410 (calculated from refractive indexes of 20-70% solns in mineral oil). uv max (ethanol): 324-325 nm ($E_{1cm}^{1\%}$ 1835). Practically insol in water or glycerol. Sol in abs alcohol, methanol, chloroform, ether, fats and oils. Exhibits a yellow-green fluorescence when irradiated with Xuv light. LD$_{50}$ (10 day) in mice (mg/kg): 1510 i.p.; 2570 orally (Kamm).

Acetate. [127-47-9] C$_{22}$H$_{32}$O$_2$. Pale yellow prismatic crystals from methanol, mp 57-58°. uv max (ethanol): 326 nm (E$_{1cm}^{1\%}$ 1550). LD$_{50}$ (10 day) orally in mice: 4100 mg/kg (Kamm).

Palmitate. [79-81-2] Arovit; Optovit-A. C$_{36}$H$_{60}$O$_2$; mol wt 524.86. Predominant storage form of vitamin A in the liver. Amorphous or cryst. mp 28-29°. uv max (ethanol): 325-328 nm (E$_{1cm}^{1\%}$ 975). LD$_{50}$ (10 day) in mice, rats (mg/kg): 6060, 7910 orally (Kamm).

13-*cis* Form see Neovitamin A.

THERAP CAT: Vitamin (antixerophthalmic).

THERAP CAT (VET): Nutritional factor.

10014. Vitamin B$_{12}$. [68-19-9] Cyanocobalamin; 5,6-dimethylbenzimidazolyl cyanocobamide; cobinamide cyanide phosphate 3'-ester with 5,6-dimethyl-1-α-D-ribofuranosylbenzimidazole inner salt; LLD factor; *Lactobacillus lactis* Dorner factor; extrinsic factor; antipernicious anemia principle; Anacobin; Bedoz; Behepan; Berubi; Betalin-12; Betolvex; Cobalin; Crystamine; Cytacon; Cytamen; Cytobion; Docémine; Docigram; Fresmin; Millevit; Redisol; Rubesol; Rubramin PC; Vitarubin. C$_{63}$H$_{88}$CoN$_{14}$O$_{14}$P; mol wt 1355.37. C 55.83%, H 6.54%, Co 4.35%, N 14.47%, O 16.53%, P 2.29%. Prototype of the family of naturally occurring cobalt coordination compds known as *corrinoids*. Analogs of vitamin B$_{12}$ which differ only in the β-ligand of the cobalt are termed *cobalamins*. Synthesized almost exclusively by bacteria. Dietary sources include fish, meat, liver, and dairy products; plants have little or no cobalamins. Also found in soil and water, the richest sources being activated sewage sludge (*see* Milorganite) or manure. Converted by the body into its bioactive forms, methylcobalamin and cobamamide, *q.q.v.*, which serve as enzyme cofactors. Severe deficiency may result in megaloblastic anemia and/or neurological impairment. Isoln from mammalian liver: E. L. Rickes *et al., Science* **107**, 396 (1948); from cultures of *Streptomyces griseus: eidem, ibid.* **108**, 634 (1948); E. L. Rickes, T. R. Wood, US 2563794 (1951 Merck & Co.). Fermentation process using *Pseudomonas denitrificans:* R. A. Long, US 3018225 (1962 to Merck & Co.). Purification from sewage sludge: P. J. Van Melle, US 3057851 (1962 to Armour). Structure: D. C. Hodgkin *et al., Nature* **176**, 325 (1955); R. Bonnett *et al., ibid.* 328. X-ray structure analysis: D. C. Hodgkin, *Fortschr. Chem. Org. Naturst.* **15**, 167-227 (1958). Stereochemistry: Stora, *Bull. Soc. Chim. Fr.* **1959**, 1421. Total synthesis: R. B. Woodward, *Pure Appl. Chem.* **33**, 145 (1973). Nomenclature: IUPAC rules, *ibid.* **48**, 497 (1976). Gastrointestinal absorption is dependent on Castle's intrinsic factor, *q.v.*, and *haptocorrin* (R-protein); transport of the absorbed vitamin is mediated by *transcobalamins:* B. Seetharam, D. H. Alpers, *Annu. Rev. Nutr.* **2**, 343-369 (1982); R. Gräsbeck, *Clin. Biochem.* **17**, 99-107 (1984). Role of Co—C bond in B$_{12}$-dependent reactions: J. M. Pratt, *Pure Appl. Chem.* **65**, 1513 (1993). Review of biosynthesis: A. I. Scott, *Angew. Chem. Int. Ed.* **32**, 1223-1243 (1993). Comprehensive description: J. Kirschbaum, *Anal. Profiles Drug Subs.* **10**, 183-288 (1981). Book: *B$_{12}$* vols. 1 and 2, D. Dolphin, Ed. (Wiley-Interscience, New York, 1982) 672 and 506 pp. *Reviews:* B. T. Golding in *Comprehensive Organic Chemistry* vol. 5, E. Haslam, Ed. (Pergamon, New York, 1979) pp 549-584; "Vitamin B$_{12}$" in *Vitamins*, W. Friedrich, Ed. (de Gruyter, Berlin, 1988) pp 837-928. Review of chemistry and enzymology: K. L. Brown, *Chem. Rev.* **105**, 2075-2149 (2005).

Hygroscopic, dark red crystals. When exposed to air, may absorb ~12% water. The hydrated crystals are stable to air. Darkens at 210-220°. Not melted at 300°. [α]$_{656}^{23}$ −59 ± 9° (dil aq soln). Absorption max (water): 278, 361, 550 nm (A$_{1cm}^{1\%}$ 115, 204, 64). Odorless and tasteless. One gram dissolves in ~80 ml water. Aq solns are neutral, maximum stability in the pH range 4.5-5. Solns in this pH range can be autoclaved for 20 min at 120°. Soluble in alc. Insol in acetone, CHCl$_3$, ether.

Zinc tannate complex. Cyanocobalamin zinc tannate; Depinar. Long acting injectable vitamin B$_{12}$ prepn. Prepn: Thompson, US 2920015 (1960 to Armour). Comparative clinical study: A. Killander, I. Werner, *Acta Haematol.* **40**, 305 (1968). Practically insol in water. On reconstitution forms a colloidal suspension.

THERAP CAT: Vitamin (hematopoietic).

THERAP CAT (VET): Vitamin (hematopoietic).

10015. Vitamin B$_{12}$, Radioactive. Radioactive cyanocobalamin; radiocyanocobalamin. Prepn of ^{60}Co labelled compound: Chaiet *et al., Science* **111**, 601 (1950). Properties identical with unlabelled vitamin B$_{12}$, except for the presence of radioactive cobalt. Evaluation of dual-isotope Schilling test for pernicious anemia: L. S. Zuckier, L. R. Chervu, *J. Nucl. Med.* **25**, 1032 (1984).

^{60}Co Vitamin B$_{12}$. [13422-53-2] Racobalamin-60; Rubratope-60. T$_{1/2}$ 5.27 years, emitting beta and gamma rays.

^{58}Co Vitamin B$_{12}$. [18195-32-9] T$_{1/2}$ 70.8 days, emitting beta, gamma and x-rays.

^{57}Co Vitamin B$_{12}$. [13115-03-2] Rubratope-57. T$_{1/2}$ 271 days, emitting gamma and x-rays.

Combination of ^{57}Co and ^{58}Co labelled Vitamin B$_{12}$. Dicopac.

THERAP CAT: Diagnostic aid (pernicious anemia).

10016. Vitamin B$_{12r}$. [14463-33-3] Vitamin B$_{12}$-Co(II); cob(II)alamin; 5,6-dimethyl-1-(3-*O*-phosphono-α-D-ribofuranosyl)-1*H*-benzimidazole monoester with cobinamide-Co(II) inner salt. C$_{62}$H$_{88}$CoN$_{13}$O$_{14}$P; mol wt 1329.35. C 56.02%, H 6.67%, Co 4.43%, N 13.70%, O 16.85%, P 2.33%. A one-electron reduction product of vitamin B$_{12}$ containing a divalent cobalt atom. Undergoes a further one-electron reduction to vitamin B$_{12s}$. Prepn: H. Diehl, R. Murie, *Iowa State Coll. J. Sci.* **26**, 555 (1952); R. O. Brady, H. A. Barker, *Biochem. Biophys. Res. Commun.* **4**, 373 (1961); H.-U. Blaser, J. Halpern, *J. Am. Chem. Soc.* **102**, 1684 (1980). Crystal structure: B. Kräutler *et al., ibid.* **111**, 8936 (1989). Valence of reduced forms of B$_{12}$: H. A. O. Hill *et al., Chem. Ind. (London)* **1964**, 197. Review of chemistry of B$_{12r}$, B$_{12s}$ and analogs: R. Bonnett, *Chem. Rev.* **63**, 573-605 (1963); of prepns: D. Dolphin, *Methods Enzymol.* **18**, (Pt. C), 34-52 (1971). Role in enzymatic reactions: J. M. Pratt, *Pure Appl. Chem.* **65**, 1513 (1993).

Dark brown amorphous solid. Oxidized by air to aquocobalamin. Absorption max (H$_2$O): 474, 404, 312, 289, 260 nm (log ε 3.99, 3.88, 4.46, 4.29, 4.25).

Vitamin B$_{12s}$. [18534-66-2] Cobinamide-Co(I) dihydrogen phosphate (ester) 3′-ester with 5,6-dimethyl-1-α-D-ribofuranosyl-1H-benzimidazole; cob(I)alamin; hydridocobalamin. C$_{62}$H$_{89}$-CoN$_{13}$O$_{14}$P; mol wt 1330.36. Obtained as a gray-green product in solution.

10017. Vitamin D$_1$. [520-91-2] C$_{56}$H$_{88}$O$_2$; mol wt 793.30. C 84.78%, H 11.18%, O 4.03%. C$_{28}$H$_{44}$O.C$_{28}$H$_{44}$O. A 1:1 molecular compd of lumisterol and vitamin D$_2$. Prepn: Windaus *et al., Ann.* **489**, 252 (1931); **493**, 259 (1932).

Crystals from acetone, mp 124-125°. Sublimes in high vacuum at 135°. Dec 180°. Soly at 16° (g/ml): 0.037 of acetone; 0.024 of petr ether (bp 35-40°); 0.020 of methanol. uv max (0.02% sol in petr ether): 265 nm (ε 1.56). [α]$_D^{20}$ +140.5° (8.9 mg in 2 ml acetone), +140.5° (ethanol), +127° (chloroform).

10018. Vitamin D$_2$. [50-14-6] (3β,5Z,7E,22E)-9,10-Secoergosta-5,7,10(19),22-tetraen-3-ol; calciferol; ergocalciferol; oleovitamin D$_2$; activated ergosterol; viosterol; Condol; Decaps; Dee-Ron; Deltalin; De-Rat Concentrate; Deratol; Detalup; Diactol; Divit Urto; Drisdol; D-Tracetten; Ergorone; Ertron; Fortodyl; Hi-Deratol; Infron; Metadee; Mina D$_2$; Mulsiferol; Mykostin; Ostelin; Radiostol; Radsterin; Shock-Ferol; Sterogyl; Uvesterol-D; Vio-D. C$_{28}$H$_{44}$O; mol wt 396.65. C 84.78%, H 11.18%, O 4.03%. The synthetic form of vitamin D. Prepd from ergosterol by uv irradiation in a suitable solvent: Askew *et al., Proc. Roy. Soc. London* **B109**, 488 (1931/32). The best wavelengths for production of vitamin D$_2$ seem to be from 275 to 300 nm: Knudson, Benford, *J. Biol. Chem.* **124**, 287 (1938); Bunker *et al., J. Am. Chem. Soc.* **62**, 508 (1940). Prepn by electron bombardment of ergosterol using longer waves: **AT 119210.** Manuf: **US 1902785** (1933); **US 2030792** (1936); **US 1680818** (1928); **US 1871136** (1932). Direct total synthesis: B. Lythgoe *et al., Tetrahedron Lett.* **1977**, 3685. Discussion of structural problems: Papers by Askew and Windaus *et al.,* beginning in 1930. Stereochemistry: Crowfoot, Dunitz, *Nature* **162**, 608 (1948); *Chem. Ind. (London)* **1957**, 1149. General review: Inhoffen, *Angew. Chem.* **72**, 875 (1960). A polar, biologically active metabolite of vitamin D$_2$, **25-hydroxyergocalciferol,** which is ~1.5 times more active in curing rickets in rats, has been isolated from pig plasma. *See* Suda *et al., Biochem. Biophys. Res. Commun.* **35**, 182 (1969); *eidem, Biochemistry* **8**, 3515 (1969).

Prisms from acetone, mp 115-118°. Sublimes in very high vacuum (0.0006 mm) without dec. [α]$_D^{25}$ +82.6° (c = 3 in acetone); [α]$_D^{20}$ +102.5° (alcohol); [α]$_D^{20}$ +52° (CHCl$_3$). uv max (hexane): 264.5 nm (E$_{1cm}^{1\%}$ 458.9 ± 7.5). Not precipitated by digitonin (diff from ergosterol). Insol in water. Sol in the usual organic solvents. 1 ml acetone dissolves 0.0695 g at 7°. Slightly sol in vegetable oils. Commercial solns are usually made with propylene glycol or sesame oil. Vitamin D$_2$ crystals have a potency of 40 units of vitamin D (U.S.P.) per μg. The behavior in storage is described under vitamin D$_3$. *See also* Huber, Barlow, *J. Biol. Chem.* **149**, 125 (1943) for stability information.

USE: Rodenticide.

THERAP CAT: Vitamin (antirachitic).

THERAP CAT (VET): Nutritional factor (antirachitic). Low activity in poultry.

10019. Vitamin D$_3$. [67-97-0] (3β,5Z,7E)-9,10-Secocholesta-5,7,10(19)-trien-3-ol; activated 7-dehydrocholesterol; oleovitamin D$_3$; cholecalciferol; colecalciferol; CC; Duphafral D$_3$ 1000; Delsterol; Deparal; Ebivit; Neo Dohyfral D$_3$; Provitina; Ricketon;

Trivitan; D$_3$-Vicotrat; Vi-De-3; Vigantol; Vigorsan. C$_{27}$H$_{44}$O; mol wt 384.64. C 84.31%, H 11.53%, O 4.16%. The vitamin that mediates intestinal calcium absorption, bone calcium metabolism and probably, muscle activity. It usually acts as a hormone precursor as it requires two stages of metabolism, first to 25-hydroxycholecalciferol and then to 1α,25-dihydroxycholecalciferol, *q.q.v.*, before reaching actual hormonal form. Occurs in and is isolated from fish liver oils. Methods of sepn include chromatography, molecular distillation, esterification and fractionation of the esters. Prepd by irradiation of its provitamin 7-dehydrocholesterol, *q.v.*: Windaus *et al., Z. Physiol. Chem.* **241**, 100 (1936); Windaus *et al., Ann.* **533**, 118 (1938); Akhtar, Gibbons, *Tetrahedron Lett.* **1965**, 509. Direct total synthesis: B. Lythgoe *et al., Tetrahedron Lett.* **1977**, 3685. Laser photochemical production: V. Malatesta *et al., Angew. Chem.* **72**, 875-881 (1960). Review of metabolism: Haussler, Rasmussen, *J. Biol. Chem.* **247**, 2328-2335 (1972); *Nature* **245**, 180-182 (1973).

Fine needles from dilute acetone, mp 84-85°. [α]$_D^{20}$ +84.8° (c = 1.6 in acetone); [α]$_D^{20}$ +51.9° (c = 1.6 in chloroform). uv max (alcohol or hexane): 264.5 nm. (E$_{1cm}^{1\%}$ 450-490): Huber *et al., J. Am. Chem. Soc.* **67**, 609 (1945). Not precipitated by digitonin (diff from 7-dehydrocholesterol). Practically insol in water; sol in the usual organic solvents; slightly sol in vegetable oils. Oxidized and inactivated by moist air within a few days. Deterioration of pure cryst vitamin D$_3$ is negligible after storage of 1 year in amber evacuated ampuls at refrigerator temps; vitamin D$_2$ may be kept for 9 months under the same conditions. Additional stability information: Huber, Barlow, *J. Biol. Chem.* **149**, 125 (1942). Generally vitamin D$_3$ is considered more stable than vitamin D$_2$.

Note: Vitamin D$_3$ is approx as effective as vitamin D$_2$ in the human and in the rat. It is also fully active in chicks. Vitamin D$_2$ is only 1-2 percent as potent for the chick as vitamin D$_3$. Because of this difference it is important that poultry feeds are supplemented with vitamin D$_3$ rather than D$_2$. One unit (U.S.P. or international) is defined as the activity of 0.025 γ of vitamin D$_3$ contained in the U.S.P. vitamin D reference standard.

THERAP CAT: Vitamin (antirachitic).

THERAP CAT (VET): Nutritional factor (antirachitic).

10020. Vitamin D$_4$. [511-28-4] (3β,5Z,7E)-9,10-Secoergosta-5,7,10(19)-trien-3-ol; 22:23-dihydrovitamin D$_2$; 22,23-dihydroergocalciferol. C$_{28}$H$_{46}$O; mol wt 398.66. C 84.36%, H 11.63%, O 4.01%. Prepd from 22:23-dihydroergosterol by irradiation with light of the magnesium arc: Windaus, Trautmann, *Z. Physiol. Chem.* **247**, 185 (1937). Synthesis: P. J. Kocienski *et al., J. Chem. Soc. Perkin Trans.* 1 **1979**, 1290.

Platelets from dil acetone, mp 96-98°. Originally given as mp 107-108°, *see* Windaus, Guntzel, *Ann.* **538**, 122 (1939). $[\alpha]_D^{18}$ +89.3° (c = 0.47 in acetone). uv max: 265 nm. Not precipitated by digitonin. Practically insol in water. Sol in the usual organic solvents except petr ether; slightly sol in vegetable oils.

10021.   Vitamin E. [1406-18-4] General term referring to 2 groups of closely related 6-chromanol derivatives known as tocopherols and tocotrienols, each comprised of four homologs (α, β, γ, and δ) that differ in the position and number of methyl substituents on the chromanol ring. All eight compounds are found in nature, occurring as the *R,R,R*- or *R,Z,Z*- forms. Dietary sources include vegetable oils and green leafy vegetables. α-Tocopherol, *q.v.*, is the most abundant and has the greatest bioactivity. Vitamin E acts as an antioxidant to prevent free radical damage to tissues and unsaturated lipids; also thought to stabilize membrane structures. Deficiency in healthy humans is rare and is characterized by peripheral neuropathy and spinocerebellar ataxia. Discovery as nutritional factor required for normal reproduction in animals: H. M. Evans, K. S. Bishop, *Science* **56**, 650 (1922). Comparison of bioactivities of tocopherols and tocotrienols: T. Leth, H. Sondergaard, *J. Nutr.* **107**, 2236 (1977). HPLC determn in infant formula: B. R. Mendoza *et al.*, *J. Chromatogr. A* **1018**, 197 (2003). Review of chemistry, nomenclature and activity: W. Friedrich, "Vitamin E" in *Vitamins* (Walter de Gruyter, Berlin, 1988) pp 217-283. Review of biological occurrence and functions: R. S. Parker, *Adv. Food Nutr. Res.* **33**, 157-232 (1989); of nutritional requirements: E. E. J. Valk, G. Hornstra, *Int. J. Vitam. Nutr. Res.* **70**, 31-42 (2000); of metabolism: F. Brigelius-Flohé, M. G. Traber, *FASEB J.* **13**, 1145-1155 (1999). Review of antioxidant functions and role in membranes: X. Wang, P. J. Quinn, *Prog. Lipid Res.* **38**, 309-336 (1999); of non-antioxidant roles: A. Azzi, A. Stocker, *ibid.* **39**, 231-255 (2000).

Note: The international unit of vitamin E is equal to one mg of standard *dl*-α-tocopheryl acetate. Activity may also be expressed as α-tocopherol equivalents (α-TE) where one α-TE is equal to the activity of 1 mg of α-tocopherol.

10022.   Vitamin K. General term referring to a group of naphthoquinone derivatives required for the bioactivation of proteins involved in hemostasis. The designation "K" was derived from the German "Koagulationsvitamin." Vitamin K compds are classified into 3 groups: phylloquinone (K_1), *q.v.*, found in green plants; menaquinones (K_2), *q.v.*, primarily produced by intestinal bacteria; and menadione (K_3), *q.v.*, and derivatives which are synthetic, lipid soluble compounds. Reduced *in vivo* to dihydrovitamin K (KH_2) which serves as a coenzyme in the conversion of glutamic acid residues to γ-carboxyglutamic acid (Gla), *q.v.*, in the post-translational modification of blood coagulation factors II, VII, IX and X, and the anticoagulant proteins C and S. Other Gla-containing proteins, such as the bone matrix protein, osteocalcin, *q.v.*, have been identified in a wide variety of tissues. This γ-carboxylation is accompanied by the oxidation of KH_2 to vitamin K epoxide which is then recycled back to vitamin K. Discovery: H. Dam, *Biochem. Z.* **215**, 475 (1929); **220**, 158 (1930); *Nature* **135**, 652 (1935). Historical survey: H. Dam, *Vitam. Horm.* **24**, 295-306 (1966). Menadione and phylloquinone are metabolized by animals to menaquinone-4: C. Martius, H. O. Esser, *Biochem. Z.* **331**, 1 (1958); H. H. W. Thijssen, M. J. Drittij-Reijnders, *Br. J. Nutr.* **72**, 415 (1994), HPLC determn in plasma: M. Kamao *et al.*, *J. Chromatogr. B* **816**, 41 (2005). Comprehensive review: W. Friedrich in *Vitamins* (de Gruyter, New York, 1988) pp 285-338. Review of metabolism and role in human nutrition: M. J. Shearer, *Blood Rev.* **6**, 92-104 (1992); J. W. Suttie, *J. Am. Diet. Assoc.* **92**, 585-590 (1992); of mechanism of action: P. Dowd *et al.*, *Nat. Prod. Rep.* **11**, 251-264 (1994); of pharmacology and therapeutic use: J. A. Thorp *et al.*, *Drugs* **49**, 376-387 (1995). Physiological review: M. J. Shearer, *Lancet* **345**, 229-234 (1995).

10023.   Vitamin K5. [83-70-5] 4-Amino-2-methyl-1-naphthalenol; 4-amino-2-methyl-1-naphthol; 2-methyl-4-amino-1-hydroxynaphthalene; 3-methyl-4-hydroxy-1-naphthylamine; Synkamin. $C_{11}H_{11}NO$; mol wt 173.21. C 76.28%, H 6.40%, N 8.09%, O 9.24%. Prepn: Sah, *Rec. Trav. Chim.* **59**, 458 (1940); **60**, 373 (1941); Veldstra, Wiardi, *ibid.* **61**, 547 (1942); **62**, 75 (1943). Insulin-mimicking effect on glucose transport: J. N. Livingston *et al.*, *Am. J. Physiol.* **234**, E484 (1978). Polargraphic determn in aq soln: K. Takamura, F. Watanabe, *Methods Enzymol.* **67**, 134 (1980).

Hydrochloride. [130-24-5] $C_{11}H_{11}NO.HCl$. Needles from dil HCl, darkens at 262°, dec 280-282°. Turns pink to dark violet on exposure to air and light. Freely sol in water; slightly sol in alc. Insol in ether.

USE: Chemical probe to study insulin-activated hexose transport.

THERAP CAT: Vitamin (prothrombogenic).

10024.   Vitamin(s) L. Factors presumably necessary for lactation. Vitamin L_1: *See* o-Aminobenzoic Acid. Vitamin L_2 was shown to be 7-[tetrahydro-3,4-dihydroxy-5-(methylmercaptomethyl)-2-furyl]adenine: Nakahara *et al.*, *Sci. Papers Inst. Phys. Chem. Res. Jpn.* **40**, 433 (1943), *C.A.* **41**, 6317c (1947). Manuf: Sato *et al.*, *JP 62 7244* (1962), *C.A.* **59**, 1746f (1963); *JP 69 16015* (1969), *C.A.* **77**, 102146j (1972).

Vitamin L2

10025.   Vitamin T. [1407-73-4] Tegotin; termitin; torutilin; factor T; vitamin T Goetsch; Goetsch's vitamin; Temina. A complex of growth-promoting substances, originally obtained from termites: Goetsch, *Oesterr. Zool. Z.* **1**, 58-85 (1946). Also obtainable from roaches, yeasts and fungi. The isoln procedure has never been described. Isoln of "vitamin T complexes" from yeast: Koch *et al.*, *DE 1000962* (1957 to Aschaffenburger Zellstoffwerke), *C.A.* **54**, 18898d (1960). Vitamin T may be a mixture of known vitamins and growth-promoting factors: Koch *et al.*, *Naturwissenschaften* **38**, 339 (1951). Polemic by Barkow, Goetsch, *ibid.* **42**, 346 (1955).

10026.   Vitronectin. Serum spreading factor; S-protein. Multifunctional adhesive glycoprotein found in serum and in various tissues. Has binding sites for integrins, collagen, heparin, complement components, and perforin, *q.q.v.* Thought to play a regulatory role in hemostasis, wound healing, tissue remodeling and cancer. Synthesized by hepatocytes as a single chain polypeptide, mol wt ~78 kDa. Binds readily to proteoglycans of the extracellular matrix and is deposited in normal loose connective tissues, in dermal elastin fibers, and in the vascular wall. Also synthesized by platelets, macrophages and megakaryocytes. Released by activated platelets in different multimeric forms. Promotes cellular attachment, spreading and migration of a wide variety of cell types and serves as a matrix-associated regulator of blood coagulation. Identification: R. Holmes, *J. Cell Biol.* **32**, 297 (1967). Isoln and comparison with fibronectin, *q.v.*: D. Barnes *et al.*, *J. Supramol. Struct.* **14**, 47 (1980). Purification and tissue distribution: E. G. Hayman *et al.*, *Proc. Natl. Acad. Sci. USA* **80**, 4003 (1983). Amino acid sequence: S. Suzuki *et al.*, *EMBO J.* **4**, 2519 (1985). Identity with S-protein: K. T. Preissner *et al.*, *Biochem. Biophys. Res. Commun.* **134**, 951 (1986); B. R. Tomasini, D. F. Mosher, *Blood* **68**, 737 (1986). Review of structure and biological function in hemostasis: K. T. Preissner, *Annu. Rev. Cell Biol.* **7**, 275-310 (1991); K. T. Preissner, D. Jenne, *Thromb. Haemostasis* **66**, 123-132; 189-194 (1991). Review of vitronectin receptors and role in cell growth and differentiation: B. Felding-Habermann, D. A. Cheresh, *Curr. Opin. Cell Biol.* **5**, 864-868 (1993).

10027.   Voacamine. [3371-85-5] 12-Methoxy-13-[(3α)-17-methoxy-17-oxovobasan-3-yl]ibogamine-18-carboxylic acid methyl ester; voacanginine. $C_{43}H_{52}N_4O_5$; mol wt 704.90. C 73.27%, H 7.44%, N 7.95%, O 11.35%. Bisindole alkaloid found in *Voacanga africana* Stapf., *V. thouarsii* R. & Sch., var *obtusa* (K. Sch.) Pichon and *V. schweinfurthii* Staph., *Apocynaceae:* Janot, Goutarel, *Compt. Rend.* **240,** 1719 (1955); Rao, *J. Org. Chem.* **23,** 1455 (1958); Janot, Goutarel, **US 2823204** (1958 to Lab. Gobey). Identity with voacanginine: LeBarre, Gillo, *Bull. Acad. R. Med. Belg.* **20,** 194 (1956). Cleaved by acid catalysis to voacangine: Winkler, *Naturwissenschaften* **48,** 694 (1961). Structure: Goutarel *et al., Compt. Rend.* **243,** 1670 (1956); Percheron, *Ann. Chim. (Paris)* **4,** 303 (1959); Büchi *et al., J. Am. Chem. Soc.* **85,** 1893 (1963). *Review:* Gorman *et al.* in *The Alkaloids* **1,** J. E. Saxton, Ed. (The Chem. Soc., London, 1971) pp 242-249.

voacangine

Prisms from acetone + methanol, dec 223°. $[\alpha]_D^{20}$ −52° (chloroform). uv max: 225, 295 nm (log ε 4.72, 4.28). Sol in chloroform, acetone; slightly sol in methanol, ethanol.

Voacangine. Carbomethoxyibogaine; 12-methoxyibogamine-18-carboxylic acid methyl ester. $C_{22}H_{28}N_2O_3$; mol wt 368.47. Structure: Bartlett *et al., J. Am. Chem. Soc.* **80,** 126 (1958). Prismatic needles from ethanol, mp 136-137°. Sublimes$_{0.01}$ 135°. $[\alpha]_D^{20}$ −42° (c = 1.26 in chloroform). pKa 7.4 (40% aq methanol); pKa 5.73 (33% DMF). uv max (methanol): 225, 287 300 nm (log ε 4.43, 3.97, 3.93). Freely sol in acetone, chloroform; slightly sol in methanol, ethanol.

10028. Vodka. Little water. Defined as ethyl alcohol obtained from grain or potatoes, filtered through charcoal, and diluted with distilled water. Manuf by "spirit flow" process: Jacobs, **US 2946687** (1960 to Heublein).

10029. Voglibose. [83480-29-9] 3,4-Dideoxy-4-[[2-hydroxy-1-(hydroxymethyl)ethyl]amino]-2-*C*-(hydroxymethyl)-D-epiinositol; *N*-(1,3-dihydroxy-2-propyl)valiolamine; AO-128; Basen. $C_{10}H_{21}NO_7$; mol wt 267.28. C 44.94%, H 7.92%, N 5.24%, O 41.90%. α-Glucosidase inhibitor. Prepn: S. Horii *et al., EP 56194; eidem,* **US 4701559** (1982, 1987 both to Takeda); and structure-activity study: *eidem et al., J. Med. Chem.* **29,** 1038 (1986). Synthesis: H. Fukase, S. Horii, *J. Org. Chem.* **57,** 3651 (1992). Enzyme inhibition and pharmacology: T. Matsuo *et al., Am. J. Clin. Nutr.* **55,** 314S (1992). Clinical pharmacology: B. Göke *et al., Digestion* **56,** 493 (1995). Clinical evaluation in hyperinsulinemia: K. Shinozaki *et al., Metabolism* **45,** 731 (1996).

Colorless crystals, mp 162-163°. $[\alpha]_D^{25}$ +26.2° (c = 1 in water).
THERAP CAT: Antidiabetic.

10030. Volicitin. [191670-18-5] N^2-[(9Z,12Z,15Z)-17-Hydroxy-1-oxo-9,12,15-octadecatrienyl]-L-glutamine; *N*-(17-hydroxylinolenoyl)-L-glutamine. $C_{23}H_{38}N_2O_5$; mol wt 422.56. C 65.37%, H 9.06%, N 6.63%, O 18.93%. Key component in plant recognition of damage from insect herbivory. Isolated from the oral secretions of the beet armyworm caterpillar, it acts as a chemical signal to corn seedlings to produce volatile compounds to attract the caterpillar predator, parasitic wasps. Isolation and structure elucidation: H. T. Alborn *et al., Science* **276,** 945 (1997). Biosynthesis: P. W. Paré *et al., Proc. Natl. Acad. Sci. USA* **95,** 13971 (1998). Stereoselective synthesis: G. Phonert *et al., Chem. Commun.* **1999,** 1087.

10031. Vomicine. [125-15-5] 4-Hydroxy-19-methyl-16,19-secostrychnidine-10,16-dione; 12-hydroxy-*N*-methylpseudostrychnine. $C_{22}H_{24}N_2O_4$; mol wt 380.44. C 69.46%, H 6.36%, N 7.36%, O 16.82%. From seed of *Strychnos nux vomica* L., *Loganiaceae:* Wieland, Oertel, *Ann.* **469,** 193 (1929). Structure: Huisgen *et al., ibid.* **573,** 121 (1951). Synthesis: Rosenmund, *Angew. Chem.* **75,** 1127 (1963). *Reviews:* R. Robinson in *Progress in Organic Chemistry* **vol. I** (Butterworths, London, 1952) pp 2-21; J. B. Hendrickson in *The Alkaloids* **vol. VI,** R. H. F. Manske, H. L. Holmes, Eds. (Academic Press, New York, 1960) pp 195-204.

Hexagonal prisms from acetone, mp 284°. $[\alpha]_D^{22}$ +80° (c = 0.5 in alc). Weak, mono-acidic base forming salts with an acid reaction. Freely sol in chloroform, sol in hot alcohol, acetone, slightly in ether, ethyl acetate.
Hydrochloride. $C_{22}H_{24}N_2O_4$·HCl. Prisms from water, dec 245°. uv max (ethanol): 222, 263, 297 nm (log ε 4.27, 3.77, 3.52). Sparingly sol in water.
Methyl ether. $C_{23}H_{26}N_2O_4$. Needles from alcohol, dec 290°. $[\alpha]_D^{20}$ +16° (c = 0.5 in alcohol).

10032. Vomitoxin. [51481-10-8] 12,13-Epoxy-3,7,15-trihydroxytrichothec-9-en-8-one; deoxynivalenol; dehydronivalenol. $C_{15}H_{20}O_6$; mol wt 296.32. C 60.80%, H 6.80%, O 32.40%. Isoln of the trichothecene mycotoxin from *Fusarium roseum* and structure: N. Morooka *et al., J. Food Hyg. Soc. Japan* **13,** 368 (1972); T. Yoshizawa, N. Morooka, *Agric. Biol. Chem.* **37,** 2933 (1973). Isoln from *F. graminearum:* R. F. Vesonder *et al., Appl. Microbiol.* **26,** 1008 (1973); *eidem, Appl. Environ. Microbiol.* **31,** 280 (1976). Emetic and refusal activity in swine: D. M. Forsyth *et al., ibid.* **34,** 547 (1977). HPLC analysis: G. A. Bennett *et al., J. Am. Oil Chem. Soc.* **58,** 1002A (1981). Implicated as a chemical warfare agent with nivalenol, *q.v.* in Southeast Asia: N. Wade, *Science* **214,** 34 (1981).

Fine needles from ethyl acetate + petr ether, mp 151-153°. $[a]_D^{25}$+6.35° (c = 0.07 in ethanol). uv max (ethanol): 218 nm (ε 4500). LD_{50} i.p. in male, female mice (mg/kg): 70.0, 76.7 (Yoshizawa, Morooka).

10033. Voriconazole. [137234-62-9] ($\alpha R,\beta S$)-α-(2,4-Difluorophenyl)-5-fluoro-β-methyl-α-(1H-1,2,4-triazol-1-ylmethyl)-4-pyrimideethanol; 2R,3S-2-(2,4-difluorophenyl)-3-(5-fluoropyrimidin-4-yl)-1-(1H-1,2,4-triazol-1-yl)butan-2-ol; UK-109496; Vfend. $C_{16}H_{14}F_3N_5O$; mol wt 349.31. C 55.01%, H 4.04%, F 16.32%, N 20.05%, O 4.58%. Ergosterol biosynthesis inhibitor. Prepn: S. J. Ray, K. Richardson, **EP 440372**; *eidem,* **US 5278175** (1991, 1994 both to Pfizer); R. P. Dickinson *et al., Bioorg. Med. Chem. Lett.* **6**, 2031 (1996). Mechanism of action: H. Sanati *et al., Antimicrob. Agents Chemother.* **41**, 2492 (1997). *In vitro* antifungal spectrum: F. Marco *et al., ibid.* **42**, 161 (1998). HPLC determn in plasma: R. Gage, D. A. Stopher, *J. Pharm. Biomed. Anal.* **17**, 1449 (1998). Review of pharmacology and clinical development: P. E. Verweij *et al., Curr. Opin. Anti-Infect. Invest. Drugs* **1**, 361-372 (1999); J. A. Sabo, S. M. Abdel-Rahman, *Ann. Pharmacother.* **34**, 1032-1043 (2000). Clinical pharmacokinetics: L. Purkins *et al., Antimicrob. Agents Chemother.* **46**, 2546 (2002). Clinical comparison with amphotericin B: T. J. Walsh *et al., N. Engl. J. Med.* **346**, 225 (2002).

mp 127°. $[\alpha]_D^{25}$ −62° (c = 1 in methanol).

THERAP CAT: Antifungal (systemic).

10034. Vorinostat. [149647-78-9] N-Hydroxy-N'-phenyloctanediamide; suberoylanilide hydroxamic acid; SAHA. $C_{14}H_{20}N_2O_3$; mol wt 264.32. C 63.62%, H 7.63%, N 10.60%, O 18.16%. Second generation hybrid polar compound; histone deacetylase (HDAC) inhibitor that induces cell cycle arrest, differentiation and apoptosis in tumor cells. Prepn: R. Breslow *et al., WO 9307148; eidem,* **US 5369108** (1993, 1994 both to Sloan-Kettering Inst.; Columbia Univ.); J. C. Stowell *et al., J. Med. Chem.* **38**, 1411 (1995). Synthesis: A. Mai *et al., Org. Prep. Proceed. Int.* **33**, 391 (2001). HTLC determn in serum: L. Du *et al., Rapid Commun. Mass Spectrom.* **19**, 1779 (2005). *In vitro* antiproliferative activity: P. N. Munster *et al., Cancer Res.* **61**, 8492 (2001). *In vivo* antineoplastic activity: L. A. Cohen *et al., Anticancer Res.* **22**, 1497 (2002). Clinical pharmacokinetics and activity in cancer patients: W. K. Kelly *et al., J. Clin. Oncol.* **23**, 3923 (2005). Review of mechanism of action: V. M. Richon *et al., Blood Cells Mol. Dis.* **27**, 260-264 (2001); of development and therapeutic potential: R. W. Johnstone, *IDrugs* **7**, 674-682 (2004).

White solid, mp 159-160.5°.

THERAP CAT: Antineoplastic.

10035. Vorozole. [129731-10-8] 6-[(S)-(4-Chlorophenyl)-1H-1,2,4-triazol-1-ylmethyl]-1-methyl-1H-benzotriazole; (+)-(S)-6-[4-chloro-α-(1H-1,2,4-triazol-1-yl)benzyl]-1-methyl-1H-benzotriazole; R-83842; Rivizor. $C_{16}H_{13}ClN_6$; mol wt 324.77. C 59.17%, H 4.03%, Cl 10.92%, N 25.88%. Nonsteroidal aromatase inhibitor. Prepn: A. H. M. Raeymaekers *et al.,* **EP 293978** (1988 to Janssen); resolution of enantiomers: A. L. A. Willemsens *et al.,* **WO 9411364** (1994 to Janssen). Aromatase inhibition by racemate: W. Wouters *et al., J. Steroid Biochem.* **32**, 781 (1989); and enantiomers: *eidem, J. Steroid Biochem. Mol. Biol.* **37**, 1049 (1990). Abs config: O. M. Peeters *et al., Acta Crystallogr.* **C49**, 1958 (1993). Clinical studies in breast cancer: S. R. D. Johnston *et al., Cancer Res.* **54**, 5875 (1994); P. E. Goss *et al., Clin. Cancer Res.* **1**, 287 (1995). Review of clinical pharmacology and pharmacokinetics: W. Wouters *et al., Breast Cancer Res. Treat.* **30**, 89-94 (1994).

Crystals from 2-propanol, mp 130-135°. $[\alpha]_D^{20}$ +8.0° (c = 10 in CH_3OH).

(±)-**Form.** [118949-22-7] R-76713. Crystals from 2-propanone/1,1-oxybisethane, mp 178.9°.

THERAP CAT: Antineoplastic.

10036. VX. [50782-69-9] Methylphosphonothioic acid S-[2-[bis(1-methylethyl)amino]ethyl] O-ethyl ester; O-ethyl S-[2-(diisopropylamino)ethyl]methylphosphonothioate; Tx 60. $C_{11}H_{26}NO_2$-PS; mol wt 267.37. C 49.41%, H 9.80%, N 5.24%, O 11.97%, P 11.58%, S 11.99%. Nerve gas. Prepn: R. V. Ley, G. L. Sainsbury, **GB 1346409**; A. W. Wardrop, C. Stratford, **GB 1346410** (both 1974 to U.K. Sec. of State for Defence), *C.A.* **81**, 4068y, 4069z (1974); S. R. Eckhaus *et al.,* **US 3911059** (1975 to U.S.A. Sec. for Army). Activity studies in humans: F. R. Sidell, W. A. Groff, *Toxicol. Appl. Pharmacol.* **27**, 241 (1974); F. N. Craig *et al., J. Invest. Dermatol.* **68**, 357 (1977). Toxicity study: J. J. Gordon, L. Leadbeater, *Toxicol. Appl. Pharmacol.* **40**, 109 (1977).

Nonvolatile, odorless liquid. pKa' 7.9. LD_{50} s.c. in rabbits: 15.4 μg/kg (Gordon, Leadbeater).

Caution: Cholinesterase inhibitor; more potent than sarin, *q.v.*

USE: Chemical warfare agent.

W

10037. Warburganal. [62994-47-2] (1S,4aS,8aS)-1,4,4a,5,-6,7,8,8a-Octahydro-1-hydroxy-5,5,8a-trimethyl-1,2-naphthalenedicarboxaldehyde. $C_{15}H_{22}O_3$; mol wt 250.33. C 71.97%, H 8.86%, O 19.17%. Drimane sesquiterpene with antifeedant activity against the African army worm. Biological activity includes plant growth regulation, cytotoxic, antimicrobial and molluscicidal properties. Isoln from *Warburgia ugandensis, Canellaceae* and structure: I. Kubo *et al., Chem. Commun.* **1976,** 1013. Relationship between structure and antifeedant activity: K. Nakanishi, I. Kubo, *Isr. J. Chem.* **16,** 28 (1977). Synthesis of (±)-warburganal: S. P. Tanis, K. Nakanishi, *J. Am. Chem. Soc.* **101,** 4398 (1979); T. Nakata *et al., ibid.* 4400; A. S. Kende, T. J. Blacklock, *Tetrahedron Lett.* **1980,** 3119; P. A. Wender, S. L. Eck, *ibid.* **1982,** 1871; D. M. Hollinshead *et al., J. Chem. Soc. Perkin Trans. 1* **1983,** 1579. *See also:* **JP Kokai 80 136238,** and **JP 80 136240** (both 1980 to Inst. Phys. Chem. Res.); **JP Kokai 81 43236** (1981 to Suntory Ltd.); **JP Kokai 83 38232** (1983 to Teikoku Zoki). Synthesis of (−)-warburganal: H. Okawara *et al., Tetrahedron Lett.* **1982,** 1087.

mp 98-99°. uv max (methanol): 224 nm (ε 6300). $[\alpha]_D^{21}$ −260° (c = 0.350 in CHCl$_3$).

10038. Warfarin. [81-81-2] 4-Hydroxy-3-(3-oxo-1-phenyl-butyl)-2*H*-1-benzopyran-2-one; 3-(α-acetonylbenzyl)-4-hydroxycoumarin; 1-(4′-hydroxy-3′-coumarinyl)-1-phenyl-3-butanone; 3-α-phenyl-β-acetylethyl-4-hydroxycoumarin; WARF compound 42; Rodex; Sakarat X; Warfotox. $C_{19}H_{16}O_4$; mol wt 308.33. C 74.01%, H 5.23%, O 20.76%. Coumarin anticoagulant. Marketed as the racemate; the S(−)-form is the more potent isomer. Prepn: M. A. Stahmann *et al., US 2427578* (1947 to Wisconsin Alumni Res. Found.). Resolution and abs configuration: B. D. West *et al., J. Am. Chem. Soc.* **83,** 2676 (1961). Effect on vitamin K metabolism: R. G. Bell *et al., Biochemistry* **11,** 1959 (1972). Conformation in soln: E. J. Valente *et al., J. Med. Chem.* **20,** 1489 (1977). Toxicity studies: E. C. Hagan, J. L. Radomski, *J. Am. Pharm. Assoc. Sci. Ed.* **42,** 379 (1953); N. Back *et al., Pharmacol. Res. Commun.* **10,** 445 (1978). Comprehensive description: S. A. Babhair *et al., Anal. Profiles Drug Subs.* **14,** 423-452 (1985). Stereospecific HPLC determn in plasma: P. R. Ring, J. M. Bostick, *J. Pharm. Biomed. Anal.* **22,** 573 (2000). Review of rodenticide mechanisms of action and resistance: H. H. W. Thijssen, *Pestic. Sci.* **43,** 73-78 (1995). Review of pharmacology and therapeutic efficacy: J. Hirsh *et al., Chest* **102,** Suppl., 312S-326S (1992); of pharmacokinetics and effect of genetic variants: H. Takahashi, H. Echizen, *Clin. Pharmacokinet.* **40,** 587-603 (2001). Clinical comparison with aspirin following myocardial infarction: M. Hurlen *et al., N. Engl. J. Med.* **347,** 969 (2002).

Crystals from alc, mp 161°. uv max (water, pH 10): 308 nm (ε 13610). Soluble in acetone, dioxane. Moderately sol in methanol, ethanol, isopropanol, some oils. Freely sol in alkaline aq solns (forms a water-soluble sodium salt). Practically insol in water, benzene, cyclohexane, Skellysolves A and B. Warfarin has an acidic enol which forms metallic salts and an acetate, mp 117-118°, and a ketone which forms an oxime, mp 182-183° and a 2,4-dinitrophenylhydrazone, mp 215-216°.

Sodium salt. [129-06-6] Coumadin; Marevan; Warfilone. $C_{19}H_{15}NaO_4$; mol wt 330.31. Slightly bitter, crystalline powder. Discolored by light. Very sol in water; freely sol in alcohol; very slightly sol in chloroform, ether. LD_{50} in male rats, female rats, mice, rabbits (mg/kg): 323, 58, 374, ~800 orally (Hagen); also reported as LD_{50} in male, female rats (mg/kg): 100.3, 8.7 orally (Back).

Caution: Potential symptoms of overexposure to warfarin are hematuria, back pain; hematoma of arms and legs; epistaxis, bleeding lips and mucous membrane hemorrhage; abdominal pain, vomiting and fecal blood; petechial rash; abnormal hematologic indices. *See NIOSH Pocket Guide to Chemical Hazards* (DHHS/NIOSH 97-140, 1997) p 334. *See also Clinical Toxicology of Commercial Products,* R. E. Gosselin *et al.,* Eds. (Williams & Wilkins, Baltimore, 5th ed., 1984) Section III, pp 395-397.

USE: Rodenticide.

THERAP CAT: Anticoagulant.

10039. Water. [7732-18-5] Hydrogen oxide. H_2O; mol wt 18.02. H 11.19%, O 88.79%. *Reviews:* N. E. Dorsey, *Properties of Ordinary Water-Substance,* A.C.S. Monograph Series no. **81,** (Reinhold, New York, 1940) 673 pp; D. Eisenberg, W. Kauzmann, *The Structure and Properties of Water* (Oxford University Press, New York, 1969) 296 pp; Ebsworth *et al.,* in *Comprehensive Inorganic Chemistry* vol. 2, J. C. Bailar, Jr. *et al.,* Eds. (Pergamon Press, Oxford, 1973) pp 741-747. *Pyrogen-free water* (water for injection) is distilled water rendered free of fever-producing proteins (bacteria and their metabolic products). Method of prepn: Ishizuka *et al., C.A.* **49,** 15177 (1955).

Liquid. mp 0°. bp 100°. Expands on freezing. Temp of max density 3.98°. $d^{3.98}$ 1.000000 g/ml (0.999972 g/cc). d_4^{25} 0.997. d^0 (ice) 0.917 g/cc; d_4^0 (liq) 0.999868. Density tables: Bigg, *Br. J. Appl. Phys.* **18,** 521 (1967); Kell, *J. Chem. Eng. Data* **12,** 66 (1967). One liter satd vapor weighs 0.5974 g at 100° and 760 mm. Crit temp 374.2°; crit pressure 218 atm. Sp. heat (liq; 14°) 1.000 cal/g/°C. Latent heat of fusion: 1.436 kcal/mole. Latent heat of vaporization: 9.717 kcal/mole. n_D^{20} 1.3330. Dielectric const (0°) 87.740. Dipole moment (25°) in benzene 1.76; in dioxane 1.86. K for pure water only (25°): 1.008×10^{-14}; at moderate concn of solutes (e.g. 1.0M KOH): K (25°) 0.971×10^{-14}. The most universal solvent known.

10040. Watermelon. Arbuse. *Citrullus vulgaris* Schrad., *Cucurbitaceae,* cultivated in hot and temperate zones the world over. Contains diuretic principles: Bliss *et al., Am. J. Pharm.* **105,** 53 (1933); Roby *et al., ibid.* **111,** 68 (1939).

10041. Wheat Germ Oil. Cav-Ecol; Myopone; Denamone. Obtained by hydraulic expression or solvent extraction of wheat germ which constitutes ~2% of a wheat grain, the seed of *Triticum aestivum* L. (*T. sativum* Lam., *T. vulgare* Vill.), *Gramineae. Constit.* (of the oil): Linoleic acid 44.1%, oleic acid 30.0%, satd acids 15.1%, linolenic acid 10.8%, unsaponifiable matter 4.7%. The unsaponifiable matter contains vitamin E-active tocopherols (reported as 0.5% of the oil) and as 2 international vitamin E units per gram of the oil), sitosterols, dihydrositosterol and other cryst alcohols and phospholipids. *Review:* E. W. Eckey, *Vegetable Fats and Oils* (Reinhold, New York, 1954) pp 291-293.

Bland yellow oil resembling corn oil. d_{25}^{25} 0.925-0.933. n_D^{40} 1.469-1.478. Acid value 6-20. Saponif value 179-190. Iodine value 115-129. Thiocyanogen value 80-85. Hydroxyl value 10-48. Reichert-Meissl value 0.3-1.4. Polenske value 0.4-2.1. Hehner value 76-95. Miscible with chloroform, ether, benzene, petr ether. Slightly sol in alc.

USE: Nutritional supplement. Source of natural vitamin E and unsatd fatty acids (vitamin F).

THERAP CAT (VET): Dietary source of vitamin E.

10042. Whisky. Whiskey. A liquid produced by distillation of the fermented mash of malted cereal grains, which has been stored in wood containers for not less than 4 years. Straight whisky contains 47-53% abs alcohol by vol, 0.05-0.16% acid calculated as acetic acid, and 0.038-0.15% esters as ethyl acetate. Whisky marked 100 proof contains 50% ethanol (v/v). It also contains small quantities of other natural constituents (congeners), which vary according to the grain used, method of fermentation, etc., and which are largely responsible for the characteristic aroma and flavor. Blended whisky contains at least 40% ethanol (v/v) and is made from at least 20% of 100 proof straight whisky mixed with neutral spirits, *q.v.* The most popular blends are made from 65 vols neutral spirits and 35 vols straight whisky.

Light to deep amber liquid; characteristic odor and taste. d 0.923-0.935 at 25°.

THERAP CAT: Sedative, vasodilator (peripheral).

10043. White Pine. Deal pine; Northern pine; Weymouth pine. The dried inner bark of *Pinus strobus* L., *Pinaceae. Constit.* Coniferin glycoside, coniferyl alcohol, tannin, oleoresin, volatile oils.

Weak yellowish-orange to light yellowish-brown when powdered, with a slightly terebinthinate odor and a slightly mucilaginous, sweet, then bitter and astringent taste.

THERAP CAT: The bark as expectorant.

10044. Wieland-Gumlich Aldehyde. [466-85-3] (17*R*)-19,20-Didehydro-17,18-epoxycuran-17-ol; 1-deacetyldiaboline; caracurine VII. $C_{19}H_{22}N_2O_2$; mol wt 310.39. C 73.52%, H 7.14%, N 9.03%, O 10.31%. Decompn product of isonitrosostrychnine: Wieland, Kaziro, *Ann.* **506**, 60 (1933). Isoln from *Strychnos toxifera* Benth., and *S. subcordata* Spruce, *Loganiaceae:* Asmis *et al., Helv. Chim. Acta* **37**, 1983 (1954); Penna *et al., Gazz. Chim. Ital.* **87**, 1163 (1957). Identity with caracurine VII: Bernauer *et al., Helv. Chim. Acta* **41**, 1405 (1958). Structure: Deyrup *et al., ibid.* **45**, 2266 (1962). Chemistry of the degradation from strychnine, *q.v.:* Hymon *et al., ibid.* **52**, 1564-1602 (1969). Synthesis: L. Szabo, O. Clauder, *Acta Chim. Acad. Sci. Hung.* **95**, 85 (1977). ^{13}C-NMR study: E. Wenkert *et al., J. Org. Chem.* **43**, 1099 (1978).

Crystals from acetone + methanol, decomp 213-214°. $[\alpha]_D^{22}$ −133.8° (c = 0.52 in methanol). Sol in methanol, ethanol, chloroform; slightly sol in acetone, ethyl acetate.

Hydrochloride hemihydrate. Crystals from ethanol, mp >300°. uv max (water): 240, 290 nm (log ε 3.80, 3.40). Sol in water, ethanol, methanol, warm chloroform; slightly sol in acetone, chloroform.

10045. Wild Cherry. Wild black cherry bark. Dried stem bark of *Prunus serotina* Ehrh., *Rosaceae,* collected in autumn. *Habit.* North America. *Constit.* Prunasin; the enzyme emulsin capable of hydrolyzing prunasin to benzaldehyde, glucose, and hydrocyanic acid; benzoic, trimethylgallic and *p*-coumaric acids; tannin, volatile oil.

USE: Flavoring in foods. Pharmaceutic aid (flavor).

10046. Wildfire Toxin. [32190-57-1] *N*-[2-Amino-4-(3-hydroxy-2-oxo-3-azetidinyl)-1-oxobutyl]-*L*-threonine. $C_{11}H_{19}N_3O_6$; mol wt 289.29. C 45.67%, H 6.62%, N 14.53%, O 33.18%. Isoln from *Pseudomonas tabaci,* the bacterium responsible for wildfire disease of tobacco: Woolley *et al., J. Biol. Chem.* **197**, 409 (1952). Highly toxic to a variety of organisms including bacteria, algae, higher plants and animals: Sinden *et al., Toxicol. Appl. Pharmacol.* **14**, 82 (1969). Mode of action: Lovrekovich *et al., Nature* **197**, 917; **198**, 710 (1963). Structural studies: Woolley *et al., J. Biol. Chem.* **215**, 485 (1955); Stewart, *J. Am. Chem. Soc.* **83**, 435 (1961). Revised structure: *idem, Nature* **229**, 174 (1971).

Colorless, very hygroscopic substance. Very soluble in water; readily sol in methanol. Moderately sol in ethanol; sparingly sol in *n*-butanol and higher alcohols. Practically insol in acetone, ethyl acetate, and less polar organic liquids. Shows marked instability. Slowly loses potency in aq soln at pH 6. Complete loss of activity at these conditions and 0° in one month. Inactivation more rapid in methanol or when pH is shifted to either side of 6, esp in alkaline range.

10047. Wilkinson's Catalyst. [14694-95-2] (*SP*-4-2)-Chlorotris(triphenylphosphine)rhodium. $C_{54}H_{45}ClP_3Rh$; mol wt 925.21. C 70.10%, H 4.90%, Cl 3.83%, P 10.04%, Rh 11.12%. Dimorphic compd exists in two forms, red and orange, both possess the same chemical properties. Prepn: J. F. Young *et al., Chem. Commun.* **1965**, 131; J. A. Osborn, G. Wilkinson, *Inorg. Synth.* **10**, 67 (1967); *eidem, ibid.* **28**, 77 (1990). Crystal structure: M. J. Bennett, P. B. Donaldson, *Inorg. Chem.* **16**, 655 (1977). Structure and properties: Y. Nishihara *et al., Organometallics* **21**, 825 (2002). Mechanistic study: S. B. Duckett *et al., J. Am. Chem. Soc.* **116**, 10548 (1994). Reduction of nitrobenzenes: H. R. Brinkman *et al., Synth. Commun.* **26**, 973 (1996); selective hydrogenation of olefins: A. Jourdant *et al., J. Org. Chem.* **67**, 3163 (2002). Comprehensive review of properties and reactions: F. H. Jardine, *Prog. Inorg. Chem.* **28**, 63-202 (1981); of hydrogenations: F. Joo, *Acc. Chem. Res.* **35**, 738-745 (2002).

Dark, burgundy-red crystals from hot ethanol. Orange crystals from < 200 ml ethanol soln refluxed for five minutes; converted to red form on further refluxing. mp 157°. Soly in chloroform, dichloromethane (25°): ~20 g/l; in benzene, toluene (25°): ~2 g/l; much less sol in acetic acid, acetone and other ketones, methanol, lower aliphatic alcohols. Virtually insol in alkanes and cyclohexane. Donor solvents such as pyridine, dimethyl sulfoxide, acetonitrile dissolve the complex with reaction. Solns are air sensitive. Orange form d 1.363; red form d 1.379.

USE: Homogeneous hydrogenation catalyst.

10048. Withaferin A. [5119-48-2] (4β,5β,6β,22*R*)-5,6-Epoxy-4,22,27-trihydroxy-1-oxoergosta-2,24-dien-26-oic acid δ-lactone; 4β,27-dihydroxy-1-oxo-5β,6β-epoxywitha-2,24-dienolide. $C_{28}H_{38}O_6$; mol wt 470.60. C 71.46%, H 8.14%, O 20.40%. Isolated from the leaves of *Withania somnifera* Dun., *Solanaceae:* Lavie, Yarden, *J. Chem. Soc.* **1962**, 2925; Kirson *et al., Tetrahedron* **26**, 2209 (1970); Subramanian, Sethi, *Indian J. Pharm.* **32**, 16 (1970); from roots of *Withania coagulans: eidem, Curr. Sci.* **38**, 267 (1969); from *Acnistus arborescens* (L.): Kupchan *et al., J. Org. Chem.* **34**, 3858 (1969). Structure: Lavie *et al., J. Chem. Soc.* **1965**, 7517; Kupchan, *loc. cit.* Crystal structure: McPhail, Sim, *J. Chem. Soc. C* **1968**, 962. Antitumor activity studies: B. Shohat *et al., Cancer Chemother. Rep.* **51**, 271 (1967); B. Shohat, H. Joshua, *Int. J. Cancer* **8**, 487 (1971). Synthetic studies: M. Hirayama *et al., J. Chem. Soc. Perkin Trans. 1* **1981**, 88. Stereoselective synthesis: *eidem, Tetrahedron Lett.* **23**, 4725 (1982).

Consult the Name Index before using this section.

White prisms from acetone-petroleum ether, mp 252-253° (Kup-chan). Also reported as mp 243-245° (ethyl acetate). $[\alpha]_D^{28}$ +125° (c = 1.30 in CHCl$_3$). uv max (ethanol): 214, 335 nm (ε 17300, 165).

10049. Woodruff. Woodward herb; petit muguet; Waldmeister (German). Leaves of *Asperula odorata* L., *Rubiaceae. Habit.* Europe, Siberia, North Africa, Australia. *Constit.* Coumarin, tannin, asperuloside, fatty oil, essential oil, bitter principle. Discussion of its fragrance, prepn of **asperule absolute**, use of *Asperula* in various fragrant formulations: *Perfum. Essent. Oil Rec.* **1963**, (June) p 382.

USE: Flavoring agent; the fresh leaves in flavoring May wine, the dried leaves in sachets.

10050. Woodward's Reagent K. [4156-16-5] 2-Ethyl-5-(3-sulfophenyl)isoxazolium inner salt; *N*-ethyl-5-phenylisoxazolium-3′-sulfonate. C$_{11}$H$_{11}$NO$_4$S; mol wt 253.27. C 52.16%, H 4.38%, N 5.53%, O 25.27%, S 12.66%. Prepd by reacting 5-phenyl-isoxazole with chlorosulfonic acid, followed by alkylation with triethyloxonium fluoroborate, and acid hydrolysis: Woodward *et al., J. Am. Chem. Soc.* **83**, 1010 (1961).

Crystals, dec 207-208°. Stable. Non-hygroscopic.

USE: Peptide-bond former.

10051. Woollins' Reagent. [122039-27-4] 2,4-Diphenyl-1,-3,2,4-diselenadiphosphetane 2,4-diselenide. C$_{12}$H$_{10}$P$_2$Se$_4$; mol wt 532.00. C 27.09%, H 1.89%, P 11.64%, Se 59.37%. [PhP(Se)(μ-Se)]$_2$. Selenium analog of Lawesson's reagent, *q.v.* Prepn: J. C. Fitzmaurice *et al., J. Chem. Soc. Chem. Commun.* **1988**, 741; P. T. Wood, J. D. Woollins, *ibid.* 1190; M. J. Pilkington *et al., Heteroatom Chem.* **1**, 351 (1990). Synthesis and characterization by ^{31}P and ^{77}Se NMR: G. Grossmann *et al., Z. Anorg. Allg. Chem.* **627**, 1269 (2001). Improved synthesis: I. P. Gray *et al., Chem. Eur. J.* **11**, 6221 (2005). X-ray crystal structure: P. Bhattacharyya *et al., J. Chem. Soc. Dalton Trans.* **2001**, 300. Synthetic applications: I. Baxter *et al., Chem. Commun.* **1997**, 2049; P. Bhattacharyya, J. D. Woollins, *Tetrahedron Lett.* **42**, 5949 (2001); *idem et al., Chem. Eur. J.* **8**, 2705 (2002); J. Bethke *et al., Tetrahedron Lett.* **44**, 6911 (2003).

Red crystals from toluene, mp 192-204°.

USE: Selenium transfer reagent.

10052. Wormwood. Absinthium; green ginger. Shrubby, aromatic perennial plant, *Artemisia absinthium* L., *Compositae.* Medicinal portions include the essential oil and the dried leaves and flowering tops. *Habit.* Europe, northern Africa, Asia, North and South America. *Constit.* Absinthin, anabsinthin, artabsine, matricine, volatile oil. Description: E. Guenther, *The Essential Oils* **V**, 487 (Van Nostrand, New York 1952). Isolation of various constituents: Cekan, Herout, *Collect. Czech. Chem. Commun.* **21**, 79 (1956); Herout *et al., ibid.* 1485. Characterization of oil: T. Sacco, F. Chialva, *Planta Med.* **54**, 93 (1988). Extraction of antioxidant components: J. M. Canadanovic-Brunet *et al., J. Sci. Food Agric.* **85**, 265 (2005). Botanical description and medicinal uses: J. Gruenwald *et al., PDR for Herbal Medicines* (Medical Economics, Montvale, 2nd Ed., 2000) pp 829-831; A. J. Skyles, B. V. Sweet, *Am. J. Health-Syst. Pharm.* **61**, 239-241 (2004).

Very strong odor, acrid taste.

Volatile oil. [8008-93-5] Oil of wormwood; artemisia oil. Obtained by steam distillation of leaves and flowering tops. *Constit.* Highly variable among different strains, chiefly thujone, *cis*-epoxyocimene, *trans*-sabinyl acetate, chrysanthenyl acetate. Brownish-green liq. d$_{15}^{15}$ 0.925-0.955. n$_D^{20}$ 1.460-1.4741. Sol in ether, in 2 vols 80% alcohol; very slightly sol in water. *Keep well closed, cool and protected from light.*

Caution: Ingestion of large doses may cause vomiting, stomach and intestinal cramps, headache, dizziness and CNS disturbances (Gruenwald).

USE: Oil as flavoring in alcoholic beverages, *e.g.* **vermouth**, which is a blend of white wines, contg traces of absinthium and other flavors; formerly in absinthe.

THERAP CAT: Aromatic bitter; anthelmintic; externally for insect bites and wound healing.

10053. Wortmannin. [19545-26-7] (1*S*,6b*R*,9a*S*,11*R*,11b*R*)-11-(Acetyloxy)-1,6b,7,8,9a,10,11,11b-octahydro-1-(methoxymethyl)-9a,11b-dimethyl-3*H*-furo[4,3,2-*de*]indeno[4,5-*h*]-2-benzo-pyran-3,6,9-trione. C$_{23}$H$_{24}$O$_8$; mol wt 428.43. C 64.48%, H 5.65%, O 29.88%. Antifungal antibiotic from *Penicillium wortmanni* Klocker: Brian *et al., Trans. Br. Mycol. Soc.* **40**, 365 (1957). Similar to viridin, *q.v.* Structure: MacMillan *et al., Chem. Commun.* **1968**, 613; *eidem, J. Chem. Soc. Perkin Trans. 1* **1972**, 2898. Absolute stereochemistry: Petcher *et al., Chem. Commun.* **1972**, 1061; MacMillan *et al., ibid.* 1063.

Neutral solid, mp 240°. Unstable in aq solns pH 3-8.

X

10054. Xaliproden. [135354-02-8] 1,2,3,6-Tetrahydro-1-[2-(2-naphthalenyl)ethyl]-4-[3-(trifluoromethyl)phenyl]pyridine. C_{24}-$H_{22}F_3N$; mol wt 381.43. C 75.57%, H 5.81%, F 14.94%, N 3.67%. Serotonin 5HT$_{1A}$-receptor agonist; enhances production of neurotrophic factors and extends motor neuron survival. Prepn: D. Nisato *et al.*, **EP 101381**; *eidem*, **US 4521428** (1984, 1985 both to Sanofi); of radiolabelled compound: N. Robic, J.-P. Noël, *J. Labelled Compd. Radiopharm.* **42**, 109 (1999). Pharmacology and receptor binding: L. Cervo *et al.*, *Eur. J. Pharmacol.* **253**, 139 (1994). Effect on neuron survival: Y. Iwasaki *et al.*, *J. Neurol. Sci.* **160**, Suppl. 1, S92 (1998). Neuroprotective effect in animal model of multiple sclerosis: B. Bourrié *et al.*, *Proc. Natl. Acad. Sci. USA* **96**, 12855 (1999). Review of pharmacology and clinical potential in treatment of amyotrophic lateral sclerosis: J. Fournier *et al.*, *CNS Drug Rev.* **3**, 148-167 (1997).

Hydrochloride. [90494-79-4] SR-57746A. $C_{24}H_{22}F_3N.HCl$; mol wt 417.89. mp 255-260°.

THERAP CAT: Neuroprotective.

10055. Xamoterol. [81801-12-9] *N*-[2-[[2-Hydroxy-3-(4-hydroxyphenoxy)propyl]amino]ethyl]-4-morpholinecarboxamide; 1-(4-hydroxyphenoxy)-3-[2-(4-morpholinocarboxamido)ethylamino]-2-propanol. $C_{16}H_{25}N_3O_5$; mol wt 339.39. C 56.62%, H 7.42%, N 12.38%, O 23.57%. β_1-Adrenoceptor partial agonist. Prepn: **BE 867376**; B. G. Main, J. J. Barlow, **US 4143140** (1978, 1979 both to ICI); prepn and adrenoceptor stimulant activity: J. J. Barlow *et al.*, *J. Med. Chem.* **24**, 315 (1981). Cardiovascular activity: A. Nuttall, H. M. Snow, *Br. J. Pharmacol.* **77**, 381 (1982). Hemodynamics, cardioselectivity and kinetics: G. Jennings *et al.*, *Clin. Pharmacol. Ther.* **35**, 594 (1984). Hemodynamic effects: J.-M. R. Detry *et al.*, *Eur. Heart J.* **4**, 584 (1983); H. Sato *et al.*, *Circulation* **75**, 213 (1987). Metabolism: T. R. Marten *et al.*, *Drug Metab. Dispos.* **12**, 652 (1984). HPLC determn in biological fluids: C. J. Oddie *et al.*, *J. Chromatogr.* **308**, 370 (1984). Clinical evaluations: F. L. Tseu *et al.*, *Br. Heart J.* **56**, 469 (1986); L. Barrios *et al.*, *Eur. J. Clin. Pharmacol.* **29**, 667 (1986). Clinical comparison with atenolol, *q.v.*, in asthmatic patients: J. W. J. Lammers *et al.*, *Br. J. Clin. Pharmacol.* **22**, 595 (1986).

Hemifumarate. [73210-73-8] ICI-118587; Corwin. $(C_{16}H_{25}$-$N_3O_5)_2.C_4H_4O_4$; mol wt 794.85. Crystals from ethanol, mp 168-169° (dec).

THERAP CAT: Cardiotonic.

10056. Xanomeline. [131986-45-3] 3-[4-(Hexyloxy)-1,2,5-thiadiazol-3-yl]-1,2,5,6-tetrahydro-1-methylpyridine. $C_{14}H_{23}N_3$-OS; mol wt 281.42. C 59.75%, H 8.24%, N 14.93%, O 5.69%, S 11.39%. Selective muscarinic M$_1$-receptor agonist. Prepn: P. Sauerberg, P. H. Olesen, **EP 384288** (1990 to Ferrosan); *eidem*, **US 5043345** (1991 to Novo Nordisk); *eidem et al.*, *J. Med. Chem.* **35**, 2274 (1992). Prepn of crystalline tartrate: L. M. Osborne *et al.*, **WO 9429303** (1994 to Novo Nordisk). Muscarinic receptor binding study: H. E. Shannon *et al.*, *J. Pharmacol. Exp. Ther.* **269**, 271 (1994). Pharmacology: F. P. Bymaster *et al.*, *ibid.* **282**. HPLC determn in plasma: C. L. Hamilton *et al.*, *J. Chromatogr.* **613**, 365 (1993).

Oxalate. [141064-23-5] $C_{14}H_{23}N_3OS.C_2H_2O_4$. Crystals from acetone, mp 148°.

(+)-L-Hydrogen tartrate. [152854-19-8] Xanomeline tartrate; LY-246708; NNC-11-0232; Lomeron; Memcor. $C_{14}H_{23}N_3OS.C_4$-H_6O_6; mol wt 431.50. Crystals from 2-propanol, mp 95.5°.

THERAP CAT: Cholinergic; nootropic.

10057. Xanthan Gum. [11138-66-2] Polysaccharide B-1459; Kelgum; Keltrol; Kelzan; Xantural. Mol wt >10^6. Polysaccharide gum produced by the bacterium *Xathomonas campestris*: A. Jeanes *et al.*, *J. Appl. Polym. Sci.* **5**, 519 (1961). Composed of D-glucosyl, D-mannosyl and D-glucosyluronic acid residues and differing proportions of *O*-acetyl and pyruvic acid acetal. The primary structure consists of a cellulose backbone with trisaccharide side chains, the repeating unit being a pentasaccharide. Structural studies: J. H. Sloneker *et al.*, *Can. J. Chem.* **40**, 2066, 2188 (1962); **42**, 1261 (1964); P. E. Jansson *et al.*, *Carbohydr. Res.* **45**, 275 (1975); L. D. Melton *et al.*, *ibid.* **46**, 245 (1976). Review of structure and use in chemically enhanced oil recovery: G. Holzwarth, *Dev. Ind. Microbiol.* **26**, 271-280 (1985); of macromolecular properties: B. T. Stokke *et al.* in *Polysaccharides*, S. Dumitriu, Ed. (Dekker, New York, 1998) pp 433-472. Review of production and industrial uses: F. Garcia-Ochoa *et al.*, *Biotechnol. Adv.* **18**, 549-579 (2000).

Cream-colored, odorless, free-flowing powder. Dissolves readily in water with stirring to give highly viscous solns at low concns. Forms strong films on evaporation of aq solns. Resistant to heat degradation. Aq solns are highly pseudoplastic.

USE: In foods, pharmaceuticals, and cosmetics as stabilizer and thickening agent. For rheology control in water-based systems. In oil and gas drilling and completion fluids.

10058. Xanthatin. [26791-73-1] [3a*R*-(3aα,7β,8aβ)]-3,3a,4,-7,8,8a-Hexahydro-7-methyl-3-methylene-6-(3-oxo-1-butenyl)-2*H*-cyclohepta[*b*]furan-2-one. $C_{15}H_{18}O_3$; mol wt 246.30. C 73.15%, H 7.37%, O 19.49%. Antimicrobial agent from *Xanthium strumarium* L., sens. lat.; *X. pennsylvanicum* Wallr., *Compositae*; *X. riparium*. Isoln: J. E. Little *et al.*, *Arch. Biochem.* **27**, 247 (1950); T. A. Geissman *et al.*, *J. Am. Chem. Soc.* **76**, 685 (1954). Structure: P. G. Deuel, T. A. Geissman, *ibid.* **79**, 3778 (1957). Evaluation as repellent of blue mussel: A. Harada *et al.*, *Agric. Biol. Chem.* **49**, 1887 (1985).

Flat needles from methanol or ethanol, mp 114.5-115°. uv max: 275, 213 nm (ε 22800, 7300). $[\alpha]_D^{30}$ -20° (ethanol). Sol in ether, acetone, alcohol; slightly sol in hot water (neutral pH). Practically insol in petr ether, 5% NaOH, 5% HCl.

10059. Xanthine. [69-89-6] 3,7-Dihydro-1*H*-purine-2,6-dione; 2,6(1*H*,3*H*)-purinedione; 2,6-dioxopurine. $C_5H_4N_4O_2$; mol wt 152.11. C 39.48%, H 2.65%, N 36.83%, O 21.04%. Occurs in animal organs, yeast, potatoes, coffee beans, tea. First isolated from urinary bladder stones: *Beilstein* **26**, 447 (1937). Prepd by treating a sulfuric acid soln of guanine with sodium nitrite: Fischer, *Ann.* **215**, 309 (1882). Several other syntheses, *cf.* Levene, Bass, *Nucleic Acids* (New York, 1931).

Scales, plates from water. Dec on heating without melting and with partial sublimation. Kb at 40° = 6.09×10^{-14}; Ka at 40° = 1.19×10^{-10}. Absorption spectrum: Kalckar, *J. Biol. Chem.* **167**, 429 (1947). One gram dissolves in 14.5 liters of water at 16°, in 1.4 liters boiling water; less sol in alcohol. Sol in mineral acids, freely sol in NH_4OH and in NaOH solns.

1,3-Dimethylxanthine *see* Theophylline.

3,7-Dimethylxanthine *see* Theobromine.

1,3,7-Trimethylxanthine *see* Caffeine.

10060. Xanthinol Niacinate. [437-74-1] 3-Pyridinecarboxylic acid compd with 3,7-dihydro-7-[2-hydroxy-3-[(2-hydroxyethyl)methylamino]propyl]-1,3-dimethyl-1*H*-purine-2,6-dione (1:1); 7-[2-hydroxy-3-[(2-hydroxyethyl)methylamino]propyl]theophylline compd with nicotinic acid; 7-[3-[*N*-(2-hydroxyethyl)amino]-2-hydroxypropyl]theophylline nicotinate; xanthinol nicotinate; SK-331-A; Complamin; Xavin. $C_{19}H_{26}N_6O_6$; mol wt 434.45. C 52.53%, H 6.03%, N 19.34%, O 22.10%. Prepn: Bestian, **DE 1102750** (1961 to Wuelfing), *C.A.* **56**, 11602i (1962). Alternate synthesis: Korbonits *et al., Acta Pharm. Hung.* **38**, 98 (1968). Pharmacology: Hemmer, Diezemann, *Arzneim.-Forsch.* **12**, 672 (1962); Lennartz, *ibid.* 675; Stamm, *ibid.* 679.

Crystals, mp 180°. Freely sol in water.

THERAP CAT: Vasodilator (peripheral).

10061. Xanthocillin. [11042-38-9] Xantocillin; Brevicid. Antibiotic complex produced by *Penicillium notatum* Westling: Rothe, *Pharmazie* **5**, 190 (1950); Barwald, **GB 898498** (1962 to Arzneimittelwerk VEB), *C.A.* **57**, 9013a (1962). Consists of at least three antibiotics, xanthocillins X, Y_1 and Y_2; the first being the major component (about 70%).

Xanthocillin X	R = H	R' = H
Xanthocillin Y_1	R = OH	R' = H
Xanthocillin Y_2	R = OH	R' = OH

Xanthocillin X. [580-74-5] 4,4'-(2,3-Diisocyano-1,3-butadiene-1,4-diyl)bisphenol; bis(*p*-hydroxybenzylidene)ethylene isocyanide; 1,4-bis(*p*-hydroxyphenyl)-2,3-diisonitrilo-1,3-butadiene. $C_{18}H_{12}N_2O_2$; mol wt 288.30. Structure: Hagedorn, Tönjes, *Pharmazie* **11**, 409 (1956); **12**, 567 (1957); Hagedorn *et al., Ber.* **93**, 1584 (1960). Synthesis: Hagedorn, Eholzer, *Angew. Chem.* **74**, 215 (1962). Biosynthetic studies: Achenbach, Grisebach, *Z. Naturforsch.* **20b**, 137 (1965); Achenbach, König, *Ber.* **105**, 784 (1972). Crystal structure: D. Britton *et al., Cryst. Struct. Commun.* **10**, 1497 (1981). Studies on antiviral activity: Takatsuki *et al., J. Antibiot.* **21**, 671 (1968); *eidem, ibid.* **22**, 151 (1969); Kitahara, *ibid.* **34**, 1556 (1981). Clusters of yellow needles from alc; yellow rhombs from ethyl acetate. Chars at about 210°. Sol (up to 1%) in alc, ether, acetone, dioxane. Freely sol in aqueous alkaline solns. Practically insol in water, petr ether, benzene, chloroform. Forms a water-sol dipotassium salt, the concd solns of which have a pH of 10.5.

Dimethyl ether. $C_{20}H_{16}N_2O_2$. Yellow needles from dioxane + alcohol, dec 181°.

Xanthocillin Y_1. [38965-69-4] 4-[4-(4-Hydroxyphenyl)-2,3-diisocyano-1,3-butadienyl]-1,2-benzenediol. $C_{18}H_{12}N_2O_3$; mol wt 304.30.

Xanthocillin Y_2. [38965-70-7] 4,4'-(2,3-Diisocyano-1,3-butadiene-1,4-diyl)bis-1,2-benzenediol. $C_{18}H_{12}N_2O_4$; mol wt 320.30.

Structure of xanthocillins Y_1 and Y_2: Achenbach *et al., Ber.* **105**, 3061 (1972).

USE: In feed supplements.

THERAP CAT: Antibacterial.

10062. Xanthone. [90-47-1] 9*H*-Xanthen-9-one; 9-oxoxanthene; diphenylene ketone oxide; dibenzo-γ-pyrone; Genicide. $C_{13}H_8O_2$; mol wt 196.20. C 79.58%, H 4.11%, O 16.31%. Prepd by heating phenyl salicylate: Graebe, *Ann.* **254**, 279 (1889); Holleman, *Org. Synth.* **coll. vol. I** (2nd ed., 1941) p 552.

Polymorphic needles from alcohol, mp 174°. bp_{730} 351°. Sparingly volatile with steam. Dipole moment 3.0. Solubility: 0.55 g/100 ml of cold alcohol; 6.71 g/100 ml of boiling alcohol. Freely sol in chloroform. Slightly sol in hot water, ether, petr ether, benzene, toluene, xylene. Dissolves in concd H_2SO_4 to a yellow soln with pale blue fluorescence.

Oxime. Xanthoxime. mp 161°.

USE: In the prepn of xanthydrol. Ovicide for codling moth eggs; less effective as larvicide.

10063. Xanthophyll. [127-40-2] β,ε-Carotene-3,3'-diol; lutein; vegetable lutein; vegetable luteol; Bo-Xan. $C_{40}H_{56}O_2$; mol wt 568.87. C 84.45%, H 9.92%, O 5.62%. One of the most widespread carotenoid alcohols in nature. Originally isolated from egg yolk, also isolated by chromatography from nettles, algae, and petals of many yellow flowers. Occurs also in colored feathers of birds: Volker, *Z. Physiol. Chem.* **288**, 20 (1951). Extraction from petals of *Tagetes patula* L., *Compositae:* Karrer *et al., Helv. Chim. Acta* **30**, 531 (1947). Occurs together with zeaxanthin, *q.v.* Dipalmitate occurs in *Helenium autumnale* L., *Compositae* and other flowers: Kuhn, Winterstein, *Naturwissenschaften* **18**, 754 (1930). Conversion to zeaxanthin with sodium alcoholate: Karrer, Jucker, *ibid.* 266. Does not possess vitamin A potency: Schumacher *et al., Poult. Sci.* **23**, 529 (1944). Stereochemistry: Zechmeister, *Chem. Rev.* **34**, 267 (1944). Structure: Karrer, *Helv. Chim. Acta* **34**, 2160 (1951). Abs config: Goodfellow *et al., Chem. Commun.* **1970**, 1578; Buchecker *et al., Chimia* **25**, 192 (1971); *eidem, Helv. Chim. Acta* **57**, 631 (1974). Synthesis: H. Mayer, A. Rüttimann, *ibid.* **63**, 1451 (1980). Sepn and determn of configurational isomers: A. Rüttiman *et al., J. High Resolut. Chromatogr. Chromatogr. Commun.* **6**, 612 (1983). *Reviews:* Zechmeister, *Carotinoide* (Berlin, 1934); Mayer, *The Chemistry of Natural Coloring Matters* (New York, 1943); Karrer, Jucker, *Carotenoids* (New York, 1950).

Yellow prisms with metallic luster from ether + methanol, mp 190° (corr), (a higher mp indicates impure material). Also reported as mp 183° [Buchecker (1974)]. $[\alpha]_{Cd}^{18}$ +165° (c = 0.7 in benzene). Absorption max (dioxane): 481, 453, 429, 333, 268 nm (ε 142000, 152000, 100000, 15500, 35000). Insol in water, sol in fats and in fat solvents. More sol in boiling methanol (1:700) than zeaxanthin.

Dipalmitate. Helenien; Adaptinol. $C_{72}H_{116}O_4$; mol wt 1045.69. Red needles from alcohol, mp 92°.

10064. Xanthopterin. [119-44-8] 2-Amino-1,5-dihydro-4,6-pteridinedione; 2-amino-4,6-pteridinediol; 2-amino-4,6-dihydroxypteridine; 2-amino-4,6-dihydroxypyrimido[4,5-*b*]pyrazine. C_6H_5-N_5O_2; mol wt 179.14. C 40.23%, H 2.81%, N 39.09%, O 17.86%. Pigment first found in wings of butterflies. Widely distributed in insects and in animals. Has been separated from urine and from the crab. Isoln and structure: Schöpf, Becker, *Ann.* **507**, 266 (1933); **524**, 55, 126 (1936); Schöpf, Kottler, *Ann.* **539**, 128 (1939); Wieland, Purrmann, *Ann.* **544**, 163 (1940). *See also* Fukushima, Shiota, *J. Biol. Chem.* **247**, 4549 (1972). Synthesis: Purrmann, *Ann.* **546**, 98 (1940); **548**, 284 (1941); Koschara, *Z. Physiol. Chem.* **277**, 159

(1943); Totter, *J. Biol. Chem.* **154**, 105 (1944); Elion *et al., J. Am. Chem. Soc.* **71**, 741 (1949); Koschara, DE **859471** (1952 to Bayer), *C.A.* **52**, 10222f (1958); Stuart, Wood, *J. Chem. Soc.* **1963**, 4186. Facile synthesis: Taylor, Jacobi, *J. Am. Chem. Soc.* **95**, 4455 (1973); Taylor *et al., J. Org. Chem.* **40**, 2341 (1975). Exhibits tumor inhibitory properties.

Monohydrate. Orange-yellow crystals, sinters around 360°, decomp above 410°. Practically insol in water. Freely sol in dil NH_4OH and NaOH giving yellow solns and in $2N$ HCl giving colorless solns. uv max at pH 11: 255, 390 nm ($E_{1cm}^{1\%}$ 0.92, 0.355). Can be converted by yeast into folic acid.

10065. Xanthosine. [146-80-5] Xanthine riboside; 9-β-D-ribofuranosyl xanthine; 9-β-D-ribofuranosyl-9*H*-purine-2,6-diol; 9-β-D-ribofuranosyl-9*H*-purine-2,6-(1*H*,3*H*)-dione. $C_{10}H_{12}N_4O_6$; mol wt 284.23. C 42.26%, H 4.26%, N 19.71%, O 33.77%. Prepd from guanosine by treatment with sodium nitrite and acetic acid: Levene, Jacobs, *Ber.* **43**, 3163 (1910); Gulland, Macrae, *J. Chem. Soc.* **1933**, 662. Synthesis: Howard *et al., ibid.* **1949**, 232. Biosynthesis: Magasanik, Brooke, *J. Biol. Chem.* **206**, 83 (1954); Korn, Buchanan, *ibid.* **217**, 183 (1955); Bolis *et al., ibid.* **219**, 917 (1956).

Dihydrate. Long prisms from water. Anhydr felted clusters (warts) from alc. Dec on heating, no distinct melting range. $[\alpha]_D^{30}$ −51.2° (p = 8 in 0.3*N* NaOH). uv max: 253 nm (ε 8.790). a_M (molar absorbancy): 11.4×10^3 at 248.5 nm in water at pH 8.0. Sparingly sol in cold water; freely sol in hot water; sol in hot dil alcohol. Easily hydrolyzed by mineral acids.

10066. Xanthoxyletin. [84-99-1] 5-Methoxy-8,8-dimethyl-2*H*,8*H*-benzo[1,2-*b*:5,4-*b'*]dipyran-2-one; 7-hydroxy-5-methoxy-2,2-dimethyl-2*H*-1-benzopyran-6-acrylic acid δ-lactone; xanthoxylin N; xanthoxyloin. $C_{15}H_{14}O_4$; mol wt 258.27. C 69.76%, H 5.46%, O 24.78%. Found in *Xanthoxylum americanum* Mill., *Melicope ternata* Forst., *M. mantelli* Buch., *Halifordia scleroxyla* F. Muell., *Rutaceae; Chloroxylon swietenia* DC., *Meliaceae.* Isoln: Staples, *Am. J. Pharm.* **1829**, 123; Witte, *Arch. Pharm.* **212**, 283 (1878); Lloyd, *Am. J. Pharm.* **1890**, 229; Gordin, *J. Am. Chem. Soc.* **28**, 1649 (1906); Bell *et al., J. Chem. Soc.* **1936**, 627; Robertson, Subramaniam, *ibid.* **1937**, 286; Dieterle, Kruta, *Arch. Pharm.* **275**, 45 (1937); Briggs, Locker, *J. Chem. Soc.* **1951**, 3131; King *et al., ibid.* **1954**, 1392; Hegarty, Lahey, *Aust. J. Chem.* **9**, 120 (1956); Cambie, *J. Chem. Soc.* **1960**, 2376. Synthesis: Joshi, Kamat, *Tetrahedron Lett.* **1966**, 5767.

Elongated prisms from methanol, mp 132-133°. uv max: 277, 269, 322, 347 nm (log ε 4.28, 4.32, 3.99, 4.05 in ethanol). Very easily sol in benzene, chloroform, hot alcohol; sol in acetone; sparingly sol in ether. Sol in 49 parts cold acetone and 25,000 parts cold water.

10067. Xanthoxylin. [90-24-6] 1-(2-Hydroxy-4,6-dimethoxyphenyl)ethanone; 2'-hydroxy-4',6'-dimethoxyacetophenone; phloracetophenone 4,6-dimethyl ether; 2,4-dimethoxy-6-hydroxyacetophenone; brevifolin. $C_{10}H_{12}O_4$; mol wt 196.20. C 61.22%, H 6.16%, O 32.62%. Found in *Xanthoxylum piperitum* DC., *X. alatum* Roxb., *Rutaceae, Artemisia brevifolia* Wallich, *Compositae, Hippomane mancinella* L., *Sapium sebiferum* Roxb., *Euphorbiaceae.* Isoln: Stenhouse, *Ann.* **89**, 251 (1854); **104**, 236 (1857); Semmler, Schossberger, *Ber.* **44**, 2885 (1911); Smith, Smith, *Pharm. J.* **119**, 688 (1927); **123**, 604, 611 (1929); Schaeffer *et al., J. Am. Pharm. Assoc.* **43**, 43 (1954); Chu *et al., C.A.* **53**, 10532g (1959). Synthesis: Kostanecki, Lambor, *Ber.* **32**, 2260 (1899); Canter *et al., J. Chem. Soc.* **1931**, 1245; Belton *et al., Sci. Proc. R. Dublin Soc.* **25**, 19 (1949); Schmid, Bolleter, *Helv. Chim. Acta* **33**, 917 (1950); MacKenzie *et al., J. Chem. Soc.* **1950**, 2965; Dean, Robertson, *ibid.* **1953**, 1244; Kawano, *Chem. Ind. (London)* **1959**, 368.

Crystals from ethanol, mp 81-83°. Practically insol in water. Sol in alcohol, ether.

10068. Xanthurenic Acid. [59-00-7] 4,8-Dihydroxy-2-quinolinecarboxylic acid; 4,8-dihydroxyquinaldic acid. $C_{10}H_7NO_4$; mol wt 205.17. C 58.54%, H 3.44%, N 6.83%, O 31.19%. Excreted by pyridoxine-deficient animals after the ingestion of tryptophan. Isoln from the urine of albino rats fed almost exclusively on fibrin: Musajo, *Gazz. Chim. Ital.* **67**, 165 (1937). Synthesis from ethyl oxalacetate and *o*-anisidine: Musajo, Minchilli, *Ber.* **74**, 1842 (1941); Mebane, Oroshnik, *J. Am. Chem. Soc.* **73**, 3520 (1951); Furst, Olsen, *J. Org. Chem.* **16**, 412 (1951).

Sulfur-yellow crystals, mp 286°. uv max (water): 243, 342 nm (ε 30000, 6500). Insol in water. Sol in aq alkali hydroxides and carbonates (yellow solns) and in hot dil HCl. It gives a red color with Millon reagent, intense ruby-red with alkali diazobenzenesulfonates, and intense green with $FeSO_4$. When the acid is dissolved in very dil $NaHCO_3$, the green color with $FeSO_4$ is still visible at a diln of 1:200,000.

Methyl ester. $C_{11}H_9NO_4$. Yellow crystals, dec 262°. Sol in NH_4OH, alkali hydroxides and carbonates.

10069. Xanthyletin. [553-19-5] 8,8-Dimethyl-2*H*,8*H*-benzo[1,2-*b*:5,4-*b'*]dipyran-2-one; 7-hydroxy-2,2-dimethyl-2*H*-1-benzopyran-6-acrylic acid δ-lactone; 2,2-dimethylchromenocoumarin. $C_{14}H_{12}O_3$; mol wt 228.24. C 73.67%, H 5.30%, O 21.03%. Linear pyranocoumarin found in *Xanthoxylum americanum* Mill., *Luvanga scandens* Ham., *Citrus acida* Roxb., *Rutaceae; Chloroxylon swietenia* DC., *Meliaceae.* Isoln: Bell, Robertson, *J. Chem. Soc.* **1936**, 1828; Bell *et al., ibid.* **1937**, 1542; Späth *et al., Ber.* **72**, 1450 (1939); Bose, Mookerjee, *J. Indian Chem. Soc.* **21**, 181 (1944); Mookerjee, *ibid.* **23**, 41 (1946); King *et al., J. Chem. Soc.* **1954**, 1392. Synthesis: Späth, Hillel, *Ber.* **72**, 2093 (1939); Steck, *Can. J. Chem.* **49**, 2297 (1971); P. Waykole *et al., Indian J. Chem.* **19B**, 238 (1980); V. K. Ahluwalia *et al., Monatsh. Chem.* **112**, 119 (1981); J. Banerji *et al., Indian J. Chem.* **21B**, 496 (1982).

Elongated flat prisms from methanol, mp 130-131°. $bp_{0.1}$ 140-145°. uv max: 266, 348 nm (log ε 4.34, 4.15).

10070. Xemilofiban. [149820-74-6] (3*S*)-3-[[4-[[4-(Amino-iminomethyl)phenyl]amino]-1,4-dioxobutyl]amino]-4-pentynoic acid ethyl ester; ethyl (3*S*)-3-[3-[(*p*-amidinophenyl)carbamoyl]pro-pionamido]-4-pentynoate. $C_{18}H_{22}N_4O_4$; mol wt 358.39. C 60.32%, H 6.19%, N 15.63%, O 17.86%. Platelet fibrinogen receptor (GPIIb/IIIa) antagonist. Prodrug converted *in vivo* to the active acid form. Prepn: P. R. Bovy *et al.*, **WO 9307867**; *eidem*, **US 5344957** (1993, 1994 both to Monsanto; Searle); J. Cossy *et al.*, *Bioorg. Med. Chem. Lett.* **7**, 1699 (1997). Structure-activity study: J. A. Zablocki *et al.*, *J. Med. Chem.* **38**, 2378 (1995). Pharmacology: N. S. Nicholson *et al.*, *Circulation* **91**, 403 (1995). Clinical pharmacokinetics: D. J. Kereiakes *et al.*, *ibid.* **94**, 906 (1996). Clinical evaluation in unstable angina: C. Simpfendorfer *et al.*, *ibid.* **96**, 76 (1997).

Hydrochloride. [156586-91-3] SC-54684A. $C_{18}H_{22}N_4O_4$.HCl; mol wt 394.85.

Acid. [149193-61-3] SC-54701A. $C_{16}H_{18}N_4O_4$; mol wt 330.34. $[\alpha]_D$ −33.7° (c = 1.45 in methanol).

THERAP CAT: Antithrombotic.

10071. Xenbucin. [959-10-4] α-Ethyl-[1,1′-biphenyl]-4-acetic acid; 2-(4-biphenylyl)butyric acid; α-(4-biphenylyl)butyric acid; α-(4-diphenylyl)butyric acid; α-(*p*-xenyl)butyric acid; 4-diphenyl-ylethylacetic acid; 4-biphenylylethylacetic acid; ethyl-*p*-xenylacetic acid; α-ethyl-*p*-phenyl-α-toluic acid; MG-1559; Liosol. $C_{16}H_{16}O_2$; mol wt 240.30. C 79.97%, H 6.71%, O 13.32%. Prepn: Blicke, Grier, *J. Am. Chem. Soc.* **65**, 1725 (1943); Cavallini, Massarani, *Farmaco Ed. Sci.* **11**, 167 (1956). Fibrinolytic activity: R. J. Gryglewski, M. Eckstein, *Nature* **214**, 626 (1967).

Crystals from glacial acetic acid, mp 123-125°. Soluble in ethanol, methanol, acetone, carbon tetrachloride, benzene, ether, dimethylformamide. Practically insol in water.

***trans*-4-Phenylcyclohexylamine salt (1:1).** [19992-80-4] Butixirate; MG-5771; Flectar. $C_{28}H_{33}NO_2$; mol wt 415.57. Prepn, analgesic and anti-inflammatory properties: G. Cantarelli *et al.*, *Farmaco Ed. Sci.* **24**, 140 (1969); **GB 1168542** (1969 to Maggioni), *C.A.* **72**, 43197 (1970). Therapeutic effectiveness: P. Croce, *Clin. Ter.* **50**, 241 (1969). Crystals, mp 224-227°. LD_{50} i.p. in mice: 183 μM/k (Cantarelli).

THERAP CAT: Free acid as antilipemic; *trans*-4-phenylcyclohexyl-amine salt as analgesic, anti-inflammatory.

10072. Xenon. [7440-63-3] Xe; at. wt 131.29; at. no. 54. Valences 2, 4, 6, 8. Group VIIIA(18), also known as Group 0. A noble gas characterized by an electronic structure in which the outer *p* subshell is entirely filled. Naturally occurring stable isotopes (mass numbers): 124 (0.10%); 126 (0.09%); 128 (1.91%); 129 (26.4%); 130 (4.1%); 131 (21.2%); 132 (26.9%); 134 (10.4%); 136 (8.9%); known artificial, radioactive isotopes: 110-123; 125; 127; 133; 135; 137-145. Discovered in the final residues obtained after evaporating liq air: Ramsay, Travers, *Proc. Roy. Soc.* **63** [A], 405 (1898). Occurs frequently in gases evolved from thermal springs; concentration in air: 0.087 ppm by vol. Obtained commercially from the atmosphere by distillation-liquefaction process. Extraction from liq air residues: Allen, Moore, *J. Am. Chem. Soc.* **53**, 2512 (1931). *Xenon platinum hexafluoride* was the first reported xenon compound: N. Bartlett, *Proc. Chem. Soc. London* **1962**, 218. Teratogenicity study: G. A. Lane *et al.*, *Science* **210**, 899 (1980). Review of biology, chemistry and anesthetic proper-

ties: R. M. Featherstone, C. A. Muelbaecher, *Pharmacol. Rev.* **15**, 97 (1963). Review of diagnostic use of radioactive compds for pulmonary studies: F. Fazio, P. Wollman, *Clin. Physiol.* **1**, 323 (1981); for cerebral blood flow: H. Yonas *et al.*, *Adv. Tech. Stand. Neurosurg.* **15**, 3 (1987). Reviews of chemistry and compds: *Noble-Gas Compounds*, H. H. Hyman, Ed. (Univ. Chicago Press, Chicago, 1963) 404 pp; J. H. Holloway, *Noble-Gas Chemistry* (Methuen, London, 1968) 213 pp; Sladky, "Noble Gases" in *MTP Int. Rev. Sci.: Inorg. Chem., Ser. One* vol. 3, V. Gutman, Ed. (Butterworths, London, 1972) pp 1-52; Cockett, Smith, "The Mona-tomic Gases" in *Comprehensive Inorganic Chemistry* vol. 1, J. C. Bailar, Jr. *et al.*, Eds. (Pergamon Press, Oxford, 1973) pp 139-211; Bartlett, Sladky, *ibid.*, pp. 213-330; S.-C. Hwang, W. R. Weltmer, Jr. in *Kirk-Othmer Encyclopedia of Chemical Technology* vol. 13 (John Wiley & Sons, 4th ed., 1995) pp 1-38; G. J. Schrobilgen, J. M. Whalen, *ibid.* pp 38-53; *Chemistry of the Elements* N. N. Greenwood, A. Earnshaw, Eds. (Pergamon Press, New York, 1984) pp 1042-1059.

Colorless, odorless, tasteless, relatively inert, monatomic gas; will form compds with highly electronegative elements such as O, F, Cl. Soly of gas in water (20°): 108.1 cm³/kg water. Triple point temp 161.35 K, press 81.66 kPa. Critical temp 289.74 K, critical press 5840 kPa, critical d 1100 kg/m³. Gas: d^0 (101.3 kPa) 5.8971 kg/m³, d (normal bp) 11 kg/m³. Liquid: normal bp −108.13°, d (normal bp) 3057 kg/m³, d (triple pt) 3084 kg/m³, heat of vapor-ization (normal bp) 12.640 kJ/mol. Solid: d (triple pt) 3540 kg/m³, heat of vaporization (triple pt) 15.1 kJ/mol, heat of fusion (triple pt) 2.3 kJ/mol. Solid form exists as face-centered cubic crystals at normal pressure. Spectrum: Collie, *Proc. Roy. Soc.* **97** [A], 349 (1920). Emission spectra: T. Jacksier, R. M. Barnes, *Appl. Spectrosc.* **48**, 65 (1994).

Xenon-133. [14932-42-4] Xeneisol Xe 133.

Hydrate. [60212-94-4] Xe.xH$_2$O, mp 24°, and a deuterate, Xe.6D$_2$O, have been prepd: R. de Forcrand, *Compt. Rend.* **176**, 355 (1923); **181**, 15 (1925); Tamman, Krige, *Z. Anorg. Chem.* **146**, 179 (1925).

Xenon difluoride. [13709-36-9] F_2Xe; mol wt 169.29. Prepd from the elements: Weeks *et al.*, *J. Am. Chem. Soc.* **84**, 4612 (1962); Hoppe *et al.*, *Z. Anorg. Allg. Chem.* **324**, 214 (1963). Colorless crystals; d 4.32. Triple pt. 129.03°: Schreiner *et al.*, *J. Phys. Chem.* **72**, 1162 (1968). Sublimes without decompn. Soly in water at 0°: 25 g/l.

Xenon tetrafluoride. [13709-61-0] F_4Xe; mol wt 207.29. First prepd by direct combination of the elements at 6 atm and 400°: Claassen *et al.*, *J. Am. Chem. Soc.* **84**, 3593 (1962). Colorless crystals; d 4.04. Triple pt 117.10°: Schreiner *et al.*, *loc. cit.* Sublimes without decompn. Hydrolyzes to form Xe, O₂, HF and XeO₃.

Xenon hexafluoride. [13693-09-9] F_6Xe; mol wt 245.28. Laboratory prepn: Chernick *et al.*, *Inorg. Synth.* **8**, 258 (1966). Colorless solid; greenish-yellow vapor; vapor press. about 30 mm at 25°. mp 49.48°; bp 75.57°; $d^{24.4}$(solid) 3.411; $d^{55.2}$(liq) 3.173: Schreiner *et al.*, *J. Chem. Phys.* **51**, 4838 (1969). Hydrolyzed by water to form XeOF$_4$ and XeO$_3$. More powerful oxidizing and fluorinating agent than XeF$_2$ and XeF$_4$. Cannot be stored in glass or quartz containers.

Xenon trioxide. [13776-58-4] O₃Xe; mol wt 179.29. Prepn: Williamson, Koch, *Science* **139**, 1046 (1963); Jaselskis *et al.*, *J. Am. Chem. Soc.* **88**, 2149 (1966). *Powerful explosive*, formed when XeF$_4$ and XeF$_6$ are hydrolyzed. Colorless, hygroscopic solid; d 4.55. Aqueous solns, *"xenic acid"*, may be prepd in concns >2*M*.

Caution: Can act as a simple asphyxiant by displacing air. *See: Matheson Gas Data Book* (Matheson Co., Inc., 4th ed., East Rutherford, NJ, 1966) pp 499-500.

USE: Gas in lamps designed to resemble natural daylight; in lamps of extremely high brilliance. Isotopes in leak detection systems for nuclear reactors.

THERAP CAT: Anesthetic (inhalation). Xenon[133] as diagnostic aid (radioactive imaging agent).

10073. *p*-Xenylcarbimide. [92-95-5] 4-Isocyanato-1,1′-bi-phenyl; isocyanic acid 4-biphenylyl ester; *p*-diphenyl isocyanate. $C_{13}H_9NO$; mol wt 195.22. C 79.98%, H 4.65%, N 7.17%, O 8.20%. Prepd from the corresponding amine and phosgene: Kaplan, *J. Chem. Eng. Data* **6**, 272 (1961).

Needles, mp 56°; bp 283° (decomp), bp$_{2-3}$ 137-140°. Very sol in ether.

USE: As a reagent for the identification of hydroxy compounds, with which it gives crystalline derivatives of definite melting point.

10074. X-gal. [7240-90-6] 5-Bromo-4-chloro-1*H*-indol-3-yl β-D-galactopyranoside. C$_{14}$H$_{15}$BrClNO$_6$; mol wt 408.63. C 41.15%, H 3.70%, Br 19.55%, Cl 8.68%, N 3.43%, O 23.49%. Chromogenic substrate of the *lacZ* gene product, β-galactosidase; produces a rich blue color when cleaved by the enzyme. Prepn: J. P. Horwitz *et al.*, *J. Med. Chem.* **7**, 574 (1964). Colorimetric reaction in tissue to localize β-galactosidase: B. Pearson *et al.*, *Lab. Invest.* **12**, 1249 (1963); Z. Lojda, *Histochemie* **23**, 266 (1970). Protocol for blue-white α-complementation screening: J. Sambrook *et al.*, *Molecular Cloning: A Laboratory Manual* (Cold Spring Harbor, New York, 2nd ed., 1989) pp 1.7-1.9, 1.85-1.87. Optimization of detection of exogenous bacterial *lacZ* expression: D. J. Weiss *et al.*, *Hum. Gene Ther.* **8**, 1545 (1997); of fixative conditions in X-gal staining: W. Ma *et al.*, *J. Histochem. Cytochem.* **50**, 1421 (2002); of blue-white screening procedure: A. L. Sherwood, *BioTechniques* **34**, 644 (2003).

Amorphous solid from methanol, mp 237-239° (dec). [α]$_D^{24}$ −69° (c = 1.0 in 50% DMF). Sol in DMF, DMSO.

USE: In histochemical staining, in blue-white selection of bacterial colonies with *lacZ* gene activity during cloning experiments.

10075. Xibenolol. [81584-06-7] 1-[(1,1-Dimethylethyl)-amino]-3-(2,3-dimethylphenoxy)-2-propanol; 3-(*tert*-butylamino)-3-(2',3'-dimethylphenoxy)-2-propanol; (±)-1-(*tert*-butylamino)-3-(2,3-xylyloxy)-2-propanol. C$_{15}$H$_{25}$NO$_2$; mol wt 251.36. C 71.67%, H 10.02%, N 5.57%, O 12.73%. Non-selective β-adrenergic blocker. Prepn: W. Kunz *et al.*, *DE 1236523* (1967 to Sanol-Arzneimittel), *C.A.* **67**, 64046k (1967); K. Tsukamoto *et al.*, *US 4018824* (1977 to Teikoku Hormone). Pharmacology in dogs: N. Himori *et al.*, *Arch. Int. Pharmacodyn.* **220**, 4 (1976); *eidem*, *Arch. Pharmacol.* **316**, 19 (1986). Metabolism in animals: S. Honma, A. Kambekawa, *Chem. Pharm. Bull.* **23**, 1045 (1975). Stereoselective metabolism and pharmacokinetics in man: S. Honma *et al.*, *ibid.* **33**, 760 (1985). Toxicology: T. Usui *et al.*, *Yakuri to Chiryo* **12**, Suppl. 6, 969, 987 (1984); *C.A.* **102**, 125280x, 125281y (1985).

Crystals from ether, mp 57°. bp$_{0.7mm}$ 134-136°. uv max (ethanol): 271.2, 274, 279.3 nm (ε 1.08×10^3, 1.07×10^3, 1.11×10^3).

Hydrochloride. [59708-57-5] D-32; Selapin; Rhythminal. C$_{15}$H$_{25}$NO$_2$.HCl; mol wt 287.83. mp 135-137°.

THERAP CAT: Antiarrhythmic.

10076. Xibornol. [13741-18-9] 6-Isobornyl-3,4-xylenol; 6-isobornyl-3,4-dimethylphenol; 6-(2-isobornyl)-3,4-xylen-1-ol; 3,4-dimethyl-6-isobornylphenol; Nanbacine. C$_{18}$H$_{26}$O; mol wt 258.40. C 83.67%, H 10.14%, O 6.19%. Syntheses: Moldovanskaya *et al.*, *C.A.* **66**, 76163p (1967); Starkov, Glushkova, *J. Appl. Chem. USSR* **40**, 209 (1967), *C.A.* **67**, 72960u (1967); *C.A.* **71**, 70225s (1969). Prepn of cryst substance: *GB 1206774* and Mardiguian, Fournier, *DE 2032170* (1970 and 1971 to MARPHA Soc. d'Etudes et d'Ex-

ploitation de Marques), *C.A.* **74**, 13299g, 88171t (1971). Activity study: Capponi, *Bull. Soc. Pathol. Exot.* **62**, 658 (1969), *C.A.* **73**, 118883a (1970).

Crystals from petr ether, mp 94-96°, bp$_3$ 165-168°. Also reported as very viscous, pale yellow liquid; bp$_9$ 185-189°. d$_4^{20}$ 1.0240. n$_D^{20}$ 1.5382 (Starkov, Glushkova).

USE: Rubber antioxidant.

THERAP CAT: Antibacterial.

10077. Ximelagatran. [192939-46-1] *N*-[(1*R*)-1-Cyclohex-yl-2-[(2*S*)-2-[[[[4-[(hydroxyamino)iminomethyl]phenyl]methyl]-amino]carbonyl]-1-azetidinyl]-2-oxoethyl]glycine; H-376/95; Exanta. C$_{24}$H$_{35}$N$_5$O$_5$; mol wt 473.57. C 60.87%, H 7.45%, N 14.79%, O 16.89%. Orally active direct thrombin inhibitor; prodrug of melagatran, *q.v.* Prepn: T. Antonsson *et al.*, *WO 9723499*; D. Gustafsson *et al.*, *US 5965692* (1997, 1999 both to Astra). CE determn in drug formulations: P. K. Owens *et al.*, *J. Pharm. Biomed. Anal.* **27**, 587 (2002). LC-MS determn in biological samples: M. Larsson *et al.*, *J. Chromatogr. B* **783**, 335 (2003). Clinical pharmacokinetics: K. Wahlander *et al.*, *Thromb. Res.* **107**, 93 (2002); in deep vein thrombosis: M. Cullberg *et al.*, *Clin. Pharmacol. Ther.* **77**, 279 (2005). Clinical study vs warfarin as thromboprophylactic: C. W. Francis *et al.*, *Ann. Intern. Med.* **137**, 648 (2002). Review of clinical experience in acute coronary syndromes: J. S. Kalus, M. F. Caron, *Expert Opin. Invest. Drugs* **13**, 465-477 (2004); of clinical development: C. J. Boos *et al.*, *Eur. J. Int. Med.* **16**, 267-278 (2005).

THERAP CAT: Antithrombotic.

10078. Ximoprofen. [56187-89-4] 4-[3-(Hydroxyimino)-cyclohexyl]-α-methylbenzeneacetic acid; *p*-(3-oxocyclohexyl)hy-dratropic acid oxime; XIFAM; 2-[4-(3-oximinocyclohexyl)phenyl]-propionic acid; 13832-JL. C$_{15}$H$_{19}$NO$_3$; mol wt 261.32. C 68.94%, H 7.33%, N 5.36%, O 18.37%. Nonsteroidal anti-inflammatory. Prepn: J. G. Maillard, *DE 2442910*; *idem*, *US 3935255* (1975, 1976 both to Lab. Jacques Logeais). Metabolism: B. C. Mayo *et al.*, *Xenobiotica* **20**, 233 (1990). Clinical pharmacokinetics: I. W. Taylor *et al.*, *Br. J. Clin. Pharmacol.* **32**, 242 (1991). GC determn in plasma: I. W. Taylor, L. F. Chasseaud, *J. Chromatogr.* **495**, 275 (1989). HPLC determn in urine: G. R. Morris *et al.*, *ibid.* **530**, 377 (1990). Clinical evaluation: M. Dougados *et al.*, *J. Rheumatol.* **16**, 1167 (1989).

Crystals from water/methanol, mp 178°.

THERAP CAT: Anti-inflammatory.

10079. Xipamide. [14293-44-8] 4-Chloro-5-sulfamoyl-2',6'-salicyloxylidide; 4-chloro-2',6'-dimethyl-5-sulfamoylsalicylanilide; 4-chloro-5-sulfamylsalicyloyl-2',6'-dimethylanilide; Bei-1293; Aquaphor; Chronexan; Diurexan; Lumitens. C$_{15}$H$_{15}$ClN$_2$O$_4$S;

mol wt 354.81. C 50.78%, H 4.26%, Cl 9.99%, N 7.90%, O 18.04%, S 9.04%. Salicylic acid derivative. Prepn: **NL 6607680**; Liebenow, **US 3567777** (1966, 1970 both to P. Beiersdorf). Clinical studies: O. Hammer, U. Dembowski, *Med. Klin.* **64**, 1862 (1969); R. Fischer, A. Lenhartz, *Med. Welt* **1970**, 270. Review of pharmacology and therapeutic efficacy: B. N. C. Prichard, R. N. Brogden, *Drugs* **30**, 313-332 (1985).

Crystals from methanol-water, mp 256°.
THERAP CAT: Diuretic; antihypertensive.

10080. Xylazine. [7361-61-7] *N*-(2,6-Dimethylphenyl)-5,6-dihydro-4*H*-1,3-thiazin-2-amine; 5,6-dihydro-2-(2,6-xylidino)-4*H*-1,3-thiazine; 2-(2,6-dimethylphenylamino)-4*H*-5,6-dihydro-1,3-thiazine; Bay 1470; Bay Va 1470; Wh-7286. C$_{12}$H$_{16}$N$_2$S; mol wt 220.33. C 65.41%, H 7.32%, N 12.71%, S 14.55%. Prepn: O. Behner *et al., BE 634552 C.A.* **61**, 4369b (1964); *eidem,* **DE 1173475** *C.A.* **61**, 13323c (1964); *eidem,* **US 3235550** (1964, 1964, 1966 all to Bayer). Pharmacology: G. Sagner *et al., Dtsch. Tieraerztl. Wochenschr.* **75**, 565 (1968); Kroneberg, Schlossman, *Arch. Pharmakol. Exp. Pathol.* **268**, 348 (1971). Metabolic studies: Duhm *et al., Berl. Muench. Tieraerztl. Wochenschr.* **82**, 104 (1969). Veterinary clinical studies: Clarke, Hall, *Vet. Rec.* **85**, 512 (1969); Burns, McMullan, *Vet. Med.* **67**, 77 (1972).

Colorless, almost tasteless crystals from benzene-ligroin, mp 140-142°. Also reported as mp 136-139°. Soluble in dilute acids, benzene, acetone, chloroform; sparingly sol in petr ether. Practically insol in water, alkalies. LD$_{50}$ in mice (mg/kg): 43 i.v.; 121 s.c.; 240 orally; LD$_{50}$ in rats (mg/kg): 130 orally (Sagner).
Hydrochloride. [23076-35-9] Narcoxyl; Rompun; Solvazine; Xylapan; Xylasol. C$_{12}$H$_{16}$N$_2$S.HCl; mol wt 256.79.
THERAP CAT (VET): Sedative, analgesic, muscle relaxant.

10081. Xylene. [1330-20-7] Dimethylbenzene; xylol. C$_8$H$_{10}$; mol wt 106.17. C 90.50%, H 9.49%. First isolated from a crude wood distillate: Cahours, *Compt. Rend.* **30**, 319 (1850). Obtained from coal tar: Fittig, *Ann.* **153**, 265 (1870). The xylene of commerce is a mixture of the three isomers *o*-, *m*- and *p*-xylene, the *m*-isomer predominating. Manuf from pseudocumene: Seubold, **US 2960545** (1960 to Union Oil); by catalytic isomerization of a hydrocarbon fraction: Berger, **US 3078318** (1963 to Universal Oil Prod.). Separation of isomers by clathration: Schaeffer, **US 3029300** (1962 to Union Oil). Use as clearing agent: K. Kubota, *J. Polym. Sci.* **5**, 1179 (1967); J. B. Matthews, *J. Clin. Pathol.* **34**, 103 (1981). Toxicity data: H. F. Smyth *et al., Am. Ind. Hyg. Assoc. J.* **23**, 95 (1962). Series of articles on toxicity: *Environ. Health Perspect.* **101**, Suppl. 6, 115-149 (1993). Review of toxicology and human exposure: *Toxicological Profile for Xylene* (PB95-264404, 1995) 298 pp; of mfg processes and properties: W. J. Cannella in *Kirk-Othmer Encyclopedia of Chemical Technology* **Suppl.** (Wiley-Interscience, New York, 4th ed., 1998) pp 831-863.

Mobile, flammable liquid; d ~0.86; bp 137-140°. Flash pt 29°C. Practically insol in water. Miscible with abs alcohol, ether, and many other organic liquids.

m-**Xylene.** [108-38-3] Colorless liquid; d$_4^{15}$ 0.8684; mp −47.4°; bp 139.3°; n$_D^{20}$ 1.4973. Flash pt, closed cup: 81°F (27°C). Insol in water. Miscible with alcohol, ether, and many other organic solvents. LD$_{50}$ orally in rats: 7.71 ml/kg (Smyth).
o-**Xylene.** [95-47-6] Colorless liquid; d$_4^{20}$ 0.8801; mp −25°; bp 144°; n$_D^{20}$ 1.5058. Flash pt, closed cup: 90°F (32°C). Insol in water. Miscible with alc, ether.
p-**Xylene.** [106-42-3] Colorless plates or prisms at low temp; d$_4^{20}$ 0.86104; mp 13-14°; bp 137-138°; n$_D^{20}$ 1.49575: Thorne *et al., Ind. Eng. Chem. Anal. Ed.* **17**, 481 (1945). Flash pt, closed cup: 81°F (27°C). Insol in water. Sol in alcohol, ether, organic solvents.
Caution: Potential symptoms of acute overexposure by inhalation to *m*-, *o*-, or *p*-isomers are flushing and reddening of the face, a feeling of increased heat due to dilation of superficial blood vessels, disturbed vision, dizziness, tremors, salivation, cardiac stress, drowsiness, incoordination and staggering gait, CNS depression, confusion, coma. Symptoms of chronic inhalation exposure may include respiratory irritation, CNS excitation followed by CNS depression, paresthesia, tremors, apprehension, impaired memory, weakness, nervous irritation, vertigo, headache, anorexia, nausea, flatulence, anemia, mucosal hemorrhage. Overexposure by ingestion may cause severe GI distress. Aspiration into lungs may cause chemical pneumonitis, pulmonary edema, hemorrhage. Direct contact may cause eye irritation, conjuctivitis, corneal burns; skin irritation and dermatitis due to defatting action. *See Patty's Industrial Hygiene and Toxicology* **vol. 2B**, G. D. Clayton, F. E. Clayton, Eds. (Wiley-Interscience, New York, 4th ed., 1994) p 1332-1339; *NIOSH Pocket Guide to Chemical Hazards* (DHHS/NIOSH 97-140, 1997) pp 334-337.
USE: As solvent; raw material for production of benzoic acid, phthalic anhydride, isophthalic and terephthalic acids as well as their dimethyl esters used in the manufacture of polyester fibers; manuf dyes and other organics; sterilizing catgut; with Canada balsam as oil-immersion in microscopy; clearing agent in microscope technique.

10082. Xylenol. [1300-71-6] Dimethylphenol. C$_8$H$_{10}$O; mol wt 122.16. C 78.66%, H 8.25%, O 13.10%. (CH$_3$)$_2$C$_6$H$_3$-OH. Constituent of "cresylic acid." There are 6 isomers of xylenol. They are only slightly sol in water but freely sol in alcohol, chloroform, ether, benzene, etc.; also sol in NaOH soln. Prepn and physical properties: R. J. L. Andon *et al., J. Chem. Soc.* **1960**, 5246.
2,3-Dimethylphenol. *vic-o*-Xylenol. Needles from water or dil alc, mp 75°, bp 218°: Thöl, *Ber.* **18**, 2561 (1885); also reported as mp 72.57 ±0.02°, bp$_{760}$ 216.87 ±0.001° (Andon).
2,4-Dimethylphenol. *as-m*-Xylenol. Crystals, bp$_{766}$ 211.5°, mp 25.4-26°: Jacobsen, *Ber.* **11**, 17 (1878); **18**, 3463 (1885); also reported as mp 24.54 ±0.01°, bp$_{760}$ 210.931 ±0.001° (Andon).
2,5-Dimethylphenol. *p*-Xylenol. Crystals from alcohol + ether, mp 74.5°, bp$_{762}$ 211.5° (Jacobsen); bp 213.5°: Würtz, *Ann.* **147**, 372 (1868); also reported as mp 74.85 ±0.02°, bp$_{760}$ 211.132 ±0.002° (Andon).
2,6-Dimethylphenol. *vic-m*-Xylenol. Needles, mp 49°, bp 203°: Gattermann, *Ann.* **357**, 313 (1907); also reported as mp 45.62 ±0.01°, bp$_{760}$ 201.030 ±0.001° (Andon).
3,4-Dimethylphenol. *as-o*-Xylenol. Needles from water, mp 62.5°, bp 225°: Jacobsen, *Ber.* **17**, 159 (1884); also reported as mp 65.11 ±0.01°, bp$_{760}$ 226.947 ±0.001° (Andon).
3,5-Dimethylphenol. *sym-m*-Xylenol. Needles from water, mp 64°, bp 219.5°: Thöl, *Ber.* **18**, 359 (1885); also reported as mp 63.27 ±0.02°, bp$_{760}$ 221.962 ±0.003° (Andon). LD$_{50}$ orally in mice: 620 mg/kg: W. A. McOmie *et al., J. Am. Pharm. Assoc.* **38**, 366 (1949).
USE: For the prepn of coal tar disinfectants; manuf of artificial resins.

10083. Xylenol Blue. [125-31-5] 4,4′-(3*H*-2,1-Benzoxathiol-3-ylidene)bis[2,5-dimethylphenol] *S,S*-dioxide; *p*-xylenolsulfone-phthalein; 1,4-dimethyl-5-hydroxybenzenesulfonephthalein; α,4,4′-trihydroxy-2,5,2′,5′-tetramethyltriphenylmethane-2″-sulfonic acid γ-sultone. C$_{23}$H$_{22}$O$_5$S; mol wt 410.48. C 67.30%, H 5.40%, O 19.49%, S 7.81%. Prepd from *o*-sulfobenzoic acid dichloride or *o*-sulfobenzoic acid anhydride and *p*-xylenol in the presence of zinc chloride: Cohen, *Biochem. J.* **16**, 31 (1922).

Brown crystals from alcohol.

USE: Indicator, used in 0.02% soln: pH 1.2 red, 2.8 yellow, 9.6 blue.

10084. Xylidine. [1300-73-8] *ar,ar*-Dimethylbenzenamine; dimethylaniline; aminodimethylbenzene. $C_8H_{11}N$; mol wt 121.18. C 79.29%, H 9.15%, N 11.56%. $(CH_3)_2C_6H_3NH_2$. There are six isomeric xylidines. Prepd by reduction of corresponding nitro-compounds: Allchin, **US 1867962** (to I.C.I.); physical properties of all six isomers also given: Birch *et al., J. Am. Chem. Soc.* **71**, 1362 (1949); van Loon *et al., Rec. Trav. Chim.* **79**, 977 (1960); Bergmann, Berkovic, *J. Org. Chem.* **26**, 919 (1961).

All except *o*-4-xylidine are liquids above 20°. d 0.97-0.99, and bp 213-226°. They are sparingly sol in water, sol in alcohol and form more or less sol salts with the strong mineral acids.

Caution: Potential symptoms of overexposure are anoxia, cyanosis, methemoglobinemia; lung, liver and kidney damage. *See NIOSH Pocket Guide to Chemical Hazards* (DHHS/NIOSH 97-140, 1997) p 336.

USE: Chiefly in the manuf of dyes.

10085. Xylitol. [87-99-0] *xylo*-Pentane-1,2,3,4,5-pentol; xylite; Eutrit; Kannit; Klinit; Kylit; Newtol; Torch; Xyliton. $C_5H_{12}O_5$; mol wt 152.15. C 39.47%, H 7.95%, O 52.58%. Intermediate in metabolism of D-glucose through glucuronate cycle in livers. Prepd by reduction of xylose: G. Bertrand, *Bull. Soc. Chim. Fr.* [3] **5**, 555 (1891); E. Fischer, R. Stahel, *Ber.* **24**, 538 (1891). Prepn of metastable crystals: M. L. Wolfrom, E. J. Kohn, *J. Am. Chem. Soc.* **64**, 1739 (1942); of stable form: J. F. Carson *et al., ibid.* **65**, 1777 (1943). Crystal structure: H. S. Kim, G. A. Jeffrey, *Acta Crystallogr.* **25B**, 2607 (1969). Use in prevention of dental caries: E. Grunberg *et al., Int. J. Vitam. Nutr. Res.* **43**, 227 (1973); A. Scheinin, K. K. Makinen, **DE 2606533** (1976 to Hoffmann-La Roche), *C.A.* **85**, 149140h (1976). Acute toxicity: S. Salminen *et al., Toxicol. Lett.* **18**, Suppl. 1, 37 (1983). Reviews of toxicity, metabolism and use as dietary additive: *International Symposium on Metabolism, Physiology and Clinical Uses of Pentoses and Pentitols,* B. L. Horecker *et al.,* Eds. (Springer-Verlag, New York, 1969) 408 pp; *Sugars in Nutrition,* H. L. Sipple, K. W. McNutt, Eds. (Academic Press, New York, 1974) *passim;* G. E. Demetrakopoulos, H. Amos, *World Rev. Nutr. Diet* **32**, 96-122 (1979); R. Ylikahri, *Adv. Food Res.* **25**, 159-180 (1979). Book: *Xylitol,* J. N. Counsel, Ed. (Applied Science, London, 1978) 191 pp.

$$CH_2OH$$
$$HC{-}OH$$
$$HO{-}CH$$
$$HC{-}OH$$
$$CH_2OH$$

Stable form: orthorhombic needles from THF, prisms from ethanol; mp 93-94.5°; d 1.52. Metastable form: colorless, monoclinic, lath-shaped crystals from anhydrous methanol; hygroscopic; mp 61-61.5°. Soly of stable form (g/100 g soln): abs methanol 6.0; abs ethanol 1.2; water 64.2. Relative sweetness equal to sucrose. LD_{50} orally in mice: approx 22 g/kg (Salminen).

USE: As oral and intravenous nutrient; in anticaries preparations.

10086. Xylometazoline. [526-36-3] 2-[[4-(1,1-Dimethylethyl)-2,6-dimethylphenyl]methyl]-4,5-dihydro-1*H*-imidazole; 2-(4-*tert*-butyl-2,6-dimethylbenzyl)-2-imidazoline. $C_{16}H_{24}N_2$; mol wt 244.38. C 78.64%, H 9.90%, N 11.46%. α-Adrenergic agonist;

topical vasoconstrictor. Prepn: Hüni, **US 2868802** (1959 to Ciba). Pharmacology: S. Morimoto, H. Tanaka, *Osaka-shiritsu Daigaku Igaku Zasshi* **18**, 211 (1969), *C.A.* **72**, 20437n (1970). Comprehensive description: Y. Golander, W. J. DeWitte, *Anal. Profiles Drug Subs.* **14**, 135-156 (1985). GC determn in plasma and urine: A. Sioufi *et al., J. Chromatogr.* **487**, 81 (1989). Clinical trial in allergic rhinitis: M. Fradis *et al., J. Laryngol. Otol.* **101**, 666 (1987); in nasal surgery: J. P. Campbell *et al., Otolaryngol. Head Neck Surg.* **107**, 697 (1992).

mp 131-133°.

Hydrochloride. [1218-35-5] Novorin; Olynth; Otrivine; Xymelin. $C_{16}H_{24}N_2 \cdot HCl$; mol wt 280.84. Soly in water: up to 3%; also sol in methanol, ethanol. Practically insol in ether, benzene.

THERAP CAT: Decongestant.

10087. Xylose. [58-86-6] D-Xylose; wood sugar; Xylomed; Xylo-Pfan. $C_5H_{10}O_5$; mol wt 150.13. C 40.00%, H 6.71%, O 53.29%. Widely distributed in plant materials, especially in wood (maple, cherry), in straw, in hulls. Not found in free state, but in form of xylan, a polysaccharide built from D-xylose units and occurring in association with cellulose. Xylose occurs also as part of glycosides. Isoln from corn cobs by boiling with 8% H_2SO_4: Monroe, *J. Am. Chem. Soc.* **41**, 1002 (1919). Peanut shells and cottonseed hulls also are practical sources of xylose: Ling, Nanji, *J. Chem. Soc.* **1923**, 620. Configuration: Hudson, Yanovsky, *J. Am. Chem. Soc.* **39**, 1029 (1917); Haworth, *Nature* **116**, 430 (1925). Review on history, constitution and prepn: Harding, *Sugar* **24**, 14 (1922).

Monoclinic needles or prisms. Very sweet taste. mp 144-145° (Wheeler, Tollens, *Ann.* **254**, 309); mp 153-154° (Hébert, *Compt. Rend.* **110**, 970). d_4^{20} 1.525. Shows mutarotation. $[\alpha]_D^{20} +92° \rightarrow +18.6°$ (16 hrs c = 10). One gram dissolves in 0.8 ml water. Sol in pyridine, hot alcohol. pKa (18°): 12.14. Reduces warm Fehling's soln. Upon heating with water in closed tube to 140° or by boiling with dil H_2SO_4, furfurol is formed.

USE: In tanning, dyeing, and as a diabetic food.

THERAP CAT: Diagnostic aid (intestinal function).

10088. Xylulose. [5962-29-8] *threo*-Pentulose. $C_5H_{10}O_5$; mol wt 150.13. C 40.00%, H 6.71%, O 53.29%. L-Form has been found in the urine of humans with pentosuria. Prepn of DL-form: Gascoigne, *Chem. Ind. (London)* **1959**, 402; of D-form: Mendicino, *J. Am. Chem. Soc.* **82**, 4975 (1960); of L-form: Wolfrom, Bennett, *J. Org. Chem.* **30**, 458 (1965). Isoln of DL-form from the acid hydrolysate of bagasse hemicellulose: Banerjee *et al., Sci. Cult.* **27**, 498 (1961), *C.A.* **56**, 11682d (1962). Enzymic prepn of L-form: Hough, Jones, *Chem. Ind. (London)* **1952**, 907; *eidem, J. Chem. Soc.* **1952**, 4047. Formation of L-form in normal humans and guinea pigs, and its utilization by guinea-pig liver prepns: Touster *et al., J. Am. Chem. Soc.* **76**, 5005 (1954). Reviews: *The Carbohydrates,* W. Pigman, Ed. (Academic Press, New York, 1957) pp 80, 86-87, 759, 795; *Methods in Carbohydrate Chemistry* vol. **1**, R. L. Whistler, M. L. Wolfrom, Eds. (Academic Press, New York, 1962) pp 94-101.

$$CH_2OH$$
$$C{=}O$$
$$HC{-}OH$$
$$HO{-}CH$$
$$CH_2OH$$

L-isomer

D-Isomer. Syrup. $[\alpha]_D^{18}$ −33° (c = 2.5).

D-Isomer p-bromophenylhydrazone. $C_{11}H_{15}BrN_2O_4$. Pale yellow crystals from abs ethanol + water, mp 128-129°. $[\alpha]_D^{20}$ +24° (15 min) → −31° (7 days, in pyridine).

L-Isomer. Syrup. $[\alpha]_D^{21}$ +31°.

L-Isomer p-bromophenylhydrazone. Yellow plates from dil alc, mp 128°. $[\alpha]_D^{20}$ −20° (10 min) → +22° (5 hrs, c = 0.5 in ethanol).

10089. 1-Xylylazo-2-naphthol. [85-82-5] 1-[(2,4-Dimethylphenyl)azo]-2-naphthalenol; C.I. Solvent Orange 7; 1-(2,4-xylylazo)-2-naphthol; FD & C Red no. 32; Oil Red XO; Ext. D & C Red no. 14; C.I. 12140. $C_{18}H_{16}N_2O$; mol wt 276.33. C 78.24%, H 5.84%, N 10.14%, O 5.79%. Once reported as 2,5-xylylazo deriv. Prepd by coupling diazotized m-xylidene with 2-naphthol: J. M. Tedder, *J. Chem. Soc.* **1957**, 4003; R. B. Smyth, G. G. McKeown, *J. Chromatogr.* **5**, 395 (1961). Metabolism: J. L. Radomski, *J. Pharmacol. Exp. Ther.* **136**, 378 (1962).

Red needles, mp 166°. Insol in water; sol in ethanol, acetone, benzene.

10090. Xylyl Bromide. C_8H_9Br; mol wt 185.06. C 51.92%, H 4.90%, Br 43.18%. Prepn of m-isomer: Wenner, *J. Org. Chem.* **17**, 523 (1952); of o-isomer: Dev, *J. Indian Chem. Soc.* **32**, 403 (1955); of p-isomer: Cockburn et al., *J. Chem. Soc.* **1960**, 3340.

m-Xylyl bromide. [620-13-3] 1-(Bromomethyl)-3-methylbenzene; α-bromo-m-xylene; m-methylbenzyl bromide; ω-bromo-m-xylene. Liquid, bp 212-215° with slight dec. d^{23} 1.371. Practically insol in water; sol in alcohol, ether.

o-Xylyl bromide. [89-92-9] Prisms, mp 21°. bp 223-234°, bp_{742} 216-217°, bp_{15} 102°. n_D^{27} 1.5730. d^{23} 1.381. Practically insol in water. Sol in alcohol, ether.

p-Xylyl bromide. [104-81-4] Needles from alcohol, mp 38°. bp_{740} 218-220°, bp_{15} 120°. d 1.324. Practically insol in water. Very sol in chloroform, hot ether.

Caution: Powerful lacrimator.

USE: In organic syntheses; in war-gas formulations.

10091. Xylyl Chloride. C_8H_9Cl; mol wt 140.61. C 68.33%, H 6.45%, Cl 25.21%. Prepn of o-isomer: Rabjohn, *J. Am. Chem. Soc.* **76**, 5479 (1954); of m-isomer: van Zanten, Nauta, *Rec. Trav. Chim.* **79**, 1211 (1960); of p-isomer: Newman, George, *J. Org. Chem.* **26**, 4306 (1961).

m-Xylyl chloride. [620-19-9] 1-(Chloromethyl)-3-methylbenzene; α-chloro-m-xylene; m-methylbenzyl chloride; ω-chloro-m-xylene. Liquid, bp 195-196°. bp_{10} 90-92°. d^{20} 1.064. Practically insol in water; miscible with abs alcohol, ether.

o-Xylyl chloride. [552-45-4] Liquid, bp 195-203°, bp_{25} 95-96°. n_D^{20} 1.5391. Practically insol in water; miscible with abs alcohol, ether.

p-Xylyl chloride. [104-82-5] Fuming liquid, characteristic odor. bp 200-202°, bp_1 48-50°. n_D^{17} 1.5360. Practically insol in water; miscible with abs alcohol, ether.

Caution: Powerful lacrimator.

Y

10092. Yam, Mexican. Giant yam; cabeza de negro. *Dioscorea macrostachya* Benth., *Dioscoreaceae* or one of ~600 other *Dioscoreae*, native to subtropical countries. The underground tubers weigh as much as 90 lbs. and contain steroidal sapogenins. Account of nature, origins, cultivation and utilization of the useful members of the *Dioscoreaceae:* D. G. Coursey, *Yams* (Longmans, London, 1967) 230 pp. *See also* Dioscorea and Barbasco.

USE: In the partial synthesis of hormones having a steroid structure.

10093. Yangonin. [500-62-9] (*E*)-4-Methoxy-6-[2-(4-methoxyphenyl)ethenyl]-2*H*-pyran-2-one; 4-methoxy-6-(*p*-methoxystyryl)-2*H*-pyran-2-one; 5-hydroxy-3-methoxy-7-(*p*-methoxyphenyl)-2,4,6-heptatrienoic acid δ-lactone; 4-methoxy-6-[β-(*p*-anisyl)-vinyl]-α-pyrone; 6-(*p*-methoxystyryl)-4-methoxy-α-pyrone. C$_{15}$-H$_{14}$O$_4$; mol wt 258.27. C 69.76%, H 5.46%, O 24.78%. From root of *Piper methysticum* Forst., *Piperaceae* (kava): Winzhermer, *Arch. Pharm.* **246**, 338 (1908); Borsche, Gerhardt, *Ber.* **47**, 2902 (1914). From *Ranunculus quelpaertensis* Nakai, *Ranunculaceae:* Shibata *et al.*, *Bull. Chem. Soc. Jpn.* **45**, 930 (1972). Structure: Chmielewska *et al.*, *Tetrahedron* **4**, 36 (1958); Bu'Lock, Smith, *J. Chem. Soc.* **1960**, 502. Synthesis: Harris, Combs, *J. Org. Chem.* **33**, 2399 (1968); R. Bacardit, *J. Heterocycl. Chem.* **19**, 157 (1982). Molecular and crystal structure: Engel, Nowacki, *Z. Kristallogr. Kristallgeom. Kristallphys. Kristallchem.* **134**, 180 (1971). Activity studies: Kretzschmar *et al.*, *Arch. Int. Pharmacodyn. Ther.* **180**, 471 (1969).

Crystals from methanol, mp 155-157°. uv max (ethanol): 360 nm (log ε 4.33). Practically insol in water; sol in hot alcohol, glacial acetic acid, ethyl acetate, acetone; slightly sol in benzene, ether.
Dihydroyangonin. C$_{15}$H$_{16}$O$_4$. Needles from alc, mp 106-107°. uv max (methanol): 274, 228 nm (log ε 3.82, 3.71).

10094. Yeast. The moist, living cells of a fungus or fungi whose usual and dominant growth form is unicellular. The term yeast is not one with an exact botanical meaning, *see Henrici's Molds, Yeasts and Actinomycetes* (New York, 1947) p 264 sqq. Normally produces alcoholic fermentation in fluids contg sugar. Moist yeast is usually combined with a starchy or absorbent base and comes on the market in the form of white or yellowish-white, soft, easily broken masses of a characteristic, slightly sour odor. Description of a modern process of manuf: Schultz, Swift, US 2717837 (1955 to Standard Brands).

The dried yeast of pharmacopoeias consists of the dry cells of any suitable strain of *Saccharomyces cerevisiae* Meyen, *Saccharomytaceae* or *Candida utilis* (Hanneberg) Lodder and Kreger-Van Rij, *Cryptococcaceae* (torula yeast), usually obtained as a by-product from the brewing of beer made from an extract of cereal grains and hops. The yeast cells are washed free of beer and dried, and may be debittered. These yeasts are commonly known as "Brewer's Dried Yeast" and "Debittered Brewer's Dried Yeast." Dried yeast may be obtained also by growing suitable strains of yeast, using media other than those required for the production of beer, and under appropriate environmental conditions. The yeast thus obtained is commonly known as "Primary Dried Yeast." Dried yeast that fulfills pharmacopeal requirements contains not less than 40% protein, and, in each gram, the equivalent of not less than 0.12 mg of thiamine hydrochloride, 0.04 mg of riboflavin, and 0.25 mg of nicotinic acid. It occurs as yellowish-white to weak yellowish-orange flakes, granules or powder, having an odor indicative of the type. It is inactive in fermenting power.

USE: Moist yeast in baking bread, brewing; producing alcohol by fermentation of sugar, molasses, and cereals; as a source of vitamins. Dried yeast as a source of vitamins; in baking.

THERAP CAT: Source of protein and vitamin B complex.
THERAP CAT (VET): Dietary source of B vitamins.

10095. Yellow AB. [85-84-7] 1-Phenylazo-2-naphthalenamine; C.I. Solvent Yellow 5; FD & C Yellow no. 3; Ext. D & C Yellow no. 9; C.I. 11380. C$_{16}$H$_{13}$N$_3$; mol wt 247.29. C 77.71%, H 5.30%, N 16.99%. Prepd from diazotized aniline and β-naphthylamine: Lawson, *Ber.* **18**, 796 (1885); *Colour Index* **vol. 4** (3rd ed., 1971) p 4021. Toxicity studies: Allmark *et al.*, *J. Pharm. Pharmacol.* **7**, 591 (1955); Hansen *et al.*, *Toxicol. Appl. Pharmacol.* **5**, 16 (1963). Formerly used in the U.S. for coloring oleomargarine.

Red platelets from abs alc, mp 102-104°. Practically insol in water. Sol in alcohol, carbon tetrachloride, acetic acid, vegetable oils. An alcoholic soln becomes redder with HCl addition, and is unaltered by NaOH addition.

10096. Yellow OB. [131-79-3] 1-[(2-Methylphenyl)azo]-2-naphthalenamine; C.I. Solvent Yellow 6; 1-*o*-tolylazo-2-naphthylamine; FD & C Yellow no. 4; Ext. D & C Yellow no. 10; C.I. 11390. C$_{17}$H$_{15}$N$_3$; mol wt 261.32. C 78.13%, H 5.79%, N 16.08%. Prepd from diazotized *o*-toluidine and β-naphthylamine: Krüss, *Z. Phys. Chem.* **51**, 270 (1905); Norman, *J. Chem. Soc.* **101**, 1913 (1912); Fischer, *J. Prakt. Chem.* **104**, 102 (1922); Hodgson, Foster, *J. Chem. Soc.* **1942**, 30. Toxicity studies: Allmark *et al.*, *J. Pharm. Pharmacol.* **7**, 591 (1955); Hansen *et al.*, *Toxicol. Appl. Pharmacol.* **5**, 16 (1963). Formerly used in the U.S. for coloring oleomargarine.

Deep red crystals from alc. Also reported as bright yellow needles (Krüss). mp 125-126° (Fischer). Practically insol in water. Sol in alc, ether, benzene, carbon tetrachloride, vegetable oils, glacial acetic acid. An alcoholic soln becomes redder with HCl addition, but is unaltered by NaOH addition.

10097. Yig. [12063-56-8] Iron yttrium oxide; yttrium iron garnet. Fe$_5$O$_{12}$Y$_3$; mol wt 737.94. Fe 37.84%, O 26.02%, Y 36.14%. Y$_3$Fe$_5$O$_{12}$. Man-made mineral. Prepn by molten salt technique: Nielsen, *Electronics*, Jan. 31, **1964**, pp 44-45. Advances in manufacture and applications: Gundlach, *ibid.*, Oct. 14, **1968**, pp 104-118. Electronic structure: Y.-N. Xu *et al.*, *J. Appl. Phys.* **87**, 4867 (2000).

Hard, brittle, garnet-type crystals. Hardness about equal to that of quartz. mp >1040°. The melt is easily amenable to doping and crystal nucleation by epitaxy. Crystals may be oriented along the simple axes (100), (110), and (111) using the natural (110) face of the crystal.

USE: In microwave tunable filters and limiters.

10098. Yingzhaosu. Family of sesquiterpenes isolated from the roots of *Yingzhao,* (*Artabotrys uncinatus* (L.) Merr.) a traditional Chinese herbal medicine for treatment of malaria. Yingzhaosu A & C contain a peroxy group which is needed for antimalarial activity. Isoln of A: X.-T. Liang *et al.*, *Acta Chim. Sin.* **37**, 215 (1979), *C.A.* **92**, 146954 (1980); of C: L. Zhang *et al.*, *J. Chem. Soc. Chem. Commun.* **1988**, 523. Structure of C: *eidem*, *Sci. China Ser. B* **32**, 800 (1989). Total synthesis of A: X.-X. Xu *et al.*, *Tetrahedron Lett.* **32**, 5785 (1991); stereocontrolled synthesis: W.-S. Zhou in *Newer Trends Essent. Oils. Flavours*, Sel. Pap. Int. Symp., K. L. Dhar *et al.*, Eds. (Tata McGraw-Hill, New Delhi, India, 1993) pp 43-50. Enantioselective synthesis of C: X.-X. Xu, H.-Q. Dong, *J. Org. Chem.* **60**, 3039 (1995).

Yingzhaosu A

Yingzhaosu A. [73301-54-9] (3S,4E)-5-[(1S,4S,5S,8R)-4,8-Dimethyl-2,3-dioxabicyclo[3.3.1]non-4-yl]-2-methyl-4-pentene-2,3-diol; (+)-yingzhosu A. $C_{15}H_{26}O_4$; mol wt 270.36. Contains a unique dioxabicyclo[3.3.1]nonane ring system. Isolated as solid, mp 95-96°. $[\alpha]_D^{25}$ +226° (in CHCl$_3$).

Yingzhaosu C. [121067-52-5] (3R,6S)-rel-α,α,6-Trimethyl-6-(4-methylphenyl)-1,2-dioxane-3-methanol. $C_{15}H_{22}O_3$; mol wt 250.33. Occurs naturally as an enantiomeric mixture of the (3R,6S), (3S,6R) with a predominance of the former. Oily substance. $[\alpha]_D^{14}$ +2.89° (c = 2.15 in methanol); (6S,3R): $[\alpha]_D$ +189.3° (c = 0.93 in CHCl$_3$); (3S,6R): $[\alpha]_D$ −185.4° (c = 0.78 in CHCl$_3$).

THERAP CAT: Antimalarial.

10099. Ylangene. [14912-44-8] 1,3-Dimethyl-8-(1-methylethyl)tricyclo[4.4.0.0^{2,7}]dec-3-ene; (1S,2R,6R,7R,8S)-(+)-8-isopropyl-1,3-dimethyltricyclo[4.4.0.0^{2,7}]dec-3-ene; α-ylangene. $C_{15}H_{24}$; mol wt 204.35. C 88.16%, H 11.84%. From ylang-ylang oil: Heraut, Dimitrov, Chem. Listy **46**, 432 (1952); from oil of birch buds: Holub et al., Collect. Czech. Chem. Commun. **24**, 3730 (1959); from oil of Juniperus oxycedrus Linn., Cupressaceae: Motl et al., ibid. **25**, 1656 (1960). Structure: Motl et al., Chem. Ind. (London) **1963**, 1759; Hunter, Brogden, J. Org. Chem. **29**, 982 (1964); Motl et al., Tetrahedron Lett. **1965**, 451. Stereoisomer of copaene, q.v. Total synthesis of (±)-form: Heathcock et al., J. Am. Chem. Soc. **89**, 4133 (1967); Corey, Watt, ibid. **95**, 2303 (1973).

Oil. d$_4^{20}$ 0.9091. n$_D^{20}$ 1.4934. $[\alpha]_D^{20}$ +15.4°.

10100. Ylang-Ylang Oil. Cananga oil. Volatile oil distilled in Madagascar, Reunion Island, Comoro Islands and the Philippine Islands from freshly picked flowers of Cananga odorata Hook & Thoms., Anonaceae. The first distillate yields the so-called "ylang-ylang extra" and is the finest oil. The first, second and third fractions follow, the first two having insignificant commercial value. Constit. Geraniol and linalool esters of acetic and benzoic acids; p-cresol methyl ether, cadinene, a sesquiterpene, a phenol.

Light yellow, very fragrant liquid. d$_{20}^{20}$ 0.930-0.950. Rotation: −27° to −50° in 100-mm tube.

USE: In delicate perfumes.

10101. Yogurt. Yoghurt; joghurt; kisselo-mleko; mazun; leben raib; dahi. Fermented whole milk. Produced by evaporating milk to ~50% of its volume and maintaining at 50°C for 3 hrs after adding "maya" a mixture of Lactobacillus bulgaricus, L. acidophilus, and Streptococcus lactis. Used as food. Contains antibacterial principles. Differentiation of yogurt and **clabber** as produced in Kentucky: J. Am. Med. Assoc. **209**, 778 (1969).

10102. Yohimbine. [146-48-5] (16α,17α)-17-Hydroxy-yohimban-16-carboxylic acid methyl ester; quebrachine; corynine; aphrodine. $C_{21}H_{26}N_2O_3$; mol wt 354.44. C 71.16%, H 7.39%, N 7.90%, O 13.54%. Indole alkaloid with α$_2$-adrenergic blocking activity. Found in Corynanthe johimbe K. Schum., Rubiaceae and related trees, also in Rauwolfia serpentina (L.) Benth., Apocynaceae: Raymond-Hamet, J. Pharm. Chim. **19**, 209 (1934); Hofmann, Helv. Chim. Acta **37**, 849 (1954); Stoll, Jucker, Ullmanns Encyklopädie der technischen Chemie vol. 3 (Munich, 3rd ed., 1953) p 266; Bader et al., J. Am. Chem. Soc. **76**, 1695 (1954). Structure: Witkop, Ann. **554**, 83 (1943); Clemo, Swan, J. Chem. Soc. **1946**, 617. Stereochemistry: Janot et al., Bull. Soc. Chim. Fr. **1952**, 1085; Godfredsen, Vandegal, Acta Chem. Scand. **10**, 1414

(1956); Van Tamelen et al., J. Am. Chem. Soc. **78**, 4628 (1956); Ban, Yonemitsu, Tetrahedron **20**, 2877 (1964). Synthesis: Van Tamelen et al., J. Am. Chem. Soc. **80**, 5006 (1958); Liljegren, Potts, J. Org. Chem. **27**, 377 (1962). Total synthesis: Van Tamelen et al., J. Am. Chem. Soc. **91**, 7315 (1969); Stork, Guthikonda, ibid. **94**, 5109 (1972); T. Kametani et al., Chem. Pharm. Bull. **24**, 2500 (1976); E. Wenkert et al., J. Am. Chem. Soc. **100**, 4894 (1978); **101**, 5370 (1979); **104**, 2244 (1982); I. Ninomiya et al., Heterocycles **14**, 631 (1980). Pharmacokinetics in humans: J. A. Owen et al., Eur. J. Clin. Pharmacol. **32**, 577 (1987). Clinical studies in impotence: K. Reid et al., Lancet **2**, 421 (1987); A. Morales et al., J. Urol. **137**, 1168 (1987). Review of pharmacology and use in molecular studies of α$_2$-adrenoreceptor: M. R. Goldberg, D. Robertson, Pharmacol. Rev. **35**, 143-180 (1987). Comprehensive description: A. G. Mekkawi, A. A. Al-Badr, Anal. Profiles Drug Subs. **16**, 731-768 (1986).

Orthorhombic needles from dil alc, mp 234°. Also mp 235-237°. $[\alpha]_D^{20}$ +50.9 to +62.2° (ethanol); $[\alpha]_D^{20}$ +108° (pyridine); $[\alpha]_{546}^{20}$ +129° (c = 0.5 in pyridine). uv max (methanol): 226, 280, 291 nm (log ε 4.56, 3.88, 3.80). Sparingly sol in water. Sol in alcohol, chloroform, hot benzene; moderately sol in ether.

Hydrochloride. [65-19-0] Antagonil; Aphrodyne; Erex; Yobine; Yocon; Yohimex; Yohydrol; Yovital. $C_{21}H_{26}N_2O_3 \cdot HCl$; mol wt 390.90. Orthorhombic plates, prisms from alc; dec 302°. $[\alpha]_D^{22}$ +105° (H$_2$O). Sol in ~120 ml water, 400 ml alc. The aq soln is about neutral.

USE: Pharmacological probe for the study of α$_2$-adrenoceptor.

THERAP CAT: Mydriatic. In treatment of impotence.

THERAP CAT (VET): Xylazine reversing agent.

10103. allo-Yohimbine. [522-94-1] 17-Hydroxyyohimban-16-carboxylic acid methyl ester; alloyohimbine; dihydroyohimbine. $C_{21}H_{26}N_2O_3$; mol wt 354.44. C 71.16%, H 7.39%, N 7.90%, O 13.54%. From bark of Corynanthe johimbe K. Schum., Rubiaceae: Warnat, Ber. **59**, 2388 (1926); Hahn, Brandenberg, ibid. **60**, 699 (1927). Identity with dihydroyohimbine: Heinemann, ibid. **67**, 15 (1934). Structure and stereochemistry: LeHir et al., Bull. Soc. Chim. Fr. **1953**, 1027; Janot et al., ibid. **1961**, 637. Revised structure and total synthesis: Töke et al., J. Org. Chem. **38**, 2496 (1973). Total synthesis: E. Wenkert et al., J. Am. Chem. Soc. **101**, 5370 (1979). Review: A. Chatterjee et al., "Rauwolfia Alkaloids" in Zechmeister, Progress in the Chemistry of Organic Natural Products vol. **XIII** (Springer Verlag, Vienna, 1956) pp 354-356.

Trihydrate, needles from 50% alcohol, mp 98-99°. After drying at 100° and 0.01 mm Hg for 24 hrs, the anhydrous form melts at 135-140°. $[\alpha]_D^{19}$ +84° (c = 0.40 in pyridine). uv max (methanol): 225, 280, 290 nm (log ε 4.52, 3.91, 3.74). Sol in ethanol, methanol, pyridine, dil acids; slightly sol in benzene. Practically insol in water.

10104. α-Yohimbine. [131-03-3] 17α-Hydroxy-20α-yohimban-16β-carboxylic acid methyl ester; corynanthidine; isoyohimbine; mesoyohimbine; rauwolscine. $C_{21}H_{26}N_2O_3$; mol wt 354.44. C 71.16%, H 7.39%, N 7.90%, O 13.54%. From bark of Corynanthe johimbe K. Schum., Rubiaceae: Hahn, Brandenburg,

Ber. **60**, 669 (1927); Wilbaut, van Gastel, *Rec. Trav. Chim.* **54**, 88 (1935); from *Rauwolfia canescens* L., *Apocynaceae:* Mookerjee, *J. Indian Chem. Soc.* **18**, 33 (1941), *C.A.* **35**, 7967 (1941); Stoll *et al., Helv. Chim. Acta* **38**, 270 (1955). Identity with corynanthidine: Janot, Goutarel, *Bull. Soc. Chim, Fr.* **1946**, 535. Identity with isoyohimbine: Heinemann, *Ber.* **60**, 15 (1934). Identity with rauwolscine: Chatterjee *et al., Chem. Ind. (London)* **1954**, 491. Structure and stereochemistry: Le Hir *et al., Bull. Soc. Chim. Fr.* **1953**, 1027; Wenkert, Liu, *Experientia* **11**, 302 (1955); Aldrich *et al., J. Am. Chem. Soc.* **81**, 2481 (1959); Janot *et al., Bull. Soc. Chim. Fr.* **1961**, 637. Total synthesis: Töke *et al., J. Org. Chem.* **38**, 2496 (1973).

Crystals, mp 243-244°. $[\alpha]_D^{19}$ −18° (pyridine); $[\alpha]_D^{19}$ −27° (abs alcohol). pKa 6.34. uv max (methanol): 227, 281 nm (log ε 4.50, 3.93). Sol in warm methanol, ethanol; slightly sol in ether, benzene; practically insol in petr ether, water.

Hydrochloride. $C_{21}H_{26}N_2O_3 \cdot HCl$. Crystals, mp 288°. $[\alpha]_D^{20}$ +55.5° (water).

10105. Ytterbium. [7440-64-4] Yb; at. wt 173.04; at. no. 70; valences 2, 3. A rare earth metal of the yttrium group; member of the lanthanide series. Naturally occurring isotopes (mass numbers): 168 (0.13%); 170 (3.05%); 171 (14.3%); 172 (21.9%); 173 (16.12%); 174 (31.8%); 176 (12.7%); known artificial radioactive isotopes: 152-167; 169; 175; 177; 178. Estimated abundance in earth's crust: 2.66-3.1 ppm. Occurs in the rare earth minerals xenotime, ytterbite (gadolinite), monazite. Discovered independently: Urbain, *Compt. Rend.* **145**, 759 (1907); and called *aldebaranium*: von Welsbach, *Monatsh. Chem.* **29**, 181 (1908); **34**, 1713 (1913). Sepn and purification: Urbain, *Congress of Applied Chemistry* [X] **94** (1909); Prandtl, *Z. Anorg. Chem.* **238**, 321 (1938); Spedding *et al., J. Am. Chem. Soc.* **74**, 2783 (1952); **76**, 2557 (1954). Spectrum: Exner, Haschek *et al.,* cited by Mellor, *A Comprehensive Treatise on Inorganic and Theoretical Chemistry* **5**, 706 (1929). Toxicity study: Haley, *J. Pharm. Sci.* **54**, 663 (1965). Reviews of prepn, properties and compds: *The Rare Earths*, F. H. Spedding, A. H. Daane, Eds. (Krieger, Huntington, N.Y., 1971, reprint of 1961 ed.) 641 pp; Hulet, Bode, "Separation Chemistry of the Lanthanides and Transplutonium Actinides", in *MTP Int. Rev. Sci.: Inorg. Chem., Ser. One* vol. 7, K. W. Bagnall, Ed. (University Park Press, Baltimore, 1972) pp 1-45; Moeller, "The Lanthanides", in *Comprehensive Inorganic Chemistry* vol. 4, J. C. Bailar Jr. *et al.,* Eds. (Pergamon Press, Oxford, 1973) pp 1-101; F. H. Spedding in *Kirk-Othmer Encyclopedia of Chemical Technology* vol. 19 (John Wiley & Sons, New York, 3rd ed., 1982) pp 833-854; *Chemistry of the Elements,* N. N. Greenwood, A. Earnshaw, Eds. (Pergamon Press, New York, 1984) pp 1423-1449. Brief review of properties: G. T. Seaborg, *Radiochim. Acta* **61**, 115-122 (1993).

Silvery, ductile metal. Crystalline forms: face-centered cubic α-form, d 6.977, transforms to β-form at 798°; body-centered cubic β-form, d 6.54, exists at >798°. mp 819°. bp 1196°. Heat of fusion: 7.657 kJ/mol. Heat of sublimation (25°): 152.1 kJ/mol. Forms both di- and trivalent salts.

Oxide. Ytterbia. O_3Yb_2. Colorless mass, sol in dil acids.

Hydroxide. $Yb(OH)_3$. Colorless gelatinous precipitate.

Chloride. $YbCl_3$. Hexahydrate, deliquescent crystals, d 2.575; mp 150-155°. LD_{50} in mice: 395 mg/kg i.p.; 6.7 g/kg orally (Haley).

Nitrate. $Yb(NO_3)_3$. Tetrahydrate, transparent hygroscopic prisms from concd nitric acid. LD_{50} (hexahydrate) in rats: 255 mg/kg i.p.; 3.1 g/kg orally (Haley).

Sulfate. $Yb_2(SO_4)_3$. Octahydrate, lustrous colorless crystals, soly decreases with rise in temp.

10106. Ytterbium Triflate. [54761-04-5] Trifluoromethanesulfonic acid ytterbium(3+) salt; ytterbium(III) trifluoromethanesulfonate. $C_3F_9O_9S_3Yb$; mol wt 620.25. C 5.81%, F 27.57%, O 23.22%, S 15.51%, Yb 27.90%. $Yb(SO_3CF_3)_3$. Recyclable, water-stable Lewis acid catalyst. Prepn: J. Massaux, G. Duyckaerts, *Anal. Chim. Acta* **73**, 416 (1974). Thermal decompn of nonahydrate: J. E. Roberts, J. S. Bykowski, *Thermochim. Acta* **25**, 233 (1978). Catalytic applications in solvent-free carbamate synthesis: M. Curini *et al., Tetrahedron Lett.* **43**, 4895 (2002); in Aldol-Grob synthesis of (*E*)-alkenes: *idem et al., Eur. J. Org. Chem.* **2003**, 1631; in imino ene reactions: M. Yamanaka *et al., J. Org. Chem.* **68**, 3112 (2003); in Fries-type rearrangements of acylanilides: W. Su, C. Jin, *J. Chem. Res.* **2004**, 611; in Friedel-Crafts reactions: *eidem, Synth. Commun.* **34**, 4199, 4249 (2004); in intramolecular Cannizzaro reactions of aryl methyl ketones: M. Curini *et al., Org. Lett.* **7**, 1331 (2005); in aqueous Michael addition reactions: E. Keller, B. L. Feringa, *Tetrahedron Lett.* **37**, 1879 (1996); R. Ding *et al., J. Org. Chem.* **71**, 352 (2006). Review of synthetic applications of lanthanide triflates: S. Kobayashi *et al., Chem. Rev.* **102**, 2227-2302 (2002).

USE: Versatile rare earth metal catalyst in organic synthesis.

10107. Yttrium. [7440-65-5] Y; at. wt 88.90585; at. no. 39; valence 3. Group IIIb (3). A rare earth metal. Naturally occurring isotope (mass number): 89; known artificial radioactive isotopes: 80-88; 90-100. Estimated abundance in earth's crust: 28.1-31 ppm. Natural sources: xenotime, fergusonite, samarskite, yttrialite, gadolinite, and other rare earth minerals. Discovered in 1794 by Gadolin; separated as yttria in 1843 by Mosander; named by Ekeberg. Sepn by fractional precipitation: Bonardi, James, *J. Am. Chem. Soc.* **37**, 2642 (1915); Willand, James, *ibid.* **38**, 1198 (1916); Wichers *et al., ibid.* **40**, 1615 (1918); by ion exchange: Spedding *et al., ibid.* **69**, 2812 (1947); Mayer, Freiling, *ibid.* **75**, 5647 (1953). Toxicity study: Cochran *et al., Arch. Ind. Hyg. Occup. Med.* **1**, 637 (1950). Reviews of prepn, properties and compds: *The Rare Earths*, F. H. Spedding, A. H. Daane, Eds. (Krieger, Huntington, N.Y., 1971, reprint of 1961 ed.) 641 pp; Vickery, "Scandium, Yttrium and Lanthanum", in *Comprehensive Inorganic Chemistry* vol. 3, J. C. Bailar Jr. *et al.,* Eds. (Pergamon Press, Oxford, 1973) pp 329-353; Moeller, "The Lanthanides", *ibid.* vol. 4, pp 1-101; F. H. Spedding in *Kirk-Othmer Encyclopedia of Chemical Technology* vol. 19 (John Wiley & Sons, New York, 3rd ed., 1982) pp 833-854; *Chemistry of the Elements* N. N. Greenwood, A. Earnshaw, Eds. (Pergamon Press, New York, 1984) pp 1102-1110, 1423-1449.

Iron-gray, lustrous powder; darkens on exposure to light. Forms hexagonal close-packed crystals. d 4.4689. mp 1522°. bp 3338°. Heat of fusion: 11.43 kJ/mol. Heat of sublimation (25°): 424.7 kJ/mol. E°(aq) Y^{3+}/Y −2.37 V (calc). Oxidizes on heating in air or oxygen; dec cold water slowly, boiling water rapidly.

Oxide. Yttria. O_3Y_2. White powder, body-centered cubic structure, d 5.03. Obtained by igniting yttrium or its salts. Sol in dil acids; readily absorbs ammonia from the air; displaces ammonia from ammonium salts. LD_{50} i.p. in rats: 500 mg/kg (Cochran).

Hydroxide. $Y(OH)_3$. White gelatinous ppt, dries to a white powder which absorbs CO_2 from the air, obtained by the action of ammonium or alkali hydroxides on a soln of an yttrium salt.

Chloride. YCl_3. Hexahydrate, colorless, deliquesc crystals. Sol in water, alc. Anhydr chloride obtained by heating in a stream of HCl.

Carbonate. $Y_2(CO_3)_3$. Trihydrate, white to reddish-white powder, prepd by hydrolysis of yttrium trichloroacetate. Insol in water. Sol in dil mineral acids.

Sulfate. $Y_2(SO_4)_3$. Octahydrate, monoclinic crystals. Sol in concd sulfuric acid with formation of $Y(HSO_4)_3$. Soly in water decreases with increase in temp. Forms double salts with alkali sulfates.

Nitrate. $Y(NO_3)_3$. Hexahydrate, deliquesc crystals, sol in water, produces basic nitrates on partial decompn. LD_{50} i.p. in rats: 350 mg/kg (Cochran).

Caution: Potential symptom of overexposure to metal is eye irritation. *See NIOSH Pocket Guide to Chemical Hazards* (DHHS/-NIOSH 97-140, 1997) p 338.

USE: Yttrium doped with rare earths as phosphors for color television receivers. Oxide for mantles in gas and acetylene lights. Chloride in prepn of pure metal. Yttrium aluminum garnets (YAGS) in lasers and for making artificial diamonds.

Z

10108. Zafirlukast. [107753-78-6] [3-[[2-Methoxy-4-[[[(2-methylphenyl)sulfonyl]amino]carbonyl]phenyl]methyl]-1-methyl-1*H*-indol-5-yl]carbamic acid cyclopentyl ester; cyclopentyl 3-[2-methoxy-4-[(*o*-tolylsulfonyl)carbamoyl]benzyl]-1-methylindole-5-carbamate; *N*-[4-[5-(cyclopentyloxycarbonyl)amino-1-methylindol-3-ylmethyl]-3-methoxybenzoyl]-2-methylbenzenesulfonamide; ICI-204219; Accolate. $C_{31}H_{33}N_3O_6S$; mol wt 575.68. C 64.68%, H 5.78%, N 7.30%, O 16.68%, S 5.57%. Cysteinyl leukotriene type 1 receptor antagonist. Prepn: F. J. Brown *et al.,* **EP 199543**; P. R. Bernstein *et al.,* **US 4859692** (1986, 1989 both to ICI); V. G. Matassa *et al., J. Med. Chem.* **33,** 1781 (1990). Improved prepn: K. Srinivas *et al., Org. Process Res. Dev.* **8,** 952 (2004). Preclinical pharmacology: R. D. Krell *et al., Am. Rev. Respir. Dis.* **141,** 978 (1990). Effect on allergen-induced bronchoconstriction: S. R. Findlay *et al., J. Allergy Clin. Immunol.* **89,** 1040 (1992); K. M. O'Shaughnessy *et al., Am. Rev. Respir. Dis.* **147,** 1431 (1993). Review of pharmacology and clinical efficacy in asthma: C. J. Dunn, K. L. Goa, *Drugs* **61,** 285-315 (2001); of clinical pharmacokinetics: P. N. R. Dekhuijzen, P. P. Koopmans, *Clin. Pharmacokinet.* **41,** 105-114 (2002).

White solid from methanol, mp 138-140°. Slightly sol in methanol; freely sol in tetrahydrofuran, acetone, DMSO. Practically insol in water.

THERAP CAT: Antiasthmatic.

10109. Zalcitabine. [7481-89-2] 2′,3′-Dideoxycytidine; dideoxycytidine; ddCyd; Hivid. $C_9H_{13}N_3O_3$; mol wt 211.22. C 51.18%, H 6.20%, N 19.89%, O 22.72%. Pyrimidine nucleoside analog with antiviral activity. Prepn: J. P. Horwitz *et al., J. Org. Chem.* **32,** 817 (1967); R. Marumoto, M. Honjo, *Chem. Pharm. Bull.* **22,** 128 (1974). Prepn and structure-activity study: T.-S. Lin *et al., J. Med. Chem.* **30,** 440 (1987). *In vitro* inhibition of viral DNA synthesis: P. C. van der Vliet, M. M. Kwant, *Biochemistry* **20,** 2628 (1981); of HIV-1 virus replication: H. Mitsuya, S. Broder, *Proc. Natl. Acad. Sci. USA* **83,** 1911 (1986). Phosphorylation by human cells: D. A. Cooney *et al., Biochem. Pharmacol.* **35,** 2065 (1986). Metabolism by human cells: M. C. Starnes, Y. Cheng, *J. Biol. Chem.* **262,** 988 (1987). Potential application in acquired immunodeficiency syndrome (AIDS): E. De Clercq, *J. Med. Chem.* **29,** 1561 (1986).

Crystals from ethanol + benzene, mp 215-217° (Horwitz); also reported as mp 209-210° (Lin). $[\alpha]_D^{25}$ +81° (c = 0.635 in water). uv max in 0.1*N* HCl: 280 nm (ε 17720); in 0.1*N* NaOH: 270 nm (ε 8410).

THERAP CAT: Antiviral.

10110. Zaldaride. [109826-26-8] 1,3-Dihydro-1-[1-[(4-methyl-4*H*,6*H*-pyrrolo[1,2-*a*][4,1]benzoxazepin-4-yl)methyl]-4-piperidinyl]-2*H*-benzimidazol-2-one. $C_{26}H_{28}N_4O_2$; mol wt 428.53. C 72.87%, H 6.59%, N 13.07%, O 7.47%. Non-specific ion channel and calmodulin blocker. Prepn: J. W. F. Wasley, J. Norman, **EP 233483**; *eidem,* **US 4758559** (1987, 1988 both to Ciba-

Geigy). Synthesis: S. Boyer *et al., J. Heterocycl. Chem.* **25,** 1003 (1988). Calmodulin inhibition: J. A. Norman *et al., Mol. Pharmacol.* **31,** 535 (1987); and ion channel inhibition: R. Neuhaus, B. F. X. Reber, *Eur. J. Pharmacol.* **226,** 183 (1992). Inhibition of gastric acid secretion: E. W. Black *et al., J. Pharmacol. Exp. Ther.* **248,** 208 (1988); of secretory diarrhea in mice and rats: J. E. Shook *et al., ibid.* **251,** 247 (1989). LC determn in human plasma: D. Chollet, M. Salanon, *J. Chromatogr.* **593,** 73 (1992). Clinical trial in travelers' diarrhea: H. L. DuPont *et al., Gastroenterology* **104,** 709 (1993).

Crystals, mp 173-175° as hydrate.

Maleate. [109826-27-9] CGS-9343B; ZY-17617B. $C_{26}H_{28}$-$N_4O_2 \cdot C_4H_4O_4$; mol wt 544.60. Crystals, mp 189-190°.

THERAP CAT: Antidiarrheal.

10111. Zaleplon. [151319-34-5] *N*-[3-(3-Cyanopyrazolo[1,-5-*a*]pyrimidin-7-yl)phenyl]-*N*-ethylacetamide; CL-284846; Sonata. $C_{17}H_{15}N_5O$; mol wt 305.33. C 66.87%, H 4.95%, N 22.94%, O 5.24%. Selective non-benzodiazepine GABA$_A$ receptor agonist. Prepn: J. P. Dusza *et al.,* **US 4626538** (1986 to Am. Cyanamid). Clinical pharmacology: D. Allen *et al., Eur. J. Clin. Pharmacol.* **45,** 313 (1993); B. Beer *et al., J. Clin. Pharmacol.* **34,** 335 (1994). Clinical pharmacokinetics: A. S. Rosen *et al., Biopharm. Drug Dispos.* **20,** 171 (1999). Clinical comparison with zolpidem, *q.v.:* R. Elie *et al., J. Clin. Psychiatry* **60,** 536 (1999). CE-LIF determn of metabolites in urine: C. Horstkötter *et al., J. Chromatogr. A* **1014,** 71 (2003). Review of pharmacology and clinical experience: W. E. Heydorn, *Expert Opin. Invest. Drugs* **9,** 841-858 (2000).

White to off-white powder. mp 186-187°. Log P (octanol/-water): 1.23 (pH 1-7). Sparingly sol in alcohol, propylene glycol. Practically insol in water.

Note: This is a controlled substance (depressant): **21 CFR,** 1308.14.

THERAP CAT: Sedative, hypnotic.

10112. Zaltoprofen. [74711-43-6] 10,11-Dihydro-α-methyl-10-oxodibenzo[*b,f*]thiepin-2-acetic acid; 2-(10,11-dihydro-10-oxodibenzo[*b,f*]thiepin-2-yl)propionic acid; CN-100; Soreton; Peon. $C_{17}H_{14}O_3S$; mol wt 298.36. C 68.43%, H 4.73%, O 16.09%, S 10.75%. Anti-inflammatory activity resides in (*S*)-enantiomer. Prepn: Y. Fujimoto, S. Yamabe, **DE 2941869**; *eidem,* **US 4247706** (1980, 1981 both to Nippon Chemiphar). Series of articles on pharmacology: *Arzneim.-Forsch.* **36,** 1796-1822 (1986). Resolution of racemate: M. Yamamoto *et al., Chirality* **2,** 280 (1990). HPLC determn in human plasma and urine; pharmacokinetics: J. Oshima *et al., J. Chromatogr.* **414,** 381 (1987).

Pale yellow crystals from benzene/*n*-hexane, mp 130.5-131.5°; also reported as mp 131-133°. Tasteless, odorless. Freely sol in acetone, chloroform; sol in methanol; slightly sol in ethanol, benzene. Practically insol in water, cyclohexane.

(S)-form. [89482-01-9] Crystals from ethylendichloride, mp 129.5-131°. $[\alpha]_D^{25}$ +32.4° (c = 1 in CHCl$_3$).

THERAP CAT: Anti-inflammatory.

10113. Zanamivir. [139110-80-8] 5-(Acetylamino)-4-[(aminoiminomethyl)amino]-2,6-anhydro-3,4,5-trideoxy-D-*glycero*-D-*galacto*-non-2-enonic acid; 4-guanidino-2,4-dideoxy-2,3-dehydro-*N*-acetylneuraminic acid; 4-guanidino-Neu5Ac2en; 5-acetamido-4-guanidino-2,3,4,5-tetradeoxy-D-*glycero*-D-*galacto*-non-2-enopyranosonic acid; GG-167; GR-121167X; Relenza. C$_{12}$H$_{20}$N$_4$-O$_7$; mol wt 332.31. C 43.37%, H 6.07%, N 16.86%, O 33.70%. Influenza viral neuraminidase inhibitor; structural analog of the sialic acids, *q.v.* Prepn: L. M. von Itzstein *et al.*, **WO 9116320**; *eidem*, **US 5360817** (1991, 1994 both to Biota); M. von Itzstein *et al.*, *Carbohydr. Res.* **259**, 301 (1994). Structure-activity study: *eidem et al.*, *Nature* **363**, 418 (1993). Inhibition of sialidase (neuraminidase) from influenza virus: M. S. Pegg, M. von Itzstein, *Biochem. Mol. Biol. Int.* **32**, 851 (1994). In vitro antiviral activity: J. M. Woods *et al.*, *Antimicrob. Agents Chemother.* **37**, 1473 (1993). HPLC determn in serum: R. J. Stubbs, A. J. Harker, *J. Chromatogr. B* **670**, 279 (1995). Clinical trial in influenza A and B infection: F. G. Hayden *et al.*, *N. Engl. J. Med.* **337**, 874 (1997); in prevention of influenza in healthy adults: A. S. Monto *et al.*, *J. Am. Med. Assoc.* **282**, 31 (1999).

Colorless crystals as the sesquihydrate, mp 256° (dec). $[\alpha]_D^{20}$ +40.9° (c = 0.9 in water). Zwitterionic at physiological pH.

THERAP CAT: Antiviral.

10114. Zaragozic Acids. Squalestatins. Family of fungal metabolites with a core 4,6,7-trihydroxy-2,8-dioxobicyclo[3.2.1]octane-3,4,5-tricarboxylic acid ring system differing among C6-O-acyl and C1-alkyl side chains. Inhibitors of squalene synthase, which catalyzes the first committed step of the sterol biosynthetic pathway. Originally isolated as zaragozic acid from a fungus found in Jalon River in Zaragosa, Spain and as squalestatins from *Phoma* sp. C2932 found in a soil sample from Armacao de Pera, Portugal. Isolation and properties of squalestatins 1, 2, and 3: M. J. Dawson *et al.*, *J. Antibiot.* **45**, 639 (1992); structure elucidation: P. J. Sidebottom *et al.*, *ibid* 648. Isolation, structure, and properties of zaragozic acids A, B, and C: J. D. Bergstrom *et al.*, *Proc. Natl. Acad. Sci. USA* **90**, 80 (1993). Review of discovery and mechanism of action: J. D. Bergstrom *et al.*, *Annu. Rev. Microbiol.* **49**, 607-639 (1995); and antihypercholesterolemia and antifungal properties: N. S. Watson, P. A. Procopiou, *Prog. Med. Chem.* **33**, 331-338 (1996); of chemistry and biology: A. Nadin, K.C. Nicolaou, *Angew. Chem. Int. Ed.* **35**, 1623-1656 (1996); of synthetic studies: A. Armstrong, T. J. Blench, *Tetrahedron* **58**, 9321-9349 (2002).

Zaragozic acid A

Zaragozic Acid A. [142561-96-4] (7*S*)-2,7-Anhydro-3,4-di-*C*-carboxy-8,9,10,12,13-pentadeoxy-10-methylene-12-(phenylmethyl)-L-*erythro*-L-*glycero*-D-*altro*-7-trideculo-7,4-furanosonic acid 11-acetate 5-[(2*E*,4*S*,6*S*)-4,6-dimethyl-2-octenoate]; squalestatin 1; squalestatin S1. C$_{35}$H$_{46}$O$_{14}$; mol wt 690.73. Absolute stereochemistry: K. E. Wilson *et al.*, *J. Org. Chem.* **57**, 7151 (1992). Biosynthesis: K. M. Byrne *et al.*, *ibid* **58**, 1019 (1993). Synthesis of bicyclic core: H. Abdel-Rahman *et al.*, *J. Chem. Soc. Chem. Commun.* **24**, 1841 (1993). Total synthesis: K. C. Nicolaou *et al.*, *Chem. Eur. J.* **1**, 467 (1995). Accumulation of farnesol-derived dicarboxylic acids in liver: S. Vaidya *et al.*, *Arch. Biochem. Biophys.* **355**, 84 (1998). Induction of CYP2B enzymes: T. A. Kocarek *et al.*, *Mol. Pharmacol.* **54**, 474 (1998). White foam. $[\alpha]_D^{22}$ +18.3° (c = 0.60 in CHCl$_3$); $[\alpha]_D^{25}$ +37° (c = 1.29 in methanol). uv max (methanol): 214 nm (log ε 4.29); uv max (MeCN): 210 nm (E$_{1cm}^{1\%}$ 314).

Zaragozic Acid B. [146389-61-9] (7*S*,10ξ,11ξ,12ξ)-2,7-Anhydro-3,4-di-*C*-carboxy-8,9,10,12,13,14,15-heptadeoxy-10,12-dimethyl-15-phenyl-L-*glycero*-D-*altro*-pentadec-14-en-7-ulo-7,4-furanosonic acid 5-[(6*E*,12*E*)-6,12-tetradecadienoate]. C$_{39}$H$_{54}$O$_{13}$; mol wt 730.84. Accumulation of farnesol contributing to antifungal activity: J. M. Hornby *et al.*, *Antimicrob. Agents Chemother.* **47**, 2366 (2003). $[\alpha]_D^{25}$ +5.9° (c = 0.27 in methanol). uv max (methanol): 205, 251 nm (log ε 4.44, 4.32).

Zaragozic Acid C. [146389-62-0] (7*S*)-2,7-Anhydro-3,4-di-*C*-carboxy-8,9,10,12,13-pentadeoxy-12-(phenylmethyl)-L-*erythro*-L-*glycero*-D-*altro*-7-trideculo-7,4-furanosonic acid 5-[(4*E*,6*R*)-6-methyl-9-phenyl-4-nonenoate]. C$_{40}$H$_{50}$O$_{14}$; mol wt 754.82. Isolation and structure elucidation: C. Dufresne *et al.*, *Tetrahedron* **48**, 10221 (1992). Synthesis of bicyclic core: I. Paterson *et al.*, *Tetrahedron Lett.* **38**, 4301 (1997). Total synthesis based on aldol approach: S. Nakamura *et al.*, *Tetrahedron* **61**, 11078 (2005). Review of syntheses: S. Nakamura, *Chem. Pharm. Bull.* **53**, 1-10 (2005). White powder. $[\alpha]_D^{20}$ +9.6° (c = 0.29 in ethanol). uv max (ethanol): 209, 259 nm (log ε 4.16, 2.81).

10115. Zatebradine. [85175-67-3] 3-[3-[[2-(3,4-Dimethoxyphenyl)ethyl]methylamino]propyl]-1,3,4,5-tetrahydro-7,8-dimethoxy-2*H*-3-benzazepin-2-one; 1-(7,8-dimethoxy-1,3,4,5-tetrahydro-2*H*-3-benzazepin-2-on-3-yl)-3-[*N*-methyl-*N*-[2-(3,4-dimethoxyphenyl)ethyl]amino]propane. C$_{26}$H$_{36}$N$_2$O$_5$; mol wt 456.57. C 68.40%, H 7.95%, N 6.14%, O 17.52%. Specific bradycardic agent; sinus node inhibitor. Prepn: M. Reiffen *et al.*, **EP 65229**; *eidem*, **US 4490369** (1982, 1984 both to Thomae); and structure-activity study: M. Reiffen *et al.*, *J. Med. Chem.* **33**, 1496 (1990). Pharmacology: W. Kobinger, C. Lillie, *Eur. J. Pharmacol.* **104**, 9 (1984). Mechanism of action study: M. Goethals *et al.*, *Circulation* **88**, 2389 (1993). Pharmacokinetics: W. Roth *et al.*, *J. Pharm. Sci.* **82**, 99 (1993). GC-MS determn in plasma: J. Schmid *et al.*, *J. Chromatogr.* **658**, 93 (1994).

Hydrochloride. [91940-87-3] UL-FS-49. C$_{26}$H$_{36}$N$_2$O$_5$.HCl; mol wt 493.04. Two crystalline modifications, mp 188° and mp 168°. Sol in water.

THERAP CAT: Antianginal.

10116. Zearalenone. [17924-92-4] (3*S*,11*E*)-3,4,5,6,9,10-Hexahydro-14,16-dihydroxy-3-methyl-1*H*-2-benzoxacyclotetradecin-1,7(8*H*)-dione; 6-(10-hydroxy-6-oxo-*trans*-1-undecenyl)-β-resorcylic acid lactone; Compd F-2; FES. C$_{18}$H$_{22}$O$_5$; mol wt 318.36. C 67.91%, H 6.97%, O 25.13%. Estrogenic mycotoxin produced by *Fusarium* fungi commonly found in grains. One of a group of compounds known as *resorcylic acid lactones*. Isoln from the mycelia of *Gibberella zeae (Fusarium graminearum)*: M. Stob *et al.*, *Nature* **196**, 1318 (1962); F. N. Andrews, M. Stob, **US 3196019** (1965 to Purdue Res. Found.). Structure: W. H. Urry *et al.*, *Tetrahedron Lett.* **1966**, 3109. Synthesis of *dl*-form: D. Taub *et al.*, *Chem. Commun.* **1967**, 225; **NL 6812148**; N. N. Girotra, N. L. Wendler, **US 3551455** (1968, 1970 both to Merck & Co.); Vlattas *et* *al., J. Org. Chem.* **33**, 4176 (1968); T. Takahashi *et al., Tetrahedron Lett.* **22**, 1363 (1981). Total synthesis and abs config: D. Taub *et al., Tetrahedron* **24**, 2443 (1968). Physicochemical data: A. E. Pohland *et al., Pure Appl. Chem.* **54**, 2219 (1982). Natural occurrence in agricultural products: T. Tanaka *et al., J. Agric. Food Chem.* **36**, 979 (1988). GC determn in cereals: K. Schwadorf, H.-M. Müller, *J. Chromatogr.* **595**, 259 (1992).

Crystals, mp 164-165°. $[\alpha]_{546}^{25}$ −170.5° (c = 1.0 in CH_3OH). uv max (CH_3OH): 236, 274, 316 nm (ε 29700; 13909; 6020). Sol in aq alkali, ether, benzene, alcohols. Practically insol in water. **dl-Form.** Crystals, mp 187-189°.

10117. Zeatin. [1637-39-4] (2*E*)-2-Methyl-4-(1*H*-purin-6-ylamino)-2-buten-1-ol; *trans*-zeatin. $C_{10}H_{13}N_5O$; mol wt 219.24. C 54.78%, H 5.98%, N 31.94%, O 7.30%. Naturally occurring plant growth hormone; cytokinin originally isolated from sweet corn kernels, *Zea mays* L. *Gramineae*. Isoln and structure determn: D. S. Letham *et al., Proc. Chem. Soc. London* **1964**, 230. Synthesis: G. Shaw, D. V. Wilson, *ibid.* 231; G. Shaw *et al., J. Chem. Soc. C* **1966**, 921; J. Corse, J. Kuhnle, *Synthesis* **1972**, 618; G. M. Gray, *ibid.* **1983**, 488; *idem,* **EP 86454** (1983 to J. T. Baker). Inhibition of mitochondrial function: C. O. Miller, *Plant Physiol.* **69**, 1274 (1982); translocation in soybean explants: L. Noodén, D. S. Letham, *J. Plant Growth Regul.* **2**, 265 (1984). *Reviews:* D. S. Letham, *Annu. Rev. Plant Physiol.* **18**, 349-363 (1967); D. S. Letham, L. M. S. Palni, *ibid.* **34**, 163-197 (1983).

Crystals from water, mp 207-208°. uv max in 0.1*M* HCl: 207, 275 nm (ε 14500, 14650); at pH 7.2: 212, 270 nm (ε 17050, 16150); in 0.1*M* NaOH: 220, 276 nm (ε 15900, 14650).

10118. Zeaxanthin. [144-68-3] β,β-Carotene-3,3'-diol; *all-trans*-β-carotene-3,3'-diol; (3*R*,3'*R*)-dihydroxy-β-carotene; zeaxanthol; anchovyxanthin. $C_{40}H_{56}O_2$; mol wt 568.87. C 84.45%, H 9.92%, O 5.62%. One of the most widespread carotenoid alcohols in nature. Occurs together and is isomeric with xanthophyll, *q.v.* It is the pigment of yellow corn *Zea mays* L., *Gramineae*. Isoln from yellow corn grits: Karrer *et al., Helv. Chim. Acta* **13**, 268 (1930). Isoln by chromatography: Kuhn, Grundmann, *Ber.* **67**, 596 (1934). Isoln from algae, bacteria: A. J. Aasen *et al., Acta Chem. Scand.* **26**, 404 (1972). Isoln of dipalmitate from *Physalis* petal: Kuhn *et al., Ber.* **63**, 1489 (1930). Does not possess vitamin A potency: Schumacher *et al., Poult. Sci.* **23**, 529 (1944). Stereochemistry: Zechmeister, *Chem. Rev.* **34**, 267 (1944). Abs config of natural zeaxanthin: T. E. de Ville *et al., Chem. Commun.* **1969**, 1311; J. R. Hlubucek *et al., J. Chem. Soc. Perkin Trans. 1* **1974**, 848. Total synthesis: Isler *et al., Helv. Chim. Acta* **39**, 2041 (1956); **40**, 456 (1957); Loeber *et al., J. Chem. Soc. C* **1971**, 404; A. Rüttimann, H. Mayer, *Helv. Chim. Acta* **63**, 1456 (1980); P. R. Ellis *et al., ibid.* **64**, 1092 (1980); E. Widmer *et al., ibid.* **65**, 944, 958 (1982). Sepn of configurational isomers by HPLC: A. Rüttimann *et al., J. High Resolut. Chromatogr. Chromatogr. Commun.* **6**, 612 (1983). First isoln of enantiomeric and *meso*-zeaxanthin in nature: T. Maoka *et al., Comp. Biochem. Physiol.* **83B**, 121 (1986). Mfg procedure: Isler *et al., US 2917539* (1959 to Hoffmann-La Roche). *Reviews:* Zechmeister, *Carotinoide* (Berlin, 1934); Mayer, *The Chemistry of Natural Coloring Matters* (New York, 1943); Karrer, Jucker, *Carotenoids* (New York, 1950).

Yellow rhombic plates with steel-blue metallic luster from ethanol, mp 207° (Zechmeister); mp 215.5° (Kuhn). Optically inactive. Absorption bands (ethanol) 483, 451.5 nm. Practically insol in water. Slightly sol in petr ether, methanol; sol in carbon disulfide, benzene, chloroform, carbon tetrachloride, pyridine, ethyl acetate; sol in glacial acetic acid upon addition of hexane. Less sol in boiling methanol (1:1550) than xanthophyll.
Dipalmitate. Physalien; physalin. $C_{72}H_{116}O_4$. Fine yellow or red needles from benzene, mp 97°.

10119. Zein. A prolamine; an alcohol-soluble protein present in amounts of 2.5-10% (dry basis) in corn *(Zea mays* L., *Gramineae)*. The greater part of zein has a mol wt of 38,000. Does not contain lysine or tryptophan. Extracted commercially from gluten meal with dil isopropanol: Swallen, *Ind. Eng. Chem.* **33**, 394 (1941). Improved method: Carter, Reck, *DE 2002337* (1971 to Nutrilite Prod.), *C.A.* **75**, 117341b (1971). *Review:* Mossé, *Ann. Physiol. Végétale* **3**, 105 (1961).

White to slightly yellow powder, d 1.226. When completely dry may be heated to 200° without visible signs of decompn. Soluble in aq alcohols, the glycols, the ethyl ether of ethylene glycol, furfuryl alcohol, tetrahydrofurfuryl alcohol, aq alkaline solns of pH 11.5 (or greater). Tends to become denatured when in soln and becomes insol. Insol in water, acetone; but readily sol in acetone-water mixtures between the limits of 60-80% acetone by volume. Insol in anhydr alcohols except methanol.

USE: Manuf plastics, paper coatings, adhesives, substitutes for shellac, laminated board, in solid color printing, films, edible coatings for foodstuffs.

10120. Zeolites. Crystalline, hydrated alkali-aluminum silicates of the general formula $M_{2/n}O.Al_2O_3.ySiO_2.wH_2O$ where M represents a group IA or IIA element, *n* is the cation valence, *y* is 2 or greater and *w* is the number of water molecules contained in the channels or interconnected voids within the zeolite. The cations are mobile and capable of undergoing ion exchange. Zeolites occur naturally in sedimentary and volcanic rocks, altered basalts, ores, clay deposits. Some 40 known zeolite minerals and a great number of synthetic zeolites are available commercially. Ref: Milton, **US 2882243** (1959 to Union Carbide). Environmentally friendly synthesis: H. Lee *et al., Nature* **425**, 385 (2003). *Reviews:* D. W. Breck, R. A. Anderson, "Molecular Sieves" in *Kirk-Othmer Encyclopedia of Chemical Technology* **vol. 15** (Wiley-Interscience, New York, 3rd ed., 1981) pp 638-669; P. L. Layman, *Chem. Eng. News* **60**, 10 (Sept. 27, 1982); J. Haggin, *ibid.* **60**, 9 (Dec. 13, 1982). *Books: Adv. Chem. Ser.* **101, 102**, entitled "Molecular Sieve Zeolites - I, II," E. M. Flanigan, Ed. (ACS, Washington DC, 1971) 526 pp, 459 pp; *Adv. Chem. Ser.* **121**, entitled "Molecular Sieves," W. M. Meier, Ed. (ACS, Washington DC, 1973) 634 pp; D. W. Breck, *Zeolite Molecular Sieves* (John Wiley, New York, 1974) 771 pp; *Natural Zeolites: Occurrence, Properties, Use,* L. B. Sand, F. A. Mumpton, Eds. (Pergamon, Oxford, 1978). Studies on fibrous zeolites as possible environmental hazards: A. N. Rohl *et al., Science* **216**, 518 (1982); Y. I. Baris, *Arch. Environ. Health* **37**, 177 (1982). Use as microscopic chemical reactor vessels: R. Pool, *Science* **263**, 1698 (1994).

USE: As molecular sieves, filters, adsorbents, catalysts, drying agents, cation exchangers, dispersing agents, detergent builders.

10121. Zeranol. [26538-44-3] (3*S*,7*R*)-3,4,5,6,7,8,9,10,11,-12-Decahydro-7,14,16-trihydroxy-3-methyl-1*H*-2-benzoxacyclo-tetradecin-1-one; 6-(6,10-dihydroxyundecyl)-β-resorcylic acid μ-lactone; α-zearalanol; MK-188; P-1496; Ralgro; Ralabol; Ralone. $C_{18}H_{26}O_5$; mol wt 322.40. C 67.06%, H 8.13%, O 24.81%. Animal growth promotant prepd from zearalenone, *q.v.:* E. B. Hodge *et al., US 3239345* (1966 to Commercial Solvents). Stereoselective prepn and abs config: G. Snatzke *et al., Helv. Chim. Acta* **69**, 734 (1986). TLC determn in plasma and tissues: M. B. Medina, N. Nagdy, *J. Chromatogr.* **614**, 315 (1993). Growth regulating and repartitioning effects in cattle: P. G. Lemieux *et al., J. Anim.*

Sci. **68,** 1702 (1990). *Review:* R. S. Baldwin *et al., Regul. Toxicol. Pharmacol.* **3,** 9-25 (1983).

Crystals from isopropanol/water, mp 182-183°; $[\alpha]_D$ +46.3° (c = 1.0 in methanol). LD_{50} in mice (mg/kg): 4400 i.p.; >40000 orally (Baldwin).

THERAP CAT (VET): Anabolic.

10122. Ziconotide. [107452-89-1] ω-Conotoxin M VIIA; ω-conopeptide MVIIA; SNX-111; CI-1009; Prialt. $C_{102}H_{172}N_{36}O_{32}$-$S_7$; mol wt 2639.13. C 46.42%, H 6.57%, N 19.11%, O 19.40%, S 8.50%. Selective antagonist of N-type voltage sensitive calcium channels (VSCC). Blocks neurotransmitter release by preventing depolarization-induced calcium influx. Synthetic, 25-residue peptide corresponding to one of the conotoxins, *q.v.,* derived from the venom of the marine cone snail, *Conus magus* L. Synthesis: B. M. Olivera *et al., Biochemistry* **26,** 2086 (1987). Structure-activity study: L. Nadasdi *et al., ibid.* **34,** 8076 (1995). Binding study and use as biochemical tool: R. Kristipati *et al., Mol. Cell. Neurosci.* **5,** 219 (1994). NMR studies: L. K. MacLachlan *et al., Methods Mol. Biol.* **60,** 337 (1997). Radioimmunoassay: C. M. Barksdale *et al., J. Clin. Ligand Assay* **19,** 229 (1996). Clinical pharmacology: D. McGuire *et al., J. Cardiovasc. Pharmacol.* **30,** 400 (1997). Clinical trial in pain relief from cancer or AIDS: P. S. Staats *et al., J. Am. Med. Assoc.* **291,** 63 (2004).

USE: Ligand for binding studies of voltage sensitive calcium channels.

THERAP CAT: Analgesic; neuroprotective.

10123. Zidovudine. [30516-87-1] 3'-Azido-3'-deoxythymidine; azidothymidine; AZT; BW-A509U; Retrovir. $C_{10}H_{13}N_5O_4$; mol wt 267.24. C 44.94%, H 4.90%, N 26.21%, O 23.95%. Pyrimidine nucleoside analog; reverse transcriptase inhibitor. Prepn: J. P. Horwitz *et al., J. Org. Chem.* **29,** 2076 (1964); R. P. Glinski *et al., ibid.* **38,** 4299 (1973). *See also:* J. L. Rideout *et al.,* US 4724232 (1988 to Burroughs Wellcome). Total synthesis: C. K. Chu *et al., Tetrahedron Lett.* **29,** 5349 (1988). *In vitro* antiviral and antitumor activity: E. De Clercq *et al., Biochem. Pharmacol.* **29,** 1849 (1980); vs HIV-1 virus: H. Mitsuya *et al., Proc. Natl. Acad. Sci. USA* **82,** 7096 (1985). Clinical pharmacokinetics: R. W. Klecker *et al., Clin. Pharmacol. Ther.* **41,** 407 (1987). Toxicology studies: K. M. Ayers, *Am. J. Med.* **85,** Suppl. 2A, 186 (1988). Comprehensive description: M. L. Sethi, *Anal. Profiles Drug Subs.* **20,** 729-765 (1991). Review of clinical experience: G. X. McLeod, S. M. Hammer, *Ann. Intern. Med.* **117,** 487-501 (1992); in prevention of perinatal HIV transmission: R. Sperling, *Infect. Dis. Obstet. Gynecol.* **6,** 197-203 (1998).

Needles from petr ether, mp 106-112° (Horwitz). Also reported as crystals from water, mp 120-122° (Glinski). $[\alpha]_D^{25}$ +99° (c = 0.5 in water). Soly in water (25°C): 25 mg/ml. uv max (water): 266.5 nm (ε 11650). LD_{50} in male, female mice, male, female rats (mg/kg): 3568, 3062, 3084, 3683 orally; >750 i.v. (all species) (Ayers).

THERAP CAT: Antiviral.

10124. Zileuton. [111406-87-2] *N*-(1-Benzo[*b*]thien-2-yl-ethyl)-*N*-hydroxyurea; (±)-*N*-hydroxy-*N*-(1-benzo[*b*]thien-2-ylethyl)urea; A-64077; Abbott 64077; Leutrol; Zyflo. $C_{11}H_{12}N_2O_2S$;

mol wt 236.29. C 55.91%, H 5.12%, N 11.86%, O 13.54%, S 13.57%. Inhibitor of 5-lipoxygenase, the initial enzyme in the biosynthesis of leukotrienes from arachidonic acid. Prepn: J. B. Summers, Jr. *et al.,* EP 279263; *eidem,* US 4873259 (1988, 1989 both to Abbott). Chromatographic resolution of enantiomers: S. B. Thomas *et al., J. Chromatogr.* **623,** 390 (1992). Inhibition of 5-lipoxygenase: G. W. Carter *et al., J. Pharmacol. Exp. Ther.* **256,** 929 (1991). Pharmacokinetics: P. Rubin *et al., Agents Actions Suppl.* **35,** 103 (1991). Clinical evaluation in rheumatoid arthritis: M. E. Weinblatt *et al., J. Rheumatol.* **19,** 1537 (1992). Clinical trial in asthma: E. Israel *et al., Ann. Intern. Med.* **119,** 1059 (1993). Reviews: R. L. Bell *et al., Int. J. Immunopharmacol.* **14,** 505-510 (1992); K. McGill, W. W. Busse, *Lancet* **348,** 519-524 (1996).

Crystals, mp 157-158°.

THERAP CAT: Antiasthmatic.

10125. Zilpaterol. [119520-05-7] (6*R*,7*R*)-*rel*-4,5,6,7-Tetra-hydro-7-hydroxy-6-[(1-methylethyl)amino]imidazo[4,5,1-*jk*][1]benzazepin-2(1*H*)-one; (±)-*trans*-4,5,6,7-tetrahydro-7 hy-droxy-6-(isopropylamino)imidazo[4,5,1-*jk*][1]benzazepin-2(1*H*)-one; RU-42173. $C_{14}H_{19}N_3O_2$; mol wt 261.32. C 64.35%, H 7.33%, N 16.08%, O 12.25%. β-Adrenergic agonist. Prepn: D. Fréchet *et al.,* FR 2534257; *eidem,* US 4585770 (1984, 1986 both to Roussel Uclaf). Effects on growth performance and carcass characteristics of steers: A. Plascencia *et al., Proc. West. Sect. Am. Soc. Anim. Sci.* **50,** 331-334 (1999). GC/MS determn in commercial feeds: B. Bocca *et al., J. Chromatogr. B* **783,** 141 (2003); in calf eye: *idem et al., J. AOAC Int.* **86,** 8 (2003). Residue analysis in cattle and pigs: C. S. Stachel *et al., Anal. Chim. Acta* **493,** 63 (2003). ELISA screening method: W. L. Shelver, D. J. Smith, *J. Agric. Food Chem.* **52,** 2159 (2004).

(*R*,*R*)-form

mp ≈166°.

Hydrochloride. [119520-06-8]; [186046-04-8] (monohydrate)]; [186046-05-9] (trihydrate). Zilmax. $C_{14}H_{19}N_3O_2$.HCl; mol wt 297.78. mp ≈270°.

THERAP CAT (VET): Growth promotant.

10126. Zimeldine. [56775-88-3] (*Z*)-3-(4-Bromophenyl)-*N,N*-dimethyl-3-(3-pyridinyl)-2-propen-1-amine; (*Z*)-3-(4'-bromo-phenyl)-3-(3''-pyridyl)dimethylallylamine; zimelidine; *cis*-H-102/09. $C_{16}H_{17}BrN_2$; mol wt 317.22. C 60.58%, H 5.40%, Br 25.19%, N 8.83%. Serotonin uptake inhibitor. Prepn: P. B. Berntsson *et al.,* ZA 7201503; *eidem,* US 3928369 (1972, 1975 both to AB Hassle). X-ray crystallographic study: S. Abrahamsson *et al., Acta Chem. Scand.* **A30,** 609 (1976). *In vivo* study in rats and humans: S. B. Ross *et al., Life Sci.* **19,** 205 (1976). Pharmacokinetics: D. Brown, *Eur. J. Clin. Pharmacol.* **17,** 111 (1980). Mode of action: K. Fuxe *et al., Neurosci. Lett.* **13,** 307 (1979). Metabolism: J. Lundström *et al., Arzneim.-Forsch.* **31,** 486 (1981). Clinical studies: A. Georgotas *et al., Am. J. Psychiatry* **139,** 1057 (1982); E. Syvalahti *et al., J. Int. Med. Res.* **10,** 250 (1982). Profile of antidepressant action: S. A. Montgomery *et al., Adv. Biochem. Psychopharmacol.* **32,** 35 (1982). Reversal of ethanol-induced memory impairment in human subjects: H. Weingartner *et al., Science* **221,** 472 (1983). Review of pharmacology and therapeutic efficacy: R. C. Heel *et al., Drugs* **24,** 169-206 (1982). Symposium on pharmacology, pharmacokinetics, metabolism, clinical studies: *Br. J. Clin. Pract.* **1982,** Suppl. 19, 1-122.

Dihydrochloride monohydrate. [61129-30-4] Normud; Zelmid. $C_{16}H_{17}BrN_2.2HCl.H_2O$; mol wt 408.16. Crystals, mp 193°.
THERAP CAT: Antidepressant.

10127. Zinc. [7440-66-6] Zn; at. wt 65.409; at. no. 30; valence 2. Group IIB (12). Essential nutritional trace element necessary for function of many metalloenzymes. Abundance in earth's crust: 0.02% by wt. Natural isotopes: 64 (48.89%); 66 (27.81%); 68 (18.57%); 67 (4.11%); 70 (0.62%); eight radioactive isotopes and two isomers. Occurs in smithsonite or zinc spar, sphalerite or zinc blende, zincite, willemite, *franklinite*, [(Zn,Mn,-Fe)O.(Fe.Mn$_2$)O$_3$] or *gahnite* (ZnAl$_2$O$_4$). Has been known since very early times. Commercial forms: ingots; lumps; sheets; wire; shot; strips; sticks; granules; mossy; powder (dust). Prepn: Gowland, Bannister, *Metallurgy of Non-Ferrous Metals* (Griffin, London, 1930); *Zinc Production, Properties and Uses* (Zinc Development Association, London, 1968). *Reviews: Zinc,* C. H. Mathewson, Ed., A.C.S. Monograph Series no. **142** (Reinhold, New York, 1959) 721 pp; Schlechter, Thompson, "Zinc and Zinc Alloys" in *Kirk-Othmer Encyclopedia of Chemical Technology* **vol. 22** (Interscience, New York, 2nd ed., 1970) pp 555-603; Aylett, "Group IIB" in *Comprehensive Inorganic Chemistry* **vol. 3,** J. C. Bailar, Jr. *et al.,* Eds. (Pergamon Press, Oxford, 1973) pp 187-328. Review of toxicology and human exposure: *Toxicological Profile for Zinc* (PB2006-100008, 2005) 352 pp.
Bluish-white, lustrous metal; distorted hexagonal close-packed structure; stable in dry air; becomes covered with a white coating of basic carbonate on exposure to moist air. mp 419.5°. bp 908°. d^{25} 7.14. Heat capacity at constant pressure (25°): 6.07 cal/mole deg. Mohs' hardness 2.5. When heated to 100-150° becomes malleable, at 210° becomes brittle and pulverizable. Burns in air with a bluish-green flame. Loses electrons in aqueous systems to form Zn^{2+} E° (aq) Zn/Zn^{2+} 0.763 V. Slowly attacked by H_2SO_4 or HCl; oxidizing agents or metal ions, e.g. Cu^{2+}, Ni^{2+}, Co^{2+}, accelerate the process. Reacts slowly with ammonia water and acetic acid; rapidly with HNO_3. Reacts with alkali hydroxides to form *"zincates"*, ZnO_2^{2-}, which are actually hydroxo complexes such as $Zn(OH)_3^-$; $Zn(OH)_4^{2-}$, $[Zn(OH)_4(H_2O)_2]^{2-}$.
Caution: Potential symptoms of overexposure by fume inhalation are metal fume fever; by acute oral overexposure are stomach cramps, nausea, vomiting; by chronic oral overexposure are anemia, pancreatic damage, decreased HDL cholesterol levels (PB2006-100008).
USE: Galvanizing sheet iron; as ingredient of alloys such as bronze, brass, Babbitt metal, German silver, and special alloys for die-casting; as a protective coating for other metals to prevent corrosion; for electrical apparatus, especially dry cell batteries, household utensils, castings, printing plates, building materials, railroad car linings, automotive equipment; as reducing agent in organic chemistry; for deoxidizing bronze; extracting gold by the cyanide process, purifying fats for soaps; bleaching bone glue; manuf sodium hydrosulfite; insulin zinc salts; as reagent in analytical chemistry, e.g., in the Marsh and Gutzeit test for arsenic; as a reducer in the determination of iron. It is a nutritional trace element.

10128. Zinc Acetate. [557-34-6] Galzin. $C_4H_6O_4Zn$; mol wt 183.50. C 26.18%, H 3.30%, O 34.88%, Zn 35.65%. $Zn(C_2-H_3O_2)_2$. Prepn of anhydr salt from zinc nitrate and acetic anhydride: Späth, *Monatsh. Chem.* **33,** 235 (1912). Clinical evaluations in Wilson's disease: G. M. Hill *et al., Hepatology* **7,** 522 (1987); G. J. Brewer *et al., J. Lab. Clin. Med.* **109,** 526 (1987). Toxicity: H. F. Smyth *et al., Am. Ind. Hyg. Assoc. J.* **30,** 470 (1969).
Dihydrate. [5970-45-6] Wilzin. $C_4H_6O_4Zn.2H_2O$; mol wt 219.53. C 21.88%, H 4.59%, O 43.73%, Zn 29.80%. Crystallizes from dil acetic acid; faint, acetous odor; astringent taste; slightly efflorescent. d 1.735; mp 237°. One gram dissolves in 2.3 ml

water, 1.6 ml boiling water, 30 ml alcohol, about 1 ml boiling alcohol. The aq soln is neutral or slightly acid to litmus; pH about 5-6. *Keep in well-closed containers.* LD_{50} orally in rats: 2.46 g/kg (Smyth).
USE: Preserving wood; as mordant in dyeing; manuf glazes for painting on porcelain. As a reagent in testing for albumin, tannin, urobilin, phosphate, blood.
THERAP CAT: Styptic, astringent. In treatment of Wilson's disease.
THERAP CAT (VET): Antiseptic, astringent, protective (topical). Has been used as an emetic.

10129. Zinc Bromide. [7699-45-8] Br_2Zn; mol wt 225.22. Br 70.96%, Zn 29.04%. $ZnBr_2$. Usually contains at least 97% $ZnBr_2$, the remainder being chiefly water.
Very hygroscopic, granular powder; sharp, metallic taste. d 4.22; mp 394°; bp 697° with partial decompn. One gram dissolves in 0.25 ml water, 0.5 ml 90% alcohol; sol in ether, solns of alkali hydroxides. The aq soln is acid to litmus; pH about 4. *Keep tightly closed.*
USE: Making silver bromide collodion emulsions for photography; in the shielding of viewing windows for nuclear reactions.

10130. Zinc Caprylate. [557-09-5] Octanoic acid zinc salt. $C_{16}H_{30}O_4Zn$; mol wt 351.82. C 54.62%, H 8.59%, O 18.19%, Zn 18.59%. $Zn(C_8H_{15}O_2)_2$. Prepd from ammonium caprylate and zinc sulfate: van Renesse, *Ann.* **171,** 380 (1874).
Lustrous scales from alc, mp 136°. Sparingly sol in boiling water; moderately sol in boiling alcohol. *Keep well closed.* Dec in moist atm giving off caprylic acid.
USE: As fungicide like zinc propionate.

10131. Zinc Carbonate. [3486-35-9] CO_3Zn; mol wt 125.42. C 9.58%, O 38.27%, Zn 52.15%. $ZnCO_3$. Occurs in nature as the minerals *smithsonite, zincspar*. Prepn: Hüttig *et al., Monatsh. Chem.* **72,** 31 (1939).
Rhombohedral structure. Solubility in water at 15° 0.001 g/100 g; sol in dil acids, alkalies, solns of NH_4^+ salts.
Basic carbonate. Zinc carbonate hydroxide; zinc subcarbonate. Variable composition, usually characterized as $3Zn(OH)_2.2ZnCO_3$. Occurs as the mineral *hydrozincite*. Reagent specification: 70% ZnO minimum.
USE: As pigment; manuf of porcelains, pottery, rubber.
THERAP CAT: Astringent, topical antiseptic.
THERAP CAT (VET): Astringent, antiseptic, protective (topical). Also used in rations to prevent Zn deficiency diseases.

10132. Zinc Chloride. [7646-85-7] Butter of zinc. Cl_2Zn; mol wt 136.32. Cl 52.01%, Zn 47.98%. $ZnCl_2$. Usually contains at least 95% $ZnCl_2$; remainder is chiefly water and oxychloride. Toxicity: Bruner, *Fed. Proc.* **9,** 260 (1950).
White, odorless, very deliquesc granules, or fused pieces or rods. d^{25} 2.907; mp ~290°; bp 732°. Solubility in H_2O: 432 g/100 g (25°); 614 g/100 g (100°). One gram dissolves in 0.25 ml of 2% HCl, in 1.3 ml alcohol, 2 ml glycerol; freely sol in acetone. With much water some zinc oxychloride is formed. The aq soln is acid to litmus; pH about 4. *Keep tightly closed.* LD i.v. in rats: 60-90 mg/kg (Bruner).
Caution: Potential symptoms of overexposure to fumes are conjunctivitis; irritation of skin, eyes, nose and throat; coughing, copious sputum; dyspnea, chest pain, pulmonary edema and bronchopneumonia; pulmonary fibrosis, cor pulmonale; fever; cyanosis; tachypnea; skin burns. *See NIOSH Pocket Guide to Chemical Hazards* (DHHS/NIOSH 97-140, 1997) p 338.
USE: Deodorant, disinfecting and embalming material; alone or with phenol and other antiseptics for preserving railway ties; fireproofing lumber; with ammonium chloride as flux for soldering; etching metals; manuf parchment paper, artificial silk, dyes, activated carbon, cold-water glues, vulcanized fiber; browning steel, galvanizing iron, copper-plating iron; in magnesia cements; petroleum oil refining; cement for metals and for facing stone; mordant in printing and dyeing textiles; carbonizing woolen goods; producing crepe and crimping fabrics; mercerizing cotton; sizing and weighting fabrics; vulcanizing rubber; solvent for cellulose; preserving anatomical specimens; in microscopy for separating silk, wool, and plant fibers; as dehydrating agent in chemical syntheses. Dentin desensitizer.

THERAP CAT: Astringent.

THERAP CAT (VET): Antiseptic, astringent. Has been used in ulcers, fistulas, pododermatitis.

10133.   Zinc Chromate(VI) Hydroxide. [13530-65-9] Zinc yellow; buttercup yellow; C.I. Pigment Yellow 36. A basic salt of somewhat variable composition. Approx $Zn_2CrO_4(OH)_2$.

Hydrate. Yellow, odorless, fine powder. Slightly sol in water; sol in dil acids, including acetic acid.

Caution: Chromium hexavalent compounds are listed as known human carcinogens: *Report on Carcinogens, Eleventh Edition* (PB2005-104914, 2004) p III-63.

USE: As pigment in paints, varnishes, oil colors, linoleum, rubber, etc.

10134.   Zinc Citrate. [546-46-3] 2-Hydroxy-1,2,3-propane-tricarboxylic acid zinc salt. $C_{12}H_{10}O_{14}Zn_3$; mol wt 574.43. C 25.09%, H 1.75% O 38.99%, Zn 34.16%. $Zn_3(C_6H_5O_7)_2$. Prepd from zinc carbonate and citric acid: Heldt, *Ann.* **47,** 157 (1843).

Dihydrate. Odorless powder. Slightly sol in water; sol in dil mineral acids, in alkali hydroxides.

USE: In toothpaste and mouthwash.

10135.   Zinc Cyanide. [557-21-1] C_2N_2Zn; mol wt 117.44. C 20.45%, N 23.85%, Zn 55.70%. $Zn(CN)_2$. Usually contains about 85% zinc cyanide, some water and oxide.

White powder. *Poison!* Insol in water; sol in solns of alkali cyanides or hydroxides; not appreciably attacked by organic acids, but readily dec by dil mineral acid with evolution of hydrogen cyanide.

USE: Electroplating; removing NH_3 from producer gas.

10136.   Zinc Fluoride. [7783-49-5] F_2Zn; mol wt 103.41. F 36.74%, Zn 63.25%. ZnF_2. Prepd from $ZnCO_3$ and HF: Ruff, *Die Chemie des Fluors* (Berlin, 1920) p 36; Emeleus in *Fluorine Chemistry* vol. **1,** J. H. Simons, Ed. (Academic Press, New York, 1950) p 38; Kwasnik in *Handbook of Preparative Inorganic Chemistry* vol. **1,** G. Brauer, Ed. (Academic Press, New York, 2nd ed., 1963) p 242.

Tetragonal needles (rutile lattice) or white cryst mass. d^{25} 5.00; Haendler *et al., J. Am. Chem. Soc.* **74,** 3167 (1952). mp 872°. bp 1500°. Soly in water: 5×10^{-5} moles/l, Kwasnik, *loc. cit.* Slightly sol in aq HF, more sol in HCl, HNO_3, NH_4OH. Zinc fluoride used for fluorinations should be slightly hydrated.

Tetrahydrate. Rhombohedral crystals, becomes anhyd at 100°. Soly in water: 1.516 g/100 ml. May be stored in glass bottles.

USE: In the fluorination of organic compds, manuf phosphors for fluorescent electric lights, glazes and enamels for porcelain, preserving wood, in electroplating baths.

10137.   Zinc Formate. [557-41-5] $C_2H_2O_4Zn$; mol wt 155.44. C 15.45%, H 1.30%, O 41.17%, Zn 42.08%. $Zn(HCOO)_2$. Forms dihydrate readily. Prepd from zinc carbonate and formic acid: Kendall, Adler, *J. Am. Chem. Soc.* **43,** 1470 (1921).

Dihydrate. Crystals. d 2.207. Solubility in H_2O (20°): 5.2 g/100 g. Practically insol in alc.

10138.   Zinc Hexafluorosilicate. [16871-71-9] Zinc fluosilicate; zinc silicofluoride. F_6SiZn; mol wt 207.48. F 54.94%, Si 13.54%, Zn 31.53%. $ZnSiF_6$.

Hexahydrate. White crystals. Soluble in water. pH of 1% aqueous solution 3.2.

USE: Mothproofing agent; laundry sour; hardener for concrete.

10139.   Zinc Iodate. [7790-37-6] Iodic acid (HIO_3) zinc salt. I_2O_6Zn; mol wt 415.21. I 61.13%, O 23.12%, Zn 15.75%. $Zn(IO_3)_2$. Prepn of dihydrate: F. Mylius, R. Funk, *Ber.* **30,** 1716 (1897). Soly studies: J. E. Ricci, G. J. Nesse, *J. Am. Chem. Soc.* **64,** 2305 (1942); J. N. Spencer *et al., J. Chem. Eng. Data* **19,** 140 (1974). X-ray, IR and Raman spectroscopic study: S. Peter *et al., Z. Anorg. Allg. Chem.* **626,** 208 (2000).

White, crystalline powder. Soly in water at 25°: 0.01542 M.

Dihydrate. [13986-19-1] $I_2O_6Zn.2H_2O$; mol wt 451.24.

10140.   Zinc Iodide. [10139-47-6] I_2Zn; mol wt 319.22. I 79.51%, Zn 20.49%. ZnI_2. Usually contains at least 98% ZnI_2.

White or almost white, odorless, hygroscopic, granular powder; sharp, saline taste; becomes brown on exposure to air and light, due to liberation of iodine. d^{25} 4.74; mp ~446°; bp ~625° with

decompn. One gram dissolves in 0.3 ml water, 0.2 ml boiling water, 2 ml glycerol; freely sol in alcohol, ether. The aq soln is acid to litmus; pH about 5. *Keep well closed and protected from light.*

THERAP CAT: Topical antiseptic, astringent.

10141.   Zinc Iodide-Starch. [9010-71-3] Trommsdorff's starch. A soln is prepd by heating 4 parts starch, 20 $ZnCl_2$, and 2 ZnI_2 with 1 liter water. Deteriorates with age and acquires a blue color.

USE: For detecting nitrites, free Cl, and other oxidizing agents.

10142.   Zinc Lactate. [16039-53-5] $C_6H_{10}O_6Zn$; mol wt 243.55. C 29.59%, H 4.14%, O 39.42%, Zn 26.86%. $Zn(C_3H_5-O_3)_2$. Prepd from zinc carbonate and lactic acid: Pederson *et al., J. Biol. Chem.* **68,** 151 (1926).

Trihydrate. Crystals. Soluble in 60 parts cold, 6 parts boiling water.

10143.   Zinc Meta-arsenite. [10326-24-6] ZMA. As_2O_4Zn; mol wt 279.25. As 53.66%, O 22.92%, Zn 23.42%. $Zn(AsO_2)_2$.

White powder. Sol in acids.

USE: Wood preservative, insecticide.

10144.   Zinc Nitrate. [7779-88-6] N_2O_6Zn; mol wt 189.42. N 14.79%, O 50.68%, Zn 34.53%.

Hexahydrate. Colorless, odorless crystals; d 2.065; mp ~36°. Sol in about 0.5 part water, freely in alcohol. The aq soln is acid to litmus; pH of 5% aq soln 5.1. *Keep well closed and in a cool place.* Also available in the form of fused pieces. In this form it contains only about 20% water. Technical flake usually contains 25.6% H_2O.

USE: As a mordant in dyeing.

10145.   Zinc Oleate. [557-07-3] 9-Octadecenoic acid zinc salt. $C_{36}H_{66}O_4Zn$; mol wt 628.32. C 68.82%, H 10.59%, O 10.19%, Zn 10.41%. $(C_{17}H_{33}CO_2)_2Zn$. Usually contains small amounts of the zinc salts of other fatty acids. Prepn: Grabner, *Monatsh. Chem.* **42,** 287 (1921).

White, dry, greasy powder. Insol in water; sol in alcohol, ether, carbon disulfide, benzene, petr ether.

10146.   Zinc Oxalate. [547-68-2] C_2O_4Zn; mol wt 153.43. C 15.66%, O 41.71%, Zn 42.63%. ZnC_2O_4. Prepn: Chatterjee, Dhar, *J. Phys. Chem.* **28,** 1020 (1924).

Dihydrate. powder. Very slightly sol in water; sol in dil mineral acids, ammonia.

10147.   Zinc Oxide. [1314-13-2] Flowers of zinc; philosopher's wool; zinc white; C.I. Pigment White 4; C.I. 77947. OZn; mol wt 81.41. O 19.65%, Zn 80.35%. ZnO. Occurs as the mineral *zincite.* Prepd by vaporization of metallic zinc and oxidation of the vapors with preheated air (French process); also from franklinite, (American process) or from zinc sulfide: *Faith, Keyes & Clark's Industrial Chemicals,* F. A. Lowenheim, M. K. Moran, Eds. (Wiley-Interscience, New York, 4th ed., 1975) pp 882-888. Purification: Depew, **US 2372367** (1945 to American Zinc, Lead & Smelting). The medicinal grade contains 99.5% or more ZnO; technical grades contain 90-99% ZnO and a few tenths of 1% of lead. *See also: Colour Index* vol. **4** (3rd ed., 1971) p 4687. Efficacy as sunblock: S. R. Pinnell *et al., Dermatol. Surg.* **26,** 309 (2000).

White or yellowish-white, odorless powder. Hexagonal crystals: d 5.67. Also reported as d_4^{20} 5.607. Sublimes at normal pressure. n_D 2.0041, 2.0203. American process zinc oxide pH 6.95. French process zinc oxide pH 7.37. Practically insol in water. Sol in dil acetic or mineral acids, ammonia, ammonium carbonate, fixed alkali hydroxide solns.

Caution: Potential symptoms of overexposure are metal fume fever (chills, muscle aches, nausea, fever, dry throat, cough, weakness, lassitude); metallic taste; headache; blurred vision; low back pain; vomiting; fatigue; malaise; tight chest, dyspnea, rales, decreased pulmonary function. *See NIOSH Pocket Guide to Chemical Hazards* (DHHS/NIOSH 97-140, 1997) p 338.

Calamine. Eczederm. Zinc oxide with a small proportion of ferric oxide as a coloring agent. Pink powder. Insol in water. Almost completely sol in mineral acids.

USE: As pigment in white paints instead of lead carbonate; in cosmetics, driers, quick-setting cements; with syrupy phosphoric acid or $ZnCl_2$ in dental cements; manuf opaque glass and certain types of transparent glass; manuf enamels, automobile tires, white glue, matches, white printing inks, porcelains, zinc green; as a reagent in analytical chemistry; in electrostatic copying paper; as flame retardant; in electronics as semiconductor.

THERAP CAT: Astringent; topical protectant; ultraviolet screen.

THERAP CAT (VET): Antiseptic; astringent; topical protectant.

10148. Zinc Perchlorate. [13637-61-1] Cl_2O_8Zn; mol wt 264.31. Cl 26.83%, O 48.43%, Zn 24.75%. $Zn(ClO_4)_2$.

Hexahydrate, deliquesc crystals, mp 106°. Freely sol in water. Sol in alcohol. Also forms a tetrahydrate.

10149. Zinc Peroxide. [1314-22-3] ZPO; zinc superoxide. O_2Zn; mol wt 97.41. O 32.85%, Zn 67.15%. ZnO_2. The peroxide of commerce contains 50-60% ZnO_2, the remainder is ZnO.

White to yellowish-white, odorless powder. Dec above 150°. Insol in, but gradually dec by, water. Sol in dil acids, liberating hydrogen peroxide.

USE: Accelerator in rubber compounding; curing agent for synthetic elastomers. Deodorant for wounds and skin diseases.

THERAP CAT: Antiseptic (topical), astringent.

10150. Zinc p-Phenolsulfonate. [127-82-2] p-Hydroxybenzenesulfonic acid zinc salt; 1-phenol-4-sulfonic acid zinc salt; zinc p-hydroxybenzenesulfonate; zinc sulfocarbolate; zinc sulfophenate; Phenozin. $C_{12}H_{10}O_8S_2Zn$; mol wt 411.74. C 35.00%, H 2.45%, O 31.09%, S 15.58%, Zn 15.89%. $Zn(HOC_6H_4SO_3)_2$. It is at least 99.5% pure. Prepn: Rojahn, *Dtsch. Apoth. Ztg.* **50**, 1095 (1935), *C.A.* **31**, 6816⁸ (1937).

Octahydrate, crystals or cryst powder; odorless. Effloresces in dry air; loses all its H_2O at about 120°. One gram dissolves in 1.6 ml water, 0.4 ml boiling water, 1.8 ml alcohol. The aq soln is acid to litmus; pH about 4.

USE: In insecticide formulations.

THERAP CAT: Astringent.

THERAP CAT (VET): Has been used as an intestinal antiseptic, and externally to promote healing of ulcers, slowly granulating wounds.

10151. Zinc Phosphate. [7779-90-0] $O_8P_2Zn_3$; mol wt 386.17. O 33.14%, P 16.04%, Zn 50.81%. $Zn_3(PO_4)_2$. The tetrahydrate occurs in nature as the mineral ***hopeite***; the article of commerce is about 98% pure.

Tetrahydrate, white, odorless powder. Insol in water or alcohol. Sol in dil mineral acids, acetic acid, ammonia, and in alkali hydroxide solns.

USE: In dental cements.

10152. Zinc Phosphide. [1314-84-7] P_2Zn_3; mol wt 258.17. P 23.99%, Zn 76.01%. Zn_3P_2. Toxicity study: L. Y. Ming, *Malays. Agric. J.* **52**, 166 (1979).

Dark gray tetragonal crystals, lustrous or dull powder; faint phosphorus odor. d 4.55. When strongly heated with the exclusion of air it melts and finally sublimes. The mp has been given as 420° and the bp as 1100°. When kept dry it is quite stable. Insol in water, alcohol. Sol in benzene, carbon disulfide; reacts with HCl, H_2SO_4 with evolution of spontaneously flammable phosphine. Reacts violently with concd H_2SO_4, HNO_3 and other oxidizing agents. *Keep dry.* LD_{50} in male, female rats (mg/kg): 12.00, 15.72 orally (Ming).

USE: Rodenticide.

10153. Zinc Propionate. [557-28-8] $C_6H_{10}O_4Zn$; mol wt 211.55. C 34.06%, H 4.76%, O 30.25%, Zn 30.92%. $Zn(C_3H_5O_2)_2$. Prepd by dissolving zinc oxide in dil propionic acid and concentrating the soln: Gaze, *Arch. Pharm.* **229**, 488 (1891).

Clusters of plates, tablets; crystallizes also in needles as the monohydrate. The soly of the anhydr salt is 32% (w/w) in water at 15°; 2.8% in alc at 15°; 17.2% in boiling alc. *Keep well closed.* Dec in moist atm, giving off propionic acid.

USE: As fungicide on adhesive tape to reduce plaster irritation caused by molds, fungi, and bacterial action.

THERAP CAT: Antifungal (topical).

10154. Zinc Pyrophosphate. [7446-26-6] Diphosphoric acid, zinc salt (1:2). $O_7P_2Zn_2$; mol wt 304.76. O 36.75%, P 20.33%, Zn 42.92%. $Zn_2P_2O_7$.

White, crystalline powder. d²³ 3.75. Insoluble in water. Soluble in dilute mineral acids.

10155. Zinc Salicylate. [16283-36-6] 2-Hydroxybenzoic acid zinc salt. $C_{14}H_{10}O_6Zn$; mol wt 339.63. C 49.51%, H 2.97%, O 28.26%, Zn 19.26%. Prepd from sodium salicylate and zinc sulfate: Clark, Kao, *J. Am. Chem. Soc.* **70**, 2151 (1948).

Trihydrate, needles or cryst powder. Sol in water, alc. The aq soln is practically neutral to litmus.

THERAP CAT: Antiseptic; astringent.

10156. Zinc Selenide. [1315-09-9] SeZn; mol wt 144.37. Se 54.69%, Zn 45.31%. ZnSe. Prepd by mixing a soln of a zinc salt and potassium selenide: Berzelius, cited in *Mellor's* **10**, 776 (1930); by passing selenium vapor over zinc heated *in vacuo*: Moser, Doctor, *Z. Anorg. Chem.* **118**, 284 (1921); by passing H_2Se into a methanol soln of zinc acetate: Nitsche, **US 2805917** (1957 to du Pont); from $ZnSe.N_2H_4$ (zinc selenide hydrazinate): Conn *et al.*, **US 3014779** (1961 to Merck & Co.).

Yellow, cubic crystals. d_4^{15} 5.42. mp >1100°. Dec in air. Insol in water. Dec in dil nitric acid.

USE: Commercial phosphor.

10157. Zinc Silicate. [13597-65-4] Zinc orthosilicate. O_4SiZn_2; mol wt 222.90. O 28.71%, Si 12.60%, Zn 58.69%. Zn_2SiO_4. Occurs in nature as the mineral ***willemite***. Prepd by heating the proper amounts of ZnO and SiO_2 at about 1200°.

White powder, insol in water or dil acids.

USE: In television screens.

10158. Zinc Stearate. [557-05-1] Octadecanoic acid zinc salt. $C_{36}H_{70}O_4Zn$; mol wt 632.35. C 68.38%, H 11.16%, O 10.12%, Zn 10.34%. $Zn(C_{18}H_{35}O_2)_2$. Usually occurs as a mixture of the zinc salts of stearic and palmitic acids, and usually with some excess of zinc oxide. Contains 13.5-15% ZnO. Prepd from stearic acid and zinc chloride: Vold, Hattiangdi, *Ind. Eng. Chem.* **41**, 2311 (1949).

Fine, soft, bulky powder; slight characteristic odor; neutral reaction. Repels water. mp about 120°. Insol in water, alcohol, ether. Sol in benzene; dec by dil acids.

Caution: Potential symptoms of overexposure are irritation of eyes, skin, upper respiratory system; cough. *See NIOSH Pocket Guide to Chemical Hazards* (DHHS/NIOSH 97-140, 1997) p 338.

USE: In tablet manuf; in cosmetic and pharmaceutical powders and ointments; as a flatting and sanding agent in lacquers; as a drying lubricant and dusting agent for rubber; as a plastic mold releasing agent; as a waterproofing agent for concrete, rock wool, paper, textiles.

THERAP CAT (VET): Antiseptic, astringent, protective (topical).

10159. Zinc Sulfate. [7733-02-0] White vitriol; zinc vitriol. O_4SZn; mol wt 161.47. O 39.63%, S 19.86%, Zn 40.51%. $ZnSO_4$. Prepn and physical properties: *Gmelins, Zink* (8th ed.) **32**, 936-960 (1956). Effects of oral zinc sulfate in acne treatment: G. Michaelsson *et al.*, *Arch. Dermatol.* **113**, 31 (1977). Clinical evaluations in Wilson's Disease: T. U. Hoogenraad, C. J. A. Van den Hamer, *Acta Neurol. Scand.* **67**, 356 (1983); T. U. Hoogenraad *et al.*, *J. Neurol. Sci.* **77**, 137 (1987).

Monohydrate. [7446-19-7] Dried zinc sulfate; Zincaps; Z Span. Powder or granules. Loses H_2O above 238°. Sol in water. Practically insol in alcohol.

Heptahydrate. [7446-20-0] Collazin; Keratol; Op-Thal-Zin; Redeema; Solvazinc; Solvezink; Virudermin; Zincate; Zincomed. Odorless crystals or granules or powder; astringent taste. Effluorescent in dry air. d 1.97. mp 100°. At 280° loses all H_2O; dec above 500°. One gram dissolves in 0.6 ml water, 2.5 ml glycerol. Insol in alcohol. The aq soln is acid to litmus; pH about 4.5. *Keep well closed.*

Note: The monohydrate does not cake as the heptahydrate does, and hence is more convenient for use during the warm season and in warm climates.

Caution: Irritating to skin, mucous membranes: H. E. Stokinger, *Patty's Industrial Hygiene and Toxicology* **2A**, G. D. Clayton, F. E. Clayton, Eds. (John Wiley & Sons, New York, 1981) pp 2033-2049.

USE: As mordant in calico-printing; preserving wood and skins; with hypochlorite for bleaching paper; manuf lithopone and other zinc salts; clarifying glue; electrodepositing Zn; also as reagent in analytical chemistry.

THERAP CAT: Ophthalmic astringent. Zinc supplement.

THERAP CAT (VET): Astringent. Has been used as an emetic.

10160. Zinc Sulfide. [1314-98-3] Zinc Blende. SZn; mol wt 97.47. S 32.90%, Zn 67.11%. ZnS.

Occurs in nature as the minerals ***wurtzite*** (hexagonal, d 4.087) and ***sphalerite*** (cubic, d 4.102). White to grayish-white or yellowish powder. When contg water, it slowly oxidizes in air to sulfate. Insol in water, alkalies. Sol in dil mineral acids. Precipitated zinc sulfide of commerce usually contains 15-20% water of hydration. The dried precipitate may have been heated to 725° in the absence of air to obtain substantial conversion to wurtzite, the form preferred by the pigment industry.

USE: Pigment for paints, oilcloths, linoleum, leather, dental rubber, etc., especially in the form of lithopone; mixed with ZnO as "mineral white." Anhydr zinc sulfide is used in x-ray screens and with a trace of a radium or mesothorium salt in luminous dials of watches; also television screens.

10161. Zinc Tartrate. [551-64-4] $C_4H_4O_6Zn$; mol wt 213.48. C 22.50%, H 1.89%, O 44.97%, Zn 30.64%. $ZnC_4H_4O_6$. Prepd from potassium tartrate and zinc chloride. Prepn and solubility in water: Cantoni, Zachoder, *Bull. Soc. Chim.* [3] **33**, 747 (1905).

Dihydrate, cryst powder.

10162. Zinc Telluride. [1315-11-3] TeZn; mol wt 193.01. Te 66.11%, Zn 33.89%. ZnTe. Prepd by fusing Zn and Te: Braithwaite, *Proc. Phys. Soc. London* **64B**, 274 (1951); Bube, *Proc. IRE* **43**, 1836 (1955), *see also* Dennis, Anderson, *J. Am. Chem. Soc.* **36**, 882 (1914). From zinc oxide and powdered tellurium in aq alkaline medium: Montignie, *Bull. Soc. Chim. Fr.* **1947**, 750.

Gray or brownish-red powder. Ruby-red crystals (cubic system) by sublimation. Stable in dry air. d_4^{15} 6.34. mp 1239°. Forms a monohydrate. Prolonged contact with water or dil HCl yields H_2 and H_2Te.

USE: In semiconductor research, as photoconductor.

10163. Zinc Thiocyanate. [557-42-6] Zinc sulfocyanate. $C_2N_2S_2Zn$; mol wt 181.57. C 13.23%, N 15.43%, S 35.32%, Zn 36.02%. $Zn(SCN)_2$.

White, deliquesc crystals. Sol in water, alcohol. The aq soln is only slightly acid to litmus. *Keep well closed and protected from light.*

USE: To assist in textile dyeing.

10164. Zinc Valerate. [556-38-7] Pentanoic acid zinc salt. $C_{10}H_{18}O_4Zn$; mol wt 267.66. C 44.87%, H 6.78%, O 23.91%, Zn 24.44%. $Zn(C_5H_9O_2)_2$. The article of commerce is usually basic. Prepd from valeric acid and zinc hydrate: Lieben, Rossi, *Ann.* **159**, 58 (1871).

Dihydrate, lustrous scales or powder; valerian odor; sweetish taste. Gradually dec on exposure to air. One gram dissolves in 70 ml water or in 22 ml alcohol when free from basic salt; dec by acid. *Keep tightly closed and in cool place.*

10165. Zineb. [12122-67-7] [[1,2-Ethanediylbis[carbamodithioato]](2−)]zinc; [ethylenebis(dithiocarbamato)]zinc; zinc ethylenebis(dithiocarbamate); ethylenebis(dithiocarbamic acid) zinc salt; ENT-14874; Tritoftorol. $(C_4H_6N_2S_4Zn)_n$. Polymeric salt of ethylenebisdithiocarbamic acid; related to maneb and mancozeb, *q.q.v.* Prepd from a zinc salt and nabam, *q.v.:* C. B. Luginbuhl, US **2690448** (1954 to du Pont). Fungicidal activity is due to degradation products, principally ***ethylenethiuram monosulfide:*** R. A. Ludwig *et al., Can. J. Bot.* **33**, 42 (1955). Activity against potato blight: B. K. De, S. B. Chattopadhyay, *Pesticides* **18**, 52 (1984).

Decomposition of zineb to ethylenebisdicarbamate and ethylene thiourea, *q.v.,* in tomatoes: B. D. Ripley, D. F. Cox, *J. Agric. Food Chem.* **26**, 1137 (1978). HPLC determn: K. Gustafsson *et al., ibid.* **29**, 729 (1981). Toxicity data: T. B. Gaines, *Toxicol. Appl. Pharmacol.* **14**, 515 (1969). Aquatic toxicology: C. J. Van Leeuwen *et al., Aquat. Toxicol.* **7**, 145 (1985).

Powder or crystals from chloroform + alcohol. Practically insol in water. The powder spreads easily on water, also forms aq suspensions. Sol in carbon disulfide, pyridine. LD_{50} orally in rats: >5000 mg/kg (Gaines).

Caution: Irritation of skin and mucous membranes has been reported. *See: Clinical Toxicology of Commercial Products,* R. E. Gosselin *et al.,* Eds. (Williams & Wilkins, Baltimore, 5th Ed., 1984) Section II, p 313.

USE: Agricultural fungicide.

10166. Zingerone. [122-48-5] 4-(4-Hydroxy-3-methoxyphenyl)-2-butanone; (4-hydroxy-3-methoxyphenyl)ethyl methyl ketone; vanillylacetone; zingherone; zingiberone. $C_{11}H_{14}O_3$; mol wt 194.23. C 68.02%, H 7.27%, O 24.71%. Isolated from ginger root or prepd from vanillin and acetone followed by catalytic hydrogenation: Nomura, *J. Chem. Soc.* **111**, 769 (1917); *idem*, **US 1263796** (1918); **US 1306710** (1919); Cotton, **US 2381210** (1945 to Penn. Coal Prod.); K. Banno, T. Mukaiyama, *Bull. Chem. Soc. Jpn.* **49**, 1453 (1976).

Crystals from acetone, petr ether, ether + petr ether, mp 40-41°. bp_{14} 187-188°. Spicy, pungent odor, characteristic of ginger. Flash point: 208°F (98°C). Sparingly sol in water, petr ether; sol in ether, dil alkalies.

USE: In fragrances, flavors and cosmetics; in artificial spice oils.

10167. Zinostatin. [9014-02-2] Neocarzinostatin; neocarcinostatin; NCS; NSC-69856; An antitumor acidic antibiotic consisting of 2 components: a protein of mol wt 10,700 containing 109 amino acid residues of 18 kinds and a labile non-protein chromophore which possesses the full biological activity of NCS. Isoln from the culture filtrate of *Streptomyces carcinostaticus* var. F-41: N. Ishida *et al., J. Antibiot.* **18A**, 68 (1965). Characterization: H. Maeda *et al., ibid.* **19A**, 253 (1966). Prodn: N. Ishida *et al.,* **US 3334022** (1967 to Empire Corp.). Amino acid sequence: J. Meienhofer *et al., Science* **178**, 875 (1972). Review of protein structural studies: *eidem, Progress in Peptide Research* vol. **II**, S. Lande, Ed. (Gordon and Breach, New York, 1972) pp 295-306. Spectral characterization and separation of the chromophore: M. A. Napier *et al., Biochem. Biophys. Res. Commun.* **89**, 635 (1979). Partial structure of the chromophore: G. Albers-Schönberg *et al., ibid.* **95**, 1351 (1980). Roles of chromophore and apo-protein in biological activity: L. S. Kappen *et al., Proc. Natl. Acad. Sci. USA* **77**, 1970 (1980). Molecular basis of action: I. H. Goldberg *et al., Mol. Biol. Biochem. Biophys.* **32**, 308 (1980). Absorption, distribution, excretion: K. Toriyama *et al., Jpn. J. Antibiot.* **28**, 64 (1975). Review of pharmacology: T. A. Beerman *et al.,* in *Advances in Enzyme Regulation* vol. **14**, G. Weber, Ed. (Pergamon Press, New York, 1976) pp 207-228.

White powder, mp 260° (dec). uv max (water): 278 nm ($E_{1cm}^{1\%}$ 15). Isoelectric pt: pH 3.26 [*Jpn. Med. Gaz.* **14**(3), 11 (1977)]. Sol in water. Insol in most common org solvents. *See* M. Kohno *et al., Jpn. J. Antibiot.* **27**, 707 (1974) for stability of aq solns. LD_{50} in mice (mg/kg): 1050 orally, 0.96 i.v. (Toriyama).

THERAP CAT: Antineoplastic.

10168. Zinpyr. Family of fluorescent sensors for Zn^{2+} in biological applications. Prepn of ZP-1: G. K. Walkup *et al., J. Am.*

Chem. Soc. **122**, 5644 (2000); and characterization of ZP-1 and ZP-2: S. C. Burdette *et al., ibid.* **123**, 7831 (2001); of ZP-4: *idem et al., ibid.* **125**, 1778 (2003).

Zinpyr-1   R = Cl
Zinpyr-2   R = H

Zinpyr-1. [288574-78-7] 4′,5′-Bis[[bis(2-pyridinylmethyl)-amino]methyl]-2′,7′-dichloro-3′,6′-dihydroxy-spiro[isobenzofuran-1(3*H*),9′-[9*H*]xanthen]-3-one; 9-(*o*-carboxyphenyl)-2,7-dichloro-4,5-bis[bis(2-pyridylmethyl)aminomethyl]-6-hydroxy-3-xanthanone; ZP-1. $C_{46}H_{36}Cl_2N_6O_5$; mol wt 823.72. C 67.07%, H 4.41%, Cl 8.61%, N 10.20%, O 9.71%. Salmon-pink solid, mp 185-187° (dec). pKa 2.8. Quantum yield 0.38.

Zinpyr-2. [357916-12-2] 9-(*o*-Carboxyphenyl)-4,5-bis[bis(2-pyridylmethyl)aminomethyl]-6-hydroxy-3-xanthanone; ZP-2. $C_{46}H_{38}N_6O_5$; mol wt 754.83. C 73.19%, H 5.07%, N 11.13%, O 10.60%. Orange solid, mp 195-197° (dec). pKa 3.9. Quantum yield 0.25.

USE: Probe for measurement of cellular Zn^{2+}.

10169. Zinquin. [151606-29-0] [[2-Methyl-8-[[(4-methylphenyl)sulfonyl]amino]-6-quinolinyl]oxy]acetic acid; Zinquin A. $C_{19}H_{18}N_2O_5S$; mol wt 386.42. C 59.06%, H 4.70%, N 7.25%, O 20.70%, S 8.30%. TSQ, *q.v.*, derived membrane permeant fluorescent probe selective for Zn^{2+} in the presence of Ca^{2+} and Mg^{2+}. Synthesis: I. B. Mahadevan *et al., Aust. J. Chem.* **49**, 561 (1996). Coordination chemistry: C. J. Fahrni, T. V. O'Halloran, *J. Am. Chem. Soc.* **121**, 11448 (1999); potentiometric coordination of fluorophore: K. M. Hendrickson *et al., ibid.* **125**, 3889 (2003). Visualization of intracellular Zn^{2+} pools in pancreatic islets: P. D. Zalewski *et al., J. Histochem. Cytochem.* **42**, 877 (1994); in apoptosis: P. J. Smith *et al., Am. J. Physiol. Cell Physiol.* **283**, C609 (2002); G. R. Sauer *et al., J. Cell Biochem.* **88**, 954 (2003).

Crystals from ethyl acetate or ethyl acetate/light petroleum, mp 198-200°. pK_1 (quinoline nitrogen): <2; pK (carboxylic acid proton): 5.77 ±0.03; pK (sulfonamide proton): 9.91 ±0.02.

Ethyl Ester. [181530-09-6] Zinquin E. $C_{21}H_{22}N_2O_5S$; mol wt 414.47. Colorless crystals from dichloromethane/light petroleum, mp 111-113°. pK_1 (quinoline nitrogen): <2; pK (sulfonamide proton): 9.32 ±0.02.

USE: Determn of intracellular Zn^{2+} and labile Zn^{2+} ions.

10170. Zipeprol. [34758-83-3] 4-(2-Methoxy-2-phenylethyl)-α-(methoxyphenylmethyl)-1-piperazineethanol; α-(α-methoxybenzyl)-4-(β-methoxyphenethyl)-1-piperazineethanol; 1-(2-hydroxy-3-methoxy-3-phenylpropyl)-4-(2-methoxy-2-phenylethyl)-piperazine; 1-(2-methoxy-2-phenylethyl)-4-(2-hydroxy-3-methoxy-

3-phenylpropyl)piperazine. $C_{23}H_{32}N_2O_3$; mol wt 384.51. C 71.84%, H 8.39%, N 7.29%, O 12.48%. Prepn: R. Y. Mauvernay *et al.,* **DE 2109366**; *eidem,* **US 3718650** (1971, 1973 both to Mauvernay). Pharmacology: G. Rispat *et al., Arzneim.-Forsch.* **26**, 523 (1976); D. Cosnier *et al., ibid.* 848. Clinical abuse potential: L. Janiri *et al., Drug Alcohol Depend.* **27**, 121 (1991). GC-MS determn in plasma and urine: P. Kintz *et al., J. Pharm. Biomed. Anal.* **11**, 335 (1993).

Crystals from abs ethanol, mp 83°.

Dihydrochloride. [34758-84-2] CERM-3024; Antituxil-Z; Citizeta; Mirsol; Respirase; Robnin; Zitoxil. $C_{23}H_{32}N_2O_3 \cdot 2HCl$; mol wt 457.43. Crystals from abs ethanol, mp 231°. Very stable in aq soln. LD_{50} orally in mice: 301 mg/kg (Rispat).

THERAP CAT: Antitussive.

10171. Ziprasidone. [146939-27-5] 5-[2-[4-(1,2-Benzisothiazol-3-yl)-1-piperazinyl]ethyl]-6-chloro-1,3-dihydro-2*H*-indol-2-one; 5-(2-(4-(1,2-benzisothiazol-3-yl)piperazinyl)ethyl)-6-chlorooxindole; CP-88059. $C_{21}H_{21}ClN_4OS$; mol wt 412.94. C 61.08%, H 5.13%, Cl 8.59%, N 13.57%, O 3.87%, S 7.77%. Combined serotonin ($5HT_2$) and dopamine (D_2) receptor antagonist. Prepn: J. A. Lowe III, A. A. Nagel, **EP 281309**; *eidem,* **US 4831031** (1988, 1989 both to Pfizer). Clinical pharmacology: C. J. Bench *et al., Psychopharmacology* **112**, 308 (1993). HPLC determn in serum: J. S. Janiszewski *et al., J. Chromatogr. B* **668**, 133 (1995). Receptor binding profile: A. W. Schmidt *et al., Eur. J. Pharmacol.* **425**, 197 (2001). Review of pharmacology and clinical experience: G. L. Stimmel *et al., Clin. Ther.* **24**, 21-37 (2002); P. D. Harvey, C. R. Bowie, *Expert Opin. Pharmacother.* **6**, 337-346 (2005).

Hydrochloride monohydrate. [138982-67-9]; [122883-93-6] (anhydrous). CP-88059-1; Geodon; Zeldox. $C_{21}H_{21}ClN_4 \cdot OS \cdot HCl \cdot H_2O$; mol wt 467.41. Prepn: D. J. M. Allen *et al.,* **EP 586191**; *eidem,* **US 5312925** (1993, 1994 both to Pfizer). White to slightly pink powder. Also prepd as the hemihydrate, mp >300°.

THERAP CAT: Antipsychotic.

10172. Ziram. [137-30-4] (*T*-4)-Bis(dimethylcarbamodithioato-*S,S′*)zinc; bis(dimethyldithiocarbamato)zinc; zinc dimethyldithiocarbamate; dimethyldithiocarbamic acid zinc salt; zinc bis(dimethylthiocarbamoyl) disulfide; methyl cymate; Crittam; Mezene; Pomarsol Z; Thionic; Triscabol. $C_6H_{12}N_2S_4Zn$; mol wt 305.84. C 23.56%, H 3.95%, N 9.16%, S 41.94%, Zn 21.39%. Prepd from zinc oxide, dimethylamine, and carbon disulfide: Olin, Deger, **US 2492314** (1949 to Sharples Chemicals). Crystal structure: Klug, *Acta Crystallogr.* **21**, 536 (1966). Toxicity study: Hodge *et al., J. Pharmacol. Exp. Ther.* **118**, 174 (1956). Field analysis of residues in air: J. E. Woodrow *et al., J. Agric. Food Chem.* **43**, 1524 (1995). Review and evaluation of toxicity studies: *IARC Monographs* **53**, 423-438 (1991).

Crystals from hot chloroform + alcohol, mp 250°. *Can form a flammable dust.* d_4^{25} 1.66. Practically insol in water. Soly per 100 ml of solvent at 25°: <0.2 g, alcohol; <0.5 g, acetone; <0.5 g, benzene; <0.2 g, carbon tetrachloride, more sol in chloroform; <0.2 g, ether; 0.5 g, naphtha. Sol in dil caustic solns. LD_{50} orally in rats: 1.4 g/kg (Hodge).

Caution: May be irritating to skin and mucous membranes. *See: Clinical Toxicology of Commercial Products,* R. E. Gosselin *et al.,* Eds. (Williams & Wilkins, Baltimore, 5th ed., 1984) Section II, p. 314.

USE: Rubber vulcanization accelerator; agricultural fungicide.

10173. Zirconium. [7440-67-7] Zr; at. wt 91.224; at. no. 40; valence 4; also 3. Group IVB (4). Five naturally occurring isotopes: 90 (51.46%); 91 (11.23%); 92 (17.11%); 94 (17.40%); 96 (2.80%); artificial radioactive isotopes: 81-89, 93, 95, 97-99. Occurrence in earth's crust: 0.023%. Occurs in the minerals zircon, malacon, baddeleyite, zirkelite, eudialyte; frequently found in the rare-earth minerals; in monazite sand. Discovered by Klaproth in 1789; prepd by Berzelius in 1824. Prepn: Fast, *Z. Anorg. Chem.* **239**, 145 (1938); purification of zirconium by ion exchange columns: Ayres, *J. Am. Chem. Soc.* **69**, 1879 (1947). Sepn of zirconium and hafnium: Fischer *et al., Angew. Chem. Int. Ed.* **5**, 15 (1966). Reviews of zirconium and its compds: W. B. Blumenthal, *The Chemical Behavior of Zirconium* (Van Nostrand, Princeton, 1958); *Gmelins, Zirconium* (8th ed.) **42**, (1958) 448 pp; Larsen, "Zirconium and Hafnium Chemistry" in *Adv. Inorg. Chem. Radiochem.* **13**, 1-333 (1970); Bradley, Thornton, "Zirconium and Hafnium" in *Comprehensive Inorganic Chemistry* vol. **3**, J. C. Bailar, Jr. *et al.,* Eds. (Pergamon Press, Oxford, 1973) pp 419-490.

Bluish-black, amorphous powder or grayish-white lustrous metal (platelets or flakes) of hexagonal lattice below 865°, body-centered cubic above 865°, mp 1857°; bp 3577°. d 6.5. Brinnell hardness: 85. Can absorb up to 10 atoms per cent of oxygen or nitrogen. Reacts with hydrofluoric acid, aqua regia, hot phosphoric acid. Not attacked by cold, very slightly attacked by hot, concd sulfuric or hydrochloric acid; not attacked by nitric acid. Attacked by fused potassium hydroxide or nitrate. On prolonged heating the compact form combines with oxygen, nitrogen, carbon, and the halogens. The powder form has a very low ignition temp and is very explosive when mixed with oxidizing agents.

Caution: Zirconium and its salts generally have low systemic toxicity. A granulomatous disease of the skin, particularly in the axilla, has been reported in users of a deodorant contg sodium zirconium lactate: *see* E. Browning, *Toxicity of Industrial Metals* (Appleton-Century-Crofts, New York, 2nd ed., 1969) pp 356-360. Consult latest Government regulations on use in aerosol antiperspirants.

USE: Pure zirconium (hafnium-free) is a valuable structural material for atomic reactors because of its low nuclear cross-section and high corrosion and heat resistance. Because of hafnium's high neutron absorption characteristics, it must be removed from zirconium which is to be used in nuclear reactors; removal unnecessary for other commercial purposes. As an ingredient of priming or explosive mixtures; flashlight powders; as deoxidizer in metallurgy; as "getter" in vacuum tubes; in constructing rayon spinnerets in lamp filaments, flash bulbs.

10174. Zirconium Chloride. [10026-11-6] Zirconium tetrachloride. Cl_4Zr; mol wt 233.04. Cl 60.85%, Zr 39.15%. $ZrCl_4$. In large-scale prepns zirconium oxide is converted to the carbide, which is chlorinated to yield the tetrachloride: Kroll *et al., J. Electrochem. Soc.* **94**, 1 (1948). Lab prepn based on the equation $ZrO_2 + 2CCl_4 \rightarrow ZrCl_4 + 2COCl_2$: Hummers *et al., Inorg. Synth.* **4**, 121 (1953). Toxicology study: N. A. Zhilova, A. A. Kasparov *Hyg. Sanit.* **31**, 328 (1966). *Review:* Blumenthal, *J. Chem. Educ.* **39**, 604-610 (1962).

Lustrous monoclinic crystals: Krebs, *Angew. Chem. Int. Ed.* **8**, 146 (1969); *idem, Z. Anorg. Allg. Chem.* **378**, 263 (1970). Tetrahedral symmetry in gas phase with the Zr-Cl distance of 2.33 Å. Lewis acid. Extremely hygroscopic, forms HCl vapor and gives off fumes in moist air. d 2.803. Sublimes at 331°. mp 437° under its own pressure which is about 25 atm at this temp. Decomposed by water to form $ZrOCl_2$ and HCl; sol in alcohol, ether. LD_{50} in mice, rats (mg/kg): 665, 1688 orally (Zhilova, Kasparov).

USE: Friedel-Crafts catalyst. Component of Ziegler-type catalysts in the condensation of ethylene. Starting material in the synthesis of a number of organic derivs of zirconium, such as alkoxides and zircocene. The alkoxides have been shown to be of value in the curing of silicone plastic films. The alkoxyzirconium carboxylates are said to be useful in the water-repellent treatment of textiles and other fibrous materials.

10175. Zirconium Fluoride. [7783-64-4] Zirconium tetrafluoride. F_4Zr; mol wt 167.22. F 45.45%, Zr 54.55%. ZrF_4. Prepd by thermal decompn of $(NH_4)_2ZrF_6$: v. Hevesy, Dullenkamp, *Z. Anorg. Allg. Chem.* **221**, 161 (1934); according to the equation $ZrCl_4 + 4HF \rightarrow ZrF_4 + 4HCl$: Wolter, *Chem. Ztg.* **51**, 607 (1908); from zirconium oxide and fluorine: Haendler *et al., J. Am. Chem. Soc.* **76**, 2177 (1954).

Strongly refractive, crystalline mass (monoclinic system). d^{16} 4.6. Sublimes above 600°. Solubility in water (20°): 1.32 g/100 ml. Does not react with water; forms stable trihydrate. Freely soluble in hydrofluoric acid.

10176. Zirconium Hydride. [7704-99-6] Ideal composition: ZrH_2. Prepd by the reduction of zirconium oxide with calcium hydride in the presence of hydrogen above 600°: Alexander, **US 2427339** (1947 to Metal Hydride).

Gray-black metallic powder. Stable, no reaction with water.

USE: Powerful reducing agent in acid solution or at high temps; hydrogenation catalyst; in the vacuum tube industry and powder metallurgy.

10177. Zirconium Hydroxide. [14475-63-9] H_4O_4Zr; mol wt 159.25. H 2.53%, O 40.19%, Zr 57.28%. $Zr(OH)_4$. Proposed structures of freshly pptd and aged compds, cyclic tetramers: Zaitsev, *Russ. J. Inorg. Chem.* **11**, 900 (1966).

White, bulky, amorphous powder; d 3.25. Insol in water; sol in mineral acids when freshly pptd; less sol when aged. It colors turmeric paper brown.

USE: In the pigment, dye, and glass industries.

10178. Zirconium Iodide. [13986-26-0] Zirconium tetraiodide. I_4Zr; mol wt 598.84. I 84.77%, Zr 15.23%. ZrI_4. Prepd from the elements at a furnace temp of 450°: Eberly, *Inorg. Synth.* **7**, 52 (1963).

Orange-colored, crystalline solid. Sublimes at 431°. mp 499° (elevated pressure). Fumes heavily in air. Dissolves in water with the liberation of steam. Heat of formation: 90 kcal/mol at 25°. Magnetic susceptibility -0.238×10^{-6} c.g.s. electromagnetic units.

10179. Zirconium Nitrate. [13746-89-9] $N_4O_{12}Zr$; mol wt 339.24. N 16.52%, O 56.59%, Zr 26.89%. $Zr(NO_3)_4$. Prepn according to the equation $ZrCl_4 + 4N_2O_5 \rightarrow Zr(NO_3)_4 + 4NO_2Cl$: Field, Hardy, *Proc. Chem. Soc. London* **1962**, 76. Pentahydrate obtained from strong nitric acid. The zirconium nitrate of commerce is usually somewhat basic.

Pentahydrate. White, very hygroscopic crystals or white pieces or scales. Very sol in water; sol in alcohol. The aq soln is acid to litmus. *Keep tightly closed.*

10180. Zirconium Oxide. [1314-23-4] Zirconia; zirconium dioxide; zirconic anhydride. O_2Zr; mol wt 123.22. O 25.97%, Zr 74.03%. ZrO_2. Occurs in nature as the mineral *baddeleyite*. Prepn: Clark, Reynolds, *Ind. Eng. Chem.* **29**, 711 (1937); Henderson, Higbie, *J. Am. Chem. Soc.* **76**, 5878 (1954).

White, heavy, amorphous, odorless, tasteless powder or monoclinic crystals. Also forms tetragonal crystals above ~1100°; cubic above ~1900°. d 5.85. mp 2680°. bp 4300°. Practically insol in water; slightly sol in HCl, HNO_3; slowly sol in HF; dissolves on heating with a mixt of 2 parts H_2SO_4 and 1 part H_2O. Fusion with sodium carbonate results in the formation of sodium zirconate which dec hydrolytically with water to form sodium hydroxide and practically insol zirconium hydroxide.

USE: Instead of lime for the oxyhydrogen light; with earths of the yttrium group in incandescent lighting (Nernst lamps); as pigment, abrasive; manuf enamels, white glass, refractory crucibles, and furnace linings.

THERAP CAT: Dermatologic.

10181. Zirconium Silicate. [10101-52-7] Zirconium ortho-silicate. O_4SiZr; mol wt 183.31. O 34.91%, Si 15.32%, Zr 49.76%. $ZrSiO_4$. Occurs in nature as the mineral *zircon*. Widely scattered in all kinds of rocks and in beach sand (South Carolina, Northeast Florida). Usually separated from sand by electrostatic and electromagnetic elutriation, yielding 99% pure $ZrSiO_4$. Prepn from SiO_2 and ZrO_2 in an arc furnace: Curtis, Sowman, *J. Am. Ceram. Soc.* **36**, 195 (1953); can also be made from solns of zirconium salts and sodium silicate.

Tetragonal, bipyramidal crystals. Should be colorless. Colors are from impurities and radioactive bombardment, often removable by calcination. Dissociates to ZrO_2 and SiO_2 when heated above 1540°. Recombines when cooled slowly, but forms a mixture of monoclinic ZrO_2 and vitreous SiO_2 when rapidly quenched. Undissociated (α-form) $ZrSiO_4$ has a high sp gr, 4.7, and a high birefringence; the dissociated, γ-form has a lower sp gr, 3.9-4.0, and a low birefringence. Hardness of α-form about the same as that of quartz (6-7.5). Very inert chemically. Unaffected by aq reagents.

USE: In refractories, ceramics, glazes, cements, coatings for casting molds, polishing materials, gem stones, catalyst in alkyl and alkenyl hydrocarbon manuf, in fritted glass filters, as stabilizer in silicone rubbers. In Europe in cosmetic creams and powders.

10182. Zirconium Sulfate. [14644-61-2] Disulfatozirconic acid. O_8S_2Zr; mol wt 283.35. O 45.17%, S 22.63%, Zr 32.19%. $Zr(SO_4)_2$. Tetrahydrate usually prepd by treating zirconium oxychloride with hot concd H_2SO_4: Blumenthal, *J. Chem. Educ.* **39**, 604 (1962). Toxicity study: Cochran *et al., Arch. Ind. Hyg. Occup. Med.* **1**, 637 (1950).

Tetrahydrate. Crystalline solid. Converted to monohydrate at 100°; to anhyd form at 380°. Soly in water (18°): 52.5 g/100 g of soln. A soln at room temp deposits a solid on standing. The more dilute the soln, the more rapid the deposition. The composition of the solid is $4ZrO_2.3SO_3.15H_2O$, known as *Hauser's salt*: Hauser, Herzfeld, *Z. Anorg. Allg. Chem.* **67**, 369 (1910). This pptn does not take place if the soln has been heated above 64°. LD_{50} in rats: 3.5 g/kg orally; 175 mg/kg i.p. (Cochran).

USE: Catalyst support; precipitation of amino acids and proteins; in the tanning industry.

10183. Zirconyl Acetate. [5153-24-2] Diacetatozirconic acid. Approx formula: $Zr(OH)_2(C_2H_3O_2)_2$. Obtained as aq soln by adding acetic acid to an aq slurry of carbonated hydrous zirconia: Blumenthal, *J. Chem. Educ.* **39**, 604 (1962). Toxicity data: Cochran *et al., Arch. Ind. Hyg. Occup. Med.* **1**, 637 (1950).

Available as 22% ZrO_2 soln. d 1.46. mp −7°. pH 3.8-4.2. Stable at room temp. Also available as 13% ZrO_2 soln. d 1.20. pH 3.3-4.0. Undergoes exchange with anion exchange resins, but not with cation exchangers. Evaporation of the solns under reduced pressure yields the solid compd. It is resinous or glue-like in appearance and amorphous under x-rays. Its properties indicate it to be a highly polymerized product. The powdered solid readily dissolves when added slowly to rapidly swirling water. On heating, the solns yield a solid hydrolyzate, which is a more basic acetate with the compn $ZrOOHC_2H_3O_2$. When the mixt is allowed to cool and stand at room temp, this ppt slowly redissolves. LD_{50} in rats: 4.1 g/kg orally; 300 mg/kg i.p. (Cochran).

USE: Precipitating agent for gelatin and starch on textiles and paper; water-repellent for textiles (especially in combination with silicones).

10184. Zirconyl Chloride. [7699-43-6] Dichlorooxozirconium; zirconium oxychloride; basic zirconium chloride. Cl_2OZr; mol wt 178.13. Cl 39.81%, O 8.98%, Zr 51.21%. $ZrOCl_2$. Prepn from $ZrCl_4$ and Cl_2O: Dehnicke, Meyer, *Z. Anorg. Allg. Chem.* **331**, 121 (1964). Octahydrate conveniently prepd by crystn of an aq soln of zirconium chloride: v. Siemens, Zander, *Wiss. Veroeff. Siemens-Werken* **2**, 484 (1922); Blumenthal, *J. Chem. Educ.* **39**, 607 (1962). Toxicity study: Cochran *et al., Arch. Ind. Hyg. Occup. Med.* **1**, 637 (1950).

Octahydrate. Tetragonal crystals from water. Crystals contain tetramers of the form $[Zr_4(OH)_8(H_2O)_{16}]^{8+}$; d 1.91: Mak, *Can. J. Chem.* **46**, 3491 (1968). Freely sol in water, alcohol. The pH is about equal to that of HCl of the same molarity. LD_{50} in rats: 400 mg/kg i.p.; 3.5 g/kg orally (Cochran).

USE: To make other zirconium compds; to precipitate acid dyes; to prepare high quality pigment toners; to improve the properties of color lakes. Aq $ZrOCl_2$ solns have considerable solvent action on sparingly sol sulfates, such as calcium sulfate. The free acid in $ZrOCl_2$ solns may be neutralized, and a sol compd $ZrOOHCl.xH_2O$ can be recovered. It is highly polymerized in soln and amorphous in the solid state; has been used in the prepn of body deodorants and antiperspirant preparations.

10185. Zoapatanol. [71117-51-6] 9-[(2S,3R,6E)-3-Hydroxy-6-(2-hydroxyethylidene)-2-methyl-2-oxepanyl]-2,6-dimethyl-2-nonen-5-one. $C_{20}H_{34}O_4$; mol wt 338.48. C 70.97%, H 10.12%, O 18.91%. Oxepane diterpenoid isolated from the leaves of the zoapatle plant, *Montanoa tomentosa, Compositeae*, which has been used by Mexican women to prepare "tea" to induce menses and labor. Isoln and structure: M. P. Wachter, R. M. Kanojia, US **4086358** (1978 to Ortho); S. D. Levine *et al., J. Am. Chem. Soc.* **101**, 3404 (1979); R. M. Kanojia *et al., J. Org. Chem.* **47**, 1310 (1982). Spasmogenic effects: J. B. Smith *et al., Life Sci.* **28**, 2743 (1981). Total syntheses of (±)-form: R. Chen, D. A. Rowand, *J. Am. Chem. Soc.* **102**, 6609 (1980); K. C. Nicolau *et al., ibid.* 6611; V. V. Kane, D. L. Doyle, *Tetrahedron Lett.* **22**, 3027, 3031 (1981). Mass spec: C. J. Shaw, *Org. Mass Spectrom.* **16**, 281 (1981). ^{13}C-NMR study: M. L. Cotter, *Org. Magn. Reson.* **17**, 14 (1981).

Pale yellow oil.

10186. Zofenopril. [81872-10-8] (4S)-1-[(2S)-3-(Benzoyl-thio)-2-methyl-1-oxopropyl]-4-(phenylthio)-L-proline; [1(S),4(S)]-1-(3-mercapto-2-methyl-1-oxopropyl)-4-phenyl-thio-L-proline-S-benzoylester. $C_{22}H_{23}NO_4S_2$; mol wt 429.55. C 61.51%, H 5.40%, N 3.26%, O 14.90%, S 14.93%. Angiotensin-converting enzyme (ACE) inhibitor; de-esterified *in vivo* to its active sulfhydryl-containing metabolite, *zofenoprilat*. Prepn: M. A. Ondetti, J. Krapcho, **GB 2028327**; *eidem*, US **4316906** (1980, 1982 both to E. R. Squibb & Sons). LC/MS/MS determn in plasma: L. Dal Bo *et al., J. Chromatogr. B* **749**, 287 (2000). Role of sulfhydryl group in improvement of endothelial dysfunction: H. Buikema *et al., Br. J. Pharmacol.* **130**, 1999 (2000); L. Cominacini *et al., Am. J. Hypertens.* **15**, 891 (2002). Clinical comparison with lisinopril of effect on post-infarction survival: C. Borghi, E. Ambrosioni, *Am. Heart J.* **145**, 80 (2003). Review of properties and pharmacokinetics: A. Subissi *et al., Cardiovasc. Drug Rev.* **17**, 115-133 (1999); of clinical efficacy in cardiovascular diseases: C. Borghi *et al., Expert Opin. Pharmacother.* **5**, 1965-1977 (2004).

Foamy solid, mp 42-44°. $[\alpha]_D^{25}$ −36.5° (c = 1 in methanol).
Calcium salt. [81938-43-4] MEN-8029; SQ-26991; Bifril; Zofenil. $C_{44}H_{44}CaN_2O_8S_4$; mol wt 897.17. White crystalline powder, mp >250°. $[\alpha]_D^{23}$ −67.6° (c = 1 in methanol/HCl). Partition coefficient (octanol/water): 3.5.

THERAP CAT: Antihypertensive.

10187. Zoledronic Acid. [118072-93-8]; [165800-06-6] (monohydrate). [1-Hydroxy-2-(1H-imidazol-1-yl)ethylidene]-bisphosphonic acid; 2-(imidazol-1-yl)-1-hydroxyethane-1,1-diphosphonic acid; CGP-42446; Zometa. $C_5H_{10}N_2O_7P_2$; mol wt 272.09. C 22.07%, H 3.70%, N 10.30%, O 41.16%, P 22.77%. Bisphosphonate antiresorptive agent. Prepn: **JP Kokai 88 150291**; K. A. Jaeggi, L. Wilder, US **4939130** (1988, 1990 both to Ciba-Geigy). Effect on bone metabolism: J. R. Green *et al., J. Bone Miner. Res.* **9**, 745 (1994). Determn in plasma by enzyme inhibition assay: F. Risser *et al., J. Pharm. Biomed. Anal.* **15**, 1877 (1997). Series of articles on pharmacology and clinical experience: *Br. J. Clin.*

Pract. Suppl. **87,** 15-22 (1996). Clinical trial in tumor-induced hypercalcemia: J. J. Body, *Cancer* **80,** 1699 (1997); of i.v. infusion in osteoporosis: I. R. Reid *et al., N. Engl. J. Med.* **346,** 653 (2002); in bone metastases of prostate cancer: F. Saad *et al., J. Natl. Cancer Inst.* **94,** 1458 (2002). Review of pharmacology and therapeutic use: J.-J. Body, *Expert Opin. Pharmacother.* **4,** 567-580 (2003).

Crystals from water, mp 239° (dec).

Disodium salt tetrahydrate. [165800-07-7] Zoledronate disodium; CGP-42446A. $C_5H_8N_2Na_2O_7P_2.4H_2O$; mol wt 388.11.

Trisodium salt hydrate. [165800-08-8] Zoledronate trisodium; CGP-42446B. $(C_5H_7N_2Na_3O_7P_2)_5.2H_2O$; mol wt 1726.21.

THERAP CAT: Bone resorption inhibitor.

10188. Zolimidine. [1222-57-7] 2-[4-(Methylsulfonyl)phenyl]imidazo[1,2-*a*]pyridine; zoliridine; Solimidin. $C_{14}H_{12}N_2O_2S$; mol wt 272.32. C 61.75%, H 4.44%, N 10.29%, O 11.75%, S 11.77%. Gastroprotective agent. Prepn: **GB 991589**; L. Almirante *et al.,* **US 3318880** (1965, 1967 both to Selvi); *eidem, J. Med. Chem.* **8,** 305 (1965). Metabolism: *eidem, Farmaco Ed. Sci.* **29,** 941 (1974). Series of articles on pharmacology: *Panminerva Med.* **16,** 301-359 (1974). Pharmacokinetics: E. Schraven, D. Trottnow, *Arzneim.-Forsch.* **26,** 213 (1976). Clinical mucopoietic activity: S. Abate *et al., Int. J. Tissue React.* **4,** 319 (1982); M. C. Parodi *et al., Scand. J. Gastroenterol.* **19,** Suppl. 92, 163 (1984). Clinical study: A. Materia *et al., Clin. Ter.* **97,** 183 (1981).

Crystals, mp 242-244°. LD_{50} orally in rats: 3710 mg/kg (Almirante, 1967).

THERAP CAT: Antiulcerative.

10189. Zolmitriptan. [139264-17-8] (4*S*)-4-[[3-[2-(Dimethylamino)ethyl]-1*H*-indol-5-yl]methyl]-2-oxazolidinone; (*S*)-*N,N*-dimethyl-2-[5-(2-oxo-1,3-oxazolidin-4-ylmethyl)-1*H*-indol-3-yl]-ethylamine; 311C90; BW-311C90; Zomig. $C_{16}H_{21}N_3O_2$; mol wt 287.36. C 66.87%, H 7.37%, N 14.62%, O 11.14%. Serotonin $5HT_{1D}$-receptor agonist. Prepn: A. D. Robertson *et al.,* **WO 9118897** (1991 to Wellcome Foundation); *eidem,* **US 5466699** (1995 to Burroughs Wellcome). Structure-activity and receptor binding study: R. C. Glen *et al., J. Med. Chem.* **38,** 3566 (1995). Pharmacology: P. J. Goadsby, L. Edvinsson, *Headache* **34,** 394 (1994). Clinical pharmacokinetics: E. Seaber *et al., Br. J. Clin. Pharmacol.* **41,** 141 (1996). Clinical trial in migraine: S. J. Tepper *et al., Curr. Med. Res. Opin.* **15,** 254 (1999). Review of clinical experience and pharmacokinetics: M. Gawel, I. Worthington, *Expert Opin. Pharmacother.* **6,** 1019-1024 (2005).

White crystals from isopropanol as the 0.9 isopropanolate hemihydrate, mp 139-141°. $[\alpha]_D^{22} -5.79°$ (c = 0.5 in methanol). pKa 9.64. Stable; nonhygroscopic. Soly in aq soln at neutral pH: >20 mg/ml.

THERAP CAT: Antimigraine.

10190. Zolpidem. [82626-48-0] *N,N,*6-Trimethyl-2-(4-methylphenyl)imidazo[1,2-*a*]pyridine-3-acetamide; *N,N,*6-trimethyl-2-*p*-tolylimidazo[1,2-*a*]pyridine-3-acetamide; SL-80.0750. C_{19}-$H_{21}N_3O$; mol wt 307.39. C 74.24%, H 6.89%, N 13.67%, O 5.20%.

Selective non-benzodiazepine $GABA_A$ receptor agonist. Prepn: J. P. Kaplan, P. George, **EP 50563**; *eidem,* **US 4382938** (1982, 1983 both to Synthelabo). Neuropharmacology: S. Arbilla *et al., Arch. Pharmacol.* **330,** 248 (1985); H. Depoortere *et al., J. Pharmacol. Exp. Ther.* **237,** 649 (1986). Neurochemical profile: B. Scatton *et al., ibid.* 659. Binding study in rat brain: S. Arbilla *et al., Eur. J. Pharmacol.* **130,** 257 (1986). HPLC determn in plasma: P. Guinebault *et al., J. Chromatogr.* **383,** 206 (1986). Clinical evaluation of hypnotic activity: A. N. Nicholson, P. A. Pascoe, *Br. J. Clin. Pharmacol.* **21,** 205 (1986). Evaluation as pre-anesthetic medication: J. N. Cashman *et al., ibid.* **24,** 85 (1987). Review of pharmacology and therapeutic potential: H. D. Langtry, P. Benfield, *Drugs* **40,** 291-313 (1990).

mp 196°. pKa 6.2.

L-(+)-Hemitartrate. [99294-93-6] SL-80.0750-23N; Ambien; Ivadal; Niotal; Stilnoct; Stilnox. $(C_{19}H_{21}N_3O)_2.C_4H_6O_6$; mol wt 764.87. Soly in water (20°): 23 mg/ml. Sparingly sol in alcohol, propylene glycol.

Note: This is a controlled substance (depressant): **21 CFR,** 1308.14.

THERAP CAT: Sedative, hypnotic.

10191. Zomepirac. [33369-31-2] 5-(4-Chlorobenzoyl)-1,4-dimethyl-1*H*-pyrrole-2-acetic acid; 1,4-dimethyl-5-(*p*-chlorobenzoyl)pyrrole-2-acetic acid. $C_{15}H_{14}ClNO_3$; mol wt 291.73. C 61.76%, H 4.84%, Cl 12.15%, N 4.80%, O 16.45%. Prepn: J. R. Carson, **DE 2102746**; *idem,* **US 3752826** (1971, 1973 both to McNeil); J. R. Carson, S. Wong, *J. Med. Chem.* **16,** 172 (1973). Pharmacology: R. Sofia *et al., Pharmacol. Res. Commun.* **11,** 179 (1979); P. O'Neill *et al., J. Pharmacol. Exp. Ther.* **209,** 366 (1979). Determn in plasma by HPLC: K.-T. Ng, T. Snyderman, *J. Chromatogr.* **178,** 241 (1979). Metabolism: J. M. Grindel *et al., Drug Metab. Dispos.* **8,** 343 (1980); W. N. Wu *et al., ibid.* 349. Pharmacokinetics: R. K. Nayak *et al., Clin. Pharmacol. Ther.* **27,** 395 (1980). Series of articles on pharmacology, kinetics, clinical studies: *J. Clin. Pharmacol.* **20,** 213-424 (1980). Preclinical narcotic abuse liability evaluation: J. H. Woods *et al., Arzneim.-Forsch.* **33,** 218 (1983). Multicenter clinical study in painful conditions: C. E. Steele, W. L. Jefferson, *Curr. Med. Res. Opin.* **8,** 382 (1983). Review of pharmacology and therapeutic efficacy: P. A. Morley *et al., Drugs* **23,** 250-275 (1982). Comprehensive description: M. Zinic *et al., Anal. Profiles Drug Subs.* **15,** 673-698 (1986).

White cryst from 2-propanol, mp 178-179°.

Sodium salt dihydrate. [64092-49-5] Zomax; Zomaxin; Zopirac. $C_{15}H_{13}ClNNaO_3.2H_2O$; mol wt 349.74. Crystals from isopropanol + water, mp 295-296°.

THERAP CAT: Analgesic; anti-inflammatory.

10192. Zonisamide. [68291-97-4] 1,2-Benzisoxazole-3-methanesulfonamide; 3-(sulfamoylmethyl)-1,2-benzisoxazole; AD-810; CI-912; Excegran; Zonegran. $C_8H_8N_2O_3S$; mol wt 212.23. C 45.27%, H 3.80%, N 13.20%, O 22.62%, S 15.11%. Sulfonamide antiseizure agent; blocks repetitive firing of voltage-sensitive sodium channels and reduces voltage-sensitive T-type calcium currents. Prepn: H. Uno *et al.,* **JP Kokai 78 77057**; *eidem,* **US 4172896** (1978, 1979 both to Dainippon); *eidem, J. Med. Chem.* **22,** 180 (1979). Pharmacology and toxicity: Y. Masuda *et al., Arzneim.-Forsch.* **30,** 477 (1980). Mode of action study: T. Ito *et* *al., ibid.* 603. HPLC determn in serum: U. Juergens, *J. Chromatogr.* **385** 233 (1987). Clinical trial in epilepsy: D. Schmidt *et al., Epilepsy Res.* **15**, 67 (1993). Review of neuropharmacology: E. J. Hammond *et al., Gen. Pharmacol.* **18**, 303 (1987); of pharmacokinetics and therapeutic potential: D. H. Peters, E. M. Sorkin, *Drugs* **45**, 760-787 (1993); of pharmacokinetics and mechanism of action: I. E. Leppik, *Seizure* **13S**, S5-S9 (2004).

White needles from ethyl acetate, mp 160-163° (Uno); also reported as mp 162-166° (Masuda, 1980). pKa 10.2. Soly (mg/ml): water 0.80; 0.1 *N* HCl 0.50. Sparingly sol in chloroform, *n*-hexane. Sol in methanol, ethanol, ethyl acetate, and acetic acid. LD_{50} in mice, rats (mg/kg): 1892, 2001 orally; 1273, 2569 s.c.; 699, 733 i.p.; 604, 748 i.v. (Masuda, 1980).

THERAP CAT: Anticonvulsant.

10193. Zopiclone. [43200-80-2] 4-Methyl-1-piperazinecarboxylic acid 6-(5-chloro-2-pyridinyl)-6,7-dihydro-7-oxo-5*H*-pyrrolo[3,4-*b*]pyrazin-5-yl ester; 6-(5-chloropyrid-2-yl)-5-(4-methylpiperazin-1-yl)carbonyloxy-7-oxo-6,7-dihydro-5*H*-pyrrolo[3,4-*b*]pyrazine; RP-27267; Amoban; Imovane; Limovan; Sopivan; Ximovan; Zimovane. $C_{17}H_{17}ClN_6O_3$; mol wt 388.81. C 52.51%, H 4.41%, Cl 9.12%, N 21.61%, O 12.34%. Cyclopyrrolone member of a family of non-benzodiazepine $GABA_A$ receptor agonists. Prepn: C. Cotrel *et al.*, **DE 2300491**; *eidem,* **US 3862149** (1973, 1975 both to Rhone-Poulenc); C. Jeanmart, C. Cotrel, *C.R. Seances Acad. Sci. Ser. C* **287**, 377 (1978). *In vitro* and *in vivo* inhibition of benzodiazepine binding: J. C. Blanchard *et al., Life Sci.* **24**, 2417 (1979); *see also* P. H. Wu *et al., ibid.* **28**, 1023 (1981). Comparative study with benzodiazepines: E. Wickström, K. E. Giercksky, *Eur. J. Clin. Pharmacol.* **17**, 93 (1980). HPLC determn of enantiomers in plasma: C. Fernandez *et al., J. Chromatogr.* **572**, 195 (1991); in urine: *eidem, ibid.* **617**, 271 (1993). Pharmacokinetics of zopiclone and enantiomers: *eidem, Drug Metab. Dispos.* **21**, 1125 (1993). Mechanism of action: A. Doble *et al., Eur. Psychiatr.* **10**, Suppl 3, 117s (1995). Sedative and anxiolytic effects of enantiomers and metabolite in rats: J. N. Carlson *et al., Eur. J. Pharmacol.* **415**, 181 (2001). Series of articles on pharmacokinetics, pharmacology and efficacy in insomnia: *Sleep* **10**, Suppl 1, 1-87 (1987). Clinical overview: B. Musch, F. Maillard, *Int. J. Clin. Psychopharmacol.* **5**, 147-158 (1990). Review of pharmacology, tolerability and therapeutic efficacy: S. Noble *et al., Drugs* **55**, 277-302 (1998).

Crystals from acetonitrile/diisopropyl ether (1:1), mp 178°.
S-Form. [138729-47-2] Eszopiclone; Estorra; Lunesta. Prepn: C. Cotrel, G. Roussel, **WO 9212980** (1992 to Rhone-Poulenc Rorer); *see also: eidem,* **US 6319926** (2001 to Sepracor). Crystals from acetonitrile, mp 206.5°. $[\alpha]_D^{20}$ +135 ±3° (c = 1.0 in acetone).
Note: This is a controlled substance (depressant): **21 CFR,** 1308.14.

THERAP CAT: Sedative, hypnotic.

10194. Zopolrestat. [110703-94-1] 3,4-Dihydro-4-oxo-3-[[5-(trifluoromethyl)-2-benzothiazolyl]methyl]-1-phthalazineacetic acid; 2-[4-oxo-3-[5-(trifluoromethyl)benzothiazol-2-ylmethyl]-3,4-dihydrophthalazin-1-yl]acetic acid; CP-73850. $C_{19}H_{12}F_3N_3O_3S$; mol wt 419.38. C 54.41%, H 2.88%, F 13.59%, N 10.02%, O 11.45%, S 7.65%. Aldose reductase inhibitor. Prepn: B. L. Myl-

ari *et al.,* **EP 222576**; E. R. Larson, B. L. Mylari, **US 4939140** (1987, 1990 both to Pfizer); B. L. Mylari *et al. J. Med. Chem.* **34**, 108 (1991). Pharmacology: B. Tesfamariam *et al., J. Cardiovasc. Pharmacol.* **21**, 205 (1993); B. Tesfamariam *et al., Am. J. Physiol.* **265**, H1189 (1993). Clinical pharmacokinetics: P. B. Inskeep *et al., J. Clin. Pharmacol.* **34**, 760 (1994).

Crystals, mp 197-198°. pKa (dioxane/water): 5.46 (1:1); 6.38 (2:1). Log P (*n*-octanol/water): 3.43.
THERAP CAT: Treatment of diabetic complications.

10195. Zorubicin. [54083-22-6] (2*S-cis*)-Benzoic acid [1-[4-[(3-amino-2,3,6-trideoxy-α-L-*lyxo*-hexopyranosyl)oxy]-1,2,3,4,6,-11-hexahydro-2,5,12-trihydroxy-7-methoxy-6,11-dioxo-2-napthacenyl]ethylidene]hydrazide; benzoic acid hydrazide 3-hydrazone with daunorubicin; RP-22050. $C_{34}H_{35}N_3O_{10}$; mol wt 645.66. C 63.25%, H 5.46%, N 6.51%, O 24.78%. Semi-synthetic antibiotic related to daunorubicin, *q.v.* Prepn: G. Jolles, **DE 2327211** (1974 to Rhone-Poulenc), *C.A.* **82**, 171381x (1975). Biological activity: R. Maral *et al., C.R. Seances Acad. Sci. Ser. D* **275**, 301 (1972); R. Maral, *Cancer Chemother. Pharmacol.* **2**, 31 (1979). Distribution and metabolism in mice: R. Baurain *et al., ibid.* 37. Mechanism of action: G. P. Sartiano *et al., J. Antibiot.* **32**, 1038 (1979). Acute cardiovascular effects in dogs: E. H. Herman, R. S. Young, *Cancer Treat. Rep.* **63**, 1771 (1979). Clinical study in breast cancer: J. N. Ingle, *ibid.* 1701.

Hydrochloride. [36508-71-1] NSC-164011; Rubidazone. $C_{34}H_{35}N_3O_{10}$·HCl; mol wt 682.12. Red-orange crystalline powder from ethanol. $[\alpha]_D^{20}$ −50° (c = 0.2 in water). uv max (methanol): 232.5, 253, 480, 495 nm (ε 40225, 35300, 10480, 10300). LD_{50} in mice (mg/kg): 13.66 s.c., 4.42 i.p., 8.50 i.v. (Maral, 1972).
THERAP CAT: Antineoplastic.

10196. Zosuquidar. [167354-41-8] (α*R*)-4-[(1aα,6α,10bα)-1,1,-Difluoro-1,1a,6,10b-tetrahyrodibenzo[*a,e*]cyclopropa[*c*]cyclohepten-6-yl]-α-[(5-quinolinyloxy)methyl]-1-piperazineethanol; (2*R*)-*anti*-5-[3-[4-(10,11-difluoromethanodibenzosuber-5-yl)piperazin-1-yl]-2-hydroxypropoxy]quinoline. $C_{32}H_{31}F_2N_3O_2$; mol wt 527.60. C 72.85%, H 5.92%, F 7.20%, N 7.96%, O 6.06%. Multidrug resistance (MDR) modulator; selective inhibitor of P-glycoprotein (P-gp), *q.v.* Prepn: J. R. Pfister, D. L. Slate, **WO 9424107**; *eidem,* **US 5654304** (1994, 1997 both to Syntex); J. R. Pfister *et al., Bioorg. Med. Chem. Lett.* **5**, 2473 (1995). Improved synthesis: C. J. Barnett *et al., J. Org. Chem.* **69**, 7653 (2004). Effect on multidrug resistant cell lines: L. J. Green *et al., Biochem. Pharmacol.* **61**, 1393 (2001). Specificity for P-gp: R. L. Shepard *et al., Int. J. Cancer* **103**, 121 (2003). Clinical pharmacology and pharmacokinetics in patients with advanced malignancies: E. H. Rubin *et al., Clin. Cancer Res.* **8**, 3710 (2002). Effect on pharmacokinetics of doxorubicin: S. Callies *et al., Cancer Chemother. Pharmacol.* **51**, 107 (2003).

action: D. H. Young, R. A. Slawecki, *Pestic. Biochem. Physiol.* **69**, 100 (2001). Laboratory resistance risk study: D. H. Young *et al.*, *Pest Manage. Sci.* **57**, 1081 (2001).

Trihydrochloride. [167465-36-3] LY-335979; RS-33295-198. $C_{32}H_{31}F_2N_3O_2 \cdot 3HCl$; mol wt 636.99. mp 190°.

THERAP CAT: Antineoplastic adjunct (chemosensitizer).

10197. Zotepine. [26615-21-4] 2-[(8-Chlorodibenzo[*b*,*f*]-thiepin-10-yl)oxy]-*N*,*N*-dimethylethanamine; 2-chloro-11-(2-dimethylaminoethoxy)dibenzo[*b*,*f*]thiepine; Lodopin; Nipolept; Setous; Zoleptil. $C_{18}H_{18}ClNOS$; mol wt 331.86. C 65.15%, H 5.47%, Cl 10.68%, N 4.22%, O 4.82%, S 9.66%. Combined dopamine (D_2) and serotonin (5-HT$_2$) receptor antagonist. Prepn: S. Umio *et al.*, **DE 1907670**; *eidem*, **US 3704245** (1969, 1972 both to Fujisawa); I. Ueda *et al.*, *Chem. Pharm. Bull.* **26**, 3058 (1978). Pharmacology: S. Uchida *et al.*, *Arzneim.-Forsch.* **29**, 1588 (1979). Pharmacokinetics and metabolism: K. Noda *et al., ibid.* 1595. Toxicology: K. Fukuhara *et al., ibid.* 1600. Effects on serotonin receptors: A. Czyrak *et al., Pharmacopsychiatry* **26**, 53 (1993). GC-MS determn in plasma: O. Tanaka *et al., Ther. Drug Monit.* **18**, 294 (1996). Clinical trials in schizophrenia: C. Barnas *et al., Int. Clin. Psychopharmacol.* **7**, 23 (1992); A. Meyer-Lindenberg *et al., Pharmacopsychiatry* **30**, 35 (1997).

Crystals from cyclohexane, mp 90-91°. uv max (95% ethanol): 266 nm. LD$_{50}$ in male mice, rats (mg/kg): 108, 458 orally; 43.3, 39.7 i.v.; 40.0, 97.0 i.p.; 84.9, 2080 s.c. (Fukuhara).

THERAP CAT: Antipsychotic.

10198. Zoxamide. [156052-68-5] 3,5-Dichloro-*N*-(3-chloro-1-ethyl-1-methyl-2-oxopropyl)-4-methylbenzamide; *N*-[3′-(1′-chloro-3′-methyl-2′-oxopentan)]-3,5-dichloro-4-methylbenzamide; RH-7281; Zoxium. $C_{14}H_{16}Cl_3NO_2$; mol wt 336.64. C 49.95%, H 4.79%, Cl 31.59%, N 4.16%, O 9.51%. Fungicide for foliar use on potatoes, vines and vegetables, targeting Oomycete fungi. Prepn: E. L. Michelotti, D. H. Young, **US 5304572** (1994 to Rohm and Haas); H. L. Rayle, L. Fellmeth, *Org. Process Res. Dev.* **3**, 172 (1999). Comprehensive description: A. R. Egan *et al., Brighton Crop Prot. Conf. - Pests Dis.* **1998**, 335-342. Mode of

White solid. mp 158-160° (Rayle); also reported as mp 159.5-160.5° (Egan). Log P (octanol/water): 3.76 (20°). Vapor pressure at 25°, 35°, 45°: $<1 \times 10^{-7}$ torr. Soly at 20° (mg/l): water 0.681. LD$_{50}$ in rats (mg/kg): >5000 orally; >2000 dermally. LC$_{50}$ in rats (mg/l): >5.3 by inhalation; in mallard ducks, bobwhite quail (mg/kg): >5250, >5250 dietary; in trout (μg/l): 160 (Egan).

USE: Agricultural fungicide.

10199. Zoxazolamine. [61-80-3] 5-Chloro-2-benzoxazolamine; 2-amino-5-chlorobenzoxazole; McN-485; Flexin. C_7H_5-ClN_2O; mol wt 168.58. C 49.87%, H 2.99%, Cl 21.03%, N 16.62%, O 9.49%. Centrally acting myorelaxant; formerly used as an antispasmodic and uricosuric. Prepn: T. Nagana *et al., J. Am. Chem. Soc.* **75**, 2770 (1953); J. Sam, **US 2780633** (1957 to McNeil). Pharmacology and structure-activity studies: C. K. Cain, A. P. Roszkowski, "Benzoxazoles, Benzothiazoles and Benzimidazoles" in *Medicinal Chemistry: A Series of Monographs* **4**, G. DeStevens, Ed. (Academic Press, New York, 1964) pp 325-357. Use in assay of microsomal oxidase activity: J. E. Tomaszeski *et al., Arch. Biochem. Biophys.* **176**, 788 (1976). GLC determn and pharmacokinetics: M van der Graaff *et al., Drug Metab. Dispos.* **14**, 331 (1986).

Crystals from benzene, mp 185-185.5°. uv max (methanol): 244, 285 nm. Slightly sol in water; sol in alcohol. LD$_{50}$ in mice, rats (mg/kg): 376, 102 i.p.; 678, 730 orally (Cain, Roszkowski).

Hydrochloride. $C_7H_5ClN_2O \cdot HCl$. Needles, mp 229° (dec).

USE: Tool for assessing hepatic cytochrome P-450 activity in rodents.

10200. Zymosan. [9010-72-4] Anticomplementary factor. Crude yeast cell wall prepns consisting chiefly of protein-carbohydrate complexes. Prepn from whole yeast cells: Pillemer, Ecker, *J. Biol. Chem.* **137**, 139 (1941); Pillemer *et al., J. Exp. Med.* **103**, 1 (1956); from yeast cell walls: Z. Holan, *Folia Microbiol.* **25**, 501 (1980). Composition of zymosan: F. J. DiCarlo, J. V. Fiore, *Science* **127**, 756 (1958). Enhances the specific defenses of an organism through the activation of the properdin system, *q.v.* Activity studies: Brade *et al., J. Immunol.* **111**, 1389 (1973); **112**, 1115 (1974). Induces aggregation and a release reaction in human platelet-rich plasma: Zucker, Grant, *ibid.* 1219. *Review:* Fitzpatrick, DiCarlo, *Ann. N.Y. Acad. Sci.* **118**, art. 4, 233 (1964).

Light gray powder. Practically insol in water, but readily disperses to give a homogeneous suspension.

USE: In the assay of properdin.

SUPPLEMENTAL TABLES

ALPHABETICAL LIST OF SUPPLEMENTAL TABLES

TABLE-1

Glossary

Listed below are brief definitions for selected terms used in the monographs and/or frequently encountered within the references cited.

abzyme Catalytic antibody; antibody that can act like an enzyme in a specific chemical reaction.

adjuvant Substance administered with an antigen to augment its immunogenicity.

adrenergic System of autonomic innervation activated by epinephrine, norepinephrine or dopamine; particularly referring to substances that mimic the actions of the sympathetic nervous system.

agonist Receptor-specific activator; also a substance that mimics the effects of an endogenous regulatory compound.

aldose reductase Aldehyde reductase, EC 1.1.1.21; an oxidoreductase that reversibly catalyzes NADPH-dependent reduction of aldehydes, ketones, trioses, and triose phosphates.

alkaloid A nitrogenous, basic, usually bitter, substance found in plants. Term also applied to synthetic structural analogs.

allomone Chemical messenger used for communication between different species. Causes a reaction in the other species which is favorable to the organism secreting the substance.

allotrope One of several possible forms of an element; each of which differs in the atom bonding pattern.

aminoglycoside Carbohydrate typically consisting of 3 or 4 rings which has primary or secondary amines as ring substituents. Classification of antibiotics derived from various species of *Streptomyces,* which interfere with the function of bacterial ribosomes, e.g. streptomycin, gentamicin.

amyloid Complex proteinaceous fibrillar material deposited in blood vessels, heart, liver, brain, and other tissues in various disease states; gives characteristic starch-like reaction with iodine.

angiogenesis The development and formation of new blood vessels; postulated that tumor growth is preceded by an increase in new capillaries which converge upon the tumor.

antagonist Receptor-specific blocker; also a compound devoid of intrinsic regulatory activity which blocks or diminishes the action of an agonist.

anti Stereodescriptor restricted to bicyclo[X.Y.Z]anes in which the Z bridge reference group is oriented toward the Y bridge. Analogous to *trans* in double-bonded nitrogen systems such as oximes.

antibiotic Substance produced and secreted by various microorganisms which in low concentrations is toxic to other species.

antibody Immunoglobulin molecule produced in vertebrates by B-cells as a response to antigenic challenge; exist in different forms, each with a different binding site specifically recognizing the antigen that induced its formation.

antigen Immunogen; an agent that elicits an immune response including the production of an antibody; also considered to be any substance to which an antibody can bind.

antisense The DNA strand which is not transcribed; therefore, it has the same oligonucleotide sequence as the mRNA which codes for the protein.

antipyretic An agent that reduces or relieves fever.

apoprotein The protein portion of a conjugated protein without its prosthetic group.

apoptosis A regulated series of events leading to the death and removal of a cell in response to specific developmental or physiological signals; also known as "programmed cell death".

aromatase EC 1.14.14.1; enzyme that catalyzes the conversion of androgens to estrogens.

atriopeptidase Neutral endopeptidase, EC 3.4.24.11; an endopeptidase that catalyzes the degradation of atrial natriuretic factor.

bacteriocin A protein produced by bacteria that is toxic to another closely related strain.

balsam Resinous plant exudate containing the aromatic substances benzoic acid or cinnamic acid or their esters resulting from either a physiological or pathological response.

biological response modifiers Agents that alter the immune response such as interleukins, interferons, colony-stimulating factors, and tumor necrosis factor.

bitter A liquid, often alcoholic, that is prepared by steeping or distilling of a bitter herb or herb part that is used medicinally.

carbene A neutral organic radical containing a divalent carbon atom having only six electrons in its outer shell (R_2C:).

carbonic anhydrase Carbonate dehydratase, EC 4.2.1.1; catalyzes interconversion (reversible hydration) of carbonic acid to carbon dioxide and water.

carcinoma A malignant tumor arising from epithelial cells.

catechol O-methyl transferase EC 2.1.1.6; a methyltransferase that catalyzes the transfer of a methyl group from S-adenosyl-L-methionine to catechol or catecholamine.

chelate The cyclic structure formed by unshared electrons on neighboring atoms complexing with a metal ion; used as a sequestrant in metal poisoning.

chemoselectivity Pertains to the preferential reaction of a reagent with one functional group of a multifunctional molecule.

chemotaxis Migration of cells or organisms within a chemical concentration gradient.

chimeric Individual organism with cell populations from genetically different sources.

chiral The arrangements of atoms in space such that the resulting molecule is nonsuperimposable on its mirror image.

cholinesterase EC 3.1.1.8; catalyzes hydrolysis of acetylcholine and other choline esters to form choline and a carboxylic acid.

chromophore The group of atoms in a molecule that absorbs light and is responsible for the color of the molecule.

cis Relative stereodescriptor limited to cyclic systems with two stereocenters. Configuration where the two groups of higher priority are on the same side of the reference plane. See also *zusammen.*

TABLE-2

clinical trial, Phase I Safety testing and pharmacological profiling in humans; usually involves 20-80 healthy volunteers and takes about one year.

clinical trial, Phase II Effectiveness testing in volunteer patients; usually involves 100-300 volunteers and takes about two years.

clinical trial, Phase III Extensive clinical testing in humans to determine efficacy and to identify adverse reactions; usually involves 1000-3000 patients and lasts about three years.

clinical trial, Phase IV Additional post-marketing studies to evaluate long term effects.

cloning Proliferation of a single cell to a large colony; replication from a single gene introduced into a host cell.

coenzyme Nonprotein molecule that is essential for the activity of an enzyme; functions as a cofactor of an enzyme.

conformers Different three-dimensional arrangements of atoms within a molecule that can be interconverted by rotation around single bonds; not usually separable. May also be referred to as conformation isomers or rotamers. (e.g. the chair, boat and twist forms of cyclohexane).

corticosteroid A 21-carbon steroid hormone produced by the adrenal cortex in response to the release of corticotropin (ACTH) or angiotensin.

cyclooxygenase An activity of prostaglandin endoperoxide synthase (EC 1.14.99.1) that catalyzes the oxidation of arachidonic acid to produce prostaglandins and thromboxanes.

cytochromes Family of colored proteins, related by the presence of a porphyrin metal (usually Fe), which undergo rapid oxidation and reduction in organisms.

cytokines Diverse group of soluble, nonantibody proteins secreted by a variety of cell types, which modulate the functional activities of individual cells by interaction with specific cell surface receptors, e.g. interferon, interleukin.

cytokinin Plant hormone that stimulates cell division and metabolism.

dative bond Semipolar linkage between two atoms where one atom contributes both electrons; also referred to as a coordinate covalent bond.

depsipeptide Polypeptide that contains ester bonds as well as peptide bonds, commonly but not necessarily alternating. Naturally occurring depsipeptides are often cyclic. Common metabolic products of microorganisms; often have antibiotic activity.

eicosanoids Collective term applied to substances such as prostaglandins, thromboxanes, leukotrienes and lipoxins, which are all derived from arachidonic acid; play an important role in inflammation.

enantioselectivity Pertains to a stereoselective reaction in which the potential products are mirror images.

endo Stereodescriptor used only for ring positions on [X.Y.Z.]anes in which X≥Y>Z>0 and the group of higher priority is on the opposite side of the ring reference plane to the Z-bridgehead.

endopeptidase Endoproteinase, proteinase; catalyzes the cleavage of non-terminal peptide bonds in a polypeptide or protein.

endorphins Naturally occurring neuropeptides that bind to opioid receptors with pain relieving action; the name is derived from endogenous morphine.

endotoxins Heat-stable lipopolysaccharide-protein complexes contained in cell walls of gram-negative bacteria including non-infectious gram-negatives; released only when the cells are disrupted.

entactogen Non-hallucinogenic psychoactive compound which is purported to facilitate communication and introspective states. Derived from the Greek roots of *en* for within or inside, *gen* to produce or originate and the Latin root *tactus* for touch.

enterotoxin Exotoxin produced by enterobacteria, which, when ingested or produced within the intestine, affects its function, inducing nausea, diarrhea, vomiting, etc.

entgegen (E) German for opposite. Relative stereodescriptor for configuration about double bonds; used when groups of higher priority are on different sides of the vertical reference plane.

epitope Structural entity on the antigen that forms the recognition site for binding.

ergot The hardened web-like mass of threads of *Claviceps purpurea* developed on rye attacked by the fungus. Ergot alkaloids are used as oxytocics and in treatment of migraine.

essential fatty acids A group of polyunsaturated fatty acids, such as linoleic acid, required for growth in mammals; they cannot be synthesized and must be obtained in the diet.

essential oil Volatile, aromatic oil physically extracted from plants.

excipient Any more or less inert substance added to a drug to give suitable consistency or form to the drug.

excitotoxin Neurotoxic analogs of glutamic acid which mimic its excitatory effects on neurons of the CNS.

exo Stereodescriptor used only for ring positions on [X.Y.Z.]anes in which X≥Y>Z>0 and the group of higher priority is on the same side of the ring reference plane to the Z-bridgehead.

exotoxins Disease-producing proteins secreted by species of certain bacteria into surrounding medium.

flavoprotein Flavin dependent enzymes which normally contain FAD or FMN as tightly bound coenzymes.

galenic Prepared from a plant rather than chemically synthesized.

geminal (*gem*) Indicates that the two substituents in a disubstituted compound are on the same carbon atom.

glioma A tumor arising from the glial tissue of the brain or spinal cord.

glucocorticoid A 21-carbon steroid hormone secreted by adrenal cortex. Acts on carbohydrate, lipid and protein metabolism and inhibits the release of corticotropin (ACTH).

α-glucosidase Maltase, glucoinvertase, EC 3.2.1.20; a glucohydrolase that catalyzes hydrolysis of terminal non-reducing 1,4-linked α-D-glucose residues to release α-D-glucose.

green chemistry Development of chemical products, procedures, and technologies with the goal of minimizing or eliminating the generation of hazardous substances.

TABLE-3

Glossary (Continued)

hapten Small nonantigenic molecule which becomes an antigen when combined with a larger carrier molecule.

herbaceous Plants or parts of plants that do not have woody stems and typically die down annually.

HMG CoA reductase β-Hydroxyl-β-methyl glutarate CoA reductase, EC 1.1.1.88; oxidoreductase that catalyzes 3-hydroxy-3-methylglutaryl CoA reduction to mevalonate with NADPH as the electron donor.

homeopathy The theory that "like cures like"; wherein small amounts of compounds which in large amounts would produce undesirable symptoms are beneficial.

hybridoma Cell line produced by fusing an antibody-secreting cell with a myeloma cell; used to produce specific monoclonal antibodies in great quantity.

hyperplasia Abnormal increase in the number of normal cells in a tissue or organ.

hypertrophy Abnormal enlargement of an organ or tissue, not due to tumor formation; caused by the increase in size of its cellular components.

idiotype The segment of an immunoglobulin molecule that determines its antigenic specificity.

immunoglobulins Proteins produced by plasma cells derived from B cells of the immune system; function as antibodies to aid in fighting infection.

immunotoxins Molecules that comprise a cytotoxic agent linked to an antibody specific for target cell antigens.

inosine monophosphate dehydrogenase IMPH; EC 1.1.1.205; NAD^+-dependent enzyme that catalyzes oxidation of inosine 5'-monophosphate (IMP) to xanthosine 5'-monophosphate (XMP); rate limiting step in *de novo* guanine nucleotide synthesis.

isoform Protein that has the same function as another protein but which is encoded by a different gene or alternative splicing of variant alleles and may have small differences in its primary structure.

kairomones Chemical messengers used for communication between different species which are either nonadaptive or actually detrimental to the organisms producing them.

ketolide Semi-synthetic derivative of the macrolide erythromycin A.

knockout mutation A mutation in which a single gene of choice is inactivated without affecting other genes.

lake Organic pigment made of an oil-soluble organic dye, a precipitant, and an absorptive inorganic substrate.

lantobiotics Polycyclic bacteriocins consisting of the thioether amino acids lanthionine and beta-methyllanthionine.

liposome Closed vesicles of lipid bilayer formed by emulsification of cell membranes; the interior may be used to encapsulate drugs for targeted cellular delivery.

5-lipoxygenase EC 1.13.11.34; actin-binding protein that initiates the synthesis of leukotrienes via the oxidation of arachidonic acid.

lymphoma A malignant tumor of the lymphoid tissue.

lymphokine Nonimmunoglobulin protein synthesized primarily by T-lymphocytes that modulates an immune response, e.g. interleukin-2, γ-interferon.

major histocompatibility complex Large, multigene cluster that encodes for the cell surface glycoproteins which are essential in the cellular immune response to distinguish "self" and "non-self".

matrix metalloproteinase Zinc-dependent endopeptidases that catalyze the hydrolysis of extracellular proteins, particularly collagen and elastin.

melanoma A malignant tumor derived from melanocytes.

meso compound Pertaining to a compound which contains equal numbers of enantiomeric groups which are identically linked. Compound having at least two chiral centers, yet no optical rotation because it contains a plane of symmetry.

mesomerism The existence of chemical structures having the same molecular arrangements that differ only in the location of electrons; the actual electronic distribution is not represented by any one structure, but is a hybrid of contributing structures.

monoamine oxidase MAO, amine oxidase, EC 1.4.3.4; flavoprotein enzyme that catalyzes oxidative deamination of monoamines to form aldehydes or ketones with the release of hydrogen peroxide and ammonia.

monoclonal antibody Antibody produced by a cloned hybridoma cell, active against a single target antigen.

mordant Substance used to fix a dyestuff on a material by combining with the dye to form an insoluble compound.

morphogens Soluble substances that control the embryonic differentiation of cells and tissues.

multidrug resistance The resistance of tumor cells to varied chemotherapeutic agents mediated by the expression of a transmembrane pump, P-glycoprotein, which actively pumps the drugs out of the cells, lowering the intracellular concentration and cytotoxic effectiveness.

mutagen Agent that causes a permanent inheritable change in the DNA of the organism.

mutein Name applied to a protein arising as a result of a mutation.

mycotoxins Fungal toxins that are harmful to other organisms.

myeloma A malignant tumor derived from hemopoietic tissue.

neuraminidase Acetyl-neuraminyl hydrolase; sialidase; EC 3.2.1.18; enzyme that catalyzes the hydrolysis of terminal sialic acid groups from glycoproteins and oligosaccharides; found on the surface of the influenza virus.

neuroleptic Agent that pharmacologically manages the manifestations of a psychotic disorder, affecting cognition and behavior; also called major tranquilizer or anti-psychotic.

nitrene Carbene analog consisting of an electron-deficient, neutral monovalent nitrogen species.

neurotrophic factors Polypeptides that support the growth and survival of specific populations of neurons.

nootropic Agent having positive effects on organically impaired cognition or nervous system function; from the Greek *noos* or *nous* for mind and *-tropic* for nourishing, stimulating.

TABLE-4

nor Originally the abbreviation for *Nitrogen ohne Radikal.* Currently a subtractive prefix for stereoparents indicating ring contraction or the loss of a methyl group from the carbon skeleton.

nucleic acids Biologically occurring polynucleotides in which the nucleotide residues are linked in a specific sequence by phosphodiester bonds; DNA and RNA.

nucleoside A purine or pyrimidine base in glycosidic linkage with a pentose sugar (e.g. adenosine, cytosine, guanosine, thymidine).

nucleotide The phosphate ester of a nucleoside.

oleoresin Plant exudate containing essential oil and resin.

orexigenic Appetite stimulating.

peptidyl dipeptidase A Angiotensin converting enzyme; EC 3.4.15.1; a zinc-containing hydrolase that catalyzes cleavage of a C-terminal dipeptide; catalyzes conversion of angiotensin I to yield the active angiotensin II.

peroxidases Oxidoreductase enzymes that catalyze oxidation of substrates by hydrogen peroxide.

pharmacodynamics Study of the biochemical and physiological effects of drugs on living systems and their mechanism of action.

pharmacognosy Study of biological and chemical properties of naturally occurring medicinal products.

pharmacokinetics Study of the action of drugs in the body over time, including absorption, biotransformation, tissue distribution, and elimination of the drugs and their metabolites.

pharmacophore An abstract concept that defines the set molecular characteristics (steric, and electronic) and chemical functionalities necessary to ensure the optimal interaction with the target site.

pheromones Chemical substances used for communication between individual organisms of the same species. Perceived primarily by the olfactory sense and to a lesser extent the gustatory sense. From the Greek *pherein* to transfer, and *hormon* to excite or stimulate.

phytosterols Sterols obtained from higher plants; differ from sterols occurring in animals by having C_1 or C_2 residues at C-24 and/or a double bond at C-22.

prebiotic Food ingredients that function by stimulating growth of beneficial bacteria of the digestive system.

primary structure (protein) Amino acid sequence.

prion A small proteinaceous infectious particle which resists inactivation by procedures that modify nucleic acids.

probiotic Beneficial bacteria of the digestive system.

prochiral Achiral compound or group that would become chiral if one of two identical substituents is replaced by a new ligand.

prodrug A drug precursor; a substance which is inactive by itself and which must undergo chemical conversion by metabolic processes to become an active pharmacological agent.

prostaglandin endoperoxide synthase Prostaglandin synthase; EC 1.14.99.1; heme-containing enzyme that with dioxygenase and peroxidase activity; catalyzes the biosynthesis of prostaglandins G and H from arachidonic acid.

prosthetic group Tightly bound non-protein portion of a conjugated protein essential for the activity of a protein or enzyme.

pyrogens Fever-producing substances; agents which produce a febrile response when administered parenterally to man and certain animals.

quaternary structure (protein) Three-dimensional structure of a protein, in particular how subunits are integrated; typically classified as fibrous, globular, or conjugated.

receptor Protein or protein complex that binds a specific ligand such as a neurotransmitter, hormone, lymphokine, etc., producing a secondary biological signal within the cell.

rectus (R)—(right) Opposite of (*S*). Absolute term describing the spatial arrangement about an asymmetric carbon when the substituent of lowest priority lies below the reference plane and the priority of the remaining substituents decreases in a clockwise direction.

5-α reductase EC 1.3.99.5; membrane-bound enzyme that catalyzes the irreversible reduction of testosterone to the more potent androgen, dihydrotestosterone.

regioselectivity Pertains to the preferential formation of one structural isomer when two or more are possible.

reverse transcriptase EC 2.7.7.49; RNA-directed DNA polymerase; required for the replication of retroviruses.

RNA interference (RNAi) Process in which short interfering RNA (siRNA) binds to specific mRNA and silences gene expression.

saponins Foaming glycoside of sterols or triterpenes that are widely distributed in plants. Causes cell lysis.

sarcoma Malignant tumor arising from connective tissue or muscle cells.

secondary structure (protein) Residue by residue conformation of the backbone of the polypeptide chain. Typical conformations include the α helices, β sheets and random coils; given rise to by the regular hydrogen-bond interactions within contiguous stretches of polypeptide chain.

semiconductor Material with electric conductivity range between metals and insulators.

sinister (S)—(left) Opposite of (*R*). Absolute term describing the spatial arrangement about an asymmetric carbon when the substituent of lowest priority lies below the reference plane and the priority of the remaining substituents decreases in a counterclockwise direction.

sol-gel process Solution process for the transformation of colloidal liquids into ultrahomogeneous ceramic and glass gels used in material science.

stereoselectivity Pertains to the preferential formation of one stereoisomer when two or more are possible.

stereospecific reaction A reaction where starting materials, which differ only in their configuration, are converted to stereoisomerically distinct products. Applies when the reaction processes are constrained to proceed in a stereochemically defined manner.

superconductors Materials that below a certain critical temperature show zero resistance to electrical current flow. Ideally if resistance is truly zero, then electrons flowing in a loop of superconducting wire would never lose any energy.

TABLE-5

syn   Stereodescriptor restricted to bicyclo[X.Y.Z]anes in which the Z bridge reference group is oriented toward the X bridge; analogous to *cis* in double-bonded nitrogen systems such as oximes.

teratogen   Agent that causes abnormal fetal development.

terpene   Hydrocarbon derived from essential oils, resins, etc., containing multiples of the C_5 isoprene unit as its carbon skeleton. Monoterpene is $C_{10}H_{16}$.

tertiary structure (protein)   Three dimensional conformation of the polypeptide chain after folding.

tocolytic   Compound to reduce uterine contractions.

topoisomerase   Enzyme that can remove (or create) supercoiling in double stranded DNA by creating transitory breaks in one (type I) or both (type II) strands of the sugar-phosphate backbone.

toxoid   A toxin which has been treated by a chemical agent or by heat to destroy its toxic properties while retaining its ability to stimulate antibody production.

trans   Relative stereodescriptor limited to cyclic systems with two stereocenters. Configuration where the two groups of highest priority are on opposite sides of the reference plane.

transduction   Transfer of genetic material from one cell to another by a viral vector.

transfection   Introduction of exogenous DNA (usually viral or bacterial) into mammalian cells or bacterial cells.

transgenic   Containing artificially introduced DNA as a result of experimental splicing of a segment of DNA from one genome into the germ line of another.

vasopeptidase inhibitor   Cardiovascular drug that simultaneously inhibits both neutral endopeptidase and angiotensin-converting enzyme.

vicinal (*vic*)   Indicates that two substituents in a disubstituted compound are on adjacent carbon atoms.

ylide   Compounds in which a carbon atom with an unshared electron pair is connected to cation from Group 15 (Va) or 16 (VIa) of the periodic table.

zusammen (Z)   German for together. Relative stereodescriptor for configuration about double bonds; used when groups of higher priority are on the same side of the vertical reference plane.

zwitterion   Dipolar ion in which positive and negative charges are physically separated.

zymogen   Inactive precursor molecule to an enzyme which is activated as a result of catalysis. Also known as a proenzyme.

TABLE-6

Acronyms

Following are the expanded meanings of acronyms or acronym-like abbreviations for chemical, agricultural, biomedical, or pharmaceutical terms, agencies, or organizations related to information found in *The Merck Index*.

AAAS	American Association for the Advancement of Science
AALAS	American Association for Laboratory Animal Science
AAPS	American Association of Pharmaceutical Scientists
AAS	Atomic absorption spectroscopy
AAV	Adeno-associated virus
AB	Aktiebolag
ABC	ATP binding cassette
ABPI	Association of the British Pharmaceutical Industry
ACAT	Acyl-CoA cholesterol transferase
ACE	Angiotensin converting enzyme
ACP	Acyl carrier protein
	American College of Physicians
ACRP	Association of Clinical Research Professionals
ACS	American Cancer Society
	American Chemical Society
	American College of Surgeons
ACTH	Adrenocorticotropic hormone
AD	Alzheimer's disease
ADA	American Dental Association
ADCC	Antibody-dependent cellular cytotoxicity
ADD	Attention deficit disorder
ADE	Adverse drug event
ADH	Alcohol dehydrogenase
ADHD	Attention deficit hyperactivity disorder
ADI	Acceptable daily intake
ADL	Activities of daily living
ADME	Absorption, distribution, metabolism, excretion
ADR	Adverse drug reaction
AE	Adverse event
AFC	Antibody forming cells
AFLP	Amplified fragment length polymorphism
AFM	Atomic force microscopy
AG	Aktiengesellschaft
AGE	Advanced glycation endproduct
AHA	American Heart Association
AHFS	American Hospital Formulary Service
AIChE	American Institute of Chemical Engineers
AIDS	Acquired immune deficiency syndrome
AIF	Apoptosis-inducing factor
AII	Angiotensin II
ALA	Aminolevulinic acid
ALG	Anti-lymphocyte globulin
ALL	Acute lymphoblastic leukemia
ALS	Amyotrophic lateral sclerosis
	Anti-lymphocyte serum
ALT	Alanine aminotransferase
AMA	American Medical Association
AMD	Age-related macular degeneration
AMI	Acute myocardial infarction
AML	Acute myeloid leukemia
ANDA	Abbreviated New Drug Application
ANOVA	Analysis of variance
ANP	Atrial natriuretic peptide
ANSI	American National Standards Institute
AOAC	Association of Official Analytical Chemists
APC	Antigen presenting cells
APhA	American Pharmaceutical Association
API	Active pharmaceutical ingredient
	American Petroleum Institute
APOE	Apolipoprotein E
APP	Amyloid precursor protein
APPI	Academy of Pharmaceutical Physicians and Investigators
APT	Alum precipitated toxoid

APTT	Activated partial thromboplastin time
ARC	AIDS-related complex
	American Red Cross
ARDS	Acute respiratory distress syndrome
	Adult respiratory distress syndrome
ARMS	Alveolar rhabdomyosarcoma
ASBMB	American Society for Biochemistry and Molecular Biology
ASHG	American Society for Human Genetics
ASHP	American Society of Hospital-System Pharmacists
ASIST	American Society for Information Science and Technology
ASM	American Society for Microbiology
ASPET	American Society for Pharmacology and Experimental Therapeutics
AST	Asparate amino transferase
ASTM	American Society for Testing and Materials
ATCC	American Type Culture Collection
AUC	Area under the curve
AV	Atrioventricular
AVMA	American Veterinary Medical Association
BAC	Bacterial artificial chromosome
BACE	Beta-site amyloid precursor protein cleaving enzyme
BACR	British Association for Cancer Research
BAL	Blood alcohol level
BAN	British Approved Name
BBB	Blood-brain barrier
BBSRC	Biotechnology and Biological Sciences Research Center (UK)
BCG	Bacillus Calmette-Guerin
BCPC	British Crop Protection Council
BCRP	Breast cancer resistance protein
BES	Balanced electrolyte solution
BGG	Bovine gamma globulin
BIBRA	British Industrial Biological Research Association
BLA	Biologics License Application (US)
BMA	British Medical Association
BMD	Bone mineral density
BMI	Body mass index
BMR	Basal metabolic rate
BNF	British National Formulary
BOD	Biochemical oxygen demand
BP	British Pharmacopeia
BPH	Benign prostatic hyperplasia
	Benign prostatic hypertrophy
BRM	Biological response modifier
BSA	Bovine serum albumin
BSE	Bovine spongiform encephalopathy
BSI	British Standard Institutes
BUN	Blood urea nitrogen
BV	Besloten Vennootschap
BVA	British Veterinary Association
CA	Chemical Abstracts
CABG	Coronary artery bypass grafts
CAD	Coronary artery disease
CAM	Cell adhesion molecules
	Complementary and alternative medicine
cAMP	Cyclic adenosine monophosphate
CAS	Chemical Abstracts Service
CAT	Computerized axial tomography
CB	Cannabinoid
CBC	Complete blood count
CBER	Center for Biologics Evaluation and Research (US)

TABLE-7

CBF	Cerebral blood flow	CVM	Center for Veterinary Medicine (US)
CCD	Charge-coupled device	DC	Dendritic cells
CCK	Cholecystokinin	DCL	Diffuse cutaneous leishmaniasis
CD	Circular dichroism	DEA	Drug Enforcement Administration (US)
	Clusters of differentiation	DEFRA	Department for Environment, Food & Rural
CDC	Centers for Disease Control and Prevention (US)		Affairs (UK)
CDER	Center for Drug Evaluation and Research (US)	DXA	Dual-energy X-ray absorptiometry
CDK	Cyclin dependent kinase	DFA	Direct fluorescent antibody
cDNA	Complementary deoxyribonucleic acid	DHA	Docosahexaenoic acid
CE	Capillary electrophoresis	DHFR	Dihydrofolate reductase
CEA	Carcinoembryonic antigen	DHHS	Department of Health and Human Services
CETP	Cholesteryl ester transfer protein		(US)
CF	Cystic fibrosis	DIC	Disseminated intravascular coagulation
CFA	Complete Freund's adjuvant	DKA	Diabetic ketoacidosis
CFC	Chlorofluorocarbon	DM	Diabetes mellitus
CFR	Code of Federal Regulations (US)	DMARD	Disease modifying antirheumatic drug
CFSAN	Center for Food Safety and Applied Nutrition	DNA	Deoxyribonucleic acid
	(US)	DOD	Department of Defense (US)
CFT	Complement fixation test	DPP	Dipeptidyl peptidase
CFTR	Cystic fibrosis transmembrane regulator	DPT	Diphtheria, pertussis, tetanus
CFU	Colony forming unit	DRG	Diagnosis related grouping
cGMP	Cyclic guanosine monophosphate	DRSP	Drug-resistant *Streptococcus pneumonia*
CHD	Coronary heart disease	ds	Double stranded
CHF	Chronic heart failure	DSC	Differential scanning calorimetry
	Congestive heart failure	DTA	Differential thermal analysis
CHO	Chinese hamster ovary (cells)	DTaP	Diphtheria-Tetanus-acellular-Pertussis
CI	Colour Index	DTC	Direct to consumer
CIMS	Chemical ionization mass spectroscopy	DTH	Delayed type hypersensitivity
CIP	Cahn-Ingol-Prelog	DVT	Deep venous thrombosis
CIR	Cosmetic Ingredient Review (US)	EAA	Excitatory amino acid
CJD	Creutzfeldt-Jakob disease	EAC	Erythrocyte coated by antibody and complement
CKD	Chronic kidney disease	EAE	Experimental allergic encephalomyelitis
CLA	Cutaneous lymphocyte antigen		Experimental autoimmune encephalomyelitis
CLL	Chronic lymphocytic leukemia	EBI	European Bioinformatics Institute
CMC	Critical micelle concentration	EBT	Electron beam tomography
CMI	Cell mediated immunity	EBV	Epstein Barr virus
CML	Cell-mediated lymphocytotoxicity	EC	Effective concentration
	Chronic myelogenous leukemia		Electron capture
CMV	Cytomegalovirus		Enzyme Commission
CNS	Central nervous system		European Commission
CoA	Coenzyme A	ECB	European Chemicals Bureau
COD	Chemical oxygen demand		European Congress on Biotechnology
COMP	Committee for Orphan Medicinal Products (EU)	ECETOC	European Center for Ecotoxicology and
COMT	Catechol-*o*-methyltransferase		Toxicology of Chemicals
COPD	Chronic obstructive pulmonary disease	ECF	Extracellular fluid
COSY	Correlation spectroscopy	ECF-A	Eosinophil chemotactic factor of anaphylaxis
COX	Cyclo-oxygenase	ECG	Electrocardiogram
CP	Canadian Pharmacopeia	ECM	Extracellular matrix
	Chemically pure	ED	Effective dose
CPAP	Continuous positive airway pressure		Erectile dysfunction
CPR	Cardiopulmonary resuscitation	EDG	Electron donating group
CRADA	Cooperative Research and Development	EDHF	Endothelial-derived hyperpolarizing factor
	Agreement (US)	EDRF	Endothelium-derived relaxing factor
CRF	Chronic renal failure	EDTA	Ethylenediaminetetraacetic acid
CRH	Corticotropin-releasing hormone	EEG	Electroencephalogram
CRO	Contract research organization	EFA	Essential fatty acids
CSF	Cerebrospinal fluid	EFB	European Federation of Biotechnology
	Colony stimulating factors	EFPIA	European Federation of Pharmaceutical
CSIRO	Commonwealth Scientific and Industrial		Industries and Associations
	Research Organization (Australia)	EGA	Evolved gas analysis
CSM	Committee on Safety of Medicines (UK)	EGF	Epidermal growth factor
CSP	Cold shock protein	EGFR	Epidermal growth factor receptor
CSPS	Canadian Society for Pharmaceutical Sciences	EHR	Electronic Health Records
CT	Charge transfer	EINECS	European Inventory of Existing Commercial
	Computed tomography		Chemical Substances
CTFA	Cosmetic, Toiletry, and Fragrance Association	EKG	Elektrokardiographie
CTL	Cytotoxic T lymphocyte	ELINCS	EHR-Lab Interoperability and Connectivity
CV	Ceiling value		Standards
CVA	Cerebral vascular accidents		European List of Notified Chemical Substances
CVD	Cardiovascular disease	ELISA	Enzyme-linked immunosorbent assay
	Chemical vapor deposition	EMBO	European Molecular Biology Organization

TABLE-8

EMEA	European Medicines Evaluation Agency		GBS	Guillain-Barré syndrome
EMG	Electromyography		GC	Gas chromatography
EMSA	Electrophoretic mobility shift assay		GCPF	Global Crop Protection Federation
ENDOR	Electron-nuclear double resonance		GEM	Genetically engineered microorganism
EORTC	European Organization for Research and Treatment of Cancer			Genetically engineered mouse
EPA	Eicosapentaenoic acid		GERD	Gastroesophageal reflux disease
	Environmental Protection Agency		GF	Growth factor
EPO	Erythropoietin		GFP	Green fluorescent protein
	European Patent Office		GFR	Glomerular filtration rate
	European Pharmacopoeia Office		GGT	Gamma glutamyl transferase
EPPO	European and Mediterranean Plant Protection Organization		GH	Growth hormone
			GHRH	Growth hormone releasing hormone
EPR	Electron paramagnetic resonance		GI	Gastrointestinal
EPS	Extracellular polysaccharide		GLA	Gamma-linolenic acid
ER	Endoplasmic reticulum		GLC	Gas-liquid chromatography
	Estrogen receptor		GLP	Glucagon like peptide
ERCP	Endoscopic retrograde cholangiopancreatography		GLP	Good laboratory practices
			GmbH	Gesellschaft mit Beschrankter Haftung
ES	Embryonic stem (cells)		GMO	Genetically modified organism
ESA	Ecological Society of America		GMP	Good manufacturing practices
	Entomological Society of America		GnRH	Gonadotropin-releasing hormone
	European Space Agency		GPC	Gel permeation chromatography
ESF	European Science Foundation		GPCR	G protein-coupled receptor
ESHG	European Society of Human Genetics		GRAS	Generally recognized as safe
ESP	End sequence profiling		GTP	Guanosine triphosphate
ESR	Electron spin resonance		GVH	Graft-versus-host
	Erythrocyte sedimentation rate		HAART	Highly active anti-retroviral therapy
ESRD	End-stage renal disease		HAT	Histone acetyl transferase
EST	Expressed sequence tag		HBV	Hepatitis B virus
EU	European Union		HC	Heavy chain
EUP	Experimental Use Permit (US)			Hematopoietic cell
EVM	European Vaccine Manufacturers		HCFC	Hydrochlorofluorocarbon
EWG	Electron withdrawing group		HCL	Hairy cell leukemia
FA	Fanconi anemia		HCV	Hepatitis C virus
FAB	Fast atom bombardment		HD	Huntington's Disease
FABP	Fatty acid binding protein		HDAC	Histone deacetylase
FACS	Fluorescence activated cell sorting		HDL	High density lipoprotein
FAO	Food and Agriculture Organization of the United Nations		HEK	Human embryonic kidney (cells)
			hESC	Human embryonic stem cell
FASEB	Federation of American Societies for Experimental Biology		HETE	Hydroxyeicosatetraenoic acid
			HFC	Hydrofluorocarbon
FCA	Freund's complete adjuvant		HGF	Hepatocyte growth factor
FCC	Food Chemicals Codex (US)		HGG	Human gamma globulin
FCS	Fetal calf serum		HGH	Human growth hormone
FDA	Food and Drug Administration (US)		HHS	Health and Human Services (US)
FEBS	Federation of European Biochemical Societies		HiB	Hemophilus influenza B
FEMS	Federation of European Microbiological Societies		HIPAA	Health Insurance Portability and Accountability Act (US)
FEV	Forced expiratory volume		HIV	Human immunodeficiency virus
FFDCA	Federal Food, Drug, and Cosmetic Act (US)		HLA	Human leukocyte antigen
FGF	Fibroblast growth factor		HLB	Hydrophilic/Lipophilic balance
FIA	Freund's incomplete adjuvant		HMO	Health maintenance organization
FIP	Fédération Internationale Pharmaceutique		HOMO	Highest occupied molecular orbital
FISH	Fluorescence in situ hybridization		HPA	Hypothalamic-pituitary-adrenal
FOI	Freedom of information		HPB	Health Protection Branch (Canada)
FP	Fusion protein		HPBL	Human peripheral blood lymphocyte
FPLC	Fast performance liquid chromatography		HPLC	High performance liquid chromatography
	Fast protein liquid chromatography			High pressure liquid chromatography
FRET	Fluorescent resonance energy transfer		HPV	Human papillomavirus
FSH	Follicle-stimulating hormone		HRT	Hormone replacement therapy
FT	Fourier transform		HSA	Human serum albumin
FTC	Federal trade commission (US)		HSC	Hematopoietic stem cell
FTIR	Fourier transform infrared (spectroscopy)		HSP	Heat shock protein
FWHM	Full width at half maximum		HSV	Herpes simplex virus
FXR	Farnesoid X receptor		HTLV	Human T lymphotropic virus
FXS	Fragile X syndrome		HUGO	Human Genome Organization
GABA	Gamma amino butyric acid		HUVEC	Human umbilical vein endothelial cell
GALT	Gut associated lymphoid tissue		IACR	International Association of Cancer Registries
GAP	Good agricultural practices		IACUC	Institutional Animal Care and Use Committee (US)
	GTPase activating protein			

TABLE-9

IAEA	International Atomic Energy Agency	LC	Lethal concentration
IARC	International Agency for Research on Cancer		Liquid chromatography
IBD	Inflammatory bowel disease	LD	Lethal dose
IBS	Irritable bowel syndrome	LDH	Lactic dehydrogenase
IC	Inhibitory concentration	LDL	Low density lipoprotein
ICAM	Intercellular adhesion molecules	LED	Light-emitting diode
ICC	Interstate Commerce Commission (US)		Lowest effective dose
ICF	Intracellular fluid	LES	Lower esophageal sphincter
ICFA	Incomplete Freund's adjuvant	LFA	Leukocyte functional age
ICGEB	International Center for Genetic Engineering	LH	Luteinizing hormone
	and Biotechnology	LHRH	Luteinizing hormone releasing hormone
ICP	Intracranial pressure	LLC	Limited Liability Company
ICSI	Intracytoplasmic sperm injection	LM	Light microscopy
ID	Inhibitory dose	LOAEL	Lowest observed adverse effect level
	Intradermal	LOEL	Lowest observed effect level
IDDM	Insulin dependent diabetes mellitus	LOH	Loss of heterozygosity
IFN	Interferon	LPS	Lipopolysaccharide
Ig	Immunoglobulin	LT	Leukotriene
IGF	Insulin-like growth factor	LTR	Long terminal repeat
IGR	Insect growth regulator	LUMO	Lowest unoccupied molecular orbital
IHD	Ischemic heart disease	LVEDD	Left ventricular end-diastolic diameter
IL	Interleukin	LVEF	Left ventricular ejection fraction
	Ionic liquids	LXR	Liver X receptor
ILD	Interstitial lung diseases	mAb	Monoclonal antibody
IM	Intramuscular	MAC	Maximum allowable concentration
IMB	Irish Medicine Board	MALDI	Matrix-assisted laser desorption/ionization
IN	Intranasal	MALT	Mucosal-associated lymphoid tissue
INCI	International Nomenclature Cosmetic Ingredient	MAOI	Monoamine oxidase inhibitor
IND	Investigational New Drug (application) (US)	MAPK	Mitogen-activated protein kinase
INN	International Nonproprietary Name	MBP	Myelin basic protein
iNOS	Inducible nitric oxide synthase	MCHC	Mean corpuscular hemoglobin concentration
INRIA	Institut National de Recherche en Informatique	MCV	Mean corpuscular volume
	et en Automatique (Fr)	MD	Muscular dystrophy
IOBC	International Organization for Biological	MDD	Major depressive disorder
	Control	MDR	Multidrug resistant
IOTF	International Obesity Task Force	MEFV	Maximal expiratory flow volume
IP	Intraperitoneal	MEL	Maximum exposure limit
IPPB	Intermittent positive pressure breathing	MF	Molecular formula
IPT	Individual perception threshold	MGD	Mouse genome database
IPV	Inactivated polio vaccine	MHC	Major histocompatibility complex
IRB	Institutional review board	MHRA	Medicines and Healthcare products Regulatory
ISO	International Organization for Standardization		Agency (UK)
ISS	Ion scattering spectroscopy	MHW	Ministry of Health and Welfare (Japan)
ITP	Idiopathic thrombocytopenic purpura	MI	Myocardial infarction
IU	International Units	MLCT	Metal to ligand charge transfer
IUPAC	International Union of Pure and Applied	MLD	Minimum lethal dose
	Chemistry	MLR	Mixed lymphocyte reaction
IV	Intravenous	MLV	Modified live virus
IVF	*in vitro* fertilization	MMP	Matrix metalloproteinase
IVP	Intravenous pyelogram	MMR	Measles-mumps-rubella (vaccine)
JAN	Japanese Accepted Name	MPL	Maximum permissible level
JCIC	Japanese Cosmetic Ingredients Codex	MPS	Mucopolysaccharidosis
JCPA	Japan Crop Protection Association	MRI	Magnetic resonance imaging
JNK	c-Jun NH2-terminal kinase	MRL	Maximum residue level
JP	Japanese Pharmacopoeia	mRNA	Messenger ribonucleic acid
JPMA	Japan Pharmaceutical Manufacturers Association	MRP	Multidrug resistance protein
JSCI	Japanese Standards of Cosmetic Ingredients	MRSA	Methicillin-resistant *Staphylococcus aureus*
JSFA	Japanese Standards of Food Additives	MS	Mass spectrometry
KG	Kommanditgesellschaft		Multiple sclerosis
KGaA	Kommanditgesellschaft auf Aktien	MSDS	Material Safety Data Sheet
KK	Kabushiki Kaishi	MTC	Maximum tolerable concentration
KLH	Keyhole limpet hemocyanin	MTD	Maximum tolerated dose
KPA	Kidney plasminogen activator	MTEL	Maximum tolerated exposure level
LAB	Lactic acid bacteria	MW	Molecular weight
LAD	Lactic acid dehydrogenase	NABR	National Association for Biomedical Research
	Left anterior descending		(US)
	Lymphocyte-activating determinant	NACHGR	National Advisory Council for Human Genome
LAIV	Live attenuated influenza vaccine		Research (US)
LAK	Lymphokine activated killer (cell)	NAD	Nicotinamide adenine dinucleotide
LAMMA	Laser microprobe mass analysis	NADH	Nicotinamide adenine dinucleotide (reduced
LATS	Long acting thyroid stimulator		form)

TABLE-10

NADP	Nicotinamide adenine dinucleotide phosphate
NADPH	Nicotinamide adenine dinucleotide phosphate (reduced form)
NAL	National Agricultural Library (US)
NAS	National Academy of Sciences (US)
NASA	National Aeronautics and Space Administration (US)
NBS	National Bureau of Standards (US)
NCBI	National Center for Biotechnology Information (US)
NCE	New Chemical Entity
NCGR	National Center for Genome Resources (US)
NCHGR	National Center for Human Genome Research (US)
NCI	National Cancer Institute (US)
NCIC	National Cancer Institute of Canada
NCID	National Center for Infectious Diseases (US)
NCTC	National Collection of Type Cultures (UK)
NDA	New Drug Application (US)
NDO	Non-digestible oligosaccharides
NEP	Neutral endopeptidase
NER	Nucleotide excision repair
NF	National Formulary (US)
NFkB	Nuclear factor kappa B
NGF	Nerve growth factor
NHGRI	National Human Genome Research Institute (US)
NICE	National Institute for Health and Clinical Excellence (UK)
NIDDM	Non-insulin dependent diabetes mellitus
NIH	National Institutes of Health (US)
NIMH	National Institute of Mental Health (US)
NIOSH	National Institute for Occupational Safety and Health (US)
NIST	National Institute for Standards and Technology (US)
NK	Natural killer (cell)
NK	Neurokinin
NLM	National Library of Medicine (US)
NMDA	N-methyl-D-aspartate
NMP	Nuclear matrix protein
NMR	Nuclear magnetic resonance
NNRTI	Non-nucleoside reverse transcriptase inhibitor
NOAEL	No observed adverse effect level
NOE	Nuclear Overhauser effect
NOEL	No observed effect level
NOS	Nitric oxide synthase
NPA	National Pharmaceutical Association (UK) National Pharmacy Association (UK)
NPY	Neuropeptide Y
NRC	National Research Council (US) Nuclear Regulatory Commission (US)
NRTI	Nucleoside reverse transcriptase inhibitor
NSAID	Nonsteroidal anti-inflammatory drug
NSCLC	Non-small-cell lung cancer
NSF	National Science Foundation (US)
NTP	National Toxicology Program (US)
OA	Osteoarthritis
OC	Oral contraceptive
OCD	Obsessive compulsive disorder
OD	Optical density
OES	Occupational exposure standard
OGTT	Oral glucose tolerance test
OPPTS	Office of Prevention, Pesticides and Toxic Substances (US)
ORD	Optical rotary dispersion
ORDA	Office of Recombinant DNA Activities (US)
ORF	Open reading frame
OSD	Oral solid dosage
OSHA	Occupational Safety and Health Administration
OTC	Over the counter

PAF	Platelet activating factor
PAGE	Polyacrylamide gel electrophoresis
PAH	Poly-aromatic hydrocarbons
PAW	Pulmonary artery wedge
PBC	Peripheral blood cell
PBS	Phosphate buffered saline
PBSC	Peripheral blood stem cell
PCA	Passive cutaneous anaphylaxis
PCB	Polychlorinated biphenyls
PCP	Pneumocystis carinii pneumonia Primary care physician Primary care provider
PCR	Polymerase chain reaction
PCT	Patent Co-operation Treaty
PCV	Packed cell volume
PD	Pharmacodynamics
PDE	Phosphodiesterase
PDGF	Platelet-derived growth factor
PDR	Physicians Desk Reference
PDT	Photodynamic therapy
PE	Phosphatidylethanolamine
PEEP	Peak end expiratory pressure
PEF	Peak expiratory flow
PEG	Polyethylene glycol
PES	Photoelectron spectroscopy
PET	Positron emission tomography
PFC	Plaque-forming cell
PFGE	Pulsed-field gel electrophoresis
PG	Prostaglandin
PGES	Prostaglandin E synthase
PHA	Phytohemagglutinin
PhRMA	Pharmaceutical Research and Manufacturers of America (US)
PI	Protease inhibitor
PID	Pelvic inflammatory disease
PK	Pharmacokinetics
PKC	Protein kinase C
PKD	Polycystic kidney disease
PKU	Phenylketonuria
PMA	Premarket Approval (US)
PMN	Polymorphonuclear leukocyte
PMS	Post-marketing surveillance Premenstrual syndrome
PNS	Peripheral nervous system
PPAR	Peroxisome proliferator-activated receptor
PPV	Positive predictive value
PSA	Prostate specific antigen
PSD	Pesticides Safety Directorate (UK)
PSVT	Paroxysmal supraventricular tachycardia
PTC	Percutaneous transhepatic cholangiography
PTCA	Percutaneous transluminal coronary angioplasty
PTFE	Polytetrafluoroethylene
PTH	Parathyroid hormone
PTK	Protein tyrosine kinase
PTO	Patent and Trademark Office (US)
PTT	Partial thromboplastin time
PUFA	Polyunsaturated fatty acids
PVC	Polyvinyl chloride
PVDF	Polyvinylidene difluoride
PVR	Peripheral vascular resistance
PVT	Pressure-volume-temperature
QED	Quod erat demonstrandum (which was to be proved)
QSAR	Quantitative structure-activity relationship
RA	Rheumatoid arthritis
RAGE	Receptor of advanced glycation endproduct
RANTES	Regulated on activation, normal T expressed and secreted
RAR	Retinoic acid receptor
RAS	Renin-angiotensin system
RBC	Red blood cell

TABLE-11

RCC	Renal cell carcinoma
RCT	Randomized clinical trial
RCVS	Royal College of Veterinary Surgeons (UK)
RDA	Recommended daily allowance
RDI	Recommended dietary intake
REM	Rapid eye movement
RFLP	Restriction fragment length polymorphism
RIA	Radioimmunoassay
RIND	Reversible ischemic neurological deficit
rINN	Recommended International Non-proprietary Name
RMR	Resting metabolic rate
RNAi	Ribonucleic acid interference
ROS	Reactive oxygen species
RRS	Resonance raman spectroscopy
RS	Raman spectroscopy
RSC	Royal Society of Chemistry (UK)
RSM	Royal Society of Medicine (UK)
RSV	Respiratory syncytical virus
	Rous sarcoma virus
RT	Room temperature
RTECS	Registry of Toxic Effects of Chemical Substances (US)
RTI	Reverse transcriptase inhibitor
RXR	Retinoid X receptor
SA	Sociedad Anónima
	Sociedade por Ações
	Societate pe Actiuni
	Société Anonyme
	Spolka Akcyjna
SAE	Society of Automotive Engineers
SAM	S-adenosyl methionine
SApA	Societá in accomandita per azioni
SAR	Structure activity relationship
SARS	Severe acute respiratory syndrome
SC	Subcutaneous
SCF	Supercritical fluid
SCFA	Short chain fatty acids
SCID	Severe combined immune deficiency
SCP	Single cell protein
SD	Standard deviation
SDH	Sorbitol dehydrogenase
SE	Standard error
SEC	Size-exclusion chromatography
SEM	Scanning electron microscopy
SERM	Selective estrogen-receptor modulator
SGGT	Serum gamma glutamyl transferase
SGOT	Serum glutamic oxaloacetic transaminase
SGPT	Serum glutamic-pyruvic transaminase
SHIV	Simian-human immunodeficiency virus
SIADH	Syndrome of inappropriate antidiuretic hormone (secretion)
SIB	Society for Industrial Biology
SIDS	Sudden infant death syndrome
SIM	Society for Industrial Microbiology
siRNA	Small interfering RNA
SIRS	Systemic inflammatory response syndrome
SIV	Simian immunodeficiency virus
SLE	Systemic lupus erythematosus
SMART	Somatic mutation and recombination test
SNP	Single nucleotide polymorphism
SNRI	Serotonin-noradrenaline reuptake inhibitor
SOCMA	Synthetic Organic Chemical Manufacturers Association
SOD	Superoxide dismutase
SP	Substance P
SpA	Società per Azioni
SPECT	Single photon emission computed tomography
SPF	Sun protection factor
SPPARM	Selective PPAR modulator
SPRM	Selective progesterone receptor modulator

SRBC	Sheep red blood cell
Src	Sociedad Regular Colectiva
Srl	Società a Responsabilità Limitata
	Societate cu Raspoudere Limitata
SRM	Standard reference material
SSEA	Stage specific embryonic antigen
SSRI	Selective serotonin reuptake inhibitor
STD	Sexually transmitted disease
STEM	Scanning transmission electron microscopy
STM	Scanning tunneling microscopy
STP	Standard temperature and pressure
STS	Sequence-tagged site
SV	Stroke volume
TB	Tuberculosis
TCA	Tricarboxylic acid
	Tricyclic antidepressants
TCTP	Translationally controlled tumor protein
TDL	Thoracic duct lymphocyte
TDN	Total digestible nutrients
TF	Transcription factor
TGF	Transforming growth factor
TIA	Transient ischemic attack
TK	Toxicokinetics
TLC	Thin-layer chromatography
TLR	Toll-like receptor
TLV	Threshold limit value
TNF	Tumor necrosis factor
TPN	Total parenteral nutrition
TRAIL	TNF related apoptosis inducing ligand
tRNA	Transfer ribonucleic acid
TSA	Tumor specific antigen
TSG	Tumor suppressor gene
TSH	Thyroid stimulating hormone
TSTA	Tumor-specific transplantation antigens
TTP	Thrombotic thrombocytopenic purpura
TUNEL	Terminal deoxynucleotidyl transferase (TdT)-mediated dUTP nick-end labeling
TZD	Thiazolidinedione
UES	Upper esophageal sphincter
UNEP	United Nations Environment Program
URI	Upper respiratory infection
USAN	United States Adopted Name
USDA	United States Department of Agriculture
USP	United States Pharmacopeia
USPHS	United States Public Health Service
USPTO	United States Patent and Trademark Office
UTI	Urinary tract infection
UTR	Untranslated region
UV	Ultraviolet
VCAM	Vascular cell adhesion molecule
VEGF	Vascular endothelial growth factor
VLA	Very late antigens
VLDL	Very low density lipoproteins
VNTR	Variable number of tandem repeats
VOC	Volatile organic compound
VPD	Ventricular premature depolarization
VSEPR	Valence shell electron pair repulsion
VUV	Vacuum ultraviolet
VZV	Varicella-zoster virus
WBC	White blood cell
WHO	World Health Organization
WIPO	World Intellectual Property Organization
WNL	Within normal limits
WNV	West Nile virus
WSSA	Weed Science Society of America
WT	Wild type
WVA	World Veterinary Association
XAFS	X-ray absorption fine structure spectroscopy
XPS	X-ray photoelectron spectroscopy
YAC	Yeast artificial chromosome
ZFP	Zinc finger protein

TABLE-12

Vaccines

The following table lists selected preparations for use in the prevention of infectious diseases by immunization.

Single vaccines

Product Name	Generic name	Manufacturer	Description
ActHIB®	Haemophilus b Conjugate Vaccine (Tetanus Toxoid Conjugate)	Sanofi Pasteur	Purified polyribose-ribitol-phosphate capsular polysaccharide of *Haemophilus influenzae* type b (strain 1482), covalently bound to tetanus toxoid
ACWY Vax®	Meningococcal Polysaccharide Vaccine (Groups A, C, W$_{135}$, Y)	GlaxoSmithKline	Purified polysaccharide antigens from *Neisseria meningitidis* groups A, C, Y, and W$_{135}$
Agrippal®	Influenza Virus Vaccine (Surface Antigen, Inactivated)	Chiron	Purified surface antigen from influenza virus types A and B propagated in embryonated chicken eggs and inactivated with formaldehyde
Ari!vax®	Yellow Fever Vaccine, Live	Chiron	Live, attenuated yellow fever virus strain 17D grown in fertilized hens eggs
Attenuvax®	Measles Virus Vaccine, Live	Merck & Co.	Attenuated measles virus derived from Enders' attenuated Edmonston strain grown in chick embryo cell culture
Avaxim®	Inactivated Hepatitis A Vaccine	Sanofi Pasteur	Hepatitis A virus inactivated by formaldehyde, adsorbed onto aluminum hydroxide
Dukoral®	Vaccine against Cholera and ETEC-Diarrhoea	SBL Vaccines	*Vibrio cholerae* O1 Inaba and Ogawa, classic and El Tor-strains (heat/formalin inactivated), cholera toxin B subunit
Encepur®	Tick-borne Encephalitis Virus Vaccine, Inactivated, Adsorbed	Chiron	Tick-borne encephalitis virus (strain K23) grown in chicken fibroblast cell culture, inactivated with formaldehyde, adsorbed onto aluminum hydroxide (adjuvant)
Engerix-B®	Hepatitis B Vaccine (Recombinant)	GlaxoSmithKline	Purified hepatitis B surface antigen produced by recombinant DNA technology in *Saccharomyces cerevisiae*, adsorbed onto aluminum hydroxide
Epaxal®	Virosomal Hepatitis A Vaccine	Berna Biotech	Hepatitis A virus antigen (RG-SB strain) anchored to a liposomal membrane
Ervevax®	Rubella Vaccine, Live	GlaxoSmithKline	Live, attenuated RA 27/3 strain of rubella virus grown in human diploid cells
Euvax B®	Hepatitis B Vaccine, Recombinant	Sanofi Pasteur	Purified hepatitis B surface antigen produced by recombinant DNA technology in *Saccharomyces cerevisiae*, adsorbed onto aluminum hydroxide
Fendrix®	Hepatitis B (rDNA) Vaccine (Adjuvanted, Adsorbed)	GlaxoSmithKline	Purified hepatitis B surface antigen produced by recombinant DNA technology in *Saccharomyces cerevisiae*, adsorbed on aluminum phosphate, adjuvanted by AS04C containing 3-*O*-desacyl-4′-monophosphoryl lipid A (MPL)
Fluad®	Adjuvanted Influenza Virus Vaccine	Chiron	Subunit antigens (hemagglutinin and neuraminidase) from influenza virus types A and B grown in embryonated chicken eggs, combined with MF59 adjuvant emulsion
Fluarix®	Influenza Vaccine (Split Virion, Inactivated)	GlaxoSmithKline	Influenza virus types A and B propagated in embryonated chicken eggs, inactivated by sodium deoxycholate and formaldehyde (split virion, trivalent)
FluMist®	Influenza Virus Vaccine, Live, Intranasal	MedImmune	Live attenuated influenza virus reassortants (types A and B) grown in specific pathogen free eggs, trivalent
Fluvirin®	Influenza Virus Vaccine, Types A and B (Surface Antigen)	Chiron	Influenza virus types A and B grown in embryonated chicken eggs, inactivated by beta-propiolactone and nonylphenol ethoxylate (split virus, trivalent)

TABLE-13

Single vaccines (continued)

Product Name	Generic name	Manufacturer	Description
Fluzone®	Influenza Virus Vaccine (Zonal Purified, Subvirion)	Sanofi Pasteur	Influenza virus types A and B grown in embryonated chicken eggs, inactivated by formaldehyde and octoxinol-9 (split virus, trivalent)
FSME-Immun®	Tick-borne Encephalitis Virus Vaccine, Inactivated, Adsorbed	Baxter	Inactivated tick-borne encephalitis virus (Neudröfl strain) grown in chick embryo fibroblast cells, adsorbed on aluminum hydroxide
Gardasil®	Quadrivalent Human Papillomavirus (Types 6, 11, 16, 18) Recombinant Vaccine	Merck & Co.	Purified virus-like particles of the major capsid (L1) protein of human papillomavirus types 6, 11, 16 and 18 produced by recombinant DNA technology in *Saccharomyces cerevisiae*.
GenHevac B®	Recombinant Hepatitis B Vaccine	Sanofi Pasteur	Recombinant hepatitis B virus surface antigen (S and pre-S_2 proteins) produced on CHO cell line
Havrix®	Hepatitis A Vaccine, Inactivated	GlaxoSmithKline	Purified hepatitis A virus strain HM 175 grown in human diploid MRC-5 cells, inactivated by formalin
Hiberix®	*Haemophilus influenzae* type b (Hib) Vaccine	GlaxoSmithKline	Purified polyribosyl-ribitol-phosphate capsular polysaccharide of Hib covalently bound to tetanus toxoid
HibTiter®	Haemophilus b Conjugate Vaccine (Diphtheria CRM_{197} Protein Conjugate)	Wyeth	Conjugate of oligosaccharides of the capsular antigen of *Haemophilus influenzae* type b and diphtheria CRM_{197} protein
Imovax® Rabies	Rabies Vaccine	Sanofi Pasteur	Wistar rabies virus strain PM-1503-3M grown in human diploid MRC-5 cells, purified and inactivated by beta-propiolactone
Inflexal®V	Virosomal Influenza Vaccine	Berna Biotech	Purified surface antigens from selected influenza virus strains, grown on allantoic fluid of chicken eggs and inactivated with β-propiolactone, anchored to a liposomal membrane
Influvac®	Influenza Vaccine (Surface Antigen, Inactivated)	Solvay	Purifed surface antigens from influenza virus types A and B, grown in chicken eggs and inactivated by formaldehyde
Invivac®	Virosomal Influenza Vaccine (Surface Antigen, Inactivated)	Solvay	Purifed surface antigens from influenza virus types A and B, grown in chicken eggs and inactivated by formaldehyde, anchored to a liposomal membrane
IPOL®	Poliovirus Vaccine Inactivated	Sanofi Pasteur	Purified, formalin-inactivated poliovirus type 1 (Mahoney), type 2 (MEF-1) and type 3 (Saukett) grown in VERO cell culture
Je-Vax®	Japanese Encephalitis Virus Vaccine Inactivated	Sanofi Pasteur	Partially purified, formaldehyde-inactivated Japanese encephalitis virus, Nakayama-NIH strain, grown in mice
Menactra®	Meningococcal (Groups A, C, Y, W-135) Polysaccharide Diphtheria Toxoid Conjugate Vaccine	Sanofi Pasteur	*Neisseria meningitidis* serogroup A, C, Y, and W-135 capsular polysaccharide antigens individually conjugated to diphtheria toxoid protein
Meningitec®	Meningococcal Group C Conjugate Vaccine, Adsorbed	Wyeth	Capsular polysaccharide antigen of *Neisseria meningitidis* group C (strain C11) conjugated to *Corynebacterium diphtheria* protein CRM_{197}, adsorbed onto aluminum phosphate
Menjugate®	Meningococcal Group C–CRM197 Conjugate Vaccine	Chiron	Meningococcal group C oligosaccharides conjugated to a protein carrier, a non-toxic mutant of diphtheria toxin, CRM197, adsorbed onto aluminum hydroxide
Menomune®	Meningococcal Polysaccharide Vaccine Groups A, C, Y, W-135 Combined	Sanofi Pasteur	Purified polysaccharide antigens from *Neisseria meningitidis* groups A, C, Y, and W-135
Meruvax® II	Rubella Virus Vaccine Live	Merck & Co.	Wistar RA 27/3 strain of live attenuated rubella virus propagated in WI-38 human diploid lung fibroblasts

TABLE-14

Vaccines (Continued)

Single vaccines (continued)

Product Name	Generic name	Manufacturer	Description
Mumpsvax®	Mumps Virus Vaccine Live	Merck & Co.	Jeryl Lynn™ (B level) strain of mumps virus propagated in chick embryo cell culture
NeisVac-C®	Meningococcal Serogroup C Polysaccharide Conjugate Vaccine	Baxter	*Neisseria meningitidis* serogroup C (strain C11) polysaccharide conjugated to tetanus toxoid, adsorbed onto aluminum hydroxide
Okavax®	Live Attenuated Varicella Virus Vaccine Biken™	Sanofi Pasteur	Attenuated live varicella zoster virus (Oka strain) grown in human diploid cells
PedvaxHIB®	Haemophilus b Conjugate Vaccine (Meningococcal Protein Conjugate)	Merck & Co.	Purified capsular polysaccharide (polyribosyl-ribitol phosphate) of *Haemophilus influenzae* type b, Ross strain, covalently bound to an outer membrane protein complex of the B11 strain of *Neisseria meningitidis* serogroup B
Pneumo 23®	Polysaccharide Pneumococcal Vaccine	Sanofi Pasteur	Polysaccharides of *Streptococcus pneumoniae* serotypes 1, 2, 3, 4, 5, 6B, 7F, 8, 9N, 9V, 10A, 11A, 12F, 14, 15B, 17F, 18C, 19A, 19F, 20, 22F, 23F, 33F
Pneumovax® 23	Pneumococcal Vaccine Polyvalent	Merck & Co.	Mixture of highly purified capsular polysaccharides from *Streptococcus pneumoniae* serotypes 1, 2, 3, 4, 5, 6B, 7F, 8, 9N, 9V, 10A, 11A, 12F, 14, 15B, 17F, 18C, 19A, 19F, 20, 22F, 23F, 33F
Polio Sabin™	Live Attenuated Poliomyelitis (Sabin) Vaccine (Oral)	GlaxoSmithKline	Mixture of poliovirus type 1 (LS-c, 2ab), type 2 (P712, Ch, 2ab), and type 3 (Leon 12a1b) live attenuated Sabin strains of poliomyelitis virus grown in VERO cell culture
Prevnar® Prevenar®	Pneumococcal 7-valent Conjugate Vaccine (Diphtheria CRM_{197} Protein Conjugate)	Wyeth	Saccharides of the capsular antigens of *Streptococcus pneumoniae* serotypes 4, 6B, 9V, 14, 18C, 19F, and 23F individually conjugated to diphtheria CRM_{197} protein
RabAvert® RabiPur®	Rabies Vaccine	Chiron	Rabies virus strain Flurry LEP grown in chicken fibroblast cultures, inactivated with beta-propiolactone, purified
Recombivax HB®	Hepatitis B Vaccine (Recombinant)	Merck & Co.	Purified hepatitis B surface antigen produced by recombinant DNA technology in *Saccharomyces cerevisiae*
RotaTeq®	Rotavirus Vaccine, Live, Oral, Pentavalent	Merck & Co.	Mixture of 5 live reassortant rotoviruses: four expressing attachment protein P7 and one of capsid proteins G1, G2, G3 or G4 and one expressing attachment protein P1A and capsid protein G6; propagated in VERO cell culture
Rouvax®	Attenuated Measles Vaccine	Sanofi Pasteur	Live attenuated measles virus (Schwarz strain) grown in chick embryo cell culture
Rudivax®	Attenuated Rubella Vaccine	Sanofi Pasteur	Live attenuated rubella virus (Wistar RA 27/3M strain) grown in human diploid cells
Stamaril®	Yellow Fever Vaccine (Live), Stabilized	Sanofi Pasteur	Live, attenuated yellow fever virus (17D strain) grown in specific pathogen free chick embryos
Tetavax®	Adsorbed Tetanus Toxoid Vaccine	Sanofi Pasteur	Tetanus toxoid adsorbed on aluminum hydroxide dihydrate
Typherix®	Typhoid Vaccine (Purified Polysaccharide Antigen)	GlaxoSmithKline	Purified Vi polysaccharide of *Salmonella typhi*
Typhim Vi®	Polysaccharide Typhoid Vaccine	Sanofi Pasteur	Purified capsular polysaccharide of *Salmonella typhi* (Ty2 strain)
Vaqta®	Hepatitis A Vaccine, Inactivated	Merck & Co.	Purified Hepatitis A virus grown in human diploid MRC-5 cells, inactivated by formalin and adsorbed onto aluminum hydroxyphosphate sulfate

TABLE-15

Single vaccines (continued)

Product Name	Generic name	Manufacturer	Description
Varilrix®	Varicella Vaccine (Adult)	GlaxoSmithKline	Live, attenuated varicella-zoster (Oka strain) virus propagated in human diploid MRC-5 cells
Varivax®	Varicella Virus Vaccine Live (Oka/Merck)	Merck & Co.	Oka/Merck strain of live, attenuated varicella virus propagated in human diploid MRC-5 cells
Vaxigrip®	Influenza Vaccine (Split Virion, Inactivated)	Sanofi Pasteur	Inactivated influenza virus types A and B, propagated in eggs (split virion)
Verorab®	Purified Inactivated Rabies Vaccine	Sanofi Pasteur	Purified, inactivated rabies virus (Wistar strain PM/WI 38-1503-3M) produced in VERO cell line
Vivotif®	Typhoid Vaccine Live Oral Ty21a	Berna Biotech	Live, attenuated *Salmonella typhi* (Ty21a strain)
YF-Vax®	Yellow Fever Vaccine	Sanofi Pasteur	Live, attenuated yellow fever virus (17D-204 strain) grown in ALV-free chick embryos
Zostavax®	Zoster Vaccine Live (Oka/Merck)	Merck & Co.	Live, attenuated varicella-zoster virus (Oka/Merck strain) propagated in human diploid MRC-5 cells

Combination vaccines

Product Name	Generic name	Manufacturer	Description
Adacel®	Tetanus Toxoid, Reduced Diphtheria Toxoid and Acellular Pertussis Vaccine Adsorbed	Sanofi Pasteur	Tetanus toxoid, diphtheria toxoid, and 5 pertussis antigens (detoxified pertussis toxin, filamentous hemagglutinin, pertactin, fimbriae types 2 and 3) individually adsorbed onto aluminum phosphate
Boostrix®	Tetanus Toxoid, Reduced Diphtheria Toxoid and Acellular Pertussis Vaccine, Adsorbed	GlaxoSmithKline	Diphtheria toxoid, tetanus toxoid, and 3 pertussis antigens (inactivated pertussis toxin, filamentous hemagglutinin, and pertactin) adsorbed onto aluminum hydroxide
Comvax®	Haemophilus b Conjugate Vaccine (Meningococcal Protein Conjugate) and Hepatitis B (Recombinant) Vaccine	Merck & Co.	Preparation containing the antigenic components used in producing PedvaxHIB® and Recombivax HB®
Daptacel®	Diphtheria and Tetanus Toxoids and Acellular Pertussis Vaccine Adsorbed	Sanofi Pasteur	Tetanus toxoid, diphtheria toxoid, and 5 pertussis antigens (detoxified pertussis toxin, filamentous hemagglutinin, pertactin, fimbriae types 2 and 3) individually adsorbed onto aluminum phosphate
Decavac®	Tetanus and Diphtheria Toxoids Adsorbed (Adult)	Sanofi Pasteur	Alum-precipitated tetanus and diphtheria toxoids
Dultavax® Revaxis®	Diphtheria, Tetanus and Inactivated Poliomyelitis Vaccine Adsorbed	Sanofi Pasteur	Diphtheria toxoid, tetanus toxoid, inactivated poliovirus types 1, 2, and 3 adsorbed on aluminum hydroxide
Hepatyrix®	Hepatitis A (Inactivated, Adsorbed) and Typhoid Polysaccharide Vaccine	GlaxoSmithKline	Inactivated Hepatitis A virus (HM175 strain) grown in MRC-5 cells plus Vi polysaccharide of *Salmonella typhi* (Ty2 strain) adsorbed on aluminum hydroxide
Imovax® d.T.	Diphtheria and Tetanus Vaccine (Adsorbed)	Sanofi Pasteur	Diphtheria toxoid and tetanus toxoid adsorbed on aluminum hydroxide dihydrate
Infanrix®	Diphtheria and Tetanus Toxoids and Acellular Pertussis Vaccine Adsorbed	GlaxoSmithKline	Diphtheria and tetanus toxoids and 3 pertussis antigens (inactivated pertussis toxin, filamentous hemagglutinin, and pertactin) adsorbed onto aluminum hydroxide
Infanrix® IPV	Diphtheria, Tetanus, Pertussis (Acelluar, Component) and Poliomyelitis (Inactivated) Vaccine (Adsorbed)	GlaxoSmithKline	Diphtheria and tetanus toxoids and 3 pertussis antigens (inactivated pertussis toxin, filamentous hemagglutinin, and pertactin) adsorbed onto aluminum hydroxide plus inactivated poliovirus types 1, 2, and 3 grown in VERO cell culture

TABLE-16

Combination vaccines (continued)

Product Name	Generic name	Manufacturer	Description
M-M-R® II	Measles, Mumps, and Rubella Virus Vaccine Live	Merck & Co.	Preparation of Attenuvax®, MumpsVax®, and Meruvax® II
M-M Vax™	Measles and Mumps Virus Vaccine Live	Merck & Co.	Preparation of Attenuvax® and MumpsVax®
Pediarix®	Diphtheria and Tetanus Toxoids and Acellular Pertussis Adsorbed, Hepatitis B (Recombinant) and Inactivated Poliovirus Vaccine Combined	GlaxoSmithKline	Preparation containing the antigenic components used in producing Infanrix® and Engerix-B®, plus purified, formaldehyde-inactivated poliovirus Type 1 (Mahoney), Type 2 (MEF-1), and Type 3 (Saukett) grown in VERO cell culture
Pentacel®	Haemophilus b Conjugate Vaccine (Tetanus Toxoid Conjugate) Reconstituted with Diphtheria and Tetanus Toxoids and Acellular Pertussis Vaccine Adsorbed Combined with Poliovirus Vaccine Inactivated	Sanofi Pasteur	Preparation of ActHIB® reconstituted with Quadracel®
Pentavac® Pentaxim®	Adsorbed Diphtheria, Tetanus, Acellular Pertussis, Inactivated Poliomyelitis Vaccine and Conjugate *Haemophilus influenzae* type b Vaccine	Sanofi Pasteur	Diphtheria toxoid, tetanus toxoid, pertussis antigens (toxoid, filamentous hemagglutinin), inactivated poliomyelitis virus types 1, 2, and 3, and Hib polysaccharide conjugated with tetanus protein
Priorix®	Measles, Mumps, and Rubella Vaccine (Live Attenuated Virus)	GlaxoSmithKline	Schwarz measles, RIT 4385 mumps and Wistar RA 27/3 rubella virus strains
Proquad®	Measles, Mumps, Rubella and Varicella (Oka/Merck) Virus Vaccine Live	Merck & Co.	Preparation containing the components of M-M-R® II, and Varivax®
Quadracel®	Component Pertussis Vaccine and Diphtheria and Tetanus Toxoids Adsorbed Combined with Inactivated Poliomyelitis Vaccine	Sanofi Pasteur	Preparation of Adacel® combined with inactivated poliomyelitis vaccine (diploid cell origin) types 1, 2, and 3
R.O.R.® Trimovax®	Live Attenuated Virus Vaccine against Measles, Mumps and Rubella	Sanofi Pasteur	Live attenuated measles virus (Schwarz strain) grown in chick embryo cells, mumps virus (Urabe AM-9 strain) grown in embryonated hens eggs, and rubella virus (Wistar RA 27/3M strain) grown in human diploid cells
Rudi-Rouvax®	Live Attenuated Virus Vaccine against Rubella and Measles	Sanofi Pasteur	Live attenuated measles virus (Schwarz strain) grown on chick embryo cell culture and rubella virus (Wistar RA 27/3M strain)
TriHIBit®	Haemophilus b Conjugate Vaccine (Tetanus Toxoid Conjugate) Reconstituted with Diphtheria and Tetanus Toxoids and Acellular Pertussis Vaccine Adsorbed	Sanofi Pasteur	Preparation of ActHIB® reconstituted with Tripedia®
Tripedia®	Diphtheria and Tetanus Toxoids and Acellular Pertussis Vaccine Adsorbed	Sanofi Pasteur	Alum adsorbed diphtheria and tetanus toxoids combined with acellular pertussis concentrate (inactivated pertussis toxin and filamentous hemagglutinin)
Twinrix®	Hepatitis A Inactivated and Hepatitis B (Recombinant) Vaccine	GlaxoSmithKline	Preparation containing the antigenic components used in producing Havrix® and Engerix-B®

TABLE-17

International Patent Country Codes

Code	Country Name	Code	Country Name
AE	United Arab Emirates	KR	Republic of Korea
AG	Antigua and Barbuda	KZ	Kazakhstan
AL	Albania	LC	Saint Lucia
AM	Armenia	LI	Liechtenstein
AR	Argentina	LK	Sri Lanka
AT	Austria	LR	Liberia
AU	Australia	LS	Lesotho
AZ	Azerbaijan	LT	Lithuania
BA	Bosnia and Herzegovina	LU	Luxembourg
BB	Barbados	LV	Latvia
BE	Belgium	LY	Libyan Arab Jamahiriya
BF	Burkina Faso	MA	Morocco
BG	Bulgaria	MC	Monaco
BJ	Benin	MD	Republic of Moldova
BR	Brazil	MG	Madagascar
BW	Botswana	MK	The former Yugoslav Republic of Macedonia
BY	Belarus	ML	Mali
BZ	Belize	MN	Mongolia
CA	Canada	MR	Mauritania
CF	Central African Republic	MW	Malawi
CG	Congo	MX	Mexico
CH	Switzerland	MZ	Mozambique
CI	Côte d'Ivoire	NA	Namibia
CM	Cameroon	NE	Niger
CN	China	NG	Nigeria
CO	Colombia	NI	Nicaragua
CR	Costa Rica	NL	Netherlands
CS	Czechoslovakia	NO	Norway
CU	Cuba	NZ	New Zealand
CY	Cyprus	OM	Oman
CZ	Czech Republic	PG	Papua New Guinea
DD	German Democratic Republic	PH	Philippines
DE	Germany	PL	Poland
DK	Denmark	PT	Portugal
DM	Dominica	RO	Romania
DZ	Algeria	RU	Russian Federation
EC	Ecuador	SC	Seychelles
EE	Estonia	SD	Sudan
EG	Egypt	SE	Sweden
EP	European Patent Office	SG	Singapore
ES	Spain	SK	Slovakia
FI	Finland	SL	Sierra Leone
FR	France	SM	San Marino
GA	Gabon	SN	Senegal
GB	United Kingdom	SU	USSR
GD	Grenada	SY	Syrian Arab Republic
GE	Georgia	SZ	Swaziland
GH	Ghana	TD	Chad
GM	Gambia	TG	Togo
GN	Guinea	TJ	Tajikistan
GQ	Equatorial Guinea	TM	Turkmenistan
GR	Greece	TN	Tunisia
GW	Guinea-Bissau	TR	Turkey
HR	Croatia	TT	Trinidad and Tobago
HU	Hungary	TW	Taiwan, Province of China
ID	Indonesia	TZ	United Republic of Tanzania
IE	Ireland	UA	Ukraine
IL	Israel	UG	Uganda
IN	India	US	United States of America
IS	Iceland	UZ	Uzbekistan
IT	Italy	VC	Saint Vincent and the Grenadines
JP	Japan	VN	Viet Nam
KE	Kenya	WO	World Intellectual Property Organization (WIPO)
KG	Kyrgyzstan	YU	Serbia and Montenegro
KM	Comoros	ZA	South Africa
KN	Saint Kitts and Nevis	ZM	Zambia
KP	Democratic People's Republic of Korea	ZW	Zimbabwe

TABLE-18

Company Register

The following table lists the full company name and location corresponding to the abbreviations given in the Name Index for companies associated with trademarks.

Abbott	Abbott Labs., Abbott Park, Illinois
ABC	Instituto Biologico Chemioterapico ABC SpA, Torino, Italy
Abello	Abello SA, Madrid, Spain
Adolor	Adolor Corp., Exton, Pennsylvania
Adroka	Adroka AG, Allschwil, Switzerland
AGIPS	AGIPS Pharmaceutici srl, Rapallo, Italy
AgrEvo	see Bayer CropScience
Air Prods. Chem.	Air Products and Chemicals, Inc., Allentown, Pennsylvania
Ajinomoto	Ajinomoto Co., Inc., Tokyo, Japan
Akorn	Akorn, Inc., Buffalo Grove, Illinois
Akzo	Akzo Nobel NV, Arnhem, The Netherlands
Alcon	Alcon Labs., Inc. (subsidiary of Nestle SA), Fort Worth, Texas
Alconox	Alconox Inc., New York, New York
Aldrich	Aldrich Chemical Co., Inc. (subsidiary of Sigma-Aldrich Corp.), Milwaukee, Wisconsin
Alfa	Alfa Wassermann SpA, Bologna, Italy
Allard	Lab. Allard SA (subsidiary of Bristol-Myers Squibb Co.), Paris, France
Allen & Hanburys	see GSK
Allergan	Allergan, Inc., Irvine, California
Allergopharma	Allergopharma Joachim Ganzer KG, Hamburg, Germany
Allied	Allied Signal, Inc. (formerly Allied Chemical Co.), Hopewell, Virginia
Almirall	Almirall-Prodesfarma SA, Barcelona, Spain
Alpharma	Alpharma, Inc., Fort Lee, New Jersey
Altana	Altana AG, Konstanz, Germany
Alza	Alza Corp., Mountain View, California
Am. Cyanamid	see Wyeth
Am. Home	see Wyeth
Amersham Biosci.	Amersham Biosciences Corp., (subsidiary of GE Healthcare), Piscataway, NJ
Amgen	Amgen Inc., Thousand Oaks, California
Amino	Amino AG, Neuenhof, Switzerland
Amsa	Amsa, srl, Rome, Italy
Andreu	see Roche
Andromaco	Labs. Andromaco, SA, Madrid, Spain
Angelini	Angelini Group, Rome, Italy
Apotex	Apotex, Toronto, Canada
Apothecon	Apothecon Products (division of Bristol-Myers Squibb Co.), Princeton, New Jersey
APS	see Teva
Ardeypharm	Ardeypharm GmbH Pharmazeutische Fabrik, Herdecke, Germany
Armour Pharm.	see Sanofi-Aventis
Arnolds	Arnolds Veterinary Products Ltd., Harlescott, Shrewsbury, UK
Artesan	Artesan Pharma GmbH & Co. KG, Lüchow, Germany
Arun	Arun Pharmaceuticals Ltd., Farnborough, Hants., UK
Asahi	Asahi Chemical Industry Co., Ltd., Tokyo, Japan
Asche	Asche AG (subsidiary of Schering AG), Hamburg, Germany
Ascher	B. F. Ascher & Co., Inc., Lenexa, Kansas
Asta	see Viatris
Astellas	Astellas Pharma Inc., Tokyo, Japan
Astier	Lab. Urpac-Astier, Paris, France
AstraZeneca	AstraZeneca UK Ltd., Kings Langley, Herts., UK
Athenstaedt	Athenstaedt Nachf. GmbH & Co. KG, Munich, Germany
Ausonia	Ausonia Farmaceutici, Pomezia (Rome), Italy
Aventis	Aventis Pharmaceuticals, Inc., (subsidiary of Sanofi-Aventis), Bridgewater, NJ
AWD	AWD.pharma GmbH & Co. KG (subsidiary of Pliva d.d.), Dresden, Germany
Axcan	Axcan Pharma Inc., Mont-Saint-Hilaire, Quebec, Canada
Ayerst	see Wyeth
Azupharma	Azupharma GmbH & Co., Gerlingen, Germany
Bailly	Lab. A. Bailly-SPEAB, Paris, France
Baker Norton	Baker Norton, London, UK
Baldacci	Labs. Baldacci, SpA, Pisa, Italy
Banyu	Banyu Pharmaceutical Co., Ltd. (subsidiary of Merck & Co., Inc.), Tokyo, Japan
Barnes-Hind	Pilkington Barnes-Hind, Inc. (subsidiary of Pilkington Brothers plc), Sunnyvale, California
BASF	BASF Group (formerly Badische Anilin- und Soda-Fabrik) Ludwigshafen, Germany
Basotherm	Basotherm GmbH (subsidiary of L'Oreal), Biberach an der Riss, Germany
Bastian	Bastian-Werk GmbH, Munich, Germany
Bausch & Lomb	Bausch & Lomb Pharmaceuticals, Inc., Tampa, Florida
Baxter	Baxter International, Inc. (formerly Baxter Travenol Labs.), Deerfield, Illinois
Bayer	Bayer AG, Leverkusen, Germany
Bayer CropSci.	Bayer CropScience AG (subsidiary of Bayer AG), Monheim am Rhein, Germany
Beiersdorf	Beiersdorf AG, Hamburg, Germany
Bellon	see Sanofi-Aventis
Belupo	Belupo, Koprivnica, Croatia
Bencard	see GSK
Bene-Arzneimittel	Bene-Arzneimittel GmbH, Munich, Germany

TABLE-19

Bengué	*see* Roche
Benzon	Benzon Pharma A/S, Copenhagen, Denmark
Bergamon	Bergamon srl, Rome, Italy
Berk	*see* Teva
Berlex	Berlex Labs. Inc. (subsidiary of Schering AG), Wayne, New Jersey
Berlin-Chemie	Berlin-Chemie AG (subsidiary of Menarini), Berlin, Germany
Berna	Berna Biotech AG, Bern, Switzerland
Besins-Iscovesco	Labs. Besins-Iscovesco, Paris, France
Beta	Lab. Biologico Chemioterapico Beta srl, Prevalle, Italy
Bial	Bial - Portela & Ca., SA, S. Mamede do Coronado, Portugal
Biochemie	Biochemie GmbH (subsidiary of Novartis), Kundl, Austria
Biocodex	Lab. Biocodex, Montrouge, France
Bioindustria	Bioindustria Farmaceutici srl, Rome, Italy
Biologici	Biologici Italia Lab. srl, Novate Milanese, Italy
Biopharma	Biopharma (Labs. Biopharmaceutiques de France) (subsidiary of Servier), Neuilly-sur-Seine, France
Biorex	Biorex Labs, Enfield, Middlesex, UK
Biosedra	*see* Fresenius
Biosintetica	Labs. Biosintetica Ltda., Sao Paulo, Brazil
Block	Block Drug Co., Inc. (subsidiary of GlaxoSmithKline), Jersey City, New Jersey
BLS	Boston Life Sciences, Inc., Boston, Massachusetts
BMS	Bristol-Myers Squibb Co., Princeton, New Jersey
Boehringer, Ing.	Boehringer Ingelheim GmbH (subsidiary of C. H. Boehringer Sohn), Ingelheim, Germany
Boehringer, Mann.	*see* Roche
Bonomelli	Bonomelli srl, Dolzago, Italy
Boots	*see* Abbott
Bottu	*see* Sanofi-Aventis
Bouchara	Lab. du Dr. E. Bouchara, Levallois-Perret, France
Bracco	Bracco SpA, Milan, Italy
Braun	B. Braun Melsungen AG, Melsungen, Germany
Brenner-Efeka	*see* Wyeth
Britannia	Britannia Pharmaceuticals Ltd., Redhill, Surrey, UK
Bruneau	Lab. Bruneau de la Salle, Paris, France
Bruschettini	Bruschettini srl, Genoa, Italy
Burroughs Wellcome	*see* GSK
Byk Gulden	*see* Altana
Caber	Farmaceutici Caber SpA, Commachio, Italy
Calbiochem	EMD Biosciences, Inc., San Diego, California
Calmic	Calmic BV, Utrecht, Netherlands
Carnrick	Carnrick Labs., Inc., Cedar Knolls, New Jersey
Carter-Wallace	*see* Wallace
Cascan	Cascan GmbH & Co. KG (subsidiary of GlaxoSmithKline plc), Hamburg, Germany
Cassella-med	Cassella-med GmbH & Co. KG, Köln, Germany
Cassenne	*see* Sanofi-Aventis
Centerchem	Centerchem, Inc., Stamford, Connecticut
Central Pharm.	Central Pharmaceuticals, Inc., Seymour, Indiana
Century	Century Pharmaceuticals, Inc., Indianapolis, Indiana
Cesra	Cesra Arzneimittel GmbH & Co. KG, Baden-Baden, Germany
CFPI	CFPI (subsidiary of Nufarm Ltd.), Gennevilliers, France
Chauvin	Labs. Chauvin SA, Montpellier, France
Chefaro	Deutsche Chefaro Pharma GmbH (subsidiary of Akzo Nobel NV), Waltrop, Germany
Chemie Linz	Chemie Linz GmbH (subsidiary of DSM NV), Linz, Austria
Chephasaar	Chephasaar, Chem.-Pharm. Fabrik GmbH, St. Ingbert, Germany
Chesebrough	Chesebrough-Ponds USA (subsidiary of Unilever, Inc.), Greenwich, Connecticut
Chevron	Chevron Chemical Co., Houston, Texas
Chibret	Labs. Merck Sharp & Dohme-Chibret SA (subsidiary of Merck & Co., Inc.), Paris, France
Chiesi	Chiesi Farmaceutici SpA, Parma, Italy
Chinoin	Chinoin Gyogyszer es Vegyeszeti Termekek Gyara, Budapest, Hungary
Chinosolfabrik	Chinosolfabrik (subsidiary of Riedel-de Haen AG), Seelze, Germany
Chugai	Chugai Pharmaceutical Co., Ltd., Tokyo, Japan
Ciba	Ciba Specialty Chemicals, Basle, Switzerland
Ciba-Geigy	*see* Novartis
Cilag	Cilag AG (subsidiary of Johnson & Johnson), Schaffhausen, Switzerland
Circle	Circle Pharmaceuticals, Inc., Indianapolis, Indiana
Cleary	Cleary Chemical Corp., Dayton, New Jersey
Combe	Combe Inc., White Plains, New York
Consolidated Chem.	Consolidated Chemicals Ltd., Wrexham, Clywd., UK
Cooper	The Cooper Cos., Inc., Irvine, California
CooperVision	CooperVision Inc., Fairport, New York
Coop. Farm.	Cooperative Farmaceutica Societa Coop., a.r.l., Milan, Italy
COR	*see* Millennium
Cox	A.H. Cox & Co. Ltd., Barnstaple, Devon, UK
CP Kelco	CP Kelco, Wilmington, Delaware
CP Pharm.	CP Pharmaceuticals Ltd., Wrexham, Clywd., UK
Crinos	Crinos Industria Farmacobiologica SpA, Como Villaguardia, Italy
Croda	Croda, Inc., Parsippany, New Jersey

TABLE-20

Crookes	Crookes Healthcare Ltd., Nottingham, UK
Crosara	Lab. Farmaco Biologico Crosara SpA, Rome, Italy
Crystal Chem.	Crystal Chemical, Inc., Chicago, Illinois
CT	C.T.-Lab. Farmaceutico srl, San Remo, Italy
Cusi	Laboratorios Cusi SA, El Masnou (Barcelona), Spain
Cutter	*see* Bayer
Daiichi	Daiichi Pharmaceutical Co., Ltd., Tokyo, Japan
Dainippon	Dainippon Pharmaceutical Co., Ltd., Osaka, Japan
Damor	Farmaceutici Damor SpA, Naples, Italy
DDSA	DDSA Pharmaceuticals, London, UK
Debat	Lab. Debat, Garches, France
Degussa	Degussa-Huls AG (subsidiary of Veba AG), Frankfurt, Germany
Dermal	Dermal Laboratories Ltd., Gosmore, Herts, UK
Dermik	Dermik Labs., Inc. (subsidiary of Sanofi-Aventis), Berwyn, Pennsylvania
Desitin	Desitin Arzneimittel GmbH, Hamburg, Germany
Dexo	Labs. Dexo, Saint-Cloud, France
Dieckmann	Dieckmann Arzneimittel GmbH (subsidiary of Merck & Co., Inc.), Haar, Germany
Dista	*see* Lilly
Doetsch, Grether	Doetsch, Grether & Cie AG, Basel, Switzerland
Dolorgiet	Dolorgiet GmbH & Co. KG, St. Augustin/Bonn, Germany
Dompé	Dompé Farmaceutici SpA, Milan, Italy
Dow	The Dow Chemical Co., Midland, Michigan
Dow AgroSci.	Dow AgroSciences LLC (subsidiary of The Dow Chemical Co.), Indianapolis, Indiana
Draco	Draco Lakemedel AB (subsidiary of AstraZeneca), Lund, Sweden
Dreluso	Dreluso Pharmazeutika, Dr. Elten & Sohn GmbH, Hessisch Oldendorf, Germany
Drossapharm	Drossapharm AG, Basel, Switzerland
DSM	Koninklijke DSM N.V., Heerlen, The Netherlands
Dumex	*see* Alpharma
Duncan	Duncan Farmaceutici SpA, Verona, Italy
Duphar	*see* Solvay
DuPont	E. I. du Pont de Nemours & Co., Inc., Wilmington, Delaware
Dura	Merck dura GmbH (formerly Durachemie) (subsidiary of Merck KGaA), Darmstadt, Germany
Eastman Kodak	Eastman Kodak Co., Rochester, New York
Eisai	Eisai Co., Ltd., Tokyo, Japan
Elan	Elan Corp. plc, Dublin, Ireland
Elanco	Elanco Animal Health Co. (division of Eli Lilly & Co.), Indianapolis, Indiana
Elf Atochem	Elf Atochem North America, Inc. (subsidiary of Elf Aquitaine), Philadelphia, Pennsylvania
Emery	Emery Industries, Inc. (subsidiary of National Distillers & Chem. Corp.), Mauldin, South Carolina
Endo	Endo Pharmaceuticals, Inc., Chadds Ford, Delaware
Engelhard KG	Engelhard Arzneimittel GmbH & Co. KG, Niederdorfelden, Germany
Errekappa	Errekappa Euroterapici SpA, Milan, Italy
Espe	Espe Dental AG, Seefeld, Germany
Esseti	Esseti Farmaceutici SpA, S. Giorgi-Cremano, Italy
Essex	Essex Pharma (subsidiary of Schering-Plough), Munich, Germany
Esteve	Esteve Group, Barcelona, Spain
Ethicon	Ethicon, Inc. (subsidiary of Johnson & Johnson), Somerville, New Jersey
Europharma	Europharma, SA, Madrid, Spain
Eutherapie	Lab. Eutherapie (subsidiary of Servier), Neuilly-sur-Seine, France
Evans	*see* Medeva
Fabre	Pierre Fabre SA, Boulogne, France
Falk	Dr. Falk Pharma GmbH, Freiburg, Germany
Farillon	Farillon Ltd., Romford, Essex, UK
Farmacologico	Laboratorio Farmacologico Milanese srl, Caronno Pertusella, Italy
Farmades	Farmades SpA, Rome, Italy
Farmetrusca	Farmetrusca s.a.s. di C. Pini e C., Tavarnuzze, Italy
Farmigea	Farmigea SpA-Industria Chimico Farmaceutica, Pisa, Italy
Farmila	Farmila-Farmaceutici Milano srl, Milan, Italy
Farmitalia	Phamacia Italia SpA (formerly Farmitalia Carlo Erba srl) (subsidiary of Pfizer, Inc.), Milan, Italy
Farmos	Orion Corp., Espoo, Finland
Fatol	Fatol Arzneimittel GmbH, Schiffweiler, Germany
Faulding	F. H. Faulding & Co. Ltd., Underdale, SA, Australia
FBA Pharm	FBA Pharmaceuticals, Inc., West Haven, Connecticut
Ferndale	Ferndale Labs., Inc., Ferndale, Michigan
Ferrer	Ferrer Internacional, Barcelona, Spain
Ferring	Ferring BV, Hoofddorp, Netherlands
Ferrosan	AB Ferrosan (subsidiary of Novo Nordisk), Malmo, Sweden
Fher	Fher SA, Laboratorios, Barcelona, Spain
Fidia	Fidia SpA (Farmaceutici Italiani Derivati Industrialie Affini SpA), Albano Terme, Italy
Firma	Firma, Fabbr. Ital. Ritrov. Medic. Aff. SpA, Florence, Italy
Firmenich	Firmenich SA, Geneva, Switzerland
FMC	FMC Corp., Chicago, Illinois
Forest	Forest Pharmaceuticals, Inc., St. Louis, Missouri
Formenti	Prodotti Formenti srl, Milan, Italy
Fort Dodge	Fort Dodge Animal Health (division of Wyeth), Overland Park, Kansas
Foscama	Biomedica Foscama SpA, Rome, Italy

TABLE-21

Fougera	E. Fougera & Co. (division of Altana, Inc.), Melville, New York
Fournier	Group Fournier, Chenove, France
Francia	Francia Farmaceutici Industria Farmaco Biologica srl, Milan, Italy
Fresenius	Fresenius Kabi AG, Bad Homburg, Germany
Frosst	Merck Frosst Canada (subsidiary of Merck & Co., Inc.), Kirkland, QC, Canada
Fujinaga	Fujinaga Pharmaceutical Co., Ltd., Tokyo, Japan
Fujisawa	see Astellas
Fumouze	Labs. Fumouze, SA, Levallois-Perret, France
Funai	Funai Corp., Osaka, Japan
Fuso	Fuso Pharmaceutical Industries, Ltd., Osaka, Japan
Gador	Gador SA, Buenos Aires, Argentina
Galderma	Galderma Pharma SA, Lausanne, Switzerland
Galen	Galen Ltd., Craigavon, Co. Armagh, Northern Ireland
Galenica	Galenica Vertretungen AG, Bern, Switzerland
Galenika	Galenika, Zemun, Yugoslavia
GE Healthcare	GE Healthcare Ltd. (subsidiary of General Electric), Little Chalfont, Buckinghamshire, UK
GEA	GEA A/S, Frederiksberg, Denmark
Geigy	see Novartis
Geistlich	Geistlich-Pharma AG, Wolhusen, Switzerland
Genentech	Genentech, Inc., South San Francisco, California
Geneva	Geneva Pharmaceuticals, Inc., Broomfield, Colorado
Gentili	Istituto Gentili SpA, Pisa, Italy
Genzyme	Genzyme Corp., Cambridge, Massachusetts
Gepepharm	Gepepharm GmbH, Siegburg, Germany
Gerot	Gerot Pharmazeutika, Vienna, Austria
Geymonat	Geymonat SpA, Anagni, Italy
Ghimas	Ghimas SpA, Casalecchio di Reno, Italy
Gilead	Gilead Sciences, Foster City, California
Giulini	Giulini Pharma GmbH (subsidiary of Solvay SA), Hannover, Germany
Givaudan	Givaudan-Roure Intl. SA (subsidiary of Hoffmann-La Roche), Vernier, Switzerland
Glaxo	see GSK
Glenwood	Glenwood Inc., Tenafly, New Jersey
Globopharm	Globopharm AG, Küsnacht, Switzerland
Gödecke	Gödecke AG, Berlin, Germany
Goldshield	Goldshield Pharmaceuticals Ltd., Croyden, Surrey, UK
Gramon	Laboratorios Gramon, Buenos Aires, Argentina
Green Cross	see Yoshitomi
Grelan	Grelan Pharmaceutical Co., Ltd., Tokyo, Japan
Grünenthal	Grünenthal GmbH, Aachen, Germany
GSK	GlaxoSmithKline plc, Uxbridge, Middlesex, UK
Guardian	Guardian Laboratories (division of United-Guardian, Inc.), Hauppauge, New York
Guerbet	Lab. Guerbet, Aulnay-sous-Bois Cedex, France
Guidotti	Laboratori Guidotti SpA, Pisa, Italy
Guilford	Guilford Pharmaceuticals, Inc., Baltimore, Maryland
Halsey	Halsey Drug Co., Rockford, Illinois
Hamilton	Hamilton Pharm. Pty. Ltd., Adelaide, Australia
Han Wha	Han Wha Pharma Co., Ltd., Seoul, South Korea
Hässle	Hässle Lakemedel AB (subsidiary of AstraZeneca), Molndal, Sweden
Hefa	Hefa Pharma Vertriebs GmbH & Co. KG, Werne, Germany
Heilit	Heilit Arzneimittel GmbH, Reinbek, Germany
Helsinn	Helsinn Healthcare SA, Lugano, Switzerland
Henkel	Henkel, Dusseldorf, Germany
Hennig	Hennig Arzneimittel GmbH & Co. KG, Florsheim am Main, Germany
Henning	Henning Berlin GmbH & Co., OHG, Berlin, Germany
Herbert	Herbert Arzn. GmbH, Wiesbaden, Germany
Herbrand	Dr. Herbrand KG Chem.-Pharm. Werk, Gengenback, Germany
Hercules	Hercules Inc., Wilmington, Delaware
Hermal	Hermal Kurt Herrmann (subsidiary of Boots Co.), Reinbek, Germany
Hermes	Hermes Arzneimittel GmbH, Grosshesselohe/Munich, Germany
Heterochemical	HeteroChemical Corp., Valley Stream, New York
Heumann	Heumann Pharma GmbH, Nurenberg, Germany
Heyl	Heyl Chem.-Pharm. Fabrik GmbH & Co. KG, Berlin, Germany
Hishiyama	Hishiyama Pharmaceutical Co., Ltd., Osaka, Japan
HMR	see Sanofi-Aventis
Hobein	Dr. Hobein & Co., GmbH Arzneimittel Nachf., Meckenheim, Germany
Hoechst	see Sanofi-Aventis
Hoei	Hoei Pharmaceutical Co., Ltd., Osaka, Japan
Hokuriku	Hokuriku Seiyaku Co., Ltd., Tokyo, Japan
Hopkins	Hopkins Agricultural Chemical Co., Madison, Wisconsin
Hor-Fer-Vit	Hor-Fer-Vit Pharmazeutische GmbH, Oldenburg, Germany
Horita	Horita Yakuhin Gosei K.K., Nagoya, Japan
Hormosan	Hormosan-Kwizda GmbH, Frankfurt/Main, Germany
Horner	Carter-Horner Corp., Mississauga, Ontario, Canada
Houdé	see Sanofi-Aventis

TABLE-22

Hoyer	Hoyer-Madaus & Co. KG, Monheim, Germany
Hyrex	Hyrex Pharmaceuticals, Memphis, Tennessee
IBI	Istituto Biochimico Italiano G. Lorenzini SpA, Milan, Italy
Ibirn	Istituto Bioterapico Nazionale srl, Rome, Italy
IBP	Istituto Biochimico Pavese SpA, Pavia, Italy
Ichthyol	Ichthyol-Gesellschaft Cordes, Hermanni & Co., Hamburg, Germany
ICI	Imperial Chemical Industries plc, London, UK
ICN	*see* Valeant
Immunex	Immunex Corporation, Seattle, Washington
Inava	Labs. Inava, Departement Médical de Pierre Fabre Médicament, Bologna, France
Innothéra	Innothéra Industrie, Arcueil, France
Interdelta	Interdelta SA, Fribourg, Switzerland
Intersan	Intersan, Institut für pharmazeutische und klinische Forschung GmbH, Ettlingen, Germany
Intervet	Intervet International bv (subsidiary of Akzo Nobel), Boxmeer, The Netherlands
Inverni	Inverni Della Beffa SpA (subsidiary of Sanofi-Aventis), Milan, Italy
Ipsen	Beaufour-Ipsen, Paris, France
Iromedica	Iromedica AG, St. Gallen, Switzerland
Isagro	Isagro SpA, Milan, Italy
Isei	Isei Co., Ltd., Yamagata, Japan
ISF	ISF SpA, Perugia, Italy
ISI	Istituto Sierovaccinogeno Italiano SpA, Castelvecchio Pascoli, Italy
Isis	*see* Alpharma
ISK Biosci	ISK Biosciences, Inc., Memphis, Tennessee
Isola-Ibi	Isola-Ibi, Genova-Quarto, Italy
ISP	International Specialty Products, Wayne, New Jersey
Ist. Chim. Inter	Istituto Chimico Internazionale di Dr. Giuseppe Rendre srl, Rome, Italy
Italchimici	Italchimici SpA, Rome, Italy
Italfarmaco	Italfarmaco SpA, Milan, Italy
Ivax	Ivax Corp., Miami, Florida
Iwaki	Iwaki Seiyaku Co., Ltd., Tokyo, Japan
J & J	Johnson & Johnson, New Brunswick, New Jersey
Janssen	Janssen Pharmaceutica NV (subsidiary of Johnson & Johnson), Beerse, Belgium
Janssen-Cilag	Janssen-Cilag Int. NV (subsidiary of Johnson & Johnson), Beerse, Belgium
Jenapharm	Jenapharm GmbH & Co., KG, Jena, Germany
Kabi	*see* Pharmacia
Kade	Dr. Kade Pharmazeutische Fabrik GmbH, Berlin, Germany
Kaigai	Kaigai Seiyaku Co., Ltd., Tokyo, Japan
Kaken	Kaken Pharmaceutical Co., Ltd., Tokyo, Japan
Kali-Chemie	Solvay Arzneimittel GmbH (formerly Kali-Chemie AG), Hannover, Germany
Kanebo	Kanebo Pharmaceuticals, Ltd., Tokyo, Japan
Kayaku	Kayaku Co., Ltd., Tokyo, Japan
Key	Key Pharmaceuticals, Inc. (subsidiary of Schering-Plough), Kenilworth, New Jersey
Kissei	Kissei Pharmaceutical Co., Ltd., Nagano, Japan
Klinge	Klinge Pharma GmbH (subsidiary of Astellas Pharma), Munich, Germany
Knoll	*see* Abbott
Kodama	Kodama Ltd., Tokyo, Japan
Kotobuki	Kotobuki Pharmaceutical Co., Ltd., Nagano, Japan
Kowa	Kowa Company Ltd., Nagoya, Japan
Kowa Yakuhin	Kowa Yakuhin Kogyo, Tokyo, Japan
Kremers-Urban	Kremers-Urban Co., Mequon, Wisconsin
Kreussler	Chemische Fabrik Kreussler & Co. GmbH, Wiesbaden, Germany
Krewel	Krewel-Meuselbach GmbH, Eitorf, Germany
Krka	Krka d.d., Novo Mesto, Slovenia
Kureha	Kureha Chemical Industry Co., Ltd. Pharmaceutical Div., Tokyo, Japan
Kwizda	F. J. Kwizda GmbH, Vienna, Austria
Kyorin	Kyorin Pharmaceutical Co., Ltd., Tokyo, Japan
Kyoritsu	Kyoritsu Pharmaceutical Co., Ltd., Nara, Japan
Kyowa	Kyowa Hakko Kogyo Co., Ltd., Tokyo, Japan
L.A.B.	Laboratories for Applied Biology, Ltd., London, UK
Labatec	Labatec-Pharma SA, Meyrin, Switzerland
Labcatal	Lab. Labcatal, Montrouge, France
Lacer	Lacer SA, Barcelona, Spain
Lafare	Lab. Farmaceutico Reggiano srl, Ercolana Resina, Italy
Lafon	Labs. L. Lafon, Maisons-Alfort, France
Lagap	Lagap Pharmaceuticals Ltd., Bordon, Hants., UK
Lampugnani	Lampugnani Farmaceutici SpA, Milan, Italy
Lannacher	Lannacher Heilmittel GmbH, Lannach, Austria
Lannett	The Lannett Co., Inc., Philadelphia, Pennsylvania
Laser	Laser, Inc., Crown Point, Indiana
Lederle	*see* Wyeth
Lek	Lek Pharmaceutical and Chemical Co., DD, Ljubljana, Slovenia
Lemmon	Lemmon Co., Sellersville, Pennsylvania
Leo Pharm	Leo Pharmaceutic Products, Ballerup, Denmark
Lepetit	Gruppo Lepetit SpA, Milan, Italy

TABLE-23

Lichtenstein	Lichtenstein Pharmazeutica GmbH, Mulheim/Karlich, Germany
Lifepharma	Lifepharma srl, Milan, Italy
Ligand	Ligand Pharmaceuticals, San Diego, California
Lilly	Eli Lilly & Co., Indianapolis, Indiana
Link	Link Pharmaceuticals Ltd., West Sussex, UK
Lipha	Lipha Santé SA, Lyon, France
Lipo	Lipo Chemicals, Inc., Paterson, New Jersey
Liposome Co.	The Liposome Company, Inc., Princeton, New Jersey
Lisapharma	Lisapharma SpA, Como, Italy
Logeais	see Chiesi
Lorex	Lorex Synthélabo, Ltd. (subsidiary of L'Oreal SA), Marlow, Bucks., UK
Lotus	Lotus Biochem. Corp., Bristol, Tennessee
Lundbeck	H. Lundbeck A/S, Copenhagen, Denmark
Lusofarmaco	Istituto Luso Farmaco d'Italia SpA, Milan, Italy
Lyocentre	Lab. Lyocentre, Aurillac, France
3M	Minnesota Mining & Manufacturing Co., St. Paul, Minnesota
3M Pharma	3M Pharmaceuticals (division of 3M), St. Paul, Minnesota
M & B	see Sanofi-Aventis
Mack, Illert.	Heinrich Mack Nachf., Gmbh & Co. KG (subsidiary of Pfizer Inc.), Illertissen, Germany
Madaus	Madaus AG, Cologne, Germany
Maggioni	Maggioni-Winthrop Farmaceutici SpA, Milan, Italy
Magis	Lab. Magis Farmaceuti SpA, Brescia, Italy
Makhteshim-Agan	Makhteshim-Agan Ind. Ltd., Omer, Israel
Malesci	Malesci Istituto Farmacobiologico, SpA, Florence, Italy
Mallinckrodt	Mallinckrodt, Inc., St. Louis, Missouri
Manetti Roberts	L. Manetti & H. Roberts & C. per Azioni, Florence, Italy
Mann	Dr. Gerhard Mann, Chem.-Pharm. Fabrik GmbH (subsidiary of Bausch & Lomb), Berlin, Germany
Maruishi	Maruishi Pharmaceutical Co., Ltd., Osaka, Japan
Maruko	Maruko Seiyaku Co., Ltd., Nagoya, Japan
Master	Master Pharma srl, Parma, Italy
Maurer	Maurer-Pharma GmbH, Saarbrücken, Germany
Mayrand	see Merz
McGaw	McGaw, Inc. (subsidiary of IVAX Corp.), Irvine, California
McNeil	McNeil Consumer Healthcare (subsidiary of Johnson & Johnson), Fort Washington, Pennsylvania
Mead Johnson	see BMS
Mect	Mect srl, Alpignano, Italy
Medac	Medac, Hamburg, Germany
Medeva	Medeva Pharma Ltd., Leatherhead, Surrey, UK
Medice	Medice, Chem.-Pharm. Fabrik Pütter GmbH & Co. KG, Iserlohn, Germany
Medichemie	Medichemie AG, Ettingen, Switzerland
Medici	Lab. Farm. Dr. Medici srl, Rome, Italy
Medicis	Medicis Pharmaceutical Corp., Scotsdale, Arizona
Medinova	Medinova AG, Zurich, Switzerland
Mediolanum	Mediolanum Farmaceutici SpA, Milan, Italy
Medi-Physics	see GE Healthcare
Medo	Medo Pharmaceuticals Ltd., Chesham, Bucks., UK
Medosan	Medosan srl Industrie Biochimiche Riunite, Cecchina, Italy
Meiji	Meiji Seika Kaisha, Ltd., Tokyo, Japan
Menarini	A. Menarini Industrie Farmaceutiche Riunite srl, Florence, Italy
Mendelejeff	Stabilimento chimico Farmaceutico Mendelejeff srl, Rome, Italy
Mepha	Mepha Pharma AG, Aesch, Switzerland
Merck & Co.	Merck & Co., Inc., Whitehouse Station, New Jersey
Merck KGaA	Merck KGaA (formerly E. Merck), Darmstadt, Germany
Merck/Schering-Plough	Merck/Schering-Plough Pharmaceuticals (joint venture of Merck & Co., Inc. and Schering-Plough Corp.), West Point, Pennsylvania
Merckle	Merckle GmbH, Blaubeuren, Germany
Merial	Merial Ltd., London, UK
Merz	Merz & Co., GmbH, Frankfurt/Main, Germany
Midy	Sterling-Midy, Paris, France
Mikasa	Mikasa Seiyaku Co., Ltd., Tokyo, Japan
Miles	see Bayer
Millennium	Millennium Pharmaceuticals, Inc., Cambridge, Massachusetts
Miquel	Laboratorios Miquel SA (subsidiary of Otsuka Pharm. Co., Ltd.), Barcelona, Spain
Misemer	Misemer Pharmaceuticals, Inc., Springfield, Missouri
Mission Pharmacal	Mission Pharmacal Co., San Antonio, Texas
Mitsubishi	Mitsubishi Tokyo Pharmaceuticals, Tokyo, Japan
Mitsui	Mitsui Pharmaceuticals, Inc., Tokyo, Japan
Mochida	Mochida Pharmaceutical Co., Ltd., Tokyo, Japan
Mohan	Mohan Medicine Research Inst., Tokyo, Japan
Molimin	Molimin Arzneimittel GmbH, Hallstadt, Germany
Molteni	Molteni L. & C. dei F. Ili Alitti Societa Esercizio SpA, Scandicci, Italy
Monsanto	Monsanto Co., St. Louis, Missouri
Morishita	Morishita Pharmaceutical Co., Ltd., Osaka, Japan
Mundipharma	Mundipharma AG, Basel, Switzerland

TABLE-24

Mylan Bertek	Mylan Bertek Pharmaceuticals Inc., Research Triangle Park, North Carolina
Nagase	Nagase & Co., Ltd., Tokyo, Japan
Napp	Napp Labs., Cambridge, UK
NEGMA	Labs. NEGMA, Toussus-le-Noble, France
Nexstar	see Gilead
Nichiiko	Nihon Iyakuhin Kogyo Co., Ltd., Toyama, Japan
Nicholas	see Roche
Nikken	Nikken Chemicals Co., Ltd., Tokyo, Japan
Nippon Chemiphar	Nippon Chemiphar Co., Ltd., Tokyo, Japan
Nippon Kayaku	Nippon Kayaku Co., Ltd., Tokyo, Japan
Nippon Shinyaku	Nippon Shinyaku Co., Ltd., Kyoto, Japan
Nippon Shoji	Nippon Shoji Kaisha, Ltd., Osaka, Japan
Nippon Soda	Nippon Soda Co., Ltd., Tokyo, Japan
Nippon Zoki	Nippon Zoki Pharmaceutical Co., Ltd., Osaka, Japan
Nissan	Nissan Chemical Industries, Ltd., Tokyo, Japan
Norbrook	Norbrook Labs. Ltd., Carlisle, Cumbria, UK
Norgine	Norgine GmbH, Marburg, Germany
Norwich	see Procter & Gamble
Novartis	Novartis Pharma AG, Basel, Switzerland
Novartis Agro	see Syngenta
Novo	Novo Nordisk A/S, Bagsvaerd, Denmark
Novus	Novus International, Inc., St. Louis, Missouri
Nuovo Cons.	Nuovo Consorzio Sanitario Nazionale srl, Rome, Italy
Nycomed	Nycomed Pharma, Roskilde, Denmark
OGS	Oxford GlycoSciences Ltd., Abingdon, Oxon, UK
Ohmeda	Ohmeda Pharm. Prods. (Div. Baxter Pharm. Prods.), New Providence, New Jersey
Ohta	Ohta Pharmaceutical Co., Ltd., Tokyo, Japan
Olin	Olin Corp., Norwalk, Connecticut
OM	OM Pharma, Geneva, Switzerland
Ono	Ono Pharmaceutical Co., Ltd., Osaka, Japan
Opfermann	Opfermann Arzneimittel GmbH, Wiehl, Germany
OPW	Oranienburger Pharmawerk GmbH, Oranienburg, Germany
Organon	Organon International BV (subsidiary of Akzo Nobel), Oss, Netherlands
Orion	Orion Pharm, Espoo, Finland
Orphan Europe	Orphan Europe SARL, Paris, France
Ortho	Ortho-McNeil Pharmaceutical Corp. (subsidiary of Johnson & Johnson), Raritan, New Jersey
Otsuka	Otsuka Pharmaceutical Co., Ltd., Tokyo, Japan
Parke-Davis	Parke-Davis (division of Warner-Lambert Co., LLC), New York, New York
Parmed	see Alpharma
Penick	Penick Corp., Newark, New Jersey
Penn	Penn Pharmaceuticals Ltd., Tradegar, Gwent, UK
Permamed	Permamed AG, Therwil, Switzerland
Person & Covey	Person & Covey, Inc., Glendale, California
Pfizer	Pfizer, Inc., New York, New York
Pfleger	Dr. R. Pfleger Chemische Fabrik GmbH, Bamberg, Germany
Pharmacia	Pharmacia (subsidiaries of Pfizer, Inc.), New York, New York
Pharmacia & Upjohn	Pharmacia & Upjohn (division of Pfizer, Inc.), New York, New York
Pharmascience	Laboratoires Pharmascience, Courbevoie, France
Pharma-Selz	Pharma-Selz GmbH, Bockenheim, Germany
Pharma-Stern	Pharma-Stern GmbH, Wedel, Germany
Pharmax	Pharmax Ltd., Bexley, Kent, UK
Pharmion	Pharmion Corp., Boulder, Colorado
Piam	Vecchi & C. Piam di G. Assereto, Genoa, Italy
Pickles	J. Pickles & Sons, Knaresborough, N. Yorks, UK
Pirri	Istituto Pirri srl, Milan, Italy
Pitman-Moore	see Schering-Plough
Pliva	Pliva d.d., Zagreb, Croatia
Pohl	G. Pohl-Boskamp GmbH & Co., Hohenlocksted, Germany
Poli	Poli Group, Milan, Italy
Polifarma	Polifarma SpA, Rome, Italy
PPG	PPG Industries, Pittsburgh, Pennsylvania
Procter & Gamble	Procter & Gamble, Cincinnati, Ohio
Promedica	see Chiesi
Proter	Proter SpA, Milan, Italy
Protina	Protina Pharmazeutische GmbH, Ismaning, Germany
Pulitzer	Pulitzer Italiana SpA, Rome, Italy
Purdue Frederick	The Purdue Frederick Co., Inc., Norwalk, Connecticut
Quinoderm	Quinoderm Ltd., Oldham, Lancs., UK
Radiumfarma	Radiumfarma srl, Milan, Italy
R.A.N.	R.A.N. Novesia AG Arzneimittel, Neuss/Rhein, Germany
Ravensberg	Ravensberg GmbH, Chemische Fabrik, Konstanz, Germany
Ravizza	Ravizza SpA (subsidiary of BASF), Muggio (Milan), Italy
Reckitt Benckiser	Reckitt Benckiser plc, Slough, Berkshire, UK
Reckitt & Colman	see Reckitt Benckiser

TABLE-25

Recordati	Recordati Industria Chimica e Farmaceutica SpA, Milan, Italy
Rentschler	Dr. Rentschler Arzneimittel GmbH & Co., Laupheim, Germany
Rexall	Rexall Group, Fort Lauderdale, Florida
Rhein-Pharma	Rhein-Pharma GmbH, Plankstadt, Germany
Rhone-Poulenc	*see* Sanofi-Aventis
Riom	Riom Labs.-CERM, Puteaux, France
Ripari-Gero	Istituto Farmaco Biologico Ripari-Gero, SpA, Monteriggioni, Italy
Ritsert	Dr. E. Ritsert, GmbH & Co. KG, Eberbach, Germany
Roberts	*see* Shire
Robins	*see* Wyeth
Robugen	Robugen GmbH Pharmazeutische Fabrik, Esslingen, Germany
Roche	F. Hoffmann-La Roche Ltd., Basel, Switzerland
Rodleben	Rodleben Pharma GmbH, Rodleben, Germany
Roemmers	Roemmers S.A.I.C.F., Buenos Aires, Argentina
Roerig	Roerig (division of Pfizer Inc.), New York, New York
Rohm & Haas	Rohm & Haas Co., Philadelphia, Pennsylvania
Romark	Romark Laboratories L.C., Tampa, Florida
Rosemont	Rosemont Pharm. Ltd., Leeds UK
Ross	Ross Products Division of Abbott Labs., Columbus, Ohio
Rotta	Rotta Research Laboratorium SpA, Monza, Milan, Italy
Roxane	Roxane Labs., Inc. (subsidiary of Boehringer, Ing.), Columbus, Ohio
RPR	*see* Sanofi-Aventis
Rystan	Rystan Co., Inc. (subsidiary of Integra Life Sciences Corp.), Plainsboro, New Jersey
Salix	Salix Pharmaceuticals, Inc., Morrisville, North Carolina
Salsbury	Salsbury Labs. Inc. (subsidiary of Cambrex Corp.), Charles City, Iowa
Salus	Salus Researches SpA, Rome, Italy
San Carlo	San Carlo Farmaceutici SpA, Rome, Italy
Sandoz	*see* Novartis
Sanko	Sanko Junyaku Co., Ltd. (subsidiary of Eisai Co., Ltd.), Tokyo, Japan
Sankyo	Sankyo Co., Ltd., Tokyo, Japan
Sanofi-Aventis	Sanofi-Aventis Group, Paris, France
Sanofi-Synthelabo	Sanofi-Synthélabo Inc., (subsidiary of Sanofi-Aventis), New York, NY
Sanofi Winthrop	*see* Sanofi-Aventis
Sanol	Sanol GmbH, Monheim, Germany
Sanorania	Sanorania GmbH (subsidiary of Pharmacia Corp.), Berlin, Germany
Santen	Santen Pharmaceutical Co., Ltd., Osaka, Japan
Sanwa	Sanwa Kagaku Kenkyusho Co., Ltd., Nagoya, Japan
Sanzen	Sanzen Pharmaceutical Co., Ltd., Ohmiya, Japan
Sarm	Sarm srl, Rome, Italy
Savage	Savage Labs. (division of Altana AG), Melville, New York
Savoma	Savoma Medicinali SpA, Parma, Italy
Sawai	Sawai Pharmaceutical Co., Ltd., Osaka, Japan
Schaper & Brummer	Schaper & Brummer GmbH & Co. KG, Salzgitter (Ringelheim), Germany
Schering AG	Schering AG, Berlin, Germany
Schering-Plough	Schering-Plough Corp., Kenilworth, New Jersey
Schiapparelli	Schiapparelli srl (subsidiary of Alfa-Wassermann SpA), Milan, Italy
Schülke & Mayr	Schülke & Mayr GmbH, Norderstedt, Germany
Schwabe	Dr. Willmar Schwabe GmbH, Karlsruhe, Germany
Schwarz	Schwarz Pharma AG, Monheim, Germany
Schwarzhaupt	Kommanditgesellschaft Schwarzhaupt GmbH & Co., Cologne, Germany
Sclavo	Sclavo SpA, Siena, Italy
Scott	O. M. Scott and Sons Co., Marysville, Ohio
Searle	G. D. Searle & Co., LLC (division of Pfizer, Inc.) New York, New York
Senju	Senju Pharmaceutical Co., Ltd., Osaka, Japan
Serono	Serono Intl. SA, Geneva, Switzerland
Serpero	Serpero, Industria Galenica Milanese SpA, Milan, Italy
Servier	Servier Institut de Recherches Internationales, Courbevoie, France
Servipharm	Servipharm Ltd. (subsidiary of Novartis AG), Basel, Switzerland
Shell	Shell Chemical Co., Houston, Texas
Shionogi	Shionogi & Co., Ltd., Osaka, Japan
Shire	Shire Pharmaceuticals Group plc, Basingstoke, UK
Showa Shinyaku	Showa Yakka, Tokyo, Japan
Showa Yakuhin	Showa Yakuhin Kako Co., Ltd., Tokyo, Japan
Sidus	Instituto Sidus I.C.S.A., Buenos Aires, Argentina
Siegfried	Siegfried Group, Zofingen, Switzerland
Sifi	Societa Industria Farmaceutica Italiana SpA, Catania, Italy
Sigma	Sigma Chemical Co. (subsidiary of Sigma-Aldrich Corp.), St. Louis, Missouri
Sigma-Tau	Sigma-Tau Industrie Farmaceutiche Riunite SpA, Rome, Italy
Sinclair	Sinclair Pharmaceuticals Ltd., Godalming, Surrey, UK
Sintyal	*see* Otsuka
SIT	Specialita Igienico Terapeutiche srl, Mede (Pavia), Italy
S&K Pharma	S&K Pharma, Schumann u. Kohl GmbH, Perl, Germany
SK & F	*see* GSK
SKB	*see* GSK

TABLE-26

SkyePharma	SkyePharma plc, London, UK
Smith & Nephew	Smith & Nephew Healthcare Ltd., Hull, North Humberside, UK
Solutia	Solutia, Inc., St. Louis, Missouri
Solvay	Solvay SA, Brussels, Belgium
SPA	Societa Prodotti Antibiotici SpA, Milan, Italy
Specia	*see* Sanofi-Aventis
Spitzner	W. Spitzner, Arzneimittelfabrik GmbH, Ettlingen, Germany
Squibb	*see* BMS
SS Pharm.	SSP Co., Ltd., Tokyo, Japan
Stada	Stada Arzneimittel AG, Bad Vilbel, Germany
Stafford-Miller	Stafford-Miller Ltd., Welwyn Garden City, Herts., UK
Steiner	Steiner & Co., Deutsche Arzneimittel Gesellschaft, Berlin, Germany
Stepan	Stepan Co., Northfield, Illinois
Sterling Winthrop	*see* Sanofi-Aventis
Stiefel	Stiefel Labs., Inc., Coral Gables, Florida
Streuli	G. Streuli & Co. AG, Uznach, Switzerland
Stroder	Ist. Farmaco Biologico Stroder srl, Florence, Italy
Sumitomo	Sumitomo Pharmaceuticals Co., Ltd., Osaka, Japan
Swedish Orphan	Swedish Orphan AB, Stockholm, Sweden
Symrise	Symrise GmbH & Co. KG, Holzminden, Germany
Syncro	Syncro Argentina S.A.Q.I.C.I.F., Buenos Aires, Argentina
Syngenta	Syngenta AG, Basel, Switzerland
Syntex	Syntex Labs., Inc. (subsidiary of F. Hoffmann-La Roche Ltd.), Palo Alto, California
Synthelabo	*see* Sanofi-Aventis
TAD	TAD Pharma GmbH, Cuxhaven, Germany
Taiho	Taiho Pharmaceutical Co., Ltd., Tokyo, Japan
Taisho	Taisho Pharmaceutical Co., Ltd., Tokyo, Japan
Taiyo	Taiyo Pharmaceutical Industry Co., Ltd., Nagoya, Japan
Takata	Takata Pharmaceutical Co., Ltd., Tokyo, Japan
Takeda	Takeda Chem. Ind. Ltd., Osaka, Japan
Tanabe Seiyaku	Tanabe Seiyaku Co., Ltd., Osaka, Japan
TAP	TAP Pharmaceuticals Inc. (subsidiary of Takeda Chem. Ind. Ltd.), Deerfield, Illinois
Taro	Taro Pharm USA, Hawthorne, New York
Tatsumi	Tatsumi Kagaku Co., Ltd., Kanazawa, Japan
Teikoku Kagaku	Teikoku Chemical Ind. Co., Ltd., Osaka, Japan
Teikoku Zoki	Teikoku Hormone Mfg. Co., Ltd., Osaka, Japan
Teisan	Teisan Seiyaku K.K., Tokyo, Japan
Temmler	Temmler Pharma GmbH & Co. KG, Marburg/Lahn, Germany
Tenneco	*see* Solvay
Teofarma	Teofarma srl, Pavia, Italy
Teva	Teva Pharmaceutical Industries Ltd., Petach Tikva, Israel
Theranol	Theranol Deglaude, Rungis, France
Théraplix	Théraplix SA (subsidiary of Sanofi-Aventis), Paris, France
Thiemann	Thiemann Arzneimittel GmbH, Waltrop, Germany
Thomae	*see* Boehringer, Ing.
Tillotts	Tillotts Labs., Henlow, Bedfordshire, UK
Toa Eiyo	Toa Eiyo Ltd., Tokyo, Japan
Tobishi	Tobishi Pharmaceutical Co., Ltd., Tokyo, Japan
Tokyo Tanabe	Tokyo Tanabe Seiyaku Co., Ltd., Tokyo, Japan
Torii	Torii & Co., Ltd., Tokyo, Japan
Tosi	Tosi Farmaceutici sas di Silvana Tosi & Co., Novara, Italy
Towa Yakuhin	Towa Yakuhin Co., Ltd., Kadoma, Japan
Toyama	Toyama Chemical Co., Ltd., Tokyo, Japan
Toyo Jozo	Toyo Jozo Co., Ltd., Tokyo, Japan
Travenol	*see* Baxter
Trommsdorff	H. Trommsdorff GmbH & Co. KG Arzneimittel, Alsdorf, Germany
Troponwerke	Tropenwerke GmbH & Co. KG, Koln, Germany
Tsuruhara	Tsuruhara Pharmaceutical Co., Ltd., Ikeda, Japan
Tubi Lux	Tubilux Pharma SpA, Rome, Italy
UCB	UCB, SA (formerly Union Chimique Belge), Brussels, Belgium
Ulmer	The Ulmer Pharmacal Co., Plymouth, Minnesota
Unimed	Unimed Pharmaceutical, Inc., Buffalo Grove, Illinois
Union Carbide	Union Carbide Corp. (subsidiary of The Dow Chemical Co.), Danbury, Connecticut
Uniroyal	Uniroyal Chemical Co., Inc., Middlebury, Connecticut
United Ther.	United Therapeutics Corp., Silver Springs, Maryland
UOP	UOP (formerly Universal Oil and Petroleum, Inc.) (unit of Union Carbide), Des Plaines, Illinois
Upjohn	*see* Pfizer
UPSA	UPSA, Agen, France
Upsher-Smith	Upsher-Smith Labs., Inc., Minneapolis, Minnesota
Uriach	Uriach Corp., Barcelona, Spain
Ursapharm	Ursapharm Arzneimittel GmbH & Co. KG, Saarbrücken, Germany
Valeant	Valeant Pharmaceuticals International, Costa Mesa, California
Valeas	Valeas SpA, Milan, Italy
Valent	Valent USA Corp. (subsidiary of Sumitomo Chemical Co., Ltd.), Walnut Creek, California

TABLE-27

Vanderbilt	R. T. Vanderbilt Co., Inc., Norwalk, Connecticut
Van Dyk	Van Dyk & Company, Inc., Belleville, New Jersey
Velsicol	Velsicol Chemical Co., Basingstoke, Hants., UK
Verla	Verla-Pharm. Arzneimittelfabrik, Tutzing, Germany
Veterinaria	Veterinaria AG, Zurich, Switzerland
Veyron-Froment	Lab. Veyron et Froment, Marseille, France
Viatris	Viatris GmbH & Co. KG, Frankfurt, Germany
Vifor	Vifor (International) AG, St. Gallen, Switzerland
Vineland	Vineland Labs. Inc. (division of IGI, Inc.), Vineland, New Jersey
Vita	Laboratorio Farmaceutici Vita srl, Milan, Italy
Viti	Marco Viti Farmaceutici SpA, Mozzate (CO), Italy
Wakamoto	Wakamoto Pharmaceutical Co., Ltd., Tokyo, Japan
Walker	Walker Corp. & Co., Inc., Syracuse, New York
Wallace	Wallace Pharmaceuticals (division of MedPointe Healthcare, Inc.) Somerset, New Jersey
Wander	Wander Healthcare AG (subsidiary of Novartis AG), Bern, Switzerland
Warner-Chilcott	Warner-Chilcott Inc., Rockaway, New Jersey
Warner-Lambert	Warner-Lambert Co., LLC (subsidiary of Pfizer, Inc.) Morris Plains, New Jersey
Watson	Watson Pharmaceuticals, Inc., Corona, California
Welcker-Lyster	Welcker-Lyster Ltd., Montreal, Canada
Wernigerode	Pharma Wernigerode GmbH, Wernigerode, Hartz, Germany
Westwood-Squibb	Westwood-Squibb Pharmaceuticals, Inc. (subsidiary of Bristol-Myers Squibb Co.), Buffalo, New York
Whitby	*see* UCB
Will-Pharma	Will-Pharma SA, Brussels, Belgium
Winthrop	*see* Sanofi-Aventis
Winzer	Dr. Winzer Pharma GmbH, Olching, Germany
WPC	WPC Brands (formerly Wisconsin Pharmacal), Jackson, Wisconsin
Woelm	Woelm Pharma GmbH & Co., Bad Honnef, Germany
Wolff	Dr. August Wolff GmbH & Co. Arzneimittel, Bielefeld, Germany
Wyeth	Wyeth, Madison, New Jersey
Wyeth-Ayerst	*see* Wyeth
Xttrium	Xttrium Labs., Inc., Chicago, Illinois
Yamanouchi	*see* Astellas
Yoshitomi	Yoshitomi Pharmaceutical Ind. Ltd., Osaka, Japan
Zambeletti	Dr. L. Zambeletti SpA (subsidiary of GlaxoSmithKline plc), Milan, Italy
Zambon	Zambon Group SpA, Milan, Italy
Zeneca	*see* AstraZeneca
Zeneca Ag Prod	*see* Syngenta
Zeria	Zeria Pharmaceutical Co., Ltd., Tokyo, Japan
ZLB Behring	ZLB Behring LLC, King of Prussia, Pennsylvania
Zyma	Zyma SA (subsidiary of Novartis AG), Nyon, Switzerland

TABLE-28

Code Letters Used by Companies for Experimental Substances

A	Abbott Laboratories, USA		CGA	Novartis AG, Switzerland
	AstraZeneca plc, UK		CGP	Novartis AG, Switzerland
	Eli Lilly & Co., USA		CGS	Novartis AG, Switzerland
	Ohmeda Pharm. Prods. Div., Inc., USA		CH	Chinoin Pharm. Chem. Works Co. Ltd., Hungary
	Sanofi-Aventis Group, France		CHX	Chemex Pharmaceuticals Inc., USA
AA	Takeda Chemical Ind. Ltd., Japan		CI	Pfizer Inc., USA
AB	Dainippon Pharmaceutical Co. Ltd., Japan		CK	Schering AG, Germany
ABT	Abbott Laboratories, USA		CL	Wyeth, USA
AC	Amylin Pharmaceuticals Inc., USA		CM	Sanofi-Aventis Group, France
	Ajinomoto Co. Ltd., Japan		CP	Cortech Inc., USA
	BASF AG, Germany			Pfizer Inc., USA
	Hercules Inc., USA		CR	Rotta Farmaceutici SpA, Italy
AD	Dainippon Pharmaceutical Co. Ltd., Japan		CRL	Labs. Lafon, France
ADL	Adolor Corp., USA		CS	Sankyo Co. Ltd., Japan
ADR	Pfizer Inc., USA		CT	Cell Therapeutics Inc., USA
AE	Bayer CropScience, USA		CV	Takeda Chemical Ind. Ltd., Japan
AF	Angelini Group, Italy		CVT	CV Therapeutics, USA
AG	Agouron Pharmaceuticals, USA		CX	Cortex Pharmaceuticals Inc., USA
AGN	Allergan, Inc., USA		CY	Epimmune Inc., USA
AH	GlaxoSmithKline plc, UK			Sanofi-Aventis Group, France
AHR	Wyeth, USA		CYC	Cyclacel Ltd., UK
AL	Alcon Labs., Inc., USA			
ALS	Advanced Life Sciences, USA		D	Asta Medica AG, Germany
ALT	Alteon Inc., USA			Daiichi Pharmaceutical Co. Ltd., Japan
AM	AMRAD Corp., Australia		DA	Dong A Pharmaceutical Co. Ltd., Korea
	Kyorin Pharmaceutical Co. Ltd., Japan		DC	Kyowa Hakko Kogyo Co. Ltd., Japan
AMA	Takeda Chemical Ind. Ltd., Japan		DE	Dow AgroSciences LLC, USA
AMD	AnorMED, Canada			Santen Pharmaceutical Co. Ltd., Japan
AMG	Amgen Inc., USA		DH	Sanofi-Aventis Group, France
AMI	Advanced Magnetics, Inc., USA		DJ	Daiichi Seiyaku Co. Ltd., Japan
AN	Elan Corp. plc, Ireland		DL	Sanofi-Aventis Group, France
ATL	Alizyme plc, UK		DPX	DuPont Crop Protection, USA
AW	Novartis AG, Switzerland		DS	Daiichi Seiyaku Co. Ltd., Japan
AY	Wyeth, USA		DU	Solvay SA, Belgium
AZ	AstraZeneca plc, UK		DUP	Bristol-Myers Squibb Co., USA
AZD	AstraZeneca plc, UK			DuPont Crop Protection, USA
			DX	Daiichi Sankyo Co. Ltd., Japan
B	Altana AG, Germany			
	Bayer CropScience, USA		E	Eisai Co. Ltd., Japan
	Bracco SpA, Italy			Laboratorios Dr. Esteve SA, Spain
Ba	Novartis AG, Switzerland		EB	Leo Pharma AS, Denmark
BAJ	Bayer AG, Germany		EF	Efamol Ltd., UK
BAS	BASF AG, Germany		EGIS	EGIS Pharmaceutical Works, Hungary
BAX	Baxter Healthcare Corp., USA		EGYT	EGIS Pharmaceutical Works, Hungary
BAY, Bay	Bayer AG, Germany		EI	Kyowa Hakko Kogyo Co. Ltd., Japan
BB	Bristol-Myers Squibb Co., USA		EL	Dow AgroSciences LLC, USA
	British Biotech plc, UK			Elan Corp. plc, Ireland
BC	Novartis AG, Switzerland		EMD	Merck KGaA, Germany
BCH	Shire BioChem Pharma Inc., Canada		EN	Essential Nutrition Ltd., UK
BDF	Eli Lilly & Co., USA		ENT	BASF AG, Germany
BG	Biogen Idec Inc., USA			Bayer CropScience, USA
BI	Boehringer Ingelheim GmbH, Germany			Dow AgroSciences LLC, USA
BIM	Beaufour-Ipsen International, France		ER	Eisai Co. Ltd., Japan
BL	Bioglan Labs Ltd., UK			Ergo Science Corp., USA
	Bristol-Myers Squibb Co., USA		ES	Sankyo Co. Ltd., Japan
BM	BioMarin Pharmaceuticals, USA		EU	The Procter & Gamble Co., USA
	F. Hoffmann-LaRoche Ltd., Switzerland			
BMS	Bristol-Myers Squibb Co., USA		F	FAES, Spain
BMY	Bristol-Myers Squibb Co., USA			Ferring AB, Sweden
BN	Beaufour-Ipsen International, France			Fujirebio, Inc., Japan
BP	Bioprojet Pharma, France			Pierre Fabre SA, France
BRL	GlaxoSmithKline plc, UK			Sankyo Co. Ltd., Japan
BTS	Abbott Laboratories, USA		FB	The Procter & Gamble Co., USA
BU	Bristol-Myers Squibb Co., USA		FBA	Bayer AG, Germany
BW	GlaxoSmithKline plc, UK		FC	Orion Corp., Finland
BX	Biorex Laboratories, UK		FCE	Pfizer Inc., USA
	Boehringer Ingelheim GmbH, Germany		FG	AB Ferrosan, Sweden
				FGene SA, France
C	Novartis AG, Switzerland		FI	Ferrer Internacional SA, Spain
	Sanofi-Aventis Group, France		FK	Astellas Pharma Inc., Japan
CC	Celgene Corp., USA		FL	Chinoin Pharm. Chem. Works Co. Ltd., Hungary
CDP	Celltech Group, UK		FLC	Labs. Delagrange, France
CDRI	Central Drug Research Inst., India		FMC	FMC Corp., USA
CERM	NV Organon, The Netherlands		FR	Astellas Pharma Inc., Japan
CG	Chemie Grunenthal GmbH, Germany		FUT	Torii & Co. Ltd., Japan
	GlaxoSmithKline plc, UK		FW	Rohm & Haas Co., USA
	Novartis AG, Switzerland			

TABLE-29

G	Genentech Inc., USA
	Genta Inc., USA
	Novartis AG, Switzerland
	Wyeth, USA
GEA	GEA A/S, Denmark
GI	GlaxoSmithKline plc, UK
Gö, Goe	Gödecke AG, Germany
GP	Novartis AG, Switzerland
GR	GlaxoSmithKline plc, UK
GS	Gilead Sciences, USA
	Novartis AG, Switzerland
GSK	GlaxoSmithKline plc, UK
GT	Gliatech Inc., USA
GW	GlaxoSmithKline plc, UK
H	AstraZeneca plc, UK
HC	Novartis AG, Switzerland
HE	Hollis-Eden Pharmaceuticals, USA
HGP	H. G. Pars Labs., USA
HMR	Sanofi-Aventis Group, France
HN	Nycomed Pharma, Norway
HOE	Bayer CropScience, USA
	Sanofi-Aventis Group, France
HP	Sanofi-Aventis Group, France
HR	Sanofi-Aventis Group, France
HSR	Hokuriku Seiyaku Co. Ltd., Japan
I	Ohmeda Pharm. Prods. Div., Inc., USA
IC	ICOS Corp., USA
ICI	AstraZeneca plc, UK
ICN	Valeant Pharmaceuticals Intl., USA
IKF	Ishikara Sangyo Kaisha Ltd., Japan
IMC	ImClone Systems Inc., USA
IMI	Pfizer Inc., USA
IMMU	Immunomedics Inc., USA
INS	Inspire Pharmaceuticals Inc., USA
ISIS	ISIS Pharmaceuticals Inc., USA
ISF	ISF SpA, Italy
ITF	Italfarmaco SpA, Italy
J	Jenapharm (Schering AG), Germany
JAU	Bayer CropScience, USA
JM	Johnson Matthey, Inc., USA
JO	Jouveinal Labs., France
K	Klinge Pharma GmbH, Germany
	Kowa Company Ltd., Japan
	Pfizer Inc., USA
KB	Kanebo Pharmaceuticals Ltd., Japan
	NV Organon, The Netherlands
KC	Chugai Pharmaceutical Co., Ltd., Japan
	Solvay SA, Belgium
KD	Kyowa Hakko Kogyo Co. Ltd., Japan
KF	Kyowa Hakko Kogyo Co. Ltd., Japan
KMD	Kissei Pharmaceutical Co. Ltd., Japan
KO	Boehringer Ingelheim GmbH, Germany
KP	Kaken Pharmaceutical Co. Ltd., Japan
KRN	Kirin Brewery Co. Ltd., Japan
KRX	Keryx Biopharmaceutical Inc., USA
KT	Kyowa Hakko Kogyo Co. Ltd., Japan
KU	Kyorin Pharmaceutical Co. Ltd., Japan
KW	Kyowa Hakko Kogyo Co. Ltd., Japan
KWD	AstraZeneca plc, UK
L	Alfa Wassermann SpA, Italy
	Sanofi-Aventis Group, France
	Wyeth, USA
LA	Lacer SA, Spain
LAS	Almirall Prodesfarma SA, Spain
LCB	Merck KGaA, Germany
LF	Groupe Fournier, France
LG	Fresenius AG, Germany
	Lab. Guidotti SpA, Italy
	Ligand Pharmaceuticals, Inc., USA
LGD	Ligand Pharmaceuticals, Inc., USA
LJC	Wyeth, USA
LJP	La Jolla Pharmaceutical Co., USA

LL	Wyeth, USA
LM	LiphaTech Inc., USA
	Menarini Ind. Farma. Riunite Srl, Italy
	Merck KGaA, Germany
	Pfizer Inc., USA
LS	Bayer CropScience, USA
	Leo Pharma AS, Denmark
	Merck KGaA, Germany
	Sanofi-Aventis Group, USA
LU	Abbott Laboratories, USA
	H. Lundbeck A/S, Denmark
LY	Eli Lilly & Co., USA
M	AstraZeneca plc, UK
	Mochida Pharm. Co. Ltd., Japan
	Reckitt & Colman Ltd., UK
M & B	Sanofi-Aventis Group, France
MBR	3M Pharmaceuticals, USA
MCI	Mitsubishi Kasei Corp., Japan
McN	Johnson & Johnson, USA
MCW	Makteshim-Agan Ind. Ltd., Israel
MD	Sanofi-Aventis Group, France
MDL	Pfizer Inc., USA
	Sanofi-Aventis Group, France
ME	Meiji Seika Kaisha Ltd., Japan
MEDI	MedImmune, Inc., USA
MF	Mediolanum Farmaceutici SpA, Italy
MG	Millennium Pfharmaceuticals Inc., USA
	Sanofi-Aventis Group, France
MGI	MGI Pharma, Inc., USA
MEN	Menarini Ind. Farma. Riunite Srl, Italy
MJ	Bristol-Myers Squibb Co., USA
MK	Merck & Co., Inc., USA
ML	Merckle GmbH, Germany
MON	Monsanto Co., USA
MP	Mallinckrodt Inc., USA
MPV	Orion Corp., Finland
MS	Mitsui Pharm., Inc., Japan
MSI	Magainin Pharmaceuticals, Inc., USA
MT	Ishihara Sangyo KK, Japan
MTI	Mitsui Chemicals Inc., Japan
MY	Mitsubishi Kasei Corp., Japan
N	Nelson Res. & Dev., USA
	Nisshin Flour Milling Co. Ltd., Japan
	UCB SA, Belgium
NA	Nippon Kayaku Co. Ltd., Japan
NBI	Neurocrine Biosciences, USA
NC	Neurochem Inc., Canada
	Nippon Chemiphar Co. Ltd., Japan
	Nycomed Amersham, plc, UK
NE	Neose Technologies Inc., USA
	The Procter & Gamble Co., USA
NF	Nippon Soda Co. Ltd., Japan
NIH	National Institutes of Health, USA
NIK	Nikken Chemical Co. Ltd., Japan
NK	Nippon Kayaku Co. Ltd., Japan
NN	Novo-Nordisk A/S, Denmark
NNC	Novo-Nordisk A/S, Denmark
NNF	BASF AG, Germany
NO	Novo-Nordisk A/S, Denmark
NP	Nippon Soda Co. Ltd., Japan
NSC	Genta Inc., USA
	National Cancer Institute, USA
NVP	Novartis AG, Switzerland
NX	NeoRX Corp., USA
	Nymox Pharmaceutical Corp., Canada
NY	Nycomed Pharma, Norway
NZ	Nippon Zoki Pharmaceutical Co. Ltd., Japan
OGT	Oxford GlycoSciences plc, UK
OM	OM Pharma, Switzerland
ONO	Ono Pharmaceutical Co. Ltd., Japan
OPC	Otsuka Pharmaceutical Co. Ltd., Japan
OR	Orion Pharma, Finland
ORF	Johnson & Johnson, USA

TABLE-30

Code Letters Used by Companies for Experimental Substances (Continued)

Org	NV Organon, The Netherlands		SPA	Societa Prodotti Antibiotici SpA, Italy
P	Leo Pharma AS, Denmark		SPC	Sphinx Pharmaceutical Corp., USA
	PhotoCure ASA, Norway		SPM	Schwarz Pharma AG, Germany
	Poli Group, Italy		SQ	Bristol-Myers Squibb Co., USA
	Sanofi-Aventis Group, France		SR	Sanofi-Aventis Group, France
	UCB SA, Belgium		SRA	Bayer CropScience, USA
PA	Pfizer Inc., USA		ST	Boehringer Ingelheim GmbH, Germany
PC	ProCyte Corporation, USA			Pierre Fabre Medicament, France
PCI	Pharmacyclics Inc., USA			Sigma Tau Ind. Farma. Riunite SpA, Italy
PD	Pfizer Inc., USA		SU	SUGEN Inc., USA
PF	Almirall Prodesfarma SA, Spain		SUN	Suntory Ltd., Japan
	Pharmos Corporation, USA		SZX	Bayer CropScience, USA
PKC	Novartis AG, Switzerland		T	Takeda Chemical Ind. Ltd., Japan
PN	Novartis AG, Switzerland			Tanabe Seiyaku Co. Ltd., Japan
PNU	Pfizer Inc., USA			Toyama Chemical Co. Ltd., Japan
PP	Syngenta AG, Switzerland		TA	Tanabe Seiyaku Co. Ltd., Japan
PPI	Praecis Pharmaceuticals Inc., USA		TAK	Takeda Pharmaceutical Co. Ltd., Japan
PT	Palatin Tehnologies Inc., USA		TAP	TAP Pharmaceuticals Inc., USA
			TBC	Encysive Pharmaceuticals, USA
R	3M Pharmaceuticals, USA		TC	Targacept Inc., USA
	F. Hoffmann-LaRoche Ltd., Switzerland		TCV	Takeda Chemical Ind. Ltd., Japan
	Johnson & Johnson, USA		TEI	Teijin Ltd., Japan
	Sankyo Co. Ltd., Japan		TER	Telik Inc., USA
Rec	Recordati Ind. Chim. Farm. SpA, Italy		TH	Boehringer Ingelheim GmbH, Germany
RG	Sanofi-Aventis Group, France		TI	Teijin Ltd., Japan
RGH	Gedeon Richter, Ltd., Hungary		TLK	Telik Inc., USA
RH	Dow AgroSciences LLC, USA		TMX	Teijin Ltd., Japan
	Rohm & Haas Co., USA		TO	Japan Tobacco Ind. Corp., Japan
RMI	Sanofi-Aventis Group, France		TR	Bayer AG, Germany
Ro	F. Hoffmann-La Roche Ltd., Switzerland		TRK	Toray Industries Inc., Japan
RP	Sanofi-Aventis Group, France		TS	Taisho Seiyaku KK, Japan
RPA	Bayer CropScience, USA		TV	Teva Pharm. Ind. Ltd., Isreal
RS	F. Hoffmann-La Roche Ltd., Switzerland		TVX	Bayer AG, Germany
	Sankyo Co. Ltd., Japan			
RU	Sanofi-Aventis Group, France		U	Pfizer Inc., USA
RWJ	Johnson & Johnson, USA		UC	Kyowa Hakko Kogyo Co. Ltd., Japan
RX	Reckitt & Colman Ltd., UK			Uniroyal Chemical Co. Inc., USA
			UCB	UCB SA, Belgium
S	Kaken Pharmaceutical Co. Ltd., Japan		UK	Pfizer Inc., USA
	Lab. Servier, France		UR	Grupo Uriach, Spain
	3M Pharmaceuticals, USA		VC	Mobil Chemical Co., USA
	Sanofi-Aventis Group, France		VCS	Velsicol Chemical Corp., USA
	Shionogi & Co. Ltd., Japan		VX	Vertex Pharmaceuticals Inc., USA
	Sumitomo Pharmaceuticals Co. Ltd., Japan			
	Valeant Pharmacetuicals Intl., USA		W	Carter-Wallace, Inc., USA
SA	Santen Pharmaceutical Co. Ltd., Japan			Pfizer Inc., USA
SAN	Syngenta AG, Switzerland		WAY	Wyeth, USA
SB	GlaxoSmithKline plc, UK		WEB	Boehringer Ingelheim GmbH, Germany
SC	Pfizer Inc., USA		WF	Astellas Pharma Inc., Japan
	Scotia Pharmaceuticals, UK		WHR	Sanofi-Aventis Group, France
SCE	Takeda Chemical Ind. Ltd., Japan		Win	Sanofi-Aventis Group, France
Sch	Schering-Plough Corp., USA		WR	Walter Reed Army Institute of Research, USA
SD	Pfizer Inc., USA		WRC	Aderis Pharmaceuticals, USA
	Santen Pharmaceutical Co. Ltd., Japan		WY	Wyeth, USA
	Shell Oil Co., USA			
SDZ	Novartis AG, Switzerland		X	Dow AgroSciences LLC, USA
SE	Bristol-Myers Squibb Co., USA			F. Hoffmann-La Roche Ltd., Switzerland
	DuPont Crop Protection, USA		XDE	Dow AgroSciences LLC, USA
SF	Meiji Seika Kaisha Ltd., Japan		XK	Kyowa Hakko Kogyo Co. Ltd., Japan
SG	Chugai Pharmaceutical Co., Ltd., Japan		XR	Xenova Group plc, UK
SGD	Siegfried Pharma AG, Switzerland		Y	Astellas Pharma Inc., Japan
SH	Schering AG, Germany			Welfide Corp., Japan
SKF	GlaxoSmithKline plc, UK		YI	Yashima Chemical Ind. Co. Ltd., Japan
SL	Sanofi-Aventis Group, France		YM	Astellas Pharma Inc., Japan
SM	Greenwich Pharmaceuticals Inc., USA		YTR	Taiho Pharmaceutical Co. Ltd., Japan
	Sumitomo Pharmaceuticals Co. Ltd., Japan		Z	Zambon Group SpA, Italy
SMS	Novartis AG, Switzerland			Zeria Pharm. Co. Ltd., Japan
SN	GlaxoSmithKline plc, UK		ZA	Syngenta AG, Switzerland
	Novartis AG, Germany		ZD	AstraZeneca plc, UK
SNK	Sanwa Kagaku Kenkyusho Co. Ltd., Japan		ZK	Schering AG, Germany
SP	Menarini Ind. Farma. Riunite Srl, Italy		ZY	Novartis AG, Switzerland
	Signal Pharmaceuticals, USA			

TABLE-31

Terms for Radicals and Groups Used for Nonproprietary Names

Listed by the United States Adopted Names (USAN) Council and the
World Health Organization (WHO) International Nonproprietary Names (INN) Programme

USAN	WHO/INN	Chemical Name
acefurate	acefurate	acetate (ester), furan-2-carboxylate (ester)
	aceglumate	*rac*-hydrogen N-acetyl-glutamate
	aceponate	acetate (ester), propanoate (ester)
acetonide	acetonide	isopropylidenedioxy
aceturate	aceturate	N-acetylglycinate
	acibutate	acetate (ester), 2-methylpropanoate (ester)
acistrate	acistrate	acetate (ester), stearate (salt) or acetate (ester), octadecanoate (salt)
acoxil	acoxil	acetoxymethyl
	alfoscerate	(2R)-2,3-dihydroxypropyl hydrogen phosphate
	amsonate	2,2'-ethene-1,2-diylbis(5-aminobenzene-1-sulfonate)
anisatil	anisatil	4-methoxyphenacyl
arbamel	arbamel	ester with N,N-dimethylglycolamide
axetil	axetil	(RS)-1-acetoxyethyl
beloxil		benzyloxy
	benetonide	N-benzoyl-2-methyl-β-alanine (ester), acetonide
besylate	besilate	benzenesulfonate
betadex		β-cyclodextrin
	bezomil	(benzoyloxy)methyl
buciclate	buciclate	*trans*-4-butylcyclohexanecarboxylate
	bunapsilate	3,7-di-*tert*-butylnaphthalene-1,5-disulfonate
camsylate	camsilate	camphorsulfonate
caproate	caproate	hexanoate
	carbesilate	4-sulfobenzoate
cilexetil	cilexetil	(RS)-1-[[(cyclohexyloxy)carbonyl]oxy]ethyl
	cituxetan	N-[4-[(2RS)-2-[bis(carboxymethyl)amino)]-3-[[2-[bis(carboxymethyl)amino]ethyl](carboxymethyl)amino)propyl]phenyl]thiocarbamoyl
	clofibrol	2-(4-chlorophenoxy)-2-methylpropyl
closylate	closilate	4-chlorobenzenesulfonate
	crobefate	*rac*-3-[(3E)-4-methoxybenzylidene]-2-(4-methoxyphenyl)chroman-6-yl phosphate (2−)
	cromacate	2-[(6-hydroxy-4-methyl-2-oxo-2H-chromen-7-yl)oxy]-acetate

USAN	WHO/INN	Chemical Name
	cromesilate	6,7-dihydroxy-2-oxo-2H-chromen-4-yl)methanesulfonate
crosfumaril	crosfumaril	(2E)-but-2-enedioyl
	cyclamate	cyclohexylsulfamate
cyclotate	ciclotate	4-methylbicyclo[2.2.2]oct-2-ene-1-carboxylate
cypionate	cipionate	cyclopentanepropanoate
	daloxate	L-alaninate (ester), (5-methyl-2-oxo-1,3-dioxol-4-yl)methyl
daropate	daropate	N,N-dimethyl-β-alaninate
	deanil	2-(dimethylamino)ethyl
detemir	detemir	tetradecanoyl
	dibudinate	2,6-di-*tert*-butylnaphthalene-1,5-disulfonate
	dibunate	2,6-di-*tert*-butylnaphthalene-1-sulfonate
	dicibate	dicyclohexylmethyl carbonate
	digolil	2-(2-hydroxyethoxy)ethyl
diolamine	diolamine	diethanolamine or 2,2'-iminodiethanol
dofosfate	dofosfate	octadecyl hydrogen phosphate
	ecamate	N-ethylcarbamate
edamine	edamine	ethylenediamine
edetate		ethylenediaminetetraacetate
edisylate	edisilate	1,2-ethanedisulfonate
enanthate	enantate	heptanoate
	enbutate	acetate (ester), butanoate (ester)
epolamine	epolamine	1-pyrrolidineethanol
erbumine	erbumine	*tert*-butylamine
estolate	estolate	propionate (ester), dodecyl sulfate (salt)
esylate	esilate	ethanesulfonate
etabonate	etabonate	ethyl carbonate
	etexilate	O-n-hexylcarbamate, ethyl ester
	farnesil	(2E,6E)-3,7,11-trimethyldodeca-2,6,10-trien-1-yl
	fendizoate	2-(6-hydroxybiphenyl-3-carbonyl)benzoate
fostedate	fostedate	tetradecyl hydrogen phosphate
	furetonide	1-benzofurane-2-carboxylate (ester), propane-2,2-diylbis(oxy)
	gamolenate	(6Z,9Z,12Z)-octadeca-6,9,12-trienoate
gluceptate	gluceptate	D-*glycero*-D-*gulo*-heptanoate
	glutamer	glutaraldehyde polymer

TABLE-32

USAN	WHO/INN	Chemical Name
	guacil	2-methoxyphenyl
hexacetonide	hexacetonide	3,3-dimethylbutyrate (ester), acetonide
hybenzate	hibenzate	2-(4-hydroxybenzoyl)benzoate
hyclate	hyclate	monohydrochloride hemiethanolate hemihydrate
	hydroxynaphthtoate	3-hydroxynaphthalene-2-carboxylate
isethionate	isetionate	2-hydroxyethanesulfonate
	lauril	dodecyl
	lisetil	L-lysinate (ester), diethyl (ester)
	lisicol	[*N*-[(5*S*)-5-carboxy-5-(3α,-7α,12α-trihydroxy-5β-cholan-24-amido)pentyl]carbamothioyl]amino
medoxomil	medoxomil	(5-methyl-2-oxo-1,3-dioxol-4-yl)methyl
	megallate	3,4,5-trimethoxybenzoate
meglumine		*N*-methylglucamine
merpentan	merpentan	4,5-bis(2-mercaptoacetamido)valeric acid
mertansine	mertansine	*N*²′-deacetyl-*N*²′-(3-mercapto-1-oxopropyl)maytansine
mesylate	mesilate	methanesulfonate
	metembonate	4,4′-methylenebis(3-methoxynaphthalene-2-carboxylate)
mofetil	mofetil	2-morpholinoethyl
	napadisilate	naphthalene-1,5-disulfonate
napsylate	napsilate	2-naphthalenesulfonate
olamine	olamine	ethanolamine or 2-aminoethanol
	oxoglurate	hydrogen 2-oxopentanedioate
pamoate	embonate	4,4′-methylenebis[3-hydroxy-2-naphthoate]
pegol	pegol	α-(2-carboxyethyl)-ω-methoxypoly(oxyethane-1,2-diyl)
pendetide		*N*⁶-[*N*-[2-[[2-[bis(carboxymethyl)amino]ethyl](carboxymethyl)amino]ethyl]-*N*-(carboxymethyl)glycyl]-*N*²-(*N*-glycyl-L-tyrosyl)-L-lysine
	pentexil	(*RS*)-1-[(2,2-dimethylpropanoyl)oxy]ethyl
phenpropionate		3-phenylpropionate
pivalate	pivalate	trimethylacetate (ester)

USAN	WHO/INN	Chemical Name
pivoxetil	pivoxetil	1-[(2-methoxy-2-methyl-propionyl)oxy]ethyl
pivoxil	pivoxil	(pivaloyloxy)methyl
poliglumex	poliglumex	L-glutamic acid homopolymer
probutate	buteprate	propionate (ester), butyrate (ester)
proxetil	proxetil	1-[(isopropoxycarbonyl)oxy]-ethyl
	soproxil	[[(propan-2-yloxy)carbonyl]-oxy]methyl
	steaglate	2-(octadecanoyloxy)acetate (ester)
	stinoprate	*N*-acetylcysteinate (salt), propanoate (ester)
	succinil	3-carboxypropanoyl
suleptanate	suleptanate	8-[methyl(2-sulfoethyl)amino]-8-oxooctanoate (ester), monosodium salt
	sulfoxylate	sulfinomethyl, monosodium salt
tebutate	tebutate	*tert*-butylacetate or 3,3-dimethylbutanoate
	tenoate	thiophene-2-carboxylate
	teoclate	8-chloro-1,3-dimethyl-2,6-dioxo-3,6-dihydro-1*H*-purin-7-(2*H*)-ide
	teprosilate	3-(1,3-dimethyl-2,6-dioxo-1,2,3,6-tetrahydro-7*H*-purin-7-yl)propane-1-sulfonate
tetraxetan	tetraxetan	[4,7,10-tris(carboxymethyl)-1,4,7,10-tetraazacyclodec-1-yl]acetyl
	tidoxil	*rac*-2-(decyloxy)-3-(dodecyl-sulfanyl)propyl
tiuxetan	tiuxetan	*N*-[4-[(2*S*)-2-[bis(carboxymethyl)amino]-3-[(2*RS*)-[2-[bis(carboxymethyl)amino]-propyl](carboxymethyl)amino]propyl]phenyl]thiocarbamoyl
	tofesilate	3-(1,3-dimethyl-2,6-dioxo-1,2,3,6-tetrahydro-7*H*-purin-7-yl)ethane-1-sulfonate
tosylate	tosilate	4-toluenesulfonate
	triclofenate	2,4,5-trichlorophenolate
triflutate	triflutate	trifluoroacetate
trolamine	trolamine	triethanolamine or 2,2′,2″-nitrilotriethanol
	troxundate	[2-(2-ethoxyethoxy)ethoxy]-acetate
xinafoate	xinafoate	1-hydroxy-2-naphthoate

TABLE-33

Radioactive Isotopes Used in Medical Diagnosis and Therapy

Name and Symbol	Principal Nuclear Properties	Form	Use
Americium ^{241}Am	Half-life 432.7y α(5.49, 5.44) γ(0.060)	Encapsulated source	Diagnostic: External radiation source for bone mineral analyzer
			Therapeutic: Antineoplastic (intracavitary radiation source)
Calcium ^{47}Ca	Half-life 4.53d β^-(0.67, 1.98) γ(1.297)	Calcium chloride	Diagnostic: Calcium metabolism studies
Cesium ^{137}Cs	Half-life 30.0y β^-(1.176, 0.514)	Cesium chloride or cesium sulfate (encased in needles or applicator cells)	Therapeutic: Antineoplastic (teletherapy source, intracavitary or interstitial radiation source)
Daughter ^{137m}Ba	Half-life 2.552min γ(0.662)		
Californium ^{252}Cf	Half-life 2.645y α(6.217)	Sealed source	Therapeutic: Antineoplastic (intracavitary or interstitial radiation source)
Chromium ^{51}Cr	Half-life 27.704d K; γ(0.32)	Chromic chloride	Diagnostic: Determn of serum protein loss into the gastrointestinal tract
		Chromium disodium edetate	Diagnostic: Determn of glomerular filtration rate
		Labeled human serum albumin	Diagnostic: Placenta localization; gastrointestinal protein loss
		Sodium chromate labeled red blood cells	Diagnostic: Determn of red cell volume or mass; red cell survival time; evaluation of blood loss; spleen imaging; placenta localization
Cobalt ^{60}Co	Half-life 5.271y β^-(0.318, 1.48) γ(1.173, 1.332)	Metallic cobalt	Therapeutic: Antineoplastic (teletherapy source, intracavitary or interstitial radiation source)
		Radioactive vitamin B_{12}	Diagnostic: In Schilling test for absence of intrinsic factor (pernicious anemia) or other defects of intestinal vitamin B_{12} absorption
^{57}Co	Half-life 271.77d K; γ(0.122)	Radioactive vitamin B_{12}	Diagnostic: In Schilling test for absence of intrinsic factor (pernicious anemia) or other defects of intestinal vitamin B_{12} absorption
^{58}Co	Half-life 71.91d K; β^+(0.48) γ(0.811)	Radioactive vitamin B_{12}	Diagnostic: In Schilling test for absence of intrinsic factor (pernicious anemia) or other defects of intestinal vitamin B_{12} absorption
Copper ^{64}Cu	Half-life 12.701h β^-(0.571), β^+(0.657), γ(1.34)	Copper versenate	Diagnostic: Brain scan
		Copper acetate	Diagnostic: Study of Wilson's disease
Fluorine ^{18}F	Half-life 1.8295h β^+(0.635)	Fludeoxyglucose (FDG)	Diagnostic: Functional brain imaging
		Sodium fluoride (reactor produced)	Diagnostic: Bone scan
Gadolinium ^{153}Gd	Half-life 241.6d K; γ(0.70, 0.097, 0.103)	Sealed source	Diagnostic: External radiation source for bone mineral analyzer
Gallium ^{67}Ga	Half-life 3.261d K; γ(0.093, 0.184, 0.300, 0.393)	Gallium citrate	Diagnostic: Detection of neoplastic and inflammatory lesions; tumor seeking agent
Gold ^{198}Au	Half-life 2.6935d β^-(1.371, 0.962) γ(0.412)	Colloidal gold	Diagnostic: Liver imaging
		Colloidal gold or seeds	Therapeutic: Antineoplastic (radiation source) in treatment of widespread abdominal carcinomatosis with ascites; carcinomatosis of pleura with effusion; lymphomas; interstitially in metastatic tumors

TABLE-34

Name and Symbol	Principal Nuclear Properties	Form	Use
Indium ^{113m}In	Half-life 1.658h $\gamma(0.393)$	Indium colloid	Diagnostic: Liver and spleen imaging
		Indium Fe(OH)$_3$	Diagnostic: Pulmonary perfusion imaging; cardiac output
		Indium labeled red blood cells	Diagnostic: Determn of blood volume
		Indium pentetate (DTPA)	Diagnostic: Brain scan; renal function studies
		Indium transferrin	Diagnostic: Static cardiovascular blood pool imaging; hepatic and placenta blood pool imaging; placenta localization
^{111}In	Half-life 2.807d K; $\gamma(0.172, 0.247)$	Indium bleomycin	Diagnostic: Tumor detection
		Indium capromab pendetide	Diagnostic: Tumor detection for prostate cancer
		Indium chloride	Diagnostic: Hematopoietic bone marrow imaging; tumor detection
		Indium oxyquinoline (oxine) labeled leukocytes	Diagnostic: Detection of abscesses, infections and inflammation
		Indium oxyquinoline (oxine) labeled platelets	Diagnostic: Detection of deep vein thrombosis; cardiac thrombosis; renal transplant rejection
		Indium oxyquinoline (oxine) labeled red blood cells	Diagnostic: Detection of gastrointestinal bleeding
		Indium pentetate (DTPA)	Diagnostic: Gastric emptying studies; cardiac output; renal scintigraphy; cisternography
		Indium pentetreotide	Diagnostic: Neuroendocrine tumor detection
		Indium satumomab pendetide	Diagnostic: Tumor detection
Iodine ^{131}I	Half-life 8.040d $\beta^-(0.607, 0.81, 0.336)$ $\gamma(0.080, 0.284, 0.364, 0.637, 0.723)$	Diiodofluorescein	Diagnostic: Brain scan
		Iobenguane (MIBG)	Diagnostic: Adrenomedullary imaging and tumor detection
			Therapeutic: Antineoplastic (radiation source) in treatment of neuroendocrine tumors
		Iodinated fats and fatty acids, e.g. oleic acid, triolein	Diagnostic: Pancreatic function; intestinal fat absorption
		Iodinated fibrinogen	Diagnostic: In vitro determn of fibrinolytic enzymes
		Iodinated human serum albumin (IHSA)	Diagnostic: Plasma volume determn; peripheral vascular flow; cardiac output; circulation time; cerebral vascular flow. Brain scan; placenta localization. Cisternography
		Iodinated human serum albumin (macroaggregated)	Diagnostic: Pulmonary perfusion imaging
		Iodinated human serum albumin (microaggregated)	Diagnostic: Hepatic blood pool imaging
		Iodinated levothyroxine	Diagnostic: Metabolic study of endogenous thyroxine. In vitro determn of thyroid function
		Iodinated liothyronine	Diagnostic: In vitro determn of thyroid function
		Iodinated povidone	Diagnostic: Protein-loss enteropathy
		Iodinated rose bengal	Diagnostic: Liver function in hepatic excretion studies
		Iodinated tositumomab	Therapeutic: Antineoplastic (radiation source) in treatment of non-Hodgkin's lymphoma
		Iodohippurate sodium	Diagnostic: Determn of renal function, renal blood flow, urinary tract obstruction; renal imaging
		Sodium iodide	Diagnostic: Thyroid function studies; thyroid imaging
			Therapeutic: Hyperthyroidism; antineoplastic (radiation source) in treatment of thyroid cancer

TABLE-35

Name and Symbol	Principal Nuclear Properties	Form	Use
Iodine ^{125}I	Half-life 60.14d K; $\gamma(0.035)$	Iodinated fats and fatty acids	Diagnostic: Pancreatic function; intestinal fat absorption
		Iodinated fibrinogen	Diagnostic: Localization of deep vein thrombosis; study of fibrinogen metabolism. *In vitro* determn of fibrinolytic enzymes
		Iodinated human serum albumin (IHSA)	Diagnostic: Determn of blood or plasma volume; circulation time; cardiac output
		Iodinated levothyroxine	Diagnostic: Metabolic study of endogenous thyroxine. *In vitro* determn of thyroid function
		Iodinated liothyronine	Diagnostic: *In vitro* determn of thyroid function
		Iodinated povidone	Diagnostic: Protein-loss enteropathy
		Iodinated rose bengal	Diagnostic: Liver function in hepatic excretion studies
		Sealed source	Diagnostic: External radiation source for bone mineral analyzer
		Sodium iodide	Diagnostic: Thyroid function studies; thyroid imaging
^{123}I	Half-life 13.2h K; $\gamma(0.159)$	IACFT	Diagnostic: SPECT cerebral imaging
		Iobenguane (MIBG)	Diagnostic: Adrenomedullary imaging and tumor detection
			Therapeutic: Antineoplastic (radiation source) in treatment of neuroendocrine tumors
		Iodohippurate sodium	Diagnostic: Determn of renal function, renal blood flow, urinary obstruction; renal imaging
		Iofetamine hydrochloride (IMP)	Diagnostic: Cerebral imaging
		Ioflupane (I-FP-CIT)	Diagnostic: SPECT cerebral imaging
		Sodium iodide	Diagnostic: Thyroid function studies; thyroid imaging
Iridium ^{192}Ir	Half-life 73.831d $\beta^-(0.67)$ $\gamma(0.296, 0.308, 0.317, 0.468, 0.589, 0.604, 0.612)$	Seed encased in nylon ribbon	Therapeutic: Antineoplastic (interstitial radiation source)
Iron ^{59}Fe	Half-life 44.496d $\beta^-(0.273, 0.475)$ $\gamma(1.095, 1.292)$	Ferric chloride Ferrous citrate Ferrous sulfate	Diagnostic: Ferrokinetics
		Labeled red blood cells	Diagnostic: Red cell maturation studies
^{55}Fe	Half-life 2.73y K	Labeled red blood cells	Diagnostic: Red cell maturation studies
Krypton ^{85}Kr	Half-life 10.72y $\beta^-(0.67)$ $\gamma(0.517)$	Gas	Diagnostic: Cardiac abnormalities; skeletal muscle, coronary or cerebral blood flow
^{81m}Kr	Half-life 13s $\gamma(0.19)$	Gas	Diagnostic: Lung ventilation studies
Lead RaD(^{210}Pb)	Half-life 22.3y $\beta^-(0.017)$ $\gamma(0.047)$	Beta ray applicator	Therapeutic: See Strontium (^{90}Sr)
Daughter RaE(^{210}Bi)	Half-life 5.013d $\beta^-(1.16)$		
Mercury ^{197}Hg	Half-life 2.6725d K; $\gamma(0.077)$	Chlormerodrin	Diagnostic: Brain scan; renal imaging
		Merisoprol	Diagnostic: Determn of renal function

TABLE-36

Name and Symbol	Principal Nuclear Properties	Form	Use
Mercury ^{203}Hg	Half-life 46.60d β^-(0.214) γ(0.279)	Chlormerodrin	Diagnostic: Brain scan; renal imaging
Phosphorous ^{32}P	Half-life 14.282d β^-(1.71)	Chromic phosphate	Therapeutic: Antineoplastic (radiation source) in treatment of peritoneal or pleural effusions caused by metastatic disease
		Labeled red blood cells	Diagnostic: Blood volume determn
		Sodium phosphate	Diagnostic: Study of peripheral vascular disease; localization of ocular, brain and skin tumors; study of breast carcinomas
			Therapeutic: Polycythemia vera; chronic myelocytic leukemia; chronic lymphocytic leukemia; skeletal metastases; antineoplastic (radiation source)
Potassium ^{43}K	Half-life 22.3h β^-(0.83, 0.46, 1.22, 1.82) γ(0.618, 0.373, 0.39, 0.59, 0.22)	Potassium chloride	Diagnostic: Myocardial scan; determn of total exchangeable potassium
^{42}K	Half-life 12.360h β^-(3.52) γ(1.524)	Potassium carbonate	Diagnostic: Localization of brain tumors; determn of intracellular fluid space
		Potassium chloride	Diagnostic: Tumor detection; renal blood flow; determn of total exchangeable potassium
Radium ^{226}Ra	Half-life 1600y α(4.78, 4.60) γ(0.187)	Radium bromide; α and β particles filtered by platinum	Therapeutic: Antineoplastic (radiation source) in interstitial treatment of malignancies such as cancer of uterine cervix and fundus, oral pharynx, urinary bladder, skin and metastatic cancer of lymph nodes
Radon (Radium Emanation) ^{222}Rn (Daughter of ^{226}Ra)	Half-life 3.825d α(5.49) γ(0.510)	Gaseous radon; α and β particles filtered by 0.3 mm of gold	Therapeutic: See Radium (^{226}Ra)
Ruthenium ^{106}Ru	Half-life 1.020y β^-(0.039)	Beta ray applicator	Therapeutic: See Strontium (^{90}Sr)
Daughter (^{106}Rh)	Half-life 29.80s β^-(3.53, 3.1, 2.4) γ(0.512, 0.622, 1.128)		
Samarium ^{153}Sm	Half life 1.946d β^-(0.81, 0.71, 0.64) γ(0.103, 0.070)	Sm-lexidronam (EDTMP)	Therapeutic: Antineoplastic (radiation source) in treatment of bone cancer
Selenium ^{75}Se	Half-life 119.77d K; γ(0.265, 0.136, 0.121, 0.280, 0.401)	Selenomethionine	Diagnostic: Imaging of pancreas and parathyroid glands
Sodium ^{24}Na	Half-life 14.659h β^-(1.389, 4.17) γ(1.369, 2.754)	Sodium chloride	Diagnostic: Determn of circulation times, sodium space, total exchangeable sodium
^{22}Na	Half-life 2.602y β^+(0.545, 1.83) K; γ(1.275)	Sodium chloride	Diagnostic: Determn of sodium space and total exchangeable sodium
Strontium ^{85}Sr	Half-life 64.84d K; γ(0.514)	Strontium chloride Strontium nitrate	Diagnostic: Bone imaging
^{87m}Sr	Half-life 2.795h γ(0.388)		

TABLE-37

Radioactive Isotopes Used in Medical Diagnosis and Therapy (Continued)

Name and Symbol	Principal Nuclear Properties	Form	Use
Strontium ^{90}Sr Daughter ^{90}Y	Half-life 28.5y β^-(0.546) Half-life 2.671d β^-(2.288) γ(2.186)	Beta ray applicator	Therapeutic: External irradiation for treatment of benign conditions of eye such as pterygia, traumatic corneal ulceration, corneal scars, vernal conjunctivitis, hemangioma of eyelid, vascularization of cornea and in preparation for a corneal transplant
Sulfur ^{35}S	Half-life 87.51d β^-(0.167)	Sodium sulfate	Diagnostic: Determn of extracellular fluid volume
Technetium ^{99m}Tc	Half-life 6.006h IT; γ(0.141)	Sodium pertechnetate	Diagnostic: Brain imaging. Cerebral angiography; thyroid imaging; salivary gland imaging; placenta localization; blood pool imaging; gastric mucosa imaging; cardiac function studies; renal blood flow studies. Urinary bladder imaging. Nasolacrimal drainage system imaging
		Sodium pertechnetate labeled red blood cells	Diagnostic: Determn of red blood cell volume, short-term survival studies. *In vitro* compatibility studies
		Tc-albumin	Diagnostic: Blood pool imaging; cardiovascular studies; placenta localization; determn of blood or plasma volumes
		Tc-albumin (aggregated)	Diagnostic: Pulmonary perfusion imaging
		Tc-albumin (microaggregated)	Diagnostic: Liver imaging
		Tc-apcitide	Diagnostic: Acute venous thrombosis imaging
		Tc-arcitumomab	Diagnostic: Tumor detection for colorectal cancer
		Tc-bicisate	Diagnostic: Brain imaging
		Tc-butedronate (DPD)	Diagnostic: Brain imaging
		Tc-depreotide	Diagnostic: Tumor detection for lung cancer
		Tc-disofenin (DISIDA)	Diagnostic: Hepatobiliary imaging
		Tc-etidronate (EHDP)	Diagnostic: Bone imaging
		Tc-exametazine (HM-PAO)	Diagnostic: Cerebral perfusion imaging
		Tc-fanolesomab	Diagnostic: Imaging and diagnosis of infections
		Tc-gluceptate	Diagnostic: Brain imaging; renal imaging; assess renal and brain perfusion
		Tc-labeled red blood cells	Diagnostic: Determn of red cell volume; short-term red cell survival studies
		Tc-lidofenin (HIDA)	Diagnostic: Hepatobiliary imaging
		Tc-mebrofenin	Diagnostic: Hepatobiliary imaging
		Tc-medronate (MDP)	Diagnostic: Bone imaging
		Tc-mertiatide (MAG3)	Diagnostic: Renal imaging
		Tc-oxidronate (HDP)	Diagnostic: Bone imaging
		Tc-pentetate (DTPA)	Diagnostic: Brain imaging; renal imaging; assess renal and brain perfusion; estimate glomerular filtration rate. Lung ventilation studies
		Tc-polyphosphates	Diagnostic: Bone imaging; myocardial imaging; blood pool imaging; detection of gastrointestinal bleeding
		Tc-pyrophosphate	Diagnostic: Bone imaging; cardiac imaging; blood pool imaging; detection of gastrointestinal bleeding
		Tc-sestamibi (HEXAMIBI)	Diagnostic: Myocardial perfusion imaging
		Tc-succimer	Diagnostic: Renal imaging
		Tc-sulesomab	Diagnostic: Detection of infections and inflammation

TABLE-38

Name and Symbol	Principal Nuclear Properties	Form	Use
Technetium ^{99m}Tc (Cont'd)		Tc-sulfur colloid	Diagnostic: Liver, spleen and bone marrow imaging. Esophageal transit studies; gastro-esophageal reflux scintigraphy; determn of pulmonary aspiration of gastric contents; detection of intrapulmonary and lower gastrointestinal bleeding. Lung ventilation imaging
		Tc-teboroxime	Diagnostic: Myocardial perfusion imaging
		Tc-tetrofosmin	Diagnostic: Myocardial perfusion imaging
Thallium ^{201}Tl	Half-life 3.046d K; γ(0.135, 0.167)	Thallous chloride	Diagnostic: Myocardial perfusion imaging; localization of sites of parathyroid hyperactivity
Xenon ^{133}Xe	Half-life 5.245d β^-(0.346) γ(0.081)	Gas	Diagnostic: Pulmonary perfusion imaging; cerebral blood flow; lung ventilation studies
		Gas in saline solution	Diagnostic: Pulmonary perfusion imaging; regional blood flow; lung ventilation studies
^{127}Xe	Half-life 36.41d K; γ(0.172, 0.203)	Gas	Diagnostic: Pulmonary perfusion imaging; lung ventilation studies
Ytterbium ^{169}Yb	Half-life 32.022d K; γ(0.063, 0.100, 0.313, 0.177, 0.198, 0.308)	Yb-pentetate (DTPA)	Diagnostic: Cisternography; brain scan
Yttrium ^{90}Y	Half life 2.671d β^-(2.288) γ(2.186)	Y-edotreotide	Therapeutic: Antineoplastic (radiation source) in treatment of neuroendocrine tumors
		Y-epratuzumab	Therapeutic: Antineoplastic (radiation source) in treatment of non-Hodgkin's lymphoma
		Y-ibritumomab tiuxetan	Therapeutic: Antineoplastic (radiation source) in treatment of non-Hodgkin's lymphoma

References
1. S. Baum, R. Bramlet, *Basic Nuclear Medicine* (Appleton-Century-Crofts, New York, 1975).
2. C. Behrns *et al., Atomic Medicine* (Williams & Wilkins Co., Baltimore, 5th ed., 1969).
3. H.M. Chilton, R. L. Witcofski, *Nuclear Pharmacy* (Lea & Febiger, Philadelphia, 1986).
4. *CRC Handbook of Radioactive Nuclides,* Y. Wang, Ed. (Chemical Rubber Co., Cleveland, Ohio, 1969).
5. *Diagnostic and Investigational Uses of Radiolabeled Blood Elements,* R. J. Davey, M. E. Wallace, Eds. (Am. Assoc. of Blood Banks, Arlington, Va., 1987).
6. *Martindale: The Complete Drug Reference,* S. C. Sweetman, Ed. (Pharmaceutical Press, London, 34th ed., 2005) pp. 1522-1526.
7. *Physician's Desk Reference for Radiology and Nuclear Medicine,* L. M. Freeman, M. D. Blaufox, Editorial Consultants (Medical Economics Co., Oradell, N.J., 4th ed., 1974/75, 5th ed., 1975/76.).
8. *Remington: The Science and Practice of Pharmacy,* A. R. Gennaro, Ed. (Lippincott Williams & Wilkins, Baltimore, MD, 20th ed., 2000) pp. 469-482.
9. D. P. Swanson *et al., Pharmaceuticals in Medical Imaging* (Macmillan Publishing Co., Inc., New York, 1990).

Notes
1. The following abbreviations for time units are used: y = years, d = days, h = hours, min = minutes, s = seconds.
2. The column for Principal Nuclear Properties lists the principal modes of disintegration and energies of the radiation in million electronvolts (MeV) for the individual isotopes. Symbols used to represent the modes of decay are: α = alpha particle emission, β^- = beta particle, β^+ = positron, γ = gamma ray, K = electron capture.

TABLE-39

Amino Acids Found in Proteins

General structure of the 20 common amino acids found in proteins except for proline, which has a 3-carbon cyclic side chain bound to the nitrogen of the backbone.

Amino Group → ^+H_3N

Carboxyl Group

Side Chain → R

α-Carbon

Name	Abbreviations		pKa Values			R Group Structure
	3 Letter	1 Letter	–COOH	–NH$_3^+$	R Group	
Alanine	Ala	A	2.34	9.69		—CH$_3$
Arginine	Arg	R	2.17	9.04	12.48	
Asparagine	Asn	N	2.02	8.80		
Aspartic Acid	Asp	D	1.88	9.60	3.65	
Cysteine	Cys	C	1.71	8.33	10.78	SH
Glutamic Acid	Glu	E	2.19	9.67	4.25	
Glutamine	Gln	Q	2.17	9.13		
Glycine	Gly	G	2.34	9.60		—H
Histidine	His	H	1.82	9.17	6.00	
Isoleucine	Ile	I	2.36	9.68		
Leucine	Leu	L	2.36	9.60		
Lysine	Lys	K	2.18	8.95	10.53	

TABLE-40

Amino Acids Found in Proteins (Continued)

Name	Abbreviations		pKa Values			R Group Structure
	3 Letter	1 Letter	–COOH	–NH$_3^+$	R Group	
Methionine	Met	M	2.28	9.21		
Phenylalanine	Phe	F	1.83	9.13		
Proline	Pro	P	1.99	10.60		
Serine	Ser	S	2.21	9.15		
Threonine	Thr	T	2.63	10.43		
Tryptophan	Trp	W	2.38	9.39		
Tyrosine	Tyr	Y	2.20	9.11	10.07	
Valine	Val	V	2.32	9.62		

TABLE-41

Chemical Terms Translator

English	French	German	Russian	Japanese
acetic acid	acide acétique	Essigsäure	уксусная кислота	酢酸
acetone	acétone	Aceton	ацетон	アセトン
acidic	acide	sauer	кислотный	酸性の
alkaline	alcalin	alkalisch	щелочной	アルカリ性の
amorphous	amorphe	amorph	аморфный	無定形の
anhydrous	anhydre	wasserfrei	безводный	無水の
aqueous	aqueux	wässrig	водный	水性の
boiling point	point d'ébullition	Siedepunkt	точка кипения	沸点
chloroform	chloroforme	Chloroform	хлороформ	クロロホルム
chromatography	chromatographie	Chromatographie	хроматография	クロマトグラフィー
cold	froid	kalt	холодный	冷たい
colorless	incolore	farblos	бесцветный	無色の
compound	composé	Verbindung	соединение	化合物
condensation	condensation	Kondensation	конденсация	凝縮
cool	refroidir	kühlen	охлаждать	冷却する
corrosive	corrosif	korrosiv; ätzend	коррозионный	腐食性の
crude	brut	roh	неочищенный	粗製の
crystal	cristal	Kristall	кристалл	結晶
crystalline	cristallin	kristallin	кристаллический	結晶性の
decomposition	décomposition	Zersetzung	разложение	分解
dehydration	déshydratation	Dehydratisierung	дегидратация	脱水
deliquescense	déliquescence	Zerfließlichkeit	расплывание	潮解
density	densité	Dichte	плотность	密度
dextrorotatory	dextrogyre	rechtsdrehend	правовращающий	右施性の
dilute (adjective)	dilué	verdünnt	разбавленный	希釈した
dilute (verb)	diluer	verdünnen	разбавлять	希釈する
dissolve	dissoudre	lösen	растворять	溶解する
distill	distiller	destillieren	дистиллировать	蒸留する
dry	sécher	trocknen	сушить	乾燥する
easily soluble	facilement soluble	leicht löslich	легкорастворимый	溶解しやすい
empirical formula	formule empirique	Summenformel	эмпирическая формула	実験式
esterification	estérification	Veresterung	эстерификация	エステル化
ethanol	éthanol	Äthanol	этанол	エタノール
ether	éther	Äther	простой эфир	エーテル
evaporation	évaporation	Verdunstung	выпаривание	蒸発
explosive	explosif	explosiv	взрывчатый	爆発性の
flammable	inflammable	entflammbar	воспламеняемый	引火性の
flash point	point d'éclair	Flammpunkt	температура вспышки	引火点
fraction	fraction	Fraktion	фракция	分画
freezing point	point de congélation	Gefrierpunkt	точка замерзания	凝固点
gas	gaz	Gas	газ	気体
heat	chauffer	erhitzen	нагревать	加熱する
hot	chaud	heiß	горячий	熱い
hydrochloric acid	acide chlorhydrique	Salzsäure	соляная кислота	塩酸
hygroscopic	hygroscopique	hygroskopisch	гигроскопический	吸湿性の
immiscible	immiscible	unmischbar	несмешивающийся	混和しない
impure	impur	unrein	нечистый	不純な
IR (infrared)	IR (infrarouge)	IR (infrarot)	ИК (инфракрасный)	IR（赤外の）
insoluble	insoluble	unlöslich	нерастворимый	不溶性の
isolation	isolation	Isolierung	выделение	単離
isomer	isomère	Isomer	изомер	異性体

TABLE-42

Chemical Terms Translator (Continued)

English	French	German	Russian	Japanese
levorotatory	lévogyre	linksdrehend	левовращающий	左施性の
light	lumière	Licht	свет	光
liquid	liquide	Flüssigkeit	жидкость	液体
lustrous	lustré	glänzend	блестящий	光沢がある
MS (mass spectrometry)	spectrométrie de masse	MS (Massenspektrometrie)	МС (масс-спектрометрия)	MS (質量分析)
maximum	maximum	Maximum	максимум	最大の
melting point	point de fusion	Schmelzpunkt	точка плавления	融点
minimum	minimum	Minimum	минимум	最小の
miscible	miscible	mischbar	смешивающийся	混合できる
mix	mélanger	mischen	смешивать	混合する
mixture	mélange	Mischung	смесь	混合物
mole	mole	Mol	моль	モル
molecular weight	poids moléculaire	Molekulargewicht	молекулярный вес	分子量
nitric acid	acide nitrique	Salpetersäure	азотная кислота	硝酸
NMR (nuclear magnetic resonance)	résonance magnétique nucléaire	NMR (kernmagnetische Resonanz)	ЯМР (ядерный магнитный резонанс)	NMR (核磁気共鳴)
normal (N)	normal (N)	normal (N)	нормальный (о растворе)	規定(N)
odorless	inodore	geruchlos	без запаха	無臭の
oil	huile	Öl	нефть	油
optical rotation	rotation optique	optische Drehung	оптическое вращение	旋光
phase	phase	Phase	фаза	相
powder	poudre	Pulver	порошок	粉末
practically insoluble	pratiquement insoluble	nahezu unlöslich	практически нерастворимый	ほとんど溶けない
precipitate (noun)	précipité	Präzipitat	осадок	沈殿
precipitate (verb)	précipiter	präzipitieren	осаждать	沈殿する
preparation	préparation	Präparat	препарат	調製
pure	pur	rein	чистый	純粋な
racemate	racémate	Razemat	рацемат	ラセミ体
recrystallize	recristalliser	umkristallisieren	перекристаллизовывать	再結晶する
residue	résidu	Rückstand	остаток	残留物
resolution	résolution	Auflösung	разрешающая способность	分解能
saturated	saturé	gesättigt	насыщенный	飽和した
slightly soluble	légèrement soluble	schwer löslich	слегка растворимый	溶けにくい
sodium hydroxide	hydroxyde de sodium	Natriumhydroxid	едкий натр	水酸化ナトリウム
solid	solide	Feststoff	твердое вещество	固体
solubility	solubilité	Löslichkeit	растворимость	溶解度
soluble	soluble	löslich	растворимый	可溶性の
solution	solution	Lösung	раствор	溶液
solvent	solvant	Lösungsmittel	растворитель	溶媒
somewhat soluble	quelque peu soluble	mäßig löslich	частично растворимый	若干可溶性の
sparingly soluble	difficilement soluble	wenig löslich	слаборастворимый	やや溶けにくい
sublime	sublimer	sublimieren	сублимировать	昇華する
synthesis	synthèse	Synthese	синтез	合成
uv (ultraviolet)	uv (ultraviolet)	UV (ultraviolett)	УФ (ультрафиолетовый)	uv (紫外線の)
vapor pressure	pression de vapeur	Dampfdruck	упругость пара	蒸気圧
very soluble	très soluble	sehr leicht löslich	высокорастворимый	非常に可溶性の
viscous	visqueux	viskos	вязкий	粘性の
volatile	volatil	flüchtig	летучий	揮発性の
warm	réchauffer	erwärmen	подогревать	温める
water	eau	Wasser	вода	水
yield	rendement	Ausbeute	выход	収量

TABLE-43

Selected Hexoses and Pentoses

Carbohydrates comprise one of the most abundant groups of naturally occurring organic compounds in living systems as well as being of great industrial importance. Presented below are various structural depictions of the common 5- and 6- carbon monosaccharides. Generally accepted carbohydrate nomenclature conventions include:

The use of D- and L-. The optical activity of the sugars is related to the reference compound glyceraldehyde which has only one D-form and one L-form. Since many of the aldoses have two or more chiral centers, the prefixes D- and L- refer to the configuration of the chiral carbon most distant from the carbonyl carbon. When the OH-group is drawn to the right in a Fischer projection, a D-sugar is designated.

Definition of the anomeric carbon. The new stereogenic center formed upon conversion from the Fischer projection to the cyclic hemiacetal is the anomeric carbon; the stereochemistry at this center is either α- or β-.

anomeric carbon

α–form   β–form

Sugar	Haworth Ring Pyranose	Haworth Ring Furanose	Chair Perspective β-form	Fischer Projection
Hexoses				**Aldohexoses**
D-Allose				
D-Altrose				
D-Glucose				
D-Gulose				
D-Galactose				
D-Idose				

TABLE-44

Sugar	Haworth Ring Pyranose	Haworth Ring Furanose	Chair Perspective β-form	Fischer Projection
D-Mannose				
D-Talose				

Ketoses

Sugar	Haworth Ring Pyranose	Haworth Ring Furanose	Chair Perspective β-form	Fischer Projection
D-Fructose β–form				
D-Sorbose β-form				

Pentoses

Aldohexoses

Sugar	Haworth Ring Pyranose	Haworth Ring Furanose	Chair Perspective β-form	Fischer Projection
D-Arabinose				
D-Lyxose				
D-Ribose				
D-Xylose				

TABLE-45

INTERNATIONAL SYSTEM OF UNITS (SI)

SI Basic and Supplementary Units

Name	Symbol	Physical Quantity
SI BASE UNITS		
meter	m	length
kilogram	kg	mass
second	s	time
ampere	A	electric current
kelvin	K	thermodynamic temperature
mole	mol	amount of substance
candela	cd	luminous intensity
SI SUPPLEMENTARY UNITS		
radian	rad	plane angle
steradian	sr	solid angle

SI Derived Units with Special Names

Formula	Symbol	Name	Physical Quantity
$kg \cdot m/s^2$	N	Newton	force
N/m^2	Pa	Pascal	pressure or stress
$N \cdot m$	J	Joule	work, energy, or quantity of heat
J/s	W	watt	power or radiant energy flux
W/A	V	volt	electric potential, potential difference or electromotive force
A/V	S	siemens	electric conductance
V/A	Ω	ohm	electric resistance
$A \cdot s$	C	Coulomb	quantity of electricity or electric charge
C/V	F	Farad	electric capacitance
$V \cdot s$	Wb	Weber	magnetic flux
Wb/A	H	Henry	inductance
Wb/m^2	T	Tesla	magnetic flux density or magnetic induction
$cd \cdot sr$	lm	lumen	luminous flux
lm/m^2	lx	lux	illuminance
J/kg	Gy	gray	absorbed dose (of ionizing radiation)
1 (disintegrations)/s	Bq	Becquerel	activity (of a radionuclide)
1 (cycle)/s	Hz	hertz	frequency (of a periodic phenomenon)
$K - 273$	°C	degree Celsius	temperature

SI Prefixes

Factor	Prefix	Symbol	Factor	Prefix	Symbol
10^{-24}	yocto	y	10	deca	da
10^{-21}	zepto	z	10^2	hecto	h
10^{-18}	atto	a	10^3	kilo	k
10^{-15}	femto	f	10^6	mega	M
10^{-12}	pico	p	10^9	giga	G
10^{-9}	nano	n	10^{12}	tera	T
10^{-6}	micro	μ	10^{15}	peta	P
10^{-3}	milli	m	10^{18}	exa	E
10^{-2}	centi	c	10^{21}	zetta	Z
10^{-1}	deci	d	10^{24}	yotta	Y

TABLE-46

Numerical Prefixes Commonly Used in Forming Chemical Names

Numeral	Prefix	Numeral	Prefix	Numeral	Prefix
$\frac{1}{2}$	hemi-	13	trideca-	28	octacosa-
1	mono-	14	tetradeca-	29	nonacosa-
$1\frac{1}{2}$	sesqui-	15	pentadeca-	30	triaconta-
2	di-, bi-	16	hexadeca-	40	tetraconta-
$2\frac{1}{2}$	hemipenta-	17	heptadeca-	50	pentaconta-
3	tri-	18	octadeca-	60	hexaconta-
4	tetra-	19	nonadeca-	70	heptaconta-
5	penta-	20	eicosa-	80	octaconta-
6	hexa-	21	heneicosa-	90	nonaconta-
7	hepta-	22	docosa-	100	hecta-
8	octa-	23	tricosa-	101	henhecta-
9	ennea, nona-	24	tetracosa-	102	dohecta-
10	deca-	25	pentacosa-	110	decahecta-
11	hendeca-, undeca-	26	hexacosa-	120	eicosahecta-
12	dodeca-	27	heptacosa-	200	dicta-

Alchemical Symbols Used in Biology and Botany

Symbol	Meaning
☉	Sun; gold; annual plant.
☉ ☉	Biennial plant.
○ or ☽	Moon; silver; *sometimes* female sex.
☿	Mercury.
♀	Venus; copper; *female sex.*
♁	Earth; terra; *sometimes* male sex.
♁ ♀	Having male and female flowers separate.
♁ — ♀	Having male and female flowers on the same plant.
♁ : ♀	Having male and female flowers on different plants.
♂	Mars; iron; *male sex.*
♂	Conjunction; mating; mated.
♃	Jupiter; tin; perennial herb.
♄	Saturn; lead.
🜍	Sulfur.
🜺	Arsenic.

Prescription Notation

The units of quantities written on prescriptions in the Apothecaries System are usually designated by symbols. Occasionally abbreviations are used. The following list provides these symbols and abbreviations.

Apothecaries' Weight

Symbol	Abbreviation	Unit
—	gr.	grain
℈	sc.	scruple
ʒ	dr.	dram
℥	oz.	ounce
℔	lb.	pound

Apothecaries' Volume

Symbol	Abbreviation	Unit
♏	min.	minim
ƒʒ	fl. dr.	fluid dram
ƒ℥	fl. oz.	fluid ounce
O.	pt.	pint
Cong.	gal.	gallon

Roman numerals (lower case) are always used following the symbol to designate the number of units required, but, if the abbreviation is used, arabic numerals are used and precede the appreviation. For example:

ʒ iv　but　4 dr.

For less than one unit, one-half may be designated by ss following the symbol, but other fractions must be designated by arabic numeral fractions. For example:

ʒ ss　but　gr. $\frac{1}{8}$

Roman numerals are also usually used to designate the number of dosage forms required. For example:

Caps. No. xiv

TABLE-47

Latin Terms

Abbreviation	Expanded form	Meaning	Abbreviation	Expanded form	Meaning
a.	ante	before	d.	dexter	right
a., aur.	auris	ear	d.	dies	a day
aa.	ana	of each	d.	dosis	a dose
a.c.	ante cibos	before meals	da.	da	give
ad	ad	to, up to	dent., d.	dentur	let be given, give
add.	adde, addantur, addendus, addendo	add, let them be added, to be added, by adding	det.	detur	let it be given
			dieb. alt.	diebus alternis	on alternate days
			dieb. secund.	diebus secundis	every second day
ad lib.	ad libitum	at pleasure	dil.	dilue	dilute
adm.	admove	apply	disp.	dispensa, dispensetur	dispense
ad man. med.	ad manus medici	(to be delivered) into the hands of the (pre-scribing) physician	div.	divide	divide
			div. in par. aeq.	dividatur in partes aequales	divide in equal parts
ad satur.	ad saturandum	to saturation			
agit.	agita	shake	d.t.d.	dentur tales doses	give such doses
alb.	albus	white	dulc.	dulcis	sweet
alt. hor.	alternis horis	every other hour	dur.	durus	hard
A.M.	ante meridiem	before noon	e.m.p.	ex modo prescripto	after the manner prescribed
ampl.	amplus	large			
ampul.	ampulla	ampul, ampule	et	et	and
applicand.	applicandus	to be applied	ex	ex	out of
aq.	aqua	water	ext.	extractum	an extract
aq. bull.	aqua bulliens	boiling water	f., ft.	fac, fiat, fiant	make, let be made
aq. dest.	aqua destillata	distilled water	ferv.	fervens	hot
aq. ferv.	aqua fervens	hot water	filt.	filtra	filter (imperative form)
aq. frig.	aqua frigida	cold water	fl.	fluidus	fluid
b.	bis	twice	flav.	flavus	yellow
ben.	bene	well	fldext.	fluidextractum	fluidextract
bib.	bibe	drink	fort.	fortis	strong
b.i.d.	bis in die	twice a day	frig.	frigidus	cold
bol.	bolus	a large pill	garg.	gargarisma	a gargle
brevis	brevis	short	Gm.	gramma	gram
bull.	bulliens, bulliat, bulliant	boiling, let boil	gr.	granum	grain
			gran.	granulatus	granulated
c̄	cum	with	gtt.	gutta	a drop
C	centum	a hundred	h.s.	hora somni	at the hour of sleep, at bedtime
cap.	capiat	let the patient take			
caps.	capsula	a capsule	hydrarg.	hydrargyrum.	mercury
cerat.	ceratum	wax ointment	i.c.	inter cibos	between meals
chart.	charta	paper, a powder in paper	juxt.	juxta	near
			Kal.	Kalium	potassium
chart. cerat.	charta cerata	waxed paper, parch-ment paper	l.a.	lege artis	according to the art
chirurg.	chirurgicalis	surgical	laev.	laevus	left
chord chirurg.	chorda chirurgicalis	surgical "catgut"	lb.	libra	pound
			lev.	levis	light
cito disp!	cito dispensetur!	let it be dispensed quickly	liq.	liquor	a liquor, a solution
			lot.	lotio	lotion
coch. amp.	cochleare amplum	a tablespoonful	m.	mane	in the morning
			M.	misce	mix
coch. mag.	cochleare magnum	a tablespoonful	m.	mitte	send
			mag.	magnus	large
coch. med.	cochleare medium	a dessertspoonful	m. dict.	more dicto	as directed
			min.	minimum	minim
coch. mod.	cochleare modicum	a dessertspoonful	mist.	mistura	mixture
			mixt.	mixtura	mixture
coch. parv.	cochleare parvum	a teaspoonful	m.p.	modo praescripto	in the manner prescribed
col.	cola	strain (imperative form)	m.t.d.	mitte tales doses	send such doses
colet.	coletur	let it be strained	n.	naris	nostril
collun.	collunarium	a nose wash	Natr.	Natrium	sodium
collut.	collutorium	a mouth wash	nebul.	nebula	a spray
collyr.	collyrium	an eye wash	n. et m.	nocte maneque	night and morning
comp.	compositus	compound, compounded	nig.	niger	black
			no.	numero	number
cong.	congius	a gallon	noct.	nocte	at night
consperg.	consperge, conspergetur	dust, sprinkle	non rep.	non repetatur	do not repeat
			O.	Octarius	a pint
			o.d.	oculus dexter	right eye
cont.	contra	against	o.l.	oculus laevus	left eye
contus.	contusus	bruised	omn. hor.	omni hora	at every hour
coq.	coque, coquatur	boil, let it boil	omn. man.	omni mane	on every morning

TABLE-48

Latin Terms (Continued)

Abbreviation	Expanded form	Meaning	Abbreviation	Expanded form	Meaning
opt.	optimus	best	s.a.	secundum artem	according to art
o.s.	oculus sinister	left eye	sat.	saturatus	saturated
o.u.	oculi uterque	both eyes	scat.	scatula	box
p. ae.	partes aequales	equal parts	scat. orig.	scatula originalis	original package, manufacturer's package (and label)
parv.	parvus	small			
p.c.	post cibos	after meals			
phial.	phiala	bottle	sic.	siccus	dried
Plumb.	Plumbum	lead	s.n.	secundum naturam	according to nature
P.M.	post meridiem	after noon			
p.o.	per os	by mouth	sol.	solubilis	soluble
pond.	ponderosus	heavy	sol.	solutio	solution
ppt.	praecipitatus	precipitated	solv.	solve	dissolve
p.r.n.	pro re nata	as occasion arises, as needed	s.o.s.	si opus sit	if there is need
			spir.	spiritus	spirit
pro rect.	pro recto	rectal	spiss.	spissus	dried
pt.	perstetur	let it be continued	ss.	semis	one half
pulv.	pulvis, pulveres	powder, powders	stat.	statim	immediately
q., qq.	quodque, quaeque	each, every	suc.	succus	juice
			sum.	sume, sumendus	take, to be taken
q.i.d.	quater in die	four times a day	S.V.R.	spiritus vini rectificatus	alcohol
qq. hor.	quaque hora	every hour			
Q.R.	quantum rectum	the quantity is correct	syr.	syrupus	syrup
			tab.	tabella	tablet
q.s.	quantum sufficiat, quantum satis	a sufficient quantity	tal.	talis, tales, talia	such
			ter.	tere	rub
			t.i.d.	ter in die	three times a day
quot. op. sit	quoties opus sit	as often as necessary	tinct., tr.	tinctura	tincture
q.v.	quantum voleris	as much as you wish	trit.	tritura	triturate
℞	recipe	you take	ult.	ultime	lastly
recen.	recens	fresh	unct.	unctus	smeared
rect.	rectificatus	rectified	ung., ungt.	unguentum	ointment
ren. sem.	renovetur semel	shall be renewed (only) once	ust.	ustus	burnt
			ut dict.	ut dictum	as directed
rept.	repetatur	let it be repeated	v.	vel	or
rub.	ruber	red	vesp.	vesper	evening
S., Sig.	signa, signetur	write, it shall be written (as instruction to the patient)	vir.	viridis, viride	green
			vol.	volatilis, volatile	volatile

TABLE-49

Greek Alphabet

Name of Letter	Capital	Lower Case	Transliteration	Name of Letter	Capital	Lower Case	Transliteration
alpha	A	α	a	nu	N	ν	n
beta	B	β	b	xi	Ξ	ξ	x
gamma	Γ	γ	g	omicron	O	o	o short
delta	Δ	δ	d	pi	Π	π	p
epsilon	H	ε	e short	rho	P	ρ	r
zeta	Z	ζ	z	sigma	Σ	σ or ς	s
eta	H	η	e long	tau	T	τ	t
theta	Θ	θ	th	upsilon	Υ	υ	y
iota	I	ι	i	phi	Φ	φ or ϕ	f
kappa	K	κ	k, c	chi	X	χ	ch as in German echt
lambda	Λ	λ	l	psi	Ψ	ψ	ps
mu	M	μ	m	omega	Ω	ω	o long

Russian Alphabet

Cyrillic Print		Transliteration	Pronunciation	Cyrillic Print		Transliteration	Pronunciation
А	а	a	*a* in far	Р	р	r	*r*
Б	б	b	*b*	С	с	s	*s* in say
В	в	v	*v*	Т	т	t	*t*
Г	г	g (h)	*g* in gay	У	у	u	*oo* in boot
Д	д	d	*d*	Ф	ф	f	*f*
Е	е	e	*e* in fell; also *ye* in yell	Х	х	kh	like German *ch*
Ж	ж	zh	*z* in azure	Ц	ц	ts	*ts* in hoots
З	з	z	*z* in zeal	Ч	ч	ch	*ch* in church
И	и	i	*i* in meet	Ш	ш	sh	*sh*
Й	й	ĭ	*y* in boy	Щ	щ	shch	*shch* as in fre*sh ch*eese
к	к	k	*k*	Ъ	ъ	″	silent*
Л	л	l	*l*	Ы	ы	y	*y* in rhythm (hard)
М	м	m	*m*	Ь	ь	′	silent* (softens preceding consonant)
Н	н	n	*n*	Э	э	ė	*e* in met
О	о	o	*o* in or	Ю	ю	iu	*u* in union
П	п	p	*p*	Я	я	ia	*ya* in yard

* Hard sign; used to separate a consonant from a soft vowel especially in foreign words; frequently replaced by an apostrophe.

Roman Numerals

I 1	II 2	III 3	IV 4	V 5	VI 6	VII 7	VIII 8	IX 9	X 10
XX 20	XXX 30	XL 40	L 50	LX 60	LXX 70	LXXX 80	XC 90	IC 99	C 100
CC 200	CCC 300	CD 400	D 500	DC 600	DCC 700	DCCC 800	CM 900	XM 990	M 1000

TABLE-50

Common Heterocyclic Ring Systems

O - Containing Rings

oxirane   furan   2*H*-pyran   4*H*-pyran   2*H*-chromene   benzo[*b*]furan

S - Containing Rings

thiophene   benzo[*b*]thiophene   parathiazine

N - Containing Rings

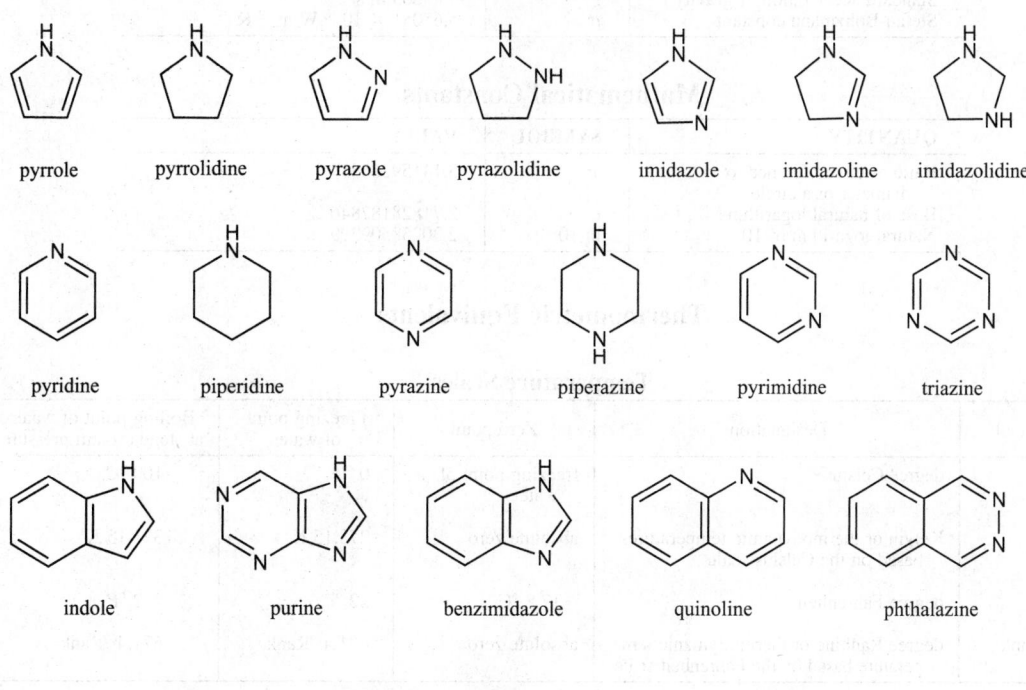

pyrrole   pyrrolidine   pyrazole   pyrazolidine   imidazole   imidazoline   imidazolidine

pyridine   piperidine   pyrazine   piperazine   pyrimidine   triazine

indole   purine   benzimidazole   quinoline   phthalazine

Other

succinimide   thiazolidine   phenothiazine   morpholine   thiomorpholine

TABLE-51

Fundamental Physical and Mathematical Constants

Physical Constants

QUANTITY	SYMBOL	VALUE
Atomic mass unit (Dalton)	amu	1.661×10^{-24} g
Avogadro constant	N_A, L	6.0221367×10^{23} mol^{-1}
Bohr magneton	μ_B	$9.2740154 \times 10^{-24}$ J T^{-1}
Boltzmann constant	k	1.380658×10^{-23} J K^{-1}
Electron mass	m_e	$9.1093897 \times 10^{-31}$ kg
Elementary charge	e	$1.60217653 \times 10^{-19}$ C
Faraday constant	F	9.6485309×10^4 C mol^{-1}
Gas constant	R	8.314510 J mol^{-1} K^{-1}
		8.314510×10^{-2} L bar mol^{-1} K^{-1}
		8.20578×10^{-2} L atm mol^{-1} K^{-1}
		6.2364 L Torr mol^{-1} K^{-1}
		1.9872 cal mol^{-1} K^{-1}
Gravitational constant	G	6.67259×10^{-11} m^3 kg^{-1} s^{-2}
Molar volume of ideal gas at STP	V_m	22.413996×10^{-3} m^3 mol^{-1}
Neutron mass	m_n	$1.6749286 \times 10^{-27}$ kg
Nuclear magneton	μ_N	$5.0507866 \times 10^{-27}$ J T^{-1}
Permeability of vacuum	μ_0	$4\pi \times 10^{-7}$ H m^{-1}
Permittivity of vacuum	ε_0	8.85419×10^{-12} J^{-1} C^2 m^{-1}
Planck constant	h	$6.6260755 \times 10^{-34}$ J s
	h	$4.13566743 \times 10^{-15}$ eV s
	$\hbar = h/2\pi$	$1.05457168 \times 10^{-34}$ J s
Proton mass	m_p	$1.6726231 \times 10^{-27}$ kg
Rydberg constant	R_∞	1.0973731534×10^7 m^{-1}
Speed of light in a vacuum	c, c_0	2.99792458×10^8 m s^{-1}
Standard acceleration of gravity	g	9.80665 m s^{-2}
Stefan-Boltzmann constant	σ	5.67051×10^{-8} W m^{-2} K^{-4}

Mathematical Constants

QUANTITY	SYMBOL	VALUE
Ratio of circumference to diameter of a circle	π	3.14159265359
Base of natural logarithms	e	2.71828182846
Natural logarithm of 10	ln 10	2.30258509299

Thermometric Equivalents

Temperature Scales

Symbol	Designation	Zero point	Freezing point of water	Boiling point of water at standard atm pressure
°C	degree Celsius	freezing point of water	0 °C	100 °C
K	Kelvin or thermodynamic temperature based on the Celsius scale	absolute zero	273.15 K	373.15 K
°F	degree Fahrenheit	−17.8 °C	32 °F	212 °F
°Rank	degree Rankine or thermodymanic temperature based on the Fahrenheit scale	absolute zero	491.4 °Rank	671.4 °Rank

The following formulas may be used to convert temperatures from one scale to another:

Temperature given in	Temperature wanted in			
	°C	K	°F	°Rank
°C	°C	°C + 273.15	1.8 °C + 32	1.8 °C + 491.4
K	K − 273.15	K	1.8 K − 459.4	1.8 K
°F	0.556 °F − 17.8	0.556 °F + 255.3	°F	°F + 459.4
°Rank	0.556 °Rank − 273.15	0.556 °Rank	°Rank − 459.4	°Rank

TABLE-52

Universal Conversion Factors

To convert units of one system into another, find the given units in the table and multiply by the appropriate conversion factor. For example:
To convert 26.5 centimeters into inches, find centimeters in the table, read across to inches and multiply by 0.3937.

$$26.5 \text{ cm} \times \frac{0.3937 \text{ inch}}{\text{cm}} = 10.4 \text{ inches}$$

To convert 8.75 inches into centimeters, find inches in the table, read across to centimeters and multiply by 2.540.

$$8.75 \text{ inches} \times \frac{2.540 \text{ cm}}{\text{inch}} = 22.2 \text{ cm}$$

TO CONVERT	INTO	MULTIPLY BY	TO CONVERT	INTO	MULTIPLY BY
A			baryes	dynes/sq cm	1.000
abcoulombs	statcoulombs	2.998×10^{10}	bolts (US cloth)	meters	36.576
acres	sq chains (Gunter's)	10	Btu	liter—atmosphere	10.409
acres	sq rods	160	Btu	ergs	1.0550×10^{10}
acres	square links		Btu	foot-lb	778.3
	(Gunter's)	1×10^5	Btu	gram-calories	252.0
acres	hectares or		Btu	horsepower-hr	3.931×10^{-4}
	sq hectometers	0.4047	Btu	joules	1,054.8
acres	sq ft	43,560.0	Btu	kilogram-calories	0.2520
acres	sq meters	4,047	Btu	kilogram-meters	107.5
acres	sq miles	1.562×10^{-3}	Btu	kilowatt-hr	2.928×10^{-4}
acres	sq yd	4,840	Btu/hr	foot-lb/sec	0.2162
acre-feet	cu ft	43,560.0	Btu/hr	gram-cal/sec	0.0700
acre-feet	gallons	3.259×10^5	Btu/hr	horsepower-hr	3.929×10^{-4}
amperes/sq cm	amps/sq in	6.452	Btu/hr	watts	0.2931
amperes/sq cm	amps/sq meter	10^4	Btu/min	foot-lb/sec	12.96
amperes/sq in	amps/sq cm	0.1550	Btu/min	horsepower	0.02356
amperes/sq in	amps/sq meter	1,550.0	Btu/min	kilowatts	0.01757
amperes/sq meter	amps/sq cm	10^{-4}	Btu/min	watts	17.57
amperes/sq meter	amps/sq in	6.452×10^{-4}	Btu/sq ft/min	watts/sq in	0.1221
ampere-hours	coulombs	3,600.0	bucket (UK dry)	cubic cm	1.818×10^4
ampere-hours	faradays	0.03731	bushels	cu ft	1.2445
ampere-turns	gilberts	1.257	bushels	cu in	2,150.42
ampere-turns/cm	amp-turns/in	2.540	bushels	cu meters	0.03524
ampere-turns/cm	amp-turns/meter	100.0	bushels	liters	35.24
ampere-turns/cm	gilberts/cm	1.257	bushels	pecks	4.0
ampere-turns/in	amp-turns/cm	0.3937	bushels	pints (dry)	64.0
ampere-turns/in	amp-turns/meter	39.37	bushels	quarts (dry)	32.0
ampere-turns/in	gilberts/cm	0.4950			
ampere-turns/meter	amp-turns/cm	0.01			
ampere-turns/meter	amp-turns/in	0.0254		**C**	
ampere-turns/meter	gilberts/cm	0.01257	calories, gram		
angstrom unit	inches	3937×10^{-9}	(mean)	Btu (mean)	3.9685×10^{-3}
angstrom unit	meters	1×10^{-10}	candle/sq cm	lamberts	3.142
angstrom unit	microns or (μ)	1×10^{-4}	candle/sq inch	lamberts	0.4870
ares	acres (US)	0.02471	Celsius	Fahrenheit	$1.8°C + 32$
ares	sq yd	119.60	centares (centiares)	sq meters	1.0
ares	acres	0.02471	centigrams	grams	0.01
ares	sq meters	100.0	centiliters	ounces (fl)	0.3382
astronomical units	kilometers	1.495×10^8	centiliters	cu in	0.6103
atmospheres	ton/sq in	0.007348	centiliters	drams	2.705
atmospheres	cm of mercury	76.0	centiliters	liters	0.01
atmospheres	mm of mercury	760.0	centimeters	feet	3.281×10^{-2}
atmospheres	torrs	760.0	centimeters	inches	0.3937
atmospheres	ft of water (at 4°C)	33.90	centimeters	kilometers	10^{-5}
atmospheres	in of mercury (at 0°C)	29.92	centimeters	meters	0.01
atmospheres	kg/sq cm	1.0333	centimeters	miles	6.214×10^{-6}
atmospheres	kg/sq meter	10,332	centimeters	millimeters	10.0
atmospheres	lb/sq in	14.70	centimeters	mils	393.7
atmospheres	tons/sq ft	1.058	centimeters	yards	1.094×10^{-2}
			centimeter-dynes	cm-grams	1.020×10^{-3}
	B		centimeter-dynes	meter-kg	1.020×10^{-8}
barrels (US, dry)	cu in	7056	centimeter-dynes	lb-ft	7.376×10^{-8}
barrels (US, dry)	quarts (dry)	105.0	centimeter-grams	cm-dynes	980.7
barrels (US, liq)	gallons	31.5	centimeter-grams	meter-kg	10^{-5}
barrels (oil)	gallons (oil)	42.0	centimeter-grams	lb-ft	7.233×10^{-5}
bars	atmospheres	0.9869	centimeters of		
bars	dynes/sq cm	10^6	mercury	atmospheres	0.01316
bars	kg/sq meter	1.020×10^4	centimeters of		
bars	lb/sq ft	2,089	mercury	ft of water	0.4461
bars	lb/sq in	14.50			

TABLE-53

TO CONVERT	INTO	MULTIPLY BY	TO CONVERT	INTO	MULTIPLY BY
centimeters of mercury	kg/sq meter	136.0	cubic inches	bushels	4.650×10^{-4}
centimeters of mercury	lb/sq ft	27.85	cubic inches	cu cm	16.39
centimeters of mercury	lb/sq in	0.1934	cubic inches	cu ft	5.787×10^{-4}
centimeters/sec	ft/min	1.1969	cubic inches	cu meters	1.639×10^{-5}
centimeters/sec	ft/sec	0.03281	cubic inches	cu yards	2.143×10^{-5}
centimeters/sec	kilometers/hr	0.036	cubic inches	drams (fl)	4.4329
centimeters/sec	knots	0.1943	cubic inches	gallons (US)	4.329×10^{-3}
centimeters/sec	meters/min	0.6	cubic inches	gallons (UK)	3.605×10^{-3}
centimeters/sec	miles/hr	0.02237	cubic inches	gills	0.1385
centimeters/sec	miles/min	3.728×10^{-4}	cubic inches	liters	0.01639
centimeters/sec/sec	ft/sec/sec	0.03281	cubic inches	milliliters	16.39
centimeters/sec/sec	km/hr/sec	0.036	cubic inches	mil-ft	1.061×10^5
centimeters/sec/sec	meters/sec/sec	0.01	cubic inches	minims	265.974
centimeters/sec/sec	miles/hr/sec	0.02237	cubic inches	ounces (fl)	0.5541
chain	inches	792.00	cubic inches	pecks	1.860×10^{-3}
chain	meters	20.12	cubic inches	pints (dry)	0.0298
chains (surveyors' or Gunter's)	yards	22.00	cubic inches	pints (liq)	0.03463
circular mils	sq cm	5.067×10^{-6}	cubic inches	quarts (dry)	0.0149
circular mils	sq mils	0.7854	cubic inches	quarts (liq)	0.01732
circular mils	sq in	7.854×10^{-7}	cubic meters	bushels	28.38
circumference	radians	6.283	cubic meters	cu cm	10^6
cords	cord ft	8	cubic meters	cu ft	35.31
cord feet	cu ft	16	cubic meters	cu in	61,023.74
coulomb	statcoulombs	2.998×10^9	cubic meters	cu yards	1.308
coulombs	faradays	1.036×10^{-5}	cubic meters	gallons (US)	264.2
coulombs/sq cm	coulombs/sq in	64.52	cubic meters	gallons (UK)	220.0
coulombs/sq cm	coulombs/sq meter	10^4	cubic meters	liters	1,000.0
coulombs/sq in	coulombs/sq cm	0.1550	cubic meters	milliliters	10^6
coulombs/sq in	coulombs/sq meter	1,550	cubic meters	pecks	113.51
coulombs/sq meter	coulombs/sq cm	10^{-4}	cubic meters	pints (dry)	1,816.166
coulombs/sq/meter	coulombs/sq in	6.452×10^{-4}	cubic meters	pints (liq)	2,113.0
cubic centimeters	cu ft	3.531×10^{-5}	cubic meters	quarts (dry)	908.083
cubic centimeters	cu in	0.06102	cubic meters	quarts (liq)	1,057
cubic centimeters	cu meters	10^{-6}	cubic yards	cu cm	7.646×10^5
cubic centimeters	cu yards	1.308×10^{-4}	cubic yards	cu ft	27.0
cubic centimeters	drams (fl)	0.2705	cubic yards	cu in	46,656.0
cubic centimeters	gallons (US)	2.642×10^{-4}	cubic yards	cu meters	0.7646
cubic centimeters	gills	8.454×10^{-3}	cubic yards	gallons (US)	202.0
cubic centimeters	liters	0.001	cubic yards	gallons (UK)	168.2
cubic centimeters	milliliters	1.0	cubic yards	liters	764.6
cubic centimeters	minims	16.231	cubic yards	milliliters	7.646×10^5
cubic centimeters	ounces (fl)	0.0338	cubic yards	pints (liq)	1,615.9
cubic centimeters	pints (liq)	2.113×10^{-3}	cubic yards	quarts (liq)	807.9
cubic centimeters	quarts (liq)	1.057×10^{-3}	cubic yards/min	cubic ft/sec	0.45
cubic feet	bushels	0.8036	cubic yards/min	gallons/sec	3.367
cubic feet	cu cm	28,316.85	cubic yards/min	liters/sec	12.74
cubic feet	cu in	1,728.0			
cubic feet	cu meters	0.02832	**D**		
cubic feet	cu yards	0.03704	Dalton	gram	1.650×10^{-24}
cubic feet	drams (fl)	7660.05	days	seconds	86,400.0
cubic feet	gallons (US)	7.48052	decigrams	grams	0.1
cubic feet	gallons (UK)	6.229	deciliters	liters	0.1
cubic feet	gills	239.38	decimeters	meters	0.1
cubic feet	liters	28.32	degrees (angle)	quadrants	0.01111
cubic feet	milliliters	28,316.85	degrees (angle)	radians	0.01745
cubic feet	minims	459,603.1	degrees (angle)	seconds	3,600.0
cubic feet	ounces (fl)	957.51	degrees/sec	radians/sec	0.01745
cubic feet	pecks	3.2143	degrees/sec	revolutions/min	0.1667
cubic feet	pints (dry)	51.428	degrees/sec	revolutions/sec	2.778×10^{-3}
cubic feet	pints (liq)	59.84	dekagrams	grams	10.0
cubic feet	quarts (dry)	25.714	dekaliters	liters	10.0
cubic feet	quarts (liq)	29.92	dekameters	meters	10.0
cubic feet/min	cu cm/sec	472.0	drams (avdp)	drams (apoth)	0.4557
cubic feet/min	gallons/sec	0.1247	drams (avdp)	grains	27.3437
cubic feet/min	liters/sec	0.4720	drams (avdp)	grams	1.7718
cubic feet/min	lb of water/min	62.43	drams (avdp)	kilograms	1.7718×10^{-3}
cubic feet/sec	million gals/day	0.646317	drams (avdp)	milligrams	1771.85
cubic feet/sec	gallons/min	448.831	drams (avdp)	ounces (apoth or troy)	0.0570
			drams (avdp)	ounces (avdp)	0.0625
			drams (avdp)	pennyweights	1.139

TABLE-54

TO CONVERT	INTO	MULTIPLY BY	TO CONVERT	INTO	MULTIPLY BY
drams (avdp)	pounds (apoth or troy)	4.747×10^{-3}	faradays	coulombs	9.649×10^{4}
drams (avdp)	pounds (avdp)	3.906×10^{-3}	fathoms	meters	1.828804
drams (avdp)	scruples	1.367	fathoms	feet	6.0
drams (apoth)	drams (avdp)	2.1943	feet	centimeters	30.48
drams (apoth)	grains	60.0	feet	inches	12.0
drams (apoth)	grams	3.8879	feet	kilometers	3.048×10^{-4}
drams (apoth)	kilograms	3.888×10^{-3}	feet	meters	0.3048
drams (apoth)	milligrams	3887.93	feet	miles (nautical)	1.645×10^{-4}
drams (apoth)	ounces (apoth or troy)	0.125	feet	miles (statute)	1.894×10^{-4}
drams (apoth)	ounces (avdp)	0.1371429	feet	millimeters	304.8
drams (apoth)	pennyweights	2.5	feet	mils	1.2×10^{4}
drams (apoth)	pounds (apoth or troy)	0.0104	feet	yards	0.333
drams (apoth)	pounds (avdp)	8.571×10^{-3}	feet of water	atmospheres	0.02950
drams (apoth)	scruples	3.0	feet of water	in of mercury	0.8826
drams (fl)	cu cm	3.6967	feet of water	kg/sq cm	0.03048
drams (fl)	cu ft	1.3055×10^{-4}	feet of water	kg/sq meter	304.8
drams (fl)	cu in	0.2256	feet of water	lb/sq ft	62.43
drams (fl)	gallons (US)	9.7656×10^{-4}	feet of water	lb/sq in	0.4335
drams (fl)	gills	0.03125	feet/min	cm/sec	0.5080
drams (fl)	liters	3.6967×10^{-3}	feet/min	feet/sec	0.01667
drams (fl)	milliliters	3.6967	feet/min	km/hr	0.01829
drams (fl)	minims	60.0	feet/min	meters/min	0.3048
drams (fl)	ounces (fl)	0.125	feet/min	miles/hr	0.01136
drams (fl)	pints (liq)	7.8125×10^{-3}	feet/sec	cm/sec	30.48
drams (fl)	quarts (liq)	3.9063×10^{-3}	feet/sec	km/hr	1.097
dynes	grams	1.020×10^{-3}	feet/sec	knots	0.5921
dynes	joules/cm	10^{-7}	feet/sec	meters/min	18.29
dynes	joules/meter (newtons)	10^{-5}	feet/sec	miles/hr	0.6818
dynes	kilograms	1.020×10^{-6}	feet/sec	miles/min	0.01136
dynes	poundals	7.233×10^{-5}	feet/sec/sec	cm/sec/sec	30.48
dynes	pounds	2.248×10^{-6}	feet/sec/sec	km/hr/sec	1.097
dynes/cm	ergs/sq mm	.01	feet/sec/sec	meters/sec/sec	0.3048
dynes/sq cm	atmospheres	9.869×10^{-7}	feet/sec/sec	miles/hr/sec	0.6818
dynes/sq cm	bars	10^{-6}	feet/100 feet	percent grade	1.0
dynes/sq cm	in of mercury at 0°C	2.953×10^{-5}	foot-candles	lumens/sq meter	10.764
dynes/sq cm	in of water at 4°C	4.015×10^{-4}	foot-pounds	Btu	1.286×10^{-3}
			foot-pounds	ergs	1.356×10^{7}
E			foot-pounds	gram-calories	0.3238
ell	cm	114.30	foot-pounds	hp-hr	5.050×10^{-7}
ell	inches	45	foot-pounds	joules	1.356
em, pica	inches	.167	foot-pounds	kg-calories	3.24×10^{-4}
em, pica	cm	.4233	foot-pounds	kg-meters	0.1383
ergs	Btu	9.480×10^{-11}	foot-pounds	kilowatt-hr	3.766×10^{-7}
ergs	dyne-centimeters	1.0	foot-pounds/min	Btu/min	1.286×10^{-3}
ergs	foot-lb	7.367×10^{-8}	foot-pounds/min	foot-lb/sec	0.01667
ergs	gram-calories	0.2389×10^{-7}	foot-pounds/min	horsepower	3.030×10^{-5}
ergs	gram-cm	1.020×10^{-3}	foot-pounds/min	kg-calories/min	3.24×10^{-4}
ergs	horsepower-hr	3.7250×10^{-14}	foot-pounds/min	kilowatts	2.260×10^{-5}
ergs	joules	10^{-7}	foot-pounds/sec	Btu/hr	4.6263
ergs	kg-calories	2.389×10^{-11}	foot-pounds/sec	Btu/min	0.07717
ergs	kg-meters	1.020×10^{-8}	foot-pounds/sec	horsepower	1.818×10^{-3}
ergs	kilowatt-hr	0.2778×10^{-13}	foot-pounds/sec	kg-calories/min	0.01945
ergs	watt-hr	0.2778×10^{-10}	foot-pounds/sec	kilowatts	1.356×10^{-3}
ergs/sec	Btu/min	5.688×10^{-6}	furlongs	miles (US)	0.125
ergs/sec	dyne-cm/sec	1.000	furlongs	rods	40.0
ergs/sec	ft-lb/min	4.427×10^{-6}	furlongs	feet	660.0
ergs/sec	ft-lb/sec	7.3756×10^{-8}			
ergs/sec	horsepower	1.341×10^{-10}	**G**		
ergs/sec	kg-calories/min	1.433×10^{-9}	gallons (US)	cu cm	3,785.0
ergs/sec	kilowatts	10^{-10}	gallons (US)	cu ft	0.1337
			gallons (US)	cu in	231.0
F			gallons (US)	cu meters	3.785×10^{-3}
Fahrenheit	Celsius	$0.556°F - 17.8$	gallons (US)	cu yards	4.951×10^{-3}
farads	microfarads	10^{6}	gallons (US)	drams (fl)	1024.0
faradays/sec	ampere (abs)	9.6500×10^{4}	gallons (US)	gallons (UK)	0.83267
faradays	ampere-hr	26.80	gallons (US)	gills	32.0
			gallons (US)	liters	3.785
			gallons (US)	milliliters	3,785.0
			gallons (US)	minims	61,440.0
			gallons (US)	ounces (fl)	128.0
			gallons (US)	pints (liq)	8.0

TABLE-55

TO CONVERT	INTO	MULTIPLY BY	TO CONVERT	INTO	MULTIPLY BY
gallons (US)	quarts (liq)	4.0	grams	tons (short)	1.102×10^{-6}
gallons (UK)	cu ft	0.1605	grams/cm	lb/in	5.600×10^{-3}
gallons (UK)	cu in	277.4	grams/cu cm	lb/cu ft	62.43
gallons (UK)	cu meters	4.546×10^{-3}	grams/cu cm	lb/cu in	0.03613
gallons (UK)	cu yards	5.946×10^{-3}	grams/cu cm	lb/mil-ft	3.405×10^{-7}
gallons (UK)	gallons (US)	1.20095	grams/liter	grains/gal	58.417
gallons (UK)	liters	4.546	grams/liter	lb/1,000 gal	8.345
gallons of water	lb of water	8.3453	grams/liter	lb/cu ft	0.062427
gallons/min	cu ft/sec	2.228×10^{-3}	grams/liter	parts/million	1,000.0
gallons/min	liters/sec	0.06308	grams/sq cm	lb/sq ft	2.0481
gallons/min	cu ft/hr	8.0208	gram-calories	Btu	3.9683×10^{-3}
gauss	lines/sq in	6.452	gram-calories	ergs	4.1868×10^{7}
gauss	webers/sq cm	10^{-8}	gram-calories	ft-lb	3.0880
gauss	webers/sq in	6.452×10^{-8}	gram-calories	horsepower-hr	1.5596×10^{-6}
gauss	webers/sq meter	10^{-4}	gram-calories	kilowatt-hr	1.1630×10^{-6}
gilberts	ampere-turns	0.7958	gram-calories	watt-hr	1.1630×10^{-3}
gilberts/cm	amp-turns/cm	0.7958	gram-calories/sec	Btu/hr	14.286
gilberts/cm	amp-turns/in	2.021	gram-centimeters	Btu	9.297×10^{-8}
gilberts/cm	amp-turns/meter	79.58	gram-centimeters	ergs	980.7
gills	cu cm	118.2941	gram-centimeters	joules	9.807×10^{-5}
gills	cu ft	4.1775×10^{-3}	gram-centimeters	kg-cal	2.343×10^{-8}
gills	cu in	7.21875	gram-centimeters	kg-meters	10^{-5}
gills	drams (fl)	32.0			
gills	gallons (US)	0.03125			
gills	liters	0.1183	**H**		
gills	milliliters	118.2941	hand	cm	10.16
gills	minims	1920.0	hectares	acres	2.471
gills	ounces (fl)	4.0	hectares	sq ft	1.076×10^{5}
gills	pints (liq)	0.25	hectograms	grams	100.0
gills	quarts (liq)	0.125	hectoliters	liters	100.0
gills (UK)	cu cm	142.07	hectometers	meters	100.0
grade	radian	0.01571	hectowatts	watts	100.0
grains	drams (apoth)	0.0167	henries	millihenries	1,000.0
grains	drams (avdp)	0.03657143	hogsheads (UK)	cu ft	10.114
grains	grams	0.0648	hogsheads (US)	cu ft	8.42184
grains	kilograms	6.479×10^{-5}	hogsheads (US)	gallons (US)	63
grains	milligrams	64.799	horsepower	Btu/min	42.44
grains	ounces (apoth or troy)	2.083×10^{-3}	horsepower	ft-lb/min	33,000
grains	ounces (avdp)	2.286×10^{-3}	horsepower	ft-lb/sec	550.0
grains	pennyweights	0.04167	horsepower	horsepower (metric)	1.014
grains	pounds (apoth or troy)	1.736×10^{-4}	horsepower	kg-calories/min	10.68
grains	pounds (avdp)	1.423×10^{-4}	horsepower	kilowatts	0.7457
grains	scruples	0.05	horsepower	watts	745.7
grains (troy)	grains (avdp)	1.0	horsepower (boiler)	Btu/hr	33,479
grains (troy)	grams	0.06480	horsepower (boiler)	kilowatts	9.803
grains (troy)	ounces (avdp)	2.286×10^{-3}	horsepower (metric)	horsepower	0.9863
grains (troy)	pennyweight (troy)	0.04167	horsepower (metric)	ft-lb/sec	542.5
grains/US gal	parts/million	17.118	horsepower-hours	Btu	2,547
grains/US gal	lb/million gal	142.86	horsepower-hours	ergs	2.6845×10^{13}
grains/UK gal	parts/million	14.286	horsepower-hours	ft-lb	1.98×10^{6}
grams	drams (apoth)	0.2572	horsepower-hours	gm-cal	641,190
grams	drams (avdp)	0.5644	horsepower-hours	joules	2.684×10^{6}
grams	dynes	980.7	horsepower-hours	kg-calories	641.1
grams	grains	15.43	horsepower-hours	kg-meters	2.737×10^{5}
grams	joules/cm	9.807×10^{-5}	horsepower-hours	kilowatt-hr	0.7457
grams	joules/meter (newtons)	9.807×10^{-3}	hours	days	4.167×10^{-2}
grams	kilograms	0.001	hours	weeks	5.952×10^{-3}
grams	milligrams	1,000.0	hundredweights (long)	cwt (short)	1.12
grams	ounces (apoth or troy)	0.03215	hundredweights (long)	kilograms	50.802
grams	ounces (avdp)	0.03527	hundredweights (long)	ounces	1792.0
grams	pennyweights	0.643	hundredweights (long)	pounds	112
grams	pounds (apoth or troy)	2.679×10^{-3}	hundredweights (long)	slugs	3.4811
grams	pounds (avdp)	2.205×10^{-3}	hundredweights (long)	tons (long)	0.05
grams	poundals	0.07093	hundredweights (long)	tons (short)	0.056
grams	scruples	0.7716			
grams	slugs	6.852×10^{-5}			

TABLE-56

TO CONVERT	INTO	MULTIPLY BY	TO CONVERT	INTO	MULTIPLY BY
hundredweights (short)	cwt (short)	0.8929	kilograms	joules/meters (newtons)	9.807
hundredweights (short)	kilograms	45.359	kilograms	milligrams	10^6
hundredweights (short)	ounces	1600.0	kilograms	ounces (apoth or troy)	32.151
hundredweights (short)	pounds	100.0	kilograms	ounces (avdp)	35.274
hundredweights (short)	slugs	3.1081	kilograms	pennyweights	643.015
hundredweights (short)	tons (metric)	0.0453592	kilograms	pounds (apoth or troy)	2.679
hundredweights (short)	tons (long)	0.0446429	kilograms	pounds (avdp)	2.205
hundredweights (short)	tons (short)	0.05	kilograms	poundals	70.93
			kilograms	scruples	771.62
			kilograms	slugs	0.0685
I			kilograms	tons (metric)	0.001
inches	centimeters	2.540	kilograms	tons (long)	9.842×10^{-4}
inches	feet	0.0833	kilograms	tons (short)	1.102×10^{-3}
inches	meters	2.540×10^{-2}	kilograms/cu meter	gm/cu cm	0.001
inches	miles	1.578×10^{-5}	kilograms/cu meter	lb/cu ft	0.06243
inches	miles (naut)	1.3715×10^{-5}	kilograms/cu meter	lb/cu in	3.613×10^{-5}
inches	millimeters	25.40	kilograms/cu meter	lb/mil-foot	3.405×10^{-10}
inches	mils	1,000.0	kilograms/meter	lb/ft	0.6720
inches	yards	2.778×10^{-2}	kilograms/sq cm	dynes	980,665
inches of mercury	atmospheres	0.03342	kilograms/sq cm	atmospheres	0.9678
inches of mercury	ft of water	1.133	kilograms/sq cm	ft of water	32.81
inches of mercury	kg/sq cm	0.03453	kilograms/sq cm	in of mercury	28.96
inches of mercury	kg/sq meter	345.3	kilograms/sq cm	lb/sq ft	2,048
inches of mercury	lb/sq ft	70.73	kilograms/sq cm	lb/sq in	14.22
inches of mercury	lb/sq in	0.4912	kilograms/sq meter	atmospheres	9.678×10^{-5}
inches of water (at 4°C)	atmospheres	2.458×10^{-3}	kilograms/sq meter	bars	9.807×10^{-5}
inches of water (at 4°C)	in of mercury	0.07355	kilograms/sq meter	ft of water	3.281×10^{-3}
inches of water (at 4°C)	kg/sq cm	2.540×10^{-3}	kilograms/sq meter	in of mercury	2.896×10^{-3}
inches of water (at 4°C)	oz/sq in	0.5781	kilograms/sq meter	lb/sq ft	0.2048
inches of water (at 4°C)	lb/sq ft	5.204	kilograms/sq meter	lb/sq in	1.422×10^{-3}
inches of water (at 4°C)	lb/sq in	0.03613	kilograms/sq mm	kg/sq meter	10^6
international ampere	ampere (abs)	.9998	kilograms-calories	Btu	3.968
international volt	volts (abs)	1.0003	kilogram-calories	ft-lb	3,088
international volt	joules	9.654×10^4	kilogram-calories	hp-hr	1.560×10^{-3}
			kilogram-calories	joules	4,186
J			kilogram-calories	kg-meters	426.9
joules	Btu	9.480×10^{-4}	kilogram-calories	kilojoules	4.186
joules	ergs	10^7	kilogram-calories	kilowatt-hr	1.163×10^{-3}
joules	ft-lb	0.7376	kilogram-meters	Btu	9.294×10^{-3}
joules	kg-calories	2.389×10^{-4}	kilogram-meters	ergs	9.804×10^7
joules	kg-meters	0.1020	kilogram-meters	ft-lb	7.233
joules	watt-hr	2.778×10^{-4}	kilogram-meters	joules	9.804
joules/cm	grams	1.020×10^4	kilogram-meters	kg-calories	2.342×10^{-3}
joules/cm	dynes	10^7	kilogram-meters	kilowatt-hr	2.723×10^{-6}
joules/cm	joules/meter (newtons)	100.0	kilolines	maxwells	1,000.0
joules/cm	poundals	723.3	kiloliters	liters	1,000.0
joules/cm	pounds	22.48	kilometers	centimeters	10^5
			kilometers	feet	3,281
K			kilometers	inches	3.937×10^4
kilograms	cwt (long)	0.0197	kilometers	meters	1,000.0
kilograms	cwt (short)	0.022	kilometers	miles	0.6214
kilograms	drams (apoth)	257.21	kilometers	millimeters	10^6
kilograms	drams (avdp)	564.38	kilometers	yards	1,094
kilograms	dynes	980,665	kilometers/hr	cm/sec	27.78
kilograms	grains	15,432.36	kilometers/hr	ft/min	54.68
kilograms	grams	1000.0	kilometers/hr	ft/sec	0.9113
kilograms	joules/cm	0.09807	kilometers/hr	knots	0.5396
			kilometers/hr	meters/min	16.67
			kilometers/hr	miles/hr	0.6214
			kilometers/hr/sec	cm/sec/sec	27.78
			kilometers/hr/sec	ft/sec/sec	0.9113
			kilometers/hr/sec	meters/sec/sec	0.2778
			kilometers/hr/sec	miles/hr/sec	0.6214
			kilowatts	Btu/min	56.92
			kilowatts	foot-lb/min	4.426×10^4
			kilowatts	foot-lb/sec	737.6
			kilowatts	horsepower	1.341
			kilowatts	kg-calories/min	14.34

TABLE-57

TO CONVERT	INTO	MULTIPLY BY	TO CONVERT	INTO	MULTIPLY BY
kilowatts	watts	1,000.0	meters	millimeters	1,000.0
kilowatt-hours	Btu	3,413	meters	rods	0.1988
kilowatt-hours	ergs	3.600×10^{13}	meters	yards	1.094
kilowatt-hours	ft-lb	2.655×10^6	meters	varas	1.179
kilowatt-hours	gram-calories	859,850	meters/min	cm/sec	1.667
kilowatt-hours	horsepower-hr	1.341	meters/min	ft/min	3.281
kilowatt-hours	joules	3.6×10^6	meters/min	ft/sec	0.05468
kilowatt-hours	kg-calories	860.5	meters/min	km/hr	0.06
kilowatt-hours	kg-meters	3.671×10^5	meters/min	knots	0.03238
kilowatt-hours	lb of water evap-		meters/min	miles/hr	0.03728
	orated from and at		meters/sec	feet/min	196.8
	212°F.	3.53	meters/sec	feet/sec	3.281
kilowatt-hours	lb of water raised		meters/sec	kilometers/hr	3.6
	from 62° to 212°F.	22.75	meters/sec	kilometers/min	0.06
knots	ft/hr	6,080	meters/sec	miles/hr	2.237
knots	kilometers/hr	1.8532	meters/sec	miles/min	0.03728
knots	nautical miles/hr	1.0	meters/sec/sec	cm/sec/sec	100.0
knots	statute miles/hr	1.151	meters/sec/sec	ft/sec/sec	3.281
knots	yd/hr	2,027	meters/sec/sec	km/hr/sec	3.6
knots	ft/sec	1.689	meters/sec/sec	miles/hr/sec	2.237
			meter-kilograms	cm-dynes	9.807×10^7
	L		meter-kilograms	cm-gm	10^5
league	miles (approx.)	3.0	meter-kilograms	lb-ft	7.233
light year	miles	5.9×10^{12}	microfarad	farads	10^{-6}
light year	kilometers	9.46091×10^{12}	micrograms	grams	10^{-6}
lines/sq cm	gauss	1.0	microhms	megohms	10^{-12}
lines/sq in	gauss	0.1550	microhms	ohms	10^{-6}
lines/sq in	webers/sq cm	1.550×10^{-9}	microliters	liters	10^{-6}
lines/sq in	webers/sq in	10^{-8}	microns	meters	1×10^{-6}
lines/sq in	webers/sq meter	1.550×10^{-5}	miles (naut)	feet	6,080.27
links(engineer's)	inches	12.0	miles (naut)	inches	7.2913×10^4
links(surveyor's)	inches	7.92	miles (naut)	kilometers	1.853
liters	bushels	0.02838	miles (naut)	meters	1,853
liters	cu cm	1,000.0	miles (naut)	miles (statute)	1.1516
liters	cu ft	0.03531	miles (naut)	yards	2,027
liters	cu in	61.024	miles (statute)	centimeters	1.609×10^5
liters	cu meters	0.001	miles (statute)	feet	5,280
liters	cu yards	1.308×10^{-3}	miles (statute)	inches	6.336×10^4
liters	drams (fl)	270.512	miles (statute)	kilometers	1.609
liters	gallons (US)	0.2642	miles (statute)	meters	1,609
liters	gallons (UK)	0.220	miles (statute)	miles (naut)	0.8684
liters	gills	8.454	miles (statute)	rods	320
liters	milliliters	1,000	miles (statute)	yards	1,760
liters	minims	16,230.73	miles/hr	cm/sec	44.70
liters	ounces (fl)	33.814	miles/hr	ft/min	88
liters	pecks	0.1135	miles/hr	ft/sec	1.467
liters	pints (dry)	1.8162	miles/hr	km/hr	1.609
liters	pints (liq)	2.113	miles/hr	km/min	0.02682
liters	quarts (dry)	0.9081	miles/hr	knots	0.8684
liters	quarts (liq)	1.057	miles/hr	meters/min	26.82
liters/min	cu ft/sec	5.886×10^{-4}	miles/hr	miles/min	0.01667
liters/min	gal/sec	4.403×10^{-3}	miles/hr/sec	cm/sec/sec	44.70
lumens/sq ft	foot-candles	1.0	miles/hr/sec	ft/sec/sec	1.467
lumen	spherical candle		miles/hr/sec	km/hr/sec	1.609
	power	0.07958	miles/hr/sec	meters/sec/sec	0.4470
lumen	watt	0.001496	miles/min	cm/sec	2,682
lumen/sq ft	lumen/sq meter	10.76	miles/min	ft/sec	88
lux	foot-candles	0.0929	miles/min	km/min	1.609
			miles/min	knots/min	0.8684
	M		miles/min	miles/hr	60.0
maxwells	kilolines	0.001	mil-feet	cu in	9.425×10^{-6}
maxwells	webers	10^{-8}	milliers	kilograms	1,000
megalines	maxwells	10^6	milligrams	drams (apoth)	2.572×10^{-4}
megohms	microhms	10^{12}	milligrams	drams (avdp)	5.644×10^{-4}
megohms	ohms	10^6	milligrams	grains	0.01543236
meters	centimeters	100.0	milligrams	grams	0.001
meters	feet	3.281	milligrams	kilograms	10^{-6}
meters	inches	39.37	milligrams	ounces (apoth or	
meters	kilometers	0.001		troy)	3.215×10^{-5}
meters	miles (naut)	5.396×10^{-4}	milligrams	ounces (avdp)	3.527×10^{-5}
meters	miles (stat)	6.214×10^{-4}	milligrams	pennyweights	6.43×10^{-4}

TABLE-58

TO CONVERT	INTO	MULTIPLY BY	TO CONVERT	INTO	MULTIPLY BY
milligrams	pounds (apoth or troy)	2.679×10^{-6}	ounces (avdp)	milligrams	28,349.5
milligrams	pounds (avdp)	2.2046×10^{-6}	ounces (avdp)	ounces (apoth or troy)	0.9115
milligrams	scruples	7.7162×10^{-4}	ounces (avdp)	pennyweights	18.23
milligrams/liter	parts/million	1.0	ounces (avdp)	pounds (apoth or troy)	0.0759
millihenries	henries	0.001			
milliliters	cu cm	1.0	ounces (avdp)	pounds (avdp)	0.0625
milliliters	cu ft	3.531×10^{-5}	ounces (avdp)	scruples	21.875
milliliters	cu in	0.06102	ounces (avdp)	slugs	1.9426×10^{-3}
milliliters	drams (fl)	0.2705	ounces (avdp)	tons (long)	2.790×10^{-5}
milliliters	gallons (US)	2.642×10^{-4}	ounces (avdp)	tons (metric)	2.835×10^{-5}
milliliters	gills	8.454×10^{-3}	ounces (avdp)	tons (short)	3.125×10^{-5}
milliliters	liters	0.001	ounces (apoth or troy)	drams (apoth)	8.0
milliliters	minims	16.231			
milliliters	ounces (fl)	0.0338	ounces (apoth or troy)	drams (avdp)	17.554
milliliters	pints (liq)	2.113×10^{-3}			
milliliters	quarts (liq)	1.057×10^{-3}	ounces (apoth or troy)	grains	480.0
millimeters	centimeters	0.1			
millimeters	feet	3.281×10^{-3}	ounces (apoth or troy)	grams	31.103481
millimeters	inches	0.03937			
millimeters	kilometers	10^{-6}	ounces (apoth or troy)	kilograms	0.0311
millimeters	meters	0.001			
millimeters	miles	6.214×10^{-7}	ounces (apoth or troy)	milligrams	31,103.48
millimeters	mils	39.37			
millimeters	yards	1.094×10^{-3}	ounces (apoth or troy)	ounces (avdp)	1.09714
millimeters of Hg	atmospheres	1.316×10^{-3}			
millimeters of Hg	torr	1.0	ounces (apoth or troy)	pennyweights	20.0
millimicrons	meters	1×10^{-9}			
million gals/day	cu ft/sec	1.54723	ounces (apoth or troy)	pounds (apoth or troy)	0.08333
mils	centimeters	2.540×10^{-3}			
mils	feet	8.333×10^{-5}	ounces (apoth or troy)	pounds (avdp)	0.0686
mils	inches	0.001			
mils	kilometers	2.540×10^{-8}	ounces (apoth or troy)	scruples	24.0
mils	yards	2.778×10^{-5}			
miner's inches	cu ft/min	1.5	ounces (fl)	cu cm	29.5735
minims (UK)	cu cm	0.059192	ounces (fl)	cu ft	1.0444×10^{-3}
minims	cu cm	0.061612	ounces (fl)	cu in	1.805
minims	cu ft	2.176×10^{-6}	ounces (fl)	drams (fl)	8.0
minims	cu in	3.7598×10^{-3}	ounces (fl)	gallons (US)	7.8125×10^{-3}
minims	drams (fl)	0.0167	ounces (fl)	gills	0.25
minims	gallons (US)	1.628×10^{-5}	ounces (fl)	liters	0.02957
minims	gills	5.208×10^{-4}	ounces (fl)	milliliters	29.5735
minims	liters	6.161×10^{-5}	ounces (fl)	minims	480.0
minims	milliliters	0.061612	ounces (fl)	pints (liq)	0.0625
minims	ounces (fl)	0.0021	ounces (fl)	quarts (liq)	0.03125
minims	pints (liq)	1.302×10^{-4}	ounces/sq in	dynes/sq cm	4309
minims (liq)	quarts (liq)	6.51×10^{-5}	ounces/sq in	pounds/sq in	0.0625
minutes (angles)	degrees	0.01667			
minutes (angles)	quadrants	1.852×10^{-4}	**P**		
minutes (angles)	radians	2.909×10^{-4}	parsecs	miles	19×10^{12}
minutes (angles)	seconds	60.0	parsecs	kilometers	3.084×10^{13}
myriagrams	kilograms	10.0	parts/million	grains/US gal	0.0584
myriameters	kilometers	10.0	parts/million	grains/UK gal	0.07016
myriawatts	kilowatts	10.0	parts/million	lb/million gal	8.345
			pecks (UK)	cu in	554.6
			pecks (UK)	liters	9.091901
N			pecks	bushels	0.25
nepers	decibels	8.686	pecks	cu ft	0.3111
newtons	dynes	1×10^5	pecks	cu in	537.605
			pecks	cu meters	8.8098×10^{-3}
O			pecks	liters	8.8098
ohm (Int)	ohm (abs)	1.0005	pecks	pints (dry)	16.0
ohms	megohms	10^{-6}	pecks	quarts (dry)	8.0
ohms	microhms	10^6	pennyweights	drams (apoth)	0.4
ounces (avdp)	cwt (long)	5.5804×10^{-4}	pennyweights	drams (avdp)	0.8777
ounces (avdp)	cwt (short)	6.25×10^{-4}	pennyweights	grains	24.0
ounces (avdp)	drams (apoth)	7.292	pennyweights	grams	1.55517
ounces (avdp)	drams (avdp)	16.0	pennyweights	kilograms	1.555×10^{-3}
ounces (avdp)	grains	437.5	pennyweights	milligrams	1,555.17
ounces (avdp)	grams	28.349527	pennyweights	ounces (apoth or troy)	0.05
ounces (avdp)	kilograms	0.0283			

TABLE-59

TO CONVERT	INTO	MULTIPLY BY	TO CONVERT	INTO	MULTIPLY BY
pennyweights	ounces (avdp)	0.0549	pounds (apoth or troy)	ounces (apoth or troy)	12.0
pennyweights	pounds (apoth or troy)	4.1667×10^{-3}	pounds (apoth or troy)	ounces (avdp)	13.1657
pennyweights	pounds (avdp)	3.428×10^{-3}	pounds (apoth or troy)	pennyweights	240.0
pennyweights	scruples	1.2	pounds (apoth or troy)	pounds (avdp)	0.822857
pints (dry)	bushels	0.0156	pounds (apoth or troy)	scruples	288.0
pints (dry)	cu ft	0.0194	pounds (apoth or troy)	tons (long)	3.6753×10^{-4}
pints (dry)	cu in	33.60			
pints (dry)	cu meters	5.506×10^{-4}	pounds (apoth or troy)	tons (metric)	3.7324×10^{-4}
pints (dry)	liters	0.5506			
pints (dry)	pecks	0.0625	pounds (apoth or troy)	tons (short)	4.1143×10^{-4}
pints (dry)	quarts (dry)	0.5	pounds of water	cu ft	0.01602
pints (liq)	cu cm	473.2	pounds of water	cu in	27.68
pints (liq)	cu ft	0.01671	pounds of water	gallons	0.1198
pints (liq)	cu in	28.875	pounds of water/min	cu ft/sec	2.670×10^{-4}
pints (liq)	cu meters	4.732×10^{-4}	pound-feet	cm-dynes	1.356×10^{7}
pints (liq)	cu yards	6.189×10^{-4}	pound-feet	cm-gm	13,825
pints (liq)	drams (fl)	128.0	pound-feet	meter-kg	0.1383
pints (liq)	gallons (US)	0.125	pounds/cu ft	gm/cu cm	0.01602
pints (liq)	gills	4.0	pounds/cu ft	kg/cu meter	16.02
pints (liq)	liters	0.4732	pounds/cu ft	lb/cu in	5.787×10^{-4}
pints (liq)	milliliters	473.2	pounds/cu ft	lb/mil-foot	5.456×10^{-9}
pints (liq)	minims	7680.0	pounds/cu in	gm/cu cm	27.68
pints (liq)	ounces (fl)	16.0	pounds/cu in	kg/cu meter	2.768×10^{4}
pints (liq)	quarts (liq)	0.5	pounds/cu in	lb/cu ft	1,728
Planck's quantum	erg-sec	6.624×10^{-27}	pounds/cu in	lb/mil-foot	9.425×10^{-6}
poise	gm/cm sec	1.00	pounds/ft	kg/meter	1.488
poundals	dynes	13,826	pounds/in	gm/cm	178.6
poundals	grams	14.10	pounds/mil-foot	gm/cu cm	2.306×10^{6}
poundals	joules/cm	1.383×10^{-3}	pounds/sq ft	atmospheres	4.725×10^{-4}
poundals	joules/meter (newtons)	0.1383	pounds/sq ft	ft of water	0.01602
poundals	kilograms	0.01410	pounds/sq ft	in of mercury	0.01414
poundals	pounds	0.03108	pounds/sq ft	kg/sq meter	4.882
pounds (avdp)	cwt (long)	8.929×10^{-3}	pounds/sq ft	lb/sq in	6.944×10^{-3}
pounds (avdp)	cwt (short)	0.01	pounds/sq in	atmospheres	0.06804
pounds (avdp)	drams (apoth)	116.67	pounds/sq in	ft of water	2.307
pounds (avdp)	drams (avdp)	256.0	pounds/sq in	in of mercury	2.036
pounds (avdp)	dynes	44.4823×10^{4}	pounds/sq in	kg/sq meter	703.1
pounds (avdp)	grains	7,000.0	pounds/sq in	lb/sq ft	144.0
pounds (avdp)	grams	453.5924			
pounds (avdp)	joules/cm	0.04448		**Q**	
pounds (avdp)	joules/meter (newtons)	4.448	quadrants (angle)	degrees	90.0
pounds (avdp)	kilograms	0.4536	quadrants (angle)	minutes	5,400.0
pounds (avdp)	milligrams	453,592.37	quadrants (angle)	radians	1.571
pounds (avdp)	ounces (apoth or troy)	14.5833	quadrants (angle)	seconds	3.24×10^{5}
pounds (avdp)	ounces (avdp)	16.0	quarts (dry)	bushels	0.0313
pounds (avdp)	pennyweights	291.667	quarts (dry)	cu ft	0.0389
pounds (avdp)	poundals	32.17	quarts (dry)	cu in	67.20
pounds (avdp)	pounds (apoth or troy)	1.21528	quarts (dry)	cu meters	1.101×10^{-3}
pounds (avdp)	scruples	350.0	quarts (dry)	liters	1.1012
pounds (avdp)	slugs	3.108×10^{-2}	quarts (dry)	pecks	0.125
pounds (avdp)	tons (long)	4.464×10^{-4}	quarts (dry)	pints (dry)	2.0
pounds (avdp)	tons (metric)	4.536×10^{-4}	quarts (liq)	cu cm	946.4
pounds (avdp)	tons (short)	5.0×10^{-4}	quarts (liq)	cu ft	0.03342
pounds (apoth or troy)	drams (apoth)	96.0	quarts (liq)	cu in	57.75
pounds (apoth or troy)	drams (avdp)	210.65	quarts (liq)	cu meters	9.464×10^{-4}
pounds (apoth or troy)	grains	5,760.0	quarts (liq)	cu yards	1.238×10^{-3}
pounds (apoth or troy)	grams	373.2417	quarts (liq)	drams (fl)	256.0
			quarts (liq)	gallons (US)	0.25
pounds (apoth or troy)	kilograms	0.3732	quarts (liq)	gills	8.0
			quarts (liq)	liters	0.9464
pounds (apoth or troy)	milligrams	373,241.72	quarts (liq)	milliliters	946.4
			quarts (liq)	minims	15,360.0
			quarts (liq)	ounces (fl)	32.0
			quarts (liq)	pints (liq)	2.0

TABLE-60

TO CONVERT	INTO	MULTIPLY BY	TO CONVERT	INTO	MULTIPLY BY
R			square feet	sq miles	3.587×10^{-8}
radians	degrees	57.30	square feet	sq mm	9.290×10^{4}
radians	minutes	3,438	square feet	sq yd	0.1111
radians	quadrants	0.6366	square inches	circular mils	1.273×10^{6}
radians	seconds	2.063×10^{5}	square inches	sq cm	6.452
radians/sec	degrees/sec	57.30	square inches	sq ft	6.944×10^{-3}
radians/sec	rev/min	9.549	square inches	sq mm	645.2
radians/sec	rev/sec	0.1592	square inches	sq mils	10^{6}
radians/sec/sec	rev/min/min	573.0	square inches	sq yd	7.716×10^{-4}
radians/sec/sec	rev/min/sec	9.549	square kilometers	acres	247.1
radians/sec/sec	rev/sec/sec	0.1592	square kilometers	sq cm	10^{10}
revolutions	degrees	360.0	square kilometers	sq ft	1.076×10^{7}
revolutions	quadrants	4.0	square kilometers	sq in	1.550×10^{9}
revolutions	radians	6.283	square kilometers	sq meters	10^{6}
revolutions/min	degrees/sec	6.0	square kilometers	sq miles	0.3861
revolutions/min	radians/sec	0.1047	square kilometers	sq yd	1.196×10^{6}
revolutions/min	rev/sec	0.01667	square meters	acres	2.471×10^{-4}
revolutions/min/min	radians/sec/sec	1.745×10^{-3}	square meters	sq cm	10^{4}
revolutions/min/min	rev/min/sec	0.01667	square meters	sq ft	10.76
revolutions/min/min	rev/sec/sec	2.778×10^{-4}	square meters	sq in	1,550
revolutions/sec	degrees/sec	360.0	square meters	sq miles	3.861×10^{-7}
revolutions/sec	radians/sec	6.283	square meters	sq mm	10^{6}
revolutions/sec	rev/min	60.0	square meters	sq yd	1.196
revolutions/sec/sec	radians/sec/sec	6.283	square miles	acres	640.0
revolutions/sec/sec	rev/min/min	3,600.0	square miles	sq ft	2.788×10^{7}
revolutions/sec/sec	rev/min/sec	60.0	square miles	sq km	2.590
rods	chain (Gunter's)	0.25	square miles	sq meters	2.590×10^{6}
rods	meters	5.029	square miles	sq yd	3.098×10^{6}
rods (surveyors' measure)	yards	5.5	square millimeters	circular mils	1,973
rods	feet	16.5	square millimeters	sq cm	0.01
			square millimeters	sq ft	1.076×10^{-5}
S			square millimeters	sq in	1.550×10^{-3}
scruples	drams (apoth)	0.3333	square mils	circular mils	1.273
scruples	drams (avdp)	0.7314	square mils	sq cm	6.452×10^{-6}
scruples	grains	20.0	square mils	sq in	10^{-6}
scruples	grams	1.296	square yards	acres	2.066×10^{-4}
scruples	kilograms	1.296×10^{-3}	square yards	sq cm	8,361
scruples	milligrams	1295.97	square yards	sq ft	9.0
scruples	ounces (apoth or troy)	0.0417	square yards	sq in	1,296
scruples	ounces (avdp)	0.0457	square yards	sq meters	0.8361
scruples	pennyweights	0.8333	square yards	sq miles	3.228×10^{-7}
scruples	pounds (apoth or troy)	3.472×10^{-3}	square yards	sq mm	8.361×10^{5}
scruples	pounds (avdp)	2.857×10^{-3}			
seconds (angle)	degrees	2.778×10^{-4}	**T**		
seconds (angle)	minutes	0.01667	temperature (°C) + 273	absolute temperature (K)	1.0
seconds (angle)	quadrants	3.087×10^{-6}	temperature (°C) + 17.78	temperature (°F)	1.8
seconds (angle)	radians	4.848×10^{-6}	temperature (°F) + 460	absolute temperature (°Rank)	1.0
slugs	cwt (long)	0.2873	temperature (°F) − 32	temperature (°C)	5/9
slugs	cwt (short)	0.3217	tons (long)	cwt (long)	20
slugs	grams	1.459×10^{4}	tons (long)	cwt (short)	22.4
slugs	kilograms	14.59	tons (long)	kilograms	1,016
slugs	ounces (avdp)	514.79	tons (long)	ounces (avdp)	35,840.0
slugs	pounds (avdp)	32.17	tons (long)	pounds (avdp)	2,240.0
slugs	tons (long)	1.436×10^{-2}	tons (long)	slugs	69.621
slugs	tons (short)	1.609×10^{-2}	tons (long)	tons (metric)	1.0160
sphere	steradians	12.57	tons (long)	tons (short)	1.120
square centimeters	circular mils	1.973×10^{5}	tons (metric)	cwt (short)	22.046
square centimeters	sq ft	1.076×10^{-3}	tons (metric)	kilograms	1,000.0
square centimeters	sq in	0.1550	tons (metric)	ounces (avdp)	35,273.96
square centimeters	sq meters	0.0001	tons (metric)	pounds (avdp)	2,205
square centimeters	sq miles	3.861×10^{-11}	tons (metric)	tons (long)	0.9842
square centimeters	sq mm	100.0	tons (metric)	tons (short)	1.1023
square centimeters	sq yd	1.196×10^{-4}	tons (short)	cwt (long)	17.857
square feet	acres	2.296×10^{-5}	tons (short)	cwt (short)	20.0
square feet	circular mils	1.833×10^{8}	tons (short)	grams	9.072×10^{5}
square feet	sq cm	929.0	tons (short)	kilograms	907.1847
square feet	sq in	144.0			
square feet	sq meters	0.09290			

TABLE-61

Universal Conversion Factors (Continued)

TO CONVERT	INTO	MULTIPLY BY	TO CONVERT	INTO	MULTIPLY BY
tons (short)	ounces (apoth or troy)	29,166.66	watts (abs)	Btu (mean)/min	0.056884
tons (short)	ounces (avdp)	32,000.0	watts (abs)	joules/sec	1
tons (short)	pounds (apoth or troy)	2,430.56	watt-hours	Btu	3.413
tons (short)	pounds (avdp)	2,000.0	watt-hours	ergs	3.60×10^{10}
tons (short)	slugs	62.16	watt-hours	ft-lb	2,656
tons (short)	tons (long)	0.89286	watt-hours	gm-cal	859.85
tons (short)	tons (metric)	0.9072	watt-hours	horsepower-hr	1.341×10^{-3}
tons (short)/sq ft	kg/sq meter	9,765	watt-hours	kg-cal	0.8605
tons (short)/sq ft	lb/sq in	2,000	watt-hours	kg-meters	367.2
tons of water/24 hr	lb of water/hr	83.333	watt-hours	kilowatt-hr	0.001
tons of water/24 hr	gal/min	0.16643	watt (int)	watt (abs)	1.0002
tons of water/24 hr	cu ft/hr	1.3349	webers	maxwells	10^8
torr	mm of mercury	1.0	webers	kilolines	10^5
torr	atmospheres	1.316×10^{-3}	webers/sq in	gauss	1.550×10^7
V			webers/sq in	lines/sq in	10^8
volt/inch	volt/cm	0.39370	webers/sq in	webers/sq cm	0.1550
volt (abs)	statvolts	0.003336	webers/sq in	webers/sq meter	1,550
W			webers/sq meter	gauss	10^4
watts	Btu/hr	3.4129	webers/sq meter	lines/sq in	6.452×10^4
watts	Btu/min	0.05688	webers/sq meter	webers/sq cm	10^{-4}
watts	ergs/sec	10^7	webers/sq meter	webers/sq in	6.452×10^{-4}
watts	ft-lb/min	44.27	**Y**		
watts	ft-lb/sec	0.7378	yards	centimeters	91.44
watts	horsepower	1.341×10^{-3}	yards	feet	3.0
watts	horsepower (metric)	1.360×10^{-3}	yards	inches	36.0
watts	kg-calories/min	0.01433	yards	kilometers	9.144×10^{-4}
watts	kilowatts	0.001	yards	meters	0.9144
			yards	miles (naut)	4.934×10^{-4}
			yards	miles (stat)	5.682×10^{-4}
			yards	millimeters	914.4

TABLE-62

Table of Minerals

Minerals are naturally occurring, homogeneous solids formed in the Earth's crust by the inorganic forces of nature, and possess definite, but generally not fixed, chemical compositions, physical characteristics, and highly ordered atomic arrangements. This table contains a group of common minerals selected for their relative importance and frequency of occurrence. Several physical properties commonly used to identify minerals have been included for each entry. The information provided here should be used with the understanding that there is a certain amount of variation in physical properties from specimen to specimen. For more information about the material presented here, consult the references cited at the end of the table.

Streak is the color of a finely powdered mineral obtained by rubbing the mineral on a streak plate, which is an unglazed piece of porcelain.

Since minerals are frequently polymorphic, the crystal system reported in the table is that of the most commonly observed form. The term amorphous (amor) is used to describe noncrystalline minerals that lack an ordered atomic arrangement. The crystal systems have been abbreviated in the table as follows:

hex	hexagonal	ortho	orthorhombic
iso	isometric	tet	tetragonal
mono	monoclinic	trig	trigonal

Hardness, which is the resistance of a smooth surface of a mineral to scratching, is expressed in terms of the Mohs' Hardness Scale. This relative scale spans from 1-9 and is defined as follows:

<2.5	can be scratched by a fingernail
>2.5-3	cannot be scratched by a fingernail; can be scratched by a copper cent
>3-5.5	cannot be scratched by a copper cent; can be scratched by a knife
>5.5-<7	cannot be scratched by a knife; can be scratched by quartz
>7	cannot be scratched by quartz

Mineral	Composition	Color	Streak	Crystal System	Hardness	Index of Refraction	Specific Gravity
Acanthite	Ag_2S	gray-black	black	mono	2-2.5	-	7.3
Actinolite	$Ca_2(Mg,Fe)_5Si_8O_{22}(OH)_2$	green	white	mono	6	1.64	3.0-3.4
Aegirine	$NaFeSi_2O_6$	dark green, brown, black	white	mono	6	1.82	3.6
Allanite	$(Ca,Ce)_3(Al,Fe)_2Si_3O_{12}(OH)$	brown to pitch-black	colorless	mono	5.5-6	1.70-1.81	3.5-4.2
Almandine	$Fe_3Al_2Si_3O_{12}$	red to black	white	iso	7-7.5	1.83	4.0-4.3
Alunite	$KAl_3(SO_4)_2(OH)_6$	white, red	colorless	hex	4	1.57	2.6-2.8
Amblygonite	$LiAlFPO_4$	white, pale green, blue	colorless	trig	6	1.60	3.0-3.1
Analcime	$NaAlSi_2O_6.H_2O$	colorless, white	colorless	iso	5-5.5	1.48-1.49	2.27
Anatase	TiO_2	brown	white	tet	5.5-6	2.6	3.9
Andalusite	Al_2SiO_5	reddish-brown, white, gray	colorless	ortho	7.5	1.64	3.16-3.20
Andradite	$Ca_3Fe_2Si_3O_{12}$	yellow, green, brown, black	white	iso	7-7.5	1.89	3.8-3.9
Anglesite	$PbSO_4$	colorless, white	colorless	ortho	3	1.88	6.2-6.4
Anhydrite	$CaSO_4$	colorless	colorless	ortho	3-3.5	1.58	2.89-2.98
Anthophyllite	$(Mg,Fe)_7Si_8O_{22}(OH)_2$	white, gray	colorless	ortho	5.5-6	1.61-1.71	2.85-3.2
Antimony	Sb	white to gray	gray	hex	3-3.5	-	6.7
Antlerite	$Cu_3(SO_4)(OH)_4$	dark emerald-green	light green	ortho	3.5-4	1.74	3.88
Apatite	$Ca_5(PO_4)_3(F,Cl,OH)$	green, blue, violet, brown, colorless	colorless	hex	5	1.63	3.15-3.20
Apophyllite	$KCa_4(Si_4O_{10})_2F.8H_2O$	colorless, white	colorless	tet	4.5-5	1.54	2.3-2.4
Aragonite	$CaCO_3$	colorless, white	colorless	ortho	3.5-4	1.68	2.95
Argentite	Ag_2S	black	dark gray-black	iso	2-2.5	-	7.2-7.4
Arsenic	As	tin-white	gray	hex	3.5	-	5.7

TABLE-63

Table of Minerals (Continued)

Mineral	Composition	Color	Streak	Crystal System	Hardness	Index of Refraction	Specific Gravity
Arsenopyrite	FeAsS	silver-white	black	mono	5.5-6	-	6.0-6.2
Atacamite	$Cu_2Cl(OH)_3$	emerald-green	light green	ortho	3-3.5	1.86	3.75-3.77
Augite	$(Ca,Na)(Mg,Fe,Al)$ $(Si,Al)_2O_6$	black, dark green	white	mono	6	1.67-1.73	3.25-3.55
Autunite	$Ca(UO_2)_2(PO_4)_2.10-12H_2O$	lemon-yellow	yellow	tet	2-2.5	1.58	3.1-3.2
Axinite	$(Ca,Fe,Mn)_3Al_2(BO_3)$ $(Si_4O_{12})(OH)$	clove-brown	colorless	trig	6.5-7	1.69	3.27-3.35
Azurite	$Cu_3(CO_3)_2(OH)_2$	azure-blue	light blue	mono	3.5-4	1.76	3.77
Barite	$BaSO_4$	colorless, white	colorless	ortho	3-3.5	1.64	4.5
Bauxite	A mixture of Al hydroxides	yellow, brown, gray, white	colorless	-	1-3	-	2.0-2.55
Beryl	$Be_3Al_2(Si_6O_{18})$	bluish-green, yellow, colorless	colorless	hex	7.5-8	1.57-1.61	2.65-2.8
Biotite	$K(Mg,Fe)_3(AlSi_3O_{10})$ $(OH)_2$	dark brown, green to black	colorless	mono	2.5-3	1.61-1.70	2.95-3
Bismuth	Bi	silver-white	silver-white	hex	2-2.5	-	9.8
Boehmite	γ-AlO(OH)	white, yellow, brown	white	ortho	3	1.65	3.0-3.1
Borax	$Na_2B_4O_5(OH)_4.8H_2O$	colorless, white	colorless	mono	2-2.5	1.47	1.71
Bornite	Cu_5FeS_4	brownish-bronze	gray-black	tet	3	-	5.1
Boulangerite	$Pb_5Sb_4S_{11}$	bluish-lead-gray	brownish-gray	mono	2.5-3	-	6.23
Bournonite	$PbCuSbS_3$	steel-gray to black	steel-gray to black	ortho	2.5-3	-	5.8-5.9
Braunite	$3Mn_2O_3.MnSiO_3$	gray to black	gray to black	tet	6-6.5	-	4.7-4.8
Brochantite	$Cu_4SO_4(OH)_6$	green	green	mono	3.5-4	1.78	4.0
Brookite	TiO_2	brown to black	white to gray	ortho	5.5-6	2.6	4.1
Brucite	$Mg(OH)_2$	white, gray, green	colorless	hex	2.5	1.57	2.39
Bustamite	$(Mn,Ca,Fe)SiO_3$			trig	5.5-6.5	1.67-1.70	3.3-3.4
Calaverite	$AuTe_2$	tin-white to brass yellow	yellowish to green-gray	mono	2.5	-	9.4
Calcite	$CaCO_3$	colorless, white	colorless	hex	3	1.66	2.71
Cancrinite	$Na_6Ca_2(AlSiO_4)_6$ $(CO_3)_2$	yellow, white, pink	white	hex	6	1.52	2.4-2.5
Carnallite	$KMgCl_3.6H_2O$	colorless, white	white	ortho	2.5	1.48	1.60
Carnotite	$K_2(UO_2)_2$ $(VO_4)_2.3 H_2O$	yellow	yellow	mono	2	1.93	4-5
Cassiterite	SnO_2	brown to black	white	tet	6-7	2.00	6.8-7.1
Celestite	$SrSO_4$	colorless, white, pale blue	colorless	ortho	3-3.5	1.62	3.95-3.97
Cerussite	$PbCO_3$	colorless, white	colorless	ortho	3-3.5	2.08	6.55
Chabazite	$Ca_2Al_2Si_4O_{12}.6H_2O$	white, flesh-red	colorless	hex	4-5	1.48	2.05-2.15
Chalcanthite	$CuSO_4.5H_2O$	blue	pale blue	trig	2.5	1.54	2.28
Chalcocite	Cu_2S	steel-gray	gray-black	ortho	2.5-3	-	5.7

TABLE-64

Table of Minerals (Continued)

Mineral	Composition	Color	Streak	Crystal System	Hardness	Index of Refraction	Specific Gravity
Chalcopyrite	$CuFeS_2$	brass-yellow	greenish-black	tet	3.5-4	-	4.1-4.3
Chlorargyrite	AgCl	pearl-gray, colorless	colorless	iso	2-3	2.07	~5.5
Chlorite	$Mg,Fe_3(Si,Al)_4O_{10}$ $(OH)_2.(Mg,Fe)_3(OH)_6$	green of various shades	colorless	mono	2-2.5	1.57-1.67	2.6-2.9
Chloritoid	$(Fe,Mg,Mn)_2(Al,Fe)$ $Al_3O_2(SiO_4)_2(OH)_4$	grassy green	white	mono	6.5	1.72-1.73	3.58-3.61
Chondrodite	$Mg_5(SiO_4)_2(F,OH)_2$	light yellow, brown	colorless	mono	6-6.5	1.60-1.63	3.1-3.2
Chromite	$FeCr_2O_4$	iron-black to brownish black	dark brown	iso	5.5	2.16	4.6
Chrysoberyl	$BeAl_2O_4$	yellowish to green	colorless	ortho	8.5	1.75	3.65-3.8
Chrysocolla	$(Cu,Al)_2H_2Si_2O_5$ $(OH)_4.nH_2O$	light green to turquoise-blue	light blue	amor	2-4	~4	2.0-2.4
Cinnabar	HgS	red to vermillion	bright red	hex	2-2.5	2.81	8.1
Clinozoisite	$Ca_2Al_3OSi_3O_{12}(OH)$	grayish-white, green	colorless	mono	6-6.5	1.67-1.72	3.25-3.37
Cobaltite	CoAsS	silver-white	gray-black	iso	5.5-6	-	6.3
Colemanite	$CaB_3O_4(OH)_3.H_2O$	colorless, white	colorless	mono	4-4.5	1.59	2.42
Columbite	$(Fe,Mn)Nb_2O_6$	black	dark brown to black	ortho	6	-	5.3-7.3
Copper	Cu	copper-red	copper-red	iso	2.5-3	-	8.9
Cordierite	$(Mg,Fe)_2Al_4Si_5$ $O_{18}.nH_2O$	blue, gray, brown	colorless	ortho	7-7.5	1.53-1.57	2.60-2.66
Corundum	Al_2O_3	gray, blue, pink, brown	white	trig	9	1.77	4.0
Covellite	CuS	indigo-blue to black	lead-gray to black	hex	1.5-2	-	4.6
Cristobalite	SiO_2	colorless, white	colorless	iso	7	1.48	2.32
Crocoite	$PbCrO_4$	red	orange-yellow	mono	2.5-3	2.36	5.9-6.1
Cryolite	Na_3AlF_6	colorless, white	colorless	mono	2.5	1.34	2.95-3.0
Cummingtonite	$(Fe,Mg,Mn)_7Si_8O_{22}$ $(OH)_2$	brown	white	mono	6	1.66-1.68	3.2-3.6
Cuprite	Cu_2O	red	brownish-red	iso	3.5-4	-	6.0
Danburite	$CaB_2(SiO_4)_2$	-	-	ortho	7	1.63	2.97-3.02
Datolite	$CaB(SiO_4)(OH)$	colorless, pale green	colorless	mono	5-5.5	1.65	2.8-3.0
Diamond	C	colorless, yellow, black	colorless	iso	10	2.42	3.5
Diaspore	AlO(OH)	white, gray	colorless	ortho	6.5-7	1.72	3.35-3.45
Diopside	$Ca(Mg,Fe)Si_2O_6$	white, green	white	mono	6	1.67	3.25-3.40
Dioptase	$CuSiO_2(OH)_2$	green		hex	5	1.65	3.3
Dolomite	$CaMg(CO_3)_2$	colorless, white, pink	colorless	hex	3.5-4	1.68	2.85
Enargite	Cu_3AsS_4	gray-black	gray-black	ortho	3	-	4.4
Enstatite	$MgSiO_3$	gray-brown, green, brown	colorless	ortho	5.5	1.65	3.2-3.5

TABLE-65

Mineral	Composition	Color	Streak	Crystal System	Hardness	Index of Refraction	Specific Gravity
Epidote	$Ca_2(Al,Fe)Al_2(SiO_4)_3$ (OH)	yellowish to blackish green	colorless	mono	6-7	1.72-1.78	3.35-3.45
Epsomite	$MgSO_4.7H_2O$	white	white	ortho	2	1.46	1.67
Erythrite	$Co_3(AsO_4)_2.8H_2O$	red to pink	pink	mono	1.5-2.5	1.66	3.06
Euclase	$BeAl(SiO_4)(OH)$	-	-	mono	7.5	1.66	3.1
Eucryptite	$LiAlSiO_4$	-	-	hex	-	1.55	2.67
Fayalite	Fe_2SiO_4	-	-	ortho	6.5	1.86	4.39
Fluorite	CaF_2	colorless, violet, green	colorless	iso	4	1.43	3.18
Franklinite	$(Fe,Zn,Mn)(Fe,Mn)_2O_4$	iron-black	dark brown	iso	6	-	5.15
Gahnite	$ZnAl_2O_4$	dark green	colorless	iso	7.5-8	1.80	4.55
Galena	PbS	lead-gray	lead-gray	iso	2.5	-	7.6
Garnet	$(Ca,Mg,Fe,Mn)_3$ $(Al,Fe,Cr)_2(SiO_4)_3$	brown to red	-	iso	6.5-7.5	1.71-1.88	3.5-4.3
Gersdorffite	$NiAsS$	silver-white	gray-black	iso	5.5	-	6.3
Gibbsite	$Al(OH)_3$	white, red, brown	white	mono	2.5-3.5	1.57	2.3-2.4
Glauconite	$(K,Na)(Fe,Mg,Al)_2$ $(Si,Al)_4O_{10}(OH)_2$	dark green to black	pale green	mono	2	1.62	2.5-2.8
Glaucophane	$Na_2Mg_3Al_2Si_8O_{22}$ $(OH)_2$	blue, blue-black	white	mono	6	1.62-1.67	3.0-3.3
Goethite	α-$FeO(OH)$	yellow-brown to dark brown	yellow-brown	ortho	5-5.5	2.39	4.37
Gold	Au	gold-yellow	gold-yellow	iso	2.5-3	-	15.0-19.3
Graphite	C	steel-gray to iron-black	black	hex	1-1.5	-	2.23
Grossular	$Ca_3Al_2Si_3O_{12}$	white, green, brown	white	iso	7-7.5	1.73	3.6
Grunerite	$Fe_7Si_8O_{22}(OH)_2$	light brown	colorless	mono	6	1.71	3.6
Gypsum	$CaSO_4.2H_2O$	colorless, white, gray	colorless	mono	2	1.52	2.32
Halite	$NaCl$	colorless, white	colorless	iso	2.5	1.54	2.1-2.3
Hausmannite	Mn_3O_4	brownish black	brown	tet	5.5-6	-	4.84
Hedenbergite	$CaFeSi_2O_6$	green to black	white	mono	5-6	1.73	3.40-3.55
Hematite	Fe_2O_3	red to vermillion	red-brown	hex	5.5-6.5	-	5.2
Hemimorphite	$Zn_4(Si_2O_7)$ $(OH)_2.H_2O$	white	colorless	ortho	4.5-5	1.62	3.4-3.5
Heulandite	$CaAl_2Si_7O_{18}.6H_2O$	colorless, white	colorless	mono	3.5-4	1.48	2.18-2.20
Hornblende	$NaCa_2(Mg,Fe,Al)_5$ $(Al,Si)_8O_{22}(OH)_2$	green, brown, black	white	mono	5-6	1.62-1.72	3.0-3.4
Humite	$(Mg,Fe)_7(SiO_4)_3$ $(F,OH)_2$	yellow, brownish red	white	ortho	6-6.5	1.64	3.15-3.35
Hypersthene	$(Mg,Fe)SiO_3$	brown, black	white	ortho	5-6	1.68-1.73	3.4-4.0
Ilmenite	$FeTiO_3$	black	black	hex	5.5-6	-	4.7
Iron	Fe	gray	gray	iso	4	-	7.8
Jadeite	$NaAlSi_2O_6$	green, white	colorless	mono	6.5-7	1.66	3.3-3.5

TABLE-66

Mineral	Composition	Color	Streak	Crystal System	Hardness	Index of Refraction	Specific Gravity
Jamesonite	$Pb_4FeSb_6S_{14}$	steel-gray to gray-black	steel-gray to gray-black	mono	2-3	-	5.5-6.0
Jarosite	$KFe_3(SO_4)_2(OH)_6$	brown	yellow	trig	3	1.82	2.9-3.3
Kainite	$KMg(Cl,SO_4).2\,3/4\,H_2O$	-	-	mono	3	1.51	2.1
Kaolinite	$Al_2Si_2O_5(OH)_4$	white	colorless	trig	2-2.5	1.55	2.6-2.63
Kernite	$Na_2B_4O_6(OH)_2.3H_2O$	colorless, white	colorless	mono	3	1.47	1.95
Kyanite	Al_2SiO_5	blue	colorless	trig	5-7	1.72	3.56-3.66
Laumontite	$CaAl_2Si_4O_{12}.4H_2O$	white	white	mono	4	1.52	2.25-2.30
Lawsonite	$CaAl_2(Si_2O_7)(OH)_2.H_2O$	colorless, gray, pink	colorless	ortho	8	1.67	3.09
Lazulite	$(Mg,Fe)Al_2(PO_4)_2(OH)_2$	azure-blue	colorless	mono	5-5.5	1.64	3.0-3.1
Lazurite	$(Na,Ca)_8(AlSiO_4)_6(SO_4,S,Cl)_2$	azure-blue, greenish-blue	colorless	iso	5-5.5	1.50	2.4-2.45
Lepidolite	$K(Li,Al)_{2-3}(AlSi_3O_{10})(O,OH,F)_2$	pink to grayish white	colorless	mono	2.5-4	1.55-1.59	2.8-3.0
Leucite	$KAlSi_2O_6$	gray, white	colorless	iso	5.5-6	1.51	2.45-2.50
Lithiophilite	$Li(Mn,Fe)PO_4$	bluish-gray	colorless	ortho	4.5-5	1.67	3.5
Magnesite	$MgCO_3$	white, yellow	colorless	hex	3.5-5	1.70	3.0-3.2
Magnetite	Fe_3O_4	black	black	iso	6	-	5.18
Malachite	$Cu_2CO_3(OH)_2$	bright green	light green	mono	3.5-4	1.88	3.9-4.03
Manganite	$MnO(OH)$	steel-gray to iron-black	dark brown	mono	4	-	4.3
Marcasite	FeS_2	pale yellow	grayish-black	iso	6-6.5	-	4.9
Margarite	$CaAl_2(Al_2Si_2O_{10})(OH)_2$	pink, gray, white	colorless	mono	3.5-5	1.65	3.0-3.1
Melanterite	$FeSO_4.7H_2O$	pale green	white	mono	2	1.48	1.90
Melilite	$Ca_2Al(AlSiO_7) - Ca_2Mg(Si_2O_7)$	nearly color-less, reddish brown, gray	white	tet	5-6	-	2.94-3.05
Microcline	$KAlSi_3O_8$	colorless, white	colorless	trig	6	1.53	2.54-2.56
Microlite	$Ca_2Ta_2O_6(O,OH,F)$	yellow, brown, black	yellow to brown	iso	5.5	1.92-1.99	5.48-5.56
Millerite	NiS	brass-yellow	greenish-black	hex	3-3.5	-	5.5
Mimetite	$Pb_5(AsO_4)_3Cl$	white, yellow	white	hex	3.5-4	2.1-2.2	7.2-7.3
Molybdenite	MoS_2	lead-gray	grayish-black	hex	1-1.5	-	4.7
Monazite	$(Ce,La,Y,Th)PO_4$	yellowish-brown	colorless	mono	5-5.5	1.79	5.0-5.3
Monticellite	$CaMgSiO_4$			ortho	5	1.65	3.2
Montmorillonite	$(Al,Mg)_2Si_4O_{10}(OH)_2.nH_2O$	white, gray, green-gray	white	mono	2	1.50-1.64	2.0-2.7
Muscovite	$KAl_2(AlSi_3)O_{10}(OH)_2$	colorless, pale tints	colorless	mono	2-2.5	1.60	2.76-2.88
Natrolite	$Na_2Al_2Si_3O_{10}.2H_2O$	colorless, white	colorless	ortho	5-5.5	1.48	2.25
Nepheline	$(Na,K)AlSiO_4$	colorless, gray, brown	colorless	hex	5.5-6	1.54	2.55-2.65

TABLE-67

Table of Minerals (Continued)

Mineral	Composition	Color	Streak	Crystal System	Hardness	Index of Refraction	Specific Gravity
Nickel Skutterudite	$(Ni,Co)As_3$	silver-white	black	iso	5.5	-	6.1-6.9
Nickeline	$NiAs$	pale copper-red	brown-black	hex	5-5.5	-	7.8
Niter	KNO_3	white	colorless	ortho	2	1.50	2.09-2.14
Nitratite	$NaNO_3$	colorless, white	colorless	hex	1-2	1.59	2.29
Olivine	$(Mg,Fe)_2SiO_4$	olive to grayish-green	colorless	ortho	6.5-7	1.69	3.27-4.37
Opal	$SiO_2.nH_2O$	colorless, white	colorless	amor	5-6	1.44	1.9-2.2
Orpiment	As_2S_3	lemon-yellow	yellow	mono	1.5-2	2.8	3.49
Orthoclase	$KAlSi_3O_8$	colorless, white	colorless	mono	6	1.52	2.54-2.56
Pectolite	$Ca_2NaH(SiO_3)_3$	white	colorless	trig	5	1.60	2.7-2.8
Pentlandite	$(Fe,Ni)_9S_8$	yellowish-bronze	bronze-brown	iso	3.5-4	-	4.6-5.0
Periclase	MgO	white	white	iso	5	1.73	3.58
Phenacite	Be_2SiO_4	white, colorless	colorless	hex	7.5-8	1.65	2.97-3.0
Phlogopite	$KMg_3(AlSi_3O_{10})(OH)_2$	pale brown	colorless	mono	2.5-3	1.56-1.64	2.86
Plagioclase	$(Na,Ca)(Al,Si)_4O_8$	colorless, white, gray	colorless	trig	6	1.53-1.59	2.62
Platinum	Pt	steel-gray	steel-gray	iso	4-4.5	-	14-19
Prehnite	$Ca_2Al(AlSi_3O_{10})(OH)_2$	apple-green, white	colorless	ortho	6-6.5	1.63	2.8-2.95
Proustite	Ag_3AsS_3	ruby-red	bright red	hex	2-2.5	3.09	5.55
Pumpellyite	$Ca_2MgAl_2(SiO_4)(Si_2O_7)(OH)_2.H_2O$	bluish green to nearly white	white	mono	5.5-6	-	3.18-3.23
Pyrargyrite	Ag_3SbS_3	red	red	hex	2.5	3.08	5.85
Pyrite	FeS_2	pale brass-yellow	brownish-black	iso	6-6.5	-	5.0
Pyrochlore	$(Ca,Na)_2(Nb,Ta)_2O_6(OH,F)$	yellow, brown, black	white	iso	5-5.5	-	4.2-6.4
Pyrolusite	MnO_2	iron-black	black	tet	1-2	-	4.7
Pyromorphite	$Pb_5(PO_4)_3Cl$	green, brown, yellow, gray	colorless	hex	3.5-4	2.06	6.5-7.1
Pyrope	$Mg_3Al_2Si_3O_{12}$	red to black	white	iso	7-7.5	1.71	3.6
Pyrophyllite	$Al_2Si_4O_{10}(OH)_2$	white, gray, green	colorless	mono	1-2	1.59	2.8-2.9
Pyrrhotite	$Fe_{1-x}S$	brownish-bronze	black	mono	4	-	4.6
Quartz	SiO_2	colorless, white, various colors	colorless	hex	7	1.54	2.65
Realgar	AsS	red	red to orange	mono	1.5-2	2.60	3.48
Rhodochrosite	$MnCO_3$	pink, rose-red, brown	colorless	hex	3.5-4.5	1.82	3.45-3.6
Rhodonite	$MnSiO_3$	pink, brown	colorless	trig	5.5-6	1.73-1.75	3.58-3.70
Riebeckite	$Na_2(Mg,Fe)_3Fe_2Si_8O_{22}(OH)_2$	dark blue, black	blue-gray	mono	6	1.66-1.71	3.3-3.6
Romanechite	$BaMn_9O_{16}(OH)_4$	black	black	ortho	5-6	-	3.7-4.7

TABLE-68

Mineral	Composition	Color	Streak	Crystal System	Hardness	Index of Refraction	Specific Gravity
Rutile	TiO_2	reddish-brown	pale brown	tet	6-6.5	2.61	4.18-4.25
Scapolite	$3NaAlSi_3O_8.NaCl - 3CaAlSi_2O_8.CaCO_3$	white, pink, gray	colorless	tet	5-6	1.55-1.60	2.65-2.74
Scheelite	$CaWO_4$	white, yellow, brown	colorless	tet	4.5-5	1.92	5.9-6.1
Serpentine	$Mg_3Si_2O_5(OH)_4$	shades of green	colorless	mono	2-5	1.55	2.3-2.66
Shattuckite	$Cu_5(SiO_3)_4(OH)_2$	blue		ortho	-	1.78	3.8
Siderite	$FeCO_3$	light to dark brown	yellow, brown	hex	3.5-4	1.88	3.83-3.88
Sillimanite	Al_2SiO_5	white, brown, gray	colorless	ortho	6-7	1.66	3.23
Silver	Ag	silver-white	silver-white	iso	2.5-3	-	10.5
Skutterudite	$(Co,Ni)As_3$	silver-white	black	iso	5.5-6	-	6.1-6.9
Smithsonite	$ZnCO_3$	green, blue, white	colorless	hex	5	1.85	4.35-4.40
Sodalite	$Na_8(AlSiO_4)_6Cl_2$	blue, white	colorless	iso	5.5-6	1.48	2.15-2.3
Sperrylite	$PtAs_2$	tin-white	black	iso	6-7	-	10.6
Spessartine	$Mn_3Al_2Si_3O_{12}$	orange, red, brown	white	iso	7-7.5	1.80	4.0-4.2
Sphalerite	ZnS	yellow-brown to black	white to yellow-brown	iso	3.5	2.37	3.9-4.1
Spinel	$MgAl_2O_4$	red, black, blue, green, brown	colorless	iso	8	1.72	3.6-4.0
Spodumene	$LiAlSi_2O_6$	white, gray, pink, green	colorless	mono	6.5-7	1.67	3.15-3.20
Staurolite	$Fe_2Al_9O_6(SiO_4)_4(O,OH)_2$	red-brown	colorless	ortho	7-7.5	1.75	3.65-3.75
Stibnite	Sb_2S_3	lead-gray to black	lead-gray to black	ortho	2	-	4.5
Stilbite	$NaCa_2Al_5Si_{13}O_{36}.14H_2O$	white	colorless	mono	3.5-4	1.50	2.1-2.2
Stilpnomelane	$K(Fe,Mg)_6Si_8Al(O,OH)_{27}.2-4H_2O$	black, yellowish to reddish brown	white	mono	3-4	1.58-1.74	2.59-2.96
Stromeyerite	$(Ag,Cu)_2S$	steel-gray	-	ortho	2.5-3	-	6.2-6.3
Strontianite	$SrCO_3$	colorless, white	colorless	ortho	3.5-4	1.67	3.7
Sulfur	S	yellow	colorless	ortho	1.5-2.5	2.04	2.05-2.09
Sylvanite	$(Au,Ag)Te_2$	tin-white	gray	mono	2	-	8-8.2
Sylvite	KCl	colorless, white	colorless	iso	2	1.49	1.99
Talc	$Mg_3Si_4O_{10}(OH)_2$	white, green, gray	colorless	mono	1	1.59	2.7-2.8
Tantalite	$(Fe,Mn)Ta_2O_6$	black	dark brown to black	ortho	6	-	5.3-7.3
Tennantite	$Cu_{12}As_4S_{13}$	black	brown to black	iso	3-4.5	-	4.6-5.1
Tetrahedrite	$Cu_{12}Sb_4S_{13}$	grayish black	black	iso	3-4.5	-	4.7-5.0
Thorite	$ThSiO_4$	brown to black	white	tet	5	1.8	5.3
Titanite	$CaTiO(SiO_4)$	brown, green, yellow	colorless	mono	5-5.5	1.91	3.4-3.55

TABLE-69

Mineral	Composition	Color	Streak	Crystal System	Hardness	Index of Refraction	Specific Gravity
Topaz	$Al_2SiO_4(F,OH)_2$	colorless, yellow, blue	colorless	ortho	8	1.61-1.63	3.4-3.6
Torbernite	$Cu(UO_2)_2(PO_4)_2.8-12H_2O$	emerald-green to apple-green	green	tet	2-2.5	1.59	3.2-3.7
Tourmaline	$(Na,Ca)(Li,Mg,Al)(Al,Fe,Mn)_6(BO_3)_3(Si_6O_{18})(OH)_4$	black, green, brown, blue, pink	colorless	hex	7-7.5	1.64-1.68	3.0-3.25
Tremolite	$Ca_2Mg_5Si_8O_{22}(OH)_2$	white	white	mono	6	1.61	3.0
Tridymite	SiO_2	colorless	colorless	hex	7	1.47	2.26
Triphylite	$Li(Fe,Mn)PO_4$	bluish-gray	colorless	ortho	4.5-5	1.69	3.42-3.56
Turquoise	$CuAl_6(PO_4)_4(OH)_8.5H_2O$	blue, bluish-green	colorless	trig	6	1.62	2.6-2.8
Ulexite	$NaCaB_5O_6(OH)_6.5 H_2O$	white	colorless	trig	1-2.5	1.50	1.96
Uraninite	UO_2	black	brownish-black	iso	5.5	-	9.0-9.7
Uvarovite	$Ca_3Cr_2Si_3O_{12}$	green	white	iso	7.5	1.87	3.90
Vanadinite	$Pb_5(VO_4)_3Cl$	ruby-red, brown, yellow	colorless	hex	3	2.25-2.42	6.7-7.1
Vermiculite	$(Mg,Fe,Al)_3(Al,Si)_4O_{10}(OH)_2.4H_2O$	yellow, brown, green	white	mono	1.5	1.55-1.58	2.4
Vesuvianite	$Ca_{10}(Mg,Fe)_2Al_4Si_9O_{34}(OH)_4$	green, brown, yellow, blue	colorless	tet	6.5	1.70-1.75	3.35-4.45
Vivianite	$Fe_3(PO_4)_2.8H_2O$	blue, blue-green	blue	mono	1-1.5	1.60	2.7
Wavellite	$Al_3(PO_4)_2(OH)_3.5 H_2O$	green, white, brown	colorless	ortho	3.5-4	1.54	2.33
Willemite	Zn_2SiO_4	yellow-green, white, brown	colorless	hex	5.5	1.69	3.9-4.2
Witherite	$BaCO_3$	colorless, white	colorless	ortho	3.5	1.68	4.3
Wolframite	$(Fe,Mn)WO_4$	brown to black	black to brown	mono	4-4.5	-	7.0-7.5
Wollastonite	$CaSiO_3$	colorless, white	colorless	trig	5-5.5	1.63	2.8-2.9
Wulfenite	$PbMoO_4$	yellow, red	colorless	tet	3	2.40	6.8
Wurtzite	ZnS	brownish black	brown	hex	3.5-4	2.35	4.09
Xenotime	YPO_4	yellowish to reddish brown	white	tet	4-5	-	4.4-5.1
Zincite	ZnO	red to orange-yellow	orange-yellow	hex	4-4.5	2.01	5.68
Zircon	$ZrSiO_4$	brown, gray, colorless	colorless	tet	7.5	1.92-1.96	4.68
Zoisite	$Ca_2Al_3Si_3O_{12}(OH)$	gray, green, pink	white	ortho	7	1.69	3.3

References

1. L. G. Berry *et al., Mineralogy: Concepts, Descriptions, Determinations* (W. H. Freeman and Co., San Francisco, 2nd ed., 1983).
2. A. M. Clark, *Hey's Mineral Index: Mineral Species, Varieties and Synonyms* (Chapman & Hall, London, 3rd ed., 1993).
3. C. Klein, C. S. Hurlbut, Jr., *Manual of Mineralogy* (John Wiley & Sons, New York, 20th ed., 1985).
4. P. G. Read, *Dictionary of Gemmology* (Butterworth, Heinemann, Oxford, 2nd ed., 1988).

TABLE-70

ORGANIC NAME REACTIONS

ORGANIC NAME REACTIONS

The Organic Name Reactions (ONR) section is intended to serve the professional chemist and student by describing organic chemical reactions which have come to be recognized and referred to by name within the chemistry community. A select group has been chosen for addition to this section. Each reaction description is designed to be informative and representative of the pertinent literature; however, it is not meant to be comprehensive. The descriptions are composed of the following: (1) name(s) associated with the reaction, (2) the original and/or primary contributor(s) connected with the discovery and/or development of the reaction, (3) a concise description of the transformation, (4) a reaction scheme, (5) key references, and (6) cross references to other ONR based on commonalities. An index to this section follows the reactions monographs.

Abbreviations

Ac	acetyl	E	electrophile
Ar	aryl	ee	enantiomeric excess
aq	aqueous	Et	ethyl
B	base	ETOH	ethanol
BBN	borabicyclo[3.3.1]nonane	EWG	electron withdrawing group
BINAP	2,2′-bix(diphenylphosphino)-1,1′-binaphthyl	HA	protic acid
BOC	t-butyloxycarbonyl	HMPT	hexamethylphosphoric triamide
Bu	butyl	LDA	lithium diisopropylamide
cat	catalytic	LHMDS	lithium hexamethyldisilazide
Cp	cyclopentadienide	Me	methyl
Δ	heat	NuH	nucleophile
dba	dibenzylideneacetone	Ph	phenyl
DCC	dicyclohexylcarbodiimide	Pr	propyl
DEAD	diethylazadicarboxylate	salen	N,N′-ethylenebis(salicylideneimine)
DME	dimethylether	Tf	trifluoromethanesulfonyl
dppf	dichloro[1,1′-bis(diphenylphosphino)ferrocene]	Ts	p-toluenesulfonyl
dppp	1,3-bis(diphenylphosphino)propane		

Organic Name Reactions

1. Acetoacetic Ester Synthesis

Base-catalyzed alkylation or arylation of β-ketoesters. Subsequent mild hydrolysis and decarboxylation yield substituted acetones. Alternately, treatment with concentrated base produces substituted esters:

$$CH_3COCH_2COOCH_2CH_3 \xrightarrow[\text{RX}]{\text{base}} H_3C-\underset{\underset{O}{\|}}{C}(R)-COOCH_2CH_3$$

$$\text{conc OH}^- \swarrow \qquad \searrow \text{H}^+ \text{ or dil OH}^-$$

$$CH_3COOH + RCH_2COOCH_2CH_3 \qquad CH_3COCH_2R$$

Synthetic applications: R. Kluger, M. Brandl, *J. Org. Chem.* **51**, 3964 (1986); T. Yamamitsu *et al., J. Chem. Soc. Perkin Trans. 1* **1989**, 1811.

2. Acyloin Condensation

L. Bouveault, R. Loquin, *Compt. Rend.* **140**, 1593 (1905).

Reductive coupling of esters by sodium to yield acyloins (α-hydroxyketones). Yields are greatly improved in the presence of trimethylchlorosilane:

K. T. Finley, *Chem. Rev.* **64**, 573 (1964); K. Ziegler, *Houben-Weyl* **4/2**, 729-822 (1955); S. M. McElvain, *Org. React.* **4**, 256 (1948); J. J. Bloomfield *et al., ibid.* **23**, 259 (1976); R. Brettle, *Comp. Org. Syn.* **3**, 613-632 (1991). *Cf.* Benzoin Condensation.

3. Akabori Amino Acid Reactions

S. Akabori, *J. Chem. Soc. Jpn.* **52**, 606 (1931); *Ber.* **66**, 143, 151 (1933); *J. Chem. Soc.* **64**, 608 (1943).

1. Formation of aldehydes by oxidative decomposition of α-amino acids when heated with sugars according to the equation:

$$RCHCOOH \ (\overset{NH_2}{|}) \xrightarrow[\text{sugar}]{O_2} RCHO + CO_2 + NH_3$$

2. Reduction of α-amino acids and esters by sodium amalgam and ethanolic hydrogen chloride to the corresponding α-amino aldehydes:

$$R-\underset{\overset{|}{NH_2}}{C}-COOEt \xrightarrow[\text{HCl/EtOH}]{\text{NaHg}} R-\underset{\overset{|}{NH_2}}{C}-CHO$$

3. Formation of alkamines by heating mixtures of aromatic aldehydes and amino acids. No reaction was observed with tertiary amino groups.

E. Takagi *et al., J. Pharm. Soc. Jpn.* **71**, 648 (1951); **72**, 812 (1952); A. Lawson, H. V. Morley, *J. Chem. Soc.* **1955**, 1695; A. Lawson, *ibid.* **1956**, 307; K. Dose, *Ber.* **90**, 1251 (1957); V. N. Belikov *et al., Izv. Akad. Nauk SSSR Ser. Khim.* **1969**, 2536.

4. Aldol Reaction (Condensation)

R. Kane, *Ann. Phys. Chem., Ser. 2,* **44**, 475 (1838); *idem, J. Prakt. Chem.* **15**, 129 (1838).

Traditionally, it is the acid- or base-catalyzed condensation of one carbonyl compound with the enolate/enol of another, which may or may not be the same, to generate a β-hydroxy carbonyl compound — an aldol. The method is compromised by self-condensation, polycondensation, generation of regioisomeric enols/enolates, and dehydration of the aldol followed by Michael addition, *q.v.* The development of methods for the preparation and use of preformed enolates or enol derivatives, that dictate specific carbon-carbon bond formation, have revolutionized the coupling of carbonyl compounds:

Organic Name Reactions

MX = LDA, LHMDS, CH₃MgBr, Bu₂BOTf/NR₃, 9-BBNCl/NR₃, LDA + ZnCl₂,
LDA + (C₅H₅)₂ZrCl₂, LDA + Ti(O-iPr)₃Cl
Lewis acid = TiCl₄, SnCl₄, AlCl₃, BF₃ • O(CH₂CH₃)₂, ZnCl₂

Historical perspective: C. H. Heathcock, *Comp. Org. Syn.* **2**, 133-179 (1991). General review: T. Mukaiyama, *Org. React.* **28**, 203-331 (1982). Application of lithium and magnesium enolates: C. H. Heathcock, *Comp. Org. Syn.* **2**, 181-238 (1991); of boron enolates: B. M. Kim *et al., ibid.* 239-275; of transition metal enolates: I. Paterson, *ibid.* 301-319. Stereoselective reactions of ester and thioester enolates: M. Braun, H. Sacha, *J. Prakt. Chem.* **335**, 653-668 (1993). Review of asymmetric methodology: A. S. Franklin, I. Paterson, *Contemp. Org. Synth.* **1**, 317-338 (1994). *Cf.* Claisen-Schmidt Condensation; Henry Reaction; Ivanov Reaction; Knoevenagel Condensation; Reformatsky Reaction; Robinson Annulation.

5. Algar-Flynn-Oyamada Reaction
J. Algar, J. P. Flynn, *Proc. R. Irish Acad.* **42B**, 1 (1934); B. Oyamada, *J. Chem. Soc. Jpn.* **55**, 1256 (1934).

Alkaline hydrogen peroxide oxidation of *o*-hydroxyphenyl styryl ketones (chalcones) to flavonols *via* the intermediate dihydroflavonols:

T. S. Wheeler, *Rec. Chem. Prog.* **18**, 133 (1957); W. P. Cullen *et al., J. Chem. Soc. C* **1971**, 2848. Mechanism: T. R. Gormley, *et al., Tetrahedron* **29**, 369 (1973); M. Bennett *et al., ibid.* **54**, 9911 (1998). Synthetic applications: H. Wagner *et al., ibid.* **33**, 1405 (1977); A. C. Jain *et al., Bull. Chem. Soc. Jpn.* **56**, 1267 (1983). *Cf.* Auwers Synthesis.

6. Allan-Robinson Reaction
J. Allan, R. Robinson, *J. Chem. Soc.* **125**, 2192 (1924).

Preparation of flavones or isoflavones by condensing *o*-hydroxyaryl ketones with anhydrides of aromatic acids and their sodium salts:

S. F. Dyke *et al., J. Org. Chem.* **26**, 2453 (1961); Seshandri in *The Chemistry of Flavonoid Compounds*, T. A. Geissman, Ed. (New York, 1962) p 182; Gripenberg, *ibid.* p 411; W. Rahman, K. T. Nasim, *J. Org. Chem.* **27**, 4215 (1962); D. L. Dreyer *et al., Tetrahedron* **20**, 2977 (1964). Synthesis applications: P. K. Dutta *et al., Indian J. Chem.* **21B**, 1037 (1982); T. Horie *et al., Chem. Pharm. Bull.* **37**, 1216 (1989); J. K. Makrandi *et al., Synth. Commun.* **19**, 1919 (1989); E. J. Corey *et al., Tetrahedron Lett.* **37**, 7162 (1996); B. P. Reddy *et al., J. Heterocycl. Chem.* **33**, 1561 (1996). *Cf.* Baker-Venkataraman Rearrangement; Kostanecki Acylation.

7. Allylic Rearrangements
L. Claisen, *Ber.* **45**, 3157 (1912).

Migration of a carbon-carbon double bond in a three carbon (allylic) system on treatment with nucleophiles under S_N1 conditions (or under S_N2 conditions when the nucleophilic attack takes place at the γ-carbon):

Reviews: J. R. DeWolfe, W. G. Young, *Chem. Rev.* **56,** 753 (1956); W. G. Young, *J. Chem. Educ.* **39,** 455 (1962); P. de la Mare in *Molecular Rearrangements* Part 1, P. de Mayo, Ed. (Wiley-Interscience, New York, 1963) pp 27-110; K. Mackenzie in *The Chemistry of Alkenes*, S. Patai, Ed. (Interscience, New York, 1964) pp 436-453; R. H. DeWolfe, W. G. Young in *ibid.* pp 681-738; J. March, *Advanced Organic Chemistry* (Wiley-Interscience, New York, 4th ed., 1992) pp 327-330.

8. Amadori Rearrangement

M. Amadori, *Atti Accad. Naz. Lincei* **2**(6), 337 (1925), *C.A.* **20,** 902 (1926); *ibid.* **9**(6), 68, 226 (1929), *C.A.* **23,** 3211, 3443 (1929).

Conversion of *N*-glycosides of aldoses to *N*-glycosides of the corresponding ketoses by acid or base catalysis:

J. E. Hodge, *Adv. Carbohydr. Chem.* **10,** 169 (1955); R. U. Lemieux in *Molecular Rearrangements* Part 2, P. de Mayo, Ed. (Wiley-Interscience, New York, 1964) p 753. ^{13}C-NMR studies: W. Funcke, *Ann.* **1978,** 2099. *Review:* K. Maruoka, H. Yamamoto, *Comp. Org. Syn.* **6,** 789-791 (1991).

9. Arens-van Dorp Synthesis; Isler Modification

D. A. van Dorp, J. F. Arens, *Nature* **160,** 189 (1947); J. F. Arens *et al., Rec. Trav. Chim.* **68,** 604, 609 (1949); O. Isler *et al., Helv. Chim. Acta* **39,** 259 (1956).

The preparation of alkoxyethynyl alcohols from ketones and ethoxyacetylene. In the **Isler modification** the tedious preparation of ethoxyacetylene is obviated by treating β-chlorovinyl ether with lithium amide to yield lithium ethoxyacetylene, which is then condensed with the ketone:

H. Heusser *et al., Helv. Chim. Acta* **33,** 370 (1950); J. F. Arens, *Adv. Org. Chem.* **2,** 117-212 (1960); H. Meerwein, *Houben-Weyl* **6/3,** 189 (1965). *Cf.* Favorskii-Babayan Synthesis; Nef Synthesis.

10. Arndt-Eistert Synthesis

F. Arndt, B. Eistert, *Ber.* **68,** 200 (1935).

Homologation of carboxylic acids:

Alternative reagent for diazomethane: T. Aoyama, *Tetrahedron Lett.* **21,** 4461 (1980). Application to synthesis of unsaturated diazoketones: T. Hudlicky *et al., ibid.* **1979,** 2667; K. Gademann *et al., Angew. Chem. Int. Ed.* **38,** 1223 (1999); via ultrasonic activation: J-Y. Winum *et al., Tetrahedron Lett.* **37,** 1781 (1996); of amino acids: R. E. Marti *et al., ibid.* **38,** 6145 (1997); R. J. DeVita *et al., Bioorg. Med. Chem. Lett.* **9,** 2621 (1999). *Reviews:* W. E. Bachmann, W. S. Struve, *Org. React.* **1,** 38-62 (1942); B. Eistert in *Newer Methods of Preparative Organic Chemistry* **vol. 1** (Interscience, New York, 1948) pp 513-570; G. B. Gill, *Comp. Org. Syn.* **3,** 888-889 (1991). *Cf.* Wolff Rearrangement.

11. Auwers Synthesis

K. v. Auwers *et al., Ber.* **41,** 4233 (1908); **48,** 85 (1915); **49,** 809 (1916); K. v. Auwers, P. Pohl, *Ann.* **405,** 243 (1914).

Expansion of coumarones to flavonols by treatment of 2-bromo-2-(α-bromobenzyl)coumarones with alcoholic alkali:

T. H. Minton, H. Stephen, *J. Chem. Soc.* **121,** 1598 (1922); J. Kalff, R. Robinson, *ibid.* **127,** 1968 (1925); B. H. Ingham *et al., ibid.* **1931,** 895; B. G. Acharya *et al., ibid.* **1940,** 817; S. Wawzonek, *Heterocycl. Compd.* **2,** 245 (1951). *Cf.* Algar-Flynn-Oyamada Reaction.

12. Baeyer-Drewson Indigo Synthesis

A. Baeyer, V. Drewson, *Ber.* **15**, 2856 (1882).

Formation of indigos by an aldol reaction, *q.v.*, of *o*-nitrobenzaldehydes to acetone, pyruvic acid or acetaldehyde; of interest mainly as a method of protecting *o*-nitrobenzaldehydes:

$$\text{o-nitrobenzaldehyde (CHO, NO}_2\text{)} + CH_3COCH_3 \xrightarrow{\text{dil NaOH}} \text{CHOHCH}_2\text{COCH}_3 \text{ (NO}_2\text{)} \longrightarrow \text{indigo}$$

K. Venkataraman, *Chemistry of Synthetic Dyes* **2**, 1008 (New York, 1952); M. Sainsbury, *Rodd's Chemistry of Carbon Compounds* **IVB**, 346, 353 (1977). Synthetic applications: J. R. Mckee *et al., J. Chem. Educ.* **68**, A242 (1991); L. Fitjer *et al., Tetrahedron* **55**, 14421 (1999).

13. Baeyer-Villiger Reaction

A. Baeyer, V. Villiger, *Ber.* **32**, 3625 (1899); **33**, 858 (1900).

The oxidation of ketones to esters or lactones by peracids:

$$\text{cyclohexyl-COCH}_3 \xrightarrow{RCO_3H} \text{cyclohexyl-O-CO-CH}_3$$

$$\text{cyclopentanone} \xrightarrow{RCO_3H} \text{lactone}$$

Reviews: P. A. S. Smith in *Molecular Rearrangements* Part 1, P. de Mayo, Ed. (Wiley-Interscience, New York, 1963) pp 577-591; J. B. Lee, B. C. Uff, *Q. Rev. Chem. Soc.* **21**, 429-457 (1967); C. H. Hassall, *Org. React.* **9**, 73 (1957); G. R. Krow, *ibid.* **43**, 251-798 (1993); *idem, Comp. Org. Syn.* **7**, 671-688 (1991); G.-J. ten Brink *et al., Chem. Rev.* **104**, 4105-4123 (2004).

14. Baker-Venkataraman Rearrangement

W. Baker, *J. Chem. Soc.* **1933**, 1381; H. S. Mahal, K. Venkataraman, *ibid.* **1934**, 1767.

Base-catalyzed rearrangement of *o*-acyloxyketones to β-diketones, important intermediates in the synthesis of chromones and flavones:

$$\text{(COCH}_3, \text{OCOC}_6H_5\text{)} \xrightarrow{\text{base}} \text{(COCH}_2\text{COC}_6H_5, \text{OH)}$$

Gripenberg in *The Chemistry of Flavonoid Compounds*, Geissman, Ed. (New York, 1962) p 410. Mechanistic studies: K. Bowden, M. Chehel-Amiran, *J. Chem. Soc. Perkin Trans. 2* **1986**, 2039. Synthetic applications: P. K. Jain *et al., Synthesis* **1982**, 221; J. Zhu *et al., Chem. Commun.* **1988**, 1549; A. V. Kalinin *et al., Tetrahedron Lett.* **39**, 4995 (1998); D. C. G. Pinto *et al., New J. Chem.* **24**, 85 (2000). *Cf.* Allan-Robinson Reaction; Kostanecki Acylation.

15. Bamberger Rearrangement

E. Bamberger, *Ber.* **27**, 1347, 1548 (1894).

Intermolecular rearrangement of *N*-phenylhydroxylamines in aqueous acid to give the corresponding 4-amino-phenols:

$$\text{C}_6H_5\text{-N(H)-OH} \xrightarrow[H_2O]{H_2SO_4} \text{HO-C}_6H_4\text{-NH}_2$$

Early review: H. J. Shine, *Aromatic Rearrangements* (Elsevier, New York, 1967) pp 182-190. Kinetic and mechanistic study: G. Kohnstam *et al., J. Chem. Soc. Perkin Trans. 2* **1984**, 423. Synthetic application: D. Johnston, D. Elder, *J. Labelled Compd. Radiopharm.* **25**, 1315 (1988). Modified conditions: A. Zoran *et al., Chem. Commun.* **1994**, 2239; M. Tordeux, C. Wakselman, *J. Fluorine Chem.* **74**, 251 (1995).

16. Bamford-Stevens Reaction; Shapiro Reaction

W. R. Bamford, T. S. Stevens, *J. Chem. Soc.* **1952**, 4735.

Formation of olefins by base-promoted decomposition of *p*-toluenesulfonylhydrazones of aldehydes and ketones:

$$R-\underset{\underset{H}{|}}{\overset{\overset{R^1}{|}}{C}}-C(R^2)=N-NHTs \xrightarrow{\underset{HOCH_2CH_2OH}{Na}} R-\underset{\underset{H}{|}}{\overset{\overset{R^1}{|}}{C}}=C-R^2$$

The formation of unrearranged alkenes, generally the less substituted isomers, by treatment of ketone derived *p*-toluenesulfonylhydrazones with alkyl lithium reagents is known as the **Shapiro reaction:** R. H. Shapiro, M. J. Heath, *J. Am. Chem. Soc.* **89,** 5734 (1967). Use of *N,N*-diethylaminosulfonylhydrazones: J. Kang *et al., Bull. Korean Chem. Soc.* **13,** 192 (1992).

Silicon directing effect: T. K. Sarkar, B. K. Ghorai, *Chem. Commun.* **1992,** 1184. *Reviews:* R. H. Shapiro, *Org. React.* **23,** 405-507 (1976); R. M. Adlington, A. G. M. Barrett, *Acc. Chem. Res.* **16,** 55-59 (1983); K. Maruka, H. Yamamoto, *Comp. Org. Syn.* **6,** 776-779 (1991); A. R. Chamberlin, D. J. Sall, *ibid.* **8,** 944-949.

17. Barbier(-type) Reaction
P. Barbier, *C.R. Hebd. Seances Acad. Sci.* **128,** 110 (1899).

One-step procedure for the preparation of alcohols from organic halides and aldehydes or ketones:

$$R-X \;+\; \underset{O}{\overset{O}{\|}} \quad \xrightarrow{M} \quad \overset{HO \; R}{\diagup\diagdown}$$

M = Mg, Li, Sm(II), Zn   R = alkyl, aryl, vinyl, allyl   X = Cl, Br, I

Review of mechanistic studies of Sm-mediated coupling: D. P. Curran *et al., Synlett* **1992,** 943-961. Book: C. Blomberg, *The Barbier Reaction and Related One-Step Processes,* K. Hafner *et al.,* Eds. (Springer-Verlag, New York, 1993) 183 pp. Zn-promoted coupling: F. Hong *et al., Chem. Commun.* **1994,** 289. Sm-mediated coupling: M. Kunishima *et al., Chem. Pharm. Bull.* **42,** 2190 (1994). Comparison with Ni(0) insertion chemistry for intramolecular cyclization: M. Kihara *et al., Tetrahedron* **48,** 67 (1992). *Cf.* Grignard Reaction.

18. Barbier-Wieland Degradation
H. Wieland, *Ber.* **45,** 484 (1912); P. Barbier, R. Locquin, *Compt. Rend.* **156,** 1443 (1913).

Stepwise carboxylic acid degradation of aliphatic acids (particularly in sterol side chains) to the next lower homolog. The ester is converted to a tertiary alcohol that is dehydrated with acetic anhydride, and the olefin oxidized with chromic acid to a lower homologous carboxylic acid:

$$RCH_2COOCH_3 \xrightarrow[\text{2. HX}]{\text{1. 2PhMgX}} RCH_2COHPh_2 \xrightarrow{Ac_2O} RCH{=}CHPh_2 \xrightarrow{CrO_3} RCOOH + Ph_2CO$$

H. Wieland *et al., Z. Physiol. Chem.* **161,** 80 (1926); C. W. Shoppee, *Ann. Repts.* (Chem. Soc., London) **44,** 184 (1947); W. Baker *et al., J. Chem. Soc.* **1958,** 1007; J. R. Dias, R. Ramachandra, *Tetrahedron Lett.* **1976,** 3685. Synthetic applications: S. C. Wilcox, J. J. Guadino, *J. Am. Chem. Soc.* **108,** 3102 (1986); C. D. Schteingart, A. E. Hofmann, *J. Lipid Res.* **29,** 1387 (1988). *Cf.* Krafft Degradation; Miescher Degradation.

19. Bart Reaction; Scheller Modification
H. Bart, **DE 250264** (1910); **DE 254092** (1910); **DE 264924** (1910); **DE 268172** (1912); *Ann.* **429,** 55 (1922); E. Scheller, **GB 261026**; A. W. Ruddy *et al., J. Am. Chem. Soc.* **64,** 828 (1942).

Formation of aromatic arsonic acids by treating aromatic diazonium compounds with alkali arsenites in the presence of cupric salts or powdered silver or copper; in the **Scheller modification** primary aromatic amines are diazotized in the presence of arsenious chloride and a trace of cuprous chloride:

$$PhN_2{}^+Cl^- + Na_3AsO_3 \longrightarrow PhAsO_3Na_2 + NaCl + N_2$$

$$PhNH_2 + HNO_2 + AsCl_3 + (H_2O) \longrightarrow PhAsO_3H_2 + N_2 + 3HCl$$

The modified Bart reaction can be applied to the formation of arylstibonic acids:

$$ArNH_2 + HNO_2 + SbCl_3 + (H_2O) \longrightarrow ArSbO_3H_2 + N_2 + 3HCl$$

C. F. Hamilton, J. F. Morgan, *Org. React.* **2,** 415 (1944); G. O. Doak, H. G. Steinman, *J. Am. Chem. Soc.* **68,** 1987 (1946); K. H. Saunders, *Aromatic Diazo-Compounds and Their Technical Applications* (London, 1949) p 330; W. A. Cowdry, D. S. Davies, *Q. Rev. Chem. Soc.* **6,** 363 (1952).

20. Bartoli Indole Synthesis
G. Bartoli *et al., Tetrahedron Lett.* **30,** 2129 (1989).

One-step reaction of *ortho*-substituted nitroarenes with vinyl Grignard reagents to yield 7-substituted indoles:

Mechanistic studies: M. Bosco *et al., J. Chem. Soc. Perkin Trans. 2* **1991,** 657. Improved protocols: A. Dobbs, *J. Org. Chem.* **66,** 638 (2001); M. C. Pirrung *et al., Synlett* **2002,** 143. Indole synthesis on solid supports: K. Knepper, S. Bräse, *Org. Lett.* **5,** 2829 (2003). *Review:* R. Dalpozzo, G. Bartoli, *Curr. Org. Synth.* **9,** 163-178 (2005).

21. Barton Decarboxylation

D. H. R. Barton *et al., Chem. Commun.* **1983**, 939; *eidem, Tetrahedron* **41**, 3901 (1985).

Radical decarboxylation of organic acids to the corresponding noralkane with tri-*n*-butyltin hydride or *t*-butyl-mercaptan:

$$RCOOH \xrightarrow{\text{DCC, DMAP}} \quad \longrightarrow \quad + CO_2 + R \cdot$$

Synthetic application: F. E. Ziegler, M. Belema, *J. Org. Chem.* **62**, 1083 (1997).

22. Barton Deoxygenation (Barton-McCombie Reaction)

D. H. R. Barton, S. W. McCombie, *J. Chem. Soc. Perkin Trans. 1* **1975**, 1574.

Deoxygenation of alcohols *via* their thiocarbonyl derivatives which undergo free radical scission upon treatment with tri-*n*-butyltin hydride:

$$\xrightarrow{n\text{-Bu}_3\text{SnH}} \quad \left[\quad \longrightarrow \quad + \cdot R^2 \right] \xrightarrow{n\text{-Bu}_3\text{SnH}} R^2 H$$

R = H, CH_3, SCH_3, Ph, OPh, imidazolyl; R^2 = alkyl

Mechanistic study: J. E. Forbes, S. Z. Zard, *Tetrahedron Lett.* **30**, 4367 (1989). *Review:* M. Pereyre *et al., Tin in Organic Synthesis* (Butterworths, Boston, 1987) pp 84-96. Review of methodological improvements, particularly the replacement of tri-*n*-butyltin hydride with silicon hydrides: C. Chatgilialoglu, C. Ferreri, *Res. Chem. Intermed.* **19**, 755-775 (1993).

23. Barton Olefin Synthesis (Barton-Kellogg Reaction)

D. H. R. Barton *et al., Chem. Commun.* **1970**, 1226; R. M. Kellogg, S. Wassenaar, *Tetrahedron Lett.* **1970**, 1987; R. M. Kellogg *et al., ibid.* 4689.

Olefin synthesis by two-fold extrusion of nitrogen and sulfur from a Δ^3-1,3,4-thiadiazoline intermediate. Particularly applicable to the synthesis of moderately hindered *tetra*-substituted ethylenes:

$$\xrightarrow{\text{PR}_3, \Delta}$$

1. H_2NNH_2
2. H_2S
3. Pb(OCOCH_3)_4

R = Bu, Ph, OCH_2CH_3, N(CH_2CH_3)_3

Scope and limitations: D. H. R. Barton *et al., J. Chem. Soc. Perkin Trans. 1* **1974**, 1794. Synthetic applications: A. P. Schaap, G. R. Faler, *J. Org. Chem.* **38**, 3061 (1973); L. K. Bee *et al., ibid.* **40**, 2212 (1975); M. D. Bachi *et al., Tetrahedron Lett.* **1978**, 4167; J. E. McMurry *et al., J. Am. Chem. Soc.* **106**, 5018 (1984); F. J. Hoogesteger *et al., J. Org. Chem.* **60**, 4375 (1995). *Cf.* McMurry Reaction.

24. Barton Reaction

D. H. R. Barton *et al., J. Am. Chem. Soc.* **82**, 2640 (1960); **83**, 4076 (1961).

Conversion of a nitrite ester to a γ-oximino alcohol by photolysis involving the homolytic cleavage of a nitrogen-oxygen bond followed by hydrogen abstraction:

$$CH_3 \quad ONO \xrightarrow{h\nu} \quad \rightleftharpoons$$

M. Akhtar, *Adv. Photochem.* **2**, 263 (1964); R. H. Hesse, *Adv. Free-Radical Chem.* **3**, 83 (1969); J. Kalvoda, *Angew. Chem. Int. Ed.* **8**, 525 (1964). Mechanism: D. H. R. Barton *et al., J. Chem. Soc. Perkin Trans. 1* **1979**, 1159. Synthetic application: A. Herzog *et al., Angew. Chem. Int. Ed.* **37**, 1552 (1998).

25. Barton-Zard Reaction

D. H. R. Barton *et al., Tetrahedron* **46,** 7587 (1990).

Formation of a pyrrole by condensation of a substituted nitroso-alkene with an isocyanoester:

Synthetic applications: T. D. Lash *et al., Tetrahedron Lett.* **35,** 2493 (1994); *idem. et al., ibid.* **38,** 2031 (1997); E. T. Pelkey *et al., Chem. Commun.* **1996,** 1909.

26. Baudisch Reaction

O. Baudisch *et al., Naturwissenschaften* **27,** 768, 769 (1939); *Science* **92,** 336 (1940); *J. Am. Chem. Soc.* **63,** 622 (1941).

Synthesis of *o*-nitrosophenols from benzene or substituted benzenes, hydroxylamine and hydrogen peroxide in the presence of copper salts:

K. Maruyama *et al., Tetrahedron Lett.* **1966,** 5889; *J. Org. Chem.* **32,** 2516 (1967); *Bull. Chem. Soc. Jpn.* **44,** 3120 (1971); W. Seidenfaden, *Houben-Weyl* **10/1,** 1025, 1027 (1971).

27. Baylis-Hillman Reaction

A. B. Baylis, M. E. D. Hillman, **DE 2155113;** *eidem,* **US 3743669** (1972, 1973 both to Celanese).

Coupling of activated vinyl systems with aldehydes, catalyzed by 1,4-diazabicyclo[2.2.2]octane (DABCO), to yield α-hydroxyalkylated or -arylated products:

EWG = COOR, COR, CN, SO$_2$R, CONR$_2$

Mechanistic studies: Y. Fort *et al., Tetrahedron* **48,** 6371 (1992); E. L. M. van Rozendaal *et al., ibid.* **49,** 6931 (1993); K. E. Price *et al., J. Org. Chem.* **70,** 3980 (2005). Rate enhancement study: J. Augé *et al., Tetrahedron Lett.* **35,** 7947 (1994). Use of chiral auxillary: S. E. Drewes *et al., Synth. Commun.* **23,** 1215 (1993). Synthetic applications: *idem et al., ibid.* 2807; P. Perlmutter, T. D. McCarthy, *Aust. J. Chem.* **46,** 253 (1993). *Reviews:* S. E. Drewes, G. H. P. Roos, *Tetrahedron* **44,** 4653-4670 (1988); D. Basavaiah *et al., Chem. Rev.* **103,** 811-891 (2003).

28. Béchamp Reduction

A. J. Béchamp, *Ann. Chim. Phys.* **42**(3), 186, (1854).

Reduction of aromatic nitro compounds to the corresponding amines by iron, ferrous salts or iron catalysts in aqueous acid:

$$ArNO_2 + 2Fe + 6HCl \longrightarrow ArNH_2 + 2H_2O + 2FeCl_3$$

J. Werner, *Ind. Eng. Chem.* **40,** 1575 (1948); **41,** 1841 (1949); S. Yagi *et al., Bull. Chem. Soc. Jpn.* **29,** 194 (1956); A. Courtin, *Helv. Chim. Acta* **62,** 2280 (1980). *Reviews:* C. S. Hamilton, J. F. Morgan, *Org. React.* **2,** 428 (1944); R. Schröter, *Houben-Weyl* **11/1,** 394-409 (1957).

29. Beckmann Rearrangement; Beckmann Fragmentation

E. Beckmann, *Ber.* **19,** 988 (1886).

Acid-mediated isomerization of oximes to amides. Oximes of cyclic ketones give ring enlargements:

Certain oximes, particularly those having a quarternary carbon *anti* to the hydroxyl, are likely to undergo the **Beckmann fragmentation** to form nitriles instead of amides:

$$Ar_2CHCR \xrightarrow{PCl_5} Ar_2CHCl + RCN$$

Application to steroidal oximes: P. Catsoulacos, D. Catsoulacos, *J. Heterocycl. Chem.* **30**, 1 (1993). Mechanistic study: A. B. Fernández *et al., Angew. Chem. Int. Ed.* **44**, 2370 (2005). *Reviews:* L. G. Donaruma, W. Z. Heldt, *Org. React.* **11**, 1-156 (1960); R. E. Gawley, *ibid.* **35**, 1-420 (1988); C. G. McCarty in *The Chemistry of the Carbon-Nitrogen Double Bond*, S. Patai, Ed. (Interscience, New York, 1970) pp 408-439; J. R. Hauske, *Comp. Org. Syn.* **1**, 98-100 (1991); K. Maruoka, H. Yamamoto, *ibid.* **6**, 763-775; D. Craig, *ibid.* **7**, 689-702. *Cf.* Schmidt Reaction; Tiemann Rearrangement.

30. Bénary Reaction

E. Bénary, *Ber.* **63**, 1573 (1930); **64**, 2543 (1931).

Action of Grignard reagents on enamino ketones or aldehydes yields β-substituted α,β-unsaturated ketones or aldehydes:

T. Cuvigny, H. Normant, *Bull. Soc. Chim. Fr.* **1960**, 515. Use of lithio derivatives instead of Grignard reagents: C. Jutz, *Ber.* **91**, 1867 (1958). Mechanism: A. Pasteur *et al., Bull. Soc. Chim. Fr.* **1965**, 2328.

31. Benkeser Reduction

R. A. Benkeser *et al., J. Am. Chem. Soc.* **74**, 5699 (1952); **77**, 3230 (1955).

Reduction of aromatic and olefinic compounds with lithium or calcium and low molecular weight amines to monounsaturated olefins, as well as the fully reduced products. The extent of reduction and selectivity can be controlled by varying the reaction conditions:

$$R = CH_3, CH_2CH_3, CH_2CH_2CH_3, CH_2CH_2NH_2$$

Selectivity study: R. A. Benkeser *et al., Tetrahedron Lett.* no. 16, 1 (1960). Comparative review: E. M. Kaiser, *Synthesis* **1972**, 391-415 *passim.* Scope and limitations: R. A. Benkeser *et al., J. Org. Chem.* **48**, 2796 (1983). Synthetic applications: C. Eaborn *et al., J. Chem. Soc. Perkin Trans. 1* **1975**, 475; R. Eckrich, D. Kuck, *Synlett* **1993**, 344. *Cf.* Birch Reduction.

32. Benzidine Rearrangement; Semidine Rearrangement

A. W. Hofmann, *Proc. Roy. Soc. London* **12**, 576 (1863); P. Jacobson *et al., Ber.* **26**, 688 (1893).

Acid-catalyzed rearrangement of hydrazobenzenes to 4,4'-diaminobiphenyls. If the hydrazobenzene contains a *para* substituent, then the favored product is *p*-aminodiphenylamine (**Semidine rearrangement**):

D. L. H. Williams, *Compr. Chem. Kinet.* vol. **13**, C. H. Bamford, C. F. H. Tipper, Eds. (Elsevier, New York, 1972) pp 437-448; R. A. Cox, E. Buncel, *The Chemistry of Hydrazo, Azo and Azoxy Groups* pt. 2, S. Patai, Ed. (Wiley, New York, 1975) pp 775-807. Mechanistic studies: H. J. Shine *et al., J. Am. Chem. Soc.* **103**, 955 (1981); **104**, 5184 (1982); **106**, 7077 (1984). Synthetic applications: T. Nozoe *et al., Chem. Lett.* **1986**, 1577; K. H. Park, J. S. Kang, *J. Org. Chem.* **62**, 3794 (1997).

33. Benzilic Acid Rearrangement (Benzil-Benzilic Acid Rearrangement)

J. Liebig, *Ann.* **25**, 27 (1838); N. Zinin, *ibid.* **31**, 329 (1939).

Base-induced rearrangement of benzil to benzylic acid *via* phenyl group migration. More commonly perceived to include the migrations of other groups in α-dicarbonyl compounds:

$$\underset{\substack{\text{O} \quad \text{O} \\ \text{C}_6\text{H}_5-\overset{\|}{\text{C}}-\overset{\|}{\text{C}}-\text{C}_6\text{H}_5}}{} \xrightarrow{\text{KOH}} \underset{\substack{\text{C}_6\text{H}_5 \\ \text{C}_6\text{H}_5-\overset{|}{\underset{|}{\text{C}}}-\text{COO}^-\ \text{K}^+ \\ \text{OH}}}{}$$

Reviews: S. Selman, J. F. Eastham, *Q. Rev. Chem. Soc.* **14**, 221 (1960); D. J. Cram, *Fundamentals of Carbanion Chemistry* (Academic Press, 1965) pp 238-243; G. B. Gill, *Comp. Org. Syn.* **3**, 821-838 (1991).

34. Benzoin Condensation
A. J. Lapworth, *J. Chem. Soc.* **83**, 995 (1903); **85**, 1206 (1904).
   Cyanide-catalyzed condensation of aromatic aldehydes to give benzoins (acyloins):

$$\text{ArCHO} + \text{Ar}^1\text{CHO} \xrightarrow{\text{KCN}} \text{ArCHOHCOAr}^1$$

H. Staudinger, *Ber.* **46**, 3530, 3535 (1913); W. S. Ide, J. S. Buck, *Org. React.* **4**, 269 (1948); H. Herlinger, *Houben-Weyl 7/2a*, 653 (1973); A. Hassner, K. M. L. Rai, *Comp. Org. Syn.* **1**, 541-577 (1991). *Cf.* Acyloin Condensation.

35. Bergius Process
F. Bergius, *Gas World* **58**, 490 (1913); **GB 18232** (1914).
   Formation of petroleum-like hydrocarbons by hydrogenation of coal at high temperatures and pressures (*e.g.,* 450°C and 300 atm) with or without catalysts; production of toluene by subjecting aromatic naphthas to cracking temperatures at 100 atm with a low partial pressure of hydrogen in the presence of a catalyst.
   B. T. Brooks, *The Chemistry of the Nonbenzenoid Hydrocarbons* (New York, 1950) p 115; *McGraw-Hill Encyclopedia of Science and Technology* **vol. 2** (New York, 1960) p 166; R. M. Baldwin in *Kirk-Othmer Encyclopedia of Chemical Technology* **vol. 6** (Wiley, New York, 4th ed., 1993) p 569. *Cf.* Fischer-Tropsch Syntheses.

36. Bergman Reaction
R. R. Jones, R. G. Bergman, *J. Am. Chem. Soc.* **94**, 660 (1972); R. G. Bergman, *Acc. Chem. Res.* **6**, 25 (1973).
   The cyclization of enediynes to generate 1,4-benzenoid diradicals:

   Application to ring annulation: J. W. Grissom *et al., Tetrahedron* **50**, 4635 (1994). Kinetic study: *idem et al., J. Org. Chem.* **59**, 5833 (1994). Reaction energetics: E. Kraka, D. Cremer, *J. Am. Chem. Soc.* **116**, 4929 (1994). Reviews of enediyne chemistry and its application to the development of antitumor agents: K. C. Nicolaou *et al., Proc. Natl. Acad. Sci. USA* **90**, 5881-5888 (1993); K. Nicolaou, *Chem. Br.* **41**, 33-36, (1994).

37. Bergmann Azlactone Peptide Synthesis
M. Bergmann *et al., Ann.* **449**, 277 (1926).
   Conversion of an acetylated amino acid and an aldehyde into an azlactone with an alkylene side chain, reaction with a second amino acid with ring opening and formation of an acylated unsaturated dipeptide, followed by catalytic hydrogenation and hydrolysis to the dipeptide:

J. S. Fruton, *Adv. Protein Chem.* **V**, 15 (1949); S. Archer in *Amino Acids and Proteins*, D. M. Greenberg, Ed. (Thomas, Springfield, IL, 1951) p 181; H. D. Springall, *The Structural Chemistry of Proteins* (New York, 1954) p 29; E. Baltazzi, *Q. Rev. Chem. Soc.* **10**, 235 (1956). *Cf.* Erlenmeyer-Plöchl Azlactone and Amino Acid Synthesis.

38. Bergmann Degradation
M. Bergmann, *Science* **79**, 439 (1934).
   Stepwise degradation of polypeptides involving benzoylation, conversion to azides and treatment of the azides with benzyl alcohol; this treatment yields, *via* rearrangement to isocyanates, carbobenzoxy compounds which undergo catalytic hydrogenation and hydrolysis to the amide of the degraded peptide:

$$R^1CONHCHRCON_3 \xrightarrow{C_6H_5CH_2OH} R^1CONHCHRNHCOOCH_2C_6H_5 \xrightarrow[H_2O]{H_2}$$

$$R^1CONH_2 + RCHO + CO_2 + C_6H_5CH_3 + NH_3$$

M. Bergmann, L. Zervas, *J. Biol. Chem.* **113**, 341 (1936); H. D. Springall, *The Structural Chemistry of Proteins* (New York, 1954) p 321. *Cf.* Curtius Rearrangement.

39. Bergmann-Zervas Carbobenzoxy Method
M. Bergmann, L. Zervas, *Ber.* **65**, 1192 (1932).

Formation of the *N*-carbobenzoxy derivative of an amino acid for use in peptide synthesis and liberation of the amino group at an appropriate stage of synthesis by hydrogenolysis of the labile carbon-oxygen bond:

C. L. A. Schmidt, *The Chemistry of the Amino Acids and Proteins* (Thomas, Springfield, IL, 1944) p 262; S. Archer in *Amino Acids and Proteins*, D. M. Greenberg, Ed. (Charles C. Thomas, Springfield, IL, 1951) p 177; G. W. Kenner, *J. Chem. Soc.* **1956**, 3689; T. W. Greene, *Protective Groups in Organic Synthesis* (Wiley, New York, 1981) p 239, *Cf.* Fischer Peptide Synthesis.

40. Bernthsen Acridine Synthesis
A. Bernthsen, *Ann.* **192**, 1 (1878); **224**, 1 (1884).

Formation of 5-substituted acridines by heating diarylamines in organic acids or anhydrides, usually in the presence of zinc chloride:

A. Albert, *The Acridines* (London, 1951) p 67; A. Albert, *Heterocycl. Compd.* **4**, 502 (1952); N. P. Buu-Hoï *et al.*, *J. Chem. Soc.* **1955**, 1082; R. M. Acheson in *The Chemistry of Heterocyclic Compounds*, A. Weissberger, Ed., *Acridines* (Interscience, New York, 1956) pp 19-25; F. D. Popp, *J. Org. Chem.* **27**, 2658 (1962). Alkyl migration: L. H. Klemm *et al.*, *Heterocyclic Chem.* **29**, 571 (1992).

41. Betti Reaction
M. Betti, *Gazz. Chim. Ital.* **30 II**, 301 (1900); **33 II**, 2 (1903); F. Pirrone, *ibid.* **66**, 518 (1936); **67**, 529 (1937).

The reaction of aromatic aldehydes, primary aromatic or heterocyclic amines and phenols leading to α-aminobenzylphenols:

R, R¹ = aryl, heterocyclic

J. P. Phillips, *Chem. Rev.* **56**, 286 (1956); J. P. Phillips, E. M. Barrall, *J. Org. Chem.* **21**, 692 (1956). *Early review:* J. P. Phillips, Leach, *Trans. K. Acad. Sci.* **24**(3-4), 95 (1964). Mechanistic study: H. Möhrle *et al.*, *Ber.* **107**, 2675 (1974). Stereoselectivity: C. Cardellicchio *et al.*, *Tetrahedron: Asymmetry* **9**, 3667 (1998). *Cf.* Mannich Reaction.

42. Biginelli Reaction
P. Biginelli, *Ber.* **24**, 1317, 2962 (1891); **26**, 447 (1893).

Synthesis of tetrahydropyrimidinones by the acid-catalyzed condensation of an aldehyde, a β-keto ester and urea:

$$CH_3COCH_2COOC_2H_5 \ + \ R{-}CHO \ + \ H_2NCONH_2 \ \longrightarrow$$

H. E. Zaugg, W. B. Martin, *Org. React.* **14**, 88 (1965); D. J. Brown, *The Pyrimidines* (Wiley, New York, 1962) p 440; *ibid.*, Suppl. I, **1970**, p 326, F. Sweet, Y. Fissekis, *J. Am. Chem. Soc.* **95**, 8741 (1973). Synthetic applications: M. V. Fernandez *et al.*, *Heterocycles* **27**, 2133 (1988); K. Singh *et al.*, *Tetrahedron* **55**, 12873 (1999); A. S. Franklin *et al.*, *J. Org. Chem.* **64**, 1512 (1999). Modified conditions: C. O. Kappe *et al.*, *Synthesis* **1999**, 1799; J. Lu, H. Ma. *Synlett* **2000**, 63. Use of cycloalkanones as starting material: Y.-L. Zhu *et al.*, *Eur. J. Org. Chem.* **2005**, 2354.

43. Birch Reduction
A. J. Birch, *J. Chem. Soc.* **1944**, 430; **1945**, 809; **1946**, 593; **1947**, 102, 1642, **1949**, 2531.

Reduction of aromatic rings by means of alkali metals in liquid ammonia to give mainly unconjugated dihydro derivatives:

R = electron-donating   R = electron-withdrawing

Reviews: A. J. Birch, H. Smith, *Q. Rev. Chem. Soc.* **12**, 17 (1958); D. Caine, *Org. React.* **23**, 1-258 (1976); P. W. Rabideau, Z. Marcinow, *ibid.* **42**, 1-334 (1992); J. M. Hook, L. N. Mander, *Nat. Prod. Rep.* **3**, 35-85 (1986); L. N. Mander, *Comp. Org. Syn.* **8**, 489-521 (1991). *Cf.* Benkeser Reduction.

44. Bischler-Möhlau Indole Synthesis
A. Bischler *et al.*, *Ber.* **25**, 2860 (1892); **26**, 1336 (1893); R. Möhlau, *ibid.* **14**, 171 (1881); **15**, 2480 (1882); E. Fischer, T. Schmitt, *ibid.* **21**, 1071 (1888).

Formation of 2-substituted indoles by heating ω-halogeno- or ω-hydroxy- ketones with excess aniline *via* cyclization of the intermediate 2-arylaminoketone:

P. L. Julian *et al.*, *Heterocycl. Compd.* **3**, 22 (1952); R. J. Sundberg, *The Chemistry of Indoles* (Academic Press, New York, 1970) p 164; R. K. Brown in *The Chemistry of Heterocyclic Compounds*, A. Weissberger, E. C. Taylor, Eds., *Indoles* **Part I**, W. J. Houlihan, Ed. (Wiley, New York, 1972) p 317; J. R. Henry, J. H. Dodd, *Tetrahedron Lett.* **38**, 8763 (1998).

45. Bischler-Napieralski Reaction
A. Bischler, B. Napieralski, *Ber.* **26**, 1903 (1893).

Cyclodehydration of β-phenethylamides to 3,4-dihydroisoquinoline derivatives by means of condensing agents such as phosphorous pentoxide or zinc chloride:

W. M. Whaley, T. R. Govindachari, *Org. React.* **6**, 74 (1951); T. Kametani *et al.*, *Tetrahedron* **27**, 5367 (1971); G. Fodor *et al.*, *Angew. Chem. Int. Ed.* **11**, 919 (1972); G. Fodor, S. Nagubandi, *Tetrahedron* **36**, 1279 (1980); *eidem, Heterocycles* **15**, 165 (1981). Review of enantioselective modifications: M. O. Rozwadowska, *ibid.* **39**, 903-931 (1994). *Cf.* Bradsher Reaction; Pechmann Condensation; Pictet-Gams Isoquinoline Synthesis; Pictet-Hubert Reaction; Skraup Reaction.

46. Blaise Ketone Synthesis; Blaise-Maire Reaction
E. E. Blaise, A. Koehler, *Bull. Soc. Chim.* [4] **7**, 215 (1910); E. E. Blaise, M. Maire, *Compt. Rend.* **145**, 73 (1907); E. E. Blaise, *Bull. Soc. Chim.* [4] **9**, 1 (1911).

Formation of ketones by treatment of acid halides with organozinc compounds; the use of β-hydroxy carbonyl chlorides to give β-hydroxy ketones, convertible into α,β-unsaturated ketones in boiling dilute sulfuric acid, is known as the **Blaise-Maire reaction:**

$$RZnCl \ + \ R^1COCl \ \longrightarrow \ RCOR^1 \ + \ ZnCl_2$$

$$AcOCH_2CHRCOCl \ + \ R^1ZnCl \ \longrightarrow \ AcOCH_2CHRCOR^1 \ \longrightarrow \ HOCH_2CHRCOR^1 \longrightarrow \ H_2C{=}CRCOR^1$$

J. Cason, *Chem. Rev.* **40**, 17 (1947); D. A. Shirley, *Org. React.* **8**, 29 (1954).

47. Blaise Reaction

E. E. Blaise, *Compt. Rend.* **132,** 478 (1901).

Formation of β-oxoesters by treatment of α-bromocarboxylic esters with zinc in the presence of nitriles. The intermediate organozinc compound reacts with the nitrile and the complex is hydrolyzed with 30% potassium hydroxide:

$$R^1R^2CBrCOOC_2H_5 + Zn \longrightarrow R^1R^2C(ZnBr)COOC_2H_5 \xrightarrow{RCN}$$

$$R^1R^2C(CR\!\!=\!\!NZnBr)COOC_2H_5 \xrightarrow{aq\ KOH} RCOCR^1R^2COOC_2H_5 + NH_3 + Zn(OH)Br$$

A. Horeau, J. Jacques, *Bull. Soc. Chim.* **1947,** Mem. 58; J. Cason *et al., J. Org. Chem.* **18,** 1594 (1953); H. Henecka, *Houben-Weyl* **7/2a,** 518 (1973); K. Nützel, *ibid.* **13/2a,** 829. Modified conditions: S. M. Hannick, Y. Kishi, *J. Org. Chem.* **48,** 3833 (1983); N. Zylber *et al., J. Organomet. Chem.* **444,** 1 (1993); K. Narkunan, B.-J. Uang, *Synthesis* **1998,** 1713. Stereoselectivity: J. J. Duffield, A. C. Regan, *Tetrahedron: Asymmetry* **7,** 663 (1996); A. S.-Y. Lee *et al., Tetrahedron Lett.* **38,** 443 (1997); J. Syed *et al., Tetrahedron: Asymmetry* **9,** 805 (1998). *Cf.* Reformatsky Reaction.

48. Blanc Reaction (Chloromethylation)

G. Blanc, *Bull. Soc. Chim. Fr.* [4], **33,** 313 (1923).

Introduction of the chloromethyl group into aromatic rings on treatment with formaldehyde and hydrogen chloride in the presence of zinc chloride:

$$ArH + CH_2O + HCl \xrightarrow{ZnCl_2} ArCH_2Cl$$

Reviews: R. C. Fuson, C. H. McKeever, *Org. React.* **1,** 63 (1942); G. Olah, W. S. Tolgyesi, in *Friedel-Crafts and Related Reactions* **vol. II,** Part 2, G. Olah, Ed. (Interscience, New York, 1963) pp 659-784. *Cf.* Quelet Reaction.

49. Blanc Reaction-Blanc Rule

H. G. Blanc, *Compt. Rend.* **144,** 1356 (1907).

Cyclization of dicarboxylic acids on heating with acetic anhydride to give either cyclic anhydrides or ketones depending on the respective positions of the carboxyl groups; 1,4- and 1,5-diacids yield anhydrides, while diacids in which the carboxy groups are in 1,6 or further removed positions yield ketones:

H. Kwart, K. King in *The Chemistry of Carboxylic Acids and Esters*, J. Patai, Ed. (Interscience, London, 1969) p 362; K. D. Bode, *Houben-Weyl* **7/2,** 640 (1973). *Cf.* Ruzicka Large Ring Synthesis.

50. Bodroux-Chichibabin Aldehyde Synthesis

F. Bodroux, *Compt. Rend.* **138,** 92 (1904); A. E. Chichibabin, *Ber.* **37,** 186, 850 (1904).

Formation of aldehydes by treatment of orthoformates with Grignard reagents:

$$HC(OC_2H_5)_3 + RMgX \longrightarrow RCH(OC_2H_5)_2 \xrightarrow[H_2O]{H^+} RCHO$$

L. I. Smith *et al., J. Org. Chem.* **6,** 437, 489 (1941); H. W. Post, *The Chemistry of the Aliphatic Orthoesters* (New York, 1943) p 96; H. Meerwein, *Houben-Weyl* **6/3,** 243 (1965); R. H. DeWolfe, *Carboxylic Orthoacid Derivatives* (Academic Press, New York, 1970) p 224. *Cf.* Bouveault Aldehyde Synthesis.

51. Bodroux Reaction

F. Bodroux, *Bull. Soc. Chim. Fr.* **33,** 831 (1905), **35,** 519 (1906); **1,** 912 (1907); *Compt. Rend.* **138,** 1427 (1904); **140,** 1108 (1905); **142,** 401 (1906).

Formation of substituted amides by reaction of a simple aliphatic or aromatic ester with an aminomagnesium halide obtained by treatment of a primary or secondary amine with a Grignard reagent at room temperature:

$$RCOOR^1 + IMgNHR^2 \longrightarrow IMgOCR(OR^1)NHR^2 \xrightarrow{IMgNHR^2} RCONHR^2$$

H. L. Bassett, C. R. Thomas, *J. Chem. Soc.* **1954,** 1188; K. Nützel, *Houben-Weyl* **13/2a,** 278 (1973).

52. Bogert-Cook Synthesis

M. T. Bogert, *Science* **77,** 289 (1933); J. W. Cook, C. L. Hewett, *J. Chem. Soc.* **1933,** 1098.

Condensation of β-phenylethylmagnesium bromide with cyclohexanones followed by cyclodehydration of the tertiary alcohol with concentrated sulfuric acid with formation of octahydrophenanthrene derivatives and a small amount of spiran:

L. F. Fieser, M. Fieser, *Natural Products Related to Phenanthrene* (New York, 1949) p 90; C. Schmidt *et al., Can. J. Chem.* **51,** 3620 (1973). For a general approach to the synthesis of phenanthrenoid compounds, *see* D. A. Evans *et al., J. Am. Chem. Soc.* **99,** 7083 (1977).

53. Bohn-Schmidt Reaction
R. Bohn, **DE 46654** (1889); R. E. Schmidt, **DE 60855** (1891).

Hydroxylation of anthraquinones containing at least one hydroxyl group by treatment with fuming sulfuric acid or sulfuric acid and boric acid in the presence of a catalyst such as mercury:

Reviews: M. Phillips, *Chem. Rev.* **6,** 168 (1929); Fieser, Fieser, *Organic Chemistry* (New York, 1956) p 903. Studies and proposed mechanism: J. Winkler, W. Jenny, *Helv. Chim. Acta* **48,** 119 (1965); B. R. Dhruva *et al., Indian J. Chem.* **14 (B),** 622 (1976).

54. Boord Olefin Synthesis
L. C. Swallen, C. E. Boord, *J. Am. Chem. Soc.* **52,** 651 (1930); **53,** 1505 (1931); **55,** 3293 (1933); H. B. Dykstra *et al., ibid.* **52,** 3396 (1930).

Regiospecific synthesis of olefins from aldehydes and Grignard reagents by zinc induced reductive elimination of halogen and alkoxy groups:

C. Niemann, C. D. Wagner, *J. Org. Chem.* **7,** 227 (1942); P. Bandart, *Bull. Soc. Chim.* **11,** 336 (1944); L. Crombie, *Q. Rev. Chem. Soc.* **6,** 131 (1952); M. Schlosser, *Houben-Weyl* **5/1b,** 213 (1972). Application to taxanes: J. S. Yadav *et al. Tetrahedron Lett.* **35,** 3617 (1994); P. H. Beusker *et al., Eur. J. Org. Chem.* **1998,** 2483.

55. Borsche-Drechsel Cyclization
E. Drechsel, *J. Prakt. Chem.* **38**(2), 69 (1858); W. Borsche, M. Feise, *Ber.* **20,** 378 (1904).

Formation of carbazole by acid-catalyzed rearrangement of cyclohexanone phenylhydrazone to tetrahydrocarbazole followed by oxidation:

N. Campbell, B. M. Barclay, *Chem. Rev.* **40,** 361 (1947); W. Freudenberg, *Heterocycl. Compd.* **3,** 298 (1952); P. Bruck, *J. Org. Chem.* **35,** 2222 (1970). *Cf.* Bucherer Carbazole Synthesis; Fischer Indole Synthesis; Piloty-Robinson Synthesis.

56. Bouveault Aldehyde Synthesis
L. Bouveault, *Bull. Soc. Chim. Fr.* **31,** 1306, 1322 (1904).

Action of Grignard or organic lithium reagents on *N,N*-disubstituted formamides yields the homologous aldehydes:

L. I. Smith, J. Nichols, *J. Org. Chem.* **6,** 489 (1941); J. Sicé *J. Am. Chem. Soc.* **75,** 3697 (1953); E. R. H. Jones *et al., J. Chem. Soc.* **1958,** 1054. Use of lithio derivatives instead of Grignard reagents: E. A. Evans, *Chem. Ind. (London)* **1957,** 1596. Synthetic applications using modified conditions: C. Pétrier *et al., Tetrahedron Lett.* **23,** 3361 (1982); J. Einhorn, J. L. Luche, *ibid.* **27,** 1791 (1986); H. Meier, H. Aust, *J. Prakt. Chem.* **341,** 466 (1999). *Cf.* Bodroux-Chichibabin Aldehyde Synthesis.

57. Bouveault-Blanc Reduction

L. Bouveault, G. Blanc, *Compt. Rend.* **136,** 1676 (1903); *Bull. Soc. Chim. Fr.* [3] **31,** 666 (1904).

Formation of alcohols by reduction of esters with sodium and an alcohol:

$$RCOOCH_3 \xrightarrow[R^1OH]{Na} RCH_2OH + CH_3OH$$

H. O. House, *Modern Synthetic Reactions* (W. A. Benjamin, Menlo Park, California, 2nd ed., 1972) p 150.

58. Boyland-Sims Oxidation

E. Boyland *et al., J. Chem. Soc.* **1953,** 3623; E. Boyland, P. Sims, *ibid.* **1954,** 980.

Alkaline persulfate oxidation of aromatic amines to yield predominantly the *o*-amino aryl sulfates. Acid-catalyzed hydrolysis generates the *o*-hydroxy aryl amines:

Regioselectivity/mechanistic study: E. J. Behrman, *J. Org. Chem.* **57,** 2266 (1992). *Review: idem, Org. React.* **35,** 421-511 (1988). *Cf.* Elbs Persulfate Oxidation.

59. Bradsher Cyclization (Bradsher Cycloaddition)

C. K. Bradsher, T. W. G. Solomons, *J. Am. Chem. Soc.* **80,** 933 (1958).

[4 + 2] addition of a common dienophile with cationic aromatic azadienes such as acridizinium or isoquinolinium:

Mechanistic study: C. K. Bradsher, J. A. Stone, *J. Org. Chem.* **33,** 519 (1968). Synthetic applications: V. Bolitt *et al., J. Am. Chem. Soc.* **113,** 6320 (1991); H. Yin *et al., J. Org. Chem.* **57,** 644 (1992); T. E. Nicolas, R. W. Franck, *ibid.* **69,** 6904 (1995). *Review:* D. L. Boger, S. M. Weinreb, *Hetero Diels-Alder Methodology* in *Organic Synthesis* (Academic Press, NY, 1987) pp 239-299.

60. Bradsher Reaction

C. K. Bradsher, *J. Am. Chem. Soc.* **62,** 486 (1940).

Acid-catalyzed cyclodehydration of *o*-acyldiarylmethanes to anthracene derivatives:

Extension to an *o*-acyldiaryl ether: H. Ishibashi *et al., Tetrahedron* **50,** 10215 (1994). Application: T. Yamato *et al., J. Chem. Soc. Perkin Trans. 1* **1997,** 1193. *Review:* C. K. Bradsher, *Chem. Rev.* **87,** 1277-1297 (1987). *Cf.* Bischler-Napieralski Reaction.

61. Brook Rearrangement

A. G. Brook, *J. Am. Chem. Soc.* **80,** 1886 (1958); *idem et al., ibid.* **81,** 981 (1959).

Base-catalyzed silicon migration from carbon to oxygen in α-, β- and γ-silyl alcohols, yielding silyl ethers:

base = NR₃, NaOH, Na/K, NaH
n = 1,2,3

Early review: A. G. Brook, *Acc. Chem. Res.* **7**, 77-84 (1974). Synthetic applications: H. J. Reich *et al., J. Am. Chem. Soc.* **112**, 5609 (1990); K. Takeda *et al., Synlett* **1993**, 841; I. Fleming, U. Ghosh *et al., J. Chem. Soc. Perkin Trans. 1* **1994**, 257.

62. Bucherer-Bergs Reaction

H. T. Bucherer, H. T. Fischbeck, *J. Prakt. Chem.* **140**, 69 (1934); H. T. Bucherer, W. Steiner, *ibid.* 291; H. Bergs, **DE 566094** (1929).

Preparation of hydantoin from carbonyl compounds by reaction with potassium cyanide and ammonium carbonate, or from the corresponding cyanohydrin and ammonium carbonate:

E. Ware, *Chem. Rev.* **46**, 422 (1950); A. Rousset *et al., Tetrahedron* **36**, 2649 (1980). Modified conditions: R. Sarges *et al., J. Med. Chem.* **33**, 1859 (1990). Synthetic applications to excitatory amino acids: K.-I. Tanaka *et al., Tetrahedron: Asymmetry* **6**, 1641, 2271 (1995); C. Domínguez *et al., ibid.* **8**, 511 (1997); J. Knabe, *Pharmazie* **52**, 912 (1997). *Cf.* Strecker Amino Acid Synthesis; Urech Cyanohydrin Method.

63. Bucherer Carbazole Synthesis

H. T. Bucherer, F. Seyde, *J. Prakt. Chem.* **77**(2), 403 (1908).

Formation of carbazoles from naphthols or naphthylamines, aryl hydrazines and sodium bisulfite:

Reviews: N. L. Drake, *Org. React.* **1**, 114 (1942); E. Enders, *Houben-Weyl* **10/2**, 250 (1967). *Cf.* Borsche-Drechsel Cyclization.

64. Bucherer Reaction

H. T. Bucherer, *J. Prakt. Chem.* [2] **69**, 49 (1904); R. Lepetit, *Bull. Soc. Ind. Mulhouse* **1903**, 326.

Reversible formation of β-naphthylamine from β-naphthol and aqueous ammonium sulfite or bisulfite *via* intermediate formation of tetralonesulfonic and tetraloneiminosulfonic acids:

N. L. Drake, *Org. React.* **1**, 105 (1942); H. Seeboth, *Angew. Chem. Int. Ed.* **6**, 307 (1967); M. S. Gibson in *The Chemistry of the Amino Group*, S. Patai, Ed. (Interscience, London, 1968) p 37; Z. Allan *et al., Tetrahedron Lett.* **1969**, 4855; W. H. Pirkle, T. C. Pochapsky, *J. Org. Chem.* **51**, 102 (1986); J. Bendig *et al., Tetrahedron* **48**, 9207 (1992).

65. Buchner-Curtius-Schlotterbeck Reaction

E. Buchner, T. Curtius, *Ber.* **18**, 2371 (1885); F. Schlotterbeck, *Ber.* **40**, 479 (1907); **42**, 2559 (1909).

Formation of ketones from aldehydes and aliphatic diazo compounds; ethylene oxides may also be formed:

$$RCHN_2 + R^1CHO \longrightarrow RCH_2COR^1 + N_2$$

B. Eistert in *Newer Methods of Preparative Organic Chemistry*, English Ed. (New York, 1948) p 521; C. D. Gutsche, *Org. React.* **8**, 364 (1954); J. B. Bastus, *Tetrahedron Lett.* **1963**, 955.

66. Buchner Method of Ring Enlargement

E. Buchner, *Ber.* **29**, 106 (1896); E. Buchner, K. Schottenhammer, *Ber.* **53**, 865 (1920).

Diazoacetic acid ester reacts with benzene and homologs to give the corresponding esters of noncaradienic acid, transformed at high temperatures to derivatives of cycloheptatriene and phenylacetic acid:

W. von F. Doering, L. H. Knox, *J. Am. Chem. Soc.* **79**, 352 (1957); W. Kirmse, *Carbene Chemistry* (Academic Press, New York, 2nd ed., 1971); A. F. Noels *et al., J. Org. Chem.* **46**, 873 (1981). *Cf.* Pfau-Plattner Azulene Synthesis.

Organic Name Reactions

67. Buchwald-Hartwig Cross Coupling Reaction
J. Louie, J. F. Hartwig, *Tetrahedron Lett.* **36**, 3609 (1995); A. S. Guram *et al., Angew. Chem. Int. Ed.* **34**, 1348 (1995).
   Metal catalyzed formation of an arylamine by a reaction of aryl halide of triflate with primary or secondary amine:

$$X = Br, I, OTf \qquad R = o\text{-}, p\text{-alkyl, CN, C(O)Ph, C(O)NEt}_2 \qquad R^1 = \text{alkyl, aryl}$$

Application: S. L. MacNeil *et al., Synlett* **1998**, 419. *Review:* J. F. Hartwig, *Angew. Chem. Int. Ed.* **37**, 2046-2067 (1998).

68. Camps Quinoline Synthesis
R. Camps, *Ber.* **22**, 3228 (1899); *Arch. Pharm.* **237**, 659 (1899); **239**, 591 (1901).
   Formation of hydroxyquinolines from *o*-acylaminoacetophenones in alcoholic sodium hydroxide. Two isomers are produced; the relative proportions are mainly determined by the residue on the amino nitrogen:

R. H. F. Manske, *Chem. Rev.* **30**, 127 (1942); B. Witkop *et al., J. Am. Chem. Soc.* **73**, 2641 (1951); J. Bornstein *et al., ibid.* **76**, 2760 (1954); R. C. Elderfield, *Heterocycl. Compd.* **4**, 60 (1952); H. Yanagisawa *et al., Chem. Pharm. Bull.* **21**, 1080 (1973).

69. Cannizzaro Reaction
S. Cannizzaro, *Ann.* **88**, 129 (1853); K. List, H. Limpricht, *Ann.* **90**, 180 (1854).
   Base-catalyzed disproportionation reaction of aromatic or aliphatic aldehydes with no α-hydrogen to corresponding acid and alcohol. If the aldehydes are different, the reaction is called the "crossed Cannizarro reaction":

$$2RCHO \xrightarrow{\text{base}} RCOO^- + RCH_2OH$$

T. A. Geissman, *Org. React.* **2**, 94 (1944); F. P. B. Van der Maeden *et al., Recl. Trav. Chim. Pays-Bas* **91**(2), 221 (1972); C. G. Swain *et al., J. Am. Chem. Soc.* **101**, 3576 (1979); R. S. McDonald, C. E. Sibley, *Can. J. Chem.* **59**, 1061 (1981). *Review:* T. Lane, A. Plagens, *Named Organic Reactions* (John Wiley & Sons, Chichester, 1998) p 40-42. *Cf.* Meerwein-Ponndorf-Verley Reduction; Oppenauer Oxidation; Tishchenko Reaction.

70. Carroll Rearrangement
M. F. Carroll, *J. Chem. Soc.* **1940**, 704; **1941**, 507; W. Kimel, A. C. Cope, *J. Am. Chem. Soc.* **65**, 1992 (1943).
   Preparation of γ,δ-unsaturated ketones by base-catalyzed reaction of allylic alcohols with β-ketoesters or thermal rearrangement of allyl acetoacetates:

Detailed experimental: S. R. Wilson, C. E. Augelli, *Org. Synth.* **68**, 210 (1990). Synthetic applications: A. V. Echavarren *et al., Tetrahedron Lett.* **32**, 6421 (1991); N. Ouvrard *et al., ibid.* **34**, 1149 (1993). *Cf.* Claisen Rearrangement.

71. Castro-Stephens Coupling (Stephens-Castro Coupling) (Castro Reaction)
C. E. Castro, R. D. Stephens, *J. Org. Chem.* **28**, 2163 (1963); R. D. Stephens, C. E. Castro, *ibid.* 3313; A. M. Sladkov *et al., Bull. Acad. Sci. USSR Div. Chem. Sci.* **1963**, 2043.
   The coupling of cuprous acetylides with aryl halides to yield arylacetylenes:

$$ArX + Cu-C\equiv C-R \xrightarrow[\Delta]{\text{Pd/pyridine}} Ar-C\equiv C-R$$

$$X = I, Br, Cl$$
$$R = \text{alkyl, aryl, vinyl}$$

Synthetic applications: J. D. Kinder *et al., Synlett* **1993**, 149; J. Kabbara *et al., Synthesis* **1995**, 299; M. S. Yu *et al., Tetrahedron Lett.* **39,** 9347 (1998). Early reviews: G. H. Posner, *Org. React.* **22,** 253-400 *passim* (1975); A. M. Sladkov, I. R. Gol'ding, *Russ. Chem. Rev.* **48,** 868-896 (1979). *Cf.* Glaser Coupling.

72. Chapman Rearrangement
O. Mumm *et al., Ber.* **48,** 379 (1915); A. W. Chapman, *J. Chem. Soc.* **127,** 1992 (1925); **1927,** 174; **1929,** 569.
   Thermal rearrangement of aryl imidates to *N,N*-diaryl amides:

$$Ar^1-C=NAr^3 \quad \xrightarrow{\Delta} \quad Ar^1-C-N{<}^{Ar^2}_{Ar^3}$$

(with OAr^2 substituent on left structure and O double bond on right)

J. W. Schulenberg *et al., Org. React.* **14,** 1 (1965); C. G. McCarty, L. Garner in *The Chemistry of Amidines and Imidates* S. Patai, Ed. (Interscience, New York, 1975) p 189. Mechanistic study: N. A. Suttle, A. Williams, *J. Chem. Soc. Perkin Trans. 2* **1983,** 1369. Synthetic applications: L. H. Peterson *et al., J. Heterocycl. Chem.* **18,** 659 (1981); N. Dubau-Assibat *et al., Bull. Soc. Chim. Fr.* **132,** 1139 (1995). Chapman-like rearrangements: F. Esser *et al., J. Chem. Soc. Perkin Trans. 1* **1988,** 3311; M. Dessolin *et al., Chem. Commun.* **1992,** 132.

73. Chichibabin Pyridine Synthesis
A. E. Chichibabin, *J. Russ. Phys. Chem. Soc.* **37,** 1229 (1906); *J. Prakt. Chem.* **107,** 122 (1924).
   Condensation of carbonyl compounds with ammonia or amines under pressure to form pyridine derivatives; the reaction is reversible and produces different pyridine derivatives along with byproducts:

$$3RCH_2CHO \ + \ NH_3 \ \longrightarrow$$

(pyridine product with R, R substituents and RH_2C group)

M. M. Sprung, *Chem. Rev.* **26,** 301 (1940); R. L. Frank, R. P. Seven, *J. Am. Chem. Soc.* **71,** 2629 (1949); H. S. Mosher, *Heterocycl. Compd.* **1,** 456 (1950); J. A. Gautier, J. Renault, *Bull. Soc. Chim. Fr.* **1955,** 588; C. P. Farley, E. L. Eliel, *J. Am. Chem. Soc.* **78,** 3477 (1956); A. T. Soldatenkov, *Zh. Org. Khim.* **16,** 188 (1980). *Cf.* Hantzsch (Dihydro)Pyridine Synthesis; Kröhnke Pyridine Synthesis.

74. Chichibabin Reaction
A. E. Chichibabin, O. A. Zeide, *J. Russ. Phys. Chem. Soc.* **46,** 1216 (1914), *C.A.* **9,** 1901 (1915).
   Amination of pyridines and other heterocyclic nitrogen compounds with alkali-metal amides:

$$\text{(pyridine)} \ + \ NaNH_2 \ \xrightarrow{100\text{-}200\,°} \ \text{(2-aminopyridine, }NH_2\text{)}$$

H. S. Mosher, *Heterocycl. Compd.* **1,** 405 (1950); A. F. Pozharskii *et al., Russ. Chem. Rev.* **47,** 1042 (1978); H. J. W. van den Haak *et al., J. Org. Chem.* **46,** 2134 (1981). Applications: N. J. Kos *et al., ibid.* **44,** 3140 (1979); H. Tondys *et al., J. Heterocycl. Chem.* **22,** 353 (1985); E. Ciganek *et al., J. Org. Chem.* **57,** 4521 (1992). *Review:* H. C. van der Plas, M. Wozniak, *Croat. Chem. Acta* **59,** 33-49 (1986). *Cf.* Kröhnke Pyridine Synthesis.

75. Chugaev Reaction (Tschugaeff Olefin Synthesis)
L. Chugaev (Tschugaeff), *Ber.* **32,** 3332 (1899).
   Formation of olefins from alcohols without rearrangement through pyrolysis of the corresponding xanthates *via cis*-elimination:

(reaction scheme: alcohol with OH → 1) CS_2 2) NaOH CH_3I → xanthate with O, SMe, S → Δ → olefin)

C. H. DePuy, R. W. King, *Chem. Rev.* **60,** 444 (1960); H. R. Nace, *Org. React.* **12,** 57 (1962); K. Harano, T. Taguchi, *Chem. Pharm. Bull.* **20,** 2357 (1972); J. March, *Advanced Organic Chemistry* (John Wiley & Sons, NY, 1992) 1014-1015. Synthetic applications: X Fu, J. M. Cook, *Tetrahedron Lett.* **31,** 3409 (1990); P. S. Ray, M. J. Manning, *Heterocycles* **33,** 1361 (1994). *Cf.* Cope Elimination Reaction.

76. Ciamician-Dennstedt Rearrangement
G. L. Ciamician, M. Dennstedt, *Ber.* **14,** 1153 (1881).
   Expansion of the pyrrole ring by heating with chloroform or other halogeno compounds in alkaline solution. The intermediate dichlorocarbene, by addition to the pyrrole, forms an unstable dihalogenocyclopropane which rearranges to a 3-halogenopyridine:

(reaction scheme: pyrrole $\xrightarrow[RO^-]{CCl_2}$ dichlorocyclopropane intermediate with Cl, Cl $\xrightarrow[RO^-]{-HCl}$ 3-chloropyridine with Cl)

A. H. Corwin, *Heterocycl. Compd.* **1**, 309 (1950); H. S. Mosher, *ibid.* 475; P. S. Skell, R. S. Sandler, *J. Am. Chem. Soc.* **80**, 2024 (1958); E. Vogel, *Angew. Chem.* **72**, 8 (1960).

77. Claisen Condensation (Acetoacetic Ester Condensation)
L. Claisen, O. Lowman, *Ber.* **20**, 651 (1887).

Base-catalyzed condensation of an ester containing an α-hydrogen atom with a molecule of the same ester or a different one to give β-keto esters:

$$CH_3COOC_2H_5 + CH_3COOC_2H_5 \xrightarrow{C_2H_5O^-} CH_3COCH_2COOC_2H_5 + C_2H_5OH$$

C. R. Hauser, B. E. Hudson, *Org. React.* **1**, 266-322 (1942); H. O. House, *Modern Synthetic Reactions* (W. A. Benjamin, Menlo Park, California, 2nd ed., 1972) pp 734-746; J. F. Garst, *J. Chem. Educ.* **56**, 721 (1979); J. E. Bartmess *et al., J. Am. Chem. Soc.* **103**, 1338 (1981); B. R. Davis, P. J. Garratt, *Comp. Org. Syn.* **2**, 795-805 (1991). *Cf.* Dieckmann Reaction.

78. Claisen Rearrangement; Eschenmoser-Claisen Rearrangement; Johnson-Claisen Rearrangement; Ireland-Claisen Rearrangement
L. Claisen, *Ber.* **45**, 3157 (1912); L. Claisen, E. Tietze, *ibid.* **58**, 275 (1925); **59**, 2344 (1926).

Highly stereoselective [3,3]-sigmatropic rearrangement of allyl vinyl or allyl aryl ethers to yield γ,δ-unsaturated carbonyl compounds or *o*-allyl substituted phenols, respectively:

When R' = NR$_2$, the reaction is referred to as the **Eschenmoser-Claisen rearrangement:** A. E. Wick *et al., Helv. Chim. Acta* **47**, 2425 (1964); M. Lautens *et al., Tetrahedron Lett.* **31**, 5829 (1990); B. Coates *et al., ibid.* **32**, 4199 (1991).

When R' = OR, the reaction is referred to as the **Johnson-Claisen rearrangement:** W. S. Johnson *et al., J. Am. Chem. Soc.* **92**, 741 (1970); R. Bao *et al., Synlett* **1992**, 217; D. Basavaiah, S. Pandiaraju, *Tetrahedron Lett.* **36**, 757 (1995).

When R' = OSiR$_3$ or OLi, the reaction is referred to as the **Ireland-Claisen rearrangement:** R. E. Ireland, R. H. Mueller, *J. Am. Chem. Soc.* **94**, 5897 (1972); R. E. Ireland *et al., J. Org. Chem.* **56**, 650 (1991); *idem et al., ibid.* 3572; K. Hattori, H. Yamamoto, *Tetrahedron* **50**, 3099 (1994).

Inclusive reviews: S. J. Rhoads, N. R. Raulins, *Org. React.* **22**, 1-252 (1975); F. E. Ziegler, *Chem. Rev.* **88**, 1423-1452 (1988); P. Wipf, *Comp. Org. Syn.* **5**, 827-873 (1991); A. M. M. Castro, *Chem. Rev.* **104**, 2939-3002 (2004). *Cf.* Carroll Rearrangement; Cope Rearrangement; Overman Rearrangement.

79. Claisen-Schmidt Condensation
L. Claisen, A. Claparède, *Ber.* **14**, 2460 (1881); J. G. Schmidt, *ibid.* 1459.

Condensation of an aromatic aldehyde with an aliphatic aldehyde or ketone in the presence of a relatively strong base (hydroxide or alkoxide ion) to form an α,β-unsaturated aldehyde or ketone:

$$C_6H_5CHO + H_3C\overset{O}{\overset{\|}{C}}-R \xrightarrow{NaOH} C_6H_5HC=CH-COR$$

A. T. Nielsen, W. J. Houlihan, *Org. React.* **16**, 1 (1968); H. O. House, *Modern Synthetic Reactions* (W. A. Benjamin, Menlo Park, California, 2nd ed., 1972) pp 632-639; J. A. Fine, P. Pulaski, *J. Org. Chem.* **38**, 1747 (1973). *Cf.* Aldol Reaction.

80. Clemmensen Reduction
E. Clemmensen, *Ber.* **46**, 1837 (1913); **47**, 51, 681 (1914).

Reduction of carbonyl groups of aldehydes and ketones to methylene groups with zinc amalgam and hydrochloric acid:

$$RCOR^1 \xrightarrow[HCl]{Zn(Hg)} RCH_2R^1$$

E. L. Martin, *Org. React.* **1**, 155 (1942); M. Smith in *Reduction*, R. L. Augustine, Ed. (M. Dekker, New York, 1968) pp 95-170; W. Reusch, *ibid.* pp 186-194; J. G. St. C. Buchanan, P. D. Woodgate, *Q. Rev. Chem. Soc.* **23**, 522 (1969); D. Straschewski, *Angew. Chem.* **71**, 726 (1959); E. Vedejs, *Org. React.* **22**, 401 (1975); S. Yamamura, S. Nishiyama, *Comp. Org. Syn.* **8**, 309-313 (1991). *Cf.* Haworth Phenanthrene Synthesis; Wolff-Kishner Reduction.

81. Combes Quinoline Synthesis

A. Combes, *Bull. Soc. Chim. Fr.* **49**, 89 (1888).

Formation of quinolines by condensation of β-diketones with primary arylamines followed by acid-catalyzed ring closure of the intermediate Schiff base:

W. S. Johnson, F. J. Matthews, *J. Am. Chem. Soc.* **66**, 210 (1944); F. W. Bergstrom, *Chem. Rev.* **35**, 156 (1944); J. C. Perche *et al., J. Chem. Soc. Perkin Trans. 1* **1972**, 260; J. Born, *J. Org. Chem.* **37**, 3952 (1972). *Cf.* Conrad-Limpach Reaction; Doebner Reaction.

82. Conrad-Limpach Cyclization

M. Conrad, L. Limpach, *Ber.* **20**, 944 (1887); **24**, 2990 (1891).

Thermal condensation of arylamines with β-ketoesters followed by cyclization of the intermediate Schiff bases to 4-hydroxyquinolines:

R. H. Manske, *Chem. Rev.* **30**, 121 (1942); R. H. Reitsema, *ibid.* **43**, 47 (1948); H. Henecka, *Chemie der Beta-Dicarbonylverbindungen* (Berlin, 1950) p 307; R. C. Elderfield, *Heterocycl. Compd.* **4**, 30 (1952); J.-C. Perche, G. Saint-Ruf, *J. Heterocycl. Chem.* **11**, 93 (1974); J. M. Barker *et al., J. Chem. Res. Synop.* **1980**, 4; J. A. Moore, T. D. Mitchell, *J. Polym. Chem.* **18**, 3029 (1980). *Cf.* Combes Quinoline Synthesis; Doebner Reaction.

83. Cope Elimination Reaction

A. C. Cope *et al., J. Am. Chem. Soc.* **71**, 3929 (1949); *idem et al., ibid.* **75**, 3212 (1953).

Formation of an olefin and a hydroxylamine by pyrolysis of an amine oxide:

Early reviews: C. H. DePuy, R. W. King, *Chem. Rev.* **60**, 448 (1960); A. C. Cope, E. R. Trumbull, *Org. React.* **11**, 317-493 *passim* (1960). Synthetic application: E. Tojo *et al., Heterocycles* **27**, 2367 (1988). Mechanistic study: R. D. Bach, M. L. Braden, *J. Org. Chem.* **56**, 7194 (1991). Methods development: A. D. Woolhouse, *J. Heterocycl. Chem.* **30**, 873 (1993). Synthetic applications of the reverse reaction (retro-Cope elimination): E. Ciganek, *J. Org. Chem.* **55**, 3007 (1990); M. B. Gravestock *et al., Chem. Commun.* **1993**, 169. *Cf.* Chugaev Reaction; Hofmann Degradation.

84. Cope Rearrangement; Oxy-Cope Rearrangement

A. C. Cope *et al., J. Am. Chem. Soc.* **62**, 441 (1940).

Highly stereoselective [3,3]-sigmatropic rearrangement of 1,5-dienes; "all-carbon" equivalent of the Claisen rearrangement, *q.v.*:

When R = OH, the transformation is referred to as the **oxy-Cope rearrangement:** J. Berson, M. Jones, *ibid.* **86**, 5019 (1964).

Reviews: S. J. Rhodds, N. R. Raulins, *Org. React.* **22**, 1-252 (1975); S. R. Wilson, *ibid.* **43**, 93-250 *passim* (1993); R. K. Hill, *Comp. Org. Syn.* **5**, 785-826 (1991). Review of hetero-Cope rearrangements: S. Blechert, *Synthesis* **1989**, 71-82. Brief review of synthetic applications: K. Durairaj, *Curr. Sci.* **66**, 917-922 (1994).

85. Corey-Bakshi-Shibata Reduction (CBS)

E. J. Corey *et al., J. Am. Chem. Soc.* **109**, 5551 (1987).

Enantioselective borane reduction of ketones catalyzed by chiral oxazaborolidines:

R_L = larger group
R_S = smaller group
R^1 = H, CH$_3$, C$_2$H$_5$, C$_4$H$_9$, etc.

Practical catalyst synthesis: D. J. Mathre *et al., J. Org. Chem.* **58**, 2880 (1993). Synthetic application: E. J. Corey *et al., J. Am. Chem. Soc.* **119**, 11769 (1997). *Reviews:* V. K. Singh, *Synthesis* **1992**, 605-617; L. Deloux, M. Srebnik, *Chem. Rev.* **93**, 763-784 (1993); E. J. Corey, C. J. Helal, *Angew. Chem. Int. Ed.* **37**, 1986-2012 (1998).

86. Corey-Kim Oxidation
E. J. Corey, C. U. Kim, *J. Am. Chem. Soc.* **94**, 7586 (1972).

Oxidation of primary and secondary alcohols *via* their alkoxysulfonium salts. Upon the addition of base, the salt rearranges intramolecularly to aldehydes and ketones, respectively:

Application to the synthesis of α-hydroxy ketones: E. J. Corey, C. U. Kim, *Tetrahedron Lett.* **1974**, 287; of 1,3-dicarbonyl compounds: S. Katayama *et al., Synthesis* **1988**, 178; J. T. Pulkkinen *et al., J. Org. Chem.* **61**, 8604 (1996). *Cf.* Pfitzner-Moffatt Oxidation; Swern Oxidation.

87. Corey-Winter Olefin Synthesis
E. J. Corey, R. A. E. Winter, *J. Am. Chem. Soc.* **85**, 2677 (1963).

Synthesis of olefins from 1,2-diols and thiocarbonyldiimidazole. Treatment of the intermediate cyclic thionocarbonate with trimethylphosphite yields the olefin by *cis*-elimination:

M. Tichy, J. Sicher, *Tetrahedron Lett.* **1969**, 4609; E. J. Corey, P. B. Hopkiss, *ibid.* **23**, 1797 (1982); S. Kaneko *et al., Chem. Pharm. Bull.* **45**, 43 (1997). Applications in nucleotide synthesis: L. W. Dudycz, *Nucleosides Nucleotides* **8**, 35 (1989); R. L. K. Carr *et al., Org. Prep. Proced. Int.* **22**, 245 (1990); in enediynes syntheses: M. F. Semmelhack, J. Gallagher, *Tetrahedron Lett.* **34**, 4121 (1993); D. Crich *et al., Synth. Commun.* **29**, 359 (1999).

88. Cornforth Rearrangement
J. W. Cornforth, *The Chemistry of Penicillin* (Princeton University Press, New Jersey, 1949) p 700.

Thermal rearrangement of 4-carbonyl substituted oxazoles to their isomeric oxazoles *via* the postulated dicarbonyl nitrile ylides:

Mechanistic study: M. J. S. Dewar, I. J. Turchi, *J. Am. Chem. Soc.* **96**, 6148 (1974). Scope and limitations: *eidem, J. Org. Chem.* **40**, 1521 (1975). Extension to the synthesis of 5-aminothiazoles: S. L. Corrao *et al., ibid.* **55**, 4484 (1990). Synthetic application: G. L'abbé *et al., J. Chem. Soc. Perkin Trans. 1* **1993**, 2259.

89. Craig Method

L. C. Craig, *J. Am. Chem. Soc.* **56**, 231 (1934).

Introduction of a halogen into the α-position of aminopyridines by treatment with sodium nitrite in hydrohalic acid followed by warming:

H. S. Mosher, *Heterocycl. Compd.* **1**, 515, 555 (1950); H. E. Mertel in *The Chemistry of Heterocyclic Compounds*, A. Weissberger, Ed., *Pyridine and Its Derivatives* **Pt. Two**, E. Klingsberg, Ed. (Interscience, New York, 1961) p 334.

90. Criegee Reaction

R. Criegee, *Ber.* **64**, 260 (1931).

Oxidative cleavage of vicinal glycols by lead tetraacetate:

Reviews: R. Criegee in *Newer Methods of Preparative Organic Chemistry* vol. **1** (Interscience, New York, 1948) pp 12-20; H. O. House, *Modern Synthetic Reactions* (W. A. Benjamin, Menlo Park, California, 2nd ed., 1972) pp 359-387; K. W. Bentley in *Elucidation of Organic Structures by Physical and Chemical Methods* pt. 2, K. W. Bentley, G. W. Kirby, Eds. (Wiley, New York, 2nd ed., 1973) pp 169-177; S. Hatakeyama, H. Akimoto, *Res. Chem. Intermed.* **20**, 503-524 (1994). Mechanism: S. Chandrasekhar, C. D. Roy, *J. Chem. Soc. Perkin Trans. 2* **1994**, 2141; R. Ponec *et al.*, *J. Org. Chem.* **62**, 2757 (1997); R. M. Goodman, Y. Kishi, *J. Am. Chem. Soc.* **120**, 9392 (1998). *Cf.* Malaprade Reaction.

91. Curtius Rearrangement; Curtius Reaction

T. Curtius, *Ber.* **23**, 3023 (1890); *idem, J. Prakt. Chem.* [2] **50**, 275 (1894).

Formation of isocyanates by thermal decomposition of acyl azides:

$$RCON_3 \xrightarrow{\Delta} R-N=C=O$$

The stepwise conversion of a carboxylic acid to an amine having one fewer carbon unit, *via* the azide and isocyanate, is referred to as the **Curtius reaction:**

$$RCOOH \longrightarrow RCON_3 \longrightarrow RNCO \longrightarrow RNH_2$$

Synthetic applications: R. Lo Scalzo *et al.*, *Gazz. Chim. Ital.* **118**, 819 (1988); N. De Kimpe *et al.*, *J. Org. Chem.* **59**, 8215 (1994). *Reviews:* P. A. S. Smith, *Org. React.* **3**, 337-449 (1946); J. H. Saunders, R. J. Slocombe, *Chem. Rev.* **43**, 205 (1948); D. V. Banthorpe in *The Chemistry of the Azido Group*, S. Patai, Ed. (Interscience, New York, 1971) pp 397-405; T. Shioiri, *Comp. Org. Syn.* **6**, 795-828 (1991). *Cf.* Bergmann Degradation; Hofmann Reaction; Lossen Rearrangement; Schmidt Reaction.

92. D-Homo Rearrangement of Steroids

L. Ruzicka, H. Meldahl, *Helv. Chim. Acta* **21**, 1760 (1938); **22**, 421 (1939).

Originally discovered in 17β-hydroxy-20-ketosteroids, but thoroughly studied in the 17α-hydroxy-20-keto series, this reaction involves an acid- or base-catalyzed acyloin rearrangement which yields a 6-membered D-ring:

R. B. Turner, *J. Am. Chem. Soc.* **75**, 3484 (1953); D. K. Fukushima *et al., ibid.* **77**, 6585 (1955); N. L. Wendler *et al., Tetrahedron* **11**, 163 (1960). *Review:* N. L. Wendler in *Molecular Rearrangements* Part 2, P. de Mayo, Ed. (Wiley-Interscience, New York, 1964) p 1114-1138. Extensive studies: D. Rabinovich *et al., Chem. Commun.* **1976**, 461; N. G. Steinberg *et al., J. Org. Chem.* **49**, 4731 (1984); L. Schor *et al., J. Chem. Soc. Perkin Trans. 1* **1990**, 163; *eidem, ibid.* **1992**, 453.

93. Dakin Reaction

H. D. Dakin, *Am. Chem. J.* **42**, 477 (1909).

Replacement of the formyl or acetyl groups in phenolic aldehydes or ketones by a hydroxyl group by means of hydrogen peroxide:

J. E. Leffler, *Chem. Rev.* **45**, 385 (1949). Mechanistic studies: M. B. Hocking, *et al., Can. J. Chem.* **55**, 102 (1977); *eidem, ibid.* **56**, 2646 (1978); M. B. Hocking *et al., J. Org. Chem.* **47**, 4208 (1982). Sodium percarbonate as oxidizing reagent: G. W. Kabalka *et al., Tetrahedron Lett.* **33**, 865 (1992).

94. Dakin-West Reaction

H. D. Dakin, R. West, *J. Biol. Chem.* **78**, 91, 745, 757 (1928).

Reaction of α-amino acids with acetic anhydride in the presence of base to give α-acetamido ketones. The reaction occurs *via* the intermediate azlactone:

Mechanism: R. Knorr, R. Huisgen, *Ber.* **103**, 2598 (1970); W. Steglich, *et al., Ber.* **104**, 3644 (1971); G. Holfe *et al., Ber.* **105**, 1718 (1972); N. Allinger *et al., J. Org. Chem.* **39**, 1730 (1974); M. Kawase *et al., Chem. Pharm. Bull.* **48**, 114 (2000). Synthetic applications: J. R. Casimir *et al., Tetrahedron Lett.* **36**, 4797 (1995); T. T. Curran, *J. Fluorine Chem.* **74**, 107 (1995). *Review:* G. L. Buchanan, *Chem. Soc. Rev.* **17**, 91 (1988).

95. Darzens Condensation (Darzens-Claisen Reaction) (Glycidic Ester Condensation)

G. Darzens, *Compt. Rend.* **139**, 1214 (1904); **141**, 766 (1905); **142**, 214 (1906).

Formation of α,β-epoxy esters (glycidic esters) by the condensation of aldehydes or ketones with esters of α-haloacids; the corresponding thermally unstable glycidic acids yield aldehydes or ketones on decarboxylation:

M. S. Newman, B. J. Magerlein, *Org. React.* **5**, 413 (1949); M. Ballester, *Chem. Rev.* **55**, 283 (1955); H. O. House, *Modern Synthetic Reactions* (W. Benjamin, Menlo Park, California, 2nd ed., 1972) pp 666-671. Intramolecular reaction: G. Fráter *et al., Tetrahedron Lett.* **34**, 2753 (1993). Enantioselectivity: D. Enders, R. Hett, *Synlett* **1998**, 961; S. Arai *et al., Tetrahedron* **55**, 6375 (1999). Modified conditions: R. F. Borch, *Tetrahedron Lett.* **1972**, 3761; I. Shibata *et al., J. Org. Chem.* **57**, 6909 (1992). Review: T. Rosen, *Comp. Org. Syn.* **2**, 409-439 (1991).

96. Darzens-Nenitzescu Synthesis of Ketones

G. Darzens, *Compt. Rend.* **150**, 707 (1910); C. D. Nenitzescu, I. P. Cantuniari, *Ann.* **510**, 269 (1934); C. D. Nenitzescu, C. Cioranescu, *Ber.* **69**, 1820 (1936).

Acylation of olefins with acid chlorides or anhydrides catalyzed by Lewis acids. When performed in the presence of a saturated hydrocarbon the product is the saturated ketone:

G. A. Olah, *Friedel-Crafts and Related Reactions* **vol. 1** (Interscience, New York, 1963) p 129; C. D. Nenitzescu, A. T. Balaban, *ibid.* **vol. 3**, Part 2, 1069 (1964); L. Ötvös *et al., Acta Chim. Acad. Sci. Hung.* **71**(2), 193 (1972); H. O. House, *Modern Synthetic Reactions* (W. A. Benjamin, Menlo Park, California, 2nd ed., 1972) p 786; J. K. Groves, *Chem. Soc. Rev.* **1**, 73 (1972). Synthetic applications: D. Villemin, B. Labiad, *Synth. Commun.* **22**, 3181 (1992); S. Nakanishi *et al., ibid.* **28**, 1967 (1998). *Cf.* Friedel-Crafts Reaction; Nencki Reaction; Nenitzescu Reductive Acylation.

97. Darzens Synthesis of Tetralin Derivatives

G. Darzens, *Compt. Rend.* **183**, 748 (1926).

Cyclization of α-benzyl-α-allylacetic acid type compounds by moderate heating in concentrated sulfuric acid to yield tetralin derivatives:

E. Bergmann, *Chem. Rev.* **29**, 536 (1941); J. N. Chatterjea *et al., Indian J. Chem.* **20B**, 264 (1981).

98. Delépine Reaction (Delépine Amine Synthesis)

M. Delépine, *Compt. Rend.* **120**, 501 (1895); **124**, 292 (1897).

Preparation of primary amines by reaction of alkyl halides with hexamethylenetetramine followed by acid hydrolysis of the formed quaternary salts:

$$RCH_2X + C_6H_{12}N_4 \longrightarrow [RCH_2C_6H_{12}N_4]^+ X^- \xrightarrow{HX} RCH_2NH_3^+ X^-$$

S. J. Angyal, *Org. React.* **8**, 197 (1954); Y. Basace *et al., Bull. Soc. Chim. Fr.* **1971**, 1468. Synthetic applications: S. N. Quessy *et al., J. Chem. Soc. Perkin Trans. 1* **1979**, 512; S. Brandänge, B. Rodriguez, *Synth. Commun.* **1988**, 347; R. A. Henry *et al., J. Org. Chem.* **55**, 1796 (1990).

99. de Mayo Reaction

P. de Mayo *et al., Proc. Chem. Soc. London* **1962**, 119; P. de Mayo, H. Takeshita, *Can. J. Chem.* **41**, 440 (1963).

Synthesis of 1,5-diketones by photoaddition of enol derivatives of 1,3-diketones to olefins, followed by a retro-aldol reaction, *q.v.*:

P. de Mayo, *Acc. Chem. Res.* **4**, 49 (1971); H. Meier, *Houben-Weyl 4/5b*, 924 (1975); W. Oppolzer, *Pure Appl. Chem.* **53**, 1189 (1981). Intramolecular reactions: A. J. Barker, G. Pattenden, *Tetrahedron Lett.* **21**, 3513 (1980); *eidem, J. Chem. Soc. Perkin Trans. 1* **1983**, 1901. Intermolecular reactions: M. Sato *et al., Chem. Lett.* **1994**, 2191; P. Galatsis, J. J. Manwell, *Tetrahedron* **51**, 665 (1995); T. M. Quevillon, A. C. Weedon, *Tetrahedron Lett.* **37**, 3939 (1996).

100. Demjanov Rearrangement

N. J. Demjanov, M. Lushnikov, *J. Russ. Phys. Chem. Soc.* **35**, 26 (1903); *Chem. Zentralbl.* **1903**, 1, 828.

Deamination of primary amines by diazotization to give rearranged alcohols. In the case of alicyclic amines, ring enlargement or contraction occurs:

P. A. S. Smith, D. R. Baer, *Org. React.* **11**, 157 (1960); H. Stetter, P. Goebel, *Ber.* **96**, 550 (1963); R. Kotani, *J. Org. Chem.* **30**, 350 (1965); V. Dave *et al., Can. J. Chem.* **57**, 1557 (1979); R. K. Murray, Jr., T. M. Ford, *J. Org. Chem.* **44**, 3504 (1979); D. Fattori, *et al., Tetrahedron* **49**, 1649 (1993). *Cf.* Tiffeneau-Demjanov Rearrangement; Wagner-Meerwein Rearrangement.

101. Dess-Martin Oxidation

D. B. Dess, J. C. Martin, *J. Org. Chem.* **48**, 4155 (1983).

Mild oxidation of primary and secondary alcohols to aldehydes and ketones, respectively, employing the triacetoxyperiodinane (the "Dess-Martin Periodinane" reagent):

Scope and limitations of fluoroalkyl-substituted carbinols as substrates: R. J. Linderman, D. M. Graves, *J. Org. Chem.* **54**, 661 (1989). Methods development: D. B. Dess, J. C. Martin, *J. Am. Chem. Soc.* **113**, 7277 (1991). Application to the synthesis of 2′- and 3′-ketonucleosides: V. Samano, M. J. Robins, *J. Org. Chem.* **55**, 5186 (1990); of substituted oxazoles: P. Wipf, C. P. Miller, *ibid.* **58**, 3604 (1993). *See* monograph: Dess-Martin Periodinane.

102. Dieckmann Reaction

W. Dieckmann, *Ber.* **27**, 102, 965 (1894); **33**, 595, 2670, (1900); *Ann.* **317**, 51, 93, (1901).

Base-catalyzed cyclization of dicarboxylic acid esters to give β-ketoesters, the intramolecular equivalent of the Claisen condensation, *q.v.*:

J. P. Schaefer, J. J. Bloomfield, *Org. React.* **15**, 1-203 (1967); H. O. House, *Modern Synthetic Reactions* (W. A. Benjamin, Menlo Park, California, 2nd ed., 1972) pp 740-743; H. Kwart, K. Sing in *The Chemistry of Carboxylic Acids and Esters*, S. Patai, Ed. (Interscience, New York, 1969) p 341; B. R. Davis, P. J. Garrett, *Comp. Org. Syn.* **2**, 806-829 (1991). *Cf.* Gabriel-Colman Rearrangement.

103. Diels-Alder Reaction

O. Diels, K. Alder, *Ann.* **460**, 98 (1928); **470**, 62 (1929); *Ber.* **62**, 2081, 2087 (1929).

The 1,4-addition of the double bond of a dienophile to a conjugated diene to generate a six-membered ring, such that up to four new stereocenters may be created simultaneously. The [4+2]-cycloaddition usually occurs with high regio- and stereoselectivity:

diene   dienophile

Heteroatomic analogs of the diene (e.g., $CHR=CR-CR=O$, $O=CR-CR=O$, and $RN=CR-CR=NR$) and dienophile (e.g., $RN=NR$, $R_2C=NR$, and $RN=O$) may also serve as reactants.

Early reviews: M. C. Kloetzel, *Org. React.* **4**, 1-59 (1948); H. L. Holmes *ibid.* 60-173; L. W. Butz, A. W. Rytina, *ibid.* **5**, 136-192 (1949). Intermolecular reactions: W. Oppolzer, *Comp. Org. Syn.* **5**, 315-399 (1991). Intramolecular reactions: E. Ciganek, *Org. React.* **32**, 1-374 (1984); W. R. Rousch, *Comp. Org. Syn.* **5**, 513-550 (1991). Use of heterodienophiles: S. M. Weinreb, *ibid.* 401-449. Use of nitroso dienophiles: J. Streith, A. DeFoin, *Synthesis* **1994**, 1107-1117. Use of heterodienes: D. L. Boger, *ibid*, 451-512. Review of diastereoselectivity: J. M. Coxon *et al.*, "Diastereofacial Selectivity in the Diels-Alder Reaction" in *Adv. Detailed React. Mech.* **3**, 131-166 (1994); T. Oh, M. Reilly, *Org. Prep. Proced. Int.* **26**, 131-158 (1994); H. Waldmann, *Synthesis* **1994**, 535-551. *Cf.* Wagner-Jauregg Reaction.

104. Dienone-Phenol Rearrangement

K. von Auwers, K. Ziegler, *Ann.* **425**, 217 (1921).

Transformation of a 4,4-disubstituted cyclohexadienone into a 3,4-disubstituted phenol upon acid treatment:

Reviews: C. J. Collins, *et al.*, in *The Chemistry of the Carbonyl Group*, S. Patai, Ed. (Interscience, New York, 1966) pp 775-778; A. J. Waring, *Adv. Alicyclic Chem.* **1**, 207 (1967); B. Miller in *Mechanisms of Molecular Migrations* vol. 1, B. S. Thyagarajan, Ed. (Interscience, New York, 1968) pp 275-285; B. Miller, *Acc. Chem. Res.* **8**, 277 (1975). Mechanism: G. Goodyear, A. J. Waring, *J. Chem. Soc. Perkin Trans. 2* **1990**, 103. Steric effects: A. G. Schultz, N. J. Green, *J. Am. Chem. Soc.* **114**, 1824 (1992); A. A. Frimer *et al.*, *J. Org. Chem.* **59**, 1831 (1994). Synthetic applications: D. J. Hart *et al.*, *Tetrahedron* **48**, 8179 (1992); R. W. Draper *et al.*, *Steroids* **63**, 135 (1998).

105. Dimroth Rearrangement

O. Dimroth, *Ann.* **364**, 183 (1909); **459**, 39 (1927).

Rearrangement whereby exo- and endocyclic heteroatoms on a heterocyclic ring are translocated:

D. J. Brown, J. S. Harper in *Pteridine Chemistry*, W. Pfleiderer, E. C. Taylor, Ed. (Macmillan, New York, 1964) pp 219-230; D. J. Brown in *Mechanisms of Molecular Migrations* vol. 1, B. S. Thyagarajan, Ed. (Wiley-Interscience, New York, 1968) p 209; D. J. Brown in *The Pyrimidines* Suppl. I (Interscience, New York, 1970) p 287; D. J. Brown, K. Lenega, *J. Chem. Soc. Perkin Trans. 1* **1974**, 372. Mechanism: K. Vaughan *et al.*, *Heterocyclic Chem.* **28**, 1709 (1991); T. Itaya *et al.*, *Chem. Pharm. Bull.* **45**, 832 (1997). Modified reaction: A. R. Katritzky *et al.*, *J. Org. Chem.* **57**, 190 (1992); A. R. Pagano *et al.*, *J. Org. Chem.* **63**, 3213 (1998). *Review:* E. S. H. El Ashry *et al.*, *Adv. Heterocycl. Chem.* **75**, 79-167 (2000).

106. Doebner-Miller Reaction; Beyer Method for Quinolines

O. Doebner, W. v. Miller, *Ber.* **16**, 2464 (1883).

Acid-catalyzed synthesis of quinolines from primary aromatic amines and α,β-unsaturated carbonyl compounds. When the latter are prepared *in situ* from two molecules of aldehyde or an aldehyde and methyl ketone, the reaction is known as the **Beyer method for quinolines:**

F. W. Bergström, *Chem. Rev.* **35**, 153 (1944); Y. Ogata *et al., J. Chem. Soc. B* **1969**, 805; G. A. Dauphinee, T. P. Forrest, *J. Chem. Soc. D* **1969**, 327; *Can. J. Chem.* **56**, 632 (1978); C. M. Leir, *J. Org. Chem.* **42**, 911 (1977). Applications: G. K. Lund *et al., J. Chem. Eng. Data* **26**, 227 (1981); W. Buchowiecki *et al., J. Prakt. Chem.* **327**, 1015 (1985); T. Blitzke *et al., ibid.* **335**, 683 (1993). *Cf.* Gould-Jacobs Reaction; Knorr Quinoline Synthesis.

107. Doebner Reaction

O. Doebner, *Ann.* **242**, 265 (1887); *Ber.* **20**, 277 (1887); **27**, 352, 2020 (1894).

Formation of substituted cinchoninic acids from aromatic amines on heating with aldehydes and pyruvic acid:

F. W. Bergström, *Chem. Rev.* **35**, 156 (1944); R. C. Elderfield, *Heterocycl. Compd.* **4**, 25 (1952); C. Centini, *Rev. Soe. Venez. Quim.* **7**(5), 265 (1970); *C.A.* **74**, 76301x (1971); G. E. Gream, A. K. Serelis, *Aust. J. Chem.* **31**, 863 (1978). *Cf.* Combes Quinoline Synthesis; Conrad-Limpach Reaction.

108. Doering-LaFlamme Allene Synthesis

W. von E. Doering, P. M. LaFlamme, *Tetrahedron* **2**, 75 (1958); *US 2933544* (1960).

Treatment of an olefin with bromoform and an alkoxide to yield the 1,1-dibromocyclopropane which reacts with an active metal to produce an allene:

Reviews: M. Murray, *Houben-Weyl* **5/2a**, 985 (1977); V. Nair, *Comp. Org. Syn.* **4**, 1009-1012 (1991).

109. Dötz Reaction

K. H. Dötz, *Angew. Chem. Int. Ed.* **14**, 644 (1975).

Three component cyclization of an aromatic or vinylic alkoxy pentacarbonyl chromium carbene complex, an alkyne, and carbon monoxide, generating a $Cr(CO)_3$ coordinated phenol:

Solvent effects: K. S. Chan *et al., J. Organomet. Chem.* **334**, 9 (1987). Methods development: S. Chamberlin *et al., Tetrahedron* **49**, 5531 (1993); S. Chamberlin, W. D. Wulff, *J. Org. Chem.* **59**, 3047 (1994). Synthetic applications: W. D. Wulff *et al., J. Am. Chem. Soc.* **110**, 7419 (1988); D. L. Boger, I. C. Jacobson, *J. Org. Chem.* **56**, 2115 (1991). *Review:* K. H. Dötz, *New J. Chem.* **14**, 433-445 (1990).

110. Dowd-Beckwith Ring Expansion Reaction

A. L. J. Beckwith *et al., J. Am. Chem. Soc.* **110**, 2565 (1988); P. Dowd, S. C. Choi, *Tetrahedron* **45**, 77 (1989).

Free radical mediated ring expansions of haloalkyl β-ketoesters:

X = Br, I, SePh

Synthetic application: M. G. Banwell, J. M. Cameron, *Tetrahedron Lett.* **37**, 525 (1996); C. Wang *et al., Tetrahedron* **54**, 8355 (1998).

111. Duff Reaction

J. C. Duff, E. J. Bills, *J. Chem. Soc.* **1932**, 1987; **1934**, 1305; **1941**, 547; **1945**, 276.

Formylation of phenols or aromatic amines with hexamethylenetetramine in the presence of an acidic catalyst. *Ortho*-substitution is usual; however in the presence of anhydrous trifluoroacetic acid (TFA) regioselective *ortho* and *para* substitutions are observed.

L. N. Ferguson, *Chem. Rev.* **38**, 230 (1946); Y. Ogata, F. Sugiura, *Tetrahedron* **24**, 5001 (1968); F. Wada *et al., Bull. Chem. Soc. Jpn.* **53**, 1473 (1980). Use of TFA: W. E. Smith, *J. Org. Chem.* **37**, 3972 (1972); J. F. Larrow *et al., ibid.* **59**, 1939 (1994); L. F. Lindoy *et al., Synthesis* **1998**, 1029. *Cf.* Reimer-Tiemann Reaction.

112. Dutt-Wormall Reaction

P. K. Dutt, H. R. Whitehead, A. Wormall, *J. Chem. Soc.* **119**, 2088 (1921); P. K. Dutt, *ibid.* **125**, 1463 (1924).

Preparation of diazoaminosulfinates by reaction of diazonium salts with aryl- or alkylsulfonamides followed by alkaline hydrolysis to yield the corresponding sulfinic acid of the sulfonamide, and the azide:

$$ArN_2Cl \xrightarrow{H_2NSO_2R} ArN=NNHSO_2R \xrightarrow{HO^-} ArN_3 + HO_2SR$$

H. Bretschneider, H. Rager, *Monatsh. Chem.* **81**. 970 (1950); I. G. Laing, *Rodd's Chemistry of Carbon Compounds* **IIIC**, 107 (1973); C. Grundmann, *Houben-Weyl* **10/3**, 808 (1965).

113. Eastwood Reaction (Eastwood Deoxygenation)

G. Grank, F. W. Eastwood, *Aust. J. Chem.* **17**, 1392 (1964).

Stereospecific conversion of vicinal diols into olefins:

Review: E. Block, *Org. React.* **30**, 478-491 (1984). *Cf.* Corey-Winter Olefin Synthesis.

114. Edman Degradation

P. Edman, *Acta Chem. Scand.* **4**, 283 (1950).

Cyclic degradation of peptides based on the reaction of phenylisothiocyanate with the free amino group of the *N*-terminal residue such that amino acids are removed one at a time and identified as their phenylthiohydantoin derivatives:

S. Bösze *et al., J. Chromatogr. A* **668**, 345 (1994). *Reviews:* R. A. Laursen *et al., Methods Biochem. Anal.* **26**, 201-284 (1980); R. L. Heinrikson, "The Edman Degradation in Protein Sequence Analysis" in *Biochemical and Biophysical Studies of Proteins and Nucleic Acids*, T.-B. Lo *et al.*, Eds. (Elsevier, New York, 1984) pp 285-302; K.-K. Han *et al., Int. J. Biochem.* **17**, 429-445 (1985); C. G. Fields *et al., Pept. Res.* **6**, 39-47 (1993).

115. Ehrlich-Sachs Reaction

P. Ehrlich, F. Sachs, *Ber.* **32**, 2341 (1899).

Formation of *N*-phenylimines by the base-catalyzed condensation of compounds containing active methylene groups with aromatic nitroso compounds; nitrones also may be formed:

$$C_6H_5CH_2CN + C_6H_5NO \longrightarrow \underset{C_6H_5}{\overset{NC}{>}}\!=\!NC_6H_5 + H_2O$$

F. Barrow, F. J. Thorneycroft, *J. Chem. Soc.* **1939**, 769; A. McGookin, *J. Appl. Chem.* **5**, 65 (1955); F. Bell, *J. Chem. Soc.* **1957**, 516; D. M. W. Anderson, F. Bell, *ibid.* **1959**, 3708; D. M. W. Anderson, J. L. Duncan, *ibid.* **1961**, 1631; W. Seidenfaden, *Houben-Weyl* **10/1**, 1079 (1971). Applications: F. Millich, M. T. El-Shoubary, *Org. Prep. Proced. Int.* **28**, 366 (1996); S. K. De *et al.*, *Can. J. Chem.* **76**, 199 (1998).

116. Einhorn-Brunner Reaction

A. Einhorn *et al.*, *Ann.* **343**, 229 (1905); K. Brunner, *Ber.* **47**, 2671 (1914); *Monatsh. Chem.* **36**, 509 (1915).

Formation of substituted 1,2,4-triazoles by acid-catalyzed condensation of hydrazines or semicarbazides with diacylamines:

M. R. Atkinson, J. B. Polya, *J. Chem. Soc.* **1952**, 3418; **1954**, 141, 3319; Theilheimer, *Synthetic Methods* **9**, No. 449 (1955); K. T. Potts, *Chem. Rev.* **61**, 103 (1961); K. Hu *et al.*, *J. Org. Chem.* **63**, 4786 (1998). *Cf.* Pellizzari Reaction.

117. Elbs Persulfate Oxidation

K. Elbs, *J. Prakt. Chem.* **48**, 179 (1893).

Hydroxylation of monophenols to predominantely *p*-diphenols or oxidation of methyl-substituted aromatics by persulfates:

S. M. Sethna, *Chem. Rev.* **49**, 91 (1951); J. B. Lee, B. C. Uff, *Q. Rev. Chem. Soc.* **21**, 453 (1967); E. J. Behrman, *Org. React.* **35**, 421-511 (1988); K. A. Parker, *et al.*, *J. Org. Chem.* **52**, 183 (1987); K. G. Watson, A. Serban, *Aust. J. Chem.* **48**, 1503 (1995). *Cf.* Boyland-Sims Oxidation.

118. Elbs Reaction

K. Elbs, E. Larsen, *Ber.* **17**, 2847 (1884).

Formation of polyaromatics (*eg.* anthracene) by intramolecular condensation of diaryl ketones containing a methyl or methylene substituent adjacent to the carbonyl group:

L. F. Fieser, *Org. React.* **1**, 129 (1942); G. N. Badger, B. J. Christie, *J. Chem. Soc.* **1956**, 3435; N. P. Buu-Hoi, D. Lavit, *Rec. Trav. Chim.* **76**, 419 (1957); Cl. Marie *et al.*, *J. Chem. Soc.* **1971**, 431; M. S. Newman, V. K. Khanna, *J. Org. Chem.* **45**, 4507 (1980).

119. Emde Degradation

H. Emde, *Ber.* **42**, 2590 (1909); *Ann.* **391**, 88 (1912).

Modification of the Hofmann degradation, *q.v.*, method for reductive cleavage of the carbon-nitrogen bond by treatment of an alcoholic or aqueous solution of a quaternary ammonium halide with sodium amalgam. Also used as a catalytic method with palladium and platinum catalysts. The method succeeds with ring compounds not degraded by the Hofmann procedure:

Reviews: A. Birch, *Org. React.* **7**, 143 278 (1953); F. Möller, *Houben-Weyl* **11/1,** 973 (1955); Z. Spialter, J. A. Pappalardo, *Acyclic Aliphatic Tertiary Amines* (Macmillan, New York, 1965) pp 79-81. Photodegradation: V. Partail, *Helv. Chim. Acta* **68,** 1952 (1985). Synthetic applications: J. G. Cannon *et al., J. Med. Chem.* **18,** 110 (1975); J. Lévy *et al., Tetrahedron: Asymmetry* **8,** 4127 (1997).

120. Emmert Reaction
B. Emmert, E. Asendorf, *Ber.* **72,** 1188 (1939); B. Emmert, E. Pirot, *ibid.* **74,** 714 (1941).
Formation of pyridyldialkylcarbinols by condensation of ketones with pyridine or its homologs in the presence of aluminum or magnesium amalgam:

C. H. Tilford *et al., J. Am. Chem. Soc.* **70,** 4001 (1948); H. L. Lochti *et al., ibid.* **75,** 4477 (1953); R. Abramovitch, R. Vinutha, *J. Chem. Soc. C* **1969,** 2104; C. A. Russell *et al., J. Chem. Soc. D* **1970,** 1406; R. Tschesche, W. Führer, *Ber.* **111,** 3502 (1978).

121. Ene Reaction (Alder-Ene Reaction); Conia-Ene Reaction
K. Alder *et al., Ber.* **76,** 27 (1943).
The addition of an alkene having an allylic hydrogen (ene) to a compound containing a multiple bond (enophile) to form a new bond between two unsaturated termini, with an allylic shift of the ene double bond, and transfer of the allylic hydrogen to the enophile. The mechanism is related to that of the Diels-Alder reaction, *q.v.*:

enophile = carbonyl and thiocarbonyl compounds, imines, alkenes, alkynes
Lewis acid = BF₃•O(CH₂CH₃)₂, SnCl₄, Al(CH₂CH₃)Cl₂, Al(CH₃)₂Cl

Lewis acid-promoted cyclization of 5-hexenals: J. A. Marshall, *Chemtracts: Org. Chem.* **5,** 1-7 (1992). Review of alkenes as enophiles: B. B. Snider, *Comp. Org. Syn.* **5,** 1-27 (1991). Review of carbonyl compounds as enophiles: *idem, ibid.* **2,** 527-561; in conjunction with asymmetric synthesis: K. Mikami, M. Shimizu, *Chem. Rev.* **92,** 1021-1050 (1992); K. Mikami *et al., Synlett* **1992,** 255-265.
The intramolecular Ene reaction of unsaturated ketones, in which the carbonyl functionality serves as the ene component, *via* its tautomer, and the olefinic moiety serves as the enophile, is known as the **Conia-Ene reaction**: F. Rouessac *et al., Tetrahedron Lett.* **6,** 3319 (1965).

A. S. Kende, R. C. Newbold, *Tetrahedron Lett.* **30,** 4329 (1989). J. J. Kennedy-Smith *et al., J. Am. Chem. Soc.* **126,** 4526 (2004). Q. Gao *et al., Org. Lett.* **7,** 2185 (2005). *Review:* J. M. Conia, P. Le Perchec, *Synthesis* **1975,** 1-19.

122. Erlenmeyer-Plöchl Azlactone and Amino Acid Synthesis
E. Erlenmeyer, *Ann.* **275,** 1 (1893); J. Plöchl, *Ber.* **17,** 1616 (1884).
Formation of azlactones by intramolecular condensation of acylglycines in the presence of acetic anhydride. The reaction of azlactones with carbonyl compounds followed by hydrolysis to the unsaturated α-acylamino acid and by reduction yields the amino acid; drastic hydrolysis gives the α-oxo acid:

C. L. A. Schmidt, *The Chemistry of the Amino Acids and Proteins* (Springfield, IL, 1944) p 54; H. E. Carter, *Org. React.* **3**, 198 (1946); M. Crawford, W. T. Little, *J. Chem. Soc.* **1959**, 729; W. Steglich, *Fortschr. Chem. Forsch.* **12**, 84 (1969); J. Cornforth, D. Ming-hui, *J. Chem. Soc. Perkin Trans. 1* **1991**, 2183; A. P. Combs, R. W. Armstrong, *Tetrahedron Lett.* **33**, 6419 (1992). *Cf.* Bergmann Azlactone Peptide Synthesis; Perkin Reaction.

123. Eschenmoser Coupling Reaction (Sulfide Contraction)

A. Fischli, A. Eschenmoser, *Angew. Chem. Int. Ed.* **6**, 866 (1967); M. Roth *et al., Helv. Chim. Acta* **54**, 710 (1971).

Formation of vinylogous amides and urethanes by alkylation of secondary or tertiary thioamides with an electrophilic agent followed by elimination of sulfur:

Synthetic applications: E. Götschi *et al., Angew. Chem. Int. Ed.* **12**, 910 (1973); O. Sakurai *et al., J. Org. Chem.* **61**, 7889 (1996), T. G. Minehan, Y. Kishi, *Tetrahedron Lett.* **38**, 6811 (1997). *Review:* K. Shiosaki, *Comp. Org. Syn.* **2**, 865-894 (1991).

124. Eschenmoser Fragmentation (Eschenmoser-Tanabe Fragmentation)

A. Eschenmoser *et al., Helv. Chim. Acta* **50**, 708 (1967); J. Schreiber *et al., ibid.* 2101; M. Tanabe *et al., Tetrahedron Lett.* **1967**, 3943.

Cleavage of α,β-epoxyketones under mild conditions, *via* sulfonylhydrazone intermediates, to yield acetylenic and carbonyl compounds:

R^5 = *p*-toluene, 2,4,6-trimethylbenzene, 2,4-dinitrobenzene
optional catalyst = C_6H_5N, $NaHCO_3$, Na_2CO_3, silica gel

Early review: D. Felix *et al., Helv. Chim. Acta* **54**, 2896-2912 (1971). Synthetic applications: C. B. Reese, H. P. Sanders, *Synthesis* **1981**, 276; W. Dai, J. A. Katzenellenbogen, *J. Org. Chem.* **58**, 1900 (1993); A. Abad *et al., Synlett* **1991**, 787. *Cf.* Grob Fragmentation; Wharton Reaction.

125. Étard Reaction

A. L. Étard, *Compt. Rend.* **90**, 534 (1880); *Ann. Chim. Phys.* **22**, 218 (1881).

Oxidation of an arylmethyl group to an aldehyde by treatment with chromyl chloride:

$$C_6H_5CH_3 \xrightarrow{CrO_2Cl_2} C_6H_5CHO$$

W. H. Hartford, M. Darrin, *Chem. Rev.* **58**, 1 (1958); H. O. House, *Modern Synthetic Reactions* (W. A. Benjamin, Menlo Park, California, 2nd ed., 1972) p 289; C. D. Nenitzescu *et al., Rev. Roum. Chim.* **14**, 1543, 1553 (1969); I. I.

Schiketanz *et al., ibid.* **22**, 1097 (1977); J. C. W. Chien, J. K. Y. Kiang, *Macromolecules* **13**, 280 (1980); F. A. Luzzio, W. J. Moore, *J. Org. Chem.* **58**, 512 (1993).

126. Evans Aldol Reaction
D. A. Evans *et al., J. Am. Chem. Soc.* **101**, 6120 (1979); **103**, 2127 (1981).

Highly enantioselective aldol condensation of the chiral *N*-acyl-oxazolidone via its dibutylboryl enolate with the appropriate aldehyde:

Mechanistic studies: D. A. Evans *et al., J. Am. Chem. Soc.* **103**, 3099 (1981). Synthetic applications: C. W. Phoon, C. Abell, *Tetrahedron Lett.* **39**, 2655 (1998); C. Pearson *et al., ibid.* **40**, 411 (1999). Inversion of product stereochemistry: K. Iseki *et al., ibid.* **34**, 8147 (1993); T. Gabriel, L. Wessjohann, *ibid.* **38**, 4387 (1997). *Review:* D. A. Evans, *Aldrichim. Acta* **15**, 23-32 (1982); B. M. Kim *et al., Comp. Org. Syn.* **2**, 239-275 (1991). *Cf.* Aldol Condensation, Mukaiyama Aldol Reaction.

127. Favorskii-Babayan Synthesis
A. E. Favorskii, *J. Russ. Phys. Chem. Soc.* **37**, 643 (1905); *Chem. Zentralbl.* **1905, II**, 1018; A. Babayan *et al., J. Gen. Chem. USSR* **9**, 1631 (1939).

Synthesis of acetylenic alcohols from ketones and terminal acetylenes in the presence of anhydrous alkali:

A. W. Johnson, *The Chemistry of Acetylenic Compounds* **vol. 1** (London, 1946) p 14; R. A. Raphael, *Acetylenic Compounds in Organic Synthesis* (New York, 1955) p 10; M. F. Shostakovskii *et al., Zh. Org. Khim.* **4**, 1747 (1968); A. V. Shchelkunov *et al., ibid.* **6**, 930 (1970); E. M. Glazunova *et al., Zh. Org. Khim.* **12**, 516 (1976); Y. M. Vilenchik *et al., ibid.* **14**, 447 (1978). *Cf.* Arens-van Dorp Synthesis; Nef Synthesis.

128. Favorskii Rearrangement; Wallach Degradation
A. E. Favorskii, *J. Prakt. Chem.* **88**(2), 658 (1913); O. Wallach, *Ann.* **414**, 296 (1918).

Base-catalyzed rearrangement of *α*-haloketones to acids or esters. The rearrangement of *α,α′*-dibromo-cyclohexanones to 1-hydroxycyclopentanecarboxylic acids, followed by oxidation to the ketones is known as the **Wallach degradation:**

Detailed experimental procedure: D. W. Goheen, W. R. Vaughan, *Org. Synth.* **coll. vol. 4**, 594 (1963). Application to the synthesis of carboxylic acids: T. Satoh *et al., Bull. Chem. Soc. Jpn.* **66**, 2339 (1993). Applications to asymmetric synthesis: *idem et al., Tetrahedron Lett.* **34**, 4823 (1993); E. Lee, C. H. Yoon, *Chem. Commun.* **1994**, 479. *Reviews:* A. S. Kende, *Org. React.* **11**, 261-316 (1960); P. J. Chenier, *J. Chem. Educ.* **55**, 286 (1978); A. Baretta, B. Waegill, "A Survey of Favorskii Rearrangement Mechanisms" in *Reactive Intermediates*, R. A. Abramovitch, Ed. (Plenum Press, New York, 1982) pp 527-585; J. Mann, *Comp. Org. Syn.* **3**, 839-859 (1991).

129. Feist-Bénary Synthesis
F. Feist, *Ber.* **35**, 1537, 1545 (1902); E. Bénary, *Ber.* **44**, 489, 493 (1911).

Formation of furans from *α*-halogenated ketones or ethers and 1,3-dicarbonyl compounds in the presence of pyridine. When ammonia is used as the condensing agent, pyrrole derivatives are always formed as secondary products:

T. Reichstein, H. Zschokke, *Helv. Chim. Acta* **14**, 1270 (1931); **15**, 268, 1105, 1112 (1932); R. C. Elderfield, T. N. Dodd, *Heterocycl. Compd.* **1**, 132 (1950); J. Kagan, K. C. Mattes, *J. Org. Chem.* **45**, 1524 (1980). Alternative substrate: R. C. Cambie *et al.*, *Synth. Commun.* **20**, 1923 (1990). Catalytic, enantioselective "interrupted" reaction: M. A. Calter *et al.*, *J. Am. Chem. Soc.* **127**, 14566 (2005). *Cf.* Hantzsch Pyrrole Synthesis.

130. Fenton Reaction

H. J. H. Fenton, *Proc. Chem. Soc. London* **9**, 113 (1893); *J. Chem. Soc.* **65**, 899 (1894).

Oxidation of α-hydroxy acids with hydrogen peroxide and ferrous salts (Fenton's reagent) to α-keto acids or of 1,2-glycols to hydroxy aldehydes:

W. A. Waters in *Organic Chemistry* vol. 4, H. Gilman, Ed. (Wiley, New York, 1953) p 1157; G. Sosnovsky, D. Rawlinson in *Organic Peroxides* **vol. 2**, D. Swern, Ed. (Interscience, New York, 1970) pp 269-336; C. Walling, *Acc. Chem. Res.* **8**, 125 (1975); T. Tezuka *et al.*, *J. Am. Chem. Soc.* **103**, 3045 (1981); C. Walling, K. Amarnath, *ibid.* **104**, 1185 (1982). Extension to additional substrates: aromatic alcohols: F. J. Benitez *et al.*, *Ind. Eng. Chem. Res.* **38**, 1341 (1999); L. Lunar *et al.*, *Water Res.* **34**, 1791 (2000); *N*-heterocyclics: M. A. Oturan *et al.*, *New J. Chem.* **23**, 793 (1999); E. L. Bier *et al.*, *Environ. Toxicol. Chem.* **18**, 1078 (1999); organometals: K. Banerjee *et al.*, *Environ. Prog.* **18**, 280 (1999).

131. Ferrier Rearrangement

R. J. Ferrier, *J. Chem. Soc. Perkin Trans. 1* **1979**, 1455.

The stereochemically controlled conversion of hex-5-enopyranosides into cyclohexanones (inosose derivatives), catalyzed by mercury(II) salts, such that the 5-hydroxyl and the 3-substituent of the product are predominantly in a *trans* relationship:

Stereochemical/mechanistic study: A. S. Machado *et al.*, *Carbohydr. Res.* **233**, C5 (1992); N. Yamauchi *et al.*, *Tetrahedron* **50**, 4125 (1994). Scope and limitations: N. Chida *et al.*, *Bull. Chem. Soc. Jpn.* **64**, 2118 (1991). Synthetic applications: D. H. R. Barton *et al.*, *Tetrahedron* **46**, 215 (1990); R. Chretien *et al.*, *Nat. Prod. Lett.* **2**, 69 (1993); A. B. Smith III *et al.*, *Org. Lett.* **1**, 909 (1999); *eidem, ibid.* 913. Modification of catalysis: J. C. López *et al.*, *J. Org. Chem.* **60**, 3851 (1995); T. Linker *et al.*, *Tetrahedron Lett.* **39**, 9637 (1998); B. S. Babu *et al.*, *Synth. Commun.* **29**, 4299 (1999); S. Hotha, A. Tripathi, *Tetrahedron Lett.* **46**, 4555 (2005).

132. Finkelstein Reaction

H. Finkelstein, *Ber.* **43**, 1528 (1910).

Reaction of alkyl halides with sodium iodide in acetone:

$$RBr + NaI \longrightarrow RI + NaBr$$

C. K. Ingold, *Structure and Mechanism in Organic Chemistry* (Cornell Univ. Press, London, 2nd ed., 1969) p 435; J. Hayami *et al.*, *Tetrahedron Lett.* **1973**, 385; S. Samaan, F. Rolla, *Phosphorus Sulfur* **4**, 145 (1978); W. B. Smith, G. D. Branum, *Tetrahedron Lett.* **22**, 2055 (1981). Modified conditions: D. Landini *et al.*, *J. Chem. Soc. Perkin Trans. 1* **1992**, 2309. Applications: A. J. Pearson, K. Lee, *J. Org. Chem.* **59**, 2304 (1994); A. Schmidt, M. K. Kindermann, *ibid.* **62**, 3910 (1997); T. Zoller *et al.*, *Tetrahedron Lett.* **39**, 8089 (1998).

133. Fischer-Hepp Rearrangement (Nitrosamine Rearrangement)

O. Fischer, E. Hepp, *Ber.* **19**, 2991 (1886).

Rearrangement of secondary aromatic nitrosamines to *p*-nitrosoarylamines:

$$R-N-NO \xrightarrow{\quad HCl \quad} R-N-H$$

H. J. Shine, *Aromatic Rearrangements* (Elsevier, New York, 1967) p 231; D. L. H. Williams in *Comprehensive Chemical Kinetics* **vol. 13** (1972) p 454; S. Johan *et al., J. Chem. Soc. Perkin Trans. 2* **1980,** 165. Mechanism: D. L. H. Williams, *ibid.* **1982,** 801. Applications: J. B. Kyziol, *J. Heterocycl. Chem.* **22,** 1301 (1985); P. Kannan *et al., J. Mol. Catal.* **118,** 189 (1997).

134. Fischer Indole Synthesis
E. Fischer, F. Jourdan, *Ber.* **16,** 2241 (1883); E. Fischer, O. Hess, *ibid.* **17,** 559 (1884).

Formation of indoles on heating aryl hydrazones of aldehydes or ketones in the presence of catalysts such as Lewis or proton acids:

Reviews: B. Robinson, *Chem. Rev.* **63,** 373 (1963); **69,** 227 (1969); H. Ishii, *Acc. Chem. Res.* **14,** 233-247 (1981); B. Robinson, *The Fischer Indole Synthesis* (Wiley, New York, 1982) 923 pp.; D. L. Hughes, *Org. Prep. Proced. Int.* **25,** 607-632 (1993). Modified conditions: S. M. Hutchins, K. T. Chapman, *Tetrahedron Lett.* **37,** 4869 (1996); O. Miyata *et al., ibid.* **40,** 3601 (1999); S. Wagaw *et al., J. Am. Chem. Soc.* **121,** 10251 (1999). *Cf.* Borsche-Drechsel Cyclization; Piloty-Robinson Synthesis.

135. Fischer Oxazole Synthesis
E. Fischer, *Ber.* **29,** 205 (1896).

Condensation of equimolar amounts of aldehyde cyanohydrins and aromatic aldehydes in dry ether in the presence of dry hydrochloric acid:

$$RCHOHCN + R^1CHO \xrightarrow{\quad ether \quad} \underset{N}{R^1}\overset{O}{\diagup}R + H_2O + H_2$$

R. H. Wiley, *Chem. Rev.* **37,** 410 (1945); J. W. Cornforth, R. H. Cornforth, *J. Chem. Soc.* **1949,** 1028; J. W. Cornforth, *Heterocycl. Compd.* **5,** 309 (1957); T. Onaka, *Tetrahedron Lett.* **1971,** 4391.

136. Fischer Peptide Synthesis
E. Fischer, *Ber.* **36,** 2982 (1903).

Formation of polypeptides by treatment of an α-chloro or α-bromo acyl chloride with an amino acid ester, hydrolysis to the acid and conversion to a new acid chloride which is again condensed with a second amino acid ester, and so on. The terminal chloride is finally converted to an amino group with ammonia:

(steps repeated)

C. L. A. Schmidt, *The Chemistry of the Amino Acids and Proteins* (Thomas, Springfield, IL, 1944) p 257; B. Rockland in *Amino Acids and Proteins,* D. M. Greenberg, Ed. (Charles C. Thomas, Springfield, IL, 1951) p 232; H. D. Springall, *The Structural Chemistry of Proteins* (New York, 1954) p 24. *Cf.* Bergmann-Zervas Carbobenzoxy Method.

137. Fischer Phenylhydrazine Synthesis
E. Fischer, *Ber.* **8,** 589 (1875).

Formation of arylhydrazines by reduction of diazo compounds with excess sodium sulfite and hydrolysis of the substituted hydrazine sulfonic acid salt with hydrochloric acid. The process is a standard industrial method for production of arylhydrazines:

$$ArN_2^+ \xrightarrow{\text{NaSO}_3^-} ArN=NSO_3Na \xrightarrow{\text{NaHSO}_3} \underset{ArNNHSO_3Na}{\overset{SO_3Na}{\diagdown}} \xrightarrow{\text{HCl}} ArNHNH_2$$

G. H. Colemann, *Org. Synth.* **coll. vol. I,** 432 (1932); K. H. Saunders, *The Aromatic Diazo-Compounds and Their Technical Applications* (London, 1949) p 183; R. Huisgen, R. Lux, *Ber.* **93,** 540 (1960).

138. Fischer Phenylhydrazone and Osazone Reaction
E. Fischer, *Ber.* **17,** 579 (1884).

Formation of phenylhydrazones and osazones by heating sugars with phenylhydrazine in dilute acetic acid:

$$\underset{\overset{|}{HCOH}}{\overset{\overset{|}{CHO}}{}} \xrightarrow{C_6H_5NHNH_2} \underset{\overset{|}{HCOH}}{\overset{\overset{|}{HC=NNHC_6H_5}}{}} \longrightarrow \underset{\overset{|}{COH}}{\overset{\overset{|}{HCNHNC_6H_5}}{\overset{\|}{}}} \xrightarrow{-C_6H_5NH_2}$$

$$\underset{\overset{|}{CO}}{\overset{\overset{|}{HC=NH}}{}} \xrightarrow{2eq.\ C_6H_5NHNH_2} \underset{\overset{|}{C=NNHC_6H_5}}{\overset{\overset{|}{HC=NNHC_6H_5}}{}}$$

E. G. V. Percival, *Adv. Carbohydr. Chem.* **3,** 23 (1948); F. Micheel, *Chemie der Zucker und Polysaccharide* (Leipzig, 1956) p 54; W. Pigman, *The Carbohydrates* **1957,** 452, 455; H. Simon *et al., Fortschr. Chem. Forsch.* **14,** 451 (1970).

139. Fischer-Speier Esterification Method
E. Fischer, A. Speier, *Ber.* **28,** 3252 (1895).

Esterification of acids by refluxing with excess alcohol in the presence of hydrogen chloride or other acid catalysts:

$$CH_3COOH + CH_3CH_2OH \xrightarrow{3\%\ HCl} CH_3COOCH_2CH_3 + H_2O$$

E. D. Hughes, *Q. Rev. Chem. Soc.* **2,** 110 (1948); A. J. Kirby in *Comprehensive Chemical Kinetics* **vol. 10,** C. H. Bamford, C. F. H. Tipper, Eds. (Elsevier, New York, 1972) p 57; E. K. Euranto in *The Chemistry of Carboxylic Acids and Esters,* S. Patai, Ed. (Interscience, New York, 1969) p 505.

140. Fischer-Tropsch Syntheses; Synthol Process; Oxo Synthesis
F. Fischer, H. Tropsch, *Ber.* **56,** 2428 (1923).

Synthesis of hydrocarbons, aliphatic alcohols, aldehydes, and ketones by the catalytic hydrogenation of carbon monoxide using enriched synthesis gas from passage of steam over heated coke. The ratio of products varies with conditions. The high pressure **Synthol process** gives mainly oxygenated products and addition of olefins in the presence of cobalt catalyst, **Oxo synthesis,** produces aldehydes. Normal pressure synthesis leads mainly to petroleum-like hydrocarbons.

C. Masters, *Adv. Organomet. Chem.* **17,** 61 (1979); C. K. Rofer-DePoorter, *Chem. Rev.* **31,** 447 (1981); W. A. Herrmann, *Angew. Chem. Int. Ed.* **21,** 117 (1982). *Reviews:* P. M. Maitlis *et al., Chem. Commun.* **1996,** 1-8; H. Schulz, *Appl. Catal.* **186,** 3-12 (1999). *Cf.* Bergius Process; Oxo Process.

141. Flood Reaction
E. A. Flood, *J. Am. Chem. Soc.* **55,** 1735 (1933).

Formation of trialkylsilyl halides from hexaalkyldisiloxanes using concentrated sulfuric acid in the presence of ammonium chloride or fluoride, or by treatment of the intermediate silane sulfates with hydrogen chloride in the presence of ammonium sulfate:

$$R_3SiOSiR_3 \xrightarrow[H_2SO_4]{NH_4Cl} R_3SiCl$$

$$R_3SiOSiR_3 \xrightarrow{H_2SO_4} (R_3Si)_2SO_2 \xrightarrow[(NH_4)_2SO_4]{HCl} R_3SiCl$$

H. W. Post, *Silicones and Other Organic Compounds* (New York, 1949) p 64; E. G. Rochow *et al., The Chemistry of Organometallic Compounds* (New York, 1957) p 158, 159. Synthetic applications: L. Birkofer, O. Stuhl, *Top. Curr. Chem.* **88,** 33 (1980).

142. Forster Diazoketone Synthesis
M. O. J. Forster, *J. Chem. Soc.* **107,** 260 (1915).

Formation of diazoketones from α-oximinoketones by reaction with chloramine:

M. P. Cava, R. L. Litle, *Chem. Ind. (London)* **1957,** 367; W. Kirmse *et al., Angew. Chem.* **69,** 106 (1957). Mechanism: J. Meinwald *et al., J. Am. Chem. Soc.* **81,** 4751 (1959). Application to steroids: M. P. Cava, B. R.

Vogt, *J. Org. Chem.* **30**, 3776 (1965). Review and applications: F. Weygand, H. J. Bestmann, *Angew. Chem.* **72**, 535 (1960); W. Rundel, *ibid.* **74**, 469 (1962).

143. Forster Reaction
M. O. J. Forster, *J. Chem. Soc.* **75**, 934 (1899); H. Decker, P. Becker, *Ann.* **395**, 362 (1913).
  Formation of secondary amines by condensation of a primary amine with an aldehyde, addition of alkyl halide to the Schiff base, and subsequent hydrolysis:

H. Glaser, *Houben-Weyl* **11/1**, 108 (1957); F. Möller, *ibid.* p 956.

144. Franchimont Reaction
A. P. N. Franchimont, *Ber.* **5**, 1048 (1872).
  Carboxylic acid dimerization to 1,2-dicarboxylic acids by treating α-bromocarboxylic acids with potassium cyanide followed by hydrolysis and decarboxylation:

$$2C_6H_5CHBrCOOR + KCN \longrightarrow \begin{matrix} CN \\ | \\ C_6H_5-CCOOR \\ | \\ C_6H_5-CHCOOR \end{matrix} \xrightarrow[\text{2. -CO}_2]{\text{1. OH}^-} \begin{matrix} C_6H_5-CHCOOH \\ | \\ C_6H_5-CHCOOH \end{matrix}$$

N. Zelinsky, *Ber.* **21**, 3160 (1888); O. Poppe, *ibid.* **23**, 113 (1890); R. C. Fuson *et al., J. Am. Chem. Soc.* **51**, 1536 (1929); **52**, 4074 (1930); **60**, 1237 (1938); H. N. Rydon, *J. Chem. Soc.* **1936**, 593; H. Henecka, *Chemie der Beta-Dicarbonylverbindungen* (Berlin, 1950) p 176.

145. Frankland-Duppa Reaction
E. Frankland, *Ann.* **126**, 109 (1863); E. Frankland, B. F. Duppa, *Ann.* **135**, 25 (1865).
  Formation of α-hydroxycarboxylic esters by reaction of dialkyl oxalates with alkyl halides in the presence of zinc, or amalgamated zinc, and acid:

$$ROOC-COOR + 2R^1I + 2Zn + 2HCl \longrightarrow R^1R^1C(OH)COOR + ROH + ZnI_2 + ZnCl_2$$

E. Krause, A. von Grosse, *Die Chemie der Metallorganischen Verbindungen* (Berlin, 1937) p 225; K. Nützel, *Houben-Weyl* **13/2a**, 741 (1973).

146. Frankland Synthesis
E. Frankland, *Ann.* **71**, 213 (1849); **85**, 3641 (1853).
  Synthesis of zinc dialkyls from alkyl halides and zinc:

$$2C_2H_5I + 2Zn \longrightarrow (C_2H_5)_2Zn + ZnI_2$$

Reviews: K. Nützel, *Houben-Weyl* **13/2a**, 570 (1973); C. R. Noller, *Org. Synth.* **coll. vol. II**, 184 (1943).

147. Freund Reaction; Gustavson Reaction; Hass Cyclopropane Process
A. Freund, *Monatsh. Chem.* **3**, 625 (1882); G. Gustavson, *J. Prakt. Chem.* [2] **36**, 300 (1887); H. B. Hass *et al., Ind. Eng. Chem.* **28**, 1178 (1936).
  Formation of alicyclic hydrocarbons by the action of sodium (Freund reaction) or zinc (**Gustavson reaction**) on open chain dihalo compounds; 1,3-dichloropropane derived from the chlorination of propane obtained from natural gas is cyclized in the **Hass cyclopropane process** by treating with zinc dust in aqueous alcohol in the presence of catalytic sodium iodide:

H. Gilman, *Organic Chemistry* **I** (New York, 1943) p 74; J. D. Bartleson *et al., J. Am. Chem. Soc.* **68**, 2513 (1946); R. N. Shortsidge *et al., ibid.* **70**, 946 (1948); B. T. Brooks, *The Chemistry of the Nonbenzenoid Hydrocarbons* (New York, 1950) p 88; H. F. Ebel, A. Lüttringhaus, *Houben-Weyl* **13/1**, 492 (1970).

148. Friedel-Crafts Reaction
C. Friedel, J. M. Crafts, *Compt. Rend.* **84**, 1392, 1450 (1877).
  The alkylation or acylation of aromatic compounds catalyzed by aluminum chloride or other Lewis acids:

RCOX = acyl halides, anhydrides
RX = alkyl halides, alkenes, alkynes, alcohols

Reviews: C. C. Price, *Org. React.* **3**, 1 (1946); G. A. Olah, *Friedel-Crafts and Related Reactions* vol. **1-4** (Interscience, New York, 1963-1965); J. K. Groves, *Chem. Soc. Rev.* **1**, 73 (1972); H. Heaney, *Comp. Org. Syn.* **2**, 733-752, 753-768 (1991); **3**, 293-339. Aliphatic version: S. C. Eyley, *ibid.* **2**, 707-731. Intramolecular reactions: H.-J. Knölker, *Angew. Chem. Int. Ed.* **38**, 2583 (1999); M.-C. P. Yeh *et al., J. Organomet. Chem.* **599**, 128 (2000); C.-L. Kao *et al., Tetrahedron Lett.* **41**, 2207 (2000). Modified conditions: U. Bierman, J. O. Metzger, *Angew. Chem. Int. Ed.* **38**, 3675 (1999). *Cf.* Darzens-Nenitzescu Synthesis of Ketones; Haworth Phenanthrene Synthesis; Nencki Reaction.

149. Friedlaender Synthesis
P. Friedlaender, *Ber.* **15**, 2572 (1882); P. Friedlaender, C. F. Gohring, *ibid.* **16**, 1833 (1883).
  Base-catalyzed condensation of 2-aminobenzaldehydes with ketones to form quinoline derivatives:

Reviews: R. H. Manske, *Chem. Rev.* **30**, 124 (1942); C. C. Cheng, S. J. Yan, *Org. React.* **28**, 37 (1982). Cyclic ketones containing S, or N: G. Kempter, S. Hirschberg, *ibid.* **98**, 419 (1965); K. Rao *et al., J. Heterocycl. Chem.* **16**, 1241 (1979). Modified conditions: I.-S. Cho *et al., J. Org. Chem.* **56**, 7288 (1991); G. Sabitha *et al., Synth. Commun.* **29**, 4403 (1999). Review: R. P. Thummel, *Synlett* **1992**, 1-12. *Cf.* Niementowski Quinoline Synthesis; Pfitzinger Reaction.

150. Fries Rearrangement
K. Fries, G. Fink, *Ber.* **41**, 4271 (1908); K. Fries, W. Pfaffendorf, *ibid.* **43**, 212 (1910).
  Rearrangement of phenolic esters to *o*- and/or *p*-phenolic ketones with Lewis acid catalysts:

A. H. Blatt, *Org. React.* **1**, 342 (1942); A. Gerecs in *Friedel-Crafts and Related Reactions* in vol. **3,** Part 1; G. Olah, Ed. (Interscience, New York, 1964) pp 499-533; F. R. Jensen, G. Goldman in *ibid.* Part 2, p 1349; R. Martin *et al., Monatsh. Chem.* **81**, 111 (1980); R. Martin, *Org. Prep. Proced. Int.* **24**, 369 (1992). Photo-rearrangement: J. C. Anderson, C. B. Reese, *Proc. Chem. Soc. London* **1960**, 217; D. Bellus, *Adv. Photochem.* **8**, 109 (1971); D. J. Crouse *et al., J. Org. Chem.* **46**, 374 (1981); W. Gu *et al., J. Am. Chem. Soc.* **121**, 9467 (1999). Modified conditions: K. J. Balkus, Jr. *et al., J. Mol. Catal. A* **134**, 137 (1998); B. Kaboudin, *Tetrahedron* **55**, 12865 (1999); B. M. Khadilkar, V. R. Madyar, *Synth. Commun.* **29**, 1195 (1999).

151. Fritsch-Buttenberg-Wiechell Rearrangement
P. Fritsch, *Ann.* **279**, 319 (1894); W. P. Buttenberg, *ibid.* 327; H. Wiechell, *ibid.* 332.
  Carbene-mediated rearrangement of 1,1-diaryl-2-haloethylenes to diaryl acetylenes:

G. Köbrich, *Angew. Chem. Int. Ed.* **4**, 49 (1965); G. Köbrich, P. Buck in *Acetylenes*, H. G. Viehe, Ed. (Marcel Dekker, New York, 1969) pp 117, 131; G. Köbrich, *Angew. Chem. Int. Ed.* **11**, 473 (1972); P. J. Stang, D. P. Fox, *J. Org. Chem.* **43**, 364 (1978). Synthetic applications: V. Mouriès *et al., Synthesis* **1998**, 271; I. Creton *et al., Tetrahedron Lett.* **40**, 1899 (1999). Substituent effects: T. Kawase *et al., Chem. Lett.* **1995**, 499; H. Rezaei *et al., Org. Lett.* **2**, 419 (2000).

152. Fujimoto-Belleau Reaction
C. I. Fujimoto, *J. Am. Chem. Soc.* **73**, 1856 (1951); B. Belleau, *ibid.* 5441.
  Synthesis of cyclic α-substituted α,β-unsaturated ketones from enol lactones and Grignard reagents prepared from primary halides:

Review: J. Weill-Raynal, *Synthesis* **1969**, 49. Modified conditions: M. Aloui *et al., Synlett* **1994**, 115.

153. Gabriel-Colman Rearrangement (Phthalimidoacetic Ester → Isoquinoline Rearrangement) (Gabriel Isoquinoline Synthesis)

S. Gabriel, J. Colman, *Ber.* **33**, 980, 996, 2630 (1900); **35**, 2421 (1902).

Formation of isoquinoline derivatives or substituted benzothiazines by the action of alkoxides on phthalimidoacetic or saccharin esters or ketones:

C. F. H. Allen, *Chem. Rev.* **47**, 284 (1950); H. Henecka, *Houben-Weyl* **8**, 578 (1952); J. H. M. Hill, *J. Org. Chem.* **30**, 620 (1965); W. C. Groutas *et al.*, *Biochem. Biophys. Res. Commun.* **194**, 1491 (1993); *idem et al.*, *Bioorg. Med. Chem.* **3**, 187 (1995); S.-K. Kwon, *J. Korean Chem. Soc.* **40**, 678 (1996). Mechanism: M. T. Ivery, J. E. Gready, *J. Chem. Res. Synop.* **9**, 349 (1993). *Cf.* Dieckmann Reaction.

154. Gabriel Ethylenimine Method (Gabriel-Marckwald Ethylenimine Synthesis)

S. Gabriel *et al.*, *Ber.* **21**, 1049 (1888); W. Marckwald *et al.*, *ibid.* **32**, 2036 (1899); **33**, 764 (1900); **34**, 3544 (1901).

Formation of ethylenimines (aziridines) by elimination of hydrogen halides from aliphatic vicinal haloamines with alkali. The method can be extended to the preparation of five- and six-membered cyclic amines:

$$H_2NCH_2CH_2Br \xrightarrow{KOH} \overset{H}{\underset{\triangle}{N}} + H_2O + KBr$$

O. C. Dermer, G. E. Ham, *Ethylenimine and Other Aziridines* (Academic Press, New York, 1969) pp 1-59; R. Bartnik *et al.*, *Pol. J. Chem.* **53**, 537 (1979); K. H. Sunwoo *et al.*, *Dyes Pigm.* **41**, 19 (1999).

155. Gabriel Synthesis

S. Gabriel, *Ber.* **20**, 2224 (1887).

Conversion of alkyl halides to primary amines by treatment with potassium phthalimide and subsequent hydrolysis:

M. S. Gibson, R. W. Bradshaw, *Angew. Chem. Int. Ed.* **7**, 919 (1968); B. Dietrich *et al.*, *J. Am. Chem. Soc.* **103**, 1282 (1981); O. Mitsunobu, *Comp. Org. Syn.* **6**, 79-85 (1991). Modified conditions: S. E. Sen, S. L. Roach, *Synthesis* **1994**, 756; M. N. Khan, *J. Org. Chem.* **61**, 8063 (1996). Stereoselectivity: A. Kubo *et al.*, *Tetrahedron Lett.* **37**, 4957 (1996).

156. Gattermann Aldehyde Synthesis

L. Gattermann, *Ber.* **31**, 1149 (1898); *Ann.* **313**, (1907).

Preparation of phenolic aldehydes, phenol ethers or heterocyclic compounds by treatment of the aromatic substrate with hydrogen cyanide and hydrogen chloride in the presence of Lewis acid catalysts:

W. E. Truce, *Org. React.* **9**, 37 (1957); E. Baltazzi, L. I. Krimen, *Chem. Rev.* **63**, 526 (1963); F. M. Aslam *et al.*, *J. Chem. Soc. Perkin Trans. 1* **1972**, 892; Y. Sato *et al.*, *J. Am. Chem. Soc.* **117**, 3037 (1995). *Cf.* Houben-Hoesch Reaction; Reimer-Tiemann Reaction.

157. Gattermann-Koch Reaction

L. Gattermann, J. A. Koch, *Ber.* **30**, 1622 (1897); L. Gattermann, *Ann.* **347**, 347 (1906).

Formylation of benzene, alkylbenzenes or polycyclic aromatic hydrocarbons with carbon monoxide and hydrogen chloride in the presence of aluminum chloride at high pressure. Addition of cuprous chloride allows the reaction to proceed at atmospheric pressure:

N. N. Crounse, *Org. React.* **5**, 290 (1949); G. A. Olah, S. J. Kuhn in *Friedel-Crafts and Related Reactions* vol. **3**, Part 2, G. Olah, Ed. (Interscience, New York, 1964) pp 1153-1156. Use of CuCl(PPh$_3$)$_n$: L. Toniolo, M. Graziani, *J. Organomet. Chem.* **194**, 221 (1980).

158. Glaser Coupling; Eglinton Reaction; Cadiot-Chodkiewicz Coupling
C. Glaser, *Ber.* **2**, 422 (1869).

Homocoupling of terminal alkynes catalyzed by cuprous salts in the presence of an oxidant and ammonium chloride:

$$R-C\equiv CH \quad \xrightarrow[NH_4Cl]{CuCl, O_2} \quad R-C\equiv C-C\equiv C-R$$

Heterocoupling may be accomplished *via* the **Cadiot-Chodkiewicz coupling** of terminal alkynes with haloalkynes, catalyzed by cuprous salts in the presence of aliphatic amines:

$$HC-C\equiv CH \ + \ Br-C\equiv C-R^1 \quad \xrightarrow[\substack{CH_3CH_2NH_2 \\ NH_2OH \cdot HCl}]{CuCl} \quad R-C\equiv C-C\equiv C-R^1$$

Synthetic applications: F. M. Menger *et al., J. Am. Chem. Soc.* **115**, 6600 (1993); L. Guo *et al., Chem. Commun.* **1994**, 243.

This coupling may also be effected by cupric salts in pyridine and is often referred to as the **Eglinton reaction.** It is particularly applicable to cyclizations: G. Eglinton, A. R. Galbraith, *Chem. Ind. (London)* **1956**, 737; N. Hébert *et al., J. Org. Chem.* **57**, 1777 (1992).

W. Chodkiewicz *et al., Compt. Rend.* **245**, 322 (1957); B. N. Ghose, *Synth. React. Inorg. Met.-Org. Chem.* **24**, 29 (1994); with supercritical CO$_2$ as solvent: J. Li, H. Jiang, *Chem. Commun.* **1999**, 2369.

Inclusive reviews: P. Cadiot, W. Chodkiewicz, "Couplings of Acetylenes" in *Chemistry of Acetylenes*, H. G. Viehe, Ed. (Marcel Dekker, New York, 1969) pp 597-647; K. Sonogashira, *Comp. Org. Syn.* **3**, 551-561 (1991). *Cf.* Castro-Stephens Coupling; Ullmann Reaction.

159. Gomberg-Bachmann Reaction
M. Gomberg, W. E. Bachmann, *J. Am. Chem. Soc.* **46**, 2339 (1924).

Alkali dependent formation of diaryl compounds from aryl diazonium salts and aromatic compounds.

$$Ar-N\overset{+}{\equiv}N \quad \xrightarrow{HO^-} \quad Ar-N=N-OH \quad \xrightarrow{-N_2} \quad Ar^\bullet \ + \ HO^\bullet$$

W. E. Bachmann, R. A. Hoffman, *Org. React.* **2**, 224 (1944); O. C. Dermer, M. T. Edmison, *Chem. Rev.* **57**, 77 (1957); D. H. Hey, *Adv. Free-Radical Chem.* **2**, 47 (1966); D. E. Rosenberg, *et al., Tetrahedron Lett.* **21**, 4141 (1980); J. R. Beadle *et al., J. Org. Chem.* **49**, 1594 (1984); T. C. McKenzie, S. M. Rolfes, *J. Heterocycl. Chem.* **24**, 859 (1987); M. Gurczynski, P. Tomasik, *Org. Prep. Proced. Int.* **23**, 438 (1991). For intramolecular version, *see* Pschorr Reaction.

160. Gomberg Free Radical Reaction
M. Gomberg, *J. Am. Chem. Soc.* **22**, 757 (1900).

Formation of free radicals by abstraction of the halogen from triarylmethyl halides with metals:

$$2(C_6H_5)_3CCl \ + \ Zn \quad \longrightarrow \quad 2(C_6H_5)_3C-Cl^{\bullet-} \quad \longrightarrow \quad 2(C_6H_5)_3C^\bullet + \ ZnCl_2$$

A. R. Forrester *et al., in Organic Chemistry of Stable Free Radicals* (Academic Press, New York, 1968); Scholle, Rozantsev, *Russ. Chem. Rev.* **42**, 1101 (1973); J. M. McBride, *Tetrahedron* **30**, 2009 (1974).

161. Gould-Jacobs Reaction
R. G. Gould, W. A. Jacobs, *J. Am. Chem. Soc.* **61**, 2890 (1939).

Synthesis of 4-hydroxyquinolines from anilines and diethyl ethoxymalonate *via* cyclization of the intermediate anilinomethylenemalonate followed by hydrolysis and decarboxylation:

R. H. Reitsema, *Chem. Rev.* **43**, 53 (1948); R. C. Elderfield, *Heterocycl. Compd.* **4**, 38 (1952); C. C. Price, R. N. Roberts, *Org. Synth.* **coll. vol. III**, 272 (New York, 1955); D. G. Markees, L. S. Schwab, *Helv. Chim. Acta* **55**, 1319 (1972); R. Albrecht, G. A. Hoyer, *Ber.* **105**, 3118 (1972); J. M. Barker *et al.*, *J. Chem. Res. Synop.* **1980**, 4; A. Pipaud *et al.*, *Synth. Commun.* **27**, 1727 (1997); C. G. Dave, R. D. Shah, *Heterocycles* **51**, 1819 (1999). *Cf.* Doebner-Miller Reaction; Knorr Quinoline Synthesis.

162. Graebe-Ullmann Synthesis
C. Graebe, F. Ullmann, *Ann.* **291**, 16 (1896); F. Ullmann, *ibid.* **332**, 82 (1904).
Formation of carbazoles by the action of nitrous acid on 2-aminodiphenylamines, followed by thermal decomposition of the resulting benzotriazoles:

O. Bremer, *Ann.* **514**, 279 (1934); S. H. Tucker *et al.*, *J. Chem. Soc.* **1942**, 500; N. Campbell, B. Barclay, *Chem. Rev.* **40**, 360 (1947); C. C. Colser *et al.*, *J. Chem. Soc.* **1951**, 110; B. W. Ashton, H. Suschitzky, *ibid.* **1957**, 4559; R. A. Abramovitch, I. D. Spenser, *Adv. Heterocycl. Chem.* **3**, 128 (1964). Photo-decomposition: L. K. Mehta *et al.*, *J. Chem. Soc. Perkin Trans. 1* **1993**, 1261. Synthetic applications: A. Molina *et al.*, *J. Org. Chem.* **61**, 5587 (1996); D. J. Hagan *et al.*, *J. Chem. Soc. Perkin Trans. 1* **1998**, 915.

163. Griess Diazo Reaction (Witt and Knoevenagel Diazotization Methods)
P. Griess, *Ann.* **106**, 123 (1858); **121**, 257 (1862); E. Knoevenagel, *Ber.* **23**, 2994 (1890); O. N. Witt, *ibid.* **42**, 2953 (1909).
Formation of aromatic diazonium salts from primary aromatic amines and nitrous acid or other nitrosating agents:

$$ArNH_2 + NaNO_2 + 2HX \longrightarrow ArN_2^+ X^- + NaX + 2H_2O$$

$$2ArNH_2 + N_2O_3 + 2HNO_3 + H_2O \longrightarrow 2ArN_2^+NO_3^- + 4H_2O \text{ (Griess reaction)}$$

$$2ArNH_2 + Na_2S_2O_5 + 4HNO_3 \longrightarrow 2ArN_2^+NO_3^- + Na_2S_2O_7 + 4H_2O \text{ (Witt method)}$$

$$ArNH_2 + RONO + HX \longrightarrow ArN_2^+ X^- + ROH + H_2O \text{ (Knoevenagel method)}$$

N. Kornblum, *Org. React.* **2**, 264 (1944); W. A. Cowdry, D. S. Davies, *Q. Rev. Chem. Soc.* **6**, 358 (1952); Ridd, *ibid.* **15**, 418 (1961); B. I. Belov, V. V. Kozlov, *Russ. Chem. Rev.* **32**, 59 (1963); K. Schank in *The Chemistry of Diazonium and Diazo Groups*, S. Patai, Ed. (Wiley, New York, 1978) p 645; J. B. Fox, Jr., *Anal. Chem.* **51**, 1493 (1979). Evaluation in determination of biological nitrogen: I. Guevara *et al.*, *Clin. Chim. Acta* **274**, 177 (1998); K. Schulz *et al.*, *Nitric Oxide: Biology & Chemistry* **3**, 225 (1999).

164. Grignard Degradation
W. Steinkopf *et al.*, *Ann.* **512**, 136 (1934); **543**, 128 (1940).
Stepwise dehalogenation of a polyhalo compound through its Grignard reagent which on treatment with water yields a product containing one halogen atom less:

V. Grignard, *Compt. Rend.* **130**, 1322 (1900); F. F. Blicke, *Heterocycl. Compd.* **1**, 222 (1950); K. Nützel, *Houben-Weyl* **13/2a**, 128 (1973).

165. Grignard Reaction
V. Grignard, *Compt. Rend.* **130**, 1322 (1900).
Traditionally, it is the addition of organomagnesium compounds (Grignard reagents) to carbonyl compounds to generate alcohols. A more modern interpretation extends the scope of the reaction to include the addition of Grignard reagents to a wide variety of electrophilic substrates:

Early review: D. A. Shirley, *Org. React.* **8**, 28-58 (1954). Preparation of Grignard reagents: Y. H. Lai, *Synthesis* **1981,** 585-604. Mechanistic study: K. Maruyama, T. Katagiri, *J. Phys. Org. Chem.* **2**, 205 (1989). Review of stereoselective addition of carbonyl compounds: D. M. Huryn, *Comp. Org. Syn.* **1**, 49-75 (1991). General review: G. S. Silverman, P. E. Rakita in *Kirk-Othmer Encyclopedia of Chemical Technology* **vol. 12** (Wiley-Interscience, New York, 4th ed., 1994) pp 768-786. *Cf.* Barbier(-type) Reaction.

166. Grob Fragmentation

C. A. Grob, W. Baumann, *Helv. Chim. Acta* **38**, 594 (1955).

Carbon-carbon bond cleavage primarily *via* a concerted process involving a five atom system:

$$X = OH_2^+, OTs, I, Br, Cl$$
$$Y = O^-, NR_2$$

The intramolecular version is useful for the preparation of medium-size rings:

M. Ochiai *et al., J. Org. Chem.* **54**, 4832 (1989); S. Nagumo *et al., Tetrahedron* **49**, 10501 (1993); J.-J. Wang *et al. ibid.* **54**, 13149 (1998). Synthetic applications: S. Schreiber, *J. Am. Chem. Soc.* **102**, 6163 (1980); J. Boivin *et al., Tetrahedron Lett.* **40**, 9239 (1999); A. Krief *et al., ibid.* **41**, 3871 (2000). *Reviews:* C. A. Grob, *Angew. Chem. Int. Ed.* **8**, 535-546 (1969); P. Weyerstahl, H. Marschall, *Comp. Org. Syn.* **6**, 1044-1065 (1991). *Cf.* Eschenmoser Fragmentation; Wharton Reaction.

167. Grundmann Aldehyde Synthesis

C. Grundmann, *Ann.* **524**, 31 (1936).

Transformation of an acid into an aldehyde of the same chain length by conversion of the acid chloride, *via* the diazo ketone, to the acetoxy ketone, reduction with aluminum isopropoxide and hydrolysis to the glycol, and cleavage with lead tetraacetete:

E. Mosetting, *Org. React.* **8**, 225 (1954); O. Bayer, *Houben-Weyl* **7/1**, 239 (1954); H. K. Mangold, *J. Org. Chem.* **24**, 405 (1959). *Cf.* Sonn-Müller Method; Stephen Aldehyde Synthesis.

168. Guareschi-Thorpe Condensation

I. Guareschi, *Mem. Reale Accad. Sci. Torino* **II**, 46, 7, 11, 25 (1896); H. Baron, *et al., J. Chem. Soc.* **85**, 1726 (1904).

Synthesis of pyridine derivatives by condensation of cyanoacetic ester with acetoacetic ester in the presence of ammonia. In a second type of synthesis a mixture of cyanoacetic ester and a ketone is treated with alcoholic ammonia:

C. Hollins, *The Synthesis of Nitrogen Ring Compounds* (New York, 1924) p 197; V. Migrdichian, *The Chemistry of Organic Cyanogen Compounds* (New York, 1947) p 322; H. S. Mosher, *Heterocycl. Compd.* **1**, 466 (1950); R. W. Holder *et al., J. Org. Chem.* **47**, 1445 (1982); D. J. Collins, A. M. James, *Aust. J. Chem.* **42**, 215 (1989). *Cf.* Hantzsch (Dihydro)Pyridine Synthesis; Kröhnke Pyridine Synthesis.

169. Guerbet Reaction

M. Guerbet, *Compt. Rend.* **128**, 511 (1899).

Condensation of 1° or 2° alcohols at high temperature and pressure in the presence of alkali metal hydroxide or alkoxide by a dehydrogenation, aldol condensation, *q.v.*, and hydrogenation sequence:

H. Machemer, *Angew. Chem.* **64**, 213 (1952); S. Veibel, J. T. Nielsen, *Tetrahedron* **23**, 1723 (1967); G. Gregorio *et al., J. Organomet. Chem.* **37**, 385 (1972); E. Klein, *et al., Ann.* **1973**, 1004. Rhodium-promoted reaction: P. L. Burk *et al., J. Mol. Catal.* **33**, 1 (1985).

170. Gutknecht Pyrazine Synthesis

H. Gutknecht, *Ber.* **12**, 2290 (1879); **13**, 1116 (1880).

Cyclization of α-amino ketones, produced by reduction of isonitroso ketones to yield the dihydropyrazines which are dehydrogenated with mercury(I) oxide or copper(II) sulfate, or sometimes with atmospheric oxygen:

$$2RCOCH_2R^1 \xrightarrow{2HNO_2} 2RCOC(=NOH)R^1 \xrightarrow{4H_2} 2RCOCH(NH_2)R^1 \longrightarrow$$

I. J. Krems, P. E. Spoerri, *Chem. Rev.* **40**, 291 (1947); Y. T. Pratt, *Heterocycl. Compd.* **6**, 379, 385 (1957).

171. Haller-Bauer Reaction

A. Haller, E. Bauer, *Compt. Rend.* **148**, 70, 127 (1909); **149**, 5 (1909).

Cleavage of non-enolizable ketones with sodium amide; frequently applied to formation of trisubstituted acetic acid:

K. E. Hamlin, A. W. Weston, *Org. React.* **9**, 1 (1957); H. M. Walborsky *et al., J. Org. Chem.* **36**, 2937 (1971); E. M. Kaiser, C. O. Warner, *Synthesis* **1975**, 395. Applications: G. Mehta, M. Praveen, *J. Org. Chem.* **60**, 279 (1995); *idem et al., Tetrahedron Lett.* **37**, 2289 (1996); A. Mittra *et al., J. Org. Chem.* **63**, 9555 (1998). Reviews and extension to amide formation: J. P. Gilday, L. A. Paquette, *Org. Prep. Proced. Int.* **22**, 167-201 (1990); G. Mahta, R. V. Venkateswaran, *Tetrahedron* **56**, 1399 (2000).

172. Hammick Reaction

P. Dyson, D. L. Hammick, *J. Chem. Soc.* **1937**, 1724.

Decarboxylation of α-picolinic or related acids in the presence of carbonyl compounds accompanied by the formation of a new carbon-carbon bond:

D. L. Hammick *et al., J. Chem. Soc.* **1939**, 809; **1949**, 659; N. H. Cantwell, E. V. Brown, *J. Am. Chem. Soc.* **75**, 1489 (1953); M. J. Betts, B. R. Brown, *J. Chem. Soc.* **1967**, 1730; E. V. Brown, M. B. Shambhu, *J. Org. Chem.* **36**, 2002 (1971). Effect of conditions on yield and products: V. P. Karandikar *et al., Indian J. Technol.* **23**, 28 (1985). Mechanism: R. Grigg *et al., J. Chem. Soc. Perkin Trans. 2* **1990**, 51; B. Bohn *et al., Heterocycles* **37**, 1731 (1994).

173. Hantzsch Dihydropyridine Synthesis (Pyridine Synthesis)

A. Hantzsch, *Ann.* **215**, 1, 72 (1882); *Ber.* **18**, 1744 (1885); **19**, 289 (1886).

Synthesis of dihydropyridines by condensation of two moles of a β-dicarbonyl compound with one mole of an aldehyde in the presence of ammonia. Dehydrogenation to the corresponding pyridine is accomplished with an oxidizing agent:

Note: if R at C-4 is benzyl then during oxidation cleavage will occur

H. S. Mosher, *Heterocycl. Compd.* **1**, 462 (1950); R. M. Kellog *et al., J. Org. Chem.* **45**, 2854 (1980); Y. Watanabe *et al., Synthesis* **1983**, 761. Mechanistic study: A. R. Katritzky *et al., Tetrahedron* **42**, 5729 (1986); **43**, 5171 (1987). Extension to the synthesis of unsymmetrical dihydropyridines: J. B. Sainani *et al., Indian J. Chem.* **34B**, 17 (1995); S. Visentin *et al., J. Med. Chem.* **42**, 1422 (1999). *Cf.* Chichibabin Pyridine Synthesis; Guareschi-Thorpe Condensation; Kröhnke Pyridine Synthesis.

174. Hantzsch Pyrrole Synthesis
   A. Hantzsch, *Ber.* **23**, 1474 (1890).
   Formation of pyrrole derivatives from α-chloromethyl ketones, β-keto esters and ammonia or amines:

   R. Elderfield, T. N. Dodd, Jr., *Heterocycl. Compd.* **1**, 132 (1950); A. H. Corwin, *ibid.* 290; M. W. Roomi, S. F. MacDonald, *Can. J. Chem.* **48**, 1689 (1970); K. Kirschke *et al., J. Prakt. Chem.* **332**, 143 (1990); A. W. Trautwein *et al., Bioorg. Med. Chem. Lett.* **8**, 2381 (1998). *Cf.* Feist-Bénary Synthesis; Knorr Pyrrole Synthesis; Paal-Knorr Pyrrole Synthesis.

175. Harries Ozonide Reaction (Ozonolysis)
   C. Harries, *Ann.* **343**, 311 (1905).
   Treatment of olefins with ozone as a method of cleaving olefinic linkages. On hydrolysis or catalytic hydrogenation the initially formed ozonide yields two molecules of carbonyl compounds:

   Reviews: P. S. Bailey, *Chem. Rev.* **58**, 925 (1958); L. J. Chinn, *Selection of Oxidants in Synthesis: Oxidation at the Carbon Atom* (Dekker, New York, 1971) pp 151-160; P. S. Bailey, *Ozonation in Organic Chemistry* **vols. 1 and 2** (Academic Press, New York, 1978, 1982). Mechanism: R. Criegee, *Rec. Chem. Prog.* **18**, 111 (1957); R. W. Murray, *Acc. Chem. Res.* **1**, 313 (1968); M. Miura *et al., J. Org. Chem.* **50**, 1504 (1985). Applications: J. Z. Gillies *et al., J. Am. Chem. Soc.* **110**, 7991 (1988); K. Griesbaum, V. Ball, *Tetrahedron Lett.* **35**, 1163 (1994).

176. Haworth Methylation
   W. N. Haworth, *J. Chem. Soc.* **107**, 13 (1915).
   Formation of methylated methyl glycosides from monosaccharides with dimethyl sulfate and 30% sodium hydroxide. The glycosidic methyl group is hydrolyzed with acid to yield the free methylated sugar:

   W. N. Haworth, H. Machemer, *J. Chem. Soc.* **1932**, 2270; C. C. Barker *et al., ibid.* **1946**, 783; E. J. Bourne, S. Peat, *Adv. Carbohydr. Chem.* **5**, 146 (1950); W. Pigman, *The Carbohydrates* **1957**, 369. *Cf.* Purdie Methylation.

177. Haworth Phenanthrene Synthesis
   R. D. Haworth, *J. Chem. Soc.* **1932**, 1125, 2717, *idem et al., ibid.* 1784, 2248, 2720; **1934**, 454.
   Preparation of phenanthrenes from naphthalenes *via* a series of steps including a Friedel-Crafts acylation and two Clemmensen or Wolff-Kishner reductions, *q.q.v.*:

   E. Berliner, *Org. React.* **5**, 229 (1949); I. Agranat, Y. S. Shih, *Synthesis* **1974**, 865; R. Menicagli, O. Piccolo, *J. Org. Chem.* **45**, 2581 (1980). *Cf.* Friedel-Crafts Reaction.

178. Hayashi Rearrangement
   M. Hayashi, *J. Chem. Soc.* **1927**, 2516; **1930**, 1513, 1520, 1524.
   Rearrangement of *o*-benzoylbenzoic acids in the presence of sulfuric acids or phosphorous pentoxide:

J. W. Cook, *J. Chem. Soc.* **1932**, 1472; M. Hayashi *et al., Bull. Chem. Soc. Jpn.* **11**, 184 (1936); R. B. Sandin, L. F. Fieser, *J. Am. Chem. Soc.* **62**, 3098 (1940); R. B. Sandin *et al., ibid.* **78**, 3817 (1956); R. Goncalves *et al., J. Org. Chem.* **17**, 705 (1952); S. Cristol, M. L. Caspar, *ibid.* **33**, 2020 (1968); M. Cushman *et al., ibid.* **45**, 5067 (1980).

179. Heck Reaction

R. F. Heck, J. P. Nolley, Jr., *J. Org. Chem.* **37**, 2320 (1972).

Stereospecific palladium-catalyzed coupling of alkenes with organic halides or triflates lacking sp^3-hybridized β-hydrogens:

R^4 = aryl, alkenyl, benzyl
X = I, Br, OSO_2CF_3
[Pd] = $Pd(OCOCH_3)_2$, $PdCl_2$, $Pd(dba)_3$, $Pd(PPh_3)_4$
L = PAr_3, dppp, binap
base = $N(CH_2CH_3)_3$, K_2CO_3, $NaOCOCH_3$

Reviews: R. F. Heck, *Org. React.* **27**, 345-390 (1982); A. de Meijere, F. E. Meyer, *Angew. Chem. Int. Ed.* **33**, 2379-2411 (1994); W. Cabri, I. Candiani, *Acc. Chem. Res.* **28**, 2-7 (1995). Review of intramolecular reactions: L. E. Overman, *Pure Appl. Chem.* **66**, 1423-1430 (1994); S. E. Gibson *et al., Contemp. Org. Synth.* **3**, 447-471 (1996); J. T. Link, L. E. Overman, *Met.-Catal. Cross-Coupling React.* **1998**, 231-269; of enantioselective syntheses: M. Shibasaki, E. M. Vogl, *J. Organomet. Chem.* **576**, 1-15 (1999); O. Loiseleur *et al., ibid.* 16-22; U. Iserloh, D. P. Curran, *Chemtracts* **12**, 289-296 (1999); of mechanism: G. T. Crisp, *Chem. Soc. Rev.* **27**, 427-436 (1998); M. Shibasaki *et al., Adv. Synth. Catal.* **346**, 1533-1552 (2004). *Cf.* Stille Coupling; Suzuki Coupling.

180. Helferich Method

B. Helferich, E. Schmitz-Hillebrecht, *Ber.* **66**, 378 (1933).

Glycosidation of an acetylated sugar by heating with a phenol in the presence of a metal halide ($ZnCl_2$, $FeCl_3$) or *p*-toluenesulfonic acid as catalyst:

W. W. Pigman, R. M. Goepp, *Chemistry of the Carbohydrates* (New York, 1948) p 194; W. W. Pigman, *The Carbohydrates* (New York, 1957) p 198; B. Helferich, J. Zirner, *Ber.* **96**, 385 (1963); A. Piskala *et al., Nucleic Acid Chem.* **1**, 455 (1978). Applications: R. Polt *et al., J. Am. Chem. Soc.* **114**, 10249 (1992); P. Kosma *et al., Carbohydr. Res.* **254**, 105 (1994); D. A. Leigh *et al., ibid.* **276**, 417 (1995); V. Křen *et al., J. Chem. Soc. Perkin Trans. 1* **1997**, 2467.

181. Hell-Volhard-Zelinsky Reaction

C. Hell, *Ber.* **14**, 891 (1881); J. Volhard, *Ann.* **242**, 141 (1887); N. Zelinsky, *Ber.* **20**, 2026 (1887).

α-Halogenation of carboxylic acids in the presence of catalytic phosphorus, presumably involving the enol form of the intermediate acyl halide:

N. O. V. Sonntag, *Chem. Rev.* **52**, 237 (1953); H. J. Harwood, *ibid.* **62**, 102 (1962); H. Kwart, E. V. Scalzi, *ibid.* **86**, 5496 (1964); A. R. Sexton *et al., J. Am. Chem. Soc.* **91**, 7098 (1969); G. L. Lange, J. A. Otulakowski, *J. Org. Chem.* **47**, 5093 (1982); R. J. Crawford, *ibid.* **48**, 1364 (1983); H.-J. Liu, W. Luo, *Synth. Commun.* **21**, 2097 (1991).

182. Henkel Reaction (Raecke Process) (Henkel Process)

B. Raecke, **DE 936036** (1952) and **DE 958920** (1952) to Henkel & Co.

Industrial scale thermal rearrangement or disproportionation of alkaline salts of aromatic acids to symmetrical diacids in the presence of cadmium or other metallic salts:

Review: B. Raecke, *Angew. Chem.* **70,** 1 (1958); Y. Ogata *et al., J. Org. Chem.* **25,** 2082 (1960); E. McNelis, *ibid.* **30,** 1209 (1965); J. Szammer, L. Otvos, *Radiochem. Radioanal. Lett.* **45,** 359 (1980).

183. Henry Reaction (Nitroaldol Reaction)

L. Henry, *Compt. Rend.* **120,** 1265 (1895); J. Kamlet, **US 2151517** (1939).

Base-catalyzed aldol-type condensation, *q.v.,* of nitroalkanes with aldehydes or ketones:

Application to sugars: R. Fernández *et al., Carbohydr. Res.* **247,** 239 (1993). Reagent controlled asymmetric induction: H. Sasai *et al., Tetrahedron Lett.* **34,** 855 (1993); R. Chinchilla *et al., Tetrahedron: Asymmetry* **5,** 1393 (1994); R. S. Varma *et al., Tetrahedron Lett.* **38,** 5131 (1997); R. Ballini, G. Bosica, *J. Org. Chem.* **62,** 425 (1997); V. J. Bulbule *et al., Tetrahedron* **55,** 9325 (1999). Catalyst effects: I. Morao, F. P. Cossio, *Tetrahedron Lett.* **38,** 6461 (1997); P. B. Kisanga, J. G. Verkade, *J. Org. Chem.* **64,** 4298 (1999); D. Simoni *et al., Tetrahedron Lett.* **41,** 1607 (2000); C. Palomo *et al, Angew. Chem. Int. Ed.* **43,** 5442 (2004). *Review:* G. Rosini, *Comp. Org. Syn.* **2,** 321-340 (1991). *Cf.* Knoevenagel Condensation.

184. HERON Rearrangement (Heteroatom Rearrangements on Nitrogen)

J. M. Buccigross *et al., Aust. J. Chem.* **48,** 353 (1995); J. M. Buccigross, S. A. Glover, *J. Chem. Soc. Perkin Trans. 2* **1995,** 595.

Rearrangement of *N*-alkoxy-*N*-aminoamides to esters and 1,1-diazenes via migration of oxygen from the nitrogen to the carbonyl carbon. Analogues of *N,N'*-diacyl-*N,N'*-dialkoxyhydrazines thermally decompose to esters and N$_2$ through two consecutive rearrangements:

Application to *N,N'*-diacyl-*N,N'*-dialkoxyhydrazines: S. A. Glover *et al., J. Chem. Soc. Perkin Trans. 2* **1999,** 2053; to mutagenic *N*-acyloxy-*N*-alkoxybenzamides: J. J. Campbell, S. A. Glover, *J. Chem. Res.* **1999,** 474. Stereochemistry and computational studies: A. Rauk, S. A. Glover, *J. Org. Chem.* **61,** 2337 (1996); *eidem, ibid.* **64,** 2340 (1999). *Review:* S. A. Glover, *Tetrahedron* **54,** 7229-7272 (1998); *idem et al., Can J. Chem.* **83,** 1492-1509 (2005).

185. Herz Reaction

R. Herz, **DE 360690** (1914 to Cassella & Co.); **US 1637023** (1928); **US 1699432** (1929).

Formation of *o*-aminothiophenols by heating aromatic amines with excess sulfur monochloride. The initial products are thiazothionium halides (Herz compounds) which will undergo chlorination if the position *para* to the amino group is unsubstituted:

W. K. Warburton, *Chem. Rev.* **57,** 1011 (1957); L. D. Huestis *et al., J. Org. Chem.* **30,** 2763 (1965); P. Hope, L. A. Wiles, *J. Chem. Soc. C* **1967,** 1642; B. K. Strelets, L. S. Efros, *Zh. Org. Khim.* **1969,** 153; S. W. Schneller, *Int. J. Sulfur Chem.* **8,** 579 (1976); B. L. Chenard, *J. Org. Chem.* **49,** 1224 (1984).

186. Hilbert-Johnson Reaction

T. B. Johnson, G. E. Hilbert, *Science* **69,** 579 (1929); G. E. Hilbert, T. B. Johnson, *J. Am. Chem. Soc.* **52,** 2001, 4489 (1930).

Reaction of 2,4-dialkoxypyrimidines with halogenated sugar to yield pyrimidine nucleosides:

W. Zorbach, *Methods Carbohydr. Chem.* **6,** 445 (1972); T. Ueda, H. Ohtsuka, *Chem. Pharm. Bull.* **21,** 1451, 1530 (1973); C.-H. Kim *et al., J. Med. Chem.* **29,** 1374 (1986); A. A. Mourabit, *Tetrahedron: Asymmetry* **7,** 3455 (1996). Modified conditions: U. Neidballa, H. Vorbrüggen, *Angew. Chem. Int. Ed.* **9,** 469 (1970); H. Vorbrüggen, *et al., Ber.* **114,** 1279 (1981); H. Kristinsson *et al., Tetrahedron* **50,** 6825 (1994); G. Liu *et al., Synth. Commun.* **26,** 2681 (1996). Review of early studies: J. Pliml, M. Prystas, *Adv. Heterocycl. Chem.* **8,** 115 (1967).

187. Hinsberg Oxindole and Oxiquinoline Synthesis

O. Hinsberg, *Ber.* **21,** 110 (1888); **25,** 2545 (1892); **41,** 1367 (1908).

Formation of oxindoles from secondary aryl amines and the acid addition compound of glyoxal; primary aryl amines give glycine or glycinamide derivatives:

O. Hinsberg, J. Rosenzweig, *ibid.* **27,** 3253 (1894); C. Hollins, *Synthesis of Nitrogen Ring Compounds* (London, 1924) p 112; H. Burton, *J. Chem. Soc.* **1932,** 546; P. L. Julian *et al., Heterocycl. Compd.* **3,** 139 (1952). Mechanistic study: M. I. Abasolo *et al., J. Heterocycl. Chem.* **29,** 1279 (1992). Applications: M. I. Abasolo *et al., ibid.* **27,** 157 (1990); G. A. Rodrigo *et al., ibid.* **34,** 505 (1997). *Cf.* Stollé Synthesis.

188. Hinsberg Sulfone Synthesis

O. Hinsberg, *Ber.* **27,** 3259 (1894); **28,** 1315 (1895).

Formation of sulfonylquinol derivatives by addition of quinones to cold dilute aqueous solutions of sulfinic acids:

R. M. Scribner, *J. Org. Chem.* **31,** 3671 (1966); H. Ulrich *et al., Houben-Weyl* **7/3a,** 661 (1977). *Cf.* Thiele Reaction.

189. Hinsberg Synthesis of Thiophene Derivatives

O. Hinsberg, *Ber.* **43**, 901 (1910).

Formation of thiophene carboxylic acids from α-diketones and dialkyl thiodiacetates:

H. Wynberg, D. J. Zwanenburg, *J. Org. Chem.* **29**, 1919 (1964); H. Wynberg, H. J. Kooreman, *J. Am. Chem. Soc.* **87**, 1739 (1965); A. Birch, D. A. Crombie, *Chem. Ind.* **1971**, 177; D. J. Chadwick *et al., J. Chem. Soc. Perkin Trans. 1* **1972**, 2079.

190. Hoch-Campbell Aziridine Synthesis

J. Hoch, *Compt. Rend.* **198**, 1865 (1934); K. N. Campbell, J. F. McKenna, *J. Org. Chem.* **4**, 198 (1939).

Formation of aziridines by treatment of ketoximes with Grignard reagents and subsequent hydrolysis of the organometallic complex:

K. N. Campbell *et al., J. Org. Chem.* **8**, 99, 103 (1943); **9**, 184 (1944); J. P. Freeman, *Chem. Rev.* **73**, 283 (1973); O. C. Dermer, G. E. Ham, *Ethylenimine and Other Aziridines* (Academic Press, New York, 1969) pp 65-68; E. Y. Takehisa *et al., Chem. Pharm. Bull.* **24**, 1691 (1976); T. Sasaki *et al., Heterocycles* **11**, 235 (1978); G. Alvernhe, A. Laurent, *J. Chem. Res. Synop.* **1978**, 28.

191. Hofmann Degradation (Exhaustive Methylation)

A. W. Hofmann, *Ber.* **14**, 659 (1881).

Formation of an olefin and a tertiary amine by pyrolysis of a quaternary ammonium hydroxide:

A. C. Cope, E. R. Trumbull, *Org. React.* **11**, 317-493 *passim* (1960); K. W. Bentley, G. W. Kirby in *Techniques of Organic Chemistry* vol. IV, Pt. 2, A. Weissberger, Ed., *Elucidation of Organic Structures by Physical and Chemical Methods* (Wiley, New York, 2nd ed., 1973) pp 255-289. Isotope effects: R. D. Bach, M. L. Braden, *J. Org. Chem.* **56**, 7194 (1991). Synthetic applications: A. D. Woolhouse *et al., J. Heterocycl. Chem.* **30**, 873 (1993); D. Berkes *et al., Synth. Commun.* **28**, 949 (1998). *Cf.* Cope Elimination Reaction; Emde Degradation.

192. Hofmann Isonitrile Synthesis (Carbylamine Reaction)

A. W. Hofmann, *Ann.* **146**, 107 (1868); *Ber.* **3**, 767 (1870).

Formation of isonitriles by the reaction of primary amines with chloroform in the presence of alkali; the odor of the isocyanide is a test for a primary amine:

$$C_2H_5NH_2 + CHCl_3 + 3NaOH \longrightarrow C_2H_5NC + 3NaCl + 3H_2O$$

P. A. S. Smith, N. W. Kalenda, *J. Org. Chem.* **23**, 1599 (1958); M. B. Frankel *et al., Tetrahedron Lett.* **1959**, 5; H. L. Jackson, B. C. McKusick, *Org. Synth.* **coll. vol. IV**, 438 (1963); W. P. Weber, G. W. Gokel, *Tetrahedron Lett.* **1972**, 1637.

193. Hofmann-Löffler-Freytag Reaction

A. W. Hofmann, *Ber.* **16**, 558 (1883); **18**, 5, 109 (1885); K. Löffler, C. Freytag, *ibid.* **42**, 3427 (1909).

Formation of pyrrolidines or piperidines by thermal or photochemical decomposition of protonated N-haloamines:

M. E. Wolff, *Chem. Rev.* **63**, 55 (1963); E. J. Corey, W. R. Hertler, *J. Am. Chem. Soc.* **82**, 1657 (1960); R. Furstoss *et al., Tetrahedron Lett.* **1970**, 1263; S. Titouani *et al., Tetrahedron* **36**, 2961 (1980).

194. Hofmann-Martius Rearrangement (Aniline Rearrangement)

A. W. Hofmann, C. A. Martius, *Ber.* **4**, 742 (1871); A. W. Hofmann, *ibid.* **5**, 720 (1872).

Thermal conversion of N-alkylaniline hydrohalides to *o*- and *p*-alkylanilines:

NHCH$_3$ • HCl $\xrightarrow{\Delta}$ [2-methylaniline] + [4-methylaniline]

H. Hart, J. R. Kosak, *J. Org. Chem.* **27**, 116 (1962); Y. Ogata *et al., Tetrahedron* **20**, 2717 (1964); *J. Org. Chem.* **35**, 1642 (1970); G. F. Grillot in *Mechanisms of Molecular Migrations* **vol. 3**, B. S. Thyagarajan, Ed. (Wiley, New York, 1971) p 237; A. G. Giumanini *et al., J. Org. Chem.* **40**, 1677 (1975); W. F. Burgoyne, D. D. Dixon, *J. Mol. Catal.* **62**, 61 (1990); M. G. Siskos *et al., Bull. Soc. Chim. Belg.* **105**, 759 (1996).

195. Hofmann Reaction
A. W. Hofmann, *Ber.* **14**, 2725 (1881).

Conversion of primary carboxylic amides to primary amines with one fewer carbon atom upon treatment with hypohalites or hydroxide *via* the intermediate isocyanate:

$$\text{RCONH}_2 \xrightarrow[\text{NaOH}]{\text{Br}_2} [\text{R-N=C=O}] \xrightarrow{\text{H}_2\text{O}} \text{RNH}_2$$

Early review: E. S. Wallis, J. F. Lane, *Org. React.* **3**, 267-306 (1949). Alternative reagents/strategies: S. Kajigaeshi *et al., Chem. Lett.* **1989**, 463; S. Jew *et al., Arch. Pharmacal Res.* **15**, 333 (1992); D. S. Rane, M. M. Sharma, *J. Chem. Technol. Biotechnol.* **59**, 271 (1994); H. Moustafa *et al., Tetrahedron* **53**, 625 (1997); Y. Matsumura *et al., J. Chem. Soc. Perkin Trans. 1* **1999**, 2057. *Review:* T. Shioiri, *Comp. Org. Syn.* **6**, 800-806 (1991). *Cf.* Curtius Rearrangement; Lossen Rearrangement; Schmidt Reaction; Weerman Degradation.

196. Hofmann-Sand Reactions
K. A. Hofmann, J. Sand, *Ber.* **33**, 1340, 1353 (1900).

Olefin mercuration with mercuric salts (halides, acetates, nitrates, or sulfates) in aqueous solution. In alcoholic solutions the accelerated reaction produces alkoxyalkyl compounds:

$$\text{H}_2\text{C=CH}_2 + \text{HgX}_2 + \text{NaOH} \xrightarrow{-\text{NaX}} \text{HOCH}_2\text{CH}_2\text{HgX} \xrightarrow[\text{NaOH}]{} \text{XHgCH}_2\text{CH}_2\text{OCH}_2\text{CH}_2\text{HgX}$$

$$\text{H}_2\text{C=CH}_2 + \text{Hg(OCOCH}_3)_2 + \text{ROH} \longrightarrow \text{ROCH}_2\text{CH}_2\text{HgOCOCH}_3 + \text{CH}_3\text{COOH}$$

J. Sand, *Ber.* **34**, 1385, 2906, 2910 (1901); *Ann.* **329**, 135 (1903); J. Chatt, *Chem. Rev.* **48**, 7 (1951); E. R. Rochow *et al., Chemistry of Organometallic Compounds* (New York, 1957) p 109; W. Kitching, *Organomet. Chem. Rev.* **3**, 35 (1968); K. P. Geller, H. Straub, *Houben-Weyl* **13/2b**, 130 (1974).

197. Hooker Reaction
S. C. Hooker, *J. Am. Chem. Soc.* **58**, 1174 (1936).

Oxidation of 2-hydroxy-3-alkyl-1,4-quinones with dilute alkaline permanganate with shortening of the alkyl side chain by a methylene group and simultaneous exchange of hydroxyl and alkyl or alkenyl group positions:

[reaction scheme: CH$_2$R quinone $\xrightarrow{\text{KMnO}_4}$ o-acyl benzoic acid $\xrightarrow{-\text{CO}_2}$ hydroxy quinone $\xrightarrow{-2\text{H}}$ 2-hydroxy-3-R-quinone]

S. C. Hooker, A. Steyermark, *J. Am. Chem. Soc.* **58**, 1179 (1936); L. F. Fieser, M. Fieser, *ibid.* **70**, 3215 (1948); L. F. Fieser, A. R. Bader, *ibid.* **73**, 681 (1951); L. F. Fieser, M. Fieser, *Advanced Organic Chemistry* (New York, 1961) p 870.

198. Houben-Fischer Synthesis
J. Houben, W. Fischer, *J. Prakt. Chem.* [2] **123**, 89, 262, 313 (1929).

Formation of aromatic nitriles by basic hydrolysis of trichloromethyl aryl ketimines. Acidic hydrolysis yields ketones:

$$\text{C}_6\text{H}_6 + \text{Cl}_3\text{CCN} \longrightarrow \text{C}_6\text{H}_5\text{C(CCl}_3)\text{=NH} \cdot \text{HCl}$$

$\xrightarrow{\text{KOH}}$ PhCN + CHCl$_3$ + KCl + H$_2$O

$\xrightarrow{\text{H}^+/\text{H}_2\text{O}}$ PhCOCCl$_3$ + NH$_4$Cl

J. Houben, W. Fischer, *Ber.* **63**, 2464 (1930); **64**, 240, 2636, 2645 (1931); **66**, 339 (1933); D. T. Mowry, *Chem. Rev.* **42**, 221 (1948); P. E. Spoerri, A. S. DuBois, *Org. React.* **5**, 390 (1949); G. Hesse, *Houben-Weyl* **4/2** 103 (1955); W. Ruske in *Friedel-Crafts and Related Reactions* **vol. III**, Part 1, G. A. Olah, Ed. (Interscience, New York, 1964) p 407. *Cf.* Houben-Hoesch Reaction.

199. Houben-Hoesch Reaction

K. Hoesch, *Ber.* **48**, 1122 (1915); J. Houben, *ibid.* **59**, 2878 (1926).

Synthesis of acylphenols from phenols or phenolic ethers by the action of organic nitriles in the presence of hydrochloric acid and aluminum chloride as catalyst:

Reviews: P. E. Spoerri, A. S. DuBois, *Org. React.* **5**, 387 (1949); Thomas, *Anhydrous Aluminum Chloride in Organic Chemistry* (New York, 1941) p 504; W. Ruske in *Friedel-Crafts and Related Reactions* **vol. III**, Part 1, G. A. Olah, Ed. (Interscience, New York, 1964) p 383; M. I. Amer *et al., J. Chem. Soc. Perkin Trans. 1* **1983**, 1075; V. V. Arkhipov *et al., Chem. Heterocycl. Compd.* **33**, 515 (1997); R. Kawecki *et al., Synthesis* **1999**, 751. *Cf.* Gatterman Aldehyde Synthesis; Houben-Fischer Synthesis.

200. Houdry Cracking Process

E. Houdry, **US 1957648** and **US 1957649** (1934).

Decomposition of petroleum or heavy petroleum fractions into more useful lower boiling materials by heating at 500° and 30 psi, over a silica-alumina-magnanese oxide catalyst.

E. Houdry *et al., Oil Gas J.* **37**, 40 (1938); A. N. Sachanen, *Chemical Constituents of Petroleum* (New York, 1945) p 260; V. Haensel, M. J. Sterba, *Ind. Eng. Chem.* **40**, 1662 (1948); *Kirk-Othmer Encyclopedia of Chemical Technology* **4**, 323, 357 (New York, 1979); E. Boye, *Chem. Ztg.* **81**, 341 (1957); S. Gussow *et al., Oil Gas J.* **78**, 96 (1980); C. G. Mosley, *J. Chem. Educ.* **61**, 655 (1984); G. A. Mills, *Chemtech* **1986**, 72; Y. Nishimura, *Petrotech* **21**, 605 (1998).

201. Hunsdiecker Reaction (Borodine Reaction)

C. Hunsdiecker *et al.*, **US 2176181** (1939); H. Hunsdiecker, C. Hunsdiecker, *Ber.* **75**, 291 (1942); A. Borodine, *Ann.* **119**, 121 (1861).

Synthesis of organic halides by thermal decarboxylation of silver salts of the corresponding carboxylic acids in the presence of halogens:

$$RCOOAg + X_2 \xrightarrow{\Delta} RX + CO_2 + AgX$$

R. G. Johnson, R. K. Ingham, *Chem. Rev.* **56**, 219 (1956); C. V. Wilson, *Org. React.* **9**, 341 (1957); S. J. Cristol, W. C. Firth, Jr., *J. Org. Chem.* **26**, 280 (1961); F. F. Knapp, Jr., *Steroids* **33**, 245 (1979); A. I. Meyers, M. P. Fleming, *J. Org. Chem.* **44**, 3405 (1979). Modified catalysis by metal salt pool: S. Chowdhury, S. Roy, *Tetrahedron Lett.* **37**, 2623 (1996); D. Naskar, S. Roy, *J. Chem. Soc. Perkin Trans. 1* **1999**, 2436; *eidem, Tetrahedron* **56**, 1369 (2000). *Cf.* Kochi Reaction; Simonini Reaction.

202. Hydroboration Reaction

H. C. Brown, B. C. Subba Rao, *J. Am. Chem. Soc.* **78**, 5694 (1956); *J. Org. Chem.* **22**, 1135, 1136 (1957).

Addition of boron hydrides to alkenes, allenes, and alkynes to form organoboranes, such that boron adds to the less substituted carbon. Attack usually takes place on the less hindered side in a *cis* fashion:

Diastereofacial and regioselectivity study: B. W. Gung *et al., Synth. Commun.* **24**, 167 (1994). Methods development for asymmetric synthesis: U. P. Dhokte, H. C. Brown, *Tetrahedron Lett.* **35**, 4715 (1994). Application to hydration: G. Zweifel, H. C. Brown, *Org. React.* **13**, 1-54 (1963). General reviews: H. O. House, *Modern Synthetic Reactions* (W. A. Benjamin, Menlo Park, California, 2nd ed., 1972) pp 106-130; K. Smith, A. Pelter, *Comp. Org. Syn.* **8**, 703-731 (1991). Reviews of asymmetric synthesis: H. C. Brown, *Tetrahedron* **37**, 3547-3587 (1981); K. Burgess, M. J. Ohlmeyer in *Adv. Chem. Ser.* **230**, entitled "Homogeneous Transition Metal Catalyzed Reactions" (ACS, Washington DC, 1992) pp 163-177. *Cf.* Suzuki Coupling.

203. Ivanov Reaction

D. Ivanov, A. Spassoff, *Bull. Soc. Chim. Fr.* **49**, 19, 375 (1931); D. Ivanov *et al., ibid.* **51**, 1321, 1325, 1331 (1932).

The addition of enediolates of aryl acetic acids (Ivanov reagents) to electrophiles, particularly carbonyl compounds:

Early reviews: B. Blagoev, D. Ivanov, *Synthesis* **1970**, 615; D. Ivanov *et al., ibid.* **1975,** 83. Synthetic application: Y. A. Zhdanov *et al., Carbohydr. Res.* **29,** 274 (1973). Kinetic and mechanistic study: J. Toullec *et al., J. Org. Chem.* **50,** 2563 (1985). Stereoselectivity: M. Mladenova *et al., Tetrahedron* **37,** 2157 (1981); M. Momtchev *et al., Bull. Soc. Chim. Fr.* **5,** 844 (1985). *Cf.* Aldol Reaction; Knoevenagel Condensation.

204. Jacobsen Epoxidation

W. Zhang *et al., J. Am. Chem. Soc.* **112,** 2801 (1990); E. N. Jacobsen *et al. ibid.* **113,** 7063 (1991).

Chiral (salen)manganese(III)-catalyzed asymmetric epoxidation of alkenes. Enantio- and diastereo- selectivity depend strongly on the nature of the substrate:

Methods development: E. N. Jacobsen *et al., Tetrahedron* **50,** 4323 (1994); S. Chang *et al., J. Am. Chem. Soc.* **116,** 6937 (1994); B. D. Brandes, E. N. Jacobsen, *J. Org. Chem.* **59,** 4378 (1994). Large-scale preparation of ligand: J. F. Larrow *et al., ibid.* 1939. *Review:* E. N. Jacobsen, "Asymmetric Catalytic Epoxidation of Unfunctionalized Olefins" in *Catalytic Asymmetric Synthesis,* I. Ojima, Ed. (VCH, New York, 1993) pp 159-202. For parallel studies, *see* N. Hosoya *et al., Synlett* **1993,** 641; H. Sasaki *et al., ibid.* **1994,** 356. Mechanistic study: D. L. Hughes *et al., J. Org. Chem.* **62,** 2222 (1997). Application: P. S. Savle *et al., Tetrahedron: Asymmetry* **9,** 1843 (1998). *Review:* T. Flessner *et al., J. Prakt. Chem.* **341,** 436-444 (1999).

205. Jacobsen Rearrangement

O. Jacobsen, *Ber.* **19,** 1209 (1886); **20,** 901 (1887).

Reaction of polymethylbenzenes with concentrated sulfuric acid to give rearranged polymethylbenzenesulfonic acids. Under identical conditions halogenated polymethylbenzenes undergo disproportionation:

L. I. Smith, *Org. React.* **1,** 370 (1942); H. Suzuki *et al., Bull. Chem. Soc. Jpn.* **36,** 1642 (1963); A. Koeberg-Telder, H. Cerfontain, *J. Chem. Soc. Perkin Trans. 2* **1977,** 717; M. Nakada *et al., Bull. Chem. Soc. Jpn.* **52,** 3671 (1979).

Mechanism: J. L. Norula, R. P. Gupta, *Chem. Era* **10**, 7 (1974). ZrCl$_4$ catalysis: E. Solari *et al., Angew. Chem. Int. Ed.* **34**, 1510 (1995).

206. Janovsky Reaction

J. V. Janovsky, L. Erb, *Ber.* **19**, 2155 (1886).

Reaction of aldehydes and ketones containing α-methylene groups with *m*-dinitrobenzenes in the presence of a strong base resulting in the formation of an intense purple coloration, used for the detection of carbonyl compounds:

Reviews: Akatsuka, *J. Pharm. Soc. Jpn.* **80**, 389 (1960); Foster, Mackie, *Tetrahedron* **18**, 1131 (1962); Pollitt, Saunders, *J. Chem. Soc.* **1965**, 4615; M. Kimura *et al., Chem. Pharm. Bull.* **17**, 531 (1969); K. Kohashi *et al., ibid.* **25**, 50 (1977). Applications: R. G. Sutherland *et al., Can. J. Chem.* **64**, 2031 (1986); J. D. Artiss *et al., Microchem. J.* **65**, 277 (2000). *Cf.* Zimmermann Reaction.

207. Japp-Klingemann Reaction

F. R. Japp, F. Klingemann, *Ann.* **247**, 190 (1888); *Ber.* **20**, 2942, 3284, 3398 (1887).

Formation of hydrazones by coupling of aryldiazonium salts with active methylene compounds in which at least one of the activating groups is acyl or carboxyl. This group usually cleaves during the process:

Review: R. R. Phillips, *Org. React.* **10**, 143 (1959); H. C. Yao, P. Resnick, *J. Am. Chem. Soc.* **84**, 3504 (1962); M. O. Lozinskii, A. A. Gershkovich, *ibid.* **8**, 785 (1972); A. Kozikowski, W. C. Floyd, *Tetrahedron Lett.* **1978**, 19. Use of brominium ion as leaving group: G. Cirrincione *et al., J. Heterocycl. Chem.* **27**, 983 (1990). Synthetic applications: F. Chetoni *et al., ibid.* **30**, 1481 (1993); B. Loubinoux *et al., J. Org. Chem.* **60**, 953 (1995); B. Pete *et al., Heterocycles* **53**, 665 (2000).

208. Jones Oxidation

K. Bowden *et al., J. Chem. Soc.* **1946**, 39.

The oxidation of primary and secondary alcohols to acids and ketones, respectively, in the presence of chromic acid, aqueous sulfuric acid, and acetone. Isolated multiple bonds are not disturbed under these conditions:

P. Bladon *et al., J. Chem. Soc.* **1951**, 2402; E. R. H. Jones *et al., ibid.* **1953**, 457, 2548, 3019; C. Djerassi *et al., J. Org. Chem.* **21**, 1547 (1956); R. N. Warriner *et al., Aust. J. Chem.* **31**, 1113 (1978); S. V. Ley, A. Madin, *Comp. Org. Syn.* **7**, 253-256 (1991). Extensive synthetic applications: R. A. Epifanio *et al., Tetrahedron Lett.* **29**, 6403 (1988); P. A. Evans *et al., Synth. Commun.* **26**, 4685 (1996); N. M. Allanson *et al., Tetrahedron Lett.* **39**, 1889 (1998); Y. Watanabe *et al., ibid.* **40**, 3411 (1999). *Cf.* Sarett Oxidation.

209. Jourdan-Ullmann-Goldberg Synthesis

F. Jourdan, *Ber.* **18**, 1444 (1885); F. Ullmann, *ibid.* **36**, 2382 (1903); I. Goldberg, *ibid.* **39**, 1691 (1906); **40**, 4541 (1907).

Synthesis of substituted diphenylamines, useful as intermediates in the synthesis of acridones:

(Jourdan)

(Ullmann)

(Goldberg)

Reviews: R. M. Acheson, *Acridines* (Interscience, New York, 1956) p 148; Schulenberg, Archer, *Org. React.* **14**, 19 (1965).

210. Julia Olefination (Julia-Lythgoe Olefination)

M. Julia, M.-M. Paris, *Tetrahedron Lett.* **1973**, 4833.

The formation of predominantly *trans*-olefins *via* the addition of phenyl sulfones to aldehydes or ketones, followed by alcohol functionalization and subsequent reductive elimination with sodium amalgam:

$$R^3 = COCH_3, X = OCOCH_3; R^3 = COPh, SO_2CH_3, X = Cl$$

Reviews: P. Kocienski, *Phosphorus Sulfur* **24**, 97-127 (1985); S. E. Kelly, *Comp. Org. Syn.* **1**, 792-806. Synthetic applications: R. Bellingham *et al., Synthesis* **1996**, 285; I. E. Markú *et al., Tetrahedron Lett.* **37**, 2089 (1996); T. Satoh *et al., ibid.* **39**, 6935 (1998); C. Charrier *et al., ibid.* **40**, 5705 (1999). Modified conditions: P. R. Blakemore *et al., Synthesis* **7**, 1209 (1999); P. J. Kocienski *et al., Synlett* **2000**, 365.

211. Kendall-Mattox Reaction

V. R. Mattox, E. C. Kendall, *J. Am. Chem. Soc.* **70**, 882 (1948); **72**, 2290 (1950); *J. Biol. Chem.* **188**, 287 (1951); E. C. Kendall, W. F. McGuckin, *J. Am. Chem. Soc.* **74**, 5811 (1952).

Formation of a conjugated ketone from an α-bromoketone *via* a phenylhydrazone or semicarbazone:

C. Djerassi, *J. Am. Chem. Soc.* **71**, 1003 (1949); B. A. Koechlin *et al., J. Biol. Chem.* **184**, 393 (1950); N. L. Wendler *et al., J. Am. Chem. Soc.* **73**, 3818 (1951); J. J. Beereboom *et al., ibid.* **75**, 3500 (1953); C. R. Engel, *ibid.* **78**, 4727 (1956); E. W. Warnhoff, *J. Org. Chem.* **28**, 887 (1963).

212. Kiliani-Fischer Synthesis

H. Kiliani, *Ber.* **18**, 3066 (1885); E. Fischer, *ibid.* **22**, 2204 (1889).

Extension of the carbon atom chain of aldoses by treatment with cyanide. Hydrolysis of the cyanohydrins followed by reduction of the lactone yields the homologous aldose:

Reviews: C. S. Hudson, *Adv. Carbohydr. Chem.* **1**, 2 (1945); T. Moury, *Chem. Rev.* **42**, 239 (1948); L. Hough, A. C. Richardson, *The Carbohydrates* **1A**, 118 (1972); R. Kuhn, P. Klesse, *Ber.* **91**, 1989 (1958); R. Varma, D. French, *Carbohydr. Res.* **25**, 71 (1972); R. Blazer, T. W. Whalen, *J. Am. Chem. Soc.* **102**, 5082 (1980). Mechanistic study: A. S. Serianni *et al., J. Org. Chem.* **45**, 3329 (1980). Modified conditions: N. Adjé *et al., Tetrahedron Lett.* **37**, 5893

(1996). Stereoselective synthesis: J. Roos, F. Effenberger, *Tetrahedron: Asymmetry* **10**, 2817 (1999). *Cf.* Urech Cyanohydrin Method.

213. Kishner Cyclopropane Synthesis
N. M. Kishner, A. Zavadovskii, *J. Russ. Phys. Chem. Soc.* **43**, 1132 (1911).

Formation of cyclopropane derivatives by decomposition of pyrazolines formed by reacting α,β-unsaturated ketones or aldehydes with hydrazine:

L. I. Smith, E. R. Rogier, *J. Am. Chem. Soc.* **73**, 3840 (1951); G. S. Hammond, R. W. Todd, *ibid.* **76**, 4081 (1954); T. L. Jacobs, *Heterocycl. Compd.* **5**, 109 (1957). Mechanistic aspects of pyrazoline decomposition to cyclopropanes: R. G. Bergman in *Free Radicals* vol. **1**, J. Kochi, Ed. (Wiley, New York, 1973) p 191; R. J. Crawford, M. Ohno, *Can. J. Chem.* **52**, 3134 (1974); R. J. Crawford, H. Tokunaga, *ibid.* 4033; J. A. Berson in *Rearrangements in Ground and Excited States* vol. **1**, P. de Mayo, Ed. (Academic Press, New York, 1980) p 326.

214. Knoevenagel Condensation; Doebner Modification
E. Knoevenagel *Ber.* **31**, 2596 (1898); O. Doebner, *Ber.* **33**, 2140 (1900).

Condensation of aldehydes or ketones with active methylene compounds in the presence of ammonia or amines; the use of malonic acid and pyridine is known as the **Doebner modification:**

$$RCHO + H_2C(COOR)_2 \xrightarrow{\text{base}} RCH=C(COOR)_2 \xrightarrow[-CO_2]{HO^-} RCH=CH-COOH$$

Early reviews: J. R. Johnson, *Org. React.* **1**, 210 (1942); G. Jones, *ibid.* **15**, 204 (1967); H. O. House, *Modern Synthetic Reactions* (W. A. Benjamin, Menlo Park, California, 2nd ed., 1972) pp 646-653. Development of enantio-selective methods: L. F. Tietze, P. Saling, *Chirality* **5**, 329 (1993). Application to the synthesis of indole alkaloids: L. F. Tietze *et al., Synthesis* **1994**, 1185. Modified conditions: J. McNulty *et al., Tetrahedron Lett.* **39**, 8013 (1998); B. M. Choudary *et al., J. Mol. Catal. A* **142**, 361 (1991). Synthetic applications: B. T. Watson, G. E. Christiansen, *Tetrahedron Lett.* **39**, 6087 (1998); R. W. Draper *et al., Tetrahedron* **56**, 1811 (2000). *Review:* L. F. Tietze, U. Beifuss, *Comp. Org. Syn.* **2**, 341-394 (1991). *Cf.* Aldol Reaction; Henry Reaction; Ivanov Reaction.

215. Knoop-Oesterlin Amino Acid Synthesis
F. Knoop, H. Oesterlin, *Z. Physiol. Chem.* **148**, 294 (1925).

Preparation of α-amino acids by catalytic hydrogenation of α-oxo acids in aqueous ammonia in the presence of platinum, palladium or Raney nickel catalysts, probably *via* an unstable iminocarboxylate ion intermediate:

$$RCOCOO^- + NH_3 \longrightarrow \overset{NH}{\underset{}{\overset{\|}{R}CCOO^-}} \xrightarrow[Pd]{H_2} \overset{NH_2}{\underset{}{\overset{|}{R}CHCOOH}}$$

H. R. V. Arnstein, R. Bentley, *Q. Rev. Chem. Soc.* **4**, 186 (1950); S. Nakamura, K. Ashida, *J. Agric. Chem. Soc. Jpn.* **24**, 185 (1950-1951); T. Wieland, *et al., Houben-Weyl* **11/2**, 311, 482 (1958); C. W. Huffman, W. G. Skelly, *Chem. Rev.* **63**, 632 (1963).

216. Knorr Pyrazole Synthesis
L. Knorr, *Ber.* **16**, 2587 (1883).

Formation of pyrazole derivatives from hydrazines, hydrazides, semicarbazides, and aminoguanidines by conden-sation with 1,3-dicarbonyl compounds; substituted hydrazines yield two structurally isomeric pyrazoles:

T. J. Jacobs, *Heterocycl. Compd.* **5**, 46 (1957); M. H. Palmer, *Structure and Reactions of Heterocyclic Compounds* (Arnold, London, 1967) pp 378-385. *Cf.* Pechmann Pyrazole Synthesis.

217. Knorr Pyrrole Synthesis
L. Knorr, *Ber.* **17**, 1635 (1884); *Ann.* **236**, 290 (1886); L. Knorr, H. Lange, *Ber.* **35**, 2998 (1902).

Formation of pyrrole derivatives by condensation of α-amino ketones as such or generated *in situ* from isonitroso-ketones with carbonyl compounds containing active α-methylene groups:

Organic Name Reactions

A. H. Corwin, *Heterocycl. Compd.* **1**, 287 (1950); H. Fischer, *Org. Synth.* **coll. vol. III**, 573 (1955); S. Hauptmann, M. Martin, *Z. Chem.* **8**, 333 (1968); A. J. Castro *et al.*, *J. Org. Chem.* **35**, 2815 (1970); Y. Tamura *et al.*, *Chem. Ind. (London)* **1971**, 767; H. Rapoport, J. Harbuck, *J. Org. Chem.* **36**, 853 (1971); E. Fabiano, B. T. Golding, *J. Chem. Soc. Perkin Trans. 1* **1991**, 3371; A. Alberola *et al.*, *Tetrahedron* **55**, 6555 (1999). Synthetic applications: J. A. Bastian, T. D. Lash, *ibid.* **54**, 6299 (1998); P. E. Harrington, M. A. Tius, *Org. Lett.* **1**, 649 (1999); L. Cheng, D. A. Lightner, *Synthesis* **1999**, 46. *Cf.* Hantzsch Pyrrole Synthesis; Paal-Knorr Pyrrole Synthesis.

218. Knorr Quinoline Synthesis

L. Knorr, *Ann.* **236**, 69 (1886); **245**, 357, 378 (1888).

Formation of α-hydroxyquinolines from β-ketoesters and arylamines above 100°. The intermediate anilide undergoes cyclization by dehydration with concentrated sulfuric acid:

F. W. Bergstrom, *Chem. Rev.* **35**, 157 (1944); C. R. Hauser, G. A. Reynolds, *J. Am. Chem. Soc.* **70**, 2402 (1948); *Org. Synth.* **coll. vol. III**, 593 (1955); R. C. Elderfield, *Heterocycl. Compd.* **4**, 30 (1952); A. J. Hodgkinson, B. Staskum, *J. Org. Chem.* **34**, 1709 (1969). Synthetic application: P. López-Alvarado *et al.*, *Synthesis* **1998**, 186. *Cf.* Doebner-Miller Reaction; Gould-Jacobs Reaction.

219. Koch-Haaf Carboxylations

H. Koch, *Brennst.-Chem.* **36**, 321 (1955); H. Koch, W. Haaf, *Ann.* **618**, 251 (1958).

Formation of tertiary carboxylic acids by treating alcohols with carbon monoxide in strong acid:

Extension to olefins:

H. Langhals *et al.*, *Tetrahedron Lett.* **22**, 2365 (1981); R. R. Rao, J. Bhattacharya, *Indian J. Chem.* **20B**, 207 (1981); *eidem, ibid.* **21B**, 405 (1982); O. Farooq *et al.*, *J. Am. Chem. Soc.* **110**, 864 (1988). *Reviews:* K. E. Möller, *Brennst.-Chem.* **47**, 10 (1966); Y. T. Eidus, *et al.*, *Russ. Chem. Rev.* **42**, 199 (1973); H. Bahrmann, "Koch Reactions" in *New Syntheses with Carbon Monoxide*, J. Falbe, Ed. (Springer-Verlag, New York, 1980) pp 372-413.

G. Olah, J. Olah in *Friedel-Crafts and Related Reactions* **vol. 3**, Part 2, G. A. Olah, Ed. (Interscience, New York, 1964) pp 1272-1296; C. W. Bird, *Chem. Rev.* **62**, 283 (1962). Extension to amides: C. Leonte, E. Carp, *Rev. Roum. Chim.* **34**, 1241 (1989).

220. Kochi Reaction

J. K. Kochi, *J. Am. Chem. Soc.* **87**, 2500 (1965).

Synthesis of organic chlorides by decarboxylation of carboxylic acids in the presence of lead tetraacetate and lithium chloride:

$$RCOOH + Pb(OAc)_4 \longrightarrow RCOOPb(OAc)_3 + AcOH \xrightarrow[\Delta]{LiCl} RCl + CO_2$$

R. A. Sheldon, J. K. Kochi, *Org. React.* **19**, 279 (1972); M. Mannier, J. P. Aycard, *Can. J. Chem.* **57**, 1257 (1979). *Cf.* Hunsdiecker Reaction.

221. Koenigs-Knorr Synthesis

W. Koenigs, E. Knorr, *Ber.* **34**, 957 (1901).

Formation of glycosides from acetylated glycosyl halides and alcohols or phenols in the presence of silver salts. The reaction proceeds with inversion of configuration:

Reviews: Evans *et al., Adv. Carbohydr. Chem.* **6**, 41-52 (1951); K. Igarashi, *ibid.* **34**, 243 (1977); H. M. Flowers, *Methods Carbohydr. Chem.* **6**, 474-480 (1972); R. R. Schmidt, *Comp. Org. Syn.* **6**, 33-64 (1991). Stereoselectivity: J.-I. Tamaru *et al., J. Carbohydr. Chem.* **12**, 893 (1993). Applications: A. Milius *et al., New J. Chem.* **15**, 337 (1991); F. W. Lichtenthaler, T. W. Metz, *Tetrahedron Lett.* **38**, 5477 (1997); S. Laszlo *et al., Chem. Commun.* **1999**, 591.

222. Kolbe Electrolytic Synthesis; Crum Brown-Walker Reaction

H. Kolbe, *Ann.* **69**, 257 (1849).

Formation of symmetrical dimers by the electrolysis of carboxylates (decarboxylative dimerization). The coupling of two distinct carboxylates yields unsymmetrical products:

$$2RCOO^- \xrightarrow{\text{electrolysis}} R{-}R + 2CO_2$$

The dimerization of half-esters is known as the **Crum Brown-Walker reaction:** A. Crum Brown, J. Walker, *ibid.* **261**, 107 (1891).

Reviews: B. C. L. Weedon, *Q. Rev. Chem. Soc.* **6**, 380 (1952); A. K. Vijh, B. E. Conway, *Chem. Rev.* **67**, 623 (1967); L. Eberson in *Organic Electrochemistry,* M. M. Baizer, Ed. (M. Dekker, New York, 1973) pp 469-507; H. J. Schäfer, *Comp. Org. Syn.* **3**, 633-658 (1991); J. Weiguny, H. J. Schäfer, *Ann.* **1994**, 225; G. Nuding *et al., Synthesis* **1996**, 71; J. Hiebl *et al., Tetrahedron* **54**, 2059 (1998); M. Sugiya, H. Noshira, *Chem. Lett.* **1998**, 479; *eidem, Bull. Chem. Soc. Jpn.* **73**, 705 (2000).

223. Kolbe-Schmitt Reaction

H. Kolbe, *Ann.* **113**, 125 (1860); R. Schmitt, *J. Prakt. Chem.* [2] **31**, 397 (1885).

Formation of aromatic hydroxy acids by carboxylation of phenolates, mostly in the *ortho* position, by carbon dioxide:

Reviews: A. S. Lindsey, H. Jeskey, *Chem. Rev.* **57**, 583 (1957); D. C. Ayres, *Carbanions in Synthesis* **1966**, 168-173; J. L. Hales *et al., J. Chem. Soc.* **1954**, 3145; J. March, *Advanced Organic Chemistry* (Wiley-Interscience, New York, 4th ed., 1992) p 546.

224. Kostanecki Acylation

S. von Kostanecki, A. Rozycki, *Ber.* **34**, 102 (1901).

Formation of chromones or coumarins by acylation of *o*-hydroxyaryl ketones with aliphatic acid anhydrides, followed by cyclization:

W. Baker, *J. Chem. Soc.* **1933**, 1381; C. R. Hauser, *Org. React.* **8**, 91 (1954); T. Szell *et al., Tetrahedron* **25**, 715 (1969); *idem et al., Helv. Chim. Acta* **52**, 2636 (1969); S. R. Save *et al., J. Indian Chem. Soc.* **48**, 675 (1971); Y. A. Shaikh, K. N. Trivedi, *ibid.* **49**, 599, 713 (1972); S. R. Save *et al., ibid.* **49**, 25 (1972). *Cf.* Allan-Robinson Reaction; Baker-Venkataraman Rearrangement.

225. Krafft Degradation

F. Krafft, *Ber.* **12**, 1664 (1879).

Conversion of carboxylic acids, especially of high molecular weight, into the next lower homolog by dry distillation of the alkaline earth salt with the corresponding acetate, followed by chromic acid oxidation of the methyl ketone:

$$(RCH_2COO)_2M + (AcO)_2M \longrightarrow RCH_2COCH_3 \xrightarrow{CrO_3} RCOOH$$

F. C. Whitmore, *Organic Chemistry* (New York, 1951) p 255; F. Klages, *Lehrbuch der organischen Chemie* **I** (Berlin, 1952) pp 262, 266, 368. *Cf.* Barbier-Wieland Degradation.

226. Krapcho Decarbalkoxylation

A. P. Krapcho *et al., Tetrahedron Lett.* **1967**, 215.

The decarbalkoxylation of malonate esters, β-keto esters, α-cyano esters and α-sulfonyl esters in dipolar aprotic solvents, at high temperatures, in the presence of water and/or salt, to yield esters, ketones, nitriles and sulfonyl derivatives, respectively:

$R^1 = CH_3, CH_2CH_3$
EWG = COOR, COR, CN, SO_2R
solvent (possibly wet) = DMSO, DMF, HMPT
MX = LiCl, NaCl, LiI, NaCN, KCN, n-Bu_4NOAc

Scope and limitations: A. P. Krapcho *et al.*, *J. Org. Chem.* **43**, 138 (1978). Mechanistic studies: A. M. Bernard *et al.*, *Tetrahedron* **46**, 3929 (1990); P. J. Gilligan, P. J. Krenitsky, *Tetrahedron Lett.* **35**, 3441 (1994). Review of synthetic applications: A. P. Krapcho, *Synthesis* **1982**, 805-822, 893-914.

227. Kröhnke Oxidation
F. Kröhnke *et al.*, *Ber.* **69**, 2006 (1936); **71**, 2583 (1938); **72**, 440 (1939).

Transformation of activated halides into aldehydes *via* their pyridinium salts, which yield nitrones upon treatment with *p*-nitrosodimethylaniline. Aldehydes or ketones are generated upon hydrolysis:

$R = Ar, R^1CO, R^1CH=CH$

A. A. Goldberg, H. A. Walker, *J. Chem. Soc.* **1954**, 2540; F. Kröhnke, *Angew. Chem. Int. Ed.* **2**, 380 (1963); A. Markovac *et al.*, *Heterocyclic Chem.* **14**, 19 (1977); I. Maeba *et al.*, *J. Chem. Soc. Perkin Trans. 1* **1991**, 939; S. N. Kilenyi, *Comp. Org. Syn.* **7**, 657-659 (1991). *Cf.* Sommelet Reaction.

228. Kröhnke Pyridine Synthesis
W. Zecher, F. Kröhnke, *Ber.* **94**, 690, 698 (1961); *eidem, Angew. Chem. Int. Ed.* **1**, 626 (1962).

1,4-Michael addition, *q.v.*, of α-pyridinium methyl ketone salts to α,β-unsaturated ketones, generating the 1,5-dicarbonyl compounds which undergo ammonium acetate-promoted ring closure, to yield substituted pyridines:

Early review: F. Kröhnke, *Synthesis* **1976**, 1-24. Synthetic applications: J. N. Chatterjea *et al.*, *Indian J. Chem.* **15B**, 430 (1977); G. R. Newkome *et al.*, *J. Org. Chem.* **51**, 850 (1986); P. Lhoták, A. Kurfürst, *Collect. Czech. Chem. Commun.* **57**, 1937 (1992); T. R. Kelly *et al.*, *J. Org. Chem.* **62**, 2774 (1997). *Cf.* Chichibabin Pyridine Synthesis; Guareschi-Thorpe Condensation; Hantzsh (Dihydro)Pyridine Synthesis.

229. Kucherov Reaction
M. Kucherov, *Ber.* **14**, 1540 (1881).

Hydration of acetylenic hydrocarbons with dilute sulfuric acid in the presence of mercuric sulfate or boron trifluoride as catalyst:

Reviews: A. D. Petrov. *Usp. Khim.* **21**, 250 (1952); M. Miocque *et al.*, *Ann. Chim. (Paris)* **8**, 157 (1963); M. M. Khan, A. E. Martell, *Homogeneous Catalysis by Metal Complexes* vol. 2 (Academic Press, New York, 1974) p 1974; B. S. Krupin, A. A. Petrov, *J. Gen. Chem. USSR* **33**, 3799 (1963); W. L. Budde, R. E. Dessy, *Tetrahedron Lett.* **1963**, 651; *J. Am. Chem. Soc.* **85**, 3964 (1963); K. G. Golodova, S. I. Yakimovich, *Zh. Org. Khim.* **8**, 2015 (1972). Extension to allenes: A. V. Fedorova, A. A. Petrov, *J. Gen. Chem. USSR* **32**, 1740 (1962).

230. Kuhn-Winterstein Reaction
R. Kuhn, A. Winterstein, *Helv. Chim. Acta* **11**, 87 (1928).

Conversion of 1,2-glycols into *trans* olefins by reaction with diphosphotetraiodide (P_2I_4) or other halogenated reagents. This reaction is useful in the preparation of polyenes:

Kuhn *et al., Ber.* **71,** 1510 (1938); **84,** 566 (1961); **88,** 309 (1965); Inhoffen *et al., Ann.* **684,** 24 (1965); H. Kessler, W. Ott, *Tetrahedron Lett.* **1974,** 1383; W. W. Win *et al., J. Org. Chem.* **59,** 2803 (1994).

231. Ladenburg Rearrangement
A. Ladenburg, *Ber.* **16,** 410 (1883); *Ann.* **247,** 1 (1888).

Thermal rearrangement of an alkyl- or benzylpyridinium halide to an alkyl- or benzylpyridine:

J. H. Brewster, E. L. Eliel, *Org. React.* **7,** 135 (1953); L. E. Tenenbau in *Pyridine and Its Derivatives* **Pt. 2,** E. Klingsberg, Ed. (Interscience, New York, 1961) p 163.

232. Lebedev Process
S. V. Lebedev, *Zh. Obshch. Khim.* **3,** 698 (1933).

Formation of butadiene from ethanol by catalytic pyrolysis. The catalysts used are mixtures of sililcates and aluminum and zinc oxides:

$$2CH_3CH_2OH \longrightarrow \diagdown\!\!\diagup\diagdown + H_2 + 2H_2O$$

S. V. Lebedev, **FR 665917** (1928); **GB 331482** (1929); **RU 24393** (1931); C. Ellis, *The Chemistry of Petroleum Derivatives* **II** (New York, 1937) p 173; G. Egloff, G. Hulla, *Chem. Rev.* **36,** 67 (1945); Y. A. Gorin, *Zh. Obshch. Khim.* **20,** 1596 (1950); *Kirk-Othmer Encyclopedia of Chemical Technology* **vol. 4** (New York, 3rd ed., 1978) p 322.

233. Lehmstedt-Tanasescu Reaction
K. Lehmstedt, *Ber.* **65,** 834 (1932); I. Tanasescu, *Bull. Soc. Chim. Fr.* **41,** 528 (1927).

Preparation of acridones (and 10-hydroxyacridones) from *o*-nitrobenzaldehyde and a halobenzene in the presence of concentrated sulfuric acid containing nitrous acid as catalyst:

I. Tanasescu, Z. Frenkel, *ibid.* **1960,** 693. Mechanism: Silberg, Frenkel, *Rev. Roum. Chim.* **10,** 1035 (1965).

234. Letts Nitrile Synthesis
E. A. Letts, *Ber.* **5,** 669 (1872).

Formation of nitriles by heating aromatic carboxylic acids with metal thiocyanates:

$$RCOOH + KSCN \xrightarrow{\Delta} RCN + CO_2 + KHS$$

G. Krüss, *Ber.* **17,** 1766 (1884); E. E. Reid, *Am. Chem. J.* **43,** 162 (1910); G. D. van Epps, E. E. Reid, *J. Am. Chem. Soc.* **38,** 2120 (1916); D. T. Mowry, *Chem. Rev.* **42,** 264 (1948); F. Klages, *Lehrbuch der organischen Chemie* **I** (Berlin, 1959) p 362.

235. Leuckart (Leukart) Reaction; Leuckart-Wallach Reaction; Eschweiler-Clarke Reaction
R. Leuckart, *Ber.* **18,** 2341 (1885).

Reductive alkylation of ammonium (or amine) salts of formic acid or formamides by aldehydes or ketones:

When the reaction is performed in the presence of excess formic acid it is referred to as the **Leuckart-Wallach reaction:** O. Wallach, *Ann.* **272,** 99 (1892). Application to steroids: W. E. Solomons, N. J. Doorenbos, *J. Pharm. Sci.* **63,** 19 (1974); A. M. Bellini *et al., Steroids* **56,** 395 (1991).

The reductive methylation of primary or secondary amines employing formaldehyde and formic acid is known as the **Eschweiler-Clarke reaction:** W. Eschweiler, *Ber.* **38,** 880 (1905); H. T. Clarke *et al., J. Am. Chem. Soc.* **55,** 4571 (1933). Synthetic applications: E. Farkas, C. J. Sunman, *J. Org. Chem.* **50,** 1110 (1985); J. Casanova, P. Devi, *Synth. Commun.* **23,** 245 (1993).

Early reviews: M. L. Moore, *Org. React.* **5**, 301-330 (1949); F. Möller, R. Schröter, *Houben-Weyl* **11/1**, 648-664 (1957). Application to deoxybenzoins: M. J. Villa *et al.*, *Heterocycles* **24**, 1943 (1986). Mechanistic study: P. I. Awachie, V. C. Agwada, *Tetrahedron* **46**, 1899 (1990); A. G. Martinez *et al.*, *Tetrahedron: Asymmetry* **10**, 1499 (1999). Optimized procedure: R. Carlson *et al.*, *Acta Chem. Scand.* **47**, 1046 (1993). Modified conditions: A. Loupy *et al.*, *Tetrahedron Lett.* **37**, 8177 (1996); I. Helland, T. Lejon, *Heterocycles* **51**, 611 (1999).

236. Leuckart Thiophenol Reaction
R. Leuckart, *J. Prakt. Chem.* [2] **41**, 179 (1890).

Decomposition of diazoxanthates, by warming gently in faintly acidic cuprous media, to the corresponding aryl xanthates which afford aryl thiols on alkaline hydrolysis and aryl thioethers on warming:

$$ArN_2Cl + KSCSOR \xrightarrow{70°} ArSCSOR$$

$$\xrightarrow{\Delta} ArSR + COS$$

$$\xrightarrow[H_2O]{alkali} ArSH + HSCOOR$$

D. S. Tarbell, D. K. Fukushima, *Org. Synth.* **coll. vol. III**, 809 (1955); K. H. Saunders, *The Aromatic Diazo-Compounds and Their Technical Applications* (London, 1949) p 325; D. S. Tarbell, M. A. McCall, *J. Am. Chem. Soc.* **74**, 48 (1952); A. R. Forrester, J. L. Wardell, *Rodd's Chemistry of Carbon Compounds* **IIIA**, 422 (1971); A. Schöberl, A. Wagner, *Houben-Weyl* **9**, 12 (1955); L. Tournier, S. Z. Zard, *Tetrahedron Lett.* **46**, 971 (2005).

237. Lieben Iodoform Reaction (Haloform Reaction)
A. Lieben, *Ann.* (Suppl.) **7**, 218 (1870).

Cleavage of methyl ketones with halogens (mostly iodine) and base to carboxylic acids and haloform:

$$RCOCH_3 + NaOI \longrightarrow RCOI_3 \xrightarrow{NaOH} CH_3I + RCOO^- Na^+$$

R. C. Fuson, B. A. Bull, *Chem. Rev.* **15**, 275 (1934); R. N. Seelye, T. A. Turney, *J. Chem. Educ.* **36**, 572 (1959); H. O. House, *Modern Synthetic Reactions* (W. A. Benjamin, Menlo Park, California, 2nd ed., 1972) pp 464-465; J. March, *Advanced Organic Chemistry* (Wiley-Interscience, New York, 4th ed., 1992) p 632.

238. Lobry de Bruyn-van Ekenstein Transformation
C. A. Lobry de Bruyn, *Rec. Trav. Chim.* **14**, 150 (1895); C. A. Lobry de Bruyn, W. A. van Ekenstein, *ibid.* 195, 203; **16**, 262 (1897).

Isomerization of carbohydrates in alkaline media, considered to embrace both epimerization of aldoses and ketoses and aldose-ketose interconversion:

Reviews: Evans, *Chem. Rev.* **31**, 544 (1942); Sattler, *Adv. Carbohydr. Chem.* **3**, 113 (1948); Pigman, *The Carbohydrates* (Academic Press, New York, 1957) p 60; Speck, *Adv. Carbohydr. Chem.* **13**, 63 (1958); Schaffer, *J. Org. Chem.* **29**, 1473 (1964); M. H. Johansson, O. Samuelson, *Chem. Scr.* **9**, 151 (1976). Synthetic applications: P. Köll, G. Papert, *Ann.* **1986**, 1568; B. Sauerbrei *et al.*, *Carbohydr. Res.* **280**, 223 (1996); P. Sedmera *et al.*, *J. Carbohydr. Chem.* **17**, 1351 (1998). Mechanistic study: B. M. Kabyemela *et al.*, *Ind. Eng. Chem. Res.* **38**, 2888 (1999).

239. Lossen Rearrangement
W. Lossen, *Ann.* **161**, 347 (1872); **175**, 271, 313 (1874).

Conversion of a hydroxamic acid to an isocyanate *via* the intermediacy of its *O*-acyl, sulfonyl, or phosphoryl derivative. In the presence of amines, ureas are formed; in the presence of water, amines containing one less carbon than the starting material, are generated:

Reviews: H. L. Yale, *Chem. Rev.* **33**, 209 (1943); L. Bauer, O. Exner, *Angew. Chem. Int. Ed.* **13**, 376 (1974); T. Shiori, *Comp. Org. Syn.* **6**, 821-825 (1991). Reaction conditions leading to the formation of ureas: J. Pihuleac, L. Bauer, *Synthesis* **1989**, 61; extention to *N*-phosphinoylhydroxylamines: J. Fawcett *et al., Chem. Commun.* **1992**, 227; C. J. Salomon, E. Breuer, *J. Org. Chem.* **62**, 3858 (1997); to sulfonyloxy imides: D. A. Casteel *et al., Heterocycles* **36**, 485 (1993). Modifications: J. A. Stafford *et al., J. Org. Chem.* **63**, 10040 (1998); R. Anilkumar *et al., Tetrahedron Lett.* **41**, 5291 (2000). *Cf.* Curtius Rearrangement; Hofmann Reaction; Schmidt Reaction.

240. Madelung Synthesis

W. Madelung, *Ber.* **45**, 1128 (1912).

Formation of indole derivatives by intramolecular cyclization of an *N*-(2-alkylphenyl)alkanamide by a strong base at high temperature:

R. K. Brown in *The Chemistry of Heterocyclic Compounds*, A. Weissberger, Ed., *Indoles* **Part I**, W. J. Houlihan, Ed. (Wiley, New York, 1972) pp 385-396; W. J. Houlihan *et al., J. Org. Chem.* **46**, 4511, 4515 (1981). Under mild conditions: W. Verboom *et al., Tetrahedron Lett.* **26**, 685 (1985); *eidem, Tetrahedron* **42**, 5053 (1986); E. O. M. Orlemans *et al., ibid.* **43**, 3817 (1987).

241. Maillard Reaction ("Browning" Reaction)

L. C. Maillard, *Compt. Rend.* **154**, 66 (1912); *Ann. Chim.* **9**, 5, 258 (1916).

The reactions of amino groups of amino acids, peptides or proteins with the "glycosidic" hydroxyl group of sugars ultimately resulting in the formation of brown pigments.

G. P. Ellis, *Adv. Carbohydr. Chem.* **14**, 63 (1959); E. F. L. Anet, *ibid.* **19**, 181 (1964). Mechanism: M. Amrani-Hemaimi *et al., J. Agric. Food Chem.* **43**, 2818 (1995); high pressure effects: M. Bristow, N. S. Isaacs, *J. Chem. Soc. Perkin Trans. 2* **1999**, 221. Crosslinking in proteins: K. J. Wells-Knecht *et al., J. Org. Chem.* **60**, 6246 (1995); M. O. Lederer, R. G. Klaiber, *Bioorg. Med. Chem.* **7**, 2499 (1999). *Reviews:* C. Eriksson, *Prog. Food Nutr. Sci.* **5**, 159-176 (1981); *The Maillard Reaction in Foods and Medicine*, J. O. O'Brien *et al.*, Eds. (Royal Soc. Chem., Cambridge, U.K., 1998) 464 pp; S. Horvat, A. Jakas, *J. Peptide Sci.* **10**, 119-137 (2004).

242. Malaprade Reaction (Periodic Acid Oxidation)

L. Malaprade, *Bull. Soc. Chim. Fr.* [4] **43**, 683 (1928); *Compt. Rend.* **186**, 382 (1928).

Compounds containing two hydroxyl groups, or a hydroxyl and an amino group, attached to adjacent carbon atoms, undergo cleavage of the carbon-carbon bond when treated with periodic acid to yield aldehydes:

$$RCHOHCHOHR^1 + HIO_4 \longrightarrow RCHO + R^1CHO + H_2O + HIO_3$$

$$RCHOHCHNH_2R^1 + HIO_4 \longrightarrow RCHO + R^1CHO + NH_3 + HIO_3$$

H. O. House, *Modern Synthetic Reactions* (W. A. Benjamin, Menlo Park, California, 2nd ed., 1972) pp 353-359; K. W. Bentley in *Elucidation of Organic Structures by Physical and Chemical Methods* **Pt. 2**, K. W. Bentley, G. W. Kirby, Eds. (Wiley, New York, 2nd ed., 1973) pp 177-185. *Cf.* Criegee Reaction.

243. Malonic Ester Syntheses

Syntheses based on the strongly activated methylene group of malonic esters which on reaction with sodium ethoxide form a resonance-stabilized ion that can be alkylated or acylated. After hydrolysis, the free alkylmalonic acids readily decarboxylate to mono- or disubstituted monocarboxylic acids:

$$H_5C_2OOCCH_2COOC_2H_5 \xrightarrow[\text{2. RX}]{\text{1. NaOC}_2\text{H}_5} H_5C_2OOCCHRCOOC_2H_5 \xrightarrow{\text{HCl}} RCH_2COOH$$

H. O. House, *Modern Synthetic Reactions* (W. A. Benjamin, Menlo Park, California, 2nd ed., 1972) pp 510-518, 756-761. Use of crown ethers as catalysts: D. H. Hunter, *et al., Synthesis* **1977**, 37. Modified conditions: M. A. Casadei *et al., J. Org. Chem.* **46**, 3127 (1981); B. K. Wilk, *Synth. Commun.* **26**, 3859 (1996). Stereoselectivity: T. Sato, J. Otera, *J. Org. Chem.* **60**, 2627 (1995); B. Klotz-Berendes *et al., Tetrahedron: Asymmetry* **8**, 1821 (1997). *Cf.* Perkin Alicyclic Synthesis.

244. Mannich Reaction

C. Mannich, W. Krosche, *Arch. Pharm.* **250**, 647 (1912).

Reaction of compounds having an active hydrogen with non-enolizable aldehydes and ammonia or primary or secondary amines to give aminomethylated products (Mannich bases):

$$(CH_3)_2NH + HCHO + CH_3COCH_3 \longrightarrow (CH_3)_2NCH_2CH_2COCH_3 + H_2O$$

Early reviews: F. F. Blicke, *Org. React.* **1**, 303 (1942); H. O. House, *Modern Synthetic Reactions* (W. A. Benjamin, Menlo Park, California, 2nd ed., 1972) pp 654-660. *p*-Substituted phenols as substrates: D. A. Leigh, P. Linnane, *Tetrahedron Lett.* **34**, 5639 (1993). In synthesis of vinylphosphonates: H. Krawczyk, *Synth. Commun.* **24**, 2263 (1994). Diastereoselectivity: P. C. B. Page *et al., J. Org. Chem.* **58**, 6902 (1993); enantioselectivity: H. Ishitani *et al.*,

J. Am. Chem. Soc. **119,** 7153 (1997); *eidem, Tetrahedron Lett.* **40,** 2161 (1999); K. Yamada, *Angew. Chem. Int. Ed.* **38,** 3504 (1999). *Reviews:* M. Tramontini *et al., Tetrahedron* **46,** 1791-1837 (1990); E. F. Kleinman, *Comp. Org. Syn.* **2,** 893-951 (1991); H. Heane, *ibid.* 953-973; L. E. Overman, D. J. Ricca, *ibid.* 1007-1046; M. Arend *et al., Angew. Chem. Int. Ed.* **37,** 1044-1070 (1998). *Cf.* Betti Reaction; Robinson-Schöpf Reaction.

245. Marschalk Reaction

C. Marschalk *et al., Bull. Soc. Chim. Fr.* **3,** 1545 (1936).

Sodium dithionite reduction of 1-hydroxy- or aminoanthraquinones to their leuco-forms, followed by condensation with aldehydes to yield the 2-alkylated anthraquinones. 2-Hydroxyanthraquinones yield 1-alkylated products:

X = OH, Y = O
X = NH$_2$, Y = NH

Scope and limitations: K. Krohn, W. Baltus, *Tetrahedron* **44,** 49 (1988). Synthetic applications: F. Suzuki *et al., J. Am. Chem. Soc.* **100,** 2272 (1978); L. M. Harwood *et al., Can. J. Chem.* **62,** 1922 (1984); M. T. Furlong *et al., Synth. Commun.* **20,** 2691 (1990); N. R. Ayyangar *et al., Indian J. Chem.* **31B,** 3 (1992); K. Krohn, S. Bernhard, *J. Prakt. Chem.* **340,** 26 (1998).

246. Martinet Dioxindole Synthesis

A. Guyot, J. Martinet, *Compt. Rend.* **156,** 1625 (1913).

Formation of derivatives of dioxindole from esters of mesoxalic acid and aromatic amines or amino quinolines:

J. Martinet, *ibid.* **166,** 851, 998 (1918); *Ann. Chim.* [9] **11,** 85 (1919); W. Langenbeck *et al., Ann.* **499,** 201 (1932); **512,** 276 (1934); W. C. Sumpter, *Chem. Rev.* **37,** 472 (1945); P. L. Julian *et al., Heterocycl. Compd.* **3,** 239 (1952).

247. McFadyen-Stevens Reaction

J. S. McFadyen, T. S. Stevens, *J. Chem. Soc.* **1936,** 584.

Base-catalyzed thermal decomposition of acylbenzenesulfonylhydrazines to aldehydes:

E. Mosettig, *Org. React.* **8,** 232-240 (1954); S. Siddappa, G. A. Bhat, *J. Chem. Soc. C* **1971,** 178; S. B. Matin *et al., J. Org. Chem.* **39,** 2285 (1974); M. Nair, H. Shechter, *Chem. Commun.* **1978,** 793. Alternative hydrazide reagent: C. C. Dudman *et al., Tetrahedron Lett.* **1980,** 4645. Synthetic applications: H. Graboyes *et al., J. Heterocycl. Chem.* **12,** 1225 (1975); R. K. Manna *et al., Synth. Commun.* **28,** 9 (1998).

248. McLafferty Rearrangement

F. W. McLafferty, *Anal. Chem.* **31,** 82 (1959).

Electron-impact-induced cleavage of carbonyl compounds having a hydrogen in the γ-position, to an enolic fragment and an olefin:

D. G. I. Kingston *et al., Chem. Rev.* **74,** 215 (1974); K. Biemann, *Mass Spectrometry* (New York, 1962) p 119; Djerassi *et al., J. Am. Chem. Soc.* **87,** 817 (1965); **91,** 2069 (1969); **94,** 473 (1972); M. J. Lacey *et al., Org. Mass Spectrom.* **5,** 1391 (1971); G. Eadon, *J. Am. Chem. Soc.* **94,** 8938 (1972); F. Turecek, V. Hanus, *Org. Mass Spectrom.* **15,** 8 (1980). *Cf.* Norrish Type Cleavage.

249. McMurry Coupling Reaction

J. E. McMurry, M. P. Fleming, *J. Am. Chem. Soc.* **96,** 4708 (1974); S. Tyrlik, I. Wolochowicz, *Bull. Soc. Chim. Fr.* **1973,** 2147; T. Mukaiyama *et al., Chem. Lett.* **1973,** 1041.

Deoxygenative coupling of carbonyl compounds to alkenes induced by low-valent titanium:

Synthetic application: A. Fürstner, D. N. Jumbam, *Tetrahedron* **48**, 5991 (1992); M. Rucker, R. Brückner, *Tetrahedron Lett.* **38**, 7353 (1997); P. Harter *et al., Polyhedron* **17**, 1141 (1998). Modified conditions: T. A. Lipski *et al., J. Org. Chem.* **62**, 4566 (1997); S. Talukdar *et al., ibid.* **63**, 4925 (1998). *Reviews:* J. E. McMurry, *Chem. Rev.* **89**, 1513-1524 (1989); G. M. Robertson, *Comp. Org. Syn.* **3**, 583-595 (1991); T. Lectka, *Act. Met.* **1996**, 85-131; M. Ephritikhine, *Chem. Commun.* **23**, 2549-2554 (1998). *Cf.* Barton Olefin Synthesis.

250. Meerwein Arylation
H. Meerwein *et al., J. Prakt. Chem.* **152**, 237 (1939).

Formation of arylated olefins on treatment of olefins with diazonium salts in the presence of cupric salts:

$$Z = C=C, C=O, \text{ Ar, CN, H}$$

Synthetic applications: P. Sutter, C. D. Weis, *J. Heterocycl. Chem.* **24**, 69 (1987); G. Wurm, H. J. Gurka, *Pharmazie* **52**, 739 (1997); enhanced stereoselectivity: H. Brunner *et al., J. Organomet. Chem.* **541**, 89 (1997). Modified conditions: M. D. Obushak *et al., Tetrahedron Lett.* **39**, 9567 (1998). *Reviews:* C. S. Rondestvedt, Jr., *Org. React.* **11**, 189 (1960); *ibid.* **24**, 225-259 (1976); C. D. Weis, *Dyes Pigm.* **9**, 1-20 (1988). *Cf.* Pschorr Reaction.

251. Meerwein-Ponndorf-Verley Reduction (Aluminum Alkoxide Reduction)
H. Meerwein, R. Schmidt, *Ann.* **444**, 221 (1925); W. Ponndorf, *Angew. Chem.* **39**, 138 (1926); A. Verley, *Bull. Soc. Chim. Fr.* **37**, 537, 871 (1925).

Reduction of aldehydes or ketones to the corresponding alcohols with aluminum alkoxides (the reverse of the Oppenauer oxidation, *q.v.*):

Reviews: A. L. Wilds, *Org. React.* **2**, 178-202 (1944); R. M. Kellogg, *Comp. Org. Syn.* **8**, 88-91 (1991); C. F. de Graauw *et al., Synthesis* **10**, 1007-1017 (1994). Enantioselectivity: D. A. Evans *et al., J. Am. Chem. Soc.* **115**, 9800 (1993); M. Node *et al., ibid.* **122**, 1927 (2000). Modified conditions: P. S. Kumbhar *et al., Chem. Commun.* **1998**, 535; T. Ooi *et al., J. Am. Chem. Soc.* **120**, 10790 (1998); Y. Nakano *et al., Tetrahedron Lett.* **41**, 1565 (2000). *Cf.* Cannizzaro Reaction; Tischenko Reaction.

252. Meisenheimer Rearrangements
J. Meisenheimer, *Ber.* **52**, 1667 (1919).

Formation of *O, N, N*-trisubstituted hydroxylamines from tertiary amine oxides *via* [1,2]-R group migration, or [2,3]-sigmatropic rearrangement when R' = allyl:

[1,2]-Rearrangements: N. Castagnoli, Jr. *et al., Tetrahedron* **26**, 4319 (1970); J. B. Bremner *et al., Aust. J. Chem.* **41**, 293 (1988); R. Yoneda *et al., Tetrahedron Lett.* **35**, 3749 (1994); *eidem, Tetrahedron* **52**, 14563 (1996). *Cf.* Stevens Rearrangement; [1,2]-Wittig Rearrangement.

[2,3]-Rearrangements: V. Rautenstrauch, *Helv. Chim. Acta* **56**, 2492 (1973); Y. Yamamato *et al., J. Org. Chem.* **41**, 303 (1976); or [1,2]: T. Kurihara *et al., Chem. Pharm. Bull.* **42**, 475 (1994). Asymmetric syntheses: D. Enders, H.

Kempen, *Synlett* **1994**, 969; S. G. Davies, G. D. Smyth, *Tetrahedron: Asymmetry* **7**, 1001 (1996); J. E. H. Buston *et al.*, *ibid.* **9**, 1995 (1998). *Cf.* Mislow-Evans Rearrangement; Sommelet-Hauser Rearrangement; [2,3]-Wittig Rearrangement.

253. Menschutkin Reaction

N. Menschutkin, *Z. Phys. Chem.* **5**, 589 (1890); **6**, 41 (1890).

Reaction of tertiary amines with alkyl halides to form quaternary salts:

$$R_3{}^1N \ + \ RX \longrightarrow R_3{}^1RN^+X^-$$

Mechanistic studies: C. K. Ingold, *Structure and Mechanism in Organic Chemistry* (Cornell Univ. Press, New York, 2nd ed., 1969) p 435; M. H. Abraham, *Prog. Phys. Org. Chem.* **11**, 1 (1974); E. M. Arnett, R. Reich, *J. Am. Chem. Soc.* **102**, 5892 (1980); S. Shaik *et al., ibid.* **116**, 262 (1994); S. H. Kim *et al., J. Phys. Org. Chem.* **11**, 254 (1998). Solvent effects: J.-L. M. Abboud *et al., J. Phys. Chem.* **93**, 214 (1989); S.-G. Kang *et al., Bull. Chem. Soc. Jpn.* **66**, 972 (1993).

254. Merrifield Solid-Phase Peptide Synthesis (SPPS)

R. B. Merrifield, *J. Am. Chem. Soc.* **85**, 2149 (1963).

Synthesis of long peptides involving the following steps: (1) attachment of the C-terminal amino acid to an insoluble polymeric support resin, (2) elongation of the peptide chain, and (3) cleavage of the peptide from the resin:

Elongation step (P = support resin):

Method for monitoring synthesis: B. D. Larsen *et al., J. Am. Chem. Soc.* **115**, 6247 (1993). Synthetic applications: D. D. Smith *et al., J. Peptide Protein Res.* **44**, 183 (1994); M. J. O'Donnell *et al., J. Am. Chem. Soc.* **118**, 6070 (1996); R. Léger *et al., Tetrahedron Lett.* **39**, 4171 (1998). *Review:* C. Birr, *Aspects of Merrifield Peptide Synthesis*, K. Hafner *et al.*, Eds. (Springer-Verlag, New York, 1978) pp 102; B. Merrifield, *Science* **232**, 341-347 (1986); G. B. Wisdom *et al., Peptide Antigens* (Oxford University Press, 1994) pp 27-81. Autobiographical account: B. Merrifield, *Life During a Golden Age of Peptide Chemistry*, J. I. Seeman, Ed. (ACS, Washington, D.C., 1993) pp 54-118.

255. Meyer Reaction

G. Meyer, *Ber.* **16**, 1439 (1883).

Preparation of alkylstannonic acids by reacting alkali stannite with an alkyl iodide. When applied to alkali arsenites or plumbites the reaction yields alkylarsonic and alkylplumbonic acids, respectively:

$$Na_2SnO_2 \ + \ RX \longrightarrow RSnO_2Na \ + \ NaX$$

$$Na_3AsO_3 \ + \ RX \longrightarrow RAsO_3Na_2 \ + \ NaX$$

W. R. Cullen, *Adv. Organomet. Chem.* **4**, 148 (1966).

256. Meyer-Schuster Rearrangement; Rupe Rearrangement

K. H. Meyer, K. Schuster, *Ber.* **55**, 819 (1922); H. Rupe, E. Kambli, *Helv. Chim. Acta* **9**, 672 (1926).

Acid-catalyzed rearrangement of secondary and tertiary α-acetylenic alcohols to α,β-unsaturated carbonyl compounds: aldehydes result when the acetylenic group is terminal, ketones when it is internal:

$$R_2\overset{\underset{\displaystyle |}{OH}}{C}C{\equiv}CR^1 \xrightarrow{\ H^+\ } R_2C{=}CHCOR^1$$

The conversion of tertiary alkylacetylenic carbinols with a terminal acetylenic group to predominantly α,β-unsaturated ketones and not the expected aldehydes, is referred to as the **Rupe rearrangement:**

$$RCH_2\overset{\underset{\displaystyle R^1}{|}}{\underset{|}{C}}C{\equiv}CH \xrightarrow[\Delta]{HCOOH} R{-}CH{=}CR^1COCH_3$$

Metal-based catalysis: P. Chabardes, *Tetrahedron Lett.* **29**, 6253 (1988); C. Y. Lorber, J. A. Osborn, *ibid.* **37**, 853 (1996). Mechanism studies: M. Edens *et al., J. Org. Chem.* **42**, 3403 (1977); J. Andres *et al., J. Am. Chem. Soc.* **110**, 666 (1988). Applications: E. A. Omar *et al., J. Heterocycl. Chem.* **29**, 947 (1992); M. Yoshimatsu *et al., J. Org. Chem.* **60**, 4798 (1995). Early reviews: R. Heilmann, R. Glenat, *Ann. Chim. (Paris)* **8**, 178 (1963); S. Swaminathan, K. V. Narayanan, *Chem. Rev.* **71**, 429 (1971).

257. Meyer Synthesis (Victor Meyer Synthesis)
V. Meyer, O. Stuber, *Ber.* **5**, 203 (1872).

Formation of aliphatic nitrites and nitro derivatives by the reaction of aliphatic halides with metal nitrites:

$$RX + MNO_2 \longrightarrow RONO + RNO_2 + MX$$

R. B. Reynolds, H. Adkins, *J. Am. Chem. Soc.* **51**, 279 (1929). *Reviews:* H. B. Hass, E. F. Riley, *Chem. Rev.* **32**, 373 (1943); N. Kornblum, *Org. React.* **12**, 101-156 (1962). Application to the synthesis of α,ω-dinitroalkanes: J. K. Stille, E. D. Vessel, *J. Org. Chem.* **25**, 478 (1960); G. Leston, *Org. Synth.* **4**, 368 (1963).

258. Meyers Aldehyde Synthesis
A. I. Meyers *et al.*, *J. Am. Chem. Soc.* **91**, 763 (1969); *eidem, J. Org. Chem.* **38**, 36 (1973).

Synthesis of aldehydes from alkylhalides and 2-lithiomethyltetrahydro-3-oxazine:

J. March, *Advanced Organic Chemistry* (Wiley-Interscience, New York, 4th ed., 1992) pp 478-479; A. I. Meyers *et al.*, *J. Org. Chem.* **46**, 783 (1981).

259. Michael Reaction (Addition) (Condensation)
A. Michael, *J. Prakt. Chem.* [2] **35**, 349 (1887).

Base-promoted conjugate addition of carbon nucleophiles (donors) to activated unsaturated systems (acceptors):

donor = malonates, cyanoacetates, acetoacetates, carboxylic esters, ketones, aldehydes, nitriles, nitro compounds, sulfones
acceptor = α,β-unsaturated ketones, esters, aldehydes, amides, carboxylic acids, nitriles sulfoxides, sulfones, nitro compounds, phosphonates, phosphoranes
base = $NaOCH_2CH_3$, $NH(CH_2CH_3)_2$, KOH, $KOC(CH_3)_3$, $N(CH_2CH_3)_3$, NaH, BuLi, LDA

Reviews: E. D. Bergmann *et al.*, *Org. React.* **10**, 179-555 (1959); H. O. House, *Modern Synthetic Reactions* (W. A. Benjamin, Menlo Park, California, 2nd ed., 1972) pp 595-623; M. E. Jung, *Comp. Org. Syn.* **4**, 1-67 (1991). Review of organometallic nucleophiles: D. A. Hunt *et al.*, *Org. Prep. Proced. Int.* **21**, 705-749 (1989); V. J. Lee, *Comp. Org. Syn.* **4**, 69-137, 139-168 (1991); J. A. Kozlowski, *ibid.* 169-198. Reviews of stereoselective synthesis: H.-G. Schmalz, *ibid.* 199-236; D. A. Oare, C. H. Heathcock, *Top. Stereochem.* **20**, 87-170 (1991); J. d'Angelo *et al.*, *Tetrahedron: Asymmetry* **3**, 459-505 (1992); J. Leonard *et al.*, *Eur. J. Org. Chem.* **1998**, 2051-2061. *Cf.* Nagata Hydrocyanation; Robinson Annulation.

260. Michaelis-Arbuzov Reaction
A. Michaelis, R. Kaehne, *Ber.* **31**, 1048 (1898); A. E. Arbuzov, *J. Russ. Phys. Chem. Soc.* **38**, 687 (1906); *Chem. Zentralbl.* **1906**, II, 1639.

Formation of monoalkylphosphonic esters from alkyl halides and trialkyl phosphites, *via* the intermediate phosphonium salt:

$$P(OR)_3 + R^1X \longrightarrow [(RO)_3PR^1]X \xrightarrow{\Delta} (RO)_2P(O)R^1$$

K. Sasse, *Houben-Weyl* **12/1**, 433 (1963); B. A. Arbuzov, *Pure Appl. Chem.* **9**, 307 (1964); G. M. Kosolapoff, *Org. React.* **6**, 276 (1951); D. Redmore, *Chem. Rev.* **71**, 317 (1971); G. Bauer, G. Haegele, *Angew. Chem. Int. Ed.* **16**, 477 (1977); A. K. Bhattacharya, G. Thyagarajan, *Chem. Rev.* **81**, 415 (1981); B. Faure *et al.*, *Chem. Commun.* **1989**, 805; V. K. Yadav, *Synth. Commun.* **20**, 239 (1990).

261. Miescher Degradation
C. Meystre *et al.*, *Helv. Chim. Acta* **27**, 1815 (1944).

Adaptation of the Barbier-Wieland degradation, *q.v.*, to permit simultaneous elimination of three carbon atoms, as in degradation of the bile acid side chain to the methyl ketone stage. Conversion of the methyl ester of the bile acid to the tertiary alcohol, followed by dehydration, bromination, dehydrohalogenation and oxidation of the diene yields the chain-shortened ketone:

$$RR^1CHCH_2CH_2COOCH_3 \xrightarrow{PhMgBr} RR^1CHCH_2CH_2C(OH)Ph_2 \xrightarrow{-H_2O}$$

$$RR^1CHCH_2CH=CPh_2 \xrightarrow{(CH_2CO)_2NBr} RR^1CHCHBrCH=CPh_2 \xrightarrow{-HBr}$$

$$RR^1C=CH-CH=CPh_2 \xrightarrow{CrO_3} RCOR^1 + OHCCH=CPh_2$$

C. W. Shoppee, *Ann. Repts.* (Chem. Soc. London) **44**, 184 (1947); F. S. Spring, *J. Chem. Soc.* **1950**, 3355; A. Wettstein, G. Anner, *Experientia* **1954**, 407; C. J. W. Brooks, *Rodd's Chemistry of Carbon Compounds* **IID**, 26 (1970); P. G. Marshall, *ibid.* 233, 253, 323.

262. Mignonac Reaction
G. Mignonac, *Compt. Rend.* **172**, 223 (1921).
Formation of amines by catalytic hydrogenation of aldehydes or ketones in liquid ammonia and absolute ethanol in the presence of a nickel catalyst:

$$RCOR^1 + NH_3 + H_2 \xrightarrow{Ni} RR^1CHNH_2 + H_2O$$

F. Randvere, *An. Farm. Bioquim.* **18**, 81 (1948); *Houben-Weyl* **4/2**, 51 (1955).

263. Milas Hydroxylation of Olefins
N. A. Milas *et al., J. Am. Chem. Soc.* **58**, 1302 (1936); **59**, 543, 2342, 2345 (1937); **61**, 1844 (1939); **62**, 1841 (1940).
Formation of *cis*-glycols by reaction of alkenes with hydrogen peroxide and either ultraviolet light or a catalytic amount of osmium, vanadium, or chromium oxide:

$$\ce{>C=C<} + H_2O_2 \xrightarrow[\text{or } h\nu]{\text{metal oxide}} \overset{HO\ \ OH}{-\underset{|}{\overset{|}{C}}-\underset{|}{\overset{|}{C}}-}$$

F. D. Gunstone, *Adv. Org. Chem.* **1**, 115 (1960); P. N. Rylander, *Organic Syntheses with Noble Metal Catalysts* (Academic Press, New York, 1973) p 60. *Cf.* Sharpless Dihydroxylation.

264. Mislow-Evans Rearrangement
P. Bickart *et al., J. Am. Chem. Soc.* **90**, 4869 (1968); D. A. Evans *et al., ibid.* **93**, 4956 (1971).
[2,3]-Sigmatropic rearrangement of allylic sulfoxides to allylic sulfenates which are captured by thiophiles to generate the allylic alcohols, thereby effecting the 1,3-transposition of sulfoxide and alcohol functions. The reverse process is accomplished by treating the alcohol with arylsulfenyl chloride, followed by thermal rearrangement of the sulfenate to generate the allylic sulfoxide:

$$R\diagdown\diagup\diagdown\underset{O}{\overset{O}{\underset{\|}{S}}}\diagdown Ar \underset{\Delta}{\overset{\Delta}{\rightleftharpoons}} \left[ArS\diagdown O\diagup\diagdown_R \right] \underset{ArSCl, N(CH_2CH_3)_3}{\overset{thiophile}{\rightleftharpoons}} HO\diagdown\diagup\diagdown_R$$

thiophile = $P(OCH_3)_3$, $(CH_3CH_2)_2NH$, piperidine, PhS^-

Early review: D. A. Evans, G. C. Andrews, *Acc. Chem. Res.* **7**, 147 (1974). Acid-catalyzed modification: Y. Masaki *et al., Chem. Pharm. Bull.* **33**, 2531 (1985). Synthetic applications: H. J. Reich, S. Wollowitz, *J. Am. Chem. Soc.* **104**, 7051 (1982); G. H. Posner *et al., J. Org. Chem.* **52**, 4836 (1987); A. Padwa *et al., ibid.* **56**, 4252 (1991). Mechanistic studies: D. K. Jones-Hertzog, W. L. Jorgensen, *ibid.* **60**, 6682 (1995); *eidem, J. Am. Chem. Soc.* **117**, 9077 (1995). *Cf.* Meisenheimer Rearrangements; [2,3]-Wittig Rearrangement.

265. Mitsunobu Reaction
O. Mitsunobu *et al., Bull. Chem. Soc. Jpn.* **40**, 935 (1967); O. Mitsunobu, Y. Yamada, *ibid.* 2380.
Condensation of alcohols and acidic components (NuH) on treatment with dialkyl azodicarboxylates and trialkyl- or triarylphosphines occurring primarily with inversion of configuration *via* the proposed intermediary oxyphosphonium salts:

$$EtOCO-N=N-COOEt + Ph_3P \xrightarrow{NuH} \left[\underset{Ph_3\overset{|+}{P}\ \overset{-}{Nu}}{EtOCO-N-NHCOOEt} \right] \xrightarrow{\overset{OH}{R^1 \diagup R^2}}$$

$$\left[\underset{R^1 \diagup R^2}{\overset{O}{}}\overset{P^+Ph_3Nu^-}{} \right] + EtOCONHNHCOOEt \longrightarrow \underset{R^1 \diagup R^2}{\overset{Nu}{|}} + Ph_3P=O$$

NuH = phosphoric mono- and diesters, carboxylic acids, phenols, imides, oximes, hydroxymates, heterocycles, thiols, thioamides, β-keto esters

Methods development: R. F. C. Brown *et al., Tetrahedron* **50,** 5469 (1994); T. Tsunoda *et al., Tetrahedron Lett.* **40,** 7355 (1999); J. C. Pelletier, S. Kincaid, *ibid.* **41,** 797 (2000). Synthetic applications: M. A. Poelert *et al., Rec. Trav. Chim.* **113,** 355 (1994); A. Viso *et al., Tetrahedron Lett.* **41,** 407 (2000); H. Schedel *et al., Tetrahedron: Asymmetry* **11,** 2125 (2000). Solid-phase synthesis: S. R. Chhabra *et al., Tetrahedron Lett.* **41,** 1099 (2000); F. Zaragoza, H. Stephensen, *ibid.* 2015; P.-P. Kung, E. Swayze, *ibid.* **40,** 5651 (1999). Mechanism: T. Watanabe *et al., Chirality* **12,** 346 (2000). *Reviews:* O. Mitsunobu, *Synthesis* **1981,** 1-28; D. L. Hughes, *Org. React.* **29,** 1-162 (1983); D. L. Hughes, *Org. Prep. Proced. Int.* **28,** 127-164 (1996); J. A. Dodge, S. A. Jones, *Recent Res. Dev. Org. Chem.* **1,** 273-283 (1997); S. Dandapani, D. P. Curran, *Chem. Eur. J.* **10,** 3130-3138 (2004); R. Dembinski, *Eur. J. Org. Chem.* **2004,** 2763-2772.

266. Moore Myers Cyclization; Moore Cyclization; Myers Cyclization

J. O. Karlsson *et al., J. Am. Chem. Soc.* **107,** 3392 (1985); A. G. Myers *et al., ibid.* **111,** 8057 (1989); R. Nagata *et al., Tetrahedron Lett.* **30,** 4995 (1989).

Thermal generation of a biradical by cyclization of enyne-ketenes (Moore) or of enyene-allenes (Myers):

A. Rahm, W. D. Wulff, *J. Am. Chem. Soc.* **118,** 1807 (1996). *Reviews:* H. W. Moore, B. R. Yerxa, *Chemtracts* **1992,** 273-313; M. E. Maier, *Synlett* **1995,** 13-26; K. K. Wang, *Chem. Rev.* **96,** 207-222 (1996). *Cf.* Bergman Reaction.

267. Mukaiyama Aldol Reaction

T. Mukaiyama *et al., Chem. Lett.* **1973,** 1011; *idem et al., ibid.* **1974,** 323; *eidem, J. Am. Chem. Soc.* **96,** 7503 (1974).

Formation of β-hydroxy ketones via reaction of silyl enol ethers or ketene silyl acetals with aldehydes in presence of a Lewis acid, such as titanium tetrachloride, tin tetrachloride or boron trifluoride etherate:

Enantioselectivity: E. M. Carreira *et al., J. Am. Chem. Soc.* **116,** 8837 (1994). Diastereoselectivity: S. E. Denmark *et al., Tetrahedron* **54,** 10389 (1998). *Reviews:* H. Gröger *et al., Chem. Eur. J.* **4,** 1137-1141 (1998); E. M. Carreira in *Comprehensive Asymmetric Catalysis I-III* vol. 3, E. N. Jacobsen *et al.,* Eds. (Springer-Verlag, Berlin, Germany, 1999) 997-1065; K. Iseki, *ACS Symp. Ser.* **746,** 38-51 (2000). *Cf.* Aldol Reaction; Evans Aldol Reaction.

268. Mukaiyama-Michael Reaction

K. Narasaka *et al., Bull. Chem. Soc. Jpn.* **49,** 779 (1976).

Formation of 1,5-dicarbonyl compounds by reaction of ketene silyl acetals with α,β-unsaturated ketones and esters:

T. Mukaiyama, S. Kobayashi, *Heterocycles* **25,** 245 (1987). Enhanced diastereoselectivity: J. Otera *et al., Tetrahedron* **52,** 9409 (1996); in tandem-aldol reaction: N. Giuseppone *et al., Tetrahedron Lett.* **39,** 7874 (1998). Synthetic application: H. Paulsen *et al., Angew. Chem. Int. Ed.* **38,** 3373 (1999).

269. Nagata Hydrocyanation

W. Nagata *et al., Tetrahedron Lett.* **1962,** 461.

Alkylaluminum-mediated 1,4-addition of hydrogen cyanide to α,β-unsaturated carbonyl compounds:

Early review: W. Nagata, M. Yoshioka, *Org. React.* **25,** 255-476 (1977). Synthetic application: T. F. Gallagher, J. L. Adams, *J. Org. Chem.* **57,** 3347 (1992). *Cf.* Michael Reaction.

270. Nametkin Rearrangement

S. S. Nametkin, *Ann.* **432,** 207 (1923).

A special case of carbonium ion rearrangement in camphene hydrochloride derivatives involving the migration of a methyl group:

H. Henecka, *Houben-Weyl* **4/2**, 16 (1955); P. S. Moervs *et al., J. Am. Chem. Soc.* **100,** 260 (1978). *Cf.* Retropinacol Rearrangement; Wagner-Meerwein Rearrangement.

271. Nazarov Cyclization Reaction

I. N. Nazarov *et al., Izv. Akad. Nauk SSSR Otd. Khim. Nauk* **1942,** 200.

Protic or Lewis acid-catalyzed electrocyclic ring closure of divinyl ketones, or their equivalents, to yield 2-cyclopentenones:

Silicon-directed cyclizations to α-methylenecyclopentanones: H. T. Kang *et al., Tetrahedron Lett.* **33,** 3495 (1992). Diastereoselectivity of interrupted reaction: J. A. Bender *et al., J. Org. Chem.* **63,** 2430 (1998); *idem et al., J. Am. Chem. Soc.* **121,** 7443 (1999); H. Hu *et al., ibid.* **121,** 9895 (1999). Lewis acid catalyzed reactions: C. Kuroda *et al., Chem. Commun.* **1997,** 1177; H. A. Buchholz, A. de Meijere, *Eur. J. Org. Chem.* **1998,** 2301. *Reviews:* S. E. Denmark, *Comp. Org. Syn.* **5,** 751-784 (1991); K. L. Habermas *et al., Org. React.* **45,** 1-158 (1994); S. Giese, F. G. West, *Tetrahedron Lett.* **39,** 8393 (1998); of interrupted reaction: D. Zuev, L. A. Paquette, *Chemtracts* **12,** 1019-1025 (1999); of methodological advances: M. A. Tius, *Eur. J. Org. Chem.* **2005,** 2193-2206.

272. Neber Rearrangement

P. W. Neber, A. v. Friedolsheim, *Ann.* **449,** 109 (1926); P. W. Neber, G. Huh, *ibid.* **515,** 283 (1935).

Formation of α-amino ketones by treatment of sulfonic esters of ketoximes with potassium ethoxide, followed by hydrolysis:

Reviews: C. O'Brien, *Chem. Rev.* **64,** 81 (1964); C. G. McCarty in *The Chemistry of the Carbon-Nitrogen Double Bond*, S. Patai, Ed. (Interscience, New York, 1970) p 447; Y. Tamura *et al., Synthesis* **1973,** 215; R. F. Parcell, J. C. Sanchez, *J. Org. Chem.* **46,** 5229 (1981); K. Maruoka, H. Yamamoto, *Comp. Org. Syn.* **6,** 786-789 (1991). Synthetic applications: I. Moldvai *et al., Heterocycles* **43,** 2377 (1996); M. J. Mphahlele, T. A. Modro, *Phosphorus Sulfur Silicon Relat. Elem.* **127,** 131 (1997); J. Y. L. Chung *et al., Tetrahedron Lett.* **40,** 6739 (1999).

273. Nef Reaction

J. U. Nef, *Ann.* **280,** 263 (1894).

Formation of aldehydes and ketones from primary and secondary nitroalkanes, respectively, by treatment of their salts with sulfuric acid:

Modified conditions: W. Adam *et al., Synlett* **1998,** 1335; P. Ceccherelli *et al., Synth. Commun.* **28,** 3057 (1998). Application to spiroketals: T. Capecchi *et al., Tetrahedron Lett.* **39,** 5429 (1998). *Reviews:* P. Salomaa in *The Chemistry of the Carbonyl Group*, S. Patai, Ed. (Interscience, N.Y., 1966) pp 177-210; H. W. Pinnick, *Org. React.* **38,** 655-792 (1990); D. S. Grierson, H.-P. Husson, *Comp. Org. Syn.* **6,** 937-944 (1991); R. Ballini, M. Petrini, *Tetrahedron* **60,** 1017-1047 (2004).

274. Nef Synthesis

J. U. Nef, *Ann.* **308,** 281 (1899).

Addition of sodium acetylides to aldehydes and ketones to yield acetylenic carbinols; occasionally and erroneously referred to as the Nef reaction, *q.v.:*

$$RCOR^1 \xrightarrow[\text{2. } H_2O/ H^+]{\text{1. } NaC\equiv CH} RR^1C(OH)C\equiv CH$$

Farbenfabriken Bayer, **DE 280226; DE 285770** (1913); J. H. Saunders, *Org. Synth.* **20**, 40 (1940); A. W. Johnson, *The Chemistry of the Acetylenic Compounds* (London, 1946) p 11; C. D. Hurd, W. D. McPhee, *J. Am. Chem. Soc.* **69**, 239 (1947); W. Oroschnik, A. O. Mebane, *ibid.* **71**, 2062 (1949); R. A. Raphael, *Acetylenic Compounds in Organic Synthesis* (London, 1955) p 10. *Cf.* Arens-van Dorp Synthesis; Favorskii-Babayan Synthesis.

275. Negishi Cross Coupling
E. Negishi *et al., J. Org. Chem.* **42**, 1821 (1977).
Formation of unsymmetric biaryls by cross coupling arylhalides with arylzinc reagents in presence of catalytic Ni or Pd:

$$R^1Y + R^2ZnX \xrightarrow{\text{Pd or Ni}} R^1\text{--}R^2 + ZnXY$$

X, Y = halogen
R^1 = alkenyl, aryl, allylic, benzylic, propargylic
R^2 = alkenyl, aryl, alkyny, alkyl, benzylic, allylic

Synthetic application: S. Superchi *et al., Tetrahedron Lett.* **37**, 6057 (1996); J. A. Miller, R. P. Farrell, *ibid.* **39**, 6441 (1998). Extension to additional functional groups: E. Negishi, *Acc. Chem. Res.* **15**, 340 (1982). *Review:* P. Knochel, R. D. Singer, *Chem. Rev.* **93**, 2117-2188 (1993); *idem et al., Ber.* **130**, 1021-1027 (1997).

276. Nencki Reaction
M. Nencki, N. Sieber, *J. Prakt. Chem.* (2) **23**, 147 (1881).
The ring acylation of phenols with acids in the presence of zinc chloride, or the modification of the Friedel-Crafts reaction, *q.v.*, by substitution of ferric chloride for aluminum chloride.
M. Nencki, W. Schmid, *ibid.* 546; M. Nencki, *ibid.* **25**, 273 (1882); U. S. Chiema, K. Venkataraman, *J. Chem. Soc.* **1932**, 918; C. W. Schellhammer, *Houben-Weyl* **7/2a,** 284 (1973); A. S. Anjaneyulu *et al., Indian J. Chem.* **33B,** 847 (1994). *Cf.* Darzens-Nenitzescu Synthesis of Ketones.

277. Nenitzescu Indole Synthesis
C. D. Nenitzescu, *Bull. Soc. Chim. Romania* **11**, 37 (1929).
Synthesis of 5-hydroxyindole derivatives by condensation of *p*-benzoquinone with *β*-aminocrotonic esters:

Reviews: R. K. Brown in *The Chemistry of Heterocyclic Compounds*, W. J. Houlihan, Ed. (Wiley, New York, 1972) p 413; G. R. Allen, Jr., *Org. React.* **20**, 337 (1973). Synthetic applications: U. Kuecklander, W. Huehnermann, *Arch. Pharm.* **312**, 515 (1979); J. L. Bernier, J. P., Henichart, *J. Org. Chem.* **46**, 4197 (1981). M. Kinugawa *et al., J. Chem. Soc. Perkin Trans. 1* **1995**, 2677; J. M. Pawlak *et al., J. Org. Chem.* **61**, 9055 (1996).

278. Nenitzescu Reductive Acylation
C. D. Nenitzescu, E. Cioranescu, *Ber.* **69**, 1820 (1936).
Hydrogenative acylation of cycloolefins with acid chlorides in the presence of aluminum chloride; with five- and six-membered rings no change in ring size occurs but with seven-membered rings rearrangement takes place with formation of a cyclohexane derivative:

C. Nenitzescu, C. N. Ionescu, *Ann.* **491**, 189 (1931); C. D. Nenitzescu, J. P. Cantuniari, *ibid.* **510**, 269 (1934); C. D. Nenitzescu, I. Chicos, *Ber.* **68**, 1584 (1935); C. A. Thomas, *Anhydrous Aluminum Chloride in Organic Chemistry* (New York, 1941) p 759; S. L. Friess, R. Pinson, *J. Am. Chem. Soc.* **73**, 3512 (1951); Olah, *Friedel-Crafts and Related Reactions* **vol. III,** Part 2 (New York, 1964) p 1069. *Cf.* Darzens-Nenitzescu Synthesis of Ketones.

279. Nicholas Reaction
R. F. Lockwood, K. M. Nicholas, *Tetrahedron Lett.* **18**, 4163 (1977).
The reaction of dicobalthexacarbonyl-stabilized propargyl cations with nucleophiles, followed by oxidative demetalation to yield propargylated products:

$R^1 = H$, SiR_3, alkyl, aryl; $R^2 = H$, CH_3
$R^3 = H$, Ph, alkyl, substituted alkyl; $R^4 =$ alkyl, substituted alkyl
$H^+ = HBF_4 \cdot O(CH_3)_2$, CF_3COOH;
Lewis acid $= BF_3 \cdot OEt_2$, $EtAlCl_2$, $TiCl_4$, $Bu_2BOSO_2CF_3$
NuH = electron rich aromatics, β-dicarbonyl compounds, ketones,
enolates, allyl silanes, hydride, amines, enamines
[O] = $Fe(NO_3)_3$, $Ce(NH_4)_2(NO_3)_6$, $(CH_3)_3NO$

Stereochemistry: S. L. Schreiber *et al., J. Am. Chem. Soc.* **109**, 5749 (1987); A. V. Muehldorf *et al., Tetrahedron Lett.* **35**, 8755 (1994). Scope and limitations: K. D. Roth, *Synlett* **1992**, 435; K. D. Roth, U. Müller, *Tetrahedron Lett.* **34**, 2919 (1993). Synthetic applications: P. A. Jacobi, W. Zheng, *ibid.* 2581, 2585; E. Tyrrell *et al., Synlett* **1993**, 769. Diastereoselective applications: J. Berge *et al., Tetrahedron Lett.* **38**, 685 (1997); A. Mann *et al., J. Chem. Soc. Perkin Trans. 1* **1998**, 1427. Enantioselective applications: S. Tanaka *et al., Tetrahedron* **50**, 12883 (1994); A. M. Montana *et al., Tetrahedron Lett.* **40**, 6499 (1999). *Reviews:* K. M. Nicholas, *Acc. Chem. Res.* **20**, 207-214 (1987); B. J. Teobald, *Tetrahedron* **58**, 4133-4170 (2002).

280. Niementowski Quinazoline Synthesis
S. v. Niementowski, *J. Prakt. Chem.* [2] **51**, 564 (1895).
    Formation of 4-oxo-3,4-dihydroquinazolines by cyclization of the reaction products of anthranilic acid and amides:

Reviews: T. A. Williamson, *Heterocycl. Compd.* **6**, 331 (1957); W. L. F. Armarego, *Adv. Heterocycl. Chem.* **1**, 253 (1963); E. Cuny *et al., Tetrahedron Lett.* **21**, 3029 (1980).

281. Niementowski Quinoline Synthesis
S. v. Niementowski, *Ber.* **27**, 1394 (1894); **28**, 2809 (1895); **38**, 2044 (1905); **40**, 4285 (1907).
    Formation of γ-hydroxyquinoline derivatives from anthranilic acids and carbonyl compounds:

R. H. Manske, *Chem. Rev.* **30**, 127 (1942); T. A. Williamson, *Heterocycl. Compd.* **6**, 331 (1957); W. L. F. Armarego, *Quinazolines* (Interscience, New York, 1967) p 74; E. Cuny *et al., Tetrahedron Lett.* **21**, 3029 (1980). Synthetic applications: B. P. Suthar, *Indian J. Chem.* **21B**, 588 (1982); R. J. Chong *et al., Tetrahedron Lett.* **27**, 5323 (1986); M. S. Khajavi *et al., Iran. J. Chem. Chem. Eng.* **17**, 29 (1988). *Review:* T. Hisano, *Org. Prep. Proced. Int.* **5**, 145-193 (1973). *Cf.* Friedlaender Synthesis; Pfitzinger Reaction.

282. Nierenstein Reaction
D. A. Clibbens, M. Nierenstein, *J. Chem. Soc.* **107**, 1491 (1915).
    Formation of ω-chloroacetophenones by reaction of diazomethane in dry ether with aroyl chlorides. Coumaranonones are obtained if an *ortho*-hydroxy group is present:

$$ArCOCl + CH_2N_2 \longrightarrow ArCOCH_2Cl + N_2$$

W. E. Bachman, W. S. Struve, *Org. React.* **1**, 38 (1942); Y. Miyahara, *J. Heterocycl. Chem.* **16**, 1147 (1979).

283. Norrish Type Cleavage
R. G. W. Norrish, C. H. Bamford, *Nature* **138**, 1016 (1936); **140**, 195 (1937).
    Norrish Type I Cleavage: Homolytic cleavage of aldehydes and ketones originating from their excited $n\pi^*$ state. Synthetically useful for the ring cleavage of cyclic ketones:

$$R^1\text{-}C\text{-}R \xrightarrow{h\nu} R^1\text{-}C^\bullet + R^\bullet$$

Norrish Type II Cleavage: Reaction originating from the $n\pi^*$ excited state of aldehydes and ketones that involves intramolecular γ-hydrogen abstraction followed by cleavage of the resulting diradical to an olefin and an enol which tautomerizes to the carbonyl compound:

Norrish Type I: D. H. R. Barton *et al., J. Am. Chem. Soc.* **107**, 3607 (1985); J. R. Hwu *et al., Chem. Commun.* **1990**, 161. Norrish Type II: J. M. Nuss, M. M. Murphy, *Tetrahedron Lett.* **35**, 37 (1994); F. Hénin *et al., Tetrahedron* **50**, 2849 (1994). *Reviews:* J. D. Coyle, H. A. J. Carless, *Chem. Soc. Rev.* **1**, 465 (1972); O. L. Chapman, D. S. Weiss, *Org. Photochem.* **3**, 197-277 (1973); J. March, *Advanced Organic Chemistry* (Wiley-Interscience, New York, 4th ed., 1992) p 242; W. M. Horspool, *Photochemistry* **25**, 67-100 (1994). *Cf.* McLafferty Rearrangement.

284. Noyori Hydrogenation
T. Ikariya *et al., Chem. Commun.* **1985**, 922; R. Noyori *et al., J. Am. Chem. Soc.* **108**, 7117 (1986).

Homogeneous asymmetric catalytic hydrogenation of olefinic and carbonyl bonds mediated by enantiopure ruthenium(II) BINAP complexes. The substrates must have coordinating functionalities in neighboring positions which serve as directing groups during the transformation:

Detailed experimental procedure: M. Kitamura *et al., Org. Synth.* **71**, 1 (1993). Methods development for enamide substrates: *idem et al., J. Org. Chem.* **59**, 297 (1994); E. Vedejs *et al., ibid.* **64**, 6724 (1999). Development and use of arene substituted BINAP catalysts: K. Mashima *et al., ibid.* **59**, 3064 (1994). *Reviews:* H. Takaya *et al.* in *Adv. Chem. Ser.* **230**, entitled "Homogeneous Transition Metal Catalyzed Reactions" (ACS, Washington DC, 1992) pp 123-142; R. Noyori, *Asymmetric Catalysis in Organic Synthesis* (John Wiley & Sons, New York, 1994) pp 16-94.

285. Nozaki-Hiyama Coupling Reaction (Nozaki-Hiyama-Kishi Reaction)
Y. Okude *et al., J. Am. Chem. Soc.* **99**, 3179 (1977); K. Takai *et al., Tetrahedron Lett.* **24**, 5281 (1983).

Chromium chloride catalyzed redox additions or organic halides to aldehydes:

R_2 = aryl, alkynyl, alkenyl, allyl, propargyl

Use of nickel salts as catalyst: H. Jin *et al., J. Am. Chem. Soc.* **108**, 5644 (1986); K. Takai *et al., ibid.* 6048; of chromium: A. Furstner, N. Shi, *ibid.* **118**, 12349 (1996). Enantioselectivity: K. Sugimoto *et al., J. Org. Chem.* **62**, 2322 (1997); M. Bandini *et al., Angew. Chem. Int. Ed.* **38**, 3357 (1999). Synthetic applications: Y. Kishi, *Pure Appl. Chem.* **64**, 354 (1992); D. P. Stamos *et al., J. Org. Chem.* **62**, 7552 (1997). *Review:* N. A. Saccomano, *Comp. Org. Syn.* **1**, 173-207 (1991).

286. Olefin Metathesis
Carbon-carbon bond rearrangements in presence of metal carbene catalyst complexes especially those of molybdenum and ruthenium:

Organic Name Reactions

Ring-opening metathesis polymerization

Ring-closing metathesis

Cross metathesis

Comprehensive accounts: R. H. Grubbs, *Comp. Organomet. Chem.* **8**, 499 (1982); R. H. Grubbs, S. Chang, *Tetrahedron* **54**, 4413-4450 (1998). Synthetic applications: A. K. Chatterjee *et al.*, *J. Am. Chem. Soc.* **122**, 3728 (2000); C. W. Lee, R. H. Grubbs, *Org. Lett.* **2**, 2145 (2000). Series of articles on syntheses, polymerizations and catalysts: *J. Mol. Catal. A.* **133**, 1-274 (1998). *Reviews:* A. Furstner, *Angew. Chem. Int. Ed.* **39**, 3012-3043 (2000); R. H. Grubbs, *Tetrahedron* **60**, 7117-7140 (2004). *See monograph* Grubbs' Catalyst.

287. Oppenauer Oxidation
R. V. Oppenauer, *Rec. Trav. Chim.* **56**, 137 (1937).
   The aluminum or potassium alkoxide-catalyzed oxidation of a secondary alcohol to the corresponding ketone (the reverse of the Meerwein-Ponndorf-Verley reduction, *q.v.*):

$$RCHOHR^1 \; + \; CH_3COCH_3 \; \rightleftharpoons \; RCOR^1 \; + \; CH_3CHOHCH_3$$

over the arrow: $M(OC_3H_7)_3$

$$M = Al \text{ or } K$$

T. Beresin in *Newer Methods of Preparative Organic Chemistry* English Ed. (Interscience, New York, 1948) p 125; C. Djerassi, *Org. React.* **6**, 207 (1951); L. Horner, U. B. Kaps, *Ann.* **1980**, 192. Intramolecular reactions: B. B. Snider, B. E. Goldman, *Tetrahedron* **42**, 2951 (1986); G. A. Molander, J. A. McKie, *J. Am. Chem. Soc.* **115**, 5821 (1993). Alternate metals: B. Byrne, M. Karras, *Tetrahedron Lett.* **28**, 769 (1987); M. L. S. Almeida *et al.*, *J. Org. Chem.* **61**, 6587 (1996); K. Krohn *et al.*, *Synthesis* **1996**, 1341; K. Ishihara *et al.*, *J. Org. Chem.* **62**, 5664 (1997). *Review:* C. F. de Graauw *et al.*, *Synthesis* **1994**, 1007-1017. *Cf.* Cannizzaro Reaction.

288. Overman Rearrangement
L. E. Overman, *J. Am. Chem. Soc.* **96**, 597 (1974); **98**, 2901 (1976).
   Formal [3,3]-sigmatropic rearrangement of the trichloroacetimidate of allylic alcohols to allylic trichloroacetamides, thereby transposing the hydroxyl and amino functions with good chirality transfer:

Early review: L. E. Overman, *Acc. Chem. Res.* **13**, 218-224 (1980). Synthetic applications: M. Isobe *et al.*, *Tetrahedron Lett.* **31**, 3327 (1990); T. Allmendinger *et al.*, *ibid.* 7301; J. Gonda *et al.*, *Synthesis* **1993**, 729; C. G. Cho *et al.*, *Synth. Commun.* **30**, 1643 (2000); A. Montero *et al.*, *Tetrahedron Lett.* **46**, 401 (2005). Use of a chiral template and mechanistic studies: T. Eguchi *et al.*, *Tetrahedron* **49**, 4527 (1993). Modification of reaction conditions: T. Nishikawa *et al.*, *J. Org. Chem.* **63**, 188 (1998). *Cf.* Claisen Rearrangement.

289. Oxo Process (Hydroformylation Reaction)
O. Roelen, US **2327066** (1943); R. H. Hasek (Eastman), *Org. Chem. Bull.* **27**, No. 1 (1955).
   Formation of alcohols from olefins, carbon monoxide and hydrogen in the liquid phase in the presence of catalysts (metallic cobalt compounds such as Raney cobalt or cobalt carbonyls) at 115-190° and high pressures (100-200 atmospheres) in a Fischer-Tropsch-type reaction, *q.v.* The process is sometimes carried out in two stages, the initial stage giving largely aldehydes which are then reduced to the alcohols.
   B. Cornils, "Hydroformylation. Oxo Synthesis, Roelen Reaction" in *New Syntheses with Carbon Monoxide*, J. Falbe, Ed. (Springer-Verlag, Berlin, 1980) pp 1-225. Reppe modification (olefin + CO + H_2O + $Fe(CO)_5$): R. Massoudi *et al.*, *J. Am. Chem. Soc.* **109**, 7428 (1987).

290. Paal-Knorr Pyrrole Synthesis
C. Paal, *Ber.* **18**, 367 (1885); L. Knorr, *ibid.* 299.
   Formation of pyrroles via cyclization of 1,4-dicarbonyl compounds with ammonia or primary amines:

H. Fischer, H. Orth, *Die Chemie des Pyrrols* **1** (Leipzig, 1934) p 34; D. M. Young, C. F. H. Allen, *Org. Synth.* **16**, 25 (1936); A. H. Corwin, *Heterocycl. Compd.* **1**, 290 (1950); N. P. Buu-Hoi *et al.*, *J. Org. Chem.* **20**, 639, 850 (1955); H. H. Wassermann *et al.*, *Tetrahedron* **32**, 1863 (1976). Mechanistic studies: V. Amarnath *et al.*, *J. Org. Chem.* **56**, 6924 (1991); *idem*, K. Amarnath, *ibid.* **60**, 301 (1995). Applications: S.-X. Yu, P. W. Le Quesne, *Tetrahedron Lett.* **36**, 6205 (1995); R. Ballini *et al.*, *Synlett* **3**, 391 (2000); G. Minetto *et al.*, *Eur. J. Org. Chem.* **2005**, 5277 (2005). *Review:* S. E. Korostova *et al.*, *Russ. J. Org. Chem.* **34**, 1691 (1998). *Cf.* Hantzsch Pyrrole Synthesis; Knorr Pyrrole Synthesis.

291. Parham Cyclization

W. E. Parham *et al., J. Org. Chem.* **40**, 2394 (1975).

Four- to seven-membered ring annulation of aryl bromides bearing *ortho* side chains having an electrophilic moiety, accomplished by halogen-metal exchange and subsequent nucleophilic ring closure:

$$E = COOH, CONR_2, epoxide, CH_2Br, CH_2Cl, OCONR_2, NCHAr, CONRCOCH_2R, POPh_2$$

Synthetic applications: M. R. Paleo *et al., J. Org. Chem.* **40**, 2029 (1975); A. Couture *et al., Chem. Commun.* **1994;** 1329; M. I. Collado *et al., Tetrahedron Lett.* **37**, 6193 (1996); S. D. Larsen, *Synlett* **1997;** 1013; A. Ardeo *et al., Tetrahedron Lett.* **41**, 5211 (2000); J. Ruiz *et al., Tetrahedron* **61**, 3311 (2005). *Review:* W. E. Parham, C. K. Bradsher, *Acc. Chem. Res.* **15**, 300-305 (1982).

292. Passerini Reaction

M. Passerini, *Gazz. Chim. Ital.* **51**, 126, 181 (1921).

Formation of α-hydroxycarboxamides on treatment of an isonitrile with a carboxylic acid and an aldehyde or ketone:

Synthetic applications: J. R. Falck, S. Manna, *Tetrahedron Lett.* **22**, 619 (1981); R. Bossio *et al., Synthesis* **1993,** 783. Modifications: W. E. Lumma, *J. Org. Chem.* **46**, 3668 (1981); T. Carofiglio *et al., Organometallics* **12**, 2726 (1993); Q. Xia, B. Ganem, *Org. Lett.* **4**, 1631 (2002); for stereoselectivity: H. Bock, I. Ugi, *J. Prakt. Chem.* **339**, 385 (1997) P. R. Andreana *et al., Org. Lett.* **6**, 4231 (2004); for combinatorial chemistry: H. Bienaymé, *Tetrahedron Lett.* **39**, 4255 (1998); S. W. Kim *Tetrahedron Lett.* **39**, 7031 (1998). Catalytic, asymmetric reactions: S. E. Denmark, Y. Fan, *J. Am. Chem. Soc.* **125**, 7825 (2003). *Reviews:* I. Ugi, *Angew. Chem. Int. Ed.* **1**, 8 (1962); I. Ugi *et al., in Isonitrile Chemistry* (Academic Press, New York, 1971) pp 133-143; I. Ugi *et al., Comp. Org. Syn.* **2**, 1083-1087 (1991). *Cf.* Ugi Reaction.

293. Paterno-Büchi Reaction

E. Paterno, G. Chieffi, *Gazz. Chim. Ital.* **39**, 341 (1909); G. Büchi *et al., J. Am. Chem. Soc.* **76**, 4327 (1954).

Formation of oxetanes by photochemical cycloaddition of carbonyl compounds to olefins:

D. R. Arnold, *Adv. Photochem.* **6**, 301 (1968); G. Jones, II, *Org. Photochem.* **5**, 1 (1981); S. C. Freilich, K. S. Peters, *J. Am. Chem. Soc.* **103**, 6255 (1981); J. A. Porco, Jr., S. L. Schreiber, *Comp. Org. Syn.* **5**, 151-192 (1991). Mechanistic studies: D. Sun *et al., J. Org. Chem.* **64**, 2250 (1999); *eidem, J. Chem. Soc. Perkin Trans. 2* **4**, 781 (1999). Stereocontrolled cycloadditions: S. A. Fleming, J. J. Gao, *Tetrahedron Lett.* **38**, 5407 (1997); G. Kollenz *et al., Tetrahedron* **55**, 2973 (1999); followed by oxetane ring opening: T. Bach *et al., Ann.* **1997**, 1529; S. R. Thopate *et al., Angew. Chem. Int. Ed.* **37**, 110 (1998). Regio- and stereoselectivity analyses: A. G. Griesbeck *et al., Acc. Chem. Res.* **37**, 919 (2004).

294. Pauson-Khand Reaction

I. U. Khand *et al., J. Chem. Soc. Perkin Trans. 1* **1973**, 977.

The formal [2+2+1] cycloaddition of an alkene, alkyne, and carbon monoxide to form cyclopentenones:

Use of a chiral auxiliary: X. Verdaguer *et al., J. Am. Chem. Soc.* **116**, 2153 (1994); V. Bernardes *et al., J. Org. Chem.* **60**, 6670 (1995); J. Adrio, J. C. Carretero, *J. Am. Chem. Soc.* **121**, 7411 (1999). Catalytic version: N. Jeong *et al., ibid.* **116**, 3159 (1994). Intramolecular cyclizations: Y.-T. Shiu *et al., ibid.* **121**, 4066 (1999); F. A. Hicks *et al., ibid.* 5881; P. M. Breczinski *et al., Tetrahedron* **55**, 6797 (1999). Reactions of alkenyl sulfones and sulfoxides: M. R. Rivero *et al., Synlett* **2005**, 26. *Reviews:* N. E. Schore, *Org. React.* **40**, 1-90 (1991); *idem, Comp. Org. Syn.* **5**, 1037-1064 (1991); S. T. Ingate, J. Marco-Contelles, *Org. Prep. Proced. Int.* **30**, 123-143 (1998); O. Geis, H.-G. Schmalz, *Angew. Chem. Int. Ed.* **37**, 911-914 (1998); J. Blanco-Urgoiti *et al., Chem. Soc. Rev.* **33**, 32-42 (2004).

295. Payne Rearrangement

G. B. Payne, *J. Org. Chem.* **27**, 3819 (1962).

Base-promoted isomerization of 2,3-epoxyalcohols. Configuration at C-2 is inverted:

R^1 = alkyl or aryl   X = H, mesyl, tosyl, etc.

In conjunction with nucleophilic ring opening: T. Katsuki *et al., ibid.* **47**, 1373 (1982); C. H. Behrens *et al., ibid.* **50**, 5687 (1985); P. C. B. Page *et al., J. Chem. Soc. Perkin Trans. 1* **1990**, 1375; T. Konosu *et al., Chem. Pharm. Bull.* **40**, 562 (1992). *Aza-Payne rearrangements:* T. Ibuka *et al., J. Org. Chem.* **60**, 2044 (1995); K. Nakai *et al., Tetrahedron Lett.* **36**, 6247 (1995). Enhanced stereoselectivity: W. C. Frank, *Tetrahedron: Asymmetry* **9**, 3745 (1998). Review of aza-Payne: T. Ibuka *et al., Chem. Soc. Rev.* **27**, 145-154 (1998).

296. Pechmann Condensation
H. v. Pechmann, C. Duisberg, *Ber.* **16**, 2119 (1883).
Synthesis of coumarins by condensation of phenols with β-keto esters in the presence of Lewis acid catalysts:

Early reviews: S. Sethna, *Chem. Rev.* **36**, 10 (1945); S. Sethna, R. Phadke, *Org. React.* **7**, 1 (1953). T. Kappe, E. Ziegler, *Org. Prep. Proced.* **1**, 61 (1969); T. Kappe, C. Mayer, *Synthesis* **1981**, 524; A. G. Osborne, *Tetrahedron* **37**, 2021 (1981); D. H. Hau *et al., Synlett* **1990**, 233; T-S. Li *et al., J. Chem. Res.* **1998**, 39. Modified conditions: J. E. T. Corrie, *J. Chem. Soc. Perkin Trans. 1* **1990**, 2151; D. H. Hua *et al., J. Org. Chem.* **57**, 399 (1992). *Cf.* Bischler-Napieralski Reaction; Simonis Chromone Cyclization.

297. Pechmann Pyrazole Synthesis
H. v. Pechmann, *Ber.* **31**, 2950 (1898).
Formation of pyrazoles from acetylenes and diazomethane. The analogous addition of diazoacetic esters to the triple bond yields pyrazolecarboxylic acid derivatives:

R. A. Raphael, *Acetylenic Compounds in Organic Synthesis* (London, 1955) p 179; T. L. Jacobs, *Heterocycl. Compd.* **5**, 70 (1957); B. Eistert *et al., Houben-Weyl* **10/4**, 840 (1968). *Cf.* Knorr Pyrazole Synthesis.

298. Pellizzari Reaction
G. Pellizzari, *Gazz. Chim. Ital.* **41**, II, 20 (1911).
Formation of substituted 1,2,4-triazoles by the condensation of amides and acyl hydrazines. When the acyl groups of the amide and the acylhydrazine are different, interchange of acyl groups may occur with formation of a mixture of triazoles:

M. R. Atkinson, J. B. Polya, *J. Chem. Soc.* **1952**, 3418; P. Karrer, *Organic Chemistry* (New York, 4th ed., 1950) p 802; C. W. Bird, C. K. Wong, *Tetrahedron Lett.* **1974**, 1251. *Cf.* Einhorn-Brunner Reaction.

299. Pelouze Synthesis
J. Pelouze, *Ann.* **10**, 249 (1834).
Formation of nitriles from alkali cyanides by alkylation with alkyl sulfates or alkyl phosphates:

$$ROSO_2OK + KCN \longrightarrow RCN + K_2SO_4$$

V. Migrdichian, *Chemistry of Organic Cyanogen Compounds* (New York, 1947) p 6; D. T. Mowry, *Chem. Rev.* **42,** 192 (1948); P. Kurtz, *Houben-Weyl* **8,** 306 (1952).

300. Perkin Alicyclic Synthesis
W. H. Perkin, Jr., *Ber.* **16,** 1793 (1883).

Synthesis of alicyclic compounds from α,ω-dihaloalkanes and compounds containing active methylene groups in the presence of sodium ethoxide:

H. O. House, *Modern Synthetic Reactions* (W. A. Benjamin, Inc., Menlo Park, California, 2nd ed, 1972) pp 492-570. *Cf.* Malonic Ester Syntheses.

301. Perkin Reaction
W. H. Perkin, *J. Chem. Soc.* **21,** 53, 181 (1868); **31,** 388 (1877).

Formation of α,β-unsaturated carboxylic acids by aldol condensation, *q.v.,* of aromatic aldehydes and acid anhydrides in the presence of an alkali salt of the acid:

Reviews: J. R. Johnson, *Org. React.* **1,** 210 (1942); H. O. House, *Modern Synthetic Reactions* (W. A. Benjamin, Menlo Park, California, 2nd ed, 1972) pp 660-663; N. Poonia *et al., Bull. Chem. Soc. Jpn.* **53,** 3338 (1980); T. Rosen, *Comp. Org. Syn.* **2,** 395-408 (1991). Applications: S. Kinastowski, A. Nowacki, *Tetrahedron Lett.* **23,** 3723 (1982); W. T. Brady *et al., J. Heterocycl. Chem.* **25,** 969 (1988). *Cf.* Erlenmeyer-Plöchl Azlactone and Amino Acid Synthesis; Stobbe Condensation.

302. Perkin Rearrangement (Coumarin-Benzofuran Ring Contraction)
W. H. Perkin, *J. Chem. Soc.* **23,** 368 (1870).

Formation of benzofuran-2-carboxylic acids and benzofurans by heating 3-halocoumarins with alkali:

R. C. Elderfield, V. B. Meyer, *Heterocycl. Compd.* **2,** 2, 5 (1951); K. Bowden, S. Battah, *J. Chem. Soc. Perkin Trans. 2* **1998,** 1604.

303. Perkow Reaction
W. Perkow *et al., Naturwissenschaften* **39,** 353 (1952).

Formation of enol phosphates on treatment of α-halocarbonyl compounds with trialkyl phosphites:

F. W. Lichtenthaler, *Chem. Rev.* **61,** 607 (1961); B. Miller in *Topics in Phosphorus Chemistry* vol. 2, M. Grayson, E. J. Griffith, Eds. (John Wiley, New York, 1965) p 178; K. Sasse, *Houben-Weyl* **12/1,** 423 (1963); A. J. Kirby, S. G. Warren, *The Organic Chemistry of Phosphorus* (Elsevier, Amsterdam, 1967) p 123; B. A. Arbuzow, *Pure Appl. Chem.* **9,** 306 (1964); I. J. Borowitz *et al., J. Org. Chem.* **38,** 1713 (1973); T. Winkler, W. L. Bencze, *Helv. Chim. Acta* **63,** 402 (1980); M. Sekine *et al., J. Org. Chem.* **46,** 4030 (1981).

304. Peterson Reaction (Olefination)
D. J. Peterson, *J. Org. Chem.* **33,** 780 (1968).

Reaction of α-silyl carbanions with carbonyl compounds yielding β-silylalkoxides which undergo instantaneous elimination to afford olefins:

L. Birkofer, O. Stiehl, *Top. Curr. Chem.* **88**, 58 (1980); E. Colvin, *Silicon in Organic Synthesis* (Butterworth, London, 1981) p 143; D. J. Ager, *Synthesis* **1984**, 384-398; *idem, Org. React.* **38**, 1-223 (1990); S. E. Kelly, *Comp. Org. Syn.* **1**, 731-737, 782-783 (1991). *Review*: L. F. van Staden *et al.*, *Chem. Soc. Rev.* **31**, 195-200 (2002). *Cf.* Tebbe Olefination; Wittig Reaction.

305. Petrenko-Kritschenko Piperidone Synthesis
P. Petrenko-Kritschenko *et al.*, *Ber.* **39**, 1358 (1906); **40**, 2882 (1907); **41**, 1692 (1908); **42**, 2020, 3683 (1909).

Formation of piperidones *via* cyclization of two moles of aldehyde and one mole each of acetonedicarboxylic ester and ammonia or a primary amine:

R. Robinson, *J. Chem. Soc.* **111**, 762, 876, (1917); C. Mannich, O. Hieronimus, *Ber.* **75**, 49 (1942); H. S. Mosher, *Heterocyclic Compounds* **1**, 659 (New York, 1950). *Cf.* Robinson-Schöpf Reaction.

306. Pfau-Plattner Azulene Synthesis
A. St. Pfau, P. A. Plattner, *Helv. Chim. Acta* **22**, 202 (1939).

Formation of azulenes by ring enlargement of indanes on addition of diazoacetic ester, hydrolysis, dehydrogenation and decarboxylation of the resulting acid:

P. A. Plattner *et al.*, *ibid.* **23**, 907 (1940); **24**, 483 (1941); **25**, 590 (1942); B. Eistert, *Newer Methods of Preparative Organic Chemistry* (Interscience, New York, 1948) p 555; D. H. Reid, *Chem. Soc. Spec. Publ.* **12**, 69 (1958); K. Hafner, *Angew. Chem.* **70**, 419 (1958). *Cf.* Buchner Method of Ring Enlargement.

307. Pfitzinger Reaction
W. Pfitzinger, *J. Prakt. Chem.* [2] **33**, 100 (1886); **38**, 582 (1888).

Formation of quinoline-4-carboxylic acids by condensation of isatic acids from isatin with α-methylene carbonyl compounds:

C. Hollins, *The Synthesis of Nitrogen Ring Compounds* (London, 1924) p 286; R. H. Manske, *Chem. Rev.* **30**, 126 (1942); F. W. Bergstrom, *ibid.* **35**, 152 (1944); R. C. Elderfield, *Heterocycl. Compd.* **4**, 47 (1952); N. P. Buu-Hoi *et al.*,

Organic Name Reactions

Bull. Soc. Chim. Fr. **1968**, 2476; M. H. Palmer, P. S. McIntyre, *J. Chem. Soc. B* **1969**, 539. *Review:* M. G.-A. Shvekhgeimer, *Chem. Heterocycl. Compd.* **40**, 257-294 (2004). *Cf.* Friedlaender Synthesis; Niementowski Quinoline Synthesis.

308. Pfitzner-Moffatt Oxidation (Moffatt Oxidation)
K. E. Pfitzner, J. G. Moffatt, *J. Am. Chem. Soc.* **85**, 3027 (1963).

Mild oxidation of primary and secondary alcohols, promoted by dicyclohexylcarbodiimide activation of dimethyl sulfoxide, evidently involving the alkoxysulfonium ylides, which rearrange intramolecularly to generate aldehydes and ketones, respectively:

Reviews: J. G. Moffatt, "Sulfoxide-Carbodiimide and Related Oxidations" in *Oxidation* **vol. 2**, R. L. Augustine, D. J. Trecker, Eds. (Dekker, New York, 1971) pp 1-64; T. T. Tidwell, *Org. React.* **39**, 297-572 *passim* (1990); T. V. Lee, *Comp. Org. Syn.* **7**, 291-303 *passim* (1991). *Cf.* Corey-Kim Oxidation; Swern Oxidation.

309. Pictet-Gams Isoquinoline Synthesis
A. Pictet, A. Gams, *Ber.* **43**, 2384 (1910).

Formation of isoquinolines by cyclization of acylated aminomethyl phenyl carbinols or their ethers with phosphorus pentoxide in toluene or xylene:

Reviews: W. M. Whaley, T. R. Govindachari, *Org. React.* **6**, 151 (1951); W. Y. Gensler, *Heterocycl. Compd.* **4**, 361 (1952); W. Herz, L. Tsai, *J. Am. Chem. Soc.* **77**, 3529 (1955); A. A. Bindra *et al.*, *Tetrahedron Lett.* **1968**, 2677; N. Ardabilchi *et al.*, *J. Chem. Soc. Perkin Trans. 1* **1979**, 539. *Cf.* Bischler-Napieralski Reaction.

310. Pictet-Hubert Reaction (Morgan-Walls Reaction)
A. Pictet, A. Hubert, *Ber.* **29**, 1182 (1896); C. T. Morgan, L. P. Walls, *J. Chem. Soc.* **1931**, 2447; **1932**, 2225.

Phenanthridine cyclization by dehydrative ring closure of acyl-*o*-aminobiphenyls on heating with zinc chloride at 250-300° (Pictet-Hubert), or with phosphorus oxychloride in boiling nitrobenzene (Morgan-Walls):

L. P. Walls, *J. Chem. Soc.* **1945**, 294; J. Cymerman, W. F. Short, *ibid.* **1949**, 703; R. S. Theobald, K. Schofield, *Chem. Rev.* **46**, 175 (1950); L. P. Walls, *Heterocycl. Compd.* **4**, 574 (1952); J. Eisch, H. Gilman, *Chem. Rev.* **57**, 525 (1957); N. Campbell, *Chemistry of Carbon Compounds* **IVA**, 691 (1957). *Cf.* Bischler-Napieralski Reaction.

311. Pictet-Spengler Isoquinoline Synthesis
A. Pictet, T. Spengler, *Ber.* **44**, 2030 (1911).

Formation of tetrahydroisoquinoline derivatives by condensation of β-arylethylamines with carbonyl compounds and cyclization of the Schiff bases formed:

Reviews: W. M. Whaley, T. R. Govindachari, *Org. React.* **6**, 151 (1951); R. A. Abramovitch, I. D. Spenser, *Adv. Heterocycl. Chem.* **3**, 79 (1964); K. Stuart, R. Woo-Ming, *Heterocycles* **3**, 223 (1975); D. Soerens *et al.*, *J. Org. Chem.* **44**, 535 (1979); H. Ernst *et al.*, *Ber.* **114**, 1894 (1981). Stereochemical study: E. Dominguez *et al.*, *Tetrahedron* **43**, 1943 (1987). Review of enantioselective modifications: M. D. Rozwadowski, *Heterocycles* **39**, 903-931 (1994).

312. Piloty-Robinson Synthesis
O. Piloty, *Ber.* **43**, 489 (1910); G. M. Robinson, R. Robinson, *J. Chem. Soc.* **43**, 639 (1918).

Formation of pyrroles by heating azines of enolizable ketones with acid catalysts, usually zinc chloride or hydrogen chloride:

Review: N. V. Sidgwick, *Organic Chemistry of Nitrogen Compounds* (Oxford, 3rd ed., 1966) pp 619-641; H. Posvic *et al., J. Org. Chem.* **39,** 2575 (1974). *Cf.* Borsche-Drechsel Cyclization; Fischer Indole Synthesis.

313. Pinacol Coupling Reaction
R. Fittig, *Ann.* **110,** 17 (1859).
Formation of pinacols by a reductive radical-radical coupling of carbonyl compounds, especially ketones:

Reviews: G. M. Robertson, *Comp. Org. Syn.* **3,** 563 (1991); H. Jendralla *et al.,* in *Transition Metals for Organic Synthesis* (Wiley-VCH, Weinheim, 1998) pp. 403-417. *Cf.* McMurry Reaction.

314. Pinacol Rearrangement
R. Fittig, *Ann.* **114,** 54 (1860).
Acid-catalyzed rearrangement of vicinal diols to aldehydes or ketones:

Reviews: C. J. Collins, *Q. Rev. Chem. Soc.* **14,** 357 (1960); C. J. Collins, J. F. Eastham in *Chemistry of the Carbonyl Group,* S. Patai, Ed. (Interscience, New York, 1966) pp 762-767; B. Rickborn, *Comp. Org. Syn.* **3,** 721-732 (1991). *Cf.* Tiffeneau-Demjanov Rearrangement.

315. Pinner Reaction (Amidine and Ortho Ester Synthesis)
A. Pinner, F. Klein, *Ber.* **10,** 1889 (1877); **11,** 4, 1475 (1878); **16,** 352, 1643 (1883).
Formation of imino esters (alkyl imidates) by addition of dry hydrogen chloride to a mixture of a nitrile and an alcohol. Treatment of alkyl imidates with ammonia or primary or secondary amines affords amidines, while treatment with alcohols yields ortho-esters:

Reviews: R. Roger, D. Neilson, *Chem. Rev.* **61,** 179 (1961); E. N. Zil'berman, *Russ. Chem. Rev.* **31,** 615 (1962); P. L. Compagnon, M. Moeque, *Ann. Chim. (Paris)* **5,** 23 (1970); B. Decroix *et al., J. Chem. Res.* **1978,** 134.

316. Pinner Triazine Synthesis
A. Pinner, *Ber.* **23,** 2919 (1890).
Preparation of 2-hydroxy-4,6-diaryl-*s*-triazines by reaction of aryl amidines and phosgene. The reaction may be extended to halogenated aliphatic amidines:

A. Pinner, *Ber.* **25,** 1414 (1892); **28,** 483 (1895); J. Ephraim, *ibid.* **26,** 2226 (1893); P. Flatow, *ibid.* **30,** 2006 (1897); T. Rappaport, *ibid.* **34,** 1990 (1901); H. Schroeder, C. Grundmann, *J. Am. Chem. Soc.* **78,** 2447 (1956); E. M. Smolin, L.

Rapoport, *The Chemistry of Heterocyclic Compounds*, A. Weissberger, Ed., *s-Triazines and Derivatives* (Interscience, New York, 1959) p 186.

317. Piria Reaction
R. Piria, *Ann.* **78**, 31 (1851).

Formation of arylsulfamic acids or sulfonation products or both by refluxing aromatic nitro compounds with a metal sulfite and boiling the mixture with dilute acid to yield the amines and sulfamic acids:

J. F. Bunnett, R. E. Zahler, *Chem. Rev.* **49**, 398 (1951); R. Schroter, *Houben-Weyl* **11/1**, 457 (1957); R. Budziarek, *Chem. Ind. (London)* **1978**, 583.

318. Polonovski Reaction; Potier-Polonovski Reaction
M. Polonovski, M. Polonovski, *Bull. Soc. Chim. Fr.* **41**, 1190 (1927).

Rearrangement of tertiary amine oxides upon treatment with acetic anhydride or acetyl chloride, in which one of the alkyl groups attached to the nitrogen is cleaved, generating the *N,N*-disubstituted acetamide and aldehyde:

Reviews: A. R. Katritzky, J. N. Lagowski, *Chemistry of Heterocyclic N-Oxides* (Academic Press, New York, 1971) p 279, 362; D. Grierson, *Org. React.* **39**, 85-295 (1990); D. S. Grierson, H.-P. Husson, *Comp. Org. Syn.* **6**, 909-924 (1991).

The reaction proceeds *via* an iminium ion intermediate which becomes the stable reaction product when trifluoroacetic anhydride is employed. This modified procedure is commonly referred to as the **Potier-Polonovski reaction:** A. Cave *et al., Tetrahedron* **23**, 4681 (1967); T. Tamminen *et al., ibid.* **45**, 2683 (1989); R. J. Sundberg, *et al., ibid.* **48**, 277 (1992).

319. Pomeranz-Fritsch Reaction (Schlittler-Müller Modification)
C. Pomeranz, *Monatsh. Chem.* **14**, 116 (1893); P. Fritsch, *Ber.* **26**, 419 (1893); E. Schlittler, J. Müller, *Helv. Chim. Acta* **31**, 914, 1119 (1948).

Formation of isoquinolines by the acid-catalyzed cyclization of benzalaminoacetals prepared from aromatic aldehydes and aminoacetal; in the **Schlittler-Müller modification** the starting materials are benzyl amines and glyoxal semiacetal:

M. J. Bevis *et al., Tetrahedron* **27**, 1253 (1971); E. V. Brown, *J. Org. Chem.* **42**, 3208 (1977); R. Hirsenkorn, *Tetrahedron Lett.* **32**, 1775 (1991). *Reviews:* W. J. Gensler, *Org. React.* **6**, 191 (1951); *idem, Heterocycl. Compd.* **4**, 368 (1952); J. M. Bobbit, A. J. Bourque, *Heterocycles* **25**, 601-614 (1987).

320. Ponzio Reaction
G. Ponzio, *Gazz. Chim. Ital.* **27, I,** 171 (1897).

Formation of dinitrophenylmethanes from benzaldoximes by oxidation with nitrogen dioxide in ether:

J. L. Riebsomer, *Chem. Rev.* **36**, 183 (1945); L. F. Fieser, W. von E. Doering, *J. Am. Chem. Soc.* **68**, 2252 (1946); L. F. Fieser, M. Fieser, *Reagents for Organic Synthesis* (New York, 1967) p 325; H. G. Padeken *et al., Houben-Weyl* **10/1**, 113 (1971). Improved procedure: H. Suzuki *et al., Bull. Chem. Soc. Jpn.* **61**, 2929 (1988).

321. Prévost Reaction
C. Prévost, *Compt. Rend.* **196**, 1129 (1933), *C.A.* **27**, 3195 (1933).
Hydroxylation of olefins with iodine and silver benzoate in an anhydrous solvent to give *trans*-glycols:

Reviews: C. V. Wilson, *Org. React.* **9**, 350 (1957); F. D. Gunstone, *Adv. Org. Chem.* **1**, 117 (1960); H. O. House, *Modern Synthetic Reactions* (W. A. Benjamin, Menlo Park, California, 2nd ed., 1972) p 438; S. Amin *et al., J. Org. Chem.* **46**, 2573 (1981). *Cf.* Woodward *cis*-Hydroxylation.

322. Prilezhaev (Prileschajew) Reaction
N. Prilezhaev, *Ber.* **42**, 4811 (1909).
Formation of epoxides by the reaction of alkenes with peracids:

Reviews: D. Swern, *Chem. Rev.* **45**, 16 (1949); *Org. React.* **7**, 378 (1953); H. O. House, *Modern Synthetic Reactions* (W. A. Benjamin, Menlo Park, California, 2nd ed., 1972) pp 302-319; D. I. Metelitra, *Russ. Chem. Rev.* **41**, 807 (1972); D. Schnurgfeil, *Z. Chem.* **20**, 445 (1980).

323. Prins Reaction
H. J. Prins, *Chem. Weekbl.* **16**, 64, 1072, 1510 (1919), *C.A.* **13**, 3155 (1919).
Acid-catalyzed addition of olefins to formaldehyde to give 1,3-diols, allylic alcohols or *meta*-dioxanes:

Reviews: R. Arundale, L. A. Mikeska, *Chem. Rev.* **51**, 505 (1952); V. I. Isagulyants *et al., Russ. Chem. Rev.* **1968**, 17; C. W. Roberts in *Friedel-Crafts and Related Reactions* **vol. 2**, Part 2, G. A. Olah, Ed. (Interscience, 1964) pp 1175-1210; D. R. Adams, S. P. Bhatnagar, *Synthesis* **1977**, 661; K. H. Schulte-Elte *et al., Helv. Chim. Acta* **62**, 2673 (1979); R. El Gharbi *et al., Synthesis* **1981**, 361; B. B. Snider, *Comp. Org. Syn.* **2**, 527-561 (1991).

324. Pschorr Reaction
R. Pschorr, *Ber.* **29**, 496 (1896).
Synthesis of phenanthrene derivatives from diazotized α-aryl-*o*-aminocinnamic acids by intramolecular arylation:

Reviews: P. H. Leake, *Chem. Rev.* **56**, 27 (1956); D. F. De Tar, *Org. React.* **9**, 409 (1957); R. A. Abramovitch, *Adv. Free-Radical Chem.* **2**, 88 (1967); T. Kametani, K. Fukumoto, *J. Heterocycl. Chem.* **8**, 341 (1971); S. Foldeak, *Tetrahedron* **27**, 3465 (1971); T. S. Kametani *et al., ibid.* **27**, 5367 (1971); F. F. Gadallah *et al., J. Org. Chem.* **38**, 2386 (1973); S. M. Kupchan *et al., ibid.* 405; G. Daidone *et al., J. Heterocycl. Chem.* **17**, 1409 (1980). Mechanistic study: P. Hanson *et al., J. Chem. Soc. Perkin Trans. 2* **1999**, 49. *Cf.* Gomberg-Bachman Reaction; Meerwein Arylation.

325. Pummerer Rearrangement

R. Pummerer, *Ber.* **43**, 1401 (1910).

Rearrangement of sulfoxides to α-acyloxythioethers in the presence of acyclic anhydrides. When nucleophiles other than those derived from the anhydride are present, different functionalization is achieved:

Diastereoselectivity in the preparation of 4-phenyl-4-butanolides: H. Su *et al., Bull. Chem. Soc. Jpn.* **66**, 2603 (1993). Application to vinyl sulfoxides (the additive Pummerer reaction): D. Craig, K. Daniels, *Tetrahedron* **49**, 11263 (1993); to oxidative cyclization of C(3) indole derivatives: K. S. Feldman *et al., J. Org. Chem.* **70**, 6429 (2005). Regiospecific cyclization: G. Majumdar, D. Mal, *Indian J. Chem.* **33B**, 700 (1994). Asymmetric synthesis: Y. Kita *et al., Tetrahedron Lett.* **35**, 3575 (1994). *Reviews:* O. DeLucchi *et al., Org. React.* **40**, 157-405 (1991); D. S. Grierson, H.-P. Husson, *Comp. Org. Syn.* **6**, 924-937 (1991); S. K. Bur, A. Padwa, *Chem. Rev.* **104**, 2401-2432 (2004).

326. Purdie Methylation (Irvine-Purdie Methylation)

T. Purdie, J. C. Irvine, *J. Chem. Soc.* **83**, 1021 (1903).

Exhaustive methylation of a methyl glycoside by repeated treatment with methyl iodide and silver oxide, followed by hydrolysis of the pentamethyl ether with dilute acid to yield the anomeric hydroxyl group:

C. C. Barker, *et al., ibid.* **1946**, 753; E. J. Bourne, S. Peat, *Adv. Carbohydr. Chem.* **5**, 146 (1950); W. Pigman, *The Carbohydrates* (New York, 1957) p 370; P. V. Kovac *et al., Carbohydr. Res.* **58**, 327 (1977). *Cf.* Haworth Methylation.

327. Quelet Reaction

R. Quelet, *Compt. Rend.* **195**, 155 (1932).

Passage of dry hydrochloric acid through a solution in ligroin of a phenolic ether and an aliphatic aldehyde in the presence or absence of a dehydration catalyst to yield α-chloroalkyl derivatives by substitution in the *para* position to the ether group or in the *ortho* position in *para*-substituted phenolic ethers:

R. Quelet, *ibid.* **196**, 1411 (1933); **198**, 102 (1934); **199**, 150 (1934); **202**, 956 (1936); *Bull. Soc. Chim. Fr.* **7**, 196 (1940); U. Neda, R. Oda, *J. Soc. Chem. Ind. Jpn.* **47**, 565 (1944). *Cf.* Blanc (Chloromethylation) Reaction.

328. Ramberg-Bäcklund Reaction

L. Ramberg, B. Bäcklund, *Arkiv Kemi Mineral. Geol.* **13A**(27), 50 (1940), *C.A.* **34**, 4725[5] (1940).

Reaction of α-halo sulfones with strong bases to yield alkenes:

Reviews: L. A. Paquette, *Acc. Chem. Res.* **1**, 209-216 (1968); F. G. Bordwell, *ibid.* **3**, 28 (1970); L. Paquette, *Org. React.* **25**, 1 (1977); G. D. Hartman, R. D. Hartman, *Synthesis* **1982**, 504; J. M. Clough, *Comp. Org. Syn.* **3**, 861-886 (1991).

329. Raschig Phenol Process

F. Raschig, **FR 698341** (1930), *C.A.* **25**, 3012 (1931).

Commercial process for the production of phenol by the hydrolysis of chlorobenzene, produced by the chlorination of benzene with hydrochloric acid and air:

$$C_6H_6 \ + \ HCl \ \xrightarrow[\text{Cu -Fe}]{230°/\text{air}} \ C_6H_5Cl \ + \ H_2O \ \xrightarrow[\text{SiO}_2]{425°} \ C_6H_5OH \ + \ HCl$$

W. H. Prahl, **US 1963761** (1934); **US 2156402** (1939); J. A. Kent, *Riegel's Industrial Chemistry* (New York, 1962) p 339; W. L. Faith, D. B. Keyes, R. L. Clark, *Industrial Chemistry* (New York, 3rd ed., 1965) p 586; R. N. Shreve,

Chemical Process Industries (New York, 3rd ed., 1967) p 105; *Kirk-Othmer Encyclopedia of Chemical Technology* **vol. 17** (New York, 1982) p 378.

330. Reed Reaction
C. F. Reed, **US 2046090** (1933); **US 2174110** (1934); **US 2174492** (1938).
 Photochemical sulfonation of paraffins and cycloparaffins by sulfur dioxide and chlorine under irradiation with ultraviolet light:

$$RH + SO_2 + Cl_2 \xrightarrow{h\nu} RSO_2Cl + HCl$$

 F. Asinger *et al., Ber.* **75,** 34, 42, 344 (1942); J. H. Helberger *et al., Ann.* **562,** 23 (1949); H. Eckoldt, *Houben-Weyl* **9,** 407-427 (1955); A. Schönberg, *Präparative Organische Photochemie* (Berlin, 1958) p 201; G. Sosnovsky, *Free Radical Reactions in Preparative Organic Chemistry* (New York, 1964) p 105.

331. Reformatsky (Reformatskii) Reaction
S. Reformatskii, *Ber.* **20,** 1210 (1887); *J. Russ. Phys. Chem. Soc.* **22,** 44 (1890).
 Condensation of aldehydes or ketones with organozinc derivatives of α-halo esters to yield β-hydroxy esters:

 Early reviews: R. L. Shriner, *Org. React.* **1,** 1 (1942); H. O. House, *Modern Synthetic Reactions* (W. A. Benjamin, Menlo Park, California, 2nd ed., 1972) pp 671-682; M. W. Rathke, *Org. React.* **22,** 423 (1975). Use of thiocarbonyl electrophiles: M. Chandrasekharam *et al., Tetrahedron Lett.* **34,** 6439 (1993). Application to the synthesis of β-keto esters: C. Kashima *et al., J. Org. Chem.* **58,** 793 (1993). Asymmetric synthesis: D. Pini *et al., Tetrahedron: Asymmetry* **5,** 1875 (1994). Methods development for the synthesis of β-lactones: H. Schick *et al., Tetrahedron* **51,** 2939 (1995). *Reviews:* A. Fürstner, *Synthesis* **1989,** 571-590; M. W. Rathke, P. Weipert, *Comp. Org. Syn.* **2,** 277-299 (1991); R. Ocampo, W. R. Dolbier, Jr., *Tetrahedron* **60,** 9325-9374 (2004). *Cf.* Aldol Reaction; Blaise Reaction.

332. Reimer-Tiemann Reaction
K. Reimer, F. Tiemann, *Ber.* **9,** 824, 1268, 1285 (1876).
 Formation of phenolic aldehydes from phenols, chloroform and alkali:

 Review: H. Wynberg, *Chem. Rev.* **60,** 169 (1960); H. Wynberg, E. W. Meijer, *Org. React.* **28,** 2 (1982); H. Wynberg, *Comp. Org. Syn.* **2,** 769-775 (1991). *Cf.* Duff Reaction; Gattermann Aldehyde Synthesis.

333. Reissert Indole Synthesis
A. Reissert, *Ber.* **30,** 1030 (1897).
 Condensation of an *o*-nitrotoluene with oxalic ester, reduction to the amine, and cyclization to the indole:

 W. O. Kermack *et al., J. Chem. Soc.* **119,** 1602 (1921); P. C. Julian *et al., Heterocycl. Compd.* **3,** 18 (1962); J. G. Cannon *et al., J. Med. Chem.* **24,** 238 (1981).

334. Reissert Reaction (Grosheintz-Fischer-Reissert Aldehyde Synthesis)
A. Reissert, *Ber.* **38,** 1603, 3415 (1905); J. M. Grosheintz, H. O. L. Fischer, *J. Am. Chem. Soc.* **63,** 2021 (1941).
 Formation of 1-acyl-2-cyano-1,2-dihydroquinoline derivatives (Reissert compounds) by reaction of acid chlorides with quinoline and potassium cyanide; hydrolysis of these compounds yields aldehydes and quinaldic acid:

 Reviews: E. Mosettig, *Org. React.* **8,** 220 (1954); W. E. McEwen, R. L. Cobb, *Chem. Rev.* **55,** 511 (1955); F. D. Popp, *Adv. Heterocycl. Chem.* **9,** 1 (1968); *idem, ibid.* **24,** 187 (1979); *idem. Bull. Soc. Chim. Belg.* **90,** 609 (1981); *idem* in *The Chemistry of Heterocyclic Compounds* **vol. 32,** Part 2, G. Jones, Ed. (Wiley, New York, 1982) p 353.

335. Reppe Chemistry
 The term designates that phase of acetylene chemistry involving the use of acetylene at high pressures in the presence of suitable catalysts to carry out the fundamental reactions of vinylation, ethynylation, cyclopolymerization and

carbonylation as developed from 1928 onward by Walter Reppe and associates in the I. G. Farbenindustrie laboratories in Ludwigshafen:

$$H_2C=CHOR \xleftarrow{\quad ROH \quad} HC\equiv CH \xrightarrow{\quad RSH \quad} H_2C=CHSR$$

$$RR^1CO + HC\equiv CH \longrightarrow RR^1C(OH)C\equiv CH \xrightarrow{\quad RR^1CO \quad} RR^1C(OH)C\equiv CC(OH)RR^1$$

$$4HC\equiv CH \longrightarrow \text{cyclooctatetraene}$$

$$4HC\equiv CH + 4C_2H_4OH + Ni(CO)_4 + 2HCl \longrightarrow 4H_2C=CHCOOC_2H_5 + NiCl_2 + H_2$$

J. W. Copenhaver, M. H. Bigelow, *Acetylene and Carbon Monoxide Chemistry* (New York, 1949) p 246; W. Reppe, *Acetylene Chemistry*, U.S. Dept. Commerce PB 18852-S (1949); *Neue Entwicklungen auf dem Gebiet des Acetylens und Kohlenoxyds* (Berlin 1949); H. Kröper, *Houben-Weyl* **4/II**, 413-422 (1955); D. W. F. Hardie, *Acetylene, Manufacture and Uses* (New York, 1965) p 67; L. F. Fieser, M. Fieser, *Reagents for Organic Synthesis* (New York, 1967) pp 61, 183, 185, 190, 519, 720, 722, 723. Review of carbonylations: A. Mullen, "Carbonylations Catalyzed by Metal Carbonyls-Reppe Reactions" in *New Syntheses with Carbon Monoxide*, J. Falbe, Ed. (Springer-Verlag, Berlin, 1980) pp 243-308. Mechanistic study of cyclooctatetraene synthesis: R. E. Colborn, K. P. C. Vollhardt, *J. Am. Chem. Soc.* **108**, 5470 (1986); C. J. Lawrie *et al., Organometallics* **8**, 2274 (1989).

336. Retro-Diels-Alder Reaction

Thermal dissociation of Diels-Alder adducts, occurring most readily when one or both fragments are particularly stable:

Early review: H. Kwart, K. King, *Chem. Rev.* **68**, 415-447 (1968). Acceleration by alkoxide substituent: O. Papies, W. Grimme, *Tetrahedron Lett.* **21**, 2799 (1980). Application to the synthesis of enethiols: Y. Vallée *et al., Synth. Commun.* **23**, 1267 (1993); of cyclopentadienyl ligands: B. Y. Lee *et al., J. Am. Chem. Soc.* **116**, 2163 (1994). Role in structure elucidation *via* mass spectrometry: F. Turecek, V. Hanus, *Mass Spectrom. Rev.* **3**, 85-152 (1984). Application to natural product synthesis: A. Ichihara, *Synthesis* **1987**, 207-222; R. W. Sweger, A. W. Czarnik, *Comp. Org. Syn.* **5**, 551-592 (1991).

337. Retropinacol Rearrangement

N. Zelinsky, J. Zelikow, *Ber.* **34**, 3249 (1901).
Conversion of an alcohol to the rearranged olefin on treatment with acid:

Application to sterols: W. F. Johns, *J. Org. Chem.* **26**, 4583 (1961); L. M. Harrison, P. V. Fennessey, *J. Steroid Biochem.* **36**, 407 (1990); to cyclohexanols: W. Hueckel, S. K. Gupte, *Ann.* **685**, 105 (1965). In conjunction with ring expansion: T. Kimura *et al., J. Org. Chem.* **43**, 1247 (1978). *Cf.* Nametkin Rearrangement; Wagner-Meerwein Rearrangement.

338. Reverdin Reaction

F. Reverdin, *Ber.* **29**, 997, 2595 (1896).
Migration of iodine during nitration of iodophenolic ethers:

F. Reverdin, *Bull. Soc. Chim. Fr.* [4] **1**, 618 (1907); G. M. Robinson, *J. Chem. Soc.* **109**, 1078 (1916); D. V. Nightingale, *Chem. Rev.* **40**, 128 (1947); M. J. S. Dewar, *Electronic Theory of Organic Chemistry* (Oxford, 1949) p 232.

339. Riehm Quinoline Synthesis

P. Riehm *et al., Ber.* **18**, 2245 (1885); **19**, 1394 (1886); *idem, Ann.* **238**, 9 (1887).
Formation of quinoline derivatives by prolonged heating of arylamine hydrochlorides with ketones with or without use of aluminum chloride or phosphorus pentachloride:

Organic Name Reactions

E. Knoevenagel *et al., Ann.* **55,** 1923, 1934 (1922); **56,** 2414 (1923); C. Hollins, *The Synthesis of Nitrogen Ring Compounds* (London, 1924) p 263; D. J. Craig, *J. Am. Chem. Soc.* **60,** 1458 (1938); R. C. Elderfield, J. R. McCarthy, *ibid.* **73,** 975 (1951); R. C. Elderfield, *Heterocycl. Compd.* **4,** 16 (1952).

340. Riemschneider Thiocarbamate Synthesis

R. Riemschneider, F. Wojahn, *Pharmazie* **4,** 460 (1949); *Chim. Ind. (Paris)* **64,** 99 (1950); *Pharm. Zentralhalle* **89,** 118 (1950).

The action of concentrated sulfuric acid followed by treatment with ice-water serves to transform arylthiocyanates into the corresponding thiocarbamates:

$$ArSCN \xrightarrow[\text{H}_2\text{O}]{\text{conc H}_2\text{SO}_4} ArS \overset{OH}{\underset{NH}{\diagdown}} \rightleftharpoons ArSCONH_2$$

R. Riemschneider, *Chim. Ind. (Milan)* **33,** 483 (1951); *idem et al., J. Am. Chem. Soc.* **73,** 5905 (1951); R. Riemschneider, G. Orlick, *Angew. Chem.* **64,** 420 (1952); R. Riemschneider, *Chim. Ind. (Milan)* **34,** 353 (1952); *idem, Z. Naturforsch.* **7b,** 277 (1952); R. Riemschneider, G. Orlick, *Monatsh. Chem.* **84,** 316 (1953); K. Schmidt, P. Kolleck-Bös, *J. Am. Chem. Soc.* **75,** 6067 (1953).

341. Riley Oxidations (Selenium Dioxide Oxidation)

H. L. Riley *et al., J. Chem. Soc.* **1932,** 1875.

Oxidations of organic compounds with selenium dioxide; *e.g.,* the oxidation of active methylene groups to carbonyl groups:

$$CH_3CH_2CHO + SeO_2 \longrightarrow CH_3COCHO + H_2O + Se$$

N. Rabjohn, *Org. React.* **5,** 331 (1949); *Oxidation,* E. N. Trachtenberg, R. L. Augustine, Eds. (Marcel Dekker, New York, 1969) pp 119-187; H. O. House, *Modern Synthetic Reactions* (W. A. Benjamin, Menlo Park, California, 2nd ed., 1972) pp 407-411.

342. Ritter Reaction

J. J. Ritter, P. P. Minieri, *J. Am. Chem. Soc.* **70,** 4045 (1948); J. J. Ritter, J. Kalish, *ibid.* 4048.

Synthesis of amides from nitriles and alcohols or alkenes in strongly acidic media:

$$\underset{H_3C}{\overset{H_3C}{\diagup}}C{=}CH_2 + R{-}C{\equiv}N \xrightarrow{H^+} \left[(H_3C)_3{-}\overset{+}{N}{\equiv}C{-}R \right] \xrightarrow{H_2O} (H_3C)_3 \overset{\displaystyle H}{\overset{\displaystyle N}{\diagdown}}\underset{O}{\overset{\diagup}{\diagdown}}R$$

Reviews: L. I. Krimen, D. J. Cota, *Org. React.* **17,** 213-325 (1969); R. C. Larock, W. W. Leong, *Comp. Org. Syn.* **4,** 292-294 (1991); R. Bishop, *ibid.* **6,** 261-300 (1991). Synthetic applications: S. Top, G. Jaouen, *J. Org. Chem.* **46,** 78 (1981); D. M. Fink, R. C. Effland, *Synth. Commun.* **24,** 2793 (1994); W. M. Samaniego *et al., Tetrahedron Lett.* **35,** 6967 (1994).

343. Robinson Annulation

W. S. Rapson, R. Robinson, *J. Chem. Soc.* **1935,** 1285.

Formation of six-membered ring α,β-unsaturated ketones by the addition of cyclohexanones to methyl vinyl ketone (or simple derivatives of methyl vinyl ketone) or its equivalents, followed by an intramolecular aldol condensation, *q.v.*:

Early review: R. E. Gawley, *Synthesis* **1976,** 777-794. Improved methodology: T. Sato *et al., Tetrahedron Lett.* **31,** 1581 (1990). Stereochemical study: C. Nussbaumer, *Helv. Chim. Acta* **73,** 1621 (1990). Synthetic applications: R. V. Bonnert *et al., J. Chem. Soc. Perkin Trans. 1* **1991,** 1225; S. Kim, P. L. Fuchs, *J. Am. Chem. Soc.* **115,** 5934 (1993). *Cf.* Michael Reaction; Wichterle Reaction.

344. Robinson-Schöpf Reaction

R. Robinson, *J. Chem. Soc.* **111,** 762, 876 (1917); C. Schöpf, *Angew. Chem.* **50,** 779, 797 (1937).

Synthesis of tropinones from a dialdehyde, methylamine and acetonedicarboxylic acid:

K. Alder *et al.*, *Ann.* **601,** 147 (1956); R. D. Guthrie, J. F. McCarthy, *J. Chem. Soc. C* **1967,** 62; R. V. Stevens, A. W. M. Lee, *J. Am. Chem. Soc.* **101,** 7032 (1979); M. Langlois *et al.*, *Synth. Commun.* **22,** 3115 (1992); T. Jarevang *et al.*, *Acta Chem. Scand.* **52,** 1350 (1998). *Cf.* Mannich Reaction; Petrenko-Kritschenko Piperidone Synthesis.

345. Rosenmund Reduction

K. W. Rosenmund, *Ber.* **51,** 585 (1918); K. W. Rosenmund, F. Zetzsche, *ibid.* **54,** 425 (1921).
Catalytic reduction of acid chlorides to aldehydes. To prevent further hydrogenation a poison is added to the catalyst:

$$RCOCl + H_2 \xrightarrow{Pd\text{-}BaSO_4} RCHO + HCl$$

Reviews: E. Mosettig, R. Mozingo, *Org. React.* **4,** 362 (1948); A. Rachlin *et al.*, *Org. Synth.* **51,** 8 (1971); J. A. Peters, H. Van Bekkum, *Rec. Trav. Chim.* **100,** 21 (1981). Investigation of reaction parameters: W. F. Maier *et al.*, *J. Am. Chem. Soc.* **108,** 2608 (1986). Modified procedure applied to the synthesis of esters: V. V. Grushin, H. Alper, *J. Org. Chem.* **56,** 5159 (1991).

346. Rosenmund-von Braun Synthesis

K. W. Rosenmund, E. Struck, *Ber.* **52,** 1749 (1916); J. von Braun, G. Manz, *Ann.* **488,** 111 (1931).
Conversion of aryl halides to aromatic nitriles in the presence of cuprous cyanide:

$$ArX + CuCN \xrightarrow{\Delta} ArCN + CuX$$

Reviews: D. T. Moury, *Chem. Rev.* **42,** 207 (1948); J. E. Callen *et al.*, *Org. Synth.* **3,** 212 (1955); M. S. Newman, *ibid.* 631; K. Takagi *et al.*, *Bull. Chem. Soc. Jpn.* **48,** 3298 (1975); P. Bouyssou *et al.*, *J. Heterocycl. Chem.* **29,** 895 (1992).

347. Rothemund Reaction

P. Rothemund, *J. Am. Chem. Soc.* **57,** 2010 (1935); **61,** 2912 (1939).
Preparation of *meso*-tetrasubstituted porphyrins by condensation of pyrrole with an aldehyde:

Ball *et al.*, *J. Am. Chem. Soc.* **68,** 2278 (1946); Thomas, Martell, *ibid.* **78,** 1335 (1956). Mechanism: Badger *et al.*, *Aust. J. Chem.* **17,** 1028 (1964); R. G. Little, *J. Heterocycl. Chem.* **18,** 833 (1981).

348. Rubottom Oxidation

A. G. Brook, D. M. Macrae, *J. Organomet. Chem.* **77,** C19 (1974); A. Hassner *et al.*, *J. Org. Chem.* **40,** 3427 (1975); G. M. Rubottom *et al.*, *Tetrahedron Lett.* **1974,** 4319.
Oxidation of enolsilanes with *m*-chloroperbenzoic acid (*m*-CPBA) to afford α-hydroxy ketones:

Synthetic applications: R. Gleiter *et al.*, *J. Org. Chem.* **57,** 252 (1992); C. R. Johnson *et al.*, *J. Am. Chem. Soc.* **114,** 9414 (1992); M. T. Crimmins *et al.*, *ibid.* **115,** 3146 (1993).

349. Ruff-Fenton Degradation

O. Ruff, *Ber.* **31,** 1573 (1898); **32,** 550 (1899); H. J. H. Fenton, *Proc. Chem. Soc. London* **9,** 113 (1893).
Shortening of the carbon chain of sugars by the oxidation of aldonic acids (as calcium salts) with hydrogen peroxide and ferric salts:

$$RCH(OH)COOH + H_2O_2 \xrightarrow{Fe^{3+}} RCHO + CO_2 + 2H_2O$$

W. Pigman, *The Carbohydrates* (Academic Press, New York, 1957) p 118; H. S. Isbell, M. A. Salam, *Carbohydr. Res.* **90,** 123 (1981).

350. Ruzicka Large Ring Synthesis

L. Ruzicka *et al.*, *Helv. Chim. Acta* **9,** 249, 339, 389, 499 (1926).
Formation of large ring alicyclic ketones from dicarboxylic acids by thermal decomposition of salts with metals of the second and fourth groups of the periodic table (Ca, Th, Ce):

$$\text{(CH}_2)_n \begin{array}{c} \text{CH}_2\text{COO} \\ \diagdown \\ \text{M} \\ \diagup \\ \text{CH}_2\text{COO} \end{array} \longrightarrow \text{(CH}_2)_n \begin{array}{c} \text{CH}_2 \\ \diagdown \\ \text{CO} \\ \diagup \\ \text{CH}_2 \end{array}$$

L. Ruzicka, *Chem. Ind. (London)* **54**, 2 (1935); H. Gilman, *Organic Chemistry* **vol. 1** (New York, 1943) p 78; K. Ziegler, *Houben-Weyl* **4/2**, 754 (1955). *Cf.* Blanc Reaction.

351. Sabatier-Senderens Reduction
P. Sabatier, J. B. Senderens, *Compt. Rend.* **128**, 1173 (1899).
  Catalytic hydrogenation of organic compounds in the vapor phase by passage over hot, finely divided nickel (the oldest of all hydrogenation methods).
  E. B. Maxted in *Handbuch der Katalyse* **vol. 7**, G. M. Schwab, Ed. (Vienna, 1943) p 624; H. Roth *et al., Houben-Weyl* **2**, 288 (1953); G. Schiller, *ibid.* **IV/2**, 284 (1955); H. O. House, *Modern Synthetic Reactions* (W. A. Benjamin, Menlo Park, California, 2nd ed., 1972) Chapter 1.

352. Saegusa Oxidation
Y. Ito *et al., J. Org. Chem.* **43**, 1011 (1978).
  Conversion of silyl enol ethers into corresponding α,β-enones using stoichiometric amounts of palladium acetate:

$$\begin{array}{c} \text{H} \quad \text{R}^1 \\ \diagdown \diagup \\ \diagup \diagdown \\ \text{RCH}_2 \quad \text{OSiMe}_3 \end{array} \xrightarrow[\text{CH}_3\text{CN}]{\text{Pd(OAc)}_2} \begin{array}{c} \text{H} \quad \text{R}^1 \\ \diagdown \diagup \\ \text{H} - \text{C} \\ \diagup \diagdown \\ \text{RCH}_2 \quad \text{O} \end{array}$$

Application: M. Kim *et al., Synth. Commun.* **20**, 989 (1990). Mechanism: S. Porth *et al., Angew. Chem. Int. Ed.* **38**, 2015 (1999).

353. Sakurai Reaction (Hosomi-Sakurai Reaction)
A. Hosomi, H. Sakurai, *Tetrahedron Lett.* **1976**, 1295; A. Hosomi *et al., Chem. Lett.* **1976**, 941.
  Lewis acid-promoted nucleophilic addition of allylic silanes to carbon electrophiles accompanied by regiospecific transposition of the allylic moiety:

$$(\text{H}_3\text{C})_3\text{Si} \underset{a \quad b}{\diagup\!\!\diagdown\!\!\diagup} \xrightarrow[\text{Lewis acid}]{\text{E}} \underset{a \quad b}{\diagup\!\!\diagdown\!\!\diagup}^{\text{E}^1}$$

E = aldehydes, ketones, enones, acid chlorides, acetals, ketals, epoxides, iminium salts
Lewis acid = TiCl_4, AlCl_3, $\text{BF}_3 \cdot \text{O(CH}_2\text{CH}_3)_2$, SnCl_4, $(\text{CH}_3\text{CH}_2)_2\text{AlCl}$, cat $(\text{CH}_3)_3\text{SiOSO}_2\text{CF}_3$

Synthetic applications: I. E. Markó, D. J. Bayston, *Tetrahedron Lett.* **34**, 6595 (1993); H. Hioki *et al., ibid.* 6131. [$\text{TiCp}_2(\text{OSO}_2\text{CF}_3)_2$] as catalyst: T. K. Hollis *et al., ibid.* 4309. *Reviews:* I. Fleming *et al., Org. React.* **37**, 57-575 (1989); Y. Yamamoto, N. Sasaki, "The Stereochemistry of the Sakurai Reaction" in *Stereochemistry of Organo-metallic and Inorganic Compounds* **vol. 3**, I. Bernal, Ed. (Elsevier, New York, 1989) pp 363-437; I. Fleming, *Comp. Org. Syn.* **2**, 563-593 (1991).

354. Sandmeyer Diphenylurea Isatin Synthesis
T. Sandmeyer, *Z. Farben Text. Chem.* **2**, 129 (1903).
  Formation of a cyanoformamidine by treatment of a symmetrical diphenylthiourea with potassium cyanide in alcohol containing lead carbonate, reduction with ammonium sulfide and ring-closure with concentrated sulfuric acid to isatin-2-anil; also formed smoothly by ring closure of the cyanoformamidine with aluminum chloride in benzene or carbon disulfide:

$$(\text{C}_6\text{H}_5\text{NH})_2\text{CS} \xrightarrow[\text{PbCO}_3]{\text{KCN}} \text{C}_6\text{H}_5\text{NHC}(=\text{NC}_6\text{H}_5)\text{CN} \xrightarrow{(\text{NH}_4)_2\text{S}} \text{C}_6\text{H}_5\text{NHC}(=\text{NC}_6\text{H}_5)\text{CSNH}_2$$

DE 115169, DE 116563 (both 1900 to J. R. Geigy & Co.); *Frdl.* **6**, 574, 575 (1900-1902); A. Reissert, *Ber.* **37**, 3708 (1904); G. Schultz *et al., J. Prakt. Chem.* [2] **74**, 74, 76 (1906); C. Hollins, *The Synthesis of Nitrogen Ring Compounds* (London, 1924) p 102; C. S. Marvel, G. S. Hiers, *Org. Synth.* **coll. vol. I**, 327 (1943); P. L. Julian *et al., Heterocycl. Compd.* **3**, 207 (1952); O. Bayer, W. Eckert, *Houben-Weyl* **7/4**, 11 (1968). *Cf.* Sandmeyer Isonitrosoacetanilide Isatin Synthesis.

355. Sandmeyer Isonitrosoacetanilide Isatin Synthesis

T. Sandmeyer, *Helv. Chim. Acta* **2**, 234 (1919).

Formation of isonitrosoacetodiphenylamidine by condensation of chloral hydrate, hydroxylamine and aniline, cyclization with concentrated sulfuric acid, and quantitative hydrolysis to isatin on dilution:

J. Martinet, P. Cousset, *Compt. Rend.* **172**, 1234 (1921); C. Hollins, *The Synthesis of Nitrogen Ring Compounds* (London, 1924) p 103; C. S. Marvel, G. S. Hiers, *Org. Synth.* **coll. vol. I**, 327 (1943); P. L. Julian *et al., Heterocyci. Compd.* **3**, 208 (1952); F. E. Sheibley, J. S. McNulty, *J. Org. Chem.* **21**, 171 (1956); O. Bayer, W. Eckert, *Houben-Weyl* **7/4**, 14 (1968); S. J. Garden *et al., Tetrahedron Lett.* **38**, 1501 (1997). *Cf.* Sandmeyer Diphenylurea Isatin Synthesis.

356. Sandmeyer Reaction (Gattermann Reaction) (Körner-Contardi Reaction)

T. Sandmeyer, *Ber.* **17**, 1633, 2650 (1884); L. Gattermann, *Ber.* **23**, 1218 (1890); G. Körner, A. Contardi, *Atti Accad. Naz. Lincei* **23 II**, 464 (1914), *C.A.* **9**, 1478 (1915).

Substitution of diazonium groups in aromatic compounds by halo or cyano groups in the presence of cuprous salts (Sandmeyer reaction), copper powder and hydrochloric or hydrobromic acid (Gattermann reaction) or cupric salts (Körner-Contardi reaction):

$$C_6H_5N_2^+ \ X^- \xrightarrow{CuCl} C_6H_5Cl$$

Early reviews: H. H. Hodgson, *Chem. Rev.* **40**, 251-277 (1947); W. A. Coudrey, D. S. Davies, *Q. Rev. Chem. Soc.* **6**, 358-379 (1952); A. Roedig, *Houben-Weyl* **5/4**, 438 (1960); R. Stroh, *ibid.* **5/3**, 846 (1962). Direct conversion of aryl amines to aryl halides: M. P. Doyle, *J. Org. Chem.* **42**, 2426 (1977). Mechanistic studies: J. K. Kochi, *J. Am. Chem. Soc.* **79**, 2942 (1957); C. Galli, *J. Chem. Soc. Perkin Trans. 2* **1984**, 897. Synthetic application: C. Corral *et al., Heterocycles* **23**, 1431 (1985). Improved methodology: N. Suzuki *et al., J. Chem. Soc. Perkin Trans. 1* **1987**, 645; A. P. Krapcho, S. N. Haydar, *Heterocycl. Commun.* **4**, 291 (1998).

357. Sarett Oxidation; Collins Oxidation

G. I. Poos, G. E. Arth, R. E. Beyler, L. H. Sarett, *J. Am. Chem. Soc.* **75**, 422 (1953).

Oxidation of primary and secondary alcohols to aldehydes (and/or carboxylic acids) and ketones by means of CrO_3-pyridine complex:

$$>\!\!C\!\!<^H_{OH} \xrightarrow[C_5H_5N]{CrO_3} \ >\!\!C\!=\!O$$

J. R. Holum, *J. Org. Chem.* **26**, 4814 (1961); E. J. Kris, *Chem. Ind. (London)* **1961**, 1834; V. I. Stenberg, R. J. Perkins, *J. Org. Chem.* **28**, 323 (1963); P. G. Gassman, P. G. Pape, *J. Org. Chem.* **29**, 160 (1964); H. O. House, *Modern Synthetic Reactions* (W. A. Benjamin, Menlo Park, California, 2nd ed., 1972) pp 264-273. Mechanistic studies: F. Hasan, J. Rocek, *J. Am. Chem. Soc.* **97**, 1444, 3762 (1975).

The **Collins oxidation** is characterized by a modified procedure (dichloromethane as solvent) that reliably oxidizes primary alcohols to aldehydes: J. C. Collins, *Tetrahedron Lett.* **1968**, 3363; J. C. Collins, W. W. Hess, *Org. Synth.* **52**, 5 (1972); R. W. Ratcliffe, *ibid.* **55**, 84 (1976). *Cf.* Jones Oxidation.

358. Schiemann Reaction (Balz-Schiemann Reaction)

G. Balz, G. Schiemann, *Ber.* **60**, 1186 (1927).

Formation of diazonium fluoroborates by diazotization of aromatic amines in the presence of fluoroborates, followed by their thermal decomposition to aryl fluorides:

$$ArNH_2 + HNO_2 + HBF_4 \longrightarrow ArN_2^+ BF_4^- \xrightarrow{\Delta} ArF + N_2 + BF_3$$

Reviews: A. Roe, *Org. React.* **5**, 193 (1949); H. Suschitzky, *Adv. Fluorine Chem.* **4**, 1 (1965); T. K. Al'sing, E. G. Sochilin, *Zh. Org. Khim.* **7**, 530 (1971); R. Bartsch *et al., J. Am. Chem. Soc.* **98**, 6753 (1976); H. G. O. Becker, G. Israel, *J. Prakt. Chem.* **321**, 579 (1979).

359. Schmidt Reaction

R. F. Schmidt, *Ber.* **57**, 704 (1924).

Acid-catalyzed addition of hydrazoic acid to carboxylic acids, aldehydes and ketones to give amines, nitriles and amides, respectively. Tertiary alcohols and substituted alkenes yield imines upon treatment with hydrazoic acid:

$$RCOOH \xrightarrow[\text{H}_2\text{SO}_4]{\text{HN}_3} RNH_2$$

$$RCHO \xrightarrow[\text{H}_2\text{SO}_4]{\text{HN}_3} RCN + RNHCHO$$

$$RCOR \xrightarrow[\text{H}_2\text{SO}_4]{\text{HN}_3} RCONHR$$

$$R_3COH \xrightarrow[\text{H}_2\text{SO}_4]{\text{HN}_3} R_2C=NR$$

$$R_2C=CR_2 \xrightarrow[\text{H}_2\text{SO}_4]{\text{HN}_3} R_2CHC=NR \atop R$$

Early reviews: H. Wolff, *Org. React.* **3,** 307-336 (1946); P. A. S. Smith in *Molecular Rearrangements* Part 1, P. de Mayo, Ed. (Wiley-Interscience, New York, 1963) pp 507-558; D. V. Banthorpe, *The Chemistry of the Azido Group*, S. Patai, Ed. (Interscience, New York, 1971) pp 405-421; G. I. Koldobskii, *Russ. Chem. Rev.* **47,** 1084 (1978). Application to cyclic ketones: A. Lévai *et al., Heterocycles* **34,** 1523 (1992); J.-Y. Mérour *et al., J. Heterocycl. Chem.* **31,** 87 (1994); to alcohols and alkenes: W. H. Pearson *et al., J. Am. Chem. Soc.* **115,** 10183 (1993). Extension to dialkyl acylphosphonates: M. Sprecher, D. Kost, *ibid.* **116,** 1016 (1994). *Review:* T. Shioiri, *Comp. Org. Syn.* **6,** 817-821 (1991). *Cf.* Beckmann Rearrangement; Curtius Rearrangement; Hofmann Reaction; Lossen Rearrangement.

360. Scholl Reaction

R. Scholl, C. Seer, *Ann.* **394,** 111 (1912).

Coupling of aromatic molecules by treatment with Lewis acid catalysts:

$$2ArH \xrightarrow[\text{H}^+]{\text{AlCl}_3} Ar-Ar + H_2$$

Review: C. D. Nenitzescu, A. T. Balaban in *Friedel-Crafts and Related Reactions* **vol. 2,** part 2, G. Olah, Ed. (Wiley, New York, 1964) pp 979-1048; G. A. Clowes, *J. Chem. Soc. C* **1968,** 2519; A. C. Buchanan *et al., J. Am. Chem. Soc.* **102,** 5262 (1980).

361. Schöllkopf Bis-Lactim Amino Acid Synthesis

U. Schöllkopf *et al., Angew. Chem. Int. Ed.* **18,** 863 (1979); **20,** 798 (1981).

Asymmetric amino acid synthesis *via* diastereoselective alkylation of the lithiated bis-lactim ether (derived from L-Val and Gly or Ala) by an electrophile. Subsequent acid hydrolysis liberates L-Val-OCH$_3$ and the *(R)*-α-substituted amino acid ester. When the bis-lactim is generated from D-Val, the *(S)*-enantiomer forms:

R = H, CH$_3$
E = alkyl halides, aldehydes, ketones, thioketones, acid chlorides, epoxides, acrylates

Synthetic applications: S. Kotha, A. Kuki, *Chem. Commun.* **1992,** 404; M. S. Allen *et al., Synth. Commun.* **22,** 2077 (1992). Isotopic labeling: N. R. Thomas, D. Gani, *Tetrahedron* **47,** 497 (1991). *Reviews:* U. Schöllkopf, *Top. Curr. Chem.* **109,** 65-84 (1983); *idem, Pure Appl. Chem.* **55,** 1799-1806 (1983); R. M. Williams, *Synthesis of Optically Active α-Amino Acids* (Pergamon, New York, 1989) pp 1-33.

362. Schotten-Baumann Reaction

C. Schotten, *Ber.* **17,** 2544 (1884); E. Baumann, *ibid.* **19,** 3218 (1886).

Acylation of alcohols or amines with acid chlorides in aqueous alkaline solution:

$$\text{ROH} + \underset{O}{\overset{R^1}{C}}X \xrightarrow{\text{NaOH}} \underset{O}{\overset{R^1}{C}}OR$$

Review: N. O. V. Sonntag, *Chem. Rev.* **52**, 272-273 (1953). Synthetic applications: M. Tsuchiya *et al., Bull. Chem. Soc. Jpn.* **42**, 1756 (1969); G. I. Georg, *Bioorg. Med. Chem. Lett.* **4**, 335 (1994).

363. Semmler-Wolff Reaction (Wolff-Semmler Aromatization) (Wolff Aromatization)

W. Semmler, *Ber.* **25**, 3352 (1892); L. Wolff, *Ann.* **322**, 351 (1902).

Rearrangement of α,β-unsaturated cyclohexenyl ketoximes into aromatic amines under acidic conditions:

Review: R. T. Conley, S. Ghosh in *Mechanisms of Molecular Migrations* **vol. 4**, B. S. Thyagarajan, Ed., (Interscience, New York, 1971) p 251; M. I. El-Sheikh, J. M. Cook, *J. Org. Chem.* **45**, 2585 (1980); Y. Tamura *et al., Synthesis* **1980**, 483.

364. Serini Reaction

A. Serini *et al., Ber.* **72**, 391 (1939).

Zinc-promoted rearrangement of 17-hydroxy-20-acetoxysterol derivatives into C-20 ketones; the reaction is applicable to other cyclic, as well as open-chain alcohols:

Reviews: C. W. Shoppe, *Chimia* **4**, 418 (1948); L. F. Fieser, M. Fieser, *Steroids* (Reinhold Publishing Corp., New York, 1959) p 628; N. L. Wendler in *Molecular Rearrangements* Part 2, P. de Mayo, Ed. (Wiley-Interscience, New York, 1964) p 1038; E. Ghera, *Chem. Commun.* **1968**, 1639; *J. Org. Chem.* **35**, 660 (1970).

365. Sharpless Dihydroxylation

E. N. Jacobsen *et al., J. Am. Chem. Soc.* **110**, 1968 (1988).

Osmium-catalyzed asymmetric *cis*-dihydroxylation of olefins:

A premix of the four reagent components is commercially available. The composition containing (DHQD)$_2$-PHAL is termed AD-mix-β; the composition containing (DHQ)$_2$-PHAL is termed AD-mix-α.

(DHQD)$_2$-PHAL = 1,4-bis(9-O-dihydroquinidine)phthalazine; (DHQ)$_2$-PHAL =1,4-bis(9-O-dihydroquinine)phthalazine.

R$_L$ = largest substituent; R$_M$ = medium-sized substituent; R$_S$ = smallest substituent.

Note: The scheme shown is an empirical mnemonic indicating olefin orientation and face selectivity. It is not to be considered an absolute predictor of new diol configurations.

Allyl and vinyl silanes as substrates: A. R. Bassindale *et al., J. Chem. Soc. Perkin Trans. 1* **1994**, 1061. Chemoselective dihydroxylation of a polyene: S. C. Sinha, E. Keinan, *J. Org. Chem.* **59**, 949 (1994). *Reviews:* R. A. Johnson, K. B. Sharpless, "Catalytic Asymmetric Dihydroxylation" in *Catalytic Asymmetric Synthesis*, I. Ojima, Ed. (VCH, New York, 1993) pp 227-272; H. C. Kolb *et al., Chem. Rev.* **94**, 2483-2547 (1994). *Cf.* Milas Hydroxylation of Olefins.

366. Sharpless Epoxidation

T. Katsuki, K. B. Sharpless, *J. Am. Chem. Soc.* **102**, 5974 (1980).

Titanium-catalyzed asymmetric epoxidation of allylic alcohols employing titanium alkoxide, an optically active tartrate ester and an alkyl hydroperoxide. A high degree of enantiomeric purity is attainable having predictable absolute stereochemistry:

D-(-)-diethyl tartrate (unnatural)

70-90% yields,
>90% ee

L-(+)-diethyl tartrate (natural)

Note: The asterisk at a chiral center denotes a preponderance of either the *R* or *S* configuration.

Mechanistic studies: S. S. Woodward *et al., J. Am. Chem. Soc.* **113**, 106 (1991); M. G. Finn, K. B. Sharpless, *ibid.* 113. Methods development for the synthesis of enantiopure allylic alcohols: D. C. Dittmer *et al., J. Org. Chem.* **58**, 718 (1993). Alkenylsilanols as substrates: T. H. Chan *et al., Can. J. Chem.* **71**, 60 (1993). *Reviews:* R. A. Johnson, K. B. Sharpless, *Comp. Org. Syn.* **7**, 389-436 (1991); E. Höft, *Top. Curr. Chem.* **164**, 63-77 (1993).

367. Sharpless Oxyamination
K. B. Sharpless *et al., J. Am. Chem. Soc.* **97**, 2305 (1975).

Osmium-mediated *cis*-addition of nitrogen and oxygen moieties to mono-, di- and tri-substituted olefins to yield vicinal amino or amido alcohols:

$$R^3 = C(CH_3)_3, \text{1-adamantyl}$$
$$R^4 = CH_2CH_3, C(CH_3)_3, CH_2Ph$$
$$R^5 = R^3, Ts, COOR^4$$

Methods development in the context of taxol synthesis: L. Mangatal *et al., Tetrahedron* **45**, 4177 (1989). Synthetic applications: S. K. Dubey, E. E. Knaus, *Can. J. Chem.* **61**, 565 (1983); M. Lemaire *et al., Synlett* **1990**, 615. Brief review: *Organic Syntheses by Oxidation with Metal Compounds*, W. J. Mijs, C. R. H. I. de Jonge, Eds. (Plenum Press, New York, 1986) pp 642-645.

368. Shi Epoxidation
Y. Tu *et al., J. Am. Chem. Soc.* **118**, 9806 (1996); Z.-X. Wang *et al., ibid.* **119**, 11224 (1997).

Enantioselective epoxidation of *trans*- and tri-substituted olefins using a fructose derived chiral ketone catalyst and potassium peroxomonosulfate or H_2O_2 as an oxidant:

Catalyst modification for epoxidation of *cis*-olefins: H. Tian *et al., J. Am. Chem. Soc.* **122**, 11551 (2000). Use of hydrogen peroxide as the primary oxidant: L. Shu, Y, Shi, *Tetrahedron* **57**, 5213 (2001). Epoxidation of terminal olefins: H. Tian *et al., Org. Lett.* **3**, 1929 (2001). Isotope effects: D. A. Singleton, Z. Wang, *J. Am. Chem. Soc.* **127**, 6679 (2005). *Reviews:* M. Frohn, Y. Shi, *Synthesis* **2000**, 1979-2000; Y. Shi, *Acc. Chem. Res.* **37**, 488-496 (2004).

369. Simmons-Smith Reaction
  H. E. Simmons, R. D. Smith, *J. Am. Chem. Soc.* **80**, 5323 (1958).
  Stereospecific synthesis of cyclopropanes by treatment of olefins with methylene iodide and zinc-copper couple:

$$\text{(olefin)} + CH_2I_2 + Zn(Cu) \xrightarrow{(C_2H_5)_2O} \text{(cyclopropane)} + ZnI_2 + Cu$$

  Synthetic applications: J. Long *et al., Tetrahedron Lett.* **46**, 2737 (2005). Mechanistic studies: M. Nakamura *et al., J. Am. Chem. Soc.* **125**, 2341 (2003). *Reviews:* H. E. Simmons *et al., Org. React.* **20**, 1 (1973); C. Girard, J. M. Conia, *J. Chem. Res. Synop.* **1978**, 182; W. Ratier *et al., ibid.* 179; A. Sele *et al., Helv. Chim. Acta* **62**, 866 (1979); J. Joska, J. Fajkos, *Collect. Czech. Chem. Commun.* **46**, 2751 (1981); V. K. Aggarwal *et al., Eur. J. Org. Chem.* **2002**, 319-326.

370. Simonini Reaction
  A. Simonini, *Monatsh. Chem.* **13**, 320 (1892); **14**, 81 (1893).
  The preparation of aliphatic esters by the reaction of the silver salt of a carboxylic acid with iodine:

$$2RCOOAg + I_2 \xrightarrow{\Delta} RCOOR + 2AgI + CO_2$$

  H. Wieland, F. G. Fischer, *Ann.* **446**, 49 (1926); J. Kleinberg, *Chem. Rev.* **40**, 381 (1947); R. G. Johnson, R. K. Ingham, *ibid.* **56**, 259 (1956); C. V. Wilson, *Org. React.* **9**, 332 (1957); N. J. Bunce, M. Hadley, *Can. J. Chem.* **54**, 2612 (1976). *Cf.* Hunsdiecker Reaction.

371. Simonis Chromone Cyclization
  E. Petschek, H. Simonis, *Ber.* **46**, 2014 (1913).
  Formation of chromones from phenol and β-keto esters in the presence of phosphorus pentoxide, phosphorus oxychloride or sulfuric acid. Coumarins may also form (Pechmann condensation, *q.v.*):

$$\text{(phenol)} + RCH_2COCH_2COOC_2H_5 \xrightarrow{P_2O_5} \text{(chromone)} + C_2H_5OH + H_2O$$

  Reviews: S. M. Sethna, N. M. Shah, *Chem. Rev.* **36**, 14 (1945); S. M. Sethna, R. Phadke, *Org. React.* **7**, 15 (1953); R. N. Lacey, *J. Chem. Soc.* **1954**, 854; O. Dann, G. Illing, *Ann.* **605**, 158 (1957); S. F. Tan, *Aust. J. Chem.* **25**, 1367 (1972).

372. Skraup Reaction
  Z. H. Skraup, *Ber.* **13**, 2086 (1880).
  Synthesis of quinolines from aromatic amines, glycerol, an oxidizing agent and sulfuric acid:

$$\text{(aniline)} + \begin{array}{c} CH_2OH \\ | \\ CHOH \\ | \\ CH_2OH \end{array} \xrightarrow[C_6H_5NO_2]{H_2SO_4} \text{(quinoline)}$$

  Early review: R. H. F. Manske, M. Kulka, *Org. React.* **7**, 80-99 (1953). G. M. Badger *et al., Aust. J. Chem.* **16**, 814, 828 (1963); M. Wahren, *Tetrahedron* **20**, 2773 (1964); E. B. Mullock *et al., J. Chem. Soc. C* **1970**, 829; N. P. Buu-Hoi *et al., J. Chem. Soc. Perkin Trans. 1* **1972**, 260, 263. *Cf.* Bischler-Napieralski Reaction.

373. Smiles Rearrangement; Truce-Smiles Rearrangement
  A. A. Levi *et al., J. Chem. Soc.* **1931**, 3264; W. J. Evans, S. Smiles, *ibid.* **1935**, 181; **1936**, 329.
  Intramolecular nucleophilic aromatic substitution in alkaline solution resulting in the migration of an aromatic system from one heteroatom to another. The two-carbon unit joining X and Y is usually part of an aromatic ring but may also be aliphatic:

$$\xrightarrow[\text{base}]{\text{strong}}$$

X = S, SO, SO$_2$, O, COO   YH = OH, NHR, SH, CH$_2$R, CONHR
Z = NO$_2$, SO$_2$R

  The conversion of *o*-methyldiaryl sulfones to *o*-benzylbenzenesulfinic acids is referred to as the **Truce-Smiles rearrangement:** W. E. Truce *et al., J. Am. Chem. Soc.* **80**, 3625 (1958); G. P. Crowther, C. R. Hauser, *J. Org. Chem.* **33**, 2228 (1968).

$$\xrightarrow{t\text{-BuLi}}$$

Early reviews: J. F. Bunnett, R. E. Zahler, *Chem. Rev.* **49**, 362 (1951); H. J. Shine, *Aromatic Rearrangements* (Elsevier, New York, 1967) pp 307-316; W. E. Truce *et al., Org. React.* **18**, 99-215 (1970). Conversion of phenols to anilines: I. G. C. Coutts, M. R. Southcott, *J. Chem. Soc. Perkin Trans. 1* **1990**, 767. Kinetic study: K. Bowden, P. R. Williams, *J. Chem. Soc. Perkin Trans. 2* **1991**, 215. Methods development for aliphatic substrates: M. Sako *et al., Chem. Pharm. Bull.* **42**, 806 (1994). Application to the synthesis of phenothiazines: S. K. Mukherjee *et al., Pharmazie* **49**, 453 (1994); J. Mukesh *et al., ibid.* 689.

374. Sommelet-Hauser Rearrangement

M. Sommelet, *Compt. Rend.* **205**, 56 (1937).

Rearrangement of benzyl quaternary ammonium salts to *ortho* substituted benzyldialkylamines on treatment with alkali metal amides:

Early reviews: H. E. Zimmerman in *Molecular Rearrangements* Part 1, P. de Mayo, Ed. (Wiley-Interscience, New York, 1963) pp 382-391; S. H. Pine, *Org. React.* **18**, 403-464 (1970). Extension to sulfur ylides: M. Yamamoto *et al., Bull. Chem. Soc. Jpn.* **62**, 958 (1989); H. Ishibashi *et al., Chem. Pharm. Bull.* **39**, 2878 (1991). Effects of aromatic substitution: T. Tanaka *et al., ibid.* **40**, 518 (1992). Selectivity studies (Sommelet-Hauser rearrangement vs Stevens rearrangement, *q.v.*): T. Kitano *et al., J. Chem. Soc. Perkin Trans. 1* **1992**, 2851; T. Tanaka *et al., J. Org. Chem.* **57**, 5034 (1992). *Cf.* Meisenheimer Rearrangements; [2,3]-Wittig Rearrangement.

375. Sommelet Reaction

M. Sommelet, *Compt. Rend.* **157**, 852 (1913); *Bull. Soc. Chim. Fr.* [4] **23**, 95 (1918).

Preparation of aldehydes from aralkyl halides by treatment with hexamethylenetetramine to yield the quaternary salt, followed by mild hydrolysis:

$$ArCH_2X + C_6H_{12}N_4 \longrightarrow [ArCH_2-C_6H_{12}N_4]^+ \, X^- \xrightarrow[H_2O]{\Delta} ArCHO$$

Early reviews: S. J. Angyal, *Org. React.* **8**, 197-217 (1954); Bayer, *Houben-Weyl* **7/1**, 194 (1954). Synthetic applications: S. Miyano *et al., Bull. Chem. Soc. Jpn.* **59**, 3285 (1986); D. Evans *et al., Heterocycles* **26**, 1569 (1987). *Cf.* Kröhnke Oxidation.

376. Sonn-Müller Method

A. Sonn, E. Müller, *Ber.* **52**, 1927 (1919).

Reaction sequence employed to convert aromatic anilides to aldehydes. Treatment of the anilide with phosphorus pentachloride generates the imidoyl chloride, which is reduced to the imine with a mixture of stannous chloride and hydrochloric acid. Subsequent hydrolysis yields the aldehyde:

$$ArCONHPh \xrightarrow{PCl_5} \underset{Cl}{\overset{Ar}{{\diagup}}} =NPh \xrightarrow[HCl]{SnCl_2} ArCH=NPh \xrightarrow{H_2O} ArCHO$$

T. Reichstein, H. Zschokke, *Helv. Chim. Acta* **15**, 1105 (1932); W. E. Bachmann, *J. Am. Chem. Soc.* **57**, 1381 (1935); T. S. Work, *J. Chem. Soc.* **1942**, 429; L. N. Ferguson, *Chem. Rev.* **38**, 244 (1946); E. Mosettig, *Org. React.* **8**, 240 (1954); L. F. Fieser, M. Fieser, *Advanced Organic Chemistry* (New York, 1961) p 832. *Cf.* Grundmann Aldehyde Synthesis; Stephen Aldehyde Synthesis.

377. Sonogashira Coupling (Sonogashira-Hagihara Coupling)

K. Sonogashira *et al., Tetrahedron Lett.* **16**, 4467 (1975).

Palladium(0)-copper(I) catalyzed cross-coupling between sp^2-hybridized organic halides and terminal acetylenes. Synthetic applications: A. S. Karpov *et al., J. Org. Chem.* **68**, 1503 (2003); M. Erdélyi, A. Gogoll, *ibid.* 6431; A. Elangovan *et al., Org. Lett.* **5**, 1841 (2003); M. S. M. Ahmed, A. Mori, *ibid.* 3057; M. Eckhardt, G. C. Fu, *J. Am. Chem. Soc.* **125**, 13642 (2003); E. Mas-Marzá *et al., Tetrahedron Lett.* **44**, 6595 (2003). Nickel catalyzed reaction: I. P. Beletskaya *et al., ibid.* 5011. Copper-free modifications: A. Soheili *et al., Org. Lett.* **5**, 4191 (2003); L. Djakovitch, P. Rollet, *Adv. Synth. Catal.* **346**, 1782 (2004). *Reviews:* K. Sonogashira, *J. Organomet. Chem.* **653**, 46-49 (2002); R. R. Tykwinski, *Angew. Chem. Int. Ed.* **42**, 1566-1568 (2003).

378. Staudinger Reaction

H. Staudinger, J. Meyer, *Helv. Chim. Acta* **2**, 635 (1919).

Synthesis of phosphazo compounds by the reaction of tertiary phosphines with organic azides:

$$R_3P \ + \ N_3R^1 \ \longrightarrow \ R_3P{=}N{-}N{=}N{-}R^1 \ \xrightarrow{\ -N_2\ } \ R_3P{=}N{-}R^1$$

phosphazide

Synthetic applications: M. Taillefer *et al., Chem. Commun.* **6,** 565 (1999); M. D. Velasco *et al., Tetrahedron* **56,** 4079 (2000); P. Vanek, P. Klán, *Synth. Commun.* **30,** 1503 (2000). Cell surface engineering: E. Saxon, C. R. Bertozzi, *Science* **287,** 2007 (2000). *Reviews:* Y. G. Gololobov *et al., Tetrahedron* **37,** 437-472 (1981); Y. G. Gololobov, L. F. Kasukhin, *ibid.* 1353-1406 (1992); M. Köhn, R. Breinbauer, *Angew. Chem. Int. Ed.* **43,** 3106-3116 (2004).

379. Stephen Aldehyde Synthesis

H. Stephen, *J. Chem. Soc.* **127,** 1874 (1925); T. Stephen, H. Stephen, *ibid.* **1956,** 4695.

Reaction sequence employed to convert nitriles to aldehydes. Treatment of the nitrile with a mixture of stannous chloride and hydrochloric acid yields the imine salt complex which is subsequently hydrolyzed to the aldehyde. Practically applied only to aromatic aldehydes:

$$RCN \ \xrightarrow[\text{HCl}]{\text{SnCl}_2} \ (RCH{=}NH \cdot HCl)_2 \ SnCl_4 \ \xrightarrow{\ H_2O\ } \ RCHO$$

L. N. Ferguson, *Chem. Rev.* **38,** 243 (1946); E. Mosettig, *Org. React.* **8,** 246 (1954); O. Bayer, *Houben-Weyl* **7/1,** 299 (1954); E. N. Zilberman, P. S. Pyryalova, *J. Gen. Chem. USSR* (Engl. trans.) **33,** 3348 (1963); C. G. Stuckwisch, *J. Org. Chem.* **37,** 318 (1972). *Cf.* Grundmann Aldehyde Synthesis; Sonn-Müller Method.

380. Stevens Rearrangement

T. S. Stevens *et al., J. Chem. Soc.* **1928,** 3193; **1930,** 2107, 2119; **1932,** 55, 1926, 1932.

Migration of an alkyl group from a sulfonium or quaternary ammonium salt to an adjacent carbanionic center on treatment with strong base. The product is a rearranged tertiary amine or sulfide:

$$R^1 \underset{R^3}{\overset{+}{\underset{|}{Y}}} R^2 \ \xrightarrow{\ \text{NaNH}_2\ } \ R^1 \underset{R^3}{\overset{-}{\underset{|}{Y}}} R^2 \ \longrightarrow \ R^1 \underset{Y}{\overset{R^2}{\diagdown}} R^3$$

Y = NR or S

Early reviews: H. E. Zimmerman in *Molecular Rearrangements* Part 1, P. de Mayo, Ed. (Wiley-Interscience, New York, 1963) pp 345-406; D. J. Cram, *Fundamentals of Carbanion Chemistry* (Academic Press, New York, 1965) pp 223-229; S. M. Pine, *Org. React.* **18,** 403-464 (1970). Selectivity studies vs Sommelet-Hauser rearrangement, *q.v.:* T. Kitano *et al., J. Chem. Soc. Perkin Trans. 1* **1992,** 2851; T. Tanaka *et al., J. Org. Chem.* **57,** 5034 (1992). *Review:* I. E. Markó, *Comp. Org. Syn.* **3,** 913-932 (1991). Comprehensive review and applications in natural product synthesis: J. A. Vanecko *et al., Tetrahedron* **62,** 1043-1062 (2006). *Cf.* Meisenheimer Rearrangements; [1,2]-Wittig Rearrangement.

381. Stieglitz Rearrangement

J. Stieglitz, P. N. Leech, *Ber.* **46,** 2147 (1913); *J. Am. Chem. Soc.* **36,** 272 (1914).

Rearrangement of trityl hydroxylamines to Schiff bases on treatment with phosphorus pentachloride:

$$Ar_3CNHOH \ \xrightarrow{\ PCl_5\ } \ Ar_2C{=}NAr \ + \ POCl_3 \ + \ 2HCl$$

Reviews: P. A. S. Smith in *Molecular Rearrangements* Part 1, P. de Mayo, Ed. (Wiley-Interscience, New York, 1963) p 479; *Trans. N.Y. Acad. Sci.* **31,** 504 (1969); N. Koga, J. P. Anselme, *Tetrahedron Lett.* **1969,** 4773; R. V. Hoffman, D. J. Poelker, *J. Org. Chem.* **44,** 2364 (1979).

382. Stille Coupling

M. Kosugi *et al., Chem. Lett.* **1977,** 301 (1977); D. Milstein, J. K. Stille, *J. Am. Chem. Soc.* **100,** 3636 (1978).

Palladium-catalyzed cross coupling reaction of organostannanes with organic halides, acetates or perfluorinated sulfonates lacking a sp^3-hybridized β-hydrogen:

$$R_3Sn{-}R^1 \ + \ R^2{-}X \ \xrightarrow{\ [Pd]\ } \ R^1{-}R^2 \ + \ R_3SnX$$

[Pd] = Pd(PPh$_3$)$_4$, PhCH$_2$Pd(PPh$_3$)$_2$Cl
R^1 = alkynyl, alkenyl, aryl, allyl, benzyl, alkyl
R^2 = acyl, alkenyl, allyl, benzyl, aryl
X = Cl, Br, I, OCOCH$_3$, OSO$_2$(C$_n$F$_{2n+1}$), n = 0,1,4

Allylic acetates as substrates: L. Del Valle *et al., J. Org. Chem.* **55,** 3019 (1990). Effect of additives: S. Gronowitz *et al., J. Organomet. Chem.* **460,** 127 (1993); V. Farina *et al., J. Org. Chem.* **59,** 5905 (1994). Synthesis of α-methylene lactones: R. M. Adlington *et al., J. Chem. Soc. Perkin Trans. 1* **1994,** 1697. Solid-phase synthesis of 1,4-benzodiazepines: M. J. Plunkett, J. A. Ellman, *J. Am. Chem. Soc.* **117,** 3306 (1995). *Reviews:* J. K. Stille, *Angew. Chem. Int. Ed.* **25,** 508-524 (1986); M. Pereyre *et al., Tin in Organic Synthesis* (Butterworths, Boston, 1987) pp 185-207 *passim.* Review of synthetic applications: T. N. Mitchell, *Synthesis* **1992,** 803-815; of mechanisms: P. Espinet, A. M. Echavarren, *Angew. Chem. Int. Ed.* **43,** 4704-4734 (2004). *Cf.* Heck Reaction; Suzuki Coupling.

383. Stobbe Condensation

H. Stobbe, *Ber.* **26,** 2312 (1893); *Ann.* **282,** 280 (1894).

Condensation of aldehydes or ketones with diethyl succinate in the presence of a strong base to form monoesters of α-alkylidene (or arylidene) succinic acids:

Reviews: W. S. Johnson, G. H. Daub, *Org. React.* **6,** 1 (1951); H. O. House, *Modern Synthetic Reactions* (W. A. Benjamin, Menlo Park, California, 2nd ed., 1972) pp 663-666; R. J. Hart, H. G. Heller, *J. Chem. Soc. Perkin Trans. 1* **1972,** 1321; N. R. El-Rayyes, *J. Prakt. Chem.* **315,** 295 (1973); V. B. Bagos *et al., Helv. Chim. Acta* **62,** 90 (1979). *Cf.* Perkin Reaction.

384. Stollé Synthesis

R. Stollé, *Ber.* **46,** 3915 (1913); **47,** 2120 (1914); *J. Prakt. Chem.* **105,** 137 (1923); **128,** 1 (1930).

Formation of indole derivatives by the reaction of arylamines with α-haloacid chlorides or oxalyl chloride, followed by cyclization of the resulting amides with aluminum chloride:

W. C. Sumpter, *Chem. Rev.* **34,** 396 (1944); **37,** 446 (1945); P. L. Julian *et al., Heterocycl. Compd.* **3,** 142, 209 (1952); A. H. Beckett *et al., Tetrahedron* **24,** 6093 (1968). *Cf.* Hinsberg Oxindole Synthesis.

385. Stork Enamine Reaction

G. Stork *et al., J. Am. Chem. Soc.* **76,** 2029 (1954); G. Stork, H. Landesman, *ibid.* **78,** 5128 (1956).

Synthesis of α-alkyl or α-acyl carbonyl compounds from enamines and alkyl or acyl halides:

Reviews: J. Szmuszkovicz, *Adv. Org. Chem.* **4,** 1 (1963); A. G. Cook, Ed., *Enamines* (Marcel Dekker, New York, 1969); H. O. House, *Modern Synthetic Reactions* (W. A. Benjamin, Menlo Park, California, 2nd ed., 1972) pp 570-580, 766-772; S. F. Dyke, *Chemistry of Enamines* (Cambridge University Press, New York, 1973); P. W. Hickmott, *Tetrahedron* **38,** 1975 (1982). Synthetic applications: C. F. Bridge, D. O'Hagan, *J. Fluorine Chem.* **82,** 21 (1997); J. J. Li *et al., Tetrahedron Lett.* **39,** 6111 (1998).

386. Strecker Amino Acid Synthesis

A. Strecker, *Ann.* **75,** 27 (1850); **91,** 349 (1854).

Synthesis of α-amino acids by reaction of aldehydes with ammonia and hydrogen cyanide followed by hydrolysis of the resulting α-aminonitriles. Safer, milder, and more selective reaction conditions have been developed, esp in regard to asymmetric synthesis. The scope of the reaction has been extended to include primary and secondary amines:

Reviews: J. P. Greenstein, M. Winitz, *Chemistry of the Amino Acids* **vol. 3** (New York, 1961) pp 698-700; G. C. Barrett, *Chemistry and Biochemistry of the Amino Acids* (Chapman and Hall, New York, 1985) pp 251, 261. Asymmetric synthesis using enantiopure sulfinimines: F. A. Davis *et al., Tetrahedron Lett.* **35**, 9351 (1994); *idem et al., J. Org. Chem.* **61**, 440 (1996). Asymmetric syntheses: M. S. Sigman, E. N. Jacobsen, *J. Am. Chem. Soc.* **120**, 4901 (1998); E. J. Corey, M. J. Grogan, *Org. Lett.* **1**, 157 (1999). Review of catalytic enantioselective syntheses: H. Gröger, *Chem. Rev.* **103**, 2795-2827 (2003). *Cf.* Bucherer-Bergs Reaction.

387. Strecker Degradation
A. Strecker, *Ann.* **123**, 363 (1862).
Interaction of an α-amino acid with a carbonyl compound in aqueous solution or suspension to give carbon dioxide and an aldehyde or ketone containing one less carbon atom. Inorganic oxidizing agents can also be used to bring about the reaction:

Early review: A. Schönberg, R. Moubacher, *Chem. Rev.* **50**, 261 (1952). Photo-promoted oxidation: Y. Ogata *et al., Bull. Chem. Soc. Jpn.* **54**, 2057 (1981). Synthetic studies: A. Schönberg *et al., J. Chem. Soc.* **1948**, 176; C.-T. Ho, G. J. Hartman, *J. Agric. Food Chem.* **1982**, 793; A. F. Ghiron *et al., ibid.* **36**, 677 (1988); J. Koch *et al., Carbohydr. Res.* **313**, 117 (1998).

388. Strecker Sulfite Alkylation
A. Strecker, *Ann.* **148**, 90 (1868).
Formation of alkyl sulfonates by reaction of alkyl halides with alkali or ammonium sulfites in aqueous solution in the presence of iodide:

$$RX + M_2SO_3 \xrightarrow{NaI} RSO_3M + MX$$

A. Collmann, *ibid.* 101; W. Hemilian, *ibid.* **168**, 145 (1873); *Ber.* **6**, 562 (1873); **CH 105845**; **CH 104907** (both 1925); F. C. Wagner, E. E. Reid, *J. Am. Chem. Soc.* **53**, 3409 (1931); C. Weygand, *Organic Preparations* (New York, 1945) p 306; M. Quaedvlieg, *Houben-Weyl* **9**, 372 (1955).

389. Suarez Reaction (Suarez Fragmentation)
J. I. Concepion *et al., Tetrahedron Lett.* **25**, 1953 (1984); *eidem, J. Org. Chem.* **51**, 402 (1986).
Photoinduced conversion of hydroxyl-containing substrates with hypervalent iodine I(III)I$_2$ to the corresponding oxygen-centered radical:

DIB = (diacetoxyiodo)benzene

P. De Armas *et al., Angew. Chem. Int. Ed.* **31**, 772 (1992). Mechanistic studies: J. L. Courtneidge *et al., Tetrahedron Lett.* **35**, 1003 (1994); T. Muraki *et al., J. Chem. Soc. Perkin Trans. 1* **1999**, 1713. Synthetic applications: C. M. Hayward *et al., Tetrahedron Lett.* **34**, 3989 (1993); A. Kittaka *et al., Tetrahedron* **55**, 5319 (1999).

390. Sugasawa Reaction
T. Sugasawa *et al., J. Am. Chem. Soc.* **100**, 4842 (1978); M. Adachi *et al., Chem. Pharm. Bull.* **33**, 1826 (1985).
Ortho acylation of anilines by nitriles in the presence of BCl$_3$ and an auxillary Lewis acid:

Mechanistic study: A. W. Douglas *et al., Tetrahedron Lett.* **35**, 6807 (1994). Synthetic application: J. N. Houpis *et al., ibid.* 6811.

391. Suzuki Coupling (Suzuki-Miyaura Cross-Coupling)

N. Miyaura *et al., Tetrahedron Lett.* **1979**, 3437; N. Miyaura, A. Suzuki, *Chem. Commun.* **1979**, 866.

Palladium-catalyzed cross coupling of organic halides or perfluorinated sulfonates with organoboron derivatives proceeding with high stereo- and regioselectivity:

$$R^1\text{-}BY_2 \ + \ R^2\text{-}X \ \xrightarrow[\text{base}]{\text{[Pd]}} \ R^1\text{-}R^2$$

$BY_2 = B(OR)_2$, 9–BBN, $B(CHCH_3CH(CH_3)_2)_2$
$X = I, Br, Cl, OSO_2(C_nF_{2n+1})$, n = 0,1,4
R^1 = aryl, alkenyl, alkyl
R^2 = aryl, alkenyl, alkynyl, benzyl, allyl, alkyl
$[Pd] = Pd(PPh_3)_4$, $Pd(dppf)Cl_2$
base = Na_2CO_3, $NaOCH_2CH_3$, $TlOH$, $N(CH_2CH_3)_3$, K_3PO_4

Competition with Heck reaction, *q.v.*, when using an alkenyl boronate ester: A. R. Hunt *et al., Tetrahedron Lett.* **34**, 3599 (1993). Alternative palladium catalysts: G. Marck *et al., ibid.* **35**, 3277 (1994); T. I. Wallow, B. M. Novak, *J. Org. Chem.* **59**, 5034 (1994). *Reviews:* A. Suzuki, *Pure Appl. Chem.* **63**, 419-422 (1991); A. R. Martin, Y. Yang, *Acta Chem. Scand.* **47**, 221-230 (1993); S. Kotha *et al., Tetrahedron* **58**, 9633-9695 (2002). *Cf.* Hydroboration Reaction; Stille Coupling.

392. Swarts Reaction

F. Swartx, *Bull. Acad. R. Belg.* **24**, 309 (1892).

Fluorination of organic polyhalides with antimony trifluoride (or zinc and mercury fluorides) in the presence of a trace of a pentavalent antimony salt:

$$ClHC{=}CClCHCl_2 \ + \ SbF_3 \ \xrightarrow{SbCl_5} \ ClHC{=}CClCF_3 \ + \ SbCl_3$$

A. L. Henne, *Org. React.* **2**, 49 (1944); M. Hudlicky, *Chemistry of Organic Fluorine Compounds* (MacMillan, New York, 1962) pp 93-98.

393. Swern Oxidation (Moffatt-Swern Oxidation)

K. Omura, D. Swern, *Tetrahedron* **34**, 1651 (1978).

Mild oxidation of primary and secondary alcohols, promoted by oxalyl chloride activation of dimethyl sulfoxide, evidently involving the dimethyl alkoxysulfonium salts. Upon the addition of base, the intermediates rearrange intramolecularly to generate aldehydes or ketones, respectively:

Reactivity/selectivity studies: M. Marx, T. T. Tidwell, *J. Org. Chem.* **49**, 788 (1984). *Reviews:* A. J. Mancuso, D. Swern, *Synthesis* **1981**, 165-185 *passim;* T. T. Tidwell, *Org. React.* **39**, 297-572 *passim* (1990). *Cf.* Corey-Kim Oxidation; Pfitzner-Moffatt Oxidation.

394. Tafel Rearrangement

J. Tafel, H. Hahl, *Ber.* **40**, 3312 (1907).

Rearrangement of the carbon skeleton of substituted acetoacetic esters to hydrocarbons with the same number of carbon atoms by electrolytic reduction at a lead cathode in alcoholic sulfuric acid:

$$CH_3COCRR^1COOC_2H_5 \Bigg\langle \begin{array}{l} CH_3CH_2CRR^1CH_3 \quad \text{(normal)} \\[2mm] CH_3CH_2CH_2CHRR^1 \quad \text{(rearranged)} \end{array}$$

J. Tafel, W. Jürgen, *ibid.* **42**, 2548 (1909); J. Tafel, *ibid.* **45**, 437 (1912); C. J. Brockman, *Electro-organic Chemistry* (New York, 1926) p 321; H. Stenzl, F. Fichter, *Helv. Chim. Acta* **17**, 669 (1934); **19**, 392 (1936); **20**, 846 (1937); F. Asinger, H. H. Vogel, *Houben-Weyl* **5/1a**, 280, 471 (1970).

395. Tebbe Olefination (Methylenation)

F. N. Tebbe *et al., J. Am. Chem. Soc.* **100**, 3611 (1978); S. H. Pine *et al., ibid.* **102**, 3270 (1980).

Exchange of the oxygen atom of a carbonyl function for the methylene group of the proposed titanium carbene complex (the Tebbe reagent) to yield terminal alkenes:

Y = H, R, OR, NR$_2$

Comparative study with Wittig reaction, *q.v.*: S. H. Pines *et al., Synthesis* **1991**, 165. *Reviews:* K. A. Brown-Wensley *et al., Pure Appl. Chem.* **55**, 1733-1744 (1983); S. E. Kelly, *Comp. Org. Syn.* **1**, 743-746 (1991); S. H. Pines, *Org. React.* **43**, 1-91 (1993). *Cf.* Peterson Reaction.

396. Thiele Reaction (Thiele-Winter Acetoxylation)

J. Thiele, *Ber.* **31**, 1247 (1898).

Formation of triacetoxy aromatic compounds by the reaction of quinones with acetic anhydride catalyzed by sulfuric acid or boron trifluoride:

Review: J. F. W. McOmie, J. N. Blatchly, *Org. React.* **19**, 199 (1972). J. M. Blatchly *et al., J. Chem. Soc. Perkin Trans. 1* **1972**, 2286; J. F. W. McOmie, S. A. Saleh, *ibid.* **1974**, 384; M. Hirama, S. Ito, *Chem. Lett.* **1977**, 627. *Cf.* Hinsberg Sulfone Synthesis.

397. Thorpe Reaction

H. Baron *et al., J. Chem. Soc.* **85**, 1726 (1904); K. Ziegler *et al., Ann.* **504**, 94 (1933).

Base-catalyzed self-condensation of nitriles to yield imines which tautomerize to enamines:

Reviews: J. P. Schaefer, J. J. Bloomfield, *Org. React.* **15**, 1 (1967); H. O. House, *Modern Synthetic Reactions* (W. Benjamin, Menlo Park, California, 2nd ed., 1972) p 742; E. C. Taylor, A. McKillop, *Chemistry of Enaminonitriles and o-Aminonitriles* (Wiley-Interscience, N.Y., 1970) pp 1-58; *eidem, Adv. Org. Chem.* **7**, 1 (1970). *Cf.* Ziegler Method.

398. Tiemann Rearrangement

F. Tiemann, *Ber.* **24**, 4162 (1891).

Rearrangement of amide oximes (available from nitriles and hydroxylamine) to monosubstituted ureas by treatment with benzenesulfonyl chloride and water:

P. A. S. Smith, *Org. React.* **3**, 366 (1946); M. W. Partridge, H. A. Turner, *J. Pharm. Pharmacol.* **5**, 103 (1953); R. F. Plapinger. O. O. Owens, *J. Org. Chem.* **21**, 1186 (1956); J. Garapon *et al., Tetrahedron Lett.* **1970**, 4905. *Cf.* Beckmann Rearrangement.

399. Tiffeneau-Demjanov Rearrangement

M. Tiffeneau *et al., Compt. Rend.* **205**, 54 (1937).

Rearrangement of β-amino alcohols upon diazotization with nitrous acid to give carbonyl compounds. Cyclic alcohols yield ring expanded or contracted products:

Reviews: P. A. S. Smith, D. R. Baer, *Org. React.* **11**, 157-188 (1960); H. Metzger, *Houben-Weyl* **10/4**, 233 (1968); D. J. Coveney, *Comp. Org. Syn.* **3**, 781-782 (1991). W. E. Parham, C. S. Roosevelt, *J. Org. Chem.* **37**, 1975 (1972); D. Fattori *et al., Tetrahedron* **49**, 1649 (1993). *Cf.* Demjanov Rearrangement; Pinacol Rearrangement.

400. Tishchenko Reaction

L. Claisen, *Ber.* **20**, 646 (1887); V. Tishchenko, *J. Russ. Phys. Chem. Soc.* **38**, 355, 482, 540, 547 (1906); *Chem. Zentralbl.* **1906 II**, 1309, 1552, 1555, 1556.

Formation of esters from aldehydes by an oxidation-reduction process in the presence of aluminum or sodium alkoxides:

$$2RCHO \xrightarrow{Al(OC_2H_5)_3} RCOOCH_2R$$

O. Kamm, W. F. Kamm, *Org. Synth.* **coll. vol. I**, 104 (1941); Y. Ogata, A. Kawasaki, *Tetrahedron* **25**, 929, 2845 (1969); P. R. Stapp, *J. Org. Chem.* **38**, 1433 (1973); G. Fouquet *et al., Ann.* **1979**, 1591. *Review:* L. Cichon, *Wiad. Chem.* **20**, 641, 783 (1966), *C.A.* **66**, 54672b, 94408b (1967). *Cf.* Cannizzaro Reaction; Meerwein-Pondorf-Verley Reduction.

401. Traube Purine Synthesis

W. Traube, *Ber.* **33**, 1371, 3035 (1900).

Preparation of 4,5-diaminopyrimidines by introduction of the amino group into the 5-position of 4-amino-6-hydroxy- or 4,6-diaminopyrimidines by nitrosation and ammonium sulfide reduction, followed by ring closure with formic acid or chlorocarbonic ester:

J. H. Davidson, *The Nucleic Acids I* (New York, 1955) p 131; A. R. Katritzky, *Q. Rev. Chem. Soc.* **10**, 397 (1956); *idem, Rev. Pure Appl. Chem.* **11**, 178 (1961); J. H. Lister, *Purines* (Wiley, New York, 1971) pp 31-90.

402. Trost Allylation (Tsuji-Trost Reaction)

J. Tsuji *et al., Tetrahedron Lett.* **1965**, 4387; B. M. Trost, T. J. Fullerton, *J. Am. Chem. Soc.* **95**, 292 (1973).

Palladium-catalyzed allylation of nucleophiles proceeding in an SN2 or SN2′ fashion depending on the catalyst, nucleophile, and substituents on the substrate:

NuH = malonates, β-diketones, β-keto esters, enamines, β-keto sulfones, bis-sulfones
X = Br, Cl, OCOOR, SO$_2$R, OCOR, OCONR$_2$, OPO(OR)$_2$, NO$_2$
[Pd]^0 = Pd(PPh$_3$)$_4$, Pd$_2$(dba)$_3$ • CHCl$_3$, + PPh$_3$, Pd(OCOCH$_3$)$_2$ + PPh$_3$
base = NaH, if necessary

Scope and limitations under neutral conditions: J. Tsuji *et al., J. Org. Chem.* **50**, 1523 (1985); in biphasic media: C. de Bellefon *et al., J. Mol. Catal. A.* **145**, 121 (1999). Application to the synthesis of polyprenoids: E. Keinan, D. Eren, *Pure Appl. Chem.* **60**, 89 (1988). Review of intramolecular applications: B. M. Trost in *Adv. Chem. Ser.* **230**, entitled "Homogeneous Transition Metal Catalyzed Reactions" (ACS, Washington DC, 1992) pp 463-478. *Review:* C. G. Frost *et al., Tetrahedron: Asymmetry* **3**, 1089-1122 (1992).

403. Trost Desymmetrization

B. M. Trost *et al., J. Am. Chem. Soc.* **114**, 9333 (1992).

Formation of an enantiomerically pure, azide or amine containing, five or six membered ring by a pallidium catalyzed desymmetrization using a nitrogen nucleophile, where the palladium complex is derived from a chiral ligand and π-allylpalladium chloride:

S. R. Pulley, B. M. Trost, *J. Am. Chem. Soc.* **117**, 10143 (1995).

404. Tscherniac-Einhorn Reaction

J. Tscherniac, **DE 134979;** A. Einhorn *et al., Ann.* **343,** 207 (1905); **361,** 113 (1908).

Introduction of the amidomethyl group into aromatic rings or activated methylene groups in the presence of sulfuric acid:

Reviews: R. Schröter, *Houben-Weyl* **11/1,** 795 (1957); Hellman *Angew. Chem.* **69,** 463 (1957); H. E. Zaugg, W. B. Martin, *Org. React.* **14,** 52 (1965); H. E. Zaugg *et al., J. Org. Chem.* **34,** 11, 14 (1969); K. Bott, *Ber.* **106,** 2513 (1973); A. R. Mitchell *et al., Tetrahedron Lett.* **1976,** 3795.

405. Twitchell Process

E. Twitchell, **US 601603; US 628503** (1898); **DE 365522; DE 385074.**

Commercial process for splitting fats to glycerol and fatty acids by heating the sulfuric-acid-washed fat 20-48 hours in an open tank with steam in a mixture of 25-50% water, 0.5% sulfuric acid and 0.75-1.25% Twitchell reagent (sulfonated petroleum products):

E. Twitchell, *J. Am. Chem. Soc.* **22,** 22 (1900); **28,** 196 (1906); J. W. Lawrie, *Glycerol and the Glycols* (New York, 1928) p 32; R. B. Trusler, *J. Oil Fat Ind.* **8,** 141 (1931); A. F. Bailey, *Industrial Oil and Fat Products* (New York, 1945) p 668; C. J. Marsel, H. D. Allen, *Chem. Eng.* **54**(6), 104 (1947); V. Mills, H. K. McClain, *Ind. Eng. Chem.* **41,** 1982 (1949); L. Lascaray, *J. Am. Oil Chem. Soc.* **29,** 362 (1952); *Faith, Keyes & Clark's Industrial Chemicals* (Wiley-Interscience, New York, 4th ed., 1975) p 431.

406. Ueno-Stork Cyclization

Y. Ueno *et al., J. Am. Chem. Soc.* **104,** 5564 (1982); G. Stork *et al., ibid.* **105,** 3741 (1983).

Radical cyclization of haloacetals. The cyclic acetal product can be converted to a lactone via Jones Oxidation, *q.v.*:

Synthetic applications: Y. Ueno *et al., J. Chem. Soc. Perkin Trans. 1* **1986,** 1351; G. Stork *et al., J. Am. Chem. Soc.* **108,** 6384 (1986); F. Villar *et al., Org. Lett.* **2,** 1061 (2000); G. K. Friestad, G. M. Fioroni, *ibid.* **7,** 2393 (2005). Stereochemistry studies: F. Villar *et al., Chem. Eur. J.* **9,** 1566 (2003); O. Corminboeuf *et al., ibid.* 1578. *Review:* X. J. Salom-Roig *et al., Synthesis* **2004,** 1903-1928.

407. Ugi Reaction (Four-Component Condensation) (4CC)

I. Ugi, *Angew. Chem. Int. Ed.* **1,** 8 (1962).

The α-addition of an iminium ion and the conjugate base of a carboxylic acid to an isocyanide, followed by spontaneous rearrangement of the α-adduct to yield an α-aminocarboxamide derivative. Carbonyl compounds and amines, or their condensation products, serve as precursors to the iminium ion. The nature of the product depends primarily on the acid component:

When four discrete reactants are used, the reaction is often referred to as the four-component condensation (4CC). Diastereoselective methods development: H. Kunz *et al., Synthesis* **1991,** 1039; M. Goebel, I. Ugi, *ibid.* 1095. Synthetic applications: T. Ziegler *et al., Tetrahedron Lett.* **39,** 5957 (1998); *eidem, Tetrahedron* **55,** 8397 (1999). *Reviews:* I. Ugi, *Proc. Est. Acad. Sci. Chem.* **40,** 1-13 (1991); I. Ugi *et al., Comp. Org. Syn.* **2,** 1083-1109 (1991).

Organic Name Reactions

408. Ullmann Reaction

F. Ullmann, *Ann.* **332**, 38 (1904); F. Ullmann, P. Sponagel, *Ber.* **38**, 2211 (1905).

Copper-mediated coupling of aryl halides. Biaryl ether synthesis is similarly accomplished with aryl halides and phenols:

$$2 \ \text{C}_6\text{H}_5\text{-I} \xrightarrow{\text{Cu}} \text{C}_6\text{H}_5\text{-C}_6\text{H}_5 + \text{CuI}_2$$

P. E. Fanta, *Chem. Rev.* **38**, 139 (1946); **64**, 613 (1964); A. A. Moroz, M. S. Shvartsberg, *Russ. Chem. Rev.* **43**, 679 (1974); P. E. Fanta, *Synthesis* **1974**, 9; M. F. Semmelhack *et al.*, *J. Am. Chem. Soc.* **103**, 6460 (1981); D. W. Knight, *Comp. Org. Syn.* **3**, 499-507 (1991). *Cf.* Glaser Coupling.

409. Urech Cyanohydrin Method (Ultee Cyanohydrin Method)

F. Urech, *Ann.* **164**, 225 (1872); A. J. Ultee, *Rec. Trav. Chim.* **28**, 1 (1909).

Cyanohydrin formation by addition of alkali cyanide to the carbonyl group in the presence of acetic acid (Urech method) or by reaction of the carbonyl compound with anhydrous hydrogen cyanide in the presence of a basic catalyst (Ultee cyanohydrin method):

$$\text{RR}^1\text{CO} + \text{KCN} + \text{CH}_3\text{COOH} \longrightarrow \text{RR}^1\text{C(OH)CN} + \text{CH}_3\text{COO}^- \text{K}^+$$

$$\text{RR}^1\text{CO} + \text{HCN} \xrightarrow{\text{HO}^-} \text{RR}^1\text{C(OH)CN}$$

A. J. Ultee, *Ber.* **39**, 1856 (1906); *Rec. Trav. Chim.* **28**, 248, 257 (1909); K. N. Welch, G. R. Clemo, *J. Chem. Soc.* **1928**, 2629; H. R. Dittmar, **US 2101823** (1937); V. Migrdichian, *The Chemistry of Organic Cyanogen Compounds* (New York, 1947) p 173; D. T. Mowry, *Chem. Rev.* **42**, 231 (1948); P. Kurz, *Houben-Weyl* **8**, 274 (1952); R. F. B. Cox, R. T. Stormont, *Org. Synth.* **coll. vol. 2**, 7 (1955). *Cf.* Bucherer-Bergs Reaction; Kiliani-Fischer Synthesis.

410. Urech Hydantoin Synthesis

F. Urech, *Ann.* **165**, 99 (1873).

Formation of hydantoins from α-amino acids by treatment with potassium cyanate in aqueous solution and heating the salt of the intermediate hydantoic acid with 25% hydrochloric acid:

H. D. Dakin, *Am. Chem. J.* **44**, 48 (1910); T. B. Johnson, *J. Am. Chem. Soc.* **35**, 780 (1913); W. J. Boyd, W. Robson, *Biochem. J.* **29**, 542, 546, 2256 (1935); E. Ware, *Chem. Rev.* **46**, 407 (1950); M. Sainsbury, R. S. Theobald, *Rodd's Chemistry of Carbon Compounds* **IVC**, 185 (1986).

411. Vilsmeier-Haack Reaction

A. Vilsmeier, A. Haack, *Ber.* **60**, 119 (1927).

Formylation of activated aromatic or heterocyclic compounds with disubstituted formamides and phosphorus oxychloride:

Reviews: M. R. de Maheas, *Bull. Soc. Chim. Fr.* **1962**, 1989; W. G. Jackson *et al.*, *J. Am. Chem. Soc.* **103**, 533 (1981); C. Jutz, *Adv. Org. Chem.* **9**, 225-342 (1976); O. Meth-Cohn, S. P. Stanforth, *Comp. Org. Syn.* **2**, 777-794 (1991).

412. Voight Amination

K. Voight, *J. Prakt. Chem.* [2] **34**, 1 (1886).

Amination of benzoins with amines in the presence of phosphorus pentoxide or hydrochloric acid:

H. H. Strain, *J. Am. Chem. Soc.* **51**, 269 (1929); R. M. Cowper, T. S. Stevens, *J. Chem. Soc.* **1940**, 347; P. L. Julian *et al.*, *J. Am. Chem. Soc.* **67**, 1203 (1945); R. E. Lutz *et al.*, *ibid.* **70**, 2016 (1948); I. A. Kaye *et al.*, *ibid.* **75**, 746 (1953); J. Iwao *et al.*, *J. Pharm. Soc. Jpn.* **74**, 551 (1954); R. E. Lutz, J. W. Baker, *J. Org. Chem.* **21**, 49 (1956).

413. Volhard-Erdmann Cyclization
J. Volhard, H. Erdmann, *Ber.* **18**, 454 (1885).

Synthesis of alkyl and aryl thiophenes by cyclization of disodium succinate or other 1,4-difunctional compounds (γ-oxo acids, 1,4-diketones, chloroacetyl-substituted esters) with phosphorus heptasulfide:

L. H. Friedburg, *J. Am. Chem. Soc.* **12**, 83 (1890); *J. Chem. Soc.* **58**, 1400 (1890); R. Phillips, *Org. Synth.* **coll. vol. II,** 578 (1943); F. F. Blicke, *Heterocycl. Compd.* **1,** 212 (1950); D. E. Wolf, K. Folkers, *Org. React.* **4,** 412 (1951); R. F. Feldkamp, B. F. Tullar, *Org. Synth.* **coll. vol. IV,** 671 (1963).

414. von Braun Amide Degradation
H. von Pechmann, *Ber.* **33,** 611 (1900); J. von Braun, *ibid.* **37,** 3210 (1904).

$$RCONHR^1 \xrightarrow{PCl_5} RCN + R^1Cl$$

Mechanistic study: B. A. Phillips *et al., Tetrahedron* **29,** 3309 (1973). Application to *N-t-*butylamides: R. B. Perni, G. W. Gribble, *Org. Prep. Proced. Int.* **15,** 297 (1983).

415. von Braun Reaction
J. von Braun, *Ber.* **40,** 3914 (1907); **42,** 2219 (1909); **44,** 1250 (1911).

Reaction of tertiary amines with cyanogen bromide to form disubstituted cyanamides and an alkyl halide:

$$R_2NR^1 + BrCN \longrightarrow R_2NCN + R^1Br$$

Mechanistic correlation with Ritter, Bischler-Napieralski, Beckmann and Schmidt reactions, *q.q.v.:* G. Fodor, S. Nagubandi, *Tetrahedron* **36,** 1279 (1980). Synthetic applications: S. Siddiqui *et al., Z. Naturforsch.* **37b,** 1481 (1982); *idem et al., Pak. J. Sci. Ind. Res.* **30,** 163 (1987). *Reviews:* H. A. Hageman, *Org. React.* **7,** 198-262 (1953); J. H. Cooley, E. J. Evain, *Synthesis* **1989,** 1-7.

416. von Richter (Cinnoline) Synthesis
V. von Richter, *Ber.* **16,** 677 (1883).

Formation of cinnoline derivatives by diazotization of *o*-aminoarylpropiolic acids or *o*-aminoarylacetylenes followed by hydration and cyclization:

M. Busch, M. Klett, *Ber.* **25,** 2847 (1892); N. J. Leonard, *Chem. Rev.* **37,** 270 (1945); K. Schofield, J. C. E. Simpson, *J. Chem. Soc.* **1945,** 512, K. Schofield, T. Swain, *ibid.* **1949,** 2393; J. C. E. Simpson, *Condensed Pyridazine and Pyrazine Rings* (New York, 1953) p 16; G. R. Ramage, J. K. Landquist, *Chemistry of Carbon Compounds* **IVB,** 1217 (1959); G. T. Rogere *et al., Tetrahedron Lett.* **9,** 1028 (1968); A. C. Ellis *et al., J. Chem. Soc. Chem. Commun.* **1977,** 152. *Cf.* Widman-Stoermer Synthesis.

417. von Richter Rearrangement
V. von Richter, *Ber.* **4,** 21, 459, 553 (1871).

Carboxylation of *para-* or *meta-*substituted aromatic nitro compounds with cyanate at 120-270°. The carboxyl group enters with cine substitution in a position *ortho* to the eliminated nitro group:

J. F. Bunnett, *Q. Rev. Chem. Soc.* **12,** 15 (1958); D. Samuel, *J. Chem. Soc.* **1960,** 1318; J. Sauer, R. Huisgen, *Angew. Chem.* **72,** 314 (1960); M. Rosenblum, *J. Am. Chem. Soc.* **82,** 3796 (1960); E. Cullen, P. L'Ecuyer, *Can. J. Chem.* **39,** 144, 154, 382, 862 (1961); E. F. Ullman, E. A. Bartkus, *Chem. Ind. (London)* **1962,** 93; K. M. Ibne-Rasa, E. Koubak, *J. Org. Chem.* **28,** 3240 (1963); G. T. Rogers, T. L. V. Ulbricht, *Tetrahedron Lett.* **9,** 1028 (1968); A. C. Ellis, I. D. Rae, *Chem. Commun.* **1977,** 152; E. Tomitori *et al., Yakugaku Zasshi* **103,** 601 (1983).

418. Vorbrüggen Glycosylation
U. Niedballa, H. Vorbrüggen, *Angew. Chem. Int. Ed.* **9,** 461 (1970).

The reaction of silylated heterocyclic bases with peracylated sugars in the presence of Lewis acids to yield natural β-nucleosides. If the sugar lacks a 2α-acyloxy substituent, an anomeric mixture forms:

R = COCH₃, COPh

Lewis acid = BF₃ • O(CH₂CH₃)₂, SnCl₄, (CH₃)₃SiOSO₂CF₃, (CH₃)₃SiClO₄, TiCl₄, AlCl₃

Scope and limitations: H. Vorbrüggen *et al., Ber.* **114**, 1234 (1981). Mechanistic study: H. Vorbrüggen, G. Höfle, *ibid.* 1256. Synthetic applications: U. Niedballa, H. Vorbrüggen, *J. Org. Chem.* **39**, 3654, 3660, 3664, 3668, 3672 (1974); R. O. Dempcy, E. B. Skibo, *ibid.* **56**, 776 (1991); S. H. Kawai, G. Just, *Nucleosides Nucleotides* **10**, 1485 (1991). *Cf.* Hilbert-Johnson Reaction.

419. Wacker Oxidation

J. Smidt *et al., Angew. Chem. Int. Ed.* **1**, 176 (1959).

The oxidation of ethylene to acetaldehyde employing palladium chloride and cupric chloride as catalysts and molecular oxygen as oxidant. The reaction has been extensively developed for the oxidation of terminal alkenes to methyl ketones:

Application to hydroxy-α,β-unsaturated esters: S. X. Auclair *et al., Tetrahedron Lett.* **33**, 7739 (1992). Use of a multicomponent catalytic system: E. Monflier *et al., ibid.* **36**, 387 (1995). Synthetic applications: M. Romero *et al., ibid.* **35**, 3255 (1994); L. A. Paquette, X. Wang, *J. Org. Chem.* **59**, 2052 (1994). *Reviews:* L. S. Hegedus, *Comp. Org. Syn.* **4**, 552-559 (1991); J. Tsuji, *ibid.* **6**, 449-468.

420. Wagner-Jauregg Reaction

T. Wagner-Jauregg, *Ber.* **63**, 3213 (1930); *Ann.* **491**, 1 (1931).

Addition of maleic anhydride to diarylethylenes with formation of *bis* adducts which can be converted to aromatic ring systems:

F. Bergmann *et al., J. Am. Chem. Soc.* **69**, 1773, 1777, 1779 (1947); K. Alder in *Newer Methods of Preparative Organic Chemistry*, English Ed. (Interscience, New York, 1948) p 425; M. C. Kloetzel, *Org. React.* **4**, 32 (1948). *Cf.* Diels-Alder Reaction.

421. Wagner-Meerwein Rearrangement

G. Wagner, *J. Russ. Phys. Chem. Soc.* **31**, 690 (1899); H. Meerwein, *Ann.* **405**, 129 (1914).

Carbon-to-carbon migration of alkyl, aryl or hydride ions. The original example is the acid-catalyzed rearrangement of camphene hydrochloride to isobornyl chloride:

C. Le Drian, P. Vogel, *Helv. Chim. Acta* **70,** 1703 (1987); M. Asaoka, H. Takei, *Tetrahedron Lett.* **28,** 6343 (1987); L. U. Román *et al., J. Org. Chem.* **56,** 1938 (1991). Review of applications to alcohols: Y. Pocker in *Molecular Rearrangements* Part 1, P. de Mayo, Ed. (Wiley-Interscience, New York, 1963) pp 6-15; to bicyclic systems: J. Berson, *ibid.* 111-231; to terpenes: J. F. King, P. de Mayo, *ibid.* 813-840; to alkaloids: E. W. Warnhof, *ibid.* 842-879; to steroids: N. L. Wendler, *ibid.* 1020-1028. *Reviews:* R. L. Cargill *et al., Acc. Chem. Res.* **7,** 106-113 (1974); H. Hogeveen, E. M. G. A. Van Kruchten, *Top. Curr. Chem.* **80,** 89-124 (1979); J. R. Hanson, *Comp. Org. Syn.* **3,** 705-719 (1991). *Cf.* Demjanov Rearrangement; Nametkin Rearrangement; Retropinacol Rearrangement.

422. Walden Inversion
P. Walden, *Ber.* **28,** 1287, 2766 (1895).
Inversion of configuration of a chiral center in bimolecular nucleophilic substitution (S$_N$2) reactions:

H. A. Bent, *Chem. Rev.* **68,** 587 (1968); D. P. G. Harmon, *J. Chem. Educ.* **47,** 398 (1970); L. Kryger *et al., Acta Chem. Scand.* **26,** 2339, 2349 (1972); C. W. Shoppee, J. Nemorin, *J. Chem. Soc. Perkin Trans. I* **1973,** 542; K.-C. To *et al., J. Chem. Phys.* **74,** 1499 (1981).

423. Wallach Rearrangement
O. Wallach, L. Belli, *Ber.* **13,** 525 (1880).
Acid-catalyzed rearrangement of azoxybenzenes to *p*-hydroxyazobenzenes:

Reviews: K. H. Schündehütte, *Houben-Weyl* **10/3,** 771-773 (1965); E. Buncel in *Mechanisms of Molecular Migrations* **vol. 1,** B. S. Thyagarajan, Ed. (Interscience, New York, 1968) p 61; R. A. Cox, E. Buncel in *The Chemistry of Hydrazo, Azo and Azoxy Groups* pt. 2, S. Patai, Ed. (Wiley, New York, 1975) pp 808-837; J. Yamamoto *et al., Tetrahedron* **36,** 3177 (1980).

424. Weerman Degradation
R. A. Weerman, *Rec. Trav. Chim.* **37,** 1, 16 (1918).
Formation of an aldose with one less carbon from an aldonic acid by a Hofmann-type reaction, *q.v.,* of the corresponding amide. This is a general reaction of α-hydroxy carboxylic acids:

W. N. Haworth *et al., J. Chem. Soc.* **1934,** 1722; **1938,** 1975; E. S. Wallis, J. F. Lane, *Org. React.* **3,** 275 (1946); J. C. Sowden in *The Carbohydrates,* W. Pigman, Ed. (New York, 1957) p 120; L. F. Fieser, M. Fieser, *Advanced Organic Chemistry* (New York, 1961) p 945. *Cf.* Hofmann Reaction.

425. Weiss Reaction
U. Weiss, J. M. Edwards, *Tetrahedron Lett.* **1968,** 4885.
Reaction of 1,2-dicarbonyl compounds with 3-oxoglutarates to yield *cis*-bicyclo[3.3.0]octane-3,7-dione or [n.3.3]propellanedione (n > 2) tetracarboxylates. Subsequent acid-catalyzed hydrolysis and decarboxylation yield the respective 2,4,6,8-unsubstituted diones:

Organic Name Reactions

$E = COOCH_3$; R^1 or $R^2 = H$, alkyl, aryl or R^1—$R^2 = (CH_2)_n$, $n > 2$

Experimental procedure: S. H. Bertz *et al., Org. Synth.* **coll. vol. VII**, 50 (1990). Review of synthetic applications: A. K. Gupta *et al., Tetrahedron* **47**, 3665-3710 (1991). *Review:* H.-U. Reissig, "The Weiss Reaction" in *Organic Synthesis Highlights*, J. Mulzer *et al.,* Eds. (VCH, New York, 1991) pp 121-125.

426. Wessely-Moser Rearrangement
F. Wessely, G. H. Moser, *Monatsh. Chem.* **56**, 97 (1930).
Rearrangement of flavones and flavanones possessing a 5-hydroxyl group, through fission of the heterocyclic ring and reclosure of the intermediate diaroylmethanes in the alternate direction:

alternate substrates: chromones, isoflavones, flavonols, xanthones, furanochromones

Reviews: Wheeler, *Rec. Chem. Prog.* **18**, 133 (1957); T. R. Seshadri, *Tetrahedron* **6**, 169 (1959); H. D. Locksley, *Fortschr. Chem. Org. Naturst.* **30**, 292 (1973).

427. Westphalen-Lettré Rearrangement
T. Westphalen, *Ber.* **48**, 1064 (1915); H. Lettré, M. Müller, *ibid.* **70**, 1947 (1937).
Dehydration of 5-hydroxycholesterol derivatives accompanied by C-10 to C-5 methyl migration in compounds with a β-substituent at C-6:

Early review: N. L. Wendler in *Molecular Rearrangements* Part 2, P. de Mayo, Ed. (Wiley-Interscience, New York, 1964) p 1027. A. T. Rowland, *J. Org. Chem.* **29**, 222 (1964); J. W. Blunt *et al., Tetrahedron* **21**, 1567 (1965); K. Kieslich, G. Schulz, *Ann.* **726**, 152 (1969); B. Marples, J. G. L. Jones, *J. Chem. Soc. C* **1970**, 2273; J. Wicha, *Tetrahedron Lett.* **1972**, 2877; P. Kocovsky *et al., Collect. Czech. Chem. Commun.* **44**, 234 (1979).

428. Wharton Reaction
P. S. Wharton, D. H. Bohlen, *J. Org. Chem.* **26**, 3615 (1961); P. S. Wharton, *ibid.* 4781.
Reduction of α,β-epoxy ketones by hydrazine to allylic alcohols:

Improved procedure: C. Dupuy, J. L. Luche, *Tetrahedron* **45**, 3437 (1989). Synthetic applications: S. Takano *et al., Synlett* **1991**, 636; T. Yoshimitsu *et al., Synthesis* **1994**, 1029; K. Yamada *et al., J. Org. Chem.* **63**, 3666 (1998). *Review:* D. Caine, *Org. Prep. Proced. Int.* **20**, 3-8 (1988); A. R. Chamberlin, D. J. Sall, *Comp. Org. Syn.* **8**, 927-929 (1991). *Cf.* Eschenmoser Fragmentation; Grob Fragmentation.

429. Whiting Reaction
P. Nayler, M. C. Whiting, *J. Chem. Soc.* **1954**, 4006.
Alkynediols are reduced by lithium aluminum hydride in ether or tertiary amines to dienes:

R. A. Raphael, *Acetylene Compounds in Organic Synthesis* (New York, 1955) p 114; O. Isler, *et al., Helv. Chim. Acta* **39,** 454 (1956); L. F. Fieser, M. Fieser, *Reagents for Organic Synthesis* (New York, 1967) p 385.

430. Wichterle Reaction

O. Wichterle *et al., Collect. Czech. Chem. Commun.* **13,** 300 (1948).

Modification of the Robinson annulation, *q.v.*, in which 1,3-dichloro-*cis*-2-butene is used instead of methyl vinyl ketone:

M. Kobayashi, T. Matsumoto, *Chem. Lett.* **1973,** 957; H. Yoshioka *et al., Tetrahedron Lett.* **1979,** 3489. *Review:* M. Hudlicky, *Collect. Czech. Chem. Commun.* **58,** 2229-2244 (1993).

431. Widman-Stoermer Synthesis

O. Widman, *Ber.* **17,** 722 (1884); R. Stoermer, H. Fincke, *Ber.* **42,** 3115 (1909).

Synthesis of cinnolines by cyclization of diazotized *o*-aminoarylethylenes at room temperature:

N. J. Leonard, *Chem. Rev.* **37,** 270 (1945); J. C. E. Simpson, *Condensed Pyridazine and Pyrazine Rings* (New York, 1953) p 6; T. L. Jacobs, *Heterocycl. Compd.* **6,** 137 (1957); G. R. Ramage, J. K. Landquist, *Chemistry of Carbon Compounds* **IVB,** 1217 (1959). *Cf.* von Richter (Cinnoline) Synthesis.

432. Willgerodt-Kindler Reaction

C. Willgerodt, *Ber.* **20,** 2467 (1887); **21,** 534 (1888); K. Kindler, *Ann.* **431,** 193 (1923).

Conversion of aryl alkyl ketones to amides and/or the ammonium salts of the corresponding acids by aqueous ammonium polysulfide or by sulfur and a primary or secondary amine:

$$ArCO(CH_2)_nCH_3 \xrightarrow[H_2O]{(NH_4)_2S_x} Ar(CH_2)_{n+1}-CONH_2 + Ar(CH_2)_{n+1}-COO^- \ NH_4^+$$

Reviews: M. Carmack, M. A. Spielman, *Org. React.* **3,** 83 (1946); R. Wegler *et al., Newer Methods of Preparative Organic Chemistry* vol. 3 (Academic Press, New York, 1964) pp 1-51; E. E. Campaigne in *The Chemistry of the Carbonyl Group,* S. Patai, Ed. (Wiley, New York, 1966) p 954; A. L. J. Beckwith, *The Chemistry of Amides,* J. Zabicky, Ed. (Interscience, London, 1970) pp 145-147; S. W. Schneller, *Int. J. Sulfur Chem.* **8,** 591 (1976); G. Purrello, *Heterocycles* **65,** 411-449 (2005).

433. Williamson Synthesis

A. W. Williamson, *J. Chem. Soc.* **4,** 229 (1852).

Synthesis of symmetrical or unsymmetrical ethers by alkylation of alkoxides with primary alkyl halides, sulfates or tosylates; usually by an S_N2 mechanism:

$$OR^- + R^1X \longrightarrow ROR^1$$

Reviews: H. Feuer, J. Hooz in *The Chemistry of the Ether Linkage,* S. Patai, Ed. (Wiley, New York, 1967) pp 446-460; H. O. Kalinowski *et al., Ber.* **114,** 477 (1981). Applications on solid support: A. Weissberg *et al., J. Comb. Chem.* **3,** 154 (2001). Catalytic synthesis of alkyl aryl ethers: E. Fuhrmann, J. Talbiersky, *Org. Process Res. Dev.* **9,** 206 (2005).

434. Wittig Reaction; Horner Reaction; Horner-Wadsworth-Emmons Reaction

G. Wittig, U. Schöllkopf, *Ber.* **87,** 1318 (1954); G. Wittig, W. Haag, *ibid.* **88,** 1654 (1955).

Alkene formation from carbonyl compounds and phosphonium ylides, proceeding primarily through the proposed betaine and/or oxaphosphetane intermediates. The stereoselectivity can be controlled by the choice of ylide, carbonyl compound, and reaction conditions:

When the ylide is replaced with a phosphine oxide carbanion, the reaction is referred to as the **Horner reaction:** L. Horner *et al., Ber.* **91,** 61 (1958); *idem et al., ibid.* **92,** 2499 (1959).

When the ylide is replaced with a phosphonate carbanion, the reaction is referred to as the **Horner-Emmons-Wadsworth reaction:** W. S. Wadsworth, Jr., W. D. Emmons, *J. Am. Chem. Soc.* **83,** 1733 (1961).

Application to the synthesis of β,γ-unsaturated amides: T. Janecki *et al., Tetrahedron* **51,** 1721 (1995). *Reviews:* A. Maercker, *Org. React.* **14,** 270-490 (1965); K. P. C. Vollhardt, *Synthesis* **1975,** 765-780; W. S. Wadsworth, Jr., *Org. React.* **25,** 73-253 (1977); I. Gosney, A. G. Rowley in *Organophosphorus Reagents in Organic Synthesis,* J. I. G. Cadogan, Ed. (Academic Press, New York, 1979) pp 17-153; B. E. Maryanoff, A. B. Reitz, *Chem. Rev.* **89,** 863-927 (1989); S. E. Kelly, *Comp. Org. Syn.* **1,** 755-782 (1991). Reviews of mechanistic studies: W. E. McEwen *et al., ACS Symp. Ser.* **486,** 149-161 (1992); E. Vedejs, M. J. Peterson, *Top. Stereochem.* **21,** 1-157 (1994). *Cf.* Peterson Reaction; Tebbe Reaction.

435. [1,2]-Wittig Rearrangement
G. Wittig, L. Löhmann, *Ann.* **550,** 260 (1942); G. Wittig, *Experientia* **14,** 389 (1958).

Rearrangement of ethers with alkyl lithiums to yield alcohols *via* a [1,2]-shift:

$$R-CH_2-O-R^1 \xrightarrow{R^2Li} R^2H + R-\underset{R^1}{CH}-O^- Li^+ \longrightarrow R-\underset{R^1}{CH}-OH$$

Reviews: H. E. Zimmerman in *Molecular Rearrangements* Part 1, P. de Mayo, Ed. (Wiley-Interscience, New York, 1963) p 372-377; L. Brandsma, J. F. Arens in *Chemistry of the Ether Linkage* S. Patai, Ed. (Interscience, New York, 1967) pp 570-580; U. Schöllkopf, *Angew. Chem.* **82,** 795 (1970); A. R. Lepley, A. G. Giumanini in *Mechanisms of Molecular Migrations* **vol. 3,** B. S. Thyagarajan, Ed. (Interscience, New York, 1971); U. Schöllkopf, *Ind. Chim. Belge* **36,** 1057 (1971); G. Tennant, *Annu. Rep. Prog. Chem. Sec. B* **68,** 241 (1972); R. W. Hoffmann, *Angew. Chem.* **91,** 625 (1979); *idem, Nachr. Chem. Tech. Lab.* **30,** 483 (1982). *Cf.* Meisenheimer Rearrangements; Stevens Rearrangement.

436. [2,3]-Wittig Rearrangement
J. Cast *et al., J. Chem. Soc.* **1960,** 3521; U. Schöllkopf, K. Fellenberger, *Ber.* **698,** 80 (1966); Y. Makisumi, S. Notzumoto, *Tetrahedron Lett.* **1966,** 6393.

[2,3]-Sigmatropic rearrangement of the conjugate bases of allylic ethers with high regioselectivity. The stereoselectivity is highly dependent on the nature of the substrate:

Y = alkynyl, alkenyl, Ph, COR, CN
base = LDA, *n*-BuLi, NaNH₂

Methods development for ring contractions generating enediynes: H. Audrain *et al., Tetrahedron* **50,** 1469 (1994). Review of stereoselectivity: K. Mikami, T. Nakai, *Synthesis* **1994,** 594. *Reviews:* J. A. Marshall, *Comp. Org. Syn.* **3,** 975-1014 (1991); T. Nakai, K. Mikami, *Org. React.* **46,** 105-209 (1994). *Cf.* Meisenheimer Rearrangements; Mislow-Evans Rearrangement; Sommelet-Hauser Rearrangement.

437. Wohl Degradation; Zemplén Modification
A. Wohl, *Ber.* **26,** 730 (1893); **32,** 3666 (1899); G. Zemplén, *Ber.* **59,** 1254, 2402 (1926).

Method for the conversion of an aldose into an aldose with one less carbon atom by the reversal of the cyanohydrin synthesis. In the Wohl method the nitrile group is eliminated by treatment with ammoniacal silver oxide; in the **Zemplén modification** sodium alkoxide is used in the elimination of the nitrile:

Reviews: V. Deulofeu, *Adv. Carbohydr. Chem.* **4,** 129, 138 (1949); R. Bognár *et al., Ann.* **680,** 118 (1964); W. W. Wendall, *Tetrahedron Lett.* **1970,** 3439; L. Hough, A. C. Richardson, *The Carbohydrates* **1A,** 128 (1972).

438. Wohl-Ziegler Reaction
A. Wohl, *Ber.* **52,** 51 (1919); K. Ziegler *et al., Ann.* **551,** 30 (1942).

Allylic bromination of olefins with *N*-bromosuccinimide. Peroxides or ultraviolet light are used as initiators:

Reviews: C. Djerassi, *Chem. Rev.* **43**, 271 (1948); L. Horner, E. M. Winkelman, *Angew. Chem.* **71**, 349 (1959); S. S. Novikov *et al., Russ. Chem. Rev.* **31**, 671 (1962); A. Nechvatal, *Adv. Free-Radical Chem.* **4**, 175-201 (1972).

439. Wolff-Kishner Reduction; Huang-Minlon Modification
N. Kishner, *J. Russ. Phys. Chem. Soc.* **43**, 582 (1911), *C.A.* **6**, 347 (1912); L. Wolff, *Ann.* **394**, 86 (1912); Huang-Minlon, *J. Am. Chem. Soc.* **68**, 2487 (1946).

Complete reduction of carbonyl compounds to methyl or methylene groups on heating with hydrazine hydrate and a base. In the **Huang-Minlon modification** diethylene glycol is used as a solvent:

Reviews: D. Todd, *Org. React.* **4**, 378 (1948); H. H. Szmant, *Angew. Chem. Int. Ed.* **7**, 120 (1968); F. Asinger, H. H. Vogel, *Houben-Weyl* **5/1a**, 251, 456 (1970); H. Balli, *ibid.* **5/1b**, 629 (1972); R. O. Hutchins, M. K. Hutchins, *Comp. Org. Syn.* **8**, 327-343 (1991). Bond cleavage: R. P. Lemieux, P. Beak, *Tetrahedron Lett.* **30**, 1353 (1989). Synthetic application: A. Srikrishna, D. Vijaykumuv, *J. Chem. Soc. Perkin Trans. 1* **1999**, 1265. *Cf.* Clemmensen Reduction; Haworth Phenanthrene Synthesis.

440. Wolff Rearrangement
L. Wolff *Ann.* **394**, 25 (1912).

Rearrangement of diazoketones to ketenes thermally, photochemically or catalytically. The rearrangement is the key step in the Arndt-Eistert synthesis, *q.v.*:

Reviews: P. A. S. Smith in *Molecular Rearrangements* Part 1, Ed. (Wiley-Interscience, New York, 1963) pp 528-550, 558-568; W. Kirmse, *Carbene Chemistry* (Academic Press, New York, 2nd ed., 1971) pp 475-492; H. Meier, K. P. Zeller, *Angew. Chem. Int. Ed.* **14**, 32 (1975); M. Torres, *Pure Appl. Chem.* **52**, 1623 (1980); C. B. Gill, *Comp. Org. Syn.* **3**, 887-912 (1991). Photo-induced mechanistic studies: T. Lippert *et al., J. Am. Chem. Soc.* **118**, 1551 (1996); Y. Chiang *et al., ibid.* **121**, 5930 (1999). Synthetic application: Y. R. Lee *et al., Tetrahedron Lett.* **40**, 8219 (1999).

441. Wolffenstein-Böters Reaction
O. Böters, R. Wolffenstein, **DE 194883** (1906); **FR 380121** (1907); **GB 17521** (1907); **US 923761** (1909).

Simultaneous oxidation and nitration of aromatic compounds to nitrophenols with nitric acid or the higher oxides of nitrogen in the presence of a mercury salt as catalyst:

R. Wolffenstein, O. Böters, *Ber.* **46**, 586 (1913); F. H. Westheimer *et al., J. Am. Chem. Soc.* **69**, 773 (1947); M. Carmack *et al., ibid.* 785; E. E. Aristoff *et al., Ind. Eng. Chem.* **40**, 1281 (1948); W. Seidenfaden, W. Pawellek, *Houben-Weyl* **10/1**, 815 (1971).

442. Woodward *cis*-Hydroxylation
R. B. Woodward, **US 2687435** (1954); R. B. Woodward, F. V. Brutcher, *J. Am. Chem. Soc.* **80**, 209 (1958).

The hydroxylation of an olefin with iodine and silver acetate in wet acetic acid to give *cis*-glycols:

L. B. Barkley, M. W. Farrar, *J. Am. Chem. Soc.* **76**, 5014, (1954); W. S. Knowles, Q. E. Thompson, *ibid.* **79**, 3212 (1957); W. F. Forbes, R. Shelton, *J. Org. Chem.* **24**, 436 (1959); F. D. Gunstone, *Adv. Org. Chem.* **1**, 117 (1960). Application to steroids: L. Mangoni, V. Dovinola, *Tetrahedron Lett.* **1969**, 5235; P. Kocovsky, V. Cerny, *Collect. Czech. Chem. Commun.* **42**, 163 (1977). Modification: L. Mangoni *et al., Gazz. Chim. Ital.* **105**, 377 (1975). *Cf.* Prévost Reaction.

443. Wurtz-Fittig Reaction

B. Tollens, R. Fittig, *Ann.* **131**, 303 (1864); R. Fittig, J. König, *ibid.* **144**, 277 (1867).
Formation of alkylated aromatic hydrocarbons on coupling of an alkyl and an aryl halide with sodium:

T. L. Kwa, C. Boelhouwer, *Tetrahedron* **25**, 5771 (1969); B. J. Wakefield, *Comp. Organometal. Chem.* **7**, 45 (1982); K. Miyoshi *et al., Chemosphere* **41**, 819 (2000).

444. Wurtz Reaction

A. Wurtz, *Ann. Chim. Phys.* [3] **44**, 275 (1855); *Ann.* **96**, 364 (1855).
Coupling of two alkyl radicals by treating two moles of alkyl halides with two moles of sodium:

$$2RX + 2Na \longrightarrow R-R + 2NaX$$

J. L. Wardell, *Comp. Organometal. Chem.* **1**, 52 (1982); W. E. Lindsell, *ibid.* 193; B. J. Wakefield, *ibid.* **7**, 45; D. C. Billington, *Comp. Org. Syn.* **3**, 413-423 (1991).

445. Ziegler Method (Thorpe-Ziegler Method)

K. Ziegler *et al., Ann.* **504**, 94 (1933).
Cyclization of dinitriles at high dilution in dialkyl ether in the presence of ether-soluble metal alkylanilide and hydrolysis of the resultant imino-nitrile with formation of macrocyclic ketones (yield is dependent on ring size):

K. Ziegler *et al., ibid.* **511**, 1 (1933); **512**, 164; **513**, 43 (1934); *idem, Ber.* **67**, 139 (1934); *idem, et al., Ann.* **528**, 114, 143 (1937); R. C. Fuson in *Organic Chemistry* **vol. I**, H. Gilman, Ed. (New York, 1943) p 89; V. Migrdichian, *The Chemistry of Organic Cyanogen Compounds* (New York, 1947) p 288; K. Ziegler, *Houben-Weyl* **4/2**, 758 (1955). *Review:* J. P. Schaefer, J. J. Bloomfield, *Org. React.* **15**, 1-203 (1967). *Cf.* Thorpe Reaction.

446. Ziegler-Natta Polymerization

K. Ziegler *et al., Angew. Chem.* **67**, 426, 541 (1955); G. Natta, *ibid.* **68**, 393 (1956).
Polymerization of vinyl monomers under mild conditions using Lewis acid catalysts to give a stereoregulated, or tactic, polymer.
K. Ziegler, *ibid.* **71**, 623 (1959); **72**, 829 (1960); C. L. Arcus in *Progress in Stereochemistry* **vol. 3**, P. B. D. de la Mare, W. Klyne, Eds. (Butterworth Inc., Washington, D.C., 1962) pp 269-288; M. N. Berger *et al., Adv. Catal.* **19**, 211 (1969); T. Keii, *Kinetics of Ziegler-Natta Polymerization* (Halsted Press, New York, 1973) pp 129-162; *Developments in Polymerization* **vol. 2**, R. N. Haward, Ed. (Burgess-Intl., Philadelphia, 1979) pp 81-148; H. J. Sinn, W. Kaminsky, *Adv. Organomet. Chem.* **18**, 207 (1980); D. M. P. Mingos, *Comp. Organometal. Chem.* **3**, 72-75 (1982); P. D. Gavens *et al., ibid.* 475-547.

447. Zimmermann Reaction

W. Zimmermann, *Z. Physiol. Chem.* **233**, 257 (1935).
The reaction that occurs between methylene ketones and aromatic polynitro compounds in the presence of alkali. When applied to 17-oxosteroids, the colored compounds formed can be used for the quantitative determination of 17-oxosteroids:

W. Zimmerman *et al., ibid.* **289**, 91 (1952); *idem. ibid.* **300**, 141 (1955). Studies on mechanism: Neunhoffer *et al., ibid.* **323**, 116 (1961); Foster, Mackie, *Tetrahedron* **18**, 1131 (1962); H. Hoffmeister, C. Rufer, *Ber.* **98**, 2376 (1965); B. T. Rudd, O. M. Galal, *Proc. Assoc. Clin. Biochem.* **4**, 175 (1967); C. S. Feldkamp *et al., Microchem. J.* **22**, 201 (1977). *Cf.* Janovsky Reaction.

448. Zincke Disulfide Cleavage

T. Zincke, *Ber.* **44**, 769 (1911).
Formation of sulfenyl halides by three essentially similar methods involving the action of chlorine or bromine on aryl disulfides, thiophenols, or arylbenzyl sulfides:

$$ArSSAr + X_2 \longrightarrow 2ArSX$$

$$ArSH + X_2 \longrightarrow ArSX + HX$$

$$ArSCH_2C_6H_5 + 2X_2 \longrightarrow ArSX + C_6H_5CHX_2 + HX$$

T. Zincke *et al., ibid.* **45,** 471 (1912); **51,** 751 (1918); *Ann.* **391,** 55 (1912); **400,** 1 (1913); **406,** 103 (1914); **416,** 86 (1918); M. H. Hubacher, *Org. Synth.* **coll. II,** 455 (1943); N. Kharasch *et al., Chem. Rev.* **39,** 283 (1946); A. Schöberl, A. Wagner, *Houben-Weyl* **9,** 268 (1955); E. Kühle, *Synthesis* **1970,** 561.

449. Zincke Nitration
T. Zincke, *J. Prakt. Chem.* **61,** 561 (1900).

Replacement of *ortho-* or *para*-bromine or iodine atoms (but not fluorine or chlorine atoms) in phenols by a nitro group on treatment with nitrous acid or a nitrite in acetic acid:

L. C. Raiford, W. Heyl, *Am. Chem. J.* **43,** 393 (1910); **44,** 209 (1911); H. H. Hodgson, J. Nixon, *J. Chem. Soc.* **1932,** 273; L. C. Raiford, G. R. Miller, *J. Am. Chem. Soc.* **55,** 2125 (1933); L. C. Raiford, A. L. LeRosen, *ibid.* **66,** 1872 (1944); W. Seidenfaden, D. Pawellek, *Houben-Weyl* **10/1,** 821 (1971).

450. Zincke-Suhl Reaction
T. Zincke, R. Suhl, *Ber.* **39,** 4148 (1906).

Phenol-dienone rearrangement of *p*-cresols by addition of carbon tetrachloride in the presence of aluminum chloride with formation of 4-methyl-4-trichloromethylcyclohexa-2,5-dienone:

M. S. Newman, A. G. Pinkus, *J. Org. Chem.* **19,** 978, 985, 992, 997 (1954); M. S. Newman, L. L. Wood, Jr., *J. Am. Chem. Soc.* **81,** 6450 (1959); G. A. Olah, *Friedel-Crafts and Related Reactions* **vol. I** (Interscience, New York, 1963) p 128.

CHEMICAL ABSTRACTS SERVICE
REGISTRY NUMBERS

CHEMICAL ABSTRACTS SERVICE REGISTRY NUMBERS

The following table provides the Chemical Abstracts Service (CAS) registry numbers for the monograph title compounds and selected derivatives. The table is ordered numerically by CAS registry number.

CHEMICAL ABSTRACTS REGISTRY NUMBERS

[50-00-0] Formaldehyde, *4235*
[50-01-1] Guanidine Hydrochloride, *4562*
[50-02-2] Dexamethasone, *2943*
[50-03-3] Hydrocortisone 21-Acetate, *4787*
[50-04-4] Cortisone 21-Acetate, *2539*
[50-06-6] Phenobarbital, *7238*
[50-07-7] Mitomycin C, *6215*
[50-09-9] Hexobarbital Sodium Salt, *4704*
[50-10-2] Oxyphenonium Bromide, *6975*
[50-11-3] Metharbital, *5961*
[50-12-4] Mephenytoin, *5853*
[50-13-5] Meperidine Hydrochloride, *5849*
[50-14-6] Vitamin D$_2$, *10018*
[50-18-0] Cyclophosphamide (anhydrous), *2747*
[50-22-6] Corticosterone, *2538*
[50-23-7] Hydrocortisone, *4787*
[50-24-8] Prednisolone, *7721*
[50-27-1] Estriol, *3707*
[50-28-2] Estradiol, *3703*
[50-29-3] DDT, *2841*
[50-32-8] Benzo[*a*]pyrene, *1103*
[50-33-9] Phenylbutazone, *7277*
[50-34-0] Propantheline Bromide, *7805*
[50-35-1] Thalidomide, *9255*
[50-36-2] Cocaine, *2455*
[50-37-3] Lysergide, *5634*
[50-39-5] Protheobromine, *7886*
[50-41-9] Clomiphene Citrate, *2386*
[50-42-0] Adiphenine Hydrochloride, *161*
[50-44-2] 6-Mercaptopurine, *5871*
[50-47-5] Desipramine, *2920*
[50-48-6] Amitriptyline, *487*
[50-49-7] Imipramine, *4920*
[50-50-0] Estradiol Benzoate, *3703*
[50-52-2] Thioridazine, *9359*
[50-53-3] Chlorpromazine, *2185*
[50-54-4] Quinidine Sulfate, *8060*
[50-55-5] Reserpine (anhydrous), *8145*
[50-56-6] Oxytocin, *6979*
[50-57-7] Lypressin, *5630*
[50-58-8] Phendimetrazine Bitartrate, *7220*
[50-59-9] Cephaloridine, *1979*
[50-60-2] Phentolamine, *7264*
[50-62-4] Hexobendine Dihydrochloride, *4705*
[50-63-5] Chloroquine Diphosphate, *2163*
[50-65-7] Niclosamide, *6519*
[50-67-9] Serotonin, *8462*
[50-69-1] D-Ribose, *8204*
[50-70-4] Sorbitol, *8725*
[50-71-5] Alloxan, *282*
[50-76-0] Dactinomycin, *2800*
[50-78-2] Aspirin, *851*
[50-81-7] Ascorbic Acid, *830*
[50-85-1] *m*-Cresotic Acid, *2580*
[50-89-5] Thymidine, *9397*

[50-91-9] Floxuridine, *4112*
[50-98-6] Ephedrine Hydrochloride, *3608*
[50-99-7] Glucose, *4459*
[51-02-5] Pronethalol Hydrochloride, *7790*
[51-03-6] Piperonyl Butoxide, *7476*
[51-05-8] Procaine Hydrochloride, *7757*
[51-12-7] Nialamide, *6491*
[51-15-0] Pralidoxime Chloride, *7703*
[51-17-2] Benzimidazole, *1081*
[51-18-3] Triethylenemelamine, *9671*
[51-20-7] 5-Bromouracil, *1440*
[51-21-8] Fluorouracil, *4181*
[51-24-1] Tiratricol, *9462*
[51-26-3] Thyropropic Acid, *9412*
[51-28-5] 2,4-Dinitrophenol, *3280*
[51-34-3] Scopolamine, *8406*
[51-35-4] Hydroxyproline, *4840*
[51-41-2] Norepinephrine, *6695*
[51-42-3] Epinephrine Bitartrate, *3619*
[51-43-4] Epinephrine, *3619*
[51-45-6] Histamine, *4719*
[51-48-9] Thyroxine, *9415*
[51-49-0] Dextrothyroxine, *9415*
[51-52-5] Propylthiouracil, *7869*
[51-55-8] Atropine, *875*
[51-56-9] Homatropine DL-Hydrobromide, *4730*
[51-57-0] Methamphetamine Hydrochloride, *5948*
[51-60-5] Neostigmine Methyl Sulfate, *6464*
[51-61-6] Dopamine, *3421*
[51-63-8] Dextroamphetamine Sulfate, *2954*
[51-64-9] Dextroamphetamine, *2954*
[51-66-1] *p*-Acetanisidine, *51*
[51-67-2] Tyramine, *9835*
[51-68-3] Meclofenoxate, *5780*
[51-71-8] Phenelzine, *7221*
[51-73-0] Tremorine, *9582*
[51-74-1] Histamine Phosphate, *4719*
[51-75-2] Mechlorethamine, *5775*
[51-77-4] Gefarnate, *4378*
[51-79-6] Urethan, *9874*
[51-83-2] Carbachol, *1779*
[51-85-4] Cystamine, *2776*
[51-98-8] Norethindrone Acetate, *6697*
[52-01-7] Spironolactone, *8760*
[52-21-1] Prednisolone 21-Acetate, *7721*
[52-24-4] Triethylenethiophosphoramide, *9673*
[52-26-6] Morphine Hydrochloride, *6276*
[52-28-8] Codeine Phosphate, *2464*
[52-31-3] Cyclobarbital, *2711*
[52-39-1] Aldosterone, *225*
[52-43-7] Allobarbital, *263*
[52-46-0] Apholate, *728*
[52-49-3] Trihexyphenidyl Hydrochloride, *9695*
[52-51-7] Bronopol, *1447*
[52-52-8] Cycloleucine, *2734*

[52-53-9] Verapamil, *9950*
[52-62-0] Pentolinium Tartrate, *7132*
[52-66-4] Penicillamine DL-Form, *7088*
[52-67-5] Penicillamine, *7088*
[52-68-6] Trichlorfon, *9623*
[52-76-6] Lynestrenol, *5629*
[52-78-8] Norethandrolone, *6696*
[52-85-7] Famphur, *3932*
[52-86-8] Haloperidol, *4598*
[52-88-0] Atropine Methylnitrate, *875*
[52-89-1] Cysteine Hydrochloride, *2781*
[52-90-4] Cysteine, *2781*
[53-03-2] Prednisone, *7722*
[53-05-4] Tetrahydrocortisone, *9210*
[53-06-5] Cortisone, *2539*
[53-10-1] Hydroxydione Sodium, *4823*
[53-16-7] Estrone, *3708*
[53-19-0] Mitotane, *6216*
[53-21-4] Cocaine Hydrochloride, *2455*
[53-33-8] Paramethasone, *7029*
[53-34-9] Fluprednisolone, *4192*
[53-36-1] Methylprednisolone 21-Acetate, *6111*
[53-39-4] Oxandrolone, *6921*
[53-41-8] Androsterone, *640*
[53-43-0] Dehydroepiandrosterone, *2871*
[53-46-3] Methantheline Bromide, *5958*
[53-57-6] NADPH, *6348*
[53-59-8] NADP, *6348*
[53-60-1] Promazine Hydrochloride, *7783*
[53-70-3] 1,2:5,6-Dibenzanthracene, *3007*
[53-73-6] Angiotensin Amide, *651*
[53-79-2] Puromycin, *7943*
[53-84-9] NAD, *6344*
[53-86-1] Indomethacin, *4968*
[53-96-3] *N*-2-Fluorenylacetamide, *4157*
[54-03-5] Hexobendine, *4705*
[54-04-6] Mescaline, *5905*
[54-05-7] Chloroquine, *2163*
[54-06-8] Adrenochrome, *172*
[54-11-5] Nicotine, *6524*
[54-21-7] Salicylic Acid Sodium Salt, *8332*
[54-25-1] 6-Azauridine, *904*
[54-28-4] γ-Tocopherol, *9497*
[54-31-9] Furosemide, *4309*
[54-32-0] Moxisylyte, *6292*
[54-36-4] Metyrapone, *6159*
[54-42-2] Idoxuridine, *4891*
[54-47-7] Pyridoxal 5-Phosphate, *7979*
[54-49-9] Metaraminol, *5932*
[54-62-6] Aminopterin, *472*
[54-64-8] Thimerosal, *9317*
[54-71-7] Pilocarpine Hydrochloride, *7424*
[54-80-8] Pronethalol, *7790*
[54-85-3] Isoniazid, *5186*
[54-91-1] Pipobroman, *7480*
[54-92-2] Iproniazid, *5078*
[54-95-5] Pentylenetetrazole, *7141*
[54-96-6] 3,4-Diaminopyridine, *2986*

[55-03-8] Levothyroxine Sodium, *9415*
[55-06-1] Liothyronine Sodium Salt, *5510*
[55-10-7] Vanilmandelic Acid, *9933*
[55-16-3] Scopolamine Hydrochloride, *8406*
[55-18-5] *N*-Nitrosodiethylamine, *6636*
[55-21-0] Benzamide, *1060*
[55-22-1] Isonicotinic Acid, *5187*
[55-31-2] Epinephrine Hydrochloride, *3619*
[55-38-9] Fenthion, *4002*
[55-43-6] *N*-(2-Chloroethyl)dibenzyl-amine Hydrochloride, *2138*
[55-48-1] Atropine Sulfate, *875*
[55-55-0] *p*-Methylaminophenol Sulfate (anhydrous), *6017*
[55-56-1] Chlorhexidine, *2091*
[55-63-0] Nitroglycerin, *6607*
[55-65-2] Guanethidine, *4560*
[55-68-5] Phenylmercuric Nitrate, *7302*
[55-73-2] Bethanidine, *1186*
[55-86-7] Mechlorethamine Hydrochloride, *5775*
[55-91-4] Isoflurophate, *5176*
[55-94-7] Succinylcholine Bromide, *8874*
[55-97-0] Hexamethonium Bromide, *4688*
[55-98-1] Busulfan, *1505*
[56-03-1] Biguanide, *1215*
[56-04-2] Methylthiouracil, *6128*
[56-06-4] 2,4-Diamino-6-hydroxypy-rimidine, *2981*
[56-10-0] AET, *178*
[56-12-2] *γ*-Aminobutyric Acid, *430*
[56-23-5] Carbon Tetrachloride, *1816*
[56-25-7] Cantharidin, *1752*
[56-29-1] Hexobarbital, *4704*
[56-34-8] Tetraethylammonium Chloride, *9200*
[56-38-2] Parathion, *7033*
[56-40-6] Glycine, *4491*
[56-41-7] Alanine, *204*
[56-45-1] Serine, *8460*
[56-47-3] Deoxycorticosterone Acetate, *2901*
[56-49-5] 3-Methylcholanthrene, *6044*
[56-53-1] Diethylstilbestrol, *3129*
[56-54-2] Quinidine, *8060*
[56-55-3] 1,2-Benzanthracene, *1062*
[56-59-7] Felypressin, *3954*
[56-65-5] Adenosine Triphosphate, *155*
[56-69-9] 5-Hydroxytryptophan, *4847*
[56-72-4] Coumaphos, *2558*
[56-73-5] Glucose-6-phosphate, *4462*
[56-75-7] Chloramphenicol, *2077*
[56-81-5] Glycerol, *4484*
[56-82-6] Glyceraldehyde, *4481*
[56-84-8] Aspartic Acid, *840*
[56-85-9] Glutamine, *4471*
[56-86-0] Glutamic Acid, *4469*
[56-87-1] Lysine, *5636*
[56-88-2] L-Cystathionine, *2777*
[56-89-3] Cystine, *2782*
[56-92-8] Histamine Dihydrochloride, *4719*
[56-94-0] Demecarium Bromide, *2885*
[56-95-1] Chlorhexidine Diacetate, *2091*
[57-00-1] Creatine, *2568*
[57-03-4] Glycerophosphoric Acid (DL-*α*-form), *4486*

[57-06-7] Allyl Isothiocyanate, *295*
[57-08-9] *ε*-Acetamidocaproic Acid, *45*
[57-09-0] Cetrimonium Bromide, *2025*
[57-10-3] Palmitic Acid, *6996*
[57-11-4] Stearic Acid, *8804*
[57-13-6] Urea, *9867*
[57-14-7] 1,1-Dimethylhydrazine, *3247*
[57-15-8] Chlorobutanol, *2129*
[57-22-7] Vincristine, *9986*
[57-24-9] Strychnine, *8855*
[57-27-2] Morphine, *6276*
[57-29-4] Nalorphine Hydrochloride, *6361*
[57-30-7] Phenobarbital Sodium Salt, *7238*
[57-33-0] Pentobarbital Sodium Salt, *7130*
[57-37-4] Benactyzine Hydrochloride, *1029*
[57-39-6] Metepa, *5936*
[57-41-0] Phenytoin, *7322*
[57-42-1] Meperidine, *5849*
[57-43-2] Amobarbital, *570*
[57-44-3] Barbital, *962*
[57-47-6] Physostigmine, *7384*
[57-48-7] Fructose, *4273*
[57-50-1] Sucrose, *8881*
[57-53-4] Meprobamate, *5862*
[57-55-6] Propylene Glycol, *7855*
[57-57-8] *β*-Propiolactone, *7820*
[57-62-5] Chlortetracycline, *2192*
[57-63-6] Ethinyl Estradiol, *3734*
[57-64-7] Physostigmine Salicylate, *7384*
[57-66-9] Probenecid, *7754*
[57-67-0] Sulfaguanidine, *8908*
[57-68-1] Sulfamethazine, *8915*
[57-74-9] Chlordan(e), *2082*
[57-83-0] Progesterone, *7773*
[57-85-2] Testosterone Propionate, *9180*
[57-87-4] Ergosterol, *3659*
[57-88-5] Cholesterol, *2201*
[57-91-0] *α*-Estradiol, *3704*
[57-92-1] Streptomycin, *8826*
[57-94-3] Tubocurarine Chloride, *9807*
[57-96-5] Sulfinpyrazone, *8949*
[57-97-6] 9,10-Dimethyl-1,2-benzan-thracene, *3235*
[58-00-4] Apomorphine, *746*
[58-05-9] Folinic Acid, *4222*
[58-08-2] Caffeine, *1636*
[58-14-0] Pyrimethamine, *7985*
[58-15-1] Aminopyrine, *474*
[58-18-4] 17-Methyltestosterone, *6125*
[58-19-5] Dromostanolone, *3448*
[58-20-8] Testosterone 17*β*-Cyclopen-tanepropionate, *9180*
[58-22-0] Testosterone, *9180*
[58-25-3] Chlordiazepoxide, *2084*
[58-27-5] Menadione, *5831*
[58-28-6] Desipramine Hydrochloride, *2920*
[58-32-2] Dipyridamole, *3346*
[58-33-3] Promethazine Hydrochloride, *7786*
[58-34-4] Thiazinamium Methylsulfate, *9306*
[58-36-6] 10,10′-Oxydiphenoxarsine, *6961*
[58-37-7] Aminopromazine, *467*
[58-38-8] Prochlorperazine, *7761*
[58-39-9] Perphenazine, *7183*
[58-40-2] Promazine, *7783*

[58-46-8] Tetrabenazine, *9182*
[58-54-8] Ethacrynic Acid, *3717*
[58-55-9] Theophylline, *9285*
[58-56-0] Pyridoxine Hydrochloride, *7982*
[58-58-2] Puromycin Dihydrochloride, *7943*
[58-61-7] Adenosine, *153*
[58-63-9] Inosine, *4975*
[58-64-0] Adenosine Diphosphate, *154*
[58-68-4] NADH, *6344*
[58-71-9] Cephalothin Sodium Salt, *1982*
[58-73-1] Diphenhydramine, *3309*
[58-74-2] Papaverine, *7019*
[58-82-2] Bradykinin, *1359*
[58-85-5] Biotin, *1231*
[58-86-6] Xylose, *10087*
[58-89-9] Lindane, *5501*
[58-93-5] Hydrochlorothiazide, *4781*
[58-94-6] Chlorothiazide, *2168*
[58-95-7] *α*-Tocopherol Acetate, *9495*
[58-96-8] Uridine, *9877*
[58-97-9] 5′-Uridylic Acid, *9881*
[58-98-0] Uridine 5′-Diphosphate, *9878*
[59-00-7] Xanthurenic Acid, *10068*
[59-01-8] Kanamycin A, *5281*
[59-02-9] *α*-Tocopherol, *9495*
[59-05-2] Methotrexate, *5985*
[59-06-3] Ethopabate, *3745*
[59-14-3] Broxuridine, *1452*
[59-23-4] D-Galactose, *4335*
[59-26-7] Nikethamide, *6543*
[59-30-3] Folic Acid, *4221*
[59-31-4] Carbostyril, *1825*
[59-32-5] Chloropyramine, *2162*
[59-33-6] Pyrilamine Maleate, *7984*
[59-39-2] Piperoxan, *7478*
[59-40-5] Sulfaquinoxaline, *8939*
[59-42-7] Phenylephrine, *7286*
[59-43-8] Thiamine, *9295*
[59-46-1] Procaine, *7757*
[59-47-2] Mephenesin, *5850*
[59-50-7] Chlorocresol, *2133*
[59-51-8] Methionine DL-Form, *5975*
[59-52-9] Dimercaprol, *3209*
[59-56-3] *α*-Glucose-1-phosphate, *4461*
[59-58-5] Prosultiamine, *7882*
[59-63-2] Isocarboxazid, *5157*
[59-66-5] Acetazolamide, *53*
[59-67-6] Nicotinic Acid, *6525*
[59-87-0] Nitrofurazone, *6600*
[59-88-1] Phenylhydrazine Hydrochloride, *7293*
[59-89-2] *N*-Nitrosomorpholine, *6640*
[59-92-7] Levodopa, *5464*
[59-96-1] Phenoxybenzamine, *7256*
[59-97-2] Tolazoline Hydrochloride, *9506*
[59-98-3] Tolazoline, *9506*
[59-99-4] Neostigmine, *6464*
[60-00-0] EDTA, *3517*
[60-01-5] Tributyrin, *9620*
[60-02-6] Guanethidine Sulfate, *4560*
[60-09-3] *p*-Aminoazobenzene, *419*
[60-10-6] Dithizone, *3377*
[60-11-7] *p*-Dimethylaminoazobenzene, *3229*
[60-12-8] Phenethyl Alcohol, *7224*
[60-13-9] Amphetamine Sulfate, *582*
[60-18-4] Tyrosine, *9839*
[60-19-5] Tyramine Hydrochloride, *9835*
[60-23-1] Cysteamine, *2779*

[60-24-2] 2-Mercaptoethanol, 5869
[60-26-4] Hexamethonium, 4688
[60-27-5] Creatinine, 2569
[60-29-7] Ethyl Ether, 3806
[60-31-1] Acetylcholine Chloride, 87
[60-32-2] ε-Aminocaproic Acid, 432
[60-33-3] Linoleic Acid, 5505
[60-34-4] Methylhydrazine, 6086
[60-35-5] Acetamide, 43
[60-39-9] Mazipredone Hydrochloride, 5763
[60-40-2] Mecamylamine, 5774
[60-41-3] Strychnine Sulfate, 8855
[60-46-8] Aminopentamide, 459
[60-51-5] Dimethoate, 3220
[60-54-8] Tetracycline, 9196
[60-56-0] Methimazole, 5971
[60-57-1] Dieldrin, 3103
[60-70-8] Veratramine, 9952
[60-79-7] Ergonovine, 3655
[60-80-0] Antipyrine, 716
[60-81-1] Phloridzin, 7327
[60-82-2] Phloretin, 7326
[60-87-7] Promethazine, 7786
[60-91-3] Diethazine, 3108
[60-92-4] Cyclic AMP, 2708
[60-93-5] Quinine Dihydrochloride, 8061
[60-99-1] Methotrimeprazine, 5986
[61-00-7] Acepromazine, 32
[61-12-1] Dibucaine Hydrochloride, 3031
[61-16-5] Methoxamine Hydrochloride, 5987
[61-19-8] 5′-Adenylic Acid, 158
[61-24-5] Cephalosporin C, 1980
[61-25-6] Papaverine Hydrochloride, 7019
[61-33-6] Penicillin G, 7094
[61-50-7] N,N-Dimethyltryptamine, 3262
[61-54-1] Tryptamine, 9796
[61-56-3] Sulthiame, 8993
[61-57-4] Niridazole, 6563
[61-68-7] Mefenamic Acid, 5798
[61-72-3] Cloxacillin, 2419
[61-73-4] Methylene Blue, 6060
[61-75-6] Bretylium Tosylate, 1371
[61-76-7] Phenylephrine Hydrochloride, 7286
[61-78-9] p-Aminohippuric Acid, 442
[61-80-3] Zoxazolamine, 10199
[61-82-5] Amitrole, 489
[61-90-5] Leucine, 5451
[61-96-1] Nordefrin Hydrochloride (R*,S*-(±)-form), 6692
[62-13-5] Adrenalone Hydrochloride, 171
[62-31-7] Dopamine Hydrochloride, 3421
[62-33-9] EDTA Calcium Disodium Salt, 3517
[62-37-3] Chlormerodrin, 2105
[62-38-4] Phenylmercuric Acetate, 7300
[62-44-2] Phenacetin, 7204
[62-46-4] Thioctic Acid, 9326
[62-49-7] Choline, 2204
[62-50-0] Ethyl Methanesulfonate, 3827
[62-51-1] Methacholine Chloride, 5940
[62-53-3] Aniline, 659
[62-54-4] Calcium Acetate, 1646
[62-55-5] Thioacetamide, 9319
[62-56-6] Thiourea, 9367

[62-57-7] α-Aminoisobutyric Acid, 445
[62-59-9] Cevadine, 2033
[62-67-9] Nalorphine, 6361
[62-73-7] Dichlorvos, 3079
[62-74-8] Fluoroacetic Acid Sodium Salt, 4167
[62-75-9] N-Nitrosodimethylamine, 6637
[62-76-0] Sodium Oxalate, 8650
[62-90-8] Nandrolone Phenpropionate, 6365
[62-97-5] Diphemanil Methylsulfate, 3306
[63-05-8] Androstenedione, 638
[63-12-7] Benzquinamide, 1119
[63-25-2] Carbaryl, 1787
[63-39-8] Uridine 5′-Triphosphate, 9880
[63-42-3] Lactose, 5343
[63-45-6] Primaquine Diphosphate, 7744
[63-56-9] Thonzylamine Hydrochloride, 9373
[63-68-3] Methionine, 5975
[63-74-1] Sulfanilamide, 8925
[63-75-2] Arecoline, 778
[63-84-3] Dopa DL-Form, 3420
[63-89-8] Colfosceril Palmitate, 2477
[63-91-2] Phenylalanine, 7271
[63-92-3] Phenoxybenzamine Hydrochloride, 7256
[63-98-9] Phenacemide, 7203
[64-02-8] EDTA Tetrasodium Salt, 3517
[64-04-0] Phenethylamine, 7225
[64-10-8] Phenylurea, 7319
[64-17-5] Ethyl Alcohol, 3760
[64-18-6] Formic Acid, 4241
[64-19-7] Acetic Acid Glacial, 55
[64-31-3] Morphine Sulfate, 6276
[64-39-1] Promedol (anhydrous), 7784
[64-43-7] Amobarbital Sodium Salt, 570
[64-47-1] Physostigmine Sulfate, 7384
[64-55-1] Mebutamate, 5773
[64-65-3] Bemegride, 1027
[64-67-5] Diethyl Sulfate, 3130
[64-69-7] Iodoacetic Acid, 5025
[64-72-2] Chlortetracycline Hydrochloride, 2192
[64-73-3] Demeclocycline Hydrochloride, 2886
[64-75-5] Tetracycline Hydrochloride, 9196
[64-77-7] Tolbutamide, 9507
[64-85-7] Deoxycorticosterone, 2900
[64-86-8] Colchicine, 2471
[64-95-9] Adiphenine, 161
[65-19-0] Yohimbine Hydrochloride, 10102
[65-28-1] Phentolamine Methanesulfonate, 7264
[65-29-2] Gallamine Triethiodide, 4343
[65-30-5] Nicotine Sulfate, 6524
[65-31-6] Nicotine Bitartrate, 6524
[65-45-2] Salicylamide, 8328
[65-46-3] Cytidine, 2786
[65-49-6] p-Aminosalicylic Acid, 477
[65-71-4] Thymine, 9398
[65-82-7] N-Acetylmethionine, 96
[65-85-0] Benzoic Acid, 1091
[65-86-1] Orotic Acid, 6876
[66-02-4] 3,5-Diiodotyrosine, 3192
[66-22-8] Uracil, 9850

[66-23-9] Acetylcholine Bromide, 86
[66-25-1] Caproic Aldehyde, 1760
[66-27-3] Methyl Methanesulfonate, 6097
[66-28-4] Strophanthidin, 8851
[66-32-0] Strychnine Nitrate, 8855
[66-71-7] o-Phenanthroline, 7214
[66-72-8] Pyridoxal, 7978
[66-75-1] Uracil Mustard, 9851
[66-76-2] Dicumarol, 3090
[66-79-5] Oxacillin, 6904
[66-81-9] Cycloheximide, 2728
[66-86-4] Neomycin C, 6454
[66-93-3] 3-Quinuclidinol dl-Form Benzoate (Ester), 8082
[66-97-7] Psoralen, 7928
[67-03-8] Thiamine Hydrochloride, 9295
[67-07-2] Phosphocreatine, 7340
[67-16-3] Thiamine Disulfide, 9297
[67-20-9] Nitrofurantoin, 6599
[67-21-0] Ethionine DL-Form, 3738
[67-28-7] Nihydrazone, 6542
[67-42-5] EGTA, 3529
[67-43-6] Pentetic Acid, 7125
[67-45-8] Furazolidone, 4300
[67-47-0] 5-(Hydroxymethyl)-2-furaldehyde, 4832
[67-48-1] Choline Chloride, 2206
[67-52-7] Barbituric Acid, 963
[67-56-1] Methanol, 5957
[67-62-9] Methoxyamine, 5989
[67-63-0] Isopropyl Alcohol, 5208
[67-64-1] Acetone, 66
[67-66-3] Chloroform, 2141
[67-68-5] Dimethyl Sulfoxide, 3259
[67-71-0] Dimethyl Sulfone, 3258
[67-72-1] Hexachloroethane, 4679
[67-73-2] Fluocinolone Acetonide, 4150
[67-78-7] Triamcinolone 16,21-Diacetate, 9595
[67-92-5] Dicyclomine Hydrochloride, 3097
[67-96-9] Dihydrotachysterol, 3180
[67-97-0] Vitamin D₃, 10019
[67-99-2] Gliotoxin, 4441
[68-04-2] Sodium Citrate, 8602
[68-11-1] Thioglycolic Acid, 9336
[68-12-2] N,N-Dimethylformamide, 3243
[68-19-9] Vitamin B₁₂, 10014
[68-22-4] Norethindrone, 6697
[68-23-5] Norethynodrel, 6698
[68-26-8] Vitamin A, 10013
[68-35-9] Sulfadiazine, 8903
[68-36-0] 1,4-Bis(trichloromethyl)-benzene, 1303
[68-41-7] Cycloserine, 2751
[68-76-8] Triaziquone, 9603
[68-81-5] Iodinin, 5021
[68-88-2] Hydroxyzine, 4849
[68-90-6] Benziodarone, 1083
[68-91-7] Trimethaphan Camsylate, 9707
[68-94-0] Hypoxanthine, 4869
[68-96-2] 17α-Hydroxyprogesterone, 4839
[69-09-0] Chlorpromazine Hydrochloride, 2185
[69-14-7] Hexestrol Bis(β-diethylaminoethyl ether) Dihydrochloride, 4702
[69-22-7] Caffeine Citrate, 1636
[69-23-8] Fluphenazine, 4189

[69-24-9] Cinchotoxine, 2289
[69-25-0] Eledoisin, 3539
[69-27-2] Chlorisondamine Chloride, 2101
[69-33-0] Tubercidin, 9804
[69-43-2] Prenylamine Lactate, 7737
[69-46-5] Calcium Acetylsalicylate, 1647
[69-52-3] Ampicillin Sodium Salt, 586
[69-53-4] Ampicillin, 586
[69-57-8] Penicillin G Sodium Salt, 7094
[69-65-8] Mannitol, 5745
[69-72-7] Salicylic Acid, 8332
[69-78-3] Ellman's Reagent, 3551
[69-79-4] Maltose, 5714
[69-81-8] Adrenochrome Monosemicarbazone, 172
[69-89-6] Xanthine, 10059
[69-91-0] α-Phenylglycine, 7291
[69-93-2] Uric Acid, 9875
[70-00-8] Trifluridine, 9687
[70-07-5] Mephenoxalone, 5851
[70-11-1] ω-Bromoacetophenone, 1402
[70-18-8] Glutathione, 4475
[70-19-9] Thurfyl Nicotinate, 9395
[70-22-4] Oxotremorine, 6951
[70-25-7] N-Methyl-N'-nitro-N-nitrosoguanidine, 6103
[70-26-8] Ornithine, 6874
[70-30-4] Hexachlorophene, 4680
[70-34-8] 1-Fluoro-2,4-dinitrobenzene, 4172
[70-43-9] Barthrin, 1003
[70-47-3] Asparagine, 837
[70-49-5] Thiomalic Acid, 9343
[70-51-9] Deferoxamine, 2860
[70-69-9] p-Aminopropiophenone, 470
[70-70-2] Paroxypropione, 7044
[70-78-0] 3-Iodotyrosine, 5047
[71-00-1] Histidine, 4720
[71-23-8] n-Propyl Alcohol, 7842
[71-27-2] Succinylcholine Chloride, 8875
[71-30-7] Cytosine, 2795
[71-36-3] n-Butyl Alcohol, 1540
[71-41-0] 1-Pentanol, 7118
[71-43-2] Benzene, 1066
[71-44-3] Spermine, 8743
[71-48-7] Cobaltous Acetate, 2433
[71-55-6] 1,1,1-Trichloroethane, 9636
[71-58-9] Medroxyprogesterone 17-Acetate, 5793
[71-62-5] Veratridine, 9954
[71-63-6] Digitoxin, 3163
[71-67-0] Sulfobromophthalein Sodium, 8954
[71-68-1] Hydromorphone Hydrochloride, 4803
[71-73-8] Thiopental Sodium, 9350
[71-78-3] Pipradrol Hydrochloride, 7484
[71-81-8] Isopropamide Iodide, 5202
[71-82-9] Levallorphan Tartrate, 5458
[71-91-0] Tetraethylammonium Bromide, 9199
[72-14-0] Sulfathiazole, 8943
[72-17-3] Sodium Lactate, 8635
[72-18-4] Valine, 9909
[72-19-5] Threonine, 9380
[72-20-8] Endrin, 3578
[72-23-1] 11-Dehydrocorticosterone, 2869
[72-33-3] Mestranol, 5917

[72-43-5] Methoxychlor, 5990
[72-44-6] Methaqualone, 5960
[72-48-0] Alizarin, 251
[72-54-8] 1,1-Dichloro-2,2-bis(p-chlorophenyl)ethane, 3061
[72-57-1] Trypan Blue, 9792
[72-63-9] Methandrostenolone, 5951
[72-69-5] Nortriptyline, 6715
[72-80-0] Chlorquinaldol, 2190
[73-03-0] Cordycepin, 2529
[73-05-2] Phentolamine Hydrochloride, 7264
[73-09-6] Etozolin, 3891
[73-22-3] Tryptophan, 9797
[73-24-5] Adenine, 152
[73-31-4] Melatonin, 5816
[73-32-5] Isoleucine, 5179
[73-40-5] Guanine, 4564
[73-48-3] Bendroflumethiazide, 1037
[73-49-4] Quinethazone, 8056
[73-67-6] Toxopyrimidine, 9561
[73-78-9] Lidocaine Hydrochloride, 5482
[74-11-3] p-Chlorobenzoic Acid, 2125
[74-31-7] N,N'-Diphenyl-p-phenylenediamine, 3329
[74-39-5] Magneson, 5695
[74-55-5] Ethambutol, 3720
[74-61-3] 2,3-Dimercapto-1-propanesulfonic Acid, 3210
[74-79-3] Arginine, 780
[74-82-8] Methane, 5952
[74-83-9] Methyl Bromide, 6029
[74-84-0] Ethane, 3723
[74-85-1] Ethylene, 3791
[74-86-2] Acetylene, 90
[74-87-3] Methyl Chloride, 6041
[74-88-4] Methyl Iodide, 6087
[74-89-5] Methylamine, 6014
[74-90-8] Hydrogen Cyanide, 4795
[74-93-1] Methanethiol, 5956
[74-95-3] Methylene Bromide, 6061
[74-96-4] Ethyl Bromide, 3771
[74-98-6] Propane, 7799
[75-00-3] Ethyl Chloride, 3782
[75-01-4] Vinyl Chloride, 9994
[75-03-6] Ethyl Iodide, 3813
[75-04-7] Ethylamine, 3762
[75-05-8] Acetonitrile, 70
[75-07-0] Acetaldehyde, 39
[75-08-1] Ethanethiol, 3726
[75-09-2] Methylene Chloride, 6063
[75-10-5] Difluoromethane, 3151
[75-11-6] Methylene Iodide, 6066
[75-12-7] Formamide, 4237
[75-13-8] Isocyanic Acid, 5165
[75-15-0] Carbon Disulfide, 1811
[75-18-3] Methyl Sulfide, 6123
[75-19-4] Cyclopropane, 2748
[75-20-7] Calcium Carbide, 1656
[75-21-8] Ethylene Oxide, 3802
[75-25-2] Bromoform, 1420
[75-26-3] Isopropyl Bromide, 5210
[75-27-4] Bromodichloromethane, 1417
[75-29-6] Isopropyl Chloride, 5211
[75-30-9] Isopropyl Iodide, 5214
[75-31-0] Isopropylamine, 5209
[75-34-3] Ethylidene Chloride, 3810
[75-35-4] Vinylidene Chloride, 9996
[75-36-5] Acetyl Chloride, 85
[75-39-8] Acetaldehyde Ammonia, 40
[75-44-5] Phosgene, 7335
[75-46-7] Fluoroform, 4173
[75-47-8] Iodoform, 5033

[75-50-3] Trimethylamine, 9710
[75-52-5] Nitromethane, 6611
[75-56-9] Propylene Oxide, 7856
[75-58-1] Tetramethylammonium Iodide, 9225
[75-59-2] Tetramethylammonium Hydroxide, 9224
[75-60-5] Cacodylic Acid, 1604
[75-64-9] tert-Butylamine, 1545
[75-65-0] tert-Butyl Alcohol, 1542
[75-66-1] tert-Butyl Mercaptan, 1579
[75-69-4] Trichlorofluoromethane, 9640
[75-71-8] Dichlorodifluoromethane, 3064
[75-73-0] Carbon Tetrafluoride, 1817
[75-75-2] Methanesulfonic Acid, 5954
[75-76-3] Tetramethylsilane, 9229
[75-84-3] Neopentyl Alcohol, 6457
[75-85-4] tert-Pentyl Alcohol, 7140
[75-86-5] Acetone Cyanohydrin, 67
[75-87-6] Trichloroacetaldehyde, 9626
[75-89-8] Trifluoroethanol, 9682
[75-91-2] tert-Butyl Hydroperoxide, 1570
[75-93-4] Methyl Sulfate, 6122
[75-96-7] Tribromoacetic Acid, 9609
[75-97-8] Pinacolone, 7440
[75-98-9] Pivalic Acid, 7511
[75-99-0] Dalapon, 2802
[76-00-6] 1,1,1-Trichloro-2-propanol, 9645
[76-01-7] Pentachloroethane, 7108
[76-03-9] Trichloroacetic Acid, 9627
[76-05-1] Trifluoroacetic Acid, 9681
[76-06-2] Chloropicrin, 2156
[76-08-4] Tribromo-tert-butyl Alcohol, 9611
[76-09-5] Pinacol, 7439
[76-14-2] Cryofluorane, 2605
[76-19-7] Perfluoropropane, 7158
[76-20-0] Sulfonethylmethane, 8958
[76-22-2] Camphor, 1732
[76-24-4] Alloxantin, 283
[76-25-5] Triamcinolone Acetonide, 9596
[76-29-9] 3-Bromo-d-camphor, 1414
[76-30-2] Dihydroxytartaric Acid, 3187
[76-36-8] α,α,β-Trichloro-n-butyraldehyde, 9633
[76-37-9] 2,2,3,3-Tetrafluoro-1-propanol, 9206
[76-38-0] Methoxyflurane, 5994
[76-41-5] Oxymorphone, 6969
[76-42-6] Oxycodone, 6959
[76-43-7] Fluoxymesterone, 4186
[76-44-8] Heptachlor, 4656
[76-45-9] Protoverine, 7900
[76-47-1] Hydrocortamate, 4786
[76-49-3] Bornyl Acetate, 1339
[76-53-9] Veatchine, 9940
[76-57-3] Codeine, 2463
[76-58-4] Ethylmorphine, 3830
[76-59-5] Bromthymol Blue, 1445
[76-60-8] Bromcresol Green, 1386
[76-61-9] Thymol Blue, 9400
[76-62-0] 3',3'',5',5''-Tetrabromophenolphthalein, 9186
[76-66-4] Rhynchophylline, 8197
[76-74-4] Pentobarbital, 7130
[76-77-7] Neoquassin, 6463
[76-78-8] Quassin, 8026
[76-80-2] Tephrosin, 9150
[76-84-6] Triphenylcarbinol, 9739
[76-87-9] Triphenyltin Hydroxide, 9745

[76-90-4] Mepenzolate Bromide, 5848
[76-93-7] Benzilic Acid, 1080
[76-99-3] Methadone, 5944
[77-02-1] Aprobarbital, 756
[77-03-2] Piperidione, 7469
[77-04-3] Pyrithyldione, 7995
[77-06-5] Gibberellic Acid, 4419
[77-07-6] Levorphanol, 5470
[77-09-8] Phenolphthalein, 7243
[77-10-1] Phencyclidine, 7219
[77-14-5] Proheptazine, 7776
[77-15-6] Ethoheptazine, 3743
[77-16-7] Plumericin, 7539
[77-19-0] Dicyclomine, 3097
[77-20-3] Alphaprodine, 310
[77-21-4] Glutethimide, 4477
[77-22-5] Caramiphen, 1776
[77-23-6] Carbetapentane, 1794
[77-25-8] Ethyl Diethylmalonate, 3789
[77-26-9] Butalbital, 1511
[77-27-0] Thiamylal, 9302
[77-28-1] Butethal, 1521
[77-32-7] Thiobarbital, 9321
[77-36-1] Chlorthalidone, 2193
[77-37-2] Procyclidine, 7763
[77-38-3] Chlorphenoxamine, 2181
[77-40-7] Bisphenol B, 1298
[77-41-8] Methsuximide, 6004
[77-42-9] β-Santalol, 8358
[77-48-5] Dibromantin, 3017
[77-51-0] Isoaminile, 5110
[77-52-1] Ursolic Acid, 9890
[77-53-2] Cedrol, 1911
[77-58-7] Dibutyltin Dilaurate, 3038
[77-59-8] Tomatidine, 9544
[77-60-1] Tigogenin, 9435
[77-65-6] Carbromal, 1831
[77-66-7] Acecarbromal, 21
[77-67-8] Ethosuximide, 3748
[77-75-8] Meparfynol, 5846
[77-78-1] Dimethyl Sulfate, 3256
[77-79-2] 3-Sulfolene, 8956
[77-81-6] Tabun, 9021
[77-86-1] Tromethamine, 9772
[77-91-8] Choline Dihydrogen Citrate, 2207
[77-92-9] Citric Acid, 2326
[77-94-1] Butyl Citrate, 1564
[77-95-2] Quinic Acid, 8059
[77-98-5] Tetraethylammonium Hydroxide, 9201
[78-00-2] Tetraethyllead, 9202
[78-05-7] Phenoctide, 7240
[78-10-4] Ethyl Silicate, 3851
[78-11-5] Pentaerythritol Tetranitrate, 7112
[78-28-4] Emylcamate, 3566
[78-30-8] Tri-o-tolyl Phosphate, 9764
[78-34-2] Dioxathion, 3301
[78-40-0] Triethyl Phosphate, 9674
[78-44-4] Carisoprodol, 1842
[78-48-8] Tribufos, 9617
[78-59-1] Isophorone, 5196
[78-67-1] 2,2'-Azobisisobutyronitrile, 918
[78-70-6] Linalool, 5495
[78-75-1] Propylene Dibromide, 7853
[78-76-2] sec-Butyl Bromide, 1554
[78-77-3] Isobutyl Bromide, 5135
[78-79-5] Isoprene, 5201
[78-81-9] Isobutylamine, 5132
[78-82-0] Isobutyronitrile, 5156
[78-83-1] Isobutyl Alcohol, 5131
[78-84-2] Isobutyraldehyde, 5154

[78-86-4] sec-Butyl Chloride, 1561
[78-87-5] Propylene Dichloride, 7854
[78-89-7] Propylene Chlorohydrin, 7850
[78-90-0] Propylenediamine, 7852
[78-91-1] 2-Aminopropanol, 468
[78-92-2] sec-Butyl Alcohol, 1541
[78-93-3] Methyl Ethyl Ketone, 6072
[78-94-4] Methyl Vinyl Ketone, 6134
[78-95-5] Chloroacetone, 2114
[78-98-8] Methylglyoxal, 6081
[78-99-9] Propylidene Chloride, 7861
[79-00-5] 1,1,2-Trichloroethane, 9637
[79-01-6] Trichloroethylene, 9639
[79-03-8] Propionyl Chloride, 7828
[79-04-9] Chloracetyl Chloride, 2067
[79-05-0] Propionamide, 7824
[79-06-1] Acrylamide, 129
[79-07-2] Chloroacetamide, 2110
[79-08-3] Bromoacetic Acid, 1400
[79-09-4] Propionic Acid, 7825
[79-10-7] Acrylic Acid, 130
[79-11-8] Chloroacetic Acid, 2112
[79-14-1] Glycolic Acid, 4498
[79-15-2] N-Bromoacetamide, 1398
[79-17-4] Aminoguanidine, 441
[79-19-6] Thiosemicarbazide, 9361
[79-20-9] Methyl Acetate, 6008
[79-21-0] Peracetic Acid, 7150
[79-22-1] Methyl Chlorocarbonate, 6043
[79-24-3] Nitroethane, 6597
[79-27-6] sym-Tetrabromoethane, 9185
[79-31-2] Isobutyric Acid, 5155
[79-33-4] L-Lactic Acid, 5337
[79-34-5] Tetrachloroethane, 9189
[79-36-7] 2,2-Dichloroacetyl Chloride, 3053
[79-37-8] Oxalyl Chloride, 6914
[79-40-3] Rubeanic Acid, 8279
[79-41-4] Methacrylic Acid, 5941
[79-42-5] Thiolactic Acid, 9340
[79-43-6] Dichloroacetic Acid, 3050
[79-46-9] 2-Nitropropane, 6628
[79-49-2] Pentabromoacetone, 7106
[79-54-9] Levopimaric Acid, 5468
[79-55-0] Pempidine, 7080
[79-57-2] Oxytetracycline, 6976
[79-58-3] Rubijervine, 8287
[79-61-8] Dichlorisone 21-Acetate, 3048
[79-63-0] Lanosterol, 5360
[79-64-1] Dimethisterone, 3219
[79-68-5] γ-Irone, 5098
[79-69-6] α-Irone, 5096
[79-70-9] β-Irone, 5097
[79-74-3] 2,5-Di-tert-pentylhydroquinone, 3304
[79-80-1] 3-Dehydroretinol, 2874
[79-81-2] Vitamin A Palmitate, 10013
[79-83-4] Pantothenic Acid, 7015
[79-85-6] Quatrimycin, 8028
[79-90-3] Triclobisonium Chloride, 9653
[79-91-4] Terebic Acid, 9161
[79-92-5] Camphene, 1730
[80-00-2] Sulphenone, 8988
[80-02-4] 2-p-Sulfanilylanilinoethanol, 8927
[80-03-5] Acediasulfone, 23
[80-05-7] Bisphenol A, 1297
[80-08-0] Dapsone, 2822
[80-11-5] p-Tolylsulfonylmethylnitrosamide, 9543

[80-12-6] Tetramethylenedisulfotetramine, 9227
[80-13-7] Halazone, 4590
[80-17-1] Porofor® BSH, 7598
[80-32-0] Sulfachlorpyridazine, 8900
[80-35-3] Sulfamethoxypyridazine, 8919
[80-40-0] Ethyl p-Toluenesulfonate, 3858
[80-46-6] p-tert-Pentylphenol, 7142
[80-49-9] Homatropine DL-Methylbromide, 4730
[80-50-2] Anisotropine Methylbromide, 671
[80-53-5] Terpin, 9169
[80-56-8] α-Pinene, 7445
[80-58-0] α-Bromobutyric Acid, 1413
[80-59-1] Tiglic Acid, 9433
[80-60-4] α-Aminobutyric Acid, 428
[80-62-6] Methacrylic Acid Methyl Ester, 5941
[80-69-3] Tartronic Acid, 9073
[80-72-8] Reductic Acid, 8127
[80-73-9] 1,3-Dimethyl-2-imidazolidinone, 3249
[80-74-0] Acetyl Sulfisoxazole, 8952
[80-77-3] Chlormezanone, 2106
[80-78-4] Solanidine, 8704
[80-92-2] Pregnanediol, 7727
[80-97-7] Cholestanol, 2200
[81-04-9] Armstrong's Acid, 788
[81-05-0] 2-Naphthylamine-5-sulfonic Acid, 6407
[81-07-2] Saccharin, 8311
[81-11-8] Amsonic Acid, 595
[81-13-0] Dexpanthenol, 2947
[81-16-3] 2-Naphthylamine-1-sulfonic Acid, 6406
[81-23-2] Dehydrocholic Acid, 2868
[81-24-3] Taurocholic Acid, 9075
[81-25-4] Cholic Acid, 2203
[81-27-6] Sennoside A, 8455
[81-38-9] Laureline, 5383
[81-54-9] Purpurin, 7945
[81-61-8] Quinalizarin, 8050
[81-64-1] Quinizarin, 8064
[81-67-4] Pukateine, 7936
[81-77-6] Indanthrene, 4934
[81-81-2] Warfarin, 10038
[81-82-3] Coumachlor, 2556
[81-88-9] Rhodamine B, 8183
[81-90-3] Phenolphthalin, 7244
[81-92-5] Phenolphthalol, 7245
[81-93-6] Phenosafranin, 7251
[82-02-0] Khellin, 5309
[82-05-3] Benzanthrone, 1063
[82-08-6] Rottlerin, 8272
[82-12-2] Rufigallol, 8292
[82-22-4] Anthrimide, 690
[82-24-6] 1-Aminoanthraquinone-2-carboxylic Acid, 418
[82-40-6] Lunacrine, 5604
[82-45-1] 1-Aminoanthraquinone, 417
[82-54-2] Cotarnine, 2552
[82-57-5] Visnagin, 10011
[82-58-6] Lysergic Acid, 5633
[82-62-2] 3,4,6-Trichloro-2-nitrophenol, 9642
[82-66-6] Diphacinone, 3305
[82-68-8] Quintozene, 8080
[82-71-3] Styphnic Acid, 8859
[82-75-7] 1-Naphthylamine-8-sulfonic Acid, 6405
[82-76-8] 1-Anilino-8-naphthalenesulfonate, 661

[82-82-6] 4-Pyridoxic Acid, 7981
[82-88-2] Phenindamine, 7233
[82-89-3] Prodigiosin, 7767
[82-92-8] Cyclizine, 2710
[82-93-9] Chlorcyclizine, 2081
[82-95-1] Buclizine, 1464
[82-98-4] Piperidolate, 7470
[82-99-5] Thiphenamil, 9370
[83-07-8] Ampyrone, 591
[83-12-5] Phenindione, 7234
[83-14-7] Pellotine, 7074
[83-25-0] Succinanil, 8867
[83-26-1] Pindone, 7444
[83-28-3] 2-Isovalerylindane-1,3-dione, 5233
[83-32-9] Acenaphthene, 28
[83-34-1] Skatole, 8560
[83-40-9] o-Cresotic Acid, 2581
[83-43-2] Methylprednisolone, 6111
[83-44-3] Deoxycholic Acid, 2899
[83-45-4] Stigmastanol, 8814
[83-46-5] β-Sitosterol, 8556
[83-47-6] γ-Sitosterol, 8557
[83-48-7] Stigmasterol, 8815
[83-49-8] Hyodeoxycholic Acid, 4857
[83-54-5] Echinopsine, 3498
[83-58-9] Lunacridine, 5603
[83-60-3] Reserpic Acid, 8143
[83-67-0] Theobromine, 9282
[83-70-5] Vitamin K₅, 10023
[83-72-7] Lawsone, 5393
[83-73-8] Iodoquinol, 5042
[83-74-9] Ibogaine, 4875
[83-79-4] Rotenone, 8271
[83-81-8] N,N,N′,N′-Tetraethylphthalamide, 9203
[83-86-3] Phytic Acid, 7387
[83-88-5] Riboflavin, 8200
[83-89-6] Quinacrine, 8044
[83-94-3] Tabernanthine, 9020
[83-95-4] Skimmianine, 8561
[83-98-7] Orphenadrine, 6879
[84-01-5] Chlorproethazine, 2183
[84-02-6] Prochlorperazine Dimaleate, 7761
[84-04-8] Pipamazine, 7454
[84-06-0] Thiopropazate, 9356
[84-11-7] Phenanthrenequinone, 7213
[84-12-8] Phanquinone, 7197
[84-16-2] Hexestrol, 4701
[84-17-3] Dienestrol, 3104
[84-19-5] Dienestrol Diacetate, 3104
[84-21-9] 3′-Adenylic Acid, 157
[84-22-0] Tetrahydrozoline, 9219
[84-24-2] Physodic Acid, 7382
[84-26-4] Rutecarpine, 8298
[84-31-1] Quininone, 8063
[84-36-6] Syrosingopine, 9017
[84-37-7] Pseudoyohimbine, 7922
[84-52-6] 3′-Cytidylic Acid, 2788
[84-54-8] 2-Methylanthraquinone, 6021
[84-55-9] Viquidil, 10003
[84-58-2] 2,3-Dichloro-5,6-dicyanobenzoquinone, 3063
[84-62-8] Phenyl Phthalate, 7306
[84-65-1] Anthraquinone, 687
[84-66-2] Phthalic Acid Ethyl Ester, 7371
[84-68-4] 2,2′-Dichlorobenzidine, 3058
[84-74-2] Dibutyl Phthalate, 3035
[84-79-7] Lapachol, 5366
[84-80-0] Phylloquinone, 7380
[84-81-1] Menaquinone 6, 5833
[84-82-2] Toxoflavin, 9559

[84-86-6] 1-Naphthylamine-4-sulfonic Acid, 6403
[84-87-7] 1-Naphthol-4-sulfonic Acid, 6391
[84-88-8] 8-Hydroxy-5-quinolinesulfonic Acid, 4844
[84-89-9] 1-Naphthylamine-5-sulfonic Acid, 6404
[84-96-8] Trimeprazine, 9704
[84-97-9] Perazine, 7151
[84-99-1] Xanthoxyletin, 10066
[85-00-7] Diquat Dibromide, 3352
[85-01-8] Phenanthrene, 7212
[85-02-9] Benzo[f]quinoline, 1105
[85-17-6] Streptidine, 8822
[85-31-4] Thioguanosine, 9338
[85-32-5] 5′-Guanylic Acid, 4570
[85-38-1] 3-Nitrosalicylic Acid, 6631
[85-41-6] Phthalimide, 7373
[85-44-9] Phthalic Anhydride, 7372
[85-47-2] 1-Naphthalenesulfonic Acid, 6376
[85-55-2] 2-(p-Toluyl)benzoic Acid, 9539
[85-61-0] Coenzyme A, 2466
[85-64-3] Laudanine, 5380
[85-66-5] Pyocyanine, 7951
[85-73-4] Phthalylsulfathiazole, 7377
[85-74-5] 1-Naphthylamine-4,6-disulfonic Acid, 6401
[85-75-6] 1-Naphthylamine-4,7-disulfonic Acid, 6402
[85-79-0] Dibucaine, 3031
[85-82-5] 1-Xylylazo-2-naphthol, 10089
[85-83-6] Scarlet Red, 8393
[85-84-7] Yellow AB, 10095
[85-86-9] Sudan III, 8884
[85-90-5] Tricromyl, 9658
[85-94-9] 2′-Cytidylic Acid, 2787
[85-97-2] 2-Phenyl-6-chlorophenol, 7279
[85-98-3] N,N′-Diethylcarbanilide, 3117
[86-00-0] o-Nitrobiphenyl, 6592
[86-12-4] Thenaldine, 9278
[86-14-6] Thiambutene, 9293
[86-21-5] Pheniramine, 7235
[86-22-6] Brompheniramine, 1443
[86-34-0] Phensuximide, 7261
[86-35-1] Ethotoin, 3749
[86-36-2] Mercumallylic Acid, 5872
[86-42-0] Amodiaquin, 572
[86-48-6] 1-Hydroxy-2-naphthoic Acid, 4834
[86-50-0] Azinphos-methyl, 913
[86-54-4] Hydralazine, 4763
[86-55-5] 1-Naphthoic Acid, 6381
[86-56-6] N,N-Dimethyl-1-naphthylamine, 3252
[86-57-7] 1-Nitronaphthalene, 6614
[86-58-8] 8-Quinolineboronic Acid, 8069
[86-59-9] 8-Quinolinecarboxylic Acid, 8070
[86-60-2] Badische Acid, 940
[86-65-7] Amido-G-Acid, 401
[86-68-0] Quininic Acid, 8062
[86-73-7] 9H-Fluorene, 4155
[86-74-8] Carbazole, 1790
[86-80-6] Dimethisoquin, 3218
[86-84-0] 1-Naphthylisocyanate, 6410
[86-87-3] 1-Naphthaleneacetic Acid, 6371

[86-88-4] ANTU, 722
[87-00-3] Homatropine, 4730
[87-08-1] Penicillin V, 7100
[87-09-2] Penicillin O, 7099
[87-10-5] Tribromsalan, 9616
[87-11-6] Thiolutin, 9342
[87-17-2] Salicylanilide, 8330
[87-18-3] 4-tert-Butylphenyl Salicylate, 1586
[87-20-7] Isoamyl Salicylate, 5125
[87-21-8] Piridocaine, 7494
[87-28-5] Glycol Salicylate, 4499
[87-29-6] Cinnamyl Anthranilate, 2303
[87-33-2] Isosorbide Dinitrate, 5225
[87-39-8] Violuric Acid, 10000
[87-40-1] 2,4,6-Trichloroanisole, 9629
[87-42-3] 6-Chloropurine, 2161
[87-44-5] Caryophyllene, 1875
[87-45-6] 4-(5-Isopropenyl-2-methyl-1-cyclopenten-1-yl)-2-butanone, 5204
[87-47-8] Pyrolan, 8002
[87-51-4] Indoleacetic Acid, 4964
[87-52-5] Gramine, 4533
[87-53-6] Penicillanic Acid, 7091
[87-56-9] Mucochloric Acid, 6297
[87-58-1] Iodopyrrole, 5041
[87-61-6] 1,2,3-Trichlorobenzene, 9630
[87-65-0] 2,6-Dichlorophenol, 3073
[87-66-1] Pyrogallol, 8000
[87-68-3] Hexachlorobutadiene, 4678
[87-69-4] L-Tartaric Acid, 9070
[87-73-0] D-Glucaric Acid, 4450
[87-74-1] Glucoheptonic Acid, 4455
[87-79-6] Sorbose, 8726
[87-81-0] D-Tagatose, 9030
[87-86-5] Pentachlorophenol, 7109
[87-88-7] Chloranilic Acid, 2079
[87-89-8] Inositol, 4978
[87-90-1] Trichloroisocyanuric Acid, 9641
[87-91-2] Ethyl Tartrate, 3855
[87-99-0] Xylitol, 10085
[88-04-0] Chloroxylenol, 2176
[88-06-2] 2,4,6-Trichlorophenol, 9644
[88-09-5] Diethylacetic Acid, 3110
[88-12-0] Povidone Monomer, 7697
[88-13-1] 3-Thenoic Acid, 9279
[88-14-2] 2-Furoic Acid, 4307
[88-21-1] Orthanilic Acid, 6882
[88-29-9] Versalide®, 9965
[88-30-2] TFM, 9253
[88-67-5] o-Iodobenzoic Acid, 5030
[88-72-2] o-Nitrotoluene, 6650
[88-73-3] o-Chloronitrobenzene, 2151
[88-74-4] o-Nitroaniline, 6583
[88-75-5] o-Nitrophenol, 6620
[88-85-7] Dinoseb, 3287
[88-88-0] Picryl Chloride, 7417
[88-89-1] Picric Acid, 7410
[88-95-9] Phthaloyl Chloride, 7375
[88-96-0] Phthalamide, 7369
[88-99-3] Phthalic Acid, 7371
[89-00-9] Quinolinic Acid, 8073
[89-01-0] 2,3-Pyrazinedicarboxylic Acid, 7958
[89-05-4] Pyromellitic Acid, 8004
[89-25-8] Norphenazone, 6713
[89-31-6] Salsoline (−)-Form, 8340
[89-38-3] Pteropterin, 7934
[89-45-2] Salicylsulfuric Acid, 8334
[89-47-4] Menthyl Valerate, 5841
[89-48-5] Menthyl Acetate, 5839
[89-56-5] p-Cresotic Acid, 2582
[89-57-6] Mesalamine, 5904

[89-65-6] Isoascorbic Acid, *5126*
[89-68-9] Chlorothymol, *2170*
[89-73-6] Salicylhydroxamic Acid, *8331*
[89-78-1] Menthol, *5837*
[89-81-6] Piperitone, *7473*
[89-82-7] Pulegone, *7937*
[89-83-8] Thymol, *9399*
[89-84-9] Resacetophenone, *8140*
[89-86-1] β-Resorcylic Acid, *8157*
[89-92-9] *o*-Xylyl Bromide, *10090*
[90-00-6] 2-Ethylphenol, *3839*
[90-01-7] Salicyl Alcohol, *8325*
[90-02-8] Salicylaldehyde, *8326*
[90-05-1] Guaiacol, *4553*
[90-11-9] 1-Bromonaphthalene, *1425*
[90-13-1] 1-Chloronaphthalene, *2149*
[90-15-3] 1-Naphthol, *6383*
[90-18-6] Quercetagetin, *8033*
[90-19-7] Rhamnetin, *8171*
[90-20-0] 1-Naphthol-8-amino-3,6-disulfonic Acid, *6385*
[90-22-2] Valethamate Bromide, *9906*
[90-24-4] Xanthoxylin, *10067*
[90-29-9] Pseudobaptigenin, *7911*
[90-33-5] Hymecromone, *4854*
[90-34-6] Primaquine, *7744*
[90-39-1] Sparteine, *8737*
[90-43-7] *o*-Phenylphenol, *7304*
[90-44-8] Anthrone, *691*
[90-45-9] Aminacrine, *407*
[90-47-1] Xanthone, *10062*
[90-49-3] Pheneturide, *7230*
[90-54-0] Etafenone, *3710*
[90-59-5] 3,5-Dibromosalicylaldehyde, *3027*
[90-64-2] Mandelic Acid, *5717*
[90-65-3] Penicillic Acid, *7092*
[90-69-7] Lobeline, *5551*
[90-74-4] Rutinose, *8305*
[90-80-2] Gluconolactone, *4457*
[90-81-3] Ephedrine *dl*-Form, *3608*
[90-82-4] Pseudoephedrine, *7916*
[90-84-6] Diethylpropion, *3127*
[90-86-8] Cinnamedrine, *2298*
[90-89-1] Diethylcarbamazine, *3116*
[90-94-8] Michler's Ketone, *6177*
[91-00-9] Benzhydrylamine, *1076*
[91-01-0] Benzohydrol, *1090*
[91-16-7] Veratrole, *9956*
[91-17-8] Decalin®, *2846*
[91-18-9] Pteridine, *7931*
[91-19-0] Quinoxaline, *8078*
[91-20-3] Naphthalene, *6370*
[91-22-5] Quinoline, *8068*
[91-23-6] *o*-Nitroanisole, *6585*
[91-33-8] Benzthiazide, *1120*
[91-40-7] *N*-Phenylanthranilic Acid, *7273*
[91-47-4] α-Phenylcinnamic Acid *cis*-Form, *7281*
[91-48-5] α-Phenylcinnamic Acid *trans*-Form, *7281*
[91-53-2] Ethoxyquin, *3753*
[91-56-5] Isatin, *5104*
[91-58-7] 2-Chloronaphthalene, *2150*
[91-59-8] 2-Naphthylamine, *6399*
[91-60-1] 2-Naphthalenethiol, *6379*
[91-63-4] Quinaldine, *8047*
[91-64-5] Coumarin, *2562*
[91-66-7] Diethylaniline, *3114*
[91-75-8] Antazoline, *680*
[91-76-9] Benzoguanamine, *1089*
[91-79-2] Thenyldiamine, *9280*

[91-80-5] Methapyrilene, *5959*
[91-81-6] Tripelennamine, *9738*
[91-82-7] Pyrrobutamine, *8012*
[91-84-9] Pyrilamine, *7984*
[91-94-1] 3,3'-Dichlorobenzidine, *3059*
[92-04-6] 4-Phenyl-2-chlorophenol, *7280*
[92-12-6] Phenyltoloxamine, *7316*
[92-13-7] Pilocarpine, *7424*
[92-24-0] Naphthacene, *6369*
[92-28-4] Amido-R-Acid, *402*
[92-31-9] Tolonium Chloride, *9520*
[92-32-0] Pyronine Y, *8007*
[92-41-1] 2,7-Naphthalenedisulfonic Acid, *6375*
[92-43-3] 1-Phenyl-3-pyrazolidinone, *7309*
[92-52-4] Diphenyl, *3314*
[92-59-1] Ethylbenzylaniline, *3769*
[92-61-5] Scopoletin, *8408*
[92-62-6] Proflavine, *7771*
[92-67-1] *p*-Biphenylamine, *1235*
[92-69-3] *p*-Phenylphenol, *7305*
[92-70-6] 3-Hydroxy-2-naphthoic Acid, *4835*
[92-82-0] Phenazine, *7217*
[92-84-2] Phenothiazine, *7252*
[92-87-5] Benzidine, *1077*
[92-93-3] *p*-Nitrobiphenyl, *6593*
[92-95-5] *p*-Xenylcarbimide, *10073*
[93-01-6] 2-Naphthol-6-sulfonic Acid, *6392*
[93-04-9] 2-Methoxynaphthalene, *5997*
[93-07-2] Veratric Acid, *9953*
[93-09-4] 2-Naphthoic Acid, *6382*
[93-10-7] Quinaldic Acid, *8046*
[93-14-1] Guaifenesin, *4555*
[93-15-2] Methyleugenol, *6073*
[93-18-5] 2-Ethoxynaphthalene, *3752*
[93-20-9] 2-(2-Naphthyloxy)ethanol, *6413*
[93-30-1] Methoxyphenamine, *5998*
[93-35-6] Umbelliferone, *9847*
[93-39-0] Skimmin, *8562*
[93-42-5] Thionalide, *9344*
[93-43-6] 2-Naphthyl Lactate, *6412*
[93-44-7] 2-Naphthyl Benzoate, *6408*
[93-51-6] Creosol, *2571*
[93-54-9] α-Ethylbenzyl Alcohol, *3768*
[93-55-0] Propiophenone, *7830*
[93-56-1] Styrene Glycol, *8861*
[93-58-3] Methyl Benzoate, *6024*
[93-59-4] Perbenzoic Acid, *7152*
[93-60-7] Methyl Nicotinate, *6100*
[93-76-5] 2,4,5-T, *9019*
[93-88-9] Phenylpropylmethylamine, *7308*
[93-89-0] Ethyl Benzoate, *3766*
[93-95-8] 5-(α-Phenylethyl)semi-oxamazide, *7289*
[93-97-0] Benzoic Anhydride, *1092*
[93-98-1] Benzanilide, *1061*
[93-99-2] Phenyl Benzoate, *7275*
[94-02-0] Ethyl Benzoylacetate, *3767*
[94-07-5] Synephrine, *9012*
[94-09-7] Benzocaine, *1086*
[94-13-3] Propylparaben, *7866*
[94-14-4] Isobutyl *p*-Aminobenzoate, *5133*
[94-15-5] Dimethocaine, *3221*
[94-16-6] *p*-Aminohippuric Acid Sodium Salt, *442*
[94-19-9] Sulfaethidole, *8907*
[94-20-2] Chlorpropamide, *2186*

[94-25-7] Butamben, *1512*
[94-26-8] Butylparaben, *1584*
[94-36-0] Benzoyl Peroxide, *1116*
[94-41-7] Chalcone, *2037*
[94-44-0] Nicotinic Acid Benzyl Ester, *6526*
[94-46-2] Isoamyl Benzoate, *5113*
[94-53-1] Piperonylic Acid, *7477*
[94-59-7] Safrole, *8317*
[94-62-2] Piperine, *7472*
[94-63-3] Pralidoxime Iodide, *7703*
[94-67-7] Salicylaldoxime, *8327*
[94-70-2] *o*-Phenetidine, *7227*
[94-74-6] MCPA, *5764*
[94-75-7] 2,4-D, *2796*
[94-78-0] Phenazopyridine, *7210*
[94-82-6] 2,4-DB, *2835*
[94-93-9] Salen (unspecified stereo), *8322*
[94-96-2] Ethohexadiol, *3744*
[95-01-2] β-Resorcylaldehyde, *8156*
[95-05-6] Sulfiram, *8950*
[95-06-7] Sulfallate, *8911*
[95-13-6] Indene, *4939*
[95-14-7] 1*H*-Benzotriazole, *1108*
[95-15-8] Thianaphthene, *9303*
[95-16-9] Benzothiazole, *1107*
[95-25-0] Chlorzoxazone, *2194*
[95-38-5] Amine 220, *408*
[95-43-2] D-Threose, *9381*
[95-44-3] L-Threose, *9382*
[95-45-4] Dimethylglyoxime, *3246*
[95-47-6] *o*-Xylene, *10081*
[95-48-7] *o*-Cresol, *2579*
[95-49-8] *o*-Chlorotoluene, *2171*
[95-50-1] *o*-Dichlorobenzene, *3056*
[95-51-2] *o*-Chloroaniline, *2118*
[95-52-3] *o*-Fluorotoluene, *4180*
[95-53-4] *o*-Toluidine, *9536*
[95-54-5] *o*-Phenylenediamine, *7284*
[95-55-6] *o*-Aminophenol, *461*
[95-56-7] *o*-Bromophenol, *1428*
[95-57-8] *o*-Chlorophenol, *2154*
[95-63-6] Pseudocumene, *7915*
[95-76-1] 3,4-Dichloroaniline, *3054*
[95-86-3] 2,4-Diaminophenol, *2983*
[95-92-1] Diethyl Oxalate, *3125*
[95-93-2] Durene, *3468*
[95-95-4] 2,4,5-Trichlorophenol, *9643*
[96-00-4] Sebacoin, *8417*
[96-01-5] Sebacil, *8416*
[96-11-7] 1,2,3-Tribromopropane, *9614*
[96-12-8] Dibromochloropropane, *3020*
[96-20-8] 2-Amino-1-butanol, *427*
[96-22-0] Diethyl Ketone, *3121*
[96-23-1] 1,3-Dichloro-2-propanol, *3074*
[96-24-2] α-Chlorohydrin, *2145*
[96-26-4] Dihydroxyacetone, *3182*
[96-27-5] Thioglycerol, *9335*
[96-33-3] Methyl Acrylate, *6011*
[96-34-4] Methyl Chloroacetate, *6042*
[96-41-3] Cyclopentanol, *2742*
[96-45-7] Ethylene Thiourea, *3803*
[96-48-0] Butyrolactone, *1596*
[96-50-4] 2-Aminothiazole, *479*
[96-64-0] Soman, *8713*
[96-77-5] Phenoldisulfonic Acid, *7242*
[96-82-2] Lactobionic Acid, *5342*
[96-83-3] Iopanoic Acid, *5058*
[96-84-4] Iophenoxic Acid, *5061*
[96-88-8] Mepivacaine, *5859*
[96-91-3] Picramic Acid, *7409*
[96-97-9] 5-Nitrosalicylic Acid, *6632*

[97-00-7] 1-Chloro-2,4-dinitrobenzene, 2136
[97-02-9] 2,4-Dinitroaniline, 3270
[97-05-2] Sulfosalicylic Acid, 8964
[97-11-0] Cyclethrin, 2706
[97-17-6] Dichlofenthion, 3043
[97-18-7] Bithionol, 1306
[97-23-4] Dichlorophen, 3071
[97-24-5] Fenticlor, 4004
[97-25-6] Urochloralic Acid, 9884
[97-26-7] Toluylene Blue, 9822
[97-30-3] α-Methylglucoside, 6080
[97-31-4] Normetanephrine, 6708
[97-44-9] Acetarsone, 52
[97-53-0] Eugenol, 3898
[97-54-1] Isoeugenol, 5171
[97-56-3] o-Aminoazotoluene, 420
[97-59-6] Allantoin, 258
[97-62-1] Ethyl Isobutyrate, 3814
[97-64-3] Ethyl Lactate, 3817
[97-65-4] Itaconic Acid, 5242
[97-67-6] Malic Acid L-(−)-Form, 5707
[97-75-6] Scopolamine N-Oxide, 8407
[97-77-8] Disulfiram, 3364
[97-85-8] Isobutyl Isobutyrate, 5145
[97-94-9] Triethylborane, 9668
[97-99-4] Tetrahydrofurfuryl Alcohol, 9213
[98-00-0] Furfuryl Alcohol, 4305
[98-01-1] Furfural, 4304
[98-04-4] Phenyltrimethylammonium Iodide, 7318
[98-05-5] Benzenearsonic Acid, 1067
[98-06-6] tert-Butylbenzene, 1551
[98-07-7] Benzotrichloride, 1109
[98-08-8] Benzotrifluoride, 1110
[98-09-9] Benzenesulfonyl Chloride, 1072
[98-11-3] Benzenesulfonic Acid, 1070
[98-50-0] Arsanilic Acid, 792
[98-54-4] p-tert-Butylphenol, 1585
[98-55-5] α-Terpineol, 9171
[98-56-6] p-Chlorobenzotrifluoride, 2126
[98-58-8] p-Bromobenzenesulfonyl Chloride, 1407
[98-59-9] p-Toluenesulfonyl Chloride, 9534
[98-61-3] Pipsyl Chloride, 7486
[98-62-4] Sulfanilyl Fluoride, 8929
[98-66-8] p-Chlorobenzenesulfonic Acid, 2122
[98-67-9] p-Phenolsulfonic Acid, 7246
[98-71-5] 4-Hydrazinobenzenesulfonic Acid, 4773
[98-72-6] Nitarsone, 6566
[98-79-3] L-Pyroglutamic Acid, 8001
[98-80-6] Benzeneboronic Acid, 1068
[98-82-8] Cumene, 2617
[98-84-0] α-Methylbenzylamine, 6026
[98-86-2] Acetophenone, 73
[98-87-3] Benzal Chloride, 1057
[98-88-4] Benzoyl Chloride, 1112
[98-89-5] Cyclohexanecarboxylic Acid, 2724
[98-92-0] Nicotinamide, 6523
[98-95-3] Nitrobenzene, 6588
[98-96-4] Pyrazinamide, 7956
[98-97-5] Pyrazinoic Acid, 7959
[98-98-6] Picolinic Acid, 7403
[99-05-8] m-Aminobenzoic Acid, 421
[99-08-1] m-Nitrotoluene, 6650
[99-09-2] m-Nitroaniline, 6582
[99-11-6] Citrazinic Acid, 2325

[99-14-9] Tricarballylic Acid, 9622
[99-17-2] Populin, 7594
[99-20-7] Trehalose, 9580
[99-24-1] Gallic Acid Methyl Ester, 4345
[99-32-1] Chelidonic Acid, 2052
[99-33-2] 3,5-Dinitrobenzoyl Chloride, 3277
[99-34-3] 3,5-Dinitrobenzoic Acid, 3276
[99-35-4] sym-Trinitrobenzene, 9726
[99-43-4] Benoxinate, 1047
[99-45-6] Adrenalone, 171
[99-49-0] Carvone, 1874
[99-50-3] Protocatechuic Acid, 7894
[99-56-9] 4-Nitro-o-phenylenediamine, 6623
[99-65-0] m-Dinitrobenzene, 3273
[99-66-1] Valproic Acid, 9913
[99-73-0] p-Bromophenacyl Bromide, 1427
[99-76-3] Methylparaben, 6107
[99-79-6] Iophendylate, 5060
[99-83-2] α-Phellandrene, 7200
[99-87-6] p-Cymene, 2763
[99-88-7] Cumidine, 2620
[99-90-1] p-Bromoacetophenone, 1403
[99-91-2] p-Chloroacetophenone, 2116
[99-96-7] p-Hydroxybenzoic Acid, 4812
[99-98-9] Dimethyl-p-phenylenediamine, 3254
[99-99-0] p-Nitrotoluene, 6650
[100-00-5] p-Chloronitrobenzene, 2151
[100-01-6] p-Nitroaniline, 6584
[100-02-7] p-Nitrophenol, 6621
[100-07-2] p-Anisoyl Chloride, 673
[100-09-4] p-Anisic Acid, 666
[100-10-7] p-Dimethylaminobenzaldehyde, 3230
[100-16-3] (4-Nitrophenyl)hydrazine, 6624
[100-17-4] p-Nitroanisole, 6585
[100-21-0] Terephthalic Acid, 9162
[100-22-1] Tetramethyl-p-phenylenediamine, 9228
[100-25-4] p-Dinitrobenzene, 3273
[100-26-5] Isocinchomeronic Acid, 5159
[100-33-4] Pentamidine, 7115
[100-37-8] 2-Diethylaminoethanol, 3112
[100-39-0] Benzyl Bromide, 1128
[100-41-4] Ethylbenzene, 3765
[100-42-5] Styrene, 8860
[100-44-7] Benzyl Chloride, 1129
[100-46-9] Benzylamine, 1125
[100-47-0] Benzonitrile, 1097
[100-49-2] Cyclohexylcarbinol, 2731
[100-51-6] Benzyl Alcohol, 1124
[100-52-7] Benzaldehyde, 1058
[100-53-8] Thiobenzyl Alcohol, 9322
[100-55-0] Nicotinyl Alcohol, 6527
[100-56-1] Phenylmercuric Chloride, 7301
[100-59-4] Phenylmagnesium Chloride, 7298
[100-61-8] Methylaniline, 6019
[100-63-0] Phenylhydrazine, 7293
[100-65-2] Phenylhydroxylamine, 7294
[100-66-3] Anisole, 669
[100-67-4] Potassium Phenoxide, 7657
[100-76-5] Quinuclidine, 8081
[100-79-8] Isopropylidene Glycerol, 5213

[100-88-9] Cyclamic Acid, 2703
[100-91-4] Eucatropine, 3897
[100-92-5] Mephentermine, 5852
[100-97-0] Methenamine, 5966
[101-05-3] Anilazine, 657
[101-14-4] 4,4′-Methylenebis[2-chloroaniline], 6059
[101-20-2] Triclocarban, 9654
[101-21-3] Chlorpropham, 2187
[101-26-8] Pyridostigmine Bromide, 7977
[101-31-5] Hyoscyamine, 4858
[101-38-2] Gibbs Reagent, 4421
[101-40-6] Propylhexedrine, 7860
[101-42-8] Fenuron, 4009
[101-53-1] p-Benzylphenol, 1143
[101-57-5] N-Phenylsulfanilic Acid, 7313
[101-60-0] Porphine, 7599
[101-61-1] Michler's Base, 6176
[101-62-2] Phenamidine, 7208
[101-64-4] N-(p-Methoxyphenyl)-p-phenylenediamine, 5999
[101-77-9] p,p′-Diaminodiphenylmethane, 2980
[101-81-5] Diphenylmethane, 3328
[101-83-7] Dicyclohexylamine, 3095
[101-84-8] Phenyl Ether, 7288
[101-91-7] 4′-Hydroxybutyranilide, 4814
[101-94-0] p-Cresyl Phenylacetate, 2585
[101-97-3] Ethyl Phenylacetate, 3840
[101-99-5] Phenylurethan(e), 7320
[102-01-2] Acetoacetanilide, 58
[102-02-3] Phenyl Biguanide, 7276
[102-06-7] 1,3-Diphenylguanidine, 3324
[102-07-8] Carbanilide, 1785
[102-08-9] sym-Diphenylthiourea, 3333
[102-09-0] Phenyl Carbonate, 7278
[102-14-7] Succinanilic Acid, 8868
[102-29-4] Resorcinol Monoacetate, 8155
[102-45-5] Cyclopentamine, 2740
[102-54-5] Ferrocene, 4037
[102-60-3] Entprol, 3599
[102-71-6] Triethanolamine, 9665
[102-76-1] Triacetin, 9589
[102-82-9] Tributylamine, 9618
[102-92-1] Cinnamoyl Chloride, 2301
[102-98-7] Phenylmercury Borate, 7303
[103-01-5] N-Phenylglycine, 7292
[103-09-3] Octyl Acetate, 6763
[103-12-8] Sulfamidochrysoidine, 8923
[103-16-2] Monobenzone, 6248
[103-26-4] Cinnamic Acid Methyl Ester, 2299
[103-29-7] Bibenzyl, 1198
[103-30-0] Stilbene trans-Form, 8817
[103-32-2] Benzylaniline, 1126
[103-33-3] Azobenzene, 917
[103-34-4] 4,4′-Dithiodimorpholine, 3372
[103-36-6] Cinnamic Acid Ethyl Ester, 2299
[103-41-3] Benzyl Cinnamate, 1130
[103-47-9] CHES, 2055
[103-49-1] Dibenzylamine, 3011
[103-50-4] Benzyl Ether, 1132
[103-65-1] n-Propylbenzene, 7844
[103-69-5] Ethylaniline, 3764
[103-70-8] Formanilide, 4238
[103-71-9] Phenyl Isocyanate, 7296

Chemical Abstracts Registry Numbers

[103-72-0] Phenyl Isothiocyanate, 7297
[103-73-1] Phenetole, 7229
[103-79-7] Phenylacetone, 7269
[103-81-1] α-Phenylacetamide, 7266
[103-82-2] Phenylacetic Acid, 7268
[103-84-4] Acetanilide, 50
[103-85-5] Phenylthiourea, 7315
[103-88-8] p-Bromoacetanilide, 1399
[103-89-9] p-Acetotoluide, 74
[103-90-2] Acetaminophen, 47
[103-97-9] Phenocoll, 7239
[104-03-0] p-Nitrophenylacetic Acid, 6622
[104-04-1] p-Nitroacetanilide, 6581
[104-06-3] Thiacetazone, 9290
[104-14-3] Octopamine, 6759
[104-15-4] p-Toluenesulfonic Acid, 9533
[104-28-9] Cinoxate, 2310
[104-29-0] Chlorphenesin, 2178
[104-31-4] Benzonatate, 1096
[104-32-5] Propamidine, 7797
[104-46-1] Anethole (unspecified stereo), 643
[104-51-8] n-Butylbenzene, 1549
[104-54-1] Cinnamyl Alcohol, 2302
[104-55-2] Cinnamaldehyde, 2297
[104-57-4] Benzyl Formate, 1134
[104-76-7] 2-Ethyl-1-hexanol, 3808
[104-80-3] 2,5-Tetrahydrofurandimethanol, 9212
[104-81-4] p-Xylyl Bromide, 10090
[104-82-5] p-Xylyl Chloride, 10091
[104-85-8] p-Tolunitrile, 9538
[104-90-5] 5-Ethyl-2-picoline, 3844
[104-91-6] 4-Nitrosophenol, 6642
[105-13-5] Anise Alcohol, 665
[105-20-4] Betazole, 1183
[105-29-3] 1-Pentol, 7131
[105-37-3] Ethyl Propionate, 3847
[105-39-5] Ethyl Chloroacetate, 3783
[105-41-9] Methylhexaneamine, 6085
[105-45-3] Methyl Acetoacetate, 6009
[105-46-4] sec-Butyl Acetate, 1536
[105-53-3] Ethyl Malonate, 3823
[105-54-4] Ethyl Butyrate, 3775
[105-56-6] Ethyl Cyanoacetate, 3786
[105-57-7] Acetal, 38
[105-58-8] Ethyl Carbonate, 3780
[105-60-2] Caprolactam, 1761
[105-61-3] Maleuric Acid, 5706
[105-66-8] Propyl Butyrate, 7846
[105-92-0] Rhodopin, 8191
[106-02-5] Exaltolide®, 3910
[106-22-9] β-Citronellol, 2330
[106-23-0] Citronellal, 2329
[106-24-1] Geraniol, 4403
[106-25-2] Nerol, 6475
[106-26-3] Neral, 2322
[106-27-4] Isoamyl Butyrate, 5115
[106-30-9] Ethyl Oenanthate, 4389
[106-31-0] Butyric Anhydride, 1594
[106-32-1] Ethyl Caprylate, 3778
[106-33-2] Ethyl Laurate, 3818
[106-34-3] Quinhydrone, 8058
[106-36-5] Propyl Propionate, 7867
[106-37-6] p-Dibromobenzene, 3019
[106-40-1] p-Bromoaniline, 1404
[106-41-2] p-Bromophenol, 1428
[106-42-3] p-Xylene, 10081
[106-43-4] p-Chlorotoluene, 2171
[106-44-5] p-Cresol, 2579
[106-45-6] p-Thiocresol, 9325
[106-46-7] p-Dichlorobenzene, 3057

[106-47-8] p-Chloroaniline, 2118
[106-48-9] p-Chlorophenol, 2154
[106-49-0] p-Toluidine, 9536
[106-50-3] p-Phenylenediamine, 7285
[106-51-4] Quinone, 8074
[106-57-0] 2,5-Piperazinedione, 7466
[106-60-5] δ-Aminolevulinic Acid, 446
[106-68-3] 3-Octanone, 6753
[106-89-8] Epichlorohydrin, 3611
[106-93-4] Ethylene Dibromide, 3796
[106-94-5] Propyl Bromide, 7845
[106-95-6] Allyl Bromide, 288
[106-97-8] Butane, 1515
[106-98-9] 1-Butene, 1519
[106-99-0] 1,3-Butadiene, 1509
[107-01-7] 2-Butene, 1520
[107-02-8] Acrolein, 128
[107-05-1] Allyl Chloride, 289
[107-06-2] Ethylene Dichloride, 3797
[107-07-3] Ethylene Chlorohydrin, 3793
[107-08-4] Propyl Iodide, 7862
[107-10-8] Propylamine, 7843
[107-11-9] Allylamine, 287
[107-12-0] Propionitrile, 7827
[107-13-1] Acrylonitrile, 131
[107-15-3] Ethylenediamine, 3795
[107-18-6] Allyl Alcohol, 286
[107-19-7] Propargyl Alcohol, 7809
[107-20-0] Chloroacetaldehyde, 2109
[107-21-1] Ethylene Glycol, 3798
[107-22-2] Glyoxal, 4509
[107-27-7] Ethylmercuric Chloride, 3826
[107-29-9] Acetaldoxime, 42
[107-30-2] Chloromethyl Methyl Ether, 2146
[107-31-3] Methyl Formate, 6077
[107-32-4] Performic Acid, 7160
[107-34-6] 1-Propanearsonic Acid, 7800
[107-35-7] Taurine, 9074
[107-36-8] Isethionic Acid, 5107
[107-38-0] Arsonoacetic Acid, 810
[107-41-5] Hexylene Glycol, 4710
[107-43-7] Betaine, 1179
[107-44-8] Sarin, 8374
[107-49-3] Tetraethyl Pyrophosphate, 9204
[107-51-7] Octamethyltrisiloxane, 6748
[107-52-8] Tetradecamethylhexasiloxane, 9197
[107-53-9] Tetracosamethylhendecasiloxane, 9194
[107-59-5] tert-Butyl Chloroacetate, 1563
[107-68-6] N-Methyltaurine, 6124
[107-73-3] Phosphorylcholine, 7362
[107-82-4] Isoamyl Bromide, 5114
[107-84-6] Isoamyl Chloride, 5116
[107-85-7] Isoamylamine, 5112
[107-86-8] Senecialdehyde, 8448
[107-87-9] Methyl Propyl Ketone, 6114
[107-88-0] 1,3-Butylene Glycol, 1567
[107-89-1] Aldol, 224
[107-91-5] Cyanoacetamide, 2688
[107-92-6] Butyric Acid, 1593
[107-93-7] Crotonic Acid, 2597
[107-94-8] β-Chloropropionic Acid, 2159
[107-95-9] β-Alanine, 205
[107-97-1] Sarcosine, 8373
[108-01-0] Deanol, 2843
[108-03-2] 1-Nitropropane, 6627

[108-05-4] Vinyl Acetate, 9992
[108-10-1] Isopropylacetone, 5207
[108-12-3] Isovaleryl Chloride, 5232
[108-18-9] Diisopropylamine, 3196
[108-19-0] Biuret, 1309
[108-20-3] Isopropyl Ether, 5212
[108-21-4] Isopropyl Acetate, 5205
[108-22-5] Isopropenyl Acetate, 5203
[108-24-7] Acetic Anhydride, 56
[108-28-1] Protoanemonin, 7892
[108-30-5] Succinic Anhydride, 8870
[108-31-6] Maleic Anhydride, 5704
[108-38-3] m-Xylene, 10081
[108-39-4] m-Cresol, 2579
[108-40-7] m-Thiocresol, 9325
[108-41-8] m-Chlorotoluene, 2171
[108-42-9] m-Chloroaniline, 2118
[108-43-0] m-Chlorophenol, 2154
[108-44-1] m-Toluidine, 9536
[108-45-2] m-Phenylenediamine, 7283
[108-46-3] Resorcinol, 8155
[108-48-5] 2,6-Lutidine, 5616
[108-56-5] Ethyl Oxalacetate, 3836
[108-59-8] Methyl Malonate, 6096
[108-64-5] Ethyl Isovalerate, 3816
[108-67-8] Mesitylene, 5907
[108-70-3] 1,3,5-Trichlorobenzene, 9632
[108-73-6] Phloroglucinol, 7328
[108-75-8] 2,4,6-Trimethylpyridine, 9718
[108-77-0] Cyanuric Chloride, 2699
[108-78-1] Melamine, 5811
[108-80-5] Cyanuric Acid, 2698
[108-85-0] Cyclohexyl Bromide, 2730
[108-86-1] Bromobenzene, 1406
[108-87-2] Methylcyclohexane, 6047
[108-88-3] Toluene, 9529
[108-89-4] γ-Picoline, 7402
[108-90-7] Chlorobenzene, 2121
[108-91-8] Cyclohexylamine, 2729
[108-93-0] Cyclohexanol, 2725
[108-94-1] Cyclohexanone, 2726
[108-95-2] Phenol, 7241
[108-98-5] Thiophenol, 9355
[108-99-6] β-Picoline, 7401
[109-06-8] α-Picoline, 7400
[109-21-7] n-Butyl n-Butyrate, 1556
[109-52-4] n-Valeric Acid, 9904
[109-57-9] Thiosinamine, 9362
[109-60-4] Propyl Acetate, 7841
[109-61-5] Propyl Chlorocarbonate, 7848
[109-63-7] Boron Trifluoride Etherate, 1350
[109-64-8] Trimethylene Bromide, 9713
[109-65-9] n-Butyl Bromide, 1553
[109-66-0] Pentane, 7116
[109-67-1] 1-Pentene, 7122
[109-68-2] 2-Pentene, 7123
[109-69-3] n-Butyl Chloride, 1560
[109-73-9] n-Butylamine, 1543
[109-74-0] Butyronitrile, 1597
[109-75-1] Allyl Cyanide, 290
[109-77-3] Malononitrile, 5711
[109-78-4] Ethylene Cyanohydrin, 3794
[109-79-5] n-Butyl Mercaptan, 1577
[109-80-8] 1,3-Propanedithiol, 7801
[109-82-0] Methyleneaminoacetonitrile, 6057
[109-83-1] 2-Methylaminoethanol, 6015
[109-86-4] Methyl Cellosolve®, 6038

REG-9

[109-87-5] Methylal, *6012*
[109-89-7] Diethylamine, *3111*
[109-93-3] Vinyl Ether, *9995*
[109-94-4] Ethyl Formate, *3807*
[109-95-5] Ethyl Nitrite, *3831*
[109-96-6] 3-Pyrroline, *8017*
[109-97-7] 1H-Pyrrole, *8014*
[109-98-8] 2-Pyrazoline, *7961*
[109-99-9] Tetrahydrofuran, *9211*
[110-00-9] Furan, *4296*
[110-01-0] Tetrahydrothiophene, *9218*
[110-02-1] Thiophene, *9353*
[110-04-3] 1,2-Ethanedisulfonic Acid, *3724*
[110-05-4] DTBP, *3461*
[110-13-4] Acetonylacetone, *71*
[110-14-5] Succinamide, *8866*
[110-15-6] Succinic Acid, *8869*
[110-16-7] Maleic Acid, *5703*
[110-17-8] Fumaric Acid, *4287*
[110-18-9] TEMED, *9134*
[110-19-0] Isobutyl Acetate, *5130*
[110-27-0] Isopropyl Myristate, *5215*
[110-38-3] Ethyl Caprate, *3776*
[110-43-0] 2-Heptanone, *4663*
[110-44-1] Sorbic Acid, *8721*
[110-45-2] Isoamyl Formate, *5119*
[110-46-3] Isoamyl Nitrite, *5123*
[110-49-6] Methyl Cellosolve® Acetate, *6039*
[110-53-2] n-Amyl Bromide, *602*
[110-54-3] n-Hexane, *4694*
[110-58-7] n-Amylamine, *598*
[110-59-8] Valeronitrile, *9905*
[110-60-1] Putrescine, *7947*
[110-61-2] Succinonitrile, *8872*
[110-62-3] n-Valeraldehyde, *9902*
[110-66-7] n-Amyl Mercaptan, *611*
[110-71-4] 1,2-Dimethoxyethane, *3224*
[110-74-7] Propyl Formate, *7858*
[110-75-8] 2-Chloroethyl Vinyl Ether, *2139*
[110-77-0] 2-(Ethylthio)ethanol, *3857*
[110-80-5] 2-Ethoxyethanol, *3750*
[110-82-7] Cyclohexane, *2723*
[110-83-8] Cyclohexene, *2727*
[110-85-0] Piperazine, *7464*
[110-86-1] Pyridine, *7970*
[110-88-3] s-Trioxane, *9734*
[110-89-4] Piperidine, *7468*
[110-91-8] Morpholine, *6277*
[110-94-1] Glutaric Acid, *4473*
[110-97-4] Diisopropanolamine, *3195*
[111-01-3] Squalane, *8767*
[111-02-4] Squalene, *8768*
[111-13-7] Hexyl Methyl Ketone, *4711*
[111-14-8] Heptanoic Acid, *4660*
[111-15-9] 2-Ethoxyethyl Acetate, *3751*
[111-16-0] Pimelic Acid, *7431*
[111-17-1] 3,3'-Thiodipropionic Acid, *9332*
[111-20-6] Sebacic Acid, *8415*
[111-27-3] 1-Hexanol, *4697*
[111-28-4] Sorbic Alcohol, *8722*
[111-29-5] 1,5-Pentanediol, *7117*
[111-30-8] Glutaraldehyde, *4472*
[111-36-4] Butyl Isocyanate, *1575*
[111-42-2] Diethanolamine, *3107*
[111-43-3] Propyl Ether, *7857*
[111-44-4] sym-Dichloroethyl Ether, *3066*
[111-46-6] Diethylene Glycol, *3119*
[111-47-7] Propyl Sulfide, *7868*
[111-48-8] 2,2'-Thiodiethanol, *9330*

[111-51-3] Tetramethyldiaminobutane, *9226*
[111-55-7] Ethylene Glycol Diacetate, *3799*
[111-65-9] Octane, *6749*
[111-66-0] Caprylene, *1764*
[111-70-6] 1-Heptanol, *4661*
[111-71-7] Heptanal, *4658*
[111-76-2] Butyl Cellosolve®, *1559*
[111-77-3] Methyl Carbitol®, *6037*
[111-83-1] n-Octyl Bromide, *6764*
[111-87-5] 1-Octanol, *6751*
[111-90-0] Carbitol®, *1800*
[111-92-2] n-Dibutylamine, *3032*
[111-96-6] Diglyme, *3165*
[112-05-0] Pelargonic Acid, *7070*
[112-12-9] Methyl Nonyl Ketone, *6104*
[112-24-3] Trientine, *9663*
[112-27-6] Triethylene Glycol, *9670*
[112-30-1] n-Decyl Alcohol, *2855*
[112-34-5] Butyl Carbitol®, *1557*
[112-36-7] Diethyl Carbitol®, *3118*
[112-38-9] Undecylenic Acid, *9848*
[112-47-0] Decamethylene Glycol, *2849*
[112-49-2] Triglyme, *9692*
[112-53-8] 1-Dodecanol, *3405*
[112-63-0] Methyl Linoleate, *6095*
[112-72-1] Myristyl Alcohol, *6335*
[112-79-8] Elaidic Acid, *3533*
[112-80-1] Oleic Acid, *6828*
[112-85-6] Behenic Acid, *1023*
[112-86-7] Erucic Acid, *3674*
[112-92-5] Stearyl Alcohol, *8805*
[113-00-8] Guanidine, *4562*
[113-15-5] Ergotamine, *3661*
[113-18-8] Ethchlorvynol, *3729*
[113-22-4] Estriol 16,17-Bis(sodium Hemisuccinate), *3707*
[113-38-2] Estradiol Dipropionate, *3703*
[113-42-8] Methylergonovine, *6070*
[113-45-1] Methylphenidate, *6110*
[113-52-0] Imipramine Hydrochloride, *4920*
[113-53-1] Dothiepin, *3429*
[113-59-7] Chlorprothixene, *2188*
[113-73-5] Gramicidin S, *4531*
[113-78-0] Deaminooxytocin, *2842*
[113-92-8] Chlorpheniramine Maleate, *2180*
[113-98-4] Penicillin G Potassium Salt, *7094*
[114-04-5] Neuraminic Acid, *6483*
[114-07-8] Erythromycin, *3681*
[114-21-6] Mandelic Acid Sodium Salt, *5717*
[114-25-0] Biliverdine, *1219*
[114-26-1] Propoxur, *7836*
[114-42-1] Flavaspidic Acid, *4090*
[114-43-2] Desaspidin BB, *2917*
[114-49-8] Scopolamine Hydrobromide Trihydrate, *8406*
[114-80-7] Neostigmine Bromide, *6464*
[114-85-2] Bethanidine Sulfate, *1186*
[114-86-3] Phenformin, *7231*
[114-90-9] Obidoxime Chloride, *6738*
[114-91-0] Metyridine, *6160*
[115-02-6] Azaserine, *899*
[115-07-1] Propylene, *7849*
[115-08-2] Thioformamide, *9333*
[115-10-6] Methyl Ether, *6071*
[115-11-7] Isobutylene, *5141*
[115-17-3] Bromal, *1383*

[115-19-5] 2-Methyl-3-butyn-2-ol, *6034*
[115-20-8] 2,2,2-Trichloroethanol, *9638*
[115-24-2] Sulfonmethane, *8960*
[115-25-3] Octafluorocyclobutane, *6745*
[115-26-4] Dimefox, *3205*
[115-27-5] Chlorendic Anhydride, *2086*
[115-29-7] Endosulfan, *3574*
[115-31-1] Isobornyl Thiocyanoacetate, *5129*
[115-32-2] Dicofol, *3086*
[115-33-3] Oxyphenisatin Acetate, *6974*
[115-37-7] Thebaine, *9276*
[115-38-8] Mephobarbital, *5854*
[115-39-9] Bromphenol Blue, *1444*
[115-40-2] Bromcresol Purple, *1387*
[115-44-6] Talbutal, *9036*
[115-51-5] Ambutonium Bromide, *387*
[115-53-7] Sinomenine, *8546*
[115-61-7] Tachysterol, *9023*
[115-63-9] Hexocyclium Methyl Sulfate, *4706*
[115-67-3] Paramethadione, *7028*
[115-68-4] Sulfadicramide, *8904*
[115-69-5] 2-Amino-2-methyl-1,3-propanediol, *448*
[115-70-8] 2-Amino-2-ethyl-1,3-propanediol, *439*
[115-71-9] α-Santalol, *8357*
[115-77-5] Pentaerythritol, *7111*
[115-79-7] Ambenonium Chloride, *379*
[115-86-6] Triphenyl Phosphate, *9742*
[115-90-2] Fensulfothion, *4000*
[115-93-5] Cythioate, *2785*
[115-95-7] Linalyl Acetate, *5496*
[116-04-1] β-Humulene, *4753*
[116-06-3] Aldicarb, *222*
[116-09-6] Acetol, *65*
[116-14-3] Tetrafluoroethylene, *9205*
[116-25-6] 1-(Hydroxymethyl)-5,5-dimethylhydantoin, *4831*
[116-26-7] Safranal, *8316*
[116-29-0] Tetradifon, *9198*
[116-30-3] Rhodoxanthin, *8195*
[116-31-4] Retinal, *8164*
[116-38-1] Edrophonium Chloride, *3516*
[116-42-7] Sulfaproxyline, *8936*
[116-43-8] Succinylsulfathiazole, *8877*
[116-44-9] Sulfapyrazine, *8937*
[116-45-0] Sulfabromomethazine, *8898*
[116-58-5] 4-Pregnene-11β,17α,20β,21-tetrol-3-one, *7730*
[116-59-6] 4-Pregnene-17α,20β,21-triol-3,11-dione, *7731*
[116-63-2] 1-Amino-2-naphthol-4-sulfonic Acid, *454*
[117-02-2] Rubiadin, *8281*
[117-10-2] Danthron, *2815*
[117-12-4] Anthrarufin, *689*
[117-34-0] Diphenylacetic Acid, *3316*
[117-37-3] Anisindione, *668*
[117-39-5] Quercetin, *8034*
[117-51-1] Synhexyl, *9013*
[117-56-6] 1-Naphthol-4,8-disulfonic Acid, *6386*
[117-68-0] 3'-Guanylic Acid, *4569*
[117-80-6] Dichlone, *3045*
[117-81-7] DEHP, *2864*
[117-89-5] Trifluoperazine, *9680*
[117-92-0] Quinaldine Red, *8049*
[118-00-3] Guanosine, *4566*
[118-08-1] Hydrastine, *4767*
[118-10-5] Cinchonine, *2287*

[118-23-0] Bromodiphenhydramine, *1418*
[118-32-1] 2-Naphthol-6,8-disulfonic Acid, *6388*
[118-34-3] Syringin, *9016*
[118-42-3] Hydroxychloroquine, *4818*
[118-52-5] 1,3-Dichloro-5,5-dimethyl-hydantoin, *3065*
[118-55-8] Phenyl Salicylate, *7310*
[118-56-9] Homosalate, *4738*
[118-57-0] Acetaminosalol, *48*
[118-58-1] Benzyl Salicylate, *1144*
[118-60-5] Octyl Salicylate, *6770*
[118-61-6] Ethyl Salicylate, *3850*
[118-65-0] Isocaryophyllene, *1875*
[118-71-8] Maltol, *5713*
[118-74-1] Hexachlorobenzene, *4677*
[118-75-2] Chloranil, *2078*
[118-78-5] Uramil, *9852*
[118-79-6] 2,4,6-Tribromophenol, *9613*
[118-91-2] *o*-Chlorobenzoic Acid, *2124*
[118-92-3] *o*-Aminobenzoic Acid, *422*
[118-96-7] 2,4,6-Trinitrotoluene, *9730*
[119-04-0] Neomycin B, *6454*
[119-13-1] δ-Tocopherol, *9498*
[119-24-4] Pteroic Acid, *7933*
[119-26-6] 2,4-Dinitrophenylhydrazine, *3283*
[119-28-8] 1,7-Cleve's Acid, *2351*
[119-36-8] Methyl Salicylate, *6120*
[119-38-0] Isolan, *5178*
[119-41-5] Efloxate, *3523*
[119-44-8] Xanthopterin, *10064*
[119-53-9] Benzoin, *1093*
[119-61-9] Benzophenone, *1098*
[119-64-2] Tetralin®, *9221*
[119-65-3] Isoquinoline, *5222*
[119-79-9] 1,6-Cleve's Acid, *2350*
[119-90-4] Dianisidine, *2991*
[119-93-7] *o*-Tolidine, *9514*
[119-96-0] Arsthinol, *812*
[119-98-2] Tocol, *9494*
[120-05-8] Sulfuretin, *8972*
[120-08-1] Scoparone, *8404*
[120-12-7] Anthracene, *682*
[120-14-9] Veratraldehyde, *9951*
[120-18-3] 2-Naphthalenesulfonic Acid, *6377*
[120-23-0] 2-Naphthoxyacetic Acid, *6397*
[120-29-6] Tropine, *9781*
[120-32-1] Clorophene, *2407*
[120-34-3] *N*-Sulfanilyl-3,4-xylamide, *8932*
[120-36-5] Dichlorprop, *3078*
[120-46-7] Dibenzoylmethane, *3009*
[120-47-8] Ethylparaben, *3837*
[120-51-4] Benzyl Benzoate, *1127*
[120-57-0] Piperonal, *7475*
[120-58-1] Isosafrole, *5223*
[120-62-7] Sulfoxide, *8967*
[120-66-1] *o*-Acetotoluide, *74*
[120-72-9] Indole, *4963*
[120-73-0] 1*H*-Purine, *7942*
[120-78-5] 2,2′-Dithiobis[benzothiazole], *3370*
[120-80-9] Pyrocatechol, *7999*
[120-82-1] 1,2,4-Trichlorobenzene, *9631*
[120-83-2] 2,4-Dichlorophenol, *3072*
[120-87-6] 9,10-Dihydroxystearic Acid, *3186*
[120-89-8] Parabanic Acid, *7022*
[120-92-3] Cyclopentanone, *2743*

[120-93-4] 2-Imidazolidinone, *4914*
[120-97-8] Dichlorphenamide, *3077*
[121-19-7] Roxarsone, *8273*
[121-20-0] Cinerin II, *2292*
[121-21-1] Pyrethrin I, *7964*
[121-25-5] Amprolium, *590*
[121-29-9] Pyrethrin II, *7964*
[121-30-2] Chloraminophenamide, *2076*
[121-32-4] Ethyl Vanillin, *3859*
[121-33-5] Vanillin, *9932*
[121-34-6] Vanillic Acid, *9931*
[121-40-4] Terreic Acid, *9172*
[121-43-7] Trimethyl Borate, *9712*
[121-44-8] Triethylamine, *9666*
[121-47-1] Metanilic Acid, *5927*
[121-54-0] Benzethonium Chloride, *1074*
[121-57-3] Sulfanilic Acid, *8926*
[121-59-5] Carbarsone, *1786*
[121-60-8] *N*-Acetylsulfanilyl Chloride, *103*
[121-61-9] *N⁴*-Acetylsulfanilamide, *8925*
[121-62-0] *N*-Acetylsulfanilic Acid, *102*
[121-66-4] 2-Amino-5-nitrothiazole, *457*
[121-69-7] *N,N*-Dimethylaniline, *3234*
[121-73-3] *m*-Chloronitrobenzene, *2151*
[121-75-5] Malathion, *5700*
[121-79-9] Propyl Gallate, *7859*
[121-81-3] Nitromide, *6612*
[121-82-4] Cyclonite, *2736*
[121-91-5] Isophthalic Acid, *5197*
[122-03-2] Cuminaldehyde, *2621*
[122-04-3] 4-Nitrobenzoyl Chloride, *6590*
[122-06-5] Stilbamidine, *8816*
[122-09-8] Phentermine, *7262*
[122-10-1] Bomyl®, *1330*
[122-11-2] Sulfadimethoxine, *8905*
[122-14-5] Fenitrothion, *3976*
[122-16-7] Sulfanitran, *8933*
[122-18-9] Cetalkonium Chloride, *2017*
[122-25-8] 5,5′-Methylenedisalicylic Acid, *6065*
[122-28-1] *m*-Nitroacetanilide, *6581*
[122-32-7] Triolein, *9732*
[122-34-9] Simazine, *8533*
[122-39-4] Diphenylamine, *3317*
[122-42-9] Propham, *7816*
[122-46-3] *m*-Cresyl Acetate, *2583*
[122-48-5] Zingerone, *10166*
[122-51-0] Orthoformic Acid Triethyl Ester, *6884*
[122-57-6] Benzylideneacetone, *1137*
[122-59-8] Phenoxyacetic Acid, *7254*
[122-62-3] Bis(2-ethylhexyl) Sebacate, *1251*
[122-69-0] Cinnamyl Cinnamate, *2304*
[122-78-1] Phenylacetaldehyde, *7265*
[122-79-2] Phenyl Acetate, *7267*
[122-80-5] *p*-Aminoacetanilide, *411*
[122-87-2] *N*-(4-Hydroxyphenyl)-glycine, *4837*
[122-99-6] 2-Phenoxyethanol, *7257*
[123-02-4] Tridecylbenzene, *9659*
[123-03-5] Cetylpyridinium Chloride, *2032*
[123-08-0] *p*-Hydroxybenzaldehyde, *4811*
[123-11-5] *p*-Anisaldehyde, *663*
[123-19-3] Dipropyl Ketone, *3345*
[123-29-5] Ethyl Pelargonate, *3838*

[123-30-8] *p*-Aminophenol, *462*
[123-31-9] Hydroquinone, *4808*
[123-33-1] Maleic Hydrazide, *5705*
[123-35-3] β-Myrcene, *6331*
[123-38-6] Propionaldehyde, *7823*
[123-39-7] *N*-Methylformamide, *6076*
[123-42-2] Diacetone Alcohol, *2964*
[123-43-3] Sulfoacetic Acid, *8953*
[123-45-5] Sulfonyldiacetic Acid, *8961*
[123-47-7] Prolonium Iodide, *7782*
[123-51-3] Isopentyl Alcohol, *5195*
[123-54-6] Acetylacetone, *81*
[123-56-8] Succinimide, *8871*
[123-62-6] Propionic Anhydride, *7826*
[123-63-7] Paraldehyde, *7027*
[123-66-0] Ethyl Caproate, *3777*
[123-72-8] Butyraldehyde, *1591*
[123-75-1] Pyrrolidine, *8015*
[123-76-2] Levulinic Acid, *5472*
[123-77-3] Azodicarbonamide, *919*
[123-78-4] Sphingosine, *8747*
[123-82-0] Tuaminoheptane, *9802*
[123-84-2] 1-[(2-Aminoethyl)amino]-2-propanol, *438*
[123-86-4] *n*-Butyl Acetate, *1535*
[123-90-0] Thiamorpholine, *9300*
[123-91-1] Dioxane, *3300*
[123-92-2] Isoamyl Acetate, *5111*
[123-93-3] Thiodiglycolic Acid, *9331*
[123-95-5] Butyl Stearate, *1589*
[123-96-6] 2-Octanol, *6752*
[123-99-9] Azelaic Acid, *905*
[124-02-7] Diallylamine, *2971*
[124-03-8] Cetyldimethylethylammonium Bromide, *2029*
[124-04-9] Adipic Acid, *162*
[124-07-2] Caprylic Acid, *1765*
[124-09-4] 1,6-Hexanediamine, *4695*
[124-13-0] Caprylic Aldehyde, *1766*
[124-20-9] Spermidine, *8742*
[124-28-7] Dymanthine, *3475*
[124-38-9] Carbon Dioxide, *1809*
[124-40-3] Dimethylamine, *3228*
[124-41-4] Sodium Methoxide, *8643*
[124-42-5] Acetamidine Hydrochloride, *44*
[124-43-6] Carbamide Peroxide, *1782*
[124-47-0] Urea Nitrate, *9869*
[124-48-1] Chlorodibromomethane, *2135*
[124-58-3] Methanearsonic Acid, *5953*
[124-63-0] Methanesulfonyl Chloride, *5955*
[124-65-2] Sodium Cacodylate, *8595*
[124-68-5] 2-Amino-2-methyl-1-propanol, *449*
[124-72-1] Teflurane, *9110*
[124-76-5] Isoborneol, *5128*
[124-87-8] Picrotoxin, *7415*
[124-90-3] Oxycodone Hydrochloride, *6959*
[124-92-5] Metopon Hydrochloride, *6150*
[124-94-7] Triamcinolone, *9595*
[124-97-0] Protoveratrine B, *7899*
[124-98-1] Cevine, *2035*
[124-99-2] Scillaren A, *8399*
[125-02-0] Prednisolone 21-Disodium Phosphate, *7721*
[125-03-1] Hydrocortamate Hydrochloride, *4786*
[125-04-2] Hydrocortisone 21-Sodium Succinate, *4787*
[125-10-0] Prednisone 21-Acetate, *7722*

[125-15-5] Vomicine, *10031*
[125-20-2] Thymolphthalein, *9401*
[125-24-6] Pseudomorphine, *7919*
[125-28-0] Dihydrocodeine, *3171*
[125-29-1] Hydrocodone, *4785*
[125-31-5] Xylenol Blue, *10083*
[125-33-7] Primidone, *7746*
[125-46-2] Usnic Acid, *9893*
[125-51-9] Pipenzolate Bromide, *7461*
[125-52-0] Oxyphencyclimine Hydrochloride, *6973*
[125-53-1] Oxyphencyclimine, *6973*
[125-60-0] Fenpiverinium Bromide, *3990*
[125-64-4] Methyprylon, *6136*
[125-65-5] Pleuromutilin, *7534*
[125-68-8] Levomethorphan Hydrobromide, *8091*
[125-69-9] Dextromethorphan Hydrobromide, *8091*
[125-73-5] Levorphanol *d*-Form, *5470*
[125-84-8] Aminoglutethimide, *440*
[125-85-9] Caramiphen Hydrochloride, *1776*
[125-86-0] Caramiphen Ethanedisulfonate, *1776*
[125-88-2] Aprobarbital Sodium Salt, *756*
[125-99-5] Tridihexethyl Iodide, *9661*
[126-00-1] Diphenolic Acid, *3312*
[126-07-8] Griseofulvin, *4549*
[126-11-4] Tris(hydroxymethyl)nitromethane, *9753*
[126-12-5] Anileridine Dihydrochloride, *658*
[126-14-7] Sucrose Octaacetate, *8882*
[126-15-8] R-11, *8088*
[126-17-0] Solasodine, *8709*
[126-18-1] Smilagenin, *8565*
[126-19-2] Sarsasapogenin, *8380*
[126-22-7] Butonate, *9623*
[126-27-2] Oxethazaine, *6933*
[126-29-4] Violaxanthin, *9998*
[126-30-7] Neopentyl Glycol, *6458*
[126-31-8] Methiodal Sodium, *5973*
[126-33-0] Sulfolane, *8955*
[126-45-4] Silver Citrate, *8511*
[126-49-8] Prephenic Acid, *7738*
[126-52-3] Ethinamate, *3733*
[126-72-7] Tris-BP, *9751*
[126-73-8] Tributyl Phosphate, *9619*
[126-81-8] 5,5-Dimethyl-1,3-cyclohexanedione, *3242*
[126-96-5] Sodium Diacetate, *8607*
[126-98-7] Methacrylonitrile, *5942*
[127-00-4] *sec*-Propylene Chlorohydrin, *7851*
[127-06-0] Acetoxime, *75*
[127-07-1] Hydroxyurea, *4848*
[127-08-2] Potassium Acetate, *7605*
[127-09-3] Sodium Acetate, *8571*
[127-17-3] Pyruvic Acid, *8021*
[127-18-4] Tetrachloroethylene, *9190*
[127-19-5] *N,N*-Dimethylacetamide, *3227*
[127-20-8] Dalapon Sodium Salt, *2802*
[127-22-0] Taraxerol, *9062*
[127-25-3] Methyl Abietate, *6006*
[127-27-5] Pimaric Acid, *7428*
[127-31-1] Fludrocortisone, *4130*
[127-33-3] Demeclocycline, *2886*
[127-35-5] Phenazocine, *7218*
[127-39-9] Diisobutyl Sodium Sulfosuccinate, *3194*

[127-40-2] Xanthophyll, *10063*
[127-47-9] Vitamin A Acetate, *10013*
[127-48-0] Trimethadione, *9706*
[127-52-6] Chloramine-B, *2074*
[127-56-0] Sulfacetamide Sodium Salt, *8899*
[127-57-1] Sulfapyridine Sodium Salt Monohydrate, *8938*
[127-58-2] Sulfamerazine Monosodium Salt, *8913*
[127-60-6] Acediasulfone Sodium Salt, *23*
[127-63-9] Diphenyl Sulfone, *3332*
[127-65-1] Chloramine-T, *2075*
[127-69-5] Sulfisoxazole, *8952*
[127-71-9] Sulfabenzamide, *8897*
[127-77-5] Sulfabenz, *8896*
[127-79-7] Sulfamerazine, *8913*
[127-82-2] Zinc *p*-Phenolsulfonate, *10150*
[127-83-3] Calcium Phenolsulfonate, *1690*
[127-85-5] Sodium Arsanilate, *8578*
[127-91-3] β-Pinene, *7446*
[127-95-7] Potassium Binoxalate, *7611*
[127-96-8] Potassium Tetraoxalate, *7689*
[128-00-7] Silver Lactate, *8517*
[128-08-5] *N*-Bromosuccinimide, *1438*
[128-09-6] *N*-Chlorosuccinimide, *2164*
[128-13-2] Ursodiol, *9889*
[128-19-8] 4-Pregnene-17α,20β,21-triol-3-one, *7732*
[128-20-1] Pregnan-3α-ol-20-one, *7729*
[128-23-4] 3,20-Pregnanedione, *7728*
[128-27-8] Pyrocalciferol, *7997*
[128-37-0] Butylated Hydroxytoluene, *1548*
[128-46-1] Dihydrostreptomycin, *3179*
[128-49-4] Docusate Calcium, *3400*
[128-50-7] Nopol ((±)-form), *6683*
[128-53-0] *N*-Ethylmaleimide, *3822*
[128-57-4] Sennoside B, *8455*
[128-62-1] Noscapine, *6718*
[128-68-7] Phenicin, *7232*
[128-71-2] Phenoltetrachlorophthalein Disodium Salt, *7248*
[128-76-7] Laurotetanine, *5388*
[128-80-3] Quinizarin Green SS, *8065*
[128-87-0] Bis(4-amino-1-anthraquinonyl)amine, *1243*
[129-00-0] Pyrene, *7963*
[129-03-3] Cyproheptadine, *2773*
[129-06-6] Warfarin Sodium Salt, *10038*
[129-16-8] Merbromin, *5867*
[129-17-9] Sulphan Blue, *8987*
[129-18-0] Phenylbutazone Sodium Salt, *7277*
[129-20-4] Oxyphenbutazone, *6972*
[129-24-8] Viridicatin, *10005*
[129-46-4] Suramin Sodium, *9006*
[129-49-7] Methysergide Hydrogen Maleate, *6137*
[129-51-1] Ergonovine Maleate, *3655*
[129-63-5] Acetrizoate Sodium, *79*
[129-64-6] Carbic Anhydride, *1796*
[129-66-8] 2,4,6-Trinitrobenzoic Acid, *9727*
[129-73-7] Leucomalachite Green, *5699*
[129-74-8] Buclizine Dihydrochloride, *1464*
[129-77-1] Piperidolate Hydrochloride, *7470*
[129-79-3] 2,4,7-Trinitrofluorenone, *9728*

[129-83-9] Phenampromid(e), *7209*
[130-01-8] Senecionine, *8451*
[130-15-4] 1,4-Naphthoquinone, *6395*
[130-16-5] Cloxyquin, *2422*
[130-22-3] Sodium Alizarinesulfonate, *8573*
[130-24-5] Vitamin K$_5$ Hydrochloride, *10023*
[130-26-7] Iodochlorhydroxyquin, *5031*
[130-37-0] Menadione Sodium Bisulfite, *5831*
[130-40-5] Riboflavin Monophosphate Monosodium Salt, *8201*
[130-61-0] Thioridazine Hydrochloride, *9359*
[130-73-4] Methestrol, *5968*
[130-79-0] Dimestrol, *3211*
[130-80-3] Diethylstilbestrol Dipropionate, *3129*
[130-85-8] Pamoic Acid, *7005*
[130-86-9] Protopine, *7896*
[130-89-2] Quinine Hydrochloride, *8061*
[130-95-0] Quinine (anhydrous), *8061*
[131-01-1] Deserpidine, *2918*
[131-02-2] Reserpiline, *8144*
[131-03-3] α-Yohimbine, *10104*
[131-11-3] Dimethyl Phthalate, *3255*
[131-12-4] Pimpinellin, *7437*
[131-13-5] Menadiol Sodium Diphosphate, *5830*
[131-28-2] Narceine, *6422*
[131-49-7] Meglumine Diatrizoate, *5807*
[131-53-3] Dioxybenzone, *3303*
[131-54-4] Benzophenone-6, *1099*
[131-56-6] Benzoresorcinol, *1106*
[131-57-7] Oxybenzone, *6954*
[131-67-9] Phthalofyne, *7409*
[131-69-1] Phthalylsulfacetamide, *7376*
[131-73-7] Dipicrylamine, *3335*
[131-74-8] Ammonium Picrate, *547*
[131-79-3] Yellow OB, *10096*
[131-89-5] 2-Cyclohexyl-4,6-dinitrophenol, *2733*
[131-91-9] 1-Nitroso-2-naphthol, *6641*
[131-99-7] Inosinic Acid, *4977*
[132-13-8] α-Ribazole, *8199*
[132-17-2] Benztropine Mesylate, *1121*
[132-18-3] Diphenylpyraline Hydrochloride, *3331*
[132-20-7] Pheniramine Maleate, *7235*
[132-21-8] Brompheniramine *d*-Form, *1443*
[132-22-9] Chlorpheniramine, *2180*
[132-27-4] *o*-Phenylphenol Sodium Salt, *7304*
[132-35-4] Proxazole Citrate, *7903*
[132-40-1] Papaverine Nitrite, *7019*
[132-49-0] Magnesium Acetylsalicylate, *5655*
[132-57-0] Croceic Acid, *2588*
[132-58-1] Cinchophen Hydrochloride, *2288*
[132-60-5] Cinchophen, *2288*
[132-66-1] Naptalam, *6418*
[132-69-4] Benzydamine Hydrochloride, *1122*
[132-73-0] Chloroquine Sulfate, *2163*
[132-86-5] Naphthoresorcinol, *6396*
[132-92-3] Methicillin Sodium, *5969*
[132-93-4] Phenethicillin Potassium, *7223*
[132-98-9] Penicillin V Potassium Salt, *7100*

[133-04-0] Asarinin, *823*
[133-06-2] Captan, *1772*
[133-07-3] Folpet, *4224*
[133-09-5] *p*-Aminosalicylic Acid Potassium Salt, *477*
[133-11-9] Phenyl Aminosalicylate, *7272*
[133-15-3] *p*-Aminosalicylic Acid Calcium Salt, *477*
[133-17-5] *o*-Iodohippurate Sodium, *5034*
[133-26-6] Peucedanin, *7191*
[133-32-4] Indolebutyric Acid, *4965*
[133-36-8] Piperazine Tartrate, *7464*
[133-37-9] DL-Tartaric Acid, *9069*
[133-51-7] *N*-Methylglucamine Antimonate, *6078*
[133-53-9] Dichloroxylenol, *3076*
[133-58-4] Nitromersol, *6610*
[133-65-3] Solasulfone, *8711*
[133-67-5] Trichlormethiazide, *9624*
[133-89-1] Uridine Diphosphate Glucose, *9879*
[133-91-5] 3,5-Diiodosalicylic Acid, *3190*
[134-01-0] Peonidin, *7143*
[134-03-2] Sodium Ascorbate, *830*
[134-04-3] Pelargonidin, *7071*
[134-09-8] Menthyl Anthranilate, *5840*
[134-20-3] Methyl Anthranilate, *6020*
[134-31-6] 8-Hydroxyquinoline Sulfate, *4843*
[134-32-7] 1-Naphthylamine, *6398*
[134-36-1] Erythromycin Propionate, *3686*
[134-49-6] Phenmetrazine, *7237*
[134-50-9] Aminacrine Hydrochloride, *407*
[134-55-4] Phenyl Acetylsalicylate, *7270*
[134-58-7] 8-Azaguanine, *896*
[134-62-3] Deet, *2856*
[134-63-4] Lobeline Hydrochloride, *5551*
[134-64-5] Lobeline Sulfate, *5551*
[134-65-6] Lobeline (±)-Form, *5551*
[134-71-4] Ephedrine *dl*-Form Hydrochloride, *3608*
[134-72-5] Ephedrine Sulfate, *3608*
[134-80-5] Diethylpropion Hydrochloride, *3127*
[134-81-6] Benzil, *1078*
[134-95-2] Mandelic Acid Calcium Salt, *5717*
[134-96-3] Syringaldehyde, *9015*
[135-07-9] Methyclothiazide, *6005*
[135-09-1] Hydroflumethiazide, *4789*
[135-19-3] 2-Naphthol, *6384*
[135-20-6] Cupferron, *2622*
[135-23-9] Methapyrilene Hydrochloride, *5959*
[135-31-9] Pyrrobutamine Diphosphate, *8012*
[135-43-3] Lauroguadine, *5386*
[135-48-8] Pentacene, *7107*
[135-58-0] Mesulfen, *5918*
[135-59-1] Thionine, *9346*
[135-67-1] Phenoxazine, *7253*
[135-68-2] 4-Amino-4′-chlorodiphenyl, *435*
[135-97-7] Pseudotropine, *7921*
[135-98-8] *sec*-Butylbenzene, *1550*
[136-25-4] Erbon, *2802*
[136-35-6] Diazoaminobenzene, *2998*

[136-40-3] Phenazopyridine Hydrochloride, *7210*
[136-44-7] Glyceryl *p*-Aminobenzoate, *4487*
[136-47-0] Tetracaine Hydrochloride, *9188*
[136-55-0] Procaine Butyrate, *7757*
[136-60-7] *n*-Butyl Benzoate, *1552*
[136-69-6] Protokylol Hydrochloride, *7895*
[136-70-9] Protokylol, *7895*
[136-72-1] Piperic Acid *(E,E)*-Form, *7467*
[136-77-6] 4-Hexylresorcinol, *4712*
[136-79-8] 5-Nitro-*o*-phenetidine, *6617*
[136-82-3] Piperocaine, *7474*
[136-95-8] 2-Aminobenzothiazole, *424*
[137-00-8] 4-Methyl-5-thiazoleethanol, *6126*
[137-05-3] Methyl Cyanoacrylate, *6046*
[137-06-4] *o*-Thiocresol, *9325*
[137-08-6] Pantothenic Acid Calcium Salt, *7015*
[137-16-6] Gardol®, *4368*
[137-26-8] Thiram, *9371*
[137-30-4] Ziram, *10172*
[137-32-6] 2-Methyl-1-butanol, *6030*
[137-40-6] Sodium Propionate, *8669*
[137-42-8] Metham Sodium, *5949*
[137-53-1] Dextrothyroxine Sodium, *9415*
[137-58-6] Lidocaine, *5482*
[137-76-8] Cetotiamine, *2023*
[137-86-0] Octotiamine, *6760*
[138-14-7] Deferoxamine Methanesulfonate, *2860*
[138-15-8] Glutamic Acid Hydrochloride, *4469*
[138-32-9] Cetrimonium Tosylate, *2025*
[138-37-4] Mafenide Hydrochloride, *5649*
[138-39-6] Mafenide, *5649*
[138-41-0] Carzenide, *1876*
[138-52-3] Salicin, *8324*
[138-53-4] Mandelonitrile Glucoside, *5720*
[138-55-6] Picrocrocin, *7411*
[138-56-7] Trimethobenzamide, *9708*
[138-59-0] Shikimic Acid, *8480*
[138-61-4] Nordefrin Hydrochloride (unspecified stereo), *6692*
[138-84-1] Potassium *p*-Aminobenzoate, *7606*
[138-86-3] Limonene, *5493*
[138-89-6] *p*-Nitroso-*N,N*-dimethylaniline, *6638*
[138-91-0] Perillaldehyde Oxime, *7167*
[138-92-1] Betazole Dihydrochloride, *1183*
[139-02-6] Phenol Sodium Salt, *7241*
[139-06-0] Calcium Cyclamate, *1665*
[139-10-6] Amphetamine Phosphate, *582*
[139-13-9] Nitrilotriacetic Acid, *6579*
[139-33-3] EDTA Disodium Salt, *3517*
[139-40-2] Propazine, *7812*
[139-42-4] Cerous Oxalate, *2001*
[139-62-8] Cyclomethycaine, *2735*
[139-66-2] Phenyl Sulfide, *7314*
[139-68-4] Phenatine, *7216*
[139-85-5] Protocatechualdehyde, *7893*
[139-88-8] Sodium Tetradecyl Sulfate, *8689*
[139-89-9] Versenol®, *9966*

[139-91-3] Furaltadone, *4294*
[139-93-5] Arsphenamine, *811*
[139-94-6] Nithiazide, *6569*
[140-11-4] Benzyl Acetate, *1123*
[140-22-7] *sym*-Diphenylcarbazide, *3321*
[140-28-3] Benzathine, *1064*
[140-29-4] Benzyl Cyanide, *1131*
[140-40-9] Aminitrozole, *410*
[140-47-6] Phenocoll Salicylate, *7239*
[140-55-6] Pseudoconhydrine, *7914*
[140-59-0] Stilbamidine Isethionate, *8816*
[140-63-6] Propamidine Isethionate, *7797*
[140-64-7] Pentamidine Isethionate, *7115*
[140-65-8] Pramoxine, *7709*
[140-67-0] Estragole, *3705*
[140-80-7] Novoldiamine, *6723*
[140-87-4] Cyacetacide, *2680*
[140-88-5] Ethyl Acrylate, *3759*
[140-89-6] Potassium Xanthogenate, *7696*
[140-93-2] Sodium Isopropyl Xanthate, *8634*
[140-95-4] Oxymethurea, *6968*
[140-99-8] Calcium Succinate, *1705*
[141-01-5] Ferrous Fumarate, *4046*
[141-05-9] Diethyl Maleate, *3123*
[141-10-6] Pseudoionone, *7917*
[141-20-8] Diethylene Glycol Monolaurate, *3120*
[141-22-0] Ricinoleic Acid, *8211*
[141-26-4] α-Citronellal, *2329*
[141-27-5] Geranial, *2322*
[141-32-2] *n*-Butyl Acrylate, *1539*
[141-43-5] Ethanolamine, *3727*
[141-52-6] Sodium Ethoxide, *8613*
[141-53-7] Sodium Formate, *8621*
[141-62-8] Decamethyltetrasiloxane, *2850*
[141-63-9] Dodecamethylpentasiloxane, *3404*
[141-66-2] Dicrotophos, *3087*
[141-75-3] *n*-Butyryl Chloride, *1598*
[141-78-6] Ethyl Acetate, *3757*
[141-79-7] Mesityl Oxide, *5908*
[141-82-2] Malonic Acid, *5710*
[141-84-4] Rhodanine, *8184*
[141-90-2] 2-Thiouracil, *9366*
[141-94-6] Hexetidine, *4703*
[141-97-9] Ethyl Acetoacetate, *3758*
[142-03-0] Aluminum Hydroxydiacetate, *344*
[142-10-9] Glyceraldehyde 3-Phosphate, *4482*
[142-17-6] Calcium Oleate, *1684*
[142-47-2] Monosodium Glutamate, *6254*
[142-59-6] Nabam, *6341*
[142-61-0] Caproyl Chloride, *1763*
[142-62-1] *n*-Caproic Acid, *1759*
[142-68-7] Tetrahydropyran, *9217*
[142-71-2] Cupric Acetate, *2624*
[142-72-3] Magnesium Acetate, *5654*
[142-73-4] Iminodiacetic Acid, *4917*
[142-82-5] *n*-Heptane, *4659*
[142-84-7] *n*-Dipropylamine, *3343*
[142-88-1] Piperazine Adipate, *7465*
[142-96-1] *n*-Butyl Ether, *1569*
[143-07-7] Lauric Acid, *5384*
[143-08-8] *n*-Nonyl Alcohol, *6679*
[143-13-5] *n*-Nonyl Acetate, *6678*

[143-15-7] Lauryl Bromide, *5389*
[143-18-0] Potassium Oleate, *7650*
[143-19-1] Oleic Acid Sodium Salt, *6828*
[143-24-8] Tetraglyme, *9208*
[143-28-2] Oleyl Alcohol, *6831*
[143-33-9] Sodium Cyanide, *8605*
[143-50-0] Chlordecone, *2083*
[143-52-2] Metopon, *6150*
[143-57-7] Protoveratrine A, *7899*
[143-62-4] Digitoxigenin, *3162*
[143-66-8] Sodium Tetraphenylborate, *8690*
[143-67-9] Vinblastine Sulfate, *9982*
[143-74-8] Phenolsulfonphthalein, *7247*
[143-76-0] Cyclobarbital Calcium Salt, *2711*
[143-81-7] Butabarbital Sodium, *1506*
[144-02-5] Barbital Sodium Salt, *962*
[144-12-7] Tiemonium Iodide, *9431*
[144-14-9] Anileridine, *658*
[144-23-0] Magnesium Citrate Dibasic, *5663*
[144-29-6] Piperazine Citrate, *7464*
[144-33-2] Citric Acid Disodium Salt, *2326*
[144-49-0] Fluoroacetic Acid, *4167*
[144-55-8] Sodium Bicarbonate, *8583*
[144-62-7] Oxalic Acid, *6911*
[144-68-3] Zeaxanthin, *10118*
[144-75-2] Sulfoxone Sodium, *8968*
[144-80-9] Sulfacetamide, *8899*
[144-82-1] Sulfamethizole, *8916*
[144-83-2] Sulfapyridine, *8938*
[145-12-0] Oxymesterone, *6965*
[145-13-1] Pregnenolone, *7733*
[145-41-5] Dehydrocholic Acid Sodium Salt, *2868*
[145-73-3] Endothall, *3575*
[146-14-5] Flavine-Adenine Dinucleotide, *4091*
[146-17-8] Riboflavin Monophosphate, *8201*
[146-22-5] Nitrazepam, *6575*
[146-28-1] Thiopropazate Dihydrochloride, *9356*
[146-37-2] Laurolinium Acetate, *5387*
[146-48-5] Yohimbine, *10102*
[146-54-3] Triflupromazine, *9685*
[146-56-5] Fluphenazine Dihydrochloride, *4189*
[146-80-5] Xanthosine, *10065*
[146-84-9] Silver Picrate, *8526*
[146-90-7] Cinnabarine, *2296*
[147-14-8] Copper Phthalocyanine, *2520*
[147-20-6] Diphenylpyraline, *3331*
[147-24-0] Diphenhydramine Hydrochloride, *3309*
[147-48-8] Penicillin V Calcium Salt, *7100*
[147-52-4] Nafcillin, *6352*
[147-61-5] Pentoxyl, *7137*
[147-71-7] D-Tartaric Acid, *9068*
[147-73-9] *meso*-Tartaric Acid, *9071*
[147-81-9] Arabinose, *761*
[147-82-0] 2,4,6-Tribromoaniline, *9610*
[147-85-3] Proline, *7780*
[147-90-0] Morpholine Salicylate, *6277*
[147-93-3] Thiosalicylic Acid, *9360*
[147-94-4] Cytarabine, *2784*
[148-01-6] Dinitolmide, *3269*
[148-03-8] β-Tocopherol (*dl*-form), *9496*

[148-18-5] Ditiocarb Sodium, *3378*
[148-24-3] 8-Hydroxyquinoline, *4843*
[148-25-4] Chromotropic Acid, *2241*
[148-56-1] Flumethiazide, *4139*
[148-64-1] Chlorothen Citrate, *2167*
[148-65-2] Chlorothen, *2167*
[148-72-1] Pilocarpine Nitrate, *7424*
[148-75-4] 2-Naphthol-3,6-disulfonic Acid, *6387*
[148-79-8] Thiabendazole, *9289*
[148-82-3] Melphalan, *5828*
[148-83-4] Ostruthin, *6896*
[149-15-5] Butacaine Sulfate, *1507*
[149-16-6] Butacaine, *1507*
[149-29-1] Patulin, *7053*
[149-30-4] 2-Mercaptobenzothiazole, *5868*
[149-32-6] Erythritol, *3675*
[149-44-0] Sodium Formaldehydesulfoxylate, *8620*
[149-45-1] Tiron, *9465*
[149-64-4] *N*-Butylscopolammonium Bromide, *1588*
[149-73-5] Orthoformic Acid Trimethyl Ester, *6884*
[149-90-6] Acetylleucine Monoethanolamine, *95*
[149-91-7] Gallic Acid, *4345*
[150-13-0] *p*-Aminobenzoic Acid, *423*
[150-25-4] Bicine, *1201*
[150-30-1] Phenylalanine DL-Form, *7271*
[150-38-9] EDTA Trisodium Salt, *3517*
[150-59-4] Alverine, *371*
[150-60-7] Dibenzyl Disulfide, *3013*
[150-61-8] 1,2-Dianilinoethane, *2990*
[150-68-5] Monuron, *6261*
[150-69-6] Dulcin, *3464*
[150-86-7] Phytol, *7390*
[150-90-3] Sodium Succinate, *8679*
[150-97-0] Mevalonic Acid, *6163*
[151-06-4] Chlorphentermine Hydrochloride, *2182*
[151-07-5] Chloroarsenol, *2119*
[151-18-8] 3-Aminopropionitrile, *469*
[151-21-3] Sodium Lauryl Sulfate, *8636*
[151-50-8] Potassium Cyanide, *7626*
[151-56-4] Ethylenimine, *3804*
[151-63-3] Aminoacetonitrile Sulfate (1:1), *412*
[151-67-7] Halothane, *4603*
[151-73-5] Betamethasone 21-Phosphate Disodium Salt, *1180*
[152-02-3] Levallorphan, *5458*
[152-11-4] Verapamil Hydrochloride, *9950*
[152-16-9] Schradan, *8395*
[152-43-2] Quinestrol, *8055*
[152-47-6] Sulfalene, *8910*
[152-58-9] 11-Desoxy-17-hydroxycorticosterone, *2932*
[152-62-5] Dydrogesterone, *3474*
[152-72-7] Acenocoumarol, *29*
[152-84-1] Ruberythric Acid, *8280*
[152-93-2] Vicine, *9975*
[152-95-4] Sophoricoside, *4391*
[152-97-6] Fluocortolone, *4153*
[153-00-4] Methenolone, *5967*
[153-18-4] Rutin, *8304*
[153-61-7] Cephalothin, *1982*
[153-77-5] 8-Hydroxyquinoline Aluminum Sulfate, *4843*
[153-87-7] Oxypertine, *6971*

[154-17-6] 2-Deoxy-D-glucose, *2904*
[154-21-2] Lincomycin, *5500*
[154-23-4] Catechin, *1902*
[154-41-6] Phenylpropanolamine Hydrochloride, *7307*
[154-42-7] Thioguanine, *9337*
[154-61-0] Primulaverin, *7749*
[154-68-7] Antazoline Phosphate, *680*
[154-69-8] Tripelennamine Hydrochloride, *9738*
[154-82-5] Simetride, *8535*
[154-87-0] Thiamine Diphosphate, *9296*
[154-93-8] Carmustine, *1845*
[154-97-2] Pralidoxime Mesylate, *7703*
[155-09-9] Tranylcypromine, *9573*
[155-38-4] Noformicin, *6670*
[155-41-9] Methscopolamine Bromide, *6003*
[155-54-4] Hydroorotic Acid, *4804*
[155-58-8] Rhapontin, *8174*
[156-08-1] Benzphetamine, *1118*
[156-10-5] *p*-Nitrosodiphenylamine, *6639*
[156-34-3] Amphetamine *l*-Form, *582*
[156-43-4] *p*-Phenetidine, *7228*
[156-51-4] Phenelzine Acid Sulfate, *7221*
[156-56-9] Hypoglycine A, *4866*
[156-59-2] Acetylene Dichloride *cis*-Form, *92*
[156-60-5] Acetylene Dichloride *trans*-Form, *92*
[156-62-7] Calcium Cyanamide, *1662*
[157-03-9] 6-Diazo-5-oxo-L-norleucine, *3002*
[191-07-1] Coronene, *2536*
[192-97-2] Benzo[*e*]pyrene, *1104*
[195-19-7] 3,4-Benzphenanthrene, *1117*
[198-55-0] Perylene, *7184*
[213-46-7] Picene, *7396*
[217-59-4] Triphenylene, *9740*
[218-01-9] Chrysene, *2255*
[222-93-5] 2,3:6,7-Dibenzphenanthrene, *3010*
[244-69-9] γ-Carboline, *1805*
[253-14-5] Twistane, *9828*
[253-52-1] Phthalazine, *7370*
[253-66-7] Cinnoline, *2306*
[253-82-7] Quinazoline, *8053*
[254-04-6] 1,2-Benzopyran, *1102*
[260-94-6] Acridine, *122*
[261-31-4] Thioxanthene, *9368*
[271-44-3] 1*H*-Indazole, *4936*
[271-89-6] Benzofuran, *1088*
[275-51-4] Azulene, *926*
[277-10-1] Cubane, *2611*
[280-57-9] Triethylenediamine, *9669*
[281-23-2] Adamantane, *149*
[286-08-8] Norcarane, *6688*
[287-23-0] Cyclobutane, *2714*
[287-92-3] Cyclopentane, *2741*
[288-13-1] Pyrazole, *7960*
[288-32-4] Imidazole, *4912*
[288-47-1] Thiazole, *9307*
[288-88-0] 1*H*-1,2,4-Triazole, *9605*
[288-99-3] 1,3,4-Oxadiazole, *6906*
[289-80-5] Pyridazine, *7969*
[289-95-2] Pyrimidine, *7987*
[290-37-9] Pyrazine, *7957*
[290-87-9] *s*-Triazine, *9602*
[292-46-6] Lenthionine, *5438*
[297-76-7] Ethynodiol Diacetate, *3860*
[297-78-9] Isobenzan, *5127*

[297-90-5] Levorphanol *dl*-Form, 5470
[298-00-0] Methyl Parathion, 6108
[298-02-2] Phorate, 7331
[298-04-4] Disulfoton, 3365
[298-12-4] Glyoxylic Acid, 4511
[298-14-6] Potassium Bicarbonate, 7609
[298-45-3] Bulbocapnine, 1481
[298-46-4] Carbamazepine, 1781
[298-55-5] Clocinizine, 2367
[298-57-7] Cinnarizine, 2305
[298-59-9] Methylphenidate Hydrochloride, 6110
[298-81-7] Methoxsalen, 5988
[298-95-3] Neotetrazolium Chloride, 6466
[298-96-4] Triphenyltetrazolium Chloride, 9744
[299-11-6] *N*-Methylphenazonium Methosulfate, 6109
[299-26-3] α-Methyltryptamine, 6131
[299-27-4] Potassium Gluconate, 4456
[299-28-5] Calcium Gluconate, 1669
[299-29-6] Ferrous Gluconate, 4047
[299-42-3] Ephedrine, 3608
[299-45-6] Hymecromone *O,O*-Diethyl Phosphorothioate, 4855
[299-84-3] Ronnel, 8256
[299-85-4] DMPA, 3392
[299-86-5] Crufomate, 2604
[299-89-8] Acetiamine, 54
[300-08-3] Arecoline Hydrobromide, 778
[300-30-1] DL-Thyroxine, 9415
[300-37-8] Iodopyracet, 5040
[300-38-9] 3,5-Dibromo-L-tyrosine, 3030
[300-48-1] 3-*O*-Methyldopa, 6056
[300-54-9] Muscarine, 6310
[300-62-9] Amphetamine, 582
[300-76-5] Naled, 6358
[300-85-6] β-Hydroxybutyric Acid, 4816
[301-04-2] Lead Acetate, 5397
[301-16-6] Scoparin, 8402
[301-19-9] Robinin, 8243
[301-21-3] Laudanidine, 5379
[302-01-2] Hydrazine, 4770
[302-17-0] Chloral Hydrate, 2071
[302-22-7] Chlormadinone Acetate, 2102
[302-27-2] Aconitine, 118
[302-40-9] Benactyzine, 1029
[302-41-0] Piritramide, 7498
[302-49-8] Uredepa, 9872
[302-66-9] Meparfynol Carbamate, 5846
[302-70-5] Mechlorethamine Oxide Hydrochloride, 5776
[302-72-7] DL-Alanine, 204
[302-79-4] Retinoic Acid, 8165
[302-84-1] Serine DL-Form, 8460
[302-91-0] Allopregnane-3α,11β,-17α,21-tetrol-20-one, 273
[302-96-5] Stanozolol (1′*H* form), 8794
[303-25-3] Cyclizine Hydrochloride, 2710
[303-34-4] Lasiocarpine, 5375
[303-40-2] Fluocortolone 21-Hexanoate, 4153
[303-42-4] Methenolone 17-Enanthate, 5967
[303-45-7] Gossypol, 4528
[303-47-9] Ochratoxin A, 6740

[303-49-1] Clomipramine, 2387
[303-53-7] Cyclobenzaprine, 2713
[303-69-5] Prothipendyl, 7888
[303-81-1] Novobiocin, 6722
[303-98-0] Ubiquinone 50, 9843
[304-20-1] Hydralazine Hydrochloride, 4763
[304-21-2] Harmaline, 4613
[304-55-2] Succimer, 8865
[304-59-6] Potassium Sodium Tartrate, 7670
[304-84-7] Ethamivan, 3721
[305-01-1] Esculetin, 3697
[305-03-3] Chlorambucil, 2073
[305-13-5] Acetamidoeugenol, 46
[305-33-9] Iproniazid Phosphate, 5078
[305-80-6] *p*-Diazobenzenesulfonic Acid, 2999
[305-84-0] Carnosine, 1850
[305-85-1] Disophenol, 3359
[305-96-4] α-Methyl-*m*-tyrosine, 6132
[306-03-6] Hyoscyamine Hydrobromide, 4858
[306-07-0] Pargyline Hydrochloride, 7038
[306-08-1] Homovanillic Acid, 4740
[306-11-6] Toliprolol Hydrochloride, 9516
[306-21-8] Hydroxyamphetamine Hydrobromide, 4810
[306-44-5] Isonitrosoacetone, 5190
[306-52-5] Triclofos, 9655
[306-60-5] Agmatine, 188
[306-61-6] Magnesium Thiocyanate, 5693
[306-94-5] Perfluorodecalin, 4183
[309-00-2] Aldrin, 226
[309-29-5] Doxapram, 3432
[309-43-3] Secobarbital Sodium, 8420
[309-88-6] Ishikawa Reagent, 5108
[311-45-5] Paraoxon, 7030
[312-10-7] Penicillamine Disulfide, 7090
[312-45-8] Hemicholinium Dibromide, 4643
[312-84-5] Serine D-Form, 8460
[313-04-2] Desmosterol, 2925
[313-05-3] Azacosterol, 892
[313-06-4] Estradiol Cypionate, 3703
[313-67-7] Aristolochic Acid, 786
[314-13-6] Evan's Blue, 3905
[314-19-2] Apomorphine Hydrochloride, 746
[314-35-2] Etamiphyllin, 3711
[314-40-9] Bromacil, 1381
[314-50-1] Orotidine, 6877
[315-22-0] Monocrotaline, 6250
[315-30-0] Allopurinol, 279
[315-37-7] Testosterone Enanthate, 9180
[315-72-0] Opipramol, 6853
[315-80-0] Dibenzepin Hydrochloride, 3008
[316-42-7] Emetine Dihydrochloride, 3559
[316-81-4] Thioproperazine, 9357
[317-34-0] Aminophylline, 465
[317-52-2] Hexafluorenium Bromide, 4684
[318-23-0] Imolamine, 4923
[318-98-9] Propranolol Hydrochloride, 7840
[319-89-1] Tetroquinone, 9249
[320-67-2] Azacitidine, 890

[321-54-0] Coroxon, 2537
[321-55-1] Haloxon, 4605
[321-64-2] Tacrine, 9024
[322-35-0] Benserazide, 1050
[322-79-2] Triflusal, 9688
[326-43-2] Phenyramidol Hydrochloride, 7321
[327-57-1] Norleucine, 6706
[327-97-9] Chlorogenic Acid, 2142
[328-42-7] Oxalacetic Acid, 6909
[328-50-7] α-Ketoglutaric Acid, 5303
[329-56-6] Norepinephrine Hydrochloride, 6695
[329-63-5] Epinephrine *dl*-Form Hydrochloride, 3619
[329-65-7] Epinephrine *dl*-Form, 3619
[329-71-5] 2,5-Dinitrophenol, 3281
[329-98-6] PMSF, 7542
[330-54-1] Diuron, 3382
[330-55-2] Linuron, 5509
[330-95-0] Nicarbazin, 6494
[331-39-5] Caffeic Acid, 1635
[333-20-0] Potassium Thiocyanate, 7691
[333-36-8] Flurothyl, 4201
[333-41-5] Diazinon, 2995
[334-20-3] Queen Substance, 8032
[334-48-5] *n*-Capric Acid, 1758
[334-88-3] Diazomethane, 3001
[337-47-3] Thiamylal Sodium Salt, 9302
[338-69-2] D-Alanine, 204
[338-83-0] Perfluorotripropylamine, 4183
[338-95-4] Isoflupredone, 5174
[338-98-7] Isoflupredone 21-Acetate, 5174
[339-43-5] Carbutamide, 1832
[339-44-6] Glymidine, 4507
[340-56-7] Methaqualone Hydrochloride, 5960
[340-57-8] Mecloqualone, 5781
[341-70-8] Diethazine Hydrochloride, 3108
[341-88-8] HQNO, 4751
[342-10-9] Kallidin, 5278
[343-65-7] Kynurenine, 5328
[345-78-8] Pseudoephedrine Hydrochloride, 7916
[346-18-9] Polythiazide, 7584
[348-67-4] Methionine D-Form, 5975
[349-46-2] Cystine D-Form, 2782
[350-03-8] Methyl Pyridyl Ketone, 6116
[350-12-9] Sulbentine, 8892
[352-21-6] 4-Amino-3-hydroxybutyric Acid, 444
[352-32-9] *p*-Fluorotoluene, 4180
[352-70-5] *m*-Fluorotoluene, 4180
[352-93-2] Ethyl Sulfide, 3854
[352-97-6] Glycocyamine, 4495
[353-50-4] Carbonyl Fluoride, 1820
[355-42-0] Perfluorohexane, 7157
[355-80-6] 2,2,3,3,4,4,5,5-Octafluoro-1-pentanol, 6746
[356-12-7] Fluocinonide, 4151
[357-07-3] Oxymorphone Hydrochloride, 6969
[357-08-4] Naloxone Hydrochloride, 6362
[357-56-2] Dextromoramide, 2955
[357-57-3] Brucine, 1455
[357-67-5] Phenetharbital, 7222
[357-70-0] Galantamine, 4340

[358-52-1] Hexapropymate, 4698
[359-83-1] Pentazocine, 7121
[360-66-7] Androisoxazole, 634
[360-68-9] Coprosterol, 2524
[360-70-3] Nandrolone Decanoate, 6365
[361-37-5] Methysergide, 6137
[362-29-8] Propiomazine, 7822
[362-74-3] Bucladesine, 1463
[363-24-6] Prostaglandin E₂, 7877
[364-62-5] Metoclopramide, 6143
[364-98-7] Diazoxide, 3004
[365-26-4] p-Hydroxyephedrine, 4824
[366-13-2] Neutral Red (free base), 6488
[366-18-7] α,α'-Dipyridyl, 3347
[366-70-1] Procarbazine Hydrochloride, 7758
[367-25-9] 2,4-Difluoroaniline, 3147
[367-51-1] Sodium Thioglycolate, 8692
[367-93-1] IPTG, 5082
[368-39-8] Meerwein's Reagent, 5796
[369-77-7] Cloflucarban, 2379
[370-14-9] Pholedrine, 7330
[371-11-9] Difluoroiodotoluene, 3150
[371-40-4] p-Fluoroaniline, 4169
[371-86-8] Mipafox, 6205
[372-09-8] Cyanoacetic Acid, 2689
[372-66-7] Heptaminol, 4657
[372-75-8] Citrulline, 2331
[373-02-4] Nickel Acetate, 6499
[378-44-9] Betamethasone, 1180
[379-93-1] Ergotamine Tartrate, 3661
[382-45-6] Adrenosterone, 176
[382-67-2] Desoximetasone, 2930
[386-17-4] Iodophthalein, 5038
[388-51-2] Metofenazate, 6145
[389-08-2] Nalidixic Acid, 6359
[390-28-3] Methoxamine, 5987
[390-64-7] Prenylamine, 7737
[392-56-3] Hexafluorobenzene, 4686
[395-28-8] Isoxsuprine, 5238
[396-01-0] Triamterene, 9599
[398-23-2] 4,4'-Difluorodiphenyl, 3149
[402-61-9] 5-Methylpyrazole-3-carboxylic Acid, 6115
[404-82-0] Fenfluramine Hydrochloride, 3973
[404-86-4] Capsaicin, 1768
[405-50-5] p-Fluorophenylacetic Acid, 4177
[406-76-8] Carnitine DL-Form, 1849
[406-90-6] Fluroxene, 4202
[407-41-0] Phosphoserine, 7363
[409-21-2] Silicon Carbide, 8492
[420-04-2] Cyanamide, 2684
[420-05-3] Cyanic Acid, 2686
[421-20-5] Methyl Fluorosulfonate, 6075
[423-55-2] Perflubron, 7156
[426-13-1] Fluorometholone, 4175
[427-00-9] Desomorphine, 2927
[427-01-0] Geissospermine, 4381
[427-51-0] Cyproterone Acetate, 2774
[429-41-4] Tetrabutylammonium Fluoride, 9187
[431-03-8] Diacetyl, 2966
[432-60-0] Allylestrenol, 291
[432-68-8] Echinenone, 3495
[434-03-7] Ethisterone, 3741
[434-05-9] Methenolone 17-Acetate, 5967
[434-07-1] Oxymetholone, 6967
[434-13-9] Lithocholic Acid, 5545

[434-16-2] (3β)-7-Dehydrocholesterol, 2867
[434-22-0] Nandrolone, 6365
[434-43-5] Pentorex, 7133
[435-97-2] Phenprocoumon, 7259
[436-05-5] Curine, 2674
[437-38-7] Fentanyl, 4001
[437-50-3] Gentisin, 4399
[437-74-1] Xanthinol Niacinate, 10060
[438-08-4] Etiocholanic Acid, 3867
[438-22-2] Androstane, 635
[438-23-3] Etiocholane, 3866
[438-41-5] Chlordiazepoxide Hydrochloride, 2084
[438-60-8] Protriptyline, 7901
[439-14-5] Diazepam, 2994
[439-89-4] Gentianine, 4394
[440-17-5] Trifluoperazine Dihydrochloride, 9680
[440-58-4] Iodamide, 5011
[441-38-3] Benzoin Oxime, 1094
[441-61-2] Ethylmethylthiambutene, 3829
[442-16-0] Ethacridine, 3716
[442-51-3] Harmine, 4616
[442-52-4] Clemizole, 2346
[443-48-1] Metronidazole, 6157
[444-27-9] Timonacic, 9445
[445-30-7] Homarine, 4729
[446-71-9] Homoeriodictyol, 4736
[446-72-0] Genistein, 4391
[446-86-6] Azathioprine, 902
[446-95-7] l-α-Isosparteine, 8737
[447-41-6] Nylidrin, 6732
[451-13-8] Homogentisic Acid, 4737
[451-71-8] Glyhexamide, 4506
[452-35-7] Ethoxzolamide, 3755
[453-17-8] Glyceraldehyde D-Form, 4481
[453-18-9] Fluoroacetic Acid Methyl Ester, 4167
[454-14-8] Cuscohygrine, 2677
[456-22-4] p-Fluorobenzoic Acid, 4171
[456-59-7] Cyclandelate, 2704
[457-60-3] Neoarsphenamine, 6447
[457-87-4] N-Ethylamphetamine, 3763
[458-24-2] Fenfluramine, 3973
[458-35-5] Coniferyl Alcohol, 2504
[458-37-7] Curcumin, 2673
[458-88-8] Coniine, 2505
[459-67-6] Hydnocarpic Acid, 4761
[459-72-3] Fluoroacetic Acid Ethyl Ester, 4167
[459-86-9] Mitoguazone, 6213
[460-19-5] Cyanogen, 2691
[461-05-2] Carnitine DL-Form Hydrochloride, 1849
[461-58-5] Dicyanodiamide, 3092
[461-72-3] Hydantoin, 4760
[461-78-9] Chlorphentermine, 2182
[461-98-3] Kyanmethin, 5326
[462-02-2] Cyamelide, 2682
[462-06-6] Fluorobenzene, 4170
[462-08-8] β-Aminopyridine, 473
[462-10-2] Homocystine, 4735
[462-94-2] Cadaverine, 1609
[463-40-1] Linolenic Acid, 5506
[463-51-4] Ketene, 5298
[463-56-9] Thiocyanic Acid, 9328
[463-58-1] Carbonyl Sulfide, 1821
[463-72-9] Carbamyl Chloride, 1783
[463-78-5] Orthoformic Acid, 6884
[463-82-1] Neopentane, 6456
[463-88-7] Neurine, 6484

[464-41-5] Bornyl Chloride, 1340
[464-48-2] Camphor L-Form, 1732
[464-49-3] Camphor D-Form, 1732
[464-72-2] Benzopinacol, 1100
[464-81-3] Bufotoxin, 1479
[465-11-2] Gamabufotalin, 4358
[465-16-7] Oleandrin, 6826
[465-21-4] Bufalin, 1471
[465-22-5] Scillarenin, 8400
[465-28-1] Carotol, 1856
[465-39-4] Resibufogenin, 8146
[465-42-9] Capsanthin, 1769
[465-65-6] Naloxone, 6362
[465-74-7] Quinovic Acid, 8075
[465-92-9] Marrubiin, 5754
[465-99-6] Hederagenin, 4624
[466-06-8] Proscillaridin, 7874
[466-07-9] Neriifolin, 6474
[466-09-1] Uzarigenin, 9897
[466-40-0] Isomethadone, 5184
[466-43-3] Atisine, 862
[466-49-9] Aspidospermine, 850
[466-61-5] Lycopodine, 5622
[466-80-8] α-Erythroidine, 3679
[466-81-9] β-Erythroidine, 3680
[466-85-3] Wieland-Gumlich Aldehyde, 10044
[466-90-0] Dihydrocodeinone Enol Acetate, 3172
[466-96-6] Pseudocodeine, 7913
[466-97-7] Normorphine, 6711
[466-99-9] Hydromorphone, 4803
[467-04-9] Oripavine, 6867
[467-14-1] Neopine, 6460
[467-15-2] Norcodeine, 6690
[467-18-5] Myrophine, 6337
[467-36-7] Thialbarbital, 9292
[467-43-6] Methitural, 5978
[467-51-6] Samandarine, 8346
[467-53-8] Diginin, 3157
[467-55-0] Hecogenin, 4622
[467-60-7] Pipradrol, 7484
[467-83-4] Dipipanone, 3337
[467-84-5] Phenadoxone, 7207
[467-85-6] Normethadone, 6709
[467-98-1] Thebainone, 9277
[468-07-5] Phenomorphan, 7249
[468-10-0] Morphinan, 6275
[468-28-0] Lupulon, 5612
[468-56-4] Hydroxypethidine, 4836
[468-61-1] Oxeladin, 6930
[468-65-5] Buthalital, 1524
[468-76-8] Cassaine, 1891
[468-89-3] Nupharidine, 6727
[469-21-6] Doxylamine, 3441
[469-32-9] Hamamelitannin, 4607
[469-36-3] Oryzanol C, 6886
[469-59-0] Jervine, 5264
[469-62-5] Propoxyphene, 7839
[469-79-4] Ketobemidone, 5301
[469-81-8] Morpheridine, 6274
[469-83-0] Cafestol, 1634
[470-40-6] Thujopsene, 9393
[470-82-6] Eucalyptol, 3895
[470-90-6] Chlorfenvinphos, 2089
[471-09-0] Felinine, 3952
[471-15-8] β-Thujone, 9392
[471-25-0] Propiolic Acid, 7821
[471-29-4] Methylguanidine, 6083
[471-34-1] Calcium Carbonate, 1657
[471-35-2] Cacodyl, 1603
[471-46-5] Oxamide, 6918
[471-47-6] Oxamic Acid, 6917
[471-53-4] Enoxolone, 3590

[471-80-7] Steviol, *8810*
[471-87-4] Stachydrine, *8771*
[471-95-4] Bufotalin, *1477*
[472-15-1] Betulinic Acid, *1190*
[472-61-7] Astaxanthin, *855*
[472-70-8] Cryptoxanthin, *2609*
[472-87-7] 3-Dehydroretinal, *2873*
[472-92-4] δ-Carotene, *1855*
[472-93-5] γ-Carotene, *1854*
[473-06-3] Chrysanthenone, *2252*
[473-30-3] Thiazolsulfone, *9309*
[473-34-7] Dichloramine T, *3047*
[473-41-6] Tolbutamide Sodium Salt, *9507*
[473-81-4] Glyceric Acid, *4483*
[473-90-5] Mesoxalic Acid, *5913*
[473-98-3] Betulin, *1189*
[474-00-0] Eburnamonine, *3487*
[474-07-7] Brazilin, *1367*
[474-25-9] Chenodiol, *2054*
[474-40-8] α₁-Sitosterol, *8555*
[474-45-3] Funtumine, *4292*
[474-62-4] Campesterol, *1729*
[474-69-1] Lumisterol, *5602*
[474-70-4] Isopyrocalciferol, *5219*
[474-73-7] 24-Hydroxycholesterol, *4820*
[474-77-1] Epicholesterol, *3613*
[474-86-2] Equilin, *3643*
[475-20-7] Longifolene, *5567*
[475-25-2] Hematein, *4634*
[475-26-3] DFDT, *2957*
[475-31-0] Glycocholic Acid, *4494*
[475-54-7] Oosporein, *6850*
[475-67-2] Isocorydine, *5162*
[475-81-0] Glaucine, *4436*
[476-28-8] Lycorine, *5626*
[476-32-4] Chelidonine (+)-Form, *2053*
[476-33-5] Homochelidonine, *4732*
[476-45-9] Javanicin, *5262*
[476-66-4] Ellagic Acid, *3547*
[476-69-7] Corydine, *2546*
[476-70-0] Boldine, *1325*
[476-71-1] Domesticine, *3413*
[477-27-0] Colchiceine, *2470*
[477-30-5] Demecolcine, *2887*
[477-32-7] Visnadine, *10010*
[477-47-4] Picropodophyllin, *7546*
[477-58-7] Chondrocurine, *2212*
[477-60-1] Bebeerine, *1016*
[477-62-3] Isochondrodendrine, *5158*
[477-67-8] Picropodophyllic Acid, *7545*
[477-75-8] Triptycene, *9749*
[478-10-4] Elliptone, *3550*
[478-43-3] Rhein, *8176*
[478-60-4] Citromycetin, *2328*
[478-61-5] Berbamine, *1153*
[478-73-9] Pseudococaine, *7912*
[478-84-2] Bromolysergide, *1423*
[478-85-3] Apo-β-erythroidine, *744*
[478-94-4] Lysergamide, *5632*
[478-95-5] Isolysergic Acid, *5180*
[479-00-5] Ergometrinine, *3654*
[479-13-0] Coumestrol, *2564*
[479-18-5] Dyphylline, *3479*
[479-20-9] Atranorin, *869*
[479-23-2] Cholanthrene, *2197*
[479-27-6] 1,8-Naphthalenediamine, *6372*
[479-36-7] Daphnoline, *2819*
[479-45-8] Nitramine, *6573*
[479-61-8] Chlorophyll A, *2155*
[479-68-5] Broparoestrol, *1448*
[479-81-2] Bietamiverine, *1205*

[479-92-5] Propyphenazone, *7871*
[479-98-1] Aucubin, *877*
[480-11-5] Oroxylin A, *6878*
[480-15-9] Datiscetin, *2830*
[480-16-0] Morin, *6269*
[480-17-1] Leucocyanidin, *5452*
[480-30-8] Dichloralphenazone, *3046*
[480-36-4] Linarin, *5498*
[480-40-0] Chrysin, *2256*
[480-41-1] Naringenin, *6424*
[480-44-4] Acacetin, *13*
[480-49-9] Filipin III, *4080*
[480-54-6] Retrorsine, *8167*
[480-64-8] *o*-Orsellinic Acid, *6881*
[480-68-2] 5-Nitrobarbituric Acid, *6586*
[480-78-4] Platyphylline, *7531*
[480-81-9] Seneciphylline, *8452*
[480-85-3] Retronecine, *8166*
[481-05-0] Artemisin, *816*
[481-06-1] α-Santonin, *8361*
[481-17-4] Chondrillasterol, *2211*
[481-18-5] α-Spinasterol, *8749*
[481-20-9] Coprostane, *2523*
[481-21-0] (5α)-Cholestane, *2199*
[481-26-5] Pregnane, *7726*
[481-29-8] Epiandrosterone, *3609*
[481-37-8] Ecgonine, *3493*
[481-39-0] Juglone, *5269*
[481-42-5] Plumbagin, *7538*
[481-49-2] Cepharanthine, *1985*
[481-72-1] Aloe-Emodin, *306*
[481-74-3] Chrysophanic Acid, *2258*
[481-85-6] Menadiol, *5830*
[481-97-0] Estrone Sulfate, *3708*
[482-05-3] Diphenic Acid, *3310*
[482-15-5] Isothipendyl, *5227*
[482-20-2] Tylophorine, *9831*
[482-28-0] Cinchonamine, *2285*
[482-44-0] Imperatorin, *4925*
[482-66-6] 1,2-Cyclopentenophenanthrene, *2744*
[482-68-8] Sarpagine, *8378*
[482-70-2] Chimaphilin, *2058*
[482-74-6] Cryptopine, *2608*
[482-89-3] Indigo, *4943*
[482-91-7] Aricine, *784*
[483-04-5] Raubasine, *8119*
[483-10-3] Corynanthine, *2548*
[483-17-0] Cephaeline, *1973*
[483-18-1] Emetine, *3559*
[483-19-2] Emetamine, *3559*
[483-55-6] Phthiocol, *7378*
[483-57-8] Fervenulin, *4066*
[483-63-6] Crotamiton, *2594*
[483-64-7] Damascenine, *2808*
[483-65-8] Retene, *8160*
[483-78-3] Cadalene, *1608*
[484-11-7] Neocuproine, *6449*
[484-12-8] Osthole, *6895*
[484-20-8] Bergapten, *1157*
[484-23-1] Dihydralazine, *3169*
[484-29-7] Dictamnine, *3089*
[484-31-1] Apiole (Dill), *733*
[484-49-1] Olivacine, *6834*
[484-89-9] Fumigatin, *4288*
[484-93-5] Ecgonidine, *3492*
[485-19-8] Reticuline, *8163*
[485-35-8] Cytisine, *2789*
[485-41-6] Sulfachrysoidine, *8901*
[485-43-8] Iridomyrmecin, *5089*
[485-47-2] Ninhydrin, *6554*
[485-49-4] Bicuculline, *1203*
[485-50-7] Capnoidine, *165*
[485-64-3] Hydrocinchonidine, *4782*

[485-65-4] Hydrocinchonine, *4783*
[485-70-1] Epicinchonine, *2287*
[485-71-2] Cinchonidine, *2286*
[485-72-3] Formononetin, *4244*
[485-89-2] Oxycinchophen, *6957*
[485-91-6] Allocryptopine, *265*
[486-12-4] Triprolidine, *9746*
[486-16-8] Carbinoxamine, *1799*
[486-17-9] Captodiamine, *1773*
[486-18-0] Flavopereirine, *4093*
[486-35-1] Daphnetin, *2817*
[486-39-5] Coclaurine, *2459*
[486-47-5] Ethaverine, *3728*
[486-54-4] 1-Naphthylamine-2,7-disulfonic Acid, *6400*
[486-55-5] Daphnin, *2818*
[486-56-6] Cotinine, *2553*
[486-66-8] Daidzein, *2801*
[486-67-9] Mersalyl Acid, *5901*
[486-70-4] Lupinine, *5609*
[486-79-3] Dipyrocetyl, *3349*
[486-84-0] Harman, *4615*
[486-86-2] Methylcytisine, *6049*
[486-87-3] α-Isolupanine, *5607*
[486-88-4] Lupanine *l*-Form, *5607*
[486-89-5] Anagyrine, *623*
[487-06-9] Limettin, *5492*
[487-21-8] Lumazine, *5596*
[487-27-4] Scopoline, *8410*
[487-41-2] Phillyrin, *7323*
[487-58-1] Hypaphorine, *4861*
[487-60-5] Indican (Plant Indican), *4942*
[487-79-6] Kainic Acid, *5276*
[487-90-1] Porphobilinogen, *7600*
[487-93-4] Bufotenine, *1478*
[487-94-5] Indican (Metabolic Indican), *4941*
[488-04-0] Holomycin, *4728*
[488-10-8] Jasmone, *5259*
[488-41-5] Mitobronitol, *6212*
[488-43-7] Glucamine, *4449*
[488-69-7] Fructose-1,6-diphosphate, *4275*
[488-73-3] *d*-Quercitol, *8036*
[488-81-3] Adonitol, *168*
[488-84-6] D-Ribulose, *8207*
[489-21-4] Sarkomycin A, *8376*
[489-32-7] Icariin, *3617*
[489-84-9] Guaiazulene, *4554*
[489-86-1] Guaiol, *4556*
[490-02-8] Aspergillic Acid, *841*
[490-03-9] Diosphenol, *3298*
[490-10-8] Nepetalactone, *6470*
[490-11-9] Cinchomeronic Acid, *2283*
[490-23-3] β-Tocotrienol, *9501*
[490-53-9] Carnegine, *1847*
[490-55-1] Amiphenazole, *483*
[490-79-9] Gentisic Acid, *4398*
[490-83-5] Dehydroascorbic Acid, *2866*
[490-98-2] Hydroxytetracaine, *4846*
[491-35-0] Lepidine, *5441*
[491-50-9] Quercimeritrin, *8035*
[491-58-7] Chrysarobin Pure Substance, *2253*
[491-59-8] Chrysarobin, *2253*
[491-67-8] Baicalein, *942*
[491-70-3] Luteolin, *5614*
[491-88-3] Isopilosine, *5199*
[491-92-9] Pamaquine, *7001*
[492-11-5] Leucopterin, *5454*
[492-17-1] 2,4'-Biphenyldiamine, *1236*
[492-18-2] Mersalyl, *5901*
[492-22-8] Thioxanthone, *9369*

[492-27-3] Kynurenic Acid, 5327
[492-38-6] Atropic Acid, 874
[492-39-7] Norpseudoephedrine, 6714
[492-70-6] Hydrobenzoin, 4777
[492-89-7] 3-Pentadecylcatechol, 7110
[492-99-9] Nioxime, 6560
[493-49-2] Corydaldine, 2543
[493-52-7] Methyl Red, 6119
[493-92-5] Prolintane, 7781
[494-03-1] Chlornaphazine, 2108
[494-08-6] Glucovanillin, 4464
[494-44-0] Cassella's Acid F, 1893
[494-47-3] Hydrofuramide, 4791
[494-52-0] Anabasine, 619
[494-55-3] Hydrohydrastinine, 4802
[494-79-1] Melarsoprol, 5815
[494-97-3] Nornicotine, 6712
[495-20-5] Conhydrine, 2500
[495-31-8] Nodakenin, 6668
[495-42-1] Halostachine, 4601
[495-45-4] Dypnone, 3480
[495-48-7] Azoxybenzene, 923
[495-54-5] Chrysoidine Free Base, 2257
[495-69-2] Hippuric Acid, 4716
[495-83-0] Tigloidine, 9434
[495-84-1] Salinazid, 8335
[495-85-2] Methysticin, 6138
[495-87-4] Piperic Acid (E,Z)-Form, 7467
[495-88-5] Piperic Acid (Z,E)-Form, 7467
[495-89-6] Piperic Acid (Z,Z)-Form, 7467
[495-91-0] Chavicine, 2049
[495-99-8] Hydroxystilbamidine, 4845
[496-00-4] Dibromopropamidine, 3024
[496-11-7] Indan, 4931
[496-16-2] Coumaran, 2559
[496-41-3] Coumarilic Acid, 2561
[496-46-8] Acetyleneurea, 93
[496-49-1] Hygrine, 4850
[496-65-1] Pantetheine, 7011
[496-67-3] Bromisovalum, 1397
[496-74-2] Toluene-3,4-dithiol, 9531
[496-77-5] Butyroin, 1595
[497-09-6] Glyceraldehyde L-Form, 4481
[497-18-7] Carbohydrazide, 1804
[497-19-8] Sodium Carbonate, 8596
[497-30-3] Ergothioneine, 3663
[497-39-2] DBMC, 2837
[497-59-6] Meconic Acid, 5782
[497-72-3] Methymycin, 6135
[497-73-4] Neomethymycin, 6453
[497-75-6] Dioxethedrine, 3302
[497-76-7] Arbutin, 773
[497-78-9] Rhododendrin, 8189
[497-92-7] Allethrin II, 260
[498-02-2] Apocynin, 741
[498-23-7] Citraconic Acid, 2321
[498-24-8] Mesaconic Acid, 5903
[498-59-9] Djenkolic Acid, 3387
[498-71-5] Sobrerol, 8567
[498-94-2] Isonipecotic Acid, 5189
[498-95-3] Nipecotic Acid, 6561
[498-96-4] Guvacine, 4584
[499-04-7] Arecaidine, 777
[499-12-7] Aconitic Acid, 117
[499-14-9] Chondrosine, 2215
[499-15-0] Hyalobiuronic Acid, 4756
[499-20-7] Dhurrin, 2958
[499-44-5] β-Thujaplicin, 9390
[499-67-2] Proparacaine, 7807

[499-75-2] Carvacrol, 1872
[499-89-8] Thujic Acid, 9391
[500-05-0] Coumalic Acid, 2557
[500-12-9] Goitrin, 4513
[500-34-5] β-Eucaine, 3894
[500-38-9] Nordihydroguaiaretic Acid (unspecified stereo), 6693
[500-44-7] Mimosine, 6199
[500-55-0] Apoatropine, 739
[500-62-9] Yangonin, 10093
[500-64-1] Kawain, 5287
[500-92-5] Chlorguanide, 2090
[501-15-5] Deoxyepinephrine, 2903
[501-30-4] Kojic Acid, 5317
[501-36-0] Resveratrol, 8158
[501-52-0] Hydrocinnamic Acid, 4784
[501-53-1] Carbobenzoxy Chloride, 1801
[501-65-5] Tolan, 9504
[501-68-8] Beclamide, 1018
[501-81-5] 3-Pyridineacetic Acid, 7971
[501-82-6] Carbanilic Acid, 1784
[501-92-8] Chavicol, 2050
[502-37-4] Hypoglycine B, 4866
[502-42-1] Cycloheptanone, 2722
[502-54-5] Glycerol 1-Octanoate, 6252
[502-55-6] Dixanthogen, 3384
[502-61-4] α-Farnesene, 3935
[502-65-8] Lycopene, 5620
[502-85-2] γ-Hydroxybutyrate Sodium Salt, 4815
[502-98-7] Chloroazodin, 2120
[503-01-5] Isometheptene, 5185
[503-07-1] Vernolic Acid (+)-Form, 9963
[503-30-0] Trimethylene Oxide, 9715
[503-38-8] Diphosgene, 3334
[503-40-2] Methionic Acid, 5974
[503-49-1] Meglutol, 5808
[503-64-0] Isocrotonic Acid, 5164
[503-66-2] Hydracrylic Acid, 4762
[503-74-2] Isovaleric Acid, 5231
[504-02-9] Dihydroresorcinol, 3178
[504-15-4] Orcinol, 6864
[504-20-1] Phorone, 7333
[504-24-5] Fampridine, 3933
[504-29-0] α-Aminopyridine, 473
[504-63-2] Trimethylene Glycol, 9714
[504-64-3] Carbon Suboxide, 1815
[505-32-8] Isophytol, 5198
[505-48-6] Suberic Acid, 8862
[505-60-2] Mustard Gas, 6316
[505-70-4] Muconic Acid, 6299
[505-75-9] Cicutoxin, 2267
[506-03-6] Chimyl Alcohol, 2060
[506-12-7] Margaric Acid, 5751
[506-25-2] Isanic Acid, 5103
[506-26-3] γ-Linolenic Acid, 5507
[506-30-9] Arachidic Acid, 764
[506-32-1] Arachidonic Acid, 765
[506-33-2] Brassidic Acid, 1364
[506-58-1] Ethylamine Hydriodide, 3762
[506-59-2] Dimethylamine Hydrochloride, 3228
[506-61-6] Potassium Silver Cyanide, 7669
[506-64-9] Silver Cyanide, 8512
[506-65-0] Gold Monocyanide, 4516
[506-66-1] Beryllium Carbide, 1165
[506-68-3] Cyanogen Bromide, 2693
[506-77-4] Cyanogen Chloride, 2694
[506-78-5] Cyanogen Iodide, 2695
[506-80-9] Carbon Diselenide, 1810

[506-82-1] Dimethylcadmium, 3239
[506-89-8] Urea Hydrochloride, 9867
[506-93-4] Guanidine Nitrate, 4562
[506-96-7] Acetyl Bromide, 82
[507-02-8] Acetyl Iodide, 94
[507-09-5] Thioacetic Acid, 9320
[507-16-4] Thionyl Bromide, 9347
[507-19-7] tert-Butyl Bromide, 1555
[507-20-0] tert-Butyl Chloride, 1562
[507-25-5] Carbon Tetraiodide, 1818
[507-27-7] Tetraphenylarsonium Bromide, 9235
[507-28-8] Tetraphenylarsonium Chloride, 9236
[507-36-8] tert-Amyl Bromide, 603
[507-40-4] tert-Butyl Hypochlorite, 1571
[507-42-6] Bromal Hydrate, 1384
[507-60-8] Scilliroside, 8401
[507-61-9] Azafrin, 895
[507-70-0] Borneol, 1338
[507-79-9] Tazettine, 9082
[508-02-1] Oleanolic Acid, 6827
[508-29-2] 3-Chloro-d-camphor, 2132
[508-44-1] Anemonin, 642
[508-52-1] Ouabagenin, 6900
[508-54-3] Hydroxycodeinone, 4822
[508-59-8] Parthenin, 7047
[508-65-6] Germine, 4412
[508-75-8] Convallatoxin, 2512
[508-77-0] Cymarin, 2761
[509-00-2] Cortisone 21-Cyclopentanepropionate, 2539
[509-14-8] Tetranitromethane, 9233
[509-15-9] Gelsemine, 4384
[509-17-1] Ajacine, 5618
[509-18-2] Delsoline, 2882
[509-20-6] Aconine, 115
[509-24-0] Songorine, 8717
[509-36-4] β-Colubrine, 2491
[509-40-0] Diaboline, 2959
[509-44-4] α-Colubrine, 2491
[509-60-4] Dihydromorphine, 3177
[509-67-1] Pholcodine, 7329
[509-71-7] Diacetyldihydromorphine, 2967
[509-74-0] Methadyl Acetate, 5945
[509-78-4] Dimenoxadol, 3208
[509-86-4] Heptabarbital, 4655
[509-93-3] Ambrosin, 385
[510-13-4] Malachite Green (carbinol base), 5699
[510-20-3] Diethylmalonic Acid, 3124
[510-35-0] Santonic Acid, 8360
[510-53-2] Racemethorphan, 8091
[510-90-7] Buthalital Sodium, 1524
[511-07-9] Ergocristine 8α-Isomer, 3649
[511-08-0] Ergocristine, 3649
[511-09-1] α-Ergocryptine, 3650
[511-10-4] Ergocryptinine, 3651
[511-12-6] Dihydroergotamine, 3174
[511-13-7] Chlophedianol Hydrochloride, 2066
[511-18-2] Norcholanic Acid, 6689
[511-20-6] Ergostane, 3657
[511-26-2] Pregnenolone Methyl Ether, 7733
[511-28-4] Vitamin D$_4$, 10020
[511-34-2] Digitogenin, 3160
[511-45-5] Pridinol, 7741
[511-89-7] Plumieride, 7540
[511-96-6] Gitogenin, 4431
[512-04-9] Diosgenin, 3295

[512-15-2] Cyclopentolate, 2746
[512-16-3] Cyclobutyrol, 2715
[512-29-8] Flavoxanthin, 4095
[512-35-6] Benzenesulfonic Anhydride, 1071
[512-48-1] Valdetamide, 9901
[512-64-1] Echinomycin, 3497
[512-69-6] Raffinose, 8096
[512-85-6] Ascaridole, 827
[513-10-0] Echothiophate Iodide, 3501
[513-15-5] Sodium β-Sulfopropionitrile, 8683
[513-29-1] Glycine Sulfate, 4492
[513-31-5] 2,3-Dibromopropene, 3025
[513-35-9] Amylene, 607
[513-36-0] Isobutyl Chloride, 5138
[513-37-1] 1-Chloro-2-methyl-1-propene, 2147
[513-38-2] Isobutyl Iodide, 5144
[513-44-0] Isobutyl Mercaptan, 5147
[513-48-4] sec-Butyl Iodide, 1574
[513-53-1] sec-Butyl Mercaptan, 1578
[513-74-6] Ammonium Dithiocarbamate, 516
[513-77-9] Barium Carbonate, 969
[513-78-0] Cadmium Carbonate, 1616
[513-79-1] Cobaltous Carbonate, 2436
[513-81-5] 2,3-Dimethyl-1,3-butadiene, 3238
[513-85-9] 2,3-Butylene Glycol, 1568
[513-86-0] Acetoin, 64
[513-88-2] 1,1-Dichloroacetone, 3051
[513-92-8] Tetraiodoethylene, 9220
[513-96-2] Chlorocyanohydrin, 2134
[514-10-3] Abietic Acid, 7
[514-17-0] Androstane-3β,11β-diol-17-one, 636
[514-36-3] Fludrocortisone 21-Acetate, 4130
[514-39-6] Periplogenin, 7176
[514-61-4] Normethandrone, 6710
[514-65-8] Biperiden, 1233
[514-73-8] Dithiazanine Iodide, 3369
[514-76-1] Astacin, 853
[514-78-3] Canthaxanthin, 1753
[514-92-1] Torularhodin, 9553
[515-30-0] Atrolactic Acid, 873
[515-40-2] Neophyl Chloride, 6459
[515-49-1] Sulfathiourea, 8944
[515-64-0] Sulfisomidine, 8951
[515-69-5] α-Bisabolol, 1241
[515-72-0] Barium Benzenesulfonate, 966
[515-82-2] Chloral Formamide, 2070
[515-83-3] Chloral Alcoholate, 2069
[515-84-4] Trichloroacetic Acid Ethyl Ester, 9627
[515-94-6] 2,3-Diaminopropionic Acid, 2984
[515-96-8] Semioxamazide, 8445
[516-02-9] Barium Oxalate, 985
[516-03-0] Ferrous Oxalate, 4051
[516-12-1] N-Iodosuccinimide, 5045
[516-16-5] Allopregnane-3β,11β,21-triol-20-one, 274
[516-18-7] Asaprol, 822
[516-21-2] Cycloguanil, 2721
[516-38-1] Cortol, 2541
[516-41-6] Hydrallostane, 4764
[516-42-7] Cortolone, 2542
[516-51-8] Uranediol, 9853
[516-53-0] Allopregnane-3β,20β-diol, 270
[516-54-1] Allopregnan-3α-ol-20-one, 275

[516-55-2] Allopregnan-3β-ol-20-one, 276
[516-58-5] Allopregnan-20β-ol-3-one, 278
[516-59-6] Allopregnan-20α-ol-3-one, 277
[516-85-8] Dehydroergosterol, 2872
[516-95-0] Epicholestanol, 3612
[516-98-3] Neoergosterol, 6451
[517-04-4] Isoestradiol, 5167
[517-06-6] 8-Isoestrone, 5168
[517-09-9] Equilenin, 3642
[517-10-2] Allocholesterol, 264
[517-21-5] Glyoxal-Sodium Bisulfite, 4510
[517-23-7] α-Acetylbutyrolactone, 83
[517-25-9] Trinitromethane, 9729
[517-28-2] Hematoxylin, 4637
[517-56-6] Corytuberine, 2550
[517-60-2] Mellitic Acid, 5825
[517-66-8] Dicentrine, 3041
[517-69-1] Actinodaphnine, 139
[517-82-8] Echinochrome A, 3496
[517-88-4] Alkannin, 257
[517-97-5] Tsuduranine, 9800
[518-05-8] Naphthalic Acid, 6380
[518-17-2] Evodiamine, 3908
[518-20-7] Cyclocumarol, 2717
[518-28-5] Podophyllotoxin, 7546
[518-29-6] β-Peltatin, 7076
[518-34-3] Tetrandrine, 9231
[518-44-5] Fluorescin, 4160
[518-47-8] Fluorescein Disodium Salt, 4159
[518-69-4] Corydaline, 2544
[518-75-2] Citrinin, 2327
[518-82-1] Emodin, 3561
[519-02-8] Matrine, 5759
[519-04-0] Anhalonine, 655
[519-05-1] Opianic Acid, 6851
[519-09-5] Benzoylecgonine, 1113
[519-21-1] Mycaminose, 6317
[519-23-3] Ellipticine, 3548
[519-26-6] Sodium Iodomethamate, 8633
[519-34-6] Maclurin, 5644
[519-37-9] Etofylline, 3878
[519-40-4] Aspidinol, 847
[519-44-8] 2,4-Dinitroresorcinol, 3284
[519-62-0] Chlorophyll B, 2155
[519-72-2] N,N-Diethylbenzhydrylamine, 3115
[519-73-3] Triphenylmethane, 9741
[519-87-9] Diphenylacetamide, 3315
[519-95-9] Florantyrone, 4107
[520-07-0] Antipyrine Salicylate, 717
[520-09-2] Dopan, 3422
[520-12-7] Pectolinarigenin, 7064
[520-18-3] Kaempferol, 5274
[520-26-3] Hesperidin, 4671
[520-27-4] Diosmin, 3297
[520-33-2] Hesperetin, 4670
[520-34-3] Diosmetin, 3296
[520-36-5] Apigenin, 730
[520-43-4] Sparassol, 8734
[520-45-6] Dehydroacetic Acid, 2865
[520-52-5] Psilocybin, 7926
[520-53-6] Psilocin, 7925
[520-77-4] Ethadione, 3718
[520-85-4] Medroxyprogesterone, 5793
[520-91-2] Vitamin D₁, 10017
[521-04-0] 7-Dehydrositosterol, 2875
[521-10-8] Methandriol, 5950
[521-11-9] Mestanolone, 5915

[521-12-0] Dromostanolone Propionate, 3448
[521-17-5] Androstenediol, 637
[521-18-6] Stanolone, 8793
[521-24-4] Sodium β-Naphthoquinone-4-sulfonate, 8646
[521-31-3] Luminol, 5600
[521-35-7] Cannabinol, 1748
[521-40-4] Narcotoline, 6423
[521-62-0] Frangulin A, 4264
[521-74-4] Broxyquinoline, 1453
[521-78-8] Trimipramine Maleate, 9722
[521-88-0] Karanjin, 5283
[522-00-9] Ethopropazine, 3747
[522-12-3] Quercitrin, 8037
[522-17-8] Deguelin, 2863
[522-18-9] Chlorbenzoxamine, 2080
[522-23-6] Metofenazate Difumarate, 6145
[522-27-0] α-Furildioxime, 4306
[522-40-7] Fosfestrol, 4253
[522-48-5] Tetrahydrozoline Hydrochloride, 9219
[522-51-0] Dequalinium Chloride, 2913
[522-57-6] Papaveraldine, 7017
[522-66-7] Hydroquinine, 4807
[522-70-3] Antimycin A₃, 715
[522-94-1] allo-Yohimbine, 10103
[522-97-4] Canadine, 1736
[523-21-7] Sodium Rhodizonate, 8670
[523-27-3] 9,10-Dibromoanthracene, 3018
[523-44-4] Orange I, 6857
[523-64-8] Flindersine, 4101
[523-80-8] Apiole (Parsley), 734
[523-87-5] Dimenhydrinate, 3207
[524-15-2] Fagarine, 3928
[524-17-4] Dauricine, 2833
[524-20-9] Armepavine, 787
[524-30-1] Fraxin, 4266
[524-34-5] Cinchophen Allyl Ester, 2288
[524-36-7] Pyridoxamine Dihydrochloride, 7980
[524-38-9] N-Hydroxyphthalimide, 4838
[524-40-3] Ricinine, 8210
[524-42-5] 1,2-Naphthoquinone, 6394
[524-46-9] Adlumine, 166
[524-63-0] Cupreine, 2623
[524-81-2] Mebhydroline, 5770
[524-83-4] Ethybenztropine, 3756
[524-84-5] Dimethylthiambutene, 3260
[524-96-9] Benzylimidobis(p-methoxyphenyl)methane, 1139
[524-97-0] Pterocarpin, 7932
[525-05-3] Nitroso-R Salt, 6644
[525-06-4] Diphenylketene, 3326
[525-37-1] 1,6-Naphthalenedisulfonic Acid, 6373
[525-52-0] Pyrogallol Triacetate, 8000
[525-57-5] Harmalol, 4614
[525-61-1] Quinocide, 8067
[525-64-4] 9H-Fluorene-2,7-diamine, 4156
[525-66-6] Propranolol, 7840
[525-79-1] Kinetin, 5311
[525-82-6] Flavone, 4092
[525-94-0] Penicillin N, 7098
[526-02-3] Actiphenol, 143
[526-07-8] Sesamolin, 8471
[526-08-9] Sulfaphenazole, 8935
[526-13-6] Meteloidine, 5935
[526-18-1] Osalmid, 6887

[526-31-8] Abrine, *10*
[526-36-3] Xylometazoline, *10086*
[526-55-6] Tryptophol, *9798*
[526-78-3] 2,3-Dibromosuccinic Acid, *3029*
[526-84-1] Dihydroxymaleic Acid, *3185*
[526-94-3] Sodium Bitartrate, *8589*
[526-95-4] Gluconic Acid, *4456*
[526-97-6] L-Gulonic Acid, *4577*
[526-98-7] 2-Keto-L-gulonic Acid, *5304*
[526-99-8] Galactaric Acid, *4331*
[527-07-1] Sodium Gluconate, *4456*
[527-09-3] Cupric Gluconate, *2640*
[527-17-3] Duroquinone, *3470*
[527-18-4] Durohydroquinone, *3469*
[527-38-8] Mycosamine, *6328*
[527-52-6] Digitoxose, *3164*
[527-53-7] Isodurene, *5166*
[527-62-8] 2-Amino-4,6-dichloro-phenol, *437*
[527-72-0] 2-Thiophenecarboxylic Acid, *9354*
[527-73-1] Azomycin, *921*
[527-84-4] *o*-Cymene, *2763*
[527-85-5] *o*-Toluamide, *9528*
[527-89-9] Dithiosalicylic Acid, *3375*
[527-93-5] Diploicin, *3339*
[528-21-2] Gallacetophenone, *4342*
[528-29-0] *o*-Dinitrobenzene, *3273*
[528-43-8] Magnolol, *5697*
[528-44-9] Trimellitic Acid, *9702*
[528-45-0] 3,4-Dinitrobenzoic Acid, *3275*
[528-48-3] Fisetin, *4088*
[528-50-7] Cellobiose, *1961*
[528-53-0] Delphinidin, *2880*
[528-58-5] Cyanidin Chloride, *2687*
[528-71-2] Hemipyocyanine, *4645*
[528-75-6] 2,4-Dinitrobenzaldehyde, *3272*
[528-76-7] 2,4-Dinitrobenzenesulfenyl Chloride, *3274*
[528-79-0] Thymol Acetate, *9399*
[528-81-4] 6-Deoxy-L-ascorbic Acid, *2898*
[528-88-1] D-Glucoascorbic Acid, *4451*
[528-94-9] Ammonium Salicylate, *550*
[529-05-5] Chamazulene, *2040*
[529-17-9] Tropane, *9777*
[529-19-1] *o*-Tolunitrile, *9537*
[529-20-4] *o*-Tolualdehyde, *9527*
[529-21-5] 3-Ethyl-4-picoline, *3842*
[529-28-2] *o*-Iodoanisole, *5028*
[529-36-2] 1-Naphthalenethiol, *6378*
[529-38-4] Cocaethylene, *2454*
[529-44-2] Myricetin, *6332*
[529-53-3] Scutellarein, *8412*
[529-59-9] Genistin, *4391*
[529-64-6] Tropic Acid, *9779*
[529-86-2] Anthranol, *686*
[530-08-5] Isoetharine, *5170*
[530-14-3] Picein, *7395*
[530-31-4] Ammonium Mandelate, *532*
[530-40-5] Isonicotinic Acid Diethyl-amide, *5188*
[530-43-8] Chloramphenicol Palmitate, *2077*
[530-44-9] *p*-Dimethylaminobenzo-phenone, *3233*
[530-45-0] 1,1-Di-*p*-tolylethane, *3379*
[530-48-3] 1,1-Diphenylethene, *3323*
[530-50-7] 1,1-Diphenylhydrazine, *3325*

[530-55-2] 2,6-Dimethoxyquinone, *3225*
[530-62-1] *N,N′*-Carbonyldiimidazole, *1819*
[530-75-6] Acetylsalicylsalicylic Acid, *100*
[530-78-9] Flufenamic Acid, *4132*
[530-85-8] *o*-Nitrophenylpropiolic Acid, *6625*
[530-91-6] Tetralol, *9222*
[530-97-2] Heptoxime, *4665*
[531-18-0] Hexamethylolmelamine, *4691*
[531-29-3] Coniferin, *2503*
[531-44-2] Scopolin, *8409*
[531-53-3] Azure A, *927*
[531-55-5] Azure B, *928*
[531-57-7] Azure C, *929*
[531-58-8] Cichoriin, *2262*
[531-72-6] Arsenamide, *793*
[531-73-7] Proflavine Dihydrochloride, *7771*
[531-75-9] Esculin, *3698*
[531-81-7] Coumarin-3-carboxylic Acid, *2563*
[531-91-9] *N,N′*-Diphenylbenzidine, *3319*
[531-95-3] Equol, *3644*
[532-03-6] Methocarbamol, *5980*
[532-05-8] 1,3-Di-6-quinolylurea, *3353*
[532-11-6] Anethole Trithione, *644*
[532-18-3] β,β′-Dinaphthylamine, *3267*
[532-27-4] ω-Chloroacetophenone, *2115*
[532-28-5] Mandelonitrile, *5719*
[532-32-1] Sodium Benzoate, *8582*
[532-40-1] Thiamine Monophosphate, *9296*
[532-43-4] Thiamine Mononitrate, *9295*
[532-48-9] Euparin, *3900*
[532-52-5] Cyclexedrine, *2707*
[532-54-7] Isonitrosoacetophenone, *5191*
[532-55-8] Benzoyl Isothiocyanate, *1114*
[532-59-2] Amylocaine Hydrochloride, *614*
[532-65-0] *ar*-Turmerone, *9825*
[532-76-3] Hexylcaine Hydrochloride, *4708*
[532-82-1] Chrysoidine, *2257*
[533-06-2] Mephenesin Carbamate, *5850*
[533-18-6] *o*-Cresyl Acetate, *2584*
[533-22-2] Hydroxystilbamidine Ise-thionate, *4845*
[533-28-8] Piperocaine Hydrochloride, *7474*
[533-30-2] 6-Aminobenzothiazole, *425*
[533-45-9] Clomethiazole, *2384*
[533-48-2] Desthiobiotin, *2934*
[533-49-3] L-Erythrose, *3691*
[533-50-6] L-Erythrulose, *3694*
[533-51-7] Silver Oxalate, *8520*
[533-58-4] *o*-Iodophenol, *5035*
[533-62-0] Hydroxyglutamic Acid, *4825*
[533-67-5] D-2-Deoxyribose, *2908*
[533-70-0] 2,4-Diiodoaniline, *3188*
[533-73-3] 1,2,4-Benzenetriol, *1073*
[533-74-4] Dazomet, *2834*
[533-76-6] Ketipic Acid, *5300*
[533-87-9] Aleuritic Acid, *231*
[533-96-0] Sodium Sesquicarbonate, *8674*

[533-98-2] α-Butylene Dibromide, *1566*
[534-00-9] *d*-Amyl Bromide, *601*
[534-07-6] 1,3-Dichloroacetone, *3052*
[534-13-4] *N,N′*-Dimethylthiourea, *3261*
[534-15-6] Dimethylacetal, *3226*
[534-16-7] Silver Carbonate, *8507*
[534-17-8] Cesium Carbonate, *2010*
[534-18-9] Sodium Thiocarbonate, *8691*
[534-26-9] Lysidine, *5635*
[534-30-5] Hercynine, *4667*
[534-46-3] Sophorose, *8719*
[534-51-0] 3,5-Diiodothyronine, *3191*
[534-52-1] Dinitrocresol, *3279*
[534-59-8] *n*-Butylmalonic Acid, *1576*
[534-64-5] Pyrithiamine, *7992*
[534-82-7] 3-Methoxy-4-hydroxy-phenylglycol, *5996*
[534-87-2] Etilefrin Hydrochloride, *3865*
[535-11-5] Ethyl α-Bromopropionate, *3772*
[535-13-7] Ethyl α-Chloropropionate, *3785*
[535-46-6] Benzenestibonic Acid, *1069*
[535-55-7] Mercuric Sodium *p*-Phenol-sulfonate, *5886*
[535-65-9] Glybuthiazol(e), *4479*
[535-75-1] Pipecolic Acid, *7458*
[535-77-3] *m*-Cymene, *2763*
[535-80-8] *m*-Chlorobenzoic Acid, *2123*
[535-83-1] Trigonelline, *9694*
[535-87-5] 3,5-Diaminobenzoic Acid, *2978*
[536-08-3] Digallic Acid, *3153*
[536-17-4] *p*-Dimethylaminobenzal-rhodanine, *3231*
[536-21-0] Norfenefrine, *6699*
[536-24-3] Ethylnorepinephrine, *3834*
[536-25-4] Orthocaine, *6883*
[536-33-4] Ethionamide, *3737*
[536-37-8] 2-Hexyldecanoic Acid So-dium Salt, *4709*
[536-38-9] *p*-Chlorophenacyl Bromide, *2153*
[536-43-6] Dyclonine Hydrochloride, *3473*
[536-50-5] *p*,α-Dimethylbenzyl Alco-hol, *3237*
[536-57-2] *p*-Toluenesulfinic Acid, *9532*
[536-60-7] Cumic Alcohol, *2619*
[536-66-3] Cumic Acid, *2618*
[536-69-6] Fusaric Acid, *4314*
[536-74-3] Ethynylbenzene, *3861*
[536-75-4] 4-Ethylpyridine, *3849*
[536-78-7] 3-Ethylpyridine, *3848*
[536-80-1] Iodosobenzene, *5044*
[536-88-9] 4-Ethyl-2-picoline, *3843*
[537-01-9] Cerous Carbonate, *1996*
[537-21-3] Chlorproguanil, *2184*
[537-26-8] Tropacocaine, *9774*
[537-45-1] 2,6-Dibromoquinone-4-chlorimide, *3026*
[537-46-2] Methamphetamine, *5948*
[537-47-3] 4-Phenylsemicarbazide, *7312*
[537-49-5] Surinamine, *9007*
[537-61-1] Cyclomethycaine Hydro-chloride, *2735*
[537-64-4] *p*-Ditolylmercury, *3381*

[537-65-5] 4,4'-Diaminodiphenylamine, 2979
[537-91-7] Nitrophenide, 6618
[537-92-8] m-Acetotoluide, 74
[538-03-4] Oxophenarsine Hydrochloride, 6948
[538-04-5] 2-Chloro-4-(hydroxymercuriphenol), 4830
[538-08-9] Diallylcyanamide, 2972
[538-17-0] Aluminum Thiocyanate, 369
[538-28-3] S-Benzylthiuronium Chloride, 1146
[538-32-9] Benzylurea, 1147
[538-37-4] Dibenzyl Chlorophosphonate, 3012
[538-39-6] 1,2-Di-p-tolylethane, 3380
[538-41-0] p-Diaminoazobenzene, 2977
[538-43-2] Phenylglyceryl Ether, 7290
[538-45-4] 3,3-Dithiodipyridine Dihydrochloride, 3373
[538-51-2] Benzylideneaniline, 1138
[538-56-7] Cinnamic Acid Anhydride, 2299
[538-58-9] Dibenzalacetone, 3006
[538-62-5] Diphenylcarbazone, 3322
[538-64-7] Benzyl Fumarate, 1135
[538-65-8] Cinnamic Acid n-Butyl Ester, 2299
[538-68-1] Amylbenzene, 600
[538-71-6] Domiphen Bromide, 3415
[538-74-9] Benzyl Sulfide, 1145
[538-75-0] Dicyclohexylcarbodiimide, 3096
[538-86-3] Benzyl Methyl Ether, 1140
[538-90-9] β-Coniceine, 2501
[538-93-2] Isobutylbenzene, 5134
[539-00-4] Isopelletierine, 7072
[539-10-6] Phenocoll Hydrochloride, 7239
[539-12-8] p-Anol, 678
[539-15-1] Hordenine, 4746
[539-30-0] Benzyl Ethyl Ether, 1133
[539-35-5] Mycobacidin, 6322
[539-47-9] 2-Furanacrylic Acid, 4297
[539-54-8] Antimony Sodium Thioglycollate, 703
[539-64-0] N,N-Dimethylglycine Hydrazide Hydrochloride, 3245
[539-68-4] Dihydroxyaluminum Sodium Carbonate, 3184
[539-82-2] n-Valeric Acid Ethyl Ester, 9904
[539-86-6] Allicin, 211
[539-88-8] Ethyl Levulinate, 3819
[539-89-9] Isobutyl Urethane, 5153
[539-90-2] Isobutyl n-Butyrate, 5136
[540-05-6] Phytofluene, 7389
[540-07-8] n-Amyl Caproate, 605
[540-10-3] Cetyl Palmitate, 2031
[540-16-9] Cupric Butyrate, 2630
[540-18-1] n-Amyl Butyrate, 604
[540-36-3] p-Difluorobenzene, 3148
[540-37-4] p-Iodoaniline, 5027
[540-38-5] p-Iodophenol, 5036
[540-42-1] Isobutyl Propionate, 5150
[540-47-6] Cyclopropyl Methyl Ether, 2749
[540-49-8] Acetylene Dibromide, 91
[540-51-2] Ethylene Bromohydrin, 3792
[540-54-5] Propyl Chloride, 7847
[540-59-0] Acetylene Dichloride, 92
[540-61-4] Aminoacetonitrile, 412
[540-63-6] 1,2-Ethanedithiol, 3725

[540-67-0] Ethyl Methyl Ether, 3828
[540-69-2] Ammonium Formate, 523
[540-72-7] Thiocyanate Sodium, 9327
[540-73-8] 1,2-Dimethylhydrazine, 3248
[540-80-7] tert-Butyl Nitrite, 1583
[540-82-9] Ethyl Sulfate, 3853
[540-84-1] Isooctane, 5193
[540-88-5] tert-Butyl Acetate, 1537
[540-92-1] Acetone Sodium Bisulfite, 69
[540-97-6] Dodecamethylcyclohexasiloxane, 3403
[541-02-6] Decamethylcyclopentasiloxane, 2848
[541-07-1] Mevaldic Acid, 6162
[541-09-3] Uranyl Acetate, 9861
[541-14-0] Carnitine D-Form, 1849
[541-15-1] Carnitine L-Form, 1849
[541-16-2] Di-tert-butyl Malonate, 3034
[541-19-5] Succinylcholine Iodide, 8876
[541-22-0] Decamethonium Bromide, 2847
[541-25-3] Dichloro(2-chlorovinyl)-arsine, 3062
[541-28-6] Isoamyl Iodide, 5120
[541-33-3] Butylidene Chloride, 1572
[541-35-5] n-Butyramide, 1592
[541-41-3] Ethyl Chloroformate, 3784
[541-42-4] Isopropyl Nitrite, 5216
[541-43-5] Barium Formate, 975
[541-46-8] Isovaleramide, 5230
[541-48-0] β-Aminobutyric Acid, 429
[541-50-4] Acetoacetic Acid, 59
[541-53-7] 2,4-Dithiobiuret, 3371
[541-64-0] Furtrethonium Iodide, 4312
[541-66-2] Oxapropanium Iodide, 6923
[541-73-1] m-Dichlorobenzene, 3055
[541-85-5] 5-Methyl-3-heptanone, 6084
[541-88-8] Chloroacetic Anhydride, 2113
[541-91-3] Muscone, 6313
[542-05-2] Acetonedicarboxylic Acid, 68
[542-08-5] Isopropyl Acetoacetate, 5206
[542-10-9] Ethylidene Diacetate, 3811
[542-18-7] Cyclohexyl Chloride, 2732
[542-32-5] α-Aminoadipic Acid, 416
[542-37-0] tert-Amyl Isovalerate, 610
[542-40-5] β-Norbixin, 1311
[542-42-7] Calcium Palmitate, 1687
[542-46-1] Civetone, 2335
[542-52-9] n-Butyl Carbonate, 1558
[542-54-1] Isoamyl Cyanide, 5117
[542-55-2] Isobutyl Formate, 5143
[542-56-3] Isobutyl Nitrite, 5149
[542-59-2] Ethylene Glycol Monoacetate, 3801
[542-62-1] Barium Cyanide, 973
[542-69-8] n-Butyl Iodide, 1573
[542-75-6] 1,3-Dichloropropene, 3075
[542-76-7] β-Chloropropionitrile, 2160
[542-78-9] Malondialdehyde, 5709
[542-83-6] Cadmium Cyanide, 1618
[542-84-7] Cobaltous Cyanide, 2439
[542-85-8] Ethyl Isothiocyanate, 3815
[542-88-1] sym-Dichloromethyl Ether, 3069
[542-91-6] Diethylsilane, 3128
[542-92-7] Cyclopentadiene, 2739
[543-15-7] Heptaminol Hydrochloride, 4657

[543-20-4] Succinyl Chloride, 8873
[543-21-5] Cellocidin, 1962
[543-24-8] Aceturic Acid, 80
[543-27-1] Isobutyl Chlorocarbonate, 5139
[543-28-2] Isobutyl Carbamate, 5137
[543-29-3] Isobutyl Nitrate, 5148
[543-38-4] Canavanine, 1737
[543-49-7] 2-Heptanol, 4662
[543-59-9] Amyl Chloride, 606
[543-63-5] n-Butylmercuric Chloride, 1580
[543-67-9] n-Propyl Nitrite, 7865
[543-80-6] Barium Acetate, 965
[543-81-7] Beryllium Acetate, 1162
[543-82-8] Octodrine, 6757
[543-83-9] Galegine, 4341
[543-87-3] Isoamyl Nitrate, 5122
[543-90-8] Cadmium Acetate, 1614
[543-94-2] Strontium Acetate, 8836
[544-00-3] Diisoamylamine, 3193
[544-01-4] Isoamyl Ether, 5118
[544-10-5] 1-Chlorohexane, 2144
[544-12-7] 3-Hexen-1-ol, 4700
[544-13-8] Glutaronitrile, 4474
[544-16-1] n-Butyl Nitrite, 1582
[544-17-2] Calcium Formate, 1668
[544-18-3] Cobaltous Formate, 2441
[544-19-4] Cupric Formate, 2639
[544-27-4] Arsenoacetic Acid, 808
[544-31-0] Palmidrol, 6995
[544-35-4] Ethyl Linoleate, 3820
[544-40-1] n-Butyl Sulfide, 1590
[544-44-5] Agrocybin, 192
[544-47-8] p-Chlorobenzylpseudothiuronium Chloride, 2128
[544-51-4] Mycomycin, 6326
[544-60-5] Ammonium Oleate, 535
[544-62-7] Batyl Alcohol, 1011
[544-63-8] Myristic Acid, 6333
[544-92-3] Cuprous Cyanide, 2661
[544-97-8] Dimethylzinc, 3263
[545-06-2] Trichloroacetonitrile, 9628
[545-26-6] Gitoxigenin, 4433
[545-47-1] Lupeol, 5608
[545-55-1] Triethylenephosphoramide, 9672
[545-56-2] Delcosine, 2882
[545-61-9] Ajaconine, 193
[545-80-2] Poldine Methylsulfate, 7554
[545-91-5] Phenadoxone Hydrochloride, 7207
[545-93-7] Propallylonal, 7796
[546-06-5] Conessine, 2497
[546-43-0] Alantolactone, 207
[546-46-3] Zinc Citrate, 10134
[546-48-5] Pempidine Tartrate, 7080
[546-62-3] Verbascose, 9958
[546-67-8] Lead Tetraacetate, 5423
[546-68-9] Titanium Tetraisopropoxide, 9480
[546-74-7] Sodium Ethyl Sulfate, 8614
[546-80-5] α-Thujone, 9392
[546-88-3] Acetohydroxamic Acid, 63
[546-89-4] Lithium Acetate, 5521
[546-97-4] Columbin, 2493
[547-25-1] Turanose, 9821
[547-36-4] Succisulfone 2,2'-Iminodiethanol Salt, 8878
[547-44-4] Sulfanilylurea, 8931
[547-52-4] N⁴-Sulfanilylsulfanilamide, 8930
[547-57-9] Tropaeolin O, 9775
[547-58-0] Methyl Orange, 6105

[547-63-7] Methyl Isobutyrate, *6088*
[547-64-8] Methyl Lactate, *6094*
[547-65-9] α-Methylene Butyrolactone, *6062*
[547-66-0] Magnesium Oxalate, *5676*
[547-67-1] Nickel Oxalate, *6514*
[547-68-2] Zinc Oxalate, *10146*
[547-77-3] Allotetrahydrocortisone, *281*
[547-81-9] 16-Epiestriol, *3616*
[547-91-1] 8-Hydroxy-7-iodo-5-quino-linesulfonic Acid, *4826*
[548-00-5] Ethyl Biscoumacetate, *3770*
[548-04-9] Hypericin, *4863*
[548-24-3] Eosine I Bluish, *3602*
[548-37-8] Verbenalin, *9959*
[548-40-3] Oxyacanthine, *6953*
[548-42-5] Agroclavine, *191*
[548-43-6] Elymoclavine, *3553*
[548-51-6] o-Thymotic Acid, *9408*
[548-54-9] Violacein, *9997*
[548-57-2] Lucanthone Hydrochloride, *5591*
[548-62-9] Gentian Violet, *4395*
[548-66-3] Drofenine Hydrochloride, *3445*
[548-68-5] Thiphenamil Hydrochloride, *9370*
[548-73-2] Droperidol, *3450*
[548-76-5] Irigenin, *5090*
[548-77-6] Tectorigenin, *9107*
[548-80-1] Chromotrope 2B, *2240*
[548-83-4] Galangin, *4339*
[548-84-5] Pyrvinium Chloride, *8022*
[548-98-1] Cholane, *2195*
[549-18-8] Amitriptyline Hydrochloride, *487*
[549-28-0] Protostephanine, *7898*
[549-38-2] 3'-Methyl-1,2-cyclopenteno-phenanthrene, *6048*
[549-56-4] Quinine Bisulfate, *8061*
[550-10-7] Hydrocotarnine (anhydrous), *4788*
[550-24-3] Embelin, *3555*
[550-33-4] Nebularine, *6433*
[550-49-2] Adlumidine, *165*
[550-54-9] Epicinchonidine, *2286*
[550-60-7] 1-Nitro-2-naphthol, *6615*
[550-74-3] Picrolonic Acid, *7412*
[550-82-3] Resazurin, *8141*
[550-83-4] Propoxycaine Hydrochloride, *7837*
[550-90-3] Lupanine d-Form, *5607*
[550-97-0] 1-Naphthyl Salicylate, *6414*
[550-99-2] Naphazoline Hydrochloride, *6368*
[551-01-9] Plasmocid, *7522*
[551-06-4] 1-Naphthylisothiocyanate, *6411*
[551-09-7] N-(1-Naphthyl)ethylene-diamine, *6409*
[551-11-1] Prostaglandin $F_{2\alpha}$, *7878*
[551-16-6] 6-Aminopenicillanic Acid, *458*
[551-27-9] Propicillin, *7817*
[551-64-4] Zinc Tartrate, *10161*
[551-68-8] D-Psicose, *7924*
[551-76-8] 2,4,6-Trichloro-m-cresol, *9634*
[551-78-0] 4,5,6-Trichloro-o-cresol, *9635*
[551-88-2] 3-Nitrophthalic Acid, *6616*
[551-92-8] Dimetridazole, *3265*
[552-21-6] Methylenedigallic Acid, *6064*

[552-23-8] 2-Nitro-4-sulfobenzoic Acid, *6645*
[552-25-0] Diampromide, *2988*
[552-30-7] Trimellitic Anhydride, *9703*
[552-32-9] o-Nitroacetanilide, *6581*
[552-45-4] o-Xylyl Chloride, *10091*
[552-58-9] Eriodictyol, *3668*
[552-59-0] Prunetin, *7909*
[552-70-5] Pseudopelletierine, *7920*
[552-79-4] N-Methylephedrine, *6068*
[552-82-9] Methyldiphenylamine, *6054*
[552-93-2] Thymol Carbonate, *9399*
[552-94-3] Salsalate, *8339*
[553-03-7] Hydrocarbostyril, *4779*
[553-12-8] Protoporphyrin IX, *7897*
[553-19-5] Xanthyletin, *10069*
[553-20-8] 5'-Nitro-2'-propoxyacetani-lide, *6629*
[553-24-2] Neutral Red, *6488*
[553-26-4] γ,γ'-Dipyridyl, *3348*
[553-27-5] Aniline Mustard, *660*
[553-30-0] Proflavine Sulfate, *7771*
[553-39-9] Allenolic Acid, *259*
[553-54-8] Lithium Benzoate, *5523*
[553-58-2] Butethamine *meta*-Isomer Hydrochloride, *1523*
[553-63-9] Dimethocaine Hydrochloride, *3221*
[553-68-4] Butethamine Hydrochloride, *1523*
[553-69-5] Phenyramidol, *7321*
[553-70-8] Magnesium Benzoate, *5657*
[553-74-2] Nitrin, *6580*
[553-79-7] 5-Nitro-2-propoxyaniline, *6630*
[553-84-4] Perilla Ketone, *7166*
[553-90-2] Methyl Oxalate, *6106*
[553-91-3] Lithium Oxalate, *5537*
[554-01-8] 5-Methylcytosine, *6050*
[554-10-9] Glyceryl Iodide, *4488*
[554-12-1] Methyl Propionate, *6112*
[554-13-2] Lithium Carbonate, *5527*
[554-15-4] N-Methylpyrroline, *6118*
[554-18-7] Glucosulfone Sodium, *4463*
[554-35-8] Linamarin, *5497*
[554-57-4] Methazolamide, *5962*
[554-70-1] Triethyl Phosphine, *9675*
[554-72-3] Tryparsamide, *9794*
[554-73-4] Tropaeolin OO, *9776*
[554-84-7] m-Nitrophenol, *6619*
[554-91-6] Gentiobiose, *4396*
[554-92-7] Trimethobenzamide Hydrochloride, *9708*
[554-99-4] N-Methylepinephrine, *6069*
[555-03-3] m-Nitroanisole, *6585*
[555-10-2] β-Phellandrene, *7201*
[555-21-5] p-Nitrobenzyl Cyanide, *6591*
[555-30-6] Methyldopa, *6055*
[555-31-7] Aluminum Isopropoxide, *347*
[555-32-8] Aluminum Benzoate, *329*
[555-35-1] Aluminum Palmitate, *357*
[555-37-3] Neburon, *6435*
[555-43-1] Tristearin, *9756*
[555-44-2] Tripalmitin, *9736*
[555-45-3] Trimyristin, *9724*
[555-54-4] Diphenylmagnesium, *3327*
[555-57-7] Pargyline, *7038*
[555-59-9] Maleanilic Acid, *5702*
[555-68-0] m-Nitrocinnamic Acid, *6595*
[555-75-9] Aluminum Ethoxide, *338*
[555-76-0] Ferric Formate, *4023*
[555-77-1] Trichlormethine, *9625*

[555-89-5] Bis(p-chlorophenoxy)meth-ane, *1247*
[555-92-0] Coniine Hydrochloride, *2505*
[556-10-5] (4-Nitrophenyl)urea, *6626*
[556-22-9] Glyodin, *4508*
[556-24-1] Methyl Isovalerate, *6093*
[556-27-4] Alliin, *262*
[556-38-7] Zinc Valerate, *10164*
[556-50-3] N-Glycylglycine, *4503*
[556-52-5] Glycidol, *4490*
[556-56-9] Allyl Iodide, *294*
[556-61-6] Methyl Isothiocyanate, *6092*
[556-63-8] Lithium Formate, *5532*
[556-64-9] Methyl Thiocyanate, *6127*
[556-67-2] Octamethylcyclotetrasilox-ane, *6747*
[556-88-7] Nitroguanidine, *6608*
[556-89-8] Nitrourea, *6651*
[556-91-2] Aluminum *tert*-Butoxide, *333*
[556-99-0] Triuret, *9766*
[557-04-0] Magnesium Stearate, *5690*
[557-05-1] Zinc Stearate, *10158*
[557-07-3] Zinc Oleate, *10145*
[557-08-4] Undecylenic Acid Zinc Salt, *9848*
[557-09-5] Zinc Caprylate, *10130*
[557-11-9] Allylurea, *298*
[557-17-5] Methyl Propyl Ether, *6113*
[557-18-6] Diethylmagnesium, *3122*
[557-19-7] Nickel Cyanide, *6506*
[557-20-0] Diethylzinc, *3131*
[557-21-1] Zinc Cyanide, *10135*
[557-24-4] Maleamic Acid, *5701*
[557-25-5] Monobutyrin, *6249*
[557-28-8] Zinc Propionate, *10153*
[557-31-3] Allyl Ethyl Ether, *293*
[557-34-6] Zinc Acetate, *10128*
[557-35-7] sec-Octyl Bromide, *6765*
[557-36-8] sec-Octyl Iodide, *6768*
[557-39-1] Magnesium Formate, *5666*
[557-40-4] Allyl Ether, *292*
[557-41-5] Zinc Formate, *10137*
[557-42-6] Zinc Thiocyanate, *10163*
[557-59-5] Lignoceric Acid, *5488*
[557-61-9] Octacosanol, *6744*
[557-66-4] Ethylamine Hydrochloride, *3762*
[559-48-8] Kopsine, *5320*
[559-49-9] Annotinine, *677*
[559-57-9] Diginatigenin, *3155*
[559-70-6] β-Amyrin, *618*
[559-74-0] Friedelin, *4271*
[560-88-3] Bornyl Salicylate, *1341*
[561-07-9] Delphinine, *2881*
[561-10-4] Isomethadone l-Form, *5184*
[561-20-6] Cacotheline, *1605*
[561-25-1] Dihydrothebaine, *3181*
[561-27-3] Diacetylmorphine, *2968*
[561-77-3] Dihexyverine, *3168*
[561-78-4] Alphaprodine Hydrochloride, *310*
[561-86-4] Brallobarbital, *1361*
[561-94-4] Ergosine, *3656*
[561-95-5] Nimbiol, *6547*
[562-09-4] Chlorphenoxamine Hydrochloride, *2181*
[562-10-7] Doxylamine Succinate, *3441*
[562-26-5] Phenoperidine, *7250*
[562-34-5] Chlorogenin, *2143*
[562-71-0] Suprasterol II, *9004*
[562-76-5] Potassium Tetracyanoplatinate(II), *7685*

[562-81-2] Barium Platinous Cyanide, 991
[562-90-3] Silicon Tetraacetate, 8498
[563-12-2] Ethion, 3736
[563-41-7] Semicarbazide Hydrochloride, 8444
[563-47-3] 3-Chloro-2-methyl-1-propene, 2148
[563-52-0] 3-Chloro-1-butene, 2131
[563-63-3] Silver Acetate, 8505
[563-68-8] Thallium Acetate, 9257
[563-72-4] Calcium Oxalate, 1685
[563-80-4] Methyl Isopropyl Ketone, 6090
[564-00-1] Erythritol Anhydride, 3676
[564-25-0] Doxycycline (anhydrous), 3440
[564-36-3] Ergocornine, 3648
[564-37-4] Ergocorninine, 3648
[565-50-4] Terpin trans-Form, 9169
[565-63-9] Angelic Acid, 646
[565-74-2] α-Bromoisovaleric Acid, 1422
[566-48-3] Formestane, 4240
[566-56-3] Allopregnane-3β,20α-diol, 269
[566-57-4] Allopregnane-3α,20β-diol, 268
[566-58-5] Allopregnane-3α,20α-diol, 267
[566-65-4] 3,20-Allopregnanedione, 272
[566-78-9] 21-Acetoxypregnenolone, 77
[567-18-0] 1-Naphthol-2-sulfonic Acid, 6390
[568-02-5] Alizarine Blue, 253
[568-21-8] Isothebaine, 5226
[568-53-6] α-Peltatin, 7075
[568-93-4] Alizarine Orange, 254
[569-31-3] Meconin, 5783
[569-57-3] Chlorotrianisene, 2174
[569-58-4] Aluminon, 322
[569-59-5] Phenindamine Hydrogen Tartrate, 7233
[569-64-2] Malachite Green, 5699
[569-65-3] Meclizine, 5777
[569-77-7] Purpurogallin, 7946
[569-84-6] Antipyrine Acetylsalicylate, 716
[570-54-7] Allopregnane-3β,17α-diol-20-one, 271
[572-09-8] Acetobromglucose, 60
[572-59-8] Epiquinidine, 3620
[572-60-1] Epiquinine, 3621
[572-76-9] Nandinine, 6364
[572-96-3] Phytonadiol, 7380
[573-01-3] Menadoxime, 5832
[573-20-6] Menadiol Diacetate, 5830
[573-35-3] Inositol Monophosphate, 4978
[573-41-1] Theophylline Ethanolamine, 9285
[573-56-8] 2,6-Dinitrophenol, 3282
[573-58-0] Congo Red, 2498
[574-12-9] Isoflavone, 5173
[574-64-1] Trypan Red, 9793
[574-65-2] Vital Red, 10012
[574-84-5] Fraxetin, 4265
[574-95-8] Aureothricin, 880
[575-19-9] 6,7-Benzomorphan, 1095
[575-47-3] Amylpenicillin Sodium Salt, 616
[575-74-6] Buclosamide, 1465

[575-75-7] Toldimfos Sodium, 9512
[576-19-2] Biocytin, 1227
[576-55-6] 3,4,5,6-Tetrabromo-o-cresol, 9184
[576-97-6] Noprylsulfamide, 6684
[577-11-7] Docusate Sodium, 3401
[577-27-5] Ledol, 5430
[577-33-3] Anthrarobin, 688
[577-37-7] Aphylline, 729
[577-91-3] Iodoalphionic Acid, 5026
[578-20-1] Thymyl N-Isoamylcarbamate, 9409
[578-36-9] Potassium Salicylate, 7665
[578-74-5] Apigetrin, 731
[578-94-9] Phenarsazine Chloride, 7215
[579-04-4] Cymarose, 2762
[579-10-2] N-Methylacetanilide, 6007
[579-13-5] Oligomycin A, 6833
[579-23-7] Cyclovalone, 2755
[579-38-4] Diloxanide, 3201
[579-56-6] Isoxsuprine Hydrochloride, 5238
[579-92-0] Diphenylamine-2,2'-dicarboxylic Acid, 3318
[580-02-9] Methyl Acetylsalicylate, 6010
[580-13-2] 2-Bromonaphthalene, 1426
[580-52-9] Oxalenediuramidoxime, 6910
[580-74-5] Xanthocillin X, 10061
[581-49-7] Anatabine, 626
[581-75-9] 2,6-Naphthalenedisulfonic Acid, 6374
[581-88-4] Debrisoquin Sulfate, 2844
[582-36-5] Oxythiamine, 6977
[582-52-5] Diacetoneglucose, 2965
[582-60-5] 5,6-Dimethylbenzimidazole, 3236
[583-03-9] Fenipentol, 3975
[583-15-3] Mercuric Benzoate, 5874
[583-39-1] 2-Benzimidazolethiol, 1082
[583-50-6] D-Erythrose, 3690
[583-52-8] Potassium Oxalate, 7651
[583-91-5] Methionine Hydroxy Analog, 5976
[584-02-1] 3-Pentanol, 7120
[584-08-7] Potassium Carbonate, 7619
[584-10-1] Potassium Tetraiodocadmate, 7687
[584-28-1] Aspidin, 846
[584-42-9] Metachrome Yellow, 5919
[584-79-2] Allethrin I, 260
[584-84-9] Toluene 2,4-Diisocyanate, 9530
[584-85-0] Anserine, 679
[585-18-2] D-Erythrose 4-Phosphate, 3692
[585-21-7] Glutamine DL-Form, 4471
[585-29-5] Triethylammonium Formate, 9667
[585-48-8] 2,6-Di-tert-butylpyridine, 3036
[585-86-4] Lactitol, 5340
[585-99-9] Melibiose, 5820
[586-02-7] Phrenosin, 7367
[586-06-1] Metaproterenol, 5931
[586-60-7] Dyclonine, 3473
[586-76-5] p-Bromobenzoic Acid, 1408
[587-23-5] Methenamine Mandelate, 5966
[587-26-8] Lanthanum Carbonate, 5364
[587-33-7] m-Tyrosine, 9840
[587-61-1] Propyliodone, 7863
[587-63-3] Dihydrokawain, 5287

[587-90-6] 4,4'-Dinitrocarbanilide, 3278
[587-98-4] Metanil Yellow, 5928
[588-59-0] Stilbene, 8817
[589-15-1] p-Bromobenzyl Bromide, 1409
[589-17-3] p-Bromobenzyl Chloride, 1410
[589-21-9] p-Bromophenylhydrazine, 1429
[589-44-6] 3-Amino-4-hydroxybutyric Acid, 443
[589-57-1] Ethyl Phosphorochloridite, 3841
[589-59-3] Isobutyl Isovalerate, 5146
[589-97-9] Potassium Percarbonate, 7652
[590-01-2] n-Butyl Propionate, 1587
[590-28-3] Potassium Cyanate, 7625
[590-29-4] Potassium Formate, 7633
[590-46-5] Betaine Hydrochloride, 1179
[590-47-6] Betaine Monohydrate, 1179
[590-63-6] Bethanechol Chloride, 1185
[590-86-3] Isovaleraldehyde, 5229
[590-92-1] β-Bromopropionic Acid, 1433
[591-01-5] Dicyanodiamidine Sulfate, 3093
[591-09-3] Acetyl Nitrate, 97
[591-20-8] m-Bromophenol, 1428
[591-27-5] m-Aminophenol, 460
[591-50-4] Iodobenzene, 5029
[591-64-0] Calcium Levulinate, 1679
[591-78-6] Methyl Butyl Ketone, 6033
[591-81-1] γ-Hydroxybutyrate, 4815
[591-87-7] Allyl acetate, 288
[591-89-9] Potassium Tetracyanomercurate(II), 7683
[591-97-9] 1-Chloro-2-butene, 2130
[592-01-8] Calcium Cyanide, 1664
[592-04-1] Mercuric Cyanide, 5877
[592-65-4] Isobutyl Sulfide, 5152
[592-85-8] Mercuric Thiocyanate, 5890
[592-87-0] Lead Thiocyanate, 5426
[592-88-1] Allyl Sulfide, 297
[593-26-0] Ammonium Palmitate, 538
[593-29-3] Potassium Stearate, 7673
[593-39-5] Petroselinic Acid, 7189
[593-50-0] 1-Triacontanol, 9591
[593-53-3] Fluoromethane, 4174
[593-74-8] Dimethylmercury, 3250
[593-81-7] Trimethylamine Hydrochloride, 9710
[594-08-1] Trithiocarbonic Acid, 9759
[595-05-1] Calycanthine, 1723
[595-33-5] Megestrol Acetate, 5805
[595-39-1] Isovaline, 5234
[595-40-4] Isovaline L-Form, 5234
[595-77-7] Algestone, 239
[596-01-0] α-Naphtholphthalein, 6389
[596-03-2] 4',5'-Dibromofluorescein, 3022
[596-27-0] o-Cresolphthalein, 2576
[596-51-0] Glycopyrrolate, 4501
[597-12-6] Melezitose, 5819
[597-71-7] Pentaerythritol Tetraacetate, 7111
[598-31-2] Bromoacetone, 1401
[598-54-9] Cuprous Acetate, 2658
[598-55-0] Methyl Carbamate, 6036
[598-58-3] Methyl Nitrate, 6101
[598-62-9] Manganese Carbonate, 5726
[598-75-4] 3-Methyl-2-butanol, 6031

[598-82-3] DL-Lactic Acid, 5336
[599-04-2] Pantolactone, 7013
[599-33-7] Prednylidene, 7724
[599-71-3] Piloty's Acid, 7426
[599-79-1] Sulfasalazine, 8942
[599-88-2] Sulfaperine, 8934
[602-09-5] BINOL, 1226
[602-41-5] Thiocolchicine 2-Glucoside Analog, 9324
[602-64-2] Anthragallol, 683
[603-00-9] Proxyphylline, 7905
[603-35-0] Triphenylphosphine, 9743
[603-45-2] Aurin, 881
[603-50-9] Bisacodyl, 1242
[603-57-6] Aminopyrine Salicylate, 474
[603-59-8] Antipyrine Salicylacetate, 716
[603-64-5] Antipyrine Mandelate, 716
[604-51-3] Deptropine, 2912
[604-75-1] Oxazepam, 6926
[605-50-5] Isoamyl Phthalate, 5124
[605-65-2] Dansyl Chloride, 2814
[606-04-2] Pamabrom, 7000
[606-17-7] Iodipamide, 5022
[606-21-3] 2-Chloro-1,3-dinitrobenzene, 2137
[606-22-4] 2,6-Dinitroaniline, 3271
[606-58-6] Toyocamycin, 9562
[606-90-6] Diphenylpyraline 8-Chlorotheophyllinate, 3331
[607-80-7] Sesamin, 8470
[607-91-0] Myristicin, 6334
[608-07-1] 5-Methoxytryptamine, 6002
[608-66-2] Galactitol, 4332
[608-89-9] Ethyl Tartrate, Acid, 3856
[609-36-9] Proline DL-Form, 7780
[609-78-9] Cycloguanil Pamoate, 2721
[610-60-6] Methyl Benzoylsalicylate, 6025
[610-88-8] Tenuazonic Acid, 9149
[611-40-5] Tectoridin, 9107
[611-75-6] Bromhexine Hydrochloride, 1391
[612-83-9] 3,3'-Dichlorobenzidine Dihydrochloride, 3059
[613-78-5] 2-Naphthyl Salicylate, 6415
[613-82-1] Phenylethanolamine Sulfate, 7287
[613-89-8] Phenacylamine, 7206
[614-39-1] Procainamide Hydrochloride, 7756
[614-87-9] Dibromopropamidine Isethionate, 3024
[615-05-4] 2,4-Diaminoanisole, 2976
[616-05-7] α-Bromo-n-caproic Acid, 1415
[616-07-9] Ornithine DL-Form, 6874
[616-38-6] Dimethyl Carbonate, 3241
[616-45-5] 2-Pyrrolidone, 8016
[616-68-2] Trimecaine, 9700
[616-91-1] Acetylcysteine, 88
[617-12-9] Chorismic Acid, 2217
[617-48-1] Malic Acid DL-Form, 5707
[617-57-2] Lactic Acid Lactate, 5339
[617-65-2] Glutamic Acid DL-Form, 4469
[618-27-9] Hydroxyproline cis-Form, 4840
[618-65-5] Helicin, 4628
[618-82-6] Sulfarsphenamine, 8941
[619-84-1] 4-(Dimethylamino)benzoic Acid, 3232
[620-13-3] m-Xylyl Bromide, 10090
[620-19-9] m-Xylyl Chloride, 10091

[620-30-4] Metyrosine DL-Form, 6161
[620-45-1] 2,6-Dichloroindophenol Sodium, 3068
[620-90-6] Phenamidine Isethionate, 7208
[620-99-5] Phenacaine Hydrochloride, 7202
[621-82-9] Cinnamic Acid, 2299
[622-91-3] Metoquinone, 6152
[623-32-5] Chaulmoogric Acid Ethyl Ester, 2048
[623-42-7] Methyl Butyrate, 6035
[623-47-2] Ethyl Propiolate, 3846
[623-73-4] Diazoacetic Ester, 2997
[624-04-4] Glycol Dilaurate, 4497
[624-65-7] Propargyl Chloride, 7810
[624-83-9] Methyl Isocyanate, 6089
[625-04-7] Diacetonamine, 2962
[625-51-4] Formicin, 4242
[626-48-2] 6-Methyluracil, 6133
[626-76-6] α-Norbixin, 1311
[627-13-4] n-Propyl Nitrate, 7864
[628-52-4] Chromous Acetate, 2242
[628-55-7] Isobutyl Ether, 5142
[628-96-6] Ethylene Glycol Dinitrate, 3800
[629-11-8] Hexamethylene Glycol, 4690
[630-08-0] Carbon Monoxide, 1813
[630-56-8] 17α-Hydroxyprogesterone Caproate, 4839
[630-60-4] Ouabain, 6901
[630-64-8] Helveticoside, 4632
[630-67-1] Prednisolone 21-m-Sulfobenzoate Sodium Salt, 7721
[630-93-3] Phenytoin Sodium Salt, 7322
[631-60-7] Mercurous Acetate, 5892
[631-61-8] Ammonium Acetate, 495
[631-69-6] β-Boswellic Acid, 1355
[632-22-4] Tetramethylurea, 9230
[632-68-8] Rose Bengal, 8262
[632-69-9] Rose Bengal Disodium Salt, 8262
[632-99-5] Magenta I, 5652
[633-03-4] Brilliant Green, 1374
[633-47-6] Cropropamide, 2591
[633-59-0] Clopenthixol Dihydrochloride, 2394
[633-96-5] Orange II, 6858
[634-03-7] Phendimetrazine, 7220
[634-25-3] Pyridoxal 5-Phosphate Oxime, 7979
[635-05-2] Pamaquine Pamoate, 7001
[635-41-6] Trimetozine, 9720
[635-65-4] Bilirubin, 1218
[636-46-4] 4-Hydroxyisophthalic Acid, 4827
[636-47-5] Stallimycin, 8772
[636-54-4] Clopamide, 2393
[636-61-3] Malic Acid D-(+)-Form, 5707
[636-65-7] L-Isoglutamine, 5177
[637-03-6] Oxophenylarsine, 6949
[637-07-0] Clofibrate, 2377
[637-12-7] Aluminum Stearate, 364
[637-32-1] Chlorguanide Hydrochloride, 2090
[637-39-8] Triethanolamine Hydrochloride, 9665
[637-49-0] Coniine Hydrobromide, 2505
[637-58-1] Pramoxine Hydrochloride, 7709

[637-92-3] Ethyl tert-Butyl Ether, 3774
[638-23-3] Carbocysteine, 1802
[638-38-0] Manganese Acetate, 5724
[638-39-1] Stannous Acetate, 8781
[638-94-8] Desonide, 2928
[638-95-9] α-Amyrin, 617
[639-43-0] Akuammicine, 199
[639-44-1] Phenoltetrachlorophthalein, 7248
[639-48-5] Nicomorphine, 6520
[639-81-6] Ergotaminine, 3662
[639-86-1] Solanocapsine, 8706
[639-97-4] Apiose, 735
[640-19-7] Fluoroacetamide, 4166
[640-67-5] Manganese Oxalate, 5734
[641-36-1] Apocodeine, 740
[641-85-0] Allopregnane, 266
[642-08-0] Ostruthol, 6897
[642-15-9] Antimycin A₁, 714
[642-18-2] Alstonine, 316
[642-44-4] Aminometradine, 451
[642-72-8] Benzydamine, 1122
[642-75-1] Adrenolutin, 174
[642-78-4] Cloxacillin Sodium Salt, 2419
[643-13-0] Fructose-6-phosphate (anhydrous), 4276
[643-22-1] Erythromycin Stearate, 3687
[643-60-7] Anhalamine, 653
[643-79-8] o-Phthalaldehyde, 7368
[643-84-5] Malvidin Chloride, 5715
[644-31-5] Acetozone, 78
[644-62-2] Meclofenamic Acid, 5779
[645-05-6] Altretamine, 320
[645-17-0] Linoleic Acid Aluminum Salt, 5505
[645-43-2] Guanethidine Monosulfate, 4560
[645-49-8] Stilbene cis-Form, 8817
[646-13-9] Isobutyl Stearate, 5151
[650-51-1] Trichloroacetic Acid Sodium Salt, 9627
[650-69-1] β-Citraurin, 2324
[651-06-9] Sulfameter, 8914
[651-48-9] Dehydroepiandrosterone Sulfate, 2871
[651-55-8] Dihydroequilin 17α-Form, 3173
[652-37-9] Acefylline, 24
[652-67-5] Isosorbide, 5224
[653-03-2] Butaperazine, 1516
[655-05-0] Thozalinone, 9379
[655-35-6] Chromonar Hydrochloride, 2239
[655-76-5] Quinaldine Sulfate, 8047
[655-86-7] 2,3-Diaminophenazine, 2982
[657-24-9] Metformin, 5938
[657-27-2] L-Lysine Monohydrochloride, 5636
[659-40-5] Hexamidine Isethionate, 4692
[659-70-1] Isoamyl Isovalerate, 5121
[660-27-5] Diisopropylamine Dichloroacetate, 3197
[660-60-6] Cupric Stearate, 2652
[661-19-8] n-Docosanol, 3399
[664-95-9] Tolcyclamide, 9511
[665-66-7] Amantadine Hydrochloride, 374
[666-99-9] Agaricic Acid, 186
[670-54-2] Tetracyanoethylene, 9195
[670-65-5] Neopterin, 6462
[671-16-9] Procarbazine, 7758
[671-95-4] Clofenamide, 2374

[672-15-1] Homoserine, *4739*
[672-87-7] Metyrosine, *6161*
[673-06-3] Phenylalanine D-Form, *7271*
[673-31-4] Phenprobamate, *7258*
[680-31-9] HMPA, *4725*
[684-16-2] Hexafluoroacetone, *4685*
[685-73-4] D-Galacturonic Acid, *4337*
[688-37-9] Aluminum Oleate, *354*
[689-13-4] Hadacidin, *4587*
[692-13-7] Buformin, *1476*
[693-30-1] Hemisulfur Mustard, *4646*
[693-65-2] *n*-Amyl Ether, *608*
[693-72-1] Vaccenic Acid, *9898*
[694-59-7] Pyridine 1-Oxide, *7972*
[695-34-1] 2-Amino-4-picoline, *466*
[695-53-4] Dimethadione, *3213*
[703-95-7] 5-Fluoroorotic Acid, *4176*
[705-16-8] Chrysanthemic Acid *dl-trans*-Form, *2251*
[709-55-7] Etilefrin, *3865*
[709-98-8] Propanil, *7804*
[716-79-0] 2-Phenyl-1*H*-benzimidazole, *7274*
[721-50-6] Prilocaine, *7743*
[723-46-6] Sulfamethoxazole, *8918*
[728-88-1] Tolperisone, *9522*
[729-99-7] Sulfamoxole, *8924*
[730-68-7] Methitural Sodium Salt, *5978*
[732-11-6] Phosmet, *7336*
[737-31-5] Diatrizoate Sodium, *2992*
[738-70-5] Trimethoprim, *9709*
[738-99-8] Dipin, *3336*
[739-71-9] Trimipramine, *9722*
[742-20-1] Cyclopenthiazide, *2745*
[745-65-3] Prostaglandin E₁, *7876*
[747-36-4] Hydroxychloroquine Sulfate, *4818*
[749-02-0] Spiperone, *8751*
[749-13-3] Trifluperidol, *9684*
[751-84-8] Penicillin G Benethamine, *7095*
[751-94-0] Fusidic Acid Sodium Salt, *4317*
[751-97-3] Rolitetracycline, *8252*
[752-56-7] Riboflavin 2′,3′,4′,5′-Tetrabutyrate, *8200*
[752-61-4] Digitalin, *3158*
[756-79-6] DMMP, *3391*
[759-73-9] *N*-Ethyl-*N*-nitrosourea, *3833*
[759-94-4] EPTC, *3640*
[764-05-6] Cyanogen Azide, *2692*
[767-21-5] Piperidine Phosphate, *7468*
[768-94-5] Amantadine, *374*
[770-05-8] Octopamine DL-Form Hydrochloride, *6759*
[770-12-7] Phenyl Dichlorophosphate, *7282*
[773-76-2] Chloroxine, *2175*
[777-11-7] Haloprogin, *4600*
[790-69-2] Loflucarban, *5559*
[791-35-5] Chlophedianol, *2066*
[795-13-1] *N*²-Formylsulfisomidine, *4248*
[795-38-0] Dihydroisocodeine, *3176*
[797-63-7] Levonorgestrel, *6704*
[797-64-8] Norgestrel (+)-Form, *6704*
[800-22-6] Chloracizine, *2068*
[800-24-8] 2,5-Bis(1-aziridinyl)-3,6-bis(2-methoxyethoxy)-1,4-benzoquinone, *1245*
[801-52-5] Porfiromycin, *7597*
[804-10-4] Chromonar, *2239*
[804-30-8] Fursultiamine, *4311*

[804-36-4] Nitrovin, *6654*
[804-53-5] Tetrabenazine Methanesulfonate, *9182*
[804-63-7] Quinine Sulfate, *8061*
[807-31-8] Aceperone, *30*
[808-71-9] Penethamate Hydriodide, *7085*
[811-54-1] Lead Formate, *5409*
[811-97-2] HFC-134a, *4714*
[813-94-5] Calcium Citrate, *1661*
[814-71-1] Calcium Thioglycollate, *1711*
[814-80-2] Calcium Lactate, *1678*
[814-87-9] Aluminum Oxalate, *355*
[814-89-1] Cobaltous Oxalate, *2445*
[814-91-5] Cupric Oxalate, *2645*
[814-93-7] Lead Oxalate, *5415*
[814-94-8] Stannous Oxalate, *8786*
[815-78-1] Aluminum Tartrate, *368*
[815-82-7] Cupric Tartrate, *2656*
[815-85-0] Stannous Tartrate, *8792*
[817-09-4] Trichlormethine Hydrochloride, *9625*
[821-33-0] 4,4′-Oxydi-2-butanol, *6960*
[822-16-2] Sodium Stearate, *8678*
[826-39-1] Mecamylamine Hydrochloride, *5774*
[828-00-2] Dimethoxane, *3223*
[829-74-3] Nordefrin (−)-Form, *6692*
[830-89-7] Albutoin, *217*
[834-12-8] Ametryn, *393*
[834-28-6] Phenformin Hydrochloride, *7231*
[835-31-4] Naphazoline, *6368*
[837-27-4] Acefylline Sodium Salt, *24*
[841-73-6] Bucolome, *1466*
[846-48-0] Boldenone, *1324*
[846-49-1] Lorazepam, *5579*
[846-50-4] Temazepam, *9133*
[846-70-8] Naphthol Yellow S, *6393*
[847-25-6] Thiamphenicol DL-Form, *9301*
[847-84-7] Normethadone Hydrochloride, *6709*
[848-21-5] Norgestrienone, *6705*
[848-53-3] Homochlorcyclizine, *4733*
[848-75-9] Lormetazepam, *5581*
[849-55-8] Nylidrin Hydrochloride, *6732*
[850-52-2] Altrenogest, *319*
[852-19-7] Sulfazamet, *8945*
[853-34-9] Kebuzone, *5288*
[855-19-6] Clostebol Acetate, *2413*
[855-96-9] Eupatorin, *3901*
[856-87-1] Dipipanone Hydrochloride, *3337*
[860-07-1] 3′,3″,5′,5″-Tetrabromophenolphthalein Disodium Salt, *9186*
[860-22-0] Indigo Carmine, *4944*
[863-61-6] Menaquinone 4, *5833*
[865-04-3] 10-Methoxydeserpidine, *2918*
[865-21-4] Vinblastine, *9982*
[865-28-1] Tyrocidine B, *9836*
[865-44-1] Iodine Trichloride, *5020*
[866-82-0] Cupric Citrate, *2636*
[866-83-1] Potassium Citrate, Monobasic, *7624*
[866-84-2] Potassium Citrate, *7623*
[867-27-6] Demeton-*O*-methyl, *6051*
[867-81-2] Pantothenic Acid Sodium Salt, *7015*
[868-14-4] Potassium Bitartrate, *7615*
[868-18-8] Sodium Tartrate, *8684*

[868-54-2] 2-Amino-1,1,3-tricyanopropene, *480*
[870-72-4] Formaldehyde Sodium Bisulfite, *4236*
[872-50-4] 1-Methylpyrrolidone, *6117*
[875-83-2] 2-Naphthol Sodium Salt, *6384*
[876-04-0] Octopamine D(−)-Form, *6759*
[877-24-7] Potassium Biphthalate, *7612*
[881-17-4] *o*-Iodohippurate Sodium ¹³¹I-Labeled Form, *5034*
[882-09-7] Clofibric Acid, *2378*
[886-38-4] Diphencyprone, *3308*
[886-65-7] 1,4-Diphenyl-1,3-butadiene, *3320*
[886-74-8] Chlorphenesin Carbamate, *2179*
[886-86-2] Tricaine, *9621*
[887-08-1] Daucol, *2831*
[894-71-3] Nortriptyline Hydrochloride, *6715*
[897-15-4] Dothiepin Hydrochloride, *3429*
[897-61-0] Penicillin O Potassium Salt, *7099*
[900-77-6] Drocarbil, *778*
[901-93-9] Estrone Acetate, *3708*
[904-04-1] Captodiamine Hydrochloride, *1773*
[908-54-3] Diminazene Aceturate, *3266*
[909-39-7] Opipramol Dihydrochloride, *6853*
[911-45-5] Clomiphene, *2386*
[911-65-9] Etonitazene, *3883*
[912-60-7] Noscapine Hydrochloride, *6718*
[914-00-1] Methacycline, *5943*
[915-30-0] Diphenoxylate, *3313*
[915-67-3] Amaranth (Dye), *375*
[917-61-3] Sodium Cyanate, *8604*
[917-69-1] Cobaltic Acetate, *2428*
[918-04-7] Acetaldehyde Sodium Bisulfite, *41*
[919-16-4] Lithium Citrate, *5530*
[919-86-8] Demeton-*S*-methyl, *6051*
[921-53-9] Potassium Tartrate, *7677*
[922-55-4] Lanthionine, *5365*
[922-80-5] Diamyl Sodium Sulfosuccinate, *2989*
[923-06-8] Bromosuccinic Acid, *1437*
[923-32-0] Cystine DL-Form, *2782*
[926-26-1] Di-*tert*-butyl Succinate, *3037*
[926-93-2] Methallibure, *5946*
[930-55-2] *N*-Nitrosopyrrolidine, *6643*
[932-53-6] 6-Azathymine, *903*
[937-13-3] Oxonic Acid, *6947*
[938-73-8] Ethenzamide, *3731*
[941-69-5] *N*-Phenylmaleimide, *7299*
[944-22-9] Fonofos, *4233*
[947-08-0] Thiobutabarbital Sodium Salt, *9323*
[950-10-7] Mephosfolan, *5855*
[950-37-8] Methidathion, *5970*
[951-78-0] Deoxyuridine, *2910*
[952-54-5] Morphazinamide, *6273*
[956-90-1] Phencyclidine Hydrochloride, *7219*
[957-51-7] Diphenamid, *3307*
[957-56-2] Fluindione, *4134*
[957-68-6] 7-Aminocephalosporanic Acid, *434*
[959-10-4] Xenbucin, *10071*

[959-14-8] Oxolamine, *6944*
[959-24-0] Sotalol Hydrochloride, *8728*
[962-02-7] Nitrodan, *6596*
[964-52-3] Moxisylyte Hydrochloride, *6292*
[965-52-6] Nifuroxazide, *6535*
[965-90-2] Ethylestrenol, *3805*
[965-93-5] Methyltrienolone, *6129*
[968-58-1] Pridinol Hydrochloride, *7741*
[968-81-0] Acetohexamide, *62*
[968-93-4] Testolactone, *9179*
[969-99-3] Opromazine, *6855*
[972-02-1] Diphenidol, *3311*
[973-21-7] Dinobuton, *3285*
[973-99-9] Prosultiamine Hydrochloride, *7882*
[975-64-4] Estrone Propionate, *3708*
[976-71-6] Canrenone, *1750*
[977-79-7] Medrogestone, *5791*
[979-32-8] Estradiol 17-Valerate, *3703*
[980-71-2] Brompheniramine Maleate, *1443*
[982-24-1] Clopenthixol, *2394*
[982-43-4] Prenoxdiazine Hydrochloride, *7736*
[982-57-0] Chloramphenicol Monosuccinate Sodium Salt, *2077*
[983-85-7] Penamecillin, *7081*
[985-12-6] Drotaverine Hydrochloride, *3455*
[985-13-7] Ethaverine Hydrochloride, *3728*
[985-16-0] Nafcillin Sodium Salt, *6352*
[985-32-0] Quinacillin Disodium Salt (anhydrous), *8043*
[987-24-6] Betamethasone 21-Acetate, *1180*
[987-65-5] Adenosine Triphosphate Disodium Salt, *155*
[987-78-0] Citicoline, *2319*
[989-51-5] EGCG, *3526*
[990-73-8] Fentanyl Citrate, *4001*
[991-42-4] Norbormide, *6687*
[992-21-2] Lymecycline, *5628*
[992-46-1] Thiamine Disulfide Phosphate, *9297*
[992-59-6] Benzopurpurine 4B, *1101*
[994-05-8] *tert*-Amyl Methyl Ether, *612*
[997-55-7] *N*-Acetyl-L-aspartic Acid, *840*
[997-68-2] L-Saccharopine, *8312*
[999-81-5] Chlormequat Chloride, *2104*
[999-97-3] Hexamethyldisilazane, *4689*
[1002-89-7] Ammonium Stearate, *553*
[1003-78-7] 2,4-Dimethylsulfolane, *3257*
[1005-24-9] Trigonellamide Chloride, *9693*
[1005-51-2] Bullvalene, *1482*
[1013-59-8] Tenuazonic Acid Sodium Salt, *9149*
[1014-70-6] Simetryn, *8536*
[1018-71-9] Pyrrolnitrin, *8018*
[1028-33-7] Pentifylline, *7127*
[1037-50-9] Sulfadimethoxine Sodium Salt, *8905*
[1041-90-3] Nalorphine Hydrobromide, *6361*
[1043-21-6] Pirenoxine, *7490*
[1045-69-8] Testosterone Acetate, *9180*
[1050-79-9] Moperone, *6263*
[1059-14-9] Taraxasterol, *9060*
[1063-55-4] Butaperazine Dimaleate, *1516*

[1063-77-0] Nomilin, *6674*
[1066-17-7] Colistin, *2479*
[1066-30-4] Chromic Acetate, *2219*
[1066-33-7] Ammonium Bicarbonate, *497*
[1069-54-1] Bis(1,2-dimethylpropyl)-borane, *1250*
[1069-55-2] Isobutyl Cyanoacrylate, *5140*
[1069-66-5] Valproic Acid Sodium Salt (1:1), *9913*
[1070-11-7] Ethambutol Dihydrochloride, *3720*
[1070-83-3] *tert*-Butylacetic Acid, *1538*
[1071-83-6] Glyphosate, *4512*
[1072-35-1] Lead Stearate, *5418*
[1077-27-6] Thioctic Acid *l*-Form, *9326*
[1077-28-7] Thioctic Acid *dl*-Form, *9326*
[1078-19-9] 6-Methoxy-α-tetralone, *6000*
[1078-21-3] 4-Amino-3-phenylbutyric Acid, *464*
[1081-34-1] α-Terthienyl, *9174*
[1082-57-1] Tramazoline, *9567*
[1083-57-4] Bucetin, *1458*
[1085-98-9] Dichlofluanid, *3044*
[1086-80-2] Lumichrome, *5598*
[1088-11-5] Nordazepam, *6691*
[1088-56-8] Lumiflavine, *5599*
[1088-92-2] Nifurtoinol, *6539*
[1091-94-7] Estrone Methyl Ether, *3708*
[1093-58-9] Clostebol, *2413*
[1094-08-2] Ethopropazine Hydrochloride, *3747*
[1094-61-7] NMN, *6663*
[1095-90-5] Methadone Hydrochloride, *5944*
[1098-60-8] Triflupromazine Hydrochloride, *9685*
[1098-97-1] Pyritinol, *7996*
[1099-87-2] Dehydroepiandrosterone Sodium Sulfate, *2871*
[1107-99-9] Prednisolone 21-Trimethylacetate, *7721*
[1108-68-5] Cinobufotalin, *2307*
[1109-15-5] Tris(pentafluorophenyl)-boron, *9755*
[1110-40-3] Cortivazol, *2540*
[1110-80-1] Pipacycline, *7453*
[1111-39-3] Acetyldigitoxins α-Form, *89*
[1111-67-7] Cuprous Thiocyanate, *2669*
[1111-78-0] Ammonium Carbamate, *507*
[1113-38-8] Ammonium Oxalate, *537*
[1113-41-3] Penicillamine L-Form, *7088*
[1114-34-7] D-Lyxose, *5641*
[1114-41-6] Muramic Acid, *6304*
[1114-71-2] Pebulate, *7061*
[1115-70-4] Metformin Hydrochloride, *5938*
[1115-84-0] *S*-Methylmethionine L-Form Chloride, *6098*
[1116-54-7] *N*-Nitrosodiethanolamine (L-form chloride), *6635*
[1118-68-9] *N,N*-Dimethylglycine, *3244*
[1119-33-1] L-Glutamic Acid 5-Ethyl Ester, *4470*
[1119-34-2] Arginine Hydrochloride, *780*
[1119-97-7] Myristyltrimethylammonium Bromide, *6336*

[1120-44-1] Cupric Oleate, *2644*
[1121-30-8] Pyrithione, *7994*
[1121-55-7] 3-Ethenylpyridine, *3730*
[1122-58-3] DMAP, *3389*
[1130-23-0] Cyclobutyrol Sodium Salt, *2715*
[1131-64-2] Debrisoquin, *2844*
[1132-61-2] MOPS, *6265*
[1134-47-0] Baclofen, *937*
[1134-98-1] Sulfarside, *8940*
[1135-24-6] Ferulic Acid, *4062*
[1135-40-6] CAPS, *1767*
[1143-38-0] Anthralin, *684*
[1146-04-9] Illudin M, *4899*
[1146-98-1] Bromindione, *1393*
[1146-99-2] Clorindione, *2406*
[1147-62-2] Pyrovalerone Hydrochloride, *8010*
[1149-99-1] Illudin S, *4899*
[1151-11-7] Ipodate Calcium Salt, *5071*
[1151-15-1] *o*-(*p*-Anisoyl)benzoic Acid, *672*
[1153-51-1] (3α,5α)-Androst-16-en-3-ol, *639*
[1154-59-2] 3,3′,4′,5-Tetrachlorosalicylanilide, *9191*
[1156-19-0] Tolazamide, *9505*
[1162-15-8] Dioxadrol *d*-Form Hydrochloride, *3299*
[1162-65-8] Aflatoxin B₁, *180*
[1163-36-6] Clemizole Hydrochloride, *2346*
[1163-37-7] Moxaverine Hydrochloride, *6288*
[1165-39-5] Aflatoxin G₁, *181*
[1165-48-6] Dimefline, *3204*
[1172-02-7] 9-Dicyanomethylene-2,4,7-trinitrofluorene, *3094*
[1172-18-5] Flurazepam Dihydrochloride, *4198*
[1172-63-0] Jasmolin II, *5258*
[1176-03-0] Pseudococaine Tartrate, *7912*
[1177-30-6] Fenbenicillin Potassium Salt, *3961*
[1177-87-3] Dexamethasone 21-Acetate, *2943*
[1178-60-5] Pentagestrone Acetate, *7114*
[1179-69-7] Thiethylperazine Dimaleate, *9315*
[1180-71-8] Limonin, *5494*
[1181-54-0] Clomocycline, *2388*
[1183-76-2] Daphnandrine, *2819*
[1184-78-7] Trimethylamine *N*-Oxide, *9711*
[1185-57-5] Ferric Ammonium Citrate, *4017*
[1187-56-0] Selenomethionine ⁷⁵Se-Injection, *8441*
[1188-38-1] Carglumic acid, *1838*
[1190-53-0] Buformin Hydrochloride, *1476*
[1191-80-6] Mercuric Oleate, *5881*
[1194-65-6] Dichlobenil, *3042*
[1195-16-0] Citiolone, *2320*
[1197-17-7] Tranexamic Acid *cis*-Form, *9569*
[1197-18-8] Tranexamic Acid, *9569*
[1197-21-3] Phentermine Hydrochloride, *7262*
[1197-55-3] *p*-Aminophenylacetic Acid, *463*
[1200-22-2] Thioctic Acid *d*-Form, *9326*

[1201-26-9] 3-Indolylacetone, *4967*
[1209-98-9] Fencamfamine, *3966*
[1210-56-6] Adrenoglomerulotropin, *173*
[1211-28-5] Prolintane Hydrochloride, *7781*
[1211-29-6] Jasmonic Acid Methyl Ester, *5260*
[1215-83-4] Clobutinol Hydrochloride, *2365*
[1218-35-5] Xylometazoline Hydrochloride, *10086*
[1219-20-1] Oxolamine Hydrochloride, *6944*
[1219-77-8] Bensuldazic Acid, *1051*
[1221-56-3] Ipodate Sodium Salt, *5071*
[1222-05-5] HHCB, *4715*
[1222-57-7] Zolimidine, *10188*
[1225-20-3] Iothalamic Acid Sodium Salt, *5064*
[1225-55-4] Protriptyline Hydrochloride, *7901*
[1225-60-1] Isothipendyl Hydrochloride, *5227*
[1225-65-6] Prothipendyl Hydrochloride, *7888*
[1229-29-4] Doxepin Hydrochloride, *3435*
[1229-35-2] Methdilazine Hydrochloride, *5964*
[1229-69-2] Bamipine Hydrochloride, *956*
[1231-93-2] Ethynodiol, *3860*
[1235-15-0] Norbolethone, *6686*
[1235-82-1] Biperiden Hydrochloride, *1233*
[1239-04-9] Phenazocine (±)-Hydrobromide, *7218*
[1239-29-8] Furazabol, *4299*
[1239-45-8] Homidium Bromide, *4731*
[1240-15-9] Propiomazine Hydrochloride, *7822*
[1242-56-4] Stenbolone Acetate, *8808*
[1245-44-9] Propicillin Potassium Salt, *7817*
[1247-42-3] Meprednisone, *5861*
[1247-71-8] Colpormon, *2489*
[1249-84-9] Azacosterol Dihydrochloride, *892*
[1253-28-7] Gestonorone Caproate, *4414*
[1255-35-2] Fluprednidene Acetate, *4191*
[1260-17-9] Carminic Acid, *1843*
[1263-79-2] Tetrandrine *l*-Form, *9231*
[1263-89-4] Paromomycin Sulfate, *7041*
[1264-72-8] Colistin Sulfate, *2479*
[1271-19-8] Titanocene Dichloride, *9482*
[1299-86-1] Aluminum Carbide, *335*
[1300-32-9] Furoyl Chloride, *4310*
[1300-51-2] Sodium Phenolsulfonate, *8658*
[1300-71-6] Xylenol, *10082*
[1300-73-8] Xylidine, *10084*
[1301-96-8] Silver(II) Oxide, *8522*
[1302-09-6] Silver Selenide, *8528*
[1302-42-7] Sodium Aluminate, *8574*
[1302-78-9] Bentonite, *1055*
[1302-81-4] Aluminum Sulfide, *367*
[1302-82-5] Aluminum Selenide, *361*
[1302-83-6] Lazurite, *5395*
[1303-00-0] Gallium Arsenide, *4347*

[1303-11-3] Indium Arsenide, *4949*
[1303-28-2] Arsenic Pentoxide, *798*
[1303-33-9] Arsenic Trisulfide, *806*
[1303-34-0] Arsenic Pentasulfide, *797*
[1303-36-2] Arsenic Triselenide, *805*
[1303-52-2] Gold Trihydroxide, *4523*
[1303-58-8] Gold Trioxide, *4524*
[1303-61-3] Gold Trisulfide, *4525*
[1303-86-2] Boric Anhydride, *1337*
[1303-94-2] Lithium Borate Pentahydrate, *5524*
[1303-96-4] Sodium Borate Decahydrate, *8590*
[1304-28-5] Barium Oxide, *986*
[1304-29-6] Barium Peroxide, *989*
[1304-39-8] Barium Selenide, *992*
[1304-40-1] Barium Silicide, *993*
[1304-54-7] Beryllium Nitride, *1171*
[1304-56-9] Beryllium Oxide, *1172*
[1304-76-3] Bismuth Oxide, *1273*
[1304-82-1] Bismuth Telluride, *1289*
[1304-85-4] Bismuth Subnitrate, *1284*
[1305-62-0] Calcium Hydroxide, *1673*
[1305-78-8] Calcium Oxide, *1686*
[1305-79-9] Calcium Peroxide, *1689*
[1305-84-6] Calcium Selenide, *1701*
[1305-99-3] Calcium Phosphide, *1695*
[1306-01-0] Thomas Phosphate, *9372*
[1306-06-5] Durapatite, *3467*
[1306-19-0] Cadmium Oxide, *1623*
[1306-23-6] Cadmium Sulfide, *1628*
[1306-24-7] Cadmium Selenide, *1626*
[1306-25-8] Cadmium Telluride, *1629*
[1306-38-3] Ceric Oxide, *1989*
[1307-52-4] Ruthenium Red, *8300*
[1307-96-6] Cobaltous Oxide, *2446*
[1308-06-1] Cobaltic-Cobaltous Oxide, *2429*
[1308-14-1] Chromic Hydroxide, *2225*
[1308-38-9] Chromium(III) Oxide, *2234*
[1308-56-1] Chalcopyrite, *2038*
[1309-37-1] Ferric Oxide, *4028*
[1309-42-8] Magnesium Hydroxide, *5670*
[1309-48-4] Magnesium Oxide, *5677*
[1309-60-0] Lead Dioxide, *5407*
[1309-64-4] Antimony Trioxide, *711*
[1310-32-3] Ferrous Selenide, *4055*
[1310-43-6] Ferrous Phosphide, *4054*
[1310-45-8] Monsel's Solution, *6256*
[1310-52-7] Magnesium Germanide, *5667*
[1310-53-8] Germanium Dioxide, *4409*
[1310-58-3] Potassium Hydroxide, *7640*
[1310-61-8] Potassium Bisulfide, *7614*
[1310-65-2] Lithium Hydroxide, *5534*
[1310-73-2] Sodium Hydroxide, *8627*
[1310-82-3] Rubidium Hydroxide, *8285*
[1311-90-6] Ammonium Phosphotungstate, *546*
[1312-15-8] Sulfur Iodide, *8975*
[1312-41-0] Indium Antimonide, *4948*
[1312-42-1] Indium Selenide, *4954*
[1312-43-2] Indium Oxide, *4952*
[1312-45-4] Indium Telluride, *4956*
[1312-46-5] Iridium Sesquioxide, *5087*
[1312-73-8] Potassium Sulfide, *7675*
[1312-74-9] Potassium Selenide, *7667*
[1312-76-1] Potassium Silicate, *7668*
[1313-04-8] Magnesium Selenide, *5686*
[1313-08-2] Magnesium Stannide, *5689*
[1313-13-9] Manganese Dioxide, *5730*

[1313-22-0] Manganese Selenide, *5736*
[1313-27-5] Molybdenum Trioxide, *6239*
[1313-29-7] Molybdenum Sesquioxide, *6238*
[1313-30-0] Sodium Phosphomolybdate, *8664*
[1313-59-3] Sodium Oxide, *8651*
[1313-60-6] Sodium Peroxide, *8655*
[1313-82-2] Sodium Sulfide, *8681*
[1313-85-5] Sodium Selenide, *8672*
[1313-96-8] Niobium Pentoxide, *6559*
[1313-99-1] Nickel Monoxide, *6512*
[1314-06-3] Nickel Sesquioxide, *6516*
[1314-08-5] Palladium Oxide, *6993*
[1314-11-0] Strontium Oxide, *8846*
[1314-12-1] Thallium Oxide, *9266*
[1314-13-2] Zinc Oxide, *10147*
[1314-15-4] Platinic Oxide, *7527*
[1314-18-7] Strontium Peroxide, *8847*
[1314-20-1] Thorium Oxide, *9377*
[1314-22-3] Zinc Peroxide, *10149*
[1314-23-4] Zirconium Oxide, *10180*
[1314-24-5] Phosphorus Trioxide, *7360*
[1314-27-8] Lead Sesquioxide, *5417*
[1314-28-9] Rhenium Trioxide, *8180*
[1314-32-5] Thallium Sesquioxide, *9268*
[1314-34-7] Vanadium Trioxide, *9923*
[1314-35-8] Tungsten Trioxide, *9817*
[1314-41-6] Lead Tetroxide, *5425*
[1314-56-3] Phosphorus Pentoxide, *7355*
[1314-60-9] Antimony Pentoxide, *698*
[1314-61-0] Tantalum Pentoxide, *9056*
[1314-62-1] Vanadium Pentoxide, *9921*
[1314-64-3] Uranyl Sulfate, *9864*
[1314-68-7] Rhenium Heptoxide, *8178*
[1314-80-3] Phosphorus Pentasulfide, *7354*
[1314-82-5] Phosphorus Pentaselenide, *7353*
[1314-84-7] Zinc Phosphide, *10152*
[1314-85-8] Tetraphosphorus Trisulfide, *9238*
[1314-86-9] Phosphorus Triselenide, *7361*
[1314-87-0] Lead Sulfide, *5421*
[1314-91-6] Lead Telluride, *5422*
[1314-95-0] Stannous Sulfide, *8791*
[1314-96-1] Strontium Sulfide, *8849*
[1314-97-2] Thallium Sulfide, *9270*
[1314-98-3] Zinc Sulfide, *10160*
[1315-01-1] Stannic Sulfide, *8780*
[1315-03-3] Vanadium Trisulfide, *9924*
[1315-04-4] Antimony Pentasulfide, *697*
[1315-05-5] Antimony Triselenide, *712*
[1315-06-6] Stannous Selenide, *8789*
[1315-09-9] Zinc Selenide, *10156*
[1315-11-3] Zinc Telluride, *10162*
[1317-33-5] Molybdenum Disulfide, *6236*
[1317-34-6] Manganese Sesquioxide, *5737*
[1317-35-7] Manganese Oxide, *5735*
[1317-36-8] Lead Monoxide, *5413*
[1317-37-9] Ferrous Sulfide, *4058*
[1317-38-0] Cupric Oxide, *2646*
[1317-39-1] Cuprous Oxide, *2664*
[1317-40-4] Cupric Sulfide, *2655*
[1317-41-5] Cupric Selenide, *2651*
[1317-42-6] Cobaltous Sulfide, *2449*
[1317-54-0] Ferrite, *4035*

Chemical Abstracts Registry Numbers

[1317-61-9] Ferrosoferric Oxide, *4040*

[1317-82-4] Sapphire, *8367*

[1317-97-1] Ultramarine, *9846*

[1318-00-9] Vermiculite, *9961*

[1318-93-0] Montmorillonite, *6260*

[1319-46-6] Basic Lead Carbonate, *1005*

[1319-77-3] Cresols, *2579*

[1320-44-1] Methylbenzethonium Chloride Monohydrate, *6023*

[1321-14-8] Potassium Guaiacolsulfonate, *7634*

[1327-39-5] Calcium Aluminosilicate, *1648*

[1327-41-9] Aluminum Hydroxychloride, *343*

[1327-53-3] Arsenic Trioxide, *804*

[1329-83-5] Tigonin, *9435*

[1330-20-7] Xylene, *10081*

[1330-43-4] Sodium Borate, *8590*

[1330-51-4] Pyrogallol Monoacetate, *8000*

[1330-78-5] Tritolyl Phosphate, *9763*

[1332-10-1] Potassium Arsenite Solution, *7608*

[1332-14-5] Cupric Sulfate, Basic, *2654*

[1332-77-0] Potassium Tetraborate, *7680*

[1333-38-6] Angelica Lactone, *647*

[1333-74-0] Hydrogen, *4792*

[1333-82-0] Chromium(VI) Oxide, *2235*

[1333-83-1] Sodium Bifluoride, *8584*

[1334-74-3] Sodium Glycerophosphate, *8622*

[1335-31-5] Mercuric Oxycyanide, *5884*

[1335-32-6] Lead Subacetate, *5419*

[1335-94-0] Irone, *5095*

[1336-20-5] Tetracycline Phosphate Complex, *9196*

[1336-29-4] Bisacodyl Complex with Tannin, *1242*

[1336-80-7] Ferrocholinate, *4038*

[1338-16-5] Iron Sorbitex, *5100*

[1338-39-2] Sorbitan Laurate, *8724*

[1338-41-6] Sorbitan Stearate, *8724*

[1338-43-8] Sorbitan Oleate, *8724*

[1338-98-3] Ethylstibamine, *3852*

[1339-92-0] Basic Aluminum Carbonate Gel, *1004*

[1340-26-7] Phenacetolin, *7205*

[1340-35-8] Urea Stibamine, *9871*

[1340-69-8] Bentoquatam, *1056*

[1341-49-7] Ammonium Bifluoride, *498*

[1343-98-2] Silicic Acid, *8490*

[1344-09-8] Sodium Silicate, *8675*

[1344-09-8] Sodium Silicate Solution, *8676*

[1344-28-1] Aluminum Oxide, *356*

[1344-48-5] Mercuric Sulfide, Black, *5888*

[1344-48-5] Mercuric Sulfide, Red, *5889*

[1344-57-6] Uranium Dioxide, *9855*

[1344-58-7] Uranium Trioxide, *9860*

[1344-95-2] Calcium Silicate, *1702*

[1345-04-6] Antimony Trisulfide, *713*

[1345-05-7] Lithopone, *5546*

[1345-07-9] Bismuth Sulfide, *1287*

[1345-24-0] Gold Stannate, *4520*

[1345-25-1] Ferrous Oxide, *4052*

[1361-49-5] Taxine A, *9078*

[1362-42-1] Absinthin, *12*

[1390-93-8] Citrullol, *2332*

[1391-14-6] Coptine, *2525*

[1391-82-8] Grisein, *4548*

[1392-21-8] Leucomycins, *5453*

[1392-46-7] Micrococcin P, *6180*

[1392-81-0] Parotin, *7042*

[1392-87-6] Phasin, *7199*

[1392-97-8] Protokosin, *5322*

[1393-12-0] Rimocidin, *8228*

[1393-25-5] Secretin, *8421*

[1393-38-0] Subtilin, *8864*

[1393-48-2] Thiostrepton, *9364*

[1393-62-0] Abrin, *9*

[1393-63-1] Annatto, *675*

[1393-64-2] Araroba, *768*

[1393-68-6] Bottromycin, *1356*

[1393-87-9] Fusafungine, *4313*

[1394-02-1] Hachimycin, *4586*

[1395-18-2] Azolitmin, *920*

[1397-74-6] Acetyltannic Acid, *104*

[1397-77-9] Actinorhodine, *142*

[1397-84-8] Alazopeptin, *208*

[1397-89-3] Amphotericin B, *585*

[1398-17-0] Bakankosin, *943*

[1398-61-4] Chitin, *2065*

[1398-78-3] Colocynthin, *2487*

[1399-57-1] Graphitic Acid, *4541*

[1399-64-0] Gymnemic Acid, *4585*

[1400-61-9] Nystatin, *6736*

[1400-62-0] Orcein, *6863*

[1401-54-3] Tanacetin, *9050*

[1401-59-8] Granaticin Tetraacetylgranaticin, *4534*

[1401-69-0] Tylosin, *9832*

[1401-79-2] Viomycin Pantothenate Sulfate, *10001*

[1401-98-5] Condurangin, *2496*

[1402-10-4] Lichenin, *5478*

[1402-37-5] Actinomycetin, *140*

[1402-44-4] Actinomycin F$_1$, *141*

[1402-82-0] Amphomycin, *584*

[1403-17-4] Candicidin, *1740*

[1403-66-3] Gentamicin, *4392*

[1403-71-0] Hamycin, *4609*

[1404-00-8] Mitomycins, *6215*

[1404-04-2] Neomycin, *6454*

[1404-15-5] Nogalamycin, *6671*

[1404-23-5] Pleurotin(e), *7535*

[1404-26-8] Polymyxin B, *7573*

[1404-52-0] Rhodomycin B, *8190*

[1404-55-3] Ristocetin, *8234*

[1404-59-7] Oligomycin D, *6833*

[1404-64-4] Sparsomycin, *8736*

[1404-74-6] Streptovaricin, *8830*

[1404-88-2] Tyrothricin, *9841*

[1404-90-6] Vancomycin, *9929*

[1404-93-9] Vancomycin Monohydrochloride, *9929*

[1405-10-3] Neomycin B Sulfate, *6454*

[1405-20-5] Polymyxin B Sulfate, *7573*

[1405-36-3] Capreomycin Disulfate, *1757*

[1405-41-0] Gentamicin C Complex Sulfate, *4392*

[1405-59-0] Ristocetin B, *8234*

[1405-76-1] Gitalin, *4430*

[1405-86-3] Glycyrrhizic Acid, *4505*

[1405-87-4] Bacitracin, *934*

[1405-88-5] Bacitracin Methylenedisalicylate, *935*

[1405-89-6] Bacitracin Zinc, *936*

[1405-90-9] Candidin, *1741*

[1406-11-7] Polymyxin, *7573*

[1406-18-4] Vitamin E, *10021*

[1406-65-1] Chlorophyll, *2155*

[1407-47-2] Angiotensin, *651*

[1407-73-4] Vitamin T, *10025*

[1407-85-8] Dextroamphetamine Tannate, *2954*

[1407-93-8] Plantisul, *7518*

[1414-39-7] Albomycin, *213*

[1414-45-5] Nisin, *6564*

[1415-94-7] Iodopsin, *5039*

[1416-60-0] Splenin, *8763*

[1420-04-8] Niclosamide Ethanolamine Salt, *6519*

[1420-53-7] Codeine Sulfate, *2463*

[1420-55-9] Thiethylperazine, *9315*

[1421-14-3] Propanidid, *7803*

[1421-68-7] Amidephrine Methanesulfonate, *399*

[1422-07-7] Codeine Hydrochloride, *2463*

[1424-00-6] Mesterolone, *5916*

[1424-27-7] Acetazolamide Sodium Salt, *53*

[1429-30-7] Petunidin, *7190*

[1435-55-8] Hydroquinidine, *4806*

[1438-30-8] Netropsin, *6481*

[1438-57-9] Grindelic Acid, *4547*

[1443-44-3] α-Methylfentanyl Hydrochloride, *6074*

[1456-55-9] Sporidesmin A, *8764*

[1464-42-2] Selenomethionine, *8441*

[1473-73-0] Morphazinamide Hydrochloride, *6273*

[1476-53-5] Novobiocin Monosodium Salt, *6722*

[1476-98-8] Hydroquinidine Hydrochloride, *4806*

[1477-10-7] Bietamiverine Hydrochloride, *1205*

[1477-39-0] Noracymethadol, *6685*

[1477-40-3] Levomethadyl Acetate, *5466*

[1477-57-2] Fertilysin, *4060*

[1480-19-9] Fluanisone, *4114*

[1481-70-5] Tyrocidine A, *9836*

[1483-07-4] Albizziin, *211*

[1491-41-4] Naftalofos, *6354*

[1491-59-4] Oxymetazoline, *6966*

[1492-02-0] Glybuzole, *4480*

[1493-02-3] Formyl Fluoride, *4247*

[1493-13-6] Triflic Acid, *9676*

[1501-84-4] Rimantadine Hydrochloride, *8224*

[1508-45-8] Podophyllinic Acid 2-Ethylhydrazide, *7545*

[1508-65-2] Oxybutynin Hydrochloride, *6955*

[1508-75-4] Tropicamide, *9780*

[1508-76-5] Procyclidine Hydrochloride, *7763*

[1511-16-6] Haloperidol Hydrochloride, *4598*

[1518-86-1] Hydroxyamphetamine, *4810*

[1524-88-5] Flurandrenolide, *4197*

[1531-12-0] Norlevorphanol, *6707*

[1538-09-6] Penicillin G Benzathine, *7096*

[1553-60-2] Ibufenac, *4880*

[1555-53-9] Magnesium Oleate, *5675*

[1562-85-2] Gallocyanine, *4355*

[1562-90-9] Celestin Blue, *1959*

[1563-66-2] Carbofuran, *1803*

[1582-09-8] Trifluralin, *9686*

[1590-87-0] Disilane, *3356*
[1592-23-0] Calcium Stearate, *1703*
[1593-77-7] Dodemorph, *3407*
[1596-63-0] Quinacillin, *8043*
[1596-70-9] Levopropoxyphene Hydrochloride, *5469*
[1596-84-5] Daminozide, *2810*
[1597-82-6] Paramethasone 21-Acetate, *7029*
[1600-27-7] Mercuric Acetate, *5873*
[1603-91-4] 2-Amino-4-methylthiazole, *450*
[1604-01-9] γ-Coniceine, *2502*
[1605-89-6] Bolasterone, *1323*
[1607-17-6] Pentrinitrol, *7138*
[1609-47-8] Pyrocarbonic Acid Diethyl Ester, *7998*
[1610-18-0] Prometon, *7788*
[1613-17-8] Dymanthine Hydrochloride, *3475*
[1617-90-9] Vincamine, *9983*
[1618-26-4] Bis[methylthio]methane, *1256*
[1619-34-7] 3-Quinuclidinol, *8082*
[1620-21-9] Chlorcyclizine Hydrochloride, *2081*
[1622-61-3] Clonazepam, *2389*
[1622-62-4] Flunitrazepam, *4146*
[1622-79-3] Melperone Hydrochloride, *5827*
[1633-05-2] Strontium Carbonate, *8838*
[1634-04-4] Methyl *tert*-Butyl Ether, *6032*
[1637-39-4] Zeatin, *10117*
[1639-43-6] Androstenediol 3-Acetate, *637*
[1639-60-7] Propoxyphene Hydrochloride, *7839*
[1641-17-4] Mexenone, *6167*
[1642-54-2] Diethylcarbamazine Citrate, *3116*
[1649-18-9] Azaperone, *898*
[1668-19-5] Doxepin, *3435*
[1672-46-4] Digoxigenin, *3166*
[1675-54-3] Bisphenol A Diglycidyl Ether, *1297*
[1679-76-1] Drofenine, *3445*
[1684-40-8] Tacrine Hydrochloride, *9024*
[1684-42-0] Acranil®, *121*
[1689-84-5] Bromoxynil, *1441*
[1689-89-0] Nitroxynil, *6656*
[1689-99-2] Bromoxynil Octanoate, *1441*
[1695-77-8] Spectinomycin, *8739*
[1702-17-6] Clopyralid, *2400*
[1702-77-8] Fusarubin, *4315*
[1707-14-8] Phenmetrazine Hydrochloride, *7237*
[1715-33-9] Prednisolone 21-Succinate Sodium Salt, *7721*
[1721-51-3] α-Tocotrienol (unspecified stereo), *9500*
[1721-69-3] Betulin Diacetate, *1189*
[1722-62-9] Mepivacaine Hydrochloride, *5859*
[1733-12-6] Cresol Red, *2578*
[1740-22-3] Pyrinoline, *7989*
[1744-22-5] Riluzole, *8223*
[1746-01-6] TCDD, *9084*
[1747-53-1] Orotic Acid Ethyl Ester, *6876*
[1762-95-4] Ammonium Thiocyanate, *561*

[1777-82-8] Dichlorobenzyl Alcohol, *3060*
[1781-78-8] Cyclooctyne, *2738*
[1783-96-6] Aspartic Acid D-Form, *840*
[1786-81-8] Prilocaine Hydrochloride, *7743*
[1787-61-7] Eriochrome® Black T, *3667*
[1794-74-7] Cethexonium Bromide, *2019*
[1803-67-4] Sporidesmolide III, *8765*
[1805-85-2] Hasubanonine, *4619*
[1805-86-3] Metaphanine, *5929*
[1808-12-4] Bromodiphenhydramine Hydrochloride, *1418*
[1812-30-2] Bromazepam, *1385*
[1821-16-5] Ethylidene Dicoumarol, *3812*
[1824-50-6] Benzylhydrochlorothiazide, *1136*
[1829-00-1] Thiazol Yellow G, *9310*
[1830-32-6] Azintamide, *914*
[1832-53-7] EMPA, *3563*
[1832-54-8] IMPA, *4924*
[1836-75-5] Nitrofen, *6598*
[1841-19-6] Fluspirilene, *4207*
[1843-05-6] Octabenzone, *6742*
[1853-37-8] Podophyllinic Acid, *7545*
[1858-47-5] *N*-Ethylamphetamine Hydrochloride, *3763*
[1859-87-6] Echinuline, *3499*
[1861-32-1] DCPA, *2839*
[1861-40-1] Benfluralin, *1040*
[1863-63-4] Ammonium Benzoate, *496*
[1867-58-9] Clomethiazole Ethanedisulfonate, *2384*
[1867-66-9] Ketamine Hydrochloride, *5295*
[1871-22-3] Tetrazolium Blue, *9244*
[1873-77-4] Tris(trimethylsilyl)silane, *9757*
[1874-54-0] Psicofuranine, *7923*
[1882-26-4] Pyridinol Carbamate, *7975*
[1891-29-8] Lactucin, *5345*
[1892-56-4] Athamantin, *860*
[1892-80-4] Fenethylline Hydrochloride, *3972*
[1893-33-0] Pipamperone, *7455*
[1897-45-6] Chlorothalonil, *2166*
[1898-66-4] 1,1-Diphenyl-2-picrylhydrazyl (Free Radical), *3330*
[1904-98-9] 2,6-Diaminopurine, *2985*
[1910-42-5] Paraquat Dichloride, *7031*
[1910-68-5] Methisazone, *5977*
[1912-24-9] Atrazine, *871*
[1912-26-1] Trietazine, *9664*
[1918-00-9] Dicamba, *3040*
[1918-02-1] Picloram, *7397*
[1918-08-7] Dipropalin, *3341*
[1918-16-7] Propachlor, *7793*
[1921-70-6] Pristane, *7752*
[1923-76-8] Bunamiodyl Sodium, *1486*
[1926-48-3] Fenbenicillin, *3961*
[1926-49-4] Clometocillin, *2385*
[1929-82-4] Nitrapyrin, *6574*
[1934-21-0] Tartrazine, *9072*
[1936-18-1] Salutaridine, *8341*
[1937-19-5] Aminoguanidine Hydrochloride, *441*
[1937-54-8] Solanone, *8707*
[1944-10-1] Fenoterol Hydrochloride, *3981*
[1944-12-3] Fenoterol Hydrobromide, *3981*

[1945-53-5] Palustric Acid, *6998*
[1949-20-8] Oxolamine Citrate, *6944*
[1949-45-7] Metrizoic Acid, *6156*
[1950-15-8] Bensuldazic Acid Sodium Salt, *1051*
[1950-39-6] Deferoxamine Hydrochloride, *2860*
[1951-25-3] Amiodarone, *482*
[1953-02-2] Tiopronin, *9453*
[1953-04-4] Galantamine Hydrobromide, *4340*
[1954-28-5] Etoglucid, *3880*
[1962-14-7] Acacic Acid, *15*
[1963-48-0] Anisomycin Hydrochloride, *670*
[1972-08-3] Δ⁹-Tetrahydrocannabinol, *9209*
[1977-10-2] Loxapine, *5587*
[1977-11-3] Perlapine, *7179*
[1981-58-4] Sulfamethazine Sodium Salt, *8915*
[1982-36-1] Homochlorcyclizine Dihydrochloride, *4733*
[1982-37-2] Methdilazine, *5964*
[1982-49-6] Siduron, *8487*
[1983-72-8] Medicagol, *5788*
[1984-15-2] Medronic Acid, *5792*
[1986-53-4] Bolandiol Dipropionate, *1322*
[1986-70-5] Calotropin, *1720*
[1987-71-9] Nicotinamide Ascorbate, *6523*
[1990-29-0] D-Altrose, *321*
[1997-15-5] Triamcinolone Acetonide 21-Disodium Phosphate, *9596*
[2001-95-8] Valinomycin, *9910*
[2002-29-1] Flumethasone 21-Pivalate, *4138*
[2002-44-0] MIF-I, *5813*
[2008-41-5] Butylate, *1546*
[2009-64-5] Neopterin D-*erythro*-Form, *6462*
[2011-67-8] Nimetazepam, *6549*
[2013-58-3] Meclocycline, *5778*
[2016-36-6] Choline Salicylate, *2209*
[2016-63-9] Bamifylline, *955*
[2022-85-7] Flucytosine, *4125*
[2030-53-7] Aporeine, *748*
[2030-63-9] Clofazimine, *2373*
[2032-59-9] Aminocarb, *433*
[2032-65-7] Methiocarb, *5972*
[2033-24-1] Meldrum's Acid, *5817*
[2037-48-1] 2-Deoxystreptamine, *2909*
[2043-38-1] Buthiazide, *1525*
[2050-87-5] Diallyl Trisulfide, *2973*
[2052-01-9] α-Bromoisobutyric Acid, *1421*
[2052-63-3] Neovitamin A, *6468*
[2055-44-9] Perisoxal, *7177*
[2058-46-0] Oxytetracycline Hydrochloride, *6976*
[2058-52-8] Clothiapine, *2415*
[2058-58-4] Asparagine D-Form, *837*
[2061-86-1] Methandriol Diacetate, *5950*
[2062-77-3] Trifluperidol Hydrochloride, *9684*
[2062-78-4] Pimozide, *7435*
[2062-84-2] Benperidol, *1048*
[2065-00-1] Filicinic Acid, *4079*
[2066-89-9] Isoniazid 4-Aminosalicylate, *5186*
[2068-78-2] Vincristine Sulfate, *9986*
[2074-50-2] Paraquat Bismethyl Sulfate, *7031*

[2078-54-8] Propofol, *7834*
[2079-00-7] Blasticidin S, *1316*
[2085-33-8] Aluminum Tris(8-hydroxy-quinoline), *370*
[2086-83-1] Berberine, *1154*
[2086-96-6] Canadine *d*-Form, *1736*
[2090-89-3] Butethamine, *1523*
[2092-16-2] Calcium Thiocyanate, *1710*
[2092-17-3] Barium Thiocyanate, *998*
[2095-57-0] Thiobutabarbital, *9323*
[2096-42-6] Gougerotin, *4529*
[2098-66-0] Cyproterone, *2774*
[2099-26-5] Androstenediol Diacetate, *637*
[2103-64-2] Gallein, *4344*
[2104-64-5] EPN, *3626*
[2104-96-3] Bromophos, *1431*
[2105-47-7] Tetrabenazine Hydrochloride, *9182*
[2111-75-3] Perillaldehyde, *7167*
[2119-75-7] Fluperolone Acetate, *4188*
[2122-29-4] Retamine, *8159*
[2124-57-4] Menaquinone 7, *5833*
[2127-01-7] Clorexolone, *2404*
[2135-17-3] Flumethasone, *4138*
[2139-25-5] Perisoxal Citrate, *7177*
[2140-46-7] 25-Hydroxycholesterol, *4821*
[2141-09-5] Magnoflorine, *5696*
[2150-48-3] Pyronine B, *8006*
[2152-34-3] Pemoline, *7079*
[2152-44-5] Betamethasone 17-Valerate, *1180*
[2152-56-9] Arabitol, *762*
[2152-76-3] Idose, *4889*
[2153-98-2] Norpseudoephedrine Hydrochloride, *6714*
[2156-27-6] Benproperine, *1049*
[2164-08-1] Lenacil, *5435*
[2164-09-2] Dicryl, *3088*
[2164-17-2] Fluometuron, *4154*
[2165-19-7] Guanoxan, *4568*
[2167-85-3] Pipazethate, *7456*
[2169-64-4] 6-Azauridine 2′,3′,5′-Triacetate, *904*
[2169-75-7] Deptropine Citrate, *2912*
[2174-16-5] Triethanolamine Salicylate, *9665*
[2179-16-0] Ninopterin, *6555*
[2179-37-5] Bencyclane, *1033*
[2180-92-9] Bupivacaine, *1495*
[2181-04-6] Canrenone Free Acid Potassium Salt, *1750*
[2182-14-1] Vindoline, *9988*
[2192-20-3] Hydroxyzine Dihydrochloride, *4849*
[2198-93-8] Trichodermol, *9647*
[2207-50-3] Aminorex, *476*
[2210-63-1] Mofebutazone, *6231*
[2210-64-2] Pyrrocaine Hydrochloride, *8013*
[2210-77-7] Pyrrocaine, *8013*
[2217-44-9] Iodophthalein Sodium, *5038*
[2218-94-2] Nitron, *6613*
[2219-30-9] Penicillamine Hydrochloride, *7088*
[2221-95-6] Fichtelite, *4076*
[2226-96-2] TEMPOL, *9141*
[2227-17-0] Dienochlor, *3105*
[2240-14-4] Fencamfamine Hydrochloride, *3966*
[2241-90-9] Cyclobuxine D, *2716*
[2243-33-6] α-Phellandrene *d*-Form, *7200*

[2243-76-7] Alizarine Yellow R, *255*
[2244-21-5] Troclosene Potassium, *9767*
[2255-39-2] Muscazone, *6311*
[2257-09-2] Phenethyl Isothiocyanate, *7226*
[2259-14-5] Chrysanthemic Acid *l-trans*-Form, *2251*
[2259-96-3] Cyclothiazide, *2754*
[2272-11-9] Ethanolamine Oleate, *3727*
[2276-90-6] Iothalamic Acid, *5064*
[2277-92-1] Oxyclozanide, *6958*
[2280-32-2] Kanamycin C, *5281*
[2284-31-3] Pratensein, *7713*
[2290-11-1] Verrucarin B, *9964*
[2292-79-7] Congressane, *2499*
[2295-58-1] Flopropione, *4106*
[2297-30-5] Androstenediol Dipropionate, *637*
[2303-01-7] Cresol Purple, *2577*
[2303-16-4] Diallate, *2970*
[2303-17-5] Triallate, *9594*
[2306-22-1] Citramalic Acid, *2323*
[2307-68-8] Solan, *8702*
[2310-17-0] Phosalone, *7334*
[2312-35-8] Propargite, *7808*
[2315-02-8] Oxymetazoline Hydrochloride, *6966*
[2315-08-4] Salazosulfadimidine, *8321*
[2319-84-8] Thioctic Acid Sodium Salt, *9326*
[2319-97-3] [2.2]Metacyclophane, *5921*
[2320-96-9] 4′,5′-Dichlorofluorescein, *3067*
[2321-07-5] Fluorescein, *4159*
[2323-36-6] (±)-Deprenyl, *8428*
[2326-89-8] Drimenin, *3444*
[2338-05-8] Ferric Citrate (undefined stoichiometry), *4021*
[2338-37-6] Levopropoxyphene, *5469*
[2347-80-0] Thioproperazine Dimethanesulfonate, *9357*
[2350-32-5] Butoxycaine Hydrochloride, *1531*
[2353-33-5] Decitabine, *2853*
[2353-45-9] Fast Green FCF, *3941*
[2363-58-8] Epitiostanol, *3624*
[2370-18-5] Galvinoxyl, *4357*
[2375-03-3] Methylprednisolone 21-Succinate Sodium Salt, *6111*
[2382-48-1] Ubichromenol 50, *9843*
[2385-81-1] Furethidine, *4303*
[2385-85-5] Mirex, *6207*
[2390-99-0] Chanoclavine, *2042*
[2391-03-9] Brompheniramine *d*-Form Maleate, *1443*
[2392-39-4] Dexamethasone 21-Phosphate Disodium Salt, *2943*
[2398-81-4] Oxiniacic Acid, *6941*
[2398-96-1] Tolnaftate, *9519*
[2410-93-7] Methopterin, *5984*
[2413-38-9] Flupentixol Dihydrochloride, *4187*
[2425-06-1] Captafol, *1771*
[2426-63-3] 5-Methoxy-*N,N*-diisopropyltryptamine Hydrochloride, *5991*
[2429-71-2] Benzo Azurine G, *1085*
[2430-27-5] Valpromide, *9914*
[2430-49-1] Vinylbital, *9993*
[2431-96-1] *N,N*-Diethylphenylacetamide, *3126*
[2435-76-9] 5-Diazouracil, *3003*
[2437-29-8] Malachite Green Oxalate Salt, *5699*

[2438-32-6] Chlorpheniramine *d*-Form Maleate, *2180*
[2438-72-4] Bufexamac, *1474*
[2438-80-4] L-Fucose, *4279*
[2439-01-2] Oxythioquinox, *6978*
[2439-10-3] Dodine, *3408*
[2440-22-4] Drometrizole, *3447*
[2447-54-3] Sanguinarine, *8356*
[2447-57-6] Sulfadoxine, *8906*
[2448-68-2] Pipamperone Dihydrochloride, *7455*
[2451-01-6] Terpin *cis*-Form Hydrate, *9169*
[2454-11-7] Formebolone, *4239*
[2466-09-3] Pyrophosphoric Acid, *8008*
[2468-21-5] Catharanthine, *1904*
[2470-73-7] Dixyrazine, *3385*
[2482-00-0] Agmatine Sulfate, *188*
[2490-97-3] Aceglutamide, *25*
[2493-02-9] *p*-Bromophenyl Isocyanate, *1430*
[2497-78-1] Iopanoic Acid Sodium Salt, *5058*
[2507-24-6] Physalaemin, *7381*
[2507-91-7] Kethoxal Bis(thiosemicarbazone), *5299*
[2508-72-7] Antazoline Hydrochloride, *680*
[2508-79-4] Methyldopa Ethyl Ester Hydrochloride, *6055*
[2517-04-6] 2-Azetidinecarboxylic Acid, *908*
[2520-21-0] Celesticetin, *1958*
[2529-45-5] Flurogestone Acetate, *4200*
[2533-89-3] Karsil, *5285*
[2537-29-3] Proxibarbal, *7904*
[2540-82-1] Formothion, *4246*
[2551-62-4] Sulfur Hexafluoride, *8973*
[2552-55-8] Ibotenic Acid, *4877*
[2557-49-5] Diflorasone, *3140*
[2564-83-2] TEMPO, *9140*
[2571-22-4] Tutin, *9827*
[2571-86-0] Coriamyrtin, *2530*
[2574-78-9] Orazamide, *6861*
[2576-92-3] Isoetharine Hydrochloride, *5170*
[2577-32-4] Sulfamethoxypyridazine Sodium Salt, *8919*
[2580-88-3] Eburnamonine (±)-Form, *3487*
[2589-47-1] Prajmaline Hydrogen Tartrate, *7702*
[2591-17-5] Firefly Luciferin, *4086*
[2595-97-3] D-Allose, *280*
[2606-93-1] Blankophor® R, *1315*
[2607-06-9] Diflucortolone, *3143*
[2608-24-4] Piposulfan, *7481*
[2609-46-3] Amiloride, *406*
[2610-10-8] Sirius Red, *8548*
[2612-33-1] Clonitrate, *2391*
[2618-25-9] Ioglycamic Acid, *5051*
[2618-26-0] Iodipamide Disodium Salt, *5022*
[2622-26-6] Pericyazine, *7164*
[2622-30-2] Carphenazine, *1860*
[2622-37-9] Trifluomeprazine, *9679*
[2624-43-3] Cyclofenil, *2720*
[2624-44-4] Ethamsylate, *3722*
[2627-69-2] Acadesine, *16*
[2630-39-9] Methyl Dihydrojasmonate (−)-(1*R*,2*R*)-Form, *6052*
[2636-26-2] Ciafos, *2261*
[2638-46-2] Cortolone 3,20,21-Triacetate, *2542*

[2642-98-0] 6-Chrysenamine, *2254*
[2652-13-3] Eicosamethylnonasiloxane, *3530*
[2667-89-2] Bisbentiamine, *1246*
[2668-66-8] Medrysone, *5794*
[2673-40-7] Perivine, *7178*
[2682-20-4] Methylisothiazolinone, *6091*
[2686-47-7] Amphenone B, *581*
[2688-77-9] Laudanosine, *5381*
[2691-41-0] Octogen, *6758*
[2691-45-4] Hexestrol Bis(β-diethylaminoethyl ether), *4702*
[2691-46-5] Bietamiverine Dihydrochloride, *1205*
[2696-92-6] Nitrosyl Chloride, *6646*
[2698-41-1] o-Chlorobenzylidenemalononitrile, *2127*
[2699-79-8] Sulfuryl Fluoride, *8981*
[2709-56-0] Flupentixol, *4187*
[2712-78-9] Phenyliodine(III) Bis(trifluoroacetate), *7295*
[2718-25-4] Rheadine, *8175*
[2730-71-4] Thiocolchicine, *9324*
[2740-04-7] Dimefline Hydrochloride, *3204*
[2746-81-8] Fluphenazine Enanthate, *4189*
[2750-76-7] Rifamide, *8215*
[2751-09-9] Troleandomycin, *9770*
[2751-68-0] Acetophenazine, *72*
[2752-65-0] Gambogic Acid, *4361*
[2753-45-9] Mebeverine Hydrochloride, *5769*
[2757-90-6] Agaritine, *187*
[2763-96-4] Muscimol, *6312*
[2765-04-0] Thioacetaldehyde, *9318*
[2768-90-3] Quinaldine Blue, *8048*
[2773-92-4] Dimethisoquin Hydrochloride, *3218*
[2779-55-7] Opiniazide, *6852*
[2783-94-0] Sunset Yellow FCF, *9001*
[2798-20-1] Gardenin B, *4366*
[2809-21-4] Etidronic Acid, *3863*
[2813-95-8] Dinoseb Acetate, *3287*
[2825-00-5] Aureothin, *879*
[2825-60-7] Formocortal, *4243*
[2834-90-4] 4-Amino-1-naphthol, *453*
[2869-83-2] Janus Green B, *5255*
[2870-71-5] Atropine Methylbromide, *875*
[2873-97-4] Diacetone Acrylamide, *2963*
[2892-51-5] Squaric Acid, *8769*
[2892-62-8] Squaric Acid Dibutylester, *8769*
[2898-11-5] Medazepam Hydrochloride, *5786*
[2898-12-6] Medazepam, *5786*
[2900-38-1] Sporidesmolide I, *8765*
[2919-66-6] Melengestrol Acetate, *5818*
[2921-88-2] Chlorpyrifos, *2189*
[2921-92-8] Propatyl Nitrate, *7811*
[2924-67-6] Fluoresone, *4161*
[2933-94-0] Toliprolol, *9516*
[2935-23-1] Chrysanthemic Acid *dl-cis-*Form, *2251*
[2945-88-2] Sophorabioside, *8718*
[2955-23-9] Olivil, *6837*
[2955-38-6] Prazepam, *7715*
[2957-21-3] Sakuranetin, *8319*
[2970-95-8] Macromerine, *5645*
[2971-90-6] Clopidol, *2397*
[2975-34-0] Carphenazine Dimaleate, *1860*

[2998-57-4] Estramustine, *3706*
[3012-65-5] Ammonium Citrate, Dibasic, *512*
[3017-60-5] Cobaltous Thiocyanate, *2450*
[3031-95-6] SAICAR, *8318*
[3040-38-8] Acetylcarnitine L-Form, *84*
[3051-09-0] Murexide, *6306*
[3054-35-1] Aspartic Acid Compound with L-Arginine, *840*
[3056-17-5] Stavudine, *8803*
[3059-97-0] Isovaline D-Form, *5234*
[3060-41-1] 4-Amino-3-phenylbutyric Acid Hydrochloride, *464*
[3060-89-7] Metobromuron, *6142*
[3092-17-9] Midodrine Hydrochloride, *6184*
[3093-35-4] Halcinonide, *4591*
[3094-09-5] Doxifluridine, *3437*
[3095-65-6] Ammonium Bitartrate, *503*
[3101-51-7] Ergoflavin, *3652*
[3102-00-9] Febuprol, *3947*
[3105-97-3] Hycanthone, *4759*
[3115-49-9] (p-Nonylphenoxy)acetic Acid, *6682*
[3116-76-5] Dicloxacillin, *3084*
[3122-01-8] Thiazesim Hydrochloride, *9305*
[3131-03-1] Pristinamycin IA, *7753*
[3144-16-9] d-Camphorsulfonic Acid, *1734*
[3147-14-6] Calmagite, *1718*
[3147-55-5] 3,5-Dibromosalicylic Acid, *3028*
[3148-09-2] Verrucarin A, *9964*
[3150-28-5] D-Chalcose, *2039*
[3155-48-4] Kawain (±)-Form, *5287*
[3155-57-5] (±)-Dihydromethysticin, *6138*
[3160-91-6] Moroxydine Hydrochloride, *6272*
[3164-34-9] Calcium Tartrate, *1709*
[3166-62-9] Benactyzine Methobromide, *1029*
[3167-49-5] 6-Aminonicotinic Acid, *456*
[3176-03-2] Drotebanol, *3456*
[3198-07-0] Ethylnorepinephrine Hydrochloride, *3834*
[3200-06-4] Nafronyl Acid Oxalate, *6353*
[3200-75-7] Sporidesmolide II, *8765*
[3202-84-4] 4-Salicyloylmorpholine, *8333*
[3207-50-9] Linoleic Acid Cyclohexylamide, *5505*
[3215-70-1] Hexoprenaline, *4707*
[3230-75-9] Oxenin, *6932*
[3230-94-2] Ornithine L-Form Aspartate, *6874*
[3232-84-6] Urazole, *9866*
[3239-44-9] Dexfenfluramine, *3973*
[3239-45-0] Dexfenfluramine Hydrochloride, *3973*
[3244-88-0] Acid Fuchsin, *107*
[3251-23-8] Cupric Nitrate, *2643*
[3252-29-7] Tyrocidine C, *9836*
[3254-66-8] Diisopropyl Paraoxon, *3198*
[3254-89-5] Diphenidol Hydrochloride, *3311*
[3264-82-2] Nickel Acetylacetonate, *6500*
[3269-83-8] Pheniramine p-Aminosalicylate, *7235*

[3279-54-7] Disodium Phenyl Phosphate, *3357*
[3286-46-2] Thiamine Disulfide O,O-Diisobutyrate, *9297*
[3306-52-3] Viridin, *10006*
[3317-61-1] DMPO, *3393*
[3326-32-7] Asenapine (5-isothiocyanate), *4089*
[3329-91-7] Dioscorine, *3294*
[3337-71-1] Asulam, *857*
[3342-61-8] Deanol Aceglumate, *2843*
[3344-18-1] Magnesium Citrate Tribasic, *5663*
[3347-22-6] Dithianon, *3368*
[3349-06-2] Nickel Formate, *6509*
[3351-86-8] Fucoxanthin, *4281*
[3354-67-4] Amidephrine, *399*
[3363-58-4] Nifurfoline, *6533*
[3366-95-8] Secnidazole, *8419*
[3368-16-9] α-Phenylcinnamic Acid, *7281*
[3371-85-5] Voacamine, *10027*
[3376-24-7] PBN, *7056*
[3376-83-8] Biotin l-Sulfoxide, *1232*
[3380-34-5] Triclosan, *9657*
[3383-96-8] Temephos, *9135*
[3385-03-3] Flunisolide, *4145*
[3397-23-7] Ornipressin, *6873*
[3416-24-8] Glucosamine, *4458*
[3416-26-0] Lidoflazine, *5484*
[3420-59-5] Isomaltol, *5181*
[3424-98-4] Telbivudine, *9117*
[3426-08-2] Prozapine, *7906*
[3440-28-6] Betamipron, *1181*
[3458-22-8] Improsulfan Hydrochloride, *4927*
[3458-28-4] D-Mannose, *5747*
[3459-06-1] Cyclopentamine Hydrochloride, *2740*
[3459-20-9] Glymidine Sodium Salt, *4507*
[3460-67-1] Furonazide, *4308*
[3463-92-1] Carpaine, *1858*
[3475-65-8] Thiamine Triphosphate, *9298*
[3483-12-3] 1,4-Dithiothreitol, *3376*
[3485-14-1] Cyclacillin, *2702*
[3485-62-9] Clidinium Bromide, *2354*
[3486-35-9] Zinc Carbonate, *10131*
[3486-66-6] Coptisine, *2527*
[3486-67-7] Palmatine, *6994*
[3493-12-7] S-Methylmethionine DL-Form Chloride, *6098*
[3505-38-2] Carbinoxamine Maleate, *1799*
[3511-16-8] Hetacillin, *4672*
[3521-62-8] Erythromycin Estolate, *3683*
[3521-84-4] Iodipamide Bis[N-methylglucamine] Salt, *5022*
[3522-50-7] Ferric Citrate (1:1 iron(III) citrate salt), *4021*
[3543-75-7] Bendamustine Hydrochloride, *1034*
[3544-35-2] Iproclozide, *5076*
[3546-03-0] Cyamemazine, *2683*
[3546-21-2] Homidium, *4731*
[3546-41-6] Pyrvinium Pamoate, *8022*
[3562-84-3] Benzbromarone, *1065*
[3562-99-0] Menbutone, *5834*
[3563-27-7] Dihydroequilin, *3173*
[3563-49-3] Pyrovalerone, *8010*
[3563-84-6] Dihydrostreptomycin Pantothenate, *3179*

[3564-09-8] Ponceau 3R, 7590
[3565-72-8] Embramine, 3556
[3568-24-9] Propionylpromazine, 7829
[3568-94-3] 4-Methylaminorex, 6018
[3569-99-1] N-(Hydroxymethyl)nicotinamide, 4833
[3571-88-8] Platonin, 7530
[3572-06-3] Cuelure, 2616
[3572-43-8] Bromhexine, 1391
[3572-52-9] Biphenamine, 1234
[3572-60-9] Amidinomycin, 400
[3572-74-5] Moxastine, 6287
[3572-80-3] Cyclazocine, 2705
[3573-82-8] Hygrophylline, 4853
[3575-80-2] Melperone, 5827
[3577-01-3] Cephaloglycin, 1976
[3583-64-0] Bumadizon, 1483
[3589-73-9] 10-Methoxyharmalan, 5995
[3590-05-4] Acetyl Sulfamethoxypyrazine, 101
[3593-85-9] Methandriol Dipropionate, 5950
[3595-11-7] Propylhexedrine dl-Form, 7860
[3598-37-6] Acepromazine Maleate, 32
[3599-32-4] Indocyanine Green, 4962
[3600-95-1] Perezone, 7155
[3604-87-3] Ecdysone, 3491
[3605-01-4] Piribedil, 7493
[3607-18-9] Doxepin trans-Form Hydrochloride, 3435
[3611-72-1] Clobenfurol, 2360
[3614-30-0] Emepronium Bromide, 3558
[3614-69-5] Dimethindene Maleate, 3216
[3615-24-5] Ramifenazone, 8102
[3615-37-0] D-Fucose, 4278
[3615-41-6] Rhamnose, 8172
[3615-44-9] D-manno-Heptulose, 4666
[3615-82-5] Phytic Acid Calcium Magnesium Salt, 7387
[3616-78-2] Fenfluramine l-Form Hydrochloride, 3973
[3621-36-1] Columbamine, 2492
[3621-38-3] Jatrorrhizine, 5261
[3625-06-7] Mebeverine, 5769
[3627-49-4] Phenoperidine Hydrochloride, 7250
[3632-91-5] Magnesium Gluconate, 4456
[3635-74-3] Deanol Acetamidobenzoate, 2843
[3639-12-1] Butethamate Citrate, 1522
[3644-61-9] Tolperisone Hydrochloride, 9522
[3650-17-7] Hirsutic Acid C, 4717
[3653-48-3] MCPA Sodium Salt, 5764
[3666-69-1] Dioxadrol Hydrochloride, 3299
[3679-64-9] Bromosalicylchloranilide, 1435
[3682-35-7] 2,4,6-Tripyridyl-s-triazine, 9750
[3684-26-2] 3-Quinuclidinol dl-Form, 8082
[3685-84-5] Meclofenoxate Hydrochloride, 5780
[3686-58-6] Tolycaine, 9541
[3688-62-8] Aminopromazine Fumarate, 467
[3689-24-5] Sulfotep, 8966
[3689-50-7] Oxomemazine, 6946

[3689-76-7] Chlormidazole, 2107
[3691-21-2] Buzepide, 1599
[3691-35-8] Chlorophacinone, 2152
[3691-74-5] Glyconiazide, 4500
[3691-81-4] Sulfoniazide, 8959
[3693-39-8] Flucloronide, 4121
[3697-42-5] Chlorhexidine Dihydrochloride, 2091
[3703-76-2] Cloperastine, 2395
[3703-79-5] Bamethan, 954
[3704-09-4] Mibolerone, 6174
[3715-90-0] Tramazoline Hydrochloride Monohydrate, 9567
[3717-88-2] Flavoxate Hydrochloride, 4096
[3724-89-8] Phosphocysteamine Sodium Salt, 7341
[3731-59-7] Moroxydine, 6272
[3734-33-6] Denatonium Benzoate, 2891
[3734-52-9] Metazocine, 5933
[3735-45-3] Vetrabutine, 9972
[3735-84-0] Reserpilic Acid Dimethylaminoethyl Ester Dihydrochloride, 8144
[3736-08-1] Fenethylline, 3972
[3736-36-5] Tropine Benzylate, 9782
[3736-81-0] Diloxanide Furoate, 3201
[3737-09-5] Disopyramide, 3360
[3738-01-0] Otobain, 6899
[3749-97-1] Laureline (±)-Form, 5383
[3750-26-3] Primocarcin, 7748
[3759-07-7] Dimetacrine Tartrate, 3212
[3763-55-1] Rubixanthin, 8289
[3772-43-8] Butoxycaine, 1531
[3772-76-7] Sulfamethomidine, 8917
[3778-73-2] Ifosfamide, 4896
[3778-76-5] Todralazine Hydrochloride, 9502
[3779-59-7] Cimigenol, 2281
[3779-61-1] Ocimene trans-β-Form, 6741
[3785-32-8] Salicylamide O-Acetic Acid Sodium Salt, 8329
[3790-78-1] Nerolidol cis-Form, 6476
[3801-06-7] Fluorometholone 17-Acetate, 4175
[3804-89-5] Isoniazid Methanesulfonate Sodium, 5186
[3810-35-3] Tenonitrozole, 9147
[3810-74-0] Streptomycin Sesquisulfate, 8826
[3810-80-8] Diphenoxylate Hydrochloride, 3313
[3811-04-9] Potassium Chlorate, 7620
[3811-20-9] Cuminaldehyde Thiosemicarbazone, 2621
[3811-25-4] Clorprenaline, 2408
[3811-56-1] Aminoquinuride, 475
[3811-75-4] Hexamidine, 4692
[3818-50-6] Bephenium Hydroxynaphthoate, 1148
[3818-62-0] Betoxycaine, 1187
[3819-00-9] Piperacetazine, 7462
[3835-52-7] O-Cinnamoyltaxicin-II triacetate, 9077
[3844-45-9] Brilliant Blue FCF, 1373
[3847-29-8] Erythromycin Lactobionate, 3685
[3856-25-5] Copaene, 2515
[3858-89-7] Chloroprocaine Hydrochloride, 2158
[3861-73-2] Anazolene Sodium, 628
[3871-82-7] Moperone Hydrochloride, 6263

[3900-31-0] Fludiazepam, 4128
[3902-71-4] Trioxsalen, 9735
[3922-90-5] Oleandomycin, 6825
[3930-19-6] Streptonigrin, 8827
[3930-20-9] Sotalol, 8728
[3947-65-7] Neamine, 6430
[3952-98-5] Sinigrin, 8545
[3963-95-9] Methacycline Hydrochloride, 5943
[3964-81-6] Azatadine, 901
[3978-86-7] Azatadine Dimaleate, 901
[3982-91-0] Phosphorus Sulfochloride, 7356
[4008-48-4] Nitroxoline, 6655
[4021-34-5] 5-Methoxy-N,N-diisopropyltryptamine, 5991
[4042-30-2] Parvaquone, 7050
[4044-65-9] Bitoscanate, 1308
[4055-39-4] Mitomycin A, 6215
[4055-40-7] Mitomycin B, 6215
[4065-45-6] Sulisobenzone, 8983
[4075-81-4] Calcium Propionate, 1698
[4076-02-2] 2,3-Dimercapto-1-propanesulfonic Acid Sodium Salt, 3210
[4080-31-3] Quaternium-15, 8027
[4091-75-2] Clomestrone, 2382
[4093-35-0] Bromopride, 1432
[4097-22-7] Dideoxyadenosine, 3101
[4098-40-2] Mitragynine, 6218
[4111-54-0] Diisopropylamine Lithium Salt, 3196
[4112-89-4] Guaiacol Phenylacetate, 4553
[4119-52-2] Ferric Thiocyanate, 4034
[4135-11-9] Polymyxin B₁, 7573
[4147-51-7] Dipropetryn, 3342
[4154-10-3] Rolitetracycline Compd with Chloramphenicol Succinate, 8252
[4154-53-4] d-Camphocarboxylic Acid Basic Bismuth Salt, 1731
[4156-16-5] Woodward's Reagent K, 10050
[4163-15-9] Cyclorphan, 2750
[4170-30-3] Crotonaldehyde, 2596
[4171-13-5] Valnoctamide, 9912
[4180-23-8] Anethole, 643
[4197-25-5] Sudan Black B, 8885
[4205-23-6] D-Gulose, 4578
[4205-90-7] Clonidine, 2390
[4205-91-8] Clonidine Hydrochloride, 2390
[4221-98-1] α-Phellandrene l-Form, 7200
[4232-99-9] 3,5-Dibromo-4-hydroxybenzenesulfonic Acid, 3023
[4245-41-4] Estradiol 3-Acetate, 3703
[4258-85-9] Clocortolone 21-Acetate, 2369
[4267-05-4] Teclothiazide, 9104
[4268-36-4] Tybamate, 9829
[4271-30-1] N-(p-Aminobenzoyl)-glutamic Acid, 426
[4282-16-0] N,N'-Dimethylcyclobuxine D, 2716
[4291-63-8] Cladribine, 2337
[4299-57-4] Plastoquinone 9, 7523
[4299-60-9] Sulfisoxazole Diethanolamine Salt, 8952
[4300-28-1] D-Ribose-5-phosphoric Acid, 8205
[4316-74-9] N-Methyltaurine Sodium Salt, 6124
[4317-14-0] Amitriptylinoxide, 488

[4320-30-3] Arginine Glutamate, *781*
[4321-58-8] ε-Aminocaproic Acid Hydrochloride, *432*
[4323-43-7] Hexoprenaline Dihydrochloride, *4707*
[4330-99-8] Trimeprazine Tartrate, *9704*
[4342-03-4] Dacarbazine, *2798*
[4345-03-3] α-Tocopherol Succinate, *9495*
[4350-07-6] 5-Hydroxytryptophan D-Form, *4847*
[4350-09-8] 5-Hydroxytryptophan L-Form, *4847*
[4353-06-4] 2-Nonyldioxolane, *6680*
[4356-43-8] Lupanine *dl*-Form, *5607*
[4360-12-7] Ajmaline, *194*
[4368-28-9] Tetrodotoxin, *9246*
[4378-36-3] Fenbutrazate, *3965*
[4386-35-0] Meralein Sodium, *5865*
[4388-82-3] Propylhexedrine *l*-Form Ethylphenylbarbiturate, *7860*
[4393-19-5] *p*-Sulfanilylbenzylamine, *8928*
[4394-00-7] Niflumic Acid, *6531*
[4396-01-4] Pelletierine, *7072*
[4403-90-1] Alizarin Cyanine Green F, *252*
[4406-22-8] Cyprenorphine, *2769*
[4412-09-3] Mucochloric Anhydride, *6298*
[4419-39-0] Beclomethasone, *1019*
[4432-31-9] MES, *5902*
[4438-22-6] Atropine *N*-Oxide, *875*
[4439-84-3] HON, *4741*
[4448-95-7] Shellolic Acid, *8479*
[4461-30-7] Chloroacetyl Isocyanate, *2117*
[4462-95-7] Truxillic Acid, *9791*
[4466-14-2] Jasmolin I, *5258*
[4468-02-4] Zinc Gluconate, *4456*
[4478-93-7] Sulforaphane (unspecified stereo), *8962*
[4481-55-4] Pentryl, *7139*
[4482-83-1] BBB, *4081*
[4493-18-9] Amylpenicillin, *616*
[4493-23-6] Dodecahedrane, *3402*
[4493-37-2] Chromous Formate, *2246*
[4498-32-2] Dibenzepin, *3008*
[4499-40-5] Choline Theophyllinate, *2210*
[4533-39-5] Nitracrine, *6571*
[4533-89-5] Flunisolide 21-Acetate, *4145*
[4544-15-4] Piperilate Hydrochloride, *7471*
[4546-39-8] Piperilate, *7471*
[4548-53-2] Ponceau SX, *7591*
[4562-36-1] Gitoxin, *4434*
[4564-87-8] Carbomycin A, *1806*
[4573-78-8] Hamamelose, *4608*
[4589-33-7] Bostrycoidin, *1354*
[4602-84-0] Farnesol, *3937*
[4611-02-3] Chlorproethazine Hydrochloride, *2183*
[4618-18-2] Lactulose, *5346*
[4619-74-3] 2,4,6-Tribromo-*m*-cresol, *9612*
[4626-00-0] Kitol, *5315*
[4630-95-9] Prifinium Bromide, *7742*
[4638-92-0] Chrysanthemic Acid *d*-*trans*-Form, *2251*
[4643-58-7] Verrucarin J, *9964*
[4663-83-6] Buramate, *1501*

[4670-05-7] Theaflavine, *9274*
[4673-18-1] Buphanitine, *1493*
[4678-44-8] Grayanotoxin II, *4543*
[4678-45-9] Grayanotoxin III, *4543*
[4680-78-8] Guinea Green B, *4575*
[4682-36-4] Orphenadrine Citrate, *6879*
[4682-48-8] Cytolipin H, *2794*
[4682-50-2] Trichodermin, *9647*
[4685-14-7] Paraquat, *7031*
[4695-62-9] *d*-Fenchone, *3968*
[4696-76-8] Kanamycin B, *5281*
[4697-14-7] Ticarcillin Disodium Salt, *9428*
[4697-36-3] Carbenicillin, *1792*
[4719-75-9] Fosfestrol Tetrasodium Salt, *4253*
[4720-09-6] Grayanotoxin I, *4543*
[4727-40-6] *S*-Methylmethionine, *6098*
[4747-99-3] Tetrahydropapaveroline, *9216*
[4757-55-5] Dimetacrine, *3212*
[4759-48-2] Isotretinoin, *5228*
[4764-17-4] MDA, *5765*
[4767-03-7] Dimethylolpropionic Acid, *3253*
[4776-06-1] Fluorosalan, *4178*
[4800-94-6] Carbenicillin Disodium Salt, *1792*
[4803-27-4] Anthramycin, *685*
[4825-86-9] Ochratoxin B, *6740*
[4826-71-5] Phosphorylcholine Calcium Salt, *7362*
[4828-27-7] Clocortolone, *2369*
[4846-91-7] Fenoxazoline, *3985*
[4850-21-9] Quebrachamine, *8030*
[4865-85-4] Ochratoxin C, *6740*
[4880-88-0] Eburnamonine (−)-Form, *3487*
[4914-30-1] Dehydroemetine, *2870*
[4936-47-4] Nifuratel, *6532*
[4940-11-8] Ethyl Maltol, *3824*
[4940-39-0] Chromocarb, *2237*
[4945-47-5] Bamipine, *956*
[4955-90-2] Gentisic Acid Sodium Salt, *4398*
[4956-37-0] Estradiol Enanthate, *3703*
[4968-09-6] Algestone Cyclic Acetal with Acetone, *239*
[4968-29-0] Guaiazulene Trinitrobenzene Deriv, *4554*
[4969-02-2] Methixene, *5979*
[4976-25-4] Tremetone, *9581*
[4991-65-5] Tioxolone, *9456*
[5001-33-2] Metanephrine, *5926*
[5002-47-1] Fluphenazine Decanoate, *4189*
[5003-47-4] Betoxycaine Monohydrochloride, *1187*
[5003-48-5] Benorylate, *1045*
[5008-52-6] Napelline, *6367*
[5011-34-7] Trimetazidine, *9705*
[5036-02-2] Tetramisole, *5459*
[5051-62-7] Guanabenz, *4558*
[5053-06-5] Fenspiride, *3999*
[5053-08-7] Fenspiride Hydrochloride, *3999*
[5060-55-9] Prednisolone 21-Stearoylglycolate, *7721*
[5072-26-4] Buthionine Sulfoximine, *1526*
[5080-50-2] Acetylcarnitine L-Form Hydrochloride, *84*
[5086-74-8] Tetramisole Hydrochloride, *5459*

[5096-57-1] Canadine *l*-Form, *1736*
[5103-42-4] Hydrindantin, *4775*
[5104-49-4] Flurbiprofen, *4199*
[5118-17-2] Furazolium Chloride, *4301*
[5118-29-6] Melitracen, *5823*
[5119-48-2] Withaferin A, *10048*
[5133-19-7] Aloin, *307*
[5141-20-8] Light Green SF Yellowish, *5485*
[5142-76-7] Bismuth Subacetate, *1281*
[5153-24-2] Zirconyl Acetate, *10183*
[5169-78-8] Tipepidine, *9457*
[5175-83-7] Bismuth Tribromophenate, *1291*
[5189-11-7] Pizotyline Malate, *7515*
[5192-84-7] Trengestone, *9584*
[5197-58-0] Stenbolone, *8808*
[5205-82-3] Bevonium Methyl Sulfate, *1193*
[5221-53-4] Dimethirimol, *3217*
[5231-60-7] Demethoxyvindoline, *9988*
[5234-68-4] Carboxin, *1827*
[5250-39-5] Floxacillin, *4111*
[5251-34-3] Cloprednol, *2398*
[5285-18-7] Piperic Acid, *7467*
[5289-74-7] 20-Hydroxyecdysone, *3491*
[5300-03-8] Alitretinoin, *249*
[5306-80-9] Teclothiazide Potassium Salt, *9104*
[5308-89-4] Taxicin-I, *9077*
[5308-90-7] Taxicin-II, *9077*
[5309-42-2] Monobutyrin *(R)*-Form, *6249*
[5318-76-3] Imidocarb Dihydrochloride, *4915*
[5321-32-4] Hetacillin Potassium Salt, *4672*
[5323-95-5] Ricinoleic Acid Sodium Salt, *8211*
[5329-14-6] Sulfamic Acid, *8921*
[5330-29-0] Sitamaquine Dihydrochloride, *8553*
[5341-61-7] Hydrazine Dihydrochloride, *4770*
[5355-16-8] Diaveridine, *2993*
[5355-48-6] β-Acetyldigoxin, *3167*
[5370-01-4] Mexiletine Hydrochloride, *6169*
[5373-42-2] Thalicarpine, *9254*
[5376-03-4] Tropylium Bromide, *9785*
[5377-20-8] Metomidate, *6148*
[5392-40-5] Citral, *2322*
[5394-83-2] Camphoric Acid, *1733*
[5408-52-6] L-Lysine L-Glutamate, *5638*
[5411-22-3] Benzphetamine Hydrochloride, *1118*
[5421-04-5] Mandelic Acid Isoamyl Ester, *5718*
[5451-09-2] δ-Aminolevulinic Acid Hydrochloride, *446*
[5466-22-8] Aminoacetonitrile Sulfate (2:1), *412*
[5466-77-3] Octyl Methoxycinnamate, *6769*
[5470-11-1] Hydroxylamine Hydrochloride, *4828*
[5486-03-3] Buquinolate, *1500*
[5490-27-7] Dihydrostreptomycin Sesquisulfate, *3179*
[5503-08-2] Phenindamine Hydrochloride, *7233*
[5508-58-7] Andrographolide, *633*
[5511-98-8] α-Acetyldigoxin, *3167*

[5522-66-7] Protoporphyrin IX Dimethyl Ester, 7897
[5534-09-8] Beclomethasone Dipropionate, 1019
[5534-95-2] Pentagastrin, 7113
[5536-17-4] Vidarabine, 9976
[5545-89-1] Chimonanthine, 2059
[5560-59-8] Alverine Citrate, 371
[5560-62-3] Biphenamine Hydrochloride, 1234
[5560-69-0] Ethyl Dibunate, 3788
[5560-72-5] Iprindole, 5075
[5560-78-1] Teclozan, 9105
[5575-21-3] Cephalonium, 1978
[5576-62-5] Chlorbenzoxamine Dihydrochloride, 2080
[5579-81-7] Aldioxa, 223
[5579-84-0] Betahistine Dihydrochloride, 1178
[5581-52-2] Thiamiprine, 9299
[5585-52-4] Pentorex Hydrochloride, 7133
[5585-73-9] Butriptyline Hydrochloride, 1533
[5585-93-3] Oxypendyl, 6970
[5586-87-8] Mefenorex Hydrochloride, 5799
[5587-89-3] Ipodate, 5071
[5588-10-3] Methoxyphenamine Hydrochloride, 5998
[5588-16-9] Althiazide, 318
[5588-22-7] Clorprenaline Hydrochloride Monohydrate, 2408
[5588-25-0] Dihexyverine Hydrochloride, 3168
[5588-33-0] Mesoridazine, 5910
[5591-29-7] Etafedrine Hydrochloride, 3709
[5591-45-7] Thiothixene, 9365
[5591-74-2] Rhodoquinone, 8193
[5593-20-4] Betamethasone 17,21-Dipropionate, 1180
[5598-13-0] Chlorpyrifos O,O-Dimethyl Analog, 2189
[5600-19-1] Theophylline Isopropanolamine, 9285
[5610-40-2] Securinine, 8422
[5611-51-8] Triamcinolone Hexacetonide, 9598
[5614-56-2] 1-Theobromineacetic Acid, 9283
[5625-37-6] PIPES, 7479
[5630-53-5] Tibolone, 9427
[5631-00-5] Benzoylpas Calcium Salt Pentahydrate, 1115
[5632-44-0] Tolpropamine, 9523
[5633-14-7] Benzetimide Hydrochloride, 1075
[5633-20-5] Oxybutynin, 6955
[5633-25-0] Noracymethadol Hydrochloride, 6685
[5634-39-9] Iodinated Glycerol, 5013
[5634-42-4] Tocamphyl, 9492
[5636-83-9] Dimethindene, 3216
[5636-92-0] Picloxydine, 7398
[5638-76-6] Betahistine, 1178
[5639-34-9] 1-Amino-2-naphthol-6-sulfonic Acid, 455
[5650-44-2] Methcathinone, 5963
[5695-98-7] Cotinine Fumarate, 2553
[5696-09-3] Proxazole, 7903
[5697-56-3] Carbenoxolone, 1793
[5704-04-1] Tricine, 9651
[5704-60-9] Nifenalol Hydrochloride, 6530

[5714-00-1] Acetophenazine Dimaleate, 72
[5714-04-5] Guanoxan Sulfate, 4568
[5714-73-8] Methenamine Hippurate, 5966
[5714-90-9] Levopropoxyphene 2-Naphthalenesulfonate, 5469
[5716-20-1] Bamethan Sulfate, 954
[5728-52-9] Felbinac, 3951
[5735-19-3] Galactoflavin, 4333
[5741-22-0] Moprolol, 6264
[5743-26-0] Calcium Acetate Monohydrate, 1646
[5743-27-1] Calcium Ascorbate, 830
[5743-34-0] Calcium Borogluconate, 1653
[5746-40-7] Phosphocysteamine, 7341
[5746-57-6] Glycerophosphoric Acid α-Acid L-Form, 4486
[5749-67-7] Calcium Acetylsalicylate Complex with Urea, 1647
[5779-39-5] Desosamine, 2929
[5785-44-4] Calcium Citrate Tetrahydrate, 1661
[5786-21-0] Clozapine, 2423
[5787-63-3] Toldimfos Sodium Trihydrate, 9512
[5793-84-0] Calcium Phenoxide, 1691
[5793-88-4] Calcium D-Saccharate, 1700
[5793-94-2] Calcium Stearyl-2 Lactylate, 1704
[5793-98-6] Calcium Thioglycollate Trihydrate, 1711
[5794-16-1] Antipyrine Methylethylglycolate, 716
[5794-88-7] 5-Bromoanthranilic Acid, 1405
[5796-17-8] Dopa D-Form, 3420
[5796-30-5] Ecgonine l-Form Monohydrate, 3493
[5796-31-6] Ecgonine Hydrochloride, 3493
[5798-41-4] Bismuth Potassium Tartrate, 1277
[5798-43-6] Bismuth Sodium Triglycollamate, 1280
[5798-45-8] Bismuth Subcarbonate Hemihydrate, 1282
[5798-49-2] Bis(1-naphthylmethyl)-amine, 1293
[5798-78-7] p-Bromobenzyl Chloroformate, 1411
[5798-79-8] α-Bromobenzyl Cyanide, 1412
[5798-94-7] 5-Bromosalicylhydroxamic Acid, 1436
[5807-87-4] Diphenylpyraline Hydrobromide, 3331
[5815-08-7] Bredereck's Reagent, 1368
[5835-26-7] Isopimaric Acid, 5200
[5843-53-8] Clobenzorex Hydrochloride, 2362
[5845-26-1] Thiazesim, 9305
[5852-98-2] Carnosine Nitrate, 1850
[5852-99-3] Carnosine Hydrochloride, 1850
[5853-00-9] Carnosine D-Form, 1850
[5853-25-8] Carnegine Hydrobromide Monohydrate, 1847
[5854-93-3] L-Alanosine, 206
[5864-18-6] Carnegine Hydrochloride Monohydrate, 1847
[5868-05-3] Niceritrol, 6497

[5868-06-4] Fentonium Bromide, 4006
[5870-29-1] Cyclopentolate Hydrochloride, 2746
[5874-97-5] Metaproterenol Sulfate, 5931
[5875-06-9] Proparacaine Hydrochloride, 7807
[5892-10-4] Bismuth Subcarbonate, 1282
[5893-64-1] DL-Lactic Acid Copper Salt Dihydrate, 5336
[5897-76-7] α-(α-Aminopropyl)benzyl Alcohol, 471
[5902-51-2] Terbacil, 9155
[5905-52-2] Ferrous Lactate, 4050
[5907-38-0] Dipyrone, 3350
[5908-63-4] Baptigenin, 958
[5908-99-6] Atropine Sulfate Monohydrate, 875
[5909-04-6] Chrysoidine Citrate, 2257
[5911-58-0] Carnegine Methyliodide, 1847
[5912-86-7] Isoeugenol cis-Form, 5171
[5913-82-6] Conessine Dihydrobromide, 2497
[5928-84-7] Penicillin V Compd with Dibenzylethylenediamine, 7100
[5932-68-3] Isoeugenol trans-Form, 5171
[5934-14-5] Succisulfone, 8878
[5936-28-7] Hydrastine Hydrochloride, 4767
[5937-72-4] Androstenediol 17-Acetate, 637
[5942-95-0] Carpipramine, 1861
[5945-50-6] Monotropein, 6255
[5945-86-8] Nimbin, 6546
[5947-49-9] Podocarpic Acid, 7543
[5949-44-0] Testosterone Undecanoate, 9180
[5953-63-9] Androstenediol 3-Acetate-17-benzoate, 637
[5957-75-5] Δ8-Tetrahydrocannabinol, 9209
[5959-52-4] 3-Amino-2-naphthoic Acid, 452
[5961-85-3] TCEP, 9085
[5962-29-8] Xylulose, 10088
[5965-09-3] Fosfestrol Disodium Salt, 4253
[5965-33-3] Antimony Potassium Oxalate, 699
[5965-49-1] Ketobemidone Hydrochloride, 5301
[5967-52-2] Metaraminol Hydrochloride, 5932
[5967-53-3] Metaraminol Oxalate Dihydrate, 5932
[5967-73-7] Methadone l-Form Hydrochloride, 5944
[5970-32-1] Mercuric Salicylate, 5885
[5970-45-6] Zinc Acetate Dihydrate, 10128
[5972-72-5] Ammonium Binoxalate, 499
[5972-76-9] Ammonium Caprylate, 506
[5973-17-1] Phenol Ammonium Salt, 7241
[5974-09-4] Vetrabutine Hydrochloride, 9972
[5978-87-0] D-Araboflavin, 763
[5984-61-2] Pelletierine Hydrochloride, 7072
[5985-04-6] Hydrohydrastinine Hydrochloride, 4802

[5985-05-7] Hydrohydrastinine Hydrobromide, *4802*

[5985-06-8] Hydrohydrastinine Platinichloride, *4802*

[5985-28-4] Synephrine Hydrochloride, *9012*

[5985-35-3] Levorphanol *dl*-Form Hydrobromide, *5470*

[5985-38-6] Levorphanol Tartrate Dihydrate, *5470*

[5986-55-0] Patchouli Alcohol, *7052*

[5987-82-6] Benoxinate Hydrochloride, *1047*

[5988-22-7] Phytonadiol Sodium Diphosphate, *7380*

[5988-51-2] Deanol Bitartrate, *2843*

[5989-43-5] Matricarin, *5758*

[5991-71-9] Clorazepic Acid Monopotassium Salt, *2403*

[5995-96-0] Eseridine Salicylate, *3699*

[5996-14-5] α-Glucose-1-phosphate Dipotassium Salt Dihydrate, *4461*

[5997-53-5] Ensulizole Sodium Salt, *3593*

[6000-74-4] Hydrocortisone 21-Phosphate Disodium Salt, *4787*

[6001-51-0] Bis(*p*-dimethylaminobenzylidene)benzidine, *1249*

[6001-74-7] Clomethiazole Hydrochloride, *2384*

[6001-97-4] Bis(1-methylamyl) Sodium Sulfosuccinate, *1255*

[6003-09-4] Aleuritic Acid Ethyl Ester, *231*

[6003-10-7] Aleuritic Acid Hydrazide, *231*

[6004-24-6] Cetylpyridinium Chloride Monohydrate, *2032*

[6006-09-3] Gravitol(e), *4542*

[6009-81-0] Morphine (monohydrate), *6276*

[6010-09-9] Ferrous Thiocyanate, *4059*

[6010-17-9] Harmalol *O*-Ethylharmalol, *4614*

[6011-14-9] Aminoacetonitrile Hydrochloride, *412*

[6011-39-8] Penicillin G Mixture with Clemizole, *7094*

[6018-19-5] *p*-Aminosalicylic Acid Sodium Salt Dihydrate, *477*

[6018-40-2] Corypalmine, *2549*

[6018-53-7] 6-Desoxy-D-glucosamine, *2931*

[6018-84-4] *p*-Aminobenzoic Acid Diethylamine Salt, *423*

[6019-02-9] Nicotine Dihydrochloride, *6524*

[6020-39-9] *meso*-Cystine, *2782*

[6024-76-6] Tetraethylammonium Chloride Tetrahydrate, *9200*

[6027-13-0] Homocysteine, *4734*

[6027-23-2] Hordenine Hydrochloride, *4746*

[6027-89-0] L-Gulose, *4579*

[6027-99-2] Harmalol Trihydrate, *4614*

[6028-01-9] Harmalol *O*-*n*-Propylharmalol, *4614*

[6028-08-6] Harmalol Lactate, *4614*

[6028-35-9] Thibenzazoline, *9312*

[6031-86-3] Racemethorphan Hydrobromide, *8091*

[6032-06-0] Cyproheptadine Hydrochloride Monohydrate, *2773*

[6032-14-0] *N*-Methylepinephrine DL-Form, *6069*

[6032-29-7] 2-Pentanol, *7119*

[6032-32-2] Methylarbutin, *773*

[6032-92-4] Mycarose, *6318*

[6033-08-5] Hematoporphyrin Hydrochloride Monohydrate, *4636*

[6033-69-8] Deserpidine Hydrochloride, *2918*

[6035-40-1] Noscapine *dl*-Form, *6718*

[6035-45-6] Folinic Acid Calcium Salt Pentahydrate, *4222*

[6035-50-3] DL-Fructose, *4274*

[6036-25-5] Narbomycin, *6421*

[6047-24-1] Ferrous Lactate Trihydrate, *4050*

[6054-98-4] Olsalazine Disodium Salt, *6841*

[6055-19-2] Cyclophosphamide, *2747*

[6055-56-7] Ergocristine Ethanesulfonate, *3649*

[6055-73-8] Adrenochrome Oxime Sesquihydrate, *172*

[6056-11-7] Pipazethate Hydrochloride, *7456*

[6056-70-8] α-Glucose-1-phosphate Barium Salt Trihydrate, *4461*

[6064-83-1] Fosfosal, *4255*

[6078-26-8] Bikhaconitine, *1216*

[6088-51-3] DDD (Analytical), *2840*

[6091-05-0] Physovenine, *7385*

[6099-90-7] Phloroglucinol Dihydrate, *7328*

[6100-05-6] Potassium Citrate Monohydrate, *7623*

[6101-04-8] Strychnine Hydrochloride Dihydrate, *8855*

[6101-32-2] Sulfanilic Acid Monohydrate, *8926*

[6101-34-4] Sulfathiourea Sodium Salt, *8944*

[6106-21-4] Sodium Succinate Hexahydrate, *8679*

[6106-22-5] Sulfanilic Acid Sodium Salt Dihydrate, *8926*

[6106-46-3] Scopolamine Methyl Nitrate, *8406*

[6106-81-6] Scopolamine *N*-Oxide Hydrobromide, *8407*

[6108-05-0] Lidocaine Hydrochloride Monohydrate, *5482*

[6108-17-4] Lithium Acetate Dihydrate (monohydrate), *5521*

[6109-70-2] 3-Quinuclidinol *dl*-Form Acetate Hydrochloride, *8082*

[6114-26-7] Pholedrine Sulfate, *7330*

[6117-91-5] Crotyl Alcohol, *2601*

[6119-47-7] Quinine Hydrochloride Dihydrate, *8061*

[6119-70-6] Quinine Sulfate Dihydrate, *8061*

[6130-64-9] Penicillin G Procaine, *7097*

[6132-04-3] Sodium Citrate Dihydrate, *8602*

[6138-23-4] Trehalose Dihydrate, *9580*

[6138-26-7] Tricarballylic Acid Trimethyl Ester, *9622*

[6138-47-2] Liothyronine Hydrochloride, *5510*

[6138-56-3] Tripelennamine Citrate, *9738*

[6138-73-4] Trilobine, *9697*

[6138-79-0] Triprolidine Hydrochloride Monohydrate, *9746*

[6147-11-1] Mangostin, *5742*

[6147-37-1] Menadione Sodium Bisulfite (trihydrate), *5831*

[6150-79-4] Magnesium Citrate Tribasic (tetradecahydrate), *5663*

[6150-97-6] Dipyrone Magnesium Salt, *3350*

[6151-25-3] Quercetin Dihydrate, *8034*

[6151-30-0] Quinacrine Dihydrochloride Dihydrate, *8044*

[6151-39-9] Quinidine Hydrogen Sulfate Tetrahydrate, *8060*

[6153-16-8] β-Phellandrene *d*-Form, *7201*

[6153-17-9] β-Phellandrene *l*-Form, *7201*

[6153-19-1] Phenacaine Hydrochloride Monohydrate, *7202*

[6153-33-9] Mebhydroline 1,5-Naphthalenedisulfonate Salt, *5770*

[6153-44-2] Orotic Acid Methyl Ester, *6876*

[6155-64-2] Salicylsulfuric Acid Monosodium Salt, *8334*

[6159-55-3] Vasicine, *9937*

[6160-12-9] Sparteine Sulfate Pentahydrate, *8737*

[6163-66-2] Di-*tert*-butyl Ether, *3033*

[6164-87-0] Nicotinyl Alcohol *d*-Tartrate, *6527*

[6164-98-3] Chlordimeform, *2085*

[6168-76-9] Crotethamide, *2595*

[6168-86-1] Isometheptene Hydrochloride, *5185*

[6170-25-8] *p*-Aminopropiophenone Hydrochloride, *470*

[6170-29-2] Aminopyrine Hydrochloride, *474*

[6170-42-9] Chloropyramine Hydrochloride, *2162*

[6183-68-2] Quinine Bisulfate Heptahydrate, *8061*

[6190-36-9] Cotarnine Phthalate, *2552*

[6190-39-2] Dihydroergotamine Methanesulfonate, *3174*

[6190-43-8] Methenamine Anhydromethylenecitrate, *5966*

[6190-60-9] Mephentermine Sulfate Dihydrate, *5852*

[6191-56-6] Apomorphine Diacetate (Ester), *746*

[6192-89-8] Procaine Dihydrate, *7757*

[6192-92-3] Procaine Nitrate, *7757*

[6192-95-6] Propylhexedrine *dl*-Form Hydrochloride, *7860*

[6192-96-7] Propylhexedrine *d*-Form Hydrochloride, *7860*

[6192-97-8] Propylhexedrine *l*-Form, *7860*

[6192-98-9] Propylhexedrine *l*-Form Hydrochloride, *7860*

[6197-30-4] Octocrylene, *6756*

[6197-42-8] Harmalol *O*-*n*-Butylharmalol, *4614*

[6199-67-3] Cucurbitacin B, *2614*

[6202-23-9] Cyclobenzaprine Hydrochloride, *2713*

[6209-17-2] Sulfacetamide Sodium Salt (monohydrate), *8899*

[6211-15-0] Morphine Sulfate Pentahydrate, *6276*

[6214-20-6] Methyl *p*-Nitrobenzenesulfonate, *6102*

[6217-54-5] Docosahexaenoic Acid, *3398*

[6223-35-4] Guaiazulene 3-Sulfonate Sodium Salt, *4554*

[6236-05-1] Nifuroxime, *6536*
[6272-74-8] Lapyrium Chloride, *5370*
[6277-14-1] Acetoxolone, *76*
[6284-40-8] *N*-Methylglucamine, *6078*
[6292-91-7] MDA Hydrochloride, *5765*
[6303-21-5] Hypophosphorous Acid, *4868*
[6314-28-9] Thionaphthene-2-carboxylic Acid, *9345*
[6341-58-8] αMNP Hydroxy Acid (unspecified stereo), *6224*
[6358-53-8] Citrus Red 2, *2333*
[6358-69-6] Pyranine, *7954*
[6363-57-1] Pseudococaine Hydrochloride, *7912*
[6365-83-9] Dinoseb Ammonium Salt, *3287*
[6372-96-9] Polar® Yellow, *7553*
[6376-26-7] Salverine, *8342*
[6377-18-0] Chartreusin, *2045*
[6379-56-2] Hygromycin, *4851*
[6379-69-7] Trichothecin, *9650*
[6384-92-5] NMDA, *6662*
[6385-58-6] Bithionol Sodium Salt, *1306*
[6385-62-2] Diquat Dibromide Monohydrate, *3352*
[6398-98-7] Amodiaquin Dihydrochloride Dihydrate, *572*
[6402-23-9] Ethacridine Lactate Monohydrate, *3716*
[6402-36-4] Traumatic Acid, *9576*
[6411-75-2] Tuaminoheptane Sulfate, *9802*
[6414-49-9] Synephrine Tartaric Acid Monoester, *9012*
[6420-47-9] Dinoseb Triethanolamine Salt, *3287*
[6424-36-8] Ergocristine Phosphate, *3649*
[6452-71-7] Oxprenolol, *6952*
[6452-73-9] Oxprenolol Hydrochloride, *6952*
[6458-13-5] Ethyldimethyl-9-octadecenylammonium Bromide, *3790*
[6469-93-8] Chlorprothixene Hydrochloride, *2188*
[6474-85-7] Fenbutrazate Hydrochloride, *3965*
[6484-52-2] Ammonium Nitrate, *534*
[6484-71-5] Phosphorylcholine Barium Salt, *7362*
[6484-74-8] Pteroylhexaglutamylglutamic Acid, *7935*
[6484-89-5] Sodium Folate, *8619*
[6489-61-8] Metampicillin Sodium Salt, *5925*
[6489-97-0] Metampicillin, *5925*
[6493-05-6] Pentoxifylline, *7136*
[6495-46-1] Dioxadrol, *3299*
[6500-81-8] Ethacrynic Acid Sodium Salt, *3717*
[6506-37-2] Nimorazole, *6552*
[6533-00-2] Norgestrel, *6704*
[6533-54-6] Dihydrostreptomycin Trihydrochloride, *3179*
[6533-73-9] Thallium Carbonate, *9259*
[6533-78-4] Antimony Thioglycollamide, *705*
[6536-18-1] Morazone, *6267*
[6538-02-9] Ergostanol, *3658*
[6539-57-7] Nordefrin (unspecified stereo), *6692*
[6556-11-2] Inositol Niacinate, *4979*

[6556-12-3] D-Glucuronic Acid, *4465*
[6556-29-2] Propylhexedrine *d*-Form, *7860*
[6569-51-3] Borazine, *1334*
[6576-51-8] Stallimycin Hydrochloride, *8772*
[6577-41-9] Cyclonium Iodide, *2737*
[6591-55-5] Bismuth Oxalate, *1272*
[6591-63-5] Quinidine Sulfate Dihydrate, *8060*
[6592-85-4] Hydrastinine, *4768*
[6598-46-5] Quinacrine Methanesulfonate Monohydrate, *8044*
[6600-40-4] Norvaline, *6716*
[6606-65-1] *n*-Butyl Cyanoacrylate, *1565*
[6620-60-6] Proglumide, *7775*
[6621-47-2] Perhexiline, *7163*
[6645-46-1] Carnitine L-Form Hydrochloride, *1849*
[6673-35-4] Practolol, *7700*
[6696-47-5] Oleandomycin Hydrochloride, *6825*
[6696-59-9] Ethylmorphine Methiodide, *3830*
[6700-39-6] Isoproterenol *dl*-Form Sulfate Dihydrate, *5217*
[6700-56-7] Ethoheptazine Citrate, *3743*
[6701-17-3] Octyl Cyanoacrylate, *6766*
[6724-53-4] Perhexiline Maleate, *7163*
[6736-85-2] Catalposide, *1901*
[6740-88-1] Ketamine, *5295*
[6745-93-3] Methotrexate Monohydrate, *5985*
[6746-59-4] Ethylmorphine Hydrochloride Dihydrate, *3830*
[6753-98-6] Humulene, *4753*
[6754-13-8] Helenalin, *4626*
[6754-20-7] Polygodial, *7570*
[6793-24-4] Buphanamine, *1492*
[6795-23-9] Aflatoxin M₁, *182*
[6795-60-4] Norvinisterone, *6717*
[6799-26-4] *d*-Camphocarboxylic Acid Ammonium Salt, *1731*
[6802-63-3] Bipiperidyl Mustard, *1237*
[6804-07-5] Carbadox, *1780*
[6805-41-0] Escin, *3696*
[6807-82-5] Diopterin, *3291*
[6809-52-5] Teprenone, *9153*
[6812-78-8] Rhodinol, *8185*
[6818-37-7] Olaflur, *6820*
[6823-79-6] Pentamidine Dimethanesulfonate, *7115*
[6829-98-7] Imipramine *N*-Oxide, *4921*
[6830-17-7] Oxamarin Dihydrochloride, *6915*
[6831-14-7] Arborescin, *771*
[6833-84-7] Nonactin, *6675*
[6834-92-0] Sodium Metasilicate, *8642*
[6834-98-6] Fungichromin, *4290*
[6835-16-1] Hyoscyamine Sulfate Dihydrate, *4858*
[6846-50-0] Texanol Isobutyrate, *9251*
[6856-31-1] Pridinol Methanesulfonate, *7741*
[6871-44-9] Echitamine, *3500*
[6873-15-0] Glycosine, *4502*
[6874-98-2] Vellosimine, *9944*
[6877-35-6] Digalogenin, *3154*
[6878-83-7] Tecomanine, *9106*
[6878-98-4] Tropacine, *9773*
[6879-02-3] Tylocrebrine, *9830*
[6882-99-1] Sempervirine, *8447*

[6885-57-0] Aflatoxin M₂, *182*
[6888-23-9] Toxiferine I, *9558*
[6893-02-3] Liothyronine, *5510*
[6893-26-1] Glutamic Acid D-Form, *4469*
[6894-38-8] Jasmonic Acid, *5260*
[6901-22-0] Lunasine, *5605*
[6903-12-4] Anabsinthin, *620*
[6909-62-2] Demanyl Phosphate, *2884*
[6915-15-7] Malic Acid, *5707*
[6915-57-7] Bibrocathol, *1199*
[6923-22-4] Monocrotophos, *6251*
[6940-50-7] *p*-Bromomandelic Acid, *1424*
[6946-29-8] *p*-Aminosalicylic Acid Hydrazide, *478*
[6961-46-2] Idrocilamide, *4893*
[6964-20-1] Tiadenol, *9416*
[6983-79-5] Bixins, *1311*
[6988-58-5] Olivomycin A, *6838*
[6990-06-3] Fusidic Acid, *4317*
[6998-60-3] Rifamycin SV, *8218*
[7001-56-1] Pentagestrone, *7114*
[7008-26-6] Dichlorisone, *3048*
[7054-25-3] Quinidine Gluconate, *8060*
[7059-23-6] Mitoguazone Dihydrochloride, *6213*
[7059-24-7] Chromomycin A₃, *2238*
[7060-74-4] Oleandomycin Phosphate, *6825*
[7067-12-1] Laserpitin, *5374*
[7075-03-8] Carpipramine Dihydrochloride Monohydrate, *1861*
[7080-50-4] Chloramine-T Trihydrate, *2075*
[7081-38-1] Oxyphenbutazone Monohydrate, *6972*
[7081-40-5] Methixene Hydrochloride Monohydrate, *5979*
[7081-44-9] Cloxacillin Sodium Monohydrate, *2419*
[7081-52-9] Piminodine Ethanesulfonate, *7433*
[7081-53-0] Doxapram Hydrochloride Monohydrate, *3432*
[7085-19-0] Mecoprop, *5784*
[7085-44-1] Chlorothiazide Sodium Salt, *2168*
[7085-55-4] Troxerutin, *9789*
[7085-85-0] Ethyl Cyanoacrylate, *3787*
[7097-60-1] Tetraglycine Hydroperiodide, *9207*
[7104-38-3] Methotrimeprazine Maleate, *5986*
[7128-64-5] BBOT, *1014*
[7168-64-1] *C*-Curarine I, *2672*
[7173-51-5] Didecyldimethylammonium Chloride, *3099*
[7177-48-2] Ampicillin Trihydrate, *586*
[7177-50-6] Nafcillin Sodium Salt Monohydrate, *6352*
[7177-54-0] Penicillin O Sodium Salt, *7099*
[7179-49-9] Lincomycin Hydrochloride Monohydrate, *5500*
[7187-01-1] 2-Furanacrylonitrile, *4298*
[7195-27-9] Mefruside, *5803*
[7199-29-3] Cyheptamide, *2759*
[7205-52-9] Phytic Acid Sodium Salt, *7387*
[7207-92-3] Nandrolone Propionate, *6365*
[7210-92-6] Tolycaine Hydrochloride, *9541*

[7212-44-4] Nerolidol, *6476*
[7220-79-3] Methylene Blue Trihydrate, *6060*
[7220-81-7] Aflatoxin B$_2$, *180*
[7225-61-8] Metrizoic Acid Sodium Salt, *6156*
[7234-48-2] ε-Acetamidocaproic Acid Sodium Salt, *45*
[7235-40-7] β-Carotene, *1853*
[7239-48-7] Colistin B, *2479*
[7240-38-2] Oxacillin Sodium Salt Monohydrate, *6904*
[7240-90-6] X-gal, *10074*
[7241-98-7] Aflatoxin G$_2$, *181*
[7242-04-8] Gitoxin Pentaacetate, *4434*
[7246-20-0] Triclofos Monosodium Salt, *9655*
[7246-21-1] Tyropanoate Sodium, *9837*
[7248-28-4] Strychnine N^6-Oxide, *8856*
[7257-29-6] C-Toxiferine II, *9558*
[7261-97-4] Dantrolene, *2816*
[7262-75-1] Lefetamine, *5431*
[7270-12-4] 8-Hydroxy-7-iodo-5-quinolinesulfonic Acid Compd with Chloroquine (2:1), *4826*
[7280-37-7] Estrone Sulfate Piperazine Salt, *3708*
[7287-19-6] Prometryn, *7789*
[7295-85-4] Catechin *dl*-Form, *1902*
[7297-25-8] Erythrityl Tetranitrate, *3677*
[7309-58-2] Helenynolic Acid, *4627*
[7320-34-5] Potassium Pyrophosphate, *7663*
[7327-87-9] Dihydralazine Sulfate, *3169*
[7361-61-7] Xylazine, *10080*
[7365-44-8] TES, *9176*
[7365-45-9] HEPES, *4654*
[7365-82-4] ACES, *36*
[7377-03-9] Octanohydroxamic Acid, *6750*
[7400-08-0] *p*-Coumaric Acid, *2560*
[7408-20-0] Iminodisuccinic Acid, *4918*
[7413-34-5] Methotrexate Disodium Salt, *5985*
[7413-36-7] Nifenalol, *6530*
[7414-83-7] Etidronic Acid Disodium Salt, *3863*
[7416-34-4] Molindone, *6233*
[7421-40-1] Carbenoxolone Disodium Salt, *1793*
[7429-90-5] Aluminum, *323*
[7429-91-6] Dysprosium, *3482*
[7429-92-7] Einsteinium, *3532*
[7432-25-9] Etaqualone, *3714*
[7439-88-5] Iridium, *5085*
[7439-89-6] Iron, *5093*
[7439-90-9] Krypton, *5325*
[7439-91-0] Lanthanum, *5363*
[7439-92-1] Lead, *5396*
[7439-93-2] Lithium, *5520*
[7439-94-3] Lutetium, *5615*
[7439-95-4] Magnesium, *5653*
[7439-96-5] Manganese, *5723*
[7439-97-6] Mercury, *5898*
[7439-98-7] Molybdenum, *6235*
[7439-99-8] Neptunium, *6471*
[7440-00-8] Neodymium, *6450*
[7440-01-9] Neon, *6455*
[7440-02-0] Nickel, *6498*
[7440-02-0] Raney® Nickel, *8107*
[7440-03-1] Niobium, *6556*

[7440-04-2] Osmium, *6891*
[7440-05-3] Palladium, *6989*
[7440-06-4] Platinum, *7529*
[7440-07-5] Plutonium, *7541*
[7440-08-6] Polonium, *7561*
[7440-09-7] Potassium, *7604*
[7440-10-0] Praseodymium, *7712*
[7440-11-1] Mendelevium, *5835*
[7440-12-2] Promethium, *7787*
[7440-13-3] Protactinium, *7883*
[7440-14-4] Radium, *8094*
[7440-15-5] Rhenium, *8177*
[7440-16-6] Rhodium, *8186*
[7440-17-7] Rubidium, *8282*
[7440-18-8] Ruthenium, *8299*
[7440-19-9] Samarium, *8347*
[7440-20-2] Scandium, *8392*
[7440-21-3] Silicon, *8491*
[7440-22-4] Silver, *8504*
[7440-23-5] Sodium, *8570*
[7440-24-6] Strontium, *8835*
[7440-25-7] Tantalum, *9053*
[7440-26-8] Technetium, *9097*
[7440-27-9] Terbium, *9157*
[7440-28-0] Thallium, *9256*
[7440-29-1] Thorium, *9374*
[7440-30-4] Thulium, *9394*
[7440-31-5] Tin, *9446*
[7440-32-6] Titanium, *9470*
[7440-33-7] Tungsten, *9814*
[7440-34-8] Actinium, *137*
[7440-35-9] Americium, *392*
[7440-36-0] Antimony, *692*
[7440-37-1] Argon, *783*
[7440-38-2] Arsenic, *794*
[7440-39-3] Barium, *964*
[7440-40-6] Berkelium, *1158*
[7440-41-7] Beryllium, *1161*
[7440-42-8] Boron, *1343*
[7440-43-9] Cadmium, *1613*
[7440-44-0] Carbon, *1807*
[7440-45-1] Cerium, *1991*
[7440-46-2] Cesium, *2008*
[7440-47-3] Chromium, *2231*
[7440-48-4] Cobalt, *2427*
[7440-50-8] Copper, *2519*
[7440-51-9] Curium, *2675*
[7440-52-0] Erbium, *3646*
[7440-53-1] Europium, *3904*
[7440-54-2] Gadolinium, *4326*
[7440-55-3] Gallium, *4346*
[7440-56-4] Germanium, *4407*
[7440-57-5] Gold, *4514*
[7440-58-6] Hafnium, *4588*
[7440-59-7] Helium, *4630*
[7440-60-0] Holmium, *4727*
[7440-61-1] Uranium, *9854*
[7440-62-2] Vanadium, *9918*
[7440-63-3] Xenon, *10072*
[7440-64-4] Ytterbium, *10105*
[7440-65-5] Yttrium, *10107*
[7440-66-6] Zinc, *10127*
[7440-67-7] Zirconium, *10173*
[7440-68-8] Astatine, *854*
[7440-69-9] Bismuth, *1257*
[7440-70-2] Calcium, *1645*
[7440-71-3] Californium, *1716*
[7440-72-4] Fermium, *4014*
[7440-73-5] Francium, *4262*
[7440-74-6] Indium, *4947*
[7446-07-3] Tellurium Dioxide, *9123*
[7446-08-4] Selenium Oxide, *8434*
[7446-09-5] Sulfur Dioxide, *8971*
[7446-11-9] Sulfur Trioxide, *8979*

[7446-14-2] Lead Sulfate, *5420*
[7446-18-6] Thallium Sulfate, *9269*
[7446-19-7] Zinc Sulfate Monohydrate, *10159*
[7446-20-0] Zinc Sulfate Heptahydrate, *10159*
[7446-26-6] Zinc Pyrophosphate, *10154*
[7446-27-7] Lead Phosphate, *5416*
[7446-32-4] Antimony Sulfate, *704*
[7446-70-0] Aluminum Chloride, *337*
[7447-39-4] Cupric Chloride, *2633*
[7447-40-7] Potassium Chloride, *7621*
[7447-41-8] Lithium Chloride, *5528*
[7449-03-8] Erythropterin, *3689*
[7455-39-2] Fonazine Methanesulfonate, *4231*
[7456-24-8] Fonazine, *4231*
[7460-12-0] Pseudoephedrine Sulfate, *7916*
[7461-02-1] Stylopine, *8858*
[7481-89-2] Zalcitabine, *10109*
[7487-81-2] Isomethadone *l*-Form Hydrochloride, *5184*
[7487-88-9] Magnesium Sulfate, *5691*
[7487-94-7] Mercuric Chloride, *5876*
[7488-55-3] Stannous Sulfate, *8790*
[7488-56-4] Selenium Disulfide, *8436*
[7488-99-5] α-Carotene, *1852*
[7491-09-0] Docusate Potassium, *3401*
[7491-74-9] Piracetam, *7487*
[7512-17-6] N-Acetylglucosamine, *4458*
[7527-91-5] Acrisorcin, *126*
[7535-00-4] D-Galactosamine, *4334*
[7542-37-2] Paromomycin, *7041*
[7550-35-8] Lithium Bromide, *5526*
[7550-45-0] Titanium Tetrachloride, *9478*
[7553-56-2] Iodine, *5014*
[7554-65-6] Fomepizole, *4226*
[7558-79-4] Sodium Phosphate, Dibasic, *8659*
[7558-80-7] Sodium Phosphate, Monobasic, *8660*
[7563-42-0] Pentobarbital Calcium Salt, *7130*
[7568-93-6] Phenylethanolamine, *7287*
[7580-67-8] Lithium Hydride, *5533*
[7601-54-9] Sodium Phosphate, Tribasic, *8662*
[7601-55-0] Metocurine Iodide, *6144*
[7601-89-0] Sodium Perchlorate, *8653*
[7601-90-3] Perchloric Acid, *7153*
[7616-22-0] γ-Tocopherol (*dl*-form), *9497*
[7616-94-6] Perchloryl Fluoride, *7154*
[7618-86-2] Furtrethonium, *4312*
[7631-86-9] Silicon Dioxide, *8493*
[7631-90-5] Sodium Bisulfite, *8588*
[7631-94-9] Sodium Dithionate, *8611*
[7631-95-0] Sodium Molybdate(VI), *8645*
[7631-99-4] Sodium Nitrate, *8647*
[7632-00-0] Sodium Nitrite, *8648*
[7632-04-4] Sodium Perborate, *8652*
[7633-29-6] Psychotrine, *7929*
[7635-51-0] Phendimetrazine Hydrochloride, *7220*
[7637-07-2] Boron Trifluoride, *1349*
[7646-69-7] Sodium Hydride, *8625*
[7646-78-8] Stannic Chloride, *8774*
[7646-79-9] Cobaltous Chloride, *2437*
[7646-85-7] Zinc Chloride, *10132*
[7646-93-7] Potassium Bisulfate, *7613*

[7647-01-0] Hydrochloric Acid, *4780*
[7647-01-0] Hydrogen Chloride, *4794*
[7647-10-1] Palladium Chloride, *6990*
[7647-14-5] Sodium Chloride, *8599*
[7647-15-6] Sodium Bromide, *8594*
[7647-17-8] Cesium Chloride, *2011*
[7647-18-9] Antimony Pentachloride, *695*
[7647-19-0] Phosphorus Pentafluoride, *7352*
[7658-08-4] Quinovose, *8077*
[7664-38-2] Phosphoric Acid, *7344*
[7664-39-3] Hydrofluoric Acid, *4790*
[7664-39-3] Hydrogen Fluoride, *4796*
[7664-41-7] Ammonia, *492*
[7664-93-9] Sulfuric Acid, *8974*
[7665-99-8] Cyclic GMP, *2709*
[7681-11-0] Potassium Iodide, *7643*
[7681-14-3] Prednisolone 2l-*tert*-Butyl-acetate, *7721*
[7681-28-9] Quinidine Polygalacturon-ate, *8060*
[7681-38-1] Sodium Bisulfate, *8586*
[7681-49-4] Sodium Fluoride, *8618*
[7681-52-9] Sodium Hypochlorite, *8628*
[7681-53-0] Sodium Hypophosphite, *8629*
[7681-55-2] Sodium Iodate, *8630*
[7681-57-4] Sodium Metabisulfite, *8638*
[7681-65-4] Cuprous Iodide, *2662*
[7681-76-7] Ronidazole, *8254*
[7681-79-0] Etafedrine, *3709*
[7681-82-5] Sodium Iodide, *8631*
[7681-93-8] Natamycin, *6427*
[7683-59-2] Isoproterenol, *5217*
[7689-03-4] Camptothecin, *1735*
[7696-12-0] Tetramethrin, *9223*
[7697-37-2] Nitric Acid, *6577*
[7699-43-6] Zirconyl Chloride, *10184*
[7699-45-8] Zinc Bromide, *10129*
[7700-17-6] Crotoxyphos, *2600*
[7704-34-9] Sulfur, *8969*
[7704-34-9] Sulfur, Pharmaceutical, *8977*
[7704-98-5] Titanium Hydride, *9473*
[7704-99-6] Zirconium Hydride, *10176*
[7705-07-9] Titanium Trichloride, *9481*
[7705-08-0] Ferric Chloride, *4019*
[7706-67-4] Dimecrotic Acid, *3203*
[7718-54-9] Nickel Chloride, *6505*
[7719-09-7] Thionyl Chloride, *9348*
[7719-12-2] Phosphorus Trichloride, *7358*
[7720-78-7] Ferrous Sulfate, *4057*
[7721-01-9] Tantalum Pentachloride, *9054*
[7722-44-3] Colistin A, *2479*
[7722-64-7] Potassium Permanganate, *7655*
[7722-76-1] Ammonium Phosphate, Monobasic, *543*
[7722-84-1] Hydrogen Peroxide, *4798*
[7722-86-3] Caro's Acid, *1851*
[7722-88-5] Tetrasodium Pyrophosphate, *9240*
[7723-14-0] Phosphorus, *7347*
[7726-95-6] Bromine, *1394*
[7727-15-3] Aluminum Bromide, *332*
[7727-18-6] Vanadyl Trichloride, *9927*
[7727-21-1] Potassium Persulfate, *7656*
[7727-37-9] Nitrogen, *6601*
[7727-43-7] Barium Sulfate, *994*

[7727-54-0] Ammonium Peroxydisulfate, *541*
[7732-18-5] Water, *10039*
[7733-02-0] Zinc Sulfate, *10159*
[7753-60-8] Anecortave Acetate, *641*
[7757-79-1] Potassium Nitrate, *7648*
[7757-82-6] Sodium Sulfate, *8680*
[7757-83-7] Sodium Sulfite, *8682*
[7757-86-0] Magnesium Phosphate, Dibasic, *5681*
[7757-87-1] Magnesium Phosphate, Tribasic, *5683*
[7757-88-2] Magnesium Sulfite, *5692*
[7757-93-9] Calcium Phosphate, Dibasic, *1692*
[7758-01-2] Potassium Bromate, *7617*
[7758-02-3] Potassium Bromide, *7618*
[7758-05-6] Potassium Iodate, *7642*
[7758-09-0] Potassium Nitrite, *7649*
[7758-11-4] Potassium Phosphate, Dibasic, *7658*
[7758-16-9] Sodium Acid Pyrophosphate, *8572*
[7758-19-2] Sodium Chlorite, *8600*
[7758-23-8] Calcium Phosphate, Monobasic, *1693*
[7758-29-4] Sodium Tripolyphosphate, *8697*
[7758-87-4] Calcium Phosphate, Tribasic, *1694*
[7758-88-5] Cerous Fluoride, *1998*
[7758-89-6] Cuprous Chloride, *2660*
[7758-94-3] Ferrous Chloride, *4043*
[7758-95-4] Lead Chloride, *5404*
[7758-97-6] Lead Chromate(VI), *5405*
[7758-98-7] Cupric Sulfate, *2653*
[7758-99-8] Cupric Sulfate Pentahydrate, *2653*
[7759-00-4] Manganese Silicate, *5738*
[7759-02-6] Strontium Sulfate, *8848*
[7759-35-5] Elcometrine, *3538*
[7761-88-8] Silver Nitrate, *8518*
[7772-98-7] Sodium Thiosulfate, *8694*
[7772-99-8] Stannous Chloride, *8783*
[7773-01-5] Manganese Chloride, *5728*
[7773-06-0] Ammonium Sulfamate, *554*
[7774-29-0] Mercuric Iodide, Red, *5879*
[7775-09-9] Sodium Chlorate, *8598*
[7775-11-3] Sodium Chromate(VI), *8601*
[7775-14-6] Sodium Hydrosulfite, *8626*
[7775-19-1] Sodium Metaborate, *8639*
[7775-27-1] Sodium Persulfate, *8656*
[7775-41-9] Silver Fluoride, *8514*
[7778-18-9] Calcium Sulfate, *1706*
[7778-39-4] Arsenic Acid, *795*
[7778-43-0] Sodium Arsenate, Dibasic, *8579*
[7778-44-1] Calcium Arsenate, *1649*
[7778-50-9] Potassium Dichromate(VI), *7627*
[7778-53-2] Potassium Phosphate, Tribasic, *7660*
[7778-54-3] Calcium Hypochlorite, *1674*
[7778-54-3] Chlorinated Lime, *2094*
[7778-74-7] Potassium Perchlorate, *7653*
[7778-77-0] Potassium Phosphate, Monobasic, *7659*
[7778-80-5] Potassium Sulfate, *7674*
[7779-25-1] Magnesium Citrate, *5663*

[7779-88-6] Zinc Nitrate, *10144*
[7779-90-0] Zinc Phosphate, *10151*
[7782-39-0] Deuterium, *2939*
[7782-40-3] Diamond, *2987*
[7782-41-4] Fluorine, *4162*
[7782-42-5] Graphite, *4539*
[7782-44-7] Oxygen, *6964*
[7782-49-2] Selenium, *8431*
[7782-50-5] Chlorine, *2095*
[7782-63-0] Ferrous Sulfate Heptahydrate, *4057*
[7782-64-1] Manganese Difluoride, *5729*
[7782-65-2] Germane, *4406*
[7782-68-5] Iodic Acid, *5012*
[7782-77-6] Nitrous Acid, *6652*
[7782-78-7] Nitrosylsulfuric Acid, *6648*
[7782-79-8] Hydrazoic Acid, *4774*
[7782-87-8] Potassium Hypophosphite, *7641*
[7782-89-0] Lithium Amide, *5522*
[7782-91-4] Molybdic(VI) Acid, *6240*
[7782-92-5] Sodium Amide, *8576*
[7782-94-7] Nitramide, *6572*
[7782-99-2] Sulfurous Acid, *8976*
[7783-00-8] Selenious Acid, *8430*
[7783-03-1] Tungstic(VI) Acid, *9818*
[7783-05-3] Pyrosulfuric Acid, *8009*
[7783-06-4] Hydrogen Sulfide, *4800*
[7783-07-5] Hydrogen Selenide, *4799*
[7783-08-6] Selenic Acid, *8429*
[7783-09-7] Hydrogen Telluride, *4801*
[7783-18-8] Ammonium Thiosulfate, *562*
[7783-19-9] Ammonium Selenite, *552*
[7783-20-2] Ammonium Sulfate, *555*
[7783-21-3] Ammonium Selenate, *551*
[7783-22-4] Ammonium Uranate(VI), *565*
[7783-26-8] Trisilane, *9754*
[7783-28-0] Ammonium Phosphate, Dibasic, *542*
[7783-29-1] Tetrasilane, *9239*
[7783-33-7] Potassium Tetraiodomercurate(II), *7688*
[7783-35-9] Mercuric Sulfate, *5887*
[7783-36-0] Mercurous Sulfate, *5897*
[7783-39-3] Mercuric Fluoride, *5878*
[7783-40-6] Magnesium Fluoride, *5665*
[7783-41-7] Fluorine Monoxide, *4164*
[7783-42-8] Thionyl Fluoride, *9349*
[7783-44-0] Fluorine Dioxide, *4163*
[7783-46-2] Lead Fluoride, *5408*
[7783-47-3] Stannous Fluoride, *8784*
[7783-48-4] Strontium Fluoride, *8842*
[7783-49-5] Zinc Fluoride, *10136*
[7783-50-8] Ferric Fluoride, *4022*
[7783-51-9] Gallium Trifluoride, *4354*
[7783-52-0] Indium Trifluoride, *4959*
[7783-53-1] Manganese Trifluoride, *5741*
[7783-54-2] Nitrogen Fluoride, *6604*
[7783-55-3] Phosphorus Trifluoride, *7359*
[7783-56-4] Antimony Trifluoride, *709*
[7783-58-6] Germanium Tetrafluoride, *4411*
[7783-59-7] Lead Tetrafluoride, *5424*
[7783-60-0] Sulfur Tetrafluoride, *8978*
[7783-61-1] Silicon Tetrafluoride, *8501*
[7783-62-2] Stannic Fluoride, *8776*
[7783-63-3] Titanium Tetrafluoride, *9479*
[7783-64-4] Zirconium Fluoride, *10175*

[7783-66-6] Iodine Pentafluoride, *5018*
[7783-68-8] Niobium Pentafluoride, *6558*
[7783-70-2] Antimony Pentafluoride, *696*
[7783-71-3] Tantalum Pentafluoride, *9055*
[7783-72-4] Vanadium Pentafluoride, *9920*
[7783-75-7] Iridium Hexafluoride, *5086*
[7783-77-9] Molybdenum Hexafluoride, *6237*
[7783-79-1] Selenium Hexafluoride, *8433*
[7783-80-4] Tellurium Hexafluoride, *9124*
[7783-81-5] Uranium Hexafluoride, *9856*
[7783-82-6] Tungsten Hexafluoride, *9816*
[7783-84-8] Ferric Hypophosphite, *4026*
[7783-86-0] Ferrous Iodide, *4049*
[7783-90-6] Silver Chloride, *8509*
[7783-92-8] Silver Chlorate, *8508*
[7783-93-9] Silver Perchlorate, *8523*
[7783-95-1] Silver Difluoride, *8513*
[7783-96-2] Silver Iodide, *8516*
[7783-97-3] Silver Iodate, *8515*
[7783-98-4] Silver Permanganate, *8524*
[7783-99-5] Silver Nitrite, *8519*
[7784-01-2] Silver Chromate(VI), *8510*
[7784-03-4] Silver Tetraiodomercurate(II), *8531*
[7784-09-0] Silver Phosphate, *8525*
[7784-13-6] Aluminum Chloride Hexahydrate, *337*
[7784-14-7] Ammonium Tetrachloroaluminate, *558*
[7784-15-8] Aluminum Chlorate Nonahydrate, *336*
[7784-16-9] Sodium Tetrachloroaluminate, *8687*
[7784-18-1] Aluminum Fluoride, *339*
[7784-19-2] Ammonium Hexafluoroaluminate, *524*
[7784-21-6] Aluminum Hydride, *341*
[7784-22-7] Aluminum Hypophosphite, *345*
[7784-23-8] Aluminum Iodide, *346*
[7784-25-0] Aluminum Ammonium Sulfate, *327*
[7784-30-7] Aluminum Phosphate, *358*
[7784-33-0] Arsenic Tribromide, *800*
[7784-34-1] Arsenic Trichloride, *801*
[7784-35-2] Arsenic Trifluoride, *802*
[7784-36-3] Arsenic Pentafluoride, *796*
[7784-40-9] Lead Arsenate, *5399*
[7784-41-0] Potassium Arsenate, *7607*
[7784-42-1] Arsine, *809*
[7784-45-4] Arsenic Triiodide, *803*
[7784-46-5] Sodium Arsenite, *8580*
[7785-20-8] Nickel Ammonium Sulfate Hexahydrate, *6501*
[7785-23-1] Silver Bromide, *8506*
[7785-24-2] Cobaltous Arsenate, *2434*
[7785-84-4] Sodium Trimetaphosphate, *8696*
[7785-87-7] Manganese Sulfate, *5739*
[7786-30-3] Magnesium Chloride, *5662*
[7786-34-7] Mevinphos, *6165*
[7786-81-4] Nickel Sulfate, *6517*
[7787-32-8] Barium Fluoride, *974*
[7787-35-1] Barium Manganate(VI), *981*

[7787-36-2] Barium Permanganate, *988*
[7787-39-5] Barium Sulfite, *997*
[7787-46-4] Beryllium Bromide, *1164*
[7787-47-5] Beryllium Chloride, *1166*
[7787-49-7] Beryllium Fluoride, *1167*
[7787-52-2] Beryllium Hydride, *1168*
[7787-55-5] Beryllium Nitrate Trihydrate, *1170*
[7787-57-7] Bismuth Bromide Oxide, *1260*
[7787-58-8] Bismuth Bromide, *1259*
[7787-59-9] Bismuth Chloride Oxide, *1263*
[7787-60-2] Bismuth Chloride, *1262*
[7787-61-3] Bismuth Fluoride, *1265*
[7787-62-4] Bismuth Pentafluoride, *1274*
[7787-63-5] Bismuth Iodide Oxide, *1270*
[7787-64-6] Bismuth Iodide, *1269*
[7787-68-0] Bismuth Sulfate, *1286*
[7787-69-1] Cesium Bromide, *2009*
[7787-70-4] Cuprous Bromide, *2659*
[7787-71-5] Bromine Trifluoride, *1396*
[7788-96-7] Chromyl Fluoride, *2249*
[7788-97-8] Chromic Fluoride, *2223*
[7788-98-9] Ammonium Chromate(VI), *510*
[7789-00-6] Potassium Chromate(VI), *7622*
[7789-04-0] Chromic Phosphate, *2227*
[7789-06-2] Strontium Chromate(VI), *8841*
[7789-09-5] Ammonium Dichromate-(VI), *515*
[7789-17-5] Cesium Iodide, *2014*
[7789-18-6] Cesium Nitrate, *2015*
[7789-19-7] Cupric Fluoride, *2638*
[7789-20-0] Deuterium Oxide, *2940*
[7789-21-1] Fluorosulfonic Acid, *4179*
[7789-23-3] Potassium Fluoride, *7632*
[7789-24-4] Lithium Fluoride, *5531*
[7789-25-5] Nitrosyl Fluoride, *6647*
[7789-26-6] Fluorine Nitrate, *4165*
[7789-27-7] Thallium Fluoride, *9262*
[7789-28-8] Ferrous Fluoride, *4045*
[7789-29-9] Potassium Bifluoride, *7610*
[7789-30-2] Bromine Pentafluoride, *1395*
[7789-31-3] Bromic Acid, *1392*
[7789-33-5] Iodine Monobromide, *5016*
[7789-38-0] Sodium Bromate, *8593*
[7789-39-1] Rubidium Bromide, *8283*
[7789-40-4] Thallium Bromide, *9258*
[7789-41-5] Calcium Bromide, *1654*
[7789-42-6] Cadmium Bromide, *1615*
[7789-43-7] Cobaltous Bromide, *2435*
[7789-45-9] Cupric Bromide, *2629*
[7789-46-0] Ferrous Bromide, *4042*
[7789-47-1] Mercuric Bromide, *5875*
[7789-48-2] Magnesium Bromide, *5659*
[7789-57-3] Tribromosilane, *9615*
[7789-59-5] Phosphorus Oxybromide, *7348*
[7789-60-8] Phosphorus Tribromide, *7357*
[7789-61-9] Antimony Tribromide, *706*
[7789-65-3] Selenium Tetrabromide, *8437*
[7789-66-4] Silicon Tetrabromide, *8499*
[7789-67-5] Stannic Bromide, *8773*
[7789-68-6] Titanium Tetrabromide, *9477*
[7789-69-7] Phosphorus Pentabromide, *7350*

[7789-75-5] Calcium Fluoride, *1667*
[7789-78-8] Calcium Hydride, *1672*
[7789-79-9] Calcium Hypophosphite, *1675*
[7789-80-2] Calcium Iodate, *1676*
[7789-82-4] Calcium Molybdate(VI), *1681*
[7790-21-8] Potassium Periodate, *7654*
[7790-26-3] Sodium Iodide, Radioactive, *8632*
[7790-28-5] Sodium Metaperiodate, *8640*
[7790-29-6] Rubidium Iodide, *8286*
[7790-30-9] Thallium Iodide, *9264*
[7790-33-2] Manganese Iodide, *5732*
[7790-37-6] Zinc Iodate, *10139*
[7790-44-5] Antimony Triiodide, *710*
[7790-47-8] Stannic Iodide, *8777*
[7790-48-9] Tellurium Tetraiodide, *9127*
[7790-53-6] Potassium Metaphosphate, *7646*
[7790-58-1] Potassium Tellurate(IV), *7678*
[7790-59-2] Potassium Selenate, *7666*
[7790-60-5] Potassium Tungstate(VI), *7694*
[7790-62-7] Potassium Pyrosulfate, *7664*
[7790-63-8] Potassium Uranate(VI), *7695*
[7790-69-4] Lithium Nitrate, *5536*
[7790-75-2] Calcium Tungstate(VI), *1712*
[7790-79-6] Cadmium Fluoride, *1619*
[7790-80-9] Cadmium Iodide, *1621*
[7790-84-3] Cadmium Sulfate Hydrate, *1627*
[7790-85-4] Cadmium Tungstate(VI), *1630*
[7790-86-5] Cerous Chloride, *1997*
[7790-87-6] Cerous Iodide, *1999*
[7790-89-8] Chlorine Monofluoride, *2098*
[7790-91-2] Chlorine Trifluoride, *2100*
[7790-92-3] Hypochlorous Acid, *4865*
[7790-93-4] Chloric Acid, *2092*
[7790-94-5] Chlorosulfonic Acid, *2165*
[7790-98-9] Ammonium Perchlorate, *540*
[7790-99-0] Iodine Monochloride, *5017*
[7791-03-9] Lithium Perchlorate, *5539*
[7791-08-4] Antimony Chloride Oxide, *693*
[7791-10-8] Strontium Chlorate, *8839*
[7791-11-9] Rubidium Chloride, *8284*
[7791-12-0] Thallium Chloride, *9260*
[7791-13-1] Cobaltous Chloride Hexahydrate, *2437*
[7791-16-4] Antimony Dichlorotrifluoride, *694*
[7791-20-0] Nickel Chloride Hexahydrate, *6505*
[7791-21-1] Chlorine Monoxide, *2099*
[7791-23-3] Selenium Oxychloride, *8435*
[7791-25-5] Sulfuryl Chloride, *8980*
[7791-26-6] Uranyl Chloride, *9862*
[7795-51-9] α-Methyltryptamine (*S*)-Form, *6131*
[7795-52-0] α-Methyltryptamine (*R*)-Form, *6131*
[7798-23-4] Cupric Phosphate, *2648*
[7803-49-8] Hydroxylamine, *4828*

[7803-51-2] Phosphine, *7338*
[7803-52-3] Stibine, *8811*
[7803-54-5] Magnesium Amide, *5656*
[7803-55-6] Ammonium Vanadate(V), *568*
[7803-57-8] Hydrazine Hydrate, *4771*
[7803-58-9] Sulfamide, *8922*
[7803-60-3] Hypophosphoric Acid, *4867*
[7803-62-5] Silane, *8488*
[7803-63-6] Ammonium Bisulfate, *500*
[7803-65-8] Ammonium Hypophosphite, *528*
[7803-68-1] Telluric(VI) Acid, *9120*
[8000-10-0] Theophylline Sodium Glycinate, *9285*
[8000-25-7] Oil of Rosemary, *8264*
[8000-28-0] Oil of Lavender, *5390*
[8000-42-8] Oil of Caraway, *1777*
[8000-48-4] Oil of Eucalyptus, *3896*
[8000-61-1] Aluminum Subacetate Solution, *365*
[8000-66-6] Oil of Cardamom, *1834*
[8000-68-8] Parsley Seed Oil, *7046*
[8000-78-0] Oil of Garlic, *4370*
[8001-08-9] Acerin, *34*
[8001-27-2] Hirudin, *4718*
[8001-35-2] Toxaphene, *9557*
[8001-39-6] Japan Wax, *5256*
[8001-40-9] Iodized Oil, *5024*
[8001-54-5] Benzalkonium Chloride, *1059*
[8001-58-9] Creosote, Coal Tar, *2572*
[8001-60-3] Coparaffinate, *2518*
[8001-61-4] Copaiba, *2516*
[8001-75-0] Ceresin, *1987*
[8001-95-4] Alseroxylon, *8120*
[8002-36-6] Ustilagic Acid, *9894*
[8002-41-3] Laurel Berry Oil, *5382*
[8002-43-5] Lecithins, *5428*
[8002-53-7] Montan Wax, *6257*
[8002-55-9] Myrtol, *6339*
[8002-65-1] Neem Fixed Oil, *6437*
[8002-66-2] German Chamomile Oil, *2041*
[8002-68-4] Oil of Juniper, *5270*
[8002-75-3] Palm Oil, *6818*
[8002-76-4] Papaveretum, *7018*
[8002-88-8] Theobromine Sodium Acetate, *9282*
[8002-89-9] Theophylline Sodium Acetate, *9285*
[8003-05-2] Phenylmercuric Nitrate, Basic, *7302*
[8003-22-3] Quinoline Yellow Spirit Soluble, *8072*
[8004-38-4] Fenbutrazate Hydrochloride Mixture with Phenmetrazine Theoclate, *3965*
[8004-92-0] Quinoline Yellow, *8071*
[8005-78-5] Bismark Brown R, *1252*
[8006-08-4] Ergotinine, *3664*
[8006-13-1] Aluminum Acetate Solution, *324*
[8006-25-5] Ergotoxine, *3665*
[8006-28-8] Soda Lime, *8569*
[8006-44-8] Candelilla Wax, *1738*
[8006-54-0] Lanolin, *5358*
[8006-64-2] Turpentine Oil, *9826*
[8006-77-7] Oil of Pimenta, *7432*
[8006-80-2] Oil of Sassafras, *8381*
[8006-82-4] Black Pepper Oil, *1313*
[8006-84-6] Oil of Fennel, *3977*
[8006-87-9] Oil of Santal, *8353*

[8006-90-4] Oil of Peppermint, *7145*
[8006-91-5] Dextri-Maltose®, *2952*
[8007-04-3] Oil of Hops, *4745*
[8007-06-5] Oil of Cascarilla, *1881*
[8007-08-7] Oil of Ginger, *4423*
[8007-14-5] Argol, *782*
[8007-20-3] Oil of Cedar Leaf, *9389*
[8007-31-6] Toughened Silver Nitrate, *8518*
[8007-44-1] Pennyroyal American Pennyroyal Oil, *7102*
[8007-56-5] Nitrohydrochloric Acid, *6609*
[8007-61-2] Verdigris, *2624*
[8007-70-3] Oil of Anise, *664*
[8007-80-5] Oil of Cassia, *2300*
[8007-87-2] Oil of Cubeb, *2612*
[8008-20-6] Kerosene, *5294*
[8008-45-5] Oil of Nutmeg, *6729*
[8008-52-4] Oil of Coriander, *2531*
[8008-53-5] Ethiodized Oil, *3735*
[8008-79-5] Oil of Spearmint, *8738*
[8008-88-6] Oil of Valerian, *9903*
[8008-93-3] Oil of Wormwood, *10052*
[8011-61-8] Tyrocidine, *9836*
[8011-62-9] Barium Sulfide, Black, *996*
[8011-63-0] Bordeaux Mixture, *1335*
[8012-89-3] Beeswax, *1020*
[8013-17-0] Invert Sugar, *5006*
[8013-43-2] Spirit of Ether, *8755*
[8013-44-3] Spirit of Ether Compound, *8756*
[8013-59-0] Spirit of Ammonia, Aromatic, *8754*
[8013-61-4] Ammonium Acetate Solution, *495*
[8013-75-0] Fusel Oil, *4316*
[8013-88-5] Calcium Cyanamide Citrated, *1663*
[8013-97-6] Oil of Copaiba, *2516*
[8013-99-8] Oil of Pennyroyal, *7102*
[8014-63-9] Seidlitz Mixture, *8423*
[8014-95-7] Sulfuric Acid, Fuming, *8974*
[8015-14-3] Lynestrenol Mixture with Mestranol, *5629*
[8015-18-7] Pfeiffer's Substance, *7194*
[8015-19-8] Dimethisterone Mixture with Ethinyl Estradiol, *3219*
[8015-30-3] Norethynodrel Mixture with Mestranol, *6698*
[8015-51-8] Cropropamide Combination with Crotethamide, *2591*
[8015-64-3] Angelica Root Oil, *645*
[8015-79-0] Oil of Calamus, *1637*
[8015-86-9] Carnauba Wax, *1846*
[8015-91-6] Oil of Cinnamon, *2300*
[8015-92-7] Roman Chamomile Oil, *2041*
[8016-69-1] Oil of Asarum, *825*
[8016-78-2] Spike Lavender Oil, *5390*
[8018-01-7] Mancozeb, *5716*
[8018-15-3] Mercumallylic Acid Sodium Salt Compd with Theophylline, *5872*
[8021-39-4] Creosote, Wood, *2573*
[8022-00-2] Methyl Demeton, *6051*
[8022-07-9] Oil of Yarrow, *105*
[8022-15-9] Lavandin Oil, *5390*
[8023-62-9] Storax, *8819*
[8023-79-8] Palm Kernel Oil, *6818*
[8024-00-8] Oil of Savin, *8387*
[8025-81-8] Spiramycin, *8752*
[8027-28-9] Sodium Phosphate, Radioactive, *8661*

[8027-33-6] Lanolin Alcohols, *5359*
[8029-68-3] Ichthammol, *4885*
[8030-30-6] Petroleum Benzin, *7188*
[8030-97-5] Pyroligneous Acid, *8003*
[8031-14-9] Oxychlorosene, *6956*
[8031-21-8] Napalm, *6366*
[8031-66-1] Osmaron B, *6890*
[8032-32-4] Ligroin, *5489*
[8038-65-1] Ambergris, *381*
[8047-13-0] Ryania, *8306*
[8047-67-4] Iron Sucrose, *5101*
[8048-16-6] Streptodornase Mixture with Streptokinase, *8823*
[8048-31-5] Theobromine Sodium Salicylate, *9282*
[8048-52-0] Acriflavine, *123*
[8049-11-4] Devarda's Metal, *2941*
[8049-20-5] Misch Metal, *6209*
[8049-47-6] Pancreatic Extract, *7006*
[8049-62-5] Zinc Insulin, *4980*
[8049-99-8] Milorganite®, *6195*
[8050-07-5] Olibanum, *6832*
[8050-81-5] Simethicone, *3215*
[8050-88-2] Celluloid, *1964*
[8051-02-3] Sabadilla, *8308*
[8052-16-2] Cactinomycin, *1606*
[8052-27-5] Kino, *5313*
[8052-41-3] Mineral Spirits Type I, *6201*
[8053-05-2] Yellow Phenolphthalein, *7243*
[8053-39-2] Horse Chestnut Seed Extract, *4748*
[8056-51-7] Norgestrel Mixture with Ethinyl Estradiol, *6704*
[8063-06-7] Curare, *2671*
[8063-07-8] Kanamycin, *5281*
[8063-16-9] Psyllium Seed Gum, *7517*
[8063-24-9] Acriflavine Dihydrochloride, *123*
[8064-12-8] Meglumine Diatrizoate Mixture with Sodium Diatrizoate, *5807*
[8064-51-5] Megestrol Acetate Mixture with Mestranol, *5805*
[8064-66-2] Megestrol Acetate Mixture with Ethinyl Estradiol, *5805*
[8064-73-1] Tioxolone Combination with Hydrocortisone, *9456*
[8064-75-3] Norgesterone Mixture with Ethinyl Estradiol, *6702*
[8064-76-4] Lynestrenol Mixture with Ethinyl Estradiol, *5629*
[8064-90-2] Sulfamethoxazole Mixture with Trimethoprim, *8918*
[8065-48-3] Demeton, *2889*
[8065-51-8] Theobromine Calcium Salicylate, *9282*
[8065-91-6] Chlormadinone Acetate Mixture with Mestranol, *2102*
[8067-24-1] Ergoloid Mesylates, *3653*
[8067-82-1] Alfaxalone Mixture with Alfadolone Acetate, *235*
[8068-28-8] Colistin Sodium Methanesulfonate, *2479*
[8069-64-5] Meralluride, *5866*
[8075-95-4] Clofibrate Mixture with Androsterone, *2377*
[8075-98-7] Ascorbigen, *831*
[9000-01-5] Acacia, *14*
[9000-02-6] Amber, *380*
[9000-03-7] Ammoniacum, *493*
[9000-04-8] Asafetida, *821*
[9000-05-9] Gum Benzoin, *4580*

[9000-07-1] Carrageenan, *1864*
[9000-14-0] Copal, *2517*
[9000-16-2] Damar, *2807*
[9000-21-9] Furcellaran, *4302*
[9000-25-3] Gamboge, *4360*
[9000-28-6] Ghatti Gum, *4416*
[9000-29-7] Guaiac, *4552*
[9000-30-0] Guaran, *4571*
[9000-30-0] Guar Gum, *4572*
[9000-32-2] Gutta-Percha, *4583*
[9000-34-4] Resin Ipomea, *8148*
[9000-35-5] Resin Jalap, *8149*
[9000-36-6] Karaya Gum, *5284*
[9000-45-7] Myrrh, *6338*
[9000-47-9] Mesquite Gum, *5914*
[9000-55-9] Podophyllin, *7547*
[9000-58-2] Resin Scammony, *8150*
[9000-59-3] Shellac, *8478*
[9000-65-1] Gum Tragacanth, *4581*
[9000-69-5] Pectin, *7063*
[9000-70-8] Gelatin, *4382*
[9000-71-9] Casein, *1883*
[9000-85-5] α-Amylase (Bacterial), *599*
[9000-88-8] D-Amino Acid Oxidase, *414*
[9000-89-9] L-Amino Acid Oxidase, *415*
[9000-90-2] α-Amylase (Porcine), *599*
[9000-91-3] β-Amylase (Sweet Potato), *599*
[9000-92-4] Amylase, *599*
[9000-95-7] Apyrase, *759*
[9001-00-7] Bromelain, *1388*
[9001-01-8] Kallikrein, *5279*
[9001-03-0] Carbonic Anhydrase, *1812*
[9001-04-1] Pyruvate Decarboxylase, *8020*
[9001-05-2] Catalase, *1900*
[9001-08-5] Choline Esterase, *2208*
[9001-09-6] Chymopapain, *2259*
[9001-12-1] Collagenase, *2481*
[9001-19-8] Taka-Diastase, *9031*
[9001-24-5] Factor V, *3919*
[9001-25-6] Factor VII, *3920*
[9001-26-7] Prothrombin, *7889*
[9001-27-8] Factor VIII, *3921*
[9001-28-9] Factor IX, *3922*
[9001-29-0] Factor X, *3923*
[9001-30-3] Factor XII, *3925*
[9001-31-4] Fibrin, *4070*
[9001-32-5] Fibrinogen, *4071*
[9001-33-6] Ficin, *4077*
[9001-37-0] Glucose Oxidase, *4460*
[9001-45-0] β-Glucuronidase, *4466*
[9001-53-0] Diamine Oxidase, *2975*
[9001-54-1] Hyaluronidases, *4758*
[9001-57-4] Invertase, *5005*
[9001-60-9] Lactate Dehydrogenase, *5334*
[9001-62-1] Lipase, *5511*
[9001-63-2] Lysozyme, *5640*
[9001-66-5] Monoamine Oxidase, *6247*
[9001-68-7] Old Yellow Enzyme, *6824*
[9001-73-4] Papain, *7016*
[9001-74-5] Penicillinase, *7093*
[9001-75-6] Pepsin, *7146*
[9001-90-5] Plasmin, *7520*
[9001-91-6] Plasminogen, *7521*
[9001-97-2] Q-Enzyme, *8023*
[9001-98-3] Rennin, *8134*
[9001-99-4] Ribonuclease, *8202*
[9002-01-1] Streptokinase, *8825*
[9002-04-4] Thrombin, *9383*
[9002-07-7] Trypsin, *9795*

[9002-10-2] Tyrosinase, *9838*
[9002-12-4] Uricase, *9876*
[9002-13-5] Urease, *9870*
[9002-18-0] Agar, *184*
[9002-60-2] ACTH, *134*
[9002-61-3] Chorionic Gonadotropin (Human), *2216*
[9002-62-4] Prolactin, *7779*
[9002-64-6] Parathyroid Hormone, *7034*
[9002-67-9] Luteinizing Hormone, *5613*
[9002-68-0] Follicle-Stimulating Hormone, *4223*
[9002-69-1] Relaxin, *8129*
[9002-70-4] Chorionic Gonadotropin (Equine), *2216*
[9002-71-5] Thyrotropin, *9414*
[9002-72-6] Somatotropin, *8716*
[9002-84-0] Polytetrafluoroethylene, *7583*
[9002-86-2] Polyvinyl Chloride, *7586*
[9002-88-4] Polyethylene, *7567*
[9002-89-5] Polyvinyl Alcohol, *7585*
[9002-91-9] Metaldehyde, *5923*
[9002-92-0] Polidocanol, *7558*
[9002-93-1] Octoxynol, *6761*
[9003-07-0] Polypropylene, *7581*
[9003-11-6] Poloxalene, *7562*
[9003-24-1] Darvan®, *2828*
[9003-39-8] Povidone, *7697*
[9003-59-2] Sodium Polystyrene Sulfonate, *8668*
[9003-97-8] Calcium Polycarbophil, *1697*
[9003-98-9] Deoxyribonuclease I, *2906*
[9004-02-8] Lipoprotein Lipase, *5512*
[9004-07-3] α-Chymotrypsin, *2260*
[9004-10-8] Insulin, *4980*
[9004-17-5] Protamine Zinc Insulin, *4980*
[9004-32-4] Carboxymethylcellulose Sodium, *1829*
[9004-34-6] Cellulose, *1965*
[9004-53-9] Dextrin, *2953*
[9004-54-0] Dextran, *2948*
[9004-57-3] Ethyl Cellulose, *3781*
[9004-58-4] Cellulose Ethyl Hydroxyethyl Ether, *1967*
[9004-61-9] Hyaluronic Acid, *4757*
[9004-62-0] Hetastarch, *4673*
[9004-64-2] Hydroxypropyl Cellulose, *4841*
[9004-65-3] Hydroxypropyl Methylcellulose, *4842*
[9004-66-4] Iron Dextran, *5094*
[9004-67-5] Methylcellulose, *6040*
[9004-70-0] Pyroxylin, *8011*
[9005-32-7] Alginic Acid, *242*
[9005-35-0] Alginic Acid Calcium Salt, *242*
[9005-38-3] Algin, *241*
[9005-48-5] Heparin Potassium Salt, *4653*
[9005-49-6] Heparin, *4653*
[9005-53-2] Lignin, *5487*
[9005-65-6] Polysorbate 80, *7582*
[9005-79-2] Glycogen, *4496*
[9005-80-5] Inulin, *5004*
[9005-84-9] Starch, Soluble, *8799*
[9005-90-7] Turpentine, *9826*
[9005-97-4] Thyroprotein, *9413*
[9006-58-0] Lysalbinic Acid, *5631*
[9006-65-9] Dimethicone, *3215*

[9007-03-8] Bifidus Factor, *1211*
[9007-12-9] Calcitonin, *1643*
[9007-20-9] Carboxypolymethylene, *1830*
[9007-28-7] Chondroitin Sulfate, *2214*
[9007-31-2] Clupeine, *2424*
[9007-40-3] Crotoxin, *2599*
[9007-41-4] CRP, *2603*
[9007-43-6] Cytochrome *c*, *2791*
[9007-57-2] Edestin, *3509*
[9007-67-4] Enterogastrone, *3597*
[9007-73-2] Ferritin, *4036*
[9007-76-5] Fibroin, *4073*
[9007-90-3] Gliadin, *4437*
[9007-92-5] Glucagon, *4446*
[9007-93-6] Glycinin, *4493*
[9008-08-6] Hypalon®, *4860*
[9008-19-9] Krebiozen, *5323*
[9008-22-4] Laminaran, *5350*
[9008-96-2] Phosvitin, *7365*
[9008-99-5] Piromen, *7504*
[9009-58-9] Porphyropsin, *7601*
[9009-72-7] Purothionin, *7944*
[9009-81-8] Rhodopsin, *8192*
[9009-86-3] Ricin, *8209*
[9010-01-9] Sodium Amylosulfate, *8577*
[9010-30-4] Taraxein, *9061*
[9010-71-3] Zinc Iodide-Starch, *10141*
[9010-72-4] Zymosan, *10200*
[9011-02-3] Policresulen, *7556*
[9011-05-6] Ureaform, *9868*
[9011-18-1] Dextran Sulfate Sodium, *2951*
[9011-93-2] Lysostaphin, *5639*
[9011-97-6] Cholecystokinin, *2198*
[9012-92-4] Oxycodone Pectinate, *6959*
[9013-55-2] Factor XI, *3924*
[9013-56-3] Factor XIII, *3926*
[9013-83-6] Insulinase, *4981*
[9014-02-2] Zinostatin, *10167*
[9014-44-2] Toxohormone, *9560*
[9014-67-9] Aloxiprin, *309*
[9015-13-8] ECTEOLA-Cellulose, *3504*
[9015-51-4] Silver Protein, *8527*
[9015-68-3] L-Asparaginase, *836*
[9015-71-8] CRF, *2586*
[9015-73-0] Detaxtran, *2936*
[9015-94-5] Renin, *8133*
[9025-41-6] Keratinase, *5292*
[9025-70-1] Dextranase, *2949*
[9025-75-6] Calcineurin, *1640*
[9031-37-2] Ceruloplasmin, *2006*
[9034-40-6] LH-RH, *5474*
[9034-50-8] Vasopressin, *9938*
[9035-55-6] Lipotropic Hormone, *5513*
[9035-58-9] Thromboplastin, *9385*
[9035-68-1] Proinsulin, *7778*
[9037-22-3] Amioca, *481*
[9037-24-5] Amberlyst 15®, *383*
[9038-41-9] Sodium Cellulose Phosphate, *8597*
[9039-53-6] Urokinase, *9887*
[9039-61-6] Batroxobin, *1010*
[9040-61-3] Staphylokinase, *8796*
[9041-08-1] Heparin Sodium Salt, *4653*
[9041-92-3] α₁-Antitrypsin, *719*
[9041-93-4] Bleomycins Sulfate, *1318*
[9044-70-6] Coherin, *2469*
[9046-56-4] Ancrod, *630*
[9048-46-8] Serum Albumin, *8468*
[9050-67-3] Sizofiran, *8559*
[9054-89-1] Superoxide Dismutase, *9002*

[9061-61-4] Nerve Growth Factor, *6477*
[9063-57-4] Tuftsin, *9809*
[9064-91-9] Detaxtran Hydrochloride, *2936*
[9064-92-0] Polidexide, *7557*
[9066-59-5] Lysozyme Hydrochloride, *5640*
[9067-32-7] Hyaluronic Acid Sodium Salt, *4757*
[9073-56-7] α-L-Iduronidase, *4894*
[9073-78-3] Thermolysin, *9286*
[9079-25-8] Amberlite®, *382*
[9083-38-9] Melanostatin, *5813*
[9087-70-1] Aprotinin, *757*
[10001-43-1] Pimefylline, *7430*
[10004-44-1] Hymexazol, *4856*
[10010-67-0] PIPES Monosodium Salt, *7479*
[10017-44-4] Carnitine D-Form Hydrochloride, *1849*
[10018-19-6] Cotarnine Chloride, *2552*
[10022-31-8] Barium Nitrate, *983*
[10022-50-1] Nitryl Fluoride, *6658*
[10023-07-1] Frenolicin, *4269*
[10024-97-2] Nitrous Oxide, *6653*
[10025-65-7] Platinous Chloride, *7528*
[10025-66-8] Radium Chloride, *8094*
[10025-67-9] Sulfur Chloride, *8970*
[10025-68-0] Selenium Chloride, *8432*
[10025-69-1] Stannous Chloride Dihydrate, *8783*
[10025-70-4] Strontium Chloride Hexahydrate, *8840*
[10025-71-5] Tellurium Dichloride, *9122*
[10025-73-7] Chromic Chloride, *2222*
[10025-78-2] Trichlorosilane, *9646*
[10025-82-8] Indium Trichloride, *4958*
[10025-83-9] Iridium Trichloride, *5088*
[10025-85-1] Nitrogen Chloride, *6602*
[10025-87-3] Phosphorus Oxychloride, *7349*
[10025-91-9] Antimony Trichloride, *707*
[10025-91-9] Antimony Trichloride Solution, *708*
[10025-93-1] Uranium Trichloride, *9859*
[10025-99-7] Potassium Tetrachloroplatinate(II), *7682*
[10026-03-6] Selenium Tetrachloride, *8438*
[10026-04-7] Silicon Tetrachloride, *8500*
[10026-07-0] Tellurium Tetrachloride, *9126*
[10026-08-1] Thorium Chloride, *9375*
[10026-10-5] Uranium Tetrachloride, *9857*
[10026-11-6] Zirconium Chloride, *10174*
[10026-12-7] Niobium Pentachloride, *6557*
[10026-13-8] Phosphorus Pentachloride, *7351*
[10026-17-2] Cobaltous Fluoride, *2440*
[10026-18-3] Cobaltic Fluoride, *2430*
[10026-22-9] Cobaltous Nitrate Hexahydrate, *2444*
[10026-24-1] Cobaltous Sulfate Heptahydrate, *2448*
[10028-14-5] Nobelium, *6664*
[10028-15-6] Ozone, *6981*
[10028-17-8] Tritium, *9762*

[10028-18-9] Nickel Fluoride, *6508*
[10028-22-5] Ferric Sulfate, *4032*
[10030-90-7] Ferrous Succinate, *4056*
[10031-13-7] Lead Arsenite, *5400*
[10031-18-2] Mercurous Bromide, *5893*
[10031-22-8] Lead Bromide, *5403*
[10031-23-9] Radium Bromide, *8094*
[10031-24-0] Stannous Bromide, *8782*
[10031-25-1] Chromic Bromide, *2220*
[10031-26-2] Ferric Bromide, *4018*
[10031-27-3] Tellurium Tetrabromide, *9125*
[10034-81-8] Magnesium Perchlorate, *5678*
[10034-85-2] Hydriodic Acid, *4776*
[10034-85-2] Hydrogen Iodide, *4797*
[10034-93-2] Hydrazine Sulfate, *4772*
[10034-94-3] Magnesium Orthosilicate, *5687*
[10034-99-8] Magnesium Sulfate Heptahydrate, *5691*
[10035-05-9] Calcium Chlorate Dihydrate, *1658*
[10035-10-6] Hydrobromic Acid, *4778*
[10035-10-6] Hydrogen Bromide, *4793*
[10038-98-9] Germanium Tetrachloride, *4410*
[10039-53-9] Sodium Chromate(VI) ^{51}Cr-Labeled Compound, *8601*
[10039-54-0] Hydroxylamine Sulfate, *4828*
[10040-45-6] Picosulfate Sodium, *7406*
[10042-76-9] Strontium Nitrate, *8845*
[10043-01-3] Aluminum Sulfate, *366*
[10043-11-5] Boron Nitride, *1346*
[10043-35-3] Boric Acid, *1336*
[10043-49-9] Gold, Radioactive, Colloidal, *4517*
[10043-52-4] Calcium Chloride, *1659*
[10043-67-1] Aluminum Potassium Sulfate, *360*
[10043-84-2] Manganese Hypophosphite, *5731*
[10043-92-2] Radon, *8095*
[10045-86-0] Ferric Phosphate, *4029*
[10045-89-3] Ammonium Ferrous Sulfate, *521*
[10045-94-0] Mercuric Nitrate, *5880*
[10048-32-5] Parasorbic Acid, *7032*
[10048-98-3] Barium Phosphate, Dibasic, *990*
[10048-99-4] Barium Mercuric Iodide, *982*
[10049-01-1] Bismuth Phosphate, *1275*
[10049-04-4] Chlorine Dioxide, *2096*
[10049-05-5] Chromous Chloride, *2244*
[10049-06-6] Titanium Dichloride, *9471*
[10049-07-7] Rhodium Chloride, *8188*
[10049-08-8] Ruthenium Trichloride, *8302*
[10049-10-2] Chromous Fluoride, *2245*
[10049-12-4] Vanadium Trifluoride, *9922*
[10049-14-6] Uranium Tetrafluoride, *9858*
[10049-17-9] Rhenium Hexafluoride, *8179*
[10049-18-0] Ferric Pyrophosphate Nonahydrate, *4030*
[10049-23-7] Tellurous Acid, *9128*
[10049-25-9] Chromous Bromide, *2243*
[10058-07-8] Pimefylline Nicotinate, *7430*

[10058-44-3] Ferric Pyrophosphate, *4030*
[10060-10-3] Ceric Fluoride, *1988*
[10060-11-4] Germanium Dichloride, *4408*
[10061-01-5] 1,3-Dichloropropene *cis*-Form, *3075*
[10061-02-6] 1,3-Dichloropropene *trans*-Form, *3075*
[10072-50-1] Polymyxin D$_1$, *7573*
[10075-24-8] Imipramine Pamoate, *4920*
[10075-36-2] Isoaminile Cyclamate, *5110*
[10075-85-1] 9,10-Bis(phenylethynyl)-anthracene, *1299*
[10085-81-1] Benzoctamine Hydrochloride, *1087*
[10088-95-6] Radicinin, *8093*
[10090-54-7] Potassium Pyroantimonate, Acid, *7662*
[10097-28-6] Silicon Monoxide, *8496*
[10097-84-4] Tetrahydropalmatine, *9215*
[10099-74-8] Lead Nitrate, *5414*
[10099-79-3] Lead Vanadate(V), *5427*
[10101-50-5] Sodium Permanganate, *8654*
[10101-52-7] Zirconium Silicate, *10181*
[10101-53-8] Chromic Sulfate, *2230*
[10101-63-0] Lead Iodide, *5411*
[10101-83-4] Sodium Tellurate(VI), *8686*
[10101-88-9] Sodium Thiophosphate, *8693*
[10101-97-0] Nickel Sulfate Hexahydrate, *6517*
[10101-98-1] Nickel Sulfate Heptahydrate, *6517*
[10102-03-1] Nitrogen Pentoxide, *6605*
[10102-05-3] Palladium Nitrate, *6992*
[10102-18-8] Sodium Selenite, *8673*
[10102-20-2] Sodium Tellurate(IV), *8685*
[10102-23-5] Sodium Selenate Decahydrate, *8671*
[10102-24-6] Lithium Silicate, *5540*
[10102-40-6] Sodium Molybdate(VI) Dihydrate, *8645*
[10102-43-9] Nitric Oxide, *6578*
[10102-44-0] Nitrogen Dioxide, *6603*
[10102-45-1] Thallium Mononitrate, *9265*
[10102-68-8] Calcium Iodide, *1677*
[10102-71-3] Aluminum Sodium Sulfate, *363*
[10108-64-2] Cadmium Chloride, *1617*
[10108-73-3] Cerous Nitrate, *2000*
[10112-91-1] Mercurous Chloride, *5894*
[10114-58-6] Bismark Brown Y, *1253*
[10116-22-0] Demegestone, *2888*
[10117-38-1] Potassium Sulfite, *7676*
[10118-56-6] Cascarillin, *1882*
[10118-76-0] Calcium Permanganate, *1688*
[10118-90-8] Minocycline, *6202*
[10124-36-4] Cadmium Sulfate, *1627*
[10124-37-5] Calcium Nitrate, *1682*
[10124-43-3] Cobaltous Sulfate, *2448*
[10124-53-5] Magnesium Thiosulfate, *5694*
[10129-92-7] Eledoisin Trifluoroacetate, *3539*
[10137-74-3] Calcium Chlorate, *1658*

[10138-04-2] Ammonium Ferric Sulfate, 518
[10139-06-7] Linatine, 5499
[10139-47-6] Zinc Iodide, 10140
[10139-51-2] Nitric Acid Ammonium Cerium Salt, 1992
[10140-70-2] Curvularin (nitric acid ammonium cerium salt), 2676
[10141-00-1] Chromic Potassium Sulfate, 2229
[10141-05-6] Cobaltous Nitrate, 2444
[10161-33-8] Trenbolone, 9583
[10161-34-9] Trenbolone Acetate, 9583
[10170-69-1] Manganese Carbonyl, 5727
[10190-55-3] Lead Molybdate(VI), 5412
[10191-41-0] dl-α-Tocopherol, 9495
[10192-30-0] Ammonium Bisulfite, 502
[10196-04-0] Ammonium Sulfite, 557
[10199-21-0] Guanidinium Aluminum Sulfate Hexahydrate, 4563
[10210-64-7] Beryllium Acetylacetonate, 1163
[10210-68-1] Dicobalt Octacarbonyl, 3085
[10212-25-6] Ancitabine Hydrochloride, 629
[10213-09-9] Vanadyl Dichloride, 9925
[10213-10-2] Sodium Tungstate(VI) Dihydrate, 8698
[10214-39-8] Lead Borate, 5402
[10236-47-2] Naringin, 6425
[10236-58-5] Selenocysteine, 8440
[10238-21-8] Glyburide, 4478
[10246-75-0] Hydroxyzine Pamoate, 4849
[10252-34-3] Sporidesmolide IV, 8765
[10257-54-2] Cupric Sulfate Monohydrate, 2653
[10257-55-3] Calcium Sulfite, 1708
[10262-69-8] Maprotiline, 5748
[10265-92-6] Methamidophos, 5947
[10290-12-7] Cupric Arsenite, 2626
[10294-26-5] Silver Sulfate, 8529
[10294-29-8] Gold Monochloride, 4515
[10294-33-4] Boron Tribromide, 1347
[10294-34-5] Boron Trichloride, 1348
[10294-40-3] Barium Chromate(VI), 972
[10294-48-1] Chlorine Heptoxide, 2097
[10294-52-7] Ferric Chromate(VI), 4020
[10294-54-9] Cesium Sulfate, 2016
[10294-64-1] Potassium Manganate-(VI), 7644
[10294-66-3] Potassium Thiosulfate, 7692
[10294-70-9] Stannous Iodide, 8785
[10297-61-7] Propylure, 7870
[10310-32-4] Tribenoside, 9608
[10318-26-0] Mitolactol, 6214
[10321-12-7] Propizepine, 7833
[10325-94-7] Cadmium Nitrate, 1622
[10326-21-3] Magnesium Chlorate, 5661
[10326-24-6] Zinc Meta-arsenite, 10143
[10326-41-7] D-Lactic Acid, 5335
[10331-57-4] Niclofolan, 6518
[10343-61-0] Titanium Sesquisulfate, 9476
[10347-81-6] Maprotiline Hydrochloride, 5748
[10352-73-5] Pseudopederin, 7065

[10361-03-2] Maddrell's Salt, 5647
[10361-29-2] Ammonium Carbonate, 508
[10361-37-2] Barium Chloride, 971
[10361-43-0] Bismuth Hydroxide, 1267
[10361-44-1] Bismuth Nitrate, 1271
[10373-81-6] 3-Hydroxycamphor, 4817
[10376-48-4] Shionone, 8481
[10377-48-7] Lithium Sulfate, 5541
[10377-51-2] Lithium Iodide, 5535
[10377-58-9] Magnesium Iodide, 5671
[10377-60-3] Magnesium Nitrate, 5674
[10377-62-5] Magnesium Permanganate, 5679
[10377-66-9] Manganese Nitrate, 5733
[10379-14-3] Tetrazepam, 9243
[10380-31-1] Barium Uranium Oxide, 1001
[10381-36-9] Nickel Phosphate, 6515
[10389-72-7] Clortermine Hydrochloride, 2410
[10389-73-8] Clortermine, 2410
[10397-75-8] Iocarmic Acid, 5009
[10402-53-6] Eprazinone Dihydrochloride, 3632
[10402-90-1] Eprazinone, 3632
[10405-02-4] Trospium Chloride, 9786
[10415-75-5] Mercurous Nitrate, 5896
[10417-94-4] Eicosapentaenoic Acid, 3531
[10418-03-8] Stanozolol (2′H form), 8794
[10421-48-4] Ferric Nitrate, 4027
[10450-55-2] Ferric Acetate, Basic, 4016
[10450-60-9] Periodic Acid, 7171
[10453-86-8] Resmethrin, 8153
[10453-89-1] Chrysanthemic Acid, 2251
[10457-66-6] Geranylhydroquinone, 4405
[10457-90-6] Bromperidol, 1442
[10476-81-0] Strontium Bromide, 8837
[10476-85-4] Strontium Chloride, 8840
[10476-86-5] Strontium Iodide, 8844
[10534-89-1] Hexaaminecobalt Trichloride, 4675
[10539-19-2] Moxaverine, 6288
[10540-29-1] Tamoxifen, 9048
[10543-57-4] TAED, 9028
[10553-31-8] Barium Bromide, 968
[10563-70-9] Melitracen Hydrochloride, 5823
[10567-69-8] Barium Iodate, 979
[10580-02-6] Ammonium Titanium Oxalate, 563
[10588-01-9] Sodium Dichromate(VI), 8609
[10592-03-7] Vincamine Hydrochloride, 9983
[10596-23-3] Clodronic Acid, 2371
[10597-89-4] N-Acetylmuramic Acid, 6304
[10605-21-7] Carbendazim, 1791
[11000-03-6] Strepogenin, 8821
[11003-38-6] Capreomycin, 1757
[11003-70-6] Scillaren, 8399
[11005-20-2] Pseudohecogenin, 4622
[11005-63-3] Strophanthin, 8852
[11006-76-1] Virginiamycin, 10004
[11006-77-2] Statolon, 8801
[11006-83-0] Thermorubin, 9287
[11015-37-5] Bambermycins, 952
[11016-07-2] Perimycin, 7169

[11016-39-0] Properdin, 7814
[11017-56-4] Strigol, 8833
[11021-66-2] Ristocetin A, 8234
[11024-24-1] Digitonin, 3161
[11028-71-0] Concanavalin A, 2495
[11030-31-2] Lanatoside D, 5354
[11030-71-0] Amanitin, 373
[11031-48-4] Sarkomycin, 8376
[11031-82-6] Streptovaricin B, 8830
[11031-85-9] Streptovaricin G, 8830
[11032-05-6] Teleocidin B₄, 9118
[11034-45-0] O-Cinnamoyltaxicin-I, 9077
[11035-08-8] Substance P, 8863
[11041-12-6] Cholestyramine Resin, 2202
[11042-38-9] Xanthocillin, 10061
[11042-64-1] γ-Oryzanol, 6886
[11050-21-8] CTX-1, 2270
[11050-94-5] Oligomycin B, 6833
[11051-71-1] Avilamycin, 887
[11052-72-5] Oligomycin C, 6833
[11061-68-0] Insulin (Human), 4980
[11061-96-4] Cardiotoxin, 1835
[11070-73-8] Insulin (Bovine), 4980
[11072-93-8] β-Escin, 3696
[11075-36-8] Tuberactinomycin, 9803
[11076-19-0] Bongkrekic Acid, 1332
[11078-21-0] Filipin, 4080
[11079-53-1] Hyperforin, 4862
[11085-36-2] HCS, 4620
[11089-65-9] Tunicamycin, 9819
[11096-26-7] Erythropoietin, 3688
[11096-49-4] Partricin, 7049
[11104-88-4] Phosphomolybdic Acid, 7342
[11110-52-4] Sodium Amalgam, 8575
[11113-63-6] Graphite Fluoride, 4540
[11113-80-7] Polyoxins, 7576
[11115-82-5] Enduracidin, 3579
[11116-31-7] Bleomycin A₂, 1318
[11120-25-5] Ammonium Tungstate-(VI), 564
[11121-16-7] Aluminum Borate, 330
[11121-32-7] Mepartricin, 5847
[11125-96-5] Burgundy Mixture, 1335
[11138-66-2] Xanthan Gum, 10057
[11141-17-6] Azadirachtin, 893
[12001-72-8] Mafenide Propionate, 5649
[12002-03-8] Cupric Acetoarsenite, 2625
[12002-30-1] Piperazine Edetate Calcium, 7464
[12002-43-6] Gilsonite, 4422
[12002-53-8] Trimedlure, 9701
[12007-25-9] Magnesium Diboride, 5664
[12007-56-6] Calcium Borate, 1652
[12007-58-8] Ammonium Borate, 504
[12007-60-2] Lithium Borate, 5524
[12016-69-2] Cobaltous Chromate(III), 2438
[12016-80-7] Cobaltic Oxide Monohydrate, 2431
[12017-68-4] Samarium Cobalt, 8348
[12018-01-8] Chromium Dioxide, 2233
[12018-10-9] Cupric Chromite, 2635
[12023-99-3] Gallium Hydroxide, 4346
[12024-20-3] Gallium Suboxide, 4346
[12024-21-4] Gallium Oxide, 4352
[12026-06-1] Thallium Hydroxide, 9263
[12026-66-3] Ammonium Phosphomolybdate, 545

[12027-06-4] Ammonium Iodide, *529*
[12027-67-7] Ammonium Molybdate-(VI), *533*
[12029-98-0] Iodine Pentoxide, *5019*
[12033-88-4] Nitrogen Selenide, *6606*
[12033-89-5] Silicon Nitride, *8497*
[12040-44-7] Alcian Blue, *218*
[12041-72-4] Formosulfathiazole, *8943*
[12047-27-7] Barium Titanate(IV), *1000*
[12048-50-9] Bismuth Tetroxide, *1290*
[12052-78-7] Samarium Cobalt (Sm$_2$Co$_{17}$), *8348*
[12054-48-7] Nickel Hydroxide, *6510*
[12057-24-8] Lithium Oxide, *5538*
[12058-66-1] Sodium Stannate(IV), *8677*
[12060-59-2] Strontium Titanate, *8850*
[12062-24-7] Cupric Hexafluorosilicate, *2641*
[12063-56-8] Yig, *10097*
[12063-98-8] Gallium Phosphide, *4353*
[12067-99-1] Phosphotungstic Acid, *7364*
[12068-69-8] Bismuth Selenide, *1278*
[12069-32-8] Boron Carbide, *1344*
[12069-69-1] Cupric Carbonate, Basic, *2631*
[12070-12-1] Tungsten Carbide, *9815*
[12071-83-9] Propineb, *7819*
[12108-13-3] MMT, *6223*
[12111-24-9] Pentetate Calcium Trisodium, *7124*
[12122-67-7] Zineb, *10165*
[12124-97-9] Ammonium Bromide, *505*
[12124-99-1] Ammonium Bisulfide, *501*
[12125-01-8] Ammonium Fluoride, *522*
[12125-02-9] Ammonium Chloride, *509*
[12125-08-5] Ammonium Osmium Chloride, *536*
[12125-09-6] Phosphonium Iodide, *7343*
[12126-59-9] Conjugated Estrogens, *2508*
[12135-22-7] Pearlman's Catalyst, *7060*
[12135-76-1] Ammonium Sulfide, *556*
[12141-46-7] Aluminum Silicate, *362*
[12142-33-5] Potassium Stannate(IV), *7672*
[12173-47-6] Hectorite, *4623*
[12192-57-3] Aurothioglucose, *883*
[12230-71-6] Barium Hydroxide Octahydrate, *977*
[12232-99-4] Sodium Bismuthate(V), *8585*
[12233-56-6] Bismuth Germanate, *1266*
[12240-15-2] Prussian Blue (unspecified formula), *7910*
[12244-26-7] Kininogens, *5312*
[12244-57-4] Gold Sodium Thiomalate, *4518*
[12279-90-2] Arsenic Sulfide, *799*
[12284-76-3] Bismuth Aluminate, *1258*
[12286-76-9] Fructose Ferric Form, *4273*
[12304-65-3] Hydrotalcite, *5660*
[12321-44-7] Calcitonin (Porcine), *1643*
[12427-38-2] Maneb, *5721*
[12505-77-0] Boron Monoxide, *1345*
[12511-31-8] Aluminum Magnesium Silicate, *350*
[12520-88-6] Silicotungstic Acid, *8502*

[12542-36-8] Gossypol Acetic Acid, *4528*
[12550-17-3] Sodium Antimonylgluconate, *701*
[12584-58-6] Insulin (Porcine), *4980*
[12584-83-7] Cobrotoxin, *2452*
[12607-70-4] Nickel Carbonate Hydroxide, *6503*
[12607-92-0] Aceglutamide Aluminum Complex, *25*
[12607-93-1] Taxine, *9078*
[12609-84-6] Thiopeptin, *9351*
[12616-24-9] Ammonium Zirconyl Carbonate, *569*
[12629-01-5] Human Growth Hormone, *8716*
[12650-69-0] Mupirocin, *6302*
[12698-96-3] Thearubigins, *9275*
[12704-90-4] Aurodox, *882*
[12740-44-2] Sodium-Lead Alloy, *8637*
[12751-04-1] Creolin, *2570*
[12758-40-6] Propagermanium, *7795*
[12771-68-5] Ancymidol, *631*
[12772-35-9] Butirosin, *1528*
[12772-57-5] Monorden, *6253*
[13002-65-8] Tamoxifen (*E*)-Form, *9048*
[13007-85-7] Glucoheptonic Acid Sodium Salt, *4455*
[13007-90-4] Bis(triphenylphosphine)dicarbonylnickel, *1304*
[13007-92-6] Chromium Carbonyl, *2232*
[13007-93-7] Cuproxoline, *2670*
[13008-73-6] L-Streptose, *8828*
[13009-99-9] Mafenide Acetate, *5649*
[13010-47-4] Lomustine, *5564*
[13040-98-7] Guamecycline Dihydrochloride, *4557*
[13042-18-7] Fendiline, *3970*
[13051-01-9] Carbazochrome Salicylate, *1788*
[13055-82-8] Reproterol Hydrochloride, *8139*
[13058-67-8] Lucensomycin, *5592*
[13071-79-9] Terbufos, *9158*
[13073-35-3] Ethionine, *3738*
[13085-08-0] Mazipredone, *5763*
[13087-53-1] Iothalamic Acid *N*-Methylglucamine Salt, *5064*
[13092-66-5] Magnesium Phosphate, Monobasic, *5682*
[13093-88-4] Perimethazine, *7168*
[13100-82-8] Cysteic Acid, *2780*
[13103-34-9] Boldenone 10-Undecenoate, *1324*
[13115-03-2] Vitamin B$_{12}$-^{57}Co, *10015*
[13121-70-5] Cyhexatin, *2760*
[13137-64-9] Periplocin, *7174*
[13138-45-9] Nickel Nitrate, *6513*
[13157-90-9] Quercetin Pentabenzyl Ether, *8034*
[13171-21-6] Phosphamidon, *7337*
[13171-25-0] Trimetazidine Dihydrochloride, *9705*
[13190-97-1] Solanesol, *8703*
[13194-48-4] Ethoprop, *3746*
[13246-02-1] Febarbamate, *3945*
[13291-74-2] Gentamicin A, *4392*
[13292-46-1] Rifampin, *8216*
[13311-84-7] Flutamide, *4208*
[13327-32-7] Beryllium Hydroxide, *1169*

[13347-42-7] Dowicide 9®, *3430*
[13356-08-6] Fenbutatin Oxide, *3964*
[13364-32-4] Clobenzorex, *2362*
[13392-18-2] Fenoterol, *3981*
[13392-28-4] Rimantadine, *8224*
[13397-24-5] Calcium Sulfate Dihydrate, *1706*
[13400-13-0] Cesium Fluoride, *2012*
[13401-40-6] Phaseolin, *7198*
[13402-08-9] Acetylpheneturide, *99*
[13405-60-2] β-Glucogallin, *4454*
[13408-56-5] Ponasterone A, *7588*
[13410-01-0] Sodium Selenate, *8671*
[13411-16-0] Nifurpirinol, *6537*
[13412-64-1] Dicloxacillin Sodium Salt Monohydrate, *3084*
[13422-51-0] Hydroxocobalamin, *4809*
[13422-52-1] Aquacobalamin, *4809*
[13422-53-2] Vitamin B$_{12}$-^{60}Co, *10015*
[13422-55-4] Methylcobalamin, *6045*
[13424-46-9] Lead Azide, *5401*
[13425-22-4] Aminorex Fumarate, *476*
[13425-39-3] Etofylline Nicotinate, *3879*
[13425-98-4] Improsulfan, *4927*
[13444-24-1] 1-Ethyl-3-piperidinol, *3845*
[13444-90-1] Nitryl Chloride, *6657*
[13445-63-1] Itramin Tosylate, *5246*
[13446-03-2] Manganese Bromide, *5725*
[13446-24-7] Magnesium Pyrophosphate, *5684*
[13446-34-9] Manganese Chloride Tetrahydrate, *5728*
[13446-49-6] Potassium Molybdate-(VI), *7647*
[13447-95-5] Isoniazid Methanesulfonate, *5186*
[13450-90-3] Gallium Chloride, *4348*
[13452-36-3] *O*-Cinnamoyltaxicin-I triacetate, *9077*
[13453-07-1] Gold Trichloride, *4521*
[13453-34-4] Thallium Cyanide, *9261*
[13454-94-9] Cerous Sulfate, *2002*
[13455-36-2] Cobaltous Phosphate, *2447*
[13457-18-6] Pyrazophos, *7962*
[13462-88-9] Nickel Bromide, *6502*
[13462-90-3] Nickel Iodide, *6511*
[13463-39-3] Nickel Carbonyl, *6504*
[13463-40-6] Iron Pentacarbonyl, *5099*
[13463-41-7] Pyrithione Zinc Derivative, *7994*
[13463-67-7] Titanium Dioxide, *9472*
[13464-35-2] Potassium Arsenite, *7608*
[13464-82-9] Indium Sulfate, *4955*
[13465-09-3] Indium Tribromide, *4957*
[13465-66-2] Selenium Tetrafluoride, *8439*
[13465-94-6] Barium Nitrite, *984*
[13465-95-7] Barium Perchlorate, *987*
[13466-78-9] 3-Carene, *1836*
[13472-45-2] Sodium Tungstate(VI), *8698*
[13473-90-0] Aluminum Nitrate, *352*
[13477-00-4] Barium Chlorate, *970*
[13478-93-8] Nickel Dimethylglyoxime, *6507*
[13479-54-4] Cupric Bisglycinate, *2627*
[13484-14-5] Sarmentose, *8377*
[13492-01-8] Tranylcypromine Sulfate, *9573*
[13492-26-7] Potassium Phosphite, *7661*

[13494-80-9] Tellurium, *9121*
[13494-90-1] Gallium Nitrate, *4350*
[13495-09-5] Piminodine, *7433*
[13510-49-1] Beryllium Sulfate, *1175*
[13510-89-9] Lead Antimonate(V), *5398*
[13523-86-9] Pindolol, *7443*
[13530-65-9] Zinc Chromate(VI) Hydroxide, *10133*
[13539-59-8] Apazone, *726*
[13548-38-4] Chromic Nitrate, *2226*
[13548-42-0] Cupric Chromate(VI), *2634*
[13548-43-1] Ammonium Chromic Sulfate, *511*
[13552-61-9] 2-Thiolhistidine, *9341*
[13553-79-2] Rifamycin S, *8217*
[13560-89-9] Dechlorane® Plus, *2851*
[13563-60-5] Norgesterone, *6702*
[13573-16-5] Reinecke Salt, *8128*
[13587-35-4] Cupric Tungstate(VI), *2657*
[13588-16-4] Senecic Acid, *8449*
[13590-82-4] Ceric Sulfate, *1990*
[13597-65-4] Zinc Silicate, *10157*
[13597-99-4] Beryllium Nitrate, *1170*
[13598-36-2] Phosphorous Acid, *7346*
[13600-98-1] Sodium Cobaltinitrite, *8603*
[13601-13-3] Cupric Ferrocyanide, *2637*
[13601-19-9] Sodium Ferrocyanide, *8616*
[13609-67-1] Hydrocortisone 17-Butyrate, *4787*
[13614-98-7] Minocycline Hydrochloride, *6202*
[13636-18-5] Fendiline Hydrochloride, *3970*
[13637-61-1] Zinc Perchlorate, *10148*
[13640-28-3] Pilosine, *5199*
[13642-52-9] Soterenol, *8729*
[13647-35-3] Trilostane, *9698*
[13655-52-2] Alprenolol, *313*
[13669-70-0] Nefopam, *6440*
[13674-87-8] TDCPP, *9087*
[13682-61-6] Potassium Tetrachloroaurate(III), *7681*
[13682-73-0] Cuprous Potassium Cyanide, *2665*
[13682-92-3] Dihydroxyaluminum Aminoacetate, *3183*
[13684-63-4] Phenmedipham, *7236*
[13693-09-9] Xenon Hexafluoride, *10072*
[13698-49-2] Delmadinone Acetate, *2878*
[13701-67-2] Diboron Tetrachloride, *3016*
[13703-82-7] Magnesium Borate, *5658*
[13707-88-5] Alprenolol Hydrochloride, *313*
[13708-85-5] Sodium Phosphite, *8663*
[13709-36-9] Xenon Difluoride, *10072*
[13709-61-0] Xenon Tetrafluoride, *10072*
[13710-19-5] Tolfenamic Acid, *9513*
[13717-04-9] Propiram Fumarate, *7831*
[13718-26-8] Sodium Vanadate(V), *8700*
[13718-50-8] Barium Iodide, *980*
[13718-94-0] Isomaltulose, *5182*
[13721-34-1] Sodium Uranate(VI), *8699*

[13739-02-1] Diacerein, *2960*
[13741-18-9] Xibornol, *10076*
[13746-66-2] Potassium Ferricyanide, *7630*
[13746-89-9] Zirconium Nitrate, *10179*
[13746-98-0] Thallium Trinitrate, *9271*
[13755-29-8] Sodium Fluoborate, *8617*
[13755-38-9] Sodium Nitroprusside Dihydrate, *8649*
[13759-10-9] Silicon Disulfide, *8494*
[13762-51-1] Potassium Borohydride, *7616*
[13765-19-0] Calcium Chromate(VI), *1660*
[13768-38-2] Osmium Hexafluoride, *6892*
[13770-18-8] Cupric Perchlorate, *2647*
[13773-81-4] Krypton Difluoride, *5325*
[13776-58-4] Xenon Trioxide, *10072*
[13776-74-4] Magnesium Metasilicate, *5687*
[13780-03-5] Calcium Bisulfite, Solution, *1651*
[13780-06-8] Calcium Nitrite, *1683*
[13782-01-9] Cobaltic Potassium Nitrite, *2432*
[13804-51-8] Juvenile Hormone I, *5273*
[13820-09-2] Trimethyl Orthovalerate, *9717*
[13820-41-2] Ammonium Platinous Chloride, *549*
[13823-29-5] Thorium Nitrate, *9376*
[13825-74-6] Titanium Oxysulfate, *9475*
[13825-86-0] Chromous Sulfate, *2247*
[13826-64-7] Angeli's Salt, *648*
[13838-08-9] Azidamfenicol, *909*
[13838-16-9] Enflurane, *3581*
[13867-82-8] Cloxotestosterone Acetate, *2421*
[13870-90-1] Cobamamide, *2451*
[13871-27-7] Beryllium Sodium Fluoride, *1174*
[13876-85-2] Cuprous Mercuric Iodide, *2663*
[13898-58-3] Benzoylpas, *1115*
[13912-77-1] Octacaine, *6743*
[13925-12-7] Myxin, *6340*
[13929-35-6] Rifamycin B, *8217*
[13930-31-9] Oxethazaine Hydrochloride, *6933*
[13931-64-1] Procymate, *7764*
[13943-58-3] Potassium Ferrocyanide, *7631*
[13952-84-6] *sec*-Butylamine, *1544*
[13956-29-1] Cannabidiol, *1747*
[13963-58-1] Potassium Hexacyanocobaltate(III), *7637*
[13967-50-5] Potassium Dicyanoaurate(I), *7628*
[13967-90-3] Barium Bromate, *967*
[13977-28-1] Embramine Hydrochloride, *3556*
[13982-53-1] Cuprous Sulfite, *2668*
[13986-19-1] Zinc Iodate Dihydrate, *10139*
[13986-26-0] Zirconium Iodide, *10178*
[13993-65-2] Metiazinic Acid, *6139*
[13997-19-8] Nequinate, *6472*
[14007-64-8] Butethamate, *1522*
[14008-44-7] Metopimazine, *6149*
[14008-48-1] Bisoxatin Acetate, *1296*
[14009-24-6] Drotaverine, *3455*
[14028-44-5] Amoxapine, *576*

[14038-43-8] Prussian Blue, *7910*
[14051-33-3] Benzetimide, *1075*
[14062-23-8] Felbinac Ethyl Ester, *3951*
[14066-79-6] Chloroprednisone 21-Acetate, *2157*
[14073-97-3] *l*-Menthone, *5838*
[14075-53-7] Potassium Tetrafluoroborate, *7686*
[14101-04-3] Frangulin B, *4264*
[14148-99-3] Lefetamine Hydrochloride, *5431*
[14176-10-4] Cetiedil, *2021*
[14188-82-0] Hexestrol Diphosphate, *4701*
[14217-01-7] Chromic Potassium Oxalate, *2228*
[14220-17-8] Potassium Tetracyanonickelate(II), *7684*
[14221-47-7] Ammonium Ferric Oxalate, *517*
[14221-48-8] Ammonium Ferricyanide, *519*
[14222-60-7] Protionamide, *7891*
[14252-80-3] Bupivacaine Hydrochloride Monohydrate, *1495*
[14255-61-9] Oxidronic Acid Sodium Salt, *6940*
[14255-87-9] Parbendazole, *7035*
[14259-45-1] Asperuloside, *844*
[14277-97-5] Domoic Acid, *3417*
[14283-05-7] Tetraamminecopper Sulfate, *9181*
[14283-07-9] Lithium Tetrafluoroborate, *5543*
[14286-84-1] Bencyclane Fumarate, *1033*
[14293-44-8] Xipamide, *10079*
[14293-70-0] Fremy's Salt, *4268*
[14297-87-1] Benzylmorphine, *1141*
[14307-33-6] Calcium Dichromate(VI), *1666*
[14307-35-8] Lithium Chromate(VI), *5529*
[14317-18-1] Ioglycamic Acid Meglumine Salt, *5051*
[14334-40-8] Pramiverin, *7707*
[14334-41-9] Pramiverin Hydrochloride, *7707*
[14338-32-0] Mukaiyama Reagent, *6301*
[14350-67-5] Ormosinine, *6871*
[14357-78-9] Diprenorphine, *3340*
[14358-43-1] Dehydroemetine (±)-Form Dihydrochloride, *2870*
[14375-45-2] Abscisic Acid (±)-*cis,trans*-Form, *11*
[14376-16-0] Sulfaloxic Acid, *8912*
[14398-53-9] Abscisic Acid (−)-*cis,trans*-Form, *11*
[14402-67-6] Potassium Titanyl Oxalate, *7693*
[14402-73-4] Lithium Tetracyanoplatinate(II), *5542*
[14402-75-6] Cadmium Potassium Cyanide, *1624*
[14402-89-2] Sodium Nitroprusside, *8649*
[14417-88-0] Melinamide, *5822*
[14429-30-2] 2-Deoxystreptamine Dihydrochloride, *2909*
[14451-99-1] Menadione Dimethylpyrimidinol Bisulfite, *5831*
[14452-57-4] Magnesium Peroxide, *5680*

[14457-87-5] Cerous Bromide, *1995*
[14459-29-1] Hematoporphyrin, *4636*
[14463-33-3] Vitamin B₁₂ᵣ, *10016*
[14475-63-9] Zirconium Hydroxide, *10177*
[14481-29-9] Ammonium Ferrocyanide, *520*
[14481-33-5] Thorium Tetracyanoplatinate(II), *9378*
[14484-47-0] Deflazacort, *2862*
[14484-64-1] Ferbam, *4013*
[14487-05-9] Rifamycin O, *8217*
[14492-68-3] Lapyrium Chloride Stearoyl Analog, *5370*
[14504-73-5] Tritoqualine, *9765*
[14521-96-1] Etorphine, *3888*
[14523-22-9] Rhodium Carbonyl Chloride, *8187*
[14556-46-8] Bupranolol, *1496*
[14559-79-6] Propizepine Hydrochloride, *7833*
[14590-13-7] Ammonium Cobaltous Phosphate, *513*
[14611-51-9] Selegiline, *8428*
[14611-52-0] Selegiline Hydrochloride, *8428*
[14613-30-0] Clofibric Acid Magnesium Salt, *2378*
[14635-75-7] Nitrosyl Tetrafluoroborate, *6649*
[14636-12-5] Terlipressin, *9167*
[14639-25-9] Chromium Picolinate, *2236*
[14639-94-2] Ammonium Hexafluorogallate, *525*
[14639-97-5] Ammonium Tetrachlorozincate, *559*
[14639-98-6] Ammonium Pentachlorozincate, *539*
[14644-61-2] Zirconium Sulfate, *10182*
[14663-23-1] Dantrolene Sodium Salt, *2816*
[14679-73-3] Todralazine (anhydrous), *9502*
[14694-95-2] Wilkinson's Catalyst, *10047*
[14698-29-4] Oxolinic Acid, *6945*
[14721-21-2] Cupric Chlorate, *2632*
[14759-06-9] Sulforidazine, *8963*
[14769-73-4] Levamisole, *5459*
[14807-96-6] Talc, *9037*
[14816-18-3] Phoxim, *7366*
[14816-67-2] Soterenol Monohydrochloride, *8729*
[14817-09-5] Decimemide, *2852*
[14838-15-4] Phenylpropanolamine, *7307*
[14855-76-6] Methyl Green, *6082*
[14860-49-2] Clobutinol, *2365*
[14871-79-5] Barium Hypophosphite, *978*
[14874-24-9] Tris(ethylenediamine)-cadmium Dihydroxide, *9752*
[14875-96-8] Heme, *4639*
[14882-18-9] Bismuth Subsalicylate, *1285*
[14885-29-1] Ipronidazole, *5079*
[14897-39-3] Rifamycin SV Sodium Salt, *8218*
[14901-08-7] Cycasin, *2701*
[14912-44-8] Ylangene, *10099*
[14918-35-5] Destomycin A, *2935*
[14919-77-8] Benserazide Hydrochloride, *1050*

[14929-11-4] Simfibrate, *8537*
[14930-96-2] Cytochalasin B, *2790*
[14932-42-4] Xenon-133, *10072*
[14940-41-1] Ferrous Phosphate, *4053*
[14959-86-5] Looplure, *5570*
[14976-57-9] Clemastine Hydrogen Fumarate, *2345*
[14977-61-8] Chromyl Chloride, *2248*
[14984-68-0] Cloperastine Hydrochloride, *2395*
[14987-04-3] Magnesium Trisilicate, *5687*
[14992-59-7] Sodium Dibunate, *8608*
[14992-62-2] DL-Acetylcarnitine, *84*
[15060-55-6] Ammonium Tetrathiomolybdate (DL-form), *560*
[15096-52-3] Cryolite, *2606*
[15123-69-0] Cupric Selenate, *2650*
[15139-76-1] Orange B, *6859*
[15148-80-8] Bupranolol Hydrochloride, *1496*
[15165-67-0] Dichlorprop (*R*)-(+)-Form, *3078*
[15176-29-1] Edoxudine, *3514*
[15180-00-4] Prednival, *7723*
[15180-03-7] Alcuronium Dichloride, *221*
[15189-51-2] Sodium Tetrachloroaurate(III), *8688*
[15238-00-3] Cobaltous Iodide, *2443*
[15263-53-3] Cartap, *1865*
[15265-28-8] Palitantin, *6987*
[15280-09-8] Sodium Dicyanoaurate(I), *8610*
[15283-45-1] Gold Sodium Thiosulfate, *4519*
[15291-75-5] Ginkgolide A, *4426*
[15291-76-6] Ginkgolide C, *4426*
[15291-77-7] Ginkgolide B, *4426*
[15299-99-7] Napropamide, *6416*
[15301-48-1] Bezitramide, *1196*
[15301-69-6] Flavoxate, *4096*
[15301-80-1] Oxamarin, *6915*
[15302-16-6] Fenozolone, *3988*
[15307-79-6] Diclofenac Sodium Salt, *3081*
[15307-81-0] Diclofenac Potassium Salt, *3081*
[15307-86-5] Diclofenac, *3081*
[15308-34-6] Norfenefrine *dl*-Form Hydrochloride, *6699*
[15318-45-3] Thiamphenicol, *9301*
[15320-30-6] Magnesium Sulfate Trihydrate, *5691*
[15328-32-2] 1-Cyanobenzotriazole, *2690*
[15351-05-0] Buzepide Methiodide, *1599*
[15356-74-8] Dihydroactinidiolide, *3170*
[15358-48-2] Hydroxylupanine, *4829*
[15385-57-6] Mercurous Iodide, *5895*
[15421-84-8] Trapidil, *9574*
[15468-10-7] Oxidronic Acid, *6940*
[15477-33-5] Aluminum Chlorate, *336*
[15489-16-4] Stibophen, *8813*
[15489-90-4] Hematin, *4635*
[15490-91-2] Struvite, *8854*
[15500-66-0] Pancuronium Bromide, *7007*
[15537-71-0] *N*-Acetylpenicillamine, *98*
[15537-76-5] Chlorproguanil Hydrochloride, *2184*
[15545-48-9] Chlorotoluron, *2172*

[15571-91-2] Potassium Tellurate(VI), *7679*
[15572-25-5] Thallium Selenide, *9267*
[15574-96-6] Pizotyline, *7515*
[15578-26-4] Stannous Pyrophosphate, *8788*
[15588-95-1] DOM, *3412*
[15589-00-1] DOM Hydrochloride, *3412*
[15590-23-5] Sodium Methylsulfinylmethylide, *8644*
[15599-39-0] Noxythiolin, *6724*
[15610-76-1] Ammonium Cupric Chloride, *514*
[15622-65-8] Molindone Hydrochloride, *6233*
[15656-28-7] Bis(pyridine)iodonium Tetrafluoroborate, *1302*
[15662-33-6] Ryanodine, *8307*
[15663-27-1] Cisplatin, *2317*
[15671-27-9] Sulfitocobalamin, *4809*
[15676-16-1] Sulpiride, *8989*
[15686-51-8] Clemastine, *2345*
[15686-61-0] Fenproporex, *3994*
[15686-71-2] Cephalexin, *1974*
[15686-83-6] Pyrantel, *7955*
[15686-91-6] Propiram, *7831*
[15687-27-1] Ibuprofen, *4881*
[15687-41-9] Oxyfedrine, *6962*
[15690-55-8] Clomiphene *cis*-Form, *2386*
[15690-57-0] Clomiphene *trans*-Form, *2386*
[15699-18-0] Nickel Ammonium Sulfate, *6501*
[15708-41-5] Ferric Sodium Edetate, *4031*
[15722-48-2] Olsalazine, *6841*
[15764-04-2] α-Vetivone, *9971*
[15823-89-9] Imolamine Hydrochloride, *4923*
[15825-70-4] D-Mannitol Hexanitrate, *5746*
[15826-37-6] Cromolyn Disodium Salt, *2590*
[15845-98-4] Iothalamic Acid ¹³¹I-Labeled Sodium Salt, *5064*
[15871-57-5] TOAC, *9488*
[15876-67-2] Distigmine Bromide, *3362*
[15879-93-3] α-Chloralose, *2072*
[15972-60-8] Alachlor, *201*
[16009-13-5] Hemin, *4644*
[16034-77-8] Iocetamic Acid, *5010*
[16037-91-5] Sodium Stibogluconate, *701*
[16039-53-5] Zinc Lactate, *10142*
[16048-96-7] Cupric Salicylate, *2649*
[16051-77-7] Isosorbide-5-mononitrate, *5225*
[16110-51-3] Cromolyn, *2590*
[16188-61-7] Talastine, *9035*
[16188-76-4] Talastine Hydrochloride, *9035*
[16283-36-6] Zinc Salicylate, *10155*
[16286-69-4] Cetiedil Citrate, *2021*
[16298-90-1] Jesaconitine, *5265*
[16320-04-0] Gestrinone, *4415*
[16330-92-0] Ammonium Tetrathiomolybdate (tetrathiomolybdate(2−)), *560*
[16357-59-8] EEDQ, *3518*
[16377-00-7] Indospicine, *4970*
[16378-21-5] Piroheptine, *7503*
[16378-22-6] Piroheptine Hydrochloride, *7503*

[16423-68-0] Erythrosine, *3693*
[16462-65-0] Plicatic Acid, *7537*
[16478-59-4] Hemicholinium, *4643*
[16506-27-7] Bendamustine, *1034*
[16545-11-2] Guamecycline, *4557*
[16550-22-4] Cyprenorphine Hydrochloride, *2769*
[16589-24-5] Synephrine Tartrate, *9012*
[16590-41-3] Naltrexone, *6363*
[16595-80-5] Levamisole Hydrochloride, *5459*
[16604-45-8] Medifoxamine Fumarate, *5790*
[16625-20-0] Haplophytine, *4611*
[16643-66-6] Menbutone Magnesium Salt, *5834*
[16648-69-4] Oxyfedrine DL-Form Hydrochloride, *6962*
[16649-79-9] Calcium *N*-Carbamoylaspartate, *1655*
[16649-82-4] Calcium *N*-Carbamoylaspartate D-Form, *1655*
[16662-46-7] Gallopamil Hydrochloride, *4356*
[16662-47-8] Gallopamil, *4356*
[16672-87-0] Ethephon, *3732*
[16674-78-5] Magnesium Acetate Tetrahydrate, *5654*
[16676-29-2] Naltrexone Hydrochloride, *6363*
[16679-58-6] Desmopressin, *2924*
[16698-35-4] β-Tocopherol, *9496*
[16721-80-5] Sodium Bisulfide, *8587*
[16731-55-8] Potassium Metabisulfite, *7645*
[16752-77-5] Methomyl, *5982*
[16755-07-0] Showdomycin, *8482*
[16773-42-5] Ornidazole, *6872*
[16774-21-3] Cerium(IV) Ammonium Nitrate, *1992*
[16777-42-7] Oxyfedrine L-Form Hydrochloride, *6962*
[16816-67-4] Pantethine, *7012*
[16830-15-2] Asiaticoside, *833*
[16833-54-8] Pinolenic Acid, *7450*
[16846-24-5] Josamycin, *5267*
[16853-85-3] Aluminum Lithium Hydride, *349*
[16871-60-6] Potassium Hexachloroosmate(IV), *7635*
[16871-71-9] Zinc Hexafluorosilicate, *10138*
[16871-90-2] Potassium Hexafluorosilicate, *7638*
[16872-11-0] Fluoboric Acid, *4149*
[16893-85-9] Sodium Hexafluorosilicate, *8624*
[16903-35-8] Gold Trichloride, Acid, *4522*
[16919-19-0] Ammonium Hexafluorosilicate, *527*
[16919-58-7] Ammonium Platinic Chloride, *548*
[16921-30-5] Potassium Hexachloroplatinate(IV), *7636*
[16921-96-3] Iodine Heptafluoride, *5015*
[16923-58-3] Sodium Hexachloroplatinate(IV), *8623*
[16923-95-8] Potassium Hexafluorozirconate(IV), *7639*
[16925-39-6] Calcium Hexafluorosilicate, *1671*
[16940-66-2] Sodium Borohydride, *8592*

[16941-10-9] Aluminum Calcium Hydride, *334*
[16941-11-0] Ammonium Hexafluorophosphate, *526*
[16941-12-1] Platinic Chloride, *7526*
[16949-15-8] Lithium Borohydride, *5525*
[16949-65-8] Magnesium Hexafluorosilicate, *5668*
[16960-16-0] Cosyntropin, *2551*
[16961-83-4] Fluosilicic Acid, *4182*
[16962-07-5] Aluminum Borohydride, *331*
[16980-89-5] Bucladesine Sodium Salt, *1463*
[17021-26-0] Calusterone, *1722*
[17032-39-2] Phosphorylcholine Magnesium Salt, *7362*
[17034-34-3] Secretin Porcine Secretin Acetate Salt, *8421*
[17034-35-4] Porcine Secretin, *8421*
[17035-90-4] *N*^G-Methylarginine, *6022*
[17086-28-1] Doxycycline (monohydrate), *3440*
[17088-37-8] Triacetone Triperoxide, *9590*
[17090-79-8] Monensin, *6246*
[17092-92-1] Dihydroactinidiolide (*R*)-Form, *3170*
[17099-70-6] Aluminum Hexafluorosilicate, *340*
[17109-49-8] Edifenphos, *3510*
[17125-80-3] Barium Hexafluorosilicate, *976*
[17140-68-0] Etamiphyllin Hydrochloride, *3711*
[17140-81-7] Nitrofurantoin Monohydrate, *6599*
[17146-95-1] Pentazocine Lactate, *7121*
[17155-31-6] Veralkamine, *9949*
[17162-36-6] Arecoline *p*-Stibonobenzoic Acid, *778*
[17169-60-7] Ferroglycine Sulfate, *4039*
[17176-77-1] Dibenzyl Phosphite, *3014*
[17181-54-3] Glycerophosphoric Acid (β-form), *4486*
[17185-29-4] Tristriphenylphosphine Rhodium Carbonyl Hydride, *9758*
[17194-00-2] Barium Hydroxide, *977*
[17230-88-5] Danazol, *2812*
[17243-38-8] Azidocillin, *910*
[17243-39-9] Benzoctamine, *1087*
[17243-57-1] Mefenorex, *5799*
[17243-64-0] Piprozolin, *7485*
[17257-71-5] Mosher's Reagent (*S*)-(−)-Form, *6280*
[17297-82-4] Oxypendyl Dihydrochloride, *6970*
[17321-77-6] Clomipramine Hydrochloride, *2387*
[17334-58-6] Pelargonidin 3,5-Diglucoside, *7071*
[17365-01-4] Etiroxate, *3872*
[17372-87-1] Eosine Yellowish—(YS), *3603*
[17375-41-6] Ferrous Sulfate Monohydrate, *4057*
[17388-17-9] Nandinine *dl*-Form, *6364*
[17388-39-5] Swertiamarin, *9010*
[17397-89-6] Cerulenin, *2004*
[17406-45-0] Tomatine, *9545*
[17440-83-4] Amiloride Hydrochloride Dihydrate, *406*

[17466-45-4] Phalloidin, *7196*
[17500-49-1] Schweizer's Reagent, *8397*
[17560-51-9] Metolazone, *6147*
[17575-20-1] Lanatoside A, *5354*
[17575-21-2] Lanatoside B, *5354*
[17575-22-3] Lanatoside C, *5354*
[17590-01-1] Amphetaminil, *583*
[17598-65-1] Deslanoside, *2921*
[17598-82-2] D-Tagatose L-Tagatose, *9030*
[17605-67-3] Fucosterol, *4280*
[17617-23-1] Flurazepam, *4198*
[17617-45-7] Picrotoxinin, *7416*
[17627-77-9] Anhalonidine, *654*
[17650-86-1] Amicetin, *397*
[17650-98-5] Ceruletide, *2005*
[17651-61-5] Adonitoxin, *169*
[17673-25-5] Phorbol, *7332*
[17692-31-8] Dropropizine, *3452*
[17692-39-6] Fomocaine, *4230*
[17692-51-2] Metergoline, *5937*
[17693-51-5] Promethazine Compd with 8-Chlorotheophylline, *7786*
[17702-41-9] Decaborane(14), *2845*
[17737-65-4] Clonixin, *2392*
[17754-44-8] Atractyloside, *867*
[17784-12-2] Sulfacytine, *8902*
[17795-21-0] Allopurinol Sodium Salt, *279*
[17804-35-2] Benomyl, *1044*
[17854-59-0] Mepixanox, *5860*
[17879-96-8] Iopanoic Acid *d*-Form, *5058*
[17879-97-9] Iopanoic Acid *l*-Form, *5058*
[17902-23-7] Tegafur, *9112*
[17924-92-4] Zearalenone, *10116*
[17946-87-1] Desacetoxymatricarin, *5758*
[17951-19-8] Justicidin B, *5272*
[17969-20-9] Fenclozic Acid, *3969*
[18005-40-8] EMPTA, *3564*
[18016-80-3] Lisuride, *5518*
[18046-21-4] Fentiazac, *4003*
[18053-31-1] Fominoben, *4228*
[18059-10-4] Imperialine, *4926*
[18059-99-9] Demexiptiline Hydrochloride, *2890*
[18077-77-5] Ammonium Uranium Carbonate, *566*
[18109-80-3] Butamirate, *1513*
[18109-81-4] Butamirate Citrate, *1513*
[18174-58-8] Pipoxolan Hydrochloride, *7483*
[18181-70-9] Iodofenphos, *5032*
[18181-80-1] Bromopropylate, *1434*
[18195-32-9] Vitamin B₁₂-⁵⁸Co, *10015*
[18198-39-5] Tetraphenylphosphonium, *9237*
[18265-54-8] Phentetiothalein Sodium, *7263*
[18282-10-5] Stannic Oxide, *8778*
[18283-93-7] Tetraborane(10), *9183*
[18286-49-2] HNE (*E*-form), *4726*
[18288-22-7] Bismuthine, *1268*
[18305-29-8] Fenproporex Hydrochloride, *3994*
[18309-32-5] *d*-Verbenone, *9960*
[18323-44-9] Clindamycin, *2356*
[18378-89-7] Plicamycin, *7536*
[18397-07-4] Geissoschizoline, *4380*
[18423-69-3] Cubebin, *2613*
[18433-40-4] Ammonium Uranium Fluoride, *567*

[18433-84-6] Pentaborane(11), *7105*
[18444-66-1] Cucurbitacin E, *2614*
[18444-79-6] β-Vetivone, *9971*
[18454-12-1] Lead Chromate(VI) Oxide, *5406*
[18456-04-7] Cephalonic Acid, *1977*
[18466-51-8] Pelargonidin 3-Glucoside, *7071*
[18467-77-1] Dikegulac, *3199*
[18470-94-5] Nandrolone Cyclohexane-carboxylate, *6365*
[18471-20-0] Ditazol, *3367*
[18472-51-0] Chlorhexidine D-Diglu-conate, *2091*
[18480-07-4] Strontium Hydroxide, *8843*
[18499-92-8] Kermesic Acid, *5293*
[18507-89-6] Decoquinate, *2854*
[18524-67-9] Mycobacillin, *6323*
[18524-94-2] Loganin, *5560*
[18530-30-8] *d*-Camphocarboxylic Acid, *1731*
[18531-94-7] BINOL (*R*)-(+)-Form, *1226*
[18531-99-2] BINOL (*S*)-(−)-Form, *1226*
[18534-66-2] Vitamin B$_{12s}$, *10016*
[18542-37-5] Vernolepin, *9962*
[18559-59-6] Tretoquinol *l*-Form Hydrochloride, *9587*
[18559-63-2] Tretoquinol *dl*-Form Hydrochloride, *9587*
[18559-94-9] Albuterol, *216*
[18598-63-5] Mecysteine Hydrochlo-ride, *5785*
[18624-44-7] Ferrous Hydroxide, *4048*
[18642-10-9] Thiamine Disulfide Hydrochloride, *9297*
[18656-21-8] Iodamide *N*-Methyl-D-glucamine Salt, *5011*
[18679-90-8] Hopantenic Acid, *4744*
[18683-91-5] Ambroxol, *386*
[18691-97-9] Methabenzthiazuron, *5939*
[18694-40-1] Epirizole, *3622*
[18696-26-9] Sinapine, *8541*
[18699-02-0] Actarit, *133*
[18700-78-2] Cervicarcin, *2007*
[18786-24-8] Serpentine (Alkaloid), *8464*
[18791-21-4] Pyridomycin, *7976*
[18794-84-8] β-Farnesene, *3936*
[18820-29-6] Manganese Sulfide, *5740*
[18829-56-6] 2-Nonenal, *6676*
[18829-70-4] Catechin *l*-Form, *1902*
[18836-50-5] Park Nucleotide (L-lysyl form), *7040*
[18836-52-7] Pellitorine, *7073*
[18837-96-2] Bucladesine Barium Salt, *1463*
[18839-90-2] Mestilbol, *3129*
[18840-45-4] Penicillamine Cysteine Disulfide, *7089*
[18840-47-6] Gepefrine, *4401*
[18861-78-4] Asenapine (6-isothiocyan-ate), *4089*
[18883-66-4] Streptozocin, *8832*
[18904-54-6] Corynantheine, *2547*
[18917-89-0] Magnesium Salicylate, *5685*
[18917-91-4] Aluminum Lactate, *348*
[18917-93-6] Magnesium Lactate, *5672*
[18968-99-5] Pemoline Magnesium Hydroxide Mixture, *7079*

[18972-56-0] Magnesium Hexafluoro-silicate Hexahydrate, *5668*
[19010-79-8] Cadmium Salicylate, *1625*
[19026-31-4] Taxodione, *9079*
[19044-88-3] Oryzalin, *6885*
[19057-60-4] Dioscin, *3292*
[19121-58-5] Solasonine, *8710*
[19130-96-2] 1-Deoxynojirimycin, *2905*
[19171-19-8] Actimid, *135*
[19172-47-5] Lawesson's Reagent, *5391*
[19216-56-9] Prazosin, *7717*
[19237-84-4] Prazosin Hydrochloride, *7717*
[19246-24-3] Telomycin, *9131*
[19262-68-1] Methylphenidate *d-threo*-Form Hydrochloride, *6110*
[19286-37-4] Convicine, *2513*
[19287-45-7] Diborane(6), *3015*
[19295-31-9] Urothion, *9888*
[19326-29-5] Etamiphyllin Camphor-sulfonate, *3711*
[19356-17-3] Calcifediol, *1638*
[19379-90-9] Benzoxonium Chloride, *1111*
[19387-91-8] Tinidazole, *9447*
[19388-87-5] Taurolidine, *9076*
[19396-03-3] Polyoxin A, *7576*
[19396-06-6] Polyoxin B, *7576*
[19428-14-9] Benproperine Trihydro-gen Phosphate, *1049*
[19457-37-5] Batrachotoxinin A, *1009*
[19504-77-9] Pecilocin, *7062*
[19545-26-7] Wortmannin, *10053*
[19554-22-4] Cytohemin, *2793*
[19562-30-2] Piromidic Acid, *7505*
[19624-22-7] Pentaborane(9), *7104*
[19625-10-6] Lactobacillic Acid, *5341*
[19660-77-6] Phytochlorin, *7388*
[19666-30-9] Oxadiazon, *6907*
[19700-21-1] Geosmin, *4400*
[19721-56-3] Picromycin, *7413*
[19728-88-2] Metitepine Maleate, *6141*
[19767-45-4] Mesna, *5909*
[19771-63-2] L-2-Oxo-4-thiazolidine-carboxylic acid, *6950*
[19774-82-4] Amiodarone Hydrochlo-ride, *482*
[19793-20-5] Bolandiol, *1322*
[19794-93-5] Trazodone, *9579*
[19803-62-4] Picloxydine Dihydrochlo-ride, *7398*
[19804-27-4] *p*-Methyldiphenhydra-mine, *6053*
[19807-27-3] Palladium Diacetate, *6991*
[19809-78-0] Uliginosin A, *9845*
[19809-79-1] Uliginosin B, *9845*
[19875-60-6] Lisuride Maleate, *5518*
[19879-03-9] Granaticin B, *4534*
[19879-06-2] Granaticin, *4534*
[19881-18-6] Nitroscanate, *6633*
[19888-56-3] Fluazacort, *4115*
[19891-74-8] Lycoxanthin, *5627*
[19891-75-9] Lycophyll, *5621*
[19973-76-3] Estrone *dl*-Form, *3708*
[19982-08-2] Memantine, *5829*
[19992-80-4] Xenbucin *trans*-4-Phenyl-cyclohexylamine Salt (1:1), *10071*
[20004-62-0] Resistomycin, *8152*
[20123-80-2] Dobesilate Calcium, *3394*
[20150-34-9] Ferrous Bisglycinate, *4041*

[20153-98-4] Dilazep Dihydrochloride, *3200*
[20170-20-1] Difenamizole, *3134*
[20187-55-7] Bendazac, *1035*
[20196-67-2] Sinalbin, *8540*
[20229-30-5] Metitepine, *6141*
[20231-81-6] Uzarin, *9897*
[20236-82-2] Dihydrocodeinone Enol Acetate Hydrochloride, *3172*
[20246-33-7] D-Gulonic Acid, *4576*
[20267-87-2] Chelidonine (±)-Form, *2053*
[20283-48-1] Chalcomycin, *2036*
[20284-40-6] Murexine, *6307*
[20287-37-0] Fenquizone, *3997*
[20300-26-9] Gossypol *S*-Form, *4528*
[20310-89-8] Saponarin, *8364*
[20311-78-8] Enanthotoxin, *3569*
[20315-46-2] β-Ergocryptine, *3650*
[20316-18-1] Lycodine, *5619*
[20338-08-3] Titanic(IV) Acid, *9469*
[20344-49-4] Ferric Hydroxide, *4025*
[20350-15-6] Brefeldin A, *1369*
[20380-58-9] Tilidine, *9437*
[20405-64-5] Cuprous Selenide, *2666*
[20408-97-3] 5-Thio-D-glucose, *9334*
[20427-56-9] Ruthenium Tetroxide, *8301*
[20427-59-2] Cupric Hydroxide, *2642*
[20432-64-8] Iprindole Hydrochloride, *5075*
[20438-98-6] Imipramine *N*-Oxide Hydrochloride, *4921*
[20445-31-2] Mosher's Reagent (*R*)-(+)-Form, *6280*
[20445-33-4] Mosher's Reagent (*S*)-(+)-Acid Chloride, *6280*
[20449-79-0] Melittin, *5824*
[20480-93-7] Methenamine Sulfosalicy-late, *5966*
[20493-41-8] Quinapyramine, *8052*
[20537-88-6] Amifostine, *404*
[20548-54-3] Calcium Sulfide, *1707*
[20554-84-1] Parthenolide, *7048*
[20559-55-1] Oxibendazole, *6936*
[20562-02-1] Solanine (α-form), *8705*
[20574-50-9] Morantel, *6266*
[20594-83-6] Nalbuphine, *6357*
[20623-13-6] Nitrocobalamin, *4809*
[20642-05-1] Potassium Diformate, *7629*
[20644-87-5] Vanadium Carbonyl, *9919*
[20667-12-3] Silver Oxide, *8521*
[20684-06-4] Bamifylline Hydrochlo-ride, *955*
[20702-77-6] Neohesperidin Dihydro-chalcone, *6452*
[20725-03-5] Fustin, *4318*
[20734-58-1] DMAN, *3388*
[20770-09-6] Stannic Selenide, *8779*
[20788-07-2] Resorantel, *8154*
[20816-12-0] Osmium Tetroxide, *6893*
[20830-75-5] Digoxin, *3167*
[20830-81-3] Daunorubicin, *2832*
[20831-76-9] Gentiopicrin, *4397*
[20846-91-7] EDDS *S,S*-Form, *3508*
[20859-73-8] Aluminum Phosphide, *359*
[20867-01-0] Fulvoplumierin, *4285*
[20902-45-8] Penicillamine Disulfide D-Form, *7090*
[20905-71-9] Pyridoxal 5-Phosphate *O*-Methyloxime, *7979*

[20972-43-4] Azoxybenzene *trans-* Form, *923*
[21018-84-8] Amarogentin, *377*
[21040-59-5] Codamine, *2462*
[21041-93-0] Cobaltous Hydroxide, *2442*
[21041-95-2] Cadmium Hydroxide, *1620*
[21056-98-4] Calcium Phosphite, *1696*
[21087-64-9] Metribuzin, *6154*
[21109-95-5] Barium Sulfide, *995*
[21133-52-8] Lycoramine, *5625*
[21133-53-9] Glucofrangulin A, *4452*
[21150-22-1] β-Amanitin, *373*
[21174-80-1] Penicillamine Disulfide DL-Form, *7090*
[21187-73-5] Gardenin A, *4366*
[21187-98-4] Gliclazide, *4439*
[21200-24-8] Indolmycin, *4966*
[21215-62-3] Calcitonin (Human Synthetic), *1643*
[21238-30-2] Carbomycin B, *1806*
[21238-33-5] Oryzanol A, *6886*
[21245-01-2] 4-(Dimethylamino)benzoic Acid 3-Methylbutyl Ester, *3232*
[21245-02-3] 4-(Dimethylamino)benzoic Acid 2-Ethylhexyl Ester, *3232*
[21256-18-8] Oxaprozin, *6924*
[21259-20-1] T-2 Toxin, *9801*
[21259-76-7] Mercaptomerin Sodium, *5870*
[21293-20-9] Isoquassin, *5220*
[21293-29-8] Abscisic Acid, *11*
[21302-79-4] Ceanothic Acid, *1909*
[21312-10-7] N^4-Acetylsulfamethoxazole, *8918*
[21351-79-1] Cesium Hydroxide, *2013*
[21361-93-3] Nicotine Hydrochloride, *6524*
[21362-69-6] Mepitiostane, *5858*
[21363-18-8] Viminol, *9981*
[21370-21-8] Fenoxazoline Hydrochloride, *3985*
[21411-53-0] Virginiamycin M₁, *10004*
[21416-53-5] Picrotin, *7414*
[21416-67-1] Razoxane, *8123*
[21462-39-5] Clindamycin Hydrochloride, *2356*
[21466-07-9] Bromofenofos, *1419*
[21498-08-8] Lofexidine Hydrochloride, *5558*
[21535-47-7] Mianserin Hydrochloride, *6172*
[21548-73-2] Silver Sulfide, *8530*
[21564-17-0] TCMTB, *9086*
[21590-92-1] Etomidoline, *3882*
[21609-90-5] Leptophos, *5445*
[21637-25-2] Isoquercitrin, *5221*
[21645-51-2] Aluminum Hydroxide, *342*
[21649-57-0] Carbenicillin Phenyl Sodium, *1792*
[21650-42-0] Tretoquinol, *9587*
[21650-65-7] Azoxybenzene *cis-*Form, *923*
[21651-19-4] Stannous Oxide, *8787*
[21651-62-7] Nepetalactone *cis-trans-* Form, *6470*
[21679-14-1] Fludarabine, *4126*
[21715-46-8] Etifoxine, *3864*
[21725-46-2] Cyanazine, *2685*
[21730-16-5] Metapramine, *5930*

[21738-42-1] Oxamniquine, *6919*
[21755-66-8] Picoperine, *7404*
[21829-25-4] Nifedipine, *6528*
[21888-96-0] Dexetimide Hydrochloride, *2945*
[21888-98-2] Dexetimide, *2945*
[21898-19-1] Clenbuterol Hydrochloride, *2347*
[21908-53-2] Mercuric Oxide, Red, *5882*
[21908-53-2] Mercuric Oxide, Yellow, *5883*
[22006-84-4] Denopterin, *2895*
[22059-60-5] Disopyramide Phosphate, *3360*
[22071-15-4] Ketoprofen, *5305*
[22089-22-1] Trofosfamide, *9768*
[22103-14-6] Bufeniode, *1472*
[22131-35-7] Butalamine, *1510*
[22131-79-9] Alclofenac, *219*
[22131-80-2] Alclofenac Monoethanolamine Complex, *219*
[22139-77-1] Pinosylvin, *7451*
[22150-76-1] Biopterin, *1229*
[22151-68-4] Methohexital Sodium, *5981*
[22154-43-4] Meglumine Acetrizoate, *5806*
[22178-11-6] Pipotiazine Undecylenic Ester, *7482*
[22189-32-8] Spectinomycin Dihydrochloride Pentahydrate, *8739*
[22195-34-2] Guanadrel Sulfate, *4559*
[22199-08-2] Sulfadiazine Silver Salt, *8903*
[22202-75-1] Cephaloglycin Dihydrate, *1976*
[22204-24-6] Pyrantel Pamoate, *7955*
[22204-53-1] Naproxen, *6417*
[22204-88-2] Tramadol Hydrochloride, *9566*
[22205-45-4] Cuprous Sulfide, *2667*
[22224-92-6] Fenamiphos, *3957*
[22232-54-8] Carbimazole, *1798*
[22232-55-9] Pentorex Hydrogen D-Tartrate, *7133*
[22232-71-9] Mazindol, *5762*
[22248-79-9] Tetrachlorvinphos, *9192*
[22254-24-6] Ipratropium Bromide, *5073*
[22260-51-1] Bromocriptine Methanesulfonate, *1416*
[22263-79-2] Antheridiol, *681*
[22298-29-9] Betamethasone 17-Benzoate, *1180*
[22304-30-9] Apazone Dihydrate, *726*
[22316-47-8] Clobazam, *2359*
[22326-55-2] Barium Hydroxide Monohydrate, *977*
[22345-47-7] Tofisopam, *9503*
[22368-82-7] Pithecolobine, *7509*
[22398-80-7] Indium Phosphide, *4953*
[22457-89-2] Benfotiamine, *1041*
[22465-48-1] Acetatocobalamin, *4809*
[22494-42-4] Diflunisal, *3146*
[22537-19-5] Lawrencium, *5392*
[22560-16-3] Lithium Triethylborohydride, *5544*
[22560-50-5] Clodronic Acid Disodium Salt, *2371*
[22572-05-0] Penicillamine DL-Form Hydrochloride, *7088*
[22573-93-9] Alexidine, *232*
[22619-35-8] Tioclomarol, *9451*

[22633-88-1] Cosyntropin Hexaacetate, *2551*
[22650-86-8] Bismuth Subgallate, *1283*
[22662-39-1] Rafoxanide, *8097*
[22664-55-7] Metipranolol, *6140*
[22668-01-5] Etanidazole, *3713*
[22672-74-8] Isocorybulbine, *5161*
[22722-98-1] SMEAH, *8564*
[22733-60-4] Siccanin, *8486*
[22760-18-5] Proquazone, *7873*
[22775-12-8] Dimetofrine Hydrochloride, *3264*
[22775-52-6] Mycelianamide, *6319*
[22781-23-3] Bendiocarb, *1036*
[22831-39-6] Magnesium Silicide, *5688*
[22832-87-7] Miconazole Nitrate, *6178*
[22839-47-0] Aspartame, *839*
[22862-76-6] Anisomycin, *670*
[22887-42-9] Prednylidene 21-Diethylaminoacetate Hydrochloride, *7724*
[22888-70-6] Silybin, *8532*
[22916-47-8] Miconazole, *6178*
[22950-29-4] Dimetofrine, *3264*
[22963-93-5] Juvenile Hormone III, *5273*
[22994-85-0] Benznidazole, *1084*
[23031-25-6] Terbutaline, *9159*
[23031-32-5] Terbutaline Sulfate, *9159*
[23031-36-9] Prallethrin, *7704*
[23047-25-8] Lofepramine, *5557*
[23049-93-6] Enfenamic Acid, *3580*
[23067-13-2] Erythromycin Glucoheptonate, *3684*
[23076-35-9] Xylazine Hydrochloride, *10080*
[23089-26-1] α-Bisabolol (−)-Form, *1241*
[23092-17-3] Halazepam, *4589*
[23093-74-5] Bunitrolol Hydrochloride, *1489*
[23103-98-2] Pirimicarb, *7496*
[23109-05-9] α-Amanitin, *373*
[23110-15-8] Fumagillin, *4286*
[23135-22-0] Oxamyl, *6920*
[23142-01-0] Carbetapentane Citrate, *1794*
[23152-29-6] Virginiamycin S₁, *10004*
[23155-02-4] Fosfomycin, *4254*
[23178-88-3] α-Bisabolol (+)-Form, *1241*
[23184-66-9] Butachlor, *1508*
[23192-42-9] Hexalure, *4687*
[23210-56-2] Ifenprodil, *4895*
[23214-92-8] Doxorubicin, *3439*
[23214-96-2] Alcuronium, *221*
[23239-37-4] Etoxadrol (+)-Hydrochloride, *3889*
[23239-41-0] Cephacetrile Sodium, *1972*
[23239-51-2] Ritodrine Hydrochloride, *8237*
[23249-97-0] Procodazole, *7762*
[23255-54-1] Dihydro-β-erythroidine, *3175*
[23255-59-6] Lunularic Acid, *5606*
[23255-93-8] Hycanthone Mesylate, *4759*
[23255-99-4] Bendazac Sodium Salt, *1035*
[23256-30-6] Nifurtimox, *6538*
[23256-40-8] Guanoxabenz Hydrochloride, *4567*
[23256-50-0] Guanabenz Monoacetate, *4558*

[23257-56-9] Levophacetoperane Hydrochloride, 5467
[23277-43-2] Nalbuphine Hydrochloride, 6357
[23282-20-4] Nivalenol, 6659
[23282-55-5] Sulfachlorpyridazine Sodium Salt, 8900
[23288-49-5] Probucol, 7755
[23288-60-0] Sodium Pertechnetate 99mTc, 8657
[23315-05-1] Elaiomycin, 3534
[23319-63-3] Vedejs Reagent, 9943
[23325-78-2] Cephalexin Monohydrate, 1974
[23327-57-3] Nefopam Hydrochloride, 6440
[23344-16-3] Streptovaricin A, 8830
[23344-17-4] Streptovaricin C, 8830
[23383-11-1] Ferrous Citrate, 4044
[23454-33-3] Trenbolone Cyclohexylmethylcarbonate, 9583
[23465-76-1] Caroverine, 1857
[23496-41-5] Verticine, 9969
[23505-41-1] Pirimiphos-ethyl, 7497
[23509-16-2] Batrachotoxin, 1009
[23509-17-3] Homobatrachotoxin, 1009
[23513-14-6] [6]-Gingerol, 4424
[23541-50-6] Daunorubicin Hydrochloride, 2832
[23560-59-0] Heptenophos, 4664
[23564-05-8] Thiophanate-methyl, 9352
[23564-06-9] Thiophanate, 9352
[23593-75-1] Clotrimazole, 2417
[23602-78-0] Benfluorex, 1039
[23642-66-2] Benfluorex Hydrochloride, 1039
[23651-95-8] Droxidopa, 3457
[23666-50-4] Rhodomycin A, 8190
[23668-11-3] Pactamycin, 6985
[23672-07-3] Levosulpiride, 8989
[23674-86-4] Difluprednate, 3152
[23694-17-9] Sultopride Hydrochloride, 8994
[23694-81-7] Mepindolol, 5856
[23696-28-8] Olaquindox, 6823
[23696-85-7] β-Damascenone (stereo unspecified), 2809
[23726-93-4] β-Damascenone, 2809
[23736-58-5] Cloxacillin Benzathine Salt, 2419
[23777-80-2] Hexaborane(10), 4676
[23779-99-9] Floctafenine, 4103
[23784-10-3] Viminol p-Hydroxybenzoate, 9981
[23795-03-1] Probenecid Sodium Salt, 7754
[23828-92-4] Ambroxol Hydrochloride, 386
[23843-52-9] Phloionic Acid, 7325
[23873-81-6] Benzil Dioxime, 1079
[23887-31-2] Clorazepic Acid, 2403
[23887-41-4] Cinepazet, 2290
[23887-46-9] Cinepazide, 2291
[23915-80-2] Chromocarb Diethylamine, 2237
[23918-98-1] Eritadenine, 3670
[23930-19-0] Alfaxalone, 235
[23930-37-2] Alfadolone Acetate, 233
[23947-60-6] Ethirimol, 3740
[23950-58-5] Propyzamide, 7872
[23964-57-0] Carticaine Hydrochloride, 1869
[23964-58-1] Carticaine, 1869
[24017-47-8] Triazophos, 9606

[24047-25-4] Guanoxabenz, 4567
[24147-36-2] Thiazole Orange Iodide, 9308
[24159-07-7] Febrifugine, 3946
[24166-13-0] Cloxazolam, 2420
[24168-96-5] Isoconazole Nitrate, 5160
[24169-02-6] Econazole Nitrate, 3502
[24219-97-4] Mianserin, 6172
[24237-54-5] Tinoridine, 9448
[24243-97-8] Tymazoline, 9834
[24279-91-2] Carboquone, 1824
[24280-93-1] Mycophenolic Acid, 6327
[24304-00-5] Aluminum Nitride, 353
[24305-27-9] TRH, 9588
[24307-26-4] Mepiquat Chloride, 5857
[24321-47-9] Uscharidin, 9892
[24345-16-2] Apamin, 725
[24356-60-3] Cephapirin Sodium, 1984
[24356-94-3] Algestone Acetophenide, 240
[24381-49-5] Orotic Acid Choline Salt, 6876
[24381-60-0] Chromic Phosphate Radioactive Form, 2227
[24382-04-5] Malondialdehyde Sodium Salt, 5709
[24390-14-5] Doxycycline Hyclate, 3440
[24394-09-0] Cnicin, 2425
[24397-89-5] Actinobolin, 138
[24424-95-1] Di-tert-butyl Tricarbonate, 3039
[24526-64-5] Nomifensine, 6673
[24527-27-3] Clospirazine, 2412
[24531-57-5] 1-Thiosorbitol, 9363
[24558-01-8] Levophacetoperane, 5467
[24579-73-5] Propamocarb, 7798
[24582-91-0] Elenolide, 3543
[24584-09-6] Razoxane (+)-Form, 8123
[24600-36-0] Fominoben Hydrochloride, 4228
[24602-86-6] Tridemorph, 9660
[24634-61-5] Potassium Sorbate, 7671
[24656-22-2] Picoperine Tripalmitate, 7404
[24697-74-3] Leonurine, 5440
[24699-40-9] Picoperine Hydrochloride, 7404
[24701-51-7] Demexiptiline, 2890
[24724-90-1] Fucosamine, 4277
[24729-96-2] Clindamycin 2-Dihydrogen Phosphate, 2356
[24730-10-7] Dihydroergocristine Methanesulfonate, 3653
[24751-69-7] Nucleocidin, 6726
[24815-24-5] Rescinnamine, 8142
[24815-25-6] Ethybenztropine Hydrobromide, 3756
[24818-79-9] Clofibric Acid Basic Aluminum Salt, 2378
[24828-59-9] Chaulmoogric Acid Methyl Ester, 2048
[24851-98-7] Methyl Dihydrojasmonate, 6052
[24868-20-0] Dantrolene Sodium Salt Hemiheptahydrate, 2816
[24870-04-0] Giractide, 4428
[24880-43-1] Mesembrine, 5906
[24916-50-5] Spiramycin I, 8752
[24916-51-6] Spiramycin II, 8752
[24916-52-7] Spiramycin III, 8752
[24934-91-6] Chlormephos, 2103
[24967-93-9] Chondroitin 4-Sulfate, 2214

[24967-94-0] Dermatan Sulfate, 2214
[25001-57-4] Justicidin A, 5272
[25013-16-5] Butylated Hydroxyanisole, 1547
[25038-54-4] Nylon 6, 6734
[25046-79-1] Glisoxepid, 4444
[25053-27-4] Lyapolate Sodium, 5617
[25057-89-0] Bentazon, 1053
[25067-29-2] Methyl Cyanoacrylate Polymer, 6046
[25067-30-5] Ethyl Cyanoacrylate Polymer, 3787
[25104-18-1] Polylysine, 7571
[25122-41-2] Clobetasol, 2363
[25122-46-7] Clobetasol 17-Propionate, 2363
[25122-57-0] Clobetasone 17-Butyrate, 2364
[25126-32-3] Sincalide, 8543
[25127-31-5] Doxepin cis-Form Hydrochloride, 3435
[25152-52-7] Aluminum Antimonide, 328
[25154-52-3] Nonyl Phenol, 6681
[25154-80-7] n-Butyl Cyanoacrylate Polymer, 1565
[25155-15-1] Cymene, 2763
[25155-18-4] Methylbenzethonium Chloride, 6023
[25155-30-0] Sodium Dodecylbenzenesulfonate, 8612
[25161-91-5] Loline, 5561
[25301-02-4] Tyloxapol, 9833
[25311-71-1] Isofenphos, 5172
[25312-65-6] Cholanic Acid, 2196
[25316-40-9] Doxorubicin Hydrochloride, 3439
[25322-46-7] Chondroitin 6-Sulfate, 2214
[25322-68-3] Polyethylene Glycol, 7568
[25332-39-2] Trazodone Hydrochloride, 9579
[25333-42-0] 3-Quinuclidinol l-Form, 8082
[25333-43-1] 3-Quinuclidinol dl-Form Hydrochloride, 8082
[25333-48-6] 3-Quinuclidinol dl-Form Benzoate Hydrochloride, 8082
[25333-79-3] Noscapine Camphorsulfonate, 6718
[25354-97-6] 2-Hexyldecanoic Acid, 4709
[25384-17-2] Allylprodine, 296
[25389-94-0] Kanamycin A Sulfate, 5281
[25389-99-5] Neomycin B Hydrochloride, 6454
[25394-57-4] Affinin, 179
[25394-75-6] Alstonidine, 315
[25395-22-6] Salicylamide O-Acetic Acid, 8329
[25395-31-7] Diacetin, 2961
[25402-06-6] Cinerin I, 2292
[25451-15-4] Felbamate, 3950
[25486-55-9] Phylloquinone 2,3-Epoxide, 7380
[25523-97-1] Chlorpheniramine d-Form, 2180
[25546-65-0] Ribostamycin, 8206
[25573-43-7] Eseridine, 3699
[25583-20-4] Titanium Nitride, 9474
[25606-41-1] Propamocarb Hydrochloride, 7798

[25614-03-3] Bromocriptine, *1416*
[25617-97-4] Gallium Nitride, *4351*
[25617-98-5] Indium Nitride, *4951*
[25655-41-8] Povidone-Iodine, *7698*
[25672-33-7] Metformin *p*-Chlorophenoxyacetate (Salt), *5938*
[25679-28-1] *cis*-Anethole, *643*
[25717-80-0] Molsidomine, *6234*
[25803-14-9] Clometacin, *2383*
[25808-74-6] Lead Hexafluorosilicate, *5410*
[25812-30-0] Gemfibrozil, *4388*
[25827-76-3] Iomeglamic Acid, *5053*
[25846-73-5] Petunidin 3,5-Diglucoside, *7190*
[25867-19-0] Lycaconitine, *5618*
[25869-00-5] Ammonium Ferric Hexacyanoferrate, *7910*
[25869-98-1] Potassium Ferric Ferrocyanide, *7910*
[25875-50-7] Robenidine Hydrochloride, *8242*
[25875-51-8] Robenidine, *8242*
[25876-10-2] Gentamicin C$_1$, *4392*
[25876-11-3] Gentamicin C$_2$, *4392*
[25895-60-7] Sodium Cyanoborohydride, *8606*
[25905-77-5] Minaprine, *6200*
[25913-34-2] Tinoridine Hydrochloride, *9448*
[25953-17-7] Minaprine Dihydrochloride, *6200*
[25953-19-9] Cefazolin, *1917*
[25956-17-6] Allura Red AC, *284*
[25967-29-7] Flutoprazepam, *4213*
[25990-43-6] Mepenzolate, *5848*
[25999-31-9] Lasalocid A, *5373*
[26000-17-9] Lycoctonine, *5618*
[26002-80-2] Phenothrin, *7211*
[26016-98-8] Fosfomycin Calcium, *4254*
[26020-55-3] Oxetorone (anhydrous), *6934*
[26023-30-3] Lactic Acid Homopolymer, *5338*
[26027-38-3] Nonoxynol, *6677*
[26082-78-0] EGTA Disodium Salt, *3529*
[26086-49-7] Deoxydihydrostreptomycin, *2902*
[26095-59-0] Otilonium Bromide, *6898*
[26097-80-3] Cambendazole, *1726*
[26098-04-4] Gentamicin C$_{1a}$, *4392*
[26155-31-7] Morantel Tartrate, *6266*
[26159-34-2] Naproxen Sodium Salt, *6417*
[26161-42-2] Lactic Acid Homopolymer (L-form), *5338*
[26171-23-3] Tolmetin, *9518*
[26172-55-4] Methylchloroisothiazolinone, *6091*
[26195-62-0] Isotrilobine, *9697*
[26225-79-6] Ethofumesate, *3742*
[26239-55-4] ADA, *147*
[26241-81-6] Coumingine, *2565*
[26296-41-3] Cassaidine, *1890*
[26299-14-9] Pyridinium Chlorochromate, *7974*
[26305-03-3] Pepstatin, *7147*
[26309-95-5] Pivampicillin Hydrochloride, *7512*
[26328-04-1] Cinepazide Maleate, *2291*
[26328-53-0] Amoscanate, *574*
[26445-03-4] Thiocresol, *9325*

[26446-35-5] Monacetin, *6242*
[26472-41-3] Humulon, *4754*
[26490-31-3] Nandrolone Dodecanoate, *6365*
[26499-65-0] Calcium Sulfate Hemihydrate, *1706*
[26530-20-1] Octhilinone, *6755*
[26531-85-1] Primeverose, *7745*
[26532-22-9] Grandisol, *4535*
[26538-44-3] Zeranol, *10121*
[26544-34-3] Apiin, *732*
[26570-10-5] Propoxyphene Napsylate Monohydrate, *7839*
[26591-04-8] COP, *2514*
[26594-41-2] Isomethadone *d*-Form, *5184*
[26598-44-7] Ethybenztropine Hydrochloride, *3756*
[26605-16-3] Nocardamin, *6665*
[26605-69-6] Carindacillin Sodium Salt, *1840*
[26608-34-4] Etioporphyrin, *3869*
[26615-21-4] Zotepine, *10197*
[26628-22-8] Sodium Azide, *8581*
[26644-46-2] Triforine, *9691*
[26652-09-5] Ritodrine, *8237*
[26657-13-6] Rolitetracycline Nitrate Sesquihydrate, *8252*
[26658-42-4] Colestipol, *2475*
[26675-46-7] Isoflurane, *5175*
[26715-00-4] PVNO, *7948*
[26750-66-3] Potassium Thiocarbonate, *7690*
[26750-81-2] Alibendol, *244*
[26774-90-3] Epicillin, *3614*
[26786-32-3] Lofepramine Hydrochloride, *5557*
[26787-78-0] Amoxicillin, *577*
[26791-73-1] Xanthatin, *10058*
[26807-65-8] Indapamide, *4935*
[26809-38-1] Isobutyl Cyanoacrylate Polymer, *5140*
[26839-75-8] Timolol, *9444*
[26844-12-2] Indoramin, *4969*
[26864-56-2] Penfluridol, *7087*
[26871-30-7] Herqueinone, *4668*
[26877-34-9] Octyl Cyanoacrylate Polymer, *6766*
[26909-33-1] Rugulovasine A, *8295*
[26909-34-2] Rugulovasine B, *8295*
[26917-25-9] Lactic Acid Homopolymer (D-form), *5338*
[26921-17-5] Timolol Hydrogen Maleate Salt, *9444*
[26944-48-9] Glibornuride, *4438*
[26952-21-6] Isooctyl Alcohol, *5194*
[26973-24-0] Ceftezole, *1948*
[27007-85-8] Clospirazine Hydrochloride, *2412*
[27013-91-8] α-Hederin, *4625*
[27025-41-8] Glutathione Disulfide, *4475*
[27031-08-9] Sulfaguanole, *8909*
[27035-30-9] Oxametacine, *6916*
[27058-84-0] Moprolol Hydrochloride, *6264*
[27060-91-9] Flutazolam, *4209*
[27072-45-3] Asenapine (isomeric mixture), *4089*
[27073-72-9] Tiliacorine, *9436*
[27107-79-5] Tilidine *trans*-(±)-Hydrochloride, *9437*
[27115-36-2] Chromic Formate, *2224*
[27126-76-7] Koser's Reagent, *5321*

[27127-62-4] Viscosin, *10009*
[27164-46-1] Cefazolin Sodium Salt, *1917*
[27167-30-2] Oxazolam, *6927*
[27200-12-0] Ampelopsin, *579*
[27203-92-5] Tramadol, *9566*
[27208-80-6] Resveratrol 3-β-Mono-D-glucoside, *8158*
[27214-00-2] Calcium Glycerophosphate, *1670*
[27220-47-9] Econazole, *3502*
[27223-35-4] Ketazolam, *5297*
[27262-47-1] Levobupivacaine, *1495*
[27262-48-2] Levobupivacaine Hydrochloride, *1495*
[27267-69-2] Collinomycin, *2482*
[27279-76-1] Stibocaptate, *8812*
[27314-13-2] Norflurazon, *6701*
[27314-97-2] Tirapazamine, *9461*
[27315-91-9] Pipebuzone, *7457*
[27367-90-4] Niaprazine, *6492*
[27469-53-0] Almitrine, *301*
[27470-51-5] Suxibuzone, *9009*
[27471-60-9] Fenoxedil Hydrochloride, *3986*
[27491-70-9] Seyferth-Gilbert Reagent, *8476*
[27503-81-7] Ensulizole, *3593*
[27511-99-5] Eterobarb, *3715*
[27519-02-4] Muscalure, *6309*
[27523-40-6] Isoconazole, *5160*
[27588-43-8] Eprozinol Dihydrochloride, *3636*
[27589-33-9] Azosemide, *922*
[27591-69-1] Tilorone Dihydrochloride, *9440*
[27591-97-5] Tilorone, *9440*
[27607-77-8] Trimethylsilyl Triflate, *9719*
[27686-84-6] Nordihydroguaiaretic Acid (*meso*-form), *6693*
[27724-96-5] Cetraxate Hydrochloride, *2024*
[27726-31-4] Pivcefalexin Hydrochloride, *7513*
[27762-78-3] Kethoxal, *5299*
[27774-13-6] Vanadyl Sulfate, *9926*
[27780-11-6] Chrysanthemaxanthin, *2250*
[27792-36-5] Etiocobalamin, *3868*
[27833-64-3] Loxapine Succinate, *5587*
[27848-84-6] Nicergoline, *6496*
[27876-94-4] Crocetin, *2589*
[27877-51-6] Tolindate, *9515*
[27885-92-3] Imidocarb, *4915*
[27905-02-8] Gallium Citrate, *4349*
[27912-14-7] Levobunolol Hydrochloride, *5462*
[27917-82-4] Nitroxynil *N*-Ethylglucamine, *6656*
[27922-80-1] Phendimetrazine Pamoate, *7220*
[27928-00-3] Pyranine (free acid), *7954*
[27958-06-1] Deacetylanisomycin, *670*
[27973-72-4] Pederin, *7065*
[28008-04-0] Acetiamine Hydrochloride, *54*
[28014-46-2] Polyestradiol Phosphate, *7566*
[28159-98-0] Irgarol®, *5084*
[28189-85-7] Etoxadrol, *3889*
[28272-18-6] Pyrethrosin, *7965*
[28289-54-5] MPTP, *6294*
[28300-74-5] Antimony Potassium Tartrate, *700*

[28319-77-9] Choline Alfoscerate, 2205
[28375-03-3] Rugulovasines Hydrochloride, 8295
[28380-24-7] Nigericin, 6541
[28384-96-5] Enterobactin, 3596
[28393-42-2] Cephalosporin P₁, 1981
[28395-03-1] Bumetanide, 1484
[28416-66-2] Isoaminile Citrate, 5110
[28434-01-7] Bioresmethrin, 1230
[28439-19-2] Norbolethone d-Form, 6686
[28510-15-8] Rugulovasines Hydrochloride, 8295
[28523-86-6] Sevoflurane, 8475
[28553-12-0] DINP, 3290
[28558-32-9] Thiabendazole Hypophosphite, 9289
[28591-01-7] F-Gitonin, 4432
[28610-84-6] Rimazolium Metilsulfate, 8225
[28633-45-6] Ferric Citrate (undefined iron(III) salt), 4021
[28657-80-9] Cinoxacin, 2309
[28704-27-0] Glatiramer, 4435
[28721-07-5] Oxcarbazepine, 6929
[28728-55-4] Hexadimethrine Bromide, 4682
[28757-47-3] Polyhexamethylene Biguanide, 7560
[28772-56-7] Bromadiolone (base), 1382
[28782-19-6] Flavoxate Succinate, 4096
[28782-42-5] Difenoxin, 3136
[28797-61-7] Pirenzepine, 7491
[28860-95-9] Carbidopa, 1797
[28905-10-4] Glucosamine β-Form, 4458
[28905-11-5] Glucosamine α-Form, 4458
[28911-01-5] Triazolam, 9604
[28947-50-4] Fencamine, 3967
[28950-34-7] Tetrasulfur Tetranitride, 9241
[28981-97-7] Alprazolam, 312
[28983-56-4] Methyl Blue, 6028
[28994-41-4] o-Benzylphenol, 1142
[29025-14-7] Butropium Bromide, 1534
[29031-19-4] Glucosamine Sulfate Salt, 4458
[29069-24-7] Prednimustine, 7720
[29074-38-2] Canadine dl-Form, 1736
[29091-21-2] Prodiamine, 7766
[29094-61-9] Glipizide, 4442
[29098-15-5] Terofenamate, 9168
[29106-32-9] Chaulmoogric Acid, 2048
[29110-47-2] Guanfacine, 4561
[29110-48-3] Guanfacine Hydrochloride, 4561
[29119-03-7] Frequentin, 4270
[29122-68-7] Atenolol, 859
[29177-84-2] Ethyl Loflazepate, 3821
[29202-00-4] Gardenin D, 4366
[29216-28-2] Mequitazine, 5864
[29218-27-7] Toloxatone, 9521
[29232-93-7] Pirimiphos-methyl, 7497
[29306-57-8] Trinitrotriazidobenzene, 9731
[29334-07-4] Sulmarin, 8984
[29342-05-0] Ciclopirox, 2266
[29342-22-1] Moore's Ketene, 6262
[29343-52-0] HNE (unspecified stereo), 4726
[29365-11-5] Giractide Hexaacetate Salt, 4428

[29393-20-2] Bacilysin, 933
[29400-42-8] Helvolic Acid, 4633
[29493-77-4] 4-Methylaminorex (±)-cis Form, 6018
[29550-05-8] Gardenin C, 4366
[29550-07-0] Gardenin E, 4366
[29560-58-5] Moricizine Hydrochloride, 6268
[29608-49-9] Almitrine Dimethanesulfonate, 301
[29684-56-8] Burgess Reagent, 1502
[29689-14-3] Chromic Carbonate, 2221
[29701-07-3] Kanamycin B Sulfate, 5281
[29714-87-2] Ocimene, 6741
[29728-34-5] Acetoxolone Aluminum Salt, 76
[29767-20-2] Teniposide, 9145
[29790-52-1] Nicotine Salicylate, 6524
[29804-22-6] Disparlure (cis-form), 3361
[29836-26-8] n-Octyl-β-D-glucoside, 6767
[29838-46-8] Roccellic Acid, 8244
[29868-97-1] Pirenzepine Dihydrochloride, 7491
[29883-15-6] Amygdalin, 597
[29899-95-4] Clobenoside, 2361
[29908-03-0] S-Adenosylmethionine, 156
[29913-86-8] Amarolide, 378
[29915-38-6] TAPS, 9058
[29952-87-2] Clofibric Acid Pyridoxine Salt, 2378
[29956-24-9] Pyridoxal 5-Phosphate Calcium Salt, 7979
[29975-16-4] Estazolam, 3702
[30042-37-6] Lankamycin, 5356
[30123-17-2] Tianeptine Sodium Salt, 9420
[30223-48-4] Fluacizine, 4113
[30272-08-3] Amineptine Hydrochloride, 409
[30286-75-0] Oxitropium Bromide, 6943
[30299-08-2] Clinofibrate, 2357
[30392-40-6] Bitolterol, 1307
[30392-41-7] Bitolterol Methanesulfonate, 1307
[30403-03-3] Gallium Citrate (unspecified stoichiometry), 4349
[30408-30-1] Nybomycin, 6731
[30452-69-8] L-Cystine S,S-Dioxide, 2783
[30484-77-6] Flunarizine Dihydrochloride, 4144
[30516-87-1] Zidovudine, 10123
[30525-89-4] Paraformaldehyde, 7025
[30544-47-9] Etofenamate, 3875
[30544-61-7] Clanobutin, 2338
[30560-19-1] Acephate, 31
[30578-37-1] Amezinium Methyl Sulfate, 394
[30652-11-0] Deferiprone, 2859
[30653-83-9] Parsalmide, 7045
[30685-43-9] β-Methyldigoxin, 3167
[30748-29-9] Feprazone, 4012
[30905-63-6] Calcium N-Carbamoyl-aspartate DL-Form, 1655
[30909-51-4] Flupentixol Decanoate, 4187
[30924-31-3] Cafaminol, 1633
[30964-13-7] Cynarin(e), 2766
[31002-79-6] Triamcinolone Benetonide, 9597

[31036-80-3] Lofexidine, 5558
[31112-62-6] Metrizamide, 6155
[31139-87-4] Tipepidine Hibenzate, 9457
[31218-83-4] Propetamphos, 7815
[31282-04-9] Hygromycin B, 4852
[31314-38-2] Prodipine, 7768
[31314-39-3] Prodipine Hydrochloride, 7768
[31329-57-4] Nafronyl, 6353
[31342-36-6] Chloramphenicol Pantothenate Calcium Complex (4:1), 2077
[31362-50-2] Bombesin, 1329
[31366-25-3] Tetrathiafulvalene, 9242
[31377-23-8] Amantadine Sulfate, 374
[31418-71-0] Coprogen, 2522
[31428-61-2] Tiamenidine, 9418
[31430-15-6] Flubendazole, 4118
[31431-39-7] Mebendazole, 5768
[31431-43-3] Cyclobendazole, 2712
[31477-60-8] Centchroman, 1971
[31566-31-1] Glyceryl Monostearate, 4489
[31570-39-5] Neocembrene, 6448
[31586-77-3] Bismuth Sodium Tartrate, 1279
[31637-97-5] Etofibrate, 3877
[31677-93-7] Bupropion Hydrochloride, 1499
[31698-14-3] Ancitabine, 629
[31721-17-2] Quinupramine, 8083
[31774-33-1] Abikoviromycin, 8
[31828-50-9] Cephradine Dihydrate, 1986
[31828-71-4] Mexiletine, 6169
[31842-61-2] Rimiterol Hydrobromide, 8227
[31853-38-0] 1,2-Naphthoquinone 2-Semicarbazone, 6394
[31868-18-5] Mexazolam, 6166
[31879-05-7] Fenoprofen, 3980
[31883-05-3] Moricizine, 6268
[31884-76-1] Sulfanilic Acid Zinc Salt Tetrahydrate, 8926
[31884-77-2] Meclizine Dihydrochloride Monohydrate, 5777
[31944-97-5] Chondrofoline, 2213
[32157-29-2] Propanethial S-Oxide, 7802
[32164-16-2] Verticillin A, 9968
[32164-26-4] Streptovaricin D, 8830
[32190-57-1] Wildfire Toxin, 10046
[32222-06-3] Calcitriol, 1644
[32245-40-2] 1-Theobromineacetic Acid Sodium Salt, 9283
[32248-43-4] Samarium Iodide, 8349
[32266-10-7] Hexoprenaline Sulfate, 4707
[32267-39-3] Divicine, 3383
[32289-58-0] Polihexanide, 7560
[32359-34-5] Medifoxamine, 5790
[32381-42-3] Vernolic Acid (−)-Form, 9963
[32383-76-9] Medicarpin, 5789
[32385-11-8] Sisomicin, 8550
[32421-46-8] Bunaftine, 1485
[32449-92-6] D-Glucuronolactone, 4467
[32467-88-2] ACV, 145
[32476-67-8] Periplocymarin, 7175
[32527-55-2] Tiaramide, 9424
[32619-42-4] Oleuropein, 6830
[32630-75-4] Pododacric Acid, 7544
[32665-36-4] Eprozinol, 3636
[32672-69-8] Mesoridazine Benzenesulfonate, 5910

[32728-78-2] Heliosupine, *4629*
[32780-64-6] Labetalol Hydrochloride, *5329*
[32784-82-0] Improsulfan Tosylate, *4927*
[32795-44-1] Acecainide, *20*
[32795-47-4] Nomifensine Maleate, *6673*
[32809-16-8] Procymidone, *7765*
[32828-81-2] Picotamide, *7407*
[32854-75-4] Lappaconitine, *5369*
[32886-97-8] Amdinocillin Pivoxil, *390*
[32887-01-7] Amdinocillin, *389*
[32887-03-9] Amdinocillin Pivoxil Hydrochloride, *390*
[32909-92-5] Sulfametrole, *8920*
[32953-89-2] Rimiterol, *8227*
[32986-56-4] Tobramycin, *9490*
[32988-50-4] Viomycin, *10001*
[33005-95-7] Tiaprofenic Acid, *9422*
[33032-12-1] Methapyrilene Fumarate, *5959*
[33069-62-4] Paclitaxel, *6982*
[33089-61-1] Amitraz, *486*
[33103-21-8] Tuberactinomycin A, *9803*
[33103-22-9] Enviomycin, *3600*
[33125-97-2] Etomidate, *3881*
[33137-73-4] Tuberactinomycin O, *9803*
[33159-27-2] Ecabet, *3489*
[33178-86-8] Alinidine, *246*
[33194-27-3] Alsactide Acetate, *314*
[33237-74-0] Aprindine Hydrochloride, *754*
[33245-39-5] Fluchloralin, *4120*
[33286-22-5] Diltiazem Hydrochloride, *3202*
[33320-16-0] Methyl Aminolevulinate, *6016*
[33342-05-1] Gliquidone, *4443*
[33368-20-6] Enduracidin A Hydrochloride, *3579*
[33369-31-2] Zomepirac, *10191*
[33386-08-2] Buspirone Hydrochloride, *1504*
[33396-37-1] Proscillaridin-4-methyl Ether, *7874*
[33401-94-4] Pyrantel Tartrate, *7955*
[33402-03-8] Metaraminol Bitartrate (Hydrogen L-Tartrate), *5932*
[33404-78-3] Negamycin, *6441*
[33419-42-0] Etoposide, *3886*
[33445-35-1] Sulfamidochrysoidine Hydrochloride, *8923*
[33490-33-4] Capreomycin IB, *1757*
[33515-32-1] S-Methylmethionine Bromide, *6098*
[33538-71-5] Venturicidin A, *9947*
[33538-72-6] Venturicidin B, *9947*
[33564-30-6] Cefoxitin Sodium Salt, *1936*
[33564-31-7] Diflorasone Diacetate, *3140*
[33570-04-6] Bilobalide, *1220*
[33579-45-2] Scotophobin, *8411*
[33580-30-2] Tertatolol Hydrochloride, *9173*
[33605-67-3] Cargutocin, *1839*
[33605-94-6] Pyrisuccideanol, *7991*
[33614-49-2] Gold Sodium Thiosulfate Dihydrate, *4519*
[33629-47-9] Butralin, *1532*
[33636-93-0] Stryker's Reagent, *8857*

[33665-90-6] Acesulfame, *37*
[33671-46-4] Clotiazepam, *2416*
[33765-68-3] Oxendolone, *6931*
[33797-51-2] Dimethyl(methylene)-ammonium Iodide, *3251*
[33817-20-8] Pivampicillin, *7512*
[33818-15-4] Citicoline Sodium Salt, *2319*
[33842-02-3] Viehe's Salt, *9977*
[33861-17-5] Phenylselenotrimethyl-silane, *7311*
[33996-33-7] Oxaceprol, *6903*
[34014-18-1] Tebuthiuron, *9095*
[34031-32-8] Auranofin, *878*
[34089-81-1] Sodium Ferric Gluconate, *8615*
[34097-16-0] Clocortolone 21-Pivalate, *2369*
[34118-92-8] Acecainide Hydrochloride, *20*
[34123-59-6] Isoproturon, *5218*
[34135-85-8] Methyl Allyl Trisulfide, *6013*
[34140-59-5] Trimebutine Maleate, *9699*
[34161-23-4] Fipexide Hydrochloride, *4084*
[34161-24-5] Fipexide, *4084*
[34167-45-8] Polymyxin D_2, *7573*
[34183-22-7] Propafenone Hydrochloride, *7794*
[34184-77-5] Promegestone, *7785*
[34195-34-1] Hydrocodone Bitartrate Hemipentahydrate, *4785*
[34214-51-2] Floxacillin Sodium Monohydrate, *4111*
[34218-61-6] Juvenile Hormone II, *5273*
[34255-08-8] Rhodoviolascin, *8194*
[34256-82-1] Acetochlor, *61*
[34272-51-0] Histrionicotoxin, *4723*
[34273-10-4] Saralasin, *8372*
[34291-02-6] Butirosin A, *1528*
[34291-03-7] Butirosin B, *1528*
[34301-55-8] Isometamidium Chloride, *5183*
[34312-10-2] Citrulline Hydrochloride, *2331*
[34316-15-9] Chelerythrine, *2051*
[34327-18-9] Chloramphenicol Monosuccinate Arginine Salt, *2077*
[34368-04-2] Dobutamine, *3395*
[34381-68-5] Acebutolol Hydrochloride, *19*
[34391-04-3] Albuterol (R)-Form, *216*
[34433-31-3] Asoxime Chloride, *835*
[34444-01-4] Cefamandole, *1914*
[34461-22-8] Metformin Embonate, *5938*
[34493-98-6] Dibekacin, *3005*
[34503-87-2] Polymyxin B_2, *7573*
[34521-09-0] Antimony Sodium Tartrate, *702*
[34522-46-8] Oxetorone Fumarate, *6934*
[34524-20-4] Boromycin, *1342*
[34552-83-5] Loperamide Hydrochloride, *5571*
[34580-13-7] Ketotifen, *5307*
[34580-14-8] Ketotifen Fumarate, *5307*
[34590-94-8] Dipropylene Glycol Monomethyl Ether, *3344*
[34633-34-6] Bifluranol, *1212*

[34642-77-8] Amoxicillin Sodium Salt, *577*
[34661-75-1] Urapidil, *9865*
[34675-84-8] Cetraxate, *2024*
[34707-92-1] Chlorothricin, *2169*
[34758-83-3] Zipeprol, *10170*
[34758-84-4] Zipeprol Dihydrochloride, *10170*
[34765-96-3] Alsactide, *314*
[34765-98-5] Enduracidin B Hydrochloride, *3579*
[34784-64-0] Tertatolol, *9173*
[34786-70-4] Nystatin A_1, *6736*
[34787-01-4] Ticarcillin, *9428*
[34816-55-2] Moxestrol, *6289*
[34866-46-1] Carbuterol Hydrochloride, *1833*
[34866-47-2] Carbuterol, *1833*
[34911-55-2] Bupropion, *1499*
[34915-68-9] Bunitrolol, *1489*
[34919-98-7] Cetamolol, *2018*
[34994-11-1] Hypusine, *4870*
[35035-05-3] Timepidium Bromide, *9442*
[35080-11-6] Prajmaline, *7702*
[35108-88-4] Bufetolol Hydrochloride, *1473*
[35112-53-9] Barium Thiosulfate, *999*
[35121-78-9] Prostacyclin, *7875*
[35124-13-1] d-cis-α-Irone, *5096*
[35189-28-7] Norgestimate, *6703*
[35212-22-7] Ipriflavone, *5074*
[35274-05-6] Cetyl Lactate, *2030*
[35287-72-0] Secalonic Acid A, *8418*
[35334-12-4] Azidocillin Sodium Salt, *910*
[35354-74-6] Honokiol, *4742*
[35367-38-5] Diflubenzuron, *3142*
[35380-71-3] Estradiol Hemihydrate, *3703*
[35400-43-2] Sulprofos, *8990*
[35405-51-7] Calcium Pyrophosphate, *1699*
[35413-63-9] Streptovaricin E, *8830*
[35455-20-0] 3-Fluoro-D-alanine, *4168*
[35457-80-8] Midecamycin A_1, *6183*
[35512-37-9] Streptovaricin F, *8830*
[35531-88-5] Carindacillin, *1840*
[35543-24-9] Buflomedil Hydrochloride, *1475*
[35554-08-6] Saxitoxin, *8389*
[35554-44-0] Enilconazole, *3583*
[35595-03-0] Centaurein, *1968*
[35597-44-5] Phosphinothricin, *7339*
[35604-67-2] Viloxazine Hydrochloride, *9980*
[35607-66-0] Cefoxitin, *1936*
[35619-65-9] Trithiozine, *9760*
[35691-65-7] 1,2-Dibromo-2,4-dicyano-butane, *3021*
[35700-21-1] Carboprost Methyl Ester, *1823*
[35700-23-3] Carboprost, *1823*
[35834-26-5] Rosaramicin, *8261*
[35836-73-8] Nopol, *6683*
[35846-53-8] Maytansine, *5761*
[35898-87-4] Dilazep, *3200*
[35941-65-2] Butriptyline, *1533*
[35941-71-0] Tiaramide Hydrochloride, *9424*
[35991-93-6] Nadoxolol Hydrochloride, *6347*
[36025-69-1] Midecamycin A_3, *6183*
[36085-73-1] Talipexole Dihydrochloride, *9039*

[36104-64-0] Micranthine, *6179*
[36104-80-0] Camazepam, *1725*
[36141-82-9] Diamfenetide, *2974*
[36167-63-2] Halofantrine Hydrochloride, *4594*
[36190-93-9] Oleandrin Desacetyl-oleandrin, *6826*
[36222-39-6] Gallopamil *l*-Form Hydrochloride, *4356*
[36289-36-8] 1-Cyanoimidazole, *2696*
[36296-31-8] Oxiniacic Acid Ethanol-amine Salt, *6941*
[36304-84-4] Dimemorfan Phosphate, *3206*
[36309-01-0] Dimemorfan, *3206*
[36322-90-4] Piroxicam, *7506*
[36330-85-5] Fenbufen, *3963*
[36338-96-2] Carthamin, *1867*
[36364-49-5] Imidazole Salicylate, *4913*
[36478-76-9] Uranyl Nitrate, *9863*
[36499-65-7] EDTA Cobalt Salt, *3517*
[36505-84-7] Buspirone, *1504*
[36508-71-1] Zorubicin Hydrochloride, *10195*
[36508-79-9] Nitroxynil D-*N*-Methyl-glucamine Salt, *6656*
[36531-26-7] Oxantel, *6922*
[36556-75-9] Bucumolol Hydrochloride, *1467*
[36590-19-9] Amocarzine, *571*
[36592-77-5] Metipranolol Hydrochloride, *6140*
[36635-61-7] Tosylmethyl Isocyanide, *9556*
[36637-18-0] Etidocaine, *3862*
[36637-19-1] Etidocaine Hydrochloride, *3862*
[36647-02-6] Cotarnine Hydrochloride, *2552*
[36653-82-4] Cetyl Alcohol, *2028*
[36703-88-5] Inosine Pranobex, *4976*
[36734-19-7] Iprodione, *5077*
[36735-22-5] Quazepam, *8029*
[36791-04-5] Ribavirin, *8198*
[36798-79-5] Budralazine, *1470*
[36861-47-9] 4-Methylbenzylidene Camphor, *6027*
[36894-69-6] Labetalol, *5329*
[37025-55-1] Carbetocin, *1795*
[37065-29-5] Miloxacin, *6196*
[37091-65-9] Azlocillin Sodium Salt, *916*
[37091-66-0] Azlocillin, *916*
[37106-97-1] Bentiromide, *1054*
[37112-31-5] Levoglucosenone, *5465*
[37115-32-5] Adinazolam, *160*
[37134-80-8] Dopastin, *3423*
[37148-27-9] Clenbuterol, *2347*
[37196-57-9] Crotamine, *2593*
[37220-17-0] Konjac Mannan, *5319*
[37221-79-7] VIP, *10002*
[37248-47-8] Validamycin A, *9908*
[37267-86-0] Phosphoric Acid, Meta, *7345*
[37270-69-2] Benserazide Combination with Levodopa, *1050*
[37270-89-6] Heparin Calcium Salt, *4653*
[37280-35-6] Capreomycin IA, *1757*
[37288-97-4] Pinguinain, *7449*
[37291-07-9] Crilanomer, *2587*
[37296-80-3] Colestipol Hydrochloride, *2475*

[37300-21-3] Pentosan Polysulfate, *7134*
[37301-55-6] Chlormadinone Acetate Mixture with Ethinyl Estradiol, *2102*
[37319-17-8] Pentosan Polysulfate Sodium Salt, *7134*
[37321-09-8] Apramycin, *752*
[37332-99-3] Avoparcin, *889*
[37338-39-9] Pyrimethamine Combination with Sulfadoxine, *7985*
[37339-90-5] Lentinan, *5439*
[37340-82-2] Streptodornase, *8823*
[37342-97-5] Schwartz's Reagent, *8396*
[37350-58-6] Metoprolol, *6151*
[37415-62-6] Mycophenolic Acid Sodium Salt, *6327*
[37517-26-3] Pipotiazine Palmitic Ester, *7482*
[37517-28-5] Amikacin, *405*
[37517-30-9] Acebutolol, *19*
[37561-27-6] Fenoverine, *3982*
[37577-24-5] Fenfluramine *l*-Form, *3973*
[37640-71-4] Aprindine, *754*
[37661-08-8] Bacampicillin Hydrochloride, *931*
[37686-84-3] Terguride, *9164*
[37686-85-4] Terguride Hydrogen Maleate, *9164*
[37693-01-9] Clofoctol, *2380*
[37758-47-7] Ganglioside G$_{m1}$, *4364*
[37764-25-3] Dichlormid, *3049*
[37878-19-6] Detoxin D$_1$, *2938*
[37883-00-4] Viomycin Sulfate, *10001*
[37895-35-5] Albofungin, *212*
[37933-66-7] Thevetin A, *9288*
[38029-10-6] Pirbuterol Dihydrochloride, *7489*
[38078-09-0] Diethylaminosulfur Trifluoride, *3113*
[38129-37-2] Bicozamycin, *1202*
[38142-58-4] *ar*-Turmerone (±)-Form, *9825*
[38176-02-2] Dexverapamil Hydrochloride, *9950*
[38176-09-9] Gallopamil *d*-Form Hydrochloride, *4356*
[38183-12-9] Fluorescamine, *4158*
[38194-50-2] Sulindac, *8982*
[38234-21-8] Fertirelin, *4061*
[38260-01-4] Trientine Dihydrochloride, *9663*
[38260-54-7] Etrimfos, *3893*
[38270-90-5] Strontium Chloride ⁸⁹Sr-Labeled Form, *8840*
[38304-91-5] Minoxidil, *6203*
[38321-02-7] Dexverapamil, *9950*
[38345-66-3] Chirald, *2062*
[38363-32-5] Penbutolol Sulfate, *7082*
[38363-40-5] Penbutolol, *7082*
[38398-32-2] Ganaxolone, *4362*
[38455-77-5] Stannic Chromate(VI), *8775*
[38562-01-5] Prostaglandin F$_{2\alpha}$ Tromethamine Salt, *7878*
[38577-97-8] 4′,5′-Diiodofluorescein, *3189*
[38640-92-5] Ampligen, *588*
[38641-94-0] Glyphosate Mono(isopropylamine) Salt, *4512*
[38677-81-5] Pirbuterol, *7489*
[38677-85-9] Flunixin, *4147*
[38721-52-7] L-Selectride, *8427*
[38748-32-2] Triptolide, *9747*

[38821-52-2] Indoramin Hydrochloride, *4969*
[38821-53-3] Cephradine, *1986*
[38916-34-6] Somatostatin, *8715*
[38932-40-0] Cephalexin Sodium Salt, *1974*
[38957-41-4] Emorfazone, *3562*
[38965-69-4] Xanthocillin Y$_1$, *10061*
[38965-70-7] Xanthocillin Y$_2$, *10061*
[38966-21-1] Aphidicolin, *727*
[39025-23-5] Z-Guggulsterone, *4573*
[39025-24-6] *E*-Guggulsterone, *4573*
[39133-31-8] Trimebutine, *9699*
[39148-24-8] Fosetyl Al, *4252*
[39156-41-7] 2,4-Diaminoanisole Sulfate, *2976*
[39236-46-9] Imidurea, *4916*
[39238-36-3] Myxin Copper(II) Complex, *6340*
[39290-85-2] Cupric Borate, *2628*
[39295-60-8] Sulfadoxine Mixture with Trimethoprim, *8906*
[39300-45-3] Dinocap, *3286*
[39366-37-5] Levonorgestrel Mixture with Ethinyl Estradiol, *6704*
[39379-15-2] Neurotensin, *6486*
[39391-39-4] Nocardicin A, *6666*
[39404-00-7] Hemozoin, *4649*
[39409-82-0] Magnesium Carbonate Hydroxide, *5660*
[39416-48-3] Pyridinium Bromide Perbromide, *7973*
[39455-18-0] Chondroitin 4-Sulfate Disodium Salt, *2214*
[39492-01-8] Gabexate, *4320*
[39515-40-7] Cyphenothrin, *2768*
[39515-41-8] Fenpropathrin, *3991*
[39543-79-8] Befunolol Hydrochloride, *1022*
[39552-01-7] Befunolol, *1022*
[39562-70-4] Nitrendipine, *6576*
[39563-28-5] Cloranolol, *2402*
[39577-19-0] Picumast, *7418*
[39577-20-3] Picumast Dihydrochloride, *7418*
[39589-98-5] Dimethyl Carbate, *3240*
[39637-99-5] Mosher's Reagent (*R*)-(−)-Acid Chloride, *6280*
[39640-15-8] Piberaline, *7392*
[39647-11-5] Methyl Dihydrojasmonate (+)-(1R,2S)-Form, *6052*
[39664-27-2] Ethylamine Oleate, *3762*
[39698-78-7] Saralasin Hydrated Acetate, *8372*
[39711-79-0] Ethyl Menthane Carboxamide, *3825*
[39715-02-1] Endralazine, *3577*
[39718-89-3] Alminoprofen, *300*
[39733-35-2] Ammonium Magnesium Chloride, *531*
[39800-16-3] Perfosfamide (unspecified stereo), *7161*
[39807-15-3] Oxadiargyl, *6905*
[39809-25-1] Penciclovir, *7083*
[39831-55-5] Amikacin Sulfate, *405*
[39860-99-6] Pipotiazine, *7482*
[39878-70-1] Talampicillin Hydrochloride, *9033*
[39937-23-0] Bixins *trans*-Form, *1311*
[39978-42-2] Nifurzide, *6540*
[40034-42-2] Rosoxacin, *8268*
[40054-69-1] Etizolam, *3873*
[40180-04-9] Ticrynafen, *9430*
[40372-00-7] Taribavirin Hydrochloride, *9063*

[40391-99-9] Pamidronic Acid, 7003
[40431-64-9] Methylphenidate d-threo-Form, 6110
[40487-42-1] Pendimethalin, 7084
[40507-23-1] Fluproquazone, 4193
[40507-78-6] Indanazoline, 4932
[40507-80-0] Indanazoline Hydrochloride, 4932
[40516-48-1] Tocoretinate, 9499
[40580-59-4] Guanadrel, 4559
[40596-69-8] Methoprene, 5983
[40665-92-7] Cloprostenol, 2399
[40666-16-8] Fluprostenol, 4194
[40716-66-3] Nerolidol trans-Form, 6476
[40762-15-0] Doxefazepam, 3434
[40816-40-8] Solanine Hydrochloride, 8705
[40819-93-0] Lorajmine Hydrochloride, 5577
[40828-46-4] Suprofen, 9005
[41096-46-2] Hydroprene, 4805
[41100-52-1] Memantine Hydrochloride, 5829
[41114-59-4] Nysted Reagent, 6737
[41136-22-5] Ceftezole Sodium Salt, 1948
[41183-64-6] ^{67}Ga Gallium Citrate, 4349
[41198-08-7] Profenofos, 7770
[41294-56-8] 1α-Hydroxycholecalciferol, 4819
[41340-25-4] Etodolac, 3874
[41342-53-4] Erythromycin Ethylsuccinate, 3681
[41354-29-4] Cyproheptadine Hydrochloride Sesquihydrate, 2773
[41372-20-7] Apomorphine Hydrochloride (hemihydrate), 746
[41394-05-2] Metamitron, 5924
[41451-75-6] Bruceantin, 1454
[41470-05-7] 11-cis-3-Dehydroretinal, 2873
[41473-08-9] Iopronic Acid, 5063
[41483-43-6] Bupirimate, 1494
[41544-24-5] Tromantadine Hydrochloride, 9771
[41567-78-6] Fumagillin Dicyclohexylamine Salt, 4286
[41570-61-0] Tulobuterol, 9811
[41575-94-4] Carboplatin, 1822
[41621-49-2] Ciclopirox Ethanolamine Salt (1:1), 2266
[41663-50-7] Isobutol, 3720
[41708-72-9] Tocainide, 9491
[41744-40-5] Sulbenicillin, 8890
[41767-29-7] Fluocortin Butyl, 4152
[41826-92-0] Trepibutone, 9585
[41859-67-0] Bezafibrate, 1195
[41906-86-9] Nitrocefin, 6594
[41944-01-8] Bismuth Potassium Iodide, 1276
[41992-22-7] Spirogermanium Dihydrochloride, 8758
[41992-23-8] Spirogermanium, 8758
[42116-76-7] Carnidazole, 1848
[42200-33-9] Nadolol, 6346
[42399-41-7] Diltiazem, 3202
[42408-82-2] Butorphanol, 1530
[42461-84-7] Flunixin Meglumine Salt, 4147
[42471-28-3] Nimustine, 6553
[42540-40-9] Cefamandole Nafate, 1914

[42542-10-9] MDMA, 5767
[42553-65-1] Crocetin Di-gentiobiose Ester, 2589
[42576-02-3] Bifenox, 1208
[42597-57-9] Ronifibrate, 8255
[42794-76-3] Midodrine, 6184
[42835-25-6] Flumequine, 4137
[42852-95-9] N-Methyl-α-L-glucosamine, 6079
[42864-78-8] Bevantolol Hydrochloride, 1192
[42874-03-3] Oxyfluorfen, 6963
[42924-53-8] Nabumetone, 6343
[42971-09-5] Vinpocetine, 9991
[43033-72-3] Levomethadyl Acetate Hydrochloride, 5466
[43121-43-3] Triadimefon, 9592
[43200-80-2] Zopiclone, 10193
[43210-67-9] Fenbendazole, 3960
[43222-48-6] Difenzoquat Methyl Sulfate, 3138
[43229-80-7] Formoterol Fumarate, 4245
[46464-11-3] Meobentine, 5843
[46817-91-8] Viloxazine, 9980
[47141-42-4] Levobunolol, 5462
[47562-08-3] Lorajmine, 5577
[47739-98-0] Clocapramine, 2366
[47747-56-8] Talampicillin, 9033
[47931-85-1] Calcitonin (Salmon Synthetic), 1643
[49562-28-9] Fenofibrate, 3978
[49564-56-9] Fazadinium Bromide, 3943
[49582-09-4] PBB, 4081
[49638-23-5] Betaprodine Hydrochloride, 310
[49642-07-1] Statine, 8800
[49656-78-2] Methcathinone Hydrochloride, 5963
[49697-38-3] Rimexolone, 8226
[49745-95-1] Dobutamine Hydrochloride, 3395
[49746-00-1] Carbinoxamine l-Form d-Tartrate, 1799
[49866-87-7] Difenzoquat, 3138
[50264-69-2] Lonidamine, 5568
[50276-98-7] Erythrocentaurin, 3678
[50291-21-9] Rose Bengal ^{131}I-Labeled Disodium Salt, 8262
[50293-90-8] Albuterol (R)-Form Hydrochloride, 216
[50321-35-2] Morazone Hydrochloride, 6267
[50327-22-5] Nylon 46, 6735
[50357-45-4] Pentamidine Dihydrochloride, 7115
[50435-25-1] Nimidane, 6550
[50471-44-8] Vinclozolin, 9984
[50594-66-6] Acifluorfen, 109
[50629-82-8] Halometasone, 4597
[50650-76-5] Piroctone, 7502
[50679-07-7] Cinepazet Maleate, 2290
[50679-08-8] Terfenadine, 9163
[50700-49-7] Acetimidoquinone, 57
[50700-72-6] Vecuronium Bromide, 9941
[50767-79-8] Prodlure, 7769
[50782-69-9] VX, 10036
[50813-16-6] Sodium Polymetaphosphate, 8667
[50838-36-3] Tolciclate, 9509
[50847-11-5] Ibudilast, 4879
[50865-01-5] Protoporphyrin IX Disodium Salt, 7897

[50887-69-9] Orotic Acid Monohydrate, 6876
[50924-49-7] Mizoribine, 6222
[50927-09-8] Sydnones, 9011
[50933-06-7] Sulfalene Mixture with Trimethoprim, 8910
[50933-33-0] Gossyplure, 4527
[50935-04-1] Carubicin, 1870
[50935-71-2] Mocimycin, 6225
[50972-17-3] Bacampicillin, 931
[51005-85-7] PBP, 4081
[51012-32-9] Tiapride, 9421
[51012-33-0] Tiapride Hydrochloride, 9421
[51016-68-3] Josamycin Propionate, 5267
[51022-69-6] Amcinonide, 388
[51022-70-9] Albuterol Sulfate, 216
[51022-71-0] Nabilone, 6342
[51022-98-1] Butirosin Sulfate Dihydrate, 1528
[51023-56-4] Centchroman Hydrochloride, 1971
[51025-85-5] Arbekacin, 770
[51037-30-0] Acipimox, 111
[51115-67-4] Trimethyl Isopropyl Butanamide, 9716
[51218-45-2] Metolachlor, 6146
[51218-49-6] Pretilachlor, 7740
[51229-78-8] Quaternium-15 cis-Form, 8027
[51235-04-2] Hexazinone, 4699
[51264-14-3] Amsacrine, 594
[51274-83-0] Tiamenidine Hydrochloride, 9418
[51276-47-2] Phosphinothricin DL-Form, 7339
[51306-35-5] DTAF, 3460
[51312-42-6] Sodium Phosphotungstate, 8665
[51322-75-9] Tizanidine, 9485
[51325-91-8] DCM, 2838
[51333-22-3] Budesonide, 1468
[51338-27-3] Diclofop-methyl, 3082
[51395-42-7] Butedronic Acid, 1517
[51410-30-1] Pirenoxine Sodium Salt, 7490
[51424-33-0] Salsoline Hydrochloride, 8340
[51460-26-5] Carbazochrome Sodium Sulfonate, 1789
[51481-10-8] Vomitoxin, 10032
[51481-60-8] Naloxone Hydrochloride (dihydrate), 6362
[51481-61-9] Cimetidine, 2279
[51481-65-3] Mezlocillin, 6171
[51484-40-3] Difenpiramide, 3137
[51503-61-8] Ammonium Phosphite, 544
[51570-36-6] Milbemycins, 6191
[51579-82-9] Amfenac, 395
[51596-10-2] Milbemycin A$_3$, 6189
[51596-11-3] Milbemycin A$_4$, 6189
[51596-16-8] Milbemycin β_1, 6191
[51598-60-8] Cimetropium Bromide, 2280
[51627-14-6] Cefatrizine, 1915
[51630-58-1] Fenvalerate, 4010
[51707-55-2] Thidiazuron, 9313
[51762-05-1] Cefroxadine, 1944
[51773-92-3] Mefloquine Hydrochloride, 5801
[51781-06-7] Carteolol, 1866
[51781-21-6] Carteolol Hydrochloride, 1866

[51803-78-2] Nimesulide, *6548*
[51805-45-9] TCEP Hydrochloride, *9085*
[51873-93-9] Azulene Sodium Sulfonate, *926*
[51888-09-6] Prochlorperazine Dimethanesulfonate, *7761*
[51938-42-2] Solanine (unspecified stereo), *8705*
[51940-44-4] Pipemidic Acid, *7460*
[51952-41-1] LH-RH Hydrochloride, *5474*
[52003-58-4] Ammonium Lactate, *530*
[52080-57-6] Chloroprednisone, *2157*
[52093-21-7] Micronomicin, *6181*
[52094-70-9] Tetrantoin, *9234*
[52109-93-0] Cyclodrine, *2719*
[52110-55-1] Strobilurin A, *8834*
[52128-35-5] Trimetrexate, *9721*
[52152-93-9] Cefsulodin Sodium Salt, *1945*
[52205-73-9] Estramustine 17-(Dihydrogenphosphate) Disodium Salt (anhydrous), *3706*
[52207-99-5] Gossyplure (Z,Z)-Form, *4527*
[52211-63-9] Viquidil Hydrochloride, *10003*
[52212-02-9] Pipecurium Bromide, *7459*
[52212-86-9] Verticillin B, *9968*
[52214-84-3] Ciprofibrate, *2313*
[52225-20-4] *dl*-α-Tocopherol Acetate, *9495*
[52239-63-1] Thiethylperazine Dimalate, *9315*
[52246-40-9] Fenquizone Monopotassium Salt, *3997*
[52260-69-2] Dicyanine, *3091*
[52275-61-3] Streptovaricin J, *8830*
[52279-57-9] Nandrolone *p*-Hexyloxyphenylpropionate, *6365*
[52304-36-6] Ethyl Butylacetylaminopropionate, *3773*
[52306-35-1] Lunacridine (±)-Form, *5603*
[52315-07-8] Cypermethrin, *2767*
[52365-63-6] Dipivefrin, *3338*
[52423-56-0] Bromopride Hydrochloride, *1432*
[52432-72-1] Oxeladin Citrate, *6930*
[52441-47-1] Semtex, *2736*
[52443-21-7] Glucametacin, *4448*
[52463-83-9] Pinazepam, *7442*
[52468-60-7] Flunarizine, *4144*
[52479-85-3] Exifone, *3915*
[52485-79-7] Buprenorphine, *1497*
[52486-78-9] Mercurophen, *5891*
[52500-59-1] Mexicain, *6168*
[52500-60-4] Thioredoxin, *9358*
[52500-61-5] β-Amino-α-methylphenethyl Alcohol, *447*
[52549-17-4] Pranoprofen, *7711*
[52589-12-5] Diginatin, *3156*
[52645-53-1] Permethrin, *7180*
[52665-69-7] Calcimycin, *1639*
[52705-43-8] α-Hydroxybenzylphosphinic Acid, *4813*
[52712-76-2] Bunazosin Hydrochloride, *1487*
[52731-38-1] Glucofrangulin, *4452*
[52740-16-6] Calcium Arsenite, *1650*
[52757-95-6] Sevelamer, *8474*
[52775-76-5] Methylenomycin A, *6067*

[52775-77-6] Methylenomycin B, *6067*
[52794-97-5] Carubicin Hydrochloride, *1870*
[52809-07-1] Quisqualic Acid, *8085*
[52906-84-0] Oxychlorosene Sodium Salt, *6956*
[52906-92-0] Motilin, *6283*
[52918-63-5] Deltamethrin, *2883*
[52942-31-1] Etoperidone, *3885*
[52951-36-7] Bisdequalinium Chloride, *1248*
[52951-37-8] Bismuth Ethyl Camphorate, *1264*
[52993-95-0] Sodium Polyanetholesulfonate, *8666*
[53003-10-4] Salinomycin, *8336*
[53005-05-3] DIDS, *3102*
[53016-31-2] Norelgestromin, *6694*
[53042-79-8] Gossyplure (Z,E)-Form, *4527*
[53078-86-7] Arogenic Acid, *790*
[53092-86-7] Lindlar Catalyst, *5502*
[53112-28-0] Pyrimethanil, *7986*
[53123-88-9] Rapamycin, *8114*
[53152-21-9] Buprenorphine Hydrochloride, *1497*
[53164-05-9] Acemetacin, *27*
[53179-09-2] Sisomicin Sulfate, *8550*
[53179-11-6] Loperamide, *5571*
[53230-10-7] Mefloquine, *5801*
[53251-94-8] Pinaverium Bromide, *7441*
[53260-52-9] Heparamine, *4652*
[53260-54-1] Fungisterol, *4291*
[53267-01-9] Cifenline, *2269*
[53308-83-1] *N*G-Methylarginine Acetate, *6022*
[53318-36-8] α-Glucogallin, *4453*
[53370-90-4] Exalamide, *3909*
[53414-68-9] Tonin, *9546*
[53447-14-6] Isocorypalmine, *5163*
[53449-58-4] Ciclonicate, *2265*
[53450-33-2] Oxalomolybdic Acid, *6913*
[53516-73-7] Quinovin, *8076*
[53558-25-1] Pyriminil, *7988*
[53567-47-8] Tiropramide Hydrochloride, *9466*
[53583-79-2] Sultopride, *8994*
[53586-99-5] Periodyl, *7172*
[53597-25-4] Salmine Sulfate, *8338*
[53597-27-6] Fendosal, *3971*
[53608-75-6] Pancrelipase, *7006*
[53608-77-8] Penicilloyl Polylysine, *7101*
[53608-96-1] Cloxotestosterone, *2421*
[53643-48-4] Vindesine, *9987*
[53643-53-1] Tuberin, *9806*
[53648-05-8] Ibuproxam, *4882*
[53648-55-8] Dezocine, *2956*
[53659-00-0] Pyrisuccideanol Dimaleate, *7991*
[53678-77-6] Muramyl Dipeptide, *6305*
[53684-48-3] Beryllium Potassium Sulfate, *1173*
[53684-49-4] Bufetolol, *1473*
[53714-56-0] Leuprolide, *5457*
[53716-44-2] Rociverine, *8245*
[53716-49-7] Carprofen, *1862*
[53716-50-0] Oxfendazole, *6935*
[53734-79-5] Metralindole Hydrochloride, *6153*
[53746-45-5] Fenoprofen Calcium Salt Dihydrate, *3980*

[53772-83-1] Clopenthixol *cis(Z)*-Form, *2394*
[53780-34-0] Mefluidide, *5802*
[53783-83-8] Tromantadine, *9771*
[53797-35-6] Ribostamycin Sulfate, *8206*
[53808-87-0] Tetroxoprim, *9250*
[53808-88-1] Lonazolac, *5566*
[53850-34-3] Thaumatin, *9273*
[53850-35-4] Dubnium, *3462*
[53850-36-5] Rutherfordium, *8303*
[53861-57-7] γ-Carboxyglutamic Acid, *1828*
[53882-12-5] Lodoxamide, *5555*
[53882-13-6] Lodoxamide Diethyl Ester, *5555*
[53885-35-1] Ticlopidine Hydrochloride, *9429*
[53897-25-9] Bismuth Butylthiolaurate, *1261*
[53902-12-8] Tranilast, *9570*
[53910-25-1] Pentostatin, *7135*
[53943-88-7] Letosteine, *5449*
[53984-74-0] Tocainide *R*-(−)-Form Hydrochloride, *9491*
[53984-76-2] Tocainide *S*-(+)-Form Hydrochloride, *9491*
[54024-22-5] Desogestrel, *2926*
[54029-12-8] Albendazole Sulfoxide, *210*
[54037-14-8] Bohrium, *1321*
[54037-57-9] Hassium, *4618*
[54038-01-6] Meitnerium, *5809*
[54038-81-2] Seaborgium, *8414*
[54048-10-1] Etonogestrel, *3884*
[54063-32-0] Clobetasone, *2364*
[54063-40-0] Fenoxedil, *3986*
[54063-51-3] Nadoxolol, *6347*
[54063-53-5] Propafenone, *7794*
[54063-54-6] Reproterol, *8139*
[54083-22-6] Zorubicin, *10195*
[54083-77-1] Darmstadtium, *2826*
[54084-26-3] Element 112, *3540*
[54085-16-4] Element 114, *3541*
[54100-71-9] Element 116, *3542*
[54110-25-7] Pirozadil, *7507*
[54120-61-5] Prostalene, *7880*
[54125-02-9] 1-Methoxy-3-(trimethylsilyloxy)-1,3-butadiene (*E*-form), *6001*
[54143-55-4] Flecainide, *4098*
[54143-56-5] Flecainide Monoacetate, *4098*
[54143-57-6] Metoclopramide Monohydrochloride Monohydrate, *6143*
[54182-58-0] Sucralfate, *8879*
[54187-04-1] Rilmenidine, *8222*
[54188-38-4] Metralindole, *6153*
[54239-37-1] Cimaterol, *2278*
[54247-25-5] Cloranolol Hydrochloride, *2402*
[54283-65-7] Dimecrotic Acid Magnesium Salt, *3203*
[54340-58-8] Meptazinol, *5863*
[54340-62-4] Bufuralol, *1480*
[54350-48-0] Etretinate, *3892*
[54386-24-2] Roentgenium, *8247*
[54397-85-2] Thromboxane B₂, *9388*
[54400-59-8] Butamisole, *1514*
[54400-62-3] Butamisole Hydrochloride, *1514*
[54464-57-2] Iso E Super® (unspecified stereo), *5169*
[54479-70-8] Heparin Magnesium Salt, *4653*

[54504-70-0] Theofibrate, 9284
[54527-84-3] Nicardipine Hydrochloride, 6495
[54530-86-8] Clometocillin Sodium Salt, 2385
[54533-85-6] Nizofenone, 6661
[54533-86-7] Nizofenone Fumarate, 6661
[54556-98-8] Propiverine Hydrochloride, 7832
[54573-75-0] Doxercalciferol, 3436
[54575-49-4] K-Selectride, 8427
[54593-83-8] Chlorethoxyfos, 2087
[54605-45-7] Iocarmic Acid Di-N-methylglucamine Salt, 5009
[54663-47-7] Tibezonium Iodide, 9426
[54739-18-3] Fluvoxamine, 4219
[54749-86-9] Phenylbutazone 2-Amino-2-thiazoline Salt, 7277
[54749-90-5] Chlorozotocin, 2177
[54761-04-5] Ytterbium Triflate, 10106
[54783-95-8] Fortimicin B, 4249
[54910-51-9] Disparlure (2S-cis-form), 3361
[54910-89-3] Fluoxetine, 4185
[54940-97-5] Citrulline Malate (Salt), 2331
[54965-21-8] Albendazole, 210
[54965-24-1] Tamoxifen Citrate, 9048
[54974-54-8] TRH Tartrate, 9588
[54983-89-0] DL-Lactic Acid Barium Salt, 5336
[55028-70-1] Arbaprostil, 769
[55028-71-2] Fluprostenol Sodium Salt, 4194
[55028-72-3] Cloprostenol Sodium Salt, 2399
[55077-30-0] Aclatonium Napadisilate, 114
[55079-83-9] Acitretin, 112
[55096-26-9] Nalmefene, 6360
[55134-13-9] Narasin, 6419
[55142-85-3] Ticlopidine, 9429
[55179-31-2] Bitertanol, 1305
[55219-65-3] Triadimenol, 9593
[55242-55-2] Propentofylline, 7813
[55268-74-1] Praziquantel, 7716
[55268-75-2] Cefuroxime, 1954
[55283-68-6] Ethalfluralin, 3719
[55285-14-8] Carbosulfan, 1826
[55285-45-5] Pirifibrate, 7495
[55290-64-7] Oxidimethiin, 6938
[55297-95-5] Tiamulin, 9419
[55297-96-6] Tiamulin Fumarate, 9419
[55327-22-5] Etiroxate Hydrochloride, 3872
[55335-06-3] Triclopyr, 9656
[55354-43-3] Arylsulfatase B, 819
[55406-53-6] IPBC, 5069
[55429-45-3] Nitracrine Dihydrochloride Monohydrate, 6571
[55453-87-7] Isoxepac, 5237
[55482-89-8] Aspirin Guaiacol Ester, 851
[55512-33-9] Pyridate, 7968
[55560-96-8] Tixocortol 21-Pivalate, 9484
[55589-62-3] Acesulfame Potassium Salt, 37
[55608-72-5] Pseudococaine n-Propyl Ester Analog, 7912
[55661-38-6] Nimustine Hydrochloride, 6553
[55721-31-8] Salinomycin Sodium Salt, 8336

[55722-12-8] S-Adenosylmethionine Disulfate Tosylate, 156
[55726-47-1] Enocitabine, 3586
[55774-33-9] Azathioprine Sodium Salt, 902
[55779-06-1] Fortimicin A, 4249
[55837-18-8] Butibufen, 1527
[55837-20-2] Halofuginone, 4596
[55837-25-7] Buflomedil, 1475
[55837-27-9] Piretanide, 7492
[55837-29-1] Tiropramide, 9466
[55837-30-4] Clonixin Lysine Salt, 2392
[55881-07-7] Miokamycin, 6204
[55893-12-4] Gephyrotoxin, 4402
[55905-53-8] Clebopride, 2344
[55965-63-4] O-(β-Hydroxyethyl)-rutinosides (mixture), 9789
[55965-84-9] Methylisothiazolinone Mixture with Methylchloroisothiazolinone, 6091
[55981-09-4] Nitazoxanide, 6567
[55985-32-5] Nicardipine, 6495
[56030-54-7] Sufentanil, 8887
[56038-13-2] Sucralose, 8880
[56073-07-5] Difenacoum, 3133
[56073-10-0] Brodifacoum, 1379
[56087-11-7] Dextranomer, 2950
[56124-62-0] Valrubicin, 9915
[56180-94-0] Acarbose, 18
[56187-47-4] Cefazedone, 1916
[56187-89-4] Ximoprofen, 10078
[56208-01-6] Pifarnine, 7420
[56211-40-6] Torsemide, 9552
[56222-04-9] Femoxetine Hydrochloride, 3955
[56238-63-2] Cefuroxime Sodium Salt, 1954
[56254-07-0] o-Iodohippurate Sodium ^{123}I-Labeled Form, 5034
[56281-36-8] Motretinide, 6284
[56281-37-9] 2C-B Hydrochloride, 1908
[56283-74-0] Laidlomycin, 5348
[56287-74-2] Afloqualone, 183
[56341-08-3] Mabuterol, 5642
[56377-79-8] Nosiheptide, 6719
[56390-09-1] Epirubicin Hydrochloride, 3623
[56391-56-1] Netilmicin, 6479
[56391-57-2] Netilmicin Sulfate, 6479
[56392-17-7] Metoprolol Tartrate, 6151
[56393-22-7] Pildralazine Dihydrochloride, 7423
[56396-94-2] Mepindolol Sulfate Salt, 5856
[56420-45-2] Epirubicin, 3623
[56425-91-3] Flurprimidol, 4204
[56430-99-0] Flumecinol, 4136
[56518-41-3] Brodimoprim, 1380
[56553-60-7] Sodium Triacetoxyborohydride, 8695
[56592-32-6] Efrotomycin, 3525
[56695-65-9] Rosaprostol, 8260
[56695-66-0] Rosaprostol Sodium Salt, 8260
[56775-88-3] Zimeldine, 10126
[56776-01-3] Tulobuterol Hydrochloride, 9811
[56776-32-0] Etifoxine Hydrochloride, 3864
[56796-20-4] Cefmetazole, 1926
[56796-39-5] Cefmetazole Sodium Salt, 1926

[56824-20-5] Amiprilose, 484
[56833-74-0] Streptovirudin, 8831
[56839-43-1] Eperisone Hydrochloride, 3606
[56974-46-0] Butalamine Hydrochloride, 1510
[56974-61-9] Gabexate Methanesulfonate, 4320
[56980-93-9] Celiprolol, 1960
[56995-20-1] Flupirtine, 4190
[57018-04-9] Tolclofos-methyl, 9510
[57021-61-1] Isonixin, 5192
[57041-67-5] Desflurane, 2919
[57109-90-7] Clorazepic Acid Dipotassium Salt, 2403
[57132-53-3] Proglumetacin, 7774
[57149-07-2] Naftopidil, 6356
[57149-08-3] Naftopidil Dihydrochloride, 6356
[57197-43-0] Sulfamoxole Mixture with Trimethoprim, 8924
[57213-69-1] Triclopyr Triethylamine Salt, 9656
[57248-88-1] Pamidronic Acid Disodium Salt, 7003
[57249-13-5] Heptaminol 5′-Adenylate, 4657
[57308-51-7] Carbidopa Combination with Levodopa, 1797
[57333-96-7] Tacalcitol, 9022
[57381-26-7] Irsogladine, 5102
[57432-61-8] Methylergonovine Maleate, 6070
[57460-41-0] Talinolol, 9038
[57469-78-0] Ketoprofen Lysine Salt, 5305
[57470-78-7] Celiprolol Hydrochloride, 1960
[57474-29-0] Nifuroquine, 6534
[57475-17-9] Brovincamine, 1451
[57524-89-7] Hydrocortisone 17-Valerate, 4787
[57526-81-5] Prenalterol, 7735
[57574-09-1] Amineptine, 409
[57576-44-0] Aclacinomycin A, 113
[57576-52-0] Thromboxane A$_2$, 9388
[57596-79-9] Aclacinomycin B, 113
[57644-54-9] Colloidal Bismuth Subcitrate, 2485
[57645-91-7] Clebopride Malate, 2344
[57648-21-2] Timiperone, 9443
[57653-27-7] Droprenilamine, 3451
[57695-04-2] Sitamaquine, 8553
[57704-10-6] Bufuralol (−)-Hydrochloride, 1480
[57704-11-7] Bufuralol (+)-Hydrochloride, 1480
[57754-85-5] Clopyralid Monoethanolamine Salt, 2400
[57760-36-8] Alborixin, 214
[57773-63-4] Triptorelin, 9748
[57773-65-6] Deslorelin, 2923
[57775-22-1] Etoperidone Hydrochloride, 3885
[57775-26-5] Sultosilic Acid, 8995
[57775-27-6] Sultosilic Acid Piperazine Salt, 8995
[57775-29-8] Carazolol, 1778
[57781-14-3] Halopredone Acetate, 4599
[57801-81-7] Brotizolam, 1450
[57808-65-8] Closantel, 2411
[57808-66-9] Domperidone, 3418
[57817-89-7] Stevioside, 8810

[57821-29-1] Sulodexide, *8986*
[57837-19-1] Metalaxyl, *5922*
[57852-57-0] Idarubicin Hydrochloride, *4886*
[57938-82-6] Adinazolam Methanesulfonate, *160*
[57960-19-7] Acequinocyl, *33*
[57966-95-7] Cymoxanil, *2765*
[57982-77-1] Buserelin, *1503*
[57982-78-2] Budipine, *1469*
[57998-68-2] Diaziquone, *2996*
[58001-44-8] Clavulanic Acid, *2341*
[58024-13-8] Isomaltulose (monohydrate), *5182*
[58045-23-1] Clopenthixol *cis(Z)*-Form Dihydrochloride, *2394*
[58066-85-6] Miltefosine, *6198*
[58095-31-1] Sulbenox, *8891*
[58138-08-2] Tridiphane, *9662*
[58152-03-7] Isepamicin, *5106*
[58186-27-9] Idebenone, *4888*
[58207-19-5] Clindamycin Hydrochloride (monohydrate), *2356*
[58306-30-2] Febantel, *3944*
[58337-35-2] Elliptinium Acetate, *3549*
[58409-52-2] Albaspidin, *209*
[58409-59-9] Bucumolol, *1467*
[58416-00-5] Protiofate, *7890*
[58473-74-8] Cinromide, *2311*
[58503-79-0] Meobentine Sulfate, *5843*
[58551-69-2] Carboprost Tromethamine Salt, *1823*
[58579-51-4] Anagrelide Hydrochloride, *622*
[58580-55-5] Dibekacin Sulfate, *3005*
[58581-89-8] Azelastine, *906*
[58670-63-6] Dinosterol, *3288*
[58694-52-3] Tertiapin, *9175*
[58712-69-9] Traxanox, *9578*
[58749-22-7] Licochalcone A, *5479*
[58749-23-8] Licochalcone B, *5479*
[58785-63-0] Lonomycin A, *5569*
[58786-99-5] Butorphanol Tartrate, *1530*
[58795-03-2] Apalcillin Sodium Salt, *724*
[58798-97-3] Berninamycin, *1160*
[58845-80-0] Lonomycin A Sodium Salt, *5569*
[58864-81-6] α-Tocotrienol, *9500*
[58880-19-6] Trichostatin A, *9649*
[58895-00-4] Trichostatin B, *9649*
[58895-64-0] Nalmefene Hydrochloride, *6360*
[58934-46-6] Lorcainide Hydrochloride, *5580*
[58944-73-3] Sinefungin, *8544*
[58957-92-9] Idarubicin, *4886*
[58970-76-6] Ubenimex, *9842*
[58994-96-0] Ranimustine, *8109*
[59017-64-0] Ioxaglic Acid, *5067*
[59056-94-9] Iso E Super® (*trans*-form), *5169*
[59092-07-8] Lycopene 15,15′-*cis*-Form, *5620*
[59122-46-2] Misoprostol, *6210*
[59128-97-1] Haloxazolam, *4604*
[59160-29-1] Lidofenin, *5483*
[59170-23-9] Bevantolol, *1192*
[59182-63-7] Droprenilamine Hydrochloride, *3451*
[59198-70-8] Diflucortolone 21-Valerate, *3143*
[59209-40-4] Proglumetacin Dimaleate, *7774*

[59227-89-3] Laurocapram, *5385*
[59263-76-2] Meptazinol Hydrochloride, *5863*
[59277-89-3] Acyclovir, *146*
[59333-67-4] Fluoxetine Hydrochloride, *4185*
[59338-87-3] Alizapride Hydrochloride, *250*
[59338-93-1] Alizapride, *250*
[59392-53-9] Maitotoxin, *5698*
[59414-23-2] 1-Methoxy-3-(trimethylsilyloxy)-1,3-butadiene (unspecified stereo), *6001*
[59467-70-8] Midazolam, *6182*
[59467-94-6] Midazolam Maleate, *6182*
[59467-96-8] Midazolam Hydrochloride, *6182*
[59512-37-7] Piketoprofen Hydrochloride, *7422*
[59598-29-7] Vernolepin (±)-Form, *9962*
[59619-81-7] Etiproston, *3871*
[59652-29-8] Bufuralol Hydrochloride, *1480*
[59669-26-0] Thiodicarb, *9329*
[59672-20-7] Sulfaloxic Acid Calcium Salt, *8912*
[59703-84-3] Piperacillin Sodium Salt, *7463*
[59708-57-5] Xibenolol Hydrochloride, *10075*
[59721-28-7] Camostat, *1728*
[59721-29-8] Camostat Methanesulfonate, *1728*
[59727-70-7] Octacaine Hydrochloride, *6743*
[59729-31-6] Lorcainide, *5580*
[59729-32-7] Citalopram Hydrobromide, *2318*
[59729-33-8] Citalopram, *2318*
[59767-13-4] Setastine Hydrochloride, *8472*
[59787-61-0] Cyclosporin C, *2752*
[59798-30-0] Mezlocillin Sodium Salt Monohydrate, *6171*
[59803-98-4] Brimonidine, *1375*
[59804-37-4] Tenoxicam, *9148*
[59859-58-4] Femoxetine, *3955*
[59865-13-3] Cyclosporin A, *2752*
[59865-23-5] MeBmt, *5771*
[59917-39-4] Vindesine Sulfate Salt, *9987*
[59937-28-9] Malotilate, *5712*
[59973-80-7] Exisulind, *3916*
[59985-21-6] Diquafosol, *3351*
[59989-18-3] Eniluracil, *3584*
[59995-64-1] Thienamycin, *9314*
[60084-10-8] Tiazofurin, *9425*
[60134-71-6] Nocardicin B, *6666*
[60142-96-3] Gabapentin, *4319*
[60166-93-0] Iopamidol, *5057*
[60168-88-9] Fenarimol, *3958*
[60200-06-8] Clorsulon, *2409*
[60202-16-6] Protein C, *7884*
[60207-31-0] Azaconazole, *891*
[60207-90-1] Propiconazole, *7818*
[60212-94-4] Xenon Hydrate, *10072*
[60282-87-3] Gestodene, *4413*
[60318-52-7] Trichosanthin, *9648*
[60325-46-4] Sulprostone, *8991*
[60414-06-4] Amiprilose Hydrochloride, *484*
[60450-21-7] Morindin, *6270*
[60477-34-1] Pifithrin-β, *7421*

[60529-33-1] Frangulin, *4264*
[60539-20-0] Dixyrazine Dihydrochloride, *3385*
[60560-33-0] Pinacidil, *7438*
[60561-17-3] Sufentanil Citrate, *8887*
[60569-19-9] Propiverine, *7832*
[60576-13-8] Piketoprofen, *7422*
[60607-34-3] Oxatomide, *6925*
[60607-68-3] Indenolol, *4940*
[60616-74-2] Magnesium Hydride, *5669*
[60628-96-8] Bifonazole, *1213*
[60643-86-9] Vigabatrin, *9978*
[60668-24-8] Alafosfalin, *202*
[60719-84-8] Amrinone, *592*
[60731-46-6] Elcatonin, *3537*
[60761-10-6] TMD, *9486*
[60763-48-6] Gepefrine Tartrate, *4401*
[60789-62-0] Clocapramine Dihydrochloride Monohydrate, *2366*
[60925-61-3] Ceforanide, *1931*
[60940-34-3] Ebselen, *3486*
[61036-64-4] Teicoplanin, *9115*
[61129-30-4] Zimeldine Dihydrochloride Monohydrate, *10126*
[61197-73-7] Loprazolam, *5574*
[61228-92-0] Periplanone B, *7173*
[61230-25-9] Aplasmomycin, *736*
[61260-05-7] Prenalterol Hydrochloride, *7735*
[61270-58-4] Cefonicid, *1929*
[61270-78-8] Cefonicid Disodium Salt, *1929*
[61318-90-9] Sulconazole, *8893*
[61318-91-0] Sulconazole Nitrate, *8893*
[61336-70-7] Amoxicillin Trihydrate, *577*
[61337-67-5] Mirtazapine, *6208*
[61379-65-5] Rifapentine, *8219*
[61380-40-3] Lofentanil, *5556*
[61380-41-4] Lofentanil Oxalate, *5556*
[61413-54-5] Rolipram, *8251*
[61422-45-5] Carmofur, *1844*
[61434-67-1] *cis*-Resveratrol, *8158*
[61477-96-1] Piperacillin, *7463*
[61512-20-7] Cord Factor(s), *2528*
[61545-06-0] Temocillin Disodium Salt, *9137*
[61570-90-9] Tioxidazole, *9455*
[61618-27-1] Amfenac Sodium Salt Monohydrate, *395*
[61622-34-2] Cefotiam, *1935*
[61676-87-7] Cymiazole, *2764*
[61717-82-6] *o*-Iodoxybenzoic Acid (cyclic tautomer), *5048*
[61718-82-9] Fluvoxamine Maleate, *4219*
[61788-48-5] Acetylated Lanolin, *5358*
[61788-49-6] Acetylated Lanolin Alcohols, *5359*
[61802-93-5] Metaclazepam Hydrochloride, *5920*
[61825-94-3] Oxaliplatin, *6912*
[61849-14-7] Prostacyclin Sodium Salt, *7875*
[61869-07-6] Domiodol, *3414*
[61869-08-7] Paroxetine, *7043*
[61891-34-7] Flufenamic Acid Aluminum Salt, *4132*
[61951-99-3] Tixocortol, *9484*
[61954-97-0] Drotaverine Acephyllinate, *3455*
[62013-04-1] Dirithromycin, *3354*
[62031-54-3] Fibroblast Growth Factor, *4072*

[62087-72-3] Pentigetide, *7128*
[62232-46-6] Bifemelane Hydrochloride, *1206*
[62265-68-3] Quinfamide, *8057*
[62288-83-9] Desmopressin Monoacetate, *2924*
[62304-98-7] Thymalfasin, *9405*
[62327-61-1] Perimycin A, *7169*
[62435-42-1] Perfosfamide, *7161*
[62499-27-8] Gastrodin, *4375*
[62534-68-3] Mepartricin A, *5847*
[62534-69-4] Mepartricin B, *5847*
[62568-57-4] DSIP, *3458*
[62571-86-2] Captopril, *1774*
[62587-73-9] Cefsulodin, *1945*
[62613-82-5] Oxiracetam, *6942*
[62637-93-8] Trimethylamine *N*-Oxide Dihydrate, *9711*
[62640-05-5] Ajugarin-I, *197*
[62640-06-6] Ajugarin-II, *197*
[62640-07-7] Ajugarin-III, *197*
[62658-63-3] Bopindolol, *1333*
[62658-64-4] Bopindolol Maleate, *1333*
[62666-20-0] Progabide, *7772*
[62774-96-3] Tilisolol Hydrochloride, *9438*
[62778-11-4] Olah's Reagent, *6821*
[62893-19-0] Cefoperazone, *1930*
[62893-20-3] Cefoperazone Sodium Salt, *1930*
[62952-06-1] Lysine Acetylsalicylate, *5637*
[62973-76-6] Azanidazole, *897*
[62989-33-7] Sapropterin, *8368*
[62994-47-2] Warburganal, *10037*
[62996-74-1] Staurosporine, *8802*
[63075-47-8] Fepradinol, *4011*
[63147-28-4] DBHBT, *2836*
[63208-82-2] Pifithrin-α, *7421*
[63251-39-8] Sulfinalol Hydrochloride, *8948*
[63329-53-3] Lobenzarit, *5552*
[63333-35-7] Bromethalin, *1389*
[63358-49-6] Aspoxicillin, *852*
[63394-05-8] Plafibride, *7516*
[63469-19-2] Apalcillin, *724*
[63516-07-4] Flutropium Bromide, *4216*
[63521-15-3] Cefazedone Sodium Salt, *1916*
[63527-52-6] Cefotaxime, *1933*
[63543-09-9] Thiarubrin(e) A, *9304*
[63547-13-7] Adrafinil, *170*
[63585-09-1] Foscarnet Sodium, *4251*
[63590-64-7] Terazosin, *9154*
[63610-08-2] Indobufen, *4961*
[63610-09-3] Lodoxamide Tromethamine Salt, *5555*
[63612-50-0] Nilutamide, *6544*
[63628-25-1] αMNP, *6224*
[63628-26-2] αMNP (−)-(*R*)-Form, *6224*
[63659-18-7] Betaxolol, *1182*
[63659-19-8] Betaxolol Hydrochloride, *1182*
[63661-61-0] Budipine Hydrochloride, *1469*
[63675-72-9] Nisoldipine, *6565*
[63717-27-1] Amifostine Monohydrate, *404*
[63739-93-5] Verrucarin K, *9964*
[63749-94-0] Sulfametrole Mixture with Trimethoprim, *8920*
[63758-79-2] Indalpine, *4930*

[63767-79-3] Ceforanide L-Lysine Salt, *1931*
[63775-95-1] Cyclosporin B, *2752*
[63775-96-2] Cyclosporin D, *2752*
[63814-06-2] Isomethadone *d*-Form Hydrochloride, *5184*
[63836-75-9] Pivcefalexin, *7513*
[63918-50-3] Fencamine Hydrochloride, *3967*
[63968-64-9] Artemisinin, *817*
[64000-73-3] Pildralazine, *7423*
[64006-44-6] Paroxetine Maleate, *7043*
[64011-61-6] Cyclexedrine Hydrochloride, *2707*
[64019-93-8] Dipivefrin Hydrochloride, *3338*
[64024-15-3] Pentazocine Hydrochloride, *7121*
[64057-70-1] MDMA Hydrochloride, *5767*
[64058-48-6] Spectinomycin Sulfate Tetrahydrate, *8739*
[64092-49-5] Zomepirac Sodium Salt Dihydrate, *10191*
[64204-55-3] Esaprazole, *3695*
[64211-46-7] Oxiconazole Nitrate, *6937*
[64217-62-5] Cefatrizine Compd with Propylene Glycol, *1915*
[64218-02-6] Plaunotol, *7532*
[64221-86-9] Imipenem (anhydrous), *4919*
[64228-81-5] Atracurium Besylate, *868*
[64238-92-2] Benproperine Pamoate, *1049*
[64241-34-5] Cadralazine, *1631*
[64285-06-9] Anatoxin a, *627*
[64294-95-7] Setastine, *8472*
[64297-64-9] *o*-Iodoxybenzoic Acid, *5048*
[64318-79-2] Gemeprost, *4387*
[64359-81-5] 4,5-Dichloro-2-octyl-3-isothiazolone, *3070*
[64461-82-1] Tizanidine Hydrochloride, *9485*
[64475-85-0] Mineral Spirits, *6201*
[64485-93-4] Cefotaxime Sodium Salt (*syn*-Isomer), *1933*
[64490-92-2] Tolmetin Sodium Salt Dihydrate, *9518*
[64506-49-6] Sofalcone, *8701*
[64536-78-3] Crabtree's Catalyst, *2566*
[64603-91-4] Gaboxadol, *4321*
[64628-44-0] Triflumuron, *9678*
[64700-56-7] Triclopyr Butoxyethyl Ester, *9656*
[64706-27-0] Salatrim, *8320*
[64706-54-3] Bepridil, *1150*
[64726-91-6] Japonilure, *5257*
[64808-48-6] Lobenzarit Disodium Salt, *5552*
[64840-90-0] Eperisone, *3606*
[64872-76-0] Butoconazole, *1529*
[64872-77-1] Butoconazole Nitrate, *1529*
[64896-28-2] (*S*,*S*)-Chiraphos, *2063*
[64902-72-3] Chlorsulfuron, *2191*
[64924-67-0] Halofuginone Hydrobromide, *4596*
[64952-97-2] Moxalactam, *6286*
[64953-12-4] Moxalactam Disodium Salt, *6286*
[65002-17-7] Bucillamine, *1460*
[65009-35-0] Lidamidine Hydrochloride, *5481*

[65035-34-9] Lineatin, *5503*
[65043-22-3] Indeloxazine Hydrochloride, *4938*
[65052-63-3] Cefetamet, *1923*
[65057-90-1] Tallysomycin A, *9043*
[65057-91-2] Tallysomycin B, *9043*
[65085-01-0] Cefmenoxime, *1925*
[65085-02-1] Cefmenoxime Sodium Salt (*syn*-Isomer), *1925*
[65141-46-0] Nicorandil, *6521*
[65154-06-5] Platelet Activating Factor, *7524*
[65189-78-8] Tropesin, *9778*
[65202-63-3] Gaboxadol Hydrobromide, *4321*
[65243-33-6] Cefetamet Pivaloyloxymethyl Ester, *1923*
[65271-80-9] Mitoxantrone, *6217*
[65277-42-1] Ketoconazole, *5302*
[65322-72-7] Endralazine Methanesulfonate, *3577*
[65472-88-0] Naftifine, *6355*
[65473-14-5] Naftifine Hydrochloride, *6355*
[65474-79-5] 3-Hydroxymethyl-β-carboline, *3779*
[65576-45-6] Asenapine, *832*
[65646-68-6] Fenretinide, *3998*
[65666-07-1] Silymarin, *8532*
[65717-97-7] Disofenin, *3358*
[65733-16-6] Methoprene (7*S*)-Form, *5983*
[65733-18-8] Hydroprene (*S*)-Form, *4805*
[65807-02-5] Goserelin, *4526*
[65847-85-0] Niflumic Acid β-Morpholinoethyl Ester, *6531*
[65884-46-0] Cyadox, *2681*
[65899-73-2] Tioconazole, *9452*
[65928-58-7] Dienogest, *3106*
[65981-49-9] Laureline (*S*)-Form, *5383*
[65988-34-3] α-Latrotoxin, *5377*
[66002-66-2] Fertirelin Monoacetate, *4061*
[66085-59-4] Nimodipine, *6551*
[66104-22-1] Pergolide, *7162*
[66104-23-2] Pergolide Mesylate, *7162*
[66108-95-0] Iohexol, *5052*
[66142-81-2] 2C-B, *1908*
[66146-62-1] Cycloleucine Hydrochloride (monohydrate), *2734*
[66148-78-5] Temocillin, *9137*
[66195-31-1] Ibopamine, *4876*
[66215-27-8] Cyromazine, *2775*
[66230-04-4] Fenvalerate (*S*,*S*)-Isomer, *4010*
[66251-18-1] Grundmann's Ketone, *4551*
[66264-77-5] Sulfinalol, *8948*
[66309-69-1] Cefotiam Dihydrochloride, *1935*
[66332-96-5] Flutolanil, *4212*
[66357-35-5] Ranitidine, *8110*
[66357-59-3] Ranitidine Hydrochloride, *8110*
[66376-36-1] Alendronic Acid, *229*
[66441-23-4] Fenoxaprop-ethyl, *3984*
[66455-27-4] PSK®, *7927*
[66508-37-0] Fosmidomycin Monosodium Salt, *4257*
[66508-53-0] Fosmidomycin, *4257*
[66532-85-2] Propacetamol, *7792*
[66532-86-3] Propacetamol Hydrochloride, *7792*

[77337-73-6] Acamprosate Calcium, *17*
[77392-58-6] Paraherquamide, *7026*
[77469-98-8] Pimobendan Hydrochloride, *7434*
[77521-29-0] AMPA, *578*
[77590-95-5] Cetamolol Hydrochloride, *2018*
[77671-31-9] Enoximone, *3589*
[77732-09-3] Oxadixyl, *6908*
[77734-91-9] Palytoxin, *6999*
[77855-81-3] Milbemycin D, *6191*
[77874-90-9] Ellman's Anion, *3551*
[77883-43-3] Doxazosin Methanesulfonate, *3433*
[77907-69-8] Interferon Alfa-2a, *4990*
[77912-79-9] Sulfazecin, *8946*
[78110-38-0] Aztreonam, *925*
[78111-17-8] Okadaic Acid, *6819*
[78113-36-7] Romurtide, *8253*
[78126-10-0] Stepronin Sodium Salt, *8809*
[78148-59-1] (−)-Epi-α-bisabolol, *1241*
[78178-41-3] Podophyllinic Acid Hydrazide, *7545*
[78186-34-2] Bisantrene, *1244*
[78213-16-8] Diclofenac Diethylammonium Salt, *3081*
[78246-49-8] Paroxetine Hydrochloride, *7043*
[78266-06-5] Mebrofenin (hydrochloride), *5772*
[78281-72-8] Nepafenac, *6469*
[78415-72-2] Milrinone, *6197*
[78439-06-2] Ceftazidime Pentahydrate, *1946*
[78473-71-9] Enterolactone, *3598*
[78474-55-2] Teleocidins, *9118*
[78491-02-8] Diazolidinyl Urea, *3000*
[78499-27-1] Bermoprofen, *1159*
[78587-05-0] Hexythiazox, *4713*
[78613-35-1] Amorolfine, *573*
[78613-38-4] Amorolfine Hydrochloride, *573*
[78628-28-1] Roxatidine Acetate, *8274*
[78628-80-5] Terbinafine Hydrochloride, *9156*
[78649-41-9] Iomeprol, *5054*
[78654-44-1] Amicoumacin A, *398*
[78664-73-0] Posatirelin, *7603*
[78697-56-0] Lophotoxin, *5572*
[78712-43-3] Ozagrel Hydrochloride, *6980*
[78718-25-9] Benexate Hydrochloride, *1038*
[78755-81-4] Flumazenil, *4135*
[78822-40-9] Pirlimycin Hydrochloride, *7500*
[78833-03-1] Pentisomide, *7129*
[78853-39-1] Cyclodrine Hydrochloride, *2719*
[78919-13-8] Iloprost, *4901*
[78948-87-5] Magnesium Monoperoxyphthalate, *5673*
[78964-85-9] Fosfomycin Tromethamine, *4254*
[78967-07-4] Mofezolac, *6232*
[78994-23-7] Centchroman (−)-Form, *1971*
[79094-20-5] Daltroban, *2806*
[79277-27-3] Thifensulfuron-methyl, *9316*
[79307-93-0] Azelastine Hydrochloride, *906*

[79350-37-1] Cefixime, *1924*
[79416-27-6] Methyl Aminolevulinate Hydrochloride, *6016*
[79455-30-4] Nicaraven, *6493*
[79483-69-5] Piritrexim Isethionate, *7499*
[79516-68-0] Levocabastine, *5463*
[79517-01-4] Octreotide Acetate, *6762*
[79538-32-2] Tefluthrin, *9111*
[79547-78-7] Levocabastine Hydrochloride, *5463*
[79548-73-5] Pirlimycin, *7500*
[79559-97-0] Sertraline Hydrochloride, *8467*
[79617-96-2] Sertraline, *8467*
[79622-59-6] Fluazinam, *4117*
[79645-27-5] Tobramycin Sulfate, *9490*
[79660-72-3] Fleroxacin, *4099*
[79704-88-4] α-Methylfentanyl, *6074*
[79770-24-4] Iotrolan, *5065*
[79778-41-9] Neridronic Acid, *6473*
[79794-75-5] Loratadine, *5578*
[79831-76-8] Castanospermine, *1896*
[79871-54-8] Norgestimate Mixture with Ethinyl Estradiol, *6703*
[79874-76-3] Delmopinol, *2879*
[79902-63-9] Simvastatin, *8539*
[79917-90-1] Butylmethylimidazolium Chloride, *1581*
[79944-56-2] Idazoxan Hydrochloride, *4887*
[79944-58-4] Idazoxan, *4887*
[79983-71-4] Hexaconazole, *4681*
[80012-43-7] Epinastine, *3618*
[80060-09-9] Diafenthiuron, *2969*
[80125-14-0] Remoxipride, *8132*
[80214-83-1] Roxithromycin, *8276*
[80370-57-6] Ceftiofur, *1950*
[80382-23-6] Loxoprofen Sodium Salt, *5589*
[80387-96-8] Difemerine, *3132*
[80409-82-1] Crabtree's Catalyst Tetrafluoroborate, *2566*
[80432-08-2] Butylmethylimidazolium, *1581*
[80433-71-2] Folinic Acid *l*-Form Calcium Salt, *4222*
[80449-31-6] Urinastatin, *9882*
[80455-68-1] Fredericamycin A, *4267*
[80471-63-2] Epostane, *3627*
[80474-14-2] Fluticasone Propionate, *4211*
[80529-93-7] Gadopentetic Acid, *4327*
[80530-63-8] Picotamide Monohydrate, *7407*
[80573-04-2] Balsalazide, *945*
[80576-83-6] Edatrexate, *3507*
[80621-81-4] Rifaximin, *8220*
[80663-95-2] Iobenguane, *5007*
[80729-79-9] Neridronic Acid Monosodium Salt, *6473*
[80734-02-7] Lenampicillin Hydrochloride, *5437*
[80755-51-7] Bunazosin, *1487*
[80844-07-1] Etofenprox, *3876*
[80863-62-3] Alitame, *248*
[81025-03-8] Lactitol Dihydrate, *5340*
[81025-04-9] Lactitol Monohydrate, *5340*
[81098-60-4] Cisapride, *2316*
[81103-11-9] Clarithromycin, *2339*
[81110-73-8] Racecadotril, *8090*
[81129-83-1] Cilastatin Sodium Salt, *2272*

[81131-70-6] Pravastatin Sodium, *7714*
[81147-92-4] Esmolol, *3700*
[81161-17-3] Esmolol Hydrochloride, *3700*
[81262-93-3] Procaterol Hydrochloride Hemihydrate, *7759*
[81290-20-2] Trifluoromethyltrimethylsilane, *9683*
[81334-34-1] Imazapyr, *4905*
[81335-37-7] Imazaquin, *4906*
[81335-77-5] Imazethapyr, *4907*
[81403-68-1] Alfuzosin Hydrochloride, *238*
[81403-80-7] Alfuzosin, *238*
[81405-85-8] Imazamethabenz, *4903*
[81406-37-3] Fluroxypyr 1-Methylheptyl Ester, *4203*
[81409-90-7] Cabergoline, *1601*
[81486-22-8] Nipradilol, *6562*
[81510-83-0] Imazapyr Isopropylamine Salt, *4905*
[81525-10-2] Nafamostat, *6350*
[81584-06-7] Xibenolol, *10075*
[81591-81-3] Glyphosate Trimethylsulfonium Salt, *4512*
[81627-83-0] Macrophage Colony-Stimulating Factor, *5646*
[81655-41-6] Mosher's Reagent, *6280*
[81669-57-0] Anistreplase, *674*
[81732-46-9] Bambuterol Hydrochloride, *953*
[81732-65-2] Bambuterol, *953*
[81777-89-1] Clomazone, *2381*
[81789-85-7] Indenolol Hydrochloride, *4940*
[81800-41-1] Dihydroactinidiolide (*S*)-Form, *3170*
[81801-12-9] Xamoterol, *10055*
[81840-15-5] Vesnarinone, *9970*
[81846-19-7] Treprostinil, *9586*
[81858-94-8] Peptide YY (porcine), *7149*
[81872-10-8] Zofenopril, *10186*
[81919-14-4] Bendazac Lysine Salt, *1035*
[81938-43-4] Zofenopril Calcium Salt, *10186*
[81982-32-3] Alpiripride, *311*
[81988-88-7] Ramoplanin A$_2$, *8104*
[82009-34-5] Cilastatin, *2272*
[82030-87-3] Methionyl Human Growth Hormone, *8716*
[82034-46-6] Loteprednol Etabonate, *5584*
[82097-50-5] Triasulfuron, *9600*
[82101-18-6] Balsalazide Disodium Salt (anhydrous), *945*
[82115-62-6] Interferon-γ, *4992*
[82159-09-9] Epalrestat, *3605*
[82186-77-4] Lumefantrine, *5597*
[82219-78-1] Cefuzonam, *1955*
[82225-47-6] Ajugarin-IV, *197*
[82231-14-9] Ajugarin-V, *197*
[82248-59-7] Atomoxetine Hydrochloride, *863*
[82310-93-8] Hypusine Dihydrochloride, *4870*
[82410-32-0] Ganciclovir, *4363*
[82413-20-5] Droloxifene, *3446*
[82419-36-1] Ofloxacin, *6771*
[82473-24-3] CHAPS Hydroxy Analog, *2044*
[82504-20-9] Asoxime Chloride Monohydrate, *835*

[82547-58-8] Cefteram, *1947*
[82547-81-7] Cefteram Pivaloyloxymethyl Ester, *1947*
[82558-50-7] Isoxaben, *5235*
[82560-54-1] Benfuracarb, *1042*
[82571-53-7] Ozagrel, *6980*
[82586-52-5] Moexipril Hydrochloride, *6229*
[82586-55-8] Quinapril Hydrochloride, *8051*
[82586-57-0] Moexiprilat Hydrochloride, *6229*
[82626-48-0] Zolpidem, *10190*
[82640-04-8] Raloxifene Hydrochloride, *8098*
[82657-04-3] Bifenthrin, *1209*
[82657-92-9] Pro-Urokinase, *7902*
[82697-16-3] Clofencet Sodium Salt, *2375*
[82697-71-0] Clofencet Potassium Salt, *2375*
[82747-56-6] Cicletanine Hydrochloride, *2264*
[82752-99-6] Nefazodone Hydrochloride, *6438*
[82768-85-2] Quinaprilat, *8051*
[82785-45-3] Neuropeptide Y, *6485*
[82801-81-8] MDE, *5766*
[82834-16-0] Perindopril, *7170*
[82855-09-2] Combretastatin, *2494*
[82857-38-3] Bopindolol Malonate, *1333*
[82952-64-5] Trimetrexate D-Glucuronate, *9721*
[82956-11-4] Nafamostat Dimethanesulfonate, *6350*
[82964-04-3] Tolrestat, *9524*
[82989-25-1] Tazanolast, *9080*
[83014-44-2] Quin2 (acid), *8042*
[83015-26-3] Atomoxetine, *863*
[83055-99-6] Bensulfuron-methyl, *1052*
[83104-85-2] Quin2 Acetoxymethyl Ester, *8042*
[83105-70-8] Sultamicillin Tosylate, *8992*
[83121-18-0] Teflubenzuron, *9109*
[83150-76-9] Octreotide, *6762*
[83164-33-4] Diflufenican, *3144*
[83314-01-6] Bryostatin 1, *1457*
[83366-66-9] Nefazodone, *6438*
[83382-98-3] Synsorbs, *9014*
[83387-25-1] Methylnaltrexonium, *6099*
[83435-66-9] Delapril (methylnaltrexonium), *2876*
[83435-67-0] Delapril Hydrochloride, *2876*
[83461-56-7] Mepact, *5844*
[83480-29-9] Voglibose, *10029*
[83602-05-5] Spiraprilat, *8753*
[83621-06-1] Omoconazole Nitrate, *6846*
[83643-88-3] L-AMPA, *578*
[83647-97-6] Spirapril, *8753*
[83657-18-5] Diniconazole (−)-Form, *3268*
[83657-19-6] Diniconazole (+)-Form, *3268*
[83657-24-3] Diniconazole, *3268*
[83712-60-1] Defibrotide, *2861*
[83729-01-5] Salvinorin A, *8344*
[83799-24-0] Fexofenadine, *4068*
[83846-83-7] Ketanserin Tartrate, *5296*
[83869-56-1] Granulocyte-Macrophage Colony-Stimulating Factor, *4538*

[83881-51-0] Cetirizine, *2022*
[83881-52-1] Cetirizine Dihydrochloride, *2022*
[83905-01-5] Azithromycin, *915*
[83915-83-7] Lisinopril, *5516*
[83919-23-7] Mometasone Furoate, *6241*
[83930-13-6] Somatoliberin, *8714*
[84031-17-4] Metaclazepam, *5920*
[84057-84-1] Lamotrigine, *5353*
[84057-95-4] Ropivacaine, *8258*
[84082-34-8] Bilberry Extract, *1217*
[84088-42-6] Roquinimex, *8259*
[84294-96-2] Enoxacin Sesquihydrate, *3587*
[84297-59-6] Cabenegrin A-I, *1600*
[84297-60-9] Cabenegrin A-II, *1600*
[84305-41-9] Cefminox, *1927*
[84371-65-3] Mifepristone, *6186*
[84449-90-1] Raloxifene, *8098*
[84504-69-8] Irsogladine Maleate, *5102*
[84611-23-4] Erdosteine, *3647*
[84625-59-2] Dotarizine, *3428*
[84625-61-6] Itraconazole, *5245*
[84799-02-0] Laidlomycin Propionate Potassium, *5348*
[84845-57-8] Ritipenem, *8236*
[84845-58-9] Ritipenem Sodium Salt, *8236*
[84878-61-5] Maduramicin, *5648*
[84880-03-5] Cefpimizole, *1938*
[84937-45-1] Gusperimus (−)-Form Trihydrochloride, *4582*
[84957-29-9] Cefpirome, *1940*
[84957-30-2] Cefquinome, *1943*
[84964-12-5] Brovincamine Hydrogen Fumarate, *1451*
[85068-76-4] Iofetamine [123]I Hydrochloride, *5049*
[85118-33-8] Gaboxadol Hydrochloride, *4321*
[85136-71-6] Tilisolol, *9438*
[85175-67-3] Zatebradine, *10115*
[85233-19-8] BAPTA, *957*
[85248-93-7] Pseudomonic Acid D, *7918*
[85287-61-2] Cefpimizole Monosodium Salt, *1938*
[85320-68-9] Amosulalol, *575*
[85329-89-1] Cabergoline Diphosphate, *1601*
[85371-64-8] Pinacidil Monohydrate, *7438*
[85441-61-8] Quinapril, *8051*
[85468-01-5] Gusperimus Trihydrochloride, *4582*
[85509-19-9] Flusilazole, *4206*
[85622-93-1] Temozolomide, *9139*
[85637-73-6] Atrial Natriuretic Peptide, *872*
[85649-12-3] Cyfluthrin *(1R,3R,αR)*-Form, *2756*
[85649-15-6] Cyfluthrin *(1R,3R,αS)*-Form, *2756*
[85649-19-0] Cyfluthrin *(1R,3S,αS)*-Form, *2756*
[85650-56-2] Asenapine Maleate, *832*
[85721-33-1] Ciprofloxacin, *2314*
[85856-54-8] Moveltipril, *6285*
[85865-74-3] Pygeum Africanum Extract, *7949*
[85898-30-2] Interleukin-2, *4994*
[85921-53-5] Moveltipril Calcium Salt, *6285*

[85960-17-4] Imipenem Combination with Cilastatin Sodium, *4919*
[86050-77-3] Gadopentetic Acid Dimeglumine Salt, *4327*
[86168-78-7] Sermorelin, *8461*
[86197-47-9] Dopexamine, *3424*
[86209-51-0] Primisulfuron-methyl, *7747*
[86220-42-0] Nafarelin Acetate Hydrate, *6351*
[86227-47-6] Eicosapentaenoic Acid Ethyl Ester, *3531*
[86273-18-9] Lenampicillin, *5437*
[86303-22-2] BIGCHAP, *1214*
[86303-23-3] Deoxy-BIGCHAP, *1214*
[86329-79-5] Cefodizime Disodium Salt, *1928*
[86340-94-5] *N*-Iodosaccharin, *5043*
[86347-14-0] Medetomidine, *5787*
[86347-15-1] Medetomidine Hydrochloride, *5787*
[86386-73-4] Fluconazole, *4122*
[86393-32-0] Ciprofloxacin Monohydrochloride Monohydrate, *2314*
[86401-95-8] Methylprednisolone Aceponate, *6111*
[86408-72-2] Ecabet Sodium Salt, *3489*
[86479-06-3] Hexaflumuron, *4683*
[86484-91-5] Dopexamine Dihydrochloride, *3424*
[86541-74-4] Benazepril Hydrochloride, *1031*
[86541-75-5] Benazepril, *1031*
[86541-78-8] Benazeprilat, *1031*
[86598-92-7] Imibenconazole, *4909*
[86697-68-9] Fasciculins, *3939*
[86767-75-1] Octenidine Disaccharin, *6754*
[86780-90-7] Aranidipine, *767*
[86832-68-0] Carumonam Disodium Salt, *1871*
[87041-58-5] Hementin, *4640*
[87051-43-2] Ritanserin, *8235*
[87056-78-8] Quinagolide, *8045*
[87081-35-4] Leptomycin B, *5444*
[87130-20-9] Diethofencarb, *3109*
[87233-61-2] Emedastine, *3557*
[87233-62-3] Emedastine Difumarate, *3557*
[87234-24-0] Piroxicam Cinnamic Acid Ester, *7506*
[87238-52-6] Ritipenem Acetoxymethyl Ester, *8236*
[87239-81-4] Cefpodoxime Proxetil, *1941*
[87333-19-5] Ramipril, *8103*
[87344-06-7] Amtolmetin Guacil, *596*
[87392-12-9] Metolachlor *S*-Form, *6146*
[87413-09-0] Dess-Martin Periodinane, *2933*
[87440-45-7] Taprostene Sodium Salt, *9057*
[87546-18-7] Flumiclorac-pentyl, *4142*
[87547-04-4] Flumiclorac, *4142*
[87625-62-5] Ptaquiloside, *7930*
[87638-04-8] Carumonam, *1871*
[87674-68-8] Dimethenamid, *3214*
[87679-37-6] Trandolapril, *9568*
[87679-71-8] Trandolaprilat, *9568*
[87726-17-8] Panipenem, *7009*
[87760-53-0] Tandospirone, *9051*
[87771-40-2] Ioversol, *5066*
[87806-31-3] Porfimer Sodium, *7596*

[87818-31-3] Cinmethylin, *2295*
[87820-88-0] Tralkoxydim, *9564*
[87848-99-5] Acrivastine, *127*
[88040-23-7] Cefepime, *1922*
[88069-49-2] Pilsicainide Hydrochloride Hemihydrate, *7427*
[88069-67-4] Pilsicainide, *7427*
[88122-99-0] Ethylhexyl Triazone, *3809*
[88150-42-9] Amlodipine, *491*
[88150-47-4] Amlodipine Maleate, *491*
[88189-03-1] Bismuth Triflate, *1292*
[88200-01-5] Chelidonine (−)-Form, *2053*
[88255-01-0] Netobimin, *6480*
[88283-41-4] Pyrifenox, *7983*
[88416-50-6] Clodronic Acid Disodium Salt (tetrahydrate), *2371*
[88426-33-9] Buparvaquone, *1491*
[88430-50-6] Beraprost, *1152*
[88475-69-8] Beraprost Sodium Salt, *1152*
[88495-63-0] Artesunate, *818*
[88671-89-0] Myclobutanil, *6321*
[88678-31-3] Liranaftate, *5515*
[88768-40-5] Cilazapril, *2273*
[88805-35-0] Prohexadione, *7777*
[88816-02-8] Belleau's Reagent, *1026*
[88889-14-9] Fosinopril Sodium Salt, *4256*
[88911-35-7] Clinprost Free Acid, *2358*
[88931-51-5] Clinprost, *2358*
[89213-87-6] Carperitide, *872*
[89226-50-6] Manidipine, *5743*
[89226-75-5] Manidipine Dihydrochloride, *5743*
[89365-50-4] Salmeterol, *8337*
[89371-37-9] Imidapril, *4911*
[89371-44-8] Imidaprilat, *4911*
[89396-94-1] Imidapril Monohydrochloride, *4911*
[89419-40-9] Mosapramine, *6278*
[89482-01-9] Zaltoprofen (S)-Form, *10112*
[89565-68-4] Tropisetron, *9783*
[89750-14-1] GLP-1, *4447*
[89750-15-2] GLP-2, *4447*
[89778-26-7] Toremifene, *9550*
[89778-27-8] Toremifene Citrate, *9550*
[89785-84-2] Tazobactam Sodium Salt, *9083*
[89786-04-9] Tazobactam, *9083*
[89796-99-6] Aceclofenac, *22*
[89797-00-2] Iopentol, *5059*
[89899-81-0] HPA-23, *4750*
[89943-82-8] Cicletanine, *2264*
[89987-06-4] Tiludronic Acid, *9441*
[90035-08-8] Flocoumafen, *4102*
[90098-04-7] Rebamipide, *8124*
[90139-06-3] Cilazaprilat, *2273*
[90141-22-3] Gossypol R-Form, *4528*
[90242-81-2] d-trans-α-Irone, *5096*
[90274-24-1] Ractopamine Hydrochloride, *8092*
[90293-01-9] Bifemelane, *1206*
[90357-06-5] Bicalutamide, *1200*
[90409-78-2] Polifeprosan, *7559*
[90494-79-4] Xaliproden Hydrochloride, *10054*
[90717-03-6] Quinmerac, *8066*
[90729-43-4] Ebastine, *3484*
[90779-69-4] Atosiban, *865*
[90803-92-2] Thymomodulin, *9402*
[90825-43-7] Mepact Sodium Salt, *5844*

[90857-62-8] Brassard's Diene (E-form), *1363*
[90881-70-2] D-Galactose Microparticulate Form, *4335*
[90961-53-8] Tedisamil, *9108*
[90965-06-3] Bestmann-Ohira Reagent, *1177*
[90982-32-4] Chlorimuron-ethyl, *2093*
[90996-54-6] Rhizoxin, *8181*
[91032-26-7] Teicoplanin A₂-2, *9115*
[91032-34-7] Teicoplanin A₂-1, *9115*
[91032-36-9] Teicoplanin A₂-3, *9115*
[91032-37-0] Teicoplanin A₂-4, *9115*
[91032-38-1] Teicoplanin A₂-5, *9115*
[91161-71-6] Terbinafine, *9156*
[91296-86-5] Difloxacin Monohydrochloride, *3141*
[91296-87-6] Sarafloxacin Monohydrochloride, *8370*
[91374-20-8] Ropinirole Hydrochloride, *8257*
[91374-21-9] Ropinirole, *8257*
[91421-42-0] Rubitecan, *8288*
[91421-43-1] 9-Aminocamptothecin, *431*
[91423-46-0] [S-(all-E)]-3-(1,3,5,7,9-Dodecapentaenyloxy)-1,2-propanediol, *3406*
[91448-99-6] Cystatin C, *2778*
[91465-08-6] λ-Cyhalothrin, *2758*
[91574-91-3] Benexate Hydrochloride Compd with β-Cyclodextrin (1:1), *1038*
[91599-74-5] Benidipine Hydrochloride, *1043*
[91618-36-9] Ibafloxacin, *4872*
[91714-93-1] Bromfenac Monosodium Salt, *1390*
[91714-94-2] Bromfenac, *1390*
[91832-40-5] Cefdinir, *1920*
[91940-87-3] Zatebradine Hydrochloride, *10115*
[92077-78-6] Cilazapril Monohydrate, *2273*
[92118-27-9] Fotemustine, *4261*
[92129-86-7] Purified Protein Derivative, *9805*
[92134-98-0] Fosphenytoin Disodium Salt, *4258*
[92284-99-6] Ajoene (E)-Form, *195*
[92285-01-3] Ajoene, *195*
[92339-11-2] Iodixanol, *5023*
[92398-48-6] Cycloleucine Hydrochloride, *2734*
[92589-98-5] Ipsapirone Hydrochloride, *5081*
[92623-85-3] Milnacipran, *6194*
[92665-29-7] Cefprozil (anhydrous), *1942*
[92676-86-3] Cefprozil E-Form, *1942*
[92761-26-7] Ecamsule, *3490*
[92823-03-5] Flomoxef Sodium Salt, *4104*
[92981-78-7] Tesmilifene Hydrochloride, *9178*
[93076-39-2] Ritanserin L-Tartrate, *8235*
[93106-60-6] Enrofloxacin, *3592*
[93227-64-6] Betaine Sodium Aspartate, *1179*
[93384-43-1] Botulin A, *1357*
[93384-44-2] Botulin B, *1357*
[93390-81-9] Fosphenytoin, *4258*

[93413-04-8] Asperlicin, *843*
[93413-05-9] Asperlicin E, *843*
[93413-06-0] Asperlicin C, *843*
[93413-07-1] Asperlicin D, *843*
[93413-08-2] Asperlicin B, *843*
[93413-69-5] Venlafaxine, *9946*
[93479-97-1] Glimepiride, *4440*
[93633-92-2] Amosulalol Monohydrochloride, *575*
[93793-83-0] Roxatidine Acetate Hydrochloride, *8274*
[93957-54-1] Fluvastatin, *4218*
[93957-55-2] Fluvastatin Sodium Salt, *4218*
[94050-52-9] Flucycloxuron (E-isomer), *4123*
[94050-53-0] Flucycloxuron (Z-isomer), *4123*
[94055-76-2] Suplatast Tosylate, *9003*
[94125-34-5] Prosulfuron, *7881*
[94134-60-8] Eburnamonine (−)-Form Phosphate, *3487*
[94157-87-6] Bunaftine Citrate, *1485*
[94359-66-7] Pavoninin-4, *7054*
[94361-06-5] Cyproconazole, *2771*
[94421-68-8] Anandamide, *624*
[94424-50-7] Quinagolide Hydrochloride, *8045*
[94426-01-4] Pavoninin-1, *7054*
[94442-12-3] Aminopyrine Bicamphorate, *474*
[94470-67-4] Cromakalim, *5460*
[94480-49-6] Pavoninins, *7054*
[94497-51-5] Tamibarotene, *9047*
[94535-50-9] Levcromakalim, *5460*
[94749-08-3] Salmeterol 1-Hydroxy-2-naphthoate, *8337*
[94841-17-5] Spirapril Hydrochloride, *8753*
[95058-81-4] Gemcitabine, *4386*
[95153-31-4] Perindoprilat, *7170*
[95233-18-4] Atovaquone, *866*
[95266-40-3] Trinexapac-ethyl, *9725*
[95343-20-7] Pirarubicin Hydrochloride, *7488*
[95382-33-5] Omeprazole Magnesium Salt, *6845*
[95399-71-6] Fosinopril Diacid, *4256*
[95465-99-9] Cadusafos, *1632*
[95522-45-5] Colestilan, *2474*
[95635-55-5] Ranolazine, *8111*
[95635-56-6] Ranolazine Dihydrochloride, *8111*
[95656-48-7] Mabuterol dl-Form Hydrochloride, *5642*
[95656-54-5] Mabuterol d-Form Hydrochloride, *5642*
[95656-55-6] Mabuterol l-Form Hydrochloride, *5642*
[95715-87-0] Garner's Aldehyde R-Form, *4371*
[95723-59-4] Lunacrine dl-Form, *5604*
[95737-68-1] Pyriproxyfen, *7990*
[95751-30-7] Charybdotoxin, *2046*
[95789-30-3] Cefotiam Hexetil Hydrochloride, *1935*
[95847-70-4] Ipsapirone, *5081*
[95896-08-5] Anaritide, *872*
[95975-55-6] Guggulsterone, *4573*
[96020-91-6] Eflornithine Hydrochloride Monohydrate, *3522*
[96036-03-2] Meropenem, *5900*
[96055-45-7] Nicotine Polacrilex, *6524*
[96125-53-0] Clentiazem, *2348*

[105462-24-6] Risedronic Acid, *8232*
[105512-06-9] Clodinafop-Propargyl, *2370*
[105613-48-7] Exametazime, *3911*
[105628-07-7] Fasudil Hydrochloride, *3942*
[105650-23-5] PhIP, *7324*
[105784-61-0] Temafloxacin Hydrochloride, *9132*
[105816-04-4] Nateglinide, *6428*
[105826-92-4] Tropisetron Monohydrochloride, *9783*
[105827-78-9] Imidacloprid, *4910*
[105851-17-0] Fludeoxyglucose F^{18}, *4127*
[105857-23-6] Alteplase, *9468*
[105879-42-3] Cephalexin Monohydrochloride Monohydrate, *1974*
[105889-45-0] Cefcapene Pivoxil, *1919*
[105956-97-6] Clinafloxacin, *2355*
[105956-99-8] Clinafloxacin Hydrochloride, *2355*
[105979-17-7] Benidipine, *1043*
[106017-08-7] Rufloxacin Hydrochloride, *8294*
[106096-92-8] Acidic Fibroblast Growth Factor, *4072*
[106096-93-9] Basic Fibroblast Growth Factor, *4072*
[106133-20-4] Tamsulosin, *9049*
[106266-06-2] Risperidone, *8233*
[106308-44-5] Rufinamide, *8293*
[106325-08-0] Epoxiconazole (unspecified stereo), *3629*
[106362-32-7] Peptide T, *7148*
[106388-42-5] Peptide YY (unspecified source), *7149*
[106392-12-5] Poloxamers, *7562*
[106463-17-6] Tamsulosin Hydrochloride, *9049*
[106486-76-4] Carzinophilin A, *1877*
[106516-24-9] Sertindole, *8466*
[106560-14-9] Faropenem, *3938*
[106602-62-4] Amylin, *609*
[106635-80-7] Tafenoquine, *9029*
[106635-81-8] Tafenoquine Succinate, *9029*
[106650-56-0] Sibutramine, *8485*
[106685-40-9] Adapalene, *150*
[106730-54-5] Loprinone, *5575*
[106819-53-8] Doxacurium Chloride, *3431*
[106861-44-3] Mivacurium Chloride, *6219*
[106941-25-7] Adefovir, *151*
[107007-99-8] Granisetron Hydrochloride, *4536*
[107091-89-4] Thiazole Orange Tosylate, *9308*
[107097-80-3] Loxiglumide, *5588*
[107133-36-8] Perindopril *tert*-Butylamine, *7170*
[107220-28-0] Cevimeline Hydrochloride, *2034*
[107233-08-9] Cevimeline (anhydrous), *2034*
[107254-86-4] NPPB, *6725*
[107452-89-1] Ziconotide, *10122*
[107534-96-3] Tebuconazole, *9092*
[107544-29-6] Cystatin A, *2778*
[107667-60-7] Polaprezinc, *7552*
[107724-20-9] Eplerenone, *3625*
[107753-78-6] Zafirlukast, *10108*
[107761-42-2] Aβ_{42}, *615*

[107793-72-6] Ioxilan, *5068*
[107868-30-4] Exemestane, *3913*
[107910-75-8] Ganciclovir Sodium Salt, *4363*
[108050-54-0] Tilmicosin, *9439*
[108050-82-4] Roxindole Hydrochloride, *8275*
[108153-74-8] Secretin Human Secretin, *8421*
[108212-75-5] Calicheamicin γ_1^I, *1715*
[108319-06-8] Temafloxacin, *9132*
[108424-49-3] Indium Gallium Aluminum Phosphide, *4950*
[108605-62-5] Teriflunomide (unspecified stereo), *9165*
[108612-45-9] Mizolastine, *6221*
[108730-13-8] Indium Gallium Aluminum Phosphide, *4950*
[108731-70-0] Fomesafen Sodium Salt, *4227*
[108736-35-2] Lanreotide, *5361*
[108778-82-1] Beractant, *1151*
[108929-04-0] Epinastine Hydrochloride, *3618*
[108945-35-3] Taprostene, *9057*
[109293-97-2] Diflufenzopyr, *3145*
[109489-77-2] Tetranectin, *9232*
[109581-73-9] Technetium ^{99m}Tc Sestamibi, *9102*
[109581-93-3] Tacrolimus Monohydrate, *9025*
[109628-27-5] TSQ, *9799*
[109784-48-7] Doisynolic Acid, *3410*
[109826-26-8] Zaldaride, *10110*
[109826-27-9] Zaldaride Maleate, *10110*
[109852-02-0] Gestodene Mixture with Ethinyl Estradiol, *4413*
[109889-09-0] Granisetron, *4536*
[110075-07-5] Captopril Combination with Hydrochlorothiazide, *1774*
[110101-66-1] Tirilazad, *9463*
[110140-89-1] Ridogrel, *8212*
[110221-44-8] Temocapril Hydrochloride, *9136*
[110221-53-9] Temocaprilat, *9136*
[110230-98-3] Talaporfin, *9034*
[110235-47-7] Mepanipyrim, *5845*
[110267-81-7] Amrubicin, *593*
[110311-30-3] Amrubicin Hydrochloride, *593*
[110429-35-1] Paroxetine Hydrochloride Hemihydrate, *7043*
[110488-70-5] Dimethomorph, *3222*
[110588-57-3] Saperconazole, *8362*
[110703-94-1] Zopolrestat, *10194*
[110871-86-8] Sparfloxacin, *8735*
[110942-02-4] Interleukin-2 Recombinant Human Interleukin-2, *4994*
[111011-53-1] Efonidipine Hydrochloride, *3524*
[111011-63-3] Efonidipine, *3524*
[111011-76-8] Efonidipine Hydrochloride Ethanol, *3524*
[111025-46-8] Pioglitazone, *7452*
[111223-26-8] Ceronapril, *1994*
[111266-55-8] Doxorubicin Citrate, *3439*
[111324-04-0] Schwesinger P$_4$ Base (doxorubicin citrate), *8398*
[111406-87-2] Zileuton, *10124*
[111470-99-6] Amlodipine Besylate, *491*
[111479-05-1] Propaquizafop, *7806*

[111686-79-4] Remacemide Hydrochloride, *8130*
[111753-73-2] Satigrel, *8383*
[111793-42-1] Tirilazad Methanesulfonate Monohydrate, *9463*
[111902-57-9] Temocapril, *9136*
[111974-69-7] Quetiapine, *8039*
[111974-72-2] Quetiapine Hemifumarate, *8039*
[111988-49-9] Thiacloprid, *9291*
[111991-09-4] Nicosulfuron, *6522*
[112132-09-9] Piretanide Monosodium Salt, *7492*
[112143-82-5] Triazamate, *9601*
[112192-04-8] Roxindole, *8275*
[112226-61-6] Halofenozide, *4595*
[112244-09-4] Tilidine *cis*-(±)-Form, *9437*
[112281-77-3] Tetraconazole, *9193*
[112347-74-7] Papuamine Dihydrochloride, *7021*
[112362-50-2] Dalfopristin, *2804*
[112373-40-7] Prodigiosin Hydrochloride, *7767*
[112398-08-0] Danofloxacin, *2813*
[112410-23-8] Tebufenozide, *9093*
[112455-84-2] Papuamine, *7021*
[112457-95-1] Tandospirone Citrate, *9051*
[112529-15-4] Pioglitazone Hydrochloride, *7452*
[112573-73-6] Racecadotril (*S*)-Form, *8090*
[112665-43-7] Seratrodast, *8459*
[112709-47-4] Periplanone A, *7173*
[112727-80-7] Renzapride, *8135*
[112809-51-5] Letrozole, *5450*
[112811-59-3] Gatifloxacin, *4376*
[112885-41-3] Mosapride, *6279*
[112885-42-4] Mosapride Citrate, *6279*
[112887-68-0] Raltitrexed, *8099*
[112901-68-5] Amifostine Trihydrate, *404*
[112924-45-5] Dexanabinol, *2944*
[112965-21-6] Calcipotriene, *1641*
[112966-96-8] Domitroban, *3416*
[113036-88-7] Flucycloxuron, *4123*
[113185-69-6] Adrenochrome Thiosemicarbazone, *172*
[113359-04-9] Cefozopran, *1937*
[113378-31-7] Semduramicin, *8443*
[113427-24-0] Epoetin Alfa, *3688*
[113482-87-4] Moprolol *l*-Form Hydrochloride, *6264*
[113507-06-5] Moxidectin, *6290*
[113617-63-3] Orbifloxacin, *6862*
[113626-33-8] Penicillamine Disulfide L-Form, *7090*
[113665-84-2] Clopidogrel, *2396*
[113775-47-6] Dexmedetomidine, *2946*
[113790-28-6] Stepronin Lysine Salt, *8809*
[113806-05-6] Olopatadine, *6840*
[113852-37-2] Cidofovir, *2268*
[114084-78-5] Ibandronic Acid, *4873*
[114311-32-9] Imazamox, *4904*
[114369-43-6] Fenbuconazole, *3962*
[114432-13-2] Fantofarone, *3934*
[114471-18-0] Brain Natriuretic Peptide, *1360*
[114798-26-4] Losartan, *5583*
[114870-03-0] Fondaparinux Sodium, *4232*
[114899-77-3] Ecteinascidin 743, *3503*

[114977-28-5] Docetaxel, *3397*
[115103-54-3] Tiagabine, *9417*
[115256-11-6] Dofetilide, *3409*
[115266-92-7] Domitroban (±)-Form, *3416*
[115436-72-1] Risedronic Acid Monosodium Salt, *8232*
[115457-83-5] Hecameg®, *4621*
[115550-35-1] Marbofloxacin, *5750*
[115575-11-6] Liarozole, *5475*
[115850-27-6] Metconazole *cis*-Form, *5934*
[115850-28-7] Metconazole *trans*-Form, *5934*
[115852-48-7] Fenoxanil, *3983*
[115956-12-2] Dolasetron, *3411*
[115956-13-3] Dolasetron Methanesulfonate, *3411*
[115964-29-9] Tosufloxacin Tosylate, *9555*
[115966-23-9] Urodilatin, *9886*
[116036-70-5] Fibrolase, *4074*
[116057-75-1] Idoxifene, *4890*
[116078-65-0] Bidisomide, *1204*
[116094-23-6] Insulin Aspart, *4982*
[116255-48-2] Bromuconazole, *1446*
[116355-83-0] Fumonisin B₁, *4289*
[116476-13-2] Semotiadil, *8446*
[116476-14-3] Semotiadil Fumarate, *8446*
[116539-59-4] Duloxetine, *3465*
[116644-53-2] Mibefradil, *6173*
[116649-85-5] Ramatroban, *8100*
[116666-63-8] Mibefradil Dihydrochloride, *6173*
[116714-46-6] Novaluron, *6720*
[116836-09-0] Isomethadone *dl*-Form, *5184*
[116876-37-0] Clavulanic Acid Combination of Potassium Salt with Ticarcillin Disodium, *2341*
[117048-59-6] Combretastatin A-4, *2494*
[117060-71-6] Sulbactam Mixture of Sodium Salt with Ampicillin Sodium, *8889*
[117091-64-2] Etoposide Phosphate, *3886*
[117149-90-3] Thymostimulin, *9407*
[117276-75-2] 4-221-Colony-stimulating Factor 1 (Human Clone p3ACSF-69 Protein Moiety Reduced), *5646*
[117279-73-9] Israpafant, *5241*
[117337-19-6] Fluthiacet-methyl, *4210*
[117381-09-6] Trimetrexate Monoacetate Monohydrate, *9721*
[117399-94-7] Endothelin, *3576*
[117428-22-5] Picoxystrobin, *7408*
[117467-28-4] Cefditoren Pivaloyloxymethyl Ester, *1921*
[117591-79-4] Remoxipride Hydrochloride Monohydrate, *8132*
[117704-25-3] Doramectin, *3425*
[117718-60-2] Thiazopyr, *9311*
[117772-70-0] Azithromycin Dihydrate, *915*
[117976-89-3] Rabeprazole, *8089*
[117976-90-6] Rabeprazole Sodium Salt, *8089*
[118072-93-8] Zoledronic Acid, *10187*
[118081-34-8] Ceftibuten Dihydrate, *1949*
[118134-30-8] Spiroxamine, *8761*
[118230-97-0] Inaperisone Hydrochloride, *4928*

[118248-94-5] Mangafodipir (free acid), *5722*
[118288-08-7] Lafutidine, *5347*
[118292-40-3] Tazarotene, *9081*
[118390-30-0] Interferon Alfacon-1, *4990*
[118443-89-3] Cefquinome Sulfate, *1943*
[118457-14-0] Nebivolol, *6432*
[118812-69-4] Ularitide, *9886*
[118949-22-7] Vorozole (±)-Form, *10035*
[118997-30-1] Peptide YY (human), *7149*
[119006-77-8] Flutrimazole, *4215*
[119068-77-8] Semduramicin Sodium Salt, *8443*
[119119-85-6] α-Glucose-1-phosphate Calcium Salt, *4461*
[119141-88-7] Omeprazole *S*-Form, *6845*
[119168-77-3] Tebufenpyrad, *9094*
[119169-78-7] Episteride, *3634*
[119257-34-0] Besipirdine, *1176*
[119257-40-8] Besipirdine Maleate, *1176*
[119302-91-9] Rocuronium Bromide, *8246*
[119356-77-3] Dapoxetine, *2821*
[119413-54-6] Topotecan Hydrochloride, *9548*
[119413-55-7] Elgodipine, *3546*
[119446-68-3] Difenoconazole, *3135*
[119478-55-6] Danofloxacin Methanesulfonate, *2813*
[119478-56-7] Meropenem Trihydrate, *5900*
[119506-01-3] Deserpidine Oxalate, *2918*
[119515-38-7] Picaridin, *7394*
[119520-05-7] Zilpaterol, *10125*
[119520-06-8] Zilpaterol Hydrochloride, *10125*
[119567-79-2] Taribavirin, *9063*
[119600-43-0] Vinconate Monohydrochloride, *9985*
[119683-68-0] Ferumoxides, *4063*
[119742-13-1] Roxindole Methanesulfonate, *8275*
[119784-94-0] Tenidap Sodium Salt, *9144*
[119817-90-2] Loxiglumide (*R*)-Form, *5588*
[119914-60-2] Grepafloxacin, *4545*
[120010-32-4] Park Nucleotide (pimelate form), *7040*
[120011-70-3] Donepezil Hydrochloride, *3419*
[120014-06-4] Donepezil, *3419*
[120066-54-8] Gadoteridol, *4328*
[120068-37-3] Fipronil, *4085*
[120103-35-7] HLö-7, *4724*
[120116-88-3] Cyazofamid, *2700*
[120138-50-3] Quinupristin, *8084*
[120162-55-2] Azimsulfuron, *912*
[120210-48-2] Tenidap, *9144*
[120279-96-1] Dorzolamide, *3426*
[120287-85-6] Cetrorelix, *2026*
[120373-24-2] Unoprostone Isopropyl Ester, *9849*
[120373-36-6] Unoprostone, *9849*
[120410-24-4] Biapenem, *1197*
[120444-71-5] Deramciclane, *2915*
[120444-72-6] Deramciclane Fumarate, *2915*

[120511-73-1] Anastrozole, *625*
[120608-46-0] Duteplase, *9468*
[120635-72-5] Cilansetron Hydrochloride, *2271*
[120635-74-7] Cilansetron, *2271*
[120638-55-3] Bromfenac Monosodium Salt Sesquihydrate, *1390*
[120685-11-2] Midostaurin, *6185*
[120895-52-5] Amphotericin B Compd with Cholesteryl Sulfate, *585*
[120923-37-7] Amidosulfuron, *403*
[120928-09-8] Fenazaquin, *3959*
[120993-53-5] Desirudin, *4718*
[121025-46-5] Sphingofungin C, *8745*
[121032-29-9] Nelarabine, *6442*
[121067-52-5] Yingzhaosu C, *10098*
[121123-17-9] Cefprozil (monohydrate), *1942*
[121124-29-6] Emamectin (major component), *3554*
[121181-53-1] Filgrastim, *4537*
[121268-17-5] Alendronic Acid Monosodium Salt Trihydrate, *229*
[121281-41-2] Technetium ⁹⁹ᵐTc Bicisate, *9099*
[121412-77-9] Cefprozil Z-Form, *1942*
[121424-52-0] Emamectin (minor component), *3554*
[121451-02-3] Noviflumuron, *6721*
[121489-04-1] Elgodipine Hydrochloride, *3546*
[121543-68-8] Lunasine (−)-Form Perchlorate, *5605*
[121547-04-4] Mirimostim, *5646*
[121552-61-2] Cyprodinil, *2772*
[121584-18-7] Valspodar, *9917*
[121652-76-4] Eptastigmine Tartrate, *3638*
[121679-13-8] Naratriptan, *6420*
[121696-62-6] Piroxicam Compd with β-Cyclodextrin, *7506*
[121808-62-6] Pidotimod, *7419*
[121961-22-6] Loracarbef, *5576*
[122007-85-6] Monteplase, *6259*
[122039-27-4] Woollins' Reagent, *10051*
[122111-03-9] Gemcitabine Hydrochloride, *4386*
[122191-40-6] Caspase-1, *1884*
[122312-54-3] Epoetin Beta, *3688*
[122312-55-4] Dosmalfate, *3427*
[122320-73-4] Rosiglitazone, *8265*
[122341-38-2] Temoporfin, *9138*
[122384-88-7] Human Amylin, *609*
[122453-73-0] Chlorfenapyr, *2088*
[122547-49-3] Faropenem Sodium Salt, *3938*
[122548-33-8] Imazosulfuron, *4908*
[122647-31-8] Ibutilide, *4883*
[122647-32-9] Ibutilide Fumarate, *4883*
[122836-35-5] Sulfentrazone, *8947*
[122841-10-5] Cefoselis, *1932*
[122841-12-7] Cefoselis Sulfate, *1932*
[122852-42-0] Alosetron, *308*
[122852-69-1] Alosetron Hydrochloride, *308*
[122883-93-6] Ziprasidone Hydrochloride, *10171*
[122892-31-3] Itopride Hydrochloride (anhydrous), *5244*
[122898-67-3] Itopride, *5244*
[122931-48-0] Rimsulfuron, *8230*
[123040-16-4] Azasetron Hydrochloride, *900*

[123040-69-7] Azasetron, *900*
[123122-54-3] Candoxatrilat, *1742*
[123122-55-4] Candoxatril, *1742*
[123171-59-5] Cefepime Hydrochloride Monohydrate, *1922*
[123258-84-4] Itasetron, *5243*
[123312-89-0] Pymetrozine, *7950*
[123318-82-1] Clofarabine, *2372*
[123342-93-8] Pyrithiobac, *7993*
[123343-16-8] Pyrithiobac Sodium Salt, *7993*
[123407-36-3] Arteflene (Z-form), *814*
[123441-03-2] Rivastigmine, *8240*
[123447-62-1] Prulifloxacin, *7908*
[123524-52-7] Azelnidipine, *907*
[123572-88-3] Furametpyr, *4295*
[123618-00-8] Fedotozine, *3949*
[123774-72-1] Sargramostim, *4538*
[123948-87-8] Topotecan, *9548*
[123997-26-2] Eprinomectin, *3633*
[124051-64-5] Asoxime, *835*
[124351-85-5] Incadronic Acid (free base), *4929*
[124495-18-7] Quinoxyfen, *8079*
[124508-66-3] Triptorelin Pamoate, *9748*
[124584-08-3] Nesiritide, *1360*
[124689-65-2] Cryptophycin-1, *2607*
[124750-99-8] Losartan Monopotassium Salt, *5583*
[124832-26-4] Valacyclovir, *9899*
[124832-27-5] Valacyclovir Hydrochloride, *9899*
[124858-35-1] Nadifloxacin, *6345*
[124904-93-4] Ganirelix, *4365*
[124937-51-5] Tolterodine, *9525*
[124937-52-6] Tolterodine Tartrate, *9525*
[125116-23-6] Metconazole, *5934*
[125224-05-7] Technetium ^{99m}Tc Mertiatide, *9101*
[125251-66-3] Arbutamine Hydrochloride, *772*
[125317-39-7] Vinorelbine Ditartrate, *9990*
[125376-11-6] DMC, *3390*
[125401-75-4] Bispyribac, *1301*
[125401-92-5] Bispyribac Sodium Salt, *1301*
[125472-02-8] Mivazerol, *6220*
[125494-59-9] Sibutramine Hydrochloride Monohydrate, *8485*
[125533-88-2] Mofarotene, *6230*
[125995-03-1] Atorvastatin Lactone, *864*
[126339-09-1] Peptide YY (3-36) (porcine), *7149*
[126535-15-7] Triflusulfuron-methyl, *9689*
[126544-47-6] Ciclesonide, *2263*
[126602-89-9] Dalfopristin Mixture with Quinupristin, *2804*
[126801-58-9] Ethoxysulfuron, *3754*
[126833-17-8] Fenhexamid, *3974*
[127000-20-8] Gadobenate Dimeglumine, *4322*
[127045-41-4] Pazufloxacin, *7055*
[127170-73-4] Mivazerol Hydrochloride, *6220*
[127254-12-0] Sitafloxacin, *8551*
[127277-53-6] Prohexadione Calcium, *7777*
[127294-70-6] Balofloxacin, *944*
[127373-66-4] Sivelestat, *8558*

[127455-27-0] Tetrofosmin ^{99m}Tc-Complex, *9247*
[127502-06-1] Tetrofosmin, *9247*
[127589-93-9] Garner's Aldehyde, *4371*
[127618-28-4] Itasetron Hydrochloride, *5243*
[127757-91-9] Regramostim, *4538*
[127779-20-8] Saquinavir, *8369*
[127786-29-2] Epinastine Hydrobromide, *3618*
[127829-86-1] Kistrin, *5314*
[127943-53-7] Discodermolide, *3355*
[127984-74-1] Lanreotide Acetate, *5361*
[128196-01-0] Citalopram *S*-(+)-Form, *2318*
[128270-60-0] Bivalirudin, *1310*
[128298-28-2] Remacemide, *8130*
[128345-62-0] Ranitidine Bismuth Citrate, *8110*
[128470-16-6] Arbutamine, *772*
[128639-02-1] Carfentrazone-ethyl, *1837*
[128794-94-5] Mycophenolate Mofetil, *6327*
[129025-54-3] Clofencet, *2375*
[129033-04-1] Cyclotheonamide A, *2753*
[129033-05-2] Cyclotheonamide B, *2753*
[129069-19-8] Poractant Alfa, *7595*
[129075-73-6] DPQ, *3442*
[129101-54-8] Rivastigmine Hydrogen Tartrate, *8240*
[129203-60-7] Iberiotoxin, *4874*
[129273-38-7] Perospirone Hydrochloride, *7182*
[129311-55-3] Ganirelix Acetate, *4365*
[129409-01-4] Salen (*E,E*-form), *8322*
[129453-61-8] Fulvestrant, *4284*
[129496-10-2] Milbemycin Oxime, *6190*
[129497-78-5] Verteporfin, *9967*
[129580-63-8] Satraplatin, *8384*
[129618-40-2] Nevirapine, *6490*
[129722-12-9] Aripiprazole, *785*
[129731-10-8] Vorozole, *10035*
[129791-92-0] Rifalazil, *8214*
[129909-90-6] Amicarbazone, *396*
[129938-20-1] Dapoxetine Hydrochloride, *2821*
[129981-36-8] Sampatrilat, *8352*
[130018-77-8] Levocetirizine, *2022*
[130018-87-0] Cetirizine (*R*)-Form Dihydrochloride, *2022*
[130167-69-0] Pegaspargase, *836*
[130209-82-4] Latanoprost, *5376*
[130370-60-4] Batimastat, *1008*
[130391-54-7] Exendin-3, *3914*
[130636-43-0] Nifekalant, *6529*
[130656-51-8] Nifekalant Hydrochloride, *6529*
[130693-82-2] Dorzolamide Hydrochloride, *3426*
[130726-68-0] Neticonazole, *6478*
[130773-02-3] Neticonazole Hydrochloride, *6478*
[130929-57-6] Entacapone, *3594*
[130939-66-1] Neurotrophin-3, *6487*
[130953-69-4] Besipirdine Hydrochloride, *1176*
[131069-91-5] Gadoversetamide, *4329*
[131179-95-8] Efaproxiral, *3520*

[131341-86-1] Fludioxonil, *4129*
[131391-55-4] Magnesium Monoperoxyphthalate Hexahydrate, *5673*
[131410-48-5] Gadodiamide, *4324*
[131410-51-0] Gadodiamide Injection, *4324*
[131438-79-4] Aβ_{40}, *615*
[131740-09-5] Flavopiridol Hydrochloride, *4094*
[131807-57-3] Famoxadone, *3931*
[131860-33-8] Azoxystrobin, *924*
[131918-61-1] Paricalcitol, *7039*
[131929-60-7] Spinosyns, *8750*
[131929-63-0] Spinosyn D, *8750*
[131986-45-3] Xanomeline, *10056*
[132036-88-5] Ramosetron, *8105*
[132068-98-5] Duthaler-Hafner Reagent, *3472*
[132112-35-7] Ropivacaine Hydrochloride Monohydrate, *8258*
[132203-70-4] Cilnidipine, *2275*
[132449-46-8] Lesopitron, *5447*
[132449-89-9] Lesopitron Dihydrochloride, *5447*
[132523-84-3] Tedisamil Dihydrochloride, *9108*
[132523-91-2] Rhod-2, *8182*
[132539-06-1] Olanzapine, *6822*
[132539-07-2] Remifentanil Hydrochloride, *8131*
[132682-98-5] Glufosfamide, *4468*
[132747-47-8] Domitroban Calcium Salt, *3416*
[132810-10-7] Blonanserin, *1319*
[132866-11-6] Lercanidipine Hydrochloride, *5446*
[132875-61-7] Remifentanil, *8131*
[132907-72-3] Ramosetron Hydrochloride, *8105*
[133040-01-4] Eprosartan, *3635*
[133099-04-4] Darifenacin, *2825*
[133099-07-7] Darifenacin Hydrobromide, *2825*
[133107-64-9] Insulin Lispro, *4987*
[133220-30-1] Indanofan, *4933*
[133242-30-5] Landiolol, *5355*
[133267-27-3] Fedotozine D(−)-Tartrate, *3949*
[133305-88-1] Eprinomectin Component B$_{1a}$, *3633*
[133305-89-2] Eprinomectin Component B$_{1b}$, *3633*
[133343-39-9] Ciliary Neurotrophic Factor (Human), *2274*
[133454-47-4] Iloperidone, *4900*
[133514-43-9] Exendin(9-39), *3914*
[133652-38-7] Reteplase, *8161*
[133737-96-9] Ranpirnase, *8112*
[133855-98-8] Epoxiconazole, *3629*
[133865-89-1] Safinamide, *8315*
[133868-46-9] Valnemulin Hydrochloride, *9911*
[134088-74-7] Nartograstim, *4537*
[134098-61-6] Fenpyroximate, *3996*
[134308-13-7] Tolcapone, *9508*
[134381-21-8] Epoxomicin, *3630*
[134404-52-7] Seocalcitol, *8456*
[134523-00-5] Atorvastatin, *864*
[134523-01-6] Atorvastatin Sodium Salt, *864*
[134523-03-8] Atorvastatin Calcium Salt, *864*
[134564-82-2] Befloxatone (anhydrous), *1021*

[134678-17-4] Lamivudine, *5352*
[134710-25-1] Calciseptine, *1642*
[134774-45-1] Rasburicase, *8117*
[135038-57-2] Fasidotril, *3940*
[135038-59-4] Fasidotril Diacid, *3940*
[135046-48-9] Clopidogrel Hydrogen Sulfate, *2396*
[135062-02-1] Repaglinide, *8136*
[135158-54-2] Acibenzolar-*S*-methyl, *106*
[135285-90-4] Hexanitrohexaazaiso-wurtzitane, *4696*
[135326-11-3] Gadoxetic Acid, *4330*
[135326-22-6] Gadoxetic Acid Sodium Salt, *4330*
[135354-02-8] Xaliproden, *10054*
[135459-87-9] Ranelic Acid Strontium Salt, *8106*
[135459-90-4] Ranelic Acid, *8106*
[135558-11-1] Lobaplatin, *5549*
[135590-91-9] Mefenpyr-diethyl, *5800*
[135729-61-2] Palonosetron, *6997*
[135729-62-3] Palonosetron Hydrochloride, *6997*
[135886-70-3] Gallium Nitrate Nonahydrate, *4350*
[135889-00-8] Cefcapene Pivoxil Free Acid, *1919*
[135968-09-1] Lenograstim, *4537*
[136087-85-9] Fidarestat, *4078*
[136236-51-6] Rasagiline, *8116*
[136279-32-8] Teceleukin, *4994*
[136310-93-5] Tiotropium Bromide, *9454*
[136426-54-5] Fluquinconazole, *4196*
[136434-34-9] Duloxetine Hydrochloride, *3465*
[136470-78-5] Abacavir, *1*
[136572-09-3] Irinotecan Hydrochloride Trihydrate, *5091*
[136705-64-1] (*R,R*)-Et-DuPHOS, *3466*
[136735-95-0] (*S,S*)-Me-DuPHOS, *3466*
[136817-59-9] Delavirdine, *2877*
[136949-58-1] Iobitridol, *5008*
[137061-46-2] Nisin Z, *6564*
[137071-32-0] Pimecrolimus, *7429*
[137159-92-3] Aptiganel, *758*
[137160-11-3] Aptiganel Hydrochloride, *758*
[137181-56-7] Systemin, *9018*
[137219-37-5] Aplidine, *738*
[137234-62-9] Voriconazole, *10033*
[137281-23-3] Pemetrexed, *7077*
[137335-79-6] Emamectin, *3554*
[137463-76-4] PIXY321, *4995*
[137512-74-4] Emamectin Benzoate, *3554*
[137641-05-5] Picolinafen, *7399*
[137862-53-4] Valsartan, *9916*
[137945-48-3] Ajulemic Acid, *198*
[138068-37-8] Lepirudin, *4718*
[138071-82-6] Gadobutrol, *4323*
[138112-76-2] Agomelatine, *190*
[138117-50-7] Leteprinim, *5448*
[138124-32-0] Jacobsen's Catalyst (*R,R*)-Form, *5252*
[138184-95-9] Caprenin, *1756*
[138199-71-0] Ofloxacin *S*-(−)-Form (hemihydrate), *6771*
[138240-65-0] Panipenem Mixture with Betamipron, *7009*
[138330-18-4] Incadronic Acid Disodium Salt, *4929*

[138402-11-6] Irbesartan, *5083*
[138531-07-4] Sinapultide, *8542*
[138661-02-6] Pentetreotide, *7126*
[138729-47-2] Zopiclone *S*-Form, *10193*
[138786-67-1] Pantoprazole Sodium Salt, *7014*
[138844-81-2] Ibandronic Acid Sodium Salt (anhydrous), *4873*
[138890-62-7] Brinzolamide, *1376*
[138926-19-9] Ibandronic Acid Sodium Salt (monohydrate), *4873*
[138955-27-8] Indium ^{111}In Satumomab Pendetide, *8385*
[138982-67-9] Ziprasidone Hydrochloride Monohydrate, *10171*
[139096-04-1] Pentetreotide ^{111}In Chelate, *7126*
[139110-80-8] Zanamivir, *10113*
[139133-26-9] Lexipafant, *5473*
[139264-17-8] Zolmitriptan, *10189*
[139341-09-6] CTX-3, *2270*
[139481-59-7] Candesartan, *1739*
[139755-83-2] Sildenafil, *8489*
[140111-52-0] Epibatidine, *3610*
[140194-24-7] Triptorelin Acetate, *9748*
[140462-73-3] Duthaler-Hafner Reagent (*S,S*)-Form, *3472*
[140462-76-6] Olopatadine Hydrochloride, *6840*
[140608-64-6] Muromonab CD3, *6308*
[140661-97-8] Bradycor, *1358*
[140678-14-4] Mangafodipir Trisodium Salt, *5722*
[140681-55-6] Selectfluor®, *8425*
[140898-91-5] Hexaminolevulinate Hydrochloride, *4693*
[140898-97-1] Hexaminolevulinate, *4693*
[140923-17-7] Iprovalicarb, *5080*
[141064-23-5] Xanomeline Oxalate, *10056*
[141112-29-0] Isoxaflutole, *5236*
[141204-94-6] Co-artemether, *5597*
[141396-28-3] Argatroban Monohydrate, *779*
[141505-32-0] Ibuprofen *S*-Form L-Lysine Salt Monohydrate, *4881*
[141505-33-1] Levosimendan, *5471*
[141517-21-7] Trifloxystrobin, *9677*
[141625-93-6] Dronedarone Hydrochloride, *3449*
[141626-36-0] Dronedarone, *3449*
[141702-36-5] Faropenem Daloxate, *3938*
[141732-76-5] Exendin-4, *3914*
[141750-63-2] Pitavastatin Lactone, *7508*
[141776-32-1] Sulfosulfuron, *8965*
[142155-43-9] Cizolirtine, *2336*
[142155-44-0] Cizolirtine Citrate, *2336*
[142185-85-1] CTX-2, *2270*
[142192-09-4] Interferon Alfa-2c, *4990*
[142217-69-4] Entecavir, *3595*
[142340-99-6] Adefovir Dipivoxil, *151*
[142373-60-2] Tirofiban Hydrochloride, *9464*
[142459-58-3] Flufenacet (hydrochloride), *4131*
[142561-96-4] Zaragozic Acids Zaragozic Acid A, *10114*
[142583-61-7] Policosanol, *7555*
[142825-10-3] Sulforaphane, *8962*

[142891-20-1] Cinidon-ethyl, *2293*
[143003-46-7] Alglucerase, *243*
[143011-72-7] Granulocyte Colony-Stimulating Factor, *4537*
[143090-92-0] Anakinra, *5001*
[143201-11-0] Cerivastatin Sodium Salt, *1993*
[143322-58-1] Eletriptan, *3544*
[143334-20-7] Carbon Nitride, *1814*
[143388-64-1] Naratriptan Hydrochloride, *6420*
[143390-89-0] Kresoxim-methyl, *5324*
[143413-84-7] Thiazole Orange Dimer, *9308*
[143491-57-0] Emtricitabine, *3565*
[143558-00-3] Rocuronium, *8246*
[143653-53-6] Abciximab, *5*
[143807-66-3] Chromafenozide, *2218*
[143831-71-4] Dornase Alfa, *2906*
[144034-80-0] Rizatriptan, *8241*
[144046-30-0] D-Galactose Transpulmonary Microparticulate Form, *4335*
[144058-40-2] Satumomab, *8385*
[144060-53-7] Febuxostat, *3948*
[144115-48-0] Dichlormid Combination with Acetochlor, *3049*
[144143-96-4] Eprosartan Mesylate, *3635*
[144171-61-9] Indoxacarb (*RS*)-Form, *4971*
[144189-66-2] 3-Nitrosobenzamide, *6634*
[144245-52-3] Fomivirsen, *4229*
[144252-71-1] Asoxime Dimethanesulfonate, *835*
[144348-08-3] Binodenoson, *1225*
[144412-49-7] Lamifiban, *5349*
[144412-50-0] Lamifiban Trifluoroacetate Salt, *5349*
[144481-98-1] Landiolol Hydrochloride, *5355*
[144494-65-5] Tirofiban, *9464*
[144506-14-9] Licochalcone C, *5479*
[144506-15-0] Licochalcone D, *5479*
[144510-96-3] Pixantrone, *7514*
[144538-83-0] Iminodisuccinic Acid Tetrasodium Salt, *4918*
[144550-36-7] Iodosulfuron-methyl-sodium, *5046*
[144665-07-6] Lubeluzole, *5590*
[144675-97-8] Pixantrone Dimalate Salt, *7514*
[144689-63-4] Olmesartan, *6839*
[144701-48-4] Telmisartan, *9129*
[144740-53-4] Flupyrsulfuron-methyl, *4195*
[144740-54-5] Flupyrsulfuron-methyl Sodium Salt, *4195*
[144875-48-9] Resiquimod, *8151*
[144980-29-0] Repinotan, *8137*
[144980-77-8] Repinotan Hydrochloride, *8137*
[145026-81-9] Propoxycarbazone, *7838*
[145026-88-6] Flucarbazone, *4119*
[145040-37-5] Candesartan Cilexetil, *1739*
[145108-58-3] Dexmedetomidine Hydrochloride, *2946*
[145137-38-8] Desmoteplase, *3459*
[145155-23-3] Interferon Beta-1b, *4991*
[145158-71-0] Tegaserod, *9113*
[145202-66-0] Rizatriptan Benzoate, *8241*
[145258-61-3] Interferon Beta-1a, *4991*

[145375-43-5] Mitiglinide, *6211*
[145464-28-4] Capromab Pendetide, *1762*
[145525-41-3] Mitiglinide Calcium, *6211*
[145599-86-6] Cerivastatin (anhydrous), *1993*
[145613-73-6] HLö-7 Dimethanesulfonate, *4724*
[145626-87-5] Bis(2-mercaptoethyl)-sulfone, *1254*
[145672-81-7] Cetrorelix Acetate, *2026*
[145701-21-9] Diclosulam, *3083*
[145701-23-1] Florasulam, *4108*
[145808-47-5] Margatoxin, *5752*
[145821-59-6] Tiagabine Hydrochloride, *9417*
[145858-50-0] Liarozole Hydrochloride, *5475*
[145858-52-2] Liarozole Fumarate, *5475*
[145918-75-8] Troxacitabine, *9788*
[145941-26-0] Oprelvekin, *5000*
[146368-15-2] Cy 5, *2679*
[146389-61-9] Zaragozic Acid B, *10114*
[146389-62-0] Zaragozic Acid C, *10114*
[146397-20-8] Cy 3, *2678*
[146426-40-6] Flavopiridol, *4094*
[146939-27-7] Ziprasidone, *10171*
[146961-34-4] Trovafloxacin Hydrochloride, *9787*
[147059-72-1] Trovafloxacin, *9787*
[147059-75-4] Trovafloxacin Methanesulfonate, *9787*
[147098-20-2] Rosuvastatin Calcium Salt, *8270*
[147127-20-6] Tenofovir, *9146*
[147149-76-6] Nolatrexed, *6672*
[147221-93-0] Delavirdine Mesylate, *2877*
[147245-92-9] Glatiramer Acetate, *4435*
[147253-67-6] (*R,R*)-Me-DuPHOS, *3466*
[147511-69-1] Pitavastatin, *7508*
[147526-32-7] Pitavastatin Calcium Salt, *7508*
[147536-97-8] Bosentan, *1353*
[147664-63-9] Pexiganan, *7193*
[148477-71-8] Spirodiclofen, *8757*
[148553-50-8] Pregabalin, *7725*
[148641-02-5] Muplestim, *4995*
[148717-90-2] Squalamine, *8766*
[148849-67-6] Ivabradine Hydrochloride, *5247*
[148883-56-1] Tifacogin, *9467*
[149003-01-0] Razoxane (+)-Form Hydrochloride, *8123*
[149152-95-4] Splendipherin, *8762*
[149193-61-3] Xemilofiban Acid, *10070*
[149204-42-2] Kahalalide F, *5275*
[149470-60-0] Ivabradine (±)-Form, *5247*
[149508-90-7] Simeconazole, *8534*
[149647-78-9] Vorinostat, *10034*
[149656-63-3] Jacobsen's Catalyst, *5252*
[149676-40-4] Pefloxacin Methanesulfonate Dihydrate, *7066*
[149820-74-6] Xemilofiban, *10070*
[149824-15-7] Ilodecakin, *4999*

[149838-22-2] FM1-43, *4220*
[149845-06-7] Saquinavir Mesylate, *8369*
[149845-07-8] Tiludronic Acid Disodium Salt, *9441*
[149877-41-8] Bifenazate, *1207*
[149888-94-8] Azimilide Dihydrochloride, *911*
[149908-53-2] Azimilide, *911*
[149920-56-9] Idraparinux Sodium, *4892*
[149979-41-9] Tepraloxydim, *9152*
[150103-82-5] Sonicated Human Serum Albumin, *8468*
[150374-95-1] Sivelestat Sodium, *8558*
[150378-17-9] Indinavir (anhydrous), *4945*
[150399-21-6] Balsalazide Disodium Salt Dihydrate, *945*
[150399-23-8] Pemetrexed Sodium Salt, *7077*
[150683-30-0] Tolvaptan, *9540*
[150726-52-6] Bosentan Sodium Salt, *1353*
[150824-47-8] Nitenpyram, *6568*
[150915-40-5] Tirofiban Hydrochloride Monohydrate, *9464*
[150915-41-6] Perospirone, *7182*
[150937-43-2] Brinzolamide Hydrochloride, *1376*
[151031-37-7] Stellar®, *8806*
[151096-09-2] Moxifloxacin, *6291*
[151126-32-8] Pramlintide, *7708*
[151319-34-5] Zaleplon, *10111*
[151438-54-9] Harpin, *4617*
[151606-29-0] Zinquin, *10169*
[151716-36-8] Methyl Dihydrojasmonate (+)-(1*S*,2*S*)-Form, *6052*
[151763-64-3] Capromab, *1762*
[151767-02-1] Montelukast Monosodium Salt, *6258*
[151879-73-1] Aprinocarsen, *755*
[151912-11-7] Amediplase, *391*
[152044-53-6] Epothilone A, *3628*
[152044-54-7] Epothilone B, *3628*
[152459-95-5] Imatinib, *4902*
[152520-56-4] Nebivolol Hydrochloride, *6432*
[152751-57-0] Sevelamer Hydrochloride, *8474*
[152811-62-6] Piboserod, *7393*
[152854-19-8] Xanomeline Tartrate, *10056*
[152923-56-3] Daclizumab, *2799*
[152923-57-4] Luteinizing Hormone Lutropin Alfa, *5613*
[152946-68-4] Nolatrexed Dihydrochloride, *6672*
[153168-05-9] Pleconaril, *7533*
[153233-91-1] Etoxazole, *3890*
[153259-65-5] Cilomilast, *2276*
[153439-40-8] Fexofenadine Hydrochloride, *4068*
[153504-70-2] Cevimeline Hydrochloride Hemihydrate, *2034*
[153507-46-1] Technetium ⁹⁹ᵐTc Apcitide Dimer, *9098*
[153531-96-5] Magnesium Citrate Tribasic (nonahydrate), *5663*
[153559-49-0] Bexarotene, *1194*
[153719-23-4] Thiamethoxam, *9294*
[153832-38-3] Ertapenem Sodium Salt, *3673*
[153832-46-3] Ertapenem, *3673*

[154039-60-8] Marimastat, *5753*
[154323-57-6] Almotriptan, *304*
[154361-48-5] Arcitumomab, *774*
[154361-49-6] Arcitumomab ⁹⁹ᵐTc-Labeled Form, *774*
[154361-50-9] Capecitabine, *1754*
[154427-83-5] Samarium ¹⁵³Sm Lexidronam, *8350*
[154598-52-4] Efavirenz, *3521*
[155030-63-0] Emodepside, *3560*
[155141-29-0] Rosiglitazone Maleate, *8265*
[155206-00-1] Bimatoprost, *1221*
[155213-67-5] Ritonavir, *8238*
[155319-91-8] Mangafodipir (hexahydrogen), *5722*
[155453-10-4] Tiludronic Acid Disodium Salt (hemihydrate), *9441*
[155773-57-2] Pegorgotein, *9002*
[155798-07-5] Ioflupane ¹²³I, *5050*
[155974-00-8] Ivabradine, *5247*
[156052-68-5] Zoxamide, *10198*
[156053-89-3] Alvimopan, *372*
[156137-99-4] Rapacuronium Bromide, *8113*
[156436-89-4] Motexafin Gadolinium (hydrate), *6281*
[156436-90-7] Motexafin Lutetium (hydrate), *6282*
[156586-89-9] Edrecolomab, *3515*
[156586-91-3] Xemilofiban Hydrochloride, *10070*
[156604-79-4] Dexketoprofen Trometamol, *5305*
[156611-76-6] Rupatadine Trihydrochloride, *8297*
[156897-06-2] Licofelone, *5480*
[156910-61-1] Phenserine Tartrate, *7260*
[157212-55-0] Bosentan Monohydrate, *1353*
[157283-68-6] Travoprost, *9577*
[157716-52-4] Perifosine, *7165*
[157810-81-6] Indinavir Sulfate, *4945*
[157856-25-2] Sulesomab ⁹⁹ᵐTc-Labeled Form, *8895*
[158062-67-0] Flonicamid, *4105*
[158113-60-1] Opebecan, *938*
[158237-07-1] Fentrazamide, *4007*
[158382-37-7] Canfosfamide, *1745*
[158440-71-2] Irofulven, *5092*
[158681-13-1] Rimonabant Hydrochloride, *8229*
[158747-02-5] Frovatriptan, *4272*
[158876-82-5] Rupatadine, *8297*
[158930-09-7] Frovatriptan Succinate (anhydrous), *4272*
[158930-17-7] Frovatriptan Succinate, *4272*
[158966-92-8] Montelukast, *6258*
[159138-80-4] Cariporide, *1841*
[159138-81-5] Cariporide Methanesulfonate, *1841*
[159351-69-6] Everolimus, *3907*
[159519-65-0] Enfuvirtide, *3582*
[159652-53-6] Phenserine (racemate), *7260*
[159752-39-3] Methoxyethylbenzeneboronic Acid (+)-*R*-Form, *5992*
[159776-70-2] Melagatran, *5810*
[159912-53-5] Sabcomeline, *8309*
[159912-58-0] Sabcomeline Hydrochloride, *8309*
[159989-64-7] Nelfinavir, *6443*

[159989-65-8] Nelfinavir Methanesulfonate, 6443
[159997-94-1] Biricodar, 1240
[160337-95-1] Insulin Glargine, 4984
[160369-77-7] Fomivirsen Sodium Salt, 4229
[160369-78-8] Samarium ^{153}Sm Lexidronam Pentasodium Salt, 8350
[160430-64-8] Acetamiprid, 49
[160970-54-7] Silodosin, 8503
[161050-58-4] Methoxyfenozide, 5993
[161326-34-7] Fenamidone, 3956
[161735-79-1] Rasagiline Methanesulfonate, 8116
[161814-49-9] Amprenavir, 589
[161832-65-1] Talampanel, 9032
[161967-81-3] Grepafloxacin Hydrochloride, 4545
[161973-10-0] Esomeprazole magnesium, 6845
[161982-62-3] Depreotide, 2911
[162011-90-7] Rofecoxib, 8248
[162359-55-9] Fingolimod, 4083
[162359-56-0] Fingolimod Hydrochloride, 4083
[162394-19-6] Palifermin, 6986
[162401-32-3] Roflumilast, 8249
[162610-17-5] Idraparinux, 4892
[162635-04-3] Temsirolimus (Idraparinux), 9142
[162652-95-1] Vinflunine, 9989
[162808-62-0] Caspofungin, 1889
[163120-03-4] Nodulisporic acid, 6669
[163222-33-1] Ezetimibe, 3918
[163252-36-6] Clevudine, 2353
[163253-35-8] Sitafloxacin Sesquihydrate, 8551
[163451-81-8] Teriflunomide, 9165
[163515-14-8] Dimethenamid P, 3214
[163515-35-3] Chlorotoxin, 2173
[163545-26-4] Ancestim, 8807
[163680-77-1] Pazufloxacin Methanesulfonate, 7055
[163706-06-7] Cangrelor, 1746
[163706-36-3] Cangrelor Tetrasodium Salt, 1746
[164656-23-9] Dutasteride, 3471
[165101-51-9] Becaplermin, 7525
[165252-70-0] Dinotefuran, 3289
[165450-17-9] Neotame, 6465
[165800-03-3] Linezolid, 5504
[165800-06-6] Zoledronic Acid (monohydrate), 10187
[165800-07-7] Zoledronic Acid Disodium Salt Tetrahydrate, 10187
[165800-08-8] Zoledronic Acid Trisodium Salt Hydrate, 10187
[166191-23-7] Methoxyethylbenzeneboronic Acid (−)-S-Form, 5992
[166518-60-1] Avasimibe, 884
[166518-61-2] Avasimibe Sodium Salt, 884
[166663-25-8] Anidulafungin, 656
[166944-16-7] Saporin-6, 8366
[167221-71-8] Clevidipine, 2352
[167305-00-2] Omapatrilat, 6843
[167354-41-8] Zosuquidar, 10196
[167465-36-3] Zosuquidar Trihydrochloride, 10196
[167747-19-5] Sulesomab, 8895
[168021-77-0] Disufenton, 3363
[168021-79-2] Disufenton Sodium Salt, 3363
[168273-06-1] Rimonabant, 8229

[168316-95-8] Spinosad, 8750
[168626-94-6] Conivaptan Hydrochloride, 2507
[169147-32-4] Abetimus Sodium, 6
[169148-63-4] Insulin Detemir, 4983
[169149-90-0] Kogenate, 3921
[169590-41-4] Deracoxib, 2914
[169590-42-5] Celecoxib, 1956
[169592-56-7] Caspase-3, 1885
[169869-90-3] Exatecan Methanesulfonate, 3912
[169939-93-9] Ruboxistaurin Hydrochloride (anhydrous), 8290
[169939-94-0] Ruboxistaurin, 8290
[170098-38-1] Alvimopan Dihydrate, 372
[170277-31-3] Infliximab, 4972
[170475-05-5] Dienogest Mixture with Ethinyl Estradiol, 3106
[170713-75-4] Nociceptin, 6667
[170729-80-3] Aprepitant, 753
[170780-00-4] Hanatoxin 1 (reduced), 4610
[170780-01-5] Hanatoxin 2 (reduced), 4610
[171099-57-3] Oritavancin, 6868
[171228-49-2] Posaconazole, 7602
[171335-80-1] Exatecan, 3912
[171500-79-1] Dalbavancin, 2803
[171543-83-2] Urocortin (rat), 9885
[171544-35-7] Ferumoxsil, 4064
[171596-29-5] Tadalafil, 9027
[171599-83-0] Sildenafil Citrate, 8489
[172222-30-9] Grubbs' Catalyst, 4550
[172339-62-7] HHCB (−)-(4S,7S)-Form, 4715
[172339-63-8] HHCB (+)-(4R,7S)-Form, 4715
[172418-32-5] Herrmann-Beller Catalyst, 4669
[172668-52-9] Thiazole Orange Methyl Sulfate, 9308
[172673-20-0] Fosaprepitant, 753
[172777-84-3] Cy 5.5 (free acid), 2679
[172820-23-4] Pexiganan Acetate, 7193
[173146-27-5] Denileukin Diftitox, 2893
[173159-57-4] Foramsulfuron, 4234
[173240-15-8] Nemifitide, 6445
[173334-57-1] Aliskiren, 247
[173334-58-2] Aliskiren Hemifumarate, 247
[173584-44-6] Indoxacarb, 4971
[173937-91-2] Atrasentan, 870
[174254-13-8] Biricodar Dicitrate, 1240
[174402-32-5] Edotecarin, 3512
[174484-41-4] Tipranavir, 9459
[174501-64-5] Butylmethylimidazolium, 1581
[174501-65-6] Butylmethylimidazolium Tetrafluoroborate, 1581
[174545-76-7] Eleutherobin, 3545
[174625-00-4] Clevudine Triphosphate, 2353
[174722-31-7] Rituximab, 8239
[175013-18-0] Pyraclostrobin, 7953
[175463-14-6] Gemifloxacin, 4389
[175481-36-4] Lacosamide, 5333
[175865-59-5] Valganciclovir Hydrochloride, 9907
[175865-60-8] Valganciclovir, 9907
[175989-38-5] Pixantrone Hydrochloride, 7514
[176591-49-4] Urocortin (human), 9885

[177036-94-1] Ambrisentan, 384
[177073-44-8] Choriogonadotropin Alfa, 2216
[177834-92-3] Eletriptan Hydrobromide, 3544
[177976-12-4] Sarizotan Dihydrochloride, 8375
[178273-87-5] Piboserod Hydrochloride, 7393
[178307-42-1] Revaprazan Hydrochloride, 8168
[178928-70-6] Prothioconazole, 7887
[178959-14-3] Technetium ^{99m}Tc Apcitide, 9098
[178979-85-6] Capravirine, 1755
[179045-86-4] Basiliximab, 1006
[179241-78-2] Caspase-8, 1886
[179324-69-7] Bortezomib, 1351
[179463-17-3] Caspofungin Acetate, 1889
[179474-81-8] Prucalopride, 7907
[180189-96-2] Caspase-9, 1887
[180200-66-2] Gatifloxacin Sesquihydrate, 4376
[180268-78-4] IACFT ^{125}I, 4871
[180288-69-1] Trastuzumab, 9575
[180384-56-9] Clazosentan, 2342
[180384-57-0] Tezosentan, 9252
[180384-58-1] Tezosentan Sodium Salt, 9252
[180468-34-2] IACFT, 4871
[181183-52-8] Almotriptan Maleate, 304
[181274-15-7] Propoxycarbazone Sodium Salt, 7838
[181274-17-9] Flucarbazone Sodium Salt, 4119
[181530-09-6] Zinquin Ethyl Ester, 10169
[181587-01-9] Ethiprole, 3739
[181630-15-9] Picoplatin, 7405
[181695-72-7] Valdecoxib, 9900
[182133-25-1] Arzoxifene, 820
[182133-27-3] Arzoxifene Hydrochloride, 820
[182136-94-3] Dysidiolide, 3481
[182349-12-8] Rupatadine Fumarate, 8297
[182485-36-5] TPMPA, 9563
[182760-06-1] Ravuconazole, 8121
[182815-44-7] Colesevelam Hydrochloride, 2473
[183319-69-9] Erlotinib Hydrochloride, 3672
[183321-74-6] Erlotinib, 3672
[183325-78-2] Calfactant, 1714
[183552-38-7] Abarelix, 3
[184036-34-8] Sitaxsentan, 8554
[184475-35-2] Gefitinib, 4379
[185229-68-9] Alicaforsen, 245
[185243-69-0] Etanercept, 3712
[185954-98-7] Eritoran Tetrasodium Salt, 3671
[185955-34-4] Eritoran, 3671
[186046-04-8] Zilpaterol Hydrochloride (monohydrate), 10125
[186046-05-9] Zilpaterol Hydrochloride (trihydrate), 10125
[186256-67-7] Cryptophycin-52, 2607
[186459-75-6] EDDS, 3508
[186826-86-8] Moxifloxacin Hydrochloride, 6291
[187269-40-5] Bimosiamose, 1222
[187269-60-9] Bimosiamose Disodium Salt, 1222

[187393-00-6] Bemotrizinol, *1028*
[187888-07-9] Endostatin, *3573*
[188039-54-5] Palivizumab, *6988*
[188062-50-2] Abacavir Sulfate, *1*
[188425-85-6] Boscalid, *1352*
[188627-80-7] Eptifibatide, *3641*
[188630-14-0] Liatermin, *4377*
[188842-14-0] Penetratin, *7086*
[189047-99-2] Ferumoxtran 10, *4065*
[189188-57-6] Tegaserod Maleate, *9113*
[189261-10-7] Natalizumab, *6426*
[189453-10-9] Epothilone D, *3628*
[189954-96-9] Firocoxib, *4087*
[190786-43-7] Bepotastine, *1149*
[190786-44-8] Bepotastine Benzenesulfonate Salt, *1149*
[190977-41-4] Oblimersen Sodium, *6739*
[191114-48-4] Telithromycin, *9119*
[191217-81-9] Pramipexole Dihydrochloride Monohydrate, *7705*
[191588-94-0] Tenecteplase, *9143*
[191670-18-5] Volicitin, *10030*
[191732-72-6] Lenalidomide, *5436*
[192050-59-2] Ruboxistaurin Methanesulfonate, *8290*
[192185-68-5] Tipifarnib (unspecified stereo), *9458*
[192185-72-1] Tipifarnib (anhydrous), *9458*
[192230-81-2] Synsorb Pk, *9014*
[192329-42-3] Prinomastat, *7751*
[192391-48-3] ^{131}I Tositumomab, *9554*
[192564-13-9] Leteprinim Potassium Salt, *5448*
[192564-14-0] Oritavancin Diphosphate, *6868*
[192725-17-0] Lopinavir, *5573*
[192939-46-1] Ximelagatran, *10077*
[193275-84-2] Lonafarnib, *5565*
[193901-90-5] Gadofosveset Trisodium Salt, *4325*
[194100-83-9] Thyrotropin Alfa, *9414*
[194468-36-5] Vinflunine Ditartrate, *9989*
[194798-83-9] Fluconazole Dihydrogen Phosphate Ester, *4122*
[194804-75-6] Garenoxacin, *4369*
[194874-06-1] Apoptolidin, *747*
[195532-12-8] Pradofloxacin, *7701*
[195733-43-8] Atrasentan Hydrochloride, *870*
[195883-09-1] 14-Succinyl Triptolide Sodium Salt, *9747*
[196597-26-9] Ramelteon, *8101*
[196618-13-0] Oseltamivir, *6889*
[197720-53-9] Exatecan Methanesulfonate Dihydrate, *3912*
[198283-73-7] Tebanicline, *9090*
[198283-74-8] Tebanicline Tosylate, *9090*
[198470-84-7] Parecoxib, *7036*
[198470-85-8] Parecoxib Sodium Salt, *7036*
[198481-32-2] Bazedoxifene, *1013*
[198481-33-3] Bazedoxifene Acetate, *1013*
[198821-22-6] Merimepodib, *5899*
[198904-31-3] Atazanavir, *858*
[199331-40-3] Etiprednol Dicloacetate, *3870*
[199396-76-4] Asoprisnil, *834*
[199463-33-7] Revaprazan, *8168*

[199612-75-4] Py-Phe, *7952*
[200393-05-1] *S*-Adenosylmethionine 1,4-Butanedisulfonate, *156*
[200815-49-2] Formoterol *R,R*-Form L-Tartrate, *4245*
[201341-05-1] Tenofovir Disoproxil, *9146*
[201530-41-8] Deferasirox, *2858*
[201677-61-4] Sivelestat Sodium Salt Tetrahydrate, *8558*
[201677-75-0] Taltirelin Tetrahydrate, *9045*
[201688-00-8] Gadofosveset, *4325*
[202138-50-9] Tenofovir Disoproxil Fumarate, *9146*
[202260-21-7] Ruboxistaurin Methanesulfonate Monohydrate, *8290*
[202289-38-1] Deoxo-Fluor®, *2897*
[202409-33-4] Etoricoxib, *3887*
[202825-46-5] Safinamide Methanesulfonate, *8315*
[203258-38-2] Brostallicin Hydrochloride, *1449*
[203258-60-0] Brostallicin, *1449*
[203564-54-9] Tebanicline Hydrochloride, *9090*
[204255-11-8] Oseltamivir Phosphate, *6889*
[204318-14-9] Edotreotide, *3513*
[204512-90-3] Tecadenoson, *9096*
[204656-20-2] Liraglutide, *5514*
[204992-09-6] Nemifitide Ditriflutate, *6445*
[205110-48-1] Cethromycin, *2020*
[205599-45-7] Cameleons, *1727*
[205599-75-3] Orexin A, *6866*
[205599-76-4] Orexin B, *6866*
[205923-56-4] Cetuximab, *2027*
[205923-57-5] Epratuzumab, *3631*
[206181-63-7] Ibritumomab Tiuxetan, *4878*
[206361-99-1] Darunavir, *2827*
[206873-63-4] Tariquidar, *9064*
[207748-29-6] Insulin Glulisine, *4985*
[207844-01-7] Mitiglinide Calcium Salt Dihydrate, *6211*
[208265-92-3] Granulocyte Colony-Stimulating Factor Pegfilgrastim, *4537*
[208465-21-8] Mesosulfuron-methyl, *5911*
[208517-65-1] IACFT ^{123}I, *4871*
[208538-73-2] Micafungin Sodium Salt, *6175*
[208921-02-2] Tositumomab, *9554*
[209216-23-9] Entecavir Monohydrate, *3595*
[209467-52-7] Ceftobiprole, *1952*
[209810-58-2] Darbepoetin Alfa, *2824*
[209859-87-0] Cilansetron Hydrochloride (monohydrate), *2271*
[210101-16-9] Conivaptan, *2507*
[210421-74-2] Sitaxsentan Sodium Salt, *8554*
[210880-92-5] Clothianidin, *2414*
[211050-90-7] Diflufenzopyr Mixture with Dicamba, *3145*
[211427-08-6] Diquafosol Tetrasodium Salt, *3351*
[211448-85-0] Denufosol, *2896*
[211914-51-1] Dabigatran, *2797*
[211915-06-9] Dabigatran Etexilate, *2797*
[212141-54-3] Vatalanib, *9939*

[212142-18-2] Vatalanib Succinate, *9939*
[213327-37-8] Oregovomab, *6865*
[214745-43-4] Efalizumab, *3519*
[216503-57-0] Alemtuzumab, *228*
[216586-46-8] Virulizin®, *10007*
[216974-75-3] Bevacizumab, *1191*
[217500-96-4] Tulathromycin A, *9810*
[218620-50-9] Pegvisomant, *7069*
[219685-50-4] Eculizumab, *3506*
[219685-93-5] Pexelizumab, *7192*
[219714-96-2] Penoxsulam, *7103*
[219861-08-2] Escitalopram Oxalate, *2318*
[219989-84-1] Ixabepilone, *5249*
[220119-17-5] Selamectin, *8424*
[220127-57-1] Imatinib Methanesulfonate, *4902*
[220201-34-3] Talaporfin Tetrasodium Salt, *9034*
[220578-59-6] Gemtuzumab Ozogamicin, *4390*
[220620-09-7] Tigecycline, *9432*
[220991-20-8] Lumiracoxib, *5601*
[222535-22-0] Alefacept, *227*
[222716-86-1] Pegaptanib Sodium, *7068*
[223652-82-2] Garenoxacin Methanesulfonate, *4369*
[223652-90-2] Garenoxacin Methanesulfonate (monohydrate), *4369*
[224785-90-4] Vardenafil, *9935*
[224785-91-5] Vardenafil Hydrochloride Trihydrate (anhydrous), *9935*
[225239-31-6] Technetium ^{99m}Tc Fanolesomab, *9100*
[226256-56-0] Cinacalcet, *2282*
[226700-79-4] Fosamprenavir, *4250*
[226700-81-8] Fosamprenavir Calcium Salt, *4250*
[229975-97-7] Atazanavir Sulfate, *858*
[231277-92-2] Lapatinib, *5367*
[235114-32-6] Micafungin, *6175*
[239076-74-5] Altrakincept, *5002*
[242138-07-4] Omalizumab, *6842*
[242478-37-1] Solifenacin, *8712*
[242478-38-2] Solifenacin Succinate, *8712*
[244015-05-2] Iseganan Hydrochloride (hydrate), *5105*
[246252-04-0] Motexafin Lutetium, *6282*
[246252-06-2] Motexafin Gadolinium, *6281*
[246539-15-1] Dibotermin Alfa, *1331*
[247184-89-0] Kalkitoxin, *5277*
[249296-44-4] Varenicline, *9936*
[250378-38-2] Alronidase, *4894*
[251565-85-2] Tesaglitazar, *9177*
[251925-26-5] drFP583, *8126*
[252188-71-9] Ceftobiprole Medocaril Sodium Salt, *1952*
[252198-49-5] Tertiapin Q, *9175*
[252332-95-9] HHCB (−)-(4*S*,7*R*)-Form, *4715*
[252332-96-0] HHCB (+)-(4*R*,7*R*)-Form, *4715*
[252870-53-4] Ispronicline, *5239*
[252870-54-5] Ispronicline Hemigalactarate, *5239*
[253687-10-4] Hanatoxins, *4610*
[254753-54-3] Monastrol, *6244*
[255881-88-0] αMNP Hydroxy Acid (*S*-(+)-form), *6224*

[256475-21-5] Iseganan Hydrochloride, *5105*

[257277-05-7] Iseganan, *5105*

[258279-04-8] Ghrelin Human Ghrelin, *4418*

[258516-87-9] Fospropofol Disodium Salt, *4259*

[258516-89-1] Fospropofol, *4259*

[259074-76-5] Alfimeprase, *237*

[262352-17-0] Torcetrapib, *9549*

[263351-82-2] Paclitaxel Poliglumex, *6983*

[265121-04-8] Fosaprepitant Dimeglumine, *753*

[267243-28-7] Canertinib, *1744*

[270076-60-3] Pristinamycin, *7753*

[274901-16-5] Vildagliptin, *9979*

[280755-12-6] Tulathromycin B, *9810*

[281212-01-9] Hanatoxin 1 (native), *4610*

[283594-90-1] Spiromesifen, *8759*

[284041-10-7] Rostaporfin, *8269*

[284461-73-0] Sorafenib, *8720*

[287714-41-4] Rosuvastatin, *8270*

[288574-78-7] Zinpyr-1, *10168*

[289030-99-5] Oleocanthal, *6829*

[289480-64-4] Treprostinil Sodium Salt, *9586*

[289499-45-2] Canertinib Dihydrochloride, *1744*

[302962-49-8] Dasatinib, *2829*

[304853-26-7] Ghrelin, *4418*

[305838-77-1] Neovastat®, *6467*

[308068-04-4] H-Kininogen, *5312*

[308081-97-2] Omega-3 Acid Ethyl Esters, *6844*

[318250-11-2] Denufosol Tetrasodium Salt, *2896*

[322407-70-5] Edotreotide ⁹⁰Y Chelate, *3513*

[325715-02-4] Indiplon, *4946*

[328538-04-1] Edifoligide Sodium, *3511*

[330808-88-3] Vardenafil Hydrochloride (trihydrate), *9935*

[331257-52-4] Alicaforsen Sodium Salt, *245*

[331257-53-5] Aprinocarsen Sodium Salt, *755*

[331731-18-1] Adalimumab, *148*

[331741-94-7] Muraglitazar, *6303*

[332348-12-6] Abatacept, *4*

[339177-26-3] Panitumumab, *7010*

[339184-10-0] Certolizumab Pegol (Fab fragment), *2003*

[341028-37-3] Alagebrium Chloride, *203*

[341031-54-7] Sunitinib Maleate, *9000*

[343798-00-5] Torcetrapib Ethanolate, *9549*

[344423-98-9] Atorvastatin Calcium Salt Trihydrate, *864*

[347396-82-1] Ranibizumab, *8108*

[350992-10-8] Bifeprunox, *1210*

[350992-13-1] Bifeprunox Methanesulfonate, *1210*

[351862-32-3] Sarizotan, *8375*

[357336-20-0] Brivaracetam, *1377*

[357916-12-2] Zinpyr-2, *10168*

[361377-29-9] Fluoxastrobin, *4184*

[364782-34-3] Cinacalcet Hydrochloride, *2282*

[371163-96-1] Epicocconone, *3615*

[372075-36-0] Cintredekin Besudotox, *2312*

[372151-71-8] Telavancin, *9116*

[375815-87-5] Varenicline Tartrate, *9936*

[375823-41-9] Tocilizumab, *9493*

[376348-65-1] Maraviroc, *5749*

[376653-43-9] Ceftobiprole Medocaril, *1952*

[384329-61-7] Hoodia P57AS3, *4743*

[388082-77-7] Lapatinib Ditoluenesulfonate, *5367*

[388082-78-8] Lapatinib Ditoluenesulfonate Monohydrate, *5367*

[396715-57-4] Norelgestromin Combination with Ethinyl Estradiol, *6694*

[420784-05-0] Alglucosidase Alfa, *108*

[428863-50-7] Certolizumab Pegol, *2003*

[439943-59-6] Canfosfamide Hydrochloride, *1745*

[448235-52-7] Pyrrolysine, *8019*

[461023-63-2] Aplaviroc Hydrochloride, *737*

[461443-59-4] Aplaviroc, *737*

[475207-59-1] Sorafenib Tosylate, *8720*

[486460-32-6] Sitagliptin, *8552*

[501423-23-0] Epratuzumab (⁹⁰Y-labeled form), *3631*

[501423-25-2] ⁹⁰Y Epratuzumab Tetraxetan, *3631*

[503271-02-1] Clazosentan Disodium Salt, *2342*

[511296-88-1] Pifithrin-β (hydrobromide), *7421*

[552858-79-4] Galsulfase, *819*

[557795-19-4] Sunitinib, *9000*

[560130-42-9] Telavancin Hydrochloride, *9116*

[618903-56-3] Tetrahydrogestrinone, *9214*

[654671-77-9] Sitagliptin Monophosphate Monohydrate, *8552*

[654671-78-0] Sitagliptin monophosphate, *8552*

[656820-32-5] Reversine (anhydrous), *8169*

[674289-55-5] Blebbistatin, *1317*

[706808-37-9] Belatacept, *1024*

[713516-99-5] Ambrisentan, *384*

THERAPEUTIC CATEGORY AND
BIOLOGICAL ACTIVITY
INDEX

THERAPEUTIC CATEGORY AND BIOLOGICAL ACTIVITY INDEX

This index is designed to serve as an additional entry point to the monographs of this edition for which a therapeutic category (THERAP CAT) has been given. It contains listings for discrete chemical entities. Plants and plant portions, *e.g.* seeds or leaves, although used medicinally, have generally been excluded. An attempt has been made to standardize the nomenclature used for index terms. Therefore, the heading under which a compound is listed may differ slightly from the therapeutic category found within the monograph.

Biological activities indicating mechanism of action have also been included as index headings. Whenever possible, cross references to appropriate therapeutic categories have been given for these listings. Cross references have also been provided for synonyms of preferred terms or, in some cases, for closely related entries. In addition, many therapeutic category headings have been subclassified according to chemical or pharmacological features.

Monographs are listed alphabetically by title under each heading. Selected derivatives and isomers of title compounds have been listed by generic or trivial name and are referenced to the appropriate monograph by number.

Therapeutic categories have been assigned to reflect the major indications listed in manufacturer's product information, reported in the clinical literature, or published by the USAN Council. Inclusion of a drug in this index does not imply efficacy or endoresement, nor does it imply that the compound is *presently* being marketed. Omission of a compound from a particular category does not imply that the substance is not in use or under investigation for that indication. Additional information on each entry can be found in the cited monograph. Reference to primary sources is encouraged.

ABORTIFACIENT/INTERCEPTIVE

Epostane, *3627*
Gemeprost, *4387*
Mifepristone, *6186*
Prostaglandin E$_2$, *7877*
Prostaglandin F$_{2\alpha}$, *7878*
Sulprostone, *8991*
Trichosanthin, *9648*

ACE-INHIBITOR *see also Antihypertensive; Vasopeptidase Inhibitor*

Alacepril, *200*
Benazepril, *1031*
Captopril, *1774*
Ceronapril, *1994*
Cilazapril, *2273*
Delapril, *2876*
Enalapril, *3567*
Enalaprilat, *3568*
Fosinopril, *4256*
Imidapril, *4911*
Lisinopril, *5516*
Moexipril, *6229*
Moveltipril, *6285*
Perindopril, *7170*
Quinapril, *8051*
Ramipril, *8103*
Spirapril, *8753*
Temocapril, *9136*
Trandolapril, *9568*
Zofenopril, *10186*

ACIDIFIER

Ammonium Chloride, *509*
Betaine Hydrochloride *see 1179*
Glutamic Acid Hydrochloride
see 4469
Methionine, *5975*

ADENOSINE RECEPTOR AGONIST

Binodenoson, *1225*
Tecadenoson, *9096*

α-ADRENERGIC AGONIST *see also Antihypotensive; Antihypertensive; Antiulcerative; Decongestant; Mydriatic*

Adrafinil, *170*
Adrenalone, *171*
Amidephrine, *399*
Apraclonidine, *751*
Budralazine, *1470*
Clonidine, *2390*
Cyclopentamine, *2740*
Dexmedetomidine, *2946*
Dimetofrine, *3264*
Dipivefrin, *3338*
Ecabapide, *3488*
Ephedrine, *3608*
Epinephrine, *3619*
Fenoxazoline, *3985*
Guanabenz, *4558*
Guanfacine, *4561*
Hydroxyamphetamine, *4810*
Ibopamine, *4876*
Indanazoline, *4932*
Isometheptene, *5185*
Mephentermine, *5852*
Metaraminol, *5932*

Methoxamine, *5987*
Methylhexaneamine, *6085*
Midodrine, *6184*
Mivazerol, *6220*
Modafinil, *6228*
Moxonidine, *6293*
Naphazoline, *6368*
Norepinephrine, *6695*
Norfenefrine, *6699*
Octodrine, *6757*
Octopamine, *6759*
Oxymetazoline, *6966*
Phenylephrine, *7286*
Phenylpropanolamine, *7307*
Phenylpropylmethylamine, *7308*
Pholedrine, *7330*
Propylhexedrine, *7860*
Pseudoephedrine, *7916*
Rilmenidine, *8222*
Synephrine, *9012*
Talipexole, *9039*
Tetrahydrozoline, *9219*
Tiamenidine, *9418*
Tramazoline, *9567*
Tuaminoheptane, *9802*
Tymazoline, *9834*
Tyramine, *9835*
Xylometazoline, *10086*

β-ADRENERGIC AGONIST *see also Bronchodilator; Cardiotonic; Tocolytic*

Albuterol, *216*
Bambuterol, *953*
Bitolterol, *1307*
Carbuterol, *1833*
Clenbuterol, *2347*
Clorprenaline, *2408*
Denopamine, *2894*
Dioxethedrine, *3302*
Dopexamine, *3424*
Ephedrine, *3608*
Epinephrine, *3619*
Etafedrine, *3709*
Ethylnorepinephrine, *3834*
Fenoterol, *3981*
Formoterol, *4245*
Hexoprenaline, *4707*
Ibopamine, *4876*
Isoetharine, *5170*
Isoproterenol, *5217*
Mabuterol, *5642*
Metaproterenol, *5931*
Methoxyphenamine, *5998*
Oxyfedrine, *6962*
Pirbuterol, *7489*
Prenalterol, *7735*
Procaterol, *7759*
Protokylol, *7895*
Reproterol, *8139*
Rimiterol, *8227*
Ritodrine, *8237*
Salmeterol, *8337*
Soterenol, *8729*
Terbutaline, *9159*
Tretoquinol, *9587*
Tulobuterol, *9811*
Xamoterol, *10055*

α-ADRENERGIC BLOCKER *see also Antihypertensive*

Alfuzosin, *238*
Amosulalol, *575*

Arotinolol, *791*
Dapiprazole, *2820*
Doxazosin, *3433*
Ergoloid Mesylates, *3653*
Fenspiride, *3999*
Idazoxan, *4887*
Indoramin, *4969*
Labetalol, *5329*
Naftopidil, *6356*
Nicergoline, *6496*
Prazosin, *7717*
Silodosin, *8503*
Tamsulosin, *9049*
Terazosin, *9154*
Tolazoline, *9506*
Yohimbine, *10102*

β-ADRENERGIC BLOCKER *see also Antianginal; Antiarrhythmic; Antiglaucoma; Antihypertensive*

Acebutolol, *19*
Alprenolol, *313*
Amosulalol, *575*
Arotinolol, *791*
Atenolol, *859*
Befunolol, *1022*
Betaxolol, *1182*
Bevantolol, *1192*
Bisoprolol, *1295*
Bopindolol, *1333*
Bucindolol, *1461*
Bucumolol, *1467*
Bufetolol, *1473*
Bufuralol, *1480*
Bunitrolol, *1489*
Bupranolol, *1496*
Carazolol, *1778*
Carteolol, *1866*
Carvedilol, *1873*
Celiprolol, *1960*
Cetamolol, *2018*
Cloranolol, *2402*
Esmolol, *3700*
Indenolol, *4940*
Labetalol, *5329*
Landiolol, *5355*
Levobunolol, *5462*
Mepindolol, *5856*
Metipranolol, *6140*
Metoprolol, *6151*
Moprolol, *6264*
Nadolol, *6346*
Nadoxolol, *6347*
Nebivolol, *6432*
Nifenalol, *6530*
Nipradilol, *6562*
Oxprenolol, *6952*
Penbutolol, *7082*
Pindolol, *7443*
Practolol, *7700*
Pronethalol, *7790*
Propranolol, *7840*
Sotalol, *8728*
Sulfinalol, *8948*
Talinolol, *9038*
Tertatolol, *9173*
Tilisolol, *9438*
Timolol, *9444*
Toliprolol, *9516*
Xibenolol, *10075*

ADRENOCORTICAL STEROID *see Glucocorticoid; Mineralocorticoid*

ADRENOCORTICAL SUPPRES-SANT

Aminoglutethimide, 440
Trilostane, 9698

ADRENOCORTICOTROPIC HOR-MONE

ACTH, 134
Giractide, 4428

ALCOHOL DEPENDENCE TREAT-MENT

Acamprosate Calcium, 17
Calcium Cyanamide Citrated, 1663
Disulfiram, 3364
Naltrexone, 6363

ALDOSE REDUCTASE INHIBITOR

Epalrestat, 3605
Fidarestat, 4078
Tolrestat, 9524
Zopolrestat, 10194

ALDOSTERONE ANTAGONIST see also *Diuretic*

Canrenone, 1750
Eplerenone, 3625
Spironolactone, 8760

ALKALINIZING AGENT

Potassium Citrate, 7623
Sodium Bicarbonate, 8583
Sodium Citrate, 8602
Sodium Lactate, 8635
Tromethamine, 9772

5-ALPHA REDUCTASE INHIBI-TOR see *5α-Reductase Inhibitor*

AMPA RECEPTOR ANTAGONIST

Talampanel, 9032

ANABOLIC

Androisoxazole, 634
Bolandiol, 1322
Clostebol, 2413
Ethylestrenol, 3805
Formebolone, 4239
Methandriol, 5950
Methenolone, 5967
Nandrolone, 6365
Oxymesterone, 6965
Pizotyline, 7515

ANALEPTIC see *CNS Stimulant*

ANALGESIC (DENTAL)

Chlorobutanol, 2129
Clove Oil see 2418
Eugenol, 3898

ANALGESIC (NARCOTIC)

Alfentanil, 236
Alphaprodine, 310
Anileridine, 658
Benzylmorphine, 1141
Bezitramide, 1196
Buprenorphine, 1497
Butorphanol, 1530
Codeine, 2463
Codeine Phosphate, 2464
Desomorphine, 2927
Dextromoramide, 2955
Dezocine, 2956
Diampromide, 2988
Dihydrocodeine, 3171
Dihydrocodeinone Enol Acetate, 3172
Dihydromorphine, 3177
Dimenoxadol, 3208
Dimethylthiambutene, 3260
Dipipanone, 3337
Eptazocine, 3639
Ethoheptazine, 3743
Ethylmethylthiambutene, 3829
Ethylmorphine, 3830
Etonitazene, 3883
Fentanyl, 4001
Hydrocodone, 4785
Hydromorphone, 4803
Hydroxypethidine, 4836
Isomethadone, 5184
Ketobemidone, 5301
Levorphanol, 5470
Lofentanil, 5556
Meperidine, 5849
Meptazinol, 5863
Metazocine, 5933
Methadone, 5944
Metopon, 6150
Morphine, 6276
Myrophine, 6337
Nalbuphine, 6357
Narceine, 6422
Nicomorphine, 6520
Norlevorphanol, 6707
Normethadone, 6709
Normorphine, 6711
Opium, 6854
Oxycodone, 6959
Oxymorphone, 6969
Papaveretum, 7018
Pentazocine, 7121
Phenadoxone, 7207
Phenazocine, 7218
Phenoperidine, 7250
Piminodine, 7433
Piritramide, 7498
Proheptazine, 7776
Promedol, 7784
Propiram, 7831
Propoxyphene, 7839
Remifentanil, 8131
Sufentanil, 8887
Tilidine, 9437

ANALGESIC (NON-NARCOTIC)

Aceclofenac, 22
Acetaminophen, 47
Acetaminosalol, 48
Acetylsalicylsalicylic Acid, 100
Alclofenac, 219
Alminoprofen, 300
Aloxiprin, 309
2-Amino-4-picoline, 466
Aminopyrine, 474

Ammonium Salicylate, 550
Amtolmetin Guacil, 596
Antipyrine, 716
Antipyrine Salicylate, 717
Apazone, 726
Aspirin, 851
Benorylate, 1045
Benzydamine, 1122
Bermoprofen, 1159
p-Bromoacetanilide, 1399
Bucetin, 1458
Bufexamac, 1474
Bumadizon, 1483
Butixirate see 10071
Calcium Acetylsalicylate, 1647
Choline Salicylate, 2209
Cinchophen, 2288
Cizolirtine, 2336
Clometacin, 2383
Clonixin, 2392
Cropropamide, 2591
Crotethamide, 2595
Dexoxadrol see 3299
Difenamizole, 3134
Diflunisal, 3146
Dipyrocetyl, 3349
Dipyrone, 3350
Emorfazone, 3562
Enfenamic Acid, 3580
Epirizole, 3622
Ethenzamide, 3731
Etodolac, 3874
Etoricoxib, 3887
Felbinac, 3951
Fenoprofen, 3980
Floctafenine, 4103
Flufenamic Acid, 4132
Fluoresone, 4161
Flupirtine, 4190
Fluproquazone, 4193
Flurbiprofen, 4199
Fosfosal, 4255
Gabapentin, 4319
Gentisic Acid, 4398
Ibufenac, 4880
Imidazole Salicylate, 4913
Indomethacin, 4968
Isonixin, 5192
Ketoprofen, 5305
Ketorolac, 5306
Lacosamide, 5333
Lefetamine, 5431
Lornoxicam, 5582
Loxoprofen, 5589
Lysine Acetylsalicylate, 5637
Magnesium Acetylsalicylate, 5655
Methotrimeprazine, 5986
Mofezolac, 6232
Morazone, 6267
Morpholine Salicylate see 6277
Naproxen, 6417
Nefopam, 6440
5'-Nitro-2'-propoxyacetanilide, 6629
Parecoxib, 7036
Parsalmide, 7045
Perisoxal, 7177
Phenacetin, 7204
Phenazopyridine, 7210
Phenocoll, 7239
Phenyl Acetylsalicylate, 7270
Phenyl Salicylate, 7310
Phenyramidol, 7321
Pipebuzone, 7457
Pregabalin, 7725
Propacetamol, 7792

Propyphenazone, *7871*
Ramifenazone, *8102*
Rimazolium Metilsulfate, *8225*
Rofecoxib, *8248*
Salicin, *8324*
Salicylamide, *8328*
Salicylamide *O*-Acetic Acid, *8329*
Salicylsulfuric Acid, *8334*
Salsalate, *8339*
Salverine, *8342*
Simetride, *8535*
Sodium Salicylate *see 8332*
Suprofen, *9005*
Talniflumate, *9044*
Tenoxicam, *9148*
Terofenamate, *9168*
Tetrandrine, *9231*
Tinoridine, *9448*
Tolfenamic Acid, *9513*
Tramadol, *9566*
Tropesin, *9778*
Valdecoxib, *9900*
Viminol, *9981*
Ziconotide, *10122*
Zomepirac, *10191*

ANDROGEN

Cloxotestosterone, *2421*
Dehydroepiandrosterone, *2871*
Fluoxymesterone, *4186*
Mesterolone, *5916*
Methandrostenolone, *5951*
17-Methyltestosterone, *6125*
Norethandrolone, *6696*
Normethandrone, *6710*
Oxandrolone, *6921*
Oxymesterone, *6965*
Oxymetholone, *6967*
Stanolone, *8793*
Stanozolol, *8794*
Testosterone, *9180*

ANESTHETIC (INHALATION)

Cyclopropane, *2748*
Desflurane, *2919*
Enflurane, *3581*
Ethylene, *3791*
Ethyl Ether, *3806*
Halothane, *4603*
Isoflurane, *5175*
Methoxyflurane, *5994*
Methyl Propyl Ether, *6113*
Nitrous Oxide, *6653*
Sevoflurane, *8475*
Teflurane, *9110*
Trichloroethylene, *9639*
Vinyl Ether, *9995*
Xenon, *10072*

ANESTHETIC (INTRAVENOUS)

Acetamidoeugenol, *46*
Alfadolone Acetate, *233*
Alfaxalone, *235*
Buthalital Sodium, *1524*
Etoxadrol, *3889*
Fospropofol, *4259*
Hexobarbital, *4704*
Hydroxydione Sodium, *4823*
Ketamine, *5295*
Methohexital Sodium, *5981*
Midazolam, *6182*
Phencyclidine, *7219*
Propanidid, *7803*

Propofol, *7834*
Sodium Oxybate *see 4815*
Thialbarbital, *9292*
Thiamylal, *9302*
Thiobutabarbital, *9323*
Thiopental Sodium, *9350*

ANESTHETIC (LOCAL)

Amylocaine Hydrochloride, *614*
Benoxinate, *1047*
Benzocaine, *1086*
Betoxycaine, *1187*
Biphenamine, *1234*
Bupivacaine, *1495*
Butacaine, *1507*
Butamben, *1512*
Butethamine, *1523*
Butoxycaine, *1531*
Carticaine, *1869*
Chloroprocaine Hydrochloride, *2158*
Cocaethylene, *2454*
Cocaine, *2455*
Cyclomethycaine, *2735*
Dibucaine, *3031*
Dimethisoquin, *3218*
Dimethocaine, *3221*
Dixyrazine, *3385*
Dyclonine, *3473*
Ecgonidine, *3492*
Ecgonine, *3493*
Ethyl Chloride, *3782*
Etidocaine, *3862*
β-Eucaine, *3894*
Fomocaine, *4230*
Hexylcaine Hydrochloride, *4708*
Hydroxytetracaine, *4846*
Isobutyl *p*-Aminobenzoate, *5133*
Levoxadrol *see 3299*
Lidocaine, *5482*
Mepivacaine, *5859*
Octacaine, *6743*
Orthocaine, *6883*
Oxethazaine, *6933*
Phenacaine Hydrochloride, *7202*
Phenol, *7241*
Piperocaine, *7474*
Piridocaine, *7494*
Polidocanol, *7558*
Pramoxine, *7709*
Prilocaine, *7743*
Procaine, *7757*
Proparacaine, *7807*
Propoxycaine Hydrochloride, *7837*
Pseudococaine, *7912*
Pyrrocaine, *8013*
Ropivacaine, *8258*
Salicyl Alcohol, *8325*
Tetracaine Hydrochloride, *9188*
Tolycaine, *9541*
Trimecaine, *9700*

ANGIOTENSIN CONVERTING ENZYME INHIBITOR *see ACE-Inhibitor*

ANGIOTENSIN II RECEPTOR ANTAGONIST *see also Antihypertensive*

Candesartan, *1739*
Eprosartan, *3635*
Irbesartan, *5083*

Losartan, *5583*
Olmesartan, *6839*
Telmisartan, *9129*
Valsartan, *9916*

ANOREXIC

Aminorex, *476*
Amphetamine, *582*
Benzphetamine, *1118*
Chlorphentermine, *2182*
Clobenzorex, *2362*
Clortermine, *2410*
Cyclexedrine, *2707*
Dextroamphetamine, *2954*
Diethylpropion, *3127*
N-Ethylamphetamine, *3763*
Fenbutrazate, *3965*
Fenfluramine, *3973*
Fenproporex, *3994*
Levophacetoperane, *5467*
Mazindol, *5762*
Mefenorex, *5799*
Methamphetamine, *5948*
Norpseudoephedrine, *6714*
Pentorex, *7133*
Phendimetrazine, *7220*
Phenmetrazine, *7237*
Phentermine, *7262*
Phenylpropanolamine, *7307*
Sibutramine, *8485*

ANTACID

Almagate, *299*
Aluminum Hydroxide, *342*
Aluminum Magnesium Silicate, *350*
Aluminum Phosphate, *358*
Azulene, *926*
Basic Aluminum Carbonate Gel, *1004*
Bismuth Aluminate, *1258*
Bismuth Phosphate, *1275*
Bismuth Subcarbonate, *1282*
Bismuth Subgallate, *1283*
Bismuth Subnitrate, *1284*
Calcium Carbonate, *1657*
Dihydroxyaluminum Aminoacetate, *3183*
Dihydroxyaluminum Sodium Carbonate, *3184*
Magaldrate, *5651*
Magnesium Carbonate Hydroxide, *5660*
Magnesium Hydroxide, *5670*
Magnesium Oxide, *5677*
Magnesium Peroxide, *5680*
Magnesium Phosphate, Tribasic, *5683*
Magnesium Silicates, *5687*
Sodium Bicarbonate, *8583*

ANTHELMINTIC (CESTODES)

Albendazole, *210*
Aspidin, *846*
Aspidinol, *847*
Dichlorophen, *3071*
Embelin, *3555*
Kosins, *5322*
Naphthalene, *6370*
Niclosamide, *6519*
Nitazoxanide, *6567*
Pelletierine, *7072*
Quinacrine, *8044*

ANTHELMINTIC (NEMATODES)

Amocarzine, *571*
Amoscanate, *574*
Ascaridole, *827*
Bephenium Hydroxynaphthoate, *1148*
Bitoscanate, *1308*
Carbon Tetrachloride, *1816*
Carvacrol, *1872*
Cyclobendazole, *2712*
Diethylcarbamazine, *3116*
Dithiazanine Iodide, *3369*
Dymanthine, *3475*
Gentian Violet, *4395*
4-Hexylresorcinol, *4712*
Ivermectin, *5248*
Kainic Acid, *5276*
Levamisole, *5459*
Mebendazole, *5768*
2-Naphthol, *6384*
Oxantel, *6922*
Papain, *7016*
Piperazine, *7464*
Piperazine Adipate, *7465*
Pyrantel, *7955*
Pyrvinium Pamoate, *8022*
α-Santonin, *8361*
Suramin Sodium, *9006*
Tetrachloroethylene, *9190*
Thiabendazole, *9289*
Thymol, *9399*
Thymyl *N*-Isoamylcarbamate, *9409*
Urea Stibamine, *9871*

ANTHELMINTIC (SCHISTOSOMA)

Amoscanate, *574*
Antimony Potassium Tartrate, *700*
Antimony Sodium Tartrate, *702*
Antimony Sodium Thioglycollate, *703*
Antimony Thioglycollamide, *705*
Hycanthone, *4759*
Lucanthone Hydrochloride, *5591*
Niridazole, *6563*
Oxamniquine, *6919*
Praziquantel, *7716*
Sodium Antimonylgluconate *see 701*
Stibocaptate, *8812*
Stibophen, *8813*
Trichlorfon, *9623*
Urea Stibamine, *9871*

ANTHELMINTIC (TREMATODES)

Tetrachloroethylene, *9190*

ANTIACNE *see also Keratolytic*

Adapalene, *150*
Algestone Acetophenide, *240*
Azelaic Acid, *905*
Benzoyl Peroxide, *1116*
Cyproterone, *2774*
Isotretinoin, *5228*
Motretinide, *6284*
Resorcinol, *8155*
Retinoic Acid, *8165*
Tazarotene, *9081*
Tioxolone, *9456*

ANTIALLERGIC *see also Antihistaminic; Decongestant; Glucocorticoid*

Amlexanox, *490*
Cromolyn, *2590*
Ibudilast, *4879*
Ketotifen, *5307*
Lodoxamide, *5555*
Nedocromil, *6436*
Omalizumab, *6842*
Oxatomide, *6925*
Pemirolast, *7078*
Pentigetide, *7128*
Picumast, *7418*
Ramatroban, *8100*
Repirinast, *8138*
Suplatast Tosylate, *9003*
Tazanolast, *9080*
Tranilast, *9570*
Traxanox, *9578*

ANTIALLERGIC (HYPOSENSITIZATION THERAPY)

Histamine, *4719*
Poison Ivy Extract *see 7549*
Poison Oak Extract *see 7550*
Poison Sumac Extract *see 7551*
Urushiol, *9891*

ANTIALLERGIC (STEROIDAL, NASAL) *see also Glucocorticoid*

Beclomethasone, *1019*
Dexamethasone, *2943*
Flunisolide, *4145*
Fluticasone Propionate, *4211*
Triamcinolone Acetonide, *9596*

ANTIALOPECIA AGENT

Diphencyprone, *3308*
Finasteride, *4082*
Minoxidil, *6203*
Squaric Acid Dibutylester *see 8769*

ANTIAMEBIC

Arsthinol, *812*
Carbarsone, *1786*
Cephaeline, *1973*
Chloroquine, *2163*
Chlortetracycline, *2192*
Dehydroemetine, *2870*
Dibromopropamidine, *3024*
Diloxanide, *3201*
Emetine, *3559*
Fumagillin, *4286*
8-Hydroxy-7-iodo-5-quinolinesulfonic Acid, *4826*
Iodochlorhydroxyquin, *5031*
Iodoquinol, *5042*
Paromomycin, *7041*
Phanquinone, *7197*
Propamidine, *7797*
Quinfamide, *8057*
Secnidazole, *8419*
Sulfarside, *8940*
Teclozan, *9105*
Tetracycline, *9196*
Tinidazole, *9447*

ANTIANDROGEN *see also Antiacne; Antialopecia Agent; Antineoplastic (Hormonal); Antiprostatic Hypertrophy*

Bicalutamide, *1200*
Bifluranol, *1212*
Cyproterone, *2774*
Flutamide, *4208*
Nilutamide, *6544*
Osaterone, *6888*
Oxendolone, *6931*

ANTIANEMIC *see Hematinic; Hematopoietic*

ANTIANGINAL *see also Vasodilator (Coronary)*

Acebutolol, *19*
Alprenolol, *313*
Amlodipine, *491*
Arotinolol, *791*
Atenolol, *859*
Barnidipine, *1002*
Bepridil, *1150*
Bevantolol, *1192*
Bucumolol, *1467*
Bufetolol, *1473*
Bufuralol, *1480*
Bunitrolol, *1489*
Bupranolol, *1496*
Carazolol, *1778*
Carteolol, *1866*
Celiprolol, *1960*
Cinepazet, *2290*
Diltiazem, *3202*
Elgodipine, *3546*
Felodipine, *3953*
Gallopamil, *4356*
Imolamine, *4923*
Indenolol, *4940*
Isosorbide Dinitrate, *5225*
Isradipine, *5240*
Ivabradine, *5247*
Limaprost, *5490*
Mepindolol, *5856*
Metoprolol, *6151*
Molsidomine, *6234*
Nadolol, *6346*
Nicardipine, *6495*
Nicorandil, *6521*
Nifedipine, *6528*
Nifenalol, *6530*
Nilvadipine, *6545*
Nipradilol, *6562*
Nisoldipine, *6565*
Nitroglycerin, *6607*
Oxprenolol, *6952*
Oxyfedrine, *6962*
Ozagrel, *6980*
Penbutolol, *7082*
Pentaerythritol Tetranitrate, *7112*
Pindolol, *7443*
Pronethalol, *7790*
Propranolol, *7840*
Ranolazine, *8111*
Semotiadil, *8446*
Sotalol, *8728*
Tedisamil, *9108*
Timolol, *9444*
Toliprolol, *9516*
Verapamil, *9950*
Zatebradine, *10115*

ANTIARRHYTHMIC

Acebutolol, *19*
Acecainide, *20*
Adenosine, *153*
Ajmaline, *194*
Alprenolol, *313*
Amiodarone, *482*
Aprindine, *754*
Arotinolol, *791*
Atenolol, *859*
Azimilide, *911*
Bevantolol, *1192*
Bidisomide, *1204*
Bretylium Tosylate, *1371*
Bucumolol, *1467*
Bufetolol, *1473*
Bunaftine, *1485*
Bunitrolol, *1489*
Bupranolol, *1496*
Carazolol, *1778*
Carteolol, *1866*
Cifenline, *2269*
Cloranolol, *2402*
Disopyramide, *3360*
Dofetilide, *3409*
Dronedarone, *3449*
Encainide, *3570*
Esmolol, *3700*
Flecainide, *4098*
Hydroquinidine, *4806*
Ibutilide, *4883*
Indecainide, *4937*
Indenolol, *4940*
Ipratropium Bromide, *5073*
Landiolol, *5355*
Lidocaine, *5482*
Lorajmine, *5577*
Lorcainide, *5580*
Meobentine, *5843*
Mexiletine, *6169*
Moricizine, *6268*
Nadoxolol, *6347*
Nifekalant, *6529*
Nifenalol, *6530*
Oxprenolol, *6952*
Penbutolol, *7082*
Pentisomide, *7129*
Pilsicainide, *7427*
Pindolol, *7443*
Pirmenol, *7501*
Practolol, *7700*
Prajmaline, *7702*
Procainamide Hydrochloride, *7756*
Pronethalol, *7790*
Propafenone, *7794*
Propranolol, *7840*
Pyrinoline, *7989*
Quinidine, *8060*
Sematilide, *8442*
Sotalol, *8728*
Talinolol, *9038*
Tecadenoson, *9096*
Tedisamil, *9108*
Tilisolol, *9438*
Timolol, *9444*
Tocainide, *9491*
Verapamil, *9950*
Xibenolol, *10075*

ANTIARTHRITIC/ANTIRHEU-
MATIC *see also Anti-inflammatory (Nonsteroidal); Glucocorticoid*

Actarit, *133*
Auranofin, *878*

Aurothioglucose, *883*
Azathioprine, *902*
Bucillamine, *1460*
Chloroquine, *2163*
Cuproxoline, *2670*
Diacerein, *2960*
Glucosamine, *4458*
Gold Sodium Thiomalate, *4518*
Gold Sodium Thiosulfate, *4519*
Hydroxychloroquine, *4818*
Kebuzone, *5288*
Leflunomide, *5432*
Lobenzarit, *5552*
Melittin, *5824*
Methotrexate, *5985*
Penicillamine, *7088*

ANTIASTHMATIC (NONBRON-
CHODILATOR) *see also Bronchodilator; Glucocorticoid*

Altrakincept *see 5002*
Amlexanox, *490*
Cilomilast, *2276*
Cromolyn, *2590*
Domitroban, *3416*
Ibudilast, *4879*
Israpafant, *5241*
Ketotifen, *5307*
Montelukast, *6258*
Nedocromil, *6436*
Omalizumab, *6842*
Oxatomide, *6925*
Pranlukast, *7710*
Ramatroban, *8100*
Roflumilast, *8249*
Seratrodast, *8459*
Suplatast Tosylate, *9003*
Tiaramide, *9424*
Traxanox, *9578*
Zafirlukast, *10108*
Zileuton, *10124*

ANTIASTHMATIC (STEROIDAL,
INHALANT) *see also Glucocorticoid*

Beclomethasone, *1019*
Budesonide, *1468*
Dexamethasone, *2943*
Flunisolide, *4145*
Fluticasone Propionate, *4211*
Triamcinolone Acetonide, *9596*

ANTIATHEROSCLEROTIC *see also
Antilipemic*

Alagebrium Chloride, *203*
Motexafin Lutetium, *6282*
Pyridinol Carbamate, *7975*
Torcetrapib, *9549*

ANTIBACTERIAL (ANTIBIOTICS)

Aminoglycosides
Amikacin, *405*
Arbekacin, *770*
Bambermycins, *952*
Butirosin, *1528*
Dibekacin, *3005*
Dihydrostreptomycin, *3179*
Fortimicins, *4249*
Gentamicin, *4392*
Isepamicin, *5106*
Kanamycin, *5281*

Micronomicin, *6181*
Neomycin, *6454*
Netilmicin, *6479*
Paromomycin, *7041*
Ribostamycin, *8206*
Sisomicin, *8550*
Spectinomycin, *8739*
Streptomycin, *8826*
Tobramycin, *9490*

Amphenicols
Azidamfenicol, *909*
Chloramphenicol, *2077*
Thiamphenicol, *9301*

Ansamycins
Rifamide, *8215*
Rifampin, *8216*
Rifamycin SV, *8218*
Rifapentine, *8219*
Rifaximin, *8220*

β-Lactams
Carbacephems
Loracarbef, *5576*

Carbapenems
Biapenem, *1197*
Ertapenem, *3673*
Imipenem, *4919*
Meropenem, *5900*
Panipenem, *7009*

Cephalosporins
Cefaclor, *1912*
Cefadroxil, *1913*
Cefamandole, *1914*
Cefatrizine, *1915*
Cefazedone, *1916*
Cefazolin, *1917*
Cefcapene Pivoxil, *1919*
Cefdinir, *1920*
Cefditoren, *1921*
Cefepime, *1922*
Cefetamet, *1923*
Cefixime, *1924*
Cefmenoxime, *1925*
Cefodizime, *1928*
Cefonicid, *1929*
Cefoperazone, *1930*
Ceforanide, *1931*
Cefoselis, *1932*
Cefotaxime, *1933*
Cefotiam, *1935*
Cefozopran, *1937*
Cefpimizole, *1938*
Cefpiramide, *1939*
Cefpirome, *1940*
Cefpodoxime Proxetil, *1941*
Cefprozil, *1942*
Cefroxadine, *1944*
Cefsulodin, *1945*
Ceftazidime, *1946*
Cefteram, *1947*
Ceftezole, *1948*
Ceftibuten, *1949*
Ceftizoxime, *1951*
Ceftobiprole Medocaril, *1952*
Ceftriaxone, *1953*
Cefuroxime, *1954*
Cefuzonam, *1955*
Cephacetrile Sodium, *1972*
Cephalexin, *1974*
Cephaloglycin, *1976*
Cephaloridine, *1979*
Cephalosporin C, *1980*
Cephalothin, *1982*

ANTIBACTERIAL (ANTIBIOTICS)
β-Lactams (*continued*)

Cephapirin Sodium, *1984*
Cephradine, *1986*
Pivcefalexin, *7513*

Cephamycins
Cefbuperazone, *1918*
Cefmetazole, *1926*
Cefminox, *1927*
Cefotetan, *1934*
Cefoxitin, *1936*

Monobactams
Aztreonam, *925*
Carumonam, *1871*

Oxacephems
Flomoxef, *4104*
Moxalactam, *6286*

Penems
Faropenem, *3938*
Ritipenem, *8236*

Penicillins
Amdinocillin, *389*
Amdinocillin Pivoxil, *390*
Amoxicillin, *577*
Ampicillin, *586*
Apalcillin, *724*
Aspoxicillin, *852*
Azidocillin, *910*
Azlocillin, *916*
Bacampicillin, *931*
Carbenicillin, *1792*
Carindacillin, *1840*
Clometocillin, *2385*
Cloxacillin, *2419*
Cyclacillin, *2702*
Dicloxacillin, *3084*
Epicillin, *3614*
Fenbenicillin, *3961*
Floxacillin, *4111*
Hetacillin, *4672*
Lenampicillin, *5437*
Metampicillin, *5925*
Methicillin Sodium, *5969*
Mezlocillin, *6171*
Nafcillin, *6352*
Oxacillin, *6904*
Penamecillin, *7081*
Penethamate Hydriodide, *7085*
Penicillin G, *7094*
Penicillin G Benzathine, *7096*
Penicillin G Procaine, *7097*
Penicillin N, *7098*
Penicillin O, *7099*
Penicillin V, *7100*
Phenethicillin Potassium, *7223*
Piperacillin, *7463*
Pivampicillin, *7512*
Propicillin, *7817*
Quinacillin, *8043*
Sulbenicillin, *8890*
Sultamicillin, *8992*
Talampicillin, *9033*
Temocillin, *9137*
Ticarcillin, *9428*

Lincosamides
Clindamycin, *2356*
Lincomycin, *5500*

Macrolides
Azithromycin, *915*
Cethromycin, *2020*

Clarithromycin, *2339*
Dirithromycin, *3354*
Erythromycin, *3681*
Erythromycin Acistrate, *3682*
Erythromycin Estolate, *3683*
Erythromycin Glucoheptonate, *3684*
Erythromycin Lactobionate, *3685*
Erythromycin Propionate, *3686*
Erythromycin Stearate, *3687*
Josamycin, *5267*
Leucomycins, *5453*
Midecamycins, *6183*
Miokamycin, *6204*
Oleandomycin, *6825*
Primycin, *7750*
Rokitamycin, *8250*
Rosaramicin, *8261*
Roxithromycin, *8276*
Spiramycin, *8752*
Telithromycin, *9119*
Troleandomycin, *9770*

Polypeptides
Amphomycin, *584*
Bacitracin, *934*
Bacitracin Zinc, *936*
Capreomycin, *1757*
Colistin, *2479*
Dalbavancin, *2803*
Daptomycin, *2823*
Enduracidin, *3579*
Enviomycin, *3600*
Fusafungine, *4313*
Gramicidin(s), *4532*
Gramicidin S, *4531*
Iseganan, *5105*
Oritavancin, *6868*
Polymyxin, *7573*
Quinupristin, *8084*
Ramoplanin, *8104*
Ristocetin, *8234*
Teicoplanin, *9115*
Telavancin, *9116*
Thiostrepton, *9364*
Tuberactinomycin, *9803*
Tyrocidine, *9836*
Tyrothricin, *9841*
Vancomycin, *9929*
Viomycin, *10001*

Tetracyclines
Chlortetracycline, *2192*
Clomocycline, *2388*
Demeclocycline, *2886*
Doxycycline, *3440*
Guamecycline, *4557*
Lymecycline, *5628*
Meclocycline, *5778*
Methacycline, *5943*
Minocycline, *6202*
Oxytetracycline, *6976*
Pipacycline, *7453*
Rolitetracycline, *8252*
Tetracycline, *9196*
Tigecycline, *9432*

Others
Cycloserine, *2751*
Dalfopristin, *2804*
Fosfomycin, *4254*
Fusidic Acid, *4317*
Mupirocin, *6302*
Pristinamycin, *7753*
Virginiamycin, *10004*

ANTIBACTERIAL (SYNTHETIC)
2,4-Diaminopyrimidines
Brodimoprim, *1380*
Tetroxoprim, *9250*
Trimethoprim, *9709*

Nitrofurans
Furaltadone, *4294*
Furazolium Chloride, *4301*
Nifuratel, *6532*
Nifurfoline, *6533*
Nifurpirinol, *6537*
Nifurtoinol, *6539*
Nitrofurantoin, *6599*

Oxazolidinones
Linezolid, *5504*

Quinolones and Analogs
Balofloxacin, *944*
Cinoxacin, *2309*
Ciprofloxacin, *2314*
Clinafloxacin, *2355*
Enoxacin, *3587*
Fleroxacin, *4099*
Flumequine, *4137*
Garenoxacin, *4369*
Gatifloxacin, *4376*
Gemifloxacin, *4389*
Grepafloxacin, *4545*
Lomefloxacin, *5562*
Miloxacin, *6196*
Moxifloxacin, *6291*
Nadifloxacin, *6345*
Nalidixic Acid, *6359*
Norfloxacin, *6700*
Ofloxacin, *6771*
Oxolinic Acid, *6945*
Pazufloxacin, *7055*
Pefloxacin, *7066*
Pipemidic Acid, *7460*
Piromidic Acid, *7505*
Prulifloxacin, *7908*
Rosoxacin, *8268*
Rufloxacin, *8294*
Sitafloxacin, *8551*
Sparfloxacin, *8735*
Tosufloxacin, *9555*
Trovafloxacin, *9787*

Sulfonamides
Acetyl Sulfamethoxypyrazine, *101*
Chloramine-B, *2074*
Chloramine-T, *2075*
Dichloramine T, *3047*
N^2-Formylsulfisomidine, *4248*
Mafenide, *5649*
Noprylsulfamide, *6684*
Phthalylsulfacetamide, *7376*
Phthalylsulfathiazole, *7377*
Salazosulfadimidine, *8321*
Succinylsulfathiazole, *8877*
Sulfabenzamide, *8897*
Sulfacetamide, *8899*
Sulfachlorpyridazine, *8900*
Sulfachrysoidine, *8901*
Sulfacytine, *8902*
Sulfadiazine, *8903*
Sulfadicramide, *8904*
Sulfadoxine, *8906*
Sulfaethidole, *8907*
Sulfaguanidine, *8908*
Sulfaguanole, *8909*
Sulfalene, *8910*
Sulfaloxic Acid, *8912*
Sulfamerazine, *8913*
Sulfameter, *8914*

Sulfamethazine, *8915*
Sulfamethizole, *8916*
Sulfamethomidine, *8917*
Sulfamethoxazole, *8918*
Sulfamethoxypyridazine, *8919*
Sulfametrole, *8920*
Sulfamidochrysoidine, *8923*
Sulfamoxole, *8924*
Sulfanilamide, *8925*
N⁴-Sulfanilylsulfanilamide, *8930*
Sulfanilylurea, *8931*
N-Sulfanilyl-3,4-xylamide, *8932*
Sulfaperine, *8934*
Sulfaphenazole, *8935*
Sulfaproxyline, *8936*
Sulfapyrazine, *8937*
Sulfapyridine, *8938*
Sulfathiazole, *8943*
Sulfathiourea, *8944*
Sulfisomidine, *8951*
Sulfisoxazole, *8952*

Sulfones
Acediasulfone, *23*
Dapsone, *2822*
Glucosulfone Sodium, *4463*
Solasulfone, *8711*
Succisulfone, *8878*
Sulfanilic Acid, *8926*
p-Sulfanilylbenzylamine, *8928*
Sulfoxone Sodium, *8968*
Thiazolsulfone, *9309*

Others
Clofoctol, *2380*
Methenamine, *5966*
Metronidazole, *6157*
Nitroxoline, *6655*
Pexiganan, *7193*
Taurolidine, *9076*
Xibornol, *10076*

ANTIBACTERIAL (LEPROSTATIC)
Clofazimine, *2373*
Dapsone, *2822*
Glucosulfone Sodium, *4463*
Hydnocarpic Acid, *4761*
Solasulfone, *8711*
Succisulfone, *8878*
Sulfoxone Sodium, *8968*

ANTIBACTERIAL (RICKETTSIA) see *Antirickettsial*

ANTIBACTERIAL (TUBERCULO-STATIC)
p-Aminosalicylic Acid, *477*
p-Aminosalicylic Acid Hydrazide, *478*
Benzoylpas, *1115*
5-Bromosalicylhydroxamic Acid, *1436*
Capreomycin, *1757*
Clofazimine, *2373*
Cyacetacide, *2680*
Cycloserine, *2751*
Dihydrostreptomycin, *3179*
Enviomycin, *3600*
Ethambutol, *3720*
Ethionamide, *3737*
Furonazide, *4308*
Glyconiazide, *4500*
Isoniazid, *5186*

Morphazinamide, *6273*
Opiniazide, *6852*
Phenyl Aminosalicylate, *7272*
Protionamide, *7891*
Pyrazinamide, *7956*
Rifabutin, *8213*
Rifalazil, *8214*
Rifampin, *8216*
Rifapentine, *8219*
Salinazid, *8335*
Streptomycin, *8826*
Sulfoniazide, *8959*
Thiacetazone, *9290*
Tuberactinomycin, *9803*
Viomycin, *10001*

ANTIBACTERIAL ADJUNCTS
β-Lactamase Inhibitors
Clavulanic Acid, *2341*
Sulbactam, *8889*
Sultamicillin, *8992*
Tazobactam, *9083*

Renal Dipeptidase Inhibitors
Cilastatin, *2272*

Renal Protectant
Betamipron, *1181*

ANTIBIOTIC see *Antibacterial (Antibiotics); Antifungal (Antibiotics); Antineoplastic*

ANTICANCER see *Antineoplastic*

ANTICHOLELITHOGENIC see *Cholelitholytic Agent*

ANTICHOLESTEREMIC see *Antilipemic*

ANTICHOLINERGIC see *Antimuscarinic*

ANTICOAGULANT see also *Antithrombotic; Thrombolytic*
Acenocoumarol, *29*
Ancrod, *630*
Anisindione, *668*
Bivalirudin, *1310*
Bromindione, *1393*
Clorindione, *2406*
Cyclocumarol, *2717*
Dextran Sulfate Sodium, *2951*
Dicumarol, *3090*
Ethyl Biscoumacetate, *3770*
Ethylidene Dicoumarol, *3812*
Fluindione, *4134*
Heparin, *4653*
Hirudin, *4718*
Lyapolate Sodium, *5617*
Pentosan Polysulfate, *7134*
Phenindione, *7234*
Phenprocoumon, *7259*
Phosvitin, *7365*
Picotamide, *7407*
Tioclomarol, *9451*
Warfarin, *10038*

ANTICONVULSANT
Acetylpheneturide, *99*
Albutoin, *217*
Aminoglutethimide, *440*
4-Amino-3-hydroxybutyric Acid, *444*
Beclamide, *1018*
Brivaracetam, *1377*
Buramate, *1501*
Calcium Bromide, *1654*
Carbamazepine, *1781*
Cinromide, *2311*
Clomethiazole, *2384*
Clonazepam, *2389*
Decimemide, *2852*
Diazepam, *2994*
Dimethadione, *3213*
Eterobarb, *3715*
Ethadione, *3718*
Ethosuximide, *3748*
Ethotoin, *3749*
Felbamate, *3950*
Fluoresone, *4161*
Fosphenytoin, *4258*
Gabapentin, *4319*
Ganaxolone, *4362*
Lacosamide, *5333*
Lamotrigine, *5353*
Levetiracetam, *5461*
Lorazepam, *5579*
Magnesium Bromide, *5659*
Magnesium Sulfate, *5691*
Mephenytoin, *5853*
Mephobarbital, *5854*
Metharbital, *5961*
Methsuximide, *6004*
Midazolam, *6182*
Nitrazepam, *6575*
Oxcarbazepine, *6929*
Paramethadione, *7028*
Phenacemide, *7203*
Phenetharbital, *7222*
Pheneturide, *7230*
Phenobarbital, *7238*
Phensuximide, *7261*
Phenytoin, *7322*
Potassium Bromide, *7618*
Pregabalin, *7725*
Primidone, *7746*
Progabide, *7772*
Rufinamide, *8293*
Safinamide, *8315*
Sodium Bromide, *8594*
Solanum, *8708*
Strontium Bromide, *8837*
Sulthiame, *8993*
Talampanel, *9032*
Tetrantoin, *9234*
Tiagabine, *9417*
Topiramate, *9547*
Trimethadione, *9706*
Valproic Acid, *9913*
Valpromide, *9914*
Vigabatrin, *9978*
Zonisamide, *10192*

ANTIDEPRESSANT see also *Antimanic*
Bicyclics
Citalopram, *2318*
Fencamine, *3967*
Indalpine, *4930*
Indeloxazine Hydrochloride, *4938*
Nefopam, *6440*
Nomifensine, *6673*

ANTIDEPRESSANT
Bicyclics (continued)
Oxitriptan see 4847
Oxypertine, 6971
Paroxetine, 7043
Sertraline, 8467
Thiazesim, 9305
Trazodone, 9579

Hydrazides/Hydrazines
Iproclozide, 5076
Iproniazid, 5078
Isocarboxazid, 5157
Nialamide, 6491
Phenelzine, 7221

Phenyloxazolidinones
Befloxatone, 1021
Toloxatone, 9521

Pyrrolidones
Cotinine, 2553

Tetracyclics
Maprotiline, 5748
Metralindole, 6153
Mianserin, 6172
Mirtazapine, 6208

Tricyclics
Adinazolam, 160
Amineptine, 409
Amitriptyline, 487
Amitriptylinoxide, 488
Amoxapine, 576
Butriptyline, 1533
Clomipramine, 2387
Demexiptiline, 2890
Desipramine, 2920
Dibenzepin, 3008
Dimetacrine, 3212
Dothiepin, 3429
Doxepin, 3435
Fluacizine, 4113
Imipramine, 4920
Imipramine N-Oxide, 4921
Iprindole, 5075
Lofepramine, 5557
Melitracen, 5823
Metapramine, 5930
Nortriptyline, 6715
Opipramol, 6853
Pizotyline, 7515
Propizepine, 7833
Protriptyline, 7901
Quinupramine, 8083
Tianeptine, 9420
Trimipramine, 9722

Others
Adrafinil, 170
Agomelatine, 190
Bupropion, 1499
Dioxadrol, 3299
Duloxetine, 3465
Etoperidone, 3885
Femoxetine, 3955
Fluoxetine, 4185
Fluvoxamine, 4219
Hematoporphyrin, 4636
Hypericin, 4863
Levophacetoperane, 5467
Medifoxamine, 5790
Milnacipran, 6194
Minaprine, 6200
Moclobemide, 6226
Nefazodone, 6438

Nemifitide, 6445
Piberaline, 7392
Prolintane, 7781
Pyrisuccideanol, 7991
Reboxetine, 8125
Ritanserin, 8235
Roxindole, 8275
Rubidium Chloride, 8284
Sulpiride, 8989
Tandospirone, 9051
Thozalinone, 9379
Tranylcypromine, 9573
Tryptophan, 9797
Venlafaxine, 9946
Viloxazine, 9980
Zimeldine, 10126

ANTIDIABETIC
Biguanides
Buformin, 1476
Metformin, 5938
Phenformin, 7231

Hormones/Analogs
Amylin, 609
Insulin, 4980
Insulin Aspart, 4982
Insulin Detemir, 4983
Insulin Glargine, 4984
Insulin Glulisine, 4985
Insulin Lispro, 4987
Liraglutide, 5514
Pramlintide, 7708

Sulfonylurea Derivatives
Acetohexamide, 62
Carbutamide, 1832
Chlorpropamide, 2186
Glibornuride, 4438
Gliclazide, 4439
Glimepiride, 4440
Glipizide, 4442
Gliquidone, 4443
Glisoxepid, 4444
Glyburide, 4478
Glybuthiazol(e), 4479
Glybuzole, 4480
Glyhexamide, 4506
Glymidine, 4507
Tolazamide, 9505
Tolbutamide, 9507
Tolcyclamide, 9511

Thiazolidinediones
Pioglitazone, 7452
Rosiglitazone, 8265
Troglitazone, 9769

Others
Acarbose, 18
Exenatide see 3914
Miglitol, 6187
Mitiglinide, 6211
Muraglitazar, 6303
Nateglinide, 6428
Repaglinide, 8136
Sitagliptin, 8552
Tesaglitazar, 9177
Vildagliptin, 9979
Voglibose, 10029

ANTIDIARRHEAL
Acetyltannic Acid, 104
Bismuth Subcarbonate, 1282
Bismuth Subsalicylate, 1285

Catechin, 1902
Difenoxin, 3136
Diphenoxylate, 3313
Lidamidine, 5481
Loperamide, 5571
Racecadotril, 8090
Trillium, 9696
Uzarin, 9897
Zaldaride, 10110

ANTIDIURETIC
Desmopressin, 2924
Felypressin, 3954
Lypressin, 5630
Ornipressin, 6873
Oxycinchophen, 6957
Pituitary, Posterior, 7510
Terlipressin, 9167
Vasopressin, 9938

ANTIDOTE (ACETAMINOPHEN POISONING)
Acetylcysteine, 88
Cysteamine, 2779
Methionine, 5975

ANTIDOTE (CURARE)
Edrophonium Chloride, 3516
Neostigmine, 6464
Tacrine, 9024

ANTIDOTE (CYANIDE)
p-Aminopropiophenone, 470
Dicobalt Edetate see 3517
Methylene Blue, 6060
Potassium Nitrite, 7649
Sodium Nitrite, 8648
Sodium Thiosulfate, 8694

ANTIDOTE (FOLIC ACID ANTAGONISTS)
Folinic Acid, 4222

ANTIDOTE (HEAVY METAL POISONING)
Albumen, 215
Deferoxamine, 2860
Dimercaprol, 3209
2,3-Dimercapto-1-propanesulfonic Acid, 3210
Ditiocarb Sodium, 3378
Prussian Blue, 7910
Succimer, 8865
Tiopronin, 9453

ANTIDOTE (METHANOL AND ETHYLENE GLYCOL POISONING)
Fomepizole, 4226

ANTIDOTE (ORGANOPHOSPHATE POISONING)
Asoxime Chloride, 835
HLö-7, 4724
Obidoxime Chloride, 6738
Pralidoxime Chloride, 7703

ANTIDYSKINETIC see also Antiparkinsonian

Amantadine, 374
Clonidine, 2390
Haloperidol, 4598
Pimozide, 7435
Sarizotan, 8375
Tetrabenazine, 9182
Tiapride, 9421

ANTIECZEMATIC

Evening Primrose Oil, 3906
γ-Linolenic Acid, 5507

ANTIEMETIC

Acetylleucine Monoethanol-
amine, 95
Alizapride, 250
Aprepitant, 753
Azasetron, 900
Benzquinamide, 1119
Bismuth Subsalicylate, 1285
Bromopride, 1432
Buclizine, 1464
Chlorpromazine, 2185
Clebopride, 2344
Cyclizine, 2710
Dimenhydrinate, 3207
Diphenidol, 3311
Dixyrazine, 3385
Dolasetron, 3411
Domperidone, 3418
Granisetron, 4536
Itasetron, 5243
Meclizine, 5777
Metoclopramide, 6143
Metopimazine, 6149
Nabilone, 6342
Ondansetron, 6848
Oxypendyl, 6970
Palonosetron, 6997
Pipamazine, 7454
Prochlorperazine, 7761
Ramosetron, 8105
Scopolamine, 8406
Sulpiride, 8989
Tetrahydrocannabinols, 9209
Thiethylperazine, 9315
Thioproperazine, 9357
Trimethobenzamide, 9708
Tropisetron, 9783

ANTIEPILEPTIC see Anticonvulsant

ANTIFIBROTIC

Potassium p-Aminobenzoate, 7606

ANTIFLATULENT

Dimethicone, 3215

ANTIFUNGAL (ANTIBIOTICS)

Echinocandins
Anidulafungin, 656
Caspofungin, 1889
Micafungin, 6175

Polyenes
Amphotericin B, 585
Candicidin, 1740

Filipin, 4080
Fungichromin, 4290
Hachimycin, 4586
Hamycin, 4609
Lucensomycin, 5592
Mepartricin, 5847
Natamycin, 6427
Nystatin, 6736
Pecilocin, 7062
Perimycin, 7169

Others
Griseofulvin, 4549
Oligomycins, 6833
Pyrrolnitrin, 8018
Siccanin, 8486
Viridin, 10006

ANTIFUNGAL (SYNTHETIC)

Allylamines
Butenafine, 1518
Naftifine, 6355
Terbinafine, 9156

Imidazoles
Bifonazole, 1213
Butoconazole, 1529
Chlormidazole, 2107
Cloconazole, 2368
Clotrimazole, 2417
Econazole, 3502
Enilconazole, 3583
Fenticonazole, 4005
Flutrimazole, 4215
Isoconazole, 5160
Ketoconazole, 5302
Lanoconazole, 5357
Miconazole, 6178
Neticonazole, 6478
Omoconazole, 6846
Oxiconazole Nitrate, 6937
Sertaconazole, 8465
Sulconazole, 8893
Tioconazole, 9452

Thiocarbamates
Liranaftate, 5515
Tolciclate, 9509
Tolindate, 9515
Tolnaftate, 9519

Triazoles
Fluconazole, 4122
Itraconazole, 5245
Posaconazole, 7602
Ravuconazole, 8121
Saperconazole, 8362
Terconazole, 9160
Voriconazole, 10033

Others
Acrisorcin, 126
Amorolfine, 573
Biphenamine, 1234
Bromosalicylchloranilide, 1435
Buclosamide, 1465
Calcium Propionate, 1698
Chlorphenesin, 2178
Ciclopirox, 2266
Cloxyquin, 2422
Coparaffinate, 2518
Exalamide, 3909
Flucytosine, 4125
Haloprogin, 4600
Hexetidine, 4703
Loflucarban, 5559

Nifuratel, 6532
Potassium Iodide, 7643
Propionic Acid, 7825
Pyrithione, 7994
Salicylanilide, 8330
Sodium Propionate, 8669
Sulbentine, 8892
Tenonitrozole, 9147
Triacetin, 9589
Undecylenic Acid, 9848
Zinc Propionate, 10153

ANTIGLAUCOMA

Acetazolamide, 53
Apraclonidine, 751
Befunolol, 1022
Betaxolol, 1182
Bimatoprost, 1221
Brimonidine, 1375
Brinzolamide, 1376
Bupranolol, 1496
Carteolol, 1866
Dapiprazole, 2820
Dichlorphenamide, 3077
Dipivefrin, 3338
Dorzolamide, 3426
Epinephrine, 3619
Latanoprost, 5376
Levobunolol, 5462
Methazolamide, 5962
Metipranolol, 6140
Pilocarpine, 7424
Pindolol, 7443
Timolol, 9444
Travoprost, 9577
Unoprostone, 9849

ANTIGONADOTROPIN

Danazol, 2812
Gestrinone, 4415
Paroxypropione, 7044

ANTIGOUT

Allopurinol, 279
Carprofen, 1862
Colchicine, 2471
Febuxostat, 3948
Probenecid, 7754
Sulfinpyrazone, 8949

ANTIHEMOPHILIC FACTOR

Factor VIII, 3921
Moroctocog Alfa, 6271

ANTIHEMORRHAGIC see Hemostatic

ANTIHISTAMINIC see also Antiallergic

Alkylamine Derivatives
Acrivastine, 127
Bamipine, 956
Brompheniramine, 1443
Chlorpheniramine, 2180
Dimethindene, 3216
Pheniramine, 7235
Pyrrobutamine, 8012
Thenaldine, 9278
Tolpropamine, 9523
Triprolidine, 9746

ANTIHISTAMINIC (continued)

Aminoalkylethers
Bromodiphenhydramine, *1418*
Carbinoxamine, *1799*
Chlorphenoxamine, *2181*
Clemastine, *2345*
Diphenhydramine, *3309*
Diphenylpyraline, *3331*
Doxylamine, *3441*
Embramine, *3556*
p-Methyldiphenhydramine, *6053*
Moxastine, *6287*
Orphenadrine, *6879*
Phenyltoloxamine, *7316*
Setastine, *8472*

Ethylenediamine Derivatives
Chloropyramine, *2162*
Chlorothen, *2167*
Methapyrilene, *5959*
Pyrilamine, *7984*
Talastine, *9035*
Thenyldiamine, *9280*
Thonzylamine Hydrochloride, *9373*
Tripelennamine, *9738*

Piperazines
Cetirizine, *2022*
Chlorcyclizine, *2081*
Cinnarizine, *2305*
Clocinizine, *2367*
Homochlorcyclizine, *4733*
Hydroxyzine, *4849*

Tricyclics
Phenothiazines
Mequitazine, *5864*
Promethazine, *7786*
Thiazinamium Methylsulfate, *9306*

Other Tricyclics
Azatadine, *901*
Cyproheptadine, *2773*
Deptropine, *2912*
Desloratadine, *2922*
Isothipendyl, *5227*
Loratadine, *5578*
Olopatadine, *6840*
Rupatadine, *8297*

Others
Antazoline, *680*
Astemizole, *856*
Azelastine, *906*
Bepotastine, *1149*
Clemizole, *2346*
Ebastine, *3484*
Emedastine, *3557*
Epinastine, *3618*
Fexofenadine, *4068*
Levocabastine, *5463*
Mebhydroline, *5770*
Mizolastine, *6221*
Phenindamine, *7233*
Terfenadine, *9163*
Tritoqualine, *9765*

ANTIHYPERCHOLESTEROLEMIC
see **Antilipemic**

ANTIHYPERLIPIDEMIC *see* **Antilipemic**

ANTIHYPERPARATHYROID
Calcitriol, *1644*
Cinacalcet, *2282*
Doxercalciferol, *3436*
Maxacalcitol, *5760*
Paricalcitol, *7039*

ANTIHYPERPHOSPHATEMIC
Aluminum Hydroxide, *342*
Aluminum Hydroxychloride, *343*
Calcium Acetate, *1646*
Lanthanum Carbonate, *5364*
Sevelamer, *8474*

ANTIHYPERTENSIVE *see also* **Diuretic**

Arylethanolamine Derivatives
Amosulalol, *575*
Bufuralol, *1480*
Labetalol, *5329*
Pronethalol, *7790*
Sotalol, *8728*
Sulfinalol, *8948*

Aryloxypropanolamine Derivatives
Acebutolol, *19*
Alprenolol, *313*
Arotinolol, *791*
Atenolol, *859*
Betaxolol, *1182*
Bevantolol, *1192*
Bisoprolol, *1295*
Bopindolol, *1333*
Bucindolol, *1461*
Bunitrolol, *1489*
Bupranolol, *1496*
Carazolol, *1778*
Carteolol, *1866*
Carvedilol, *1873*
Celiprolol, *1960*
Cetamolol, *2018*
Indenolol, *4940*
Mepindolol, *5856*
Metipranolol, *6140*
Metoprolol, *6151*
Moprolol, *6264*
Nadolol, *6346*
Nebivolol, *6432*
Nipradilol, *6562*
Oxprenolol, *6952*
Penbutolol, *7082*
Pindolol, *7443*
Propranolol, *7840*
Talinolol, *9038*
Tertatolol, *9173*
Tilisolol, *9438*
Timolol, *9444*
Toliprolol, *9516*

Biphenyltetrazole Derivatives
Candesartan, *1739*
Irbesartan, *5083*
Losartan, *5583*
Olmesartan, *6839*
Valsartan, *9916*

N-Carboxyalkyl (peptide/lactam) Derivatives
Alacepril, *200*
Benazepril, *1031*
Captopril, *1774*
Ceronapril, *1994*
Cilazapril, *2273*
Delapril, *2876*
Enalapril, *3567*
Enalaprilat, *3568*
Fosinopril, *4256*
Imidapril, *4911*
Lisinopril, *5516*
Moexipril, *6229*
Moveltipril, *6285*
Perindopril, *7170*
Quinapril, *8051*
Ramipril, *8103*
Spirapril, *8753*
Temocapril, *9136*
Trandolapril, *9568*
Zofenopril, *10186*

Dihydropyridine Derivatives
Amlodipine, *491*
Aranidipine, *767*
Azelnidipine, *907*
Barnidipine, *1002*
Benidipine, *1043*
Cilnidipine, *2275*
Clevidipine, *2352*
Efonidipine, *3524*
Felodipine, *3953*
Isradipine, *5240*
Lacidipine, *5331*
Lercanidipine, *5446*
Manidipine, *5743*
Nicardipine, *6495*
Nifedipine, *6528*
Nilvadipine, *6545*
Nisoldipine, *6565*
Nitrendipine, *6576*

Guanidine Derivatives
Bethanidine, *1186*
Debrisoquin, *2844*
Guanabenz, *4558*
Guanadrel, *4559*
Guanethidine, *4560*
Guanfacine, *4561*
Guanoxabenz, *4567*
Guanoxan, *4568*
Pinacidil, *7438*

Hydrazines/Phthalazines
Budralazine, *1470*
Cadralazine, *1631*
Dihydralazine, *3169*
Endralazine, *3577*
Hydralazine, *4763*
Pildralazine, *7423*
Todralazine, *9502*

Imidazoleacrylic Acid Derivatives
Eprosartan, *3635*

Imidazole Derivatives
Clonidine, *2390*
Lofexidine, *5558*
Moxonidine, *6293*
Phentolamine, *7264*
Tiamenidine, *9418*

Quaternary Ammonium Compounds
Hexamethonium, *4688*
Pentolinium Tartrate, *7132*

Quinazoline Derivatives
Alfuzosin, *238*
Bunazosin, *1487*
Doxazosin, *3433*
Prazosin, *7717*
Terazosin, *9154*

Reserpine Derivatives
Deserpidine, *2918*
Rescinnamine, *8142*
Reserpine, *8145*
Syrosingopine, *9017*

Sulfonamide Derivatives
Clopamide, *2393*
Furosemide, *4309*
Tripamide, *9737*
Xipamide, *10079*

Thiazides and Analogs
Althiazide, *318*
Bendroflumethiazide, *1037*
Benzthiazide, *1120*
Benzylhydrochlorothiazide, *1136*
Buthiazide, *1525*
Chlorothiazide, *2168*
Chlorthalidone, *2193*
Cyclopenthiazide, *2745*
Cyclothiazide, *2754*
Diazoxide, *3004*
Fenquizone, *3997*
Hydrochlorothiazide, *4781*
Hydroflumethiazide, *4789*
Indapamide, *4935*
Methyclothiazide, *6005*
Metolazone, *6147*
Polythiazide, *7584*
Quinethazone, *8056*
Teclothiazide, *9104*
Trichlormethiazide, *9624*

Others
Ajmaline, *194*
Aliskiren, *247*
Ambrisentan, *384*
γ-Aminobutyric Acid, *430*
Atrial Natriuretic Peptide, *872*
Bosentan, *1353*
Bufeniode, *1472*
Cicletanine, *2264*
Clentiazem, *2348*
Eplerenone, *3625*
Fantofarone, *3934*
Fasidotril, *3940*
Fenoldopam, *3979*
Flosequinan, *4110*
Indoramin, *4969*
Ketanserin, *5296*
Levcromakalim, *5460*
Mebutamate, *5773*
Mecamylamine, *5774*
Methyldopa, *6055*
Mibefradil, *6173*
Minoxidil, *6203*
Naftopidil, *6356*
Omapatrilat, *6843*
Pargyline, *7038*
Pempidine, *7080*
Piperoxan, *7478*
Protoveratrines, *7899*
Raubasine, *8119*
Rilmenidine, *8222*
Sampatrilat, *8352*
Saralasin, *8372*
Semotiadil, *8446*
Sildenafil, *8489*
Sitaxsentan, *8554*
Sodium Nitroprusside, *8649*
Telmisartan, *9129*
Ticrynafen, *9430*
Treprostinil, *9586*
Trimethaphan Camsylate, *9707*
Tyrosinase, *9838*
Urapidil, *9865*

ANTIHYPERTHYROID
2-Aminothiazole, *479*
Carbimazole, *1798*
3,5-Dibromo-L-tyrosine, *3030*
3,5-Diiodotyrosine, *3192*
Iodine, *5014*
Methimazole, *5971*
Methylthiouracil, *6128*
Propylthiouracil, *7869*
Sodium Perchlorate, *8653*
Thibenzazoline, *9312*
Thiobarbital, *9321*
2-Thiouracil, *9366*

ANTIHYPOGLYCEMIC
Diazoxide, *3004*
Glucagon, *4446*
Glucose, *4459*

ANTIHYPOTENSIVE
Amezinium Methyl Sulfate, *394*
Angiotensin Amide *see 651*
Dimetofrine, *3264*
Dopamine, *3421*
Etilefrin, *3865*
Gepefrine, *4401*
Metaraminol, *5932*
Methoxamine, *5987*
Midodrine, *6184*
Norepinephrine, *6695*
Pholedrine, *7330*
Synephrine, *9012*

ANTIHYPOTHYROID
Liothyronine, *5510*
Thyroid, *9410*
Thyroidin, *9411*
Thyroxine, *9415*
Tiratricol, *9462*

ANTI-INFECTIVE *see Antiseptic/Disinfectant*

ANTI-INFLAMMATORY (BIOLOGICAL RESPONSE MODIFIER)
Adalimumab, *148*
Alicaforsen, *245*
Anakinra *see 5001*
Bimosiamose, *1222*
Certolizumab Pegol, *2003*
Eculizumab, *3506*
Etanercept, *3712*
Infliximab, *4972*
Natalizumab, *6426*
Pexelizumab, *7192*
Tocilizumab, *9493*

ANTI-INFLAMMATORY (GASTROINTESTINAL)
Alicaforsen, *245*
Balsalazide, *945*
Infliximab, *4972*
Mesalamine, *5904*
Natalizumab, *6426*
Olsalazine, *6841*
Sulfasalazine, *8942*

ANTI-INFLAMMATORY (NONSTEROIDAL) *see also* **Antiarthritic/Antirheumatic**

Aminoarylcarboxylic Acid Derivatives
Enfenamic Acid, *3580*
Etofenamate, *3875*
Flufenamic Acid, *4132*
Isonixin, *5192*
Meclofenamic Acid, *5779*
Mefenamic Acid, *5798*
Niflumic Acid, *6531*
Talniflumate, *9044*
Terofenamate, *9168*
Tolfenamic Acid, *9513*

Arylacetic Acid Derivatives
Aceclofenac, *22*
Acemetacin, *27*
Alclofenac, *219*
Amfenac, *395*
Amtolmetin Guacil, *596*
Bromfenac, *1390*
Bufexamac, *1474*
Diclofenac, *3081*
Etodolac, *3874*
Felbinac, *3951*
Fenclozic Acid, *3969*
Fentiazac, *4003*
Glucametacin, *4448*
Ibufenac, *4880*
Indomethacin, *4968*
Isoxepac, *5237*
Lonazolac, *5566*
Metiazinic Acid, *6139*
Mofezolac, *6232*
Nepafenac, *6469*
Oxametacine, *6916*
Proglumetacin, *7774*
Sulindac, *8982*
Tiaramide, *9424*
Tolmetin, *9518*
Tropesin, *9778*
Zomepirac, *10191*

Arylbutyric Acid Derivatives
Bumadizon, *1483*
Butibufen, *1527*
Butixirate *see 10071*
Fenbufen, *3963*

Arylcarboxylic Acids
Ketorolac, *5306*
Tinoridine, *9448*

Arylpropionic Acid Derivatives
Alminoprofen, *300*
Bermoprofen, *1159*
Carprofen, *1862*
Fenoprofen, *3980*
Flunoxaprofen, *4148*
Flurbiprofen, *4199*
Ibuprofen, *4881*
Ibuproxam, *4882*
Ketoprofen, *5305*
Loxoprofen, *5589*
Naproxen, *6417*
Oxaprozin, *6924*
Piketoprofen, *7422*
Pranoprofen, *7711*
Suprofen, *8830*
Tiaprofenic Acid, *9422*
Ximoprofen, *10078*
Zaltoprofen, *10112*

Pyrazoles
Difenamizole, *3134*
Epirizole, *3622*

ANTI-INFLAMMATORY (NONSTE-ROIDAL) (continued)

Pyrazolones
Apazone, 726
Feprazone, 4012
Mofebutazone, 6231
Morazone, 6267
Oxyphenbutazone, 6972
Phenylbutazone, 7277
Pipebuzone, 7457
Propyphenazone, 7871
Ramifenazone, 8102
Suxibuzone, 9009

Salicylic Acid Derivatives
Acetaminosalol, 48
Aspirin, 851
Balsalazide, 945
Benorylate, 1045
Calcium Acetylsalicylate, 1647
Diflunisal, 3146
Fendosal, 3971
Gentisic Acid, 4398
Glycol Salicylate, 4499
Imidazole Salicylate, 4913
Lysine Acetylsalicylate, 5637
Mesalamine, 5904
Morpholine Salicylate see 6277
1-Naphthyl Salicylate, 6414
Olsalazine, 6841
Parsalmide, 7045
Phenyl Acetylsalicylate, 7270
Phenyl Salicylate, 7310
Salicylamide O-Acetic Acid, 8329
Salicylsulfuric Acid, 8334
Salsalate, 8339
Sodium Salicylate see 8332
Sulfasalazine, 8942

Thiazinecarboxamides
Ampiroxicam, 587
Lornoxicam, 5582
Meloxicam, 5826
Piroxicam, 7506
Tenoxicam, 9148

Others
ε-Acetamidocaproic Acid, 45
S-Adenosylmethionine, 156
Ajulemic Acid, 198
3-Amino-4-hydroxybutyric Acid, 443
Bendazac, 1035
Benzydamine, 1122
α-Bisabolol, 1241
Bucolome, 1466
Celecoxib, 1956
Difenpiramide, 3137
Ditazol, 3367
Emorfazone, 3562
Etoricoxib, 3887
Fepradinol, 4011
Guaiazulene, 4554
Lexipafant, 5473
Licofelone, 5480
Lumiracoxib, 5601
Nabumetone, 6343
Nimesulide, 6548
Oxaceprol, 6903
Parecoxib, 7036
Perisoxal, 7177
Proquazone, 7873
Rofecoxib, 8248
Superoxide Dismutase, 9002
Tenidap, 9144
Valdecoxib, 9900

ANTI-INFLAMMATORY (STEROI-DAL) see Glucocorticoid

ANTILEPROTIC see Antibacterial (Leprostatic)

ANTILEUKEMIC see Antineoplastic

ANTILIPEMIC

Bile Acid Sequestrants
Cholestyramine Resin, 2202
Colesevelam Hydrochloride, 2473
Colestilan, 2474
Colestipol, 2475
Polidexide, 7557

Fibrates
Bezafibrate, 1195
Binifibrate, 1224
Ciprofibrate, 2313
Clinofibrate, 2357
Clofibrate, 2377
Clofibric Acid, 2378
Etofibrate, 3877
Fenofibrate, 3978
Gemfibrozil, 4388
Pirifibrate, 7495
Ronifibrate, 8255
Simfibrate, 8537
Theofibrate, 9284

HMG CoA Reductase Inhibitors
Atorvastatin, 864
Cerivastatin, 1993
Fluvastatin, 4218
Lovastatin, 5586
Pitavastatin, 7508
Pravastatin Sodium, 7714
Rosuvastatin, 8270
Simvastatin, 8539

Nicotinic Acid Derivatives
Acipimox, 111
Aluminum Nicotinate, 351
Niceritrol, 6497
Oxiniacic Acid, 6941

Thyroid Hormones/Analogs
Dextrothyroxine see 9415
Etiroxate, 3872
Thyropropic Acid, 9412

Others
Acifran, 110
Avasimibe, 884
Benfluorex, 1039
Detaxtran, 2936
Eicosapentaenoic Acid, 3531
Ezetimibe, 3918
Meglutol, 5808
Melinamide, 5822
Omega-3 Acid Ethyl Esters, 6844
γ-Oryzanol, 6886
Pantethine, 7012
Pirozadil, 7507
Policosanol, 7555
Probucol, 7755
β-Sitosterol, 8556
Sultosilic Acid, 8995
Tiadenol, 9416
Torcetrapib, 9549
Xenbucin, 10071

ANTILIPIDEMIC see Antilipemic

ANTIMALARIAL
Amodiaquin, 572
Arteether, 813
Arteflene, 814
Artemether, 815
Artemisinin, 817
Artesunate, 818
Bebeerine, 1016
Berberine, 1154
Chirata, 2064
Chlorguanide, 2090
Chloroquine, 2163
Chlorproguanil, 2184
Cinchona, 2284
Cinchonidine, 2286
Cinchonine, 2287
Cycloguanil, 2721
Fosmidomycin, 4257
Gentiopicrin, 4397
Halofantrine, 4594
Hydroxychloroquine, 4818
Lumefantrine, 5597
Mefloquine, 5801
Pamaquine, 7001
Plasmocid, 7522
Primaquine, 7744
Pyrimethamine, 7985
Pyronaridine, 8005
Quinacrine, 8044
Quinidine, 8060
Quinine, 8061
Quinocide, 8067
Quinoline, 8068
Sodium Arsenate, Dibasic, 8579
Sulfadoxine, 8906
Tafenoquine, 9029

ANTIMANIC
Lithium Acetate, 5521
Lithium Carbonate, 5527
Lithium Chloride, 5528
Lithium Citrate, 5530
Lithium Sulfate, 5541
Valproic Acid, 9913

ANTIMETHEMOGLOBINEMIC
Methylene Blue, 6060

ANTIMIGRAINE
Almotriptan, 304
Alpiropride, 311
Dihydroergotamine, 3174
Dotarizine, 3428
Eletriptan, 3544
Ergocryptine, 3650
Ergot, 3660
Ergotamine, 3661
Fonazine, 4231
Frovatriptan, 4272
Ganaxolone, 4362
Lisuride, 5518
Lomerizine, 5563
Methysergide, 6137
Naratriptan, 6420
Oxetorone, 6934
Pizotyline, 7515
Rizatriptan, 8241
Sumatriptan, 8997

Topiramate, *9547*
Valproic Acid, *9913*
Zolmitriptan, *10189*

ANTIMUSCARINIC see also *Antiparkinsonian; Antispasmodic; Mydriatic*

Adiphenine, *161*
Ambutonium Bromide, *387*
Aminopentamide, *459*
Anisotropine Methylbromide, *671*
Atropine, *875*
Benactyzine, *1029*
Benzetimide, *1075*
Benztropine Mesylate, *1121*
Bevonium Methyl Sulfate, *1193*
Biperiden, *1233*
Butropium Bromide, *1534*
N-Butylscopolammonium Bromide, *1588*
Buzepide, *1599*
Chlorbenzoxamine, *2080*
Cimetropium Bromide, *2280*
Clidinium Bromide, *2354*
Cyclodrine, *2719*
Cyclopentolate, *2746*
Darifenacin, *2825*
Dexetimide, *2945*
Dicyclomine, *3097*
Diethazine, *3108*
Difemerine, *3132*
Dihexyverine, *3168*
Diphemanil Methylsulfate, *3306*
Emepronium Bromide, *3558*
Ethopropazine, *3747*
Ethybenztropine, *3756*
Eucatropine, *3897*
Fenpiverinium Bromide, *3990*
Fentonium Bromide, *4006*
Flavoxate, *4096*
Flutropium Bromide, *4216*
Glycopyrrolate, *4501*
Hexocyclium Methyl Sulfate, *4706*
Homatropine, *4730*
Hyoscyamine, *4858*
Ipratropium Bromide, *5073*
Isopropamide Iodide, *5202*
Mepenzolate Bromide, *5848*
Methantheline Bromide, *5958*
Methixene, *5979*
Methscopolamine Bromide, *6003*
Otilonium Bromide, *6898*
Oxitropium Bromide, *6943*
Oxybutynin, *6955*
Oxyphencyclimine, *6973*
Oxyphenonium Bromide, *6975*
Pipenzolate Bromide, *7461*
Piperidolate, *7470*
Piperilate, *7471*
Poldine Methylsulfate, *7554*
Prifinium Bromide, *7742*
Procyclidine, *7763*
Propantheline Bromide, *7805*
Propiverine, *7832*
Scopolamine, *8406*
Scopolamine N-Oxide, *8407*
Solifenacin, *8712*
Tiemonium Iodide, *9431*
Timepidium Bromide, *9442*
Tiotropium Bromide, *9454*
Tiquizium Bromide, *9460*
Tolterodine, *9525*
Tridihexethyl Iodide, *9661*
Trihexyphenidyl Hydrochloride, *9695*

Tropicamide, *9780*
Trospium Chloride, *9786*
Valethamate Bromide, *9906*

ANTIMYCOTIC see *Antifungal (Antibiotics); Antifungal (Synthetic)*

ANTINAUSEANT see *Antiemetic*

ANTINEOPLASTIC
Alkaloids/Natural Products

Camptothecin Derivatives
9-Aminocamptothecin, *431*
Exatecan, *3912*
Irinotecan, *5091*
Rubitecan, *8288*
Topotecan, *9548*

Podophyllum Derivatives
Etoposide, *3886*
Teniposide, *9145*

Taxanes
Docetaxel, *3397*
Paclitaxel, *6982*
Paclitaxel Poliglumex, *6983*

Vinca Alkaloids
Vinblastine, *9982*
Vincristine, *9986*
Vindesine, *9987*
Vinflunine, *9989*
Vinorelbine, *9990*

Others
Aplidine, *738*
Elliptinium Acetate, *3549*
Irofulven, *5092*
Ixabepilone, *5249*
Kahalalide F, *5275*
Midostaurin, *6185*
Trabectedin see *3503*

Alkylating Agents
Alkyl Sulfonates
Busulfan, *1505*
Improsulfan, *4927*
Piposulfan, *7481*

Aziridines
Carboquone, *1824*
Diaziquone, *2996*
Uredepa, *9872*

Ethylenimines and Methylmelamines
Altretamine, *320*
Triethylenemelamine, *9671*
Triethylenephosphoramide, *9672*
Triethylenethiophosphoramide, *9673*

Nitrogen Mustards
Bendamustine, *1034*
Canfosfamide, *1745*
Chlorambucil, *2073*
Chlornaphazine, *2108*
Cyclophosphamide, *2747*
Estramustine, *3706*
Glufosfamide, *4468*
Ifosfamide, *4896*
Mechlorethamine, *5775*
Mechlorethamine Oxide Hydrochloride, *5776*

Melphalan, *5828*
Perfosfamide, *7161*
Prednimustine, *7720*
Trichlormethine, *9625*
Trofosfamide, *9768*
Uracil Mustard, *9851*

Nitrosoureas
Carmustine, *1845*
Chlorozotocin, *2177*
Fotemustine, *4261*
Lomustine, *5564*
Nimustine, *6553*
Ranimustine, *8109*

Others
Dacarbazine, *2798*
Etoglucid, *3880*
Mitobronitol, *6212*
Mitolactol, *6214*
Pipobroman, *7480*
Procarbazine, *7758*
Temozolomide, *9139*

Antibiotics and Analogs
Actinomycins
Cactinomycin, *1606*
Dactinomycin, *2800*

Anthracyclines
Aclacinomycins, *113*
Amrubicin, *593*
Carubicin, *1870*
Daunorubicin, *2832*
Doxorubicin, *3439*
Epirubicin, *3623*
Idarubicin, *4886*
Pirarubicin, *7488*
Valrubicin, *9915*
Zorubicin, *10195*

Others
Bleomycins, *1318*
Mitomycins, *6215*
Peplomycin, *7144*
Plicamycin, *7536*
Porfiromycin, *7597*
Streptozocin, *8832*
Temsirolimus, *9142*
Zinostatin, *10167*

Antimetabolites
Folic Acid Analogs/Antagonists
Denopterin, *2895*
Edatrexate, *3507*
Methotrexate, *5985*
Nolatrexed, *6672*
Pemetrexed, *7077*
Piritrexim, *7499*
Pteropterin, *7934*
Raltitrexed, *8099*
Trimetrexate, *9721*

Purine Analogs
Cladribine, *2337*
Clofarabine, *2372*
Fludarabine, *4126*
6-Mercaptopurine, *5871*
Nelarabine, *6442*
Thiamiprine, *9299*
Thioguanine, *9337*
Tiazofurin, *9425*

Pyrimidine Analogs
Ancitabine, *629*
Azacitidine, *890*
6-Azauridine, *904*

ANTINEOPLASTIC

Antimetabolites (*continued*)
Capecitabine, *1754*
Carmofur, *1844*
Cytarabine, *2784*
Decitabine, *2853*
Doxifluridine, *3437*
Enocitabine, *3586*
Floxuridine, *4112*
Fluorouracil, *4181*
Gemcitabine, *4386*
Tegafur, *9112*
Troxacitabine, *9788*

Enzymes
L-Asparaginase, *836*
Ranpirnase, *8112*

Farnesyl Transferase Inhibitors
Lonafarnib, *5565*
Tipifarnib, *9458*

Immunomodulators
Aldesleukin *see 4994*
Interferon-α, *4990*
Interferon-γ, *4992*
Lentinan, *5439*
Mepact, *5844*
Oregovomab, *6865*
Propagermanium, *7795*
PSK®, *7927*
Roquinimex, *8259*
Sipuleucel-T, *8547*
Sizofiran, *8559*
Teceleukin *see 4994*
Ubenimex, *9842*

Immunotoxins
Cintredekin Besudotox, *2312*
Denileukin Diftitox, *2893*

Monoclonal Antibodies
Alemtuzumab, *228*
Bevacizumab, *1191*
Cetuximab, *2027*
Edrecolomab, *3515*
Epratuzumab, *3631*
Gemtuzumab Ozogamicin, *4390*
Oregovomab, *6865*
Panitumumab, *7010*
Rituximab, *8239*
Tositumomab [131]I *see 9554*
Trastuzumab, *9575*

Oligonucleotides
Aprinocarsen, *755*
Oblimersen Sodium, *6739*

Platinum Complexes
Carboplatin, *1822*
Cisplatin, *2317*
Lobaplatin, *5549*
Oxaliplatin, *6912*
Picoplatin, *7405*
Satraplatin, *8384*

Retinoids and Analogs
Alitretinoin, *249*
Bexarotene, *1194*
Fenretinide, *3998*
Mofarotene, *6230*
Tamibarotene, *9047*

Tyrosine Kinase Inhibitors
Canertinib, *1744*
Dasatinib, *2829*
Erlotinib, *3672*
Gefitinib, *4379*
Imatinib, *4902*
Lapatinib, *5367*
Sorafenib, *8720*
Sunitinib, *9000*
Vatalanib, *9939*

Others
Amsacrine, *594*
Arsenic Trioxide, *804*
Atrasentan, *870*
Bisantrene, *1244*
Bortezomib, *1351*
Brostallicin, *1449*
Calcitriol, *1644*
Edotecarin, *3512*
Eflornithine, *3522*
Flavopiridol, *4094*
Gallium Nitrate, *4350*
Hydroxyurea, *4848*
Liarozole, *5475*
Lonidamine, *5568*
Miltefosine, *6198*
Mitoguazone, *6213*
Mitoxantrone, *6217*
Nitracrine, *6571*
Pentostatin, *7135*
Perifosine, *7165*
Pixantrone, *7514*
Razoxane, *8123*
Seocalcitol, *8456*
Sobuzoxane, *8568*
Spirogermanium, *8758*
Tirapazamine, *9461*
Vorinostat, *10034*

ANTINEOPLASTIC (HORMONAL)

Androgens
Dromostanolone, *3448*
Epitiostanol, *3624*
Mepitiostane, *5858*
Testolactone, *9179*

Antiadrenals
Aminoglutethimide, *440*
Mitotane, *6216*
Trilostane, *9698*

Antiandrogens
Bicalutamide, *1200*
Flutamide, *4208*
Nilutamide, *6544*

Antiestrogens
Arzoxifene, *820*
Droloxifene, *3446*
Fulvestrant, *4284*
Idoxifene, *4890*
Tamoxifen, *9048*
Toremifene, *9550*

Antiprogestins
Onapristone, *6847*

Aromatase Inhibitors
Aminoglutethimide, *440*
Anastrozole, *625*
Exemestane, *3913*
Fadrozole, *3927*
Formestane, *4240*
Letrozole, *5450*
Vorozole, *10035*

Estrogens
Diethylstilbestrol, *3129*
Fosfestrol, *4253*
Hexestrol, *4701*
Polyestradiol Phosphate, *7566*

LH-RH Analogs
Abarelix, *3*
Buserelin, *1503*
Cetrorelix, *2026*
Goserelin, *4526*
Leuprolide, *5457*
Triptorelin, *9748*

Progestogens
Chlormadinone Acetate, *2102*
Medroxyprogesterone, *5793*
Megestrol Acetate, *5805*

Somatostatin Analog
Lanreotide, *5361*

ANTINEOPLASTIC (PHOTOSENSI-TIZER)

δ-Aminolevulinic Acid, *446*
Methyl Aminolevulinate, *6016*
Motexafin Lutetium, *6282*
Porfimer Sodium, *7596*
Talaporfin, *9034*
Temoporfin, *9138*

ANTINEOPLASTIC (RADIATION SOURCE)

Americium [241]Am *see 392*
Californium [252]Cf *see 1716*
Chromic Phosphate [32]P *see 2227*
Cobalt [60]Co *see 2427*
Edotreotide [90]Y Chelate *see 3513*
Epratuzumab Tetraxetan [90]Y *see 3631*
Ethiodized Oil [131]I *see 3735*
Gold, Radioactive, Colloidal, *4517*
Ibritumomab Tiuxetan [90]Y *see 4878*
Iobenguane [131]I *see 5007*
Radium, *8094*
Radon, *8095*
Samarium [153]Sm Lexidronam, *8350*
Sodium Iodide, Radioactive, *8632*
Sodium Phosphate, Radioactive, *8661*
Strontium [89]Sr *see 8835*
Strontium [89]Sr Chloride *see 8840*
Tositumomab [131]I *see 9554*

ANTINEOPLASTIC ADJUNCT

Antimetastatic Agent
Batimastat, *1008*
Marimastat, *5753*
Prinomastat, *7751*

Chemomodulator
Eniluracil, *3584*

Chemosensitizer
Biricodar, *1240*
Tariquidar, *9064*
Tesmilifene, *9178*
Valspodar, *9917*
Zosuquidar, *10196*

Folic Acid Replenisher
Folinic Acid, *4222*

Radioprotective
Amifostine, *404*
Palifermin, *6986*

Radiosensitizer
Broxuridine, *1452*
Efaproxiral, *3520*
Etanidazole, *3713*
Motexafin Gadolinium, *6281*

Uroprotective
Mesna, *5909*

ANTINEUTROPENIC
Granulocyte Colony-Stimulating
Factor, *4537*
Granulocyte-Macrophage Col-
ony-Stimulating Factor, *4538*
Interleukin-3, *4995*

ANTIOBESITY AGENT *see also An-orexic*
Orlistat, *6869*
Rimonabant, *8229*
Sibutramine, *8485*

ANTIOBSESSIONAL
Clomipramine, *2387*
Fluoxetine, *4185*
Fluvoxamine, *4219*
Paroxetine, *7043*
Sertraline, *8467*

ANTIOSTEOPOROTIC *see also Bone Resorption Inhibitor; Calcium Regulator*
Alendronic Acid, *229*
Bazedoxifene, *1013*
Clodronic Acid, *2371*
Etidronic Acid, *3863*
Ibandronic Acid, *4873*
Incadronic Acid, *4929*
Neridronic Acid, *6473*
Pamidronic Acid, *7003*
Raloxifene, *8098*
Risedronic Acid, *8232*
Sodium Fluoride, *8618*
Strontium Ranelate *see 8106*
Teriparatide Acetate, *9166*
Zoledronic Acid, *10187*

ANTIPAGETIC *see also Bone Re-sorption Inhibitor; Calcium Regula-tor*
Alendronic Acid, *229*
Elcatonin, *3537*
Gallium Nitrate, *4350*
Neridronic Acid, *6473*
Pamidronic Acid, *7003*
Risedronic Acid, *8232*
Tiludronic Acid, *9441*
Zoledronic Acid, *10187*

ANTIPARKINSONIAN
Amantadine, *374*
Apomorphine, *746*
Benserazide, *1050*
Benzetimide, *1075*

Benztropine Mesylate, *1121*
Biperiden, *1233*
Bromocriptine, *1416*
Budipine, *1469*
Cabergoline, *1601*
Carbidopa, *1797*
Dexetimide, *2945*
Diethazine, *3108*
Droxidopa, *3457*
Entacapone, *3594*
Ethopropazine, *3747*
Ethybenztropine, *3756*
Idazoxan, *4887*
Lazabemide, *5394*
Levodopa, *5464*
Memantine, *5829*
Methixene, *5979*
Pergolide, *7162*
Piroheptine, *7503*
Pramipexole, *7705*
Pridinol Hydrochloride *see 7741*
Procyclidine, *7763*
Prodipine, *7768*
Rasagiline, *8116*
Ropinirole, *8257*
Safinamide, *8315*
Scopolamine *N*-Oxide, *8407*
Selegiline, *8428*
Talipexole, *9039*
Terguride, *9164*
Tolcapone, *9508*
Trihexyphenidyl Hydrochloride, *9695*
Tropacine, *9773*

ANTIPERISTALTIC *see Anti-diarrheal*

ANTIPHEOCHROMOCYTOMA
Metyrosine, *6161*
Phenoxybenzamine, *7256*
Phentolamine, *7264*

ANTIPNEUMOCYSTIC
Atovaquone, *866*
Eflornithine, *3522*
Pentamidine, *7115*
Sulfamethoxazole, *8918*

ANTIPROGESTIN *see also Selective Progesterone Receptor Modulator*
Onapristone, *6847*

ANTIPROSTATIC HYPERTROPHY
Alfuzosin, *238*
Doxazosin, *3433*
Dutasteride, *3471*
Epristeride, *3634*
Finasteride, *4082*
Gestonorone Caproate, *4414*
Mepartricin, *5847*
Osaterone, *6888*
Oxendolone, *6931*
Tamsulosin, *9049*
Terazosin, *9154*

ANTIPROTOZOAL (AMEBA) *see Antiamebic*

ANTIPROTOZOAL (CRYPTOSPO-RIDIUM)
Nitazoxanide, *6567*

ANTIPROTOZOAL (GIARDIA)
Acranil®, *121*
Tinidazole, *9447*

ANTIPROTOZOAL (LEISHMANIA)
Ethylstibamine, *3852*
Hydroxystilbamidine, *4845*
N-Methylglucamine, *6078*
Miltefosine, *6198*
Pentamidine, *7115*
Sitamaquine, *8553*
Sodium Stibogluconate *see 701*
Stilbamidine, *8816*
Urea Stibamine, *9871*

ANTIPROTOZOAL (MALARIA) *see Antimalarial*

ANTIPROTOZOAL (PNEUMOCYS-TIS) *see Antipneumocystic*

ANTIPROTOZOAL (TOXO-PLASMA)
Pyrimethamine, *7985*

ANTIPROTOZOAL (TRICHO-MONAS)
Acetarsone, *52*
Aminitrozole, *410*
Azanidazole, *897*
Furazolidone, *4300*
Hachimycin, *4586*
Lauroguadine, *5386*
Mepartricin, *5847*
Metronidazole, *6157*
Nifuratel, *6532*
Nifuroxime, *6536*
Nimorazole, *6552*
Secnidazole, *8419*
Silver Picrate, *8526*
Tenonitrozole, *9147*
Tinidazole, *9447*

ANTIPROTOZOAL (TRYPANO-SOMA)
Benznidazole, *1084*
Eflornithine, *3522*
Melarsoprol, *5815*
Nifurtimox, *6538*
Oxophenarsine Hydrochloride, *6948*
Pentamidine, *7115*
Propamidine, *7797*
Quinapyramine, *8052*
Stilbamidine, *8816*
Suramin Sodium, *9006*
Trypan Red, *9793*
Tryparsamide, *9794*

ANTIPRURITIC
Camphor, *1732*
Cyproheptadine, *2773*

ANTIPRURITIC (continued)

Dichlorisone, 3048
Halometasone, 4597
3-Hydroxycamphor, 4817
Menthol, 5837
Mesulfen, 5918
Methdilazine, 5964
Phenol, 7241
Polidocanol, 7558
Thenaldine, 9278
Tolpropamine, 9523
Trimeprazine, 9704

ANTIPSORIATIC

Abatacept, 4
Acitretin, 112
Alefacept, 227
Ammonium Salicylate, 550
Anthralin, 684
6-Azauridine, 904
Bergapten, 1157
Calcipotriene, 1641
Calcitriol, 1644
Chrysarobin, 2253
Efalizumab, 3519
Etanercept, 3712
Etretinate, 3892
Flurandrenolide, 4197
Maxacalcitol, 5760
Pyrogallol, 8000
Tacalcitol, 9022
Tazarotene, 9081

ANTIPSYCHOTIC

Benzamides

Amisulpride, 485
Nemonapride, 6446
Remoxipride, 8132
Sulpiride, 8989
Sultopride, 8994

Benzisoxazoles

Iloperidone, 4900
Risperidone, 8233

Butyrophenones

Benperidol, 1048
Bromperidol, 1442
Droperidol, 3450
Fluanisone, 4114
Haloperidol, 4598
Melperone, 5827
Moperone, 6263
Pipamperone, 7455
Spiperone, 8751
Timiperone, 9443
Trifluperidol, 9684

Phenothiazines

Acetophenazine, 72
Butaperazine, 1516
Carphenazine, 1860
Chlorpromazine, 2185
Clospirazine, 2412
Cyamemazine, 2683
Dixyrazine, 3385
Fluphenazine, 4189
Mesoridazine, 5910
Metofenazate, 6145
Perazine, 7151
Pericyazine, 7164
Perimethazine, 7168
Perphenazine, 7183
Piperacetazine, 7462

Pipotiazine, 7482
Prochlorperazine, 7761
Promazine, 7783
Sulforidazine, 8963
Thiopropazate, 9356
Thioproperazine, 9357
Thioridazine, 9359
Trifluoperazine, 9680
Triflupromazine, 9685

Thioxanthenes

Chlorprothixene, 2188
Clopenthixol, 2394
Flupentixol, 4187
Thiothixene, 9365

Other Tricyclics

Asenapine, 832
Benzquinamide, 1119
Carpipramine, 1861
Clocapramine, 2366
Clothiapine, 2415
Clozapine, 2423
Mosapramine, 6278
Olanzapine, 6822
Opipramol, 6853
Prothipendyl, 7888
Quetiapine, 8039
Tetrabenazine, 9182
Zotepine, 10197

Others

Aripiprazole, 785
Bifeprunox, 1210
Blonanserin, 1319
Buramate, 1501
Fluspirilene, 4207
Molindone, 6233
Penfluridol, 7087
Perospirone, 7182
Pimozide, 7435
Sertindole, 8466
Ziprasidone, 10171

ANTIPYRETIC

Acetaminophen, 47
Acetaminosalol, 48
Alclofenac, 219
Aminopyrine, 474
Aspirin, 851
Benorylate, 1045
Benzydamine, 1122
Berberine, 1154
Bermoprofen, 1159
p-Bromoacetanilide, 1399
Bufexamac, 1474
Bumadizon, 1483
Calcium Acetylsalicylate, 1647
Choline Salicylate, 2209
Dipyrocetyl, 3349
Dipyrone, 3350
Epirizole, 3622
Imidazole Salicylate, 4913
Lysine Acetylsalicylate, 5637
Magnesium Acetylsalicylate, 5655
Meclofenamic Acid, 5779
Morazone, 6267
Morpholine Salicylate see 6277
Naproxen, 6417
5′-Nitro-2′-propoxyacetanilide, 6629
Phenacetin, 7204
Phenocoll, 7239
Phenyl Acetylsalicylate, 7270
Phenyl Salicylate, 7310

Pipebuzone, 7457
Propacetamol, 7792
Propyphenazone, 7871
Ramifenazone, 8102
Salicylamide O-Acetic Acid, 8329
Sodium Salicylate see 8332
Tetrandrine, 9231
Tinoridine, 9448

ANTIRESTENOTIC

Paclitaxel, 6982
Rapamycin, 8114

ANTIRHEUMATIC see Antiarthritic/Antirheumatic

ANTIRICKETTSIAL

p-Aminobenzoic Acid, 423
Chloramphenicol, 2077
Tetracycline, 9196

ANTISEBORRHEIC

Chloroxine, 2175
Piroctone, 7502
Pyrithione, 7994
Resorcinol, 8155
Selenium Sulfides, 8436
Tioxolone, 9456

ANTISEPSIS

Drotecogin Alfa see 7884
Eritoran, 3671
Opebacan see 938

ANTISEPTIC/DISINFECTANT

Alcohols

Dichlorobenzyl Alcohol, 3060
Ethyl Alcohol, 3760
Isopropyl Alcohol, 5208

Aldehydes

Formaldehyde Solution see 4235
Glutaraldehyde, 4472

Dyes

Acriflavine, 123
Aminacrine, 407
Brilliant Green, 1374
Ethacridine, 3716
Gentian Violet, 4395
Magenta I, 5652
Methyl Blue, 6028

Guanidines

Alexidine, 232
Chlorhexidine, 2091
Picloxydine, 7398
Polihexanide, 7560

Halogens/Halogen Containing Compounds

Bibrocathol, 1199
Bismuth Iodide Oxide, 1270
Bismuth Tribromophenate, 1291
Bornyl Chloride, 1340
Calcium Iodate, 1676
Chlorinated Lime, 2094
Cloflucarban, 2379

Fluorosalan, *4178*
Iodic Acid, *5012*
Iodine, *5014*
Iodine Monochloride, *5017*
Iodine Trichloride, *5020*
Iodoform, *5033*
Oxychlorosene, *6956*
Povidone-Iodine, *7698*
Sodium Hypochlorite, *8628*
Sodium Iodate, *8630*
Trichloroisocyanuric Acid, *9641*
Triclocarban, *9654*
Triclosan, *9657*
Troclosene Potassium, *9767*

Mercurial compounds
Meralein Sodium, *5865*
Merbromin, *5867*
Mercuric Chloride, *5876*
Mercuric Sodium *p*-Phenolsul-
fonate, *5886*
Mercuric Sulfide, Red, *5889*
Mercurophen, *5891*
Mercurous Acetate, *5892*
Mercurous Chloride, *5894*
Nitromersol, *6610*
Potassium Tetraiodomercur-
ate(II), *7688*
Thimerosal, *9317*

Nitrofurans
Furazolidone, *4300*
Nifuroxime, *6536*
Nifurzide, *6540*
Nitrofurazone, *6600*

Peroxides/Permanganates
Calcium Peroxide, *1689*
Carbamide Peroxide, *1782*
Hydrogen Peroxide, *4798*
Magnesium Peroxide, *5680*
Potassium Permanganate, *7655*
Strontium Peroxide, *8847*

Phenols
Bithionol, *1306*
Cadmium Salicylate, *1625*
Carvacrol, *1872*
Chlorocresol, *2133*
Chloroxylenol, *2176*
Creosote, Wood, *2573*
Cresols, *2579*
Fenticlor, *4004*
Hexachlorophene, *4680*
1-Naphthyl Salicylate, *6414*
2-Naphthyl Salicylate, *6415*
2,4,6-Tribromo-*m*-cresol, *9612*

**Quaternary Ammonium Com-
pounds**
Benzalkonium Chloride, *1059*
Benzethonium Chloride, *1074*
Benzoxonium Chloride, *1111*
Bisdequalinium Chloride, *1248*
Cetalkonium Chloride, *2017*
Cethexonium Bromide, *2019*
Cetrimonium Bromide, *2025*
Cetylpyridinium Chloride, *2032*
Dequalinium Chloride, *2913*
Domiphen Bromide, *3415*
Lapyrium Chloride, *5370*
Laurolinium Acetate, *5387*
Methylbenzethonium Chloride,
6023
Phenoctide, *7240*
Tibezonium Iodide, *9426*
Triclobisonium Chloride, *9653*

Quinolines
Aminoquinuride, *475*
Broxyquinoline, *1453*
Chloroxine, *2175*
Chlorquinaldol, *2190*
Cloxyquin, *2422*
Hydrastine, *4767*
8-Hydroxyquinoline, *4843*
Iodochlorhydroxyquin, *5031*

Silver compounds
Silver Bromide, *8506*
Silver Fluoride, *8514*
Silver Lactate, *8517*
Silver Nitrate, *8518*
Silver Protein, *8527*

Others
Aluminum Acetate Solution, *324*
Aluminum Lactate, *348*
Aluminum Subacetate Solution,
365
Aluminum Sulfate, *366*
3-Amino-4-hydroxybutyric Acid,
443
Boric Acid, *1336*
Chloroazodin, *2120*
m-Cresyl Acetate, *2583*
Cupric Sulfate, *2653*
Dibromopropamidine, *3024*
Hexamidine, *4692*
Ichthammol, *4885*
Noxythiolin, *6724*
Octenidine, *6754*
Ornidazole, *6872*
Policresulen, *7556*
Polynoxylin, *7574*
β-Propiolactone, *7820*
α-Terpineol, *9171*

ANTISPASMODIC *see also **Antimuscarinic***

Adiphenine, *161*
Alibendol, *244*
Alverine, *371*
Ambutonium Bromide, *387*
Aminopentamide, *459*
Aminopromazine, *467*
Anisotropine Methylbromide, *671*
Atropine, *875*
Benactyzine, *1029*
Bevonium Methyl Sulfate, *1193*
Bietamiverine, *1205*
Butropium Bromide, *1534*
N-Butylscopolammonium Bro-
mide, *1588*
Buzepide, *1599*
Caroverine, *1857*
Chlorbenzoxamine, *2080*
Cimetropium Bromide, *2280*
Cinnamedrine, *2298*
Clebopride, *2344*
Clidinium Bromide, *2354*
Cyclonium Iodide, *2737*
Darifenacin, *2825*
Dicyclomine, *3097*
Difemerine, *3132*
Dihexyverine, *3168*
Drofenine, *3445*
Drotaverine, *3455*
Emepronium Bromide, *3558*
Ethaverine, *3728*
Etomidoline, *3882*
Fenoverine, *3982*
Fenpiverinium Bromide, *3990*
Fentonium Bromide, *4006*

Flavoxate, *4096*
Flopropione, *4106*
Glycopyrrolate, *4501*
Hymecromone, *4854*
Hyoscyamine, *4858*
Isopropamide Iodide, *5202*
Mebeverine, *5769*
Memantine, *5829*
Mepenzolate Bromide, *5848*
Methantheline Bromide, *5958*
Methscopolamine Bromide, *6003*
Moxaverine, *6288*
Otilonium Bromide, *6898*
Oxyphencyclimine, *6973*
Oxyphenonium Bromide, *6975*
Phloroglucinol, *7328*
Pinaverium Bromide, *7441*
Pipenzolate Bromide, *7461*
Piperidolate, *7470*
Piperilate, *7471*
Pipoxolan Hydrochloride, *7483*
Poldine Methylsulfate, *7554*
Pramiverin, *7707*
Prifinium Bromide, *7742*
Propantheline Bromide, *7805*
Proxazole, *7903*
Prozapine, *7906*
Rociverine, *8245*
Scopolamine, *8406*
Tiemonium Iodide, *9431*
Tigloidine, *9434*
Timepidium Bromide, *9442*
Tiquizium Bromide, *9460*
Tiropramide, *9466*
Trepibutone, *9585*
Tricromyl, *9658*
Tridihexethyl Iodide, *9661*
Trimebutine, *9699*
Trospium Chloride, *9786*
Valethamate Bromide, *9906*

ANTITHROMBOCYTHEMIC
Anagrelide, *622*

ANTITHROMBOTIC *see also **Anticoagulant; Thrombolytic***

Abciximab, *5*
Ardeparin, *775*
Argatroban, *779*
Aspirin, *851*
Beraprost, *1152*
Bivalirudin, *1310*
Cangrelor, *1746*
Cilostazol, *2277*
Clinprost, *2358*
Clopidogrel, *2396*
Cloricromen, *2405*
Dabigatran, *2797*
Dalteparin, *2805*
Daltroban, *2806*
Danaparoid, *2811*
Defibrotide, *2861*
Dipyridamole, *3346*
Enoxaparin, *3588*
Eptifibatide, *3641*
Fondaparinux Sodium, *4232*
Idraparinux Sodium, *4892*
Iloprost, *4901*
Indobufen, *4961*
Lamifiban, *5349*
Melagatran, *5810*
Nadroparin, *6349*
Ozagrel, *6980*
Pamicogrel, *7002*

ANTITHROMBOTIC (continued)

Picotamide, 7407
Plafibride, 7516
Reviparin Sodium, 8170
Ridogrel, 8212
Satigrel, 8383
Sulfinpyrazone, 8949
Sulodexide, 8986
Taprostene, 9057
Ticlopidine, 9429
Tifacogin see 9467
Tinzaparin, 9450
Tirofiban, 9464
Triflusal, 9688
Xemilofiban, 10070
Ximelagatran, 10077

ANTITUBERCULAR see Antibacterial (Tuberculostatic)

ANTITUMOR see Antineoplastic

ANTITUSSIVE

Benproperine, 1049
Benzonatate, 1096
Bromoform, 1420
Butamirate, 1513
Butethamate, 1522
Caramiphen, 1776
Carbetapentane, 1794
Chlophedianol, 2066
Clobutinol, 2365
Cloperastine, 2395
Codeine, 2463
Codeine Phosphate, 2464
Dextromethorphan see 8091
Dihydrocodeine, 3171
Dihydrocodeinone Enol Acetate, 3172
Dimemorfan, 3206
Dropropizine, 3452
Drotebanol, 3456
Eprazinone, 3632
Ethyl Dibunate, 3788
Ethylmorphine, 3830
Fominoben, 4228
Hydrocodone, 4785
Isoaminile, 5110
Levopropoxyphene, 5469
Narceine, 6422
Normethadone, 6709
Noscapine, 6718
Oxeladin, 6930
Oxolamine, 6944
Pholcodine, 7329
Picoperine, 7404
Pipazethate, 7456
Piperidione, 7469
Prenoxdiazine Hydrochloride, 7736
Racemethorphan, 8091
Sodium Dibunate, 8608
Tipepidine, 9457
Zipeprol, 10170

ANTIULCERATIVE see also Antacid

Aceglutamide Aluminum Complex see 25
Acetoxolone, 76
Aldioxa, 223
Benexate Hydrochloride, 1038
Bismuth Subnitrate, 1284

Carbenoxolone, 1793
Cetraxate, 2024
Cimetidine, 2279
Colloidal Bismuth Subcitrate, 2485
Ebrotidine, 3485
Ecabapide, 3488
Ecabet, 3489
Enprostil, 3591
Esaprazole, 3695
Famotidine, 3930
Gefarnate, 4378
Guaiazulene, 4554
Irsogladine, 5102
Lafutidine, 5347
Lansoprazole, 5362
S-Methylmethionine, 6098
Misoprostol, 6210
Nizatidine, 6660
Omeprazole, 6845
Ornoprostil, 6875
γ-Oryzanol, 6886
Pantoprazole, 7014
Pifarnine, 7420
Pirenzepine, 7491
Plaunotol, 7532
Polaprezinc, 7552
Rabeprazole, 8089
Ranitidine, 8110
Rebamipide, 8124
Revaprazan, 8168
Rioprostil, 8231
Rosaprostol, 8260
Roxatidine Acetate, 8274
Sofalcone, 8701
Sucralfate, 8879
Teprenone, 9153
Trimoprostil, 9723
Trithiozine, 9760
Troxipide, 9790
Zinc Acexamate see 45
Zolimidine, 10188

ANTIUROLITHIC

Acetohydroxamic Acid, 63
Allopurinol, 279
Potassium Citrate, 7623
Succinimide, 8871

ANTIVENIN

Antivenin (Latrodectus mactans), 721

ANTIVERTIGO see Antiemetic

ANTIVIRAL

Imidazoquinolines
Imiquimod, 4922
Resiquimod, 8151

Monoclonal Antibodies
Palivizumab, 6988

Peptidomimetics
Amprenavir, 589
Atazanavir, 858
Darunavir, 2827
Fosamprenavir, 4250
Indinavir, 4945
Lopinavir, 5573
Nelfinavir, 6443
Ritonavir, 8238
Saquinavir, 8369

Polynucleotides
Ampligen, 588
Fomivirsen, 4229

Purines/Pyrimidinones
Abacavir, 1
Acyclovir, 146
Adefovir, 151
Brivudine, 1378
Cidofovir, 2268
Clevudine, 2353
Didanosine, 3098
Dideoxyadenosine, 3101
Edoxudine, 3514
Emtricitabine, 3565
Entecavir, 3595
Famciclovir, 3929
Floxuridine, 4112
Ganciclovir, 4363
Idoxuridine, 4891
Inosine Pranobex, 4976
Lamivudine, 5352
Penciclovir, 7083
Sorivudine, 8727
Stavudine, 8803
Taribavirin, 9063
Telbivudine, 9117
Tenofovir, 9146
Trifluridine, 9687
Valacyclovir, 9899
Valganciclovir, 9907
Vidarabine, 9976
Zalcitabine, 10109
Zidovudine, 10123

Sialic Acid Analogs
Oseltamivir, 6889
Zanamivir, 10113

Others
Acemannan, 26
Acetylleucine Monoethanolamine, 95
Amantadine, 374
Amidinomycin, 400
Aplaviroc, 737
Capravirine, 1755
Delavirdine, 2877
n-Docosanol, 3399
Efavirenz, 3521
Enfuvirtide, 3582
Foscarnet Sodium, 4251
Interferon-α, 4990
Interferon-β, 4991
Interferon-γ, 4992
Kethoxal, 5299
Lysozyme, 5640
Maraviroc, 5749
Merimepodib, 5899
Methisazone, 5977
Moroxydine, 6272
Nevirapine, 6490
Pleconaril, 7533
Podophyllotoxin, 7546
Ribavirin, 8198
Rimantadine, 8224
Stallimycin, 8772
Statolon, 8801
Tipranavir, 9459
Tromantadine, 9771

ANXIOLYTIC

Arylpiperazines
Buspirone, 1504
Flesinoxan, 4100
Ipsapirone, 5081

Lesopitron, *5447*
Tandospirone, *9051*

Benzodiazepine Derivatives
Alprazolam, *312*
Bromazepam, *1385*
Camazepam, *1725*
Chlordiazepoxide, *2084*
Clobazam, *2359*
Clorazepic Acid, *2403*
Clotiazepam, *2416*
Cloxazolam, *2420*
Diazepam, *2994*
Ethyl Loflazepate, *3821*
Etizolam, *3873*
Fludiazepam, *4128*
Flutazolam, *4209*
Flutoprazepam, *4213*
Halazepam, *4589*
Ketazolam, *5297*
Lorazepam, *5579*
Medazepam, *5786*
Metaclazepam, *5920*
Mexazolam, *6166*
Nordazepam, *6691*
Oxazepam, *6926*
Oxazolam, *6927*
Pinazepam, *7442*
Prazepam, *7715*
Tofisopam, *9503*

Carbamates
Emylcamate, *3566*
Meprobamate, *5862*
Tybamate, *9829*

Others
Benzoctamine, *1087*
Captodiamine, *1773*
Chlormezanone, *2106*
Deramciclane, *2915*
Etifoxine, *3864*
Fluoresone, *4161*
Hydroxyzine, *4849*
Loxapine, *5587*
Phenibut *see 464*
Pregabalin, *7725*
Valnoctamide, *9912*

AROMATASE INHIBITORS *see also*
Antineoplastic (Hormonal)
Aminoglutethimide, *440*
Anastrozole, *625*
Exemestane, *3913*
Fadrozole, *3927*
Formestane, *4240*
Letrozole, *5450*
Vorozole, *10035*

ASTRINGENT
Alkannin, *257*
Aluminum Acetate Solution, *324*
Aluminum Acetotartrate, *325*
Aluminum Ammonium Sulfate, *327*
Aluminum Chlorate, *336*
Aluminum Chloride, *337*
Aluminum Hydroxychloride, *343*
Aluminum Potassium Sulfate, *360*
Aluminum Sodium Sulfate, *363*
Aluminum Subacetate Solution, *365*
Ammonium Ferric Sulfate, *518*

Baicalein, *942*
Bismuth Oxide, *1273*
Bismuth Subgallate, *1283*
Bismuth Tannate, *1288*
Boric Acid, *1336*
Calcium Hydroxide, *1673*
Cupric Citrate, *2636*
Dichloroacetic Acid, *3050*
Ferric Chloride, *4019*
Gallic Acid, *4345*
Iodic Acid, *5012*
Lead Acetate, *5397*
Methionic Acid, *5974*
Silver Bromide, *8506*
Silver Lactate, *8517*
Silver Nitrate, *8518*
Sodium Formate, *8621*
Tannic Acid, *9052*
Zinc Acetate, *10128*
Zinc Carbonate, *10131*
Zinc Chloride, *10132*
Zinc Iodide, *10140*
Zinc Oxide, *10147*
Zinc Peroxide, *10149*
Zinc *p*-Phenolsulfonate, *10150*
Zinc Salicylate, *10155*
Zinc Sulfate, *10159*

BENZODIAZEPINE ANTAGONIST
Flumazenil, *4135*

BETA-BLOCKER *see β-Adrenergic Blocker*

BLOOD SUBSTITUTE
Fluosol DA, *4183*
Polymerized Pyridoxylated Hemoglobin, *7572*

BONE RESORPTION INHIBITOR
see also ***Calcium Regulator***
Alendronic Acid, *229*
Clodronic Acid, *2371*
Etidronic Acid, *3863*
Gallium Nitrate, *4350*
Ibandronic Acid, *4873*
Incadronic Acid, *4929*
Neridronic Acid, *6473*
Pamidronic Acid, *7003*
Risedronic Acid, *8232*
Strontium Ranelate *see 8106*
Tiludronic Acid, *9441*
Zoledronic Acid, *10187*

BRADYCARDIC AGENT *see also*
Antianginal
Tedisamil, *9108*
Zatebradine, *10115*

BRADYKININ ANTAGONIST
Bradycor, *1358*

BRONCHODILATOR *see also An-
tiasthmatic; Glucocorticoid*
Ephedrine Derivatives
Albuterol, *216*
Bambuterol, *953*

Bitolterol, *1307*
Carbuterol, *1833*
Clenbuterol, *2347*
Clorprenaline, *2408*
Dioxethedrine, *3302*
Ephedrine, *3608*
Epinephrine, *3619*
Eprozinol, *3636*
Etafedrine, *3709*
Ethylnorepinephrine, *3834*
Fenoterol, *3981*
Formoterol, *4245*
Hexoprenaline, *4707*
Isoetharine, *5170*
Isoproterenol, *5217*
Mabuterol, *5642*
Metaproterenol, *5931*
N-Methylephedrine, *6068*
Pirbuterol, *7489*
Procaterol, *7759*
Protokylol, *7895*
Reproterol, *8139*
Rimiterol, *8227*
Salmeterol, *8337*
Soterenol, *8729*
Terbutaline, *9159*
Tulobuterol, *9811*

**Quaternary Ammonium Com-
pounds**
Flutropium Bromide, *4216*
Ipratropium Bromide, *5073*
Oxitropium Bromide, *6943*
Tiotropium Bromide, *9454*

Xanthine Derivatives
Acefylline, *24*
Aminophylline, *465*
Bamifylline, *955*
Choline Theophyllinate, *2210*
Doxofylline, *3438*
Dyphylline, *3479*
Etamiphyllin, *3711*
Etofylline, *3878*
Guaithylline *see 4555*
Proxyphylline, *7905*
Theobromine, *9282*
1-Theobromineacetic Acid, *9283*
Theophylline, *9285*

Others
Fenspiride, *3999*
Methoxyphenamine, *5998*
Tretoquinol, *9587*

CALCIUM CHANNEL BLOCKER
see also ***Antianginal; Antihyperten-
sive; Vasodilator (Coronary)***
Arylalkylamines
Bepridil, *1150*
Fendiline, *3970*
Gallopamil, *4356*
Mibefradil, *6173*
Prenylamine, *7737*
Semotiadil, *8446*
Verapamil, *9950*

Benzothiazepines
Clentiazem, *2348*
Diltiazem, *3202*

Dihydropyridine Derivatives
Amlodipine, *491*
Aranidipine, *767*
Barnidipine, *1002*
Benidipine, *1043*

CALCIUM CHANNEL BLOCKER
Dihydropyridine Derivatives
(*continued*)

Cilnidipine, *2275*
Clevidipine, *2352*
Efonidipine, *3524*
Elgodipine, *3546*
Felodipine, *3953*
Isradipine, *5240*
Lacidipine, *5331*
Lercanidipine, *5446*
Manidipine, *5743*
Nicardipine, *6495*
Nifedipine, *6528*
Nilvadipine, *6545*
Nimodipine, *6551*
Nisoldipine, *6565*
Nitrendipine, *6576*

Piperazine Derivatives
Cinnarizine, *2305*
Dotarizine, *3428*
Flunarizine, *4144*
Lidoflazine, *5484*
Lomerizine, *5563*

Others
Bencyclane, *1033*
Etafenone, *3710*
Fantofarone, *3934*
Perhexiline, *7163*

CALCIUM REGULATOR

Calcifediol, *1638*
Calcitonin, *1643*
Calcitriol, *1644*
Dihydrotachysterol, *3180*
Elcatonin, *3537*
Ipriflavone, *5074*
Parathyroid Hormone, *7034*
Teriparatide Acetate, *9166*

CALCIUM SUPPLEMENT *see Replenishers/Supplements*

CANCER CHEMOTHERAPY *see Antineoplastic*

CAPILLARY PROTECTANT *see Vasoprotectant*

CARBONIC ANHYDRASE INHIBITOR *see also Antiglaucoma; Diuretic*

Acetazolamide, *53*
Brinzolamide, *1376*
Dichlorphenamide, *3077*
Dorzolamide, *3426*
Ethoxzolamide, *3755*
Flumethiazide, *4139*
Methazolamide, *5962*

CARDIAC DEPRESSANT (ANTIARRHYTHMIC) *see Antiarrhythmic*

CARDIOPROTECTIVE

Acadesine, *16*
Cariporide, *1841*
Dexrazoxane *see 8123*

CARDIOTONIC

Acetyldigitoxins, *89*
2-Amino-4-picoline, *466*
Amrinone, *592*
Bucladesine, *1463*
Convallatoxin, *2512*
Cymarin, *2761*
Denopamine, *2894*
Deslanoside, *2921*
Digitalin, *3158*
Digitalis, *3159*
Digitoxin, *3163*
Digoxin, *3167*
Dobutamine, *3395*
Docarpamine, *3396*
Dopamine, *3421*
Dopexamine, *3424*
Enoximone, *3589*
Gitalin, *4430*
Gitoxin, *4434*
Glycocyamine, *4495*
Heptaminol, *4657*
Hydrastinine, *4768*
Ibopamine, *4876*
Lanatosides, *5354*
Levosimendan, *5471*
Loprinone, *5575*
Milrinone, *6197*
Neriifolin, *6474*
Oleandrin, *6826*
Ouabain, *6901*
Oxyfedrine, *6962*
Pimobendan, *7434*
Prenalterol, *7735*
Proscillaridin, *7874*
Resibufogenin, *8146*
Scillaren, *8399*
Scillarenin, *8400*
Strophanthin, *8852*
Sulmazole, *8985*
Theobromine, *9282*
Vesnarinone, *9970*
Xamoterol, *10055*

CATHARTIC *see Laxative/Cathartic*

CATION-EXCHANGE RESIN *see Ion-exchange Resin*

CCK ANTAGONIST

Loxiglumide, *5588*
Proglumide, *7775*

CENTRAL STIMULANT *see CNS Stimulant*

CEREBRAL VASODILATOR *see Vasodilator (Cerebral)*

CETP INHIBITOR *see also Antiatherosclerotic; Antilipemic*

Torcetrapib, *9549*

CHELATING AGENT

Ammonium Tetrathiomolybdate, *560*
Deferasirox, *2858*
Deferiprone, *2859*
Deferoxamine, *2860*
Ditiocarb Sodium, *3378*
EDTA, *3517*
Penicillamine, *7088*
Pentetate Calcium Trisodium, *7124*
Pentetic Acid, *7125*
Succimer, *8865*
Trientine, *9663*

CHOLECYSTOKININ ANTAGONIST *see CCK Antagonist*

CHOLELITHOLYTIC AGENT

Chenodiol, *2054*
Methyl *tert*-Butyl Ether, *6032*
Monoctanoin, *6252*
Ursodiol, *9889*

CHOLERETIC

Alibendol, *244*
Anethole Trithione, *644*
Azintamide, *914*
Cholic Acid, *2203*
Clanobutin, *2338*
Cyclobutyrol, *2715*
Cyclovalone, *2755*
Cynarin(e), *2766*
Dehydrocholic Acid, *2868*
Deoxycholic Acid, *2899*
Dimecrotic Acid, *3203*
α-Ethylbenzyl Alcohol, *3768*
Febuprol, *3947*
Fenipentol, *3975*
Florantyrone, *4107*
Hymecromone, *4854*
Menbutone, *5834*
Osalmid, *6887*
Ox Bile Extract, *6928*
4,4′-Oxydi-2-butanol, *6960*
Piprozolin, *7485*
4-Salicyloylmorpholine, *8333*
Sincalide, *8543*
Taurocholic Acid, *9075*
Tocamphyl, *9492*
Trepibutone, *9585*

CHOLINERGIC

Aceclidine *see 8082*
Acetylcholine Bromide, *86*
Acetylcholine Chloride, *87*
Aclatonium Napadisilate, *114*
Bethanechol Chloride, *1185*
Carbachol, *1779*
Demecarium Bromide, *2885*
Dexpanthenol, *2947*
Diisopropyl Paraoxon, *3198*
Echothiophate Iodide, *3501*
Edrophonium Chloride, *3516*
Eptastigmine, *3638*
Eseridine, *3699*
Furtrethonium, *4312*
Guanidine, *4562*
Isoflurophate, *5176*
Methacholine Chloride, *5940*
Muscarine, *6310*
Neostigmine, *6464*
Oxapropanium Iodide, *6923*
Physostigmine, *7384*
Pyridostigmine Bromide, *7977*
Xanomeline, *10056*

CHOLINESTERASE INHIBITOR

Ambenonium Chloride, *379*
Distigmine Bromide, *3362*
Eptastigmine, *3638*
Galantamine, *4340*
Phenserine, *7260*
Rivastigmine, *8240*
Tacrine, *9024*

CHOLINESTERASE REACTIVA-TOR

Asoxime Chloride, *835*
HLö-7, *4724*
Obidoxime Chloride, *6738*
Pralidoxime Chloride, *7703*

CNS STIMULANT

Amphetamine, *582*
Amphetaminil, *583*
Bemegride, *1027*
Benzphetamine, *1118*
Brucine, *1455*
Caffeine, *1636*
Chlorphentermine, *2182*
Clortermine, *2410*
Coca, *2453*
Deanol, *2843*
Demanyl Phosphate, *2884*
Dexoxadrol *see 3299*
Dextroamphetamine, *2954*
Diethylpropion, *3127*
Ethamivan, *3721*
N-Ethylamphetamine, *3763*
Fencamfamine, *3966*
Fenethylline, *3972*
Fenozolone, *3988*
Flurothyl, *4201*
Lobeline, *5551*
Mazindol, *5762*
Methamphetamine, *5948*
Methylphenidate, *6110*
Modafinil, *6228*
Nikethamide, *6543*
Pemoline, *7079*
Pentylenetetrazole, *7141*
Phendimetrazine, *7220*
Phenmetrazine, *7237*
Phentermine, *7262*
Picrotoxin, *7415*
Pipradrol, *7484*
Prolintane, *7781*
Pyrovalerone, *8010*

COGNITION ACTIVATOR *see Nootropic*

COMT INHIBITOR

Entacapone, *3594*
Tolcapone, *9508*

CONTRACEPTIVE (IMPLANTABLE)

Elcometrine, *3538*
Etonogestrel, *3884*
Levonorgestrel *see 6704*

CONTRACEPTIVE (INJECTABLE)

Medroxyprogesterone, *5793*
Norethindrone, *6697*

CONTRACEPTIVE (ORAL)

Centchroman, *1971*
Desogestrel, *2926*
Dienogest, *3106*
Drospirenone, *3454*
Ethinyl Estradiol, *3734*
Ethynodiol, *3860*
Gestodene, *4413*
Lynestrenol, *5629*
Mestranol, *5917*
Norethindrone, *6697*
Norethynodrel, *6698*
Norgestimate, *6703*
Norgestrel, *6704*

CONTRACEPTIVE (TRANSDERMAL)

Norelgestromin, *6694*

CONVERTING ENZYME INHIBITOR *see ACE-Inhibitor*

CORONARY VASODILATOR *see Vasodilator (Coronary)*

CYCLOOXYGENASE-2 SELECTIVE INHIBITOR *see also Antiinflammatory (Nonsteroidal)*

Celecoxib, *1956*
Etoricoxib, *3887*
Lumiracoxib, *5601*
Parecoxib, *7036*
Rofecoxib, *8248*
Valdecoxib, *9900*

CYTOPROTECTANT (GASTRIC) *see also Antiulcerative*

Aceglutamide Aluminum Complex *see 25*
Acetoxolone, *76*
Benexate Hydrochloride, *1038*
Carbenoxolone, *1793*
Cetraxate, *2024*
Dosmalfate, *3427*
Guaiazulene, *4554*
Irsogladine, *5102*
Plaunotol, *7532*
Polaprezinc, *7552*
Rebamipide, *8124*
Sofalcone, *8701*
Sucralfate, *8879*
Teprenone, *9153*
Troxipide, *9790*
Zolimidine, *10188*

DEBRIDING AGENT

Collagenase, *2481*
Deoxyribonuclease I, *2906*
Papain, *7016*
Streptodornase, *8823*

DECONGESTANT

Amidephrine, *399*
Cafaminol, *1633*
Cyclopentamine, *2740*
Ephedrine, *3608*
Epinephrine, *3619*
Fenoxazoline, *3985*
Indanazoline, *4932*
Naphazoline, *6368*
Nordefrin, *6692*
Octodrine, *6757*
Oxymetazoline, *6966*
Phenylephrine, *7286*
Phenylpropanolamine, *7307*
Phenylpropylmethylamine, *7308*
Propylhexedrine, *7860*
Pseudoephedrine, *7916*
Tetrahydrozoline, *9219*
Tramazoline, *9567*
Tuaminoheptane, *9802*
Tymazoline, *9834*
Xylometazoline, *10086*

DENTAL PLAQUE INHIBITOR

Delmopinol, *2879*

DEPIGMENTOR

Hydroquinine, *4807*
Hydroquinone, *4808*
Monobenzone, *6248*

DERMATITIS HERPETIFORMIS SUPPRESSANT

Dapsone, *2822*
Sulfapyridine, *8938*

DIAGNOSTIC AID

Alsactide, *314*
Americium ^{241}Am *see 392*
p-Aminohippuric Acid, *442*
Anazolene Sodium, *628*
Arbutamine, *772*
Arginine, *780*
Bentiromide, *1054*
Betazole, *1183*
Binodenoson, *1225*
Broxuridine, *1452*
Ceruletide, *2005*
Colfosceril Palmitate, *2477*
Congo Red, *2498*
Cosyntropin, *2551*
Cystatin C *see 2778*
Dexamethasone, *2943*
Dipyridamole, *3346*
Edrophonium Chloride, *3516*
Evan's Blue, *3905*
Fluorescein, *4159*
D-Galactose, *4335*
Glycerol, *4484*
Gold Sodium Thiosulfate, *4519*
Hexaminolevulinate, *4693*
Histamine, *4719*
Ibopamine, *4876*
Indocyanine Green, *4962*
Inulin, *5004*
Iodinated Serum Albumin *see 8468*
Isosulphan Blue *see 8987*
Mannitol, *5745*
Methacholine Chloride, *5940*
Metyrapone, *6159*
Nickel Sulfate, *6517*
Oleic Acid, *6828*
Penicilloyl Polylysine, *7101*
3-Pentadecylcatechol, *7110*
Pentagastrin, *7113*
Phenolsulfonphthalein, *7247*

Phenoltetrachlorophthalein, 7248
Phentolamine, 7264
Piperoxan, 7478
Porfimer Sodium, 7596
Rose Bengal, 8262
Saralasin, 8372
Secretin, 8421
Sodium Benzoate, 8582
Sodium Chromate(VI), Radioactive see 8601
Sodium Iodide, Radioactive, 8632
Sulfobromophthalein Sodium, 8954
Teriparatide Acetate, 9166
Thyrotropin, 9414
Tolonium Chloride, 9520
Tuberculin, 9805
Vitamin B_{12}, Radioactive, 10015
Xylose, 10087

DIAGNOSTIC AID (MRI CONTRAST AGENT)

Ferumoxides, 4063
Ferumoxsil, 4064
Ferumoxtran 10, 4065
Gadobenate Dimeglumine, 4322
Gadobutrol, 4323
Gadodiamide, 4324
Gadofosveset, 4325
Gadopentetic Acid, 4327
Gadoteridol, 4328
Gadoversetamide, 4329
Gadoxetic Acid, 4330
Mangafodipir, 5722
Perflubron, 7156

DIAGNOSTIC AID (RADIOACTIVE IMAGING AGENT)

Arcitumomab Complex with ^{99m}Tc see 774
Butedronic Acid Complex with ^{99m}Tc see 1517
Capromab Pendetide ^{111}In see 1762
Depreotide Complex with ^{99m}Tc see 2911
Disofenin Complex with ^{99m}Tc see 3358
Exametazime Complex with ^{99m}Tc see 3911
Fludeoxyglucose F^{18}, 4127
Gallium Citrate, 4349
IACFT ^{123}I see 4871
Iobenguane ^{123}I see 5007
o-Iodohippurate Sodium ^{123}I see 5034
o-Iodohippurate Sodium ^{131}I see 5034
Iofetamine ^{123}I, 5049
Ioflupane ^{123}I, 5050
Krypton ^{81m}Kr see 5325
Lidofenin Complex with ^{99m}Tc see 5483
Mebrofenin Complex with ^{99m}Tc see 5772
Medronic Acid Complex with ^{99m}Tc see 5792
Oxidronic Acid Complex with ^{99m}Tc see 6940
Pentetreotide Chelate with ^{111}In see 7126

Satumomab Pendetide ^{111}In see 8385
Selenomethionine ^{75}Se see 8441
Sodium Pertechnetate ^{99m}Tc, 8657
Sodium Phosphate, Radioactive, 8661
Stannous Pyrophosphate Complex with ^{99m}Tc see 8788
Succimer Complex with ^{99m}Tc see 8865
Sulesomab Complex with ^{99m}Tc see 8895
Technetium, 9097
Technetium ^{99m}Tc Apcitide, 9098
Technetium ^{99m}Tc Bicisate, 9099
Technetium ^{99m}Tc Fanolesomab, 9100
Technetium ^{99m}Tc Gluceptate see 4455
Technetium ^{99m}Tc Mertiatide, 9101
Technetium ^{99m}Tc Sestamibi, 9102
Technetium ^{99m}Tc Teboroxime, 9103
Tetrofosmin Complex with ^{99m}Tc see 9247
Xenon ^{133}Xe see 10072

DIAGNOSTIC AID (RADIOPAQUE MEDIUM)

Acetrizoate Sodium, 79
Barium Sulfate, 994
Bunamiodyl Sodium, 1486
Diatrizoate Sodium, 2992
Ethiodized Oil, 3735
Iobitridol, 5008
Iocarmic Acid, 5009
Iocetamic Acid, 5010
Iodamide, 5011
Iodipamide, 5022
Iodixanol, 5023
Iodized Oil, 5024
Iodoalphionic Acid, 5026
o-Iodohippurate Sodium, 5034
Iodophthalein Sodium, 5038
Iodopyracet, 5040
Ioglycamic Acid, 5051
Iohexol, 5052
Iomeglamic Acid, 5053
Iomeprol, 5054
Iopamidol, 5057
Iopanoic Acid, 5058
Iopentol, 5059
Iophendylate, 5060
Iophenoxic Acid, 5061
Iopromide, 5062
Iopronic Acid, 5063
Iothalamic Acid, 5064
Iotrolan, 5065
Ioversol, 5066
Ioxaglic Acid, 5067
Ioxilan, 5068
Ipodate, 5071
Meglumine Acetrizoate, 5806
Meglumine Diatrizoate, 5807
Methiodal Sodium, 5973
Metrizamide, 6155
Metrizoic Acid, 6156
Phentetiothalein Sodium, 7263
Propyliodone, 7863
Sodium Iodomethamate, 8633
3′,3″,5′,5″-Tetrabromophenolphthalein, 9186

Thorium Oxide, 9377
Tyropanoate Sodium, 9837

DIAGNOSTIC AID (ULTRASOUND CONTRAST AGENT)

Perfluorohexane, 7157
Perfluoropropane, 7158
Serum Albumin, 8468

DIGESTIVE AID

Amylase, 599
Lipase, 5511
Papain, 7016
Pepsin, 7146
Rennin, 8134

DIPEPTIDYL PEPTIDASE IV INHIBITOR

Sitagliptin, 8552
Vildagliptin, 9979

DISINFECTANT see Antiseptic/Disinfectant

DIURETIC

Organomercurials
Chlormerodrin, 2105
Meralluride, 5866
Mercaptomerin Sodium, 5870
Mercumatilin Sodium see 5872
Mercurous Chloride, 5894
Mersalyl, 5901

Purines
Pamabrom, 7000
Protheobromine, 7886
Theobromine, 9282

Steroids
Canrenone, 1750
Oleandrin, 6826
Spironolactone, 8760

Sulfonamide Derivatives
Acetazolamide, 53
Azosemide, 922
Bumetanide, 1484
Chloraminophenamide, 2076
Clofenamide, 2374
Clopamide, 2393
Clorexolone, 2404
Ethoxzolamide, 3755
Furosemide, 4309
Mefruside, 5803
Methazolamide, 5962
Piretanide, 7492
Torsemide, 9552
Tripamide, 9737
Xipamide, 10079

Thiazides and Analogs
Althiazide, 318
Bendroflumethiazide, 1037
Benzthiazide, 1120
Benzylhydrochlorothiazide, 1136
Buthiazide, 1525
Chlorothiazide, 2168
Chlorthalidone, 2193
Cyclopenthiazide, 2745
Cyclothiazide, 2754
Fenquizone, 3997

Hydrochlorothiazide, *4781*
Hydroflumethiazide, *4789*
Indapamide, *4935*
Methyclothiazide, *6005*
Metolazone, *6147*
Polythiazide, *7584*
Quinethazone, *8056*
Teclothiazide, *9104*
Trichlormethiazide, *9624*

Uracils
Aminometradine, *451*

Others
Amiloride, *406*
Ethacrynic Acid, *3717*
Etozolin, *3891*
Isosorbide, *5224*
Mannitol, *5745*
Perhexiline, *7163*
Ticrynafen, *9430*
Triamterene, *9599*
Urea, *9867*

DOPAMINE RECEPTOR AGONIST
see also ***Antihypertensive; Antimigraine; Antiparkinsonian; Prolactin Inhibitor***

Apomorphine, *746*
Bromocriptine, *1416*
Cabergoline, *1601*
Dopexamine, *3424*
Fenoldopam, *3979*
Ibopamine, *4876*
Lisuride, *5518*
Pergolide, *7162*
Pramipexole, *7705*
Quinagolide, *8045*
Ropinirole, *8257*
Roxindole, *8275*
Talipexole, *9039*

DOPAMINE RECEPTOR ANTAGONIST *see also* ***Antiemetic; Antipsychotic***

Amisulpride, *485*
Clebopride, *2344*
Domperidone, *3418*
Metoclopramide, *6143*
Mosapramine, *6278*
Nemonapride, *6446*
Remoxipride, *8132*
Sarizotan, *8375*
Sulpiride, *8989*
Sultopride, *8994*

DOPAMINE-SEROTONIN SYSTEM STABILIZER

Aripiprazole, *785*
Bifeprunox, *1210*

ECTOPARASITICIDE

Benzyl Benzoate, *1127*
Carbaryl, *1787*
Crotamiton, *2594*
Dixanthogen, *3384*
Lindane, *5501*
Malathion, *5700*
Mercuric Oleate, *5881*
Mesulfen, *5918*
Permethrin, *7180*

Sulfiram, *8950*
Sulfur, Pharmaceutical, *8977*

ELECTROLYTE REPLENISHER
see ***Replenishers/Supplements***

EMETIC

Apocodeine, *740*
Apomorphine, *746*
Cephaeline, *1973*
Ipecac, *5070*
Sodium Chloride, *8599*
Zinc Acetate, *10128*

ENDOTHELIN RECEPTOR ANTAGONIST *see also* ***Antineoplastic; Vasodilator (Peripheral)***

Ambrisentan, *384*
Atrasentan, *870*
Bosentan, *1353*
Clazosentan, *2342*
Sitaxsentan, *8554*
Tezosentan, *9252*

ENKEPHALINASE INHIBITOR *see* ***Neutral Endopeptidase Inhibitor***

ENZYME
Digestive
Amylase, *599*
Lipase, *5511*
Pepsin, *7146*
Rennin, *8134*

Mucolytic
Lysozyme, *5640*

Penicillin Inactivating
Penicillinase, *7093*

Proteolytic
Chymopapain, *2259*
Chymotrypsins, *2260*
Collagenase, *2481*
Papain, *7016*
Trypsin, *9795*

ENZYME COFACTOR *see also* ***Vitamin***

Acetiamine, *54*
Benfotiamine, *1041*
Bisbentiamine, *1246*
Carnitine, *1849*
Cetotiamine, *2023*
Dexpanthenol, *2947*
Fursultiamine, *4311*
Nicotinamide, *6523*
Nicotinic Acid, *6525*
Octotiamine, *6760*
Pantothenic Acid, *7015*
Prosultiamine, *7882*
Pyridoxal 5-Phosphate, *7979*
Pyridoxine Hydrochloride, *7982*
Riboflavin, *8200*
Riboflavin Monophosphate, *8201*
Sapropterin, *8368*
Thiamine, *9295*
Thiamine Diphosphate, *9296*
Thiamine Disulfide, *9297*

ENZYME INDUCER (HEPATIC)
Flumecinol, *4136*

ENZYME REPLACEMENT THERAPY
Acid α-Glucosidase, *108*
Alglucerase, *243*
$α_1$-Antitrypsin, *719*
Arylsulfatase B, *819*
α-Galactosidase A, *4336*
α-L-Iduronidase, *4894*
Pancreatic Extract, *7006*

ESTROGEN
Nonsteroidal
Broparoestrol, *1448*
Chlorotrianisene, *2174*
Dienestrol, *3104*
Diethylstilbestrol, *3129*
Fosfestrol, *4253*
Hexestrol, *4701*
Methestrol, *5968*

Steroidal
Colpormon, *2489*
Conjugated Estrogens, *2508*
Equilenin, *3642*
Equilin, *3643*
Estradiol, *3703*
Estriol, *3707*
Estrone, *3708*
Ethinyl Estradiol, *3734*
Mestranol, *5917*
Moxestrol, *6289*
Quinestrol, *8055*

ESTROGEN ANTAGONIST *see* ***Antiestrogen***

EXPECTORANT
Ambroxol, *386*
Ammonium Bicarbonate, *497*
Ammonium Carbonate, *508*
Bromhexine, *1391*
Calcium Iodide, *1677*
Carbocysteine, *1802*
Guaiacol, *4553*
Guaifenesin, *4555*
Guaithylline, *4555*
Hydriodic Acid, *4776*
Potassium Guaiacolsulfonate, *7634*
Potassium Iodide, *7643*
Sodium Iodide, *8631*
Storax, *8819*
Terpin, *9169*

FIBRINOGEN RECEPTOR ANTAGONIST *see also* ***Antithrombotic***

Lamifiban, *5349*
Tirofiban, *9464*
Xemilofiban, *10070*

GASTRIC AND PANCREATIC SECRETION STIMULANT

Ceruletide, *2005*
Sincalide, *8543*

GASTRIC PROTON PUMP INHIBITOR see also Antiulcerative

Lansoprazole, 5362
Omeprazole, 6845
Pantoprazole, 7014
Rabeprazole, 8089

GASTRIC SECRETION INHIBITOR

Enterogastrone, 3597
Octreotide, 6762

GASTROPROKINETIC

Alvimopan, 372
Cinitapride, 2294
Cisapride, 2316
Fedotozine, 3949
Itopride, 5244
Loxiglumide, 5588
Mosapride, 6279
Piboserod, 7393
Prucalopride, 7907
Renzapride, 8135
Tegaserod, 9113

GLUCOCORTICOID

21-Acetoxypregnenolone, 77
Alclometasone, 220
Algestone, 239
Amcinonide, 388
Beclomethasone, 1019
Betamethasone, 1180
Budesonide, 1468
Chloroprednisone, 2157
Ciclesonide, 2263
Clobetasol, 2363
Clobetasone, 2364
Clocortolone, 2369
Cloprednol, 2398
Cortisone, 2539
Cortivazol, 2540
Deflazacort, 2862
Desonide, 2928
Desoximetasone, 2930
Dexamethasone, 2943
Diflorasone, 3140
Diflucortolone, 3143
Difluprednate, 3152
Enoxolone, 3590
Etiprednol Dicloacetate, 3870
Fluazacort, 4115
Flucloronide, 4121
Flumethasone, 4138
Flunisolide, 4145
Fluocinolone Acetonide, 4150
Fluocinonide, 4151
Fluocortin Butyl, 4152
Fluocortolone, 4153
Fluorometholone, 4175
Fluperolone Acetate, 4188
Fluprednidene Acetate, 4191
Fluprednisolone, 4192
Flurandrenolide, 4197
Fluticasone Propionate, 4211
Formocortal, 4243
Halcinonide, 4591
Halobetasol Propionate, 4593
Halometasone, 4597
Halopredone Acetate, 4599
Hydrocortamate, 4786
Hydrocortisone, 4787
Loteprednol Etabonate, 5584
Mazipredone, 5763

Medrysone, 5794
Meprednisone, 5861
Methylprednisolone, 6111
Mometasone Furoate, 6241
Paramethasone, 7029
Prednicarbate, 7719
Prednisolone, 7721
Prednisone, 7722
Prednival, 7723
Prednylidene, 7724
Rimexolone, 8226
Tixocortol, 9484
Triamcinolone, 9595
Triamcinolone Acetonide, 9596
Triamcinolone Benetonide, 9597
Triamcinolone Hexacetonide, 9598

α-GLUCOSIDASE INHIBITOR see also Antidiabetic

Acarbose, 18
Miglitol, 6187
Voglibose, 10029

GONAD-STIMULATING PRINCIPLE

Buserelin, 1503
Chorionic Gonadotropin, 2216
Clomiphene, 2386
Cyclofenil, 2720
Follicle-Stimulating Hormone, 4223
LH-RH, 5474
Luteinizing Hormone, 5613

GOUT SUPPRESSANT see Antigout

GROWTH HORMONE ANTAGONIST/INHIBITOR

Octreotide, 6762
Pegvisomant, 7069
Somatostatin, 8715

GROWTH HORMONE RELEASING FACTOR

Sermorelin, 8461

GROWTH STIMULANT

Somatotropin, 8716

HEMATINIC

Cobaltous Chloride, 2437
Ferric Ammonium Citrate, 4017
Ferric Citrate, 4021
Ferric Fructose see 4273
Ferric Pyrophosphate, 4030
Ferric Sodium Edetate, 4031
Ferritin, 4036
Ferroglycine Sulfate, 4039
Ferrous Bisglycinate, 4041
Ferrous Citrate, 4044
Ferrous Fumarate, 4046
Ferrous Gluconate, 4047
Ferrous Lactate, 4050
Ferrous Succinate, 4056
Ferrous Sulfate, 4057
Iron Dextran, 5094

Iron Sorbitex, 5100
Iron Sucrose, 5101
Sodium Ferric Gluconate, 8615

HEMATOPOIETIC

Darbepoetin Alfa, 2824
Erythropoietin, 3688
Granulocyte Colony-Stimulating Factor, 4537
Granulocyte-Macrophage Colony-Stimulating Factor, 4538
Interleukin-3, 4995
Oprelvekin see 5000
Stem Cell Factor, 8807

HEMOLYTIC

Phenylhydrazine, 7293

HEMORHEOLOGIC AGENT

Pentoxifylline, 7136
Poloxamer 188 see 7562

HEMOSTATIC

Adrenalone, 171
Adrenochrome, 172
Algin, 241
Alginic Acid, 242
ε-Aminocaproic Acid, 432
Aminochromes, 436
Batroxobin, 1010
Carbazochrome Salicylate, 1788
Carbazochrome Sodium Sulfonate, 1789
Cephalins, 1975
Cotarnine, 2552
Desmopressin, 2924
Ellagic Acid, 3547
Ethamsylate, 3722
Factor IX, 3922
Factor VIII, 3921
Factor XIII, 3926
Fibrinogen, 4071
Gelatin, 4382
Monsel's Solution, 6256
1,2-Naphthoquinone, 6394
1-Naphthylamine-4-sulfonic Acid, 6403
Oxamarin, 6915
Oxidized Cellulose, 6939
Styptic Collodion see 2484
Sulmarin, 8984
Thrombin, 9383
Thromboplastin, 9385
Tolonium Chloride, 9520
Tranexamic Acid, 9569
Vapreotide, 9934
Vasopressin, 9938

HEPARIN ANTAGONIST

Hexadimethrine Bromide, 4682

HEPATOPROTECTANT

S-Adenosylmethionine, 156
Betaine, 1179
Catechin, 1902
Citiolone, 2320
Malotilate, 5712
Methionine, 5975

Orazamide, *6861*
Phosphorylcholine, *7362*
Protoporphyrin IX, *7897*
Silymarin, *8532*
Thioctic Acid, *9326*
Timonacic, *9445*
Tiopronin, *9453*

HISTAMINE H₁-RECEPTOR ANTAGONIST *see Antihistaminic*

HISTAMINE H₂-RECEPTOR ANTAGONIST *see also Antiulcerative*

Cimetidine, *2279*
Ebrotidine, *3485*
Famotidine, *3930*
Lafutidine, *5347*
Nizatidine, *6660*
Ranitidine, *8110*
Roxatidine Acetate, *8274*

HIV FUSION INHIBITOR *see also Antiviral*

Enfuvirtide, *3582*

HIV PROTEASE INHIBITOR *see also Antiviral*

Amprenavir, *589*
Darunavir, *2827*
Fosamprenavir, *4250*
Indinavir, *4945*
Lopinavir, *5573*
Nelfinavir, *6443*
Ritonavir, *8238*
Saquinavir, *8369*

HMG COA REDUCTASE INHIBITOR *see also Antilipemic*

Atorvastatin, *864*
Cerivastatin, *1993*
Fluvastatin, *4218*
Lovastatin, *5586*
Pitavastatin, *7508*
Pravastatin Sodium, *7714*
Rosuvastatin, *8270*
Simvastatin, *8539*

HYPNOTIC *see Sedative/Hypnotic*

HYPOCHOLESTEREMIC *see Antilipemic*

HYPOLIPIDEMIC *see Antilipemic*

HYPOTENSIVE *see Antihypertensive*

IMMUNOMODULATOR

Acemannan, *26*
Actimid, *135*
Aldesleukin *see 4994*
Amiprilose, *484*
Ampligen, *588*
Bucillamine, *1460*
Ditiocarb Sodium, *3378*

Glatiramer, *4435*
Imiquimod, *4922*
Inosine Pranobex, *4976*
Interferon-β, *4991*
Interferon-γ, *4992*
Leflunomide, *5432*
Lenalidomide, *5436*
Lentinan, *5439*
Levamisole, *5459*
Lisofylline, *5517*
Macrophage Colony-Stimulating
  Factor, *5646*
Mitoxantrone, *6217*
Pidotimod, *7419*
Platonin, *7530*
Polyoxidonium, *7575*
Procodazole, *7762*
Propagermanium, *7795*
Resiquimod, *8151*
Romurtide, *8253*
Teriflunomide, *9165*
Thalidomide, *9255*
Thymalfasin *see 9405*
Thymomodulin, *9402*
Thymopentin, *9403*
Thymostimulin, *9407*
Ubenimex, *9842*
Virulizin®, *10007*

IMMUNOSUPPRESSANT

Abatacept, *4*
Abetimus Sodium, *6*
Alefacept, *227*
Alemtuzumab, *228*
Azathioprine, *902*
Basiliximab, *1006*
Belatacept, *1024*
Brequinar, *1370*
Cyclosporins, *2752*
Daclizumab, *2799*
Everolimus, *3907*
Fingolimod, *4083*
Gusperimus, *4582*
6-Mercaptopurine, *5871*
Mizoribine, *6222*
Muromonab CD3, *6308*
Mycophenolic Acid, *6327*
Pimecrolimus, *7429*
Rapamycin, *8114*
Tacrolimus, *9025*

IMPDH INHIBITOR

Mycophenolic Acid, *6327*
Ribavirin, *8198*
Tiazofurin, *9425*

IMPOTENCE THERAPY

Apomorphine, *746*
Sildenafil, *8489*
Tadalafil, *9027*
Vardenafil, *9935*

INOTROPIC AGENT *see Cardiotonic*

INSULIN SENSITIZER *see also Antidiabetic*

Pioglitazone, *7452*
Rosiglitazone, *8265*
Troglitazone, *9769*

ION-EXCHANGE RESIN

Cholestyramine Resin, *2202*
Colestilan, *2474*
Colestipol, *2475*
Polidexide, *7557*
Sodium Polystyrene Sulfonate,
  8668

KERATOLYTIC *see also Antiacne*

Benzoyl Peroxide, *1116*
Dichloroacetic Acid, *3050*
Glutaraldehyde, *4472*
Resorcinol, *8155*
Retinoic Acid, *8165*
Salicylic Acid, *8332*
Sulfur, Pharmaceutical, *8977*

LACTATION STIMULATING HORMONE

Prolactin, *7779*

LAXATIVE/CATHARTIC

Agar, *184*
Aloe-Emodin, *306*
Aloin, *307*
Bisacodyl, *1242*
Bisoxatin Acetate, *1296*
Calcium Polycarbophil, *1697*
Casanthranol, *1878*
Castor Oil, *1898*
Cellulose Ethyl Hydroxyethyl
  Ether, *1967*
Colocynthin, *2487*
Danthron, *2815*
Docusate Calcium, *3400*
Docusate Sodium, *3401*
Emodin, *3561*
Frangulin, *4264*
Glucofrangulin, *4452*
Lactitol, *5340*
Lactulose, *5346*
Magnesium Carbonate Hydroxide, *5660*
Magnesium Chloride, *5662*
Magnesium Citrate, *5663*
Magnesium Hydroxide, *5670*
Magnesium Lactate, *5672*
Magnesium Phosphate, Dibasic,
  5681
Magnesium Sulfate, *5691*
Mercurous Chloride, *5894*
Methylcellulose, *6040*
Oxyphenisatin Acetate, *6974*
Petrolatum, Liquid, *7186*
Phenolphthalein, *7243*
Phenolphthalol, *7245*
Phenoltetrachlorophthalein, *7248*
Picosulfate Sodium, *7406*
Polyethylene Glycol, *7568*
Potassium Bisulfate, *7613*
Potassium Bitartrate, *7615*
Potassium Phosphate, Dibasic,
  7658
Potassium Sodium Tartrate, *7670*
Potassium Sulfate, *7674*
Potassium Sulfite, *7676*
Potassium Tartrate, *7677*
Seidlitz Mixture, *8423*
Senna, *8454*
Sennosides, *8455*
Sodium Phosphate, Dibasic,
  8659

LAXATIVE/CATHARTIC
(*continued*)

Sodium Sulfate, *8680*
Sodium Tartrate, *8684*
Sorbitol, *8725*

LEUKOTRIENE ANTAGONIST *see also Antiasthmatic*

Ibudilast, *4879*
Montelukast, *6258*
Pranlukast, *7710*
Zafirlukast, *10108*

LH-RH AGONIST *see also Antineoplastic; Gonad-Stimulating Principle*

Buserelin, *1503*
Deslorelin, *2923*
Goserelin, *4526*
Histrelin, *4722*
Leuprolide, *5457*
Nafarelin, *6351*
Triptorelin, *9748*

LH-RH ANTAGONIST *see also Antineoplastic*

Cetrorelix, *2026*
Ganirelix, *4365*

LIPOTROPIC

N-Acetylmethionine, *96*
Choline Chloride, *2206*
Choline Dihydrogen Citrate, *2207*
Inositol, *4978*
Lecithins, *5428*

5-LIPOXYGENASE INHIBITOR *see also Antiallergic; Antiasthmatic; Anti-inflammatory; Antipsoriatic*

Amlexanox, *490*
Tenidap, *9144*
Zileuton, *10124*

LOCAL ANESTHETIC *see Anesthetic (Local)*

LUPUS ERYTHEMATOSUS SUPPRESSANT

Bismuth Sodium Triglycollamate, *1280*
Chloroquine, *2163*
Hydroxychloroquine, *4818*

MACULAR DEGENERATION TREATMENT

Anecortave Acetate, *641*
Motexafin Lutetium, *6282*
Pegaptanib Sodium, *7068*
Ranibizumab, *8108*
Rostaporfin, *8269*
Verteporfin, *9967*

MAJOR TRANQUILIZER *see Antipsychotic*

MATRIX METALLOPROTEINASE INHIBITOR

Batimastat, *1008*
Prinomastat, *7751*

MELATONIN RECEPTOR AGONIST

Ramelteon, *8101*

MINERALOCORTICOID

Aldosterone, *225*
Deoxycorticosterone, *2900*
Deoxycorticosterone Acetate, *2901*
Fludrocortisone, *4130*

MINOR TRANQUILIZER *see Anxiolytic*

MIOTIC

Carbachol, *1779*
Neostigmine, *6464*
Physostigmine, *7384*
Pilocarpine, *7424*

MONOAMINE OXIDASE INHIBITOR *see also Antidepressant; Antihypertensive; Antiparkinsonian*

Befloxatone, *1021*
Iproclozide, *5076*
Iproniazid, *5078*
Isocarboxazid, *5157*
Lazabemide, *5394*
Moclobemide, *6226*
Pargyline, *7038*
Phenelzine, *7221*
Prodipine, *7768*
Safinamide, *8315*
Selegiline, *8428*
Toloxatone, *9521*
Tranylcypromine, *9573*

MUCOLYTIC

Acetylcysteine, *88*
Bromhexine, *1391*
Carbocysteine, *1802*
Domiodol, *3414*
Erdosteine, *3647*
Letosteine, *5449*
Lysozyme, *5640*
Mecysteine Hydrochloride, *5785*
Mesna, *5909*
Sobrerol, *8567*
Stepronin, *8809*
Tiopronin, *9453*
Tyloxapol, *9833*

MUSCLE RELAXANT (SKELETAL) *see also Neuromuscular Blocking Agent*

Afloqualone, *183*
Baclofen, *937*
Botulin Toxins, *1357*
Carisoprodol, *1842*
Chlormezanone, *2106*
Chlorphenesin Carbamate, *2179*
Chlorzoxazone, *2194*
Cyclobenzaprine, *2713*

Dantrolene, *2816*
Diazepam, *2994*
Eperisone, *3606*
Idrocilamide, *4893*
Inaperisone, *4928*
Mephenesin, *5850*
Mephenoxalone, *5851*
Methocarbamol, *5980*
Mivacurium Chloride, *6219*
Orphenadrine, *6879*
Phenprobamate, *7258*
Pridinol Mesylate *see 7741*
Quinine, *8061*
Tetrazepam, *9243*
Thiocolchicoside *see 9324*
Tizanidine, *9485*
Tolperisone, *9522*

MUSCLE RELAXANT (SMOOTH) *see Antimuscarinic*

MYDRIATIC

Atropine, *875*
Cyclodrine, *2719*
Cyclopentolate, *2746*
Epinephrine, *3619*
Eucatropine, *3897*
Homatropine, *4730*
Hydroxyamphetamine, *4810*
Phenylephrine, *7286*
Scopolamine, *8406*
Tropicamide, *9780*
Yohimbine, *10102*

NARCOTIC ANALGESIC *see Analgesic (Narcotic)*

NARCOTIC ANTAGONIST

Amiphenazole, *483*
Cyclazocine, *2705*
Levallorphan, *5458*
Methylnaltrexone Bromide, *6099*
Nalmefene, *6360*
Nalorphine, *6361*
Naloxone, *6362*
Naltrexone, *6363*

NASAL DECONGESTANT *see Decongestant*

NEURAMINIDASE INHIBITOR *see also Antiviral*

Oseltamivir, *6889*
Zanamivir, *10113*

NEUROKININ RECEPTOR ANTAGONIST *see also Antiemetic*

Aprepitant, *753*

NEUROLEPTIC *see Antipsychotic*

NEUROMUSCULAR BLOCKING AGENT

Depolarizing Agents
Decamethonium Bromide, *2847*
Succinylcholine Bromide, *8874*

Succinylcholine Chloride, *8875*
Succinylcholine Iodide, *8876*

Nondepolarizing Agents
Alcuronium, *221*
Atracurium Besylate, *868*
Curare, *2671*
Doxacurium Chloride, *3431*
Fazadinium Bromide, *3943*
Gallamine Triethiodide, *4343*
Metocurine Iodide, *6144*
Pancuronium Bromide, *7007*
Pipecurium Bromide, *7459*
Rapacuronium Bromide, *8113*
Rocuronium, *8246*
Tubocurarine Chloride, *9807*
Vecuronium Bromide, *9941*

**NEUTRAL ENDOPEPTIDASE IN-
HIBITOR** *see also Antihypertensive;
Antidiarrheal; Vasopeptidase Inhibi-
tor*
Candoxatril, *1742*
Racecadotril, *8090*

NEUROPROTECTIVE
Aptiganel, *758*
Citicoline, *2319*
Dexanabinol, *2944*
Disufenton, *3363*
Lubeluzole, *5590*
Memantine, *5829*
Remacemide, *8130*
Repinotan, *8137*
Riluzole, *8223*
Xaliproden, *10054*
Ziconotide, *10122*

NMDA RECEPTOR ANTAGONIST
see also Neuroprotective
Aptiganel, *758*
Dexanabinol, *2944*
Memantine, *5829*
Remacemide, *8130*

NOOTROPIC
Aceglutamide, *25*
Acetylcarnitine, *84*
Aniracetam, *662*
Besipirdine, *1176*
Bifemelane, *1206*
Choline Alfoscerate, *2205*
Donepezil, *3419*
Exifone, *3915*
Fipexide, *4084*
Idebenone, *4888*
Indeloxazine Hydrochloride,
4938
Ispronicline, *5239*
Leteprinim, *5448*
Nefiracetam, *6439*
Nizofenone, *6661*
Oxiracetam, *6942*
Piracetam, *7487*
Posatirelin, *7603*
Pramiracetam, *7706*
Propentofylline, *7813*
Pyritinol, *7996*
Rivastigmine, *8240*
Sabcomeline, *8309*
Sabeluzole, *8310*

Tacrine, *9024*
Vinconate, *9985*
Xanomeline, *10056*

NSAID *see Anti-inflammatory (Nonsteroidal)*

OPIOID ANALGESIC *see Analgesic
(Narcotic)*

ORAL CONTRACEPTIVE *see Contraceptive (Oral)*

OSTEOINDUCTIVE AGENT
Bone Morphogenetic Proteins,
1331

OVARIAN HORMONE
Relaxin, *8129*

OXYTOCIC
Carboprost, *1823*
Cargutocin, *1839*
Deaminooxytocin, *2842*
Ergonovine, *3655*
Gemeprost, *4387*
Methylergonovine, *6070*
Oxytocin, *6979*
Pituitary, Posterior, *7510*
Prostaglandin E$_2$, *7877*
Prostaglandin F$_{2\alpha}$, *7878*

PARASYMPATHOMIMETIC *see
Cholinergic*

PEDICULICIDE *see Ectoparasiticide*

PEPSIN INHIBITOR
Sodium Amylosulfate, *8577*

PERIPHERAL VASODILATOR *see
Vasodilator (Peripheral)*

PERISTALTIC STIMULANT *see
Gastroprokinetic*

**PHOSPHODIESTERASE INHIBI-
TOR** *see also Antiasthmatic; Anti-
thrombotic*
Cilomilast, *2276*
Cilostazol, *2277*
Dipyridamole, *3346*
Roflumilast, *8249*
Satigrel, *8383*
Sildenafil, *8489*
Tadalafil, *9027*
Vardenafil, *9935*

PIGMENTATION AGENT
Methoxsalen, *5988*
Trioxsalen, *9735*

PLASMA VOLUME EXPANDER
Dextran, *2948*
Hetastarch, *4673*
Serum Albumin, *8468*

**PLATELET ACTIVATING FAC-
TOR ANTAGONIST**
Israpafant, *5241*
Lexipafant, *5473*
Rupatadine, *8297*

**POTASSIUM CHANNEL ACTIVA-
TOR/OPENER** *see also Antihyper-
tensive; Antianginal*
Levcromakalim, *5460*
Nicorandil, *6521*
Pinacidil, *7438*

POTASSIUM CHANNEL BLOCKER
see also Antiarrhythmic
Azimilide, *911*
Dofetilide, *3409*
Fampridine, *3933*
Nifekalant, *6529*
Tedisamil, *9108*

PRESSOR AGENT *see Antihypotensive*

PROGESTOGEN
Allylestrenol, *291*
Chlormadinone Acetate, *2102*
Delmadinone Acetate, *2878*
Demegestone, *2888*
Desogestrel, *2926*
Dienogest, *3106*
Dimethisterone, *3219*
Drospirenone, *3454*
Dydrogesterone, *3474*
Elcometrine, *3538*
Ethynodiol, *3860*
Etonogestrel, *3884*
Flurogestone Acetate, *4200*
Gestodene, *4413*
Gestonorone Caproate, *4414*
17α-Hydroxyprogesterone, *4839*
Lynestrenol, *5629*
Medrogestone, *5791*
Medroxyprogesterone, *5793*
Megestrol Acetate, *5805*
Norelgestromin, *6694*
Norethindrone, *6697*
Norethynodrel, *6698*
Norgesterone, *6702*
Norgestimate, *6703*
Norgestrel, *6704*
Norgestrienone, *6705*
Norvinisterone, *6717*
Pentagestrone, *7114*
Progesterone, *7773*
Promegestone, *7785*
Trengestone, *9584*

PROLACTIN INHIBITOR
Bromocriptine, *1416*
Cabergoline, *1601*
Lisuride, *5518*
Metergoline, *5937*

PROLACTIN INHIBITOR
(*continued*)

Quinagolide, *8045*
Terguride, *9164*

PROSTAGLANDIN/PROSTAGLANDIN ANALOG *see also Abortifacient/Interceptive; Antiglaucoma; Antithrombotic; Antiulcerative; Oxytocic*

Beraprost, *1152*
Bimatoprost, *1221*
Carboprost, *1823*
Clinprost, *2358*
Enprostil, *3591*
Gemeprost, *4387*
Latanoprost, *5376*
Limaprost, *5490*
Misoprostol, *6210*
Ornoprostil, *6875*
Prostacyclin, *7875*
Prostaglandin E$_1$, *7876*
Prostaglandin E$_2$, *7877*
Prostaglandin F$_{2\alpha}$, *7878*
Rioprostil, *8231*
Rosaprostol, *8260*
Sulprostone, *8991*
Trimoprostil, *9723*
Unoprostone, *9849*

PROTEASE INHIBITOR *see also HIV Protease Inhibitor*

Aprotinin, *757*
Camostat, *1728*
Gabexate, *4320*
Nafamostat, *6350*
Tipranavir, *9459*
Urinastatin, *9882*

PROTON PUMP INHIBITOR *see Gastric Proton Pump Inhibitor*

PULMONARY SURFACTANT

Beractant, *1151*
Calfactant, *1714*
Colfosceril Palmitate, *2477*
Exosurf®, *3917*
Lucinactant *see 8542*
Poractant Alfa, *7595*
Pumactant, *7939*

PURINOCEPTOR P2Y AGONIST

Denufosol, *2896*
Diquafosol, *3351*

5α-REDUCTASE INHIBITOR *see also Antiprostatic Hypertrophy*

Dutasteride, *3471*
Epristeride, *3634*
Finasteride, *4082*

RENIN INHIBITOR

Aliskiren, *247*

REPLENISHERS/SUPPLEMENTS

Calcium
Calcium Carbonate, *1657*
Calcium Citrate, *1661*

Calcium Gluconate, *1669*
Calcium Hypophosphite, *1675*
Calcium Lactate, *1678*
Calcium Levulinate, *1679*
Calcium Phosphate, Dibasic, *1692*
Calcium Phosphate, Tribasic, *1694*

Chromium
Chromium Picolinate, *2236*

Copper
Cupric Bisglycinate, *2627*
Cupric Gluconate, *2640*
Cupric Oxide, *2646*
Cupric Sulfate, *2653*

Electrolyte
Calcium Chloride, *1659*
Potassium Acetate, *7605*
Potassium Chloride, *7621*
Sodium Chloride, *8599*
Sodium Lactate, *8635*

Iodine
Periodyl, *7172*
Potassium Iodide, *7643*
Prolonium Iodide, *7782*
Rubidium Iodide, *8286*
Sodium Iodide, *8631*
Strontium Iodide, *8844*

Magnesium
Magnesium Gluconate *see 4456*
Magnesium Sulfate, *5691*

Nutrient
Glucose, *4459*
Glutamic Acid, *4469*
Protein Hydrolysates, *7885*

Phosphorus
Calcium Glycerophosphate, *1670*
Durapatite, *3467*

Potassium
Potassium Acetate, *7605*
Potassium Bicarbonate, *7609*
Potassium Gluconate *see 4456*

Selenium
Sodium Selenite, *8673*

Zinc
Zinc Gluconate *see 4456*
Zinc Sulfate, *10159*

RESPIRATORY STIMULANT

Almitrine, *301*
Bemegride, *1027*
Carbon Dioxide, *1809*
Cropropamide, *2591*
Crotethamide, *2595*
Dimefline, *3204*
Doxapram, *3432*
Ethamivan, *3721*
Fominoben, *4228*
Lobeline, *5551*
Mepixanox, *5860*
Nikethamide, *6543*
Picrotoxin, *7415*
Tacrine, *9024*

RETROVIRAL PROTEASE INHIBITOR *see HIV Protease Inhibitor*

REVERSE TRANSCRIPTASE INHIBITOR *see also Antiviral*

Abacavir, *1*
Capravirine, *1755*
Delavirdine, *2877*
Didanosine, *3098*
Dideoxyadenosine, *3101*
Efavirenz, *3521*
Emtricitabine, *3565*
Foscarnet Sodium, *4251*
Lamivudine, *5352*
Nevirapine, *6490*
Stavudine, *8803*
Suramin Sodium, *9006*
Tenofovir, *9146*
Zalcitabine, *10109*
Zidovudine, *10123*

SCABICIDE *see Ectoparasiticide*

SCLEROSING AGENT

Ethanolamine, *3727*
Ethylamine, *3762*
2-Hexyldecanoic Acid, *4709*
Polidocanol, *7558*
Sodium Ricinoleate *see 8211*
Sodium Tetradecyl Sulfate, *8689*
Tribenoside, *9608*

SEDATIVE/HYPNOTIC *see also Anxiolytic*

Acylic Ureides
Acecarbromal, *21*
Bromisovalum, *1397*
Carbromal, *1831*

Alcohols
Ethchlorvynol, *3729*
Meparfynol, *5846*
tert-Pentyl Alcohol, *7140*
2,2,2-Trichloroethanol, *9638*

Amides
Niaprazine, *6492*
Trimetozine, *9720*
Valdetamide, *9901*

Barbituric Acid Derivatives
Allobarbital, *263*
Amobarbital, *570*
Aprobarbital, *756*
Barbital, *962*
Brallobarbital, *1361*
Butabarbital Sodium, *1506*
Butalbital, *1511*
Butethal, *1521*
Cyclobarbital, *2711*
Febarbamate, *3945*
Heptabarbital, *4655*
Hexobarbital, *4704*
Mephobarbital, *5854*
Methitural, *5978*
Pentobarbital, *7130*
Phenobarbital, *7238*
Propallylonal, *7796*
Proxibarbal, *7904*
Secobarbital Sodium, *8420*
Talbutal, *9036*
Vinylbital, *9993*

Benzodiazepine Derivatives
Brotizolam, *1450*
Cinolazepam, *2308*

Doxefazepam, *3434*
Estazolam, *3702*
Flunitrazepam, *4146*
Flurazepam, *4198*
Haloxazolam, *4604*
Loprazolam, *5574*
Lormetazepam, *5581*
Midazolam, *6182*
Nimetazepam, *6549*
Nitrazepam, *6575*
Quazepam, *8029*
Temazepam, *9133*
Triazolam, *9604*

Bromides
Ammonium Bromide, *505*
Calcium Bromide, *1654*
Lithium Bromide, *5526*
Magnesium Bromide, *5659*
Potassium Bromide, *7618*
Sodium Bromide, *8594*

Carbamates
Ethinamate, *3733*
Hexapropymate, *4698*

Chloral Derivatives
Chloral Formamide, *2070*
Chloral Hydrate, *2071*
Dichloralphenazone, *3046*
Triclofos, *9655*

Imidazopyridines
Indiplon, *4946*
Zaleplon, *10111*
Zolpidem, *10190*

Piperidinediones
Glutethimide, *4477*
Methyprylon, *6136*
Piperidione, *7469*
Pyrithyldione, *7995*
Thalidomide, *9255*

Quinazolone Derivatives
Etaqualone, *3714*
Mecloqualone, *5781*

Others
Bromoform, *1420*
α-Chloralose, *2072*
Clomethiazole, *2384*
Cypripedium, *2770*
Dexmedetomidine, *2946*
Diphenhydramine, *3309*
Doxylamine, *3441*
Etomidate, *3881*
Gaboxadol, *4321*
Hydrobromic Acid, *4778*
Menthyl Valerate, *5841*
Opium, *6854*
Paraldehyde, *7027*
Perlapine, *7179*
Propiomazine, *7822*
Ramelteon, *8101*
Rilmazafone, *8221*
Sulfonethylmethane, *8958*
Sulfonmethane, *8960*
Zopiclone, *10193*

**SELECTIVE ESTROGEN RECEP-
TOR MODULATOR (SERM)** *see
also **Antineoplastic (Hormonal);
Antiosteoporotic***
Arzoxifene, *820*
Bazedoxifene, *1013*

Droloxifene, *3446*
Idoxifene, *4890*
Raloxifene, *8098*
Tamoxifen, *9048*
Toremifene, *9550*

**SELECTIVE PROGESTERONE RE-
CEPTOR MODULATOR (SPRM)**
Asoprisnil, *834*

SERENIC
Eltoprazine, *3552*

**SEROTONIN-DOPAMINE ANTAG-
ONIST** *see also **Antipsychotic***
Asenapine, *832*
Blonanserin, *1319*
Clozapine, *2423*
Iloperidone, *4900*
Olanzapine, *6822*
Perospirone, *7182*
Quetiapine, *8039*
Risperidone, *8233*
Sertindole, *8466*
Ziprasidone, *10171*
Zotepine, *10197*

**SEROTONIN NORADRENALINE
REUPTAKE INHIBITOR (SNRI)**
*see also **Antidepressant; Antiobesity
Agent***
Duloxetine, *3465*
Milnacipran, *6194*
Sibutramine, *8485*
Venlafaxine, *9946*

**SEROTONIN RECEPTOR AGO-
NIST** *see also **Anxiolytic; Anti-
depressant; Antimigraine; Neuro-
protective; Serenic***
Almotriptan, *304*
Buspirone, *1504*
Dihydroergotamine, *3174*
Eletriptan, *3544*
Eltoprazine, *3552*
Ergotamine, *3661*
Flesinoxan, *4100*
Frovatriptan, *4272*
Ipsapirone, *5081*
Lesopitron, *5447*
Methysergide, *6137*
Naratriptan, *6420*
Repinotan, *8137*
Rizatriptan, *8241*
Sarizotan, *8375*
Sumatriptan, *8997*
Tandospirone, *9051*
Tegaserod, *9113*
Xaliproden, *10054*
Zolmitriptan, *10189*

**SEROTONIN RECEPTOR ANTAG-
ONIST** *see also **Antidepressant;
Antiemetic; Antihypertensive; Anti-
migraine; Anxiolytic***
Agomelatine, *190*
Alosetron, *308*
Azasetron, *900*
Cilansetron, *2271*

Deramciclane, *2915*
Dolasetron, *3411*
Dotarizine, *3428*
Granisetron, *4536*
Itasetron, *5243*
Ketanserin, *5296*
Methysergide, *6137*
Nefazodone, *6438*
Ondansetron, *6848*
Oxetorone, *6934*
Palonosetron, *6997*
Piboserod, *7393*
Ramosetron, *8105*
Ritanserin, *8235*
Tropisetron, *9783*

SEROTONIN UPTAKE INHIBITOR
*see also **Antidepressant; Antiobses-
sional***
Citalopram, *2318*
Dapoxetine, *2821*
Femoxetine, *3955*
Fluoxetine, *4185*
Fluvoxamine, *4219*
Indalpine, *4930*
Indeloxazine Hydrochloride,
4938
Milnacipran, *6194*
Paroxetine, *7043*
Sertraline, *8467*
Zimeldine, *10126*

SIALAGOGUE
Anethole Trithione, *644*
Cevimeline, *2034*
Pilocarpine, *7424*

SKELETAL MUSCLE RELAXANT
*see **Muscle Relaxant (Skeletal)***

SNRI *see **Serotonin Noradrenaline
Reuptake Inhibitor (SNRI)***

SOMATOSTATIN ANALOG
Edotreotide, *3513*
Lanreotide, *5361*
Octreotide, *6762*
Pentetreotide, *7126*
Vapreotide, *9934*

SPASMOLYTIC *see **Antispasmodic***

STOOL SOFTENER *see **Laxative/
Cathartic***

SUCCINYLCHOLINE SYNERGIST
Hexafluorenium Bromide, *4684*

SYMPATHOMIMETIC *see **α-Adrenergic Agonist; β-Adrenergic Agonist***

THROMBOLYTIC *see also **Anticoag-
ulant; Antithrombotic***
Alfimeprase, *237*
Alteplase *see 9468*

THROMBOLYTIC (continued)

Amediplase, *391*
Anistreplase, *674*
Desmoteplase *see 3459*
Duteplase *see 9468*
Monteplase, *6259*
Pamiteplase, *7004*
Plasmin, *7520*
Pro-Urokinase, *7902*
Reteplase, *8161*
Staphylokinase, *8796*
Streptokinase, *8825*
Tenecteplase, *9143*
Tissue Plasminogen Activator, *9468*
Urokinase, *9887*

THROMBOXANE A₂-RECEPTOR ANTAGONIST *see also Antithrombotic; Antiasthmatic*

Daltroban, *2806*
Domitroban, *3416*
Ramatroban, *8100*
Ridogrel, *8212*
Seratrodast, *8459*

THROMBOXANE A₂-SYTHETASE INHIBITOR *see also Antithrombotic*

Ozagrel, *6980*
Ridogrel, *8212*

THYROID HORMONE *see also Antihypothyroid*

Liothyronine, *5510*
Thyroid, *9410*
Thyroidin, *9411*
Thyroxine, *9415*

THYROID INHIBITOR *see Antihyperthyroid*

THYROTROPIC HORMONE

TRH, *9588*

TISSUE ADHESIVE

n-Butyl Cyanoacrylate, *1565*
Isobutyl Cyanoacrylate, *5140*
Methyl Cyanoacrylate, *6046*
Octyl Cyanoacrylate, *6766*

TOCOLYTIC

Albuterol, *216*
Atosiban, *865*
Fenoterol, *3981*
Hexoprenaline, *4707*
Ritodrine, *8237*
Terbutaline, *9159*

TOPICAL PROTECTANT

Allantoin, *258*
Balsam Peru, *949*
Balsam Traumatic, *951*
Bismuth Phosphate, *1275*
Bismuth Subgallate, *1283*
Bismuth Tannate, *1288*

Collodion, *2484*
Gum Benzoin, *4580*
Hydroxypropyl Cellulose, *4841*
Pyroxylin, *8011*
Shark Liver Oil, *8477*
Storax, *8819*
Titanium Dioxide, *9472*
Zinc Oxide, *10147*

TOPOISOMERASE I INHIBITOR *see also Antineoplastic*

9-Aminocamptothecin, *431*
Edotecarin, *3512*
Exatecan, *3912*
Irinotecan, *5091*
Topotecan, *9548*

TOPOISOMERASE II INHIBITOR *see also Antineoplastic*

Amrubicin, *593*
Amsacrine, *594*
Daunorubicin, *2832*
Doxorubicin, *3439*
Epirubicin, *3623*
Etoposide, *3886*
Garenoxacin, *4369*
Idarubicin, *4886*
Mitoxantrone, *6217*
Pirarubicin, *7488*
Pixantrone, *7514*
Razoxane, *8123*
Sobuzoxane, *8568*
Teniposide, *9145*

TRANQUILIZER *see Antipsychotic; Anxiolytic*

ULTRAVIOLET SCREEN

p-Aminobenzoic Acid, *423*
Avobenzone, *888*
Bemotrizinol, *1028*
Bisoctrizole, *1294*
β-Carotene, *1853*
Cinoxate, *2310*
4-(Dimethylamino)benzoic Acid, *3232*
Dioxybenzone, *3303*
Drometrizole, *3447*
Ecamsule, *3490*
Ensulizole, *3593*
Ethylhexyl Triazone, *3809*
Homosalate, *4738*
Lawsone, *5393*
Menthyl Anthranilate, *5840*
4-Methylbenzylidene Camphor, *6027*
Mexenone, *6167*
Octabenzone, *6742*
Octocrylene, *6756*
Octyl Methoxycinnamate, *6769*
Octyl Salicylate, *6770*
Oxybenzone, *6954*
Sulisobenzone, *8983*
Zinc Oxide, *10147*

URICOSURIC *see also Antigout*

Benzbromarone, *1065*
Benziodarone, *1083*
Orotic Acid, *6876*
Oxycinchophen, *6957*

Probenecid, *7754*
Sulfinpyrazone, *8949*
Ticrynafen, *9430*

VASODILATOR (CEREBRAL)

Bencyclane, *1033*
Ciclonicate, *2265*
Cinnarizine, *2305*
Cyclandelate, *2704*
Diisopropylamine Dichloroacetate, *3197*
Eburnamonine, *3487*
Fasudil, *3942*
Fenoxedil, *3986*
Flunarizine, *4144*
Ibudilast, *4879*
Ifenprodil, *4895*
Lomerizine, *5563*
Nafronyl, *6353*
Nicergoline, *6496*
Nimodipine, *6551*
Papaverine, *7019*
Pentifylline, *7127*
Vincamine, *9983*
Vinpocetine, *9991*
Viquidil, *10003*

VASODILATOR (CORONARY)

Binodenoson, *1225*
Chloracizine, *2068*
Chromonar, *2239*
Clobenfurol, *2360*
Clonitrate, *2391*
Cloricromen, *2405*
Dilazep, *3200*
Droprenilamine, *3451*
Efloxate, *3523*
Erythrityl Tetranitrate, *3677*
Etafenone, *3710*
Fendiline, *3970*
Hexestrol Bis(β-diethylaminoethyl ether), *4702*
Hexobendine, *4705*
Itramin Tosylate, *5246*
Khellin, *5309*
Lidoflazine, *5484*
D-Mannitol Hexanitrate, *5746*
Nitroglycerin, *6607*
Pentaerythritol Tetranitrate, *7112*
Pentrinitrol, *7138*
Perhexiline, *7163*
Pimefylline, *7430*
Prenylamine, *7737*
Propatyl Nitrate, *7811*
Trapidil, *9574*
Tricromyl, *9658*
Trimetazidine, *9705*
Visnadine, *10010*

VASODILATOR (PERIPHERAL)

Bamethan, *954*
Bencyclane, *1033*
Beraprost, *1152*
Betahistine, *1178*
Bradykinin, *1359*
Brovincamine, *1451*
Bufeniode, *1472*
Buflomedil, *1475*
Butalamine, *1510*
Cetiedil, *2021*
Ciclonicate, *2265*

Cinepazide, *2291*
Cinnarizine, *2305*
Cyclandelate, *2704*
Diisopropylamine Dichloroace-
tate, *3197*
Eledoisin, *3539*
Fenoxedil, *3986*
Flunarizine, *4144*
Ifenprodil, *4895*
Iloprost, *4901*
Inositol Niacinate, *4979*
Isoxsuprine, *5238*
Kallidin, *5278*
Kallikrein, *5279*
Moxisylyte, *6292*
Nafronyl, *6353*
Nebivolol, *6432*
Nicergoline, *6496*
Nicotinyl Alcohol, *6527*
Nylidrin, *6732*
Pentifylline, *7127*
Piribedil, *7493*
Prostaglandin E₁, *7876*
Tolazoline, *9506*
Xanthinol Niacinate, *10060*

VASOPEPTIDASE INHIBITOR *see
also **Angiotensin Converting Enzyme
Inhibitor; Neutral Endopeptidase In-
hibitor***
Fasidotril, *3940*
Omapatrilat, *6843*
Sampatrilat, *8352*

**VASOPRESSIN RECEPTOR AN-
TAGONIST**
Conivaptan, *2507*
Tolvaptan, *9540*

VASOPRESSOR *see **Antihypotensive***

VASOPROTECTANT
Bioflavonoids, *1228*
Chromocarb, *2237*
Clazosentan, *2342*
Clobenoside, *2361*
Diosmin, *3297*

Dobesilate Calcium, *3394*
Escin, *3696*
Leucocyanidin, *5452*
Quercetin, *8034*
Rutin, *8304*
Troxerutin, *9789*

VITAMIN/VITAMIN SOURCE *see
also **Enzyme Cofactor***
Vitamin A
α-Carotene, *1852*
β-Carotene, *1853*
γ-Carotene, *1854*
Vitamin A, *10013*

Vitamin B₁
Acetiamine, *54*
Benfotiamine, *1041*
Bisbentiamine, *1246*
Cetotiamine, *2023*
Fursultiamine, *4311*
Octotiamine, *6760*
Prosultiamine, *7882*
Thiamine, *9295*
Thiamine Diphosphate, *9296*
Thiamine Disulfide, *9297*

Vitamin B₂
Riboflavin, *8200*
Riboflavin Monophosphate, *8201*

Vitamin B₃ (Niacin)
Nicotinamide, *6523*
Nicotinic Acid, *6525*

Vitamin B₅
Dexpanthenol, *2947*
Pantothenic Acid, *7015*

Vitamin B₆
Pyridoxal 5-Phosphate, *7979*
Pyridoxine Hydrochloride, *7982*

Vitamin B₁₂
Cobamamide, *2451*
Hydroxocobalamin, *4809*
Methylcobalamin, *6045*
Vitamin B₁₂, *10014*

Vitamin C
Ascorbic Acid, *830*

Vitamin D
Calcipotriene, *1641*
Calcitriol, *1644*
Ergosterol, *3659*
1α-Hydroxycholecalciferol, *4819*
Vitamin D₂, *10018*
Vitamin D₃, *10019*

Vitamin E
α-Tocopherol, *9495*

Vitamin K
Menadiol, *5830*
Menadione, *5831*
Menadoxime, *5832*
Menaquinones, *5833*
Phylloquinone, *7380*
Vitamin K₅, *10023*

Others
Biotin, *1231*
Carnitine, *1849*
Folic Acid, *4221*
Inositol, *4978*
Sodium Folate, *8619*

VULNERARY
Acetylcysteine, *88*
Allantoin, *258*
Becaplermin *see 7525*
Cadexomer Iodine, *1610*
Chitin, *2065*
Dextranomer, *2950*
Oxaceprol, *6903*
Tocoretinate, *9499*

WILSON'S DISEASE TREATMENT
Ammonium Tetrathiomolybdate,
560
Ditiocarb Sodium, *3378*
Penicillamine, *7088*
Trientine, *9663*

XANTHINE OXIDASE INHIBITOR
*see also **Antigout***
Allopurinol, *279*
Febuxostat, *3948*

FORMULA INDEX

FORMULA INDEX

A

AgBr
Silver Bromide, 8506
AgCl
Silver Chloride, 8509
AgClO₃
Silver Chlorate, 8508
AgClO₄
Silver Perchlorate, 8523
AgF
Silver Fluoride, 8514
AgF₂
Silver Difluoride, 8513
AgI
Silver Iodide, 8516
AgIO₃
Silver Iodate, 8515
AgMnO₄
Silver Permanganate, 8524
AgNO₂
Silver Nitrite, 8519
AgNO₃
Silver Nitrate, 8518
AgO
Silver(II) Oxide, 8522
Ag₂CrO₄
Silver Chromate(VI), 8510
Ag₂HgI₄
Silver Tetraiodomercurate(II), 8531
Ag₂O
Silver Oxide, 8521
Ag₂O₄S
Silver Sulfate, 8529
Ag₂S
Silver Sulfide, 8530
Ag₂Se
Silver Selenide, 8528
Ag₃O₄P
Silver Phosphate, 8525
AlB₃H₁₂
Aluminum Borohydride, 331
AlBr₃
Aluminum Bromide, 332
AlCl₃
Aluminum Chloride, 337
AlCl₃O₉
Aluminum Chlorate, 336
AlCl₄H₄N
Ammonium Tetrachloroaluminate, 558
AlCl₄Na
Sodium Tetrachloroaluminate, 8687
AlF₃
Aluminum Fluoride, 339
AlF₆H₁₂N₃
Ammonium Hexafluoroaluminate, 524
AlF₆Na₃
Cryolite, 2606
AlH₃
Aluminum Hydride, 341
AlH₃O₃
Aluminum Hydroxide, 342

AlH₄Li
Aluminum Lithium Hydride, 349
AlH₄NO₈S₂
Aluminum Ammonium Sulfate, 327
AlH₆O₆P₃
Aluminum Hypophosphite, 345
AlI₃
Aluminum Iodide, 346
AlKO₈S₂
Aluminum Potassium Sulfate, 360
AlN
Aluminum Nitride, 353
AlN₃O₉
Aluminum Nitrate, 352
AlNaO₂
Sodium Aluminate, 8574
AlNaO₈S₂
Aluminum Sodium Sulfate, 363
AlO₄P
Aluminum Phosphate, 358
AlP
Aluminum Phosphide, 359
AlSb
Aluminum Antimonide, 328
Al₂CaH₈
Aluminum Calcium Hydride, 334
Al₂F₁₈Si₃
Aluminum Hexafluorosilicate, 340
Al₂MgO₈Si₂
Aluminum Magnesium Silicate, 350
Al₂O₃
Aluminum Oxide, 356
Al₂O₅Si
Aluminum Silicate, 362
Al₂O₁₂S₃
Aluminum Sulfate, 366
Al₂S₃
Aluminum Sulfide, 367
Al₂Se₃
Aluminum Selenide, 361
Al₆Bi₂O₁₂
Bismuth Aluminate, 1258
AsBr₃
Arsenic Tribromide, 800
AsCl₃
Arsenic Trichloride, 801
AsF₃
Arsenic Trifluoride, 802
AsF₅
Arsenic Pentafluoride, 796
AsGa
Gallium Arsenide, 4347
AsHNaO₂
Sodium Arsenite, 8580
AsHNa₂O₄
Sodium Arsenate, Dibasic, 8579
AsH₂KO₄
Potassium Arsenate, 7607
AsH₃
Arsine, 809
AsH₃O₄
Arsenic Acid, 795
AsI₃
Arsenic Triiodide, 803

AsIn
Indium Arsenide, 4949
As₂Ca₃O₈
Calcium Arsenate, 1649
As₂Co₃O₈
Cobaltous Arsenate, 2434
As₂O₃
Arsenic Trioxide, 804
As₂O₄Zn
Zinc Meta-arsenite, 10143
As₂O₅
Arsenic Pentoxide, 798
As₂S₃
Arsenic Trisulfide, 806
As₂S₅
Arsenic Pentasulfide, 797
As₂Se₃
Arsenic Triselenide, 805
As₄S₄
Arsenic Sulfide, 799
AuCl
Gold Monochloride, 4515
AuCl₃
Gold Trichloride, 4521
AuCl₄H
Gold Trichloride, Acid, 4522
AuCl₄K
Potassium Tetrachloroaurate(III), 7681
AuCl₄Na
Sodium Tetrachloroaurate(III), 8688
AuH₃O₃
Gold Trihydroxide, 4523
AuNa₃O₆S₄
Gold Sodium Thiosulfate, 4519
Au₂O₃
Gold Trioxide, 4524
Au₂S₃
Gold Trisulfide, 4525

B

BBr₃
Boron Tribromide, 1347
BCl₃
Boron Trichloride, 1348
BF₃
Boron Trifluoride, 1349
BF₄H
Fluoboric Acid, 4149
BF₄K
Potassium Tetrafluoroborate, 7686
BF₄Li
Lithium Tetrafluoroborate, 5543
BF₄NO
Nitrosyl Tetrafluoroborate, 6649
BF₄Na
Sodium Fluoborate, 8617
BH₃O₃
Boric Acid, 1336
BH₄K
Potassium Borohydride, 7616

BH₄Li
Lithium Borohydride, 5525
BH₄Na
Sodium Borohydride, 8592
BN
Boron Nitride, 1346
BNaO₂
Sodium Metaborate, 8639
BNaO₃
Sodium Perborate, 8652
BO
Boron Monoxide, 1345
B₂Cl₄
Diboron Tetrachloride, 3016
B₂H₆
Diborane(6), 3015
B₂Mg
Magnesium Diboride, 5664
B₂MgO₄
Magnesium Borate, 5658
B₂O₃
Boric Anhydride, 1337
B₃H₆N₃
Borazine, 1334
B₄CaO₇
Calcium Borate, 1652
B₄H₈N₂O₇
Ammonium Borate, 504
B₄H₁₀
Tetraborane(10), 9183
B₄K₂O₇
Potassium Tetraborate, 7680
B₄Li₂O₇
Lithium Borate, 5524
B₄Na₂O₇
Sodium Borate, 8590
B₅H₉
Pentaborane(9), 7104
B₅H₁₁
Pentaborane(11), 7105
B₆H₁₀
Hexaborane(10), 4676
B₁₀H₁₄
Decaborane(14), 2845
BaBr₂
Barium Bromide, 968
BaBr₂O₆
Barium Bromate, 967
BaCl₂
Barium Chloride, 971
BaCl₂O₆
Barium Chlorate, 970
BaCl₂O₈
Barium Perchlorate, 987
BaCrO₄
Barium Chromate(VI), 972
BaF₂
Barium Fluoride, 974
BaF₆Si
Barium Hexafluorosilicate, 976
BaHO₄P
Barium Phosphate, Dibasic, 990
BaH₂O₂
Barium Hydroxide, 977
BaH₂O₂.H₂O
Barium Hydroxide Monohydrate, 977
BaH₂O₂.8H₂O
Barium Hydroxide Octahydrate, 977
BaH₄O₄P₂
Barium Hypophosphite, 978
BaHgI₄
Barium Mercuric Iodide, 982
BaI₂
Barium Iodide, 980
BaI₂O₆
Barium Iodate, 979

BaMnO₄
Barium Manganate(VI), 981
BaMn₂O₈
Barium Permanganate, 988
BaN₂O₄
Barium Nitrite, 984
BaN₂O₆
Barium Nitrate, 983
BaO
Barium Oxide, 986
BaO₂
Barium Peroxide, 989
BaO₃S
Barium Sulfite, 997
BaO₃S₂
Barium Thiosulfate, 999
BaO₃Ti
Barium Titanate(IV), 1000
BaO₄S
Barium Sulfate, 994
BaO₇U₂
Barium Uranium Oxide, 1001
BaS
Barium Sulfide, 995
BaSe
Barium Selenide, 992
BaSi₂
Barium Silicide, 993
BeBr₂
Beryllium Bromide, 1164
BeCl₂
Beryllium Chloride, 1166
BeF₂
Beryllium Fluoride, 1167
BeF₄Na₂
Beryllium Sodium Fluoride, 1174
BeH₂
Beryllium Hydride, 1168
BeH₂O₂
Beryllium Hydroxide, 1169
BeK₂O₈S₂
Beryllium Potassium Sulfate, 1173
BeN₂O₆
Beryllium Nitrate, 1170
BeO
Beryllium Oxide, 1172
BeO₄S
Beryllium Sulfate, 1175
Be₃N₂
Beryllium Nitride, 1171
BiBrO
Bismuth Bromide Oxide, 1260
BiBr₃
Bismuth Bromide, 1259
BiClO
Bismuth Chloride Oxide, 1263
BiCl₃
Bismuth Chloride, 1262
BiF₃
Bismuth Fluoride, 1265
BiF₅
Bismuth Pentafluoride, 1274
BiH₃
Bismuthine, 1268
BiH₃O₃
Bismuth Hydroxide, 1267
BiIO
Bismuth Iodide Oxide, 1270
BiI₃
Bismuth Iodide, 1269
BiI₃K₄
Bismuth Potassium Iodide, 1276
BiN₃O₉
Bismuth Nitrate, 1271
BiNaO₃
Sodium Bismuthate(V), 8585

BiO₄P
Bismuth Phosphate, 1275
Bi₂O₃
Bismuth Oxide, 1273
Bi₂O₄
Bismuth Tetroxide, 1290
Bi₂O₁₂S₃
Bismuth Sulfate, 1286
Bi₂S₃
Bismuth Sulfide, 1287
Bi₂Se₃
Bismuth Selenide, 1278
Bi₂Te₃
Bismuth Telluride, 1289
Bi₄Ge₃O₁₂
Bismuth Germanate, 1266
Bi₅H₉N₄O₂₂
Bismuth Subnitrate, 1284
BrCs
Cesium Bromide, 2009
BrCu
Cuprous Bromide, 2659
BrF₃
Bromine Trifluoride, 1396
BrF₅
Bromine Pentafluoride, 1395
BrH
Hydrogen Bromide, 4793
BrHO₃
Bromic Acid, 1392
BrH₄N
Ammonium Bromide, 505
BrI
Iodine Monobromide, 5016
BrK
Potassium Bromide, 7618
BrKO₃
Potassium Bromate, 7617
BrLi
Lithium Bromide, 5526
BrNa
Sodium Bromide, 8594
BrNaO₃
Sodium Bromate, 8593
BrRb
Rubidium Bromide, 8283
BrTl
Thallium Bromide, 9258
Br₂Ca
Calcium Bromide, 1654
Br₂Cd
Cadmium Bromide, 1615
Br₂Co
Cobaltous Bromide, 2435
Br₂Cr
Chromous Bromide, 2243
Br₂Cu
Cupric Bromide, 2629
Br₂Fe
Ferrous Bromide, 4042
Br₂Hg
Mercuric Bromide, 5875
Br₂Hg₂
Mercurous Bromide, 5893
Br₂Mg
Magnesium Bromide, 5659
Br₂Mn
Manganese Bromide, 5725
Br₂Ni
Nickel Bromide, 6502
Br₂OS
Thionyl Bromide, 9347
Br₂Pb
Lead Bromide, 5403
Br₂Sn
Stannous Bromide, 8782

Br₂Sr
Strontium Bromide, 8837
Br₂Zn
Zinc Bromide, 10129
Br₃Ce
Cerous Bromide, 1995
Br₃Cr
Chromic Bromide, 2220
Br₃Fe
Ferric Bromide, 4018
Br₃HSi
Tribromosilane, 9615
Br₃In
Indium Tribromide, 4957
Br₃OP
Phosphorus Oxybromide, 7348
Br₃P
Phosphorus Tribromide, 7357
Br₃Sb
Antimony Tribromide, 706
Br₄Se
Selenium Tetrabromide, 8437
Br₄Si
Silicon Tetrabromide, 8499
Br₄Sn
Stannic Bromide, 8773
Br₄Te
Tellurium Tetrabromide, 9125
Br₄Ti
Titanium Tetrabromide, 9477
Br₅P
Phosphorus Pentabromide, 7350

C

CAgN
Silver Cyanide, 8512
CAg₂O₃
Silver Carbonate, 8507
CAuN
Gold Monocyanide, 4516
CB₄
Boron Carbide, 1344
CBaO₃
Barium Carbonate, 969
CBe₂
Beryllium Carbide, 1165
CBi₂O₅
Bismuth Subcarbonate, 1282
CBrN
Cyanogen Bromide, 2693
CCaN₂
Calcium Cyanamide, 1662
CCaO₃
Calcium Carbonate, 1657
CCdO₃
Cadmium Carbonate, 1616
CClN
Cyanogen Chloride, 2694
CCl₂F₂
Dichlorodifluoromethane, 3064
CCl₂O
Phosgene, 7335
CCl₃F
Trichlorofluoromethane, 9640
CCl₃NO₂
Chloropicrin, 2156
CCl₄
Carbon Tetrachloride, 1816
CCoO₃
Cobaltous Carbonate, 2436
CCs₂O₃
Cesium Carbonate, 2010

CCuN
Cuprous Cyanide, 2661
CCuNS
Cuprous Thiocyanate, 2669
CF₂O
Carbonyl Fluoride, 1820
CF₄
Carbon Tetrafluoride, 1817
CHBrCl₂
Bromodichloromethane, 1417
CHBr₂Cl
Chlorodibromomethane, 2135
CHBr₃
Bromoform, 1420
CHCl₃
Chloroform, 2141
CHFO
Formyl Fluoride, 4247
CHF₃
Fluoroform, 4173
CHF₃O₃S
Triflic Acid, 9676
CHI₃
Iodoform, 5033
CHKO₂
Potassium Formate, 7633
CHKO₃
Potassium Bicarbonate, 7609
CHLiO₂
Lithium Formate, 5532
CHN
Hydrogen Cyanide, 4795
CHNO
Cyanic Acid, 2686
Isocyanic Acid, 5165
CHNS
Thiocyanic Acid, 9328
CHN₃O₆
Trinitromethane, 9729
CHNaO₂
Sodium Formate, 8621
CHNaO₃
Sodium Bicarbonate, 8583
CH₂AlNaO₅
Dihydroxyaluminum Sodium Carbonate, 3184
CH₂Br₂
Methylene Bromide, 6061
CH₂ClNO
Carbamyl Chloride, 1783
CH₂Cl₂
Methylene Chloride, 6063
CH₂Cl₂Na₂O₆P₂
Clodronic Acid Disodium Salt, 2371
CH₂Cu₂O₅
Cupric Carbonate, Basic, 2631
CH₂F₂
Difluoromethane, 3151
CH₂INaO₃S
Methiodal Sodium, 5973
CH₂I₂
Methylene Iodide, 6066
CH₂N₂
Cyanamide, 2684
Diazomethane, 3001
CH₂O
Formaldehyde, 4235
CH₂O₂
Formic Acid, 4241
CH₂O₃
Performic Acid, 7160
CH₂S₃
Trithiocarbonic Acid, 9759
CH₃AsNa₂O₃
Methanearsonic Acid Disodium Salt, 5953

CH₃BNNa
Sodium Cyanoborohydride, 8606
CH₃Br
Methyl Bromide, 6029
CH₃Cl
Methyl Chloride, 6041
CH₃ClO₂S
Methanesulfonyl Chloride, 5955
CH₃F
Fluoromethane, 4174
CH₃FO₃S
Methyl Fluorosulfonate, 6075
CH₃I
Methyl Iodide, 6087
CH₃NO
Formamide, 4237
CH₃NO₂
Nitromethane, 6611
CH₃NO₃
Methyl Nitrate, 6101
CH₃NS
Thioformamide, 9333
CH₃N₃O₃
Nitrourea, 6651
CH₃NaO
Sodium Methoxide, 8643
CH₃NaO₃S
Sodium Formaldehydesulfoxylate, 8620
CH₃NaO₄S
Formaldehyde Sodium Bisulfite, 4236
CH₃O₃Re
Methyltrioxorhenium, 6130
CH₄
Methane, 5952
CH₄AsNaO₃
Methanearsonic Acid Monosodium Salt, 5953
CH₄Cl₂O₆P₂
Clodronic Acid, 2371
CH₄N₂O
Urea, 9867
CH₄N₂O₂
Hydroxyurea, 4848
CH₄N₂S
Ammonium Thiocyanate, 561
Thiourea, 9367
CH₄N₄O₂
Nitroguanidine, 6608
CH₄Ni₃O₇
Nickel Carbonate Hydroxide, 6503
CH₄O
Methanol, 5957
CH₄O₃
Orthoformic Acid, 6884
CH₄O₃S
Methanesulfonic Acid, 5954
CH₄O₄S
Methyl Sulfate, 6122
CH₄O₆S₂
Methionic Acid, 5974
CH₄S
Methanethiol, 5956
CH₅AsO₃
Methanearsonic Acid, 5953
CH₅N
Methylamine, 6014
CH₅NO
Methoxyamine, 5989
CH₅NO₂
Ammonium Formate, 523
CH₅NO₃
Ammonium Bicarbonate, 497
CH₅N₃
Guanidine, 4562

CH$_5$N$_3$O$_4$
Urea Nitrate, 9869
CH$_5$N$_5$S
Thiosemicarbazide, 9361
CH$_6$ClN$_3$O
Semicarbazide Hydrochloride, 8444
CH$_6$N$_2$
Methylhydrazine, 6086
CH$_6$N$_2$O$_2$
Ammonium Carbamate, 507
CH$_6$N$_2$O$_3$
Carbamide Peroxide, 1782
CH$_6$N$_2$S$_2$
Ammonium Dithiocarbamate, 516
CH$_6$N$_4$
Aminoguanidine, 441
CH$_6$N$_4$O
Carbohydrazide, 1804
CH$_6$O$_6$P$_2$
Medronic Acid, 5792
CH$_6$O$_7$P$_2$
Oxidronic Acid, 6940
CH$_{18}$AlN$_3$O$_{14}$S$_2$
Guanidinium Aluminum Sulfate Hexa-
hydrate, 4563
CIN
Cyanogen Iodide, 2695
CI$_4$
Carbon Tetraiodide, 1818
CKN
Potassium Cyanide, 7626
CKNO
Potassium Cyanate, 7625
CKNS
Potassium Thiocyanate, 7691
CK$_2$O$_3$
Potassium Carbonate, 7619
CK$_2$S$_3$
Potassium Thiocarbonate, 7690
CLi$_2$O$_3$
Lithium Carbonate, 5527
CMnO$_3$
Manganese Carbonate, 5726
CNNa
Sodium Cyanide, 8605
CNNaO
Sodium Cyanate, 8604
CNNaS
Thiocyanate Sodium, 9327
CNTl
Thallium Cyanide, 9261
CN$_4$
Cyanogen Azide, 2692
CN$_4$O$_8$
Tetranitromethane, 9233
CNa$_2$O$_3$
Sodium Carbonate, 8596
CNa$_2$S$_3$
Sodium Thiocarbonate, 8691
CNa$_3$O$_5$P
Foscarnet Sodium, 4251
CO
Carbon Monoxide, 1813
COS
Carbonyl Sulfide, 1821
CO$_2$
Carbon Dioxide, 1809
CO$_3$Sr
Strontium Carbonate, 8838
CO$_3$Tl$_2$
Thallium Carbonate, 9259
CO$_3$Zn
Zinc Carbonate, 10131
CS$_2$
Carbon Disulfide, 1811

CSe$_2$
Carbon Diselenide, 1810
CSi
Silicon Carbide, 8492
CW
Tungsten Carbide, 9815
C$_2$AgKN$_2$
Potassium Silver Cyanide, 7669
C$_2$Ag$_2$O$_4$
Silver Oxalate, 8520
C$_2$AuKN$_2$
Potassium Dicyanoaurate(I), 7628
C$_2$AuN$_2$Na
Sodium Dicyanoaurate(I), 8610
C$_2$BaN$_2$
Barium Cyanide, 973
C$_2$BaN$_2$S$_2$
Barium Thiocyanate, 998
C$_2$BaO$_4$
Barium Oxalate, 985
C$_2$Ca
Calcium Carbide, 1656
C$_2$CaN$_2$
Calcium Cyanide, 1664
C$_2$CaN$_2$S$_2$
Calcium Thiocyanate, 1710
C$_2$CaO$_4$
Calcium Oxalate, 1685
C$_2$CdN$_2$
Cadmium Cyanide, 1618
C$_2$Cl$_2$F$_4$
Cryofluorane, 2605
C$_2$Cl$_2$O$_2$
Oxalyl Chloride, 6914
C$_2$Cl$_3$N
Trichloroacetonitrile, 9628
C$_2$Cl$_3$NS$_2$
Appel's Salt, 749
C$_2$Cl$_4$
Tetrachloroethylene, 9190
C$_2$Cl$_4$O$_2$
Diphosgene, 3334
C$_2$Cl$_6$
Hexachloroethane, 4679
C$_2$CoN$_2$
Cobaltous Cyanide, 2439
C$_2$CoN$_2$S$_2$
Cobaltous Thiocyanate, 2450
C$_2$CoO$_4$
Cobaltous Oxalate, 2445
C$_2$CuKN$_2$
Cuprous Potassium Cyanide, 2665
C$_2$CuO$_4$
Cupric Oxalate, 2645
C$_2$F$_4$
Tetrafluoroethylene, 9205
C$_2$FeN$_2$S$_2$
Ferrous Thiocyanate, 4059
C$_2$FeO$_4$
Ferrous Oxalate, 4051
C$_2$HBrClF$_3$
Halothane, 4603
C$_2$HBrF$_4$
Teflurane, 9110
C$_2$HBr$_3$O
Bromal, 1383
C$_2$HBr$_3$O$_2$
Tribromoacetic Acid, 9609
C$_2$HCl$_3$
Trichloroethylene, 9639
C$_2$HCl$_3$O
2,2-Dichloroacetyl Chloride, 3053
Trichloroacetaldehyde, 9626
C$_2$HCl$_3$O$_2$
Trichloroacetic Acid, 9627

C$_2$HCl$_5$
Pentachloroethane, 7108
C$_2$HF$_3$O$_2$
Trifluoroacetic Acid, 9681
C$_2$HKO$_4$
Potassium Binoxalate, 7611
C$_2$HNa$_3$O$_6$
Sodium Sesquicarbonate, 8674
C$_2$H$_2$
Acetylene, 90
C$_2$H$_2$AsCl$_3$
Dichloro(2-chlorovinyl)arsine, 3062
C$_2$H$_2$BaO$_4$
Barium Formate, 975
C$_2$H$_2$Br$_2$
Acetylene Dibromide, 91
C$_2$H$_2$Br$_4$
sym-Tetrabromoethane, 9185
C$_2$H$_2$CaO$_4$
Calcium Formate, 1668
C$_2$H$_2$ClNaO$_2$
Chloroacetic Acid Sodium Salt, 2112
C$_2$H$_2$Cl$_2$
Acetylene Dichloride, 92
Vinylidene Chloride, 9996
C$_2$H$_2$Cl$_2$O
Chloracetyl Chloride, 2067
C$_2$H$_2$Cl$_2$O$_2$
Dichloroacetic Acid, 3050
C$_2$H$_2$Cl$_4$
Tetrachloroethane, 9189
C$_2$H$_2$CoO$_4$
Cobaltous Formate, 2441
C$_2$H$_2$CrO$_4$
Chromous Formate, 2246
C$_2$H$_2$CuO$_4$
Cupric Formate, 2639
C$_2$H$_2$FNaO$_2$
Fluoroacetic Acid Sodium Salt, 4167
C$_2$H$_2$F$_4$
HFC-134a, 4714
C$_2$H$_2$MgO$_4$
Magnesium Formate, 5666
C$_2$H$_2$MoO$_7$
Oxalomolybdic Acid, 6913
C$_2$H$_2$N$_2$O
1,3,4-Oxadiazole, 6906
C$_2$H$_2$NiO$_4$
Nickel Formate, 6509
C$_2$H$_2$O
Ketene, 5298
C$_2$H$_2$O$_2$
Glyoxal, 4509
C$_2$H$_2$O$_3$
Glyoxylic Acid, 4511
C$_2$H$_2$O$_4$
Oxalic Acid, 6911
C$_2$H$_2$O$_4$Pb
Lead Formate, 5409
C$_2$H$_2$O$_4$Zn
Zinc Formate, 10137
C$_2$H$_2$O$_8$Pb$_3$
Basic Lead Carbonate, 1005
C$_2$H$_3$AgO$_2$
Silver Acetate, 8505
C$_2$H$_3$BiO$_3$
Bismuth Subacetate, 1281
C$_2$H$_3$BrO
Acetyl Bromide, 82
C$_2$H$_3$BrO$_2$
Bromoacetic Acid, 1400
C$_2$H$_3$Br$_3$O$_2$
Bromal Hydrate, 1384
C$_2$H$_3$Cl
Vinyl Chloride, 9994

C₂H₃ClO
Acetyl Chloride, 85
Chloroacetaldehyde, 2109
C₂H₃ClO₂
Chloroacetic Acid, 2112
Methyl Chlorocarbonate, 6043
C₂H₃Cl₃
1,1,1-Trichloroethane, 9636
1,1,2-Trichloroethane, 9637
C₂H₃Cl₃NaO₄P
Triclofos Monosodium Salt, 9655
C₂H₃Cl₃O
2,2,2-Trichloroethanol, 9638
C₂H₃Cl₃O₂
Chloral Hydrate, 2071
C₂H₃CuO₂
Cuprous Acetate, 2658
C₂H₃FO₂
Fluoroacetic Acid, 4167
C₂H₃F₃O
Trifluoroethanol, 9682
C₂H₃IO
Acetyl Iodide, 94
C₂H₃IO₂
Iodoacetic Acid, 5025
C₂H₃KO₂
Potassium Acetate, 7605
C₂H₃KO₄
Potassium Diformate, 7629
C₂H₃LiO₂
Lithium Acetate, 5521
C₂H₃N
Acetonitrile, 70
C₂H₃NO
Methyl Isocyanate, 6089
C₂H₃NO₃
Oxamic Acid, 6917
C₂H₃NO₄
Acetyl Nitrate, 97
C₂H₃NS
Methyl Isothiocyanate, 6092
Methyl Thiocyanate, 6127
C₂H₃N₃
1H-1,2,4-Triazole, 9605
C₂H₃N₃O₂
Urazole, 9866
C₂H₃NaO₂
Sodium Acetate, 8571
C₂H₃NaO₂S
Sodium Thioglycolate, 8692
C₂H₃O₂Tl
Thallium Acetate, 9257
C₂H₄
Ethylene, 3791
C₂H₄BrNO
N-Bromoacetamide, 1398
C₂H₄Br₂
Ethylene Dibromide, 3796
C₂H₄ClNO
Chloroacetamide, 2110
C₂H₄Cl₂
Ethylene Dichloride, 3797
Ethylidene Chloride, 3810
C₂H₄Cl₂N₆
Chloroazodin, 2120
C₂H₄Cl₂O
sym-Dichloromethyl Ether, 3069
C₂H₄Cl₃O₄P
Triclofos, 9655
C₂H₄FNO
Fluoroacetamide, 4166
C₂H₄NNaS₂
Metham Sodium, 5949
C₂H₄N₂
Aminoacetonitrile, 412

C₂H₄N₂O₂
Oxamide, 6918
C₂H₄N₂O₆
Ethylene Glycol Dinitrate, 3800
C₂H₄N₂S₂
Rubeanic Acid, 8279
C₂H₄N₄
Amitrole, 489
Dicyanodiamide, 3092
C₂H₄N₄O₂
Azodicarbonamide, 919
C₂H₄Na₂O₈S₂
Glyoxal-Sodium Bisulfite, 4510
C₂H₄O
Acetaldehyde, 39
Ethylene Oxide, 3802
C₂H₄OS
Thioacetic Acid, 9320
C₂H₄O₂
Acetic Acid Glacial, 55
Methyl Formate, 6077
C₂H₄O₂S
Thioglycolic Acid, 9336
C₂H₄O₃
Glycolic Acid, 4498
Peracetic Acid, 7150
C₂H₄O₅S
Sulfoacetic Acid, 8953
C₂H₄S₅
Lenthionine, 5438
C₂H₅AsO₅
Arsonoacetic Acid, 810
C₂H₅Br
Ethyl Bromide, 3771
C₂H₅BrO
Ethylene Bromohydrin, 3792
C₂H₅Cl
Ethyl Chloride, 3782
C₂H₅ClHg
Ethylmercuric Chloride, 3826
C₂H₅ClO
Chloromethyl Methyl Ether, 2146
Ethylene Chlorohydrin, 3793
C₂H₅FeNO₆S
Ferroglycine Sulfate, 4039
C₂H₅I
Ethyl Iodide, 3813
C₂H₅N
Ethylenimine, 3804
C₂H₅NO
Acetaldoxime, 42
Acetamide, 43
N-Methylformamide, 6076
C₂H₅NO₂
Acetohydroxamic Acid, 63
Ethyl Nitrite, 3831
Glycine, 4491
Methyl Carbamate, 6036
Nitroethane, 6597
C₂H₅NO₄
Ammonium Binoxalate, 499
C₂H₅NS
Thioacetamide, 9319
C₂H₅N₃O₂
Biuret, 1309
Semioxamazide, 8445
C₂H₅N₃S₂
2,4-Dithiobiuret, 3371
C₂H₅N₅O₃
N-Methyl-N'-nitro-N-nitrosoguanidine, 6103
C₂H₅NaO
Sodium Ethoxide, 8613
C₂H₅NaOS
Sodium Methylsulfinylmethylide, 8644

C₂H₅NaO₃S₂
Mesna, 5909
C₂H₅NaO₄S
Acetaldehyde Sodium Bisulfite, 41
Sodium Ethyl Sulfate, 8614
C₂H₆
Ethane, 3723
C₂H₆AlNO₄
Dihydroxyaluminum Aminoacetate, 3183
C₂H₆AsNaO₂
Sodium Cacodylate, 8595
C₂H₆BaO₈S₂
Methyl Sulfate Barium Salt, 6122
C₂H₆CaO₈S₂
Methyl Sulfate Calcium Salt, 6122
C₂H₆Cd
Dimethylcadmium, 3239
C₂H₆ClO₃P
Ethephon, 3732
C₂H₆Co₅O₁₂
Cobaltous Carbonate Basic, 2436
C₂H₆Hg
Dimethylmercury, 3250
C₂H₆N₂O
N-Nitrosodimethylamine, 6637
C₂H₆Na₂O₇P₂
Etidronic Acid Disodium Salt, 3863
C₂H₆O
Ethyl Alcohol, 3760
Methyl Ether, 6071
C₂H₆OS
Dimethyl Sulfoxide, 3259
2-Mercaptoethanol, 5869
C₂H₆O₂
Ethylene Glycol, 3798
C₂H₆O₂S
Dimethyl Sulfone, 3258
C₂H₆O₃S
Methyl Methanesulfonate, 6097
C₂H₆O₄S
Dimethyl Sulfate, 3256
Ethyl Sulfate, 3853
Isethionic Acid, 5107
C₂H₆O₆S₂
1,2-Ethanedisulfonic Acid, 3724
C₂H₆S
Ethanethiol, 3726
Methyl Sulfide, 6123
C₂H₆S₂
1,2-Ethanedithiol, 3725
C₂H₆Zn
Dimethylzinc, 3263
C₂H₇AsO₂
Cacodylic Acid, 1604
C₂H₇ClN₂
Acetamidine Hydrochloride, 44
C₂H₇N
Dimethylamine, 3228
Ethylamine, 3762
C₂H₇NO
Acetaldehyde Ammonia, 40
Ethanolamine, 3727
C₂H₇NO₂
Ammonium Acetate, 495
C₂H₇NO₃S
Taurine, 9074
C₂H₇NS
Cysteamine, 2779
C₂H₇N₃
Methylguanidine, 6083
C₂H₇N₅
Biguanide, 1215
C₂H₈NO₂PS
Methamidophos, 5947

C₂H₈NO₃PS
Phosphocysteamine, 7341

C₂H₈N₂
1,1-Dimethylhydrazine, 3247
1,2-Dimethylhydrazine, 3248
Ethylenediamine, 3795

C₂H₈N₂O₄
Ammonium Oxalate, 537

C₂H₈O₇P₂
Etidronic Acid, 3863

C₂H₁₄Al₂Mg₆O₂₀.4H₂O
Almagate, 299

C₂HgN₂
Mercuric Cyanide, 5877

C₂HgN₂S₂
Mercuric Thiocyanate, 5890

C₂Hg₂N₂O
Mercuric Oxycyanide, 5884

C₂I₄
Tetraiodoethylene, 9220

C₂K₂O₄
Potassium Oxalate, 7651

C₂K₂O₆
Potassium Percarbonate, 7652

C₂Li₂O₄
Lithium Oxalate, 5537

C₂MgN₂S₂
Magnesium Thiocyanate, 5693

C₂MgO₄
Magnesium Oxalate, 5676

C₂MnO₄
Manganese Oxalate, 5734

C₂N₂
Cyanogen, 2691

C₂N₂Ni
Nickel Cyanide, 6506

C₂N₂PbS₂
Lead Thiocyanate, 5426

C₂N₂S₂Zn
Zinc Thiocyanate, 10163

C₂N₂Zn
Zinc Cyanide, 10135

C₂Na₂O₄
Sodium Oxalate, 8650

C₂NiO₄
Nickel Oxalate, 6514

C₂O₄Pb
Lead Oxalate, 5415

C₂O₄Sn
Stannous Oxalate, 8786

C₂O₄Zn
Zinc Oxalate, 10146

C₃AlN₃S₃
Aluminum Thiocyanate, 369

C₃Al₄
Aluminum Carbide, 335

C₃BiF₉O₉S₃
Bismuth Triflate, 1292

C₃Ce₂O₉
Cerous Carbonate, 1996

C₃Cl₂KN₃O₃
Troclosene Potassium, 9767

C₃Cl₃N₃
Cyanuric Chloride, 2699

C₃Cl₃N₃O₃
Trichloroisocyanuric Acid, 9641

C₃F₆O
Hexafluoroacetone, 4685

C₃F₈
Perfluoropropane, 7158

C₃F₉O₉S₃Yb
Ytterbium Triflate, 10106

C₃FeN₃S₃
Ferric Thiocyanate, 4034

C₃HBr₅O
Pentabromoacetone, 7106

C₃H₂ClF₅O
Enflurane, 3581
Isoflurane, 5175

C₃H₂ClNO₂
Chloroacetyl Isocyanate, 2117

C₃H₂Cl₃NO
Chlorocyanohydrin, 2134

C₃H₂F₆O
Desflurane, 2919

C₃H₂N₂
Malononitrile, 5711

C₃H₂N₂O₃
Parabanic Acid, 7022

C₃H₂O₂
Propiolic Acid, 7821

C₃H₂O₅
Mesoxalic Acid, 5913

C₃H₃Cl
Propargyl Chloride, 7810

C₃H₃Cl₂NaO₂
Dalapon Sodium Salt, 2802

C₃H₃CrO₆
Chromic Formate, 2224

C₃H₃FeO₆
Ferric Formate, 4023

C₃H₃N
Acrylonitrile, 131

C₃H₃NOS
Rhodanine, 8184

C₃H₃NO₂
Cyanoacetic Acid, 2689

C₃H₃NS
Thiazole, 9307

C₃H₃N₃
s-Triazine, 9602

C₃H₃N₃O₂
Azomycin, 921

C₃H₃N₃O₂S
2-Amino-5-nitrothiazole, 457

C₃H₃N₃O₃
Cyamelide, 2682
Cyanuric Acid, 2698

C₃H₄Br₂
2,3-Dibromopropene, 3025

C₃H₄ClN
β-Chloropropionitrile, 2160

C₃H₄Cl₂
1,3-Dichloropropene, 3075

C₃H₄Cl₂F₂O
Methoxyflurane, 5994

C₃H₄Cl₂O
1,1-Dichloroacetone, 3051
1,3-Dichloroacetone, 3052

C₃H₄Cl₂O₂
Dalapon, 2802

C₃H₄Cl₃NO₂
Chloral Formamide, 2070

C₃H₄F₄O
2,2,3,3-Tetrafluoro-1-propanol, 9206

C₃H₄NNaO₃S
Sodium β-Sulfopropionitrile, 8683

C₃H₄N₂
Imidazole, 4912
Methyleneaminoacetonitrile, 6057
Pyrazole, 7960

C₃H₄N₂O
Cyanoacetamide, 2688

C₃H₄N₂O₂
Hydantoin, 4760

C₃H₄N₂S
2-Aminothiazole, 479

C₃H₄N₄O₆
TNAZ, 9487

C₃H₄O
Acrolein, 128
Propargyl Alcohol, 7809

C₃H₄O₂
Acrylic Acid, 130
Malondialdehyde, 5709
Methylglyoxal, 6081
β-Propiolactone, 7820

C₃H₄O₃
Pyruvic Acid, 8021

C₃H₄O₄
Malonic Acid, 5710

C₃H₄O₅
Tartronic Acid, 9073

C₃H₅AgO₃
Silver Lactate, 8517

C₃H₅Br
Allyl Bromide, 288

C₃H₅BrO
Bromoacetone, 1401

C₃H₅BrO₂
β-Bromopropionic Acid, 1433

C₃H₅Br₂Cl
Dibromochloropropane, 3020

C₃H₅Br₃
1,2,3-Tribromopropane, 9614

C₃H₅CaO₄P.H₂O
Fosfomycin Calcium Salt Monohydrate, 4254

C₃H₅Cl
Allyl Chloride, 289

C₃H₅ClN₂O₆
Clonitrate, 2391

C₃H₅ClO
Chloroacetone, 2114
Epichlorohydrin, 3611
Propionyl Chloride, 7828

C₃H₅ClO₂
β-Chloropropionic Acid, 2159
Ethyl Chloroformate, 3784
Methyl Chloroacetate, 6042

C₃H₅Cl₃O
1,1,1-Trichloro-2-propanol, 9645

C₃H₅I
Allyl Iodide, 294

C₃H₅KOS₂
Potassium Xanthogenate, 7696

C₃H₅N
Propionitrile, 7827

C₃H₅NO
Acrylamide, 129
Ethylene Cyanohydrin, 3794

C₃H₅NO₂
Isonitrosoacetone, 5190

C₃H₅NO₄
Hadacidin, 4587

C₃H₅NS
Ethyl Isothiocyanate, 3815
Thiocyanic Acid Ethyl Ester, 9328

C₃H₅N₃O
Cyacetacide, 2680

C₃H₅N₃O₉
Nitroglycerin, 6607

C₃H₅NaO₂
Sodium Propionate, 8669

C₃H₅NaO₃
Sodium Lactate, 8635

C₃H₆
Cyclopropane, 2748
Propylene, 7849

C₃H₆BrNO₄
Bronopol, 1447

C₃H₆Br₂
Propylene Dibromide, 7853
Trimethylene Bromide, 9713

C₃H₆Cl₂
Propylene Dichloride, 7854
Propylidene Chloride, 7861

C₃H₆Cl₂O
$C_3H_6Cl_2O$
1,3-Dichloro-2-propanol, 3074

$C_3H_6Cl_3N$
Viehe's Salt, 9977

$C_3H_6FNO_2$
3-Fluoro-D-alanine, 4168

$C_3H_6N_2$
3-Aminopropionitrile, 469
2-Pyrazoline, 7961

$C_3H_6N_2O$
2-Imidazolidinone, 4914

$C_3H_6N_2O_2$
Cycloserine, 2751

$C_3H_6N_2S$
Ethylene Thiourea, 3803

$C_3H_6N_4O_3$
Triuret, 9766

$C_3H_6N_6$
Melamine, 5811

$C_3H_6N_6O_6$
Cyclonite, 2736

C_3H_6O
Acetone, 66
Allyl Alcohol, 286
Propionaldehyde, 7823
Propylene Oxide, 7856
Trimethylene Oxide, 9715

C_3H_6OS
Propanethial S-Oxide, 7802

$C_3H_6O_2$
Acetol, 65
Ethyl Formate, 3807
Glycidol, 4490
Methyl Acetate, 6008
Propionic Acid, 7825

$C_3H_6O_2S$
Thiolactic Acid, 9340

$C_3H_6O_3$
Dihydroxyacetone, 3182
Dimethyl Carbonate, 3241
Glyceraldehyde, 4481
Hydracrylic Acid, 4762
D-Lactic Acid, 5335
DL-Lactic Acid, 5336
L-Lactic Acid, 5337
s-Trioxane, 9734

$C_3H_6O_4$
Glyceric Acid, 4483

C_3H_7Br
Isopropyl Bromide, 5210
Propyl Bromide, 7845

$C_3H_7CaO_6P$
Calcium Glycerophosphate, 1670

C_3H_7Cl
Isopropyl Chloride, 5211
Propyl Chloride, 7847

C_3H_7ClO
Propylene Chlorohydrin, 7850
sec-Propylene Chlorohydrin, 7851

$C_3H_7ClO_2$
α-Chlorohydrin, 2145

C_3H_7I
Isopropyl Iodide, 5214
Propyl Iodide, 7862

$C_3H_7IO_2$
Glyceryl Iodide, 4488

C_3H_7N
Allylamine, 287

C_3H_7NO
Acetoxime, 75
N,N-Dimethylformamide, 3243
Propionamide, 7824

$C_3H_7NO_2$
Alanine, 204
β-Alanine, 205
Formicin, 4242

Isopropyl Nitrite, 5216
1-Nitropropane, 6627
2-Nitropropane, 6628
n-Propyl Nitrite, 7865
Sarcosine, 8373
Urethan, 9874

$C_3H_7NO_2S$
Cysteine, 2781

$C_3H_7NO_2Se$
Selenocysteine, 8440

$C_3H_7NO_3$
n-Propyl Nitrate, 7864
Serine, 8460

$C_3H_7NO_5S$
Cysteic Acid, 2780

$C_3H_7N_2O_3P$
Seyferth-Gilbert Reagent, 8476

$C_3H_7N_3O_2$
N-Ethyl-N-nitrosourea, 3833
Glycocyamine, 4495

$C_3H_7N_3O_4$
L-Alanosine, 206

$C_3H_7NaO_3S_3$
2,3-Dimercapto-1-propanesulfonic
Acid Sodium Salt, 3210

$C_3H_7NaO_4S$
Acetone Sodium Bisulfite, 69

$C_3H_7Na_2O_6P$
Sodium Glycerophosphate, 8622

$C_3H_7O_4P$
Fosfomycin, 4254

$C_3H_7O_6P$
Glyceraldehyde 3-Phosphate, 4482

C_3H_8
Propane, 7799

C_3H_8IN
Dimethyl(methylene)ammonium
Iodide, 3251

$C_3H_8NO_5P$
Glyphosate, 4512

$C_3H_8NO_6P$
Phosphoserine, 7363

$C_3H_8N_2OS$
Noxythiolin, 6724

$C_3H_8N_2O_2$
2,3-Diaminopropionic Acid, 2984

$C_3H_8N_2O_3$
Oxymethurea, 6968

$C_3H_8N_2S$
N,N'-Dimethylthiourea, 3261

C_3H_8O
Ethyl Methyl Ether, 3828
Isopropyl Alcohol, 5208
n-Propyl Alcohol, 7842

$C_3H_8OS_2$
Dimercaprol, 3209

$C_3H_8O_2$
Methylal, 6012
Methyl Cellosolve®, 6038
Propylene Glycol, 7855
Trimethylene Glycol, 9714

$C_3H_8O_2S$
Thioglycerol, 9335

$C_3H_8O_3$
Glycerol, 4484

$C_3H_8O_3S$
Ethyl Methanesulfonate, 3827

$C_3H_8O_3S_3$
2,3-Dimercapto-1-propanesulfonic
Acid, 3210

$C_3H_8S_2$
Bis[methylthio]methane, 1256
1,3-Propanedithiol, 7801

$C_3H_9AsO_3$
1-Propanearsonic Acid, 7800

$C_3H_9BO_3$
Trimethyl Borate, 9712

C_3H_9N
Isopropylamine, 5209
Propylamine, 7843
Trimethylamine, 9710

$C_3H_9NNa_2O_7P_2$
Pamidronic Acid Disodium Salt, 7003

$C_3H_9NO_3$
Ammonium Lactate, 530

$C_3H_9NO_3S$
N-Methyltaurine, 6124

$C_3H_9O_2PS$
EMPTA, 3564

$C_3H_9O_3P$
DMMP, 3391
EMPA, 3563

$C_3H_9O_6P$
Glycerophosphoric Acid, 4486

$C_3H_{10}N_2$
Propylenediamine, 7852

$C_3H_{11}Br_2N_3S$
AET, 178

$C_3H_{11}NO_7P_2$
Pamidronic Acid, 7003

$C_3H_{13}N_3O_{10}Zr$
Ammonium Zirconyl Carbonate, 569

$C_3H_{16}N_4O_{11}U$
Ammonium Uranium Carbonate, 566

$C_3La_2O_9$
Lanthanum Carbonate Octahydrate, 5363
Lanthanum Carbonate, 5364

C_3N_4
Carbon Nitride, 1814

C_3O_2
Carbon Suboxide, 1815

C_4BaN_4Pt
Barium Platinous Cyanide, 991

$C_4CdK_2N_4$
Cadmium Potassium Cyanide, 1624

$C_4Cl_2O_4Rh_2$
Rhodium Carbonyl Chloride, 8187

C_4Cl_6
Hexachlorobutadiene, 4678

C_4F_8
Octafluorocyclobutane, 6745

C_4HCoO_4
Cobalt Carbonyl Hydride, 3085

C_4HI_4N
Iodopyrrole, 5041

$C_4H_2Cl_2O_3$
Mucochloric Acid, 6297

$C_4H_2FeO_4$
Ferrous Fumarate, 4046

$C_4H_2N_2O_4$
Alloxan, 282

$C_4H_2N_4O_2$
5-Diazouracil, 3003

$C_4H_2O_3$
Maleic Anhydride, 5704

$C_4H_2O_4$
Squaric Acid, 8769

$C_4H_3AuNa_2O_4S$
Gold Sodium Thiomalate, 4518

$C_4H_3BrN_2O_2$
5-Bromouracil, 1440

$C_4H_3FN_2O_2$
Fluorouracil, 4181

$C_4H_3F_7O$
Sevoflurane, 8475

$C_4H_3KO_8$
Potassium Tetroxalate, 7689

$C_4H_3N_3$
1-Cyanoimidazole, 2696

C₄H₃N₃O₄
Oxonic Acid, 6947
Violuric Acid, 10000

C₄H₃N₃O₅
5-Nitrobarbituric Acid, 6586

C₄H₄As₂Na₂O₄
Arsenoacetic Acid Disodium Salt, 808

C₄H₄AuNaO₄S
Gold Sodium Thiomalate, 4518

C₄H₄BrNO₂
N-Bromosuccinimide, 1438

C₄H₄Br₂O₄
2,3-Dibromosuccinic Acid, 3029

C₄H₄CaO₄
Calcium Succinate, 1705

C₄H₄CaO₆
Calcium Tartrate, 1709

C₄H₄ClNO₂
N-Chlorosuccinimide, 2164

C₄H₄Cl₂O₂
Succinyl Chloride, 8873

C₄H₄Cl₂O₃
Chloroacetic Anhydride, 2113

C₄H₄CuO₆
Cupric Tartrate, 2656

C₄H₄FN₃O
Flucytosine, 4125

C₄H₄F₆O
Flurothyl, 4201

C₄H₄FeO₄
Ferrous Succinate, 4056

C₄H₄INO₂
N-Iodosuccinimide, 5045

C₄H₄KNO₄S
Acesulfame Potassium Salt, 37

C₄H₄KNaO₆
Potassium Sodium Tartrate, 7670

C₄H₄K₂O₄.3H₂O
Succinic Acid Potassium Salt Trihydrate, 8869

C₄H₄K₂O₆
Potassium Tartrate, 7677

C₄H₄N₂
Pyrazine, 7957
Pyridazine, 7969
Pyrimidine, 7987
Succinonitrile, 8872

C₄H₄N₂OS
2-Thiouracil, 9366

C₄H₄N₂O₂
Cellocidin, 1962
Maleic Hydrazide, 5705
Uracil, 9850

C₄H₄N₂O₃
Barbituric Acid, 963

C₄H₄N₆O
8-Azaguanine, 896

C₄H₄NaO₄S₂Sb
Antimony Sodium Thioglycollate, 703

C₄H₄NaO₇Sb
Antimony Sodium Tartrate, 702

C₄H₄Na₂O₄
Sodium Succinate, 8679

C₄H₄Na₂O₄.6H₂O
Sodium Succinate Hexahydrate, 8679

C₄H₄Na₂O₆
Sodium Tartrate, 8684

C₄H₄O
Furan, 4296

C₄H₄O₃
Succinic Anhydride, 8870

C₄H₄O₄
Fumaric Acid, 4287
Maleic Acid, 5703

C₄H₄O₅
Oxalacetic Acid, 6909

C₄H₄O₆
Dihydroxymaleic Acid, 3185

C₄H₄O₆Sn
Stannous Tartrate, 8792

C₄H₄O₆Zn
Zinc Tartrate, 10161

C₄H₄S
Thiophene, 9353

C₄H₅BrO₄
Bromosuccinic Acid, 1437

C₄H₅Cl₃O
α,α,β-Trichloro-n-butyraldehyde, 9633

C₄H₅Cl₃O₂
Trichloroacetic Acid Ethyl Ester, 9627

C₄H₅F₃O
Fluroxene, 4202

C₄H₅KO₆
Potassium Bitartrate, 7615

C₄H₅N
Allyl Cyanide, 290
Methacrylonitrile, 5942
1H-Pyrrole, 8014

C₄H₅NOS
Methylisothiazolinone, 6091

C₄H₅NO₂
Hymexazol, 4856
Succinimide, 8871

C₄H₅NO₃
Maleamic Acid, 5701

C₄H₅NO₃S
L-2-Oxo-4-thiazolidinecarboxylic acid, 6950

C₄H₅NO₄S
Acesulfame, 37

C₄H₅NS
Allyl Isothiocyanate, 295

C₄H₅N₃O
Cytosine, 2795

C₄H₅N₃O₂
6-Azathymine, 903
Mizoribine Aglycone, 6222

C₄H₅N₃O₃
Uramil, 9852

C₄H₅NaO₆
Sodium Bitartrate, 8589

C₄H₆
1,3-Butadiene, 1509

C₄H₆As₂O₄
Arsenoacetic Acid, 808

C₄H₆As₂Cu₄O₁₆
Cupric Acetoarsenite, 2625

C₄H₆BaO₄
Barium Acetate, 965

C₄H₆BeO₄
Beryllium Acetate, 1162

C₄H₆CaO₄
Calcium Acetate, 1646

C₄H₆CaO₄S₂
Calcium Thioglycollate, 1711

C₄H₆CdO₄
Cadmium Acetate, 1614

C₄H₆CoO₄
Cobaltous Acetate, 2433

C₄H₆CrO₄
Chromous Acetate, 2242

C₄H₆CuO₄
Cupric Acetate, 2624

C₄H₆HgO₄
Mercuric Acetate, 5873

C₄H₆Hg₂O₄
Mercurous Acetate, 5892

C₄H₆MgO₄
Magnesium Acetate, 5654

C₄H₆MnO₄
Manganese Acetate, 5724

C₄H₆N₂
Fomepizole, 4226

C₄H₆N₂Na₂S₄
Nabam, 6341

C₄H₆N₂O₂
Diazoacetic Ester, 2997
Muscimol, 6312
2,5-Piperazinedione, 7466

C₄H₆N₂S
2-Amino-4-methylthiazole, 450
Methimazole, 5971

C₄H₆N₄O
2,4-Diamino-6-hydroxypyrimidine, 2981

C₄H₆N₄O₂
Acetyleneurea, 93
Divicine, 3383

C₄H₆N₄O₃
Allantoin, 258

C₄H₆N₄O₃S₂
Acetazolamide, 53

C₄H₆N₄O₁₂
Erythrityl Tetranitrate, 3677

C₄H₆NiO₄
Nickel Acetate, 6499

C₄H₆O
Crotonaldehyde, 2596
Methyl Vinyl Ketone, 6134
Vinyl Ether, 9995

C₄H₆O₂
Butyrolactone, 1596
Crotonic Acid, 2597
Diacetyl, 2966
Erythritol Anhydride, 3676
Isocrotonic Acid, 5164
Methacrylic Acid, 5941
Methyl Acrylate, 6011
Vinyl Acetate, 9992

C₄H₆O₂S
3-Sulfolene, 8956

C₄H₆O₃
Acetic Anhydride, 56
Acetoacetic Acid, 59

C₄H₆O₄
Methyl Oxalate, 6106
Succinic Acid, 8869

C₄H₆O₄Pb
Lead Acetate, 5397

C₄H₆O₄Pd
Palladium Diacetate, 6991

C₄H₆O₄S
Thiodiglycolic Acid, 9331
Thiomalic Acid, 9343

C₄H₆O₄S₂
Succimer, 8865

C₄H₆O₄Sn
Stannous Acetate, 8781

C₄H₆O₄Sr
Strontium Acetate, 8836

C₄H₆O₄Zn
Zinc Acetate, 10128

C₄H₆O₄Zn.2H₂O
Zinc Acetate Dihydrate, 10128

C₄H₆O₅
Malic Acid, 5707

C₄H₆O₆
D-Tartaric Acid, 9068
DL-Tartaric Acid, 9069
L-Tartaric Acid, 9070
meso-Tartaric Acid, 9071

C₄H₆O₆S
Sulfonyldiacetic Acid, 8961

C₅H₇NO₃
Dimethadione, 3213
L-Pyroglutamic Acid, 8001

C₅H₇N₃
3,4-Diaminopyridine, 2986

C₅H₇N₃O
5-Methylcytosine, 6050

C₅H₇N₃O₂
Dimetridazole, 3265

C₅H₇N₃O₄
Azaserine, 899

C₅H₇N₃O₅
Quisqualic Acid, 8085

C₅H₈
Isoprene, 5201

C₅H₈Cl₂N₂
DMC, 3390

C₅H₈NNaO₄
Monosodium Glutamate, 6254

C₅H₈N₂S₄Zn
Propineb, 7819

C₅H₈N₄O₃S₂
Methazolamide, 5962

C₅H₈N₄O₁₂
Pentaerythritol Tetranitrate, 7112

C₅H₈O
Cyclopentanone, 2743
2-Methyl-3-butyn-2-ol, 6034
Senecialdehyde, 8448

C₅H₈O₂
Acetylacetone, 81
Allyl acetate, 285
Angelic Acid, 646
Ethyl Acrylate, 3759
Glutaraldehyde, 4472
Isopropenyl Acetate, 5203
Tiglic Acid, 9433

C₅H₈O₃
Levulinic Acid, 5472
Methyl Acetoacetate, 6009

C₅H₈O₄
Glutaric Acid, 4473
Methyl Malonate, 6096

C₅H₈O₅
Citramalic Acid, 2323

C₅H₉BrO₂
α-Bromoisovaleric Acid, 1422
Ethyl α-Bromopropionate, 3772

C₅H₉ClO
Isovaleryl Chloride, 5232

C₅H₉ClO₂
Ethyl α-Chloropropionate, 3785
Isobutyl Chlorocarbonate, 5139

C₅H₉Cl₂N₃O₂
Carmustine, 1845

C₅H₉IO₃
Domiodol, 3414

C₅H₉N
N-Methylpyrroline, 6118
Valeronitrile, 9905

C₅H₉NO
Butyl Isocyanate, 1575
1-Methylpyrrolidone, 6117

C₅H₉NO₂
Proline, 7780

C₅H₉NO₃
δ-Aminolevulinic Acid, 446
Hydroxyproline, 4840

C₅H₉NO₃S
Acetylcysteine, 88
Tiopronin, 9453

C₅H₉NO₄
Glutamic Acid, 4469
HON, 4741
NMDA, 6662

C₅H₉NO₄S
Carbocysteine, 1802

C₅H₉NO₅
Hydroxyglutamic Acid, 4825

C₅H₉N₂O₄P
Bestmann-Ohira Reagent, 1177

C₅H₉N₃
Betazole, 1183
Histamine, 4719

C₅H₉N₃O₁₀
Pentrinitrol, 7138

C₅H₁₀
Amylene, 607
Cyclopentane, 2741
1-Pentene, 7122
2-Pentene, 7123

C₅H₁₀NNaS₂
Ditiocarb Sodium, 3378

C₅H₁₀N₂O
1,3-Dimethyl-2-imidazolidinone, 3249

C₅H₁₀N₂O₂S
Methomyl, 5982

C₅H₁₀N₂O₃
Glutamine, 4471
L-Isoglutamine, 5177

C₅H₁₀N₂O₇P₂
Zoledronic Acid, 10187

C₅H₁₀N₂S₂
Dazomet, 2834

C₅H₁₀O
Allyl Ethyl Ether, 293
Cyclopentanol, 2742
Diethyl Ketone, 3121
Isovaleraldehyde, 5229
Methyl Isopropyl Ketone, 6090
Methyl Propyl Ketone, 6114
Tetrahydropyran, 9217
n-Valeraldehyde, 9902

C₅H₁₀O₂
Ethyl Propionate, 3847
Isobutyl Formate, 5143
Isopropyl Acetate, 5205
Isovaleric Acid, 5231
Methyl Butyrate, 6035
Methyl Isobutyrate, 6088
Pivalic Acid, 7511
Propyl Acetate, 7841
Tetrahydrofurfuryl Alcohol, 9213
n-Valeric Acid, 9904

C₅H₁₀O₃
Ethyl Carbonate, 3780
Ethyl Lactate, 3817
Methyl Cellosolve® Acetate, 6039

C₅H₁₀O₃S
Methionine Hydroxy Analog, 5976

C₅H₁₀O₄
D-2-Deoxyribose, 2908
Dimethylolpropionic Acid, 3253
Monacetin, 6242

C₅H₁₀O₅
Apiose, 735
Arabinose, 761
D-Lyxose, 5641
D-Ribose, 8204
D-Ribulose, 8207
Xylose, 10087
Xylulose, 10088

C₅H₁₀O₁₀P₂
Butedronic Acid, 1517

C₅H₁₁Br
d-Amyl Bromide, 601
n-Amyl Bromide, 602
tert-Amyl Bromide, 603
Isoamyl Bromide, 5114

C₅H₁₁Cl
Amyl Chloride, 606
Isoamyl Chloride, 5116

C₅H₁₁ClHgN₂O₂
Chlormerodrin, 2105

C₅H₁₁Cl₂N
Mechlorethamine, 5775

C₅H₁₁I
Isoamyl Iodide, 5120

C₅H₁₁N
Piperidine, 7468

C₅H₁₁NO
Isovaleramide, 5230

C₅H₁₁NO₂
Betaine, 1179
Isoamyl Nitrite, 5123
Isobutyl Carbamate, 5137
Isovaline, 5234
3-Nitropentane, 6616
Norvaline, 6716
Valine, 9909

C₅H₁₁NO₂S
Methionine, 5975
Penicillamine, 7088

C₅H₁₁NO₂Se
Selenomethionine, 8441

C₅H₁₁NO₃
Isoamyl Nitrate, 5122

C₅H₁₁N₂O₂P
Tabun, 9021

C₅H₁₁O₈P
D-Ribose-5-phosphoric Acid, 8205

C₅H₁₂
Neopentane, 6456
Pentane, 7116

C₅H₁₂ClO₂PS₂
Chlormephos, 2103

C₅H₁₂Cl₃NO
Mechlorethamine Oxide Hydrochloride, 5776

C₅H₁₂NO₃PS₂
Dimethoate, 3220

C₅H₁₂NO₄P
Phosphinothricin, 7339

C₅H₁₂N₂O
Tetramethylurea, 9230

C₅H₁₂N₂O₂
Ornithine, 6874

C₅H₁₂N₄O₃
Canavanine, 1737

C₅H₁₂N₈
Mitoguazone, 6213

C₅H₁₂O
Isopentyl Alcohol, 5195
2-Methyl-1-butanol, 6030
3-Methyl-2-butanol, 6031
Methyl tert-Butyl Ether, 6032
Neopentyl Alcohol, 6457
1-Pentanol, 7118
2-Pentanol, 7119
3-Pentanol, 7120
tert-Pentyl Alcohol, 7140

C₅H₁₂O₂
Neopentyl Glycol, 6458
1,5-Pentanediol, 7117

C₅H₁₂O₃
Methyl Carbitol®, 6037

C₅H₁₂O₄
Pentaerythritol, 7111

C₅H₁₂O₅
Adonitol, 168
Arabitol, 762
Xylitol, 10085

C₅H₁₂S
n-Amyl Mercaptan, 611

$C_5H_{13}CaClNO_4P$
Phosphorylcholine Calcium Salt, 7362

$C_5H_{13}ClMgNO_4P$
Phosphorylcholine Magnesium Salt, 7362

$C_5H_{13}Cl_2N$
Chlormequat Chloride, 2104

$C_5H_{13}N$
n-Amylamine, 598
Isoamylamine, 5112

$C_5H_{13}NO$
Neurine, 6484

$C_5H_{13}NO_2$
2-Amino-2-ethyl-1,3-propanediol, 439

$C_5H_{13}N_2O_4P$
Alafosfalin, 202

$C_5H_{14}ClNO$
Choline Chloride, 2206

$C_5H_{14}ClN_3O$
Girard Reagent T, 4429

$C_5H_{14}NO^+$
Choline, 2204

$C_5H_{14}N_2$
Cadaverine, 1609

$C_5H_{14}N_2O$
1-[(2-Aminoethyl)amino]-2-propanol, 438

$C_5H_{14}N_4$
Agmatine, 188

$C_5H_{15}ClNO_4P$
Phosphorylcholine, 7362

$C_5H_{15}NO_2$
Choline Hydroxide, 2204

$C_5H_{15}N_2O_3PS$
Amifostine, 404

$C_5H_{15}N_2O_4P$
Phosphinothricin DL-Form Monoammonium Salt, 7339

$C_6Al_2O_{12}$
Aluminum Oxalate, 355

$C_6Bi_2O_{12}$
Bismuth Oxalate, 1272

C_6N_4
Tetracyanoethylene, 9195

$C_6Ce_2O_{12}$
Cerous Oxalate, 2001

$C_6Cl_4O_2$
Chloranil, 2078

$C_6Cl_5NO_2$
Quintozene, 8080

C_6Cl_6
Hexachlorobenzene, 4677

$C_6CoK_3N_6$
Potassium Hexacyanocobaltate(III), 7637

$C_6CrK_3O_{12}$
Chromic Potassium Oxalate, 2228

C_6CrO_6
Chromium Carbonyl, 2232

$C_6Cu_2FeN_6$
Cupric Ferrocyanide, 2637

C_6F_6
Hexafluorobenzene, 4686

C_6F_{14}
Perfluorohexane, 7157

$C_6FeK_3N_6$
Potassium Ferricyanide, 7630

$C_6FeK_4N_6$
Potassium Ferrocyanide, 7631

$C_6FeN_6Na_4$
Sodium Ferrocyanide, 8616

$C_6HBiBr_4O_3$
Bibrocathol, 1199

C_6HCl_5O
Pentachlorophenol, 7109

$C_6H_2AgN_3O_7$
Silver Picrate, 8526

$C_6H_2Br_2ClNO$
2,6-Dibromoquinone-4-chlorimide, 3026

$C_6H_2ClN_3O_6$
Picryl Chloride, 7417

$C_6H_2Cl_2O_4$
Chloranilic Acid, 2079

$C_6H_2Cl_3NO$
Gibbs Reagent, 4421

$C_6H_2Cl_3NO_3$
3,4,6-Trichloro-2-nitrophenol, 9642

$C_6H_3Br_2NaO_4S.2H_2O$
3,5-Dibromo-4-hydroxybenzenesulfonic Acid Sodium Salt Dihydrate, 3023

$C_6H_3Br_3O$
2,4,6-Tribromophenol, 9613

$C_6H_3ClN_2O_4$
1-Chloro-2,4-dinitrobenzene, 2136
2-Chloro-1,3-dinitrobenzene, 2137

$C_6H_3ClN_2O_4S$
2,4-Dinitrobenzenesulfenyl Chloride, 3274

$C_6H_3Cl_2NO_2$
Clopyralid, 2400

$C_6H_3Cl_3$
1,2,3-Trichlorobenzene, 9630
1,2,4-Trichlorobenzene, 9631
1,3,5-Trichlorobenzene, 9632

$C_6H_3Cl_3N_2O_2$
Picloram, 7397

$C_6H_3Cl_3O$
2,4,5-Trichlorophenol, 9643
2,4,6-Trichlorophenol, 9644

$C_6H_3Cl_4N$
Nitrapyrin, 6574

$C_6H_3FN_2O_4$
1-Fluoro-2,4-dinitrobenzene, 4172

$C_6H_3I_2NO_3$
Disophenol, 3359

$C_6H_3N_3O_6$
sym-Trinitrobenzene, 9726

$C_6H_3N_3O_7$
Picric Acid, 7410

$C_6H_3N_3O_8$
Styphnic Acid, 8859

$C_6H_4BrClO_2S$
p-Bromobenzenesulfonyl Chloride, 1407

$C_6H_4Br_2$
p-Dibromobenzene, 3019

$C_6H_4Br_2O_4S$
3,5-Dibromo-4-hydroxybenzenesulfonic Acid, 3023

$C_6H_4Br_3N$
2,4,6-Tribromoaniline, 9610

$C_6H_4ClNO_2$
Chloronitrobenzene, 2151

$C_6H_4Cl_2$
m-Dichlorobenzene, 3055
o-Dichlorobenzene, 3056
p-Dichlorobenzene, 3057

$C_6H_4Cl_2O$
2,4-Dichlorophenol, 3072
2,6-Dichlorophenol, 3073

$C_6H_4Cu_2O_7$
Cupric Citrate, 2636

$C_6H_4F_2$
p-Difluorobenzene, 3148

$C_6H_4HgNNaO_4$
Mercurophen, 5891

$C_6H_4N_2O_2$
Eniluracil, 3584

$C_6H_4N_2O_3S$
p-Diazobenzenesulfonic Acid, 2999

$C_6H_4N_2O_4$
Dinitrobenzene, 3273
2,3-Pyrazinedicarboxylic Acid, 7958

$C_6H_4N_2O_5$
2,4-Dinitrophenol, 3280

$C_6H_4N_2O_6$
2,4-Dinitroresorcinol, 3284

$C_6H_4N_4$
2-Amino-1,1,3-tricyanopropene, 480
Pteridine, 7931

$C_6H_4N_4O_2$
Lumazine, 5596

$C_6H_4Na_2O_8S_2$
Tiron, 9465

$C_6H_4O_2$
Quinone, 8074

$C_6H_4O_4$
Coumalic Acid, 2557

$C_6H_4O_6$
Tetroquinone, 9249

$C_6H_4S_4$
Tetrathiafulvalene, 9242

$C_6H_5Ag_3O_7$
Silver Citrate, 8511

C_6H_5AsO
Oxophenylarsine, 6949

C_6H_5Br
Bromobenzene, 1406

C_6H_5BrO
Bromophenol, 1428

C_6H_5Cl
Chlorobenzene, 2121

C_6H_5ClHg
Phenylmercuric Chloride, 7301

$C_6H_5ClHgO_2$
2-Chloro-4-(hydroxymercuriphenol), 4830

C_6H_5ClMg
Phenylmagnesium Chloride, 7298

$C_6H_5ClNNaO_2S$
Chloramine-B, 2074

C_6H_5ClO
Chlorophenols, 2154

$C_6H_5ClO_2S$
Benzenesulfonyl Chloride, 1072

$C_6H_5ClO_3S$
p-Chlorobenzenesulfonic Acid, 2122

$C_6H_5Cl_2N$
3,4-Dichloroaniline, 3054

$C_6H_5Cl_2NO$
2-Amino-4,6-dichlorophenol, 437

$C_6H_5Cl_2O_2P$
Phenyl Dichlorophosphate, 7282

C_6H_5F
Fluorobenzene, 4170

$C_6H_5F_2N$
2,4-Difluoroaniline, 3147

$C_6H_5GaO_7$
Gallium Citrate, 4349

$C_6H_5HgNO_3$
Phenylmercuric Nitrate, 7302

C_6H_5I
Iodobenzene, 5029

C_6H_5IO
o-Iodophenol, 5035
p-Iodophenol, 5036
Iodosobenzene, 5044

$C_6H_5I_2N$
2,4-Diiodoaniline, 3188

C_6H_5KO
Potassium Phenoxide, 7657

$C_6H_5K_3O_7$
Potassium Citrate, 7623

C₇H₄Br₂O₂
3,5-Dibromosalicylaldehyde, 3027
C₇H₄Br₂O₃
3,5-Dibromosalicylic Acid, 3028
C₇H₄Br₄O
3,4,5,6-Tetrabromo-o-cresol, 9184
C₇H₄ClF₃
p-Chlorobenzotrifluoride, 2126
C₇H₄ClNO₂
Chlorzoxazone, 2194
C₇H₄ClNO₃
4-Nitrobenzoyl Chloride, 6590
C₇H₄Cl₃NO₃
Triclopyr, 9656
C₇H₄F₃NO₃
TFM, 9253
C₇H₄HgO₃
Mercuric Salicylate, 5885
C₇H₄INO₃S
N-Iodosaccharin, 5043
C₇H₄I₂O₃
3,5-Diiodosalicylic Acid, 3190
C₇H₄N₂O₅
2,4-Dinitrobenzaldehyde, 3272
C₇H₄N₂O₆
3,4-Dinitrobenzoic Acid, 3275
3,5-Dinitrobenzoic Acid, 3276
C₇H₄N₄
1-Cyanobenzotriazole, 2690
C₇H₄O₃S
Tioxolone, 9456
C₇H₄O₆
Chelidonic Acid, 2052
C₇H₄O₇
Meconic Acid, 5782
C₇H₅AgO₂
Benzoic Acid Silver Salt, 1091
C₇H₅BiO₄
Bismuth Subsalicylate, 1285
C₇H₅BiO₆
Bismuth Subgallate, 1283
C₇H₅BrO₂
p-Bromobenzoic Acid, 1408
C₇H₅Br₃
2,4,6-Tribromo-m-cresol, 9612
C₇H₅ClN₂O
Zoxazolamine, 10199
C₇H₅ClN₃NaO₄S₂
Chlorothiazide Sodium Salt, 2168
C₇H₅ClO
Benzoyl Chloride, 1112
C₇H₅ClO₂
m-Chlorobenzoic Acid, 2123
o-Chlorobenzoic Acid, 2124
p-Chlorobenzoic Acid, 2125
C₇H₅Cl₂FN₂O₃
Fluroxypyr, 4203
C₇H₅Cl₂NO₄S
Halazone, 4590
C₇H₅Cl₃
Benzotrichloride, 1109
C₇H₅Cl₃O
2,4,6-Trichloroanisole, 9629
2,4,6-Trichloro-m-cresol, 9634
C₇H₅FO₂
p-Fluorobenzoic Acid, 4171
C₇H₅F₃
Benzotrifluoride, 1110
C₇H₅HgNO₃
Nitromersol, 6610
C₇H₅IO₂
o-Iodobenzoic Acid, 5030
C₇H₅IO₄
o-Iodoxybenzoic Acid, 5048

C₇H₅KO₂.3H₂O
Benzoic Acid Potassium Salt Trihydrate, 1091
C₇H₅KO₃
Potassium Salicylate, 7665
C₇H₅LiO₂
Lithium Benzoate, 5523
C₇H₅N
Benzonitrile, 1097
C₇H₅NO
2-Furanacrylonitrile, 4298
Phenyl Isocyanate, 7296
C₇H₅NO₃
Nitrobenzaldehyde, 6587
C₇H₅NO₃S
Saccharin, 8311
C₇H₅NO₄
Cinchomeronic Acid, 2283
Isocinchomeronic Acid, 5159
Nitrobenzoic Acid, 6589
Quinolinic Acid, 8073
C₇H₅NO₅
3-Nitrosalicylic Acid, 6631
5-Nitrosalicylic Acid, 6632
C₇H₅NO₇S
2-Nitro-4-sulfobenzoic Acid, 6645
C₇H₅NS
Benzothiazole, 1107
Phenyl Isothiocyanate, 7297
C₇H₅NS₂
2-Mercaptobenzothiazole, 5868
C₇H₅N₃O₅
Nitromide, 6612
C₇H₅N₃O₆
2,4,6-Trinitrotoluene, 9730
C₇H₅N₅O₈
Nitramine, 6573
C₇H₅NaO₂
Sodium Benzoate, 8582
C₇H₅NaO₂S
Thiosalicylic Acid Sodium Salt, 9360
C₇H₅NaO₄
Gentisic Acid Sodium Salt, 4398
C₇H₆BrCl
p-Bromobenzyl Chloride, 1410
C₇H₆BrNO₂
5-Bromoanthranilic Acid, 1405
C₇H₆BrNO₃
5-Bromosalicylhydroxamic Acid, 1436
C₇H₆Br₂
p-Bromobenzyl Bromide, 1409
C₇H₆ClN₃O₄S₂
Chlorothiazide, 2168
C₇H₆Cl₂
Benzal Chloride, 1057
C₇H₆Cl₂O
Dichlorobenzyl Alcohol, 3060
C₇H₆KNO₂
Potassium p-Aminobenzoate, 7606
C₇H₆NNaO₃.2H₂O
p-Aminosalicylic Acid Sodium Salt Dihydrate, 477
C₇H₆NO₃K
p-Aminosalicylic Acid Potassium Salt, 477
C₇H₆N₂
Benzimidazole, 1081
1H-Indazole, 4936
C₇H₆N₂O₂
3-Nitrosobenzamide, 6634
C₇H₆N₂O₂S₂
Holomycin, 4728
C₇H₆N₂O₅
Dinitrocresol, 3279

C₇H₆N₂S
2-Aminobenzothiazole, 424
6-Aminobenzothiazole, 425
2-Benzimidazolethiol, 1082
C₇H₆N₄O
N,N′-Carbonyldiimidazole, 1819
C₇H₆N₄O₂
Tirapazamine, 9461
C₇H₆O
Benzaldehyde, 1058
C₇H₆OS₂
Dithiosalicylic Acid, 3375
C₇H₆O₂
Benzoic Acid, 1091
p-Hydroxybenzaldehyde, 4811
Salicylaldehyde, 8326
C₇H₆O₂S
Thiosalicylic Acid, 9360
C₇H₆O₃
2-Furanacrylic Acid, 4297
p-Hydroxybenzoic Acid, 4812
Perbenzoic Acid, 7152
Protocatechualdehyde, 7893
β-Resorcylaldehyde, 8156
Salicylic Acid, 8332
C₇H₆O₄
Gentisic Acid, 4398
Patulin, 7053
Protocatechuic Acid, 7894
β-Resorcylic Acid, 8157
Terreic Acid, 9172
C₇H₆O₅
Gallic Acid, 4345
C₇H₆O₆S
Salicylsulfuric Acid, 8334
Sulfosalicylic Acid, 8964
C₇H₇Br
Benzyl Bromide, 1128
Bromotoluene, 1439
Tropylium Bromide, 9785
C₇H₇BrO
Bromophenol p-Form Methyl Ether, 1428
C₇H₇Cl
Benzyl Chloride, 1129
Chlorotoluene, 2171
C₇H₇ClNNaO₂S
Chloramine-T, 2075
C₇H₇ClNa₂O₆P₂S
Tiludronic Acid Disodium Salt, 9441
C₇H₇ClO
Chlorocresol, 2133
C₇H₇ClO₂S
p-Toluenesulfonyl Chloride, 9534
C₇H₇Cl₂NO
Clopidol, 2397
C₇H₇Cl₂NO₂S
Dichloramine T, 3047
C₇H₇Cl₃NO₃PS
Chlorpyrifos O,O-Dimethyl Analog, 2189
C₇H₇F
Fluorotoluene, 4180
C₇H₇FO₂S
PMSF, 7542
C₇H₇F₂I
Difluoroiodotoluene, 3150
C₇H₇IO
o-Iodoanisole, 5028
C₇H₇KO₅S
Potassium Guaiacolsulfonate, 7634
C₇H₇N
3-Ethenylpyridine, 3730

C₇H₁₄N₃O₃P
Uredepa, 9872
C₇H₁₄N₄O₃
Dinotefuran, 3289
C₇H₁₄N₄S₂
Methallibure, 5946
C₇H₁₄O
Cyclohexylcarbinol, 2731
Dipropyl Ketone, 3345
Heptanal, 4658
2-Heptanone, 4663
C₇H₁₄O₂
n-Butyl Propionate, 1587
Ethyl Isovalerate, 3816
Heptanoic Acid, 4660
Isoamyl Acetate, 5111
Isobutyl Propionate, 5150
Propyl Butyrate, 7846
n-Valeric Acid Ethyl Ester, 9904
C₇H₁₄O₄
D-Chalcose, 2039
Cymarose, 2762
Monobutyrin, 6249
Mycarose, 6318
Sarmentose, 8377
C₇H₁₄O₆
α-Methylglucoside, 6080
C₇H₁₄O₇
D-manno-Heptulose, 4666
C₇H₁₄O₈
Glucoheptonic Acid, 4455
C₇H₁₅Cl₂N₂O₂P
Ifosfamide, 4896
C₇H₁₅Cl₂N₂O₂P.H₂O
Cyclophosphamide, 2747
C₇H₁₅Cl₂N₂O₄P
Perfosfamide, 7161
C₇H₁₅NO
1-Ethyl-3-piperidinol, 3845
C₇H₁₅NO₂
Emylcamate, 3566
Isobutyl Urethane, 5153
C₇H₁₅NO₃
Carnitine, 1849
C₇H₁₅NO₄S
MOPS, 6265
C₇H₁₅NO₅
N-Methyl-α-L-glucosamine, 6079
C₇H₁₅N₃O₂
Indospicine, 4970
C₇H₁₅N₃O₂S₂
Cartap, 1865
C₇H₁₆
n-Heptane, 4659
C₇H₁₆BrNO₂
Acetylcholine Bromide, 86
C₇H₁₆ClN
Mepiquat Chloride, 5857
C₇H₁₆ClNO₂
Acetylcholine Chloride, 87
C₇H₁₆ClN₃O₂S₂
Cartap Monohydrochloride, 1865
C₇H₁₆FO₂P
Soman, 8713
C₇H₁₆INO₂
Oxapropanium Iodide, 6923
C₇H₁₆N₄O₂
Nᴳ-Methylarginine, 6022
C₇H₁₆N₄O₄S₂
Taurolidine, 9076
C₇H₁₆O
1-Heptanol, 4661
2-Heptanol, 4662
C₇H₁₆O₃
Dipropylene Glycol Monomethyl
Ether, 3344

Orthoformic Acid Triethyl Ester,
6884
C₇H₁₆O₄S₂
Sulfonmethane, 8960
C₇H₁₇AsClNO₃
Chloroarsenol Ammonium Salt, 2119
C₇H₁₇ClN₂O₂
Bethanechol Chloride, 1185
C₇H₁₇N
Methylhexaneamine, 6085
Tuaminoheptane, 9802
C₇H₁₇NO₂
Triethylammonium Formate, 9667
C₇H₁₇NO₅
N-Methylglucamine, 6078
C₇H₁₇NO₆S
TAPS, 9058
C₇H₁₇N₄O₄P
Anatoxin A(s), 627
C₇H₁₇O₂PS₃
Phorate, 7331
C₇H₁₈NO₇P
Fosfomycin Tromethamine, 4254
C₇H₁₉N₃
Spermidine, 8742
C₈BrF₁₇
Perflubron, 7156
C₈Cl₂N₂O₂
2,3-Dichloro-5,6-dicyanobenzoqui-
none, 3063
C₈Cl₄N₂
Chlorothalonil, 2166
C₈Co₂O₈
Dicobalt Octacarbonyl, 3085
C₈H₂Cl₄O₅
Mucochloric Anhydride, 6298
C₈H₃I₂NNa₂O₅
Sodium Iodomethamate, 8633
C₈H₄Cl₂O₂
Phthaloyl Chloride, 7375
C₈H₄Cl₆
1,4-Bis(trichloromethyl)benzene,
1303
C₈H₄K₂O₁₂Sb₂.3H₂O
Antimony Potassium Tartrate, 700
C₈H₄N₂S₂
Bitoscanate, 1308
C₈H₄O₃
Phthalic Anhydride, 7372
C₈H₅Cl₃O₃
2,4,5-T, 9019
C₈H₅F₃N₂OS
Riluzole, 8223
C₈H₅KO₄
Potassium Biphthalate, 7612
C₈H₅NOS
Benzoyl Isothiocyanate, 1114
C₈H₅NO₂
Agrocybin, 192
Isatin, 5104
Phthalimide, 7373
C₈H₅NO₃
N-Hydroxyphthalimide, 4838
C₈H₅N₃O₃S₂
Tenonitrozole, 9147
C₈H₆
Ethynylbenzene, 3861
C₈H₆BrClO
p-Chlorophenacyl Bromide, 2153
C₈H₆BrClO₂
p-Bromobenzyl Chloroformate, 1411
C₈H₆BrN
α-Bromobenzyl Cyanide, 1412
C₈H₆Br₂O
p-Bromophenacyl Bromide, 1427

C₈H₆Cl₂O₃
2,4-D, 2796
Dicamba, 3040
C₈H₆F₃N₃O₄S₂
Flumethiazide, 4139
C₈H₆KNO₄S
Indican (Metabolic Indican) Potas-
sium Salt, 4941
C₈H₆N₂
Cinnoline, 2306
Phthalazine, 7370
Quinazoline, 8053
Quinoxaline, 8078
C₈H₆N₂OS₂
Acibenzolar-S-methyl, 106
C₈H₆N₂O₂
p-Nitrobenzyl Cyanide, 6591
C₈H₆N₄O₅
Nitrofurantoin, 6599
C₈H₆N₄O₈
Alloxantin, 283
C₈H₆N₆O₁₁
Pentryl, 7139
C₈H₆O
Benzofuran, 1088
C₈H₆O₂
o-Phthalaldehyde, 7368
C₈H₆O₃
Piperonal, 7475
C₈H₆O₄
Isophthalic Acid, 5197
Phthalic Acid, 7371
Piperonylic Acid, 7477
Terephthalic Acid, 9162
C₈H₆O₅
Fomecin B, 4225
4-Hydroxyisophthalic Acid, 4827
C₈H₆S
Thianaphthene, 9303
C₈H₇BrO
ω-Bromoacetophenone, 1402
p-Bromoacetophenone, 1403
C₈H₇BrO₃
p-Bromomandelic Acid, 1424
C₈H₇ClN₂O₂S
Diazoxide, 3004
C₈H₇ClO
ω-Chloroacetophenone, 2115
p-Chloroacetophenone, 2116
C₈H₇ClO₂
p-Anisoyl Chloride, 673
Carbobenzoxy Chloride, 1801
m-Chlorobenzoic Acid Methyl Ester,
2123
p-Chlorobenzoic Acid Methyl Ester,
2125
C₈H₇Cl₄N₃O₄S₂
Teclothiazide, 9104
C₈H₇FO₂
p-Fluorophenylacetic Acid, 4177
C₈H₇N
Benzyl Cyanide, 1131
Indole, 4963
o-Tolunitrile, 9537
C₈H₇NO
Mandelonitrile, 5719
C₈H₇NO₂
Acetimidoquinone, 57
Isonitrosoacetophenone, 5191
C₈H₇NO₃
4-Pyridoxic Acid Lactone, 7981
C₈H₇NO₄
p-Nitrophenylacetic Acid, 6622
C₈H₇NO₄S
Indican (Metabolic Indican), 4941

C₈H₇N₃O₂
Luminol, 5600
C₈H₇N₃O₅
Dinitolmide, 3269
Furazolidone, 4300
C₈H₇NaO₃
Mandelic Acid Sodium Salt, 5717
C₈H₇NaO₄·H₂O
Dehydroacetic Acid Sodium Salt
Hydrate, 2865
C₈H₈
Cubane, 2611
Styrene, 8860
C₈H₈BrCl₂O₃PS
Bromophos, 1431
C₈H₈BrNO
p-Bromoacetanilide, 1399
C₈H₈ClNO
Chloroacetanilide, 2111
C₈H₈ClNO₃S
N-Acetylsulfanilyl Chloride, 103
C₈H₈Cl₂IO₃PS
Iodofenphos, 5032
C₈H₈Cl₂N₄
Guanabenz, 4558
C₈H₈Cl₂N₄O
Guanoxabenz, 4567
C₈H₈Cl₂O
Dichloroxylenol, 3076
C₈H₈Cl₃N₃O₄S₂
Clorsulon, 2409
Trichlormethiazide, 9624
C₈H₈Cl₃O₃PS
Ronnel, 8256
C₈H₈F₃N₃O₄S₂
Hydroflumethiazide, 4789
C₈H₈HgO₂
Phenylmercuric Acetate, 7300
C₈H₈K₂O₅
Endothall Dipotassium Salt, 3575
C₈H₈NNaO₄S
N-Acetylsulfanilic Acid Sodium Salt,
102
C₈H₈N₂O₂
Phthalamide, 7369
Ricinine, 8210
C₈H₈N₂O₂S₂
Thiolutin, 9342
C₈H₈N₂O₃
Nitroacetanilide, 6581
C₈H₈N₂O₃S
Zonisamide, 10192
C₈H₈N₃Na₂O₆S⁹⁹ᵐTc
Technetium ⁹⁹ᵐTc Mertiatide, 9101
C₈H₈N₄
Hydralazine, 4763
C₈H₈N₆O₆
Murexide, 6306
C₈H₈O
Acetophenone, 73
Coumaran, 2559
Phenylacetaldehyde, 7265
o-Tolualdehyde, 9527
C₈H₈O₂
p-Anisaldehyde, 663
Benzyl Formate, 1134
Methyl Benzoate, 6024
Phenyl Acetate, 7267
Phenylacetic Acid, 7268
Toluic Acid, 9535
C₈H₈O₃
p-Anisic Acid, 666
m-Cresotic Acid, 2580
o-Cresotic Acid, 2581
p-Cresotic Acid, 2582
Mandelic Acid, 5717

Methylparaben, 6107
Methyl Salicylate, 6120
Phenoxyacetic Acid, 7254
Resacetophenone, 8140
Resorcinol Monoacetate, 8155
Vanillin, 9932
C₈H₈O₄
Dehydroacetic Acid, 2865
2,6-Dimethoxyquinone, 3225
Fumigatin, 4288
Gallacetophenone, 4342
Homogentisic Acid, 4737
o-Orsellinic Acid, 6881
Pyrogallol Monoacetate, 8000
Vanillic Acid, 9931
C₈H₈O₅
Fomecin A, 4225
Gallic Acid Methyl Ester, 4345
C₈H₉Br
Xylyl Bromide, 10090
C₈H₉BrO
Bromophenol p-Form Ethyl Ether,
1428
C₈H₉Cl
Xylyl Chloride, 10091
C₈H₉ClO
Chloroxylenol, 2176
C₈H₉FN₂O₃
Tegafur, 9112
C₈H₉FO₂S
Fluoresone, 4161
C₈H₉NO
Acetanilide, 50
Aminoacetophenone, 413
Phenacylamine, 7206
α-Phenylacetamide, 7266
o-Toluamide, 9528
C₈H₉NO₂
Acetaminophen, 47
p-Aminophenylacetic Acid, 463
Methyl Anthranilate, 6020
α-Phenylglycine, 7291
N-Phenylglycine, 7292
C₈H₉NO₃
N-(4-Hydroxyphenyl)glycine, 4837
Orthocaine, 6883
Pyridoxal, 7978
C₈H₉NO₄
4-Pyridoxic Acid, 7981
C₈H₉NO₄S
N-Acetylsulfanilic Acid, 102
C₈H₉NO₅
Clavulanic Acid, 2341
C₈H₉N₂NaO₃S
Sulfacetamide Sodium Salt, 8899
C₈H₉N₃O₄
Nicorandil, 6521
C₈H₁₀
Ethylbenzene, 3765
Xylene, 10081
C₈H₁₀AsNO₅
Acetarsone, 52
C₈H₁₀AsN₂NaO₄
Tryparsamide, 9794
C₈H₁₀ClN₃O
Lazabemide, 5394
C₈H₁₀ClN₃S
Tiamenidine, 9418
C₈H₁₀ClN₅O₃S
Thiamethoxam, 9294
C₈H₁₀Cl₂N₂S
p-Chlorobenzylpseudothiuronium
Chloride, 2128
C₈H₁₀FN₃O₃S
Emtricitabine, 3565

C₈H₁₀IN₃
Iobenguane, 5007
C₈H₁₀NNaO₅S
Sulbactam Sodium Salt, 8889
C₈H₁₀NO₅PS
Methyl Parathion, 6108
C₈H₁₀NO₆P
Pyridoxal 5-Phosphate, 7979
C₈H₁₀N₂O
p-Aminoacetanilide, 411
Benzylurea, 1147
p-Nitroso-N,N-dimethylaniline,
6638
C₈H₁₀N₂O₃
5-Nitro-o-phenetidine, 6617
C₈H₁₀N₂O₃S
N⁴-Acetylsulfanilamide, 8925
Sulfacetamide, 8899
p-Tolylsulfonylmethylnitrosamide,
9543
C₈H₁₀N₂O₄
Mimosine, 6199
C₈H₁₀N₂O₄S
Asulam, 857
C₈H₁₀N₂S
Ethionamide, 3737
C₈H₁₀N₄O₂
Caffeine, 1636
C₈H₁₀N₆
Dihydralazine, 3169
C₈H₁₀O
Benzyl Methyl Ether, 1140
2-Ethylphenol, 3839
Methylenomycin B, 6067
Phenethyl Alcohol, 7224
Phenetole, 7229
Xylenol, 10082
C₈H₁₀O₂
Anise Alcohol, 665
Creosol, 2571
2-Phenoxyethanol, 7257
Styrene Glycol, 8861
Veratrole, 9956
C₈H₁₀O₃
Filicinic Acid, 4079
C₈H₁₀O₃S
Benzenesulfonic Acid Ethyl Ester,
1070
C₈H₁₀O₄
Penicillic Acid, 7092
C₈H₁₀O₅
Endothall, 3575
C₈H₁₁ClN₂S
S-Benzylthiuronium Chloride, 1146
C₈H₁₁Cl₂NO
Dichlormid, 3049
C₈H₁₁Cl₂N₃O₂
Uracil Mustard, 9851
C₈H₁₁Cl₃O₆
α-Chloralose, 2072
C₈H₁₁Cl₃O₇
Urochloralic Acid, 9884
C₈H₁₁N
N,N-Dimethylaniline, 3234
Ethylaniline, 3764
3-Ethyl-4-picoline, 3842
4-Ethyl-2-picoline, 3843
5-Ethyl-2-picoline, 3844
α-Methylbenzylamine, 6026
Phenethylamine, 7225
2,4,6-Trimethylpyridine, 9718
Xylidine, 10084
C₈H₁₁NO
Metyridine, 6160
o-Phenetidine, 7227
p-Phenetidine, 7228

C₁₀H₄Cl₂O₂
Dichlone, 3045

C₁₀H₄N₂Na₂O₈S
Naphthol Yellow S, 6393

C₁₀H₅ClN₂
o-Chlorobenzylidenemalononitrile, 2127

C₁₀H₅Cl₇
Heptachlor, 4656

C₁₀H₅NNa₂O₈S₂
Nitroso-R Salt, 6644

C₁₀H₅NaO₅S
Sodium β-Naphthoquinone-4-sulfonate, 8646

C₁₀H₆ClN₅O
Triazoxide, 9607

C₁₀H₆Cl₂N₂O₂
Pyrrolnitrin, 8018

C₁₀H₆Cl₄O₄
DCPA, 2839

C₁₀H₆Cl₈
Chlordan(e), 2082

C₁₀H₆N₂OS₂
Oxythioquinox, 6978

C₁₀H₆O₂
1,2-Naphthoquinone, 6394
1,4-Naphthoquinone, 6395

C₁₀H₆O₃
Juglone, 5269
Lawsone, 5393

C₁₀H₆O₄
Chromocarb, 2237
Coumarin-3-carboxylic Acid, 2563

C₁₀H₆O₈
Pyromellitic Acid, 8004

C₁₀H₇Br
1-Bromonaphthalene, 1425
2-Bromonaphthalene, 1426

C₁₀H₇Cl
1-Chloronaphthalene, 2149
2-Chloronaphthalene, 2150

C₁₀H₇Cl₂NO
Chlorquinaldol, 2190

C₁₀H₇Cl₂N₃O
Anagrelide, 622

C₁₀H₇Cl₅O
Tridiphane, 9662

C₁₀H₇F₃O₄
Triflusal, 9688

C₁₀H₇KN₆O
Pemirolast Potassium Salt, 7078

C₁₀H₇NO₂
1-Nitronaphthalene, 6614
1-Nitroso-2-naphthol, 6641
N-Phenylmaleimide, 7299
Quinaldic Acid, 8046
8-Quinolinecarboxylic Acid, 8070

C₁₀H₇NO₃
Kynurenic Acid, 5327
1-Nitro-2-naphthol, 6615

C₁₀H₇NO₄
Xanthurenic Acid, 10068

C₁₀H₇N₃S
Thiabendazole, 9289

C₁₀H₇NaO
2-Naphthol Sodium Salt, 6384

C₁₀H₇NaO₄S
2-Naphthol-6-sulfonic Acid Sodium Salt, 6392

C₁₀H₈
Azulene, 926
Naphthalene, 6370

C₁₀H₈ClN₄NaO₂S
Sulfachlorpyridazine Sodium Salt, 8900

C₁₀H₈F₂N₄O
Rufinamide, 8293

C₁₀H₈NNaO₄S.2½H₂O
1-Amino-2-naphthol-6-sulfonic Acid Sodium Salt Hemipentahydrate, 455

C₁₀H₈NNaO₃S.4H₂O
1-Naphthylamine-4-sulfonic Acid Sodium Salt Tetrahydrate, 6403

C₁₀H₈N₂
α,α'-Dipyridyl, 3347
γ,γ'-Dipyridyl, 3348

C₁₀H₈N₂O₂S₂
Pyrithione Dimer, 7994

C₁₀H₈N₂O₂S₂Zn
Pyrithione Zinc Derivative, 7994

C₁₀H₈N₂O₄
α-Furildioxime, 4306

C₁₀H₈N₄O₃S₂
Nitrodan, 6596

C₁₀H₈N₄O₅
Picrolonic Acid, 7412

C₁₀H₈N₆O
Pemirolast, 7078

C₁₀H₈O
1-Naphthol, 6383
2-Naphthol, 6384

C₁₀H₈OS₃
Anethole Trithione, 644

C₁₀H₈O₂
Naphthoresorcinol, 6396
Tricromyl, 9658

C₁₀H₈O₃
Erythrocentaurin, 3678
Hymecromone, 4854

C₁₀H₈O₃S
1-Naphthalenesulfonic Acid, 6376
2-Naphthalenesulfonic Acid, 6377

C₁₀H₈O₄
Anemonin, 642
Scopoletin, 8408

C₁₀H₈O₄S
Cassella's Acid, 1892
Croceic Acid, 2588
1-Naphthol-2-sulfonic Acid, 6390
1-Naphthol-4-sulfonic Acid, 6391
2-Naphthol-6-sulfonic Acid, 6392

C₁₀H₈O₅
Fraxetin, 4265

C₁₀H₈O₆S₂
Armstrong's Acid, 788
1,6-Naphthalenedisulfonic Acid, 6373
2,6-Naphthalenedisulfonic Acid, 6374
2,7-Naphthalenedisulfonic Acid, 6375

C₁₀H₈O₇S₂
1-Naphthol-4,8-disulfonic Acid, 6386
2-Naphthol-3,6-disulfonic Acid, 6387
2-Naphthol-6,8-disulfonic Acid, 6388

C₁₀H₈O₈S₂
Chromotropic Acid, 2241

C₁₀H₈O₁₀S₂
Sulmarin, 8984

C₁₀H₈S
1-Naphthalenethiol, 6378
2-Naphthalenethiol, 6379

C₁₀H₉ClN₄O₂S
Sulfachlorpyridazine, 8900

C₁₀H₉ClN₄S
Thiacloprid, 9291

C₁₀H₉Cl₂NO
Dicryl, 3088

C₁₀H₉Cl₂NaO₃
2,4-DB Sodium Salt, 2835

C₁₀H₉Cl₄NO₂S
Captafol, 1771

C₁₀H₉Cl₄O₄P
Tetrachlorvinphos, 9192

C₁₀H₉F₃O₃
Mosher's Reagent, 6280

C₁₀H₉N
Lepidine, 5441
1-Naphthylamine, 6398
2-Naphthylamine, 6399
Quinaldine, 8047

C₁₀H₉NO
4-Amino-1-naphthol, 453
Echinopsine, 3498

C₁₀H₉NO₂
Gentianine, 4394
Indoleacetic Acid, 4964
Succinanil, 8867

C₁₀H₉NO₃
Maleanilic Acid, 5702

C₁₀H₉NO₃S
Badische Acid, 940
Cassella's Acid F, 1893
1,6-Cleve's Acid, 2350
1,7-Cleve's Acid, 2351
1-Naphthylamine-4-sulfonic Acid, 6403
1-Naphthylamine-5-sulfonic Acid, 6404
1-Naphthylamine-8-sulfonic Acid, 6405
2-Naphthylamine-1-sulfonic Acid, 6406
2-Naphthylamine-5-sulfonic Acid, 6407

C₁₀H₉NO₄S
1-Amino-2-naphthol-4-sulfonic Acid, 454
1-Amino-2-naphthol-6-sulfonic Acid, 455

C₁₀H₉NO₆S₂
Amido-G-Acid, 401
Amido-R-Acid, 402
1-Naphthylamine-2,7-disulfonic Acid, 6400
1-Naphthylamine-4,6-disulfonic Acid, 6401
1-Naphthylamine-4,7-disulfonic Acid, 6402

C₁₀H₉NO₇S₂
1-Naphthol-8-amino-3,6-disulfonic Acid, 6385

C₁₀H₉N₃O
Amrinone, 592

C₁₀H₉N₄NaO₂S
Sulfadiazine Sodium Salt, 8903

C₁₀H₉N₅O
Kinetin, 5311

C₁₀H₁₀
Bullvalene, 1482

C₁₀H₁₀CaO₅
Prohexadione Calcium Salt, 7777

C₁₀H₁₀Cl₂N₂S₂
3,3-Dithiodipyridine Dihydrochloride, 3373

C₁₀H₁₀Cl₂O₃
2,4-DB, 2835

C₁₀H₁₀Cl₂Ti
Titanocene Dichloride, 9482

C₁₀H₁₀Fe
Ferrocene, 4037

C₁₀H₁₀IN₂.BF₄
Bis(pyridine)iodonium Tetrafluoroborate, 1302

C₁₀H₁₀NNaO₄S₂
Stepronin Sodium Salt, 8809

C₁₀H₁₀N₂
1,8-Naphthalenediamine, 6372

$C_{10}H_{10}N_2O$
Norphenazone, 6713

$C_{10}H_{10}N_2O_2$
Procodazole, 7762

$C_{10}H_{10}N_2O_3$
Imidazole Salicylate, 4913

$C_{10}H_{10}N_4O$
Metamitron, 5924

$C_{10}H_{10}N_4OS$
Methisazone, 5977

$C_{10}H_{10}N_4O_2S$
Sulfadiazine, 8903
Sulfapyrazine, 8937

$C_{10}H_{10}N_6O_2$
Azanidazole, 897

$C_{10}H_{10}O$
Benzylideneacetone, 1137

$C_{10}H_{10}O_2$
Isosafrole, 5223
Safrole, 8317

$C_{10}H_{10}O_4$
Dimethyl Phthalate, 3255
Ferulic Acid, 4062
Meconin, 5783
Methyl Acetylsalicylate, 6010
Terephthalic Acid Dimethyl Ester, 9162

$C_{10}H_{10}O_5$
Opianic Acid, 6851

$C_{10}H_{10}O_6$
Chorismic Acid, 2217
Prephenic Acid, 7738

$C_{10}H_{11}BrN_2O_3$
Brallobarbital, 1361

$C_{10}H_{11}ClFN_5O_3$
Clofarabine, 2372

$C_{10}H_{11}ClKO_3$
Mecoprop Potassium Salt, 5784

$C_{10}H_{11}ClN_4$
Acetamiprid, 49

$C_{10}H_{11}ClO_3$
Clofibric Acid, 2378
Mecoprop, 5784

$C_{10}H_{11}ClZr$
Schwartz's Reagent, 8396

$C_{10}H_{11}F_3N_2O$
Fluometuron, 4154

$C_{10}H_{11}F_3N_2O_5$
Trifluridine, 9687

$C_{10}H_{11}I_2NO_3$
Propyliodone, 7863

$C_{10}H_{11}NO$
Abikoviromycin, 8
Tryptophol, 9798

$C_{10}H_{11}NO_2$
Acetoacetanilide, 58
Tuberin, 9806

$C_{10}H_{11}NO_3$
Actarit, 133
Betamipron, 1181
Succinanilic Acid, 8868

$C_{10}H_{11}NO_4S_2$
Stepronin, 8809

$C_{10}H_{11}N_3OS$
Methabenzthiazuron, 5939

$C_{10}H_{11}N_3O_3S$
Sulfamethoxazole, 8918

$C_{10}H_{11}N_3O_5S$
Nifuratel, 6532

$C_{10}H_{11}N_4NaO_5S$
Carbazochrome Sodium Sulfonate, 1789
Tazobactam Sodium Salt, 9083

$C_{10}H_{11}N_5O$
Pymetrozine, 7950

$C_{10}H_{12}$
Tetralin®, 9221

$C_{10}H_{12}BrCl_2O_3PS$
Bromophos O,O-Diethyl Analog, 1431

$C_{10}H_{12}ClNO$
Beclamide, 1018

$C_{10}H_{12}ClNO_2$
Baclofen, 937
Chlorpropham, 2187

$C_{10}H_{12}ClNO_4$
Chlorphenesin Carbamate, 2179

$C_{10}H_{12}ClN_3O_3S$
Quinethazone, 8056

$C_{10}H_{12}ClN_5O_3$
Cladribine, 2337

$C_{10}H_{12}Cl_2N_4O_2$
Guanabenz Monoacetate, 4558

$C_{10}H_{12}FN_5O_4$
Fludarabine, 4126

$C_{10}H_{12}FeN_2NaO_8$
Ferric Sodium Edetate, 4031

$C_{10}H_{12}N_2$
Anatabine, 626
Tolazoline, 9506
Tryptamine, 9796

$C_{10}H_{12}N_2O$
Cotinine, 2553
4-Methylaminorex, 6018
Serotonin, 8462

$C_{10}H_{12}N_2O_3$
Allobarbital, 263
Kynurenine, 5328

$C_{10}H_{12}N_2O_3S$
Bentazon, 1053

$C_{10}H_{12}N_2O_4$
Stavudine, 8803

$C_{10}H_{12}N_2O_5$
Dinoseb, 3287

$C_{10}H_{12}N_2O_5S$
7-Aminocephalosporanic Acid, 434

$C_{10}H_{12}N_2O_6S$
Ritipenem, 8236

$C_{10}H_{12}N_2O_8$
Orotidine, 6877

$C_{10}H_{12}N_3O_3PS_2$
Azinphos-methyl, 913

$C_{10}H_{12}N_4OS$
Thiacetazone, 9290

$C_{10}H_{12}N_4O_2S_2$
Sulfaethidole, 8907

$C_{10}H_{12}N_4O_3$
Adrenochrome Monosemicarbazone, 172
Didanosine, 3098

$C_{10}H_{12}N_4O_4$
Nebularine, 6433

$C_{10}H_{12}N_4O_5$
Inosine, 4975

$C_{10}H_{12}N_4O_5S$
Tazobactam, 9083

$C_{10}H_{12}N_4O_6$
Xanthosine, 10065

$C_{10}H_{12}N_5O_6P$
Cyclic AMP, 2708

$C_{10}H_{12}N_5O_7P$
Cyclic GMP, 2709

$C_{10}H_{12}O$
Anethole, 643
Cuminaldehyde, 2621
Estragole, 3705
Tetralol, 9222

$C_{10}H_{12}O_2$
Cumic Acid, 2618
Duroquinone, 3470
Ethyl Phenylacetate, 3840

Eugenol, 3898
Isoeugenol, 5171
β-Thujaplicin, 9390
Thujic Acid, 9391

$C_{10}H_{12}O_3$
Coniferyl Alcohol, 2504
Propylparaben, 7866

$C_{10}H_{12}O_4$
Cantharidin, 1752
Sparassol, 8734
Xanthoxylin, 10067

$C_{10}H_{12}O_5$
Prohexadione, 7777
Propyl Gallate, 7859

$C_{10}H_{13}BrN_2O_3$
Propallylonal, 7796

$C_{10}H_{13}Cl$
Neophyl Chloride, 6459

$C_{10}H_{13}ClN_2$
Chlordimeform, 2085

$C_{10}H_{13}ClN_2O$
Chlorotoluron, 2172

$C_{10}H_{13}ClN_2O_3S$
Chlorpropamide, 2186

$C_{10}H_{13}ClO$
Chlorothymol, 2170

$C_{10}H_{13}Cl_2N$
Aniline Mustard, 660

$C_{10}H_{13}Cl_2O_3PS$
Dichlofenthion, 3043

$C_{10}H_{13}FN_2O_5$
Clevudine, 2353

$C_{10}H_{13}FN_5O_7P$
Fludarabine 5′-Monophosphate, 4126

$C_{10}H_{13}FN_6O_6S$
Nucleocidin, 6726

$C_{10}H_{13}NO$
Methcathinone, 5963

$C_{10}H_{13}NO_2$
4-Amino-3-phenylbutyric Acid, 464
Fusaric Acid, 4314
4′-Hydroxybutyranilide, 4814
MDA, 5765
Phenacetin, 7204
Phenprobamate, 7258
Propham, 7816

$C_{10}H_{13}NO_3$
Buramate, 1501
Damascenine, 2808
α-Methyl-m-tyrosine, 6132
Metyrosine, 6161
Surinamine, 9007

$C_{10}H_{13}NO_4$
Glyceryl p-Aminobenzoate, 4487
Methyldopa, 6055
3-O-Methyldopa, 6056

$C_{10}H_{13}NO_5$
Arogenic Acid, 790

$C_{10}H_{13}N_2NaO_3$
Aprobarbital Sodium Salt, 756

$C_{10}H_{13}N_3$
Debrisoquin, 2844

$C_{10}H_{13}N_3O_2$
Guanoxan, 4568
5-(α-Phenylethyl)semioxamazide, 7289

$C_{10}H_{13}N_3O_5S$
Nifurtimox, 6538

$C_{10}H_{13}N_4O_8P$
Inosinic Acid, 4977

$C_{10}H_{13}N_5O$
Zeatin, 10117

$C_{10}H_{13}N_5O_2$
Dideoxyadenosine, 3101

$C_{10}H_{13}N_5O_3$
Cordycepin, 2529

C₁₀H₁₃N₅O₄
Adenosine, 153
Zidovudine, 10123

C₁₀H₁₃N₅O₄·H₂O
Vidarabine, 9976

C₁₀H₁₃N₅O₄S
Thioguanosine, 9338

C₁₀H₁₃N₅O₅
Guanosine, 4566

C₁₀H₁₃N₅O₁₂P₃
Cordycepin Triphosphate, 2529

C₁₀H₁₄
n-Butylbenzene, 1549
sec-Butylbenzene, 1550
tert-Butylbenzene, 1551
Cymene, 2763
Durene, 3468
Isobutylbenzene, 5134
Isodurene, 5166

C₁₀H₁₄BeO₄
Beryllium Acetylacetonate, 1163

C₁₀H₁₄BrNO₂
2C-B, 1908

C₁₀H₁₄CaO₆
Calcium Levulinate, 1679

C₁₀H₁₄ClN
Chlorphentermine, 2182
Clortermine, 2410

C₁₀H₁₄ClNO₃
Pyridoxal Monoethylacetal Hydrochloride, 7978

C₁₀H₁₄ClN₃OS
Azintamide, 914

C₁₀H₁₄Cl₂NO₂PS
DMPA, 3392

C₁₀H₁₄Cl₃N₂O₃
Fenuron Trichloroacetate, 4009

C₁₀H₁₄Cl₆N₄O₂
Triforine, 9691

C₁₀H₁₄NNaO₃
Tenuazonic Acid Sodium Salt, 9149

C₁₀H₁₄NO₅PS
Parathion, 7033

C₁₀H₁₄NO₆P
Paraoxon, 7030

C₁₀H₁₄N₂
Anabasine, 619
Nicotine, 6524

C₁₀H₁₄N₂O
Isonicotinic Acid Diethylamide, 5188
Nikethamide, 6543

C₁₀H₁₄N₂O₂
Phenocoll, 7239

C₁₀H₁₄N₂O₃
Aprobarbital, 756

C₁₀H₁₄N₂O₄
Porphobilinogen, 7600
Proxibarbal, 7904

C₁₀H₁₄N₂O₄·H₂O
Carbidopa, 1797

C₁₀H₁₄N₂O₄S₂
Sulthiame, 8993

C₁₀H₁₄N₂O₅
Telbivudine, 9117
Thymidine, 9397

C₁₀H₁₄N₄O₂
Morphazinamide, 6273

C₁₀H₁₄N₄O₃
Protheobromine, 7886
Proxyphylline, 7905

C₁₀H₁₄N₄O₄
Dyphylline, 3479

C₁₀H₁₄N₅O₇P
3'-Adenylic Acid, 157
5'-Adenylic Acid, 158

C₁₀H₁₄N₅O₈P
3'-Guanylic Acid, 4569
5'-Guanylic Acid, 4570

C₁₀H₁₄NiO₄
Nickel Acetylacetonate, 6500

C₁₀H₁₄O
p-tert-Butylphenol, 1585
Carvacrol, 1872
Carvone, 1874
Chrysanthenone, 2252
Cumic Alcohol, 2619
Perillaldehyde, 7167
Safranal, 8316
Thymol, 9399
d-Verbenone, 9960

C₁₀H₁₄O₂
Durohydroquinone, 3469
Nepetalactone, 6470
Perilla Ketone, 7166

C₁₀H₁₄O₃
Mephenesin, 5850

C₁₀H₁₄O₄
Guaifenesin, 4555

C₁₀H₁₅BrO
3-Bromo-d-camphor, 1414

C₁₀H₁₅ClO
3-Chloro-d-camphor, 2132

C₁₀H₁₅N
Diethylaniline, 3114
Methamphetamine, 5948
Phentermine, 7262
Phenylpropylmethylamine, 7308

C₁₀H₁₅NO
α-(α-Aminopropyl)benzyl Alcohol,
471
Anatoxin A, 627
Ephedrine, 3608
Hordenine, 4746
Perillaldehyde Oxime, 7167
Pholedrine, 7330
Pseudoephedrine, 7916

C₁₀H₁₅NO₂
Etilefrin, 3865
Hexapropymate, 4698
p-Hydroxyephedrine, 4824

C₁₀H₁₅NO₃
Ethylnorepinephrine, 3834
Metanephrine, 5926
N-Methylepinephrine, 6069
Tenuazonic Acid, 9149

C₁₀H₁₅NO₄
Kainic Acid, 5276

C₁₀H₁₅NO₅S
Tricaine, 9621

C₁₀H₁₅N₂NaO₂S
Thiobutabarbital Sodium Salt, 9323

C₁₀H₁₅N₂NaO₃
Butabarbital Sodium, 1506

C₁₀H₁₅N₂Na₃O₇
Versenol®, 9966

C₁₀H₁₅N₃
Bethanidine, 1186

C₁₀H₁₅N₃O
Sabcomeline, 8309

C₁₀H₁₅N₃O₅
Benserazide, 1050
Dinoseb Ammonium Salt, 3287

C₁₀H₁₅N₃O₈
Convicine, 2513

C₁₀H₁₅N₃S
Talipexole, 9039

C₁₀H₁₅N₅
Phenformin, 7231
Trapidil, 9574

C₁₀H₁₅N₅O₃
Penciclovir, 7083

C₁₀H₁₅N₅O₁₀P₂
Adenosine Diphosphate, 154

C₁₀H₁₅OPS₂
Fonofos, 4233

C₁₀H₁₅O₃PS₂
Fenthion, 4002

C₁₀H₁₆
Adamantane, 149
Camphene, 1730
3-Carene, 1836
Limonene, 5493
β-Myrcene, 6331
Ocimene, 6741
α-Phellandrene, 7200
β-Phellandrene, 7201
α-Pinene, 7445
β-Pinene, 7446
Terpinene, 9170
Twistane, 9828

C₁₀H₁₆BrNO
Edrophonium Bromide, 3516

C₁₀H₁₆Br₂N₂O₂
Pipobroman, 7480

C₁₀H₁₆ClNO
Edrophonium Chloride, 3516

C₁₀H₁₆Cl₃NOS
Triallate, 9594

C₁₀H₁₆KNO₉S₂
Sinigrin, 8545

C₁₀H₁₆NO₅PS₂
Famphur, 3932

C₁₀H₁₆N₂
Tetramethyl-p-phenylenediamine, 9228

C₁₀H₁₆N₂O
Rilmenidine, 8222

C₁₀H₁₆N₂OS
Albutoin, 217

C₁₀H₁₆N₂O₂S
Thiobutabarbital, 9323

C₁₀H₁₆N₂O₃
Butethal, 1521

C₁₀H₁₆N₂O₃S
Amidephrine, 399
Biotin, 1231

C₁₀H₁₆N₂O₄
TAED, 9028

C₁₀H₁₆N₂O₄S
Biotin l-Sulfoxide, 1232

C₁₀H₁₆N₂O₄S₃
Dorzolamide, 3426

C₁₀H₁₆N₂O₈
EDDS, 3508
EDTA, 3517

C₁₀H₁₆N₄O₃
Anserine, 679

C₁₀H₁₆N₄O₇
Vicine, 9975

C₁₀H₁₆N₅O₁₃P₃
Adenosine Triphosphate, 155

C₁₀H₁₆N₆S
Cimetidine, 2279

C₁₀H₁₆O
Camphor, 1732
Citral, 2322
d-Fenchone, 3968
Piperitone, 7473
Pulegone, 7937
Thujone, 9392

C₁₀H₁₆O₂
Ascaridole, 827
Chrysanthemic Acid, 2251
Diosphenol, 3298
3-Hydroxycamphor, 4817
Iridomyrmecin, 5089
Lineatin, 5503
Sebacil, 8416

C₁₁H₉NaO₅S
  Menadione Sodium Bisulfite, 5831
C₁₁H₁₀BrN₅
  Brimonidine, 1375
C₁₁H₁₀Cl₂F₂N₄O₃S
  Sulfentrazone, 8947
C₁₁H₁₀FNO₂S
  Flosequinan, 4110
C₁₁H₁₀N₂S
  ANTU, 722
C₁₁H₁₀N₃NaO₂S.H₂O
  Sulfapyridine Sodium Salt Monohy-
    drate, 8938
C₁₁H₁₀N₄O₄
  Carbadox, 1780
C₁₁H₁₀O
  2-Methoxynaphthalene, 5997
C₁₁H₁₀O₂
  Menadiol, 5830
C₁₁H₁₀O₄
  Limettin, 5492
  Scoparone, 8404
C₁₁H₁₀O₆
  Dipyrocetyl, 3349
C₁₁H₁₁ClO₃
  Alclofenac, 219
C₁₁H₁₁Cl₂NO₂
  Benoxacor, 1046
C₁₁H₁₁F₃N₂O₃
  Flutamide, 4208
C₁₁H₁₁I₃O₃
  Iophenoxic Acid, 5061
C₁₁H₁₁NO
  3-Indolylacetone, 4967
  Vitamin K₅, 10023
C₁₁H₁₁NO₂
  Phensuximide, 7261
C₁₁H₁₁NO₄S
  Woodward's Reagent K, 10050
C₁₁H₁₁N₃O₂
  Mivazerol, 6220
C₁₁H₁₁N₃O₂S
  Sulfapyridine, 8938
C₁₁H₁₁N₄NaO₂S
  Sulfamerazine Monosodium Salt,
    8913
C₁₁H₁₁N₄NaO₃S
  Sulfamethoxypyridazine Sodium Salt,
    8919
C₁₁H₁₁N₅
  Phenazopyridine, 7210
C₁₁H₁₁N₅O₃S₂
  Urothion, 9888
C₁₁H₁₂AsNO₅S₂
  Arsenamide, 793
C₁₁H₁₂BrNO
  Cinromide, 2311
C₁₁H₁₂ClNO₃S
  Chlormezanone, 2106
C₁₁H₁₂Cl₂N₂O
  Lofexidine, 5558
C₁₁H₁₂Cl₂N₂O₅
  Chloramphenicol, 2077
C₁₁H₁₂Cl₂O₃
  2,4-D Isopropyl Ester, 2796
C₁₁H₁₂I₃NO₂
  Iopanoic Acid, 5058
C₁₁H₁₂NO₄PS₂
  Phosmet, 7336
C₁₁H₁₂N₂O
  Antipyrine, 716
  Vasicine, 9937
C₁₁H₁₂N₂O₂
  Ethotoin, 3749
  Fenozolone, 3988

Idazoxan, 4887
Thozalinone, 9379
Tryptophan, 9797
C₁₁H₁₂N₂O₂S
  Zileuton, 10124
C₁₁H₁₂N₂O₃
  5-Hydroxytryptophan, 4847
C₁₁H₁₂N₂S
  Levamisole, 5459
C₁₁H₁₂N₄O₂
  Todralazine, 9502
C₁₁H₁₂N₄O₂S
  Sulfamerazine, 8913
  Sulfaperine, 8934
C₁₁H₁₂N₄O₃S
  Sulfalene, 8910
  Sulfameter, 8914
  Sulfamethoxypyridazine, 8919
C₁₁H₁₂O₂
  Cinnamic Acid Ethyl Ester, 2299
  6-Methoxy-α-tetralone, 6000
C₁₁H₁₂O₃
  Ethyl Benzoylacetate, 3767
  Myristicin, 6334
C₁₁H₁₂O₅
  Elenolide, 3543
C₁₁H₁₃BrN₂O₅
  Brivudine, 1378
C₁₁H₁₃BrN₂O₆
  Sorivudine, 8727
C₁₁H₁₃ClF₃N₃O₄S₃
  Polythiazide, 7584
C₁₁H₁₃ClN₂
  Epibatidine, 3610
C₁₁H₁₃ClO
  Dowicide 9®, 3430
C₁₁H₁₃F₃N₂O₃S
  Mefluidide, 5802
C₁₁H₁₃N
  Pargyline, 7038
C₁₁H₁₃NO₂
  Hydrohydrastinine, 4802
  Idrocilamide, 4893
C₁₁H₁₃NO₃
  Corydaldine, 2543
  Hydrastinine, 4768
  4-Salicyloylmorpholine, 8333
  Thurfyl Nicotinate, 9395
  Toloxatone, 9521
C₁₁H₁₃NO₄
  Bendiocarb, 1036
  Mephenoxalone, 5851
C₁₁H₁₃N₃O
  Ampyrone, 591
C₁₁H₁₃N₃O₃S
  Sulfamoxole, 8924
  Sulfisoxazole, 8952
C₁₁H₁₃N₅O₅
  Azidamfenicol, 909
C₁₁H₁₄AsNO₃S₂
  Arsthinol, 812
C₁₁H₁₄ClNO
  Propachlor, 7793
C₁₁H₁₄ClNO₂
  Buclosamide, 1465
C₁₁H₁₄ClN₃O₄S₃
  Althiazide, 318
C₁₁H₁₄ClN₅
  Cycloguanil, 2721
C₁₁H₁₄N₂
  Gramine, 4533
  α-Methyltryptamine, 6131
C₁₁H₁₄N₂O
  Cytisine, 2789
  5-Methoxytryptamine, 6002

C₁₁H₁₄N₂O₂
  Levulinic Acid Phenylhydrazone,
    5472
  Pheneturide, 7230
C₁₁H₁₄N₂O₃S
  Sulfadicramide, 8904
C₁₁H₁₄N₂O₄
  Felbamate, 3950
  5′-Nitro-2′-propoxyacetanilide,
    6629
C₁₁H₁₄N₂S
  Pyrantel, 7955
C₁₁H₁₄N₄O₂
  Epirizole, 3622
C₁₁H₁₄N₄O₄
  Doxofylline, 3438
  Tubercidin, 9804
C₁₁H₁₄O₂
  n-Butyl Benzoate, 1552
  Methyleugenol, 6073
C₁₁H₁₄O₃
  Butylparaben, 1584
  o-Thymotic Acid, 9408
  Zingerone, 10166
C₁₁H₁₄O₄
  Dimethyl Carbate, 3240
C₁₁H₁₅BrClO₃PS
  Profenofos, 7770
C₁₁H₁₅ClN₂O₂
  Iproclozide, 5076
C₁₁H₁₅ClN₄O₂
  Nitenpyram, 6568
C₁₁H₁₅Cl₂N₅
  Chlorproguanil, 2184
C₁₁H₁₅NO
  PBN, 7056
  Phenmetrazine, 7237
C₁₁H₁₅NO₂
  Butamben, 1512
  Isobutyl p-Aminobenzoate, 5133
  MDMA, 5767
  Salsoline, 8340
C₁₁H₁₅NO₂S
  Methiocarb, 5972
C₁₁H₁₅NO₃
  Anhalamine, 653
  Propoxur, 7836
C₁₁H₁₅NO₄
  Mephenesin Carbamate, 5850
C₁₁H₁₅NO₅
  Methocarbamol, 5980
C₁₁H₁₅NO₇S₂
  Disufenton, 3363
C₁₁H₁₅N₂NaO₂S
  Buthalital Sodium, 1524
C₁₁H₁₅N₂O₈P
  NMN, 6663
C₁₁H₁₅N₃O₄
  Pyridinol Carbamate, 7975
C₁₁H₁₅N₅O₅
  Nelarabine, 6442
  Psicofuranine, 7923
C₁₁H₁₆
  Amylbenzene, 600
C₁₁H₁₆ClNO
  Clorprenaline, 2408
C₁₁H₁₆ClN₃O₄S₂
  Buthiazide, 1525
C₁₁H₁₆ClN₅
  Chlorguanide, 2090
C₁₁H₁₆FN₃O₃
  Carmofur, 1844
C₁₁H₁₆I₂N₂O₅
  Iodopyracet, 5040
C₁₁H₁₆N₂O
  Tocainide, 9491

C₁₂H₉Cl₂NO₃
Vinclozolin, 9984

C₁₂H₉F₂N₅O₂S
Flumetsulam, 4141

C₁₂H₉F₃N₂O₂
Leflunomide, 5432
Teriflunomide, 9165

C₁₂H₉N
Carbazole, 1790

C₁₂H₉NO
Phenoxazine, 7253

C₁₂H₉NO₂
Dictamnine, 3089
o-Nitrobiphenyl, 6592
p-Nitrobiphenyl, 6593

C₁₂H₉NO₆
Miloxacin, 6196

C₁₂H₉NS
Phenothiazine, 7252

C₁₂H₉N₂NaO₅S
Tropaeolin O, 9775

C₁₂H₉N₃O
Milrinone, 6197

C₁₂H₉N₃O₄
Magneson, 5695

C₁₂H₉N₃O₅
Nifuroxazide, 6535

C₁₂H₉N₃O₅S
Nitazoxanide, 6567

C₁₂H₉N₅O₃
Cyadox, 2681

C₁₂H₉NaO
o-Phenylphenol Sodium Salt, 7304

C₁₂H₁₀
Acenaphthene, 28
Diphenyl, 3314

C₁₂H₁₀BaO₆S₂
Barium Benzenesulfonate, 966

C₁₂H₁₀BaO₈S₂
p-Phenolsulfonic Acid Barium Salt, 7246

C₁₂H₁₀Ba₃O₁₄.7H₂O
Citric Acid Barium Salt Heptahydrate, 2326

C₁₂H₁₀CaO₂
Calcium Phenoxide, 1691

C₁₂H₁₀CaO₈S₂
Calcium Phenolsulfonate, 1690

C₁₂H₁₀CaO₁₀S₂
Dobesilate Calcium, 3394

C₁₂H₁₀Ca₃O₁₄
Calcium Citrate, 1661

C₁₂H₁₀ClN
4-Amino-4'-chlorodiphenyl, 435

C₁₂H₁₀ClN₃S
Thionine, 9346

C₁₂H₁₀Cl₂N₂
2,2'-Dichlorobenzidine, 3058
3,3'-Dichlorobenzidine, 3059

C₁₂H₁₀FN₃O₄
Fidarestat, 4078

C₁₂H₁₀F₃N₃O₄
Nilutamide, 6544

C₁₂H₁₀Mg
Diphenylmagnesium, 3327

C₁₂H₁₀Mg₃O₁₄
Magnesium Citrate, 5663

C₁₂H₁₀N₂
Azobenzene, 917
Harman, 4615

C₁₂H₁₀N₂O
Azoxybenzene, 923
3-Hydroxymethyl-β-carboline, 3779
p-Nitrosodiphenylamine, 6639

C₁₂H₁₀N₂O₄
Nifurpirinol, 6537

C₁₂H₁₀N₂O₅
Cinoxacin, 2309

C₁₂H₁₀N₂O₈S
Ranelic Acid, 8106

C₁₂H₁₀N₄
2,3-Diaminophenazine, 2982

C₁₂H₁₀N₄O₂
Lumichrome, 5598

C₁₂H₁₀O
Phenyl Ether, 7288
o-Phenylphenol, 7304

C₁₂H₁₀O₂
Chimaphilin, 2058
1-Naphthaleneacetic Acid, 6371

C₁₂H₁₀O₂S
Diphenyl Sulfone, 3332

C₁₂H₁₀O₃
2-Naphthoxyacetic Acid, 6397

C₁₂H₁₀O₄
Acifran, 110
Piperic Acid, 7467
Quinhydrone, 8058

C₁₂H₁₀O₅S₂
Benzenesulfonic Anhydride, 1071

C₁₂H₁₀O₇
Echinochrome A, 3496

C₁₂H₁₀O₈S₂Zn
Zinc p-Phenolsulfonate, 10150

C₁₂H₁₀O₁₄Zn₃
Zinc Citrate, 10134

C₁₂H₁₀P₂Se₄
Woollins' Reagent, 10051

C₁₂H₁₀S
Phenyl Sulfide, 7314

C₁₂H₁₁ClN₂O₅S
Furosemide, 4309

C₁₂H₁₁ClN₆O₂S₂
Azosemide, 922

C₁₂H₁₁Cl₂NO
Propyzamide, 7872

C₁₂H₁₁Cl₂N₃O₂
Anecortave Acetate, 891

C₁₂H₁₁F₃N₄O₆S
Flucarbazone, 4119

C₁₂H₁₁I₃N₂O₄
Iodamide, 5011
Metrizoic Acid, 6156

C₁₂H₁₁N
p-Biphenylamine, 1235
Diphenylamine, 3317

C₁₂H₁₁NOS
Thionalide, 9344

C₁₂H₁₁NO₂
4-Amino-1-naphthol N-Acetyl Deriv, 453
Carbaryl, 1787

C₁₂H₁₁NO₃S
N-Phenylsulfanilic Acid, 7313

C₁₂H₁₁N₂NaO₃
Phenobarbital Sodium Salt, 7238

C₁₂H₁₁N₃
p-Aminoazobenzene, 419
Diazoaminobenzene, 2998

C₁₂H₁₁N₃O₂
Furonazide, 4308

C₁₂H₁₁N₇
Triamterene, 9599

C₁₂H₁₂Al₂O₁₈
Aluminum Tartrate, 368

C₁₂H₁₂BrN₄NaO₂S.H₂O
Sulfabromomethazine Sodium Salt Monohydrate, 8898

C₁₂H₁₂Br₂N₂
Diquat Dibromide, 3352

C₁₂H₁₂ClNO₂S
Dansyl Chloride, 2814

C₁₂H₁₂ClN₅O₄S
Chlorsulfuron, 2191

C₁₂H₁₂I₃N₃NaO₂
Ipodate Sodium Salt, 5071

C₁₂H₁₂N₂
Benzidine, 1077
2,4'-Biphenyldiamine, 1236
1,1-Diphenylhydrazine, 3325

C₁₂H₁₂N₂O
Harmalol, 4614

C₁₂H₁₂N₂OS₂
p-Dimethylaminobenzalrhodanine, 3231

C₁₂H₁₂N₂O₂
Tetrantoin, 9234

C₁₂H₁₂N₂O₂S
Dapsone, 2822
Enoximone, 3589
Sulfabenz, 8896

C₁₂H₁₂N₂O₃
Nalidixic Acid, 6359
Phenobarbital, 7238

C₁₂H₁₂N₄
Chrysoidine Free Base, 2257
p-Diaminoazobenzene, 2977

C₁₂H₁₂N₄O₃
Benznidazole, 1084

C₁₂H₁₂N₆Na₂O₁₀S₂
Carumonam Disodium Salt, 1871

C₁₂H₁₂O
2-Ethoxynaphthalene, 3752

C₁₂H₁₂O₂
2-(2-Naphthyloxy)ethanol, 6413

C₁₂H₁₂O₅
Fraxetin Dimethyl Ether, 4265
Radicinin, 8093

C₁₂H₁₂O₆
Pyrogallol Triacetate, 8000

C₁₂H₁₃BrN₄O₂S
Sulfabromomethazine, 8898

C₁₂H₁₃ClF₃N₃O₄
Fluchloralin, 4120

C₁₂H₁₃ClN₄
Chrysoidine, 2257
Pyrimethamine, 7985

C₁₂H₁₃Cl₂N₃
Alinidine, 246

C₁₂H₁₃I₃N₂O₂
Ipodate, 5071

C₁₂H₁₃I₃N₂O₃
Iocetamic Acid, 5010
Iomeglamic Acid, 5053

C₁₂H₁₃N
N,N-Dimethyl-1-naphthylamine, 3252
Rasagiline, 8116

C₁₂H₁₃NO₂
Indolebutyric Acid, 4965
Methsuximide, 6004

C₁₂H₁₃NO₂S
Carboxin, 1827

C₁₂H₁₃NO₃
Aniracetam, 662

C₁₂H₁₃N₂NaO₂S₂
Bensuldazic Acid Sodium Salt, 1051

C₁₂H₁₃N₂NaO₅
2-Cyclohexyl-4,6-dinitrophenol Sodium Salt, 2733

C₁₂H₁₃N₃
4,4'-Diaminodiphenylamine, 2979
Pyrimethanil, 7986

C₁₂H₁₃N₃O₂
Isocarboxazid, 5157
Triaziquone, 9603

C₁₂H₁₃N₃O₄
Olaquindox, 6823

$C_{12}H_{13}N_3O_4S_2$
N^4-Sulfanilylsulfanilamide, 8930
$C_{12}H_{13}N_3O_6$
Glyconiazide, 4500
$C_{12}H_{13}N_4NaO_2S$
Sulfamethazine Sodium Salt, 8915
$C_{12}H_{13}N_5O_2S$
Sulfamidochrysoidine, 8923
$C_{12}H_{13}N_5O_4$
Toyocamycin, 9562
$C_{12}H_{13}N_5O_6S_2$
Thifensulfuron-methyl, 9316
$C_{12}H_{14}ClNO_2$
Clomazone, 2381
$C_{12}H_{14}ClNO_3$
Cotarnine Chloride, 2552
$C_{12}H_{14}Cl_2FNO_4S$
Florfenicol, 4109
$C_{12}H_{14}Cl_2N_2$
Paraquat Dichloride, 7031
$C_{12}H_{14}Cl_2O_3$
2,4-D Butyl Ester, 2796
$C_{12}H_{14}Cl_3O_4P$
Chlorfenvinphos, 2089
$C_{12}H_{14}N_2$
Detomidine, 2937
N-(1-Naphthyl)ethylenediamine, 6409
$C_{12}H_{14}N_2^{2+}$
Paraquat, 7031
$C_{12}H_{14}N_2O_2$
Abrine, 10
Mephenytoin, 5853
Primidone, 7746
$C_{12}H_{14}N_2O_2S_2$
Bensuldazic Acid, 1051
$C_{12}H_{14}N_2O_3S$
Tioxidazole, 9455
$C_{12}H_{14}N_2O_5$
N-(p-Aminobenzoyl)glutamic Acid, 426
2-Cyclohexyl-4,6-dinitrophenol, 2733
$C_{12}H_{14}N_2O_6$
Dinoseb Acetate, 3287
$C_{12}H_{14}N_2S$
Cymiazole, 2764
$C_{12}H_{14}N_4O_2S$
Sulfamethazine, 8915
Sulfisomidine, 8951
$C_{12}H_{14}N_4O_3S$
Sulfacytine, 8902
Sulfamethomidine, 8917
$C_{12}H_{14}N_4O_4S$
Sulfadimethoxine, 8905
Sulfadoxine, 8906
$C_{12}H_{14}N_4O_4S_2$
Thiophanate O,O-Dimethyl Analog, 9352
$C_{12}H_{14}N_6O_{10}S_2$
Carumonam, 1871
$C_{12}H_{14}O_2$
Precocene I, 7718
$C_{12}H_{14}O_3$
Cuelure, 2616
$C_{12}H_{14}O_4$
Apiole (Dill), 733
Apiole (Parsley), 734
Dimecrotic Acid, 3203
Phthalic Acid Ethyl Ester, 7371
$C_{12}H_{15}AsN_6OS_2$
Melarsoprol, 5815
$C_{12}H_{15}ClNO_4PS_2$
Phosalone, 7334
$C_{12}H_{15}ClO_3$
Clofibrate, 2377
$C_{12}H_{15}Cl_2NO$
Karsil, 5285

$C_{12}H_{15}Cl_2NO_5S$
Thiamphenicol, 9301
$C_{12}H_{15}N$
6,7-Benzomorphan, 1095
MPTP, 6294
$C_{12}H_{15}NNaO_5S$
Faropenem Sodium Salt, 3938
$C_{12}H_{15}NO_3$
Anhalonine, 655
Carbofuran, 1803
Hydrocotarnine, 4788
$C_{12}H_{15}NO_4$
Cotarnine, 2552
Ethopabate, 3745
$C_{12}H_{15}NO_5S$
Faropenem, 3938
$C_{12}H_{15}N_2NaO_3$
Hexobarbital Sodium Salt, 4704
$C_{12}H_{15}N_2O_3PS$
Phoxim, 7366
$C_{12}H_{15}N_3$
Indanazoline, 4932
$C_{12}H_{15}N_3O_2S$
Albendazole, 210
$C_{12}H_{15}N_3O_2S_2$
Glybuzole, 4480
$C_{12}H_{15}N_3O_3$
Oxibendazole, 6936
$C_{12}H_{15}N_3O_5S$
Amezinium Methyl Sulfate, 394
$C_{12}H_{15}N_5O_3$
Entecavir, 3595
$C_{12}H_{15}N_5O_3S$
Sulfaguanole, 8909
$C_{12}H_{16}ClNO_3$
Meclofenoxate, 5780
$C_{12}H_{16}ClN_3O_2S$
Oxythiamine, 6977
$C_{12}H_{16}Cl_2N_2O$
Neburon, 6435
$C_{12}H_{16}F_3N$
Fenfluramine, 3973
$C_{12}H_{16}N_2$
N,N-Dimethyltryptamine, 3262
Fenproporex, 3994
$C_{12}H_{16}N_2O$
Bufotenine, 1478
Methylcytisine, 6049
Psilocin, 7925
$C_{12}H_{16}N_2O_2$
Eltoprazine, 3552
$C_{12}H_{16}N_2O_3$
Cyclobarbital, 2711
Hexobarbital, 4704
$C_{12}H_{16}N_2S$
Morantel, 6266
Xylazine, 10080
$C_{12}H_{16}N_3O_3PS$
Triazophos, 9606
$C_{12}H_{16}N_3O_3PS_2$
Azinphos-methyl O,O-Diethyl Analog, 913
$C_{12}H_{16}N_4O_2S_2$
Glybuthiazol(e), 4479
$C_{12}H_{16}O_2$
Ibufenac, 4880
Isoamyl Benzoate, 5113
Thymol Acetate, 9399
$C_{12}H_{16}O_3$
Asarones, 824
Isoamyl Salicylate, 5125
$C_{12}H_{16}O_4$
Aspidinol, 847
$C_{12}H_{16}O_4S_2$
Malotilate, 5712

$C_{12}H_{16}O_6S$
Protiofate, 7890
$C_{12}H_{16}O_7$
Arbutin, 773
$C_{12}H_{17}ClN_4OS$
Thiamine, 9295
$C_{12}H_{17}Cl_2NO_3$
2,4-DB Dimethylamine Salt, 2835
$C_{12}H_{17}NO$
Deet, 2856
N,N-Diethylphenylacetamide, 3126
Phendimetrazine, 7220
$C_{12}H_{17}NO_2$
Ciclopirox, 2266
MDE, 5766
$C_{12}H_{17}NO_3$
Anhalonidine, 654
Bucetin, 1458
Bufexamac, 1474
Cerulenin, 2004
Deacetylanisomycin, 670
Ethamivan, 3721
Rimiterol, 8227
$C_{12}H_{17}N_2NaO_2S$
Thiamylal Sodium Salt, 9302
$C_{12}H_{17}N_2NaO_3$
Secobarbital Sodium, 8420
$C_{12}H_{17}N_2O_4P$
Psilocybin, 7926
$C_{12}H_{17}N_3O$
Cimaterol, 2278
$C_{12}H_{17}N_3O_3S$
Cariporide, 1841
$C_{12}H_{17}N_3O_4$
Agaritine, 187
$C_{12}H_{17}N_3O_4S.H_2O$
Imipenem, 4919
$C_{12}H_{17}N_5O_4S$
Thiamine Mononitrate, 9295
$C_{12}H_{17}NaO_7$
Dikegulac Sodium Salt, 3199
$C_{12}H_{17}Na_3O_{17}Sb_2.9H_2O$
Sodium Stibogluconate, 701
$C_{12}H_{18}ClN$
Mefenorex, 5799
$C_{12}H_{18}ClNO$
Tulobuterol, 9811
$C_{12}H_{18}ClNO_2S$
Dimethenamid, 3214
$C_{12}H_{18}ClNO_4$
Methyldopa Ethyl Ester Hydrochloride, 6055
$C_{12}H_{18}ClN_4O_4PS$
Thiamine Monophosphate, 9296
$C_{12}H_{18}Cl_2N_2O$
Clenbuterol, 2347
$C_{12}H_{18}{}^{123}IN$
Iofetamine ^{123}I, 5049
$C_{12}H_{18}NO_6P$
Diisopropyl Paraoxon, 3198
$C_{12}H_{18}N_2O$
Isoproturon, 5218
Oxotremorine, 6951
$C_{12}H_{18}N_2O_2S$
Thiamylal, 9302
$C_{12}H_{18}N_2O_3S$
Tolbutamide, 9507
$C_{12}H_{18}N_2O_4$
Midodrine, 6184
$C_{12}H_{18}N_2O_5$
Bacilysin, 933
Hypoglycine B, 4866
$C_{12}H_{18}N_2O_7$
Bicozamycin, 1202
$C_{12}H_{18}N_4O_6S$
Oryzalin, 6885

C₁₂H₁₈O
Propofol, 7834

$C_{12}H_{18}O$
Propofol, 7834

$C_{12}H_{18}O_2$
4-Hexylresorcinol, 4712

$C_{12}H_{18}O_3$
Jasmonic Acid, 5260

$C_{12}H_{18}O_7$
Dikegulac, 3199

$C_{12}H_{19}BrN_2O_2$
Neostigmine Bromide, 6464

$C_{12}H_{19}ClNO_3P$
Crufomate, 2604

$C_{12}H_{19}ClN_4O_7P_2S$
Thiamine Diphosphate, 9296

$C_{12}H_{19}Cl_3O_8$
Sucralose, 8880

$C_{12}H_{19}NO$
Etafedrine, 3709

$C_{12}H_{19}NO_2$
Bamethan, 954
DOM, 3412
Fepradinol, 4011
Octyl Cyanoacrylate, 6766

$C_{12}H_{19}NO_3$
Macromerine, 5645
Prenalterol, 7735
Terbutaline, 9159

$C_{12}H_{19}NO_4$
Choline Salicylate, 2209

$C_{12}H_{19}N_2NaO_2S_2$
Methitural Sodium Salt, 5978

$C_{12}H_{19}N_2O_2{}^+$
Neostigmine, 6464

$C_{12}H_{19}N_3O$
Procarbazine, 7758

$C_{12}H_{19}N_4O_{10}P_3S$
Thiamine Triphosphate, 9298

$C_{12}H_{19}O_2PS_3$
Sulprofos, 8990

$C_{12}H_{20}B_2CaO_{16}$
Calcium Borogluconate, 1653

$C_{12}H_{20}Cl_4N_2O_2$
Fertilysin, 4060

$C_{12}H_{20}N_2$
Tremorine, 9582

$C_{12}H_{20}N_2O_2$
Aspergillic Acid, 841

$C_{12}H_{20}N_2O_2S_2$
Methitural, 5978

$C_{12}H_{20}N_2O_3$
Pirbuterol, 7489

$C_{12}H_{20}N_2O_3S$
Sotalol, 8728

$C_{12}H_{20}N_2O_4S$
Soterenol, 8729

$C_{12}H_{20}N_4O_2$
Hexazinone, 4699

$C_{12}H_{20}N_4O_7$
Zanamivir, 10113

$C_{12}H_{20}N_4O_9S$
Sulfazecin, 8946

$C_{12}H_{20}O_2$
Bornyl Acetate, 1339
Linalyl Acetate, 5496

$C_{12}H_{20}O_4$
Traumatic Acid, 9576

$C_{12}H_{20}O_6$
Diacetoneglucose, 2965

$C_{12}H_{20}O_7$
Citric Acid Ethyl Ester, 2326

$C_{12}H_{21}ClO_2$
Trimedlure, 9701

$C_{12}H_{21}N$
Memantine, 5829
Rimantadine, 8224

$C_{12}H_{21}NO_8S$
Topiramate, 9547

$C_{12}H_{21}NO_{11}$
Chondrosine, 2215
Hyalobiuronic Acid, 4756

$C_{12}H_{21}N_2O_3PS$
Diazinon, 2995

$C_{12}H_{21}N_2O_5S_2{}^{99m}Tc$
Technetium ^{99m}Tc Bicisate, 9099

$C_{12}H_{21}N_3O_3$
Pyrrolysine, 8019

$C_{12}H_{21}N_3O_5S_3$
Brinzolamide, 1376

$C_{12}H_{21}N_5O_2S_2$
Nizatidine, 6660

$C_{12}H_{21}N_5O_3$
Cadralazine, 1631
Choline Theophyllinate, 2210

$C_{12}H_{21}NaO_7S$
Diisobutyl Sodium Sulfosuccinate, 3194

$C_{12}H_{22}CaO_{14}$
Calcium Gluconate, 1669

$C_{12}H_{22}Cl_2N_2O_3$
Pirbuterol Dihydrochloride, 7489

$C_{12}H_{22}CuO_{14}$
Cupric Gluconate, 2640

$C_{12}H_{22}FeO_{14}$
Ferrous Gluconate, 4047

$C_{12}H_{22}MgO_{14}$
Gluconic Acid Magnesium Salt, 4456

$C_{12}H_{22}N_2O_2$
Crotethamide, 2595

$C_{12}H_{22}N_2O_8S_2$
Piposulfan, 7481

$C_{12}H_{22}O$
Geosmin, 4400

$C_{12}H_{22}O_2$
Menthyl Acetate, 5839

$C_{12}H_{22}O_4$
Di-*tert*-butyl Succinate, 3037

$C_{12}H_{22}O_6$
Etoglucid, 3880

$C_{12}H_{22}O_{10}$
Rutinose, 8305

$C_{12}H_{22}O_{11}$
Cellobiose, 1961
Gentiobiose, 4396
Isomaltulose, 5182
Lactose, 5343
Lactulose, 5346
Maltose, 5714
Melibiose, 5820
Sophorose, 8719
Sucrose, 8881
Trehalose, 9580
Turanose, 9821

$C_{12}H_{22}O_{12}$
Lactobionic Acid, 5342

$C_{12}H_{22}O_{14}Zn$
Gluconic Acid Zinc Complex, 4456

$C_{12}H_{23}N$
Dicyclohexylamine, 3095

$C_{12}H_{23}NO_3$
Picaridin, 7394

$C_{12}H_{23}N_3O$
Esaprazole, 3695

$C_{12}H_{24}B_2O_4$
Bis(pinacolato)diborane, 1300

$C_{12}H_{24}CaN_2O_6S_2$
Calcium Cyclamate, 1665

$C_{12}H_{24}N_2O_4$
Carisoprodol, 1842

$C_{12}H_{24}N_6O_2P_2$
Dipin, 3336

$C_{12}H_{24}N_9P_3$
Apholate, 728

$C_{12}H_{24}O_2$
Ethyl Caprate, 3776
Lauric Acid, 5384
2-Nonyldioxolane, 6680

$C_{12}H_{24}O_6$
18-Crown-6, 2602

$C_{12}H_{24}O_{11}$
Lactitol, 5340

$C_{12}H_{25}Br$
Lauryl Bromide, 5389

$C_{12}H_{25}NaO_4S$
Sodium Lauryl Sulfate, 8636

$C_{12}H_{26}N_4O_6$
Neamine, 6430

$C_{12}H_{26}O$
1-Dodecanol, 3405

$C_{12}H_{26}O_6P_2S_4$
Dioxathion, 3301

$C_{12}H_{27}AlO_3$
Aluminum *tert*-Butoxide, 333

$C_{12}H_{27}N$
Tributylamine, 9618

$C_{12}H_{27}OPS_3$
Tribufos, 9617

$C_{12}H_{27}O_4P$
Tributyl Phosphate, 9619

$C_{12}H_{28}BK$
K-Selectride, 8427

$C_{12}H_{28}BLi$
L-Selectride, 8427

$C_{12}H_{28}O_4Ti$
Titanium Tetraisopropoxide, 9480

$C_{12}H_{30}Br_2N_2$
Hexamethonium Bromide, 4688

$C_{12}H_{30}Cl_2N_2$
Hexamethonium Chloride, 4688

$C_{12}H_{30}I_2N_2$
Hexamethonium Iodide, 4688

$C_{12}H_{30}N_2{}^{2+}$
Hexamethonium, 4688

$C_{12}H_{36}O_4Si_5$
Dodecamethylpentasiloxane, 3404

$C_{12}H_{36}O_6Si_6$
Dodecamethylcyclohexasiloxane, 3403

$C_{12}H_{54}Al_{16}O_{75}S_8$
Sucralfate, 8879

$C_{13}H_4Cl_2F_6N_4O_4$
Fluazinam, 4117

$C_{13}H_5ClN_5NaO_2.5H_2O$
Traxanox Sodium Salt Pentahydrate, 9578

$C_{13}H_5N_3O_7$
2,4,7-Trinitrofluorenone, 9728

$C_{13}H_6ClN_5O_2$
Traxanox, 9578

$C_{13}H_6Cl_5NO_3$
Oxyclozanide, 6958

$C_{13}H_6Cl_6O_2$
Hexachlorophene, 4680

$C_{13}H_7Cl_4NO_2$
3,3′,4′,5-Tetrachlorosalicylanilide, 9191

$C_{13}H_8Br_3NO_2$
Tribromsalan, 9616

$C_{13}H_8Cl_2N_2O_4$
Niclosamide, 6519

$C_{13}H_8Cl_2O_4S$
Ticrynafen, 9430

$C_{13}H_8F_2O_3$
Diflunisal, 3146

$C_{13}H_8N_2O_3S$
Nitroscanate, 6633

C₁₃H₁₄N₂O₃
  Mephobarbital, 5854
C₁₃H₁₄N₂O₄
  Menadoxime, 5832
C₁₃H₁₄N₂O₄S₂
  Gliotoxin, 4441
C₁₃H₁₄N₃NaO₄S
  Glymidine Sodium Salt, 4507
C₁₃H₁₄N₄O
  sym-Diphenylcarbazide, 3321
C₁₃H₁₄N₄O₃S
  N²-Formylsulfisomidine, 4248
C₁₃H₁₄N₄O₄S
  Acetyl Sulfamethoxypyrazine, 101
C₁₃H₁₄O₂
  Tremetone, 9581
C₁₃H₁₄O₅
  Citrinin, 2327
C₁₃H₁₅BrN₄O₂
  Brodimoprim, 1380
C₁₃H₁₅ClN₆O₇S
  Halosulfuron-methyl, 4602
C₁₃H₁₅NO₂
  Glutethimide, 4477
  Securinine, 8422
C₁₃H₁₅N₃O₂
  Pyrolan, 8002
C₁₃H₁₅N₃O₃
  Imazapyr, 4905
C₁₃H₁₅N₃O₄S
  Acetyl Sulfisoxazole, 8952
  Glymidine, 4507
C₁₃H₁₅N₅O₃
  Tazanolast, 9080
C₁₃H₁₅N₅O₆
  Nifurfoline, 6533
C₁₃H₁₆ClNO
  Ketamine, 5295
C₁₃H₁₆F₃N₃O₄
  Benfluralin, 1040
  Trifluralin, 9686
C₁₃H₁₆HgNNaO₆
  Mersalyl, 5901
C₁₃H₁₆N₂
  Dexmedetomidine, 2946
  Medetomidine, 5787
  Tetrahydrozoline, 9219
C₁₃H₁₆N₂O
  Adrenoglomerulotropin, 173
  Oxantel, 6922
C₁₃H₁₆N₂O₂
  Aminoglutethimide, 440
  Melatonin, 5816
  Mofebutazone, 6231
C₁₃H₁₆N₂O₂S
  Thialbarbital, 9292
C₁₃H₁₆N₂O₃
  Acetylpheneturide, 99
C₁₃H₁₆N₃NaO₄S.H₂O
  Dipyrone, 3350
C₁₃H₁₆N₄O₂
  Diaveridine, 2993
C₁₃H₁₆N₄O₆
  Furaltadone, 4294
C₁₃H₁₆N₁₀O₅S
  Azimsulfuron, 912
C₁₃H₁₆O₂
  Cinnamic Acid *n*-Butyl Ester, 2299
  Dihydrotremetone, 9581
  R-11, 8088
C₁₃H₁₆O₃
  Precocene II, 7718
C₁₃H₁₆O₅
  Trinexapac-ethyl, 9725
C₁₃H₁₆O₇
  Helicin, 4628

C₁₃H₁₆O₁₀
  α-Glucogallin, 4453
  β-Glucogallin, 4454
C₁₃H₁₇ClN₂O₂
  Moclobemide, 6226
C₁₃H₁₇F₃N₄O₄
  Prodiamine, 7766
C₁₃H₁₇HgNO₆
  Mersalyl Acid, 5901
C₁₃H₁₇N
  Selegiline, 8428
C₁₃H₁₇NO
  Crotamiton, 2594
C₁₃H₁₇NO₂
  Alminoprofen, 300
C₁₃H₁₇NO₄
  Alibendol, 244
C₁₃H₁₇NO₇
  Synephrine Tartaric Acid Monoester, 9012
C₁₃H₁₇N₂NaO₄S₂
  Penicillin O Sodium Salt, 7099
C₁₃H₁₇N₃
  Tramazoline, 9567
C₁₃H₁₇N₃O
  Aminopyrine, 474
C₁₃H₁₇N₃O₂
  Parbendazole, 7035
C₁₃H₁₇N₅O₈S₂
  Aztreonam, 925
C₁₃H₁₈AlClTi
  Tebbe Reagent, 9091
C₁₃H₁₈Br₂N₂O
  Ambroxol, 386
C₁₃H₁₈ClF₃N₂O
  Mabuterol, 5642
C₁₃H₁₈ClNO
  Bupropion, 1499
  Solan, 8702
C₁₃H₁₈ClNO₄
  Alclofenac Monoethanolamine Complex, 219
C₁₃H₁₈ClN₃O₄S₂
  Cyclopenthiazide, 2745
C₁₃H₁₈Cl₂N₂O₂
  Melphalan, 5828
C₁₃H₁₈NNaO₄S
  Probenecid Sodium Salt, 7754
C₁₃H₁₈N₂O
  Fenoxazoline, 3985
C₁₃H₁₈N₂O₂
  Lenacil, 5435
C₁₃H₁₈N₂O₃
  Heptabarbital, 4655
  Lacosamide, 5333
C₁₃H₁₈N₂O₄S₂
  Penicillin O, 7099
C₁₃H₁₈N₄O₃
  Pentoxifylline, 7136
C₁₃H₁₈O
  β-Damascenone, 2809
C₁₃H₁₈O₂
  Ibuprofen, 4881
C₁₃H₁₈O₃
  Mandelic Acid Isoamyl Ester, 5718
C₁₃H₁₈O₅S
  Ethofumesate, 3742
C₁₃H₁₈O₇
  Gastrodin, 4375
  Salicin, 8324
C₁₃H₁₉ClN₂O₅S₂
  Mefruside, 5803
C₁₃H₁₉Cl₂NO₂
  Cloranolol, 2402
C₁₃H₁₉NO
  Diethylpropion, 3127

C₁₃H₁₉NO₂
  Carnegine, 1847
  Dioscorine, 3294
  Exalamide, 3909
  Ibuproxam, 4882
C₁₃H₁₉NO₂S
  Isobornyl Thiocyanoacetate, 5129
C₁₃H₁₉NO₃
  Pellotine, 7074
  Viloxazine, 9980
C₁₃H₁₉NO₄S
  Probenecid, 7754
C₁₃H₁₉NO₈
  Metaraminol Bitartrate (Hydrogen L-Tartrate), 5932
C₁₃H₁₉N₃O₄
  Dipropalin, 3341
  Pendimethalin, 7084
C₁₃H₁₉N₃O₅S₂
  Sparsomycin, 8736
C₁₃H₁₉N₄O₁₂P
  SAICAR, 8318
C₁₃H₁₉N₅
  Pinacidil, 7438
C₁₃H₂₀Cl₂N₂O₂
  Chloroprocaine Hydrochloride, 2158
C₁₃H₂₀N₂O
  Prilocaine, 7743
C₁₃H₂₀N₂O₂
  Butethamine, 1523
  Dropropizine, 3452
  Procaine, 7757
C₁₃H₂₀N₂O₃S
  Carticaine, 1869
  Etozolin, 3891
C₁₃H₂₀N₂O₆
  Actinobolin, 138
C₁₃H₂₀N₄O₂
  Pentifylline, 7127
C₁₃H₂₀N₄O₃
  Lisofylline, 5517
C₁₃H₂₀N₆O₄
  Valacyclovir, 9899
C₁₃H₂₀O
  Ionone, 5056
  4-(5-Isopropenyl-2-methyl-1-cyclopenten-1-yl)-2-butanone, 5204
  Pseudoionone, 7917
C₁₃H₂₀O₃
  Febuprol, 3947
C₁₃H₂₁N
  2,6-Di-*tert*-butylpyridine, 3036
C₁₃H₂₁NO₂
  Tigloidine, 9434
  Toliprolol, 9516
C₁₃H₂₁NO₃
  Albuterol, 216
  Isoetharine, 5170
  Moprolol, 6264
C₁₃H₂₁NO₄
  Meteloidine, 5935
C₁₃H₂₁N₃O₃
  Carbuterol, 1833
C₁₃H₂₁N₅O₂
  Etamiphyllin, 3711
C₁₃H₂₁O₅P
  Fospropofol, 4259
C₁₃H₂₂ClN₃O
  Procainamide Hydrochloride, 7756
C₁₃H₂₂NO₃PS
  Fenamiphos, 3957
C₁₃H₂₂N₂
  Dicyclohexylcarbodiimide, 3096
C₁₃H₂₂N₂O₄
  Salicylamide *O*-Acetic Acid Diethylamine Salt, 8329

$C_{14}H_{12}N_2O_2S$
Zolimidine, 10188
$C_{14}H_{12}N_4OS$
Nolatrexed, 6672
$C_{14}H_{12}N_4O_2S$
Sulfaquinoxaline, 8939
$C_{14}H_{12}N_6O$
Levosimendan, 5471
$C_{14}H_{12}N_6O_3$
Pteroic Acid, 7933
$C_{14}H_{12}N_6O_6$
Nitrovin, 6654
$C_{14}H_{12}O$
Phenyl Tolyl Ketone, 7317
$C_{14}H_{12}O_2$
Benzoin, 1093
Benzyl Benzoate, 1127
Diphenylacetic Acid, 3316
Felbinac, 3951
Pinosylvin, 7451
$C_{14}H_{12}O_3$
Benzilic Acid, 1080
Benzyl Salicylate, 1144
Oxybenzone, 6954
Resveratrol, 8158
Trioxsalen, 9735
Xanthyletin, 10069
$C_{14}H_{12}O_3S$
Suprofen, 9005
Tiaprofenic Acid, 9422
$C_{14}H_{12}O_4$
Dioxybenzone, 3303
Fulvoplumierin, 4285
$C_{14}H_{12}O_5$
Khellin, 5309
$C_{14}H_{12}O_6S$
Sulisobenzone, 8983
$C_{14}H_{12}S_2$
Mesulfen, 5918
$C_{14}H_{13}ClN_6O_5S$
Imazosulfuron, 4908
$C_{14}H_{13}ClO_5S$
Sulcotrione, 8894
$C_{14}H_{13}F_4N_3O_2S$
Flufenacet, 4131
$C_{14}H_{13}IN_5NaO_6S$
Iodosulfuron-methyl-sodium, 5046
$C_{14}H_{13}NO$
Diphenylacetamide, 3315
$C_{14}H_{13}NO_2$
Benzoin Oxime, 1094
Flindersine, 4101
$C_{14}H_{13}NO_4$
Skimmianine, 8561
$C_{14}H_{13}NO_7S$
Mesotrione, 5912
$C_{14}H_{13}N_2NaO_4S$
Acediasulfone Sodium Salt, 23
$C_{14}H_{13}N_3$
Fadrozole, 3927
Mepanipyrim, 5845
$C_{14}H_{13}N_3O_2S$
Sulmazole, 8985
$C_{14}H_{13}N_3O_4S_2$
Meloxicam, 5826
$C_{14}H_{13}N_3O_5S$
Sulfanitran, 8933
$C_{14}H_{13}N_5O_5S_2$
Cefdinir, 1920
$C_{14}H_{13}N_8NaO_4S_3$
Cefazolin Sodium Salt, 1917
$C_{14}H_{13}NaO_3$
Naproxen Sodium Salt, 6417
$C_{14}H_{14}$
Bibenzyl, 1198

$C_{14}H_{14}As_2N_2Na_2O_8S_2$
Sulfarsphenamine, 8941
$C_{14}H_{14}ClNS$
Ticlopidine, 9429
$C_{14}H_{14}ClN_3O_4S_2$
Benzylhydrochlorothiazide, 1136
$C_{14}H_{14}ClN_3S$
Azure A, 927
$C_{14}H_{14}ClO_3P$
Dibenzyl Chlorophosphonate, 3012
$C_{14}H_{14}Cl_2N_2O$
Enilconazole, 3583
$C_{14}H_{14}Cl_3O_6P$
Haloxon, 4605
$C_{14}H_{14}Hg$
p-Ditolylmercury, 3381
$C_{14}H_{14}HgO_6$
Mercumallylic Acid, 5872
$C_{14}H_{14}NO_4PS$
EPN, 3626
$C_{14}H_{14}N_2$
Naphazoline, 6368
$C_{14}H_{14}N_2Na_2O_6S_3$
Sulfoxone Sodium, 8968
$C_{14}H_{14}N_2O$
Metyrapone, 6159
$C_{14}H_{14}N_2O_2$
Isonixin, 5192
$C_{14}H_{14}N_2O_4S$
Acediasulfone, 23
N-Methylphenazonium Methosulfate, 6109
$C_{14}H_{14}N_2O_6S_2$
Amsonic Acid, 595
$C_{14}H_{14}N_3NaO_3S$
Methyl Orange, 6105
$C_{14}H_{14}N_4O$
Phenamidine, 7208
$C_{14}H_{14}N_4O_2S$
Cambendazole, 1726
$C_{14}H_{14}N_8O_4S_3$
Cefazolin, 1917
$C_{14}H_{14}O$
Benzyl Ether, 1132
$C_{14}H_{14}O_2$
Hydrobenzoin, 4777
$C_{14}H_{14}O_2P_2S_4$
Lawesson's Reagent, 5391
$C_{14}H_{14}O_3$
Euparin O-Methyl Deriv, 3900
2-Isovalerylindane-1,3-dione, 5233
Kawain, 5287
αMNP, 6224
Naproxen, 6417
Pindone, 7444
$C_{14}H_{14}O_4$
Phthalofyne, 7374
$C_{14}H_{14}S$
Benzyl Sulfide, 1145
$C_{14}H_{14}S_2$
Dibenzyl Disulfide, 3013
$C_{14}H_{15}BrClNO_6$
X-gal, 10074
$C_{14}H_{15}Cl_2N$
Chlornaphazine, 2108
$C_{14}H_{15}Cl_2N_3OS$
Prothioconazole, 7887
$C_{14}H_{15}N$
Dibenzylamine, 3011
$C_{14}H_{15}N_3$
o-Aminoazotoluene, 420
Cyprodinil, 2772
p-Dimethylaminoazobenzene, 3229
$C_{14}H_{15}N_3O_2$
Indolmycin, 4966

$C_{14}H_{15}N_3O_5$
Entacapone, 3594
$C_{14}H_{15}N_5O$
Endralazine, 3577
$C_{14}H_{15}N_5O_5S_2$
Cefetamet, 1923
$C_{14}H_{15}N_5O_6S$
Metsulfuron-methyl, 6158
$C_{14}H_{15}O_2PS_2$
Edifenphos, 3510
$C_{14}H_{15}O_3P$
Dibenzyl Phosphite, 3014
$C_{14}H_{16}$
Chamazulene, 2040
$C_{14}H_{16}ClN_3O_2$
Triadimefon, 9592
$C_{14}H_{16}ClN_3O_4S_2$
Cyclothiazide, 2754
$C_{14}H_{16}ClN_5O_5S$
Triasulfuron, 9600
$C_{14}H_{16}ClO_5PS$
Coumaphos, 2558
$C_{14}H_{16}ClO_6P$
Coroxon, 2537
$C_{14}H_{16}Cl_2N_4O_3$
Asoxime Chloride, 835
Obidoxime Chloride, 6738
$C_{14}H_{16}Cl_3NO_2$
Zoxamide, 10198
$C_{14}H_{16}N_2$
Atipamezole, 861
1,2-Dianilinoethane, 2990
o-Tolidine, 9514
$C_{14}H_{16}N_2O$
Harmalol O-Ethylharmalol, 4614
$C_{14}H_{16}N_2O_2$
Dianisidine, 2991
Etomidate, 3881
$C_{14}H_{16}N_2O_3$
Nadoxolol, 6347
Phenetharbital, 7222
$C_{14}H_{16}N_2O_3S$
Monastrol, 6244
2-p-Sulfanilylanilinoethanol, 8927
$C_{14}H_{16}N_4$
Budralazine, 1470
Imiquimod, 4922
$C_{14}H_{16}N_4O_3$
Piromidic Acid, 7505
$C_{14}H_{16}O_3$
Dihydrokawain, 5287
$C_{14}H_{17}BrN_6O_2S_3$
Ebrotidine, 3485
$C_{14}H_{17}ClN_2O_3S$
Clorexolone, 2404
$C_{14}H_{17}Cl_2NO_2$
Fenhexamid, 3974
$C_{14}H_{17}Cl_2N_3O$
Hexaconazole, 4681
$C_{14}H_{17}I_3N_2O_2$
Ipodate Ethyl Ester, 5071
$C_{14}H_{17}NO_2$
3-Quinuclidinol dl-Form Benzoate (Ester), 8082
$C_{14}H_{17}NO_3$
EEDQ, 3518
$C_{14}H_{17}NO_4$
Chromocarb Diethylamine, 2237
$C_{14}H_{17}NO_6$
Indican (Plant Indican), 4942
Mandelonitrile Glucoside, 5720
$C_{14}H_{17}NO_7$
Dhurrin, 2958
$C_{14}H_{17}NS_2$
Dimethylthiambutene, 3260

C14H17N2NaO3
  Methohexital Sodium, 5981
C14H17N3O
  Frovatriptan, 4272
C14H17N3O2S
  Fasudil, 3942
C14H17N3O9
  6-Azauridine 2′,3′,5′-Triacetate, 904
C14H17N5O3
  Pipemidic Acid, 7460
C14H17N5O7S2
  Rimsulfuron, 8230
C14H17O5PS
  Hymecromone O,O-Diethyl Phos-
    phorothioate, 4855
C14H18CaN3Na3O10
  Pentetate Calcium Trisodium, 7124
C14H18ClNO2
  Indeloxazine Hydrochloride, 4938
C14H18ClN3O2
  Triadimenol, 9593
C14H18ClN3S
  Chlorothen, 2167
C14H18N2
  DMAN, 3388
C14H18N2O
  Ibudilast, 4879
  Propyphenazone, 7871
C14H18N2O2
  Hypaphorine, 4861
  Nefiracetam, 6439
  Parsalmide, 7045
C14H18N2O3
  Physovenine, 7385
C14H18N2O4
  Oxadixyl, 6908
  α-Ribazole, 8199
C14H18N2O5
  Aspartame, 839
  Lidofenin, 5483
C14H18N2O6S
  Carpetimycin A, 1859
C14H18N2O7
  Dinobuton, 3285
C14H18N2O9S2
  Carpetimycin B, 1859
C14H18N4O3
  Benomyl, 1044
  Trimethoprim, 9709
C14H18N4O4S2
  Thiophanate, 9352
C14H18N6O
  Abacavir, 1
C14H18O4
  Cinoxate, 2310
C14H18O7
  Picein, 7395
C14H18O8
  Glucovanillin, 4464
C14H19BrO9
  Acetobromglucose, 60
C14H19ClN4
  Amprolium, 590
C14H19Cl2NO2
  Chlorambucil, 2073
C14H19NO
  Ethoxyquin, 3753
C14H19NO2
  Levophacetoperane, 5467
  Methylphenidate, 6110
  Piperoxan, 7478
C14H19NO4
  Anisomycin, 670
C14H19NO4S
  Furtrethonium Benzenesulfonate, 4312
  Trithiozine, 9760

C14H19NO5
  Trimetozine, 9720
C14H19N3O
  Oxolamine, 6944
  Ramifenazone, 8102
C14H19N3O2
  Zilpaterol, 10125
C14H19N3S
  Methapyrilene, 5959
  Thenyldiamine, 9280
C14H19N5O4
  Famciclovir, 3929
C14H19N5O5
  Tecadenoson, 9096
C14H19O6P
  Crotoxyphos, 2600
C14H20
  Congressane, 2499
C14H20Br2N2
  Bromhexine, 1391
C14H20Br2N4O
  Pyrithiamine, 7992
C14H20ClNO2
  Acetochlor, 61
  Alachlor, 201
C14H20ClN3O3S
  Clopamide, 2393
C14H20Cl6N2
  Chlorisondamine Chloride, 2101
C14H20FN3OSi
  Simeconazole, 8534
C14H20GdN3O10
  Gadopentetic Acid, 4327
C14H20IN3O8
  Nitroxynil D-N-Methylglucamine Salt,
    6656
C14H20N2O
  Pyrrocaine, 8013
  Siduron, 8487
  Tymazoline, 9834
C14H20N2O2
  Bunitrolol, 1489
  Pindolol, 7443
  Piridocaine, 7494
C14H20N2O3
  Propacetamol, 7792
  Vorinostat, 10034
C14H20N2O3S
  Tolcyclamide, 9511
C14H20N2O6S
  p-Methylaminophenol Sulfate, 6017
C14H20N2O8S2
  Paraquat Bismethyl Sulfate, 7031
C14H20N3O5PS
  Pyrazophos, 7962
C14H20N4O
  Imolamine, 4923
C14H20N4O7S2
  Netobimin, 6480
C14H20O2
  Butibufen, 1527
C14H20O7
  Frequentin, 4270
C14H21NO2
  4-(Dimethylamino)benzoic Acid 3-
    Methylbutyl Ester, 3232
C14H21NO3
  Diethofencarb, 3109
C14H21NO4
  1,3,4-Tri-O-acetyl-N-acetyl-6-desoxy-
    β-D-glucosamine, 2931
C14H21N3O2S
  Sumatriptan, 8997
C14H21N3O3
  Oxamniquine, 6919

C14H21N3O3S
  Tolazamide, 9505
C14H21N3O4
  Butralin, 1532
C14H21N3O5
  Leonurine, 5440
C14H21N3O6S
  Penicillin N, 7098
C14H21N5O6S.H2O
  Serotonin Complex with Creatinine
    Sulfate, Monohydrate, 8462
C14H22BrN3O2
  Bromopride, 1432
C14H22ClNO
  Clobutinol, 2365
C14H22ClNO2
  Amylocaine Hydrochloride, 614
  Bupranolol, 1496
C14H22ClNO3
  Mecoprop Diethylamine Salt, 5784
C14H22ClN3O2
  Metoclopramide, 6143
C14H22Cl2N2O6S4
  Clomethiazole Ethanedisulfonate,
    2384
C14H22N2O
  Ispronicline, 5239
  Lidocaine, 5482
  Octacaine, 6743
C14H22N2O2
  Rivastigmine, 8240
C14H22N2O3
  Atenolol, 859
  Bucolome, 1466
  Practolol, 7700
  Trimetazidine, 9705
C14H22N2O3S
  Piprozolin, 7485
C14H22N2O4S
  Amylpenicillin, 616
C14H22N2O7S
  Rimazolium Metilsulfate, 8225
C14H22N6O5
  Valganciclovir, 9907
C14H22O
  Irone, 5095
  α-Irone, 5096
  β-Irone, 5097
  γ-Irone, 5098
C14H22O4
  Palitantin, 6987
C14H23NO
  Affinin, 179
C14H23NO2
  Piroctone, 7502
C14H23N3OS
  Xanomeline, 10056
C14H23N3O3S
  Sematilide, 8442
C14H23N3O10
  Pentetic Acid, 7125
C14H24CaN4O8
  Piperazine Edetate Calcium, 7464
C14H24N2O3
  Ciclopirox Ethanolamine Salt (1:1),
    2266
C14H24N2O5
  Pirbuterol Monoacetate, 7489
C14H24N2O7
  Spectinomycin, 8739
C14H24N2O10
  EGTA, 3529
C14H24O2
  Japonilure, 5257
C14H25NO
  Pellitorine, 7073

$C_{16}H_5N_5O_6$
9-Dicyanomethylene-2,4,7-trinitrofluor-
ene, 3094
$C_{16}H_7N_2NaO_5$
Pirenoxine Sodium Salt, 7490
$C_{16}H_7Na_3O_{10}S_3$
Pyranine, 7954
$C_{16}H_8Cl_2FN_5O$
Fluquinconazole, 4196
$C_{16}H_8Cl_2F_6N_2O_3$
Hexaflumuron, 4683
$C_{16}H_8N_2Na_2O_8S_2$
Indigo Carmine, 4944
$C_{16}H_8N_2O_5$
Pirenoxine, 7490
$C_{16}H_8O_6$
Medicagol, 5788
$C_{16}H_9N_3Na_2O_{10}S_2$
Chromotrope 2B, 2240
$C_{16}H_9N_4Na_3O_9S_2$
Tartrazine, 9072
$C_{16}H_{10}$
Pyrene, 7963
$C_{16}H_{10}ClKN_2O_4$
Clorazepic Acid Monopotassium Salt,
2403
$C_{16}H_{10}ClN_3$
Lotrifen, 5585
$C_{16}H_{10}Cl_4O_5$
Diploicin, 3339
$C_{16}H_{10}MgO_{10}$
Magnesium Monoperoxyphthalate,
5673
$C_{16}H_{10}N_2Na_2O_7S_2$
Sunset Yellow FCF, 9001
$C_{16}H_{10}N_2O_2$
Indigo, 4943
$C_{16}H_{10}N_2O_6S_4$
DIDS, 3102
$C_{16}H_{10}O_5$
Pseudobaptigenin, 7911
$C_{16}H_{10}O_7$
Laccaic Acid D, 5330
$C_{16}H_{10}O_8$
Kermesic Acid, 5293
$C_{16}H_{11}ClK_2N_2O_4$
Clorazepic Acid Dipotassium Salt, 2403
$C_{16}H_{11}ClN_2O_3$
Clorazepic Acid, 2403
$C_{16}H_{11}ClN_4$
Estazolam, 3702
$C_{16}H_{11}NO_2$
Cinchophen, 2288
$C_{16}H_{11}NO_3$
Oxycinchophen, 6957
$C_{16}H_{11}N_2NaO_4S$
Orange I, 6857
Orange II, 6858
$C_{16}H_{12}ClFN_2O$
Fludiazepam, 4128
$C_{16}H_{12}Cl_2N_2O_2$
Lormetazepam, 5581
$C_{16}H_{12}FNO_3$
Flunoxaprofen, 4148
$C_{16}H_{12}FN_3O_3$
Flubendazole, 4118
Flunitrazepam, 4146
$C_{16}H_{12}O_3$
Anisindione, 668
$C_{16}H_{12}O_4$
Chrysin Methylchrysin, 2256
Formononetin, 4244
Isoxepac, 5237
$C_{16}H_{12}O_5$
Acacetin, 13
Emodin 3-Methyl Ether, 3561

Olmelin, 4391
Oroxylin A, 6878
Prunetin, 7909
$C_{16}H_{12}O_6$
Acetylsalicylsalicylic Acid, 100
Diosmetin, 3296
Hematein, 4634
Pratensein, 7713
Tectorigenin, 9107
$C_{16}H_{12}O_7$
Rhamnetin, 8171
$C_{16}H_{13}ClFNO_5$
Flumiclorac, 4142
$C_{16}H_{13}ClN_2O$
Diazepam, 2994
Mazindol, 5762
$C_{16}H_{13}ClN_2O_2$
Clobazam, 2359
Temazepam, 9133
$C_{16}H_{13}ClN_6$
Vorozole, 10035
$C_{16}H_{13}ClO_6$
Peonidin, 7143
$C_{16}H_{13}ClO_7$
Petunidin, 7190
$C_{16}H_{13}Cl_2NO_4$
Aceclofenac, 22
Quinfamide, 8057
$C_{16}H_{13}Cl_3N_2OS$
Tioconazole, 9452
$C_{16}H_{13}F_2N_3O$
Flutriafol, 4214
$C_{16}H_{13}NO_3S$
1-Anilino-8-naphthalenesulfonate,
661
$C_{16}H_{13}N_2NaO_3$
Bendazac Sodium Salt, 1035
$C_{16}H_{13}N_2Na_2O_6P$
Fosphenytoin Disodium Salt, 4258
$C_{16}H_{13}N_3$
Yellow AB, 10095
$C_{16}H_{13}N_3O_3$
Mebendazole, 5768
Nimetazepam, 6549
$C_{16}H_{14}$
1,4-Diphenyl-1,3-butadiene, 3320
$C_{16}H_{14}CaO_6$
Mandelic Acid Calcium Salt, 5717
$C_{16}H_{14}ClN_3O$
Chlordiazepoxide, 2084
$C_{16}H_{14}Cl_2O_4$
Diclofop-methyl, 3082
$C_{16}H_{14}FN_3O$
Afloqualone, 183
$C_{16}H_{14}F_2N_3NaO_4S$
Pantoprazole Sodium Salt, 7014
$C_{16}H_{14}F_3NO_3S$
Tolrestat, 9524
$C_{16}H_{14}F_3N_3O_2S$
Lansoprazole, 5362
$C_{16}H_{14}F_3N_5O$
Voriconazole, 10033
$C_{16}H_{14}F_5N_5O_5S$
Penoxsulam, 7103
$C_{16}H_{14}N_2O$
Glycosine, 4502
Methaqualone, 5960
$C_{16}H_{14}N_2O_2S$
Mefenacet, 5797
$C_{16}H_{14}N_2O_3$
Bendazac, 1035
$C_{16}H_{14}N_2O_3S$
Valdecoxib, 9900
$C_{16}H_{14}N_2O_4$
Amlexanox, 490
Nybomycin, 6731

$C_{16}H_{14}N_2O_6S$
Phthalylsulfacetamide, 7376
$C_{16}H_{14}N_7NaO_5S_4.2H_2O$
Cefuzonam Sodium Salt Dihydrate,
1955
$C_{16}H_{14}O$
Dypnone, 3480
$C_{16}H_{14}O_2$
Benzyl Cinnamate, 1130
$C_{16}H_{14}O_3$
Fenbufen, 3963
Ketoprofen, 5305
$C_{16}H_{14}O_4$
Imperatorin, 4925
Medicarpin, 5789
$C_{16}H_{14}O_5$
Aspirin Guaiacol Ester, 851
Brazilin, 1367
Licochalcone B, 5479
Sakuranetin, 8319
$C_{16}H_{14}O_6$
Hematoxylin, 4637
Hesperetin, 4670
Homoeriodictyol, 4736
$C_{16}H_{15}ClN_2$
Medazepam, 5786
$C_{16}H_{15}ClN_2OS$
Clotiazepam, 2416
$C_{16}H_{15}Cl_3O_2$
Methoxychlor, 5990
$C_{16}H_{15}FN_2O_4$
Pazufloxacin, 7055
$C_{16}H_{15}F_2N_3O_4S$
Pantoprazole, 7014
$C_{16}H_{15}F_2N_3Si$
Flusilazole, 4206
$C_{16}H_{15}F_3O$
Flumecinol, 4136
$C_{16}H_{15}F_6N_5O$
Sitagliptin, 8552
$C_{16}H_{15}N$
Dizocilpine, 3386
$C_{16}H_{15}NO$
Cyheptamide, 2759
$C_{16}H_{15}N_2NaO_5S_2$
Cephalothin Sodium Salt, 1982
$C_{16}H_{15}N_2O_6P$
Fosphenytoin, 4258
$C_{16}H_{15}N_3$
Epinastine, 3618
$C_{16}H_{15}N_3O_5$
Opiniazide, 6852
$C_{16}H_{15}N_3O_7S$
Sulfaloxic Acid, 8912
$C_{16}H_{15}N_4NaO_8S$
Cefuroxime Sodium Salt, 1954
$C_{16}H_{15}N_5O_7S_2$
Cefixime, 1924
$C_{16}H_{15}N_7O_5S_4$
Cefuzonam, 1955
$C_{16}H_{16}$
[2.2]Metacyclophane, 5921
$C_{16}H_{16}ClNO_2S$
Clopidogrel, 2396
$C_{16}H_{16}ClNO_3$
Fenoldopam, 3979
$C_{16}H_{16}ClNO_4S$
Daltroban, 2806
$C_{16}H_{16}ClN_3O_3S$
Indapamide, 4935
Metolazone, 6147
$C_{16}H_{16}ClN_3O_4.H_2O$
Loracarbef, 5576
$C_{16}H_{16}NO_4P$
Naftalofos, 6354

C₁₆H₂₁N₃
$C_{16}H_{21}N_3$
Tripelennamine, 9738

$C_{16}H_{21}N_3O_2$
Zolmitriptan, 10189

$C_{16}H_{21}N_3O_4S$
Epicillin, 3614

$C_{16}H_{21}N_3O_8S$
Cephalosporin C, 1980

$C_{16}H_{21}N_5O_2$
Alizapride, 250

$C_{16}H_{21}N_7O_7S_3$
Cefminox, 1927

$C_{16}H_{22}ClN_3O$
Tebuconazole, 9092

$C_{16}H_{22}ClN_3O_2$
Renzapride, 8135

$C_{16}H_{22}ClN_3O_4$
Plafibride, 7516

$C_{16}H_{22}FNO$
Melperone, 5827

$C_{16}H_{22}N_2$
Lycodine, 5619

$C_{16}H_{22}N_2O_3$
Procaterol, 7759

$C_{16}H_{22}N_2O_3S$
Glyhexamide, 4506

$C_{16}H_{22}N_2O_4$
Antipyrine Methylethylglycolate, 716

$C_{16}H_{22}N_2O_6$
2,5-Bis(1-aziridinyl)-3,6-bis(2-methoxy-ethoxy)-1,4-benzoquinone, 1245

$C_{16}H_{22}N_4O_4$
Tetroxoprim, 9250

$C_{16}H_{22}N_4O_4S$
Acetiamine, 54

$C_{16}H_{22}N_6O_4$
TRH, 9588

$C_{16}H_{22}O_2$
Geranylhydroquinone, 4405

$C_{16}H_{22}O_3$
Homosalate, 4738

$C_{16}H_{22}O_4$
Dibutyl Phthalate, 3035

$C_{16}H_{22}O_6$
Trepibutone, 9585

$C_{16}H_{22}O_8$
Coniferin, 2503

$C_{16}H_{22}O_{10}$
Swertiamarin, 9010

$C_{16}H_{22}O_{11}$
Monotropein, 6255

$C_{16}H_{23}BrN_2O_3$
Remoxipride, 8132

$C_{16}H_{23}ClN_4O$
Thonzylamine Hydrochloride, 9373

$C_{16}H_{23}HgN_6NaO_8$
Meralluride, 5866

$C_{16}H_{23}I_3N_2O_8$
Meglumine Acetrizoate, 5806

$C_{16}H_{23}NO$
Dezocine, 2956
Inaperisone, 4928
Pyrovalerone, 8010
Tolperisone, 9522

$C_{16}H_{23}NO_2$
Alphaprodine, 310
Bufuralol, 1480
Ethoheptazine, 3743
Etoxadrol, 3889
Piperocaine, 7474

$C_{16}H_{23}NO_3$
Acetamidoeugenol, 46

$C_{16}H_{23}NO_6$
Monocrotaline, 6250

$C_{16}H_{23}NO_8$
Bakankosin, 943

$C_{16}H_{23}N_3OS$
Buprofezin, 1498

$C_{16}H_{23}N_3O_4$
Gabexate, 4320

$C_{16}H_{23}N_5O$
Tegaserod, 9113

$C_{16}H_{24}ClNO_2$
Hexylcaine Hydrochloride, 4708

$C_{16}H_{24}NO_5^+$
Sinapine, 8541

$C_{16}H_{24}N_2$
Isoaminile, 5110
Xylometazoline, 10086

$C_{16}H_{24}N_2O$
Oxymetazoline, 6966
Ropinirole, 8257

$C_{16}H_{24}N_2O_2$
Molindone, 6233
N,N,N',N'-Tetraethylphthalamide, 9203

$C_{16}H_{24}N_2O_3$
Carteolol, 1866

$C_{16}H_{24}N_2O_4$
Ubenimex, 9842

$C_{16}H_{24}N_2O_6$
Pyrisuccideanol, 7991

$C_{16}H_{24}N_{10}O_4$
Aminophylline, 465

$C_{16}H_{24}O_5$
Brefeldin A, 1369

$C_{16}H_{24}O_7$
Rhododendrin, 8189

$C_{16}H_{25}HgNNa_2O_6S$
Mercaptomerin Sodium, 5870

$C_{16}H_{25}NO$
Lycopodine, 5622

$C_{16}H_{25}NO_2$
Butethamate, 1522
Gravitol(e), 4542
Thymyl N-Isoamylcarbamate, 9409
Tramadol, 9566

$C_{16}H_{25}NO_2S$
Tertatolol, 9173

$C_{16}H_{25}NO_3$
Moxisylyte, 6292

$C_{16}H_{25}NO_4$
Esmolol, 3700

$C_{16}H_{25}N_2NaO_5S$
Cilastatin Sodium Salt, 2272

$C_{16}H_{25}N_3O$
Propiram, 7831

$C_{16}H_{25}N_3O_5$
Xamoterol, 10055

$C_{16}H_{25}N_7O_8$
Gougerotin, 4529

$C_{16}H_{26}GdN_5O_8$
Gadodiamide, 4324

$C_{16}H_{26}NO_4S.C_7H_7O_3S$
Suplatast Tosylate, 9003

$C_{16}H_{26}N_2O_2$
Dimethocaine, 3221

$C_{16}H_{26}N_2O_3$
Proparacaine, 7807

$C_{16}H_{26}N_2O_4$
Cetamolol, 2018

$C_{16}H_{26}N_2O_5S$
Cilastatin, 2272

$C_{16}H_{26}O$
Iso E Super®, 5169

$C_{16}H_{26}O_2$
2,5-Di-*tert*-pentylhydroquinone, 3304

$C_{16}H_{26}O_3$
Juvenile Hormone III, 5273

$C_{16}H_{26}O_5$
Artemether, 815

$C_{16}H_{26}O_7$
Picrocrocin, 7411

$C_{16}H_{27}ClN_2O_3$
Propoxycaine Hydrochloride, 7837

$C_{16}H_{27}N_3O_8$
Dinoseb Triethanolamine Salt, 3287

$C_{16}H_{28}N_2O_2$
Tromantadine, 9771

$C_{16}H_{28}N_2O_4$
Oseltamivir, 6889

$C_{16}H_{28}N_2O_6Zn$
ε-Acetamidocaproic Acid Zinc Salt, 45

$C_{16}H_{28}N_4O_4S$
Biocytin, 1227

$C_{16}H_{28}O_2$
Hydnocarpic Acid, 4761
Prodlure, 7769

$C_{16}H_{29}NaO_7S$
Bis(1-methylamyl) Sodium Sulfosuccinate, 1255

$C_{16}H_{30}N_2O_3$
Piroctone Ethanolamine Salt (1:1), 7502

$C_{16}H_{30}O$
Muscone, 6313

$C_{16}H_{30}O_4$
Texanol Isobutyrate, 9251

$C_{16}H_{30}O_4Zn$
Zinc Caprylate, 10130

$C_{16}H_{32}O_2$
2-Hexyldecanoic Acid, 4709
Myristic Acid Ethyl Ester, 6333
Palmitic Acid, 6996

$C_{16}H_{32}O_4$
Diethylene Glycol Monolaurate, 3120

$C_{16}H_{32}O_5$
Aleuritic Acid, 231

$C_{16}H_{33}BiO_4S$
Bismuth Butylthiolaurate, 1261

$C_{16}H_{33}NO_2$
Delmopinol, 2879

$C_{16}H_{34}O$
Cetyl Alcohol, 2028

$C_{16}H_{35}NO_2$
Ammonium Palmitate, 538

$C_{16}H_{36}FN$
Tetrabutylammonium Fluoride, 9187

$C_{16}H_{38}Br_2N_2$
Decamethonium Bromide, 2847

$C_{16}H_{42}I_7N_8O_{16}$
Tetraglycine Hydroperiodide, 9207

$C_{17}H_{14}$
1,2-Cyclopentenophenanthrene, 2744

$C_{17}H_7Cl_2F_9N_2O_3$
Noviflumuron, 6721

$C_{17}H_8Cl_2F_8N_2O_3$
Lufenuron, 5595

$C_{17}H_9ClF_8N_2O_4$
Novaluron, 6720

$C_{17}H_9Cl_3N_4O_2$
Diclazuril, 3080

$C_{17}H_9NO_4$
Alizarine Blue, 253

$C_{17}H_{10}Cl_2N_4O_2$
Clazuril, 2343

$C_{17}H_{10}O$
Benzanthrone, 1063

$C_{17}H_{10}O_4$
Fluorescamine, 4158

$C_{17}H_{11}ClF_4N_2S$
Quazepam, 8029

$C_{17}H_{11}NO_7$
Aristolochic Acid, 786

$C_{17}H_{11}N_5$
Letrozole, 5450

$C_{17}H_{12}Br_2O_3$
  Benzbromarone, 1065
$C_{17}H_{12}ClF_3N_2O$
  Halazepam, 4589
$C_{17}H_{12}ClNO_2S$
  Fentiazac, 4003
$C_{17}H_{12}Cl_2N_2O$
  Fenarimol, 3958
$C_{17}H_{12}Cl_2N_4$
  Triazolam, 9604
$C_{17}H_{12}I_2O_3$
  Benziodarone, 1083
$C_{17}H_{12}O_2$
  2-Naphthyl Benzoate, 6408
$C_{17}H_{12}O_3$
  1-Naphthyl Salicylate, 6414
  2-Naphthyl Salicylate, 6415
$C_{17}H_{12}O_6$
  Aflatoxin B$_1$, 180
$C_{17}H_{12}O_7$
  Aflatoxin G$_1$, 181
  Aflatoxin M$_1$, 182
$C_{17}H_{13}ClFNO_4$
  Clodinafop-Propargyl, 2370
$C_{17}H_{13}ClFN_3O$
  Epoxiconazole, 3629
$C_{17}H_{13}ClN_2O_2$
  Lonazolac, 5566
$C_{17}H_{13}ClN_4$
  Alprazolam, 312
  Liarozole, 5475
$C_{17}H_{13}Cl_3N_4S$
  Imibenconazole, 4909
$C_{17}H_{13}N_3Na_2O_6.2H_2O$
  Balsalazide Disodium Salt Dihydrate,
  945
$C_{17}H_{13}N_3O_5S_2$
  Phthalylsulfathiazole, 7377
$C_{17}H_{14}BrFN_2O_2$
  Haloxazolam, 4604
$C_{17}H_{14}ClFN_2O_3$
  Doxefazepam, 3434
$C_{17}H_{14}ClF_7O_2$
  Tefluthrin, 9111
$C_{17}H_{14}Cl_2F_2N_2O_3$
  Roflumilast, 8249
$C_{17}H_{14}Cl_2N_2O$
  Cloxazolam, 2420
$C_{17}H_{14}F_3N_3O_2S$
  Celecoxib, 1956
$C_{17}H_{14}F_3N_3O_3S$
  Deracoxib, 2914
$C_{17}H_{14}N_2$
  Ellipticine, 3548
  Flavopereirine, 4093
  Olivacine, 6834
$C_{17}H_{14}N_2O_3$
  Rosoxacin, 8268
$C_{17}H_{14}N_2O_5S$
  Calmagite, 1718
$C_{17}H_{14}O$
  Dibenzalacetone, 3006
$C_{17}H_{14}O_3S$
  Zaltoprofen, 10112
$C_{17}H_{14}O_4S$
  Rofecoxib, 8248
$C_{17}H_{14}O_5$
  Pterocarpin, 7932
$C_{17}H_{14}O_6$
  Aflatoxin B$_2$, 180
  Pectolinarigenin, 7064
$C_{17}H_{14}O_7$
  Aflatoxin G$_2$, 181
  Aflatoxin M$_2$, 182
$C_{17}H_{15}ClN_4S$
  Etizolam, 3873

$C_{17}H_{15}ClO_7$
  Malvidin Chloride, 5715
$C_{17}H_{15}NO_5$
  Benorylate, 1045
$C_{17}H_{15}N_3$
  Yellow OB, 10096
$C_{17}H_{15}N_3O_6$
  Balsalazide, 945
$C_{17}H_{15}N_5O$
  Zaleplon, 10111
$C_{17}H_{15}N_7Na_2O_8S_4$
  Cefotetan Disodium Salt, 1934
$C_{17}H_{16}Br_2O_3$
  Bromopropylate, 1434
$C_{17}H_{16}ClFN_2O_2$
  Progabide, 7772
$C_{17}H_{16}ClN_3O$
  Amoxapine, 576
$C_{17}H_{16}F_3NO_2$
  Flutolanil, 4212
$C_{17}H_{16}F_6N_2O$
  Mefloquine, 5801
$C_{17}H_{16}N_2Na_2O_6S$
  Carbenicillin Disodium Salt, 1792
$C_{17}H_{16}N_2O$
  Etaqualone, 3714
$C_{17}H_{16}N_2O_3S$
  TSQ, 9799
$C_{17}H_{16}N_3NaO_6S_2$
  Cephapirin Sodium, 1984
$C_{17}H_{16}O_3$
  Eugenol Benzoate, 3898
$C_{17}H_{17}ClFN_3O_3$
  Clinafloxacin, 2355
$C_{17}H_{17}ClN_2O$
  Etifoxine, 3864
$C_{17}H_{17}ClN_6O_3$
  Zopiclone, 10193
$C_{17}H_{17}ClO_6$
  Griseofulvin, 4549
$C_{17}H_{17}Cl_2N$
  Sertraline, 8467
$C_{17}H_{17}Cl_2NO_3$
  Terofenamate, 9168
$C_{17}H_{17}Cl_2N_2NaO_5S$
  Clometocillin Sodium Salt, 2385
$C_{17}H_{17}NO_2$
  Apomorphine, 746
$C_{17}H_{17}N_2^+$
  Difenzoquat, 3138
$C_{17}H_{17}N_2NaO_5S$
  Piretanide Monosodium Salt, 7492
$C_{17}H_{17}N_3O$
  Ramosetron, 8105
$C_{17}H_{17}N_3OS$
  Fenamidone, 3956
$C_{17}H_{17}N_3O_3$
  Imazaquin, 4906
$C_{17}H_{17}N_4NaO_6$
  Carbazochrome Salicylate, 1788
$C_{17}H_{17}N_7O_8S_4$
  Cefotetan, 1934
$C_{17}H_{18}Br_2N_4O_2$
  Dibromopropamidine, 3024
$C_{17}H_{18}ClNO_4$
  Pirifibrate, 7495
$C_{17}H_{18}ClN_3O_4$
  Celestin Blue, 1959
$C_{17}H_{18}Cl_2N_2O_5S$
  Clometocillin, 2385
$C_{17}H_{18}FN_3O_3$
  Ciprofloxacin, 2314
$C_{17}H_{18}FN_3O_3S$
  Rufloxacin, 8294

$C_{17}H_{18}F_2O_2$
  Bifluranol, 1212
$C_{17}H_{18}F_3NO$
  Fluoxetine, 4185
$C_{17}H_{18}F_3N_3O_3$
  Fleroxacin, 4099
$C_{17}H_{18}N_2$
  Amphetaminil, 583
$C_{17}H_{18}N_2O_5S$
  Piretanide, 7492
$C_{17}H_{18}N_2O_6$
  Nifedipine, 6528
$C_{17}H_{18}N_2O_6S$
  Carbenicillin, 1792
  Menadione Dimethylpyrimidinol
    Bisulfite, 5831
$C_{17}H_{18}N_2S_2$
  Sulbentine, 8892
$C_{17}H_{18}N_3NaO_4S$
  Metampicillin Sodium Salt, 5925
$C_{17}H_{18}N_4O$
  Alosetron, 308
$C_{17}H_{18}N_4O_3S$
  Enviroxime, 3601
$C_{17}H_{18}O_3$
  4-tert-Butylphenyl Salicylate, 1586
$C_{17}H_{18}O_4$
  Diphenolic Acid, 3312
$C_{17}H_{19}ClN_2O$
  Pyronine Y, 8007
$C_{17}H_{19}ClN_2OS$
  Opromazine, 6855
$C_{17}H_{19}ClN_2S$
  Chlorpromazine, 2185
$C_{17}H_{19}FN_2O_2$
  Safinamide, 8315
$C_{17}H_{19}FN_4O_4$
  Marbofloxacin, 5750
$C_{17}H_{19}F_2N_3O_3$
  Lomefloxacin, 5562
$C_{17}H_{19}F_3N_6O_5$
  Triflusulfuron-methyl, 9689
$C_{17}H_{19}KN_2O_5S$
  Phenethicillin Potassium, 7223
$C_{17}H_{19}NO$
  Nefopam, 6440
$C_{17}H_{19}NO_3$
  Chavicine, 2049
  Coclaurine, 2459
  Hydromorphone, 4803
  Morphine, 6276
  Norcodeine, 6690
  Piperine, 7472
$C_{17}H_{19}NO_4$
  Buphanamine, 1492
  Fenoxycarb, 3987
  Oxymorphone, 6969
$C_{17}H_{19}N_2NaO_6S$
  Methicillin Sodium, 5969
$C_{17}H_{19}N_3$
  Antazoline, 680
  Mirtazapine, 6208
$C_{17}H_{19}N_3O$
  Phentolamine, 7264
  Piberaline, 7392
$C_{17}H_{19}N_3O_3S$
  Omeprazole, 6845
$C_{17}H_{19}N_3O_4S$
  Metampicillin, 5925
$C_{17}H_{19}N_5$
  Anastrozole, 625
$C_{17}H_{19}N_5O_2$
  Piritrexim, 7499
  Pixantrone, 7514
$C_{17}H_{20}BrNO$
  Bromodiphenhydramine, 1418

C₁₇H₂₀ClNO
Chlophedianol, 2066

C₁₇H₂₀ClN₃O₂
Furametpyr, 4295

C₁₇H₂₀ClN₃O₃
Azasetron, 900

C₁₇H₂₀FN₃O₃
Pefloxacin, 7066

C₁₇H₂₀F₆N₂O₃
Flecainide, 4098

C₁₇H₂₀N₂O
N,N'-Diethylcarbanilide, 3117
Michler's Ketone, 6177
Remacemide, 8130

C₁₇H₂₀N₂O₂
Tropicamide, 9780
Tropisetron, 9783

C₁₇H₂₀N₂O₂S
Tinoridine, 9448

C₁₇H₂₀N₂O₃
Bifenazate, 1207
Nicotine Salicylate, 6524

C₁₇H₂₀N₂O₅S
Bumetanide, 1484

C₁₇H₂₀N₂S
Promazine, 7783
Promethazine, 7786

C₁₇H₂₀N₄O
Propizepine, 7833

C₁₇H₂₀N₄O₂
Propamidine, 7797

C₁₇H₂₀N₄O₃
Imazaquin Ammonium Salt, 4906

C₁₇H₂₀N₄O₆
D-Araboflavin, 763
Riboflavin, 8200

C₁₇H₂₀N₄S
Olanzapine, 6822

C₁₇H₂₀N₆O₇S
Foramsulfuron, 4234

C₁₇H₂₀O₅
Matricarin, 5758
Oleocanthal, 6829

C₁₇H₂₀O₅S
Firocoxib, 4087

C₁₇H₂₀O₆
Mycophenolic Acid, 6327

C₁₇H₂₀O₉
Chlorogenic Acid 3'-Methyl Ether, 2142

C₁₇H₂₁ClN₂O₂S
Hexythiazox, 4713

C₁₇H₂₁N
Benzphetamine, 1118
N,N-Diethylbenzhydrylamine, 3115

C₁₇H₂₁NO
Atomoxetine, 863
Diphenhydramine, 3309
Phenyltoloxamine, 7316

C₁₇H₂₁NO₂
Apoatropine, 739
Desomorphine, 2927
Napropamide, 6416

C₁₇H₂₁NO₃
Dihydromorphine, 3177
Etodolac, 3874
Galantamine, 4340
Ritodrine, 8237

C₁₇H₂₁NO₄
Cocaine, 2455
Fenoterol, 3981
Pseudococaine, 7912
Scopolamine, 8406

C₁₇H₂₁NO₅
Buphanitine, 1493
Scopolamine N-Oxide, 8407

C₁₇H₂₁N₄O₉P
Riboflavin Monophosphate, 8201

C₁₇H₂₁N₅O₉S₂
Mesosulfuron-methyl, 5911

C₁₇H₂₂BrNOS₂
Timepidium Bromide, 9442

C₁₇H₂₂ClN₃O
Metconazole, 5934

C₁₇H₂₂I₃N₃O₈
Iomeprol, 5054
Iopamidol, 5057

C₁₇H₂₂NO₃⁺
Lunasine, 5605

C₁₇H₂₂N₂
Michler's Base, 6176

C₁₇H₂₂N₂O
Doxylamine, 3441

C₁₇H₂₂N₂OS
Neticonazole, 6478

C₁₇H₂₂N₂O₃
Trichostatin A, 9649

C₁₇H₂₂N₂S
Thenaldine, 9278

C₁₇H₂₂N₄O
Minaprine, 6200

C₁₇H₂₂N₄O₂
Resiquimod, 8151

C₁₇H₂₂O₂
Cicutoxin, 2267
Enanthotoxin, 3569

C₁₇H₂₂O₃
Bornyl Salicylate, 1341
Podocarpic Acid, 7543

C₁₇H₂₂O₅
Pyrethrosin, 7965

C₁₇H₂₃NO
Levorphanol, 5470

C₁₇H₂₃NO₂
Tilidine, 9437

C₁₇H₂₃NO₃
Atropine, 875
Hyoscyamine, 4858
Lycoramine, 5625
Mesembrine, 5906

C₁₇H₂₃NO₄
Atropine N-Oxide, 875
Bucumolol, 1467
Cetraxate, 2024
Lunacridine, 5603

C₁₇H₂₃N₃O
Pyrilamine, 7984

C₁₇H₂₃N₇O₅
Taltirelin, 9045

C₁₇H₂₄ClNO₄
Tepraloxydim, 9152

C₁₇H₂₄N₂O
Dimethisoquin, 3218
Pilsicainide, 7427

C₁₇H₂₄N₂O₃
Tilisolol, 9438

C₁₇H₂₄O₃
Cyclandelate, 2704

C₁₇H₂₄O₄
Trichodermin, 9647

C₁₇H₂₄O₉
Syringin, 9016

C₁₇H₂₄O₁₀
Verbenalin, 9959

C₁₇H₂₅Cl₂F₃N₅O₁₂P₃S₂
Cangrelor, 1746

C₁₇H₂₅N
Phencyclidine, 7219

C₁₇H₂₅NO
Eperisone, 3606

C₁₇H₂₅NO₂
Menthyl Anthranilate, 5840
Proheptazine, 7776
Promedol, 7784

C₁₇H₂₅NO₃
Cyclopentolate, 2746
Eucatropine, 3897
Levobunolol, 5462
Pecilocin, 7062

C₁₇H₂₅NO₄
Buflomedil, 1475
Ibopamine, 4876

C₁₇H₂₅N₃O
Plasmocid, 7522
Proxazole, 7903

C₁₇H₂₅N₃O₂
Vildagliptin, 9979

C₁₇H₂₅N₃O₂S
Almotriptan, 304
Naratriptan, 6420

C₁₇H₂₅N₃O₅S
Meropenem, 5900
Veralipride, 9948

C₁₇H₂₅N₅O₁₃
Polyoxin B, 7576

C₁₇H₂₅N₇O₄
Binodenoson, 1225

C₁₇H₂₆ClN
Sibutramine, 8485

C₁₇H₂₆ClNO₂
Butachlor, 1508
Pretilachlor, 7740

C₁₇H₂₆ClNO₃S
Clethodim, 2349

C₁₇H₂₆N₂O
5-Methoxy-N,N-diisopropyltrypt-amine, 5991
Phenampromid(e), 7209
Ropivacaine, 8258

C₁₇H₂₆N₂O₄S
Sultopride, 8994

C₁₇H₂₆N₄O
Emedastine, 3557

C₁₇H₂₆N₄O₃S₂
Fursultiamine, 4311

C₁₇H₂₆N₄O₄S
Alpiropride, 311

C₁₇H₂₆N₈O₅
Blasticidin S, 1316

C₁₇H₂₆O₃
(p-Nonylphenoxy)acetic Acid, 6682

C₁₇H₂₆O₃S
DBHBT, 2836

C₁₇H₂₆O₄
Embelin, 3555
[6]-Gingerol, 4424

C₁₇H₂₆O₁₀
Loganin, 5560

C₁₇H₂₇NO₂
4-(Dimethylamino)benzoic Acid 2-Ethylhexyl Ester, 3232
Venlafaxine, 9946

C₁₇H₂₇NO₃
Butoxycaine, 1531
Pramoxine, 7709

C₁₇H₂₇NO₄
Metipranolol, 6140
Nadolol, 6346

C₁₇H₂₇N₃O₄S
Amisulpride, 485

C₁₇H₂₈N₂O
Etidocaine, 3862

C₁₇H₂₈N₂O₃
Benoxinate, 1047

C₁₇H₂₈N₂O₅
Perindopril Diacid Form, 7170

C₁₇H₂₈N₄O₄
Posatirelin, 7603

C₁₇H₂₈O₃
Juvenile Hormone II, 5273

C₁₇H₂₈O₅
Arteether, 813

C₁₇H₂₉GdN₄O₇
Gadoteridol, 4328

C₁₇H₂₉NO₃S
Sethoxydim, 8473

C₁₇H₃₀O
Civetone, 2335

C₁₇H₃₀O₂
Hydroprene, 4805

C₁₇H₃₁ClN₂O₅S
Pirlimycin, 7500

C₁₇H₃₂BrNO₂
Anisotropine Methylbromide, 671

C₁₇H₃₂O₄
Roccellic Acid, 8244

C₁₇H₃₄N₂O₄
Embelin Diammonium Salt, 3555

C₁₇H₃₄N₄O₁₀
Ribostamycin, 8206

C₁₇H₃₄O₂
Isopropyl Myristate, 5215
Margaric Acid, 5751

C₁₇H₃₅N₅O₆
Fortimicin A, 4249

C₁₇H₃₆GeN₂
Spirogermanium, 8758

C₁₇H₃₇N₇O₃
Gusperimus, 4582

C₁₇H₃₈BrN
Myristyltrimethylammonium Bromide, 6336

C₁₈BF₁₅
Tris(pentafluorophenyl)boron, 9755

C₁₈Fe₇N₁₈
Prussian Blue, 7910

C₁₈H₆BiBr₉O₃
Bismuth Tribromophenate, 1291

C₁₈H₁₀I₆N₂O₇
Ioglycamic Acid, 5051

C₁₈H₁₀O₆
Hydrindantin, 4775

C₁₈H₁₂
1,2-Benzanthracene, 1062
3,4-Benzphenanthrene, 1117
Chrysene, 2255
Naphthacene, 6369
Triphenylene, 9740

C₁₈H₁₂Cl₂N₂O
Boscalid, 1352

C₁₈H₁₂Cl₁₂
Dechlorane® Plus, 2851

C₁₈H₁₂CrN₃O₆
Chromium Picolinate, 2236

C₁₈H₁₂NNaO₃
Naptalam Sodium Salt, 6418

C₁₈H₁₂N₂O₂
Xanthocillin X, 10061

C₁₈H₁₂N₂O₃
Xanthocillin Y₁, 10061

C₁₈H₁₂N₂O₄
Xanthocillin Y₂, 10061

C₁₈H₁₂N₆
2,4,6-Tripyridyl-s-triazine, 9750

C₁₈H₁₂O₄
Karanjin, 5283

C₁₈H₁₃ClFN₃
Midazolam, 6182

C₁₈H₁₃ClFN₃O₂
Cinolazepam, 2308

C₁₈H₁₃ClN₂O
Pinazepam, 7442

C₁₈H₁₃N
6-Chrysenamine, 2254

C₁₈H₁₃NNa₂O₈S₂
Picosulfate Sodium, 7406

C₁₈H₁₃NO₃
Naptalam, 6418

C₁₈H₁₃N₃O
Rutecarpine, 8298

C₁₈H₁₄CaO₈
Calcium Acetylsalicylate, 1647

C₁₈H₁₄ClFN₂O₃
Ethyl Loflazepate, 3821

C₁₈H₁₄Cl₂N₅NaO₅S₃
Cefazedone Sodium Salt, 1916

C₁₈H₁₄Cl₄N₂O
Isoconazole, 5160
Miconazole, 6178

C₁₈H₁₄Cl₄N₄O₄
Oxiconazole Nitrate, 6937

C₁₈H₁₄F₃NO₂
Flurtamone, 4205

C₁₈H₁₄F₃N₃O₄S
Toltrazuril, 9526

C₁₈H₁₄F₃N₃O₆S
Ponazuril, 7589

C₁₈H₁₄F₄N₂O₄S
Bicalutamide, 1200

C₁₈H₁₄MgO₈
Magnesium Acetylsalicylate, 5655

C₁₈H₁₄N₂Na₂O₇S₂
Ponceau SX, 7591

C₁₈H₁₄N₂Na₂O₈S₂
Allura Red AC, 284

C₁₈H₁₄N₃NaO₃S
Metanil Yellow, 5928
Tropaeolin OO, 9776

C₁₈H₁₄N₄O₅S
Sulfasalazine, 8942

C₁₈H₁₄O₃
Cinnamic Acid Anhydride, 2299

C₁₈H₁₅ClN₂O
Cloconazole, 2368

C₁₈H₁₅ClN₂O₂S
Etoricoxib, 3887

C₁₈H₁₅ClN₂O₆S₂
Sitaxsentan, 8554

C₁₈H₁₅ClN₄
Phenosafranin, 7251

C₁₈H₁₅Cl₂N₅O₅S₃
Cefazedone, 1916

C₁₈H₁₅Cl₃N₂O
Econazole, 3502

C₁₈H₁₅Cl₃N₂S
Sulconazole, 8893

C₁₈H₁₅NO₃
Oxaprozin, 6924

C₁₈H₁₅O₄P
Triphenyl Phosphate, 9742

C₁₈H₁₅P
Triphenylphosphine, 9743

C₁₈H₁₆
3′-Methyl-1,2-cyclopentenophenanthrene, 6048

C₁₈H₁₆ClNO₅
Fenoxaprop-ethyl, 3984

C₁₈H₁₆Cl₂N₂O₂
Mexazolam, 6166

C₁₈H₁₆F₃NO₄
Picoxystrobin, 7408

C₁₈H₁₆N₂
N,N′-Diphenyl-p-phenylenediamine, 3329

C₁₈H₁₆N₂O
1-Xylylazo-2-naphthol, 10089

C₁₈H₁₆N₂O₂
Blebbistatin, 1317

C₁₈H₁₆N₂O₃
Citrus Red 2, 2333
Roquinimex, 8259

C₁₈H₁₆N₄O₆S
Quinacillin, 8043

C₁₈H₁₆N₆Na₂O₈S₃
Cefonicid Disodium Salt, 1929

C₁₈H₁₆N₈Na₂O₇S₃·3½H₂O
Ceftriaxone Disodium Salt Hemiheptahydrate, 1953

C₁₈H₁₆OSn
Triphenyltin Hydroxide, 9745

C₁₈H₁₆O₂
Cinnamyl Cinnamate, 2304

C₁₈H₁₆O₃
Ipriflavone, 5074
Phenprocoumon, 7259

C₁₈H₁₆O₄
Benzyl Fumarate, 1135
Bermoprofen, 1159
Truxillic Acid, 9791

C₁₈H₁₆O₇
Eupatorin, 3901
Usnic Acid, 9893

C₁₈H₁₆O₈
Irigenin, 5090

C₁₈H₁₇ClN₂O₂
Oxazolam, 6927

C₁₈H₁₇ClO₆
Monorden, 6253

C₁₈H₁₇FN₂O
Fluproquazone, 4193

C₁₈H₁₇F₃N₂O₃
Ridogrel, 8212

C₁₈H₁₇I₄NO₄
Etiroxate, 3872

C₁₈H₁₇NO₂
Aporeine, 748

C₁₈H₁₇NO₃
Indobufen, 4961
Pukateine, 7936

C₁₈H₁₇NO₄
Actinodaphnine, 139

C₁₈H₁₇NO₅
Tranilast, 9570

C₁₈H₁₈
Retene, 8160

C₁₈H₁₈BrClN₂O
Metaclazepam, 5920

C₁₈H₁₈ClNOS
Zotepine, 10197

C₁₈H₁₈ClNO₄
Clanobutin, 2338

C₁₈H₁₈ClNO₅
Etofibrate, 3877

C₁₈H₁₈ClNS
Chlorprothixene, 2188

C₁₈H₁₈ClN₃O
Loxapine, 5587

C₁₈H₁₈ClN₃S
Clothiapine, 2415

C₁₈H₁₈F₃NO₂
Flufenamic Acid Butyl Ester, 4132

C₁₈H₁₈F₃NO₄
Etofenamate, 3875

C₁₈H₁₈F₃N₃O₃
Pleconaril, 7533

C₁₈H₁₈N₂
Cifenline, 2269

C₁₈H₁₈N₂O
Demexiptiline, 2890
Proquazone, 7873

C₁₈H₁₈N₂O₄
Antipyrine Salicylate, 717

C$_{19}$H$_{16}$O$_4$
Warfarin, 10038
C$_{19}$H$_{16}$O$_5$
Efloxate, 3523
C$_{19}$H$_{17}$ClFN$_3$O$_5$S
Floxacillin, 4111
C$_{19}$H$_{17}$ClN$_2$O
Prazepam, 7715
C$_{19}$H$_{17}$ClN$_2$O$_4$
Oxametacine, 6916
Quizalofop-ethyl, 8086
C$_{19}$H$_{17}$ClN$_3$NaO$_5$S.H$_2$O
Cloxacillin Sodium Monohydrate, 2419
C$_{19}$H$_{17}$ClN$_4$
Fenbuconazole, 3962
C$_{19}$H$_{17}$Cl$_2$NO$_4$
Cinidon-ethyl, 2293
C$_{19}$H$_{17}$Cl$_2$N$_3$O$_3$
Difenoconazole, 3135
C$_{19}$H$_{17}$Cl$_2$N$_3$O$_5$S
Dicloxacillin, 3084
C$_{19}$H$_{17}$Cl$_3$N$_2$S
Butoconazole, 1529
C$_{19}$H$_{17}$NOS
Tolnaftate, 9519
C$_{19}$H$_{17}$NO$_4$
Stylopine, 8858
C$_{19}$H$_{17}$NO$_5$
Mofezolac, 6232
C$_{19}$H$_{17}$NO$_7$
Nedocromil, 6436
C$_{19}$H$_{17}$N$_2$S$^+$
Thiazole Orange, 9308
C$_{19}$H$_{17}$N$_3$O
DCM, 2838
Evodiamine, 3908
C$_{19}$H$_{17}$N$_3$O$_4$S$_2$
Cephaloridine, 1979
C$_{19}$H$_{17}$N$_5$O$_2$
Nafamostat, 6350
C$_{19}$H$_{17}$N$_5$O$_5$S
Salazosulfadimidine, 8321
C$_{19}$H$_{17}$N$_5$O$_7$S$_3$
Ceftiofur, 1950
C$_{19}$H$_{17}$N$_6$NaO$_5$S$_3$.1½H$_2$O
Cefditoren Sodium Salt, Sesquihydrate, 1921
C$_{19}$H$_{17}$N$_6$NaO$_6$S$_2$
Cefamandole Nafate, 1914
C$_{19}$H$_{17}$N$_9$O$_5$S$_2$
Cefozopran, 1937
C$_{19}$H$_{18}$CaN$_2$O$_9$
Calcium Acetylsalicylate Complex with Urea, 1647
C$_{19}$H$_{18}$ClFN$_2$O$_3$
Flutazolam, 4209
C$_{19}$H$_{18}$ClF$_2$N$_3$O$_3$
Sitafloxacin, 8551
C$_{19}$H$_{18}$ClN$_3$O$_3$
Camazepam, 1725
C$_{19}$H$_{18}$ClN$_3$O$_4$
Pyraclostrobin, 7953
C$_{19}$H$_{18}$ClN$_3$O$_5$S
Cloxacillin, 2419
C$_{19}$H$_{18}$ClN$_5$
Adinazolam, 160
C$_{19}$H$_{18}$N$_2$O$_3$
Kebuzone, 5288
C$_{19}$H$_{18}$N$_2$O$_4$S
Parecoxib, 7036
C$_{19}$H$_{18}$N$_2$O$_5$S
Zinquin, 10169
C$_{19}$H$_{18}$N$_3$NaO$_5$S.H$_2$O
Oxacillin Sodium Salt Monohydrate, 6904

C$_{19}$H$_{18}$N$_4$O$_2$
Pimobendan, 7434
C$_{19}$H$_{18}$N$_4$O$_8$
Bispyribac, 1301
C$_{19}$H$_{18}$N$_6$O$_5$S$_3$
Cefditoren, 1921
C$_{19}$H$_{18}$N$_6$O$_6$
Nicarbazin, 6494
C$_{19}$H$_{18}$N$_7$NaO$_6$
Sodium Folate, 8619
C$_{19}$H$_{18}$O$_7$
Gardenin B, 4366
C$_{19}$H$_{18}$O$_8$
Atranorin, 869
Gardenin D, 4366
C$_{19}$H$_{18}$O$_9$
Gardenin E, 4366
C$_{19}$H$_{19}$ClN$_2$
Desloratadine, 2922
C$_{19}$H$_{19}$N
Phenindamine, 7233
C$_{19}$H$_{19}$NOS
Ketotifen, 5307
C$_{19}$H$_{19}$NO$_3$
Laureline, 5383
C$_{19}$H$_{19}$NO$_4$
Bulbocapnine, 1481
Domesticine, 3413
Nandinine, 6364
C$_{19}$H$_{19}$N$_2$NaO$_2$
Phenylbutazone Sodium Salt, 7277
C$_{19}$H$_{19}$N$_3$O$_3$
Talampanel, 9032
C$_{19}$H$_{19}$N$_3$O$_5$S
Oxacillin, 6904
C$_{19}$H$_{19}$N$_3$O$_6$
Nilvadipine, 6545
C$_{19}$H$_{19}$N$_7$O$_6$
Folic Acid, 4221
C$_{19}$H$_{20}$ClNO$_4$
Bezafibrate, 1195
C$_{19}$H$_{20}$ClNO$_5$
Ronifibrate, 8255
C$_{19}$H$_{20}$ClN$_3$
Clemizole, 2346
C$_{19}$H$_{20}$FNO$_3$
Paroxetine, 7043
C$_{19}$H$_{20}$FN$_3$O$_3$
Danofloxacin, 2813
C$_{19}$H$_{20}$F$_3$NO$_2$
Benfluorex, 1039
C$_{19}$H$_{20}$F$_3$NO$_4$
Fluazifop-butyl, 4116
C$_{19}$H$_{20}$F$_3$N$_3$O$_3$
Niflumic Acid β-Morpholinoethyl Ester, 6531
Orbifloxacin, 6862
C$_{19}$H$_{20}$N$_2$
Mebhydroline, 5770
C$_{19}$H$_{20}$N$_2$O
Vellosimine, 9944
C$_{19}$H$_{20}$N$_2$O$_2$
Phenylbutazone, 7277
C$_{19}$H$_{20}$N$_2$O$_3$
Ditazol, 3367
Dolasetron, 3411
Oxyphenbutazone, 6972
C$_{19}$H$_{20}$N$_2$O$_3$S
Pioglitazone, 7452
C$_{19}$H$_{20}$N$_2$O$_7$
Aranidipine, 767
C$_{19}$H$_{20}$N$_6$O
Imidocarb, 4915
C$_{19}$H$_{20}$N$_8$O$_5$
Aminopterin, 472

C$_{19}$H$_{20}$O$_2$
Cyclofenil Free Diol, 2720
C$_{19}$H$_{20}$O$_9$
Cervicarcin, 2007
C$_{19}$H$_{21}$ClN$_2$OS
Chloracizine, 2068
C$_{19}$H$_{21}$ClN$_4$O$_5$
Theofibrate, 9284
C$_{19}$H$_{21}$FN$_2$O$_4$
Nadifloxacin, 6345
C$_{19}$H$_{21}$F$_3$N$_2$S
Trifluomeprazine, 9679
C$_{19}$H$_{21}$N
Nortriptyline, 6715
Protriptyline, 7901
C$_{19}$H$_{21}$NO
Doxepin, 3435
C$_{19}$H$_{21}$NO$_3$
Isothebaine, 5226
Nalorphine, 6361
Thebaine, 9276
C$_{19}$H$_{21}$NO$_4$
Boldine, 1325
Corytuberine, 2550
Laurotetanine, 5388
Naloxone, 6362
Salutaridine, 8341
C$_{19}$H$_{21}$NS
Dothiepin, 3429
Pizotyline, 7515
C$_{19}$H$_{21}$N$_3$
Perlapine, 7179
C$_{19}$H$_{21}$N$_3$O
Talastine, 9035
Zolpidem, 10190
C$_{19}$H$_{21}$N$_3$O$_5$
Isradipine, 5240
C$_{19}$H$_{21}$N$_3$S
Cyamemazine, 2683
C$_{19}$H$_{21}$N$_5$O$_2$
Pirenzepine, 7491
C$_{19}$H$_{21}$N$_5$O$_4$
Prazosin, 7717
C$_{19}$H$_{22}$BrNO$_4$S$_2$
Tiotropium Bromide, 9454
C$_{19}$H$_{22}$ClN$_5$O
Trazodone, 9579
C$_{19}$H$_{22}$FN$_3$O
Azaperone, 898
C$_{19}$H$_{22}$FN$_3$O$_3$
Enrofloxacin, 3592
Grepafloxacin, 4545
C$_{19}$H$_{22}$FN$_3$O$_4$
Gatifloxacin, 4376
C$_{19}$H$_{22}$F$_2$N$_4$O$_3$
Sparfloxacin, 8735
C$_{19}$H$_{22}$KN$_3$O$_4$S
Hetacillin Potassium Salt, 4672
C$_{19}$H$_{22}$N$_2$
Triprolidine, 9746
C$_{19}$H$_{22}$N$_2$O
Cinchonidine, 2286
Cinchonine, 2287
Cinchotoxine, 2289
Eburnamonine, 3487
C$_{19}$H$_{22}$N$_2$OS
Acepromazine, 32
Thiazesim, 9305
C$_{19}$H$_{22}$N$_2$O$_2$
Cupreine, 2623
Sarpagine, 8378
Wieland-Gumlich Aldehyde, 10044
C$_{19}$H$_{22}$N$_2$O$_3$
Bumadizon, 1483
C$_{19}$H$_{22}$N$_2$O$_6$S
Penamecillin, 7081

C$_{19}$H$_{31}$NO$_2$
Samandarine, 8346
C$_{19}$H$_{31}$NO$_4$
Decimemide, 2852
C$_{19}$H$_{32}$
Androstane, 635
Etiocholane, 3866
Tridecylbenzene, 9659
C$_{19}$H$_{32}$BrNO$_2$
Valethamate Bromide, 9906
C$_{19}$H$_{32}$N$_2$
Tedisamil, 9108
C$_{19}$H$_{32}$N$_2$O$_4$
Betoxycaine, 1187
C$_{19}$H$_{32}$N$_2$O$_5$
Perindopril, 7170
C$_{19}$H$_{32}$N$_4$O$_{11}$
Muramyl Dipeptide, 6305
C$_{19}$H$_{33}$NO$_2$
Fingolimod, 4083
C$_{19}$H$_{33}$N$_3$O
Pentisomide, 7129
C$_{19}$H$_{34}$
Fichtelite, 4076
C$_{19}$H$_{34}$N$_8$O$_8$
Streptothricin F, 8829
C$_{19}$H$_{34}$O$_2$
Methyl Linoleate, 6095
C$_{19}$H$_{34}$O$_3$
Methoprene, 5983
C$_{19}$H$_{35}$N
Perhexiline, 7163
C$_{19}$H$_{35}$NO$_2$
Dicyclomine, 3097
C$_{19}$H$_{36}$O$_2$
Lactobacillic Acid, 5341
Oleic Acid Methyl Ester, 6828
C$_{19}$H$_{37}$NO
Lactobacillic Acid Amide, 5341
C$_{19}$H$_{37}$N$_5$O$_7$
Sisomicin, 8550
C$_{19}$H$_{38}$O
Disparlure, 3361
C$_{19}$H$_{38}$O$_2$
Stearic Acid Methyl Ester, 8804
C$_{19}$H$_{38}$O$_3$
Cetyl Lactate, 2030
C$_{19}$H$_{39}$NO
Tridemorph, 9660
C$_{19}$H$_{39}$N$_5$O$_7$
Gentamicin C$_{1a}$, 4392
C$_{19}$H$_{40}$
Pristane, 7752
C$_{19}$H$_{40}$O$_3$
Chimyl Alcohol, 2060
C$_{19}$H$_{42}$BrN
Cetrimonium Bromide, 2025
C$_{20}$H$_{12}$
Benzo[a]pyrene, 1103
C$_{20}$H$_2$Cl$_4$I$_4$K$_2$O$_5$
Rose Bengal, 8262
C$_{20}$H$_2$Cl$_4$I$_4$Na$_2$O$_5$
Rose Bengal Disodium Salt, 8262
C$_{20}$H$_6$Br$_2$N$_2$Na$_2$O$_9$
Eosine I Bluish, 3602
C$_{20}$H$_6$Br$_4$Na$_2$O$_5$
Eosine Yellowish—(YS), 3603
C$_{20}$H$_6$I$_4$Na$_2$O$_5$
Erythrosine, 3693
C$_{20}$H$_8$Br$_2$HgNa$_2$O$_6$
Merbromin, 5867
C$_{20}$H$_8$Br$_2$Na$_2$O$_5$
4′,5′-Dibromofluorescein Disodium Salt, 3022

C$_{20}$H$_8$Br$_4$Na$_2$O$_4$
3′,3″,5′,5″-Tetrabromophenolphthalein Disodium Salt, 9186
C$_{20}$H$_8$Br$_4$Na$_2$O$_{10}$S$_2$
Sulfobromophthalein Sodium, 8954
C$_{20}$H$_8$Br$_4$O$_5$
Eosine Yellowish—(YS) Free Acid, 3603
C$_{20}$H$_8$Cl$_2$Na$_2$O$_5$
4′,5′-Dichlorofluorescein Disodium Salt, 3067
C$_{20}$H$_8$Cl$_4$Na$_2$O$_4$
Phenoltetrachlorophthalein Disodium Salt, 7248
C$_{20}$H$_8$I$_2$Na$_2$O$_5$
4′,5′-Diiodofluorescein Sodium Salt, 3189
C$_{20}$H$_8$I$_4$Na$_2$O$_4$
Iodophthalein Sodium, 5038
Phentetiothalein Sodium, 7263
C$_{20}$H$_{10}$Br$_2$O$_5$
4′,5′-Dibromofluorescein, 3022
C$_{20}$H$_{10}$Br$_4$O$_4$
3′,3″,5′,5″-Tetrabromophenolphthalein, 9186
C$_{20}$H$_{10}$Cl$_2$O$_5$
4′,5′-Dichlorofluorescein, 3067
C$_{20}$H$_{10}$Cl$_4$O$_4$
Phenoltetrachlorophthalein, 7248
C$_{20}$H$_{10}$I$_2$O$_5$
4′,5′-Diiodofluorescein, 3189
C$_{20}$H$_{10}$I$_4$O$_4$
Iodophthalein Sodium Free Acid, 5038
C$_{20}$H$_{10}$Na$_2$O$_5$
Fluorescein Disodium Salt, 4159
C$_{20}$H$_{10}$Na$_2$O$_7$
Gallein Disodium Salt, 4344
C$_{20}$H$_{11}$N$_2$Na$_3$O$_{10}$S$_3$
Amaranth (Dye), 375
C$_{20}$H$_{12}$
Benzo[e]pyrene, 1104
Perylene, 7184
C$_{20}$H$_{12}$Li$_2$N$_2$O$_{10}$S$_3$
Lucifer Yellow VS, 5594
C$_{20}$H$_{12}$N$_3$NaO$_7$S
Eriochrome® Black T, 3667
C$_{20}$H$_{12}$O$_5$
Fluorescein, 4159
C$_{20}$H$_{12}$O$_7$
Gallein, 4344
C$_{20}$H$_{13}$N$_3$O$_3$
Violacein, 9997
C$_{20}$H$_{14}$
Cholanthrene, 2197
Triptycene, 9749
C$_{20}$H$_{14}$CaO$_8$S$_2$
Asaprol, 822
C$_{20}$H$_{14}$ClNO$_4$
Sanguinarine Chloride, 8356
C$_{20}$H$_{14}$I$_6$N$_2$O$_6$
Iodipamide, 5022
C$_{20}$H$_{14}$NO$_4$$^+$
Sanguinarine, 8356
C$_{20}$H$_{14}$N$_4$
Porphine, 7599
C$_{20}$H$_{14}$O$_2$
BINOL, 1226
C$_{20}$H$_{14}$O$_2$S$_2$
DDD (Analytical), 2840
C$_{20}$H$_{14}$O$_3$
Florantyrone, 4107
C$_{20}$H$_{14}$O$_4$
Phenolphthalein, 7243
Phenyl Phthalate, 7306
C$_{20}$H$_{14}$O$_5$
Fluorescin, 4160

C$_{20}$H$_{14}$O$_6$
Ethylidene Dicoumarol, 3812
C$_{20}$H$_{15}$ClN$_4$
Vatalanib, 9939
C$_{20}$H$_{15}$Cl$_3$N$_2$OS
Sertaconazole, 8465
C$_{20}$H$_{15}$F$_3$N$_4$O$_3$
Trovafloxacin, 9787
C$_{20}$H$_{15}$N
β,β′-Dinaphthylamine, 3267
C$_{20}$H$_{15}$N$_3$O$_6$
Rubitecan, 8288
C$_{20}$H$_{16}$
9,10-Dimethyl-1,2-benzanthracene, 3235
C$_{20}$H$_{16}$N$_2$O$_4$
Camptothecin, 1735
C$_{20}$H$_{16}$N$_4$
Nitron, 6613
C$_{20}$H$_{16}$N$_4$O$_2$S
Indiplon, 4946
C$_{20}$H$_{16}$O$_6$
Elliptone, 3550
Viridin, 10006
C$_{20}$H$_{17}$ClN$_2$O$_3$
Ketazolam, 5297
C$_{20}$H$_{17}$ClO$_3$
Indanofan, 4933
C$_{20}$H$_{17}$Cl$_3$N$_2$O$_2$
Omoconazole, 6846
C$_{20}$H$_{17}$FO$_3$S
Sulindac, 8982
C$_{20}$H$_{17}$FO$_4$S
Exisulind, 3916
C$_{20}$H$_{17}$F$_2$N$_3$O$_3$
Sarafloxacin, 8370
C$_{20}$H$_{17}$F$_3$N$_2$O
Floctafenine, 4103
C$_{20}$H$_{17}$NO$_6$
Adlumidine, 165
Bicuculline, 1203
C$_{20}$H$_{17}$N$_3$Na$_2$O$_9$S$_3$
Acid Fuchsin, 107
C$_{20}$H$_{17}$N$_3$O$_4$
9-Aminocamptothecin, 431
C$_{20}$H$_{18}$ClNO$_6$
Ochratoxin A, 6740
C$_{20}$H$_{18}$NO$_4$$^+$
Berberine, 1154
C$_{20}$H$_{18}$N$_4$O$_5$S$_2$
Cephalonium, 1978
C$_{20}$H$_{18}$N$_6$Na$_2$O$_7$S$_4$
Cefodizime Disodium Salt, 1928
C$_{20}$H$_{18}$N$_6$Na$_2$O$_9$S
Moxalactam Disodium Salt, 6286
C$_{20}$H$_{18}$O$_2$Sn
Triphenyltin Hydroxide Acetate, 9745
C$_{20}$H$_{18}$O$_3$
Phenolphthalol, 7245
C$_{20}$H$_{18}$O$_4$
Cyclocumarol, 2717
Phaseolin, 7198
C$_{20}$H$_{18}$O$_6$
Asarinin, 823
Sesamin, 8470
C$_{20}$H$_{18}$O$_7$
Sesamolin, 8471
C$_{20}$H$_{18}$O$_9$
Frangulin B, 4264
C$_{20}$H$_{19}$F$_3$N$_2$O$_4$
Trifloxystrobin, 9677
C$_{20}$H$_{19}$NO$_3$
Pyriproxyfen, 7990
C$_{20}$H$_{19}$NO$_4$
Satigrel, 8383

C₂₀H₁₉NO₅
Chelidonine, 2053
Papaveraldine, 7017
Protopine, 7896

C₂₀H₁₉NO₆
Ochratoxin B, 6740

C₂₀H₁₉NO₈S
Berberine Acid Sulfate, 1154

C₂₀H₂₀
Dodecahedrane, 3402

C₂₀H₂₀ClN₃
Magenta I, 5652

C₂₀H₂₀ClN₃O₃
Tepoxalin, 9151

C₂₀H₂₀Cl₂MgO₆
Clofibric Acid Magnesium Salt, 2378

C₂₀H₂₀Cl₂N₄O₂S
Capravirine, 1755

C₂₀H₂₀NO₄⁺
Columbamine, 2492
Jatrorrhizine, 5261

C₂₀H₂₀N₂O₂
Feprazone, 4012

C₂₀H₂₀N₂O₃
Elliptinium Acetate, 3549

C₂₀H₂₀N₂O₅
Antipyrine Acetylsalicylate, 716

C₂₀H₂₀N₂O₆
Antipyrine Salicylacetate, 716

C₂₀H₂₀N₆O₇S₄
Cefodizime, 1928

C₂₀H₂₀N₆O₉S
Moxalactam, 6286

C₂₀H₂₀N₈Na₂O₅
Methotrexate Disodium Salt, 5985

C₂₀H₂₀O₄
Otobain, 6899

C₂₀H₂₀O₆
Cubebin, 2613

C₂₀H₂₀O₇
Herqueinone, 4668

C₂₀H₂₀O₉
Gardenin C, 4366

C₂₀H₂₀O₁₄
Hamamelitannin, 4607

C₂₀H₂₁AlCl₂O₇
Clofibric Acid Basic Aluminum Salt, 2378

C₂₀H₂₁CaN₇O₇.5H₂O
Folinic Acid Calcium Salt Pentahydrate, 4222

C₂₀H₂₁ClN₂O₄
Fipexide, 4084

C₂₀H₂₁ClO₄
Fenofibrate, 3978

C₂₀H₂₁FN₂O
Citalopram, 2318

C₂₀H₂₁F₃N₂OS
Fluacizine, 4113

C₂₀H₂₁N
Cyclobenzaprine, 2713

C₂₀H₂₁NOS
Tolciclate, 9509

C₂₀H₂₁NO₂
Moxaverine, 6288

C₂₀H₂₁NO₃
Dimefline, 3204
Mepixanox, 5860

C₂₀H₂₁NO₄
Canadine, 1736
Dicentrine, 3041
Papaverine, 7019

C₂₀H₂₁NO₅
Repirinast, 8138

C₂₀H₂₁N₃
Aptiganel, 758

C₂₀H₂₁N₃O
Cilansetron, 2271

C₂₀H₂₁N₃O₇S
Ampiroxicam, 587

C₂₀H₂₁N₅O₆
Pemetrexed, 7077

C₂₀H₂₁N₇O₆
Methopterin, 5984
Ninopterin, 6555

C₂₀H₂₁N₇O₆S₂
Ceforanide, 1931

C₂₀H₂₂ClN
Pyrrobutamine, 8012

C₂₀H₂₂ClN₃O
Amodiaquin, 572

C₂₀H₂₂N₂
Azatadine, 901

C₂₀H₂₂N₂O
Fenazaquin, 3959

C₂₀H₂₂N₂O₂
Akuammicine, 199
Gelsemine, 4384
Quininone, 8063

C₂₀H₂₂N₂O₃
Perivine, 7178

C₂₀H₂₂N₂O₇S
Sivelestat, 8558

C₂₀H₂₂N₂S
Mequitazine, 5864

C₂₀H₂₂N₄O
Difenamizole, 3134

C₂₀H₂₂N₄O₅
Camostat, 1728

C₂₀H₂₂N₄O₆S
Febantel, 3944

C₂₀H₂₂N₄O₁₀S
Cefuroxime 1-Acetoxyethyl Ester, 1954

C₂₀H₂₂N₅NaO₆S
Azlocillin Sodium Salt, 916

C₂₀H₂₂N₈O₅
Methotrexate, 5985

C₂₀H₂₂N₈O₆S₂
Ceftobiprole, 1952

C₂₀H₂₂O₂
Norgestrienone, 6705

C₂₀H₂₂O₃
Avobenzone, 888

C₂₀H₂₂O₆
Columbin, 2493

C₂₀H₂₂O₈
Populin, 7594

C₂₀H₂₂O₁₀
Plicatic Acid, 7537

C₂₀H₂₃N
Amitriptyline, 487
Maprotiline, 5748

C₂₀H₂₃NO
Amitriptylinoxide, 488

C₂₀H₂₃NO₂
Dioxadrol, 3299

C₂₀H₂₃NO₃
Benalaxyl, 1030

C₂₀H₂₃NO₄
Corydine, 2546
Corypalmine, 2549
Dihydrocodeinone Enol Acetate, 3172
Efaproxiral, 3520
Isocorydine, 5162
Isocorypalmine, 5163
Naltrexone, 6363

C₂₀H₂₃NS
Methixene, 5979

C₂₀H₂₃N₃O₂
Bitertanol, 1305
Phenserine, 7260

C₂₀H₂₃N₅O₆S
Azlocillin, 916

C₂₀H₂₃N₇O₇
Folinic Acid, 4222

C₂₀H₂₄BrN₃O
Bromolysergide, 1423

C₂₀H₂₄ClNO
Cloperastine, 2395

C₂₀H₂₄ClN₃O₂
Clebopride, 2344

C₂₀H₂₄ClN₃S
Prochlorperazine, 7761

C₂₀H₂₄Cl₂N₁₀
Picloxydine, 7398

C₂₀H₂₄FN₃O₄
Balofloxacin, 944

C₂₀H₂₄NO₄⁺
Magnoflorine, 5696

C₂₀H₂₄N₂
Dimethindene, 3216

C₂₀H₂₄N₂O
Indecainide, 4937

C₂₀H₂₄N₂OS
Propiomazine, 7822
Propionylpromazine, 7829

C₂₀H₂₄N₂O₂
Epiquinidine, 3620
Epiquinine, 3621
Quinidine, 8060
Quinine, 8061
Viquidil, 10003

C₂₀H₂₄N₂O₂S
Hycanthone, 4759

C₂₀H₂₄N₂O₄
Metoquinone, 6152

C₂₀H₂₄N₂O₅
Diamfenetide, 2974

C₂₀H₂₄N₂O₆
Nisoldipine, 6565

C₂₀H₂₄N₂S₂
Metitepine, 6141

C₂₀H₂₄O₂
Dimestrol, 3211
Ethinyl Estradiol, 3734
Exemestane, 3913

C₂₀H₂₄O₃
Estrone Acetate, 3708
Trenbolone Acetate, 9583

C₂₀H₂₄O₄
Crocetin, 2589

C₂₀H₂₄O₆
Dibenzo-18-crown-6, 2602
Triptolide, 9747

C₂₀H₂₄O₇
Olivil, 6837

C₂₀H₂₄O₇S
Tesaglitazar, 9177

C₂₀H₂₄O₉
Ginkgolide A, 4426
Nodakenin, 6668

C₂₀H₂₄O₁₀
Ginkgolide B, 4426

C₂₀H₂₄O₁₁
Ginkgolide C, 4426

C₂₀H₂₅ClN₂OS
Lucanthone Hydrochloride, 5591

C₂₀H₂₅ClN₂O₅
Amlodipine, 491

C₂₀H₂₅ClO₄
Osaterone, 6888

C₂₀H₂₅FN₄O
Niaprazine, 6492

C₂₀H₂₅N
Prodipine, 7768

C$_{20}$H$_{25}$NO
Normethadone, 6709
Pridinol, 7741
C$_{20}$H$_{25}$NOS
Thiphenamil, 9370
C$_{20}$H$_{25}$NO$_2$
Adiphenine, 161
Dienogest, 3106
Femoxetine, 3955
Fomocaine, 4230
C$_{20}$H$_{25}$NO$_2$S$_2$
Tiagabine, 9417
C$_{20}$H$_{25}$NO$_3$
Benactyzine, 1029
Difemerine, 3132
Dimenoxadol, 3208
C$_{20}$H$_{25}$NO$_4$
Cilomilast, 2276
Codamine, 2462
Laudanidine, 5379
Laudanine, 5380
C$_{20}$H$_{25}$N$_3$O
Lysergide, 5634
Prodigiosin, 7767
C$_{20}$H$_{25}$N$_3$O$_2$
Methylergonovine, 6070
C$_{20}$H$_{25}$N$_3$O$_4$
Ecabapide, 3488
C$_{20}$H$_{25}$N$_3$S
Perazine, 7151
C$_{20}$H$_{25}$N$_5$O$_7$S$_2$
Cefetamet Pivaloyloxymethyl Ester, 1923
C$_{20}$H$_{26}$ClNO$_5$
Cloricromen, 2405
C$_{20}$H$_{26}$N$_2$
Dimetacrine, 3212
Trimipramine, 9722
C$_{20}$H$_{26}$N$_2$O
Ibogaine, 4875
Tabernanthine, 9020
C$_{20}$H$_{26}$N$_2$O$_2$
Ajmaline, 194
Epsiprantel, 3637
Hydroquinidine, 4806
Hydroquinine, 4807
C$_{20}$H$_{26}$N$_2$O$_4$
Itopride, 5244
C$_{20}$H$_{26}$N$_2$O$_5$S
Alacepril, 200
C$_{20}$H$_{26}$N$_2$O$_5$S$_2$
Spirapril Diacid, 8753
C$_{20}$H$_{26}$N$_4$O
Lisuride, 5518
C$_{20}$H$_{26}$N$_4$OS
Oxypendyl, 6970
C$_{20}$H$_{26}$N$_4$O$_2$
Hexamidine, 4692
C$_{20}$H$_{26}$O
3-Dehydroretinal, 2873
C$_{20}$H$_{26}$O$_2$
Methestrol, 5968
Norethindrone, 6697
Norethynodrel, 6698
C$_{20}$H$_{26}$O$_5$
Allethrin II, 260
C$_{20}$H$_{26}$O$_7$
Cnicin, 2425
C$_{20}$H$_{27}$BrN$_2$O
Ambutonium Bromide, 387
C$_{20}$H$_{27}$N
Alverine, 371
C$_{20}$H$_{27}$NO
Cyclorphan, 2750
C$_{20}$H$_{27}$NO$_2$
Vetrabutine, 9972

C$_{20}$H$_{27}$NO$_3$
Tralkoxydim, 9564
Trilostane, 9698
C$_{20}$H$_{27}$NO$_4$
Bevantolol, 1192
C$_{20}$H$_{27}$NO$_4$S
Domitroban, 3416
Sulfinalol, 8948
C$_{20}$H$_{27}$NO$_5$
Buquinolate, 1500
Chromonar, 2239
C$_{20}$H$_{27}$NO$_{11}$
Amygdalin, 597
C$_{20}$H$_{27}$N$_3$O$_5$
Cilazapril Diacid, 2273
C$_{20}$H$_{27}$N$_3$O$_6$
Febarbamate, 3945
Imidapril, 4911
C$_{20}$H$_{27}$N$_3$O$_7$S
Succisulfone 2,2'-Iminodiethanol Salt, 8878
C$_{20}$H$_{27}$N$_5$O$_2$
Cilostazol, 2277
C$_{20}$H$_{27}$N$_5$O$_3$
Bamifylline, 955
C$_{20}$H$_{27}$N$_5$O$_5$S
Glisoxepid, 4444
C$_{20}$H$_{28}$BrN
Emepronium Bromide, 3558
C$_{20}$H$_{28}$Cl$_4$N$_2$O$_4$
Teclozan, 9105
C$_{20}$H$_{28}$I$_3$N$_3$O$_9$
Iobitridol, 5008
Iopentol, 5059
C$_{20}$H$_{28}$N$_2$O$_3$
Oxyphencyclimine, 6973
C$_{20}$H$_{28}$N$_2$O$_5$
Enalapril, 3567
Remifentanil, 8131
C$_{20}$H$_{28}$N$_2$O$_5$S
Tamsulosin, 9049
C$_{20}$H$_{28}$N$_2$O$_6$
Cinepazet, 2290
C$_{20}$H$_{28}$N$_4$O
Terguride, 9164
C$_{20}$H$_{28}$N$_4$O$_8$S$_2$
Stilbamidine Isethionate, 8816
C$_{20}$H$_{28}$N$_6$O$_2$
Fencamine, 3967
C$_{20}$H$_{28}$O
3-Dehydroretinol, 2874
Lynestrenol, 5629
Retinal, 8164
C$_{20}$H$_{28}$O$_2$
Alitretinoin, 249
Ethynodiol, 3860
Isotretinoin, 5228
Methandrostenolone, 5951
Norgesterone, 6702
Norvinisterone, 6717
Retinoic Acid, 8165
C$_{20}$H$_{28}$O$_3$
Cafestol, 1634
Cinerin I, 2292
C$_{20}$H$_{28}$O$_3$S
Ethyl Dibunate, 3788
C$_{20}$H$_{28}$O$_4$
Marrubiin, 5754
C$_{20}$H$_{28}$O$_5$
Pododacric Acid, 7544
C$_{20}$H$_{28}$O$_5$S
Ecabet, 3489
C$_{20}$H$_{28}$O$_6$
Amarolide, 378
Phorbol, 7332

C$_{20}$H$_{28}$O$_6$S
Tiaprost, 9423
C$_{20}$H$_{28}$O$_{13}$
Primulaverin, 7749
C$_{20}$H$_{29}$FO$_3$
Fluoxymesterone, 4186
C$_{20}$H$_{29}$NO$_5$S
Latrunculin B, 5378
C$_{20}$H$_{29}$N$_3$O$_2$
Dibucaine, 3031
C$_{20}$H$_{29}$N$_3$O$_5$
Propiram Fumarate, 7831
C$_{20}$H$_{29}$N$_3$O$_7$
Amicoumacin A, 398
C$_{20}$H$_{29}$N$_5$O$_3$
Urapidil, 9865
C$_{20}$H$_{30}$BrNO$_3$
Ipratropium Bromide, 5073
C$_{20}$H$_{30}$N$_2$O$_2$
Furazabol, 4299
C$_{20}$H$_{30}$N$_2$O$_3$
Morpheridine, 6274
C$_{20}$H$_{30}$N$_2$O$_5$
Neotame, 6465
C$_{20}$H$_{30}$N$_2$O$_5$S
Benfuracarb, 1042
C$_{20}$H$_{30}$O
Neovitamin A, 6468
Vitamin A, 10013
C$_{20}$H$_{30}$O$_2$
Abietic Acid, 7
Eicosapentaenoic Acid, 3531
Isopimaric Acid, 5200
Levopimaric Acid, 5468
Methenolone, 5967
17-Methyltestosterone, 6125
Mibolerone, 6174
Norethandrolone, 6696
Oxendolone, 6931
Oxenin, 6932
Palustric Acid, 6998
Pimaric Acid, 7428
Stenbolone, 8808
C$_{20}$H$_{30}$O$_3$
Leukotriene A$_4$, 5455
Oxymesterone, 6965
C$_{20}$H$_{30}$O$_5$
Andrographolide, 633
Taxicin-II, 9077
C$_{20}$H$_{30}$O$_6$
Taxicin-I, 9077
C$_{20}$H$_{30}$O$_8$
Ptaquiloside, 7930
C$_{20}$H$_{31}$NO
Deramciclane, 2915
C$_{20}$H$_{31}$NO$_2$
Drofenine, 3445
C$_{20}$H$_{31}$NO$_2$S
Cetiedil, 2021
C$_{20}$H$_{31}$NO$_3$
Carbetapentane, 1794
C$_{20}$H$_{31}$NO$_7$
Heliosupine, 4629
C$_{20}$H$_{31}$NaO$_5$
Prostacyclin Sodium Salt, 7875
C$_{20}$H$_{32}$
Neocembrene, 6448
C$_{20}$H$_{32}$ClNO
Trihexyphenidyl Hydrochloride, 9695
C$_{20}$H$_{32}$N$_2$O$_3$S
Carbosulfan, 1826
C$_{20}$H$_{32}$N$_5$O$_8$P
Adefovir Di(pivaloyloxymethyl) Ester, 151
C$_{20}$H$_{32}$N$_6$O$_{12}$S$_2$
Glutathione Disulfide, 4475

$C_{20}H_{32}O$
Ethylestrenol, 3805
$C_{20}H_{32}O_2$
Arachidonic Acid, 765
Dromostanolone, 3448
Etiocholanic Acid, 3867
Mestanolone, 5915
Mesterolone, 5916
Methandriol, 5950
$C_{20}H_{32}O_3$
Grindelic Acid, 4547
5-HETE, 4674
$C_{20}H_{32}O_4$
Leukotriene B_4, 5455
$C_{20}H_{32}O_5$
Grayanotoxin II, 4543
Prostacyclin, 7875
Prostaglandin E_2, 7877
Thromboxane A_2, 9388
$C_{20}H_{33}NO$
Fenpropimorph, 3993
$C_{20}H_{33}NO_3$
Oxeladin, 6930
$C_{20}H_{33}NO_7$
Candoxatril Diacid, 1742
$C_{20}H_{33}N_3O_3$
Talinolol, 9038
$C_{20}H_{33}N_3O_3S$
Quinagolide, 8045
$C_{20}H_{33}N_3O_4$
Celiprolol, 1960
$C_{20}H_{34}AuO_9PS$
Auranofin, 878
$C_{20}H_{34}GdN_5O_{10}$
Gadoversetamide, 4329
$C_{20}H_{34}O_2$
Plaunotol, 7532
$C_{20}H_{34}O_4$
Aphidicolin, 727
Zoapatanol, 10185
$C_{20}H_{34}O_5$
Prostaglandin E_1, 7876
Prostaglandin $F_{2\alpha}$, 7878
$C_{20}H_{34}O_6$
Grayanotoxin III, 4543
Thromboxane B_2, 9388
$C_{20}H_{35}ClO_4S$
Oxychlorosene, 6956
$C_{20}H_{35}NO_2$
Dihexyverine, 3168
$C_{20}H_{35}NO_{13}$
Validamycin A, 9908
$C_{20}H_{36}CaNO_5.\frac{1}{2}H_2O$
Hopantenic Acid Calcium Salt Hemi-
hydrate, 4744
$C_{20}H_{36}N_2O_3S$
Ibutilide, 4883
$C_{20}H_{36}N_6O$
Lauroguadine, 5386
$C_{20}H_{36}O_2$
Ethyl Linoleate, 3820
$C_{20}H_{36}O_6$
Dicyclohexano-18-crown-6, 2602
$C_{20}H_{37}KO_7S$
Docusate Potassium, 3401
$C_{20}H_{37}NO_3$
Rociverine, 8245
$C_{20}H_{37}N_3O_{13}$
Destomycin A, 2935
Hygromycin B, 4852
$C_{20}H_{37}NaO_7S$
Docusate Sodium, 3401
$C_{20}H_{38}O_2$
Oleic Acid Ethyl Ester, 6828
$C_{20}H_{40}N_2O_{12}$
Hexamethonium Tartrate, 4688

$C_{20}H_{40}O$
Isophytol, 5198
Phytol, 7390
$C_{20}H_{40}O_2$
Arachidic Acid, 764
Stearic Acid Ethyl Ester, 8804
$C_{20}H_{41}N_5O_7$
Gentamicin C_2, 4392
Micronomicin, 6181
$C_{20}H_{42}O_3$
Phytantriol, 7386
$C_{20}H_{43}N$
Dymanthine, 3475
$C_{20}H_{44}BrN$
Cetyldimethylethylammonium Bro-
mide, 2029
$C_{20}H_{60}O_8Si_9$
Eicosamethylnonasiloxane, 3530
$C_{21}H_{11}ClF_6N_2O_3$
Flufenoxuron, 4133
$C_{21}H_{11}NO_5S$
Asenapine, 4089
$C_{21}H_{13}F_3N_2O_4$
Talniflumate, 9044
$C_{21}H_{14}Br_4O_5S$
Bromcresol Green, 1386
$C_{21}H_{15}AlO_6$
Aluminum Benzoate, 329
$C_{21}H_{15}CeO_6.3H_2O$
Benzoic Acid Cerium Salt Trihydrate,
1091
$C_{21}H_{15}N_3O_4$
Deferasirox, 2858
$C_{21}H_{16}$
3-Methylcholanthrene, 6044
$C_{21}H_{16}Br_2O_5S$
Bromcresol Purple, 1387
$C_{21}H_{16}ClFN_4O_5$
Fluoxastrobin, 4184
$C_{21}H_{16}ClF_3N_4O_3$
Sorafenib, 8720
$C_{21}H_{16}N_4O_8S_2$
Nitrocefin, 6594
$C_{21}H_{16}O_6$
Justicidin B, 5272
$C_{21}H_{18}ClNO_6$
Acemetacin, 27
$C_{21}H_{18}F_3N_3O_3$
Temafloxacin, 9132
$C_{21}H_{18}NO_4^+$
Chelerythrine, 2051
$C_{21}H_{18}O_5S$
Cresol Purple, 2577
Cresol Red, 2578
$C_{21}H_{18}O_{12}$
Scutellarein Glucuronide, 8412
$C_{21}H_{19}F_2N_3O_3$
Difloxacin, 3141
$C_{21}H_{19}N_3O_3S$
Amsacrine, 594
$C_{21}H_{20}BrN_3$
Homidium Bromide, 4731
$C_{21}H_{20}ClNO_5$
Flavopiridol, 4094
$C_{21}H_{20}Cl_2N_6O_3$
Rilmazafone, 8221
$C_{21}H_{20}Cl_2O_3$
Permethrin, 7180
$C_{21}H_{20}FN_3O_6S$
Prulifloxacin, 7908
$C_{21}H_{20}N_2O_3$
Alstonine, 316
Serpentine (Alkaloid), 8464
$C_{21}H_{20}N_3^+$
Homidium, 4731

$C_{21}H_{20}N_4O_3$
Picotamide, 7407
$C_{21}H_{20}N_6O$
Aminoquinuride, 475
$C_{21}H_{20}O_6$
Cabenegrin A-I, 1600
Curcumin, 2673
$C_{21}H_{20}O_8$
α-Peltatin, 7075
$C_{21}H_{20}O_9$
Chrysophanic Acid Glucoside,
2258
Daidzein 7-Glucoside, 2801
Frangulin A, 4264
$C_{21}H_{20}O_{10}$
Apigetrin, 731
Genistin, 4391
$C_{21}H_{20}O_{11}$
Kaempferol 3-Glucoside, 5274
Luteolin 5-Glucoside, 5614
Quercitrin, 8037
$C_{21}H_{20}O_{12}$
Isoquercitrin, 5221
Myricetin 3-Rhamnoside, 6332
Quercimeritrin, 8035
$C_{21}H_{20}O_{12}.2\frac{1}{2}H_2O$
Quercetin 3-β-D-Galactoside Hemi-
pentahydrate, 8034
$C_{21}H_{20}O_{13}$
Gossypitrin, 8035
Quercetagetin 7-Glucoside, 8033
$C_{21}H_{21}ClN_2O_8$
Demeclocycline, 2886
$C_{21}H_{21}ClN_4OS$
Ziprasidone, 10171
$C_{21}H_{21}ClN_4O_3$
Nizofenone, 6661
$C_{21}H_{21}ClO_{10}$
Pelargonidin 3-Glucoside, 7071
$C_{21}H_{21}ClO_{11}$
Cyanidin Chloride 3-Glucoside,
2687
$C_{21}H_{21}ClO_{12}$
Delphinidin 3-Glucoside, 2880
$C_{21}H_{21}FN_2O_4S$
Ramatroban, 8100
$C_{21}H_{21}FN_4O_3$
Pradofloxacin, 7701
$C_{21}H_{21}HgN_4NaO_8$
Mercumallylic Acid Sodium Salt
Compd with Theophylline, 5872
$C_{21}H_{21}N$
Cyproheptadine, 2773
Naftifine, 6355
$C_{21}H_{21}NO_2$
Oxetorone, 6934
$C_{21}H_{21}NO_2S$
Tazarotene, 9081
$C_{21}H_{21}NO_6$
Adlumine, 166
Hydrastine, 4767
Rheadine, 8175
$C_{21}H_{21}NO_7$
Narcotoline, 6423
$C_{21}H_{21}N_2NaO_5S.H_2O$
Nafcillin Sodium Salt Monohydrate,
6352
$C_{21}H_{21}N_3O_7$
Cacotheline, 1605
$C_{21}H_{21}O_4P$
Tritolyl Phosphate, 9763
Tri-o-tolyl Phosphate, 9764
$C_{21}H_{22}ClNO_4$
Dimethomorph, 3222
$C_{21}H_{22}NO_4^+$
Palmatine, 6994

$C_{21}H_{27}N_7O_{14}P_2$
 NAD, 6344

$C_{21}H_{27}Na_2O_8P$
 Prednisolone 21-Disodium Phosphate, 7721

$C_{21}H_{28}BrNO_4$
 Cimetropium Bromide, 2280

$C_{21}H_{28}Cl_3N_3O_2$
 Acranil®, 121

$C_{21}H_{28}N_2O$
 Diampromide, 2988

$C_{21}H_{28}N_2O_2$
 Aspidospermine N-Formyl-N-deacetylaspidospermine, 850

$C_{21}H_{28}N_2O_5$
 Trimethobenzamide, 9708

$C_{21}H_{28}N_7O_{17}P_3$
 NADP, 6348

$C_{21}H_{28}O_2$
 Demegestone, 2888
 Dydrogesterone, 3474
 Ethisterone, 3741
 Guggulsterone, 4573
 Norgestrel, 6704
 Tetrahydrogestrinone, 9214
 Tibolone, 9427

$C_{21}H_{28}O_3$
 Cyclethrin, 2706
 Pyrethrin I, 7964

$C_{21}H_{28}O_4$
 11-Dehydrocorticosterone, 2869
 Formebolone, 4239

$C_{21}H_{28}O_5$
 Aldosterone, 225
 Cinerin II, 2292
 Cortisone, 2539
 Prednisolone, 7721

$C_{21}H_{29}ClO_3$
 Clostebol Acetate, 2413

$C_{21}H_{29}ClO_6S$
 Luprostiol, 5610

$C_{21}H_{29}Cl_3O_3$
 Cloxotestosterone, 2421

$C_{21}H_{29}FO_5$
 Fludrocortisone, 4130

$C_{21}H_{29}NO$
 Biperiden, 1233

$C_{21}H_{29}NO_2$
 Butorphanol, 1530
 Norelgestromin, 6694

$C_{21}H_{29}NS_2$
 Captodiamine, 1773

$C_{21}H_{29}N_3O$
 Disopyramide, 3360

$C_{21}H_{29}N_5O_2$
 Tandospirone, 9051

$C_{21}H_{29}N_5O_4$
 Pfeiffer's Substance, 7194

$C_{21}H_{29}N_7O_{14}P_2$
 NAD Reduced Form, 6344

$C_{21}H_{29}Na_2O_8P$
 Hydrocortisone 21-Phosphate Disodium Salt, 4787

$C_{21}H_{30}BrNO_4$
 N-Butylscopolammonium Bromide, 1588

$C_{21}H_{30}Br_2N_4O_{10}S_2$
 Dibromopropamidine Isethionate, 3024

$C_{21}H_{30}Cl_2N_2O_5$
 Loxiglumide, 5588

$C_{21}H_{30}Cl_2N_6O_{10}$
 Chloramphenicol Monosuccinate Arginine Salt, 2077

$C_{21}H_{30}FN_3O_2$
 Pipamperone, 7455

$C_{21}H_{30}N_2O$
 Bunaftine, 1485

$C_{21}H_{30}N_2O_8S$
 Docarpamine, 3396

$C_{21}H_{30}N_4O_4$
 Cinitapride, 2294

$C_{21}H_{30}N_7O_{17}P_3$
 NADP Reduced Form, 6348

$C_{21}H_{30}O_2$
 Cannabidiol, 1747
 Progesterone, 7773
 Tetrahydrocannabinols, 9209

$C_{21}H_{30}O_3$
 Deoxycorticosterone, 2900
 17α-Hydroxyprogesterone, 4839
 Jasmolin I, 5258
 Nandrolone Propionate, 6365

$C_{21}H_{30}O_4$
 Algestone, 239
 Corticosterone, 2538
 11-Desoxy-17-hydroxycorticosterone, 2932

$C_{21}H_{30}O_4S$
 Tixocortol, 9484

$C_{21}H_{30}O_5$
 Humulon, 4754
 Hydrocortisone, 4787
 4-Pregnene-17α,20β,21-triol-3,11-dione, 7731

$C_{21}H_{31}ClN_2O$
 Viminol, 9981

$C_{21}H_{31}ClN_6O_3$
 PPACK, 7699

$C_{21}H_{31}NO_2$
 Androisoxazole, 634

$C_{21}H_{31}NO_4$
 Furethidine, 4303

$C_{21}H_{31}N_3O_5.2H_2O$
 Lisinopril, 5516

$C_{21}H_{31}N_5O_2$
 Buspirone, 1504

$C_{21}H_{32}N_2O$
 Stanozolol, 8794

$C_{21}H_{32}N_4O_{10}S_2$
 Propamidine Isethionate, 7797

$C_{21}H_{32}N_6O_3$
 Alfentanil, 236

$C_{21}H_{32}O$
 Allylestrenol, 291

$C_{21}H_{32}O_2$
 3,20-Allopregnanedione, 272
 Bolasterone, 1323
 Calusterone, 1722
 Methyl Abietate, 6006
 Norbolethone, 6686
 3,20-Pregnanedione, 7728
 Pregnenolone, 7733

$C_{21}H_{32}O_3$
 Alfaxalone, 235
 Oxymetholone, 6967

$C_{21}H_{32}O_4$
 4-Pregnene-17α,20β,21-triol-3-one, 7732

$C_{21}H_{32}O_5$
 Allotetrahydrocortisone, 281
 Hydrallostane, 4764
 4-Pregnene-11β,17α,20β,21-tetrol-3-one, 7730
 Tetrahydrocortisone, 9210

$C_{21}H_{33}NO_7$
 Lasiocarpine, 5375

$C_{21}H_{33}N_2O_6P$
 Ceronapril, 1994

$C_{21}H_{33}N_3O$
 Sitamaquine, 8553

$C_{21}H_{33}N_3O_2$
 Eptastigmine, 3638

$C_{21}H_{33}N_3O_5S$
 Amdinocillin Pivoxil, 390

$C_{21}H_{34}BrNO_3$
 Oxyphenonium Bromide, 6975

$C_{21}H_{34}O_2$
 Allopregnan-3α-ol-20-one, 275
 Allopregnan-3β-ol-20-one, 276
 Allopregnan-20α-ol-3-one, 277
 Allopregnan-20β-ol-3-one, 278
 Pregnan-3α-ol-20-one, 7729

$C_{21}H_{34}O_3$
 Allopregnane-3β,17α-diol-20-one, 271

$C_{21}H_{34}O_4$
 Allopregnane-3β,11β,21-triol-20-one, 274

$C_{21}H_{34}O_5$
 Allopregnane-3α,11β,17α,21-tetrol-20-one, 273
 Arbaprostil, 769
 Cortolone, 2542

$C_{21}H_{35}ClN_2O_3$
 Lapyrium Chloride, 5370

$C_{21}H_{35}NO$
 Amorolfine, 573
 Funtumine, 4292

$C_{21}H_{35}NO_5S$
 Procyclidine Methosulfate, 7763

$C_{21}H_{36}$
 Allopregnane, 266
 Pregnane, 7726

$C_{21}H_{36}INO$
 Tridihexethyl Iodide, 9661

$C_{21}H_{36}N_2O_5S$
 Hexocyclium Methyl Sulfate, 4706

$C_{21}H_{36}N_7O_{16}P_3S$
 Coenzyme A, 2466

$C_{21}H_{36}O_2$
 Allopregnane-3α,20α-diol, 267
 Allopregnane-3α,20β-diol, 268
 Allopregnane-3β,20α-diol, 269
 Allopregnane-3β,20β-diol, 270
 3-Pentadecylcatechol, 7110
 Pregnanediol, 7727
 Uranediol, 9853

$C_{21}H_{36}O_5$
 Carboprost, 1823
 Cortol, 2541

$C_{21}H_{38}ClN$
 Cetylpyridinium Chloride, 2032

$C_{21}H_{38}N_2OS$
 Kalkitoxin, 5277

$C_{21}H_{38}O_4$
 Rioprostil, 8231

$C_{21}H_{39}N_7O_{12}$
 Streptomycin, 8826

$C_{21}H_{40}N_8O_6$
 Tuftsin, 9809

$C_{21}H_{41}N_5O_7$
 Netilmicin, 6479

$C_{21}H_{41}N_5O_{11}$
 Apramycin, 752

$C_{21}H_{41}N_5O_{12}$
 Butirosin, 1528

$C_{21}H_{41}N_7O_{11}$
 Deoxydihydrostreptomycin, 2902

$C_{21}H_{41}N_7O_{12}$
 Dihydrostreptomycin, 3179

$C_{21}H_{43}N_5O_7$
 Gentamicin C_1, 4392

$C_{21}H_{44}O_3$
 Batyl Alcohol, 1011

$C_{21}H_{45}N_3$
 Hexetidine, 4703

$C_{24}H_{20}I_6N_4O_8$
Iocarmic Acid, 5009
$C_{24}H_{20}N_2$
N,N'-Diphenylbenzidine, 3319
$C_{24}H_{20}N_4O$
Scarlet Red, 8393
$C_{24}H_{20}N_6O_3$
Candesartan, 1739
$C_{24}H_{20}P^+$
Tetraphenylphosphonium, 9237
$C_{24}H_{21}F_2NO_3$
Ezetimibe, 3918
$C_{24}H_{21}I_6N_5O_8$
Ioxaglic Acid, 5067
$C_{24}H_{22}FN_3O_4$
Exatecan, 3912
$C_{24}H_{22}F_3N$
Xaliproden, 10054
$C_{24}H_{23}N_3O_2$
Bifeprunox, 1210
$C_{24}H_{23}N_3O_6S$
Talampicillin, 9033
$C_{24}H_{24}CaI_6N_4O_4$
Ipodate Calcium Salt, 5071
$C_{24}H_{24}N_2O_5$
Amtolmetin Guacil, 596
$C_{24}H_{25}ClFN_5O_3$
Canertinib, 1744
$C_{24}H_{25}FNNaO_4$
Fluvastatin Sodium Salt, 4218
$C_{24}H_{25}FN_6O$
Mizolastine, 6221
$C_{24}H_{25}NO_3$
Benzylmorphine, 1141
Cyphenothrin, 2768
$C_{24}H_{25}NO_4$
Flavoxate, 4096
$C_{24}H_{26}BrN_3O_3$
Nicergoline, 6496
$C_{24}H_{26}ClFN_4O$
Sertindole, 8466
$C_{24}H_{26}FNO_4$
Fluvastatin, 4218
$C_{24}H_{26}MgO_8$
Dimecrotic Acid Magnesium Salt,
3203
$C_{24}H_{26}N_2O_4$
Carvedilol, 1873
$C_{24}H_{26}N_2O_6$
Suxibuzone, 9009
$C_{24}H_{26}N_8O_9$
Diopterin, 3291
$C_{24}H_{26}O_6$
Mangostin, 5742
$C_{24}H_{26}O_{13}$
Centaurein, 1968
Irigenin 7-Glucoside, 5090
$C_{24}H_{27}FN_2O_4$
Iloperidone, 4900
$C_{24}H_{27}N$
Prenylamine, 7737
$C_{24}H_{27}NO_2$
Octocrylene, 6756
$C_{24}H_{27}NO_4$
Tylocrebrine, 9830
Tylophorine, 9831
$C_{24}H_{27}NO_5S$
Troglitazone, 9769
$C_{24}H_{27}N_3O_4$
Fenpyroximate, 3996
$C_{24}H_{28}BiN_4Na_7O_{25}$
Bismuth Sodium Triglycollamate,
1280
$C_{24}H_{28}ClN_5O_3$
Dimenhydrinate, 3207

$C_{24}H_{28}F_3N_3O_3$
Tafenoquine, 9029
$C_{24}H_{28}N_2O_3$
Naftopidil, 6356
$C_{24}H_{28}N_2O_5$
Benazepril, 1031
$C_{24}H_{28}N_4O_6$
Lamifiban, 5349
$C_{24}H_{28}O_2$
Bexarotene, 1194
$C_{24}H_{28}O_4$
Diethylstilbestrol Dipropionate, 3129
$C_{24}H_{29}BrFNO_3$
Flutropium Bromide, 4216
$C_{24}H_{29}ClO_4$
Cyproterone Acetate, 2774
$C_{24}H_{29}Cl_2FO_5$
Flucloronide, 4121
$C_{24}H_{29}FN_2O_2$
Aceperone, 30
$C_{24}H_{29}FO_6$
Fluprednidene Acetate, 4191
$C_{24}H_{29}NO$
Phenomorphan, 7249
$C_{24}H_{29}NO_3$
Donepezil, 3419
$C_{24}H_{29}NO_4$
Ethaverine, 3728
$C_{24}H_{29}N_5O_3$
Valsartan, 9916
$C_{24}H_{29}NaO_5$
Beraprost Sodium Salt, 1152
Taprostene Sodium Salt, 9057
$C_{24}H_{30}CaN_4O_6$
Cyclobarbital Calcium Salt, 2711
$C_{24}H_{30}ClFO_5$
Clocortolone 21-Acetate, 2369
$C_{24}H_{30}Cl_2O_6$
Etiprednol Dicloacetate, 3870
$C_{24}H_{30}FNa_2O_9P$
Triamcinolone Acetonide 21-Diso-
dium Phosphate, 9596
$C_{24}H_{30}F_2O_6$
Fluocinolone Acetonide, 4150
$C_{24}H_{30}N_2O_2$
Doxapram, 3432
$C_{24}H_{30}N_2O_2S$
Piperacetazine, 7462
$C_{24}H_{30}N_2O_3$
Chromafenozide, 2218
$C_{24}H_{30}N_2O_5$
Demethoxyvindoline, 9988
$C_{24}H_{30}O_3$
Drospirenone, 3454
$C_{24}H_{30}O_5$
Beraprost, 1152
Taprostene, 9057
$C_{24}H_{30}O_6$
Eplerenone, 3625
$C_{24}H_{30}O_7$
Athamantin, 860
$C_{24}H_{30}O_8$
Desaspidin BB, 2917
Flavaspidic Acid, 4090
$C_{24}H_{31}ClO_7$
Loteprednol Etabonate, 5584
$C_{24}H_{31}FO_6$
Betamethasone 21-Acetate, 1180
Dexamethasone 21-Acetate, 2943
Flunisolide, 4145
Fluperolone Acetate, 4188
Paramethasone 21-Acetate, 7029
Triamcinolone Acetonide, 9596
$C_{24}H_{31}NO$
Dipipanone, 3337

$C_{24}H_{31}NO_4$
Drotaverine, 3455
$C_{24}H_{31}N_3OS$
Butaperazine, 1516
$C_{24}H_{31}N_3O_2S$
Carphenazine, 1860
$C_{24}H_{32}ClFO_5$
Halcinonide, 4591
$C_{24}H_{32}N_2O_2$
Eprazinone, 3632
$C_{24}H_{32}O_4$
Acequinocyl, 33
Estradiol Dipropionate, 3703
Ethynodiol Diacetate, 3860
Megestrol Acetate, 5805
Resibufogenin, 8146
Scillarenin, 8400
$C_{24}H_{32}O_4S$
Spironolactone, 8760
$C_{24}H_{32}O_6$
Desonide, 2928
Methylprednisolone 21-Acetate, 6111
$C_{24}H_{32}O_7$
Etiproston, 3871
$C_{24}H_{33}FO_6$
Flurandrenolide, 4197
$C_{24}H_{33}N$
Droprenilamine, 3451
$C_{24}H_{33}NO_3$
Nafronyl, 6353
$C_{24}H_{33}N_3O_2S$
Dixyrazine, 3385
$C_{24}H_{33}N_3O_3S_2$
Pipotiazine, 7482
$C_{24}H_{33}N_3O_4$
Ranolazine, 8111
$C_{24}H_{33}NaO_5$
Dehydrocholic Acid Sodium Salt,
2868
$C_{24}H_{33}NaO_7S$
Bufalin Sodium Sulfate, 1471
$C_{24}H_{34}Br_2N_2O_4$
Hemicholinium Dibromide, 4643
$C_{24}H_{34}N_2Na_2O_{18}S_3$
Glucosulfone Sodium, 4463
$C_{24}H_{34}N_2O$
Bepridil, 1150
$C_{24}H_{34}N_2O_4^{2+}$
Hemicholinium, 4643
$C_{24}H_{34}N_2O_5$
Trandolapril, 9568
$C_{24}H_{34}N_4O_5S$
Glimepiride, 4440
$C_{24}H_{34}N_8O_4S_2$
Thiamine Disulfide, 9297
$C_{24}H_{34}O_3$
Rimexolone, 8226
$C_{24}H_{34}O_4$
Algestone Cyclic Acetal with Ace-
tone, 239
Bufalin, 1471
Medroxyprogesterone 17-Acetate,
5793
$C_{24}H_{34}O_5$
Dehydrocholic Acid, 2868
Gamabufotalin, 4358
$C_{24}H_{34}O_7$
Ajugarin-I, 197
$C_{24}H_{34}O_9$
T-2 Toxin, 9801
$C_{24}H_{35}NO_5$
Decoquinate, 2854
$C_{24}H_{35}N_5O_5$
Ximelagatran, 10077
$C_{24}H_{36}N_2O_9S$
Celesticetin, 1958

C$_{25}$H$_{40}$N$_2$
Papuamine, 7021
C$_{25}$H$_{40}$N$_2$O$_6$S
Leukotriene D$_4$, 5455
C$_{25}$H$_{40}$O$_2$S
Mepitiostane, 5858
C$_{25}$H$_{40}$O$_4$
Pregnanediol Diacetate, 7727
C$_{25}$H$_{41}$NO$_7$
Delsoline, 2882
Lycoctonine, 5618
C$_{25}$H$_{41}$NO$_9$
Aconine, 115
C$_{25}$H$_{42}$N$_2$O
Cyclobuxine D, 2716
C$_{25}$H$_{43}$NO$_7$
Methymycin, 6135
Neomethymycin, 6453
C$_{25}$H$_{43}$NO$_{18}$
Acarbose, 18
C$_{25}$H$_{43}$N$_{13}$O$_9$
Tuberactinomycin O, 9803
C$_{25}$H$_{43}$N$_{13}$O$_{10}$
Enviomycin, 3600
Viomycin, 10001
C$_{25}$H$_{43}$N$_{13}$O$_{11}$
Tuberactinomycin A, 9803
C$_{25}$H$_{44}$N$_2$O
Azacosterol, 892
C$_{25}$H$_{44}$N$_{14}$O$_7$
Capreomycin IB, 1757
C$_{25}$H$_{44}$N$_{14}$O$_8$
Capreomycin IA, 1757
C$_{25}$H$_{44}$O$_5$
Unoprostone Isopropyl Ester, 9849
C$_{25}$H$_{45}$FeN$_6$O$_8$
Deferoxamine Iron Complex, 2860
C$_{25}$H$_{45}$NO$_9$
Pederin, 7065
C$_{25}$H$_{46}$ClN
Cetalkonium Chloride, 2017
C$_{25}$H$_{47}$NO$_8$
Carboprost Tromethamine Salt, 1823
C$_{25}$H$_{48}$N$_6$O$_8$
Deferoxamine, 2860
C$_{25}$H$_{52}$NO$_4$P
Perifosine, 7165
C$_{26}$H$_{16}$N$_3$Na$_3$O$_{10}$S$_3$
Anazolene Sodium, 628
C$_{26}$H$_{18}$CuN$_4$O$_8$
Myxin Copper(II) Complex, 6340
C$_{26}$H$_{19}$NO$_{12}$
Laccaic Acid A, 5330
C$_{26}$H$_{21}$F$_6$NO$_5$
Acrinathrin, 125
C$_{26}$H$_{22}$ClF$_3$N$_2$O$_3$
Fluvalinate, 4217
C$_{26}$H$_{22}$O$_2$
Benzopinacol, 1100
C$_{26}$H$_{23}$F$_2$NO$_4$
Flucythrinate, 4124
C$_{26}$H$_{23}$K$_4$N$_3$O$_{10}$
Quin2, 8042
C$_{26}$H$_{25}$ClN$_2$O$_3$
Tolvaptan, 9540
C$_{26}$H$_{25}$F$_9$N$_2$O$_4$
Torcetrapib, 9549
C$_{26}$H$_{25}$N$_2$NaO$_6$S
Carindacillin Sodium Salt, 1840
C$_{26}$H$_{25}$N$_3$O$_3$S
Fenoverine, 3982
C$_{26}$H$_{25}$N$_3$O$_{11}$
Tunichrome B-1, 9820
C$_{26}$H$_{25}$N$_8$NaO$_{11}$S$_2$
Ceftobiprole Medocaril Sodium Salt, 1952

C$_{26}$H$_{26}$ClN$_3$
Rupatadine, 8297
C$_{26}$H$_{26}$F$_2$N$_2$
Flunarizine, 4144
C$_{26}$H$_{26}$N$_2$O$_2$S
BBOT, 1014
C$_{26}$H$_{26}$N$_2$O$_6$S
Carindacillin, 1840
C$_{26}$H$_{26}$N$_8$O$_{11}$S$_2$
Ceftobiprole Medocaril, 1952
C$_{26}$H$_{27}$ClN$_2$
Clocinizine, 2367
C$_{26}$H$_{27}$ClN$_2$O
Lofepramine, 5557
C$_{26}$H$_{27}$NO$_9$
Idarubicin, 4886
C$_{26}$H$_{27}$NO$_{10}$
Carubicin, 1870
C$_{26}$H$_{28}$ClNO
Clomiphene, 2386
Toremifene, 9550
C$_{26}$H$_{28}$ClN$_3$
Pyrvinium Chloride, 8022
C$_{26}$H$_{28}$Cl$_2$N$_4$O$_4$
Ketoconazole, 5302
C$_{26}$H$_{28}$N$_2$
Cinnarizine, 2305
C$_{26}$H$_{28}$N$_4$O$_2$
Zaldaride, 10110
C$_{26}$H$_{28}$O$_{14}$
Apiin, 732
C$_{26}$H$_{29}$FN$_2$O$_2$
Levocabastine, 5463
C$_{26}$H$_{29}$F$_2$N$_7$
Almitrine, 301
C$_{26}$H$_{29}$NO
Tamoxifen, 9048
C$_{26}$H$_{29}$NO$_2$
Droloxifene, 3446
C$_{26}$H$_{29}$N$_3$O$_6$
Nicardipine, 6495
C$_{26}$H$_{30}$Cl$_2$F$_3$NO
Halofantrine, 4594
C$_{26}$H$_{30}$Na$_2$O$_9$
Estriol 16,17-Bis(sodium Hemisuccinate), 3707
C$_{26}$H$_{30}$O$_8$
Limonin, 5494
Physodic Acid, 7382
C$_{26}$H$_{31}$Cl$_2$N$_5$O$_3$
Terconazole, 9160
C$_{26}$H$_{31}$N$_5$O$_2$
Physostigmine, 7384
C$_{26}$H$_{32}$ClFO$_5$
Clobetasone 17-Butyrate, 2364
C$_{26}$H$_{32}$F$_2$O$_7$
Diflorasone Diacetate, 3140
Fluocinonide, 4151
C$_{26}$H$_{32}$MgN$_6$O$_8$S$_2$
Dipyrone Magnesium Salt, 3350
C$_{26}$H$_{32}$N$_2$O$_5$
Delapril, 2876
C$_{26}$H$_{32}$N$_2$O$_8$
Tritoqualine, 9765
C$_{26}$H$_{33}$FNNaO$_5$
Cerivastatin Sodium Salt, 1993
C$_{26}$H$_{33}$FO$_7$
Flunisolide 21-Acetate, 4145
C$_{26}$H$_{33}$NO$_2$
Fenretinide, 3998
C$_{26}$H$_{33}$NO$_4$
Cyprenorphine, 2769
C$_{26}$H$_{33}$NO$_6$
Lacidipine, 5331

C$_{26}$H$_{33}$NaO$_8$
Methylprednisolone 21-Succinate Sodium Salt, 6111
C$_{26}$H$_{34}$FNO$_5$
Cerivastatin, 1993
C$_{26}$H$_{34}$O$_4$
Methestrol Dipropionate, 5968
C$_{26}$H$_{34}$O$_7$
Cinobufotalin, 2307
Fumagillin, 4286
C$_{26}$H$_{35}$FO$_5$
Fluocortin Butyl, 4152
C$_{26}$H$_{35}$F$_3$O$_6$
Travoprost, 9577
C$_{26}$H$_{35}$NO$_4$
Diprenorphine, 3340
C$_{26}$H$_{36}$N$_2$O$_5$
Zatebradine, 10115
C$_{26}$H$_{36}$N$_2$O$_9$
Antimycin A$_3$, 715
Quinidine Gluconate, 8060
C$_{26}$H$_{36}$O$_3$
Estradiol 17β-Cyclopentanepropanoate, 3703
C$_{26}$H$_{36}$O$_6$
Bufotalin, 1477
Prednisolone 21-Trimethylacetate, 7721
Prednival, 7723
C$_{26}$H$_{37}$ClN$_4$O$_6$S$_2$.H$_2$O
Penicillin O 2-Chloroprocaine Salt Monohydrate, 7099
C$_{26}$H$_{37}$N$_5$O$_2$
Cabergoline, 1601
C$_{26}$H$_{38}$N$_2$O$_4$
Mazipredone, 5763
C$_{26}$H$_{38}$O$_3$
Pentagestrone, 7114
C$_{26}$H$_{38}$O$_4$
Gestonorone Caproate, 4414
Lupulon, 5612
C$_{26}$H$_{38}$O$_5$S
Tixocortol 21-Pivalate, 9484
C$_{26}$H$_{38}$O$_6$
Hydrocortisone 17-Valerate, 4787
C$_{26}$H$_{39}$NO$_6$S
Epothilone A, 3628
C$_{26}$H$_{40}$Cl$_4$N$_5$O$_{10}$PS
Canfosfamide, 1745
C$_{26}$H$_{40}$N$_4$O$_9$S
Sampatrilat, 8352
C$_{26}$H$_{40}$O$_3$
Testosterone Enanthate, 9180
C$_{26}$H$_{40}$O$_4$
Methandriol Dipropionate, 5950
C$_{26}$H$_{40}$O$_5$
Latanoprost, 5376
C$_{26}$H$_{41}$Br$_2$NO$_4$
Pinaverium Bromide, 7441
C$_{26}$H$_{41}$NO
Melinamide, 5822
C$_{26}$H$_{42}$O$_4$
DINP, 3290
Maxacalcitol, 5760
C$_{26}$H$_{42}$O$_9$
Pseudomonic Acid D, 7918
C$_{26}$H$_{43}$NO$_6$
Glycocholic Acid, 4494
C$_{26}$H$_{44}$NNaO$_7$S
Taurocholic Acid Sodium Salt, 9075
C$_{26}$H$_{44}$O$_2$
Tocol, 9494
C$_{26}$H$_{44}$O$_8$
Pseudomonic Acid C, 7918
C$_{26}$H$_{44}$O$_9$
Mupirocin, 6302

$C_{27}H_{46}N_2O_2$
Solanocapsine, 8706
$C_{27}H_{46}O$
Allocholesterol, 264
Cholesterol, 2201
Epicholesterol, 3613
$C_{27}H_{46}O_2$
24-Hydroxycholesterol, 4820
25-Hydroxycholesterol, 4821
δ-Tocopherol, 9498
$C_{27}H_{47}ClN_2O_3$
Lapyrium Chloride Stearoyl Analog, 5370
$C_{27}H_{48}$
(5α)-Cholestane, 2199
Coprostane, 2523
$C_{27}H_{48}N_6O_9$
Nocardamin, 6665
$C_{27}H_{48}O$
Cholestanol, 2200
Coprosterol, 2524
Epicholestanol, 3612
$C_{27}H_{50}N_6O_9$
Deferoxamine N-Acetyl Derivative, 2860
$C_{27}H_{58}N_2O_3.2HF$
Olaflur, 6820
$C_{28}H_{14}N_2O_4$
Indanthrene, 4934
$C_{28}H_{15}NO_4$
Anthrimide, 690
$C_{28}H_{17}N_3O_4$
Bis(4-amino-1-anthraquinonyl)amine, 1243
$C_{28}H_{18}O_4$
α-Naphtholphthalein, 6389
$C_{28}H_{19}N_5Na_2O_6S_4$
Thiazol Yellow G, 9310
$C_{28}H_{20}CaN_2O_8.5H_2O$
Benzoylpas Calcium Salt Pentahydrate, 1115
$C_{28}H_{20}N_2Na_2O_8S_2$
Alizarin Cyanine Green F, 252
$C_{28}H_{22}Cl_2FNO_3$
Flumethrin, 4140
$C_{28}H_{22}N_2O_2$
Quinizarin Green SS, 8065
$C_{28}H_{22}N_4Na_2O_8S_2$
Blankophor® R, 1315
$C_{28}H_{24}Br_2N_6$
Fazadinium Bromide, 3943
$C_{28}H_{24}ClNO_6$
Tropesin, 9778
$C_{28}H_{25}N_6NaO_{10}S_2$
Cefpimizole Monosodium Salt, 1938
$C_{28}H_{26}ClN_7$
Isometamidium Chloride, 5183
$C_{28}H_{26}N_4O_3$
Staurosporine, 8802
$C_{28}H_{26}N_6O_{10}S_2$
Cefpimizole, 1938
$C_{28}H_{27}ClF_5NO$
Penfluridol, 7087
$C_{28}H_{27}NO_4S$
Raloxifene, 8098
$C_{28}H_{28}N_2O_2$
Difenoxin, 3136
$C_{28}H_{28}N_4O_3$
Ruboxistaurin, 8290
$C_{28}H_{28}O_3$
Adapalene, 150
$C_{28}H_{28}O_{11}$
Aloeresin A, 305
$C_{28}H_{28}P_2$
(S,S)-Chiraphos, 2063

$C_{28}H_{29}ClN_4S$
Israpafant, 5241
$C_{28}H_{29}F_2N_3O$
Pimozide, 7435
$C_{28}H_{29}NO_4$
Bephenium Hydroxynaphthoate, 1148
$C_{28}H_{29}NO_4S$
Arzoxifene, 820
$C_{28}H_{30}INO$
Idoxifene, 4890
$C_{28}H_{30}N_2O_2$
Darifenacin, 2825
$C_{28}H_{30}O_4$
Thymolphthalein, 9401
$C_{28}H_{30}O_{14}.3H_2O$
Pseudobaptigenin 7-Rhamnoglucoside Trihydrate, 7911
$C_{28}H_{31}ClN_2O_3$
Rhodamine B, 8183
$C_{28}H_{31}FN_4O$
Astemizole, 856
$C_{28}H_{31}NO_5$
Bitolterol, 1307
$C_{28}H_{31}NO_9$
Rhodomycin B, 8190
$C_{28}H_{31}N_3O_6$
Benidipine, 1043
$C_{28}H_{31}NaO_9S$
Prednisolone 21-m-Sulfobenzoate Sodium Salt, 7721
$C_{28}H_{32}FNO_6$
Dexamethasone 21-Isonicotinate, 2943
$C_{28}H_{32}IN_3S_2$
Tibezonium Iodide, 9426
$C_{28}H_{32}O_{14}$
Acacetin 7-Rhamnoglucoside, 13
Linarin, 5498
$C_{28}H_{32}O_{15}$
Diosmin, 3297
$C_{28}H_{33}ClN_2$
Buclizine, 1464
$C_{28}H_{33}ClO_{16}$
Peonidin 3,5-Diglucoside, 7143
$C_{28}H_{33}ClO_{17}$
Petunidin 3,5-Diglucoside, 7190
$C_{28}H_{33}NO_2$
Xenbucin trans-4-Phenylcyclohexylamine Salt (1:1), 10071
$C_{28}H_{34}N_2O_3$
Denatonium Benzoate, 2891
$C_{28}H_{34}O_8$
Uliginosin B, 9845
$C_{28}H_{34}O_8S_2$
Ecamsule, 3490
$C_{28}H_{34}O_9$
Nomilin, 6674
$C_{28}H_{34}O_{15}$
Hesperidin, 4671
$C_{28}H_{35}ClN_4O$
Mosapramine, 6278
$C_{28}H_{35}FO_7$
Amcinonide, 388
$C_{28}H_{35}FO_9$
Triamcinolone Acetonide 21-Hemisuccinate, 9596
$C_{28}H_{35}NO_4$
Asoprisnil, 834
$C_{28}H_{35}N_3O_5$
Paraherquamide, 7026
$C_{28}H_{35}N_3O_7$
Virginiamycin M_1, 10004
$C_{28}H_{36}N_2O_4$
Psychotrine, 7929
$C_{28}H_{36}O_6$
Clinofibrate, 2357

$C_{28}H_{36}O_8$
Uliginosin A, 9845
$C_{28}H_{36}O_{11}$
Bruceantin, 1454
$C_{28}H_{36}O_{15}$
Neohesperidin Dihydrochalcone, 6452
$C_{28}H_{37}ClN_4O$
Clocapramine, 2366
$C_{28}H_{37}ClO_7$
Alclometasone 17,21-Dipropionate, 220
Beclomethasone Dipropionate, 1019
$C_{28}H_{37}FO_7$
Betamethasone 17,21-Dipropionate, 1180
Dexamethasone 17,21-Dipropionate, 2943
$C_{28}H_{37}N_5O_7$
Leu⁵-Enkephalin, 3572
$C_{28}H_{38}BrNO_4$
Butropium Bromide, 1534
$C_{28}H_{38}N_2O_4$
Cephaeline, 1973
$C_{28}H_{38}N_2O_6$
Simetride, 8535
$C_{28}H_{38}N_4O$
Carpipramine, 1861
$C_{28}H_{38}N_4O_8$
Pactamycin, 6985
$C_{28}H_{38}O_6$
Withaferin A, 10048
$C_{28}H_{38}O_7$
Bongkrekic Acid, 1332
Prednival 21-Acetate, 7723
$C_{28}H_{38}O_{19}$
Octaacetyl-aldehydo-cellobiose, 1961
Sucrose Octaacetate, 8882
$C_{28}H_{39}FO_5$
Fluocortolone 21-Hexanoate, 4153
$C_{28}H_{40}N_2O_5$
Gallopamil, 4356
$C_{28}H_{40}N_2O_9$
Antimycin A_1, 714
$C_{28}H_{40}O_4$
Pentagestrone Acetate, 7114
$C_{28}H_{40}O_7$
Diginin, 3157
$C_{28}H_{41}N_3O_2$
Teleocidin B_4, 9118
$C_{28}H_{41}N_3O_3$
Oxethazaine, 6933
Tiropramide, 9466
$C_{28}H_{41}N_3O_8$
Detoxin D_1, 2938
$C_{28}H_{42}Cl_4N_4O_2$
Ambenonium Chloride, 379
$C_{28}H_{42}N_2O_5$
Fenoxedil, 3986
$C_{28}H_{42}O$
Dehydroergosterol, 2872
$C_{28}H_{42}O_2$
β-Tocotrienol, 9501
$C_{28}H_{44}ClNO_2$
Methylbenzethonium Chloride, 6023
$C_{28}H_{44}O$
Ergosterol, 3659
Fungisterol, 4291
Isopyrocalciferol, 5219
Lumisterol, 5602
Pyrocalciferol, 7997
Suprasterol II, 9004
Tachysterol, 9023
Vitamin D_2, 10018

$C_{28}H_{44}O_2$
Doxercalciferol, 3436

$C_{28}H_{44}O_3$
Nandrolone Decanoate, 6365

$C_{28}H_{46}O$
Dihydrotachysterol, 3180
Ergosterol 22,23-Dihydro Analog, 3659
Vitamin D_4, 10020

$C_{28}H_{47}NO_4S$
Tiamulin, 9419

$C_{28}H_{47}NO_7$
Narbomycin, 6421

$C_{28}H_{47}NO_8$
Picromycin, 7413

$C_{28}H_{48}O$
Campesterol, 1729

$C_{28}H_{48}O_2$
β-Tocopherol, 9496
γ-Tocopherol, 9497

$C_{28}H_{48}O_6$
Brassinolide, 1365

$C_{28}H_{50}$
Ergostane, 3657

$C_{28}H_{50}N_2O_4$
Carpaine, 1858

$C_{28}H_{50}N_4O_7$
Epoxomicin, 3630

$C_{28}H_{50}O$
Ergostanol, 3658

$C_{28}H_{54}GdN_5O_{20}$
Gadopentetic Acid Dimeglumine Salt, 4327

$C_{28}H_{58}NO_7P$
1-O-Octadecyl-PAF, 7524

$C_{28}H_{58}O$
Octacosanol, 6744

$C_{28}H_{60}Al_{14}O_{71}S_7$
Dosmalfate, 3427

$C_{29}H_{24}N_4O_8$
Niceritrol, 6497

$C_{29}H_{24}N_6$
Sudan Black B, 8885

$C_{29}H_{24}O_{12}$
Theaflavine, 9274

$C_{29}H_{25}NO_3$
Py-Phe, 7952

$C_{29}H_{25}N_3O_5$
Nicomorphine, 6520

$C_{29}H_{26}ClFN_4O_4S$
Lapatinib, 5367

$C_{29}H_{27}ClN_2O_{14}S$
Meclocycline 5-Sulfosalicylate, 5778

$C_{29}H_{27}NO_4S_2$
Tipepidine Hibenzate, 9457

$C_{29}H_{27}N_3O_{14}$
Fura-2, 4293

$C_{29}H_{28}N_2O_7$
Muraglitazar, 6303

$C_{29}H_{28}N_4O_{11}$
Edotecarin, 3512

$C_{29}H_{30}N_6O_6$
Olmesartan, 6839

$C_{29}H_{30}O_{13}$
Amarogentin, 377

$C_{29}H_{31}F_2N_3O$
Fluspirilene, 4207

$C_{29}H_{31}N_7O$
Imatinib, 4902

$C_{29}H_{32}ClN_5O_2$
Pyronaridine, 8005

$C_{29}H_{32}N_2O_6S$
Semotiadil, 8446

$C_{29}H_{32}O_{13}$
Etoposide, 3886

$C_{29}H_{33}ClN_2O_2$
Loperamide, 5571

$C_{29}H_{33}FN_2O_6$
Elgodipine, 3546

$C_{29}H_{33}FO_6$
Betamethasone 17-Benzoate, 1180

$C_{29}H_{33}N_9O_{12}$
Pteropterin, 7934

$C_{29}H_{33}O_{16}P$
Etoposide Phosphate, 3886

$C_{29}H_{34}N_2O_2$
Dotarizine, 3428

$C_{29}H_{34}O_6$
Tribenoside, 9608

$C_{29}H_{34}O_{15}$
Pectolinarigenin 7-Rutinoside, 7064

$C_{29}H_{35}ClO_{17}$
Malvidin Chloride 3,5-Diglucoside, 5715

$C_{29}H_{35}NO_2$
Mifepristone, 6186

$C_{29}H_{36}N_2O_4$
Emetamine, 3559

$C_{29}H_{36}O_4$
Algestone Acetophenide, 240

$C_{29}H_{36}O_7$
O-Cinnamoyltaxicin-I, 9077

$C_{29}H_{37}NO_5$
Cytochalasin B, 2790

$C_{29}H_{37}N_3O_6$
Calcimycin, 1639

$C_{29}H_{38}ClFO_8$
Formocortal, 4243

$C_{29}H_{38}FN_3O_3$
Mibefradil, 6173

$C_{29}H_{38}F_3N_3O_2S$
Fluphenazine Enanthate, 4189

$C_{29}H_{38}N_2O_4$
Dehydroemetine, 2870

$C_{29}H_{38}N_2O_6$
Atrasentan, 870

$C_{29}H_{38}N_4O_6S.H_2O$
Penicillin G Procaine, 7097

$C_{29}H_{38}N_4O_9$
Pipacycline, 7453

$C_{29}H_{38}N_4O_{10}$
Lymecycline, 5628

$C_{29}H_{38}N_8O_8$
Guamecycline, 4557

$C_{29}H_{38}O_9$
Uscharidin, 9892

$C_{29}H_{39}NO_2$
Mofarotene, 6230

$C_{29}H_{39}NO_3$
Onapristone, 6847

$C_{29}H_{39}N_3O_2$
Echinuline, 3499

$C_{29}H_{39}N_5O_8$
Tigecycline, 9432

$C_{29}H_{40}N_2O_4$
Emetine, 3559

$C_{29}H_{40}O_6$
Cortisone 21-Cyclopentanepropionate, 2539

$C_{29}H_{40}O_9$
Calotropin, 1720

$C_{29}H_{41}F_2N_5O$
Maraviroc, 5749

$C_{29}H_{41}NO_4$
Buprenorphine, 1497

$C_{29}H_{41}NO_7$
Candoxatril, 1742

$C_{29}H_{41}O_2$
Galvinoxyl, 4357

$C_{29}H_{42}N_6O_9$
Amicetin, 397

$C_{29}H_{42}O_5$
Antheridiol, 681

$C_{29}H_{42}O_9$
Helveticoside, 4632

$C_{29}H_{42}O_{10}$
Adonitoxin, 169
Convallatoxin, 2512

$C_{29}H_{43}BrN_2O_4$
Otilonium Bromide, 6898

$C_{29}H_{43}NO_4S$
Avasimibe, 884

$C_{29}H_{44}O_2$
α-Tocotrienol, 9500

$C_{29}H_{44}O_{12}$
Ouabain, 6901

$C_{29}H_{47}NO_6$
Coumingine, 2565

$C_{29}H_{48}O$
Chondrillasterol, 2211
7-Dehydrositosterol, 2875
Fucosterol, 4280
α-Spinasterol, 8749
Stigmasterol, 8815

$C_{29}H_{50}O_2$
α-Tocopherol, 9495

$C_{29}H_{52}O$
Stigmastanol, 8814

$C_{29}H_{53}NO_5$
Orlistat, 6869

$C_{30}H_{16}O_8$
Hypericin, 4863

$C_{30}H_{18}$
9,10-Bis(phenylethynyl)anthracene, 1299

$C_{30}H_{21}FeN_3O_{15}{}^{3-}$
Ferric Enterobactin, 3596

$C_{30}H_{21}NO_9$
Fredericamycin A, 4267

$C_{30}H_{23}BrO_4$
Bromadiolone, 1382

$C_{30}H_{26}CaO_6.2H_2O$
Fenoprofen Calcium Salt Dihydrate, 3980

$C_{30}H_{26}MgO_8$
Menbutone Magnesium Salt, 5834

$C_{30}H_{26}O_{14}$
Ergoflavin, 3652

$C_{30}H_{27}N_3O_{15}$
Enterobactin, 3596

$C_{30}H_{28}N_2Na_4O_{14}S_5$
Solasulfone, 8711

$C_{30}H_{28}N_6O_6S_4$
Verticillin A, 9968

$C_{30}H_{28}N_6O_7S_4$
Verticillin B, 9968

$C_{30}H_{28}N_6O_7S_5$
Verticillin C, 9968

$C_{30}H_{28}O_8$
Rottlerin, 8272

$C_{30}H_{30}N_4$
Bis(p-dimethylaminobenzylidene)-benzidine, 1249

$C_{30}H_{30}O_8$
Gossypol, 4528

$C_{30}H_{31}ClN_6$
Janus Green B, 5255

$C_{30}H_{32}Cl_3NO$
Lumefantrine, 5597

$C_{30}H_{32}N_2O_2$
Diphenoxylate, 3313

$C_{30}H_{34}N_2O_3$
Bazedoxifene, 1013

$C_{30}H_{34}O_{13}$
Picrotoxin, 7415

$C_{30}H_{35}BrN_{12}O_5$
Brostallicin, 1449

C$_{32}$H$_{45}$NO$_7$
  Milbemycin Oxime, 6190
C$_{32}$H$_{45}$N$_3$O$_4$S
  Nelfinavir, 6443
C$_{32}$H$_{46}$N$_8$O$_6$S$_2$
  Thiamine Disulfide O,O-Diisobutyrate, 9297
C$_{32}$H$_{46}$O$_7$
  Milbemycin A$_4$, 6189
C$_{32}$H$_{46}$O$_8$
  Cucurbitacin B, 2614
C$_{32}$H$_{47}$F$_5$O$_3$S
  Fulvestrant, 4284
C$_{32}$H$_{48}$O$_5$
  Acetoxolone, 76
C$_{32}$H$_{48}$O$_7$
  Milbemycin β_1, 6191
C$_{32}$H$_{48}$O$_9$
  Neriifolin 2′-Acetate, 6474
  Oleandrin, 6826
C$_{32}$H$_{49}$NO$_9$
  Cevadine, 2033
C$_{32}$H$_{51}$NO$_8$S
  Tiamulin Fumarate, 9419
C$_{32}$H$_{52}$Br$_2$N$_4$O$_4$
  Demecarium Bromide, 2885
C$_{32}$H$_{52}$O$_2$
  Taraxasterol Acetate, 9060
C$_{32}$H$_{53}$N$_2$O$_4$$^+$
  Rocuronium, 8246
C$_{32}$H$_{56}$N$_4$O$_8$
  Sporidesmolide III, 8765
C$_{32}$H$_{58}$N$_2$O$_7$S
  CHAPS, 2044
C$_{32}$H$_{58}$N$_2$O$_8$S
  CHAPS Hydroxy Analog, 2044
C$_{32}$H$_{62}$CaO$_4$
  Calcium Palmitate, 1687
C$_{32}$H$_{64}$O$_2$
  Cetyl Palmitate, 2031
C$_{32}$H$_{64}$O$_4$Sn
  Dibutyltin Dilaurate, 3038
C$_{33}$H$_{25}$F$_3$O$_4$
  Flocoumafen, 4102
C$_{33}$H$_{25}$N$_3$O$_3$
  Norbormide, 6687
C$_{33}$H$_{30}$N$_4$O$_2$
  Telmisartan, 9129
C$_{33}$H$_{34}$N$_4$O$_6$
  Azelnidipine, 907
  Biliverdine, 1219
C$_{33}$H$_{34}$N$_6$O$_6$
  Candesartan 1-[[(Cyclohexyloxy)-carbonyl]oxy]ethyl Ester, 1739
C$_{33}$H$_{35}$FN$_2$O$_5$
  Atorvastatin, 864
C$_{33}$H$_{35}$N$_5$O$_5$
  Ergotamine, 3661
  Ergotaminine, 3662
C$_{33}$H$_{36}$N$_4$O$_6$
  Bilirubin, 1218
C$_{33}$H$_{37}$N$_5$O$_5$
  Dihydroergotamine, 3174
C$_{33}$H$_{38}$GdN$_3$Na$_3$O$_{14}$P
  Gadofosveset Trisodium Salt, 4325
C$_{33}$H$_{38}$N$_4$O$_6$
  Irinotecan, 5091
C$_{33}$H$_{40}$N$_2$O$_9$
  Deserpidine 10-Methoxy Deriv, 2918
  Reserpine, 8145
C$_{33}$H$_{40}$O$_{15}$
  Icariin, 3617
C$_{33}$H$_{40}$O$_{19}$
  Robinin, 8243

C$_{33}$H$_{41}$GdN$_3$O$_{14}$P
  Gadofosveset, 4325
C$_{33}$H$_{42}$O$_{19}$
  Troxerutin, 9789
C$_{33}$H$_{43}$FN$_{10}$O$_6$
  Nemifitide, 6445
C$_{33}$H$_{43}$N$_3$O$_6$
  Aplaviroc, 737
C$_{33}$H$_{44}$N$_4$O$_{10}$
  Riboflavin 2′,3′,4′,5′-Tetrabutyrate, 8200
C$_{33}$H$_{44}$O$_8$
  Helvolic Acid, 4633
C$_{33}$H$_{45}$NO$_9$
  Delphinine, 2881
C$_{33}$H$_{46}$Bi$_2$O$_{11}$
  d-Camphocarboxylic Acid Basic Bismuth Salt, 1731
C$_{33}$H$_{46}$O$_4$
  Nandrolone p-Hexyloxyphenylpropionate, 6365
C$_{33}$H$_{47}$NO$_{13}$
  Natamycin, 6427
C$_{33}$H$_{48}$O$_6$
  Leptomycin B, 5444
C$_{33}$H$_{48}$O$_7$
  Milbemycin D, 6191
C$_{33}$H$_{50}$O$_8$
  Cephalosporin P$_1$, 1981
C$_{33}$H$_{53}$NO$_8$
  Imperialine β-D-Glucopyranoside, 4926
C$_{33}$H$_{55}$NO$_8$
  Discodermolide, 3355
  Verticine 3-Glucoside, 9969
C$_{33}$H$_{57}$N$_3$O$_9$
  Enniatin B, 3585
C$_{33}$H$_{58}$N$_4$O$_8$
  Sporidesmolide I, 8765
C$_{34}$H$_{24}$CaCl$_2$N$_4$O$_4$
  Lonazolac Calcium Salt, 5566
C$_{34}$H$_{24}$N$_4$Na$_2$O$_{10}$S$_2$
  Benzo Azurine G, 1085
C$_{34}$H$_{24}$N$_6$Na$_4$O$_{14}$S$_4$
  Evan's Blue, 3905
  Trypan Blue, 9792
C$_{34}$H$_{25}$N$_6$Na$_3$O$_9$S$_3$
  Vital Red, 10012
C$_{34}$H$_{26}$N$_6$Na$_2$O$_6$S$_2$
  Benzopurpurine 4B, 1101
C$_{34}$H$_{32}$ClFeN$_4$O$_4$
  Hemin, 4644
C$_{34}$H$_{33}$FeN$_4$O$_4$
  Heme, 4639
C$_{34}$H$_{32}$N$_2$O$_5$
  Micranthine, 6179
C$_{34}$H$_{32}$N$_4$Na$_2$O$_4$
  Protoporphyrin IX Disodium Salt, 7897
C$_{34}$H$_{32}$N$_6$O$_4$
  1,3-Diphenylguanidine Phthalate, 3324
C$_{34}$H$_{33}$FeN$_4$O$_5$
  Hematin, 4635
C$_{34}$H$_{34}$N$_4$O$_4$
  Protoporphyrin IX, 7897
C$_{34}$H$_{35}$N$_3$O$_{10}$
  Zorubicin, 10195
C$_{34}$H$_{36}$F$_3$NO$_{13}$
  Valrubicin, 9915
C$_{34}$H$_{36}$N$_2$O$_6$
  Pseudomorphine, 7919
C$_{34}$H$_{36}$N$_4$O$_6$
  Phytochlorin, 7388
C$_{34}$H$_{38}$N$_3$O$_7$P
  Efonidipine, 3524

C$_{34}$H$_{38}$N$_4$O$_6$
  Hematoporphyrin, 4636
C$_{34}$H$_{40}$O$_{12}$
  PBP, 4081
C$_{34}$H$_{41}$N$_3$O$_7$
  Biricodar, 1240
C$_{34}$H$_{46}$ClN$_3$O$_{10}$
  Maytansine, 5761
C$_{34}$H$_{46}$O$_8$
  Helvolic Acid Methyl Ester, 4633
C$_{34}$H$_{47}$NO$_{11}$
  Aconitine, 118
C$_{34}$H$_{48}$I$_6$N$_4$O$_{16}$
  Iodipamide Bis[N-methylglucamine] Salt, 5022
C$_{34}$H$_{48}$N$_2$O$_9$
  Ajacine, 5618
C$_{34}$H$_{48}$Na$_2$O$_7$
  Carbenoxolone Disodium Salt, 1793
C$_{34}$H$_{50}$N$_4$O$_9$S
  Dalfopristin, 2804
C$_{34}$H$_{50}$O$_7$
  Carbenoxolone, 1793
C$_{34}$H$_{50}$O$_{12}$
  Thapsigargin, 9272
C$_{34}$H$_{51}$NO$_{13}$
  Tetrin A, 9245
C$_{34}$H$_{51}$NO$_{14}$
  Tetrin B, 9245
C$_{34}$H$_{53}$NaO$_8$
  Lasalocid A Sodium Salt, 5373
C$_{34}$H$_{54}$O$_8$
  Lasalocid A, 5373
C$_{34}$H$_{56}$CuN$_6$O$_{14}$S$_4$
  Cuproxoline, 2670
C$_{34}$H$_{57}$BrN$_2$O$_4$
  Vecuronium Bromide, 9941
C$_{34}$H$_{59}$NO$_{15}$
  Fumonisin B$_1$, 4289
C$_{34}$H$_{60}$N$_4$O$_8$
  Sporidesmolide II, 8765
C$_{34}$H$_{63}$N$_5$O$_9$
  Pepstatin, 7147
C$_{34}$H$_{67}$N$_3$O$_5$S
  Squalamine, 8766
C$_{35}$H$_{30}$N$_4$O$_4$
  Midostaurin, 6185
C$_{35}$H$_{34}$N$_2$O$_5$
  Trilobine, 9697
C$_{35}$H$_{35}$ClNNaO$_3$S
  Montelukast Monosodium Salt, 6258
C$_{35}$H$_{36}$ClNO$_3$S
  Montelukast, 6258
C$_{35}$H$_{36}$N$_2$O$_6$
  Daphnoline, 2819
C$_{35}$H$_{38}$Cl$_2$N$_8$O$_4$
  Itraconazole, 5245
C$_{35}$H$_{38}$F$_2$N$_8$O$_4$
  Saperconazole, 8362
C$_{35}$H$_{38}$N$_4$O$_6$
  Manidipine, 5743
C$_{35}$H$_{39}$N$_5$O$_5$
  Ergocristine, 3649
C$_{35}$H$_{42}$FNO$_8$
  Triamcinolone Benetonide, 9597
C$_{35}$H$_{42}$N$_2$O$_9$
  Rescinnamine, 8142
C$_{35}$H$_{42}$N$_2$O$_{11}$
  Syrosingopine, 9017
C$_{35}$H$_{42}$O$_9$
  O-Cinnamoyltaxicin-II Triacetate, 9077
C$_{35}$H$_{42}$O$_{10}$
  O-Cinnamoyltaxicin-I Triacetate, 9077

$C_{38}H_{44}O_8$
Gambogic Acid, 4361
$C_{38}H_{49}N_3O_5$
Bemotrizinol, 1028
$C_{38}H_{50}N_6O_5$
Saquinavir, 8369
$C_{38}H_{51}NO_4$
Myrophine, 6337
$C_{38}H_{52}N_6O_2$
Tirilazad, 9463
$C_{38}H_{52}N_6O_7$
Atazanavir, 858
$C_{38}H_{54}I_6N_6O_{18}$
Iocarmic Acid Di-N-methylglucamine
Salt, 5009
$C_{38}H_{54}O_{13}$
Colocynthin, 2487
$C_{38}H_{55}Na_9O_{49}S_7$
Idraparinux Sodium, 4892
$C_{38}H_{58}CaN_4O_{10}S_2$
Moveltipril Calcium Salt, 6285
$C_{38}H_{60}O_{18}$
Stevioside, 8810
$C_{38}H_{61}I_2N_3S_3$
Platonin, 7530
$C_{38}H_{69}NO_{13}$
Clarithromycin, 2339
$C_{38}H_{72}N_2O_{12}$
Azithromycin, 915
$C_{39}H_{43}N_3O_{11}S$
Ecteinascidin 743, 3503
$C_{39}H_{47}NO_{14}$
Rifamycin O, 8217
Streptovaricin F, 8830
$C_{39}H_{49}NO_{14}$
Rifamycin B, 8217
$C_{39}H_{49}NO_{16}$
Nogalamycin, 6671
$C_{39}H_{53}N_9O_{15}S$
β-Amanitin, 373
$C_{39}H_{54}N_{10}O_{14}S$
α-Amanitin, 373
$C_{39}H_{54}O_{13}$
Zaragozic Acid B, 10114
$C_{39}H_{61}NO_{14}$
Rimocidin, 8228
$C_{40}H_{32}Cl_2N_8O_2$
Tetrazolium Blue, 9244
$C_{40}H_{43}ClN_4O_{11}$
Rhod-2, 8182
$C_{40}H_{44}N_4O^{2+}$
C-Curarine I, 2672
$C_{40}H_{46}N_4O_2^{2+}$
Toxiferine I, 9558
$C_{40}H_{48}I_2N_2O_6$
Metocurine Iodide, 6144
$C_{40}H_{48}N_4O_2^{2+}$
C-Toxiferine II, 9558
$C_{40}H_{48}N_4O_3$
Geissospermine, 4381
$C_{40}H_{48}O_4$
Astacin, 853
$C_{40}H_{49}NO_{14}$
Streptovaricin E, 8830
$C_{40}H_{50}O_2$
Rhodoxanthin, 8195
$C_{40}H_{50}O_{14}$
Zaragozic Acid C, 10114
$C_{40}H_{51}NO_{13}$
Streptovaricin D, 8830
$C_{40}H_{51}NO_{14}$
Streptovaricin C, 8830
$C_{40}H_{51}NO_{15}$
Streptovaricin G, 8830
$C_{40}H_{52}CaN_2O_8S_2$
Domitroban Calcium Salt, 3416

$C_{40}H_{52}O_2$
Canthaxanthin, 1753
Torularhodin, 9553
$C_{40}H_{52}O_4$
Astaxanthin, 855
$C_{40}H_{54}O$
Echinenone, 3495
$C_{40}H_{56}$
α-Carotene, 1852
β-Carotene, 1853
γ-Carotene, 1854
δ-Carotene, 1855
Lycopene, 5620
$C_{40}H_{56}O$
Cryptoxanthin, 2609
Lycoxanthin, 5627
Rubixanthin, 8289
$C_{40}H_{56}O_2$
Lycophyll, 5621
Xanthophyll, 10063
Zeaxanthin, 10118
$C_{40}H_{56}O_3$
Capsanthin, 1769
Chrysanthemaxanthin, 2250
Flavoxanthin, 4095
$C_{40}H_{56}O_4$
Violaxanthin, 9998
$C_{40}H_{58}Cl_2N_4$
Bisdequalinium Chloride, 1248
$C_{40}H_{58}O$
Rhodopin, 8191
$C_{40}H_{58}O_4$
Oryzanol A, 6886
$C_{40}H_{60}BNaO_{14}$
Aplasmomycin, 736
$C_{40}H_{60}N_4O_{10}$
Bufotoxin, 1479
$C_{40}H_{60}O_2$
Kitol, 5315
$C_{40}H_{63}N_3O_4S_2$
Pipotiazine Palmitic Ester, 7482
$C_{40}H_{64}O_{12}$
Nonactin, 6675
$C_{40}H_{66}N_6$
Ormosinine, 6871
$C_{40}H_{66}O_{10}$
Venturicidin B, 9947
$C_{40}H_{67}NO_{14}$
Leucomycin A_1, 5453
$C_{40}H_{68}$
Phytofluene, 7389
$C_{40}H_{68}O_{11}$
Nigericin, 6541
$C_{40}H_{71}NO_{14}$
Erythromycin Propionate, 3686
$C_{40}H_{74}CaO_{14}S_2$
Docusate Calcium, 3400
$C_{40}H_{80}NO_8P$
Colfosceril Palmitate, 2477
$C_{41}H_{39}ClO_{21}$
Delphinidin Compound with Glucose
+ Hydroxybenzoic Acid, 2880
$C_{41}H_{42}N_4O_8$
Verteporfin, 9967
$C_{41}H_{48}N_2O_8$
Thalicarpine, 9254
$C_{41}H_{50}N_6O_2$
Bisoctrizole, 1294
$C_{41}H_{52}N_6O_7$
Ergonovine Hydracrylate, 3655
$C_{41}H_{56}O_2$
Menaquinone 6, 5833
$C_{41}H_{58}FeN_9O_{20}$
Ferrichrome A, 4024
$C_{41}H_{60}O_4$
Oryzanol C, 6886

$C_{41}H_{63}NO_{14}$
Protoveratrine A, 7899
$C_{41}H_{63}NO_{15}$
Protoveratrine B, 7899
$C_{41}H_{64}O_8$
Prednisolone 21-Stearoylglycolate,
7721
$C_{41}H_{64}O_{13}$
Digitoxin, 3163
$C_{41}H_{64}O_{14}$
Digoxin, 3167
Gitoxin, 4434
$C_{41}H_{64}O_{15}$
Diginatin, 3156
$C_{41}H_{65}NO_{10}$
Spinosyn A, 8750
$C_{41}H_{65}NO_{15}$
Midecamycin A_3, 6183
$C_{41}H_{66}O_{12}$
α-Hederin, 4625
$C_{41}H_{67}NO_{11}$
Venturicidin A, 9947
$C_{41}H_{67}NO_{15}$
Midecamycin A_1, 6183
Troleandomycin, 9770
$C_{41}H_{76}N_2O_{15}$
Roxithromycin, 8276
$C_{41}H_{79}N_3O_{12}$
Tulathromycin, 9810
$C_{42}H_{27}AlF_9N_3O_6$
Flufenamic Acid Aluminum Salt,
4132
$C_{42}H_{30}N_6O_{12}$
Inositol Niacinate, 4979
$C_{42}H_{38}O_{20}$
Sennosides, 8455
$C_{42}H_{51}NO_{15}$
Aclacinomycin B, 113
$C_{42}H_{53}NO_{15}$
Aclacinomycin A, 113
Streptovaricin J, 8830
$C_{42}H_{53}NO_{16}$
Streptovaricin A, 8830
$C_{42}H_{58}O_6$
Fucoxanthin, 4281
$C_{42}H_{59}N_3O_{10}$
Cethromycin, 2020
$C_{42}H_{60}K_2O_{16}$
Glycyrrhizic Acid Dipotassium Salt,
4505
$C_{42}H_{60}O_2$
Rhodoviolascin, 8194
$C_{42}H_{62}N_8O_7S$
Bottromycin A_2, 1356
$C_{42}H_{62}O_{16}$
Glycyrrhizic Acid, 4505
$C_{42}H_{64}O_{19}$
Thevetin A, 9288
$C_{42}H_{65}N_{11}O_{12}$
Cargutocin, 1839
$C_{42}H_{65}N_{13}O_{10}$
Saralasin, 8372
$C_{42}H_{66}O_{14}$
β-Methyldigoxin, 3167
$C_{42}H_{67}NO_{10}$
Spinosyn D, 8750
$C_{42}H_{67}NO_{15}$
Carbomycin B, 1806
$C_{42}H_{67}NO_{16}$
Carbomycin A, 1806
$C_{42}H_{69}NO_{15}$
Josamycin, 5267
Rokitamycin, 8250
$C_{42}H_{69}NaO_{11}$
Salinomycin Sodium Salt, 8336

$C_{61}H_{90}Cl_2O_{32}$
Avilamycin C, 887
$C_{61}H_{109}N_{11}O_{12}$
Cyclosporin B, 2752
$C_{62}H_{42}O_6Ru_2$
Shvo Catalyst, 8483
$C_{62}H_{80}CaCl_8N_{10}O_{30}$
Chloramphenicol Pantothenate Calcium Complex (4:1), 2077
$C_{62}H_{86}N_{12}O_{16}$
Dactinomycin, 2800
$C_{62}H_{88}CoN_{13}O_{14}P$
Vitamin B_{12r}, 10016
$C_{62}H_{88}CoN_{14}O_{16}P$
Nitrocobalamin, 4809
$C_{62}H_{89}CoN_{13}O_{15}P$
Hydroxocobalamin, 4809
$C_{62}H_{89}CoN_{13}O_{17}PS$
Sulfitocobalamin, 4809
$C_{62}H_{90}CoN_{13}O_{15}P.OH$
Aquacobalamin, 4809
$C_{62}H_{97}N_{23}O_{26}$
Scotophobin, 8411
$C_{62}H_{98}N_{20}O_{26}S_2$
Tallysomycin B, 9043
$C_{62}H_{111}N_{11}O_{12}$
Cyclosporin A, 2752
$C_{62}H_{111}N_{11}O_{13}$
Cyclosporin C, 2752
$C_{68}H_{84}{}^{111}InN_{13}O_{19}S_2$
Pentetreotide ^{111}In Chelate, 7126
$C_{63}H_{87}N_{13}O_{19}S_2$
Pentetreotide, 7126
$C_{63}H_{88}CoN_{14}O_{14}P$
Vitamin B_{12}, 10014
$C_{63}H_{88}N_{12}O_{16}$
Actinomycin C_2, 1606
$C_{63}H_{91}CoN_{13}O_{14}P$
Methylcobalamin, 6045
$C_{63}H_{98}N_{18}O_{13}S$
Substance P, 8863
$C_{63}H_{111}N_{11}O_{12}$
Valspodar, 9917
$C_{63}H_{113}N_{11}O_{12}$
Cyclosporin D, 2752
$C_{64}H_{82}N_{18}O_{13}$
Triptorelin, 9748
$C_{64}H_{83}N_{17}O_{12}$
Deslorelin, 2923
$C_{64}H_{90}N_{12}O_{16}$
Actinomycin C_3, 1606
$C_{64}H_{91}CoN_{13}O_{16}P$
Acetatocobalamin, 4809
$C_{65}H_{82}N_2O_{18}S_2$
Atracurium Besylate, 868
$C_{65}H_{85}N_{13}O_{30}$
Mycobacillin, 6323
$C_{65}H_{92}N_{14}O_{18}S_2$
Edotreotide, 3513
$C_{65}H_{96}N_{16}O_{12}S_2$
Depreotide, 2911
$C_{65}H_{98}ClN_3O_{39}$
Benexate Hydrochloride Compd with β-Cyclodextrin (1:1), 1038
$C_{66}H_{68}CaF_2N_4O_{10}\cdot 3H_2O$
Atorvastatin Calcium Salt Trihydrate, 864
$C_{66}H_{75}Cl_2N_9O_{24}$
Vancomycin, 9929
$C_{66}H_{83}N_{17}O_{13}$
Nafarelin, 6351
$C_{66}H_{86}N_{18}O_{12}$
Histrelin, 4722
$C_{66}H_{87}N_{13}O_{13}$
Tyrocidine A, 9836

$C_{66}H_{126}N_2O_{19}P_2$
Eritoran, 3671
$C_{68}H_{88}N_{14}O_{13}$
Tyrocidine B, 9836
$C_{68}H_{110}N_{22}O_{27}S_2$
Tallysomycin A, 9043
$C_{70}H_{89}N_{15}O_{13}$
Tyrocidine C, 9836
$C_{70}H_{92}ClN_{17}O_{14}$
Cetrorelix, 2026
$C_{71}H_{110}N_{24}O_{18}S$
Bombesin, 1329
$C_{72}H_{85}N_{19}O_{18}S_5$
Thiostrepton, 9364
$C_{72}H_{95}ClN_{17}O_{14}$
Abarelix, 3
$C_{72}H_{100}CoN_{18}O_{17}P$
Cobamamide, 2451
$C_{72}H_{101}N_{17}O_{26}$
Daptomycin, 2823
$C_{72}H_{116}O_4$
Xanthophyll Dipalmitate, 10063
Zeaxanthin Dipalmitate, 10118
$C_{73}H_{131}N_3O_{31}$
Ganglioside G_{M1}, 4364
$C_{75}H_{70}N_6O_6$
Pyrvinium Pamoate, 8022
$C_{75}H_{124}N_{14}O_{16}$
Kahalalide F, 5275
$C_{75}H_{126}N_{24}O_{15}$
Dynorphin$_{1-13}$, 3478
$C_{76}H_{52}O_{46}$
Tannic Acid, 9052
$C_{76}H_{104}N_{18}O_{19}S_2$
Somatostatin, 8715
$C_{78}H_{111}N_{21}O_{19}$
Melanotan, 5814
$C_{78}H_{126}N_{30}O_{18}S_4$
Iseganan, 5105
$C_{79}H_{129}N_{27}O_{22}$
Nociceptin, 6667
$C_{79}H_{131}N_{31}O_{24}S_4$
Apamin, 725
$C_{80}H_{106}Cl_2N_{11}O_{27}P$
Telavancin, 9116
$C_{80}H_{113}ClN_{18}O_{13}$
Ganirelix, 4365
$C_{84}H_{92}N_8O_{35}$
Ristocetin B, 8234
$C_{84}H_{133}N_{21}O_{26}.6H_2O$
Bovine Neurotensin Triacetate Hexahydrate, 6486
$C_{86}H_{97}Cl_3N_{10}O_{26}$
Oritavancin, 6868
$C_{88}H_{95}Cl_2N_9O_{33}$
Teicoplanin A_2-1, 9115
$C_{88}H_{97}Cl_2N_9O_{33}$
Teicoplanin A_2-3, 9115
$C_{88}H_{100}Cl_2N_{10}O_{28}$
Dalbavancin, 2803
$C_{89}H_{99}Cl_2N_9O_{33}$
Teicoplanin A_2-4, 9115
$C_{89}H_{101}Cl_2N_9O_{36}$
β-Avoparcin, 889
$C_{89}H_{102}ClN_9O_{36}$
α-Avoparcin, 889
$C_{95}H_{110}N_8O_{44}$
Ristocetin A, 8234
$C_{96}H_{141}AlO_{15}$
Acetoxolone Aluminum Salt, 76
$C_{98}H_{138}N_{24}O_{33}$
Bivalirudin, 1310
$C_{99}H_{155}N_{29}O_{21}S$
Alsactide, 314
$C_{100}H_{156}N_{34}O_{22}S$
Giractide, 4428

$C_{102}H_{172}N_{36}O_{32}S_7$
Ziconotide, 10122
$C_{104}H_{168}N_{34}O_{20}S$
Penetratin, 7086
$C_{108}H_{96}Cu_6P_6$
Stryker's Reagent, 8857
$C_{112}H_{162}N_{36}O_{43}S_{10}$
Technetium ^{99m}Tc Apcitide Dimer, 9098
$C_{119}H_{154}ClN_{21}O_{40}$
Ramoplanin A_2, 8104
$C_{122}H_{210}N_{32}O_{22}$
Pexiganan, 7193
$C_{126}H_{238}N_{26}O_{22}$
Sinapultide, 8542
$C_{128}H_{194}N_{40}O_{28}S_2$
Bradycor, 1358
$C_{129}H_{223}N_3O_{54}$
Palytoxin, 6999
$C_{130}H_{220}N_{44}O_{41}$
Porcine Secretin, 8421
$C_{131}H_{229}N_{39}O_{31}$
Melittin, 5824
$C_{136}H_{210}N_{40}O_{31}S$
Cosyntropin, 2551
$C_{143}H_{230}N_{42}O_{37}S_7$
Nisin, 6564
$C_{145}H_{234}N_{52}O_{44}S_3$
Ularitide, 9886
$C_{148}H_{244}N_{42}O_{47}$
Elcatonin, 3537
$C_{149}H_{246}N_{44}O_{42}S$
Sermorelin, 8461
$C_{164}H_{256}Na_2O_{68}S_2$
Maitotoxin, 5698
$C_{171}H_{267}N_{51}O_{53}S_2$
Pramlintide, 7708
$C_{172}H_{265}N_{43}O_{51}$
Liraglutide, 5514
$C_{176}H_{277}N_{57}O_{55}S_7$
Charybdotoxin, 2046
$C_{178}H_{286}N_{52}O_{50}S_7$
Margatoxin, 5752
$C_{198}H_{340}N_{68}O_{56}S_8$
α_1-Purothionin, 7944
$C_{202}H_{348}N_{68}O_{59}S_8$
α_2-Purothionin, 7944
$C_{203}H_{339}N_{67}O_{59}S_8$
β-Purothionin, 7944
$C_{204}H_{243}N_{63}Na_{20}O_{114}P_{20}S_{20}$
Fomivirsen Sodium Salt, 4229
$C_{204}H_{263}N_{63}O_{114}P_{20}S_{20}$
Fomivirsen, 4229
$C_{204}H_{301}N_{51}O_{64}$
Enfuvirtide, 3582
$C_{258}H_{384}N_{64}O_{78}S_6$
Insulin Glulisine, 4985
$C_{267}H_{402}N_{64}O_{76}S_6$
Insulin Detemir, 4983
$C_{284}H_{432}N_{84}O_{79}S_7$
Aprotinin, 757
$C_{331}H_{512}N_{94}O_{101}S_7$
Mecasermin, 4986
$C_{938}H_{1465}N_{257}O_{278}S_6$
Somatotropin, 8716
$C_{938}H_{1469}N_{255}O_{275}S_7$
Somatotropin, 8716
$C_{976}H_{1533}N_{265}O_{286}S_8$
Somatotropin, 8716
$C_{977}H_{1527}N_{265}O_{287}S_7$
Somatotropin, 8716
$C_{978}H_{1537}N_{265}O_{286}S_9$
Somatotropin, 8716
$C_{979}H_{1527}N_{265}O_{287}S_8$
Somatotropin, 8716

Cl₂S₂
Sulfur Chloride, 8970
Cl₂Se₂
Selenium Chloride, 8432
Cl₂Sn
Stannous Chloride, 8783
Cl₂Sr
Strontium Chloride, 8840
Cl₂Te
Tellurium Dichloride, 9122
Cl₂Ti
Titanium Dichloride, 9471
Cl₂Zn
Zinc Chloride, 10132
Cl₃CoH₁₈N₆
Hexaaminecobalt Trichloride, 4675
Cl₃Cr
Chromic Chloride, 2222
Cl₃Fe
Ferric Chloride, 4019
Cl₃Ga
Gallium Chloride, 4348
Cl₃HSi
Trichlorosilane, 9646
Cl₃H₄MgN
Ammonium Magnesium Chloride, 531
Cl₃I
Iodine Trichloride, 5020
Cl₃In
Indium Trichloride, 4958
Cl₃Ir
Iridium Trichloride, 5088
Cl₃N
Nitrogen Chloride, 6602
Cl₃OP
Phosphorus Oxychloride, 7349
Cl₃OV
Vanadyl Trichloride, 9927
Cl₃P
Phosphorus Trichloride, 7358
Cl₃PS
Phosphorus Sulfochloride, 7356
Cl₃Rh
Rhodium Chloride, 8188
Cl₃Ru
Ruthenium Trichloride, 8302
Cl₃Sb
Antimony Trichloride, 707
Cl₃Ti
Titanium Trichloride, 9481
Cl₃U
Uranium Trichloride, 9859
Cl₄CuH₈N₂
Ammonium Cupric Chloride, 514
Cl₄Ge
Germanium Tetrachloride, 4410
Cl₄H₈N₂Pt
Ammonium Platinous Chloride, 549
Cl₄H₈N₂Zn
Ammonium Tetrachlorozincate, 559
Cl₄K₂Pt
Potassium Tetrachloroplatinate(II), 7682
Cl₄Se
Selenium Tetrachloride, 8438
Cl₄Si
Silicon Tetrachloride, 8500
Cl₄Sn
Stannic Chloride, 8774
Cl₄Te
Tellurium Tetrachloride, 9126
Cl₄Th
Thorium Chloride, 9375
Cl₄Ti
Titanium Tetrachloride, 9478

Cl₄U
Uranium Tetrachloride, 9857
Cl₄Zr
Zirconium Chloride, 10174
Cl₅H₁₂N₃Zn
Ammonium Pentachlorozincate, 539
Cl₅Nb
Niobium Pentachloride, 6557
Cl₅P
Phosphorus Pentachloride, 7351
Cl₅Sb
Antimony Pentachloride, 695
Cl₅Ta
Tantalum Pentachloride, 9054
Cl₆H₂Pt
Platinic Chloride, 7526
Cl₆H₈N₂Os
Ammonium Osmium Chloride, 536
Cl₆H₈N₂Pt
Ammonium Platinic Chloride, 548
Cl₆H₄₂N₁₄O₂Ru₃
Ruthenium Red, 8300
Cl₆K₂Os
Potassium Hexachloroosmate(IV), 7635
Cl₆K₂Pt
Potassium Hexachloroplatinate(IV), 7636
Cl₆Na₂Pt
Sodium Hexachloroplatinate(IV), 8623
CoCr₂O₄
Cobaltous Chromate(III), 2438
CoF₂
Cobaltous Fluoride, 2440
CoF₃
Cobaltic Fluoride, 2430
CoHO₂
Cobaltic Oxide Monohydrate, 2431
CoH₂O₂
Cobaltous Hydroxide, 2442
CoH₄NO₄P
Ammonium Cobaltous Phosphate, 513
CoI₂
Cobaltous Iodide, 2443
CoK₃N₆O₁₂
Cobaltic Potassium Nitrite, 2432
CoN₂O₆
Cobaltous Nitrate, 2444
CoN₆Na₃O₁₂
Sodium Cobaltinitrite, 8603
CoO
Cobaltous Oxide, 2446
CoO₄S
Cobaltous Sulfate, 2448
CoS
Cobaltous Sulfide, 2449
Co₃O₄
Cobaltic-Cobaltous Oxide, 2429
Co₃O₈P₂
Cobaltous Phosphate, 2447
Co₅Sm
Samarium Cobalt, 8348
Co₁₇Sm₂
Samarium Cobalt (Sm₂Co₁₇), 8348
CrCuO₄
Cupric Chromate(VI), 2634
CrF₂
Chromous Fluoride, 2245
CrF₂O₂
Chromyl Fluoride, 2249
CrF₃
Chromic Fluoride, 2223
CrH₃O₃
Chromic Hydroxide, 2225

CrH₄NO₈S₂
Ammonium Chromic Sulfate, 511
CrH₈N₂O₄
Ammonium Chromate(VI), 510
CrKO₈S₂
Chromic Potassium Sulfate, 2229
CrK₂O₄
Potassium Chromate(VI), 7622
CrLi₂O₄
Lithium Chromate(VI), 5529
CrN₃O₉
Chromic Nitrate, 2226
CrNa₂O₄
Sodium Chromate(VI), 8601
CrO₂
Chromium Dioxide, 2233
CrO₃
Chromium(VI) Oxide, 2235
CrO₄P
Chromic Phosphate, 2227
CrO₄Pb
Lead Chromate(VI), 5405
CrO₄S
Chromous Sulfate, 2247
CrO₄Sr
Strontium Chromate(VI), 8841
CrPb₂O₅
Lead Chromate(VI) Oxide, 5406
Cr₂CuO₄
Cupric Chromite, 2635
Cr₂H₈N₂O₇
Ammonium Dichromate(VI), 515
Cr₂K₂O₇
Potassium Dichromate(VI), 7627
Cr₂Na₂O₇
Sodium Dichromate(VI), 8609
Cr₂O₃
Chromium(III) Oxide, 2234
Cr₂O₈Sn
Stannic Chromate(VI), 8775
Cr₂O₁₂S₃
Chromic Sulfate, 2230
Cr₃Fe₂O₁₂
Ferric Chromate(VI), 4020
CsF
Cesium Fluoride, 2012
CsHO
Cesium Hydroxide, 2013
CsI
Cesium Iodide, 2014
CsNO₃
Cesium Nitrate, 2015
Cs₂O₄S
Cesium Sulfate, 2016
CuF₂
Cupric Fluoride, 2638
CuF₆Si
Cupric Hexafluorosilicate, 2641
CuFeS₂
Chalcopyrite, 2038
CuH₂O₂
Cupric Hydroxide, 2642
CuH₁₂N₄O₄S
Tetraamminecopper Sulfate, 9181
CuI
Cuprous Iodide, 2662
CuN₂O₆
Cupric Nitrate, 2643
CuO
Cupric Oxide, 2646
CuO₄S
Cupric Sulfate, 2653
CuO₄Se
Cupric Selenate, 2650
CuO₄W
Cupric Tungstate(VI), 2657

G

GaN
Gallium Nitride, 4351
GaN₃O₉

GaN
Gallium Nitride, 4351
GaN3O9
Gallium Nitrate, 4350
GaP
Gallium Phosphide, 4353
Gd2O3
Gadolinium Oxide, 4326
GeH4
Germane, 4406
GeMg2
Magnesium Germanide, 5667
GeO2
Germanium Dioxide, 4409

H

HBr
Hydrobromic Acid, 4778
HCl
Hydrochloric Acid, 4780
HF
Hydrofluoric Acid, 4790
HI
Hydriodic Acid, 4776
Hydrogen Iodide, 4797
HIO3
Iodic Acid, 5012
HKO
Potassium Hydroxide, 7640
HKO4S
Potassium Bisulfate, 7613
HKS
Potassium Bisulfide, 7614
HK2O3P
Potassium Phosphite, 7661
HK2O4P
Potassium Phosphate, Dibasic, 7658
HLi
Lithium Hydride, 5533
HLiO
Lithium Hydroxide, 5534
HMgO4P
Magnesium Phosphate, Dibasic, 5681
HNO2
Nitrous Acid, 6652
HNO3
Nitric Acid, 6577
HNO5S
Nitrosylsulfuric Acid, 6648
HN3
Hydrazoic Acid, 4774
HNa
Sodium Hydride, 8625
HNaO
Sodium Hydroxide, 8627
HNaO3S
Sodium Bisulfite, 8588
HNaO4S
Sodium Bisulfate, 8586
HNaS
Sodium Bisulfide, 8587
HNa2O3P
Sodium Phosphite, 8663
HNa2O4P
Sodium Phosphate, Dibasic, 8659
HORb
Rubidium Hydroxide, 8285

HOTl
Thallium Hydroxide, 9263
H2KO2P
Potassium Hypophosphite, 7641
H2KO4P
Potassium Phosphate, Monobasic, 7659
H2LiN
Lithium Amide, 5522
H2Mg
Magnesium Hydride, 5669
H2MgO2
Magnesium Hydroxide, 5670
H2MoO4
Molybdic(VI) Acid, 6240
H2NNa
Sodium Amide, 8576
H2N2O2
Nitramide, 6572
H2NaO2P
Sodium Hypophosphite, 8629
H2NaO4P
Sodium Phosphate, Monobasic, 8660
H2Na2O7P2
Sodium Acid Pyrophosphate, 8572
H2NiO2
Nickel Hydroxide, 6510
H2O
Water, 10039
²H2O
Deuterium Oxide, 2940
H2O2
Hydrogen Peroxide, 4798
H2O2Pd
Pearlman's Catalyst, 7060
H2O2Sr
Strontium Hydroxide, 8843
H2O3Se
Selenious Acid, 8430
H2O3Te
Tellurous Acid, 9128
H2O4S
Sulfuric Acid, 8974
H2O4Se
Selenic Acid, 8429
H2O4W
Tungstic(VI) Acid, 9818
H2O5S
Caro's Acid, 1851
H2O7S2
Pyrosulfuric Acid, 8009
H2S
Hydrogen Sulfide, 4800
H2Se
Hydrogen Selenide, 4799
H2Te
Hydrogen Telluride, 4801
H2Ti
Titanium Hydride, 9473
H3N
Ammonia, 492
H3NO
Hydroxylamine, 4828
H3NO3S
Sulfamic Acid, 8921
H3O2P
Hypophosphorous Acid, 4868
H3O3P
Phosphorous Acid, 7346
H3O4P
Phosphoric Acid, 7344
H3P
Phosphine, 7338
H3Sb
Stibine, 8811

H4IN
Ammonium Iodide, 529
H4IP
Phosphonium Iodide, 7343
H4MgN2
Magnesium Amide, 5656
H4MgO8P2
Magnesium Phosphate, Monobasic, 5682
H4MnO4P2
Manganese Hypophosphite, 5731
H4NO3V
Ammonium Vanadate(V), 568
H4N2
Hydrazine, 4770
H4N2O2S
Sulfamide, 8922
H4N2O3
Ammonium Nitrate, 534
H4O4Zr
Zirconium Hydroxide, 10177
H4O6P2
Hypophosphoric Acid, 4867
H4O7P2
Pyrophosphoric Acid, 8008
H4O40SiW12
Silicotungstic Acid, 8502
H4Si
Silane, 8488
H5IO6
Periodic Acid, 7171
H5NO3S
Ammonium Bisulfite, 502
H5NO4S
Ammonium Bisulfate, 500
H5NS
Ammonium Bisulfide, 501
H6MgNO5P.6H2O
Struvite, 8854
H6NO2P
Ammonium Hypophosphite, 528
H6NO4P
Ammonium Phosphate, Monobasic, 543
H6N2O
Hydrazine Hydrate, 4771
H6N2O3S
Ammonium Sulfamate, 554
H6N2O4S
Hydrazine Sulfate, 4772
H6O6Te
Telluric(VI) Acid, 9120
H6Si2
Disilane, 3356
H8MoN2S4
Ammonium Tetrathiomolybdate, 560
H8N2NiO8S2
Nickel Ammonium Sulfate, 6501
H8N2O3S
Ammonium Sulfite, 557
H8N2O3S2
Ammonium Thiosulfate, 562
H8N2O3Se
Ammonium Selenite, 552
H8N2O4S
Ammonium Sulfate, 555
H8N2O4Se
Ammonium Selenate, 551
H8N2O7U2
Ammonium Uranate(VI), 565
H8N2O8S2
Ammonium Peroxydisulfate, 541
H8N2S
Ammonium Sulfide, 556
H8Si3
Trisilane, 9754

$H_9N_2O_3P$
Ammonium Phosphite, 544
$H_9N_2O_4P$
Ammonium Phosphate, Dibasic, 542
$H_{10}Si_4$
Tetrasilane, 9239
$H_{12}Mo_{12}N_3O_{40}P$
Ammonium Phosphomolybdate, 545
$H_{12}N_3O_{40}PW_{12}$
Ammonium Phosphotungstate, 546
$H_{24}Mo_7N_6O_{24}$
Ammonium Molybdate(VI), 533
$H_{40}N_{10}O_{41}W_{12}$
Ammonium Tungstate(VI), 564
$H_{68}Na_2N_{17}O_{86}Sb_9W_{21}$
HPA-23, 4750
HgI_2
Mercuric Iodide, Red, 5879
HgI_4K_2
Potassium Tetraiodomercurate(II), 7688
HgN_2O_6
Mercuric Nitrate, 5880
HgO
Mercuric Oxide, Red, 5882
Mercuric Oxide, Yellow, 5883
HgO_4S
Mercuric Sulfate, 5887
HgS
Mercuric Sulfide, Black, 5888
Mercuric Sulfide, Red, 5889
Hg_2I_2
Mercurous Iodide, 5895
$Hg_2N_2O_6$
Mercurous Nitrate, 5896
Hg_2O_4S
Mercurous Sulfate, 5897
Ho_2O_3
Holmium Oxide, 4727

I

IK
Potassium Iodide, 7643
IKO_3
Potassium Iodate, 7642
IKO_4
Potassium Periodate, 7654
ILi
Lithium Iodide, 5535
INa
Sodium Iodide, 8631
$INaO_3$
Sodium Iodate, 8630
$INaO_4$
Sodium Metaperiodate, 8640
IRb
Rubidium Iodide, 8286
ITl
Thallium Iodide, 9264
I_2Mg
Magnesium Iodide, 5671
I_2Mn
Manganese Iodide, 5732
I_2Ni
Nickel Iodide, 6511
I_2O_5
Iodine Pentoxide, 5019
I_2O_6Zn
Zinc Iodate, 10139
I_2Pb
Lead Iodide, 5411

I_2Sm
Samarium Iodide, 8349
I_2Sn
Stannous Iodide, 8785
I_2Sr
Strontium Iodide, 8844
I_2Zn
Zinc Iodide, 10140
I_3Sb
Antimony Triiodide, 710
I_4Sn
Stannic Iodide, 8777
I_4Te
Tellurium Tetraiodide, 9127
I_4Zr
Zirconium Iodide, 10178
InN
Indium Nitride, 4951
InP
Indium Phosphide, 4953
$InSb$
Indium Antimonide, 4948
$InSe$
Indium Selenide, 4954
In_2O_3
Indium Oxide, 4952
$In_2O_{12}S_3$
Indium Sulfate, 4955
In_2Te_3
Indium Telluride, 4956
Ir_2O_3
Iridium Sesquioxide, 5087

K

$KMnO_4$
Potassium Permanganate, 7655
KNO_2
Potassium Nitrite, 7649
KNO_3
Potassium Nitrate, 7648
K_2MnO_4
Potassium Manganate(VI), 7644
K_2MoO_4
Potassium Molybdate(VI), 7647
$K_2NO_7S_2$
Fremy's Salt, 4268
K_2O_3S
Potassium Sulfite, 7676
$K_2O_3S_2$
Potassium Thiosulfate, 7692
K_2O_3Sn
Potassium Stannate(IV), 7672
K_2O_3Te
Potassium Tellurate(IV), 7678
K_2O_4S
Potassium Sulfate, 7674
K_2O_4Se
Potassium Selenate, 7666
K_2O_4Te
Potassium Tellurate(VI), 7679
K_2O_4W
Potassium Tungstate(VI), 7694
$K_2O_5S_2$
Potassium Metabisulfite, 7645
$K_2O_7S_2$
Potassium Pyrosulfate, 7664
$K_2O_7U_2$
Potassium Uranate(VI), 7695
$K_2O_8S_2$
Potassium Persulfate, 7656
K_2S
Potassium Sulfide, 7675

K_2Se
Potassium Selenide, 7667
K_3O_4P
Potassium Phosphate, Tribasic, 7660
$K_4O_7P_2$
Potassium Pyrophosphate, 7663

L

La_2O_3
Lanthanum Oxide, 5363
$LiNO_3$
Lithium Nitrate, 5536
Li_2O
Lithium Oxide, 5538
Li_2O_3Si
Lithium Silicate, 5540
Li_2O_4S
Lithium Sulfate, 5541

M

$MgMn_2O_8$
Magnesium Permanganate, 5679
MgN_2O_6
Magnesium Nitrate, 5674
MgO
Magnesium Oxide, 5677
MgO_2
Magnesium Peroxide, 5680
MgO_3S
Magnesium Sulfite, 5692
MgO_3S_2
Magnesium Thiosulfate, 5694
MgO_4S
Magnesium Sulfate, 5691
$MgSe$
Magnesium Selenide, 5686
$MgSiO_3$
Magnesium Metasilicate, 5687
$Mg_2O_7P_2$
Magnesium Pyrophosphate, 5684
Mg_2Si
Magnesium Silicide, 5688
Mg_2SiO_4
Magnesium Orthosilicate, 5687
$Mg_2Si_3O_8$
Magnesium Trisilicate, 5687
Mg_2Sn
Magnesium Stannide, 5689
$Mg_3O_7Si_2$
Serpentine (Mineral), 5687
$Mg_3O_8P_2$
Magnesium Phosphate, Tribasic, 5683
MnN_2O_6
Manganese Nitrate, 5733
$MnNaO_4$
Sodium Permanganate, 8654
MnO_2
Manganese Dioxide, 5730
MnO_4S
Manganese Sulfate, 5739
MnS
Manganese Sulfide, 5740
$MnSe$
Manganese Selenide, 5736
Mn_2O_3
Manganese Sesquioxide, 5737
Mn_3O_4
Manganese Oxide, 5735

NAME INDEX

NAME INDEX

The Name Index refers the reader to monograph numbers with three types of citations:

Ethacrynic Acid, 3643 (format for titles)
Ethacrynate Sodium *see* 3643 (format for all synonyms)

Company name included in citation denotes trademark owner or its subsidiary, affiliate, licensee or distributor.

Edecrin [Merck & Co.] *see* 3643

1C50 *see* 3829
02-115 *see* 9038
2-5410-3A *see* 5023
4A65 *see* 4915
4-C-32 *see* 9429
6-12 [Union Carbide] *see* 3744
6-H.E.S. [Morishita] *see* 4673
7E3 *see* 5
7E11-C5.3-glycyl-tyrosyl-(*N*-ε-diethyl-enetriaminepentaacetic Acid)-lysine *see* 1762
7E11-C5.3-GYK-DTPA *see* 1762
8-AL *see* 6497
15AU81 *see* 9586
17-1A Antibody *see* 3515
27-400 *see* 2752
51W89 *see* 868
53-32 C *see* 9429
84L *see* 3116
87/312 *see* 6594
96-H-60 *see* 4605
101-E *see* 6403
101-G *see* 6403
106-7 *see* 2751
141W94 *see* 589
191C49 *see* 9293
217-MI *see* 3501
256U *see* 9899
264-EUP-99 *see* 5236
295C51 *see* 9746
311C90 *see* 10189
338C48 *see* 3260
378C48 *see* 3337
501-P *see* 4463
506U *see* 6442
516-MD *see* 2305
524W91 *see* 3565
566C80 *see* 866
683-M *see* 6944
688-A *see* 7256
710-F *see* 7522
722 D *see* 7507
746-CE *see* 3632
776C85 *see* 3584
864T *see* 4927
921 C *see* 9661
1080 [Tull] *see* 4167
1081 *see* 4166
1162-F *see* 8925
1314-Th *see* 3737
1358F *see* 2822
1489-RB *see* 7460
1497-CB *see* 7829
1522-CB *see* 32
1589mRB *see* 7066
1589RB *see* 7066
1592U89 *see* 1
1600 Antibiotic *see* 7041
1609-RB *see* 7488
1633 Labaz *see* 8608
1665-RB *see* 770
1703-18B *see* 4851
2249-F *see* 6923
2329 Labaz *see* 1083

2601-A *see* 2185
3123-L *see* 7943
5512-M *see* 680
6063 *see* 53
6315-S *see* 4104
6720 CDRI *see* 1971
7432-S *see* 1949
8053CB *see* 9301
8102 CB *see* 955
10040 *see* 2091
10275-S *see* 3624
10364-S *see* 5858
13832-JL *see* 10078
29060-LE *see* 9982
47657 *see* 752
81723 hfu *see* 9419
450191-S *see* 8221
710674-S *see* 2368
A-21 *see* 5217
A-41-304 *see* 2930
A-65 *see* 7498
A-66 *see* 7237
A-101 *see* 6691
A-145 *see* 7783
A-272 *see* 6833
A-300-I *see* 9649
A-363 *see* 433
A-585 *see* 8995
A-820 *see* 1532
A-3823A *see* 6246
A-4166 *see* 6428
A-4696 *see* 132
A-4942 *see* 4896
A-5610 *see* 906
A-8103 *see* 7480
A-9145 *see* 8544
A-16686 *see* 8104
A-19120 *see* 7038
A-20968 *see* 7481
A-23187 *see* 1639
A-29622 *see* 4251
A-33547 *see* 8132
A-35957 *see* 319
A-38414 *see* 630
A-40926 *see* 2803
A-43818 *see* 5457
A-46745 *see* 4415
A-56268 *see* 2339
A-56619 *see* 3141
A-56620 *see* 8370
A-60386X *see* 1151
A-60969 *see* 9555
A-61827 *see* 9555
A-62254 *see* 9132
A-63004 *see* 9132
A-64077 *see* 10124
A-64730 *see* 9555
A-65006 *see* 5362
A-70569 *see* 9417
A-83543A *see* 8750
A-83543D *see* 8750
A-84538 *see* 8238
(+)-A-127722 *see* 870
A-147627.1 *see* 870

A-157378 *see* 5573
A-195773 *see* 2020
A-771726 *see* 9165
Aα *see* 4010
Aβ *see* 615
β/A4 *see* 615
AA-149 *see* 9585
AA-673 *see* 490
AA-2414 *see* 8459
Aa-5648 *see* 8957
Aacifemine [Aaciphar] *see* 3707
AAF *see* 4157
AAT *see* 719
A1AT *see* 719
AAtrex [Syngenta] *see* 871
AB-021 *see* 9485
AB-100 *see* 9872
AB-206 *see* 6196
ABA *see* 11
AB-A-663 *see* 2278
Abacavir, 1
Abacin [Benedetti] *see* 8918
Abadol [Specia] *see* 479
Abalyn *see* 6006
Abamectin, 2
Abar [Velsicol] *see* 5445
Abarelix, 3
Abasin [Bayer] *see* 21
Abatacept, 4
Abate [BASF] *see* 9135
Abbocillin [Abbott] *see* 7097
Abboflox [Abbott] *see* 4111
Abbokinase [Abbott] *see* 9887
Abboticine [Abbott] *see* 3687
Abbott 16900 *see* 9110
Abbott 30400 *see* 7079
Abbott 35616 *see* 2403
Abbott 36581 *see* 1513
Abbott 43326 *see* 1866
Abbott 43818 *see* 5457
Abbott 44747 *see* 4249
Abbott 45975 *see* 9154
Abbott 46811 *see* 1945
Abbott 48999 *see* 1935
Abbott 50192 *see* 1925
Abbott 50711 *see* 9913
Abbott 56619 *see* 3141
Abbott 56620 *see* 8370
Abbott 64077 *see* 10124
Abbott 73001 *see* 8459
Abbott 84538 *see* 8238
Abbsa [Sanko] *see* 9522
ABC-12/3 *see* 3438
ABCD *see* 585
Abciximab, 5
ABDP *see* 229
Abelcet [Liposome Co.] *see* 585
Abequito [Am. Cyanamid] *see* 6550
Aberel [Janssen-Cilag] *see* 8165
Abetimus Sodium, 6
ABG-6215 *see* 3987
Abicoviromycin *see* 8
Δ^{6,8(14)}-Abietadienoic Acid *see* 5468
Abietic Acid, 7

Abietic Anhydride *see* 8266
Abietin *see* 2503
Abikoviromycin, 8
Abil [Goldschmidt Chem.] *see* 8495
Abilify [BMS] *see* 785
Abilit [Sumitomo] *see* 8989
Abilitat [BMS] *see* 785
Abimasten 100 [ABIC] *see* 6534
Abiocine [Lepetit] *see* 3179
Abiol [3V Inc.] *see* 4916
Abitilguanide *see* 6272
Abitylguanide *see* 6272
ABLC *see* 585
Abminthic [Pfizer] *see* 3369
ABOB *see* 6272
Abomasal Enzyme *see* 8134
Aboren [Promeco] *see* 6183
Abovis [Toyama] *see* 114
Abramen [Mepha] *see* 386
Abrastol *see* 822
Abreva [GSK] *see* 3399
Abrial Lavandin Oil *see* 5390
Abrifam [Abbott] *see* 8216
Abrin, 9
Abrine, 10
Abrodil [Schering] *see* 5973
Abrus Agglutinin *see* 9
Abscisic Acid, 11
(*R*)-(−)-Abscisic Acid *see* 11
Abscisin II *see* 11
Absentol [Nourypharma] *see* 9706
Absinthiin *see* 12
Absinthin, 12
Absinthium *see* 10052
Absolute Alcohol *see* 3760
Absonal [Boehringer, Ing.] *see* 1111
Absorbable Cellulose *see* 6939
Abstem *see* 1663
Absynthin *see* 12
ABT-378 *see* 5573
ABT-538 *see* 8238
ABT-594 *see* 9090
ABT-627 *see* 870
ABT-773 *see* 2020
Abufène [Théraplix] *see* 205
Abuphenine *see* 1522
Aburamycin B *see* 2238
ABX-EGF *see* 7010
9-AC *see* 431
AC-001 *see* 609
AC-17 *see* 1789
AC-137 *see* 7708
AC-145 *see* 33
AC-223 *see* 5822
AC-293 *see* 4903
AC-528 *see* 3301
AC-601 *see* 1501
AC-1198 *see* 3213
AC-1370 *see* 1938
AC-1802 *see* 754
AC-2993 *see* 3914
AC-3422 *see* 7033
AC-3810 *see* 955
AC-3911 *see* 7331
AC-4464 *see* 9552
AC-5223 *see* 3408
AC-38555 *see* 2104
AC-47300 *see* 3976
AC-52160 *see* 9135
AC-84633 *see* 6550
AC-84777 *see* 3138
AC-92100 *see* 9158
AC-92553 *see* 7084
AC-217300 *see* 4765
AC-222293 *see* 4903

AC-222705 *see* 4124
AC-252214 *see* 4906
AC-252925 *see* 4905
AC-263499 *see* 4907
AC-263780 *see* 2278
AC-299263 *see* 4904
AC-303630 *see* 2088
AC-382042 *see* 3983
AC-900001 *see* 7399
7-ACA *see* 434
Acabel [Grünenthal] *see* 1193
Acacetin, 13
Acacetin-*β*-rutinoside *see* 5498
Acacia, 14
Acacic Acid, 15
Acaciin *see* 13
Acadesine, 16
Acadione [Cassenne] *see* 9453
Acamol [Teva] *see* 47
Acamprosate Calcium, 17
Acanto [Syngenta] *see* 7408
Acapodene [GTx] *see* 9550
Acaprin *see* 3353
Acarbose, 18
Acariflor [Sipcam] *see* 4713
Acarin [Makhteshim-Agan] *see* 3086
Acarol [Syngenta] *see* 1434
Acarosan [Allergopharma] *see* 1127
ACC-9653 *see* 4258
Accelerator Globulin *see* 3919
Accelerin *see* 3919
Accelerine *see* 6638
Accent [Underwood] *see* 6254
Accent [DuPont] *see* 6522
Acclaim *see* 3984
Accolate [AstraZeneca] *see* 10108
Accord [Dow AgroSci.] *see* 4512
Accothion *see* 3976
Accupril [Parke-Davis] *see* 8051
Accuprin [Pfizer] *see* 8051
Accupro [Pfizer] *see* 8051
Accuretic [Parke-Davis] *see* 8051
Accutane [Roche] *see* 5228
Acdeam [Grelan] *see* 5640
Ac-Di-Sol [FMC] *see* 2592
Acea Gel [Ferndale] *see* 6157
Acebutolol, 19
Acecainide, 20
Acecarbromal, 21
Aceclidine *see* 8082
Aceclofenac, 22
Acecol [Sankyo] *see* 9136
Acecoline [Lematte et Boinot] *see* 87
Acecor [SPA] *see* 19
Acediamine Hydrochloride *see* 44
Acediasulfone, 23
Acedicon [Boehringer, Ing.] *see* 3172
Acedist [Chemiefarma] *see* 1419
Acediur [Guidotti] *see* 1774
Acef [Tiber] *see* 1917
Acefylline, 24
Acefylline Piperazine *see* 24
Aceglutamide, 25
Aceglutamide Aluminum *see* 25
Acemannan, 26
Acemetacin, 27
Acemethadone *see* 5945
Acemix [Bioprogress] *see* 27
Acenalin [Janssen Kyowa] *see* 2316
Acenaphthene, 28
Acenocoumarin *see* 29
Acenocoumarol, 29
Aceon [Solvay] *see* 7170
Aceperone, 30
Acephate, 31

Acephen *see* 5780
Acepifylline *see* 24
Aceplus [BMS] *see* 1774
Acepress [Guidotti] *see* 1774
Acepreval *see* 7723
Acepril [Duncan Flockhart] *see* 1774
Acepromazine, 32
Acequide [Recordati] *see* 8051
Acequin [Recordati] *see* 8051
Acequinocyl, 33
Acerbon [AstraZeneca] *see* 5516
Acerin, 34
Acerola, 35
Aceroxatidine *see* 8274
ACES, 36
Acesistem [Sigma-Tau] *see* 3567
Acesulfame, 37
Acesulfame-K *see* 37
Acetabutone *see* 30
Acetadote [Cumberland] *see* 88
Acetal, 38
Acetaldehyde, 39
Acetaldehyde Ammonia, 40
Acetaldehyde Diethyl Acetal *see* 38
Acetaldehyde Dimethyl Acetal *see* 3226
Acetaldehyde Oxime *see* 42
Acetaldehyde Sodium Bisulfite, 41
Acetaldol *see* 224
Acetaldoxime, 42
Acetamide, 43
Acetamidine Hydrochloride, 44
3-Acetamido-5-(acetamidomethyl)-2,4,6-
   triiodobenzoic Acid *see* 5011
Acetamidoacetic Acid *see* 80
N-(2-Acetamido)-2-aminoethanesulfonic
   Acid *see* 36
p-Acetamidobenzaldehyde Thiosemicarbazone *see* 9290
4-Acetamidobenzenesulfonic Acid *see*
   102
p-Acetamidobenzenesulfonyl Chloride
   see 103
ε-Acetamidocaproic Acid, 45
2-Acetamido-2-deoxy-3-*O*-(D-2-propion-
   yl-L-alanyl-D-isoglutamine)-D-gluco-
   pyranose *see* 6305
(−)-(*S*)-2-Acetamido-*N*-(3,4-dihydroxy-
   phenethyl)-4-(methylthio)butyram-
   ide Bis(ethylcarbonate) (Ester) *see*
   3396
5-Acetamido-2,4-dimethyltrifluoro-
   methanesulfonanilide *see* 5802
6-Acetamido-1,2-dithiolo[4,3-*b*]pyrrol-
   5(4*H*)-one *see* 4728
4-Acetamido-2-ethoxybenzoic Acid
   Methyl Ester *see* 3745
Acetamidoeugenol, 46
5-Acetamido-4-guanidino-2,3,4,5-tetra-
   deoxy-D-*glycero*-D-*galacto*-non-2-eno-
   pyranosonic Acid *see* 10113
6-Acetamidohexanoic Acid *see* 45
3-Acetamido-4-hydroxybenzenearsonic
   Acid *see* 52
3-Acetamido-4-hydroxydithiobenzene-
   arsonous Acid, Cyclic (Hydroxymethyl)ethylene Ester *see* 812
3-Acetamido-4-hydroxydithiobenzene-
   arsonous Acid Cyclic 3-Hydroxypro-
   pylene Ester *see* 812
3-Acetamido-4-hydroxyphenylarsonic
   Acid *see* 52
2-(3′-Acetamido-4′-hydroxyphenyl)-1,3-
   dithia-2-arsacyclopentane-4-metha-
   nol *see* 812

7-Acetamido-10-hydroxy-1,2,3-trimeth-oxy-6,7-dihydrobenzo[*a*]heptalen-9(5*H*)-one *see* 2470

N-(2-Acetamido)iminodiacetic Acid *see* 147

2-Acetamido-4-mercaptobutyric Acid γ-Thiolactone *see* 2320

L-α-Acetamido-β-mercaptopropionic Acid *see* 88

6-(Acetamido)-4-methyl-1,2-dithiolo-[4,3-*b*]pyrrol-5(4*H*)-one *see* 9342

3-Acetamido-5-methylpyrrolin-4-one-[4,3-*d*]-1,2-dithiole *see* 9342

4-Acetamido-1-naphthol *see* 453

2-Acetamido-5-nitrothiazole *see* 410

4-Acetamido-4-penten-3-one-1-carbox-amide *see* 7748

p-Acetamidophenol *see* 47

1-(4-Acetamidophenoxy)-3-isopropyl-amino-2-propanol *see* 7700

(*p*-Acetamidophenyl)acetic Acid *see* 133

4′-(Acetamido)phenyl-2-acetoxybenzoate *see* 1045

p-Acetamidophenyl Acetylsalicylate *see* 1045

4-Acetamidophenyl (Diethylamino)ace-tate *see* 7792

p-Acetamidophenyl Salicylate *see* 48

1-Acetamido-2-pyrrolidinone *see* 7487

5-Acetamido-1,3,4-thiadiazole-2-sulfon-amide *see* 53

α-Acetamido-γ-thiobutyrolactone *see* 2320

3-Acetamido-2,4,6-triiodobenzoic Acid Methylglucamine Salt *see* 5806

3-Acetamido-2,4,6-triiodobenzoic Acid Sodium Salt *see* 79

2-[3-Acetamido-2,4,6-triiodo-5-(*N*-methylacetamido)benzamido]-2-de-oxy-D-glucopyranose *see* 6155

2-[3-Acetamido-2,4,6-triiodo-5-(*N*-methylacetamido)benzamido]-2-de-oxy-D-glucose *see* 6155

3-Acetamido-2,4,6-triiodo-5-(*N*-methyl-acetamido)benzoic Acid *see* 6156

5-Acetamido-2,4,6-triiodo-*N*-methyliso-phthalamic Acid *see* 5064

(±)-2-[[2-(3-Acetamido-2,4,6-triiodo-phenoxy)ethoxy]methyl]butyric Acid *see* 5063

4-Acetaminobenzenesulfon-4′-nitroani-lide *see* 8933

p-Acetaminobenzenesulfonyl Chloride *see* 103

p-Acetaminobenzylidenethiosemicarba-zone *see* 9290

Acetaminocaproic Acid *see* 45

Acetaminophen, 47

p-Acetaminophenol *see* 47

Acetaminosalol, 48

Acetamiprid, 49

Acetamox [Tobishi-Santen] *see* 53

Acetanilide, 50

Acetanilide-*p*-sulfonyl Chloride *see* 103

Acetanilidsulfonic Acid *see* 102

p-Acetanisidide *see* 51

p-Acetanisidine, 51

Acetannin *see* 104

Acetanol [RPR] *see* 19

Acetarsol *see* 52

Acetarsone, 52

Acetarsonic Acid Disodium Salt *see* 810

Acetasol *see* 716

Acetate C-9 *see* 6678

Acetate Replacing Factor *see* 9326

Acetatocobalamin *see* 4809

(Acetato)phenylmercury *see* 7300

(Acetato)trimetaarsenitodicopper *see* 2625

Acetazine *see* 32

Acetazolamide, 53

Acetexa [Lilly] *see* 6715

Acethropan [Hoechst] *see* 134

Acetiamine, 54

Acetic Acid Amide *see* 43

Acetic Acid Ammonium Salt *see* 495

Acetic Acid Anhydride with Nitric Acid *see* 97

Acetic Acid Basic Bismuth Salt *see* 1281

Acetic Acid Benzyl Ester *see* 1123

Acetic Acid Beryllium Salt *see* 1162

Acetic Acid Butyl Ester *see* 1535

Acetic Acid *sec*-Butyl Ester *see* 1536

Acetic Acid *tert*-Butyl Ester *see* 1537

Acetic Acid, Calcium Magnesium Salt *see* 1680

Acetic Acid Calcium Salt *see* 1646

Acetic Acid Copper(1+) Salt *see* 2658

Acetic Acid Copper (2+) Salt *see* 2624

Acetic Acid *m*-Cresol Ester *see* 2583

Acetic Acid Dimethylamide *see* 3227

Acetic Acid 1,1-Dimethylethyl Ester *see* 1537

Acetic Acid Ethenyl Ester *see* 9992

Acetic Acid Ethyl Ester *see* 3757

Acetic Acid 2-Ethylhexyl Ester *see* 6763

Acetic Acid Glacial, 55

Acetic Acid 2-Methylphenyl Ester *see* 2584

Acetic Acid 3-Methylphenyl Ester *see* 2583

Acetic Acid 1-Methylpropyl Ester *see* 1536

Acetic Acid [(5-Nitro-2-furanyl)methyl-ene]hydrazide *see* 6542

Acetic Acid 5-(Nitrofurfurylidene)hydra-zide *see* 6542

Acetic Acid *n*-Nonyl Ester *see* 6678

Acetic Acid Oxime *see* 63

Acetic Acid Palladium Salt *see* 6991

Acetic Acid Phenyl Ester *see* 7267

Acetic Acid Phenylmethyl Ester *see* 1123

Acetic Acid α-Phenyl-2-piperidylmethyl Ester *see* 5467

Acetic Acid 2-Propenyl Ester *see* 285

Acetic Acid *n*-Propyl Ester *see* 7841

Acetic Acid Tetraanhydride with Silicic Acid *see* 8498

Acetic Acid *o*-Tolyl Ester *see* 2584

Acetic Acid Vinyl Ester *see* 9992

Acetic Aldehyde *see* 39

Acetic Anhydride, 56

Acetic Ether *see* 3757

Acetic Oxide *see* 56

Acetimidoquinone, 57

(+)-(5*R*,6*S*)-3-[[(*S*)-1-Acetimidoyl-3-pyr-rolidinyl]thio]-6-[(*R*)-1-hydroxyethyl]-7-oxo-1-azabicyclo[3.2.0]hept-2-ene-2-carboxylic Acid *see* 7009

Acetin *see* 6242

Acetoacetanilide, 58

Acetoacetic Acid, 59

Acetoacetic Acid Ethyl Ester *see* 3758

Acetoacetic Anilide *see* 58

Acetoacetic Ester *see* 3758

Aceto-*m*-aminotoluene *see* 74

Acetobromamide *see* 1398

Acetobromglucose, 60

α-Acetobromoglucose *see* 60

Acetobuton *see* 30

α-Acetobutyrolactone *see* 83

Acetochlor, 61

Acetocinnamone *see* 1137

Acetohexamide, 62

Acetohydroxamic Acid, 63

Acetoin, 64

Acetol, 65

Acetomenaphthone *see* 5830

Acetomethoxane *see* 3223

Acetomethylanilide *see* 6007

Acetomorphine *see* 2968

Acetone, 66

Acetone Alcohol *see* 65

Acetone Bis(3,5-di-*tert*-butyl-4-hydroxy-phenyl)mercaptole *see* 7755

Acetone-bromoform *see* 9611

Acetonecarboxylic Acid *see* 59

Acetone Chloroform *see* 2129

Acetone Cyanohydrin, 67

Acetonedicarboxylic Acid, 68

Acetone Glycerol *see* 5213

Acetone Oxime *see* 75

Acetone Sodium Bisulfite, 69

Acetone Sulfite *see* 69

Acetonitrile, 70

Acetonylacetone, 71

3-(α-Acetonylbenzyl)-4-hydroxycou-marin *see* 10038

Acetonyl Chloride *see* 2114

3-(α-Acetonyl-*p*-chlorobenzyl)-4-hydr-oxycoumarin *see* 2556

3-Acetonyl-5,8-dihydroxy-2-(hydroxy-methyl)-6-methoxy-1,4-naphthoqui-none *see* 4315

3-Acetonyl-5,8-dihydroxy-6-methoxy-2-methyl-1,4-naphthoquinone *see* 5262

(±)-Acetonyl Methyl 1,4-Dihydro-2,6-dimethyl-4-(*o*-nitrophenyl)-3,5-pyri-dinedicarboxylate *see* 767

3-(α-Acetonyl-*p*-nitrobenzyl)-4-hydroxy-coumarin *see* 29

2-Acetonylpiperidine *see* 7072

Acetophenazine, 72

p-Acetophenetide *see* 7204

p-Acetophenetidide *see* 7204

Acetophenetidin *see* 7204

Acetophenetidin *see* 7204

Acetophenone, 73

Acetopromazine *see* 32

Acetopyrine *see* 716

Acetopyrrothine *see* 9342

Acetoquat CDAC *see* 2017

Acetorphan *see* 8090

Acetorphine *see* 3888

Acetosulfam *see* 37

Acetotoluide, 74

m-Acetotoluide *see* 74

o-Acetotoluide *see* 74

p-Acetotoluide *see* 74

m-Acetotoluidide *see* 74

Acetovanillon *see* 741

Acetoxanon [Organon] *see* 77

Acetoxime, 75

Acetoxolone, 76

2-Acetoxy-4′-(acetamino)phenylbenzoate *see* 1045

9-[4-Acetoxy-3-(acetoxymethyl)but-1-yl]-2-aminopurine *see* 3929

5-Acetoxy-3-acetylthio-2-[(4-amino-2-methyl-5-pyrimidinyl)methyl-*N*-for-mylamino]-2-pentene *see* 54

2-(2′-Acetoxy)benzamido-5-nitrothiazole *see* 6567

2-Acetoxybenzoic Acid *see* 851

17α-Acetoxy-6-chloro-6,7-dehydropro-gesterone *see* 2102

2-Acetoxy-3-(*N*,*N*-diethylcarboxamido)-9,10-dimethoxy-1,2,3,4,6,7-hexahydro-11b*H*-benzopyridocoline *see* 1119

21-Acetoxy-6α,9α-difluoro-11β-hydroxy-16α,17α-isopropylidenedioxy-1,4-pregnadiene-3,20-dione *see* 4151

3-Acetoxy-6-dimethylamino-4,4-diphenylheptane *see* 5945

5-Acetoxy-2-dimethylamino-4,4-diphenylheptane *see* 5945

6-Acetoxy-2,4-dimethyl-*m*-dioxane *see* 3223

α-*dl*-3-Acetoxy-4,4-diphenyl-6-methylaminoheptane *see* 6685

cis-1-Acetoxy-7-dodecene *see* 5570

7β-Acetoxy-8,13-epoxy-1α,6β,9α-trihydroxylabd-14-en-11-one *see* 2476

17β-Acetoxyestra-4,9,11-trien-3-one *see* 9583

1-(2-Acetoxyethyl)-4-[3-(2-chloro-10-phenothiazinyl)propyl]piperazine *see* 9356

N-(β-Acetoxyethyl)-*N'*-[γ-(2'-chloro-10'-phenothiazinyl)propyl]piperazine *see* 9356

17α-Acetoxy-13-ethyl-17-ethynylgon-4-en-3-one Oxime *see* 6703

10-[3-[1-(2-Acetoxyethyl)-4-piperazinyl]propyl]-2-chlorophenothiazine *see* 9356

17α-Acetoxy-9α-fluoro-11β-hydroxyprogesterone *see* 4200

cis-1-Acetoxy-7-hexadecene *see* 4687

21-Acetoxy-3α-hydroxy-5α-pregnane-11,-20-dione *see* 233

Acetoxyl [Stiefel] *see* 1116

3-Acetoxymethyl-7-aminoceph-3-em-4-oic Acid *see* 434

α-*dl*-3-Acetoxy-6-methylamino-4,4-diphenylheptane *see* 6685

17β-Acetoxy-1α-methyl-5α-androstan-3-one *see* 5916

Acetoxymethyl Benzylpenicillinate *see* 7081

4'-Acetoxy-3'-(α-methylbutyryloxy)-2',2'-dimethyldihydropyrano(7,8:6',5')-coumarin *see* 10010

17α-Acetoxy-6-methylpregna-4,6-diene-3,20-dione *see* 5805

17α-Acetoxy-6α-methylprogesterone *see* 5793

17β-Acetoxy-3-oxoestra-4,9,11-triene *see* 9583

Acetoxyphenylmercury *see* 7300

threo-1-Acetoxy-1-phenyl-1-(2-piperidyl)methane *see* 5467

3α-Acetoxypregnan-20α-ol *see* 7727

20α-Acetoxypregnan-3α-ol *see* 7727

21-Acetoxypregnenolone, 77

21-Acetoxy-5-pregnen-3-ol-20-one *see* 77

17α-Acetoxyprogesterone *see* 4839

17α-Acetoxyprogesterone 3-Cyclopentyl Enol Ether *see* 7114

3-Acetoxy-1-propene *see* 285

17β-[2-Acetoxypropionyl]-9α-fluoro-11β,17-dihydroxyandrosta-1,4-dien-3-one *see* 4188

trans-1-Acetoxy-10-(*n*-propyl)trideca-5,-9-diene *see* 7870

(2-Acetoxypropyl)trimethylammonium Chloride *see* 5940

3-Acetoxyquinuclidine *see* 8082

6-Acetoxythymol 2-(Dimethylamino)ethyl Ether *see* 6292

(6-Acetoxythymoxy)ethyldimethylamine *see* 6292

Acetoxytriphenyltin *see* 9745

Acetozone, 78

Acetphenarsine *see* 52

Acet-*p*-phenetidin *see* 7204

para-Acetphenetidin *see* 7204

Acetphenolisatin *see* 6974

Acetpyrogall *see* 8000

Acetrizoate Sodium, 79

Acetrizoic Acid Sodium Salt *see* 79

Acetulan [Amerchol] *see* 5359

Aceturic Acid, 80

α-Acetylacetanilide *see* 58

Acetylacetic Acid *see* 59

Acetylacetone, 81

Acetylaminoacetic Acid *see* 80

3-(Acetylamino)-5-[(acetylamino)methyl]-2,4,6-triiodobenzoic Acid *see* 5011

3-(Acetylamino)-5-(acetylmethylamino)-2,4,6-triiodobenzoic Acid *see* 6156

2-[[3-(Acetylamino)-5-(acetylmethylamino)-2,4,6-triiodobenzoyl]amino]-2-deoxy-D-glucose *see* 6155

(3*R*,4*R*,5*S*)-4-(Acetylamino)-5-amino-3-(1-ethylpropoxy)-1-cyclohexene-1-carboxylic Acid Ethyl Ester *see* 6889

5-(Acetylamino)-4-[(aminoiminomethyl)-amino]-2,6-anhydro-3,4,5-trideoxy-D-*glycero*-D-*galacto*-non-2-enonic Acid *see* 10113

p-Acetylaminobenzaldehyde Thiosemicarbazone *see* 9290

Acetylaminobenzene *see* 50

4-(Acetylamino)benzeneacetic Acid *see* 133

4-(Acetylamino)benzenesulfonic Acid *see* 102

4-(Acetylamino)benzenesulfonyl Chloride *see* 103

N-(*p*-Acetylaminobenzene Sulfonyl)-*p*-nitroaniline *see* 8933

N-[(Acetylamino)carbonyl]-2-bromo-2-ethylbutanamide *see* 21

N-[(Acetylamino)carbonyl]-α-ethylbenzeneacetamide *see* 99

(*R*)-2-(Acetylamino)-3-*O*-(1-carboxyethyl)-2-deoxy-D-glucose *see* 6304

(4''*R*)-4''-(Acetylamino)-5-*O*-demethyl-25-de(1-methylpropyl)-4''-deoxy-25-(1-methylethyl)avermectin A$_{1a}$ *see* 3633

(4''*R*)-4''-(Acetylamino)-5-*O*-demethyl-4''-deoxyavermectin A$_{1a}$ *see* 3633

(4''*R*)-4''-(Acetylamino)-4''-deoxyavermectin B$_1$ *see* 3633

(7α,25*R*)-7-[[2-(Acetylamino)-2-deoxy-β-D-glucopyranosyl]oxy]-26-(acetyloxy)-cholest-4-en-3-one *see* 7054

(7*S*,9*S*)-9-Acetyl-9-amino-7-[(2-deoxy-β-D-*erythro*-pentopyranosyl)oxy]-7,8,9,-10-tetrahydro-6,11-dihydroxy-5,12-naphthacenedione *see* 593

5-(Acetylamino)-3,5-dideoxy-D-*glycero*-D-*galacto*-2-nonulosonic Acid *see* 8484

4-(Acetylamino)-*N*-[2-(diethylamino)ethyl]benzamide *see* 20

(5*R*,6*R*)-3-[(*R*)-[(1*E*)-2-(Acetylamino)ethenyl]sulfinyl]-6-(1-hydroxy-1-methylethyl)-7-oxo-1-azabicyclo[3.2.0]hept-2-ene-2-carboxylic Acid *see* 1859

2-Acetylaminofluorene *see* 4157

6-(Acetylamino)hexanoic Acid *see* 45

N-Acetyl-6-aminohexanoic Acid *see* 45

[3-(Acetylamino)-4-hydroxyphenyl]arsonic Acid *see* 52

(2*R*)-2-(Acetylamino)-3-methoxy-*N*-(phenylmethyl)propanamide *see* 5333

2-Acetylamino-4-(methylolcycloethylene-dimercaptoarsine)phenol *see* 812

5-Acetylamino-4-methyl-Δ^2-1,3,4-thiadiazoline-2-sulfonamide *see* 5962

4-[2-[[(2*S*)-2-(Acetylamino)-4-(methylthio)-1-oxobutyl]amino]ethyl]-1,2-phenylene Diethyl Ester *see* 3396

2-Acetylamino-5-nitrothiazole *see* 410

5-(Acetylamino)-4-oxo-5-hexenamide *see* 7748

N-Acetyl-*p*-aminophenol *see* 47

p-Acetylaminophenol *see* 47

p-Acetylaminophenol Salicylic Acid Ester *see* 48

(8*R*)-7-Acetyl-5-(4-aminophenyl)-8,9-dihydro-8-methyl-7*H*-1,3-dioxolo[4,5-*h*][2,3]benzodiazepine *see* 9032

2-[[4-(Acetylamino)phenyl]methylene]-hydrazinecarbothioamide *see* 9290

Acetylaminophenyl Salicylate *see* 48

3-(Acetylamino)-1-propanesulfonic Acid Calcium Salt (2:1) *see* 17

Acetyl-*p*-aminosalol *see* 48

2-[[[4-[(Acetylamino)sulfonyl]phenyl]-amino]carbonyl]benzoic Acid *see* 7376

2-Acetylamino-1,3,4-thiadiazole-5-sulfonamide *see* 53

(8*S*-*cis*)-Acetyl-10-[(3-amino-2,3,6-trideoxy-α-L-*lyxo*-hexopyranosyl)oxy]-7,8,9,10-tetrahydro-1,6,8,11-tetrahydroxy-5,12-naphthacenedione *see* 1870

(8*S*-*cis*)-8-Acetyl-10-[(3-amino-2,3,6-trideoxy-α-L-*lyxo*-hexopyranosyl)oxy]-7,8,9,10-tetrahydro-6,8,11-trihydroxy-1-methoxy-5,12-naphthacenedione *see* 2832

(7*S*,9*S*)-9-Acetyl-7-[(3-amino-2,3,6-trideoxy-α-L-*lyxo*-hexopyranosyl)oxy]-7,8,9,10-tetrahydro-6,9,11-trihydroxy-5,12-naphthacenedione *see* 4886

3-Acetylamino-2,4,6-triiodobenzoate of Methylglucamine *see* 5806

3-(Acetylamino)-2,4,6-triiodobenzoic Acid Sodium Salt *see* 79

3-(Acetylamino)-2,4,6-triiodo-5-[(methylamino)carbonyl]benzoic Acid *see* 5064

3-[2-(3-Acetylamino-2,4,6-triiodophenoxy)ethoxy]-2-ethylpropionic Acid *see* 5063

2-[[2-[3-(Acetylamino)-2,4,6-triiodophenoxy]ethoxy]methyl]butanoic Acid *see* 5063

3-[Acetyl-(3-amino-2,4,6-triiodophenyl)amino]-2-methylpropanoic Acid *see* 5010

N-Acetyl-*N*-(3-amino-2,4,6-triiodophenyl)-2-methyl-β-alanine *see* 5010

Acetylandromedol *see* 4543

Acetylaniline *see* 50

N-*p*-Acetylanilinosulfonic Acid *see* 102

N-Acetylanthranilic Acid Ester *see* 5618

N-Acetyl-L-aspartic Acid *see* 840

Acetylated Lanolin *see* 5358

Acetylated Lanolin Alcohols *see* 5359

2-Acetyl-9-azabicyclo[4.2.1]non-2ene *see* 627

Acetylazide [Specia] *see* 101

Acetylbenzene *see* 73

N-(*p*-Acetylbenzenesulfonyl)-*N'*-cyclohexylurea *see* 62

N-Acetyl-*p*-benzoquinonimine *see* 57

Acetyl Benzoyl Peroxide *see* 78

Acetyl Bromide, 82

Acetylbromodiethylacetylcarbamide *see* 21

N-Acetyl-*N*-bromodiethylacetylurea *see* 21

N-Acetyl-*N'*-α-bromo-α-ethylbutyrylcarbamide *see* 21

N-Acetyl-*N*-butyl-β-alanine Ethyl Ester *see* 3773

N-[3-Acetyl-4-(3'-*tert*-butylamino-2'-hydroxy)propoxy]phenyl-*N'*-diethylurea *see* 1960

L-3-Acetyl-5-*sec*-butyl-4-hydroxy-3-pyrrolin-2-one *see* 9149

L-3-Acetyl-5-*sec*-butyltetramic Acid *see* 9149

1-(2-Acetyl-4-*n*-butyramidophenoxy)-2-hydroxy-3-isopropylaminopropane *see* 19

α-Acetylbutyrolactone, 83

Acetylcarbinol *see* 65

Acetylcarbromal *see* 21

Acetylcarnitine, 84

Acetyl-L-carnitine *see* 84

Acetyl-L-carnitine Chloride *see* 84

Acetyl Chloride, 85

Acetylcholine Bromide, 86

Acetylcholine Chloride, 87

Acetylcholinesterase *see* 2208

Acetyl-*o*-cresol *see* 2584

4-Acetyl-*N*-[(cyclohexylamino)carbonyl]-benzenesulfonamide *see* 62

Acetylcysteine, 88

N-Acetyl-L-cysteine *see* 88

N-Acetyldeferoxamine *see* 2860

Acetyldemethyldihydrothebaine *see* 3172

N-Acetyldesferrioxamine B *see* 2860

cis-1-Acetyl-4-[4-[[2-(2,4-dichlorophenyl)-2-(1*H*-imidazol-1-ylmethyl)-1,3-dioxolan-4-yl]methoxy]phenyl]piperazine *see* 5302

1-Acetyl-19,20-didehydro-17,18-epoxycuran-17-ol *see* 2959

(1*S*)-1-*C*-[(2*S*,3*S*)-7-[[4-*O*-Acetyl-2,6-dideoxy-3-*O*-(2,6-dideoxy-4-*O*-methyl-α-D-*lyxo*-hexopyranosyl)-β-D-*lyxo*-hexopyranosyl]oxy]-3-[[*O*-4-*O*-acetyl-2,6-dideoxy-3-*C*-methyl-α-L-*arabino*-hexopyranosyl-(1 → 3)-*O*-2,6-dideoxy-β-D-*arabino*-hexopyranosyl-(1 → 3)-2,-6-dideoxy-β-D-*arabino*-hexopyranosyl]oxy]-1,2,3,4-tetrahydro-5,10-dihydroxy-6-methyl-4-oxo-2-anthracenyl]-5-deoxy-1-*O*-methyl-D-*threo*-2-pentulose *see* 2238

3^D-*O*-(4-*O*-Acetyl-2,6-dideoxy-3-*C*-methyl-α-L-*arabino*-hexopyranosyl)-7-methylolivomycin D *see* 2238

Acetyldigitoxins, 89

α-Acetyldigoxin *see* 3167

β-Acetyldigoxin *see* 3167

Acetyldihydrocodeinone *see* 3172

3-Acetyldihydro-2(3*H*)-furanone *see* 83

O^3-Acetyl-7,8-dihydro-7α-[1(*R*)-hydroxy-1-methylbutyl]-*O*^6-methyl-6,14-*endo*-ethenomorphine *see* 3888

(5*S*)-3-Acetyl-1,5-dihydro-4-hydroxy-5-[(1*S*)-1-methylpropyl]-2*H*-pyrrol-2-one *see* 9149

5-[Acetyl(2,3-dihydroxypropyl)amino]-*N*,*N'*-bis(2,3-dihydroxypropyl)-2,4,6-triiodo-1,3-benzenedicarboxamide *see* 5052

5-[Acetyl(2,3-dihydroxypropyl)amino]-*N*-(2,3-dihydroxypropyl)-*N'*-(2-hydr-oxyethyl)-2,4,6-triiodo-1,3-benzene-dicarboxamide *see* 5068

O-Acetyl-6-dimethylamino-4,4-diphenyl-3-heptanol *see* 5945

2-Acetyl-10-(3-dimethylaminopropyl)-phenothiazine *see* 32

3-Acetyl-10-(3-dimethylaminopropyl)-phenothiazine *see* 32

N'-[3-Acetyl-4-[3-[(1,1-dimethylethyl)-amino]-2-hydroxypropoxy]phenyl]-*N*,*N*-diethylurea *see* 1960

Acetyldiphenylamine *see* 3315

Acetylene, 90

Acetylene Carbamide *see* 93

Acetylenecarboxylic Acid *see* 7821

Acetylene Dibromide, 91

Acetylenedicarboxamide *see* 1962

Acetylenedicarboxylic Acid Diamide *see* 1962

Acetylene Dichloride, 92

Acetylenediureine *see* 93

Acetylene Tetrabromide *see* 9185

Acetylene Tetrachloride *see* 9189

Acetyleneurea, 93

Acetylenogen *see* 1656

2'-Acetylerythromycin Stearate *see* 3682

Acetyl Ethylene *see* 6134

Acetylformaldehyde *see* 6081

Acetylformic Acid *see* 8021

Acetylgalactosamine 4-Sulfatase *see* 819

Acetylgalactosamine 4-Sulfatase (Human CSL4S-342 Cell) *see* 819

α-*N*-Acetyl-L-glutamine *see* 25

N^2-Acetyl-L-glutamine *see* 25

Acetyl Glyceryl Ether Phosphorylcholine *see* 7524

N-Acetylglycine *see* 80

N-Acetylglycine Compd with 4,4'-(Diazoamino)dibenzamidine *see* 3266

N-Acetylglycine Compd with 4,4'-(1-Triazene-1,3-diyl)bis(benzenecarboximidamide) (2:1) *see* 3266

Acetylglycocoll *see* 80

3-*O*-Acetyl-18β-glycyrrhetic Acid *see* 76

Acetylglycyrrhetinic Acid *see* 76

(1*S*,3*S*)-3-Acetyl-1,2,3,4,6,11-hexahydro-3,5,10,12-tetrahydroxy-6,11-dioxo-1-naphthacenyl 3-Amino-2,3,6-trideoxy-α-L-*lyxo*-hexopyranoside *see* 1870

(1*S*,3*S*)-3-Acetyl-1,2,3,4,6,11-hexahydro-3,5,12-trihydroxy-6,11-dioxo-1-naphthacenyl-3-amino-2,3,6-trideoxy-α-L-*lyxo*-hexopyranoside *see* 4886

N-Acetylhomocysteinethiolactone *see* 2320

Acetyl Hydroperoxide *see* 7150

N'-[5-[[4-[[5-(Acetylhydroxyamino)pentyl]amino]-1,4-dioxobutyl]hydroxyamino]pentyl]-*N*-(5-aminopentyl)-*N*-hydroxybutanediamide *see* 2860

N-Acetyl-4-hydroxy-*m*-arsanilic Acid *see* 52

α-Acetyl-γ-hydroxybutyric Acid γ-Lactone *see* 83

17β-Acetyl-17-hydroxyestr-4-ene-3-one Hexanoate *see* 4414

2-Acetyl-10-[3-[4-(β-hydroxyethyl)piperazinyl]propyl]phenothiazine *see* 72

2-Acetyl-10-[3-[γ-(2-hydroxyethyl)piperidino]propyl]phenothiazine *see* 7462

2-Acetyl-10-[3-[4-(β-hydroxyethyl)piperidino]propyl]phenothiazine *see* 7462

5-Acetyl-6-hydroxy-2-isopropenylbenzofuran *see* 3900

2-Acetyl-7-(2-hydroxy-3-isopropylaminopropoxy)benzofuran *see* 1022

3'-Acetyl-4'-[2-hydroxy-3-(isopropylamino)propoxy]butyranilide *see* 19

N-Acetylhydroxylamine *see* 63

5-[Acetyl(2-hydroxy-3-methoxypropyl)amino]-*N*,*N'*-bis(2,3-dihydroxypropyl)-2,4,6-triiodo-1,3-benzenedicarboxamide *see* 5059

3-*O*-Acetyl-7α-[1(*R*)-hydroxy-1-methylbutyl]-6,14-*endo*-ethenotetrahydrooripavine *see* 3888

N-[3-Acetyl-4-[2-hydroxy-3-[(1-methylethyl)amino]propoxy]phenyl]butanamide *see* 19

2-Acetyl-5-hydroxy-3-oxo-4-hexenoic Acid δ-Lactone *see* 2865

(4*R*)-1-Acetyl-4-hydroxy-L-proline *see* 6903

1-Acetyl-4-hydroxy-2-pyrrolidinecarboxylic Acid *see* 6903

N-Acetylimidoquinone *see* 57

Acetyl Iodide, 94

Acetyllactoylcholine 1,5-Naphthalenedisulfonate *see* 114

N-Acetyl-DL-leucine Compd with 2-Aminoethanol (1:1) *see* 95

Acetylleucine Monoethanolamine, 95

DL-Acetylleucine Monoethanolamine Salt *see* 95

N-Acetyl-3-mercaptoalanine *see* 88

N-Acetyl-3-mercapto-D-valine *see* 98

Acetylmetacresol *see* 2583

Acetylmethadol *see* 5945

α-*l*-Acetylmethadol *see* 5466

levo-α-Acetylmethadol *see* 5466

Acetylmethanol *see* 65

N-Acetylmethionine, 96

N-(*N*-Acetyl-L-methionyl)-*O*,*O*-bis(ethoxycarbonyl)dopamine *see* 3396

N-(*N*-Acetyl-L-methionyl)-3,4-diethoxycarboxyphenethylamine *see* 3396

1-Acetyl-17-methoxyaspidospermidine *see* 850

N^1-Acetyl-*N*^1-(3-methoxypyrazinyl)sulfanilamide *see* 101

N-Acetyl-5-methoxytryptamine *see* 5816

3-[[[[3-(Acetylmethylamino)-2,4,6-triiodo-5-[(methylamino)carbonyl]benzoyl]amino]acetyl]amino]-5-[[(2-hydroxyethyl)amino]carbonyl]-2,4,6-triiodobenzoic Acid *see* 5067

Acetyl Methyl Carbinol *see* 64

Acetyl-β-methylcholine Chloride *see* 5940

O-Acetyl-β-methylcholine Chloride *see* 5940

α-[2-[Acetyl(1-methylethyl)amino]ethyl]-α-(2-chlorophenyl)-1-piperidinebutanamide *see* 1204

N-Acetyl-*N*-methyl-L-isoleucyl-L-isoleucyl-*N*-[(1*S*)-3-methyl-1[[(2*R*)-2-methyloxiranyl]carbonyl]butyl]-L-threoninamide *see* 3630

3-Acetyl-6-methyl-2*H*-pyran-2,4(3*H*)-dione *see* 2865

N-Acetylmuramic Acid *see* 6304

N-Acetylmuramide Glycanohydrolase *see* 5640

N-(*N*-Acetylmuramoyl)-L-alanyl-D-α-glutamine *see* 6305

N-(*N*-Acetylmuramoyl)-L-alanyl-D-α-glutaminyl-*N*-[(7*R*)-4-hydroxy-4-oxido-10-oxo-7-[(1-oxohexadecyl)oxy]-3,5,9-trioxa-4-phosphapentacos-1-yl]-L-alaninamide *see* 5844

Acid Rubin *see* 107
Acid Sodium Phosphate *see* 8660
Acid Trypaflavine *see* 123
Acidulin [Lilly] *see* 4469
Acidum Fenclozicum *see* 3969
Acid Yellow 3 *see* 8071
Acid Yellow D *see* 9776
Acid Yellow S *see* 6393
Acifluorfen, 109
Acifran, 110
Aci-Jel [Ortho] *see* 55
Aciloc [Orion] *see* 2279
Acimethin [Gry] *see* 5975
Acinil [GEA] *see* 2279
Acinitrazole *see* 410
Acino [IMA] *see* 3973
Acintol C *see* 9040
Aciphex [Eisai] *see* 8089
Acipimox, 111
Acitretin, 112
ACL-59 *see* 9767
ACL-85 *see* 9641
Aclacin [Lundbeck] *see* 113
Aclacinomycin A *see* 113
Aclacinomycin B *see* 113
Aclacinomycins, 113
Aclacinon [Yamanouchi] *see* 113
Aclame [Danisco] *see* 248
Aclaplastin [Medac] *see* 113
Aclarubicin *see* 113
Aclarubicin Hydrochloride *see* 113
Aclatonium Napadisilate, 114
Aclosone [Schering] *see* 220
Aclovate [GSK] *see* 220
[*N*-Ac-D-Nal(2)¹-D-*p*Cl-Phe²-D-Pal(3)³-D-hArg(Et₂)⁶-hArg(Et₂)⁸-D-Ala¹⁰]-GnRH *see* 4365
Ac-D-Nal¹-4-Cl-D-Phe²-D-Pal³-*N*-Me-Tyr⁵-D-Asn⁶-Lys(iPr)⁸-D-Ala¹⁰-LH-RH *see* 3
Ac-D-Nal(2)¹-D-Phe(4Cl)²-D-Pal(3)³-D-Cit⁶-D-Ala¹⁰-LH-RH *see* 2026
Acnegel [Stiefel] *see* 1116
Acnestrol [Dermik] *see* 1448
Acnisal [Euroderma] *see* 8332
ACNU [Baxter] *see* 6553
Acocantherin *see* 6901
Acodeen [Hommel] *see* 1513
Acolen *see* 2868
Acomplia [Sanofi-Synthelabo] *see* 8229
Aconine, 115
Aconite, 116
Aconitic Acid, 117
Aconitine, 118
Aconitine, Amorphous, 119
Aconitum Ferox, 120
Acopyrine *see* 716
"Acorn Sugar" *see* 8036
Acortan [Ferring] *see* 134
Acozid [ACO] *see* 8335
ACP-332 *see* 6418
ACPC *see* 2734
ACPMD *see* 9441
Acquat CDAC *see* 2017
Acquinite *see* 2156
ACR-3453A *see* 7983
Acraldehyde *see* 128
Acranil [Bayer], 121
Acrasin *see* 2708
Acrex [Murphy] *see* 3285
9-Acridinamine *see* 407
Acridine, 122
3,6-Acridinediamine *see* 7771
4′-(9-Acridinylamino)methanesulfon-*m*-anisidide *see* 594

N-[4-(9-Acridinylamino)-3-methoxy-phenyl]methanesulfonamide *see* 594
Acriflavine, 123
Acriflavine Hydrochloride *see* 123
Acrilan [Solutia], 124
Acrinathrin, 125
Acrinol *see* 3716
Acrisorcin, 126
Acrivastine, 127
Acrobat [BASF] *see* 3222
Acrol *see* 2983
Acrolactine *see* 3716
Acrolein, 128
Acronize [Am. Cyanamid] *see* 2192
α-Acrose *see* 4274
Acrosoxacin *see* 8268
Acrp30 *see* 163
Acrylaldehyde *see* 128
Acrylamide, 129
Acrylic Acid, 130
Acrylic Acid *n*-Butyl Ester *see* 1539
Acrylic Acid Ethyl Ester *see* 3759
Acrylic Acid Methyl Ester *see* 6011
Acrylic Aldehyde *see* 128
Acrylonitrile, 131
ACS *see* 718
Actaplanins, 132
Actara [Syngenta] *see* 9294
Actarit, 133
Actasal [Purdue Frederick] *see* 2209
Actase [Ortho] *see* 7520
Actellic [Syngenta] *see* 7497
Actellifog [Zeneca] *see* 7497
Actemin [Lazar] *see* 582
Actemra [Chugai] *see* 9493
ACTH, 134
Acthar [RPR] *see* 134
ACTH-β-lipotropin Common Precursor *see* 7791
Acthormon [Shionogi] *see* 4428
Acticolin [Upsamedica] *see* 2319
Actidil [Wellcome] *see* 9746
Actidilon [Wellcome] *see* 9746
Actidione *see* 2728
Actigall [Novartis] *see* 9889
Actigam [Daltan] *see* 4461
Actilin *see* 6454
Actilyse [Boehringer, Ing.] *see* 9468
Actimax [Sankyo] *see* 6291
Actimid [Celgene], 135
Actimide [Tobishi] *see* 2451
Actimmune [Genentech] *see* 4992
Actin, 136
α-Actin *see* 136
β-Actin *see* 136
γ-Actin *see* 136
F-Actin *see* 136
G-Actin *see* 136
Actinex [Schwarz] *see* 6693
Actinium, 137
Actinium X *see* 8094
Actinobolin, 138
Actinodaphnine, 139
Actinolite *see* 826
Actinomycetin, 140
Actinomycin IV *see* 2800
Actinomycin A_IV *see* 2800
Actinomycin C *see* 1606
Actinomycin C₁ *see* 2800
Actinomycin C₂ *see* 1606
Actinomycin C₃ *see* 1606
Actinomycin D *see* 2800
Actinomycin F₁, 141
Actinomycin I₁ *see* 2800
Actinomycin KS4 *see* 141

Actinomycin-[thr-val-pro-sar-meval] *see* 2800
Actinomycin X₁ *see* 2800
Actinon *see* 8095
Actinorhodine, 142
Actinospectacin *see* 8739
Actinum K *see* 4262
Action [Kumiai] *see* 4210
Actiphenol, 143
Actiplas [Dompé] *see* 9468
Actiq [Cephalon] *see* 4001
Actira [Bayer] *see* 6291
Actithiazic Acid *see* 6322
Activase [Genentech] *see* 9468
Activated Barium Hydroxide *see* 977
Activated Carbon *see* 1808
Activated Charcoal *see* 1808
Activated 7-Dehydrocholesterol *see* 10019
Activated Dimethicone *see* 3215
Activated Ergosterol *see* 10018
Active Amyl Alcohol *see* 6030
Active Methionine *see* 156
Activin, 144
Activin A *see* 144
Activin AB *see* 144
Activol [Zeneca] *see* 4419
Actol [Fournier] *see* 6531
Actomyosin *see* 136
Acton [Ferring] *see* 134
Actonel [Procter & Gamble] *see* 8232
Actos [Takeda] *see* 7452
Actosin [Daiichi Seiyaku] *see* 1463
Actosolv [HMR] *see* 9887
Actriol [Organon] *see* 3616
Acuatim [Otsuka] *see* 6345
Acuitel [Pfizer] *see* 8051
Acular [Allergan] *see* 5306
Acupan [3M] *see* 6440
AcuTect [Diatide] *see* 9098
Acutil-S [ISF] *see* 25
ACV, 145
Acycloguanosine *see* 146
Acyclovir, 146
Acylan [Croda] *see* 5358
Acylanid [Sandoz] *see* 89
N-(Acylcolaminoformylmethyl)pyridinium Chloride *see* 5370
Acylpyrin [Slovakofarma] *see* 851
AD₆ *see* 2405
AD-32 *see* 9915
AD-810 *see* 10192
AD-1590 *see* 1159
AD-4833 *see* 7452
AD-5423 *see* 1319
ADA, 147
Ada *see* 3183
Adage [Syngenta] *see* 9294
ADAH *see* 1244
Adalat(e) [Bayer] *see* 6528
Adalimumab, 148
Adalin [Bayer] *see* 1831
"Adam" *see* 5767
1-Adamantanamine *see* 374
Adamantane, 149
N-1-Adamantyl-*N*-[2-(dimethylamino)-ethoxy]acetamide *see* 9771
6-[3-(1-Adamantyl)-4-methoxyphenyl]-2-naphthoic Acid *see* 150
Adams' Catalyst *see* 7527
Adamsite *see* 7215
Adancor [Merck-Clévenot] *see* 6521
Adapalene, 150
Adapin [Lotus] *see* 3435
Adaptinol [Bayer] *see* 10063

ADCA see 1244
Adcortyl [BMS] see 9596
ADD-03055 see 3950
ADD-234037 see 5333
Addisomnol [Synochem] see 1831
Adecut [Takeda] see 2876
Adefovir, 151
Adefovir Dipivoxil see 151
Adekin [Desitin] see 374
Adelir [Merck KGaA] see 9843
Ademetionine see 156
Ademide [Toyo Jozo] see 2451
Ademin(e) see 9599
Ademol [BMS] see 4139
Adenaron [Kowa] see 1789
Adenine, 152
Adenine Arabinoside see 9976
Adenine Riboside see 153
Adenocard [Fujisawa] see 153
Adenock [Mitsubishi] see 279
Adenocor [Sanofi Winthrop] see 153
Adenogen see 1788
Adenohypophyseal Growth Hormone see 8716
Adenohypophysial Luteotropin see 7779
Adenoscan [Fujisawa] see 153
Adenosine, 153
Adenosine Cyclic 3′,5′-(Hydrogen Phosphate) see 2708
Adenosine 3′,5′-Cyclic Monophosphate see 2708
Adenosine 3′,5′-Cyclic Phosphate see 2708
Adenosine Diphosphate, 154
Adenosinediphosphoric Acid see 154
Adenosine 3′-Monophosphate see 157
Adenosine 3′,5′-Monophosphate see 2708
Adenosine 5′-Monophosphate see 158
Adenosine-3′-monophosphoric Acid see 157
Adenosine-5′-monophosphoric Acid see 158
Adenosine Phosphate see 158
Adenosine 3′,5′-Phosphate see 2708
Adenosine-3′-phosphoric Acid see 157
Adenosine-5′-phosphoric Acid see 158
Adenosine 5′-Pyrophosphoric Acid see 154
Adenosine 5′-(Tetrahydrogen Triphosphate) see 155
Adenosine 5′-(Trihydrogen Diphosphate) see 154
Adenosine 5′-(Trihydrogen Diphosphate) 2′-(Dihydrogen Phosphate) P′ → 5′-Ester with 3-(Aminocarbonyl)-1-β-D-ribofuranosylpyridinium Inner Salt see 6348
Adenosine 5′-(Trihydrogen Diphosphate) P′ → 5′-Ester with 3-(Aminocarbonyl)-1-β-D-ribofuranosylpyridinium Inner Salt see 6344
Adenosine 5′-(Trihydrogen Diphosphate) 5′ → 5′-Ester with Riboflavine see 4091
Adenosine Triphosphate, 155
Adenosine 5′-Triphosphoric Acid see 155
Adenosyl-B₁₂ see 2451
S-Adenosylmethionine, 156
Adényl [Am. Home] see 158
Adenylate Cyclase see 2708
3′-Adenylic Acid, 157
5′-Adenylic Acid, 158
Adenylic Acid b see 157
5′-Adenylphosphoric Acid see 154
Adepril [Teofarma] see 487

Adeps see 5371
Adepsine Oil see 7186
Adermine Hydrochloride see 7982
Adermykon see 2178
Aderoxal see 7979
Adesitrin [Pharmacia] see 6607
Adetol [Kyowa] see 155
Adetphos [Kowa] see 155
Adfeed [Lead Chem.] see 4199
Adhatoda, 159
Adhatodai see 159
Adiaben see 2186
Adiazine [Recordati] see 8903
Adicillin see 7098
Adifax [Servier] see 3973
Adigal [Beiersdorf] see 5354
Adinazolam, 160
Adinazolam Mesylate see 160
Adipex-P [Gate] see 7262
Adiphenine, 161
Adipic Acid, 162
Adipic Acid Di(3-carboxy-2,4,6-triiodo-anilide) see 5022
Adipic Ketone see 2743
Adipine [Chiesi] see 6528
Adipiodone see 5022
Adipogenesis Inhibitory Factor see 5000
Adipokinetic Hormone see 5513
Adipomin [Streuli] see 3973
Adiponectin, 163
AdipoQ see 163
Adiposetten [Reiss] see 6714
3,3′-(Adipoyldiimino)bis[2,4,6-triiodo-benzoic Acid] see 5022
5,5′-(Adipoyldiimino)bis[2,4,6-triiodo-N-methylisophthalamic Acid] see 5009
Adipsin, 164
N,N′-Adipylbis(3-amino-2,4,6-triiodo-benzoic Acid) see 5022
Adiuretin SD see 2924
Adizem [Napp] see 3202
ADL-8-2698 see 372
Adlone [Pharmascience] see 3915
Adlumidine, 165
Adlumine, 166
Admire [Bayer CropSci.] see 4910
Admon [Esteve] see 6551
A-DNA see 2907
Adnexol [Protina] see 4885
Adobiol [Yoshitomi] see 1473
Adofen [Ferrer] see 4185
Adomal [Malesci] see 3146
AdoMet see 156
Adona [Tanabe Seiyaku] see 1789
Adonis Vernalis, 167
Adonite see 168
Adonitol, 168
Adonitoxin, 169
D-Adonose see 8207
ADP see 154, 7003
Adphen [Ferndale] see 7220
ADR-033 see 9737
ADR-529 see 8123
Adrafinil, 170
Adral [Lifepharma] see 6535
Adrenalin [Monarch] see 3619
Adrenaline see 3619
Adrenaline Oxidase see 6247
Adrenalone, 171
Adrenochrome, 172
Adrenochrome Monosemicarbazone Sodium Salicylate Complex see 1788
Adrenochrome Semicarbazone Compd with Sodium Salicylate see 1788
Adrenocorticotrop(h)ic Hormone of the Pituitary Gland see 134

Adrenocorticotrop(h)in see 134
Adrenoglomerulotropin, 173
Adrenolutin, 174
Adrenomedullin, 175
Adrenone see 171
Adrenor see 6695
Adrenosterone, 176
Adrenoxyl [Sanofi Winthrop] see 172
Adrestat-F [Organon] see 1788
Adrevil [Zyma] see 1510
Adriacin [Pfizer] see 3439
Adriamicina [Farmochim. Ital.] see 5943
Adriamycin [Pfizer] see 3439
Adriamycinone see 3439
Adriblastina [Pfizer] see 3439
Adronat [Neopharmed] see 229
Adroyd [Parke-Davis] see 6967
Adrucil [Adria] see 4181
ADT see 644
Adulsa see 159
Adumbran [Boehringer, Ing.] see 6926
Adurix [Nycomed] see 2393
Advantage [Bayer] see 4910
Advantan [Schering AG] see 6111
Advil [Wyeth] see 4881
Advocin [Pfizer] see 2813
AE-17 see 9009
AE-941 see 6467
AE-B066752 see 7798
AE-F107892 see 5800
AE-F115008 see 5046
AE-F130060 see 5911
AE-F130360 see 4234
Aedurid [Robugen] see 3514
Aequamen [Promonta] see 1178
Aequorin, 177
Aerobec [3M Pharma] see 1019
Aerobid [Forest] see 4145
Aerobin [Farmasan] see 9285
Aerolate [Fleming] see 9285
Aerolin [3M Pharma] see 216
Aerolone [Lilly] see 5217
Aeromatt see 1657
Aeroseb-Dex [Allergan] see 2943
Aeroseb-HC [Allergan] see 4787
Aerosol AY see 2989
Aerosol IB see 3194
Aerosol MA see 1255
Aerosol OT [Cyanamid] see 3401
Aerosporin [Burroughs Wellcome] see 7573
Aerotrol [Abbott] see 5217
Aerrane [Baxter] see 5175
Aescin see 3696
Aescorin [Steigerwald] see 4748
Aescusan [Jenapharm] see 4748
AET, 178
Aether Oenanthicus see 3835
Aethone [Sopar] see 6884
Aethoxysklerol [Kreussler] see 7558
Aethylis Chloridum see 3782
Aetina see 3737
Aetiocholanic Acid see 3867
Aetoxisclerol [Dexo] see 7558
AF-102B see 2034
AF-438 see 6944
AF-634 see 7903
AF-983 see 1035
AF-1161 see 9579
AF-1191 see 3885
AF-1890 see 5568
AF-2139 see 2820
Afalon [Hoechst] see 5509
Afema [Novartis] see 3927
Affinin, 179

Affinitac [Lilly] *see* 755
Affinitak [Lilly] *see* 755
Affinitins *see* 5429
Affirm [Novartis] *see* 3554
Affront [Wellmark] *see* 2189
aFGF *see* 4072
aFGF-1 *see* 4072
aFGF-2 *see* 4072
AFI-phyllin *see* 3479
AFI-Tiazin *see* 7252
Aflatoxicol *see* 180
Aflatoxin B$_1$ *see* 180
Aflatoxin B$_2$ *see* 180
Aflatoxin G$_1$ *see* 181
Aflatoxin G$_2$ *see* 181
Aflatoxin M$_1$ *see* 182
Aflatoxin M$_2$ *see* 182
Aflatoxins B, 180
Aflatoxins G, 181
Aflatoxins M, 182
Aflix [Sandoz] *see* 4246
Afloben [Esseti] *see* 1122
Aflodac [Janus] *see* 8982
Afloqualone, 183
Aflorix [Gramon] *see* 6178
Afloxan [Rottapharm] *see* 7774
Afluon [Viatris] *see* 906
Afongan [Galderma] *see* 6846
Afonilum [Knoll] *see* 465
Afonilum *see* 9285
Afos [Salus] *see* 4254
Afrazine [Schering-Plough] *see* 6966
African Oil Palm *see* 6818
African Saffron *see* 1868
Afrin [Schering-Plough] *see* 6966
Afrinol [Schering] *see* 7916
Aftate [Schering-Plough] *see* 9519
Afugan [Hoechst] *see* 7962
Afwillite *see* 1702
Afzelechin *see* 1902
AG-337 *see* 6672
AG-1343 *see* 6443
AG-1346 *see* 6443
AG-1549 *see* 1755
AG-1749 *see* 5362
AG-3340 *see* 7751
Agar, 184
Agar-agar *see* 184
Agaric, 185
Agaric Acid *see* 186
Agaricic Acid, 186
Agaricin *see* 186
Agaricinic Acid *see* 186
Agarin *see* 6312
Agaritine, 187
Agaropectin *see* 184
Agarose *see* 184
Agate *see* 8493
Agbayun *see* 6206
Agedoite *see* 837
AG-EE-623 ZW *see* 8136
Agene *see* 6602
Agenerase [GSK] *see* 589
Agent Orange *see* 9084
AGEPC *see* 7524
Ageratochromene *see* 7718
Agerite *see* 6248
Ageroplas [Serono] *see* 3367
Agglutinin *see* 9
Agglutinins *see* 5429
Aggrastat [Merck & Co.] *see* 9464
Aggrenox [Boehringer, Ing.] *see* 3346
AGIF *see* 5000
Agifutol S [Kyorin] *see* 4475
Agilect [Teva] *see* 8116

Agilene [Am. Agile] *see* 7567
Agit [Sanofi Winthrop] *see* 3174
Agkistrodon rhodostoma Venom Protein-
    ase *see* 630
Agkistrodon Serine Proteinase *see* 630
Aglumin *see* 3722
Agmatine, 188
AGN-1135 *see* 8116
AGN-190168 *see* 9081
AGN-190342 *see* 1375
AGN-190342-LF *see* 1375
AGN-191622 *see* 1357
AGN-192024 *see* 1221
Agnolyt [Madaus] *see* 189
Agnus Castus, 189
Agofollin [Biotika] *see* 3703
Agomelatine, 190
Agon [TheraPharm] *see* 3953
Agoniadin *see* 7540
Agontan [Knoll] *see* 3192
Agopton [Takeda] *see* 5362
Agotan *see* 2288
Agr-1240 *see* 6200
Agradil [Synthelabo] *see* 9948
Agram [Fabre] *see* 577
Agréal [Delagrange] *see* 9948
Agricultural Limestone *see* 5491
Agri-Mek [Syngenta] *see* 2
AgriStrep [Merck & Co.] *see* 8826
Agritox [Nufarm] *see* 5764
Agroclavine, 191
Agrocybin, 192
Agropyrum *see* 9761
Agrosan [Zeneca] *see* 7300
Agroxone [Zeneca] *see* 5764
Agrylin [Shire] *see* 622
Agrypnal [Eggochemia] *see* 7238
Agstone *see* 5491
Ague Tree *see* 8381
AH-42 *see* 5959
AH-289 *see* 2081
AH-2250 *see* 1495
AH-3365 *see* 216
AH-5158A *see* 5329
AH-8165 *see* 3943
AH-19065 *see* 8110
AHA *see* 63
Ahanon [Rodleben] *see* 9035
AHCTL *see* 2320
AHF *see* 3921
AHG *see* 3921
AHMHA *see* 8800
AHP-200 *see* 6903
AHPrBP *see* 7003
AHR-85 *see* 5980
AHR-233 *see* 5851
AHR-504 *see* 4501
AHR-619 *see* 3432
AHR-857 *see* 8914
AHR-3018 *see* 726
AHR-3053 *see* 1802
AHR-3070-C *see* 6143
AHR-5850D *see* 395
AHR-9434 *see* 6469
AHR-10282 *see* 1390
AHR-10282B *see* 1390
A-hydroCort [Abbott] *see* 4787
AI-27303 *see* 2018
AIBN *see* 918
Aicamin [Crinos] *see* 6861
AICA Orotate *see* 6861
AICA-riboside *see* 16
Aicorat [Mack, Illert.] *see* 6861
Aida [Paraphar] *see* 4808
Aiglonyl [Fumouze] *see* 8989

Aimax [Ayerst] *see* 5946
Airol [Pierre Fabre] *see* 8165
Airtal [Prodes] *see* 22
Airum [Promeco] *see* 3981
Aisemide *see* 4309
AIT-082 *see* 5448
Aizumycin *see* 1202
AJ-1590 *see* 1159
Ajacine *see* 5618
Ajaconine, 193
Ajan [3M] *see* 6440
Ajicef [Ajinomoto] *see* 1938
Aji-no-moto [Suzuki] *see* 6254
Ajmalan-17,21-diol *see* 194
(17*R*,21α)-Ajmalan-17,21-diol 17-
    (Chloroacetate) *see* 5577
Ajmalicine *see* 8119
Ajmaline, 194
Ajoene, 195
Ajowan Oil, 196
Ajugarin-I *see* 197
Ajugarin-II *see* 197
Ajugarin-III *see* 197
Ajugarin-IV *see* 197
Ajugarin-V *see* 197
Ajugarins, 197
Ajulemic Acid, 198
AK-33X *see* 6223
AK-602 *see* 737
Akarpine [Akorn] *see* 7424
Akatinol [Merz] *see* 5829
Ak-Con [Akorn] *see* 6368
AKD-2023 *see* 33
Ak-Dex [Akorn] *see* 2943
Ak-Dilate [Akorn] *see* 7286
Akermanite *see* 1702
Ak-Fluor [Akorn] *see* 4159
Akineton [Knoll] *see* 1233
Akinophyl [Knoll] *see* 1233
Akistin [Nycomed] *see* 8329
Aklavinone *see* 113
Ak-Nefrin [Akorn] *see* 7286
Aknemycin [Hermal] *see* 3681
Akneroxid L [Lubapharm] *see* 1116
Aknin [Lichtenstein] *see* 3681
Ak-Pentolate [Akorn] *see* 2746
Akrinol [Schering] *see* 126
Akrochem ETU-22 [Akron Chem.] *see*
    3803
Ak-Sulf [Akorn] *see* 8899
Ak-Taine [Akorn] *see* 7807
Aktamin *see* 6695
Ak-Tate [Akorn] *see* 7721
Aktedron [Chinoin] *see* 582
Aktivin [Kobayashi] *see* 9297
Ak-Tracin [Akorn] *see* 934
Akuammicine, 199
Akwa Tears [Akorn] *see* 7585
AL-1241 *see* 7762
AL-4682 *see* 1376
AL-4943A *see* 6840
AL-6221 *see* 9577
AL-6515 *see* 6469
Ala *see* 204
ALA *see* 446
Alabandite *see* 5740
Alabaster *see* 1706
Alacepril, 200
Alachlor, 201
Ala-Cort [Del-Ray] *see* 4787
ALAcortril [Pfizer] *see* 4188
Ala²-cyclosporine *see* 2752
Aladotril *see* 3940
Alafosfalin, 202
Alagebrium Chloride, 203

[**β-Ala^1,lys^{17}**]ACTH$^{1-17}$-4-amino-*N*-bu-
  tylamide *see* 314
[**β-Ala^1,lys^{17}**]corticotropin-(1-17)-hep-
  tadecapeptide-4-amino-*N*-butylamide
  see 314
Alamine *see* 3183
Alamon [Grelan] *see* 4849
Alamycin [Norbrook] *see* 6976
Alanap *see* 6418
Alanetorin [Takata; Nippon Kayaku] *see*
  223
Alanex [Makhteshim-Agan] *see* 201
Alanine, 204
L-**Alanine** *see* 204
L-*α*-**Alanine** *see* 204
β-**Alanine,** 205
1-*β*-**Alanine-17-[*N*-(4-aminobutyl)-L-ly-**
  sinamide]-*α*$^{1-17}$-corticotropin *see* 314
1-*β*-**Alanine-17-[L-2,6-diamino-*N*-(4-**
  aminobutyl)hexanamide]-*α*$^{1-17}$-cortico-
  tropin *see* 314
Alanine Nitrogen Mustard *see* 5828
L-**Alanosine,** 206
Alant Camphor *see* 207
Alantin *see* 5004
Alantolactone, 207
Alant Starch *see* 5004
1*R*-1-(L-**Alanylamino)ethylphosphonic**
  Acid *see* 202
N-L-**Alanyl-blood Coagulation Factor**
  LACI (Human Clone λP9 Protein
  Moiety Reduced) *see* 9467
L-**Alanyl-(6-diazo-5-oxo)-L-norleucyl-(6-**
  diazo-5-oxo)-L-norleucine *see* 208
[*N*-*β*-**Alanyl-L-histidinato(2−)-*N*,*N*^{N},-**
  ***O*^{α}]zinc** *see* 7552
β-**Alanyl-L-histidinato Zinc** *see* 7552
β-**Alanyl-L-histidine** *see* 1850
N-*β*-**Alanyl-3-methyl-L-histidine** *see* 679
[1*R*-(1*α*,2*β*,6*α*)]-*N*-L-**Alanyl-3-(5-oxo-7-**
  oxabicyclo[4.1.0]hept-2-yl)-L-alanine
  see 933
L-**Alanyl-L-valyl-L-glutaminyl-L-seryl-**
  L-lysyl-L-prolyl-L-prolyl-L-seryl-L-ly-
  syl-L-argininyl-L-*α*-aspartyl-L-prolyl-
  L-prolyl-L-lysyl-L-methionyl-L-gluta-
  minyl-L-threonyl-L-aspartic Acid *see*
  9018
[D-**Ala^1**] **Peptide T Amide** *see* 7148
Alaphosphin *see* 202
Alapril [Mediolanum] *see* 5516
Alar [Uniroyal] *see* 2810
Alathon [DuPont] *see* 7567
Alatriopril *see* 3940
Alatrioprilat *see* 3940
Alavert [Wyeth] *see* 5578
Alazopeptin, 208
Albac [Alpharma] *see* 936
Albacar *see* 1657
Albalon [Allergan] *see* 6368
Albamycin [Pharmacia & Upjohn] *see*
  6722
Albasil C *see* 8930
Albaspidin, 209
Albaspidin-BB *see* 209
Albego [Boehringer, Ing.] *see* 1725
Albendazole, 210
Albendazole Oxide *see* 210
Albenza [GSK] *see* 210
Albert-285 *see* 7813
Albiotic [Pharmacia] *see* 5500
Albipen [Intervet] *see* 586
Albistat [Ortho] *see* 6178
Albizziin, 211
Albocresil [Altana] *see* 7556

Albofungin, 212
Alboline *see* 7186
Albomycetin *see* 7413
Albomycin, 213
Albon [Pfizer] *see* 8905
Albone *see* 4798
Alborixin, 214
Albothyl [Altana] *see* 7556
Albucid [Ankerpharm] *see* 8899
Albumen, 215
Albuminar [ZLB Behring] *see* 8468
Albumose Silver *see* 8527
Albumotope-^{131}I [Bracco] *see* 8468
Albunex [Molecular Biosystems] *see* 8468
Albuterol, 216
Albutest [Miles] *see* 1444
Albutoin, 217
Alcacyl [Novartis] *see* 1647
Alcaine [Alcon] *see* 7807
ALCAR *see* 84
Alchloquin *see* 5031
Alcian Blue, 218
Alcian Blue 8GX *see* 218
Alclofenac, 219
Alclometasone, 220
Alcobon [Roche] *see* 4125
Alcodin [Alcon] *see* 1217
Alcohol *see* 3760
95% Alcohol *see* 3760
Alcohol Ethoxylates *see* 7577
Alcohol, USP *see* 3760
Alcomicin [Alcon] *see* 4392
Alconefrin [Polymedica] *see* 7286
Alcopan-250 *see* 2947
Alcuronium, 221
Aldactazine [Searle] *see* 318
Aldactone [Pharmacia & Upjohn] *see* 8760
Aldanil *see* 8620
Aldara [3M Pharma] *see* 4922
Aldazine [Alphapharm] *see* 9359
Aldebaranium *see* 10105
Aldecin [Schering-Plough] *see* 1019
"Aldehyde" *see* 39
Aldehyde Ammonia *see* 40
Aldehyde C-7 *see* 4658
Aldehyde-collidine *see* 3844
Aldehydine *see* 3844
Alder Buckthorn *see* 4263
Alderlin [Zeneca] *see* 7790
Aldesleukin *see* 4994
Aldesulfone Sodium *see* 8968
Aldicarb, 222
Aldifen *see* 3280
Aldioxa, 223
Aldipin [Helvepharm] *see* 6528
Aldocorten [Novartis] *see* 225
Aldol, 224
Aldomet [Merck & Co.] *see* 6055
Aldomin [Merck & Co.] *see* 6055
Aldomycin *see* 6600
Aldosterone, 225
Aldosterone-stimulating Hormone *see*
  173
Aldoxime *see* 42
Aldrin, 226
Aldrox [Am. Home] *see* 342
Aldurazyme [BioMarin] *see* 4894
ALEC *see* 7939
Alecor [Andromaco] *see* 3636
Alefacept, 227
Alemtuzumab, 228
Alendronate Sodium *see* 229
Alendronic Acid, 229
Alendros [Abiogen] *see* 229
Aleppo-galls *see* 6728

Alergicide *see* 2081
Alerlisin [Prodes] *see* 2022
Alesion [Boehringer, Ing.] *see* 3618
Aletris, 230
Aleudrin [Lewis] *see* 5217
Aleuritic Acid, 231
Alevaire [Sanofi Winthrop] *see* 9833
Aleve [Procter & Gamble] *see* 6417
Alexan [Ebewe] *see* 2784
Alexidine, 232
Alfacalcidol *see* 4819
Alfacet [Galenika] *see* 1912
Alfadil [Pfizer] *see* 3433
Alfadione *see* 235
Alfadryl [Leciva] *see* 6287
Alfa-interferon *see* 4990
Alfamedin [Kade] *see* 3433
Alfamox [Teofarma] *see* 577
Alfaprostol, 234
Alfarol [Chugai] *see* 4819
Alfason [Yamanouchi] *see* 4787
Alfaspoven [Alfa] *see* 1974
Alfatésin [Glaxo] *see* 235
Alfatil [Lilly] *see* 1912
Alfavet [Roche] *see* 234
Alfaxalone, 235
Alfenamin *see* 4132
Alfenta [Janssen] *see* 236
Alfentanil, 236
Alfentanil Hydrochloride *see* 236
Alferon [Interferon Sciences] *see* 4990
Alficetin [BMS] *see* 2479
Alfimeprase, 237
Alfonic [Vista] *see* 7577
Alfospas [Rorer] *see* 9466
Alfuzosin, 238
Alganex [Roche] *see* 9148
Algeril [Bayer] *see* 7831
Algestone, 239
Algestone Acetonide *see* 239
Algestone Acetophenide, 240
Algil [Maggioni] *see* 5849
Algin, 241
Alginic Acid, 242
Alginic Acid Sodium Salt *see* 241
Alginodia [Beta] *see* 3350
Alginor [De Angeli] *see* 2280
Alglucerase, 243
Alglucosidase Alfa *see* 108
Algobaz [Labaz] *see* 6045
Algocalmin *see* 3350
Algocetil [Francia] *see* 8982
Algocor [Ravizza] *see* 4356
Algylen *see* 9639
Alibendol, 244
Alicaforsen, 245
Alidase [Searle] *see* 4758
Aliette [Bayer CropSci.] *see* 4252
Alimemazine *see* 9704
Alimet [Novus] *see* 5976
Alimix [Janssen-Cilag] *see* 2316
Alimta [Lilly] *see* 7077
Alinam [Lucien] *see* 2106
Alinamin [Takeda] *see* 7882
Alinamin F [Takeda] *see* 4311
Alindapril *see* 2876
Alinia [Romark] *see* 6567
Alinidine, 246
Alisactide *see* 314
Aliskiren, 247
Alisobumal *see* 1511
Alitame, 248
Alitretinoin, 249
Alival [Hoechst] *see* 6673

Alizapride, 250
Alizarin, 251
Alizarin Blue R *see* 253
Alizarin Bordeaux B *see* 8050
Alizarin Cyanine Green F, 252
Alizarine Blue, 253
Alizarine Carmine *see* 8573
Alizarine Orange, 254
Alizarine S *see* 8573
Alizarine Yellow C *see* 4342
Alizarine Yellow GG *see* 5919
Alizarine Yellow R, 255
Alizarine Yellow RW *see* 255
β-2-Alizarin Primeveroside *see* 8280
Alizarin Violet *see* 4344
Alkacitron [PDH] *see* 2326
Alkalovert [Klein] *see* 7387
Alkamuls SML [Alkaril] *see* 8724
Alkamuls SMO [Alkaril] *see* 8724
Alkamuls SMS [Alkaril] *see* 8724
Alkanet, 256
Alkanet Extract *see* 257
Alkanna *see* 256
Alkanna Red *see* 257
Alkannin, 257
Alkannin Paper *see* 256
Alkathene [ICI] *see* 7567
Alkavervir *see* 9957
Alkeran [GSK] *see* 5828
Alkiron *see* 6128
Alkron *see* 7033
1-*O*-Alkyl-2-acetyl-*sn*-glycero-3-phos-phorylcholine *see* 7524
Alkylaluminum Halide *see* 326
Alkylaluminum Sesquihalide *see* 326
Alkylbenzyldimethyl Quaternary Am-monium Compounds Chlorides *see* 1059
Alkyldimethyl(phenylmethyl)ammonium Chloride *see* 1059
Allantoin, 258
(Allantoinato)dihydroxyaluminum *see* 223
Allantoxanic Acid *see* 6947
All-*trans* Bixin *see* 1311
Allegra [Aventis] *see* 4068
Allegron [Dista] *see* 6715
Allenolic Acid, 259
Alleoside A *see* 4632
Allercur [Schering AG] *see* 2346
Allergefon [Lafon] *see* 1799
Allergina [Boehringer, Ing.] *see* 3309
Allergisan [Pharmacia] *see* 2180
Allergocrom [Ursapharm] *see* 2590
Allergodil [Viatris] *see* 906
Allethrin I *see* 260
Allethrin II *see* 260
Allethrins, 260
Allethrolone Ester of Chrysanthemum-dicarboxylic Acid Monomethyl Ester *see* 260
Allethrolone Ester of Chrysanthemum-monocarboxylic Acid *see* 260
Allicin, 261
Allie [DuPont] *see* 6158
Alliin, 262
Allitridium *see* 2973
Allium *see* 4370
Allobarbital, 263
Allobarbitone *see* 263
Alloca [Pharmacia & Upjohn] *see* 6875
Allocholesterol, 264
Allocor [Kwizda] *see* 5354
Allocryptopine, 265

Allodihydro F *see* 4764
Allodihydrohydrocortisone *see* 4764
Alloferin [Roche] *see* 221
Allohydroxyproline *see* 4840
Alloid [Kyosei] *see* 241
L(+)-Alloisoleucine *see* 5179
2-D-Alloisoleucine Sporidesmolide I *see* 8765
Allomaleic Acid *see* 4287
Allomelanins *see* 5812
Allophycocyanins *see* 7379
Allopregnane, 266
Allopregnane-3α,20α-diol, 267
Allopregnane-3α,20β-diol, 268
Allopregnane-3β,20α-diol, 269
Allopregnane-3β,20β-diol, 270
Allopregnane-3β,17α-diol-20-one, 271
3,20-Allopregnanedione, 272
Allopregnane-3α,11β,17α,21-tetrol-20-one, 273
Allopregnane-3α,17α,21-triol-11,20-di-one *see* 281
Allopregnane-11β,17α,21-triol-3,20-di-one *see* 4764
Allopregnane-3β,11β,21-triol-20-one, 274
Allopregnan-3α-ol-20-one, 275
Allopregnan-3β-ol-20-one, 276
Allopregnan-20α-ol-3-one, 277
Allopregnan-20β-ol-3-one, 278
Alloptrex [Fabre] *see* 2590
Allo-Puren [Isis] *see* 279
Allopurinol, 279
Allopydin [Chugai] *see* 219
β-D-Allopyranose *see* 280
Allorphine *see* 6361
D-Allose, 280
Allose [Kyosei] *see* 241
Allotelluric Acid *see* 9120
3α-Allotetrahydrocortisol *see* 273
Allotetrahydrocortisone, 281
Allotetrahydroprogesterone *see* 275
Allotropal [Heyl] *see* 5846
Alloxan, 282
Alloxan 5-Oxime *see* 10000
Alloxantin, 283
Alloyohimbine *see* 10103
Allozym [Sawai] *see* 279
Allspice *see* 7432
Allspice Berry Oil *see* 7432
(All-*E*)-4,8,13,17-tetramethyl-2,4,6,8,-10,12,14,16,18-eicosanonaenedioic Acid *see* 1311
Alltox *see* 9557
All-trans Norbixin *see* 1311
D-Allulose *see* 7924
Allural [Rovi] *see* 279
Allura Red AC, 284
Allurit [Aventis] *see* 279
Alluval [Berlin-Chemie] *see* 1397
Allvoran [TAD] *see* 3081
Ally [DuPont] *see* 6158
Allyl Acetate, 285
Allyl Alcohol, 286
Allylamine, 287
Allylamine-epichlorohydrin Copolymer *see* 8474
Allylamine Polymer with 1-Chloro-2,3-epoxypropane *see* 8474
1-Allyl-6-amino-3-ethyl-2,4(1*H*,3*H*)-pyr-imidinedione *see* 451
1-Allyl-6-amino-3-ethyluracil *see* 451
6-Allyl-2-amino-5,6,7,8-tetrahydro-4*H*-thiazolo[4,5-*d*]azepine *see* 9039
p-Allylanisole *see* 3705

Allylbarbital *see* 1511
Allyl Bromide, 288
5-Allyl-5-(2-bromoallyl)barbituric Acid *see* 1361
5-Allyl-5-*sec*-butylbarbituric Acid *see* 9036
3-Allyl-5-*sec*-butyl-2-thiohydantoin *see* 217
Allylcarbamide *see* 298
Allylcatechol Methylene Ether *see* 8317
Allyl Chloride, 289
Allyl Cinerins *see* 260
Allyl Cyanide, 290
5-Allyl-5-(2-cyclohexen-1-yl)-2-thiobar-bituric Acid *see* 9292
S-Allyl-L-cysteine Sulfoxide *see* 262
2-(*N*-Allyl-2,6-dichloroanilino)-2-imi-dazoline *see* 246
2-[*N*-Allyl-*N*-(2,6-dichlorophenyl)ami-no]-2-imidazoline *see* 246
17-Allyl-1,14-dihydroxy-12-[2-(4-hydr-oxy-3-methoxycyclohexyl)-1-methyl-vinyl]-23,25-dimethoxy-13,19,21,27-tetramethyl-11,28-dioxa-4-azatricy-clo[22.3.1.0^{4,9}]octacos-18-ene-2,3,-10,16-tetraone *see* 9025
1-Allyl-1-(3α,17β-dihydroxy-2β-mor-pholino-5α-androstan-16β-yl)pyrrol-idinium 17-Acetate *see* 8246
1-Allyl-2-(3α,17β-dihydroxy-2β-piperi-dino-5α-androstan-16β-yl)piperidi-nium Bromide 3-Acetate 17-Propi-onate *see* 8113
1-Allyl-2,3-dimethoxy-4,5-(methylene-dioxy)benzene *see* 733
1-Allyl-2,5-dimethoxy-3,4-methylene-dioxybenzene *see* 734
4-Allyl-1,2-dimethoxybenzene *see* 6073
Allyldioxybenzene Methylene Ether *see* 8317
17-Allyl-4,5α-epoxy-3,14-dihydroxy-morphinan-6-one *see* 6362
1-[(6-Allylergoline-8β-yl)carbonyl]-1-[3-(dimethylamino)propyl]-3-ethylurea *see* 1601
Allylestrenol, 291
17-Allylestr-4-en-17β-ol *see* 291
Allyl Ether, 292
1-Allyl-3-ethyl-6-amino-1,2,3,4-tetrahy-dro-2,4-pyrimidinedione *see* 451
Allyl Ethyl Ether, 293
Allyl Glucosinolate *see* 8545
Allylguaiacol *see* 3898
Allyl 1,5-Hexadienyltrisulfide *see* 195
17α-Allyl-17-hydroxyestra-4,9,11-trien-3-one *see* 319
5-Allyl-2-hydroxy-*N*-(2-hydroxyethyl)-*m*-anisamide *see* 244
l,*N*-Allyl-3-hydroxymorphinan *see* 5458
17α-Allyl-17-hydroxy-19-nor-4-andro-stene *see* 291
(−)-*N*-Allyl-14-hydroxynordihydromor-phinone *see* 6362
5-Allyl-5-(β-hydroxypropyl)barbituric Acid *see* 7904
5-Allyl-5-(2-hydroxypropyl)barbituric Acid *see* 7904
5-Allyl-5-(β-hydroxypropyl)malonylurea *see* 7904
Allyl Iodide, 294
5-Allyl-5-isobutylbarbituric Acid *see* 1511
5-Allyl-5-isobutyl-2-thiobarbituric Acid Sodium Salt *see* 1524
3-Allyl-5-isobutyl-2-thiohydantoin *see* 217

5-Allyl-5-isopropylbarbituric Acid *see* 756

Allyl Isosulfocyanate *see* 295

Allyl Isothiocyanate, 295

Allylmercaptomethylpenicillin *see* 7099

Allylmercaptomethylpenicillinic Acid *see* 7099

5-Allyl-1-methoxy-2,3-(methylenedioxy)benzene *see* 6334

4-Allyl-2-methoxyphenol *see* 3898

2-(4-Allyl-2-methoxyphenoxy)-*N*,*N*-diethylacetamide *see* 46

2-(2-Allyl-6-methoxyphenoxy)triethylamine *see* 4542

5-Allyl-5-(1-methylbutyl)barbituric Acid Sodium Salt *see* 8420

5-Allyl-5-(1-methylbutyl)malonylurea Sodium Salt *see* 8420

5-Allyl-5-(1-methylbutyl)-2-thiobarbituric Acid *see* 9302

4-Allyl-1,2-methylenedioxybenzene *see* 8317

5-Allyl-5-methyl-5-(1-methyl-2-pentynyl)barbituric Acid Sodium Salt *see* 5981

α-3-Allyl-1-methyl-4-phenyl-4-piperidinol Propionate *see* 296

α-3-Allyl-1-methyl-4-phenyl-4-propionoxypiperidine *see* 296

5-Allyl-5-(1-methylpropyl)barbituric Acid *see* 9036

5-Allyl-5-(2-methylpropyl)barbituric Acid *see* 1511

5-Allyl-5-(2-methylpropyl)-2-thiobarbituric Acid Sodium Salt *see* 1524

Allyl Methyl Trisulfide *see* 6013

Allyl Mustard Oil *see* 295

N-Allylnormorphine *see* 6361

N-Allylnoroxymorphone *see* 6362

[4-(Allyloxy)-3-chlorophenyl]acetic Acid *see* 219

(±)-1-[β-(Allyloxy)-2,4-dichlorophenethyl]imidazole *see* 3583

1-[*o*-(Allyloxy)phenoxy]-3-(isopropylamino)-2-propanol *see* 6952

p-Allylphenol *see* 2050

1-(*o*-Allylphenoxy)-3-(isopropylamino)-2-propanol *see* 313

Allyl 2-Phenylcinchoninate *see* 2288

α-Allylpiperidine *see* 2501

Allylprodine, 296

m-Allylpyrocatechin Methylene Ether *see* 8317

(±)-*N*-[(1-Allyl-2-pyrrolidinyl)methyl]-4-amino-5-(methylsulfamoyl)-*o*-anisamide *see* 311

N-(1-Allyl-2-pyrrolidinylmethyl)-2-methoxy-4-amino-5-methylsulfamoylbenzamide *see* 311

N-[(1-Allyl-2-pyrrolidinyl)methyl]-6-methoxy-1*H*-benzotriazole-5-carboxamide *see* 250

N-[(1-Allyl-2-pyrrolidinyl)methyl]-5-sulfamoyl-*o*-veratramide *see* 9948

Allyl Sulfide, 297

3-((*S*)-Allylsulfinyl)-L-alanine *see* 262

Allylthiocarbamide *see* 9362

3-[(Allylthio)methyl]-6-chloro-3,4-dihydro-2*H*-1,2,4-benzothiadiazine-7-sulfonamide 1,1-Dioxide *see* 318

3-Allylthiomethyl-6-chloro-7-sulfamoyl-3,4-dihydrobenzothiadiazine 1,1-Dioxide *see* 318

[(Allylthio)methyl] Penicillin *see* 7099

Allyl Thiourea *see* 9362

Allyl Tribromide *see* 9614

Allyl Trisulfide *see* 2973

Allylurea, 298

4-Allylveratrole *see* 6073

Allypropymal *see* 756

Allytrenbolone *see* 319

Almacet [Celtia] *see* 76

Almagate, 299

Alman [Kyosei] *see* 241

Almarl [Sumitomo] *see* 791

Almarytm [Synthelabo] *see* 4098

Almax [Almirall] *see* 299

Almeta [Shionogi] *see* 220

Aminoprofen, 300

Almitrine, 301

Almitrine Dimesylate *see* 301

Almocarpine [Ayerst] *see* 7424

Almogran [Almirall] *see* 304

Almond, Bitter, 302

Almond, Sweet, 303

Almora [Forest] *see* 4456

Almotriptan, 304

Almuth *see* 1258

Alnert [Fujisawa] *see* 1206

Alnide [Cusi] *see* 2746

Alnovin [Hoechst] *see* 3971

Alnulin *see* 9062

ALO-2145 *see* 751

Alodan [Gerot] *see* 5849

Aloe, 305

Aloe-Emodin, 306

Aloeresin A *see* 305

Aloginan [Tobishi] *see* 2345

Aloin, 307

Alomide [Alcon] *see* 5555

Aloperidin *see* 4598

Alopexil [Fabre] *see* 6203

Alopresin [Alonga] *see* 1774

Aloprim [Nabi] *see* 279

Aloral [Lagap] *see* 279

Alosetron, 308

Alositol [Tanabe] *see* 279

Alostil [Pfizer] *see* 6203

Alotec [Boehringer, Ing.] *see* 5931

Aloxi [Helsinn] *see* 6997

Aloxiprin, 309

Aloxyn *see* 4843

ALP-201 *see* 3938

Alpha₁-antitrypsin *see* 719

Alphacept [SKB] *see* 234

Alphacetylmethadol *see* 5945

Alpha-Chymocutan [Hasenclever] *see* 2260

Alpha D₃ [Teva] *see* 4819

Alphadione *see* 235

Alphadolone Acetate *see* 233

Alphagan [Allergan] *see* 1375

Alpha-hypophamine *see* 6979

Alpha-interferon *see* 4990

Alphakil [Rentokil] *see* 2072

Alphamide *see* 8928

Alphamin [SS Pharm.] *see* 2345

Alpha-naphthol *see* 6383

Alphanate [Alpha Ther.] *see* 3921

AlphaNine [Alpha Ther.] *see* 3922

Alpha-pipradrol *see* 7484

Alphapress [Alphapharm] *see* 4763

Alphaprodine, 310

Alphasol AY *see* 2989

Alphasol IB *see* 3194

Alphasol MA *see* 1255

Alphasone *see* 239

Alphasone Acetonide *see* 239

Alphasone Acetophenide *see* 240

Alphaxalone *see* 235

Alphol *see* 6414

Alpiny [SS Pharm.] *see* 47

Alpiropride, 311

Alplax [Gador] *see* 312

Alprazolam, 312

Alprenolol, 313

Alpress LP [Pfizer] *see* 7717

Alprostadil *see* 7876

Alq₃ *see* 370

Alredase [Am. Home] *see* 9524

Alreumat [Bayer] *see* 5305

Alrex [Bausch & Lomb] *see* 5584

Alrheumun [Bayer] *see* 5305

Alronidase *see* 4894

ALRT-1057 *see* 249

ALS-357 *see* 1190

Alsactide, 314

Alsanate [Dainippon] *see* 4378

Alseroxylon *see* 8120

Alsol [Athenstaedt] *see* 325

Alstonia Cortex *see* 3366

Alstonidine, 315

Alstonine, 316

Alsystin [Bayer] *see* 9678

ALT-711 *see* 203

Altabactina *see* 4294

Altace [Aventis] *see* 8103

Altacite [HMR] *see* 5660

Altafur [Norwich] *see* 4294

Altaite *see* 5422

Altan *see* 2815

Altat [Teikoku Hormone] *see* 8274

Alteplase *see* 9468

ALternaGEL [J & J-Merck] *see* 342

Althea, 317

Altheine *see* 837

Althesin [Glaxo] *see* 235

Althiazide, 318

Altiazem [Lusofarmaco] *see* 3202

Altim [Roussel Diamant] *see* 2540

Altimina [Miquel] *see* 3967

Altinil [BMS] *see* 9305

Altiopril *see* 6285

Altizide *see* 318

Alto [Kyosei] *see* 241

Alto [Syngenta] *see* 2771

Altodor [Synthelabo] *see* 3722

Altosid [Wellmark] *see* 5983

Altrenogest, 319

Altretamine, 320

Altropane [Organix] *see* 4871

D-Altropyranose *see* 321

D-Altrose, 321

Alubasine *see* 3183

Aludex [Intervet] *see* 486

Aludrin [Boehringer, Ing.] *see* 5217

Aludrine *see* 5217

Aludyal [Sandoz] *see* 342

Alufibrate *see* 2378

Alum *see* 360

Alum Flour *see* 360

Alumina *see* 356

Aluminium *see* 323

Aluminon, 322

Aluminum, 323

Aluminum Acetate Solution, 324

Aluminum Acetotartrate, 325

Aluminum Alkyls, 326

Aluminum Aminoacetate (Basic) *see* 3183

Aluminum Ammonium Chloride *see* 558

Aluminum Ammonium Sulfate, 327

Aluminum Antimonide, 328

Aluminum Benzoate, 329

Aluminum Bismuth Oxide *see* 1258

Aluminum Borate, 330

Aluminum Borohydride, 331
Aluminum Bromide, 332
Aluminum *tert*-Butoxide, 333
Aluminum Calcium Hydride, 334
Aluminum Calcium Silicate *see* 1648
Aluminum Carbide, 335
Aluminum Chlorate, 336
Aluminum Chloride, 337
Aluminum Chlorohydrate *see* 343
Aluminum Chlorohydroxide *see* 343
Aluminum Diacetate *see* 344
Aluminum Dihydroxy Allantoinate *see* 223
Aluminum Dihydroxyaminoacetate *see* 3183
Aluminum Ethoxide, 338
Aluminum Ethylate *see* 338
Aluminum Flufenamate *see* 4132
Aluminum Fluoride, 339
Aluminum Fluosilicate *see* 340
Aluminum Glycinate *see* 3183
Aluminum Hexafluorosilicate, 340
Aluminum Hydrate *see* 342
Aluminum Hydride, 341
Aluminum Hydroxide, 342
Aluminum Hydroxyacetate *see* 344
Aluminum Hydroxychloride, 343
Aluminum Hydroxydiacetate, 344
Aluminum Hypophosphite, 345
Aluminum Iodide, 346
Aluminum Isopropoxide, 347
Aluminum Isopropylate *see* 347
Aluminum Lactate, 348
Aluminum Lithium Hydride, 349
Aluminum Magnesium Hydroxide Sulfate (Al$_5$Mg$_{10}$(OH)$_{31}$(SO$_4$)$_2$) Hydrate *see* 5651
Aluminum Magnesium Silicate, 350
Aluminum Nicotinate, 351
Aluminum Nitrate, 352
Aluminum Nitride, 353
Aluminum Oleate, 354
Aluminum Orthophosphate *see* 358
Aluminum Oxalate, 355
Aluminum Oxide, 356
Aluminum Oxide Silicate [Al$_2$O(SiO$_4$)] *see* 362
Aluminum Palmitate, 357
Aluminum Phosphate, 358
Aluminum Phosphide, 359
Aluminum Potassium Sulfate, 360
Aluminum Selenide, 361
Aluminum Silicate, 362
Aluminum Silicofluoride *see* 340
Aluminum Sodium Carbonate Hydroxide *see* 3184
Aluminum Sodium Chloride *see* 8687
Aluminum Sodium Oxide *see* 8574
Aluminum Sodium Sulfate, 363
Aluminum Stearate, 364
Aluminum Subacetate *see* 344
Aluminum Subacetate Solution, 365
Aluminum Sulfate, 366
Aluminum Sulfide, 367
Aluminum Sulfocyanate *see* 369
Aluminum Tartrate, 368
Aluminum Tetrahydroborate *see* 331
Aluminum Thiocyanate, 369
Aluminum Trifluoride *see* 339
Aluminum Trihydrate *see* 342
Aluminum Tris(ethyl Phosphite) *see* 4252
Aluminum Tris(*O*-ethylphosphonate) *see* 4252
Aluminum Tris(8-hydroxyquinoline), 370
Aluminum Tristearate *see* 364

Alum Meal *see* 360
Alum Root *see* 4404
Alundum *see* 356
Alunogenite *see* 366
Alupent [Boehringer, Ing.] *see* 5931
Alurate [Roche] *see* 756
Alusa [Towa Yakuhin] *see* 223
"Alutiae" *see* 7529
Alutyl *see* 2288
Alven [Firma] *see* 9608
Alveograf *see* 3467
Alverine, 371
Alvesco [Altana] *see* 2263
Alvimopan, 372
Alvo [Taisho] *see* 6924
Alvodine [Winthrop] *see* 7433
Alvonal MR [Gödecke] *see* 2761
Alyrane [Baxter] *see* 3581
Alzinox [Berlex] *see* 3183
AM-80 *see* 9047
AM-109 *see* 5978
AM-715 *see* 6700
AM-725 *see* 7066
AM-833 *see* 4099
AM-1091 *see* 2355
AM-1155 *see* 4376
AM-2282 *see* 8802
AMA-1080 *see* 1871
Amabevan *see* 1786
Amacetam *see* 7706
Amadol [TAD] *see* 9566
Amadou *see* 185
Amal [Knoll] *see* 570
Amanin *see* 373
Amanitin, 373
α-Amanitin *see* 373
β-Amanitin *see* 373
Amantadine, 374
Amaranth (Dye), 375
Amaranth (Plant), 376
Amarogentin, 377
Amarolide, 378
Amaromycin *see* 7413
Amaryl [Aventis] *see* 4440
Amarylline *see* 5626
Amasulin [Takeda] *see* 1871
Amasust [Knoll] *see* 570
Amatine [Roberts] *see* 6184
Amaze *see* 5172
Ambacamp [Pharmacia & Upjohn] *see* 931
Ambamide *see* 5649
Ambaxin [Pharmacia] *see* 931
Ambene [Merckle] *see* 7277
Ambenonium Chloride, 379
Amber, 380
Amber [Syngenta] *see* 9600
Amber Acid *see* 8869
Ambergris, 381
Amberlite [Rohm & Haas], 382
Amberlyst 15 [Rohm & Haas], 383
Ambien [Sanofi-Aventis] *see* 10190
Ambilhar [Novartis] *see* 6563
AmBisome [Nexstar] *see* 585
Ambivalon [Nattermann] *see* 488
Amblosin [Hoechst] *see* 586
Amblygonite *see* 5520
Ambodryl [Parke-Davis] *see* 1418
Ambramicina [Lepetit] *see* 9196
Ambra-Vena [Lepetit] *see* 7453
Ambril [Cascan] *see* 386
Ambrisentan, 384
Ambrocef [Lusofarmaco] *see* 1984
Ambrosia *see* 6785
Ambrosin, 385
Ambroxol, 386

Ambush [Syngenta] *see* 7180
Ambuterol *see* 5642
Ambutonium Bromide, 387
Ambutyrosin *see* 1528
AMCHA *see* 9569
Amchem 70-25 *see* 1532
Amciderm [Hermal] *see* 388
Amcinonide, 388
Amco [Am. Mfg.] *see* 7581
AMD *see* 6055
AMD-473 *see* 7405
Amdinocillin, 389
Amdinocillin Pivoxil, 390
Amdray [Novartis] *see* 9917
Amdro [BASF] *see* 4765
Ameban *see* 1786
Amebarsone [Lilly] *see* 1786
Amebil *see* 5031
Amechol [Moorsfields] *see* 5940
Amedel [Dainippon] *see* 7480
Amediplase, 391
Ameisensäure (German) *see* 4241
Amekrin [Warner-Lambert] *see* 594
Ameliaroside *see* 7395
Amen [Elan] *see* 5793
Amenide [Sterling Winthrop] *see* 8057
Amenox [Sanofi Winthrop] *see* 8057
Amenyl *see* 2102
Amerchol 400 [Amerchol] *see* 5359
Amerfil [Am. Thermoplastic] *see* 7581
Amerge [GSK] *see* 6420
Americaine [Medeva] *see* 1086
American Cyanamid 12880 *see* 3220
American Cyanamid 38023 *see* 3932
American Elder *see* 8351
American Hellebore *see* 9957
American Horsemint *see* 6243
American Indian Hemp *see* 743
American Mandrake *see* 7547
American Nightshade Root *see* 7391
American Oil Palm *see* 6818
American Pennyroyal *see* 7102
American Saffron *see* 1868
American Spikenard *see* 766
American Valerian *see* 2770
American Veratrum *see* 9957
American Wormseed *see* 6785
Americium, 392
Amerscan MDP [Amersham] *see* 5792
Ametazole *see* 1183
Amethocaine Hydrochloride *see* 9188
Amethopterin *see* 5985
Amethyst *see* 8493
Ametox *see* 8694
Ametrex [Makhteshim-Agan] *see* 393
Ametriodinic Acid *see* 5011
Ametryn, 393
Ametryne *see* 393
Ametycine [Sanofi Winthrop] *see* 6215
Amevive [Biogen] *see* 227
Amexine [CFPI] *see* 1532
Amezinium Methyl Sulfate, 394
AmF 297 *see* 6820
Amfamox [Merck & Co.] *see* 3930
Amfebutamone *see* 1499
Amfenac, 395
Amfepramone *see* 3127
Amfipen [Yamanouchi] *see* 586
Amfomycin *see* 584
AMG-073 *see* 2282
AMG-412 *see* 3631
AMI-25 *see* 4063
AMI-121 *see* 4064
AMI-227 *see* 4065
Amianthus *see* 826

Amias [Takeda] *see* 1739
Amibiarson *see* 1786
Amicar [Wyeth] *see* 432
Amicarbazone, 396
Amicetin, 397
Amicos [Banyu] *see* 2344
Amicoumacin A, 398
Amidate [Abbott] *see* 3881
Amidazine *see* 3737
Amidazophen *see* 474
Amidephrine, 399
Amidephrine Mesylate *see* 399
[[1-[*N*-(*p*-Amidinobenzoyl)-L-tyrosyl]-4-
    piperidinyl]oxy]acetic Acid *see* 5349
N-[(*R*)-[[(2*S*)-2-[[*p*-Amidinobenzyl]car-
    bamoyl]-1-azetidinyl]carbonyl]cyclo-
    hexylmethyl]glycine *see* 5810
N-Amidino-3,5-diamino-6-chloropyra-
    zinamide *see* 406
N-Amidino-3,5-diamino-6-chloropyra-
    zinecarboxamide *see* 406
N-Amidino-2-(2,6-dichlorophenyl)acet-
    amide *see* 4561
N-(2'-Amidinoethyl)-3-aminocyclopen-
    tanecarboxamide *see* 400
2-[*N*-(2-Amidinoethyl)carbamoyl]-5-imi-
    nopyrrolidine *see* 6670
N'-(2-Amidinoethyl)-4-(2-guanidinoacet-
    amido)-1,1'-dimethyl-*N*,4'-bi[pyrrole-
    2-carboxamide] *see* 6481
N-(2-Amidinoethyl)-5-imino-2-pyrroli-
    dinecarboxamide *see* 6670
N-Amidinoglycine *see* 4495
Amidinoguanidine *see* 1215
Amidinomycin, 400
6-Amidino-2-naphthyl-4-guanidinoben-
    zoate *see* 6350
L-6-Amidinonorleucine *see* 4970
7-*m*-Amidinophenyldiazoamino-2-ami-
    no-10-ethyl-9-phenylphenanthridin-
    ium Chloride *see* 5183
8-[3-(*m*-Amidinophenyl)-2-triazeno]-3-
    amino-5-ethyl-6-phenylphenanthridin-
    ium Chloride *see* 5183
N-Amidinosarcosine *see* 2568
*N*¹-Amidinosulfanilamide *see* 8908
2-Amidino-1,2,3,4-tetrahydroisoquino-
    line *see* 2844
Amidocyanogen *see* 2684
Amido-G-Acid, 401
Amidol *see* 2983
Amidolacetate *see* 5945
Amidonal [PCR Arzneimittel] *see* 754
Amidopyrine *see* 474
Amido-R-Acid, 402
Amidosulfonic Acid *see* 8921
1-(*p*-Amidosulfonylphenyl)-2-thiapiperi-
    dine 2,2-Dioxide *see* 8993
Amidosulfuron, 403
Amifostine, 404
Amifur [Norwich] *see* 6600
Amiglyde-V [Fort Dodge] *see* 405
Amikacin, 405
Amikal [GEA] *see* 406
Amikin [BMS] *see* 405
Amiklin [BMS] *see* 405
Amilan [Toyo] *see* 6734
Amilar [DuPont] *see* 7569
Amil-Co [Baker Norton] *see* 406
Amiloride, 406
Amimetilina *see* 7901
Amimycin *see* 6825
Aminacrine, 407
Aminacyl [Wander] *see* 477
Aminarsone *see* 1786

Amindan [Desitin] *see* 8428
Amine 220, 408
Amine Fluoride 297 *see* 6820
Amine Oxidase *see* 6247
Amineptine, 409
Amineurin [Hexal] *see* 487
Aminitrozole, 410
p-Aminoacetanilide, 411
4'-Aminoacetanilide *see* 411
Aminoacetic Acid *see* 4491
Aminoacetonitrile, 412
α-Amino-*p*-acetophenetide *see* 7239
2-Amino-*p*-acetophenetidide *see* 7239
Aminoacetophenetidine *see* 7239
Aminoacetophenone, 413
α-Aminoacetophenone *see* 7206
ω-Aminoacetophenone *see* 7206
m-Aminoacetophenone *see* 413
o-Aminoacetophenone *see* 413
p-Aminoacetophenone *see* 413
2-Aminoacetophenone *see* 7206
3'-Aminoacetophenone *see* 413
5-[[(Aminoacetyl)amino]methyl]-1-[4-
    chloro-2-(2-chlorobenzoyl)phenyl]-
    N,*N*-dimethyl-1*H*-1,2,4-triazole-3-
    carboxamide *see* 8221
m-Aminoacetylbenzene *see* 413
D-Amino Acid Oxidase, 414
L-Amino Acid Oxidase, 415
5-Aminoacridine *see* 407
9-Aminoacridine *see* 407
9-Aminoacridine Compd with 4-Hexyl-
    resorcinol *see* 126
9-Aminoacridinium 4-Hexylresorcinolate
    see 126
1-Aminoadamantane *see* 374
α-Aminoadipic Acid, 416
δ-(L-α-Aminoadipyl)-L-cysteinyl-D-val-
    ine *see* 145
3-Aminoalanine *see* 2984
L-α-Amino-ε-amidinocaproic Acid *see*
    4970
L-2-Amino-6-amidinohexanoic Acid *see*
    4970
4-Amino-1-[(aminoacetyl)methylamino]-
    1,4-dideoxy-3-*O*-(2,6-diamino-2,3,4,-
    6,7-pentadeoxy-β-L-*lyxo*-heptopyran-
    osyl)-6-*O*-methyl-D-*chiro*-inositol *see*
    4249
*N*¹-[4-Amino-6-[[3-[(4-aminobutyl)ami-
    no]propyl]amino]-6-oxohexyl]-13-[(4-
    amino-4,6-dideoxy-α-L-talopyrano-
    syl)oxy]-19-demethyl-12-hydroxybleo-
    mycinamide *see* 9043
4-Amino-*N*-(aminocarbonyl)benzenesul-
    fonamide *see* 8931
5-[[2-Amino-5-*O*-(aminocarbonyl)-2-de-
    oxy-L-xylonoyl]amino]-1,5-dideoxy-1-
    [3,4-dihydro-5-(hydroxymethyl)-2,4-
    dioxo-1(2*H*)-pyrimidinyl]-β-D-*allo*-
    furanuronic Acid *see* 7576
[*S*-(*Z*)]-1-[5-[[2-Amino-5-*O*-(aminocar-
    bonyl)-2-deoxy-L-xylonoyl]amino]-1,-
    5-dideoxy-1-[3,4-dihydro-5-(hydr-
    oxymethyl)2,4-dioxo-1(2*H*)-pyrimi-
    dinyl]-β-D-allofuranuronoyl]-3-ethyli-
    dene-2-azetidinecarboxylic Acid *see*
    7576
[1a*S*-(1aα,8β,8aα,8bα)]-6-Amino-8-
    [[(aminocarbonyl)oxy]methyl]-1,-
    1a,2,8,8a,8b-hexahydro-8a-methoxy-
    1,5-dimethylazirino[2',3':3,4]pyr-
    rolo[1,2-*a*]indole-4,7-dione *see* 7597
[1a*S*-(1aα,8β,8aα,8bα)]-6-Amino-8-
    [[(aminocarbonyl)oxy]methyl]-1,1a,-

2,8,8a,8b-hexahydro-8a-methoxy-5-
    methylazirino[2',3':3,4]pyrrolo[1,2-
    a]indole-4,7-dione *see* 6215
L-2-Amino-4-[(2-amino-2-carboxyethyl)-
    thio]butyric Acid *see* 2777
4-*O*-[3α-Amino-6α-[(4-amino-4-deoxy-α-
    D-glucopyranosyl)oxy]-2,3,4,4aβ,6,-
    7,8aα-octahydro-8β-hydroxy-7β-
    (methylamino)pyranopyrano[3,2-*b*]-
    pyran-2α-yl]-2-deoxy-D-streptamine
    see 752
5-Amino-6-(7-amino-5,8-dihydro-6-
    methoxy-5,8-dioxo-2-quinolyl)-4-(2-
    hydroxy-3,4-dimethoxyphenyl)-3-
    methylpicolinic Acid *see* 8827
5-Amino-6-(7-amino-5,8-dihydro-6-
    methoxy-5,8-dioxo-2-quinolyl)-4-(2-
    hydroxy-3,4-dimethoxyphenyl)-3-
    methyl-2-pyridinecarboxylic Acid
    see 8827
(α*S*,γ*S*,δ*S*,ζ*S*)-δ-Amino-*N*-(3-amino-2,2-
    dimethyl-3-oxopropyl)-γ-hydroxy-4-
    methoxy-3-(3-methoxypropoxy)-α,ζ-
    bis(1-methylethyl)benzeneoctanam-
    ide *see* 247
4-Amino-6-[(2-amino-1,6-dimethyl-4-
    pyrimidinyl)amino]-1,2-dimethyl-
    quinoline Salts *see* 8052
4-Amino-6-[(2-amino-1,6-dimethyl-
    4(1*H*)-pyrimidinylidene)amino]-1,2-
    dimethylquinolinium Conjugate
    Monoacid *see* 8052
(*S*)-4-Amino-1-[4-[(2-amino-3-hydroxy-
    1-oxopropyl)amino]-9-[(aminoimino-
    methyl)amino]-6-*C*-carboxy-2,3,4,7,9-
    pentadeoxy-α-L-*talo*-non-2-enopyran-
    osyl]-5-(hydroxymethyl)-2(1*H*)-pyrimi-
    dinone *see* 6192
(*S*)-2-Amino-5-[(aminoiminomethyl)ami-
    no]pentanoic Acid *see* 780
4-Amino-*N*-(aminoiminomethyl)benzene-
    sulfonamide *see* 8908
4-[[3-Amino-5-[(aminoiminomethyl)-
    methylamino]-1-oxopentyl]amino]-1-
    (4-amino-2-oxo-1(2*H*)-pyrimidinyl)-1,-
    2,3,4-tetradeoxy-β-*erythro*-hex-2-
    enopyranuronic Acid *see* 1316
3-Amino-8-[3-[3-(aminoiminomethyl)-
    phenyl]-1-triazenyl]-5-ethyl-6-phenyl-
    phenanthridinium Chloride *see* 5183
3-Amino-*N*-(3-amino-3-iminopropyl)cy-
    clopentanecarboxamide *see* 400
5-Amino-*N*-(3-amino-3-iminopropyl)-3,-
    4-dihydro-2*H*-pyrrole-2-carboxamide
    see 6670
(2*S*-*cis*)-4-*O*-[3-Amino-6-(aminomethyl)-
    3,4-dihydro-2*H*-pyran-2-yl]-2-deoxy-
    6-*O*-[3-deoxy-4-*C*-methyl-3-(methyl-
    amino)-β-L-arabinopyranosyl]-*N*¹-eth-
    yl-D-streptamine *see* 6479
(2*S*-*cis*)-4-*O*-[3-Amino-6-(aminomethyl)-
    3,4-dihydro-2*H*-pyran-2-yl]-2-deoxy-
    6-*O*-[3-deoxy-4-*C*-methyl-3-(methyl-
    amino)-β-L-arabinopyranosyl]-D-
    streptamine *see* 8550
4-Amino-6-(2-amino-6-methyl-4-pyrimi-
    dinyl)amino]-1-methylquinaldinium
    Methosalts *see* 8052
4-Amino-6-(2-amino-6-methyl-4-pyrim-
    idylamino)quinaldine-1,1'-dimetho-
    salts *see* 8052
3-Amino-4-[[4'-[(2-amino-6-sulfo-1-
    naphthalenyl)azo]-3,3'-dimethyl[1,1'-
    biphenyl]-4-yl]azo]-2,7-naphthalene-
    disulfonic Acid Trisodium Salt *see*
    10012

4-Amino-2-chlorobenzoic Acid 2-(Diethylamino)ethyl Ester Monohydrochloride *see* 2158

2-Amino-5-chlorobenzoxazole *see* 10199

p-Amino-*p*'-chlorobiphenyl *see* 435

4-Amino-5-chloro-*N*-[2-(diethylamino)ethyl]-*o*-anisamide *see* 6143

4-Amino-5-chloro-*N*-[(2-diethylamino)ethyl]-2-methoxybenzamide *see* 6143

4-Amino-5-chloro-2,3-dihydro-*N*-[1-(3-methoxypropyl)-4-piperidinyl]-7-benzofurancarboxamide *see* 7907

4-Amino-3-chloro-α-[[(1,1-dimethylethyl)amino]methyl]-5-(trifluoromethyl)benzenemethanol *see* 5642

4-Amino-4'-chlorodiphenyl, 435

(±)-4-Amino-5-chloro-*N*-[[4-(4-fluorobenzyl)-2-morpholinyl]methyl]benzamide *see* 6279

4-Amino-5-chloro-2-ethoxy-*N*-[[4-[(4-fluorophenyl)methyl]-2-morpholinyl]methyl]benzamide *see* 6279

cis-4-Amino-5-chloro-*N*-[1-[3-(*p*-fluorophenoxy)propyl]-3-methoxy-4-piperidinyl]-*o*-anisamide *see* 2316

cis-4-Amino-5-chloro-*N*-[1-[3-(4-fluorophenoxy)propyl]-3-methoxy-4-piperidinyl]-2-methoxybenzamide *see* 2316

(±)-*endo*-4-Amino-5-chloro-2-methoxy-*N*-(1-azabicyclo[3.3.1]non-4-yl)benzamide *see* 8135

4-Amino-5-chloro-2-methoxy-*N*-(β-diethylaminoethyl)benzamide *see* 6143

4-Amino-5-chloro-2-methoxy-*N*-[1-(phenylmethyl)-4-piperidinyl]benzamide *see* 2344

γ-Amino-β-(*p*-chlorophenyl)butyric Acid *see* 937

6-[(*R*)-Amino(4-chlorophenyl)(1-methyl-1*H*-imidazol-5-yl)methyl]-4-(3-chlorophenyl)-1-methyl-2(1*H*)-quinolinone *see* 9458

4-Amino-*N*-(6-chloro-3-pyridazinyl)benzenesulfonamide *see* 8900

1-(4'-Amino-3'-chloro-5'-trifluoromethylphenyl)-2-*tert*-butylaminoethanol *see* 5642

Aminochromes, 436

6-Aminochrysene *see* 2254

o-Aminocinnamic Acid Lactam *see* 1825

p-Aminoclonidine *see* 751

4-Aminocumene *see* 2620

5-Amino-3-cyano-1-(2,6-dichloro-4-trifluoromethylphenyl)-4-ethylsulfinylpyrazole *see* 3739

5-Amino-3-cyano-1-(2,6-dichloro-4-trifluoromethylphenyl)-4-trifluoromethylsulfinylpyrazole *see* 4085

1-(4-Amino-3-cyanophenyl)-2-isopropylaminoethanol *see* 2278

4-Amino-5-cyano-7-(D-ribofuranosyl)-7*H*-pyrrolo[2,3-*d*]pyrimidine *see* 9562

7-[D-2-Amino-2-(1,4-cyclohexadienyl)acetamide]-3-methoxy-3-cephem-4-carboxylic Acid *see* 1944

7-[D-2-Amino-2-(1,4-cyclohexadienyl)acetamido]desacetoxycephalosporanic Acid *see* 1986

6-[D-α-Amino-2-(1,4-cyclohexadien-1-yl)acetamido]penicillanic Acid *see* 3614

(2*S*,5*R*,6*R*)-6-[[(2*R*)-Amino-1,4-cyclohexadien-1-ylacetyl]amino]-3,3-dimethyl-7-oxo-4-thia-1-azabicyclo[3.2.0]heptane-2-carboxylic Acid *see* 3614

(6*R*,7*R*)-7-[[(2*R*)-Amino-1,4-cyclohexadien-1-ylacetyl]amino]-3-methoxy-8-oxo-5-thia-1-azabicyclo[4.2.0]oct-2-ene-2-carboxylic Acid *see* 1944

(6*R*,7*R*)-7-[[(2*R*)-Amino-1,4-cyclohexadien-1-ylacetyl]amino]-3-methyl-8-oxo-5-thia-1-azabicyclo[4.2.0]oct-2-ene-2-carboxylic Acid *see* 1986

D-α-Amino-(1,4-cyclohexadien-1-yl)methylpenicillin *see* 3614

Aminocyclohexane *see* 2729

6-(1-Aminocyclohexanecarboxamido)penicillanic Acid *see* 2702

4-Amino-*N*-[1-(3-cyclohexen-1-ylmethyl)-4-piperidinyl]-2-ethoxy-5-nitrobenzamide *see* 2294

(2*S*,5*R*,6*R*)-6-[[(1-Aminocyclohexyl)carbonyl]amino]-3,3-dimethyl-7-oxo-4-thia-1-azabicyclo[3.2.0]heptane-2-carboxylic Acid *see* 2702

(1-Aminocyclohexyl)penicillin *see* 2702

1-Aminocyclopentanecarboxylic Acid *see* 2734

(1*S*,4*R*)-4-[2-Amino-6-(cyclopropylamino)-9*H*-purin-9-yl]-2-cyclopentene-1-methanol *see* 1

(−)-*cis*-4-[2-Amino-6-(cyclopropylamino)-9*H*-purin-9-yl]-2-cyclopentene-1-methanol *see* 1

rel-5-Amino-1-cyclopropyl-7-[(3*R*,5*S*)-3,5-dimethyl-1-piperazinyl]-6,8-difluoro-1,4-dihydro-4-oxo-3-quinolinecarboxylic Acid *see* 8735

(3*S*)-10-(1-Aminocyclopropyl)-9-fluoro-2,3-dihydro-3-methyl-7-oxo-7*H*-pyrido[1,2,3-*de*]-1,4-benzoxazine-6-carboxylic Acid *see* 7055

4'-Amino-3'-deamino-18-decarboxy-40-demethyl-4'-deoxy-3,7-dideoxo-3,3',7-trihydroxy-*N*47,18,dimethyl-5-oxocandicidin D Cyclic 15,19-Hemiacetal *see* 7169

2-Amino-5-(3,7,11,15,19,23,27,31,35,39-decamethyl-2,6,10,14,18,22,26,30,34,38-tetracontadecaenyl)-3-methoxy-6-methyl-2,5-cyclohexadiene-1,4-dione *see* 8193

(+)-9-Amino-4-demethoxy-9-deoxy-7-*O*-(2-deoxy-β-D-*erythro*-pentopyranosyl)-daunomycinone *see* 593

2-Amino-2-deoxy-D-galactose *see* 4334

1-Amino-1-deoxy-D-glucitol *see* 4449

O-3-Amino-3-deoxy-α-D-glucopyranosyl-(1 → 6)-*O*-[6-amino-6-deoxy-α-D-glucopyranosyl-(1 → 4)]-*N*[1]-[(2*S*)-4-amino-2-hydroxy-1-oxobutyl]-2-deoxy-D-streptamine *see* 405

O-3-Amino-3-deoxy-α-D-glucopyranosyl-(1 → 6)-*O*-[6-amino-6-deoxy-α-D-glucopyranosyl-(1 → 4)]-2-deoxy-D-streptamine *see* 5281

O-4-Amino-4-deoxy-α-D-glucopyranosyl-(1 → 8)-*O*-(8*R*)-2-amino-2,3,7-trideoxy-7-(methylamino)-D-glycero-α-D-*allo*-octodialdo-1,5:8,4-dipyranosyl-(1 → 4)-2-deoxy-D-streptamine *see* 752

O-2-Amino-2-deoxy-α-D-glucopyranosyl-(1 → 4)-*O*-[3-deoxy-3-(methylamino)-α-D-xylopyranosyl-(1 → 6)]-2-deoxy-D-streptamine *see* 4392

O-6-Amino-6-deoxy-α-D-glucopyranosyl-(1 → 4)-*O*-[3-deoxy-4-*C*-methyl-3-(methylamino)-β-L-arabinopyranosyl-(1 → 6)]-*N*[1]-[(2*S*)-3-amino-2-hydroxy-1-oxopropyl]-2-deoxy-D-streptamine *see* 5106

O-2-Amino-2-deoxy-α-D-glucopyranosyl-(1 → 4)-*O*-[*O*-2,6-diamino-2,6-dideoxy-β-L-idopyranosyl-(1 → 3)-β-D-ribofuranosyl-(1 → 5)]-2-deoxy-D-streptamine *see* 7041

O-3-Amino-3-deoxy-α-D-glucopyranosyl-(1 → 6)-*O*-[2,6-diamino-2,3,4,6-tetradeoxy-α-D-*erythro*-hexopyranosyl-(1 → 4)]-*N*[1]-[(2*S*)-4-amino-2-hydroxy-1-oxobutyl]-2-deoxy-D-streptamine *see* 770

O-3-Amino-3-deoxy-α-D-glucopyranosyl-(1 → 6)-*O*-[2,6-diamino-2,3,4,6-tetradeoxy-α-D-*erythro*-hexopyranosyl-(1 → 4)]-2-deoxy-D-streptamine *see* 3005

O-3-Amino-3-deoxy-α-D-glucopyranosyl-(1 → 6)-*O*-[2,6-diamino-2,3,6-trideoxy-α-D-*ribo*-hexopyranosyl-(1 → 4)]-2-deoxy-D-streptamine *see* 9490

2-Amino-2-deoxy-3-*O*-β-D-glucopyranuronosyl-D-glucose *see* 4756

2-Amino-2-deoxy-3-*O*-β-D-glucopyranurosyl-D-galactose *see* 2215

2-Amino-2-deoxy-D-glucose *see* 4458

O-6-Amino-6-deoxy-L-*glycero*-D-*galacto*-heptopyranosylidene-(1 → 2-3)-*O*-β-D-talopyranosyl-(1 → 5)-2-deoxy-*N*'-methyl-D-streptamine *see* 2935

O-6-Amino-6-deoxy-L-*glycero*-D-*galacto*-heptopyranosylidene-(1 → 2-3)-*O*-β-D-talopyranosyl-(1 → 5)-2-deoxy-*N*[3]-methyl-D-streptamine *see* 4852

Aminodeoxykanamycin *see* 5281

4-Amino-1-(2-deoxy-β-*erythro*-pentofuranosyl)-1,3,5-triazin-2(1*H*)-one *see* 2853

3-Amino-3-deoxyrhamnose *see* 6328

1-Amino-1-deoxysorbitol *see* 4449

1-Aminodiamantane (obsolete) *see* 374

[1-Amino-3-[[[2-[(diaminomethylene)amino]-4-thiazolyl]methyl]thio]propylidene]sulfamide *see* 3930

4-Amino-*N*-(diaminomethylene)benzenesulfonamide *see* 8908

N-(2-Amino-3,5-dibromobenzyl)-*N*-methylcyclohexylammonium *see* 1391

2-Amino-3,5-dibromo-*N*-cyclohexyl-*N*-methylbenzenemethanamine *see* 1391

4-[[(2-Amino-3,5-dibromophenyl)methyl]amino]cyclohexanol *see* 386

5-Amino-*N*-(1,2-dicarboxyethyl)-1-ribofuranosylimidazole-4-carboxamide 5'-Phosphate *see* 8318

4-Amino-3,5-dichloro-α-[[(1,1-dimethylethyl)amino]methyl]benzenemethanol *see* 2347

[(4-Amino-3,5-dichloro-6-fluoro-2-pyridinyl)oxy]acetic Acid *see* 4203

2-Amino-4,6-dichlorophenol, 437

2-[(4-Amino-2,6-dichlorophenyl)imino]imidazolidine *see* 751

5-Amino-1-[2,6-dichloro-4-(trifluoromethyl)phenyl]-4-(ethylsulfinyl)-1*H*-pyrazole-3-carbonitrile *see* 3739

5-Amino-1-[2,6-dichloro-4-(trifluoromethyl)phenyl]-4-[(trifluoromethyl)sulfinyl]-1*H*-pyrazole-3-carbonitrile *see* 4085

(±)-5-Amino-1-(2,6-dichloro-α,α,α-trifluoro-*p*-tolyl)-4-trifluoromethylsulfinylpyrazole-3-carbonitrile *see* 4085

3-Amino-3,6-dideoxy-D-aldohexose *see* 6328

4-Amino-1,4-dideoxy-3-*O*-(2,6-diamino-2,3,4,6,7-pentadeoxy-β-L-*lyxo*-

4-[(Aminoiminomethyl)amino]benzoic
Acid 6-(Aminoiminomethyl)-2-naph-
thalenyl Ester *see* 6350

4-[[4-[(Aminoiminomethyl)amino]benz-
oyl]oxy]benzeneacetic Acid 2-(Dimethylamino)-2-oxoethyl Ester *see* 1728

N-[5-[[[5-[[[2-[(Aminoiminomethyl)ami-
no]ethyl]amino]carbonyl]-1-methyl-
1*H*-pyrrol-3-yl]amino]carbonyl]-1-
methyl-1*H*-pyrrol-3-yl]-4-[[[4-[(2-
bromo-1-oxo-2-propenyl)amino]-1-
methyl-1*H*-pyrrol-2-yl]carbonyl]-
amino]-1-methyl-1*H*-pyrrole-2-carbox-
amide *see* 1449

O-[(Aminoiminomethyl)amino]homo-
serine *see* 1737

[4*S*-(4α,4aα,5aα,6β,12aα)]-*N*-[[4-[[(Aminoiminomethyl)amino]iminomethyl]-
1-piperazinyl]methyl]-4-(dimethylamino)-1,4,4a,5,5a,6,11,12a-octahy-
dro-3,6,10,12,12a-pentahydroxy-6-
methyl-1,11-dioxo-2-naphthacene-
carboxamide *see* 4557

2-[[[*trans*-4-[[(Aminoiminomethyl)ami-
no]methyl]cyclohexyl]carbonyl]oxy]-
benzoic Acid Phenylmethyl Ester
Monohydrochloride *see* 1038

4-[[6-[(Aminoiminomethyl)amino]-1-oxo-
hexyl]oxy]benzoic Acid Ethyl Ester *see*
4320

(2*R*,4*R*)-1-[(2*S*)-5-[(Aminoiminomethyl)-
amino]-1-oxo-2-[[(1,2,3,4-tetrahydro-
3-methyl-8-quinolinyl)sulfonyl]ami-
no]pentyl]-4-methyl-2-piperidine-
carboxylic Acid *see* 779

3-[[[2-[(Aminoiminomethyl)amino]-4-
thiazolyl]methyl]thio]-*N*-(aminosulfonyl)propanimidamide *see* 3930

N-[[[2-[[[2-[(Aminoiminomethyl)amino]-
4-thiazolyl]methyl]thio]ethyl]amino]-
methylene]-4-bromobenzenesulfon-
amide *see* 3485

(*S*)-[[1-[2-[[4-(Aminoiminomethyl)ben-
zoyl]amino]-3-(4-hydroxyphenyl)-1-
oxopropyl]-4-piperidinyl]oxy]acetic
Acid *see* 5349

N-(Aminoiminomethyl)-2,6-dichloro-
benzeneacetamide *see* 4561

N-(Aminoiminomethyl)glycine *see* 4495

*N*⁶-(Aminoiminomethyl)-*N*²-(3-mercap-
to-1-oxopropyl)-L-lysylglycyl-L-α-as-
partyl-L-tryptophyl-L-prolyl-L-cys-
teinamide, Cyclic (1 → 6)-Disulfide *see*
3641

N-(Aminoiminomethyl)-4-(1-methyl-
ethyl)-3-(methylsulfonyl)benzamide
see 1841

N-(Aminoiminomethyl)-*N*-methylglycine
see 2568

N-(Aminoiminomethyl)-4-morpholine-
carboximidamide *see* 6272

(3*S*)-3-[[4-[[4-(Aminoiminomethyl)phen-
yl]amino]-1,4-dioxobutyl]amino]-4-
pentynoic Acid Ethyl Ester *see* 10070

N-[[2-[[[4-(Aminoiminomethyl)phenyl]-
amino]methyl]-1-methyl-1*H*-benzimid-
azol-5-yl]carbonyl]-*N*-2-pyridinyl-β-
alanine *see* 2797

4-[2-[4-(Aminoiminomethyl)phenyl]-
ethenyl]-3-hydroxybenzenecarbox-
imidamide *see* 4845

N-[(1*R*)-2-[(2*S*)-2-[[[[4-(Aminoiminomethyl)phenyl]methyl]amino]car-
bonyl]-1-azetidinyl]-1-cyclohexyl-2-
oxoethyl]glycine *see* 5810

(Aminoiminomethyl)urea Sulfate (2:1)
see 3093

3β-Amino-22,26-imino-16β,23-oxido-
5α,22α,23β,25α-cholestan-23-ol *see*
8706

3β-Amino-22,26-imino-16β,23-oxido-
5α,22*R*,23*S*,25*R*-cholestan-23-ol *see*
8706

N-[5-[[(3-Amino-3-iminopropyl)amino]-
carbonyl]-1-methyl-1*H*-pyrrol-3-yl]-4-
[[[4-(formylamino)-1-methyl-1*H*-pyr-
rol-2-yl]carbonyl]amino]-1-methyl-
1*H*-pyrrole-2-carboxamide *see* 8772

(*S*)-α-Amino-1*H*-indole-3-propanoic Acid
see 9797

l-α-Aminoindole-3-propionic Acid *see*
9797

l-α-Amino-3-indolepropionic Acid *see*
9797

2-Amino-3-indolylpropanoic Acid *see*
9797

2-Aminoisobutane *see* 1545

4-Amino-1-isobutyl-1*H*-imidazo[4,5-*c*]-
quinoline *see* 4922

α-Aminoisobutyric Acid, 445

2-Aminoisobutyric Acid *see* 445

α-Aminoisocaproic Acid *see* 5451

3-Aminoisonaphthoic Acid *see* 452

2-Amino-7-isopropyl-1-azaxanthone-3-
carboxylic Acid *see* 490

4-Amino-1-isopropylbenzene *see* 2620

2-Amino-7-isopropyl-5-oxo-5*H*-[1]benzo-
pyrano[2,3-b]pyridine-3-carboxylic
Acid *see* 490

anti-2-Amino-1-(isopropylsulfonyl)-6-
(α-hydroxyiminobenzyl)benzimidazole
see 3601

α-Aminoisovaleric Acid *see* 9909

2-Aminoisovaleric Acid *see* 9909

D-4-Amino-3-isoxazolidinone *see* 2751

D-4-Amino-3-isoxazolidone *see* 2751

Aminokinuride *see* 475

δ-Aminolevulinic Acid, 446

5-Aminolevulinic Acid Hexyl Ester *see*
4693

2-Amino-4-mercaptobutyric Acid *see*
4734

α-Amino-2-mercapto-4-imidazole-
propionic Acid *see* 9341

(*R*)-2-Amino-3-mercaptopropanoic Acid
see 2781

2-Amino-3-mercaptopropionic Acid *see*
2781

2-Amino-6-mercapto-9-β-D-ribofurano-
sylpurine *see* 9338

Aminomethanamide *see* 4562

Aminomethane *see* 6014

Aminomethiazole *see* 450

4-Amino-4'-methoxydiphenylamine *see*
5999

L-3'-(α-Amino-*p*-methoxyhydrocinnam-
amido)-3'-deoxy-*N*,*N*-dimethyladeno-
sine *see* 7943

4-Amino-2-methoxy-5-[(methylamino)-
sulfonyl]-*N*-[[1-(2-propenyl)-2-pyrroli-
dinyl]methyl]benzamide *see* 311

4-Amino-*N*-(6-methoxy-2-methyl-4-pyri-
midinyl)benzenesulfonamide *see* 8917

3'-[[(2*S*)-2-Amino-3-(4-methoxyphenyl)-
1-oxopropyl]amino]-3'-deoxy-*N*,*N*-
dimethyladenosine *see* 7943

4-Amino-6-methoxy-1-phenylpyrid-
azinium Methyl Sulfate *see* 394

4-Amino-*N*-(3-methoxypyrazinyl)-
benzenesulfonamide *see* 8910

4-Amino-*N*-(6-methoxy-3-pyridazinyl)-
benzenesulfonamide *see* 8919

4-Amino-*N*-(5-methoxy-2-pyrimidinyl)-
benzenesulfonamide *see* 8914

4-Amino-*N*-(4-methoxy-1,2,5-thiadiazol-
3-yl)benzenesulfonamide *see* 8920

4-Aminomethyl-4'-aminodiphenyl
Sulfone *see* 8928

3-Amino-7-methylaminophenaza-
thonium Chloride *see* 929

3-Amino-7-(methylamino)phenothiazin-
5-ium Chloride *see* 929

β-Amino-α-methylbenzeneethanol *see*
447

α-(Aminomethyl)benzenemethanol *see*
7287

β-(Aminomethyl)benzenepropanoic Acid
see 464

p-(Aminomethyl)benzenesulfonamide *see*
5649

4-(Aminomethyl)benzenesulfonamide *see*
5649

α-(Aminomethyl)benzyl Alcohol *see* 7287

(*S*)-2-Amino-3-methylbutanoic Acid *see*
9909

8-[(4-Amino-1-methylbutyl)amino]-2,6-
dimethoxy-4-methyl-5-[3-(trifluoromethyl)phenoxy]quinoline *see* 9029

8-(4-Amino-1-methylbutylamino)-6-
methoxyquinoline *see* 7744

8-[(4-Amino-4-methylbutyl)amino]-6-
methoxyquinoline *see* 8067

α-Amino-α-methylbutyric Acid *see* 5234

DL-2-Amino-2-methylbutyric Acid *see*
5234

2-Amino-3-methylbutyric Acid *see* 9909

14-*O*-[1-(D-2-Amino-3-methylbutyryl-
amino)-2-methylpropan-2-ylthio-
acetyl]mutilin *see* 9911

(2*S*,5*R*,6*R*)-6-[(2*R*)-2-[(2*R*)-2-Amino-3-
(methylcarbamoyl)propionamido]-2-
(*p*-hydroxyphenyl)acetamido]-3,3-di-
methyl-7-oxo-4-thia-1-azabicyclo-
[3.2.0]heptane-2-carboxylic Acid *see*
852

6-[D-2-(D-2-Amino-3-*N*-methylcarba-
moylpropionamido)-2-*p*-hydroxyphen-
ylacetamido]penicillanic Acid *see* 852

5-(Aminomethyl)-4-(carboxymethyl)-1*H*-
pyrrole-3-propanoic Acid *see* 7600

β-(Aminomethyl)-4-chlorobenzenepropa-
noic Acid *see* 937

β-(Aminomethyl)-*p*-chlorohydrocin-
namic Acid *see* 937

1-(Aminomethyl)cyclohexaneacetic Acid
see 4319

trans-4-(Aminomethyl)cyclohexanecar-
boxylic Acid *see* 9569

4-[[[*trans*-4-(Aminomethyl)cyclohexyl]-
carbonyl]oxy]benzenepropanoic Acid
see 2024

(1*R*,2*S*)-*rel*-2-(Aminomethyl)-*N*,*N*-di-
ethyl-1-phenylcyclopropanecarbox-
amide *see* 6194

(−)-α-(Aminomethyl)-3,4-dihydroxy-
benzyl Alcohol *see* 6695

L-2-Amino-2-methyl-3-(3,4-dihydroxy-
phenyl)propionic Acid *see* 6055

2-Amino-*N*-(1-methyl-1,2-diphenyl-
ethyl)acetamide *see* 8130

(α*S*,1*R*)-α-Amino-2-methylenecyclo-
propanepropanoic Acid *see* 4866

α-Amino-β-(2-methylenecyclopropyl)-
propionic Acid *see* 4866

2-Amino-4,5-methylenehex-5-enoic
Acid *see* 4866

Ammate [DuPont] *see* 554
Ammidin *see* 4925
(*SP*-4-3)-Amminedichloro(2-methyl-
  pyridine)platinum *see* 7405
cis-Amminedichloro(2-methyl-
  pyridine)platinum(II) *see* 7405
Amminosidin *see* 7041
Ammivin *see* 5309
Ammo [FMC] *see* 2767
Ammoidin *see* 5988
Ammonia, 492
Ammoniacum, 493
Ammonia Soap *see* 535
Ammonia Water, 494
Ammonia Water—10% *see* 494
2-Ammonio-4-methylphosphinico-
  butyrate *see* 7339
Ammonium Acetate, 495
Ammonium Acetate Solution *see* 495
Ammonium Acid Oxalate *see* 499
Ammonium Acid Tartrate *see* 503
Ammonium Alum *see* 327
Ammonium Aluminum Fluoride *see* 524
Ammonium Aminoformate *see* 507
Ammonium Antimony Tungsten Oxide
  see 4750
Ammonium Benzoate, 496
Ammonium Biborate *see* 504
Ammonium Bicarbonate, 497
Ammonium Bichromate *see* 515
Ammonium Bifluoride, 498
Ammonium Binoxalate, 499
Ammonium Biphosphate *see* 543
Ammonium Bisulfate, 500
Ammonium Bisulfide, 501
Ammonium Bisulfite, 502
Ammonium Bitartrate, 503
Ammonium Bithiolicum *see* 4885
Ammonium Bituminosulfonate *see* 4885
Ammonium Borate, 504
Ammonium Bromide, 505
Ammonium Caprylate, 506
Ammonium Carbamate, 507
Ammonium Carbazoate *see* 547
Ammonium Carbolate *see* 7241
Ammonium Carbonate, 508
Ammonium Ceric Nitrate *see* 1992
Ammonium Chloride, 509
Ammonium Chloroaluminate *see* 558
Ammonium Chlorocuprate *see* 514
Ammonium Chloroheptenearsonate *see*
  2119
Ammonium Chloroosmate *see* 536
Ammonium Chloroplatinate *see* 548
Ammonium Chloroplatinite *see* 549
Ammonium Chromate(VI), 510
Ammonium Chromic Sulfate, 511
Ammonium Citrate, Dibasic, 512
Ammonium Cobaltous Phosphate, 513
Ammonium Cryolite *see* 524
Ammonium Cupric Chloride, 514
Ammonium Cupric Sulfate *see* 9181
Ammonium Diamminetetrakis(thiocyan-
  ato-*N*)chromate(1−) *see* 8128
Ammonium Dichromate(VI), 515
Ammonium Dihydrogen Phosphate *see*
  543
Ammonium Dioxopentafluoroura-
  nate(VI) *see* 567
Ammonium Dioxotricarbonatoura-
  nate(VI) *see* 566
Ammonium Disulfatochromate(III) *see*
  511
Ammonium Dithiocarbamate, 516
Ammonium Diuranate *see* 565

Ammonium Embelate *see* 3555
Ammonium Ferric Citrate *see* 4017
Ammonium Ferric Oxalate, 517
Ammonium Ferric Sulfate, 518
Ammonium Ferricyanide, 519
Ammonium Ferrocyanide, 520
Ammonium Ferrous Sulfate, 521
Ammonium Fluoaluminate *see* 524
Ammonium Fluoride, 522
Ammonium Fluosilicate *see* 527
Ammonium Formate, 523
Ammonium Hexachloroosmate(IV) *see*
  536
Ammonium Hexachloroplatinate(IV) *see*
  548
Ammonium Hexacyanoferrate (II) *see*
  520
Ammonium Hexacyanoferrate(III) *see*
  519
Ammonium Hexafluogallate *see* 525
Ammonium Hexafluophosphate *see* 526
Ammonium Hexafluoroaluminate, 524
Ammonium Hexafluorogallate, 525
Ammonium Hexafluorophosphate, 526
Ammonium Hexafluorosilicate, 527
Ammonium Hexanitratocerate *see* 1992
Ammonium DL-Homoalanine-4-yl-
  (methyl)phosphinate *see* 7339
Ammonium Hydrogen Carbonate *see* 497
Ammonium Hydrogen Fluoride *see* 498
Ammonium Hydrogen Oxalate *see* 499
Ammonium Hydrogen Sulfate *see* 500
Ammonium Hydrogen Sulfide *see* 501
Ammonium Hydrogen Tartrate *see* 503
Ammonium Hydrosulfide *see* 501
Ammonium Hydroxide *see* 494
Ammonium Hypophosphite, 528
Ammonium Hyposulfite *see* 562
Ammonium Ichthosulfonate *see* 4885
Ammonium Iodide, 529
Ammonium Lactate, 530
Ammonium Magnesium Chloride, 531
Ammonium Mandelate, 532
Ammonium Metaborate *see* 504
Ammonium Metavanadate *see* 568
Ammonium Molybdate(VI), 533
Ammonium Molybdophosphate *see* 545
Ammonium Muriate *see* 509
Ammonium Nickel Sulfate *see* 6501
Ammonium Nitrate, 534
Ammonium Nitratocerate *see* 1992
Ammonium Oleate, 535
Ammonium Osmium Chloride, 536
Ammonium Oxalate, 537
Ammonium Oxodioxalatotitanate(IV) *see*
  563
Ammonium Palmitate, 538
Ammonium Paramolybdate *see* 533
Ammonium Paratungstate *see* 564
Ammonium Pentachlorozincate, 539
Ammonium Perchlorate, 540
Ammonium Peroxydisulfate, 541
Ammonium Persulfate *see* 541
Ammonium Phenate *see* 7241
Ammonium *p*-Phenolsulfonate *see* 7246
Ammonium Phosphate, Dibasic, 542
Ammonium Phosphate, Monobasic, 543
Ammonium Phosphite, 544
Ammonium Phosphomolybdate, 545
Ammonium Phosphorus Hexafluoride
  see 526
Ammonium Phosphotungstate, 546
Ammonium Phosphowolframate *see* 546
Ammonium Picrate, 547
Ammonium Picronitrate *see* 547

Ammonium Platinic Chloride, 548
Ammonium Platinochloride *see* 549
Ammonium Platinous Chloride, 549
Ammonium Purpurate *see* 6306
Ammonium Reineckate *see* 8128
Ammonium Rhodanide *see* 561
Ammonium Salicylate, 550
Ammonium Salt of Aurintricarboxylic
  Acid *see* 322
Ammonium Selenate, 551
Ammonium Selenite, 552
Ammonium Silicofluoride *see* 527
Ammonium Stearate, 553
Ammonium Sulfamate, 554
Ammonium Sulfate, 555
Ammonium Sulfhydrate *see* 501
Ammonium Sulfide, 556
Ammonium Sulfite, 557
Ammonium Sulfobituminate *see* 4885
Ammonium Sulfocarbamate *see* 516
Ammonium Sulfocyanate *see* 561
Ammonium Sulfocyanide *see* 561
Ammonium Sulfoichthyolate *see* 4885
Ammonium Tetraborate *see* 504
Ammonium Tetrachloroaluminate, 558
Ammonium Tetrachlorocuprate(II) *see*
  514
Ammonium Tetrachlorodiaquo-
  cuprate(II) *see* 514
Ammonium Tetrachloroplatinate(II) *see*
  549
Ammonium Tetrachlorozincate, 559
Ammonium Tetrathiocyanodiammono-
  chromate *see* 8128
Ammonium Tetrathiomolybdate, 560
Ammonium Thiocyanate, 561
Ammonium Thiosulfate, 562
Ammonium Titanium Oxalate, 563
Ammonium Tricarbonatozirconate *see*
  569
Ammonium Trioxalatoferrate(III) *see*
  517
Ammonium Tungstate(VI), 564
Ammonium 5-Tungsto-2-antimonate *see*
  4750
Ammonium Tungstophosphate *see* 546
Ammonium Uranate(VI), 565
Ammonium Uranium Carbonate, 566
Ammonium Uranium Fluoride, 567
Ammonium Uranium Oxide ((NH$_4$)
  2U$_2$O$_7$) *see* 565
Ammonium Vanadate(V), 568
Ammonium Zirconyl Carbonate, 569
Ammonyx DME [Onyx] *see* 2029
Ammonyx G *see* 2017
Ammonyx T *see* 2017
Amoban [Aventis] *see* 10193
Amobarbital, 570
Amocarzine, 571
Amocilline [Inpharzam] *see* 577
Amodex [Bouchara] *see* 577
Amodiaquin, 572
Amoenol *see* 5031
Amoksiklav [Lek] *see* 2341
Amoram [Eastern] *see* 577
Amorolfine, 573
Amorphan [Heumann] *see* 6714
Amoscanate, 574
Amosite *see* 826
Amosulalol, 575
Amosyt [Abigo] *see* 3207
Amotril *see* 2377
Amoxanox *see* 490
Amoxapine, 576
Amoxicillin, 577

Amoxidin [Lagap] *see* 577
Amoxil [GSK] *see* 577
Amoxillat [Novartis] *see* 577
Amoxycillin *see* 577
Amoxypen [Grünenthal] *see* 577
AMP *see* 158, 449
3′,5′-AMP *see* 2708
AMPA, 578
S-AMPA *see* 578
AMPC *see* 577
AMPD *see* 448
Ampecyclal [Sarget] *see* 4657
Ampelopsin, 579
Ampeloptin *see* 579
Amperozide, 580
Amphedroxyn [Lilly] *see* 5948
Amphenone *see* 581
Amphenone B, 581
Amphetamine, 582
d-Amphetamine *see* 2954
Amphetaminil, 583
Amphibole *see* 826
Amphihydroxynaphthyl-*β*-propionic
   Acid *see* 259
Amphocil [Zeneca] *see* 585
Amphojel [Wyeth-Ayerst] *see* 342
Ampho-Moronal [BMS] *see* 585
Amphomycin, 584
Amphotericin B, 585
Amphotericin B Colloidal Dispersion *see*
   585
Amphotericin B Compd with (3*β*)-Cho-
   lest-5-en-3-yl Hydrogen Sulfate (1:1)
   see 585
Amphotericin B Lipid Complex *see* 585
Ampicillin, 586
Ampicillin (5-Methyl-2-oxo-1,3-dioxo-
   len-4-yl)methyl Ester *see* 5437
Ampicillin 1-Oxo-1,3-dihydroisobenzo-
   furan-3-yl Ester *see* 9033
Ampicillin Pivaloyloxymethyl Ester *see*
   7512
Ampicin [BMS] *see* 586
Ampilar [Sandoz] *see* 586
Ampiroxicam, 587
Ampitab [Vétoquinol] *see* 586
Ampliactil [Aventis] *see* 2185
Amplicain *see* 6743
Amplictil [Aventis] *see* 2185
Ampligen, 588
Ampligram [Hermes] *see* 1979
Amplit [Daiichi] *see* 5557
Amplital *see* 586
Amplivix [1083]
Amprace [Merck & Co.] *see* 3567
Amprenavir, 589
Amprol [Merck & Co.] *see* 590
Amprol Plus [Merck & Co.] *see* 3745
Amprolium, 590
Ampyrone, 591
Amrinone, 592
Amrubicin, 593
AMS *see* 554
m-AMSA *see* 594
Amsacrine, 594
Amsidine [Parke-Davis] *see* 594
Amsidyl [Pfizer] *see* 594
Amsonic Acid, 595
Amsubit *see* 4885
Amsulosin *see* 9049
AMT *see* 6131
Amtolmetin Guacil, 596
Amudane *see* 4549
Amycor [Lipha] *see* 1213
Amygdalic Acid *see* 5717

Amygdalin, 597
Amygdalinic Acid *see* 5717
Amygdalose *see* 4396
Amygdaloside *see* 597
Amylacetic Ester *see* 5111
dl-sec-Amyl Alcohol *see* 7119
n-Amyl Alcohol *see* 7118
tert-Amyl Alcohol *see* 7140
n-Amylamine, 598
Amylase, 599
α-Amylase (*Aspergillus oryzae*) *see* 9031
γ-Amylases *see* 599
Amylbenzene, 600
n-Amylbenzene *see* 600
d-Amyl Bromide, 601
d-pri-act-Amyl Bromide *see* 601
n-Amyl Bromide, 602
tert-Amyl Bromide, 603
n-Amyl Butyrate, 604
n-Amyl Caproate, 605
Amylcarbinol *see* 4697
Amyl Chloride, 606
n-Amyl Chloride *see* 606
Amyleine Hydrochloride *see* 614
Amylene, 607
α-n-Amylene *see* 7122
β-n-Amylene *see* 7123
Amylene Hydrate *see* 7140
n-Amyl Ether, 608
Amyl Ethyl Ketone *see* 6084
3-Amyl-1-hydroxy-6,6,9-trimethyl-6*H*-
   dibenzo[*b,d*]pyran *see* 1748
Amylin, 609
Amyl Isovalerate *see* 5121
tert-Amyl Isovalerate, 610
n-Amyl Mercaptan, 611
Amylmethylcarbinol *see* 4662
tert-Amyl Methyl Ether, 612
Amyl Nitrite, 613
Amylobarbitone *see* 570
Amylocaine Hydrochloride, 614
Amylodextrin *see* 8799
Amylogen *see* 8799
Amyloid *β* Peptide, 615
Amyloid Precursor Protein *see* 615,
   7739
β-Amyloid Protein *see* 615
Amylopectin *see* 481
Amylose *see* 8798
Amyl Oxide *see* 608
Amylpenicillin, 616
p-tert-Amylphenol *see* 7142
cis-4-[3-(4-*tert*-Amylphenyl)-2-methyl-
   propyl]-2,6-dimethylmorpholine *see*
   573
Amyl Phthalate *see* 5124
Amyl Thioalcohol *see* 611
Amylum *see* 8798
Amyl Valerate *see* 5121
α-Amyrenol *see* 617
β-Amyrenol *see* 618
α-Amyrin, 617
β-Amyrin, 618
Amytal [Flynn] *see* 570
AN 1 [Krugmann] *see* 583
AN-148 *see* 5944
AN-1317 *see* 7168
AN-1324 *see* 4480
Anabact [Cambridge Healthcare] *see* 6157
Anabasine, 619
Anabiol [Searle] *see* 1322
Anabo [Hokuriku] *see* 5915
Anabolex [Samil] *see* 8793
Anabsinthin, 620
Anabsynthin *see* 620

Anacardic Acid, 621
Anacardone *see* 6543
Anacobin *see* 10014
Anadonis Green *see* 2234
Anadrol [Syntex] *see* 6967
Anaesthesin [Ritsert] *see* 1086
Anaflex [Geistlich] *see* 7574
Anaflon [GSK] *see* 47
Anafranil [Novartis] *see* 2387
Anagregal [Gentili] *see* 9429
Anagrelide, 622
Anagyrine, 623
Anahist [Warner-Lambert] *see* 9373
Anakinra *see* 5001
Analate [Winston] *see* 5685
Analeptin *see* 9012
Analetil *see* 9203
Analgesine *see* 716
Analgin *see* 3350
Analud [Unifa] *see* 4012
Analux [Polfa] *see* 5780
Anamidol [Iwaki] *see* 6965
Anamycin [Chephasaar] *see* 3681
Ananase [Rorer] *see* 1388
Anandamide, 624
Anandron [Cassenne] *see* 6544
Anapen [Celltech] *see* 3619
Anapolon [Syntex] *see* 6967
Anaprox [Syntex] *see* 6417
Anaptivan [Help] *see* 1954
Anaritide *see* 872
Anasterone *see* 6967
Anastil [Eberth] *see* 4553
Anastrozole, 625
Anatabine, 626
Anatase *see* 9472, 9475
Anatensol [BMS] *see* 4189
Anatoxin a *see* 627
Anatoxin a(s) *see* 627
Anatoxins, 627
Anatran [Tobishi] *see* 9624
Anaus [Molteni] *see* 9708
Anautine *see* 3207
Anauxite *see* 362
Anavar [Searle] *see* 6921
Anayodin *see* 8631
Anazolene Sodium, 628
Anboxan [Shionogi] *see* 3416
Ancaron [Taisho] *see* 482
Ancef [GSK] *see* 1917
Anceron [Schering-Plough] *see* 1019
Ancestim *see* 8807
Anchoic Acid *see* 905
Anchorin *see* 676
Anchovyxanthin *see* 10118
Anchusa *see* 256
Anchusa Acid *see* 257
Anchusin *see* 257
Anchusin Paper *see* 256
Ancitabine, 629
Ancobon [Roche] *see* 4125
Ancolan [Boots] *see* 5777
Ancotil [Roche] *see* 4125
Ancrod, 630
Ancylol [Am. Cyanamid] *see* 3359
Ancymidol, 631
Ancytabine *see* 629
Ancyte [Abbott] *see* 7481
Andalin [Solvay Duphar] *see* 4123
Andalusite *see* 362
Andantol [Sumitomo] *see* 5227
Andanton [Lacer] *see* 5227
Andaxin [EGYT] *see* 5862
Andere [Toyama] *see* 1476
Andergin [ISOM] *see* 6178

Anhydrous Sulfate of Lime see 1706
Anidulafungin, 656
Anifed [Formenti] see 6528
Anilazine, 657
Anileridine, 658
Aniline, 659
Aniline Green see 5699
Aniline Mustard, 660
Aniline Oil see 659
p-Anilinesulfonamide see 8925
Aniline-m-sulfonic Acid see 5927
o-Anilinesulfonic Acid see 6882
p-Anilinesulfonic Acid see 8926
Aniline Tribromide see 9610
Aniline Violet see 4395
Aniline Yellow see 419
Anilinoacetic Acid see 7292
Anilinoazobenzene see 2998
Anilinobenzene see 1235
p-Anilinobenzenesulfonic Acid see 7313
2-Anilinobenzoic Acid see 7273
2-Anilino-4,6-dimethylpyrimidine see 7986
Anilinoformylhydrazine see 7312
4'-Anilino-8-hydroxy-1,1'-azonaphtha-lene-3,5',6-trisulfonic Acid Trisodium Salt see 628
(S)-1-Anilino-4-methyl-2-methylthio-4-phenylimidazolin-5-one see 3956
3-Anilino-5-methyl-5-(4-phenoxyphen-yl)-1,3-oxazolidine-2,4-dione see 3931
2-Anilino-4-methyl-6-(1-propynyl)-pyrimidine see 5845
1-Anilino-8-naphthalenesulfonate, 661
8-Anilino-1-naphthalenesulfonic Acid see 661
m-[(p-Anilinophenyl)azo]benzenesulfonic Acid Sodium Salt see 5928
p-[(p-Anilinophenyl)azo]benzenesulfonic Acid Sodium Salt see 9776
1-(3-Anilinopropyl)-4-phenylisonipecotic Acid Ethyl Ester see 7433
Anilotic Acid see 6632
Animal Charcoal see 1808
Animal Coniine see 1609
Animal Galactose Factor see 6876
Animal Starch see 4496
Animar [Pfizer] see 8906
Anime (Soft Copal) see 2517
Aniprime [Syntex Diamond] see 4138
Anipryl [Deprenyl] see 8428
Aniracetam, 662
p-Anisaldehyde, 663
Anise, 664
Anise Alcohol, 665
Anise Camphor see 643
Aniseed, 664
Aniseed Oil see 664
p-Anisic Acid, 666
Anisic Aldehyde see 663
Anisidine, 667
m-Anisidine see 667
o-Anisidine see 667
p-Anisidine see 667
Anisindione, 668
Anisole, 669
Anisomycin, 670
Anisotropine Methylbromide, 671
Anisoylated Plasminogen Streptokinase Activator Complex see 674
o-(p-Anisoyl)benzoic Acid, 672
p-Anisoyl Chloride, 673
1-p-Anisoyl-2-pyrrolidinone see 662
Anistadin [Maruko] see 9624
Anistreplase, 674

Anisyl Alcohol see 665
Anisyldithiophosphinic Anhydride see 5391
2-p-Anisyl-1,3-indandione see 668
trans-1-p-Anisylpropene see 643
3-(p-Anisyl)trithione see 644
ANIT see 6411
Ankebin [Volpino] see 3978
Ankilostin see 9190
Ankyrin see 8740
Annalin see 1706
Annatto, 675
Annexins, 676
Annotinine, 677
Annotta see 675
Anobesina see 2733
Anodynine see 716
Anodynon see 3782
p-Anol, 678
Anone see 2726
Anoprenol [Azwell] see 279
Anorex [Crinex] see 3127
Anorthite see 1648
Anovlar [Schering AG] see 6697
ANP see 872
ANP 95-126 see 9886
ANP-235 see 5780
ANP-3624 see 9430
Anparton [Sanwa] see 2377
Anprolene see 3802
Anquil [Janssen-Cilag] see 1048
ANRL see 5795
ANS see 661
ANS-118 see 2218
Ansaid [Pfizer] see 4199
Ansar 6.6 [ISK Biosci] see 5953
Ansar 8100 [ISK Biosci] see 5953
Ansatin [Ono] see 4132
Ansatipine [Farmitalia] see 8213
Anseren [Novartis] see 5297
Anserine, 679
Ansiacal [Beolet] see 2084
Ansial [Vita] see 1504
Ansiced [Abello] see 1504
Ansilan [Lek] see 5786
Ansimar [ABC] see 3438
Ansiven [Abbott] see 7834
Ansmin [SS Pharm.] see 3311
Ansolysen Bitartrate [Wyeth] see 7132
Ansolysen Tartrate [Wyeth] see 7132
Antabuse [Odyssey] see 3364
Antacal [Errekappa] see 491
Antadys [Théramex] see 4199
Antagon [Organon] see 4365
Antagonil [Novartis] see 6495
Antagonil [Wildlife Pharm.] see 10102
Antagosan [HMR] see 757
Antalgin [Syntex] see 6417
Antallin see 3517
Antalone [Kobayashi] see 5915
Antalzyme see 5640
Antamine [Grove] see 7984
Antapentan [Ayerst] see 7220
Antasten [Novartis] see 680
Antaxone [Zambon] see 6363
Antazoline, 680
Antébor [Biologiques] see 8899
Antees [Oriental] see 1794
Antegan [Frosst] see 2773
Antegren [Elan] see 6426
Antemin [Streuli] see 3207
Antemovis [Vister] see 8462
Antepan [Henning] see 9588
Antepar [Glaxo Wellcome] see 7464
Antepsin [Wyeth] see 8879

Anterior Pituitary Growth Hormone see 8716
Anterior Pituitary Luteotropin see 7779
Antevas [Chugai] see 6493
Anthelcide EQ [Pfizer] see 6936
Anthelin see 778
Anthelone see 3527
Anthelone E see 3597
Anthelone U see 3527
Anthen [Byk Gulden] see 7768
Antheridiol, 681
Anthesterin see 9060
Anthio see 4246
Anthion see 7656
Anthiphen see 3071
Anthisan [M & B] see 7984
Anthophyllite see 826
Anthorine see 862
Anthracene, 682
Anthracene Brown see 683
9,10-Anthracenedicarboxaldehyde Bis[(4,5-dihydro-1H-imidazol-2-yl)-hydrazone] see 1244
9,10-Anthracenedicarboxaldehyde Bis(2-imidazolin-2-ylhydrazone) see 1244
9,10-Anthracenedione see 687
1,2,10-Anthracenetriol see 688
9-Anthracenol see 686
9(10H)-Anthracenone see 691
Anthraforte [Stiefel] see 684
Anthragallic Acid see 683
Anthragallol, 683
Anthralin, 684
Anthramycin, 685
Anthranilic Acid see 422
Anthranilic Acid Cinnamyl Ester see 2303
Anthranilic Acid p-Menth-3-yl Ester see 5840
Anthranilic Acid 2-(2-Piperidyl)ethyl Ester see 7494
3-Anthraniloylalanine see 5328
Anthranol [Stiefel] see 684
Anthranol, 686
Anthraquinone, 687
9,10-Anthraquinone see 687
6,6'-(1,4-Anthraquinonylene-diimino)di-m-toluenesulfonic Acid Disodium Salt see 252
Anthrarobin, 688
Anthrarufin, 689
Anthrascalp [Stiefel] see 684
1,2,10-Anthratriol see 688
Anthrimide, 690
9-Anthrol see 686
Anthrone, 691
Anthropodesoxycholic Acid see 2054
Antiangor [I.S.O.M.] see 2239
Anti-B1 Antibody see 9554
Antibason see 6128
Antibiocin [Orion] see 7100
3C Antibiotic see 6340
Antibiotic 67-694 see 8261
Antibiotic 1037 see 9562
Antibiotic 5879 see 1202
Antibiotic 6640 see 8550
Antibiotic 32232RP see 8544
Antibiotic A 246 see 4290
Antibiotic A-300 see 9649
Antibiotic A 5283 see 6427
Antibiotic A-23187 see 1639
Antibiotic A-28086 Factor A see 6419
Antibiotic AB 206 see 6196
Antibiotic Ab 651 see 1859

Antimony Glance *see* 713
Antimony Hydride *see* 8811
Antimony Oxychloride *see* 693
Antimony Pentachloride, 695
Antimony Pentafluoride, 696
Antimony Pentasulfide, 697
Antimony Pentoxide, 698
Antimony Potassium Oxalate, 699
Antimony Potassium Tartrate, 700
Antimony Pyrocatechol Sodium
    Disulfonate Heptahydrate *see* 8813
Antimony Red *see* 697
"Antimony Salt" *see* 699
Antimony Selenide *see* 712
Antimony Sodium Gluconate, 701
Antimony Sodium Oxide L(+)-Tartrate
    see 702
Antimony Sodium Tartrate, 702
Antimony Sodium Thioacetate *see* 703
Antimony Sodium Thioglycollate, 703
Antimony Sulfate, 704
Antimony Sulfide *see* 713
Antimony Thioglycollamide, 705
Antimony Thioglycollic Acid Triamide
    see 705
Antimony Tribromide, 706
Antimony Trichloride, 707
Antimony Trifluoride, 709
Antimony Trifluorodichloride *see* 694
Antimony Triiodide, 710
Antimony Trioxide, 711
Antimony Triselenide, 712
Antimony Trisulfate *see* 704
Antimony Trisulfide, 713
Antimosan *see* 8813
Antimycin *see* 2327
Antimycin A$_1$, 714
Antimycin A$_3$, 715
Antin *see* 7316
Antinonnin *see* 3279
Antinosin *see* 5038
Antipar [Farmitalia] *see* 3108
Antiparkin [Viatris] *see* 8428
Antipellagra Vitamin *see* 6525
Antipernicious Anemia Principle *see*
    10014
α_2-Antiplasmin *see* 7520
Antipyrine, 716
Antipyrine Amygdalate *see* 716
Antipyrine 2-Hydroxy-2-methylbutyrate
    see 716
Antipyrine Salicylate, 717
(Antipyrinylmethylamino)methane-
    sulfonic Acid Sodium Salt *see* 3350
Antiradon *see* 178
Anti-(Respiratory Syncytial Virus
    Protein F) Immunoglobulin G1
    (Human-Mouse Monoclonal MEDI-
    493 γ_1-Chain) Disulfide with Human-
    Mouse Monoclonal MEDI-493 κ-
    Chain, Dimer *see* 6988
Antireticular Cytotoxic Serum, 718
Antirex [Kyorin] *see* 3516
Antirobe *see* 2356
Antirrhinin *see* 2687
Antiscabiosum [Strathmann] *see* 1127
Antiscorbutic Vitamin *see* 830
Antisedan [Pfizer] *see* 861
Antisepsin *see* 1399
Antistine [Novartis] *see* 680
Anti-Stress [Sintyal] *see* 5846
Antitanil *see* 3180
Anti-tetany Substance 10 *see* 3180
Antithermin *see* 5472
Antithrombin III *see* 4653

α_1-Antitrypsin, 719
Antituxil-Z [Ghimas] *see* 10170
Antivariz *see* 3727
Antivenin [Merck & Co.] *see* 721
Antivenin (Crotalidae) Polyvalent, 720
Antivenin (*Latrodectus Mactans*), 721
Antiverm *see* 7252
Antivert [Pfizer] *see* 5777
Antiweinsäure (German) *see* 9071
Antixerophthalmic Vitamin *see* 10013
Antizol [Orphan Med.] *see* 4226
Antlerite *see* 2519, 2654
Antocin *see* 865
Antodyne *see* 7290
Antoral [Recordati] *see* 9426
Antorphine *see* 6361
Antra [AstraZeneca] *see* 6845
Antracol [Bayer] *see* 7819
Antraderm [Protea] *see* 684
Antrancine 8 [Jandekker] *see* 1548
Antrancine 12 [Jandekker] *see* 1547
Antrapurol *see* 2815
Antrenyl [Novartis] *see* 6975
Antrin [Pharmacyclics] *see* 6282
Antrycide *see* 8052
Antrypol [AstraZeneca] *see* 9006
ANTU, 722
Antulcus *see* 6973
Anturan [Novartis] *see* 8949
Anturane [Novartis] *see* 8949
Anturano [Novartis] *see* 8949
Anturat *see* 722
(+)-ANTX-a *see* 627
ANTX-a(s) *see* 627
ANTXS *see* 627
Anvil [Syngenta] *see* 4681
Anvirzel *see* 6826
Anvitoff [Abbott] *see* 9569
Anydrous Lanolin *see* 5358
Anymol *see* 1241
Anzatax [Faulding] *see* 6982
Anzemet [Aventis] *see* 3411
Anzief [Nippon Chemiphar] *see* 279
AO-128 *see* 10029
Aolan [Beiersdorf] *see* 3714
Aolept [Bayer] *see* 7164
A.O.P. *see* 77
Aotal [Merck KGaA] *see* 17
4-AP *see* 3933
AP2 *see* 8535
AP-14 *see* 3134
A-5MP *see* 158
6-APA *see* 458
Apache [FMC] *see* 1632
Apacizin *see* 478
Apacizina [Farmitalia] *see* 478
Apafant, 723
Apalcillin, 724
Apamide [Bayer] *see* 47
Apamin, 725
Aparkane [ICN] *see* 9695
Aparkazin *see* 3108
Apatef [AstraZeneca] *see* 1934
Apaurin [Krka] *see* 2994
Apazone, 726
APC *see* 7204
APC-8015 *see* 8547
Apegmone [Lipha] *see* 9451
Aperdor [Tokyo Tanabe] *see* 9502
Apertase *see* 4758
Apetinil-Depo [Drossapharm] *see* 3763
Apex 462-5 *see* 9751
APF-1 *see* 9844
Aphanin *see* 3495
Aphidicolin, 727

Aphilan [UCB] *see* 1464
Aphistar [Dow AgroSci.] *see* 9601
Apholate, 728
Aphox [Zeneca] *see* 7496
Aphoxide *see* 9672
Aphrodine *see* 10102
Aphrodyne [Star] *see* 10102
Aphthasol [Block] *see* 490
Aphtiria [Debat] *see* 5501
Aphylline, 729
A1PI *see* 719
Apidra [Sanofi-Aventis] *see* 4985
Apigenin, 730
Apigenin-7-apiosylglucoside *see* 732
Apigenin-7-D-glucoside *see* 731
Apigenin-4'-methyl Ether *see* 13
Apigetrin, 731
Apihepar [Viatris] *see* 8532
Apiin, 732
Apilak *see* 8277
Apinol *see* 5838
7-[(2-*O*-D-Apio-β-D-furanosyl-β-D-
    glucopyranosyl)oxy]-5-hydroxy-2-
    (4-hydroxyphenyl)-4*H*-1-benzopyran-
    4-one *see* 732
6-*O*-(D-Apiofuranosyl)-1,6,8-trihydr-
    oxy-3-methylanthraquinone *see* 4264
Apiol *see* 734
Apiole (Dill), 733
Apiole (Parsley), 734
Apioline *see* 734
Apiose, 735
D-Apiose *see* 735
Apioside *see* 732
Apiquel [McNeil] *see* 476
Apiracohl [Kyowa] *see* 9502
Aplace [Kyorin] *see* 9790
Aplactan [Eisai] *see* 2305
Aplasmomycin, 736
Aplaviroc, 737
Aplexal [Taiyo] *see* 2305
Aplidin [PharmaMar] *see* 738
Aplidine, 738
Aplisol [Parke-Davis] *see* 9805
Apllobal [Fujisawa] *see* 313
Aplonidine *see* 751
APM *see* 839
APNPS *see* 8933
APO *see* 9672
Apoaequorin *see* 177
Apoatropine, 739
Apocard [Esteve] *see* 4098
Apocodeine, 740
Apocynamarin *see* 8851
Apocynin, 741
Apocynum Androsaemifolium, 742
Apocynum Cannabinum, 743
Apocytochrome *c* *see* 2791
Apodel [Meiji] *see* 5518
ApoE *see* 745
Apo-β-erythroidine, 744
Apoferritin *see* 4036
Apohemocyanin *see* 4647
Apokinon [Aguettant] *see* 746
Apokyn [Mylan Bertek] *see* 746
Apolan [Stockli] *see* 2377
Apolipoprotein E, 745
Apollo [FBC] *see* 2376
Apomine [Faulding] *see* 746
Apomorphine, 746
Aponal [Boehringer, Mann.] *see* 3435
Aponeuron [Apogepha] *see* 583
Aponorin [Kodama] *see* 9624
Apopain *see* 1885
Apophedrin *see* 7287

Apoptolidin, 747
Aporeine, 748
Aporheine *see* 748
6αβ-Aporphine-10,11-diol *see* 746
Apo-Sulfatrim [Apotex] *see* 8918
Apotomin [Kowa] *see* 2305
3α,16α-Apovincaminic Acid Ethyl
    Ester *see* 9991
A-Poxide [Abbott] *see* 2084
Appel's Salt, 749
Appertex [Janssen] *see* 2343
Appetize [Source Food Technology], 750
Applaud [Nihon Nohyaku] *see* 1498
Apple Acid *see* 5707
Apple of Peru *see* 8820
Apple Oil *see* 5121
Apraclonidine, 751
Apralan [Elanco] *see* 752
Apramycin, 752
Apranax [Syntex] *see* 6417
Aprecon *see* 5110
Aprepitant, 753
Apresoline [Novartis] *see* 4763
Aprical [Shire] *see* 6528
Apride [Kodama] *see* 9502
Apridol *see* 5846
Aprindine, 754
Aprinocarsen, 755
Aprinox [Sovereign] *see* 1037
APRL *see* 7524
Aprobarbital, 756
Aprobarbital Sodium *see* 756
Aprocarb *see* 7836
Apron [Syngenta] *see* 5922
Aprotinin, 757
Aprovel [Sanofi-Synthelabo] *see* 5083
APSAC *see* 674
Apsolol [APS] *see* 7840
Apstil [APS] *see* 3129
Aptaguanal *see* 758
Aptiganel, 758
Aptine [Astra] *see* 313
Aptivus [Boehringer, Ing.] *see* 9459
Aptol Duriles [Astra] *see* 313
Aptosyn [Cell Pathways] *see* 3916
Apulonga [Dorsch] *see* 279
Apurin [GEA] *see* 279
Apurol [Siegfried] *see* 279
Apurone [3M Pharma] *see* 4137
APY-606 *see* 2412
Apyrase, 759
Apyron [Wülfing] *see* 5655
AQ-110 *see* 9587
AQP1 *see* 760
AQP2 *see* 760
AQP.At1 *see* 760
AQP-CD *see* 760
AQP-CHIP *see* 760
Aqua Ammonia *see* 494
Aquacare [Allergan] *see* 9867
Aquacobalamin *see* 4809
Aquadrate [Procter & Gamble] *see* 9867
Aquafen [Schering-Plough] *see* 4109
Aquaflor [Schering-Plough] *see* 4109
Aqua Fortis *see* 6577
Aqualin [Shell] *see* 128
Aquamarine *see* 1161
AquaMephyton [Merck & Co.] *see* 7380
Aquamox [Lederle] *see* 8056
Aquamycetin [Winzer] *see* 2077
Aquamycin *see* 1962
Aquanil [Selena] *see* 9444
Aquaphor [Lilly] *see* 10079
Aquaporin-CHIP *see* 760
Aquaporins, 760

Aquareduct [Azupharma] *see* 8760
Aqua Regia *see* 6609
Aquaretic [Azupharma] *see* 406
Aquarius [Frosst] *see* 4781
Aquasept [Hough, Hoseason] *see* 9657
Aquasol A [AAI] *see* 10013
Aquatensen [Mallinckrodt] *see* 6005
Aquathol [Elf Atochem] *see* 3575
Aquathol K [Elf Atochem] *see* 3575
Aquavan [Guilford] *see* 4259
Aquedux [Delagrange] *see* 2374
Aquirel *see* 2754
Aquocobalamin *see* 4809
Aquo-Trinitrosan [Merck KGaA] *see* 6607
AR-12008 *see* 9574
Ara-A *see* 9976
Arabinitol *see* 762
9-β-D-Arabinofuranosyladenine
    Monohydrate *see* 9976
1-β-D-Arabinofuranosyl-5-[(1E)-2-
    bromoethenyl]-2,4(1H,3H)-pyrimi-
    dinedione *see* 8727
1-β-D-Arabinofuranosyl-(E)-5-(2-bromo-
    vinyl)uracil *see* 8727
1-β-D-Arabinofuranosylcytosine *see* 2784
N-(1-β-D-Arabinofuranosyl-1,2-dihy-
    dro-2-oxo-4-pyrimidinyl)docosan-
    amide *see* 3586
9-β-D-Arabinofuranosyl-2-fluoroadenine
    see 4126
9-β-D-Arabinofuranosyl-2-fluoro-9H-
    purin-6-amine *see* 4126
9-β-D-Arabinofuranosyl-6-methoxy-9H-
    purin-2-amine *see* 6442
9-β-D-Arabinofuranosyl-9H-purine-6-
    amine Monohydrate *see* 9976
L-Arabinose *see* 761
Arabinose, 761
Arabinosyladenine *see* 9976
Arabite *see* 762
Arabitol, 762
D-Araboascorbic Acid *see* 5126
D-Araboflavin, 763
Ara-C *see* 2784
Arachic Acid *see* 764
Arachidic Acid, 764
Arachidonic Acid, 765
Arachidonylethanolamide *see* 624
Arachis Oil *see* 7059
AraCTP *see* 2784
Aracytidine *see* 2784
Aracytine [Pfizer] *see* 2784
Aragonite *see* 1657
Aralast [Baxter] *see* 719
Aralen [Sanofi-Synthelabo] *see* 2163
Aralia, 766
Aramine [Merck & Co.] *see* 5932
Araminon [Banyu] *see* 5932
Aramo [BASF] *see* 9152
Arantoick [Ohta] *see* 9522
Aranesp [Amgen] *see* 2824
Aranidipine, 767
"Arariba" *see* 768
Araroba, 768
Arasan [DuPont] *see* 9371
Arasena-A [Mochida] *see* 9976
Arasine [Gensia] *see* 16
Arava [Sanofi-Aventis] *see* 5432
Arbaprostil, 769
Arbekacin, 770
Arbelic [Theravance] *see* 9116
Arborescin, 771
Arborine *see* 4502
Arbor Vitae *see* 9389
Arbotect [Syngenta] *see* 9289

Arbuse *see* 10040
Arbutamine, 772
Arbutin, 773
Arbutoside *see* 773
Arbuz *see* 7016
AR-C69931MX *see* 1746
AR-C69931XX *see* 1746
Arcalion [Servier] *see* 9297
Arcanum Duplicatum *see* 7674
Arcasin [Meda] *see* 7100
Archil *see* 6863
Archin *see* 3561
Arcilla *see* 782
Arcitumomab, 774
Arcomonol Tablets *see* 6231
Arcosolv DPM [Arco] *see* 3344
Arcoxia [Merck & Co.] *see* 3887
Arcton [ICI] *see* 2140
Arcton 11 [ICI] *see* 9640
Arcton 12 [ICI] *see* 3064
Arcton 114 [ICI] *see* 2605
Arctuvan [Klinge] *see* 9896
Ardeparin, 775
Ardeytropin [Ardeypharm] *see* 9797
AR-DF 26 *see* 4443
Ardine [Antibioticos] *see* 577
Arduan [Organon] *see* 7459
Areca, 776
Arecaidine, 777
Arecaine *see* 777
Arecaline *see* 778
Arechin [Polfa] *see* 2163
Arecholine *see* 778
Arecoline, 778
Arecoline-acetarsol *see* 778
Arecoline-acetarsone *see* 778
Arecoline p-Stibonobenzoic Acid *see* 778
Aredia [Novartis] *see* 7003
Arelix [HMR] *see* 7492
Arelon [Griffin] *see* 5218
Arena [Arvesta] *see* 2414
A-Rest [SePRO] *see* 631
Arestin [OroPharma] *see* 6202
Aretit [Hoechst] *see* 3287
Arfen [Lisapharma] *see* 4881
Arfonad [Roche] *see* 9707
Arformoterol *see* 4245
Arformoterol Tartrate *see* 4245
Arg *see* 780
Argatroban, 779
Argentic Fluoride *see* 8513
Argentic Oxide *see* 8522
Argentite *see* 8504, 8530
Argentoproteinum *see* 8527
Argentous Chlorate *see* 8508
Argentous Fluoride *see* 8514
Argentous Oxide *see* 8521
Argentous Sulfide *see* 8530
Argentum Vitellinum *see* 8527
Argil *see* 782
Argilla *see* 5282
Argilla Vini *see* 782
Arginine, 780
L-Arginine *see* 780
Arginine L-Aspartate *see* 840
Arginine Glutamate, 781
5-L-Arginine-27-glycine-33-L-isoleucine-
    34-L-serine-42-glycine-purothionin A I
    (Reduced) *see* 7944
[199-Arginine, 223-Histidine]prepro-α-
    glucosidase (Human) *see* 108
8-D-Arginine-1-(3-mercaptopropanoic
    Acid) Vasopressin *see* 2924
5-L-Arginine-6-L-threonine-18-L-serine-
    26-L-serine-27-L-threonine-42-

glycine-purothionin A I (Reduced) *see* 7944
Arginine Vasopressin *see* 9938
N-(*N*-(*N*²-L-Arginyl-L-lysyl)-L-α-aspartyl)-L-valyl)-L-tyrosine *see* 9403
Argipidine *see* 779
Argipressin *see* 9938
Argobyl [Specia] *see* 4106
Argol, 782
Argon, 783
Argun L [Merckle] *see* 5566
Argyrol [J & J] *see* 8527
Aria [FMC] *see* 4105
Arial [Dompé] *see* 8337
Aribine *see* 4615
Aricept [Eisai] *see* 3419
Aricine, 784
Ariclaim [Lilly] *see* 3465
Aricyl [Winthrop] *see* 810
Ariflo [GSK] *see* 2276
Arilin [Wolff] *see* 6157
Arimidex [AstraZeneca] *see* 625
Aripiprazole, 785
Aristamid [Nordmark] *see* 8951
Aristocort [Lederle] *see* 9595
Aristolochic Acid, 786
Aristolochic Acid-I *see* 786
Aristolochine *see* 786
Aristololactams *see* 786
Aristosol [Lederle] *see* 9596
Aristospan [Fujisawa] *see* 9598
Aritmina [Altana] *see* 194
Arixtra [GSK] *see* 4232
Arkin [Otsuka] *see* 9970
Arkitropin *see* 4730
ARL *see* 791
AR-L 115BS *see* 8985
ARL-16556 *see* 3363
Arlacel 20 [ICI] *see* 8724
Arlacel 60 [ICI] *see* 8724
Arlacel 80 [ICI] *see* 8724
Arlanto [Nichiiko] *see* 223
Arlef [Parke-Davis] *see* 4132
Arlidin [USV] *see* 6732
Arliflav *see* 1228
Arlitene [Viatris] *see* 6292
Armazal *see* 2680
Armepavine, 787
Armol *see* 6017
Armstrong's Acid, 788
Arnaudon's Green *see* 2227
Arnica, 789
Arnica Flowers *see* 789
Arnold's Base *see* 6176
Arnotta *see* 675
Arobon *see* 5554
Aroclor [Monsanto] *see* 7564
Aroclor 1242 *see* 7564
Aroclor 1254 *see* 7564
Aroclor 1260 *see* 7564
Arofuto [Tanabe] *see* 183
Arogenate *see* 790
Arogenic Acid, 790
Aromasin [Pharmacia & Upjohn] *see* 3913
Aropax [GSK] *see* 7043
Arotinolol, 791
Arovit [Roche] *see* 10013
Arpicolin [Rosemont] *see* 7763
Arpimycin [Rosemont] *see* 3681
Arquel [Parke-Davis] *see* 5779
Arranon [GSK] *see* 6442
Arret [Janssen] *see* 5571
Arrhenal [Cleary] *see* 5953
Arrivo [FMC] *see* 2767
Arrow Wood *see* 4263

Arsacol [Zambon] *see* 9889
Arsambide *see* 1786
Arsamin *see* 8578
Arsanilic Acid, 792
Arsanilic Acid Sodium Salt *see* 8578
Arsanyl [Taiyo] *see* 4378
Arsecodile *see* 8595
Arsenal [BASF] *see* 4905
Arsenamide, 793
Arsen (German) *see* 794
Arsenic, 794
Arsenic Acid, 795
Arsenic Acid Anhydride *see* 798
Arsenical Solution *see* 7608
Arsenic Chloride Solution *see* 807
Arsenic Pentafluoride, 796
Arsenic Pentasulfide, 797
Arsenic Pentoxide, 798
Arsenic Sesquioxide *see* 804
Arsenic Sulfide, 799
Arsenic Tribromide, 800
Arsenic Trichloride, 801
Arsenic Trifluoride, 802
Arsenic Trihydride *see* 809
Arsenic Triiodide, 803
Arsenic Trioxide, 804
Arsenic Triselenide, 805
Arsenic Trisulfide, 806
Arsenic Yellow *see* 806
Arsenik *see* 794
Arsenious Acid Copper(2+) Salt (1:1) *see* 2626
Arsenious Acid Solution, 807
Arsenious Selenide *see* 805
Arseno 39 *see* 6948
Arsenoacetic Acid, 808
Arsenodiacetic Acid *see* 808
Arsenolite *see* 804
Arsenosan *see* 6948
Arsenosobenzene *see* 6949
Arsenous Acid *see* 804
Arsenous Acid Anhydride *see* 804
Arsenous Oxide *see* 804
Arsenous Selenide *see* 805
Arsenoxide *see* 6948
Arsevan *see* 6447
Arsicodile *see* 8595
Arsine, 809
Arsinyl [Cleary] *see* 5953
Arsobal [Specia] *see* 5815
Arsonic Acid Copper(2+) Salt (1:1) *see* 2626
Arsonoacetic Acid, 810
p-Arsonophenylurea *see* 1786
Arsphenamine, 811
Arsphenamine Methylenesulfoxylic Acid Sodium Salt *see* 6447
Arsthinol, 812
Arsycodile *see* 8595
Artabotrine *see* 5162
Artam *see* 2288
Artane [Wyeth] *see* 9695
Artate [Nippon Chemiphar] *see* 2305
Arteannuin *see* 817
Arteether, 813
Arteflene, 814
Artegodan [Artesan] *see* 7019
Artelac [Mann] *see* 4842
Artemether, 815
Artemin *see* 4377
Artemisia Oil *see* 10052
Artemisin, 816
Artemisine *see* 817
Artemisinin, 817
Artemotil *see* 813

Arteoptic [Novartis] *see* 1866
Arterenol [HMR] *see* 6695
Arteriohom [Weisskopf] *see* 2378
Arteriovinca [Farma-Lepori] *see* 9983
Arterocoline *see* 87
Arterolo [Nuovo Cons.] *see* 2382
Artes [Sumitomo] *see* 5822
Artesunate, 818
Artesunic Acid *see* 818
Arteven [Boehringer, Ing. Italia] *see* 4653
Artevil *see* 2377
Artex [Servier] *see* 9173
Artexal [Servier] *see* 9173
Arthaxan [GSK] *see* 6343
Arthrocine [Merck & Co.] *see* 8982
Arthrodont [Veyron-Froment] *see* 3590
Arthropan [Purdue Frederick] *see* 2209
Arthrosetten [Hotz] *see* 2942
Arthrotabs [Duopharm] *see* 2942
Articaine *see* 1869
Artificial Cognac Essence *see* 3835
Artificial Essential Oil of Almond *see* 1058
Artificial Ethyl Oenanthate *see* 3835
Artificial Lanthanite *see* 5363
Artificial Oil of Ants *see* 4304
Artil [Hoechst] *see* 5237
Artisone Acetate [Wyeth] *see* 77
Artolon [Roter] *see* 5862
Artosin [Roche] *see* 9507
Artribid [Merck & Co.] *see* 8982
Artrizin [Leo Pharm] *see* 7277
Artrobione *see* 2209
Artrodar [Proter] *see* 2960
Artrolasi [Lenza] *see* 9002
Artromialgina *see* 3349
Artrosilene [Dompé] *see* 5305
Artroxicam [Coli] *see* 7506
Artume *see* 1705
ARTZ [Seikagaku] *see* 4757
Arumel [SS Pharm.] *see* 4181
Arusa *see* 159
Arvigol [Zyma] *see* 2361
Arvin [Knoll] *see* 630
Arvynol [Pfizer] *see* 3729
Arwin [Knoll] *see* 630
Arxxant [Lilly] *see* 8290
Arylsulfatase B, 819
Aryplase *see* 819
Arythmol [Abbott] *see* 7794
Arzene *see* 6949
Arzoxifene, 820
AS-101 *see* 792
AS-4370 *see* 6279
5-ASA *see* 5904
Asabaine *see* 5958
Asacol [Tillotts] *see* 5904
Asacolitin [Tillotts] *see* 5904
Asafetida, 821
Asafoetida *see* 821
Asamedol [Maruko] *see* 3710
Asant *see* 821
Asaprol, 822
Asarabacca Camphor *see* 824
Asarin *see* 824
Asarinin, 823
l-Asarinin *see* 823
α-Asarone *see* 824
β-Asarone *see* 824
Asarones, 824
Asarum, 825
Asarum Camphor *see* 824
Asatard [Boehringer, Ing.] *see* 851
Asbestos, 826
ASC *see* 103

ASC-66824 *see* 4260
Ascabiol [RPR] *see* 1127
Ascal [Viatris] *see* 1647
Ascaridil [Cilag] *see* 5459
Ascaridole, 827
Ascarite [Baker] *see* 826
Ascaryl [Wander] *see* 4712
Asceptichrome *see* 5867
Ascharite *see* 5658
Asclepias, 828
Asclepias Syriaca, 829
Ascomp [Nippon Chemiphar] *see* 223
Ascorbic Acid, 830
L-Ascorbic Acid *see* 830
L-*xylo*-Ascorbic Acid *see* 830
Ascorbicap [Valeant] *see* 830
Ascorbigen, 831
Ascorbigen A *see* 831
Ascorbigen B *see* 831
Ascorbin [Montavit] *see* 830
Ascorvit [Jenapharm] *see* 830
Ascotoxin *see* 1369
AS-E 136 *see* 3354
Asebotoxin *see* 4543
Asenapine, 832
Asendin [Lederle] *see* 576
Asendis [Wyeth] *see* 576
Asepsin *see* 1399
ASH *see* 173
Asiatic Acid *see* 833
Asiaticoside, 833
Asil *see* 4885
Asiprenol *see* 5217
Aska-Rid *see* 1623
Askensil [Atmos] *see* 466
ASL-279 *see* 3421
ASL-601 *see* 20
ASL-8052 *see* 3700
Asmalar *see* 5217
Asmanex [Schering-Plough] *see* 6241
Asmaten [3M Pharma] *see* 8227
Asmaterolo [Lusofarmaco] *see* 8139
Asmaven [APS] *see* 216
Asn *see* 837
L-Asnase *see* 836
Asoprisnil, 834
Asoxime Chloride, 835
Asp *see* 840
D-Asp *see* 840
ASP-47 *see* 8966
Asparagic Acid *see* 840
L-Asparaginase, 836
Asparagine, 837
L-Asparagine *see* 837
L-*β*-Asparagine *see* 837
L-Asparagine Amidohydrolase *see* 836
103-L-Asparagine-117-L-glutamine-296-
    L-alanine-297-L-alanine-298-L-ala-
    nine-299-L-alanineplasminogen Acti-
    vator (Human Tissue-type) *see* 9143
27-L-Asparagine-nisin *see* 6564
[30-Asparagine,32-threonine,87-val-
    ine,88-asparagine,90-threonine]-
    erythropoietin (Human) *see* 2824
1-Asparagine-5-valine-angiotensin II *see*
    651
Asparaginic Acid *see* 840
Asparaginsäure (German) *see* 840
Asparagus, 838
Asparamide *see* 837
Aspartame, 839
Aspartic Acid, 840
L-Aspartic Acid *see* 840
Aspartic Acid *β*-Amide *see* 837
28[B]-L-Aspartic Acid-insulin (Human) *see*
    4982

3-(L-Aspartyl-D-alaninamido)-2,2,4,4-
    tetramethylthietane *see* 248
L-Aspartyl-D-alanine-*N*-(2,2,4,4-tetra-
    methylthietan-3-yl)amide *see* 248
N-L-*α*-Aspartyl-L-phenylalanine 1-
    Methyl Ester *see* 839
N^2-[1-[*N*-(*N*-L-*α*-Aspartyl-L-seryl)-L-*α*-
    aspartyl]-L-prolyl]-L-arginine *see*
    7128
L-*α*-Aspartyl-*N*-(2,2,4,4-tetramethyl-3-
    thietanyl)-D-alaninamide *see* 248
AspB28-insulin (Human) *see* 4982
ASPC *see* 852
Aspenon [Mitsui] *see* 754
Aspergillic Acid, 841
Aspergillin, 842
Aspergillus Diastase *see* 9031
Asperlicin, 843
Asperlicin B *see* 843
Asperlicin C *see* 843
Asperlicin D *see* 843
Asperlicin E *see* 843
Asperule Absolute *see* 10049
Asperuloside, 844
Asphalt, 845
Asphaltum *see* 845
Asphocalcium *see* 830
Aspiculamycin *see* 4529
Aspidin, 846
Aspidinol, 847
Aspidium, 848
Aspidol [Piam] *see* 5637
Aspidosperma, 849
Aspidospermine, 850
Aspirin, 851
Aspirin Lysine Salt *see* 5637
Aspisol [Bayer] *see* 5637
Aspogen [Eaton] *see* 3183
Aspoxicillin, 852
Aspro [Roche] *see* 851
Assail [Bayer] *see* 49
Assert [BASF] *see* 4903
Assiprenol *see* 5217
Assoral [Glaxo] *see* 8276
Assugrin *see* 2703
Assure [DuPont] *see* 8086
Asta C 4898 *see* 3200
Asta Z-4942 *see* 4896
Astacene *see* 853
Astacin, 853
Astaril *see* 3852
Astat [Nihon Nohyaku] *see* 5357
Astatine, 854
Astaxanthin, 855
Astelin [Wallace] *see* 906
Astemisan [Zdravlje] *see* 856
Astemizole, 856
Astenile [Recordati] *see* 2871
Asterin *see* 2687
Asteromycin *see* 4529
Asthmahaler [Menley & James] *see* 3619
Asthma Weed *see* 5550
Asthmolysin [Kade] *see* 3479
Astiban [Roche] *see* 8812
Astix CMPP [Agrotec] *see* 5784
Astmamasit [Showa Yakuhin] *see* 3479
Astomin [Yamanouchi] *see* 3206
Astonin H [Merck KGaA] *see* 4130
Astragalin *see* 5274
Astrocar *see* 6543
Astroderm [Medix] *see* 3048
Astrolin *see* 716
Astromicin *see* 4249
Astrophyllin *see* 3479
Asturidon [Cilag] *see* 1506

Asuccin *see* 8869
Asucrol *see* 2186
[ASU[1,7]]-ECT *see* 3537
Asulam, 857
Asulox [RP Agr.] *see* 857
Asuntol [Bayer] *see* 2558
Asuro [Nippon Kayaku] *see* 2951
Asverin [Tanabe Seiyaku] *see* 9457
Asymmetrical Trimethylbenzene *see*
    7915
AT-7 *see* 4680
AT 10 *see* 3180
AT-17 *see* 3206
AT-101 *see* 5224
AT-327 *see* 9457
AT-877 *see* 3942
AT-2266 *see* 3587
AT-4140 *see* 8735
ATA *see* 489
Atabrine Hydrochloride [Sanofi Win-
    throp] *see* 8044
Atacand [AstraZeneca] *see* 1739
Atapren [Sumitomo] *see* 9502
Atarax [Pfizer] *see* 4849
Atazanavir, 858
ATC *see* 9445
Ateben [Chem-Sintyal] *see* 6715
Ateculon [Nippon Chemiphar] *see* 2377
Atehexal [Hexal] *see* 859
Atelec [Morishita] *see* 2275
Atem [Chiesi] *see* 5073
Atemi [Syngenta] *see* 2771
Atemorin *see* 5846
Atempol [Norgine] *see* 5846
Atenen [Tsuruhara] *see* 155
Atenezol [Tsuruhara] *see* 53
Ateno Basan [Schoenenberger] *see* 859
Atenol [AstraZeneca] *see* 859
Atenolol, 859
Atenos [UCB] *see* 9811
Atensil *see* 7423
Atensin *see* 5850
Aterax *see* 4849
Ateriosan *see* 2377
Ateromixol [Dalmer] *see* 7555
Aterosan [Aanderson] *see* 7975
Atgard [Boehringer, Ing.] *see* 3079
Athamantin, 860
Atheran *see* 2382
Atheroitin *see* 2214
Atherolip *see* 2378
Atherolipin [Schwarz] *see* 2378
Atheropront [Mack, Illert.] *see* 2377
Athymil [Organon] *see* 6172
Athyromazole *see* 1798
Atipamezole, 861
Atirin [Intersint] *see* 1917
Atisine, 862
Ativan [Wyeth] *see* 5579
ATL-1251 *see* 8135
Atlacide [Chipman] *see* 8598
Atlas G-4829 [ICI] *see* 7558
Atlizumab *see* 9493
Atmosgen [Maruko] *see* 9522
Atocin *see* 2288
Atock [Yamanouchi] *see* 4245
Atolant [Takeda] *see* 6478
Atomoxetine, 863
Atophan [Warner-Chilcott] *see* 2288
Atopica [Novartis] *see* 2752
Atoquinol *see* 2288
Atorvastatin, 864
Atosiban, 865
Atosil [Bayer] *see* 7786
Atovaquone, 866

Atover [Recordati] *see* 7975
Atoxyl *see* 8578
Atoxylic Acid *see* 792
ATP *see* 155
ATP-dependent Proteolytic Factor *see* 9844
Atractyl *see* 5718
Atractylin (C$_{30}$ Glucoside) *see* 867
Atractyloside, 867
Atracurium Besylate, 868
Atral *see* 3353
Atranex [Makhteshim-Agan] *see* 871
Atranoric Acid *see* 869
Atranorin, 869
Atrasentan, 870
Atravet [Wyeth-Ayerst] *see* 32
Atraxin [Daiichi] *see* 5862
Atrazine, 871
Atrial Natriuretic Factor *see* 872
Atrial Natriuretic Peptide, 872
Atrican [Innotech] *see* 9147
Atridox [Atrix] *see* 3440
Atrilon 5 [Winthrop] *see* 7811
Atrimycon [Bioindustria] *see* 7890
Atrinal [Roche] *see* 3199
Atriopeptidase *see* 872
Atriopeptin *see* 872
Atriphos [Biochimica] *see* 155
Atrolactic Acid, 873
Atromid [Ayerst] *see* 2377
Atromidin *see* 2377
Atromid-S [Ayerst] *see* 2377
Atropamine *see* 739
Atropic Acid, 874
Atropine, 875
Atropine Aminoxide *see* 875
Atropisol [Novartis] *see* 875
Atropt [Sigma] *see* 875
Atropyltropeine *see* 739
Atroscine *see* 8406
Atrovent [Boehringer, Ing.] *see* 5073
Attacins, 876
Attar of Rose *see* 6811
Attenace [Cephalon] *see* 6228
Attentil [Ravizza] *see* 4084
Attribut [Bayer CropSci.] *see* 7838
Aturgyl [Dausse] *see* 3985
Atysmal [Schaefer] *see* 3748
Aubépine *see* 2567
Aucubin, 877
Aucuboside *see* 877
Audax [Napp] *see* 2209
Augmentin [SKB] *see* 2341
Augmerosen *see* 6739
Auligen *see* 3384
Aulin [Boehringer, Mann.] *see* 6548
Aulinogen [Boehringer, Ing.] *see* 3384
Auranofin, 878
Aurantiin *see* 6425
Aurantin [Pfizer] *see* 7322
Aurcoloid-198 [Abbott] *see* 4517
Aurcoscan-198 [Abbott] *see* 4517
Aureine *see* 8451
Aurelic Acid *see* 7536
Aureociclina *see* 2192
Aureocina *see* 2192
Aureolic Acid *see* 7536
Aureomycin [Lederle] *see* 2192
Aureotan [Byk Gulden] *see* 883
Aureothin, 879
Aureothricin, 880
Aureotope [BMS] *see* 4517
Auric Chloride *see* 4521
Auric Hydroxide *see* 4523
Auric Oxide *see* 4524

Auric Sulfide *see* 4525
Auriculin [Scios] *see* 872
Aurin, 881
Aurinol *see* 4367
Auripigment *see* 806
Aurochlorohydric Acid *see* 4522
Aurocidin *see* 4519
Aurodox, 882
Aurolin [UCB] *see* 4519
Aurora [FMC] *see* 1837
Aurorix [Roche] *see* 6226
Aurothioglucose, 883
Aurous Chloride *see* 4515
Aurous Cyanide *see* 4516
Aurous Stannate *see* 4520
Aurum Paradoxum *see* 9121
Ausocef [Ausonia] *see* 7513
Australian Fever Bark *see* 3366
Austrawolf [Commonwealth] *see* 8120
Austrian Cinnabar *see* 5406
Auteral [Boehringer, Mann.] *see* 7418
Authority [FMC] *see* 8947
Autoprothrombin II *see* 3922
Autoprothrombin II-A *see* 7884
Autoworm [Schering-Plough] *see* 6935
Autumn Crocus *see* 2472
Auxisone [Boehringer, Ing.] *see* 2943
Auxit [BMS] *see* 1391
Auxura [Merz] *see* 5829
AV-290 *see* 889
Ava-ava *see* 5286
Avadex *see* 2970
Avadex BW [Monsanto] *see* 9594
Avagal *see* 5958
Avage [Allergan] *see* 9081
Avalox [Bayer] *see* 6291
Avan [Takeda] *see* 4888
Avandia [GSK] *see* 8265
Avans-330 *see* 4512
Avantrin [Inverni] *see* 9574
Avantyl *see* 6715
Avapro [Sanofi-Synthelabo] *see* 5083
Avasimibe, 884
Avastin [Genentech] *see* 1191
Avatec [Roche] *see* 5373
Avazyme *see* 2260
Avelox [Bayer] *see* 6291
Avenein *see* 4464
Avenge [BASF] *see* 3138
Avenin *see* 1883
Aventox [Dow AgroSci.] *see* 9664
Aventyl [Lilly] *see* 6715
Avermectin A$_{1a/b}$ *see* 885
Avermectin A$_{2a/b}$ *see* 885
Avermectin B$_1$ *see* 2
Avermectin B$_{1a/b}$ *see* 2
Avermectin B$_{2a/b}$ *see* 885
Avermectins, 885
Averon-1 [Alfar] *see* 1982
Aviax [Pfizer] *see* 8443
Avibon [Aventis] *see* 10013
Avicel [Syngenta] *see* 2
Avid [Syngenta] *see* 2
Avidin, 886
Avigilen [Riemser] *see* 7487
Avil *see* 7235
Avilamycin, 887
Avilamycin A *see* 887
Avilamycin C *see* 887
Avinar [Armour Pharm.] *see* 9872
Avinza [Ligand] *see* 6276
Aviochina [Agrimont-Vetem] *see* 8939
Aviral [Medici Domus] *see* 4976
Avirase [Lampugnani] *see* 146
Avisco Rayon [FMC] *see* 8122

Avishot [Kanebo] *see* 6356
Avita [Bertek] *see* 8165
Avitol [Lannacher] *see* 10013
Avlocardyl [AstraZeneca] *see* 7840
Avloclor [AstraZeneca] *see* 2163
Avlosulfon [Wyeth-Ayerst] *see* 2822
AVM *see* 885
Avobenzone, 888
Avodart [GSK] *see* 3471
Avogadrite *see* 7686
Avolin *see* 3255
Avolve [GSK] *see* 3471
Avomine [Sanofi-Aventis] *see* 7786
Avonex [Biogen] *see* 4991
Avoparcin, 889
Avornin *see* 4264
Avosyl *see* 5850
Avotan [Roche] *see* 889
Avoxyl *see* 5850
AVS *see* 6493
AW-14'2333 *see* 7179
AW-105-843 *see* 6355
Axeen [Hommel] *see* 7904
Axepim [BMS] *see* 1922
Axer Alfa [Alfa] *see* 6417
Axerophthal *see* 8164
Axerophthol *see* 10013
Axert [Pharmacia & Upjohn] *see* 304
Axid [Lilly] *see* 6660
Axil [Boehringer, Mann.] *see* 7419
Axiomin [Promeco] *see* 3885
Axiquel [McNeil] *see* 9912
Axiten *see* 5773
Axonyl [Pfizer] *see* 7487
Axoren [Glaxo Wellcome] *see* 1504
Axsain [Bioglan] *see* 1768
Axungia Porci *see* 5371
Axuris [Fournier] *see* 4395
AXV-034343 *see* 2342
AY-4166 *see* 6428
AY-5406-1 *see* 1029
AY-5710 *see* 5651
AY-6108 *see* 586
AY-6608 *see* 7113
AY-8682 *see* 2759
AY-21011 *see* 7700
AY-22989 *see* 8114
AY-24031 *see* 5474
AY-24236 *see* 3874
AY-25650 *see* 9748
AY-25712 *see* 110
AY-27773 *see* 9524
AY-62014 *see* 1533
AY-62021 *see* 2394
AY-62022 *see* 5791
AY-64043 *see* 7840
Ayermicina [Ayerst] *see* 5453
Ayfactin *see* 7049
Aygestin [Barr] *see* 6697
AZ 8 [Millet Roux] *see* 4554
AZ 8 Beris [Weimer] *see* 4554
AZ-242 *see* 9177
10-Azaanthracene *see* 122
5-Aza-10-arsenaanthracene Chloride *see* 7215
1-(1*R*,6*R*)-9-Azabicyclo[4.2.1]non-2-en-2-ylethanone *see* 627
1-Azabicyclo[2.2.2]octane *see* 8081
1-Azabicyclo[2.2.2]octan-3-ol *see* 8082
N-1-Azabicyclo[2.2.2]oct-3-yl-6-chloro-3,4-dihydro-4-methyl-3-oxo-2*H*-1,4-benzoxazine-8-carboxamide *see* 900
5-(1-Azabicyclo[2.2.2]oct-3-yl)-10,11-di-hydro-5*H*-dibenz[*b*,*f*]azepine *see* 8083

(3a*S*)-2-(3*S*)-1-Azabicyclo[2.2.2]oct-3-yl-2,3,3a,4,5,6-hexahydro-1*H*-benz[*de*]-isoquinolin-1-one *see* 6997
10-(1-Azabicyclo[2.2.2]oct-3-ylmethyl)-10*H*-phenothiazine *see* 5864
1-(3-Azabicyclo[3.3.0]oct-3-yl)-3-(*p*-tolyl-sulfonyl)urea *see* 4439
5-AzaC *see* 890
Azacitidine, 890
Azacort *see* 2862
Azacortid [Lepetit] *see* 4115
Azacosterol, 892
Azactam [BMS] *see* 925
2-(1′-Azacyclooctyl)ethylguanidine *see* 4560
Azacyclopropane *see* 3804
5-Azacytidine *see* 890
5-Aza-2′-deoxycytidine *see* 2853
Azadirachtin, 893
Azaepothilone B *see* 5249
Azafenidin, 894
9-Azafluorene *see* 1790
Azafrin, 895
8-Azaguanine, 896
Azalomycin M *see* 6541
Azameno [Wyeth] *see* 6846
4-Aza-5-(*N*-methyl-4-piperidinylidene)-10,11-dihydro-5*H*-dibenzo[*a,d*]cyclo-heptene *see* 901
6-Azamianserin *see* 6208
Azamin 4B *see* 1101
Azanidazole, 897
Azanin [Tanabe] *see* 902
Azantac [GSK] *see* 8110
5-Azaorotic Acid *see* 6947
Azapen [Pfizer] *see* 5969
Azaperone, 898
1-Azaphenothiazine-10-carboxylic Acid 2-(2-Piperidinoethoxy)ethyl Ester *see* 7456
Azapropazone *see* 726
Azaribine *see* 904
Azaron [Chefaro] *see* 9738
Azaserine, 899
Azasetron, 900
5α,20β_F,22α_F,25β_F,27-Azaspirostan-3β-ol *see* 9544
Δ⁵-20β_F,22α_F,25α_F,27-Azaspirosten-3β-ol *see* 8709
Azatadine, 901
Azathioprine, 902
6-Azathymine, 903
6-Azauracil Riboside *see* 904
6-Azauridine, 904
Azelaic Acid, 905
Azelastine, 906
Azelex [Allergan] *see* 905
Azelnidipine, 907
Azene [Endo] *see* 2403
1-[4-(2-Azepan-1-ylethoxy)benzyl]-2-(4-hydroxyphenyl)-3-methyl-1*H*-indol-5-ol *see* 1013
Azeptin [Eisai] *see* 906
2-Azetidinecarboxylic Acid, 908
5-[(2*R*)-2-Azetidinylmethoxy]-2-chloro-pyridine *see* 9090
Azidamfenicol, 909
D-(−)-*threo*-2-Azidoacetamido-1-*p*-nitrophenyl-1,3-propanediol *see* 909
Azidoamphenicol *see* 909
α-Azidobenzylpenicillin *see* 910
Azidocillin, 910
3′-Azido-3′-deoxythymidine *see* 10123
2-Azido-*N*-[2-hydroxy-1-(hydroxymeth-yl)-2-(4-nitrophenyl)ethyl]acetamide *see* 909

6-[D-α-Azidophenylacetamido]penicil-lanic Acid *see* 910
(2*S*,5*R*,6*R*)-6-[[(2*R*)-Azidophenylacetyl]-amino]-3,3-dimethyl-7-oxo-4-thia-1-azabicyclo[3.2.0]heptane-2-carbox-ylic Acid *see* 910
Azidothymidine *see* 10123
Azilect [Teva] *see* 8116
Azimethylene *see* 3001
Azimidobenzene *see* 1108
Azimilide, 911
Azimsulfuron, 912
Azindole *see* 1081
Azinepurine *see* 7931
Azinomycin B *see* 1877
Azinphos-ethyl *see* 913
Azinphos-methyl, 913
Azintamide, 914
Aziridine *see* 3804
Aziridinylbenzoquinone *see* 2996
1-Aziridinylphosphonitrile Trimer *see* 728
Azithromycin, 915
Azitrocin *see* 915
Azlin [Bayer] *see* 916
Azlocillin, 916
Azmacort [Aventis] *see* 9596
Azoangin [Ursapharm] *see* 2257
p-Azoaniline *see* 2977
Azobenzene, 917
Azobenzide *see* 917
Azobenzol *see* 917
4,4′-Azobisbenzenamine *see* 2977
1,1′-Azobiscarbamide *see* 919
Azobiscarbonamide *see* 919
Azobiscarboxamide *see* 919
α,α′-Azobis[chloroformamidine] *see* 2120
1,1′-Azobisformamide *see* 919
3,3′-Azobis(6-hydroxybenzoic Acid) *see* 6841
2,2′-Azobisisobutyronitrile, 918
1,1′-Azobis[3-methyl-2-phenylimidazo-[1,2-*a*]pyridinium] Dibromide *see* 3943
2,2′-Azobis[2-methylpropanenitrile] *see* 918
5,5′-Azobis(salicylic Acid) *see* 6841
Azochloramide *see* 2120
Azo Compd No. 4 *see* 8901
4,4′-Azodianiline *see* 2977
Azodicarbonamide, 919
Azodicarboxamide *see* 919
α,α′-Azodiisobutyronitrile *see* 918
Azodisal *see* 6841
Azodisal Sodium *see* 6841
Azohel [Ursapharm] *see* 2257
Azol *see* 462
Azole *see* 8014
Azolid [USV] *see* 7277
Azolitmin, 920
Azolmen [Menarini] *see* 1213
Azomycin, 921
Azone [Nelson] *see* 5385
Azoniaspiro(3α-benziloyloxynortropane-8,1′-pyrrolidine) Chloride *see* 9786
Azoniaspiro(3α-diphenylglycoloyloxy-nortropan-8,1′-pyrrolidine) Chloride *see* 9786
Azophenylene *see* 7217
Azopt [Alcon] *see* 1376
Azosemide, 922
Azothioprine *see* 902
Azotic Acid *see* 6577
Azovan Blue *see* 3905
Azoxodone *see* 7079

Azoxybenzene, 923
Azoxybenzide *see* 923
Azoxystrobin, 924
AZQ *see* 2996
AZT *see* 10123
Aztec [BASF] *see* 9601
Azthreonam *see* 925
Aztreonam, 925
Azubromaron [Azupharma] *see* 1065
Azudimidine [Pharmacia] *see* 8321
Azudoxat [Azupharma] *see* 3440
Azuglucon [Azupharma] *see* 4478
Azulene, 926
Azulfidine [Pfizer] *see* 8942
Azulon [Rorer] *see* 4554
Azunol [Nippon Shinyaku] *see* 926
Azupentat [Azupharma] *see* 7136
AzUR *see* 904
Azure I *see* 6058
Azure II *see* 6058
Azure II Eosin *see* 6058
Azure A, 927
Azure B, 928
Azure Blue II *see* 6058
Azure C, 929
Azurene [Cilag-Chemie] *see* 1442
Azurite *see* 2631
Azusalen [Ohta] *see* 926
Azusaleon [Towa Yakuhin] *see* 3618
Azutranquil [Azupharma] *see* 6926
B-9 *see* 2810
B72.3 *see* 8385
B72.3-Glycyl-tyrosyl-*N*-ε-diethylenetri-aminepentaacetic Acid-In-111 *see* 8385
B-360 *see* 7044
B-436 *see* 7737
B-518 *see* 2747
B-577 *see* 3875
B-663 *see* 2373
B-995 *see* 2810
B-1287 *see* 3671
B-1500 *see* 5803
B-1776 *see* 9617
B2036-PEG *see* 7069
B-2310 *see* 6273
B-2311 *see* 6273
B-11420 *see* 5063
B-15000 *see* 5057
B-16880 *see* 5054
B-19036/7 *see* 4322
B-66256 *see* 9865
B-68138 *see* 3957
BA *see* 1332
Ba-168 *see* 5558
Ba-253 *see* 6943
Ba-253-BR-L *see* 6943
Ba-598Br *see* 4216
Ba-679 *see* 9454
Ba-679 BR *see* 9454
Ba-2758 *see* 2904
Ba-5473 *see* 6975
Ba-7205 *see* 2362
BA-7602-06 *see* 9044
Ba-10370 *see* 8900
Ba-21401 *see* 9608
Ba-29038 *see* 1324
Ba-29837 *see* 2860
Ba-30803 *see* 1087
Ba-32644 *see* 6563
Ba-34276 *see* 5748
Ba-34647 *see* 937
Ba-39089 *see* 6952
Ba-180265 *see* 212
Babbitt Metal, 930
Babesan *see* 3353

Babidium *see* 4731
Baburan *see* 3353
Bacacil [Rottapharm] *see* 931
Bacampicillin, 931
Bacampicine [Pharmacia & Upjohn] *see* 931
Bacancosin *see* 943
Bacarate [Tutag] *see* 7220
Baccara [Aventis] *see* 4205
Baccidal [Kyorin] *see* 6700
Bacfeed [Fujisawa] *see* 1202
Bachelor's Buttons *see* 6730
Baciferm [Roche] *see* 936
Bacifurane [Meram] *see* 6535
Baciim [Pharma-Tek] *see* 934
Bacillin *see* 933
Bacillus Calmette-Guérin *see* 1015
Bacillus Thermoproteolyticus Neutral Proteinase *see* 9286
Bacillus Thuringiensis, 932
Bacilysin, 933
Bacimex [Alter] *see* 8992
Bacitracin, 934
Bacitracin A *see* 934
Bacitracin Methylenebis[2-hydroxy-benzoate] (Salt) *see* 935
Bacitracin Methylenedisalicylate, 935
Bacitracin Methylenedisalicylic Acid *see* 935
Bacitracin Zinc, 936
Baclofen, 937
Baclon [Leiras] *see* 937
Bacterial Vitamin H[1] *see* 423
Bactericidal Permeability-Increasing Protein, 938
1-193-Bactericidal/permeability-increasing Protein [132-Alanine] (Human Reduced) *see* 938
Bacterio-opsin *see* 939
Bacteriopsins *see* 6856
Bacteriorhodopsin, 939
Bacticlens [Smith & Nephew] *see* 2091
Bactidan *see* 3587
Bactocill [SKB] *see* 6904
Bactoderm [Pfizer] *see* 6302
Bactofen [HMR] *see* 1111
Bactol *see* 5031
Bactox [Innotech] *see* 577
Bactramin [Roche] *see* 8918
Bactramyl [Carrion] *see* 7505
Bactrim [Roche] *see* 8918
Bactroban [GSK] *see* 6302
Baddeleyite *see* 10180
BADGE *see* 1297
Badil [Bayer] *see* 4395
Badional *see* 8944
Badische Acid, 940
BAF *see* 4993
Bagasse, 941
Bahama White Wood *see* 1743
Baicalein, 942
BAJ2740 *see* 8757
Bajaten [Merck KGaA] *see* 4935
Bakankoside *see* 943
Bakankosin, 943
Bakash *see* 159
Baking Soda *see* 8583
Baktar [Shionogi] *see* 8918
Baktonium [Bode] *see* 1059
BAL *see* 3209
BAL-5788 *see* 1952
BAL-9141 *see* 1952
Balan [Dow AgroSci.] *see* 1040
Balance [Yamanouchi] *see* 2084
Balance [Bayer CropSci.] *see* 5236

Balanophorin *see* 618
Balarsen *see* 812
Balfin [Dow AgroSci.] *see* 1040
"Balm of Gilead" *see* 946
Balm of Gilead *see* 948
Balmox [GSK] *see* 6343
Balofloxacin, 944
Baloxin [Chugai] *see* 944
Balsalazide, 945
Balsam Canada, 946
Balsam Capivi *see* 2516
Balsam Copaiba *see* 2516
Balsam Gurjun, 947
Balsam Mecca, 948
Balsam of Fir *see* 946
Balsam of Gilead *see* 948
Balsam Peru, 949
Balsam Tolu, 950
Balsam Traumatic, 951
Balsam Tree *see* 5755
Balsán-Katél *see* 948
Baltic Amber *see* 380
Bambec [AstraZeneca] *see* 953
Bambermycins, 952
Bamboo Curare *see* 2671
Bambuterol, 953
Bamethan, 954
Bamifylline, 955
Bamiphylline *see* 955
Bamipine, 956
Banabins *see* 7518
Banabin-Sintyal *see* 2106
Banamine [Schering-Plough] *see* 4147
Banana Oil *see* 5111
Banewort *see* 1025
Banflex [Forest] *see* 6879
Banicol *see* 2017
Banisterine *see* 4616
Banistyl [M & B] *see* 4231
Ban-kakari *see* 7547
Banminth [Pfizer] *see* 7955
Bannal *see* 8403
Banner [Syngenta] *see* 7818
Banocide [Wellcome] *see* 3116
Banol [Bayer CropSci.] *see* 7798
Bantenol [Janssen] *see* 5768
Bantex *see* 5868
Banthine Bromide [Searle] *see* 5958
Banthionine [Banyu] *see* 5975
Bantu *see* 722
Banvel [BASF] *see* 3040
BAPTA, 957
Baptigenin, 958
Baptisia, 959
Baptitoxine *see* 2789
BAQD-10 *see* 2913
Baraclude [BMS] *see* 3595
Barakshin *see* 4885
Baratol [Wyeth] *see* 4969
Barazan [Merck & Co.] *see* 6700
Barbaloin *see* 307
Barbamil *see* 570
Barbasco, 960
Barberry Bark, 961
Barbexaclone *see* 7860
Barbiphenyl [Lääkefarmos] *see* 7238
Barbipil [Conal] *see* 7238
Barbital, 962
Barbital Sodium *see* 962
Barbitone *see* 962
Barbitone Sodium *see* 962
Barbituric Acid, 963
Barbonin [Knoll] *see* 3728
Barbosec [Rowell] *see* 8420
Barbourin *see* 3641

Bardac 2250/2280 [Lonza] *see* 3099
Bardana *see* 5368
Bareon [Hokuriku] *see* 5562
Barite *see* 994
Baritop [Sakai] *see* 994
Barium, 964
Barium Acetate, 965
Barium Benzenesulfonate, 966
Barium Benzoate *see* 1091
Barium Bromate, 967
Barium Bromide, 968
Barium Carbonate, 969
Barium Chlorate, 970
Barium Chloride, 971
Barium Chromate(VI), 972
Barium Citrate *see* 2326
Barium Cyanide, 973
Barium Cyanoplatinate(II) *see* 991
Barium Dihydroxide *see* 977
Barium Dioxide *see* 989
Barium Diuranate *see* 1001
Barium Ethyl Sulfate *see* 3853
Barium Fluoride, 974
Barium Fluosilicate *see* 976
Barium Formate, 975
Barium Hexafluorosilicate, 976
Barium Hydroxide, 977
Barium Hypophosphite, 978
Barium Hyposulfite *see* 999
Barium Iodate, 979
Barium Iodide, 980
Barium Lactate *see* 5336
Barium Manganate(VI), 981
Barium Manganate(VII) *see* 988
Barium Mercuric Iodide, 982
Barium Metatitanate *see* 1000
Barium Methyl Sulfate *see* 6122
Barium Monoxide *see* 986
Barium Nitrate, 983
Barium Nitrite, 984
Barium Oleate *see* 6828
Barium Oxalate, 985
Barium Oxide, 986
Barium Perchlorate, 987
Barium Permanganate, 988
Barium Peroxide, 989
Barium *p*-Phenolsulfonate *see* 7246
Barium Phosphate, Dibasic, 990
Barium Platinocyanide *see* 991
Barium Platinous Cyanide, 991
Barium Propionate *see* 7825
Barium Protoxide *see* 986
Barium Rhodanide *see* 998
Barium Selenide, 992
Barium Silicide, 993
Barium Silicofluoride *see* 976
Barium Sulfate, 994
Barium Sulfide, 995
Barium Sulfide, Black, 996
Barium Sulfite, 997
Barium Sulfocyanate *see* 998
Barium Sulfocyanide *see* 998
Barium Superoxide *see* 989
Barium Taurocholate *see* 9075
Barium Tetracyanoplatinate(II) *see* 991
Barium Tetraiodomercurate(II) *see* 982
Barium Thiocyanate, 998
Barium Thiosulfate, 999
Barium Titanate(IV), 1000
Barium Titanium Oxide (BaTiO$_3$) *see* 1000
Barium Uranate(VI) *see* 1001
Barium Uranium Oxide, 1001
Barizin [Lek] *see* 6495
Barluenga's Reagent *see* 1302

Barnetil [Delagrange] *see* 8994
Barnidipine, 1002
Barnotil [Vita] *see* 8994
Baron *see* 2802
Baroque [Yashima] *see* 3890
Baros [Horii] *see* 3215
Baros Camphor *see* 1338
Barosma Camphor *see* 3298
Barosmin *see* 3297
Barosperse [Mallinckrodt] *see* 994
Barquinol *see* 5031
Barricade [BASF] *see* 2767
Barricade [Syngenta] *see* 7766
Barthrin, 1003
Baryta Yellow *see* 972
Barytes *see* 994
BAS-083 *see* 5857
BAS-238F *see* 3407
BAS-352F *see* 9984
BAS-392H *see* 4120
BAS-480-F *see* 3629
BAS-490 F *see* 5324
BAS-490-02F *see* 5324
BAS-500F *see* 7953
BAS-510F *see* 1352
BAS-518 *see* 8066
BAS-518H *see* 8066
BAS-615H *see* 2293
BAS-620H *see* 9152
BAS-656H *see* 3214
BAS-662 *see* 3145
BAS-3460 *see* 1791
BAS-9052 *see* 8473
BAS-42100F *see* 3993
BAS-67054 *see* 1791
BAS-85559X *see* 5857
Basagran [BASF] *see* 1053
Basalin [BASF] *see* 4120
Basaljel [Wyeth] *see* 1004
Basanite [BASF] *see* 3287
Basathrin [BASF] *see* 2767
Basecil *see* 6128
Basedol *see* 479
Basen [Takeda] *see* 10029
Basergin *see* 3655
Basethyrin *see* 6128
Basfapon *see* 2802
Basforin [BASF] *see* 9691
Basicaina [Galenica] *see* 5482
Basic Aluminum Acetate *see* 344
Basic Aluminum Carbonate Gel, 1004
Basic Aluminum Chloride *see* 343
Basic Antimony Chloride *see* 693
Basic Bismuth Bromide *see* 1260
Basic Bismuth Chloride *see* 1263
Basic Bismuth Iodide *see* 1270
Basic Bismuth Salicylate *see* 1285
Basic Chromic Sulfates *see* 2230
Basic Cupric Acetate *see* 2624
Basic Cupric Chromates *see* 2634
Basic Dextran *see* 2936
Basic Fibroblast Growth Factor *see* 4072
Basic Iron(III) Acetate *see* 4016
Basic Lead Carbonate, 1005
Basic Lead Chromate *see* 5406
Basi-Cop *see* 2654
Basic Phenylmercuric Nitrate *see* 7302
Basic Zirconium Chloride *see* 10184
Basiliximab, 1006
Basodexan [Hermal] *see* 9867
Basofortina [Novartis] *see* 6070
Basolan *see* 5971
B28-asp-insulin *see* 4982
Bassado [Pharmacia] *see* 3440
Basswood, 1007

Basta [Bayer CropSci.] *see* 7339
Bastard Saffron *see* 1868
Bastiverit [Bastian-Werk] *see* 4478
Bastnaesite *see* 6209
Basudin [Syngenta] *see* 2995
BAT *see* 9782
Batimastat, 1008
Batixim [So.Se.] *see* 5482
BatPA *see* 3459
Batrachotoxin, 1009
Batrachotoxinin A *see* 1009
Batrachotoxinin A 20-(2,4-Dimethyl-
  1*H*-pyrrole-3-carboxylate) *see* 1009
Batrafen [HMR] *see* 2266
Batroxobin, 1010
Batyl Alcohol, 1011
Baum's Acid *see* 6390
Bauxite *see* 356
Bavenite *see* 1648
Bavistin [BASF] *see* 1791
BAX-1400Z *see* 3213
BAX-1526 *see* 2259
BAX-2739Z *see* 955
Baxacor [Mack, Illert.] *see* 3710
Baxan [BMS] *see* 1913
Baxo [Toyama] *see* 7506
Bay-12-8039 *see* 6291
Bay-38-9456 *see* 9935
Bay-43-9006 *see* 8720
Bay-44-4400 *see* 3560
Bay-56-6854 *see* 3938
Bay 1470 *see* 10080
Bay 2502 *see* 6538
Bay 4503 *see* 7831
Bay 5621 *see* 7366
Bay 9002 *see* 6354
Bay 9010 *see* 7836
Bay 19639 *see* 3365
Bay 25141 *see* 4000
Bay 34727 *see* 2261
Bay 39007 *see* 7836
Bay 44646 *see* 433
Bay 68138 *see* 3957
Bay 70143 *see* 1803
Bay 77488 *see* 7366
Bay 92114 *see* 5172
Bay 94337 *see* 6154
Bay a 1040 *see* 6528
Bay b 4343 b *see* 1861
Bay b 5097 *see* 2417
Bay e 5009 *see* 6576
Bay e 6905 *see* 916
Bay e 9736 *see* 6551
Bay f 1353 *see* 6171
Bay g 5421 *see* 18
Bay h 4502 *see* 1213
Bay h 5757 *see* 3944
Bay k 5552 *see* 6565
Bay m 1099 *see* 6187
Bay n 5595 *see* 2905
Bay o 6893 *see* 8231
Bay o 9867 *see* 2314
Bay q 3939 *see* 2314
Bay q 7821 *see* 5081
Bay u 3405 *see* 8100
Bay Va 1470 *see* 10080
Bay Va 9391 *see* 6823
Bay Vh 5757 *see* 3944
Bay Vi 9142 *see* 9526
Bay Vi 9143 *see* 7589
Bay Vp 2674 *see* 3592
Bay w 6628 *see* 1993
Bay x 3702 *see* 8137
Bay-y-7432 *see* 8090
BAY DRW 1139 *see* 5924

BAY FCR 1272 *see* 2756
BAY FOE-5043 *see* 4131
BAY HWG 1608 *see* 9092
BAY KWG 0519 *see* 9593
BAY KWG 0599 *see* 1305
BAY MEB 6447 *see* 9592
BAY MKH 3586 *see* 396
BAY MKH 6561 *see* 7838
BAY MKH 6562 *see* 4119
BAY NTN 9306 *see* 8990
BAY NTN 33893 *see* 4910
BAY SAS 9244 *see* 9607
BAY SIR 8514 *see* 9678
BAY-YRC-2388 *see* 4007
Bayberry Bark, 1012
Baycain [Bayer] *see* 9541
Baycaron [Bayer] *see* 5803
Baycid [Bayer] *see* 4002
Baycidal [Bayer] *see* 9678
Baycillin [Bayer] *see* 7817
Baycip [Bayer] *see* 2314
Baycipen [Bayer] *see* 6171
Baycol [Bayer] *see* 1993
Baycor [Bayer] *see* 1305
Baycovin *see* 7998
Baycox [Bayer] *see* 9526
Bayer 21/116 *see* 6051
Bayer 21/199 *see* 2558
Bayer 205 *see* 9006
Bayer 693 *see* 3852
Bayer 1219 *see* 9704
Bayer 1362 *see* 1516
Bayer 1420 *see* 7803
Bayer 2353 *see* 6519
Bayer 3231 *see* 9603
Bayer 5312 *see* 3737
Bayer 5630 *see* 6157
Bayer 5633 *see* 5939
Bayer 8169 *see* 2889
Bayer 9015 *see* 6518
Bayer 9051 *see* 5459
Bayer 16259 *see* 913
Bayer 17147 *see* 913
Bayer 25820 *see* 6354
Bayer 29493 *see* 4002
Bayer 36205 *see* 6978
Bayer 37344 *see* 5972
Bayer 41831 *see* 3976
Bayer 46131 *see* 7819
Bayer 47531 *see* 3044
Bayer 68138 *see* 3957
Bayer 71628 *see* 5947
Bayer 74283 *see* 5939
Bayer 78418 *see* 3510
Bayer A 128 *see* 757
Bayer A 173 *see* 7761
Bayer E 39 Soluble *see* 1245
Bayer E 393 *see* 8966
Bayer L 1359 *see* 9623
Bayer S 5660 *see* 3976
Bayerite *see* 356
Bayer's Acid *see* 2588
Bayfidan [Bayer] *see* 9593
Baygon [Bayer] *see* 7836
Bay Laurel *see* 5382
Bay Leaf Oil *see* 5382
Bayleton [Bayer] *see* 9592
Bayluscid [Bayer] *see* 6519
Baymicin [Bayer] *see* 8550
Baymix [Chemagro] *see* 2558
Baymycard [Bayer] *see* 6565
Baynas [Bayer] *see* 8100
Bay-o-nox [Bayer] *see* 6823
Bayotensin [Bayer] *see* 6565
Baypen [Bayer] *see* 6171

Baypress [Bayer] see 6576
Baypure CX 100 [Bayer] see 4918
Bayrena [Bayer] see 8914
Bayrepel [Bayer] see 7394
Bayrogel [Bayropharm] see 3875
Baytan [Bayer] see 9593
Baytex [Parke-Davis] see 4002
Baythion [Bayer] see 7366
Baythroid [Bayer CropSci.] see 2756
Bayticol [Bayer] see 4140
Baytinal [Bayer] see 1524
Baytril [Bayer] see 3592
Bayvarol [Provet] see 4140
Bazedoxifene, 1013
Bazoton [Abbott] see 6482
BB-94 see 1008
BB-882 see 5473
BB-2516 see 5753
BBB see 4081
B.B.C. see 1412
BB-K8 [BMS] see 405
BBOT, 1014
BB Powder see 7671
BBR-2778 see 7514
BBS-1067 see 1942
BC-48 see 2885
BC-51 see 3362
BC-105 see 7515
BC-681 see 3518
BC-757 see 7534
levo-BC-2627 see 1530
Bc Conjugate see 7935
B-cell Activating Factor see 4993
B-cell Growth Factor see 4996
B-cell Growth Factor II see 4997
B-cell Stimulatory Factor-1 see 4996
B-cell Stimulatory Factor-2 see 4998
BCG, 1015
BCGF-1 see 4996
BCGFII see 4997
(−)-BCH-189 see 5352
(−)-BCH-204 see 9788
BCH-4556 see 9788
BCM see 1791
BCME see 3069
BCNU see 1845
BCP see 1466
BD-40A see 4245
BDCM see 1417
BDF-5895 see 6293
BDH-312 see 5850
BDMPEA see 1908
B-DNA see 2907
BDNF see 6487
B.D.P.E. see 1448
Beacillin [EGYT] see 7096
Beacon [Syngenta] see 7747
Beamette [Dawbarn] see 7581
Bearberry see 9896
Bearberry Bark see 1880
Bear's Weed see 3669
Bearwood see 1880
Bebate see 1180
Bebeerine see 1016
d-Bebeerine see 1016
l-Bebeerine see 2674
Bebeeru Bark, 1017
Beben [Pfizer] see 1180
Becantal see 8608
Becantex see 8608
Becaplermin see 7525
Becaptan [Labaz] see 2779
Becenun [BMS] see 1845
Bécilan see 7982
Beclacin [Kaigai] see 1019

Beclamide, 1018
Becloforte [GSK] see 1019
Beclomet [Orion] see 1019
Beclomethasone, 1019
Beclorhinol [Lindopharm] see 1019
Beclovent [GSK] see 1019
Becodisks [GSK] see 1019
Beconase [GSK] see 1019
Beconasol [GSK] see 1019
Becort [Rachelle] see 1180
Becotide [GSK] see 1019
Bedermin [Damor] see 1180
Bedoz see 10014
Bedranol [Lagap] see 7840
Bedriol [Andromaco] see 1213
Beechwood Creosote see 2573
Bee Glue see 7835
Beeswax, 1020
Beet Sugar see 8881
Befaprost see 1152
Befizal [Oberval] see 1195
Beflavin [Roche] see 8200
Befloxatone, 1021
Befunolol, 1022
Behenic Acid, 1023
Behenic Alcohol see 3399
N(4)-Behenoyl-1-β-D-arabinofuranosyl-
    cytosine see 3586
Behenoylcytosine Arabinoside see 3586
Behenyl Alcohol see 3399
Behepan [Pfizer] see 10014
Behyd [Kyorin] see 1136
Bei-1293 see 10079
Bekadid see 4785
Bekanamycin see 5281
Belamarine see 5626
Belatacept, 1024
Belcomycine [Sanofi-Aventis] see 2479
Belfacillin see 5969
Belivon [Organon] see 8233
Belladonna, 1025
Bellaradine see 2677
Bellasthman see 5217
Belleau's Reagent, 1026
Belmark [Shell] see 4010
Beloc [AstraZeneca] see 6151
Belseren [BMS] see 2403
Belt see 2082
Belustine [Bellon] see 5564
Bemarside see 8940
Bemegride, 1027
Bemidone see 4836
Bemotrizinol, 1028
BEMT see 1028
Benactyzine, 1029
Benadon [Roche] see 7982
Benadryl [Pfizer] see 3309
Benalaxyl, 1030
Benazepril, 1031
Benazeprilat see 1031
Bencef [Fargal-Pharmasint] see 7513
Bence-Jones Proteins, 1032
Bencyclane, 1033
Bendalina [Angelini] see 1035
Bendaline see 1035
Bendamustine, 1034
Bendazac, 1035
Bendazac Lysine see 1035
Bendazolic Acid see 1035
Bendectin [Duchesnay] see 3441
Bendiocarb, 1036
Bendioxide see 1053
Bendogen [Lagap] see 1186
Bendopa [ICN] see 5464
Bendrofluazide see 1037

Bendroflumethiazide, 1037
Benecel M [Hercules] see 6040
Benecel MP [Hercules] see 4842
Benedorm see 7995
Benefex [Makhteshim-Agan] see 1040
Benefin see 1040
Benemid [Merck & Co.] see 7754
Benerva [Roche] see 9295
Benethamine Penicillin G see 7095
Benexate-CD see 1038
Benexate Hydrochloride, 1038
dl-Benflumelol see 5597
Benflumetol see 5597
Benfluorex, 1039
Benfluralin, 1040
Benfluramate see 1039
Benfofen [Sanofi-Synthelabo] see 3081
Benfotiamine, 1041
Benfuracarb, 1042
Benfuran [Kaken] see 1022
Bengal Isinglass see 184
Benicar [Sankyo] see 6839
Benidipine, 1043
Benirol [Linobion] see 1059
Benisone [Warner-Chilcott] see 1180
Benitoite see 9470
Benlate [DuPont] see 1044
Benne Oil see 8469
Benocten [Medinova] see 3309
Benodaine [Merck & Co.] see 7478
Benomyl, 1044
Benoquin see 6248
Benoral [Sanofi Winthrop] see 1045
Benortan [Sanofi Winthrop] see 1045
Benorylate, 1045
Benoxacor, 1046
Benoxil [Santen] see 1047
Benoxinate, 1047
Benoxyl [Stiefel] see 1116
Benozil [Kyowa] see 4198
Benperidol, 1048
Benproperine, 1049
Benserazide, 1050
Bensuldazic Acid, 1051
Bensulfuron-methyl, 1052
Bensylyt see 7256
Bentazon, 1053
Bentazone see 1053
Bentelan [GSK] see 1180
Bentiromide, 1054
Bentone 34 [Rheox] see 1056
Bentonite, 1055
Bentoquatam, 1056
Bentos [Kaken] see 1022
Bentrofene [Cilag-Chemie] see 23
Bentyl [Aventis] see 3097
Bentylol [Aventis] see 3097
Benur [Pfizer] see 3433
Benuride [Bengue] see 7230
Ben-u-ron [Bene-Arzneimittel] see 47
Benylin [Warner-Lambert] see 8091
Benzac [Galderma] see 1116
Benzagel [RPR] see 1116
Benzaidin see 1186
Benzaknen [Galderma] see 1116
Benzalacetone see 1137
Benzalacetophenone see 2037
Benzalaniline see 1138
Benzal Chloride, 1057
Benzaldehyde, 1058
Benzaldehyde Cyanohydrin see 5719
Benzaldehyde FFC see 1058
Benzaldehyde Green see 5699
Benzal Green see 5699
Benzalin [Shionogi] see 6575

Benzalkonium Chloride, 1059
Benzamide, 1060
Benzamidoacetic Acid *see* 4716
DL-α-Benzamido-*p*-[2-(diethylamino)-
ethoxy]-*N,N*-dipropylhydrocinnam-
amide *see* 9466
DL-4-Benzamido-*N,N*-dipropylglutar-
amic Acid *see* 7775
(*S*)-*p*-(α-Benzamido-*p*-hydroxyhydrocin-
namamido)benzoic Acid *see* 1054
3-[2-(4-Benzamidopiperidino)ethyl]-
indole *see* 4969
β-Benzamidopropionic Acid *see* 1181
4-Benzamidosalicylic Acid *see* 1115
Benzamine *see* 3894
Benzamine Blue *see* 9792
Benzamizole *see* 5235
Benzamon *see* 4312
Benzanilide, 1061
Benz[*a*]anthracene *see* 1062
1,2-Benzanthracene, 1062
2,3-Benzanthracene *see* 6369
7*H*-Benz[*de*]anthracen-7-one *see* 1063
Benzanthrene *see* 1062
Benzanthrone, 1063
Benzathine, 1064
Benzathine Benzylpenicillin *see* 7100
Benzathine Penicillin G *see* 7096
Benzathine Penicillin V *see* 7100
1-Benzazine *see* 8068
2-Benzazine *see* 5222
Benzazoline *see* 9506
Benzbromarone, 1065
Benzchlorpropamide *see* 1018
3,4-Benzchrysene *see* 7396
Benzcurine Iodide *see* 4343
Benzcyclan *see* 1033
Benzedrex [SK & F] *see* 7860
Benzedrine [SKB] *see* 582
Benzelmin [Fort Dodge] *see* 6935
Benzenamine *see* 659
Benzene, 1066
Benzeneacetaldehyde *see* 7265
Benzeneacetamide *see* 7266
Benzeneacetic Acid *see* 7268
Benzeneacetic Acid α-Ethyl-2-(diethyl-
amino)ethyl Ester *see* 1522
Benzeneacetic Acid Ethyl Ester *see* 3840
Benzeneacetic Acid 4-Methylphenyl
Ester *see* 2585
Benzeneacetonitrile *see* 1131
Benzenearsonic Acid, 1067
Benzeneazoaniline *see* 2998
Benzeneazobenzene *see* 917
Benzeneboronic Acid, 1068
Benzene Boronic Anhydride *see* 1068
Benzenecarbonyl Chloride *see* 1112
Benzenecarboperoxoic Acid *see* 7152
Benzenecarbothioic Acid *S*-[2-[[(4-
Amino-2-methyl-5-pyrimidinyl)meth-
yl]formylamino]-1-[2-(phosphonooxy)-
ethyl]-1-propenyl] Ester *see* 1041
Benzenecarboxylic Acid *see* 1091
Benzene Chloride *see* 2121
1,2-Benzenediamine *see* 7284
1,3-Benzenediamine *see* 7283
1,4-Benzenediamine *see* 7285
1,2-Benzenedicarbonyl Dichloride *see*
7375
1,2-Benzenedicarboxaldehyde *see* 7368
1,2-Benzenedicarboxamide *see* 7369
1,2-Benzenedicarboxylic Acid *see* 7371
1,3-Benzenedicarboxylic Acid *see* 5197
1,4-Benzenedicarboxylic Acid *see* 9162
1,2-Benzenedicarboxylic Acid Bis-
(2-ethylhexyl) Ester *see* 2864

1,2-Benzenedicarboxylic Acid Bis-
(3-methylbutyl) Ester *see* 5124
1,2-Benzenedicarboxylic Acid Dibutyl
Ester *see* 3035
1,2-Benzenedicarboxylic Acid Diisononyl Ester *see* 3290
1,2-Benzenedicarboxylic Acid
Dimethyl Ester *see* 3255
1,2-Benzenedicarboxylic Acid
Diphenyl Ester *see* 7306
1,2-Benzenedicarboxylic Acid Mono-
(1-ethyl-1-methyl-2-propynyl) Ester
see 7374
1,2-Benzenediol *see* 7999
1,3-Benzenediol *see* 8155
1,4-Benzenediol *see* 4808
Benzeneethanamine *see* 7225
Benzeneethanol *see* 7224
Benzenehexacarboxylic Acid *see* 5825
γ-Benzene Hexachloride *see* 5501
Benzenemethanamine *see* 1125
Benzenemethanesulfonyl Fluoride *see*
7542
Benzenemethanethiol *see* 9322
Benzenemethanol *see* 1124
Benzenepropanoic Acid *see* 4784
Benzenepropanol Carbamate *see* 7258
Benzenestibonic Acid, 1069
4-(2-Benzenesulfinylethyl)-1,2-diphenyl-
pyrazolidine-3,5-dione *see* 8949
Benzenesulfohydrazide *see* 7598
Benzenesulfohydroxamic Acid *see* 7426
2-Benzenesulfonamido-5-*tert*-butyl-1,3,4-
thiadiazole *see* 4480
2-Benzenesulfonamido-5-(β-methoxy-
ethoxy)pyrimidine *see* 4507
Benzene Sulfonechloride *see* 1072
Benzenesulfonic Acid, 1070
Benzenesulfonic Acid Barium Salt *see*
966
Benzenesulfonic (Acid) Chloride *see* 1072
Benzenesulfonic Acid Hydrazide *see* 7598
Benzenesulfonic Anhydride, 1071
Benzenesulfonyl Chloride, 1072
5-[2-(Benzenesulfonyl)ethyl]-3-(1-meth-
ylpyrrolidin-2(*R*)-ylmethyl)-1*H*-indole
see 3544
1,2,4,5-Benzenetetracarboxylic Acid
see 8004
Benzenethiol *see* 9355
1,2,4-Benzenetricarboxylic Acid *see*
9702
1,2,3-Benzenetriol *see* 8000
1,2,4-Benzenetriol, 1073
1,3,5-Benzenetriol *see* 7328
2,2′,2″-[1,2,3-Benzenetriyltris(oxy)]-
tris[*N,N,N*-triethylethanaminium]
Triiodide *see* 4343
N,N′-Benzenyl-*o*-phenylenediamine *see*
7274
Benzenyl Trichloride *see* 1109
Benzerial [Houdé] *see* 4567
Benzetamophylline *see* 955
Benzethacil *see* 7096
Benzethonium Chloride, 1074
Benzetimide, 1075
Benzhexol Chloride *see* 9695
Benzhydramine *see* 3309
Benzhydrol *see* 1090
Benzhydrylamine, 1076
N-Benzhydryl-*N*′-*trans*-cinnamylpiper-
azine *see* 2305
O-Benzhydryldimethylaminoethanol *see*
3309
O-Benzhydryldimethylaminoethanol 8-
Chlorotheophyllinate *see* 3207

2-Benzhydryl β-Dimethylaminoethyl
Ether *see* 7316
(*N*-Benzhydryl)(*N*′-methyl)diethylene-
diamine *see* 2710
N-Benzhydryl-*N*′-methylpiperazine *see*
2710
2-(Benzhydryloxy)-*N,N*-dimethylethyl-
amine *see* 3309
2-(Benzhydryloxy)-*N,N*-dimethylethyl-
amine 8-Chlorotheophyllinate *see* 3207
4-Benzhydryloxy-*N*-methylpiperidine *see*
3331
2-(Benzhydrylsulfinyl)acetamide *see*
6228
2-(Benzhydrylsulfinyl)acetohydroxamic
Acid *see* 170
Benzidine, 1077
Benzil, 1078
Benzil Dioxime, 1079
Benzilic Acid, 1080
Benzilic Acid β-Diethylaminoethyl Ester
see 1029
Benzilic Acid Ester with 2-(Hydroxymethyl)-1,1-dimethylpiperidinium
Methyl Sulfate *see* 1193
Benzilic Acid 1-Ethyl-3-piperidyl Ester
Methyl Bromide *see* 7461
Benzilic Acid *N*-β-Fluoroethylnortropine
Ester Methobromide *see* 4216
Benzilic Acid 1-Piperidineethanol Ester
see 7471
Benzilic Acid 3α-Tropanyl Ester *see* 9782
3-Benziloyloxy-1-azabicyclo[2.2.2]octane
Methobromide *see* 2354
(8*r*)-3α-Benziloyloxy-8-(2-fluoroethyl)-8-
methyl-8-azoniabicyclo[3.2.1]octane
Bromide *see* 4216
2-Benziloyloxymethyl-1,1-dimethylpyr-
rolidinium Methyl Sulfate *see* 7554
3α-Benziloyloxyspiro(nortropane-8,1′-
pyrrolidinium) Chloride *see* 9786
Benzimidazole, 1081
2-Benzimidazolecarbamic Acid Methyl
Ester *see* 1791
1*H*-Benzimidazole-2-propanoic Acid *see*
7762
2-Benzimidazolethiol, 1082
1*H*-Benzimidazol-2-ylcarbamic Acid
Methyl Ester *see* 1791
β-(2-Benzimidazolyl)propionic Acid *see*
7762
(1*S*,2*S*)-2-[2-[[3-(2-Benzimidazolyl)pro-
pyl]methylamino]ethyl]-6-fluoro-1,2,-
3,4-tetrahydro-1-isopropyl-2-naph-
thyl Methoxyacetate *see* 6173
2-(2-Benzimidazolylsulfinylmethyl)-3-
methyl-4-(2,2,2-trifluoroethoxy)pyri-
dine *see* 5362
4-(2-Benzimidazolyl)thiazole *see* 9289
Benziminazole *see* 1081
Benzin *see* 7188
Benzindamine *see* 1122
Benzin (German) *see* 4372
Benzinoform [Mallinckrodt] *see* 1816
Benziodarone, 1083
1,2-Benzisothiazol-3(2*H*)-one 1,1-
Dioxide *see* 8311
cis-*N*-[4-[4-(1,2-Benzisothiazol-3-yl)-1-
piperazinyl]butyl]-1,2-cyclohexane-
dicarboximide *see* 7182
(3a*R*,7a*S*)-*rel*-2-[4-[4-(1,2-Benzisothia-
zol-3-yl)-1-piperazinyl]butyl]hexa-
hydro-1*H*-isoindole-1,3(2*H*)-dione *see*
7182

Benzotrichloride, 1109
Benzotrifluoride, 1110
4-(2,1,3-Benzoxadiazol-4-yl)-2,6-di-
methyl-1,4-dihydro-3-isopropyloxy-
carbonylpyridine-5-carboxylic Acid
Methyl Ester *see* 5240
4,4′-(3*H*-2,1-Benzoxathiol-3-ylidene)-
bis[2-bromo-3-methyl-6-(1-methyl-
ethyl)phenol] *S*,*S*-Dioxide *see* 1445
4,4′-(3*H*-2,1-Benzoxathiol-3-ylidene)-
bis[2-bromo-6-methylphenol] *S*,*S*-
Dioxide *see* 1387
4,4′-(3*H*-2,1-Benzoxathiol-3-ylidene)-
bis[2,6-dibromo-3-methylphenol]
S,*S*-Dioxide *see* 1386
4,4′-(3*H*-2,1-Benzoxathiol-3-ylidene)-
bis[2,6-dibromophenol] *S*,*S*-Dioxide
see 1444
4,4′-(3*H*-2,1-Benzoxathiol-3-ylidene)-
bis[2,5-dimethylphenol] *S*,*S*-Dioxide
see 10083
4,4′-(3*H*-2,1-Benzoxathiol-3-ylidene)-
bis[5-methyl-2-(1-methylethyl)-
phenol] *S*,*S*-Dioxide *see* 9400
4,4′-(3*H*-2,1-Benzoxathiol-3-ylidene)-
bisphenol *S*,*S*-Dioxide *see* 7247
Benzoxine [Sanwa] *see* 1186
Benzoxonium Chloride, 1111
3-Benzoxy-1-(2-methylpiperidino)-
propane *see* 7474
ω-Benzoylacetophenone *see* 3009
Benzoyl Acetyl Peroxide *see* 78
N-Benzoyl-*β*-alanine *see* 1181
Benzoylamide *see* 1060
Benzoylaminoacetic Acid *see* 4716
(1*R*,2*S*)-2-(Benzoylamino)-1-[[[(2a*R*,-
4*S*,4a*S*,6*R*,9*S*,11*S*,12*S*,12a*R*,12b*S*)-6,-
12b-bis(acetyloxy)-12-(benzoyloxy)-
2a,3,4,4a,5,6,9,10,11,12,12a,12b-do-
decahydro-4,11-dihydroxy-4a,8,13,-
13-tetramethyl-5-oxo-7,11-methano-
1*H*-cyclodeca[3,4]benz[1,2-*b*]oxet-9-
yl]oxy]carbonyl]-2-phenylethyl Ester
L-Glutamic Acid Homopolymer *see*
6983
α-(Benzoylamino)-4-[2-(diethylamino)-
ethoxy]-*N*,*N*-dipropylbenzenepropan-
amide *see* 9466
4-(Benzoylamino)-5-(dipropylamino)-5-
oxopentanoic Acid *see* 7775
(*αR*,*βS*)-*β*-(Benzoylamino)-*α*-hydroxy-
benzenepropanoic Acid (2a*R*,4*S*,4a*S*,-
6*R*,9*S*,11*S*,12*S*,12a*R*,12b*S*)-6,12b-Bis-
(acetyloxy)-12-(benzoyloxy)-2a,3,4,-
4a,5,6,9,10,11,12,12a,12b-dodecahy-
dro-4,11-dihydroxy-4a,8,13,13-tetra-
methyl-5-oxo-7,11-methano-1*H*-cy-
clodeca[3,4]benz[1,2-*b*]oxet-9-yl Ester
see 6982
4-(Benzoylamino)-2-hydroxybenzoic
Acid *see* 1115
4-[[(2*S*)-2-(Benzoylamino)-3-(4-hydroxy-
phenyl)-1-oxopropyl]amino]benzoic
Acid *see* 1054
(11*β*,16*α*)-21-[3-(Benzoylamino)-2-
methyl-1-oxopropoxy]-9-fluoro-11-
hydroxy-16,17-[(1-methylethyli-
dene)bis(oxy)]pregna-1,4-diene-3,20-
dione *see* 9597
3-(Benzoylamino)propionic Acid *see* 1181
N-Benzoyl-*p*-aminosalicylic Acid *see* 1115
N-Benzoylaniline *see* 1061
Benzoylbenzene *see* 1098
5-Benzoyl-2-benzimidazolecarbamic
Acid Methyl Ester *see* 5768

(5-Benzoyl-1*H*-benzimidazol-2-yl)car-
bamic Acid Methyl Ester *see* 5768
Benzoyl Chloride, 1112
5-Benzoyl-2,3-dihydro-1*H*-pyrrolizine-
1-carboxylic Acid *see* 5306
5-Benzoyl-1,2-dihydro-3*H*-pyrrolo[1,2-
a]pyrrole-1-carboxylic Acid *see* 5306
N-Benzoyl-*N*′,*N*′-di-*n*-propyl-DL-iso-
glutamine *see* 7775
Benzoylecgonine, 1113
O-Benzoyl-*l*-ecgonine Ethyl Ester *see*
2454
O-Benzoyleugenol *see* 3898
Benzoylformaldoxime *see* 5191
N-Benzoylglycine *see* 4716
m-Benzoylhydratropic Acid *see* 5305
6-Benzoyl-3-hydrazino-5,6,7,8-tetrahy-
dropyrido[4,3-*c*]pyridazine *see* 3577
Benzoyl Hydroperoxide *see* 7152
3-Benzoyl-4-hydroxy-6-methoxybenzene-
sulfonic Acid *see* 8983
5-Benzoyl-4-hydroxy-2-methoxybenzene-
sulfonic Acid *see* 8983
Benzoyl Isothiocyanate, 1114
2-Benzoyl-5-methoxy-1-phenol-4-sulfonic
Acid *see* 8983
3-Benzoyl-*α*-methylbenzeneacetic Acid
see 5305
Benzoylmethylecgonine *see* 2455
3-Benzoyl-*α*-methyl-*N*-(4-methyl-2-pyri-
dinyl)benzeneacetamide *see* 7422
Benzoyl-*γ*-(2-methylpiperidino)propanol
see 7474
m-Benzoyl-*N*-(4-methyl-2-pyridyl)hydra-
tropamide *see* 7422
5-Benzoyl-*α*-methyl-2-thiopheneacetic
Acid *see* 9422
Benzoylnaphthol *see* 6408
2-(Benzoyloxy)benzoic Acid Methyl Ester
see 6025
N-(2-Benzoyloxyethyl)norfenfluramine
see 1039
3-(Benzoyloxy)-8-methyl-8-azabicyclo-
[3.2.1]octane-2-carboxylic Acid *see*
1113
[1*R*-(*exo*,*exo*)]-3-(Benzoyloxy)-8-methyl-
8-azabicyclo[3.2.1]octane-2-carboxylic
Acid Ethyl Ester *see* 2454
[1*R*-(2-*endo*,3-*exo*)]-3-(Benzoyloxy)-8-
methyl-8-azabicyclo[3.2.1]octane-2-
carboxylic Acid Methyl Ester *see* 7912
[1*R*-(*exo*,*exo*)]-3-(Benzoyloxy)-8-methyl-
8-azabicyclo[3.2.1]octane-2-carboxylic
Acid Methyl Ester *see* 2455
3-Benzoyloxyquinuclidine *see* 8082
α-4-Benzoyloxy-2,2,6-trimethylpiperi-
dine *see* 3894
Benzoylpas, 1115
Benzoylpas Calcium *see* 1115
Benzoyl Peroxide, 1116
Benzoylphenylcarbinol *see* 1093
2-(3-Benzoylphenyl)-*N*-(4-methyl-2-
pyridyl)propionamide *see* 7422
2-(3-Benzoylphenyl)propionic Acid *see*
5305
Benzoylpseudotropeine *see* 9774
4-Benzoylresorcinol *see* 1106
N-Benzoylstaurosporine *see* 6185
*N*¹-Benzoylsulfanilamide *see* 8897
Benzoyl Superoxide *see* 1116
6-Benzoyl-5,6,7,8-tetrahydropyrido-
[4,3-*c*]pyridazin-3(2*H*)-one Hydrazone
see 3577
O-Benzoylthiamine Disulfide *see* 1246
S-Benzoylthiamine Monophosphate *see*
1041

Benzoylthiocarbimide *see* 1114
(4*S*)-1-[(2*S*)-3-(Benzoylthio)-2-methyl-1-
oxopropyl]-4-(phenylthio)-L-proline
see 10186
α-Benzoyltriethylamine *see* 3127
Benzoyl-*ψ*-tropeine *see* 9774
N-Benzoyl-L-tyrosyl-*p*-aminobenzoic
Acid *see* 1054
Benzozone *see* 78
Benzperidol *see* 1048
1,2-Benzphenanthrene *see* 2255
2,3-Benzphenanthrene *see* 1062
3,4-Benzphenanthrene, 1117
9,10-Benzphenanthrene *see* 9740
Benzphetamine, 1118
Benzpinacone *see* 1100
Benzproperine Embonate *see* 1049
1,2-Benzpyrene *see* 1103, 1104
3,4-Benzpyrene *see* 1103
4,5-Benzpyrene *see* 1104
Benzquinamide, 1119
Benzthiazide, 1120
Benztriazole *see* 1108
Benztropine Mesylate, 1121
Benztropine Methanesulfonate *see* 1121
Benzydamine, 1122
Benzydroflumethiazide *see* 1037
(*R*)-*N*-Benzyl-2-acetamido-3-methoxy-
propionamide *see* 5333
Benzyl Acetate, 1123
Benzylacetic Acid *see* 4784
Benzyl Alcohol, 1124
Benzylamine, 1125
Benzylamine Oxidase *see* 2975
Benzylaniline, 1126
2-(*N*-Benzylanilino)ethyl (±)-1,4-Dihy-
dro-2,6-dimethyl-4-(*m*-nitrophenyl)-
5-phosphononicotinate, Cyclic 2,2-
Dimethyltrimethylene Ester *see* 3524
1-[2-(*N*-Benzylanilino)-1-(isobutoxy-
methyl)ethyl]pyrrolidine *see* 1150
2-(*N*-Benzylanilinomethyl)-2-imidazoline
see 680
4-*N*-Benzylanilino-1-methylpiperidine
see 956
Benzylbenzene *see* 3328
Benzylbenzenecarboxylate *see* 1127
Benzyl Benzoate, 1127
Benzyl Bromide, 1128
(*αR*,*γS*,2*S*)-*α*-Benzyl-2-(*tert*-butylcarba-
moyl)-*γ*-hydroxy-*N*-[(1*S*,2*R*)-2-hy-
droxy-1-indanyl]-4-(3-pyridylmethyl)-
1-piperazinevaleramide *see* 4945
Benzylcarbamic Acid 2-Hydroxyethyl
Ester *see* 1501
Benzylcarbamide *see* 1147
1-[2-(Benzylcarbamoyl)ethyl]-2-iso-
nicotinoylhydrazide *see* 6491
N-[2-(Benzylcarbamyl)ethylamino]iso-
nicotinamide *see* 6491
Benzyl Carbinol *see* 7224
Benzylcarbonyl Chloride *see* 1801
Benzyl Chloride, 1129
3-Benzyl-6-chloro-3,4-dihydro-2*H*-1,2,-
4-benzothiadiazine-7-sulfonamide
1,1-Dioxide *see* 1136
3-Benzyl-6-chloro-3,4-dihydro-7-sulfa-
moyl-1,2,4-benzothiadiazine 1,1-
Dioxide *see* 1136
Benzyl Chloroformate *see* 1801
o-Benzyl-*p*-chlorophenol *see* 2407
2-Benzyl-4-chlorophenol *see* 2407
N-Benzyl-*β*-chloropropanamide *see* 1018
N-Benzyl-3-chloropropionamide *see* 1018
Benzyl Cinnamate, 1130

Bepotastine Besilate see 1149
Beprane [Biotherapie] see 7840
Bepridil, 1150
Béprocin see 1246
Berachin [Tokyo Tanabe] see 9811
Beractant, 1151
Béradia see 4405
Beraprost, 1152
Beraunite see 4029
Berbamine, 1153
Berbenine see 1153
Berberine, 1154
Berberine Bisulfate see 1154
Berberis, 1155
Berberis Aristata, 1156
Berberis Bark see 961
Berenil [Intervet] see 3266
Beret [Syngenta] see 3989
Bergacef [Bergamon] see 1914
Bergamol [Synfleur] see 5496
Bergaptan see 1157
Bergapten, 1157
Bergaptene see 1157
Berkatens [Berk] see 9950
Berkelium, 1158
Berkfurin [Berk] see 6599
Berkmycen [APS] see 6976
Berkolol [Berk] see 7840
Berkozide [APS] see 1037
Berlicetin [Chauvin ankerpharm] see 909
Berlin Blue see 7910
Bermoprofen, 1159
Berninamycin, 1160
Berninamycin A see 1160
Berninamycin B see 1160
Bernstein see 380
Bernsteinsäure (German) see 8869
Bernsteinsäureanhydrid (German) see 8870
Berofor [Boehringer, Ing.] see 4990
Berolase [Roche] see 9296
Beronald [Kowa] see 4309
Berotec [Boehringer, Ing.] see 3981
Berry Alder see 4263
Berry Wax see 1012
Bertholite see 2095
Bertrandite see 1161
Berubi [Cesra] see 10014
Beryl see 1161
Beryllia see 1172
Beryllium, 1161
Beryllium Acetate, 1162
Beryllium Acetylacetonate, 1163
Beryllium Bromide, 1164
Beryllium Carbide, 1165
Beryllium Chloride, 1166
Beryllium Fluoride, 1167
Beryllium Hydride, 1168
Beryllium Hydroxide, 1169
Beryllium Nitrate, 1170
Beryllium Nitride, 1171
Beryllium Oxide, 1172
Beryllium Potassium Sulfate, 1173
Beryllium Sodium Fluoride, 1174
Beryllium Sulfate, 1175
Berzelianite see 2666
Berzeline see 2666
Besipirdine, 1176
Besnoline [Kotobuki] see 9522
Bespar [BMS] see 1504
Bessisterol see 8749
Bestatin [Nippon Kayaku] see 9842
Bestcall [Takeda] see 1925
Bestguard [Takeda] see 6568
Bestmann-Ohira Reagent, 1177

Beston [Tanabe Seiyaku] see 1246
Betabactyl [SKB] see 2341
Betabion [Merck KGaA] see 9295
Betacaine see 3894
Beta-Cardone [Evans] see 8728
Betacef [Firma] see 1936
Betacetylmethadol see 5945
Betacor [Ayerst] see 2018
Beta-Corlan see 1180
Betadexamethasone see 1180
Betadid see 1458
Betadine [Purdue Frederick] see 7698
Betadran [Logeais] see 1496
Betadrenol [Schwarz] see 1496
Betaferon [Schering AG] see 4991
Betafluorene [Lepetit] see 1180
Betagan [Allergan] see 5462
Betagon [Schering AG] see 5856
Betahistine, 1178
Beta-hypophamine see 9938
Betaine, 1179
Betaine Hydrazide Hydrochloride see 4429
Betaine Viologen see 9999
Beta-interferon see 4991
Betaisodona [Mundipharma] see 7698
Betalin S [Lilly] see 9295
Betalin-12 [Lilly] see 10014
Betaling [Tanabe] see 1186
Betaloc [AstraZeneca] see 6151
Betalone [Lepetit] see 5861
Betamann [Mann] see 6140
Betamaze [Pfizer] see 8889
Betamet [Pharmaquest] see 6140
Betamethasone, 1180
Betamethasone 21-(Dihydrogen Phosphate) Disodium Salt see 1180
Betamipron, 1181
Betamox [Norbrook] see 577
Betanal [Bayer CropSci.] see 7236
Beta-naphthol see 6384
Betanaphthol Benzoate see 6408
Betanaphthoxyethanol see 6413
Betanidol [Tanabe Seiyaku] see 1186
Betanol [Dulcis] see 6140
Betapace [Berlex] see 8728
Betapar [Parke-Davis] see 5861
Betapindol [Helvepharm] see 7443
Betapred [Schering] see 5861
Betapressin [HMR] see 7082
Betaprodine see 310
Betaprodine Hydrochloride see 310
Betaprone [Forest] see 7820
Betarin [Beta] see 2451
Betaserc [Duphar] see 1178
Betaseron [Schering AG] see 4991
Betasolon see 1180
Beta-Tablinen [Sanorania] see 7840
Beta-Timelets [Temmler] see 7840
Betavel [Sanofi Winthrop] see 2420
Betaxin [Sterling Winthrop] see 9295
Betaxina [Terap. M. R.] see 6359
Betaxolol, 1182
Betazole, 1183
BETE see 9782
Betel, 1184
Betel Nuts see 776
Bethanechol Chloride, 1185
Bethanidine, 1186
Bethrodine see 1040
Beth Root see 9696
Betim [Leo Pharm] see 9444
Betimol [Santen] see 9444
Betnelan [GSK] see 1180
Betnesol [GSK] see 1180

Betnesol-V [GSK] see 1180
Betneval [GSK] see 1180
Betnovate [GSK] see 1180
Betol see 6415
Betolvex [Dumex] see 10014
Betoptic [Alcon] see 1182
Betoptima [Alcon] see 1182
Betotastine see 1149
Betoxycaine, 1187
Betriol [Boehringer, Ing.] see 1489
Betula, 1188
Betula Oil see 6120
Betulic Acid see 1190
Betulin, 1189
Betulinic Acid, 1190
Betulinol see 1189
Betulol see 1189
Betuloside see 8189
Bevacizumab, 1191
Bevantolol, 1192
Beveno [Fischer] see 2755
Bevonium Methyl Sulfate, 1193
Bewon [Wyeth] see 9295
Bexarotene, 1194
Bexedan [Smit] see 2081
Bexide see 3384
Bexol see 3302
Bextasol [GSK] see 1180
Bextra [Pharmacia & Upjohn] see 9900
Bexxar [Coulter] see 9554
Bezafibrate, 1195
Bezalip [Boehringer, Mann.] see 1195
Bezatol [Kissei] see 1195
Bezitramide, 1196
BFE-60 see 1022
bFGF see 4072
des 1-15 bFGF see 4072
BFL see 5597
BG-8301 see 4994
BG-8967 see 1310
BG-9273 see 227
BG-9712 see 227
BGO see 1266
BGP see 6894
α-Bgt see 1488
6R-BH$_4$ see 8368
BH-6 see 6738
BHA see 1547
BH-AC see 3586
Bhang see 1749
BHB see 1534
γ-BHC see 5501
Bhimsaim Camphor see 1338
B Hormone see 6295
BHT see 1548
B-HT-920 see 9039
BI 61.012 see 4538
BI-397 see 2803
Biacetyl see 2966
Bialaphos see 7339
Bialcol [Novartis] see 1111
Bialzepam [Bial] see 2994
Biapenem, 1197
Biarison [Sandoz-Wander] see 7873
Biaxin [Abbott] see 2339
Biazolina [Panthox & Burck] see 1917
Bibapcitide see 9098
Bibenzal see 8817
Bibenzene see 3314
o,o'-Bibenzoic Acid see 3310
Bibenzoyl see 1078
Bibenzyl, 1198
Bibenzylidene see 8817
Bibiru Bark see 1017
BIBR 277 see 9129

BIBR-953 *see* 2797
BIBR-1048 *see* 2797
Bibrocathin *see* 1199
Bibrocathol, 1199
BIC *see* 1575
Bicalutamide, 1200
Bicarbamimide *see* 9866
2,2'-Bichavicol *see* 5697
Bichloracetic Acid *see* 3050
Bichromate of Soda *see* 8609
Bicillin L-A [Wyeth-Ayerst] *see* 7096
Bicine, 1201
Biciron [Basotherm] *see* 9567
Bicnu [BMS] *see* 1845
Bicolorin *see* 3698
Bicozamycin, 1202
Bicuculline, 1203
Bicyclo[4.4.0]decane *see* 2846
Bicyclo-[0.3.5]-deca-1,3,5,7,9-pentaene
   see 926
Bicyclo-[5.3.0]-deca-2,4,6,8,10-pentaene
   see 926
Bicyclo[4.1.0]heptane *see* 6688
(*endo,endo*)-Bicyclo[2.2.1]hept-5-ene-2,-
   3-dicarboxylic Acid Dimethyl Ester
   see 3240
endo-cis-Bicyclo[2.2.1]hept-5-ene-2,3-
   dicarboxylic Anhydride *see* 1796
3-Bicyclo[2.2.1]hept-5-en-2-yl-6-chloro-
   3,4-dihydro-2*H*-1,2,4-benzothiadi-
   azine-7-sulfonamide 1,1-Dioxide *see*
   2754
α-Bicyclo[2.2.1]hept-5-en-2-yl-α-phenyl-
   1-piperidinepropanol *see* 1233
1-Bicycloheptenyl-1-phenyl-3-piperi-
   dinopropanol *see* 1233
Bicyclohexylammonium Fumagillin *see*
   4286
[1,1'-Bicyclohexyl]-1-carboxylic Acid
   2-(Diethylamino)ethyl Ester *see* 3097
[1,1'-Bicyclohexyl]-1-carboxylic Acid
   2-(1-Piperidinyl)ethyl Ester *see* 3168
Bicyclomycin *see* 1202
BID *see* 1886
Bidien [IDI] *see* 1468
Bidisomide, 1204
Δ 2,2'-Bi-1,3-dithiole *see* 9242
Bidocef [BMS] *see* 1913
Bidrin [Amvac] *see* 3087
Bieberite *see* 2448
Biebrich Scarlet Red *see* 8393
Bietamiverine, 1205
Biethylene *see* 1509
Bifemelane, 1206
Bifenazate, 1207
Bifenox, 1208
Bifenthrin, 1209
Bifeprunox, 1210
Bifeprunox Mesylate *see* 1210
Bifex [Provet] *see* 7836
Bifidus Factor, 1211
Bifluranol, 1212
Bifonazole, 1213
Biformyl *see* 4509
Biforon [Meiji] *see* 1476
Bifril [Menarini] *see* 10186
BIGCHAP, 1214
Bigitalin *see* 4434
Biguanide, 1215
Bigunal [Nikken] *see* 1476
[Δ²,²'-Biindoline]-3,3'-dione *see* 4943
Bijosal *see* 3190
Bi-Ketolan *see* 6928
Bikhaconitine, 1216
Bikhroot *see* 120

Biklin [BMS] *see* 405
Bikunin Trypsin Inhibitor *see* 9882
Bilamid(e) [Cilag-Chemie] *see* 4833
Bilarcil [Bayer] *see* 9623
Bilberry, 1217
Bilcolic [Unifa] *see* 4854
Bilein *see* 6928
Biletan [Gador] *see* 9326
Bilevon *see* 4680
Bilevon-M *see* 6518
Bilicholan *see* 6928
Bilidren *see* 2868
Biligrafin [Schering AG] *see* 5022
Biligram [Schering AG] *see* 5051
Bilijodon-Natrium *see* 5058
Bilimiro [Bracco] *see* 5063
Bilimiron [Bracco] *see* 5063
Bilimix [Gero] *see* 2715
Bilineurine *see* 2204
Biliognost *see* 5026
Biliphorine [Couvreur] *see* 9492
Bilirubin, 1218
Bilirubin IXα *see* 1218
Biliselectan *see* 5026
Biliton H [Berlin-Chemie] *see* 4854
Bilitrast *see* 5038
Biliverdine, 1219
Bilobalide, 1220
Bilopaque [Sterling Winthrop] *see* 9837
Biloptin [Schering AG] *see* 5071
Biloxazol *see* 1305
Biltricide [Bayer] *see* 7716
BIM-23014 *see* 5361
BIM-23014C *see* 5361
Δ²,²'-Bimalononitrile *see* 9195
Bimaran [Roux-Ocefa] *see* 9579
Bimatoprost, 1221
Bimethyl *see* 3723
2,2'-Bimorphine *see* 7919
Bimosiamose, 1222
Bimotrim [Vetpharma] *see* 8906
BINAP, 1223
[1,1'-Binaphthalene]-2,2'-diol *see* 1226
[1,1'-Binaphthalene]-2,2'-diylbis-
   [diphenylphosphine] *see* 1223
β-Binaphthol *see* 1226
β,β-Binaphthyleneethene *see* 7396
Binazin [Polfa] *see* 9502
Bindan *see* 7234
Bindazac *see* 1035
Bingo [BASF] *see* 2293
Binifibrate, 1224
Biniwas [Wassermann] *see* 1224
Binixin [Bayer] *see* 4147
Binodenoson, 1225
Binodrenal *see* 6695
BINOL, 1226
Binotal [Grünenthal] *see* 586
Binova [Gentili] *see* 7882
Binovum [Ortho-Cilag] *see* 6697
Biobenzyfuroline [Sumitomo] *see* 1230
Biocefalin [Benvegna] *see* 7996
Biochanin A *see* 4391
Biochanin B *see* 4244
Biociclin [Del Saz & Filippini] *see* 1954
Biocidan [Clin-Comar-Byla] *see* 2019
Biocin [Ibirn] *see* 4254
Biocolina *see* 2206
Bio-Cox [Alpharma] *see* 8336
Biocytin, 1227
Biodermatin [Lafare] *see* 1231
Biofanal [Pfleger] *see* 6736
Bioflavonoids, 1228
Biofurex [Lenza] *see* 1954

Biofusal *see* 4313
Biohulin [Biobras] *see* 4980
BIOLF-62 *see* 4363
Biomag [Pulitzer] *see* 2279
Biomioran *see* 2194
Biomitsin *see* 2192
Bion [Syngenta] *see* 106
Bionicard [Bioindustria] *see* 6495
Biopal CVL-10 *see* 5037
Bioperazone [Biopharma] *see* 1930
Bioperidolo [Firma] *see* 4598
Bioplex [Thames] *see* 1793
Biopten [Maruho] *see* 8368
Biopterin, 1229
Biopure 100 [Biophil] *see* 4916
Bioral [SKB] *see* 1793
Bioresmethrin, 1230
Biorphen *see* 6879
Bioscleran [Pfleger] *see* 2377
Bios I *see* 4978
Bios II *see* 1231
Biosinon [Farmakhim] *see* 3722
Bio Soft [Stepan] *see* 7577
Biosol [Biokema] *see* 6454
Biosone [Berk] *see* 3590
Biosynthetic Human Insulin *see* 4980
Biotamin [Sankyo] *see* 1041
Bioterciclin *see* 2886
Biotertussin [Lisapharma] *see* 2365
Bi(OTf)₃ *see* 1292
Biothion *see* 9135
Biotin, 1231
Biotin Complex of Yeast *see* 1227
Biotinin [Sankyo] *see* 9297
Biotin *l*-Sulfoxide, 1232
ε-N-Biotinyl-L-lysine *see* 1227
Biotiren [Benvegna] *see* 3030
Bioxima [Ital. Suisse] *see* 1954
Bioxiran *see* 3676
(2*R*,2'*S*)-*rel*-2,2'-Bioxirane *see* 3676
Biozate [Ind. Bioquim] *see* 2765
Biozolene [Bioindustria] *see* 4122
Biperiden, 1233
Biphenal *see* 4836
Biphenamine, 1234
Biphenate *see* 1209
Biphenthrin *see* 1209
Biphentrin *see* 1209
1,1'-Biphenyl *see* 3314
(1,1'-Biphenyl)-4-acetic Acid *see* 3951
4-Biphenylacetic Acid *see* 3951
p-Biphenylamine, 1235
[1,1'-Biphenyl]-4-amine *see* 1235
[1,1'-Biphenyl]-4,4'-diamine *see* 1077
2,4'-Biphenyldiamine, 1236
[1,1'-Biphenyl]-2,2'-dicarboxylic Acid
   see 3310
3,3'-[[1,1'-Biphenyl]-4,4'-diylbis(azo)]-
   bis[4-amino-1-naphthalenesulfonic
   Acid] Disodium Salt *see* 2498
3,3'-[1,1'-Biphenyl]-4,4'-diylbis[2,5-di-
   phenyl-2*H*-tetrazolium] Dichloride *see*
   6466
2,2'-[1,1'-Biphenyl]-4,4'-diylbis[2-hy-
   droxy-4,4-dimethylmorpholinium]
   see 4643
3,3'-[4,4'-Biphenylene]bis[2,5-diphen-
   yl-2*H*-tetrazolium] Dichloride *see* 6466
o-Biphenylenemethane *see* 4155
(1,1'-Biphenyl)-2-ol *see* 7304
[1,1'-Biphenyl]-4-ol *see* 7305
2-Biphenylol *see* 7304
3-(3-*p*-Biphenyl-1,2,3,4-tetrahydro-
   naphth-1-yl)-4-hydroxycoumarin *see*
   3133

2-[Bis(4-hydroxyphenyl)methyl]benzene-
methanol *see* 7245
2-[Bis(4-hydroxyphenyl)methyl]benzoic
Acid *see* 7244
o-[Bis(*p*-hydroxyphenyl)methyl]benzyl
Alcohol *see* 7245
4-[Bis(4-hydroxyphenyl)methylene]-2,5-
cyclohexadien-1-one *see* 881
N,N'-Bis[(2-hydroxyphenyl)methylene]-
1,2-ethanediamine *see* 8322
4,4-Bis[4'-hydroxyphenyl]pentanoic
Acid *see* 3312
3,3-Bis(*p*-hydroxyphenyl)phthalide *see*
7243
2,2-Bis(4-hydroxyphenyl)propane *see*
1297
3,3-Bis(4-hydroxyphenyl)-4,5,6,7-tet-
raiodo-1(3*H*)-isobenzofuranone
Disodium Salt *see* 7263
4-[3,5-Bis(2-hydroxyphenyl)-1*H*-1,2,4-
triazol-1-yl]benzoic Acid *see* 2858
γ,γ-Bis(*p*-hydroxyphenyl)valeric Acid
see 3312
1,4-Bis(3-hydroxypropionyl)piperazine
Dimethanesulfonate *see* 7481
Bis(2-hydroxypropyl)amine *see* 3195
N,N'-(Bis-ω-hydroxypropyl)homopipera-
zine 3,4,5-Trimethoxybenzoate
(Diester) *see* 3200
Bis-(1-hydroxy-2(1*H*)-pyridinethionato-
O,S)zinc *see* 7994
Bisibutiamine *see* 9297
1,2-Bis(4-isobutoxycarbonyloxymeth-
yl-3,5-dioxopiperazin-1-yl)ethane
see 8568
Bis(isonicotinaldoxime 1-Methyl) Ether
Dichloride *see* 6738
2,4-Bis(isopropylamino)-6-chloro-*s*-
triazine *see* 7812
Bis(isopropylamino)fluorophosphine
Oxide *see* 6205
2,4-Bis(isopropylamino)-6-methoxy-*s*-
triazine *see* 7788
2,4-Bis(isopropylamino)-6-(methyl-
thio)-*s*-triazine *see* 7789
Bismark Brown 53 *see* 1252
Bismark Brown R, 1252
Bismark Brown Y, 1253
Bismed [Technilab] *see* 1285
Bis(2-mercaptoethyl)sulfone, 1254
Bis(3-mesyloxypropyl)amine *see* 4927
1,4-Bis(methanesulfonoxy)butane *see*
1505
N,N'-Bis(3-methanesulfonyloxypro-
pionyl)piperazine *see* 7481
Bismethomyl Thioether *see* 9329
Bis(2-methoxyethyl)aminosulfur
Trifluoride *see* 2897
[*N,N''*-Bis[*N*-(2-methoxyethyl)-carbamo-
ylmethyl]diethylenetriamine-*N,N'*,-
N''-triaceto]gadolinium (III) *see* 4329
Bis(2-methoxyethyl) Ether *see* 3165
(*T*-4)-Bis[5-methoxy-2-[(*S*)-[(4-methoxy-
3,5-dimethyl-2-pyridinyl)methyl]-
sulfinyl]-1*H*-benzimidazolato]mag-
nesium *see* 6845
2,4-Bis(4-methoxyphenyl)-1,3,2,4-di-
thiadiphosphetane 2,4-Disulfide *see*
5391
(*E*)-3,4-Bis(*p*-methoxyphenyl)-3-hexene
see 3211
3,4-Bis(4-methoxyphenyl)-5-isoxazole-
acetic Acid *see* 6232
N-[Bis(4-methoxyphenyl)methylene]-
benzenemethanamine *see* 1139

2-[4,5-Bis(4-methoxyphenyl)-2-thiazol-
yl]-1*H*-pyrrole-1-acetic Acid Ethyl Ester *see* 7002
1,4-Bis[(2-methoxy-4-propylphenoxy)-
acetyl]piperazine *see* 8535
Bis(2-methyl-4-amino-6-quinolyl)urea
see 475
Bis(1-methylamyl) Sodium Sulfosuccinate, 1255
Bis(3-methyl-2-butyl)borane *see* 1250
2,3:9,10-Bis(methylenedioxy)-13a-ber-
bine *see* 8858
2,6-Bis(3,4-methylenedioxyphenyl)-3,-
7-dioxabicyclo[3.3.0]octane *see* 8470
Bis[methylenedioxy]protoberberine *see*
2527
α-[2-[Bis(1-methylethyl)amino]ethyl]-α-
(2-methylpropyl)-2-pyridineacetamide
see 7129
N-[2-[Bis(1-methylethyl)amino]ethyl]-2-
oxo-1-pyrrolidineacetamide *see* 7706
α-[2-[Bis(1-methylethyl)amino]ethyl]-α-
phenyl-2-pyridineacetamide *see* 3360
2-[(1*R*)-3-[Bis(1-methylethyl)amino]-1-
phenylpropyl]-4-methylphenol *see*
9525
Bis(1-methylethyl)carbamothioic Acid *S*-
(2,3-Dichloro-2-propenyl) Ester *see*
2970
Bis(1-methylethyl)carbamothioic Acid *S*-
(2,3,3-Trichloro-2-propenyl) Ester
see 9594
2,3:4,5-Bis-*O*-(1-methylethylidene)-β-D-
fructopyranose Sulfamate *see* 9547
1,2:5,6-Bis-*O*-(1-methylethylidene)-D-
glucofuranose *see* 2965
2,3:4,6-Bis-*O*-(methylethylidene)-α-L-
xylo-2-hexulofuranosonic Acid *see*
3199
N,N'-Bis(1-methylethyl)-6-methylthio-1,-
3,5-triazine-2,4-diamine *see* 7789
2,6-Bis(1-methylethyl)phenol *see* 7834
[2,6-Bis(1-methylethyl)phenoxy]meth-
anol Dihydrogen Phosphate *see* 4259
N-[2,6-Bis(1-methylethyl)-4-phenoxy-
phenyl]-*N'*-(1,1-dimethylethyl)thio-
urea *see* 2969
N-[2-[[2,6-Bis(1-methylethyl)phenyl]-
amino]2-oxoethyl]-*N*-(carboxymethyl)glycine *see* 3358
Bis(1-methylethyl)phosphoric Acid 4-
Nitrophenyl Ester *see* 3198
N,N'-Bis(1-methylethyl)phosphorodi-
amidic Fluoride *see* 6205
3,4-Bis(3-methyl-4-hydroxyphenyl)-
hexane *see* 5968
Bis[methylmercapto]methane *see* 1256
1,4-Bis[(4-methylphenyl)amino]-9,10-
anthracenedione *see* 8065
N,N-Bis[*N*-methyl-*N*-phenyl-*tert*-butyl-
acetamido]-β-hydroxyethylamine *see*
6933
Bis(4-methylphenyl)mercury *see* 3381
α-[[Bis(1-methylpropyl)amino]methyl]-1-
[(2-chlorophenyl)methyl]-1*H*-pyrrole-
2-methanol *see* 9981
Bis(2-methylpropyl)carbamothioic Acid
S-Ethyl Ester *see* 1546
1,3-Bis(1-methyl-2-pyrrolidinyl)-2-
propanone *see* 2677
1,4-Bis[3-[(methylsulfonyl)oxy]-1-oxo-
propyl]piperazine *see* 7481
N,N'-Bis(3-methylsulfonyloxypropionyl)-
piperazine *see* 7481
N,N-Bis(3-methylsulfonyloxypropyl)-
amine *see* 4927

(−)-(*R*)-1-[4,4-Bis(3-methyl-2-thienyl)-
3-butenyl]nipecotic Acid *see* 9417
(3*R*)-1-[4,4-Bis(3-methyl-2-thienyl)-3-
butenyl]-3-piperidinecarboxylic
Acid *see* 9417
N,N'-Bis[1-methylthioacetaldehyde *O*-
(*N*-Methylcarbamoyl)oxime]sulfide *see*
9329
Bis-[*O*-(1-methylthioethylimino)-*N*-meth-
ylcarbamic Acid]-*N,N'*-sulfide *see* 9329
Bis[methylthio]methane, 1256
N,N'-Bis[1-methyl-3-(2,2,6-trimethylcy-
clohexyl)propyl]-*N,N'*-dimethyl-1,6-
hexanediamine Bis(methochloride)
see 9653
Bismetin [Mect] *see* 7737
Bisminat [Hek] *see* 1258
Bismite *see* 1273
Bismugel [Biothrax] *see* 1275
Bismutan *see* 1268
Bismuth, 1257
Bismuth Acetate Basic *see* 1281
Bismuth Acetate Oxide *see* 1281
Bismuth Aluminate, 1258
Bismuth Bromide, 1259
Bismuth Bromide Oxide, 1260
Bismuth Butylthiolaurate, 1261
Bismuth Carbonate Oxide (Bi$_2$(CO$_3$)O$_2$)
see 1282
Bismuth Chloride, 1262
Bismuth Chloride Oxide, 1263
Bismuth Ethyl Camphorate, 1264
Bismuth Fluoride, 1265
Bismuth Gallate, Basic *see* 1283
Bismuth Germanate, 1266
Bismuth Germanium Oxide (Bi$_4$Ge$_3$O$_{12}$)
see 1266
Bismuth Hydrate *see* 1267
Bismuth Hydroxide, 1267
Bismuth Hydroxide Nitrate Oxide
(Bi$_5$(OH)$_9$(NO$_3$)$_4$O) *see* 1284
Bismuth(III) Tris(trifluoromethane-
sulfonate) *see* 1292
Bismuthine, 1268
Bismuthinite *see* 1287
Bismuth Iodide, 1269
Bismuth Iodide Oxide, 1270
Bismuth Nitrate, 1271
Bismuth Nitrate Basic *see* 1284
Bismuthous Oxide *see* 1273
Bismuth Oxalate, 1272
Bismuth Oxide, 1273
Bismuth Oxide Acetate *see* 1281
Bismuth Oxybromide *see* 1260
Bismuth Oxycarbonate *see* 1282
Bismuth Oxychloride *see* 1263
Bismuth Oxyiodide *see* 1270
Bismuth Oxynitrate *see* 1284
Bismuth Oxysalicylate *see* 1285
Bismuth Pentafluoride, 1274
"Bismuth Peroxide" *see* 1290
Bismuth Phosphate, 1275
Bismuth Potassium Iodide, 1276
Bismuth Potassium Tartrate, 1277
Bismuth(III) Salt of *d*-Camphoric Acid
Monoethyl Ester *see* 1264
Bismuth Selenide, 1278
Bismuth Sodium Tartrate, 1279
Bismuth Sodium Triglycollamate, 1280
Bismuth Subacetate, 1281
Bismuth "Subbromide" *see* 1260
Bismuth Subcarbonate, 1282
Bismuth "Subchloride" *see* 1263
Bismuth Subgallate, 1283
Bismuth "Subiodide" *see* 1270

Bismuth Subnitrate, 1284
Bismuth Subnitricum *see* 1284
Bismuth Subsalicylate, 1285
Bismuth Sulfate, 1286
Bismuth Sulfide, 1287
Bismuth Tannate, 1288
Bismuth Telluride, 1289
Bismuth Tetrabromopyrocatechol *see* 1199
Bismuth Tetroxide, 1290
Bismuth Tribromide *see* 1259
Bismuth Tribromophenate, 1291
Bismuth Tribromophenol *see* 1291
Bismuth Trichloride *see* 1262
Bismuth Triflate, 1292
Bismuth Trifluoride *see* 1265
Bismuth Trihydride *see* 1268
Bismuth Triiodide *see* 1269
Bismuth Trinitrate *see* 1271
Bismuth Trioxide *see* 1273
Bismuth Triselenide *see* 1278
Bismuth White *see* 1284
Bismuth Yellow *see* 1273
Bismuthyl Acetate *see* 1281
Bismuthyl Bromide *see* 1260
Bismuthyl Chloride *see* 1263
Bismuthyl Iodide *see* 1270
Bismuthyl Nitrate *see* 1284
Bismutite *see* 1282
Bis(1-naphthylmethyl)amine, 1293
1,2-Bis(nicotinamido)propane *see* 6493
sym-Bis(5-nitro-2-furfurylidene)acetone Guanylhydrazone *see* 6654
1,5-Bis(5-nitro-2-furyl)-3-pentadien-one Amidinohydrazone *see* 6654
1,5-Bis(5-nitro-2-furyl)-3-pentadien-one Guanylhydrazone *see* 6654
2,2-Bis[(nitrooxy)methyl]-1,3-propane-diol Dinitrate (Ester) *see* 7112
2,2-Bis[(nitrooxy)methyl]-1,3-propane-diol Mononitrate (Ester) *see* 7138
Bis(3-nitrophenyl)disulfide *see* 6618
N,*N*′-Bis(4-nitrophenyl)urea *see* 3278
N,*N*′-Bis(4-nitrophenyl)urea, Compd with 4,6-Dimethyl-2(1*H*)-pyrimidi-none (1:1) *see* 6494
Bisoctrizole, 1294
1,10-Bis-[4-(octylamino)-1-pyridi-nium]decane *see* 6754
Bisolvon [Thomae] *see* 1391
Bisoprolol, 1295
Bisoxatin Acetate, 1296
D-Bis(*N*-pantothenyl-β-aminoethyl) Disulfide *see* 7012
Bispecia *see* 1261
Bis(pentachloro-2,4-cyclopentadien-1-yl) *see* 3105
Bis(2,4-pentanedionato-*O*,*O*′)nickel *see* 6500
(*T*-4)-Bis(2,4-pentanedionato-O,O′)-beryllium *see* 1163
Bis(2,4-pentanediono)nickel(II) *see* 6500
p-Bis(perchloromethyl)benzene *see* 1303
Bisphenol A, 1297
Bisphenol B, 1298
Bis(phenoxarsin-10-yl)ether *see* 6961
Bis(10-phenoxarsinyl)oxide *see* 6961
Bis(10-phenoxarsyl)oxide *see* 6961
2,4-Bis(4-phenoxyphenyl)-1,3,2,4-di-thiadiphosphetane 2,4-Disulfide *see* 1026
9,10-Bis(phenylethynyl)anthracene, 1299
1,1′-Bis(phenylmethyl)-4,4′-bipyridi-nium *see* 9999

Bis(phenylmethyl) Disulfide *see* 3013
N,*N*′-Bis(phenylmethyl)-1,2-ethanedi-amine *see* 1064
Bis(γ-phenylpropyl)ethylamine *see* 371
4,4′-Bis(3-phenylureido)-2,2′-stilbene-disulfonic Acid Disodium Salt *see* 1315
Bisphonal [Yamanouchi] *see* 4929
N,*N*′-Bis(3-picolyl)-4-methoxyisophthal-amide *see* 7407
Bis(pinacolato)diborane, 1300
(*R*)-Bis(POC)PMPA *see* 9146
Bis(POM)-PMEA *see* 151
Bispyribac, 1301
Bis(pyridine)iodine(1+) Tetrafluorobor-ate(1−) *see* 1302
Bis(pyridine)iodonium Tetrafluorobor-ate, 1302
Bis(2-pyridylthio)zinc 1,1′-Dioxide *see* 7994
Bis(6-quinolyl)urea *see* 3353
[[4-[Bis[4-(sulfophenyl)amino]phenyl]-methylene]-2,5-cyclohexadien-1-yli-dene]amino]benzenesulfonic Acid Disodium Salt *see* 6028
Bissy Nuts *see* 5318
Bis-*N*,*N*,*N*′,*N*′-tetramethylphosphorodi-amidic Anhydride *see* 8395
Biston [Slovakofarma] *see* 1781
Bis(3,5,6-trichloro-2-hydroxyphenyl)-methane *see* 4680
1,4-Bis(trichloromethyl)benzene, 1303
Bis(trifluoroacetoxy)iodobenzene *see* 7295
Bis(trifluoroethyl) Ether *see* 4201
Bis(2,2,2-trifluoroethyl) Ether *see* 4201
(2*R*,4*S*)-4-[(3,5-Bis-trifluoromethyl-benzyl)methoxycarbonylamino]-2-ethyl-6-trifluoromethyl-3,4-dihydro-2*H*-quinoline-1-carboxylic Acid Ethyl Ester *see* 9549
17β-*N*-[2,5-Bis(trifluoromethyl)phen-yl]carbamoyl-4-aza-5α-androst-1-en-3-one *see* 3471
[1*S*-[1α,4β(*Z*),5α,8β]]-4-[2-[2,4-Bis(tri-fluoromethyl)phenyl]ethenyl]-4,8-di-methyl-2,3-dioxabicyclo[3.3.1]-nonan-7-one *see* 814
5-[[(2*R*,3*S*)-2-[(1*R*)-1-[3,5-Bis(trifluoro-methyl)phenyl]ethoxy]-3-(4-fluoro-phenyl)-4-morpholinyl]methyl]-1,2-dihydro-3*H*-1,2,4-triazol-3-one *see* 753
(2*R*)-[(1*R*)-3,5-Bis(trifluoromethyl)-phenylethoxy]-(3*S*)-(4-fluoro)phenyl-4-(3-oxo-1,2,4-triazol-5-yl)methyl-morpholine *see* 753
(2*R*,4*S*)-4-[[[3,5-Bis(trifluoromethyl)-phenyl]methyl](methoxycarbonyl)-amino]-2-ethyl-3,4-dihydro-6-(tri-fluoromethyl)-1(2*H*)-quinolinecar-boxylic Acid Ethyl Ester *see* 9549
(4a*R*,4b*S*,6a*S*,7*S*,9a*S*,9b*S*,11a*R*)-*N*-[2,5-Bis(trifluoromethyl)phenyl]-2,4a,-4b,5,6,6a,7,8,9,9a,9b,10,11,11a-tetra-decahydro-4a,6a-dimethyl-2-oxo-1*H*-indeno[5,4-*f*]quinoline-7-carbox-amide *see* 3471
(1*S*,4*R*,5*R*,8*S*)-4-[(*Z*)-2,4-Bis(trifluoro-methyl)styryl]-4,8-dimethyl-2,3-di-oxabicyclo[3.3.1]nonan-7-one *see* 814
1,5-Bis(α,α,α-trifluoro-*p*-tolyl)-1,4-pentadiene-3-one (1,4,5,6-Tetrahy-dro-5,5-dimethyl-2-pyrimidinyl)-hydrazone *see* 4765

2,2′-Bis[1,6,7-trihydroxy-3-methyl-5-isopropyl-8-aldehydonaphthalene] *see* 4528
Bistrimate [SM & P] *see* 1280
N,*N*′-Bis[3-(3,4,5-trimethoxybenzoyl-oxy)propyl]homopiperazine *see* 3200
1,4-Bis[3-(3,4,5-trimethoxybenzoyl-oxy)propyl]perhydro-1,4-diazepine *see* 3200
1,3-Bis(trimethylamino)-2-propanol Diiodide *see* 7782
α,ω-Bis(trimethylammonium)hexane *see* 4688
N,*N*′-Bis[3-trimethylammoniumphen-oxycarbonyl]-*N*,*N*′-dimethyldeca-methylenediamine Dibromide *see* 2885
Bistrimin *see* 7316
Bis(triphenylphosphine)dicarbonyl-nickel, 1304
Bistrium Bromide [BMS] *see* 4688
Bistrium Chloride [BMS] *see* 4688
Bistyryl *see* 3320
Biterol [Winthrop] *see* 1307
Bitertanol, 1305
Bithin *see* 1306
Bithiodine *see* 9457
Bithionol, 1306
Bithionolate Sodium *see* 1306
Bitin-S [Tanabe Seiyaku] *see* 1306
Bitolterol, 1307
Bitolterol Mesylate *see* 1307
Bitoscanate, 1308
Bitrex [Macfarlan Smith] *see* 2891
Bitriben *see* 1303
Bitrop [Boehringer, Ing.] *see* 5073
α-Bitter Acid *see* 4754
β-Bitter Acid *see* 5612
Bitter-almond-oil Camphor *see* 1093
Bitter Apple *see* 2486
Bitter Ash *see* 3899, 8025
Bitter-bloom *see* 1970
Bitter Cucumber *see* 2486
Bitter Gourd *see* 2486
Bitter Herb *see* 1969
Bitter Orange Peel *see* 6860
Bitter Root *see* 742, 4393
Bitter Salts *see* 5691
Bitter Stick *see* 2064
Bittersweet *see* 3463
Bitter Wintergreen *see* 2057
Bitter Wood *see* 8025
Bitulan [Adroka] *see* 4885
Bitumen *see* 845
Bituminol *see* 4885
Bitumol *see* 4885
Bituvitan [Hishiyama] *see* 8200
Biuret, 1309
Biuretamidine Sulfate *see* 3093
Bivalirudin, 1310
Bivinyl *see* 1509
Bivitasi [ISI] *see* 9296
α-Bixin *see* 1311
β-Bixin *see* 1311
Bixins, 1311
Bizolin [Boehringer, Ing.] *see* 7277
BL-5 *see* 2717
BL-139 *see* 459
BL-191 *see* 7136
BL-4162A *see* 622
BL-5583 *see* 9345
Black and White Bleaching Cream [Plough] *see* 4808
Black Ash *see* 996
Black Balsam *see* 949
Blackberry Bark *see* 8291

Black Cohosh, 1312
Black Copper Oxide *see* 2646
Black Dogwood *see* 4263
Black Hawk *see* 9974
Black Henbane *see* 4859
Black Indian Hemp *see* 743
Black Iron Oxide *see* 4040
Black Lead *see* 4539
Black Leaf 40 *see* 6524
Black Manganese Oxide *see* 5730
Black Mustard *see* 6315
Black Nickel Oxide *see* 6516
Black Pepper, 1313
Black Pepper Oil *see* 1313
Black Phosphorus *see* 7347
Black Root *see* 5442
Black Sea Sterol *see* 3288
Black Snake Root *see* 1312
Blackstrap Molasses, 1314
Black-tang *see* 4282
Black Tea *see* 9088
Black Uranium Oxide *see* 9855
Bladafum [Bayer] *see* 8966
Bladan [Bayer] *see* 9204
Bladder Fucus *see* 4282
Bladderon [Nippon Shinyaku] *see* 4096
Bladder Pod *see* 5550
Bladder-wrack *see* 4282
Bladex [Shell] *see* 2685
Blanc de Perle *see* 1263
Blanc d'Espagne *see* 1263
Blanc Fixe *see* 994
Blancol C *see* 1315
Blankophor R [Bayer], 1315
Blascorid [Guidotti] *see* 1049
Blasticidin S, 1316
Blasting Gelatin *see* 6607
Blasting Oil *see* 6607
Blastmycin *see* 715
Blattanex [Bayer] *see* 7836
Blätteralkohol *see* 4700
Blazer [BASF] *see* 109
Blazing Star *see* 230, 4631
Bleached Beeswax *see* 1020
Bleached Yellow Wax *see* 1020
Bleaching Powder *see* 2094
Blebbistatin, 1317
(−)-Blebbistatin *see* 1317
Bled [Poli] *see* 2265
Bleiweiss (German) *see* 1005
Bleminol [Gepepharm] *see* 279
Blenoxane [BMS] *see* 1318
Bleo [Nippon Kayaku] *see* 1318
Bleomycin A$_2$ *see* 1318
Bleomycins, 1318
Bleph-10 [Allergan] *see* 8899
Blex [Zeneca] *see* 7497
Blistering Beetle *see* 1751
Blistering Fly *see* 1751
Bloat Guard [Phibro] *see* 7562
Blocadren [Merck & Co.] *see* 9444
Blockain Hydrochloride [Sterling Winthrop] *see* 7837
Blocklin L [Shionogi] *see* 7443
Blonanserin, 1319
Blood-coagulation Factor II *see* 7889
Blood-coagulation Factor IIa *see* 9383
Blood-coagulation Factor III *see* 9385
Blood-coagulation Factor V *see* 3919
Blood-coagulation Factor VII *see* 3920
Blood-coagulation Factor VIII *see* 3921
(1-742)-(1637-1648)-Blood Coagulation Factor VIII (Human Reduced) Complex with 1649-2332-Blood Coagulation Factor VIII (Human Reduced) *see* 6271

Blood-coagulation Factor IX *see* 3922
Blood-coagulation Factor X *see* 3923
Blood-coagulation Factor XI *see* 3924
Blood-coagulation Factor XII *see* 3925
Blood-coagulation Factor XIII *see* 3926
Blood-coagulation Factor XIV *see* 7884
Bloodroot *see* 8355
Blood Sugar *see* 4459
Blox [Biomed. Foscama] *see* 5571
BL-P-1322 *see* 1984
BL-S578 *see* 1913
BL-S640 *see* 1915
BL-S786 *see* 1931
Blue Asbestos *see* 826
Blue Cohosh, 1320
Bluestone *see* 2653
Blue Tetrazolium *see* 9244
Blue Vitriol *see* 2653
Blusalt *see* 8599
Blutene [Abbott] *see* 9520
BM-21.0955 *see* 4873
BM-102 *see* 819
BM-02015 *see* 9552
BM-06022 *see* 8161
BM-13505 *see* 2806
BM-14190 *see* 1873
BM-15075 *see* 1195
BM-15100 *see* 7418
BM-51052 *see* 1778
BMC *see* 1791
BMD [Alpharma] *see* 935
BMIM *see* 1581
BMP-2A *see* 1331
BMP-7 *see* 1331
BMPs *see* 1331
BMS *see* 1254
BMS-180549 *see* 4065
BMS-181173 *see* 4582
BMS-182751 *see* 8384
BMS-186295 *see* 5083
BMS-186716 *see* 6843
BMS-188667 *see* 4
BMS-200475 *see* 3595
BMS-207147 *see* 8121
BMS-217380-01 *see* 9178
BMS-224818 *see* 1024
BMS-232632 *see* 858
BMS-247550 *see* 5249
BMS-284756 *see* 4369
BMS-298585 *see* 6303
BMS-354825 *see* 2829
BMY-13754 *see* 6438
BMY-26517 *see* 7078
BMY-26538-01 *see* 622
BMY-27857 *see* 8803
BMY-28100 *see* 1942
BMY-28100-03-800 *see* 1942
BMY-28142 *see* 1922
BMY-28167 *see* 1942
BMY-28488 *see* 1920
BMY-30056 *see* 4593
BMY-33419 *see* 9178
BMY-40481 *see* 3886
BMY-40900 *see* 3098
BMY-41606 *see* 9934
BMY-45594 *see* 8384
B-mycin *see* 1356
BN-1270 *see* 2264
BN-52020 *see* 4426
BN-52021 *see* 4426
BN-52022 *see* 4426
B-Nine [Uniroyal] *see* 2810
BNP *see* 1360
BNP-166 *see* 3870
BO-714 *see* 2320

Bobierrite *see* 5683
Boc-β-Ala-Trp-Met-Asp-Phe(NH$_2$) *see* 7113
B.O.E.A. *see* 3770
Boehmite *see* 356
Boettger's Paper *see* 256
Boforsin (obsolete) *see* 2476
Bog Bean *see* 5842
Bogomolets' Serum *see* 718
Bohrium, 1321
BOL-148 *see* 1423
Bolandiol, 1322
Bolasterone, 1323
Boldea *see* 1326
Boldenone, 1324
Boldenone Undecylenate *see* 1324
Boldine, 1325
Boldine Dimethyl Ether *see* 4436
Boldo, 1326
Boldoa *see* 1326
Boldu *see* 1326
Boldus *see* 1326
Bole, Armenian, 1327
Bolecic Acid *see* 5103
Boleko Oil, 1328
Boletic Acid *see* 4287
Bolstar [Miles] *see* 8990
Bolus Alba *see* 5282
Bolus Armena *see* 1327
Bolus Rubra *see* 1327
Bolvidon [Organon] *see* 6172
Bombesin, 1329
Bomyl [Hopkins], 1330
Bonadorm [Smith & Nephew] *see* 3046
Bonaid [Norwich] *see* 1500
Bonalon [Merck & Co.] *see* 229
Bonamid [Heilmittelwerke] *see* 901
Bonamine [Pfizer] *see* 5777
Bonanza [Novartis Agro] *see* 2771
Bonasanit [Weimer] *see* 7982
Bondou *see* 8382
Bondronat [Roche] *see* 4873
Bonealfa [Teijin] *see* 9022
"Bone Ash" *see* 1694
Bonefos [Schering AG] *see* 2371
Bone Gla Protein *see* 6894
Bone Morphogenetic Protein 2 (Human Recombinant RhBMP-2) *see* 1331
Bone Morphogenetic Proteins, 1331
Bone Morphogenic Factors *see* 1331
Bone Morphogenic Proteins *see* 1331
Boneset *see* 3902
Bongast *see* 1283
Bongkrekic Acid, 1332
Bonicor [Farmetrusca] *see* 7886
Bonidon [Mepha] *see* 4968
Bonifen [Merck KGaA] *see* 7996
Bonine [Insight] *see* 5777
Boniva [Roche] *see* 4873
Bonoform *see* 9189
Bonopen [Belupo] *see* 5925
Bonpac [Hoei] *see* 4231
Bonpyrin [Takeda] *see* 3350
Bonviva [Roche] *see* 4873
Bonyl [Erco] *see* 6417
Bonzi [Syngenta] *see* 6984
Bonzol [Tokyo Tanabe] *see* 2812
Bopindolol, 1333
Boracic Acid *see* 1336
Borax *see* 8590
Borax Glass *see* 8590
Borazane *see* 1334
Borazine, 1334
Borazole *see* 1334
Borazon *see* 1346

Bor-Cefazol [Proter] *see* 1917
Bordeaux Mixture, 1335
Borgal [Intervet] *see* 8906
Boric Acid, 1336
Boric Acid Trimethyl Ester *see* 9712
Boric Anhydride, 1337
Boric Oxide *see* 1337
endo-2-Bornanol *see* 1338
exo-2-Bornanol *see* 5128
2-Bornanone *see* 1732
Borneo Camphor *see* 1338
Borneol, 1338
Borneol Acetate *see* 1339
Borneol Salicylate *see* 1341
Bornite *see* 2038, 2519
Bornyl Acetate, 1339
Bornyl Alcohol *see* 1338
Bornyl Chloride, 1340
Bornyl Salicylate, 1341
Borobutane *see* 9183
Boroethane *see* 3015
Borofax [Burroughs Wellcome] *see* 1336
Borofluoric Acid *see* 4149
Borohexane *see* 4676
Boromycin, 1342
Boron, 1343
Boron Carbide, 1344
Boron Chloride *see* 3016
Boron Fluoride Etherate *see* 1350
Boron Fluoride Ethyl Ether *see* 1350
Boron Lithium Oxide ($B_4Li_2O_7$) *see* 5524
Boron Monoxide, 1345
Boron Nitride, 1346
Boron Oxide *see* 1337
Boron Oxide (BO) *see* 1345
Boron Sesquioxide *see* 1337
Boron Sodium Oxide ($B_4Na_2O_7$) *see* 8590
Boron Tribromide, 1347
Boron Trichloride, 1348
Boron Trifluoride, 1349
Boron Trifluoride Etherate, 1350
Boron Trioxide *see* 1337
Bortezomib, 1351
Boscalid, 1352
Bosentan, 1353
Bostrycoidin, 1354
β-Boswellic Acid, 1355
Bothrops atrox Serine Proteinase *see* 1010
Bothrops Venom Proteinase *see* 1010
BoTox [Allergan] *see* 1357
Botrilex [Bayer] *see* 8080
Botropase [Ravizza] *see* 1010
Bottromycin A$_2$ Acid Methyl Ester *see* 1356
Bottromycin, 1356
Bottromycin A$_2$ *see* 1356
Botulin A *see* 1357
Botulin B *see* 1357
Botulin Toxins, 1357
Botulinum Toxins *see* 1357
Botulinum Toxin Type A *see* 1357
Botulinum Toxin Type B *see* 1357
Botulinus Toxins *see* 1357
Bouncing Bet *see* 8363
Bourbonal *see* 3859
Bovatec *see* 5373
Bovilene [Syntex] *see* 3995
Bovine Somatotropin *see* 8716
Bovine Thymosin α1 *see* 9405
Bo-Xan *see* 10063
Boxer [Dow AgroSci.] *see* 4108
Boxogetten [Cheplapharm] *see* 7307
Boxol [Pharmacia & Upjohn] *see* 2805
BP-662 *see* 4084

BP-1137 *see* 3940
BPAA *see* 3951
BPD-MA *see* 9967
BPEA *see* 1299
BPI *see* 938
B$_2$pin$_2$ *see* 1300
BPM *see* 1237
BPPS *see* 7808
BQ 22-708 *see* 3577
BQC Reagent *see* 3026
BR *see* 939
BR-18 *see* 7483
BR-700 *see* 4003
BRA *see* 8157
Bradosol [Novartis] *see* 1059, 3415
Bradycor [Cortech], 1358
Bradykinin, 1359
Bradyl [Lafon] *see* 6347
Brain-derived Neurotrophic Factor *see* 6487
Brain Natriuretic Factor *see* 1360
Brain Natriuretic Peptide, 1360
Brain Sugar *see* 4335
Brallobarbital, 1361
Branching Factor *see* 8023
Brandy, 1362
Brandy Mint *see* 7145
Branigen [GSK] *see* 84
Brantur [Dong-A] *see* 6200
Brasilin *see* 1367
Brassard's Diene, 1363
Brassel [Searle] *see* 2319
Brassicol [Hoechst] *see* 8080
Brassidic Acid, 1364
Brassinolide, 1365
Bratenol [Elmu] *see* 7495
Braunite *see* 5723
Braunol [Braun Melsungen] *see* 7698
Braunosan H [Braun Melsungen] *see* 7698
Bravo [Syngenta] *see* 2166
Braxin C *see* 7930
Brayera, 1366
Brazilin, 1367
Brazil Powder *see* 768
Brazil Wax *see* 1846
Brazil Wood *see* 7181
Brazzos [Spiess-Urania] *see* 4908
BrdUrd *see* 1452
Bredereck's Reagent, 1368
Bredinin [Toyo Jozo] *see* 6222
Bredon [Organon] *see* 6944
Brefeldin A, 1369
Brek [Irbi] *see* 5571
Brelomax [Abbott] *see* 9811
Bremax [Abbott] *see* 9811
Bremen Blue *see* 2631
Bremen Green *see* 2631
Bremfol *see* 6555
Bremil *see* 4781
Brenal [Tanabe Seiyaku] *see* 5780
Brendil [Daiichi] *see* 2291
Brentan [Janssen] *see* 6178
Brenzschleimsäure (German) *see* 4307
Brenztraubensäure (German) *see* 8021
Breokinase [Sanofi Winthrop] *see* 9887
Breon *see* 7586
Brequinar, 1370
Brestan [Hoechst] *see* 9745
Brethaire [Novartis] *see* 9159
Brethine [Novartis] *see* 9159
Bretylate [GSK] *see* 1371
Bretylium Tosylate, 1371
Bretylol [GSK] *see* 1371
Brevetoxin A *see* 1372
Brevetoxin B *see* 1372

Brevetoxin C *see* 1372
Brevetoxins, 1372
Brevibloc [Ohmeda] *see* 3700
Brevicid [AWD] *see* 10061
Brevicidin *see* 9836
Brevicon [Watson] *see* 6697
Brevidil M [M & B] *see* 8874
Brevifolin *see* 10067
Brevimytal Sodium [Lilly] *see* 5981
Brevinarcon [Heyden] *see* 9323
Brevital [Lilly] *see* 5981
Brevital Sodium [Lilly] *see* 5981
Brevium *see* 7883
Brevoxyl [Stiefel] *see* 1116
Brexin [Chiesi] *see* 7506
Brezal [Novartis] *see* 2205
Bricanyl [AstraZeneca] *see* 9159
Bricef [BMS] *see* 1915
Briem [Fabre] *see* 1031
Brietal Sodium [Lilly] *see* 5981
Brigade [FMC] *see* 1209
Brigham Tea *see* 3607
Brij [ICI] *see* 7577
Brij 58 [ICI] *see* 7577
Brilliant Blue FCF, 1373
Brilliant Congo R *see* 10012
Brilliant Cotton Blue *see* 6028
Brilliant Green, 1374
Brilliant Vital Red *see* 10012
Brimonidine, 1375
Brimstone *see* 8969
Brinaldix [Novartis] *see* 2393
Brinzolamide, 1376
Briofil [Alfa] *see* 955
Bripadon *see* 4161
Briplatin [BMS] *see* 2317
Brisfirina [BMS] *see* 1984
Brispen *see* 3084
Bristacin [BMS] *see* 8252
Bristamox [BMS] *see* 577
Bristamycin [BMS] *see* 3687
Bristocef [BMS] *see* 1984
Bristopen [BMS] *see* 6904
Britaject [Britannia] *see* 746
British Anti-lewisite *see* 3209
British Gum *see* 2953
BritLofex [Britannia] *see* 5558
Brivaracetam, 1377
Brivex [Menarini] *see* 1378
Brivirac [Menarini] *see* 1378
Brivudin *see* 1378
Brivudine, 1378
BRL-284 *see* 7817
BRL-804 *see* 4672
BRL-1241 *see* 5969
BRL-1341 *see* 586
BRL-1400 *see* 6904
BRL-1621 *see* 2419
BRL-1702 *see* 3084
BRL-2039 *see* 4111
BRL-2064 *see* 1792
BRL-2288 *see* 9428
BRL-2333 *see* 577
BRL-2351 *see* 910
BRL-3475 *see* 1792
BRL-4910A *see* 6302
BRL-8988 *see* 9033
BRL-14777 *see* 6343
BRL-17421 *see* 9137
BRL-24924 *see* 8135
BRL-26921 *see* 674
BRL-29060 *see* 7043
BRL-34915 *see* 5460
BRL-38227 *see* 5460
BRL-38705 *see* 3637

BRL-39123 *see* 7083
BRL-39123A *see* 7083
BRL-42810 *see* 3929
BRL-43694A *see* 4536
BRL-49653 *see* 8265
BRL-49653c *see* 8265
Broact [Shionogi] *see* 1940
Broadstrike [Dow AgroSci.] *see* 4141
Brocasipal *see* 6879
Brochantite *see* 2654
Brocide *see* 3797
Brocillin *see* 7817
Brockmann Aluminum Oxide *see* 356
Brodiar [Intervet] *see* 1453
Brodifacoum, 1379
Brodimoprim, 1380
Broflex [Bioglan] *see* 9695
Brolene Drops [RPR] *see* 7797
Brolene Ointment [RPR] *see* 3024
Brolitène [Lab. Medicia] *see* 4893
Bromacil, 1381
Bromadal *see* 1831
Bromadiolone, 1382
Bromadryl [Spofa] *see* 3556
Bromal, 1383
Bromal Hydrate, 1384
Bromallylene *see* 288
Bromanautine *see* 1418
Bromat *see* 2025
Bromated Camphor *see* 1414
Bromazepam, 1385
Bromazine *see* 1418
Bromchlophos *see* 6358
Bromcholitin *see* 4436
Bromcresol Green, 1386
Bromcresol Purple, 1387
Bromdiphenhydramine *see* 1418
Bromelain, 1388
Bromelia *see* 3752
Bromelin *see* 1388
Brometazepam *see* 5920
Bromethalin, 1389
Brometone *see* 9611
Bromex *see* 6358
Bromfenac, 1390
Bromhexine, 1391
Bromic Acid, 1392
Bromic Ether *see* 3771
Brominal *see* 1441
Brominated Biphenyls *see* 7563
Bromindione, 1393
Bromine, 1394
Bromine Cyanide *see* 2693
Bromine Pentafluoride, 1395
Bromine Trifluoride, 1396
Bromisoval *see* 1397
Bromisovalum, 1397
N-Bromoacetamide, 1398
p-Bromoacetanilide, 1399
4'-Bromoacetanilide *see* 1399
Bromoacetic Acid, 1400
Bromoacetone, 1401
ω-Bromoacetophenone, 1402
p-Bromoacetophenone, 1403
α-Bromoallyl Bromide *see* 3025
2-Bromoallyl Bromide *see* 3025
5-(2-Bromoallyl)-5-isopropylbarbituric
   Acid *see* 7796
5-Bromo-2-aminobenzoic Acid *see* 1405
Bromoanilide *see* 1399
p-Bromoaniline, 1404
4-Bromoaniline *see* 1404
p-Bromoanisole *see* 1428
5-Bromoanthranilic Acid, 1405
Bromoantifebrin *see* 1399

Bromo-Benadryl *see* 1418
Bromobenzene, 1406
α-Bromobenzeneacetonitrile *see* 1412
4-Bromobenzeneamine *see* 1404
N-p-Bromobenzenesulfonyl-*N'*-[2-[[[2-
   [(aminoiminomethyl)amino]-4-thi-
   azolyl]methyl]thio]ethyl]formamidine
   see 3485
p-Bromobenzenesulfonyl Chloride, 1407
β-(*p*-Bromobenzhydryloxy)ethyldi-
   methylamine *see* 1418
p-Bromobenzoic Acid, 1408
p-Bromobenzyl Bromide, 1409
p-Bromobenzyl Chloride, 1410
p-Bromobenzyl Chloroformate, 1411
α-Bromobenzyl Cyanide, 1412
(*o*-Bromobenzyl)ethyldimethylam-
   monium *p*-Toluenesulfonate *see* 1371
3-[3-(4'-Bromo[1,1'-biphenyl]-4-yl)-3-
   hydroxy-1-phenylpropyl]-4-hydr-
   oxy-2*H*-1-benzopyran-2-one *see* 1382
3-[3-(4'-Bromo[1,1'-biphenyl]-4-yl)-1,2,-
   3,4-tetrahydro-1-naphthalenyl]-4-
   hydroxy-2*H*-1-benzopyran-2-one *see*
   1379
3-[3-(4'-Bromo[1,1'-biphenyl]-4-yl)-1,2,-
   3,4-tetrahydro-1-naphthalenyl]-4-
   hydroxy-2*H*-1-benzothiopyran-2-one
   see 3139
3-[3-(4'-Bromobiphenyl-4-yl)-1,2,3,4-tet-
   rahydro-1-naphthyl]-4-hydroxy-
   coumarin *see* 1379
3-Bromo-*d*-2-bornanone *see* 1414
1-Bromo-4-(bromomethyl)benzene *see*
   1409
2-Bromo-2-(bromomethyl)glutaronitrile
   see 3021
2-Bromo-2-(bromomethyl)pentanedi-
   nitrile *see* 3021
2-Bromo-1-(4-bromophenyl)ethanone *see*
   1427
4-Bromo-α-(4-bromophenyl)-α-hydroxy-
   benzeneacetic Acid 1-Methyl Ethyl
   Ester *see* 1434
1-Bromobutane *see* 1553
2-Bromobutane *see* 1554
Bromobutanedioic Acid *see* 1437
2-Bromobutanoic Acid *see* 1413
5-Bromo-3-*sec*-butyl-6-methyluracil *see*
   1381
α-Bromobutyric Acid, 1413
dl-2-Bromobutyric Acid *see* 1413
α-Bromo-*d*-camphor *see* 1414
α'-Bromo-*d*-camphor *see* 1414
3-Bromo-*d*-camphor, 1414
3α-Bromo-*d*-camphor *see* 1414
3β-Bromo-*d*-camphor *see* 1414
α-Bromo-*n*-caproic Acid, 1415
p-Bromocarbanil *see* 1430
α-Bromo-*p*-chloroacetophenone *see* 2153
2-Bromo-4'-chloroacetophenone *see* 2153
7-Bromo-6-chlorofebrifugine *see* 4596
rel-7-Bromo-6-chloro-3-[3-[(2*R*,3*S*)-3-
   hydroxy-2-piperidinyl]-2-oxopropyl]-
   4(3*H*)-quinazolinone *see* 4596
(±)-*trans*-7-Bromo-6-chloro-3-[3-(3-
   hydroxy-2-piperidyl)acetonyl]-4(3*H*)-
   quinazolinone *see* 4596
5-Bromo-4-chloro-1*H*-indol-3-yl β-D-
   Galactopyranoside *see* 10074
1-Bromo-4-(chloromethyl)benzene *see*
   1410
7-Bromo-5-(2-chlorophenyl)-2,3-dihy-
   dro-2-(methoxymethyl)-1-methyl-
   1*H*-1,4-benzodiazepine *see* 5920

2-Bromo-1-(4-chlorophenyl)ethanone *see*
   2153
4-Bromo-2-(4-chlorophenyl)-1-(ethoxymethyl)-5-(trifluoromethyl)-1*H*-pyr-
   role-3-carbonitrile *see* 2088
5-Bromo-*N*-(4-chlorophenyl)-2-hydroxy-
   benzamide *see* 1435
2-Bromo-4-(*o*-chlorophenyl)-9-methyl-
   6*H*-thieno[3,2-f]-*s*-triazolo[4,3-*a*][1,4]-
   diazepine *see* 1450
2-Bromo-4-(*o*-chlorophenyl)-9-methyl-
   6*H*-thieno[3,2-*f*][1,2,4]triazolo[4,3-*a*]-
   [1,4]diazepine *see* 1450
8-Bromo-6-(*o*-chlorophenyl)-1-methyl-
   4*H*-*s*-triazolo[3,4-*c*]thieno[2,3-*e*]-1,4-
   diazepine *see* 1450
O-(4-Bromo-2-chlorophenyl)phosphoro-
   thioic Acid *O*-Ethyl *S*-Propyl Ester *see*
   7770
5-Bromo-4'-chlorosalicylanilide *see* 1435
p-Bromo-α-chlorotoluene *see* 1410
Bromochlorotrifluoroethane *see* 4603
2-Bromo-2-chloro-1,1,1-trifluoroethane
   see 4603
Bromocriptine, 1416
Bromocyclohexane *see* 2730
Bromocyl *see* 1436
5-Bromo-2'-deoxyuridine *see* 1452
p-Bromo-*N*-[[[2-[[[2-[(diaminomethylene)amino]-4-thiazolyl]methyl]thio]-
   ethyl]amino]methylene]benzenesulfon-
   amide *see* 3485
Bromodichloromethane, 1417
O-(4-Bromo-2,5-dichlorophenyl)-*O,O*-
   dimethylphosphorothioate *see* 1431
O-(4-Bromo-2,5-dichlorophenyl) *O*-
   Methyl Phenylphosphonothioate *see*
   5445
1-[[4-Bromo-2-(2,4-dichlorophenyl)-
   tetrahydro-2-furanyl]methyl]-1*H*-
   1,2,4-triazole *see* 1446
1-[(2*RS*,4*RS*;2*RS*,4*SR*)-4-Bromo-2-(2,4-
   dichlorophenyl)tetrahydrofurfuryl]-
   1*H*-1,2,4-triazole *see* 1446
(8β)-2-Bromo-9,10-didehydro-*N,N*-di-
   ethyl-6-methylergoline-8-carboxamide
   see 1423
Bromodiethylacetylcarbamide *see* 1831
Bromodiethylacetylurea *see* 1831
2-Bromo-*N,N*-diethyl-D-lysergamide *see*
   1423
2-Bromo-6β,9-difluoro-11β,17,21-trihy-
   droxypregna-1,4-diene-3,20-dione
   17,21-Diacetate *see* 4599
8-Bromo-3,7-dihydro-1,3-dimethyl-1*H*-
   purine-2,6-dione Compd with 2-
   Amino-2-methyl-1-propanol (1:1)
   see 7000
(3α,14β,16α)-11-Bromo-14,15-dihydro-
   14-hydroxyeburnamenine-14-car-
   boxylic Acid Methyl Ester *see* 1451
5-Bromo-*N*-(4,5-dihydro-1*H*-imidazol-
   2-yl)-6-quinoxalinamine *see* 1375
7-Bromo-1,3-dihydro-5-(2-pyridinyl)-
   2*H*-1,4-benzodiazepin-2-one *see* 1385
5-Bromo-*N*,2-dihydroxybenzamide *see*
   1436
4'-Bromo-2,6-dihydroxybenzanilide *see*
   8154
4-Bromo-2,5-dimethoxybenzene-
   ethanamine *see* 1908
4-Bromo-2,5-dimethoxyphenethyl-
   amine *see* 1908
4-[(2-Bromo-4,5-dimethoxyphenyl)-
   methyl]-4-[2-[2-(6,6-dimethylbicy-

clo[3.1.1]hept-2-yl)ethoxy]ethyl]-
morpholinium Bromide *see* 7441

5-[(4-Bromo-3,5-dimethoxyphenyl)-
methyl]-2,4-pyrimidinediamine *see*
1380

2-[*p*-Bromo-α-(2-dimethylaminoethyl)-
benzyl]pyridine *see* 1443

α-Bromo-β-dimethylpropanoylurea *see*
1397

*N*¹-(5-Bromo-4,6-dimethyl-2-pyrimidi-
nyl)sulfanilamide *see* 8898

5-Bromo-4,6-dimethyl-2-sulfanilamido-
pyrimidine *see* 8898

Bromodiphenhydramine, 1418

1-(2-Bromo-1,2-diphenylethenyl)-4-
ethylbenzene *see* 1448

2-[1-(4-Bromodiphenyl)ethoxy]-*N*,*N*-
dimethylethylamine *see* 3556

α-Bromo-α,β-diphenyl-β-(*p*-ethyl-
phenyl)ethylene *see* 1448

1-Bromododecane *see* 5389

Bromoeosine *see* 3603

2-Bromoergocryptine *see* 1416

α-Bromo-α-ergokryptin *see* 1416

Bromoethane *see* 3771

2-Bromoethanol *see* 3792

5-[(1*E*)-2-Bromoethenyl]-2′-deoxyuridine
see 1378

β-Bromoethyl Alcohol *see* 3792

(α-Bromo-α-ethylbutyryl)carbamide *see*
1831

(α-Bromo-α-ethylbutyryl)urea *see* 1831

trans-3-Bromo-*N*-ethylcinnamamide *see*
2311

2-Bromo-*N*-ethyl-*N*,*N*-dimethylbenzene-
methanaminium Salt with 4-Methyl-
benzenesulfonic Acid (1:1) *see* 1371

1-Bromo-2-(4-ethylphenyl)-1,2-diphen-
ylethene *see* 1448

1-Bromo-2-(*p*-ethylphenyl)-1,2-diphen-
ylethylene *see* 1448

3-Bromo-*N*-[[(2*S*)-1-ethyl-2-pyrrolidin-
yl]methyl]-2,6-dimethoxybenzamide
see 8132

Bromofenofos, 1419

Bromofluoresceic Acid *see* 3603

10-Bromo-11b-(2-fluorophenyl)-2,3,7,-
11b-tetrahydrooxazolo[3,2-*d*][1,4]-
benzodiazepin-6(5*H*)-one *see* 4604

Bromoform, 1420

1-Bromo-1,1,2,2,3,3,4,4,5,5,6,6,7,7,8,8,-
8-heptadecafluorooctane *see* 7156

2-Bromohexanoic Acid *see* 1415

4-Bromo-α-hydroxybenzeneacetic Acid
see 1424

(5′α)-2-Bromo-12′-hydroxy-2′-(1-methyl-
ethyl)-5′-(2-methylpropyl)ergotaman-
3′,6′,18-trione *see* 1416

α-(3-Bromo-4-hydroxy-*m*-tolyl)-α-(3-
bromo-5-methyl-4-oxo-2,5-cyclohexa-
dien-1-ylidene)-*o*-toluenesulfonic
Acid *see* 1387

5-Bromo-6-(2-imidazolin-2-ylamino)-
quinoxaline *see* 1375

2-Bromoisobutane *see* 1555

α-Bromoisobutyric Acid, 1421

1-Bromo-4-isocyanatobenzene *see* 1430

2-Bromoisopentane *see* 603

α-Bromoisovaleric Acid, 1422

(α-Bromoisovaleryl)urea *see* 1397

Bromol *see* 9613

Bromo-LSD *see* 1423

ᴅ-2-Bromolysergic Acid Diethylamide
see 1423

Bromolysergide, 1423

p-Bromomandelic Acid, 1424

[[[(3-Bromomesityl)carbamoyl]methyl]-
imino]diacetic Acid *see* 5772

Bromomethane 6029

(Bromomethyl)benzene *see* 1128

1-Bromo-3-methylbenzene *see* 1439

p-Bromo-α-methylbenzhydryl 2-Dimeth-
ylaminoethyl Ether *see* 3556

1-Bromo-2-methylbutane *see* 601

ʟ-1-Bromo-2-methylbutane *see* 601

1-Bromo-3-methylbutane *see* 5114

2-Bromo-2-methylbutane *see* 603

2-Bromo-3-methylbutanoic Acid *see* 1422

1-(Bromomethyl)-3-methylbenzene *see*
10090

5-Bromo-6-methyl-3-(1-methylpropyl)-
2,4(1*H*,3*H*)-pyrimidinedione *see* 1381

5-Bromo-6-methyl-3-(1-methylpropyl)-
uracil *see* 1381

2-[(*p*-Bromo-α-methyl-α-phenylbenzyl)-
oxy]-*N*,*N*-dimethylethylamine *see* 3556

1-Bromo-2-methylpropane *see* 5135

2-Bromo-2-methylpropane *see* 1555

2-Bromo-2-methylpropanoic Acid *see*
1421

α-Bromonaphthalene *see* 1425

β-Bromonaphthalene *see* 1426

1-Bromonaphthalene, 1425

2-Bromonaphthalene, 1426

Bromone [Lipha] *see* 1382

8β-[(5-Bromonicotinoyloxy)methyl]-1,6-
dimethyl-10α-methoxyergoline *see*
6496

2-Bromo-2-nitro-1,3-propanediol *see*
1447

β-Bromo-β-nitrotrimethyleneglycol *see*
1447

1-Bromooctane *see* 6764

2-Bromooctane *see* 6765

1-Bromopentane *see* 602

Bromoperfluorooctane *see* 7156

p-Bromophenacyl Bromide, 1427

p-Bromophenetole *see* 1428

Bromophenol, 1428

m-Bromophenol *see* 1428

o-Bromophenol *see* 1428

p-Bromophenol *see* 1428

Bromophenophos, 1419

N-(4-Bromophenyl)acetamide *see* 1399

α-Bromophenylacetonitrile *see* 1412

2-(*p*-Bromo-α-phenylbenzyloxy)-*N*,*N*-
dimethylethylamine *see* 1418

4-Bromophenylcarbimide *see* 1430

p-Bromophenylcarbonimide *see* 1430

N-(4-Bromophenyl)-2,6-dihydroxybenz-
amide *see* 8154

γ-(4-Bromophenyl)-*N*,*N*-dimethyl-2-pyri-
dinepropanamine *see* 1443

(*Z*)-3-(4-Bromophenyl)-*N*,*N*-dimethyl-3-
(3-pyridinyl)-2-propen-1-amine *see*
10126

2-(4-Bromophenyl)-1,3-dioxohydrin-
dene *see* 1393

1-(4-Bromophenyl)ethanone *see* 1403

2-Bromo-1-phenylethanone *see* 1402

(2*E*)-3-(3-Bromophenyl)-*N*-ethyl-2-
propenamide *see* 2311

p-Bromophenylglycolic Acid *see* 1424

p-Bromophenylhydrazine, 1429

3-[α-[*p*-(*p*-Bromophenyl)-β-hydroxy-
phenethyl]benzyl]-4-hydroxycoumarin
see 1382

4-[4-(*p*-Bromophenyl)-4-hydroxypiperi-
dino]-4′-fluorobutyrophenone *see* 1442

4-[4-(4-Bromophenyl)-4-hydroxy-1-pip-
eridinyl]-1-(4-fluorophenyl)-1-buta-
none *see* 1442

2-(4-Bromophenyl)-1*H*-indene-1,3(2*H*)-
dione *see* 1393

p-Bromophenyl Isocyanate, 1430

3-(*p*-Bromophenyl)-1-methoxy-1-methyl-
urea *see* 6142

N′-(4-Bromophenyl)-*N*-methoxy-*N*-meth-
ylurea *see* 6142

1-(*p*-Bromophenyl)-1-phenyl-1-(2-di-
methylaminoethoxy)ethane *see* 3556

2-[1-(4-Bromophenyl)-1-phenylethoxy]-
N,*N*-dimethylethanamine *see* 3556

[2-(1-*p*-Bromophenyl-1-phenylethoxy)-
ethyl]dimethylamine *see* 3556

2-[(4-Bromophenyl)phenylmethoxy]-
N,*N*-dimethylethanamine *see* 1418

(*Z*)-3-(4′-Bromophenyl)-3-(3″-pyridyl)-
dimethylallylamine *see* 10126

1-(*p*-Bromophenyl)-1-(2-pyridyl)-3-
dimethylaminopropane *see* 1443

3-(*p*-Bromophenyl)-3-(2-pyridyl)-*N*,*N*-
dimethylpropylamine *see* 1443

Bromophos, 1431

Bromophos-ethyl *see* 1431

Bromophos-methyl *see* 1431

Bromopride, 1432

1-Bromopropane *see* 7845

2-Bromopropane *see* 5210

3-Bromopropanoic Acid *see* 1433

2-Bromopropanoic Acid Ethyl Ester *see*
3772

1-Bromo-2-propanone *see* 1401

3-Bromo-1-propene *see* 288

5-(2-Bromo-2-propenyl)-5-(1-methyl-
ethyl)-2,4,6(1*H*,3*H*,5*H*)pyrimidine-
trione *see* 7796

5-(2-Bromo-2-propenyl)-5-(2-propenyl)-
2,4,6(1*H*,3*H*,5*H*)-pyrimidinetrione *see*
1361

β-Bromopropionic Acid, 1433

Bromopropylate, 1434

3-Bromopropylene *see* 288

7-Bromo-5-(2-pyridyl)-3*H*-1,4-benzodi-
azepin-2(1*H*)-one *see* 1385

5-Bromo-2,4(1*H*,3*H*)-pyrimidinedione
see 1440

1-Bromo-2,5-pyrrolidinedione *see* 1438

4′-Bromo-γ-resorcylanilide *see* 8154

Bromosalicylchloranilide, 1435

5-Bromosalicylhydroxamic Acid, 1436

N-5-Bromosalicyloyl-*p*-chloroaniline *see*
1435

Bromosuccinic Acid, 1437

N-Bromosuccinimide, 1438

5-Bromosulfamethazine *see* 8898

Bromosulfophthalein *see* 8954

2-Bromo-1,1,1,2-tetrafluoroethane *see*
9110

8-Bromotheophylline Compd with 2-
Amino-2-methyl-1-propanol (1:1) *see*
7000

Bromotiren *see* 3030

Bromotoluene, 1439

α-Bromotoluene *see* 1128

ω-Bromotoluene *see* 1128

m-Bromotoluene *see* 1439

o-Bromotoluene *see* 1439

p-Bromotoluene *see* 1439

3-Bromotoluene *see* 1439

α-Bromo-α-tolunitrile *see* 1412

N-(3-Bromo-2,4,6-trimethylacetani-
lide)iminodiacetic Acid *see* 5772

3-Bromo-1,7,7-trimethylbicyclo[2.2.1]-
heptan-2-one *see* 1414

N-[2-[(3-Bromo-2,4,6-trimethylphenyl)-amino]-2-oxoethyl]-N-(carboxymethyl)glycine *see* 5772
5-Bromouracil, 1440
5-Bromouracil Deoxyriboside *see* 1452
4-(6-Bromoveratryl)-4-[2-[2-(6,6-dimethyl-2-norpinyl)ethoxy]ethyl]-morpholinium Bromide *see* 7441
cis-11-Bromovincamine *see* 1451
5-Bromovinyl-araU *see* 8727
(*E*)-5-(2-Bromovinyl)-2'-deoxyuridine *see* 1378
α-Bromo-*m*-xylene *see* 10090
ω-Bromo-*m*-xylene *see* 10090
Bromoxynil, 1441
Bromperidol, 1442
Brompheniramine, 1443
Bromphenol Blue, 1444
Bromphenphos *see* 1419
Bromsulphalein [Becton Dickinson] *see* 8954
Brom-Tetragnost *see* 9186
Bromthalein [Merck KGaA] *see* 8954
Bromthymol Blue, 1445
Bromuconazole, 1446
Bromural [Knoll] *see* 1397
Bromuvan *see* 1397
Bromvaletone *see* 1397
Bronalide [Syntex] *see* 4145
Bronalin [Byk-Liprandi] *see* 4707
Broncatar [Pulitzer] *see* 6944
Bronchocillin [Bellon] *see* 7085
Bronchodil [Viatris] *see* 8139
Broncholin [Kaken] *see* 5642
Bronchopront [Mack, Illert.] *see* 386
Bronchoretard [Astellas] *see* 9285
Bronchospasmin [Viatris] *see* 8139
Broncon [Wakamoto] *see* 2408
Broncoplus [Sigma-Tau] *see* 8809
Bronica [Takeda] *see* 8459
Bronkephrine [Sterling Winthrop] *see* 3834
Bronner's Acid *see* 1893
Bronopol, 1447
Bronosol [Green Cross] *see* 1447
Bronsecur [SK & F] *see* 1833
Brontine [Yamanouchi] *see* 2912
Brontyl [Reckitt Benckiser] *see* 7905
Brookite *see* 9472
Broom *see* 8403
Broparoestrol, 1448
Brosalamid *see* 1436
Brostallicin, 1449
Brotizolam, 1450
Brotopon [Pfizer Taito] *see* 4598
Brovalurea *see* 1397
Brovavir *see* 8727
Brovel [Lepetit] *see* 3636
Brovincamine, 1451
Brown Acetate of Lime *see* 1646
Brown Mustard *see* 6315
Broxine [NeoPharm] *see* 1452
Broxuridine, 1452
Broxykinolin, 1453
Broxynil *see* 1441
Broxyquinoline, 1453
BRS-640 *see* 1359
Bruceantin, 1454
Brucine, 1455
Brucite *see* 5670
Brufen [Abbott] *see* 4881
Brufort [Lampugnani] *see* 4881
Bruisewort *see* 8363
Brulidine [M & B] *see* 3024
Brumetidina [Bruschettini] *see* 2279

Brumixol [Bruschettini] *see* 2266
Brunac [Bruschettini] *see* 88
Bruneomycin *see* 8827
Brunet Saxifrage *see* 7436
Brushite *see* 1692
Bruxicam [Bruschettini] *see* 7506
Bryamycin [BMS] *see* 9364
Bryonia, 1456
Bryony *see* 1456
Bryostatins, 1457
BS-100-141 *see* 4561
BS-572 *see* 2704
BS-4231 *see* 4444
BS-5930 *see* 6879
BS-6987 *see* 2912
BSF-208075 *see* 384
BSF-1 *see* 4996
BSF-2 *see* 4998
B.S.G. [Lemmon] *see* 1283
BSN-2060 *see* 8759
BSO *see* 1526
BSP *see* 8954
Bt *see* 932
BT *see* 9244
BT-621 *see* 9502
BTC-1010 [Onyx] *see* 3099
BTE *see* 9782
BTMP *see* 1041
BTPABA *see* 1054
BTS *see* 1306
BTS-18322 *see* 4199
BTS-27419 *see* 486
BTS-40542 *see* 7760
BTS-49465 *see* 4110
BTS-54524 *see* 8485
BTX *see* 1372
BTX-B *see* 1372
BTX-C *see* 1372
B-type Natriuretic Peptide *see* 1360
BU-2231 *see* 9043
BU-2231A *see* 9043
BU-2231B *see* 9043
BU-4061T *see* 3630
Bubarbital Sodium [Philips Roxane] *see* 1506
Bucarban [Chinoin] *see* 1832
Buccalsone [Will-Pharma] *see* 4787
Buccastem [Reckitt Benckiser] *see* 7761
Bucco *see* 1459
Bucetalon [Isei] *see* 1458
Bucetin, 1458
Buchu, 1459
Buchu Camphor *see* 3298
Buchu Resin *see* 3297
Bucillamine, 1460
Bucindolol, 1461
Buck Bean *see* 5842
Buckminsterfullerene, 1462
Buckthorn Bark *see* 4263, 8173
Bucku *see* 1459
Buckyball *see* 1462
Bucladesine, 1463
Buclina [Sanofi-Synthelabo] *see* 1464
Buclizine, 1464
Buclosamide, 1465
Bucolome, 1466
Bucrilate *see* 5140
Bucrylate *see* 5140
Buctril [Bayer CropSci.] *see* 1441
Bucumarol [Sankyo] *see* 1467
Bucumolol, 1467
Buddleoflavonoloside *see* 5498
Budeprion [Teva] *see* 1499
Budeson [Fujisawa] *see* 1468
Budesonide, 1468

Budipine, 1469
Budirol [Fher] *see* 7871
Budoform [Dolder] *see* 5031
BUdR *see* 1452
Budralazine, 1470
Bueno [ISK Biosci] *see* 5953
Bufalin, 1471
Bufedil [Abbott] *see* 1475
Bufedon [Cosmopharma] *see* 6732
Bufemid [Lederle] *see* 3963
Bufeniode, 1472
Bufetolol, 1473
Bufexamac, 1474
Buflan [Fournier] *see* 1475
Buflocit [CT] *see* 1475
Buflomedil, 1475
Buflonat [Nattermann] *see* 1475
Bufonamin [Kaken] *see* 1476
Bufopto Homatrocel [Softcon] *see* 4730
Bufor [Bofors] *see* 6497
Buformin, 1476
Bufotalin, 1477
Bufotalin 3-Suberoylarginine Ester *see* 1479
Bufotenine, 1478
Bufotoxin, 1479
Bufuralol, 1480
Bugbane *see* 1312
Bugleweed *see* 5624
Bugwort *see* 1312
Buksamin *see* 444
Buku *see* 1459
Bulab 6009 [Bulab] *see* 9086
Bulbocapnine, 1481
Bulbold [Sandoz-Wander] *see* 4484
Bulbonin [Sankyo] *see* 1476
Bulbus Scillae *see* 8770
Bull Nettle *see* 8708
Bullvalene, 1482
Bumadizon, 1483
Bumaflex [Byk-Liprandi] *see* 1483
Bumetanide, 1484
Bumex [Roche] *see* 1484
Buminate [Baxter] *see* 8468
Bunaftine, 1485
Bunaiod *see* 1486
Bunamiodyl Sodium, 1486
Bunaphtide *see* 1485
Bunaphtine *see* 1485
Buna S [I. G. Farben] *see* 8390
Bunazosin, 1487
α-Bungarotoxin *see* 1488
β-Bungarotoxin *see* 1488
Bungarotoxins, 1488
Buniodyl *see* 1486
Bunitrolol, 1489
l-Bunolol *see* 5462
Bunsenite *see* 6512
Bunt-cure *see* 4677
Bunte Salts, 1490
Bunt-no-more *see* 4677
t-Bu-P$_4$ *see* 8398
Buparvaquone, 1491
Bupatol [Gedeon Richter] *see* 954
Buphanamine, 1492
Buphanitine, 1493
Buphedrin [Tatsumi] *see* 6732
Buphenine *see* 6732
Bupirimate, 1494
Bupivacaine, 1495
(*S*)-Bupivacaine *see* 1495
Bupranol *see* 1496
Bupranolol, 1496
Buprenex [Reckitt Benckiser] *see* 1497
Buprenorphine, 1497

Buprofezin, 1498
Bupropion, 1499
Buquinolate, 1500
Buramate, 1501
Burdock *see* 5368
Burgess Reagent, 1502
Burgodin [Janssen] *see* 1196
Burgundy Mixture *see* 1335
Burinex [Leo Pharm] *see* 1484
Burning Bush *see* 3899
Burnt Alum *see* 360
Burnt Ammonium Alum *see* 327
Burnt Lime *see* 1686
Burnt Sugar *see* 1775
Burnt Sugar Coloring *see* 1775
Buronil [Ferrosan] *see* 5827
Burow's Solution *see* 324
Bursine *see* 2204
Burtonite 44 *see* 4302
Burtonite V-7-E *see* 4572
Busan 72 [Buckman Labs] *see* 9086
Busan 1118 [Buckman Labs] *see* 9086
Buscapina *see* 1588
Buscol *see* 1588
Buscolysin [Pharmachim] *see* 1588
Buscopan [Boehringer, Ing.] *see* 1588
Buserelin, 1503
Busodium [Truxton] *see* 1506
Busotran [Galen] *see* 1506
Buspar [BMS] *see* 1504
Buspimen [Menarini] *see* 1504
Buspinol [Zdravlje] *see* 1504
Buspirone, 1504
Buspisal [Lesvi] *see* 1504
Busulfan, 1505
Busulfex [Orphan Med.] *see* 1505
Busulphan *see* 1505
Butabar [Flar] *see* 1506
Butabarbital Sodium, 1506
Butabarbitone Sodium *see* 1506
Butabon *see* 1506
Butacaine, 1507
Butachlor, 1508
Butacide [Roussel Uclaf] *see* 7476
Butacote [Novartis] *see* 7277
α,γ-Butadiene *see* 1509
1,3-Butadiene, 1509
1,3-Butadiene-1,4-dicarboxylic Acid
    see 6299
Butadiene Diepoxide *see* 3676
Butadiene Dioxide *see* 3676
1,1′-(1,3-Butadiene-1,4-diyl)bisbenzene
    see 3320
Butadiene Sulfone *see* 8956
Butadion [Streuli] *see* 7277
Butadiona [Miquel-Otsuka] *see* 7277
Butak [Lemmon] *see* 1506
Buta-Kay [King] *see* 1506
Butalamine, 1510
Butalan [Lannett] *see* 1506
Butalbital, 1511
Butalex [Coopers] *see* 1491
Butaliret [Fatol] *see* 9159
Butamben, 1512
Butamirate, 1513
Butamisole, 1514
Butamyrate *see* 1513
Butanal *see* 1591
Butanamide *see* 1592
1-Butanamine *see* 1543
2-Butanamine *see* 1544
Butane, 1515
n-Butane *see* 1515
Butanediamide *see* 8866
1,4-Butanediamine *see* 7947

1,4-Butanedicarboxylic Acid *see* 162
Butanedinitrile *see* 8872
Butanedioic Acid *see* 8869
Butanedioic Acid Bis(1,1-dimethylethyl)
    Ester *see* 3037
Butanedioic Acid Calcium Salt *see* 1705
Butanedioic Acid 2-(Dimethylamino)-
    ethyl [5-Hydroxy-4-(hydroxymethyl)-
    6-methyl-3-pyridinyl]methyl Ester *see*
    7991
Butanedioic Acid Mono[(4-butyl-3,5-di-
    oxo-1,2-diphenyl-4-pyrazolidinyl)-
    methyl] Ester *see* 9009
Butanedioic Acid Mono[(3R,5aS,6R,-
    8aS,9R,10R,12R,12aR)-decahydro-
    3,6,9-trimethyl-3,12-epoxy-12H-pyr-
    ano[4,3-*j*]-1,2-benzodioxepin-10-yl]
    Ester *see* 818
Butanedioic Acid Mono(2,2-dimethyl-
    hydrazide) *see* 2810
Butanedioic Anhydride *see* 8870
1,3-Butanediol *see* 1567
Butane-1,3-diol *see* 1567
2,3-Butanediol *see* 1568
1,4-Butanediol Dimethanesulfonate
    Esters *see* 1505
Butanedione *see* 3676
2,3-Butanedione *see* 2966
2,3-Butanedionedioxime *see* 3246
Butanedioyl Chloride *see* 8873
Butanenitrile *see* 1597
(2R,3S)-*rel*-1,2,3,4-Butanetetrol *see*
    3675
(2R,3S)-*rel*-1,2,3,4-Butanetetroltetra-
    nitrate *see* 3677
1-Butanethiol *see* 1577
2-Butanethiol *see* 1578
Butanex [Makhteshim-Agan] *see* 1508
Butanimide *see* 8871
Butanoic Acid *see* 1593
Butanoic Acid Anhydride *see* 1594
Butanoic Acid Butyl Ester *see* 1556
1-Butanoic Acid 1,7-Dicarbacalcitonin
    (Eel) *see* 3537
Butanoic Acid 2,3-Dihydroxypropyl
    Ester *see* 6249
Butanoic Acid Ethyl Ester *see* 3775
1-Butanoic Acid-7-glycine-1,6-dicarba-
    oxytocin *see* 1839
Butanoic Acid Methyl Ester *see* 6035
1-Butanoic Acid-2-(*O*-methyl-L-tyro-
    sine)-1-carbaoxytocin *see* 1795
Butanoic Acid Pentyl Ester *see* 604
Butanoic Acid 1,2,3-Propanetriyl Ester
    see 9620
Butanoic Acid Propyl Ester *see* 7846
1-Butanol *see* 1540
2-Butanol *see* 1541
1,2-Butanolide *see* 1596
1,4-Butanolide *see* 1596
2,3-Butanolone *see* 64
2-Butanone *see* 6072
Butanotic [Medical Arts] *see* 1506
Butanoyl Chloride *see* 1598
L-α-Butanoyl Glycerol *see* 6249
Butaperazine, 1516
Butapirazol [Polfa] *see* 7277
Butased [Schlicksup] *see* 1506
Butatensin [Benvegna] *see* 5773
Butatran [Palmedico] *see* 1506
Butatron [Sanofi] *see* 7277
Butazem [Zemmer] *see* 1506
Butazolidin [Novartis] *see* 7277
Butedronic Acid, 1517
Butelline *see* 1507

Butenafine, 1518
2-Butenal *see* 2596
1-Butene, 1519
2-Butene, 1520
(Z)-2-Butenedioic Acid *see* 5703
(2E)-2-Butenedioic Acid *see* 4287
(E)-2-Butenedioic Acid Bis(phenyl-
    methyl) Ester *see* 1135
(2Z)-2-Butenedioic Acid, Diethyl Ester
    see 3123
(2E)-2-Butenedioic Acid Iron(2+) Salt
    (1:1) *see* 4046
cis-Butenedioic Anhydride *see* 5704
3-Butenenitrile *see* 290
cis-2-Butenoic Acid *see* 5164
(2E)-2-Butenoic Acid *see* 2597
(2Z)-2-Butenoic Acid *see* 5164
2-Buten-1-ol *see* 2601
Δ³-2-Butenone *see* 6134
3-Buten-2-one *see* 6134
β-Butenonitrile *see* 290
(4R)-4-[(E)-2-Butenyl]-4,N-dimethyl-L-
    threonine *see* 5771
3-(2-Butenylidene)-2-carboxy-α-(hydr-
    oxymethylene)-1,4-cyclopentadiene-
    1-acetic Acid δ-Lactone Methyl Es-
    ter *see* 4285
(7E)-7-(2E)-Butenylidene-1,7-dihydro-1-
    oxocyclopenta[c]pyran-4-carboxylic
    Acid Methyl Ester *see* 4285
3-(3-Buten-1-ynyl)-6-(1,3-pentadiynyl)-
    1,2-dithiin *see* 9304
(2S,6R,7S,8S)-7-(1Z)-1-Buten-3-ynyl-2-
    (2Z)-2-penten-4-ynyl-1-azaspiro[5.5]-
    undecan-8-ol *see* 4723
Buterazine [Daiichi] *see* 1470
Butesin [Abbott] *see* 1512
Butethal, 1521
Butethamate, 1522
Butethamine, 1523
Butex [Phillips] *see* 1506
Butformin *see* 1476
Buthalital Sodium, 1524
Buthalitone Sodium *see* 1524
Buthiazide, 1525
Buthionine Sulfoximine, 1526
Butibufen, 1527
Buticaps [McNeil] *see* 1506
Butilate *see* 1546
Butilopan [Juste] *see* 1527
Butinat [Gramon] *see* 1484
Butirosin, 1528
Butirosin A *see* 1528
Butirosin B *see* 1528
Butisol Sodium [McNeil] *see* 1506
Butix [Fabre] *see* 5864
Butixirate *see* 10071
Butizide *see* 1525
Butobarbital *see* 1521
Butobarbitone *see* 1521
Butoconazole, 1529
Butoform *see* 1512
Butonate *see* 9623
Butopamine Hydrochloride *see* 8092
Butorphanol, 1530
Butox [Intervet] *see* 2883
Butoxone *see* 2835
3-Butoxy-4-aminobenzoic Acid 2-
    (Diethylamino)ethyl Ester *see* 1047
4-Butoxybenzoic Acid 2-(Diethylamino)-
    ethyl Ester *see* 1531
8-(*p*-Butoxybenzyl)-3α-hydroxy-1αH,-
    5αH-tropanium Bromide (−)-Tropate
    see 1534
l-[1-(*p-n*-Butoxybenzyl)hyoscyaminium]
    Bromide *see* 1534

tert-Butoxybis(dimethylamino)methane
see 1368
Butoxycaine, 1531
1-(3-Butoxy-2-carbamoyloxypropyl)-5-
phenyl-5-ethylbarbituric Acid *see* 3945
N-[*N*-[*N*-[*N*-(*N-tert*-Butoxycarbonyl-β-
alanyl)-L-tryptophanyl]-L-methionyl]-
L-aspartyl]-L-phenylalaninamide *see*
7113
2-Butoxy-*N*-(2-diethylaminoethyl)cincho-
ninamide *see* 3031
2-Butoxy-*N*-[2-(diethylamino)ethyl]-4-
quinolinecarboxamide *see* 3031
2-Butoxyethanol *see* 1559
2-(2-Butoxyethoxy)ethanol *see* 1557
α-[2-(2-Butoxyethoxy)ethoxy]-4,5-meth-
ylenedioxy-2-propyltoluene *see* 7476
5-[[2-(2-Butoxyethoxy)ethoxy]methyl]-6-
propyl-1,3-benzodioxole *see* 7476
4-Butoxy-*N*-hydroxybenzeneacetamide
see 1474
1-(3-Butoxy-2-hydroxypropyl)-5-ethyl-5-
phenylbarbituric Acid Carbamate *see*
3945
N-(Butoxymethyl)-2-chloro-2′,6′-diethyl-
acetanilide *see* 1508
N-(Butoxymethyl)-2-chloro-*N*-(2,6-dieth-
ylphenyl)acetamide *see* 1508
2-(4-Butoxyphenoxy)-*N*-(2,5-diethoxy-
phenyl)-*N*-[2-(diethylamino)ethyl]-
acetamide *see* 3986
1-Butoxy-3-phenoxy-2-propanol *see* 3947
4-[3-(4-Butoxyphenoxy)propyl]morpho-
line *see* 7709
2-(*p*-Butoxyphenyl)acetohydroxamic
Acid *see* 1474
2-(*p*-Butoxyphenyl)-*N*-[2-(diethylamino)-
ethyl]-2′,5′-diethoxyacetanilide *see*
3986
[3(*S*)-*endo*]-8-[(4-Butoxyphenyl)methyl]-
3-(3-hydroxy-1-oxo-2-phenylpropoxy)-
8-methyl-8-azoniabicyclo[3.2.1]octane
Bromide *see* 1534
p-Butoxyphenyl γ-Morpholinopropyl
Ether *see* 7709
4-Butoxyphenyl Piperidineethyl Ketone
see 3473
1-(4-Butoxyphenyl)-3-(1-piperidinyl)-1-
propanone *see* 3473
4-Butoxy-β-piperidinopropiophenone *see*
3473
4-*n*-Butoxy-β-(1-piperidyl)propiophe-
none *see* 3473
tert-Butoxy-*N*,*N*,*N*′,*N*′-tetramethyl-
methanediamine *see* 1368
Butoz [Hamilton] *see* 7277
Butralin, 1532
Butrate [Kay] *see* 1506
Butriptylene *see* 1533
Butriptyline, 1533
Butropium Bromide, 1534
Butte [Scrip] *see* 1506
Buttercup Yellow *see* 10133
Butterfly Weed *see* 828
Butternut *see* 5268
Butter of Antimony *see* 707
Butter of Arsenic *see* 801
Butter of Zinc *see* 10132
Butter Yellow *see* 3229
β-BuTX *see* 1488
Butyl Chemosept *see* 1584
Butyl Diicinol [ICI] *see* 1557
Butyl Parasept *see* 1584
n-Butyl Acetate, 1535
sec-Butyl Acetate, 1536

tert-Butyl Acetate, 1537
21-*tert*-Butylacetate-9α-fluoro-11β-hy-
droxy-16α,17α-(isopropylidenedioxy)pregna-1,4-diene-3,20-dione *see*
9598
tert-Butylacetic Acid, 1538
3-(*N*-Butyl-*N*-acetyl)-aminopropionic
Acid Ethyl Ester *see* 3773
n-Butyl Acrylate, 1539
Butyl Alcohol *see* 1540
n-Butyl Alcohol, 1540
sec-Butyl Alcohol, 1541
tert-Butyl Alcohol, 1542
n-Butylamine, 1543
sec-Butylamine, 1544
tert-Butylamine, 1545
Butyl Aminobenzoate *see* 1512
n-Butyl *p*-Aminobenzoate *see* 1512
4-(Butylamino)benzoic Acid 2-(Dimethylamino)ethyl Ester Monohydrochloride
see 9188
p-Butylaminobenzoic Acid ω-*O*-Methyl-
nonaethyleneglycol Ester *see* 1096
4-(Butylamino)benzoic Acid 3,6,9,12,15,-
18,21,24,27-Nonaoxaoctacos-1-yl
Ester *see* 1096
p-Butylaminobenzoyl-2-dimethylamino-
ethanol Hydrochloride *see* 9188
[1-[(Butylamino)carbonyl]-1*H*-benzimid-
azol-2-yl]carbamic Acid Methyl Ester
see 1044
N-[(Butylamino)carbonyl]-4-methyl-
benzenesulfonamide *see* 9507
1-*tert*-Butylamino-3-(2-chloro-5-methyl-
phenoxy)-2-propanol *see* 1496
(±)-2-(*tert*-Butylamino)-3′-chloropropio-
phenone *see* 1499
1-(*tert*-Butylamino)-3-[(6-chloro-*m*-
tolyl)oxy]-2-propanol *see* 1496
(*S*)-1-(*tert*-Butylamino)-3-(*o*-cyclopentyl-
phenoxy)-2-propanol *see* 7082
2-(*tert*-Butylamino)-4-(cyclopropylamino)-6-(methylthio)-*s*-triazine *see*
5084
1-(*tert*-Butylamino)-3-(2,5-dichloro-
phenoxy)-2-propanol *see* 2402
3-(*tert*-Butylamino)-1-(2′,3′-dimethyl-
phenoxy)-2-propanol *see* 10075
4-Butylamino-2-hydroxybenzoic Acid 2-
Dimethylaminoethyl Ester *see* 4846
(−)-1-*tert*-Butylamino-2-hydroxy-3-(2′-
cyclopentylphenoxy)propane *see* 7082
2-(2-*tert*-Butylamino-1-hydroxyethyl)-7-
ethylbenzofuran *see* 1480
(±)-5-[2-(*tert*-Butylamino)-1-hydroxy-
ethyl]-*m*-phenylene Bis(dimethylcarbamate) *see* 953
2-(*tert*-Butylamino)-1-(4-hydroxy-3-hy-
droxymethylphenyl)ethanol *see* 216
2-Butylamino-1-*p*-hydroxyphenylethanol
see 954
o-[3-(*tert*-Butylamino)-2-hydroxypro-
poxy]benzonitrile *see* 1489
5-[3-(*tert*-Butylamino)-2-hydroxypro-
poxy]-3,4-dihydrocarbostyril *see*
1866
(−)-5-[3-(*tert*-Butylamino)-2-hydroxy-
propoxy]-3,4-dihydro-1(2*H*)-naphtha-
lenone *see* 5462
(±)-8-[3-(*t*-Butylamino)-2-hydroxypro-
poxy]-5-methylcoumarin *see* 1467
4-[3-(*tert*-Butylamino)-2-hydroxypro-
poxy]-*N*-methylisocarbostyril *see* 9438
S-(−)-3-(3-*tert*-Butylamino-2-hydroxy-
propoxy)-4-morpholino-1,2,5-thiadi-
azole *see* 9444

2-[*o*-[3-(*t*-Butylamino)-2-hydroxypro-
poxy]phenoxy]-*N*-methylacetamide *see*
2018
(±)-1-[*p*-[3-(*tert*-Butylamino)-2-hydroxy-
propoxy]phenyl]-3-cyclohexylurea *see*
9038
(2*R*,3*S*)-5-[3-(*tert*-Butylamino)-2-hy-
droxypropoxy]-1,2,3,4-tetrahydro-
naphthalene-2,3-diol *see* 6346
2-(3′-*tert*-Butylamino-2′-hydroxypropyl-
thio)-4-(5′-carbamoyl-2′-thienyl)thi-
azole *see* 791
(±)-1-*t*-Butylamino-3-(*o*-*N*-methylcarba-
moylmethoxyphenoxy)propan-2-ol *see*
2018
α-[(*tert*-Butylamino)methyl]-*o*-chloro-
benzyl Alcohol *see* 9811
α-[(*tert*-Butylamino)methyl]-3,5-dihy-
droxybenzyl Alcohol *see* 9159
α-[(*tert*-Butylamino)methyl]-3,4-dihy-
droxybenzyl Alcohol 3,4-Di-*p*-toluate
see 1307
α-[(*tert*-Butylamino)methyl]-7-ethyl-2-
benzofuranmethanol *see* 1480
α-[(Butylamino)methyl]-4-hydroxy-
benzenemethanol *see* 954
α-[(Butylamino)methyl]-*p*-hydroxybenzyl
Alcohol *see* 954
α-(*t*-Butylaminomethyl)-4-hydroxy-3-
ureidobenzyl Alcohol *see* 1833
α¹-[*tert*-Butylamino)methyl]-4-hydroxy-
m-xylene-α,α′-diol *see* 216
(±)-1-(*tert*-Butylamino)-3-[(2-methylin-
dol-4-yl)oxy]-2-propanol Benzoate
(Ester) *see* 1333
3-(Butylamino)-4-phenoxy-5-sulfamoyl-
benzoic Acid *see* 1484
p-Butylaminosalicylic Acid 2-Dimethyl-
aminoethyl Ester *see* 4846
1-(*tert*-Butylamino)-3-[(5,6,7,8-tetrahy-
dro-*cis*-6,7-dihydroxy-1-naphthyl)-
oxy]-2-propanol *see* 6346
1-(*tert*-Butylamino)-3-[*o*-[(tetrahydrofurfuryl)oxy]phenoxy]-2-propanol *see*
1473
(±)-1-*tert*-Butylamino-3-(1-thiachro-
man-8-yloxy)-2-propanol *see* 9173
(±)-1-(*tert*-Butylamino)-3-(2,3-xylyl-
oxy)-2-propanol *see* 10075
Butylate, 1546
Butylated Hydroxyanisole, 1547
Butylated Hydroxytoluene, 1548
n-Butylbenzene, 1549
sec-Butylbenzene, 1550
tert-Butylbenzene, 1551
α-Butylbenzenemethanol *see* 3975
(5-Butyl-1*H*-benzimidazol-2-yl)carbamic
Acid Methyl Ester *see* 7035
n-Butyl Benzoate, 1552
2-Butyl-3-benzofuranyl-4-[2-(diethylamino)ethoxy]-3,5-diiodophenyl
Ketone *see* 482
(2-Butyl-3-benzofuranyl)[4-[2-(diethylamino)ethoxy]-3,5-diiodophenyl]-
methanone *see* 482
α-Butylbenzyl Alcohol *see* 3975
1-(*p-tert*-Butylbenzyl)-4-(*p*-chlorodi-
phenylmethyl)piperazine *see* 1464
N-(4-*t*-Butylbenzyl)-4-chloro-3-ethyl-1-
methylpyrazole-5-carboxamide *see*
9094
1-(*p-tert*-Butylbenzyl)-4-(*p*-chloro-α-
phenylbenzyl)piperazine *see* 1464
N-(*p-tert*-Butylbenzyl)-*N*-methyl-1-naph-
thalenemethylamine *see* 1518

Calcipen [Leo Pharm] *see* 7100
Calcipotriene, 1641
Calcipotriol *see* 1641
Calciseptine, 1642
Calcisorb [3M Pharma] *see* 8597
Calcitar(e) [RPR] *see* 1643
Calcite *see* 1657
Calcitonin, 1643
Calcitonin Gene Related Peptide *see* 609
Calcitriol, 1644
Calcium, 1645
Calcium Acetate, 1646
Calcium Acetyl Homotaurinate *see* 17
Calcium Acetylsalicylate, 1647
Calcium Acetylsalicylate Carbamide *see* 1647
Calcium Aluminosilicate, 1648
Calcium Aluminum Hydride *see* 334
Calcium Arsenate, 1649
Calcium Arsenite, 1650
Calcium Ascorbate *see* 830
Calcium Aspirin *see* 1647
Calcium Benzoate *see* 1091
Calcium Bichromate *see* 1666
Calcium Biphosphate *see* 1693
Calcium Bisacetyl Homotaurine *see* 17
Calcium Bisulfite, Solution, 1651
Calcium Borate, 1652
Calcium Borogluconate, 1653
Calcium Bromide, 1654
Calcium *N*-Carbamoylaspartate, 1655
Calcium Carbide, 1656
Calcium Carbimide *see* 1662
Calcium Carbolate *see* 1691
Calcium Carbonate, 1657
Calcium Chel 330 [Geigy] *see* 7124
Calcium Chlorate, 1658
Calcium Chloride, 1659
Calcium Chromate(VI), 1660
Calcium Chrome Yellow *see* 1660
Calcium Citrate, 1661
Calcium Cyanamide, 1662
Calcium Cyanamide Citrated, 1663
Calcium Cyanide, 1664
Calcium Cyclamate, 1665
Calcium Cyclohexanesulfamate *see* 1665
Calcium Cyclohexylsulfamate *see* 1665
Calcium-dependent Regulator Protein *see* 1719
Calcium Diborogluconate *see* 1653
Calcium Dichromate(VI), 1666
Calcium Dioctyl Sulfosuccinate *see* 3400
Calcium Dioxide *see* 1689
Calcium Diphosphate *see* 1699
Calcium Disodium Versenate *see* 3517
Calcium Diuretin *see* 9282
Calcium Dobesilate *see* 3394
Calcium Ethyl Sulfate *see* 3853
Calcium Fluoride, 1667
Calcium Fluosilicate *see* 1671
Calcium Folinate *see* 4222
Calcium (6S)-Folinate *see* 4222
Calcium Formate, 1668
Calcium Glucoheptonate *see* 4455
Calcium Glucomonocarbonate *see* 4455
Calcium Gluconate, 1669
Calcium Glucosemonocarbonate *see* 4455
Calcium Glycerinophosphate *see* 1670
Calcium Glycerophosphate, 1670
Calcium Homopantothenate *see* 4744
Calcium Hexafluorosilicate, 1671
Calcium Hydrate *see* 1673
Calcium Hydride, 1672
Calcium Hydroxide, 1673
Calcium 2-Hydroxy-1-naphthalene-
    sulfonate *see* 822

Calcium Hypochlorite, 1674
Calcium Hypophosphite, 1675
Calcium Iodate, 1676
Calcium Iodide, 1677
Calcium Ipodate *see* 5071
Calcium Lactate, 1678
Calcium Lactobionate *see* 5342
Calcium Levofolinate *see* 4222
Calcium Levulinate, 1679
Calcium Magnesium Acetate, 1680
Calcium Mandelate *see* 5717
Calcium Methyl Sulfate *see* 6122
Calcium Molybdate(VI), 1681
(*T*-4)-Calcium (1:1) Molybdate (MoO$_4^{2-}$) *see* 1681
Calcium Molybdenum Oxide *see* 1681
Calcium Monohydrogen Phosphate *see* 1692
Calcium β-Naphthol-α-monosulfonate *see* 822
Calcium 2-Naphthol-1-sulfonate *see* 822
Calcium Nitrate, 1682
Calcium Nitrite, 1683
Calcium Oleate, 1684
Calcium Orthophosphate Basic *see* 3467
Calcium Oxalate, 1685
Calcium Oxide, 1686
"Calcium Oxychloride" *see* 2094
Calcium Palmitate, 1687
Calcium Pectolith *see* 1702
Calcium Permanganate, 1688
Calcium Peroxide, 1689
Calcium Phenate *see* 1691
Calcium Phenolate *see* 1691
Calcium Phenolsulfonate, 1690
Calcium Phenoxide, 1691
Calcium Phenylate *see* 1691
Calcium Phosphate, Dibasic, 1692
Calcium Phosphate Hydroxide *see* 3467
Calcium Phosphate, Monobasic, 1693
Calcium Phosphate, Tetrabasic *see* 9372
Calcium Phosphate, Tribasic, 1694
Calcium Phosphide, 1695
Calcium Phosphite, 1696
Calcium Phosphoglycerate *see* 1670
Calcium Polycarbophil, 1697
Calcium Propionate, 1698
Calcium Pyroborate *see* 1652
Calcium Pyrophosphate, 1699
Calcium Rhodanate *see* 1710
Calcium D-Saccharate, 1700
Calcium Selenide, 1701
Calcium Silicate, 1702
Calcium Silicofluoride *see* 1671
Calcium Stearate, 1703
Calcium Stearyl-2 Lactylate, 1704
Calcium Stelate *see* 1704
Calcium Succinate, 1705
Calcium Sulfate, 1706
Calcium Sulfide, 1707
Calcium Sulfite, 1708
Calcium Sulfocarbolate *see* 1690
Calcium Sulfocyanate *see* 1710
Calcium Sulfomethylate *see* 6122
Calcium Sulfophenolate *see* 1690
Calcium Sulfovinate *see* 3853
"Calcium Superphosphate" *see* 1693
Calcium Tartrate, 1709
Calcium Tetraborate *see* 1652
Calcium Tetrahydroaluminate *see* 334
Calcium Thiocyanate, 1710
Calcium Thioglycollate, 1711
Calcium Trisodium Pentetate *see* 7124
Calcium Tungstate(VI), 1712
Calcium Ureidosuccinate *see* 1655

Calcort [Aventis] *see* 2862
Caldine [Boehringer, Ing.] *see* 5331
Caldon [Hoechst] *see* 3287
C-Calebassine *see* 9558
Calendula, 1713
Calepsin [Orion] *see* 1781
Calfactant, 1714
Calglucon *see* 1669
Calgon *see* 8667
Calheptose *see* 4455
Calibène [Delalande] *see* 9009
Calicheamicin γ$_1^I$ *see* 1715
Calicheamicins, 1715
Calico Yellow *see* 6269
Californit [Merckle] *see* 6972
Californium, 1716
Caliment [Apotex] *see* 7506
Calisaya Bark *see* 2284
Calixarenes, 1717
Calixin [BASF] *see* 9660
Callicrein *see* 5279
Callidin I *see* 1359
Callistephin *see* 7071
Callisto [Syngenta] *see* 5912
Callusolve [Dermal] *see* 1059
Calmactin [Solvay] *see* 2271
Calmagite, 1718
Calmatel (Aerosol) [Almirall-Omega] *see* 7422
Calmatel (Cream) [Almirall-Omega] *see* 7422
Calmaxid [Lilly] *see* 6660
Calmday [Will-Pharma] *see* 6691
Calmivet [Stricker] *see* 32
Calmodid *see* 4785
Calmodulin, 1719
Calmonal [BMS] *see* 5777
Calmpose [Ranbaxy] *see* 2994
Calmus *see* 1637
Calnathal *see* 1794
Calogreen [Mallinckrodt] *see* 5894
Calomel *see* 5894
Calomide [Yamanouchi] *see* 2451
Calorose *see* 5006
Calotropin, 1720
Caloxydim *see* 9152
Calpactin *see* 676
Calpanate [Consumers Vitamin] *see* 7015
Calphosan [Carlton] *see* 1670
Calpol [Pfizer] *see* 47
Calscorbat [Aerocid] *see* 830
Calsed [Sumitomo] *see* 593
Calsekin [Mect] *see* 4231
Calslot [Takeda] *see* 5743
Calsmin [Sumitomo] *see* 6575
Calsol *see* 3517
Calsyn [RPR] *see* 1643
Calsynar [RPR] *see* 1643
Calthor [Ayerst] *see* 2702
Caltrate [Wyeth] *see* 1657
Calumba, 1721
Calurin [Dorsey] *see* 1647
Calusterone, 1722
Calx *see* 1686
Calycanthine, 1723
Calyculin A, 1724
(−)-Calyculin A *see* 1724
Calypso [Bayer CropSci.] *see* 9291
Calystigine *see* 6994
CaM *see* 1719
CAM-AQ1 *see* 572
Camazepam, 1725
Cambendazole, 1726
Cambogia *see* 4360
Camcolit [Norgine] *see* 5527

Camdelate see 5717
Cameleons, 1727
Camila [Barr] see 6697
Camilol [Maybrook] see 1241
Camite see 1412
Camleed [Tanabe Seiyaku] see 3591
Camolar [Parke-Davis] see 2721
Camomile see 2041
Camoquin [Parke-Davis] see 572
Camostat, 1728
Camostat Mesylate see 1728
cAMP see 2708
Campath [Schering AG] see 228
Campath-1H see 228
Campel [Farmitalia] see 2237
Campesterol, 1729
endo-2-Camphanol see 1338
exo-2-Camphanol see 5128
2-Camphanone see 1732
Camphechlor see 9557
Camphene, 1730
d-Camphocarboxylic Acid, 1731
Camphol see 1338
Camphor, 1732
(1R)-(+)-Camphor see 1732
(1S)-(−)-Camphor see 1732
d-3-Camphorcarboxylic Acid see 1731
Camphoric Acid, 1733
Camphoric Acid 1-(p,α-Dimethylbenzyl)
   Ester, Compd with 2,2′-Imidodieth-
   anol (1:1) see 9492
d-Camphoric Acid Ethyl Ester Bismuth
   Salt see 1264
Camphor Monobromated see 1414
Camphor Monochlorated see 2132
Camphor Solubilized see 1731
β-Camphorsulfonic Acid see 1734
d-Camphorsulfonic Acid, 1734
10-Camphorsulfonic Acid see 1734
Camphostyl see 1734
Camphydryl see 1731
Camporit see 1674
Camposan see 3732
Campoviton 6 see 7982
Campral [Merck Santé] see 17
Campto [Sanofi-Aventis] see 5091
Camptosar [Pharmacia & Upjohn] see
   5091
Camptothecin, 1735
Camsellite see 5658
Camsylate see 1734
Camvet [Merck & Co.] see 1726
Camyna [Nycomed] see 9456
Canada Snakeroot see 825
Canada Turpentine see 946
Canadian Hemp see 743
Canadine, 1736
Canadol see 5489
Cananga Oil see 10100
Canary Dextrin see 2953
Canavanine, 1737
Canchalagua see 1969
Cancidas [Merck & Co.] see 1889
Candelilla Wax, 1738
Candesartan, 1739
Candesartan Cilexetil see 1739
Candex [Miles] see 6736
Candicidin, 1740
Candicidin D see 1740
Candidin, 1741
Candidinin see 1741
Candidoin see 1741
Candio-Hermal [Hermal] see 6736
Candit [BASF] see 5324
Candleberry Bark see 1012

Candoxatril, 1742
Candoxatrilat see 1742
Canella, 1743
Canertinib, 1744
Canescine see 2918
Canesten [Bayer] see 2417
Cane Sugar see 8881
Canex [Mallinckrodt Vet.] see 8271
Canferon [Takeda] see 4990
Canfodion [Gentili] see 8091
Canfosfamide, 1745
Canfoxil [Gentili] see 1731
Cangrelor, 1746
Canifug [Wolff] see 2417
Caniphedrin [Streuli] see 3608
Cannabidiol, 1747
Cannabinol, 1748
Cannabis, 1749
Cannabiscetin see 6332
Cannoc [Takeda] see 3702
Canocenta [Byk Gulden] see 5585
Canrenone, 1750
Cantabilin [Formenti] see 4854
Cantabiline see 4854
Cantan [Aventis] see 830
Cantharides, 1751
Cantharides Camphor see 1752
Cantharidin, 1752
Canthaxanthin, 1753
Cantil [Aventis] see 5848
Canton's Phosphorus see 1707
Cantor [Sanofi Winthrop] see 6200
Cantralax [Ferrosan] see 1878
Cantrex see 5281
Cantricin [Corvi] see 4290
Cantrodifene (obsolete) see 6633
Cantus [BASF] see 1352
Caomet [AstraZeneca] see 9843
Caoutchouc see 8278
CAP-440 see 865
Caparlem see 5271
Caparol [Syngenta] see 7789
Caparside see 793
Caparsolate [Abbott] see 793
Capastat [Lilly] see 1757
Capecitabine, 1754
Capen [Phoenix] see 9453
Caperase see 1900
Capisten [Pierre Fabre] see 8388
Capisten [Kissei] see 5305
Capitol [Dermal] see 1059
Capitrol [Westwood] see 2175
Capitus [Berk] see 3748
Capla [Wallace Labs.] see 5773
Caplenal [Teva] see 279
Capmul 8210 [Stokely-Van Camp] see
   6252
Capmul O [Capital City Prod.] see 8724
Capnoidine see 165
Capoten [BMS] see 1774
Capozide [BMS] see 1774
Capravirine, 1755
Caprenin, 1756
Capreomycin, 1757
Capreomycin IA see 1757
Capreomycin IB see 1757
Capreomycin IIA see 1757
Capreomycin IIB see 1757
n-Capric Acid, 1758
Caprine see 6706
Caproaldehyde see 1760
Caprocin [Lilly] see 1757
n-Caproic Acid, 1759
n-Caproic Acid n-Amyl Ester see 605
Caproic Aldehyde, 1760

Caprokol [Merck & Co.] see 4712
Caprolactam, 1761
ε-Caprolactam see 1761
Caprolan [AlliedSignal] see 6734
Capromab, 1762
Capromab Pendetide see 1762
Caprosem [A. B. Leo] see 2421
Caproyl Chloride, 1763
Caprylaldehyde see 1766
Capryl α-Cyanoacrylate see 6766
Caprylene, 1764
Caprylic Acid, 1765
Caprylic Acid Ammonium Salt see 506
Caprylic Acid α-Monoglyceride see 6252
Caprylic Alcohol see 6751
Caprylic Aldehyde, 1766
Caprylohydroxamic Acid see 6750
CAPS, 1767
Capsaicin, 1768
Capsanthin, 1769
Capsebon [Pitman-Moore] see 1628
Capsicum, 1770
Capstar [Novartis] see 6568
Captafol, 1771
Captagon [Viatris] see 3972
Captan, 1772
Captax see 5868
Captea [Théraplix] see 1774
Captin [Krewel] see 47
Captodiam see 1773
Captodiamine, 1773
Captodramin see 1773
Captolane [Théraplix] see 1774
Captopril, 1774
Captoril [Sankyo] see 1774
Capture [FMC] see 1209
Capval [Dreluso] see 6718
Carace [BMS] see 5516
Carachol see 2868
Caracurine VII see 10044
Caradrin [AWD] see 7874
Carafate [Aventis] see 8879
Caramba see 5934
Caramel, 1775
Caramiphen, 1776
Caraway, 1777
Carazolol, 1778
Carbacefaclor see 5576
Carbachol, 1779
Carbadipimidine see 1861
Carbadox, 1780
Carbaglu [Orphan Europe] see 1838
Carbaldehyde see 4237
Carbamamidine see 4562
Carbamate see 4013
Carbamate of 2-(Hydroxymethyl)-2-
   methylpentyl Ester of Butylcarbamic
   Acid see 9829
Carbamazepine, 1781
Carbamazine see 3116
Carbamic Acid 2-sec-Butyl-2-methyltri-
   methylene Ester see 5773
Carbamic Acid 3-(p-Chlorophenoxy)-2-
   hydroxypropyl Ester see 2179
Carbamic Acid 1-Cyclohexylpropyl Ester
   see 7764
Carbamic Acid Ethyl Ester see 9874
Carbamic Acid 1-Ethynylcyclohexyl
   Ester see 3733
Carbamic Acid (1-Methyl-5-nitroimid-
   azol-2-yl)methyl Ester see 8254
Carbamic Acid 2-Methyl-2-propyltri-
   methylene Ester see 5862
Carbamic Acid 3-Phenylpropyl Ester see
   7258

Carbamic Acid 2-Phenyltrimethylene Ester *see* 3950
Carbamic Acid 1-(2-Propynyl)cyclohexyl Ester *see* 4698
Carbamic Chloride *see* 1783
Carbamidal *see* 6543
Carbamide *see* 9867
Carbamide Peroxide, 1782
Carbamidine *see* 4562
p-Carbamidobenzenearsonic Acid *see* 1786
Carbamimidothioic Acid 2-Aminoethyl Ester Dihydrobromide *see* 178
Carbamimidothioic Acid (4-Chlorophenyl)methyl Ester Monohydrochloride *see* 2128
Carbamimidothioic Acid Phenylmethyl Ester Monohydrochloride *see* 1146
3-[[2-[(4-Carbamimidoylphenylamino)methyl]-1-methyl-1*H*-benzoimidazole-5-carbonyl]pyridin-2-ylamino]propionic Acid *see* 2797
Carbamothioic Acid, *S*,*S'*-[2-(Dimethylamino)-1,3-propanediyl] Ester *see* 1865
N-Carbamoylarsanilic Acid *see* 1786
N-Carbamoylaspartic Acid Calcium Salt *see* 1655
(6*R*,7*S*)-7-[4-(Carbamoylcarboxymethylene)-1,3-dithietane-2-carboxamido]-7-methoxy-3-[[(1-methyl-1*H*-tetrazol-5-yl)thio]methyl]-8-oxo-5-thia-1-azabicyclo[4.2.0]oct-2-ene-2-carboxylic Acid *see* 1934
5-Carbamoyl-5*H*-dibenz[*b*,*f*]azepine *see* 1781
1-Carbamoyl-7-(diethylamino)-3,4-dihydroxyphenazoxonium Chloride *see* 1959
3-(*S*)-(−)-(1-Carbamoyl-1,1-diphenylmethyl)-1-[2-(2,3-dihydrobenzofuran-5-yl)ethyl]pyrrolidine *see* 2825
(3-Carbamoyl-3,3-diphenylpropyl)diisopropylmethylammonium Iodide *see* 5202
3-(Carbamoyl-3,3-diphenylpropyl)ethyldimethylammonium Bromide *see* 387
1-(3-Carbamoyl-3,3-diphenylpropyl)hexahydro-1-methylazepinium Iodide *see* 1599
1-(3-Carbamoyl-3,3-diphenylpropyl)-1-methylpiperidinium Bromide *see* 3990
4'-Carbamoyl-2-formyl-1,1'-(oxydimethylene)dipyridinium Chloride 2-Oxime *see* 835
N-Carbamoyl-L-glutamic Acid *see* 1838
4-Carbamoyl-5-hydroxyimidazole *see* 6222
4-Carbamoylimidazolium-5-olate *see* 6222
9-Carbamoyl-9-(3-isopropylaminopropyl)fluorene *see* 4937
N-Carbamoylmaleamic Acid *see* 5706
N-(Carbamoylmethyl)arsanilic Acid Monosodium Salt *see* 9794
8-Carbamoyl-3-methylimidazo[5,1-*d*]-1,2,3,5-tetrazin-4(3*H*)-one *see* 9139
1-*p*-Carbamoylmethylphenoxy-3-isopropylamino-2-propanol *see* 859
N-(Carbamoylmethyl)taurine *see* 36
2-Carbamoyloxymethyl-5-(3,5-dichlorophenylthio)-4-isopropyl-1-(pyridin-4-yl)methyl-1*H*-imidazole *see* 1755

(6*R*,7*R*)-3-Carbamoyloxymethyl-7-[2-(2-furyl)-2-(methoxyimino)acetamido]-ceph-3-em-4-carboxylic Acid *see* 1954
(6*R*,7*R*)-3-Carbamoyloxymethyl-7-[2-(2-furyl)-2-(methoxyimino)acetamido]-8-oxo-5-thia-1-azabicyclo[4.2.0]oct-2-ene-2-carboxylic Acid *see* 1954
3-Carbamoyloxymethyl-7α-methoxy-7-[2-(2-thienyl)acetamido]-3-cephem-4-carboxylic Acid *see* 1936
1-Carbamoyloxy-3-phenylpropane *see* 7258
2-Carbamoyloxypropyltrimethylammonium Chloride *see* 1185
1-Carbamoyloxy-1-(2-propynyl)cyclohexane *see* 4698
N-(α-Carbamoylphenethyl)-3-[2-[2-[3-(carboxyamino)propionamido]-3-indol-3-ylpropionamido]-4-(methylthio)butyramido]succinamic Acid *N*-*tert*-Butyl Ester *see* 7113
α-(2-Carbamoylphenoxy)acetic Acid *see* 8329
[[(*p*-Carbamoylphenyl)arsylene]dithio]diacetic Acid *see* 793
10-[3-(4-Carbamoylpiperidino)propyl]-2-chlorophenothiazine *see* 7454
10-[3-(4-Carbamoylpiperidino)propyl]-2-(methanesulfonyl)phenothiazine *see* 6149
10-[3-(4-Carbamoylpiperidin-1-yl)propyl]-2-chlorophenothiazine *see* 7454
(2*S*)-*N*-[(1*S*)-1-[[(2*S*)-2-Carbamoyl-1-pyrrolidinyl]carbonyl]-3-methylbutyl]-6-oxopipecolamide *see* 7603
4-Carbamoyl-1-β-D-ribofuranosylimidazolium-5-olate *see* 6222
3-Carbamoyl-1-β-D-ribofuranosylpyridinium Hydroxide 5'-(Dihydrogen Phosphate) Inner Salt *see* 6663
3-Carbamoyl-1-β-D-ribofuranosylpyridinium Hydroxide 5' → 5'-Ester with Adenosine 2'-(Dihydrogen Phosphate) 5'-(Trihydrogen Pyrophosphate) Inner Salt *see* 6348
3-Carbamoyl-1-β-D-ribofuranosylpyridinium Hydroxide 5' → 5'-Ester with Adenosine 5'-(Trihydrogen Pyrophosphate) Inner Salt *see* 6344
4'-(Carbamoylsulfamoyl)-*N*-(hydroxymethyl)phthalanilic Acid *see* 8912
4'-(Carbamoylsulfamoyl)phthalanilic Acid Hydroxymethyl Derivative *see* 8912
4-Carbamylaminophenylarsonic Acid *see* 1786
N-Carbamylarsanilic Acid *see* 1786
Carbamyl Chloride, 1783
Carbamylcholine Chloride *see* 1779
Carbamylglutamic Acid *see* 1838
Carbamylguanidine Sulfate *see* 3093
Carbamylhydrazine Hydrochloride *see* 8444
Carbamylmethylcholine Chloride *see* 1185
*N*δ-Carbamylornithine *see* 2331
o-(Carbamylphenoxy)acetic Acid *see* 8329
4-Carbamylphenyl Bis[carboxymethylthio]arsenite *see* 793
Carbamylurea *see* 1309
Carbanil *see* 7296
Carbanilic Acid, 1784
Carbanilic Acid Isopropyl Ester *see* 7816
Carbanilide, 1785

Carbapen [Commonwealth] *see* 1792
Carbarsone, 1786
Carbaryl, 1787
Carbasalate Calcium *see* 1647
Carbaspirin Calcium *see* 1647
Carbathiin *see* 1827
Carbathione *see* 5949
Carbatrol [Shire] *see* 1781
Carbazilquinone *see* 1824
Carbazochrome *see* 172
Carbazochrome Salicylate, 1788
Carbazochrome Sodium Sulfonate, 1789
Carbazole, 1790
9*H*-Carbazole *see* 1790
1-(9*H*-Carbazol-4-yloxy)-3-[[2-(2-methoxyphenoxy)ethyl]amino]-2-propanol *see* 1873
1-(9*H*-Carbazol-4-yloxy)-3-[(1-methylethyl)amino]-2-propanol *see* 1778
Carbazon [Hokuriku] *see* 1789
Carbazotic Acid *see* 7410
Carbecin [Sanfer] *see* 1792
Carbendazim, 1791
Carbendazole *see* 1791
Carbenicillin, 1792
Carbenicillin Disodium *see* 1792
Carbenicillin Indanyl Ester *see* 1840
Carbenin [Sankyo] *see* 7009
Carbenoxalone *see* 1793
Carbenoxolone, 1793
Carbetane [Toyo Jozo] *see* 1794
Carbetapentane, 1794
(2*S*)-2-[(1*S*)-1-Carbethoxybutylamino]-1-oxopropyl-(2*S*,3a*S*,7a*S*)-perhydroindole-2-carboxylic Acid *see* 7170
N-Carbethoxy-2-ethoxy-1,2-dihydroquinoline *see* 3518
3-(2-Carbethoxyhydrazino)-6-[*N*-(2-hydroxypropyl)ethylamino]pyridazine *see* 1631
2-Carbethoxymethylene-3-methyl-5-piperidino-4-thiazolidone *see* 3891
4-Carbethoxy-1-methyl-4-phenylazacycloheptane *see* 3743
4-Carbethoxy-1-methyl-4-phenylhexamethylenimine *see* 3743
p-Carbethoxyphenyl ε-Guanidinocaproate *see* 4320
3-(4-Carbethoxy-4-phenylpiperidino)-1-phenyl-1-propanol *see* 7250
*N*¹-Carbethoxy-*N*²-phthalazinehydrazine *see* 9502
Carbethoxysyringoyl Methyl Reserpate *see* 9017
Carbetocin, 1795
Carbex [Endo] *see* 8428
Carbic Anhydride, 1796
Carbidopa, 1797
Carbilazine *see* 3116
Carbimazole, 1798
Carbimide *see* 1663, 2684
Carbimide *see* 5165
Carbinol *see* 5957
Carbinoxamine, 1799
Carbitol [Union Carbide], 1800
D-8β-[(Carbobenzoxyamino)methyl]-1,6-dimethyl-10α-ergoline *see* 5937
Carbobenzoxy Chloride, 1801
D-*N*-Carbobenzoxydihydro-1-methyllysergamine I *see* 5937
Carbocaina [Astra] *see* 5859
Carbocaine Hydrochloride [Winthrop] *see* 5859
Carbocalcitonin *see* 3537
Carbocholine *see* 1779

[4R,5S,6S]-3-[[(3S,5S)-5-[[(3-Carboxy-phenyl)amino]carbonyl]-3-pyrrolidin-yl]thio]-6-[(1R)-1-hydroxyethyl]-4-methyl-7-oxo-1-azabicyclo[3.2.0]hept-2-ene-2-carboxylic Acid *see* 3673

2-[(2-Carboxyphenyl)amino]-4-chloro-benzoic Acid *see* 5552

9-(*o*-Carboxyphenyl)-4,5-bis[bis(2-pyr-idylmethyl)aminomethyl]-6-hydr-oxy-3-xanthanone *see* 10168

9-(2-Carboxyphenyl)-3,6-bis(diethyl-amino)xanthylium Chloride *see* 8183

(1R,5S,6S,8R,2′S,4′S)-2-(2-(3-Carboxy-phenylcarbamoyl)pyrrolidin-4-ylthio)-6-(1-hydroxyethyl)-1-methylcarba-penem-3-carboxylic Acid *see* 3673

N-(2-Carboxyphenyl)-4-chloroanthra-nilic Acid *see* 5552

9-(*o*-Carboxyphenyl)-2,7-dichloro-4,5-bis[bis(2-pyridylmethyl)aminometh-yl]-6-hydroxy-3-xanthanone *see* 10168

N-[9-(2-Carboxyphenyl)-6-(diethylami-no)-3*H*-xanthen-3-ylidene]-*N*-ethyl-ethanaminium Chloride *see* 8183

9-(*o*-Carboxyphenyl)-6-hydroxy-3-iso-xanthenone *see* 4159

9-(*o*-Carboxyphenyl)-6-hydroxy-3*H*-xanthen-3-one *see* 4159

o-Carboxyphenyl Phosphate *see* 4255

4-Carboxy-4-(*N*-phenylpropionamido)-1-piperidinepropionic Acid Dimethyl Ester *see* 8131

(8S)-7-[(S)-*N*-[(S)-1-Carboxy-3-phenyl-propyl]alanyl]-1,4-dithia-7-azaspiro-[4.4]nonane-8-carboxylic Acid 1-Ethyl Ester *see* 8753

(2S,3aR,7aS)-1-[(S)-*N*-[(S)-1-Carboxy-3-phenylpropyl]alanyl]hexahydro-2-in-dolinecarboxylic Acid 1-Ethyl Ester *see* 9568

(2S,3aS,6aS)-1-[(S)-*N*-[(S)-1-Carboxy-3-phenylpropyl]alanyl]octahydrocyclo-penta[*b*]pyrrole-2-carboxylic Acid 1-Ethyl Ester *see* 8103

N-[(1S)-1-Carboxy-3-phenylpropyl]-L-alanyl-L-proline Dihydrate *see* 3568

1-[*N*-[(S)-1-Carboxy-3-phenylpropyl]-L-alanyl]-L-proline 1′-Ethyl Ester *see* 3567

(S)-2-[(S)-*N*-[(S)-1-Carboxy-3-phenyl-propyl]alanyl]-1,2,3,4-tetrahydro-3-isoquinolinecarboxylic Acid 1-Ethyl Ester *see* 8051

(1S,9S)-9-[[(S)-1-Carboxy-3-phenylpro-pyl]amino]octahydro-10-oxo-6*H*-pyridazino[1,2-*a*][1,2]diazepine-1-carboxylic Acid 9-Ethyl Ester *see* 2273

(3S)-3-[[(1S)-1-Carboxy-3-phenylpro-pyl]amino]-2,3,4,5-tetrahydro-2-oxo-1*H*-1-benzazepine-1-acetic Acid 3-Ethyl Ester *see* 1031

(+)-(2S,6R)-6-[[(1S)-1-Carboxy-3-phenyl-propyl]amino]tetrahydro-5-oxo-2-(2-thienyl)-1,4-thiazepine-4(5*H*)-acetic Acid, 6-Ethyl Ester *see* 9136

(S)-1-[*N*²-(1-Carboxy-3-phenylpropyl)-L-lysyl]-L-proline Dihydrate *see* 5516

[(*o*-Carboxyphenyl)thio]ethylmercury Sodium Salt *see* 9317

Carboxypolymethylene, 1830

4-(β-Carboxypropionylamino)-4′-amino-diphenyl Sulfone *see* 8878

3-*O*-(β-Carboxypropionyl)-11-oxo-18β-olean-12-en-30-oic Acid *see* 1793

2-[4-(1-Carboxypropyl)phenyl]-1-isoin-dolinone *see* 4961

3-Carboxypyridine *N*-Oxide *see* 6941

N-(D-2-Carboxy-1-pyrrolidinyl)-L-gluta-mine *see* 5499

(2S,5R,6R)-6-[[(3-Carboxy-2-quinoxalin-yl)carbonyl]amino]-3,3-dimethyl-7-oxo-4-thia-1-azabicyclo[3.2.0]hep-tane-2-carboxylic Acid *see* 8043

3-Carboxy-2-quinoxalinylpenicillin *see* 8043

Carboxysulfamidochrysoidine *see* 8901

Carboxyterfenadine *see* 4068

3-Carboxy-6,7,8,9-tetrahydro-1,6-di-methyl-4-oxo-4*H*-pyrido[1,2-*a*]pyri-midinium Methyl Sulfate, Ethyl Ester *see* 8225

(6S)-6-[2-Carboxy-2-(3-thienyl)acet-amido]-6-methoxypenicillanic Acid *see* 9137

6-[D(−)-α-Carboxy-3-thienylacet-amido]penicillanic Acid *see* 9428

(2S,5R,6R)-6-[[(2R)-Carboxy-3-thienyl-acetyl]amino]-3,3-dimethyl-7-oxo-4-thia-1-azabicyclo[3.2.0]heptane-2-carboxylic Acid *see* 9428

(2S,5R,6S)-6-[(Carboxy-3-thienylacet-yl)amino]-6-methoxy-3,3-dimethyl-7-oxo-4-thia-1-azabicyclo[3.2.0]hep-tane-2-carboxylic Acid *see* 9137

α-Carboxy-3-thienylmethylpenicillin *see* 9428

(αS)-α-Carboxy-*N*,*N*,*N*-trimethyl-1*H*-imidazole-4-ethanaminium Inner Salt *see* 4667

(αS)-α-Carboxy-*N*,*N*,*N*-trimethyl-1*H*-in-dole-3-ethanaminium Inner Salt *see* 4861

1-Carboxy-*N*,*N*,*N*-trimethylmethanami-nium Chloride *see* 1179

1-Carboxy-*N*,*N*,*N*-trimethylmethanami-nium Inner Salt *see* 1179

6-Carboxyuridine *see* 6877

4-[*o*-[(E)-2-Carboxyvinyl]phenyl]-1,4-di-hydro-2,6-dimethyl-3,5-pyridinedi-carboxylic Acid 4-*tert*-Butyl Diethyl Ester *see* 5331

Carboxyvinyl Polymer *see* 1830

Carbrital [Parke-Davis] *see* 7130

Carbromal, 1831

Carbutamide, 1832

Carbuten [Kalopharma] *see* 5773

Carbuterol, 1833

Carcinil [Abbott] *see* 5457

Cardace [Aventis] *see* 8103

Cardamine *see* 6543

Cardamom, 1834

Cardanat [Temmler] *see* 3865

Cardenalin [Pfizer] *see* 3433

Cardene [Syntex] *see* 6495

Cardiacap [Consolidated Chem.] *see* 7112

Cardiamid *see* 6543

Cardiazol [Knoll] *see* 7141

Cardibeltin [Schwarz] *see* 9950

Cardilate [Burroughs Wellcome] *see* 3677

Cardilate [Ivax] *see* 6528

Cardiloid *see* 3677

Cardimon *see* 6543

Cardine [Marshall] *see* 10010

Cardinol [CP Protea] *see* 7840

Cardinophyllin *see* 1877

Cardioaspirin [Bayer] *see* 851

Cardiogen *see* 1849

Cardiografin [BMS] *see* 5807

Cardio-Green [Becton Dickinson] *see* 4962

Cardiolan [Tosi] *see* 3167

Cardiolite [DuPont] *see* 9102

Cardionatrin *see* 872

Cardioquin [Purdue Frederick] *see* 8060

Cardiosolupsan [BMS] *see* 1647

Cardiosteril [Fresenius] *see* 3421

Cardiotec [BMS] *see* 9103

Cardiotoxin, 1835

Cardiovanil *see* 3721

Cardiovet [Intervet] *see* 3567

Cardioxane [Chiron] *see* 8123

Cardiprin [Reckitt Benckiser] *see* 851

Cardisan *see* 5246

Carditin-Same [Savoma] *see* 7737

Carditoxin [Gedeon Richter] *see* 3163

Cardizem [Biovail] *see* 3202

Cardophylin [Rhône-Poulenc] *see* 465

Cardoxin [RAFA] *see* 3346

Carduben [Madaus] *see* 10010

Cardular [Pfizer] *see* 3433

Cardura [Pfizer] *see* 3433

Carduran [Pfizer] *see* 3433

Carebastine *see* 3484

Carecin [Zensei Yakuhin] *see* 2305

Δ³-Carene *see* 1836

3-Carene, 1836

Carfecillin Sodium *see* 1792

Carfenil [Chugai] *see* 5552

Carfentrazone-ethyl, 1837

Carglumic Acid, 1838

Carguto [Tanabe Seiyaku] *see* 2894

Cargutocin, 1839

Carica *see* 7020

Caricaxanthin *see* 2609

Caricide [Am. Cyanamid] *see* 3116

Caridan *see* 6973

Carindacillin, 1840

Carindapen [Pfizer] *see* 1840

Cariporide, 1841

Cariporide Mesylate *see* 1841

Carisoma [Pharmax] *see* 1842

Carisoprodate *see* 1842

Carisoprodol, 1842

Carlytene [Viatris] *see* 6292

Carmilax [Pfizer] *see* 5670

Carmine *see* 1843

Carminic Acid, 1843

Carminomycin *see* 1870

Carminomycin I *see* 1870

Carmofur, 1844

Carmubris [BMS] *see* 1845

Carmustine, 1845

Carnacid-Cor [TAD] *see* 4434

Carnallite *see* 5653, 7604

Carnauba Wax, 1846

Carnegine, 1847

Carnicor [Sigma-Tau] *see* 1849

Carnidazole, 1848

Carnigen [Albert Roussel] *see* 4824

Carnitine, 1849

L-Carnitine *see* 1849

Carnitor [Sigma-Tau] *see* 1849

Carnosine, 1850

Carnotite *see* 9918

Carob Flour *see* 5554

Carolina Pink *see* 8748

Carony Bark *see* 652

Carophyll Red [Roche] *see* 1753

Caro's Acid, 1851

Carotaben [Hermal] *see* 1853

Carotaben Plus [Hermal] *see* 1753

α-Carotene, 1852

β-Carotene, 1853

β,β-Carotene *see* 1853

γ-Carotene, 1854

δ-Carotene, 1855
ε,ψ-Carotene *see* 1855
ψ,ψ-Carotene *see* 5620
β,β-Carotene-3,3'-diol *see* 10118
β,ε-Carotene-3,3'-diol *see* 10063
all-trans-β-Carotene-3,3'-diol *see* 10118
ψ,ψ-Carotene-16,16'-diol *see* 5621
β,β-Carotene-4,4'-dione *see* 1753
ψ,ψ-Carotene-16-ol *see* 5627
β,β-Carotene-3,3',4,4'-tetrone *see* 853
β-Caroten-3-ol *see* 2609
(3*R*)-β,β-Caroten-3-ol *see* 2609
(3*R*)-β,ψ-Caroten-3-ol *see* 8289
β,β-Caroten-4-one *see* 3495
Carotol, 1856
Caroverine, 1857
Carpaine, 1858
Carpene [Isagro] *see* 3408
Carperitide *see* 872
Carpetimycin A *see* 1859
Carpetimycin B *see* 1859
Carpetimycins, 1859
Carphenazine, 1860
Carpidine *see* 5199
Carpiline *see* 5199
Carpipramine, 1861
Carprofen, 1862
Carpropamid, 1863
Carrageen *see* 1864
Carrageenan, 1864
Carrageenin *see* 1864
Carrbutabarb [Century] *see* 1506
Carrisyn [Carrington] *see* 26
Cartap, 1865
Carteol [Otsuka] *see* 1866
Carteolol, 1866
Carthamic Acid *see* 1867
Carthamin, 1867
Carthamus, 1868
Carthamus Red *see* 1867
Carticaine, 1869
Cartonic [Yamanouchi] *see* 592
Cartric [Sanwa] *see* 8142
Cartrophen [Univet] *see* 7134
Carubicin, 1870
Carubinose *see* 5747
Carudol [Fher] *see* 7277
Carumonam, 1871
Carvacrol, 1872
Carvacron [Taiyo] *see* 9624
Carvasin [Teofarma] *see* 5225
Carvedilol, 1873
Carvol *see* 1874
6,8-Carvomenthenediol *see* 8567
Carvone, 1874
Carylderm [Mundipharma] *see* 1787
Caryolysine [Sanofi-Synthelabo] *see* 5775
Caryophyllene, 1875
α-Caryophyllene *see* 4753
β-Caryophyllene *see* 1875
γ-Caryophyllene *see* 1875
cis-Caryophyllene *see* 1875
trans-Caryophyllene *see* 1875
Caryophyllic Acid *see* 3898
Caryophyllin *see* 6827
Caryophyllus *see* 2418
Carzenide, 1876
Carzinophilin A, 1877
Casakol [Upjohn] *see* 1878
Casamino Acids *see* 1883
Casanthranol, 1878
Casanthranol A *see* 1878
Casanthranol B *see* 1878
Casca Bark *see* 8382
Cascade [BASF] *see* 4133

Cascapride [Cascan] *see* 1432
Cascara Amara, 1879
Cascara Sagrada, 1880
Cascarilla, 1881
Cascarillin, 1882
Cascarin *see* 4264
Cascarosides *see* 1880
Caseanine *see* 9215
Casein, 1883
Cas-Evac *see* 1880
Cashoo *see* 1903
Casodex [AstraZeneca] *see* 1200
Casoron [Solvay Duphar] *see* 3042
Caspase-1, 1884
Caspase-3, 1885
Caspase-8, 1886
Caspase-9, 1887
Caspase-activated DNase *see* 1885
Caspases, 1888
Caspofungin, 1889
Cassadan [Temmler] *see* 312
Cassaidine, 1890
Cassaine, 1891
Cassella 4489 *see* 2239
Cassella's Acid, 1892
Cassella's Acid F, 1893
Cassel's Green *see* 981
Cassia *see* 2300
Cassia Fistula, 1894
Cassia Pods *see* 1894
Cassia Pulp *see* 1894
Cassic Acid *see* 8176
Cassiopeium *see* 5615
Cassiterite *see* 8778
Castanea, 1895
Castanospermine, 1896
Castellan [AgrEvo] *see* 4196
Castle's Intrinsic Factor, 1897
Castor Oil, 1898
Castor Oil, Hydrogenated, 1899
Castorwax *see* 1899
Cat *see* 5963
Cataclot [Ono] *see* 6980
Cataflam [Novartis] *see* 3081
Catalase, 1900
Catalin [Senju] *see* 7490
Catalpin *see* 1901
Catalposide, 1901
Catalyst [Wellmark] *see* 7815
Catanil [DeAngeli] *see* 2186
Catapres [Boehringer, Ing.] *see* 2390
Catapresan [Boehringer, Ing.] *see* 2390
Catarase [Cooper] *see* 2260
Cataria *see* 1907
Catechin, 1902
Catechinic Acid *see* 1902
Catechol *see* 1902, 7999
Catecholase *see* 9838
Catechu *see* 4359
Catechu Black, 1903
Catechuic Acid *see* 1902
Catenins *see* 1611
Catenulin *see* 7041
Catergen [Zyma] *see* 1902
Catharanthine, 1904
Cathepsin C *see* 1905
Cathepsin D *see* 1905
Cathepsin G *see* 1905
Cathepsins, 1905
Cathine *see* 6714
Cathinone, 1906
Catlep [Sumitomo] *see* 4968
Catmint *see* 1907
Catnep, 1907
Catnip *see* 1907

Catonin [Magis] *see* 1643
Cat's Hair *see* 3903
Cattlyst [Syntex] *see* 5348
Caudaline [Exa] *see* 9429
Caulophylline *see* 6049
Caulophyllum *see* 1320
Caulosapogenin *see* 4624
Caustic Alcohol *see* 8613
Caustic Barley *see* 8308
Caustic Baryta *see* 977
Caustic Potash *see* 7640
Caustic Soda *see* 8627
Causyth [Inverni] *see* 7871
Cav-Ecol *see* 10041
Caverject [Pharmacia & Upjohn] *see* 7876
Cavinton [Thiemann] *see* 9991
Cavitands *see* 2340
Cavonyl *see* 2711
Cayenne Pepper *see* 1770
Caytine *see* 7895
CB-11 *see* 7207
CB-154 *see* 1416
CB-154 Mesylate *see* 1416
CB-302 *see* 4273
CB-304 *see* 904
CB-311 *see* 8716
CB-313 *see* 6216
CB-337 *see* 5808
CB-1048 *see* 2108
CB-1348 *see* 2073
CB-1639 *see* 2734
CB-1678 *see* 7822
CB-2041 *see* 1505
CB-3025 *see* 5828
CB-3026 *see* 5828
CB-4261 *see* 9243
CB-4306 *see* 2403
CB-4311 *see* 2403
CB-7432 *see* 4890
CB-8061 *see* 7134
CB-30038 *see* 6200
2C-B, 1908
CBA-93626 *see* 2392
CBDCA *see* 1822
CBN *see* 1748
CBS *see* 2485
CC *see* 10019
CC-2481 *see* 2712
CC-4047 *see* 135
CC-5013 *see* 5436
CCA *see* 5552
CCC *see* 1663, 2104
CCD-1042 *see* 4362
β-CCE *see* 3779
CCI-779 *see* 9142
CCI-15641 *see* 1954
CCI-18781 *see* 4211
CCK-179 *see* 3653
CCK-PZ *see* 2198
CCK *C*-Terminal Octapeptide *see* 8543
CCNU [Lundbeck] *see* 5564
CCP *see* 2366
CCRG-81045 *see* 9139
CD-68 *see* 2082
CD-271 *see* 150
CDA *see* 2029
2-CdA *see* 2337
CDC *see* 2054
CDD 95-126 *see* 9886
CDDD-5604 *see* 5584
CDEC *see* 8911
CDM *see* 2085
CDO-MeB *see* 9103
CDP-771 *see* 4390
CDP-870 *see* 2003

CDP-choline *see* 2319
CDR *see* 1719
CE-3624 *see* 9430
Ceanothic Acid, 1909
CEA-Scan [Immunomedics] *see* 774
Cebera [Irex] *see* 244
Cebesine [Chauvin] *see* 1047
Cebion [Merck KGaA] *see* 830
Cebrogen [Walker] *see* 4471
Cebrum [SIFA] *see* 2084
Cebutid [Boots] *see* 4199
Cecenu [Medac] *see* 5564
Ceclor [Lilly] *see* 1912
Cecon [Abbott] *see* 830
Cecropins, 1910
CED-3 *see* 1888
Cedad [Recordati] *see* 1029
Cedar Camphor *see* 1911
Cedar Leaf Oil *see* 9389
Cedax [Schering-Plough] *see* 1949
Cedilanid [Sandoz] *see* 5354
Cedilanide [Novartis] *see* 2921
Cedocard [Pharmacia] *see* 5225
Cedol [Tiber] *see* 1914
8βH-Cedran-8-ol *see* 1911
Cedrol, 1911
Cedro Oil *see* 6798
Cedur [Boehringer, Mann.] *see* 1195
CEE *see* 2508
CeeNU [BMS] *see* 5564
Ceepryn [J. B. Williams] *see* 2032
Cefacidal [Allard] *see* 1917
Cefaclor, 1912
Cefadol [Nippon Shinyaku] *see* 3311
Cefa-Drops [Fort Dodge] *see* 1913
Cefadros [Proter] *see* 1974
Cefadroxil, 1913
Cefadyl [BMS] *see* 1984
Cefa-Iskia [Iskia] *see* 1974
Cefa-Lak [Fort Dodge] *see* 1984
Cefalen [Lenza] *see* 7513
Cefalex [Von Boch] *see* 7513
Cefalonium *see* 1978
Cefaloridin *see* 1979
Cefalotin *see* 1982
Cefaloto [Lifepharma] *see* 1974
Cefam [Magis] *see* 1914
Cefamandole, 1914
Cefamar [Firma] *see* 1954
Cefamedin [Fujisawa] *see* 1917
Cefamezin [Fujisawa] *see* 1917
Cefamox [BMS] *see* 1913
Cefanex [Apothecon] *see* 1974
Cefaperos [Allard] *see* 1915
Cefaseptin [Chassot] *see* 1974
Cefatriaxone *see* 1953
Cefatrizine, 1915
Cefazedone, 1916
Cefazil [Giustini] *see* 1917
Cefazina [Chemil] *see* 1917
Cefazolin, 1917
Cefazone [Firma] *see* 1930
Cefbon-C₂F [Central Glass] *see* 4540
Cefbon-CF [Central Glass] *see* 4540
Cefbuperazone, 1918
Cefcapene Pivoxil, 1919
Cefdinir, 1920
Cefditoren, 1921
Cefditoren Pivoxil *see* 1921
Cefepime, 1922
Cefepime Hydrochloride *see* 1922
Cefetamet, 1923
Cefetamet Pivoxil *see* 1923
Cefibacter [Rubio] *see* 1974
Cefiran [Poli] *see* 1914

Cefixime, 1924
Cefixoral [Menarini] *see* 1924
Cefizox [Fujisawa] *see* 1951
Ceflorin [Glaxo] *see* 1979
Cefmax [TAP] *see* 1925
Cefmenoxime, 1925
Cefmetazole, 1926
Cefmetazon [Sankyo] *see* 1926
Cefminox, 1927
Cefobid [Pfizer] *see* 1930
Cefobine [Pfizer] *see* 1930
Cefobis [Pfizer] *see* 1930
Cefodie [SKB] *see* 1929
Cefodizime, 1928
Cefodox [Scharper] *see* 1941
Cefogram [Metapharma] *see* 1930
Cefomonil [TAP] *see* 1945
Cefoneg [Tosi] *see* 1930
Cefonicid, 1929
Cefoperazone, 1930
Cefoprim [Esseti] *see* 1954
Ceforal [Farmoffer] *see* 1913
Ceforanide, 1931
Cefoselis, 1932
Cefosint [Proter] *see* 1930
Cefotan [AstraZeneca] *see* 1934
Cefotax [Chugai] *see* 1933
Cefotaxime, 1933
Cefotetan, 1934
Cefotiam, 1935
Cefotiam Hexetil Hydrochloride *see* 1935
Cefotrizin [Firma] *see* 1915
Cefoxitin, 1936
Cefozopran, 1937
Cefpimizole, 1938
Cefpiramide, 1939
Cefpiran [Sumitomo] *see* 1939
Cefpirome, 1940
Cefpodoxime *see* 1941
Cefpodoxime Proxetil, 1941
Cefprozil, 1942
Cefquinome, 1943
Cefradine *see* 1986
Cefro [Sankyo] *see* 1986
Cefrom [HMR] *see* 1940
Cefroxadine, 1944
Cefspan [Fujisawa] *see* 1924
Cefsulodin, 1945
Ceftazidime, 1946
Ceftenon [Biochemie] *see* 1934
Cefteram, 1947
Cefteram Pivoxil *see* 1947
Ceftetrame *see* 1947
Ceftezole, 1948
Ceftibuten, 1949
Ceftin [GSK] *see* 1954
Ceftiofur, 1950
Ceftix [Boehringer, Mann.] *see* 1951
Ceftizon [Bago] *see* 1951
Ceftizoxime, 1951
Ceftobiprole *see* 1952
Ceftobiprole Medocaril, 1952
Ceftriaxone, 1953
Cefumax [Locatelli] *see* 1954
Cefurax [Betapharm] *see* 1954
Cefurex [Sarm] *see* 1954
Cefurin [Magis] *see* 1954
Cefuroxime, 1954
Cefuroxime Axetil *see* 1954
Cefuzonam, 1955
Cefyl [Takeda] *see* 1923
Cefzil [BMS] *see* 1942
Ceglunat [DDR] *see* 5354
Cekufon [Cequisa] *see* 9623
Cela W-524 *see* 9691

Celadigal [Beiersdorf] *see* 5354
Celance [Lilly] *see* 7162
Celaskon [Leciva] *see* 830
Celbenin [SKB] *see* 5969
Celebrex [Pfizer] *see* 1956
Celecoxib, 1956
Celectol [Sanofi-Aventis] *see* 1960
Celeport [Eisai] *see* 1206
Celery Seed, 1957
Celest [Syngenta] *see* 4129
Celestan [Essex] *see* 1180
Celestan-V [Essex] *see* 1180
Celestene [Schering-Plough] *see* 1180
Celesticetin, 1958
Celestin Blue, 1959
Celestine *see* 8835, 8848
Celestite *see* 8848
Celestoderm-V [Schering-Plough] *see* 1180
Celestone [Schering-Plough] *see* 1180
Celestovet [Biokema] *see* 1180
Celevac [Shire] *see* 6040
Celexa [Forest] *see* 2318
Celin [GSK] *see* 830
Célio [Novartis] *see* 2401
Celiomycin *see* 10001
Celiprolol, 1960
Celiptium [Sanofi-Aventis] *see* 3549
Celite *see* 4973
Cellative [Tobishi] *see* 5780
CellCept [Roche] *see* 6327
Cellidrin [Hennig] *see* 279
Cellobiose, 1961
β-Cellobiose *see* 1961
Cellocidin, 1962
Celloidin *see* 8011
Cellolax *see* 1829
Cellon *see* 9189
Cellophane, 1963
Cellose *see* 1961
Cellosolve *see* 3750
Cellosolve Acetate *see* 3751
Cellucon [Medo] *see* 6040
Celluflex 179 [Celanese] *see* 9763
Celluloid, 1964
Cellulose, 1965
Cellulose Acetates, 1966
Cellulose-ECTEOLA *see* 3504
Cellulose Ethyl Ether *see* 3781
Cellulose Ethyl Hydroxyethyl Ether, 1967
Cellulose 2-Hydroxypropyl Ether *see* 4841
Cellulose 2-Hydroxypropyl Methyl Ether *see* 4842
Cellulose Methyl Ether *see* 6040
Cellulose Nitrate *see* 8011
Cellulose Phenoxyacetate *see* 7255
Cellulosic Acid *see* 6939
Celmidol [Tobishi] *see* 3311
Cel-O-Brandt *see* 1829
Celocurine [Pfizer] *see* 8876
Celontin [Parke-Davis] *see* 6004
Celoslin [Hoechst] *see* 1948
Celospor [Novartis] *see* 1972
Celphos [Excel] *see* 359
Celpillina *see* 5969
Celtect [Kyowa] *see* 6925
Celupan [Lacer] *see* 6363
Cemado [Francia] *see* 1914
Cemandil [SIT] *see* 1914
Cemastin [Ist. Vitamine] *see* 1982
Cembrene A *see* 6448
Cemirit [Bayer] *see* 851
Cemix [Takeda] *see* 1925
Cenalene-M [Central Pharm.] *see* 7141

Cenazol *see* 7141
Cenocort [Central Pharm.] *see* 9595
Cenolate [Abbott] *see* 830
Cenomycin [Daiichi] *see* 1936
Centaurein, 1968
Centaurin *see* 2425
Centaury, American, 1970
Centaury, American, 1970
Centchroman, 1971
trans-Centchroman *see* 1971
Centedrin [Gedeon Richter] *see* 6110
Centralgin [Amino] *see* 5849
Centralgol [Zyma] *see* 7904
Centralgyl *see* 7904
Centralite I *see* 3117
Centrallasite *see* 1702
Centraureo [Central] *see* 2192
Centrax [Warner-Lambert] *see* 7715
Centrine [Fort Dodge] *see* 459
Centron [Torrent] *see* 1971
Centrophenoxine *see* 5780
Centroton [Wander] *see* 8010
Centyl [Leo Pharm] *see* 1037
Ceosunin [Kyowa] *see* 2005
CEPA *see* 3732
Cepacilina [CEPA] *see* 7096
Cepaloridin [Glaxo] *see* 1979
Cepalorin *see* 1979
Cepan [IBI] *see* 1934
Cepaverin [Globopharm] *see* 7019
Cepazine [Sanofi-Synthelabo] *see* 1954
CEPH *see* 9502
Cephacetrile Sodium, 1972
Cephaeline, 1973
Cephaeline Methyl Ether *see* 3559
Cephalexin, 1974
Cephalins, 1975
Cephaloglycin, 1976
Cephalonic Acid, 1977
Cephalonium, 1978
Cephaloridine, 1979
Cephalosporin C, 1980
Cephalosporin C$_A$ *see* 1980
Cephalosporin C$_C$ *see* 1980
Cephalosporin N *see* 7098
Cephalosporin P$_1$, 1981
Cephalothin, 1982
Cephamycins, 1983
Cephapirin Sodium, 1984
Cepharanthine, 1985
Cephation [Meiji] *see* 1982
Cephoral [Merck KGaA] *see* 1924
Cephos [CT] *see* 1913
Cephradine, 1986
Cephrol *see* 2330
Cephulac *see* 5346
Cepimex [Mead Johnson] *see* 1922
Ceporacin [Torii] *see* 1982
Ceporan [Glaxo] *see* 1979
Ceporex [GSK] *see* 1974
Ceporexin [GSK] *see* 1974
Ceporin [Glaxo] *see* 1979
Cepovenin [Hoechst; Glaxo] *see* 1982
Cepravin Dry Cow [Schering-Plough] *see* 1978
Cepticol [Banyu] *see* 1915
Cer [Nippon Glaxo] *see* 1979
Ceralan [Amerchol] *see* 5359
Ceramide-β-lactoside *see* 2794
Ceramide Trihexosidase *see* 4336
Ceranapril *see* 1994
Ceraphyl 28 *see* 2030
Cerargyrite *see* 8504
Ceraxon [Ferrer] *see* 2319
Cerazette [Organon] *see* 2926

Cerberigenin *see* 3162
Cerberin *see* 6474
Cercobin [Nippon Soda] *see* 9352
Cercobin-M [Nippon Soda] *see* 9352
Cerebid [Saron] *see* 7019
Cerebolan [Tobishi] *see* 2305
Cerebroforte [Azupharma] *see* 7487
Cerebronylsphingosylglucosidogalacto-
side *see* 2794
Cerebrose *see* 4335
Cerebrostenediol *see* 4820
Cerebrosterol *see* 4820
Cerebyx [Pfizer] *see* 4258
Cereclor *see* 7024
Ceredase [Genzyme] *see* 243
Ceredist [Tanabe Seiyaku] *see* 9045
Ceregulart [Kaken] *see* 2994
Cerekinon [Tanabe] *see* 9699
Cerepar [Mepha] *see* 2305
Ceresan [Bayer AG] *see* 7300
Ceresan Wet *see* 3826
Ceresin, 1987
Cerespan [USV] *see* 7019
Cerestat [Cambridge Neurosci.] *see* 758
Ceretec [Amersham] *see* 3911
Cerevon *see* 4056
Cerezyme [Genzyme] *see* 243
Cergem [Searle] *see* 4387
Cergodum [Duncan] *see* 6496
Ceria *see* 1989
Ceric Fluoride, 1988
Ceric Oxide, 1989
Ceric Sulfate, 1990
Cerin *see* 1987
Cerium, 1991
Cerium(IV) Ammonium Nitrate, 1992
Cerivastatin, 1993
CERM-1978 *see* 1150
CERM-3024 *see* 10170
CERM-10202 *see* 9942
Cer-O-Cillin Sodium [Upjohn] *see* 7099
Cerocral [Funai] *see* 4895
Ceronapril, 1994
Cerone [Bayer CropSci.] *see* 3732
Cerosin *see* 1987
Cerous Benzoate *see* 1091
Cerous Bromide, 1995
Cerous Carbonate, 1996
Cerous Chloride, 1997
Cerous Fluoride, 1998
Cerous Iodide, 1999
Cerous Nitrate, 2000
Cerous Oxalate, 2001
Cerous Sulfate, 2002
Cerovive [AstraZeneca] *see* 3363
Certican [Novartis] *see* 3907
Certolizumab Pegol, 2003
Certomycin [Essex] *see* 6479
Certostat [Jenapharm] *see* 3106
Cerubidin [M & B] *see* 2832
Cérubidine [Rhône-Poulenc] *see* 2832
Cerucal [Temmler] *see* 6143
Cerulein *see* 2005
Cerulenin, 2004
Ceruletide, 2005
Ceruloplasmin, 2006
Ceruse *see* 1005
Cerussa *see* 1005
Cerussite *see* 5396
Cervagem(e) [M & B] *see* 4387
Cervicarcin, 2007
Cervilaxin *see* 8129
Cervonic Acid *see* 3398
Cervoxan [Sorbio] *see* 3487
Cesamet [Lilly] *see* 6342

Cesar [AgrEvo] *see* 4713
Cescan-131 [Abbott] *see* 2011
Cesium, 2008
Cesium Bromide, 2009
Cesium Carbonate, 2010
Cesium Chloride, 2011
Cesium Fluoride, 2012
Cesium Hydrate *see* 2013
Cesium Hydroxide, 2013
Cesium Iodide, 2014
Cesium Nitrate, 2015
Cesium Sulfate, 2016
Cesol [Merck KGaA] *see* 7716
Cesplon [Esteve] *see* 1774
Cestex [SKB] *see* 3637
Cestocide [Bayer] *see* 6519
Cetab *see* 2025
Cetaceum *see* 8741
Cetacillin *see* 7817
Cetacort [Galderma] *see* 4787
Cetal [Warner-Lambert] *see* 9983
Cetalkonium Chloride, 2017
Cetamide [Alcon] *see* 8899
Cetamolol, 2018
Cetapril [Dainippon] *see* 200
Cetats [Zeeland] *see* 2025
Cetavlon [Ayerst] *see* 2025
Ceteareth *see* 7577
Cetebe [GSK] *see* 830
Ceteth *see* 7577
Ceteth 20 *see* 7577
Cethexonium Bromide, 2019
Cethromycin, 2020
Cethylose [Ascher] *see* 1829
Cetiedil, 2021
Cetiprin [Kabi] *see* 3558
Cetirizine, 2022
(−)-Cetirizine *see* 2022
Cetol *see* 2017
Cetosanol [Sanol] *see* 5354
Cetotiamine, 2023
Cetraxate, 2024
Cetrexin [Leciva] *see* 5780
Cetrimide *see* 2025
Cetrimonium Bromide, 2025
Cetrimonium Tosylate *see* 2025
Cetrorelix, 2026
Cetrotide [Serono] *see* 2026
Cetuximab, 2027
Cetyl Alcohol, 2028
Cetylamine *see* 2025
α-Cetylcitric Acid *see* 186
Cetyldimethylbenzylammonium Chlor-
ide *see* 2017
N-Cetyl-*N,N*-dimethyl-2-cyclohexanol-
ammonium Bromide *see* 2019
Cetyldimethylethylammonium Bromide,
2029
Cetyldimethyl(2-hydroxycyclohexyl)-
ammonium Bromide *see* 2019
Cetylic Acid *see* 6996
Cetyl Lactate, 2030
Cetyl Palmitate, 2031
Cetylpyridinium Chloride, 2032
Cetyltrimethylammonium Bromide *see*
2025
Cevadilla *see* 8308
Cevadine, 2033
Cevalin [Lilly] *see* 830
(3β,5α,6α)-Cevane-3,6,20-triol *see* 9969
Cevimeline, 2034
Cevine, 2035
Ce-Vi-Sol [BMS] *see* 830
Cevitamic Acid *see* 830
Cevitan [Aventis] *see* 830

Cewin [Sanofi-Synthelabo] see 830
Cex [Nippon Glaxo] see 1974
Ceylon Cinnamon see 2300
Ceylon Isinglass see 184
CEZ see 1917
CF see 4222
CFCs see 2140
C-Film [Arun] see 6677
C₃-Fluoroalcohol see 9206
CFPQ see 3592
CG see 2216
CG-113 see 7740
CG-201 see 1193
CG-315E see 9566
CG-635 see 3872
CG-1283 see 6207
CG-4203 see 9057
CG-4509 see 7902
CGA-15324 see 7770
CGA-18731 see 5218
CGA-23654 see 6633
CGA-24705 see 6146
CGA-26423 see 7740
CGA-45156 see 9329
CGA-48988 see 5922
CGA-50439 see 2764
CGA-64250 see 7818
CGA-72662 see 2775
CGA-89317 see 9652
CGA-106630 see 2969
CGA-131036 see 9600
CGA-136872 see 7747
CGA-142705 see 3989
CGA-152005 see 7881
CGA-154281 see 1046
CGA-163935 see 9725
CGA-169374 see 3135
CGA-173506 see 4129
CGA-179246 see 6190
CGA-184699 see 5595
CGA-184927 see 2370
CGA-185072 see 2401
CGA-215944 see 7950
CGA-219417 see 2772
CGA-245704 see 106
CGA-248757 see 4210
CGA-279202 see 9677
CGA-293343 see 9294
CGA-329351 see 5922
CG-B3Q see 1948
cGMP see 2709
CGP see 4620
CGP-2175 see 6151
CGP-4540 see 574
CGP-6140 see 571
CGP-7174/E see 1945
CGP-7760B see 7735
CGP-9000 see 1944
CGP-14221/E see 1935
CGP-14458 see 4593
CGP-19835 see 5844
CGP-19835A see 5844
CGP-30083 see 3625
CGP-30694 see 3507
CGP-32349 see 4240
CGP-33101 see 8293
CGP-39360 see 8802
CGP-39393 see 4718
CGP-41251 see 6185
CGP-42446 see 10187
CGP-42446A see 10187
CGP-42446B see 10187
CGP-42935 see 391
CGP-45840B see 3081
CGP-48933 see 9916

CGP-51901 see 6842
CGP-57148B see 4902
CGP-60536 see 247
CGP-60536B see 247
CGP-64128A see 755
CGP-72670 see 2858
CGP-73547 see 858
CGP-79787 see 9939
CGP-79787D see 9939
CGS-9343B see 10110
CGS-14824A see 1031
CGS-14831 see 1031
CGS-16949A see 3927
CGS-20267 see 5450
CGT-003 see 3511
CH-800 see 4003
CH-846 see 3487
CH-3635 see 9657
Chaetomidin see 6850
Chalcanthite see 2653
Chalcedony see 8493
Chalcocite see 2519, 2667
Chalcomycin, 2036
Chalcone, 2037
Chalcopyrite, 2038
D-Chalcose, 2039
Chalkone see 2037
Chalkopyrite see 2038
Chamazulene, 2040
Chamber Crystals see 6648
Chameleon Mineral see 7655
Chamomile, 2041
Champaca Camphor see 4556
Champacol see 4556
Champix [Pfizer] see 9936
Chanchalagua see 1969
Channel Black see 1808
Channel Forming Integral Protein see
    760
Chanoclavin-I see 2042
Chanoclavine, 2042
Chanoclavine II see 2042
Chanodesethylapovincamine see 9985
Chaperonins, 2043
CHAPS, 2044
CHAPSO see 2044
Charas see 1749
Charcot-Neumann Crystals see 8743
Chartarin see 2045
Chartreusin, 2045
Charybdotoxin, 2046
Chasteberry see 189
Chaste Tree see 189
Chat see 5308
Chaulmestrol see 2048
Chaulmoogra Oil, 2047
Chaulmoogric Acid, 2048
Chavicine, 2049
Chavicinic Acid see 7467
Chavicol, 2050
Chavicol Methyl Ether see 3705
Chebutan see 5288
Cheeseflower see 5708
Chelafer see 4038
Chelaplex III see 3517
Chelatran [Serb] see 3517
Chelen see 3782
Chelerythrine, 2051
ψ-Chelerythrine see 8356
Chelidonic Acid, 2052
Chelidonine, 2053
Chel-Iron see 4038
Chemcef [Chemil] see 1933
Chemet [McNeil] see 8865
Chem-Fish [Tifa] see 7476

Chemical 109 see 722
Chemical Mace see 2115
Chemifluor [Chemipharm] see 8618
Chemiofuran [Italfarmaco] see 6599
Chemofuran see 6600
Chemotrim [Rosemont] see 8918
Chemox DN [Blue Spruce] see 3287
Chemox PE [Blue Spruce] see 3287
Chemox Selective [Blue Spruce] see 3287
Chendol [CP Pharm.] see 2054
Chenic Acid see 2054
Chenocol [Astellas] see 2054
Chenodeoxycholic Acid see 2054
Chenodiol, 2054
Chenofalk [Falk] see 2054
Chenopodiol [Pohl] see 6785
Chenoposan see 6785
Chenoposetten see 6785
Chenossil [Sanofi-Aventis] see 2054
Chephalotin [Lilly] see 1982
Chepirol see 5288
Cheque see 6174
CHES, 2055
Chessylite see 2631
Chestnut see 1895
Chetazolidin [Zeria] see 5288
Chetil see 5288
Chevreul's Salt see 2668
Chibro Pilocarpine [Chibret] see 7424
Chibro-Proscar [Chibret] see 4082
Chibroxin(e) [Merck & Co.] see 6700
Chibroxol [Merck & Co.] see 6700
Chick Antidermatitis Factor see 7015
Chicle, 2056
Chi-jian see 4374
Chilean Centaury see 1969
Chile Saltpeter see 8647
Chimaphila, 2057
Chimaphilin, 2058
Chimeric A2 Antibody see 4972
Chimonanthine, 2059
Chimono [Lusofarmaco] see 5562
Chimyl Alcohol, 2060
China Bark see 8040
China Clay see 5282
China Green see 5699
China Oil see 949
"China White" see 2968
China Wood Oil see 9813
Chinese Anise see 8797
Chinese Blistering Flies see 6329
Chinese Blue see 7910
Chinese Cantharides see 6329
Chinese Cinnamon see 2300
Chinese Ginger see 4338
Chinese Isinglass see 184
Chinese Pea see 8730
Chinese Red see 5889
Chinese Seasoning see 6254
Chinese Wax, 2061
Chinic Acid see 8059
Chinicine see 10003
Chinidin-Duriles [Astra] see 8060
Chiniofon see 4826
Chinocide see 8067
Chinoform see 5031
Chinofungin [Chinoin] see 9519
Chinoleine see 8068
Chinomethionat(e) see 6978
Chinosol [Chinosolfabrik] see 4843
Chinova Acid see 8075
Chinovic Acid see 8075
Chinovin see 8076
Chinovose see 8077
CHIP28 see 760

CHIPCO-26019 [Bayer CropSci.] *see* 5077
Chiptox [Rhône-Poulenc] *see* 5764
(*S*,*S*)-Chiraphos, 2063
Chirata, 2064
Chirayita *see* 2064
Chiretta *see* 2064
Chirocaine [Abbott] *see* 1495
Chitin, 2065
Chitosamine *see* 4458
Chitosan *see* 2065
Chittem Bark *see* 1880
Chittim Bark *see* 1880
Chlochinate *see* 4826
Chlokale [Sawai] *see* 223
Chloor-hexaviet *see* 4688
Chlophedianol, 2066
Chlophenadione *see* 2406
Chloquinate *see* 4826
Chloracetone *see* 2114
Chloracetyl Chloride, 2067
Chloracizine, 2068
Chloractil [DDSA] *see* 2185
Chloracysin *see* 2068
Chloral *see* 9626
Chloral Alcoholate, 2069
Chloralamide *see* 2070
Chloraldurat [Pohl] *see* 2071
Chloral Ethylalcoholate *see* 2069
Chloral Formamide, 2070
Chloral Hydrate, 2071
Chloral Hydrocyanide *see* 2134
Chlorallylene *see* 289
Chloralosane *see* 2072
α-Chloralose, 2072
β-Chloralose *see* 2072
Chlorambucil, 2073
Chloramide *see* 2070
Chloramine *see* 2075
Chloramine-B, 2074
Chloramine-T, 2075
Chloraminophenamide, 2076
Chloraminophene *see* 2073
Chloramiphene *see* 2386
Chloramphenicol, 2077
Chloramphenicol Arginine Succinate *see* 2077
Chloramphenicol Pantothenate *see* 2077
Chloranautine *see* 3207
Chloranil, 2078
Chloranilic Acid, 2079
Chloranocryl *see* 3088
Chlorapatite *see* 7347
Chlorasept 2000 [Baxter] *see* 2091
Chlorazene [WPC] *see* 2075
Chlorazin [Streuli] *see* 2185
Chlorazine (Russian) *see* 2721
Chlorazodin *see* 2120
Chlorazol Yellow 2G *see* 9310
Chlorbenzoxamine, 2080
5-Chlorbenzoxazolin-2-one *see* 2194
Chlorbenzoxyethamine *see* 2080
Chlorbismol *see* 1263
Chlorbutol *see* 2129
Chlorcosane *see* 7024
Chlorcyclizine, 2081
Chlordan(e), 2082
Chlordecone, 2083
Chlordiazepoxide, 2084
Chlordimeform, 2085
Chloreal *see* 9641
Chlorendic Anhydride, 2086
Chloresium [Rystan] *see* 2155
Chlorethiazol *see* 2384
Chlorethoxyfos, 2087
Chlorethyl *see* 3782

Chloretone [Parke-Davis] *see* 2129
Chlorex *see* 3066
Chlorfenapyr, 2088
Chlorfenvinphos, 2089
Chlorguanide, 2090
Chlorguanide Triazine *see* 2721
Chlorhexamed [Blendax-Richardson] *see* 2091
Chlorhexidine, 2091
Chlorhydrol [Reheis] *see* 343
Chloric Acid, 2092
Chloric Acid, Aluminum Salt *see* 336
"Chloride of Lime" *see* 2094
Chlor-IFC *see* 2187
Chlorimipramine *see* 2387
Chlorimuron-ethyl, 2093
Chlorin e$_6$ *see* 7388
Chlorinated Biphenyls *see* 7564
Chlorinated Camphene *see* 9557
Chlorinated Lime, 2094
Chlorine, 2095
Chlorine Dioxide, 2096
Chlorine Fluoride *see* 2098
Chlorine Heptoxide, 2097
Chlorine Monofluoride, 2098
Chlorine Monoxide, 2099
Chlorine Nitride *see* 6602
Chlorine Peroxide *see* 2096
Chlorine Trifluoride, 2100
Chlorins *see* 7599
Chlorisept [Chinosolfabrik] *see* 2422
Chlorisondamine Chloride, 2101
Chlorisondamine Dimethochloride *see* 2101
Chlormadinone Acetate, 2102
Δ^1-Chlormadinone Acetate *see* 2878
Chlormephos, 2103
Chlormeprazine *see* 7761
Chlormequat Chloride, 2104
Chlormerodrin, 2105
Chlormeroprin *see* 2105
Chlormethazanone *see* 2106
Chlormethiazole *see* 2384
Chlormethine *see* 5775
Chlormethylenecycline *see* 2388
Chlormethylfos *see* 2103
Chlormezanone, 2106
Chlormidazole, 2107
Chlornaphazine, 2108
Chloroacetaldehyde, 2109
Chloroacetamide, 2110
2-Chloroacetamide *see* 2110
Chloroacetanilide, 2111
m-Chloroacetanilide *see* 2111
o-Chloroacetanilide *see* 2111
p-Chloroacetanilide *see* 2111
3′-Chloroacetanilide *see* 2111
Chloroacetic Acid, 2112
Chloroacetic Acid Anhydride *see* 2113
Chloroacetic Acid Anhydride with Isocyanic Acid *see* 2117
Chloroacetic Acid *tert*-Butyl Ester *see* 1563
Chloroacetic Acid 1,1-Dimethyl Ester *see* 1563
Chloroacetic Acid Ethyl Ester *see* 3783
Chloroacetic Acid Methyl Ester *see* 6042
Chloroacetic Anhydride, 2113
Chloroacetone, 2114
α-Chloroacetophenone *see* 2115
ω-Chloroacetophenone, 2115
p-Chloroacetophenone, 2116
2-Chloroacetophenone *see* 2115
4′-Chloroacetophenone *see* 2116

2-Chloro-10-[3-[1-(2-acetoxyethyl)-4-piperazinyl]propyl]phenothiazine *see* 9356
5-Chloro-8-acetoxyquinoline *see* 2422
17-Chloroacetylajmaline *see* 5577
Chloroacetyl Isocyanate, 2117
γ-Chloroallyl Chloride *see* 3075
2-Chloroallyl Diethyldithiocarbamate *see* 8911
N-(3-Chloroallyl)hexaminium Chloride *see* 8027
(±)-2-[(*E*)-1-[(*E*)-3-Chloroallyloxyimino]propyl]-5-[2-(ethylthio)propyl]-3-hydroxycyclohex-2-enone *see* 2349
2-[1-[(2*E*)-3-Chloroallyloxyimino]propyl]-3-hydroxy-5-perhydropyran-4-ylcyclohex-2-en-1-one *see* 9152
1-(3-Chloroallyl)-3,5,7-triaza-1-azonia-adamantane Chloride *see* 8027
Chloroambucil *see* 2073
2-Chloro-4-aminobenzoic Acid Diethylaminoethyl Ester Hydrochloride *see* 2158
2-Chloro-6-amino-9-(2-deoxy-β-D-erythro-pentofuranosyl)purine *see* 2337
4′-Chloro-4-aminodiphenyl *see* 435
Chloroaniline, 2118
m-Chloroaniline *see* 2118
o-Chloroaniline *see* 2118
p-Chloroaniline *see* 2118
2-*p*-Chloroanilino-5-*p*-chlorophenyl-3,5-dihydro-3-isopropyliminophenazine *see* 2373
3-(*p*-Chloroanilino)-10-(*p*-chlorophenyl)-2,10-dihydro-2-(isopropylimino)-phenazine *see* 2373
(*o*-Chloroanilino)dichlorotriazine *see* 657
2-(4-Chloroanilino)-3-isopropylimino-5-(4-chlorophenyl)-3,5-dihydrophenazine *see* 2373
1-(4-Chloroanilino)-4-(4-pyridylmethyl)phthalazine *see* 9939
1-[[*p*-[2-(5-Chloro-*o*-anisamido)ethyl]phenyl]sulfonyl]-3-cyclohexylurea *see* 4478
2-Chloro-2′-arabinofluoro-2′-deoxy-adenosine *see* 2372
Chloroarsenol, 2119
Chloroauric Acid *see* 4522
Chloroazodin, 2120
Chloroazotic Acid *see* 6609
o-Chlorobenzalmalononitrile *see* 2127
(±)-α-(*p*-Chlorobenzamido)-1,2-dihydro-2-oxo-4-quinolinepropionic Acid *see* 8124
2-[*p*-[2-(*p*-Chlorobenzamido)ethyl]phenoxy]-2-methylpropionic Acid *see* 1195
3-Chlorobenzenamine *see* 2118
Chlorobenzene, 2121
1-Chlorobenzene-2,4-disulfonamide *see* 2374
4-Chloro-*m*-benzenedisulfonamide *see* 2374
4-Chloro-1,3-benzenedisulfonamide *see* 2374
N-Chlorobenzenesulfonamide Sodium Salt *see* 2074
[*p*-[2-(*p*-Chlorobenzenesulfonamido)-ethyl]phenyl]acetic Acid *see* 2806
(*N*-Chlorobenzenesulfonamido)sodium *see* 2074
p-Chlorobenzenesulfonic Acid, 2122
4-Chlorobenzenesulfonic Acid *see* 2122
1-(*p*-Chlorobenzenesulfonyl)-3-propyl-urea *see* 2186

6-Chloro-3-(chloromethyl)-3,4-dihydro-2-methyl-2*H*-1,2,4-benzothiadiazine-7-sulfonamide 1,1-Dioxide *see* 6005

6-Chloro-3-chloromethyl-3,4-dihydro-2-methyl-7-sulfamoyl-1,2,4-benzothiadiazine 1,1-Dioxide *see* 6005

6-Chloro-3-chloromethyl-2-methyl-7-sulfamyl-3,4-dihydro-1,2,4-benzothiadiazine 1,1-Dioxide *see* 6005

5-Chloro-*N*-(2-chloro-4-nitrophenyl)-2-hydroxybenzamide *see* 6519

3-Chloro-4-(3-chloro-2-nitrophenyl)pyrrole *see* 8018

5-Chloro-*N*-(2′-chloro-4′-nitrophenyl)-salicylamide *see* 6519

3′-Chloro-4′-(*p*-chlorophenoxy)-3,5-diiodosalicylanilide *see* 8097

N-[3-Chloro-4-(4-chlorophenoxy)phenyl]-2-hydroxy-3,5-diiodobenzamide *see* 8097

1-[[2-[2-Chloro-4-(4-chlorophenoxy)-phenyl]-4-methyl-1,3-dioxolan-2-yl]-methyl]-1*H*-1,2,4-triazole *see* 3135

N-[5-Chloro-4-[(4-chlorophenyl)cyano-methyl]amino]sulfonyl]phenyl]-2-hydroxy-3,5-diiodobenzamide *see* 2411

2-Chloro-α-(4-chlorophenyl)-4-(4,5-dihydro-3,5-dioxo-1,2,4-triazin-2(3*H*)-yl)-benzeneacetonitrile *see* 2343

7-Chloro-5-(2-chlorophenyl)-1,3-dihydro-3-hydroxy-2*H*-1,4-benzodiazepin-2-one *see* 5579

7-Chloro-5-(2-chlorophenyl)-1,3-dihydro-3-hydroxy-1-methyl-2*H*-1,4-benzodiazepin-2-one *see* 5581

3-[2-Chloro-2-(4-chlorophenyl)ethenyl]-2,2-dimethylcyclopropanecarboxylic Acid Cyano(4-fluoro-3-phenoxyphenyl)methyl Ester *see* 4140

10-Chloro-11b-(2-chlorophenyl)-2,3,5,6,-7,11b-hexahydrobenzo[6,7]-1,4-diazepino[5,4-*b*]oxazol-6-one *see* 2420

8-Chloro-6-(*o*-chlorophenyl)-1-methyl-4*H*-*s*-triazolo[4,3-*a*][1,4]benzodiazepine *see* 9604

8-Chloro-6-(2-chlorophenyl)-1-methyl-4*H*-[1,2,4]triazolo[4,3-*a*][1,4]benzo-diazepine *see* 9604

10-Chloro-11b-(2-chlorophenyl)-6-oxo-2,3,5,6,7,11b-hexahydrooxazolo[3,2-*d*][1,4]benzodiazepine *see* 2420

10-Chloro-11b-(2-chlorophenyl)-2,3,7,-11b-tetrahydro-3-methyloxazolo-[3,2-*d*][1,4]benzodiazepin-6(5*H*)-one *see* 6166

10-Chloro-11b-(*o*-chlorophenyl)-2,3,7,-11b-tetrahydro-3-methyloxazolo-[3,2-*d*][1,4]benzodiazepin-6(5*H*)-one *see* 6166

10-Chloro-11b-(2-chlorophenyl)-2,3,7,-11b-tetrahydrooxazolo[3,2-*d*][1,4]-benzodiazepin-6(5*H*)-one *see* 2420

7-Chloro-5-(2-chlorophenyl)tetrahydro-oxazolo[5,4-*b*]-2,3,4,5-tetrahydro-1*H*-1,4-benzodiazepin-2-one *see* 2420

4-Chloro-α-(4-chlorophenyl)-α-(trichloromethyl)benzenemethanol *see* 3086

3-Chloro-*N*-(3-chloro-5-trifluoromethyl-2-pyridinyl)-α,α,α-trifluoro-2,6-dinitro-*p*-toluidine *see* 4117

Chlorocholine Chloride *see* 2104

Chlorocid [Egis] *see* 2077

Chlorocizin *see* 2068

Chlorocresol, 2133

4-Chloro-*m*-cresol *see* 2133

6-Chloro-*m*-cresol *see* 2133

4-Chloro-2-cyano-*N*,*N*-dimethyl-5-(4-methylphenyl)-1*H*-imidazole-1-sulfonamide *see* 2700

4-Chloro-2-cyano-*N*,*N*-dimethyl-5-*p*-tolylimidazole-1-sulfonamide *see* 2700

Chlorocyanohydrin, 2134

2,2′-[(2-Chloro-5-cyano-1,3-phenyl-ene)diimino]bis(2-oxoacetic Acid) *see* 5555

N,*N*′-(2-Chloro-5-cyano-*m*-phenylene)-dioxamic Acid *see* 5555

Chlorocyclizine *see* 2081

Chlorocyclohexane *see* 2732

(*SP*-5-13)-Chloro[[*rel*-2,2′-[(1*R*,2*R*)-1,2-cyclohexanediylbis[(nitrilo-κ*N*)-methylidyne]]bis[4,6-bis(1,1′-dimethylethyl)phenolato-κ*O*]](2−)]-manganese *see* 5252

[2-Chloro-5-(cyclohex-1-ene-1,2-dicarboximido)-4-fluorophenoxy]acetic Acid *see* 4142

7-Chloro-5-(1-cyclohexen-1-yl)-1,3-dihydro-1-methyl-2*H*-1,4-benzodiazepin-2-one *see* 9243

7-Chloro-5-(1-cyclohexenyl)-1-methyl-2-oxo-2,3-dihydro-1*H*-[1,4]benzo[*f*]diazepine *see* 9243

5-Chloro-*N*-[2-[4-[[[(cyclohexylamino)-carbonyl]amino]sulfonyl]phenyl]ethyl]-2-methoxybenzamide *see* 4478

6-Chloro-2-cyclohexyl-2,3-dihydro-3-oxo-1*H*-isoindole-5-sulfonamide *see* 2404

6-Chloro-2-cyclohexyl-3-oxo-5-isoindolinesulfonamide *see* 2404

5-Chloro-2-cyclohexyl-1-oxo-6-sulfamoylisoindoline *see* 2404

5-Chloro-2-cyclohexylphthalimidine-6-sulfonamide *see* 2404

5-Chloro-2-cyclohexyl-6-sulfamoylisoindolin-1-one *see* 2404

Chloro(η⁵-2,4-cyclopentadien-1-yl)-[(4*R*,5*R*)-2,2-dimethyl-α,α,α′,α′-tetraphenyl-1,3-dioxolane-4,5-dimethanolato(2−)-κ*O*⁴,κ*O*⁵]titanium *see* 3472

6-Chloro-3-(cyclopentylmethyl)-3,4-dihydro-2*H*-1,2,4-benzothiadiazine-7-sulfonamide 1,1-Dioxide *see* 2745

6-Chloro-3-cyclopentylmethyl-3,4-dihydro-7-sulfamoyl-2*H*-1,2,4-benzothiadiazine 1,1-Dioxide *see* 2745

4-Chloro-2-cyclopentylphenol *see* 3430

1-[α-(4-Chloro-α-cyclopropylbenzylideneaminooxy)-*p*-tolyl]-3-(2,6-difluorobenzoyl)urea *see* 4123

2-[2-(1-Chlorocyclopropyl)-3-(2-chlorophenyl)-2-hydroxypropyl]-1,2-dihydro-3*H*-1,2,4-triazole-3-thione *see* 7887

2-(1-Chlorocyclopropyl)-1-(2-chlorophenyl)-3-(5-mercapto-1,2,4-triazol-1-yl)propan-2-ol *see* 7887

(4*S*)-6-Chloro-4-(cyclopropylethynyl)-1,4-dihydro-4-(trifluoromethyl)-2*H*-3,1-benzoxazin-2-one *see* 3521

7-Chloro-1-(cyclopropylmethyl)-1,3-dihydro-5-phenyl-2*H*-1,4-benzodiazepin-2-one *see* 7715

7-Chloro-1-(cyclopropylmethyl)-5-(2-fluorophenyl)-1,3-dihydro-2*H*-1,4-benzodiazepin-2-one *see* 4213

Chlorocyzine *see* 2068

6-Chloro-6-dehydro-17α-acetoxyprogesterone *see* 2102

21-Chloro-11-dehydrobetamethasone *see* 2364

6-Chloro-6-dehydro-17α-hydroxy-1,2α-methyleneprogesterone *see* 2774

6-Chloro-6-dehydro-17α-hydroxyprogesterone Acetate *see* 2102

7-Chloro-6-demethyltetracycline *see* 2886

2-Chlorodeoxyadenosine *see* 2337

2-Chloro-2′-deoxyadenosine *see* 2337

2-Chloro-9-(2-deoxy-2-fluoro-β-D-arabinofuranosyl)adenine *see* 2372

2-Chloro-9-(2-deoxy-2-fluoro-β-D-arabinofuranosyl)-9*H*-purin-6-amine *see* 2372

7(*S*)-Chloro-7-deoxylincomycin *see* 2356

33-*epi*-Chloro-33-desoxyascomycin *see* 7429

2-[(8-Chlorodibenzo[*b*,*f*]thiepin-10-yl)-oxy]-*N*,*N*-dimethylethanamine *see* 10197

Chlorodibromomethane, 2135

3-Chloro-1,2-dibromopropane *see* 3020

Chlorodicarbonylrhodium(I) Dimer *see* 8187

1-Chloro-2-[2,2-dichloro-1-(4-chlorophenyl)ethyl]benzene *see* 6216

6-Chloro-3-(dichloromethyl)-3,4-dihydro-2*H*-1,2,4-benzothiadiazine-7-sulfonamide 1,1-Dioxide *see* 9624

6-Chloro-3-dichloromethyl-7-sulfamyl-3,4-dihydro-1,2,4-benzothiadiazine 1,1-Dioxide *see* 9624

5-Chloro-6-(2,3-dichlorophenoxy)-2-methylthio-1*H*-benzimidazole *see* 9652

5-Chloro-2-(2,4-dichlorophenoxy)-phenol *see* 9657

7-Chloro-3-[1-(2,4-dichlorophenyl)-2-(1*H*-imidazol-1-yl)ethoxy-methyl]-benzo[*b*]thiophene *see* 8465

6-Chloro-1,6-didehydroretroprogesterone *see* 9584

(*SP*-5-13)-Chloro[7,12-diethenyl-3,8,-13,17-tetramethyl-21*H*,23*H*-porphine-2,18-dipropanoato(4−)-*N*²¹,-*N*²²,*N*²³,*N*²⁴]ferrate(2−) Dihydrogen *see* 4644

2-Chloro-10-(*N*,*N*-diethyl-β-alanyl)-phenothiazine *see* 2068

Chlorodiethylaluminum *see* 326

2-Chloro-4-diethylamino-6-ethylamino-*s*-triazine *see* 9664

7-Chloro-1-[2-(diethylamino)ethyl]-5-(2-fluorophenyl)-1,3-dihydro-2*H*-1,4-benzodiazepin-2-one *see* 4198

[[8-Chloro-3-[2-(diethylamino)ethyl]-4-methyl-2-oxo-2*H*-1-benzopyran-7-yl]-oxy]acetic Acid Ethyl Ester *see* 2405

2-Chloro-5-(ω-diethylamino-α-methylbutylamino)-7-methoxyacridine *see* 8044

6-Chloro-9-[[4-(diethylamino)-1-methylbutyl]amino]-2-methoxyacridine *see* 8044

7-Chloro-4-(4-diethylamino-1-methylbutylamino)quinoline *see* 2163

7-Chloro-4-(3-diethylaminomethyl-4-hydroxyanilino)quinoline *see* 572

7-Chloro-4-(3-diethylaminomethyl-4-hydroxyphenylamino)quinoline *see* 572

2′-Chloro-2-[2-[(diethylamino)methyl]-imidazol-1-yl]-5-nitrobenzophenone *see* 6661

2-Chloro-10-[3-(diethylamino)-1-oxo-propyl]-10*H*-phenothiazine *see* 2068

fonyl]-1-methyl-1*H*-pyrazole-4-car-
boxylic Acid Methyl Ester *see* 4602

2-Chloro-*N*-[[(4,6-dimethoxy-2-pyrimi-
dinyl)amino]carbonyl]imidazo[1,2-
a]pyridine-3-sulfonamide *see* 4908

2-Chloro-6-[(4,6-dimethoxy-2-pyrimi-
dinyl)thio]benzoic Acid *see* 7993

2-[*p*-Chloro-α-(2-dimethylaminoethoxy)-
benzyl]pyridine *see* 1799

2-Chloro-11-(2-dimethylaminoethoxy)-
dibenzo[*b*,*f*]thiepine *see* 10197

2-Chloro-α-(2-dimethylaminoethyl)benz-
hydrol *see* 2066

2-[*p*-Chloro-α-(2-dimethylaminoethyl)-
benzyl]pyridine *see* 2180

(+)-(2*S*,3*S*)-8-Chloro-5-[2-(dimethylamino)ethyl]-2,3-dihydro-3-hydroxy-2-
(*p*-methoxyphenyl)-1,5-benzothiaze-
pin-4(5*H*)-one Acetate (Ester) *see* 2348

2-Chloro-α-[2-(dimethylamino)ethyl]-α-
phenylbenzenemethanol *see* 2066

4-Chloro-α-[2-(dimethylamino)-1-meth-
ylethyl]-α-methylbenzeneethanol *see*
2365

p-Chloro-α-[2-(dimethylamino)-1-meth-
ylethyl]-α-methylphenethyl Alcohol *see*
2365

8-Chloro-1-[(dimethylamino)methyl]-6-
phenyl-4*H*-s-triazolo[4,3-*a*][1,4]-
benzodiazepine *see* 160

[4*S*-(4α,4aα,5aα,6β,12aα)]-7-Chloro-4-
(dimethylamino)-1,4,4a,5,5a,6,11,-
12a-octahydro-3,6,10,12,12a-penta-
hydroxy-1,11-dioxo-2-naphthacene-
carboxamide *see* 2886

7-Chloro-4-(dimethylamino)-1,4,4a,5,-
5a,6,11,12a-octahydro-3,6,10,12,12a-
pentahydroxy-*N*-(hydroxymethyl)-6-
methyl-1,11-dioxo-2-naphthacene-
carboxamide *see* 2388

[4*S*-(4α,4aα,5aα,6β,12aα)]-7-Chloro-4-
dimethylamino-1,4,4a,5,5a,6,11,12a-
octahydro-3,6,10,12,12a-pentahy-
droxy-6-methyl-1,11-dioxo-2-naph-
thacenecarboxamide *see* 2192

[4*S*-(4α,4aα,5α,5aα,12aα)]-7-Chloro-4-
(dimethylamino)-1,4,4a,5,5a,6,11,-
12a-octahydro-3,5,10,12,12a-penta-
hydroxy-6-methylene-1,11-dioxo-2-
naphthacenecarboxamide *see* 5778

3-Chloro-5-[3-(dimethylamino)propyl]-
10,11-dihydro-5*H*-dibenz[*b*,*f*]azepine
see 2387

α-2-Chloro-10-(3-dimethylaminopropyl-
idene)thiaxanthene *see* 2188

2-Chloro-10-(3-dimethylaminopropyl)-
phenothiazine *see* 2185

3-Chloro-10-(3-dimethylaminopropyl)-
phenothiazine *see* 2185

2-Chloro-10-[3-(dimethylamino)propyl]-
phenothiazine 5-Oxide *see* 6855

2-Chloro-α,α-dimethylbenzeneethan-
amine *see* 2410

4-Chloro-α,α-dimethylbenzeneethan-
amine *see* 2182

Chlorodimethyl Ether *see* 2146

2-Chloro-α-[[(1,1-dimethylethyl)ami-
no]methyl]benzenemethanol *see* 9811

(2-Chloro-1,1-dimethylethyl)benzene
see 6459

4-Chloro-2-(1,1-dimethylethyl)-5-[[[4-
(1,1-dimethylethyl)phenyl]methyl]-
thio]-3(2*H*)-pyridazinone *see* 7967

5-Chloro-3-(1,1-dimethylethyl)-6-meth-
yl-2,4(1*H*,3*H*)-pyrimidinedione *see*
9155

4-Chloro-*N*-[[4-(1,1-dimethylethyl)-
phenyl]methyl]-3-ethyl-1-methyl-
1*H*-pyrazole-5-carboxamide *see* 9094

2-Chloro-1,3-dimethylimidazolium
Chloride *see* 3390

o-Chloro-α,α-dimethylphenethylamine
see 2410

4-Chloro-α,α-dimethylphenethylamine
see 2182

4-Chloro-3,5-dimethylphenol *see* 2176

2-Chloro-*N*,*N*-dimethyl-10*H*-phenothia-
zine-10-propanamine *see* 2185

2-Chloro-*N*,*N*-dimethyl-10*H*-phenothia-
zine-10-propanamine 5-Oxide *see* 6855

8-Chloro-*N*,*N*-dimethyl-6-phenyl-4*H*-
[1,2,4]triazolo[4,3-*a*][1,4]benzodi-
azepine-1-methanamine *see* 160

cis-4-Chloro-*N*-(2',6'-dimethyl-1'-piper-
idyl)-3-sulfamoylbenzamide *see* 2393

4-Chloro-2',6'-dimethyl-5-sulfamoyl-
salicylanilide *see* 10079

2-Chloro-*N*-(2,4-dimethyl-3-thienyl)-*N*-
(2-methoxy-1-methylethyl)acetamide
see 3214

(*Z*)-2-Chloro-*N*,*N*-dimethylthioxanthene-
Δ[9,γ]-propylamine *see* 2188

cis-2-Chloro-*N*,*N*-dimethyl-3-thioxan-
then-9-ylidenepropylamine *see* 2188

1-Chloro-2,4-dinitrobenzene, 2136

1-Chloro-2,6-dinitrobenzene *see* 2137

2-Chloro-1,3-dinitrobenzene, 2137

4-Chloro-1,3-dinitrobenzene *see* 2136

6-Chloro-1,3-dinitrobenzene *see* 2136

1-(*o*-Chloro-α,α-diphenylbenzyl)imid-
azole *see* 2417

2-[4-[(1*Z*)-4-Chloro-1,2-diphenyl-1-bu-
tenyl]phenoxy]-*N*,*N*-dimethylethan-
amine *see* 9550

(*Z*)-4-Chloro-1,2-diphenyl-1-[4-[2-(*N*,*N*-
dimethylamino)ethoxy]phenyl]-1-bu-
tene *see* 9550

2-[4-(2-Chloro-1,2-diphenylethenyl)-
phenoxy]-*N*,*N*-diethylethanamine *see*
2386

1-(*p*-Chlorodiphenylmethyl)-4-[2-(2-hy-
droxyethoxy)ethyl]piperazine *see* 4849

1-(4-Chlorodiphenylmethyl)-4-methyl-
2,3,4,5,6,7-hexahydro-1,4-diazepine
see 4733

4-Chlorodiphenyl Sulfone *see* 8988

2-[*p*-(2-Chloro-1,2-diphenylvinyl)phen-
oxy]triethylamine *see* 2386

5-Chloro-2,4-disulfamylaniline *see* 2076

4-Chloro-*N*-1,3-dithietan-2-ylidene-2-
methylbenzeneamine *see* 6550

Chlorodracylic Acid *see* 2125

5-Chloro-6-(7,8-epoxy-10-hydroxy-2-
oxo-3,5-undecadienyl)-β-resorcylic
Acid μ-Lactone *see* 6253

1-Chloro-2,3-epoxypropane *see* 3611

16α-Chloroestrone 3-Methyl Ether *see*
2382

2-Chloro-1-ethanal *see* 2109

Chloroethane *see* 3782

2-Chloroethanephosphonic Acid *see* 3732

Chloroethanoic Acid *see* 2112

2-Chloroethanol *see* 3793

Chloroethene Homopolymer *see* 7586

(2-Chloroethenyl)arsonous Dichloride
see 3062

(*SP*-5-13)-Chloro[(4*E*,8*E*)-7-ethenyl-17-
formyl-12-(1-hydroxy-5,9,13-trimeth-
yl-4,8,12-tetradecatrienyl)-3,8,13-tri-
methyl-21*H*,23*H*-porphine-2,18-di-
propanoato(4−)-κ*N*[21],κ*N*[22],κ*N*[23],-
κ*N*[24]]ferrate(2−) Dihydrogen *see* 2793

1,1',1"-(1-Chloro-1-ethenyl-2-ylidene)-
tris[4-methoxybenzene] *see* 2174

(2-Chloroethoxy)ethene *see* 2139

3-(2-Chloroethoxy)-9α-fluoro-6-formyl-
11β,21-dihydroxy-16α,17α-isopropyl-
idenedioxypregna-3,5-dien-20-one
see 4243

3-(2-Chloroethoxy)-9-fluoro-11β,16α,-
17,21-tetrahydroxy-20-oxopregna-
3,5-diene-6-carboxaldehyde, Cyclic
16,17-Acetal with Acetone, 21-Ace-
tate *see* 4243

3-(2-Chloroethoxy)-6-formyl-9α-fluoro-
pregna-3,5-diene-11β,16α,17,21-tet-
rol-20-one 21-Acetate 16α,17α-Ace-
tonide *see* 4243

2-(2-Chloroethoxy)-*N*-[[(4-methoxy-6-
methyl-1,3,5-triazin-2-yl)amino]car-
bonyl]benzenesulfonamide *see* 9600

2-Chloro-*N*-(ethoxymethyl)-6'-ethyl-*o*-
acetotoluidide *see* 61

2-Chloro-*N*-(ethoxymethyl)-*N*-(2-ethyl-6-
methylphenyl)acetamide *see* 61

2-Chloro-1-(3-ethoxy-4-nitrophenoxy)-4-
(trifluoromethyl)benzene *see* 6963

1-[2-(2-Chloroethoxy)phenylsulfonyl]-3-
(4-methoxy-6-methyl-1,3,5-triazin-2-
yl)urea *see* 9600

2-Chloroethyl Alcohol *see* 3793

2-Chloro-4-ethylamino-6-isopropyl-
amine-s-triazine *see* 871

6-Chloro-2-(ethylamino)-4-methyl-4-
phenyl-4*H*-3,1-benzoxazine *see* 3864

2-[[4-Chloro-6-(ethylamino)-1,3,5-tria-
zin-2-yl]amino]-2-methylpropane-
nitrile *see* 2685

2-[[4-Chloro-6-(ethylamino)-s-triazin-2-
yl]amino]-2-methylpropionitrile *see*
2685

3-(2-Chloroethyl)-2-[(2-chloroethyl)ami-
no]tetrahydro-2*H*-1,3,2-oxazaphos-
phorin-2-oxide *see* 4896

1-(2-Chloroethyl)-3-cyclohexyl-1-nitroso-
urea *see* 5564

N-(2-Chloroethyl)-*N'*-cyclohexyl-*N*-
nitrosourea *see* 5564

N-(2-Chloroethyl)dibenzylamine Hydrochloride, 2138

N-(2-Chloroethyl)-2,6-dinitro-*N*-propyl-
4-(trifluoromethyl)benzenamine *see*
4120

Chloroethylene *see* 9994

Chloroethylene Polymer *see* 7586

7-Chloro-4-[4-(*N*-ethyl-*N*-β-hydroxyeth-
ylamino)-1-methylbutylamino]quino-
line *see* 4818

7-Chloro-4-[4-[ethyl(2-hydroxyethyl)am-
ino]-1-methylbutylamino]quinoline *see*
4818

7-Chloro-4-[5-(*N*-ethyl-*N*-2-hydroxyeth-
ylamino)-2-pentyl]aminoquinoline *see*
4818

2-Chloroethyl 2-Hydroxyethyl Sulfide *see*
4646

β-Chloroethyl β-Hydroxyethyl Thioether
see 4646

Chloroethylmercury *see* 3826

2-Chloro-6'-ethyl-*N*-(2-methoxy-1-meth-
ylethyl)acet-*o*-toluidide *see* 6146

6-Chloro-*N*-ethyl-*N'*-(1-methylethyl)-
1,3,5-triazine-2,4-diamine *see* 871

α-Chloro-2'-ethyl-6'-methyl-*N*-(1-methyl-
2-methoxyethyl)acetanilide *see* 6146

N-(2-Chloroethyl)-*N*-(1-methyl-2-phen-
oxyethyl)benzenemethanamine *see*
7256

N-(2-Chloroethyl)-N-(1-methyl-2-phen-oxyethyl)benzylamine *see* 7256

6-Chloro-N-ethyl-4-methyl-4-phenyl-4H-3,1-benzoxazin-2-amine *see* 3864

2-Chloro-N-(2-ethyl-6-methylphenyl)-N-(2-methoxy-1-methylethyl)acetamide *see* 6146

5-(2-Chloroethyl)-4-methylthiazole *see* 2384

2-[[[(2-Chloroethyl)nitrosoamino]carbonyl]amino]-2-deoxy-D-glucose *see* 2177

[1-[[[(2-Chloroethyl)nitrosoamino]carbonyl]amino]ethyl]phosphonic Acid Diethyl Ester *see* 4261

1-(2-Chloroethyl)-1-nitroso-3-(D-glucos-2-yl)urea *see* 2177

2-[3-(2-Chloroethyl)-3-nitrosoureido]-2-deoxy-D-glucopyranose *see* 2177

6-[3-(2-Chloroethyl)-3-nitrosoureido]-6-deoxy-α-D-glucopyranoside *see* 8109

1-[N-(2-Chloroethyl)-N-nitrosoureido]-ethylphosphonic Acid Diethyl Ester *see* 4261

1-(2-Chloroethyl)-3-ethyl-1-penten-4-yl-3-ol *see* 3729

5-Chloro-3-ethylpent-1-yn-4-en-3-ol *see* 3729

Chloroethylphenamide *see* 1018

N-(2-Chloroethyl)-N-(phenylmethyl)benzenemethanamine Hydrochloride *see* 2138

(2-Chloroethyl)phosphonic Acid *see* 3732

7-Chloro-2-ethyl-6-sulfamoyl-1,2,3,4-tetrahydro-4-quinazolinone *see* 8056

7-Chloro-2-ethyl-1,2,3,4-tetrahydro-4-oxo-6-quinazolinesulfonamide *see* 8056

7-Chloro-2-ethyl-1,2,3,4-tetrahydro-4-oxo-6-sulfamoylquinazoline *see* 8056

2-(2-Chloroethylthio)ethanol *see* 4646

N-(2-Chloroethyl)-α,α,α-trifluoro-2,6-dinitro-N-propyl-p-toluidine *see* 4120

(2-Chloroethyl)trimethylammonium Chloride *see* 2104

2-Chloroethyl Vinyl Ether, 2139

2-Chloroflumethasone *see* 4597

4-(3′-Chloro-4′-fluoroanilino)-7-methoxy-6-(3-morpholinopropoxy)quinazoline *see* 4379

Chlorofluorocarbons, 2140

(6α,11β,16α)-9-Chloro-6-fluoro-11,21-dihydroxy-16-methylpregna-1,4-diene-3,20-dione *see* 2369

(11β,16β)-21-Chloro-9-fluoro-11,17-dihydroxy-16-methylpregna-1,4-diene-3,20-dione *see* 2363

[2-Chloro-4-fluoro-5-(1,3,4,5,6,7-hexahydro-1,3-dioxo-2H-isoindol-2-yl)-phenoxy]acetic Acid *see* 4142

21-Chloro-9α-fluoro-11β-hydroxy-16α,17α-isopropylidenedioxy-4-pregnene-3,20-dione *see* 4591

(11β,16α)-21-Chloro-9-fluoro-11-hydroxy-16,17-[(1-methylethylidene)-bis(oxy)]pregn-4-ene-3,20-dione *see* 4591

(16β)-21-Chloro-9-fluoro-17-hydroxy-16-methylpregna-1,4-diene-3,11,20-trione *see* 2364

9-(4-Chloro-2-fluoro-5-methoxycarbonylmethylthiophenylimino)-8-thia-1,6-diazabicyclo-[4.3.0]nonane-7-one *see* 4210

9-Chloro-6α-fluoro-16α-methyl-1,4-pregnadiene-11β,21-diol-3,20-dione *see* 2369

2-[(2-Chloro-6-fluorophenyl)amino]-5-methylbenzeneacetic Acid *see* 5601

N-[4-(3-Chloro-4-fluorophenylamino)-7-(3-morpholin-4-ylpropoxy)quinazolin-6-yl]acrylamide *see* 1744

N-[4-[(3-Chloro-4-fluorophenyl)amino]-7-[3-(4-morpholinyl)propoxy]-6-quinazolinyl]-2-propenamide *see* 1744

7-Chloro-5-(2-fluorophenyl)-1,3-dihydro-3-hydroxy-1-(2-hydroxyethyl)-2H-1,4-benzodiazepin-2-one *see* 3434

7-Chloro-5-(2-fluorophenyl)-2,3-dihydro-3-hydroxy-2-oxo-1H-1,4-benzodiazepine-1-propanenitrile *see* 2308

7-Chloro-5-(2-fluorophenyl)-1,3-dihydro-1-methyl-2H-1,4-benzodiazepin-2-one *see* 4128

7-Chloro-5-(2-fluorophenyl)-2,3-dihydro-2-oxo-1H-1,4-benzodiazepine-3-carboxylic Acid Ethyl Ester *see* 3821

7-Chloro-5-(2-fluorophenyl)-1,3-dihydro-1-(2,2,2-trifluoroethyl)-2H-1,4-benzodiazepine-2-thione *see* 8029

5-Chloro-1-(4-fluorophenyl)-3-[1-[2-(2-imidazolidinon-1-yl)ethyl]-4-piperidyl]-1H-indole *see* 8466

1-[2-[4-[5-Chloro-1-(4-fluorophenyl)-1H-indol-3-yl]-1-piperidinyl]ethyl]-2-imidazolidinone *see* 8466

N-(3-Chloro-4-fluorophenyl)-7-methoxy-6-[3-(4-morpholinyl)propoxy]-4-quinazolinamine *see* 4379

N-[3-Chloro-4-[(3-fluorophenyl)methoxy]phenyl]-6-[5[[[2-(methylsulfonyl)ethyl]amino]methyl]-2-furanyl]-4-quinazolinamine *see* 5367

8-Chloro-6-(2-fluorophenyl)-1-methyl-4H-imidazo[1,5-a][1,4]benzodiazepine *see* 6182

6-[3-(2-Chloro-6-fluorophenyl)-5-methyl-4-isoxazolecarboxamido]penicillanic Acid *see* 4111

(2S,5R,6R)-6-[[[3-(2-Chloro-6-fluorophenyl)-5-methyl-4-isoxazolyl]carbonyl]amino]-3,3-dimethyl-7-oxo-4-thia-1-azabicyclo[3.2.0]heptane-2-carboxylic Acid *see* 4111

3-(2-Chloro-6-fluorophenyl)-5-methyl-4-isoxazolylpenicillin *see* 4111

10-Chloro-11b-(2-fluorophenyl)-2,3,7,-11b-tetrahydro-7-(2-hydroxyethyl)-oxazolo[3,2-d][1,4]benzodiazepin-6(5H)-one *see* 4209

(2R)-2-[4-[(5-Chloro-3-fluoro-2-pyridinyl)oxy]phenoxy]propanoic Acid 2-Propynyl Ester *see* 2370

[[2-Chloro-4-fluoro-5-[(tetrahydro-3-oxo-1H,3H-[1,3,4]thiadiazolo[3,4-a]-pyridazin-1-ylidene)amino]phenyl]-thio]acetic Acid Methyl Ester *see* 4210

2-Chloro-4-fluoro-5-[(3,4,5,6-tetrahydro)phthalimido]phenoxyacetic Acid *see* 4142

21-Chloro-9-fluoro-11β,16α,17-trihydroxypregn-4-ene-3,20-dione Cyclic 16,17-Acetal with Acetone *see* 4591

Chlorofolin *see* 2155

Chloroform, 2141

Chloroformamide *see* 1783

Chloroformic Acid Benzyl Ester *see* 1801

Chloroformic Acid p-Bromobenzyl Ester *see* 1411

Chloroformic Acid Ethyl Ester *see* 3784

Chloroformic Acid Trichloromethyl Ester *see* 3334

Chloroformyl Chloride *see* 7335

Chlorofos *see* 9623

4-Chloro-N-furfuryl-5-sulfamoylanthranilic Acid *see* 4309

4-Chloro-N-(2-furylmethyl)-5-sulfamoylanthranilic Acid *see* 4309

Chlorogenic Acid, 2142

Chlorogenin, 2143

Chloroguanide *see* 2090

Chlorohemin *see* 4644

2-Chloro-1-heptene-1-arsonic Acid *see* 2119

(2-Chloro-1-heptenyl)arsonic Acid *see* 2119

(3α,5aα,10bα,11β,11aα)-9-Chloro-2,3,-5a,6,10b,11-hexahydro-10b,11-dihydroxy-7,8-dimethoxy-2,3,6-trimethyl-3,11a-epidithio-11aH-pyrazino-[1′,2′:1,5]pyrrolo[2,3-b]indole-1,4-dione *see* 8764

4-Chloro-N-(endo-hexahydro-4,7-methanoisoindolin-2-yl)-3-sulfamoylbenzamide *see* 9737

10-Chloro-2,3,5,6,7,11b-hexahydro-2-methyl-11b-phenylbenzo[6,7]-1,4-diazepino[5,4-b]oxazol-6-one *see* 6927

1-Chlorohexane, 2144

α-Chlorohydrin, 2145

(17β)-4-Chloro-17-hydroxyandrost-4-en-3-one *see* 2413

4-Chloro-2-hydroxybenzoic Acid n-Butylamide *see* 1465

5-Chloro-4-hydroxybenzoxazole *see* 2194

2-Chloro-2′-hydroxydiethyl Sulfide *see* 4646

2-Chloro-5-hydroxy-1,3-dimethylbenzene *see* 2176

5-Chloro-2-hydroxydiphenylmethane *see* 2407

5-Chloro-3-[4-(2-hydroxyethyl)-1-piperazinyl]carbonylmethyl-2-benzothiazolinone *see* 9424

2-Chloro-9-[3-[4-(2-hydroxyethyl)-1-piperazinyl]propylidene]thiaxanthene *see* 2394

2-Chloro-10-[3-[1-(2-hydroxyethyl)-4-piperazinyl]propyl]phenothiazine *see* 7183

5-Chloro-8-hydroxy-7-iodoquinoline *see* 5031

2-Chloro-4-(hydroxymercuriphenol) *see* 4830

3-Chloro-7-hydroxy-4-methyl-2H-1-benzopyran-2-one Bis(chloroethyl) Phosphate *see* 4605

3-Chloro-7-hydroxy-4-methylcoumarin Bis(2-chloroethyl) Phosphate *see* 4605

3-Chloro-7-hydroxy-4-methylcoumarin Diethyl Phosphate *see* 2537

3-Chloro-7-hydroxy-4-methylcoumarin O-Ester with O,O-Diethyl Phosphorothioate *see* 2558

6-Chloro-17-hydroxy-1α,2α-methylenepregna-4,6-diene-3,20-dione *see* 2774

7-Chloro-5-hydroxy-1-[2-methyl-4-(2-methylbenzoylamino)benzoyl]-2,3,4,5-tetrahydro-1H-1-benzazepine *see* 9540

6-Chloro-4-hydroxy-2-methyl-N-2-pyridinyl-2H-thieno[2,3-e]-1,2-thiazine-3-carboxamide 1,1-Dioxide *see* 5582

6-Chloro-4-hydroxy-2-methyl-3-(2-pyridylcarbamoyl)-2H-thieno[2,3-e]-1,2-thiazine-1,1-dioxide *see* 5582

6-Chloro-17-hydroxy-2-oxapregna-4,6-diene-3,20-dione *see* 6888

8-Chloro-11-(4-methyl-1-piperazinyl)-
5H-dibenzo[b,e][1,4]diazepine *see*
2423
2-Chloro-11-(4-methyl-1-piperazinyl)di-
benzo[b,f][1,4]thiazepine *see* 2415
2-Chloro-11-(4-methyl-1-piperazinyl)di-
benz[b,f][1,4]oxazepine *see* 5587
2-Chloro-10-[3-(1-methyl-4-piperazinyl)-
propyl]phenothiazine *see* 7761
2-Chloro-10-[3-(4-methyl-1-piperazinyl)-
propyl]-10H-phenothiazine *see* 7761
3-Chloro-10-[3-(4-methyl-1-piperazinyl)-
propyl]phenothiazine *see* 7761
7α-Chloro-16α-methylprednisolone *see*
220
9α-Chloro-16β-methylprednisolone *see*
1019
9α-Chloro-16β-methyl-1,4-pregnadiene-
11β,17α,21-triol-3,20-dione *see* 1019
1-Chloro-2-methylpropane *see* 5138
2-Chloro-2-methylpropane *see* 1562
2-Chloro-3-methylpropane *see* 1561
1-Chloro-2-methyl-1-propene, 2147
3-Chloro-2-methyl-1-propene, 2148
2-Chloro-1-methylpyridinium Iodide *see*
6301
7-Chloro-3-methyl-8-quinolinecarboxylic
Acid *see* 8066
2-[(4-Chloro-N¹-methyl-3-sulfamoyl-
benzenesulfonamido)methyl]-2-meth-
yltetrahydrofuran *see* 5803
2-[2-Chloro-4-(methylsulfonyl)benzoyl]-
1,3-cyclohexanedione *see* 8894
5-Chloro-3-(4-methylsulfonyl)phenyl-2-
(2-methyl-5-pyridinyl)pyridine *see*
3887
4-Chloro-N¹-methyl-N¹-[(tetrahydro-2-
methyl-2-furanyl)methyl]-1,3-ben-
zenedisulfonamide *see* 5803
4-Chloro-N¹-methyl-N¹-(tetrahydro-2-
methylfurfuryl)-m-benzenedisulfon-
amide *see* 5803
2-[(2-Chloro-4-methyl-3-thienyl)amino]-
2-imidazoline *see* 9418
N-(2-Chloro-4-methyl-3-thienyl)-4,5-di-
hydro-1H-imidazol-2-amine *see* 9418
cis,trans-3-Chloro-4-[4-methyl-2-(1H-1,-
2,4-triazol-1-ylmethyl)-1,3-dioxolan-
2-yl]phenyl 4-Chlorophenyl Ether
see 3135
3-Chloro-4-methylumbelliferone Di-
(2-chloroethyl) Phosphate *see* 4605
3-Chloro-4-methylumbelliferone Diethyl
Phosphate *see* 2537
3-Chloro-4-methylumbelliferone O-Ester
with O,O-Diethyl Phosphorothioate *see*
2558
3'-Chloro-2-methyl-p-valerotoluidide *see*
8702
p-Chloro-N-(2-morpholinoethyl)benzam-
ide *see* 6226
4-Chloro-N-[2-(4-morpholinyl)ethyl]-
benzamide *see* 6226
Chloromycetin [Warner-Lambert] *see*
2077
α-Chloronaphthalene *see* 2149
β-Chloronaphthalene *see* 2150
1-Chloronaphthalene, 2149
2-Chloronaphthalene, 2150
Chloronase [Hoechst] *see* 2186
Chloronitrobenzene, 2151
m-Chloronitrobenzene *see* 2151
o-Chloronitrobenzene *see* 2151
p-Chloronitrobenzene *see* 2151
1-Chloro-3-nitrobenzene *see* 2151

3-Chloro-4-(2'-nitro-3'-chlorophenyl)pyr-
role *see* 8018
N-(2'-Chloro-4'-nitrophenyl)-5-chloro-
salicylamide *see* 6519
Chloronitrous Acid *see* 6609
6-Chloro-3-(2-norbornen-5-yl)-7-sul-
famyl-3,4-dihydro-1,2,4-benzothia-
diazine 1,1-Dioxide *see* 2754
5-Chloro-1-[1-[3-(2-oxo-1-benzimidazol-
inyl)propyl]-4-piperidyl]-2-benzimida-
zolinone *see* 3418
4-[(5-Chloro-2-oxo-3(2H)-benzothiazol-
yl)acetyl]-1-piperazineethanol *see* 9424
S-(6-Chloro-2-oxobenzoxazolin-3-yl)-
methyl Diethyl Phosphorothiolothionate *see* 7334
3-Chloro-5-[3-(2-oxo-1,2,3,5,6,7,8,8a-oc-
tahydroimidazo[1,2-a]-pyridine-3-
spiro-4'-piperidino)propyl]-10,11-di-
hydro-5H-dibenz[b,f]azepine *see* 6278
1-Chloro-2-oxopropane *see* 2114
5-Chloro-8-oxychinolin *see* 2422
Chloropal [Graeub] *see* 2077
Chloropentaaquochromium Dichloride
Monohydrate *see* 2222
1-Chloropentane *see* 606
m-Chloroperoxybenzoic Acid *see* 5673
Chlorophacinone, 2152
p-Chlorophenacyl Bromide, 2153
Chlorophenamidine *see* 2085
m-Chlorophenol *see* 2154
o-Chlorophenol *see* 2154
p-Chlorophenol *see* 2154
2-Chlorophenol *see* 2154
3-Chlorophenol *see* 2154
4-Chlorophenol *see* 2154
Chlorophenols, 2154
Chlorophenothane *see* 2841
1-[3-(2-Chlorophenothiazin-10-yl)pro-
pyl]isonipecotamide *see* 7454
8-[3-(2-Chloro-10-phenothiazinyl)pro-
pyl]-3-oxo-1-thia-4,8-diazaspiro[4.5]-
decane *see* 2412
4-[3-(2-Chloro-10H-phenothiazin-10-yl)-
propyl]-1-piperazineethanol *see* 7183
4-[3-(2-Chlorophenothiazin-10-yl)pro-
pyl]-1-piperazineethanol Acetate *see*
9356
2-[4-[3-(2-Chlorophenothiazin-10-yl)-
propyl]-1-piperazinyl]ethyl 3,4,5-Tri-
methoxybenzoate *see* 6145
1-[3-(2-Chloro-10H-phenothiazin-10-yl)-
propyl]-4-piperidinecarboxamide *see*
7454
8-[3-(2-Chloro-10H-phenothiazin-10-yl)-
propyl]-1-thia-4,8-diazaspiro[4.5]-
decan-3-one *see* 2412
(4-Chlorophenoxy)acetic Acid 2-(Dimethylamino)ethyl Ester *see* 5780
4-(Chlorophenoxy)acetic Acid 2-(1-
Methylethyl)hydrazide *see* 5076
1-[2-(4-Chlorophenoxy)acetyl]-4-(3,4-
methylenedioxybenzyl)piperazine
see 4084
1-[(p-Chlorophenoxy)acetyl]-4-piperon-
ylpiperazine *see* 4084
β-(4-Chlorophenoxy)-α-(1,1-dimethyl-
ethyl)-1H-1,2,4-triazole-1-ethanol
see 9593
1-(4-Chlorophenoxy)-3,3-dimethyl-1-
(1H-1,2,4-triazol-1-yl)butan-2-ol *see*
9593
1-(4-Chlorophenoxy)-3,3-dimethyl-1-
(1H-1,2,4-triazol-1-yl)-2-butanone
see 9592

1-[(1Z)-2-[2-(4-Chlorophenoxy)ethoxy]-
2-(2,4-dichlorophenyl)-1-methyl-
ethenyl]-1H-imidazole *see* 6846
(1E)-[2-[[6-(2-Chlorophenoxy)-5-fluoro-
4-pyrimidinyl]oxy]phenyl](5,6-dihy-
dro-1,4,2-dioxazin-3-yl)methanone
O-Methyloxime *see* 4184
(5Z)-rel-7-[(1R,2R,3R,5S)-2-[(1E,3R)-4-
(3-Chlorophenoxy)-3-hydroxy-1-bu-
tenyl]-3,5-dihydroxycyclopentyl]-5-
heptenoic Acid *see* 2399
3-(p-Chlorophenoxy)-2-hydroxypropyl
Carbamate *see* 2179
(5Z)-7-[(1S,2R,3R,5S)-2-[[(2S)-3-(3-
Chlorophenoxy)-2-hydroxypropyl]-
thio]-3,5-dihydroxycyclopentyl]-5-
heptenoic Acid *see* 5610
α-(p-Chlorophenoxy)isobutyric Acid *see*
2378
α-[(p-Chlorophenoxy)isobutyroyl]-β-
(nicotinoyl)glycol *see* 2377
N-2-(p-Chlorophenoxy)isobutyryl-N'-
morpholinomethylurea *see* 7516
3-[α-(p-Chlorophenoxy)isobutyryloxy]-
propyl Nicotinate *see* 8255
2-(4-Chlorophenoxy)-2-methyl-N-[[(4-
morpholinylmethyl)amino]carbonyl]-
propanamide *see* 7516
2-(4-Chlorophenoxy)-2-methylpropanoic
Acid *see* 2378
2-(4-Chlorophenoxy)-2-methylpropanoic
Acid Ethyl Ester *see* 2377
2-(4-Chlorophenoxy)-2-methylpropanoic
Acid [6-(Hydroxymethyl)-2-pyridinyl]-
methyl Ester *see* 7495
2-(4-Chlorophenoxy)-2-methylpropanoic
Acid 1,3-Propanediyl Ester *see* 8537
2-(4-Chlorophenoxy)-2-methylpropanoic
Acid 2-(1,2,3,6-Tetrahydro-1,3-di-
methyl-2,6-dioxo-7H-purin-7-yl)ethyl
Ester *see* 9284
2-(p-Chlorophenoxy)-2-methylpropionic
Acid *see* 2378
2-(p-Chlorophenoxy)-2-methylpropionic
Acid Ester with 1,3-Dinicotinoyloxy-
2-propanol *see* 1224
2-(p-Chlorophenoxy)-2-methylpropionic
Acid Ester with 7-(2-Hydroxyethyl)-
theophylline *see* 9284
2-(p-Chlorophenoxy)-2-methylpropionic
Acid Trimethylene Ester *see* 8537
3-(4-Chlorophenoxy)-1,2-propanediol
see 2178
3-(4-Chlorophenoxy)-1,2-propanediol-
1-carbamate *see* 2179
N-(3-Chlorophenyl)acetamide *see* 2111
3-(α-p-Chlorophenyl-β-acetylethyl)-4-hy-
droxycoumarin *see* 2556
N-[[(4-Chlorophenyl)amino]carbonyl]-
2,6-difluorobenzamide *see* 3142
p'-Chloro-p-phenylaniline *see* 435
1-[α-(2-Chlorophenyl)benzhydryl]imid-
azole *see* 2417
α-(4-Chlorophenyl)-2-benzofuranmetha-
nol *see* 2360
1-(p-Chloro-α-phenylbenzyl)-4-cinnamyl-
piperazine *see* 2367
1-(p-Chloro-α-phenylbenzyl)-4-(2-hy-
droxyethoxyethyl)piperazine *see* 4849
1-(p-Chloro-α-phenylbenzyl)-4-(m-meth-
ylbenzyl)piperazine *see* 5777
1-(p-Chloro-α-phenylbenzyl)-4-methyl-
homopiperazine *see* 4733
1-(p-Chloro-α-phenylbenzyl)-4-methyl-
piperazine *see* 2081

Cholic Acid, 2203
Choligen see 4833
Cholimil [Takeda] see 5010
Choline, 2204
Choline Alfoscerate, 2205
Choline Chloride, 2206
Choline Chloride Carbamate see 1779
Choline Chloride Dihydrogen Phosphate see 7362
Choline Chloride Phosphate see 7362
Choline Chloride Succinate (2:1) see 8875
Choline Cytidine 5′-Pyrophosphate (Ester) see 2319
Choline Dichloride see 2104
Choline Dihydrogen Citrate, 2207
Choline Esterase, 2208
D-Choline Hydroxide 2,3-Dihydroxypropyl Hydrogen Phosphate Inner Salt see 2205
Choline 1,5-Naphthalenedisulfonate (2:1), Dilactate, Diacetate see 114
Choline Orotate see 6876
Choline Phosphate Chloride see 7362
Choline Phosphate Hexadecyl Ester, Hydroxide, Inner Salt see 6198
Choline Phosphoric Acid Ester (Chloride) see 7362
"Choline Plasmalogen" see 7519
Choline Salicylate, 2209
Choline Salicylic Acid Salt see 2209
Choline Succinate Dichloride see 8875
Choline Theophyllinate, 2210
Cholinfall [Tanabe Seiyaku] see 5979
Cholinophylline see 2210
Cholit-Ursan [Fresenius] see 9889
Chologon see 2868
Cholografin [BMS] see 5022
Cholonerton [Dolorgiet] see 4854
Cholospect see 5022
Choloxin [Knoll] see 9415
N-Choloyltaurine see 9075
Cholspasmin [Lipha] see 4854
Cholumbrin see 5038
Cholybar [Warner-Lambert] see 2202
N-Cholylglycine see 4494
Cholyltaurine see 9075
d-Chondocurine see 2212
Chondodendrine see 1016
Chondrillasterol, 2211
Chondrocurine, 2212
Chondrofoline, 2213
Chondroitin Sulfate, 2214
Chondroitin 4-Sulfate see 2214
Chondroitin 4-Sulfate Disodium Salt see 2214
Chondroitin 6-Sulfate see 2214
Chondroitin Sulfate A see 2214
Chondroitin Sulfate B see 2214
Chondroitin Sulfate C see 2214
Chondroitinsulfuric Acid see 2214
Chondrosamine see 4334
Chondrosine, 2215
Chonsurid see 2214
Chop Nut see 7383
Chopper [BASF] see 4905
Choragon [Ferring] see 2216
Choriogonadotropin see 2216
Choriogonadotropin Alfa see 2216
Chorionic Gonadotropin, 2216
Chorionic Gonadotropin (Human α-Subunit Protein Moiety Reduced) Complex with Chorionic Gonadotropin (Human β-Subunit Protein Moiety Reduced) see 2216
Chorionic Growth Hormone-prolactin see 4620

Chorismic Acid, 2217
Chorus [Syngenta] see 2772
Chothyn [Tilden-Yates] see 2207
chRFT5 see 1006
Christmas Factor see 3922
Chromafenozide, 2218
R-(−)-2-[4-[(Chroman-2-ylmethyl)-amino]butyl]-1,1-dioxobenzo[d]isothiazolone see 8137
Chromargyre see 5867
Chromatophorotropic Hormone see 6295
Chromax [Nutrition 21] see 2236
Chrome Alum see 2229
Chrome Alum Ammonium see 511
Chrome Green see 2234
1,2-Chromene see 1102
3-Chromene see 1102
Chrome Ocher see 2234
Chrome Oxide Green see 2234
Chrome Red see 5406
Chrome Yellow see 5405
Chromia see 2234
Chromic Acetate, 2219
Chromic Acid Iron(3+) Salt (3:2) see 4020
Chromic Acid Lead(2+) Salt (1:2) see 5406
Chromic Ammonium Sulfate see 511
Chromic Anhydride see 2235
Chromic Bromide, 2220
Chromic Carbonate, 2221
Chromic Chloride, 2222
Chromic Fluoride, 2223
Chromic Formate, 2224
Chromic Hydroxide, 2225
Chromic Nitrate, 2226
Chromic Oxide see 2234
Chromic Oxide Gel see 2225
Chromic Oxide, Hydrous see 2225
Chromic Phosphate, 2227
Chromic Potassium Oxalate, 2228
Chromic Potassium Sulfate, 2229
Chromic Sulfate, 2230
Chromite see 2231
Chromitope Sodium [BMS] see 8601
Chromium, 2231
Chromium Carbonyl, 2232
Chromium Cobalt Oxide (Cr$_2$CoO$_4$) see 2438
Chromium Dioxide, 2233
Chromium Dioxychloride see 2248
Chromium Hexacarbonyl see 2232
Chromium Hydroxide see 2225
Chromium Lead Oxide see 5406
Chromium(III) Nitrate see 2226
Chromium(III) Oxide, 2234
Chromium(VI) Oxide, 2235
Chromium Oxide (CrO$_3$) see 2235
Chromium Oxide (Cr$_2$O$_3$) see 2234
Chromium Oxyfluoride see 2249
Chromium Picolinate, 2236
Chromium Sesquioxide see 2234
Chromium(III) Sulfate see 2230
Chromium Trioxide see 2235
Chromium Tripicolinate see 2236
Chromium(III) Trispicolinate see 2236
Chromocarb, 2237
Chromomycin A$_3$, 2238
Chromomycinone see 2238, 7536
Chromonar, 2239
2-Chromonecarboxylic Acid see 2237
Chromosorb P [Celite Corp.] see 9014
Chromotrichia Factor see 423
Chromotrope 2B, 2240
Chromotropic Acid, 2241
Chromous Acetate, 2242

Chromous Bromide, 2243
Chromous Chloride, 2244
Chromous Fluoride, 2245
Chromous Formate, 2246
Chromous Sulfate, 2247
Chromyl Chloride, 2248
Chromyl Fluoride, 2249
Chronadalate [Bayer] see 6528
Chronexan [Viatris] see 10079
Chronogest [Intervet] see 4200
Chrono-Indocid [Merck & Co.] see 4968
Chronosyn [Veterinaria] see 2102
Chrysanthemaxanthin, 2250
Chrysanthemic Acid, 2251
Chrysanthemin see 2687
N-(Chrysanthemoxymethyl)-1-cyclohexene-1,2-dicarboximide see 9223
Chrysanthemumdicarboxylic Acid Monomethyl Ester Pyrethrolone Ester see 7964
Chrysanthemumic Acid see 2251
Chrysanthemummonocarboxylic Acid see 2251
Chrysanthemummonocarboxylic Acid 6-Chloropiperonyl Ester see 1003
Chrysanthemummonocarboxylic Acid Ester with 3-(2-Cyclopenten-1-yl)-2-methyl-4-oxo-2-cyclopenten-1-ol see 2706
Chrysanthemummonocarboxylic Acid Pyrethrolone Ester see 7964
Chrysanthenone, 2252
Chrysarobin, 2253
Chrysatropic Acid see 8408
Chrysazin, 2815
Chrysazin-3-carboxylic Acid see 8176
6-Chrysenamine, 2254
Chrysene, 2255
Chrysenex see 2254
6-Chrysenylamine see 2254
Chrysidenon 1438 see 2256
Chrysin, 2256
Chrysoberyl see 1161
Chrysogen see 6369
Chrysoidine, 2257
Chrysoidine Orange see 2257
Chrysoidine Y see 2257
Chrysoine see 9775
Chrysomykine see 2192
Chryson [Sumitomo] see 8153
Chrysophanein see 2258
Chrysophanic Acid, 2258
Chrysophaniin see 2258
Chrysophanol see 2258
Chrysotile see 826, 5687
6-Chrysylamine see 2254
Chrytemin [Fujinaga] see 4920
ChTX see 2046
Chuan-xin-lian see 632
Chugaev's Reagent see 3246
CHX-100 see 6693
CHX-3101 see 8739
CHX-3311 see 2784
CHX-3673 see 490
Chymetin [BDH] see 2260
Chymex [Savage] see 1054
Chymodiactin [Smith] see 2259
Chymolase see 2260
Chymopapain, 2259
Chymosin see 8134
Chymotase (Tabl.) see 2260
Chymotrypsins, 2260
Chymozym [Teikoku Hormone] see 2260
CI-395 see 7219
CI-440 see 4132

C.I. Direct Blue 14 *see* 9792
C.I. Direct Blue 53 *see* 3905
C.I. Direct Red 2 *see* 1101
C.I. Direct Red 28 *see* 2498
C.I. Direct Red 34 *see* 10012
C.I. Direct Red 80 *see* 8548
C.I. Fluorescent Brightener 30 *see* 1315
C.I. Fluorescent Brightener 184 *see* 1014
C.I. Food Blue 1 *see* 4944
C.I. Food Blue 2 *see* 1373
C.I. Food Blue 3 *see* 8987
C.I. Food Green 1 *see* 4575
C.I. Food Green 3 *see* 3941
C.I. Food Red 1 *see* 7591
C.I. Food Red 6 *see* 7590
C.I. Food Red 14 *see* 3693
C.I. Food Red 17 *see* 284
C.I. Food Yellow 3 *see* 9001
C.I. Food Yellow 4 *see* 9072
C.I. Food Yellow 8 *see* 9775
C.I. Ingrain Blue 1 *see* 218
C.I. Mordant Black 11 *see* 3667
C.I. Mordant Blue 10 *see* 4355
C.I. Mordant Blue 14 *see* 1959
C.I. Mordant Orange 1 *see* 255
C.I. Mordant Orange 14 *see* 254
C.I. Mordant Red 3 *see* 8573
C.I. Mordant Red 11 *see* 251
C.I. Mordant Violet 26 *see* 8050
C.I. Mordant Yellow 1 *see* 5919
C.I. Mordant Yellow 5 *see* 6841
C.I. Natural Brown 1 *see* 4088
C.I. Natural Brown 7 *see* 5269
C.I. Natural Orange 4 *see* 675
C.I. Natural Red 3 *see* 5293
C.I. Natural Red 4 *see* 1843
C.I. Natural Red 8 *see* 7945
C.I. Natural Red 16 *see* 7945
C.I. Natural Red 20 *see* 257
C.I. Natural Red 24 *see* 1367
C.I. Natural Red 25 *see* 5330
C.I. Natural Red 26 *see* 1867
C.I. Natural Yellow 3 *see* 2673
C.I. Natural Yellow 8 *see* 6269
C.I. Natural Yellow 11 *see* 5644, 269
C.I. Oxidation Base 12 *see* 2976
C.I. Pigment Black 15 *see* 2646
C.I. Pigment Blue 15 *see* 2520
C.I. Pigment Blue 27 *see* 7910
C.I. Pigment Blue 29 *see* 9846
C.I. Pigment Blue 66 *see* 4943
C.I. Pigment Brown 9 *see* 2637
C.I. Pigment Green 17 *see* 2234
C.I. Pigment Green 20 *see* 2624
C.I. Pigment Green 21 *see* 2625
C.I. Pigment Red 83 *see* 251
C.I. Pigment Red 105 *see* 5425
C.I. Pigment Red 106 *see* 5889
C.I. Pigment Red 109 *see* 4520
C.I. Pigment Violet 14 *see* 2447
C.I. Pigment White 1 *see* 1005
C.I. Pigment White 4 *see* 10147
C.I. Pigment White 5 *see* 5546
C.I. Pigment White 6 *see* 9472
C.I. Pigment Yellow 31 *see* 972
C.I. Pigment Yellow 33 *see* 1660
C.I. Pigment Yellow 34 *see* 5405
C.I. Pigment Yellow 36 *see* 10133
C.I. Pigment Yellow 39 *see* 799
C.I. Pigment Yellow 40 *see* 2432
C.I. Pigment Yellow 45 *see* 4020
C.I. Solvent Black 3 *see* 8885
C.I. Solvent Blue 8 *see* 6060
C.I. Solvent Brown 12 *see* 1252

C.I. Solvent Green 3 *see* 8065
C.I. Solvent Green 7 *see* 7954
C.I. Solvent Orange 3 *see* 2257
C.I. Solvent Orange 7 *see* 10089
C.I. Solvent Orange 32 *see* 3067
C.I. Solvent Red 23 *see* 8884
C.I. Solvent Red 24 *see* 8393
C.I. Solvent Red 43 *see* 3603
C.I. Solvent Red 72 *see* 3022
C.I. Solvent Red 73 *see* 3189
C.I. Solvent Red 80 *see* 2333
C.I. Solvent Yellow 1 *see* 419
C.I. Solvent Yellow 2 *see* 3229
C.I. Solvent Yellow 3 *see* 420
C.I. Solvent Yellow 5 *see* 10095
C.I. Solvent Yellow 6 *see* 10096
C.I. Solvent Yellow 33 *see* 8072
C.I. Solvent Yellow 94 *see* 4159
C.I. Vat Blue 1 *see* 4943
Ciafos, 2261
Cialis [Lilly] *see* 9027
Cianatil *see* 2683
Cianurina *see* 5877
Ciatyl [Troponwerke] *see* 2394
Ciba 570 *see* 7337
Ciba 2059 *see* 4154
Ciba 3126 *see* 6142
Ciba 4311b *see* 6110
Ciba 5968 *see* 4763
Ciba 8514 *see* 2085
Ciba 10370 *see* 8900
Ciba 11925 *see* 7197
Ciba 32644-Ba *see* 6563
Ciba 36278-Ba *see* 1972
Cibacalcin [Novartis] *see* 1643
Cibacen [Novartis] *see* 1031
Cibazol [Novartis] *see* 8943
Cibenol [Fujisawa] *see* 2269
Cibenzoline *see* 2269
Ciberon [Taisho] *see* 1799
Ciblor [Inava] *see* 2341
Cichorigenin *see* 3697
Cichoriin, 2262
Ciclacillin *see* 2702
Cicladol [Master] *see* 7506
Ciclesonide, 2263
Ciclesonide-active Principle *see* 2263
Cicletanide *see* 2264
Cicletanine, 2264
Ciclobendazole *see* 2712
Ciclobiotic [Beta] *see* 5943
Ciclochem [Novag] *see* 2266
Ciclonicate, 2265
Ciclonium Iodide *see* 2737
Ciclopirox, 2266
Ciclopirox Olamine *see* 2266
Ciclosporin *see* 2752
Cicloven [AGIPS] *see* 7975
Cicutine *see* 2505
Cicutoxin, 2267
Cidal [CID] *see* 8328
Cidandopa [Cidán] *see* 5464
Cidecin [Cubist] *see* 2823
Cidex [J & J] *see* 4472
Cidex OPA [J & J] *see* 7368
Cidine [Almirall] *see* 2294
Cidofovir, 2268
Cidomycin [Aventis] *see* 4392
Cidoxepin Hydrochloride *see* 3435
Cidrex *see* 4781
Cifenline, 2269
Ciflox [Bayer] *see* 2314
CIFN *see* 4990
CIG *see* 4075
Cignolin [Bayer] *see* 684

Ciguatoxins, 2270
Cilansetron, 2271
Cilantro *see* 2531
Cilastatin, 2272
Cilastatin Sodium *see* 2272
Cilazapril, 2273
Cilazaprilat *see* 2273
Cilest [Cilag] *see* 6703
Ciliary Neurotrophic Factor, 2274
Cilicaine [Sigma] *see* 7097
Cilifor [C.E.P.A.] *see* 1979
Cilleral [BMS] *see* 586
Cilligen [Sigma] *see* 7101
Cilnidipine, 2275
Cilomilast, 2276
Ciloprost *see* 4901
Cilostazol, 2277
Ciloxan [Alcon] *see* 2314
Cimadronate Sodium *see* 4929
Cimal [AL] *see* 2279
Cimaterol, 2278
Cimectacarb *see* 9725
Cimedone [Specia] *see* 8711
Cimetag [Cehasol] *see* 2279
Cimetidine, 2279
Cimetropium Bromide, 2280
Cimetum [Sintyal] *see* 2279
Cimicifuga *see* 1312
Cimicifugol *see* 2281
Cimigenol, 2281
Cimzia [UCB] *see* 2003
Cinacalcet, 2282
Cinalong [Fujirebio] *see* 2275
Cinaperazine [Yakult] *see* 2305
Cinarine *see* 2766
Cinazyn [Italchimici] *see* 2305
Cinch [DuPont] *see* 2295
Cinchamidine *see* 4782
Cinchocaine *see* 3031
Cinchol *see* 8556
Cincholepidine *see* 5441
Cincholic Acid β-D-Quinovoside *see* 8076
Cinchomeronic Acid, 2283
Cinchona, 2284
Cinchona Bark *see* 2284
Cinchonamine, 2285
(8α,9R)-Cinchonan-6′,9-diol *see* 2623
(8α,9R)-Cinchonan-9-ol *see* 2286
(8α,9S)-Cinchonan-9-ol *see* 2286
(9R)-Cinchonan-9-ol *see* 2287
(9S)-Cinchonan-9-ol *see* 2287
Cinchonicine *see* 2289
Cinchonidine, 2286
Cinchonine, 2287
Cinchophen, 2288
Cinchotine *see* 4783
Cinchotoxine, 2289
Cinchovatine *see* 784, 2286
Cincofarm [Lepori] *see* 4847
Cinconal *see* 2288
Cinconifine *see* 4783
Cinene *see* 5493
Cineole *see* 3895
Cinepazet, 2290
Cinepazic Acid Ethyl Ester *see* 2290
Cinepazide, 2291
Cinerin I *see* 2292
Cinerin II *see* 2292
Cinerins, 2292
Cinidon-ethyl, 2293
Cinitapride, 2294
Cinmethylin, 2295
Cinnabar *see* 5889
Cinnabarine, 2296
Cinnacet [Schwarzhaupt] *see* 2305

Cinnageron [Streuli] see 2305
Cinnaloid [Pfizer] see 8142
Cinnamal see 2297
Cinnamaldehyde, 2297
Cinnamedrine, 2298
Cinnamein see 1130
Cinnamene see 8860
Cinnamic Acid, 2299
trans-Cinnamic Acid Benzyl Ester see 1130
Cinnamic Acid Cinnamyl Ester see 2304
Cinnamic Alcohol see 2302
Cinnamic Aldehyde see 2297
Cinnamic Anhydride see 2299
Cinnamin [Nippon Chemiphar] see 726
Cinnamol see 8860
Cinnamon, 2300
Cinnamonin see 6322
Cinnamon Wood see 8381
Cinnamoyl Chloride, 2301
Cinnamyl Alcohol, 2302
Cinnamyl o-Aminobenzoate see 2303
Cinnamyl Anthranilate, 2303
1-Cinnamyl-4-benzhydrylpiperazine see 2305
1-Cinnamyl-4-(4-chlorobenzhydryl)-piperazine see 2367
Cinnamyl Cinnamate, 2304
1-Cinnamyl-4-(di-p-fluorobenzhydryl)-piperazine see 4144
1-Cinnamyl-4-diphenylmethylpiperazine see 2305
1-trans-Cinnamyl-4-diphenylmethyl-piperazine see 2305
N-Cinnamylephedrine see 2298
(±)-(E)-Cinnamyl 2-Methoxyethyl 1,4-Dihydro-2,6-dimethyl-4-(m-nitro-phenyl)-3,5-pyridinedicarboxylate see 2275
α-[1-(N-Cinnamyl-N-methylamino)-ethyl]benzyl Alcohol see 2298
Cinnamyl Methyl Ketone see 1137
(E)-N-Cinnamyl-N-methyl-1-naphtha-lenemethylamine see 6355
Cinnarizine, 2305
Cinnipirine see 2305
Cinnoline, 2306
Cinnoxicam see 7506
Cinnyl Cinnamate see 2304
CINO-40 [Tutag] see 9595
Cinobac [Lilly] see 2309
Cinobufotalin, 2307
Cinolazepam, 2308
Cinopal [Lederle] see 3963
Cinopenil [Hoechst] see 5969
Cinopol [Lederle] see 3963
Cinoxacin, 2309
Cinoxate, 2310
Cin-Quin [Rowell] see 8060
Cinromide, 2311
Cintredekin Besudotox, 2312
CiNU [BMS] see 5564
Ciodrin [Shell] see 2600
CIPC see 2187
Cipractin [Andromaco] see 2773
Cipralan [Roche] see 2269
Cipralex [Lundbeck] see 2318
Cipramil [Lundbeck] see 2318
Cipril [Italchimici] see 2316
Cipro [Bayer] see 2314
Ciprobay [Bayer] see 2314
Ciprofibrate, 2313
Ciprofloxacin, 2314
Ciprol [Sterling] see 2313
Ciproxan [Bayer] see 2314

Ciproxin [Bayer] see 2314
Cirantin see 4671
Circair [Circle] see 3479
Circanol [3M] see 3653
Circolene [Inverni] see 8119
Circo-Maren [Krewel] see 6496
Circubid [W. F. Merchant] see 3728
Circulen [Kyorin] see 155
Circuletin see 5279
Circulin A see 2315
Circulin B see 2315
Circulins, 2315
Circupon [Gepepharm] see 3865
Cirotyl [Parke-Davis] see 6974
Cirrocolina see 2207
Cisapride, 2316
Cisatracurium Besylate see 868
Cismaplat [Mack, Illert.] see 2317
Cisordinol [Lundbeck] see 2394
Cisplatin, 2317
Cisplatyl [Bellon] see 2317
Cistobil [Bracco] see 5058
Citalopram, 2318
Citanest [AstraZeneca] see 7743
Citicoline, 2319
Citiolase [HMR] see 2320
Citiolone, 2320
Citireuma [CT] see 8982
Citizeta [CT] see 10170
Citodon see 4704
Citofur [Lusofarmaco] see 9112
Citogel [Zyma] see 8879
Citopan see 4704
Citoplatino [Rhône-Poulenc] see 2317
Citosarin [Toyo Jozo] see 2702
Citoxid [Disprovent] see 6353
Citracal [Mission Pharmacal] see 1661
Citracholine see 2207
Citraconic Acid, 2321
Citral, 2322
cis-Citral see 2322
Citral A see 2322
Citral B see 2322
Citramag [Sanochemia] see 5663
Citramalic Acid, 2323
Citrated Caffeine see 1636
Citrated Calcium Carbimide see 1663
Citraurin see 2324
β-Citraurin, 2324
Citrazinic Acid, 2325
Citric Acid, 2326
Citric Acid Diammonium Salt see 512
Citric Acid Tributyl Ester see 1564
Citric Acid Trilithium Salt see 5530
Citrical [Shire] see 1657
Citridic Acid see 117
Citrinin, 2327
Citromycetin, 2328
Citronellal, 2329
α-Citronellal see 2329
Citronellol, 2330
α-Citronellol see 8185
β-Citronellol, 2330
1-Citronellol see 8185
Citronin A see 6393
Citrophen see 7228
Citropten see 5492
Citrosodine [GSK] see 8602
Citrostadienol see 8555
Citrovorum Factor see 4222
Citrucel [GSK] see 6040
Citrulline, 2331
Citrullol, 2332
Citrus Flavonoid Compounds see 1228
Citrus Red 2, 2333

Citrylideneacetone see 7917
Civet, 2334
Civetone, 2335
Cizolirtine, 2336
CJ-91B see 6841
CK-1752 see 8442
CK-1752A see 8442
CL-20 see 4696
CL-68 see 2369
CL-337 see 899
CL-636 see 8902
CL-1025 see 2507
CL-1388R see 4559
CL-1848C see 3889
CL-1957A see 5444
CL-11344 see 7968
CL-12625 see 6427
CL-13494 see 8919
CL-13900 see 7943
CL-14377 see 5985
CL-19823 see 9595
CL-26691 see 2785
CL-34433 see 9598
CL-34699 see 388
CL-36010 see 8056
CL-62362 see 5587
CL-67772 see 576
CL-71563 see 5587
CL-81588 see 889
CL-82204 see 3963
CL-84777 see 3138
CL-112302 see 1497
CL-118523 see 1955
CL-184116 see 7596
CL-186815 see 1197
CL-206214 see 1514
CL-206576 see 8891
CL-216942 see 1244
CL-222293 see 4903
CL-227193 see 7463
CL-232315 see 6217
CL-251931 see 1955
CL-252925 see 4905
CL-263499 see 4907
CL-263780 see 2278
CL-273703 see 5648
CL-284635 see 1924
CL-284846 see 10111
CL-285489 see 4946
CL-287088 see 6444
CL-291894 see 8716
CL-298741 see 9083
CL-299263 see 4904
CL-301423 see 6290
CL-303630 see 2088
CL-307579 see 9083
CL-318952 see 9967
CL-67310465 see 7135
Clabber see 10101
Cladinose see 6318
Cladribine, 2337
Claforan [Aventis] see 1933
Clamoxyl [GSK] see 577
Clam Poison see 8389
Clanobutin, 2338
Clanzol [Orfi Farma] see 2344
Claragine [Nicholas] see 851
Claramid [Jouveinal] see 8276
Claresan see 2378
Clarified Butter see 4417
Clarin (formerly) [Pfizer] see 4653
Clarinex [Schering-Plough] see 2922
Claripex [Usafarma] see 2377
Clarithromycin, 2339
Claritin [Schering-Plough] see 5578

Clarity [BASF] see 3040
Clarityn [Schering-Plough] see 5578
Clarosip [Grünenthal] see 2339
Clarvisan [Allergan] see 7490
Clarytin [Schering-Plough] see 5578
Classic [DuPont] see 2093
Clast [Meiji Seika] see 2344
Clasteon [Abiogen] see 2371
Clastoban [RPR] see 2371
Clathrates, 2340
Clathromycin [Taisho] see 2339
Claudetite see 804
Clausthalite see 8431
Clavacin see 7053
Clavamox [Pfizer] see 2341
Clavatin see 7053
Claversal [Merckle] see 5904
Claviformin see 7053
Clavitol see 4542
Claviton see 9661
Clavulanic Acid, 2341
Clavulin [SKB] see 2341
Clayton Yellow see 9310
Clazosentan, 2342
Clazuril, 2343
CldAdo see 2337
Cleactor [Eisai] see 6259
Clearing Factor see 5512
Clearnal [Yoshitomi] see 9578
Clearteck [Penreco] see 7186
Clebopride, 2344
Cleboril [Almirall-Omega] see 2344
Clédial [Anphar-Rolland] see 5790
Cleiton [Sankyo Zoki] see 4787
Cleland's Reagent see 3376
Clemastine, 2345
Clemizole, 2346
Clemizole-penicillin see 7094
Clenbuterol, 2347
Clenil-A [Chiesi] see 1019
Clentiazem, 2348
Cleocin [Pharmacia & Upjohn] see 2356
Cleprid [Recordati] see 2344
Clera [Person & Covey] see 6368
Clérégil [Merck-Clévenot] see 2843
Cleridium [Marcofina] see 3346
Clethodim, 2349
Clevelox [AstraZeneca] see 2352
1,6-Cleve's Acid, 2350
1,7-Cleve's Acid, 2351
Clevidipine, 2352
Clevudine, 2353
Clexane [Aventis] see 3588
Clexon [Wellcome] see 7050
Cl-F-ara-A see 2372
Cliacil [Aventis] see 7100
Clidinium Bromide, 2354
Clift [Abbott] see 7874
Climara [Berlex] see 3703
Climaval [Novartis] see 3703
Clinacox [Janssen] see 3080
Clinafarm [Janssen] see 3583
Clinafloxacin, 2355
Clinagel [Schering] see 2587
Clindamycin, 2356
Clinimycin (rescinded) see 2356
Clinitar [Smith & Nephew] see 2426
Clinium [McNeil] see 5484
Clinoenstatite see 5687
Clinofibrate, 2357
Clinofug [Wolff] see 3440
Clinolamide see 5505
Clinoril [Merck & Co.] see 8982
Clinovir [Pharmacia] see 5793
Clinozoisite see 1648

Clinprost, 2358
Clinsol [Virbac] see 2356
Clintabs [Virbac] see 2356
Cliocinizine see 2367
Clionasterol see 8557
Clioquinol see 5031
CLIP see 7791
Cliquinol see 5031
Cliradon [Novartis] see 5301
Clistin [McNeil] see 1799
Clisundac [Lagap] see 8982
Clitizina see 4308
Clivarin(e) [Knoll] see 8170
Clivoten [Lifepharma] see 5240
CLL see 1714
CLM see 1715
CLM $\gamma_1{}^I$ see 1715
Cl$_2$MDP see 2371
Clobazam, 2359
Clobenfurol, 2360
Clobenoside, 2361
Clobenzorex, 2362
Clobesol [GSK] see 2363
Clobetasol, 2363
Clobetasone, 2364
Clobren-SF [Morishita] see 2377
Clobutinol, 2365
Clocapramine, 2366
Clocarpramine see 2366
Clocete [Toyama] see 5780
Clocinizine, 2367
Cloconazole, 2368
Clocortolone, 2369
Cloderm [Ortho] see 2369
Clodinafop-Propargyl, 2370
Clodronate Disodium see 2371
Clodronic Acid, 2371
Clofarabine, 2372
Clofazimine, 2373
Clofedanol see 2066
Clofekton [Yoshitomi] see 2366
Clofen [Alphapharm] see 937
Clofenamide, 2374
Clofencet, 2375
Clofenotane see 2841
Clofentezine, 2376
Clofibrate, 2377
Clofibric Acid, 2378
Clofinit [Gentili] see 2377
Cloflucarban, 2379
Clofoctol, 2380
Clolar [Genzyme] see 2372
Clomag see 2378
Clomazone, 2381
Clomestrone, 2382
Clometacillin see 2385
Clometacin, 2383
Clometazin see 2383
Clomethacillin see 2385
Clomethiazole, 2384
Clometocillin, 2385
Clomicalm [Novartis] see 2387
Clomid [Aventis] see 2386
Clomidazole see 2107
Clomifene see 2386
Clomiphene, 2386
Clomipramine, 2387
Clomocycline, 2388
Clonazepam, 2389
Clonidine, 2390
Clonistada [Stadapharm] see 2390
Clonitrate, 2391
Clonitrilide see 6519
Clonix [Medicamenta] see 2392
Clonixic Acid see 2392

Clonixin, 2392
Clonopin [Roche] see 2389
Clont [Infectopharm] see 6157
Clopamide, 2393
Clopane [Lilly] see 2740
Clopenthixol, 2394
α-Clopenthixol see 2394
Cloperastine, 2395
Clophen [Bayer] see 7564
Clopidogrel, 2396
Clopidol, 2397
Clopindol see 2397
Clopinerin [Nippon Shoji] see 2408
Clopixol [HMR] see 2394
Clopoxide see 2084
Cloprane [Luitpold] see 8255
Cloprednol, 2398
Clopromate [Purdue Frederick] see 6143
Cloprostenol, 2399
Clopyralid, 2400
Cloquinate see 4826
Cloquintocet-Mexyl, 2401
Cloradryn [Recordati] see 2398
Cloranolol, 2402
Clorazepate Dipotassium see 2403
Clorazepic Acid, 2403
Clorazolam see 9604
Clorevan [Bago] see 2181
Clorexolone, 2404
Clorfentermina see 2182
Cloricromen, 2405
Clorindione, 2406
Clorociclin [Panthox & Burck] see 8252
Cloronaftina see 2108
Clorophene, 2407
Clorpactin [Guardian] see 6956
Clorpactin WCS [Guardian] see 6956
Clorpactin XCB [Guardian] see 6956
Clorprenaline, 2408
Clorsulon, 2409
Clortermine, 2410
Clortetrin [Fargal] see 2886
Closantel, 2411
Closina see 2751
Clospipramine see 6278
Clospirazine, 2412
Clostebol, 2413
Clostilbegyt [Egis] see 2386
Clostridiopeptidase A see 2481
Closylate see 2122
Clotam [GEA] see 9513
Clotbur see 5368
Clothianidin, 2414
Clothiapine, 2415
Clotiazepam, 2416
Clotrimazole, 2417
Clout [Scott] see 5953
Clove, 2418
Clove Oil see 2418
Cloxacillin, 2419
Cloxapen [GSK] see 2419
Cloxazolam, 2420
Cloxiquine see 2422
Cloxotestosterone, 2421
Cloxypen [BMS] see 2419
Cloxyquin, 2422
Clozan [Roerig] see 2416
Clozapine, 2423
Clozaril [Novartis] see 2423
CLSE see 1714
Cl-TMBP see 9441
ClTx see 2173
Club-moss Spores see 5623
Clupeine, 2424
CLY-503 see 8537

Cogomycin *see* 4290
Coherin, 2469
Co I *see* 6344
Co II *see* 6348
Cola *see* 5318
Colace [Roberts] *see* 3401
Colalin *see* 2203
Colamine *see* 3727
Colaspase *see* 836
Colazal [Salix] *see* 945
Colazide [Shire] *see* 945
Colcemid *see* 2887
Colchamine *see* 2887
Colchiceine, 2470
Colchicine, 2471
Colchicine-binding Protein *see* 9808
Colchicum Corm, 2472
Coldan *see* 6368
Coldrin [Nippon Shinyaku] *see* 2066
Colecalciferol *see* 10019
Coleflux [Finadiet] *see* 7485
Colemanite *see* 1652
Colenormol *see* 6960
Colepan [Panther-Osfa] *see* 2715
Colepax *see* 5058
Colepur [Draco] *see* 1453
Colerainite *see* 350
Colesevelam Hydrochloride, 2473
Colesterinex [Galenica] *see* 7975
Colestid [Pfizer] *see* 2475
Colestilan, 2474
Colestimide *see* 2474
Colestipol, 2475
Colestyramin *see* 2202
Coletrast *see* 5026
Colforsin, 2476
Colfosceril Palmitate, 2477
Colicine *see* 2478
Colicins, 2478
Colicon [Resse] *see* 3215
Colicort [Merck & Co.] *see* 7721
Colic Root *see* 230, 3293, 4338
Colidosan *see* 8211
Colifoam [Stafford-Miller] *see* 4787
Colifos *see* 7362
Colimicina [UCB] *see* 2479
Colimune [Sanofi-Aventis] *see* 2590
Colimycine [Sanofi-Aventis] *see* 2479
Coliopan [Eisai] *see* 1534
Coliquifilm [Allergan] *see* 2129
Colisone [Frosst] *see* 7722
Colistimethate Sodium *see* 2479
Colistin, 2479
Colistin B *see* 2479
Collagen, 2480
Collagenase, 2481
Collazin [Vitaplex] *see* 10159
α-Collidine *see* 3843
α,γ,α'-Collidine *see* 9718
β-Collidine *see* 3842
γ-Collidine *see* 9718
sym-Collidine *see* 9718
2,4,6-Collidine *see* 9718
Collinomycin, 2482
Collinsonia, 2483
Collodion, 2484
Collodion Cotton *see* 8011
Collodion Wool *see* 8011
Colloidal Bismuth Subcitrate, 2485
Colloidal Gold *see* 5631
Colloidal Gold ^{198}Au *see* 4517
Colloxylin *see* 8011
Collunosol *see* 9643
Collunovar *see* 6447
Colme [Lasa] *see* 1663

Colocynth, 2486
Colocynthin, 2487
Colofac [Duphar] *see* 5769
Colofoam [Stafford-Miller] *see* 4787
Cologel [Lilly] *see* 6040
Cologne Yellow *see* 5405
Colombo *see* 1721
Colomycin [Forest] *see* 2479
Colomycin (Tabl.) [Forest] *see* 2479
Colonorm [Mundipharma] *see* 8455
Colony-stimulating Factor 1 *see* 5646
1-214-Colony-stimulating Factor 1
    (Human Clone p3ACSF-69 Protein
    Moiety Reduced) Homodimer *see* 5646
4-221-Colony-stimulating Factor 1
    (Human Clone p3ACSF-69 Protein
    Moiety Reduced) *see* 5646
Colony-stimulating Factor-2 *see* 4538
Colony-stimulating Factor 2 (Human
    Clone pCSF-1 Protein Moiety
    Reduced) Glycoform GMC 89-107 *see*
    4538
Colony-stimulating Factor 2 (Human
    Clone pHG25 Protein Moiety Reduced)
    see 4538
Colony Stimulating Factors, 2488
Colophony *see* 8266
Colo-Pleon [Henning] *see* 8942
Colpermin [Pharmacia] *see* 7145
Colpogyn [Angelini] *see* 3707
Colpogynon *see* 2489
Colpormon, 2489
Colpro [Dagra] *see* 5791
Colprone [Ayerst] *see* 5791
Colrex [Solvay] *see* 4555
Coltericin [Quimica Argentia] *see* 5281
Coltramyl [Roussel Diamant] *see* 9324
Coltrax [HMR] *see* 9324
Coltsfoot, 2490
α-Colubrine *see* 2491
β-Colubrine *see* 2491
Colubrines, 2491
Columbamine, 2492
Columbin, 2493
Columbite *see* 6556, 9053
Columbium *see* 6556
Columbium Pentachloride *see* 6557
Columbium Pentafluoride *see* 6558
Columbium Pentoxide *see* 6559
Coly-Mycin M [Monarch] *see* 2479
Colyonal [Mochida] *see* 2951
Colza Oil *see* 8115
Combantrin [Pfizer] *see* 7955
Combat *see* 4765
Combec [Tokyo Tanabe] *see* 4132
Combidex [Advanced Magnetics] *see* 4065
Combot [Miles] *see* 9623
Combretastatin *see* 2494
(−)-Combretastatin *see* 2494
Combretastatin A-4 *see* 2494
Combretastatins, 2494
Comelian [Kowa] *see* 3200
Comet [BASF] *see* 7953
Comfolax [Searle] *see* 3401
Comite [Uniroyal] *see* 7808
Command [FMC] *see* 2381
Commando [Boehringer, Ing.] *see* 3736
Common Mallow *see* 5708
Common Salt *see* 8599
Common Sundew *see* 3453
Compactin *see* 6164
Compass [Bayer] *see* 9677
Compazine [GSK] *see* 7761
Compd 3-120 *see* 8939
Compd 43-663 *see* 4567

Compd 47-83 *see* 2710
Compd 47-282 *see* 2081
Compd 48/268 *see* 8874
Compd 118 *see* 226
Compd 180/442 *see* 3598
Compd 269 *see* 3578
Compd 347 *see* 3581
Compd 469 *see* 5175
Compd 497 *see* 3103
Compd 545 *see* 5052
Compd 711 *see* 226
Compd 933F *see* 7478
Compd 4072 *see* 2089
Compd 57926 *see* 8544
Compd 64716 *see* 2309
Compd 72500 *see* 4204
Compd 79891 *see* 6419
Compd 83405 *see* 1914
Compd 83846 *see* 754
Compd 99170 *see* 754
Compd 99638 *see* 1912
Compd B *see* 2538
Compd F-2 *see* 10116
Compendium [Polifarma] *see* 1385
Compitox [M & B] *see* 5784
Compitox Plus [M & B] *see* 5784
Complamin [3M Pharma] *see* 10060
Complexone *see* 3517
Comply [Syngenta] *see* 3987
Component B$_{1a}$ *see* 5248
Component B$_{1b}$ *see* 5248
Compound 1080 *see* 4167
Compound 81929 *see* 3395
Compound 112531 *see* 9987
Comprecin [Parke-Davis] *see* 3587
Comtan [Orion] *see* 3594
Comtess [Orion] *see* 3594
ConA *see* 2495
Conalbumin *see* 9571
Concanavalin A, 2495
"Concentrated Opium" *see* 7018
Conceptrol [Ortho] *see* 6677
Conceral [Takeda] *see* 4061
Concerta [Alza] *see* 6110
Conco NI [Continental Chem.] *see* 6677
Conco NI-90 [Continental Chem.] *see* 6677
Conco NIX-100 [Continental Chem.] *see*
    6761
Concor [Merck KGaA] *see* 1295
Concordin [Merck & Co.] *see* 7901
Condol *see* 10018
Condor Vine *see* 2496
Condrosulf [IBSA] *see* 2214
Conducton [Klinge] *see* 1778
Condurangin, 2496
Condurangogenin A *see* 2496
Condyline [Nycomed] *see* 7546
Condylox [Oclassen] *see* 7546
Conessine, 2497
Confidor [Bayer CropSci.] *see* 4910
Confirm [Dow AgroSci.] *see* 9093
Confortid [Alpharma] *see* 4968
Congo Blue *see* 9792
Congocidine *see* 6481
Congo Red, 2498
Congressane, 2499
Conhydrine, 2500
β-Coniceine, 2501
γ-Coniceine, 2502
Conicine *see* 2505
Coniel [Kyowa] *see* 1043
Coniferin, 2503
Coniferyl Alcohol, 2504
Coniine, 2505
Conium Fruit, 2506

Conivaptan, 2507
Conjugated Equine Estrogens *see* 2508
Conjugated Estrogens, 2508
Conjugol *see* 3708
Conjuncain [Mann] *see* 1047
Conludag [Searle] *see* 6697
Conmel [Winthrop] *see* 3350
Connectin 9483
Connettivina [Fidia] *see* 4757
Connexins, 2509
Connexon *see* 2509
Conoco C-50 *see* 8612
Conoco C-60 *see* 8612
Conoco SD 40 *see* 8612
Conoderm [C-Vet] *see* 6178
Conofite [Mallinckrodt] *see* 6178
ω-Conopeptide MVIIA *see* 10122
ω-Conotoxin M VIIA *see* 10122
Conotoxins, 2510
Conova [Gold Cross] *see* 3860
Conovid E [Searle] *see* 6698
Conquinine *see* 8060
Conray [Mallinckrodt] *see* 5064
Conray-400 [Mallinckrodt] *see* 5064
Conselt [Sana] *see* 2408
Conserve [Dow AgroSci.] *see* 8750
Consesus Interferon *see* 4990
Consolan [Novo] *see* 6343
Constilac [Alra] *see* 5346
Consult [Dow AgroSci.] *see* 4683
Consumptive's Weed *see* 3669
Contalax [3M Pharma] *see* 1242
Contax *see* 6974
Conteben [Bayer] *see* 9290
Contergan *see* 9255
Contomin [Takeda] *see* 2185
Contralac [Virbac] *see* 5937
Contramal [Grünenthal] *see* 9566
Contrapar [Burroughs Wellcome] *see* 5299
Contrathion [RPR] *see* 7703
Contratuss *see* 5469
Contrix "28" *see* 5064
Control-Om [OM] *see* 5851
Convacard [Madaus] *see* 2511
Convallan [Gödecke] *see* 2511
Convallaria, 2511
Convallaria Glycosides *see* 2511
Convallaton *see* 2512
Convallatoxigenin *see* 8851
Convallatoxin, 2512
Convallen *see* 2511
Convalyt *see* 2511
Convasid *see* 2511
Convenil [Hommel] *see* 1522
Convicine, 2513
Convulex [Pharmacia] *see* 9913
Coolspan [Hishiyama] *see* 8989
Coomassie Blue RL [BASF] *see* 628
Cooper-Sandoz [Syngenta] *see* 2664
Coopex *see* 2537
Coopex [Bayer CropSci.] *see* 7180
CO-ORD [Baxter] *see* 217
COP, 2514
COP 1 *see* 4435
COP 1 (Polyamide) *see* 4435
Copaene, 2515
α-Copaene *see* 2515
Copaiba, 2516
Copal, 2517
Coparaffinate, 2518
Coparogin [Nippon Chemiphar] *see* 9112
Copaxone [Teva] *see* 4435
Copegus [Roche] *see* 8198
Copinal [Vinas] *see* 45
Copirene *see* 5288

Copolymer 1 *see* 4435
Copper, 2519
Copper Chelazome [Albion] *see* 2627
Copper Acetate Arsenite *see* 2625
Copperas *see* 4057
Copper Carbonate Hydroxide *see* 2631
Copper-chromium Oxide *see* 2635
Copper DOS *see* 2670
Copper Glance *see* 2667
Copper(II) Gluconate *see* 2640
Copper Hydrate *see* 2642
Copper Hydroxide Sulfate *see* 2654
Copper(I) Iodomercurate(II) *see* 2663
Copper(II) Oxide *see* 2646
Copper Oxide (CuO) *see* 2646
Copper Phthalocyanine, 2520
Copper Pyrites *see* 2038
Copper(II) Sulfate *see* 2653
Copper Sulfate Dibasic *see* 2654
Copper Sulfate Tribasic *see* 2654
Copper(I) Thiophene-2-carboxylate, 2521
Coppinger's Radical *see* 4357
Copra Oil *see* 2461
Copren [Fuso] *see* 4475
COP Resist *see* 2514
Coprogen, 2522
Coprola [Dunster] *see* 3401
Coprostane, 2523
3β-Coprostanol *see* 2524
Coprostenol *see* 264
4:5-Coprosten-3-ol *see* 264
Coprosterol, 2524
Coptine, 2525
Coptis, 2526
Coptisine, 2527
CoQ₁₀ *see* 9843
Coracon *see* 6543
Coracten [UCB] *see* 6528
Coractiv N [Phyteia] *see* 6543
Corail [Bayer CropSci.] *see* 9092
Co-ral [Chemagro] *see* 2558
Coralgil *see* 4702
Coralgina *see* 4702
Corallin *see* 881
Coralox *see* 2537
Coramedan [Medice] *see* 3163
Coramine [Novartis] *see* 6543
Corangin [Novartis] *see* 5225
Coranormol *see* 7141
Corathiem [Ohta] *see* 2305
Corax [Empire] *see* 2084
Corazole *see* 7141
Corbadrine *see* 6692
Corbasil *see* 6692
Corbel [BASF] *see* 3993
Corchorgenin *see* 8851
Corchorin *see* 8851
Corchsularin *see* 8851
Cordan [IBI] *see* 3970
Cordanum [AWD] *see* 9038
Cordarex [Sanofi Winthrop] *see* 482
Cordarone [Wyeth] *see* 482
Cordes [Ichthyol] *see* 4787
Cord Factor(s), 2528
Cordiamin *see* 6543
Cordianine *see* 258
Cordicant [Mundipharma] *see* 6528
Cordilan [Roche] *see* 6528
Cordipatch [Schwarz] *see* 6607
Corditrine [Aventis] *see* 6607
Cordium [Riom] *see* 1150
Cordoval [Tempelhof] *see* 4434
Cordran [Watson] *see* 4197
Cordycepic Acid *see* 5745

Cordycepin, 2529
Cordycepin-5'-triphosphate *see* 2529
9-Cordyceposidoadenine *see* 2529
Coredamin [Meiji] *see* 7737
Corediol [Meiji] *see* 6543
Coreg [GSK] *see* 1873
Coreminal [Mitsui] *see* 4209
Co-Renitec [Merck & Co.] *see* 3567
Coretal [Polfa] *see* 6952
Corflazine [Daltan] *see* 5484
Corgard [King] *see* 6346
Corglykon *see* 2512
Coriamyrtin, 2530
Coriander, 2531
Coriandrol *see* 5495
Coriantin [Lepetit] *see* 2216
Coriban [Burroughs Wellcome] *see* 2974
Coric [BMS] *see* 5516
Corid [Merck & Co.] *see* 590
Coridil [Delalande] *see* 3346
Cori Ester *see* 4461
Corilagin *see* 9052
Corindolan [Schering AG] *see* 5856
Coriphate [Tokyo Tanabe] *see* 4150
Coristin [San Carlo] *see* 3653
Coritat [Green Cross] *see* 6699
Cork, 2532
Corlan [Evans] *see* 4787
Corlentor [Servier] *see* 5247
Corliprol [Pharmacia & Upjohn] *see* 1960
Corlopam [SKB] *see* 3979
Cormed [Reiss] *see* 6543
Cormelian [Viatris] *see* 3200
Cormid *see* 6543
Cornetite *see* 2648
Cornin *see* 9959
Cornocentin *see* 3655
Corn Oil, 2533
Cornox [Boots] *see* 5764
Corn Steep Liquor, 2534
Corn Steep Water *see* 2534
Corn Sugar *see* 4459
Cornus, 2535
Corodane *see* 2082
Corodilan [Meiji] *see* 3710
Coronarin *see* 3479
Coronarine [NEGMA] *see* 3346
Coronene, 2536
Corontin [Chinoin] *see* 7737
Corotrend [Siegfried] *see* 6528
Corotrope [Sanofi-Synthelabo] *see* 6197
Corovliss [Roche] *see* 5225
Coroxon, 2537
Corps De Pfeiffer *see* 7194
Corpus Luteum Hormone *see* 7773
Correctol [Schering-Plough] *see* 1242
Corrigast [Searle] *see* 7805
Corrigen *see* 6826
Corrinoids *see* 10014
Corrosive Mercury Chloride *see* 5876
Corrosive Sublimate *see* 5876
Corsodyl [Fink] *see* 2091
Cortaid [Pfizer] *see* 4787
Cortancyl [Aventis] *see* 7722
Cortate [Schering] *see* 2901
Cort-Dome [Miles] *see* 4787
Cortef [Pfizer] *see* 4787
Cortenema [Solvay] *see* 4787
Cortensor *see* 4657
Cortex Angosturae *see* 652
Cortex Cuspariae *see* 652
Cortexilar [Veterinaria] *see* 4138
Cortexolone *see* 2932
Cortexone *see* 2900

Cortexone Acetate *see* 2901
Cor-Theophyllin [Paramedical] *see* 3479
Corticoliberin(e) *see* 2586
Corticosteroid-binding Globulin *see* 4787
Corticosterone, 2538
Corticotrophin *see* 134
Corticotrophin Zinc Hydroxide Suspension *see* 134
Corticotropin *see* 134
α^{1-24}-Corticotropin *see* 2551
α^{1-24}-Corticotropin Hexaacetate (Salt) *see* 2551
β^{1-24}-Corticotropin *see* 2551
Corticotropin-like Intermediate Lobe Peptide *see* 7791
Corticotropin-releasing Factor *see* 2586
Corticotropin-releasing Hormone *see* 2586
Cortidene [Syntex Latino] *see* 7029
Cortifoam [Schwarz] *see* 4787
Cortiphyson [Promonta] *see* 134
Cortiplastol [Medici] *see* 4150
Cortiron [Schering AG] *see* 2901
Cortisol *see* 4787
Cortisol 21-(*N,N*-Diethyl)glycinate *see* 4786
Cortisol 21-Ester with *N,N*-Diethylglycine *see* 4786
Cortisone, 2539
Δ^1-Cortisone *see* 7722
Cortisone Acetate *see* 2539
Cortistab [Abbott] *see* 2539
Cortisyl *see* 2539
Cortivazol, 2540
Cortivent [Leiras] *see* 1468
Cortocin-F [Eisai] *see* 4243
Cortogen *see* 2539
Cortol, 2541
α-Cortol *see* 2541
β-Cortol *see* 2541
Cortolone, 2542
Cortone [Merck & Co.] *see* 2539
Cortril [Pfizer] *see* 4787
Cortrophin [Organon] *see* 134
Cortrophine-Z [Organon] *see* 134
Cortrosyn [Amphastar] *see* 2551
Corulon [Intervet] *see* 2216
Corundum *see* 356
Corvasal [Aventis] *see* 6234
Corvasol [Rieswerke] *see* 7141
Corvasymton *see* 9012
Corvaton [Aventis] *see* 6234
Corvert [Pfizer] *see* 4883
Corvitol *see* 6543
Corvotone *see* 6543
Corwin [Zeneca] *see* 10055
Corydaldine, 2543
Corydaline, 2544
d-Corydaline *see* 2544
Corydalis, 2545
Corydine, 2546
Corylophyline *see* 4460
Corynantheine, 2547
Corynanthidine *see* 10104
Corynanthine, 2548
Corynine *see* 10102
Corynomycolic Acids *see* 6325
Corypalmine, 2549
Corytuberine, 2550
Cosaldon [HMR] *see* 7127
Cosaprin *see* 102
Cosbiol [Laserson & Sabetay] *see* 8767
CoSept 200 [RDT HallStar] *see* 8027
Cosmegen [Merck & Co.] *see* 2800
Cosmocil CQ [Arch] *see* 7560

Cosmoline [E. F. Houghton] *see* 7185
Cosmos *see* 5963
Cosmosin [Nippon Lederle] *see* 1955
Cospanon [Eisai] *see* 4106
Cossmetin *see* 731
Cossym [Egnaro] *see* 1794
Costilate [Green Cross] *see* 5646
Costimulator *see* 4994
Cosumix [Novartis] *see* 8900
Cosuric [DDSA] *see* 279
Cosylan [Parke-Davis] *see* 8091
Cosyntropin, 2551
Cotarnine, 2552
Cotarnine Chloride *see* 2552
Cotarninium Chloride *see* 2552
Co-tetroxazine *see* 9250
Co-thromboplastin *see* 3920
Cotinine, 2553
Cotnion-methyl [Makhteshim-Agan] *see* 913
Cotoran [Griffin] *see* 4154
Co-trifamole *see* 8924
Co-trimazine *see* 8903
Co-trimoxazole *see* 8918
Cotton Red 4B *see* 1101
Cottonex [Makhteshim-Agan] *see* 4154
Cotton-root Bark, 2554
Cottonseed Oil, 2555
Cotunnite *see* 5404
Couch Grass *see* 9761
Coughwort *see* 2490
Coumachlor, 2556
Coumadin [BMS] *see* 10038
Coumafos *see* 2558
Coumalic Acid, 2557
Coumaphos, 2558
Coumaphos Oxygen Analog *see* 2537
Coumaran, 2559
p-Coumaric Acid, 2560
Coumarilic Acid, 2561
Coumarin, 2562
Coumarin-3-carboxylic Acid, 2563
cis-o-Coumarinic Acid Lactone *see* 2562
Coumarinic Anhydride *see* 2562
Coumarone *see* 1088
Coumarone-2-carboxylic Acid *see* 2561
Coumestrol, 2564
Coumingine, 2565
Counter [BASF] *see* 9158
Courlene [Courtaulds] *see* 7567
Courlene PY [Courtaulds] *see* 7581
Cousso *see* 1366
Covatine [Bailly] *see* 1773
Covatix [Gödecke] *see* 1773
Covellite *see* 2655
Covera-HS [Searle] *see* 9950
Coverine [Astier] *see* 2264
Coversum [Servier] *see* 7170
Coversyl [Servier] *see* 7170
Coviracil [Triangle] *see* 3565
Co-waldenase *see* 9879
Cow Clover *see* 9690
Cowrie *see* 2517
Cow's Milk *see* 6193
COX-189 *see* 5601
Coxistat *see* 6600
Coyden [Dow] *see* 2397
Cozaar [DuPont] *see* 5583
Cozymase *see* 6344
Cozyme [Travenol] *see* 2947
CP-20 *see* 2859
CP-0127 *see* 1358
CP-1001 *see* 2254
CP-1044-J3 *see* 1474
CP-4742 *see* 8911

CP-10423-16 *see* 7955
CP-10423-18 *see* 7955
CP-12009-18 *see* 6266
CP-12299-1 *see* 7717
CP-12574 *see* 9447
CP-14445 *see* 6922
CP-14445-16 *see* 6922
CP-15336 *see* 2970
CP-15464 *see* 1840
CP-15464-2 *see* 1840
CP-15639-2 *see* 1792
CP-16171 *see* 7506
CP-23426 *see* 9594
CP-24314-1 *see* 7489
CP-31393 *see* 7793
CP-34089 *see* 8991
CP-45634 *see* 8723
CP-45899 *see* 8889
CP-45899-2 *see* 8889
CP-49952 *see* 8992
CP-50144 *see* 201
CP-51974-1 *see* 8467
CP-52640-2 *see* 1930
CP-53619 *see* 1508
CP-54802 *see* 248
CP-62993 *see* 915
CP-65703 *see* 587
CP-66248 *see* 9144
CP-66248-2 *see* 9144
CP-73850 *see* 10194
CP-76136-27 *see* 2813
CP-88059 *see* 10171
CP-88059-1 *see* 10171
CP-99219 *see* 9787
CP-104594 *see* 6862
CP-358774 *see* 3672
CP-472295 *see* 9810
CP-526555 *see* 9936
CP-529414 *see* 9549
CP-547272 *see* 9810
CP-99219-27 *see* 9787
CPA *see* 2774
C_{16}-PAF *see* 7524
C_{18}-PAF *see* 7524
CPDC *see* 2317
CPG-56695 *see* 5597
CPG-56697 *see* 5597
CPI-22 *see* 3363
α_1-CPI *see* 5312
α_2-CPI *see* 5312
CPI-A *see* 2778
CPI-B *see* 2778
CPIB *see* 2377
Cpns *see* 2043
CPP32 *see* 1885
CPT-11 *see* 5091
C-Quens *see* 2102
CR-242 *see* 7775
CR-604 *see* 7774
CR-605 *see* 9466
CR-662 *see* 9457
CR-1505 *see* 5588
CR-1639 *see* 3286
CR-2017 *see* 5588
Crab-E-Rad [Vineland] *see* 5953
Crabtree's Catalyst, 2566
Crag 974 *see* 2834
Crag Fruit Fungicide 341 [Union Carbide] *see* 4508
Cramp Bark *see* 9973
Crampol [Dainippon] *see* 99
Cranberry Tree *see* 9973
Cranesbill *see* 4404
Crapinon [Sanzen] *see* 7470
Crasnitin [Bayer] *see* 836

Crataegus, 2567
Crataegus-Kreussler *see* 2567
Cravit [Daiichi] *see* 6771
CRD-401 *see* 3202
C-Reactive Protein *see* 2603
Cream of Tartar *see* 7615
Creasote *see* 2573
Creatergyl [Sanofi-Synthelabo] *see* 7340
Creatine, 2568
Creatine Phosphate *see* 7340
Creatinephosphoric Acid *see* 7340
Creatinine, 2569
C9-related Protein *see* 7159
Cremin [Yoshitomi] *see* 6278
Cremorin [Sanofi Winthrop] *see* 342
Cremor Tartari *see* 7615
Creolin, 2570
Creon [Solvay] *see* 7006
Creosedin [Osiris] *see* 1385
Creosol, 2571
Creosote, Coal Tar, 2572
Creosote, Wood, 2573
Creosotic Acid, 2574
Crepasin [Hoei] *see* 7737
Cresatin *see* 2583
Crescefel [Ayerst] *see* 6928
Crescormon [Pharmacia] *see* 8716
Creslan [Am. Cyanamid], 2575
m-Cresol *see* 2579
o-Cresol *see* 2579
p-Cresol *see* 2579
o-Cresol Acetate *see* 2584
m-Cresol Acetic Acid Ester *see* 2583
Cresolase *see* 9838
o-Cresolphthalein, 2576
Cresol Purple, 2577
Cresol Red, 2578
Cresols, 2579
m-Cresolsulfonphthalein *see* 2577
o-Cresolsulfonphthalein *see* 2578
γ-Cresotic Acid *see* 2580
m-Cresotic Acid, 2580
o-Cresotic Acid, 2581
p-Cresotic Acid, 2582
2,3-Cresotic Acid *see* 2581
2,4-Cresotic Acid *see* 2580
2,5-Cresotic Acid *see* 2582
m-Cresotinic Acid *see* 2580
o-Cresotinic Acid *see* 2581
p-Cresotinic Acid *see* 2582
Cresoxydiol *see* 5850
Cresoxypropanediol *see* 5850
Crestabolic *see* 5950
Crestmoreite *see* 1702
Crestomycin *see* 7041
Crestor [AstraZeneca] *see* 8270
m-Cresyl Acetate, 2583
o-Cresyl Acetate, 2584
o-Cresyl Glycerol Ether *see* 5850
o-Cresylic Acetate *see* 2584
Cresylic Acid *see* 2579
o-Cresylic Acid *see* 2579
Cresylol *see* 2579
p-Cresyl Phenylacetate, 2585
CRF, 2586
CRH *see* 2586
Crilanomer, 2587
Crinone [Serono] *see* 7773
Crinovaryl *see* 3708
Crinovyl [Rhovyl] *see* 7586
Crinuryl [Assia] *see* 3717
Crisalbine *see* 4519
Crisinor [Rubio] *see* 878
Crisofin [Allergan] *see* 878
Crispin [Kowa] *see* 9566

Cristal [Vifor] *see* 4484
Cristallovar *see* 3708
Cristalomicina *see* 5281
Cristaloxine *see* 4430
Cristapen [Glaxo Wellcome] *see* 7094
Cristapurat *see* 3163
Cristobalite *see* 8493
Crithidia Factor *see* 6462
Crittam [Caffaro] *see* 10172
Crixivan [Merck & Co.] *see* 4945
CRL-40028 *see* 170
CRL-40476 *see* 6228
Croceic Acid, 2588
Crocetin, 2589
trans-Crocetin *see* 2589
Crocidolite *see* 826
Crocin *see* 2589
Croconazole *see* 2368
Crocus *see* 8314
Cromabak [Théa] *see* 2590
Cromadoses [Théa] *see* 2590
Cromakalim *see* 5460
(−)-Cromakalim *see* 5460
Cromedil [Europhta] *see* 2590
Cromocap [Fidia] *see* 2405
Cromogen [Ivax] *see* 2590
Cromoglycic Acid *see* 2590
Cromolyn, 2590
Cromolyn Sodium *see* 2590
Cromonalgina [Ceccarelli] *see* 9658
Cromoptic [Chauvin] *see* 2590
Cromosan *see* 5654
Cromosil [Zambeletti] *see* 172
Cronassial [Fidia] *see* 4364
Cronaze [Ivax] *see* 3870
Cronizat [Caber] *see* 6660
Cronodione *see* 7234
Cronolone [Searle] *see* 4200
Cropropamide, 2591
Croscarmellose Sodium, 2592
Crospovidone *see* 7697
Crotaline *see* 6250
Crotamine, 2593
Crotamitex [Troponwerke] *see* 2594
Crotamiton, 2594
Crotethamide, 2595
Crotonaldehyde, 2596
Crotonchloral *see* 9633
Crotonic Acid, 2597
α-Crotonic Acid *see* 2597
cis-Crotonic Acid *see* 5164
trans-Crotonic Acid *see* 2597
Crotonic Aldehyde *see* 2596
Croton Oil, 2598
Croton Oil Factor A₁ *see* 7332
Crotonyl Alcohol *see* 2601
α-(*N'*-Crotonyl-*N'*-ethyl)amino-*N,N*-di-
  methylbutyramide *see* 2595
Crotonyl-*N*-ethyl-*o*-toluidine *see* 2594
α-(*N'*-Crotonyl-*N'*-propyl)amino-*N,N*-di-
  methylbutyramide *see* 2591
Crotoxin, 2599
Crotoxyphos, 2600
Crottle *see* 2615
Crotyl Alcohol, 2601
Crotyl Chloride *see* 2130
Crovaril *see* 6972
Crovicina [Viti] *see* 8252
18-Crown-6 *see* 2602
Crown Compounds *see* 2602
Crown Ethers, 2602
Croysulfone *see* 2822
CRP, 2603
Crude Chrysarobin *see* 768
Crude Cream of Tartar *see* 782

Crude Oil *see* 7187
Crude Opium *see* 6854
Crude Potassium Bitartrate *see* 782
Cruex [Novartis] *see* 9848
Crufomate, 2604
Cruiser [Syngenta] *see* 9294
Crustecdysone *see* 3491
Cryofluorane, 2605
Cryolite, 2606
Cryptates *see* 2602
Cryptaz [Romark] *see* 6567
Cryptocavine *see* 2608
Cryptocillin [Hoechst] *see* 6904
Cryptohalite *see* 527
Cryptophycin-1 *see* 2607
Cryptophycin-52 *see* 2607
Cryptophycin A *see* 2607
Cryptophycins, 2607
Cryptopine, 2608
Cryptoxanthin, 2609
all-trans-Cryptoxanthin *see* 2609
Cryptoxanthol *see* 2609
Crystallinic Acid *see* 6722
Crystallins, 2610
Crystallose [Tenneco] *see* 8311
Crystal Violet *see* 4395
Crystamine *see* 10014
Crystapen [Britannia] *see* 7094
Crystex *see* 8969
Crysticillin [BMS] *see* 7097
Crystodigin [Lilly] *see* 3163
Crystoids [Merck & Co.] *see* 4712
CS *see* 2127
CS-045 *see* 9769
CS-359 *see* 1467
CS-370 *see* 2420
CS-386 *see* 6166
CS-430 *see* 4604
CS-443 *see* 1181
CS-500 *see* 6164
CS-514 *see* 7714
CS-533 *see* 7009
CS-600 *see* 5589
CS-622 *see* 9136
CS-684 *see* 7532
CS-807 *see* 1941
CS-866 *see* 6839
CS-905 *see* 907
CS-976 *see* 7009
CS-1170 *see* 1926
CSA *see* 2214
CS-A4 *see* 2494
CSFα *see* 4538
CSF-β *see* 4537
γ-CSF *see* 2778
CSF-1 *see* 5646
CSF-2 *see* 4538
CSFs *see* 2488
CSIF *see* 4999
CSP *see* 4075
C-Stuff *see* 4771
CT-3 *see* 198
CT-848 *see* 6942
CT-1341 *see* 235
CT-1501R *see* 5517
CT-2103 *see* 6983
C.T.A.B. *see* 2025
CTAC *see* 8027
CTLA-4Ig *see* 4
CTR-6110 *see* 6596
CTR-6669 *see* 1791
CTX *see* 2046, 2270
Ctx *see* 2173, 2510
CTX-1 *see* 2270
CTX-2 *see* 2270

CTX-3 *see* 2270
CTZ *see* 1948
Cubane, 2611
Cube Alum *see* 360
Cubeb, 2612
Cubebin, 2613
Cubicin [Cubist] *see* 2823
Cubic Niter *see* 8647
Cuca *see* 2453
Cucoline *see* 8546
Cucurbitacin B *see* 2614
Cucurbitacin E *see* 2614
Cucurbitacins, 2614
Cudbear, 2615
Cuelure, 2616
Cuemid [Merck & Co.] *see* 2202
Cuivasil [IDC] *see* 5482
Cujec [Mallinckrodt] *see* 2670
Culpen [Fujisawa] *see* 4111
Cultar [Zeneca Ag Prod] *see* 6984
Culver's Root *see* 5442
Cu-lyt *see* 2660
Cumaldehyde *see* 2621
Cumaran *see* 2559
Cumarin *see* 2562
Cumarone *see* 1088
Cumarote C [Towa Yakuhin] *see* 4854
Cumene, 2617
3-*p*-Cumenyl-1,1-dimethylurea *see* 5218
2-[(*o*-Cumenyloxy)methyl]-2-imidazoline
    see 3985
Cumertilin Sodium [Endo] *see* 5872
Cumic Acid, 2618
Cumic Alcohol, 2619
Cumidine, 2620
Cuminal *see* 2621
Cuminaldehyde, 2621
Cuminic Acid *see* 2618
Cuminol *see* 2619
Cuminyl Alcohol *see* 2619
Cumol *see* 2617
Cumopyran [Abbott] *see* 2717
Cumopyrin *see* 2717
Cumotocopherol *see* 9496
Cupferron, 2622
Cuprammonium Sulfate *see* 9181
Cupreine, 2623
Cupreol *see* 8556
Cupressin [Takeda] *see* 2876
Cuprex [Merck KGaA] *see* 2644
Cupric Acetate, 2624
Cupric Acetoarsenite, 2625
Cupric Aminoacetate *see* 2627
Cupric Ammonium Chloride *see* 514
Cupric Arsenite, 2626
Cupric Benzoate *see* 1091
Cupric Bisglycinate, 2627
Cupric Bis[8-hydroxyquinoline Di(di-
    ethylammonium Sulfonate)] *see* 2670
Cupric Borate, 2628
Cupric Bromide, 2629
Cupric Butyrate, 2630
Cupric Carbonate, Basic, 2631
Cupric Chlorate, 2632
Cupric Chloride, 2633
Cupric Chromate(III) *see* 2635
Cupric Chromate(VI), 2634
Cupric Chromite, 2635
Cupric Citrate, 2636
Cupric Ferrocyanide, 2637
Cupric Ferrous Sulfide *see* 2038
Cupric Fluoride, 2638
Cupric Fluosilicate *see* 2641
Cupric Formate, 2639
Cupric Gluconate, 2640

Cupric Hexacyanoferrate(II) *see* 2637
Cupric Hexafluorosilicate, 2641
Cupric Hydroxide, 2642
Cupricin *see* 2661
Cupric Lactate *see* 5336
Cupric Nitrate, 2643
Cupric Oleate, 2644
Cupric Oxalate, 2645
Cupric Oxide, 2646
Cupric Perchlorate, 2647
Cupric Phosphate, 2648
Cupric Salicylate, 2649
Cupric Selenate, 2650
Cupric Selenide, 2651
Cupric Silicofluoride *see* 2641
Cupric Stearate, 2652
Cupric Subcarbonate *see* 2631
Cupric Subsulfate *see* 2654
Cupric Sulfate, 2653
Cupric Sulfate, Ammoniated *see* 9181
Cupric Sulfate, Basic, 2654
Cupric Sulfide, 2655
Cupric Tartrate, 2656
Cupric Tungstate(VI), 2657
Cupric Wolframate *see* 2657
Cuprimine [Merck & Co.] *see* 7088
Cuprimyl [M & B] *see* 2670
Cuprimyxin *see* 6340
Cupripen [Rubio] *see* 7088
Cuprite *see* 2664
Cuprocitrol *see* 2636
Cupro-cupric Sulfate *see* 2668
Cupron [Ayerst] *see* 1094
Cuprous Acetate, 2658
Cuprous Bromide, 2659
Cuprous Chloride, 2660
Cuprous Cyanide, 2661
Cuprous Iodide, 2662
Cuprous Mercuric Iodide, 2663
Cuprous Oxide, 2664
Cuprous Potassium Cyanide, 2665
Cuprous Selenide, 2666
Cuprous Sulfide, 2667
Cuprous Sulfite, 2668
Cuprous Sulfocyanate *see* 2669
Cuprous Sulfocyanide *see* 2669
Cuprous Tetraiodomercurate(II) *see*
    2663
Cuprous Thiocyanate, 2669
Cuproxat [Agrolinz] *see* 2654
Cuproxoline, 2670
Curacron [Syngenta] *see* 7770
Curamil [Hoechst] *see* 7962
Curan-17-ol *see* 4380
Curantyl [Berlin-Chemie] *see* 3346
Curare, 2671
C-Curarine I, 2672
Curatin [Pfizer] *see* 3435
Curatoderm [Merck KGaA] *see* 9022
Curatrem [Merial] *see* 2409
Curbix [Bayer CropSci.] *see* 3739
Curcuma Longa *see* 9824
Curcumin, 2673
Curfew [Dow AgroSci.] *see* 3075
Curine, 2674
Curium, 2675
Curled Dock *see* 8296
Curled Mint *see* 8738
Curling Factor *see* 4549
Curocef [GSK] *see* 1954
Curosajin *see* 4733
Curosurf [Chiesi] *see* 7595
Curoxim [Elan] *see* 1954
Curtacrat *see* 2567
Curvularin, 2676

Curythan *see* 5850
Curzate [DuPont] *see* 2765
Cuscohygrine, 2677
Cus Cus Oil *see* 6816
Cuskhygrine *see* 2677
Cusparia Bark *see* 652
Cusso *see* 1366
CuTC *see* 2521
Cutch *see* 1903
Cutheparine [Biosedra] *see* 4653
Cutisan [Boots] *see* 9654
Cutisterol [Farmitalia] *see* 4243
Cutivate [GSK] *see* 4211
Cutless [SePRO] *see* 4204
Cuttle-fish Bone *see* 8457
Cut-weed *see* 4282
Cuvalit [Schering AG] *see* 5518
Cuxacillin [TAD] *see* 577
Cuxanorm [TAD] *see* 859
CV-205-502 *see* 8045
CV-2619 *see* 4888
CV-3317 *see* 2876
CV-4093 *see* 5743
CV-11974 *see* 1739
C-Vimin [AstraZeneca] *see* 830
CVP *see* 2089
C.V.P. [USV] *see* 1228
CVT-510 *see* 9096
CXY-059 *see* 3363
Cy 3, 2678
Cy 5, 2679
Cy 5.5 *see* 2679
CY-116 *see* 432
CY-216 *see* 6349
Cyacetacide, 2680
Cyadox, 2681
Cyalume [Omniglow] *see* 1299
Cyamelide, 2682
Cyamemazine, 2683
Cyamepromazine *see* 2683
Cyamopsis Gum *see* 4572
Cyanacethydrazide *see* 2680
Cyanacethydrazine *see* 2680
Cyanacetylhydrazide *see* 2680
"Cyanamide" *see* 1662
Cyanamide, 2684
Cyanazide *see* 2680
Cyanazine, 2685
Cyanein *see* 1369
Cyanic Acid, 2686
Cyanic Acid Sodium Salt *see* 8604
(+)-Cyanidanol-3 *see* 1902
Cyanidanon-3-methyl Ether 1625 *see*
    4736
Cyanidanon 4'-Methyl Ether 1626 *see*
    4670
Cyanidenolon 1522 *see* 8034
Cyanidenolon-7-methyl Ether 1537 *see*
    8171
Cyanidenon 1470 *see* 5614
Cyanidenon-4'-methyl Ether 1479 *see*
    3296
Cyanidin Chloride, 2687
Cyanidol *see* 1902
Cyanin *see* 2687
Cyanite *see* 362
Cyanizide *see* 2680
Cyanoacetamide, 2688
Cyanoacetic Acid, 2689
Cyanoacetic Acid Ethyl Ester *see* 3786
Cyanoacetic Acid Hydrazide *see* 2680
Cyanoacetic Ester *see* 3786
Cyanoacetohydrazide *see* 2680
Cyanoacetonitrile *see* 5711
2-Cyanoacrylic Acid Isobutyl Ester *see*
    5140

2-Cyanoacrylic Acid Methyl Ester *see* 6046

Cyanobenzene *see* 1097

1-Cyanobenzotriazole, 2690

4-Cyano-5,5-bis(4-methoxyphenyl)-4-pentenoic Acid *see* 8383

1-Cyanobutane *see* 9905

N-Cyano-*N*′-(2-chloro-5-pyridylmethyl)-*N*′-methylacetamidine *see* 49

Cyanocobalamin *see* 10014

Cyanocobalamin Zinc Tannate *see* 10014

cis-4-Cyano-4-[3-(cyclopentyloxy)-4-methoxyphenyl]cyclohexanecarboxylic Acid *see* 2276

8-Cyano-1-cyclopropyl-7-((1*S*,6*S*)-2,8-diazabicyclo[4.3.0]nonan-8-yl)-6-fluoro-1,4-dihydro-4-oxo-3-quinolinecarboxylic Acid *see* 7701

8-Cyano-1-cyclopropyl-6-fluoro-1,4-dihydro-7-[(4a*S*,7a*S*)-octahydro-6*H*-pyrrolo[3,4-*b*]pyridin-6-yl]-4-oxo-3-quinolinecarboxylic Acid *see* 7701

N-Cyanodiallylamine *see* 2972

4-Cyano-3-(2,3-dichlorophenyl)pyrrole *see* 3989

(*E*)-α-Cyano-*N*,*N*-diethyl-3,4-dihydroxy-5-nitrocinnamamide *see* 3594

(*E*)-2-Cyano-*N*,*N*-diethyl-3-(3,4-dihydroxy-5-nitrophenyl)acrylamide *see* 3594

(−)-6-Cyano-3,4-dihydro-2,2-dimethyl-*trans*-4-(2-oxo-1-pyrrolidinyl)-2*H*-benzo[*b*]pyran-3-ol *see* 5460

2-Cyano-1,4-dihydro-6-methyl-4-(3-nitrophenyl)-3,5-pyridinedicarboxylic Acid 3-Methyl 5-(1-Methylethyl) Ester *see* 6545

N-[(3*S*)-3-[4-[(1*E*)-3-[(2*R*,3*R*,5*R*,7*S*,8*S*,-9*R*)-2-[(1*S*,3*S*,4*S*,5*R*,6*R*,7*E*,9*E*,11*E*,-13*Z*)-14-Cyano-3,5-dihydroxy-1-methoxy-4,6,8,9,13-pentamethyl-7,9,11,13-tetradecatetraenyl]-9-hydroxy-4,4,8-trimethyl-3-(phosphonooxy)-1,6-dioxaspiro[4.5]dec-7-yl]-1-propenyl]-2-oxazolyl]butyl]-4-deoxy-4-(dimethylamino)-5-*O*-methyl-L-ribonamide *see* 1724

(2*E*)-2-Cyano-3-(3,4-dihydroxy-5-nitrophenyl)-*N*,*N*-diethyl-2-propenamide *see* 3594

2-Cyano-10-(3-dimethylamino-2-methylpropyl)phenothiazine *see* 2683

3-Cyano-5-dimethylamino-3-phenyl-2-methylhexane *see* 5110

N-(1-Cyano-1,2-dimethylpropyl)-2-(2,4-dichlorophenoxy)propanamide *see* 3983

α-Cyanodiphenylmethane *see* 3316

2-Cyano-3,3-diphenyl-2-propenoic Acid 2-Ethylhexyl Ester *see* 6756

1′-(3-Cyano-3,3-diphenylpropyl)-[1,4′-bipiperidine]-4′-carboxamide *see* 7498

1-(3-Cyano-3,3-diphenylpropyl)-4-(2-oxo-3-propionyl-1-benzimidazolinyl)piperidine *see* 1196

1-(3-Cyano-3,3-diphenylpropyl)-4-phenylisonipecotic Acid *see* 3136

1-(3-Cyano-3,3-diphenylpropyl)-4-phenylisonipecotic Acid Ethyl Ester *see* 3313

1-(3-Cyano-3,3-diphenylpropyl)-4-phenyl-4-piperidinecarboxylic Acid *see* 3136

1-(3-Cyano-3,3-diphenylpropyl)-4-phenyl-4-piperidinecarboxylic Acid Ethyl Ester *see* 3313

1-[1-(3-Cyano-3,3-diphenylpropyl)-4-piperidinyl]-1,3-dihydro-3-(1-oxopropyl)-2*H*-benzimidazol-2-one *see* 1196

1-[1-(3-Cyano-3,3-diphenylpropyl)-4-piperidyl]-3-propionyl-2-benzimidazolinone *see* 1196

2α-Cyano-4α,5α-epoxyandrostan-17β-ol-3-one *see* 9698

2-Cyanoethanesulfonic Acid Sodium Salt *see* 8683

Cyanoethydrazide *see* 2680

2-Cyano-*N*-[(ethylamino)carbonyl]-2-(methoxyimino)acetamide *see* 2765

(±)-*N*-2-Cyanoethylamphetamine *see* 3994

2-Cyano-*N*-ethylcarbamoyl-2-methoxyiminoacetamide *see* 2765

1-(2-Cyanoethyl)-7-chloro-3-hydroxy-5-(2′-fluorophenyl)-1,3-dihydro-2*H*-1,4-benzodiazepin-2-one *see* 2308

Cyanoethylene *see* 131

(*R*,*S*)-α-Cyano-4-fluoro-3-phenoxybenzyl-(1*R*,*S*)-*cis*,*trans*-3-(2,2-dichlorovinyl)-2,2-dimethylcyclopropanecarboxylate *see* 2756

(−)-*trans*-1-[*cis*-4-Cyano-4-(*p*-fluorophenyl)cyclohexyl]-3-methyl-4-phenylisonipecotic Acid *see* 5463

[3*S*-[1(*cis*),3α,4β]]-1-[4-Cyano-4-(4-fluorophenyl)cyclohexyl]-3-methyl-4-phenyl-4-piperidinecarboxylic Acid *see* 5463

Cyanogas *see* 1664

Cyanogen, 2691

Cyanogenamide *see* 2684

Cyanogen Azide, 2692

Cyanogen Bromide, 2693

Cyanogen Chloride, 2694

Cyanogen Iodide, 2695

Cyanogran *see* 8605

Cyanoguanidine *see* 3092

2-Cyano-10-[3-(4-hydroxypiperidino)-propyl]phenothiazine *see* 7164

(2*Z*)-2-Cyano-3-hydroxy-*N*-[4-(trifluoromethyl)phenyl]-2-butenamide *see* 9165

N-Cyanoimidazole *see* 2696

1-Cyanoimidazole, 2696

2-(3-Cyano-4-isobutyloxyphenyl)-4-methyl-5-thiazolecarboxylic Acid *see* 3948

Cyanomethane *see* 70

1-(2-Cyano-2-methoxyiminoacetyl)-3-ethylurea *see* 2765

Cyanomethylamine *see* 412

17α-Cyanomethyl-17β-hydroxy-4,9-estradien-3-one *see* 3106

17α-Cyanomethyl-17β-hydroxy-13β-methylgona-4,9-dien-3-one *see* 3106

N-Cyano-*N*′-methyl-*N*″-[2-[[(5-methyl-1*H*-imidazol-4-yl)methyl]thio]ethyl]-guanidine *see* 2279

2-[3-Cyano-4-(2-methylpropoxy)phenyl]-4-methyl-5-thiazolecarboxylic Acid *see* 3948

(6*R*,7*S*)-7-[[[(Cyanomethyl)thio]acetyl]-amino]-7-methoxy-3-[[(1-methyl-1*H*-tetrazol-5-yl)thio]methyl]-8-oxo-5-thia-1-azabicyclo[4.2.0]oct-2-ene-2-carboxylic Acid *see* 1926

N-(Cyanomethyl)-4-(trifluoromethyl)-nicotinamide *see* 4105

N-(Cyanomethyl)-4-(trifluoromethyl)-3-pyridinecarboxamide *see* 4105

α-Cyano-3-phenoxybenzyl α-(4-Chlorophenyl)isovalerate *see* 4010

α-Cyano-3-phenoxybenzyl-2-(4-chlorophenyl)-3-methylbutyrate *see* 4010

(±)-α-Cyano-3-phenoxybenzyl 3-(2-Chloro-3,3,3-trifluoroprop-1-enyl)-2,2-dimethylcyclopropane Carboxylate *see* 2758

(*RS*)-α-Cyano-3-phenoxybenzyl (1*R*)-*cis*,-*trans*-Chrysanthemate *see* 2768

(*S*)-α-Cyano-3-phenoxybenzyl-(1*R*)-*cis*-3-(2,2-dibromovinyl)-2,2-dimethylcyclopropane Carboxylate *see* 2883

(±)-α-Cyano-3-phenoxybenzyl-(±)-*cis*,-*trans*-3-(2,2-dichlorovinyl)-2,2-dimethylcyclopropane Carboxylate *see* 2767

α-Cyano-*m*-phenoxybenzyl 2,2-Dimethyl-3-(2-methylpropenyl)cyclopropanecarboxylate *see* 2768

(*S*)-α-Cyano-3-phenoxybenzyl (1*R*-*cis*)-2,2-Dimethyl-3-[(*Z*)-3-oxo-3-[2-(1,1,-1,3,3,3-hexafluoropropoxy)]-1-propenyl]cyclopropanecarboxylate *see* 125

(*S*)-α-Cyano-3-phenoxybenzyl (1*R*)-*cis*-2,2-Dimethyl-3-[(*RS*)-1,2,2,2-tetrabromoethyl]cyclopropanecarboxylate *see* 9565

α-Cyano-3-phenoxybenzyl 2,2,3,3-Tetramethylcyclopropanecarboxylate *see* 3991

1-(2-Cyanophenoxy)-2-hydroxy-3-*tert*-butylaminopropane *see* 1489

Cyano(3-phenoxyphenyl)methyl 4-Chloro-α-(1-methylethyl)benzeneacetate *see* 4010

(±)-Cyano-(3-phenoxyphenyl)methyl (+)-4-(Difluoromethoxy)-α-(1-methylethyl)benzeneacetate *see* 4124

(α*E*)-2-[[6-(2-Cyanophenoxy)-4-pyrimidinyl]oxy]-α-(methoxymethylene)benzeneacetic Acid Methyl Ester *see* 924

5-*p*-Cyanophenyl-5,6,7,8-tetrahydroimidazo[1,5-*a*]pyridine *see* 3927

(2*R*,3*R*)-3-[4-(4-Cyanophenyl)thiazol-2-yl]-2-(2,4-difluorophenyl)-1-(1*H*-1,2,-4-triazol-1-yl)-2-butanol *see* 8121

4-[1-(4-Cyanophenyl)-1-(1,2,4-triazol-1-yl)methyl]benzonitrile *see* 5450

Cyanophos *see* 2261

2-Cyanopropane *see* 5156

2-Cyano-2-propenoic Acid Butyl Ester *see* 1565

2-Cyano-2-propenoic Acid Ethyl Ester *see* 3787

2-Cyano-2-propenoic Acid Methyl Ester *see* 6046

2-Cyano-2-propenoic Acid 2-Methylpropyl Ester *see* 5140

2-Cyano-2-propenoic Acid Octyl Ester *see* 6766

Cyanopsin, 2697

N-[3-(3-Cyanopyrazolo[1,5-*a*]pyrimidin-7-yl)phenyl]-*N*-ethylacetamide *see* 10111

N-Cyano-*N*′-4-pyridinyl-*N*″-(1,2,2-trimethylpropyl)guanidine *see* 7438

ω-Cyanotoluene *see* 1131

o-Cyanotoluene *see* 9537

(±)-4′-Cyano-α,α,α-trifluoro-3-[(*p*-fluorophenyl)sulfonyl]-2-methyl-*m*-lactotoluidide *see* 1200

21-Cyclopropyl-6,7,8,14-tetrahydro-7α-(1-hydroxy-1-methylethyl)-6,14-*endo*-ethanooripavine *see* 3340
N-Cyclopropyl-1,3,5-triazine-2,4,6-triamine *see* 2775
1-Cyclopropyl-5,6,8-trifluoro-(*cis*-3,5-dimethyl-1-piperazinyl)-1,4-dihydro-4-oxoquinoline-3-carboxylic Acid *see* 6862
Cyclorphan, 2750
Cyclosa [Nourypharma] *see* 2926
Cycloserine, 2751
Cyclospasmol [Wyeth-Ayerst] *see* 2704
Cyclosporin A *see* 2752
Cyclosporin B *see* 2752
Cyclosporin C *see* 2752
Cyclosporin D *see* 2752
Cyclosporin G *see* 2752
Cyclosporine *see* 2752
Cyclosporins, 2752
Cyclostin [Pharmacia] *see* 2747
Cyclosulfyne *see* 7808
Cyclotetramethylene Tetranitramine *see* 6758
Cyclotheonamide A *see* 2753
Cyclotheonamide B *see* 2753
Cyclotheonamides, 2753
Cyclothiazide, 2754
Cyclotrimethylenetrinitramine *see* 2736
Cyclotriphosphazenes *see* 2340
Cyclovalone, 2755
Cycloviran [Sigma-Tau] *see* 146
Cycocel [BASF] *see* 2104
Cycogan [Makhteshim-Agan] *see* 2104
Cycostat [Am. Cyanamid] *see* 8242
Cycrin [Wyeth] *see* 5793
Cydectin [Fort Dodge] *see* 6290
Cydonia Seed *see* 8054
Cyfen *see* 3976
Cyfluthrin, 2756
Cyfoxylate *see* 2756
Cygon *see* 3220
Cygro [Am. Cyanamid] *see* 5648
Cyhalothrin, 2757
λ-Cyhalothrin, 2758
Cyheptamide, 2759
Cyhexatin, 2760
Cyklodorm *see* 2711
Cyklokapron [Pfizer] *see* 9569
Cyklosal *see* 2740
Cylert [Abbott] *see* 7079
Cyllind [Abbott] *see* 2339
Cymarigenin *see* 8851
Cymarin, 2761
Cymarose, 2762
Cymbalta [Lilly] *see* 3465
Cymbi [Dolorgiet] *see* 586
Cymbush [Syngenta] *see* 2767
Cymene, 2763
m-Cymene *see* 2763
o-Cymene *see* 2763
p-Cymene *see* 2763
2-*p*-Cymenol *see* 1872
3-*p*-Cymenol *see* 9399
Cymerin [Tokyo Tanabe] *see* 8109
Cymeval [Roche] *see* 9907
Cymevan [Syntex] *see* 4363
Cymevene [Syntex] *see* 4363
Cymiazole, 2764
Cymidon *see* 5301
Cymoxanil, 2765
Cynarin(e), 2766
Cynaroside *see* 5614
Cynisin *see* 2425
Cynoff [FMC] *see* 2767

Cynoglossophine *see* 4629
Cynomel [GSK] *see* 5510
Cynotoxin *see* 8851
Cynt [Beiersdorf] *see* 6293
Cypermethrin, 2767
Cyphenothrin, 2768
Cypip [Am. Cyanamid] *see* 3116
Cyprenorphine, 2769
Cypress Camphor *see* 1911
Cypripedium, 2770
Cyproconazole, 2771
Cyprodinil, 2772
Cyproheptadine, 2773
Cyprome Ether *see* 2749
Cyprostat [Schering AG] *see* 2774
Cyproterone, 2774
Cyren A [Bayer] *see* 3129
Cyren B [Bayer] *see* 3129
Cyromazine, 2775
Cyrpon [Bayer] *see* 5862
Cys *see* 2781
Cystadane [Orphan Med.] *see* 1179
Cystafos *see* 7341
Cystamine, 2776
Cystaphos *see* 7341
L-Cystathionine, 2777
Cystatin A *see* 2778
Cystatin B *see* 2778
Cystatin C *see* 2778
Cystatins, 2778
Cysteamine, 2779
Cysteamine-S-phosphate *see* 7341
Cysteic Acid, 2780
Cysteine, 2781
L-Cysteine, 2781
L-Cysteine Methyl Ester Hydrochloride *see* 5785
Cysteine Protease P32 *see* 1885
α₁-Cysteine Proteinase Inhibitor *see* 5312
α₂-Cysteine Proteinase Inhibitor *see* 5312
L-Cysteine Thioacetal of Formaldehyde *see* 3387
*N*²-[*N*-(*N*-L-Cysteinyl-L-tyrosyl)-L-cysteinyl]-interferon γ (Human Lymphocyte Protein Moiety Reduced) *see* 4992
Cystemme [Abbott] *see* 8602
Cystine, 2782
L-Cystine, 2782
Cystine *S,S'*-Dioxide *see* 2783
L-Cystine *S,S*-Dioxide, 2783
L-Cystine Thiosulfonate *see* 2783
Cystit [BMS] *see* 6599
Cysto-Conray [Mallinckrodt] *see* 5064
Cystografin [BMS] *see* 5807
Cystokon [Mallinckrodt] *see* 79
Cystorelin [Abbott] *see* 5474
Cystospaz [Alcon] *see* 4858
Cystrin [Sanofi-Synthelabo] *see* 6955
Cys-Tyr-Cys-interferon γ *see* 4992
CYT-099 *see* 8385
CYT-356 *see* 1762
CYT-424 *see* 8350
Cytacon [Goldshield] *see* 10014
Cytadren [Novartis] *see* 440
Cytamen [UCB] *see* 10014
Cytarabine, 2784
Cyten *see* 3976
Cythioate, 2785
Cythion *see* 5700
Cytidine, 2786
Cytidine Diphosphate Choline Ester *see* 2319
Cytidine-2'-monophosphate *see* 2787
Cytidine-3'-monophosphate *see* 2788
Cytidine-2'-phosphate *see* 2787

Cytidine-3'-phosphate *see* 2788
2'-Cytidinephosphoric Acid *see* 2787
3'-Cytidinephosphoric Acid *see* 2788
Cytidine 5'-(Trihydrogen Diphosphate) *P*'-[2-(Trimethylammonio)ethyl] Ester Inner Salt *see* 2319
Cytidylic Acid *a* *see* 2787
Cytidylic Acid *b* *see* 2788
2'-Cytidylic Acid, 2787
3'-Cytidylic Acid, 2788
Cytisine, 2789
Cytiton [USSR] *see* 2789
Cytoadhesins *see* 4988
Cytobin [Pfizer] *see* 5510
Cytobion [Merck KGaA] *see* 10014
Cytochalasin B *see* 2790
Cytochalasins, 2790
Cytochrome *c*, 2791
Cytochromes P₄₅₀, 2792
Cytohemin, 2793
Cytokine Synthesis Inhibitory Factor *see* 4999
Cytolipin H, 2794
Cytolysin *see* 7159
Cytomel [GSK] *see* 5510
Cytophosphane *see* 2747
Cytorest [Mochida] *see* 2791
Cytosar [Pharmacia & Upjohn] *see* 2784
Cytosine, 2795
β-Cytosine Arabinoside *see* 2784
Cytosine Riboside *see* 2786
1-(1'-Cytosinyl)-4-[L-3'-amino-5'-(1"-*N*-methylguanidino)-valerylamino]-1,2,-3,4-tetradeoxy-β-D-*erythro*-hex-2-enuronic Acid *see* 1316
Cytostasan *see* 1034
Cytostatin *see* 4701
2'-Cytosylic Acid *see* 2787
3'-Cytosylic Acid *see* 2788
Cytotec [Pfizer] *see* 6210
Cytovene [Syntex] *see* 4363
Cytoxan [BMS] *see* 2747
Cytoxin-anticytotoxin Serum *see* 718
Cytozyme *see* 9385
Cytrol *see* 489
Cytrolane [BASF] *see* 5855
CZ *see* 1877
1,3-D *see* 3075
2,4-D, 2796
D₅ *see* 2848
D & C Blue No. 6 *see* 4943
D & C Green No. 5 *see* 252
D & C Green No. 6 *see* 8065
D & C Orange No. 4 *see* 6858
D & C Orange No. 5 *see* 3022
D & C Orange No. 8 *see* 3067
D & C Orange No. 10 *see* 3189
D & C Orange No. 11 *see* 3189
D & C Red No. 17 *see* 8884
D & C Red No. 19 *see* 8183
D & C Red No. 21 *see* 3603
D & C Red No. 22 *see* 3603
D & C Yellow No. 7 *see* 4159
D & C Yellow No. 8 *see* 4159
D & C Yellow No. 10 *see* 8071
D & C Yellow No. 11 *see* 8072
D2E7 *see* 148
D4T *see* 8803
D-20 *see* 2721
D-32 *see* 10075
D-40 *see* 8633
D-40TA *see* 3702
D-41 *see* 9771
D-50 *see* 7956
D-65MT *see* 312

D-109 *see* 4708
D-138 *see* 6703
D-145 *see* 5829
D-201 *see* 5227
D-206 *see* 7888
D-254 *see* 7456
D-301 *see* 1111
D-365 *see* 9950
D-563 *see* 6962
D-600 *see* 4356
D-706 *see* 6970
D-860 *see* 9507
D-1959 *see* 8139
D-2083 *see* 2928
D-2341 *see* 1207
D-4720 *see* 1051
D-7093 *see* 5909
D-9998 *see* 4190
D-18506 *see* 6198
D-19466 *see* 5549
D-19575 *see* 4468
D-20761 *see* 2026
D-21266 *see* 7165
DA-398 *see* 3622
DA-688 *see* 4378
DA-708 *see* 9110
DA-759 *see* 5994
DA-2370 *see* 4012
DA-3177 *see* 2280
2,4-DAA *see* 2976
DAAO *see* 414
Dabco [Air Prods.] *see* 9669
Dabigatran, 2797
DAB₃₈₉IL2 *see* 2893
Dabroson [Hoyer] *see* 279
DABS *see* 2999
DAC-2787 *see* 2166
Dacarbazine, 2798
Dacarel [Roemmers] *see* 6495
Dacatic [Lääkefarmos] *see* 2798
Dacliximab *see* 2799
Daclizumab, 2799
Dacogen [SuperGen] *see* 2853
Daconate [ISK Biosci] *see* 5953
Daconil 2787 [Syngenta] *see* 2166
Dacoren [Nattermann] *see* 3653
Dacortilen [Merck KGaA] *see* 7724
Dacortin [Merck KGaA] *see* 7722
DACPM *see* 6059
Dacron [DuPont] *see* 7569
Dacthal *see* 2839
Dactil [RPR] *see* 7470
Dactin *see* 3065
Dactinomycin, 2800
DADA *see* 3197
DADPS *see* 2822
Dafalgan [UPSA] *see* 47
Daflon [Servier] *see* 3297
Dafnegin [Poli] *see* 2266
Dagenan *see* 8938
Dagger [BASF] *see* 4903
Dagutan *see* 8311
Dahi *see* 10101
Dahlin *see* 5004
Dahl's Acid *see* 6407
Dahl's Acid II *see* 6401
Dahl's Acid III *see* 6402
Daidzein, 2801
Daidzin *see* 2801
Daipisate [Taisho] *see* 7471
Daitec [Lederle] *see* 3951
Daivonex [Leo Pharm] *see* 1641
Dakin's Solution *see* 8628
Daktar [Janssen] *see* 6178
Daktarin [Janssen] *see* 6178

Dalacin C [Pharmacia & Upjohn] *see* 2356
Dalacin T [Pharmacia & Upjohn] *see* 2356
Dalalone [Forest] *see* 2943
Dalapon, 2802
Dalbavancin, 2803
Dal-E-Rad [Vineland] *see* 5953
Dalfopristin, 2804
Dalgan [Wyeth] *see* 2956
Dalgen [Elmu] *see* 4011
Dalgol *see* 5846
Dalmadorm [Roche] *see* 4198
Dalmane [Roche] *see* 4198
Dalmate [Roche] *see* 4198
Dalmatian Insect Powder *see* 7966
Dalnate [USV] *see* 9515
Dalpac *see* 1548
Dalteparin, 2805
Daltroban, 2806
Dalysep [Syntex] *see* 8910
Dalzic [Zeneca] *see* 7700
Damar, 2807
Damascenine, 2808
β-Damascenone, 2809
Dambose *see* 4978
Damide *see* 4935
Daminozide, 2810
Dammar, 2807
DAN-2163 *see* 485
Danabol *see* 5951
Danantizol *see* 5971
Danaparoid, 2811
Danatrol [Sanofi-Synthelabo] *see* 2812
Danazol, 2812
Dandelion *see* 9059
Daneral [Aventis] *see* 7235
Danex [Makhteshim-Agan] *see* 9623
Danilon [Esteve] *see* 9009
Danish Agar *see* 4302
Danishefsky's Diene *see* 6001
Danitol [Sumitomo] *see* 3991
Danka [Mediolanum] *see* 3452
Danocrine [Sanofi-Synthelabo] *see* 2812
Danofloxacin, 2813
Danol [Sanofi-Synthelabo] *see* 2812
Danoval [Krka] *see* 2812
Dansyl Chloride, 2814
Dantamacrin [Procter & Gamble] *see* 2816
Danthron, 2815
Dantrium [Bago] *see* 1033
Dantrium [Procter & Gamble] *see* 2816
Dantrolene, 2816
Dantron *see* 2815
DAO *see* 2975
Daonil [Sanofi-Aventis] *see* 4478
3,4-DAP *see* 2986
Daphnandrine *see* 2819
Daphnetin, 2817
Daphnetin 7-β-D-Glucoside *see* 2818
Daphnin, 2818
Daphnoline, 2819
Dapiprazole, 2820
Dapotum [BMS] *see* 4189
Dapoxetine, 2821
Dapropterin *see* 8368
Dapsone, 2822
DAPT *see* 483
Daptazile *see* 483
Daptazole [Nicholas] *see* 483
Daptomycin, 2823
DAR *see* 2960
Daramin *see* 8311
Daranide [Merck & Co.] *see* 3077
Daraprim [GSK] *see* 7985
Darbepoetin Alfa, 2824
Darbid [SK & F] *see* 5202

D'Arcet Metal-fusible *see* 1257
Dardum [Lisapharma] *see* 1930
Daricol *see* 6973
Daricon [Pfizer] *see* 6973
Darifenacin, 2825
Darlan *see* 2828
Darmstadtium, 2826
Darob [Knoll] *see* 8728
Darotol *see* 2155
Dartal [Searle] *see* 9356
Dartalan [Searle] *see* 9356
Daruma [Takeda] *see* 4888
Darunavir, 2827
Darvan [Celanese], 2828
Darvilen [Schering AG] *see* 1934
Darvisul [Burroughs Wellcome] *see* 2993
Darvon [AAI Pharma] *see* 7839
Darvon Alcohol *see* 2062
Darvon-N [AAI Pharma] *see* 7839
Darvyl *see* 5636
Dasanit [Bayer] *see* 4000
Dasatinib, 2829
Daserol *see* 5850
Dasovas [Erba] *see* 2861
DAST *see* 3113
Dasten [Duncan] *see* 6925
D.A.T. *see* 54
DATC *see* 2970
Datiscetin, 2830
Datril [BMS] *see* 47
DATS *see* 2973
DaTSCAN [GE Healthcare] *see* 5050
Daturine *see* 4858
DAU 6215 *see* 5243
Daucol, 2831
Daunoblastina [Farmitalia] *see* 2832
Daunomycin *see* 2832
Daunomycinone *see* 2832
Daunorubicin, 2832
Daunosamine *see* 2832, 3439
Dauricine, 2833
Davainex *see* 3038
Davosin [Pharmacia] *see* 8919
Daxas [Altana] *see* 8249
Daxauten [3M Pharma] *see* 7737
Dayfen [3M Pharma] *see* 3331
Daypro [Pfizer] *see* 6924
Dazomet, 2834
2,4-DB, 2835
DB-32 *see* 8930
DBC *see* 2451
DBcAMP *see* 1463
DBCM *see* 2135
DBCP *see* 3020
DBD *see* 6214
DBDMH *see* 3017
DBED *see* 1064
DBED-penicillin *see* 7096
DBH *see* 3017
DBHBT, 3017
DBM *see* 6212
DBMC, 2837
DBP *see* 3035
DBPCl *see* 3012
DC 13-116 *see* 5361
DC-826 *see* 1631
DC-2797 *see* 1463
DCA *see* 2901, 3050
D(C-A-C-A-C-A-C-A-C-A-C-A-C-A-C-
     A-C-A-C-A)-DNA 5'-Ester with 1,2-
     Ethanediylbis(oxy-2,1-ethanediyl)
     Bis[2-(21,21-dihydroxy-21-oxido-
     4,11-dioxo-20-oxa-13-thia-3,10-di-
     aza-21-phophaheneicos-1-yl)-23,23-
     dihydroxy-23-oxido-6,13-dioxo-22-

oxa-15-thia-2,5,12-triaza-23-phos-
phatricosanoate] (4:1) Complex with
D(T-G-T-G-T-G-T-G-T-G-T-G-
T-G-T-G-T-G)-DNA (1:1) Hexa-
pentacontahectasodium Salt *see* 6
DCB *see* 3059
DCC *see* 3096
DCCI *see* 3096
DCCK [Rentschler] *see* 3653
DCEE *see* 3066
DCET *see* 2023
DCF *see* 7135
2′-dCF *see* 7135
DCM, 2838
DCMO *see* 1827
DCMX *see* 3076
DCNU *see* 2177
DCOI *see* 3070
d(COMOT) *see* 1795
3,6-DCP *see* 2400
DCPA, 2839
DCPM *see* 1247
DD-3480 *see* 9443
DDA *see* 3101
ddAdo *see* 3101
DDAVP [Ferring] *see* 2924
DDB *see* 738
DDC *see* 3378
ddCyd *see* 10109
DDD *see* 3061
o,p′-DDD *see* 6216
p,p′-DDD *see* 3061
DDD (Analytical), 2840
ddI *see* 3098
ddIno *see* 3098
DDP *see* 2317
cis-DDP *see* 2317
DDQ *see* 1487, 3063
DDS *see* 2822
DDT, 2841
p,p′-DDT *see* 2841
DDTC *see* 3378
DDVP *see* 3079
DE-019 *see* 1460
DE-105 *see* 8750
DE-436 *see* 3959
DE-473 *see* 4683
DE-498 *see* 4141
DE-638 *see* 7103
DE-795 *see* 8079
Deacetoxycefotaxime *see* 1923
Deacetoxy Ligstroside Aglycon *see* 6829
Deacetylandromedotoxin *see* 4543
Deacetylanhydroandromedotoxin *see*
4543
Deacetylanisomycin *see* 670
10-Deacetylbaccatin III *see* 3397
1-Deacetyldiaboline *see* 10044
Deacetyllanatoside C *see* 2921
N-Deacetyl-*N*-methylcolchicine *see* 2887
17-Deacetylnorgestimate *see* 6694
Deacylated Gellan Gum *see* 4383
Deacylated PS-60 *see* 4383
Dead-burned Gypsum *see* 1706
Deadly Nightshade *see* 1025
Deadopa [DeAngeli] *see* 5464
DEAE-cellulose *see* 1965
DEAE-dextran *see* 2936
DEAE-Sephadex [Amersham] *see* 7557
Dealgic [Pharmacia] *see* 3081
Deal Pine *see* 10043
Deamino-2-*O*-methyltyrosine-1-carba-
oxytocin *see* 1795
Deaminooxytocin, 2842
1-Deamino-D-tyr-(OEt)-4-thr-8-orn-
oxytocin *see* 865

Deanase [Consolidated Chem.] *see* 2906
Deaner [3M Pharma] *see* 2843
Deanol, 2843
Death-inducing Signaling Complex
(DISC) *see* 1886
Death's Herb *see* 1025
7-Deazaadenosine *see* 9804
Debecacin *see* 3005
Débékacyl [Bellon] *see* 3005
N-Debenzoyl-*N*-(*tert*-butoxycarbonyl)-
10-deacetyltaxol *see* 3397
Debeone [Armstrong] *see* 5938
Debetrol [Sanofi] *see* 9415
Deblaston [Madaus] *see* 7460
Debricin [J & J] *see* 4077
Debridat [Pfizer] *see* 9699
Debrisan [Pharmacia] *see* 2950
Debrisorb [Pharmacia] *see* 2950
Debrisoquin, 2844
Debrox [SKB] *see* 1782
Debroxide [Alcon] *see* 1116
Debut [DuPont] *see* 9689
Dec [Wendt] *see* 3116
Decabid [Lilly] *see* 4937
Decaborane(14), 2845
Decaboron Tetradecahydride *see* 2845
Decacarbonyldimanganese *see* 5727
Decachlor *see* 3105
1,1′,2,2′,3,3′,4,4′,5,5′-Decachlorobi-2,4-
cyclopentadien-1-yl *see* 3105
1,1a,3,3a,4,5,5,5a,5b,6-Decachloroocta-
hydro-1,3,4-metheno-2*H*-cyclobuta-
[*cd*]pentalen-2-one *see* 2083
Decadron [Merck & Co.] *see* 2943
Decadronal [Merck & Co.] *see* 2943
Decadron-LA [Merck & Co.] *see* 2943
Deca-Durabolin [Organon] *see* 6365
Decafar [Lafare] *see* 9843
Decahydro-3,5,1,7-[1,2,3,4]butanetetra-
ylnaphthalene *see* 2499
[3a*S*-(3α,5aβ,6β,9aα,9bβ)]-Decahydro-
6,9a-dihydroxy-5a-methyl-3,9-bis-
(methylene)naphtho[1,2-*b*]furan-
2(3*H*)-one *see* 9050
1,6,7,8,9,11a,12,13,14,14a-Decahydro-
1,13-dihydroxy-6-methyl-4*H*-cyclo-
pent[*f*]oxacyclotridecin-4-one *see* 1369
[1*R*-(1α,4aβ,4bα,10aα)]-1,2,3,4,4a,4b,5,-
6,10,10a-Decahydro-1,4a-dimethyl-
7-(1-methylethyl)-1-phenanthrene-
carboxylic Acid *see* 7
[1*R*-(1α,4aβ,4bα,10aα)]-1,2,3,4,4a,4b,5,-
9,10,10a-Decahydro-1,4a-dimethyl-
7-(1-methylethyl)-1-phenanthrene-
carboxylic Acid *see* 5468
[1*R*-(1α,4aβ,10aα)]-1,2,3,4,4a,5,6,9,10,-
10a-Decahydro-1,4a-dimethyl-7-(1-
methylethyl)-1-phenanthrenecar-
boxylic Acid *see* 6998
(4a*S*,4b*R*,10a*R*,10b*S*,12a*S*)-3,4,4a,5,6,-
10a,10b,11,12,12a-Decahydro-10a,-
12a-dimethyl-2*H*-phenanthro[2,1-b]-
pyran-2,8(4b*H*)-dione *see* 9179
3a,4,5,6a,7,7a,8,11a,11b,11c-Decahy-
dro-5-hydroxy-2,10-dimethoxy-3,8,-
11a,11c-tetramethylphenanthro[10,-
1-*bc*]pyran-1,11-dione *see* 6463
(1a*R*,2*R*,3a*R*,3b*R*,5*S*,6a*R*,7a*S*)-Decahy-
dro-2-hydroxy-3a,5-dimethyl-3-meth-
ylenecyclopenta[4,5]pentaleno[1,6a-
b]oxirene-5-carboxylic Acid *see* 4717
1,2,3,4,4a,4b,7,9,10,10a-Decahydro-2-
hydroxy-2,4b-dimethyl-7-oxo-1-
phenanthrenepropionic Acid
δ-Lactone *see* 9179

(3*E*,4*S*)-3-[2-[((1*R*,4a*S*,5*R*,6*R*,8a*S*)-Deca-
hydro-6-hydroxy-5-(hydroxymethyl)-
5,8a-dimethyl-2-methylene-1-naph-
thalenyl]ethylidene]dihydro-4-hydr-
oxy-2(3*H*)-furanone *see* 633
(3b*S*,4a*S*,5a*S*,6*R*,6a*R*,7a*S*,7b*S*,8a*S*,-
8b*S*)-3b,4,4a,6,6a,7a,7b,8b,9,10-
Decahydro-6-hydroxy-8b-methyl-
6a-(1-methylethyl)trisoxireno[4b,5:
6,7:8a,9]phenanthro[1,2-*c*]furan-
1(3*H*)-one *see* 9747
(3*R*,5a*S*,6*R*,8a*S*,9*R*,10*S*,12*R*,12a*R*)-
Decahydro-10-methoxy-3,6,9-trimeth-
yl-3,12-epoxy-12*H*-pyrano[4,3-*j*]-1,2-
benzodioxepin *see* 815
(2aα,4aβ,5β,6β,8aα,12bβ,12cβ,12dβ)-
(−)-2a,3,4,4a,5,6,7,8a,12b,12c-Deca-
hydro-6-methyl-2*H*-5,12d-ethano-
furo[4′,3′,2′:4,10]anthra[9,1-*bc*]oxe-
pin-2,9,12-trione *see* 7535
Decahydronaphthalene *see* 2846
Decahydro-2-oxo-1,3-bis(phenylmethyl)thieno[1′,2′:1,2]thieno[3,4-*d*]imid-
azol-5-ium Salt with (1*S*)-7,7-Dimeth-
yl-2-oxobicyclo[2.2.1]heptane-1-
methanesulfonic Acid (1:1) *see* 9707
[3*S*-(3α,4aα,5α,6α,11β,12α,12aβ)]-1,3,4,-
4a,5,6,7,11,12,12a-Decahydro-3,5,6,-
11,12-pentahydroxy-9,12a,13,13-tet-
ramethyl-4-methylene-6,10-meth-
anobenzocyclodecen-8(2*H*)-one *see*
9077
[1a*R*-(1aα,1bβ,4aβ,7aα,7bα,8α,9β,9aα)]-
1,1a,1b,4,4a,7a,7b,8,9,9a-Decahydro-
4a,7b,9,9a-tetrahydroxy-3-(hydroxymethyl)-1,1,6,8-tetramethyl-5*H*-cy-
clopropa[3,4]benz[1,2-*e*]azulen-5-one
see 7332
(4a*S*,6a*S*,11b*R*,13a*S*,13b*S*)-1,2,3,4,4a,-
5,6,6a,11b,13b-Decahydro-4,4,6a,9-
tetramethyl-13*H*-benzo[*a*]furo[2,3,4-
mn]xanthen-11-ol *see* 8486
[1a*R*-(1aα,4α,4aβ,7α,7aβ,7bα)]-Decahy-
dro-1,1,4,7-tetramethyl-1*H*-cyclo-
prop[*e*]azulen-4-ol *see* 5430
(3*S*,7*R*)-3,4,5,6,7,8,9,10,11,12-Decahy-
dro-7,14,16-trihydroxy-3-methyl-
1*H*-2-benzoxacyclotetradecin-1-one
see 10121
[2*R*-(2α,4aβ,5aβ,6β,7β,8β,9α,9aα,-
10aβ)]-Decahydro-4a,7,9-trihydr-
oxy-2-methyl-6,8-bis(methylamino)-
4*H*-pyrano[2,3-*b*][1,4]benzodioxin-4-
one *see* 8739
[1*S*-(1α,3aβ,4α,8aβ)]-Decahydro-4,8,8-
trimethyl-9-methylene-1,4-methano-
azulene *see* 5567
3-[[(1*R*,2*S*,4a*S*,8a*S*)-Decahydro-1,2,4a-
trimethyl-5-methylene-1-naphtha-
lenyl]methyl]-2-hydroxy-5-methoxy-
2,5-cyclohexadiene-1,4-dione *see*
4898
Decahydro-1,1,4a-trimethyl-2-naph-
thalenol *see* 9486
Decalin [DuPont], 2846
Decamethonium Bromide, 2847
Decamethrin *see* 2883
Decamethylcyclopentasiloxane, 2848
1,1′-Decamethylenebis[4-aminoquin-
aldinium Chloride] *see* 2913
Decamethylenebis[*m*-dimethylamino-
phenyl *N*-Methylcarbamate] Dimethobromide *see* 2885
Decamethylenebis[*N*-methylcarbamic
Acid *m*-Dimethylaminophenyl Ester]
Bromomethylate *see* 2885

Decamethylenebis[trimethylammonium Bromide] *see* 2847

$N^1,N^{1'}$-Decamethylene-$N^4,N^{4'}$-decamethylenebis[4-aminoquinaldinium Chloride] *see* 1248

1,1'-Decamethylene-4,4'-(1,10-decamethylenediimino)bis[quinaldinium Chloride] *see* 1248

2,2'-(Decamethylenedithio)diethanol *see* 9416

Decamethylene Glycol, 2849

Decamethyltetrasiloxane, 2850

Decamine *see* 2913

Decanedioic Acid *see* 8415

Decanedioic Acid Bis(2-ethylhexyl) Ester *see* 1251

Decanedioic Acid Polymer with 4,4'-[1,3-Propanediylbis(oxy)]bis[benzoic Acid] *see* 7559

1,10-Decanediol *see* 2849

1,1'-(1,10-Decanediyl)bis-[4-amino-2-methylquinolinium Chloride] *see* 2913

3,3'-[1,10-Decanediylbis[(methylimino)carbonyloxy]bis[N,N,N-trimethylbenzenaminium]dibromide *see* 2885

2,2'-[1,10-Decanediylbis(thio)]bisethanol *see* 9416

N,N'-(1,10-Decanediyldi-1(4H)-pyridinyl-4-ylidene)bis[1-octanamine] *see* 6754

Decanoic Acid *see* 1758

Decanoic Acid Ethyl Ester *see* 3776

1-Decanol *see* 2855

Decapeptyl [Ipsen] *see* 9748

Decapinol [Biosurface] *see* 2879

Decaprednil [Galen] *see* 7721

Decaps *see* 10018

(3-Decarbamoyloxy)-3-hydroxyventuricidin A *see* 9947

Decarboxycysteine *see* 2779

Decarboxycystine *see* 2776

Decaris [Janssen] *see* 5459

Decaserpyl *see* 2918

Decaspir [Pulitzer] *see* 3999

Decaspiride *see* 3999

2,4,6,8-Decatetraenedioic Acid Mono-[4-(1,2-epoxy-1,5-dimethyl-4-hexenyl)-5-methoxy-1-oxaspiro[2.5]oct-6-yl] Ester *see* 4286

(2E,4E,6E,8E)-2,4,6,8-Decatetraenedioic Acid Mono[(3R,4S,5S,6R)-5-methoxy-4-[(2R,3R)-2-methyl-3-(3-methyl-2-butenyl)oxiranyl]-1-oxaspiro[2.5]oct-6-yl] Ester *see* 4286

Decatylen [Mepha] *see* 2913

Deccotane *see* 1544

Deccox [Merial] *see* 2854

1-Decene-1,10-dicarboxylic Acid *see* 9576

Decentan [Merck KGaA] *see* 7183

[R-(Z)]-5-(1-Decenyl)dihydro-2(3H)-furanone *see* 5257

(R,Z)-5-(Dec-1-enyl)oxacyclopentan-2-one *see* 5257

Dechlorane [Occidental] *see* 6207

Dechlorane Plus [Occidental], 2851

Decholin [Miles] *see* 2868

Decicain [Winthrop] *see* 9188

Decimemide, 2852

Decis [Bayer CropSci.] *see* 2883

Decitabine, 2853

Declinax [Roche] *see* 2844

Declomycin [Wyeth] *see* 2886

Decme [Spitzner] *see* 3653

Decoderm [Merck KGaA] *see* 4191

Decolorized Phenolphthalein *see* 7244

Decolorizing Carbon *see* 1808

Decomoton [Aesculaap] *see* 1795

Decontractyl *see* 5850

Decoquinate, 2854

Decorenone [Italfarmaco] *see* 9843

Decorpa [Norgine] *see* 4572

Decortilen [Merck KGaA] *see* 7724

Decortilen Soluble [Merck KGaA] *see* 7724

Decortin [Merck KGaA] *see* 7722

Decortin H [Merck KGaA] *see* 7721

Decosteron [Kwizda] *see* 2901

Decree [Arvesta] *see* 3974

Decrelip [Ferrer] *see* 4388

Decreten [Dumex] *see* 7443

Decril [Mediolanum] *see* 3653

Dectancyl [Sanofi-Aventis] *see* 2943

Dectomax [Pfizer] *see* 3425

Decumbin *see* 1369

n-Decyl Alcohol, 2855

$N^{3''}$-[2-(Decylamino)ethyl]-29-[[(phosphonomethyl)amino]methyl]vancomycin *see* 9116

3-O-Decyl-2-deoxy-6-O-[2-deoxy-3-O-[(3R)-3-methoxydecyl]-6-O-methyl-2-[[(11Z)-1-oxo-11-octadecenyl]amino]-4-O-phosphono-β-D-glucopyranosyl]-2-[(1,3-dioxotetradecyl)amino]-α-D-glucopyranose 1-(Dihydrogen Phosphate) *see* 3671

N-Decyl-N,N-dimethyl-1-decanaminium Chloride *see* 3099

(2S-*cis*)-2-Decyl-3-(5-methylhexyl)oxirane *see* 3361

4-(Decyloxy)-3,5-dimethoxybenzamide *see* 2852

6-Decyloxy-7-ethoxy-4-hydroxy-3-quinolinecarboxylic Acid Ethyl Ester *see* 2854

DEDC *see* 3378

Dedevap [Bayer CropSci.] *see* 3079

4^A-O-De(2,6-dideoxy-3-C-methyl-α-L-*ribo*-hexopyranosyl)-20-deoxo-20-(3,5-dimethyl-1-piperidinyl)tylosin *see* 9439

3-De[[(2,6-dideoxy-3-C-methyl-3-O-methyl-α-L-ribohexopyranosyl)oxy]-11,12-dideoxy-6-O-methyl-3-oxo-12,-11-[oxycarbonyl[[4-[4-(3-pyridinyl)-1H-imidazol-1-yl]butyl]imino]]erythromycin *see* 9119

Dedrogyl [DESMA] *see* 1638

DeDTC *see* 3378

DeeO *see* 4460

Deep Purple [Amersham Biosci.] *see* 3615

9,10-Deepithio-9,10-didehydroacanthifolicin *see* 6819

12,13-Deepoxy-12,13-didehydroverrucarin A *see* 9964

Dee-Ron *see* 10018

Deer's Tongue *see* 5476

Deet, 2856

16-Deethyl-3-O-demethyl-16-methyl-3-O-(1-oxopropyl)monensin *see* 5348

Def [Bayer CropSci.] *see* 9617

Defanyl [Lederle] *see* 576

Defekton [Yoshitomi] *see* 1861

Defenidol *see* 3311

Defensins, 2857

Deferasirox, 2858

Deferiprone, 2859

Deferoxamine, 2860

Defibrase [Gerot] *see* 1010

Defibrinotide *see* 2861

Defibrotide, 2861

Défiltran [Gallier] *see* 53

Define [Bayer CropSci.] *see* 4131

Definity [BMS] *see* 7158

Deflamat [Sankyo] *see* 3081

Deflamene [Farmitalia] *see* 4243

Deflamon [SPA] *see* 6157

Deflan [Guidotti] *see* 2862

Deflazacort, 2862

Deflorin [Glaxo] *see* 1979

Defluina [Simes] *see* 3653

Defol [Drexel] *see* 8598

Defungit [Hoechst] *see* 1051

Deganol *see* 2886

Degener's Indicator *see* 7205

Deguelia Root *see* 2916

Deguelin, 2863

Dehacodin *see* 3171

Dehistin [EGYT] *see* 9738

DEHP, 2864

Dehychol [Rexall] *see* 2868

Dehydol [Henkel] *see* 7577

Dehydrated Alcohol *see* 3760

Dehydrite *see* 5678

Dehydroacetic Acid, 2865

trans-Dehydroandrosterone *see* 2871

Dehydroascorbic Acid, 2866

Dehydrobenzperidol [Janssen] *see* 3450

Dehydrobilirubin *see* 1219

11-Dehydro C *see* 281

(3β)-7-Dehydrocholesterol, 2867

24-Dehydrocholesterol *see* 2925

Dehydrocholic Acid, 2868

Dehydrocollinusin *see* 5272

11-Dehydrocorticosterone, 2869

Δ^1-Dehydrocortisol *see* 7721

Δ^1-Dehydrocortisone *see* 7722

Dehydrodichavicol *see* 5697

Dehydrodidemnin B *see* 738

Dehydroemetine, 2870

2-Dehydroemetine *see* 2870

2,3-Dehydroemetine *see* 2870

Dehydroepiandrosterone, 2871

Dehydroergosterol, 2872

1-Dehydro-9α-fluorohydrocortisone *see* 5174

Δ^1-Dehydrohydrocortisone *see* 7721

11-Dehydro-17-hydroxycorticosterone *see* 2539

Dehydroisoandrosterone *see* 2871

2,3-Dehydroisoemetine *see* 2870

6-Dehydro-6-methyl-17α-acetoxyprogesterone *see* 5805

1-Dehydro-16α-methyl-9α-fluorohydrocortisone *see* 2943

1-Dehydro-6α-methylhydrocortisone *see* 6111

1-Dehydro-17α-methyltestosterone *see* 5951

Dehydronivalenol *see* 10032

Dehydroperillic Acid *see* 9391

6-Dehydro-*retro*-progesterone *see* 3474

3-Dehydroretinal, 2873

all-trans-3,4-Dehydroretinal *see* 2873

3-Dehydroretinol, 2874

all-trans-3-Dehydroretinol *see* 2874

7-Dehydrositosterol, 2875

Dehydro-6-sulfoabietic Acid *see* 3489

1-Dehydrotestololactone *see* 9179

Dehydrotestosterone *see* 1324

6-Dehydrotestosterone-17α-propionic Acid γ-Lactone *see* 1750

Deidrocolico Vita *see* 2868

Deiten [ABC] *see* 6576

Dejo *see* 3369
Dekadin *see* 2913
DeKalin *see* 2846
Dekamin *see* 2913
Dekamin [Monico] *see* 7885
Dekelmin 6160
Dekrysil *see* 3279
DEL-1267 *see* 6143
Deladroxone (obsolete) [BMS] *see* 240
Delan [BASF] *see* 3368
Delaprem [Savage] *see* 4707
Delapril, 2876
Delatestryl [BMS] *see* 9180
Delavirdine, 2877
Delavirdine Mesylate *see* 2877
Delaxin [Ferndale] *see* 5980
Delcaine *see* 7912
Delcosine *see* 2882
Delecit [LPB] *see* 2205
Delestrogen [Monarch] *see* 3703
Delfen [Ortho] *see* 6677
Delgesic [Karlspharma] *see* 5637
Delimmun [Newport] *see* 4976
Delipid [Coop. Farm.] *see* 9416
Deliver [Certis] *see* 932
Delix [Aventis] *see* 8103
Delmadinone Acetate, 2878
Delmeson [Aventis] *see* 4175
Delminal [Rhône-Mérieux] *see* 2878
Delmopinol, 2879
Delnav [Hercules] *see* 3301
Delonal [Essex] *see* 220
m-Delphene *see* 2856
Delphicort [Lederle] *see* 9596
Delphidenolon 1575 *see* 6332
Delphin *see* 2880
Delphinac [Riemser] *see* 3081
Delphinic Acid *see* 5231
Delphinidin, 2880
Delphinidol *see* 2880
Delphinin *see* 2880
Delphinine, 2881
Delphinium *see* 5372
Delphoside *see* 2880
Delpregnin [Novo] *see* 5805
Delsene [DuPont] *see* 1791
Delsoline, 2882
Delsterol *see* 10019
Delta Goal [Dow AgroSci.] *see* 6963
Deltacortene [Bruno] *see* 7722
Deltacortisone *see* 7722
Deltacortone [Merck & Co.] *see* 7722
Deltacortril [Pfizer] *see* 7721
Delta E *see* 7722
Delta F *see* 7721
Delta Gluconolactone *see* 4457
Deltalin [Lilly] *see* 10018
Deltamethrin, 2883
Deltamycin A₄ *see* 1806
Deltan [Berna] *see* 3259
Deltar [Osiris] *see* 2392
Delta Sleep Factor *see* 3458
Delta Sleep-inducing Peptide (Rabbit) *see* 3458
Delta Sleep Peptide *see* 3458
Deltasone [Upjohn] *see* 7722
Deltastab *see* 7721
Delta-1-testololactone *see* 9179
Deltathione [Tobishi] *see* 4475
Deltazen [Sanofi-Aventis] *see* 3202
Deltison [Ferring] *see* 7722
Deltisona B *see* 5861
Delursan [Houdé] *see* 9889
Delvex [Lilly] *see* 3369
Delvomycin 6225

Demadex [Roche] *see* 9552
Demanyl Phosphate, 2884
Demecarium Bromide, 2885
Demeclocycline, 2886
Demecolcine, 2887
Demegestone, 2888
Demerol Hydrochloride [Sanofi Winthrop] *see* 5849
6-Demethoxyageratochromene *see* 7718
4-Demethoxydaunomycin *see* 4886
4-Demethoxydaunorubicin *see* 4886
2-Demethoxy-2-glucosidoxythiocolchicine *see* 9324
Demethoxyvindoline *see* 9988
5-*O*-Demethylavermectin A₁ₐ and 5-*O*-Demethyl-25-de(1-methylpropyl)-25-(1-methylethyl)avermectin A₁ₐ (4:1) *see* 2
1-Demethylcalycanthidine *see* 2059
Demethylchlortetracycline (obsolete) *see* 2886
4-*O*-Demethyldaunorubicin *see* 1870
[6*R*,23*S*,25*S*(*E*)]-5-*O*-Demethyl-28-deoxy-25-(1,3-dimethyl-1-butenyl)-6,-28-epoxy-23-hydroxymilbemycin B *see* 6444
(6*R*,23*E*,25*S*)-5-*O*-Demethyl-28-deoxy-25-[(1*E*)-1,3-dimethyl-1-butenyl]-6,-28-epoxy-23-(methoxyimino)milbemycin B *see* 6290
(6*R*,25*R*)-5-*O*-Demethyl-28-deoxy-6,28-epoxy-25-(1-methylethyl)milbemycin B *see* 6191
(6*R*,25*R*)-5-*O*-Demethyl-28-deoxy-6,28-epoxy-25-methylmilbemycin *see* 6189
(4″*R*)-5-*O*-Demethyl-4″-deoxy-4″-(methylamino)avermectin A₁ₐ and (4″*R*)-5-*O*-Demethyl-25-de(1-methylpropyl)-4″-deoxy-4″-(methylamino)-25-(1-methylethyl)avermectin A₁ₐ (9:1) *see* 3554
S-Demethyl-3′-depropyl-*S*-[2-[(2-hydroxybenzoyl)oxy]ethyl]-7-*O*-methyllincomycin *see* 1958
40-Demethyl-3,7-dideoxo-3,7-dihydroxy-*N*⁴⁷-methyl-5-oxocandicidin D Methyl Ester Cyclic 15,19-Hemiacetal *see* 5847
5-*O*-Demethyl-22,23-dihydroavermectin A₁ₐ *see* 5248
Demethyldihydrothebaine Acetate (Ester) *see* 3172
Demethyldopan *see* 9851
4′-Demethylepipodophyllotoxin 9-[4,6-*O*-Ethylidene-β-D-glucopyranoside] *see* 3886
4′-Demethylepipodophyllotoxin 9-(4,6-*O*-2-Thenylidene-β-D-glucopyranoside) *see* 9145
4′-Demethylepipodophyllotoxin-β-D-thenylidene Glucoside *see* 9145
N-Demethyl-*N*-heptylphysostigmine *see* 3638
Demethylhomopterocarpin *see* 5789
5-*O*-Demethyl-25-*de*(1-methylpropyl)-22,23-dihydro-25-(1-methylethyl)-avermectin A₁ₐ *see* 5248
6-Demethylmevinolin *see* 6164
26-Demethyloligomycin A *see* 6833
4-Demethyl-3-oxovobasan-17-oic Acid Methyl Ester *see* 7178
*O*³-Demethylthebaine *see* 6867
N-Demethylthiolutin *see* 4728
Demeton, 2889
Demeton-methyl *see* 6051
Demetraciclina [Bios] *see* 2886

Demetrin [Parke-Davis] *see* 7715
Demexiptiline, 2890
Demidone *see* 4836
Demolox [Am. Cyanamid] *see* 576
Demon [Syngenta] *see* 2767
Demorphan Hydrobromide *see* 8091
Demoxytocin *see* 2842
Demser [Merck & Co.] *see* 6161
Demulen [Searle] *see* 3860
DEN *see* 6636
DENA *see* 6636
Denagard [Novartis] *see* 9419
Denamone *see* 10041
Denan [Boehringer, Ing.] *see* 8539
Denapol [Nagase] *see* 2305
"Denarcotized" Opium *see* 6854
Denatonium Benzoate, 2891
Denatured Alcohol *see* 3761
Denavir [SKB] *see* 7083
Dendrid [Alcon] *see* 4891
Dendrotoxins, 2892
Denegyt *see* 2852
Deniban [Synthelabo] *see* 485
Denileukin Diftitox, 2893
De-Nol [Yamanouchi] *see* 2485
De-Noltab [Yamanouchi] *see* 2485
Denopamine, 2894
Denopterin, 2895
Denosine [Syntex] *see* 4363
Denufosol, 2896
Deobase *see* 5294
[9*S*(*R*)]-9-Deoxo-11-deoxy-9,11-[imino-[2-(2-methoxyethoxy)ethylidene]-oxy]erythromycin *see* 3354
20-Deoxo-20-(3,5-dimethylpiperidin-1-yl)desmycosin *see* 9439
9-Deoxo-9a-methyl-9a-aza-9a-homo-erythromycin A *see* 915
1-De(5-oxo-L-proline)-2-*de*-L-glutamine-5-L-methioninecaerulein *see* 8543
4-Deoxo-3,4-[2-spiro-(*N*-isobutyl-4-piperidyl)]-(1*H*)-imidazo-(2,5-dihydro)rifamycin S *see* 8213
3′-Deoxyadenosine *see* 2529
3′-Deoxyadenosine-5′-(tetrahydrogen Triphosphate) *see* 2529
5′-Deoxyadenosyl-B₁₂ *see* 2451
5′-Deoxyadenosylcobalamine *see* 2451
D-2-Deoxyarabinose *see* 2908
6-Deoxy-L-ascorbic Acid, 2898
3′-Deoxy ATP *see* 2529
Deoxy-BIGCHAP *see* 1214
7-Deoxy-7(*S*)-chlorolincomycin *see* 2356
Deoxycholic Acid, 2899
4′-Deoxycirramycin A₁ *see* 8261
2′-Deoxycoformycin *see* 7135
Deoxycorticosterone, 2900
11-Deoxycorticosterone *see* 2900
Deoxycorticosterone Acetate, 2901
11-Deoxycorticosterone Acetate *see* 2901
Deoxycortone Acetate *see* 2901
31-*O*-[6-Deoxy-4-*O*-(6-deoxy-2,4-di-*O*-methylhexopyranosyl)-3-*O*-methyl-hexopyranosyl]-1-methylmocimycin *see* 3525
31-*O*-[6-Deoxy-4-*O*-(6-deoxy-2,4-di-*O*-methyl-α-L-mannopyranosyl)-3-*O*-methyl-β-D-allopyranosyl]-1-methyl-mocimycin *see* 3525
(*E*)-5-Deoxy-5-[[3-[4-[(6-deoxy-β-D-*arabino*-hexofuranos-5-ulos-1-yl)oxy]-3-hydroxyphenyl]-2-methyl-1-oxo-2-propenyl]amino]-1,2-*O*-methylene-D-*neo*-inositol *see* 4851

10-[[6-Deoxy-2-O-(6-deoxy-3-O-methyl-α-D-galactopyranosyl)-β-D-galacto-pyranosyl]oxy]-6-hydroxy-1-methyl-benzo[h][1]benzopyrano[5,4,3-cde][1]-benzopyran-5,12-dione see 2045

2-Deoxy-4-O-(2,6-diamino-2,6-dideoxy-α-D-glucopyranosyl)-D-streptamine see 6430

2'-Deoxy-2',2'-difluorocytidine see 4386

4'-Deoxy-20',20'-difluoro-8'-norvinca-leukoblastine see 9989

1-Deoxy-1-(3,4-dihydro-7,8-dimethyl-2,4-dioxobenzo[g]pteridin-10(2H)-yl)-D-arabinitol see 763

1-Deoxy-1-(3,4-dihydro-7,8-dimethyl-2,4-dioxobenzo[g]pteridin-10(2H)-yl)-D-galactitol see 4333

6-Deoxy-7,8-dihydro-14-hydroxy-3-O-methyl-6-oxomorphine see 6959

Deoxydihydrostreptomycin, 2902

Deoxydihydrothebacodine see 8091

25-Deoxyecdysterone see 7588

d-Deoxyephedrine see 5948

Deoxyepinephrine, 2903

(12S,13S)-9-Deoxy-12,13-epoxy-12,13-dihydro-9-oxoleucomycin V 3-Ace-tate 4B-(3-Methylbutanoate) see 1806

(5Z)-9-Deoxy-6,9α-epoxy-Δ5-PGF1α see 7875

(2'S,3'R)-2'-Deoxy-2',3'-epoxyverru-carin A see 9964

15-Deoxy-15,15-ethylenedioxy-16-phenoxy-17,18,19,20-tetranor-prostaglandin F2α see 3871

2'-Deoxy-5-ethyluridine see 3514

1-(2-Deoxy-2-fluoro-β-D-arabinofurano-syl)-5-iodo-2,4(1H,3H)-pyrimidine-dione see 4069

1-(2-Deoxy-2-fluoro-β-D-arabinofurano-syl)-5-iodouracil see 4069

1-(2-Deoxy-2-fluoro-β-L-arabinofurano-syl)-5-methyl-2,4(1H,3H)-pyrimidine-dione see 2353

1-(2-Deoxy-2-fluoro-β-D-arabinofurano-syl)thymine see 2353

2-Deoxy-2-(fluoro-18F)-α-D-glucopyran-ose see 4127

5'-Deoxy-5-fluoro-N-[(pentyloxy)carbo-nyl]cytidine see 1754

2'-Deoxy-5-fluorouridine see 4112

5'-Deoxy-5-fluorouridine see 3437

5-Deoxy-3-C-formyl-L-lyxose see 8828

6-Deoxy-D-galactose see 4278

6-Deoxy-L-galactose see 4279

(3β)-3-[(6-Deoxy-4-O-β-D-glucopyrano-syl-α-L-mannopyranosyl)oxy]-14-hy-droxybufa-4,20,22-trienolide see 8399

(3β,5β,16β)-3-[(6-Deoxy-4-O-β-D-gluco-pyranosyl-β-D-galacto-pyranosyl)oxy]-14,16-dihydroxycard-20(22)-enolide see 3158

6-Deoxy-D-glucosamine see 2931

2-Deoxyglucose see 2904

2-Deoxy-D-glucose, 2904

6-Deoxy-D-glucose see 8077

Deoxyhemocyanin see 4647

2-Deoxy-D-arabino-hexose see 2904

25-Deoxy-20-hydroxyecdysone see 7588

(±)-15-Deoxy-(16RS)-16-hydroxy-16-methyl-PGE1 Methyl Ester see 6210

(12R)-10-Deoxy-12-hydroxymethymycin see 6453

α-6-Deoxy-5-hydroxytetracycline Mono-hydrate see 3440

2-Deoxy-1,3-myo-inosadiamine see 2909

D-1-Deoxy-muco-inositol see 8036

2-Deoxy-D-chiro-inositol see 8036

2'-Deoxy-5-iodouridine see 4891

α-2'-Deoxy-5-iodouridine see 4891

15-Deoxylagosin see 4080

3-[[6-O-(6-Deoxy-α-L-mannopyranosyl)-β-D-galactopyranosyl]oxy]-7-[(6-de-oxy-α-L-mannopyranosyl)oxy]-5-hy-droxy-2-(4-hydroxyphenyl)-4H-1-ben-zopyran-4-one see 8243

(2S)-7-[[6-O-(6-Deoxy-α-L-mannopyra-nosyl)-β-D-glucopyranosyl]oxy]-2,3-dihydro-5-hydroxy-2-(3-hydroxy-4-methoxyphenyl)-4H-1-benzopyran-4-one see 4671

7-[[2-O-(6-Deoxy-α-L-mannopyranosyl)-β-D-glucopyranosyl]oxy]-2,3-dihydro-5-hydroxy-2-(4-hydroxyphenyl)-4H-1-benzopyran-4-one see 6425

2-[[6-O-(6-Deoxy-α-L-mannopyranosyl)-β-D-glucopyranosyl]oxy]-1,5-dihy-droxy-6-methyl-9,10-anthracene-dione see 6270

3-[[6-O-(6-Deoxy-α-L-mannopyranosyl)-β-D-glucopyranosyl]oxy]-2-(3,4-dihy-droxyphenyl)-5,7-dihydroxy-4H-1-benzopyran-4-one see 8304

1-[4-[[2-O-(6-Deoxy-α-L-mannopyrano-syl)-β-D-glucopyranosyl]oxy]-2,6-di-hydroxyphenyl]-3-(3-hydroxy-4-methoxyphenyl)-1-propanone see 6452

7-[[6-O-(6-Deoxy-α-L-mannopyranosyl)-β-D-glucopyranosyl]oxy]-5-hydroxy-2-(3-hydroxy-4-methoxyphenyl)-4H-1-benzopyran-4-one see 3297

7-[[6-O-(6-Deoxy-α-L-mannopyranosyl)-β-D-glucopyranosyl]oxy]-5-hydroxy-2-(4-methoxyphenyl)-4H-1-benzopyran-4-one see 5498

3-[4-[[2-O-(6-Deoxy-α-L-mannopyrano-syl)-β-D-glucopyranosyl]oxy]phenyl]-5,7-dihydroxy-4H-1-benzopyran-4-one see 8718

6-O-(6-Deoxy-α-L-mannopyranosyl)-D-glucose see 8305

(3β,5β)-3-[(6-Deoxy-α-L-mannopyrano-syl)oxy]-5,14-dihydroxy-19-oxocard-20(22)-enolide see 2512

(3β,5β,16β)-3-[(6-Deoxy-α-L-manno-pyranosyl)oxy]-14,16-dihydroxy-19-oxocard-20(22)-enolide see 169

3-[(6-Deoxy-α-L-mannopyranosyl)oxy]-2-(3,4-dihydroxyphenyl)-5,7-dihy-droxy-4H-1-benzopyran-4-one see 8037

3-[(6-Deoxy-α-L-mannopyranosyl)oxy]-7-(β-D-glucopyranosyloxy)-5-hydroxy-2-(4-methoxyphenyl)-8-(3-methyl-2-butenyl)-4H-1-benzopyran-4-one see 3617

3-[(6-Deoxy-α-L-mannopyranosyl)oxy]-1-(β-D-glucopyranosyloxy)-8-hydroxy-6-methyl-9,10-anthracenedione see 4452

(3β)-3-[(6-Deoxy-α-L-mannopyranosyl)-oxy]-14-hydroxybufa-4,20,22-trieno-lide see 7874

(1β,3β,5β,11α)-3-[(6-Deoxy-α-L-manno-pyranosyl)oxy]-1,5,11,14,19-pentahy-droxycard-20(22)-enolide see 6901

6-Deoxy-L-mannose see 8172

Deoxymatrine see 5759

9-Deoxy-2',9α-methano-3-oxa-4,5,6-tri-nor-3,7-(1',3'-interphenylene)-13,14-dihydroprostaglandin F1 see 9586

4''-Deoxy-4''-epi-N-methylaminoavermec-tin B1 Benzoate see 3554

1-Deoxy-1-(methylamino)-D-glucitol see 6078

1-Deoxy-1-(methylamino)-D-glucitol 3-(Acetylamino)-2,4,6-triiodobenzoate (Salt) see 5806

1-Deoxy-1-(methylamino)-D-glucitol 3,5-Bis(acetylamino)-2,4,6-triiodobenzo-ate Salt see 5807

1-Deoxy-1-(methylamino)-D-glucitol [3-[[(2R,3S)-2-[(1R)-1-[Bis(trifluoromethyl)phenyl]ethoxy]-3-(4-fluorophenyl)-4-morpholinyl]methyl]-2,5-dihydro-5-oxo-1H-1,2,4-triazol-1-yl]phosphon-ate (2:1) (Salt) see 753

1-Deoxy-1-(methylamino)-D-glucitol [4-(Carboxy-κO)-5,8,11-tris[(carboxy-κO)methyl]-1-phenyl-2-oxa-5,8,11-tri-azatridecan-13-oato(5−)-κN5,κN8,-κN11,κN13]gadolinate(2−) (2:1) see 4322

O-2-Deoxy-2-(methylamino)-α-L-gluco-pyranosyl-(1 → 2)-O-5-deoxy-3-C-form-yl-α-L-lyxofuranosyl-(1 → 4)-N,N'-bis-(aminoiminomethyl)-D-streptamine see 8826

O-2-Deoxy-2-(methylamino)-α-L-gluco-pyranosyl-(1 → 2)-O-5-deoxy-3-C-(hy-droxymethyl)-α-L-lyxofuranosyl-(1 → 4)-N,N'-bis(aminoiminomethyl)-D-streptamine see 3179

O-2-Deoxy-2-(methylamino)-α-L-gluco-pyranosyl-(1 → 2)-O-3,5-dideoxy-3-(hydroxymethyl)-α-L-arabinofurano-syl-(1 → 4)-N,N'-bis(aminoiminometh-yl)-D-streptamine see 2902

(3β,12β,14β)-3-[(O-6-Deoxy-3-O-meth-yl-β-D-glucopyranosyl-(1 → 4)-O-2,6-dideoxy-3-O-methyl-β-D-ribo-hexo-pyranosyl-(1 → 4)-2,6-dideoxy-3-O-methyl-β-D-ribo-hexopyranosyl)oxy]-14-hydroxy-12-[[(2E)-2-methyl-1-oxo-2-butenyl]oxy]pregn-5-en-20-one see 4743

(3β,5β)-3-[(6-Deoxy-3-O-methyl-α-L-glucopyranosyl)oxy]-14-hydroxycard-20(22)-enolide see 6474

O-3-Deoxy-4-C-methyl-3-(methylamino)-β-L-arabinopyranosyl-(1 → 6)-O-[2,6-diamino-2,3,4,6-tetradeoxy-α-D-glyc-ero-hex-4-enopyranosyl-(1 → 4)]-2-de-oxy-N1-ethyl-D-streptamine see 6479

O-3-Deoxy-4-C-methyl-3-(methylamino)-β-L-arabinopyranosyl-(1 → 6)-O-[2,6-diamino-2,3,4,6-tetradeoxy-α-D-glyc-ero-hex-4-enopyranosyl-(1 → 4)]-2-de-oxy-D-streptamine see 8550

O-3-Deoxy-4-C-methyl-3-(methylamino)-β-L-arabinopyranosyl-(1 → 6)-O-[2,6-diamino-2,3,4,6-tetradeoxy-α-D-erythro-hexopyranosyl-(1 → 4)]-2-de-oxy-D-streptamine see 4392

2-Deoxy-2-[[(methylnitrosoamino)carbo-nyl]amino]-D-glucopyranose see 8832

2-Deoxy-2-(3-methyl-3-nitrosoureido)-D-glucopyranose see 8832

4-Deoxy-4'-methylpyrido[1',2'-1,2]imid-azo[5,4-c]rifamycin SV see 8220

[2R-(2α,3β,4α,5β,6α,11β,13α,14α)]-11-[(6-Deoxy-3-C-methyl-2,3,4-tri-O-methyl-α-L-mannopyranosyl)oxy]-4-(dimethylamino)-3,4,5,6,9,11,12,13,-14,16-decahydro-3,5,8,10,13-penta-hydroxy-6,13-dimethyl-9,16-dioxo-

Desflurane, 2919
Desglucotransvaaline *see* 7874
Des-Gly[10]-NH₂-LH-RH-ethylamide *see* 4061
Desicol [Parke-Davis] *see* 6928
Desipramine, 2920
Desirudin *see* 4718
Desitriptilina *see* 6715
Deslanoside, 2921
Desloratadine, 2922
Deslorelin, 2923
Desmesterol *see* 2925
11-Desmethoxyreserpine *see* 2918
Desmethylamitriptyline *see* 6715
N-Desmethylcodeine *see* 6690
Desmethyldiazepam *see* 6691
α-Desmethyl DOB *see* 1908
Desmethyldopan *see* 9851
Desmethylemetine *see* 1973
Desmethylimipramine *see* 2920
Desmethylmethadone *see* 6709
Desmethylmorphine *see* 6711
Desmethylnarcotine *see* 6423
5-*O*-Desmethyltangeretin *see* 4366
Desmocollins *see* 1611
Desmogleins *see* 1611
Desmopressin, 2924
Desmospray [Ferring] *see* 2924
Desmosterol, 2925
Desmoteplase *see* 3459
Desmycosin *see* 9832
Desocort [Bausch & Lomb] *see* 2943
Desogen [Organon] *see* 2926
Desogestrel, 2926
Desol [CT] *see* 9889
Desomedine [Chauvin] *see* 4692
Desomorphine, 2927
Desonide, 2928
Desopan [Mochida] *see* 9698
Desosamine, 2929
Desoximetasone, 2930
Desoxiribon *see* 2907
Desoxostrophanthidin *see* 7176
S-(5′-Desoxyadenosin-5′-yl)-L-methionine *see* 156
Desoxyalizarin *see* 688
2-Desoxy-D-altromethylose *see* 3164
Desoxycholic Acid *see* 2899
Desoxycorticosterone *see* 2900
Desoxycorticosterone Acetate *see* 2901
11-Desoxycortisone *see* 2932
Desoxycortone *see* 2900
Desoxycortone Acetate *see* 2901
14-Desoxy-14-[(2-diethylaminoethyl)-mercaptoacetoxy]mutilin *see* 9419
d-Desoxyephedrine *see* 5948
Desoxyepothilone B *see* 3628
Desoxyfed *see* 5948
21-Desoxy-9α-fluoro-6α-methylprednisolone *see* 4175
6-Desoxy-D-glucosamine, 2931
D-*arabino*-2-Desoxyhexose *see* 2904
11-Desoxy-17-hydroxycorticosterone, 2932
Desoxymethasone *see* 2930
6-Desoxy-6-methylenenaltrexone *see* 6360
21-Desoxy-6α-methyl-9α-fluoroprednisolone *see* 4175
Desoxymycin [Kaken] *see* 2902
Desoxyn [Abbott] *see* 5948
(±)-Desoxynorephedrine *see* 582
3-Desoxynorlutin *see* 5629
[3′-Desoxy-3′-oxo-MeBmt]¹-[Val]²-cyclosporin *see* 9917

2-Desoxyphenobarbital *see* 7746
5-Desoxyquercetin *see* 4088
Desoxyribonucleic Acid *see* 2907
Desoxyribose *see* 2908
DESP *see* 3999
Desquaman [Hermal] *see* 7994
Dessin [Union Carbide] *see* 3285
Dess-Martin Periodinane, 2933
Desthiobiotin, 2934
Destim [Central Pharm.] *see* 5948
Destolit [Norgine] *see* 9889
Destomycin A, 2935
Destonate 20 [Meiji] *see* 2935
Destriol *see* 3707
Destrone *see* 3708
N-Desulfoheparin *see* 4652
63-Desulfohirudin (*Hirudo medicinalis* Isoform HV1) *see* 4718
Desuric [Sanofi Winthrop] *see* 1065
Desyrel [Apothecon] *see* 9579
m-DETA *see* 2856
Detal *see* 3279
Detalup [Bayer] *see* 10018
Detamide *see* 2856
Detantol [Eisai] *see* 1487
Detaxtran, 2936
Detensiel [Merck-Clévenot] *see* 1295
Detergent Alkylate #5 *see* 9659
Dethylandiamine *see* 9280
Dethyrona [Abbott] *see* 9415
Deticene [Bellon] *see* 2798
DET MS [Rentschler] *see* 3174
Detomidine, 2937
Detoxepa [Wyeth-Ayerst] *see* 9445
Detoxin C₁ *see* 2938
Detoxin C_{d1} *see* 2938
Detoxin Complex, 2938
Detoxin D₁ *see* 2938
Detoxinine *see* 2938
Detravis [Vis] *see* 2886
Detrol [Pharmacia & Upjohn] *see* 9525
Detrovel [Geigy] *see* 46
Detrunorm [Schering] *see* 7832
Detrusitol [Pharmacia & Upjohn] *see* 9525
Détryptoréline *see* 9748
Dettol [Reckitt & Colman] *see* 2176
Detulin [Woelm] *see* 9495
Deumacard [Jenapharm] *see* 7141
Deursil [Midy] *see* 9889
Deuterium, 2939
Deuterium Oxide, 2940
Devarda's Alloy *see* 2941
Devarda's Metal, 2941
Devaricin *see* 4709
Develin [Gödecke] *see* 7839
Developer Z *see* 6713
Devil's Apple *see* 8820
Devil's Claw, 2942
Devil's Dung *see* 821
Devrinol [Stauffer] *see* 6416
Dewaxed Lanolin *see* 5358
Dexabene [Merckle] *see* 2943
Dexacilina [BMS] *see* 3614
Dexacillin [BMS] *see* 3614
Dexacortal [Organon] *see* 2943
Dexacortin [Streuli] *see* 2943
Dexambutol [L'Arguenon] *see* 3720
Dexamethasone, 2943
Dexamethasone 21-(Dihydrogen Phosphate) Disodium Salt *see* 2943
Dexamethasone 21-(4-Pyridinecarboxylate) *see* 2943
Dexamethasone Sodium Phosphate *see* 2943
Dexamin [Streuli] *see* 2954

Dexamisole *see* 5459
Dexamonozon [Medice] *see* 2943
Dexamphetamine *see* 2954
Dexanabinol, 2944
Dexapos [Ursapharm] *see* 2943
Dexa-sine [Alcon] *see* 2943
Dexasone [Valeant] *see* 2943
Dexawin [Winthrop] *see* 9301
Dexbenzetimide *see* 2945
Dexbrompheniramine *see* 1443
Dexchlorpheniramine *see* 2180
Dexcyanidanol *see* 1902
Dexedrine [GSK] *see* 2954
Dexef [Dexo] *see* 1986
Dexetimide, 2945
Dexfenfluramine *see* 3973
DexFerrum [American Regent] *see* 5094
Dexibuprofen Lysine *see* 4881
Dexide [Sanofi-Synthelabo] *see* 2936
Dexium [Delalande] *see* 3394
Dexivacaine *see* 5859
Dexketoprofen Trometamol *see* 5305
Dexloxiglumide *see* 5588
Dexmedetomidine, 2946
Dexmethylphenidate *see* 6110
Dexmethylphenidate Hydrochloride *see* 6110
Dexnorgestrel Acetime *see* 6703
Dexnorgestrel (obsolete) *see* 6704
Dexol *see* 8652
Dexoxadrol Hydrochloride *see* 3299
Dexpanthenol, 2947
Dexrazoxane *see* 8123
Dextran, 2948
Dextran 40 *see* 2948
Dextran 70 *see* 2948
Dextranase, 2949
Dextran 2-(Diethylamino)ethyl 2-[[2-(Diethylamino)ethyl]diethylammonio]-ethyl Ether Chloride Hydrochloride Epichlorohydrin Crosslinked *see* 7557
Dextran 2-(Diethylamino)ethyl Ether *see* 2936
Dextran 2,3-Dihydroxypropyl 2-Hydroxy-1,3-propanediyl Ethers *see* 2950
Dextran Iron Complex *see* 5094
Dextranomer, 2950
Dextran Sulfate Sodium, 2951
Dextran Sulfuric Acid Ester Sodium Salt *see* 2951
Dextrarine *see* 2951
Dextri-Maltose [Mead Johnson], 2952
Dextrin, 2953
Dextroamphetamine, 2954
Dextrobenzetimide *see* 2945
Dextrocaine *see* 7912
Dextrocamphoric Acid *see* 1733
Dextrofenfluramine *see* 3973
Dextroid [Baxter] *see* 9415
Dextromethorphan Hydrobromide *see* 8091
Dextromoramide, 2955
Dextronic Acid *see* 4456
Dextronorgestrel *see* 6704
Dextropimaric Acid *see* 7428
Dextropropoxyphene *see* 7839
Dextropur *see* 4459
Dextrorotatory Lactic Acid *see* 5337
Dextrorphan *see* 5470
Dextrose *see* 4459
Dextrosol *see* 4459
Dextrostat [Shire] *see* 2954
Dextrosulphenidol *see* 9301
Dextrotartaric Acid *see* 9070
Dextrothyroxine *see* 9415

Dextrothyroxine Sodium *see* 9415
Dextrotubocurarine Chloride *see* 9807
Dexulate *see* 2951
Dexverapamil Hydrochloride *see* 9950
Dezacor [HMR] *see* 2862
Dezocine, 2956
DF 118 *see* 3171
dFdC *see* 4386
dFdCyd *see* 4386
DFDT, 2957
DFMO *see* 3522
DFOM *see* 2860
DFP *see* 5176
5'-DFUR *see* 3437
5'-dFUrd *see* 3437
2-DG *see* 2904
DG-6 [Craveri] *see* 5370
DH-245 *see* 4299
DH-581 *see* 7755
DHA *see* 2865, 3398
DHAD *see* 6217
DHAQ *see* 6217
DHA-S [Dow] *see* 2865
DHBE *see* 6960
DHC [Napp] *see* 3171
1,25-DHCC *see* 1644
DH-codeine *see* 3171
D.H.E. 45 [Novartis] *see* 3174
DHEA *see* 2871
DHEAS *see* 2871
DHIC *see* 3176
D-homo-17a-oxaandrosta-1,4-diene-
   3,17-dione *see* 9179
DHPG *see* 4363
DHSM *see* 3179
Dhurrin, 2958
Diabasan [Biofarma] *see* 4478
Diabechlor *see* 2186
Diaben [Chugai] *see* 9507
Diabenal *see* 2186
Diabeta [Sanofi-Aventis] *see* 4478
Diabetes-associated Peptide *see* 609
Diabetoral [Boehringer, Mann.] *see* 2186
Diabex [Merck KGaA] *see* 5938
Diabinese [Pfizer] *see* 2186
Diaboline, 2959
Diaboral [Pharmacia] *see* 9511
Diabrin [USV] *see* 1476
Diacepin *see* 2994
Diacerein, 2960
Diacerhein *see* 2960
3,5-Diacetamido-2,4,6-triiodobenzoic
   Acid Methylglucamine Salt *see* 5807
3,5-Diacetamido-2,4,6-triiodobenzoic
   Acid Sodium Salt *see* 2992
α,5-Diacetamido-2,4,6-triiodo-*m*-toluic
   Acid *see* 5011
trans-Di(μ-acetato)bis[*o*-(di-*o*-tolylphos-
   phino)benzyl]dipalladium(II) *see* 4669
Diacetatopalladium(II) *see* 6991
Diacetatozirconic Acid *see* 10183
Diacethiamine *see* 54
Diacetic Acid *see* 59
Diacetin, 2961
1,2-Diacetin *see* 2961
1,3-Diacetin *see* 2961
Diacetonamine, 2962
Diacetone Acrylamide, 2963
Diacetone Alcohol, 2964
Diacetoneglucose, 2965
Diacetone-2-ketogulonic Acid *see* 3199
Diacetone-2-oxo-L-gulonic Acid *see* 3199
4,4'-Diacetoxybenzhydrylidenecyclo-
   hexane *see* 2720
2,3-Diacetoxybenzoic Acid *see* 3349

1,8-Diacetoxy-3-carboxyanthraqui-
   none *see* 2960
Diacetoxydiphenylisatin *see* 6974
2-(4,4'-Diacetoxydiphenylmethyl)pyri-
   dine *see* 1242
(4,4'-Diacetoxydiphenyl)(2-pyridyl)-
   methane *see* 1242
3α,17β-Diacetoxy-2β,16β-dipiperidino-
   5α-androstane Dimethobromide *see*
   7007
3,16α-Diacetoxy-Δ¹,³,⁵-estratrien-17-
   one *see* 2489
1,1-Diacetoxyethane *see* 3811
3β,17β-Diacetoxy-17α-ethynyl-4-es-
   trene *see* 3860
16α,21-Diacetoxy-9α-fluoro-11β,17α-
   dihydroxy-1,4-pregnadiene-3,20-di-
   one *see* 9595
1,4-Diacetoxy-2-methylnaphthalene
   see 5830
Di(acetoxyphenyl)oxindole *see* 6974
3α,20α-Diacetoxypregnane *see* 7727
Diacetyl, 2966
Diacetylapomorphine *see* 746
Diacetylcholine Dichloride *see* 8875
Diacetylcholine Diiodide *see* 8876
Diacetylcholine Iodide *see* 8876
Diacetyldihydromorphine, 2967
2,6-Diacetyl-7,9-dihydroxy-8,9b-di-
   methyl-1,3(2*H*,9b*H*)-dibenzofuran-
   dione *see* 9893
Diacetyldihydroxydiphenylisatin *see*
   6974
Diacetyldioxime *see* 3246
Diacetyldioxyphenylisatin *see* 6974
Diacetyldiphenolisatin *see* 6974
α,β-Diacetylethane *see* 71
Diacetylhydroxyphenylisatin *see* 6974
Diacetylmethane *see* 81
9,3''-Diacetylmidecamycin *see* 6204
Diacetylmorphine, 2968
Diacetylpyrocatechol-3-carboxylic Acid
   see 3349
Diacetylrhein *see* 2960
Diacetyltannic Acid *see* 104
O,S-Diacetylthiamine *see* 54
Diacid [Daro] *see* 1831
α,γ-Diacipiperazine *see* 7466
Diacort [Pfizer] *see* 3140
Diacta [Nicholas] *see* 8908
Di-Actane [Menarini] *see* 6353
Diactol *see* 10018
Diacylglycerol Lipase *see* 5512
Di-Adreson [Organon] *see* 7722
Diafen [3M Pharma] *see* 3331
Diafenthiuron, 2969
Diafusor [Fabre] *see* 6607
Diaginol [M & B] *see* 79
Diagnorenol *see* 5973
Dialar [Novartis] *see* 2994
Dialicor [Kissei] *see* 3710
Diallate, 2970
Diallylamine, 2971
5,5-Diallylbarbituric Acid *see* 263
3',5-Diallyl-2,4'-biphenyldiol *see* 4742
5,5'-Diallyl-2,2'-biphenyldiol *see* 5697
Diallylbis(nortoxiferine) *see* 221
Diallylcyanamide, 2972
N,N-Diallyl-2,2-dichloroacetamide *see*
   3049
5,3'-Diallyl-2,4'-dihydroxydiphenyl *see*
   4742
Diallyl Disulfide-oxide *see* 261
Diallyl Ether *see* 292
Diallylnortoxiferine *see* 221

N,N'-Diallylnortoxiferinium *see* 221
N,N'-Diallylnortoxiferinium Dichloride
   see 221
Diallyl Sulfide *see* 297
Diallyltoxiferine *see* 221
Diallyl Trisulfide, 2973
Dialuramide *see* 9852
Diamantane *see* 2499
Diamantane (obsolete) *see* 149
Diamarin *see* 3207
Diamfenetide, 2974
Diamicron [Servier] *see* 4439
4,4'-Diamidinodiazoaminobenzene
   Diaceturate *see* 3266
4,4'-Diamidino-α,ω-diphenoxyhexane
   see 4692
4,4'-Diamidino-α,ω-diphenoxypentane
   see 7115
4,4'-Diamidino-α,ω-diphenoxypropane
   see 7797
4,4'-Diamidinodiphenyl Ether *see* 7208
4,4'-Diamidinostilbene *see* 8816
N,N'-Diamidinostreptamine *see* 8822
Diamine Blue 9792
2,6-Diamine-5-hydroxy-4(3*H*)-pyrimi-
   dinone *see* 3383
Diamine Oxidase, 2975
2,8-Diaminoacridine *see* 7771
3,6-Diaminoacridine *see* 7771
3,5-Diamino-*N*-(aminoiminomethyl)-6-
   chloropyrazinecarboxamide *see* 406
6,9-Diamino-1-(6-amino-9*H*-purin-9-
   yl)-1,5,6,7,8,9-hexadeoxy-D-glycero-
   α-L-*talo*-decofuranuronic Acid *see*
   8544
3,5-Diamino-2-[[4-(aminosulfonyl)-
   phenyl]azo]benzoic Acid *see* 8901
2,4-Diaminoanisole, 2976
4,4'-Diamino-1,1'-anthrimide *see* 1243
p-Diaminoazobenzene, 2977
4,4'-Diaminoazobenzene *see* 2977
2,4-Diaminoazobenzene Hydrochloride *see* 2257
2,4-Diaminoazobenzene Hydrochloride Citrate *see* 2257
2,4-Diaminoazobenzene-4'-sulfon-
   amide *see* 8923
m-Diaminobenzene *see* 7283
o-Diaminobenzene *see* 7284
p-Diaminobenzene *see* 7285
3,5-Diaminobenzoic Acid, 2978
2,4-Diamino-5-(4-bromo-3,5-dimeth-
   oxybenzyl)pyrimidine *see* 1380
α,ε-Diaminocaproic Acid *see* 5636
2,4-Diamino-1-*p*-chlorophenyl-1,6-dihy-
   dro-6,6-dimethyl-1,3,5-triazine *see*
   2721
4,6-Diamino-1-(*p*-chlorophenyl)-1,2-di-
   hydro-2,2-dimethyl-*s*-triazine *see*
   2721
2,4-Diamino-5-(*p*-chlorophenyl)-6-ethyl-
   pyrimidine *see* 7985
Di-(4-amino-3-chlorophenyl)methane *see*
   6059
1-(3,5-Diamino-6-chloropyrazinecar-
   boxyl)guanidine *see* 406
1-(3,5-Diamino-6-chloropyrazinoyl)-
   guanidine *see* 406
4,4'-Diamino-1,1'-dianthraquinonyl-
   amine *see* 1243
1,8-Diamino-3,6-diazaoctane *see* 9663
β,β'-Diamino-β,β'-dicarboxydiethyl
   Disulfide *see* 2782
4,4'-Diamino-3,3'-dichlorodiphenyl-
   methane *see* 6059

2,4-Diamino-6-(2,5-dichlorophenyl)-*s*-triazine *see* 5102

3,5-Diamino-6-(2,3-dichlorophenyl)-1,2,4-triazine *see* 5353

O-2,6-Diamino-2,6-dideoxy-α-D-glucopyranosyl-(1 → 4)-*O*-[β-D-ribofuranosyl-(1 → 5)]-2-deoxy-D-streptamine *see* 8206

(*S*)-*O*-2,6-Diamino-2,6-dideoxy-α-D-glucopyranosyl-(1 → 4)-*O*-[β-D-xylofuranosyl-(1 → 5)]-*N*[1]-(4-amino-2-hydroxy-1-oxobutyl)-2-deoxystreptamine *see* 1528

O-2,6-Diamino-2,6-dideoxy-β-L-idopyranosyl-(1 → 3)-*O*-β-D-ribofuranosyl-(1 → 5)-*O*-[2-amino-2-deoxy-α-D-glucopyranosyl-(1 → 4)]-2-deoxystreptamine *see* 7041

β,β′-Diaminodiethyl Disulfide *see* 2776

2,6-Diamino-1,6-dihydro-4,5-pyrimidinedione *see* 3383

3,3′-Diamino-4,4′-dihydroxyarsenobenzenemethylenesulfoxylate Sodium *see* 6447

2,4-Diamino-5,6-dihydroxypyrimidine *see* 3383

2,4-Diamino-6-(2,5-dimethoxybenzoyl)-5-methylpyrido[2,3-*d*]pyrimidine *see* 7499

2,4-Diamino-5-(3′,4′-dimethoxybenzyl)pyrimidine *see* 2993

2,4-Diamino-5-[3,5-dimethoxy-4-(2-methoxyethoxy)benzyl]pyrimidine *see* 9250

4,4′-Diamino-3,3′-dimethylbiphenyl *see* 9514

1,6-Diamino-5-5-dimethyl-3,4-dithiahexane-1,6-dicarboxylic Acid *see* 7089

p-Diaminodiphenyl *see* 1077

2,4′-Diaminodiphenyl *see* 1236

p-*p*′-Diaminodiphenylamine *see* 2979

4,4′-Diaminodiphenylamine, 2979

p,*p*′-Diaminodiphenylmethane, 2980

4,4′-Diaminodiphenyl Sulfone *see* 2822

Diaminodiphenylsulfone-*N*-acetic Acid *see* 23

p,*p*′-Diaminodiphenylsulfone-*N*,*N*′-di-(dextrose Sodium Sulfonate) *see* 4463

4,4′-Diaminodiphenylsulfone Disodium Formaldehyde Sulfoxylate *see* 8968

α-Diamino-β-dithiolactic Acid *see* 2782

1,2-Diaminoethane *see* 3795

2,5-Diamino-7-ethoxyacridine *see* 3716

6,9-Diamino-2-ethoxyacridine *see* 3716

2,7-Diamino-10-ethyl-9-phenylphenanthridinium *see* 4731

3,8-Diamino-5-ethyl-6-phenylphenanthridinium *see* 4731

2,7-Diaminofluorene *see* 4156

2,6-Diamino-5-(β-D-glucopyranosyloxy)-4(1*H*)-pyrimidinone *see* 9975

1,6-Diaminohexane *see* 4695

(*S*)-2,6-Diaminohexanoic Acid *see* 5636

(2*S*,9*R*)-2,11-Diamino-9-hydroxy-7-azaundecanoic Acid *see* 4870

3,6-Diamino-5-hydroxyhexanoic Acid 2-(Carboxymethyl)-2-methylhydrazide *see* 6441

[2-(3,6-Diamino-5-hydroxy-1-oxohexyl)-1-methylhydrazino]acetic Acid *see* 6441

2,4-Diamino-6-hydroxypyrimidine, 2981

4,4′-Diamino-1,1′-iminobisanthraquinone *see* 1243

(2*S*)-2,7-Diamino-7-iminoheptanoic Acid *see* 4970

3,6-Diamino-10-methylacridinium Chloride Mixt with 3,6-Acridinediamine *see* 123

N-[4-[(2,4-Diamino-5-methylphenyl)imino]-2,5-cyclohexadien-1-ylidene]-*N*-methylmethanaminium Chloride *see* 9822

2,4-Diamino-5-methyl-6-[(3,4,5-trimethoxyanilino)methyl]quinazoline *see* 9721

1,8-Diaminonaphthalene *see* 6372

1,2-Diamino-4-nitrobenzene *see* 6623

α,2-Diamino-γ-oxobenzenebutanoic Acid *see* 5328

(*S*)-2,4-Diamino-4-oxobutanoic Acid *see* 837

(*S*)-2,5-Diamino-5-oxopentanoic Acid *see* 4471

(4*S*)-4,5-Diamino-5-oxopentanoic Acid *see* 5177

2,4-Diamino-6-oxypyrimidine-5-(β-D-glucopyranoside) *see* 9975

2,5-Diaminopentanoic Acid *see* 6874

2,3-Diaminophenazine, 2982

2,4-Diaminophenol, 2983

3,7-Diaminophenothiazin-5-ium Chloride *see* 9346

4-[(2,4-Diaminophenyl)azo]benzenesulfonamide *see* 8923

2,6-Diamino-3-phenylazopyridine *see* 7210

2,7-Diamino-9-phenyl-10-ethylphenanthridinium *see* 4731

3,7-Diamino-5-phenylphenazinium Chloride *see* 7251

2,4-Diamino-5-phenylthiazole *see* 483

2,4-Diamino-6-phenyl-*s*-triazine *see* 1089

4,6-Diamino-2-phenyl-*s*-triazine *see* 1089

2,4-Diamino-6-piperidinopyrimidine 3-Oxide *see* 9822

2,3-Diaminopropanoic Acid *see* 2984

α,β-Diaminopropionic Acid *see* 2984

2,3-Diaminopropionic Acid, 2984

N-[4-[[(2,4-Diamino-6-pteridinyl)methyl]amino]benzoyl]-L-glutamic Acid *see* 472

N-[4-[[(2,4-Diamino-6-pteridinyl)methyl]methylamino]benzoyl]-L-glutamic Acid *see* 5985

N-[4-[1-[(2,4-Diamino-6-pteridinyl)methyl]propyl]benzoyl]-L-glutamic Acid *see* 3507

2,6-Diaminopurine, 2985

2,6-Diamino-9*H*-purine *see* 2985

3,4-Diaminopyridine, 2986

2,6-Diamino-4,5-pyrimidinediol *see* 3383

2,6-Diamino-4(1*H*)-pyrimidinone *see* 2981

Di-(4-aminoquinald-6-yl)urea *see* 475

4,4′-Diamino-2,2′-stilbenedisulfonic Acid *see* 595

3,5-Diamino-2-[*p*-(sulfamoylphenyl)azo]benzoic Acid *see* 8901

3,6-Diamino-2,3,4,6-tetradeoxy-L-*threo*-hexonic Acid 2-(Carboxymethyl)-2-methylhydrazide *see* 6441

[4-(4,6-Diamino-*m*-tolyl)imino-2,5-cyclohexadien-1-ylidene]dimethylammonium Chloride *see* 9822

p-[(4,6-Diamino-*s*-triazin-2-yl)amino]dithiobenzenearsonous Acid 3-Hydroxypropylene Ester *see* 5815

2-[4-[(4,6-Diamino-1,3,5-triazin-2-yl)amino]phenyl]-1,3,2-dithiarsolane-4-methanol *see* 5815

2-*p*-(4,6-Diamino-*s*-triazin-2-ylamino)phenyl-4-hydroxymethyl-1,3,2-dithiarsoline *see* 5815

4-[2,6-Diamino-2,3,6-trideoxy-α-D-glycopyranosyl]-6-[3-amino-3-deoxy-α-D-glycopyranosyl]-2-deoxystreptamine *see* 9490

1,3-Diamino-4,5,6-trihydroxycyclohexane *see* 2909

2,4-Diamino-5-(3,4,5-trimethoxybenzyl)pyrimidine *see* 9709

1,3-Diaminourea *see* 1804

α,δ-Diaminovaleric Acid *see* 6874

2,4-Diamino-5-veratrylpyrimidine *see* 2993

(*SP*-4-2)-Diammine[1,1-cyclobutanedi-(carboxylato-κ*O*)(2−)]platinum *see* 1822

cis-Diammine(1,1-cyclobutanedicarboxylato)platinum(II) *see* 1822

cis-Diamminedichloroplatinum *see* 2317

(*SP*-4-2)-Diamminedichloroplatinum *see* 2317

Diammonium Citrate *see* 512

Diammonium Hexafluorosilicate(2−) *see* 527

Diammonium Hydrogen Phosphate *see* 542

Diammonium Nickel Disulfate *see* 6501

(*T*-4)-Diammonium Tetrathioxomolybdate(2−) *see* 560

Diamond, 2987

Diamond Green B *see* 5699

Diamond Green Bx *see* 5699

Diamond Green G *see* 1374

Diamond Green P Extra *see* 5699

Diamorphine *see* 2968

Diamox [Barr] *see* 53

Diamphenethide *see* 2974

Diampromide, 2988

Diamyceline [Diamant] *see* 2107

Diamyl Ether *see* 608

2,5-Di-*tert*-amylhydroquinone *see* 3304

Diamyl Sodium Sulfosuccinate, 2989

Dianabol [Novartis] *see* 5951

Dianat *see* 3040

Diane 35 [Schering AG] *see* 2774

Dianette [Schering AG] *see* 2774

1,4:3,6-Dianhydro-D-glucitol *see* 5224

1,4:3,6-Dianhydro-D-glucitol Dinitrate *see* 5225

1,4:3,6-Dianhydrosorbitol *see* 5224

1,4:3,6-Dianhydrosorbitol 2,5-Dinitrate *see* 5225

Dianil Blue *see* 9792

o,*p*′-Dianiline *see* 1236

1,4-Dianilinobenzene *see* 3329

1,2-Dianilinoethane, 2990

Dianisidine, 2991

3,3′-Dianisolebis[4,4′-(3,5-diphenyl)-tetrazolium Chloride] *see* 9244

(*E*)-3,4-Dianisyl-3-hexene *see* 3211

2,2-Di-*p*-anisyl-1,1,1-trichloroethane *see* 5990

Dianthraquinonylamine *see* 690

Dianthrimide *see* 690

Diantimony Trioxide *see* 711

Diaparene [Sterling Winthrop] *see* 6023

Diaphenylsulfone *see* 2822
Diapid [Sandoz] *see* 5630
6,6'-Diapo-ψ,ψ-carotenedioic Acid *see* 1311
8,8'-Diapo-ψ,ψ-carotenedioic Acid *see* 2589
9-*cis*-6,6'-Diapo-ψ,ψ-carotenedioic Acid *see* 1311
9-*cis*-6,6'-Diapo-ψ,ψ-carotenedioic Acid Monomethyl Ester *see* 1311
Diaquone *see* 2815
Diarconal [Recordati] *see* 9571
Diarlidan [Vinas] *see* 6535
Diarsed [Sanofi Winthrop] *see* 3313
2,2'-(1,2-Diarsenediyl)bisacetic Acid *see* 808
4,4'-(1,2-Diarsenediyl)bis[2-amino-phenol] Dihydrochloride *see* 811
[1,2-Diarsenediylbis[(6-hydroxy-3,1-phenylene)imino]]bismethanesul-fonic Acid Disodium Salt *see* 8941
Diarsenic Pentasulfide *see* 797
Diarsenoacetic Acid *see* 808
Diart [Boehringer, Mann.] *see* 922
Diasone [Abbott] *see* 8968
Diaspore *see* 356
Diastabol [Sanofi-Synthelabo] *see* 6187
Diastal [Bayropharm] *see* 1472
Diastat [Xcel] *see* 2994
Diastatin *see* 6736
Diaster [Roussel Diamant] *see* 2540
Diatomaceous Earth *see* 4973
Diatrast *see* 5040
Diatrizoate Meglumine *see* 5807
Diatrizoate Methylglucamine *see* 5807
Diatrizoate Sodium, 2992
Diaveridine, 2993
1,4-Diazabicyclo[2.2.2]octane *see* 9669
20,25-Diazacholesterol *see* 892
1,3-Diaza-2,4-cyclopentadiene *see* 4912
8,10-Diaza-6-hydroxy-5-methylene-1-(2-methyl-1,2,3-trihydroxypropyl)-2-oxabicyclo[4.2.2]decan-7,9-dione *see* 1202
Diazald [Aldrich] *see* 9543
Diazamine Golden Yellow T *see* 9310
1,2-Diazanaphthalene *see* 2306
3,6-Diazaoctane-1,8-diamine *see* 9663
Diazasterol *see* 892
(*RR,SS*)-4,8-Diaza-3,6,6,9-tetramethyl-undecane-2,10-dione Bisoxime *see* 3911
Diazemuls [Alpharma] *see* 2994
Diazenedicarboxamide *see* 919
Diazepam, 2994
Diazil [Bracco] *see* 8915
1,2-Diazine *see* 7969
1,3-Diazine *see* 7987
1,4-Diazine *see* 7957
Diazinon, 2995
Diaziquone, 2996
2,5-Diaziridinyl-3,6-bis(ethoxycarbo-nylamino)-1,4-benzoquinone *see* 2996
Diazoacetic Ester, 2997
O-Diazoacetyl-L-serine *see* 899
Diazoaminobenzene, 2998
4,4'-(Diazoamino)dibenzamidine Diaceturate *see* 3266
2,2'-[(Diazoamino)di-*p*-phenylene]bis[6-methyl-7-benzothiazolesulfonic Acid] Disodium Salt *see* 9310
p-Diazobenzenesulfonic Acid, 2999
5-Diazo-2,4-dioxopyrimidine *see* 3003
Diazol [Makhteshim-Agan] *see* 2995

1,2-Diazole *see* 7960
1,3-Diazole *see* 4912
Diazolidinyl Urea, 3000
Diazoline *see* 5770
Diazomethane, 3001
(Diazomethyl)phosphonic Acid Dimethyl Ester *see* 8476
Diazon *see* 8968
6-Diazo-5-oxo-L-norleucine, 3002
(1-Diazo-2-oxopropyl)phosphonic Acid Dimethyl Ester *see* 1177
5-Diazo-2,4(1*H*,3*H*)-pyrimidinedione *see* 3003
"Diazoresorcinol" *see* 8141
Diazotized Sulfanilic Acid *see* 2999
5-Diazouracil, 3003
Diazoxide, 3004
Dibactil [Roemmers] *see* 8924
Dibasic Sodium Phosphate *see* 8659
Dibekacin, 3005
Dibenamine Hydrochloride [SK & F] *see* 2138
Dibencozide *see* 2451
Dibenon [Dainippon] *see* 1159
Dibenyline [SKB] *see* 7256
Dibenzalacetone, 3006
Dibenz[*a,h*]anthracene *see* 3007
Dibenz[*de,kl*]anthracene *see* 7184
1,2:5,6-Dibenzanthracene, 3007
5*H*-Dibenz[*b,f*]azepine-5-carboxamide *see* 1781
4-[3-(5*H*-Dibenz[*b,f*]azepin-5-yl)propyl]-1-piperazineethanol *see* 6853
Dibenzcozamide *see* 2451
Dibenzepin, 3008
Dibenzheptropine *see* 2912
1,2,3,4-Dibenznaphthalene *see* 9740
2,3:6,7-Dibenzoanthracene *see* 7107
4-[3-(5*H*-Dibenzo[*b,f*]azepin-5-yl)pro-pyl]-1-(2-hydroxyethyl)piperazine *see* 6853
Dibenzo-18-crown-6 *see* 2602
Dibenzo[*a,d*][1,4]cycloheptadiene-5-carboxamide *see* 2759
5*H*-Dibenzo[*a,d*]cyclohepten-5-one *O*-[2-(Methylamino)ethyl]oxime *see* 2890
3-(5*H*-Dibenzo[*a,d*]cyclohepten-5-yli-dene)-*N,N*-dimethyl-1-propanamine *see* 2713
4-(5*H*-Dibenzo[*a,d*]cyclohepten-5-yli-dene)-1-methylpiperidine *see* 2773
2,3,11,12-Dibenzo-1,4,7,10,13,16-hexa-oxacyclooctadeca-2,11-diene *see* 2602
Dibenzoparadiazine *see* 7217
Dibenzopenthiophene *see* 9368
Dibenzo[*a,i*]phenanthrene *see* 7396
Dibenzo[*b,h*]phenanthrene *see* 3010
Dibenzopyrazine *see* 7217
Dibenzo[*b,e*]pyridine *see* 122
Dibenzo-γ-pyrone *see* 10062
Dibenzopyrrole *see* 1790
2-[2-[4-(Dibenzo[*b,f*][1,4]thiazepin-11-yl-1-piperazinyl)ethoxy]ethanol *see* 8039
Dibenzothiazine *see* 7252
2,2'-Dibenzothiazyl Disulfide *see* 3370
3-Dibenzo[*b,e*]thiepin-11(6*H*)-ylidene-*N,N*-dimethyl-1-propanamine *see* 3429
Dibenzothiopyran *see* 9368
3-Dibenz[*b,e*]oxepin-11(6*H*)-ylidene-*N,N*-dimethyl-1-propanamine *see* 3435
Dibenzoyl *see* 1078
Dibenzoylmethane, 3009
Dibenzoyl Peroxide *see* 1116
β,β'-Dibenzphenanthrene *see* 3010

1,2,7,8-Dibenzphenanthrene *see* 7396
2,3:6,7-Dibenzphenanthrene, 3010
Dibenzthiazyl Disulfide *see* 3370
Dibenzthione *see* 8892
Dibenzyl *see* 1198
Dibenzylamine, 3011
N,N-Dibenzylaminoethyl Chloride Hydrochloride *see* 2138
N,N-Dibenzyl-β-chloroethylamine Hydrochloride *see* 2138
Dibenzylchlorophosphate *see* 3012
Dibenzyl Chlorophosphonate, 3012
N,N'-Dibenzyl-γ,γ'-dipyridylium *see* 9999
Dibenzyl Disulfide, 3013
Dibenzyl Ether *see* 1132
N,N'-Dibenzylethylenediamine *see* 1064
N,N'-Dibenzylethylenediamine Bis[ben-zylpenicillin] *see* 7096
Dibenzylethylenediamine Dipenicillin G *see* 7096
Dibenzyl Fumarate *see* 1135
Dibenzyl Hydrogen Phosphite *see* 3014
Dibenzylidene Acetone *see* 3006
Dibenzyline [SKB] *see* 7256
d-3,4-(1',3'-Dibenzyl-2'-ketoimidazo-lido)-1,2-trimethylenethiophanium *d*-Camphorsulfonate *see* 9707
4,6-Dibenzyl-5-oxo-1-thia-4,6-diazatri-cyclo[6.3.0.0³·⁷]undecanium (+)-β-Camphorsulfonate *see* 9707
Dibenzyl Phosphite, 3014
Dibenzylphosphoryl Chloride *see* 3012
Dibenzylsulfide *see* 1145
3,5-Dibenzyltetrahydro-2*H*-1,3,5-thia-diazine-2-thione *see* 8892
Dibenzyran [Procter & Gamble] *see* 7256
Dibestil [Sterling Winthrop] *see* 3129
N,N'-Dibetaine-γ,γ'-dipyridylium *see* 9999
Dibetos [Kodama] *see* 1476
Diblocin [AstraZeneca] *see* 3433
Dibondrin [Montavit] *see* 3309
Diborane(6), 3015
Diboron Hexahydride *see* 3015
Diboron Tetrachloride *see* 3016
Dibotermin Alfa *see* 1331
Dibrom [Amvac] *see* 6358
Dibromantin, 3017
p,α-Dibromoacetophenone *see* 1427
2,4'-Dibromoacetophenone *see* 1427
9,10-Dibromoanthracene, 3018
p-Dibromobenzene, 3019
4,4'-Dibromobenzilic Acid Isopropyl Ester *see* 1434
3,5-Dibromo-*N*-(4-bromophenyl)-2-hy-droxybenzamide *see* 9616
1,2-Dibromobutane *see* 1566
2,3-Dibromobutanedioic Acid *see* 3029
[2,7-Dibromo-9-(*o*-carboxyphenyl)-6-hydroxy-3-oxo-3*H*-xanthen-4-yl]hy-droxymercury Disodium Salt *see* 5867
2,6-Dibromo-*N*-chloro-*p*-benzoquinone-imine *see* 3026
4-[2-[4-[(11*R*)-3,10-Dibromo-8-chloro-6,11-dihydro-5*H*-benzo[5,6]cyclohep-ta[1,2-*b*]pyridin-11-yl]-1-piperidinyl]-2-oxoethyl]-1-piperidinecarboxamide *see* 5565
2,6-Dibromo-4-(chloroimino)-2,5-cyclohexadien-1-one *see* 3026
Dibromochloromethane *see* 2135
Dibromochloropropane, 3020
1,2-Dibromo-3-chloropropane *see* 3020
2,6-Dibromo-*N*-chloroquinonimine *see* 3026

5,5'-Dibromo-*o*-cresolsulfonphthalein *see* 1387

2,6-Dibromo-4-cyanophenol *see* 1441

3,5-Dibromo-*N*^α-cyclohexyl-*N*^α-methyl-toluene-α,2-diamine *see* 1391

2',2''-Dibromo-4',4''-diamidino-1,3-diphenoxypropane *see* 3024

1,2-Dibromo-2,4-dicyanobutane, 3021

1,6-Dibromo-1,6-dideoxydulcitol *see* 6214

1,6-Dibromo-1,6-dideoxygalactitol *see* 6214

1,6-Dibromo-1,6-dideoxy-D-mannitol *see* 6212

4',5'-Dibromo-3',6'-dihydroxy-2',7'-dinitrospiro[isobenzofuran-1(3*H*),9'-[9*H*]xanthen]-3-one Disodium Salt *see* 3602

(2'7'-Dibromo-3',6'-dihydroxy-3-oxospiro[isobenzofuran-1(3*H*),9'-[9*H*]-xanthen]-4'-yl)hydroxymercury Disodium Salt *see* 5867

4',5'-Dibromo-3',6'-dihydroxyspiro[isobenzofuran-1(3*H*),9'-[9*H*]xanthen]-3-one *see* 3022

1,3-Dibromo-5,5-dimethylhydantoin *see* 3017

1,3-Dibromo-5,5-dimethyl-2,4-imidazolidinedione *see* 3017

4',5'-Dibromo-2',7'-dinitrofluorescein Disodium Salt *see* 3602

Dibromodulcit *see* 6214

Dibromodulcitol *see* 6214

sym-Dibromoethane *see* 3796

1,2-Dibromoethane *see* 3796

1,2-Dibromoethene *see* 91

(1*R*,3*R*)-3-(2,2-Dibromoethenyl)-2,2-dimethylcyclopropanecarboxylic Acid (*S*)-Cyano(3-phenoxyphenyl)methyl Ester *see* 2883

sym-Dibromoethylene *see* 91

1,2-Dibromoethylene *see* 91

4,5-Dibromo-3,6-fluorandiol *see* 3022

4',5'-Dibromofluorescein, 3022

3,5-Dibromo-2-hydroxybenzaldehyde *see* 3027

3,5-Dibromo-4-hydroxybenzenesulfonic Acid, 3023

3,5-Dibromo-2-hydroxybenzoic Acid *see* 3028

3,5-Dibromo-4-hydroxybenzonitrile *see* 1441

3-(3,5-Dibromo-4-hydroxybenzoyl)-2-ethylbenzofuran *see* 1065

Dibromohydroxymercurifluorescein Disodium Salt *see* 5867

β-(3,5-Dibromo-4-hydroxyphenyl)alanine *see* 3030

3,5-Dibromo-4-hydroxyphenyl Cyanide *see* 1441

3,5-Dibromo-4-hydroxyphenyl 2-Ethyl-3-benzofuranyl Ketone *see* 1065

(3,5-Dibromo-4-hydroxyphenyl)(2-ethyl-3-benzofuranyl)methanone *see* 1065

5,7-Dibromo-8-hydroxyquinoline *see* 1453

3,5-Dibromo-2-hydroxy-*N*-[3-(trifluoromethyl)phenyl]benzamide *see* 4178

Dibromol [Trommsdorff] *see* 3023

Dibromomannitol *see* 6212

Dibromomethane *see* 6061

2,6-Dibromophenol-4-sulfonic Acid *see* 3023

Dibromopropamidine, 3024

α,γ-Dibromopropane *see* 9713

ω,ω'-Dibromopropane *see* 9713

1,2-Dibromopropane *see* 7853

1,3-Dibromopropane *see* 9713

2,3-Dibromo-1-propanol Phosphate-(3:1) *see* 9751

2,3-Dibromopropene, 3025

2,3-Dibromopropylene *see* 3025

5,7-Dibromo-8-quinolinol *see* 1453

2,6-Dibromoquinone-4-chlorimide, 3026

3,5-Dibromosalicylaldehyde, 3027

3,5-Dibromosalicylic Acid, 3028

α,α'-Dibromosuccinic Acid *see* 3029

sym-Dibromosuccinic Acid *see* 3029

2,3-Dibromosuccinic Acid, 3029

erythro-2,3-Dibromosuccinic Acid *see* 3029

threo-2,3-Dibromosuccinic Acid *see* 3029

Dibromotetraaquochromium Bromide Dihydrate *see* 2220

3,3'-Dibromothymolsulfonphthalein *see* 1445

p,α-Dibromotoluene *see* 1409

3,5-Dibromo-3'-trifluoromethylsalicylanilide *see* 4178

3,5-Dibromo-α,α,α-trifluoro-*m*-salicylotoluidide *see* 4178

3,5-Dibromo-L-tyrosine, 3030

Dibucaine, 3031

Dibunafon *see* 8608

Dibunate Ethyl *see* 3788

Dibutalin *see* 1532

Dibutil [Bayer] *see* 3747

3,4-Dibutoxy-3-cyclobutene-1,2-dione *see* 8769

n-Dibutylamine, 3032

2-Dibutylamino-1-[2,7-dichloro-9-(4-chlorobenzylidene)-9,11-fluoren-4-yl]ethanol *see* 5597

γ-(Dibutylamino)-1,3-dichloro-6-(trifluoromethyl)-9-phenanthrenepropanol *see* 4594

5-[[2-(Dibutylamino)ethyl]amino]-3-phenyl-1,2,4-oxadiazole *see* 1510

4-[2-[4-(Dibutylamino)phenyl]ethenyl]-1-[3-(triethylammonio)propyl]pyridinium Dibromide *see* 4220

3-(Dibutylamino)-1-propanol 4-Aminobenzoate *see* 1507

Dibutylaminopropyl-*p*-aminobenzoate *see* 1507

[(Dibutylamino)thio]methylcarbamic Acid 2,3-Dihydro-2,2-dimethyl-7-benzofuranyl Ester *see* 1826

Dibutylbis(lauroyloxy)tin *see* 3038

Dibutylbis[(1-oxodecyl)oxy]stannane *see* 3038

N,*N*-Dibutyl-1-butanamine *see* 9618

N,*N*-Dibutyl-3-[4-[(2-butyl-5-methylsulfonamido)benzofuran-3-ylcarbonyl]phenoxy]propylamine *see* 3449

Dibutyl Carbonate *see* 1558

2,6-Di-*tert*-butyl-*p*-cresol *see* 1548

4,6-Di-*tert*-butyl-*m*-cresol *see* 2837

2,6-Di-*tert*-butyl-α-(3,5-di-*tert*-butyl-4-oxo-2,5-cyclohexadiene-1-ylidene)-*p*-tolyloxy Radical *see* 4357

n-Dibutyl Ether *see* 1569

Di-*tert*-butyl Ether, 3033

S,*S*-Di-*sec*-butyl *O*-Ethyl Phosphorodithioate *see* 1632

3,5-Di-*tert*-butyl-4-hydroxybenzylthioglycollate *see* 2836

Di-*tert*-butyl Malonate, 3034

2,6-Di-*tert*-butyl-4-methylphenol *see* 1548

2,7-Di-*tert*-butylnaphthalene-4-sulfonic Acid Ethyl Ester *see* 3788

3,6-Di-*tert*-butyl-1-naphthalenesulfonic Acid Ethyl Ester *see* 3788

Di-*tert*-butyl Peroxide *see* 3461

N,*N*-Dibutyl-*N*'-(3-phenyl-1,2,4-oxadiazol-5-yl)-1,2-ethanediamine *see* 1510

Dibutyl Phthalate, 3035

2,6-Di-*tert*-butylpyridine, 3036

Dibutyl Squarate *see* 8769

Di-*tert*-butyl Succinate, 3037

Dibutyl Sulfide *see* 1590

Dibutyltin Dilaurate, 3038

Di-*tert*-butyl Tricarbonate, 3039

*N*⁶,2'-*O*-Dibutyryladenosine 3',5'-Cyclic Monophosphate *see* 1463

*N*⁶,2'-*O*-Dibutyryl cAMP *see* 1463

DIC *see* 2798

DICA *see* 5568

Dicacodyl *see* 1603

1,3-Dicaffeoylquinic Acid *see* 2766

1,5-Dicaffeylquinic Acid *see* 2766

Dicain *see* 9188

Dicalcium Orthophosphate *see* 1692

Dicamba, 3040

Dicamoylmethane *see* 5773

Dicaptol [Chinoin] *see* 3209

2,2-Dicarbamoyloxymethyl-3-methyl-pentane *see* 5773

2,2-Di(carbamoyloxymethyl)pentane *see* 5862

1,3-Dicarbamylurea *see* 9766

S-(1,2-Dicarbethoxyethyl) *O*,*O*-Dimethyldithiophosphate *see* 5700

O,*S*-Dicarbethoxythiamine *see* 2023

Dicarbonic Acid Diethyl Ester *see* 7998

Dicarbonylbis(triphenylphosphine)nickel *see* 1304

Dicarbonyldi(triphenylphosphino)nickel *see* 1304

Di-μ-carbonylhexacarbonyldicobalt *see* 3085

Dicarbosulf *see* 9329

3,3'-Dicarboxy-4,4'-dihydroxyazobenzene *see* 6841

2,2'-[(1,2-Dicarboxy-1,2-ethanediyl)-bis(thio)]bis-1,3,2-dithiastibolane-4,5-dicarboxylic Acid Hexasodium Salt *see* 8812

N-[(1*S*)-1,2-Dicarboxyethyl]-L-aspartic Acid *see* 4918

4,5-Di(2-carboxyethyl)-1,3,6,7-tetramethyl-2,8-divinylbilatriene *see* 1219

2-[*N*,*N*-Di(carboxymethyl)amino]-3-cyano-4-carboxymethylthiophene-5-carboxylic Acid *see* 8106

1,3-Di(2-carboxy-4-oxochromen-5-yloxy)propan-2-ol *see* 2590

2,3-Dicarboxypropane-1,1-diphosphonic Acid *see* 1517

Dicentrine, 3041

Diceplon [Yoshitomi] *see* 2412

Dicestal *see* 3071

Dicetamin [Shionogi] *see* 2023

Dicetel [Latema] *see* 7441

Dicethiamin *see* 2023

Dichlobenil, 3042

Dichlofenthion, 3043

Dichlofluanid, 3044

Dichlone, 3045

Dichloralantipyrine *see* 3046

Dichloralphenazone, 3046

Dichloramine T, 3047
Dichlorethanoic Acid *see* 3050
Di-chloricide *see* 3057
Dichlorine Heptoxide *see* 2097
Dichlorine Monoxide *see* 2099
Dichlorisone, 3048
Dichlormid, 3049
D-*d-threo*-2-Dichloroacetamido-1-(4-methylsulfonyl)phenyl-1,3-propanediol *see* 9301
D-(−)-*threo*-2-Dichloroacetamido-1-*p*-nitrophenyl-1,3-propanediol *see* 2077
N-Dichloroacet-4-hydroxy-*N*-methylanilide *see* 3201
Dichloroacetic Acid, 3050
Dichloroacetic Acid Compd with *N*-(1-Methylethyl)-2-propanamine (1:1) *see* 3197
Dichloroacetic Acid Diisopropylammonium Salt *see* 3197
sym-Dichloroacetic Anhydride *see* 2113
α,α-Dichloroacetone *see* 3051
α,γ-Dichloroacetone *see* 3052
sym-Dichloroacetone *see* 3052
uns-Dichloroacetone *see* 3051
1,1-Dichloroacetone, 3051
1,3-Dichloroacetone, 3052
2,2-Dichloroacetyl Chloride, 3053
4-(Dichloroacetyl)-3,4-dihydro-3-methyl-2*H*-1,4-benzoxazine *see* 1046
1-(Dichloroacetyl)-6-(2-furoyloxy)-1,2,3,-4-tetrahydroquinoline *see* 8057
D-*threo*-*N*-Dichloroacetyl-1-*p*-nitrophenyl-2-amino-1,3-propanediol *see* 2077
(11β,17α)-17-[(Dichloroacetyl)oxy]-11-hydroxy-3-oxoandrosta-1,4-diene-17-carboxylic Acid Ethyl Ester *see* 3870
S-2,3-Dichloroallyl Diisopropylthiocarbamate *see* 2970
2,4-Dichloro-6-aminophenol *see* 437
4,6-Dichloro-*o*-aminophenol *see* 437
4-[(Dichloroamino)sulfonyl]benzoic Acid *see* 4590
9α,11β-Dichloro Analog of Prednisolone *see* 3048
3,4-Dichloroaniline, 3054
2-(2,6-Dichloroanilino)-1,3-diazacyclopentene-(2) *see* 2390
2-(2,6-Dichloroanilino)-2-imidazoline *see* 2390
[*o*-(2,6-Dichloroanilino)phenyl]acetic Acid *see* 3081
3,6-Dichloro-*o*-anisic Acid *see* 3040
Dichloroazodicarbonamidine *see* 2120
(±)-4-(3,4-Dichlorobenzamido)-*N*-(3-methoxypropyl)-*N*-pentylglutaramic Acid *see* 5588
m-Dichlorobenzene, 3055
o-Dichlorobenzene, 3056
p-Dichlorobenzene, 3057
1,2-Dichlorobenzene *see* 3056
1,3-Dichlorobenzene *see* 3055
3,4-Dichlorobenzeneamine *see* 3054
4,5-Dichloro-1,3-benzenedisulfonamide *see* 3077
2,4-Dichlorobenzenemethanol *see* 3060
2,2′-Dichlorobenzidine, 3058
3,3′-Dichlorobenzidine, 3059
2,6-Dichlorobenzonitrile *see* 3042
2,6-Dichloro-*p*-benzoquinone-4-chloroimine *see* 4421
2,6-Dichloro-1,4-benzoquinone-4-(4-hydroxyanil) Sodium *see* 3068

4-[(3,4-Dichlorobenzoyl)amino]-5-[(3-methoxypropyl)pentylamino]-5-oxopentanoic Acid *see* 5588
Dichlorobenzyl Alcohol, 3060
N-(2,6-Dichlorobenzylidene)-*N*′-amidinohydrazine *see* 4558
[(2,6-Dichlorobenzylidene)amino]-guanidine *see* 4558
1-[(2,6-Dichlorobenzylidene)amino]-3-hydroxyguanidine *see* 4567
1-(2,4-Dichlorobenzyl)-1*H*-indazole-3-carboxylic Acid *see* 5568
2,2′-Dichloro[1,1′-biphenyl]-4,4′-diamine *see* 3058
3,3-Dichloro-(1,1′-biphenyl)-4,4′-diamine *see* 3059
3,3′-Dichloro-4,4′-biphenyldiamine *see* 3059
1,1-Dichloro-2,2-bis(*p*-chlorophenyl)-ethane, 3061
Dichlorobis(η^5-2,4-cyclopentadien-1-yl)titanium *see* 9482
Dichlorobromomethane *see* 1417
1,1-Dichlorobutane *see* 1572
2,4-Dichloro-6-(*o*-chloroanilino)-*s*-triazine *see* 657
(±)-1-[2,4-Dichloro-β-[(7-chlorobenzo[*b*]thien-3-yl)methoxy]phenethyl]-imidazole *see* 8465
1-[2,4-Dichloro-β-[(*p*-chlorobenzyl)-oxy]phenethyl]imidazole *see* 3502
(±)-1-[2,4-Dichloro-β-[(*p*-chlorobenzyl)thio]phenethyl]imidazole *see* 8893
3,5-Dichloro-*N*-(3-chloro-1-ethyl-1-methyl-2-oxopropyl)-4-methylbenzamide *see* 10198
2,6-Dichloro-4-(chloroimino)-2,5-cyclohexadien-1-one *see* 4421
2,4-Dichloro-α-(chloromethylene)benzyl Alcohol Diethyl Phosphate *see* 2089
(*Z*)-1-[2,4-Dichloro-β-[2-(*p*-chlorophenoxy)ethoxy]-α-methylstyryl]imidazole *see* 6846
1,1-Dichloro-2-(*o*-chlorophenyl)-2-(*p*-chlorophenyl)ethane *see* 6216
2,6-Dichloro-α-(4-chlorophenyl)-4-(4,5-dihydro-3,5-dioxo-1,2,4-triazin-2(3*H*)-yl)benzeneacetonitrile *see* 3080
2,2-Dichloro-*N*-[1-(4-chlorophenyl)-ethyl]-1-ethyl-3-methylcyclopropane-carboxamide *see* 1863
(9*Z*)-2,7-Dichloro-9-[(4-chlorophenyl)-methylene]-α-[(dibutylamino)methyl]-9*H*-fluorene-4-methanol *see* 5597
4,6-Dichloro-*N*-(2-chlorophenyl)-1,3,5-triazin-2-amine *see* 657
1-[2,4-Dichloro-β-[(2-chloro-3-thenyl)-oxy]phenethyl]imidazole *see* 9452
Dichloro(2-chlorovinyl)arsine, 3062
2-[4-(2,2-Dichlorocyclopropyl)phenoxy]isobutyric Acid *see* 2313
2-[4-(2,2-Dichlorocyclopropyl)phenoxy]-2-methylpropanoic Acid *see* 2313
5,31-Dichloro-38-de(methoxycarbonyl)-7-demethyl-19-deoxy-56-*O*-[2-deoxy-2-[(10-methyl-1-oxoundecyl)amino]-β-D-glucopyranuronosyl]-38-[[[3-(dimethylamino)propyl]amino]carbonyl]-42-*O*-α-D-mannopyranosyl-*N*¹⁵-methylristomycin A Aglycone *see* 2803
N,*N*″-Dichlorodiazenedicarboximidamide *see* 2120

1,3-Dichloro-α-[2-(dibutylamino)ethyl]-6-(trifluoromethyl)-9-phenanthrenemethanol *see* 4594
1-[2,4-Dichloro-β-[(2,4-dichlorobenzyl)oxy]phenethyl]imidazole *see* 6178
1-[2,4-Dichloro-β-[(2,6-dichlorobenzyl)oxy]phenethyl]imidazole *see* 5160
3,5-Dichloro-6-[(3,5-dichloro-6-hydroxy-4-methoxy-*o*-tolyl)oxy]-4,2-cresotic Acid ε-Lactone *see* 3339
3,5-Dichloro-*N*-(3,4-dichlorophenyl)-2-hydroxybenzamide *see* 9191
2,3-Dichloro-5,6-dicyanobenzoquinone, 3063
Dichlorodi-π-cyclopentadienyltitanium *see* 9482
1,6-Dichloro-1,6-dideoxy-β-D-fructofuranosyl-4-chloro-4-deoxy-α-D-galactopyranoside *see* 8880
β,β′-Dichlorodiethylaniline *see* 660
2,2′-Dichlorodiethyl Sulfide *see* 6316
2,2-Dichloro-1,1-difluoroethyl Methyl Ether *see* 5994
Dichlorodifluoromethane, 3064
2,2-Dichloro-1,1-difluoro-1-methoxyethane *see* 5994
α-2-Dichloro-5-[4-(difluoromethyl)-4,5-dihydro-3-methyl-5-oxo-1*H*-1,2,4-triazol-1-yl]-4-fluorobenzenepropanoic Acid Ethyl Ester *see* 1837
2′,4′-Dichloro-5′-(4-difluoromethyl-4,5-dihydro-3-methyl-5-oxo-1*H*-1,2,4-triazol-1-yl)methanesulfonanilide *see* 8947
N-[2,4-Dichloro-5-[4-(difluoromethyl)-4,5-dihydro-3-methyl-5-oxo-1*H*-1,-2,4-triazol-1-yl]phenyl]methanesulfonamide *see* 8947
N-[[(3,5-Dichloro-2,4-difluorophenyl)-amino]carbonyl]-2,6-difluorobenzamide *see* 9109
1-(3,5-Dichloro-2,4-difluorophenyl)-3-(2,6-difluorobenzoyl)urea *see* 9109
2,6-Dichloro-*N*¹-(4,5-dihydro-1*H*-imidazol-2-yl)-1,4-benzenediamine *see* 751
6,7-Dichloro-1,5-dihydroimidazo[2,1-*b*]quinazolin-2(3*H*)-one *see* 622
2,5-Dichloro-3,6-dihydroxy-*p*-benzoquinone *see* 2079
2,5-Dichloro-3,6-dihydroxy-2,5-cyclohexadiene-1,4-dione *see* 2079
5,5′-Dichloro-2,2′-dihydroxy-3,3′-dinitrobiphenyl *see* 6518
5,5′-Dichloro-2,2′-dihydroxydiphenylmethane *see* 3071
9,21-Dichloro-11β,17-dihydroxy-16α-methylpregna-1,4-diene-3,20-dione 17-(2-Furoate) *see* 6241
(11β)-9,11-Dichloro-17,21-dihydroxypregna-1,4-diene-3,20-dione *see* 3048
4′,5′-Dichloro-3′,6′-dihydroxyspiro[isobenzofuran-1(3*H*),9′-[9*H*]xanthen]-3-one *see* 3067
1,1-Dichloro-*N*-[(dimethylamino)sulfonyl]-1-fluoro-*N*-phenylmethanesulfenamide *see* 3044
2′,5-Dichloro-2-(3-dimethylcarbamoyl-5-glycylaminomethyl-1*H*-1,2,4-triazol-1-yl)benzophenone *see* 8221
1,3-Dichloro-5,5-dimethylhydantoin, 3065
1,3-Dichloro-5,5-dimethyl-2,4-imidazolidinedione *see* 3065
2,4-Dichloro-3,5-dimethylphenol *see* 3076

1,3-Dichloro-2-propanol Phosphate
(3:1) *see* 9087
1,1-Dichloro-2-propanone *see* 3051
1,3-Dichloro-2-propanone *see* 3052
1,3-Dichloropropene, 3075
3′,4′-Dichloropropionanilide *see* 7804
α,α-Dichloropropionic Acid *see* 2802
α,γ-Dichloropropylene *see* 3075
1,3-Dichloropropylene *see* 3075
3-[2,4-Dichloro-5-(2-propynyloxy)-
phenyl]-5-(1,1-dimethylethyl)-1,3,4-
oxadiazol-2(3*H*)-one *see* 6905
2-[2,4-Dichloro-5-(2-propynyloxy)-
phenyl]-5,6,7,8-tetrahydro-1,2,4-tri-
azolo[4,3-*a*]pyridin-3(2*H*)-one *see* 894
3,6-Dichloro-2-pyridinecarboxylic
Acid *see* 2400
2′,4′-Dichloro-2-(3-pyridyl)aceto-
phenone *O*-Methyloxime *see* 7983
2,4′-Dichloro-α-(pyrimidin-5-yl)benz-
hydryl Alcohol *see* 3958
5,7-Dichloro-8-quinaldinol *see* 2190
5,7-Dichloro-8-quinolinol *see* 2175
2,6-Dichloroquinone Chloroimide *see*
4421
Dichlorosal *see* 4781
p-(Dichlorosulfamoyl)benzoic Acid *see*
4590
Dichlorotetraaquochromium Chloride
Dihydrate *see* 2222
Dichlorotetracarbonyldirhodium *see*
8187
1,2-Dichloro-1,1,2,2-tetrafluoroethane
see 2605
N-[[[3,5-Dichloro-4-(1,1,2,2-tetrafluo-
roethoxy)phenyl]amino]carbonyl]-
2,6-difluorobenzamide *see* 4683
1-[3,5-Dichloro-4-(1,1,2,2-tetrafluoro-
ethoxy)phenyl]-(2,6-difluoroben-
zoyl)urea *see* 4683
6,7-Dichloro-1,2,3,5-tetrahydroimid-
azo[2,1-*b*]quinazolin-2-one *see* 622
3,5-Dichlorotetrahydro-2,4,6-trioxo-*s*-
triazin-1(2*H*)-yl Potassium *see* 9767
[2,3-Dichloro-4-(2-thenoyl)phenoxy]-
acetic Acid *see* 9430
[2,3-Dichloro-4-(2-thienylcarbonyl)-
phenoxy]acetic Acid *see* 9430
[2,3-Dichloro-4-(2-thiophenecarbonyl)-
phenoxy]acetic Acid *see* 9430
α,α-Dichlorotoluene *see* 1057
N,*N*-Dichloro-*p*-toluenesulfonamide *see*
3047
N-(2,6-Dichloro-*m*-tolyl)anthranilic
Acid *see* 5779
N-(2,6-Dichloro-*m*-tolyl)anthranilic
Acid Ethoxymethyl Ester *see* 9168
O-(2,6-Dichloro-*p*-tolyl) *O*,*O*-Dimethyl
Phosphorothioate *see* 9510
1,3-Dichloro-1,3,5-triazine-2,4,6(1*H*,-
3*H*,5*H*)-trione Potassium Salt *see* 9767
5-[(4,6-Dichloro-1,3,5-triazin-2-yl)ami-
no]-3′,6′-dihydroxyspiro[isobenzo-
furan-1(3*H*),9′-[9*H*]xanthen]-3-one
see 3460
5-(4,6-Dichlorotriazinyl)aminofluores-
cein *see* 3460
4,4′-Dichloro-α-(trichloromethyl)benz-
hydrol *see* 3086
4,4′-Dichloro-3-(trifluoromethyl)car-
banilide *see* 2379
1-(1,3-Dichloro-6-trifluoromethyl-9-
phenanthryl)-3-di(*n*-butyl)aminopro-
panol *see* 4594
Dichlorovos *see* 3079

Dichloroxide *see* 2099
Dichloroxylenol, 3076
2,4-Dichloro-3,5-xylenol *see* 3076
Dichlorphenamide, 3077
Dichlorprop, 3078
Dichlorprop-P *see* 3078
Dichlor-Stapenor [Bayer] *see* 3084
Dichlorvos, 3079
Dichlotride [Merck & Co.] *see* 4781
β-Dichroine *see* 3946
Dichystrolum *see* 3180
Dickite *see* 362
Diclazuril, 3080
Diclectin [Duchesnay] *see* 3441
Diclocil [BMS] *see* 3084
Diclofenac, 3081
Dicloflex [Dexcel] *see* 3081
Diclofop-methyl, 3082
Dicloguamine *see* 5102
Diclomax [Provalis] *see* 3081
Diclondazolic Acid *see* 5568
Diclophlogont [Azupharma] *see* 3081
Dicloreum [Alfa] *see* 3081
Diclosulam, 3083
Diclotride [Merck & Co.] *see* 4781
Dicloxacillin, 3084
Dico *see* 3171
Dicobalt Edetate *see* 3517
Dicobalt Octacarbonyl, 3085
Dicodid [Knoll] *see* 4785
Dicoferin *see* 6535
Dicofol, 3086
Dicopac [Amersham] *see* 10015
Dicophane *see* 2841
(*T*-4)-Dicopper(1+) Tetraiodomer-
curate(2−) *see* 2663
Dicopur DP [Nufarm] *see* 3078
Dicorantil [Aventis] *see* 3360
Dicoumarin *see* 3090
Dicoumarol *see* 3090
Dicromil [Organon] *see* 2926
Dicrotalic Acid *see* 5808
Dicrotophos, 3087
Dicryl, 3088
Dictamine, 3089
Dictamnine, 3089
Dictycide [Fort Dodge] *see* 2680
Dictyzide *see* 2680
Dicumacyl *see* 3770
Dicumarol, 3090
Dicumol *see* 3090
Dicuprene [UCB] *see* 2670
Dicural [Fort Dodge] *see* 3141
Dicuran [Syngenta] *see* 2172
Dicurone *see* 4467
Dicyan *see* 2691
Dicyanine, 3091
2,2′-Dicyano-2,2′-azopropane *see* 918
β,β-Dicyano-*o*-chlorostyrene *see* 2127
Dicyanodiamide, 3092
Dicyanodiamidine Sulfate, 3093
2,3-Dicyano-1,4-dithiaanthraquinone
see 3368
sym-Dicyanoethane *see* 8872
Dicyanomethane *see* 5711
4-Dicyanomethylene-2-methyl-6-*p*-di-
methylaminostyryl-4*H*-pyran *see* 2838
9-Dicyanomethylene-2,4,7-trinitrofluor-
ene, 3094
1,3-Dicyano-2,4,5,6-tetrachloroben-
zene *see* 2166
Dicyclidine *see* 7765
Dicyclohexano-18-crown-6 *see* 2602
Dicyclohexylacetic Acid 2-Piperidino-
ethyl Ester *see* 3168

Dicyclohexylamine, 3095
Dicyclohexylcarbodiimide, 3096
Dicyclohexyl-18-crown-6 *see* 2602
2-(2,2-Dicyclohexylethyl)piperidine *see*
7163
1,1-Dicyclohexyl-2-(2-piperidyl)ethane
see 7163
Dicyclomine, 3097
Dicyclopentadiene *see* 2739
Dicyclopentadienyliron *see* 4037
2-[*N*-(Dicyclopropylmethyl)amino]oxazo-
line *see* 8222
N-(Dicyclopropylmethyl)-4,5-dihydro-2-
oxazolamine *see* 8222
(2α,7α,8*R*,19α,22*E*)-7,19:8,19-Dicyclo-
9,10-secoergosta-5(10),22-dien-2-ol
see 9004
Dicycloverin *see* 3097
Dicynene [Lorex] *see* 3722
Dicynone [OM] *see* 3722
Dicysteine *see* 2782
Didakene *see* 9190
Didanosine, 3098
Didecyldimethylammonium Chloride,
3099
4′,5′-Didehydro-4,5-*retro*-β,β-carotene-
3,3′-dione *see* 8195
3′,4′-Didehydro-β,ψ-caroten-16′-oic
Acid *see* 9553
1′,4-Didehydro-1-deoxy-1,4-dihydro-
3′-hydroxy-5′-[4-(2-methylpropyl)-1-
piperazinyl]-1-oxorifamycin VIII *see*
8214
1′,4-Didehydro-1-deoxy-1,4-dihydro-
5′-(2-methylpropyl)-1-oxorifamycin
XIV *see* 8213
(16*R*,19*E*)-19,20-Didehydro-16-[(10β,-
13β,21β)-23-deoxy-21,22-dihydro-
11-oxa-12,14-secostrychnidin-10-yl]-
corynan-17-oic Acid Methyl Ester
see 4381
3′,4′-Didehydro-4′-deoxy-*C*′-norvinca-
leukoblastine *see* 9990
2′,3′-Didehydro-3′-deoxythymidine *see*
8803
(2′*E*)-2′,3′-Didehydro-2′-deoxyverru-
carin A *see* 9964
9,10-Didehydro-*N*,*N*-diethyl-6-methyl-
ergoline-8β-carboxamide *see* 5634
12,13-Didehydro-13,14-dihydro-α-
erythroidine *see* 3680
11,12-Didehydro-7,10-dihydro-10-hy-
droxyretinol *see* 6932
(3β)-1,6-Didehydro-14,17-dihydro-3-
methoxy-16(15*H*)-oxaerythrinan-15-
one *see* 3175
(16*E*,20β)-16,17-Didehydro-9,17-di-
methoxycorynan-16-carboxylic Acid
Methyl Ester *see* 6218
(3β,19α,20α)-16,17-Didehydro-10,11-
dimethoxy-19-methyloxayohimban-
16-carboxylic Acid Methyl Ester *see*
8144
(*E*)-16,17-Didehydro-9,17-dimethoxy-
17,18-seco-20α-yohimban-16-car-
boxylic Acid Methyl Ester *see* 6218
8,9-Didehydro-6,8-dimethylergoline
see 191
(5α,7α,6,7α,12β,19α)-2,3-Didehydro-6,7-
epoxyaspidospermidine-3-carboxylic
Acid Methyl Ester *see* 5553
(17*R*)-19,20-Didehydro-17,18-epoxy-
curan-17-ol *see* 10044
(5α)-6,7-Didehydro-4,5-epoxy-3,6-di-
methoxy-17-methylmorphinan *see*
3181

Diethyl Carbitol [Union Carbide], 3118
Diethyl Carbonate *see* 3780
Diethyl *N*,*N*'-(2-Chloro-5-cyano-*m*-phenylene)dioxamate *see* 5555
O,*O*-Diethyl *O*-[2-Chloro-1-(2,4-dichlorophenyl)vinyl] Phosphate *see* 2089
(±)-Diethyl [1-[3-(2-Chloroethyl)-3-nitrosoureido]ethyl]phosphonate *see* 4261
O,*O*-Diethyl *O*-(3-Chloro-4-methyl-7-coumarinyl) Phosphate *see* 2537
O,*O*-Diethyl *O*-(3-Chloro-4-methyl-7-coumarinyl) Phosphorothioate *see* 2558
O,*O*-Diethyl *S*-(Chloromethyl)dithiophosphate *see* 2103
O,*O*-Diethyl *O*-7-(3-Chloro-4-methylumbelliferone) Phosphate *see* 2537
O,*O*-Diethyl *O*-(3-Chloro-4-methylumbelliferone) Thiophosphate *see* 2558
Diethylchlorophosphinate *see* 3841
Diethylchlorophosphonate *see* 3841
N,*N*-Diethyl-2-[6-(3-chloropyridazinyl)mercapto]acetamide *see* 914
N,*N*-Diethyl-2-[6-(3-chloropyridazinyl)thio]acetamide *see* 914
O,*O*-Diethyl *O*-(α-Cyanobenzylideneamino)phosphorothioate *see* 7366
Diethyl 1-(2,4-Dichlorophenyl)-5-methyl-2-pyrazoline-3,5-dicarboxylate *see* 5800
O,*O*-Diethyl *O*-2,4-Dichlorophenyl Phosphorothioate *see* 3043
O,*O*-Diethyl *O*-[2-(Diethylamino)-6-methyl-4-pyrimidinyl]phosphorothioate *see* 7497
5,5-Diethyldihydro-2-thioxo-4,6(1*H*,-5*H*)-pyrimidinedione *see* 9321
Diethyldihydroxystilbene Diphosphate *see* 4253
(*E*)-α,α'-Diethyl-4,4'-dimethoxystilbene *see* 3211
8,8-Diethyl-*N*,*N*-dimethyl-2-aza-8-germaspiro[4.5]decane-2-propanamine *see* 8758
4,5-Diethyl-10,23-dimethyl-9,24-bis(3-hydroxypropyl)-16,17-bis[2-[2-(2-methoxyethoxy)ethoxy]ethoxy]pentaazapentacyclo[20.2.1.1³,⁶.1⁸,¹¹.-0¹⁴,¹⁹]Heptacosa-1,3,5,7,9,11(27),12,-14,16,18,20,22(25),23-tridecaene Gadolinium(III) Complex *see* 6281
4,5-Diethyl-10,23-dimethyl-9,24-bis(3-hydroxypropyl)-16,17-bis[2-[2-(2-methoxyethoxy)ethoxy]ethoxy]pentaazapentacyclo[20.2.1.1³,⁶.1⁸,¹¹. -0¹⁴,¹⁹]Heptacosa-1,3,5,7,9,11(27),12,-14,16,18,20,22(25),23-tridecaene Lutetium(III) Complex *see* 6282
3,3-Diethyl-2,4-dioxo-5-methylpiperidine *see* 6136
3,3-Diethyl-2,4-dioxopiperidine *see* 7469
3,3-Diethyl-2,4-dioxotetrahydropyridine *see* 7995
N,*N*'-Diethyl-*N*,*N*'-diphenylurea *see* 3117
sym-Diethyldiphenylurea *see* 3117
N,*N*'-Diethyl-γ,γ'-dipyridylium *see* 9999
O,*O*-Diethyl Dithiobis[thioformate] *see* 3384
Diethyldithiocarbamate Sodium *see* 3378
Diethyldithiocarbamic Acid 2-Chloroallyl Ester *see* 8911
Diethyldithiocarbamic Acid Sodium Salt *see* 3378

3-(*O*,*O*-Diethyldithiophosphorylmethyl)-6-chlorobenzoxazolinone *see* 7334
Diethylenediamine *see* 7464
Diethylenediamine Sultosylate *see* 8995
1,4-Diethylene Dioxide *see* 3300
Diethylene Glycol, 3119
Diethylene Glycol Diethyl Ether *see* 3118
Diethylene Glycol Dimethyl Ether *see* 3165
Diethylene Glycol Laurate *see* 3120
Diethylene Glycol Monobutyl Ether *see* 1557
Diethylene Glycol Monoethyl Ether *see* 1800
Diethylene Glycol Monolaurate, 3120
Diethylene Glycol Monomethyl Ether *see* 6037
Diethylene Imidoxide *see* 6277
Diethylene Oxide *see* 9211
Diethylene Oximide *see* 6277
Diethylenetriamine Pentaacetic Acid *see* 7125
N,*N*-Diethylethanamine *see* 9666
Diethyl Ethanedioate *see* 3125
(*SP*-5-35)-[[Diethyl-*N*,*N*'-1,2-ethanediyl-bis[L-cysteinato]](3−)-*N*,*N*',*S*,*S*']oxo-technetium-⁹⁹ᵐTc *see* 9099
4,4'-(1,2-Diethyl-1,2-ethanediyl)bis[2-methylphenol] *see* 5968
4,4'-(1,2-Diethyl-1,2-ethanediyl)bisphenol *see* 4701
2,2'-[(1,2-Diethyl-1,2-ethanediyl)bis(4,-1-phenyleneoxy)]bis[*N*,*N*-diethylethanamine] *see* 4702
2,2-Diethylethanolamine *see* 449
1,1'-[(1*E*)-1,2-Diethyl-1,2-ethenediyl]-bis[4-methoxybenzene] *see* 3211
4,4'-[(1*E*)-1,2-Diethyl-1,2-ethenediyl]-bisphenol *see* 3129
4,4'-[(1*E*)-1,2-Diethyl-1,2-ethenediyl]-bisphenol Bis(dihydrogen Phosphate) *see* 4253
Diethyl Ether *see* 3806
2,2'''-[(1,2-Diethylethylene)bis(*p*-phenyleneoxy)]bis(triethylamine) *see* 4702
4,4'-(1,2-Diethylethylene)di-*o*-cresol *see* 5968
4,4'-(1,2-Diethylethylene)diphenol *see* 4701
O,*O*-Diethyl-*S*-ethylmercaptoethyl Dithiophosphate *see* 3365
O,*O*-Diethyl *S*-Ethylmercaptomethyl Dithiophosphate *see* 7331
O,*O*-Diethyl *S*-(Ethylthio)methyl Phosphorodithioate *see* 7331
N,*N*-Diethylglycine 4-(Acetylamino)-phenyl Ester *see* 7792
N,*N*-Diethylglycine (11β)-11,17-Dihydroxy-3,20-dioxopregn-4-en-21-yl Ester *see* 4786
N,*N*-Diethylglycine Ester with 4'-Hydroxyacetanilide *see* 7792
N,*N*-Diethyl-1,1,2,3,3,3-hexafluoro-1-propanamine *see* 5108
N,*N*-Diethyl-1,3,4,6,7,11b-hexahydro-2-hydroxy-9,10-dimethoxy-2*H*-benzo-[*a*]quinolizine-3-carboxamide Acetate *see* 1119
Di(2-ethylhexyl) Phthalate *see* 2864
Di(2-ethylhexyl) Sebacate *see* 1251
Diethyl(2-hydroxyethyl)methylammonium Bromide Xanthene-9-carboxylate *see* 5958
Diethyl(2-hydroxyethyl)methylammonium 3-Methyl-2-phenylvalerate Bromide *see* 9906

Diethyl(2-hydroxyethyl)methylammonium α-Phenylcyclohexaneglycolate Bromide *see* 6975
dl-13β,17α-Diethyl-17β-hydroxygon-4-en-3-one *see* 6686
N,*N*-Diethyl-4-hydroxy-3-methoxybenzamide *see* 3721
(+)-(4*S*)-4,11-Diethyl-4-hydroxy-9-[(4-piperidinopiperidino)carbonyloxy]-1*H*-pyrano[3',4':6,7]indolizino[1,2-*b*]-quinoline-3,14-(4*H*,12*H*)-dione *see* 5091
4,4'-(1,2-Diethylidene-1,2-ethanediyl)-bisphenol *see* 3104
4,4'-(Diethylideneethylene)diphenol *see* 3104
N,*N*-Diethyl-*N*'-2-indanyl-*N*'-phenyl-1,3-propanediamine *see* 754
N,*N*-Diethylisonicotinamide *see* 5188
Diethyl 2-Isopropyl-4-methyl-6-pyrimidyl Thionophosphate *see* 2995
O,*O*-Diethyl *O*-2-Isopropyl-4-methyl-6-pyrimidyl Thiophosphate *see* 2995
Diethyl Ketone, 3121
N,*N*-Diethyl-D-lysergamide *see* 5634
Diethylmagnesium, 3122
Diethyl Maleate, 3123
Diethyl Malonate *see* 3823
Diethylmalonic Acid, 3124
Diethylmalonylurea *see* 962
Diethyl Mercaptosuccinate *S*-Ester with *O*,*O*-Dimethyl Phosphorothioate *see* 5700
N,*N*-Diethyl-2-methoxy-4-allylphenoxy-acetamide *see* 46
N,*N*-Diethyl-*N*-[[(methoxycarbonyl)amino]sulfonyl]ethanaminium Inner Salt *see* 1502
N,*N*-Diethyl-*N*'-(6-methoxy-4-methyl-8-quinolinyl)-1,6-hexanediamine *see* 8553
N,*N*-Diethyl-2-[2-methoxy-4-(2-propenyl)phenoxy]acetamide *see* 46
*N*¹,*N*¹-Diethyl-*N*⁴-(6-methoxy-8-quinolinyl)-1,4-pentanediamine *see* 7001
N,*N*-Diethyl-*N*'-(6-methoxy-8-quinolinyl)-1,3-propanediamine *see* 7522
5,5-Diethyl-1-methylbarbituric Acid *see* 5961
N,*N*-Diethyl-3-methylbenzamide *see* 2856
Diethyl Methyl Carbinol Urethan *see* 3566
O,*O*-Diethyl *O*-(4-Methyl-7-coumarinyl) Phosphorothioate *see* 4855
O,*O*-Diethyl *O*-(4-Methyl-7-coumarinyl) Thiophosphate *see* 4855
N,*N*-Diethyl-1-methyl-3,3-di-2-thienyl-allylamine *see* 9293
N,*N*-Diethyl-*N*'-[(8α)-6-methylergolin-8-yl]urea *see* 9164
1,1-Diethyl-3-(D-6-methylisoergolen-8-yl)urea *see* 5518
N,*N*-Diethyl-*N*-methyl-2-[(3-methyl-1-oxo-2-phenylpentyl)oxy]ethanaminium Bromide *see* 9906
N,*N*-Diethyl-*N*-methyl-2-[[4-[2-(octyloxy)benzoyl]amino]benzoyl]oxy]ethanaminium Bromide *see* 6898
N,*N*-Diethyl-α-methyl-10*H*-phenothiazine-10-ethanamine *see* 3747
N,*N*-Diethyl-*N*-methyl-2-[[4-[4-(phenylthio)phenyl]-3*H*-1,5-benzodiazepin-2-yl]thio]ethanaminium Iodide *see* 9426

Diethylmethyl[2-[[4-[*p*-(phenylthio)phen-yl]-3*H*-1,5-benzodiazepin-2-yl]thio]-ethyl]ammonium Iodide *see* 9426

N,*N*-Diethyl-4-methyl-1-piperazinecar-boxamide *see* 3116

3,3-Diethyl-5-methyl-2,4-piperidine-dione *see* 6136

5,5-Diethyl-1-methyl-2,4,6(1*H*,3*H*,5*H*)-pyrimidinetrione *see* 5961

O,*O*-Diethyl *O*-[*p*-(Methylsulfinyl)phen-yl] Phosphorothioate *see* 4000

N,*N'*-Diethyl-6-(methylthio)-1,3,5-tria-zine-2,4-diamine *see* 8536

N,*N*-Diethyl-5-methyl-[1,2,4]triazolo-[1,5-*a*]pyrimidin-7-amine *see* 9574

O,*O*-Diethyl *O*-(4-Methylumbelliferone) Phosphorothioate *see* 4855

N,*N*-Diethyl-*N*-methyl-2-[(9*H*-xanthen-9-ylcarbonyl)oxy]ethanaminium Bromide *see* 5958

N,*N*-Diethyl-2-(1-naphthalenyloxy)pro-panamide *see* 6416

O,*O*-Diethyl *O*-Naphthaloximide Phos-phate *see* 6354

N,*N*-Diethyl-2-(1-naphthyloxy)propion-amide *see* 6416

N,*N*-Diethylnicotinamide *see* 6543

Diethyl-*p*-nitrophenyl Monothiophos-phate *see* 7033

Diethyl *p*-Nitrophenyl Phosphate *see* 7030

O,*O*-Diethyl *O*-*p*-Nitrophenyl Phos-phorothioate *see* 7033

Diethylnitrosamine *see* 6636

(3*R*,4a*R*,10a*S*)-*rel*-*N*,*N*-Diethyl-*N'*-(1,2,-3,4,4a,5,10,10a-octahydro-6-hydr-oxy-1-propylbenzo[*g*]quinolin-3-yl)-sulfamide *see* 8045

Diethylolamine 3107

Diethylolglycine *see* 1201

Diethyl Oxalacetate *see* 3836

Diethyl Oxalate, 3125

Diethyl Oxide *see* 3806

Diethyl Oxydiformate *see* 7998

*N*¹,*N*¹-Diethyl-1,4-pentanediamine *see* 6723

2,2-Diethyl-4-pentenamide *see* 9901

N,*N*-Diethyl-10*H*-phenothiazine-10-ethanamine *see* 3108

N,*N*-Diethylphenylacetamide *see* 3126

α,α-Diethylphenylacetic Acid 2-(2-Di-ethylaminoethoxy)ethyl Ester *see* 6930

5,5-Diethyl-1-phenylbarbituric Acid *see* 7222

N,*N*-Diethyl-α-phenylbenzenemethan-amine *see* 3115

N,*N*-Diethyl-2-[4-(phenylmethyl)phen-oxy]ethanamine *see* 9178

N,*N*-Diethyl-3-phenyl-1,2,4-oxadiazole-5-ethanamine *see* 6944

N,*N*-Diethyl-3-(1-phenylpropyl)-1,2,4-oxadiazole-5-ethanamine *see* 7903

5,5-Diethyl-1-phenyl-2,4,6(1*H*,3*H*,5*H*)-pyrimidinetrione *see* 7222

Diethylphosphorous Acid Chloride *see* 3841

Diethyl Phthalate *see* 7371

3,3-Diethyl-2,4-piperidinedione *see* 7469

Diethylpropanedioic Acid *see* 3124

Diethylpropanedioic Acid Diethyl Ester *see* 3789

Diethylpropion, 3127

2,6-Diethyl-*N*-(2'-*n*-propoxyethyl)chlo-roacetanilide *see* 7740

N,*N*-Diethyl-3-pyridinecarboxamide *see* 6543

3,3-Diethyl-2,4-(1*H*,3*H*)pyridinedione *see* 7995

5,5-Diethyl-2,4,6(1*H*,3*H*,5*H*)-pyrimi-dinetrione *see* 962

5,5-Diethyl-2,4,6(1*H*,3*H*,5*H*)-pyrimi-dinetrione Mixture with 4-(Dimethyl-amino)-1,2-dihydro-1,5-dimethyl-2-phenyl-3*H*-pyrazol-3-one *see* 7194

Diethyl Pyrocarbonate *see* 7998

N,*N*-Diethylrifomycin B Amide *see* 8215

Diethyl Sebacate *see* 8415

Diethylsilane, 3128

(*E*)-α,α'-Diethyl-4,4'-stilbenediol *see* 3129

α,α'-Diethyl-4,4'-stilbenediol Diphos-phoric Acid Ester *see* 4253

Diethylstilbestrol, 3129

Diethylstilbestrol Diphosphate *see* 4253

Diethylstilbestryl Diphosphate *see* 4253

Diethyl Sulfate, 3130

Diethyl Sulfide *see* 3854

Diethyl Sulfide 2,2'-Dicarboxylic Acid *see* 9332

Diethylsulfondimethylmethane *see* 8960

Diethylsulfonmethylethylmethane *see* 8958

Diethyl Tartrate, 3855

O,*O*-Diethyl *O*-(1,2,2,2-Tetrachloroeth-yl)thionophosphate *see* 2087

1,8-Diethyl-1,3,4,9-tetrahydropyrano-[3,4-*b*]indole-1-acetic Acid *see* 3874

N,*N*-Diethyl-*N*-[2-[4-(1,1,3,3-tetrameth-ylbutyl)phenoxy]ethyl]benzenemeth-anaminium Chloride *see* 7240

3,3'-Diethylthiadicarbocyanine Iodide *see* 3369

Diethylthiambutene *see* 9293

5,5-Diethyl-2-thiobarbituric Acid *see* 9321

N,*N*-Diethyl-*m*-toluamide *see* 2856

O,*O*-Diethyl *O*-3,5,6-Trichloro-2-pyri-dyl Phosphorothioate *see* 2189

1,1'-Diethyl-2,2'-trimethinequinocya-nine Chloride *see* 8048

O,*O*-Diethyl *S*-(2-Trimethylammonium-ethyl)phosphorothioate Iodide *see* 3501

5,5-Diethyl-2,4,6-trioxo-1-phenylhexa-hydropyrimidine *see* 7222

9-(3,3-Diethylureido)-4,6,6a,7,8,9-hexahydro-7-methylindolo[4,3-*f*,*g*]-quinoline *see* 5518

N,*N*-Diethylvanillamide *see* 3721

Diethyl Xanthogenate *see* 3384

Diethylzinc, 3131

2-Difarnesyl-3-methyl-1,4-naphthoqui-none *see* 5833

Difaterol [Andreu] *see* 1195

Difemerine, 3132

Difenacoum, 3133

Difenamizole, 3134

Difenax [Zambeletti] *see* 3137

Difenidolin [Taiyo] *see* 3311

Difenoconazole, 3135

Difenoxilic Acid *see* 3136

Difenoxin, 3136

Difenoxylic Acid *see* 3136

Difenpiramide, 3137

Difenzoquat, 3138

Diferuloylmethane *see* 2673

Difethialone, 3139

Differin [Galderma] *see* 150

Difflam [3M Pharma] *see* 1122

Diffu-K [UCB] *see* 7621

Diffumal [Malesci] *see* 9285

Diffusin [Ortho] *see* 4758

Diffusing Factor *see* 4758

Diflorasone, 3140

Difloxacin, 3141

Diflubenzuron, 3142

Diflucan [Pfizer] *see* 4122

Diflucortolone, 3143

Difludol [Edmond] *see* 3146

Diflufenican, 3144

Diflufenzopyr, 3145

Diflunisal, 3146

N,*N'*-Di-9*H*-fluoren-9-yl-*N*,*N*,*N'*,*N'*-tetramethyl-1,6-hexanediaminium Dibromide *see* 4684

2,4-Difluoroaniline, 3147

2,4-Difluorobenzenamine *see* 3147

p-Difluorobenzene, 3148

3-(2,2-Difluorobenzodioxol-4-yl)-4-cyanopyrrole *see* 4129

4-(2,2-Difluoro-1,3-benzodioxol-4-yl)-1*H*-pyrrole-3-carbonitrile *see* 4129

N-(2,6-Difluorobenzoyl)-*N'*-(2-fluoro-4-[2-chloro-4-(trifluoromethyl)phenoxy]-phenylurea) *see* 4133

1-(2,6-Difluorobenzyl)-1*H*-1,2,3-tria-zole-4-carboxamide *see* 8293

4,4'-Difluoro-1,1'-biphenyl *see* 3149

2,4-Difluoro-α,α-bis(1*H*-1,2,4-triazol-1-ylmethyl)benzyl Alcohol *see* 4122

1,1-Difluoro-2,2-dichloroethyl Methyl Ether *see* 5994

Difluorodichloromethane *see* 3064

20',20'-Difluoro-3',4'-dihydrovinorel-bine *see* 9989

erythro-3,3'-Difluoro-4,4'-dihydroxy-α-ethyl-α'-methyldibenzyl *see* 1212

(6α,11β,16α)-6,9-Difluoro-11,21-dihy-droxy-16,17-[(1-methylethylidene)-bis(oxy)]-pregna-1,4-diene-3,20-di-one *see* 4150

(6α, 11β, 16α)-6,9-Difluoro-11,21-dihy-droxy-16-methylpregna-1,4-diene-3,20-dione *see* 3143

Difluorodioxochromium *see* 2249

4,4'-Difluorodiphenyl, 3149

Difluorodiphenyltrichloroethane *see* 2957

2-(2,2-Difluoroethoxy)-*N*-(5,8-dimeth-oxy[1,2,4]triazolo[1,5-*c*]pyrimidin-2-yl)-6-(trifluoromethyl)benzenesulfon-amide *see* 7103

6,8-Difluoro-1-(2-fluoroethyl)-1,4-di-hydro-7-(4-methyl-1-piperazinyl)-4-oxo-3-quinolinecarboxylic Acid *see* 4099

2',4'-Difluoro-4-hydroxy-[1,1'-biphen-yl]-3-carboxylic Acid *see* 3146

2',4'-Difluoro-4-hydroxy-3-biphenyl-carboxylic Acid *see* 3146

2',4'-Difluoro-4-hydroxy-[1',1-diphen-yl]-3-carboxylic Acid *see* 3146

(6α,11β,16α,17α)-6,9-Difluoro-11-hydr-oxy-16-methyl-3-oxo-17-(1-oxopro-poxy)androsta-1,4-diene-17-carbo-thioic Acid *S*-(Fluoromethyl) Ester *see* 4211

6α,9α-Difluoro-16α-hydroxypredniso-lone 16,17-Acetonide *see* 4150

Difluoroiodotoluene *see* 3150

6α,9α-Difluoro-16α,17α-isopropyli-denedioxy-1,4-pregnadiene-3,20-di-one *see* 4150

Difluoromethane, 3151

(2*R*)-*anti*-5-[3-[4-(10,11-Difluorometh-anodibenzosuber-5-yl)piperazin-1-

yl]-2-hydroxypropoxy]quinoline *see* 10196

5-(Difluoromethoxy)-2-[[(3,4-dimethoxy-2-pyridinyl)methyl]sulfinyl]-1*H*-benzimidazole *see* 7014

4-(Difluoromethoxy)-α-(1-methylethyl)-benzeneacetic Acid Cyano(3-phenoxyphenyl)methyl Ester *see* 4124

2-(Difluoromethoxy)-1,1,1,2-tetrafluoroethane *see* 2919

6α,9α-Difluoro-16α-methyl-1-dehydrocorticosterone *see* 3143

2-(Difluoromethyl)-5-(4,5-dihydro-2-thiazolyl)-4-(2-methylpropyl)-6-(trifluoromethyl)-3-pyridinecarboxylic Acid Methyl Ester *see* 9311

4-[3-(Difluoromethyl)-5-(3-fluoro-4-methoxyphenyl)-1*H*-pyrazol-1-yl]-benzenesulfonamide *see* 2914

4,4-Difluoro-*N*-[(1*S*)-3-[(3-*exo*)-3-[3-methyl-5-(1-methylethyl)-4*H*-1,2,4-triazol-4-yl]-8-azabicyclo[3.2.1]oct-8-yl]-1-phenylpropyl]-cyclohexanecarboxamide *see* 5749

2-(Difluoromethyl)-4-(2-methylpropyl)-6-(trifluoromethyl)-3,5-pyridinedicarbothioic Acid *S,S*-Dimethyl Ester *see* 3374

α-Difluoromethylornithine *see* 3522

2-(Difluoromethyl)-DL-ornithine *see* 3522

Difluoro(4-methylphenyl)iodine *see* 3150

6α,9α-Difluoro-16α-methylprednisolone *see* 4138

6α,9α-Difluoro-16β-methylprednisolone *see* 3140

6α,9α-Difluoro-16α-methyl-1,4-pregnadiene-11β,21-diol-3,20-dione *see* 3143

6α,9α-Difluoro-16β-methyl-Δ^{1,4}-pregnadiene-11β,17α,21-triol-3,20-dione *see* 3140

(±)-2-Difluoromethyl 1,2,2,2-Tetrafluoroethyl Ether *see* 2919

7-β-Difluoromethylthioacetamido-7α-methoxy-3-[[1-(2-hydroxyethyl)-1*H*-tetrazol-5-yl]thiomethyl]-1-oxa-3-cephem-4-carboxylic Acid *see* 4104

(6*R-cis*)-7-[[[(Difluoromethyl)thio]acetyl]amino]-3-[[[1-(2-hydroxyethyl)-1*H*-tetrazol-5-yl]thio]methyl]-7-methoxy-8-oxo-5-oxa-1-azabicyclo[4.2.0]oct-2-ene-2-carboxylic Acid *see* 4104

2-[1-[[[(3,5-Difluorophenyl)amino]carbonyl]hydrazono]ethyl]-3-pyridinecarboxylic Acid *see* 3145

2-(2,4-Difluorophenyl)-1,3-bis(1*H*-1,2,-4-triazol-1-yl)propan-2-ol *see* 4122

2-(2,4-Difluorophenyl)-1,3-bis(1*H*-1,2,-4-triazol-1-yl)propyl Dihydrogen Phosphate *see* 4122

1-[4,4-Di(4-fluorophenyl)butyl]-4-[(2,-6-dimethylanilinocarbonyl)methyl]-piperazine *see* 5484

1-[4,4-Di-(4-fluorophenyl)butyl]-4-(2-oxo-1-benzimidazolinyl)piperidine *see* 7435

2-(2,6-Difluorophenyl)-4-[4-(1,1-dimethylethyl)-2-ethoxyphenyl]-4,5-dihydrooxazole *see* 3890

2-(2,6-Difluorophenyl)-4-(2-ethoxy-4-*tert*-butylphenyl)-2-oxazoline *see* 3890

1-(2,4-Difluorophenyl)-6-fluoro-1,4-dihydro-7-(3-methyl-1-piperazinyl)-4-oxo-3-quinolinecarboxylic Acid *see* 9132

N-(2,6-Difluorophenyl)-8-fluoro-5-methoxy-[1,2,4]triazolo[l,5-c]pyrimidine-2-sulfonamide *see* 4108

(α*R*,β*S*)-α-(2,4-Difluorophenyl)-5-fluoro-β-methyl-α-(1*H*-1,2,4-triazol-1-yl-methyl)-4-pyrimideethanol *see* 10033

2*R*,3*S*-2-(2,4-Difluorophenyl)-3-(5-fluoropyrimidin-4-yl)-1-(1*H*-1,2,4-triazol-1-yl)butan-2-ol *see* 10033

4-[2-[(1*R*,2*R*)-2-(2,4-Difluorophenyl)-2-hydroxy-1-methyl-3-(1*H*-1,2,4-triazol-1-yl)propyl]-4-thiazolyl]benzonitrile *see* 8121

1-[(2,6-Difluorophenyl)methyl]-1*H*-1,-2,3-triazole-4-carboxamide *see* 8293

N-(2,6-Difluorophenyl)-5-methyl[1,2,-4]triazolo-[1,5-*a*]pyrimidine-2-sulfonamide *see* 4141

5-(2,4-Difluorophenyl)salicylic Acid *see* 3146

2-[1-[4-(3,5-Difluorophenyl)semicarbazono]ethyl]nicotinic Acid *see* 3145

4-[4-[4-[4-[[2-(2,4-Difluorophenyl)-2-(1*H*-1,2,4-triazol-1-ylmethyl)-1,3-dioxolan-4-yl]methoxy]phenyl]-1-piperazinyl]phenyl]-2,4-dihydro-2-(1-methylpropyl)-3*H*-1,2,4-triazol-3-one *see* 8362

(3*R-cis*)-4-[4-[4-[4-[5-(2,4-Difluorophenyl)-5-(1,2,4-triazol-1-ylmethyl)tetrahydrofuran-3-ylmethoxy]phenyl]-piperazin-1-yl]phenyl]-2-[1(*S*)-ethyl-2(*S*)-hydroxypropyl]-3,4-dihydro-2*H*-1,2,4-triazol-3-one *see* 7602

α-(2,4-Difluorophenyl)-α-(1*H*-1,2,4-triazol-1-ylmethyl)-1*H*-1,2,4-triazole-1-ethanol *see* 4122

N-(2,4-Difluorophenyl)-2-(3-trifluoromethylphenoxy)nicotinamide *see* 3144

N-(2,4-Difluorophenyl)-2-[3-(trifluoromethyl)phenoxy]-3-pyridinecarboxamide *see* 3144

6α,9α-Difluoroprednisolone-21-acetate-17-butyrate *see* 3152

6α,9α-Difluoro-11β,16α,17,21-tetrahydroxypregna-1,4-diene-3,20-dione Cyclic 16,17-Acetal with Acetone *see* 4150

6α,9-Difluoro-11β,16α,17,21-tetrahydroxypregna-1,4-diene-3,20-dione, Cyclic 16,17-Acetal with Acetone, 21-Acetate *see* 4151

(α*R*)-4-[(1aα,6α,10bα)-1,1,-Difluoro-1,-1a,6,10b-tetrahyrodibenzo[*a,e*]cyclopropa[*c*]cyclohepten-6-yl]-α-[(5-quinolinyloxy)methyl]-1-piperazineethanol *see* 10196

(*RS*)-2,4'-Difluoro-α-(1*H*-1,2,4-triazol-1-ylmethyl)benzhydryl Alcohol *see* 4214

2',4'-Difluoro-2-(α,α,α-trifluoro-*m*-tolyloxy)nicotinanilide *see* 3144

(6α,11β,16α)-6,9-Difluoro-11,17,21-trihydroxy-16-methylpregna-1,4-diene-3,20-dione *see* 4138

(6α,11β,16β)-6,9-Difluoro-11,17,21-trihydroxy-16-methylpregna-1,4-diene-3,20-dione *see* 3140

6α,9-Difluoro-11β,17,21-trihydroxypregna-1,4-diene-3,20-dione 21-Acetate 17-Butyrate *see* 3152

Difluprednate, 3152

Diflupyl *see* 5176

Diflurex [Anphar-Rolland] *see* 9430

Difluron *see* 3142

Difolatan *see* 1771

Diformyl *see* 4509

1,3-Diformylpropane *see* 4472

Difosfocin [Magis] *see* 2319

Difosfonal [SPA] *see* 2371

Difrarel [Sigma-Tau] *see* 1217

Di-2-furanylethanedione Dioxime *see* 4306

N,N'-Difurfurylidene-2-furanmethanediamine *see* 4791

Digacin [Beiersdorf-Lilly] *see* 3167

Digallic Acid, 3153

"Digallic Acid" *see* 9052

m-Digallic Acid *see* 3153

Digalogenin, 3154

Digenic Acid *see* 5276

Digenin *see* 5276

Digerent [Polifarma] *see* 9699

Digicor [Hennig] *see* 3163

Digilanide A *see* 5354

Digilanide B *see* 5354

Digilanide C *see* 5354

Digilanide D *see* 5354

Digilong [Boehringer, Mann.] *see* 3163

Digimed [Trommsdorff] *see* 3163

Digimerck [Merck KGaA] *see* 3163

Digin *see* 4431

Diginatigenin, 3155

Diginatin, 3156

Diginigenin *see* 3157

Diginin, 3157

Diginorgin *see* 3158

Diginose *see* 3157

3β-(Diginosyloxy)-12α,20α-epoxy-14β,-17α-pregn-5-ene-11,15-dione *see* 3157

Digipural [Schaper & Brümmer] *see* 3163

Digitalin, 3158

Digitalin, Crystalline *see* 3163

Digitalinum True *see* 3158

Digitalinum Verum *see* 3158

Digitalis, 3159

Digitin *see* 3161

Digitoflavone *see* 5614

Digitogenin, 3160

Digitonin, 3161

Digitophyllin *see* 3163

Digitoxigenin, 3162

Digitoxin, 3163

Digitoxose, 3164

Diglycine *see* 4917

Diglycolic Acid Bis(2,4,6-triiodo-3-carboxanilide) *see* 5051

Diglycol Laurate *see* 3120

3,3'-(Diglycoloyldiimino)bis(2,4,6-triiodobenzoic Acid) *see* 5051

Diglycolyldiamide *see* 7466

Diglyme, 3165

Dignonitrat [Sankyo] *see* 5225

Dignover [Sankyo] *see* 9950

Digoxigenin, 3166

Digoxin, 3167

Diguanide *see* 1215

2,4-Diguanidino-1-dodecyloxybenzene *see* 5386

2,4-Diguanidino-1-lauryloxybenzene *see* 5386

2,4-Diguanidinophenyl Dodecyl Ether *see* 5386

2,4-Diguanidinophenyl Lauryl Ether *see* 5386

1,3-Diguanido-2,4,5,6-cyclohexanetetrol *see* 8822

p,p'-Diguanyldiazoaminobenzene Diaceturate *see* 3266

Dihexiverine *see* 3168
Dihexyl Sodium Sulfosuccinate *see* 1255
Dihexyverine, 3168
Di-Hydan *see* 7322
Dihydergot [Novartis] *see* 3174
1,4-Dihydracryloylpiperazine Dimeth-
    anesulfonate *see* 7481
Dihydral [Duphar] *see* 3180
Dihydralazine, 3169
Dihydralazine Mesylate *see* 3169
1,4-Dihydrazinophthalazine *see* 3169
o-Dihydric Phenolase *see* 9838
Dihydrin *see* 3171
Dihydrite *see* 2648
22,23-Dihydroabamectin *see* 5248
1,2-Dihydroacenaphthylene *see* 28
Dihydroactinidiolide, 3170
N,N'-Dihydro-1,2,1',2'-anthraquinon-
    azine *see* 4934
6,15-Dihydro-5,9,14,18-anthrazine-
    tetrone *see* 4934
Dihydroartemisinin *see* 817
Dihydroartemisinin Ethyl Ether *see* 813
Dihydroartemisinin Methyl Ether *see* 815
22,23-Dihydroavermectin B$_1$ *see* 5248
22,23-Dihydroavermectin B$_{1a}$ *see* 5248
22,23-Dihydroavermectin B$_{1b}$ *see* 5248
Dihydrobaikiaine *see* 7458
1,2-Dihydrobenz[*j*]aceanthrylene *see*
    2197
9,10-Dihydro-9,10-*o*-benzenoanthra-
    cene *see* 9749
(*S*)-2-[1-[2-(2,3,-Dihydrobenzfuran-5-
    yl)ethyl]-3-pyrrolidinyl]-2,2-diphen-
    ylacetamide *see* 2825
1,3-Dihydro-2*H*-benzimidazole-2-thione
    see 1082
cis-(+)-7,11b-Dihydrobenz[*b*]indeno-
    [1,2-*d*]pyran-3,4,6a,9,10(6*H*)-pentol
    see 4637
(6a*S*-*cis*)-7,11b-Dihydrobenz[*b*]indeno-
    [1,2-*d*]pyran-3,6a,9,10(6*H*)-tetrol *see*
    1367
4-(9,10-Dihydro-4*H*-benzo[4,5]cyclo-
    hepta[1,2-*b*]thien-4-ylidene)-1-methyl-
    piperidine *see* 7515
2-(2,3-Dihydro-1,4-benzodioxin-2-yl)-
    4,5-dihydro-1*H*-imidazole *see* 4887
[(2,3-Dihydro-1,4-benzodioxin-2-yl)-
    methyl]guanidine *see* 4568
1-[(2,3-Dihydro-1,4-benzodioxin-2-yl)-
    methyl]piperidine *see* 7478
1-(2,3-Dihydro-1,4-benzodioxin-5-yl)-
    piperazine *see* 3552
2,3-Dihydrobenzofuran *see* 2559
(3*S*)-1-[2-(2,3-Dihydro-5-benzofuran-
    yl)ethyl]-α,α-diphenyl-3-pyrrolidine-
    acetamide *see* 2825
2-[4-[[[(2*R*)-3,4-Dihydro-2*H*-1-benzo-
    pyran-2-yl]methyl]amino]butyl]-1,2-
    benzisothiazol-3(2*H*)-one 1,1-Dioxide
    see 8137
N-[[(2*R*)-3,4-Dihydro-2*H*-1-benzopyran-
    2-yl]methyl]-5-(4-fluorophenyl)-3-pyri-
    dinemethanamine *see* 8375
1-[(3,4-Dihydro-2*H*-1-benzothiopyran-
    8-yl)oxy]-3-[(1,1-dimethylethyl)ami-
    no]-2-propanol *see* 9173
6,7-Dihydrobis[1,3]benzodioxolo[5,6-
    a:4',5'-*g*]quinolizinium *see* 2527
1,3-Dihydro-1,3-bis(hydroxymethyl)-
    2*H*-benzimidazole-2-thione *see* 9312
(3*R*,4*R*)-*rel*-Dihydro-3,4-bis[(3-hydroxy-
    phenyl)methyl]-2(3*H*)-furanone *see*
    3598

Dihydrobis(2-methoxyethanolato-*O,O'*)-
    aluminate(1−) Sodium *see* 8564
22,23-Dihydro C-076B$_1$ *see* 5248
22,23-Dihydro C-076B$_{1a}$ *see* 5248
3,4-Dihydrocarbostyril *see* 4779
2,3-Dihydro-5-carboxanilido-6-meth-
    yl-1,4-oxathiin *see* 1827
1,3-Dihydro-3-(4-chlorophenyl)-7-hy-
    droxy-6-methylfuro[3,4-*c*]pyridine
    see 2264
3,4-Dihydrochlorothiazide *see* 4781
Dihydrocholesterol *see* 2200
(8α,9*R*)-10,11-Dihydrocinchonan-9-ol
    see 4782
(9*S*)-10,11-Dihydrocinchonan-9-ol *see*
    4783
(−)-Dihydrocinchonidine *see* 4782
(+)-Dihydrocinchonine *see* 4783
Dihydrocodehydrogenase II *see* 6348
Dihydrocodeine, 3171
Dihydrocodeinone *see* 4785
Dihydrocodeinone Enol Acetate, 3172
4,5α-Dihydrocortisol *see* 4764
Dihydrocoumarone *see* 2559
Dihydrodeoxystreptomycin *see* 2902
Dihydrodesoxymorphine-D *see* 2927
1'-[3-(10,11-Dihydro-5*H*-dibenz[*b,f*]-
    azepin-5-yl)propyl]-[1,4'-bipiperi-
    dine]-4'-carboxamide *see* 1861
9,13b-Dihydro-1*H*-dibenz[*c,f*]imid-
    azo[1,5-*a*]azepin-3-amine *see* 3618
10,11-Dihydro-5*H*-dibenzo[*a,d*]cyclo-
    heptene-5-carboxamide *see* 2759
7-[(10,11-Dihydro-5*H*-dibenzo[*a,d*]-
    cyclohepten-5-yl)amino]heptanoic
    Acid *see* 409
3-(10,11-Dihydro-5*H*-dibenzo[*a,d*]-
    cyclohepten-5-ylidene)-*N,N*-dimethyl-
    1-propanamine *see* 487
3-(10,11-Dihydro-5*H*-dibenzo[*a,d*]-
    cyclohepten-5-ylidene)-*N,N*-dimethyl-
    1-propanamine *N*-Oxide *see* 488
3-(10,11-Dihydro-5*H*-dibenzo[*a,d*]-
    cyclohepten-5-ylidene)-1-ethyl-2-meth-
    ylpyrrolidine *see* 7503
3-(10,11-Dihydro-5*H*-dibenzo[*a,d*]cyclo-
    hepten-5-ylidene)-*N*-methyl-1-propan-
    amine *see* 6715
3-(10,11-Dihydro-5*H*-dibenzo[*a,d*]cyclo-
    hepten-5-ylidene)-*N*-methylpropyl-
    amine *see* 6715
endo-3-[(10,11-Dihydro-5*H*-dibenzo-
    [*a,d*]cyclohepten-5-yl)oxy]-8-methyl-8-
    azabicyclo[3.2.1]octane *see* 2912
3α-[(10,11-Dihydro-5*H*-dibenzo[*a,d*]-
    cyclohepten-5-yl)oxy]-1α*H*,5α*H*-tro-
    pane *see* 2912
Dihydrodiethylstilbestrol *see* 4701
(5*R*,6*R*)-5,6-Dihydro-5,6-dihydroxy-
    10'-*apo*-β,ψ-carotenoic Acid *see* 895
9,10-Dihydro-3,4-dihydroxy-9,10-di-
    oxo-2-anthracenecarboxylic Acid *see*
    8176
9,10-Dihydro-3,4-dihydroxy-9,10-di-
    oxo-2-anthracenesulfonic Acid
    Monosodium Salt *see* 8573
9,10-Dihydro-4,5-dihydroxy-9,10-di-
    oxo-2-anthroic Acid Diacetate *see*
    2960
(2*S*)-2,3-Dihydro-5,7-dihydroxy-2-(3-
    hydroxy-4-methoxyphenyl)-4*H*-1-
    benzopyran-4-one *see* 4670
2,3-Dihydro-5,7-dihydroxy-2-(4-hydr-
    oxy-3-methoxyphenyl)-4*H*-1-benzo-
    pyran-4-one *see* 4736

2,3-Dihydro-3,4-dihydroxy-2-(1-hydr-
    oxy-1-methylethyl)-5-benzofuran-
    acrylic Acid δ-Lactone Diisovalerate
    see 860
[2'*S*-(2'α,3'β,6'α)]-2',3'-Dihydro-3',6'-di-
    hydroxy-2'-(hydroxymethyl)-2',4',6'-
    trimethylspiro[cyclopropane-1,5'-
    [5*H*]inden]-7'(6'*H*)-one *see* 4899
2,3-Dihydro-5,7-dihydroxy-2-(4-hydr-
    oxyphenyl)-4*H*-1-benzopyran-4-one
    see 6424
(13α,14α)-14,19-Dihydro-12,13-dihydr-
    oxy-20-norcrotolanan-11,15-dione
    see 6250
(1α,14α)-1,2-Dihydro-12,14-dihydroxy-
    senecionan-11,16-dione *see* 4853
(3'*S-trans*)-2',3'-Dihydro-3,6-dihydroxy-
    2',2',4',6'-tetramethylspiro[cyclopro-
    pane-1,5'-[5*H*]inden]-7'(6'*H*)-one *see*
    4899
1,4-Dihydro-3,5-diiodo-1-methyl-4-
    oxo-2,6-pyridinedicarboxylic Acid
    Disodium Salt *see* 8633
3,6-Dihydro-2,6-diketo-3,7-dimethyl-
    1(2)-purineacetic Acid *see* 9283
1,4-Dihydro-1,4-diketonaphthalene *see*
    6395
5,6-Dihydro-9,10-dimethoxybenzo[*g*]-
    1,3-benzodioxolo[5,6-*a*]quinolizinium
    see 1154
12,12a-Dihydro-8,9-dimethoxy[1]ben-
    zopyrano[3,4-*b*]furo[2,3-*h*][1]benzo-
    pyran-6(6a*H*)-one *see* 3550
3,4-Dihydro-6-[4-(3,4-dimethoxyben-
    zoyl)-1-piperazinyl]-2(1*H*)-quinoli-
    none *see* 9970
(7a*S-cis*)-13,13a-Dihydro-9,10-dimeth-
    oxy-3,3-dimethyl-3*H*-bis[1]benzo-
    pyrano[3,4-*b*:6',5'-*e*]pyran-7(7a*H*)-one
    see 2863
3,4-Dihydro-6,7-dimethoxyisocarbo-
    styril *see* 2543
3,4-Dihydro-6,7-dimethoxy-1(2*H*)-iso-
    quinolinone *see* 2543
N-[2-[[[4-[2-(3,4-Dihydro-6,7-dimeth-
    oxy-2(1*H*)-isoquinolinyl)ethyl]phen-
    yl]amino]carbonyl]-4,5-dimethoxy-
    phenyl]-3-quinolinecarboxamide *see*
    9064
(2*R*)-2,3-Dihydro-4,8-dimethoxy-9-
    methyl-2-(1-methylethyl)furo[2,3-
    b]quinolinium *see* 5605
2,3-Dihydro-5,6-dimethoxy-2-[[1-
    (phenylmethyl)-4-piperidinyl]-
    methyl]-1*H*-inden-1-one *see* 3419
6,11-Dihydro-6-[2-(dimethylamino)-2-
    methylethyl]-5*H*-pyrido[2,3-*b*][1,5]-
    benzodiazepin-5-one *see* 7833
10,11-Dihydro-5-(γ-dimethylamino-
    propylidene)-5*H*-dibenzo[*a,d*]cyclo-
    heptene *see* 487
2,3-Dihydro-2,2-dimethyl-7-benzofur-
    anol Methylcarbamate *see* 1803
2,3-Dihydro-2,2-dimethyl-7-benzofur-
    anyl *N*-[*N*-[2-(Ethoxycarbonyl)ethyl]-
    N-isopropylsulfenamoyl]-*N*-methylcar-
    bamate *see* 1042
2,3-Dihydro-2,2-dimethylbenzofuran-
    7-yl *N*-(*N*-Isopropyl-*N*-ethoxycarbon-
    ylethylaminosulfenyl)-*N*-methylcarba-
    mate *see* 1042
N-[[[[(2,3-Dihydro-2,2-dimethyl-7-ben-
    zofuranyl)oxy]carbonyl]methylami-
    no]thio]-*N*-(1-methylethyl)-β-alanine
    Ethyl Ester *see* 1042

16,17-Dihydro-17-methyl-15*H*-cyclo-penta[*a*]phenanthrene *see* 6048

10,11-Dihydro-*N*-methyl-5*H*-dibenz-[*b,f*]azepine-5-propanamine *see* 2920

10,11-Dihydro-*N*-methyl-5*H*-dibenzo-[*a,d*]cycloheptene-Δ⁵,γ-propylamine *see* 6715

10,11-Dihydro-5-methyl-5*H*-dibenzo-[*a,d*]cyclohepten-5,10-imine *see* 3386

5,6-Dihydro-1-methyl-5,6-dioxo-2-in-dolinesulfonic Acid 5-Semicarba-zone Sodium Salt *see* 1789

4,5-Dihydro-3-methylene-2(3*H*)-fura-none *see* 6062

Dihydro-5-methylene-2(3*H*)-furanone *see* 647

1-[2,3-Dihydro-2-(1-methylethenyl)-5-benzofuranyl]ethanone *see* 9581

(*R*)-1-[2,3-Dihydro-2-(1-methylethyl)-5-benzofuranyl]ethanone *see* 9581

4,5-Dihydro-2-[[2-(1-methylethyl)-phenoxy]methyl]-1*H*-imidazole *see* 3985

N-[4-[(4,5-Dihydro-2-methylimidazo-[4,5-*d*][1]benzazepin-6(1*H*)-yl)carbo-nyl]phenyl][1,1'-biphenyl]-2-carbox-amide *see* 2507

4,5-Dihydro-2-methyl-1*H*-imidazole *see* 5635

1,3-Dihydro-1-methyl-2*H*-imidazole-2-thione *see* 5971

4-(3,4-Dihydro-1-methyl-2(1*H*)-isoqui-nolinyl)-*N*-(4-fluorophenyl)-5,6-di-methyl-2-pyrimidinamine *see* 8168

10,11-Dihydro-5-methyl-10-(methyl-amino)-5*H*-dibenz[*b,f*]azepine *see* 5930

cis-(±)-3,4-Dihydro-4'-methyl-4-(meth-ylamino)spiro[benz[*cd*]indole-5(1*H*),-2'(5'*H*)-furan]-5'-one *see* 8295

2-[4,5-Dihydro-4-methyl-4-(1-methyl-ethyl)-5-oxo-1*H*-imidazol-2-yl]-4(and 5)-Methylbenzoic Acid Methyl Ester *see* 4903

2-[4,5-Dihydro-4-methyl-4-(1-methyl-ethyl)-5-oxo-1*H*-imidazol-2-yl]-5-eth-yl-3-pyridinecarboxylic Acid *see* 4907

2-[4,5-Dihydro-4-methyl-4-(1-methyl-ethyl)-5-oxo-1*H*-imidazol-2-yl]-5-(methoxymethyl)-3-pyridinedicarbox-ylic Acid *see* 4904

2-[4,5-Dihydro-4-methyl-4-(1-methyl-ethyl)-5-oxo-1*H*-imidazol-2-yl]-3-pyr-idinecarboxylic Acid *see* 4905

2-[4,5-Dihydro-4-methyl-4-(1-methyl-ethyl)-5-oxo-1*H*-imidazol-2-yl]-3-qui-nolinecarboxylic Acid *see* 4906

4,5-Dihydro-2-[[5-methyl-2-(1-methyl-ethyl)phenoxy]methyl]-1*H*-imidazole *see* 9834

1,3-Dihydro-4-methyl-5-[4-(methyl-thio)benzoyl]-2*H*-imidazol-2-one *see* 3589

(5*S*)-3,5-Dihydro-5-methyl-2-(methyl-thio)-5-phenyl-3-(phenylamino)-4*H*-imidazol-4-one *see* 3956

2,4-Dihydro-5-methyl-4-nitro-2-(4-ni-trophenyl)-3*H*-pyrazol-3-one *see* 7412

1,3-Dihydro-1-methyl-7-nitro-5-phen-yl-2*H*-1,4-benzodiazepin-2-one *see* 6549

2,3-Dihydro-8-methylnortropidine *see* 9777

1,6-Dihydro-2-methyl-6-oxo-(3,4'-bi-pyridine)-5-carbonitrile *see* 6197

10,11-Dihydro-α-methyl-10-oxodiben-zo[*b,f*]thiepin-2-acetic Acid *see* 10112

N-(4,5-Dihydro-4-methyl-5-oxo-1,2-di-thiolo[4,3-*b*]pyrrol-6-yl)acetamide *see* 9342

N-(4,5-Dihydro-4-methyl-5-oxo-1,2-di-thiolo[4,3-*b*]pyrrol-6-yl)propanamide *see* 880

(3*E*,3a*R*,5*S*,8b*S*)-3-[[[(2*R*)-2,5-Dihydro-4-methyl-5-oxo-2-furanyl]oxy]meth-ylene]-3,3a,4,5,6,7,8,8b-octahydro-5-hydroxy-8,8-dimethyl-2*H*-indeno[1,-2-*b*]furan-2-one *see* 8833

3,7-Dihydro-3-methyl-1-(5-oxohexyl)-7-propyl-1*H*-purine-2,6-dione *see* 7813

3,4-Dihydro-3-methyl-4-oxoimidazo-[5,1-*d*]-1,2,3,5-tetrazine-8-carbox-amide *see* 9139

2-(1,2-Dihydro-1-methyl-2-oxo-3*H*-indol-3-ylidene)hydrazinecarbothio-amide *see* 5977

4,5-Dihydro-5-methyl-4-oxo-5-phenyl-2-furancarboxylic Acid *see* 110

2-[[[(4,5-Dihydro-5-methyl-5-oxo-3-propoxy-1*H*-1,2,4-triazol-1-yl)car-bonyl]amino]sulfonyl]benzoic Acid Methyl Ester *see* 7838

1-[[3-(1,4-Dihydro-5-methyl-4-oxo-7-propylimidazo[5,1-*f*][1,2,4]triazin-2-yl)-4-ethoxyphenyl]sulfonyl]-4-ethyl-piperazine *see* 9935

1-[[3-(4,7-Dihydro-5-methyl-7-oxo-3-propyl-1*H*-pyrazolo[4,3-*d*]pyrimidin-5-yl)-4-ethoxyphenyl]sulfonyl]-4-meth-ylpiperazine *see* 8489

(2*E*,5*S*,6*R*,7*S*,9*R*,10*E*,12*E*,15*R*,16*Z*,-18*E*)-19-[(2*S*,3*S*)-3,6-Dihydro-3-methyl-6-oxo-2*H*-pyran-2-yl]-17-eth-yl-6-hydroxy-3,5,7,9,11,15-hexameth-yl-8-oxo-2,10,12,16,18-nonadecapen-taenoic Acid *see* 5444

1,2-Dihydro-6-methyl-2-oxo-5-(4-pyri-dinyl)nicotinonitrile *see* 6197

3,4-Dihydro-2-methyl-4-oxo-*N*-2-pyr-idyl-2*H*-1,2-benzothiazine-3-carbox-amide 1,1-Dioxide *see* 7506

3-[(1,4-Dihydro-2-methyl-4-oxo-5-pyri-midinyl)methyl]-5-(2-hydroxyethyl)-4-methylthiazolium Chloride *see* 6977

N-(5-[*N*-(3,4-Dihydro-2-methyl-4-oxo-quinazolin-6-ylmethyl)-*N*-methyl-amino]-2-thenoyl)-L-glutamic Acid *see* 8099

N-[[5-[[((1,4-Dihydro-2-methyl-4-oxo-6-quinazolinyl))methyl]methylamino]-2-thienyl]carbonyl]-L-glutamic Acid *see* 8099

1,4-Dihydro-1-methyl-4-oxoquinoline *see* 3498

3,4-Dihydro-2-methyl-4-oxo-3-*o*-tolyl-quinazoline *see* 5960

5,6-Dihydro-2-methyl-*N*-phenyl-1,4-oxathiin-3-carboxamide *see* 1827

4,5-Dihydro-4-methyl-5-phenyl-2-oxa-zolamine *see* 6018

2,4-Dihydro-5-methyl-2-phenyl-3*H*-pyrazol-3-one *see* 6713

5,11-Dihydro-11-[(4-methyl-1-pipera-zinyl)acetyl]-6*H*-pyrido[2,3-*b*][1,4]-benzodiazepin-6-one *see* 7491

6,11-Dihydro-11-(1-methyl-4-piperi-dinylidene)-5*H*-benzo[5,6]cyclo-hepta[1,2-*b*]pyridine *see* 901

4,9-Dihydro-4-(1-methyl-4-piperidin-ylidene)-10*H*-benzo[4,5]cyclohepta-[1,2-*b*]thiophen-10-one *see* 5307

Dihydro-5-(2-methylpropyl)-5-(2-pro-penyl)-2-thioxo-4,6(1*H*,5*H*)-pyrimi-dinedione Monosodium Salt *see* 1524

(6*S*)-5,6-Dihydro-6-methyl-2*H*-pyran-2-one *see* 7032

(*E*)-4,5-Dihydro-6-methyl-4-[(3-pyri-dinylmethylene)amino]-1,2,4-tria-zin-3(2H)-one *see* 7950

3,4-Dihydro-1-methyl-9*H*-pyrido[3,4-*b*]indol-7-ol *see* 4614

4,9-Dihydro-1-methyl-3*H*-pyrido[3,4-*b*]indol-7-ol *see* 4614

1,3-Dihydro-1-[1-[(4-methyl-4*H*,6*H*-pyrrolo[1,2-*a*][4,1]benzoxazepin-4-yl)methyl]-4-piperidinyl]-2H-benz-imidazol-2-one *see* 10110

1-[10,11-Dihydro-8-(methylthio)diben-zo[*b,f*]thiepin-10-yl]-4-methylpipera-zine *see* 6141

2,3-Dihydro-3-methyl-2-thioxo-1*H*-imi-dazole-1-carboxylic Acid Ethyl Ester *see* 1798

2,3-Dihydro-6-methyl-2-thioxo-4(1*H*)-pyrimidinone *see* 6128

3,4-Dihydro-2-methyl-2-(4,8,12-tri-methyltridecyl)-2*H*-1-benzopyran-6-ol *see* 9494

5,6-Dihydromocimycin *see* 6225

Dihydromorphine, 3177

Dihydromorphinone *see* 4803

Dihydromyricetin *see* 579

4,5-Dihydro-2-(1-naphthalenyl-methyl)-1*H*-imidazole *see* 6368

Dihydrone *see* 6959

Dihydroneopine *see* 3171

1,4-Dihydronicotinamide Adenine Di-nucleotide *see* 6344

Dihydronicotinamide Adenine Dinucleo-tide Phosphate Diaphorase *see* 6824

2,3-Dihydro-4-nitro-3,4-dioxo-9,10-se-costrychnidin-10-oic Acid *see* 1605

6,7-Dihydro-3-(5-nitro-2-furanyl)-5*H*-imidazo[2,1-*b*]thiazol-4-ium Chloride *see* 4301

1,3-Dihydro-7-nitro-5-phenyl-2*H*-1,4-benzodiazepin-2-one *see* 6575

4,5-Dihydroorotic Acid *see* 4804

9,10-Dihydro-9-oxoanthracene *see* 691

2,3-Dihydro-3-oxobenzisosulfonazole *see* 8311

3,4-Dihydro-1-oxo-1*H*-2-benzopyran-5-carboxaldehyde *see* 3678

10,11-Dihydro-10-oxo-5*H*-dibenz[*b,f*]-azepine-5-carboxamide *see* 6929

2-(10,11-Dihydro-10-oxodibenzo[*b,f*]-thiepin-2-yl)propionic Acid *see* 10112

6,11-Dihydro-11-oxodibenz[*b,e*]oxepin-2-acetic Acid *see* 5237

N-(4,5-Dihydro-5-oxo-1,2-dithiolo[4,3-*b*]pyrrol-6-yl)acetamide *see* 4728

N-(4,5-Dihydro-5-oxo-1,2-dithiolo[4,3-*b*]pyrrol-6-yl)-*N*-methylformamide *see* 4728

2-(1,3-Dihydro-3-oxo-2*H*-indol-2-yli-dene)-1,2-dihydro-3*H*-indol-3-one *see* 4943

4-(1,3-Dihydro-1-oxo-2*H*-isoindol-2-yl)-α-ethylbenzeneacetic Acid *see* 4961

4-[[3-(1,6-Dihydro-6-oxo-9*H*-purin-9-yl)-1-oxopropyl]amino]benzoic Acid *see* 5448

2-(1,3-Dihydro-3-oxo-5-sulfo-2*H*-indol-2-ylidene)-2,3-dihydro-3-oxo-1*H*-in-

4-[[(2*R*)-2,4-Dihydroxy-3,3-dimethyl-1-oxobutyl]amino]butanoic Acid *see* 4744

3,5-Dihydroxy-4,4-dimethyl-2-(1-oxobutyl)-6-[[2,4,6-trihydroxy-3-methyl-5-(1-oxobutyl)phenyl]methyl]-2,5-cyclohexadien-1-one *see* 4090

(2*E*,11α,13*E*,15*S*,17*S*)-11,15-Dihydroxy-17,20-dimethyl-9-oxoprosta-2,13-dien-1-oic Acid *see* 5490

(2*E*,11α,13*E*,15*R*)-11,15-Dihydroxy-16,16-dimethyl-9-oxoprosta-2,13-dien-1-oic Acid Methyl Ester *see* 4387

5,7-Dihydroxy-2,2-dimethyl-6-(2,4,6-trihydroxy-3-methyl-5-acetylbenzyl)-8-cinnamoyl-1,2-chromene *see* 8272

2,2'-Dihydroxy-6,6'-dinaphthyl Disulfide *see* 2840

2,2'-Dihydroxy-1,1'-dinaphthylmethane-3,3'-dicarboxylic Acid *see* 7005

11β,17α-Dihydroxy-3,20-dioxo-21-(4-methyl-1-piperazinyl)pregna-1,4-diene *see* 5763

(*Z*)-6β,16β-Dihydroxy-3,7-dioxo-29-nor-8α,9β,13α,14β-dammara-1,-17(20),24-trien-21-oic Acid Diacetate *see* 4633

(11β)-11,21-Dihydroxy-3,20-dioxopregn-4-en-18-al *see* 225

4,4'-Dihydroxy-γ,δ-diphenyl-β,δ-hexadiene *see* 3104

4,4'-Dihydroxy-γ,δ-diphenylhexane *see* 4701

4,4'-Dihydroxydiphenylmethane-3,3'-dicarboxylic Acid *see* 6065

2,2'-Dihydroxy-*N*-(4,5-diphenyloxazol-2-yl)diethylamine *see* 3367

threo-2,3-Dihydroxy-1,4-dithiolbutane *see* 3376

Dihydroxydurene *see* 3469

(5*S*,6*Z*,8*E*,10*E*,12*R*,14*Z*)-5,12-Dihydroxy-6,8,10,14-eicosatetraenoic Acid *see* 5455

3,17-Dihydroxyestratriene *see* 3704

3,16α-Dihydroxyestra-1,3,5(10)-trien-17-one Diacetate *see* 2489

3β,17β-Dihydroxyestr-4-ene *see* 1322

Dihydroxyestrin *see* 3703

1,2-Dihydroxy-1,2-ethanedisulfonic Acid Disodium Salt *see* 4510

N,*N*-Di(hydroxyethyl)aminoacetic Acid *see* 1201

17-(1,2-Dihydroxyethyl)androsten-3-one-11,17-diol *see* 7730

17-(1,2-Dihydroxyethyl)-Δ⁴-androsten-3-on-17α-ol *see* 7732

α,β-Dihydroxyethylbenzene *see* 8861

1,2-Dihydroxyethylenedicarboxylic Acid *see* 3185

(5*Z*,13*E*)-(8*R*,9*S*,11*R*,12*R*)-9,11-Dihydroxy-15,15-ethylenedioxy-16-phenoxy-17,18,19,20-tetranorprostadienoic Acid *see* 3871

Di(hydroxyethyl)glycine *see* 1201

1(*S*),3(*R*)-Dihydroxy-20(*R*)-(5'-ethyl-5'-hydroxyhepta-1'(*E*),3'(*E*)-dien-1'-yl)-9,10-secopregna-5(*Z*),7(*E*),10(19)-triene *see* 8456

Di-(2-hydroxyethyl)nitrosamine *see* 6635

5,7-Dihydroxyflavone *see* 2256

3',6'-Dihydroxyfluoran *see* 4159

11β,17β-Dihydroxy-9α-fluoro-17α-methyl-4-androsten-3-one *see* 4186

(3β,5α,25*R*)-3,26-Dihydroxyfurost-20(22)-en-12-one *see* 4622

(1α,7β)-1,7-Dihydroxyginkgolide A *see* 4426

4,6-Dihydroxy-2-(β-D-glucosido)-β-(*p*-hydroxyphenyl)propiophenone *see* 7327

Dihydroxy(glycinato)aluminum *see* 3183

2,2'-Dihydroxy-3,3',5,5',6,6'-hexachlorodiphenylmethane *see* 4680

1,6-Dihydroxyhexane *see* 4690

5,7-Dihydroxy-3-(3-hydroxy-4,5-dimethoxyphenyl)-6-methoxy-4*H*-1-benzopyran-4-one *see* 5090

γ,4-Dihydroxy-2-(6-hydroxy-1-heptenyl)-4-cyclopentanecrotonic Acid λ-Lactone *see* 1369

3,5-Dihydroxy-4-(3-hydroxy-4-methoxyhydrocinnamoyl)phenyl-2-*O*-(6-deoxy-α-L-mannopyranosyl)-β-D-glucopyranoside *see* 6452

5,7-Dihydroxy-2-(3-hydroxy-4-methoxyphenyl)-4*H*-1-benzopyran-4-one *see* 3296

5,7-Dihydroxy-3-(3-hydroxy-4-methoxyphenyl)-4*H*-1-benzopyran-4-one *see* 7713

l-3,4-Dihydroxy-1-[1-hydroxy-2-(methylamino)ethyl]benzene *see* 3619

1,8-Dihydroxy-3-(hydroxymethyl)-9,-10-anthracenedione *see* 306

1,8-Dihydroxy-3-(hydroxymethyl)anthraquinone *see* 306

1,8-Dihydroxy-3-hydroxymethyl-10-(6-hydroxymethyl-3,4,5-trihydroxy-2-pyranyl)anthrone *see* 307

5,8-Dihydroxy-2-(hydroxymethyl)-6-methoxy-3-(2-oxopropyl)-1,4-naphthalenedione *see* 4315

7-[3,5-Dihydroxy-2-(3-hydroxy-3-methyl-1-octenyl)cyclopentyl]-5-heptenoic Acid *see* 1823

5,8-Dihydroxy-2-[(1*S*)-1-hydroxy-4-methyl-3-pentenyl]-1,4-naphthalenedione *see* 257

(−)-5,8-Dihydroxy-2-(1-hydroxy-4-methyl-3-pentenyl)-1,4-naphthoquinone *see* 257

3,5-Dihydroxy-α-[[(*p*-hydroxy-α-methylphenethyl)amino]methyl]benzyl Alcohol *see* 3981

[10-[2,3-Dihydroxy-1-(hydroxymethyl)propyl]-1,4,7,10-tetraazacyclododecane-1,4,7-triacetato(3−)-*N*¹,*N*⁴,-*N*⁷,*N*¹⁰,*O*¹,*O*⁴,*O*⁷]gadolinium *see* 4323

7-[3,5-Dihydroxy-2-(3-hydroxy-1-octenyl)cyclopentyl]-5-heptenoic Acid *see* 7878

(4*S*)-*rel*-7-[(1*R*,2*R*,3*R*,5*S*)-3,5-Dihydroxy-2-[(1*E*,3*R*)-3-hydroxy-4-phenoxy-1-butenyl]cyclopentyl]-4,5-heptadienoic Acid Methyl Ester *see* 3995

5,7-Dihydroxy-2-(4-hydroxyphenyl)-4*H*-1-benzopyran-4-one *see* 730

5,7-Dihydroxy-3-(4-hydroxyphenyl)-4*H*-1-benzopyran-4-one *see* 4391

(*R*)-3,4-Dihydroxy-α-[[[4-(*p*-hydroxyphenyl)butyl]amino]methyl]benzyl Alcohol *see* 772

5,7-Dihydroxy-3-(4-hydroxyphenyl)-6-methoxy-4*H*-1-benzopyran-4-one *see* 9107

3,4-Dihydroxy-*N*-[3-(4-hydroxyphenyl)-1-methylpropyl]-β-phenylethylamine *see* 3395

(5*Z*)-7-[(1*R*,2*R*,3*R*,5*S*)-3,5-Dihydroxy-2-[(1*E*,3*S*)-3-hydroxy-5-phenyl-1-pentenyl]cyclopentyl]-*N*-ethyl-5-heptenamide *see* 1221

(5*Z*)-7-[(1*R*,2*R*,3*R*,5*S*)-3,5-Dihydroxy-2-[(3*R*)-3-hydroxy-5-phenylpentyl]cyclopentyl]-5-heptenoic Acid 1-Methylethyl Ester *see* 5376

2,4-Dihydroxy-*N*-(3-hydroxypropyl)-3,-3-dimethylbutanamide *see* 2947

D(+)-α,γ-Dihydroxy-*N*-(3-hydroxypropyl)-β,β-dimethylbutyramide *see* 2947

7-[3,5-Dihydroxy-2-[3-hydroxy-4-(3-thienyloxy)-1-butenyl]cyclopentyl]-5-heptenoic Acid *see* 9423

(5*Z*)-*rel*-7-[(1*R*,2*R*,3*R*,5*S*)-3,5-Dihydroxy-2-[(1*E*,3*R*)-3-hydroxy-4-[3-(trifluoromethyl)phenoxy]-1-butenyl]cyclopentyl]-5-heptenoic Acid *see* 4194

(5*Z*)-7-[(1*R*,2*R*,3*R*,5*S*)-3,5-Dihydroxy-2-[(1*E*,3*R*)-3-hydroxy-4-[3-(trifluoromethyl)phenoxy]-1-butenyl]cyclopentyl]-5-heptenoic Acid 1-Methylethyl Ester *see* 9577

2,2-Dihydroxy-1,3-indanedione *see* 6554

2,2-Dihydroxy-1*H*-indene-1,3(2*H*)-dione *see* 6554

4',7-Dihydroxyisoflavan *see* 3644

4',7-Dihydroxyisoflavone *see* 2801

2,6-Dihydroxyisonicotinic Acid *see* 2325

3,4-Dihydroxy-α-[(isopropylamino)methyl]benzyl Alcohol *see* 5217

3,5-Dihydroxy-α-[(isopropylamino)methyl]benzyl Alcohol *see* 5931

3,4-Dihydroxy-α-[1-(isopropylamino)propyl]benzyl Alcohol *see* 5170

β,β'-Dihydroxyisopropyl Chloride *see* 2145

11β,21-Dihydroxy-16α,17-isopropylidenedioxy-1,4-pregnadiene-3,20-dione *see* 2928

5,6-Dihydro-2-(2,6-xylidino)-4*H*-1,3-thiazine *see* 10080

Dihydroxymaleic Acid, 3185

Dihydroxymalonic Acid *see* 5913

2,4-Dihydroxy-*N*-[3-[(2-mercaptoethyl)amino]-3-oxopropyl]-3,3-dimethylbutanamide *see* 7011

2,4-Dihydroxy-*N*-[2-[(2-mercaptoethyl)carbamoyl]ethyl]-3,3-dimethylbutyramide *see* 7011

(11β)-11,17-Dihydroxy-21-mercaptopregn-4-ene-3,20-dione *see* 9484

α,4-Dihydroxy-3-methoxybenzeneacetic Acid *see* 9933

2,2'-Dihydroxy-4-methoxybenzophenone *see* 3303

7,8-Dihydroxy-6-methoxy-2*H*-1-benzopyran-2-one *see* 4265

(3β,16*R*)-3,17-Dihydroxy-16-(methoxycarbonyl)-4-methyl-2,4(1*H*)-cyclo-3,4-secoakuammilanium *see* 3500

7,8-Dihydroxy-6-methoxycoumarin *see* 4265

7,8-Dihydroxy-6-methoxycoumarin-8-β-D-glucoside *see* 4266

4',5-Dihydroxy-7-methoxyflavanone *see* 8319

4',5-Dihydroxy-7-methoxyflavanone 5-Glucoside *see* 8319

5,7-Dihydroxy-4'-methoxyflavone *see* 13

2,5-Diketopiperazine see 7466
2,5-Diketopyrrolidine see 8871
Diketosuccinic Acid see 3187
2,5-Diketotetrahydrofuran see 8870
3,5-Diketotriazolidine see 9866
Dikol see 5026
Dilabar [Vita] see 1774
Dilabron [Sterling Winthrop] see 5170
Dilacor XR [Watson] see 3202
Diladel [Polifarma] see 3202
Dilafurane see 1083
Dilanacin [AWD] see 3167
Dilangil see 5746
Dilangio [Fournier] see 1033
Dilantin [Pfizer] see 7322
Dilar [Cassenne] see 7029
Dilasenil [Celtia] see 6496
Dilaster [Hoechst] see 2540
Dilatal see 6732
Dilatol [Troponwerke] see 6732
Dilatrate [Schwarz] see 5225
Dilatrend [Roche] see 1873
Dilatropon [Draco] see 6732
Dilaudid [Knoll] see 4803
Dilavase [Organon] see 5238
Dilazep, 3200
Dilcit see 4979
Dilcoran-80 [Gödecke] see 7112
Dilevalol Hydrochloride see 5329
Dilexpal [Winthrop] see 4979
Dilituric Acid see 6586
Dill Apiole see 733
Dillar [Sarva-Syntex] see 7029
Dill Fruit Oil see 6790
Dill Seed Oil see 6790
Diloderm [Schering] see 3048
Dilombrin [Pfizer] see 3369
Dilongifolylborane see 5567
Dilor [Savage] see 3479
Dilosyn see 5964
Diloxanide, 3201
Diloxanide 2-Furoic Acid Ester see 3201
Dilpral [Orion] see 3202
Dilrene [Sanofi-Aventis] see 3202
Diltiazem, 3202
Diluted Alcohol see 3760
Dilvasene see 6923
Dilvax [Promeco] see 4895
Dilydrin [Medichemie] see 6732
Dilzem [Gödecke] see 3202
Dilzene [Sigma-Tau] see 3202
Dimalone see 3240
Dimantine see 3475
Dimate [Tutag] see 3207
Dimaten [Promeco] see 9448
Dimaval [Heyl] see 3210
Dimazine see 3247
Dimebenzcozamide see 2451
Dimecrotic Acid, 3203
Dimedone see 3242
Dimefline, 3204
Dimefox, 3205
Dimegan [Dexo] see 1443
Dimeglumine Iocarmate see 5009
Dimeglumine Ioglycamide see 5051
Dimeline [Shionogi] see 62
Dimelor [Lilly] see 62
Dimemorfan, 3206
Dimene see 2715
Dimenhydrinate, 3207
Dimenoxadol, 3208
Dimension [Dow AgroSci.] see 3374
Dimepheprimine see 7776
Diméprotane see 7839
Dimeray [Mallinckrodt] see 5009

Dimercaprol, 3209
(2R,3S)-rel-2,3-Dimercaptobutanedioic
    Acid see 8865
(2R,3R)-rel-1,4-Dimercapto-2,3-butane-
    diol see 3376
1,2-Dimercapto-4-methylbenzene see
    9531
1,3-Dimercaptopropane see 7801
2,3-Dimercapto-1-propanesulfonic
    Acid, 3210
2,3-Dimercapto-1-propanol see 3209
meso-2,3-Dimercaptosuccinic Acid see
    8865
2,3-Dimercaptosuccinic Acid Cyclic
    Ester with Antimonic Acid, Diester
    with 2,3-Dimercaptosuccinic Acid
    Hexasodium Salt see 8812
2,3-Dimercaptosuccinic Acid Cyclic
    Thioantimonate (III) S,S-Diester with
    2,3-Dimercaptosuccinate Hexa-
    sodium Salt see 8812
Dimerin see 6136
Dimer-X [Byk Gulden] see 5009
Dimestrol, 3211
Dimetacrine, 3212
Dimetane [Robins] see 1443
Dimetfol see 2895
Dimethacrine see 3212
Dimethadione, 3213
1,4-Di(methanesulfonyloxy)butane see
    1505
Dimethazone see 2381
Dimethenamid, 3214
Dimethenamid P see 3214
Dimethibutin see 3260
Dimethicone, 3215
Dimethicone 350 see 3215
Dimethicone Copolyols see 8495
Dimethindene, 3216
Dimethiotazine see 4231
Dimethirimol, 3217
Dimethisoquin, 3218
Dimethisterone, 3219
Dimethoate, 3220
Dimethocaine, 3221
Dimethomorph, 3222
Dimethophrine see 3264
Dimethothiazine see 4231
Dimethothiazine Mesylate see 4231
Di-Methox [AgriLabs] see 8905
Dimethoxane, 3223
3,4-Dimethoxyallylbenzene see 6073
2,6-Dimethoxy-4-(p-aminobenzenesul-
    fonamido)pyrimidine see 8905
1,10-Dimethoxy-6aα-aporphine-2,9-
    diol see 1325
2,10-Dimethoxy-6aα-aporphine-1,11-
    diol see 2550
2,11-Dimethoxy-6aα-aporphin-1-ol see
    5226
3,4-Dimethoxybenzaldehyde see 9951
6-(2,6-Dimethoxybenzamido)penicil-
    lanic Acid Sodium Salt see 5969
o-Dimethoxybenzene see 9956
1,2-Dimethoxybenzene see 9956
3,4-Dimethoxybenzenecarbonal see
    9951
3,3'-Dimethoxybenzidine see 2991
3,4-Dimethoxybenzoic Acid see 9953
3,4-Dimethoxybenzoic Acid 4-[Ethyl(p-
    methoxy-α-methylphenethyl)amino]-
    butyl Ester see 5769
3,4-Dimethoxybenzoic Acid 4-[Ethyl[2-
    (4-methoxyphenyl)-1-methylethyl]-
    amino]butyl Ester see 5769

5,7-Dimethoxy-2H-1-benzopyran-2-one
    see 5492
6,7-Dimethoxy-2H-1-benzopyran-2-one
    see 8404
2,6-Dimethoxybenzoquinone see 3225
(2S,5R,6R)-6-[(2,6-Dimethoxybenzoyl)-
    amino]-3,3-dimethyl-7-oxo-4-thia-1-
    azabicyclo[3.2.0]heptane-2-carbox-
    ylic Acid Monosodium Salt see 5969
2,6-Dimethoxybenzoylpenin Sodium
    Salt see 5969
6-[4-(3,4-Dimethoxybenzoyl)-1-pipera-
    zinyl]-3,4-dihydrocarbostyril see
    9970
1-(3,4-Dimethoxybenzoyl)-4-(1,2,3,4-
    tetrahydro-2-oxo-6-quinolinyl)piper-
    azine see 9970
3-[3-[[[(7S)-3,4-Dimethoxybicyclo-
    [4.2.0]octa-1,3,5-trien-7-yl]methyl]-
    methylamino]propyl]-1,3,4,5-tetra-
    hydro-7,8-dimethoxy-2H-3-benzaze-
    pin-2-one see 5247
3,3'-Dimethoxy-[1,1'-biphenyl]-4,4'-di-
    amine see 2991
3,3'-[(3,3'-Dimethoxy[1,1'-biphenyl]-4,-
    4'-diyl)bis(azo)]bis[4-hydroxy-1-
    naphthalenesulfonic Acid] Disodium
    Salt see 1085
3,3'-(3,3'-Dimethoxy[1,1'-biphenyl]-4,-
    4'-diyl)bis[2,5-diphenyl-2H-tetrazo-
    lium] Dichloride see 9244
[[(1E)-1,3-Dimethoxy-1,3-butadienyl]-
    oxy]trimethylsilane see 1363
N-(3',4'-Dimethoxycinnamoyl)anthra-
    nilic Acid see 9570
5,7-Dimethoxycoumarin see 5492
6,7-Dimethoxycoumarin see 8404
2,6-Dimethoxy-2,5-cyclohexadiene-1,4-
    dione see 3225
3,3'-Dimethoxy-4,4'-diaminobiphenyl
    see 2991
7,8-Dimethoxydictamnine see 8561
1,10-Dimethoxy-2,9-dihydroxyapor-
    phine see 1325
7,8-Dimethoxy-3-[3-[[(1S)-(4,5-dimeth-
    oxybenzocyclobutan-1-yl)methyl]-
    methylamino]propyl]-1,3,4,5-tetra-
    hydro-2H-benzazepin-2-one see 5247
3,4-Dimethoxy-α-[(dimethylamino)-
    methyl]benzyl Alcohol see 5645
2,5-Dimethoxy-α,4-dimethylbenzene-
    ethanamine see 3412
6,7-Dimethoxy-2,2-dimethyl-2H-1-ben-
    zopyran see 7718
6,7-Dimethoxy-2,2-dimethylchromene
    see 7718
6',12'-Dimethoxy-2,2'-dimethyl-6,7-
    [methylenebis(oxy)]oxyacanthan see
    1985
2,5-Dimethoxy-α,4-dimethylphenethyl-
    amine see 3412
3,4-Dimethoxy-N,N-dimethyl-α-(3-
    phenylpropyl)benzylamine see 9972
6,7-Dimethoxy-1,2-dimethyl-1,2,3,4-
    tetrahydroisoquinoline see 1847
1'α-6,6'-Dimethoxy-2,2'-dimethyltubo-
    curaran-7',12'-diol see 1016
(1β)-6,6'-Dimethoxy-2,2'-dimethyltubo-
    curaran-7',12'-diol see 2674
6,6'-Dimethoxy-2,2'-dimethyltubo-
    curaran-7',12'-diol see 2212
α,β-Dimethoxyethane see 3224
1,1-Dimethoxyethane see 3226
1,2-Dimethoxyethane see 3224
5,6-Dimethoxy-2H-furo[2,3-h]-1-benzo-
    pyran-2-one see 7437

N-[[(4,6-Dimethoxy-2-pyrimidinyl)-
  amino]carbonyl]-3-(ethylsulfonyl)-2-
  pyridinesulfonamide *see* 8230
N-[[(4,6-Dimethoxy-2-pyrimidinyl)-
  amino]carbonyl]-1-methyl-4-(2-
  methyl-2*H*-tetrazol-5-yl)-1*H*-pyra-
  zole-5-sulfonamide *see* 912
[[(4,6-Dimethoxy-2-pyrimidinyl)ami-
  no]carbonyl]sulfamic Acid 2-Eth-
  oxyphenyl Ester *see* 3754
N-[[(4,6-Dimethoxy-2-pyrimidinyl)-
  amino]carbonyl]-3-(trifluoromethyl)-2-pyridinesulfonamide *see* 4097
3-(4,6-Dimethoxypyrimidin-2-yl)-1-(2-
  ethoxyphenoxysulfonylurea) *see* 3754
N-(4,6-Dimethoxy-2-pyrimidinyl)-3-
  methyl-2,4-dithia-3,5-diazahexan-6-
  amide 2,2,4,4-Tetraoxide *see* 403
3-(4,6-Dimethoxypyrimidin-2-yl-)-1-
  (N-methyl-N-methyl-sulfonyl)urea *see*
  403
1-(4,6-Dimethoxypyrimidin-2-yl)-3-[1-
  methyl-4-(2-methyl-2*H*-tetrazol-5-
  yl)-pyrazol-5-ylsulfonyl]urea *see* 912
N[1]-(2,6-Dimethoxy-4-pyrimidinyl)sul-
  fanilamide *see* 8905
N′-(5,6-Dimethoxy-4-pyrimidinyl)sul-
  fanilamide *see* 8906
1-(4,6-Dimethoxypyrimidin-2-yl)-3-(3-
  trifluoromethyl-2-pyridylsulfonyl)-
  urea *see* 4097
2,6-Dimethoxyquinone, 3225
2,3-Dimethoxystrychnidin-10-one *see*
  1455
10,11-Dimethoxystrychnine *see* 1455
2,4-Dimethoxy-6-sulfanilamido-1,3-di-
  azine *see* 8905
2,6-Dimethoxy-4-sulfanilamidopyrimi-
  dine *see* 8905
Dimethoxytetraethylene Glycol *see* 9208
1-(7,8-Dimethoxy-1,3,4,5-tetrahydro-
  2*H*-3-benzazepin-2-on-3-yl)-3-[*N*-
  methyl-*N*-[2-(3,4-dimethoxyphenyl)-
  ethyl]amino]propane *see* 10115
(6a*S*)-9-[4,5-Dimethoxy-2-[[(1*S*)-1,2,3,-
  4-tetrahydro-6,7-dimethoxy-2-meth-
  yl-1-isoquinolinyl]methyl]phenoxy]-
  5,6,6a,7-tetrahydro-1,2,10-trimeth-
  oxy-6-methyl-4*H*-dibenzo[*de,g*]quino-
  line *see* 9254
(3*S*)-6,7-Dimethoxy-3-[(5*R*)-5,6,7,8-tet-
  rahydro-4-hydroxy-6-methyl-1,3-di-
  oxolo[4,5-*g*]isoquinolin-5-yl]-1(3*H*)-
  isobenzofuranone *see* 6423
(3*S*)-6,7-Dimethoxy-3-[(5*R*)-5,6,7,8-tet-
  rahydro-4-methoxy-6-methyl-1,3-di-
  oxolo[4,5-*g*]isoquinolin-5-yl]-1(3*H*)-
  isobenzofuranone *see* 6718
(3*S*)-6,7-Dimethoxy-3-[(5*R*)-5,6,7,8-tet-
  rahydro-6-methyl-1,3-dioxolo[4,5-*g*]-
  isoquinolin-5-yl]-1(3*H*)-isobenzofura-
  none *see* 4767
(3β,16β,17α,18β,20α)-11,17-Dimeth-
  oxy-18-[(3,4,5-trimethoxybenzoyl)-
  oxy]yohimban-16-carboxylic Acid
  Methyl Ester *see* 8145
1,3-Dimethoxy-1-trimethylsiloxy-1,3-
  butadiene *see* 1363
6,7-Dimethoxy-1-veratroylisoquinoline
  see 7017
6,7-Dimethoxy-1-veratrylisoquinoline
  see 7019
Dimethpyrindene *see* 3216
Dimethulene *see* 2040
Dimethyl *see* 3723

Dimethyl Cellosolve *see* 3224
Dimethylacetal, 3226
N,N-Dimethylacetamide, 3227
N-(2,6-Dimethylacetanilide)iminodi-
  acetic Acid *see* 5483
Dimethylacetone *see* 3121
β,β-Dimethylacrolein *see* 8448
3,3-Dimethylacrolein *see* 8448
N[1]-Dimethylacroylsulfanilamide *see* 8904
cis-2,3-Dimethylacrylic Acid *see* 646
trans-2,3-Dimethylacrylic Acid *see* 9433
3,5-Dimethyl-1-adamantanamine *see*
  5829
6,7-Dimethylalloxazine *see* 5598
7,8-Dimethylalloxazine *see* 5598
2-Dimethylallyl-5,9-dimethyl-2′-
  hydroxybenzomorphan *see* 7121
N-3,3-Dimethylallylguanidine *see* 4341
Dimethylamidoethoxyphosphoryl Cyanide *see* 9021
Dimethylamine, 3228
(Dimethylamino)acetaldehyde Diphenyl
  Acetal *see* 5790
(Dimethylamino)acetic Acid *see* 3244
4-(Dimethylamino)antipyrine *see* 474
4-(Dimethylamino)antipyrine Compd
  with 5,5-Diethylbarbituric Acid (1:1)
  see 7194
p-Dimethylaminoazobenzene, 3229
p-Dimethylaminobenzaldehyde, 3230
p-Dimethylaminobenzalrhodanine, 3231
4-Dimethylaminobenzenecarbonal *see*
  3230
4-(Dimethylamino)benzoic Acid, 3232
p-Dimethylaminobenzophenone, 3233
5-[*p*-(Dimethylamino)benzylidene]rhoda-
  nine *see* 3231
3-Dimethylamino-1,1-bis(2-thienyl)-1-
  butene *see* 3260
[[1-[(Dimethylamino)carbonyl]-3-(1,1-di-
  methylethyl)-1*H*-1,2,4-triazol-5-yl]-
  thio]acetic Acid Ethyl Ester *see* 9601
3-[[(Dimethylamino)carbonyl]oxy]-1-
  methylpyridinium Bromide *see* 7977
3-[[(Dimethylamino)carbonyl]oxy]-*N,N,-*
  N-trimethylbenzenaminium *see* 6464
N-[1-[(Dimethylamino)carbonyl]propyl]-
  N-ethyl-2-butenamide *see* 2595
N-[1-[(Dimethylamino)carbonyl]propyl]-
  N-propyl-2-butenamide *see* 2591
(1*R*,5*S*,6*S*)-2-[(3*S*,5*S*)-5-(Dimethylaminocarbonyl)pyrrolidin-3-ylthio]-6-[(*R*)-1-
  hydroxyethyl]-1-methylcarbapen-2-
  em-3-carboxylic Acid *see* 5900
(4*R*,5*S*,6*S*)-3-[[(3*S*,5*S*)-5-[(Dimethylamino)carbonyl]-3-pyrrolidinyl]thio]-6-
  [(1*R*)-1-hydroxyethyl]-4-methyl-7-oxo-
  1-azabicyclo[3.2.0]hept-2-ene-2-car-
  boxylic Acid *see* 5900
3β-(Dimethylamino)con-5-enine *see* 2497
7-Dimethylamino-6-demethyl-6-deoxy-
  tetracycline *see* 6202
6-Dimethylamino-9-[3-deoxy-3-(*p*-meth-
  oxy-L-phenylalanylamino)-β,D-ribo-
  furanosyl]-β-purine *see* 7943
4-(Dimethylamino)-1,2-dihydro-1,5-di-
  methyl-2-phenyl-3*H*-pyrazol-3-one
  see 474
2-(Dimethylamino)-1,1-dimethylethyl
  Benzilate *see* 3132
4-Dimethylamino-2,3-dimethyl-1-phen-
  yl-3-pyrazolin-5-one *see* 474
6-(Dimethylamino)-2-[2-(2,5-dimethyl-
  1-phenyl-1*H*-pyrrol-3-yl)ethenyl]-1-
  methylquinolinium Salt with 4,4′-

Methylenebis[3-hydroxy-2-naphtha-
  lenecarboxylic Acid] (2:1) *see* 8022
6-(Dimethylamino)-2-[2-(2,5-dimethyl-
  1-phenyl-3-pyrryl)vinyl]-1-methyl-
  quinolinium Salt of 2,2′-Dihydroxy-
  1,1′-dinaphthylmethane-3,3′-dicar-
  boxylic Acid *see* 8022
2-(Dimethylamino)-5,6-dimethyl-4-pyri-
  midinyl Dimethylcarbamate *see* 7496
1-Dimethylamino-2,3-dioxamethylene-
  propane Methiodide *see* 6923
4-Dimethylamino-2,2-diphenylbutyr-
  amide Ethyl Bromide *see* 387
(−)-6-(Dimethylamino)-4,4-diphenyl-3-
  heptanol Acetate (Ester) *see* 5466
6-(Dimethylamino)-4,4-diphenyl-3-hep-
  tanol Acetate (Ester) *see* 5945
6-Dimethylamino-4,4-diphenyl-3-hepta-
  none *see* 5944
1-Dimethylamino-3,3-diphenyl-4-hexa-
  none *see* 6709
6-(Dimethylamino)-4,4-diphenyl-3-hex-
  anone *see* 6709
α-*l*-4-Dimethylamino-1,2-diphenyl-3-
  methyl-2-butanol Propionate *see*
  5469
6-(Dimethylamino)-4,4-diphenyl-5-
  methyl-3-hexanone *see* 5184
(+)-4-Dimethylamino-1,2-diphenyl-3-
  methyl-2-propionyloxybutane *see*
  7839
2-(Dimethylamino)-*N*-(1,3-diphenyl-1*H*-
  pyrazol-5-yl)propanamide *see* 3134
4-Dimethylamino-2,2-diphenylvalera-
  mide *see* 459
3-Dimethylamino-1,1-di(2′-thienyl)but-
  1-ene *see* 3260
2-(Dimethylamino)ethanol *see* 2843
2-Dimethylaminoethanol Dihydrogen
  Phosphate *see* 2884
β-Dimethylaminoethanol Diphenylmethyl Ether *see* 3309
1-(Dimethylaminoethoxyacetamido)ada-
  mantane *see* 9771
N-[(2-Dimethylaminoethoxy)benzyl]-3,-
  4,5-trimethoxybenzamide *see* 9708
N-[*p*-[2-(Dimethylamino)ethoxy]benzyl]-
  veratramide *see* 5244
1-(β-Dimethylaminoethoxy)-3-*n*-butyl-
  isoquinoline *see* 3218
5-(2-Dimethylaminoethoxy)carvacrol
  Acetate *see* 6292
α-(2-Dimethylaminoethoxy)diphenyl-
  methane *see* 3309
2-(2-Dimethylaminoethoxy)diphenyl-
  methane *see* 7316
4-(2-Dimethylaminoethoxy)-5-isopropyl-
  2-methylphenyl Acetate *see* 6292
2-α-(2-Dimethylaminoethoxy)-α-methyl-
  benzyl]pyridine *see* 3441
4-[2-(Dimethylamino)ethoxy]-2-methyl-
  5-(1-methylethyl)phenol Acetate (Ester) *see* 6292
1-*p*-β-Dimethylaminoethoxyphenyl-
  trans-1,2-diphenylbut-1-ene *see* 9048
(*E*)-α-[*p*-[2-(Dimethylamino)ethoxy]-
  phenyl]-α′-ethyl-3-stilbenol *see* 3446
(*E*)-1-[4′-(2-Dimethylaminoethoxy)-
  phenyl]-1-(3-hydroxyphenyl)-2-phenyl-
  but-1-ene *see* 3446
N-[[4-[2-(Dimethylamino)ethoxy]phen-
  yl]methyl]-3,4-dimethoxy Benzamide
  see 5244
2-Dimethylaminoethoxyphenylmethyl-2-
  picoline *see* 3441

cyclo[2.2.2]oct-3-yl]thio]methyl]-4-oxo-2-piperidinecarboxylic Acid]virginiamycin S1 *see* 8084
10-(3-Dimethylamino-2-methylpropyl)-3-cyanophenothiazine *see* 2683
5-[3-(Dimethylamino)-2-methylpropyl]-10,11-dihydro-5*H*-dibenz[*b,f*]azepine *see* 9722
5-(3-Dimethylamino-2-methylpropyl)-10,11-dihydro-5*H*-dibenzo[*a,d*]cycloheptene *see* 1533
5-(3-Dimethylamino-2-methylpropyl)iminodibenzyl *see* 9722
3-Dimethylamino-7-methyl-1,2-(*n*-propylmalonyl)-1,2-dihydro-1,2,4-benzotriazine *see* 726
(−)-10-(3-Dimethylamino-2-methylpropyl)-2-methoxyphenothiazine *see* 5986
10-[3-(Dimethylamino)-2-methylpropyl]-phenothiazine *see* 9704
10-[3-(Dimethylamino)-2-methylpropyl]-10*H*-phenothiazine-2-carbonitrile *see* 2683
10-(3-Dimethylamino-2-methylpropyl)-phenothiazine 5,5-Dioxide *see* 6946
5-(Dimethylamino)-9-methyl-2-propyl-1*H*-pyrazolo[1,2-*a*][1,2,-4]benzotriazine-1,3(2*H*)-dione *see* 726
10-[3-(Dimethylamino)-2-methylpropyl]-2-(trifluoromethyl)phenothiazine *see* 9679
α-(Dimethylaminomethyl)protocatechuyl Alcohol *see* 6069
(9*S*)-9-[(Dimethylamino)methyl]-6,7,10,-11-tetrahydro-9*H*,18*H*-5,21:12,17-dimethenodibenzo[*e,k*]pyrrolo[3,4*h*][1,-4,13]oxadiazacyclohexadecine-18,-20(19*H*)-dione *see* 8290
N-[2-[[[2-[(Dimethylamino)methyl]-4-thiazolyl]methyl]thio]ethyl]-*N*′-methyl-2-nitro-1,1-ethenediamine *see* 6660
α-[(Dimethylamino)methyl]veratryl Alcohol *see* 5645
1-Dimethylaminonaphthalene *see* 3252
5-(Dimethylamino)-1-naphthalenesulfonyl Chloride *see* 2814
[4*S*-(4α,4aα,5α,5aα,6β,12aα)]-4-(Dimethylamino)-1,4,4a,5,5a,6,11,12a-octahydro-3,5,6,10,12,12a-hexahydroxy-6-methyl-1,11-dioxo-2-naphthacenecarboxamide *see* 6976
[4*S*-(4α,4aα,5α,6β,12aα)]-4-(Dimethylamino)-1,4,4a,5,5a,6,11,12a-octahydro-3,6,10,12,12a-pentahydroxy-*N*-[[4-(2-hydroxyethyl)-1-piperazinyl]methyl]-6-methyl-1,11-dioxo-2-naphthacenecarboxamide *see* 7453
[4*R*-(4α,4aβ,5aβ,6α,12aβ)]-4-(Dimethylamino)-1,4,4a,5,5a,6,11,12a-octahydro-3,6,10,12,12a-pentahydroxy-6-methyl-1,11-dioxo-2-naphthacenecarboxamide *see* 8028
[4*S*-(4α,4aα,5aα,6β,12aα)]-4-(Dimethylamino)-1,4,4a,5,5a,6-11,12a-octahydro-3,6,10,12,12a-pentahydroxy-6-methyl-1,11-dioxo-2-naphthacenecarboxamide *see* 9196
[4*S*-(4α,4aα,5α,5aα,6α,12aα)]-4-(Dimethylamino)-1,4,4a,5,5a,6,11,12a-octahydro-3,5,10,12,12a-pentahydroxy-6-methyl-1,11-dioxo-2-naphthacenecarboxamide Monohydrate *see* 3440
*N*⁶-[[[[(4*S*,4a*S*,5a*S*,6*S*,12a*S*)-4-(Dimethylamino)-1,4,4a,5,5a,6,11,12a-octahydro-3,6,10,12,12a-pentahydroxy-6-methyl-1,11-dioxo-2-naphthacenyl]-carbonyl]amino]methyl]-L-lysine *see* 5628
[4*S*-(4α,4aα,5aα,6β,12aα)]-4-(Dimethylamino)-1,4,4a,5,5a,6,11,12a-octahydro-3,6,10,12,12a-pentahydroxy-6-methyl-1,11-dioxo-*N*-(1-pyrrolidinylmethyl)-2-naphthacenecarboxamide *see* 8252
[4*S*-(4α,4aα,5α,5aα,12aα)]-4-Dimethylamino-1,4,4a,5,5a,6,11,12a-octahydro-3,5,10,12,12a-pentahydroxy-6-methylene-1,11-dioxo-2-naphthacenecarboxamide *see* 5943
Dimethylaminophenazone *see* 474
4-[[(4-Dimethylamino)phenyl]azo]benzenesulfonic Acid Sodium Salt *see* 6105
2-[[4-(Dimethylamino)phenyl]azo]benzoic Acid *see* 6119
3-*trans*-Dimethylamino-4-phenyl-4-*trans*-carbethoxy-Δ¹-cyclohexene *see* 9437
(1*R*,2*S*)-*rel*-2-(Dimethylamino)-1-phenyl-3-cyclohexene-1-carboxylic Acid Ethyl Ester *see* 9437
4-[[4-(Dimethylamino)phenyl][4-(dimethylimino)-2,5-cyclohexadien-1-ylidene]methyl]-*N*-ethyl-*N,N*-dimethylbenzenaminium Bromide Chloride *see* 6082
Dimethylaminophenyldimethylpyrazolone *see* 474
2-[2-[4-(Dimethylamino)phenyl]ethenyl]-1-ethylquinolinium Iodide *see* 8049
[2-[2-[4-(Dimethylamino)phenyl]ethenyl]-6-methyl-4*H*-pyran-4-ylidene]-propanedinitrile *see* 2838
α-(*p*-Dimethylaminophenylethylene)quinoline Ethiodide *see* 8049
7-[4-(Dimethylamino)phenyl]-*N*-(β-D-glucopyranosyloxy)-4,6-dimethyl-7-oxo-2,4-heptadienamide *see* 9649
[*R*-(*E,E*)]-7-[4-(Dimethylamino)phenyl]-*N*-hydroxy-4,6-dimethyl-7-oxo-2,4-heptadienamide *see* 9649
(11β,13α,17α)-11-[4-(Dimethylamino)phenyl]-17-hydroxy-17-(3-hydroxypropyl)estra-4,9-dien-3-one *see* 6847
11β-(4-Dimethylaminophenyl)-17α-hydroxy-17β-(3-hydroxypropyl)-13α-methyl-4,9-gonadien-3-one *see* 6847
(11β,17β)-11-[4-(Dimethylamino)phenyl]-17-hydroxy-17-(1-propynyl)estra-4,9-dien-3-one *see* 6186
5-[[4-(Dimethylamino)phenyl]methylene]-2-thioxo-4-thiazolidinone *see* 3231
2-(Dimethylamino)-5-phenyl-2-oxazolin-4-one *see* 9379
2-(Dimethylamino)-5-phenyl-4(5*H*)-oxazolone *see* 9379
[4-(Dimethylamino)phenyl]phenylmethanone *see* 3233
N-[4-[[4-(Dimethylamino)phenyl]phenylmethylene]-2,5-cyclohexadien-1-ylidene]-*N*-methylmethanaminium Chloride *see* 5699
2-Dimethylamino-1-phenylpropanol *see* 6068
11β-[4-(*N,N*-Dimethylamino)phenyl]-17α-(prop-1-ynyl)-Δ⁴,⁹-estradiene-17β-ol-3-one *see* 6186
3-Dimethylamino-1-phenyl-1-*p*-tolylpropane *see* 9523
9-[[3-(Dimethylamino)propyl]amino]-1-nitroacridine *see* 6571

10-(γ-Dimethylaminopropyl)-1-azaphenothiazine *see* 7888
10-(2-Dimethylaminopropyl)-1-azaphenothiazine *see* 5227
[3-(Dimethylamino)propyl]carbamic Acid Propyl Ester *see* 7798
5-(γ-Dimethylaminopropyl)-3-chloroiminodibenzyl *see* 2387
N-(3-Dimethylaminopropyl)-3-chlorophenothiazine *see* 2185
10-(γ-Dimethylaminopropyl)-3-chlorphenothiazine 9-Oxide *see* 6855
2-[3-(Dimethylamino)propyl]-8,8-diethyl-2-aza-8-germaspiro[4.5]decane *see* 8758
5-(3-Dimethylamino)propyl]-10,11-dihydro-5*H*-dibenz[*b,f*]azepine *see* 4920
5-[3-(Dimethylamino)propyl]-10,11-dihydro-5*H*-dibenz[*b,f*]azepine *N*-Oxide *see* 4921
6-[2-(Dimethylamino)ethyl]-1,6-dihydro-5*H*-pyrido[2,3-*b*][1,5]benzodiazepin-5-one *see* 7833
10-[3-(Dimethylamino)propyl]-9,9-dimethylacridan *see* 3212
10-[2-(Dimethylamino)propyl]-*N,N*-dimethyl-10*H*-phenothiazine-2-sulfonamide *see* 4231
10-(2-Dimethylaminopropyl)-3-dimethylsulfamidophenothiazine *see* 4231
(8β)-*N*-[3-(Dimethylamino)propyl]-*N*-[(ethylamino)carbonyl]-6-(2-propenyl)ergoline-8-carboxamide *see* 1601
β-[2-(Dimethylamino)propyl]-α-ethyl-β-phenylbenzeneethanol Acetate (Ester) *see* 5945
(α*S*)-β-[(2*S*)-2-(Dimethylamino)propyl]-α-ethyl-β-phenylbenzeneethanol Acetate (Ester) *see* 5466
1-[3-(Dimethylamino)propyl]-1-(4-fluorophenyl)-1,3-dihydro-5-isobenzofurancarbonitrile *see* 2318
1-[3-(Dimethylamino)propyl]-1-(4-fluorophenyl)-5-phthalancarbonitrile *see* 2318
5-[3-(Dimethylamino)propyl]-6,7,8,9,-10,11-hexahydro-5*H*-cyclooct[*b*]indole *see* 5075
1-(3-Dimethylaminopropyl)-2,3-hexamethyleneindole *see* 5075
6-(3-Dimethylaminopropylidene)benzo[*b*]benzofurano[2,3-*e*]oxepine *see* 6934
5-(3-Dimethylaminopropylidene)dibenzo[*a,d*][1,4]cycloheptadiene *see* 487
5-(3-Dimethylaminopropylidene)dibenzo[*a,e*]cycloheptatriene *see* 2713
5-(γ-Dimethylaminopropylidene)-5*H*-dibenzo[*a,d*]-10,11-dihydrocycloheptene *see* 487
1-(3-Dimethylaminopropylidene)-2,3:6,-7-dibenzo-4-suberene *see* 2713
11-(3-Dimethylaminopropylidene)-6,11-dihydrodibenzo[*b,e*]thiepin *see* 3429
11-(3-Dimethylaminopropylidene)-6,11-dihydrodibenz[*b,e*]oxepin *see* 3435
(11*Z*)-11-[3-(Dimethylamino)propylidene]-6,11-dihydrodibenz[*b,e*]oxepin-2-acetic Acid *see* 6840
9-[3-(Dimethylamino)propylidene]-10,-10-dimethyl-9,10-dihydroanthracene *see* 5823
N-(γ-Dimethylaminopropyl)iminodibenzyl *see* 4920
N-(γ-Dimethylaminopropyl)iminodibenzyl *N*-Oxide *see* 4921

α-(β-Dimethylaminopropyl)-α-isopropyl-
phenylacetonitrile *see* 5110
(3β,17β)-17-[[3-(Dimethylamino)pro-
pyl]methylamino]androst-5-en-3-ol
see 892
α-[2-(Dimethylamino)propyl]-α-(1-meth-
ylethyl)benzeneacetonitrile *see* 5110
3-*O*-[3-(Dimethylamino)propyl]-1,2-*O*-
(1-methylethylidene)-α-D-glucofura-
nose *see* 484
10-(2-Dimethylaminopropyl)phenothia-
zine *see* 7786
10-(3-Dimethylaminopropyl)phenothia-
zine *see* 7783
10-(3-Dimethylaminopropyl)phenothia-
zine-3-ethylone *see* 32
1-[10-[3-(Dimethylamino)propyl]-10*H*-
phenothiazin-2-yl]ethanone *see* 32
10-[3-(Dimethylamino)propyl]phenothia-
zin-2-yl Methyl Ketone *see* 32
1-[10-[2-(Dimethylamino)propyl]-10*H*-
phenothiazin-2-yl]-1-propanone *see*
7822
1-[10-[3-(Dimethylamino)propyl]-10*H*-
phenothiazin-2-yl]-1-propanone *see*
7829
α-[2-(Dimethylamino)propyl]-α-phenyl-
benzeneacetamide *see* 459
10-(3-Dimethylaminopropyl)-2-propio-
nylphenothiazine *see* 7829
10-(3-Dimethylaminopropyl)-10*H*-pyr-
ido[3,2-*b*][1,4]benzothiazine *see* 7888
N-(3-Dimethylaminopropyl)thiophenyl-
pyridylamine *see* 7888
10-[3-(Dimethylamino)propyl]-2-trifluo-
romethylphenothiazine *see* 9685
4-(Dimethylamino)pyridine *see* 3389
2-[*p*-(Dimethylamino)styryl]-1-ethylqui-
nolinium Iodide *see* 8049
2-(*p*-Dimethylaminostyryl)quinoline
Ethiodide *see* 8049
N-(Dimethylamino)succinamic Acid *see*
2810
2-[1-[3-[2-[(Dimethylamino)sulfonyl]-
10*H*-phenothiazin-10-yl]propyl]-4-
piperidinyl]ethanol *see* 7482
4-Dimethylaminotetrahydro-6-methyl-
pyran-2,3-diol *see* 2929
p-Dimethylamino-*o*-toluenephosphonous
Acid Sodium Salt *see* 9512
4-Dimethylamino-*m*-tolyl Methylcarbamate *see* 433
(4-Dimethylamino-*o*-tolyl)phosphonous
Acid Sodium Salt *see* 9512
2-[[[[[4-(Dimethylamino)-6-(2,2,2-tri-
fluoroethoxy)-1,3,5-triazin-2-yl]ami-
no]carbonyl]amino]sulfonyl]-3-
methyl Benzoic Acid Methyl Ester
see 9689
N-[6-(Dimethylamino)-3*H*-xanthene-3-
ylidene]-*N*-methylmethanaminium
Chloride *see* 8007
[6-(Dimethylamino)-3*H*-xanthen-3-yl-
idene]dimethylammonium Chloride
see 8007
N-[(2-Dimethylammonium)ethyl]-4,5,6,-
7-tetrachloroisoindolinium Dimethochloride *see* 2101
1,3-Dimethylamylamine *see* 6085
Dimethylaniline *see* 10084
N,*N*-Dimethylaniline, 3234
2-4-[[(3,5-Dimethylanilino)carbonyl]-
methyl]phenoxy-2-methylpropionic
Acid *see* 3520

3-(10,10-Dimethyl-9(10*H*)-anthracenyli-
dene)-*N*,*N*-dimethyl-1-propanamine
see 5823
7,8-Dimethyl-10-(arabino-2,3,4,5-tet-
rahydroxypentyl)benzo[*g*]pteridine-
2,4(3*H*,10*H*)-dione *see* 763
6,7-Dimethyl-9-D-araboflavin *see* 763
Dimethylarsinic Acid *see* 1604
[(Dimethylarsino)oxy]sodium As-oxide
see 8595
1,3-Dimethylazalumazine *see* 4066
7,12-Dimethylbenz[*a*]anthracene *see*
3235
9,10-Dimethyl-1,2-benzanthracene,
3235
ar,*ar*-Dimethylbenzenamine *see* 10084
N,*N*-Dimethylbenzenamine *see* 3234
Dimethylbenzene *see* 10081
N,*N*-Dimethyl-1,4-benzenediamine *see*
3254
Dimethyl 1,2-Benzenedicarboxylate *see*
3255
α,α-Dimethylbenzeneethanamine *see*
7262
N,β-Dimethylbenzeneethanamine *see*
7308
(α*S*)-*N*,α-Dimethylbenzeneethanamine
see 5948
α,4-Dimethylbenzenemethanol *see* 3237
3,3′-Dimethylbenzidine *see* 9514
5,6-Dimethylbenzimidazole, 3236
5,6-Dimethylbenzimidazolylcobamide
Coenzyme *see* 2451
5,6-Dimethylbenzimidazolylcobamide
5′-Deoxyadenosine *see* 2451
5,6-Dimethylbenzimidazolyl Cyanocobamide *see* 10014
α-(5,6-Dimethylbenzimidazolyl)hy-
droxocobamide *see* 4809
N,α-Dimethyl-1,3-benzodioxole-5-
ethanamine *see* 5767
2,2-Dimethyl-1,3-benzodioxol-4-ol
Methylcarbamate *see* 1036
8,8-Dimethyl-2*H*,8*H*-benzo[1,2-*b*:5,4-
b′]dipyran-2-one *see* 10069
N,*N*-Dimethylbenzofuro[3,2-*c*][1]benz-
oxepin-Δ$^{6(12H),γ}$-propylamine *see* 6934
3,5-Dimethylbenzoic Acid 1-(1,1-Di-
methylethyl)-2-(4-ethylbenzoyl)hy-
drazide *see* 9093
7,8-Dimethylbenzo[*g*]pteridine-2,4-
(1*H*,3*H*)-dione *see* 5598
N^1-(3,4-Dimethylbenzoyl)sulfanilamide
see 8932
1,4-Dimethyl-2,3-benzphenanthrene
see 3235
p,α-Dimethylbenzyl Alcohol, 3237
p,α-Dimethylbenzyl Camphorate Diethanolamine Salt *see* 9492
4-(2′,3′-Dimethylbenzyl)imidazole *see*
2937
N,*N*-Dimethyl-*N*′-benzyl-*N*′-(α-pyridyl)-
ethylenediamine *see* 9738
(1*R*,5*S*)-6,6-Dimethylbicyclo[3.1.1]-
hept-2-ene-2-ethanol *see* 6683
1,1-Dimethylbiguanide *see* 5938
3,3′-Dimethyl-[1,1′-biphenyl]-4,4′-dia-
mine *see* 9514
3,3′-[(3,3′-Dimethyl[1,1′-biphenyl]-4,4′-
diyl)bis(azo)]bis[5-amino-4-hydr-
oxy-2,7-naphthalenedisulfonic Acid]
Tetrasodium Salt *see* 9792
6,6′-[(3,3′-Dimethyl[1,1′-biphenyl]-4,4′-
diyl)bis(azo)]bis[4-amino-5-hydr-
oxy-1,3-naphthalenedisulfonic Acid]
Tetrasodium Salt *see* 3905

3,3′-[(3,3′-Dimethyl[1,1′-biphenyl]-4,4′-
diyl)bis(azo)]bis[4-amino-1-naph-
thalenesulfonic Acid] Disodium Salt
see 1101
3,3′-[(3,3′-Dimethyl-4,4′-biphenylene)-
bis(azo)]bis(5-amino-4-hydroxy-2,7-
naphthalenedisulfonic Acid) Tetrasodium Salt *see* 9792
1,1′-Dimethyl-4,4′-bipyridinium *see*
7031
Dimethyl 1,3-Bis(carbomethoxy)-1-
propen-2-yl Phosphate *see* 1330
β,γ-Dimethyl-α,δ-bis(3,4-dihydroxy-
phenyl)butane *see* 6693
N,*N*′-Dimethyl-*N*,*N*′-bis[3-(3′,4′,5′-tri-
methoxybenzoxy)propyl]ethylenedi-
amine *see* 4705
β,γ-Dimethyl-Δ-α,γ-butadiene *see* 3238
2,3-Dimethyl-1,3-butadiene, 3238
2,3-Dimethyl-2,3-butanediol *see* 7439
(*R**,*S**)-4,4′-(2,3-Dimethyl-1,4-butane-
diyl)bis[1,2-benzenediol] *see* 6693
3,3-Dimethylbutanoic Acid *see* 1538
2,2-Dimethylbutanoic Acid 3-(2,4-Di-
chlorophenyl)-2-oxo-1-oxaspiro-
[4,5]dec-3-en-4-yl Ester *see* 8757
2,2-Dimethylbutanoic Acid (1*S*,3*R*,7*S*,-
8*S*,8a*R*)-1,2,3,7,8,8a-Hexahydro-3,7-
dimethyl-8-[2-[(2*R*,4*R*)-tetrahydro-4-
hydroxy-6-oxo-2*H*-pyran-2-yl]ethyl]-1-
naphthalenyl Ester *see* 8539
3,3-Dimethyl Butanoic Acid 2-Oxo-3-
(2,4,6-trimethylphenyl)-1-oxaspiro-
[4.4]non-3-en-4-yl Ester *see* 8759
3,3-Dimethyl-2-butanone *see* 7440
(2a*E*,4*E*,5′*R*,6*R*,6′*S*,8*E*,11*R*,13*S*,15*S*,-
17a*R*,20*R*,20a*R*,20b*S*)-6′-[(*E*)-1,3-Di-
methyl-1-butenyl]-5′,6,6′,7,10,11,14,-
15,17a,20,20a,20b-dodecahydro-20,-
20b-dihydroxy-5′,6,8,19-tetrameth-
ylspiro[11,15-methano-2*H*,13*H*,17*H*-
furo[4,3,2-*pq*]benzodioxacycloocta-
decin-13,2′-[2*H*]pyran]-4′,17(3′*H*)-di-
one 4′-(*E*)-(*O*-Methyloxime) *see* 6290
N-[*N*-(3,3-Dimethylbutyl)-L-α-aspar-
tyl]-L-phenylalanine 1-Methyl Ester
see 6465
N-(3,3-Dimethylbutyl)-L-α-aspartyl-L-
phenylalanine 2-Methyl Ester *see* 6465
3,3-Dimethylbutyric Acid *see* 1538
2,2-Dimethylbutyric Acid 8-Ester with
(4*R*,6*R*)-6-[2-[(1*S*,2*S*,6*R*,8*S*,8a*R*)-1,2,-
6,7,8,8a-Hexahydro-8-hydroxy-2,6-
dimethyl-1-naphthyl]ethyl]tetrahy-
dro-4-hydroxy-2*H*-pyran-2-one *see*
8539
21-(3,3-Dimethylbutyryloxy)-9α-fluo-
ro-11β-hydroxy-16α,17α-(isopropylidenedioxy)pregna-1,4-diene-3,20-di-
one *see* 9598
Dimethylcadmium, 3239
Dimethylcarbamic Acid 7-Chloro-2,3-di-
hydro-1-methyl-2-oxo-5-phenyl-1*H*-
1,4-benzodiazepin-3-yl Ester *see* 1725
Dimethylcarbamic Acid 2-(Dimethylamino)-5,6-dimethyl-4-pyrimidinyl Ester
see 7496
Dimethylcarbamic Acid 5-[2-[(1,1-Di-
methylethyl)amino]-1-hydroxyeth-
yl]-1,3-phenylene Ester *see* 953
Dimethylcarbamic Acid 3-Methyl-1-(1-
methylethyl)-1*H*-pyrazol-5-yl Ester *see*
5178
Dimethylcarbamic Acid 3-Methyl-1-
phenyl-1*H*-pyrazol-5-yl Ester *see* 8002

Name Index

2-(2,2-Dimethyl-1-oxopropyl)-1*H*-indene-1,3(2*H*)-dione *see* 7444

endo-8,8-Dimethyl-3-[(1-oxo-2-propylpentyl)oxy]-8-azoniabicyclo[3.2.1]octane Bromide *see* 671

(11*β*)-21-[(2,2-Dimethyl-1-oxopropyl)-thio]-11,17-dihydroxypregn-4-ene-3,20-dione *see* 9484

17*S*,20-Dimethyl-6-oxoprostaglandin E₁ Methyl Ester *see* 6875

(2*S*,5*R*)-3,3-Dimethyl-7-oxo-4-thia-1-azabicyclo[3.2.0]heptane-2-carboxylic Acid *see* 7091

(2*S*,5*R*)-3,3-Dimethyl-7-oxo-4-thia-1-azabicyclo[3.2.0]heptane-2-carboxylic Acid 4,4-Dioxide *see* 8889

(1*R*,3*S*)-2,2-Dimethyl-3-[(1*Z*)-3-oxo-3-[2,2,2-trifluoro-1-(trifluoromethyl)-ethoxy]-1-propenyl]cyclopropanecarboxylic Acid (*S*)-Cyano(3-phenoxyphenyl)methyl Ester *see* 125

Dimethyloxychinizin *see* 716

Dimethyloxyquinazine *see* 716

Dimethyl Parathion *see* 6108

7,8-Dimethyl-10-(D-*galacto*-2,3,4,5,6-pentahydroxyhexyl)benzo[g]pteridine-2,4(3*H*,10*H*)-dione *see* 4333

7,8-Dimethyl-10-(D-*galacto*-2,3,4,5,6-pentahydroxyhexyl)isoalloxazine *see* 4333

16,16-Dimethyl-*trans*-Δ²-PGE₁ Methyl Ester *see* 4387

2,9-Dimethyl-*o*-phenanthroline *see* 6449

2,9-Dimethyl-1,10-phenanthroline *see* 6449

α,*α*-Dimethylphenethylamine *see* 7262

dl-N,*β*-Dimethylphenethylamine *see* 7308

(*S*)-(+)-N,*α*-Dimethylphenethylamine *see* 5948

Dimethylphenol *see* 10082

3,3′-Dimethylphenolphthalein *see* 2576

N,N-Dimethyl-10*H*-phenothiazine-10-propanamine *see* 7783

(*αS*)-N-[(1*S*,3*S*,4*S*)-4-[[(2,6-Dimethylphenoxy)acetyl]amino]-3-hydroxy-5-phenyl-1-(phenylmethyl)pentyl]tetrahydro-*α*-(1-methylethyl)-2-oxo-1(2*H*)-pyrimidineacetamide *see* 5573

(2*S*,3*S*,5*S*)-2-(2,6-Dimethylphenoxyacetyl)amino-3-hydroxy-5-[2*S*-(1-tetrahydropyrimid-2-onyl)-3-methylbutanoyl]amino-1,6-diphenylhexane *see* 5573

1-(2′,6′-Dimethylphenoxy)-2-aminopropane *see* 6169

5-(2,5-Dimethylphenoxy)-2,2-dimethylpentanoic Acid *see* 4388

N,N-Dimethyl-N-(2-phenoxyethyl)benzenemethanaminium Salt with 3-Hydroxy-2-naphthalene Carboxylic Acid (1:1) *see* 1148

N,N-Dimethyl-N-(2-phenoxyethyl)-1-dodecanaminium Bromide *see* 3415

1-(2,6-Dimethylphenoxy)-2-propanamine *see* 6169

4-[[[(*E*)-[(1,3-Dimethyl-5-phenoxy-1*H*-pyrazol-4-yl)methylene]amino]oxy]methyl]benzoic Acid 1,1-Dimethylethyl Ester *see* 3996

Dimethylphenylamine *see* 3234

2-[(2,3-Dimethylphenyl)amino]benzoic Acid *see* 5798

2-(2,6-Dimethylphenylamino)-4*H*-5,6-dihydro-1,3-thiazine *see* 10080

N-[2-[(2,6-Dimethylphenyl)amino]-2-oxoethyl]-N,N-diethylbenzenemethanaminium Benzoate *see* 2891

2-[4-[2-[(3,5-Dimethylphenyl)amino]-2-oxoethyl]phenoxy]-2-methylpropanoic Acid *see* 3520

1,5-Dimethyl-2-phenyl-4-aminopyrazolone *see* 591

N,N-Dimethyl-4-(phenylazo)benzenamine *see* 3229

1-[(2,4-Dimethylphenyl)azo]-2-naphthalenol *see* 10089

N,N-Dimethyl-*α*-phenylbenzeneacetamide *see* 3307

(*αR*)-N,N-Dimethyl-*α*-phenylbenzeneethanamine *see* 5431

N-(2,6-Dimethylphenylcarbamoylmethyl)iminodiacetic Acid *see* 5483

N-(2,6-Dimethylphenyl)-N-(1-carbomethoxyethyl)phenylacetamide *see* 1030

N-(2,6-Dimethylphenyl)-1,2-dihydro-2-oxo-3-pyridinecarboxamide *see* 5192

N-(2,6-Dimethylphenyl)-5,6-dihydro-4*H*-1,3-thiazin-2-amine *see* 10080

N′-(2,4-Dimethylphenyl)-N-[[(2,4-dimethylphenyl)imino]methyl]-N-methylmethanimidamide *see* 486

1,3-Dimethyl-3-phenyl-2,5-dioxopyrrolidine *see* 6004

Dimethyl-*p*-phenylenediamine, 3254

8-[2-(N,*α*-Dimethyl-*β*-phenyl)ethylamino]-1,3,7-trimethyl-2,6-dioxopurine *see* 3967

4-[(1*S*)-1-(2,3-Dimethylphenyl)ethyl]-1*H*-imidazole *see* 2946

4-[1-(2,3-Dimethylphenyl)ethyl]-1*H*-imidazole *see* 5787

N-(2,6-Dimethylphenyl)-2-(ethylpropylamino)butanamide *see* 3862

N-(2,6-Dimethylphenyl)-4-[2-hydroxy-3-(2-methoxyphenoxy)propyl]-1-piperazineacetamide *see* 8111

N-(2,6-Dimethylphenyl)-N′-[imino(methylamino)methyl]urea *see* 5481

2-(2′,4′-Dimethylphenylimino)-3-methylthiazoline *see* 2764

2,3-Dimethyl-1-phenyl-4-isopropylpyrazolone *see* 7871

N-(2,6-Dimethylphenyl)-N-(methoxyacetyl)-DL-alanine Methyl Ester *see* 5922

N-(2,6-Dimethylphenyl)-N-(methoxyacetyl)-D-alanine Methyl Ester *see* 5922

(*R*)-[(2,6-Dimethylphenyl)methoxyacetylamino]propionic Acid Methyl Ester *see* 5922

N-(2,6-Dimethylphenyl)-2-methoxy-N-(2-oxo-3-oxazolidinyl)acetamide *see* 6908

1-(2,6-Dimethylphenyl)-3-methylamidinourea *see* 5481

(*αS*)-N,*α*-Dimethyl-N-(phenylmethyl)benzeneethanamine *see* 1118

N,N-Dimethyl-3-[[1-(phenylmethyl)cycloheptyl]oxy]-1-propanamine *see* 1033

N,N′-Dimethyl-N″-(phenylmethyl)guanidine *see* 1186

4-[(2,3-Dimethylphenyl)methyl]-1*H*-imidazole *see* 2937

N,N-Dimethyl-3-[[1-(phenylmethyl)-1*H*-indazol-3-yl]oxy]-1-propanamine *see* 1122

N,N-Dimethyl-2-[2-(phenylmethyl)phenoxy]ethanamine *see* 7316

N-(2,6-Dimethylphenyl)-1-methyl-2-piperidinecarboxamide *see* 5859

N,N-Dimethyl-N′-(phenylmethyl)-N′-2-pyridinyl-1,2-ethanediamine *see* 9738

3,4-Dimethyl-2-phenylmorpholine *see* 7220

(+)-N,N-Dimethyl-1-phenyl-3-(1-naphthalenyloxy)propanamine *see* 2821

N-(2,6-Dimethylphenyl)-2-oxo-1-pyrrolidineacetamide *see* 6439

(−)-N,N-Dimethyl-*α*-phenylphenethylamine *see* 5431

N-(2,6-Dimethylphenyl)-N-(phenylacetyl)-DL-alanine Methyl Ester *see* 1030

(*cis*)-1,3-Dimethyl-4-phenyl-4-piperidinol Propanoate *see* 310

(±)-*α*-1,3-Dimethyl-4-phenyl-4-piperidinyl Propionate *see* 310

DL-*α*-1,3-Dimethyl-4-phenyl-4-propionoxyazacycloheptane *see* 7776

1,3-Dimethyl-4-phenyl-4-propionoxyhexamethylenimine *see* 7776

dl-*α*-1,3-Dimethyl-4-phenyl-4-propionoxypiperidine *see* 310

1,1-Dimethyl-2-phenylpropylamine *see* 7133

(2*S*)-N-(2,6-Dimethylphenyl)-1-propyl-2-piperidinecarboxamide *see* 8258

N,N-Dimethyl-*α*-(3-phenylpropyl)veratrylamine *see* 9972

2,3-Dimethyl-1-phenyl-3-pyrazolin-5-one *see* 716

1,5-Dimethyl-2-phenyl-3-pyrazolone *see* 716

N,N-Dimethyl-*γ*-phenyl-2-pyridinepropanamine *see* 7235

N,N-Dimethyl-2-[1-phenyl-1-(2-pyridinyl)ethoxy]ethanamine *see* 3441

(±)-*cis*-2,6-Dimethyl-*α*-phenyl-*α*-2-pyridyl-1-piperidinebutanol *see* 7501

4,6-Dimethyl-N-phenyl-2-pyrimidinamine *see* 7986

N-(2,6-Dimethylphenyl)-1-pyrrolidineacetamide *see* 8013

1,3-Dimethyl-3-phenyl-2,5-pyrrolidinedione *see* 6004

3,4-*trans*-2,2-Dimethyl-3-phenyl-4-[*p*-(*β*-pyrrolidinoethoxy)phenyl]-7-methoxychroman *see* 1971

N-(2,6-Dimethylphenyl)-8-pyrrolizidineacetamide *see* 7427

N,2-Dimethyl-2-phenylsuccinimide *see* 6004

3,4-Dimethyl-2-phenyltetrahydro-1,4-oxazine *see* 7220

N-(2,6-Dimethylphenyl)tetrahydro-1*H*-pyrrolizine-7a(5*H*)-acetamide *see* 7427

N,N-Dimethyl-2-(*α*-phenyl-*o*-toloxy)ethylamine *see* 7316

N,N-Dimethyl-2-(*α*-phenyl-*o*-tolyloxy)-ethylamine *see* 7316

N,N-Dimethyl-3-phenyl-3-*p*-tolylpropylamine *see* 9523

N,N-Dimethyl-N-phenylurea *see* 4009

gem-Dimethylphloroglucinol *see* 4079

N,N-Dimethylphosgeniminium Chloride *see* 9977

Dimethyl Phosphate of 3-Hydroxy-N-methyl-*cis*-crotonamide *see* 6251

5,6-Dimethyl-1-(3-*O*-phosphono-*α*-D-ribofuranosyl)-1*H*-benzimidazole Monoester with Cobinamide-Co(II) Inner Salt *see* 10016

Dimethylphosphoramidocyanidic Acid, Ethyl Ester *see* 9021

O,S-Dimethyl Phosphoramidothioate *see* 5947

Dimethyl Phthalate, 3255

O,O-Dimethyl *S*-Phthalimidomethyl Phosphorothionate *see* 7336

1,1-Dimethylpiperidinium Chloride *see* 5857

2,4'-Dimethyl-3-piperidinopropiophenone *see* 9522

cis-(±)-α-[3-(2,6-Dimethyl-1-piperidinyl)propyl]-α-phenyl-2-pyridinemethanol *see* 7501

N,N-Dimethyl-4-piperidylidene-1,1-diphenylmethane Methylsulfate *see* 3306

cis-*N*-(2',6'-Dimethyl-1'-piperidyl)-3-sulfamoyl-4-chlorobenzamide *see* 2393

Dimethyl Polysiloxane *see* 3215

6,17-Dimethylpregna-4,6-diene-3,20-dione *see* 5791

2,2-Dimethylpropane *see* 6456

2,2-Dimethyl-1,3-propanediol *see* 6458

(2*E*,2'*E*,3*R*,3'*R*)-*rel*-3,3'-[(2,2-Dimethyl-1,3-propanediyl)diimino]bis-2-butanone Dioxime *see* 3911

2,2-Dimethylpropanoic Acid *see* 7511

2,2-Dimethylpropanoic Acid 4-[1-Hydroxy-2-(methylamino)ethyl]-1,2-phenylene Ester *see* 3338

2,2-Dimethyl-1-propanol *see* 6457

(3*S*-*cis*)-3-[[2-(1,1-Dimethyl-2-propenyl)-5,7-bis(3-methyl-2-butenyl)-1*H*-indol-3-yl]methyl]-6-methyl-2,5-piperazinedione *see* 3499

(2*E*)-3-[5-(1,1-Dimethyl-2-propenyl)-4-hydroxy-2-methoxyphenyl]-1-(4-hydroxyphenyl)-2-propen-1-one *see* 5479

α,α-Dimethylpropionic Acid *see* 7511

N-[2-[4-(2,2-Dimethylpropionyloxy)-phenylsulfonylamino]benzoyl]aminoacetic Acid *see* 8558

4'-[(1,4'-Dimethyl-2'-propyl[2,6'-bi-1*H*-benzimidazol]-1'-yl)methyl][1,1'-biphenyl]-2-carboxylic Acid *see* 9129

1,1-Dimethylpropyl Methyl Ether *see* 612

4-(1,1-Dimethylpropyl)phenol *see* 7142

cis-4-[3-[4-(1,1-Dimethylpropyl)phenyl]-2-methylpropyl]-2,6-dimethylmorpholine *see* 573

(α*R*)-*N*,α-Dimethyl-*N*-2-propynylbenzeneethanamine *see* 8428

L-(−)-*N*,α-Dimethyl-*N*-2-propynylphenethylamine *see* 8428

Dimethylprotocatechuic Acid *see* 9953

9,10-Dimethylpteroylglutamic Acid *see* 2895

2,2'-Dimethyl-α-pyrano(5',6',3,4)-2(1*H*)-quinolone *see* 4101

N,N-Dimethyl-4-pyridinamine *see* 3389

2,6-Dimethylpyridine *see* 5616

N,N-Dimethyl-3-[1-(2-pyridinyl)ethyl]-1*H*-indene-2-ethanamine *see* 3216

N,N-Dimethyl-*N*'-2-pyridinyl-*N*'-(2-thienylmethyl)-1,2-ethanediamine *see* 5959

N,N-Dimethyl-*N*'-2-pyridinyl-*N*'-(3-thienylmethyl)-1,2-ethanediamine *see* 9280

N,N-Dimethyl-10*H*-pyrido[3,2-*b*][1,4]-benzothiazine-10-propanamine *see* 7888

1,5-Dimethyl-6*H*-pyrido[4,3-*b*]carbazole *see* 6834

5,11-Dimethyl-6*H*-pyrido[4,3-*b*]carbazole *see* 3548

N,N-Dimethyl-*N*'-(2-pyridyl)-*N*'-(5-chloro-2-thenyl)ethylenediamine *see* 2167

N,N-Dimethyl-*N*'-(α-pyridyl)-*N*'-(2-methyl-5-chlorothienyl)ethylenediamine *see* 2167

N,N-Dimethyl-*N*'-(α-pyridyl)-*N*'-(2-methylthienyl)ethylenediamine *see* 5959

N,N-Dimethyl-*N*'-(α-pyridyl)-*N*'-(3-methylthienyl)ethylenediamine *see* 9280

N,N-Dimethyl-*N*'-(2-pyridyl)-*N*'-(2-thenyl)ethylenediamine *see* 5959

2,6-Dimethyl-4-pyrimidinamine *see* 5326

2-[[[[(4,6-Dimethyl-2-pyrimidinyl)amino]carbonyl]amino]sulfonyl]benzoic Acid Methyl Ester *see* 8957

N-[(4,6-Dimethylpyrimidin-2-yl)aminocarbonyl]-2-methoxycarbonylbenzenesulfonamide *see* 8957

5-[[4-[[(4,6-Dimethyl-2-pyrimidinyl)amino]sulfonyl]phenyl]azo]-2-hydroxybenzoic Acid *see* 8321

5-[*p*-[(4,6-Dimethyl-2-pyrimidinyl)aminosulfonyl]phenylazo]salicylic Acid *see* 8321

N-[4-[[(2,6-Dimethyl-4-pyrimidinyl)amino]sulfonyl]phenyl]formamide *see* 4248

N-(4,6-Dimethylpyrimidin-2-yl)aniline *see* 7986

N-(2,6-Dimethyl-4-pyrimidinyl)-4-(formylamino)benzenesulfonamide *see* 4248

(α*S*)-α-[(4,6-Dimethyl-2-pyrimidinyl)oxy]-β-methoxy-β-phenylbenzenepropanoic Acid *see* 384

4'-[(2,6-Dimethyl-4-pyrimidinyl)sulfamoyl]formanilide *see* 4248

4'-(4,6-Dimethylpyrimidin-2-ylsulfamoyl)-4-hydroxyazobenzene-3-carboxylic Acid *see* 8321

5-[*p*-[(4,6-Dimethyl-2-pyrimidinyl)sulfamoyl]phenylazo]salicylic Acid *see* 8321

*N*¹-(2,6-Dimethyl-4-pyrimidinyl)sulfanilamide *see* 8951

*N*¹-(4,6-Dimethyl-2-pyrimidinyl)sulfanilamide *see* 8915

2-[3-(4,6-Dimethylpyrimidin-2-yl)ureidosulfonyl]benzoic Acid Methyl Ester *see* 8957

1,6-Dimethylpyrimido[5,4-*e*]-1,2,4-triazine-5,7(1*H*,6*H*)-dione *see* 9559

6,8-Dimethylpyrimido[5,4-*e*]-1,2,4-triazine-5,7-(6*H*,8*H*)-dione *see* 4066

*N*¹-(4,6-Dimethyl-2-pyrimidyl)sulfanilamide *see* 8915

5,5-Dimethyl-1-pyrroline 1-Oxide *see* 3393

Dimethyl Quinolyl Methylsulfate Urea *see* 3353

7,8-Dimethyl-10-ribitylisoalloxazine *see* 8200

5,6-Dimethyl-1-α-D-ribofuranosyl-1*H*-benzimidazole *see* 8199

N,N-Dimethylserotonin *see* 1478

2,3-Dimethyl-5-solanesyl-1,4-benzoquinone *see* 7523

[1*R*-(1α,4aα,5α)]-2,4,4'-Dimethylspiro[2-azabicyclo[2.2.2]octane-5,2'-[2*H*]-pyran]-6'(3'*H*)-one *see* 3294

Dimethylsulfamic Acid 5-Butyl-2-(ethylamino)-6-methyl-4-pyrimidinyl Ester *see* 1494

3-Dimethylsulfamido-10-(2-dimethylaminopropyl)phenothiazine *see* 4231

3-Dimethylsulfamoyl-10-[3-(4-methylpiperazino)propyl]phenothiazine *see* 9357

O,O-Dimethyl *O*-*p*-Sulfamoylphenylphosphorothioate *see* 2785

2-Dimethylsulfamoyl-10-[3'-(4″-piperazino)propyl]phenothiazine *see* 9357

3,4-Dimethyl-5-sulfanilamidoisoxazole *see* 8952

4,5-Dimethyl-2-sulfanilamidooxazole *see* 8924

2,6-Dimethyl-4-sulfanilamidopyrimidine *see* 8951

4,6-Dimethyl-2-sulfanilamidopyrimidine *see* 8915

Dimethyl Sulfate, 3256

Dimethyl Sulfide *see* 6123

Dimethylsulfide-α,α'-dicarboxylic Acid *see* 9331

as-Dimethyl Sulfite *see* 6097

2,4-Dimethylsulfolane, 3257

Dimethyl Sulfone, 3258

*N*¹-[3-(Dimethylsulfonio)propyl]bleomycinamide *see* 1318

1,4-Di(methylsulfonoxy)butane *see* 1505

3-[(2,4-Dimethyl-5-sulfophenyl)azo]-4-hydroxy-1-naphthalenesulfonic Acid Disodium Salt *see* 7591

N,N-Dimethyl-*N*-(3-sulfopropyl)-3-[[(3α,-5β,7α,12α)-3,7,12-trihydroxy-24-oxocholan-24-yl]amino]-1-propanaminium Inner Salt *see* 2044

Dimethyl Sulfoxide, 3259

Dimethyl Terephthalate *see* 9162

7α,17α-Dimethyltestosterone *see* 1323

7β,17α-Dimethyltestosterone *see* 1722

2,2-Dimethyl-3-(1,2,2,2-tetrabromoethyl)cyclopropanecarboxylic Acid Cyano(3-phenoxyphenyl)methyl Ester *see* 9565

Dimethyl 2,3,5,6-Tetrachloroterephthalate *see* 2839

7,8-Dimethyl-10-(D-*ribo*-2,3,4,5-tetrahydroxypentyl)isoalloxazine *see* 8200

N,N-Dimethyl-*N*-[2-[2-[4-(1,1,3,3-tetramethylbutyl)phenoxy]ethoxy]ethyl]benzenemethanaminium Chloride *see* 1074

meso-4,4'-(2,3-Dimethyltetramethylene)dipyrocatechol *see* 6693

2,4-Dimethyltetramethylene Sulfone *see* 3257

2,4-Dimethylthiacyclopentane 1,1-Dioxide *see* 3257

Dimethylthiambutene, 3260

2,6-Dimethylthianthrene *see* 5918

2,7-Dimethylthianthrene *see* 5918

Dimethylthiocarbamide *see* 3261

m,N-Dimethylthiocarbanilic Acid *O*-5-Indanyl Ester *see* 9515

m,N-Dimethylthiocarbanilic Acid *O*-2-Naphthyl Ester *see* 9519

asym-Dimethylthionine Chloride *see* 927

3,5-Dimethyl-2-thionotetrahydro-1,3,-5-thiadiazine *see* 2834

N,N'-Dimethylthiourea, 3261

5,8-Dimethyltocol *see* 9496

7,8-Dimethyltocol *see* 9497

Dimethyltoluthionine Chloride *see* 9520

Diphenylacetic Acid 1-Ethyl-3-piperidyl Ester *see* 7470
Diphenylacetic Acid 3α-Tropanyl Ester *see* 9773
Diphenylacetonitrile *see* 3316
Diphenylacetyldiethylaminoethanol *see* 161
2-Diphenylacetyl-1,3-diketohydrindene *see* 3305
Diphenylacetylene *see* 9504
2-Diphenylacetyl-1,3-indandione *see* 3305
2-(Diphenylacetyl)-1*H*-indene-1,3(2*H*)-dione *see* 3305
2,3-Diphenylacrylic Acid *see* 7281
Diphenylamine, 3317
Diphenylamine-2-carboxylic Acid *see* 7273
Diphenylaminechlorarsine *see* 7215
Diphenylamine-2,2′-dicarboxylic Acid, 3318
Diphenylamine Orange *see* 9776
4-Diphenylaminesulfonic Acid *see* 7313
N,N-Diphenyl-1,4-benzenediamine *see* 3329
N,N′-Diphenylbenzidine, 3319
(±)-1-(*p,α*-Diphenylbenzyl)imidazole *see* 1213
N,N′-Diphenyl-[1,1′-biphenyl]-4,4′-diamine *see* 3319
1,4-Diphenyl-1,3-butadiene, 3320
1,3-Diphenyl-2-buten-1-one *see* 3480
(Z)-2-[4-(1,2-Diphenyl-1-butenyl)phenoxy]-*N,N*-dimethylethanamine *see* 9048
1,2-Diphenyl-4-*n*-butyl-4-hydroxymethyl-3,5-dioxopyrazolidine Hemisuccinate *see* 9009
Diphenylcarbamide *see* 1785
N-(3,3-Diphenyl-3-carbamoylpropyl)-*N*-methylperhydroazepinium Iodide *see* 1599
sym-Diphenylcarbazide, 3321
Diphenylcarbazone, 3322
2,2-Diphenyl-4-(4-carbethoxy-4-phenylpiperidino)butyronitrile *see* 3313
Diphenylcarbinol *see* 1090
Diphenyl Carbonate *see* 7278
2,2′-Diphenylcarbonic Dihydrazide *see* 3321
Diphenyl-(2-chlorophenyl)-1-imidazolylmethane *see* 2417
1-(3,3-Diphenyl-3-cyanopropyl)-4-piperidino-4-piperidinecarboxamide *see* 7498
2,4-Diphenyl-1,3-cyclobutanedicarboxylic Acid *see* 9791
1,2-Diphenylcyclopropenone *see* 3308
2,3-Diphenyl-2-cyclopropen-1-one *see* 3308
2-(2,2-Diphenylcyclopropyl)-4,5-dihydro-1*H*-imidazole *see* 2269
(±)-2-(2,2-Diphenylcyclopropyl)-2-imidazoline *see* 2269
2,4′-Diphenyldiamine *see* 1236
N,N′-Diphenyl-α,ω-diaminoethane *see* 2990
Diphenyldiazene *see* 917
Diphenyldiazene 1-Oxide *see* 923
Diphenyl Diimide *see* 917
2,2-Diphenyl-4-diisopropylaminobutyramide Methiodide *see* 5202
Diphenyl-α,β-diketone *see* 1078
2,2-Diphenyl-*N,N*-dimethylacetamide *see* 3307

1,1-Diphenyl-1-(2-dimethylaminoethyl)-2-butanone *see* 6709
4,4-Diphenyl-6-dimethylamino-3-heptanone *see* 5944
1,3-Diphenyl-5-(2-dimethylaminopropionamido)pyrazole *see* 3134
1,1-Diphenyl-1-(2-dimethylaminopropyl)-2-butanone *see* 5944
α,α-Diphenyl-γ-dimethylaminovaleramide *see* 459
2-(2,2-Diphenyl-1,3-dioxolan-4-yl)-piperidine *see* 3299
1,2-Diphenyl-3,5-dioxo-4-[(4-methyl-1-piperazinyl)methyl]-4-butylpyrazolidine *see* 7457
1,2-Diphenyl-3,5-dioxo-4-(2-phenylsulfinylethyl)pyrazolidine *see* 8949
2,4-Diphenyl-1,3,2,4-diselenadiphosphetane 2,4-Diselenide *see* 10051
2,2′-(*p*-Diphenylene)-bis[3,5-diphenyl]-ditetrazolium Chloride *see* 6466
Diphenylene Ketone Oxide *see* 10062
Diphenylenemethane *see* 4155
Diphenylenemethane Sulfide *see* 9368
Diphenylenimine *see* 1790
1,4-Diphenylerythrene *see* 3320
sym-Diphenylethane *see* 1198
1,2-Diphenylethane *see* 1198
N,N-Diphenyl-1,2-ethanediamine *see* 2990
1,2-Diphenyl-1,2-ethanediol *see* 4777
Diphenylethanedione *see* 1078
Diphenylethanedione Dioxime *see* 1079
1,1-Diphenylethene, 3323
Diphenylethenone *see* 3326
Diphenyl Ether *see* 7288
α,α-Diphenyl-α-ethoxyacetic Acid β-Dimethylaminoethyl Ester *see* 3208
2-(1,1-Diphenylethoxy)-*N,N*-dimethylethanamine *see* 6287
α,α-Diphenylethylene *see* 3323
α,β-Diphenylethylene *see* 8817
unsym-Diphenylethylene *see* 3323
N,N′-Diphenylethylenediamine *see* 2990
sym-Diphenylethylenediamine *see* 2990
Diphenylethyleneglycol *see* 4777
1-[2-[3-(2,2-Diphenylethyl)-1,2,4-oxadiazol-5-yl]ethyl]piperidine Monohydrochloride *see* 7736
3-(β,β-Diphenylethyl)-5-(β-piperidinoethyl)-1,2,4-oxadiazole Hydrochloride *see* 7736
Diphenylethyne *see* 9504
Diphenylglycolic Acid *see* 1080
Diphenylglyoxal *see* 1078
Diphenylglyoxime *see* 1079
N,N′-Diphenylguanidine *see* 3324
sym-Diphenylguanidine *see* 3324
1,3-Diphenylguanidine, 3324
2,2-Diphenyl-4-hexamethyleneiminobutyramide *see* 1599
1,1-Diphenyl-3-hexamethyleneiminopropane *see* 7906
Diphenylhydantoin *see* 7322
1,1-Diphenylhydrazine, 3325
5,5-Diphenyl-2,4-imidazolidinedione *see* 7322
Diphenyline *see* 1236
p-Diphenyl Isocyanate *see* 10073
Diphenylketene, 3326
1,2-Diphenyl-4-(γ-ketobutyl)-3,5-pyrazolidinedione *see* 5288
Diphenyl Ketone *see* 1098
Diphenylmagnesium, 3327
Diphenylmethane, 3328

Diphenylmethane-α-carboxylic Acid *see* 3316
Diphenylmethanone *see* 1098
4-Diphenylmethoxy-1-[3-(4-*tert*-butylbenzoyl)propyl]piperidine *see* 3484
2-Diphenylmethoxy-*N,N*-dimethylethanamine *see* 3309
(3-*endo*-)-3-(Diphenylmethoxy)-8-ethyl-8-azabicyclo[3.2.1]octane *see* 3756
3α-(Diphenylmethoxy)-8-ethyl-1α*H*,5α*H*-nortropane *see* 3756
3-(Diphenylmethoxy)-8-methyl-8-azabicyclo[3.2.1]octane Methanesulfonate *see* 1121
4-(Diphenylmethoxy)-1-methylpiperidine *see* 3331
3α-(Diphenylmethoxy)-1α*H*,5α*H*-tropane Methanesulfonate *see* 1121
Diphenylmethylamine *see* 6054
1,1-Diphenylmethylamine *see* 1076
α-*dl*-4,4-Diphenyl-6-methylamino-3-heptanol Acetate *see* 6685
(±)-3-(1-Diphenylmethylazetidin-3-yl) 5-Isopropyl 2-Amino-1,4-dihydro-6-methyl-4-(3-nitrophenyl)-3,5-pyridinedicarboxylate *see* 907
1-Diphenylmethyl-4-*trans*-cinnamyl-piperazine *see* 2305
Di(phenylmethyl)disulfide *see* 3013
3-(Diphenylmethylene)-1,1-diethyl-2-methylpyrrolidinium Bromide *see* 7742
4-(Diphenylmethylene)-1,1-dimethylpiperidinium Methyl Sulfate *see* 3306
3-(Diphenylmethylene)-1-ethyl-2-methylpyrrolidine Ethyl Bromide *see* 7742
1-Diphenylmethyl-4-methylpiperazine *see* 2710
d-2,2-Diphenyl-3-methyl-4-morpholinobutyrylpyrrolidine *see* 2955
1-(Diphenylmethyl)-4-[3-(2-phenyl-1,3-dioxolan-2-yl)propyl]piperazine *see* 3428
1-(Diphenylmethyl)-4-(3-phenyl-2-propenyl)piperazine *see* 2305
2-[4-(Diphenylmethyl)-1-piperazinyl]-ethyl Methyl (±)-1,4-Dihydro-2,6-dimethyl-4-(*m*-nitrophenyl)-3,5-pyridinecarboxylate *see* 5743
1-[3-[4-(Diphenylmethyl)-1-piperazinyl]-propyl]-2-benzimidazolinone *see* 6925
1-[3-[4-(Diphenylmethyl)-1-piperazinyl]-propyl]-1,3-dihydro-2*H*-benzimidazol-2-one *see* 6925
2-[(Diphenylmethyl)sulfinyl]acetamide *see* 6228
2-[(Diphenylmethyl)sulfinyl]-*N*-hydroxyacetamide *see* 170
4,5-Diphenyl-2-oxazolepropanoic Acid *see* 6924
N-(4,5-Diphenyloxazol-2-yl)diethanolamine *see* 3367
2,2′-[(4,5-Diphenyl-2-oxazolyl)imino]-bisethanol *see* 3367
β-(4,5-Diphenyloxazol-2-yl)propionic Acid *see* 6924
Diphenyl Oxide *see* 7288
1,2-Diphenyl-4-(3′-oxobutyl)-3,5-dioxopyrazolidine *see* 5288
Diphenyl-4-γ-oxo-γ-butyric Acid *see* 3963
1,5-Diphenyl-1,4-pentadien-3-one *see* 3006
1,4-Diphenyl-3-(phenylamino)-1*H*-1,2,4-triazolium Inner Salt *see* 6613

Name Index

Diquafosol, 3351
Diquat Dibromide, 3352
Diquinol [Parke-Davis] see 3728
N,N'-Di-6-quinolinylurea see 3353
1,3-Di-6-quinolylurea, 3353
sym-Di-(6-quinolyl)urea see 3353
6,6'-Diquinolylurea see 3353
Dirax [Daiichi] see 5009
Direktan [Gerot] see 6525
Direma see 4781
Direxiode [Delalande] see 5042
Dirgotarl [Horita] see 3174
Dirhenium Heptoxide see 8178
Dirithromycin, 3354
Dirocide [Solvay] see 3116
Dironyl [Schering AG] see 9164
Dirox [Gramon] see 47
Dirythmin SA [AstraZeneca] see 3360
Disadine D.P. [Stuart] see 7698
Disalcid [3M] see 8339
Disalgesic [3M] see 8339
Disalicylic Acid see 8339
Disalunil see 4781
Disarim [Bial] see 2084
Discase [Boots] see 2259
Dis-Cinil [Lusofarmaco] see 6960
Discodermolide, 3355
Discoid [Sagitta] see 4309
Discotrine [3M Pharma] see 6607
Disdolen [Uriach] see 4255
Disepron [Yoshitomi] see 2412
Diseptal C see 8930
Disgren [Uriach] see 9688
Disiamylborane see 1250
DISIDA see 3358
Disilane, 3356
Disilicane see 3356
Disilicoethane see 3356
Disilicon Hexahydride see 3356
Disintegrins see 5314
Disipal [Doetsch, Grether] see 6879
Di-Sipidin see 7510
Diskin see 6960
Dismutec [Sterling Winthrop] see 9002
Disoderm [Schering] see 3048
Disodium Acetarsenate see 810
Disodium Arsenate see 8579
Disodium Arsenoacetate see 808
Disodium Arsonoacetate see 810
Disodium Azodisalicylate see 6841
Disodium 4-[(tert-Butylimino)meth-
  yl]benzene-1,3-disulfonate N-Oxide
  see 3363
Disodium Cromoglycate see 2590
Disodium 3,3'-Diamino-4,4'-dihydroxy-
  arsenobenzene N-Dimethylenesulfo-
  nate see 8941
Disodium p,p'-Diaminodiphenylsulfone-
  N,N'-diglucose Sulfonate see 4463
Disodium o-Dianisidinediazobis(1-naph-
  thol-4-sulfonate) see 1085
Disodium Dihydrogen (1-Hydroxyethyli-
  dene)bis[phosphonate] see 3863
Disodium Dihydrogen Pyrophosphate see
  8572
Disodium-1,2-dihydroxybenzene-3,5-
  disulfonate see 9465
N⁴-(Disodium 1,3-Disulfo-3-phenylpro-
  pyl)sulfanilamide see 6684
Disodium 4,4'-Disulfoxydiphenyl-(2-
  pyridyl)methane see 7406
Disodium Ethylenebis[dithiocarbamate]
  see 6341
Disodium Formaldehydesulfoxylate-di-
  aminodiphenylsulfone see 8968

Disodium Hexachloroplatinate(2−) see
  8623
Disodium Hydrogen Citrate see 2326
Disodium Hydrogen Phosphate see 8659
Disodium 5,5'-Indigotin Disulfonate see
  4944
Disodium N-Methyl-3,5-diiodo-4-pyri-
  done-2,6-dicarboxylate see 8633
(T-4)-Disodium Molybdate (MoO₄²⁻) see
  8645
Disodium Monohydroxy Methylene Di-
  phosphonate see 6940
Disodium Monomethanearsonate see
  5953
Disodium Orthophosphate see 8659
Disodium Phenoltetrabromophthalein
  Sulfonate see 8954
Disodium Phenyl Phosphate, 3357
Disodium p-(γ-Phenylpropylamino)ben-
  zenesulfonamide-α,γ-disulfonate see
  6684
Disodium 1-Phenyl-3-p-sulfamoylanilino-
  1,3-propanedisulfonate see 6684
Disodium Phosphate see 8659
Disodium Pyrocatechol-3,5-disulfonate
  see 9465
Disodium Succinate see 8679
Disodium[sulfonylbis(p-phenylenimino)]-
  dimethanesulfinate see 8968
Disodium o-Tolidinediazobis(1-naphthyl-
  amine-4-sulfonate) see 1101
(T-4)-Disodium Tungstate (WO₄²⁻) see
  8698
Diso-Duriles [AstraZeneca] see 3360
Disofenin, 3358
Disomer [Schering] see 1443
Disonate [Lannett] see 3401
Disophenol, 3359
Disoprivan [AstraZeneca] see 7834
Disoprofol see 7834
Disopyramide, 3360
Disoquin see 5042
Disorat [Boehringer, Mann.] see 6140
Distotat [Isis] see 3197
Dispadol [Specia] see 5849
Disparlure, 3361
Dispas [Ankerfarm] see 3168
Dispril see 1647
Disprin see 1647
Disprol [Reckitt Benckiser] see 47
Disrupt [Hercon] see 3361
Dissenten [SPA] see 5571
Distaclor [Lilly] see 1912
Distamine [Dista] see 7088
Distamycin A see 8772
Distaxid see 6660
Distigmine Bromide, 3362
Distilbène [Gerda] see 3129
Distinct [BASF] see 3145
Disto-5 [Cogla] see 1306
Distol 8 see 3517
Distraneurin [AstraZeneca] see 2384
Distyryl see 3320
Distyryl Ketone see 3006
Disufenton, 3363
1,3-Disulfamyl-4,5-dichlorobenzene
  see 3077
Disulfan see 8930
Disulfatozirconic Acid see 10182
Disulfiram, 3364
2,4-Disulfonyl-α-phenyl-tert-butyl-
  nitrone see 3363
Disulfoton, 3365
Disulfur Dichloride see 8970
Disulfuric Acid see 8009

Disulfuric Acid Dipotassium Salt see 7664
Disulon [Specia] see 8930
Disulone [Specia] see 2822
Disulphine Blue [Zeneca] see 8987
Disyncran see 5964
Disynformon see 3708
Di-Syston [Bayer CropSci.] see 3365
Dita Bark, 3366
Ditaine see 3500
Ditan see 3328
Ditaven [Cascan] see 3163
Ditazol, 3367
Diteftin see 4311
Ditetrazolium Chloride see 9244
Dithane D-14 [Rohm & Haas] see 6341
Dithane M-22 [Dow AgroSci.] see 5721
Dithane M-45 [Dow AgroSci.] see 5716
1,4-Dithiaanthraquinone-2,3-dicarbo-
  nitrile see 3368
δ-[3-(1,2-Dithiacyclopentyl)]pentanoic
  Acid see 9326
Dithianon, 3368
1,2-Dithia-5,8,11,14,17-pentaazacyclo-
  eicosane Cyclic Peptide Deriv see
  6762
2,6-Dithia-1,3,5,7-tetraazaadamantane
  2,2,6,6-Tetraoxide see 9227
2,6-Dithia-1,3,5,7-tetraazatricyclo-
  [3.3.1.1³,⁷]decane 2,2,6,6-Tetraoxide
  see 9227
Dithiazanine Iodide, 3369
3-(Di-2-thienylmethylene)-5-methoxy-
  1,1-dimethylpiperidinium Bromide
  see 9442
3-(Di-2-thienylmethylene)-1-methyl-
  piperidine see 9457
3-(Di-2-thienylmethylene)-5-methyl-
  trans-quinolizidinium Bromide see
  9460
(5R,9aR)-rel-3-(Di-2-thienylmethylene)-
  octahydro-5-methyl-2H-quinolizinium
  Bromide see 9460
Dithio see 8966
4,4'-Dithiobis[2-aminobutanoic Acid]
  see 4735
4,4'-Dithiobis[2-aminobutyric Acid]
  see 4735
[R-(R*,R*)]-3,3'-Dithiobis[2-aminopro-
  panoic Acid] see 2782
2,2'-Dithiobis[benzothiazole], 3370
N,N'-[Dithiobis[2-(2-benzoyloxy)ethyl]-
  1-methyl-2,1-ethenediyl]]bis[N-[(4-
  amino-2-methyl-5-pyrimidinyl)meth-
  yl]formamide] see 1246
N,N'-[Dithiobis[1-[(carboxymethyl)car-
  bamoyl]ethylene]diglutamine see 4475
2,2'-Dithiobisethanamine see 2776
N,N'-[Dithiobis[2,1-ethanediylimino(3-
  oxo-3,1-propanediyl)]]bis[2,4-dihy-
  droxy-3,3-dimethylbutanamide] see
  7012
2,2'-Dithiobis[ethylamine] see 2776
N,N'-[Dithiobis(ethyleneiminocarbonyl-
  ethylene)]bis(2,4-dihydroxy-3,3-di-
  methylbutyramide) see 7012
N,N'-[Dithiobis[2-(2-hydroxyethyl)-1-
  methyl-2,1-ethenediyl]]bis[N-[(4-
  amino-2-methyl-5-pyrimidinyl)-
  methyl]formamide] see 9297
N,N'-[Dithiobis[2-(2-hydroxyethyl)-1-
  methylvinylene]]bis[N-[(4-amino-2-
  methyl-5-pyrimidinyl)methyl]forma-
  mide] Dibenzoate see 1246
3,3'-[Dithiobis(methylene)]bis[5-hy-
  droxy-6-methyl-4-pyridinemetha-
  nol] see 7996

4,4'-Dithiobis[morpholine] *see* 3372
6,6'-Dithiobis-2-naphthalenol *see* 2840
6,6'-Dithiobis(2-naphthol) *see* 2840
3,3'-Dithiobis[6-nitrobenzoic Acid] *see* 3551
5,5'-Dithiobis[2-nitrobenzoic Acid] *see* 3551
3,3'-Dithiobis[pyridine] Dihydrochloride *see* 3373
2,2'-Dithiobispyridine 1,1'-Dioxide *see* 7994
Dithiobis[thioformic Acid] *O,O*-Diethyl Ester *see* 3384
3,3'-Dithiobisvaline *see* 7090
2,4-Dithiobiuret, 3371
Dithiocarb *see* 3378
Dithiocarbamic Acid Monoammonium Salt *see* 516
Dithiocarbonic Acid Cyclic *S,S*-(6-Methyl-2,3-quinoxalinediyl) Ester *see* 6978
Dithiocarbonic Anhydride *see* 1811
Dithiodemeton *see* 3365
β,β'-Dithiodialanine *see* 2782
4,4'-Dithiodimorpholine, 3372
6,6'-Dithiodi-2-naphthol *see* 2840
3,3-Dithiodipyridine Dihydrochloride, 3373
3,3'-Dithiodivaline *see* 7090
Dithioethyleneglycol *see* 3725
1,2-Dithioglycerol *see* 3209
Dithioglycolyl *p*-Arsenobenzamide *see* 793
"Dithiol" *see* 9531
1,2-Dithiolane-3-pentanoic Acid *see* 9326
1,2-Dithiolane-3-valeric Acid *see* 9326
5-[3-(1,2-Dithiolanyl)]pentanoic Acid *see* 9326
5-(1,2-Dithiolan-3-yl)valeric Acid *see* 9326
2,3-Dithiolpropanesulfonic Acid *see* 3210
2-(1,3-Dithiol-2-ylidene)-1,3-dithiole *see* 9242
1,3-Dithiol-2-ylidenepropanedioic Acid Bis(1-methylethyl) Ester *see* 5712
Dithione *see* 8966
Dithionous Acid Disodium Salt *see* 8611
Dithiooxamide *see* 8279
Dithiophos *see* 8966
Dithiophosphoric Acid *O,O'*-Dimethyl-*S*-[(5-methoxy-1,3,4-thiadiazol-2(3*H*)-one-3-yl)methyl] Ester *see* 5970
Dithiopropylthiamine *see* 7882
Dithiopyr, 3374
Dithiosalicylic Acid, 3375
Dithiosteine *see* 3647
1,4-Dithiothreitol, 3376
Dithiotrimethyleneglycol *see* 7801
Dithizone, 3377
Dithranol *see* 684
Dithrocream [Dermal] *see* 684
Ditin Diphosphate *see* 8788
Ditin Pyrophosphate *see* 8788
Ditiocarb Sodium, 3378
1,4-Di-*p*-toluidinoanthraquinone *see* 8065
Ditolyldiazo-3,6-disulfo-β-naphthylamine-β-naphthylamine-6-sulfonic Acid Sodium Salt *see* 10012
α,α-Di-*p*-tolylethane *see* 3379
α,β-Di-*p*-tolylethane *see* 3380
asym-Di-*p*-tolylethane *see* 3379
sym-Di-*p*-tolylethane *see* 3380
1,1-Di-*p*-tolylethane, 3379

1,2-Di-*p*-tolylethane, 3380
p-Ditolylmercury, 3381
Ditrac [Bell] *see* 3305
Ditrazin *see* 3116
1,4-Di(2,2,2-trichloro-1-formamidoethyl)piperazine *see* 9691
Di[tri-(2-methyl-2-phenylpropyl)tin]-oxide *see* 3964
Ditripentat [Heyl] *see* 7124
Ditropan [Sanofi-Synthelabo] *see* 6955
Ditrosol *see* 3279
Diucardin [Ayerst] *see* 4789
Diucardyn Sodium [Ayerst] *see* 5870
Diumax [Cusi-Norte] *see* 7492
Diu-melusin [Schwarz] *see* 4781
Diural [Apothokermes] *see* 4309
Diurese [Am. Urologicals] *see* 9624
Diuretin [Knoll] *see* 9282
Diurex [Makhteshim-Agan] *see* 3382
Diurexan [Viatris] *see* 10079
P[1],*P*[4]-Diuridine 5'-Tetraphosphate *see* 3351
Diuril [Merck & Co.] *see* 2168
Diuriwas [IFI] *see* 53
Diuron, 3382
Diurone *see* 2105
Divalproex Sodium *see* 9913
Divanil *see* 2755
Divanillalcyclohexanone *see* 2755
2,6-Divanillylidenecyclohexanone *see* 2755
Divanon (obsolete) *see* 2755
Divarine [Tutag] *see* 3350
Divasil *see* 8522
Divegal [Waldheim] *see* 3174
Divergan [BASF] *see* 7697
Diverine [Courtois] *see* 3168
Divicine, 3383
Divicine-β-glucoside *see* 9975
Divicine 5-Glucoside *see* 9975
Dividend [Syngenta] *see* 3135
Dividol [Zambon] *see* 9981
Diviminol *see* 9981
Divinorin A *see* 8344
Divinorins *see* 8344
Divinyl *see* 1509
Divinylene Oxide *see* 4296
Divinylene Sulfide *see* 9353
Divinylenimine *see* 8014
Divinyl Ether *see* 9995
Divinyl Oxide *see* 9995
Divipan [Makhteshim-Agan] *see* 3079
Divit Urto *see* 10018
Dixanthogen, 3384
Dixarit [Boehringer, Ing.] *see* 2390
Dixeran [Lundbeck] *see* 5823
Dixnalate [Sana] *see* 4378
Di-*m*-xylylene *see* 5921
m-Dixylylene *see* 5921
N,N-Di-(2,4-xylyliminomethyl)methylamine *see* 486
Dixyrazine, 3385
Dizan [Elanco] *see* 3369
Dizocilpine, 3386
Dizol *see* 483
DJ-1461 *see* 1470
DJ-7041 *see* 8253
Djenkolic Acid, 3387
DK-7419 *see* 779
DKB *see* 3005
DKP *see* 7658
DL-458-IT *see* 2862
DL-473 *see* 8219
DL-717-IT *see* 5585
DL-832 *see* 4436

DL-3117 *see* 5065
DL-8280 *see* 6771
DLP [Dawbarn] *see* 7581
DLP-787 *see* 7988
DM *see* 7215
DM-9384 *see* 6439
DMAA *see* 5829
DMAC *see* 3227
DMAN, 3388
DMAP, 3389
DMC, 3390, 7088
DMDL Protein *see* 9895
DMDP *see* 2371
DMDR *see* 4886
DMDT *see* 5990
DMDZ *see* 6691
DMF *see* 3243
DMFA *see* 3243
DMG *see* 3244
DMGG *see* 5938
DMHP *see* 2859
DMI *see* 3249
DMMP, 3391
DMMPA *see* 6439
DMN *see* 6637
DMNA *see* 6637
DMO *see* 3213
DMP *see* 3255
DMP-115 *see* 7158
DMP-266 *see* 3521
DMPA [Geo] *see* 3253
DMPA, 3392
DMPO, 3393
DMPS *see* 3210
DMS *see* 3256, 8865
DMSA *see* 8865
DMSO *see* 3259
DMSO[2] *see* 3258
DMSP *see* 4000
DMT *see* 3262, 9162
DMTA-P *see* 3214
DMTT *see* 2834
DMX-115 *see* 7158
DN *see* 3279
DN-289 *see* 3287
DNA *see* 2907
DNA D(*P*-Thio)(C-T-A-G-A-T-T-T-C-C-C-G-C-G) Complex with DNA D(*P*-thio)(G-A-T-C-C-G-C-G-G-G-A-A-A-T)(1:1) Hexacosasodium Salt *see* 3511
DNase I *see* 2906
DNBP *see* 3287
DNC *see* 3278, 3279
DNFB *see* 4172
DNOC *see* 3279
DNOCHP *see* 2733
DNOCP *see* 3286
DNP *see* 3359
DNTP *see* 7033
DO-14 *see* 7808
Dobell's Soln *see* 8591
Dobendan [Cassella-med] *see* 2032
Doberol [Boehringer, Ing.] *see* 9516
Dobesilate Calcium, 3394
Dobesin [Abigo] *see* 3127
Dobren [Ravizza] *see* 8989
Doburil [Boehringer, Ing.] *see* 2754
Dobutamine, 3395
Dobutrex [Lilly] *see* 3395
Doca [Organon] *see* 2901
Docarpamine, 3396
Docelan [Aventis] *see* 4809
Docémine [Roussel Uclaf] *see* 10014
Docetaxel, 3397
Docigram [UCB] *see* 10014

Dociton [AstraZeneca] *see* 7840
Doconexent *see* 3398
Docosahexaenoic Acid, 3398
(4Z,7Z,10Z,13Z,16Z,19Z)-4,7,10,13,16,-
19-Docosahexaenoic Acid *see* 3398
(4aS,5aR,10aR,11aS,15aR,15bS,16E,-
18E,19aS,19bR)-2,3,4,4a,5,5a,6,7,8,-
9,10,10a,11,11a,12,13,14,15,15a,15b,-
19a,19b-Docosahydro-1H-diindeno-
[2,1-f:1′,2′-1][1,5]diazacyclotridecine
see 7021
6,7,8,9,10,11,12,13,14,15,16,17,24,25,-
26,27,28,29,30,31,32,33-Docosahy-
dro-35,37-dimethyl-5,34:18,23-dieth-
enodibenzo[b,r][1,5,16,20]tetraaza-
cyclotriacontine-23,34-diium Dichloride *see* 1248
Docosanoic Acid *see* 1023
n-Docosanol, 3399
1-Docosanol *see* 3399
Δ¹³-*cis*-Docosenoic Acid *see* 3674
(Z)-13-Docosenoic Acid *see* 3674
(13E)-13-Docosenoic Acid *see* 1364
Docosyl Alcohol *see* 3399
Docusate Calcium, 3400
Docusate Potassium *see* 3401
Docusate Sodium, 3401
1,2,3,4,7,8,9,10,13,13,14,14-Dodeca-
chloro-1,4,4a,5,6,6a,7,10,10a,11,12,-
12a-dodecahydro-1,4:7,10-dimeth-
anodibenzo[a,e]cyclooctene *see* 2851
1,1a,2,2,3,3a,4,5,5,5a,5b,6-Dodeca-
chlorooctahydro-1,3,4-metheno-1H-
cyclobuta[cd]pentalene *see* 6207
Dodecahedrane, 3402
[1R-(1α,2E,4aα,4bβ,7β,8aα,10β,10aβ)]-
(Dodecahydro-7,10-dihydroxy-1,4b,-
8,8-tetramethyl-2(1H)-phenanthren-
ylidene)acetic Acid 2-(Dimethylamino)ethyl Ester *see* 1890
1,2,3,3a,3b,7,10,10a,10b,11,12,12a-Do-
decahydro-1,11-dihydroxy-2,5,10a,-
12a-tetramethyl-7-phenylcyclopen-
ta[7,8]phenanthro[2,3-c]pyrazol-1-yl
Hydroxymethyl Ketone Acetate *see*
2540
Dodecahydrodiphenylamine *see* 3095
Dodecahydro-3-hydroxy-6-(hydroxymethyl)-3,3a,6-trimethyl-1H-benz-
[e]indene-7-acetic Acid δ-Lactone *see*
6921
[2S-(2α,7β,7aβ,14β,14aα)]-Dodecahy-
dro-2-hydroxy-7,14-methano-2H,-
11H-dipyrido[1,2-a:1′,2′-e][1,5]di-
azocin-11-one *see* 4829
[3bS-(3bα,5aβ,7β,8β,8aα,10bβ)]-3b,4,-
5,6,7,8,9,10,10a,10b,11,12-Dodecahy-
dro-7-hydroxy-10b-methyl-5a,8-
methano-5aH-cyclohepta[5,6]naph-
tho[2,1-b]furan-7-methanol *see* 1634
[1R-(1α,2E,4aα,4bβ,7β,8aα,10aβ)]-(Do-
decahydro-7-hydroxy-1,4b,8,8-tetra-
methyl-10-oxo-2(1H)-phenanthrenyli-
dene)acetic Acid 2-(Dimethylamino)-
ethyl Ester *see* 1891
5,6,7,8,9,10,10′,9′,8′,7′,6′,5′-Dodecahy-
drolycopene *see* 7389
[7S-(7α,7aα,14α,14aβ)]-Dodecahydro-
7,14-methano-2H,6H-dipyrido[1,2-
a:1′,2′-e][1,5]diazocine *see* 8737
Dodecahydro-7,14-methano-2H,6H-di-
pyrido[1,2-a:1′,2′-e][1,5]diazocin-1-ol
see 8159
[7R-(7α,7aβ,14α,14aα)]-Dodecahydro-
7,14-methano-2H,6H-dipyrido[1,2-
a:1′,2′-e][1,5]diazocin-6-one *see* 729

(7α,7aα,14α,14aβ)-Dodecahydro-7,14-
methano-2H,11H-dipyrido[1,2-a:1′,-
2′-e][1,5]diazocin-11-one *see* 5607
Dodecahydro-7,14-methano-4H,6H-di-
pyrido[1,2-a:1′,2′-e][1,5]diazocin-4-
one *see* 5607
(1R,3aR,5aR,6R,9aS)-Dodecahydro-6-
(2Z)-2-penten-4-ynyl-pyrrolo[1,2-a]-
quinoline-1-ethanol *see* 4402
Dodecahydrosqualene *see* 8767
Dodecamethylcyclohexasiloxane, 3403
Dodecamethylpentasiloxane, 3404
Dodecamolybdophosphoric Acid *see* 7342
Dodecanoic Acid *see* 5384
Dodecanoic Acid 1,2-Ethanediyl Ester
see 4497
Dodecanoic Acid Ethyl Ester *see* 3818
Dodecanoic Acid 2-(2-Hydroxyethoxy)-
ethyl Ester *see* 3120
1-Dodecanol, 3405
1-[(2-Dodecanoyloxyethylcarbamoyl)-
methyl]pyridinium Chloride *see* 5370
[S-(all-E)]-3-(1,3,5,7,9-Dodecapentaen-
yloxy)-1,2-propanediol, 3406
Dodécavit [Serb] *see* 4809
2-Dodecenedioic Acid *see* 9576
(Z)-7-Dodecen-1-ol Acetate *see* 5570
cis-7-Dodecenyl Acetate *see* 5570
Dodecoic Acid *see* 5384
Dodecyl Alcohol *see* 3405
Dodecyl Alcohol Polyoxyethylene Ether
see 7558
1-Dodecyl-4-aminoquinaldinium Acetate
see 5387
1-Dodecylazacycloheptan-2-one *see* 5385
Dodecylbenzene Sodium Sulfonate *see*
8612
Dodecylbenzenesulfonic Acid Sodium
Salt *see* 8612
N-Dodecyl-N,N-bis(2-hydroxyethyl)ben-
zenemethanaminium Chloride *see* 1111
Dodecyl Bromide *see* 5389
N-Dodecyl-ε-caprolactam *see* 5385
Dodecyl 2,4-Diguanidinophenyl Ether
see 5386
Dodecyldi(β-hydroxyethyl)benzylam-
monium Chloride *see* 1111
Dodecyldimethyl(2-phenoxyethyl)am-
monium Bromide *see* 3415
Dodecylguanidine Monoacetate *see* 3408
1-Dodecylhexahydro-2H-azepin-2-one
see 5385
α-Dodecyl-ω-hydroxypoly(oxy-1,2-eth-
anediyl) *see* 7558
(2R,3S)-2-Dodecyl-3-methylbutanedioic
Acid *see* 8244
d-α-Dodecyl-β-methylsuccinic Acid *see*
8244
(2R,3S)-2-Dodecyl-3-methylsuccinic Acid
see 8244
N,N‴-[4-(Dodecyloxy)-1,3-phenylene]-
bisguanidine *see* 5386
1,1′-[4-(Dodecyloxy)-m-phenylene]di-
guanidine *see* 5386
Dodemorph, 3407
Dodigen 1881 [Hoechst] *see* 3099
Dodine, 3408
Dofetilide, 3409
Dogalina [Angelini] *see* 1035
Dogbane *see* 742
Dog Buttons *see* 6730
Dog Grass *see* 9761
Dogmatil [Synthelabo] *see* 8989
Dogmatyl [Fujisawa] *see* 8989
Dogwood *see* 2535

Doisynolic Acid, 3410
Doktacillin *see* 586
Dolac [Syntex] *see* 5306
Doladene *see* 5958
Dolalgial [Pharmainvesti] *see* 2392
Dolantin [HMR] *see* 5849
Dolasetron, 3411
Dolasetron Mesylate *see* 3411
Dolazon [Graeub] *see* 3350
Dolcidium [Galephar] *see* 4968
Dolcol [Dainippon] *see* 7460
Dolcontin *see* 6276
Dolcuran [Szabo] *see* 8225
Dolcymene *see* 2763
Dolerophane *see* 2654
Dolestan [Krewel] *see* 3309
Dolestine [Teva] *see* 5849
Dolgit [Dolorgiet] *see* 4881
Dolicur [Schering AG] *see* 3259
Dolipol [Aventis] *see* 9507
Doliprane [Théraplix] *see* 47
Dolisal [Merck & Co.] *see* 3146
Dolisina *see* 3108
Dolmatil [Lorex] *see* 8989
Dolmen [Sigma-Tau] *see* 9148
Dolobid [Merck & Co.] *see* 3146
Dolobis [Merck & Co.] *see* 3146
Dolocyl [Novartis] *see* 4881
Dolomite *see* 5653
Dolonevran [Dausse] *see* 2451
Dolophine [Lilly] *see* 5944
Dolosal [Specia] *see* 5849
Doloteffin [Ardeypharm] *see* 2942
Dolprone [Bottu] *see* 47
DOM, 3412
Domain *see* 8951
Domar [Zambeletti] *see* 7442
Domark [Isagro] *see* 9193
Domeboro [Bayer] *see* 324
Domesticine, 3413
Domestine *see* 3413
D.O.M.F. *see* 5867
Domical [Berk] *see* 487
Domin [Boehringer, Ing.] *see* 9039
Dominal [AWD] *see* 7888
Dominator [Schering] *see* 7497
Domiodol, 3414
Domiphen Bromide, 3415
Domitor [Pfizer] *see* 5787
Domitroban, 3416
Domoic Acid, 3417
Domosedan [Farmos] *see* 2937¹
Domoso [Syntex] *see* 3259
Domperidone, 3418
DON *see* 3002
Dona [Rottapharm] *see* 4458
Donamet *see* 156
Donaseven [Yakult] *see* 1789
Donaxine *see* 4533
Donepezil, 3419
Donmox [Horita] *see* 53
Donopon *see* 1588
Donorest [Wyeth] *see* 4003
Doom [United Phosphorus] *see* 3079
Doom Bark *see* 8382
DOP *see* 2864
Dopa, 3420
L-Dopa *see* 5464
Dopacard *see* 3424
Dopaflex [Medimpex] *see* 5464
Dopaidan [DeAngeli] *see* 5464
Dopal [Kyowa] *see* 5464
Dopalina [Lepetit] *see* 5464
Dopamet [Dumex] *see* 6055
Dopamine, 3421

Dopan, 3422
Dopar *see* 5464
Doparkine [Armstrong] *see* 5464
Doparl [Kyowa] *see* 5464
threo-Dopaserine *see* 3457
Dopasol [Daiichi] *see* 5464
Dopastat [Parke-Davis] *see* 3421
Dopastin, 3423
Dopaston [Sankyo] *see* 5464
Dopastral [Astra] *see* 5464
Dopegyt [Egis] *see* 6055
Dopergin [Schering AG] *see* 5518
Dopexamine, 3424
Dopexamine Hydrochloride *see* 3424
Dopram [Robins] *see* 3432
Doprin [SK & F] *see* 5464
Dops [Sumitomo] *see* 3457
L-DOPS *see* 3457
L-*threo*-DOPS *see* 3457
Dorado [Syngenta] *see* 7983
Doral [Wallace] *see* 8029
Doralese [GSK] *see* 4969
Doralin [Menarini] *see* 6898
Doramectin, 3425
Dorantamin [Dorsey] *see* 7984
Doraxamin [Dorsey] *see* 3183
Dorcalm [Frere] *see* 2072
Dorcostrin [Dorsey] *see* 2901
Doricenone [Firmenich] *see* 2809
Dorico *see* 4704
Dorico Soluble *see* 4704
Doridamina [Angelini] *see* 5568
Doriden [Novartis] *see* 4477
Dorison *see* 5846
Dorixina [Roemmers] *see* 2392
Dormalest *see* 5846
Dormalin [Schering-Plough] *see* 8029
Dormate [Wallace] *see* 5773
Dormicum [Roche] *see* 6182
Dormidin *see* 5846
Dormigen *see* 5846
Dormigene [Pharmacobel] *see* 1397
Dormin *see* 11
Dormiphen *see* 5846
Dormison [Schering] *see* 5846
Dormodor [Roche] *see* 4198
Dormonoct [Hoechst] *see* 5574
Dormosan *see* 5846
Dormwell [Smith & Nephew] *see* 3046
Dornase Alfa *see* 2906
Dornavac [Merck & Co.] *see* 2906
Dorner [Toray] *see* 1152
Dorsiflex [Drossapharm] *see* 5851
Doryl [Merck KGaA] *see* 1779
Doryx [Faulding] *see* 3440
Dorzolamide, 3426
Dosberotec [Boehringer, Ing.] *see* 3981
Dostinex [Pharmacia & Upjohn] *see* 1601
Dosulepin *see* 3429
Dotan [Calliope S.A.] *see* 2103
(DOTA D-Phe¹,Tyr³)octreotide *see* 3513
Dotarizine, 3428
DOTATOC *see* 3513
Dothiepin, 3429
Double-mycin [Heyl] *see* 3179
Dovenix [Specia] *see* 6656
Dovonex [Westwood-Squibb] *see* 1641
Dow 1329 *see* 3392
Dow General [Dow] *see* 3287
Dow Selective [Dow] *see* 3287
Dow Shield [Dow AgroSci.] *see* 2400
Dowanol DPM [Dow] *see* 3344
Dowco 118 *see* 3392
Dowco 132 *see* 2604

Dowco 179 *see* 2189
Dowco 213 [Dow] *see* 2760
Dowco 214 *see* 2189
Dowco 233 *see* 9656
Dowco 290 *see* 2400
Dowco 356 *see* 9662
Dowco 433 *see* 4203
Dowex 1-X2-Cl *see* 2202
Dowfax 9N [Dow] *see* 6677
Dowfax 9N9 [Dow] *see* 6677
Dowfume W 85 *see* 3796
Dowicide 1 [Dow] *see* 7304
Dowicide 2 [Dow] *see* 9643
Dowicide 2S [Dow] *see* 9644
Dowicide 9 [Dow], 3430
Dowicide A [Dow] *see* 7304
Dowicide B [Dow] *see* 9643
Dowicide G [Dow] *see* 7109
Dowicil 75 [Dow] *see* 8027
Dowicil 200 [Dow] *see* 8027
Dowlap *see* 9642
Dowmycin E [Dow] *see* 3687
Dowpon *see* 2802
Doxacurium Chloride, 3431
Doxamax [Esparma] *see* 3433
Doxans [Schiapparelli] *see* 3434
Doxapram, 3432
Doxapril [Erba] *see* 3432
Doxazosin, 3433
Doxazosin Mesylate *see* 3433
Doxefazepam, 3434
Doxephrin *see* 5948
Doxepin, 3435
Doxercalciferol, 3436
Doxergan *see* 6946
Doxicrisol [Quimifar] *see* 3440
Doxidan [HMR] *see* 3400
Doxifluridine, 3437
Doxil [Ortho Biotech] *see* 3439
Doxinate [Hoechst] *see* 3401
Doxirobe [Pharmacia & Upjohn] *see* 3440
Doxium [Carrion] *see* 3394
Doxofylline, 3438
Doxol [Blair] *see* 3401
Doxophylline *see* 3438
Doxorubicin, 3439
Doxychol *see* 6928
Doxycycline, 3440
Doxycycline Hyclate *see* 3440
Doxylamine, 3441
Doxylar [Sandoz] *see* 3440
Doyle [Tanabe Seiyaku] *see* 852
Dozic [Rosemont] *see* 4598
2,4-DP *see* 3078
DP-178 *see* 3582
DPA *see* 3312, 7804
DPC *see* 3308
DPD *see* 1517
DPE *see* 3338
D-Penamine [Dista] *see* 7088
DPGME *see* 3344
DPM *see* 3344
DPN *see* 6344
DPNH *see* 6344
DPPC *see* 2477
DPPD *see* 3329
DPPE *see* 9178
DPPH *see* 3330
DPQ, 3442
D-Pron [Minnesota Pharm.] *see* 3350
d(P-Thio)(T-C-T-C-C-A-G-C-G-T-G-
 C-G-C-C-A-T)DNA *see* 6739
DPX-1410 *see* 6920
DPX-3217 *see* 2765
DPX-3674 *see* 4699

DPX-3792 *see* 33
DPX-4189 *see* 2191
DPX-5648 *see* 8957
DPX-43898 *see* 2087
DPX-66037 *see* 9689
DPX-A8947 *see* 912
DPX-E9636 *see* 8230
DPX EY-059 *see* 4133
DPX-F5384 *see* 1052
DPX-F6025 *see* 2093
DPX-H6573 *see* 4206
DPX-JE874 *see* 3931
DPX-JW062 *see* 4971
DPX-KE459 *see* 4195
DPX-KN128 *see* 4971
DPX-M6316 *see* 9316
DPX-MP062 *see* 4971
DPX-PE350 *see* 7993
DPX-R6447 *see* 894
DPX-T3792 *see* 33
DPX-T6376 *see* 6158
DPX-V9360 *see* 6522
DPX-Y6202 *see* 8086
DPX-Y5893-9 *see* 4713
DQ-2466 *see* 1873
DQ-2511 *see* 3488
DQ-2805 *see* 5091
DR-3355 *see* 6771
DRA *see* 3455
Dracylic Acid *see* 1091
Draganon [Roche] *see* 662
Dragnet [FMC] *see* 7180
Dragon's Blood, 3443
Dragosantol [Dragoco] *see* 1241
Drainasept [Geistlich] *see* 9076
Drakeol [Penreco] *see* 7186
Dramamine [Searle] *see* 3207
Dramarin *see* 3207
Dramocen [Central Pharm.] *see* 3207
Dramyl *see* 3207
Drat [M & B] *see* 2152
Draxxin [Pfizer] *see* 9810
Draza [Bayer CropSci.] *see* 5972
DRC-1201 *see* 5010
Drenison [Lilly] *see* 4197
Drenusil [Pfizer] *see* 7584
DrFP583 *see* 8126
Driclor [Stiefel] *see* 337
Dridase [Sanofi-Synthelabo] *see* 6955
Dridol *see* 3450
Dried Barium Hydroxide *see* 977
Dried Calcium Sulfate *see* 1706
Dried Cupric Sulfate *see* 2653
Dried Egg White *see* 215
Dried Ferrous Sulfate *see* 4057
Dried Gypsum *see* 1706
Dried Magnesium Sulfate *see* 5691
Dried Zinc Sulfate *see* 10159
Drierite *see* 1706
Drimenin, 3444
Dri-Na *see* 8637
Drinalfa [Squibb] *see* 5948
Drinox *see* 4656
Driol [Sanofi] *see* 6887
Drisdol [Winthrop] *see* 10018
Drithocreme [Dermik] *see* 684
Dritho-Scalp [Dermik] *see* 684
Drixin *see* 6966
Drocarbil *see* 778
Drocode *see* 3171
Drocort [Lilly] *see* 4197
Drofenine, 3445
Drogenil [Schering] *see* 4208
Drolban [Lilly] *see* 3448
Droleptan [Le Brun] *see* 3450

Droloxifene, 3446
Drometrizole, 3447
Dromilac see 4731
Dromoran [Roche] see 5470
Dromostanolone, 3448
Dronabinol see 9209
Dronal [Sigma-Tau] see 229
Droncit [Bayer] see 7716
Dronedarone, 3449
Drop Chalk see 1657
Dropp [Bayer CropSci.] see 9313
Droprenilamine, 3451
Droprenylamine see 3451
Dropropizine, 3452
Drosera, 3453
Drosophilin B see 7534
Drospirenone, 3454
Drostanolone see 3448
Drotaverine, 3455
Drotaverine Theophylline-7-acetic Acid
    see 3455
Drotebanol, 3456
Drotrecogin Alfa see 7884
Droxarol [Pharmos] see 1474
Droxaryl [Continental Pharma] see 1474
Droxia [BMS] see 4848
Droxidopa, 3457
Droxone (obsolete) [BMS] see 240
DRP see 9895
Drumstick see 1894
Dry Clox [Wyeth] see 2419
Dry Ice see 1809
Drylin [Merckle] see 8918
Drynap [Wako] see 8637
Dryobalanops Camphor see 1338
Dryophantin see 7946
Dryptal [Berk] see 4309
Drysol [Person & Covey] see 337
DS-103-282 see 9485
DS-4823 see 8446
DSCG see 2590
ds-Hirudin see 4718
DSIP, 3458
DSMA see 5953
DSP see 8659
DSPA, 3459
DsRed see 8126
DSS see 3401
DST see 3179
DT-327 see 2393
LDT see 9117
DTAF, 3460
DTBP, 3461
DTC see 3378
DTF see 3094
d[(R)-P-Thio](G-C-C-A-A-G-C-T-G-
    G-C-A-T-C-C-G-T-C-A)deoxyribonu-
    cleic Acid see 245
d(P-Thio)(G-C-G-T-T-T-G-C-T-C-T-T-C-
    T-T-C-T-T-G-C-G)deoxyribonucleic
    acid see 4229
d(P-Thio)(G-T-T-C-T-C-G-C-T-G-G-T-
    G-A-G-T-T-T-C-A)deoxyribonucleic
    Acid see 755
DTIC see 2798
DTIC-Dome [Bayer] see 2798
DTMC see 3086
DTNB see 3551
DTPA see 7125
[DTPA-D-Phe¹]-octreotide see 7126
DTPA-SMS see 7126
DTPT see 7882
D-Tracetten see 10018
dTVT see 865

DTX see 2892
DU see 3003
Du Pont 634 see 5435
Du Pont 753 see 5583
Du Pont Herbicide 326 see 5509
Du Pont Herbicide 732 see 9155
Du Pont Herbicide 976 see 1381
DU-1219 see 200
DU-6859 see 8551
DU-6859a see 8551
DU-21220 see 8237
DU-23000 see 4219
DU-28853 see 3552
DU-29373 see 4100
DU-112307 see 3142
DU-127090 see 1210
DU-319722 see 4123
Duact [Glaxo Wellcome] see 127
Dual [Syngenta] see 6146
Dual Gold [Syngenta] see 6146
Duatok [Am. Cyanamid] see 8943
Dubimax [Oberval] see 6353
Dubnium, 3462
Duboisine see 4858
"Dubos Crude Crystals" see 9841
Dufaston [ISM] see 3474
Dufrenite see 4029
Duhnul-balsan see 948
Dulcamara, 3463
Dulcin, 3464
Dulcion [Dulcis] see 3653
Dulcite see 4332
Dulcitol see 4332
Dulcivac [Harvey] see 3401
Dulcolan [Boehringer, Ing.] see 1242
Dulcolax [Boehringer, Ing.] see 1242
Dulcose see 4332
Duloxetine, 3465
Dumirox [Solvay] see 4219
Dumitone see 2822
Duna [Tedec Zambeletti] see 7442
Duodin see 4785
Duofilm [Schering] see 8332
Duogastral [ISM] see 7491
Duolip [Merckle] see 9284
Duoplant [Schering] see 8332
Duosan see 3597
Duosol [Interdelta] see 2485
DUP-453 see 3713
DUP-753 see 5583
DUP-785 see 1370
Dupéran [Cassenne] see 2383
Duphacid [Duphar] see 3142
Duphacycline [Solvay Duphar] see 6976
Duphafral D₃ 1000 see 10019
Duphalac [Solvay] see 5346
Duphaston [Roxane] see 3474
DuPHOS, 3466
Duplosan DP [BASF] see 3078
Duplosan KV [BASF] see 5784
Duponol see 4367
Duprene see 6461
Durabetason [Durachemie] see 1180
Durabolin [Organon] see 6365
Durabolin-O [Organon] see 3805
Duracebrol [Durachemie] see 6496
Duracef [BMS] see 1913
Duracide [Endura] see 7476
Duracillin [Lilly] see 7097
Duraclamid [Durachemie] see 6143
Duraclon [Roxane] see 2390
Duracreme [LRC] see 6677
Duracroman see 2590
Duract see 1390
Duradoce [Atlantis] see 4809

Duradoxal [Merck KGaA] see 3440
Durafurid [Durachemie] see 4309
Duragel [LRC] see 6677
Duragentam [Merck KGaA] see 4392
Duragesic see 4001
Duraglucon [Dura] see 4478
Duralease [Merial] see 3703
Duramin [Fuji] see 5915
Duramipress [Durachemie] see 7717
Duramucal [Durachemie] see 386
Duranest [Astra] see 3862
Durango [Dow AgroSci.] see 4512
Duranifin [Merck dura] see 6528
Duranol [Elan] see 7840
Durapatite, 3467
Durapental [Durachemie] see 7136
Duraphat [Woelm] see 8618
Duraphyllin [Merck KGaA] see 9285
Durapirenz [Durachemie] see 7491
Duraquin [Warner-Chilcott] see 8060
Duravolten [Dura] see 3081
Durazanil [Durachemie] see 1385
Durazepam [Merck KGaA] see 6926
Durenat [Schering AG] see 8914
Durene, 3468
Duretic see 6005
Duricef [BMS] see 1913
Durogesic [J & J] see 4001
Durohydroquinone, 3469
Durol see 3468
Durolax [Boehringer, Ing.] see 1242
Duromine [3M Pharma] see 7262
Duroprocin [Minerva] see 8917
Duroquinone, 3470
Durrax [Dermik] see 4849
Dursban [Dow AgroSci.] see 2189
Dusodril [Roland] see 6353
Duspatal [Duphar] see 5769
Duspatalin [Duphar] see 5769
Dutasteride, 3471
Dutch Liquid see 3797
Duteplase see 9468
Du-Ter [Duphar] see 9745
Duthaler-Hafner Reagent, 3472
Dutonin [BMS] see 6438
Duvadilan [Duphar] see 5238
Duvaline [Almirall] see 7975
Duviculine [Duphar] see 5238
Duvoid [Shire] see 1185
Duxima [Dukron] see 1954
DV [HMR] see 3104
DV-1006 see 2024
DVC see 2755
D₃-Vicotrat see 10019
DW-61 see 4096
DW-3418 see 2685
Dwale see 1025
Dwarf Bay see 6170
DX-8951 see 3912
DX-8951f see 3912
DX.C see 2938
Dya-Tron [Myers-Carter] see 3350
Dybar [DuPont] see 4009
Dybenal see 3060
Dycholium see 2868
Dycill [SKB] see 3084
Dyclone [Dow] see 3473
Dyclonine, 3473
Dydrogesterone, 3474
Dyer's Alkanet see 256
Dyer's Saffron see 1868
Dyflos see 5176
Dyfonate [Stauffer] see 4233
Dygratyl [Ferrosan] see 3180
Dykon see 8607

Dylate [Unimed] *see* 2391
Dylene [Arco] *see* 8860
Dylox [Bayer] *see* 9623
Dymanthine, 3475
Dymelor [Lilly] *see* 62
Dymid [Lilly] *see* 3307
Dymion [Pulitzer] *see* 9843
Dynabac [Lilly] *see* 3354
Dynacaine *see* 8013
Dynacil [Schwarz] *see* 4256
Dynacin [Medicis] *see* 6202
DynaCirc [Novartis] *see* 5240
Dynacoryl *see* 6543
Dynamin, 3476
Dynamite *see* 6607
Dynamutilin [Novartis] *see* 9419
Dynapen [Apothecon] *see* 3084
Dynaphylline [Welcker-Lyster] *see* 24
Dynastat [Pfizer] *see* 7036
Dynatra [Simes] *see* 3421
Dynel, 3477
Dynel [Union Carbide] *see* 6227
Dynese [Galen] *see* 5651
Dynexan [Kreussler] *see* 5482
Dynorm [Roche] *see* 2273
Dynorphin, 3478
Dynorphin₁₋₁₃ *see* 3478
1-13-Dynorphin (Pig) *see* 3478
Dynothel [Henning] *see* 9415
Dynovas [Mayrand] *see* 7019
Dyodin *see* 5042
Dyphylline, 3479
Dypnone, 3480
Dyprin [Lincoln] *see* 5975
Dyren [Sejin] *see* 9599
Dyrene [Bayer] *see* 657
Dyrenium [SKB] *see* 9599
Dyscural *see* 3728
Dysedon *see* 6946
Dysidiolide, 3481
(−)-Dysidiolide *see* 3481
Dyskinébyl [Saunier] *see* 6960
Dysmenalgit [Krewel] *see* 6417
Dyspamet [Bridge] *see* 2279
Dysport [Ipsen] *see* 1357
Dysprosia *see* 3482
Dysprosium, 3482
Dystrophin, 3483
Dystrophin-related Protein *see* 9895
Dytac [Bridge] *see* 9599
Dytransin *see* 4880
DZL-221 *see* 6439
"E" *see* 5767
E2FD *see* 3511
E2F Decoy *see* 3511
E36U31 *see* 9153
E-141 *see* 3722
E-187 *see* 6189
E-212 *see* 9562
E-250 *see* 8428
E-265 *see* 9566
E-600 *see* 7030
E-601 *see* 6108
E-605 *see* 7033
E-607 *see* 5370
E-614 *see* 9737
E-643 *see* 1487
E-646 *see* 3606
E-0659 *see* 906
E-0671 *see* 9153
E-0687 *see* 1206
E-838 *see* 4855
E-1020 *see* 5575
E-1059 *see* 2889
E-2020 *see* 3419

E-2663 *see* 1054
E-3314 *see* 4656
E-3710 *see* 2336
E-3810 *see* 8089
E-4018 *see* 2336
E-4424 *see* 5447
E-5510 *see* 8383
E-5564 *see* 3671
E-6010 *see* 6259
EA-1299 *see* 5765
EACA *see* 432
Eagle [Aventis] *see* 403
Eagle [Dow AgroSci.] *see* 6321
Eagle Vine *see* 2496
EAK *see* 6084
Eaklite *see* 1702
Earthnut *see* 7058
Earthnut Oil *see* 7059
Earth Wax *see* 1987
Easter Flower *see* 7938
Eastern Poison Oak *see* 7550
East Indian Balmony *see* 2064
"East Indian Copaiba" *see* 947
East India Root *see* 4338
Eastman No. 1361 *see* 8049
Eatan [Desitin] *see* 6575
Eau Celeste *see* 9181
Eau de Javelle *see* 4865
Eazaminum *see* 3108
EB-382 *see* 300
EB-1089 *see* 8456
EB-1856 *see* 244
Ebalin [Allergopharma] *see* 1443
E-Base *see* 3681
Ebastel [Almirall] *see* 3484
Ebastine, 3484
Ebert-Merz α-Acid *see* 6375
Ebert-Merz β-Acid *see* 6374
Ebivit *see* 10019
Ebixa [Lundbeck] *see* 5829
Ebrantil [Byk Gulden] *see* 9865
Ebrocit [Ferrer] *see* 3485
Ebrodin [Ferrer] *see* 3485
Ebrotidine, 3485
Ebselen, 3486
Ebucin *see* 1669
Ebufos *see* 1632
Eburnal [Chiesi] *see* 3487
(3α,16α)-Eburnamenine-14-carboxylic
     Acid Ethyl Ester *see* 9991
(3α,16α)-Eburnamenin-14(15H)-one *see*
     3487
Eburnamenin-14(15H)-one *see* 3487
(±)-Eburnamenin-14(15H)-one *see* 3487
Eburnamonine, 3487
(+)-cis-Eburnamonine *see* 3487
Ebutol [Kaken] *see* 3720
EC 1.4.3.6 *see* 2975
EC 3.1.6.12 *see* 819
EC 3.2.1.11 *see* 2949
EC 3.4.21.5 *see* 9383
EC 3.4.24.27 *see* 9286
EC 3.5.1.1 *see* 836
ECA *see* 3787
Ecabamide *see* 3488
Ecabapide, 3488
Ecabet, 3489
Ecamsule, 3490
Ecarazine *see* 9502
Ecasolv [Lepetit] *see* 4653
Ecazide [BMS] *see* 1774
Ecboline *see* 3665
Eccothal [Centerchem] *see* 9269
Ecdysone *see* 3491
α-Ecdysone *see* 3491

β-Ecdysone *see* 3491
Ecdysteroids, 3491
Ecdysterone *see* 3491
ECGF *see* 4072
Ecgonidine, 3492
Ecgonine, 3493
Ecgonine Benzoate *see* 1113
Ecgonine Ethyl Ester Benzoate (Ester)
     see 2454
Ecgonine Methyl Ester Benzoate *see* 2455
Echinacea, 3494
Echinacein *see* 3494
Echinacoside *see* 3494
Echinatin *see* 5479
Echinenone, 3495
Echinochrome A, 3496
Echinomycin, 3497
Echinopsine, 3498
Echinuline, 3499
Echitamine, 3500
Echothiophate Iodide, 3501
Echovist [Schering] *see* 4335
Echujetin *see* 3162
Eclipse Red *see* 1101
Ecobutazone [Empire] *see* 7277
Ecodipin [Ecosol] *see* 6528
Ecodurex [Ecosol] *see* 406
Ecofenac [Ecosol] *see* 3081
Ecolid *see* 2101
Econazole, 3502
Econor [Novartis] *see* 9911
EcoPLA [Cargill Dow] *see* 5338
Ecothiopate Iodide *see* 3501
Ecotrin [GSK] *see* 851
Ecoval 70 *see* 1180
Ecovent [Ecosol] *see* 216
ECP *see* 3703
Ecrinal [Pharma Investi] *see* 4098
Ecristidine *see* 4720
"Ecstasy" *see* 5767
Ecteinascidin 743 *see* 3503
Ecteinascidins, 3503
ECTEOLA-Cellulose, 3504
Ectiban [Schering-Plough] *see* 7180
Ectodex [Intervet] *see* 486
Ectoin *see* 3505
Ectoine, 3505
Ecuanil [Wyeth-Ayerst] *see* 5862
Eculizumab, 3506
Eczecidin *see* 5031
Eczederm [Quinoderm] *see* 10147
ED *see* 3860
ED-749 *see* 3512
10-EDAAM *see* 3507
Edalene [Rhône-Poulenc] *see* 2279
10-EdAM *see* 3507
Edathamil *see* 3517
Edatrexate, 3507
EDB *see* 3796
EDC *see* 3797
EDDP *see* 3510
EDDS, 3508
Edecril [Merck & Co.] *see* 3717
Edecrin [Merck & Co.] *see* 3717
Edemox [Wassermann] *see* 53
Edestin, 3509
Edetate Calcium Disodium *see* 3517
Edetate Disodium *see* 3517
Edetate Sodium *see* 3517
Edetate Trisodium *see* 3517
Edetic Acid *see* 3517
Edetic Acid Sodium Iron Salt *see* 4031
Edex [Schwarz] *see* 7876
EDF *see* 4997
EDGF-II *see* 4072

Edifenphos, 3510
Edifoligide Sodium, 3511
Ediphenphos *see* 3510
Edornat [Albert-Roussel] *see* 4824
Edotecarin, 3512
Edotreotide, 3513
Edoxudine, 3514
Edpetiline *see* 4926
Edrecolomab, 3515
EDRF *see* 6578
Edronax [Pharmacia & Upjohn] *see* 8125
Edrophone Bromide *see* 3516
Edrophonium Bromide *see* 3516
Edrophonium Chloride, 3516
EDTA, 3517
EDU *see* 3514
Edurid [Robugen] *see* 3514
EEDQ, 3518
E.E.S. [Abbott] *see* 3681
EF-9 *see* 9138
Efalexin [Maipe] *see* 1974
Efalizumab, 3519
Efamast [Scotia] *see* 3906
Efamol [Efamol Res.] *see* 3906
Efaproxiral, 3520
Efavirenz, 3521
Efcortelan [GSK] *see* 4787
Efcortelan Soluble [GSK] *see* 4787
Efcortesol [GSK] *see* 4787
Efektolol [Brenner-Efeka] *see* 7840
Eferox [Wyeth] *see* 9415
Effectin [Winthrop] *see* 1307
Effekton [Teofarma] *see* 3081
Effer-Syllium [J & J-Merck] *see* 7517
Effexor [Wyeth] *see* 9946
Effluderm [Allergan] *see* 4181
Efflumidex [Allergan] *see* 4175
Effontil [Boehringer, Ing.] *see* 3865
Effortil [Boehringer, Ing.] *see* 3865
Effusan *see* 3279
Efisol [Roland] *see* 2913
Eflone [Novartis] *see* 4175
Eflornithine, 3522
Efloxate, 3523
Efodine [Fougera] *see* 7698
Efonidipine, 3524
Efortil [Boehringer, Ing.] *see* 3865
Efosite Al *see* 4252
Efrane [Abbott] *see* 3581
Efrotomycin, 3525
Eftapan [Merckle] *see* 3632
Efudex [Roche] *see* 4181
Efudix [Roche] *see* 4181
Eg5 *see* 6244
Egacene *see* 4858
Egalin [Dainippon] *see* 8120
Egazil Duretter *see* 4858
EGb 761 *see* 4425
EGCG, 3526
EGDN *see* 3800
EGF *see* 3527
EGF-URO *see* 3527
EGF-Urogastrone, 3527
Egg Albumin *see* 6902
Egg Oil, 3528
Egg White *see* 215
Egibren [Chiesi] *see* 8428
EGIS-2062 *see* 8472
EGIS-3886 *see* 2915
Eglen [Tatsumi] *see* 2305
Egmol *see* 7245
Egressin *see* 9409
EGTA, 3529
EGYT-201 *see* 1033
EGYT-341 *see* 9503

EGYT-475 *see* 7392
EGYT-1050 *see* 2852
EGYT-2062 *see* 8472
Ehrlich 5 *see* 6948
Ehrlich 594 *see* 52
Ehrlich 606 *see* 811
Ehrlich's Reagent *see* 3230
EHS-laminin *see* 5351
EI-546 *see* 8558
EI-3911 *see* 7331
EI-47470 *see* 5855
Eicosamethylnonasiloxane, 3530
Eicosanoic Acid *see* 764
Eicosapentaenoic Acid, 3531
(*all-Z*)-5,8,11,14,17-Eicosapentaenoic
   Acid *see* 3531
(5Z,8Z,11Z,14Z,17Z)-5,8,11,14,17-Eico-
   sapentaenoic Acid *see* 3531
(5Z,8Z,11Z,14Z)-5,8,11,14-Eicosatetra-
   enoic Acid *see* 765
Eikonogen *see* 455
Einalon S [Kodama] *see* 4598
EinsAlpha [Thomae] *see* 4819
Einsteinium, 3532
Ejibil *see* 3768
Eka-cesium *see* 4262
Ekamet [Sandoz] *see* 3893
Ekonal [Yoshitomi] *see* 6661
Eksmin [Sumitomo] *see* 7180
Ektebin [Hefa] *see* 7891
Ekvacillin [AstraZeneca] *see* 2419
EL-103 *see* 9095
EL-107 *see* 5235
EL-110 *see* 1040
EL-119 *see* 6885
EL-161 *see* 3719
EL-222 *see* 3958
EL-349 *see* 8716
EL-436 *see* 3959
EL-466 *see* 7495
EL-500 *see* 4204
EL-531 *see* 631
EL-614 *see* 1389
EL-737 *see* 8092
EL-857 *see* 752
EL-857/820 *see* 752
EL-870 *see* 9439
EL-970 *see* 3933
Elactocin *see* 5444
Elaidic Acid, 3533
Elaiomycin, 3534
ELAM-1 *see* 8426
Elan [Schwarz] *see* 5225
Elanpres [Elan] *see* 6055
Elantan [Schwarz] *see* 5225
Elarzone [Alcon] *see* 7457
Elaspol [Ono] *see* 8558
Elastase, 3535
Elasterin [Phoenix] *see* 3978
Elastin, 3536
Elaszym [Eisai] *see* 3535
α-Elaterin *see* 2614
Elavil [AstraZeneca] *see* 487
Elayl *see* 3791
Elazor [Sigma-Tau] *see* 4122
Elbrol [Pfleger] *see* 7840
Elcatonin, 3537
Elcitonin [Toyo Jozo] *see* 3537
Elcometrine, 3538
Elcosal *see* 3183
Elcosine *see* 8951
Eldepryl [Somerset] *see* 8428
Elder *see* 8351
Elderfield Pyrimidine Mustard *see* 3422
Eldisine [Lilly] *see* 9987

Eldopal [Yamanouchi] *see* 5464
Eldopaque [Valeant] *see* 4808
Eldopar [Weifa] *see* 5464
Eldopatec [Labatec] *see* 5464
Eldoquin [Valeant] *see* 4808
Eldrin *see* 8304
Elecampane *see* 5003
Elecampane Camphor *see* 207
Elecor [Galenica] *see* 7737
Eledoisin, 3539
Element 104 *see* 8303
Element 105 *see* 3462
Element 106 *see* 8414
Element 107 *see* 1321
Element 108 *see* 4618
Element 109 *see* 5809
Element 110 *see* 2826
Element 111 *see* 8247
Element 112, 3540
Element 114, 3541
Element 116, 3542
Elen [Yamanouchi] *see* 4938
Elenium [Polfa] *see* 2084
Elenolide, 3543
Elestat [Allergan] *see* 3618
Eletriptan, 3544
Eleuthera Bark *see* 1881
Eleutherobin, 3545
Elevate [Arvesta] *see* 3974
Elfwort *see* 5003
Elgetol *see* 3279
Elgodipine, 3546
Elics [Senju] *see* 490
Elidel [Novartis] *see* 7429
Elidiur [BMS] *see* 4256
Elieten [Nippon Kayaku] *see* 6143
Eligard [Sanofi-Aventis] *see* 5457
Eliminoxy *see* 2299
Elimite [Allergan] *see* 7180
Elisal [Specia] *see* 8993
Elisor [BMS] *see* 7714
Elite [Bayer CropSci.] *see* 9092
Elitek [Sanofi-Aventis] *see* 8117
Elixophyllin [Forest] *see* 9285
Elkapin [Gödecke] *see* 3891
Elkosil *see* 8951
Elkosin [Novartis] *see* 8951
Ellagic Acid, 3547
Ellatun [Basotherm] *see* 9567
Ellence [Pharmacia & Upjohn] *see* 3623
Ellipticine, 3548
Elliptinium Acetate, 3549
Elliptone, 3550
Ellman's Reagent, 3551
Elmedal [Thiemann] *see* 7277
Elmetacin [Sankyo] *see* 4968
Elmiron [Baker Norton] *see* 7134
Elobact [Cascan] *see* 1954
Elobromol [Chinoin] *see* 6214
Elocon [Schering-Plough] *see* 6241
Elodrine *see* 4789
Eloisin [Farmitalia] *see* 3539
Elon *see* 6017
Elopram [Recordati] *see* 2318
Eloxatin [Sanofi-Aventis] *see* 6912
Elplat [Debiopharm] *see* 6912
Elrodorm *see* 4477
Elspar [Merck & Co.] *see* 836
Eltanolone *see* 7729
Eltoprazine, 3552
Eltroxin [GSK] *see* 9415
Elvanol [DuPont] *see* 7585
Elvaron [Bayer] *see* 3044
Elvorine [Lederle] *see* 4222
Elymoclavine, 3553

Elyzol [Dumex] see 6157
Elzogram [Lilly] see 1917
Emadine [Alcon] see 3557
Emamectin, 3554
Emanation see 8095
Emanil see 4891
EMB see 3720
Embafume see 6029
Embanox see 1547
Embarin [Merckle] see 279
Embark [3M] see 5802
EMBAY 8440 see 7716
Embden Ester see 4276
"Embelic Acid" see 3555
Embelin, 3555
Embequin [M & B] see 5042
Embonic Acid see 7005
Embramine, 3556
Embutox see 2835
Emcol E-607 [Witco] see 5370
Emcol E-607S [Witco] see 5370
Emconcor [Merck KGaA] see 1295
Emcor [Merck KGaA] see 1295
Emcyt [Pfizer] see 3706
EMD-9806 see 7707
EMD-30087 see 1916
EMD-33512 see 1295
EMD-34946 see 5610
EMD-38362 see 8275
EMD-49980 see 8275
EMD-77697 see 8375
EMD-128130 see 8375
Emdisterone see 3448
Emedastine, 3557
Emedyl see 3207
Emend [Merck & Co.] see 753
Emepride [Roche] see 1432
Emepronium Bromide, 3558
Emerald see 1161
Emerald Green see 1374, 2625
Emerest [Emery] see 7578
Emerest 2711 [Emery] see 7578
Emergil [Labaz] see 4187
Emericid see 5569
Emersol 132 [Emery] see 8804
Emery 1600 [Henkel] see 5358
Emery 1780 [Henkel] see 5359
Emes see 3207
Emesazine see 2305
Emeside [L.A.B.] see 3748
Emetamine see 3559
Emete-Con [Roerig] see 1119
Emethibutin see 3829
Emetic Herb see 5550
Emetid [Virbac] see 6143
Emetine, 3559
Emetine Hydrochloride see 3559
Emex [Archifar] see 1789
Emflex [Merck KGaA] see 27
Emgel [GSK] see 3681
Emgesan [Kabi] see 5670
Emilace [Yamanouchi] see 6446
Emilene see 5649
Eminase [SKB] see 674
Eminent [Isagro] see 9193
Emivan [USV] see 3721
Emmolic Acid see 1909
Emodepside see 3560
Emodin, 3561
Emodin-l-rhamnoside see 4264
Emonapride see 6446
Emoren [Wassermann] see 6933
Emorfazone, 3562
Emoril [Roemmers] see 1432

Emotival [Armstrong] see 5579
Emovate [GSK] see 2364
EMPA, 3563
Empecid [Bayer-Takeda] see 2417
Emperal [Orion] see 6143
Empire [Dow AgroSci.] see 2189
Empirin [GSK] see 851
EMPP see 3606
EMPTA, 3564
Empyreumatic Oil of Juniper see 5271
EMQ see 3753
EMS see 3827
Emselex [Novartis] see 2825
Emsorb 2500 [Henkel] see 8724
Emsorb 2515 [Henkel] see 8724
Emsorb 6900 [Emery] see 7582
Emtricitabine, 3565
Emtriva [Gilead] see 3565
Emtryl [Rhône-Poulenc] see 3265
Emulsept (obsolete) see 5370
Emulsynt [Van Dyk] see 7578
E-Mycin see 3681
Emylcamate, 3566
EN-141 see 5267
EN-313 see 6268
EN-1010 see 8013
EN-1639A see 6363
EN-1733A see 6233
EN-2234A see 6357
EN-15304 see 6362
ENA-713 see 8240
Enable [Dow AgroSci.] see 3962
Enablex [Novartis] see 2825
Enacard [Merial] see 3567
Enadel [Pfizer] see 2420
Enalapril, 3567
Enalaprilat, 3568
Enalaprilic Acid see 3568
Enallachrome see 3698
Enaloc [Leiras] see 3567
Enanthal see 4658
Enanthaldehyde see 4658
Enanthic Acid see 4660
Enanthic Alcohol see 4661
Enanthotoxin, 3569
Enantone [Takeda] see 5457
Enantyum [Menarini] see 5305
Enapren [Merck & Co.] see 3567
Enargite see 2519
Enarmon [Teikoku Zoki] see 9180
Enavid [Searle] see 6698
Enbol [Chugai] see 7996
Enbrel [Wyeth] see 3712
Enbucrilate see 1565
Encainide, 3570
Encaprin [Procter & Gamble] see 851
Encare [Norwich] see 6677
Encephabol [Merck KGaA] see 7996
Encetrop [Alpharma] see 7487
Enclomiphene see 2386
Encorton [Polfa] see 7722
Endak [Madaus] see 1866
Endep [Roche] see 487
Endiandric Acid A see 3571
Endiandric Acid B see 3571
Endiandric Acid C see 3571
Endiandric Acids, 3571
Endoamylases see 599
Endocaine [Endo] see 8013
Endociclina [Del Saz & Filippini] see 4254
Endocistobil [Bracco] see 5022
Endocorion [ELEA] see 2216
Endodextranases see 2949
Endofolliculina see 3708
Endogenous Pyrogen see 4993

Endografin [Schering AG] see 5022
Endojodin [Bayer] see 7782
Endometrion [Jenapharm] see 3106
Endomixin [Lusofarmaco] see 6454
Endo-Paractol [Temmler] see 3215
Endophenolphthalein see 6974
Endophleban [Rentschler] see 3174
Endoprost [Italfarmaco] see 4901
Endorem [Guerbet] see 4063
α-Endorphin see 3572
β-Endorphin see 3572
γ-Endorphin see 3572
α-neo-Endorphin see 3572
β-neo-Endorphin see 3572
Endorphins, 3572
Endostatin, 3573
Endosulfan, 3574
Endothal see 3575
Endothall, 3575
Endothelial Cell Growth Factor see 4072
Endothelial-Leukocyte Adhesion Molecule-1 see 8426
Endothelin, 3576
Endothelin-1 see 3576
Endothelin-2 see 3576
Endothelin-3 see 3576
Endothium-derived Relaxing Factor see 6578
Endoxan [Baxter] see 2747
3,6-Endoxohexahydrophthalic Acid see 3575
Endralazine, 3577
Endralazine Mesylate see 3577
Endrate Disodium [Abbott] see 3517
Endrate Tetrasodium [Abbott] see 3517
Endrin, 3578
Endura [BASF] see 1352
Enduracidin, 3579
Enduracidin A Hydrochloride see 3579
Enduracidin B Hydrochloride see 3579
Endurance [Syngenta] see 7766
Enduron [Abbott] see 6005
Enduronum [Abbott] see 6005
E.N.E. see 3834
Enelfa [Dolorgiet] see 47
Enerbol [Polfa] see 7996
Energona [Maurer] see 6699
Enfenamic Acid, 3580
Enflurane, 3581
Enfuvirtide, 3582
Engemycin [Intervet] see 6976
English Chamomile see 2041
English Hawthorn see 2567
English White see 1657
Enheptin [Am. Cyanamid] see 457
Enheptin-A [Am. Cyanamid] see 410
Enhexymal see 4704
Enide [Tuco] see 3307
Enidin see 5715
Enilconazole, 3583
Eniluracil, 3584
Enin see 5715
Enirant [Desitin] see 3653
Enisyl [Person & Covey] see 5636
Enkaid [Mead Johnson] see 3570
Enkalene [Kunstzijde] see 7569
Enkalon [Am. Enka] see 6734
Enkephalinase see 872
Enkephalins see 3572
Enlon [Ohmeda] see 3516
Ennds see 2155
Enniatin A see 3585
Enniatin B see 3585
Enniatin C see 3585
Enniatins, 3585

Enocitabine, 3586
3-Enolpyruvic Ether of *trans*-3,4-Dihy-
droxycyclohexa-1,5-diene Carbox-
ylic Acid *see* 2217
Enovid *see* 6698
Enoxacin, 3587
Enoxaparin, 3588
Enoxen [Dainippon] *see* 3587
Enoximone, 3589
Enoxolone, 3590
Enoxor [Fabre] *see* 3587
Enpro [Kobayashi] *see* 7757
Enprostil, 3591
Enradin [Takeda] *see* 3579
Enramycin *see* 3579
Enrofloxacin, 3592
Enrumay [Cooper] *see* 7984
E.N.S. *see* 3834
Ensidon [Novartis] *see* 6853
Enstatite *see* 5687
Ensulizole, 3593
ENT-987 *see* 9371
ENT-1122 *see* 3287
ENT-7796 *see* 5501
ENT-14250 *see* 7476
ENT-14874 *see* 10165
ENT-15108 *see* 7033
ENT-16225 *see* 3103
ENT-16273 *see* 8966
ENT-17034 *see* 5700
ENT-17251 *see* 3578
ENT-17292 *see* 6108
ENT-17510 *see* 260
ENT-17588 *see* 8002
ENT-20218 *see* 2856
ENT-20852 *see* 1441
ENT-22014 *see* 913
ENT-22374 *see* 6165
ENT-22879 *see* 3301
ENT-23233 *see* 913
ENT-23347 *see* 3365
ENT-23648 *see* 3086
ENT-23969 *see* 1787
ENT-24042 *see* 7331
ENT-24105 *see* 3736
ENT-24482 *see* 3087
ENT-24717 *see* 2600
ENT-24727 *see* 3286
ENT-24833 *see* 1330
ENT-24988 *see* 6358
ENT-25445 *see* 489
ENT-25515 *see* 7337
ENT-25540 *see* 4002
ENT-25567 *see* 6354
ENT-25640 *see* 2785
ENT-25644 *see* 3932
ENT-25647 *see* 3392
ENT-25705 *see* 7336
ENT-25715 *see* 3976
ENT-025719 *see* 6207
ENT-25784 *see* 433
ENT-25841 *see* 9192
ENT-25991 *see* 5855
ENT-26398 *see* 4176
ENT-26538 *see* 1772
ENT-27129 *see* 6251
ENT-27162 *see* 1431
ENT-27165 *see* 9135
ENT-27226 *see* 7808
ENT-27258 *see* 1431
ENT-27311 *see* 2189
ENT-27395 *see* 2760
ENT-27396 *see* 5947
ENT-27520 *see* 2189
ENT-27552 *see* 1434

ENT-27766 *see* 7496
ENT-27967 *see* 486
ENT-29054 *see* 3142
ENT-29106 *see* 6550
ENT-33266 *see* 5570
ENT-34886 *see* 3361
ENT-50852 *see* 320
ENT-50882 *see* 4725
Entacapone, 3594
Entacyl [BDH] *see* 7465
Entamide [Boots] *see* 3201
Entecavir, 3595
Enteramine *see* 8462
Entereg [Adolor] *see* 372
Enterfram *see* 6454
Enteroanthelone *see* 3597
Enterobactin, 3596
Enterobiocine [Rousselot] *see* 8943
Enterochelin *see* 3596
Enterocid [Schering] *see* 7376
Enterocol *see* 6655
Enterocura [Nordmark] *see* 8909
Enterogastrone, 3597
Enterokanacin [Sidus] *see* 5281
Enterol [Lenza] *see* 7505
Enterolactone, 3598
Enteromide [Consolidated Chem.] *see*
8912
Enteroquinol *see* 5031
Enterosalicyl [Delalande] *see* 8332
Enterosalil [Farmabraz] *see* 8332
Enterosept *see* 5042
Entero-Septol *see* 5031
Enterosulfamid [Katwijk] *see* 7376
Enterosulfon [CMC] *see* 7376
Enterozol *see* 5031
Entex (obsolete) *see* 4002
Entobex *see* 7197
Entocort [AstraZeneca] *see* 1468
Entothein *see* 8418
Entprol, 3599
Entrokin *see* 5031
Entumine [Wander] *see* 2415
Enturen [Novartis] *see* 8949
Entyderma [Taiyo] *see* 1019
ENU *see* 3833
Envacar [Pfizer] *see* 4568
Envidor [Bayer] *see* 8757
Envilon [Toyo] *see* 7586
Enviomycin, 3600
Enviroxime, 3601
Enzactin [Ayerst] *see* 9589
Enzamin [Kowa] *see* 1122
Enzaprost F [Ceva] *see* 7878
Enzicoba [Farmasa] *see* 2451
Enzodase [Squibb] *see* 4758
Enzorb-A [Regis] *see* 7255
Enzyme Q *see* 8023
Eoden [Woelm] *see* 4657
Eosin *see* 3603
Eosine *see* 3603
Eosine Acid *see* 3603
Eosine I Bluish, 3602
Eosine Yellowish—(YS), 3603
Eosinophil Differentiation Factor *see*
4997
Eosin Y *see* 3603
Eosote *see* 2573
Eotaxin, 3604
Eovist [Schering AG] *see* 4330
Ep *see* 3688
3-EP *see* 3730
EPA 3531, 7230
Epa-Bon [Sierochimica] *see* 2715
Epadel [Mochida] *see* 3531

Epafosforil [Coli] *see* 7362
Epalons *see* 275
Epalrestat, 3605
Epanutin [Pfizer] *see* 7322
Epatec [Nissan] *see* 5305
Epatiol [Medici] *see* 9453
EPEG *see* 3886
Eperisone, 3606
Epha [Woelm] *see* 3207
Ephedra, 3607
Ephedrine, 3608
d-ψ-Ephedrine *see* 7916
l-Ephedrine *see* 3608
Ephedrone *see* 5963
Ephicillin Hydriodide *see* 7085
Ephynal [Roche] *see* 9495
Epi-Aberel [Janssen-Cilag] *see* 8165
4′-Epiadriamycin *see* 3623
Epiallopregnanolone *see* 275
5-Epiandrostane *see* 3866
Epiandrosterone, 3609
Epibatidine, 3610
Epibloc [Pestcon] *see* 2145
(−)-Epicatechin *see* 1902
Epichlorohydrin, 3611
dl-α-Epichlorohydrin *see* 3611
Epicholestanol, 3612
Epicholesterol, 3613
Epicillin, 3614
Epicinchonidine *see* 2286
Epicinchonine *see* 2287
Epiclase [Bellon] *see* 7203
Epicocconone, 3615
Epicure [Novartis Agro] *see* 2771
Epidermal Growth Factor *see* 3527
α-Epidibromohydrin *see* 3025
Epidicentrine *see* 3413
3,17-Epidihydroxyestratriene *see* 3703
Epidione [Bellon] *see* 9706
Epidosin [Solvay] *see* 9906
4′-Epidoxorubicin *see* 3623
Epidropal [Teofarma] *see* 279
4′-Epi-DX *see* 3623
Epi-echinuline *see* 3499
8-Epiestradiol *see* 5167
Δ¹,³,⁵-8α-Epiestratriene-3,17β-diol *see*
5167
Δ¹,³,⁵-8-Epiestratrien-3-ol-17-one *see*
5168
16-Epiestriol, 3616
8-Epiestrone *see* 5168
Epifrin [Allergan] *see* 3619
Epifucose *see* 8077
(−)-Epigallocatechin 3-*O*-Gallate *see*
3526
(−)-Epigallocatechol Gallate *see* 3526
Epihetacillin *see* 4672
3-Epihydroxyetioallocholan-17-one *see*
640
Epileo Petitmal [Eisai] *see* 3748
Epilim [Sanofi-Aventis] *see* 9913
Epimedii Herba, 3617
(17*S*:12*S*:25*S*)-22,26-Epimino-18
(13 → 17)-*abeo*-cholesta-5,12-diene-
3β,16β-diol *see* 9949
(22*S*:25*S*)-12,26-Epimino-17β-methyl-
18-norcholesta-5,12-diene-3β,16β-
diol *see* 9949
Epi-Monistat [Cilag] *see* 6178
Epinal [Kyorin] *see* 219
Epinastine, 3618
Epinephrine, 3619
Epinephrine Isopropyl Homolog *see* 5217
Epinine *see* 2903
Epinochrome-2-sulfonic Acid 5-Mono-
semicarbazone Sodium Salt *see* 1789

Epinyl [Nordic] *see* 3718
16-Epioestriol *see* 3616
EpiPen [Dey] *see* 3619
Epi-Pevaryl [Cilag-Chemie] *see* 3502
Epiphenethicillin Potassium *see* 7223
Epiquinidine, 3620
Epiquinine, 3621
Epirenor [Byk Gulden] *see* 6759
D-Epirhamnose *see* 8077
Epirizole, 3622
Epirubicin, 3623
Episesamin *see* 823
(−)-Episesamin *see* 823
(+)-Episesamin *see* 823
Epistilbite *see* 1648
Epitetracycline *see* 8028
Epithienamycins *see* 6835
(2α,3α,5α,17β)-2,3-Epithioandrostan-
17-ol *see* 3624
(2α,3α,5α,17β)-2,3-Epithio-17-[(1-
methoxycyclopentyl)oxy]androstane
see 5858
Epitiostanol, 3624
Epitol [Teva] *see* 1781
Epitopic [Gerda] *see* 3152
Epivir [GSK] *see* 5352
Epizizanal *see* 6816
Eplerenone, 3625
EPN, 3626
Epo *see* 3688
EPO *see* 3906
EPO-906 *see* 3628
Epobron [Ono] *see* 4881
Epocan [Merck KGaA] *see* 7996
Epocelin [Fujisawa] *see* 1951
Epodyl [Ayerst] *see* 3880
Epoetin Alfa *see* 3688
Epoetin Beta *see* 3688
Epogam [Scotia] *see* 3906
Epogen [Amgen] *see* 3688
Epogin [Chugai] *see* 3688
Epontol [Bayer] *see* 7803
Epoprostenol *see* 7875
Eporal *see* 2822
Eposerin [Farmitalia] *see* 1951
Epostane, 3627
Epothilone A *see* 3628
Epothilone B *see* 3628
Epothilone D *see* 3628
Epothilones, 3628
Epoxiconazole, 3629
Epoxomicin, 3630
1α,4α-Epoxy-3-aza-A-homoandrostan-
16β-ol *see* 8346
(3β,4α,7α,15α,16β)-4,9-Epoxycevane-
3,4,7,14,15,16,20-heptol *see* 4412
(3α,4α,16β)-4,9-Epoxycevane-3,4,12,-
14,16,17,20-heptol *see* 2035
(3β,4α,16β)-4,9-Epoxycevane-3,4,12,-
14,16,17,20-heptol 3-(3,4-Dimeth-
oxybenzoate) *see* 9954
[3β(Z),4α,16β]-4,9-Epoxycevane-3,4,-
12,14,16,17,20-heptol 3-(2-Methyl-2-
butenoate) *see* 2033
(3β,4α,6α,7α,15α,16β)-4,9-Epoxycev-
ane-3,4,6,7,14,15,16,20-octol *see* 7900
[3β(2R,3R),4α,6α,7α,15α(R),16β]-4,9-
Epoxycevane-3,4,6,7,14,15,16,20-oc-
tol 6,7-Diacetate 3-(2,3-Dihydroxy-2-
methylbutanoate) 15-(2-Methylbu-
tanoate) *see* 7899
[3β(S),4α,6α,7α,15α(R),16β]-4,9-Epoxy-
cevane-3,4,6,7,14,15,16,20-octol 6,7-
Diacetate 3-(2,3-Dihydroxy-2-methyl-
butanoate) 15-(2-Methylbutanoate)
see 7899

6β,6aβ-Epoxy-2,3,3aα,3b,4,5,6,6a,7,-
7aα-decahydro-5β-hydroxy-2β,3bβ-
dimethyl-4-methylene-1H-cyclopen-
ta[a]pentalene-2-carboxylic Acid *see*
4717
(3S,3'R,5R,6'R,8R)-5,8-Epoxy-5,8-dihy-
dro-β,ε-carotene-3,3'-diol *see* 4095
(3S,3'R,5R,6'R,8S)-5,8-Epoxy-5,8-dihy-
dro-β,ε-carotene-3,3'-diol *see* 2250
(4α,5α,17β)-4,5-Epoxy-3,17-dihydroxy-
androst-2-ene-2-carbonitrile *see* 9698
(4α,5α,17β)-4,5-Epoxy-3,17-dihydroxy-
4,17-dimethylandrost-2-ene-2-car-
bonitrile *see* 3627
1,10-Epoxy-6,8-dihydroxygermacra-
4,11(13)-dien-12-oic Acid 12,8-Lac-
tone Acetate *see* 7965
15,16-Epoxy-6β,9-dihydroxy-8βH-
labda-13(16),14-dien-19-oic Acid γ-
Lactone *see* 5754
(5α)-4,5-Epoxy-3,14-dihydroxy-17-
methylmorphinan-6-one *see* 6969
(5α)-4,5-Epoxy-3,14-dihydroxy-17-(2-
propenyl)morphinan-6-one *see* 6362
(5Z,9α,11α,13E,15S)-6,9-Epoxy-11,15-
dihydroxyprosta-5,13-dien-1-oic
Acid *see* 7875
(1'α)-6',7-Epoxy-6,12'-dimethoxy-2'-
methyloxyacanthan *see* 9697
4a,9a-Epoxy-3-(2,3-epoxybutyryl)-1,2,-
3,4,4a,9a-hexahydro-1,3,4,5,10-pen-
tahydroxy-2-methylanthrone *see*
2007
3α,9α-Epoxy-14β,18β-(epoxyethano-N-
methylimino)-5β-pregna-7,16-diene-
3β,11α,20α-triol 20α-Ester with 2,4-
Dimethylpyrrole-3-carboxylic Acid
see 1009
(8r)-6β,7β-Epoxy-8-ethyl-3α-hydroxy-
1αH,5αH-tropanium Bromide (−)-
Tropate *see* 6943
β,17-Epoxy-α-(3-ethylidene-1,2,3,4,6,-
7,12,12b-octahydroindole[2,3-a]qui-
nolizin-2-yl)-curan-1-propanoic
Acid Methyl Ester *see* 4381
4,4a-Epoxy-5-ethylidene-2,3,4,4a-tet-
rahydro-5H-1-pyridine *see* 8
5β,20-Epoxy-1,2α,4,7β,10β,13α-hexa-
hydroxytax-11-en-9-one 4,10-Diace-
tate 2-Benzoate 13-Ester with (2R,-
3S)-N-Benzoyl-3-phenylisoserine *see*
6982
(3β,5β,15β)-14,15-Epoxy-3-hydroxy-5-
bufa-20,22-dienolide *see* 8146
(8β,10β)-8,10-Epoxy-8-hydroxy-3,4-di-
methoxy-17-methylhasubanan-7-one
see 5929
(5α)-4,5-Epoxy-3-hydroxy-5,17-di-
methylmorphinan-6-one *see* 6150
(2α,4α,5α,17β)-4,5-Epoxy-17-hydroxy-
4,17-dimethyl-3-oxoandrostane-2-
carbonitrile *see* 3627
4,5α-Epoxy-6β-hydroxy-germacra-
1(10),11(13)-dien-12-oic Acid γ-Lactone *see* 7048
1,10-Epoxy-6β-hydroxy-1β,5β,7α-
guaiai-3-en-12-oic Acid γ-Lactone *see*
771
[5α,7α(R)]-4,5-Epoxy-3-hydroxy-6-
methoxy-α,17-dimethyl-α-propyl-6,-
14-ethenomorphinan-7-methanol *see*
3888
(5α)-4,5-Epoxy-14-hydroxy-3-methoxy-
17-methylmorphinan-6-one *see* 6959
4,5-Epoxy-3-hydroxy-17-methylmor-
phinan-6-one *see* 4803

6β,7β-Epoxy-3β-hydroxy-8-methyl-
1αH,5αH-tropanium Bromide, Di-2-
thienylglycolate *see* 9454
6β,7β-Epoxy-3α-hydroxy-8-methyl-
1αH,5αH-tropanium Bromide Tropate
(Ester) *see* 6003
4,5-Epoxy-17-hydroxy-3-oxoandrost-
ane-2-carbonitrile *see* 9698
(7α,11α,17α)-9,11-Epoxy-17-hydroxy-
3-oxopregn-4-ene-7,21-dicarboxylic
Acid γ-Lactone Methyl Ester *see*
3625
(5Z,9α,11α,13E,15S)-9,11-Epoxy-15-hy-
droxythromboxa-5,13-dien-1-oic
Acid *see* 9388
5,6-Epoxy-3-hydroxy-p-toluquinone *see*
9172
12,13-Epoxy-4-hydroxytrichothec-9-
en-8-one Crotonate *see* 9650
3α,6α-Epoxy-7β-hydroxytropane *see*
8410
(3β,23β)-17,23-Epoxy-3-hydroxyvera-
traman-11-one *see* 5264
9,13-Epoxylabd-7-en-15-oic Acid *see*
4547
1,8-Epoxy-p-menthane *see* 3895
Epoxymethamine Bromide *see* 6003
9α,11-Epoxy-7α-(methoxycarbonyl)-3-
oxo-17α-pregn-4-ene-21,17-carbo-
lactone *see* 3625
9α,11α-Epoxy-7α-methoxycarbonyl-20-
spirox-4-ene-3,21-dione *see* 3625
(5α,6α)-4,5-Epoxy-3-methoxy-17-meth-
ylmorphinan-6-ol *see* 3171
(5α,6β)-4,5-Epoxy-3-methoxy-17-meth-
ylmorphinan-6-ol *see* 3176
4,5-Epoxy-3-methoxy-17-methylmor-
phinan-6-one *see* 4785
6',7-Epoxy-6-methoxy-2-methyl-oxy-
acanthan-12'-ol *see* 6179
(5α,6α)-4,5-Epoxy-17-methylmorphin-
an-3,6-diol *see* 3177
(5α,6α)-4,5-Epoxy-17-methylmorphin-
an-3,6-diol Diacetate (Ester) *see* 2967
4,5a-Epoxy-17-methylmorphinan-3-ol
see 2927
cis-7,8-Epoxy-2-methyloctadecane *see*
3361
Epoxymexrenone *see* 3625
cis-12,13-Epoxyoctadec-cis-9-enoic Acid
see 9963
12,13-Epoxyoleic Acid *see* 9963
(12R,13S)-(−)-12,13-Epoxyoleic Acid
see 9963
(12S,13R)-(+)-12,13-Epoxyoleic Acid *see*
9963
[4β(Z)]-12,13-Epoxy-4-[(1-oxo-2-buten-
yl)oxy]trichothec-9-en-8-one *see*
9650
2,3-Epoxy-4-oxo-7,10-dodecadienam-
ide *see* 2004
2,3-Epoxy-4-oxo-7,10-dodecadienoyl-
amide *see* 2004
1,3-Epoxypropane *see* 9715
2,3-Epoxy-1-propanol *see* 4490
(−)-(1R,2S)-(1,2-Epoxypropyl)phos-
phonic Acid *see* 4254
(3α,4β,7α)-12,13-Epoxy-3,4,7,15-tetra-
hydroxytrichothec-9-en-8-one *see*
6659
(3α,4β,8α)-12,13-Epoxytrichothec-9-
ene-3,4,8,15-tetrol 4,15-Diacetate 8-
(3-Methylbutanoate) *see* 9801
12,13-Epoxytrichothec-9-en-4-ol Acetate *see* 9647

Erythrocentaurin, 3678
Erythrocin [Abbott] see 3687
Erythrocin Lactobionate [Abbott] see 3685
Erythrocuprein see 9002
Erythrogenic Acid see 5103
Erythroglucin see 3675
D-Erythrohexulose see 7924
α-Erythroidine, 3679
β-Erythroidine, 3680
Erythrol see 3675
Erythrol Tetranitrate see 3677
Erythromid [Abbott] see 3681
Erythromycin, 3681
Erythromycin A see 3681
Erythromycin 2′-Acetate Octadecanoate (Salt) see 3682
Erythromycin Acistrate, 3682
Erythromycin Estolate, 3683
Erythromycin Gluceptate see 3684
Erythromycin Glucoheptonate, 3684
Erythromycin Glucoheptonic Acid Salt see 3684
Erythromycin Lactobionate, 3685
Erythromycin 9-[O-[(2-Methoxyethoxy)-methyl]oxime] see 8276
Erythromycin Octadecanoate (Salt) see 3687
Erythromycin 2′-Propanoate see 3686
Erythromycin 2′-Propanoate Dodecyl Sulfate (Salt) see 3683
Erythromycin Propionate, 3686
Erythromycin Propionate Lauryl Sulfate see 3683
Erythromycin Stearate, 3687
Erythroped [Abbott] see 3681
Erythropoiesis Stimulating Factor see 3688
Erythropoietin, 3688
Erythropterin, 3689
D-Erythrose, 3690
L-Erythrose, 3691
D-Erythrose 4-Phosphate, 3692
4-D-Erythrosephosphoric Acid see 3692
Erythrosine, 3693
Erythrosine B see 3693
Erythrosine BS see 3693
Erythrosine Extra Yellowish see 3189
Erythroxylon see 2453
L-Erythrulose, 3694
Erytrarsin see 1603
ES-771 see 7430
ES-902 see 7430
Esafosfina [Foscama] see 4275
Esametina see 4688
Esantene see 4979
Esaprazole, 3695
Esbatal [Burroughs Wellcome] see 1186
Esbecythrin see 2883
Esbericard [Schaper & Brümmer] see 2567
Esberidin [Schaper & Brümmer] see 9983
Esberiven [Schaper & Brümmer] see 5821
Esbuphon [Schaper & Brümmer] see 6699
Escalol 106 [Van Dyk] see 4487
Escalol 506 [Van Dyk] see 3232
Escalol 507 [Van Dyk] see 3232
Eschenmoser's Salt see 3251
Escin, 3696
α-Escin see 3696
β-Escin see 3696
Escitalopram see 2318
Escitalopram Oxalate see 2318
Esclama [Montedison] see 6552
Esclerosina see 3727
Escobedin see 895

Escor [Merck KGaA] see 6545
Escosyl see 3698
Escre [SS Pharm.] see 2071
Esculetin, 3697
Esculetin Dimethyl Ether see 8404
Esculin, 3698
Esculoside see 3698
Esdragol see 3705
E-Selectin see 8426
Eseridine, 3699
Eserine see 7384
Eserine Aminoxide see 3699
Eserine Blue see 7384
Eserine Oxide see 3699
(−)-Eseroline Phenylcarbamate see 7260
ESF see 3688
Esfenvalerate see 4010
Esiclene [LPB Braglia] see 4239
Esidrex [Novartis] see 4781
Esidrix [Novartis] see 4781
Esilgan [Takeda] see 3702
Esinol [Toyama] see 3681
Eskacef [GSK] see 1986
Eskalin [SKB] see 10004
Eskalith [GSK] see 5527
Eskazine [GSK] see 9680
Eskazinyl [SK & F] see 9680
Eskazole [GSK] see 210
Esmarin [Merck KGaA] see 9624
Esmeron [Organon] see 8246
Esmolol, 3700
Esomeprazole see 6845
Esomeprazole Magnesium see 6845
Esophotrast [RPR] see 994
Esparon [Orion] see 312
Esparto Wax, 3701
Espectinomicina see 8739
Esperal [Sanofi-Synthelabo] see 3364
Esperan [Toyama] see 2737
Esperson [HMR] see 2930
Espinomycin A see 6183
Espril see 6491
Espyre [SS Pharm.] see 3350
Esquinon [Sankyo] see 1824
Esradin [Sigma-Tau] see 5240
Essaven [Cassella-med] see 4748
Essence de Niobe see 3766
Essence of Mirbane see 6588
Essence of Niobe see 6024
Essence of Rose see 6811
"Essential Oil of Birch Wood" see 1239
Essential Salt of Lemons see 7689
Essigsäure Tonerde see 365
Essitol [Athenstaedt] see 325
Estazolam, 3702
Ester 25 see 7030
Estergel [Merck & Co.] see 5215
Esteron 44 [Dow] see 2796
Esteron 245 [Dow] see 9019
Estil [Reiss] see 46
Estima [EFFIK] see 7773
Estimulocel [Alonga] see 7762
Estinyl [Schering-Plough] see 3734
Estivan [Almirall] see 3484
Estomicina [Bergamon] see 3683
Estomycin see 7041
Estopen see 7085
Estorra [Sepracor] see 10193
Estrace [Warner-Chilcott] see 3703
Estracyt [Pfizer] see 3706
Estraderm [Novartis] see 3703
Estradiol, 3703
α-Estradiol, 3704
β-Estradiol see 3703
cis-Estradiol see 3703

8α-Estradiol see 5167
Estradiol Benzoate see 3703
Estradiol 3-Bis(2-chloroethyl)carbamate see 3706
Estradiol Cypionate see 3703
Estradiol Enanthate see 3703
Estradiol Phosphate Polymer see 7566
Estradot [Novartis] see 3703
Estradurin [Kabi] see 7566
Estragole, 3705
Estragon see 9067
Estragon Oil see 3705
Estramustine, 3706
1,3,5:10,6,8-Estrapentaen-3-ol-17-one see 3642
(17β)-Estra-1,3,5(10),7-tetraene-3,17-diol see 3173
1,3,5,7-Estratetraen-3-ol-17-one see 3643
1,3,5-Estratriene-3,17α-diol see 3704
(8α,17β)-Estra-1,3,5(10)-triene-3,17-diol see 5167
(17α)-Estra-1,3,5(10)-triene-3,17-diol see 3704
(17β)-Estra-1,3,5(10)-triene-3,17-diol see 3703
Estra-1,3,5(10)triene-3,17β-diol 3-[N,-N-Bis(2-chloroethyl)carbamate] see 3706
(17β)-Estra-1,3,5(10)-triene-3,17-diol 3-[Bis(2-chloroethyl)carbamate] see 3706
1,3,5-Estratriene-3β,16α,17β-triol see 3707
Δ1,3,5-Estratriene-3,16β,17β-triol see 3616
(16α,17β)-Estra-1,3,5(10)-triene-3,16,-17-triol see 3707
(16β,17β)-Estra-1,3,5(10)-triene-3,16,-17-triol see 3616
1,3,5-Estratrien-3-ol-17-one 3708
4,9,11-Estratrien-17β-ol-3-one see 9583
(3β,17β)-Estr-4-ene-3,17-diol see 1322
4-Estren-17β-ol-3-one see 6365
Estreptocarbocaftiazol [Bago] see 7377
Estrex [Syntex] see 2878
Estring [Pharmacia & Upjohn] see 3703
Estriol, 3707
Estriol Succinate see 3707
Estroclim [Sigma-Tau] see 3703
Estrodienol see 3104
Estrofem see 3703
Estrogel [Solvay] see 3703
Estrol see 3708
Estrone, 3708
8α-Estrone see 5168
Estropipate see 3708
Estroral see 3104
Estrostep [Warner-Lambert] see 6697
Estrovis [Gödecke] see 8055
Estrugenone [Kremers-Urban] see 3708
Estrumate [Mallinckrodt] see 2399
Estrusol [Cooper] see 3708
Estulic [Novartis] see 4561
Esucos [UCB] see 3385
Eszopiclone see 10193
ET-1 see 3576
ET-495 see 7493
ET-743 see 3503
Etabus [Ferring] see 3364
Etacortin [Hermal] see 4191
Etadrol [Farmitalia] see 4192
Etafedrine, 3709
Etafenone, 3710
Etafillina [Delalande] see 24

4-Ethenylpyridine 1-Oxide Homopolymer *see* 7948
1-Ethenyl-2-pyrrolidinone *see* 7697
1-Ethenyl-2-pyrrolidinone Homopolymer *see* 7697
1-Ethenyl-2-pyrrolidinone Homopolymer Compd with Iodine *see* 7698
Ethenzamide, 3731
Etheophyl [Lindopharm] *see* 9285
Ethephon, 3732
Ether *see* 3806
Ether Chloratus *see* 3782
Ether Hydrochloric *see* 3782
Ether Muriatic *see* 3782
Ethidium *see* 4731
Ethimide *see* 3737
Ethinamate, 3733
Ethinazone *see* 3714
Ethine *see* 90
Ethinyl Estradiol, 3734
17-Ethinylestradiol *see* 3734
17α-Ethinylestradiol 3-Cyclopentyl Ether *see* 8055
Ethinylestrenol *see* 5629
17α-Ethinyl-17β-hydroxyestr-4-ene *see* 5629
17α-Ethinyltestosterone *see* 3741
Ethinyl Trichloride *see* 9639
Ethiodan *see* 5060
Ethiodized Oil, 3735
Ethiodol [Savage] *see* 3735
Ethiofos *see* 404
Ethion, 3736
Ethionamide, 3737
Ethioniamide *see* 3737
Ethionine, 3738
Ethiops Iron *see* 4040
Ethiops Mineral *see* 5888
Ethiprole, 3739
Ethirimol, 3740
Ethisterone, 3741
Ethmosine *see* 6268
Ethmozin *see* 6268
Ethmozine [Roberts] *see* 6268
Ethnine [Allen & Hanburys] *see* 7329
Ethocel *see* 3781
Ethodin [Winthrop] *see* 3716
Ethodryl [BDH] *see* 3116
Ethofat [Akzo] *see* 7578
Ethofenprox *see* 3876
Ethofibrate *see* 3877
Ethofumesate, 3742
Ethoglucid *see* 3880
Ethoheptazine, 3743
Ethohexadiol, 3744
Ethol *see* 2028
Ethopabate, 3745
Ethoprop, 3746
Ethopropazine, 3747
Ethoprophos *see* 3746
Ethoproxyfen *see* 3876
Ethosperse [Lonza] *see* 7577
Ethosuximide, 3748
Ethotoin, 3749
Ethovan *see* 3859
2-Ethoxy-4-acetamidobenzoic Acid Methyl Ester *see* 3745
p-Ethoxyacetanilide *see* 7204
7-Ethoxy-3,9-acridinediamine *see* 3716
1-Ethoxy-2-amino-4-nitrobenzene *see* 6617
4-Ethoxyaniline *see* 7228
2-Ethoxybenzamide *see* 3731
2-Ethoxybenzenamine *see* 7227
4-Ethoxybenzenamine *see* 7228

Ethoxybenzene *see* 7229
2-Ethoxybenzenecarbonamide *see* 3731
6-Ethoxy-2-benzothiazolesulfonamide *see* 3755
2-*p*-Ethoxybenzyl-1-(2-diethylaminoethyl)-5-nitrobenzimidazole *see* 3883
(2*S*,3a*S*,7a*S*)-1-[(2*S*)-2-[[(1*S*)-1-(Ethoxycarbonyl)butyl]amino]-1-oxopropyl]-octahydro-1*H*-indole-2-carboxylic Acid *see* 7170
N-Ethoxycarbonyl-2-ethoxy-1,2-dihydroquinoline *see* 3518
1-Ethoxycarbonyl-3-methyl-2-thio-4-imidazoline *see* 1798
N-(Ethoxycarbonyl)-3-(4-morpholinyl)-sydnone Imine *see* 6234
17α-Ethoxycarbonyloxy-Δ'-cortienic Acid Chloromethyl Ester *see* 5584
18-[[4-[(Ethoxycarbonyl)oxy]-3,5-dimethoxybenzoyl]oxy]-11,17-dimethoxyyohimban-16-carboxylic Acid Methyl Ester *see* 9017
4-[1-(Ethoxycarbonyloxy)ethoxy]-2-methyl-*N*-(2-pyridyl)-2*H*-1,2-benzothiazine-3-carboxamide 1,1-Dioxide *see* 587
1'-Ethoxycarbonyloxyethyl 6-(D-α-Aminophenylacetamido)penicillanate *see* 931
(11β,17α)-17-[(Ethoxycarbonyl)oxy]-11-hydroxy-3-oxoandrosta-1,4-diene-17-carboxylic Acid Chloromethyl Ester *see* 5584
(11β)-17-[(Ethoxycarbonyl)oxy]-11-hydroxy-21-(1-oxopropoxy)pregna-1,4-diene-3,20-dione *see* 7719
N-[(1*S*)-1-(Ethoxycarbonyl)-3-phenylpropyl]-L-alanyl-*N*-(2,3-dihydro-1*H*-inden-2-yl)glycine *see* 2876
N-[*N*-[(*S*)-1-(Ethoxycarbonyl)-3-phenylpropyl]-L-alanyl]-*N*-(indan-2-yl)glycine *see* 2876
(3a*R*,7a*S*)-1-[*N*-[1-(*S*)-(Ethoxycarbonyl)-3-phenylpropyl]-(*S*)-alanyl]octahydroindole-2(*S*)-carboxylic Acid *see* 9568
N-[(1*S*)-1-(Ethoxycarbonyl)-3-phenylpropyl]-L-alanyl-L-proline *see* 3567
(1*S*,9*S*)-9-[[(1*S*)-1-(Ethoxycarbonyl)-3-phenylpropyl]amino]octahydro-10-oxo-6*H*-pyridazino[1,2-*a*][1,2]diazepine-1-carboxylic Acid *see* 2273
(8*S*)-7-[(2*S*)-2-[[(1*S*)-1-(Ethoxycarbonyl)-3-phenylpropyl]amino]-1-oxopropyl]-1,4-dithia-7-azaspiro[4.4]nonane-8-carboxylic Acid *see* 8753
(4*S*)-3-[(2*S*)-2-[[(1*S*)-1-(Ethoxycarbonyl)-3-phenylpropyl]amino]-1-oxopropyl]-1-methyl-2-oxo-4-imidazolidinecarboxylic Acid *see* 4911
[2*S*,3a*S*,6a*S*]-1-[(2*S*)-2-[[(1*S*)-1-(Ethoxycarbonyl)-3-phenylpropyl]amino]-1-oxopropyl]octahydrocyclopenta[*b*]pyrrole-2-carboxylic Acid *see* 8103
(2*S*,3a*R*,7a*S*)-1-[(2*S*)-2-[[(1*S*)-1-(Ethoxycarbonyl)-3-phenylpropyl]amino]-1-oxopropyl]octahydro-1*H*-indole-2-carboxylic Acid *see* 9568
(3*S*)-2-[(2*S*)-2-[[(1*S*)-1-(Ethoxycarbonyl)-3-phenylpropyl]amino]-1-oxopropyl]-1,2,3,4-tetrahydro-6,7-dimethoxy-3-isoquinolinecarboxylic Acid *see* 6229
(3*S*)-2-[(2*S*)-2-[[(1*S*)-1-(Ethoxycarbonyl)-3-phenylpropyl]amino]-1-oxopropyl]-1,2,3,4-tetrahydro-3-isoquinolinecarboxylic Acid *see* 8051

(4*S*)-3-[(2*S*)-2-[*N*-[(1*S*)-1-(Ethoxycarbonyl)-3-phenylpropyl]amino]propionyl]-1-methyl-2-oxoimidazolidine-4-carboxylic Acid *see* 4911
(3*S*)-3-[[(1*S*)-1-(Ethoxycarbonyl)-3-phenylpropyl]amino]-2,3,4,5-tetrahydro-2-oxo-1*H*-1-benzazepine-1-acetic Acid *see* 1031
(2*S*,6*R*)-6-[[(1*S*)-1-(Ethoxycarbonyl)-3-phenylpropyl]amino]tetrahydro-5-oxo-2-(2-thienyl)-1,4-thiazepine-4(5*H*)-acetic Acid *see* 9136
11-[*N*-(Ethoxycarbonyl)-4-piperidylidene]-8-chloro-6,11-dihydro-5*H*-benzo[5,6]cyclohepta[1,2-*b*]pyridine *see* 5578
3-(Ethoxycarbonyl)-6,7,8,9-tetrahydro-1,6-dimethyl-4-oxo-4*H*-pyrido[1,2-*a*]-pyrimidinium Methyl Sulfate *see* 8225
(3*R*,5a*S*,6*R*,8a*S*,9*R*,10*S*,12*R*,12a*R*)-10-Ethoxydecahydro-3,6,9-trimethyl-3,-12-epoxy-12*H*-pyrano[4,3-*j*]-1,2-benzodioxepin *see* 813
2-Ethoxy-6,9-diaminoacridine *see* 3716
2-Ethoxy-2,3-dihydro-3,3-dimethyl-5-benzofuranol Methanesulfonate *see* 3742
6-Ethoxy-1,2-dihydro-2,2,4-trimethyl-quinoline *see* 3753
3-Ethoxy-1,1-dihydroxy-2-butanone *see* 5299
(*S*)-3,4-[(*N*,*N*',1,1'-((2"-Ethoxy)-3"'(*O*)-4"'-(*N*,*N*-dimethylamino)butane)-bis-(3,3'-indolyl))]-1(*H*)-pyrrole-2,3-dione *see* 8290
Ethoxydiphenylacetic Acid 2-Dimethylaminoethyl Ester *see* 3208
Ethoxyethane *see* 3806
2-Ethoxyethanol, 3750
2-Ethoxyethanol Acetate *see* 3751
2-(2-Ethoxyethoxy)ethanol *see* 1800
2-Ethoxyethyl Acetate, 3751
2,2'-[1-(1-Ethoxyethyl)-1,2-ethanediylidene]bishydrazinecarbothioamide *see* 5299
1-(2-Ethoxyethyl)-2-(hexahydro-4-methyl-1*H*-1,4-diazepin-1-yl)-1*H*-benzimidazole *see* 3557
2-Ethoxyethyl *p*-Methoxycinnamate *see* 2310
1-[2-(Ethoxy)ethyl]-2-(4-methyl-1-homopiperazinyl)benzimidazole *see* 3557
O-(6-Ethoxy-2-ethyl-4-pyrimidinyl)phosphorothioic Acid *O*,*O*-Dimethyl Ester *see* 3893
3-Ethoxy-4-hydroxybenzaldehyde *see* 3859
p-Ethoxy-*N*-(β-hydroxybutyryl)aniline *see* 1458
[3-[[4-(3-Ethoxy-2-hydroxypropoxy)-phenyl]amino]-3-oxopropyl]dimethylsulfonium Salt with 4-Methylbenzenesulfonic Acid *see* 9003
(±)-[2-[[*p*-(3-Ethoxy-2-hydroxypropoxy)phenyl]carbamoyl]ethyl]dimethylsulfonium *p*-Toluenesulfonate *see* 9003
2-[1-(Ethoxyimino)butyl]-5-[2-(ethylthio)propyl]-3-hydroxy-2-cyclohexen-1-one *see* 8473
2-[1-(Ethoxyimino)propyl]-3-hydroxy-5-mesitylcyclohex-2-en-1-one *see* 9564
2-[1-(Ethoxyimino)propyl]-3-hydroxy-5-(2,4,6-trimethylphenyl)-2-cyclohexen-1-one *see* 9564

13β-Ethyl-17α-ethynyl-17β-hydroxygon-4-en-3-one *see* 6704
Ethyl Ethynyl Methyl Carbinol *see* 5846
17β-Ethyletiocholane *see* 7726
Ethyl 7-Flavonoxyacetate *see* 3523
Ethyl Flavon-7-yloxyacetate *see* 3523
Ethyl-8-fluoro-5,6-dihydro-5-methyl-6-oxo-4*H*-imidazo[1,5-*a*][1,4]benzo-diazepine-3-carboxylate *see* 4135
1-Ethyl-6-fluoro-1,4-dihydro-7-(4-methyl-1-piperazinyl)-4-oxo-3-qui-nolinecarboxylic Acid *see* 7066
1-Ethyl-6-fluoro-1,4-dihydro-4-oxo-7-(1-piperazinyl)-1,8-naphthyridine-3-carboxylic Acid *see* 3587
1-Ethyl-6-fluoro-1,4-dihydro-4-oxo-7-(1-piperazinyl)-3-quinolinecarbox-ylic Acid *see* 6700
Ethyl *p*-Fluorophenyl Sulfone *see* 4161
Ethyl Formate, 3807
Ethylformic Acid *see* 7825
Ethyl Furoate *see* 4307
γ-Ethyl L-Glutamate *see* 4470
Ethyl Green *see* 6082
Ethyl Heptanoate *see* 3835
Ethyl Heptazine *see* 3743
Ethyl *n*-Heptoate *see* 3835
N-[4-[4-(Ethylheptylamino)-1-hydroxy-butyl]phenyl]methanesulfonamide *see* 4883
Ethylhexadecyldimethylammonium Bro-mide *see* 2029
3-(3-Ethylhexahydro-1-methyl-1*H*-aze-pin-3-yl)phenol *see* 5863
[1*R*-(1α,2β,4β)]-2-Ethyl-1,2,3,4,6,11-hexahydro-2,5,7-trihydroxy-6,11-di-oxo-4-[[2,3,6-trideoxy-4-*O*-[2,6-di-deoxy-4-*O*-[(2*R*-*trans*)-tetrahydro-6-methyl-5-oxo-2*H*-pyran-2-yl]-α-L-*lyxo*-hexopyranosyl]-3-(dimethylamino)-α-L-*lyxo*-hexopyranosyl]oxy]-1-naphtha-cenecarboxylic Acid Methyl Ester *see* 113
2-Ethyl-1,3-hexanediol *see* 3744
Ethyl Hexanoate *see* 3777
2-Ethyl-1-hexanol, 3808
Ethylhexedrine *see* 2707
2-Ethylhexyl Acetate *see* 6763
2-Ethylhexyl Alcohol *see* 3808
2-Ethylhexyl-2-cyano-3,3-diphenyl-acrylate *see* 6756
2-Ethylhexyl *p*-Methoxycinnamate *see* 6769
Ethyl 3-[[[2-[[[4-[[[(Hexyloxy)carbonyl]-amino]iminomethyl]phenyl]amino]-methyl]-1-methyl-1*H*-benzimidazol-5-yl]carbonyl](pyridin-2-yl)amino]pro-panoate *see* 2797
2-Ethylhexyl Salicylate *see* 6770
Ethylhexyl Triazone, 3809
S-Ethyl-L-homocysteine *see* 3738
Ethyl Hydrate *see* 3760
Ethyl Hydride *see* 3723
Ethyl Hydrogen Sulfate *see* 3853
Ethyl Hydroxide *see* 3760
Ethyl *p*-Hydroxybenzoate *see* 3837
7-Ethyl-10-hydroxycamptothecin *see* 5091
(+)-7-Ethyl-10-hydroxycamptothecine 10-[1,4′-Bipiperidine]-1′-carboxylate *see* 5091
α-Ethyl-1-hydroxycyclohexaneacetic Acid *see* 2715
2-Ethyl-3-(4-hydroxy-3,5-diiodoben-zoyl)benzofuran *see* 1083
N-Ethyl-3-hydroxy-*N*,*N*-dimethylben-zenaminium Chloride *see* 3516

(17α)-13-Ethyl-17-hydroxy-18,19-dinor-pregna-4,15-dien-20-yn-3-one *see* 4413
(17α)-13-Ethyl-17-hydroxy-18,19-dinor-pregna-4,9,11-trien-3-one *see* 9214
(17α)-13-Ethyl-17-hydroxy-18,19-dinor-pregna-4,9,11-trien-20-yn-3-one *see* 4415
(17α)-(±)-13-Ethyl-17-hydroxy-18,19-di-norpregn-4-en-3-one *see* 6686
(8α,9β,10α,13α,14β)-13-Ethyl-17-hydr-oxy-18,19-dinorpregn-4-en-20-yn-3-one *see* 6704
(17α)-(±)-13-Ethyl-17-hydroxy-18,19-di-norpregn-4-en-20-yn-3-one *see* 6704
(17α)-13-Ethyl-17-hydroxy-18,19-dinor-pregn-4-en-20-yn-3-one Oxime *see* 6694
(+)-13-Ethyl-17-hydroxy-18,19-dinor-17α-pregn-4-en-20-yn-3-one Oxime Acetate (Ester) *see* 6703
1-Ethyl-3-[(hydroxydiphenylacetyl)oxy]-1-methylpiperidinium Bromide *see* 7461
17α-Ethyl-17β-hydroxy-4-estrene *see* 3805
(16β,17β)-16-Ethyl-17-hydroxyestr-4-en-3-one *see* 6931
7-[2-[Ethyl(2-hydroxyethyl)amino]ethyl]-3,7-dihydro-1,3-dimethyl-8-(phenyl-methyl)-1*H*-purine-2,6-dione *see* 955
Ethyl Hydroxyethyl Cellulose *see* 1967
Ethyl 2-Hydroxyethyl Ether Cellulose *see* 1967
(17α)-13-Ethyl-17-hydroxy-11-methyl-ene-18,19-dinorpregn-4-en-20-yn-3-one *see* 3884
(1*R*,3*S*,5*Z*)-5-[(2*E*)-[(1*R*,3a*S*,7a*R*)-1-[(1*R*,2*E*,4*E*)-6-Ethyl-6-hydroxy-1-methyl-2,4-octadienyl]octahydro-7a-methyl-4*H*-inden-4-ylidene]ethyli-dene]-4-methylene-1,3-cyclohexane-diol *see* 8456
1-Ethyl-3-hydroxy-1-methylpiperidinium Bromide Benzilate *see* 7461
2-Ethyl-2-(hydroxymethyl)-1,3-propane-diol Trinitrate *see* 7811
N-Ethyl-α-(hydroxymethyl)-*N*-(4-pyri-dinylmethyl)benzeneacetamide *see* 9780
(1α,6β,14α,16β)-20-Ethyl-4-(hydroxy-methyl)-1,6,14,16-tetramethoxy-aconitane-7,8-diol *see* 5618
(4*S*)-4-Ethyl-4-hydroxy-10-nitro-1*H*-py-rano[3′,4′:6,7]indolizino[1,2-*b*]quino-line-3,14(4*H*,12*H*)-dione *see* 8288
17α-Ethyl-17-hydroxy-4-norandrosten-3-one *see* 6696
17α-Ethyl-17-hydroxy-19-norandrost-4-en-3-one *see* 6696
[7(*S*)-(1α,2β,4β,5α,7β)]-9-Ethyl-7-(3-hy-droxy-1-oxo-2-phenylpropoxy)-9-methyl-3-oxa-9-azoniatricyclo-[3.3.1.0^{2,4}]nonane Bromide *see* 6943
(*E*)-14-Ethyl-13-hydroxy-3,5,7,9,13-pen-tamethyl-6-[[3,4,6-trideoxy-3-(di-methylamino)-β-D-*xylo*-hexopyrano-side]oxy]oxacyclotetradec-11-ene-2,4,-10-trione *see* 7413
Ethyl(*m*-hydroxyphenyl)dimethylammo-nium Chloride *see* 3516
Ethyl *p*-Hydroxyphenyl Ketone *see* 7044
Ethyl 4-(*m*-Hydroxyphenyl)-1-methyliso-nipecotate *see* 4836
1-Ethyl-3-hydroxypiperidine *see* 3845
Ethyl α-Hydroxypropionate *see* 3817

2-[6-[Ethyl(2-hydroxypropyl)amino]-3-pyridazinyl]hydrazinecarboxylic Acid Ethyl Ester *see* 1631
(*S*)-4-Ethyl-4-hydroxy-1*H*-pyrano[3′,4′:6,7]indolizino[1,2-*b*]quinoline-3,14-(4*H*,12*H*)-dione *see* 1735
2-Ethyl-3-hydroxy-4*H*-pyran-4-one *see* 3824
3-Ethyl-7-hydroxy-2,8,12,16-tetrameth-yl-5,13-dioxo-9-[[3,4,6-trideoxy-3-(dimethylamino)-β-D-*xylo*-hexopyra-nosyl]oxy]-4,17-dioxabicyclo[14.1.0]-heptadec-14-ene-10-acetaldehyde *see* 8261
α-Ethyl-3-hydroxy-2,4,6-triiodoben-zenepropanoic Acid *see* 5061
α-Ethyl-3-hydroxy-2,4,6-triiodohydro-cinnamic Acid *see* 5061
α-Ethyl-β-(3-hydroxy-2,4,6-triiodophen-yl)propionic Acid *see* 5061
3,3′-Ethylidenebis[4-hydroxy-2*H*-1-benzopyran-2-one] *see* 3812
3,3′-Ethylidenebis(4-hydroxycouma-rin) *see* 3812
1,1′-Ethylidenebis[4-methylbenzene] *see* 3379
3,3-Ethylidenebis(4-oxycoumarin) *see* 3812
Ethylidene Chloride, 3810
24-Ethylidenecholest-5-en-3β-ol *see* 4280
Ethylidene Diacetate, 3811
Ethylidene Dicoumarol, 3812
Ethylidene Diethyl Ether *see* 38
Ethylidene Dimethyl Ether *see* 3226
[2*S*-(2α,3*E*,4β)]-3-Ethylidene-2-(β-D-glucopyranosyloxy)-3,4-dihydro-5-(methoxycarbonyl)-2*H*-pyran-4-ace-tic Acid 2-(3,4-Dihydroxyphenyl)-ethyl Ester *see* 6830
9-[(4,6-*O*-Ethylidene-β-D-glucopyrano-syl)oxy]-5,8,8a,9-tetrahydro-5-(4-hy-droxy-3,5-dimethoxyphenyl)furo[3′,-4′:6,7]naphtho[2,3-*d*]-1,3-dioxol-6(5a*H*)-one *see* 3886
(2*R*,3*R*,5*Z*)-5-Ethylidene-2-hydroxy-2,3-dimethylhexanedioic Acid *see* 8449
Ethylidenehydroxylamine *see* 42
7-Ethylidene-1a,2,3,7-tetrahydrocyclo-pent[*b*]oxireno[*c*]pyridine *see* 8
(3*E*,3a*S*,4a*R*,7a*S*,9a*S*,9b*S*)-3-Ethyli-dene-3,3a,7a,9b-tetrahydro-2-oxo-2*H*,4a*H*-1,4,5-trioxadicyclopent-[*a*,*hi*]indene-7-carboxylic Acid Methyl Ester *see* 7533
4(5)-(2-Ethyl-2-indanyl)imidazole *see* 861
3-Ethyl-12*H*-indolo[2,3-a]quinolizin-5-ium Inner Salt *see* 4093
Ethyl Iodide, 3813
Ethyl 10-(*p*-Iodophenyl)hendecanoate *see* 5060
1-[2-[*p*-[(*E*)-β-Ethyl-α-(*p*-iodophenyl)-styryl]phenoxy]ethyl]pyrrolidine *see* 4890
Ethyl 10-(*p*-Iodophenyl)undecylate *see* 5060
5-Ethyl-5-isoamylbarbituric Acid *see* 570
Ethyl Isobutyrate, 3814
α-Ethylisonicotinoylthioamide *see* 3737
5-Ethyl-5-isopentylbarbituric Acid *see* 570
O-Ethyl *O*-2-Isopropoxycarbonylphenyl Isopropylphosphoramidothioate *see* 5172
(±)-5-Ethyl-2-(4-isopropyl-4-methyl-5-oxo-1*H*-imidazolin-2-yl)nicotinic Acid *see* 4907
Ethyl Isothiocyanate, 3815
2-Ethylisothionicotinamide *see* 3737

Etydion [Nordic] *see* 3718
Etylon *see* 9199
Etyprenaline *see* 5170
5-EU *see* 3584
EU-1806 *see* 6353
EU-4200 *see* 7493
EU-5306 *see* 7066
EU4EA *see* 6018
Eubine [Chiesi] *see* 6959
β-Eucaine, 3894
Eucaine B *see* 3894
Eucalyptol, 3895
Eucalyptus, 3896
Eucardic [Roche] *see* 1873
Eucardion [Dompé] *see* 8123
Eucatropine, 3897
Eucazulen *see* 4554
Eucerin [Beiersdorf] *see* 5359
Eucil [Farmasa] *see* 6143
Eucistin [San Carlo] *see* 6359
Euciton [Roux-Ocefa] *see* 3418
Euclorina [Bracco] *see* 2075
Eucoran *see* 6543
Eucytol *see* 2907
Eudatin [Abbott] *see* 7038
Eudemine Injection [Schering] *see* 3004
Eudermol *see* 6524
Eudigox [Simes] *see* 3167
EUDR *see* 3514
Eudyna [BASF] *see* 8165
Eufans [Sigma-Tau] *see* 596
Eufibron [Berlin-Chemie] *see* 7871
Eufin *see* 3780
Euflavine *see* 123
Euflex [Schering] *see* 4208
Eugallol [Knoll] *see* 8000
Eugenic Acid *see* 3898
Eugenol, 3898
Eugenol Methyl Ether *see* 6073
Euglucon [Sanofi-Aventis] *see* 4478
Euhypnos [Sigma] *see* 9133
Euipnos [Farmitalia] *see* 9133
Eukodal [Merck KGaA] *see* 6959
Eukraton [Nordmark] *see* 1027
Eukystol [Merckle] *see* 4598
Eulexin [Schering] *see* 4208
Eulip [SIT] *see* 9416
Eulipos [Boehringer, Mann.] *see* 9415
Eumelanins *see* 5812
Euminex [Lacer] *see* 4448
Eumotol [Byk Gulden] *see* 1483
Eumovate [GSK] *see* 2364
Eumulgin [Henkel] *see* 7577
Eumydrin [SKB] *see* 875
Eunades [Pfizer] *see* 9990
Eunal [Schering] *see* 5518
Eunatrol *see* 6828
Eunephran [Servier] *see* 1525
Eunerpan [Nordmark] *see* 5827
Eunoctal [Houdé] *see* 570
Eunoctin [Gedeon Richter] *see* 6575
Euonymit *see* 4332
Euonymus, 3899
Eupantol [Altana] *see* 7014
Euparen(e) [Bayer] *see* 3044
Euparin, 3900
Eupatorin, 3901
Eupatorium, 3902
Eupaverin [Merck KGaA] *see* 6288
Eupaverina [Bracco] *see* 6288
Euphorbia, 3903
Euphthalmine [Warner-Chilcott] *see* 3897
Euphyllina [Byk Gulden] *see* 465
Euphylline [Altana] *see* 9285
Euphylong [Altana] *see* 9285

Euplit [Desitin] *see* 487
Eupnéron [Lyocentre] *see* 3636
Eupractone [Baxter] *see* 3213
Eupragin [Alcon-Thilo] *see* 3683
Euprax [Baxter] *see* 217
Eupressyl [Byk Gulden] *see* 9865
Euprovasin [Magis] *see* 7840
Euradal [Lacer] *see* 1295
Eurax [Novartis] *see* 2594
Euraxil [Thomae] *see* 2594
Eureceptor [Zambon] *see* 2279
Eurelix [Hoechst] *see* 7492
Euresol [Knoll] *see* 8155
Eurex [Labaz] *see* 7717
Eurodin [Takeda] *see* 3702
Eurodopa [Europharma] *see* 5464
European Blueberry *see* 1217
European Pennyroyal *see* 7102
European White Birch *see* 1188
Europia *see* 3904
Europium, 3904
Eurosan [Mepha] *see* 2994
Eusaprim [GSK] *see* 8918
Eusmanid *see* 1186
Eusolex 232 [Merck KGaA] *see* 3593
Eusolex 2292 [Merck KGaA] *see* 6769
Eusolex 4360 [Merck KGaA] *see* 6954
Eusolex 6300 [Merck KGaA] *see* 6027
Eusolex 9020 [Merck KGaA] *see* 888
Eusolex HMS [Merck KGaA] *see* 4738
Eusolex OCR [Merck KGaA] *see* 6756
Eusolex OS [Merck KGaA] *see* 6770
Eusovit [Strathmann] *see* 9495
Euspiran *see* 5217
Eutensin [Aventis] *see* 4309
Euthyrox [Merck KGaA] *see* 9415
Eutonyl [Abbott] *see* 7038
Eutrit [Takeda] *see* 10085
Euvaderm [Gödecke] *see* 1180
Euvernil [Heyden] *see* 8931
Euvitol [Allen & Hanburys] *see* 3966
E-VA-16 *see* 4932
Evacort [Evans] *see* 4787
Evadene [Ayerst] *see* 1533
Evadyne [Ayerst] *see* 1533
Evan's Blue, 3905
Evansite *see* 358
Evastel [Almirall] *see* 3484
Evazol [Ravensberg] *see* 2913
"Eve" *see* 5766
Evening Primrose Oil, 3906
Eventin [Minden] *see* 2707
Everest [Bayer] *see* 4119
Everfree [Cooper] *see* 6596
Everninic Acid Methyl Ester *see* 8734
Everolimus, 3907
Everone [Hyrex] *see* 9180
Evik [Syngenta] *see* 393
Evion [Merck KGaA] *see* 9495
Evipal [Winthrop] *see* 4704
Evipal Sodium [Winthrop] *see* 4704
Evipan [Bayer] *see* 4704
Evipan Sodium [Bayer] *see* 4704
Evista [Lilly] *see* 8098
Evodiamine, 3908
Evolus [DuPont] *see* 894
Evonogenin *see* 3162
Evorel [Janssen-Cilag] *see* 3703
Evoxac [Daiichi] *see* 2034
Evoxin [Sterling Winthrop] *see* 3418
Evra [Janssen-Cilag] *see* 6694
Evramycin [Wyeth] *see* 9770
Ewer-Pick Acid *see* 6373
Ex-12-095 *see* 3715
Exacin [Schering] *see* 5106

Exacor [Searle] *see* 2269
Exacyl [Sanofi-Synthelabo] *see* 9569
Exal [Nippon Kayaku] *see* 9982
Exalamide, 3909
Exalgin *see* 6007
Exaltolide [Firmenich], 3910
Exametazime, 3911
Exangit *see* 1096
Exanta [AstraZeneca] *see* 10077
Exaprazole *see* 3695
Exatecan, 3912
Exatecan Mesylate *see* 3912
Excede [Pfizer] *see* 1950
Excegran [Dainippon] *see* 10192
Excenel [Pfizer] *see* 1950
EXD *see* 3384
Exelderm [Syntex] *see* 8893
Exelon [Novartis] *see* 8240
Exemestane, 3913
Exenatide *see* 3914
Exendin-3 *see* 3914
Exendin-4 *see* 3914
Exendin (9-39) *see* 3914
Exendin (9-39) Amide *see* 3914
9-39-Exendin 3 (Heloderma horridum)
   see 3914
9-39-Exendin 4 *see* 3914
Exendins, 3914
Exhelm [Pfizer] *see* 6266
Exhirud [Sanofi Winthrop] *see* 4718
Exifone, 3915
Exisulind, 3916
Exitelite *see* 711
Exjade [Novartis] *see* 2858
Exlan *see* 2575
Ex-Lax Ultra [Novartis] *see* 1242
Exlutena [Organon] *see* 5629
Exluton(a) [Organon] *see* 5629
Exna [Wyeth] *see* 1120
Exoamylases *see* 599
Exocin [Allergan] *see* 6771
Exocorpol [Green Cross] *see* 7562
Exoderil [Rentschler] *see* 6355
Exodextranases *see* 2949
Exodor-Grun *see* 2155
Exofene *see* 4680
(±)-2-Exo-(2-methylbenzyloxy)-1-
   methyl-4-isopropyl-7-oxabicyclo-
   [2.2.1]heptane *see* 2295
Exonal [Toyama] *see* 9112
Exosulfonyl [Théraplix] *see* 8878
Exosurf [Glaxo Wellcome], 3917
Exosurf Neonatal [GSK] *see* 2477
EXP-105-1 *see* 374
EXP-126 *see* 8224
EXP-999 *see* 6149
EXP-3174 *see* 5583
Expansine *see* 7053
Experimental Insecticide No. 269 *see*
   3578
Exponcit N [Salutas Fahlberg-List] *see*
   6714
Expressed Almond Oil *see* 6813
Exrheudon N [Optimed] *see* 7277
Exsel [Herbert] *see* 8436
Exsiccated Alum *see* 360
Exsiccated Ammonium Alum *see* 327
Exsiccated Ferrous Sulfate *see* 4057
Exsiccated Sodium Phosphate *see* 8659
Extacol [Nikken] *see* 7258
Ext. D & C Orange 3 *see* 6857
Ext. D & C Red No. 14 *see* 10089
Ext. D & C Red No. 15 *see* 7590
Ext. D & C Yellow No. 1 *see* 5928
Ext. D & C Yellow No. 7 *see* 6393

Ext. D & C Yellow No. 9 *see* 10095
Ext. D & C Yellow No. 10 *see* 10096
Extencilline [RPR] *see* 7096
Exterol [Dermal] *see* 1782
Extinguish [Wellmark] *see* 5983
Extracort [Basotherm] *see* 9596
Extractum *Ginkgo Biloba* **761** *see* 4425
Extramycin [Bayer] *see* 8550
Extranase [Rorer] *see* 1388
Extrinsic Factor *see* 10014
Extrinsic Plasminogen Activator *see* 9468
EYE-001 *see* 7068
Eye-derived Growth Factor-II *see* 4072
Eyekas [Showa Shinyaku] *see* 8200
Ezetimibe, 3918
Ezetrol [Merck/Schering-Plough] *see* 3918
E-Z-Paque [E-Z-Em] *see* 994
F-4 *see* 897
F-155 *see* 8534
F-190 *see* 52
F-314 *see* 865
F-319 *see* 4856
F-440 *see* 2816
F-1500 *see* 8878
F-1785 *see* 4105
F-1983 *see* 8010
F-1991 *see* 1044
F-2207 *see* 6194
F-2559 *see* 4343
F-3616 *see* 3427
F-6060 *see* 2720
F-6066 *see* 2720
F-6285 *see* 8947
F8426 *see* 1837
F-28249α *see* 6444
FA *see* 4168
FA-402 *see* 4006
FA-2071 *see* 5077
2-FAA *see* 4157
Fabahistin [Bayer] *see* 5770
Fabrazyme [Genzyme] *see* 4336
Fabrol [Zyma] *see* 88
F Acid *see* 1892
Factitious Air *see* 6653
Factor [Syngenta] *see* 7766
Factor I *see* 4071
Factor II *see* 7889
Factor IIa *see* 9383
Factor III *see* 9385
Factor V, 3919
Factor VII, 3920
Factor VIII, 3921
Factor IX, 3922
Factor IX Complex (Human) *see* 3922
Factor X, 3923
Factor XI, 3924
Factor XII, 3925
Factor XIII, 3926
Factor B *see* 3868
Factor T *see* 10025
Factrel [Ayerst] *see* 5474
FAD *see* 4091
FADD-like ICE *see* 1886
Fademin [Chugai] *see* 4091
Fado [Errekappa] *see* 1914
Fadrozole, 3927
Fadul [Hexal] *see* 3930
Faecla *see* 7615
Faecula *see* 7615
Fagarasterol *see* 5608
Fagarine, 3928
α-Fagarine *see* 265
β-Fagarine *see* 8561
γ-Fagarine *see* 3928
Fagarol *see* 8470

Fagine *see* 2204
Fairy Gloves *see* 3159
FAK III *see* 4248
Falapen [Frosst] *see* 7094
Falcol [Bayer] *see* 22
Falicard [AWD] *see* 9950
Falignost [Hexal] *see* 5053
Falimint *see* 6629
Falithrom [Hexal] *see* 7259
Falmonox [Winthrop] *see* 9105
Falomesin [Chugai] *see* 1948
False Hellebore *see* 167
False Indigo *see* 959
False Saffron *see* 1868
False Unicorn *see* 4631
False Winter's Bark *see* 1743
Falvin [Farmades] *see* 4005
Famciclovir, 3929
Famodil [Sigma-Tau] *see* 3930
Famophos *see* 3932
Famosan [ProMed] *see* 3930
Famosept [Spofa] *see* 7303
Famotidine, 3930
Famoxadone, 3931
Famoxal [Silanes] *see* 3930
Famoxate [DuPont] *see* 3931
Famphur, 3932
Fampridine, 3933
Famvir [SKB] *see* 3929
Fanasil [Roche] *see* 8906
Fancol ACEL [Fanning] *see* 5358
Fancol ALA [Fanning] *see* 5359
Fancol LA [Fanning] *see* 5359
Fandango [Bayer CropSci.] *see* 4184
Fanodormo *see* 2711
Fansidar [Roche] *see* 7985
Fansidol [Brocchieri] *see* 6548
Fantacin [Kyowa Hakko] *see* 4137
Fantofarone, 3934
Fantorin [Glaxo] *see* 8813
2-F-araA *see* 4126
2-F-ara-AMP *see* 4126
Farecef [Lafare] *see* 1930
Faredina [Lafare] *see* 1979
Faremicin [Lafare] *see* 4254
Fareston [Farmos] *see* 9550
Faretrizin [Lafare] *see* 1915
Farexin [Lafare] *see* 1974
Fargan [Pfizer] *see* 7786
Farganesse [Pfizer] *see* 7786
Far-Go [Monsanto] *see* 9594
Farial [Riemser] *see* 4932
Farlutal [Pharmacia] *see* 5793
Farmaproina [CEPA] *see* 7097
Farmidril [Farmitalia] *see* 5386
Farmiglucin [Farmitalia] *see* 7041
Farminosidin [Farmitalia] *see* 7041
Farmiserina [Farmitalia] *see* 2751
Farmitalia 204/122 *see* 8910
Farmolisina [Centralvet] *see* 3350
Farmorubicina [Pharmacia] *see* 3623
Farmoxin [Erba] *see* 1936
Farnesene *see* 3935
α-Farnesene, 3935
β-Farnesene, 3936
Farnesol, 3937
Farnoquinone *see* 5833
Farom [Daiichi] *see* 3938
Faropenem, 3938
Faropenem Medoxomil *see* 3938
FAS *see* 3939
Fasciculins, 3939
Fasidotril, 3940
Fasidotrilat *see* 3940
Fasigin [Pfizer] *see* 9447

Fasigyn [Pfizer] *see* 9447
Fasinex [Novartis] *see* 9652
Faslodex [AstraZeneca] *see* 4284
Fast Green *see* 5699
Fast Green FCF, 3941
Fast Green J *see* 1374
Fastic [Ajinomoto] *see* 6428
Fastin [SKB] *see* 7262
Faston [Duphar] *see* 3207
Fast Scarlet *see* 1101
Fastum [Menarini] *see* 5305
Fasturtec [Sanofi-Aventis] *see* 8117
Fast Yellow *see* 9776
Fasudil, 3942
Fasupond [Eu Rho Pharma] *see* 6714
Fat Ponceau R *see* 8393
Fatroximin [Fatro] *see* 8220
all-cis-Fatty Acid 20:5 Omega-3 *see* 3531
Faustan [Temmler] *see* 2994
Faverin [Solvay] *see* 4219
Favistan [Temmler] *see* 5971
Fazadinium Bromide, 3943
Fazadon [Glaxo Wellcome] *see* 3943
Fazol [Schering] *see* 5160
Fazor *see* 5705
FB₁ *see* 4289
FB/2 *see* 3352
FB-5097 *see* 2417
FBA-1420 *see* 7803
FBA-4503 *see* 7831
5F-BAPTA *see* 957
5-FC *see* 4125
FC 11 *see* 9640
FC-54 *see* 244
FC-1157a *see* 9550
FC-3001 *see* 9422
FCCs *see* 2140
FCE-20124 *see* 8125
FCE-21336 *see* 1601
FCE-22101 *see* 8236
FCE-22891 *see* 8236
FCE-24304 *see* 3913
FCE-26743 *see* 8315
FCR-1272 *see* 2756
FCRC-A48 *see* 4267
FCV *see* 3929
FDA-20 *see* 4183
FDA-1541 *see* 3640
FDC *see* 4183
FD & C Blue No. 1 *see* 1373
FD & C Blue No. 2 *see* 4944
FD & C Green 1 *see* 4575
FD & C Green No. 2 *see* 5485
FD & C Green No. 3 *see* 3941
FD & C Orange I *see* 6857
FD & C Red No. 1 *see* 7590
FD & C Red No. 2 *see* 375
FD & C Red No. 3 *see* 3693
FD & C Red No. 4 *see* 7591
FD & C Red No. 32 *see* 10089
FD & C Red No. 40 *see* 284
FD & C Yellow No. 1 *see* 6393
FD & C Yellow No. 3 *see* 10095
FD & C Yellow No. 4 *see* 10096
FD & C Yellow No. 5 *see* 9072
FD & C Yellow No. 6 *see* 9001
¹⁸FDG *see* 4127
FDNB *see* 4172
F3TDR *see* 9687
Featherfew *see* 4067
Featherfoil *see* 4067
Febantel, 3944
Febarbamate, 3945
Febrifugine, 3946
Febuprol, 3947

Febuxostat, 3948
Fecapentaene 12 see 3406
Fectrim [DDSA] see 8918
Fedacilina [Fedal] see 5925
Fedan [ICI] see 6823
Fedibaretta see 7222
Fedotozine, 3949
Feinalmin [Sanko] see 4920
Felacrinos see 2868
Felbamate, 3950
Felbamyl [Wallace] see 3950
Felbatol [Carter-Wallace] see 3950
Felbinac, 3951
Feldene [Pfizer] see 7506
Felicur [Asche] see 3768
Felinine, 3952
(−)-Felinine see 3952
Felison [Sigurta] see 4198
Felitrope see 3768
Felkin-Crabtree Catalyst see 2566
Felmane see 4198
Feloday [Novartis] see 3953
Felodipine, 3953
Felosan see 4833
Felviten [Grünenthal] see 644
Felypressin, 3954
Femara [Novartis] see 5450
Femestrone Inj see 3708
Femidyn see 3708
Feminone [Pharmacia & Upjohn] see 3734
Femodene [Schering AG] see 4413
Femovan [Schering AG] see 4413
Femoxetine, 3955
Fempress [Schwarz] see 6229
Femring [Warner-Chilcott] see 3703
Femstat [Syntex] see 1529
Femtrace [Warner-Chilcott] see 3703
Femulen [Searle] see 3860
Fenactil [Jelfa] see 2185
Fenadone see 5944
Fenamidone, 3956
Fenamiphos, 3957
Fenamisal see 7272
Fenamizol see 483
Fenarimol, 3958
Fenarol [Winthrop] see 2106
Fenarsone see 1786
Fenasprate see 1045
Fenatin see 7216
Fenazaquin, 3959
Fenazil [Sella] see 7786
Fenazol [Hokuriku Seiyaku] see 4132
Fenazox [Meiji] see 395
Fenazoxine see 6440
Fenbendazole, 3960
Fenbenicillin, 3961
Fenbid [Goldshield] see 4881
Fenbuconazole, 3962
Fenbufen, 3963
Fenbutatin Oxide, 3964
Fenbutrazate, 3965
Fencamfamine, 3966
Fencamine, 3967
Fenchlorphos see 8256
d-Fenchone, 3968
Fenclor [Caffaro] see 7564
Fenclozic Acid, 3969
Fendilar [SPA] see 3970
Fendiline, 3970
Fendosal, 3971
Fenethanil see 3962
Fenethylline, 3972
Fenetrazole see 9092
Fenfluramine, 3973
Fenformin see 7231

Fenhexamid, 3974
Fenhydren see 7234
Fenibut see 464
Fenibutazona see 7277
Fenibutol [Atral] see 7277
Fenican [Rhone-Poulenc] see 3144
Fenicol [Alcon] see 2077
Fenidrone see 6957
Fenilin see 7234
Fenilor [UCB] see 1453
Fenipentol, 3975
Fenistil [Novartis] see 3216
Fenitrothion, 3976
Fennel, 3977
Fenobrate [Gramon] see 3978
Fenofibrate, 3978
Fenoldopam, 3979
Fenoldopam Mesylate see 3979
Fenolovo see 9745
Fenopron [Dista] see 3980
Fenoprofen, 3980
Fenormin see 7231
Fenospen [Pharmacia] see 7100
Fenotard [Virbac] see 3978
Fenoterol, 3981
Fenoverine, 3982
Fenoxanil, 3983
Fenoxaprop-ethyl, 3984
Fenoxaprop-P-ethyl see 3984
Fenoxazoline, 3985
Fenoxedil, 3986
Fenoximone see 3589
Fenoxycarb, 3987
Fenoxypen [Novo] see 7100
Fenozolone, 3988
Fenpiclonil, 3989
Fenpidon see 3337
Fenpipramide Methobromide see 3990
Fenpiverinium Bromide, 3990
Fenpropanate see 3991
Fenpropathrin, 3991
Fenpropidin, 3992
Fenpropimorph, 3993
Fenproporex, 3994
Fenprostalene, 3995
Fenpyrate see 7968
Fenpyroximate, 3996
Fenquizone, 3997
Fenretinide, 3998
Fenspiride, 3999
Fensulfothion, 4000
Fental [Kanebo] see 9112
Fentanest [Pharmacia] see 4001
Fentanyl, 4001
Fentazin [Allen & Hanburys] see 7183
Fenthion, 4002
Fentiazac, 4003
Fentiazin see 7252
Fenticlor, 4004
Fenticonazole, 4005
Fentiderm [Zyma] see 4005
Fentigyn [Novartis] see 4005
Fentin Acetate see 9745
Fentin Hydroxide see 9745
Fentonium Bromide, 4006
Fentrazamide, 4007
Fentrinol [Frika] see 399
Fenugreek, 4008
Fenuron, 4009
Fenuron TCA see 4009
Fenvalerate, 4010
Fenyramidol see 7321
Feosol [SK & F] see 4057
Feospan [SK & F] see 4057
Fepradinol, 4011

Feprazone, 4012
Fepron [Lilly] see 3980
Feprona [Lilly] see 3980
Ferbam, 4013
Ferbeck see 4013
Fergon [Miles] see 4047
Fergon 500 [Alfar] see 1974
Feridex [Advanced Magnetics] see 4063
Fer-in-Sol [Mead Johnson] see 4057
Ferlixit [Aventis] see 8615
Ferlucon see 4047
Fermate see 4013
Fermcozyme see 4460
Fermentation Amyl Alcohol see 5195
Fermentation Butyl Alcohol see 5131
Fermentation L. casei Factor see 7934
Fermine see 3255
Fermium, 4014
Fernambuco see 7181
Fernasan [Zeneca] see 9371
Fernos [Zeneca] see 7496
Fero-Gradumet [Abbott] see 4057
Ferolactan [Bioindustria] see 7779
Feromax see 4057
Feron [Toray] see 4991
Feroritard [Nikken] see 4057
Ferradow see 4013
Ferredoxins, 4015
Ferric Acetate, Basic, 4016
Ferric Alum see 518
Ferric Ammonium Citrate, 4017
Ferric Ammonium Ferrocyanide see 7910
Ferric Ammonium Oxalate see 517
Ferric Ammonium Sulfate see 518
Ferric Bromide, 4018
Ferric Chloride, 4019
Ferric Chromate(VI), 4020
Ferric Citrate, 4021
Ferric Dimethyldithiocarbamate see 4013
Ferric Enterobactin see 3596
Ferric Ferrocyanide see 7910
Ferric Ferrous Oxide see 4040
Ferric Fluoride, 4022
Ferric Formate, 4023
Ferric Gallotannate see 4033
Ferric Hexacyanoferrate(II) see 7910
Ferrichrome, 4024
Ferrichrome A see 4024
Ferrichromes, 4024
Ferrichrysin see 4024
Ferric Hydroxide, 4025
Ferric Hydroxide Oxide see 4025
Ferric Hypophosphite, 4026
Ferric Monosodium Ethylenediamine-
    tetraacetate see 4031
Ferric Nitrate, 4027
Ferric Oxide, 4028
Ferric Persulfate see 4032
Ferric Phosphate, 4029
Ferric Pyrophosphate, 4030
Ferricrocin see 4024
Ferric Sesquioxide see 4028
Ferric Sesquisulfate see 4032
Ferric Sodium Edetate, 4031
Ferric Subsulfate Solution see 6256
Ferric Sulfate, 4032
Ferric Sulfocyanate see 4034
Ferric Sulfocyanide see 4034
Ferric Tannate, 4033
Ferric Tersulfate see 4032
Ferric Thiocyanate, 4034
Ferricytochrome c see 2791
Ferriheme Chloride see 4644
Ferriheme Hydroxide see 4635
Ferrihemoglobin see 5965

Ferrimycins see 2860
Ferrioxamine B see 2860
Ferriporphyrin Chloride see 4644
Ferriporphyrin Hydroxide see 4635
Ferriprotoporphyrin Basic see 4635
Ferriprotoporphyrin Chloride see 4644
Ferrirhodin see 4024
Ferrirubin see 4024
FerriSeltz [Otsuka] see 4017
Ferrite, 4035
Ferritin, 4036
Ferritose [Calbiochem] see 4273
Ferrivenin [Fresenius] see 5101
Ferrlecit [Watson] see 8615
Ferro Angelini [Angelini] see 4030
Ferrocene, 4037
Ferrochel [Albion] see 4041
Ferrocholinate, 4038
Ferrocontin [Napp] see 4039
Ferrocytochrome c see 2791
Ferrofolin [Schering AG] see 4036
Ferroglycine Sulfate, 4039
Ferro-Gradumet [Abbott] see 4057
Ferroheme see 4639
Ferroin see 7214
Ferrol [UCB] see 4036
Ferrolip see 4038
Ferromyn [Calmic] see 4056
Ferron see 4826
Ferronat [Galena] see 4046
Ferronicum [Sandoz] see 4047
Ferroprotoporphyrin see 4639
Ferrosanol [Schwarz] see 4039
Ferrosoferric Oxide, 4040
Ferrospinel see 4035
Ferrosprint [Pfizer] see 4036, 8615
Ferrostar [Mediolanum] see 4036
Ferrostrane see 4031
Ferrostrene see 4031
Ferrotemp [Medix] see 4046
Ferrous Aminoacetosulfate see 4039
Ferrous Ammonium Sulfate see 521
Ferrous Bisglycinate, 4041
Ferrous Bromide, 4042
Ferrous Chloride, 4043
Ferrous Citrate, 4044
Ferrous Fluoride, 4045
Ferrous Fumarate, 4046
Ferrous Gluconate, 4047
Ferrous Hydroxide, 4048
Ferrous Iodide, 4049
Ferrous Lactate, 4050
Ferrous Oxalate, 4051
Ferrous Oxide, 4052
Ferrous Phosphate, 4053
Ferrous Phosphide, 4054
Ferrous Selenide, 4055
Ferrous Succinate, 4056
Ferrous Sulfate, 4057
Ferrous Sulfide, 4058
Ferrous Sulfocyanate see 4059
Ferrous Sulfocyanide see 4059
Ferrous Thiocyanate, 4059
Ferrox see 4051
Ferroxidase see 2006
Fersaday [Goldshield] see 4046
Fersamal [Goldshield] see 4046
Fertagyl [Intervet] see 5474
Fertiletten [Chassot] see 2102
Fertilysin, 4060
Fertinorm [Serono] see 4223
Fertiral [HMR] see 5474
Fertirelin, 4061
Fertodur [Schering AG] see 2720
Ferulic Acid, 4062

3-Feruloylquinic Acid see 2142
Ferumoxides, 4063
Ferumoxsil, 4064
Ferumoxtran 10, 4065
Fervenulin, 4066
FES see 10116
Fesofor [SK & F] see 4057
Fespan [SK & F] see 4057
Festamoxin [Shionogi] see 6286
Festucine see 5561
Fétizon's Reagent see 8507
Fevarin [Solvay] see 4219
Feverall see 3350
Feverfew, 4067
Fevonil [Century] see 3350
Feximac [Nicholas] see 1474
Fexofenadine, 4068
FG-4963 see 3955
FG-5111 see 5827
FG-5606 see 580
FG-7051 see 7043
FGF see 4072
FGN-1 see 3916
FI-106 see 3439
FI-1163 see 5592
FI-3542 see 3485
FI-5853 see 7041
FI-6026 see 3428
FI-6341 see 4243
F.I. 6426 see 8772
FI-6714 see 6496
FI-6934 see 2005
FI-7045 see 8465
FI-7056 see 8465
Fialuridine, 4069
FIAU see 4069
Fiber A see 6870
Fiber V [DuPont] see 7569
Fiber X-51 see 2575
Fiber X-54 see 2575
Fiberall [Novartis] see 7517
Fiblaferon [Rentschler] see 4991
Fiboran [Christiaens] see 754
Fibrase [SK & F] see 7134
Fibravyl [Rhovyl] see 7586
Fibrezym [Bene-Arzneimittel] see 7134
Fibrin, 4070
Fibrinase see 3926
Fibrin-i see 4070
Fibrinogen, 4071
Fibrinogenase see 9383
Fibrinokinase see 9468
Fibrinolysin see 7520
Fibrin-s see 4070
Fibrin-stabilizing Factor see 3926
Fibroblast Growth Factor, 4072
24-163-Fibroblast Growth Factor 7
    (Human) see 6986
Fibroblast Interferon see 4991
Fibrogammin [Centeon] see 3926
Fibroin, 4073
Fibrolase, 4074
3-203-Fibrolase [3-Serine] (Agkistrodon
    contortrix contortrix Recombinant) see
    237
Fibrolax [Gipharmex] see 7517
Fibronectins, 4075
Ficam [Bayer CropSci.] see 1036
Fichtelite, 4076
Ficin, 4077
Ficoid [Fisons] see 4153
Ficortril [Pfizer] see 4787
Ficusin see 7928
Ficus Protease see 4077
Ficus Proteinase see 4077

Fidarestat, 4078
FIF see 4991
Filaribits [SKB] see 3116
Filazine see 3116
Fildesin [Shionogi] see 9987
Filgrastim see 4537
Filicic Acid see 4081
Filicin see 4081
Filicinic Acid, 4079
Filicinsäure (German) see 4079
Filimarisin see 4080
Filipin, 4080
Filipin III see 4080
Filixic Acids, 4081
Filix Mas (B.P.) see 848
Filixsäure (German) see 4081
Filon [Berk] see 3965
Filoral see 2210
Filtrax [Biomed. Foscama] see 7460
Finaceae [Schering AG] see 905
Finadyne [Fisons] see 4147
Finaplix [Intervet] see 9583
Finasteride, 4082
Finastid [Neopharmed] see 4082
Finaten [Finadiet] see 4228
Finaven [BASF] see 3138
Fingolimod, 4083
Finlepsin [AWD] see 1781
Finquel [Argent] see 9621
Finuret see 4789
Fipexide, 4084
Fiproles see 4085
Fipronil, 4085
Firefly Luciferin, 4086
Firemaster BP-6 see 7563
Firemaster LV-T 23P [Michigan Chem.]
    see 9751
Firemaster T 23P [Michigan Chem.] see
    9751
Firmacef [Firma] see 1917
Firocoxib, 4087
Firstcin [Takeda] see 1937
Fir-wood Oil see 6810
Fisalamine see 5904
Fischer's Yellow see 2432
Fisetin, 4088
Fish-berry see 2456
Fish Glue see 5109
Fisidenolon 1521 see 4088
Fisiobil [S.A.L.V.A.T.] see 3203
Fisiodar [Abiogen] see 2960
Fisostina see 4312
Fixed Oil see 6315
Fixical [Pharmascience] see 1657
FK-027 see 1924
FK-037 see 1932
FK-235 see 6545
FK-435 see 3446
FK-463 see 6175
FK-482 see 1920
FK-506 see 9025
FK-749 see 1951
FK-1160 see 9424
FL-113 see 5074
FL-1039 see 390
FL-1060 see 389
FLA-731 see 8132
Flabelline see 5969
Flagentyl [Rhône-Poulenc] see 8419
Flagyl [Searle] see 6157
Flake Lead see 1005
Flamazine [Smith & Nephew] see 8903
Flamitajin [Teisan; Iwaki] see 4091
Flammazine [Solvay] see 8903
Flammex AP see 9751

Flammex T 23P *see* 9751
Flamon [Mepha] *see* 9950
Flanax [Syntex] *see* 6417
Flanin F [Tokyo Tanabe] *see* 4091
Flantadin [Lepetit] *see* 2862
Flatistine *see* 1849
Flavacidin *see* 616
Flavalfate *see* 3427
Flavamed [Berlin-Chemie] *see* 1086
Flavan [Pharmafarm] *see* 5452
3,3′,4,4′,5,7-Flavanhexol *see* 5452
3,3′,4′,5,7-Flavanpentol *see* 1902
Flavaspidic Acid, 4090
Flavaxin [Winthrop] *see* 8200
Flavianic Acid *see* 6393
Flavicin *see* 616
Flavine-Adenine Dinucleotide, 4091
Flavine Yellow Shade *see* 8037
Flavin Mononucleotide *see* 8201
Flavitan *see* 4091
Flavomycin [Hoechst] *see* 952
Flavone, 4092
7-Flavone Ethyl Hydroxyacetate *see* 3523
7-Flavonoxyacetic Acid Ethyl Ester *see* 3523
Flavopereirine, 4093
Flavophospholipol *see* 952
Flavopiridol, 4094
Flavoquine [Aventis] *see* 572
Flavoxanthin, 4095
Flavoxate, 4096
Flavurol *see* 5867
Flaxedil *see* 4343
Flaxseed *see* 5508
Flazasulfuron, 4097
FLC-1374 *see* 9421
Fleabane *see* 3666
Flea Seed *see* 7517
Flebopex [Profarma] *see* 3297
Flebosan [Dukron] *see* 9608
Flebosmil [Bouchara] *see* 3297
Flebosten [Bonomelli] *see* 3297
Flebotropin [Bago] *see* 3297
Flécaine [3M Pharma] *see* 4098
Flecainide, 4098
Flectadol [Maggioni] *see* 5637
Flectar [Maggioni] *see* 10071
Flectron [BASF] *see* 2767
Fleishmilchsäure *see* 5337
Flemoxine [Yamanouchi] *see* 577
Fleroxacin, 4099
Flesinoxan, 4100
Flex [Syngenta] *see* 4227
Flexartal [Sanofi Winthrop] *see* 1842
Flexazone *see* 7277
Flexeril [Merck & Co.] *see* 2713
Flexiban [Merck & Co.] *see* 2713
Flexible Collodion *see* 2484
Flexidol [Daker-Farmasimes] *see* 4011
Flexidor [Dow AgroSci.] *see* 5235
Flexin [McNeil] *see* 10199
Flexstar [Syngenta] *see* 4227
FLICE *see* 1886
Flight Control [DCV] *see* 687
Flindersine, 4101
Flint *see* 8493
Flint [Bayer CropSci.] *see* 9677
Flivas [Asahi] *see* 6356
Flixonase [GSK] *see* 4211
Flixotide [GSK] *see* 4211
Flobacin [Sigma-Tau] *see* 6771
Flociprin [IBI] *see* 2314
Flocor [CytRx] *see* 7562
Flocoumafen, 4102
Floctafenine, 4103

Flodil [AstraZeneca] *see* 3953
Floganol [Zyma] *see* 2361
Flogar [UCB] *see* 6916
Flogencyl [Expanpharm] *see* 3696
Flogene [Polifarma] *see* 4003
Floginax [Lifepharma] *see* 6417
Flogitolo *see* 6972
Flogobene [Farge] *see* 7506
Flogobron [Intersint] *see* 6944
Flogoril *see* 6972
Flogos [Gentili] *see* 9009
Flogovital [Bago] *see* 6548
Flogozen [SPA] *see* 4913
Floionic Acid *see* 7325
Flolan [GSK] *see* 7875
Flomax [Chiesi] *see* 6531
Flomax [Astellas] *see* 9049
Flomaxtra [Astellas] *see* 9049
Flomoxef, 4104
Flonase [GSK] *see* 4211
Flonatril [Specia] *see* 2404
Flonicamid, 4105
Flonorm [Schering-Plough] *see* 8220
Flopion [Kyoritsu] *see* 4106
Flopropione, 4106
Floramite [Uniroyal] *see* 1207
Florantyrone, 4107
Floraquin [Searle] *see* 5042
Florasulam, 4108
Flores Martis *see* 4019
Florfenicol, 4109
Florid [Mochida] *see* 6178
Floridin *see* 4283
Floridin [Coli] *see* 1979
Florimycin *see* 10001
Florinef [BMS] *see* 4130
Floripavine *see* 8341
Florisil *see* 5687
Florocid *see* 8618
Florocol [Schering-Plough] *see* 4109
Florone [Pfizer] *see* 3140
Floropipamide *see* 7455
Floropryl [Merck & Co.] *see* 5176
Flosequinan, 4110
Flosequinon *see* 4110
Flou [ELEA] *see* 7903
Flovacil [Andromaco] *see* 3146
Flovent [GSK] *see* 4211
Flowering Dogwood *see* 2535
Flowers of Antimony *see* 711
Flowers of Sulfur *see* 8977
Flowers of Tin *see* 8778
Flowers of Zinc *see* 10147
Flowery-headed Spurge *see* 3903
Floxacillin, 4111
Floxacin [Merck & Co.] *see* 6700
Floxapen [GSK] *see* 4111
Floxil [Janssen-Cilag] *see* 6771
Floxin [Ortho-McNeil] *see* 6771
Floxuridine, 4112
Floxyfral [Solvay] *see* 4219
Fluacizine, 4113
Fluanisone, 4114
Fluanxol [Lundbeck] *see* 4187
Fluanxol Dépôt [Lundbeck] *see* 4187
Fluaton [Tubi Lux] *see* 4175
Fluazacort, 4115
Fluazifop-butyl, 4116
Fluazinam, 4117
Flubendazole, 4118
Flubenisolone *see* 1180
Flubenol [J & J] *see* 4118
Flubron [SS Pharm.] *see* 4216
Flubuperone *see* 5827
Flucam [Pfizer] *see* 587

Flucarbazone, 4119
Fluchloralin, 4120
Flucinom [Schering] *see* 4208
Fluclorolone Acetonide *see* 4121
Flucloronide, 4121
Flucloxacillin *see* 4111
Fluconazole, 4122
Flucort [Syntex] *see* 4138
Fluctin [Lilly] *see* 4185
Flucycloxuron, 4123
Flucythrinate, 4124
Flucytosine, 4125
Fludara [Schering AG] *see* 4126
Fludarabine, 4126
Fludarene [Merck & Co.] *see* 2237
Fludemil *see* 4139
Fludeoxyglucose F[18], 4127
Fluderma [Farmitalia] *see* 4243
Fludestrin [BMS] *see* 9179
Fludex [Eutherapie] *see* 4935
Fludiazepam, 4128
Fludilat [Thiemann] *see* 1033
Fludioxonil, 4129
Fludrocortisone, 4130
Fludroxycortide *see* 4197
Fluellite *see* 339
Flufenacet, 4131
Flufenamic Acid, 4132
Flufenoxuron, 4133
Flugeral [Italfarmaco] *see* 4144
Flugestone Acetate *see* 4200
Fluibil [Zambon] *see* 2054
Fluibron [Chiesi] *see* 386
Fluidane *see* 1393
Fluiden [Lafare] *see* 3999
Fluidil [Adria] *see* 2754
Fluifort [Dompé] *see* 1802
Fluimucil [Zambon] *see* 88
Fluindione, 4134
Fluindostatin *see* 4218
Fluitran [Shionogi] *see* 9624
Fluixol [Ripari-Gero] *see* 386
Flukanide [Merck & Co.] *see* 8097
Flukiver [Janssen] *see* 2411
Flumadine [Roche] *see* 8224
Flumarin [Shionogi] *see* 4104
Flumark [Dainippon] *see* 3587
Flumax [Shionogi] *see* 1919
Flumazenil, 4135
Flumazepil *see* 4135
Flumecinol, 4136
Flumequine, 4137
Flumethasone, 4138
Flumethiazide, 4139
Flumetholon [Santen] *see* 4175
Flumethrin, 4140
Flumetsulam, 4141
Flumiclorac, 4142
Flumidin [Kabi] *see* 6272
Flumioxazin, 4143
Flumoperone *see* 9684
Flumoxal [Janssen] *see* 4118
Flunagen [Gentili] *see* 4144
Flunarizine, 4144
Flunarl [Kyowa Hakko] *see* 4144
Flunase [GSK] *see* 4211
Fluniget [Merck & Co.] *see* 3146
Flunisolide, 4145
Flunitrazepam, 4146
Flunixin, 4147
Flunoxaprofen, 4148
Fluoboric Acid, 4149
Fluocinolide (obsolete) *see* 4151
Fluocinolide Acetate (obsolete) *see* 4151
Fluocinolone Acetonide, 4150

9-Fluoro-11β,21-dihydroxy-2′-methyl-5′βH-pregna-1,4-dieno[17,16-d]ox-azole-3,20-dione 21-Acetate see 4115

9-Fluoro-11β,17-dihydroxypregn-4-ene-3,20-dione-17-acetate see 4200

9-Fluoro-11β,17-dihydroxyprogester-one 17-Acetate see 4200

1-Fluoro-2,4-dinitrobenzene, 4172

(2S,4S)-6-Fluoro-2′,5′-dioxospiro[chro-man-4,4′-imidazolidine]-2-carbox-amide see 4078

Fluoroethanoic Acid see 4167

(endo,syn)-8-(2-Fluoroethyl)-3-[(hydr-oxydiphenylacetyl)oxy]-8-methyl-8-azoniabicyclo[3.2.1]octane Bromide see 4216

(8r)-8-(2-Fluoroethyl)-3α-hydroxy-1αH,-5αH-tropanium Bromide Benzilate see 4216

N-β-Fluoroethylnortropine Benzilate Methobromide see 4216

6-Fluoro-2-(2′-fluoro[1,1′-biphenyl]-4-yl)-3-methyl-4-quinolinecarboxylic Acid see 1370

6-Fluoro-1-(4-fluorophenyl)-1,4-dihy-dro-7-(4-methyl-1-piperazinyl)-4-oxo-3-quinolinecarboxylic Acid see 3141

6-Fluoro-1-(4-fluorophenyl)-1,4-dihy-dro-4-oxo-7-(1-piperazinyl)-3-quino-linecarboxylic Acid see 8370

1-[o-Fluoro-α-(p-fluorophenyl)-α-phenyl-benzyl]imidazole see 4215

Fluoroform, 4173

Fluoroformylon see 4243

Fluorogesarol see 2957

5-Fluoro-N-hexyl-3,4-dihydro-2,4-di-oxo-1(2H)-pyrimidinecarboxamide see 1844

9α-Fluorohydrocortisone see 4130

4′-Fluoro-4-(4-hydroxy-4-p-chlorophen-ylpiperidino)butyrophenone see 4598

9α-Fluoro-17-hydroxycorticosterone see 4130

Δ¹-9α-Fluoro-16α-hydroxyhydrocorti-sone see 9595

(+)-(S)-p-Fluoro-N-[2-[4-[2-(hydroxy-methyl)-1,4-benzodioxan-5-yl]-1-pi-perazinyl]ethyl]benzamide see 4100

(6α,11β,16α)-6-Fluoro-11-hydroxy-16-methyl-3,20-dioxopregna-1,4-dien-21-oic Acid Butyl Ester see 4152

(−)-(2R,5S)-5-Fluoro-1-[2-(hydroxy-methyl)-1,3-oxathiolan-5-yl]cytosine see 3565

p-Fluoro-4-(4′-hydroxy-4′-p-methylphen-ylpiperidino)butyrophenone see 6263

9α-Fluoro-11β-hydroxy-17α-methyltes-tosterone see 4186

9α-Fluoro-16α-hydroxyprednisolone see 9595

9α-Fluoro-16α-hydroxyprednisolone Acetonide see 9596

9α-Fluoro-16α-hydroxyprednisolone 16α,-17α-Acetonide 21-(β-Benzoylamino)-isobutyrate see 9597

p-Fluoro-4-(4′-hydroxy-4′-p-tolylpiperi-dino)butyrophenone see 6263

p-Fluoro-4-[4′-hydroxy-4′-[(3″-trifluoro-methyl)phenyl]piperidinobutyrophe-none see 9684

4′-Fluoro-4-[4-hydroxy-4-(α,α,α-trifluo-ro-m-tolyl)piperidino]butyrophenone see 9684

9α-Fluoro-16α,17-isopropylidenedioxy-prednisolone see 9596

6α-Fluoro-16α,17α-isopropylidenedi-oxy-4-pregnene-11β,21-diol-3,20-di-one see 4197

Fluoromar (formerly) [Ohio Med.] see 4202

Fluoromethane, 4174

Fluorometholone, 4175

4′-Fluoro-4-[4-(o-methoxyphenyl)-1-pi-perazinyl]butyrophenone see 4114

2′-Fluoro-5-methyl-β-L-arabinofurano-syluridine see 2353

Fluoromethylbenzene see 4180

1-Fluoro-2-methylbenzene see 4180

2-Fluoro-α-methyl[1,1′-biphenyl]-4-ace-tic Acid see 4199

9α-Fluoro-16α-methyl-Δ¹-corticosterone see 2930

6α-Fluoro-16α-methyl-1-dehydrocortico-sterone see 4153

9α-Fluoro-16α-methyl-17-desoxypredni-solone see 2930

S-Fluoromethyl 6α,9α-Difluoro-11β-hy-droxy-16α-methyl-17α-propionyl-oxy-3-oxoandrosta-1,4-diene-17β-carbothioate see 4211

9α-Fluoro-16-methyleneprednisolone 21-Acetate see 4191

9α-Fluoro-16-methylene-Δ¹,⁴-pregna-diene-11β,17,21-triol-3,20-dione 21-Acetate see 4191

Fluoromethyl 1,1,1,3,3,3-Hexafluoro-2-propyl Ether see 8475

6-Fluoro-1-methyl-7-[4-[(5-methyl-2-oxo-1,3-dioxol-4-yl)methyl]-1-piper-azinyl]-4-oxo-1H,4H-[1,3]thiazeto-[3,2-a]quinoline-3-carboxylic Acid see 7908

cis-5-Fluoro-2-methyl-1-[p-(methylsulfi-nyl)benzylidene]indene-3-acetic Acid see 8982

(1Z)-5-Fluoro-2-methyl-1-[[4-(methylsul-finyl)phenyl]methylene]-1H-indene-3-acetic Acid see 8982

7-Fluoro-1-methyl-3-(methylsulfinyl)-4(1H)-quinolinone see 4110

cis-5-Fluoro-2-methyl-1-(p-methylsulfo-nylbenzylidene)-3-acetic Acid see 3916

(1Z)-5-Fluoro-2-methyl-1-[[4-(methylsul-fonyl)phenyl]methylene]-1H-indene-3-acetic Acid see 3916

4′-Fluoro-4-(4-methylpiperidino)butyro-phenone see 5827

6α-Fluoro-16α-methylprednisolone see 7029

9α-Fluoro-16α-methylprednisolone see 2943

9α-Fluoro-16β-methylprednisolone see 1180

6α-Fluoro-16α-methyl-Δ¹,⁴-pregna-diene-11β,21-diol-3,20-dione see 4153

Fluoromethyl 2,2,2-Trifluoro-1-(tri-fluoromethyl)ethyl Ether see 8475

N-[[(5S)-3-[3-Fluoro-4-(4-morpholinyl)-phenyl]-2-oxo-5-oxazolidinyl]methyl]-acetamide see 5504

5-Fluoroorotate see 4176

5-Fluoroorotic Acid, 4176

5-[5-Fluoro-2-oxo-1,2-dihydroindol-(3Z)-ylidenemethyl]-2,4-dimethyl-1H-pyrrole-3-carboxylic Acid (2-Diethyl-aminoethyl)amide see 9000

Fluor-Op [Novartis] see 4175

Fluorophene [Stecker] see 4178

p-Fluorophenylacetic Acid, 4177

4-Fluoro-L-phenylalanyl-(4R)-4-hy-droxy-L-prolyl-L-arginylglycyl-L-tryptophanamide see 6445

5-(2-Fluorophenyl)-1,3-dihydro-1-meth-yl-7-nitro-2H-1,4-benzodiazepin-2-one see 4146

(βR,δR)-2-(4-Fluorophenyl)-β,δ-dihy-droxy-5-(1-methylethyl)-3-phenyl-4-[(phenylamino)carbonyl]-1H-pyr-role-1-heptanoic Acid see 864

(3R,5S,6E)-7-[4-(p-Fluorophenyl)-2,6-diisopropyl-5-(methoxymethyl)-3-pyridyl]-3,5-dihydroxy-6-heptenoic Acid see 1993

p-Fluorophenyl Ethyl Sulfone see 4161

(3R,4S)-1-(4-Fluorophenyl)-3-[(3S)-3-(4-fluorophenyl)-3-hydroxypropyl]-4-(4-hydroxyphenyl)-2-azetidinone see 3918

1-[(2-Fluorophenyl)(4-fluorophenyl)-phenylmethyl]-1H-imidazole see 4215

α-(2-Fluorophenyl)-α-(4-fluorophenyl)-1H-1,2,4-triazole-1-ethanol see 4214

3-Fluoro-4-phenylhydratropic Acid see 4199

1-(4-Fluorophenyl)-4-[hydroxy-4-(4-methylphenyl)-1-piperidinyl]-1-buta-none see 6263

1-(4-Fluorophenyl)-4-[4-hydroxy-4-[3-(trifluoromethyl)phenyl]-1-piperi-dinyl]-1-butanone see 9684

2-(p-Fluorophenyl)-1,3-indandione see 4134

2-(4-Fluorophenyl)-1H-indene-1,3(2H)-dione see 4134

(1R,2S,3S,5S)-3-(4-Fluorophenyl)-8-[(2E)-3-(iodo-2-propenyl)-8-azabicy-clo[3.2.1]octane-2-carboxylic Acid Methyl Ester see 4871

(±)-(3R*,5S*,6E)-7-[3-(p-Fluorophenyl)-1-isopropylindol-2-yl]-3,5-dihydroxy-6-heptenoate see 4218

(3R,5S,6E)-7-[4-(4-Fluorophenyl)-5-(methoxymethyl)-2,6-bis(1-methyl-ethyl)-3-pyridinyl]-3,5-dihydroxy-6-heptenoic Acid see 1993

(2S)-2-[[[4-[(3-Fluorophenyl)methoxy]-phenyl]methyl]amino]propanamide see 8315

1-(4-Fluorophenyl)-4-[4-(2-methoxy-phenyl)-1-piperazinyl]-1-butanone see 4114

2-[[1-[1-[(4-Fluorophenyl)methyl]-1H-benzimidazol-2-yl]-4-piperidinyl]-methylamino]-4(1H)-pyrimidinone see 6221

(αS)-2-(4-Fluorophenyl)-α-methyl-5-benzoxazoleacetic Acid see 4148

(−)-trans-4-(p-Fluorophenyl)-3-[[3,4-(methylenedioxy)phenoxy]methyl]-piperidine see 7043

5-(4-Fluorophenyl)-2-(1-methylethyl)-N,-4-diphenyl-1-[2-[(2R,4R)-tetrahydro-4-hydroxy-6-oxo-2H-pyran-2-yl]ethyl]-1H-pyrrole-3-carboxamide see 864

(3R,5S,6E)-rel-7-[3-(4-Fluorophenyl)-1-(1-methylethyl)-1H-indol-2-yl]-3,5-di-hydroxy-6-heptenoic Acid see 4218

(3R,5S,6E)-7-[4-(4-Fluorophenyl)-6-(1-methylethyl)-2-[methyl(methylsulfo-nyl)amino]-5-pyrimidinyl]-3,5-dihy-droxy-6-heptenoic Acid see 8270

N-(4-Fluorophenyl)-N-(1-methylethyl)-2-[[5-(trifluoromethyl)-1,3,4-thiadiazol-2-yl]oxy]acetamide see 4131

1-[(4-Fluorophenyl)methyl]-*N*-[1-[2-(4-methoxyphenyl)ethyl]-4-piperidinyl]-1*H*-benzimidazol-2-amine *see* 856

4-(4-Fluorophenyl)-7-methyl-1-(1-methylethyl)-2(1*H*)-quinazolinone *see* 4193

1-(4-Fluorophenyl)-4-(4-methyl-1-piperidinyl)-1-butanone *see* 5827

1′-[4-(4-Fluorophenyl)-4-oxobutyl]-[1,4′-bipiperidine]-4′-carboxamide *see* 7455

N-[[1-[4-(4-Fluorophenyl)-4-oxobutyl]-4-phenyl-4-piperidinyl]methyl]acetamide *see* 30

8-[4-(4-Fluorophenyl)-4-oxobutyl]-1-phenyl-1,3,8-triazaspiro[4.5]decan-4-one *see* 8751

1-[1-[4-(*p*-Fluorophenyl)-4-oxobutyl]piperidin-4-yl]-2-benzimidazolinone *see* 1048

1-[1-[4-(4-Fluorophenyl)-4-oxobutyl]-4-piperidinyl]-1,3-dihydro-2*H*-benzimidazol-2-one *see* 1048

1-[1-[4-(4-Fluorophenyl)-4-oxobutyl]-1,2,3,6-tetrahydro-4-pyridinyl]-1,3-dihydro-2*H*-benzimidazol-2-one *see* 3450

1-[1-[4-(*p*-Fluorophenyl)-4-oxobutyl]-1,2,3,6-tetrahydro-4-pyridyl]-2-benzimidazolinone *see* 3450

1-(*p*-Fluorophenyl)-4-(4-phenyl-4-acetamidomethylpiperidino)-1-butanone *see* 30

N-[3-[4-(*p*-Fluorophenyl)-1-piperazinyl]-1-methylpropyl]nicotinamide *see* 6492

N-[3-[4-(4-Fluorophenyl)-1-piperazinyl]-1-methylpropyl]-3-pyridinecarboxamide *see* 6492

1-(*p*-Fluorophenyl)-4-(4-piperidino-4-carbamoylpiperidino)-1-butanone *see* 7455

1-(4-Fluorophenyl)-4-[4-(2-pyridinyl)-1-piperazinyl]-1-butanone *see* 898

(*R*)-(−)-2-[5-(4-Fluorophenyl)-3-pyridylmethylaminomethyl]chromane *see* 8375

(*R*)-(−)-1-*N*-[5-(4-Fluorophenyl)-3-pyridylmethyl]-*N*-2-chromanylmethylamine *see* 8375

(+)-3-(4-Fluorophenylsulfonamido)-9-(2-carboxyethyl)-1,2,3,4-tetrahydrocarbazole *see* 8100

(3*R*)-3-[[(4-Fluorophenyl)sulfonyl]amino]-1,2,3,4-tetrahydro-9*H*-carbazole-9-propanoic Acid *see* 8100

2-(4-Fluorophenyl)-1-(1*H*-1,2,4-triazol-1-yl)-3-trimethylsilylpropan-2-ol *see* 8534

N-(4-Fluorophenyl)-6-[3-(trifluoromethyl)phenoxy]-2-pyridinecarboxamide *see* 7399

α-(4-Fluorophenyl)-α-[(trimethylsilyl)methyl]-1*H*-1,2,4-triazole-1-ethanol *see* 8534

4′-Fluoro-4-[*N*-[4-(*N*-piperidino)-4-carbamido]piperidino]butyrophenone *see* 7455

Fluoroplex [Allergan] *see* 4181

6α-Fluoroprednisolone *see* 4192

9-Fluoroprednisolone *see* 5174

6α-Fluoro-1,4-pregnadiene-11β,17α,21-triol-3,20-dione *see* 4192

N-(3-Fluoropropyl)-2β-carbomethoxy-3β-(4-¹²³I-iodophenyl)nortropane *see* 5050

[1*R*-(*exo,exo*)]-8-(3-Fluoropropyl)-3-[4-(iodo¹²³I)phenyl]-8-azabicyclo[3.2.1]-

octane-2-carboxylic Acid Methyl Ester *see* 5050

4′-Fluoro-4-[4-(2-pyridyl)-1-piperazinyl]butyrophenone *see* 898

5-Fluoro-2,4(1*H*,3*H*)-pyrimidinedione *see* 4181

Fluoros [Dieckmann] *see* 8618

Fluorosalan, 4178

Fluorosilicic Acid *see* 4182

(+)-(4*S*)-6-Fluorospiro[chroman-4,4′-imidazolidine]-2′,5′-dione *see* 8723

4′-Fluoro-5′-*O*-sulfamoyladenosine *see* 6726

9-(4-Fluoro-5-*O*-sulfamoylpentofuranosyl)adenine *see* 6726

Fluorosulfonic Acid, 4179

Fluorosulfuric Acid, 4179

Fluorosulfuric Acid Methyl Ester *see* 6075

5-Fluoro-1,2,3,6-tetrahydro-2,6-dioxo-4-pyrimidinecarboxylic Acid *see* 4176

5-Fluoro-1-(tetrahydro-2-furanyl)-2,4-(1*H*,3*H*)-pyrimidinedione *see* 9112

5-Fluoro-1-(tetrahydro-2-furyl)uracil *see* 9112

(11β, 16α)-9-Fluoro-11,16,17,21-tetrahydroxypregna-1,4-diene-3,20-dione *see* 9595

6α-Fluoro-11β,16α,17,21-tetrahydroxypregna-1,4-diene-3,20-dione Cyclic 16,17-Acetal with Acetone *see* 4145

9α-Fluoro-11β,16α,17,21-tetrahydroxypregna-1,4-diene-3,20-dione Cyclic 16,17-Acetal with Acetone *see* 9596

9-Fluoro-11β,16α,17,21-tetrahydroxypregna-1,4-diene-3,20-dione Cyclic 16,17-Acetal with Acetone, 21-(3,3-Dimethylbutyrate) *see* 9598

9-Fluoro-11β,16α,17,21-tetrahydroxypregna-1,4-diene-3,20-dione Cyclic 16,17-Acetal with Acetone 21-Ester with *N*-Benzoyl-2-methyl-β-alanine *see* 9597

9-Fluoro-11β,16α,17,21-tetrahydroxypregna-1,4-diene-3,20-dione Cyclic 16,17-Acetal with Cyclopentanone 21-Acetate *see* 388

6α-Fluoro-11β,16α,17,21-tetrahydroxypregn-4-ene-3,20-dione Cyclic 16,17-Acetal with Acetone *see* 4197

6α-Fluoro-11β,16α,17,21-tetrahydroxyprogesterone Cyclic 16,17-Acetal with Acetone *see* 4197

Fluorothiamphenicol *see* 4109

4-Fluoro-4-[4-(2-thioxo-1-benzimidazolinyl)piperidino]butyrophenone *see* 9443

Fluorotoluene, 4180

m-Fluorotoluene *see* 4180

o-Fluorotoluene *see* 4180

p-Fluorotoluene *see* 4180

Fluorotrichloromethane *see* 9640

4′-Fluoro-6-[(α,α,α-trifluoro-*m*-tolyl)oxy]picolinanilide *see* 7399

9α-Fluoro-11β,17,21-trihydroxy-16-methylenepregna-1,4-diene-3,20-dione 21-Acetate *see* 4191

(6α,11β,16α)-6-Fluoro-11,17,21-trihydroxy-16-methylpregna-1,4-diene-3,20-dione *see* 7029

(11β,16α)-9-Fluoro-11,17,21-trihydroxy-16-methylpregna-1,4-diene-3,20-dione *see* 2943

(11β,16β)-9-Fluoro-11,17,21-trihydroxy-16-methylpregna-1,4-diene-3,20-dione *see* 1180

9α-Fluoro-11β,17α,21-trihydroxy-21-methylpregna-1,4-diene-3,20-dione 21-Acetate *see* 4188

(6α,11β)-6-Fluoro-11,17,21-trihydroxypregna-1,4-diene-3,20-dione *see* 4192

(11β)-9-Fluoro-11,17,21-trihydroxypregna-1,4-diene-3,20-dione *see* 5174

(11β)-9-Fluoro-11,17,21-trihydroxypregn-4-ene-3,20-dione *see* 4130

Fluorouracil, 4181

2-Fluorovidarabine *see* 4126

Fluorspar *see* 1667

Fluosilicic Acid, 4182

Fluosol DA, 4183

Fluostigmine *see* 5176

Fluosulfonic Acid *see* 4179

Fluothane [Ayerst] *see* 4603

Fluovitef [Italfarmaco] *see* 4150

Fluoxastrobin, 4184

Fluoxeren [Menarini] *see* 4185

Fluoxetine, 4185

Fluoxymesterone, 4186

Flupenthixol *see* 4187

Flupentixol, 4187

Fluperolone Acetate, 4188

Fluphenacur *see* 5595

Fluphenazine, 4189

Flupirtine, 4190

Fluprednidene Acetate, 4191

Fluprednisolone, 4192

Fluprednylidene 21-Acetate *see* 4191

Fluproquazone, 4193

Fluprostenol, 4194

Fluprowit [Thiemann] *see* 88

Flupyrsulfuron-methyl, 4195

Fluquinconazole, 4196

Fluracil *see* 4181

Flura-Drops *see* 8618

Fluram [Roche] *see* 4158

Flurandrenolide, 4197

Flurandrenolone *see* 4197

Flurandrenolone Acetonide *see* 4197

Flurazepam, 4198

Flurazepam Hydrochloride *see* 4198

Flurbiprofen, 4199

Fluril *see* 4181

Flurinol [Boehringer, Ing.] *see* 3618

Fluro Uracil *see* 4181

Flurobate [Texas Pharmacal] *see* 1180

Fluroblastin [Farmitalia] *see* 4181

Flurofen [Boots] *see* 4199

Flurogestone Acetate, 4200

Fluropryl *see* 5176

Flurothyl, 4201

Fluroxene, 4202

Fluroxypyr, 4203

Fluroxypyr-meptyl *see* 4203

Flurprimidol, 4204

Flurtamone, 4205

Flusilazole, 4206

Fluspirilene, 4207

Flustar [Firma] *see* 3146

Flutamide, 4208

Flutamin [Merck KGaA] *see* 4208

Flutazolam, 4209

Fluthiacet-methyl, 4210

Fluticasone Propionate, 4211

Flutolanil, 4212

Flutoprazepam, 4213

Flutra [Schering] *see* 9624

Flutriafen *see* 4214

Flutriafol, 4214

Flutrimazole, 4215
Flutron [Roche] *see* 3437
Flutropium Bromide, 4216
Fluvalinate, 4217
Fluvastatin, 4218
Fluvean [Kowa] *see* 4150
Fluvermal [Janssen] *see* 4118
Fluvin *see* 4781
Fluvoxamine, 4219
Fluxarten [SKB] *see* 4144
Fluxema [Italfarmaco] *see* 1033
Fluzilazol *see* 4206
Fluzon [Taisho] *see* 4150
Flypel *see* 2856
FM1-43, 4220
L-FMAU *see* 2353
L-FMAU-TP *see* 2353
FMC-1240 *see* 3736
FMC-9260 *see* 9223
FMC-17370 *see* 8153
FMC-30980 *see* 2767
FMC-33297 *see* 7180
FMC-35001 *see* 1826
FMC-45498 *see* 2883
FMC-54800 *see* 1209
FMC-57020 *see* 2381
FMC-67825 *see* 1632
FMC-97285 *see* 8947
FML [Allergan] *see* 4175
FMN *see* 8201
5-FOA *see* 4176
Focalin [Novartis] *see* 6110
Fodrin *see* 8740
FOE-1976 *see* 5797
FOE-5043 *see* 4131
Foipan [Ono] *see* 1728
Folacin *see* 4221
Folaren [Ist. Chim. Inter.] *see* 4222
Folbex VA [Syngenta] *see* 1434
Folcodal [Syncro] *see* 2305
Foldine [Specia] *see* 4221
Folettes [Fawns & McAllan] *see* 4221
Folex [Pfizer] *see* 5985
Foliamin *see* 4221
Foliben [Firma] *see* 4222
Folic Acid, 4221
Folic Acid Sodium Salt *see* 8619
Folicet [Mission Pharmacal] *see* 4221
Folicur [Bayer CropSci.] *see* 9092
Folidol *see* 7033
Folidol-M [Bayer CropSci.] *see* 6108
Foligan [DESMA] *see* 279
Folikrin *see* 3708
Folinerin *see* 6826
Folinic Acid, 4222
Folipac *see* 4221
Folipex *see* 3708
Folisan *see* 3708
Folithion *see* 3976
Follestrine *see* 3708
Follicle-Stimulating Hormone, 4223
Follicular Hormone *see* 3708
Follicular Hormone Hydrate *see* 3707
Folliculin *see* 3708
Follicunodis *see* 3708
Follidrin (Tablets) *see* 3708
Follistim [Organon] *see* 4223
Follitropin *see* 4223
Follitropin Alfa *see* 4223
Follitropin Beta *see* 4223
Folosan [Uniroyal] *see* 8080
Folpet, 4224
Folsan [Kali-Chemie] *see* 4221
Folsäure *see* 4221
Folvite [Lederle] *see* 4221

Fomecin A *see* 4225
Fomecin B *see* 4225
Fomecins, 4225
Fomepizole, 4226
Fomesafen, 4227
Fominoben, 4228
Fomivirsen, 4229
Fomocaine, 4230
Fonazine, 4231
Fonazine Mesylate *see* 4231
Fondaparin Sodium *see* 4232
Fondaparinux Sodium, 4232
Fonderma [Biosedra] *see* 7994
Fongamil [Biorga] *see* 6846
Fonlipol [Recordati] *see* 9416
Fonofos, 4233
Fonofos [Pulitzer] *see* 4254
Fontamide *see* 8944
Fontarsan *see* 6948
Fontego [Polifarma] *see* 1484
Fontex [Lilly] *see* 4185
Fonurit [Chinoin] *see* 53
Fonzylane [Orsymonde] *see* 1475
Food of the Gods *see* 821
Food Orange 8 *see* 1753
Food Yellow 13 *see* 8071
Foradil [Novartis] *see* 4245
Foramsulfuron, 4234
Forane [Ohmeda] *see* 5175
Forapin [Mack, Illert.] *see* 5824
Forbina [Novartis] *see* 8943
Force [Syngenta] *see* 9111
Fordiuran [Thomae] *see* 1484
Fordonal [Almirall] *see* 7277
Fore [Dow AgroSci.] *see* 5716
Forene [Abbott] *see* 5175
Forenol [Roemmers] *see* 6531
Forilin [Novo] *see* 8276
Foriod *see* 5038
Forit *see* 6971
Forlax [Ipsen] *see* 7568
Formagene *see* 7025
Formal *see* 6012
Formaldehyde, 4235
Formaldehyde Acetamide *see* 4242
Formaldehyde Dimethyl Acetal *see* 6012
α,α′-Formaldehyde Glycerol *see* 4485
α,β-Formaldehyde Glycerol *see* 4485
Formaldehyde Semicarbazone *see* 4235
Formaldehyde Sodium Bisulfite, 4236
Formaldehyde Sodium Sulfoxylate *see* 8620
Formaldehyde Solution *see* 4235
Formaldehyde-sulfathiazole *see* 8943
Formaldehydesulfoxylic Acid Sodium Salt *see* 8620
Formalin *see* 4235
Formamide, 4237
Formanilide, 4238
Formebolone, 4239
Formestane, 4240
Formi [BASF] *see* 7629
Formic Acid, 4241
Formic Acid Ammonium Salt *see* 523
Formic Acid Benzyl Ester *see* 1134
Formic Acid Ethyl Ester *see* 3807
Formic Acid Methyl Ester *see* 6077
Formic Acid Phenylmethyl Ester *see* 1134
Formic Acid Potassium Salt *see* 7633
Formic Acid Potassium Salt (2:1) *see* 7629
Formic Acid Propyl Ester *see* 7858
Formic Aldehyde *see* 4235
Formicin, 4242
N-Formimidoylthienamycin Monohydrate *see* 4919

Formison *see* 5846
Formistin [Formenti] *see* 2022
Formocortal, 4243
Formol *see* 4235
Formononetin, 4244
Formononetol *see* 4244
Formophthaloylsulfanilyl Urea *see* 8912
Formosa Camphor *see* 1732
Formosa Oil of Camphor *see* 6780
Formosulfathiazole *see* 8943
Formoterol, 4245
Formothion, 4246
Formula 1 *see* 3761
Formula 2B *see* 3761
Formula 3A *see* 3761
Formula 6B *see* 3761
Formula 12A *see* 3761
Formula 13A *see* 3761
Formula 19 *see* 3761
Formula 20 *see* 3761
Formula 23A *see* 3761
Formula 28 *see* 3761
Formula 28A *see* 3761
Formula 30 *see* 3761
Formula 32 *see* 3761
Formula 33 *see* 3761
Formula 35A *see* 3761
Formula 39C *see* 3761
Formula 44 *see* 3761
4′-Formylacetanilide Thiosemicarbazone *see* 9290
3-Formylamino-4-hydroxy-α-[*N*-[1-methyl-2-(*p*-methoxyphenyl)ethyl]aminomethyl]benzyl Alcohol *see* 4245
Formylaniline *see* 4238
3-*C*-Formyl-5-deoxy-L-lyxofuranose *see* 8828
Formyldienolone *see* 4239
5-Formyl-3,4-dihydro-1*H*-2-benzopyran-1-one *see* 3678
5-Formyl-3,4-dihydroisocoumarin *see* 3678
3-Formyl-2,4-dihydroxy-6-methylbenzoic Acid 3-Hydroxy-4-(methoxycarbonyl)-2,5-dimethylphenyl Ester *see* 869
6-Formyl-2,3-dimethoxybenzoic Acid *see* 6851
4-Formyl-2,2-dimethyl-3-oxazolidinecarboxylic Acid 1,1-Dimethylethyl Ester *see* 4371
Formyl Fluoride, 4247
Formylformic Acid *see* 4511
16-Formylgitoxin *see* 4430
Formyl Hydroperoxide *see* 7160
N-Formyl-*N*-hydroxyaminoacetic Acid *see* 4587
[3-(Formylhydroxyamino)propyl]phosphonic Acid *see* 4257
N-Formyl-*N*-hydroxyglycine *see* 4587
2-Formyl-11α-hydroxy-Δ[1]-methyltestosterone *see* 4239
N-Formyl-L-leucine Ester with (3*S*,4*S*)-3-Hexyl-4-[(2*S*)-2-hydroxytridecyl]-2-oxetanone *see* 6869
N-Formyl-L-leucine (1*S*)-1-[[(2*S*,3*S*)-3-Hexyl-4-oxo-2-oxetanyl]methyl]dodecyl Ester *see* 6869
*N*ᵅ-Formyl Melittin *see* 5824
N-Formyl *trans-p*-Methoxystyrylamine *see* 9806
2-Formyl-17α-methylandrosta-1,4-diene-11α,17β-diol-3-one *see* 4239
S-(*N*-Formyl-*N*-methylcarbamoylmethyl) *O*,*O*-Dimethyl Phosphorodithioate *see* 4246

β-D-**Fructofuranosyl**-α-D-**glucopyrano-**
side *see* 8881
β-D-**Fructofuranosyl**-α-D-**glucopyrano-**
side Octakis(hydrogen Sulfate) Alumi-
num Complex *see* 8879
Fructose, 4273
D-**Fructose** *see* 4273
DL-**Fructose,** 4274
β-D-**Fructose** *see* 4273
D-**Fructose 1,6-Bis(dihydrogen Phos-**
phate) *see* 4275
D-**Fructose 6-(Dihydrogen Phosphate)**
see 4276
Fructose-1,6-diphosphate, 4275
1,6-D-Fructosediphosphoric Acid *see*
4275
Fructose Monophosphate *see* 4276
Fructose-6-phosphate, 4276
D-**Fructose-6-phosphoric Acid** *see* 4276
β-h-**Fructosidases** *see* 5005
Fructosteril *see* 4273
Fruitone-N [Rhone-Poulenc] *see* 6371
Fruit Sugar *see* 4273
Frupica [Kumiai] *see* 5845
Frusemide *see* 4309
Frusetic [Unimed] *see* 4309
Frusid [DDSA] *see* 4309
FS-069 *see* 7158
FSF *see* 3926
FSH *see* 4223
FSR-3 *see* 5186
FT-207 *see* 9112
Ftalicetimida *see* 7376
Ftalofyne *see* 7374
(−)-**FTC** *see* 3565
F-TEDA-BF₄ *see* 8425
Ftoracizine *see* 4113
Ftorafur [Grünenthal] *see* 9112
Ftorocort [Gedeon Richter] *see* 9596
FTPA *see* 4183
FTY-720 *see* 4083
5-FU *see* 4181
FU-40A *see* 747
Fuadin [Winthrop] *see* 8813
Fua-Med [Med. Fabrik] *see* 6599
Fuchsine *see* 5652
Fuchsin(e) Acid *see* 107
Fucidin [Leo Pharm] *see* 4317
Fucidine [Leo Pharm] *see* 4317
Fucithalmic [Leo Pharm] *see* 4317
Fucosamine, 4277
D-**Fucose,** 4278
L-**Fucose,** 4279
Fucostanol *see* 8814
Fucosterol, 4280
Fucoxanthin, 4281
all-trans-**Fucoxanthin** *see* 4281
Fucus, 4282
FUDR [Roche] *see* 4112
Fugerel [Schering] *see* 4208
Fugu Poison *see* 9246
Fujiglucon [Fujisawa] *see* 4457
Fulaid [Takeda] *see* 9112
Fulcin [Zeneca] *see* 4549
Fuldazin [Sumitomo] *see* 6196
Fulfeel [Kyorin] *see* 9112
Fulfill [Syngenta] *see* 7950
Ful-Glo [Sola-Barnes-Hinds] *see* 4159
Fulgram [ABC] *see* 6700
[5,6]Fullerene-C₆₀-Ih *see* 1462
Fullerenes *see* 1462
Fuller's Earth, 4283
Fuller's Herb *see* 8363
Fullsafe [Ohta] *see* 4132
Fulsix [Tatsumi] *see* 4309

Fuluminol [Tatsumi] *see* 2345
Fuluvamide [Mect] *see* 4309
Fulvestrant, 4284
Fulvicin [Schering] *see* 4549
Fulvoplumierin, 4285
Fumafer [Sanofi-Synthelabo] *see* 4046
Fumagillin, 4286
Fumaric Acid, 4287
Fumaric Acid Dibenzyl Ester *see* 1135
Fumarine *see* 7896
Fumazone *see* 3020
Fumidil B [Sanofi] *see* 4286
Fumigacin *see* 4633
Fumigatin, 4288
Fuming Liquid Arsenic *see* 801
Fuming Spirit of Libavius *see* 8774
Fumiron [Sanofi-Synthelabo] *see* 4046
Fumonisin B₁, 4289
Fundal [Schering] *see* 2085
Funduscein [IOLAB] *see* 4159
Fungacetin [Harvey] *see* 9589
Fungarest [Janssen] *see* 5302
Fungex [Streuli] *see* 9848
Fungibacid [Asche] *see* 9452
Fungichromin, 4290
Fungicidin *see* 6736
Fungiderm [Janssen] *see* 6178
Fungifos [S & K Pharma] *see* 9509
Fungilin [BMS] *see* 585
Fungimycin *see* 7169
Funginex [Shell] *see* 9691
Fungiplex [Hermal] *see* 8892
Fungisan [Galderma] *see* 6846
Fungisdin [Isdin] *see* 6178
Fungistat [Cilag] *see* 9160
Fungisterol, 4291
Fungistop [Essex] *see* 9519
Fungizone [BMS] *see* 585
Fungoid Solution [Pedinol] *see* 9848
Fungoral [Janssen] *see* 5302
Funtumine, 4292
Fura-2, 4293
Fura-2/AM *see* 4293
Furachel [Rachelle] *see* 6599
Furacin [Eaton] *see* 6600
Furacinetten *see* 6600
Furacoccid *see* 6600
Furacrylic Acid *see* 4297
Furadan [FMC] *see* 1803
Furadantin [Dura Pharm.] *see* 6599
Furadantine MC [Procter & Gamble] *see*
6599
Furadoin [Eaton] *see* 6599
Furafluor [Green Cross] *see* 9112
2-Furalacetic Acid *see* 4297
Furalan [Lannett] *see* 6599
2-Furaldehyde *see* 4304
Furaltadone, 4294
Furametpyr, 4295
Furamide [Knoll] *see* 3201
Furamon *see* 4312
Furan, 4296
Furanace [Dainippon] *see* 6537
2-Furanacrylic Acid, 4297
2-Furanacrylonitrile *see* 4298
2-Furancarbinol *see* 4305
Furancarbonyl Chloride *see* 4310
2-Furancarboxaldehyde *see* 4304
2-Furancarboxylic Acid *see* 4307
2-Furancarboxylic Acid 1-(Dichloroace-
tyl)-1,2,3,4-tetrahydro-6-quinolinyl
Ester *see* 8057
2,5-Furandione *see* 5704
N₁-(2′-Furanidyl)-5-fluorouracil *see* 9112
2-Furanmethanol *see* 4305

Furanol *see* 4312
Furantoina [Uriach] *see* 6599
1-(2-Furanyl)-N,N′-bis(2-furanylmethyl-
ene)methanediamine *see* 4791
9-(3-Furanyl)decahydro-4-hydroxy-
4a,10a-dimethyl-1,4-etheno-3H,7H-
benzo[1,2-c:3,4-c′]dipyran-3,7-dione
see 2493
[2aS-(2aα,5aβ,6α,7α,8aα,8bα)]-6-[2-(3-
Furanyl)ethyl]decahydro-6-hydr-
oxy-2a,5a,7-trimethyl-2H-naphtho-
[1,8-bc]furan-2-one *see* 5754
2-[(2-Furanylmethyl)(1H-imidazol-1-yl-
carbonyl)amino]butanoic Acid 4-Pen-
tenyl Ester *see* 7067
1-(3-Furanyl)-4-methyl-1-pentanone *see*
7166
N-(2-Furanylmethyl)-1H-purin-6-amine
see 5311
2-[(2-Furanylmethyl)sulfinyl]-N-[(2Z)-4-
[[4-(1-piperidinylmethyl)-2-pyridinyl]-
oxy]-2-butenyl]-acetamide *see* 5347
[1R-(1α,4β,5α,7β,9aα)]-4-(3-Furanyl)-
octahydro-1,7-dimethyl-2H-quinoli-
zine 5-Oxide *see* 6727
3-(2-Furanyl)-2-propenenitrile *see* 4298
3-(2-Furanyl)-2-propenoic Acid *see* 4297
Furaplast *see* 6600
Furazabol, 4299
Furazalon *see* 4299
Furazol W *see* 6600
Furazolidone, 4300
Furazolin [USSR] *see* 4294
Furazolium Chloride, 4301
Furazosin *see* 7717
Furcellaran, 4302
Furcellaria Gum *see* 4302
Furesis [BMS] *see* 4309
Furesol *see* 6600
Furethidine, 4303
Furfural, 4304
Furfuralcohol *see* 4305
Furfuramide *see* 4791
Furfuran *see* 4296
"Furfurol" *see* 4304
N⁶-Furfuryladenine *see* 5311
Furfuryl Alcohol, 4305
6-Furfurylaminopurine *see* 5311
Furfurylidene Acetic Acid *see* 4297
2-(Furfurylsulfinyl)-N-[(Z)-4-[[4-(piperi-
dinomethyl)-2-pyridyl]oxy]-2-butenyl]-
acetamide *see* 5347
Furfuryltrimethylammonium *see* 4312
Furilazone *see* 4308
α-Furildioxime, 4306
Furiton *see* 6542
Furloe [PPG] *see* 2187
Furmethide [SK & F] *see* 4312
Furmethonol *see* 4294
Furnace Black *see* 1808
Furobactina [Esteve] *see* 6599
7H-Furo[3,2-g][1]benzopyran-7-one *see*
7928
Furo[3,2-g]coumarin *see* 7928
Furofutran [Taiyo] *see* 9112
α-Furoic Acid *see* 4307
2-Furoic Acid, 4307
2-Furoic Acid Ester with 1-(Dichloroacet-
yl)-1,2,3,4-tetrahydro-6-quinolinol
see 8057
Furonazide, 4308
Furopenem *see* 3938
Furophen T-Caps [Krewel] *see* 6599
Furo-Puren [Klinge-Nattermann] *see* 4309
Furore Super [Bayer CropSci.] *see* 3984

Furosedon [Santen] *see* 4309
Furosemide, 4309
Furovag *see* 4300
Furoxane *see* 4300
Furoxone [Eaton] *see* 4300
Furoyl Chloride, 4310
2-[4-(2-Furoyl)piperazin-1-yl]-4-amino-6,7-dimethoxyquinazoline *see* 7717
Furpirinol *see* 6537
Furpyrinol *see* 6537
Fursemide *see* 4309
Fursultiamine, 4311
Furtrethonium, 4312
Furtrimethonium *see* 4312
Furtulon [Roche] *see* 3437
β-2-Furylacrylic Acid *see* 4297
3-(2-Furyl)acrylonitrile *see* 4298
α-Furylcarbinol *see* 4305
2-Furylcarbinol *see* 4305
1-(3-Furyl)decahydro-11-hydroxy-4b,7,-7-11a,13a-pentamethyloxireno(4,-4a)-2-benzopyrano[6,5-g](2)benz-oxepin-3,5,9(3aH,4bH,6H)-trione Ace-tate *see* 6674
8-(3-Furyl)decahydro-2,2,4a,8a-tetra-methyl-11H,13H-oxireno[d]pyrano-[4′,3′:3,3a]isobenzofuro[5,4-f][2]ben-zopyran-4,6,13(2H,5aH)-trione *see* 5494
5-[2-(3-Furyl)ethyl]decahydro-5,8-dihy-droxy-1,4a,6-trimethyl-1-naphthoic Acid γ-Lactone *see* 5754
β-Furyl Isoamyl Ketone *see* 7166
2-Furyl Methyl Ketone Isonicotinoyl-hydrazone *see* 4308
1-(3-Furyl)-4-methyl-1-pentanone *see* 7166
Fusafungine, 4313
Fusaloyos *see* 4313
Fusaric Acid, 4314
Fusarine *see* 4313
Fusariotoxin T-2 *see* 9801
Fusarubin, 4315
Fusca [Hoei] *see* 2408
Fused Borax *see* 8590
Fused Boric Acid *see* 1337
Fusel Alcohols *see* 4316
Fusel Oil, 4316
Fusidic Acid, 4317
Fusilade [Syngenta] *see* 4116
Fussol [Sankyo] *see* 4166
Fustin, 4318
Fustpentane *see* 1794
FUT-175 *see* 6350
Futhan [Torii] *see* 6350
Futraful [Taiho] *see* 9112
Futrican [Astra] *see* 2107
Fuzeon [Roche] *see* 3582
FW-293 *see* 3086
FW-734 *see* 7804
FW-925 *see* 6598
Fybogel [Reckitt Benckiser] *see* 7517
Fybozest [Reckitt Benckiser] *see* 7517
Fyracyl *see* 5655
Fyrex *see* 542
Fyrol FR-2, 9087
Fyrol HB 32 [Stauffer] *see* 9751
Fysionorm [Nourypharma] *see* 5629

G-I *see* 4543
G-II *see* 4543
G-III *see* 4543
G-4 *see* 3071
G-11 *see* 4680
G-020 *see* 2068
G-137 *see* 7407

G-277 *see* 4882
G-605 *see* 8959
G-3139 *see* 6739
G-13871 *see* 7277
G-21133 *see* 2556
G-22008 *see* 8002
G-22355 *see* 4920
G-23350 *see* 29
G-23611 *see* 5178
G-24480 *see* 2995
G-25766 *see* 2406
G-27202 *see* 6972
G-27692 *see* 8533
G-27901 *see* 9664
G-28315 *see* 8949
G-29505 *see* 46
G-30027 *see* 871
G-30028 *see* 7812
G-30320 *see* 2373
G-31435 *see* 7788
G-32883 *see* 1781
G-32911 *see* 8536
G-33182 *see* 2193
G-34161 *see* 7789
G-34162 *see* 393
G-34586 *see* 2387
G-35020 *see* 2920
G-704650 *see* 229
GA *see* 9021
GAA *see* 108
GABA *see* 430
Gabacet [Sanofi-Synthelabo] *see* 7487
Gabapentin, 4319
Gabbromicina [Farmitalia] *see* 7041
Gabbromycin [Farmitalia] *see* 7041
Gabbroral [Farmitalia] *see* 7041
Gabexate, 4320
Gabexate Mesylate *see* 4320
Gabitril [Novo Nordisk] *see* 9417
GABOB *see* 444
Gabomade [Knoll] *see* 444
Gaboxadol, 4321
Gabren(e) [Synthelabo] *see* 7772
G Acid *see* 6388
Gacilin [Andromaco] *see* 3994
Gadobenate Dimeglumine, 4322
Gadobutrol, 4323
Gadodiamide, 4324
Gadofosveset, 4325
Gadolinia *see* 4326
Gadolinium, 4326
Gadolinium Benzyloxypropionictetra-acetate Dimeglumine *see* 4322
Gadolinium Diethylenetriaminepenta-acetic Acid *see* 4327
Gadolinium Diethylenetriamine Penta-acetic Acid Bismethylamide *see* 4324
Gadolinium Diethylenetriamine Penta-acetic Acid Bis(methyoxyethylamide) *see* 4329
Gadolinium Ethoxybenzyldiethylenetri-aminepentaacetic Acid *see* 4330
Gadolinium Texaphyrin *see* 6281
Gadolinium(III) 1,4,7-Tris(carboxy-methyl)-10-(2′-hydroxypropyl)-1,4,7,-10-tetraazacyclododecane *see* 4328
Gadopentetic Acid, 4327
Gadoteridol, 4328
Gadoversetamide, 4329
Gadovist [Schering AG] *see* 4323
Gadoxetate *see* 4330
Gadoxetic Acid, 4330
Gaduol *see* 2465
Gahnite *see* 10127
Gainex *see* 7274

Galactaric Acid, 4331
Galactin *see* 7779
Galactitol, 4332
Galactoflavin, 4333
D-Galactomethylose *see* 4278
L-Galactomethylose *see* 4279
4-D-Galactopyranosyl-4-D-fructofura-nose *see* 5346
4-O-β-D-Galactopyranosyl-D-fructose *see* 5346
O-α-D-Galactopyranosyl-(1 → 6)-[O-α-D-galactopyranosyl-(1 → 6)-]₂-O-α-D-glu-copyranosyl-(1 → 2)-β-D-fructofurano-side *see* 9958
4-O-β-D-Galactopyranosyl-D-glucitol *see* 5340
4-O-β-D-Galactopyranosyl-D-gluconic Acid *see* 5342
4-O-β-D-Galactopyranosyl-D-gluconic Acid Compd with Erythromycin (1:1) *see* 3685
1-O-(4-O-β-D-Galactopyranosyl-β-D-glu-copyranosyl)ceramide *see* 2794
4-O-β-D-Galactopyranosyl-D-glucose *see* 5343
6-O-α-D-Galactopyranosyl-D-glucose *see* 5820
(2R)-N-[(1S,2R,3E)-1-[(β-D-Galacto-pyranosyloxy)methyl]-2-hydroxy-3-heptadecenyl]-2-hydroxytetracosan-amide *see* 7367
Galactoquin [Mundipharma] *see* 8060
Galactosaccharic Acid *see* 4331
D-Galactosamine, 4334
D-Galactose, 4335
α-Galactosidase A, 4336
α-Galactosidase (Human Clone λAG18 Isoenzyme A Subunit Protein Moiety Reduced) *see* 4336
β-Galactoside Sorbitol *see* 5340
4-β-D-Galactosido-D-fructose *see* 5346
4-(β-D-Galactosido)-D-gluconic Acid *see* 5342
4-(β-D-Galactosido)-D-glucose *see* 5343
6-(α-D-Galactosido)-D-glucose *see* 5820
4-O-β-D-Galactosyl-D-fructose *see* 5346
D-Galacturonic Acid, 4337
Galanga, 4338
Galangal *see* 4338
Galangin, 4339
Galantamine, 4340
Galanthamine *see* 4340
Galanthidine *see* 5626
Galatone *see* 4500
Galatur [Wyeth] *see* 5075
Galaxolide [Int. Flavors & Fragrances] *see* 4715
Galbas *see* 3989
Galben [Isagro] *see* 1030
Galcodine [Galen] *see* 2464
Galecron *see* 2085
Galegine, 4341
Galena *see* 5396, 5421
Galenphol [Galen] *see* 7329
Galfer [Thornton & Ross] *see* 4046
Galβ1 → 4Glcβ1 → 1cer *see* 2794
Galida [AstraZeneca] *see* 9177
Galla *see* 6728
Gallacetophenone, 4342
Gallaldehyde 3,5-Dimethyl Ether *see* 9015
Gallamine Triethiodide, 4343
Gallein, 4344
Gallepronin [Taiyo] *see* 4106
Gallery [Dow AgroSci.] *see* 5235

Gallia *see* 4352
Gallic Acid, 4345
Gallic Acid Bismuth Basic Salt *see* 1283
Gallic Acid 5,6-Dihydroxy-3-carboxy-
phenyl Ester *see* 3153
Gallic Acid 3-Monogallate *see* 3153
Gallic Acid Propyl Ester *see* 7859
Gallicin *see* 4345
Gallimycin [Bimeda] *see* 3681
Gallimycin [Abbott] *see* 3687
Gallium, 4346
Gallium Arsenide, 4347
Gallium Chloride, 4348
Gallium Citrate, 4349
Gallium Mononitride *see* 4351
Gallium Nitrate, 4350
Gallium Nitride, 4351
Gallium Oxide, 4352
Gallium(III) Oxide *see* 4352
Gallium Phosphide, 4353
Gallium Sesquioxide *see* 4352
Gallium Trichloride *see* 4348
Gallium Trifluoride, 4354
Gallium Trinitrate *see* 4350
Gallocatechin *see* 1902
Gallochrome *see* 5867
Gallocyanine, 4355
Gallodesoxycholic Acid *see* 2054
Gallopamil, 4356
Gallotannic Acid *see* 9052
Gallotannin *see* 9052
Galloxon *see* 4605
m-Galloylgallic Acid *see* 3153
1-Galloyl-α-D-glucose *see* 4453
1-Galloyl-β-D-glucose *see* 4454
4-Galloylpyrogallol *see* 3915
Galls *see* 6728
GalN *see* 4334
Galoxone *see* 4605
Galphol [Galen] *see* 7329
Galpseud [Galen] *see* 7916
Galsulfase *see* 819
Galuteolin *see* 5614
Galvinoxyl, 4357
Galvus [Novartis] *see* 9979
Galzin [Lemmon] *see* 10128
Gamabufagin *see* 4358
Gamabufogenin *see* 4358
Gamabufotalin, 4358
Gamanil [Merck KGaA] *see* 5557
Gamaquil [Siegfried] *see* 7258
Gambir, 4359
Gambir Catechu *see* 4359
Gambit [Syngenta] *see* 3989
Gamboge, 4360
Gambogic Acid, 4361
Gamibetal [SIT] *see* 444
Gamma Benzene Hexachloride *see* 5501
Gamma-Col [Zeneca] *see* 5501
Gamma Hexachlor *see* 5501
Gamma-hydroxybutyrate *see* 4815
Gamma-interferon *see* 4992
Gammajust 50 [Horita] *see* 6886
Gammalon [Daiichi] *see* 430
Gamma-OH [Clintec Nutrition] *see* 4815
Gamma-OZ [Kanebo] *see* 6886
Gammaphos *see* 404
Gammariza [Toyo] *see* 6886
Gammatsul [Nippon Chemiphar] *see* 6886
Gamma-vinyl GABA *see* 9978
Gammexane [Zeneca] *see* 5501
Gamolenic Acid *see* 5507
Gamonil [Merck KGaA] *see* 5557
Gamophen [J & J] *see* 9657
Ganaton [Abbott] *see* 5244

Ganaxolone, 4362
Ganciclovir, 4363
Gangliosides, 4364
Gangliostat *see* 4688
Gangliovet [Fidia] *see* 4364
Ganidan [Specia] *see* 8908
Ganirelix, 4365
Ganite [Genta] *see* 4350
Ganja *see* 1749
Ganor [Boehringer, Ing.] *see* 3930
Gantanol [Roche] *see* 8918
Gantaprim [Lenza] *see* 8918
Gantrim [Geymonat] *see* 8918
Gantrisin [Roche] *see* 8952
GAP A *see* 4075
GAR-936 *see* 9432
Garamycin [Schering-Plough] *see* 4392
Garantose *see* 8311
Garasin [Wakamoto] *see* 1974
Garasol [Schering-Plough] *see* 4392
Gardenal [Specia] *see* 7238
Garden Chamomile *see* 2041
Gardenin A *see* 4366
Gardenin B *see* 4366
Gardenin C *see* 4366
Gardenin D *see* 4366
Gardenin E *see* 4366
Gardenins, 4366
Garden Lavender *see* 5390
Gardinol *see* 4367
Gardinol Type Detergents, 4367
Gardol, 4368
Gardona [Shell] *see* 9192
Gardrin(e) [Syntex] *see* 3591
Garenoxacin, 4369
Garenoxacin Mesylate *see* 4369
Garget *see* 7391
Gargilon *see* 2913
Garlic, 4370
Garlon [Dow AgroSci.] *see* 9656
Garmian [Fuso] *see* 954
(*R*)-Garner Aldehyde *see* 4371
(*S*)-Garner Aldehyde *see* 4371
Garner's Aldehyde, 4371
Garnierite *see* 6498
Garranil [Aristegui] *see* 1774
GAs *see* 4420
Gas Black *see* 1808
GASH *see* 4563
Gaslon [Nippon Shinyaku] *see* 5102
Gasmotin [Dainippon] *see* 6279
Gasoline, 4372
Gasstenon [Tatsumi] *see* 4106
Gaster [Yamanouchi] *see* 3930
Gasteril [Ripari-Gero] *see* 7491
Gastomax [Brocchieri] *see* 2080
Gastracid [AWD] *see* 6845
Gastralgin [De Angeli] *see* 8274
Gastramine *see* 1183
Gastrax [Asche] *see* 6660
Gastrese [Wyeth] *see* 6143
Gastrhéma *see* 1897
Gastridin [Merck & Co.] *see* 3930
Gastrins, 4373
Gastrobid [Napp] *see* 6143
Gastrodia, 4374
Gastrodiagnost [Merck KGaA] *see* 7113
Gastrodin, 4375
Gastrofrenal [Sigma-Tau] *see* 2590
Gastrogard [Merial] *see* 6845
Gastrografin [BMS] *see* 5807
Gastroloc *see* 6845
GastroMARK [Mallinckrodt] *see* 4064
Gastromax [Farmitalia] *see* 6143
Gastromet [Bayropharm] *see* 2279

Gastron [Tanabe] *see* 3489
Gastron [Winthrop] *see* 5958
Gastronerton [Dolorgiet] *see* 6143
Gastronorm [Janssen] *see* 3418
Gastropen [Schwarz] *see* 3930
Gastrosedan *see* 5958
Gastrosil [Heumann] *see* 6143
Gastro-Tablinen [Sanorania] *see* 6143
Gastrozepin [Thomae] *see* 7491
Gastrurol [Gibipharma] *see* 7505
Gas-X [Sandoz] *see* 3215
Gatalone [Barnes-Hind] *see* 4500
Gatifloxacin, 4376
Gaucho [Gustafson] *see* 4910
Gaudium [Recordati] *see* 2318
GB *see* 8374
GB-1 *see* 1372
GB-2 *see* 1372
GB-94 *see* 6172
GBP28 *see* 163
GC-1189 *see* 2083
GC-2466 *see* 6298
GC-3707 *see* 1330
GCP-23339A *see* 7003
G-CSF *see* 4537
GD *see* 8713
Gd-BOPTA/Dimeg *see* 4322
Gd-DO3A-butrol *see* 4323
Gd-DTPA *see* 4327
Gd-DTPA-BMA *see* 4324
Gd-DTPA-BMEA *see* 4329
Gd-EOB-DTPA *see* 4330
Gd(HP-DO3A) *see* 4328
GDNF, 4377
Gd-T2BET *see* 6281
Gd-Tex *see* 6281
GE-132 *see* 7795
GEA-6414 *see* 9513
Geangin [GEA] *see* 9950
Gebutox [Hoechst] *see* 3287
Gedamycin Methyl Ester *see* 5847
Gefanil [Sumitomo] *see* 4378
Gefarnate, 4378
Gefarnil *see* 4378
Gefarnyl *see* 4378
Gefitinib, 4379
Gefulcer [Ohta] *see* 4378
Gehlenite, 1648
Geigy 867 *see* 8932
Geissoschizoline, 4380
Geissospermine, 4381
Gelatin, 4382
Gelbin *see* 1660
Geldene [Pfizer] *see* 7506
Gelée Royale (French) *see* 8277
Gelfilm [Pfizer] *see* 4382
Gelfoam [Pfizer] *see* 4382
Gellan Gum, 4383
Gelocatil [Gelos] *see* 47
Gelomyrtol [Pohl] *see* 6339
Gelose *see* 184
Gelovermin *see* 4712
Gelrite [CP Kelco] *see* 4383
Gelsemine, 4384
Gelseminic Acid *see* 8408
Gelsemium, 4385
Gelthix [Kerfoot] *see* 9133
Gelucystine [Parke-Davis] *see* 2782
Gelvatol [Monsanto] *see* 7585
Gem [Bayer CropSci.] *see* 9677
Gemalgene *see* 9639
Gemcitabine, 4386
Gemeprost, 4387
Gemfibrozil, 4388
Gemifloxacin, 4389

Gemonil [Abbott] see 5961
Gemtuzumab Ozogamicin, 4390
Gemzar [Lilly] see 4386
Genasense [Genta] see 6739
Genatropine see 875
Gencor [Zoecon] see 4805
Gendon [Organon] see 8120
Generation [LiphaTech] see 3139
Generlac [Morton Grove] see 5346
GenESA [Gensia] see 772
Génésérine 3 [Amido] see 3699
Genesis [Monsanto] see 2375
Genetron [AlliedSignal] see 2140
Genetron 12 [AlliedSignal] see 3064
Genetron 32 [Honeywell] see 3151
Genicide see 10062
Geniphene see 9557
Genistein, 4391
Genisteine (Alkaloid) see 8737
Genistein-4′-glucoside see 4391
Genistein-7-O-β-D-glucoside see 4391
Genistein-4′-glucosidorhamnoside see 8718
Genisteol see 4391
Genistin see 4391
Genlip [Teofarma] see 4388
Genol see 6017
Genoptic [Allergan] see 4392
Genoscopolamine [Amido] see 8407
Genostrychnine see 8856
Genotropin [Pharmacia & Upjohn] see 8716
Gentacin [Schering-Plough] see 4392
Gent-Ak [Akorn] see 4392
Gentalline [Schering-Plough] see 4392
Gentalyn [Essex] see 4392
Gentamicin, 4392
Gentamicin A see 4392
Gentamicin C$_1$ see 4392
Gentamicin C$_{1a}$ see 4392
Gentamicin C$_2$ see 4392
Gentamicin C$_{2b}$ see 6181
Gentamicin D see 4392
Gentamycin see 4392
GenTeal [Novartis] see 4842
Gentersal [Ortho] see 6677
Gentian, 4393
Gentianic Acid see 4399
Gentianin see 4399
Gentianine, 4394
Gentian Violet, 4395
Gentiaverm [Berlin-Chemie] see 4395
Gentibioptal [Farmila] see 4392
Genticin [Roche] see 4392
Gentiin see 4399
Gentinatre see 4398
Gentiobiose, 4396
Gentiopicrin, 4397
Gentiopicroside see 4397
Gentisic Acid, 4398
Gentisin, 4399
Gentisine U.C.B. see 4398
Gentisod see 4398
Gentlax [Purdue Frederick] see 1242
Gentocin [Schering-Plough] see 4392
Gentogram [Merck-Sante] see 4392
Gent-Ophtal [Winzer] see 4392
Gentran [Baxter] see 2948
Gentran 40 [Baxter] see 2948
Gentran 70 [Baxter] see 2948
Gentrol [Wellmark] see 4805
Genurin [Recordati] see 4096
Geocillin [Roerig] see 1840
Geodon [Pfizer] see 10171
Geoffroyine see 9007

Geomycin [Pliva] see 6976
Geon [Goodrich] see 7586
Geopen [Roerig] see 1792
Geosmin, 4400
Gepefrine, 4401
Gephyrotoxin, 4402
GER-11 see 441
Geram [UCB] see 7487
Geranial see 2322
Geraniol, 4403
Geranium, 4404
Geranyl-1,4-benzenediol see 4405
Geranyl Farnesylacetate see 4378
Geranylgeranylacetone see 9153
Geranylhydroquinone, 4405
Gerbin [Sanofi Winthrop] see 22
Gerdaxyl [Gerda] see 5790
Geref [Serono] see 8461
Gerfil [G. F. Chem.] see 7581
Gerhardite see 2643
Germalgene see 9639
Germall II [Sutton] see 3000
Germall 115 [Sutton] see 4916
German Chamomile see 2041
German Chamomile Oil see 2041
Germane, 4406
German Fungus see 185
Germanin [Bayer] see 9006
Germanium, 4407
Germanium(IV) Chloride see 4410
Germanium Dichloride, 4408
Germanium Dioxide, 4409
Germanium Hydride see 4406
Germanium(IV) Oxide see 4409
Germanium Oxide (GeO$_2$) see 4409
Germanium Tetrachloride, 4410
Germanium Tetrafluoride, 4411
Germapect [Thiemann] see 1794
Germiciclin [Mendelejeff] see 5943
Germine, 4412
Gernebcin [Lilly] see 9490
Gero [URPAC] see 7757
Gerobit [Gerot] see 5948
Gerodorm [Gerot] see 2308
Gerontine see 8743
Geroquinol see 4405
Gerostop [Merckle] see 6760
Gerot-Epilan [Gerot] see 5853
Gesafram [Syngenta] see 7788
Gesagard [Syngenta] see 7789
Gesapax [Syngenta] see 393
Gesapon see 2841
Gesaprim [Syngenta] see 871
Gesarex see 2841
Gesarol see 2841
Gesatop [Syngenta] see 8533
Gestafortin [Merck KGaA] see 2102
Gestamestrol [Hermal] see 2102
Gestanin [Organon] see 291
Gestanon [Organon] see 291
Gestanyn [Organon] see 291
Gestodene, 4413
Gestone [Nordic] see 7773
Gestonorone Caproate, 4414
Gestoral [Novartis] see 5793
Gestovis see 7114
Gestrinone, 4415
Gestronol Caproate see 4414
Gevatran [Anphar-Rolland] see 6353
Gevilon [Pfizer] see 4388
Gewacalm [Nycomed] see 2994
Gewalan [Lannacher] see 6520
Gewazol see 7141
GEWO-399 see 5186
GF-196960 see 9027

GFP see 4544
GG-167 see 10113
GG-745 see 3471
GGA see 9153
GH see 8716
Ghatti Gum, 4416
GHB see 4815
Ghee see 4417
Ghi, 4417
Ghrelin, 4418
Ghrelin (Human Clone CTB-187P1 Gene GHRELIN) see 4418
GH-RF see 8714
GH-RH see 8714
GH-RIF see 8715
GI-87084 see 8131
GI-87084B see 8131
GI-198745 see 3471
Giant Yam see 10092
Giardil see 4300
Giarlam see 4300
Gibbane see 4420
Gibberellane see 4420
Gibberellic Acid, 4419
Gibberellin A$_3$ see 4419
Gibberellin X see 4419
Gibberellins, 4420
Gibbsite see 356
Gibbs Reagent, 4421
Gibicef [Metapharma] see 1954
Gibrel [AgriDyne] see 4419
Gichtex [Gerot] see 279
Gifblaar Poison see 4167
Giganten [Troponwerke] see 2305
Gilemal [Chinoin] see 4478
Gilsonite, 4422
Giltex see 8667
Gilurytmal [Solvay] see 194
Gina [Winthrop] see 7811
Ginapect [Winthrop] see 7811
Gindarine see 9215
Ginger, 4423
[6]-Gingerol, 4424
Gingilli Oil see 8469
Gingisan [Chassot] see 2091
Ginkgo, 4425
Ginkgoic Acid see 621
Ginkgolide A see 4426
Ginkgolide B see 4426
Ginkgolide C see 4426
Ginkgolides, 4426
Ginoden [Schering AG] see 4413
Ginorite see 1652
Ginseng, 4427
Ginsenosides see 4427
Ginstar [Bayer CropSci.] see 9313
Giractide, 4428
Girard Reagent P see 4429
Girard Reagents, 4429
Girard Reagent T see 4429
Girard's Reagent D see 3245
Gismondite see 1648
Gitaligin [Schering] see 4430
Gitalin, 4430
Gitaloxin see 4430
Gitogenin, 4431
Gitogenin β-Lycotetraoside see 4432
Gitonin see 4432
F-Gitonin, 4432
Gitoxigenin, 4433
Gitoxin, 4434
Gittalun [Boehringer, Ing.] see 3441
Give-Tan [Givaudan] see 2310
Giv-Gard DXN [Givaudan] see 3223
Gix see 2957

Gjellebaekite *see* 1702
GL-7 *see* 4499
Gla *see* 1828
GLA *see* 5507
Glacial Phosphoric Acid *see* 7345
Glamidolo [Angelini] *see* 2820
Glandubolin *see* 3708
Glanil [Janssen] *see* 2305
Glasel [Troponwerke] *see* 3875
Glassy Sodium Metaphosphate *see* 8667
Glatiramer, 4435
Glauber's Salt *see* 8680
Glaucine, 4436
Glaucon [Alcon] *see* 3619
Glauconex [Alcon] *see* 1022
Glaucostat [Merck & Co.] *see* 8082
Glaucotat [Chibret] *see* 8082
Glaucotensil [Farmila] *see* 3755
Glaudin [Sifi] *see* 8082
Glauline [Smith & Nephew] *see* 6140
Glaupax [Erco] *see* 53
Glaurin *see* 3120
Glausyn [Novartis] *see* 6140
Glauvent *see* 4436
Glazidim [GSK] *see* 1946
Glean [DuPont] *see* 2191
Gleevec [Novartis] *see* 4902
Gliadel *see* 7559
Gliadin, 4437
Glial Cell Line-derived Neurotrophic
    Factor *see* 4377
Glianimon [Bayer] *see* 1048
Gliatilin [Italfarmaco] *see* 2205
Glibenclamide *see* 4478
Glibenese [Pfizer] *see* 4442
Glibornuride, 4438
Glicerinformal [Calipe] *see* 4485
Gliclazide, 4439
Glimepiride, 4440
Glimicron [Dainippon] *see* 4439
Glimidstada [Stada] *see* 4478
Glioten [Armstrong] *see* 3567
Gliotoxin, 4441
Glipasol *see* 4479
Glipizide, 4442
Gliporal [Grossmann] *see* 1476
Gliquidone, 4443
Glisoxepid, 4444
Glivec [Novartis] *see* 4902
Gln *see* 4471
Globacillin [Astra] *see* 910
Globaline [Arapahoe] *see* 9207
Globenicol [Yamanouchi] *see* 2077
Globin, 4445
Globocef [Roche] *see* 1923
Globularicitrin *see* 8304
Globulin G₁ *see* 5640
Glofil-131 [Abbott] *see* 5064
Glomycin *see* 6976
Glonoin *see* 6607
Gloxazone *see* 5299
GLP-1 *see* 4447
GLP-2 *see* 4447
GLQ223 [Genelabs] *see* 9648
Glu *see* 4469
Gluborid [Grünenthal] *see* 4438
Glucagon, 4446
Glucagon-Like Peptide I *see* 4447
Glucagon-Like Peptide II *see* 4447
Glucagon-Like Peptides, 4447
Glucagon-related Peptide I *see* 4447
Glucagon-related Peptide II *see* 4447
Glucal *see* 1669
Glucametacin, 4448
Glucametacine *see* 4448

Glucamethacin *see* 4448
Glucamine, 4449
D-Glucamine *see* 4449
α-Glucan Branching Glycosyltransferase
    see 8023
α-1,6-Glucan 6-Glucanohydrolase *see*
    2949
α-1,4-Glucan 4-Glucanohydrolases *see*
    599
α-1,4-Glucan Maltohydrolases *see* 599
Glucantim [Farmitalia] *see* 6078
Glucantime [Specia] *see* 6078
D-Glucaric Acid, 4450
D-Glucaric Acid Calcium Salt *see* 1700
Glucazide *see* 4500
Gluceptate Calcium *see* 4455
Gluceptate Sodium *see* 4455
Glucid *see* 8311
Glucidoral [Servier] *see* 1832
Glucinan [Merck KGaA] *see* 5938
Glucinium *see* 1161
D-Glucitol *see* 8725
Glucitol Iron Complex, Compd with
    Citric Acid *see* 5100
Glucoamylases *see* 599
D-Glucoascorbic Acid, 4451
Glucobay [Bayer] *see* 18
Glucobiogen *see* 1669
Glucochloral *see* 2072
α-D-Glucochloralose *see* 2072
Glucofrangulin, 4452
Glucofrangulin A *see* 4452
Glucofren [Cophar] *see* 1832
D-Glucofuranurono-6,3-lactone *see* 4467
Glucogallic Acid *see* 4454
α-Glucogallin, 4453
β-Glucogallin, 4454
Glucoheptonic Acid, 4455
α-Glucoheptonic Acid *see* 4455
Glucolin *see* 4459
D-Glucomethylose *see* 8077
Glucomonocarbonic Acid *see* 4455
Gluconasturtiin *see* 7226
Gluconiazide *see* 4500
D-Gluconic Acid *see* 4456
Gluconic Acid, 4456
D-Gluconic Acid Calcium Salt (2:1) *see*
    1669
D-Gluconic Acid Cyclic 4,5-Ester with
    Boric Acid Calcium Salt (2:1) *see*
    1653
D-Gluconic Acid Iron(3+) Sodium Salt
    see 8615
D-Gluconic Acid δ-Lactone *see* 4457
Gluconic Acid Quinidine Salt *see* 8060
Glucono Delta Lactone *see* 4457
Gluconolactone, 4457
Gluconsan K [Kayaku] *see* 4456
Glucoperiplocymarin *see* 7174
Glucophage [Merck KGaA] *see* 5938
Glucoproscillaridin A *see* 8399
β-D-Glucopyranose Aerodehydrogenase
    see 4460
α-D-Glucopyranose 1-Dihydrogenphos-
    phate *see* 4461
α-D-Glucopyranose-1-gallate *see* 4453
β-D-Glucopyranose-1-gallate *see* 4454
α-D-Glucopyranose-1-phosphate *see* 4461
α-D-Glucopyranose 1-(3,4,5-Trihy-
    droxybenzoate) *see* 4453
β-D-Glucopyranose 1-(3,4,5-Trihy-
    droxybenzoate) *see* 4454
(3β,5β,12β)-3-[(O-β-D-Glucopyranosyl-
    (1 → 4)-O-3-O-acetyl-2,6-dideoxy-β-D-
    ribo-hexopyranosyl-(1 → 4)-O-2,6-dide-

oxy-β-D-*ribo*-hexopyranosyl-(1 → 4)-2,-
    6-dideoxy-β-D-*ribo*-hexopyranosyl)-
    oxy]-12,14-dihydroxycard-20(22)-
    enolide *see* 5354
(3β,5β,16β)-3-[(O-β-D-Glucopyranosyl-
    (1 → 4)-O-3-O-acetyl-2,6-dideoxy-β-D-
    ribo-hexopyranosyl-(1 → 4)-O-2,6-di-
    deoxy-β-D-*ribo*-hexopyranosyl-(1 → 4)-
    2,6-dideoxy-β-D-*ribo*-hexopyranosyl)-
    oxy]-14,16-dihydroxycard-20(22)-
    enolide *see* 5354
(3β,5β)-3-[(O-β-D-Glucopyranosyl-
    (1 → 4)-O-3-O-acetyl-2,6-dideoxy-β-D-
    ribo-hexopyranosyl-(1 → 4)-O-2,6-di-
    deoxy-β-D-*ribo*-hexopyranosyl-(1 → 4)-
    2,6-dideoxy-β-D-*ribo*-hexopyranosyl)-
    oxy]-14-hydroxycard-20(22)-enolide
    see 5354
(3β,5β,12β,16β)-3-[(O-β-D-Glucopyra-
    nosyl-(1 → 4)-O-3-O-acetyl-2,6-dide-
    oxy-β-D-*ribo*-hexopyranosyl-(1 → 4)-O-
    2,6-dideoxy-β-D-*ribo*-hexopyranosyl-
    (1 → 4)-2,6-dideoxy-β-D-*ribo*-hexopy-
    ranosyl)oxy]-12,14,16-trihydroxy-
    card-20(22)-enolide *see* 5354
α-D-Glucopyranosyl Bromide 2,3,4,6-
    Tetraacetate *see* 60
2-O-β-D-Glucopyranosylcucurbitacin E
    see 2487
β-D-Glucopyranosyl N,N'-Di(2-chloro-
    ethyl) Phosphoric Acid Diamide *see*
    4468
(3β,5β,12β)-3-[(O-β-D-Glucopyranosyl-
    (1 → 4)-O-2,6-dideoxy-β-D-*ribo*-hexo-
    pyranosyl-(1 → 4)-O-2,6-dideoxy-β-D-
    ribo-hexopyranosyl-(1 → 4)-2,6-dide-
    oxy-β-D-*ribo*-hexopyranosyl)oxy]-12,-
    14-dihydroxycard-20(22)-enolide *see*
    2921
12-β-D-Glucopyranosyl-12,13-dihydro-
    2,10-dihydroxy-6-[[2-hydroxy-1-(hy-
    droxymethyl)ethyl]amino]-5H-indo-
    lo[2,3-a]pyrrolo[3,4-c]carbazole-5,7-
    (6H)-dione *see* 3512
7-α-D-Glucopyranosyl-9,10-dihydro-3,-
    5,6,8-tetrahydroxy-1-methyl-9,10-di-
    oxo-2-anthracenecarboxylic Acid *see*
    1843
8-β-D-Glucopyranosyl-5,7-dihydroxy-2-
    (4-hydroxy-3-methoxyphenyl)-4H-1-
    benzopyran-4-one *see* 8402
10-Glucopyranosyl-1,8-dihydroxy-3-
    (hydroxymethyl)-9(10H)-anthracen-
    one *see* 307
6-O-α-D-Glucopyranosyl-D-fructofura-
    nose *see* 5182
α-D-Glucopyranosyl-β-D-fructofurano-
    side *see* 8881
O-α-D-Glucopyranosyl-(1 → 3)-β-D-fruc-
    tofuranosyl-α-D-glucopyranoside *see*
    5819
3-O-α-D-Glucopyranosyl-D-fructose *see*
    9821
6-O-α-D-Glucopyranosyl-D-fructose *see*
    5182
α-D-Glucopyranosyl-α-D-glucopyrano-
    side *see* 9580
(3β,5β)-3-[(O-β-D-Glucopyranosyl-
    (1 → 6)-O-D-glucopyranosyl-(1 → 4)-6-
    deoxy-3-O-methyl-α-L-glucopyrano-
    syl)oxy]-14-hydroxy-19-oxocard-20-
    (22)-enolide *see* 9288
[(6-O-β-D-Glucopyranosyl-β-D-gluco-
    pyranosyl)oxy]benzeneacetonitrile *see*
    597

(3β,5α)-3-[(2-O-β-D-Glucopyranosyl-β-
D-glucopyranosyl)oxy]-14-hydroxy-
card-20(22)-enolide *see* 9897
6-β-D-Glucopyranosyl-7-(β-D-glucopyranosyloxy)-5-hydroxy-2-(4-hydroxy-
phenyl)-4*H*-1-benzopyran-4-one *see*
8364
(4α)-13-[(2-O-β-D-Glucopyranosyl-β-D-
glucopyranosyl)oxy]kaur-16-en-18-oic
Acid β-D-Glucopyranosyl Ester *see*
8810
(2Z,6S)-6-β-D-Glucopyranosyl-2-[[(3S)-
3-β-D-glucopyranosyl-2,3,4-trihydr-
oxy-5-[(2E)-3-(4-hydroxyphenyl)-1-
oxo-2-propenyl]-6-oxo-1,4-cyclohexa-
dien-1-yl]methylene]-5,6-dihydroxy-
4-[(2E)-3-(4-hydroxyphenyl)-1-oxo-2-
propenyl]-4-cyclohexene-1,3-dione *see*
1867
2-O-β-D-Glucopyranosyl-α-D-glucose *see*
8719
4-O-α-D-Glucopyranosyl-D-glucose *see*
5714
4-O-β-D-Glucopyranosyl-D-glucose *see*
1961
6-O-β-D-Glucopyranosyl-D-glucose *see*
4396
4′-(β-D-Glucopyranosyloxy)acetophe-
none *see* 7395
2-(β-D-Glucopyranosyloxy)benzaldehyde
see 4628
α-(β-D-Glucopyranosyloxy)benzene-
acetonitrile *see* 5720
7-(β-D-Glucopyranosyloxy)-2*H*-1-benzo-
pyran-2-one *see* 8562
4-(β-D-Glucopyranosyloxy)benzyl Alcohol *see* 4375
(1S,2′R,4aS,7aS)-1-(β-D-Glucopyranosyloxy)-4a,7a-dihydro-4′-[(1S)-1-hy-
droxyethyl]-5′-oxospiro[cyclopenta[c]-
pyran-7(1H),2′(5′H)-furan]-4-carbox-
ylic Acid Methyl Ester *see* 7540
3-(β-D-Glucopyranosyloxy)-5,7-dihy-
droxy-2-(4-hydroxyphenyl)-1-benzo-
pyrylium Chloride *see* 7071
1-[2-(β-D-Glucopyranosyloxy)-4,6-dihy-
droxyphenyl]-3-(4-hydroxyphenyl)-
1-propanone *see* 7327
1-(β-D-Glucopyranosyloxy)-1,4a,5,6,7,-
7a-hexahydro-6-hydroxy-7-methyl-
cyclopenta[c]pyran-4-carboxylic Acid
Methyl Ester *see* 5560
[1S-(1α,4aα,7α,7aα)]-1-(β-D-Glucopyranosyloxy)-1,4a,5,6,7,7a-hexahydro-
7-methyl-5-oxocyclopenta[c]pyran-
4-carboxylic Acid Methyl Ester *see*
9959
(αS)-α-(β-D-Glucopyranosyloxy)-4-hydr-
oxybenzeneacetonitrile *see* 2958
6-(β-D-Glucopyranosyloxy)-7-hydroxy-
2H-1-benzopyran-2-one *see* 3698
7-(β-D-Glucopyranosyloxy)-6-hydroxy-
2H-1-benzopyran-2-one *see* 2262
7-β-D-Glucopyranosyloxy-8-hydroxy-
2H-1-benzopyran-2-one *see* 2818
7-(β-D-Glucopyranosyloxy)-5-hydroxy-
2-(3-hydroxy-4-methoxyphenyl)-3,6-
dimethoxy-4H-1-benzopyran-4-one
see 1968
7-(β-D-Glucopyranosyloxy)-5-hydroxy-
2-(4-hydroxyphenyl)-4H-1-benzo-
pyran-4-one *see* 731
β-D-Glucopyranosyloxy-L-*p*-hydroxy-
mandelonitrile *see* 2958

8-(β-D-Glucopyranosyloxy)-7-hydroxy-
6-methoxy-2H-1-benzopyran-2-one *see*
4266
4-(β-D-Glucopyranosyloxy)-3-methoxy-
benzaldehyde *see* 4464
7-(β-D-Glucopyranosyloxy)-6-methoxy-
2H-1-benzopyran-2-one *see* 8409
2-[1-(β-D-Glucopyranosyloxy)-1-methyl-
ethyl]-2,3-dihydro-7H-furo[3,2-g][1]-
benzopyran-7-one *see* 6668
2-(β-D-Glucopyranosyloxy)-2-methyl-
propanenitrile *see* 5497
1-[4-(β-D-Glucopyranosyloxy)phenyl]-
ethanone *see* 7395
[1S-(1α,4aα,7β,7aα)]-1-(β-D-Glucopyranosyloxy)-1,4a,7,7a-tetrahydro-7-hy-
droxy-7-(hydroxymethyl)cyclopen-
ta[c]pyran-4-carboxylic Acid *see* 6255
7′A-(β-D-Glucopyranosyloxy)-1′,3′a,4′,-
7′a-tetrahydro-4′-hydroxy-2′,4′,6′-
trimethyl-(2′R,3′aR,4′S,7′aR)-spiro-
[cyclopropane-1,5′-[5H]inden]-3′(2′H)-
one *see* 7930
(4R)-4-(β-D-Glucopyranosyloxy)-2,6,6-
trimethyl-1-cyclohexene-1-carboxal-
dehyde *see* 7411
3-O-(β-D-Glucopyranosyluronic Acid)-2-
amino-2-deoxy-D-glucose *see* 4756
β-D-Glucopyranosyluronic Acid 2-De-
oxy-2-amino-D-galactose *see* 2215
D-Glucosaccharic Acid *see* 4450
Glucosaccharonic Acid *see* 5126
Glucosamine, 4458
Glucosan Transglycosylase *see* 8023
Glucoscan [DuPont] *see* 4455
Glucose, 4459
D-Glucose *see* 4459
D-Glucose 6-(Dihydrogen Phosphate) *see*
4462
Glucosemonocarboxylic Acid *see* 4455
Glucose Oxidase, 4460
α-Glucose-1-phosphate, 4461
Glucose-6-phosphate, 4462
α-Glucose-1-phosphoric Acid *see* 4461
Glucose-6-phosphoric Acid *see* 4462
α-Glucosidases *see* 5005
3-(α-Glucosido)-D-fructose *see* 9821
4-(α-Glucosido)-D-glucose *see* 5714
4-(β-Glucosido)-D-glucose *see* 1961
6-(β-Glucosido)-D-glucose *see* 4396
7-Glucosido-8-hydroxycoumarin *see*
2818
3-(β-Glucosido)indole *see* 4942
α-*n*-Glucosidoinvertases *see* 5005
Glucosulfone Sodium, 4463
Glucosylceramidase (Human Placental
Isoenzyme Protein Moiety Reduced)
see 243
β-D-Glucosylisophosphoramide Mustard
see 4468
β-D-Glucosyloxyazoxymethane *see* 2701
7-(Glucosyloxy)coumarin *see* 8562
7-(Glucosyloxy)-3′,5-dihydroxy-4′,5′,6-
trimethoxyisoflavone *see* 5090
8-(Glucosyloxy)-6-methoxyumbelliferone
see 4266
3-(Glucosyloxy)-4′,5,7-trihydroxy-3′,5′-
dimethoxyflavylium Chloride *see*
5715
(1-D-Glucosylthio)gold *see* 883
Glucotard [Boehringer, Mann.] *see* 4572
α-D-Glucothiopyranose *see* 9334
Glucotrol [Pfizer] *see* 4442
Glucovanillin, 4464
Glucoxy *see* 4467

Glucurolactone *see* 4467
Glucurone *see* 4467
D-Glucuronic Acid, 4465
D-Glucuronic Acid γ-Lactone *see* 4467
D-Glucuronic Acid γ-Lactone 1-[(4-Pyri-
dinylcarboxyl)hydrazone] *see* 4500
β-Glucuronidase, 4466
D-Glucuronolactone, 4467
D-Glucuronolactone Isonicotinoylhydra-
zone *see* 4500
Glucuronylglucosamineglicane Sulfate
see 8986
Gludiase [Bellon] *see* 4480
Glufast [Kissei] *see* 6211
Glufosfamide, 4468
Glufosinate *see* 7339
Glufosinate-ammonium *see* 7339
Glukagon *see* 4446
Glumal [Kyowa] *see* 25
Glumamycin *see* 584
Glumin *see* 4471
Glumorin *see* 5279
Glurenorm [Thomae] *see* 4443
Gluronazide *see* 4500
Gluside *see* 8311
Glusulase [Endo] *see* 4466
Glutacid [Schering-Plough] *see* 4469
Glutamed [Boehringer, Mann.] *see* 4475
Glutamic Acid, 4469
L-Glutamic Acid *see* 4469
Glutamic Acid α-Amide *see* 5177
Glutamic Acid 5-Amide *see* 4471
L-Glutamic Acid Compd with L-Argi-
nine *see* 781
L-Glutamic Acid γ-Ethyl Ester *see* 4470
L-Glutamic Acid 5-Ethyl Ester, 4470
15-L-Glutamic Acid-16-glycine-secretin
(Pig) *see* 8421
L-Glutamic Acid 5-[2-[4-(Hydroxymeth-
yl)phenyl]hydrazide] *see* 187
Glutamic Acid Lactam *see* 8001
L-Glutamic Acid L-Lysine Salt *see* 5638
L-Glutamic Acid Monosodium Salt *see*
6254
275-L-Glutamic Acid (1-91)-(174-527)-
Plasminogen Activator (Human Tis-
sue-type Protein Moiety) *see* 7004
L-Glutamic Acid Polymer with L-Alanine, L-Lysine and L-Tyrosine *see* 4435
Glutamine, 4471
L-Glutamine *see* 4471
2-L-Glutamine-6-L-asparaginealytesin
see 1329
Glutaminic Acid *see* 4469
Glutaminol [Syntex] *see* 4469
3-γ-D-Glutamyl-D-alanylamino-3-meth-
oxyazetidin-2-one-1-sulfonic Acid *see*
8946
(3R)-3-(γ-D-Glutamyl-D-alanylamino)-3-
methoxy-2-oxoazetidine-1-sulfonic
Acid *see* 8946
γ-Glutamyl-α-amino-β-((2-ethyl-N,N,N′,-
N′-tetrakis(2-chloro)ethylphosphor-
amidate)sulfonyl)propionyl-(R)-(−)-
phenylglycine *see* 1745
1-[N-(γ-L-Glutamyl)amino]-D-proline
see 5499
(2R)-L-γ-Glutamyl-3-[[2-[[bis[bis(2-
chloroethyl)amino]phosphinyl]oxy]-
ethyl]sulfonyl]-L-alanyl-2-phenylgly-
cine *see* 1745
L-γ-Glutamyl-S-[(1R,2E,4E,6Z,9Z)-1-
[(1S)-4-carboxy-1-hydroxybutyl]-2,4,-
6,9-pentadecatetraenyl]-L-cysteinyl-
glycine *see* 5455

N-(*N*-L-γ-Glutamyl-L-cysteinyl)glycine
  see 4475
L-γ-Glutamyl-L-cysteinyl-glycine Disul-
  fide *see* 4475
β-*N*-γ-L(+)-Glutamyl)-4-hydroxymeth-
  ylphenylhydrazine *see* 187
γ-L-Glutamylhypoglycine *see* 4866
D-γ-Glutamyl-*N*-[(3*R*)-3-methoxy-2-oxo-
  1-sulfo-3-azetidinyl]-D-alaninamide
  see 8946
N-L-γ-Glutamyl-3-(2-methylenecyclo-
  propyl)alanine *see* 4866
Glutaral *see* 4472
Glutaraldehyde, 4472
Glutaric Acid, 4473
Glutaric Acid Dinitrile *see* 4474
Glutaric Dialdehyde *see* 4472
Glutarol [Dermal] *see* 4472
Glutaronitrile, 4474
ε-*N*-(L-Glutar-2-yl)-L-lysine *see* 8312
Glutasan [Sancarlo] *see* 4475
Glutathin [Mochida] *see* 4475
Glutathiol *see* 4475
Glutathion [Nichiiko] *see* 4475
L-**Glutathione** *see* 4475
Glutathione, 4475
Glutathione-SH *see* 4475
Gluten, 4476
Glutestere *see* 4470
Glutethimide, 4477
Glutimic Acid *see* 8001
Glutiminic Acid *see* 8001
Glutinal [Sankyo] *see* 4475
Glutril [Roche] *see* 4438
Gly *see* 4491
[**Gly**(A21),Arg(B31),Arg(B32)]insulin
  (Human) *see* 4984
[**Gly**[7],Asu[1,6]]oxytocin *see* 1839
Glybenzcyclamide *see* 4478
Glyburide, 4478
Glybuthiazol(e), 4479
Glybuthizol *see* 4479
Glybuzole, 4480
Glycacil [Lonza] *see* 5069
Glycamine *see* 4449
Glyceol [Chugai] *see* 4484
DL-**Glyceraldehyde** *see* 4481
Glyceraldehyde, 4481
Glyceraldehyde 3-Phosphate, 4482
Glyceric Acid, 4483
Glyceric Aldehyde *see* 4481
Glycerin *see* 4484
Glycerine *see* 4484
Glycerol, 4484
Glycerol Diacetate *see* 2961
Glycerol α,γ-**Dichlorohydrin** *see* 3074
sym-**Glycerol Dichlorohydrin** *see* 3074
Glycerol Dimethylketal *see* 5213
Glycerol Formal, 4485
Glycerol Guaiacolate *see* 4555
Glycerol α-(2-Methoxyphenyl) Ether *see*
  4555
Glycerol α-**Monobutyrate** *see* 6249
Glycerol α-**Monochlorohydrin** *see* 2145
Glycerol Mono(2-methoxyphenyl) Ether
  see 4555
Glycerol Nitric Acid Triester *see* 6607
Glycerol 1-Octanoate *see* 6252
Glycerol Tribromohydrin *see* 9614
Glycerophosphoric Acid, 4486
α-**Glycerophosphoric Acid** *see* 4486
β-**Glycerophosphoric Acid** *see* 4486
α-**Glycerophosphoric Acid Calcium Salt**
  see 1670
β-**Glycerophosphoric Acid Calcium Salt**
  see 1670

sn-**Glycero-3-phosphorylcholine** *see* 2205
Glycerose *see* 4481
Glyceryl *p*-**Aminobenzoate,** 4487
Glyceryl 2-*p*-Chlorophenoxyisobutyrate-
  1,3-dinicotinate *see* 1224
Glyceryl Diacetate *see* 2961
α-**Glyceryl Guaiacol Ether** *see* 4555
Glyceryl Guaiacyl Ether *see* 4555
Glyceryl Iodide, 4488
Glyceryl Monoacetate *see* 6242
Glyceryl 3-Monobutyrate *see* 6249
Glyceryl Monostearate, 4489
L-α-**Glycerylphosphorylcholine** *see* 2205
Glyceryl *o*-**Tolyl Ether** *see* 5850
Glyceryl Triacetate *see* 9589
Glyceryl Tributyrate *see* 9620
Glyceryl Trimyristate *see* 9724
Glyceryl Trinitrate *see* 6607
Glyceryl Trioleate *see* 9732
Glyceryl Tripalmitate *see* 9736
Glyceryl Tripetroselinate *see* 7189
Glyceryl Tristearate *see* 9756
Glycidol, 4490
Glycidyl Methacrylate-ethyl Acrylate
  Polymer *see* 2514
Glycin *see* 4837
(Glycinato-*N*,*O*)dihydroxyaluminum *see*
  3183
Glycine, 4491
Glycine, Aluminum Salt *see* 3183
7-Glycine-1,6-aminosuberic Acid-oxy-
  tocin *see* 1839
Glycine Anhydride *see* 7466
1-Glycine-18-L-argininamide-α[(1-18)]**-**
  corticotropin *see* 4428
21[A]-**Glycine-30**[B]**a-L-arginine-30**[B]**b-L-**
  arginine-insulin (Human) *see* 4984
Glycine Betaine *see* 1179
Glycine Nitrile *see* 412
Glycine *p*-**Phenetidide** *see* 7239
Glycine Sulfate, 4492
Glycinin, 4493
Glycinonitrile *see* 412
Glycocholic Acid, 4494
Glycocoll *see* 4491
Glycocoll Betaine *see* 1179
Glycocoll-copper *see* 2627
Glycocoll-*p*-phenetidide *see* 7239
Glycocyamine, 4495
Glycodiazine *see* 4507
Glycogen, 4496
Glycogenic Acid *see* 4456
Glycolande [Sanofi-Synthelabo] *see* 4478
Glycol Benzylcarbamate *see* 1501
Glycol Bromohydrin *see* 3792
Glycol Chlorohydrin *see* 3793
Glycol Cyanohydrin *see* 3794
Glycol Diacetate *see* 3799
Glycol Dilaurate, 4497
Glycol Dinitrate *see* 3800
Glycoleucine *see* 6706
Glycolic Acid, 4498
Glycolic Acid [*o*-(2,6-Dichloroanilino)-
  phenyl]acetate Ester *see* 22
Glycolic Acid 8-Ester with Octahydro-5,-
  8-dihydroxy-4,6,9,10-tetramethyl-6-
  vinyl-3a,9-propano-3a*H*-cyclopenta-
  cycloocten-1(4*H*)-one *see* 7534
Glycol-monoacetin *see* 3801
3-Glycoloyl-1,2,3,4,6,11-hexahydro-3,-
  5,12-trihydroxy-10-methoxy-6,11-di-
  oxo-1-naphthacenyl-3-amino-2,3,6-
  tridioxy-α-L-arabino-hexopyranoside
  see 3623
Glycol Salicylate, 4499

Glycoluril *see* 93
Glycolylurea *see* 4760
Glycomul L [Lonza] *see* 8724
Glycomul O [Lonza] *see* 8724
Glycomul S [Lonza] *see* 8724
Glyconiazide, 4500
Glyconic Acid *see* 4456
Glyconormal *see* 4507
Glycophene *see* 5077
Glycoprotein G *see* 9387
Glycoprotein-P *see* 7195
Glycopyrrolate, 4501
Glycopyrronium Bromide *see* 4501
Glycosine, 4502
7-D-Glycosylapigenin *see* 731
8-Glycosyl-4′,5,7-trihydroxy-3′-meth-
  oxyflavone *see* 8402
Glycyclamide *see* 9511
4-Glycylaminophenetol *see* 7239
4-Glycylaminophenol Ethyl Ether *see*
  7239
N-**Glycylglycine,** 4503
Glycylglycine Lactam *see* 7466
N-[*N*-(*N*-Glycylglycyl)glycyl]-8-L-lysine-
  vasopressin *see* 9167
*N*α-**Glycylglycylglycylvasopressin** *see*
  9167
Glycylpressin [Ferring] *see* 9167
Glycyl-L-seryl-*O*-(1-oxooctyl)-L-seryl-L-
  phenylalanyl-L-leucyl-L-seryl-L-pro-
  lyl-L-α-glutamyl-L-histidyl-L-gluta-
  minyl-L-arginyl-L-valyl-L-glutaminyl-
  L-glutaminyl-L-arginyl-L-lysyl-L-α-
  glutamyl-L-seryl-L-lysyl-L-lysyl-L-
  prolyl-L-prolyl-L-alanyl-L-lysyl-L-
  leucyl-L-glutaminyl-L-prolyl-L-argi-
  nine *see* 4418
Glycyrrhetic Acid *see* 3590
Glycyrrhetic Acid Acetate *see* 76
18β-Glycyrrhetic Acid Hydrogen Succi-
  nate *see* 1793
18β-Glycyrrhetinic Acid *see* 3590
Glycyrrhetinic Acid Glycoside *see* 4505
Glycyrrhiza, 4504
Glycyrrhizic Acid, 4505
Glycyrrhizin *see* 4505
Glycyrrhizinic Acid *see* 4505
Glydiazinamide *see* 4442
Glyfyllin *see* 3479
Glyhexamide, 4506
Glykin *see* 9782
Glykocellon *see* 1829
Glykresin *see* 5850
Glyme *see* 3224
Glymidine, 4507
Glymol *see* 7186
Glyodin, 4508
Glyotol *see* 5850
Glyoxal, 4509
Glyoxal Compd with Sodium Bisulfite *see*
  4510
Glyoxaldiureine *see* 93
Glyoxalic Acid *see* 4511
Glyoxaline *see* 4912
Glyoxaline-5-alanine *see* 4720
Glyoxal-Sodium Bisulfite, 4510
Gly-Oxide [SKB] *see* 1782
Glyoxyldiureide *see* 258
Glyoxylic Acid, 4511
Glypesin [Stada] *see* 4703
Glyphenarsine *see* 9794
Glyphomax [Dow AgroSci.] *see* 4512
Glyphosate, 4512
Glyphosate-trimesium *see* 4512
Glyphylline *see* 3479

Glypolix [Stroder] *see* 3973
Glypressin [Ferring] *see* 9167
Glypro [Dow AgroSci.] *see* 4512
Glysal *see* 4499
Glysennid [Dorsey] *see* 8455
Glyset [Pfizer] *see* 6187
Glyvenol [Novartis] *see* 9608
GM-CSF *see* 4538
GM-CSF/IL-3 Fusion Protein *see* 4995
GM-DF *see* 4537
GMP *see* 4570
3′,5′-GMP *see* 2709
GMP-140 *see* 8426
Gnoscopine *see* 6718
Gö-560 *see* 3945
Gö-687 *see* 3891
Gö-919 *see* 7485
Gö-1261C *see* 9437
Gö-3450 *see* 4319
Goal [Dow AgroSci.] *see* 6963
Goa Powder *see* 768
GOBAB *see* 443
Gödecke 3282 *see* 3891
GOE-3450 *see* 4319
Goethite *see* 4025
Goetsch's Vitamin *see* 10025
Goitrin, 4513
Gokilaht [Sumitomo] *see* 2768
Gold, 4514
Gold-bloom *see* 1713
Gold Colloid ¹⁹⁸Au *see* 4517
Gold Cyanide *see* 4516
Golden Antimony Sulfide *see* 697
Golden Apple Seed *see* 8054
Golden Ragwort *see* 8450
Golden Seal *see* 4769
Goldinodox *see* 882
Goldinomycin *see* 882
Gold Monochloride, 4515
Gold Monocyanide, 4516
Gold Orange *see* 6105
Gold Oxide *see* 4524
Gold Potassium Chloride *see* 7681
Gold Potassium Cyanide *see* 7628
Gold, Radioactive, Colloidal, 4517
Gold Sesquioxide *see* 4524
Gold Sodium Chloride *see* 8688
Gold Sodium Cyanide *see* 8610
Gold Sodium Thiomalate, 4518
Gold Sodium Thiosulfate, 4519
Gold Stannate, 4520
Gold Thioglucose *see* 883
Goldthread *see* 2526
Gold-tin Precipitate *see* 4520
Gold-tin Purple *see* 4520
Gold Trichloride, 4521
Gold Trichloride, Acid, 4522
Gold Trihydroxide, 4523
Gold Trioxide, 4524
Gold Trisulfide, 4525
Gold Yellow *see* 9775
Goltix [Bayer] *see* 5924
Gonacrine *see* 123
Gonadoliberin *see* 5474
Gonadorelin *see* 5474
Gonadorelin Acetate *see* 5474
Gonadotropin-Releasing Factor *see* 5474
Gonak [Akorn] *see* 4842
Gonal-F [Serono] *see* 4223
Gonapeptyl [Ferring] *see* 9748
Gondafon [Schering] *see* 4507
Goniosol [Novartis] *see* 4842
Gonorcin [Farmas] *see* 6700
Gonosan *see* 5287
Gonyaulax Toxin *see* 8389

Good Buffers *see* 4654, 5902
Good-Rite Nix *see* 8634
Gooroo Nuts *see* 5318
Gopten [Abbott] *see* 9568
Goserelin, 4526
Gossypine *see* 2204
Gossypitrin *see* 8035
Gossyplure, 4527
Gossypol, 4528
(−)-Gossypol *see* 4528
(+)-Gossypol *see* 4528
Gossypose *see* 8096
Gougerotin, 4529
Gourd Curare *see* 2671
Govern [Dow AgroSci.] *see* 3962
Government Rubber Styrene *see* 8390
GP-2-121-3 *see* 772
GP-26872 *see* 7277
GP-45840 *see* 3081
GP-47680 *see* 6929
GPIIb-IIIa *see* 4988
L-α-GPC *see* 2205
GPI-15715 *see* 4259
G-Proteins, 4530
GR-2/234 *see* 235
GR-2/925 *see* 2363
GR-2/1214 *see* 2364
GR-2/1574 *see* 233
GR-20263 *see* 1946
GR-33343G *see* 8337
GR-33343X *see* 8337
GR-38032F *see* 6848
GR-43175 *see* 8997
GR-43175C *see* 8997
GR-43659X *see* 5331
GR-68755 *see* 308
GR-68755C *see* 308
GR-85548A *see* 6420
GR-109714X *see* 5352
GR-121167X *see* 10113
GR-122311X *see* 8110
Gradient [Polifarma] *see* 4144
Gradocycline *see* 8252
Graham's Salt *see* 8667
Gramalil [Fujisawa] *see* 9421
Gramaxin [Boehringer, Mann.] *see* 1917
Gramicidin C (Soviet) *see* 4531
Gramicidin D (Dubos) *see* 4532
Gramicidin S, 4531
Gramicidin(s), 4532
Gramicidin S (Soviet) *see* 4531
Gramidil [Dexo] *see* 577
Gramine, 4533
Graminis *see* 9761
Gramipan [Mayoly-Spindler] *see* 2913
Gram-Micina [Lagap] *see* 4254
Grammite *see* 1702
Gramoderm [Schering] *see* 4532
Gramoxone [Syngenta] *see* 7031
Gramplus [Chiesi] *see* 2380
Granaticin, 4534
Granaticin B *see* 4534
Granatum *see* 7587
Grandaxin [EGYT] *see* 9503
Grandisol, 4535
Grandlure *see* 4535
Grandstand [Dow AgroSci.] *see* 9656
Granisetron, 4536
Granit [Rhône-Poulenc] *see* 1446
Granite [Dow AgroSci.] *see* 7103
Granocyte [Chugai] *see* 4537
Granosan *see* 3826
Granudoxy [Pierre Fabre] *see* 3440
α-Granule Membrane Protein 140 *see* 8426

Granulestin *see* 5428
Granulocyte Colony-Stimulating Factor, 4537
Granulocyte Elastase *see* 3535
Granulocyte-Macrophage Colony-Stimulating Factor, 4538
Granzymes *see* 7159
Grape Sugar *see* 4459
Graphite, 4539
Graphite Fluoride, 4540
Graphite Oxide *see* 4541
Graphitic Acid, 4541
Graphitic Oxide *see* 4541
Graphol *see* 6017
Graslan [Dow AgroSci.] *see* 9095
Grasp [Dow AgroSci.] *see* 7103
Grasp [Syngenta] *see* 9564
Gratil [Aventis] *see* 403
Gratus Strophanthin *see* 6901
Gravitol(e), 4542
Gravol [Horner] *see* 3207
Gray Acetate of Lime *see* 1646
(3β,6β,14R)-Grayanotoxane-3,5,6,10,-14,16-hexol *see* 4543
(3β,6β,14R)-Grayanotoxane-3,5,6,10,-14,16-hexol 14-Acetate *see* 4543
(3β,6β,14R)-Grayanotox-10(20)-ene-3,-5,6,14,16-pentol *see* 4543
Grayanotoxin I *see* 4543
Grayanotoxin II *see* 4543
Grayanotoxin III *see* 4543
Grayanotoxins, 4543
GR-C507/75 *see* 6848
Greek Hay *see* 4008
Green Broom *see* 8403
Green Cinnabar *see* 2234
Green Fluorescent Protein, 4544
Green Ginger *see* 10052
Greenhartin *see* 5366
Greenheart *see* 1017
Green Hellebore *see* 9957
Green Hydroquinone *see* 8058
Green Mint *see* 8738
"Green Nickel Oxide" *see* 6510
Greenockite *see* 1628
Green Oxide of Chromium *see* 2234
Green Rouge *see* 2234
Green Tea *see* 9088
Green Vitriol *see* 4057
Grenade [Zeneca] *see* 2757
Grepafloxacin, 4545
Grey Arsenic *see* 794
GRF *see* 8714
GRF(1-29)NH₂ *see* 8461
Griffith's Zinc White *see* 5546
Grifulvin [McNeil] *see* 4549
Grilon [Fibron] *see* 6734
Grindelia, 4546
Grindelic Acid, 4547
Gripenin-O [Fujisawa] *see* 1792
Grisactin [Ayerst] *see* 4549
Griséfuline [Sanofi Winthrop] *see* 4549
Grisein, 4548
Griseofulvin, 4549
Grisovin [GSK] *see* 4549
Gris-PEG [Herbert] *see* 4549
GR-M *see* 6461
Grocreme [Grossmann] *see* 2913
Grodurex [Grossmann] *see* 406
Grolean [Pitman-Moore] *see* 8716
Groliberin [Kabi] *see* 8461
Grorm [Serono] *see* 8716
Grossularite *see* 1648
Ground Holly *see* 2057
Ground Lily *see* 9696

Groundnut see 7058
Groundnut Oil see 7059
Grovex [Groves] see 7476
Growth Hormone see 8716
Growth Hormone-Release Inhibiting
    Factor see 8715
Growth Hormone-Releasing Factor see
    8714
Growth Hormone-Releasing Hormone
    see 8714
GR-S see 8390
Grubbs' Catalyst, 4550
Grundmann's Ketone, 4551
Grysio [Ayerst] see 4549
GS-95 see 9315
GS-393 see 151
GS-504 see 2268
GS-840 see 151
GS-1278 see 9146
GS-1339 see 3475
GS-2989 see 5778
GS-3065 see 3440
GS-4071 see 6889
GS-4104 see 6889
GS-4331-05 see 9146
GS-6244 see 1780
GS-13005 see 5970
GS-16068 see 3342
GS-19851 see 1434
GS-23654 see 6633
G Salt see 6388
GSH see 4475
GSSG see 4475
G-strophanthidin see 6900
G-strophanthin see 6901
GT16-026A see 8474
GT-31-104 see 2473
GT-41 see 1505
GT-92 see 2719
GT-1012 see 7702
GTP Binding Proteins see 4530
G-Tril see 3945
Guacetisal see 851
Guaiac, 4552
Guaiac Alcohol see 4556
Guaiacol, 4553
Guaiacol Glyceryl Ether see 4555
Guaiacol Glyceryl Ether Carbamate see
    5980
Guaiacum see 4552
Guaiacuran see 4555
Guaiacyl Glyceryl Ether see 4555
Guaiaspir [Lampugnani] see 851
Guaiazulene, 4554
S-Guaiazulene see 4554
Guaiazulene Soluble see 4554
Guaifenesin, 4555
Guaiol, 4556
Guaiphenesin see 4555
Guajol see 4556
Guamecycline, 4557
Guanabenz, 4558
Guanadrel, 4559
Guanamprazine see 406
Guanazolo see 896
Guaneran [Burroughs Wellcome] see 9299
Guanethidine, 4560
Guanfacine, 4561
Guanicil [Cilag] see 8908
Guanidine, 4562
Guanidineacetic Acid see 4495
Guanidinium Aluminum Sulfate Hexa-
    hydrate, 4563
4-Guanidino-1-butanol Syringate see
    5440

4-Guanidino-2,4-dideoxy-2,3-dehydro-
    N-acetylneuraminic Acid see 10113
1-(2-Guanidinoethyl)octahydroazocine
    see 4560
2-Guanidinomethyl-1,4-benzodioxan
    see 4568
4-Guanidino-Neu5Ac2en see 10113
Guanidoacetic Acid see 4495
Guanine, 4564
Guanine Nucleotide Binding Proteins see
    4530
Guanine Riboside see 4566
Guanine Riboside-3-phosphoric Acid see
    4569
Guanine Riboside-5-phosphoric Acid see
    4570
Guanite see 8854
Guano, 4565
Guanosine, 4566
Guanosine Cyclic 3',5'-(Hydrogen Phos-
    phate) see 2709
Guanosine 3',5'-Cyclic Monophosphate
    see 2709
Guanosine 3',5'-Cyclic Phosphate see
    2709
Guanosine 3'-Monophosphate see 4569
Guanosine 3',5'-Monophosphate see
    2709
Guanosine 5'-Monophosphate see 4570
Guanosine 5'-Phosphate see 4570
Guanoxabenz, 4567
Guanoxan, 4568
Guantal see 3324
Guanylate Cyclase see 2709
Guanylguanidine see 1215
Guanylhydrazine see 441
3'-Guanylic Acid, 4569
5'-Guanylic Acid, 4570
Guanylic Acid B see 4569
N^1-Guanylsulfanilamide see 8908
Guanylurea Sulfate see 3093
Guaran, 4571
Guaranine see 1636
Guardian see 4124
Guardsman [BASF] see 3214
Guarem [Shire] see 4572
Guar Flour see 4572
Guar Gum, 4572
Guarina [Norgine] see 4572
Guastil [Uriach] see 8989
Guatambuinine see 6834
Guayule see 8278
Gubernal [Novartis] see 313
Guggul see 4574
Guggulsterone, 4573
Guggulu, 4574
Guglip [Cipla] see 4574
Gugulipid see 4574
Guidazide see 4500
Guinea Green B, 4575
Guinea-pig-anti-stiffness Factor see 8815
Gujaphenyl [DDD] see 4553
L-Gulitol see 8725
Gulliostin [Taiyo] see 3346
D-Gulonic Acid, 4576
L-Gulonic Acid, 4577
D-Gulose, 4578
L-Gulose, 4579
Gum Ammoniac see 493
Gum Arabic see 14
Gumbaral [AWD] see 156
Gum Benjamin see 4580
Gum Benzoin, 4580
Gum Camphor see 1732
Gum Copal see 2517

Gum Cyamopsis see 4572
Gum Damar see 2807
Gum Ghatti see 4416
Gum Guaiac see 4552
Gum Guggul see 4574
Gum Guggulu see 4574
Gum Karaya see 5284
Gum Kino see 5313
Gum Opium see 6854
Gum Plant see 3669
Gum-plant (of California) see 4546
Gum Quince Seed see 8054
Gum-resin Myrrh see 6338
Gum Thus see 6832, 9826
Gum Tragacanth, 4581
Guntrin [Zensei] see 6886
Gunyl [Hogapharm] see 4553
G.U.-Pen [Pfizer] see 1840
Guronsan see 4467
Guru Nuts see 5318
Gusathion M [Bayer CropSci.] see 913
Gusperimus, 4582
Guthion [Bayer CropSci.] see 913
Gutron [Nycomed] see 6184
Guttalax-Fher [Boehringer, Ing., Italia] see
    7406
Gutta-Percha, 4583
Guvacine, 4584
GVG see 9978
GW-506U78 see 6442
GW-1000 see 1749
GW-433908G see 4250
GW-572016 see 5367
GW-572016F see 5367
GW-873140 see 737
GX-1048 see 5331
Gy-bon [Ciba-Geigy] see 8536
GYKI-41099 see 2402
Gymnemic Acid, 4585
Gymnemin see 4585
Gynäsan [Bastian] see 3707
Gynefollin see 3104
Gyne-Lotrimin [Schering-Plough] see
    2417
Gynera [Schering AG] see 4413
Gynergen [Novartis] see 3661
Gynesine see 9694
Gynestrel [Recordati] see 6417
Gyn-Hydralin [Lefrancq] see 4491
Gynipral [Chemie Linz] see 4707
Gynocardia Oil see 2047
Gynochrome see 5867
Gyno-Daktarin [Janssen] see 6178
Gynofug [Wolff] see 4881
Gynol II [Ortho-Cilag] see 6677
Gyno-Monistat [Cilag-Chemie] see 6178
Gyno-Myfungar [Klinge] see 6937
Gynomyk [Cassenne] see 1529
Gyno-Pevaryl [Cilag-Chemie] see 3502
Gynoplix [Théraplix] see 52
Gynorest [Mead Johnson] see 3474
Gyno-Terazol [Cilag] see 9160
Gynotherax [Pfizer] see 2190
Gyno-Travogen [Schering AG] see 5160
Gyno-Trosyd [Pfizer] see 9452
Gynovlar [Schering AG] see 6697
Gypsum see 1706
Gyramid [Warner-Lambert] see 3587
Gyrolite see 1702

h5G1.1 Fab see 3506
h5G1.1-scFv see 7192
h5G1.1VHC + h5G1.1VLC see 3506
H-33 see 3947
H48 see 5673
H-56/28 see 313

(−)H-80/62 *see* 7735
H-93/26 *see* 6151
cis-H-102/09 *see* 10126
H-115 *see* 2107
H-133 *see* 3042
H-133/22 *see* 7735
H-154/82 *see* 3953
H-168/68 *see* 6845
H-199/18 *see* 6845
H-319/68 *see* 5810
H-321 *see* 5972
H-365 *see* 7044
H-376/95 *see* 10077
H-610 *see* 3966
H-814 *see* 3972
H-990 *see* 6966
H-3292 *see* 3360
H-3452 *see* 2720
H-3625 *see* 2540
H-3749 *see* 7975
H-3774 *see* 244
H-4723 *see* 2359
HA-1077 *see* 3942
Habekacin [Meiji Seika] *see* 770
Habitrol [Novartis] *see* 6524
Hachimycin, 4586
H Acid *see* 6385
Hadacidin, 4587
h-Adenylic Acid *see* 157
Haemofort *see* 4057
Haemostop Injection *see* 6394
Haemozoin *see* 4649
Haenal [Strathmann] *see* 3218
Haertolan *see* 6408
Haflutan *see* 2374
Hafnium, 4588
Hagan Phosphate *see* 8667
Hageman Factor *see* 3925
Hahnium *see* 3462
HAL *see* 4596
Halamid [Akzo] *see* 2075
Halamid [Viatris] *see* 6436
Halane *see* 3065
Halazepam, 4589
Halazone, 4590
Halbmond [Wyeth] *see* 3309
Halciderm [BMS] *see* 4591
Halcimat [BMS] *see* 4591
Halcinonide, 4591
Halcion [Pharmacia & Upjohn] *see* 9604
Haldol [McNeil] *see* 4598
Haldol Decanoate [Janssen] *see* 4598
Haldrate [Lilly] *see* 7029
Haldrone [Lilly] *see* 7029
Halfan [SKB] *see* 4594
Halfa Wax *see* 3701
Half-cystine *see* 2781
Halibut Liver Oil, 4592
Halidor [Sumitomo] *see* 1033
Halinone [USV] *see* 1393
Halite *see* 8599
Halloysite *see* 4283
Haloanisone *see* 4114
Haloart [Taiho] *see* 4599
Halobetasol Propionate, 4593
Halochondrine A *see* 6819
Halofantrine, 4594
Halofenozide, 4595
Halofuginone, 4596
Halog [BMS] *see* 4591
Halogabide *see* 7772
Halometasone, 4597
Halomonth [Dainippon] *see* 4598
Halon *see* 3064
Haloperidol, 4598

Halopredone Acetate, 4599
Haloprogin, 4600
Halopyramine *see* 2162
Halospor [Novartis] *see* 1935
Halostachine, 4601
Halosten [Shionogi] *see* 4598
Halosulfuron-methyl, 4602
Halotestin [Pfizer] *see* 4186
Halotex [BMS] *see* 4600
Halothane, 4603
Haloxazolam, 4604
Haloxon, 4605
Halset [Strohschein] *see* 2032
Hamaméliode P [Oberlin] *see* 5452
Hamamelis, 4606
Hamamelitannin, 4607
Hamamelose, 4608
Hamarin [Roche] *see* 279
Hamburg Blue *see* 7910
Hämovannid [Bastian] *see* 4979
Hamycin, 4609
Hamycin A *see* 4609
Hanatoxins, 4610
Hanp [Zeria] *see* 872
α-HANP *see* 872
HAPA-B *see* 5106
Hapadex [Schering] *see* 6480
Haplophytine, 4611
Haptocil [Cilag-Chemie] *see* 2712
Haptocorrin *see* 10014
Haptoglobins, 4612
Harden-Young Ester *see* 4275
Hard Paraffin *see* 7023
Harkoseride *see* 5333
Harlem Oil *see* 5271
Harmaline, 4613
Harmalol, 4614
Harmalol Methyl Ether *see* 4613
Harman, 4615
Harmidine *see* 4613
Harmine, 4616
Harmogen [Abbott] *see* 3708
Harmonet [Wyeth] *see* 4413
Harmony [DuPont] *see* 9316
Harmonyl [Abbott] *see* 2918
Harnal [Astellas] *see* 9049
Harness [Monsanto] *see* 61
Harodase *see* 4758
Harpin, 4617
Hartolan [Croda] *see* 5359
Hartshorn *see* 508
Harvade [Uniroyal] *see* 6938
Harzol [Hoyer] *see* 8556
Hasethrol *see* 7112
Hashish *see* 1749
Hassium, 4618
Hasubanan *see* 4619
Hasubanonine, 4619
HAT *see* 2799
Hatchett's Brown *see* 2637
HaTx *see* 4610
HaTx₁ *see* 4610
HaTx₂ *see* 4610
Hauser's Salt *see* 10182
Hausmannite *see* 5735
Havapen [Wyeth] *see* 7081
Havlane [Roussel Diamant] *see* 5574
Haw Apple *see* 2567
Haworth Lignan *see* 5486
Haws *see* 2567
Hawthorn *see* 2567
Hay-Crom [Ivax] *see* 2590
Haynon [Rosemont] *see* 2180
Hayo *see* 2453
Hazol *see* 6966

HB-419 *see* 4478
HBA *see* 3909
HBBL *see* 3598
HBF-386 *see* 1606
HBK *see* 770
HBW-023 *see* 4718
4-HC *see* 7161
HC-3 *see* 4643
Hc45 [Crookes] *see* 4787
HC-58 *see* 3537
HC-064 *see* 6542
HC-803 *see* 5244
HC-20511 *see* 5307
25-HCC *see* 1638
HCFU *see* 1844
HCG *see* 2216
γ-HCH *see* 5501
HCS, 4620
HDNF *see* 6487
HDP *see* 6940
HE-69 *see* 6222
HE-781 *see* 9250
Headline [BASF] *see* 7953
Healon [Pfizer] *see* 4757
Healonid [Pfizer] *see* 4757
Healthied [Hokko] *see* 7067
Heartcin [Ohta] *see* 9843
Heartgard 30 [Merial] *see* 5248
Heavy Hydrogen *see* 2939
Heavy Spar *see* 994
Heavy Water *see* 2940
Hebucol *see* 2715
HEC-5725 *see* 4184
Hecameg [Vegatec], 4621
Hecogenin, 4622
Hectorite, 4623
Hectorol [Bone Care] *see* 3436
Hederagenin, 4624
α-Hederin, 4625
Hedex [GSK] *see* 47
Hedione [Firmenich] *see* 6052
Hedonal MCPP [Bayer] *see* 5784
HEDTA *see* 9966
Hefasolon i.v. [Sanavita] *see* 7721
Heferol [Alkaloid] *see* 4046
Heidelberry *see* 1217
Heitrin [Abbott] *see* 9154
Helenalin, 4626
Helenien *see* 10063
Helenin *see* 207
Helenynolic Acid, 4627
HelfaCat [Helvepharm] *see* 2995
HelfaDog [Helvepharm] *see* 2995
Helfergin [Promonta] *see* 5780
Helianthine B *see* 6105
Helicin, 4628
Helicocerin *see* 2004
Heliosupine, 4629
Heliotropin *see* 7475
Helium, 4630
Helixin C *see* 6541
Helixin (The Saponin) *see* 4625
Helmatac [SK & F] *see* 7035
Helmet Flower *see* 8413
Helmetina *see* 7252
Helmex [Infectopharm] *see* 7955
Helmezine [Allen & Hanburys] *see* 7464
Helmifren *see* 7464
Helminal *see* 5276
Helmintox [Innothéra] *see* 7955
Helmirone *see* 4605
Helmitol [Bayer] *see* 5966
Helodermin *see* 3914
Helogaphen [Spitzner] *see* 2084
Helonias, 4631

Helospectin *see* 3914
Helothion [Bayer] *see* 8990
Helvamox [Helvepharm] *see* 577
Helvecyclin [Helvepharm] *see* 9196
Helvetia Blue *see* 6028
Helveticoside, 4632
Helvolic Acid, 4633
Hem *see* 4639
Hemabate [Pfizer] *see* 1823
Hemanthine *see* 1493
Hematein, 4634
Hematin, 4635
β-Hematin *see* 4649
Hematin-protein *see* 2791
Hematite *see* 4028
Hematoporphyrin, 4636
Hematoporphyrin IX *see* 4636
Hematoxiline *see* 4637
Hematoxylin, 4637
Hematoxylon, 4638
Heme, 4639
Hemel *see* 320
Hementin, 4640
Hemerven [Interdelta] *see* 3297
Hemerythrin, 4641
Hemicelluloses, 4642
Hemicholinium, 4643
Hemicholinium-3 *see* 4643
Hemiglobin *see* 5965
Hemin, 4644
Hemineurin [AstraZeneca] *see* 2384
Heminevrin [AstraZeneca] *see* 2384
Hemipyocyanine, 4645
Hemisulfur Mustard, 4646
Hemlock *see* 2506
Hemocaprol [Sanofi-Aventis] *see* 432
Hémoclar [Sanofi Winthrop] *see* 7134
Hemocoagulase *see* 1010
Hemocuprein *see* 9002
Hemocuron [Takeda] *see* 9608
Hemocyanins, 4647
Hemodex [Alstoe] *see* 2948
Hemofil-M [Baxter] *see* 3921
Hemoglobin, 4648
Hemokine [Novartis] *see* 4995
Hemolidione [Sintetico] *see* 7234
Hemometina [Cusi] *see* 3559
Hemo-Pak [J & J] *see* 6939
Hemopoietine *see* 3688
Hemotrope [Andromaco] *see* 1510
Hemozoin, 4649
Hemp *see* 1749
Hempa *see* 4725
Henbane *see* 4859
2-Hendecanone *see* 6104
10-Hendecenoic Acid *see* 9848
Hendrickson's Reagent, 4650
Heneicosafluorotripropylamine *see* 4183
Henequem *see* 8549
Henna, 4651
HEOD *see* 3103
Hepacholine *see* 2206
Hepadial [Biocodex] *see* 3203
Hepadist *see* 4680
Hepagin *see* 7207
Hepalande [Delalande] *see* 5834
Hepalidine [3M Pharma] *see* 9445
Hepa-Merz [Merz] *see* 6874
Heparamine *see* 4652
Hepar Calcis *see* 1707
Heparegen [Syntex] *see* 9445
Heparexine *see* 7362
Heparides *see* 4652
Heparin, 4653
β-Heparin *see* 2214

Heparinic Acid *see* 4653
Heparin Sodium *see* 4653
Hepation [Nippon Chemiphar] *see* 5712
Hepatocatalase *see* 1900
Hepatocyte Stimulating Factor *see* 4998
Hepatolite [DuPont] *see* 3358
Hepatoxane [Pharm. l'Esplanade] *see* 9492
HEPES, 4654
HEPP *see* 7128
Hepsal [Weddel] *see* 4653
Hepsera [Gilead] *see* 151
Heptabarb *see* 4655
Heptabarbital, 4655
Heptachlor, 4656
1*H*-1,4,5,6,7,8,8-Heptachloro-3a,4,7,-
    7a-tetrahydro-4,7-methanoindene
    see 4656
Heptadecanoic Acid *see* 5751
(2*E*,8*E*,10*E*)-2,8,10-Heptadecatriene-4,-
    6-diyne-1,14-diol *see* 3569
(8*E*,10*E*,12*E*,14*R*)-8,10,12-Heptadeca-
    triene-4,6-diyne-1,14-diol *see* 2267
2-(8-Heptadecenyl)-4,5-dihydro-1*H*-imi-
    dazole-1-ethanol *see* 408
2-(8-Heptadecenyl)-2-imidazoline-1-
    ethanol *see* 408
2-Heptadecyl-4,5-dihydro-1*H*-imidazole
    Monoacetate *see* 4508
5-Heptadecylene-1-carboxylic Acid *see*
    7189
2-Heptadecylglyoxalidine Acetate *see*
    4508
(2*R*,3*S*,5*R*,6*R*)-*rel*-3-(1*E*,3*E*)-1,3-Hepta-
    dienyl-5,6-dihydroxy-2-(hydroxy-
    methyl)cyclohexanone *see* 6987
6-(1,3-Heptadienyl)-3,4-dihydroxy-2-
    oxocyclohexanecarboxaldehyde *see*
    4270
Heptadon [Ebewe] *see* 5944
Heptadorm *see* 4655
1,1,2,2,3,3,3-Heptafluoro-*N*,*N*-bis(hep-
    tafluoropropyl)-1-propanamine *see*
    4183
Heptaldehyde *see* 4658
Heptalgin *see* 7207
Heptalin *see* 7207
2-(1-*N*,*N*-Heptamethylenimino)ethylgua-
    nidine *see* 4560
(*all-E*)-2-(3,7,11,15,19,23,27-Hepta-
    methyl-2,6,10,14,18,22,26-octacosa-
    heptaenyl)-3-methyl-1,4-naphtha-
    lenedione *see* 5833
Heptaminol, 4657
Heptamul *see* 4656
Hept-a-myl [Delalande] *see* 4657
Heptanal, 4658
2-Heptanamine *see* 9802
n-Heptane, 4659
1,7-Heptanedicarboxylic Acid *see* 905
Heptanedioic Acid *see* 7431
Heptanoic Acid, 4660
Heptanoic Acid Ethyl Ester *see* 3835
1-Heptanol, 4661
2-Heptanol, 4662
Heptanon [Pliva] *see* 5944
2-Heptanone, 4663
4-Heptanone *see* 3345
17β-Heptanoyloxy-1-methyl-5α-androst-
    1-en-3-one *see* 5967
Heptazone *see* 7207
Heptedrine [Bellon] *see* 9802
D-*arabino*-Hept-2-enonic Acid γ-Lactone
    see 4451
Heptenophos, 4664
n-Heptoic Acid *see* 4660

Heptone *see* 7207
D-*glycero*-D-*gulo*-Heptonic Acid *see* 4455
D-*glycero*-D-*gulo*-Heptonic Acid Compd
    with Erythromycin (1:1) *see* 3684
Heptoxime, 4665
D-*manno*-Heptulose, 4666
n-Heptyl Alcohol *see* 4661
Heptylaldehyde *see* 4658
6-*O*-(*N*-Heptylcarbamoyl)-methyl-α-D-
    glucopyranoside *see* 4621
2-Heptyl-4-hydroxyquinoline *N*-Oxide
    see 4751
19-Heptyl-10-hydroxy-1,5,10,14-tetra-
    azacyclononadecan-15-one *see* 7509
n-Heptylic Acid *see* 4660
2,2′-[3-[(3-Heptyl-4-methyl-2(3*H*)-thia-
    zolylidene)ethylidene]-1-propene-1,3-
    diyl]bis(3-heptyl-4-methylthiazo-
    lium) Diiodide *see* 7530
Heptylon [Delalande] *see* 4657
Heptylphysostigmine *see* 3638
2-Heptyl-4-quinolinol 1-Oxide *see* 4751
Heptylstigmine *see* 3638
Hepzide [Merck & Co.] *see* 6569
Héraclène [Mauchant] *see* 2451
Heraclin *see* 1157
Herbadon [Mavena] *see* 2942
Herbadox [BASF] *see* 7084
Herbisan [Roberts Chemicals] *see* 3384
Herceptin [Genentech] *see* 9575
Hercules 528 *see* 3301
Hercules 3956 *see* 9557
Herculon [Hercules] *see* 7581
Hercynine, 4667
Heritage [Syngenta] *see* 924
Hermesetas *see* 8311
Hermophényl *see* 5886
Heroin *see* 2968
Herperal [Farmitalia] *see* 8772
Herpes-Gel [Master] *see* 4891
Herplex [Allergan] *see* 4891
Herqueinone, 4668
Herrmann-Beller Catalyst, 4669
Herrmann's Palladacycle *see* 4669
Herzberg's Paper *see* 2498
HES *see* 4673
Hesofen *see* 5846
Hesotanol *see* 3879
Hesotin *see* 3879
Hespan [BMS] *see* 4673
Hespander [Kyorin] *see* 4673
Hesperetin, 4670
Hesperetin 7-Rhamnoglucoside *see* 4671
Hesperetin-7-rutinoside *see* 4671
Hesperidin, 4671
Hestar [Pisa] *see* 4673
Hestrium Chloride *see* 4688
Hetacillin, 4672
Hetacin-K [Fort Dodge] *see* 4672
Hetaphenone *see* 3710
Hetastarch, 4673
5-HETE, 4674
Heteroauxin *see* 4964
Heterophylline *see* 784
Hetol *see* 1303
Hetoxol [Heterene Chem.] *see* 7577
Hetoxol CS-20 [Heterene Chem.] *see* 7577
Hetoxol L-9 [Heterene Chem.] *see* 7558
Hetrazan [Lederle] *see* 3116
Hetrazeen [Heterochemical] *see* 5831
Heulandite *see* 1648
Hevyteck [Penreco] *see* 7186
Heweneural [Hevert] *see* 5482
Hexaaminecobalt Trichloride, 4675
Hexaammonium Molybdate (Mo$_7$O$_{24}^{6-}$)
    see 533

d,l-Hexamethylpropyleneamine Oxime *see* 3911

Hexamethyl-*p*-rosaniline Chloride *see* 4395

(*all-E*)-2,6,10,15,19,23-Hexamethyl-2,-6,10,14,18,22-tetracosahexaene *see* 8768

(*all-E*)-2-(3,7,11,15,19,23-Hexamethyl-2,6,10,14,18,22-tetracosahexaenyl)-3-methyl-1,4-naphthalenedione *see* 5833

2,6,10,15,19,23-Hexamethyltetracosane *see* 8767

N,N,N',N',N'',N''-Hexamethyl-1,3,5-triazine-2,4,6-triamine *see* 320

1,1,1,3,3,3-Hexamethyl-2-(trimethylsilyl)trisilane *see* 9757

Hexameton Bromide [Burroughs Wellcome] *see* 4688

Hexameton Chloride [Burroughs Wellcome] *see* 4688

Hexamic Acid [Abbott] *see* 2703

Hexamidine, 4692

Hexamine *see* 5966

Hexaminolevulinate, 4693

Hexammino-cobalt Chloride *see* 4675

Hexanal *see* 1760

Hexanaphthene *see* 2723

Hexanastab *see* 4704

Hexanastab Oral *see* 4704

n-Hexane, 4694

1,6-Hexanediamine, 4695

1,6-Hexanedicarboxylic Acid *see* 8862

Hexanedioic Acid *see* 162

Hexanedioic Acid Compd with Piperazine (1:1) *see* 7465

1,6-Hexanediol *see* 4690

2,5-Hexanedione *see* 71

4,4'-[1,6-Hexanediylbis[imino(1-hydroxy-2,1-ethanediyl)]]bis-1,2-benzenediol *see* 4707

3',3'''-(1,6-Hexanediyl)bis[6'-(α-D-mannopyranosyloxy)[1,1'-biphenyl]]-3-acetic Acid *see* 1222

3,3'-[1,6-Hexanediylbis[(methylimino)-carbonyl]oxy]bis[1-methylpyridinium]dibromide *see* 3362

4,4'-[1,6-Hexanediylbis(oxy)]bisbenzenecarboximidamide *see* 4692

Hexanicit [Bastian] *see* 4979

Hexanicotinoyl Inositol *see* 4979

Hexanicotinyl *cis*-1,2,3,5-*trans*-4,6-Cyclohexane *see* 4979

2,4,6,2',4',6'-Hexanitrodiphenylamine *see* 3335

Hexanitrohexaazaisowurtzitane, 4696

2,4,6,8,10,12-Hexanitro-2,4,6,8,10,12-hexaazatetracyclo[5.5.0.0^{5,9}.0^{3,11}]-dodecane *see* 4696

Hexanium Bromide [Adrian-Marinier] *see* 4688

Hexanoestrol *see* 4701

Hexanoic Acid *see* 1759

Hexanoic Acid Ethyl Ester *see* 3777

Hexanoic Acid Pentyl Ester *see* 605

1-Hexanol, 4697

tert-Hexanol Carbamate *see* 3566

2-Hexanone *see* 6033

Hexanoyl Chloride *see* 1763

Hexanoylpenicillin *see* 616

Hexanurat [Durascan] *see* 279

Hexaoctacontaoxononaantimonateheneicosatungstate(19−) Heptadecaammonium Disodium *see* 4750

1,4,7,10,13,16-Hexaoxacyclooctadecane *see* 2602

Hexaprazol(e) *see* 3695

Hexapropymate, 4698

Hexarese [Durascan] *see* 406

Hexasodium *sym*-Bis(*m*-aminobenzoyl-*m*-amino-*p*-methylbenzoyl-1-naphthyl-amino-4,6,8-trisulfonate) Carbamide *see* 9006

Hexastat [Bellon] *see* 320

Hexathide [Allen & Hanburys] *see* 4688

Hexathonide *see* 4688

Hexatrione [Lederle] *see* 9598

Hexavibex [Parke-Davis] *see* 7982

Hexazinone, 4699

Hexemal *see* 2711

Hexemal Calcium *see* 2711

Hexenal *see* 4704

3-(5-Hexene-1,3-diynyl)-6-(1-propynyl)-1,2-dithiin *see* 9304

Hexene-Ol *see* 8722

3-Hexen-1-ol, 4700

δ-Δ^{α,β}-Hexenolactone *see* 7032

2-Hexen-5,1-olide *see* 7032

D-*erythro*-Hex-2-enonic Acid γ-Lactone *see* 5126

L-*threo*-Hex-2-enonic Acid γ-Lactone *see* 830

Hexermin *see* 7982

Hexestrol, 4701

Hexestrol Bis(β-diethylaminoethyl Ether), 4702

Hexestrol 4,4'-Diphosphoric Ester *see* 4701

Hexetidine, 4703

Hexigel [Warner-Lambert] *see* 4703

Hexobarbital, 4704

Hexobarbital Soluble *see* 4704

Hexobarbitone *see* 4704

Hexobendine, 4705

Hexobion [Merck KGaA] *see* 7982

Hexocil [Pharmacia] *see* 4703

Hexocyclium Methyl Sulfate, 4706

L-*threo*-2,3-Hexodiulosonic Acid γ-Lactone *see* 2866

Hexoestrol *see* 4701

Hexofen *see* 5846

Hexogen *see* 2736

Hexomedin [Sanofi-Aventis] *see* 4692

Hexone *see* 5207

Hexone Chloride *see* 4688

Hexopal [Winthrop] *see* 4979

Hexoprenaline, 4707

Hexopropynate *see* 4698

Hexoral [Pfizer] *see* 4703

Hexosan *see* 4680

Hexose Diphosphate *see* 4275

Hexose Monophosphate *see* 4276

Hexose Phosphate *see* 4276

Hextol [Hoechst] *see* 7813

Hextril [Pfizer] *see* 4703

D-*lyxo*-Hexulose *see* 9030

L-*xylo*-2-Hexulosonic Acid *see* 5304

Hexvix [PhotoCure] *see* 4693

n-Hexyl Alcohol *see* 4697

Hexyl 5-Aminolevulinate *see* 4693

4-Hexyl-1,3-benzenediol *see* 4712

4-Hexyl-1,3-benzenediol Compd with 9-Acridinamine (1:1) *see* 126

Hexylcaine Hydrochloride, 4708

1-(*n*-Hexylcarbamoyl)-5-fluorouracil *see* 1844

n-Hexyl Chloride *see* 2144

2-Hexylcyclopropanedecanoic Acid *see* 5341

2-Hexyldecanoic Acid, 4709

1-Hexyl-3,7-dihydro-3,7-dimethyl-1*H*-purine-2,6-dione *see* 7127

4-Hexyl-1,3-dihydroxybenzene *see* 4712

1-Hexyl-3,7-dimethylxanthine *see* 7127

Hexylene Glycol, 4710

2-Hexyl-5-hydroxycyclopentaheptanoic Acid *see* 8260

Hexylmethylcarbinol *see* 6752

Hexyl Methyl Ketone, 4711

2-(Hexyloxy)benzamide *see* 3909

N-[[2-[[[4-[[[(Hexyloxy)carbonyl]amino]-iminomethyl]phenyl]amino]methyl]-1-methyl-1*H*-benzimidazol-5-yl]carbonyl]-*N*-2-pyridinyl-β-alanine Ethyl Ester *see* 2797

3-[4-(Hexyloxy)-1,2,5-thiadiazol-3-yl]-1,2,5,6-tetrahydro-1-methylpyridine *see* 10056

4-Hexylresorcinol, 4712

3-Hexyl-7,8,9,10-tetrahydro-6,6,9-trimethyl-6*H*-dibenzo[*b,d*]pyran-1-ol *see* 9013

1-Hexyltheobromine *see* 7127

Hexythiazox, 4713

Heyden 611 *see* 8813

HF *see* 3925

HF-1854 *see* 2423

HF-1927 *see* 3008

HF-2333 *see* 7179

HF-6305 *see* 4909

HF-8505 *see* 4909

HFA-134a *see* 4714

HFC-32 *see* 3151

HFC-134a, 4714

HGF *see* 4446

HG-factor *see* 4446

HGH *see* 8716

HGP-1 *see* 5584

hGRF *see* 8714

HH-184 *see* 7904

HH-197 *see* 1513

HHCB, 4715

HHDN *see* 226

HI-6 *see* 835

Hi-Alarzin [Yamanouchi] *see* 9519

Hializan [Pharma Investi] *see* 6927

Hiberna [Mitsubishi] *see* 7786

Hibernal [Aventis] *see* 2185

Hibiclens [Zeneca] *see* 2091

Hibident [SKB] *see* 2091

Hibidil [Zeneca] *see* 2091

Hibiscrub [Zeneca] *see* 2091

Hibital [Zeneca] *see* 2091

Hibitane [Zeneca] *see* 2091

Hibon [Tokyo Tanabe] *see* 8200

Hibschite *see* 1648

Hicee [Takeda] *see* 830

Hiconcil [BMS] *see* 577

Hicoseen [Klimitschek] *see* 1522

HIDA *see* 5483

Hidacian *see* 2680

Hi-Deratol *see* 10018

Hidrasec [GSK] *see* 8090

Hidroferol [FAES] *see* 1638

Hidroronol *see* 4781

Hi-Enterol *see* 5031

Hiestrone *see* 3708

Hi-Fresmin [Takeda] *see* 2451

High Acyl Gellan Gum *see* 4383

High Bush Cranberry *see* 9973

High Mallow *see* 5708

High Molecular Weight Kininogen *see* 5312

Higroton [Novartis] *see* 2193

Higueroxyl Delabarre *see* 4077

Hihustan [Maruko] *see* 8091

Hilactan [Kyoritsu] *see* 2305

Hillebrandite *see* 1702
Hilong [Wyeth] *see* 6926
Himecol [Kissei] *see* 4854
Hinochloa [Bayer] *see* 5797
Hinokitiol *see* 9390
Hinosan [Bayer] *see* 3510
Hiochic Acid *see* 6163
Hiohex Chloride [Keith-Victor] *see* 4688
Hioxyl [Quinoderm] *see* 4798
Hipberries *see* 8263
Hipertan [Gramon] *see* 6184
Hipertil [Normal] *see* 1774
Hiphyllin *see* 3479
Hipoartel [Ipsen] *see* 3567
Hippocampal-derived Neurotrophic
    Factor *see* 6487
Hippodin *see* 5034
Hippuran I 131 [Mallinckrodt] *see* 5034
Hippuric Acid, 4716
Hipputope [BMS] *see* 5034
Hiprex [3M Pharma] *see* 5966
Hirathiol *see* 4885
Hiropon *see* 5948
Hirsutic Acid C, 4717
Hirudex [Cooper] *see* 4718
Hirudin, 4718
Hirulog [Medicines Co.] *see* 1310
Hirulog-1 *see* 1310
Hirulog-8 *see* 1310
His *see* 4720
Hismanal [Janssen] *see* 856
Hispril [SKB] *see* 3331
Histabromamine *see* 1418
Histabutizine *see* 1464
Histabutyzine *see* 1464
Histadyl (formerly) [Lilly] *see* 5959
Histalog [Lilly] *see* 1183
Histalon [Hance] *see* 7984
Histamen [Polifarma] *see* 856
Histaminase *see* 2975
Histamine, 4719
Histamine Deaminase *see* 2975
Histamine Oxidase *see* 2975
Histaminos [Lesvi] *see* 856
Histan [Cooper] *see* 7984
Histantin [Burroughs Wellcome] *see* 2081
Histapyran [Horton & Converse] *see* 7984
Histatex [Medix] *see* 7984
Histidine, 4720
L-Histidine *see* 4720
Histidine-betaine *see* 4667
Histidine Trimethylbetaine *see* 4667
Histimin *see* 1183
Histoacryl [Braun] *see* 1565
Histocarb [Rohm & Haas] *see* 1786
Histones, 4721
Histrelin, 4722
Histrionicotoxin, 4723
(−)-Histrionicotoxin *see* 4723
Histrionicotoxin D *see* 4402
Histryl [SKB] *see* 3331
Histyn [Hässle] *see* 3331
Hi-Ti [Kyowa] *see* 5660
Hitocobamin-M [Hishiyama] *see* 6045
Hitodesterol *see* 8749
Hittorf's Phosphorus *see* 7347
Hivid [Roche] *see* 10109
Hiwolfia [Bowman] *see* 8120
Hi-Z [Otsuka] *see* 6886
HK-137 *see* 3970
HK-256 *see* 7736
H-Kininogen *see* 5312
HL-255 *see* 1393
HL-362 *see* 2476
HL-2186 *see* 9035

HL-5746 *see* 2185
HLL2 *see* 3631
HLö-7, 4724
HLoe-7 *see* 4724
HMAF *see* 5092
3-HMC *see* 3779
HMD *see* 1797
HMDP *see* 6940
HMDS *see* 4689
HME *see* 3549
HMF *see* 4832
HMG *see* 5808
HMGA *see* 5808
HMM *see* 320
HMPA, 4725
d,l-HM-PAO *see* 3911
HMPT *see* 4725
HMR-1275 *see* 4094
HMR-1964 *see* 4985
HMR-3647 *see* 9119
HMS [Allergan] *see* 5794
HMT *see* 5966
HMTA *see* 5966
HMX *see* 6758
HN2 *see* 5775
HN-3 *see* 9625
HNE, 4726
4-HNE *see* 4726
HNIW *see* 4696
αHNP *see* 6224
HO-2474 *see* 2957
Hoarhound *see* 4747
HOE-39-893d *see* 7082
HOE-045 *see* 1869
HOE-095K *see* 37
HOE-111 *see* 1943
HOE-118 *see* 7492
HOE-144 *see* 6725
HOE-280 *see* 6771
HOE-285 *see* 7813
HOE-296 *see* 2266
HOE-296V *see* 8154
HOE-304 *see* 2930
HOE-433 *see* 314
HOE-440 *see* 9418
HOE-490 *see* 4440
HOE-498 *see* 8103
HOE-555-02A *see* 3996
HOE-642 *see* 1841
HOE-661 *see* 7339
HOE-760 *see* 8274
HOE-766 *see* 1503
HOE-777 *see* 7719
HOE-881v *see* 3960
HOE-893d *see* 7082
HOE-901 *see* 4984
HOE-984 *see* 6673
HOE-2770 *see* 9253
HOE-2810 *see* 5509
HOE-2873 *see* 7962
HOE-2904 *see* 3287
HOE-2960 *see* 9606
HOE-2982 *see* 4664
HOE-16410 *see* 5218
HOE-17411 *see* 1791
HOE-23408 *see* 3082
HOE-33171 *see* 3984
HOE-36801 *see* 3864
HOE-39866 *see* 7339
HOE-40045 *see* 1869
HOE-46360 *see* 3984
HOE-75032 *see* 403
HOE-095404 *see* 3754
HOE-102791 *see* 7798
HOE-107892 *see* 5800

Hoechst 10446 *see* 4836
Hoechst 10582 *see* 6709
Hoechst 10600 *see* 7207
Hoechst 10720 *see* 5301
Hoechst 10805 *see* 3337
Hoechst 10820 *see* 5944
Hoechst 12494 *see* 3990
Hoegrass [Bayer CropSci.] *see* 3082
Hoelon [Bayer CropSci.] *see* 3082
Hoffmann's Anodyne *see* 8756
Hoffmann's Drops *see* 8755
HOG *see* 7219
Hoggar [Stada] *see* 3441
Hogival *see* 3708
Hogpax [Ferrosan] *see* 580
Hog's Bean *see* 4859
Hogweed *see* 8403
Hokunalin [Hokuriku] *see* 9811
Holland Balsam *see* 5271
Holligold *see* 1713
Holly-leaved Barberry *see* 1155
Holmia *see* 4727
Holmium, 4727
Holocaine Hydrochloride [Winthrop] *see*
    7202
Holomycin, 4728
Holopon [Altana] *see* 6003
Holoxan [Baxter] *see* 4896
Homapin [Mission Pharmacal] *see* 4730
Homarine, 4729
Homatrisol [Cooper] *see* 4730
Homatropine, 4730
Hombre [LiphaTech] *see* 3139
Homidium, 4731
Homoarterenol *see* 6692
Homobatrachotoxin *see* 1009
Homocaine *see* 2454
Homochelidonine, 4732
α-Homochelidonine *see* 4732
Homochlorcyclizine, 4733
Homoclomin [Eisai] *see* 4733
Homocodeine *see* 7329
Homocysteine, 4734
Homocysteine *S*-Ethyl Ether *see* 3738
Homocystine, 4735
Homoeriodictyol, 4736
Homogentisic Acid, 4737
Homomenthyl Salicylate *see* 4738
Homomycin *see* 4851
Homonal [SS Pharm.] *see* 5649
D-Homopantothenic Acid *see* 4744
18a-Homo-pregna-4,9,11-trien-17β-ol-
    3-one *see* 9214
Homoproline *see* 7458
Homosalate, 4738
m-Homosalicylic Acid *see* 2580
o-Homosalicylic Acid *see* 2581
p-Homosalicylic Acid *see* 2582
Homoserine, 4739
Homosulfamine *see* 5649
4-Homosulfanilamide *see* 5649
Homotrilobine *see* 9697
Homovanillic Acid, 4740
HON, 4741
Honduras Balsam *see* 949
Honduras Bark *see* 1879
Honokiol, 4742
Honvan [Baxter] *see* 4253
Honvol [Horner] *see* 4253
Hoodia, 4743
Hopantenate Calcium *see* 4744
Hopantenic Acid, 4744
Hopate [Tanabe] *see* 4744
Hopeite *see* 10151
Hops, 4745

Hordenine, 4746
Horehound, 4747
Horizon [Bayer CropSci.] see 9092
Horizon [Novartis] see 2401
Hormezon [Tobishi] see 1180
Hormoestrol see 4701
Hormofemin [Medo] see 3104
Hormofollin see 3708
Hormomed [Merckle] see 3707
Hormonisene [Temis Lostalo] see 2174
Hormovarine [Clin-Comar-Byla] see 3708
Horn Silver see 8504
Horse Balm see 2483
Horse Chestnut, 4748
Horse Chestnut Seed Extract see 4748
Horseheal see 5003
Horse Nettle see 8708
Horse-radish, 4749
Horseweed see 3666
Hostacortin [Hoechst] see 7722
Hostacyclin [Hoechst] see 9196
Hostaginan [Hoechst] see 7737
Hostalival [Hoechst] see 6673
Hostaquick [Hoechst] see 4664
Hostathion [Hoechst] see 9606
Houpo see 5697
HP-129 see 3971
HP-549 see 5237
HP-749 see 1176
HP-873 see 4900
HPA-23, 4750
HPC see 6198, 6957
HPEK-1 see 9249
5-HPETE see 4674
hpGRF see 8714
hpGRF(1-29)NH$_2$ see 8461
HPL see 4620
HPMC see 4842
HPMF see 3598
(S)-HPMPC see 2268
HPP see 279
4-HPR see 3998
hPTH 1-34 acetate see 9166
HPTS see 7954
HQ-495 see 183
HQNO, 4751
HR see 9789
HR-111V see 1943
HR-158 see 5574
HR-221 see 1928
HR-376 see 2359
HR-756 see 1933
HR-810 see 1940
HRF [Ayerst] see 5474
HRS-16 see 3105
HS-592 see 2345
HS-902 see 9460
HSA see 8468
H$_2$sal$_2$en see 8322
HSP-2986 see 7707
HSR-770 see 4928
HSR-803 see 5244
HSR-902 see 9460
5-HT see 8462
HTH see 1674
HTIB see 5321
L-5HTP see 4847
5-HTP see 4847
HTX see 4723
(−)-HTX 1 see 4723
HTX D see 4402
HTZ see 4713
HU-211 see 2944
Hu1124 see 3519
Huanghuahaosu see 817

Huckleberry see 1217
Humagel [Parke-Davis] see 7041
Humalog [Lilly] see 4987
Human Amylin see 609
Human β-Amyloid Peptide (1-40) see 615
Human β-Amyloid Peptide (1-42) see 615
Human α-ANP see 872
Human α-ANP (4-28) see 872
Human Atriopeptin (1-28) see 872
Human Atriopeptin (4-28) see 872
Human Atriopeptin (102-126) see 872
Human Brain Natriuretic Peptide-32 see 1360
Human Chorionic Gonadotropin see 2216
Human Chorionic Gonadotropin, Glycoform α see 2216
Human Chorionic Somatomammotropin see 4620
Human EGF-URO see 3527
Human Growth Hormone see 8716
Human Growth Hormone-releasing Factor(1-29)amide see 8461
Human IgE Pentapeptide see 7128
Human Insulin-like Growth Factor I see 4986
Humanized Anti-Tac see 2799
Human LFA-3-IgG$_1$ Fusion Protein see 227
Human Menopausal Gonadotropins see 4223
Human Pancreatic Somatoliberin(1-29)-amide see 8461
Human Placental Lactogen see 4620
Human Serum Albumin see 8468
Human Thymosin α1 see 9405
Human Tumor Necrosis Factor Receptor p75 Fc Fusion Protein see 3712
Human Urodilatin see 9886
Humate-P [Centeon] see 3921
Humatin [Parke-Davis] see 7041
Humatrope [Lilly] see 8716
Humegon [Organon] see 4223
Humic Acids, 4752
Huminsulin [Lilly] see 4980
Humira [Abbott] see 148
Humorsol [Merck & Co.] see 2885
Humoryl [Delalande] see 9521
Humulene, 4753
α-Humulene see 4753
β-Humulene see 4753
Humulin [Lilly] see 4980
Humulina [Lilly] see 4980
Humulon, 4754
Humulone see 4754
Hungarian Chamomile see 2041
HUP see 4755
Huperzine A, 4755
Hurler Corrective Factor see 4894
Husar [Bayer CropSci.] see 5046
Hussar [Bayer CropSci.] see 5046
Hustazol [Yoshitomi] see 2395
HWA-285 see 7813
HWA-486 see 5432
HWG-1608 see 9092
2-HxG see 1201
HY-770 see 4928
Hyacid [Scanvet] see 4757
Hyacin see 2880
Hyacinthin see 7265
Hyalase [C.P. Pharm.] see 4758
Hyalgan [Fidia] see 4757
Hyalidase see 4758
Hyalobiuronic Acid, 4756
Hyalovet [Fidia] see 4757

Hyalozima see 4758
Hyaluronic Acid, 4757
Hyaluronidases, 4758
Hyamate [Xttrium] see 1501
Hyamine 10X [Rohm & Haas] see 6023
Hyamine 1622 [Rohm & Haas] see 1074
Hyanit [Wölfer] see 9867
Hyasmonta see 4758
Hyason see 4758
Hyazyme [Abbott] see 4758
Hybridoma Growth Factor see 4998
Hybrin [Pfizer] see 830
Hycamptamine see 9548
Hycamtin [GSK] see 9548
Hycanthone, 4759
Hyclorate [Funai] see 2377
Hycobal [Eisai] see 2451
Hydac [Aventis] see 3953
Hydagen B [Henkel] see 1241
Hydantin [Orion] see 7322
Hydantoin, 4760
Hydantol [Fujinaga] see 7322
Hydergine [Sandoz] see 3653
Hydnocarpate Sodium see 4761
Hydnocarpic Acid, 4761
Hydnocarpus Oil see 2047
Hydnocarpylacetic Acid see 2048
Hydol see 4789
Hydracort [Galderma] see 4787
Hydracrylic Acid, 4762
Hydracrylic Acid β-Lactone see 7820
Hydracrylonitrile see 3794
Hydralazine, 4763
Hydrallostane, 4764
Hydramethylnon, 4765
Hydrangea, 4766
Hydrangin see 9847
Hydrargyrum see 5898
Hydrastine, 4767
l-β-Hydrastine see 4767
Hydrastinine, 4768
Hydrastis, 4769
Hydrated Alumina see 342
Hydrated Cupric Oxide see 2642
Hydrated Ferric Oxide see 4025
Hydrated Magnesium-aluminum-iron Silicate see 9961
Hydrazine, 4770
Hydrazine Anhydrous see 4770
Hydrazinecarbothioamide see 9361
Hydrazinecarboxamide Monohydrochloride see 441
Hydrazinecarboximidamide see 441
Hydrazine Hydrate, 4771
Hydrazine Sulfate, 4772
Hydrazine Yellow see 9072
Hydrazinium Sulfate see 4772
Hydrazinobenzene see 7293
4-Hydrazinobenzenesulfonic Acid, 4773
(αS)-α-Hydrazino-3,4-dihydroxy-α-methylbenzenepropanoic Acid Monohydrate see 1797
(−)-L-α-Hydrazino-3,4-dihydroxy-α-methylhydrocinnamic Acid Monohydrate see 1797
3-Hydrazino-6-[(2-hydroxypropyl)methylamino]pyridazine see 7423
α-Hydrazino-α-methyl-β-(3,4-dihydroxyphenyl)propionic Acid Monohydrate see 1797
1-(2-Hydrazino-2-oxoethyl)pyridinium Chloride see 4429
1-Hydrazinophthalazine see 4763
(±)-1-[(6-Hydrazino-3-pyridazinyl)-methylamino]-2-propanol see 7423

2-Hydrazino-*N*,*N*,*N*-trimethyl-2-oxo-ethanaminium Chloride *see* 4429
Hydrazodicarbonimide *see* 9866
Hydrazoic Acid, 4774
Hydrazonium Sulfate *see* 4772
Hydrea [BMS] *see* 4848
Hydrenox [Boots] *see* 4789
Hydridocarbonyltris(triphenylphos-phine)rhodium(I) *see* 9758
Hydridocobalamin *see* 10016
Hydril *see* 4781
Hydrindantin, 4775
Hydrindene *see* 4931
Hydriodic Acid, 4776
Hydro-Adreson [Organon] *see* 4787
Hydro-Aquil *see* 4781
Hydrobenzoin, 4777
Hydrobromic Acid, 4778
Hydrobromic Ether *see* 3771
Hydrocal [Bioglan] *see* 4787
Hydrocarbostyril, 4779
Hydrocerussite *see* 1005
Hydrochloric Acid, 4780
Hydrochloroauric Acid *see* 4522
Hydrochlorothiazide, 4781
Hydrocinchonidine, 4782
Hydrocinchonine, 4783
Hydrocinnamic Acid, 4784
Hydrocodin *see* 3171
Hydrocodone, 4785
Hydroconchinine *see* 4806
Hydrocort [Pharmagalen] *see* 4787
Hydrocortamate, 4786
Hydrocortisone, 4787
Δ¹-Hydrocortisone *see* 7721
Hydrocortisone 21-Diethylaminoacetate *see* 4786
Hydrocortisone Hemisuccinate Sodium Salt *see* 4787
Hydrocortisone Sodium Phosphate *see* 4787
Hydrocortisone Valerate *see* 4787
Hydrocortistab [Boots] *see* 4787
Hydrocortisyl [Aventis] *see* 4787
Hydrocortone [Merck & Co.] *see* 4787
Hydrocotarnine, 4788
Hydrocupreine *see* 2623
Hydrocyanic Acid *see* 4795
Hydrocyanite *see* 2653
HydroDiuril [Merck & Co.] *see* 4781
Hydroflumethiazide, 4789
Hydrofluoboric Acid *see* 4149
Hydrofluoric Acid, 4790
Hydrofluoric Acid Gas *see* 4796
Hydrofluoric Acid Homopolymer Compd with Pyridine *see* 6821
Hydrofluosilicic Acid *see* 4182
α-Hydroformamine Cyanide *see* 6057
Hydrofuramide, 4791
Hydrogen, 4792
Hydrogen Arsenide *see* 809
Hydrogen Azide *see* 4774
Hydrogen Bromide, 4793
Hydrogen Chloride, 4794
[Hydrogen Citrato(3−)]triaquoiron, Choline Salt *see* 4038
Hydrogen Cyanamide *see* 2684
Hydrogen Cyanate *see* 2686
Hydrogen Cyanide, 4795
Hydrogen Dioxide *see* 4798
Hydrogen Fluoride, 4796
(*T*-4)-Hydrogen (Glycinato-κ*N*,κ*O*) [Sulfato(2−)-κ*O*,κ*O*′-ferrate(1−) *see* 4039
Hydrogen Hexachloroplatinate(IV) *see* 7526

Hydrogen Hexafluorosilicate *see* 4182
Hydrogen Iodide, 4797
Hydrogen Oxide *see* 10039
Hydrogen Peroxide, 4798
Hydrogen Selenide, 4799
Hydrogen Sulfide, 4800
Hydrogen Telluride, 4801
(*SP*-4-1)-Hydrogen Tetrachloro-aurate(1−) *see* 4522
Hydrogen Tetrafluoroborate *see* 4149
Hydrogen Thiocyanate *see* 9328
Hydrogen Tribromide Compd with Pyridine (1:1) *see* 7973
Hydrogen Trioxooxalatomolybdate(VI) *see* 6913
Hydro-Giene [Water Science] *see* 2662
Hydrohydrastinine, 4802
α-Hydro-ω-hydroxypoly(oxy-1,2-ethane-diyl) *see* 7568
α-Hydro-ω-hydroxypoly(oxyethylene)-poly(oxypropylene)poly(oxyethylene) Block Copolymer *see* 7562
Hydrokon *see* 4785
Hydro-long [Sanorania] *see* 2193
Hydromedin [Merck & Co.] *see* 3717
Hydromorphone, 4803
Hydromox [Lederle] *see* 8056
Hydronitric Acid *see* 4774
Hydronol [Stuart] *see* 5224
Hydronsan *see* 4500
Hydroorotic Acid, 4804
Hydroperoxide *see* 4798
cis-4-Hydroperoxycyclophosphamide *see* 7161
5-Hydroperoxy-6,8,11,14-eicosatetra-enoic Acid *see* 4674
Hydroprene, 4805
Hydroquinidine, 4806
Hydroquinol *see* 4808
Hydroquinone, 4808
Hydroquinone Benzyl Ether *see* 6248
Hydroquinone Calcium Sulfonate *see* 3394
Hydroquinone-β-D-glucopyranoside *see* 773
Hydroquinone Glucose *see* 773
Hydroquinone Monobenzyl Ether *see* 6248
Hydro-rapid [Sanorania] *see* 4309
Hydroresorcinol *see* 3178
Hydroretrocortine *see* 7721
Hydrorhombinine *see* 5607
Hydrosaluric [Merck & Co.] *see* 4781
Hydrosarpan [Eutherapie] *see* 8119
Hydrosilicofluoric Acid *see* 4182
"Hydrosulfuric Acid" *see* 4800
Hydrotalcite *see* 5660
Hydrothide *see* 4781
Hydrotrichlorothiazide *see* 9624
Hydrotricine [RPR] *see* 9841
Hydrourushiol *see* 7110
Hydrous Lanolin *see* 5358
Hydroxamethocaine *see* 4846
Hydroxocobalamin, 4809
Hydroxocobemine *see* 4809
N-Hydroxyacetamide *see* 63
p-Hydroxyacetanilide *see* 47
4′-Hydroxyacetanilide *see* 47
Hydroxyacetic Acid *see* 4498
Hydroxyacetic Acid (3a*S*,4*R*,5*S*,6*S*,8*R*,-9*R*,9a*R*,10*R*)-6-Ethenyldecahydro-5-hydroxy-4,6,9,10-tetramethyl-1-oxo-3a,9-propano-3a*H*-cyclopentacyclo-octen-8-yl Ester *see* 7534

Hydroxyacetone *see* 65
p-Hydroxyacetophenone-D-glucoside *see* 7395
3-Hydroxy-21-acetoxy-5-pregnen-20-one *see* 77
4-Hydroxy-*N*-acetylproline *see* 6903
1-[[(3-Hydroxy-1-adamantyl)amino]-acetyl]-2-cyano-(*S*)-pyrrolidine *see* 9979
(2α,3β)-3-Hydroxy-A(1),28-dinorlup-20(29)-ene-2,17-dicarboxylic Acid *see* 1909
4-Hydroxyaflatoxin B₁ *see* 182
4-Hydroxyaflatoxin B₂ *see* 182
β-Hydroxyalanine *see* 8460
2-Hydroxy-6-alkylbenzoic Acids *see* 621
17-Hydroxy-17α-allyl-4-estrene *see* 291
l-3-Hydroxy-*N*-allylmorphinan *see* 5458
α-Hydroxy-δ-aminobutylidenediphos-phonic Acid *see* 229
γ-Hydroxy-β-aminobutyric Acid *see* 443
m-Hydroxy-α-(1-aminoethyl)benzyl Alcohol *see* 5932
5-Hydroxy-3-(β-aminoethyl)indole *see* 8462
[4-(*N*-Hydroxyamino)-2*R*-isobutyl-3*S*-(2-thienylthiomethyl)succinyl]-L-phenyl-alanine-*N*-methylamide *see* 1008
3-Hydroxy-5-aminomethylisoxazole *see* 6312
6-(*p*-Hydroxy-α-aminophenylacetamido)-penicillanic Acid *see* 577
Hydroxyamphetamine, 4810
p-Hydroxyampicillin *see* 577
(17β)-17-Hydroxyandrosta-1,4-dien-3-one *see* 1324
(3α,5α)-3-Hydroxyandrostan-17-one *see* 640
(3β,5α)-3-Hydroxyandrostan-17-one *see* 3609
3α-Hydroxy-17-androstanone *see* 640
3β-Hydroxy-17-androstanone *see* 3609
(5α,17β)-17-Hydroxyandrostan-3-one *see* 8793
17β-Hydroxy-3-androstanone *see* 8793
3α-Hydroxy-5α-androst-16-ene *see* 639
4-Hydroxyandrost-4-ene-3,17-dione *see* 4240
(3β)-3-Hydroxyandrost-5-en-17-one *see* 2871
(17β)-17-Hydroxyandrost-4-en-3-one *see* 9180
p-Hydroxyaniline *see* 462
2-Hydroxyaniline *see* 461
3-Hydroxyaniline *see* 460
p-Hydroxyanilinoacetic Acid *see* 4837
o-Hydroxyanisole *see* 4553
9-Hydroxyanthracene *see* 686
1-Hydroxy-2-anthraquinonyl 6-*O*-β-D-Xylopyranosyl-β-D-glucopyranoside *see* 8280
Hydroxyapatite *see* 3467
3-Hydroxy-8′-apo-β,ψ-carotenal *see* 2324
p-Hydroxybenzaldehyde, 4811
2-Hydroxybenzaldehyde *see* 8326
2-Hydroxybenzaldehyde Oxime *see* 8327
o-Hydroxybenzal Isonicotinylhydrazone *see* 8335
2-Hydroxybenzamide *see* 8328
N-Hydroxybenzenamine *see* 7294
Hydroxybenzene *see* 7241
α-Hydroxybenzeneacetic Acid *see* 5717
endo-(±)-α-Hydroxybenzeneacetic Acid 8-Methyl-8-azabicyclo[3.2.1]oct-3-yl Ester *see* 4730

4-Hydroxy-2-pentenoic Acid γ-Lactone *see* 647

4-Hydroxy-3-pentenoic Acid γ-Lactone *see* 647

Hydroxypethidine, 4836

α-Hydroxyphenazine *see* 4645

β-Hydroxyphenethylamine *see* 7287

4-Hydroxyphenethylamine *see* 9835

2-(β-Hydroxyphenethylamino)pyridine *see* 7321

2'-Hydroxy-2-(*N*,β-phenethyl)-5,9-dimethyl-6,7-benzomorphan *see* 7218

2-[6-(β-Hydroxyphenethyl)-1-methyl-2-piperidyl]acetophenone *see* 5551

6-(*p*-Hydroxyphenethyl)salicylic Acid *see* 5606

7-Hydroxy-3*H*-phenoxazin-3-one 10-Oxide *see* 8141

3-[4-(*p*-Hydroxyphenoxy)-3,5-diiodophenyl]alanine *see* 3191

1-Hydroxy-2-phenoxyethane *see* 7257

(−)-(*S*)-1-(*p*-Hydroxyphenoxy)-3-(isopropylamino)-2-propanol *see* 7735

1-(4-Hydroxyphenoxy)-3-[2-(4-morpholinocarboxamido)ethylamino]-2-propanol *see* 10055

N-(4-Hydroxyphenyl)acetamide *see* 47

α-Hydroxyphenylacetic Acid *see* 5717

α-Hydroxy-α-phenylacetophenone *see* 1093

2-Hydroxy-2-phenylacetophenone Oxime *see* 1094

(6*R*,7*R*)-7-[[(2*R*)-Hydroxyphenylacetyl]-amino]-3-[[(1-methyl-1*H*-tetrazol-5-yl)thio]methyl]-8-oxo-5-thia-1-azabicyclo[4.2.0]oct-2-ene-2-carboxylic Acid *see* 1914

(6*R*,7*R*)-7-[[(2*R*)-Hydroxyphenylacetyl]-amino]-8-oxo-3-[[[1-(sulfomethyl)-1*H*-tetrazol-5-yl]thio]methyl]-5-thia-1-azabicyclo[4.2.0]oct-2-ene-2-carboxylic Acid *see* 1929

β-[4-Hydroxyphenyl]acrylic Acid *see* 2560

β-(*p*-Hydroxyphenyl)alanine *see* 9839

3-Hydroxy-L-phenylalanine *see* 9840

p-Hydroxyphenylaminoacetic Acid *see* 4837

α-(4-Hydroxyphenyl)-β-aminoethane *see* 9835

1-(*m*-Hydroxyphenyl)-2-aminoethanol *see* 6699

1-(*p*-Hydroxyphenyl)-2-aminoethanol *see* 6759

α-(*m*-Hydroxyphenyl)-β-aminopropanol *see* 5932

1-(*m*-Hydroxyphenyl)-2-amino-1-propanol *see* 5932

4-Hydroxy-5-[[4-(phenylamino)-5-sulfo-1-naphthalenyl]azo]-2,7-naphthalene-disulfonic Acid Trisodium Salt *see* 628

2-Hydroxy-*N*-phenylbenzamide *see* 8330

α-Hydroxy-α-phenylbenzeneacetic Acid *see* 1080

α-Hydroxy-α-phenylbenzeneacetic Acid 2-(Diethylamino)ethyl Ester *see* 1029

α-Hydroxy-α-phenylbenzeneacetic Acid 2-(Dimethylamino)-2-methylpropyl Ester *see* 3132

endo-α-Hydroxy-α-phenylbenzeneacetic Acid 8-Methyl-8-azabicyclo[3.2.1]oct-3-yl Ester *see* 9782

α-Hydroxy-α-phenylbenzeneacetic Acid 2-(1-Piperidinyl)ethyl Ester *see* 7471

p-Hydroxyphenyl Benzyl Ether *see* 6248

N-(4-Hydroxyphenyl)butanamide *see* 4814

4-(*p*-Hydroxyphenyl)-2-butanone Acetate *see* 2616

p-Hydroxyphenylbutazone *see* 6972

4-Hydroxy-α¹-[[[6-(4-phenylbutoxy)hexyl]amino]methyl]-1,3-benzenedimethanol *see* 8337

(±)-4-Hydroxy-α¹-[[[6-(4-phenylbutoxy)-hexyl]amino]methyl]-*m*-xylene-α,α¹-diol *see* 8337

1-(*p*-Hydroxyphenyl)-2-butylaminoethanol *see* 954

3-Hydroxy-4-phenylcarbostyril *see* 10005

3-Hydroxy-2-phenylcinchoninic Acid *see* 6957

1-Hydroxy-α-phenylcyclopentaneacetic Acid 2-Diethylaminoethyl Ester *see* 2719

1-Hydroxy-α-phenylcyclopentaneacetic Acid 2-(Dimethylamino)ethyl Ester *see* 2746

2-(*p*-Hydroxyphenyl)-5,7-dihydroxychromone *see* 730

O-(4-Hydroxyphenyl)-3,5-diiodotyrosine *see* 3191

4-[4-(4-Hydroxyphenyl)-2,3-diisocyano-1,3-butadienyl]-1,2-benzenediol *see* 10061

(−)-(*R*)-1-(4-Hydroxyphenyl)-2-(3,4-dimethoxyphenethylamino)ethanol *see* 2894

(3-Hydroxyphenyl)dimethylethylammonium Chloride *see* 3516

[[2(*S*)-[[4(*R*)-(3-Hydroxyphenyl)-3(*R*),4-dimethyl-1-piperidinyl]methyl]-1-oxo-3-phenylpropyl]amino]acetic Acid *see* 372

N-[(2*S*)-2-[[(3*R*,4*R*)-4-(3-Hydroxyphenyl)-3,4-dimethyl-1-piperidinyl]methyl]-1-oxo-3-phenylpropyl]glycine *see* 372

m-Hydroxyphenylethanolamine *see* 6699

p-Hydroxyphenylethanolamine *see* 6759

5-[(1*E*)-2-(4-Hydroxyphenyl)ethenyl]-1,3-benzenediol *see* 8158

2-*p*-Hydroxyphenylethylamine *see* 9835

α-(*m*-Hydroxyphenyl)-β-(ethylamino)-ethanol *see* 3865

N-(*p*-Hydroxyphenylethyl)-4-hydroxynorephedrine *see* 8237

N-[2-(*p*-Hydroxyphenyl)ethyl]-*N*-[2-(*p*-hydroxyphenyl)-2-hydroxy-1-methylethyl]amine *see* 8237

2-[(2*R*,6*S*)-6-[(2*S*)-2-Hydroxy-2-phenyl-ethyl]-1-methyl-2-piperidinyl]-1-phenylethanone *see* 5551

3-Hydroxy-*N*-(2-phenylethyl)morphinan *see* 7249

4-Hydroxyphenyl-β-D-glucopyranoside *see* 773

N-(4-Hydroxyphenyl)glycine, 4837

1-(4-Hydroxyphenyl)-1-hydroxy-2-butylaminoethane *see* 954

1-(*p*-Hydroxyphenyl)-2-[β-hydroxy-β-(3',5'-dihydroxyphenyl)]ethyl]amino-propane *see* 3981

N-[2-(4-Hydroxyphenyl)-2-hydroxyethyl]-1-methyl-3-(4-hydroxyphenyl)propylamine *see* 8092

1-(4-Hydroxyphenyl)-2-[2-(4-hydroxyphenyl)ethylamino]propanol *see* 8237

p-Hydroxyphenylisopropylamine *see* 4810

β-(*p*-Hydroxyphenyl)isopropylmethylamine *see* 7330

Hydroxyphenylmercury Mixt with (Nitrato-*O*)phenylmercury *see* 7302

1-Hydroxy-1-phenyl-2-methylaminoethane *see* 4601

l-1-(*m*-Hydroxyphenyl)-2-methylaminoethanol *see* 7286

1-(4-Hydroxyphenyl)-2-methylaminoethanol *see* 9012

α-(*p*-Hydroxyphenyl)-β-methylaminopropane *see* 7330

1-(4-Hydroxyphenyl)-2-methylaminopropanol *see* 4824

[(2-Hydroxyphenyl)methylene]hydrazide 4-Pyridinecarboxylic Acid *see* 8335

1-(4-Hydroxyphenyl)-2-[1-methyl-3-(4-hydroxyphenyl)-propylamino]ethanol *see* 8092

4-(*m*-Hydroxyphenyl)-1-methylisonipecotic Acid Ethyl Ester *see* 4836

1-(*p*-Hydroxyphenyl)-2-(1-methyl-2-phenoxyethylamino)-1-propanol *see* 5238

α-(4-Hydroxyphenyl)-β-methyl-4-(phenylmethyl)-1-piperidineethanol *see* 4895

1-(*p*-Hydroxyphenyl)-2-(1'-methyl-3'-phenylpropylamino)-1-propanol *see* 6732

4-(3-Hydroxyphenyl)-1-methyl-4-piperidinecarboxylic Acid Ethyl Ester *see* 4836

4-(*m*-Hydroxyphenyl)-1-methyl-4-piperidyl Ethyl Ketone *see* 5301

1-[4-(3-Hydroxyphenyl)-1-methyl-4-piperidyl]-1-propanone *see* 5301

4-[2-[[3-(4-Hydroxyphenyl)-1-methylpropyl]amino]ethyl]-1,2-benzenediol *see* 3395

(±)-4-[2-[[3-(*p*-Hydroxyphenyl)-1-methylpropyl]amino]ethyl]pyrocatechol *see* 3395

3-(4-Hydroxyphenyl)-1-methylpropyl β-D-Glucopyranoside *see* 8189

N-Hydroxy-*N*'-phenyloctanediamide *see* 10034

α-(*p*-Hydroxyphenyl)-α-(4-oxo-2,5-cyclohexadien-1-ylidine)-*o*-toluic Acid *see* 7243

3α-Hydroxy-8-(*p*-phenylphenacyl)-1α*H*,-5α*H*-tropanium Bromide (−)-Tropate *see* 4006

1-(*p*-Hydroxyphenyl)-2-phenyl-4-butyl-pyrazolidine-3,5-dione *see* 6972

β-(*p*-Hydroxyphenyl)phloropropiophenone *see* 7326

m-Hydroxyphenylpropanolamine *see* 5932

1-(4-Hydroxyphenyl)-1-propanone *see* 7044

3-(4-Hydroxyphenyl)-2-propenoic Acid *see* 2560

α-Hydroxy-α-phenylpropionic Acid *see* 873

2-Hydroxy-2-phenylpropionic Acid *see* 873

dl-1-*p*-Hydroxyphenyl-2-propylamine *see* 4810

L-(1-Hydroxy-1-phenyl-2-propylamino)-1-(*m*-methoxyphenyl)-1-propanone *see* 6962

4-Hydroxy-3-(1-phenylpropyl)-2*H*-1-benzopyran-2-one *see* 7259

γ-(*p*-Hydroxyphenyl)-α-propylene *see* 2050

(3β)-3-Hydroxyurs-12-ene-27,28-dioic
  Acid see 8075
(3β)-3-Hydroxyurs-12-en-28-oic Acid see
  9890
(3α,4β)-3-Hydroxyurs-12-en-23-oic
  Acid see 1355
17-Hydroxy-17α-vinyl-4-estren-3-one see
  6717
17β-Hydroxy-17α-vinylestr-5(10)-en-3-
  one see 6702
1α-Hydroxyvitamin D₂ see 3436
1α-Hydroxyvitamin D₃ see 4819
1β-Hydroxyvitamin D₃ see 4819
25-Hydroxyvitamin D₃ see 1638
8-Hydroxyxanthine see 9875
1-Hydroxy-2-[(6-O-β-D-xylopyranosyl-β-
  D-glucopyranosyl)oxy]-9,10-anthra-
  cenedione see 8280
(3β,16α,17α)-17-Hydroxyyohimban-16-
  carboxylic Acid Methyl Ester see
  7922
(16α,17α)-17-Hydroxyyohimban-16-
  carboxylic Acid Methyl Ester see
  10102
(16β,17α)-17-Hydroxyyohimban-16-
  carboxylic Acid Methyl Ester see
  2548
17-Hydroxyyohimban-16-carboxylic
  Acid Methyl Ester see 10103
17α-Hydroxy-20α-yohimban-16β-carbox-
  ylic Acid Methyl Ester see 10104
Hydroxyzine, 4849
Hydrozide [Merial] see 4781
Hydrozincite see 10131
Hygric Acid Methylbetaine see 8771
Hygrine, 4850
Hygromix [Elanco] see 4852
Hygromycin, 4851
Hygromycin A see 4851
Hygromycin B, 4852
Hygrophylline, 4853
Hygroton [Novartis] see 2193
Hykinone [Abbott] see 5831
Hylorel [Aventis] see 4559
Hymecromone, 4854
Hymecromone O,O-Diethyl Phosphoro-
  thioate, 4855
Hymexazol, 4856
Hymorphan [Endo] see 4803
Hyndarin see 9215
Hyodeoxycholic Acid, 4857
α-Hyodeoxycholic Acid see 4857
Hyodesoxycholic Acid see 4857
Hyonate [Bayer] see 4757
Hyoper [Bordet] see 1792
Hyoscine see 8406
Hyoscine-N-butyl Bromide see 1588
Hyoscine Methyl Bromide see 6003
Hyoscyamine, 4858
dl-Hyoscyamine see 875
l-Hyoscyamine see 4858
Hyoscyamus, 4859
Hyp see 4840
Hypadil [Kowa] see 6562
Hypalon [DuPont], 4860
Hypaphorine, 4861
Hypaque Cysto [Winthrop] see 5807
Hypaque Meglumine [Winthrop] see 5807
Hypaque Sodium [Winthrop] see 2992
Hyperan [SS Pharm.] see 3909
Hyperdrol [Britcair] see 343
Hyperforin, 4862
Hyperglycemic-Glycogenolytic Factor
  see 4446
Hyperici Herba see 4864

Hypericin, 4863
Hypericum, 4864
Hypericum Red see 4863
Hyperin see 8034
Hyperium [Biopharma] see 8222
Hyperol [Gedeon Richter] see 1782
Hyperoside see 8034
Hypersin [Zeria] see 1186
Hyperstat [Schering] see 3004
Hypertensin see 651
Hypertensin [Novartis] see 651
Hypertensinogen see 651
Hypertonalum [Essex] see 3004
Hy-Phos see 8667
Hyphylline see 3479
Hypnodil [Janssen] see 6148
Hypnodin [Takeda] see 7179
Hypnomidate [Janssen] see 3881
Hypnone see 73
Hypnorex [Sanofi-Synthelabo] see 5527
Hypnovel [Roche] see 6182
"Hypo" see 8694
Hypoca [Yamanouchi] see 1002
Hypochlorous Acid, 4865
Hypochlorous Acid 1,1-Dimethylethyl
  Ester see 1571
Hypochlorous Anhydride see 2099
Hypochylin [Recip] see 4469
Hypocretin-1 see 6866
Hypocretin-2 see 6866
Hypocretins see 6866
Hypocrine [Tanabe Seiyaku] see 5474
Hypoglycin see 4866
Hypoglycin A see 4866
Hypoglycine A, 4866
Hypoglycine B see 4866
Hyponitric Acid Disodium Salt see 648
Hyponitrous Acid Anhydride see 6653
β-Hypophamine see 9938
Hypophosphoric Acid, 4867
Hypophosphorous Acid, 4868
Hypophyseal Growth Hormone see 8716
Hypostamine [Promedica] see 9765
Hypostat [Herbrand] see 7044
Hyposulfite of Gold and Sodium see 4519
Hypothiazide see 4781
Hypovase [Pfizer] see 7717
Hypoxanthine, 4869
Hypoxanthine Riboside see 4975
Hypoxanthine Riboside-5-phosphoric
  Acid see 4977
Hypoxanthosine see 4975
Hyprenan [Astra] see 7735
Hypromellose see 4842
Hypurin [CP Pharm.] see 4980
Hypusine, 4870
Hyrazin [Kowa] see 9301
Hyryl see 8201
Hyskon [Pharmacia] see 2948
Hysron [Kyowa] see 5793
Hytakerol [Winthrop] see 3180
Hytone [Dermik] see 4787
Hytracin [Dainabot-Dainippon] see 9154
Hytrin [Abbott] see 9154
Hytrinex [Abbott] see 9154
Hytrol O see 2726
Hyvar [DuPont] see 1381
Hyzaar [DuPont] see 5583
HZ see 4649
I-612 see 8255
I-653 see 2919
I-2586 see 8914
IAA see 4964
IACFT, 4871
Ial [Fidia] see 4757

IAPP see 609
IB-367 see 5105
IB-367-03 see 5105
Ibafloxacin, 4872
Ibandronate Sodium see 4873
Ibandronic Acid, 4873
IBC see 5140
IBCA see 5140
Ibenzmethyzin see 7758
Iberiotoxin, 4874
Ibiamox [IBI] see 577
IBI-C83 see 8260
Ibidomide see 5329
Ibifur see 4294
Ibilex [IBI] see 1974
Ibistacin [IBI] see 8206
Ibition [IBI] see 9321
Ibogaine, 4875
Ibopamine, 4876
Ibotenic Acid, 4877
Ibritumomab Tiuxetan, 4878
IbTX see 4874
Ibudilast, 4879
Ibudros [Manetti Roberts] see 4882
Ibufenac, 4880
Ibumetin [Nycomed] see 4881
Ibunac [Kaken] see 4880
Ibuprofen, 4881
Ibuproxam, 4882
Ibustrin [Pharmacia] see 4961
Ibutilide, 4883
Ibutop [Dolorgiet] see 4881
IBX see 5048
Ibylcaine see 1523
IC-351 see 9027
IC-851589 see 4232
Icacine [BMS] see 3005
ICAD see 1885
Icaridin see 7394
Icariin see 3617
Icavex [Viatris] see 6292
"Ice" see 5948
Ice see 6018
ICE see 1884
Ice-B-Gon [Chevron] see 1680
Iceland Moss, 4884
ICE-LAP6 see 1887
Ice Spar see 2606
Ichden see 4885
Ichtammon see 4885
Ichthadone see 4885
Ichthalum see 4885
Ichthammol, 4885
Ichthammonium see 4885
Ichthium see 4885
Ichthosan see 4885
Ichthosauran see 4885
Ichthosulfol see 4885
Ichthymall [Mallinckrodt] see 4885
Ichthynat [Tenneco] see 4885
Ichthyocolla see 5109
Ichthyol [Stiefel] see 4885
Ichthyopon see 4885
Ichthysalle see 4885
Ichtopur [Ichthyol] see 4885
ICI-32865 see 3880
ICI-33828 see 5946
ICI-35868 see 7834
ICI-38174 see 7790
ICI-45520 see 7840
ICI-45763 see 9516
ICI-46474 see 9048
ICI-47699 see 9048
ICI-48213 see 2720
ICI-50123 see 7113

ICI-50172 *see* 7700
ICI-54450 *see* 3969
ICI-55052 *see* 6472
ICI-58834 *see* 9980
ICI-59118 *see* 8123
ICI-66082 *see* 859
ICI-69653 *see* 727
ICI-72222 *see* 2018
ICI-80008 *see* 4194
ICI-80996 *see* 2399
ICI-81008 *see* 4194
ICI-118587 *see* 10055
ICI-118630 *see* 4526
ICI-122378 *see* 736
ICI-139603 *see* 9248
ICI-156834 *see* 1934
ICI-176334 *see* 1200
ICI-182780 *see* 4284
ICI-194660 *see* 5900
ICI-204219 *see* 10108
ICI-204636 *see* 8039
ICI-A-0051 *see* 8894
ICI-A-192 *see* 4117
ICI-A-0224 *see* 4512
ICI-A-0523 *see* 4681
ICI-A-5504 *see* 924
ICI-D-1033 *see* 625
ICI-D-1694 *see* 8099
ICI-PP-333 *see* 6984
ICL-670 *see* 2858
ICL-670A *see* 2858
ICN-1229 *see* 8198
Iconyl *see* 4837
Icosapent *see* 3531
ICRF-159 *see* 8123
ICRF-187 *see* 8123
ICS-205-930 *see* 9783
ICSH *see* 5613
Ictéryl *see* 5834
ID-540 *see* 4128
ID-1937 *see* 4213
IDA *see* 4917
Idaein *see* 2687
Idalon [HMR] *see* 4103
Idamycin [Pharmacia & Upjohn] *see* 4886
Idarac [HMR] *see* 4103
Idarubicin, 4886
Idazoxan, 4887
Idebenone, 4888
IDEC-C2B8 *see* 8239
IDEC-Y2B8 *see* 4878
Idein *see* 2687
Idexur *see* 4891
Idocyl [Ferrosan] *see* 8332
Idomethine [Kowa] *see* 4968
Idonor [Roger] *see* 7516
Idonyx *see* 5037
Idorese *see* 2076
Idose, 4889
Idoxene [Spodefell] *see* 4891
Idoxifene, 4890
Idoxuridine, 4891
Idraparinux Sodium, 4892
Idro P$_2$ [Maggioni] *see* 8984
Idro P$_3$ [Maggioni] *see* 6915
Idrocilamide, 4893
Idrolax [Schwarz] *see* 7568
Idrolone [Maggioni] *see* 3997
IdU *see* 4891
IDUA *see* 4894
Idulea *see* 4891
Idulian [Schering] *see* 901
IdUR *see* 4891
IdUrd *see* 4891
Iduridin [Ferring] *see* 4891

L-Iduronic Acid *see* 4465
α-L-Iduronidase, 4894
α-L-Iduronide Iduronohydrolase *see* 4894
IF *see* 1897
Ifenec [Italfarmaco] *see* 3502
Ifenprodil, 4895
Ifex [BMS] *see* 4896
IFN *see* 4989
IFN-α *see* 4990
IFN-α$_2$ *see* 4990
IFN-αA *see* 4990
IFN-β *see* 4991
IFN-β$_1$ *see* 4991
IFN-β$_2$ *see* 4998
IFN-γ *see* 4992
IFN-beta$_{ser}$ *see* 4991
Ifomide [Shionogi] *see* 4896
Ifosfamide, 4896
IFP *see* 4484
^{123}I-FP-CIT *see* 5050
Ifrasarl [Showa Shinyaku] *see* 2773
Igepal CA [Rhone-Poulenc] *see* 6761
Igepal CA-630 [Rhone-Poulenc] *see* 6761
Igepal CO [Rhone-Poulenc] *see* 6677
Igepal CO-630 [Rhone-Poulenc] *see* 6677
IGF-I *see* 4986
IGF-II *see* 4986
IGF Binding Proteins *see* 4986
IGFBP *see* 4986
IGFs *see* 4986
Ignatia, 4897
Ignatius Bean *see* 4897
Ignotine *see* 1850
Igralin [Zeria] *see* 9301
^{131}I HSA *see* 8468
[^{123}I](±)-N-Isopropyl-*p*-iodoamphetamine *see* 5049
Ikaran [Fabre] *see* 3174
IKF-916 *see* 2700
IKF-1216 *see* 4117
IKI-220 *see* 4105
IKI-1145 *see* 4260
Ikorel [RPR] *see* 6521
Iktorivil [Roche] *see* 2389
IL-1 *see* 4993
IL-1β *see* 1884
IL-1β Converting Enzyme *see* 1884
IL-1ra *see* 5001
IL-2 *see* 4994
IL-3 *see* 4995
IL-4 *see* 4996
IL-4R *see* 5002
IL-5 *see* 4997
IL-6 *see* 4998
IL-10 *see* 4999
IL-11 *see* 5000
IL-13PE38 *see* 2312
IL-18 *see* 1884
IL-17803A *see* 19
^{123}I Labeled IMP *see* 5049
Ildamen [Viatris] *see* 6962
Ile *see* 5179
α-Ile *see* 5179
Ileogastrone *see* 3597
Iletin II [Lilly] *see* 4980
Iliadin [Meda] *see* 6966
Ilimaquinone, 4898
Iliren [Provet] *see* 9423
Ilixathin *see* 8304
Illcut [Nippon Zoki] *see* 9502
Illoxan [Bayer CropSci.] *see* 3082
Illudin M *see* 4899
Illudins, 4899
Illudin S *see* 4899

Ilmenite *see* 9472
ILO-522 *see* 4900
Ilodecakin *see* 4999
Ilomedin [Schering AG] *see* 4901
Ilopan [Warren-Teed] *see* 2947
Iloperidone, 4900
Iloprost, 4901
Ilosone [Lilly] *see* 3683
Ilotycin [Lilly] *see* 3681
Ilotycin Gluceptate [Lilly] *see* 3684
Ilvin [Merck KGaA] *see* 1443
^{123}I-M123 *see* 5049
Imadyl [Roche] *see* 1862
Imagent [Alliance] *see* 7156
Imagopaque [GE Healthcare] *see* 5059
Imagotan [Sandoz] *see* 8963
Imakol [Rhône-Poulenc] *see* 6946
Imap [McNeil] *see* 4207
Imatinib, 4902
Imaverol [Janssen] *see* 3583
Imavist [Schering AG] *see* 7157
Imazalil *see* 3583
Imazamethabenz, 4903
Imazamethabenz Methyl *see* 4903
Imazamox, 4904
Imazapyr, 4905
Imazaquin, 4906
Imazethabenz *see* 4903
Imazethapyr, 4907
Imazosulfuron, 4908
Imbun [Merckle] *see* 4881, 6972
[(Im-Bzl)-D-His^6,Pro^9-NEt]-gonadotropin-releasing Hormone *see* 4722
IMC-C225 *see* 2027
Imdur [Key] *see* 5225
Imecromone *see* 4854
Imeron [Bracco] *see* 5054
Imeson [Taurus] *see* 6575
IMET-3393 *see* 1034
Imex [Merz] *see* 9196
Imexim [Cimex] *see* 8918
Imferon [Fisons] *see* 5094
IMI-28 *see* 3623
IMI-30 *see* 4886
Imibenconazole, 4909
Imidacloprid, 4910
Imidamine *see* 680
Imidan [Stauffer] *see* 7336
Imidapril, 4911
Imidaprilat *see* 4911
Imidazole, 4912
1*H*-Imidazole-1-carbonitrile *see* 2696
2,4-(3*H*,5*H*)-Imidazoledione *see* 4760
1*H*-Imidazole-4-ethanamine *see* 4719
4-Imidazoleethylamine *see* 4719
5-Imidazoleethylamine *see* 4719
Imidazole Salicylate, 4913
Imidazoletrione *see* 7022
2,4-Imidazolidinedione *see* 4760
2-Imidazolidinethione *see* 3803
Imidazolidinetrione *see* 7022
2-Imidazolidinone, 4914
D-α-[(Imidazolidin-2-on-1-yl)carbonylamino]benzylpenicillin *see* 916
Imidazolidinyl Urea *see* 4916
2-Imidazolidone, 4914
Imidazoline-2-thiol *see* 3803
1-(2-Δ^2-Imidazolinyl)-2,2-diphenylcyclopropane *see* 2269
N-(2-Imidazolin-2-yl)-N-(4-indanyl)-amine *see* 4932
β-(4-Imidazolyl)acrylcholine *see* 6307
3-(Imidazol-1-yl)-7-chlorobenzo-1,2,4-triazine-1-oxide *see* 9607
α-Imidazol-4-yl-2,3-cresotamide *see* 6220

Indinavir, 4945
Indiplon, 4946
Indium, 4947
Indium Antimonide, 4948
Indium Arsenide, 4949
Indium Bromide (InBr₃) see 4957
Indium Chloride see 4958
Indium Fluoride see 4959
Indium Gallium Aluminum Phosphide, 4950
Indium ¹¹¹In Satumomab Pendetide see 8385
Indium Mononitride see 4951
Indium Nitride, 4951
Indium Oxide, 4952
Indium Phosphide, 4953
Indium Selenide, 4954
Indium Sesquioxide see 4952
Indium Sulfate, 4955
Indium Telluride, 4956
Indium Tribromide, 4957
Indium Trichloride, 4958
Indium Trifluoride, 4959
Indo-1, 4960
Indobufen, 4961
Indocid [Merck & Co.] see 4968
Indocid PDA [Merck & Co.] see 4968
Indocin [Merck & Co.] see 4968
Indocin I.V. [Merck & Co.] see 4968
Indocyanine Green, 4962
Indocybin [Sandoz] see 7926
Indoklon [Ohio Med.] see 4201
Indole, 4963
Indoleacetic Acid, 4964
1*H*-Indole-3-acetic Acid see 4964
1*H*-Indole-3-butanoic Acid see 4965
Indolebutyric Acid, 4965
Indole-3-butyric Acid see 4965
1*H*-Indole-3-carboxylic Acid (3-*endo*)-8-Methyl-8-azabicyclo[3.2.1]oct-3-yl Ester see 9783
1*H*-Indole-3-carboxylic Acid (2α,6α,8α,-9αβ)-Octahydro-3-oxo-2,6-methano-2*H*-quinolizin-8-yl Ester see 3411
Indole-2,3-dione see 5104
1*H*-Indole-3-ethanamine see 9796
3-Indoleethanol see 9798
2,3-Indolinedione see 5104
Indolmycin, 4966
1*H*-Indol-3-ol Hydrogen Sulfate Ester see 4941
3-Indolylacetone, 4967
l-β-3-Indolylalanine see 9797
4-(3-Indolyl)butyric Acid see 4965
2-Indolyl(3)-ethanol see 9798
β-Indolylethyl Alcohol see 9798
2-(3-Indolyl)ethyl Alcohol see 9798
2-(3-Indolyl)ethylamine see 9796
(1*R*,5*S*)-5-(1-Indol-3-ylethyl)-2-(methyl-amino)-2-oxazolin-4-one see 4966
(5*S*)-5-[(1*R*)-1-(1*H*-Indol-3-yl)ethyl]-2-(methylamino)-4(5*H*)-oxazolone see 4966
4-[2-(3-Indolyl)ethyl]piperidine see 4930
N-[1-[2-(1*H*-Indol-3-yl)ethyl]-4-piperidi-nyl]benzamide see 4969
1*H*-Indol-3-yl-β-D-glucopyranoside see 4942
2-*C*-(1*H*-Indol-3-ylmethyl)-β-L-*lyxo*-3-hexulofuranosonic Acid γ-Lactone Mixt with 2-*C*-(1*H*-Indol-3-ylmethyl)-β-L-*xylo*-3-hexulofuranosonic Acid γ-Lactone see 831
1-(1*H*-Indol-4-yloxy)-3-[(1-methylethyl)-amino]-2-propanol see 7443

Indol-3-yl Potassium Sulfate see 4941
Indol-3-yl-2-propanone see 4967
Indol-3-yl Sulfate see 4941
Indomed [Merck & Co.] see 4968
Indomee [Merck & Co.] see 4968
Indometacin see 4968
Indomethacin, 4968
Indomethacin Glucosamide see 4448
Indomod [Pfizer] see 4968
Indon [Parke-Davis] see 7234
Indonaphthene see 4939
Indoptic [Merck & Co.] see 4968
Indoptol [Merck & Co.] see 4968
Indoramin, 4969
Indorm [Wyeth] see 7822
Indospicine, 4970
Indoxacarb, 4971
Indoxamic Acid see 6916
Indoxen [Sigma-Tau] see 4968
Indoxyl-β-D-glucoside see 4942
3-Indoxylsulfuric Acid see 4941
[¹¹¹In-DTPA-D-Phe¹]-octreotide see 7126
Indusil [Diamant; Recordati] see 2451
INF see 4308
INF-1837 see 4132
INF-3355 see 5798
INF-4668 see 5779
Infacol [Pharmax] see 3215
Infasurf [Forest] see 1714
INFeD [Watson] see 5094
Infergen [Amgen] see 4990
Inflamase [Novartis] see 7721
Inflamen [Hokuriku] see 1388
Inflanefran [Allergan] see 7721
Inflatine see 5551
Inflazon [Taisho] see 4968
Infliximab, 4972
Informational RNA see 8203
Infron [Whittier] see 10018
Infusorial Earth, 4973
InGaAlP see 4950
INH see 5186
INH-G see 4500
Inhibace [Roche] see 2273
Inhibins, 4974
Inhibitor of CAD see 1885
Inhibostamin [Zyma] see 9765
Inhiston [Biomed. Foscama] see 7235
Inicardio see 6543
Inimur [ICN] see 6532
Iniprol [Sanofi Winthrop] see 757
Initiss see 2273
INN-00835 see 6445
Innohep [Leo Pharm] see 9450
Innovace [Merck & Co.] see 3567
Innovar see 3450
Innoxalon [Sanko] see 6359
Innozide [Merck & Co.] see 3567
Inocor [Sanofi Winthrop] see 592
Inofal see 8963
Inokiten [Nippon Yakuhin] see 9843
Inolin [Tanabe Seiyaku] see 9587
Inopamil [Simes] see 4876
Inorganic Benzene see 1334
Inosie [Morishita] see 4975
Inosine, 4975
Inosine:dimethylaminoisopropanol Acet-amidobenzoate (1:3) see 4976
Inosine Mono[4-(acetylamino)benzoate] (Salt) Compd with 1-(Dimethylamino)-2-propanol (1:3) see 4976
Inosine Pranobex, 4976
Inosinic Acid, 4977
5-Inosinic Acid see 4977
5′-Inosinic Acid see 4977

5′-Inosinic Acid Homopolymer Complex with 5′-Cytidylic Acid Polymer with 5′-Uridylic Acid (1:1) see 588
Inosiplex see 4976
Inosite see 4978
Inositol, 4978
i-Inositol see 4978
meso-Inositol see 4978
myo-Inositol see 4978
myo-Inositol Hexakis(dihydrogen Phosphate) see 7387
Inositol Hexanicotinate see 4979
meso-Inositol Hexanicotinate see 4979
Inositolhexaphosphoric Acid see 7387
myo-Inositol Hexa-3-pyridinecarboxylate see 4979
Inositol Niacinate, 4979
Inotrex (obsolete) [Lilly] see 3395
Inotropin [Bago] see 3421
Inovan [Kyowa] see 3421
Inovelon [Eisai] see 8293
Inoxyl [Debat] see 6945
INPC see 7816
INPEA see 6530
Inpea [Selvi] see 6530
¹¹¹In Pentetreotide see 7126
INS-365 see 3351
INS-37217 see 2896
Insane Root see 4859
Insariotoxin see 9801
Insecticide 1179 see 5982
Insecticide No. 497 see 3103
Insecticide No. 4049 see 5700
Insect Repellent 3535 see 3773
Insegar [Syngenta] see 3987
Insibrin [Byk-Liprandi] see 3653
Insidon [Novartis] see 6853
Insoluble Anhydrite see 1706
Insoluble Cyanuric Acid see 2682
Insoluble Prussian Blue see 7910
Insoral [Spofa] see 7231
Inspra [Pfizer] see 3625
Instalac [Virbac] see 9709
Insubeta see 5006
Insulamin [Iwaki] see 1476
Insulin, 4980
Insulinase, 4981
Insulin Aspart, 4982
Insulin Detemir, 4983
Insulin (emp) see 4980
Insulin Glargine, 4984
Insulin Glulisine, 4985
Insulin ¹³¹I see 4980
Insulin-like Growth Factor I see 4986
Insulin-like Growth Factor II see 4986
Insulin-like Growth Factors, 4986
Insulin Lispro, 4987
Insulinoma Amyloid Peptide see 609
Insulin (prb) see 4980
Insulton see 5853
Insumin [Kyorin] see 4198
Insuven [Berenguer] see 3297
In-Synch [ProLabs] see 7878
Intal [Sanofi-Aventis] see 2590
Inteban [Sumitomo] see 4968
Integerrimine see 8451
Integrilin [COR] see 3641
Integrin (formerly) [Sterling] see 6971
Integrins, 4988
Intenkordin [Polfa] see 2239
Intensain [HMR] see 2239
Intensopan [Sandoz] see 1453
Intercept [Ortho] see 6677
Interceptor [Novartis] see 6190
Intercron [Zambon] see 2590

Interferon, 4989
Interferon-α, 4990
Interferon α2 (Human Clone pAD19B-IFN Protein Moiety Reduced) see 4990
Interferon α2 (Human Leukocyte Clone Hif-SN206 Protein Moiety Reduced) see 4990
Interferon α2 (Human Leukocyte Clone pM21 Protein Moiety Reduced) see 4990
Interferon-β, 4991
Interferon-β₂ see 4998
Interferon-γ, 4992
Interferon Alfa-2a see 4990
Interferon Alfa-2b see 4990
Interferon Alfa-2c see 4990
Interferon Alfacon-1 see 4990
Interferon Alfa-n1 see 4990
Interferon Alfa-n3 see 4990
Interferon Beta-1a see 4991
Interferon Beta-1b see 4991
Interferon Beta (Human) see 4991
Interferon Gamma-1a see 4992
Interferon Gamma-1b see 4992
Interferon Gamma-2a see 4992
Interferon-γ-inducing Factor see 1884
Intergravin-orales [Werfft-Chemie] see 1659
Interleukin-1, 4993
Interleukin-1β see 1884
Interleukin-2, 4994
Interleukin-3, 4995
Interleukin-4, 4996
Interleukin-5, 4997
Interleukin-6, 4998
Interleukin-10, 4999
Interleukin-10 (Human Clone pH15C) see 4999
Interleukin-11, 5000
2-178-Interleukin 11 (Human Clone pXM/IL-11) see 5000
Interleukin-18 see 1884
Interleukin-1 Inhibitor Protein see 5001
Interleukin-1 Receptor Antagonist, 5001
Interleukin-1β Converting Enzyme see 1884
Interleukin 1β Precursor Proteinase see 1884
Interleukin-4 Receptor, 5002
Intermedin(e) see 6295
Internally Compensated Tartaric Acid see 9071
Interstitial Cell Stimulating Hormone see 5613
Intertocine-S [Veterinaria] see 6979
Intestibar [Spofa] see 994
Intestin-Euvernil [Heyden] see 8912
Intrabilix see 5022
Intrabutazone [Organon] see 7277
Intradex [Dextran Prod. Ltd.] see 2948
Intradine [Norbrook] see 8915
Intrapan [USV] see 2947
Intrasite [Fisch] see 2587
Intrasporin [Torlan] see 1979
Intrastigmina [Lusofarmaco] see 6464
Intraval Sodium [RPR] see 9350
Intrazone [Arnolds] see 7277
Intrepid [Dow AgroSci.] see 5993
Intrinsic Factor see 1897
Intromene [Teikoku] see 9624
Intron A [Schering-Plough] see 4990
Introna [Schering-Plough] see 4990
Intybin see 5345
Inula, 5003
Inula Camphor see 207

Inulin, 5004
Invanz [Merck & Co.] see 3673
Invasin see 4758
Invenol [Hoechst] see 1832
Inversine [Targacept] see 5774
Invertase, 5005
Invertin see 5005
Invert Sugar, 5006
Invesol see 5006
Invirase [Roche] see 8369
Inyoite see 1652
Iobac [West Chemical] see 5037
Iobenguane, 5007
Iobitridol, 5008
Iocarmic Acid, 5009
Iocetamic Acid, 5010
Iodamide, 5011
Iodamide Meglumine see 5011
Iodeikon [Mallinckrodt] see 5038
Iodic Acid, 5012
Iodic Acid (HIO₃) Zinc Salt see 10139
Iodic Anhydride see 5019
Iodinated Glycerol, 5013
Iodinated (¹³¹I) Human Serum Albumin see 8468
Iodine, 5014
Iodine Cyanide see 2695
Iodine Heptafluoride, 5015
Iodine Monobromide, 5016
Iodine Monochloride, 5017
Iodine Pentafluoride, 5018
Iodine Pentoxide, 5019
Iodine-polyvinylpyrrolidone Complex see 7698
Iodine Trichloride, 5020
Iodinin, 5021
Iodipamide, 5022
Iodipamide Meglumine see 5022
Iodisan see 7782
Iodixanol, 5023
Iodized Oil, 5024
Iodoacetic Acid, 5025
Iodoalphionic Acid, 5026
p-Iodoaniline, 5027
o-Iodoanisole, 5028
Iodobenzene, 5029
Iodobenzene Ditrifluoroacetate see 7295
4-Iodobenzenesulfonyl Chloride see 7486
2-Iodo-1,2-benzisothiazol-3(2H)-one 1,1-Dioxide see 5043
o-Iodobenzoic Acid, 5030
N-(2-Iodobenzoyl)glycine Monosodium Salt see 5034
m-Iodobenzylguanidine see 5007
Iodobil see 5026
1-Iodobutane see 1573
2-Iodobutane see 1574
Iodochlorhydroxyquin, 5031
Iodochlorohydroxyquinoline see 5031
Iodochloroxyquinoline see 5031
5-Iodo-2′-deoxyuridine see 4891
3-Iodo-1,2-dihydroxypropane see 4488
Iodoenterol see 5031
Iodoethane see 3813
2-(1-Iodoethyl)-1,3-dioxolane-4-methanol see 5013
2-(2-Iodoethyl)-1,3-dioxolane-4-methanol see 5013
Iodofenphos, 5032
5-Iodo-2′-fluoroarauracil see 4069
Iodoform, 5033
Iodognost see 5038
Iodogorgoic Acid see 3192
o-Iodohippurate Sodium, 5034
4-(3-Iodo-4-hydroxyphenoxy)-3,5-diiodophenylalanine see 5510

β-[4-(3′-Iodo-4′-hydroxyphenoxy)-3,5-diiodophenyl]propionic Acid see 9412
m-Iodo-o-hydroxyquinolineanasulfonic Acid see 4826
7-Iodo-8-hydroxyquinoline-5-sulfonic Acid see 4826
(±)-p-Iodo-¹²³I-N-isopropyl-α-methyl-phenethylamine see 5049
4-(Iodo-¹²³I)-α-methyl-N-(1-methyleth-yl)benzeneethanamine see 5049
Iodol see 5041
Iodomethane see 6087
Iodomethanesulfonic Acid Sodium Salt see 5973
4-Iodo-2-[[[[(4-methoxy-6-methyl-1,3,5-triazin-2-yl)amino]carbonyl]amino]-sulfonyl]benzoic Acid Methyl Ester Monosodium Salt see 5046
4-Iodo-ʟ-methylbenzenedecanoic Acid Ethyl Ester see 5060
1-Iodo-3-methylbutane see 5120
2-(Iodomethyl)-1,3-dioxolane-4-metha-nol see 3414
1-Iodo-2-methylpropane see 5144
2-Iodooctane see 6768
Iodopanoic Acid see 5058
Iodophene see 5038
Iodophene Sodium see 5038
o-Iodophenol, 5035
p-Iodophenol, 5036
[(3-Iodophenyl)methyl]guanidine see 5007
1-[2-[4-[(1E)-1-(4-Iodophenyl)-2-phenyl-1-butenyl]phenoxy]ethyl]pyrrolidine see 4890
p-Iodophenyl Sulfonyl Chloride see 7486
Iodophors, 5037
Iodophthalein see 5038
Iodophthalein Sodium, 5038
1-Iodopropane see 7862
2-Iodopropane see 5214
3-Iodo-1,2-propanediol see 4488
3-Iodo-1-propene see 294
3-Iodopropylene see 294
γ-Iodopropyleneglycol see 4488
2,3-(2-Iodopropylidenedioxy)propanol see 5013
2,3-(3-Iodopropylidenedioxy)propanol see 5013
Iodopropylidene Glycerol see 5013
3-Iodo-2-propynyl Butylcarbamate see 5069
3-Iodo-2-propynyl 2,4,5-Trichlorophen-yl Ether see 4600
Iodopsin, 5039
Iodopyracet, 5040
Iodopyracet Compound Solution see 5040
Iodopyracet Concentrated Solution see 5040
Iodopyracet Injection see 5040
Iodopyrrole, 5041
Iodoquinol, 5042
Iodorayoral see 5038
N-Iodosaccharin, 5043
Iodosobenzene, 5044
Iodosorb [Perstorp] see 1610
N-Iodosuccinimide, 5045
Iodosulfane see 8975
Iodosulfuron-methyl-sodium, 5046
Iodosylbenzene see 5044
Iodothyrin see 9411
4-Iodotoluene Difluoride see 3150
Iodotope [BMS] see 8632
3-Iodotyrosine, 5047

o-**Iodoxybenzoic Acid,** 5048
2-**Iodoxybenzoic Acid** *see* 5048
Iodoxyl *see* 8633
Iodtetragnost *see* 5038
Ioduril *see* 8631
2-**Iodylbenzoic Acid** *see* 5048
Iofetamine ^{123}**I,** 5049
Ioflupane ^{123}**I,** 5050
Ioglycamic Acid, 5051
Iohexol, 5052
Iomapidol *see* 5057
Iomeglamic Acid, 5053
Iomeprol, 5054
Iomeron [Bracco] *see* 5054
Ionamin [Lipha] *see* 7262
Ionic Liquids, 5055
Ionol CP [Shell] *see* 1548
Ionone, 5056
Ionophore X-4537A *see* 5373
Iopamidol, 5057
Iopamiro [Bracco] *see* 5057
Iopamiron [Bracco] *see* 5057
Iopanoic Acid, 5058
Iopentol, 5059
Iophendylate, 5060
Iophenoxic Acid, 5061
Iopidine [Alcon] *see* 751
Ioprep [J & J] *see* 5037
Iopromide, 5062
Iopronic Acid, 5063
Iopyracil *see* 5040
Ioquin [Abbott] *see* 5042
Iosalide [Schering] *see* 5267
Iosan [West Chemical] *see* 5037
Iothalamic Acid, 5064
Iotrol *see* 5065
Iotrolan, 5065
Ioversol, 5066
Ioxaglic Acid, 5067
Ioxilan, 5068
Ioxitol *see* 5068
IP-751 *see* 198
Ipacef [IPA] *see* 1954
Ipado *see* 2453
Ipamicina [IPA] *see* 4254
Ipamix [Gentili] *see* 4935
IPC *see* 7816
IPD [Taiho] *see* 9003
IPD-1151T *see* 9003
Ipecac, 5070
Ipecacuanha *see* 5070
Ipertrofan [SPA] *see* 5847
Iphosphamid(e) *see* 4896
IPI-1040 *see* 8554
IPNO *see* 4921
Ipodate, 5071
Ipolab [Finmedical] *see* 5329
Ipomea, 5072
Ipotensivo *see* 5773
Ipradol [CL Pharma] *see* 4707
Ipratropium Bromide, 5073
Ipren [Pharmacia] *see* 4881
Ipriflavone, 5074
Iprindole, 5075
Iproclozide, 5076
Iprodione, 5077
Ipronal [Biosedra] *see* 7904
Iproniazid, 5078
Ipronidazole, 5079
Ipropran [Roche] *see* 5079
Iprosten [Takeda] *see* 5074
Iprovalicarb, 5080
Iproveratril *see* 9950
Ipsapirone, 5081
IPTG, 5082

I.P.U. *see* 5218
IPy$_2$BF$_4$ *see* 1302
IQ *see* 4898
IQB-875 *see* 3546
IR 3535 [Merck KGaA] *see* 3773
IRAP *see* 5001
Irbesartan, 5083
Ircon [Kenwood] *see* 4046
Irenat [Troponwerke] *see* 8653
Irescein [Americal] *see* 4159
Iressa [AstraZeneca] *see* 4379
Irgafen *see* 8932
Irgalax [Novartis] *see* 4452
Irgamide [Dispersa] *see* 8904
Irgarol 1051 [Ciba], 5084
Irgasan BS200 *see* 9191
Irgasan CF3 *see* 2379
Irgasan DP 300 [Ciba] *see* 9657
Iridin *see* 5090
Iridina Due [Montefarmaco] *see* 6368
Iridine *see* 5090
Iridium, 5085
Iridium Hexafluoride, 5086
Iridium Sesquioxide, 5087
Iridium Trichloride, 5088
Iridocin [Bayer] *see* 3737
Iridomyrmecin, 5089
Iridomyrmexin *see* 5089
Irifan *see* 2711
Irigenin, 5090
Irinotecan, 5091
Iris Blue B *see* 5332
Irish Broom *see* 8403
Irisone [Givaudan] *see* 5056
Irium *see* 8636
Irofulven, 5092
Iromon [Gador] *see* 4047
Iron, 5093
Iron Alum *see* 518
Iron(III) Ammonium Citrate *see* 4017
Ironate [Wyeth] *see* 4057
Iron Blue *see* 7910
Iron Carbonyl *see* 5099
Iron Choline Citrate Complex *see* 4038
Iron Dextran, 5094
Irone, 5095
α-**Irone,** 5096
β-**Irone,** 5097
γ-**Irone,** 5098
Iron Hemiphosphide *see* 4054
Iron(III) Hexacyanoferrate(4−) *see* 7910
(OC-6-11)-**Iron(3+) (3:4) Hexakis(cyano-κC) Ferrate(4−)** *see* 7910
Iron(III) Hydroxide Sucrose Complex *see* 5101
Iron Pentacarbonyl, 5099
Iron Phosphide *see* 4054
Iron(III) Potassium Hexacyanoferrate(4−) *see* 7910
Iron Saccharate *see* 5101
Iron Sorbitex, 5100
Iron Sorbitol *see* 5100
Iron Sorbitol Citrate *see* 5100
Iron Sucrose, 5101
Iron Sulfate-glycine Complex *see* 4039
Iron Sulfuret *see* 4058
Iron Tetracarbonyl *see* 5099
Iron Vitriol *see* 4057
Iron Yttrium Oxide *see* 10097
Irox *see* 4047
Irrigor [Merck KGaA] *see* 4923
Irritren [Byk Gulden] *see* 5566
Irrodan [Biomed. Foscama] *see* 1475
Irrorin *see* 7737
Irsogladine, 5102

Irtan [Aventis] *see* 6436
Irtonin [Takeda] *see* 9588
Iruxol [Knoll] *see* 2481
IS-370 *see* 8874
IS-401 *see* 3197
IS-499 *see* 7554
Isacen *see* 6974
Isactid [Ferring] *see* 134
Isalon [Grelan] *see* 223
Isanic Acid, 5103
Isano Oil *see* 1328
Isaphen *see* 6974
Isapirone *see* 5081
Isatidine *see* 8167
Isatin, 5104
γ-**Isatropaic Acid** *see* 9791
ε-**Isatropaic Acid** *see* 9791
Iseganan, 5105
Isepacin [Toyo Jozo] *see* 5106
Isépalline [Schering] *see* 5106
Isepamicin, 5106
Isethion [Mect] *see* 4475
Isethionic Acid, 5107
ISF-2001 *see* 9760
ISF-2123 *see* 7423
ISF-2469 *see* 1631
ISF-2522 *see* 6942
ISF-09334 *see* 8294
Ishikawa Reagent, 5108
ISI-641A *see* 755
Isicom [Desitin] *see* 1797
Isinglass, 5109
Isipen [Krka] *see* 7463
ISIS-2302 *see* 245
ISIS-2922 *see* 4229
ISIS-3521 *see* 755
Islet Amyloid Polypeptide *see* 609
Ismelin [Novartis] *see* 4560
Ismo [Roche] *see* 5225
Ismotic [Alcon] *see* 5224
Isoacetophorone *see* 5196
Isoadanone *see* 5184
Isoadrenaline *see* 6692
Isoalloxazine-adenine Dinucleotide *see* 4091
Isoamidone *see* 5184
Isoamidone I *see* 6709
Isoaminile, 5110
Isoamyl Acetate, 5111
Isoamyl Alcohol *see* 5195
dl-sec-**Isoamyl Alcohol** *see* 6031
Isoamylamine, 5112
Isoamyl Benzoate, 5113
Isoamyl Bromide, 5114
Isoamyl Butyrate, 5115
Isoamylcarbamic Acid Thymyl Ester *see* 9409
Isoamyl Chloride, 5116
Isoamyl Cyanide, 5117
β-**Isoamylene** *see* 607
Isoamyleneguanidine *see* 4341
8-**Isoamylenoxypsoralen** *see* 4925
4-(β-**Isoamylenyl)-1,2-diphenyl-3,5-pyrazolidinedione** *see* 4012
Isoamyl Ether, 5118
5-**Isoamyl-5-ethylbarbituric Acid** *see* 570
Isoamyl Formate, 5119
Isoamyl Iodide, 5120
Isoamyl Isovalerate, 5121
Isoamyl Mandelate *see* 5718
Isoamyl Nitrate, 5122
Isoamyl Nitrite, 5123
Isoamyl Oxide *see* 5118
Isoamyl Phthalate, 5124
Isoamyl Salicylate, 5125

Isoamyl Valerianate *see* 5121
Isoandrosterone *see* 3609
Isoarteril [Isola-Ibi] *see* 8119
Isoascorbic Acid, 5126
Isobamate *see* 1842
Isobatrachotoxin *see* 1009
Isobebeerine *see* 5158
Iso-Benzacyl [Novartis] *see* 1115
Isobenzan, 5127
1,3-Isobenzofurandione *see* 7372
Isobide [Nikken] *see* 5224
Isobixin *see* 1311
Isoborneol, 5128
6-Isobornyl-3,4-dimethylphenol *see* 10076
Isobornyl Thiocyanoacetate, 5129
6-(2-Isobornyl)-3,4-xylen-1-ol *see* 10076
6-Isobornyl-3,4-xylenol *see* 10076
Isobromyl [Clin-Comar-Byla] *see* 1397
Isobutene *see* 5141
Isobutol *see* 3720
1-Isobutoxy-2-pyrrolidino-3-*N*-benzyl-anilinopropane *see* 1150
3-Isobutoxy-2-pyrrolidino-*N*-phenyl-*N*-benzylpropylamine *see* 1150
Isobutyl Acetate, 5130
Isobutyl Alcohol, 5131
Isobutylaldehyde *see* 5154
5-Isobutyl-5-allylbarbituric Acid *see* 1511
Isobutylamine, 5132
Isobutyl *p*-Aminobenzoate, 5133
(*S*)-(+)-3-Isobutyl-*γ*-aminobutyric Acid *see* 7725
2-(Isobutylamino)ethanol *p*-Aminobenzoate (Ester) *see* 1523
2-(Isobutylamino)ethyl *p*-Aminobenzoate *see* 1523
Isobutylbenzene, 5134
Isobutyl Bromide, 5135
3-Isobutyl-6-*sec*-butyl-2-hydroxypyrazine 1-Oxide *see* 841
Isobutyl *n*-Butyrate, 5136
Isobutyl Carbamate, 5137
Isobutyl Carbinol *see* 5195
Isobutylcarbylamine *see* 5112
Isobutyl Chloride, 5138
Isobutyl Chlorocarbonate, 5139
Isobutyl Chloroformate *see* 5139
Isobutyl Cyanoacrylate, 5140
(*E,E*)-*N*-Isobutyl-2,4-decadienamide *see* 7073
(*E,E,Z*)-*N*-Isobutyl-2,6,8-decatrienamide *see* 179
N-Isobutyldeca-*trans*-2-*cis*-6-*trans*-8-trienamide *see* 179
Isobutyl 1,4-Dihydro-5-methoxycarbonyl-2,6-dimethyl-4-(2-nitrophenyl)-3-pyridinecarboxylate *see* 6565
Isobutylene, 5141
Isobutyl Ether, 5142
Isobutyl Formate, 5143
p-Isobutylhydratropic Acid *see* 4881
Isobutylhydrochlorothiazide *see* 1525
Isobutyl Iodide, 5144
Isobutyl Isobutyrate, 5145
Isobutyl Isovalerate, 5146
Isobutyl Kelo-form *see* 5133
Isobutyl Mercaptan, 5147
Isobutyl Methyl 1,4-Dihydro-2,6-dimethyl-4-(*o*-nitrophenyl)-3,5-pyridinedicarboxylate *see* 6565
Isobutyl Nitrate, 5148
Isobutyl Nitrite, 5149
(*p*-Isobutylphenyl)acetic Acid *see* 4880

2-(4-Isobutylphenyl)butyric Acid *see* 1527
(±)-2-(4-Isobutylphenyl)propionic Acid *see* 4881
dl-2-(4-Isobutylphenyl)propionohydroxamic Acid *see* 4882
Isobutyl Propionate, 5150
4-*N*-Isobutylspiropiperidylrifamycin S *see* 8213
Isobutyl Stearate, 5151
Isobutyl Sulfide, 5152
p-Isobutyl-*α*-toluic Acid *see* 4880
Isobutyltrimethylmethane *see* 5193
Isobutyl Urethane, 5153
Isobutyl Valerate, 5146
Isobutyraldehyde, 5154
Isobutyric Acid, 5155
Isobutyric Aldehyde *see* 5154
Isobutyronitrile, 5156
3-Isobutyryl-2-isopropylpyrazolo-[1,5-*a*]pyridine *see* 4879
O-Isobutyrylthiamine Disulfide *see* 9297
Isocaine [Columbus] *see* 5133
Isocalm [Kaken] *see* 9522
Isocapronitrile *see* 5117
Isocaramidine *see* 2844
Isocarbacyclin *see* 2358
Isocarbacyclin Methyl Ester *see* 2358
Isocarboxazid, 5157
Isocard [Schwarz] *see* 5225
Isocaryophyllene *see* 1875
Isocef [Schering-Plough] *see* 1949
Isochavicine *see* 7472
Isochavicinic Acid *see* 7467
Isochinol [Schwarzhaupt] *see* 3218
Isochondrodendrine, 5158
Isochrysene *see* 9740
Isocillin [Aventis] *see* 7100
Isocinchomeronic Acid, 5159
Isococaine *see* 7912
Isocolin [Isola-Ibi] *see* 7362
Isocolumbin *see* 2493
Isoconazole, 5160
Iso-Cornox [FBC] *see* 5784
Isocorybulbine, 5161
Isocorydine, 5162
Isocorypalmine, 5163
Isocrin [Warner-Chilcott] *see* 6974
Isocrotonic Acid, 5164
Isocrotyl Chloride *see* 2147
Isocyanatobenzene *see* 7296
4-Isocyanato-1,1′-biphenyl *see* 10073
1-Isocyanatobutane *see* 1575
Isocyanatomethane *see* 6089
1-Isocyanatonaphthalene *see* 6410
Isocyanic Acid, 5165
Isocyanic Acid 4-Biphenylyl Ester *see* 10073
Isocyanic Acid Butyl Ester *see* 1575
Isocyanic Acid Methyl Ester *see* 6089
1-[(Isocyanomethyl)sulfonyl]-4-methyl-benzene *see* 9556
Isocyanuric Acid *see* 2698
Isodiamylamine *see* 3193
Isodihydroperparine *see* 3455
Isodine [Blair] *see* 7698
Isodiprene *see* 1836
Isodrin *see* 226
Isodulcit *see* 8172
Isodurene, 5166
Isoendoxan *see* 4896
d-Isoephedrine *see* 7916
Isoestradiol, 5167
8-Isoestradiol-17*β* *see* 5167
Isoestragole *see* 643

8-Isoestrone, 5168
Iso E Super [Int. Flavors & Fragrances], 5169
Isoetam [Ferrer] *see* 3720
Isoetarine *see* 5170
Isoetharine, 5170
Isoeugenol, 5171
Isofedrol [Boehringer, Mann.] *see* 3608
Isofenphos, 5172
4′,7-Isoflavandiol *see* 3644
Isoflavone, 5173
Isofluorphate *see* 5176
Isoflupredone, 5174
Isoflurane, 5175
Isoflurophate, 5176
Isoforon *see* 5196
Isogel [Charwell] *see* 7517
Isoglaucon [Boehringer, Ing.] *see* 2390
L-Isoglutamine, 5177
Isoindazole *see* 4936
1*H*-Isoindole-1,3(2*H*)-dione *see* 7373
Isoinokosterone *see* 3491
Iso-Iodeikon *see* 7263
Iso-JH 0 *see* 5273
Iso-K [San Carlo] *see* 5305
Isoket [Schwarz] *see* 5225
Isolan, 5178
Isoleucine, 5179
L-Isoleucine *see* 5179
Isolevin *see* 5217
α-Isolupanine *see* 5607
Isolysergic Acid, 5180
IsoMack [Mack, Illert.] *see* 5225
Isomaltol, 5181
Isomaltulose, 5182
Isomenyl [Kaken] *see* 5217
Isomeride [Ardix] *see* 3973
Isometamidium Chloride, 5183
Isomethadone, 5184
Isomethadone, 5184
Isomist *see* 5217
Isomonat [Roche] *see* 5225
Isomycin [Werfft] *see* 7892
Isomycomycin *see* 6326
Isomytal [Nippon Shinyaku] *see* 570
Isonaphthoic Acid *see* 6382
Isonaphthol *see* 6384
Isonex [Pfizer] *see* 5186
Isoniazid, 5186
Isonicotinic Acid, 5187
Isonicotinic Acid 2-[2-(Benzylcarbamoyl)ethyl]hydrazide *see* 6491
Isonicotinic Acid Diethylamide, 5188
Isonicotinic Acid Hydrazide *see* 5186
Isonicotinic Acid Hydrazide Hydrazone with Glucuronic Acid Lactone *see* 4500
Isonicotinic Acid 2-Isopropylhydrazide *see* 5078
Isonicotinic Acid *α*-Methylfurfurylidenehydrazide *see* 4308
Isonicotinic Acid Salicylidenehydrazide *see* 8335
Isonicotinic Acid *m*-Sulfobenzylidene Hydrazide *see* 8959
N-Isonicotinoyl-*N*′-*β*-(*N*-benzylcarboxamido)ethyl]hydrazide *see* 6491
Isonicotinoylhydrazine *see* 5186
Isonicotinoylhydrazone of D-Glucuronic Acid Lactone *see* 4500
1-Isonicotinoyl-2-isopropylhydrazine *see* 5078
1-Isonicotinoyl-2-salicylidenehydrazine *see* 8335
Isonicotinylhydrazine *see* 5186
Isonicotinyl Hydrazonotoluene-*m*-sulfonic Acid *see* 8959

1-Isonicotinyl-2-isopropylhydrazine *see* 5078
Isonipecaine *see* 5849
Isonipecotic Acid, 5189
Isonitrosoacetone, 5190
Isonitrosoacetophenone, 5191
5-Isonitrosobarbituric Acid *see* 10000
β-Isonitrosopropane *see* 75
Isonixin, 5192
Isonootkatone *see* 9971
Isonorin [SM & P] *see* 5217
Isonovobiocin *see* 6722
Isooctane, 5193
Isooctyl Alcohol, 5194
p-Isooctylpolyoxyethylenephenol Formaldehyde Polymer *see* 9833
Isoolean-14-en-3β-ol *see* 9062
Iso-oosporein *see* 6850
Isopaque [Winthrop] *see* 6156
Isopar *see* 2518
Isopelletierine *see* 7072
4-(2-Isopentenyl)-1,2-diphenyl-3,5-pyrazolidinedione *see* 4012
Isopentyl Alcohol, 5195
sec-Isopentyl Alcohol *see* 6031
Isopentylamine *see* 5112
Isopentyl 5,6-Dihydro-7,8-dimethyl-4,5-dioxo-4H-pyrano[3,2-c]quinoline-2-carboxylate *see* 8138
Isopentyl Nitrite *see* 5123
Isophane Insulin *see* 4980
Isophen [Knoll] *see* 5948
Isophenethanol *see* 6530
Isophenphos *see* 5172
Isophorone, 5196
α-Isophorone *see* 5196
Isophosphamide *see* 4896
Isophthalic Acid, 5197
Isophytol, 5198
Isopilocarpine *see* 7424
Isopilosine, 5199
Isopimaric Acid, 5200
Isopiperine *see* 7472
Isopiperinic Acid *see* 7467
IsoPPC *see* 7816
Isopral *see* 9645
10α-Isopregnenone *see* 3474
Isoprenaline *see* 5217
Isoprene, 5201
Isoprinosin [Newport] *see* 4976
Isoprinosina [Newport] *see* 4976
Isoprinosine [Newport] *see* 4976
Isoprochin P [Merckle] *see* 7871
Isoprofenamine *see* 2408
Isopromedol *see* 7784
Isopropamide Iodide, 5202
Isopropanol *see* 5208
Isopropene Cyanide *see* 5942
Isopropenyl Acetate, 5203
4-Isopropenyl-1-cyclohexene-1-carboxaldehyde *see* 7167
2-Isopropenyl-2,3-dihydro-5-acetylbenzofuran *see* 9581
2-Isopropenyl-6-methoxy-5-benzofuranyl Methyl Ketone *see* 3900
cis-(+)-2-Isopropenyl-1-methylcyclobutaneethanol *see* 4535
4-(5-Isopropenyl-2-methyl-1-cyclopenten-1-yl)-2-butanone, 5204
Isopropenylnitrile *see* 5942
Isoprophenamine *see* 2408
N¹-(4-Isopropoxybenzoyl)-p-aminobenzenesulfonamide *see* 8936
N¹-(p-Isopropoxybenzoyl)sulfanilamide *see* 8936

5-Isopropoxycarbonylaminothiabendazole *see* 1726
5-Isopropoxycarbonylamino-2-(4-thiazolyl)benzimidazole *see* 1726
(E)-O-2-Isopropoxycarbonyl-1-methylvinyl O-Methyl Ethylphosphoramidothioate *see* 7815
1-(Isopropoxycarbonyloxy)ethyl (6R,7R)-7-[2-(2-Amino-4-thiazolyl)-(Z)-2-(methoxyimino)acetamido]-3-methoxymethyl-3-cephem-4-carboxylate *see* 1941
(±)-1-[p-(2-Isopropoxyethoxymethyl)-phenoxy]-3-(isopropylamino)-2-propanol *see* 1295
(±)-1-[α-(2-Isopropoxyethoxy)-p-tolyl]-oxy]-3-(isopropylamino)-2-propanol *see* 1295
7-Isopropoxyisoflavone *see* 5074
Isopropoxymethylphosphoryl Fluoride *see* 8374
7-Isopropoxy-3-phenyl-4H-1-benzo-pyran-4-one *see* 5074
7-Isopropoxy-3-phenylchromone *see* 5074
o-Isopropoxyphenyl N-Methylcarbamate *see* 7836
2-Isopropoxypropane *see* 5212
p-Isopropoxy-N-sulfanilylbenzamide *see* 8936
Isopropydrin *see* 5217
Isopropyl Acetate, 5205
Isopropylacetic Acid *see* 5231
Isopropyl Acetoacetate, 5206
Isopropylacetone, 5207
Isopropyl Alcohol, 5208
Isopropylamine, 5209
4-Isopropylaminoantipyrine *see* 8102
(±)-1-(Isopropylamino)-3-[p-(cyclopropylmethoxyethyl)phenoxy]-2-propanol *see* 1182
4-Isopropylamino-2,3-dimethyl-1-phenyl-3-pyrazolin-5-one *see* 8102
1-(Isopropylamino)-2-hydroxy-3-[o-(allyloxy)phenoxy]propane *see* 6952
(±)-1-(Isopropylamino)-3-[p-(β-methoxyethyl)phenoxy]-2-propanol *see* 6151
1-(Isopropylamino)-3-(o-methoxyphenoxy)-2-propanol *see* 6264
Isopropylaminomethyl-(3,4-dihydroxyphenyl)carbinol *see* 5217
1-(Isopropylamino)-3-[(2-methylindol-4-yl)oxy]-2-propanol *see* 5856
α-[(Isopropylamino)methyl]-2-naphthalenemethanol *see* 7790
α-[(Isopropylamino)methyl]-p-nitrobenzyl Alcohol *see* 6530
α-(Isopropylaminomethyl)protocatechuyl Alcohol *see* 5217
2-Isopropylamino-1-(2-naphthyl)ethanol *see* 7790
1-(Isopropylamino)-3-(1-naphthyloxy)-2-propanol *see* 7840
Isopropylaminophenazone *see* 8102
9-[3-(Isopropylamino)propyl]-9-(aminocarboyl)fluorene *see* 4937
α-(1-Isopropylaminopropyl)protocatechuyl Alcohol *see* 5170
1-[3-(Isopropylamino)-2-pyridyl]-4-[(5-methanesulfonamidoindol-2-yl)carbonyl]piperazine *see* 2877
1-(Isopropylamino)-3-(m-tolyloxy)-2-propanol *see* 9516
p-Isopropylaniline *see* 2620

4-Isopropylantipyrine *see* 7871
Isopropylarterenol *see* 5217
p-Isopropylbenzaldehyde *see* 2621
Isopropylbenzene *see* 2617
p-Isopropylbenzoic Acid *see* 2618
3-Isopropyl-1H-2,1,3-benzothiadiazin-4(3H)-one 2,2-Dioxide *see* 1053
Isopropyl 4-(2,1,3-Benzoxadiazol-4-yl)-1,4-dihydro-5-methoxycarbonyl-2,6-dimethyl-3-pyridinecarboxylate *see* 5240
p-Isopropylbenzyl Alcohol *see* 2619
Isopropyl Bromide, 5210
N-4-Isopropylcarbamoylbenzyl-N'-methylhydrazine *see* 7758
3-Isopropylcarbamylsulfonamido-4-(3'-methylphenyl)aminopyridine *see* 9552
Isopropyl Carbanilate *see* 7816
Isopropylcarbinol *see* 5131
Isopropyl Chloride, 5211
N-Isopropyl-α-chloroacetanilide *see* 7793
Isopropyl [4'-(p-Chlorobenzoyl)-2-phenoxy-2-methyl]propionate *see* 3978
Isopropyl-m-chlorocarbanilate *see* 2187
Isopropyl N-(3-Chlorophenyl)carbamate *see* 2187
Isopropyl-o-cresol *see* 1872
Isopropyl-m-cresyl Ester of Isoamylcarbamic Acid *see* 9409
Isopropyl Cyanide *see* 5156
Isopropyl 6-Cyano-5-methoxycarbonyl-2-methyl-4-(3-nitrophenyl)-1,4-dihydropyridine-3-carboxylate *see* 6545
(−)-N-(trans-4-Isopropylcyclohexyl-1-carbonyl)-D-phenylalanine *see* 6428
Isopropyl 4,4'-Dibromobenzilate *see* 1434
Isopropyl 3,4-Diethoxycarbanilate *see* 3109
Isopropyl N-(3,4-Diethoxyphenyl)carbamate *see* 3109
Isopropyl (Z)-7-[(1R,2R,3R,5S)-3,5-Dihydroxy-2-[(3R)-3-hydroxy-5-phenylpentyl]cyclopentyl]-5-heptenoate *see* 5376
N-Isopropyl-β-dihydroxyphenyl-β-hydroxyethylamine *see* 5217
7-Isopropyl-1,4-dimethylazulene *see* 4554
5-Isopropyl-3,8-dimethyl-1-azulenesulfonic Acid Sodium Salt *see* 4554
2-Isopropyl-N,2,3-dimethylbutanamide *see* 9716
4-Isopropyl-1,6-dimethylnaphthalene *see* 1608
4-Isopropyl-2,3-dimethyl-1-phenyl-3-pyrazolin-5-one *see* 7871
(1R,2S,6S,7S,8S)-(−)-8-Isopropyl-1,3-dimethyltricyclo[4.4.0.0²,⁷]dec-3-ene *see* 2515
(1S,2R,6R,7R,8S)-(+)-8-Isopropyl-1,3-dimethyltricyclo[4.4.0.0²,⁷]dec-3-ene *see* 10099
Isopropyl 2,4-Dinitro-6-sec-butylphenyl Carbonate *see* 3285
N-Isopropyl-4,4-diphenylcyclohexylamine *see* 7707
1-Isopropyl-4,4-diphenylpiperidine *see* 7768
Isopropyl Ether, 5212
N-Isopropylethylnorepinephrine *see* 5170
Isopropyl Fluophosphate *see* 5176
Isopropylformic Acid *see* 5155
Isopropylhexedrine *see* 2707
Isopropylideneacetone *see* 5908

2-Isopropylideneaminooxyethyl (*R*)-2-[4-(6-Chloroquinoxalin-2-yloxy)phenoxy]propionate *see* 7806
1,2-*O*-Isopropylidene-3-*O*-[3′-(*N*,*N*-dimethylamino)propyl]-α-D-glucofuranose *see* 484
2-Isopropylidene-6,10-dimethylspiro-[4.5]dec-6-en-8-one *see* 9971
16α,17α-Isopropylidenedioxyprednisolone *see* 2928
16α,17α-Isopropylidenedioxyprogesterone *see* 239
4,4′-Isopropylidenediphenol *see* 1297
4,4′-(Isopropylidenedithio)bis[2,6-di-*tert*-butylphenol] *see* 7755
16α,17α-Isopropylidene-6α-fluorotriamcinolone 21-Acetate *see* 4151
Isopropylidene Glycerol, 5213
Isopropylidene Malonate *see* 5817
Isopropyl Iodide, 5214
Isopropyl Meprobamate *see* 1842
4-Isopropyl-3-(methanesulfonylbenzoyl)-guanidine *see* 1841
Isopropyl 3-(4-Methoxy-3-biphenylyl)-carbazate *see* 1207
Isopropyl 2-Methoxyethyl 1,4-Dihydro-2,6-dimethyl-4-(3-nitrophenyl)-3,5-pyridinedicarboxylate *see* 6551
Isopropyl (2*E*,4*E*,7*RS*)-11-Methoxy-3,-7,11-trimethyl-2,4-dodecadienoate *see* 5983
Isopropyl Methyl Carbinol *see* 6031
5-Isopropyl-3-methyl-2-cyano-1,4-dihydro-6-methyl-4-(*m*-nitrophenyl)-3,5-pyridinedicarboxylate *see* 6545
4-Isopropyl-1-methyl-1,5-cyclohexadiene *see* 7200
5-Isopropyl-2-methyl-1,3-cyclohexadiene *see* 7200
4-Isopropyl-1-methyl-1-cyclohexen-3-one *see* 7473
2-Isopropyl-1-[4-[3-[*N*-methyl-*N*-(3,4-dimethoxy-β-phenethyl)amino]propyloxy]benzenesulfonyl]indolizine *see* 3934
3-Isopropyl-6-methylene-1-cyclohexene *see* 7201
4-Isopropyl-1-methylene-2-cyclohexene *see* 7201
1-Isopropyl-7-methyl-4-(*p*-fluorophenyl)-2(1*H*)-quinazolinone *see* 4193
α-Isopropyl-α-[(*N*-methyl-*N*-homoveratryl)-γ-aminopropyl]-3,4-dimethoxyphenylacetonitrile *see* 9950
α-Isopropyl-α-[(*N*-methyl-*N*-homoveratryl)-γ-aminopropyl]-3,4,5-trimethoxyphenylacetonitrile *see* 4356
N-Isopropyl-α-(2-methylhydrazino)-*p*-toluamide *see* 7758
2-Isopropyl-1-methyl-5-nitroimidazole *see* 5079
2-(4-Isopropyl)-4-methyl-5-oxo-2-imidazolin-2-yl-5-(methoxymethyl)nicotinic Acid *see* 4904
2-(4-Isopropyl-4-methyl-5-oxo-2-imidazolin-2-yl)nicotinic Acid *see* 4905
2-(5-Isopropyl-5-methyl-4-oxo-2-imidazolin-2-yl)-3-quinolinecarboxylic Acid *see* 4906
1-Isopropyl-7-methyl-4-phenyl-2(1*H*)-quinazolinone *see* 7873
O-Isopropyl Methyl Phosphonic Acid *see* 4924
Isopropylmethylphosphonofluoridate *see* 8374

N-Isopropyl-2-methyl-2-propyl-1,3-propanediol Dicarbamate *see* 1842
1-Isopropyl-3-methyl-5-pyrazolyl Dimethylcarbamate *see* 5178
Isopropyl-2-methyl-1-[(1-*p*-tolyethyl)-carbamoyl]-(*S*)-propylcarbamate *see* 5080
N-[(1*S*)-3-[3-(3-Isopropyl-5-methyl-4*H*-1,2,4-triazol-4-yl)-*exo*-8-azabicyclo-[3.2.1]oct-8-yl]-1-phenylpropyl]-4,4-difluorocyclohexanecarboxamide *see* 5749
Isopropyl Myristate, 5215
Isopropyl Nitrite, 5216
N-Isopropylnoradrenaline *see* 5217
8-Isopropylnoratropine Methobromide *see* 5073
N-Isopropylnoratropinium Bromomethylate *see* 5073
N-(Isopropyloxycarbonyl)-L-valine-4-methylphenylethylamide *see* 5080
Isopropylphenazone *see* 7871
2-(*o*-Isopropylphenoxymethyl)-2-imidazoline *see* 3985
O-Isopropyl *N*-Phenyl Carbamate *see* 7816
N-(4-Isopropylphenyl)-*N*′,*N*′-dimethylurea *see* 5218
Isopropylphosphoramidic Acid Ethyl 4-(Methylthio)-*m*-tolyl Ester *see* 3957
Isopropylphosphoramidothioic Acid *O*-2,4-(Dichlorophenyl) *O*-Methyl Ester *see* 3392
13-Isopropylpodocarpa-7,13-dien-15-oic Acid *see* 7
13-Isopropylpodocarpa-8,13-dien-15-oic Acid *see* 6998
13-Isopropylpodocarpa-8(14),12-dien-15-oic Acid *see* 5468
5-Isopropylpyridine-2-sulfonic Acid 6-(2-Hydroxyethoxy)-5-(2-methoxyphenoxy)-2-(2-1*H*-tetrazol-5-ylpyridin-4-yl)pyrimidin-4-ylamide *see* 9252
Isopropyl 2-(4-Thiazolyl)-5-benzimidazolecarbamate *see* 1726
Isopropyl β-D-Thiogalactopyranoside *see* 5082
Isopropyl Titanate(IV) *see* 9480
Isopropyltoluene *see* 2763
1-Isopropyl-3-[(4-*m*-toluidino-3-pyridyl)-sulfonyl]urea *see* 9552
α-Isopropyl-α-[*p*-(trifluoromethoxy)-phenyl]-5-pyrimidinemethanol *see* 4204
N-Isopropyl-(5-trifluoromethyl-1,3,4-thiadiazol-2-yl)-(4′-fluorooxyacet-anilide) *see* 4131
4-Isopropyltropolone *see* 9390
Isopropylxanthic Acid Sodium Salt *see* 8634
Isoproterenol, 5217
Isoproturon, 5218
Isoptin [Abbott] *see* 9950
Isopto Carbachol [Alcon] *see* 1779
Isopto Carpine [Alcon] *see* 7424
Isopto-Dex [Alcon] *see* 2943
Isopyrin *see* 8102
Isopyrocalciferol, 5219
Isoquassin, 5220
Isoquercitrin, 5221
Isoquinoline, 5222
1-(5-Isoquinolinesulfonyl)homopiperazine *see* 3942
N-(5-Isoquinolinesulfonyl)-1,4-perhydrodiazepine *see* 3942

Isorbid [Wyeth] *see* 5225
Isordil [Wyeth] *see* 5225
Isorenin *see* 5217
D-Isorhamnose *see* 8077
Isorhodeose *see* 8077
Isorythm [Merck KGaA] *see* 3360
Isosafrole, 5223
Isosarsasapogenin *see* 8565
Isosorbide, 5224
Isosorbide Dinitrate, 5225
Isosorbide-5-mononitrate *see* 5225
l-α-Isospartaine *see* 8737
Isostenase [Azupharma] *see* 5225
Isosulfamerazine *see* 8934
Isosulfan Blue *see* 8987
Isosystox *see* 2889
Isotamine [Valeant] *see* 5186
Isoten [Lederle] *see* 1295
Isotense [Nicholas] *see* 9017
Isothazine *see* 3747
Isothebaine, 5226
Isothiazine *see* 3747
Isothiocyanatobenzene *see* 7297
Isothiocyanatoethane *see* 3815
(2-Isothiocyanatoethyl)benzene *see* 7226
Isothiocyanatomethane *see* 6092
(*R*)-1-Isothiocyanato-4-(methylsulfinyl)-butane *see* 8962
1-Isothiocyanatonaphthalene *see* 6411
4-Isothiocyanato-4′-nitrodiphenylamine *see* 574
1-Isothiocyanato-4-(4-nitrophenoxy)benzene *see* 6633
4-Isothiocyanato-*N*-(4-nitrophenyl)benzeneamine *see* 574
1-(4-Isothiocyanatophenoxy)-4-nitrobenzene *see* 6633
3-Isothiocyanato-1-propene *see* 295
Isothiocyanic Acid *see* 9328
Isothiocyanic Acid Allyl Ester *see* 295
Isothiocyanic Acid *p*-(*p*-Nitroanilino)-phenyl Ester *see* 574
Isothiocyanic Acid *p*-(*p*-Nitrophenoxy)-phenyl Ester *see* 6633
Isothiocyanic Acid *p*-Phenylene Ester *see* 1308
Isothiocyanic Acid Phenyl Ester *see* 7297
Isothipendyl, 5227
d-Isothujone *see* 9392
Isothymol *see* 1872
Isotrate [Warner-Chilcott] *see* 5225
Isotretinoin, 5228
Isotrex [Stiefel] *see* 5228
Isotrifoliin *see* 5221
Isotrilobine *see* 9697
Isotron 2 *see* 3064
Isovaleral *see* 5229
Isovaleraldehyde, 5229
Isovaleramide, 5230
Isovalerianic Acid *see* 5231
Isovaleric Acid, 5231
Isovaleric Acid *tert*-Amyl Ester *see* 610
Isovaleric Acid Diester with 8,9-Dihydro-9-hydroxy-8-(1-hydroxy-1-methylethyl)-2*H*-furo[2,3-*h*]-1-benzopyran-2-one *see* 860
Isovaleric Acid 8-Ester with *N*-(7-Butyl-8-hydroxy-4,9-dimethyl-2,6-dioxo-1,5-dioxonan-3-yl)-3-formamidosalicylamide *see* 715
Isovaleric Acid 8-Ester with 3-Formamido-*N*-(7-hexyl-8-hydroxy-4,9-dimethyl-2,6-dioxo-1,5-dioxonan-3-yl)-salicylamide *see* 714
Isovaleric Acid *p*-Menth-3-yl Ester *see* 5841

Isovaleric Acid *tert*-Pentyl Ester *see* 610
Isovaleric Aldehyde *see* 5229
Isovaleryl Chloride, 5232
2-Isovalerylindane-1,3-dione, 5233
N-Isovaleryl-L-valyl-L-valyl-3-hydroxy-
  6-methyl-γ-aminoheptanoyl-L-alanyl-
  3-hydroxy-6-methyl-γ-aminoheptanoic
  Acid *see* 7147
Isovaline, 5234
Isovex *see* 3728
Isoviral [Lenza] *see* 4976
Isovist [Schering AG] *see* 5065
Isovitamin C *see* 5126
Isovon *see* 5217
Isovue [BMS] *see* 5057
Isovyl [Rhovyl] *see* 7586
Isoxaben, 5235
Isoxaflutole, 5236
Isoxal [Shionogi] *see* 7177
Isoxepac, 5237
Isoxsuprine, 5238
Isoyohimbine *see* 10104
Isozid [Fatol] *see* 5186
ISP-1 *see* 4083
Ispaghula Husk *see* 7517
Ispan [Scott Med. Prod.] *see* 7158
Ispenoral [Rosen] *see* 7100
Isphamycin *see* 2192
Ispronicline, 5239
Isradipine, 5240
Israpafant, 5241
Isrodipine *see* 5240
Issium [Lifepharma] *see* 4144
Isteropac E.R. [Bracco] *see* 5011
Istin [Pfizer] *see* 491
Istizin [Winthrop] *see* 2815
Istonil [Siegfried] *see* 3212
Isuprel [Winthrop] *see* 5217
Isupren *see* 5217
IT-290 *see* 6131
IT-931 *see* 3368
ITA-104 *see* 7516
Itaconic Acid, 5242
Italprid [Teofarma] *see* 9421
Itasetron, 5243
Itavastatin *see* 7508
Itax [Axcan] *see* 5244
ITF-182 *see* 4913
Itobarbital *see* 1511
Itopride, 5244
Itraconazole, 5245
Itramin Tosylate, 5246
Itridal *see* 2711
Itrin [Abbott] *see* 9154
Itrizole [Janssen] *see* 5245
Itrol *see* 8511
Itrop [Boehringer, Ing.] *see* 5073
Ituran [Promonta] *see* 6599
IUdR *see* 4891
Iuvacor [Sanofi-Synthelabo] *see* 9843
Ivabradine, 5247
Ivadal [Sanofi-Aventis] *see* 10190
Ivaugan [Voigt] *see* 4781
Ivermectin, 5248
Ivomec [Merial] *see* 5248
Ivosit [Hoechst] *see* 3287
Ivy Block [Enviroderm] *see* 1056
Iwalexin [Iwaki] *see* 1974
Ixabepilone, 5249
Ixbut, 5250
Ixel [Fabre] *see* 6194
Ixense [Takeda] *see* 746
Ixertol [Rottendorf] *see* 2305
Ixodin, 5251
Ixoten [Baxter] *see* 9768

J-38 *see* 4246
J-867 *see* 834
J-107088 *see* 3512
JA *see* 5260
Jaborandi *see* 7425
Jaclacin [Medac] *see* 113
Jacobsen's Catalyst, 5252
Jacodine *see* 8452
Jacutin [Hermal] *see* 5501
Jadit [Hoechst] *see* 1465
Jaikin [Basotherm] *see* 8590
Jalap, 5253
Jalovis *see* 4758
Jamaica Pepper *see* 7432
Jamboo *see* 5254
Jambul, 5254
JA-ME *see* 5260
Jamestown Weed *see* 8820
Jamylène [Théraplix] *see* 3401
Janimine [Abbott] *see* 4920
Janus Green B, 5255
Januvia [Merck & Co.] *see* 8552
Japan Agar *see* 184
Japan Camphor *see* 1732
Japanese Oil of Camphor *see* 6780
Japan Isinglass *see* 184
Japan Tallow *see* 5256
Japan Wax, 5256
Japonilure, 5257
Jasmolin I *see* 5258
Jasmolin II *see* 5258
Jasmolins, 5258
Jasmone, 5259
Jasmonic Acid, 5260
Jateorrhizine *see* 5261
Jatroneural [Procter & Gamble] *see* 9680
Jatropur [Procter & Gamble] *see* 9599
Jatrorrhizine, 5261
Jatrox [Procter & Gamble] *see* 1285
JAU-6476 *see* 7887
Jaundice Berry *see* 961
Jaune Brilliant *see* 1628
Javanicin, 5262
Java Pepper *see* 2612
Java Plum *see* 5254
Javelin [Certis] *see* 932
Javelle Water *see* 4865
Javlor [Fabre] *see* 9989
JB-11 *see* 9721
JB-251 *see* 7895
JB-305 *see* 7470
JB-323 *see* 7461
JB-8181 *see* 2920
JD-91 *see* 3566
JDL-464 *see* 9552
Jectofer [AstraZeneca] *see* 5100
Jecto-Sal [Mallard] *see* 9360
Jee Cocktail *see* 5963
Jeff *see* 5963
Jellin [Grünenthal] *see* 4150
Jenacaine *see* 7757
Jequirity *see* 9
Jeremejevite *see* 330
Jerusalem Artichoke, 5263
Jerusalem Tea *see* 6785
Jerva Acid *see* 2052
Jervasic Acid *see* 2052
Jervine, 5264
Jesaconitine, 5265
Jestmin [Kyowa] *see* 6887
Jestryl [Ankerpharm] *see* 1779
Jesuit's Balsam *see* 2516
Jesuit's Bark *see* 2284
Jesuit's Tea *see* 5756
Jetrium [Hek] *see* 2955

Jeweler's Rouge *see* 4028
Jexin [Evans] *see* 9807
JF-6064 *see* 9111
JH *see* 5273
JH 0 *see* 5273
JH III Bisepoxide *see* 5273
Jimpson Weed *see* 8820
Jimson Weed *see* 8820
Jinofloxacin *see* 6345
JL-1078 *see* 3168
JM-8 *see* 1822
JM-216 *see* 8384
JM-473 *see* 7405
JO-1016 *see* 9484
JO-1196 *see* 3949
Jockey [AgrEvo] *see* 4196
Jodairol *see* 5034
Jodid [Merck KGaA] *see* 7643
Jodobil *see* 5026
Jodomiron [Bracco] *see* 5011
Jodozoat Meglumin [Dagra] *see* 5806
Joghurt *see* 10101
Johannisbrotmehl *see* 5554
Jojoba Oil, 5266
Jomezol *see* 5971
Jomybel [Sarva] *see* 5267
Jonctum [Hoechst] *see* 6903
Jonit [Hoechst] *see* 1308
Jopamiro [Bracco] *see* 5057
Jordan Almond *see* 303
Joristen *see* 7172
Josacine [Bellon] *see* 5267
Josamina [Novag] *see* 5267
Josamy [Yamanouchi] *see* 5267
Josamycin, 5267
Josaxin [Boots] *see* 5267
JP-992 *see* 1039
Judean Pitch *see* 845
Judolor [Woelm] *see* 4311
Juglans, 5268
Juglone, 5269
Julin's Carbon Chloride *see* 4677
Julodin [Takeda] *see* 3702
Jumbul *see* 5254
Jumex [Chiesi] *see* 8428
Junipene *see* 5567
Juniper, 5270
Juniperberry Oil *see* 5270
Juniper Tar, 5271
Junovan [IDM] *see* 5844
Justamil [Anphar-Rolland] *see* 8924
Justar [Intersan] *see* 2264
Justice [Dow AgroSci.] *see* 8750
Justicidin A *see* 5272
Justicidin B *see* 5272
Justicidins, 5272
Justor [Chiesi] *see* 2273
Juvastigmin (Amp.) [Dolder] *see* 6464
Juvastigmin (Tabl.) [Dolder] *see* 6464
Juvenile Hormones, 5273
Juvenimicin A_3 *see* 8261
K III *see* 3279
K IV *see* 3279
K-17 *see* 9255
K-33 *see* 9104
K-218 *see* 7158
K-351 *see* 6562
K-386 *see* 9511
K-1875 *see* 1247
K-1900 *see* 6552
K-2680 *see* 3882
K-3917 *see* 9133
K-3920 *see* 4961
K-4024 *see* 4442
K-9321 *see* 111

K-10033 *see* 3947
K-11941 *see* 234
K-21060E *see* 3446
K-22023 *see* 3392
Ka-2547 *see* 5920
Kabi 925 *see* 3566
Kabi 2165 *see* 2805
Kabi 2213 *see* 7729
Kabi 2234 *see* 9525
Kabikinase [Pharmacia] *see* 8825
KAD-1229 *see* 6211
Kadaya *see* 5284
Kadian [Alpharma] *see* 6276
Kaemferitrin *see* 5274
Kaempferol, 5274
Kaempferol 3-Robinoside 7-Rhamnoside
    see 8243
Kafocin [Lilly] *see* 1976
Kahalalide F, 5275
Kainic Acid, 5276
α-Kainic Acid *see* 5276
L_S-xylo-Kainic Acid *see* 5276
Kalazaquine *see* 8553
Kaleorid [Leo Pharm] *see* 7621
Kaletra [Abbott] *see* 5573
Kalgut [Tanabe Seiyaku] *see* 2894
Kalignost *see* 8690
Kalimozan [Nikken] *see* 4456
Kalinite *see* 360
Kalirechin [Toho] *see* 5279
Kalitabs [Leo Pharm] *see* 7621
Kalium *see* 7604
Kalkitoxin, 5277
Kalle's Acid *see* 6400
Kallidin, 5278
Kallidin I *see* 1359
Kallidin II *see* 5278
Kallidin-9 *see* 1359
Kallidin-10 *see* 5278
Kallidinogenase *see* 5279
Kallikrein, 5279
Kallinin *see* 5351
Kalma [Fresenius] *see* 9797
Kalmegh *see* 632
Kalmopyrin *see* 1647
Kalodil [Fidia] *see* 3197
Kalsetal *see* 1647
Kalutein [Tatsumi] *see* 2408
Kalymin [Temmler] *see* 7977
Kamala, 5280
Kamassin *see* 8030
Kameela *see* 5280
Kamila *see* 5280
Kammerer's Porphyrin *see* 7897
Kamoran [Lilly] *see* 132
Kampfstoff "Lost" *see* 6316
Kamycine [BMS] *see* 5281
Kamynex *see* 5281
Kanacedin *see* 5281
Kanamycin, 5281
Kanamycin A *see* 5281
Kanamycin B *see* 5281
Kanamycin C *see* 5281
Kanamytrex [Basotherm] *see* 5281
Kanaqua [Andromaco] *see* 5281
Kanasig *see* 5281
Kanatrol [Lusofarmaco] *see* 5281
Kanechlor [Kanegafuchi] *see* 7564
Kanemite [Agro-Kanesho] *see* 33
Kanendomycin [Meiji] *see* 5281
Kanendos [Crinos] *see* 5281
Kanescin [Torlan] *see* 5281
Kanicin *see* 5281
Kankohso 101 *see* 7530
Kannasyn *see* 5281

Kannit [Mect] *see* 10085
Kanochol [Taiyo] *see* 6887
Kanrenol [SPA] *see* 1750
Kantec [Daiichi] *see* 5712
Kantrex [Apothecon] *see* 5281
Kaolin, 5282
Kaolinite *see* 362, 4283
Kaon [Altana] *see* 4456
Kaon-Cl [Altana] *see* 7621
Kapanol [GSK] *see* 6276
Kaparlem *see* 5271
Kapilin [Glaxo] *see* 5830
Kapilon Injectable *see* 5832
Kappadione [Lilly] *see* 5830
Kappaxin [Sterling Winthrop] *see* 5831
Kapron [Klin] *see* 6734
Karanjin, 5283
Karate [Syngenta] *see* 2758
Karathane [Dow AgroSci.] *see* 3286
Karaya Gum, 5284
Karbam Black *see* 4013
Karbinon [Badrial] *see* 6394
Kardiamed [Medice] *see* 3167
Karidium *see* 8618
Karil [Novartis] *see* 1643
Karmex *see* 3382
Karmex Monuron Herbicide *see* 6261
Karminomycin *see* 1870
Karsil, 5285
Karsivan [Provet] *see* 7813
Karstenite *see* 1706
Karsulphan *see* 8941
"Kastle-Meyer Reagent" *see* 7244
KAT-256 *see* 2365
Katadolon [AWD] *see* 4190
Katana [Ishihara] *see* 4097
Katchung Oil *see* 7059
Kathon [Rohm & Haas] *see* 6755
Kathon CG [Rohm & Haas] *see* 6091
Katilo *see* 5284
Katine *see* 6714
Katlex [Iwaki] *see* 4309
Katonil [Kali-Chemie] *see* 2105
Katoseran [Hishiyama] *see* 2305
Katovit [Thomae] *see* 7781
Kaurie *see* 2517
Kautschin *see* 5493
Kava, 5286
Kavahin *see* 6138
Kavain *see* 5287
Kava-kava *see* 5286
Kavatin *see* 6138
Kawa *see* 5286
Kawain, 5287
Kay-Cee-L [Geistlich] *see* 7621
Kaydol [Sonneborn] *see* 7186
Kayexalate [Sanofi Winthrop] *see* 8668
Kayhydrin *see* 7380
Kayquinone [Abbott] *see* 5831
Kaytwo [Eisai] *see* 5833
KB-227 *see* 9567
KB-509 *see* 4213
KB-1585 *see* 5437
KB-2413 *see* 3557
KB-2796 *see* 5563
KB-3022 *see* 7002
KBR-2738 *see* 3974
KBR 3023 *see* 7394
KBT-1585 *see* 5437
KBT-3022 *see* 7002
KC-404 *see* 4879
KC-2547 *see* 5920
KC-8857 *see* 9108
KC-9147 *see* 9509
KC-9946 *see* 2271

K-CIT-V [V.E.T.] *see* 7623
K-Contin [Mundipharma] *see* 7621
KD-136 *see* 4598
K-Dur [Schering-Plough] *see* 7621
Keal [Sinbio] *see* 8879
Kebuzone, 5288
Kedacillina [Bracco] *see* 8890
Kefadim [Lilly] *see* 1946
Kefadol [Lilly] *see* 1914
Kefamin [Lilly] *see* 1946
Kefandol [Lilly] *see* 1914
Kefazim [Lilly] *see* 1946
Kefazon [Esseti] *see* 1930
Kefglycin [Lilly] *see* 1976
Kefir Fungi, 5289
Kefir Grains *see* 5289
Kefir Seeds *see* 5289
Keflet [Lilly] *see* 1974
Keflex [Lilly] *see* 1974
Keflin [Lilly] *see* 1982
Keflodin [Lilly] *see* 1979
Keflordin (obsolete) [Lilly] *see* 1979
Keforal [Lilly] *see* 1974
Kefoxina [CT] *see* 1915
Kefroxil [Torre] *see* 1913
Kefspor [Lilly] *see* 1979
Keftab [Lilly] *see* 1974
Kefurox [Lilly] *see* 1954
Kefzol [Lilly] *see* 1917
Keiperazon [Kaken] *see* 1918
Keitin [Chugai] *see* 1940
Kelcogel [CP Kelco] *see* 4383
Kelecin *see* 5428
Kelene *see* 3782
Kelfer [Cipla] *see* 2859
Kelfiprim [Farmitalia] *see* 8910
Kelfizina [Farmitalia] *see* 8910
Kelfizine W [Farmitalia] *see* 8910
Kelgum [CP Kelco] *see* 10057
Kelnac [Sankyo] *see* 7532
Kelocyanor [Serb] *see* 3517
Kelp [Omni] *see* 856
Kelpware *see* 4282
Kelthane [Dow AgroSci.] *see* 3086
Keltrol [CP Kelco] *see* 10057
Kelzan [CP Kelco] *see* 10057
Kemadrin [Glaxo Wellcome] *see* 7763
Kemicetine *see* 2077
Kemi S [Otsuka] *see* 7840
Kemithal *see* 9292
Kemsol [Carter Horner] *see* 3259
Kenacort [BMS] *see* 9595
Kenacort-A [BMS] *see* 9596
Kenaf, 5290
Kenalog [Apothecon] *see* 9596
Kendall's Compound A *see* 2869
Kendall's Compound B *see* 2538
Kendall's Compound C *see* 273
Kendall's Compound E *see* 2539
Kendall's Compound F *see* 4787
Kendall's Desoxy Compound B *see* 2900
Kenicef [Taiho] *see* 1928
Kentera [UCB] *see* 6955
Kenzen [Takeda] *see* 1739
Keoxifene *see* 8098
Kephalins *see* 1975
Kepinol [Pfleger] *see* 8918
Kepivance [Amgen] *see* 6986
Kepone [Allied Chemical] *see* 2083
Keppra [UCB] *see* 5461
Keracyanin *see* 2687
Keral [Menarini] *see* 5305
Keralyt [BMS] *see* 8332
Keraphen *see* 5038
Keratin, 5291

Name Index

Keratinamin [Kowa] *see* 9867
Keratinase, 5292
24-163-Keratinocyte Growth Factor
　(Human) *see* 6986
Keratol [Streuli] *see* 10159
Kerb [Dow AgroSci.] *see* 7872
Kerecid *see* 4891
Kerlocal [Pierre Fabre] *see* 8165
Kerlone [Synthelabo] *see* 1182
Kermesic Acid, 5293
Kernechtrot *see* 6488
Kerosene, 5294
Kerosine *see* 5294
Kertasin [Merck KGaA] *see* 3865
Keselan [Sumitomo] *see* 4598
Kesint [Proter] *see* 1954
Kessar [Pharmacia] *see* 9048
Kessazulen *see* 4554
Kestin [Almirall] *see* 3484
Kestine [Almirall] *see* 3484
Kestrone [Cooper] *see* 3708
Ket [Irbi] *see* 5296
Ketalar [Pfizer] *see* 5295
Ketalgin [Amino] *see* 5944
Ketamine, 5295
Ketanest [Pfizer] *see* 5295
Ketanrift [Ohta] *see* 279
Ketanserin, 5296
Ketas [Kyorin] *see* 4879
Ketaset [Fort Dodge] *see* 5295
Ketason *see* 5288
Ketavet [Gellini] *see* 5295
Ketazolam, 5297
Ketazone [Beytout] *see* 5288
Ketek [Aventis] *see* 9119
Ketene, 5298
Ketensin [Janssen] *see* 5296
Kethoxal, 5299
Ketipic Acid, 5300
Ketobemidone, 5301
[3′-Keto-Bmt1]-[Val2]-cyclosporin *see*
　9917
β-Ketobutyranilide *see* 58
2-Ketobutyric Acid *see* 59
3-Ketobutyric Acid *see* 59
4-Keto-β-carotene *see* 3495
Ketochromin *see* 3182
Ketoconazole, 5302
Ketocycloheptane *see* 2722
Ketocyclopentane *see* 2743
Ketoderm [Janssen] *see* 5302
3-Ketodesogestrel *see* 3884
Ketodestrin *see* 3708
(dl)-9-Keto-11α,15α-dihydroxy-16-
　phenoxy-17,18,19,20-tetranorprosta-
　4,5,13-*trans*-trienoic Acid Methyl
　Ester *see* 3591
17-(1-Ketoethyl)androstane-3,17-diol *see*
　271
17β-(1-Ketoethyl)-Δ⁵-androsten-3β-ol *see*
　7733
Ketofen [Fort Dodge] *see* 5305
Ketogan [Lundbeck] *see* 5301
Ketogin [Lundbeck] *see* 5301
3-Keto-D-glucoheptonofuranolactone *see*
　4451
α-Ketoglutaric Acid, 5303
β-Ketoglutaric Acid *see* 68
2-Keto-L-gulonic Acid, 5304
Ketoheptamethylene *see* 2722
D-*manno*-Ketoheptose *see* 4666
Ketohexamethylene *see* 2726
2-Ketohexamethylenimine *see* 1761
D-*erythro*-3-Ketohexonic Acid Lactone
　see 5126

D-*ribo*-2-Ketohexose *see* 7924
L-3-Keto-*threo*-hexuronic Acid Lactone
　see 830
Ketohydroxyestrin *see* 3708
17-(1-Keto-2-hydroxyethyl)androstane-
　3,11,17-triol *see* 273
17-(1-Keto-2-hydroxyethyl)-Δ⁴-andro-
　sten-3,11-dione *see* 2869
17-(1-Keto-2-hydroxyethyl)-4-androsten-
　17α-ol-3-one *see* 2932
3-β-Keto-γ-(3-hydroxy-2-piperidyl)pro-
　pyl]-4-quinazolone *see* 3946
Ketoisdin [Isdin] *see* 5302
Ketomalonic Acid *see* 5913
γ-Keto-β-methoxy-δ-methylene-Δᵅ-hex-
　enoic Acid *see* 7092
1-Keto-6-methoxy-1,2,3,4-tetrahydro-
　naphthalene *see* 6000
5-Keto-2-methoxy-5,6,7,8-tetrahydro-
　naphthalene *see* 6000
Ketopentamethylene *see* 2743
D-*erythro*-2-Ketopentose *see* 8207
Ketophenylbutazone *see* 5288
L-6-Ketopiperidine-2-carbonyl-L-leucyl-
　L-proline Amide *see* 7603
Ketoprofen, 5305
Ketopron [Alcon] *see* 5305
β-Ketopropane *see* 66
2-Ketopropionaldehyde *see* 6081
α-Ketopropionic Acid *see* 8021
2-Ketopyrrolidine *see* 8016
2-Ketopyrrolidine-1-ylacetamide *see*
　7487
Ketorolac, 5306
Ketoscilium [Zambon] *see* 4006
Ketosuccinic Acid *see* 6909
1-Keto-3-(3′-sulfamyl-4′-chlorophenyl)-
　3-hydroxyisoindoline *see* 2193
Ketotifen, 5307
17-Ketotrilostane *see* 9698
2-Keto-1,7,7-trimethylnorcamphane
　see 1732
Keuten *see* 8608
Kevopril [Rhone-Poulenc] *see* 8083
Kew Tree *see* 4425
Keyhole-limpet Hemocyanin *see* 4647
Keypyrone [Key] *see* 3350
KF-868 *see* 5642
Khas Khas Oil *see* 6816
Khat, 5308
Khellin, 5309
Khinocyde *see* 8067
Khloratsizin *see* 2068
Khus Oil *see* 6816
Kiditard [Belga] *see* 8060
Kidrolase [RPR] *see* 836
Kieselguhr *see* 4973
Kieserite *see* 5653, 5691
KIF-3535 *see* 5845
KIH-2023 *see* 1301
KIH-2031 *see* 7993
KIH-8921 *see* 7993
KIH-9201 *see* 4210
Kiku Oil, 5310
Killax *see* 9204
Kilmicen [Farmitalia] *see* 9509
Kilmite 40 *see* 9204
KIM-112 *see* 7777
Kimopsin [Eisai] *see* 2260
Kimoral [Nippon Chemiphar] *see* 2260
Kinaden *see* 4758
Kinadon [United Phosphorus] *see* 7337
Kinecid [Schering AG] *see* 8914
Kinedak [Ono] *see* 3605
Kineorl [Showa Shinyaku] *see* 9522

Kineret [Amgen] *see* 5001
Kinetin [Schering] *see* 4758
Kinetin, 5311
Kinevac [BMS] *see* 8543
King's Gold *see* 806
King's Yellow *see* 806, 5405
Kinic Acid *see* 8059
Kinichron [Biochimica] *see* 8060
Kinidin Durules [Astra] *see* 8060
Kininogens, 5312
Kino, 5313
Kinotomin [Toa Eiyo] *see* 2345
Kino-yellow *see* 5644
Kinupril [Bellon] *see* 8083
Kinzalmono [Bayer] *see* 9129
Kir Richter [Lepetit] *see* 757
Kirappu [Bayer CropSci.] *see* 3739
Kirocid [Schering AG] *see* 8914
Kiron [Schering AG] *see* 8914
Kirromycin *see* 6225
Kisselo-mleko *see* 10101
Kistrin, 5314
Kistrin (*Agkistrodon rhodostoma* Re-
　duced) *see* 5314
Kitasamycin *see* 5453
Kit Ligand *see* 8807
Kitol, 5315
KL4 *see* 8542
KL-255 *see* 1496
KL-373 *see* 1233
Klacid [Abbott] *see* 2339
Klaricid [Abbott] *see* 2339
Klavocin [Pliva] *see* 2341
Klebcil [SKB] *see* 5281
Kleenodyne *see* 5037
KLH *see* 4647
Klimax E [Fink] *see* 3707
Klimicin [Lek] *see* 2356
Klinit [Eisai] *see* 10085
Klinium [Janssen] *see* 5484
Klinomycin [Valeant] *see* 6202
Klion [Gedeon Richter] *see* 6157
Klismacort [Novartis] *see* 7721
Kloben Neburon [DuPont] *see* 6435
Klockmannite *see* 2651
Klonopin [Roche] *see* 2389
Klot [Warren-Teed] *see* 9520
Klotogen [Abbott] *see* 5831
KL₄-surfactant *see* 8542
Klucel [Hercules] *see* 4841
K-Lyte [Apothecon] *see* 7609
KMD-3213 *see* 8503
Knight's Spur *see* 5372
Knob Root *see* 2483
Knoll H₇₅ *see* 7330
Ko-592 *see* 9516
Ko-1173 *see* 6169
Ko-1366 *see* 1489
Koate-HP [Bayer] *see* 3921
Kobaton *see* 3260
Kochite *see* 362
Kodel [Eastman-Kodak], 5316
Kodocytochalasin-1 *see* 2790
Kofler's Quinone *see* 7523
Kogenate [Bayer] *see* 3921
Koglucoid [Panray] *see* 8120
Koji *see* 9031
Kojic Acid, 5317
Kola, 5318
Kolikodal *see* 4785
Kollateral [Ursapharm] *see* 6288
Kollerdormfix *see* 2711
Kollidon [BASF] *see* 7697
Kollidon CL [BASF] *see* 7697
Kolpon [Organon] *see* 3708

Kolton [Promonta] *see* 3331
Kombetin [Boehringer, Mann.] *see* 8852
Kombiquens [Novo] *see* 5805
Komet [Zeneca Ag Prod] *see* 9111
Kompensan [Roerig] *see* 3184
Konakion [Roche] *see* 7380
Kondurangin *see* 2496
Konesta [Akzo] *see* 9627
Koninckite *see* 4029
Konjac, 5319
Konjac Glucomannan *see* 5319
Konjac Mannan *see* 5319
Konlax [Nippon Shinyaku] *see* 7741
Konnyaku *see* 5319
Kon Oil *see* 5643
Kontexin [Pfizer] *see* 7307
Konyne [Miles] *see* 3922
Kopsine, 5320
Korazol *see* 7141
Korbutone [Nippon Glaxo] *see* 1019
Korec [Sanofi-Aventis] *see* 8051
Koretic [Sanofi-Aventis] *see* 8051
Korglykon *see* 2512
Korlan [Dow] *see* 8256
Koromite [Sankyo] *see* 6189
Koroseal [Goodrich] *see* 7586
KOS-862 *see* 3628
Koser's Reagent, 5321
Kosins, 5322
Koso *see* 1366
Kosso *see* 1366
K-Othrine [Bayer CropSci.] *see* 2883
Kotoite *see* 5658
Kouso *see* 1366
Kousso *see* 1366
KP-363 *see* 1518
KPABA *see* 7606
KPB *see* 5288
Kraton [Shell] *see* 8390
Krazy Glue [Toagosei] *see* 3787
Krebiozen, 5323
Krebon *see* 1476
Kredex [GSK] *see* 1873
Kremol [Sonneborn] *see* 7186
Kren *see* 4749
Kresoxim-methyl, 5324
KRESTIN [Kureha] *see* 7927
Kristallose *see* 8311
KRM-1648 *see* 8214
KRN-1493 *see* 2282
KRN-8601 *see* 4537
Kronitex TCP [FMC] *see* 9763
KRX-101 *see* 8986
KRX-0401 *see* 7165
Kryolith *see* 2606
Kryptocur [HMR] *see* 5474
Krypton, 5325
Krypton Difluoride *see* 5325
Kryptosterol *see* 5360
Krysid *see* 722
KS4 *see* 141
K-Selectride *see* 8427
K-Strophanthin *see* 8852
K-Strophanthin-α *see* 2761
K-Strophanthoside *see* 8852
KT-611 *see* 6356
KT-3777 *see* 5576
K-Thrombin [Fawns & McAllan] *see* 5831
KTU 3616 *see* 1863
K₂tu-PA *see* 391
KU-54 *see* 9790
Kubacron [Kayaku] *see* 9624
KUE 13032c *see* 3044
KUF-6201 *see* 5845
KUH-833 *see* 7777

KUH-911 *see* 1301
Kujimycin B *see* 5356
Kukoline *see* 8546
Kullo *see* 5284
Kupferkies *see* 2038
Kurchatovium *see* 8303
Kurnakovite *see* 5658
Kuromanin *see* 2687
Kuromatsunine *see* 5567
Kusso *see* 1366
Kusum Oil *see* 5643
Kuteera *see* 5284
Kutkasin [Lääkefarmos] *see* 8950
Ku-Zyme [Schwarz] *see* 7006
KVX-478 *see* 589
KW-110 *see* 25
KW-1062 *see* 6181
KW-2228 *see* 4537
KW-2307 *see* 9990
KW-3049 *see* 1043
KW-4679 *see* 6840
KWD-2183 *see* 953
Kwell [Reedco] *see* 5501
KWG-4168 *see* 8761
Kyamepromazine *see* 2683
Kyanmethin, 5326
Kyanol *see* 659
Kylar [Uniroyal] *see* 2810
Kylit [Taiho] *see* 10085
Kymo-trypure *see* 2260
Kynurenic Acid, 5327
Kynurenine, 5328
Kyocristine [Kyorin] *see* 9986
Kyorin AP2 *see* 8535
Kytril [SKB] *see* 4536
Kyurinett [Zensei] *see* 9705
L1 *see* 2859
L-67 *see* 7743
L-86-8275 *see* 4094
L-104 *see* 2392
L-105 *see* 8220
L-105 (Lederle) *see* 1955
L-141 *see* 3951
L-300 *see* 9499
L-554 *see* 9765
L-627 *see* 1197
L-1102 *see* 8333
L-1573 *see* 2779
L-1633 *see* 8608
L-1913 *see* 7156
L-2103 *see* 4698
L-2214 *see* 1065
L-2329 *see* 1083
L-3428 *see* 482
L-5458 *see* 2862
L-6257 *see* 6934
L-6400 *see* 4115
L-12717 *see* 5585
L-34314 *see* 3307
L-35355 *see* 3341
L-36352 *see* 9686
LA-1 *see* 6575
LA-956 *see* 7079
LA-1211 *see* 4923
LA-1221 *see* 1510
LA-6023 *see* 5938
LA-III *see* 2994
LAAM *see* 5466
LAAO *see* 415
Lab *see* 8134
Labelol [ELEA] *see* 5329
Labetalol, 5329
Lab Ferment (German) *see* 8134
Labican [Boniscontro] *see* 2084
Labile Bixin *see* 1311

Labile Factor *see* 3919
Labitan [Labinca] *see* 3200
Labosept [L.A.B.] *see* 2913
Labrocol [Lagap] *see* 5329
Labroda [Specia] *see* 4106
Labrodax [Specia] *see* 4106
Labyrin *see* 2305
Lac *see* 8478
LAC-43 *see* 1495
Lacca *see* 8478
Lacca Coerulea *see* 5547
Laccaic Acid, 5330
Laccaic Acid A *see* 5330
Laccaic Acid A₁ *see* 5330
Laccaic Acid B *see* 5330
Laccaic Acid C *see* 5330
Laccaic Acid D *see* 5330
Lacca Musica *see* 5547
Lac Dye *see* 5330
Lacea [Mitsui Toatsu] *see* 5338
Lacflavin [Towa Yakuhin] *see* 8200
LACI *see* 9467
Lacidipine, 5331
Lacimen [Menarini] *see* 5331
Lacipil [GSK] *see* 5331
Lacirex [Guidotti] *see* 5331
Lacmoid, 5332
Lacmus *see* 5547
Lacolin *see* 8635
Lacosamide, 5333
Lacretin [Tokyo Tanabe] *see* 2345
Lacrimin [Santen] *see* 1047
Lacrisert [Merck & Co.] *see* 4841
Lacrypos [Alcon] *see* 2214
Lactacidogen *see* 4276
β-Lactamase *see* 7093
Lactamin [Teisan] *see* 7737
Lactaminic Acid *see* 8484
Lactate Dehydrogenase, 5334
D-Lactic Acid, 5335
D(−)-Lactic Acid *see* 5335
DL-Lactic Acid, 5336
L-Lactic Acid, 5337
L(+)-Lactic Acid *see* 5337
d-Lactic Acid *see* 5337
l-Lactic Acid *see* 5335
DL-Lactic Acid Ammonium Salt *see* 530
Lactic Acid Cetyl Ester *see* 2030
Lactic Acid Hexadecyl Ester *see* 2030
Lactic Acid Homopolymer, 5338
Lactic Acid Lactate, 5339
Lactic Acid β-Naphthyl Ester *see* 6412
Lacticare-HC [Stiefel] *see* 4787
Lactic Dehydrogenase *see* 5334
Lactinium [Roland] *see* 6876
Lactit *see* 5340
Lactite *see* 5340
Lactit M *see* 5340
Lactitol, 5340
Lactobacillamide *see* 5341
Lactobacillic Acid, 5341
Lactobacillus bifidus Factor *see* 1211
Lactobacillus bifidus Growth Factor *see* 1211
Lactobacillus lactis Dorner Factor *see* 10014
Lactobionic Acid, 5342
Lactobionic δ-Lactone *see* 5342
Lactobiosit *see* 5340
Lactoferrin *see* 9571
Lactoflavine *see* 8200
Lactogen *see* 7779
Lactogen (Human Placental) *see* 4620
Lactogenic Hormone (Placental Human) *see* 4620

Lactol see 6412
Lactonaphthol see 6412
Lactose, 5343
Lactosit see 5340
Lactositol see 5340
Lactosylceramide see 2794
Lactotransferrin see 9571
Lactovagan [Schwartzhaupt] see 5336
2-(Lactoyloxy)propanoic Acid see 5339
Lactron [Kanebo] see 5338
Lactucarium, 5344
Lactucerin see 9060
α-Lactucerol see 9060
Lactucin, 5345
Lactucon see 9060
Lactucopicrin see 5345
Lactuflor [Chephasaar] see 5346
Lactulose, 5346
Lacty [Shimadzu] see 5338
Lacty [CCA Biochem] see 5340
Ladakamycin see 890
Ladogal [Sanofi-Synthelabo] see 2812
Ladropen [Berk] see 4111
Lady's Slipper see 2770
Laetrile see 597
Laevilac [Fresenius] see 5346
Laevoral [Laevosan] see 4273
Laevosan [Laevosan] see 4273
Laevulinic Acid see 5472
LAF see 4993
LAF-237 see 9979
Lafutidine, 5347
Lagistase [Labaz] see 3547
Lagosin see 4290
Laguncurin see 5644
Laidlomycin, 5348
Laki-Lorand Factor see 3926
LAM-1 see 8426
Lamar [Tokyo Tanabe] see 9112
Lambdamycin see 2045
Lambeth [Lambeth Rope] see 7581
Lamb Mint see 7145
Lambral [Maggioni] see 9506
Lambratene (formerly) [Cilag Italiano]
    see 2779
Lamictal [GSK] see 5353
Lamifiban, 5349
Laminaran, 5350
Laminaran Hydrogen Sulfate see 5350
Laminarin see 5350
Laminin, 5351
Laminin M see 5351
Lamisil [Novartis] see 9156
Lamivudine, 5352
Lamoryl [Leo Pharm] see 4549
Lamotrigine, 5353
Lamoxactam see 6286
Lamp Black see 1808
Lampit [Bayer] see 6538
Lampocef [Lampugnani] see 1917
Lampomandol [AGIPS] see 1914
Lamprecid [Clariant] see 9253
Lampren(e) [Novartis] see 2373
Lampsporin [Von Boch] see 1954
Lampterol see 4899
Lamra [Merckle] see 2994
Lamuran [Boehringer, Mann.] see 8119
Lanacort [Combe] see 4787
Lanadigenin see 3166
Lanarkite see 5420
Lanatilin [Wabosan] see 3167
Lanatosides, 5354
Lanatoxin [Beiersdorf] see 3163
Lancetina [Farma Uno] see 4254
Landamycine [Delalande] see 8206

Landel [Zeria] see 3524
Landiolol, 5355
Landomycin see 6825
Landruma [Landerln] see 6531
Landsen [Sumitomo] see 2389
Laneth see 7577
Lanexat [Roche] see 4135
Lanfrax [Henkel] see 5358
Langite see 2654
Langoran [Aventis] see 5225
Lanicor [Roche] see 3167
Lanimerck [Merck KGaA] see 5354
Lanirapid [Roche] see 3167
Lanitop [Roche] see 3167
Lankamycin, 5356
Lankavose see 2039
Lannate [DuPont] see 5982
Lanoconazole, 5357
Lanogene [Amerchol] see 5358
Lanolin, 5358
Lanolin Alcohols, 5359
Lanolin Oil see 5358
Lanolin Wax see 5358
(3β)-Lanosta-8,24-dien-3-ol see 5360
Lanosterol, 5360
Lanoxicaps [GSK] see 3167
Lanoxin [GSK] see 3167
Lanreotide, 5361
Lansfordite see 5660
Lansoprazole, 5362
Lansox [Takeda] see 5362
Lantadin [Lepetit] see 2862
Lantanon [Ravasini] see 6172
Lanthana see 5363
Lanthanum, 5363
Lanthanum Carbonate, 5364
Lanthanum Sesquicarbonate see 5364
Lanthanum Sesquioxide see 5363
Lanthanum Trioxide see 5363
Lanthionine, 5365
L-Lanthionine see 5365
Lantrol 1673 [Henkel] see 5358
Lantus [Aventis] see 4984
Lanvis [GSK] see 9337
Lanzor [Aventis] see 5362
Lanzyme [Nissui] see 5640
Lapachic Acid see 5366
Lapachol, 5366
Lapatinib, 5367
Lapatinib Ditosylate see 5367
Lapis Lazuli see 5395
Lappa, 5368
Lappaconitine, 5369
Lapudrine [Zeneca] see 2184
Lapyrium Chloride, 5370
Laracor [Lagap] see 6952
Laradopa [Roche] see 5464
Laraflex [Lagap] see 6417
Laragon [Roemmers] see 8532
Larapam [Lagap] see 7506
Laratrim [Lagap] see 8918
Larch Agaric see 185
Larch Turpentine see 9945
Lard, 5371
Lard-factor see 10013
Lard Oil see 5371
Laredo [Dow AgroSci.] see 6321
Larex [Geistlich] see 7574
Largactil [Aventis] see 2185
Large Fennel see 3977
Large-flowered Cereus see 1607
Largon [Wyeth] see 7822
Lariam [Roche] see 5801
Laricic Acid see 186
Laricin see 2503

Laridal [Elfar-Drag] see 856
Laristine [Roche] see 4720
Larixin [Toyama] see 1974
Larixinic Acid see 5713
Lark's-claw see 5372
Lark's-heel see 5372
Larkspur, 5372
Larnite see 1702
Larocaine [Roche] see 3221
Larodopa [Roche] see 5464
Laroféron [Roche] see 4990
Laronidase see 4894
Laroscorbine [Roche] see 830
Larostidin [Roche] see 4720
Larotid [Roche] see 577
Laroxyl [Roche] see 487
Larvacide 100 see 2156
Larvadex [Novartis] see 2775
Larvin [Bayer CropSci.] see 9329
LAS see 5637
LAS-11871 see 7277
LAS-17177 see 2294
LAS-31416 see 304
Lasalocid A, 5373
Laser [Tosi] see 6417
Laserphyrin [Meiji] see 9034
Laserpitin, 5374
Lasilix [Aventis] see 4309
Lasiocarpine, 5375
Lasix [Aventis] see 4309
Lasma [Pharmax] see 9285
Lasso [Monsanto] see 201
Lastet [Nippon Kayaku] see 3886
Lasurite see 5395
LAS-W-090 see 3484
LAT-1717 see 7441
LAT-A see 5378
Latamoxef see 6286
Latanoprost, 5376
LAT-B see 5378
Latibon [Bayer] see 3108
Laticort [Medphano] see 4787
Latocillin [Chassot] see 2419
Latoconazole see 5357
α-Latrotoxin, 5377
Latrunculin A see 5378
Latrunculin B see 5378
Latrunculins, 5378
Latumcidin see 8
Laubanite see 1648
Laudamonium [Henkel] see 1059
Laudanidine, 5379
dl-Laudanidine see 5380
Laudanine, 5380
l-Laudanine see 5379
Laudanosine, 5381
Laudicon see 4803
Laughing Gas see 6653
Laumontite see 1648
Laurabolin [Intervet] see 6365
Laurel, 5382
Laurel Berry Oil see 5382
Laurel Camphor see 1732
Laureline, 5383
Laurel Leaf Oil see 5382
Laurent's Acid see 6404
Laureth see 7577
Laureth 9 see 7558
Lauric Acid, 5384
Laurocapram, 5385
Laurodin see 5387
Lauroguadine, 5386
Laurolinium Acetate, 5387
Lauromicina [Dukron] see 3683
Laurostearic Acid see 5384

Laurotetanine, 5388
N-(Lauroylcolaminoformylmethyl)pyri-
  dinium Chloride *see* 5370
N-Lauroylsarcosine Sodium Salt *see* 4368
Lauryl Alcohol *see* 3405
Lauryl Bromide, 5389
Lauryl Sulfate Salt of the Propionic Acid
  Ester of Erythromycin *see* 3683
Lautarite, 1676
Lauth's Violet *see* 9346
Lavandin *see* 5390
Lavandin Oil *see* 5390
Lavasept [Fresenius] *see* 7560
Lavender, 5390
Lavender Oil *see* 5390
Laverin [Lemmon] *see* 3728
Lawesson's Reagent, 5391
Lawrencite *see* 4043
Lawrencium, 5392
Lawsone, 5393
Lawsonite *see* 1648
Laxadin [Teva] *see* 1242
Laxoberal [Boehringer, Ing.] *see* 7406
Laxoberon [Ferrosan] *see* 7406
Laxo-Isatin *see* 6974
Laxonalin *see* 1296
Layor Carang *see* 184
Lazabemide, 5394
Lazaroids *see* 9463
Lazurite, 5395
LB-46 *see* 7443
LB-502 *see* 4309
LB-20304 *see* 4389
LC-33 *see* 5439
LC-44 *see* 4187
L-Carn [Sigma-Tau] *see* 1849
LCB-29 *see* 4893
LCR *see* 9986
LD-3394 *see* 3988
LD-4644 *see* 7457
LDA *see* 3196
LDP-03 *see* 228
LEA-103 *see* 8258
LEA29Y *see* 1024
Lead, 5396
Lead Acetate, 5397
Lead Antimonate(V), 5398
Lead Arsenate, 5399
Lead Arsenite, 5400
Lead Azide, 5401
Lead Benzoate *see* 1091
Lead Borate, 5402
Lead Bromide, 5403
Lead Chloride, 5404
Lead Chromate(VI), 5405
Lead Chromate(VI) Oxide, 5406
Lead Difluoride *see* 5408
Lead Dioxide, 5407
Lead Distearate *see* 5418
Lead Fluoride, 5408
Lead Fluosilicate *see* 5410
Lead Formate, 5409
Lead Hexafluorosilicate, 5410
Lead Iodide, 5411
Lead Metavanadate *see* 5427
Lead Molybdate(VI), 5412
Lead Monosubacetate *see* 5419
Lead Monoxide, 5413
Lead Nitrate, 5414
Lead Orthoplumbate *see* 5425
Lead Oxalate, 5415
Lead (II) Oxide *see* 5413
Lead (IV) Oxide *see* 5407
Lead Oxide Brown *see* 5407
Lead Oxide (PbO) *see* 5413

Lead Oxide (PbO$_2$) *see* 5407
Lead Oxide Red *see* 5425
Lead Oxide Yellow *see* 5413
Lead Peroxide *see* 5407
Lead Phosphate, 5416
Lead Protoxide *see* 5413
Lead Sesquioxide, 5417
Lead Silicofluoride *see* 5410
Lead-sodium Alloy *see* 8637
Lead Stearate, 5418
Lead Subacetate, 5419
Lead Subcarbonate *see* 1005
Lead Sulfate, 5420
Lead Sulfide, 5421
Lead Sulfocyanate *see* 5426
Lead Superoxide *see* 5407
Lead Telluride, 5422
Lead Tetraacetate, 5423
Lead Tetraethyl *see* 9202
Lead Tetrafluoride, 5424
Lead Tetroxide, 5425
Lead Thiocyanate, 5426
Lead Trioxide *see* 5417
Lead Vanadate(V), 5427
Leaf Alcohol *see* 4700
Leaf Green *see* 2234
Lealgin [Janssen] *see* 7250
Leandin *see* 2680
Leanol [Yoshitomi] *see* 4707
Leanstar [Pitman-Moore] *see* 8716
Lebaycid *see* 4002
Leben Raib *see* 10101
Leblon [De Angeli] *see* 7491
LECAM-1 *see* 8426
Lecasol [Kaken] *see* 2345
Lecedil [Zdravlje] *see* 3930
Lecibis [Columbia] *see* 1148
Lecibral [Nezel] *see* 6495
Lecithins, 5428
Lecithol *see* 5428
Lecs [Bayer CropSci.] *see* 4007
Lectins, 5429
Lectopam [Roche] *see* 1385
Ledakrin [Polfa] *see* 6571
Ledclair [Sinclair] *see* 3517
Ledercort (Tabl.) [Lederle] *see* 9595
Ledercort Cream [Lederle] *see* 9596
Lederfen [Am. Cyanamid] *see* 3963
Lederfolat [Lederle] *see* 4222
Lederfolin [Lederle] *see* 4222
Lederkyn [Wyeth] *see* 8919
Lederlon [Lederle] *see* 9598
Ledermycin [Wyeth] *see* 2886
Lederplatin [Lederle] *see* 2317
Lederspan [Lederle] *see* 9598
Ledertrexate [Wyeth] *see* 5985
Ledol, 5430
Ledopa [Lepetit] *see* 5464
"Ledum Camphor" *see* 5430
Lefax [Asche] *see* 3215
Lefcar [GSK] *see* 1849
Lefetamine, 5431
Leflunomide, 5432
Leftose [Nippon Shinyaku] *see* 5640
Legalon [Madaus] *see* 8532
Legederm [Schering] *see* 220
Legential *see* 4398
Leghemoglobin, 5433
Legoglobin *see* 5433
Legumex D *see* 2835
Legumin *see* 1883
Lehydan [Abigo] *see* 7322
LeIF *see* 4990
Leipzig Yellow *see* 5405
Lemakalim *see* 5460

Lemoflur *see* 8618
Lemonol *see* 4403
Lemon Peel, 5434
Lemon Walnut *see* 5268
Lemon Yellow *see* 972
Lemoran *see* 5470
Lenacil, 5435
Lenalidomide, 5436
Lenampicillin, 5437
Lenamycin *see* 1962
Lendorm [Boehringer, Ing.] *see* 1450
Lendormin [Boehringer, Ing.] *see* 1450
Lenicet *see* 344
Lenidolor [Menarini] *see* 5779
Lenigallol [Knoll] *see* 8000
Lenirit [Bonomelli] *see* 4787
Lenisarin *see* 3384
Lenitral [Besins-Iscovesco] *see* 6607
Lenograstim *see* 4537
Lenopect [Draco] *see* 7456
Lenoxin [GSK] *see* 3167
Lensan A [CIBA Vision] *see* 4798
Lentagran [Syngenta] *see* 7968
Lentaron [Novartis] *see* 4240
Lenthionine, 5438
Lentinacin *see* 3670
Lentinan, 5439
Lentisk *see* 5755
Lentizol [Lundbeck] *see* 487
Lentogest [Amsa] *see* 4839
Lento-Kalium [Teofarma] *see* 7621
Lentopenil [Grossman] *see* 7096
Lentotran [Farmopatria] *see* 2084
Lentrat *see* 7112
Lentysine *see* 3670
Leo 640 *see* 5557
Leo-1031 *see* 7720
Leocillin [Leo Pharm] *see* 7085
Leodrine [Leo Pharm] *see* 4789
Leonurine, 5440
Leopard's Bane *see* 789
Leparan [Italfarmaco] *see* 4653
Lepargylic Acid *see* 905
Lepetan [Otsuka] *see* 1497
Lepicidin A *see* 8750
Lepidine, 5441
Lepidocrocite *see* 4025
Lepidolite *see* 2008, 5520, 8282
Lepidopterans *see* 1910
Lepirudin *see* 4718
Leponex [Novartis] *see* 2423
Leptandra, 5442
Leptilan [Dolorgiet] *see* 9913
Leptin, 5443
Leptomycin B, 5444
Leptophos, 5445
Leptospermone *see* 5912
Leptryl [Bellon] *see* 7168
Lercanidipine, 5446
Lerdip [Recordati] *see* 5446
Lergefin [Larma] *see* 1799
Lergigan [Recip] *see* 7786
Lergine *see* 7763
Lergoban [3M Pharma] *see* 3331
Lergobine [3M Pharma] *see* 3331
Leritine [Merck & Co.] *see* 658
Lescodil [Zdravlje] *see* 6495
Lescol [Novartis] *see* 4218
Lesopitron, 5447
Lespedin *see* 5274
Lesser Centaury *see* 1969
Lestid [Pfizer] *see* 2475
Leteprinim, 5448
Lethelmin *see* 7252

Lethidrone [Burroughs Wellcome] *see* 6361

Letosteine, 5449

Letrozole, 5450

LETS *see* 4075

Lettuce Opium *see* 5344

Letusin *see* 5469

Leu *see* 5451

Leu-8 *see* 8426

Leucaenine *see* 6199

Leucaenol *see* 6199

Leu-Cam Proteins *see* 4988

Leucarsone *see* 1786

Leucenine *see* 6199

Leucenol *see* 6199

Leuchtenbergite *see* 350

Leucine, 5451

L-Leucine *see* 5451

23-L-Leucinecolony-Stimulating Factor 2 (Human Clone pHG25 Protein Moiety) *see* 4538

Leucine[5]-enkephalin *see* 3572

6-D-Leucine-9-(*N*-ethyl-L-prolinamide)-10-deglycinamideluteinizing Hormone-releasing Factor (Pig) *see* 5457

6-L-Leucine Sporidesmolide I *see* 8765

1-L-Leucine-2-L-threonine-63-desulfohirudin (*Hirudo Medicinalis* Isoform HV1) *see* 4718

Leuco-4 *see* 152

Leucoalizarin *see* 688

Leucocyanidin, 5452

Leucocyanidol *see* 5452

Leucodinine *see* 6337

Leucoharmine *see* 4616

Leucokinin *see* 9809

Leucoline *see* 8068

Leucomalachite Green *see* 5699

Leucomax [Schering-Plough] *see* 4538

Leucomycin A$_1$ *see* 5453

Leucomycin A$_3$ *see* 5267

Leucomycins, 5453

Leucomycin V 3-Acetate 4^B-(3-Methylbutanoate) *see* 5267

Leucomycin V 4B-Butanoate 3B-Propanoate *see* 8250

Leucomycin V 3^B,9-Diacetate 3,4^B-Dipropanoate *see* 6204

Leucomycin V 3,4^B-Dipropanoate *see* 6183

Leucophor R *see* 1315

Leucopterin, 5454

Leucosar [Adria] *see* 4222

Leucotrofina [Ellem] *see* 9402

Leucovorin *see* 4222

Leucovorin [Lederle] *see* 4222

(D-Leu^6)-des-Gly^{10}-LH-RH-ethylamide *see* 5457

Leu^5-E *see* 3572

Leu^5-Enkephalin *see* 3572

Leukaemomycin C *see* 2832

Leukeran [GSK] *see* 2073

Leukerin *see* 5871

Leukine [Immunex] *see* 4538

Leukochthol *see* 4885

Leukocyte Adhesion Molecules *see* 4988

Leukocyte Elastase *see* 3535

Leukocyte-Endothelial Cell Adhesion Molecule-1 *see* 8426

Leukocyte Integrins *see* 4988

Leukocyte Interferon *see* 4990

Leukocytic Endogenous Mediator *see* 4993

Leukomycin-N [Bayer] *see* 909

Leukoprol [Morinaga] *see* 5646

LeukoScan [Immunomedics] *see* 8895

Leukotriene A *see* 5455

Leukotriene A$_4$ *see* 5455

Leukotriene B *see* 5455

Leukotriene B$_4$ *see* 5455

Leukotriene C *see* 5455

Leukotriene C$_1$ *see* 5455

Leukotriene C$_4$ *see* 5455

Leukotriene D *see* 5455

Leukotriene D$_4$ *see* 5455

Leukotriene E *see* 5455

Leukotriene E$_4$ *see* 5455

Leukotrienes, 5455

Leunase [Kyowa] *see* 836

Leupeptin Ac-LL *see* 5456

Leupeptin Pr-LL *see* 5456

Leupeptins, 5456

Leuplin [Takeda] *see* 5457

Leuprolide, 5457

Leuprolide Acetate *see* 5457

Leuprorelin *see* 5457

Leurocristine *see* 9986

Leustatin [Ortho Biotech] *see* 2337

LeuTech [Palatin] *see* 9100

Leutrol [Abbott] *see* 10124

Levacecarnine Hydrochloride *see* 84

Levacide [Norbrook] *see* 5459

Levadin [Univet] *see* 5459

Levalbuterol *see* 216

Levallorphan, 5458

Levamfetamine *see* 582

Levamisole, 5459

Levamphetamine *see* 582

Levant Wormseed *see* 8359

Levanxene [Montedison] *see* 9133

Levanxol [Montedison] *see* 9133

Levaquin [Ortho-McNeil] *see* 6771

Levarterenol *see* 6695

Levarterenol Bitartrate *see* 6695

Levasole [Mallinckrodt] *see* 5459

Levatol [Schwarz] *see* 7082

Levaxin [Nycomed] *see* 9415

Levcromakalim, 5460

Levemir [Novo] *see* 4983

Levetiracetam, 5461

Levitra [Bayer] *see* 9935

Levlen [Berlex] *see* 6704

Levobren [Knoll] *see* 8989

Levobunolol, 5462

Levobupivacaine *see* 1495

Levocabastine, 5463

Levocarbinoxamine *see* 1799

Levocarnil [Sigma-Tau] *see* 1849

Levocarnitine *see* 1849

Levocarnitine Chloride *see* 1849

Levocetirizine *see* 2022

Levocetirizine Hydrochloride *see* 2022

Levocitrol [Firmenich] *see* 2330

Levocycline *see* 8252

Levodopa, 5464

Levo-Dromoran *see* 5470

Levodropropizine *see* 3452

Levoglucosenone, 5465

Levoglutamina *see* 4471

Levoleucovorin Calcium *see* 4222

Levomenol *see* 1241

Levomeprazine *see* 5986

Levomepromazine *see* 5986

Levomethadone Hydrochloride *see* 5944

Levomethadyl Acetate, 5466

Levomethorphan Hydrobromide *see* 8091

Levomoprolol *see* 6264

Levonelle [Schering AG] *see* 6704

Levonordefrin *see* 6692

Levonorgestrel *see* 6704

Levonorgestrel 3-Oxime *see* 6694

Levonova [Schering AG] *see* 6704

Levopa [ICN] *see* 5464

Levophacetoperane, 5467

Levophed [Winthrop] *see* 6695

Levophta [Chauvin] *see* 5463

Levopimaric Acid, 5468

Levopraid [Ravizza] *see* 8989

Levoprome [Lederle] *see* 5986

Levopropoxyphene, 5469

Levopropoxyphene Napsylate *see* 5469

Levopropylcillin *see* 7817

Levorenin *see* 3619

Levorin *see* 1740

Levorin A$_2$ *see* 1740

Levormeloxifene *see* 1971

Levorotatory Lactic Acid *see* 5335

Levorphan *see* 5470

Levorphanol, 5470

Levosalbutamol *see* 216

Levosimendan, 5471

Levosulpiride *see* 8989

Levotartaric Acid *see* 9068

Levotensin [Simes] *see* 6264

Levothroid [Forest] *see* 9415

Levothym [Lundbeck] *see* 4847

Levothyrox [Merck-Clévenot] *see* 9415

Levothyroxine *see* 9415

Levothyroxine Sodium *see* 9415

Lévotonine [Pan Medica] *see* 4847

Levotuss [Dompé] *see* 3452

Levovermax [Virbac] *see* 5459

Levovist [Schering] *see* 4335

Levoxadrol Hydrochloride *see* 3299

Levoxan [Cutter] *see* 3299

Levoxyl [Jones] *see* 9415

Levsin [Kremers-Urban] *see* 4858

Levugen *see* 4273

Levulan [Dusa] *see* 446

Levulinic Acid, 5472

Levulinic Acid Calcium Salt *see* 1679

Levulose *see* 4273

Levynite *see* 1648

Lewisite *see* 3062

Lexapro [Forest] *see* 2318

Lexibiotico [Llano] *see* 1974

Lexinor [Astra] *see* 6700

Lexipafant, 5473

Lexiva [GSK] *see* 4250

Lexobene [Merckle] *see* 3081

Lexomil [Roche] *see* 1385

Lexone [DuPont] *see* 6154

Lexotan [Roche] *see* 1385

Lexotanil [Roche] *see* 1385

Lexus [DuPont] *see* 4195

LF-178 *see* 3978

LFA-2043 *see* 5077

1-92-LFA-3 (Antigen) (Human) Fusion Protein with Immunoglobulin G1 (Human Hinge-C$_H$2-C$_H$3 γ1-Chain), Dimer *see* 227

LFA3TIP *see* 227

LG-152 *see* 5790

LG-11457 *see* 3710

LG-30158 *see* 8245

LGD-1057 *see* 249

LGD-1069 *see* 1194

LH *see* 5613
LH-RF *see* 5474
LH-RH, 5474
LH-RH/FSH-RH *see* 5474
Liarozole, 5475
Liatris, 5476
Liazal [Janssen] *see* 5475
Libanil [APS] *see* 4478
Libeprosta [Pierre Fabre] *see* 8388
Liberty [Bayer CropSci.] *see* 7339
Libethenite *see* 2648
Libexin [Chinoin] *see* 7736
Libratar [UCB] *see* 2080
Libritabs [Roche] *see* 2084
Librium [Roche] *see* 2084
Licain [DeltaSelect] *see* 5482
Licareol *see* 5495
Licarpin [Allergan] *see* 7424
Licheniformins, 5477
Lichenin, 5478
Licochalcone A *see* 5479
Licochalcone B *see* 5479
Licochalcone C *see* 5479
Licochalcone D *see* 5479
Licochalcones, 5479
Licofelone, 5480
Licorice *see* 4504
Lidakol [Avanir] *see* 3399
Lidamidine, 5481
Lidanar [Sandoz] *see* 5910
Lidanil [Sandoz] *see* 5910
Lidaprim [Nycomed] *see* 8920
Lidarral [Rorer] *see* 5481
Liden *see* 5184
Lidepran *see* 5467
Lidesthesin [Ritsert] *see* 5482
Lidex [Syntex] *see* 4151
Lidocaine, 5482
Lidoderm [Hind] *see* 5482
Lidofast [Angelini] *see* 5482
Lidofenin, 5483
Lidoflazine, 5484
Lidoject [Hexal] *see* 5482
Lidone [Abbott] *see* 6233
LidoPosterine [Kade] *see* 5482
Lidrian [Baxter] *see* 5482
Life [SIT] *see* 7996
Life Root *see* 8450
Lifril [Kissei] *see* 9112
Lighter [Sanonda] *see* 5172
Light Green N *see* 5699
Light Green SF Yellowish, 5485
Lightning Fast *see* 3615
Light Oil of Camphor *see* 6780
Light Spar *see* 1706
Lignans, 5486
Lignin, 5487
Lignite Wax *see* 6257
Lignocaine *see* 5482
Lignocaine Benzyl Benzoate *see* 2891
Lignoceric Acid, 5488
Lignum Vitae *see* 4552
Ligroin, 5489
Ligustrin *see* 9016
Likinozym [Kaigai] *see* 5640
Likuden [HMR] *see* 4549
Lilacillin [Takeda] *see* 8890
Lilacin *see* 9016
Lilly 35483 *see* 2754
Lilly 36352 *see* 9686
Lilly 53838 *see* 3980
Lilly 69323 *see* 3980
Lilly 99170 *see* 754
Lily of the Valley *see* 2511
Liman [Kali-Chemie] *see* 9148

Limaprost, 5490
Limas [Taisho] *see* 5527
Lima Wood *see* 7181
Limber [Sumitomo] *see* 4295
Limbial [Chiesi] *see* 6926
Limclair [Sinclair] *see* 3517
Lime *see* 1686
Limestone, 5491
Limettin, 5492
Limonene, 5493
Limonin, 5494
Limonite *see* 4025
Limonoic Acid Di-δ-lactone *see* 5494
Limonoic Acid 3,19:16,17-Dilactone *see* 5494
Limovan [Aventis] *see* 10193
Limpidex [Sigma-Tau] *see* 5362
LIN-1418 *see* 8994
Linalol *see* 5495
Linalool, 5495
Linalyl Acetate, 5496
Linamarin, 5497
Linarigenin-glucoside *see* 5498
Linarin, 5498
Linaris [R.A.N.] *see* 8918
Linatine, 5499
Lincocin [Pharmacia & Upjohn] *see* 5500
Lincoln Bean *see* 8730
Lincolnensin *see* 5500
Lincomix [Pharmacia & Upjohn] *see* 5500
Lincomycin, 5500
Linctussal *see* 8608
Lindane, 5501
Linden Tree *see* 1007
Lindlar Catalyst, 5502
Lindol [Stauffer] *see* 9763
Lindoxyl [Lindopharm] *see* 386
Linear Gramicidins *see* 4532
Lineatin, 5503
4,6,6-Lineatin *see* 5503
Linezolid, 5504
Lingraine [Sanofi-Synthelabo] *see* 3661
Linnaeite *see* 2427
Linodil [Sanofi Winthrop] *see* 4979
Linoleic Acid, 5505
9,12-Linoleic Acid *see* 5505
Linolenic Acid, 5506
α-Linolenic Acid *see* 5506
γ-Linolenic Acid, 5507
Linolexamide *see* 5505
Linolic Acid *see* 5505
Linomide [Pfizer] *see* 8259
Linseed, 5508
Linton [Yoshitomi] *see* 4598
Lintox [Siapa] *see* 5501
Lintrin *see* 6408
Linum *see* 5508
Linurex [Makhteshim-Agan] *see* 5509
Linuron, 5509
Linyl [Roussel Diamant] *see* 7262
Liometacen [Chiesi] *see* 4968
Lion's Tooth *see* 9059
Lioresal [Novartis] *see* 937
Liosol [Maggioni] *see* 10071
Liothyronine, 5510
Liothyronine Sodium *see* 5510
Lioxone *see* 7971
Lipamone *see* 3104
Lipan *see* 3279
Lipanor [Winthrop] *see* 2313
Lipanthyl [Fournier] *see* 3978
Lipantil [Fournier] *see* 3978
Liparon [Finadiet] *see* 2843
Lipase, 5511
Lipaxan [Italfarmaco] *see* 4218

Lipex [Elea] *see* 7555
Liphadione [Lipha] *see* 2152
Lipidil [Ibirn] *see* 3978
Lipid-mobilizing Hormone *see* 5513
Lipiodol [Guerbet] *see* 5024
Lipitor [Parke-Davis] *see* 864
Liple [Mitsubishi] *see* 7876
Lipobay [Bayer] *see* 1993
Lipoclar [Crinos] *see* 3978
Lipoclin [Sumitomo] *see* 2357
Lipocol [Lipo] *see* 7577
Lipocol C-20 [Lipo] *see* 7577
Lipocortin *see* 676
Lipodel [Delalande] *see* 7012
Lipofene [Teofarma] *see* 3978
Lipoglutaren [Ausonia] *see* 5808
Lipo-Hepin [3M Pharma] *see* 4653
α-Lipoic Acid *see* 9326
Lipolytic Hormone *see* 5513
Lipo-Merz [Merz] *see* 3877
Liponorm [Gentili] *see* 8539
Lipopeg [Lipo] *see* 7578
Lipopeg 4-S [Lipo] *see* 7578
Lipoprotein-associated Coagulation Inhibitor *see* 9467
Lipoprotein Lipase, 5512
Liposit [SIT] *see* 3978
Liposolvin [Tosi] *see* 8537
Liposorb O-20 [Lipo] *see* 7582
Lipostat [BMS] *see* 7714
Lipotril *see* 2206
Lipotrophin *see* 5513
Lipotropic Hormone, 5513
Lipotropin *see* 5513
β-Lipotropin (61-91) *see* 3572
β-Lipotropin C-fragment *see* 3572
Lipozid [Pfizer] *see* 4388
Liprevil [Schwarz] *see* 7714
Liprinal [BMS] *see* 2377
Liprodène [Farlamedia] *see* 7133
Liprostin [Endovasc] *see* 7876
Lipsin [Fournier] *see* 3978
Lipur [Pfizer] *see* 4388
Liquaemin Sodium [Organon] *see* 4653
Liquamar [Organon] *see* 7259
Liquamycin [Pfizer] *see* 6976, 9196
Liquémin [Roche] *see* 4653
Liquiband [Medlogic] *see* 1565
Liquid Butter of Antimony *see* 708
Liquid Lanolin *see* 5358
Liquid Paraffin *see* 7186
Liquid Rosin *see* 9040
Liquid Silver *see* 5898
Liquifilm [Allergan] *see* 7585
LiquiVent [Alliance] *see* 7156
Liquorice *see* 4504
LIR-1660 *see* 9948
Liraglutide, 5514
Liranaftate, 5515
Liranol [Wyeth] *see* 7783
Lironox *see* 2796
Lisagal *see* 6974
Liserdol [Farmitalia] *see* 5937
Lisino [Essex] *see* 5578
Lisinopril, 5516
Lisium [Brunton] *see* 2091
Liskantin [Desitin] *see* 7746
Liskonum [GSK] *see* 5527
Lisofylline, 5517
Lisomucil [Sanofi-Synthelabo] *see* 1802
Lisozima [SPA] *see* 5640
Lispamol [Specia] *see* 467
Lispine [Nippon Chemiphar] *see* 3360
Lissamine Green SF [Zeneca] *see* 5485
Lissapol *see* 4367

Lissephen [Abbott] see 5850
Lissolamine V see 2025
Listenon see 8875
Listrocol [Farmitalia] see 2766
Lisuride, 5518
Lita [Opta], 5519
Litalir [BMS] see 4848
Litarex [Dumex] see 5530
Litec [Novartis] see 7515
Litesse [Pfizer] see 7565
Lithamide see 5522
Lithane [Bayer] see 5527
Litharge see 5413
Lithicarb [Aspen] see 5527
Lithiodiisopropylamine see 3196
Lithiophor [Vifor] see 5541
Lithium, 5520
Lithium Acetate, 5521
Lithium Alanate see 349
Lithium Aluminohydride see 349
Lithium Aluminum Hydride see 349
Lithium Amide, 5522
Lithium Benzoate, 5523
Lithium Biborate see 5524
Lithium Borate, 5524
Lithium Borohydride, 5525
Lithium Bromide, 5526
Lithium Carbonate, 5527
Lithium Chloride, 5528
Lithium Chromate(VI), 5529
Lithium Citrate, 5530
Lithium Diisopropylamide see 3196
Lithium-Duriles [Pharma-Stern] see 5541
Lithium Fluoborate see 5543
Lithium Fluoride, 5531
Lithium Fluoroboride see 5543
Lithium Formate, 5532
Lithium Hydrate see 5534
Lithium Hydride, 5533
Lithium (T-4)-Hydrotris(1-methylpro-
    pyl)borate(1−) see 8427
Lithium Hydroxide, 5534
Lithium Iodide, 5535
Lithium Metasilicate see 5540
Lithium Nitrate, 5536
Lithium Oxalate, 5537
Lithium Oxide, 5538
Lithium Perchlorate, 5539
Lithium Platinocyanide see 5542
Lithium Silicate, 5540
Lithium Sulfate, 5541
Lithium Tetraborate see 5524
Lithium Tetracyanoplatinate(II), 5542
Lithium Tetrafluoroborate, 5543
Lithium Tetrahydroaluminate see 349
Lithium Tetrahydroborate see 5525
Lithium Tri-sec-butylborohydride see
    8427
Lithium Triethylborohydride, 5544
(T-4)-Lithium Triethylhydroborate(1−)
    see 5544
Lithobid [Solvay] see 5527
Lithocholic Acid, 5545
Lithographic Stone see 5491
Lithol see 4885
Lithonate S [Rowell] see 5530
Lithopone, 5546
Lithostat [Mission Pharmacal] see 63
Liticon [Lagap] see 7121
Litlure A see 7769
Litmomycin see 4534
Litmus, 5547
Litosmil [Evans] see 3297
Litsoeine see 5388
Little Water see 10028

Litursol [Alfa] see 9889
Livalfa [Mitsubishi] see 9765
Livalo [Kowa] see 7508
Livazone [Specia] see 9290
Liver Lactobacillus Casei Factor see 4221
Liver of Lime see 1707
Liver of Sulfur see 8977
Liver Starch see 4496
Livetins, 5548
Livial [Organon] see 9427
Liviclina [Sierochimica] see 1917
Livonal see 3768
Livostin [Novartis] see 5463
Lixacol [Schering-Plough] see 5904
Lixidol [Farmitalia] see 5306
LJ-48 see 5785
LJ-206 see 1802
LJC-10141 see 3951
LJC-10305 see 1955
LJC-10627 see 1197
LJP-394 see 6
L-Kininogen see 5312
LL-1530 see 6347
LL-1558 see 9416
LL-1656 see 1475
LL-AV290 see 889
LLD Factor see 10014
LL-E33288 see 1715
LLF see 3926
LL-F-28249α see 6444
Lloncefal [Castillon] see 1979
Llonexina [Castillon] see 1974
LM-001 see 3951
LM-91 see 2152
LM-123 see 4134
LM-192 see 10003
LM-208 see 8083
LM-209 see 5864
LM-280 see 5009
LM-427 see 8213
LM-637 see 1382
LM-2219 see 3139
LM-2717 see 2359
LM-2909 see 2890
LM-5008 see 4930
LMD see 2948
LMWD see 2948
LN-107 see 1448
Lobak see 2106
Lobamine [Lobica] see 5975
Lobaplatin, 5549
Lobelia, 5550
Lobelidine see 5551
Lobeline, 5551
α-Lobeline see 5551
Lobenzarit, 5552
Lobivon [Menarini] see 6432
Locabiotal [Servier] see 4313
Locacorten [Novartis] see 4138
Localyn [Syntex] see 4150
Locapred [Fabre] see 2928
Locatop [Fabre] see 2928
Loceryl [Roche] see 573
Lochnericine, 5553
Locilex [Magainin] see 7193
Lock-On [Dow AgroSci.] see 2189
Locoid [Yamanouchi] see 4787
Locorten [Novartis] see 4138
Locron [Hoechst] see 343
Locust Bean Gum, 5554
Lodalès [Sanofi-Synthelabo] see 8539
Loderix [Egis] see 8472
Lodine [Wyeth] see 3874
Lodopin [Fujisawa] see 10197
Lodosyn [Merck & Co.] see 1797

Lodoxamide, 5555
Lodoxamide Ethyl see 5555
Lodoxamide Trometamol see 5555
Lodoxamide Tromethamine see 5555
Loestrin [Warner-Lambert] see 6697
Lofentanil, 5556
Lofepramine, 5557
Lofetensin [Nattermann] see 5558
Lofexidine, 5558
Loflucarban, 5559
Lofoxin [Locatelli] see 4254
Loftan [GSK] see 216
Lofton [Abbott] see 1475
Loftyl [Abbott] see 1475
Loganin, 5560
Logiparin [Novo] see 9450
Logna [Tanabe] see 2348
Logran [Syngenta] see 9600
Logwood see 4638
Logynon [Schering AG] see 6704
Lokarin see 3208
Loline, 5561
Lomadine [M & B] see 7208
Lomapect [TAD] see 7736
Lomebact [Shionogi] see 5562
Lomefloxacin, 5562
Lomerizine, 5563
Lomeron [Lilly] see 10056
Lomexin [Recordati] see 4005
Lomir [Novartis] see 5240
Lomotil [Searle] see 3313
Lomper [Esteve] see 5768
Lomudal [Sanofi-Aventis] see 2590
Lomupren [Sanofi-Aventis] see 2590
Lomusol [Sanofi-Aventis] see 2590
Lomustine, 5564
LON-798 see 4561
Lonafarnib, 5565
Lonasen [Dainippon] see 1319
Lonavar [Searle] see 6921
Lonazolac, 5566
Londax [DuPont] see 1052
Londomin [Taiyo] see 9017
Londomycin see 5943
Longastatin [Italfarmaco] see 6762
Longatren [Bayer] see 910
Longdigox [Trommsdorff] see 3167
Longestrol [Syntex] see 1448
Longheparin see 4653
Longicid [Chassot] see 3116
Longifene [UCB] see 1464
Longifolene, 5567
α-Longilobine see 8452
β-Longilobine see 8167
Longum [Farmitalia] see 8910
Lonidamine, 5568
Loniten [Pfizer] see 6203
Lonmiel [Teikoku] see 1038
Lonolox [Pfizer] see 6203
Lonomycins, 5569
Lontermin [Lek] see 7759
Lontrel [Dow AgroSci.] see 2400
Looplure, 5570
Looser [Kaken] see 1496
Lo/Ovral [Wyeth] see 6704
Lopantrol [Janssen] see 5580
Lopatol [Novartis] see 6633
Lopemid [Gentili] see 5571
Lopemin [Dainippon] see 5571
Loperamide, 5571
Loperyl [Zambeletti] see 5571
Lophotoxin, 5572
Lopid [Pfizer] see 4388
Lopinavir, 5573
Lopirin [BMS] see 1774

Luteolas [Serono] *see* 3860
Luteolin, 5614
Luteolin-4'-methyl Ether *see* 3296
Luteonorm [Serono] *see* 3860
Luteotropic Hormone *see* 7779
Luteotropin *see* 7779
Luteran [Cassenne] *see* 2102
Lutestral [Cassenne] *see* 2102
Lutetium, 5615
Lutetium Texaphyrin *see* 6282
Lu-Tex *see* 6282
α,α'-Lutidin *see* 5616
"β-Lutidine" *see* 3848
2,6-Lutidine, 5616
Lutionex [Roussel Diamant] *see* 2888
Luto-Metrodiol *see* 3860
Lutrelef [Ferring] *see* 5474
Lutrepulse [Ortho] *see* 5474
Lutrin [Pharmacyclics] *see* 6282
Luvatren [Cilag-Chemie] *see* 6263
Luveris [Serono] *see* 5613
Luviskol [BASF] *see* 7697
Luvox [Solvay] *see* 4219
Luxazone [Allergan] *see* 2943
Luxoben [Chinoin] *see* 9421
Luxon *see* 4605
LVD *see* 2948
LY-141B *see* 7162
LY-12735 *see* 6286
LY-031537 *see* 8092
LY-048740 *see* 887
LY-61017 *see* 3951
LY-061188 *see* 1974
LY-097964 *see* 1923
LY-099094 *see* 9987
LY-109514 *see* 6342
LY-110140 *see* 4185
LY-122772 *see* 3601
LY-127809 *see* 7162
LY-135837 *see* 4937
LY-139037 *see* 6660
LY-139481 *see* 8098
LY-139603 *see* 863
LY-146032 *see* 2823
LY-156758 *see* 8098
LY-163892 Monohydrate *see* 5576
LY-170053 *see* 6822
LY-177370 *see* 9439
LY-177837 *see* 8716
LY-188011 *see* 4386
LY-188695 *see* 3557
LY-210448 *see* 2821
LY-231514 *see* 7077
LY-232105 *see* 8750
LY-237216 *see* 3354
LY-246708 *see* 10056
LY-246736 *see* 372
LY-248686 *see* 3465
LY-253351 *see* 9049
LY-275585 *see* 4987
LY-300164 *see* 9032
LY-303366 *see* 656
LY-333328 *see* 6868
LY-333531 *see* 8290
LY-335348 *see* 2893
LY-335979 *see* 10196
LY-353381 *see* 820
LY-355703 *see* 2607
LY-900003 *see* 755
LY-2148568 *see* 3914
Lyapolate Sodium, 5617
Lycaconitine *see* 5618
Lycanol *see* 4507
Lycine *see* 1179
Lycoctonine, 5618

Lycodine, 5619
Lycopene, 5620
(*all-trans*)-Lycopene *see* 5620
(*all-trans*)-Lycopene-16,16'-diol *see* 5621
(*all-trans*)-Lycopen-16-ol *see* 5627
Lycopersicin *see* 9545
Lycophyll, 5621
Lycopodine, 5622
Lycopodium, 5623
Lycopodium Seed (Spores) *see* 5623
Lycopus, 5624
Lycoramine, 5625
Lycoremine *see* 4340
Lycorine, 5626
Lycoxanthin, 5627
Lycra [DuPont] *see* 8733
Lyeton [Leben's] *see* 9889
Lyman [Drossapharm] *see* 309
Lymecycline, 5628
Lymphazurin [Pharmascience] *see* 8987
Lymphoblastoid Interferon *see* 4990
LymphoCide [Immunomedics] *see* 3631
Lymphocyte Activating Factor *see* 4993
Lymphocyte Adhesion Molecule-1 *see* 8426
Lymphocyte Mitogenic Factor *see* 4994
Lymphotoxin 9812
Lynamine [Memphis] *see* 5309
Lyndiol [Organon] *see* 5629
Lynestrenol, 5629
Lynoral [Organon] *see* 3734
Lynx [Bayer CropSci.] *see* 9092
Lyogen [Promonta Lundbeck] *see* 4189
Lyphocin [Fujisawa] *see* 9929
Lypressin, 5630
Lyrica [Pfizer] *see* 7725
Lys *see* 5636
Lysal [Gellini] *see* 5637
Lysalbinic Acid, 5631
Lysalgo [SIT] *see* 5798
Lysanxia [Lynapharm] *see* 7715
[Lys(B3),Glu(B29)]-insulin (Human) *see* 4985
[Lys(B28),Pro(B29)]-insulin (Human) *see* 4987
Lyseen [Novartis] *see* 7741
Lysenyl [Spofa] *see* 5518
Lysergamide, 5632
Lysergic Acid, 5633
Lysergic Acid Amide *see* 5632
D-Lysergic Acid (+)-Butanolamide-(2) *see* 6070
D-Lysergic Acid Diethylamide *see* 5634
d-Lysergic Acid-*d*-1-hydroxybutylamide-2 *see* 6070
D-Lysergic Acid D-Propanolamide *see* 3654
D-Lysergic Acid L-2-Propanolamide *see* 3655
Lysergide, 5634
Lysergin [Toa Eiyo] *see* 3653
Lysergsäure Diethylamid *see* 5634
Lys²⁶(*N*ε-(γ-glutamyl-(*N*α-hexadecanoyl)), Arg³⁴-GLP-1(7-37) *see* 5514
Lysidine, 5635
L-Lysine *see* 5636
Lysine, 5636
Lysine Acetylsalicylate, 5637
L-Lysine L-Glutamate, 5638
3ᴮ-L-Lysine-29ᴮ-L-glutamic Acid-insulin (Human) *see* 4985
L-Lysine, Homopolymer *see* 7571
7-L-Lysine-8-L-lysine-10-L-lysine-18-L-lysine-19-*de*-L-glutamic Acid-21-L-leucine-23-L-lysinamide Magainin I *see* 7193

DL-Lysine Mono[2-(acetyloxy)benzoate] *see* 5637
Lysine Monosalicylate Acetate *see* 5637
28ᴮ-L-Lysine-29ᴮ-L-prolineinsulin (Human) *see* 4987
8-L-Lysinevasopressin *see* 5630
N-Lysinomethyltetracycline *see* 5628
Lysivane [M & B] *see* 3747
Lysmucol [Schering] *see* 8567
Lysodren [Calbiochem] *see* 6216
Lysofon [Lafon] *see* 322
"Lysophosphatidal Choline" *see* 7519
"Lysophosphatidal Ethanolamine" *see* 7519
Lysoplasmalogens *see* 7519
Lysortine [Adrian-Marinier] *see* 5636
Lysosomal α-Glucosidase *see* 108
Lysostaphin, 5639
Lysovir [Alliance] *see* 374
Lysozyme, 5640
Lyspafen [Cilag-Chemie] *see* 3136
Lysᴮ²⁹-tetradecanoyl, Des(B30)-insulin *see* 4983
Lysthenon [Nycomed] *see* 8875
Lysuride *see* 5518
Lysuron [Roche] *see* 279
*N*²-L-Lysylbradykinin *see* 5278
Lytos [Boehringer, Mann.] *see* 2371
D-Lyxose, 5641
α-D-Lyxose *see* 5641
M & B 693 *see* 8938
M & B 736 *see* 7208
M & B 744 *see* 8816
M & B 760 *see* 8943
M & B 782 *see* 7797
M & B 800 *see* 7115
M & B 2050A *see* 7132
M & B 2207 *see* 8874
M & B 4180 A *see* 5183
M & B 4486 *see* 7080
M & B 8430 *see* 2404
M & B 9057 *see* 857
M & B 15497 *see* 2854
M & B 17803A *see* 19
M & B 38544 *see* 3144
M & B 39831 *see* 9139
M-14 *see* 8215
M-19-Q *see* 8250
M-99 *see* 3888
M-141 *see* 8739
M-183 *see* 3888
M-285 *see* 2769
M-732 *see* 5515
M-1028 *see* 4600
M-1650 *see* 2879
M-4209 *see* 1806
M-4365A2 *see* 8261
M-4888 *see* 2090
M-5050 *see* 3340
M-5943 *see* 2184
M-7555 *see* 8052
M-9834 *see* 1030
M-10580 *see* 2721
M-14360 *see* 9193
M-73101 *see* 3562
M-139603 *see* 9248
2-M-4-A *see* 46
Maalox Quick Dissolve [Novartis] *see* 1657
Maalox Regular Strength [Novartis] *see* 1657
MabCampath [Schering AG] *see* 228
Mabthera [Roche] *see* 8239
Mabuterol, 5642
Macasirool [Hishiyama] *see* 4309

Macassar Oil, 5643
Mace *see* 6729
MACH *see* 1886
Mach 2 [Dow AgroSci.] *see* 4595
Machete [Monsanto] *see* 1508
Machiline 2459
Mackreazid *see* 2680
Macladin [Guidotti] *see* 2339
Macleyine *see* 7896
Maclicine [Christiaens] *see* 3084
Maclurin, 5644
Macmiror [Poli] *see* 6532
Macol [PPG] *see* 7577
Macquer's Salt *see* 7607
Macrobid [Procter & Gamble] *see* 6599
Macrobin *see* 2413
Macrodantin [Eaton] *see* 6599
Macrodex [Pharmacia] *see* 2948
Macrofusine *see* 4289
Macrogol *see* 7568
Macrogol Ester 400 *see* 7578
Macrogol Fatty Acid Esters *see* 7578
Macrogol Fatty Alcohol Ethers *see* 7577
Macrogol Nonylphenyl Ether *see* 6677
Macromerine, 5645
Macrophage Colony-Stimulating Factor, 5646
Macrophage-derived Growth Factor *see* 4072
Macrophage-targeted β-Glucocerebrosidase *see* 243
Macugen [Eyetech] *see* 7068
Maculotoxin *see* 9246
MAD *see* 5950
Madar [Ravizza] *see* 6691
Maddrell's Salt, 5647
Madelen [Finadiet] *see* 6872
Maderan [Nycomed] *see* 8920
Madlexin [Meiji] *see* 1974
Madopar [Roche] *see* 1050
Madopark [Roche] *see* 1050
Madrine [Langley] *see* 5948
Maduramicin, 5648
Maduramycin *see* 5648
Mafatate [Torii] *see* 5649
Mafenide, 5649
Magainins, 5650
Magaldrate, 5651
Magan [Warren-Teed] *see* 5685
Magcal *see* 5677
Magell *see* 6170
Magenta *see* 5652
Magenta I, 5652
Maghemite *see* 4028
Maghen [Savio] *see* 7491
Magic Methyl [Aldrich] *see* 6075
Magic Acid [Cationics] *see* 4179
Magic Tan *see* 3182
Magisal *see* 5655
Magister [Margarita] *see* 3959
Magistery of Bismuth *see* 1284
Maglite [Marine Magnesium] *see* 5677
Magmilor [Poli] *see* 6532
Magnacide [Baker] *see* 128
Magnacort [Pfizer] *see* 4786
Magnafodipir Trisodium *see* 5722
Magnesia *see* 5677
Magnesia Usta *see* 5677
Magnesite *see* 5653, 5660
Magnesium, 5653
Magnesium Acetate, 5654
Magnesium Acetylsalicylate, 5655
Magnesium Aluminate Hydrate *see* 5651
Magnesium Aluminum Silicate *see* 350
Magnesium Amide, 5656

Magnesium Ammonium Chloride *see* 531
Magnesium Ammonium Phosphate Hexahydrate *see* 8854
Magnesium Aspirin *see* 5655
Magnesium Benzoate, 5657
Magnesium Biphosphate *see* 5682
Magnesium Bis(monoperoxyphthalate) *see* 5673
Magnesium Borate, 5658
Magnesium Bromide, 5659
Magnesium Bromoglutamate *see* 4469
Magnesium Butyrate *see* 1593
Magnesium Carbonate Hydroxide, 5660
Magnesium Chlorate, 5661
Magnesium Chloride, 5662
Magnesium Citrate, 5663
Magnesium Clofibrate *see* 2378
Magnesium Diamide *see* 5656
Magnesium Diboride, 5664
Magnesium Diethyl *see* 3122
Magnesium Dioxide *see* 5680
Magnesium Diphenyl *see* 3327
Magnesium Fluoride, 5665
Magnesium Fluosilicate *see* 5668
Magnesium Formate, 5666
Magnesium Germanide, 5667
Magnesium Glucoheptonate *see* 4455
Magnesium Glucomonocarbonate *see* 4455
Magnesium Gluconate *see* 4456
Magnesium Glucosemonocarbonate *see* 4455
Magnesium Glutamate Hydrobromide *see* 4469
Magnesium Heparinate *see* 4653
Magnesium Hexafluorosilicate, 5668
Magnesium Hydrate *see* 5670
Magnesium Hydride, 5669
Magnesium Hydrogen Citrate *see* 5663
Magnesium Hydrogen Phosphate *see* 5681
Magnesium Hydroxide, 5670
Magnesium Hyposulfite *see* 5694
Magnesium Iodide, 5671
Magnesium Lactate, 5672
Magnesium Mesotrisilicate *see* 5687
Magnesium Metasilicate *see* 5687
Magnesium Monoperoxyphthalate, 5673
Magnesium Nitrate, 5674
Magnesium Oleate, 5675
Magnesium Orthosilicate *see* 5687
Magnesium Oxalate, 5676
Magnesium Oxide, 5677
Magnesium Pemoline *see* 7079
Magnesium Perchlorate, 5678
Magnesium Perhydrol *see* 5680
Magnesium Permanganate, 5679
Magnesium Peroxide, 5680
Magnesium Phosphate, Dibasic, 5681
Magnesium Phosphate, Monobasic, 5682
Magnesium Phosphate, Tribasic, 5683
Magnesium Pyrophosphate, 5684
Magnesium Salicylate, 5685
Magnesium Selenide, 5686
Magnesium Silicates, 5687
Magnesium Silicide, 5688
Magnesium Silicofluoride *see* 5668
Magnesium Stannide, 5689
Magnesium Stearate, 5690
Magnesium Sulfate, 5691
Magnesium Sulfite, 5692
Magnesium Sulfocyanate *see* 5693
Magnesium Superoxol *see* 5680
Magnesium Thiocyanate, 5693
Magnesium Thiosulfate, 5694

Magnesium Trisilicate *see* 5687
Magneson, 5695
Magnespirin *see* 5655
Magnetic Iron Oxide *see* 4040
Magnetite *see* 4040
Magnetkies *see* 4058
Magnevist [Schering AG] *see* 4327
Magnipen [Clin-Comar-Byla] *see* 5925
Magnofenyl *see* 6957
Magnoflorine, 5696
Magnogene *see* 5662
Magnolol, 5697
Magnophenyl *see* 6957
Magnopyrol [Abbott] *see* 3350
Magnosil [Polfa] *see* 5687
Magnosulf [Normark] *see* 5694
Magrilon [Sintyal] *see* 5762
Ma Huang *see* 3607
Maidenhair Tree *see* 4425
Maikohis [Nichiiko] *see* 2345
Maiorad [Rottapharm] *see* 9466
Maipedopa [Maipe] *see* 5464
Maitansine *see* 5761
Maitotoxin, 5698
Maize Oil *see* 2533
Maizena [CPC] *see* 8798
Majeptil [RPR] *see* 9357
Majudin *see* 1157
Maki [Lipha] *see* 1382
Makon *see* 6677
Malabar Nut *see* 159
Malachite *see* 2631
Malachite Green, 5699
Malachite Green G *see* 1374
Malamar 50 *see* 5700
Malaquin [Ahn Gook] *see* 2163
Malaria Pigment *see* 4649
Malaridine *see* 8005
Malaspray *see* 5700
Malathion, 5700
Malathon (obsolete) *see* 5700
Malayan Camphor *see* 1338
Malazide *see* 5705
Malcotran [Fisons] *see* 4730
Maleamic Acid, 5701
Maleanilic Acid, 5702
Male Fern *see* 848
Maleic Acid, 5703
Maleic Acid, Diethyl Ester *see* 3123
Maleic Acid Hydrazide *see* 5705
Maleic Acid Monoamide *see* 5701
Maleic Anhydride, 5704
Maleic Hydrazide, 5705
Male Shield-fern *see* 848
Maleuric Acid, 5706
Malexil [Ferrosan] *see* 3955
Malexin [BASF] *see* 6417
Maleylurea *see* 5706
Maliasin [Knoll] *see* 7860
Malic Acid, 5707
Maliner Kren *see* 4749
Malipuran [Heumann] *see* 1474
Malix [Bayer CropSci.] *see* 3574
Mallebrin [Krewel] *see* 336
Mallermin-F [Taiyo] *see* 2345
Mallorol [Novartis] *see* 9359
Mallotoxin *see* 8272
Mallow, 5708
Malocide [Aventis] *see* 7985
Malol *see* 9890
Malonaldehyde *see* 5709
Malonamide Nitrile *see* 2688
Malondialdehyde, 5709
Malonic Acid, 5710
Malonic Acid Cyclic Isopropylidene Ester *see* 5817

Malonic Acid Di-*tert*-butyl Ester *see* 3034
Malonic Acid Ethyl Ester Nitrile *see* 3786
Malonic Ester *see* 3823
Malonic Mononitrile *see* 2689
Malononitrile, 5711
Malononitrile Dimer *see* 480
Malononitrile Hydrazide *see* 2680
5,5'-[Malonylbis(methylimino)]bis-
    [*N*,*N*'-bis[2,3-dihydroxy-1-(hydroxy-
    methyl)propyl]-2,4,6-triiodo-
    isophthalamide] *see* 5065
Malonylurea *see* 963
Malotilate, 5712
Maltobiose *see* 5714
Maltol, 5713
Maltonic Acid *see* 4456
Maltos [Otsuka] *see* 5714
Maltose, 5714
Malt Sugar *see* 5714
Malvidin Chloride, 5715
Malvin *see* 5715
Malvoside *see* 5715
Mamalexin [Showa Yakuhin] *see* 1974
Mamallet-A [Showa] *see* 474
Mammacillin [Stricker] *see* 7097
Mammex *see* 6600
Mammotropin *see* 7779
Mamyzin [Boehringer, Ing.] *see* 7085
Manage [Monsanto] *see* 4602
Manage [Hokko] *see* 4909
Manchurian Bean *see* 8730
Mancona Bark *see* 8382
Mancozeb, 5716
Mandarin G *see* 6858
Mandate [Dow AgroSci.] *see* 9311
7-D-Mandelamido-3-(1-methyl-1,2,3,4-
    tetrazole-5-thiomethyl)-Δ³-cephem-
    4-carboxylic Acid *see* 1914
7-D-Mandelamido-3-[[(1-methyl-1*H*-tet-
    razol-5-yl)thio]methyl]-3-cephem-4-
    carboxylic Acid *see* 1914
7-Mandelamido-3-[[(1-methyl-1*H*-tetra-
    zol-5-yl)thio]methyl]-8-oxo-5-thia-1-
    azabicyclo[4.2.0]oct-2-ene-2-carboxylic
    Acid *see* 1914
(6*R*,7*R*)-7-[(*R*)-Mandelamido]-8-oxo-3-
    [[[1-(sulfomethyl)-1*H*-tetrazol-5-yl]-
    thio]methyl]-5-thia-1-azabicyclo-
    [4.2.0]oct-2-ene-2-carboxylic Acid *see*
    1929
Mandelamine [Warner-Chilcott] *see* 5966
Mandelic Acid, 5717
dl-Mandelic Acid *see* 5717
Mandelic Acid Ammonium Salt *see* 532
Mandelic Acid Isoamyl Ester, 5718
Mandelic Acid Isopentyl Ester *see* 5718
Mandelic Acid Nitrile *see* 5719
Mandelic Acid β-1,2,2,6-Tetramethyl-4-
    piperidyl Ester *see* 3897
Mandelic Acid 3,3,5-Trimethylcyclo-
    hexyl Ester *see* 2704
Mandelonitrile, 5719
Mandelonitrile-β-gentiobioside *see* 597
Mandelonitrile Glucoside, 5720
D-Mandelonitrile-β-D-glucosido-6-β-D-
    glucoside *see* 597
Mandelonitrile β-Glucuronide *see* 597
β-4-Mandeloyloxy-1,2,2,6-tetramethyl-
    piperidine *see* 3897
Mandelyltropeine *see* 4730
Mandenol *see* 3820
Mandokef [Lilly] *see* 1914
Mandol [Lilly] *see* 1914
Mandolsan [San Carlo] *see* 1914
Maneb, 5721

Maneon [Poli] *see* 409
Manerix [Roche] *see* 6226
Manex [Griffin] *see* 5721
Manexin *see* 5746
Mangafodipir, 5722
Manganblende *see* 5740
Manganese, 5723
Manganese Acetate, 5724
Manganese Benzoate *see* 1091
Manganese Binoxide *see* 5730
Manganese Bromide, 5725
Manganese Carbonate, 5726
Manganese Carbonyl, 5727
Manganese Chloride, 5728
Manganese Dibromide *see* 5725
Manganese Dichloride *see* 5728
Manganese Difluoride, 5729
Manganese Diiodide *see* 5732
Manganese Dioxide, 5730
Manganese Dipyridoxal Diphosphate *see*
    5722
Manganese(II)-*N*,*N*'-dipyridoxylethyl-
    enediamine-*N*,*N*'-diacetate-5,5-bis-
    (phosphonate) *see* 5722
Manganese Ethylenebis(dithiocar-
    bamate) (Polymeric) Complex with
    Zinc Salt *see* 5716
Manganese Fluoride *see* 5729
Manganese Green *see* 981
Manganese Hypophosphite, 5731
Manganese Iodide, 5732
Manganese Monosulfide *see* 5740
Manganese Nitrate, 5733
Manganese Oxalate, 5734
Manganese Oxide, 5735
Manganese Peroxide *see* 5730
Manganese Selenide, 5736
Manganese Sesquioxide, 5737
Manganese Silicate, 5738
Manganese Sulfate, 5739
Manganese Sulfide, 5740
Manganese Superoxide *see* 5730
Manganese Tetroxide *see* 5735
Manganese Trifluoride, 5741
Manganic Fluoride *see* 5741
Manganite *see* 5737
Manganjustite *see* 5738
Manganomanganic Oxide *see* 5735
Manganosite *see* 5723
Manganous Chloride *see* 5728
Manganous Ethylenebis[dithiocar-
    bamate] *see* 5721
Manganous Fluoride *see* 5729
Mangostin, 5742
Manicol *see* 5745
Manidipine, 5743
Maninil [Berlin-Chemie] *see* 4478
Maniol [Morishita] *see* 3311
Manna, 5744
Manna Sugar *see* 5745
Mannidex *see* 5745
Mannite *see* 5745
Mannitol, 5745
D-Mannitol *see* 5745
D-Mannitol Hexanitrate, 5746
Mannitol Nitrate *see* 5746
Mannitrin *see* 5746
L-Mannomethylose *see* 8172
D-Mannose, 5747
Mannose-terminated Human Placental
    Glucocerebrosidase *see* 243
Manoplax [Boots] *see* 4110
Mansil [Pfizer] *see* 6919
Mantadan [Boehringer, Ing.] *see* 374
Mantadine [Endo] *see* 374

Mantadix [BMS] *see* 374
Man-Tan *see* 3182
Manzate [Griffin] *see* 5716
Manzeb *see* 5716
Manzin [Crystal Chem.] *see* 5716
MAO *see* 6247
Maolate [Upjohn] *see* 2179
MAP *see* 5793
Mapeg [PPG] *see* 7578
Mapeg 400 MS [PPG] *see* 7578
Mapharsal *see* 6948
Mapharsen [Parke-Davis] *see* 6948
Mapharside *see* 6948
Maphenide *see* 5649
MAPO *see* 5936
Maposol [Procida] *see* 5949
Mappine *see* 1478
Maprofix *see* 4367
Maprotiline, 5748
Maratan [Ravizza] *see* 1296
Marathon [Olympic] *see* 4910
Maraviroc, 5749
Marbocyl [Vétoquinol] *see* 5750
Marbofloxacin, 5750
Marboran *see* 5977
Marcaine [AstraZeneca] *see* 1495
Marcoeritrex *see* 3683
Marcoumar [Roche] *see* 7259
Marcumar [Roche] *see* 7259
Maretin [Bayer] *see* 6354
Marevan [Goldshield] *see* 10038
Marezine [Himmel] *see* 2710
Marfanil *see* 5649
Margaric Acid, 5751
Margarite *see* 1648
Margatoxin, 5752
Margosa Tree *see* 6437
Maricolene *see* 2715
Marigold *see* 1713
Marijuana *see* 1749
Marimastat, 5753
Marinco C *see* 5660
Marinco H *see* 5670
Marindinin *see* 5287
Mariner [DuPont] *see* 1052
Marinol [Unimed] *see* 9209
Maripen [Biogal] *see* 7081
Markweed *see* 7549
Marlate [DuPont] *see* 5990
Marmelosin *see* 4925
Marme's Reagent *see* 7687
Marograstim *see* 4537
Marplan [Roche] *see* 5157
Marquis [Bayer] *see* 7589
Marrubiin, 5754
Marshal [FMC] *see* 1826
Marsh Gas *see* 5952
Marshite *see* 2662
Marshmallow *see* 317
Marsh Trefoil *see* 5842
Marsilid [Roche] *see* 5078
Marsin [Ikapharm] *see* 7237
Marsthine [Towa Yakuhin] *see* 2345
Martos-10 [Otsuka] *see* 5714
Marucotol [Maruko] *see* 5780
Marvelon 150/30 [Akzo] *see* 2926
Marvinol [Naugatuck] *see* 7586
Mary-bud *see* 1713
Maryland Pink *see* 8748
Marzine [GlaxoWellcome] *see* 2710
Masacin [Otsuka] *see* 7759
Mascagnite *see* 555
Maschitt [Showa Shinyaku] *see* 4781
Masdil [Esteve] *see* 3202
Masdiol *see* 5950

Masletine [Sioe] *see* 2345
Masmoran [Pfizer] *see* 4849
Masnidipine *see* 5446
Masoprocol *see* 6693
Masor [Formenti] *see* 8809
Maspiron [Sawai] *see* 6886
Massicot *see* 5413
Mast Cell Growth Factor *see* 8807
Masterfen [Dompé] *see* 9005
Masterid [Grünenthal] *see* 3448
Masteril [Syntex] *see* 3448
Masterone [Syntex] *see* 3448
Mastic, 5755
Mastiche *see* 5755
Mastimyxin [Chassot] *see* 7573
Mastisol *see* 5755
Mastix *see* 5755
Maté, 5756
Matacil [Bayer] *see* 433
Mataperro *see* 2496
Matico, 5757
Matric [Sankyou Agro] *see* 2218
Matricaria *see* 2041
Matricaria Oil *see* 2041
Matricarin, 5758
Matridine *see* 5759
Matridin-15-one *see* 5759
Matrine, 5759
Matrix [DuPont] *see* 8230
Matrol *see* 2102
Matromycin [Pfizer] *see* 6825
MATS *see* 6013
Matulane [Roche] *see* 7758
Maveral [Farmades] *see* 4219
Maverick [Monsanto] *see* 8965
Mavik [Abbott] *see* 9568
Mavrik [Zoecon] *see* 4217
4-MAX *see* 6018
Maxacalcitol, 5760
Maxair [3M Pharma] *see* 7489
Maxalt [Merck & Co.] *see* 8241
Maxamine [Maxim] *see* 4719
Maxaquin [Pharmacia] *see* 5562
Maxeran [Aventis] *see* 6143
Maxforce *see* 4765
Maxibolin [Organon] *see* 3805
Maxidex [Alcon] *see* 2943
Maxiflor [Allergan] *see* 3140
Maxilase [Sanofi Winthrop] *see* 599
Maxim [Syngenta] *see* 4129
Maxipen [Pfizer] *see* 7223
Maxipime [BMS] *see* 1922
Maxivate [Westwood] *see* 1180
Maxivent *see* 3438
Maxolon [GSK] *see* 6143
Maxtrex [Pharmacia] *see* 5985
Max-Uric [Labinca] *see* 1065
Maxus [Elanco] *see* 887
Mayapple *see* 7547
May Blossom *see* 2511
Maycor [Parke-Davis] *see* 5225
Maydol *see* 2533
Maygace [BMS] *see* 5805
May Lily *see* 2511
Maynar [Ferrer] *see* 146
May Pops *see* 7051
Maytansine, 5761
Mazicon [Roche] *see* 4135
Mazildene [Farmochim. Ital.] *see* 5762
Mazindol, 5762
Mazipredone, 5763
Mazola [CPC] *see* 2533
Mazun *see* 10101
MB-10064 *see* 1441
MB-10731 *see* 1441

MB-46030 *see* 4085
MBA *see* 5775
MBBT *see* 1294
MBC *see* 1791
4-MBC *see* 6027
MBLA *see* 5822
MBOCA *see* 6059
MBR-12325 *see* 5802
MBT *see* 5868
MBTS *see* 3370
MBU *see* 5939
3-MC *see* 6044
MC-838 *see* 6285
MC-903 *see* 1641
MC-1275 *see* 5760
MC-2188 *see* 2103
MC-4379 *see* 1208
MCA *see* 2112, 6046
MCAA *see* 5577
Mch5 *see* 1886
Mch6 *see* 1887
MCI *see* 6091
MCI-186 *see* 6713
MCI-196 *see* 2474
MCI-2016 *see* 1206
MCI-9038 *see* 779
MCMN *see* 8254
MCMT *see* 6223
McN-485 *see* 10199
McN-742 *see* 476
McN-822 *see* 6018
McN-1025 *see* 6687
McN-1210 *see* 7989
McN-2559 *see* 9518
McN-2559-21-98 *see* 9518
McN-4853 *see* 9547
McN-A-2833 *see* 7170
McN-A-2833-109 *see* 7170
McN-JR-4584 *see* 1048
McN-JR-7094 *see* 5484
McN-JR-8299 *see* 5459
McN-JR-15403-11 *see* 3136
McN-R-73-Z *see* 1799
McN-R-726-47 *see* 7554
McN-R-1967 *see* 3998
McN-X-181 *see* 9912
MCNU *see* 8109
MCP *see* 5764
MCPA, 5764
MCPBA *see* 5673
MCPP *see* 5784
M-CSF *see* 5646
MCT *see* 6250
MCW-275 *see* 6720
MD-76 *see* 5807
MD-141 *see* 3722
MD-805 *see* 779
MD-6753 *see* 2290
MD-67350 *see* 2291
MD-69276 *see* 9521
MD-370503 *see* 1021
MDA, 5765
MDE, 5766
MDEA *see* 5766
M-Det *see* 2856
MDGF *see* 4072
MDL-473 *see* 8219
MDL-507 *see* 9115
MDL-9918 *see* 9163
MDL-14042A *see* 5558
MDL-16455 *see* 4068
MDL-17043 *see* 3589
MDL-62198 *see* 8104
MDL-63397 *see* 2803
MDL-71754 *see* 9978

MDL-73147 *see* 3411
MDL-73147EF *see* 3411
MDMA, 5767
MDMH *see* 4831
MDP *see* 5792, 6305
MDP-Lys (L18) *see* 8253
MDS *see* 2951
ME-1206 *see* 1921
ME-1207 *see* 1921
ME-2906 *see* 9034
ME-3202 *see* 7129
ME-3625 *see* 6518
ME-3737 *see* 9441
MEA *see* 2779
Meadow Anemone *see* 7938
Meadow Clover *see* 9690
Meadow Crocus *see* 2472
Meadow Saffron *see* 2472
MEAP *see* 7341
Meat Sugar *see* 4978
Meaverin [Woelm] *see* 5859
Mebadin [Glaxo] *see* 2870
Meballymal Sodium *see* 8420
Mebaral [Winthrop] *see* 5854
Mebendazole, 5768
Mebenvet [Janssen] *see* 5768
Meberyt *see* 3687
Mebeverine, 5769
Mebhydroline, 5770
MeBmt, 5771
Mebonat [Boehringer, Mann.] *see* 2371
Mebrofenin, 5772
Mebron [Daiichi] *see* 3622
Mebrophenhydramine *see* 3556
Mebryl *see* 3556
Mebubarbital *see* 7130
Mebutamate, 5773
Mebutina [Formenti] *see* 5773
3-MECA *see* 6044
Mecadox [Pfizer] *see* 1780
Mecalmin [Yoshitomi] *see* 3311
Mecamine *see* 5774
Mecamylamine, 5774
Mecasermin *see* 4986
MeCbl *see* 6045
Mecca-galls *see* 6728
Mechiaron [Choseido] *see* 5915
Mechlorethamine, 5775
Mechlorethamine Oxide Hydrochloride, 5776
Mechlorprop *see* 5784
Meciclin [Citobios] *see* 2886
Mecilex [C.E.P.A.] *see* 1974
Mecillinam *see* 389
Meclan [Ortho] *see* 5778
Meclastine *see* 2345
Meclizine, 5777
Meclocycline, 5778
Mecloderm *see* 5778
Meclodol [Parke-Davis] *see* 5779
Meclofenamic Acid, 5779
Meclofenoxane *see* 5780
Meclofenoxate, 5780
Meclomen [Parke-Davis] *see* 5779
Meclophenamic Acid *see* 5779
Meclopran [Lagap] *see* 6143
Mecloqualone, 5781
Meclosorb [Basotherm] *see* 5778
Meclozine *see* 5777
Meclutin [ABC] *see* 5778
Mecobalamin *see* 6045
Mecocyanin *see* 2687
Mecomec [PBI/Gordon] *see* 5784
Meconic Acid, 5782
Meconin, 5783

Meconinic Acid Lactone *see* 5783
Mecopar *see* 5784
Mecoprop, 5784
Mecoprop-P *see* 5784
Mecrilate *see* 6046
Mecrylate *see* 6046
Mectizan [Merck & Co.] *see* 5248
Mecysteine Hydrochloride, 5785
MED-15 *see* 596
Medaject [Neda] *see* 7757
Medallion [Syngenta] *see* 4129
Medan [Kowa] *see* 1178
Medaron *see* 4300
Medax [BASF] *see* 7777
Medazepam, 5786
Medazepol [Farmasa] *see* 5786
Medemanol *see* 5746
Medemycin [Meiji] *see* 6183
Mederantil [Boehringer, Ing.] *see* 1450
Medetomidine, 5787
d-Medetomidine *see* 2946
MEDI-493 *see* 6988
Medialan LL-33 *see* 4368
Medialan LL-99 *see* 4368
Mediator [Biopharma] *see* 1039
Mediaven [Syntex] *see* 6394
Mediaxal [Servier] *see* 1039
Medicagol, 5788
Medicarpin, 5789
"Medicinal Chrysophanic Acid" *see* 2253
Medicoal [Lundbeck] *see* 1808
Medicort [Care] *see* 4787
Medifoxamine, 5790
Medifuran *see* 4294
Medigoxin *see* 3167
Medihaler-Epi [3M Pharma] *see* 3619
Medilave [Farillon] *see* 2032
Medilla [Omega] *see* 4854
Medinal *see* 962
Medio-Contrix "38" *see* 5064
Medomin [Novartis] *see* 4655
Medopren [Malesci] *see* 6055
Medoxim [Medici] *see* 1954
Medphalan *see* 5828
Medrate [Pharmacia & Upjohn] *see* 6111
Medrogestone, 5791
Medroglutaric Acid *see* 5808
Medrol [Pharmacia & Upjohn] *see* 6111
Medrone [Pharmacia] *see* 6111
Medronic Acid, 5792
Medroxyprogesterone, 5793
Medrysone, 5794
Medullipin, 5795
Medullipin I *see* 5795
Medullipin II *see* 5795
(*R*,*R*)-Me-DuPHOS *see* 3466
(*S*,*S*)-Me-DuPHOS *see* 3466
Meerschaum *see* 5687
Meerwein's Reagent, 5796
Meerzwiebel *see* 8770
Mefamide [Bayer] *see* 5649
Mefedina [Farmitalia] *see* 5849
Mefenacet, 5797
Mefenacid [Streuli] *see* 5798
Mefenamic Acid, 5798
Mefenorex, 5799
Mefenoxam *see* 5922
Mefenpyr-diethyl, 5800
Mefloquine, 5801
Mefluidide, 5802
Mefoxin [Merck & Co.] *see* 1936
Mefoxitin [Merck & Co.] *see* 1936
Mefruside, 5803
Mega *see* 5773
Megabion (Japanese) *see* 5950

Megace [BMS] *see* 5805
Megacert [Wakamoto] *see* 4320
Megacillin [Grünenthal] *see* 7100
Megacillin (susp.) [Frosst] *see* 7096
Megacillin (tabl.) [Frosst] *see* 7094
Megacins, 5804
Megaclor [Pharmax] *see* 2388
Megakaryocyte Potentiating Factor *see* 9386
Megalocin [Roche] *see* 4099
Megalone [Roche] *see* 4099
Megasedan [DIF] *see* 5786
Megasul [Am. Cyanamid] *see* 6618
Megestat [BMS] *see* 5805
Megestil [Boehringer, Mann.] *see* 5805
Megestrol Acetate, 5805
Megimide [Inibsa] *see* 1027
Meglum [Bago] *see* 5459
Meglumine *see* 6078
Meglumine Acetrizoate, 5806
Meglumine Amidotrizoate *see* 5807
Meglumine Diatrizoate, 5807
Meglumine Iothalamate *see* 5064
Meglutol, 5808
Meiact [Meiji Seika] *see* 1921
Meicelin [Meiji Seika] *see* 1927
Meilax [Meiji Seika] *see* 3821
Meionite *see* 1648
Meitnerium, 5809
MeJA *see* 5260
MEK *see* 6072
Meksamin *see* 6002
Mel B *see* 5815
Meladinine [DB Pharma] *see* 5988
Melagatran, 5810
Melaleuca Oil *see* 9089
Melamine, 5811
2-(4-Melamin-2-ylphenyl)-4-hydroxy-methyl-1,3-dithia-2-arsolane *see* 5815
Melampyrin *see* 4332
Melampyrite *see* 4332
Melampyrum *see* 4332
Melaniline *see* 3324
Melanins, 5812
Melanocyte-stimulating Hormone *see* 6295
Melanocyte-stimulating Hormone Release-inhibiting Factor *see* 5813
Melanophore-affecting Hormone *see* 6295
Melanophore Dilating Hormone *see* 6295
Melanophore Expanding Hormone *see* 6295
Melanophore Hormone *see* 6295
Melanophore-stimulating Hormone *see* 6295
Melanosome-dispersing Hormone *see* 6295
Melanostatin, 5813
Melanostatin I (Ox) *see* 5813
Melanotan, 5814
Melanotan-1 *see* 5814
Melanotropic Hormone *see* 6295
Melanotropin *see* 6295
α-Melanotropin *see* 6295
β-Melanotropin *see* 6295
γ-Melanotropin *see* 6295
Melanotropin Inhibiting Factor *see* 5813
Melanterite *see* 4057
Melanthigenin *see* 4624
Melarsoprol, 5815
Melatonin, 5816
Meldane [Chemagro] *see* 2558
Meldrum's Acid, 5817
Melengestrol Acetate, 5818

Meletin *see* 8034
Melex [Sankyo] *see* 6166
Melezitose, 5819
Melfalan *see* 5828
Melfax [Apotex] *see* 8110
Meliane [Schering AG] *see* 4413
Melibiose, 5820
Melilot, 5821
Melin *see* 8304
Melinamide, 5822
Melinonine G *see* 4093
Melipramine [EGYT] *see* 4920
Melissyl Alcohol *see* 9591
Melitase [Berk] *see* 2186
Melitose *see* 8096
Melitoxin *see* 3090
Melitracen, 5823
Melitriose *see* 8096
Melittin, 5824
Melittin I *see* 5824
Melium [Han Wha] *see* 6166
Melixeran [Lusofarmaco] *see* 5823
Mellaril [Novartis] *see* 9359
Melleretten [Novartis] *see* 9359
Melleril [Novartis] *see* 9359
Mellic Acid *see* 5825
Mellitic Acid, 5825
Mellitin *see* 5824
Melody [Bayer CropSci.] *see* 5080
Melon Tree *see* 7020
Melopat [Medopharm] *see* 1178
Meloxicam, 5826
Melperone, 5827
Melphalan, 5828
Melprex [Chimac-Agriphar] *see* 3408
Meltatox [BASF] *see* 3407
Melysin [Takeda] *see* 390
Memantine, 5829
Memcor [Lilly] *see* 10056
Memento 400 [Volpino] *see* 7460
MeMet *see* 6098
Memine [Macfarlan Smith] *see* 7329
Memoq [Gödecke] *see* 6496
Memphenesin *see* 5850
Memric [GSK] *see* 8309
MEN-8029 *see* 10186
MEN-9063 *see* 391
Menacor [Menarini] *see* 2360
Menadiol, 5830
Menadione, 5831
Menadione Carboxymethoxime Ammonium Salt *see* 5832
Menadoxime, 5832
Menaelle [Théramex] *see* 7773
Menamin [RPR] *see* 5305
Menaphthone *see* 5831
Menaphthone Carboxymethoxime Ammonium Salt *see* 5832
Menaquinone 4 *see* 5833
Menaquinone 6 *see* 5833
Menaquinone 7 *see* 5833
Menaquinones, 5833
Menatetrenone *see* 5833
Menazone *see* 4308
Menbutone, 5834
Mendelevium, 5835
Mendiaxon [Roland] *see* 4854
Mendon [Dainippon] *see* 2403
Mendrin *see* 3578
Menetryl *see* 3709
Menformon [Organon] *see* 3708
Menhaden Oil, 5836
Menhydrinate *see* 3207
Menichlopholan *see* 6518
Menitazine [Towa Yakuhin] *see* 1178

Menocil [Cilag-Chemie] see 476
Menoctyl [Dong Wha] see 6898
Menoflavin [Melbrosin] see 9690
Menogon [Ferring] see 4223
Menopatol [Chemiphar] see 9522
Menophase [Syntex] see 5917
Menorest see 3703
Menostar [Berlex] see 3703
Menotrophin see 4223
Menotropins see 4223
Menova [Merck KGaA] see 2102
Mensiso [Menarini] see 8550
Menstridyl see 2102
Mentax [Kaken] see 1518
p-Mentha-1,5-diene see 7200
p-Mentha-1(7),2-diene see 7201
p-Mentha-1,8-diene see 5493
p-Mentha-6,8-dien-2-one see 1874
trans-(−)-2-*p*-Mentha-1,8-dien-3-yl-5-
    pentylresorcinol see 1747
p-Menthane-1,8-diol see 9169
3-*p*-Menthanol see 5837
(1*R*,4*S*)-(−)-*p*-Menthan-3-one see 5838
2-[(*p*-Mentha-1,3,5-trien-2-yloxy)-
    methyl]-2-imidazoline see 9834
1-*p*-Menthene-6,8-diol see 8567
p-Menth-6-ene-2,8-diol see 8567
p-Menth-1-en-8-ol see 9171
1-*p*-Menthen-2-ol-3-one see 3298
p-Menth-1-en-3-one see 7473
R-(+)-*p*-Menth-4(8)-en-3-one see 7937
Menthol, 5837
l-Menthol see 5837
l-Menthone, 5838
Menthyl Acetate, 5839
Menthyl *o*-Aminobenzoate see 5840
Menthyl Anthranilate, 5840
Menthyl Valerate, 5841
Mentium [Guidotti] see 7991
Menyanthes, 5842
Menzol [Schwarz] see 6697
Meobentine, 5843
5-MeO-DIPT see 5991
Meothrin [Shell] see 3991
MEP see 3976
Mepacrine see 8044
Mepact, 5844
Mepanipyrim, 5845
Meparfynol, 5846
Mepartricin, 5847
Mepartricin A see 5847
Mepartricin B see 5847
Mepavlon [Zeneca] see 5862
Mepedyl [Glaxo] see 3331
Mepenzolate Bromide, 5848
Meperidine, 5849
Mepha-Butazon [Mepha] see 7277
Mephenamin [Boehringer, Mann.] see
    6879
Mephenesin, 5850
Mephenhydramine see 6287
Mephenon [Federa] see 5944
Mephenoxalone, 5851
Mephentermine, 5852
Mephenytoin, 5853
Mepherol see 5850
Mephesin see 5850
Mephine see 5852
Mephobarbital, 5854
Mephosfolan, 5855
Mephson see 5850
Mephyton [Merck & Co.] see 7380
Mepicaton [Pharmaton] see 5859
Mepiciclina see 7453
Mepicor [Corvi] see 5856

Mepicycline see 7453
Mepident [Parke-Davis] see 5859
Mepidium [Recordati] see 9442
Mepindolol, 5856
Mepiquat Chloride, 5857
Mepirizole see 3622
Mepirodipine see 1002
Mepirzepine see 6208
Mepitiostane, 5858
Mepivacaine, 5859
Mepivastesin [Espe] see 5859
Mepixanox, 5860
Mepixanthone see 5860
Meprane Dipropionate [Reed & Carnrick]
    see 5968
Meprednisone, 5861
Meprobamate, 5862
Meprodil [Streuli] see 5862
Meprofen [AGIPS] see 5305
Mepron [GSK] see 866
Meproscillarin see 7874
Meprospan [Wallace Labs.] see 5862
Meprotabs [Wallace Labs.] see 5862
Meptazinol, 5863
Meptid [Wyeth] see 5863
Meptin [Otsuka] see 7759
Mepyramine see 7984
Mepyrapone see 6159
Mequitazine, 5864
Mequiverine see 10003
Meractinomycin see 2800
Meradan(e) [USSR] see 8224
Meradimate see 5840
Meraklon [Montecatini] see 7581
Meralein Sodium, 5865
Meralen [HMR] see 4132
Meralluride, 5866
Meralop [ISF] see 2687
Meralops [Dulcis] see 2687
Meratran see 7484
Merbentul [HMR] see 2174
Merbentyl [Aventis] see 3097
Merbromin, 5867
Mercaleukin see 5871
Mercamine see 2779
Mercaptamine see 2779
Mercaptoacetamide Antimony Deriva-
    tive see 705
Mercaptoacetic Acid see 9336
Mercaptoacetic Acid Antimony Deriva-
    tive Sodium Salt see 703
Mercaptoacetic Acid [3,5-Bis(1,1-di-
    methylethyl)-4-hydroxyphenyl]-
    methyl Ester see 2836
Mercaptoacetic Acid Calcium Salt (2:1)
    see 1711
Mercaptoacetic Acid Sodium Salt see
    8692
(*SP*-5-25)-[*N*-[*N*-[*N*-(Mercaptoacetyl)gly-
    cyl]glycyl]glycinato(5−)-*N*,*N′*,*N″*,*S*]-
    oxotechnetate(2−)-⁹⁹ᵐTc Disodium
    see 9101
β-Mercaptoalanine see 2781
2-Mercaptobenzimidazole see 1082
2-Mercaptobenzimidazole-1,3-dimethyl-
    ol see 9312
2-Mercaptobenzoic Acid see 9360
2-Mercaptobenzothiazole, 5868
Mercaptobenzthiazyl Ether see 3370
Mercaptobutanedioic Acid see 9343
Mercaptobutanedioic Acid Mono-
    gold(1+) Sodium Salt see 4518
Mercaptodiacetic Acid see 9331
Mercaptodimethur see 5972
Mercaptoethane see 3726

2-Mercaptoethanesulfonic Acid Sodium
    Salt see 5909
β-Mercaptoethanol see 5869
2-Mercaptoethanol, 5869
β-Mercaptoethylamine see 2779
(2-Mercaptoethyl)trimethylammonium
    Iodide *O*,*O*-Diethyl Phosphorothioate
    see 3501
2-Mercaptohistidine see 9341
2-Mercapto-4-hydroxypyrimidine see
    9366
2-Mercaptoimidazoline see 3803
N-(2-Mercaptoisobutyryl)-L-cysteine see
    1460
Mercaptomerin Sodium, 5870
Mercaptomethane see 5956
N-[(*S*)-α-(Mercaptomethyl)-3,4-(methyl-
    enedioxy)-hydrocinnamoyl]-L-ala-
    nine, Benzyl Ester Acetate (Ester) see
    3940
N-(2-Mercapto-2-methyl-1-oxopropyl)-
    L-cysteine see 1460
[1(*S*),4(*S*)]-1-(3-Mercapto-2-methyl-1-
    oxopropyl)-4-phenyl-thio-L-proline-*S*-
    benzoylester see 10186
1-[(2*S*)-3-Mercapto-2-methyl-1-oxopro-
    pyl]-L-proline see 1774
N-(Mercaptomethyl)phthalimide *S*-(*O*,*O*-
    Dimethyl Phosphorodithioate) see 7336
N-(2-Mercapto-2-methylpropanoyl)-L-
    cysteine see 1460
(2*S*)-1-(3-Mercapto-2-methylpropionyl)-
    L-proline see 1774
N-[1-[(*S*)-3-Mercapto-2-methylpro-
    pionyl]-L-prolyl]-3-phenyl-L-alanine
    Acetate (Ester) see 200
1-Mercaptonaphthalene see 6378
2-Mercapto-*N*-2-naphthalenylacetamide
    see 9344
2-Mercaptonapthalene see 6379
5-Mercapto-2-nitrobenzoic Acid Ion
    (2−) see 3551
N-(2-Mercapto-1-oxopropyl)glycine see
    9453
Mercaptophos see 2889
Mercaptophos [Bayer] see 4002
3-Mercapto-1,2-propanediol see 9335
α-Mercaptopropanoic Acid see 9340
2-Mercaptopropanoic Acid see 9340
1-(3-Mercaptopropanoic Acid)-8-D-argi-
    nine Vasopressin see 2924
1-(3-Mercaptopropanoic Acid)-2-(*O*-
    ethyl-D-tyrosine)-4-L-threonine-8-L-
    ornithineoxytocin see 865
1-(3-Mercaptopropanoic Acid)oxytocin
    see 2842
2-Mercaptopropionic Acid see 9340
1-(3-Mercaptopropionic Acid)-2-[3-(*p*-
    ethoxyphenyl)-D-alanine]-4-L-threo-
    nine-8-L-ornithineoxytocin see 865
α-Mercaptopropionylglycine see 9453
N-(2-Mercaptopropionyl)glycine see 9453
N-(2-Mercaptopropionyl)glycine 2-Thio-
    phenecarboxylate (Ester) see 8809
6-Mercaptopurine, 5871
2-Mercaptopyridine 1-Oxide see 7994
2-Mercapto-4(1*H*)-pyrimidinone see 9366
2-Mercapto-4-pyrimidone see 9366
Mercaptosuccinic Acid see 9343
Mercaptothion see 5700
3-Mercapto-D-valine see 7088
Mercaptyl [Knoll] see 7088
Mercate "5" see 5126
Mercate "20" see 5126
Mercazole see 5971

Mercazolyl see 5971
Mercilon [Organon] see 2926
Mercloran [Parke-Davis] see 2105
Mercodinone see 4785
Mercol [Exakta] see 7555
Mercoral see 2105
Mercuhydrin see 5866
Mercumallylic Acid, 5872
Mercumatilin Sodium see 5872
Mercuramide see 5901
Mercuranine see 5867
Mercuretin see 5866
Mercuric Acetate, 5873
Mercuric Barium Iodide see 982
Mercuric Benzoate, 5874
Mercuric Bromide, 5875
Mercuric Cacodylate see 1604
Mercuric Chloride, 5876
Mercuric Cuprous Iodide see 2663
Mercuric Cyanide, 5877
Mercuric Fluoride, 5878
Mercuric Iodide, Red, 5879
Mercuric Nitrate, 5880
Mercuric Oleate, 5881
Mercuric Oxide, Red, 5882
Mercuric Oxide, Yellow, 5883
Mercuric Oxycyanide, 5884
Mercuric Potassium Cyanide see 7683
Mercuric Potassium Iodide see 7688
Mercuric Salicylate, 5885
Mercuric Silver Iodide see 8531
Mercuric Sodium p-Phenolsulfonate,
    5886
Mercuric Sulfate, 5887
Mercuric Sulfide, Black, 5888
Mercuric Sulfide, Red, 5889
Mercuric Sulfocyanate see 5890
Mercuric Sulfocyanide see 5890
Mercuric Thiocyanate, 5890
Mercuriphenoldisulfonate Sodium see
    5886
Mercurius Vitae see 693
Mercurochrome see 5867
Mercurocol see 5867
Mercurome see 5867
Mercurophage see 5867
Mercurophen, 5891
Mercurothiolate see 9317
Mercurous Acetate, 5892
Mercurous Bromide, 5893
Mercurous Chloride, 5894
Mercurous Iodide, 5895
Mercurous Nitrate, 5896
Mercurous Sulfate, 5897
Mercury, 5898
Mercury and Sodium Phenolsulfonate see
    5886
Mercury Bichloride see 5876
Mercury Biniodide see 5879
Mercury Bisulfate see 5887
Mercury Cyanide Oxide see 5884
Mercury Difluoride see 5878
Mercury, Dimethyl see 3250
Mercury Monochloride see 5894
Mercury Perchloride see 5876
Mercury Pernitrate see 5880
Mercury Protochloride see 5894
Mercury Protoiodide see 5895
Mercury Protonitrate see 5896
Mercury Subchloride see 5894
Mercury Subsalicylate see 5885
Meregon [Malesci] see 1485
Mereprine [Cassella-med] see 3441
Meresa [Dolorgiet] see 8989
Merfen [Zyma] see 7303

Mergamma [Zeneca] see 7300
Meridia [Knoll] see 8485
Merilid see 2105
Merimepodib, 5899
Merinax see 4698
Merislon [Eisai] see 1178
Merit [Bayer CropSci.] see 4910
Merital [Hoechst] see 6673
Merlin [Bayer CropSci.] see 5236
Merocet [HMR] see 2032
Merodicein [Becton Dickinson] see 5865
Meronem [AstraZeneca] see 5900
Meropen [Sumitomo] see 5900
Meropenem, 5900
Merosin see 5351
Merpan see 1772
Merphalan see 5828
Merphenyl Nitrate see 7302
Merrem [AstraZeneca] see 5900
Mersalyl, 5901
Mersalyl Acid see 5901
Mertax see 5868
Mertect [Syngenta] see 9289
Mertestate [Sterling Winthrop] see 9180
Merthiolate [Lilly] see 9317
Mervaldin [Lannett] see 5850
Mervan [Continental Pharma] see 219
Mervastrept see 2902
Merzonin [Takeda] see 9317
MES, 5902
Mesaconic Acid, 5903
Mesalamine, 5904
Mesalazine see 5904
Mesantoin [Sandoz] see 5853
Mesasal [Sanofi-Synthelabo] see 5904
Mescaline, 5905
Mescaline Oxidase see 6247
Mesembrine, 5906
Mesentol see 3748
Mesidicaine see 9700
Mesitylene, 5907
Mesityl Oxide, 5908
Mesityl Oxide (1-Phthalazinyl)hydrazone
    see 1470
Mesna, 5909
Mesnex [Baxter] see 5909
Mesocaine see 9700
Mesoetioporphyrin see 3869
Mesoinosite see 4978
Mesokain see 9700
Mesonex see 4979
Mesontoin see 5853
Mesopin [Endo] see 4730
Mesoridazine, 5910
Mesoridazine Besylate see 5910
Mesosulfuron-methyl, 5911
Mesotal [Galma] see 4979
Mesotartaric Acid see 9071
Mesothorium I see 8094
Mesothorium II see 137
Mesotrione, 5912
Mesoxalic Acid, 5913
Mesoxalylcarbamide see 282
Mesoxalylurea see 282
Mesoyohimbine see 10104
Mespafin [Merckle] see 3440
Mesquite Gum, 5914
Messenger [Eden Bioscience] see 4617
Messenger RNA see 8203
Mestanolone, 5915
Mestenediol see 5950
Mesterolone, 5916
Mestilbol see 3129
Mestinon [Roche] see 7977
Mestoranum [Schering AG] see 5916

Mestranol, 5917
Mesudin see 5649
Mesudrin see 5649
Mesulfa [Triosol] see 8913
Mesulfen, 5918
Mesulid [LPB] see 6548
Mesulphen see 5918
Mesurol [Bayer CropSci.] see 5972
Mesuximide see 6004
Mesyl Chloride see 5955
Met see 5975
Metab-Auxil see 7111
Metabenzthiazuron see 5939
Metabolin [Takeda] see 9295
Metabutethamine Hydrochloride see
    1523
Metacam [Boehringer, Ing.] see 5826
Metacetaldehyde see 5923
Metachlor see 201
Metachloral see 9626
Metachrome Yellow, 5919
Metacide [Bayer CropSci.] see 6108
Metaclazepam, 5920
Metacortandracin see 7722
Metacortandralone see 7721
Metacresol Acetate see 2583
Metacycline see 5943
[2.2]Metacyclophane, 5921
Metadate [Medeva] see 6110
Metadee see 10018
Metadelphene [Hercules] see 2856
Metadiazine see 7987
Metadomus [Med. Domus] see 5943
Metafar [Lafare] see 1926
Metaformaldehyde see 9734
Metahydrin [HMR] see 9624
Metalaxyl, 5922
Metalaxyl-M see 5922
Metalcaptase [Heyl] see 7088
β_1-Metal-combining Protein see 9571
Metaldehyde, 5923
Metallibure see 5946
Metallic Arsenic see 794
Metallum Problematum see 9121
Metalutin [Parke-Davis] see 6710
Metalyse [Boehringer, Ing.] see 9143
Metamide [Protea] see 6143
Metamin [Takeda] see 4187
Metamitron, 5924
Metamizol see 3350
Metampicillin, 5925
Metam Sodium see 5949
Metamucil [Procter & Gamble] see 7517
Metandiol see 5950
Metandren [Novartis] see 6125
Metanephrine, 5926
Metanilic Acid, 5927
Metanil Yellow, 5928
Metanyl see 5958
Metaoxedrin see 7286
Metaphanine, 5929
Metaphen [Abbott] see 6610
Metaphos see 6108
Metaphosphoric Acid see 7345
Metaphosphoric Acid Trisodium Salt see
    8696
Metaplexan [Rhône-Poulenc] see 5864
Metapramine, 5930
Metaprel [Dorsey] see 5931
Metaproterenol, 5931
Metaradrine see 5932
Metaraminol, 5932
Metarsenobillon see 8941
Metaspas [Leeming] see 3168
Metastigmin [Star] see 6464

Metastron [Amersham] *see* 8840
Meta-Systox *see* 6051
Metathion *see* 3976
Metatyrosine *see* 9840
Metavariscite *see* 358
Metaxan *see* 5958
Metaxanin *see* 5922
Metazepium Iodide *see* 1599
Metazocine, 5933
Metazolo *see* 5971
Metconazole, 5934
Met⁵-E *see* 3572
Metebanyl [Sankyo] *see* 3456
Metelilachlor *see* 6146
Meteloidine, 5935
Metenarin [Teikoku Zoki] *see* 6070
Metendiol *see* 5950
Metenix [Sanofi-Aventis] *see* 6147
Met⁵-Enkephalin *see* 3572
Méténolone *see* 5967
Metepa, 5936
Meterazine *see* 7761
Meterfer [Sinclair] *see* 4046
Metergoline, 5937
Metflorylthiazidine *see* 4789
Metformin, 5938
Metformin Pamoate *see* 5938
"Meth" *see* 5948
Methabenzthiazuron, 5939
Methacetin *see* 51
Methacetone *see* 3121
Methacholine Chloride, 5940
Methacide *see* 9529
Methacolimycin [Kayaku] *see* 2479
Methacrylic Acid, 5941
Methacrylonitrile, 5942
Methacycline, 5943
Methaderm [Taiho] *see* 2943
Methadone, 5944
Methadose [Mallinckrodt] *see* 5944
Methadren(e) *see* 6069
Methadyl Acetate, 5945
Methafluoridamid *see* 5802
Methaform *see* 2129
Methagon [Corvel] *see* 4138
Methallibure, 5946
Methallylchloride *see* 2148
α-Methallyl Chloride *see* 2131
β-Methallyl Chloride *see* 2148
γ-Methallyl Chloride *see* 2130
Methalutin *see* 6710
Methamidophos, 5947
Methaminodiazepoxide *see* 2084
Metampex [Lemmon] *see* 5948
Methamphetamine, 5948
Methampicillin *see* 5925
Methampyrone *see* 3350
Metham Sodium, 5949
Methanabol *see* 5950
Methanal *see* 4235
Methanamide *see* 4237
Methanamine *see* 6014
Methandienone *see* 5951
Methandiol *see* 5950
Methandriol *see* 5950
Methandrostenolone, 5951
Methane, 5952
Methanearsonic Acid, 5953
Methanebisphosphonic Acid *see* 5792
Methanebis[N,N'-(5-ureido-2,4-diketo-tetrahydroimidazole)-N,N-dimethylol] *see* 4916
Methanedicarboxylic Acid *see* 5710
Methanediphosphonic Acid *see* 5792
Methanedisulfonic Acid *see* 5974

Methaneperoxoic Acid *see* 7160
1-(5-Methanesulfonamido-1*H*-indol-2-yl-carbonyl)-4-[3-(1-methylethylamino)-pyridinyl]piperazine *see* 2877
1-(4-Methanesulfonamidophenoxy)-2-[*N*-(4-methanesulfonamidophenethyl)-*N*-methylamino]ethane *see* 3409
Methanesulfonic Acid, 5954
Methanesulfonic Acid Ethyl Ester *see* 3827
Methanesulfonic Acid Methyl Ester *see* 6097
Methanesulfonic Acid Tetramethylene Ester *see* 1505
Methanesulfonyl Chloride, 5955
N,N'-Methanetetraylbiscyclohexanamine *see* 3096
Methanethioamide *see* 9333
Methanethiol, 5956
Methanetriol *see* 6884
Methaniazide *see* 5186
Methanide *see* 5958
Methanol, 5957
9(*O*)-Methano-Δ⁶⁽⁹⁾-prostaglandin I₁ *see* 2358
O-(1,4-Methano-1,2,3,4-tetrahydro-6-naphthyl)-*N*-methyl-*N*-(*m*-tolyl)thiocarbamate *see* 9509
Methantheline Bromide, 5958
Methanthine Bromide *see* 5958
Methapoxide *see* 5936
Methapyrilene, 5959
Methaqualone, 5960
Metharbital, 5961
β-Methasone *see* 1180
Methazolamide, 5962
Methazolastone *see* 9139
Met Hb *see* 5965
Methbipyranone *see* 6159
Methcathinone, 5963
Methdilazine, 5964
Methedrine [Burroughs Wellcome] *see* 5948
Methemoglobin, 5965
Methenamine, 5966
Methenolone, 5967
Methenolone Enanthate *see* 5967
N,N'-Methenyl-*o*-phenylenediamine *see* 1081
Metheph [Napp] *see* 6068
Methergin [Novartis] *see* 6070
Methergine [Novartis] *see* 6070
Methergoline *see* 5937
Methestrol, 5968
Methetharimide *see* 1027
Methexenyl *see* 4704
Methexenyl Sodium *see* 4704
Methforylthiazidine *see* 4789
Met-HGH *see* 8716
Methiacil *see* 6128
Methiazic Acid *see* 6139
Methiazinic Acid *see* 6139
Methicil *see* 6128
Methicillin Sodium, 5969
Methidathion, 5970
Methimazole, 5971
Methiocarb, 5972
Methiocil *see* 6128
Methiodal Sodium, 5973
Methionamine *see* 96
Methionic Acid, 5974
Methionine, 5975
L-Methionine *see* 5975
Methionine⁵-enkephalin *see* 3572
Methionine Hydroxy Analog, 5976

245-L-Methionine-plasminogen Activator (Human Tissue-type 2-Chain Form Protein Moiety) *see* 9468
1-(*N*-L-Methionyl-L-alanine)-3-L-threonine-4-L-tyrosine-5-L-arginine-17-L-serinecolony-stimulating Factor (Human Clone 1034) *see* 4537
N-L-Methionyl-22-L-arginine-76-L-alanine-78-L-aspartic Acid-79-L-glutamic Acid-86-L-tyrosine-90-L-tyrosine-156-L-threonine-157-L-asparagine-158-L-leucine-interferon α1 (Human Lymphoblast Reduced) *see* 4990
N-L-Methionylcolony-stimulating Factor (Human Clone 1034) *see* 4537
N-L-Methionyl-1-165-hematopoietic Cell Growth Factor KL (Human Clone V19.8:hSCF162) Dimer *see* 8807
N-L-Methionyl-387-L-histidine-388-L-alanine-1-388-toxin (*Corynebacterium diphtheriae* strain C7) (388 → 2')-protein with 2-133-interleukin 2 (Human Clone pTIL2-21a) *see* 2893
Methionyl Human Growth Hormone *see* 8716
*N*²-L-Methionyl-1-139-interferon γ (Human Lymphocyte Protein Moiety Reduced) *see* 4992
N-L-Methionylinterleukin 2 (Human) *see* 4994
*N*²-L-Methionyl-interleukin 1 Receptor Antagonist (Human Isoform X Reduced) *see* 5001
Methionyl Neurotrophic Factor (Human Glial-derived), Dimer *see* 4377
Methioplegium *see* 9707
Methiothepin *see* 6141
Methiothepine *see* 6141
Methioturiate *see* 5978
Methisazone, 5977
Methisoprinol *see* 4976
Methitural, 5978
Methium Chloride *see* 4688
Methixart [Fuso] *see* 5979
Methixene, 5979
Methobenzmorphan *see* 5933
Methocarbamol, 5980
Methocel [Dow] *see* 4842
Methocel A [Dow] *see* 6040
Methocillin-S [Meiji] *see* 2419
Methofadin [Tanabe] *see* 8917
Methohexital Sodium, 5981
Methohexitone Sodium *see* 5981
Methoin *see* 5853
Methomidate *see* 6148
Methomyl, 5982
Methone *see* 3242
Methophenazine *see* 6145
Methoplain [Kowa Yakuhin] *see* 6055
Methoprene, 5983
S-Methoprene *see* 5983
Methopterin, 5984
Methopyrapone *see* 6159
Methorphan *see* 8091
Methorphinan *see* 5470
Methosarb *see* 1722
Methose *see* 4274
Methoserpidine *see* 2918
Methostan [Schering] *see* 5950
Methotrexate, 5985
Methotrimeprazine, 5986
Methoxadone *see* 5851
Methoxamine, 5987
Methoxone [Zeneca] *see* 5764
Methoxsalen, 5988

6-Methoxyacacetin *see* 7064

p-Methoxyacetanilide *see* 51

Methoxyacetic Acid (1*S*,2*S*)-2-[2-[[3-(1*H*-Benzimidazol-2-yl)propyl]methylamino]ethyl]-6-fluoro-1,2,3,4-tetrahydro-1-(1-methylethyl)-2-naphthalenyl Ester *see* 6173

[[2-[(Methoxyacetyl)amino]-4-(phenylthio)phenyl]carbonimidoyl]biscarbamic Acid Dimethyl Ester *see* 3944

5-Methoxyacetylamino-2,4,6-triiodoisophthalic Acid [[(2,3-Dihydroxy-*N*-methylpropyl)-(2,3-dihydroxypropyl)]diamide *see* 5062

2-Methoxy-6-allylphenol Diethylaminoethyl Ether *see* 4542

2-Methoxy-4-allylphenoxyacetic Acid *N*,*N*-Diethylamide *see* 46

Methoxyamine, 5989

3-Methoxy-4-(4′-aminobenzenesulfonamido)-1,2,5-thiadiazole *see* 8920

4-Methoxy-4′-aminodiphenylamine *see* 5999

6-Methoxy-8-(4-aminopentylamino)quinoline *see* 8067

2,2′-[3-Methoxy-4′-amyl-5′-methyl-5-(2″-pyrryl)]dipyrrylmethene *see* 7767

3-Methoxyaniline *see* 667

4-Methoxy-6-β-(*p*-anisyl)vinyl]-α-pyrone *see* 10093

10-Methoxy-6aβ-aporphin-11-ol *see* 740

4-Methoxybenzaldehyde *see* 663

2-Methoxybenzenamine *see* 667

3-Methoxybenzenamine *see* 667

4-Methoxybenzenamine *see* 667

Methoxybenzene *see* 669

4-Methoxy-1,3-benzenediamine *see* 2976

4-Methoxybenzenemethanol *see* 665

4-Methoxybenzoic Acid *see* 666

2-(4-Methoxybenzoyl)benzoic Acid *see* 672

4-Methoxybenzoyl Chloride *see* 673

1-(4-Methoxybenzoyl)-2-pyrrolidinone *see* 662

p-Methoxybenzyl Alcohol *see* 665

1-(*p*-Methoxybenzyl)-2,3-dimethylguanidine *see* 5843

N-*p*-Methoxybenzyl-*N*′,*N*′-dimethyl-*N*-α-pyridylethylenediamine *see* 7984

α-(α-Methoxybenzyl)-4-(β-methoxyphenethyl)-1-piperazineethanol *see* 10170

2-(4-Methoxy[1,1′-biphenyl]-3-yl)hydrazinecarboxylic Acid 1-Methylethyl Ester *see* 1207

2-Methoxy-4,6-bis(isopropylamino)-*s*-triazine *see* 7788

5-Methoxy-*N*,*N*-bis(1-methylethyl)-1*H*-indole-3-ethanamine *see* 5991

6-Methoxy-*N*,*N*′-bis(1-methylethyl)-1,3,5-triazine-2,4-diamine *see* 7788

4-Methoxy-*N*,*N*′-bis(3-pyridinylmethyl)-1,3-benzenedicarboxamide *see* 7407

4-Methoxy-*N*,*N*′-bis(3-pyridylmethyl)-isophthalamide *see* 7407

2-(Methoxycarbonylamino)benzimidazole *see* 1791

2-[[[(Methoxycarbonyl)amino][[2-nitro-5-(propylthio)phenyl]amino]methylene]amino]ethanesulfonic Acid *see* 6480

2-[[[(Methoxycarbonyl)amino][[2-nitro-5-(propylthio)phenyl]imino]methyl]amino]ethanesulfonic Acid *see* 6480

3-Methoxycarbonyl-6-*n*-butyl-7-benzyloxy-4-oxoquinoline *see* 6472

N-Methoxycarbonyl-*N*′-[2-nitro-5-(propylthio)phenyl]-*N*″-2-(ethylsulfonic Acid)guanidine *see* 6480

4-(Methoxycarbonyl)-4-[(1-oxopropyl)-phenylamino]-1-piperidinepropanoic Acid Methyl Ester *see* 8131

N-(2-Methoxycarbonylphenylsulfonyl)-*N*′-[4,6-bis(difluoromethoxy)pyrimidin-2-yl]urea *see* 7747

1-Methoxycarbonyl-1-propen-2-yl Dimethyl Phosphate *see* 6165

(Methoxycarbonylsulfamoyl)triethylammonium Hydroxide Inner Salt *see* 1502

*N*¹-Methoxycarbonylsulfanilamide *see* 857

Methoxychlor, 5990

N-[4-(β-(2-Methoxy-5-chlorobenzamido)ethyl)benzosulfonyl]-*N*′-cyclohexylurea *see* 4478

*N*¹-[4-β-(2-Methoxy-5-chlorobenzoylamino)ethyl]benzenesulfonyl]-*N*²-cyclohexylurea *see* 4478

(8α,9*R*)-6′-Methoxycinchonan-9-ol *see* 8061

(8α,9*S*)-6′-Methoxycinchonan-9-ol *see* 3621

(9*R*)-6′-Methoxycinchonan-9-ol *see* 3620

(9*S*)-6′-Methoxycinchonan-9-ol *see* 8060

(8α)-6′-Methoxycinchonan-9-one *see* 8063

6-Methoxycinchoninic Acid *see* 8062

p-Methoxycinnamic Acid 2-Ethoxyethyl Ester *see* 2310

Methoxyconiferine *see* 9016

9-Methoxycorynantheidine *see* 6218

2-Methoxy-*p*-cresol *see* 2571

4-Methoxy-2,6-cresotic Acid Methyl Ester *see* 8734

(1α,3α)-7-Methoxycrinan-1,3-diol *see* 1493

Methoxycyclopropane *see* 2749

Methoxy-DDT *see* 5990

10-Methoxydeserpidine *see* 2918

Methoxydichlorobenzoate *see* 3040

2-Methoxy-3,6-dichlorobenzoic Acid *see* 3040

6-(α-Methoxy-3,4-dichlorophenylacetamido)penicillanic Acid *see* 2385

8-Methoxydictamnine *see* 3928

6-Methoxy-8-(6-diethylaminohexylamine)-4-methylquinoline *see* 8553

6-Methoxy-8-(3-diethylaminopropylamino)quinoline *see* 7522

[3-Methoxy-4-[(*N*,*N*-diethylcarbamido)-methoxy]phenyl]acetic Acid *n*-Propyl Ester *see* 7803

6-Methoxy-3,4-dihydro-1(2*H*)-naphthalenone *see* 6000

4-Methoxy-2,2′-dihydroxybenzophenone *see* 3303

5-Methoxy-*N*,*N*-diisopropyltryptamine, 5991

2-Methoxy-*N*,α-dimethylbenzeneethanamime *see* 5998

5-Methoxy-8,8-dimethyl-2*H*,8*H*-benzo-[1,2-*b*:5,4-*b*′]dipyran-2-one *see* 10066

7-Methoxy-2,2-dimethyl-2*H*-1-benzopyran *see* 7718

7-Methoxy-2,2-dimethylchromene *see* 7718

(8β)-10-Methoxy-1,6-dimethylergoline-8-methanol 5-Bromo-3-pyridinecarboxylate (Ester) *see* 6496

o-Methoxy-*N*,α-dimethylphenethylamine *see* 5998

(*trans*)-1-[2-[*p*-(7-Methoxy-2,2-dimethyl-3-phenyl-4-chromanyl)phenoxy]ethyl]pyrrolidine *see* 1971

(*Z*,*E*)-2-Methoxy-3,5-dimethyl-6-[tetrahydro-4-[2-methyl-3-(4-nitrophenyl)-2-propenylidene]-2-furanyl]-4*H*-pyran-4-one *see* 879

Methoxydiuron *see* 5509

Methoxydon(e) *see* 5851

Methoxyethane *see* 3828

2-Methoxyethanol *see* 6038

2-Methoxyethanol Acetate *see* 6039

2-(2-Methoxyethoxy)ethanol *see* 6037

N-[5-(2-Methoxyethoxy)-2-pyrimidinyl]-benzenesulfonamide *see* 4507

Methoxyethylbenzeneboronic Acid, 5992

2-Methoxyethyl 1,4-Dihydro-5-(isopropoxycarbonyl)-2,6-dimethyl-4-(3-nitrophenyl)-3-pyridinecarboxylate *see* 6551

1-[4-(2-Methoxyethyl)phenoxy]-3-[(1-methylethyl)amino]-2-propanol *see* 6151

[2-[(1*R*)-1-Methoxyethyl]phenyl]boronic Acid *see* 5992

2-(β-Methoxyethyl)pyridine *see* 6160

11β-Methoxy-17α-ethynylestradiol *see* 6289

11β-Methoxy-17α-ethynyl-Δ¹,³,⁵(¹⁰)-estratriene-3,17β-diol *see* 6289

Methoxyfenozide, 5993

Methoxyflurane, 5994

"Methoxy Foxy" *see* 5991

8-Methoxy[furano-3′,2′:6,7-coumarin] *see* 5988

4-Methoxy-7*H*-furo[3,2-*g*][1]benzopyran-7-one *see* 1157

9-Methoxy-7*H*-furo[3,2-*g*][1]benzopyran-7-one *see* 5988

8-Methoxy-4′,5′:6,7-furocoumarin *see* 5988

4-Methoxyfuro[2,3-*b*]quinoline *see* 3089

10-Methoxyharmalan, 5995

Methoxyhydrastine *see* 6718

4-Methoxy-2-hydroxybenzophenone *see* 6954

3-Methoxy-4-hydroxycinnamic Acid *see* 4062

3-Methoxy-4-hydroxymandelic Acid *see* 9933

8-(2-Methoxy-3-hydroxymercuripropyl)-coumarin-3-carboxylic Acid *see* 5872

L-3-Methoxy-4-hydroxyphenylalanine *see* 6056

3-Methoxy-4-hydroxyphenylglycol, 5996

3-Methoxy-10-[3-(4-hydroxypiperidyl)-2-methylpropyl]phenothiazine *see* 7168

3-Methoxy-4-hydroxytoluene *see* 2571

12-Methoxyibogamine *see* 4875

13-Methoxyibogamine *see* 9020

12-Methoxyibogamine-18-carboxylic Acid Methyl Ester *see* 10027

R-(*Z*)-α-(Methoxyimino)-1-azabicyclo-[2.2.2]octane-3-acetonitrile *see* 8309

(α*E*)-α-(Methoxyimino)-2-[(2-methylphenoxy)methyl]benzeneacetic Acid Methyl Ester *see* 5324

(α*E*)-α-(Methoxyimino)-2-[[[(*E*)-1-[3-(trifluoromethyl)phenyl]ethylidene]-amino]oxy]methyl]benzeneacetic Acid Methyl Ester *see* 9677

(*E*,*E*)-Methoxyimino-[2-[1-(3-trifluoromethylphenyl)ethylideneaminooxymethyl]phenyl]acetic Acid Methyl Ester *see* 9677

Methrazone [Boehringer, Ing.] *see* 4012
Methscopolamine Bromide, 6003
Methscopolamine Nitrate *see* 8406
Methsuximide, 6004
Methural *see* 6968
Methyclothiazide, 6005
Methycobal [Eisai] *see* 6045
Methyl Abietate, 6006
Methylacetaldehyde *see* 7823
Methyl 4-Acetamido-2-ethoxybenzoate *see* 3745
m-Methylacetanilide *see* 74
N-Methylacetanilide, 6007
Methyl Acetate, 6008
Methylacetic Acid *see* 7825
Methylacetic Anhydride *see* 7826
Methyl Acetoacetate, 6009
(+)-*N*-Methyl-2-acetonylpyrrolidine *see* 4850
Methylacetopyronone *see* 2865
6-α-Methyl-17α-acetoxyprogesterone *see* 5793
Methyl Acetylsalicylate, 6010
β-Methylacrolein *see* 2596
Methyl Acrylate, 6011
α-Methylacrylic Acid *see* 5941
β-Methylacrylic Acid *see* 2597
α-Methylacrylonitrile *see* 5942
α-Methyl-1-adamantanemethylamine *see* 8224
N-Methyladrenaline *see* 6069
3-*O*-Methyladrenaline *see* 5926
Methylal, 6012
Methylal Acetamide *see* 4242
2-Methylalanine *see* 445
3-Methyl-*N*,α-(β-alanyl)-L-histidine *see* 679
Methyl Alcohol *see* 5957
Methyl Aldehyde *see* 4235
2-(*p*-Methylallylaminophenyl)propionic Acid *see* 300
α-Methylallyl Chloride *see* 2131
β-Methylallylchloride *see* 2148
γ-Methylallyl Chloride *see* 2130
13β-Methyl-17α-allyl-Δ4,9,11-gonatriene-17β-ol-3-one *see* 319
α-*dl*-1-Methyl-5-allyl-5-(1-methyl-2-pentynyl)barbituric Acid Sodium Salt *see* 5981
Methyl Allyl Trisulfide, 6013
Methylamine, 6014
N-Methylaminoacetic Acid *see* 8373
2-(Methylamino)-*m*-anisic Acid Methyl Ester *see* 2808
Methyl *p*-Aminobenzenesulfonylcarbamate *see* 857
Methyl 2-Aminobenzoate *see* 6020
2-(4-Methylaminobutoxy)diphenylmethane *see* 1206
N-[[(Methylamino)carbonyl]oxy]ethanimidothioic Acid Methyl Ester *see* 5982
3-Methylamino-6-carboxamido-1,2,3,4-tetrahydrocarbazole *see* 4272
4-Methylaminocetopyrocatechol *see* 171
4″-*epi*-(Methylamino)-4″-deoxyavermectin B₁ₐ *see* 3554
4″-*epi*-(Methylamino)-4″-deoxyavermectin B₁ᵦ *see* 3554
2-(Methylamino)-2-deoxy-α-L-glucopyranose *see* 6079
3-Methylamino-7-dimethylaminophenazathonium Chloride *see* 928
4-Methylamino-1,5-dimethyl-2-phenyl-3-pyrazolone Sodium Methanesulfonate *see* 3350

α-*dl*-6-(Methylamino)-4,4-diphenyl-3-heptanol Acetate *see* 6685
N-Methylaminodithioformic Acid Sodium Salt *see* 5949
N-Methylaminoethane Sodium Sulfonate *see* 6124
β-Methylaminoethane-α-sulfonic Acid *see* 6124
2-Methylaminoethanesulfonic Acid *see* 6124
Methylaminoethanoic Acid *see* 8373
2-Methylaminoethanol, 6015
l-Methylaminoethanolcatechol *see* 3619
m-Methylaminoethanolphenol *see* 7286
p-Methylaminoethanolphenol *see* 9012
p-Methylaminoethanolphenol Tartrate *see* 9012
4-[2-(Methylamino)ethyl]-1,2-benzenediol *see* 2903
(α*R*)-α-[(1*S*)-1-(Methylamino)ethyl]benzenemethanol *see* 3608
(α*S*)-α-[(1*S*)-1-(Methylamino)ethyl]benzenemethanol *see* 7916
α-(1-Methylaminoethyl)-*p*-hydroxybenzyl Alcohol *see* 4824
4-[2-(Methylamino)ethyl]-*o*-phenylene Diisobutyrate *see* 4876
2-[2-(Methylamino)ethyl]pyridine *see* 1178
4-[2-(Methylamino)ethyl]pyrocatechol *see* 2903
2-Methyl-6-aminoheptane *see* 6757
2-Methyl-6-amino-2-heptanol *see* 4657
6-Methyl-2-amino-6-heptanol *see* 4657
Methyl 3-Amino-4-hydroxybenzoate *see* 6883
2-Methyl-4-amino-1-hydroxynaphthalene *see* 10023
β-Methylamino-α-(4-hydroxyphenyl)-ethyl Alcohol *see* 9012
α-Methylamino-β-(3-indole)propionic Acid *see* 10
2-Methylamino-5α-(β-indolyl)ethyl-2-oxazolin-4-one *see* 4966
2-Methylaminoisocamphane *see* 5774
3-Methylaminoisocamphane *see* 5774
Methyl Aminolevulinate, 6016
Methyl α-Amino-β-mercaptopropionate Hydrochloride *see* 5785
(α*R*)-α-[(Methylamino)methyl]benzenemethanol *see* 4601
(−)-α-(Methylaminomethyl)benzyl Alcohol *see* 4601
1-(Methylaminomethyl)dibenzo[*b,e*]bicyclo[2.2.2]octadiene *see* 1087
9-(Methylaminomethyl)-9,10-dihydro-9,10-ethanoanthracene *see* 1087
6-Methylamino-2-methylheptene *see* 5185
Methylaminomethyl 4-Hydroxyphenyl Carbinol *see* 9012
1-(Methylamino)-2-methyl-2-phenylethane *see* 7308
2-Methylamino-2-methyl-1-phenylpropane *see* 5852
α-(Methylaminomethyl)vanillyl Alcohol *see* 5926
N-[4-(6-Methylamino-7-nitro-2-thia-5-aza-6-heptene-1-yl)-2-thiazolylmethyl]-*N*,*N*-dimethylamine *see* 6660
p-Methylaminophenol Sulfate, 6017
4-(Methylamino)phenol Sulfate Salt (2:1) *see* 6017
2-Methylamino-1-phenylethanol *see* 4601
1-Methylamino-2-phenylpropane *see* 7308

(1*R*,2*S*)-2-Methylamino-1-phenylpropan-1-ol *see* 3608
(1*S*,2*S*)-2-Methylamino-1-phenylpropan-1-ol *see* 7916
L-*erythro*-2-(Methylamino)-1-phenylpropan-1-ol *see* 3608
2-(Methylamino)-1-phenyl-1-propanone *see* 5963
1-Methyl-4-amino-*N*-phenyl-*N*-(2-thenyl)piperidine *see* 9278
5-(Methylamino)-2-phenyl-4-[3-(trifluoromethyl)phenyl]-3(2*H*)-furanone *see* 4205
5-Methylamino-2-phenyl-4-(α,α,α-trifluoro-*m*-tolyl)furan-3(2*H*)-one *see* 4205
α-Methylaminopropiophenone *see* 5963
β-(Methylamino)propylcyclopentane *see* 2740
1-(3-Methylaminopropyl)dibenzo[*b,e*]bicyclo[2.2.2]octadiene *see* 5748
7-(3-Methylaminopropyl)-1,2:5,6-dibenzocycloheptatriene *see* 7901
5-(3-Methylaminopropyl)-5*H*-dibenzo-[*a,d*]cycloheptene *see* 7901
9-(γ-Methylaminopropyl)-9,10-dihydro-9,10-ethanoanthracene *see* 5748
5-(α-Methylaminopropylidene)dibenzo-[*a,d*]cyclohepta[1,4]diene *see* 6715
N-(3-Methylaminopropyl)iminobibenzyl *see* 2920
5-(γ-Methylaminopropyl)iminodibenzyl *see* 2920
4-[2-(Methylamino)propyl]phenol *see* 7330
Methylaminopterin *see* 5985
4-Methyl-2-aminopyridine *see* 466
2-(2-Methyl-4-aminopyrimidin-5-yl)-methylformamido-5-hydroxy-2-penten-3-yl Propyl Disulfide *see* 7882
1-(2-Methyl-4-amino-5-pyrimidyl)methyl-2-methyl-3-hydroxyethylpyridinium Bromide Hydrobromide *see* 7992
4-Methylaminorex, 6018
N-Methyl-*N*-(3-amino-2,4,6-triiodophenyl)glutaramic Acid *see* 5053
3β-Methylamino-2,2,3-trimethylbicyclo[2.2.1]heptane *see* 5774
5-(Methylamino)-2-[[(2*R*,3*R*,6*S*,8*S*,9*R*,11*R*)-3,9,11-trimethyl-8-[(1*S*)-1-methyl-2-oxo-2-(1*H*-pyrrol-2-yl)ethyl]-1,7-dioxaspiro[5.5]undec-2-yl]methyl]-4-benzoxazolecarboxylic Acid *see* 1639
2-Methylamino-2,3,3-trimethylnorbornane *see* 5774
d-*N*-Methylamphetamine *see* 5948
Methyl *tert*-Amyl Ether *see* 612
Methyl Amyl Ketone *see* 4663
17α-Methylandrostan[3,2-*c*]isoxazol-17β-ol *see* 634
(5α,17β)-17-Methylandrostano[3,2-*c*]-isoxazol-17-ol *see* 634
1α-Methyl-5α-androstan-17β-ol-3-one *see* 5916
2α-Methylandrostan-17β-ol-3-one *see* 3448
17α-Methylandrostan-17β-ol-3-one *see* 5915
17α-Methylandrostan-3-on-17β-ol *see* 5915
(5α,17β)-17-Methylandrostano[2,3-*c*]-[1,2,5]oxadiazol-17-ol *see* 4299
Methylandrostenediol *see* 5950
(3β,17β)-17-Methylandrost-5-ene-3,17-diol *see* 5950

17α-Methyl-4-androstene-4,17β-diol-3-one *see* 6965
1-Methyl-Δ¹-androsten-17β-ol-3-one *see* 5967
2-Methyl-5α-androst-1-en-17β-ol-3-one *see* 8808
17α-Methyl-Δ⁴-androsten-17β-ol-3-one *see* 6125
(5α,17β)-17-Methyl-2′*H*-androst-2-eno-[3,2-*c*]pyrazol-17-ol *see* 8794
N-Methylanhalonidine *see* 7074
Methylaniline, 6019
2-Methylaniline *see* 9536
3-Methylaniline *see* 9536
4-Methylaniline *see* 9536
2-Methyl-9,10-anthracenedione *see* 6021
3-Methyl-1,8,9-anthracenetriol *see* 2253
Methyl Anthranilate, 6020
β-Methylanthraquinone *see* 6021
2-Methylanthraquinone, 6021
Methyl Aphoxide *see* 5936
Methylarbutin *see* 773
Methylarbutoside *see* 773
Methylarecaidin *see* 778
*N*ᴳ-Methylarginine, 6022
Methylarsinic Acid *see* 5953
Methylarsonic Acid *see* 5953
3-*O*-Methylarterenol *see* 6708
N-Methyl-D-asparaginsaure (German) *see* 6662
*N*⁴-Methyl-D-asparaginylamoxicillin *see* 852
(2*R*)-*N*-Methyl-D-asparaginyl-*N*-[(2*S*,5*R*,6*R*)-2-carboxy-3,3-dimethyl-7-oxo-4-thia-1-azabicyclo[3.2.0]hept-6-yl]-D-2-(4-hydroxyphenyl)glycinamide *see* 852
N-Methyl-D-aspartate *see* 6662
N-Methyl-D-aspartic Acid *see* 6662
Methylaspirin *see* 6010
Methylatropine Bromide *see* 875
Methylatropine Nitrate *see* 875
9-Methyl-9-azabicyclo[3.3.1]nonan-3-one *see* 7920
8-Methyl-8-azabicyclo[3.2.1]octane *see* 9777
endo-8-Methyl-8-azabicyclo[3.2.1]octan-3-ol *see* 9781
exo-8-Methyl-8-azabicyclo[3.2.1]octan-3-ol *see* 7921
exo-8-Methyl-8-azabicyclo[3.2.1]octan-3-ol Benzoate (Ester) *see* 9774
(1*R*)-8-Methyl-8-azabicyclo[3.2.1]oct-2-ene-2-carboxylic Acid *see* 3492
1-Methylazacyclopentan-2-one *see* 6117
N-Methyl-11-aza-10-deoxo-10-dihydro-erythromycin A *see* 915
5-Methyl-6-azauracil *see* 903
Methylazoxymethanol *see* 2701
Methylazoxymethanol β-D-Glucoside *see* 2701
(Methyl-*ONN*-azoxy)methyl β-D-Glucopyranoside *see* 2701
(*R*,*R*)-7-*O*-Methylbebeerine *see* 2213
2-Methylbenzaldehyde *see* 9527
2-Methylbenzamide *see* 9528
2-Methylbenzamine *see* 9536
3-Methylbenzamine *see* 9536
4-Methylbenzamine *see* 9536
N-Methylbenzenamine *see* 6019
Methylbenzene *see* 9529
2-Methylbenzenecarbonitrile *see* 9537
5-Methyl-1,3-benzenediol *see* 6864
α-Methylbenzeneethanamine *see* 582

(α*S*)-α-Methylbenzeneethanamine *see* 2954
α-Methylbenzenemethanamine *see* 6026
4-Methylbenzenesulfonic Acid *see* 9533
4-Methylbenzenesulfonic Acid Ethyl Ester *see* 3858
N-(4-Methylbenzenesulfonyl)-*N*′-(3-azabicyclo[3.3.0]oct-3-yl)urea *see* 4439
N′-4-Methylbenzenesulfonyl-*N*″-butyl-urea *see* 9507
Methylbenzenethiol *see* 9325
Methylbenzethonium Chloride, 6023
α-Methylbenzhydryl 2-Dimethylamino-ethyl Ether *see* 6287
p-Methylbenzhydryl 2-Dimethylamino-ethyl Ether *see* 6053
N-Methyl-*N*′-benzhydrylpiperazine *see* 2710
1-Methyl-3-benziloyloxyquinuclidinium Bromide *see* 2354
Methyl 2-Benzimidazolecarbamate *see* 1791
Methyl Benzoate, 6024
α-Methyl-1,3-benzodioxole-5-ethanamine *see* 5765
13-Methyl[1,3]benzodioxolo[5,6-*c*]-1,3-dioxolo[4,5-*i*]phenanthridinium *see* 8356
Methylbenzoic Acid *see* 9535
4-Methylbenzoic Acid 4-[2-[(1,1-Dimeth-ylethyl)amino]-1-hydroxyethyl]-1,2-phenylene Ester *see* 1307
o-Methylbenzonitrile *see* 9537
2-Methylbenzonitrile *see* 9537
2-Methylbenzophenone *see* 7317
4-Methylbenzophenone *see* 7317
4′-Methylbenzophenone-2-carboxylic Acid *see* 9539
3-Methyl-4*H*-1-benzopyran-4-one *see* 9658
α-Methyl-5*H*-[1]benzopyrano[2,3-*b*]pyri-dine-7-acetic Acid *see* 7711
3-Methyl-γ-benzopyrone *see* 9658
Methyl Benzoquate *see* 6472
Methyl 5-Benzoyl-2-benzimidazolecarba-mate *see* 5768
Methyl Benzoylsalicylate, 6025
α-Methyl-5-benzoyl-2-thienylacetic Acid *see* 9422
α-Methylbenzylamine, 6026
*N*¹-[3-[[(*S*)-α-Methylbenzyl]amino]pro-pyl]bleomycinamide *see* 7144
m-Methylbenzyl Bromide *see* 10090
m-Methylbenzyl Chloride *see* 10091
Methyl Benzyl Ether *see* 1140
3-(4′-Methylbenzylidene)camphor *see* 6027
4-Methylbenzylidene Camphor, 6027
(*R*)-(+)-1-(α-Methylbenzyl)imidazole-5-carboxylic Acid Ethyl Ester *see* 3881
1-(α-Methylbenzyl)imidazole-5-carbox-ylic Acid Methyl Ester *see* 6148
N-(α-Methylbenzyl)linoleamide *see* 5822
d-*N*-Methyl-*N*-benzyl-β-phenylisopropyl-amine *see* 1118
5-(α-Methylbenzyl)semioxamazide *see* 7289
3-Methyl-9-benzyl-1,2,3,4-tetrahydro-γ-carboline *see* 5770
N-Methyl-9-benzyltetrahydro-γ-carbo-line *see* 5770
2-Methylbiphenyl-3-ylmethyl-(*Z*)-(1*RS*)-*cis*-3-(2-chloro-3,3,3-trifluoroprop-1-enyl)-2,2-dimethylcyclopropanecar-boxylate *see* 1209

Methylbis(β-chloroethyl)amine *see* 5775
Methylbis(β-chloroethyl)amine *N*-Oxide Hydrochloride 5776
γ-[1-Methyl-5-[bis(β-chloroethyl)amino]-2-benzimidazolyl]butyric Acid *see* 1034
4-Methyl-5-[bis(β-chloroethyl)amino]-uracil *see* 3422
6-Methyl-5-[bis(2-chloroethyl)amino]-uracil *see* 3422
(3β,5α,16α,20*S*)-14-Methyl-3,20-bis-(methylamino)-4-methylene-9,19-cyclopregnan-16-ol *see* 2716
7-Methyl-2,3:9,10-bis(methylenedioxy)-7,13a-secoberbin-13a-one *see* 7896
2-Methyl-1,2-bis(3-pyridyl)-1-propa-none *see* 6159
4-Methyl-6,7-bis(sulfooxy)-2*H*-1-benzo-pyran-2-one *see* 8984
N-Methylbis(2,4-xylyliminomethyl)-amine *see* 486
Methyl Blue, 6028
Methyl Borate *see* 9712
Methyl Bromide, 6029
Methyl *p*-Bromophenyl Ketone *see* 1403
2-Methyl-1,3-butadiene *see* 5201
3-Methylbutanal *see* 5229
3-Methyl-1-butanamine *see* 5112
3-Methylbutanoic Acid *see* 5231
(2*R*)-2-Methylbutanoic Acid (9*R*,10*R*)-10-(Acetyloxy)-9,10-dihydro-8,8-di-methyl-2-oxo-2*H*,8*H*-benzo[1,2-b:3,4-b′]dipyran-9-yl Ester *see* 10010
[2*R*-(2*R**,3*S**,6*S**,7*R**,8*R**)]-3-Methyl-butanoic Acid 8-Butyl-3-[[3-(formyl-amino)-2-hydroxybenzoyl]amino]-2,6-dimethyl-4,9-dioxo-1,5-dioxonan-7-yl Ester *see* 715
(8*S*-*cis*)-3-Methylbutanoic Acid 8,9-Di-hydro-8-[1-methyl-1-(3-methyl-1-oxobutoxy)ethyl]-2-oxo-2*H*-furo[2,3-*h*]-1-benzopyran-9-yl Ester *see* 860
3-Methylbutanoic Acid 1,1-Dimethyl-propyl Ester *see* 610
3-Methylbutanoic Acid Ethyl Ester *see* 3816
3-Methylbutanoic Acid 3-[[3-(Formyl-amino)-2-hydroxybenzoyl]amino]-8-hexyl-2,6-dimethyl-4,9-dioxo-1,5-di-oxonan-7-yl Ester *see* 714
(2*S*)-2-Methylbutanoic Acid (1*S*,3*R*,7*S*,-8*S*,8a*R*)-1,2,3,7,8,8a-Hexahydro-3,7-dimethyl-8-[2-[(2*R*,4*R*)-tetrahydro-4-hydroxy-6-oxo-2*H*-pyran-2-yl]ethyl]-1-naphthalenyl Ester *see* 5586
(2*S*)-2-Methylbutanoic Acid (1*S*,7*S*,8*S*,-8a*R*)-1,2,3,7,8,8a-Hexahydro-7-methyl-8-[2-[(2*R*,4*R*)-tetrahydro-4-hydroxy-6-oxo-2*H*-pyran-2-yl]ethyl]-1-naphthalenyl Ester *see* 6164
3-Methylbutanoic Acid Methyl Ester *see* 6093
(1α,2β,5α)-3-Methylbutanoic Acid 5-Methyl-2-(1-methylethyl)cyclohexyl Ester *see* 5841
2-Methyl-1-butanol, 6030
2-Methyl-2-butanol *see* 7140
3-Methyl-1-butanol *see* 5195
3-Methyl-2-butanol, 6031
3-Methyl-1-butanol Nitrate *see* 5122
3-Methyl-2-butanone *see* 6090
2-Methyl-2-butenal *see* 8448
2-Methyl-2-butene *see* 607
(*E*)-2-Methyl-2-butenedioic Acid *see* 5903
(*Z*)-2-Methyl-2-butenedioic Acid *see* 2321
(*Z*)-2-Methyl-2-butenoic Acid *see* 646

N,*N*″-Methylenebis[*N*′-[3-(hydroxymethyl)-2,5-dioxo-4-imidazolidinyl]urea] *see* 4916

4,4′-Methylenebis[3-hydroxy-2-naphthalenecarboxylic Acid] *see* 7005

4,4′-Methylenebis(3-hydroxy-2-naphthoic Acid) *see* 7005

Methylenebis(hydroxytoluenesulfonic Acid) Polymer *see* 7556

Methylenebis[methyl Sulfide] *see* 1256

1,1′-[Methylenebis(oxy)]bis[4-chloro]-benzene *see* 1247

4,4′-Methylenebis(perhydro-1,2,4-thiadiazine 1,1-Dioxide) *see* 9076

Methylenebisphosphonic Acid *see* 5792

4,4′-Methylenebis(tetrahydro-1,2,4-thiadiazine) 1,1,1′,1′-Tetraoxide *see* 9076

2,2′-Methylenebis[3,4,6-trichlorophenol] *see* 4680

2,2′-Methylenebis[3,4,5-trihydroxybenzoic Acid] *see* 6064

Methylene Blue, 6060

Methylene Bromide, 6061

α-Methylene Butyrolactone, 6062

γ-Methylene-γ-butyrolactone *see* 647

[4-(Methylenebutyryl)-2,3-dichlorophenoxy]acetic Acid *see* 3717

Methylene Chloride, 6063

μ-Methylene-μ-chlorobis(η⁵-2,4-cyclopentadien-1-yl)(dimethylaluminum)-titanium *see* 9091

Methylene Cyanide *see* 5711

24-Methylenecycloartanyl Ferulate *see* 6886

1,2-Methylenecyclohexane *see* 6688

(3β)-24-Methylene-9,19-cyclolanostan-3-ol 3-(4-Hydroxy-3-methoxyphenyl)-2-propenoate *see* 6886

2-Methylenecyclopropanealanine *see* 4866

4,4′-Methylenedianiline *see* 2980

Methylene Dichloride *see* 6063

Methylene Difluoride *see* 3151

Methylenedigallic Acid, 6064

4,4′-Methylenedi(3-hydroxy-2-naphthoic Acid) *see* 7005

3,4-Methylenedioxyamphetamine *see* 5765

1,2-Methylenedioxyaporphine *see* 748

1,2-(Methylenedioxy)-6aβ-aporphin-11-ol *see* 7936

3,4-(Methylenedioxy)benzaldehyde *see* 7475

3,4-Methylenedioxybenzoic Acid *see* 7477

2-[4-(3,4-Methylenedioxybenzyl)piperazino]pyrimidine *see* 7493

1,2-Methylenedioxy-9,10-dimethoxyaporphine *see* 3041

5,6-Methylenedioxy-2,3-dimethyl-4-(3′,4′-methylenedioxyphenyl)-1,2,3,4-tetrahydronaphthalene *see* 6899

3,4-Methylenedioxyethamphetamine *see* 5766

1,2-Methylenedioxy-9-hydroxy-10-methoxynoraporphine *see* 139

(±)-3,4-Methylenedioxymethamphetamine *see* 5767

3,4-Methylenedioxy-8-methoxy-10-nitro-1-phenanthrenecarboxylic Acid *see* 786

6,7-Methylenedioxy-1-methoxy-4-oxo-1,4-dihydroquinoline-3-carboxylic Acid *see* 6196

3,4-Methylenedioxy-α-methyl-β-phenylethylamine *see* 5765

1,2-(Methylenedioxy)-4-[2-(octylsulfinyl)propyl]benzene *see* 8967

3,4-Methylenedioxyphenylisopropylamine *see* 5765

N-β-(3,4-Methylenedioxyphenyl)isopropyl]-β-(3,4-dihydroxyphenyl)-β-hydroxyethylamine *see* 7895

N-[2-(3,4-Methylenedioxyphenylisopropyl)]norepinephrine *see* 7895

5-(3,4-Methylenedioxyphenyl)-2,4-pentadienoic Acid *see* 7467

1,2-(Methylenedioxy)-4-propenylbenzene *see* 5223

[3,4-(Methylenedioxy)-6-propylbenzyl] Butyl Diethyleneglycol Ether *see* 7476

6-(3′,4′-Methylenedioxystyryl)-4-methoxy-5,6-dihydro-2*H*-pyran-2-one *see* 6138

α-Methylene-diphenylmethane *see* 3323

Methylenediphosphonic Acid *see* 5792

5,5′-Methylenedisalicylic Acid, 6065

3,3′-Methylenedithiobis(2-aminopropanoic Acid) *see* 3387

3,3′-(Methylenedithio)dialanine *see* 3387

16-Methylene-9α-fluoroprednisolone 21-Acetate *see* 4191

5-Methylene-2(5*H*)-furanone *see* 7892

α,α′-Methylene Glycerin *see* 4485

α,β-Methylene Glycerin *see* 4485

16-Methylene-17α-hydroxy-19-nor-4-pregnene-3,20-dione 17-Acetate *see* 3538

6-Methylene-5-hydroxytetracycline *see* 5943

Methylene Iodide, 6066

Methylenemalononitrile Copolymer with Vinyl Acetate *see* 2828

3-Methylene-6-(1-methylethyl)cyclohexene *see* 7201

(3*S*,6*S*,7*E*,11*Z*)-9-Methylene-6-(1-methylethyl)-1-oxaspiro[2.9]dodeca-7,11-dien-4-one *see* 7173

(1*R*,2*R*,5*S*,6*E*,10*R*)-8-Methylene-5-(1-methylethyl)spiro[11-oxabicyclo-[8.1.0]undec-6-ene-2,2′-oxiran]-3-one *see* 7173

11,12-Methyleneoctadecanoic Acid *see* 5341

(1*R*,3*S*,5*Z*)-4-Methylene-5-[(2*E*)-[(1*S*,-3a*S*,7a*S*)-octahydro-1-[(1*S*)-1-(3-hydroxy-3-methylbutoxy)ethyl]-7a-methyl-4*H*-inden-4-ylidene]ethylidene]-1,3-cyclohexanediol *see* 5760

Methylene Oxide *see* 4235

(*R*)-2-Methylene-3-oxocyclopentanecarboxylic Acid *see* 8376

5-Methylene-2-oxodihydrofuran *see* 7892

6-Methyleneoxytetracycline *see* 5943

16-Methyleneprednisolone *see* 7724

Methylenesuccinic Acid *see* 5242

cis-3,6-endo-Methylene-Δ⁴-tetrahydrophthalic Acid Dimethyl Ester *see* 3240

3,6-endo-Methylene-Δ⁴-tetrahydrophthalic Anhydride *see* 1796

3,6-endo-Methylene-1,2,3,6-tetrahydro-cis-phthalic Anhydride *see* 1796

16-Methylene-11β,17α,21-trihydroxypregna-1,4-diene-3,20-dione *see* 7724

Methylenomycin A *see* 6067

Methylenomycin B *see* 6067

Methylenomycins, 6067

N-Methylephedrine, 6068

N-Methylephedrine Camsylate *see* 6068

N-Methylepinephrine, 6069

3-*O*-Methylepinephrine *see* 5926

Methyl (2*E*,6*E*,10*R*,11*S*)-10,11-Epoxy-7-ethyl-3,11-dimethyl-2,6-tridecadienoate *see* 5273

Methyl (2*E*,6*E*,10*R*)-10,11-Epoxy-3,7,-11-trimethyl-2,6-dodecadienoate *see* 5273

Methyl (2*E*,6*E*,10*R*,11*S*)-10,11-Epoxy-3,7,11-trimethyl-2,6-tridecadienoate *see* 5273

Methylergobasine *see* 6070

Methylergobrevin [Wernigerode] *see* 6070

Methylergol Carbamide *see* 5518

Methylergometrine *see* 6070

Methylergonovine, 6070

6-*O*-Methylerythromycin *see* 2339

β-Methylesculetin *see* 8408

4-Methylesculetin Bis(hydrogen Sulfate) *see* 8984

4-Methylesculetindisulfonic Acid *see* 8984

4-Methylesculetin-6,7-disulfuric Ester *see* 8984

17α-Methyl-4,9,11-estratrien-17β-ol-3-one *see* 6129

Methylestrenolone *see* 6710

[[(1-Methyl-1,2-ethanediyl)bis[carbamodithioato]](2−)]zinc *see* 7819

4,4′-(1-Methyl-1,2-ethanediyl)bis-2,6-piperazinedione *see* 8123

N,*N*′-(1-Methyl-1,2-ethanediyl)bis-3-pyridinecarboxamide *see* 6493

2,2′-(1-Methyl-1,2-ethanediylidene)-bis[hydrazinecarboximidamide] *see* 6213

1,1′-[(Methylethanediylidene)dinitrilo]diguanidine *see* 6213

N-Methyl-9,10-ethanoanthracene-9(10*H*)-methanamine *see* 1087

N-Methyl-9,10-ethanoanthracene-9(10*H*)-propanamine *see* 5748

Methylethene *see* 7849

4-(1-Methylethenyl)-1-cyclohexene-1-carboxaldehyde *see* 7167

Methyl Ether, 6071

4′-Methyl Ether *see* 4391

1-[4-[[2-(1-Methylethoxy)ethoxy]methyl]phenoxy]-3-[(1-methylethyl)amino]-2-propanol *see* 1295

2-(1-Methylethoxy)phenol Methylcarbamate *see* 7836

7-(1-Methylethoxy)-3-phenyl-4*H*-1-benzopyran-4-one *see* 5074

N-[3-(1-Methylethoxy)phenyl]-2-(trifluoromethyl)benzamide *see* 4212

N-[[(1-Methylethyl)amino]carbonyl]-4-[(3-methylphenyl)amino]-3-pyridinesulfonamide *see* 9552

1-[(1-Methylethyl)amino]-3-[(2-methyl-1*H*-indol-4-yl)oxy]-2-propanol *see* 5856

α-[[(1-Methylethyl)amino]methyl]-2-naphthalenemethanol *see* 7790

α-[[(1-Methylethyl)amino]methyl]-4-nitrobenzenemethanol *see* 6530

1-[(1-Methylethyl)amino]-3-(3-methylphenoxy)-2-propanol *see* 9516

1-[(1-Methylethyl)amino]-3-(1-naphthalenyloxy)-2-propanol *see* 7840

2-Methylethylamino-1-phenyl-1-propanol *see* 3709

1-[(1-Methylethyl)amino]-3-[2-(2-propenyloxy)phenoxy]-2-propanol *see* 6952

1-[(1-Methylethyl)amino]-3-[2-(2-propenyl)phenoxy]-2-propanol *see* 313

9-[3-[(1-Methylethyl)amino]propyl]-9*H*-fluorene-9-carboxamide *see* 4937

(±)-Methyl-(1*R*,2*R*,3*R*)-3-hydroxy-2-
[(*E*)-(4*RS*)-4-hydroxy-4-methyl-1-oc-
tenyl]-5-oxocyclopentaneheptanoate
see 6210
1-Methyl-2-hydroxy-2-(4-hydroxyphen-
yl)ethyl-1-(4-benzylpiperidine) *see*
4895
Methyl *p*-[2-Hydroxy-3-(isopropylamino)propoxy]hydrocinnamate *see* 3700
(±)-Methyl 3-[4-[2-Hydroxy-3-(isopropylamino)propoxy]phenyl]propionate
see 3700
1-Methyl-3-hydroxy-4-isopropylbenzene
see 9399
1-Methyl-3-hydroxy-4-isopropyl-6-chlo-
robenzene *see* 2170
α-Methylhydroxylamine *see* 5989
O-Methylhydroxylamine *see* 5989
2-Methyl-7-hydroxy-6-methoxy-1-(3-hy-
droxy-4-methoxybenzyl)-1,2,3,4-tetra-
hydroisoquinoline *see* 8163
4-Methyl-5-hydroxymethyluracil *see*
7137
3-Methyl-4-hydroxy-1-naphthylamine
see 10023
4-(4-Methyl-L-2-hydroxypentanoic Acid)
Sporidesmolide I *see* 8765
α-Methyl-3-(*m*-hydroxyphenyl)alanine
see 6132
α-Methyl-3-(*p*-hydroxyphenyl)alanine *see*
6161
2-Methyl-2-*p*-hydroxyphenylbutane *see*
7142
N-Methyl-*N*-[3-hydroxy-3-phenyl-3-(α-
thienyl)propyl]morpholinium Iodide
see 9431
1-Methyl-4-hydroxypiperidine Benzhydryl Ether *see* 3331
6α-Methyl-11β-hydroxyprogesterone *see*
5794
6α-Methyl-17α-hydroxyprogesterone *see*
5793
1-Methyl-3-hydroxypyridinium Bromide
Dimethylcarbamate *see* 7977
1-Methyl-2-hydroxy-3,4,5-trichloroben-
zene *see* 9635
Methyl Hygrate Betaine *see* 8771
N-Methylhyoscyaminium Bromide *see*
4858
1,1′,1″-Methylidenetris[benzene] *see* 9741
Methylidinoglycerol *see* 4485
1,1′,1″-[Methylidynetris(oxy)]tris-
[ethane] *see* 6884
2-Methylimidazole Polymer with 1-Chlo-
ro-2,3-epoxypropane *see* 2474
2-Methyl-1*H*-imidazole Polymer with
(Chloromethyl)oxirane *see* 2474
1-Methylimidazole-2-thiol *see* 5971
ε-(4-Methyl-5-imidazolidone-2)-caproic
Acid *see* 2934
2-Methyl-2-imidazoline *see* 5635
l-10[(2-Methyl-1*H*-imidazol-1-yl)meth-
yl]-5,6,8,9,10,11-hexahydro-4*H*-pyr-
ido[3,2,1-jk]carbazol-11-one *see* 2271
2-Methyl-4,4′-[(4-imino-2,5-cyclohexa-
dien-1-ylidene)methylene]dianiline
Hydrochloride *see* 5652
3-Methyl-1*H*-indole *see* 8560
1-Methylindole-2,3-dione 3-Thiosemi-
carbazone *see* 5977
α-Methyl-1*H*-indole-3-ethanamine *see*
6131
1-Methyl-1*H*-indole-3,5,6-triol *see* 174
(*R*)-5-[(1-Methylindol-3-yl)carbonyl]-
4,5,6,7-tetrahydrobenzimidazole *see*
8105

(1-Methyl-1*H*-indol-3-yl)[(5*R*)-4,5,6,7-
tetrahydro-1*H*-benzimidazol-5-yl]-
methanone *see* 8105
Methyl Iodide, 6087
Methyl 4-Iodo-2-[3-(4-methoxy-6-meth-
yl-1,3,5-triazin-2-yl)ureidosulfonyl]-
benzoate Sodium Salt *see* 5046
6-Methylionone *see* 5095
N-Methylisatin 3-Thiosemicarbazone *see*
5977
Methyl Isobutyl Ketone *see* 5207
Methyl Isobutyrate, 6088
N-Methyl-2-isocamphanamine *see* 5774
2-Methylisocrotonic Acid *see* 646
Methyl Isocyanate, 6089
N-(D-6-Methyl-8-isoergolenyl)-*N*,*N*-di-
ethylurea *see* 5518
N-(D-6-Methyl-8-isoergolin-1-yl)-*N*′,*N*′-
diethylurea *see* 9164
Methylisomyn *see* 5948
Methylisooctenylamine *see* 5185
1-Methyl-4-isopropenyl-Δ⁶-cyclohexen-
2-one *see* 1874
4-(2-Methyl-5-isopropenyl-1-cyclopen-
ten-1-yl)-2-butanone *see* 5204
Methylisopropylbenzene *see* 2763
1-Methyl-4-isopropylcyclohexan-3-one
see 5838
1-Methyl-4-isopropyl-1-cyclohexen-2-ol-
3-one *see* 3298
1-Methyl-4-isopropylidene-3-cyclohexa-
none *see* 7937
Methyl Isopropyl Ketone, 6090
Methyl 2-(4-Isopropyl-4-methyl-5-oxo-2-
imidazolin-2-yl)-*p*-toluate *see* 4903
Methyl 6-(4-Isopropyl-4-methyl-5-oxo-2-
imidazolin-2-yl)-*m*-toluate *see* 4903
L-(+)-2-Methyl-5-isopropyl-1,3-nona-
dien-8-one *see* 8707
5-Methyl-2-isopropyl-1-phenol *see* 9399
6-Methyl-3-isopropylsalicylic Acid *see*
9408
(2*S*,3*S*,5*S*)-5-[*N*-[*N*-[[*N*-Methyl-*N*-[(2-iso-
propyl-4-thiazolyl)methyl]amino]car-
bonyl]valinyl]amino]-2-[*N*-[(5-thiazol-
yl)methoxycarbonyl]amino]-1,6-di-
phenyl-3-hydroxyhexane *see* 8238
Methylisothiazolinone, 6091
2-Methyl-3(2*H*)-isothiazolone *see* 6091
Methyl Isothiocyanate, 6092
Methyl Isovalerate, 6093
4-[4-β-(5-Methylisoxazole-3-carboxami-
do)ethyl]phenylsulfonyl]-1,1-hexa-
methylenesemicarbazide *see* 4444
5-Methyl-3-isoxazolecarboxylic Acid 2-
Benzylhydrazide *see* 5157
5-Methylisoxazole-4-carboxylic Acid Trifluoromethylanilide *see* 5432
5-Methyl-3(2*H*)-isoxazolone *see* 4856
*N*¹-(5-Methyl-3-isoxazolyl)sulfanilamide
see 8918
Methyl Jasmonate *see* 5260
Methyl Lactate, 6094
2-Methyllactonitrile *see* 67
Methyl Linoleate, 6095
N-Methyllorazepam *see* 5581
1-Methyllumilysergol 8-(5-Bromonico-
tinate) 10-Methyl Ether *see* 6496
(15*R*)-15-Methyllycopodan-5-one *see*
5622
1-Methyl-*d*-lysergic Acid Butanolamide
see 6137
1-Methyl-*d*-lysergic Acid (+)-1-Hydroxy-
2-butylamide *see* 6137
Methylmaleic Acid *see* 2321
2-Methylmalic Acid *see* 2323

Methyl Malonate, 6096
α-Methylmandelic Acid *see* 873
Methylmelubrin *see* 3350
Methylmercadone *see* 6532
Methyl Mercaptan *see* 5956
Methyl β-Mercaptoalanine Hydrochloride *see* 5785
1-Methyl-2-mercaptoimidazole *see* 5971
5-(Methylmercaptomethyl)-3-(5-nitro-2-
furfurylideneamino)-2-oxazolidinone
see 6532
4-Methylmercapto-3-methylphenyl Di-
methyl Thiophosphate *see* 4002
2-Methylmercapto-10-[2-(*N*-methyl-2-
piperidyl)ethyl]phenothiazine *see* 9359
3-Methylmercapto-*N*-[2′-(*N*′-methyl-2-
piperidyl)ethyl]phenothiazine *see* 9359
Methyl-mercaptophos *see* 6051
D-2-Methyl-3-mercaptopropanoyl-L-
proline *see* 1774
Methyl Mercury *see* 3250
Methyl Mesylate *see* 6097
Methyl Methacrylate *see* 5941
N-Methylmethanamine *see* 3228
Methylmethane *see* 3723
Methyl Methanesulfonate, 6097
Methyl Methanesulfonic Acid *see* 6097
S-Methylmethionine, 6098
S-Methyl-L-methionine *see* 6098
Methylmethioninesulfonium Bromide *see*
6098
Methylmethioninesulfonium Chloride *see*
6098
Methyl *N*-(2-Methoxyacetyl)-*N*-(2,6-
xylyl)-DL-alaninate *see* 5922
1-Methyl-6-methoxy-3,4-dihydro-2-car-
boline *see* 5995
1-Methyl-7-methoxy-3,4-dihydro-β-car-
boline *see* 4613
Methyl-(*E*)-methoxyiminoα-(*o*-tolyloxy)-
o-tolyl]acetate *see* 5324
l-α-2-Methyl-8-methoxy-6,7-methylene-
dioxy-1-(6,7-dimethoxy-3-phthalid-
yl)-1,2,3,4-tetrahydroisoquinoline
see 6718
Methyl 3-(3-(4-Methoxy-6-methyl-1,3,5-
triazin-2-yl)ureidosulfonyl)thio-
phene-2-carboxylate *see* 9316
(+)-*trans*-1-Methyl-3-[*p*-(methoxy)phen-
oxymethyl]-4-phenylpiperidine *see*
3955
3,4-(2′-Methyl-2′-methoxy-4′-phenyl)-
dihydropyranocoumarin *see* 2717
2-Methyl-2-methoxy-4-phenyl-5-oxodi-
hydropyrano[3,2-*c*][1]benzopyran *see*
2717
2-(3-Methyl-5-methoxy-1-pyrazolyl)-4-
methoxy-6-methylpyrimidine *see* 3622
2-Methyl-4-methoxy-6-sulfanilamido-
1,3-diazine *see* 8917
2-Methyl-4-methoxy-6-sulfanilamidopyr-
imidine *see* 8917
1-Methyl-6-methoxy-1,2,3,4-tetrahydro-
2-carboline *see* 173
3-Methyl-8-methoxy-3*H*-1,2,5,6-tetrahy-
dropyrazino[1,2,3-*ab*]-β-carboline *see*
6153
1-Methyl-6-(1-methylallyl)-2,5-dithiobi-
urea *see* 5946
2-Methyl-6-methylamino-2-heptene *see*
5185
Methyl 2-(Methylamino)-3-methoxyben-
zoate *see* 2808
6-[(2*S*,4*R*,6*E*)-4-Methyl-2-(methylamino)-3-oxo-6-octenoic Acid]cyclosporin
D *see* 9917

Methylnaltrexone Bromide, 6099

2-Methyl-1,4-naphthalenediol see 5830

2-Methyl-1,4-naphthalenediol Diphosphoric Acid Ester Tetrasodium Salt see 5830

2-Methyl-1,4-naphthalenedione see 5831

(+)-*N*-Methyl-3-(1-naphthalenyloxy)-3-(2-thienyl)propanamine see 3465

(γ*S*)-*N*-Methyl-γ-(1-naphthalenyloxy)-2-thiophenepropanamine see 3465

2-Methyl-1,4-naphthohydroquinone see 5830

2-Methyl-1,4-naphthoquinol see 5830

2-Methyl-1,4-naphthoquinone see 5831

Methyl β-Naphthyl Ether see 5997

trans-*N*-Methyl-*N*-(1-naphthylmethyl)-6,6-dimethylhept-2-en-4-ynyl-1-amine see 9156

N-Methyl-*N*-(1-naphthylmethyl)-3-phenylpropen-1-amine see 6355

(+)-(*S*)-*N*-Methyl-γ-(1-naphthyloxy)-2-thiophenepropylamine see 3465

N[1]-Methylnicotinamide Chloride see 9693

Methyl Nicotinate, 6100

Methyl Nitrate, 6101

1-Methylnitrazepam see 6549

Methylnitrobenzene see 6650

Methyl *p*-Nitrobenzenesulfonate, 6102

1-Methyl-7-nitro-5-(2-fluorophenyl)-3*H*-1,4-benzodiazepin-2(1*H*)-one see 4146

3-Methyl-*N*-[(5-nitro-2-furanyl)methylene]-4-thiomorpholinamine 1,1-Dioxide see 6538

2-Methyl-5-nitroimidazole-1-ethanol see 6157

1-Methyl-5-nitroimidazole-2-methanol Carbamate (Ester) see 8254

(1-Methyl-5-nitroimidazol-2-yl)methyl Carbamate see 8254

(*E*)-4-[2-(1-Methyl-5-nitro-1*H*-imidazol-2-yl)ethenyl]-2-pyrimidinamine see 897

[2-(2-Methyl-5-nitro-1*H*-imidazol-1-yl)ethyl]carbamothioic Acid *O*-Methyl Ester see 1848

6-(1-Methyl-4-nitro-5-imidazolyl)mercaptopurine see 902

1-(2-Methyl-5-nitroimidazol-1-yl)-2-propanol see 8419

6-[(1-Methyl-4-nitro-1*H*-imidazol-5-yl)thio]-1*H*-purin-2-amine see 9299

6-[(1-Methyl-4-nitro-1*H*-imidazol-5-yl)thio]-1*H*-purine see 902

3-Methyl-4-nitro-1-(*p*-nitrophenyl)-2-pyrazolin-5-one see 7412

N-Methyl-*N*′-nitro-*N*-nitrosoguanidine, 6103

5-Methyl-2-nitro-7-oxa-8-mercurabicyclo[4.2.0]octa-1,3,5-triene see 6610

[2-Methyl-5-nitrophenolato(2−)-*C*[6],-*O*[1]]mercury see 6610

4-Methyl-*N*-[4-[(4-nitrophenyl)amino]phenyl]-1-piperazinecarbothioamide see 571

3-Methyl-5-[(*p*-nitrophenyl)azo]rhodanine see 6596

3-Methyl-5-[(*p*-nitrophenyl)azo]-2-thio-2,4-thiazolidinedione see 6596

3-Methyl-5-[(4-nitrophenyl)azo]-2-thioxo-4-thiazolidinone see 6596

Methyl [*N*′-[2-Nitro-5-(propylthio)phenyl]-*N*-(2-sulfoethyl)amidino]carbamate see 6480

N-Methyl-*N*-nitrosomethanamine see 6637

N-Methyl-*N*-nitroso-*N*′-nitroguanidine see 6103

N-Methyl-*N*-nitroso-*p*-toluenesulfonamide see 9543

N-Methyl-*N*′-nitro-*N*″-[(tetrahydro-3-furanyl)methyl]guanidine see 3289

1-Methyl-2-nitro-3-[(3-tetrahydrofuryl)methyl]guanidine see 3289

2-Methyl-*N*-[4-nitro-3-(trifluoromethyl)phenyl]propanamide see 4208

Methyl Nonyl Ketone, 6104

α-Methylnoradrenaline see 6692

3-*O*-Methylnoradrenaline see 6708

α-Methylnorepinephrine see 6692

3-*O*-Methylnorepinephrine see 6708

18-Methylnorethindrone see 6694

17α-Methyl-19-nor-Δ[4,9]-pregnadiene-3,20-dione see 2888

17-Methyl-19-norpregna-4,9-diene-3,20-dione see 2888

17α-Methyl-Δ[9]-19-norprogesterone see 2888

(3β,16β,17α,22α)-17-Methyl-18-nor-16,28-secosolanida-5,12-diene-3,16-diol see 9949

Methylnortestosterone see 6710

17α-Methyl-19-nortestosterone see 6710

Methyloctenylamine see 5185

N-Methyl-7-chlortetracycline see 2388

Methylol Dimethylhydantoin see 4831

Methyl Oleate see 6828

Methylolsulfonic Acid Sodium Salt see 4236

Methyl Orange, 6105

Methyl Orthoformate see 6884

Methyl Orthovalerate see 9717

Methyl Oxalate, 6106

Methyloxan [Nippon Shoji] see 5979

6-Methyl-1,2,3-oxathiazin-4(3*H*)-one 2,2-Dioxide see 37

N-Methyloxazepam see 9133

23-Methyloxime LL-F282249α see 6290

Methyloxirane see 7856

Methyloxirane Block Polymer with Oxirane see 7562

(2*R*-*cis*)-(3-Methyloxiranyl)phosphonic Acid see 4254

(2*R*-*cis*)-(3-Methyloxiranyl)-phosphonic Acid Compd with 2-Amino-2-(hydroxymethyl)-1,3-propanediol (1:1) see 4254

2-(3-Methyl-1-oxobutyl)-1*H*-indene-1,3-(2*H*)-dione see 5233

N-(2-Methyl-1-oxobutyl)-L-phenylalanine (1*S*)-1-[(2*S*,3*R*)-3-(Acetyloxy)-1-[(2*S*)-2-amino-3-methyl-1-oxobutyl]-2-pyrrolidinyl]-2-carboxyethyl Ester see 2938

N-(3-Methyl-1-oxobutyl)-L-valyl-L-valyl-(3*S*,4*S*)-4-amino-3-hydroxy-6-methylheptanoyl-*N*-[(1*S*)-1-[(1*S*)-2-carboxy-1-hydroxyethyl]-3-methylbutyl]-L-alaninamide see 7147

α-Methyl-4-[(2-oxocyclopentyl)methyl]benzeneacetic Acid see 5589

(5-Methyl-2-oxo-1,3-dioxolen-4-yl)methyl 4-(1-Hydroxy-1-methylethyl)-2-propyl-1-[4-[2-(tetrazol-5-yl)phenyl]phenyl]methylimidazole-5-carboxylate see 6839

4-[2-Methyl-4-oxo-3,3-diphenyl-4-(1-pyrrolidinyl)butyl]morpholine see 2955

6-Methyl-2-oxo-1,3-dithio[4,5-*b*]quinoxaline see 6978

N-Methyl-*N*-(1-oxododecyl)glycine Sodium Salt see 4368

3-Methyl-1-(5-oxohexyl)-7-propylxanthine see 7813

5-Methyl-2-oxo-4-imidazolidinecaproic Acid see 2934

(4*R*-*cis*)-5-Methyl-2-oxo-4-imidazolidinehexanoic Acid see 2934

[[(3-Methyl-4-oxo-1(4*H*)-naphthalenylidene)amino]oxy]acetic Acid Ammonium Salt see 5832

N-[2-(2-Methyl-4-oxopentyl)]acrylamide see 2963

3-Methyl-4-oxo-2-phenyl-4*H*-1-benzopyran-8-carboxylic Acid 2-(1-Piperidinyl)ethyl Ester see 7813

[(1*R*)-3-Methyl-1-[[(2*S*)-1-oxo-3-phenyl-2-[(pyrazinylcarbonyl)amino]propyl]amino]butyl]boronic Acid see 1351

3-Methyl-4-oxo-5-piperidino-Δ[2,α]-thiazolidineacetic Acid Ethyl Ester see 3891

[3-Methyl-4-oxo-5-(1-piperidinyl)-2-thiazolidinylidene]acetic Acid Ethyl Ester see 3891

4-Methyl-3-[[1-oxo-2-(propylamino)propyl]amino]-2-thiophenecarboxylic Acid Methyl Ester see 1869

(±)-Methyl 2-Oxopropyl 1,4-Dihydro-2,6-dimethyl-4-(2-nitrophenyl)-3,5-pyridinedicarboxylate see 767

(17β)-17-Methyl-17-(1-oxopropyl)estra-4,9-dien-3-one see 7785

cis-(−)-3-Methyl-4-[(1-oxopropyl)phenylamino)]-1-(2-phenylethyl)-4-piperidinecarboxylic Acid Methyl Ester see 5556

(*S*)-2-Methyl-4-oxo-3-(2-propynyl)cyclopent-2-enyl (1*R*)-*cis*-*trans*-Chrysanthemate see 7704

(2*S*,3*S*,5*R*)-3-Methyl-7-oxo-3-(1*H*-1,2,3-triazol-1-ylmethyl)-4-thia-1-azabicyclo[3.2.0]heptane-2-carboxylic Acid 4,4-Dioxide see 9083

Methylparaben, 6107

Methylparafynol see 5846

Methyl Parasept [Tenneco] see 6107

Methyl Parathion, 6108

Methylpartricin see 5847

2-Methyl-2,4-pentanediol see 4710

4-Methylpentanenitrile see 5117

3-Methyl-3-pentanol Carbamate see 3566

4-Methyl-2-pentanone see 5207

4-Methyl-3-penten-2-one see 5908

4-Methyl-3-penten-2-one (1-Phthalazinyl)hydrazone see 1470

3-Methyl-2-(2-pentenyl)-2-cyclopenten-1-one see 5259

(−)-Methyl *cis*-2-Pent-2′-enyl-3-oxocyclopentylacetate see 5260

3-Methyl-2-penten-4-yn-1-ol see 7131

3-Methyl-3-pentyl Carbamate see 3566

Methyl *tert*-Pentyl Ether see 612

Methyl 2-Pentyl-3-oxocyclopentyl-1-acetate see 6052

Methylpentynol see 5846

3-Methyl-1-pentyn-3-ol see 5846

3-Methyl-1-pentyn-3-yl Acid Phthalate see 7374

Methylperidol see 6263

Methylperone see 5827

(15*R*)-15-Methyl-PGE$_2$ see 769

(15*S*)-15-Methyl PGF$_{2α}$ see 1823

5-Methylphenazinium Methyl Sulfate see 6109

5-Methyl-1(5*H*)-phenazinone see 7951

Methylphosphoramidic Acid 4-*tert*-Butyl-2-chlorophenyl Methyl Ester *see* 2604

Methylphosphoramidic Acid 2-Chloro-4-(1,1-dimethylethyl)phenyl Methyl Ester *see* 2604

Methyl Phthalate *see* 3255

2-Methyl-2-phytyl-6-chromanol *see* 9494

2-Methyl-2-phytyl-6-hydroxychroman *see* 9494

2-Methyl-3-phytyl-1,4-naphthoquinone *see* 7380

N-Methylpicolinic Acid *see* 4729

dl-*N*-Methylpipecolic Acid 2,6-Dimethylanilide *see* 5859

1-Methyl-2′,6′-pipecoloxylidide *see* 5859

4-Methyl-1-piperazinecarboxylic Acid 6-(5-Chloro-2-pyridinyl)-6,7-dihydro-7-oxo-5*H*-pyrrolo[3,4-*b*]pyrazin-5-yl Ester *see* 10193

N-[5-[4-(4-Methylpiperazinomethyl)benzoylamido]-2-methylphenyl]-4-(3-pyridyl)-2-pyrimidineamine *see* 4902

10-(γ-Methylpiperazinopropyl)phenothiazine *see* 7151

6-(4-Methyl-1-piperazinyl)-11*H*-dibenz-[*b*,*e*]azepine *see* 7179

3-[[(4-Methyl-1-piperazinyl)imino]methyl]rifamycin *see* 8216

4-[(4-Methyl-1-piperazinyl)methyl]-*N*-[4-methyl-3-[[4-(3-pyridinyl)-2-pyrimidinyl]amino]phenyl]benzamide *see* 4902

6-(4-Methyl-1-piperazinyl)morphanthridine *see* 7179

N-γ-(4′-Methyl-1′-piperazinyl)propyl]-3-butyrylphenothiazine *see* 1516

N-γ-(4′-Methylpiperazinyl-1′)propyl]-3-chlorophenothiazine *see* 7761

cis-9-[3-(4-Methyl-1-piperazinyl)propylidene]-2-(dimethylsulfonamido)thioxanthene *see* 9365

N-Methylpiperazinyl-*N*′-propylphenothiazine *see* 7151

10-[3-(4-Methyl-1-piperazinyl)propyl]-10*H*-phenothiazine *see* 7151

1-[10-[3-(4-Methyl-1-piperazinyl)propyl]-10*H*-phenothiazin-2-yl]-1-butanone *see* 1516

10-[3-(4-Methyl-1-piperazinyl)propyl]-2-(trifluoromethyl)-10*H*-phenothiazine *see* 9680

2-Methyl-1-piperidinepropanol Benzoate *see* 7474

N-(1-Methyl-2-piperidinoethyl)propionanilide *see* 7209

N-(1-Methyl-2-piperidinoethyl)-*N*-2-pyridylpropionamide *see* 7831

γ-(4-Methylpiperidino)-*p*-fluorobutyrophenone *see* 5827

(2-Methylpiperidino)propyl Benzoate *see* 7474

3-(2-Methylpiperidino)propyl *p*-Cyclohexyloxybenzoate *see* 2735

2-Methyl-3-piperidino-1-*p*-tolylpropan-1-one *see* 9522

10-[2-(1-Methyl-2-piperidinyl)ethyl]-2-(methylsulfinyl)-10*H*-phenothiazine *see* 5910

10-[2-(1-Methyl-2-piperidinyl)ethyl]-2-(methylsulfonyl)-10*H*-phenothiazine *see* 8963

10-[2-(1-Methyl-2-piperidinyl)ethyl]-2-(methylthio)-10*H*-phenothiazine *see* 9359

N-[1-Methyl-2-(1-piperidinyl)ethyl]-*N*-phenylpropanamide *see* 7209

N-[1-Methyl-2-(1-piperidinyl)ethyl]-*N*-2-pyridinylpropanamide *see* 7831

1-Methyl-4-piperidyl Benzhydryl Ether *see* 3331

N-Methyl-3-piperidyl Benzilate Methyl Bromide *see* 5848

N-Methyl-3-piperidyl Diphenylglycolate Methobromide *see* 5848

1-Methyl-4-piperidyl Diphenylpropoxyacetate *see* 7832

(±)-2′-[2-(1-Methyl-2-piperidyl)ethyl]-*p*-anisanilide *see* 3570

5-(1-Methylpiperidylidene-4)-5*H*-dibenzo[*a*,*d*]cycloheptene *see* 2773

4-(1-Methyl-4-piperidylidene)-9,10-dihydro-4*H*-benzo[4,5]cyclohepta[1,2-*b*]-thiophene *see* 7515

1-Methyl-3-piperidylidenedi(2-thienyl)-methane *see* 9457

9-(*N*-Methyl-3-piperidylmethyl)thioxanthene *see* 5979

γ-(2-Methylpiperidyl)propyl Benzoate *see* 7474

2-Methyl-3-*all-trans*-polyprenyl-1,4-naphthoquinones *see* 5833

Methylprednisolone, 6111

16β-Methylprednisone *see* 5861

6-Methyl-Δ[4,6]-pregnadien-17α-ol-3,20-dione Acetate *see* 5805

6α-Methyl-4-pregnen-17α-ol-3,20-dione *see* 5793

Methylpromazine *see* 9704

2-Methylpropanal *see* 5154

2-Methyl-1-propanamine *see* 5132

2-Methyl-2-propanamine *see* 1545

2-Methylpropanenitrile *see* 5156

2-Methyl-1-propanethiol *see* 5147

2-Methyl-2-propanethiol *see* 1579

2-Methylpropanoic Acid *see* 5155

2-Methylpropanoic Acid 2,2-Dimethyl-1-(1-methylethyl)-1,3-propanediyl Ester *see* 9251

2-Methylpropanoic Acid Ethyl Ester *see* 3814

2-Methylpropanoic Acid 4-[2-(Methylamino)ethyl]-1,2-phenylene Ester *see* 4876

2-Methylpropanoic Acid Methyl Ester *see* 6088

2-Methylpropanoic Acid 2-Methylpropyl Ester *see* 5145

2-Methyl-1-propanol *see* 5131

2-Methyl-2-propanol *see* 1542

2-Methyl-2-propanol Aluminum Salt *see* 333

N-Methyl-*N*-propargylbenzylamine *see* 7038

2-Methylpropene *see* 5141

2-Methyl-2-propenenitrile *see* 5942

2-Methyl-2-propenoic Acid *see* 5941

2-Methyl-2-propenoic Acid Oxiranylmethyl Ester Polymer with Ethyl 2-Propenoate *see* 2514

2-Methyl-1-propenyl Chloride *see* 2147

Methyl 2-Propenyl Trisulfane *see* 6013

Methyl-2-propenyl Trisulfide *see* 6013

4-Methyl-6-propionamido-1,2-dithiolo-[4,3-*b*]pyrrol-5(4*H*)-one *see* 880

5-Methyl-3-propionamidopyrrolin-4-one[4,3-*d*]-1,2-dithiole *see* 880

Methyl Propionate, 6112

17α-Methyl-17-propionylestra-4,9-dien-3-one *see* 7785

17α-Methyl-17β-propionyl-19-nor-4,9-androstadien-3-one *see* 7785

Methyl 6-Propoxy-2-benzothiazolylcarbamate *see* 9455

β-[(2-Methylpropoxy)methyl]-*N*-phenyl-*N*-(phenylmethyl)-1-pyrrolidineethanamine *see* 1150

2-Methylpropylamine *see* 5132

2-[(2-Methylpropyl)amino]ethanol 4-Aminobenzoate (Ester) *see* 1523

(1-Methylpropyl)benzene *see* 1550

(2-Methylpropyl)benzene *see* 5134

4-(2-Methylpropyl)benzeneacetic Acid *see* 4880

(2-Methylpropyl)carbamic Acid Ethyl Ester *see* 5153

Methyl Propyl Carbinol *see* 7119

(2*E*,4*E*)-*N*-(2-Methylpropyl)-2,4-decadienamide *see* 7073

(2*E*,6*Z*,8*E*)-*N*-(2-Methylpropyl)-2,6,8-decatrienamide *see* 179

2-(1-Methylpropyl)-4,6-dinitrophenol *see* 3287

Methyl Propyl Ether, 6113

1-Methylpropyl 2-(2-Hydroxyethyl)-piperidine-1-carboxylate *see* 7394

4,4′-(1-Methylpropylidene)bisphenol *see* 1298

1-(2-Methylpropyl)-1*H*-imidazo[4,5-*c*]-quinolin-4-amine *see* 4922

Methyl Propyl Ketone, 6114

1-Methylpropyl 3-(Methylthio)-2-propenyl Disulfide *see* 821

8-Methyl-3-(2-propylpentanoyloxy)-tropinium Bromide *see* 671

2-Methyl-2-propyl-1,3-propanediol Dicarbamate *see* 5862

1-Methylpropyl 1-Propenyl Disulfide *see* 821

5-(1-Methylpropyl)-5-(2-propenyl)-2,4,6-(1*H*,3*H*,5*H*)-pyrimidinetrione *see* 9036

5-(1-Methylpropyl)-5-(2-propenyl)-2,4,6-(1*H*,3*H*,5*H*)-pyrimidinetrione *see* 1511

5-(2-Methylpropyl)-5-(2-propenyl)-2-thioxo-4-imidazolidinone *see* 217

Methyl 5-(Propylthio)-2-benzimidazolecarbamate *see* 210

2-Methyl-2-propyltrimethylene Butylcarbamate Carbamate *see* 9829

2-Methyl-2-propyltrimethylene Carbamate *see* 5862

N-Methyl-*N*-2-propynylbenzenemethanamine *see* 7038

N-Methyl-*N*-2-propynylbenzylamine *see* 7038

N-(4-Methyl-6-prop-1-ynylpyrimidin-2-yl)aniline *see* 5845

6α-Methyl-17-(1-propynyl)testosterone *see* 3219

(15*R*)-15-Methylprostaglandin E$_2$ *see* 769

Methylprotocatechuic Aldehyde *see* 9932

O-Methylpsychotrine *see* 7929

9-Methylpteroylglutamic Acid *see* 6555

10-Methylpteroylglutamic Acid *see* 5984

(2*E*)-2-Methyl-4-(1*H*-purin-6-ylamino)-2-buten-1-ol *see* 10117

5-Methylpyrazinecarboxylic Acid 4-Oxide *see* 111

4-Methyl-1*H*-pyrazole *see* 4226

5-Methylpyrazole-3-carboxylic Acid, 6115

4-Methyl-2-pyridinamine *see* 466

2-Methylpyridine *see* 7400

3-Methylpyridine *see* 7401

4-Methylpyridine *see* 7402

1-Methylpyridine-3-carboxylic Acid Amide Chloride *see* 9693

Metocurine Iodide, 6144
Metodik [Labinca] *see* 856
Metofane [Vericore] *see* 5994
Metofenazate, 6145
Metol *see* 6017
Metolachlor, 6146
Metolazone, 6147
Metolquizolone *see* 5960
Metomidate, 6148
Meton *see* 4688
Metopimazine, 6149
Metopiron(e) [Novartis] *see* 6159
Metopon, 6150
Metoprolol, 6151
Metopyrone *see* 6159
Metoquinone, 6152
Metosomin [Maruishi] *see* 9522
Metosyn [Zeneca] *see* 4151
Metoxadone *see* 5851
Metralindole, 6153
Metramid [Nicholas] *see* 6143
Metranil *see* 7112
Metrazol [Knoll] *see* 7141
Metribolone *see* 6129
Metribuzin, 6154
Metrifonate *see* 9623
Metrizamide, 6155
Metrizoate Sodium *see* 6156
Metrizoic Acid, 6156
Metrodin [Serono] *see* 4223
Metrodiol [Clin-Comar-Byla] *see* 3860
MetroGel [Galderma] *see* 6157
Metrolag [Lagap] *see* 6157
Metrolyl [Sandoz] *see* 6157
Metronidazole, 6157
Metrosa [Linderma] *see* 6157
Metrotop [Medlock] *see* 6157
Metrulen *see* 3860
Metsulfuron-methyl, 6158
Metubine Iodide [Lilly] *see* 6144
Metuclazepam *see* 5920
Metvix [PhotoCure] *see* 6016
Metyrapone, 6159
Metyridine, 6160
Metyrosine, 6161
Mevacor [Merck & Co.] *see* 5586
Mevaldic Acid, 6162
Mevalolactone *see* 6163
Mevalon [Guidotti] *see* 5808
Mevalonic Acid, 6163
Mevalonic Lactone *see* 6163
Mevalotin [Sankyo] *see* 7714
Mevastatin, 6164
Mevinacor [Merck & Co.] *see* 5586
Mevinolin *see* 5586
Mevinphos, 6165
Mevlor [Merck & Co.] *see* 5586
Mexamine *see* 6002
Mexate [BMS] *see* 5985
Mexazolam, 6166
Mexenone, 6167
Mexicain, 6168
Mexican Scammony (Root) *see* 5072
Mexican Tea *see* 6785
Mexiletine, 6169
Mexitil [Boehringer, Ing.] *see* 6169
Mexocine [Specia] *see* 2886
Mexoryl SX [L'Oreal] *see* 3490
Meyerhofferite *see* 1652
Mezcaline *see* 5905
Mezene [Isagro] *see* 10172
Mezereon *see* 6170
Mezereum, 6170
Mezineb *see* 7819
Mezlin [Miles] *see* 6171

Mezlocillin, 6171
MF-201 *see* 3638
MF-934 *see* 8294
MFT *see* 1908
Mg 5-Sulfat [Artesan] *see* 5691
MG-02 *see* 61
MG-143 *see* 8984
MG-341 *see* 1351
MG-652 *see* 6915
MG-1559 *see* 10071
MG-2552 *see* 2406
MG-2555 *see* 1393
MG-5771 *see* 10071
MG-8926 *see* 3451
MG-13054 *see* 3997
MG-13608 *see* 3414
MG-19973 *see* 3763
MGA *see* 5818
MGI-114 *see* 5092
MGI-2 *see* 4537
MGK-11 *see* 8088
MGK Repellent 11 [McLaughlin] *see* 8088
MgTX *see* 5752
MH *see* 5705
MH-532 *see* 7258
MHA [Novus] *see* 5976
MHIP *see* 9516
MHPG *see* 5996
MI *see* 6091
MI-85 *see* 726
MI-85Di *see* 726
Miacalcic [Novartis] *see* 1643
Miacalcin [Novartis] *see* 1643
Miadenil [Francia] *see* 1643
Mianserin, 6172
Miarsenol *see* 6447
Miazine *see* 7987
Miazole *see* 4912
Mibefradil, 6173
MIBG *see* 5007
Mibolerone, 6174
MIC *see* 6089
Micafungin, 6175
Micanol [Bioglan] *see* 684
Micardis [Boehringer, Ing.] *see* 9129
Micatex [Andromaco] *see* 9612
Micatin [J & J] *see* 6178
Micetal [Uriach] *see* 4215
Michler's Base, 6176
Michler's Ketone, 6177
Michrome No. 24 *see* 218
Michrome No. 66 *see* 1959
Michrome No. 226 *see* 6488
Micinovo [Andreu] *see* 5925
Micofugal [Biopharma] *see* 3502
Micofur [Norwich] *see* 6536
Micogin [Crosara] *see* 3502
Micol *see* 2025
Miconal Ecobi [Ecobi] *see* 6178
Miconazole, 6178
Micoren [Novartis] *see* 2591
Micoserina *see* 2751
Micotef [LPB] *see* 6178
Micotil [Elanco] *see* 9439
Micoxolamina [Dompé] *see* 2266
Micranthine, 6179
Micrin *see* 2913
Micro-Cell *see* 1702
Microcide *see* 4460
Microcidin *see* 6384
Microcillin [Bayer] *see* 1792
Microcline *see* 7604
Micrococcin *see* 6180
Micrococcin P, 6180
Microgynon [Schering AG] *see* 6704

Microlite *see* 9053
Microlut [Schering AG] *see* 6704
Micromerol *see* 9890
Micromet *see* 8667
Micromite [Uniroyal] *see* 3142
Micronase [Pharmacia & Upjohn] *see* 4478
Micronomicin, 6181
Micronor [Ortho] *see* 6697
Micronovum [Janssen-Cilag] *see* 6697
Micropaque [Guerbet] *see* 994
Micropenin [Kabi] *see* 6904
Microtrast [Guerbet] *see* 994
Microtrim [Chephasaar] *see* 8918
Microtubules *see* 9808
Microval [Wyeth] *see* 6704
Mictine [Searle] *see* 451
Mictonetten [Apogepha] *see* 7832
Mictonorm [Apogepha] *see* 7832
Midafenone *see* 6661
Midalcipran *see* 6194
Midalgan *see* 6100
Midamor [Merck & Co.] *see* 406
Midarine [GSK] *see* 8875
Midazolam, 6182
Midecamycin A_1 *see* 6183
Midecamycin A_3 *see* 6183
Midecamycins, 6183
Midecin [Farmaka] *see* 6183
Midicel [Warner-Lambert] *see* 8919
Midikel [Parke-Davis] *see* 8919
Midodrine, 6184
Midol PMS [Miles] *see* 7000
Midostaurin, 6185
Midotens [Boehringer, Ing.] *see* 5331
Midronal [Delalande] *see* 2305
Midsummer Daisy *see* 4067
MIF *see* 5813
Mifegyne [HMR] *see* 6186
Mifepristone, 6186
MIF-I *see* 5813
Mifurol [Mitsui] *see* 1844
Migard [Vernalis] *see* 4272
Miglitol, 6187
Miglustat, 6188
Migranal [Novartis] *see* 3174
Migristène [Specia] *see* 4231
Miguard [Vernalis] *see* 4272
MIH *see* 7758
Mikado [Bayer CropSci.] *see* 8894
Mikametan [Mikasa] *see* 4968
Mikamycin IA *see* 7753
Mikavir [Salus] *see* 405
Mikelan [Otsuka] *see* 1866
Miketorin [Schering] *see* 487
Mikrotsid *see* 4460
Milban [Mallinckrodt] *see* 3407
Milbeknock [Sankyo] *see* 6189
Milbemectin, 6189
Milbemycin α_1 *see* 6189
Milbemycin α_3 *see* 6189
Milbemycin β_1 *see* 6191
Milbemycin A_3 *see* 6189
Milbemycin A_3 5-Oxime *see* 6190
Milbemycin A_4 *see* 6189
Milbemycin A_4 5-Oxime *see* 6190
Milbemycin D *see* 6191
Milbemycin Oxime *see* 6190
Milbemycins, 6191
Milchsäure (German) *see* 5336
D-Milchsäure (German) *see* 5335
L-Milchsäure (German) *see* 5337
Milcopen [Leiras] *see* 7100
Milcurb [Zeneca] *see* 3217
Milcurb Super [Zeneca] *see* 3740
Mild Aconitine *see* 119

Mildiomycin, 6192
Mildison [Yamanouchi] see 4787
Mild Mercury Chloride see 5894
Mild Silver Protein see 8527
Milestone [DuPont] see 894
Milezin [Spofa] see 5986
Milfoil see 105
Milgo [Zeneca] see 3740
Milid [Opfermann] see 7775
Milide [Beytout] see 7775
Milk, 6193
Milk Ipecac see 742
Milk of Sulfur see 8977
Milk Sugar see 5343
Milkweed see 829
Millafol [Parke-Davis] see 4221
Millenium [DuPont] see 4195
Millerite see 6498
Millevit [Abbott] see 10014
Millicaine [Corbiere] see 1187
Milligynon [Schering AG] see 6697
Millinese [Lampugnani] see 2186
Millisrol [Nippon Kayaku] see 6607
Millon's Base see 5898
Millophyline [Arnolds] see 3711
Milnacipran, 6194
Milontin [Warner-Lambert] see 7261
Milorganite [Milwaukee Met. Sewer. Dist.], 6195
Milori Blue see 7910
Miloxacin, 6196
Milrila [Yamanouchi] see 6197
Milrinone, 6197
Milstem [Zeneca] see 3740
Miltaun [Wallace Labs.] see 5862
Miltefosine, 6198
Miltex [Baxter] see 6198
Miltown [Wallace Labs.] see 5862
Milvane [Schering AG] see 4413
Mimedran [Esteve] see 8995
Mimetite see 5396
Mimic [Dow AgroSci.] see 9093
Mimosine, 6199
Mimpara [Amgen] see 2282
Mina D$_2$ see 10018
Minacalm [Tobishi] see 9522
Minalfene [Bouchara] see 300
Minalgin [Streuli] see 3350
Minaprine, 6200
Mincard [Searle] see 451
Mindiab [Pfizer] see 4442
Mindolic Acid see 2383
Minedil [Formenti] see 7971
Mineral Carbon see 4539
Mineral Green see 2625
Mineral Oil see 7186, 7187
Mineral Orange see 5425
Mineral Pitch see 845
Mineral Red see 5425
Mineral Spirits, 6201
Mineral Wax see 1987
Mineral White see 1706
Mingin see 9882
Minicid see 3184
Minidiab [Pfizer] see 4442
Minihep [Leo Pharm] see 4653
Miniluteolas [Serono] see 3860
Minilyn [Organon] see 5629
Mini-Pe [Searle] see 6697
"Mini-pill" see 6697
Miniplanor [Galen] see 279
Minipress [Pfizer] see 7717
Minirin [Ferring] see 2924
Mini-Sintrom [Novartis] see 29
Minitran [3M Pharma] see 6607

Minium see 5425
Minocin [Wyeth] see 6202
Minocycline, 6202
Minolip [Master] see 1039
Minor Centaury see 1969
Minovlar [Schering AG] see 6697
Minoxidil, 6203
Minoximen [Menarini] see 6203
Minozinan see 5986
Minprog [Pharmacia] see 7876
Minprostin E$_2$ [Pharmacia] see 7877
Mintacol see 7030
Mintec [Shire] see 7145
Mintezol [Merck & Co.] see 9289
Mintic [Ayerst] see 6160
Minulet [Wyeth] see 4413
Minuric [R & C] see 1065
Minusin [Doetsch, Grether] see 6714
Mioblock [Sankyo] see 7007
Miocamycin [Meiji] see 6204
Miochol [Cooper] see 87
Miocor [Ecobi] see 1849
Miokamycin, 6204
Miolaxene [Lepetit] see 5980
Miolene [Lusofarmaco] see 8237
Mional [Eisai] see 3606
Miorel [Lederle] see 9324
Mio-Sed see 2106
Miostat [Alcon] see 1779
Mioticol see 3198
Miotisal A see 7030
Miotolon [Daiichi] see 4299
Mioton [Pharmakhim] see 1768
Miotonal [Caber] see 1849
MIP see 760
Mipafox, 6205
Mipax see 3255
Mirabilite see 8680
Miracil D see 5591
Miracle Fruit see 6206
Miraclid [Mochida] see 9882
Miracol see 5591
Miraculin, 6206
Miradol [Mitsui] see 8989
Miradon [Schering] see 668
Miralin [Miralin] see 6206
Miranax [Syntex] see 6417
Mirapex [Boehringer, Ing.] see 7705
Mirapexin [Boehringer, Ing.] see 7705
Mirapront [Mack, Illert.] see 7262
Mirasept [CIBA Vision] see 4798
Mirbanil [Boehringer, Ing.] see 8989
Mircol [Rhône-Poulenc] see 5864
Mirena [Schering AG] see 6704
Miretilan [Sandoz] see 3577
Mirex, 6207
Mirfat [Merckle] see 4309
Miridacin [Taiho] see 7774
Mirimostim see 5646
Mirlon see 6734
Miropinic Acid see 5200
Mirsol [Permamed] see 10170
Mirtazapine, 6208
Mirvan [Continental Pharma] see 219
Misch Metal, 6209
Miso see 8730
Misoprostol, 6210
Mistabron [UCB] see 5909
Mistabronco [UCB] see 5909
Mistarel see 5217
Mistral [M & B] see 3993
Misulban [Nuovo ISM] see 1505
Misulvan [Bernabo] see 8989
MIT see 6091
Mitaban [Pharmacia & Upjohn] see 486

Mitac [Bayer CropSci.] see 486
Mithracin see 7536
Mithramycin see 7536
Mitigal see 5918
Mitigan [Makhteshim-Agan] see 3086
Mitiglinide, 6211
Mitis Green see 2625
Mitobronitol, 6212
Mitochondrial Ferritin see 4036
Mitocin-C [BMS] see 6215
Mitocor [Zambon] see 9843
Mitoguazone, 6213
Mitolactol, 6214
Mitomen see 5776
Mitomycin A see 6215
Mitomycin B see 6215
Mitomycin C see 6215
Mitomycins, 6215
Mitoquinones see 9843
Mitotane, 6216
Mitoxana [Baxter] see 4896
Mitoxantrone, 6217
Mitragynine, 6218
Mitramycin see 7536
Mitrinermine see 8197
Mitrolan [Robins] see 1697
Mitronal [Searle] see 2305
Mittoval [Schering AG] see 238
Mivacron [GSK] see 6219
Mivacurium Chloride, 6219
Mivazerol, 6220
Mixobar [Byk Gulden] see 994
Miyaura's Reagent see 1300
Mizolastine, 6221
Mizollen [Lorex] see 6221
Mizoribine, 6222
MJ-505 see 7321
MJ-1992 see 8729
MJ-1996 see 399
MJ-1999 see 8728
MJ-4309-1 see 6955
MJ-5190 see 399
MJ-9067 see 3570
MJ-10061 see 1065
MJ-13105-1 see 1461
MJ-13754-1 see 6438
MJF-9325 see 4896
MJF-11567-3 see 1913
MJF-12264 see 9112
MK 4 see 5833
MK 6 see 5833
MK-130 see 2713
MK-135 see 2202
MK-188 see 10121
MK-191 see 7512
MK-208 see 3930
MK-217 see 229
MK-223 see 4881
MK-231 see 8982
MK-239 see 9094
MK-240 see 7901
MK-243 see 4933
MK-244 see 3554
MK-264 see 4219
MK-306 see 1936
MK-351 see 6055
MK-360 see 9289
MK-366 see 6700
MK-383 see 9464
MK-397 see 3633
MK-401 see 2409
MK-421 see 3567
MK-422 see 3568
MK-0431 see 8552
MK-462 see 8241

MK-0462 *see* 8241
MK-476 *see* 6258
MK-486 *see* 1797
MK-507 *see* 3426
MK-0517 *see* 753
MK-521 *see* 5516
MK-595 *see* 3717
MK-621 *see* 3525
MK-639 *see* 4945
MK-647 *see* 3146
MK-650 *see* 2540
MK-663 *see* 3887
MK-0663 *see* 3887
MK-733 *see* 8539
MK-781 *see* 6161
MK-787 *see* 4919
MK-791 *see* 2272
MK-801 *see* 3386
MK-803 *see* 5586
MK-826 *see* 3673
MK-0869 *see* 753
MK-870 *see* 406
MK-905 *see* 1726
MK-906 *see* 4082
MK-0928 *see* 4321
MK-933 *see* 5248
MK-936 *see* 2
MK-950 *see* 9444
MK-954 *see* 5583
MK-955 *see* 4254
MK-965 *see* 836
MK-0966 *see* 8248
MK-990 *see* 8097
MK-0991 *see* 1889
MKH 6562 *see* 4119
ML-236 B *see* 6164
ML-1024 *see* 9284
ML-1129 *see* 1152
ML-1229 *see* 1152
ML-3000 *see* 5480
ML-1785713 *see* 4087
MM 4550 *see* 6835
MM 13902 *see* 6835
MM 14151 *see* 2341
MM 17880 *see* 6835
MM 22380 *see* 6835
MM 22381 *see* 6835
MM 22382 *see* 6835
MM 22383 *see* 6835
MMC *see* 6215
MMF *see* 6076
MMH *see* 6086
4-MMPD *see* 2976
4-MMPDS *see* 2976
MMPP *see* 5673
MMS *see* 6097
MMSC *see* 6098
MMT, 6223
α-MMT *see* 6132
MN-10T *see* 9166
MN-1695 *see* 5102
MnDPDP *see* 5722
MNE *see* 6496
Mnesis [Takeda] *see* 4888
MNNG *see* 6103
αMNP, 6224
MNPA *see* 6417
MO-911 *see* 7038
MOB *see* 6954
Mobactam [Takeda] *see* 1871
Moban [Endo] *see* 6233
Mobec [Boehringer, Ing.] *see* 5826
Mobenol [Church & Dwight] *see* 9507
Mobic [Boehringer, Ing.] *see* 5826
Mobicox [Boehringer, Ing.] *see* 5826

Mobidin [Ascher] *see* 5685
Mobiflex [Roche] *see* 9148
Mobisyl [Ascher] *see* 9665
Mobutazon *see* 6231
Mobuzon *see* 6231
MOCA *see* 6059
Mocap [Bayer CropSci.] *see* 3746
Mocimycin, 6225
Moclamine [Roche] *see* 6226
Moclobemide, 6226
Moctanin [Ethitek] *see* 6252
Mod [Irbi] *see* 3418
Modacin [GSK] *see* 1946
Modacor [Houdé] *see* 6962
Modacrylic Fibers, 6227
Modafinil, 6228
Modalim [Sanofi] *see* 2313
Modalina [Sanofi-Synthelabo] *see* 9680
Modamide [Merck & Co.] *see* 406
Modane [Adria] *see* 2815
Modatrop [Nordmark] *see* 7133
Modecate [Sanofi Winthrop] *see* 4189
Modenol *see* 1525
Moderatan [Theranol] *see* 3127
Modicare *see* 3415
Modicon [Ortho] *see* 6697
Modimmunal [Ravizza] *see* 4976
Modinal *see* 4367
Modirax *see* 4698
Moditen [Sanofi Winthrop] *see* 4189
Modown [Mobil; Rhône-Poulenc] *see* 1208
Modrasone [Schering] *see* 220
Modrastane [Winthrop] *see* 9698
Modrenal [Winthrop] *see* 9698
Modulan [Amerchol] *see* 5358
Modulon [Pfizer] *see* 9699
Modumate [Abbott] *see* 781
Moduretic [Merck & Co.] *see* 406
Moduretik [Merck & Co.] *see* 406
Modustatina [Midy] *see* 8715
Moenocinol *see* 952
Moenomycin *see* 952
Moenomycin A *see* 952
Moexipril, 6229
Moexiprilat Hydrochloride *see* 6229
Mofarotene, 6230
Mofebutazone, 6231
Mofenar [C.E.P.A.] *see* 1474
Mofesal [Medice] *see* 6231
Mofezolac, 6232
Mogadan [Valeant] *see* 6575
Mogadon [Valeant] *see* 6575
Mohr's Salt *see* 521
Molatoc *see* 3401
Molcer [Wallace] *see* 3401
Molded Silver Nitrate *see* 8518
Molecular Sieves *see* 2340
Molevac [Parke-Davis] *see* 8022
Molgramostim *see* 4538
Molindone, 6233
Molipaxin [HMR] *see* 9579
Mol-Iron [Schering] *see* 4057
Mol-Iron (obsolete) *see* 6238
Moloid [Südmedica] *see* 5746
Molsidolat [Aventis] *see* 6234
Molsidomine, 6234
Molybdenite *see* 6236
Molybdenum, 6235
Molybdenum Disulfide, 6236
Molybdenum Hexafluoride, 6237
Molybdenum(VI) Oxide *see* 6239
Molybdenum Oxide (MoO_3) *see* 6239
Molybdenum Sesquioxide, 6238
Molybdenum Trioxide, 6239
Molybdic(VI) Acid, 6240

Molybdic Anhydride *see* 6239
Molybdophosphoric Acid *see* 7342
Molycor-R [Mepha] *see* 6699
Molyhibit 100 [Amax] *see* 8645
Molysite *see* 4019
MOM *see* 6204
Momentum [Wyeth] *see* 47
Mometasone Furoate, 6241
Momicine [Morrith] *see* 6183
MON-097 *see* 61
MON-0573 *see* 4512
MON-2139 *see* 4512
MON-7200 *see* 3374
MON-12000 *see* 4602
MON-12037 *see* 4602
MON-13200 *see* 9311
MON-15100 *see* 3374
MON-21200 *see* 2375
MON-21233 *see* 2375
MON-37500 *see* 8965
Monacetin, 6242
Monacolin K *see* 5586
Monacrin [Sterling Winthrop] *see* 407
Monactin *see* 6675
Monalium Hydrate *see* 5651
Monapen [Fujisawa] *see* 9428
Monarch [SS Pharm.] *see* 279
Monarda, 6243
Monardin *see* 7071
Monasirup [RPR] *see* 643
Monaspor [Novartis] *see* 1945
Monastrol, 6244
Monazan *see* 6231
Monazol *see* 4837
Moncut [Nihon Nohyaku] *see* 4212
Mondamin [CPC] *see* 8798
Mondus [Labinca] *see* 4144
Monellins, 6245
Monensic Acid (obsolete) *see* 6246
Monensin, 6246
Monetite *see* 1692
Mongarit [Sankyo] *see* 8534
Monicor [Fabre] *see* 5225
Moniflagon [Dieetzout] *see* 9147
Monistat [Cilag-Chemie] *see* 6178
Monit [Lorex] *see* 5225
Monitan [Ives] *see* 7582
Monitor [Bayer CropSci.] *see* 5947
Monitor [Monsanto] *see* 8965
Monkshood *see* 116
Monk's Pepper *see* 189
Monoacetin *see* 6242
Monoacetylneriifolin *see* 6474
N^1-Monoacetyl Sulfisoxazole *see* 8952
Monoamine Oxidase, 6247
Mono-L-aspartyl Chlorin E_6 *see* 9034
Monobasic Lead Acetate *see* 5419
Mono-Baycuten *see* 2417
Monobenzone, 6248
Monobenzyl Hydroquinone *see* 6248
Monobromoacetanilide *see* 1399
Monobromobenzene *see* 1406
Monobromoethane *see* 3771
2-Monobromoisovalerylurea *see* 1397
Monobromomethane *see* 6029
Monobromosuccinic Acid *see* 1437
Monobutyl *see* 6231
Monobutyrin, 6249
α-Monobutyrin *see* 6249
Monocaine [Novocol] *see* 1523
Monocalcium Bis[(3*R*,5*S*,6*E*)-7-[2-cyclo-propyl-4-(4-fluorophenyl)-3-quinolin-yl]-3,5-dihydroxy-6-heptenoate] *see* 7508
Monocalcium Orthophosphate *see* 1693

Monocalcium Phosphate see 1693
α-Monocaprylin see 6252
Mono-Cedocard [Altana] see 5225
Monochloracetone see 2114
Monochlorethane see 3782
Monochloroacetaldehyde see 2109
Monochloroacetic Acid see 2112
Monochloroacetic Acid Anhydride see 2113
Monochloroacetone see 2114
17-Monochloroacetylajmaline see 5577
Monochlorobenzene see 2121
Monochlorodibromomethane see 2135
8-Monochloro-3-(β-diethylaminoethyl)-4-methyl-7-ethoxycarbonylmethoxy-coumarin see 2405
α-Monochlorohydrin see 2145
Monochloromethyl Ether see 2146
Monochlorphenamide see 2374
Monocid [SKB] see 1929
Monocidur [SKB] see 1929
Monocillin [Chassot] see 7097
Monoclair [Hennig] see 5225
Monoclate-P [Centeon] see 3921
Monoclonal Antibody B72.3-GYK-DTPA-In-111 see 8385
Monocor [Am. Cyanamid] see 1295
Monocortin [Grünenthal] see 7029
Monocrotaline, 6250
Monocrotophos, 6251
Monoctanoin, 6252
Mono[2-(dimethylamino)ethyl]phosphoric Acid Ester 2884
Monoethanolamine see 3727
Monoethanolamine DL-Acetylleucinate see 95
Monoethanolamine Salt of α-Acetamidoisocaproic Acid see 95
Monoethylamine see 3762
Monoethyl Tartrate see 3856
Monoferrous Acid Citrate Monohydrate see 4044
Monoflocet [Aventis] see 6771
Monofluoroacetamide see 4166
Mono-Gesic [Central] see 8339
Monoglycerol p-Aminobenzoate see 4487
Monoglycol Salicylate see 4499
Monoglyme see 3224
Monogynol B see 5608
Monohydrated Selenium Dioxide see 8430
Mono(2-hydroxybenzoate)-1H-imidazole see 4913
Monohydroxymercuridiiodoresorcinsulfonphthalein Sodium Salt see 5865
Monoiodotyrosine see 5047
Mono-Kay [Abbott] see 7380
Monoket [Schwarz] see 5225
Monolene see 438
Monolupine see 623
Mono Mack [Mack, Illert.] see 5225
(Monomethoxypolyethylene Glycol Succinimidyl)74-L-asparaginase see 836
Monomethylamine see 6014
Monomethyl-p-aminophenol Sulfate see 6017
Monomethylaniline see 6019
NG-Monomethyl-L-arginine see 6022
Monomethylarsinic Acid see 5953
Monomethyldiaminodiphenazothionium Chloride see 929
o-Monomethyldiphenhydramine see 6879
N-Monomethylformamide see 6076
Monomethylhydrazine see 6086
Monomethyl Mercury see 3250

Monomethyloldimethylhydantoin see 4831
Monomethylpropion see 5963
Monomethyl Sulfate see 6122
Monomethylthionine Chloride see 929
Monomycin [Grünenthal] see 3681
Monomycin A see 7041
Mononine [ZLB Behring] see 3922
Mononitrogen Monoxide see 6578
Mononuclear Cell Factor see 4993
Monooctadecyl Ether of Glycerol see 1011
Monooctanoin see 6252
Monoparin [CP Pharm.] see 4653
Monophenolase see 9838
Monophenoloxidase see 9838
Monophenylbutazone see 6231
Monopina [Bioindustria] see 491
Monopotassium Citrate see 7624
Monopotassium Phosphate see 7659
Monopril [BMS] see 4256
Monopropionylerythromycin see 3686
Monorden, 6253
Monores [Valeas] see 2347
Monorhein see 8176
Monorheumetten [Benzon] see 6231
Monos [SKB] see 8294
Monosilane see 8488
Monosodium Glutamate, 6254
Monosodium Methanearsonate see 5953
Monosodium Orthophosphate see 8660
Monosodium N-Phenylglycinamide-p-arsonate see 9794
Monosorb [Dexcel] see 5225
Monospan [Santen] see 1588
Monostearin see 4489
Monosulfiram see 8950
Monothioethyleneglycol see 5869
α-Monothioglycerol see 9335
Monotrim [Duphar] see 9709
Monotropein, 6255
Monovent [Lagap] see 9159
Monoverin [Merck KGaA] see 7707
Monoxychlorosene see 6956
Monsel's Solution, 6256
Montan Wax, 6257
Monteban [Elanco] see 6419
Montelukast, 6258
Monteplase, 6259
Montmorillonite, 6260
Montrel [Dow] see 2604
Montricin [SPA] see 5847
Monuril [Zambon] see 4254
Monurol [Zambon] see 4254
Monuron, 6261
Monuron TCA see 6261
Monydrin [AstraZeneca] see 7307
Monzal [Boehringer, Ing.] see 9972
Monzaldon [Boehringer, Ing.] see 9972
Moogrol [Burroughs Wellcome] see 2048
MoOPH see 9943
Moore's Ketene, 6262
5-MOP see 1157
8-MOP [Valeant] see 5988
Moperone, 6263
Moplen [Montecatini] see 7581
Mopral [AstraZeneca] see 6845
Moprolol, 6264
MOPS, 6265
Moracizine see 6268
d-Moramid(e) see 2955
Moranoline see 2905
Morantel, 6266
Moranyl [Specia] see 9006
Morazone, 6267

Morbicid see 4235
Morcap [Mayne] see 6276
Mordant Rouge see 344
Mordant Violet 25 see 4344
Mordant Yellow 3R see 255
Morestan [Bayer] see 6978
Morfazinamide see 6273
Morial [Takeda] see 6234
Moricizine, 6268
Morin, 6269
Morinamide see 6273
Morindin, 6270
β-Morindin see 6270
Morindone see 6270
Moringine see 1125
Morintannic Acid see 5644
Moriperan [Morishita] see 6143
Morison's Paste see 5691
Moritannic Acid see 5644
Morman Tea see 3607
Mornidine [Searle] see 7454
Morniflumate see 6531
Morning-glory see 5072
Moroctocog Alfa, 6271
Moronal [BMS] see 6736
Moroxydine, 6272
Morpan T [A.B.M. Chem.] see 6336
Morphazinamide, 6273
Morpheridine, 6274
Morphia see 6276
Morphinan, 6275
Morphinan-3-ol see 6707
Morphine, 6276
Morphine Bis(nicotinate) see 6520
Morphine Bis(pyridine-3-carboxylate) see 6520
Morphine Dinicotinate see 6520
Morphine Ester with Nicotinic Acid see 6520
Morphine Hemisulfate see 6276
Morphine 3-Methyl Ether see 2463
Morphine Monomethyl Ether see 2463
Morphium see 6276
Morphodone see 7207
Morpholine, 6277
4-Morpholinecarboximidoylguanidine see 6272
Morpholine N,N'-Disulfide see 3372
4-Morpholineethanesulfonic Acid see 5902
4-Morpholinepropanesulfonic Acid see 6265
2-(4-Morpholinoanilino)-N6-cyclohexyladenine see 8169
2-(4-Morpholinoanilino)-6-cyclohexylaminopurine see 8169
(−)-3-Morpholino-4-(3-tert-butylamino-2-hydroxypropoxy)-1,2,5-thiadiazole see 9444
2-(N-Morpholino)ethanesulfonic Acid see 5902
3-(2-Morpholinoethyl)morphine see 7329
N-2-Morpholinoethyl-5-nitroimidazole see 6552
Morpholinoethyl Norpethidine see 6274
1-(2-Morpholinoethyl)-4-phenylisonipecotic Acid Ethyl Ester see 6274
2-(4-Morpholino)ethyl Sulfonate see 5902
3-(Morpholinomethyl)-1-[(5-nitrofurfurylidene)amino]hydantoin see 6533
5-Morpholinomethyl-3-(5-nitrofurfurylideneamino)-2-oxazolidinone see 4294
N-Morpholinomethylpyrazinamide see 6273
3-(N-Morpholino)propanesulfonic Acid see 6265

10-(3-Morpholinopropionyl)phenothia-zine-2-carbamic Acid Ethyl Ester *see* 6268

γ-Morpholinopropyl 4-*n*-Butoxyphenyl Ether *see* 7709

6-(4-Morpholinyl)-4,4-diphenyl-3-hep-tanone *see* 7207

β-Morpholinylethylmorphine *see* 7329

3-[2-(4-Morpholinyl)ethyl]morphine *see* 7329

1-(2-*N*-Morpholinylethyl)-5-nitroimida-zole *see* 6552

1-[2-(Morpholinyl)ethyl]-4-phenyl-4-pip-eridinecarboxylic Acid Ethyl Ester *see* 6274

3-(4-Morpholinylmethyl)-1-[[(5-nitro-2-furanyl)methylene]amino]-2,4-imida-zolidinedione *see* 6533

5-(4-Morpholinylmethyl)-3-[[(5-nitro-2-furanyl)methylene]amino]-2-oxazoli-dinone *see* 4294

N-(4-Morpholinylmethyl)pyrazinecar-boxamide *see* 6273

[10-[3-(4-Morpholinyl)-1-oxopropyl]-10*H*-phenothiazin-2-yl]carbamic Acid Ethyl Ester *see* 6268

Morsydomine *see* 6234

MORT1-associated CED-3 Homolog *see* 1886

Mortopal *see* 9204

Mosaic Gold *see* 8780

Mosapramine, 6278

Mosapride, 6279

Mosatil *see* 3517

Moscontin [Mundipharma] *see* 6276

Mosegor [Novartis] *see* 7515

(±)-Mosher's Acid *see* 6280

Mosher's Reagent, 6280

Mospilan [Nippon Soda] *see* 49

Mossbunker Oil *see* 5836

Moss Starch *see* 5478

Motazomin [Takeda] *see* 6234

Motens [Boehringer, Ing.] *see* 5331

Motexafin Gadolinium, 6281

Motexafin Lutetium, 6282

Mother-of-Pearl Sulfur *see* 8969

Motiax [Neopharmed] *see* 3930

Motifene [Sankyo] *see* 3081

Motilex [Guidotti] *see* 2344

Motilin, 6283

Motilium [Janssen] *see* 3418

Motilyn [Abbott] *see* 2947

Motosol [Europharma] *see* 386

Motox [Tenneco] *see* 9557

Motretinide, 6284

Motrin [McNeil] *see* 4881

Mountain Balm *see* 3669

Mountain Grape *see* 1155

Mountain Tobacco *see* 789

Mouse Antialopecia Factor *see* 4978

Mouse-bane *see* 116

Mouse EGF-URO *see* 3527

Movalis [Boehringer, Ing.] *see* 5826

Movatec [Boehringer, Ing.] *see* 5826

Movecil [Farmitalia] *see* 7975

Moveltipril, 6285

Movens [Inverni] *see* 5779

Mover [Mitsubishi Kasei] *see* 133

Movergan [Orion] *see* 8428

Movirene *see* 3349

Movyl [Montecatini] *see* 7586

Mowiol [Hoechst] *see* 7585

Moxadil [Lederle] *see* 576

Moxalactam [Lilly], 6286

Moxam [Lilly] *see* 6286

Moxastine, 6287

Moxaverine, 6288

Moxestrol, 6289

Moxidectin, 6290

Moxifloxacin, 6291

Moxisylyte, 6292

Moxonidine, 6293

MP *see* 6117

4-MP *see* 4226

6MP *see* 5871

8-MP *see* 5988

MP-11 *see* 7179

MP-302 *see* 5067

MP-328 *see* 5066

MP-620 *see* 5010

MP-1177 *see* 4329

MP-1727 *see* 7126

MPC-1304 *see* 767

MPP+ *see* 6294

α-MPT *see* 6161

MPTP, 6294

MPV-785 *see* 5787

MPV-1248 *see* 861

MPV-1440 *see* 2946

M-Pyrol [ISP] *see* 6117

MQPA *see* 779

MRA *see* 9493

MRD-108 *see* 7484

MRE-0470 *see* 1225

MRIH *see* 5813

MRL-41 *see* 2386

MRNA *see* 8203

MRX-115 *see* 7158

MS Contin [Purdue Frederick] *see* 6276

MS-222 *see* 9621

MS-325 *see* 4325

MS-551 *see* 6529

MS-752 *see* 5591

MS-932 *see* 133

MS-1144 *see* 2753

MS-4101 *see* 4209

MSA III-2 *see* 4986

MSG *see* 6254

MSH, 6295

MSH Release-inhibiting Factor I *see* 5813

MSH Release-inhibiting Hormone *see* 5813

MSI-78 *see* 7193

MSIR [Purdue Frederick] *see* 6276

MSMA *see* 5953

MST Continus [Mundipharma] *see* 6276

MST-16 *see* 8568

L-α-MT *see* 6161

MT-141 *see* 1927

MTB-51 *see* 5958

MTBE *see* 6032

MTI-446 *see* 3289

MTI-500 *see* 3876

MTO *see* 6130

L-3-MTO *see* 6056

MTPA *see* 6280

(*R*)-MTPA-chloride *see* 6280

MTP-cephalin *see* 5844

MTP-PE *see* 5844

MTU *see* 6128

MTX *see* 5698, 5985

4-MU *see* 4854

MU-495 *see* 6522

Mucalan *see* 5110

Mucara *see* 5284

Mucic Acid *see* 4331

Muciclar [Pfizer] *see* 1802

Mucidin *see* 8834

Mucinex [Adams] *see* 4555

Mucinol [Sanofi Winthrop] *see* 644

Mucins, 6296

Mucitux [Riom] *see* 3632

Muclox [Sigma-Tau] *see* 3930

Mucocedyl [3M] *see* 88

Mucochloric Acid, 6297

Mucochloric Anhydride, 6298

Mucocis [So.Se.] *see* 1802

Mucoclear [Mundipharma] *see* 386

Mucodil [Valeas] *see* 8809

Mucodyne [Sanofi-Aventis] *see* 1802

Mucofar [Farmakos] *see* 386

Mucofluid [UCB] *see* 5909

Mucoglucoronan *see* 2811

Mucolase [Lampugnani] *see* 1802

Mucolator [Abbott] *see* 88

Mucolex [Warner-Lambert] *see* 1802

Mucolitico [Maggioni] *see* 3414

Mucolysin [Proter] *see* 9453

Mucomyst [BMS] *see* 88

Muconic Acid, 6299

Muconomycin A *see* 9964

Muconomycin B *see* 9964

Mucopront [Mack, Illert.] *see* 1802

Mucosan [Fher] *see* 386

Muco Sanigen [Thiemann] *see* 88

Mucosil [Dey] *see* 88

Mucosolvan [Thomae] *see* 386

Mucosta [Otsuka] *see* 8124

Mucovent [Byk Gulden] *see* 386

Mucret [Pharma-Stern] *see* 88

Muira Puama, 6300

Mukaiyama Reagent, 6301

Mulka *see* 5963

Mullite *see* 362

Mulsiferol *see* 10018

Mulsopaque [Alcon] *see* 5060

Multergan [Specia] *see* 9306

Multhiomycin *see* 6719

Multicrom [Menarini] *see* 2590

Multi-CSF *see* 4995

Multifungin [Knoll] *see* 1435

MultiHance [Bracco] *see* 4322

Multilase [Sigma-Tau] *see* 674

Multiplication-stimulating Activity III-2 *see* 4986

Multipotent Colony Stimulating Factor *see* 4995

Multum [Chephasaar] *see* 2084

Mundisal [Purdue Frederick] *see* 2209

Munobal [Aventis] *see* 3953

Muphoran [Servier] *see* 4261

Mupirocin, 6302

Muplestim *see* 4995

Muracil [Organon] *see* 6128

Muraglitazar, 6303

Muramic Acid, 6304

Muramidase *see* 5640

Muramyl Dipeptide, 6305

Muramyl Tripeptide Phosphatidyletha-nolamine *see* 5844

Murazyme [Prospa] *see* 5640

Murexide, 6306

Murexine, 6307

Muriacite *see* 1706

Muriatic Acid *see* 4780

Murillo Bark *see* 8040

Muroctasin *see* 8253

Muromonab CD3, 6308

Murrayin *see* 8409

Musaril [Sanofi-Synthelabo] *see* 9243

Muscalm [Nippon Kayaku] *see* 9522

Muscalure, 6309

Muscarine, 6310

Muscatox [Bayer] *see* 2558

Muscazone, 6311

Muscimol, 6312
Muscle Adenylic Acid see 158
Muscle Inosinic Acid see 4977
Muscone, 6313
Musco-Ril [Inverni] see 9324
Musculamine see 8743
Musculax [Nippon Organon] see 9941
Muse [Meda] see 7876
Mushroom Sugar see 9580
Muskelat [Azupharma] see 9243
Muskone see 6313
Musk Root see 8998
Musks, 6314
Mussel Poison see 8389
Mustard, 6315
Mustard Chlorohydrin see 4646
Mustard Gas, 6316
"Mustard Oil" see 295
Mustargen [Merck & Co.] see 5775
Mustine Hydrochloride see 5775
Mustron see 5776
Mutabase [Schering] see 3004
Mutamycin [BMS] see 6215
Mutesa [Wyeth] see 6933
Muthesa [Wyeth] see 6933
Muthmann's Liquid see 9185
Mutton Suet see 8886
MV-119A see 3368
MX-70906 see 4933
MY-41-6 see 7045
MY-301 see 4555
MY-5116 see 8138
Myacine see 6454
Myalex [ICI] see 3969
Myambutol [Wyeth] see 3720
Myanesin [BDH] see 5850
Myanol see 5850
Myarsenol see 8941
MYC-8003 see 6225
Mycamine [Astellas] see 6175
Mycaminose, 6317
Mycanden [Schering AG] see 4600
Mycardol [Winthrop] see 7112
Mycarose, 6318
Mycelex-G [Miles] see 2417
Mycelianamide, 6319
Mycetins, 6320
Mycifradin [Upjohn] see 6454
Mycil [BDH] see 2178
Myclobutanil, 6321
Mycobacidin, 6322
Mycobacillin, 6323
Mycobactic Acid see 6324
Mycobactin P see 6324
Mycobactins, 6324
Mycobactyl see 4500
Mycobutin [Farmitalia] see 8213
Mycobutol [Cadila] see 3720
Mycodécyl Solution [Doms-Adrian] see 9848
Mycofug [Hermal] see 2417
Mycoin C₃ see 7053
Mycolic Acids, 6325
Mycolutein see 879
(6-O-Mycolyl-α-D-glucopyranosyl)-6-O-mycolyl-α-D-glucopyranoside see 2528
Mycomycin, 6326
Mycophenolate Mofetil see 6327
Mycophenolate Sodium see 6327
Mycophenolic Acid, 6327
Mycophyt [Mycofarm] see 6427
Myco-protein see 8087
Mycosamine, 6328
Mycose see 9580
Mycospor [Bayer] see 1213

Mycosporan [Bayer] see 1213
Mycosporin [Bayer] see 2417
Mycostatin [BMS] see 6736
Mycoster [Fabre] see 2266
Mycotoxin T-2 see 9801
Mydecamycin see 6183
Mydetone see 9522
Mydfrin [Alcon] see 7286
Mydocalm [Labatec] see 9522
Mydplegic [Cooper] see 2746
Mydriacyl [Alcon] see 9780
Mydrial [Winzer] see 9835
Mydriaticum [Merck & Co.] see 9780
Mydrilate [Boehringer, Ing.] see 2746
Myebrol [Kyorin] see 6212
Myelobromol [Enzypharm] see 6212
Myelotrast [Winthrop] see 5009
Myfortic [Novartis] see 6327
Myfungar [Wyeth] see 6937
Mygdalon [DDSA] see 6143
Myk [Cassenne] see 8893
Mykostin see 10018
Mykrox [Celltech] see 6147
Mylabris, 6329
Mylar [DuPont] see 7569
Mylaxen see 4684
Mylepsinum [AWD] see 7746
Myleran [GSK] see 1505
Mylicon [J & J-Merck] see 3215
Mylis [Kanebo] see 2871
Mylodorm [G.P.] see 570
Mylofanol see 2288
Mylone see 2834
Mylosar (formerly) see 890
Mylotarg [Wyeth] see 4390
Myocet [Elan] see 3439
Myocholine [Glenwood] see 1185
Myochrysine [Merck & Co.] see 4518
Myocord [Ivax] see 859
Myodetensine see 5850
Myodigin see 3163
Myodil see 5060
Myoflex [Novartis] see 9665
Myohematin see 2791
Myolastan [Sanofi-Synthelabo] see 9243
Myolysin see 5850
Myonal [Eisai] see 3606
Myopan see 5850
Myopone see 10041
Myorexon [AstraZeneca] see 5225
Myosalvarsan see 8941
Myoscain [Sanochemia] see 4555
Myoserol see 5850
Myosin, 6330
Myoson [Strathmann] see 7741
Myoten [Central Pharm.] see 5850
Myotonine [Glenwood] see 1185
Myotrophin [Cephalon] see 4986
Myoview [GE Healthcare] see 9247
Myoxam [Menarini] see 6183
Myoxanthin see 3495
Myozyme [Genzyme] see 108
Myprozine [Am. Cyanamid] see 6427
α-Myrcene see 6331
β-Myrcene, 6331
Myreth see 7577
Myrica see 1012
Myricetin, 6332
Myricitrin see 6332
Myricodine see 6337
Myricyl Alcohol see 9591
Myriocin see 4083
Myristica see 6729
Myristic Acid, 6333
Myristicin, 6334

Myristin see 9724
29ᴮ-(N⁶-Myristoyl-L-lysine)-30ᴮ-de-L-threonineinsulin (Human) see 4983
Myristyl Alcohol, 6335
Myristyl Benzylmorphine see 6337
Myristyltrimethylammonium Bromide, 6336
Myrizone [Squibb] see 9290
Myrj [ICI] see 7578
Myrj 45 [ICI] see 7578
Myrj 52 [ICI] see 7578
Myrj 52S [ICI] see 7578
Myrocodine see 6337
Myronate Potassium see 8545
Myrophine, 6337
Myrophinium see 6337
Myrrh, 6338
Myrticolorin see 8304
Myrtillin-a see 2880
Myrtle Wax see 1012
Myrtol, 6339
Mysalfon [Spofa] see 9164
Myser [Nikken] see 3152
Mysoline [Acorus] see 7746
Mytab [Zeeland] see 6336
Mytelase [Sanofi Winthrop] see 379
Myxin, 6340
Myxoviromycin see 400
MZ-144 see 8225
MZ-0780 see 8225
M-Zyme see 5292
N-5' see 9570
N-021 see 9499
N-22 see 6232
N-0252 see 5385
N-553 see 9522
N-696 see 9438
N-714 see 2188
N-746 see 2394
N-869 see 5949
N-2790 see 4233
N-7009 see 4187
NA 22 [DuPont] see 3803
NA-73 see 4713
NA-97 see 7007
NA-274 see 1391
NA-872 see 386
NA-8318 see 5235
NAA see 840, 6371
N.A.B. see 6447
NAB-365 see 2347
NAB-365Cl see 2347
Nabadial see 5950
Nabam, 6341
Nabilone, 6342
Nabolin see 5951
Nabumetone, 6343
Nabuser [Geymonat] see 6343
Nacconate 100 [Allied] see 9530
Nacenyl [Syntex] see 6351
Nacid [Shionogi] see 5660
NaClex [Glaxo] see 4789
Nacom [Merck & Co.] see 1797
Nactate see 7554
Nacton [McNeil] see 7554
NAD, 6344
NAD⁺ see 6344
β-NAD see 6344
Nadeine see 3171
Nadex [Zyma-Galen] see 7991
NADH see 6344
Nadic Anhydride see 1796
Nadide see 6344
Nadifloxacin, 6345
Nadisan [Boehringer, Mann.] see 1832

Nadolol, 6346
Nadone *see* 2726
Nadoxolol, 6347
NADP, 6348
NADPH *see* 6348
NADPH$_2$ *see* 6348
NADPH$_2$ Diaphorase *see* 6824
Nadroparin, 6349
Nafamostat, 6350
Nafamostat Mesylate *see* 6350
Nafamstat *see* 6350
Nafarelin, 6351
Nafcil [Apothecon] *see* 6352
Nafcillin, 6352
Naferon [Sclavo] *see* 4991
Nafrine *see* 6966
Nafronyl, 6353
Naftalofos, 6354
Naftazone *see* 6394
Naftidrofuryl *see* 6353
Naftifine, 6355
Naftifungin *see* 6355
Naftin [Allergan] *see* 6355
Naftopidil, 6356
NAG *see* 6351
Naganol *see* 9006
Nagemid [Dexo] *see* 1443
Naglazyme [BioMarin] *see* 819
Na^{131}I *see* 8632
Naismeritin [Hishiyama] *see* 9522
Naixan [Tanabe] *see* 6417
Nalador [Schering AG] *see* 8991
Nalbuphine, 6357
Nalcrom [Sanofi-Aventis] *see* 2590
Nalcron [Sanofi-Aventis] *see* 2590
Naled, 6358
Nalfon [Lilly] *see* 3980
Nalgesic [Lilly] *see* 3980
Nalidicron [Toyo Shinyaku] *see* 6359
Nalidixic Acid, 6359
Nalitucsan [Hishiyama] *see* 6359
D-Nal(2)⁶-LHRH *see* 6351
Nalline [Merck & Co.] *see* 6361
Nallpen [SKB] *see* 6352
Nalmefene, 6360
Nalmetrene *see* 6360
Nalone [BMS] *see* 6362
Nalorex [DuPont Pharma] *see* 6363
Nalorphine, 6361
Naloxone, 6362
Naltrexone, 6363
Naltrexone Methobromide *see* 6099
Namenda [Forest] *see* 5829
Namuron *see* 2711
NAN *see* 8484
NANA *see* 8484
Nanbacine [Bellon] *see* 10076
Nancimycin *see* 8217
Nandinine, 6364
Nandrolin [Intervet] *see* 6365
Nandrolone, 6365
Nandrolone Laurate *see* 6365
Nandron [Morishita] *see* 3562
Nankor [Dow] *see* 8256
NANM *see* 6361
Nanormon [Novo] *see* 8716
Nantenine *see* 3413
Nantokite *see* 2660
NAPA *see* 20
Napacetin [Toyama] *see* 4881
Napageln [Lederle] *see* 3951
Napalm, 6366
Napelline, 6367
Napellonine *see* 8717
Naphazoline, 6368

Naphcon [Alcon] *see* 6368
Naphtha *see* 7188
Naphthacene, 6369
Naphthacetol *see* 453
Naphthalane *see* 2846
1-Naphthalenamine *see* 6398
2-Naphthalenamine *see* 6399
Naphthalene, 6370
α-Naphthaleneacetic Acid *see* 6371
1-Naphthaleneacetic Acid, 6371
1-Naphthalenecarboxylic Acid *see* 6381
2-Naphthalenecarboxylic Acid *see* 6382
1,8-Naphthalenediamine, 6372
1,8-Naphthalenedicarboxylic Acid *see* 6380
1,3-Naphthalenediol *see* 6396
1,2-Naphthalenedione *see* 6394
1,4-Naphthalenedione *see* 6395
1,5-Naphthalenedisulfonic Acid *see* 788
1,6-Naphthalenedisulfonic Acid, 6373
2,6-Naphthalenedisulfonic Acid, 6374
2,7-Naphthalenedisulfonic Acid, 6375
1,5-Naphthalenedisulfonic Acid Bis [2-[2-(Acetyloxy)-1-oxopropoxy]-N,N,-N-trimethylethanaminium]ion (2⁻) *see* 114
α-Naphthalenesulfonic Acid *see* 6376
β-Naphthalenesulfonic Acid *see* 6377
1-Naphthalenesulfonic Acid, 6376
2-Naphthalenesulfonic Acid, 6377
1-Naphthalenethiol, 6378
2-Naphthalenethiol, 6379
1-Naphthalenol *see* 6383
2-Naphthalenol *see* 6384
2-Naphthalenol Benzoate *see* 6408
1-Naphthalenol Methylcarbamate *see* 1787
6-[3-(2-Naphthalenyl)-D-alanine]luteinizing Hormone-releasing Factor(pig) *see* 6351
3-(2-Naphthalenyl)-D-alanyl-L-cysteinyl-L-tyrosyl-D-tryptophyl-L-lysyl-L-valyl-L-cysteinyl-L-threoninamide Cyclic (2 → 7)-Disulfide *see* 5361
2-[(1-Naphthalenylamino)carbonyl]benzoic Acid *see* 6416
N-1-Naphthalenyl-1,2-ethanediamine *see* 6409
N-(1-Naphthalenylmethyl)-1-naphthalenemethanamine *see* 1293
N-2-Naphthalenyl-2-naphthalenamine *see* 3267
2-Naphthalenyloxyacetic Acid *see* 6397
2-(2-Naphthalenyloxy)ethanol *see* 6413
1-Naphthalenylthiourea *see* 722
Naphthalic Acid, 6380
Naphthalidine *see* 6398
Naphthalin *see* 6370
Naphthalol *see* 6415
Naphthalophos *see* 6354
Naphthane *see* 2846
Naphthanthracene *see* 1062
Naphthene *see* 6370
Naphthionic Acid *see* 6403
Naphthionine *see* 6403
Naphthionine N-Glucoside *see* 6403
lin-Naphthoanthracene *see* 7107
Naphtho-2′,3′-1,2-anthracene *see* 3010
α-Naphthoic Acid *see* 6381
β-Naphthoic Acid *see* 6382
1-Naphthoic Acid, 6381
2-Naphthoic Acid, 6382
α-Naphthol *see* 6383
β-Naphthol *see* 6384
1-Naphthol, 6383

2-Naphthol, 6384
1-Naphthol-8-amino-3,6-disulfonic Acid, 6385
1-Naphthol-2-carboxylic Acid *see* 4834
3-Naphthol-2-carboxylic Acid *see* 4835
1-Naphthol-4,8-disulfonic Acid, 6386
2-Naphthol-3,6-disulfonic Acid, 6387
2-Naphthol-6,8-disulfonic Acid, 6388
1-Naphthol-3,6-disulfonic Acid-8-azo-4′-[N-phenyl-1′-naphthylamine]-8′-sulfonic Acid Trisodium Salt *see* 628
α-Naphtholdisulfonic Acid S *see* 6386
β-Naphthol-δ-monosulfonic Acid *see* 1892
α-Naphthol Orange *see* 6857
β-Naphthol Orange *see* 6858
α-Naphtholphthalein, 6389
p-α-Naphtholphthalein *see* 6389
α-Naphthol Salicylate *see* 6414
β-Naphthol Salicylate *see* 6415
1-Naphthol-2-sulfonic Acid, 6390
1-Naphthol-4-sulfonic Acid, 6391
2-Naphthol-6-sulfonic Acid, 6392
2-Naphthol-7-sulfonic Acid *see* 1892
2-Naphthol-8-sulfonic Acid *see* 2588
2-Naphthol-1-sulfonic Acid Calcium Salt *see* 822
β-Naphtholsulfonic Acid F *see* 1892
Naphthol Yellow S, 6393
Naphthopyridine *see* 1105
β-Naphthoquinoline *see* 1105
α-Naphthoquinone *see* 6395
β-Naphthoquinone *see* 6394
1,2-Naphthoquinone, 6394
1,4-Naphthoquinone, 6395
1,2-Naphthoquinone-4-sulfonic Acid Sodium Salt *see* 8646
β-Naphthoquinone-4-sulfonic Acid Sodium Salt *see* 8646
Naphthoresorcinol, 6396
Naphthosalol *see* 6415
β-Naphthoxyacetic Acid *see* 6397
2-Naphthoxyacetic Acid, 6397
2-(α-Naphthoxy)-N,N-diethylpropionamide *see* 6416
β-Naphthoxyethanol *see* 6413
Naphthylacetic Acid *see* 6371
[6-[3-(2-Naphthyl)-D-alanine]] LHRH *see* 6351
α-Naphthylamine *see* 6398
β-Naphthylamine *see* 6399
1-Naphthylamine, 6398
2-Naphthylamine, 6399
Naphthylamine Blue *see* 9792
1-Naphthylamine-2,7-disulfonic Acid, 6400
1-Naphthylamine-4,6-disulfonic Acid, 6401
1-Naphthylamine-4,7-disulfonic Acid, 6402
2-Naphthylamine-3,6-disulfonic Acid *see* 402
2-Naphthylamine-6,8-disulfonic Acid *see* 401
β-Naphthylamine-δ-sulfonic Acid *see* 1893
1-Naphthylamine-4-sulfonic Acid, 6403
1-Naphthylamine-5-sulfonic Acid, 6404
1-Naphthylamine-6-sulfonic Acid *see* 2350
1-Naphthylamine-7-sulfonic Acid *see* 2351
1-Naphthylamine-8-sulfonic Acid, 6405
2-Naphthylamine-1-sulfonic Acid, 6406
2-Naphthylamine-5-sulfonic Acid, 6407

2-Naphthylamine-6-sulfonic Acid *see* 1893

2-Naphthylamine-7-sulfonic Acid *see* 1893

2-Naphthylamine-8-sulfonic Acid *see* 940

2-Naphthyl Benzoate, 6408

β-Naphthylbis(β-chloroethyl)amine *see* 2108

β-Naphthyldi(2-chloroethyl)amine *see* 2108

O-2-Naphthyl *m,N*-Dimethylthiocarbanilate *see* 9519

N-(1-Naphthyl)ethylenediamine, 6409

β-Naphthyl Ethyl Ether *see* 3752

N-(1-Naphthyl)-*N′*-(3-ethylphenyl)-*N′*-methylguanidine *see* 758

O-(2-Naphthyl)glycolic Acid *see* 6397

1-Naphthylisocyanate, 6410

1-(2′-Naphthyl)-2-isopropylaminoethanol *see* 7790

1-Naphthylisothiocyanate, 6411

2-Naphthyl Lactate, 6412

1-Naphthyl Mercaptan *see* 6378

2-Naphthyl Mercaptan *see* 6379

1-Naphthyl *N*-Methylcarbamate *see* 1787

2-(1-Naphthylmethyl)imidazoline *see* 6368

2-Naphthyl *N*-Methyl-*N*-(3-tolyl)thionocarbamate *see* 9519

2-(2-Naphthyloxy)ethanol, 6413

4-(α-Naphthyloxy)-3-hydroxybutyramidoxime *see* 6347

α-Naphthylphthalamic Acid *see* 6418

N-1-Naphthylphthalamic Acid *see* 6418

α-Naphthyl Salicylate *see* 6414

1-Naphthyl Salicylate, 6414

2-Naphthyl Salicylate, 6415

3-(1-Naphthyl)-2-tetrahydrofurfurylpropionic Acid 2-(Diethylamino)ethyl Ester *see* 6353

α-Naphthylthiocarbamide *see* 722

α-Naphthylthiourea *see* 722

N-1-Naphthylthiourea *see* 722

1-(1-Naphthyl)-2-thiourea *see* 722

Naphuride *see* 9006

Naples Yellow *see* 5398

NAPQI *see* 57

Naprelan [Wyeth-Ayerst] *see* 6417

Napren [Nycomed] *see* 6417

Naprilene [Sigma-Tau] *see* 3567

Naprius [Magis] *see* 6417

Napropamide, 6416

Naprosyn [Syntex] *see* 6417

Naprosyne [Syntex] *see* 6417

Naproxen, 6417

Naprux [Andromaco] *see* 6417

Naptalam, 6418

Naqua [Schering] *see* 9624

Naramig [GSK] *see* 6420

Naramycin A *see* 2728

Narasin, 6419

Narasin A *see* 6419

Naratriptan, 6420

Narbivolol *see* 6432

Narbomycin, 6421

Narbonolide *see* 6421

Narcan [Endo] *see* 6362

Narcanti [BMS] *see* 6362

Narcaricin [Heumann] *see* 1065

Narceine, 6422

Narcissine *see* 5626

Narcoren [Veterinaria] *see* 7130

Narcosan Soluble *see* 4704

Narcosine *see* 6718

Narcotile *see* 3782

Narcotine *see* 6718

dl-Narcotine *see* 6718

l-α-Narcotine *see* 6718

Narcotoline, 6423

Narcoxyl [Veterinaria] *see* 10080

Narcozep [Roche] *see* 4146

Narcyl *see* 6422

Nardelzine [Warner-Lambert] *see* 7221

Nardil [Warner-Lambert] *see* 7221

Naridan *see* 6973

Narigix [Taiyo] *see* 6359

Narilet [Boehringer, Ing.] *see* 5073

Naringenin, 6424

Naringenin-7-rhamnoglucoside *see* 6425

Naringen 7-Methyl Ether *see* 8319

Naringetol *see* 6424

Naringin, 6425

Narol [Almirall] *see* 1504

Narone [Ulmer] *see* 3350

Naropin [AstraZeneca] *see* 8258

Narphen [Smith & Nephew] *see* 7218

Narsis [Sumitomo] *see* 5786

Nartate *see* 3350

Nartograstim *see* 4537

Nasacort [Aventis] *see* 9596

Nasalcrom [Pharmacia & Upjohn] *see* 2590

Nasalide [Syntex] *see* 4145

Nasanyl [Yamanouchi] *see* 6351

Nasea [Yamanouchi] *see* 8105

Nasivin [Merck KGaA] *see* 6966

Nasonex [Schering-Plough] *see* 6241

Nastenon *see* 6967

NAT-333 *see* 3999

Natacillin [Banyu] *see* 4672

Natacyn [Alcon] *see* 6427

Natalizumab, 6426

Natamycin, 6427

Nateglinide, 6428

Naticardina [Viatris] *see* 8060

Natil [3M] *see* 2704

Native Calcium Sulfate *see* 1706

Native Gellan Gum *see* 4383

Natrecor [Scios] *see* 1360

Natrilix [Servier] *see* 4935

Natriphene *see* 7304

Natrite *see* 8596

Natrium *see* 8570

Natriuretic Factor-32 (Human Brain Clone λhBNP57) *see* 1360

Natrol *see* 1279

Natron *see* 8596

Natto *see* 8730

Natulan [Roche] *see* 7758

Natural Calcium Carbonate *see* 5491

Natural Gas, 6429

Natural Tartaric Acid *see* 9070

Naturalyte [Dow AgroSci.] *see* 8750

Naturetin [BMS] *see* 1037

Naturlose [Spherix] *see* 9030

Naturon *see* 6005

Natyl [Interdelta] *see* 3346

Naucaine *see* 7757

Naumannite *see* 8431

Nausidol [SK & F] *see* 7454

Nausilen [Baldacci] *see* 250

Nauzelin [Janssen] *see* 3418

Navadel [Hercules] *see* 3301

Navane [Roerig] *see* 9365

Navelbine [Fabre] *see* 9990

Navidrex [Goldshield] *see* 2745

Navilox [Univet] *see* 5238

Navisin *see* 6966

Navoban [Novartis] *see* 9783

Navolin *see* 4455

Naxcel [Pfizer] *see* 1950

Naxen [Syntex] *see* 6417

Naxofem [Farmitalia] *see* 6552

Naxogin [Erba] *see* 6552

Naxy [Sanofi Winthrop] *see* 2339

Nazasetron *see* 900

NBA-061 *see* 4007

NBCA *see* 1565

NBI-34060 *see* 4946

NBS *see* 1438

9-NC *see* 8288

NC-14 *see* 751

NC-45 *see* 9941

NC-123 *see* 5910

NC-129 *see* 7967

NC-302 *see* 8086

NC-319 *see* 4602

NC-1667 *see* 9664

NC-1968 *see* 7169

NC-6897 *see* 1036

NC-8438 *see* 3742

NC-21314 *see* 2376

NCI-129 *see* 7967

NCI-96683 *see* 8086

NCI-C55243 *see* 1417

NCI-C55254 *see* 2135

NCI-C56462 *see* 6250

NCPI *see* 2778

NCS *see* 10167

NDEA *see* 6636

NDELA *see* 6635

2′NDG *see* 4363

NDGA *see* 6693

NDR-304 *see* 3788

NDR-5998A *see* 3999

NE-10064 *see* 911

NE-58095 *see* 8232

Neamine, 6430

Neantine [Givaudan] *see* 7371

Neatsfoot Oil, 6431

Neazina [Centralvet] *see* 8915

Nebcin [Lilly] *see* 9490

Neberk [Morishita] *see* 9112

Nebicina [Lilly] *see* 9490

Nebilet *see* 6432

Nebilox [GSK] *see* 6432

Nebivolol, 6432

dl-Nebivolol *see* 6432

Nebramycin *see* 9490

Nebramycin Factor 2 *see* 752

Nebramycin Factor 6 *see* 9490

Nebularine, 6433

Nebulin, 6434

NebuPent [Astellas] *see* 7115

Neburon, 6435

Necatorina *see* 1816

Necic Acids *see* 8449

"Necine" Bases *see* 8166

Nectocyd [Pfizer] *see* 3369

Nedocromil, 6436

Needle Antimony *see* 713

Neem, 6437

Nefazodone, 6438

Nefco *see* 6600

Nefiracetam, 6439

Nefopam, 6440

Nefrix *see* 4781

Nefrocarnit [Medice] *see* 1849

Nefrolan [M & B] *see* 2404

Neftin *see* 4300

Negamycin, 6441

Negatol [Altana] *see* 7556

NegGram [Sanofi Winthrop] *see* 6359

Negram [Sanofi Winthrop] *see* 6359

Neguvon [Bayer] *see* 9623

Nehydrin [TAD] *see* 3653

Nelarabine, 6442
Nelbon [Sankyo] see 6575
Nelfinavir, 6443
Nelfinavir Mesylate see 6443
Nema [Parke-Davis] see 9190
Nemacur [Bayer CropSci.] see 3957
Nemadectin, 6444
Nemafax [Rhône-Mérieux] see 9352
Nemafume see 3020
Nemagon see 3020
Nemasol Sodium [Valeant] see 477
Nemathorin [Ishihara Sangyo] see 4260
Nematolyt see 7016
Nemazine see 7252
Nembutal [Abbott] see 7130
Nemestran [HMR] see 4415
Nemex [Pfizer] see 7955
Nemicide [Coopers] see 5459
Nemifitide, 6445
Nemifitide Ditriflutate see 6445
Nemispor [Isagro] see 5716
Nemonapride, 6446
Nemural see 778
Nemurel [Takeda] see 3702
Nendrin see 3578
Neo Heliopan 303 [Symrise] see 6756
Neo Heliopan 357 [Symrise] see 888
Neo Heliopan AV [Symrise] see 6769
Neo Heliopan BB [Symrise] see 6954
Neo Heliopan HMS [Symrise] see 4738
Neo Heliopan Hydro [Symrise] see 3593
Neo Heliopan MA [Symrise] see 5840
Neo Heliopan OS [Symrise] see 6770
Neo-Absentol see 3718
Neoamyl Alcohol see 6457
Neo-Antergan [Poulenc] see 7984
Neoantimosan see 8813
Neo-Arsoluin see 6447
Neoarsphenamine, 6447
Neo-Atromid see 2377
Neobar [Merck KGaA] see 994
Neo-Benodine see 6053
Neobiosamine B see 6454
Neobiosamine C see 6454
Neo-Bradoral [Novartis] see 3415
Neobrettin [Norbrook] see 6454
Neocaine see 7757
Neocarcinostatin see 10167
Neo-Cardiamine see 9203
Neocardyl see 1261
Neocarzinostatin see 10167
Neo-Cebicure see 5126
Neo-Cebitate see 5126
Neocefal [Metapharma] see 1914
Neocembrene, 6448
Neocembrene A see 6448
Neochanin see 4244
Neocidol [Novartis] see 2995
Neoclym [Poli] see 2720
Neo-Cobefrin [Cook-Waite] see 6692
Neo-Codema see 4781
Neocon 1/35 [Ortho-Cilag] see 6697
Neo-Corovas see 7112
Neocuproine, 6449
Neo-Cytamen [Medeva] see 4809
Neodaian [Nichiiko] see 9297
Neodalit [Hässle] see 3008
Neo-Dioxanin [Boehringer, Ing.] see 3167
Neo Dohyfral D₃ see 10019
Neodorm [Minden] see 7130
Neo-Douxan see 6617
Neodrenal see 5217
Neo-Duplamox [ISF] see 2341
Neodymium, 6450
Neodyne see 3788

Neo-Epinine [Burroughs Wellcome] see 5217
Neoergosterol, 6451
Neo-Erycinum [Schering AG] see 3683
Neoesserin [Ankerpharm] see 6464
Neofamid see 5649
Neo-Farmadol see 6972
Neofemergen see 3655
Neo-Fluimucil [Zambon] see 88
Neoflumen see 4781
Neofocin [Medici] see 4254
Neogama [Hormosan] see 8989
Neogel [Hexal] see 1793
Neogest [Schering AG] see 6704
Neo-Gilurytmal [Kali-Chemie] see 7702
Neo H2 [Boehringer, Ing.] see 8274
Neohesperidin DHC see 6452
Neohesperidin Dihydrochalcone, 6452
Neo-Hombreol (Amp.) [Organon] see 9180
Neohombreol M [Organon] see 6125
Neohydrazid see 2680
Neo-Iopax [Schering] see 8633
Neoisocodeine see 7913
Neoisuprel see 5170
Neo Kodan [Schülke & Mayr] see 6754
Neolamin [Nippon Kayaku] see 9297
Neolate see 6454
Neolignans see 5486
Neolinarin see 7064
Neoloid [Lederle] see 1898
Neolone 950 [Rohm & Haas] see 6091
Neo-Lotan [Neopharmed] see 5583
Neolutin Depositum [Medici] see 240
Neomagnol [Chinoin] see 2074
Neomark [NeoPharm] see 1452
Neomas see 6454
Neo-mercazole [Roche] see 1798
Neomestine [Taiyo] see 4231
Neo-Metantyl [Zambon] see 7805
Neo-Methiodal see 5040
Neomethymycin, 6453
Neomethynolide see 6453
Neomin see 6454
Neomix [Tuco] see 6454
Neomycin, 6454
Neomycin A see 6430
Neomycin B see 6454
Neomycin C see 6454
Neomycin E see 7041
Neomyson [Eisai] see 9301
Neon, 6455
Neo-Naclex [Goldshield] see 1037
Neonal [Abbott] see 1521
Neonicotine see 619
Neo-Nilorex [A.V.P.] see 7220
Neopax [Janssen] see 7406
Neo-Penil see 7085
Neopentane, 6456
Neopentanol see 6457
Neopentyl Alcohol, 6457
Neopentyl Glycol, 6458
Neopenyl [Grünenthal] see 7094
Neoperidole [Kyowa Hakko] see 4598
Neophyl Chloride, 6459
Neopine, 6460
Neoplatin [BMS] see 2317
Neo-Ponden [Serono] see 634
Neoprene, 6461
Neoprotoveratrine see 7899
Neopsicaine see 7912
Neopterin, 6462
Neo-Pynamin [Sumitomo] see 9223
Neopyrithiamine see 7992
Neoquassin, 6463

Neoral [Novartis] see 2752
Neoron [Syngenta] see 1434
Neosalvarsan [Hoechst] see 6447
Neosanamid II see 8930
Neo-Skiodan see 5040
Neosorexa [Sorex] see 3133
Neospasmina [Biofarmacoterapico] see 3168
Neospiran see 9203
Neostene [SM & P] see 5950
Neostenovasan see 3479
Neosteron see 5950
Neostibosan see 3852
Neostigmin (Inj.) [Ferrosan] see 6464
Neostigmin (Tabl.) [Ferrosan] see 6464
Neostigmine, 6464
Neosulf see 6454
Neosulfine see 5918
Neo-Synephrine see 7286
Neo-T see 6466
Neotame, 6465
Neoteben [Bayer] see 5186
NeoTect [Diatide] see 2911
Neo-Tenebryl see 5040
Neotetrazolium Blue see 6466
Neotetrazolium Chloride, 6466
Neo-thyl see 6113
Neothylline [Lemmon] see 3479
Neo-Thyreostat [Herbrand] see 1798
Neotigason [Roche] see 112
Neotilina see 3479
Neotocopherol see 9496
Neoton [Alfa] see 7340
Neotran see 1247
Neotrofin [Spectrum] see 5448
Neo-Vasophylline see 3479
Neovastat [AEterna], 6467
Neovitamin A, 6468
Neovitamin A Acid see 5228
Neozine [Rhône-Poulenc] see 5986
Neo-Zine [Neo] see 7237
Nepafenac, 6469
Nepetalactone, 6470
Nepetalic Acid see 6470
Nephril [Pfizer] see 7584
Nephroflow [Medi-Physics] see 5034
Nephrotest [Biolog. Arbeitsgem.] see 442
Neporex [Novartis] see 2775
Nepresol [Novartis] see 3169
Nepresol Inject [Novartis] see 3169
Népressol [Novartis] see 3169
Neprotin see 5261
Neptal [Procter & Gamble] see 19
Neptazane [Wyeth] see 5962
Neptunium, 6471
Nequinate, 6472
Neral see 2322
Neraval [Schering] see 5978
Neravan [Promonta] see 1506
Nerbowdine see 1493
Nerdipina [Ferrer] see 6495
Neribas [Schering AG] see 3143
Nericur [Schering] see 1116
Neridronate Sodium see 6473
Neridronic Acid, 6473
Neriforte [Schering AG] see 3143
Neriifolin, 6474
Neriine see 2497
Neriodin [Nagase] see 3081
Neriolin see 6826
Nerisona [Schering AG] see 3143
Nerisone [Schering AG] see 3143
Nerixia [Abiogen] see 6473
Nerobol see 5951
Nerol, 6475

Nerolidol, 6476
Nerolin "New" see 3752
Nerolin "Old" see 5997
Neroli Oil (Artificial) see 6020
Nervanaid B see 3517
Nerve Growth Factor, 6477
Nerve Growth Factor-2 see 6487
Nerve Root see 2770
Nervinex [Menarini] see 1378
Nervonus [Orion] see 5862
Nesacaine [Astra] see 2158
Nesdonal Sodium [RPR] see 9350
Nesiritide see 1360
NESP see 2824
Nestorone [Pop. Council] see 3538
Netamifide see 6445
Nethalide see 7790
Nethamine [HMR] see 3709
Neticonazole, 6478
Netillin [Schering] see 6479
Netilmicin, 6479
Netilyn [Schering] see 6479
Netobimin, 6480
Netromicine [Schering] see 6479
Netromycin [Schering] see 6479
Netropsin, 6481
Netsusarin [Ohta] see 474
Nettacin [Schering] see 6479
Nettle, 6482
Neuberg Ester see 4276
Neucef [HMR] see 1928
Neuer [Daiichi] see 2024
Neulactil [M & B] see 7164
Neulasta [Amgen] see 4537
Neuleptil [Aventis] see 7164
Neumega [Genetics Inst.] see 5000
Neupentedrin see 9012
Neupogen [Amgen] see 4537
Neuprex [Xoma] see 938
Neuquinon [Eisai] see 9843
Neuracen [Byk Gulden] see 1018
Neuractil see 5986
Neuractiv [Novartis] see 6942
Neuraminic Acid, 6483
Neuraxin see 5980
Neuridine see 8743
Neurine, 6484
Neuriplege [Génévrier] see 2183
NeuroBloc [Elan] see 1357
Neurocil [Bayer] see 5986
Neurodye GH1-43 see 4220
Neurolene [Magis] see 6673
Neurolite [BMS] see 9099
Neuromet [SKB] see 6942
Neuronotrophin-3 see 6487
Neurontin [Parke-Davis] see 4319
Neuropeptide Tyrosine see 6485
Neuropeptide Y, 6485
Neurosedyn see 9255
Neurosin see 1670
Neurotensin, 6486
Neurotensin (Ox) Triacetate (Salt) see
6486
Neuroton [Berlin-Chemie] see 2319
Neurotoxin see 2599
Neurotrast see 5060
Neurotrophin-3 see 6487
Neurotrophins, 6487
Neurturin see 4377
Neustab [Boots] see 9290
Neutase [Sawai] see 5640
Neuthion [Senju] see 4475
Neutrafil see 3479
Neutral Acriflavine see 123
Neutral Ammonium Chromate see 510

Neutral Ammonium Fluoride see 522
Neutral Cupric Chromate see 2634
Neutral Cysteine Proteinase Inhibitor see
2778
Neutral Endopeptidase see 872
Neutralized Sarin see 4924
Neutral Lead Acetate see 5397
"Neutral" Magnesium Phosphate see
5683
Neutral Potassium Chromate see 7622
Neutral Proflavine Sulfate see 7771
Neutral Protein Hagedorn Insulin see
4980
Neutral Red, 6488
Neutral Red Chloride see 6488
Neutral Sodium Chromate see 8601
Neutral Spirits, 6489
Neutral Verdigris see 2624
Neutrapen [3M Pharma] see 7093
Neutraphylline [Dorsey] see 3479
Neutrexin [MedImmune] see 9721
Neutroflavine see 123
Neutrogin [Chugai] see 4537
Neutronyx 600's [Onyx] see 6677
Neutronyx 605 [Onyx] see 6761
Neutronyx 611 [Onyx] see 6677
Neutrormone see 5950
NeutroSpec [Palatin] see 9100
Neutrosteron see 5950
Neu-up [Kyowa] see 4537
Neuvitan [Fujisawa] see 6760
Neuzyme [Eisai] see 5640
Nevanac [Alcon] see 6469
Nevax see 3401
Nevergor see 5577
Nevigramon [Chinoin] see 6359
Nevile and Winther's Acid see 6391
Nevin [Grünenthal] see 8924
Nevirapine, 6490
Nevite see 8596
Nevralgina [Climax] see 3350
Nevriton [RPR] see 54
Newberyite see 5681
Newtol [Mohan] see 10085
Newtonite see 362
New Victoria Green Extra I see 5699
New Victoria Green Extra II see 5699
New Victoria Green Extra O see 5699
Nexaband [Closure Medical] see 6766
Nexagan [Boehringer, Ing.] see 1431
Nexavar [Bayer] see 8720
Nexion [Boehringer, Ing.] see 1431
Nexium [AstraZeneca] see 6845
Nexter [BASF] see 7967
Nexus see 1908
Nezeril [Draco] see 6966
NF 6 see 9490
NF-64 see 6542
NF-180 see 4300
NF-260 see 4294
NF-963 see 4301
NGF see 6477
β-NGF see 6477
NGF-2 see 6487
NH-502 see 4933
NHDC see 6452
NHPI see 4838
NI-25 see 49
Nia [Novo] see 5805
NIA-10242 see 1803
NIA-18739 see 1230
NIA-33297 see 7180
Niacin see 6525
Niacinamide see 6523
Niacor [Upsher-Smith] see 6525

Niagara 1240 see 3736
Niagara 4512 see 8702
Niagara 4556 see 3088
Niagara 4562 see 5285
Niagara 5006 see 3042
Niagara Blue see 9792
Niagestin [Novo] see 5805
Nialamide, 6491
Niamid [Pfizer] see 6491
Niamidal see 6491
Niamine see 6543
Niaprazine, 6492
Niaquitil see 6491
Niaspan [Kos] see 6525
Niazol see 6368
Nibiol see 6655
Nicabate [GSK] see 6524
Nicalex see 351
Nicamide see 6543
Nicangin [AstraZeneca] see 6525
Nicant [Piam] see 6495
Nicapress [Boehringer, Ing.] see 6495
Nicaragua Wood see 7181
Nicaraven, 6493
Nicarb [Merck & Co.] see 6494
Nicarbazin, 6494
Nicardal [Italfarmaco] see 6495
Nicardipine, 6495
Nicarpin [San Carlo] see 6495
Niccolite see 6498
Nicein see 5351
Nicelate [Toyo Jozo] see 6359
Nicergolent [Ramon] see 6496
Nicergoline, 6496
Niceritrol, 6497
Nicetile [Sigma-Tau] see 84
Nicholin [Wyeth] see 2319
Nicizina [Pharmacia] see 5186
Nickel, 6498
Nickel Acetate, 6499
Nickel Acetylacetonate, 6500
Nickel Ammonium Sulfate, 6501
Nickel Benzoate see 1091
Nickel Bromide, 6502
Nickel Carbonate Hydroxide, 6503
Nickel Carbonyl, 6504
Nickel Chloride, 6505
Nickel Cyanide, 6506
Nickel Dibromide see 6502
Nickel Dichloride see 6505
Nickel Difluoride see 6508
Nickel Diiodide see 6511
Nickel Dimethylglyoxime, 6507
Nickel Fluoride, 6508
Nickel Formate, 6509
Nickel Hydroxide, 6510
Nickelic Oxide see 6516
Nickel Iodide, 6511
Nickel Monoxide, 6512
Nickel Nitrate, 6513
Nickelous Fluoride see 6508
Nickelous Oxide see 6512
Nickel Oxalate, 6514
Nickel Oxide (NiO) see 6512
Nickel(II) Oxide see 6512
Nickel Phosphate, 6515
Nickel Potassium Cyanide see 7684
Nickel Protoxide see 6512
Nickel Sesquioxide, 6516
Nickel Sulfate, 6517
Nickel Tetracarbonyl see 6504
Niclocide [Miles] see 6519
Niclofolan, 6518
Niclosamide, 6519
Nicopatch [Fabre] see 6524

Nicobid [Aventis] *see* 6525
Nicobifen *see* 1352
Nicobion [Merck KGaA] *see* 6523
Nicodel [Mitsui] *see* 6495
Nicoderm CQ [GSK] *see* 6524
Nicolan [Elan] *see* 6524
Nicolar [Aventis] *see* 6525
Nicolen *see* 4300
Nicomorphine, 6520
Niconacid [Novartis] *see* 6525
Nicor *see* 6543
Nicorandil, 6521
Nicorette [GSK] *see* 6524
Nicorine *see* 6543
Nicorol [Lundbeck] *see* 4309
Nicoscorbine *see* 6523
Nicosulfuron, 6522
Nicotafuryl *see* 9395
Nicotergoline *see* 6496
Nicotinamide, 6523
Nicotinamide-adenine Dinucleotide *see* 6344
Nicotinamide-adenine Dinucleotide Phosphate *see* 6348
Nicotinamide Ascorbate *see* 6523
Nicotinamide Chloromethylate *see* 9693
Nicotinamide Methyl Chloride *see* 9693
Nicotinamide Mononucleotide *see* 6663
Nicotine, 6524
Nicotinell [Novartis] *see* 6524
Nicotine Neutral Sulfate *see* 6524
Nicotine Tartrate *see* 6524
Nicotinic Acid, 6525
Nicotinic Acid Amide *see* 6523
Nicotinic Acid Benzyl Ester, 6526
Nicotinic Acid Diethylamide *see* 6543
Nicotinic Acid Ester with 7-(2-Hydroxy-ethyl)theophylline *see* 3879
Nicotinic Acid 2-Hydroxyethyl Ester 2-(*p*-Chlorophenoxy)-2-methylpropion-ate (Ester) *see* 3877
Nicotinic Acid *N*-Methylbetaine *see* 9694
Nicotinic Acid Methyl Ester *see* 6100
Nicotinic Acid Morphine Ester *see* 6520
Nicotinic Acid Neopentanetetrayl Ester *see* 6497
Nicotinic Acid 1-Oxide *see* 6941
Nicotinic Acid β-Phenylisopropylamide *see* 7216
Nicotinic Acid Tetrahydrofurfuryl Ester *see* 9395
Nicotinic Alcohol *see* 6527
3-(Nicotinoyloxy)propyl *p*-Chlorophen-oxyisobutyrate *see* 8255
Nicotinoyl-β-phenylisopropylamine *see* 7216
Nicotinyl Alcohol, 6527
Nicoumalone *see* 29
Nicoxin *see* 6494
Nicozid [Piam] *see* 5186
Nicrazin [Merck & Co.] *see* 6494
Nidanthel [Cooper] *see* 6596
Nidantin [Warner-Lambert] *see* 6945
Nide [Ibirn] *see* 6548
Nidol [Tosi] *see* 6548
Nidrafur *see* 6542
Nidran [Sankyo] *see* 6553
Nidrane [Phoenix] *see* 1018
Nidrel [Specia] *see* 6576
Nielsbohrium *see* 1321, 3462
Nifedicor [Alfa] *see* 6528
Nifedipine, 6528
Nifekalant, 6529
Nifelan [Elan] *see* 6528
Nifelat [TAD] *see* 6528

Nifenalol, 6530
Nifensar [Aventis] *see* 6528
Niflan [Yoshitomi] *see* 7711
Niflumic Acid, 6531
Nifluril *see* 6531
Nifluril (Suppositories) [UPSA] *see* 6531
Nifos T [Monsanto] *see* 9204
NIF-T *see* 4538
Niftolid *see* 4208
Nifulidone *see* 4300
Nifuratel, 6532
Nifurfoline, 6533
Nifuroquine, 6534
Nifuroxazide, 6535
Nifuroxime, 6536
Nifurpirinol, 6537
Nifurtimox, 6538
Nifurtoinol, 6539
Nifurzide, 6540
Nifuzon *see* 6600
Nigakilactone D *see* 8026
Nigelline *see* 2808
Nigericin, 6541
Night-blooming Cereus *see* 1607
NIH-4185 *see* 9293
NIH-4542 *see* 3260
NIH-5145 *see* 3829
NIH-7274 *see* 7249
NIH-7440 *see* 296
NIH-7519 *see* 7218
NIH-7539 *see* 6707
NIH-7590 *see* 7433
NIH-7667 *see* 6685
NIH-8805 *see* 1497
Nihydrazone, 6542
Nikardin *see* 6543
Nikethamide, 6543
Nikoform *see* 4833
Nikos [Dow AgroSci.] *see* 4108
Nilandron [Aventis] *see* 6544
Nilatil [USV] *see* 5246
Nilergex *see* 5227
Nilevar [Searle] *see* 6696
Nilodin *see* 5591
Niltuvin [EGYT] *see* 6527
Nilutamide, 6544
Nilvadipine, 6545
Nilverm [Mallinckrodt] *see* 5459
Nim *see* 6437
Nimbecetin *see* 5274
Nimbex [GSK] *see* 868
Nimbin, 6546
Nimbiol, 6547
Nimbisan [Solvay] *see* 1450
Nimergoline *see* 6496
Nimesulide, 6548
Nimetazepam, 6549
Nimicor [Formenti] *see* 6495
Nimidane, 6550
Nimodipine, 6551
Nimorazole, 6552
Nimotop [Bayer] *see* 6551
Nimrod [Syngenta] *see* 1494
Nimustine, 6553
Ninhydrin, 6554
Ninopterin, 6555
Niobium, 6556
Niobium Chloride (NbCl$_5$) *see* 6557
Niobium(V) Chloride *see* 6557
Niobium Oxide (Nb$_2$O$_5$) *see* 6559
Niobium(V) Oxide *see* 6559
Niobium Pentachloride, 6557
Niobium Pentafluoride, 6558
Niobium Pentoxide, 6559
Nioform *see* 5031

Nionate [Nion] *see* 4047
Niopam [Bracco] *see* 5057
Niotal [Sanofi-Synthelabo] *see* 10190
Nioxime, 6560
Nip [Nichay] *see* 7586
Nipagin A *see* 3837
Nipagin M *see* 6107
Nipantiox 1-F [Nipa] *see* 1547
Nipasol M [Nipa] *see* 7866
Nipaxon [Pharmacia] *see* 6718
Nipecotic Acid, 6561
Nipent [SuperGen] *see* 7135
Niperyt *see* 7112
Nipolept [Aventis] *see* 10197
Nippas Calcium [Tanabe] *see* 477
Nipradilol, 6562
Nipradolol *see* 6562
Nipride [Roche] *see* 8649
Nipruss [Schwarz] *see* 8649
NiQuitin CQ [GSK] *see* 6524
Niran [Tamogan] *see* 2082
Niridazole, 6563
Nirvan *see* 5986
Nirvanil [SKB] *see* 9912
NIS *see* 5045
NISac *see* 5043
Nisaplin [Aplin & Barrett] *see* 6564
Nische [Kodama] *see* 223
Nisentil [Roche] *see* 310
Nisin, 6564
Nisin A *see* 6564
Nisin Z *see* 6564
Nisoldipine, 6565
Nisotin *see* 3737
Nissorun [Nippon Soda] *see* 4713
Nisulid [Wyeth] *see* 6548
Nisvastatin *see* 7508
Nitalapram *see* 2318
Nitarsone, 6566
Nitazoxanide, 6567
Nitenpyram, 6568
Niter *see* 7648
Nithiamide *see* 410
Nithiazide, 6569
Nithiocyamine *see* 574
Nitisinone, 6570
Nitobanil [Kyowa Yakuhin] *see* 9112
Nitogenin *see* 3295
Nitoman [Roche] *see* 9182
Niton *see* 8095
Nitorol [Eisai] *see* 5225
Nitossil [Zyma] *see* 2395
Nitracrine, 6571
Nitradisc [Pfizer] *see* 6607
Nitrados [APS] *see* 6575
Nitraldone *see* 4294
Nitramide, 6572
Nitramine, 6573
m-Nitranilide *see* 6582
o-Nitraniline *see* 6583
p-Nitraniline *see* 6584
Nitraphen *see* 6598
Nitrapyrin, 6574
2-Nitratoethylaminotoluene-*p*-sulfonate *see* 5246
(Nitrato-*O*)phenylmercury *see* 7302
Nitrazepam, 6575
Nitrendipine, 6576
Nitric Acid, 6577
Nitric Acid Chromium(3+) Salt *see* 2226
Nitric Acid, Fuming *see* 6577
Nitric Acid Gallium Salt *see* 4350
Nitric Acid Methyl Ester *see* 6101
Nitric Acid Potassium Salt *see* 7648
Nitric Acid Propyl Ester *see* 7864

Nitric Acid Silver(1+) Salt *see* 8518
Nitric Acid Silver (1+) Salt Mixt with Silver Chloride (AgCl) *see* 8518
Nitric Acid Thallium(1+) Salt *see* 9265
Nitric Acid Thallium (3+) Salt *see* 9271
Nitric Anhydride *see* 6605
Nitric Oxide, 6578
Nitric Oxide Synthase *see* 6578
5,5′-Nitrilodibarbituric Acid Monoammonium Salt *see* 6306
Nitrilotriacetic Acid, 6579
Nitrilotriacetic Acid Bismuth Complex Sodium Salt *see* 1280
2,2′,2″-Nitrilotrisethanol *see* 9665
Nitrimidazine *see* 6552
Nitrin, 6580
Nitritocobalamin *see* 4809
Nitroacetanilide, 6581
m-Nitroacetanilide *see* 6581
o-Nitroacetanilide *see* 6581
p-Nitroacetanilide *see* 6581
Nitro Acid Sulfite *see* 6648
3-Nitroalizarin *see* 254
4-Nitro-2-aminophenetole *see* 6617
1-Nitro-3-amino-4-phenyl Ethyl Ether *see* 6617
m-Nitroaniline, 6582
o-Nitroaniline, 6583
p-Nitroaniline, 6584
Nitroanisole, 6585
m-Nitroanisole *see* 6585
o-Nitroanisole *see* 6585
p-Nitroanisole *see* 6585
5-Nitrobarbituric Acid, 6586
Nitrobenzaldehyde, 6587
m-Nitrobenzaldehyde *see* 6587
o-Nitrobenzaldehyde *see* 6587
p-Nitrobenzaldehyde *see* 6587
3-Nitrobenzenamine *see* 6582
Nitrobenzene, 6588
4-Nitrobenzeneacetic Acid *see* 6622
4-Nitrobenzeneacetonitrile *see* 6591
p-Nitrobenzenearsonic Acid *see* 6566
p-Nitrobenzeneazochromotropic Acid Sodium Salt *see* 2240
p-Nitrobenzeneazosalicylic Acid *see* 255
4-Nitro-1,2-benzenediamine *see* 6623
p-Nitrobenzenesulfonic Acid Methyl Ester *see* 6102
Nitrobenzoic Acid, 6589
m-Nitrobenzoic Acid *see* 6589
o-Nitrobenzoic Acid *see* 6589
p-Nitrobenzoic Acid *see* 6589
Nitrobenzol *see* 6588
4-Nitrobenzoyl Chloride, 6590
p-Nitrobenzyl Cyanide, 6591
Nitro-Bid [Altana] *see* 6607
o-Nitrobiphenyl, 6592
p-Nitrobiphenyl, 6593
2-Nitro-1,1′-biphenyl *see* 6592
4-Nitrobiphenyl *see* 6593
4-Nitro-1,1′-biphenyl *see* 6593
9-Nitrocamptothecin *see* 8288
9-Nitro-(20*S*)-camptothecin *see* 8288
N-Nitrocarbamide *see* 6651
Nitrocarbol *see* 6611
Nitrocefin, 6594
Nitrocellulose *see* 8011
Nitrochlorobenzene *see* 2151
m-Nitrochlorobenzene *see* 2151
Nitrochloroform *see* 2156
7-Nitro-5-(2-chlorophenyl)-3*H*-1,4-benzodiazepin-2(1*H*)-one *see* 2389
Nitrocine [Schwarz] *see* 6607
m-Nitrocinnamic Acid, 6595

Nitrocobalamin *see* 4809
Nitrocontin [Mundipharma] *see* 6607
Nitrodan, 6596
Nitroderm [Novartis] *see* 6607
4-Nitro-1,2-diaminobenzene *see* 6623
o-Nitrodiphenyl *see* 6592
p-Nitrodiphenyl *see* 6593
Nitrodulcitol *see* 4332
Nitro-Dur [Schering-Plough] *see* 6607
Nitroerythrite *see* 3677
Nitroethane, 6597
5-Nitro-2-ethoxyaniline *see* 6617
Nitrofen, 6598
Nitrofene *see* 6598
Nitroform *see* 9729
Nitrofural *see* 6600
5-Nitro-2-furaldehyde Acetylhydrazone *see* 6542
5-Nitro-2-furaldehyde *p*-Hydroxybenzoylhydrazone *see* 6535
5-Nitro-2-furaldehyde Semicarbazone *see* 6600
anti-5-Nitro-2-furaldoxime *see* 6536
5-Nitro-2-furancarboxaldehyde Oxime *see* 6536
Nitrofurantoin, 6599
6-[2-(5-Nitro-2-furanyl)ethenyl]-2-pyridinemethanol *see* 6537
1-[[(5-Nitro-2-furanyl)methylene]amino]-2,4-imidazolidinedione *see* 6599
3-[[(5-Nitro-2-furanyl)methylene]amino]-2-oxazolidinone *see* 4300
2-[(5-Nitro-2-furanyl)methylene]hydrazinecarboxamide *see* 6600
2-[3-(5-Nitro-2-furanyl)-1-[2-(5-nitro-2-furanyl)ethenyl]-2-propenylidene]-hydrazinecarboximidamide *see* 6654
4-(5-Nitro-2-furanyl)-2-quinolinecarboxylic Acid 1-Oxide *see* 6534
Nitrofurazone, 6600
1-(5-Nitro-2-furfurylidene)-2-acetylhydrazine *see* 6542
1-(5-Nitro-2-furfurylideneamino)hydantoin *see* 6599
N-(5-Nitro-2-furfurylidene)-1-aminohydantoin *see* 6539
1-[(5-Nitrofurfurylidene)amino]-3-(hydroxymethyl)hydantoin *see* 6539
1-[(5-Nitrofurfurylidene)amino]-2-methyltetrahydro-1,4-thiazine 4,4-Dioxide *see* 6538
4-[(5-Nitrofurfurylidene)amino]-3-methylthiomorpholine-1,1-dioxide *see* 6538
3-(5-Nitrofurfurylideneamino)-5-(4-morpholinomethyl)-2-oxazolidone *see* 4294
3-(5-Nitrofurfurylideneamino)-2-oxazolidinone *see* 4300
N-(5-Nitro-2-furfurylidene)-3-amino-2-oxazolidone *see* 4300
Nitrofurmethone *see* 4294
*N*¹-(5-Nitro-2-furylacrylidene)-*N*²-(5-nitro-2-thenoyl)hydrazine *see* 6540
[[3-(5-Nitro-2-furyl)-1-[2-(5-nitro-2-furyl)vinyl]allylidene]amino]guanidine *see* 6654
4-(5-Nitro-2-furyl)quinaldic Acid 1-Oxide *see* 6534
6-[2-(5-Nitro-2-furyl)vinyl]-2-pyridinemethanol *see* 6537
Nitrogard [Forest] *see* 6607
Nitrogen, 6601
Nitrogen Chloride, 6602
Nitrogen Dioxide, 6603
Nitrogen Fluoride, 6604

Nitrogen Monoxide *see* 6578
Nitrogen Mustard *see* 5775
Nitrogen Oxide (NO) *see* 6578
Nitrogen Oxyfluoride *see* 6647
Nitrogen Pentoxide, 6605
Nitrogen Selenide, 6606
Nitrogen Tetroxide *see* 6603
Nitrogen Trichloride *see* 6602
Nitrogen Trifluoride *see* 6604
Nitrogen Trioxyfluoride *see* 4165
Nitroglin [Stada] *see* 6607
Nitroglycerin, 6607
Nitroglycerol *see* 6607
Nitroglycol *see* 3800
Nitroglyn [Bradley] *see* 6607
Nitrogranulogen [Pliva] *see* 5775
Nitroguanidine, 6608
Nitrohydrochloric Acid, 6609
2-Nitro-1-hydroxybenzene-4-arsonic Acid *see* 8273
2-Nitro-2-(hydroxymethyl)-1,3-propanediol *see* 9753
1-Nitro-2-hydroxynaphthalene *see* 6615
3-Nitro-4-hydroxyphenylarsonic Acid *see* 8273
5-Nitro-8-hydroxyquinoline *see* 6655
2-Nitro-1*H*-imidazole *see* 921
4-[2-(5-Nitro-1*H*-imidazol-1-yl)ethyl]-morpholine *see* 6552
4-Nitro-4′-isothiocyanodiphenyl Ether *see* 6633
Nitrol [Altana] *see* 5225
Nitrolime *see* 1662
Nitrolingual [Pohl] *see* 6607
Nitromagnesite *see* 5674
Nitromannite *see* 5746
Nitromannitol *see* 5746
Nitromersol, 6610
Nitromethane, 6611
4-Nitro-4′-[(*N*-methylpiperazinyl)thiocarbonylamino]diphenylamine *see* 571
Nitromex [Alpharma] *see* 6607
Nitromide, 6612
Nitromidine *see* 897
Nitromin *see* 5776
Nitromuriatic Acid *see* 6609
Nitron, 6613
Nitronal [Merck KGaA] *see* 6607
α-Nitronaphthalene *see* 6614
1-Nitronaphthalene, 6614
1-Nitro-2-naphthalenol *see* 6615
α-Nitro-β-naphthol *see* 6615
1-Nitro-2-naphthol, 6615
Nitrong [Lavipharm] *see* 6607
N-[2-(Nitrooxy)ethyl]-3-pyridinecarboxamide *see* 6521
Nitropenta *see* 7112
Nitropentaerythritol *see* 7112
3-Nitropentane, 6616
Nitropenton *see* 7112
Nitrophen *see* 6598
5-Nitro-*o*-phenetidine *see* 6617
Nitrophenide, 6618
m-Nitrophenol, 6619
o-Nitrophenol, 6620
p-Nitrophenol, 6621
2-Nitrophenol *see* 6620
3-Nitrophenol *see* 6619
4-Nitrophenol *see* 6621
Nitrophenolarsonic Acid *see* 8273
4-Nitro-2-phenoxymethanesulfonanilide *see* 6548
p-(*p*-Nitrophenoxy)phenyl Isothiocyanate *see* 6633
N-(4-Nitro-2-phenoxyphenyl)methanesulfonamide *see* 6548

Noctivane see 4704
Noctivane Sodium see 4704
Noctomin [Medichemie] see 3309
Noctone [GEA] see 8110
Noctosom see 4198
Nodakenetin Glucoside see 6668
Nodakenin, 6668
Nodapton see 4501
No-Doz [BMS] see 1636
Nodulisporic Acid, 6669
Nodulisporic Acid A see 6669
Noflo [Merck & Co.] see 6700
Noformicin, 6670
Noformycin see 6670
Nogalamycin, 6671
L-Nogalose see 6679
Nogram [Sanofi Winthrop] see 6359
Noin [Schering] see 4938
Nolatrexed, 6672
Noleptan [Thomae] see 4228
Nolicin [Krka] see 6700
Nolipax [Foscama] see 3978
Nolotil [Boehringer, Ing.] see 3350
Noludar [Roche] see 6136
Nolvadex [AstraZeneca] see 9048
Nolvasan [Fort Dodge] see 2091
Nomersan [Zeneca] see 9371
Nometan see 7465
Nomifensine, 6673
Nominee [Kumiai] see 1301
Nomolt [BASF] see 9109
Nonactic Acid see 6675
Nonactin, 6675
Nonaethyleneglycol Monomethyl Ether
    p-n-Butylaminobenzoate see 1096
Nonaisoprenol see 8703
Nonalol see 6679
(2E,6E,10E,14E,18E,22E,26E,30E,)-3,7,-
    11,15,19,23,27,31,35-Nonamethyl-2,-
    6,10,14,18,22,26,30,34-hexatriacon-
    tanonaen-1-ol see 8703
Nonanedioic Acid see 905
Nonanoic Acid see 7070
Nonanoic Acid Ethyl Ester see 3838
1-Nonanol see 6679
Nonanol Acetate see 6678
2-Nonenal, 6676
(E)-2-Nonenal see 6676
trans-2-Nonenaldehyde see 6676
Nonflamin [Yoshitomi] see 9448
Nonipol NO [Sankyo] see 6677
Nonoic Acid see 7070
Nonoxinol see 6677
Nonoxynol, 6677
Nonoxynol-9 see 6677
Nonoxynol-11 see 6677
Nonulosaminic Acids see 8484
n-Nonyl Acetate, 6678
n-Nonyl Alcohol, 6679
Nonylcarbinol see 2855
2-Nonyldioxolane, 6680
2-Nonyl-1,3-dioxolane see 6680
n-Nonyl Ethanoate see 6678
Nonylic Acid see 7070
Nonyl Phenol, 6681
(p-Nonylphenoxy)acetic Acid, 6682
Nonylphenoxypolyethoxyethanol see
    6677
α-(4-Nonylphenyl)-ω-hydroxypoly(oxy-
    1,2-ethanediyl) see 6677
Nonylphenyl Polyethyleneglycol Ether
    see 6677
Nootrop [UCB] see 7487
Nootropil [UCB] see 7487

Nootropyl [UCB] see 7487
Nopalcol [Henkel] see 7578
Nopar [Lilly] see 7162
Nopia [Daiichi] see 8253
Nopil [Mepha] see 8918
Nopinene see 7446
Nopol, 6683
No-Press see 5773
Nopron [Carrion] see 6492
Noprylsulfamide, 6684
NO-PYR see 6643
18-Norabietane see 4076
Noracin [Chew] see 6700
Noracymethadol, 6685
Noradrenaline see 6695
Noraminopyrine Methanesulfonate
    Sodium see 3350
Noranat [Novartis] see 4935
19-Norandrosta-4,9,11-trien-17β-ol-3-
    one see 9583
Nor-5'-anhydrovinblastine see 9990
Norantipyrine see 6713
Noravid [HMR] see 2861
Norbide see 1344
Norbiline [Bellon] see 7906
Norbolethone, 6686
Norbormide, 6687
cis-5-Norbornene-2,3-dicarboxylic Acid
    Dimethyl Ester see 3240
cis-endo-5-Norbornene-2,3-dicarboxylic
    Anhydride see 1796
α-5-Norbornen-2-yl-α-phenyl-1-piperi-
    dinepropanol see 1233
Norcarane, 6688
Norcholanic Acid, 6689
(5β)-24-Norcholan-23-oic Acid see 6689
Norcodeine, 6690
Norcolut [Gedeon Richter] see 6697
Norcuron [Organon] see 9941
Nordaz [Bouchara] see 6691
Nordazepam, 6691
Nordefrin, 6692
Norden see 6759
2'-Nor-2'-deoxyguanosine see 4363
Nordette [Wyeth] see 6704
Nordialex [Pharmacodex] see 4439
Nordiazepam see 6691
Nordihydroguaiaretic Acid, 6693
19-Nor-1α,25-dihydroxyvitamin D₂ see
    7039
Nordiocto [Nordisk] see 3921
Norditropin [Novo] see 8716
Norelgestromin, 6694
d-ψ-Norephedrine see 6714
Nor-d-ψ-ephedrine see 6714
dl-Norephedrine see 7307
Norephedrone see 1906
Norepinephrine, 6695
(3β,22E)-19-Norergosta-5,7,9,22-
    tetraen-3-ol see 6451
Norethandrolone, 6696
Norethindrone, 6697
19-Norethisterone see 6697
Norethynodrel, 6698
19-Nor-17α-ethynylandrosten-17β-ol-3-
    one see 6697
19-Nor-17α-ethynyl-17β-hydroxy-4-an-
    drosten-3-one see 6697
19-Nor-17α-ethynyltestosterone see 6697
Norfemac [HMR] see 1474
Norfen [Morishita] see 6759
Norfenefrine, 6699
Norfin [Lusofarmaco] see 6361
Norflex [3M Pharma] see 6879
Norfloxacin, 6700

Norflurazon, 6701
Norgamen see 9445
Norgan see 4785
Norgesterone, 6702
Norgestimate, 6703
Norgeston [Schering AG] see 6704
Norgestrel, 6704
D-Norgestrel see 6704
Norgestrienone, 6705
Norgine see 242
Norhomoepinephrine see 6692
Noriclan [Lilly] see 3354
Noriday [Searle] see 6697
Norimin [Searle] see 6697
Norimipramine see 2920
Norinyl 1+35 [Watson] see 6697
Norinyl-1+50 [Watson] see 6697
Norisodrine [Abbott] see 5217
d-Norisoephedrine see 6714
dl-Norisoephedrine see 447
Noristerat [Schering AG] see 6697
Norit [Norit N.V.] see 1808
Noritren [Lundbeck] see 6715
Norizalpinin see 4339
Norlaudanosoline see 9216
Norlestrin [Warner-Lambert] see 6697
Norleucine, 6706
4-L-Norleucine-7-D-phenylalanine-α-
    melanotropin (Swine) see 5814
Norlevo [HRA Pharma] see 6704
Norlevorphanol, 6707
Norlutate [Warner-Lambert] see 6697
Normabraïn [UCB] see 7487
Normal Butyl Thioalcohol see 1577
Normal Lead Acetate see 5397
Normase [Molteni] see 5346
Normastigmin (Amp.) [Sigmapharm] see
    6464
Normastigmin (Tabl.) [Sigmapharm] see
    6464
Normenon [Syntex] see 2102
Normet [Gedeon Richter] see 2377
Normetandrone see 6710
Normetanephrine, 6708
Normethadone, 6709
Normethandrolone see 6710
Normethandrone, 6710
Normetic [Abbott] see 406
Normicina [Meiji Seika] see 6183
Normiflo [Wyeth-Ayerst] see 775
Normison [Wyeth] see 9133
Normix [Alfa] see 8220
Normobren [Medosan] see 84
Normoc [Merckle] see 1385
Normodyne [Schering] see 5329
Normolipol [Delagrange] see 2377
Normonal [Eisai] see 9737
Normorix [Nycomed] see 406
Normorphine, 6711
Normorphine 3-Methyl Ether see 6690
Normoson see 3729
Normoxidil [Medosan] see 6203
Normud [Astra] see 10126
Normurat [Grünenthal] see 1065
Nornicotine, 6712
Norocin [Merck & Co.] see 6700
Noroclox [Norbrook] see 2419
Norodin [Endo] see 5948
Norodine [Norbrook] see 8903
Noromectin [Norbrook] see 5248
Noroxin(e) [Merck & Co.] see 6700
Noroxylin see 942
Norpace [Pfizer] see 3360
Norphen (Ampules) [Byk Gulden] see
    6759

Norphenazone, 6713
Norphenylephrine *see* 6699
Norphytane *see* 7752
Norplant [Wyeth] *see* 6704
Norpramin [Aventis] *see* 2920
(17α)-19-Norpregna-1,3,5(10)-trien-20-yne-3,17-diol *see* 3734
Norpregneninolone *see* 6697
(17α)-19-Norpregn-4-en-17-ol *see* 3805
(3β,17α)-19-Norpregn-4-en-20-yne-3,17-diol *see* 3860
(17α)-19-Norpregn-4-en-20-yn-17-ol *see* 5629
Nor-Progestelea *see* 6717
Norprolac [Novartis] *see* 8045
Norpropandrolate *see* 1322
Norpseudoephedrine, 6714
Norquen [Syntex] *see* 5917
(1α,3β,7E,22E)-19-Nor-9,10-seco-ergosta-5,7,22-triene-1,3,25-triol *see* 7039
Norsulfazole *see* 8943
Norsympatol *see* 6759
Norsynephrine *see* 6759
19-Nortestosterone *see* 6365
19-Nortestosterone Decanoate *see* 6365
19-Nortestosterone Hexahydrobenzoate *see* 6365
19-Nortestosterone-3-(*p*-hexyloxyphen-yl)propionate *see* 6365
19-Nortestosterone β-Phenylpropionate *see* 6365
19-Nortestosterone Propionate *see* 6365
North American Sumach *see* 8996
North and South American Antisnake-bite Serum *see* 720
Northern Pine *see* 10043
Norticon [Nihon] *see* 7471
Nortimil [Chiesi] *see* 2920
Nortran [Norden] *see* 9679
Nortrilen [Troponwerke] *see* 6715
Nortriptyline, 6715
Nortron [Lilly] *see* 3354
Nortron [Bayer CropSci.] *see* 3742
Norval [Bencard] *see* 6172
Norvaline, 6716
7-L-Norvaline Cyclosporin A *see* 2752
Norvasc [Pfizer] *see* 491
Norvedan [Wyeth] *see* 4003
Norvinisterone, 6717
Norvinodrel *see* 6702
Norvir [Abbott] *see* 8238
Norxacin [Siam Bheasach] *see* 6700
Nor-YM-060 *see* 8105
Norzepine *see* 6715
Norzetam [UCB] *see* 7487
Noscal [Sankyo] *see* 9769
Noscapine, 6718
Nosiheptide, 6719
Nosophen *see* 5038
Nosophene Sodium *see* 5038
No-Spa [Chinoin] *see* 3455
Nospan [Johnsons] *see* 9829
Nostoc [Ipesa] *see* 6522
Nostril [Novartis] *see* 7286
Nosydrast *see* 5040
Nosylan *see* 5040
Notandron *see* 5950
Notatin *see* 4460
Notézine [Specia] *see* 3116
Notul [Eurofarmaco] *see* 2279
Nova [Dow AgroSci.] *see* 6321
Novaban [Novartis] *see* 9783
Novacetyl *see* 5655
Novacid *see* 3350

Novacort [Syntex] *see* 2398
Novacyl [Astra] *see* 6941
Novadral [Diwag] *see* 6699
Novafed [HMR] *see* 7916
Noval [Yamanouchi] *see* 5805
Novaldin [Winthrop] *see* 3350
Novalgin [HMR] *see* 3350
Novaloc [Schering AG] *see* 4911
Novaluron, 6720
Novamin [BMS] *see* 405
Novamin [Shionogi] *see* 7761
Novantrone [Immunex] *see* 6217
Novapirina [Novartis] *see* 3081
Novarsan *see* 6447
Novarsenobenzol *see* 6447
Novarsenobillon *see* 6447
Novaruca [Bioglan] *see* 4472
Novasin [Danisco] *see* 6564
Novasmasol [Zambeletti] *see* 5931
Novastan [Tokyo Tanabe] *see* 779
Novastat W [Salsbury] *see* 8933
Novatec [Merck & Co.] *see* 5516
Novatrin [Ayerst] *see* 4730
Novatropine *see* 4730
Novazam [Génévrier] *see* 2994
Novedrin *see* 3709
Novel Erythropoiesis Stimulating Protein *see* 2824
Novemina [Lazar] *see* 3350
Noveril [Morishita] *see* 3008
Noverme [J & J] *see* 5768
Novesine [CIBA Vision] *see* 1047
Novex *see* 4004
Noviben [Merck & Co.] *see* 1726
Novicodin *see* 3171
Novidium *see* 4731
Novidroxin [Fatol] *see* 4809
Noviflumuron, 6721
Noviform [Dispersa] *see* 1199
Novil *see* 3350
Novismuth *see* 1284
Novobiocin, 6722
Novobiocyl [Francia] *see* 1930
Novocain [Sanofi Winthrop] *see* 7757
Novocamid [Hoechst] *see* 7756
Novocef [Pliva] *see* 1954
Novodigal [Beiersdorf-Lilly] *see* 3167
Novodil [Augot] *see* 2704
Novodolan [HMR] *see* 4103
Novodrin *see* 5217
Novofluen [Engelhard KG] *see* 3653
Novogent [Temmler] *see* 4881
Novolaudon *see* 4803
Novoldiamine, 6723
Novolin [Novo] *see* 4980
Novol Ketone *see* 6723
Novon *see* 2802
Novonal [Hoechst] *see* 9901
Novo-Nastizol A [Bago] *see* 856
Novonorm [Novo Nordisk] *see* 8136
Novophone *see* 2822
Novopulmon [Viatris] *see* 1468
Novorapid [Novo Nordisk] *see* 4982
Novoridazine [Novopharm] *see* 9359
Novorin [Polfa] *see* 10086
Novosparol [Merck KGaA] *see* 1205
Novotrone *see* 8968
Novotusil [Inpharzam] *see* 2395
Novrad [Lilly] *see* 5469
Noxaben [Unifa] *see* 3084
Noxafil [Schering-Plough] *see* 7602
Noxfire [AgrEvo] *see* 8271
Noxibiol *see* 6655
Noxigram [Firma] *see* 2309
Noxiurotan *see* 7464

Noxyflex-S [Geistlich] *see* 6724
Noxythiolin, 6724
Noxytiolin *see* 6724
Nozinan [Rhône-Poulenc] *see* 5986
NP *see* 6618
NP-13 *see* 1027
NP-55 *see* 8473
NP-113 *see* 4976
NPA-3 *see* 6418
NPAB *see* 7702
NPe6 *see* 9034
NPH-1320 *see* 1441
NPH Insulin *see* 4980
NPPB, 6725
NPT-10381 *see* 4976
NPY *see* 6485
NPYR *see* 6643
NRC-910 *see* 5077
NRDC-107 *see* 1230
NRDC-143 *see* 7180
NRDC-149 *see* 2767
NRDC-161 *see* 2883
NsA A *see* 6669
NSC-185 *see* 2728
NSC-1026 *see* 2734
NSC-1771 *see* 9371
NSC-2101 *see* 8273
NSC-3051 *see* 6076
NSC-3053 *see* 2800
NSC-3364 *see* 4080
NSC-3590 *see* 4222
NSC-5159 *see* 2045
NSC-5366 *see* 6718
NSC-5547 *see* 3475
NSC-8806 *see* 5828
NSC-9706 *see* 9671
NSC-10023 *see* 7722
NSC-11905 *see* 5366
NSC-12198 *see* 3448
NSC-13875 *see* 320
NSC-15200 *see* 4350
NSC-15780 *see* 597
NSC-17777 *see* 7321
NSC-19893 *see* 4181
NSC-20264 *see* 158
NSC-21626 *see* 7820
NSC-23436 *see* 3422
NSC-23759 *see* 9179
NSC-25154 *see* 7480
NSC-25614 *see* 7374
NSC-25855 *see* 9445
NSC-26805 *see* 3827
NSC-27640 *see* 4112
NSC-28693 *see* 6250
NSC-30152 *see* 3213
NSC-31712 *see* 4176
NSC-32946 *see* 6213
NSC-34462 *see* 9851
NSC-35051 *see* 5828
NSC-37095 *see* 9872
NSC-38297 *see* 1452
NSC-39084 *see* 902
NSC-39415 *see* 3415
NSC-39470 *see* 1180
NSC-40725 *see* 5224
NSC-43193 *see* 8794
NSC-45383 *see* 8827
NSC-45388 *see* 2798
NSC-47439 *see* 4192
NSC-47774 *see* 7481
NSC-49171 *see* 8339
NSC-52644 *see* 8013
NSC-52947 *see* 6985
NSC-59729 *see* 8736
NSC-60584 *see* 8983

NSC-64375 *see* 1119
NSC-68982 *see* 4558
NSC-69856 *see* 10167
NSC-70731 *see* 5500
NSC-70845 *see* 6671
NSC-71047 *see* 9735
NSC-75520 *see* 9687
NSC-77518 *see* 2994
NSC-77625 *see* 9599
NSC-78502 *see* 5778
NSC-79037 *see* 5564
NSC-82116 *see* 5299
NSC-83653 *see* 374
NSC-84223 *see* 4815
NSC-85998 *see* 8832
NSC-91523 *see* 7840
NSC-102627 *see* 4927
NSC-102816 *see* 890
NSC-104800 *see* 6214
NSC-105014-F *see* 2337
NSC-107429 *see* 2705
NSC-107430 *see* 7121
NSC-107433 *see* 9105
NSC-108166 *see* 9770
NSC-109229 *see* 836
NSC-109723 *see* 9768
NSC-109724 *see* 4896
NSC-112931 *see* 9249
NSC-114901 *see* 2920
NSC-115944 *see* 3581
NSC-118218 *see* 4126
NSC-118218-H *see* 4126
NSC-119875 *see* 2317
NSC-122819 *see* 9145
NSC-123127 *see* 3439
NSC-125066 *see* 1318
NSC-125973 *see* 6982
NSC-127716 *see* 2853
NSC-129943 *see* 8123
NSC-130044 *see* 9315
NSC-130181 *see* 9461
NSC-138780 *see* 9801
NSC-140117 *see* 4927
NSC-140865 *see* 9843
NSC-141540 *see* 3886
NSC-141549 *see* 594
NSC-145668 *see* 629
NSC-148958 *see* 9112
NSC-153858 *see* 5761
NSC-156303 *see* 594
NSC-164011 *see* 10195
NSC-165563 *see* 1454
NSC-169780 *see* 8123
NSC-178248 *see* 2177
NSC-180024 *see* 1870
NSC-181815 *see* 7161
NSC-182986 *see* 2996
NSC-192965 *see* 8758
NSC-208734 *see* 113
NSC-218321 *see* 7135
NSC-226080 *see* 8114
NSC-234714 *see* 727
NSC-239336 *see* 3586
NSC-241240 *see* 1822
NSC-245382 *see* 6553
NSC-245467 *see* 9987
NSC-246131 *see* 9915
NSC-249008 *see* 9721
NSC-249992 *see* 594
NSC-256439 *see* 4886
NSC-264137 *see* 3549
NSC-266046 *see* 6912
NSC-0270516 *see* 8109
NSC-279836 *see* 6217
NSC-286193 *see* 9425

NSC-296961 *see* 404
NSC-301467 *see* 3713
NSC-301739 *see* 6217
NSC-305263 *see* 4267
NSC-312887 *see* 4126
NSC-325319 *see* 3100
NSC-328002 *see* 4126
NSC-332598 *see* 8181
NSC-337766 *see* 1244
NSC-339140 *see* 4990
NSC-351521 *see* 7499
NSC-352122 *see* 9721
NSC-356894 *see* 4582
NSC-362856 *see* 9139
NSC-364372 *see* 5444
NSC-368390 *see* 1370
NSC-409962 *see* 1845
NSC-515776 *see* 3346
NSC-609669 *see* 9548
NSC-612049 *see* 3098
NSC-628503 *see* 3397
NSC-639966 *see* 7165
NSC-649890 *see* 4094
NSC-683863 *see* 5092
NSC-695238 *see* 6281
NSC-710428 *see* 5249
N-Serve [Dow AgroSci.] *see* 6574
NSILA-S *see* 4986
NT-3 *see* 6487
NTA *see* 6579
NTA-194 *see* 9424
NTANa₃ *see* 6579
NTBC *see* 6570
NTC *see* 6466
NTD-2 *see* 1865
NTN-801 *see* 5797
Nu-1196 *see* 310
Nu-1504 *see* 7233
Nu-1779 *see* 310
Nu-2121 *see* 6527
Nu-2206 *see* 5470
Nu-2222 *see* 9707
Nuarsol *see* 8578
Nubain [Endo] *see* 6357
Nubarene *see* 5781
Nucin *see* 5269
Nucite *see* 4978
Nuclear Fast Red (Acid Dye) *see* 6488
Nuclear Fast Red (Basic Dye) *see* 6488
Nucleocidin *see* 6726
Nuctalon [Takeda; Cassenne] *see* 3702
Nudrin [Shell] *see* 5982
Nuelin [3M] *see* 9285
Nuflor [Schering-Plough] *see* 4109
Nujol [Schering] *see* 7186
Nullapon *see* 3517
Nullatuss *see* 5110
Nullo Chlorophyll [DePree] *see* 2155
Nulomoline *see* 5006
Numidan [Coop. Farm.] *see* 6417
Numorphan [Endo] *see* 6969
Numotac [3M Pharma] *see* 5170
Nuncital [Kabi] *see* 3566
Nuodex 84 *see* 5868
Nupa-Sal [Smith & Nephew] *see* 8335
Nupercainal [Novartis] *see* 3031
Nupharidine *see* 6727
Nuprin [BMS] *see* 4881
Nuran [Frosst] *see* 2773
Nuredal *see* 6491
Nurofen [Boots] *see* 4881
Nuromax [Glaxo Wellcome] *see* 3431
Nustar [DuPont] *see* 4206
Nutgall, 6728
Nutinal [Boots] *see* 1029

Nutmeg, 6729
Nutmeg Butter *see* 6729
Nutracort [Galderma] *see* 4787
Nutraplus [Galderma] *see* 9867
Nutrase [Kyorin] *see* 9296
NutraSweet [NutraSweet Co.] *see* 839
Nutropin [Genentech] *see* 8716
Nutropinaq [Ipsen] *see* 8716
Nuvacon [BDH] *see* 5805
Nuvan [Syngenta] *see* 3079
Nuvance [Immunex] *see* 5002
Nuvanol N [Novartis Agro] *see* 5032
Nuviva [Bayer] *see* 9935
Nux Vomica, 6730
Nva²-cyclosporine *see* 2752
NVB *see* 9990
NVP *see* 7697
NVP-LAF237 *see* 9979
NW-1015 *see* 8315
NX-473 *see* 7405
NX-1838 *see* 7068
NXY-059 *see* 3363
NY-198 *see* 5562
Nyazin *see* 6491
Nybomycin, 6731
Nycopren [Nycomed] *see* 6417
Nyctal *see* 1831
Nycton *see* 2071
Nydrazid [BMS] *see* 5186
Nylidrin, 6732
Nylon, 6733
Nylon 6, 6734
Nylon 46, 6735
Nystan [BMS] *see* 6736
Nystatin, 6736
Nystatin A₁ *see* 6736
Nysted Reagent, 6737
Nytilax [Rohto] *see* 8455
Nytol [GSK] *see* 3309
Nyxolan *see* 4843
NZ-105 *see* 3524
Oakite *see* 8662
Oasil [Astra] *see* 5862
Obedrex [Beta] *see* 3973
Obepar [Parmed] *see* 7220
Oberon [Bayer CropSci.] *see* 8759
Obidoxime Chloride, 6738
Oblimersen Sodium, 6739
Oblivon *see* 5846
Oblivon C *see* 5846
OBPA *see* 6961
OB Protein *see* 5443
Obracin [Lilly] *see* 9490
OC-340 *see* 9985
Occlusal [Euroderma] *see* 8332
Ocelina [Roux-Ocefa] *see* 5925
Ocenol *see* 6831
Oceral [Roche] *see* 6937
Ochratoxin A *see* 6740
Ochratoxin B *see* 6740
Ochratoxin C *see* 6740
Ochratoxins, 6740
Ocimene, 6741
O.C.M. [Gobbi-Novag] *see* 2084
Ocrilate *see* 6766
Ocrylate *see* 6766
Octaacetyl-aldehydro-cellobiose *see* 1961
Octaacetyl-α-cellobiose *see* 1961
Octaacetyl-β-cellobiose *see* 1961
Octabenzone, 6742
Octacaine, 6743
Octacarbonyldicobalt *see* 3085
Octachlor *see* 2082
1,3,4,5,6,7,10,10-Octachloro-4,7-endo-
    methylene-4,7,8,9-tetrahydro-
    phthalan *see* 5127

1,2,4,5,6,7,8,8-Octachloro-2,3,3a,4,7,-
7a-hexahydro-4,7-methano-1*H*-in-
dene *see* 2082
1,3,4,5,6,7,8,8-Octachloro-1,3,3a,4,7,-
7a-hexahydro-4,7-methanoisobenzo-
furan *see* 5127
1,2,4,5,6,7,8,8-Octachloro-4,7-meth-
ane-3a,4,7,7a-tetrahydroindane *see*
2082
1,2,4,5,6,7,8,8-Octachloro-3a,4,7,7a-
tetrahydro-4,7-methanoindan *see*
2082
Octacosanol, 6744
n-Octacosanol *see* 6744
1-Octacosanol *see* 6744
Octacosyl Alcohol *see* 6744
(*Z,Z*)-9,12-Octadecadienoic Acid *see*
5505
(*Z,Z*)-9,12-Octadecadienoic Acid Ethyl
Ester *see* 3820
9,12-Octadecadienoic Acid Methyl Ester *see* 6095
Octadecafluorodecahydronaphthalene
see 4183
Octadecanoic Acid *see* 8804
Octadecanoic Acid Aluminum Salt *see*
364
Octadecanoic Acid Ammonium Salt *see*
553
Octadecanoic Acid Butyl Ester *see* 1589
Octadecanoic Acid Calcium Salt *see* 1703
Octadecanoic Acid 2-(1-Carboxyethoxy)-
1-methyl-2-oxoethyl Ester, Calcium
Salt *see* 1704
Octadecanoic Acid Compd with Erythro-
mycin 2′-Acetate *see* 3682
Octadecanoic Acid Copper Salt *see* 2652
Octadecanoic Acid Lead (2+) Salt *see*
5418
Octadecanoic Acid Magnesium Salt *see*
5690
Octadecanoic Acid Monoester with 1,2,3-
Propanetriol *see* 4489
Octadecanoic Acid 1,2,3-Propanetriyl
Ester *see* 9756
Octadecanoic Acid Zinc Salt *see* 10158
1-Octadecanol *see* 8805
(5*Z*,9*Z*,12*Z*)-5,9,12-Octadecatrienoic
Acid *see* 7450
cis-6,*cis*-9,*cis*-12-Octadecatrienoic Acid
see 5507
(6*Z*,9*Z*,12*Z*)-6,9,12-Octadecatrienoic
Acid *see* 5507
(*Z,Z,Z*)-9,12,15-Octadecatrienoic Acid
see 5506
(*E*)-D-*erythro*-4-Octadecene-1,3-diol *see*
8747
17-Octadecene-9,11-diynoic Acid *see*
5103
trans-Δ¹¹-Octadecenoic Acid *see* 9898
cis-6-Octadecenoic Acid *see* 7189
(*E*)-9-Octadecenoic Acid *see* 3533
(*Z*)-9-Octadecenoic Acid *see* 6828
(11*E*)-11-Octadecenoic Acid *see* 9898
(9*Z*)-9-Octadecenoic Acid Aluminum Salt
see 354
(*Z*)-9-Octadecenoic Acid Ammonium Salt
see 535
9-Octadecenoic Acid Calcium Salt *see*
1684
9-Octadecenoic Acid Copper Salt *see*
2644
(*Z*)-9-Octadecenoic Acid Ethyl Ester *see*
6828
9-Octadecenoic Acid Magnesium Salt *see*
5675

9-Octadecenoic Acid Mercury Salt *see*
5881
9-Octadecenoic Acid 1,2,3-Propanetriyl
Ester *see* 9732
9-Octadecenoic Acid Zinc Salt *see* 10145
cis-9-Octadecen-1-ol *see* 6831
(*Z*)-9-Octadecen-1-ol *see* 6831
Octadec-*cis*-12,13-epoxy-*cis*-9-enoic
Acid *see* 9963
Octadecyl-(1,1-dimethylpiperidinio-4-
yl)phosphate *see* 7165
Δ⁵-Octadecylenic Acid *see* 7189
3-(Octadecyloxy)-1,2-propanediol *see*
1011
3,4,5,6,14,15,20,21-Octadehydro-
yohimbanium *see* 8447
Octafluorocyclobutane, 6745
1*H*,1*H*,5*H*-Octafluoropentanol *see* 6746
2,2,3,3,4,4,5,5-Octafluoro-1-pentanol,
6746
Octafluoropropane *see* 7158
1,1,1,2,2,3,3,3-Octafluoropropane *see*
7158
Octahedrite *see* 9472
Octahedrohexa-*μ*³-hydrohexakis(triphenylphosphine)hexacopper *see* 8857
[2-(Octahydro-1-azocinyl)ethyl]guani-
dine *see* 4560
(13*aR*,25*aR*)-2,3,13a,14,15,16,25,25a-
Octahydro-18,29-dimethoxy-1,14-
dimethyl-13*H*-4,6:21,24-dietheno-8,-
12-metheno-1*H*-pyrido[3′,2′:14,15]-
[1,11]dioxacycloeicosino[2,3,4-*ij*]iso-
quinoline-9,19-diol *see* 2674
(13*aS*,25*aR*)-2,3,13a,14,15,16,25,25a-
Octahydro-18,29-dimethoxy-1,14-
dimethyl-13*H*-4,6:21,24-dietheno-8,-
12-metheno-1*H*-pyrido[3′,2′:14,15]-
[1,11]dioxacycloeicosino[2,3,4-*ij*]iso-
quinoline-9,19-diol *see* 1016
3a*β*,6a*β*,7,7a*α*,8,11a,11b*α*,11c-Octahy-
dro-2,10-dimethoxy-3,8*α*,11a*β*,11c*β*-
tetramethylphenanthro[10,1-*bc*]-
pyran-1,5,11(4*H*)-trione *see* 8026
D-[(4,6,6a,7,8,9,10,10a-Octahydro-4,7-
dimethyl-10a*α*-indolo[4,3-*fg*]quino-
lin-9*β*-yl)methyl]carbamic Acid Benzyl
Ester *see* 5937
3,3a,4,5,6,6a,9a,9b-Octahydro-6,9a-di-
methyl-3-methyleneazuleno[4,5-*b*]-
furan-2,9-dione *see* 385
[3a*R*-(3a*α*,5*β*,8a*β*,9a*α*)]-3a,5,6,7,8,8a,-
9a-Octahydro-5,8a-dimethyl-3-
methylenenaphtho[2,3-*b*]furan-
2(3*H*)-one *see* 207
(1a*R*,4*E*,7a*S*,10a*S*,10b*S*)-2,3,6,7,7a,8,-
10a,10b-Octahydro-1a,5-dimethyl-8-
methyleneoxireno[9,10]cyclodeca-
[1,2-*b*]furan-9(1a*H*)-one *see* 7048
Octahydro-6,8a-dimethyl-3-(1-methyl-
ethyl)-1*H*-3a,6-epoxyazulen-7-ol *see*
2831
(1*R*,4a*S*,10a*R*)-1,2,3,4,4a,9,10,10a-
Octahydro-1,4a-dimethyl-7-(1-meth-
ylethyl)-6-sulfo-1-phenanthrene-
carboxylic Acid *see* 3489
[4*S*-(4*α*,4a*α*,8*β*)]-Octahydro-4,8a-di-
methyl-4a(2*H*)-naphthalenol *see* 4400
Octahydro-4*α*,8a*β*-dimethyl-4a*α*(2*H*)-
naphthol *see* 4400
(1*S*,1′*S*,3*S*,3′*S*,4*S*,4′*S*,4a*S*,4′*S*,9a*R*,-
9′a*R*)-1,1′,3,3′,4,4′,9a,9′a-Octahydro-
4,4′,8,8′,9a,9′a-hexahydroxy-3,3′-di-
methyl-[7,7′-bi-1,4a-(epoxymethano)-4a*H*-xanthene]-9,9′,11,11′(2*H*,-
2′*H*)-tetrone *see* 3652

(3*R*,3′*R*,4*S*,4′*S*,4a*S*,4′a*S*)-2,2′,3,3′,4,4′,-
9,9′-Octahydro-1,1′,4,4′,8,8′-hexahy-
droxy-3,3′-dimethyl-9,9′-dioxo-[7,7′-
bi-4a*H*-xanthene]-4a,4′a-dicarboxylic
Acid Dimethyl Ester *see* 8418
Octahydro-1,3,4,7,8,10-hexanitro-5,2,6-
(iminomethenimino)-1*H*-imidazo-
[4,5-*b*]pyrazine *see* 4696
[3a*S*-(3a*α*,4*α*,4a*β*,7a*α*,8*α*,9a*α*)]-3,3a,4,-
4a,7a,8,9,9a-Octahydro-4-hydroxy-
4a,8-dimethyl-3-methyleneazuleno-
[6,5-*b*]furan-2,5-dione *see* 4626
[3a*S*-(3a*α*,6*β*,6a*α*,9a*β*,9b*α*)]-3,3a,4,5,6,-
6a,9a,9b-Octahydro-6a-hydroxy-
6,9a-dimethyl-3-methyleneazuleno-
[4,5-*b*]furan-2,9-dione *see* 7047
[1*S*-(1*α*,4a*α*,10a*β*)]-1,2,3,4,4a,9,10,10a-
Octahydro-6-hydroxy-1,4a-dimeth-
yl-1-phenanthrenecarboxylic Acid
see 7543
[1*S*-(1*α*,4a*α*,10a*β*)]-1,2,3,4,4a,9,10,10a-
Octahydro-6-hydroxy-7-[2-hydroxy-
1-(hydroxymethyl)ethyl]-1,4a-di-
methyl-1-phenanthrenecarboxylic
Acid *see* 7544
Octahydro-12-(hydroxymethyl)-2-imino-
5,9:7,10a-dimethano-10a*H*-[1,3]di-
oxocino[6,5-*d*]pyrimidine-4,7,10,11,-
12-pentol *see* 9246
(1*S*,4a*S*,8a*S*)-1,4,4a,5,6,7,8,8a-Octahy-
dro-1-hydroxy-5,5,8a-trimethyl-1,2-
naphthalenedicarboxaldehyde *see*
10037
(1*S*,6*S*,7*R*,8*R*,8a*R*)-Octahydro-1,6,7,8-
indolizinetetrol *see* 1896
2,3,4,5,6,7a,8,8a-Octahydro-3-isopro-
pyl-6,8a-dimethyl-1*H*-3a,6-epoxy-
azulen-7-ol *see* 2831
(4*S*,7*S*,10a*S*)-Octahydro-4-[[(2*S*)-2-mer-
capto-1-oxo-3-phenylpropyl]amino]-5-
oxo-7*H*-pyrido[2,1-*b*][1,3]thiazepine-
7-carboxylic Acid *see* 6843
[7*R*-(7*α*,7a*β*,14*α*)]-7,7a,8,9,10,11,13,14-
Octahydro-7,14-methano-4*H*,6*H*-di-
pyrido[1,2-*a*:1′,2′-*e*][1,5]diazocin-4-
one *see* 623
4,6,6a,7,8,9,10,10a-Octahydro-10a*α*-
methoxy-4,7-dimethylindolo[4,3-*fg*]-
quinoline-9-methanol 5-Bromonico-
tinate *see* 6496
[(4*R*,4a*S*,5*Z*,7*R*,10*S*,11*S*,12a*R*)-3,4,4a,7,-
10,11,12,12a-Octahydro-7-methoxy-
1,10-dimethyl-4-(1-methylethyl)-11-
[[(2*E*)-3-(1-methyl-1*H*-imidazol-4-yl)-
1-oxo-2-propenyl]oxy]-7,10-epoxyben-
zocyclodecen-6-yl]methyl-*β*-D-arabi-
nopyranoside 2-Acetate *see* 3545
(*αS*,3a*R*,7a*S*)-Octahydro-*γ*-oxo-*α*-(phenylmethyl)-2*H*-isoindole-2-butanoic
Acid *see* 6211
(1′*R*,4′*S*,5*S*,8′a*S*)-4,4′a,5,5′,6′,7′,8′,8′a-
Octahydro-2′,5,5′,5′,8′a-pentameth-
ylspiro[furan-2(3*H*),1′(4′*H*)-naphtha-
lene]-5-acetic Acid *see* 4547
(1*R*,1a*R*,2a*R*,5*S*,5a*S*,7a*S*,7b*R*,7c*R*)-*rel*-
1a,2,2a,5,5a,7a,7b,7c-Octahydro-5-
phenyl-1*H*-cyclobut[*bc*]acenaphth-
ylene-1-acetic Acid *see* 3571
(2*E*)-*rel*-4-[(1*R*,1a*R*,2a*R*,5*S*,5a*S*,7a*S*,-
7b*R*,7c*R*)-1a,2,2a,5,5a,7a,7b,7c-Octa-
hydro-5-phenyl-1*H*-cyclobut[*bc*]ace-
naphthylen-1-yl]-2-butenoic Acid *see*
3571
(1*R*,1a*R*,3*S*,3a*R*,6*S*,6a*S*,6b*R*,7*S*)-*rel*-1,-
1a,2,3,3a,6,6a,6b-Octahydro-1-[(2*E*,-

Oil of Cassia see 2300
Oil of Cedar Wood, 6782
Oil of Celery, 6783
Oil of Champaca, 6784
Oil of Chenopodium, 6785
Oil of Cherry Laurel, 6786
Oil of Chinese Cinnamon see 2300
Oil of Cinnamon, Ceylon see 2300
Oil of Cinnamon Leaf see 2300
Oil of Citronella, 6787
Oil of Clove see 2418
Oil of Copaiba see 2516
Oil of Cumin, 6788
Oil of Cypress, 6789
Oil of Dill, 6790
Oil of Dwarf Pine Needles, 6791
Oil of Egg Yolk see 3528
Oil of Erigeron see 6794
Oil of Eucalyptus see 3896
Oil of Fennel see 3977
Oil of Fir, 6792
Oil of Fir—Siberian, 6793
Oil of Fleabane, 6794
Oil of Geranium, 6795
Oil of Geranium—East Indian, 6796
Oil of Ginger see 4423
Oil of Grapes see 3835
Oil of Hedeoma see 7102
Oil of Hops see 4745
Oil of Hyssop, 6797
Oil of Jojoba see 5266
Oil of Juniper see 5270
Oil of Juniper Tar see 5271
Oil of Lavender see 5390
Oil of Lemon, 6798
Oil of Lemon Balm see 6774
Oil of Lemon Grass, 6799
Oil of Levant Wormseed, 6800
Oil of Linaloe, 6801
Oil of Marjoram, 6802
Oil of Melissa Balm see 6774
Oil of Mirbane see 6588
Oil of Monarda see 6243
Oil of Mountain Pine see 6791
Oil of Myrcia see 6776
Oil of Myrtle, 6803
Oil of Neem see 6437
Oil of Neroli see 6806
Oil of Niaouli, 6804
Oil of Niobe see 6024
Oil of Nutmeg see 6729
Oil of Orange, 6805
Oil of Orange Flowers, 6806
Oil of Origanum, 6807
Oil of Palma Christi see 1898
Oil of Patchouli, 6808
Oil of Pelargonium Geranium see 6795
Oil of Pennyroyal see 7102
Oil of Pepper see 1313
Oil of Peppermint see 7145
Oil of Pettigrain, 6809
Oil of Pimenta see 7432
Oil of Pine see 6793
Oil of Pine Needles, 6810
Oil of Pulegium see 7102
Oil of Rice Bran see 8208
Oil of Rose, 6811
Oil of Rose Geranium see 6795
Oil of Rosemary see 8264
Oil of Rue, 6812
Oil of Sassafras see 8381
Oil of Savin see 8387
Oil of Scotch Fir see 6810
Oil of Silver Fir see 6792
Oil of Silver Pine see 6792

Oil of Spearmint see 8738
Oil of Spike see 5390
Oil of Sweet Almond, 6813
Oil of Sweet Bay see 5382
Oil of Sweet Flag see 1637
Oil of Sweetwood Bark see 1881
Oil of Tansy, 6814
Oil of Thuja see 9389
Oil of Thyme, 6815
Oil of Turpentine see 9826
Oil of Valerian see 9903
Oil of Vetiver, 6816
Oil of Vitriol see 8974
Oil of White Cedar see 9389
Oil of Wild Marjoram see 6807
Oil of Wine see 3835
Oil of Wine, "Heavy", 6817
Oil of Wormwood see 10052
Oil of Yarrow see 105
Oil Palm, 6818
Oil Red XO see 10089
Oil Sweet Orange see 6805
Oil White Birch see 1238
Oizine see 7969
OK-174 see 1042
OK-1166 see 4097
Okacin [Novartis] see 5562
Okacyn [Novartis] see 5562
Okadaic Acid, 6819
Okenite see 1702
Oksafenamide see 6887
Oksilidin see 8082
OKT3 see 6308
Oktadin see 4560
Oktatenzin see 4560
OKY-046 see 6980
Olaflur, 6820
Olah's Reagent, 6821
Olamin [Sigamed] see 2305
Olane [Avi-Sun] see 7581
Olanzapine, 6822
Olaquindox, 6823
Olbemox [Pharmacia] see 111
Olbetam [Pharmacia] see 111
Olcadil [Sandoz] see 2420
Olcenon [Lederle] see 9499
Old Tuberculin see 9805
Old Yellow Enzyme, 6824
Olean [Procter & Gamble] see 8883
Oleandomycin, 6825
Oleandomycin Triacetate Ester see 9770
Oleandrin, 6826
(3β)-Olean-12-en-3-ol see 618
Oleanol see 6827
Oleanolic Acid, 6827
Oleate of Mercury see 5881
Olefiant Gas see 3791
Oleic Acid, 6828
Oleic Acid Aluminum Salt see 354
Oleic Acid Ammonium Salt see 535
Oleic Acid Calcium Salt see 1684
Oleic Acid Potassium Salt see 7650
Olein see 9732
Oleocanthal, 6829
Oleocreosote see 2573
Oleo Stock see 9041
Oleovitamin A see 10013
Oleovitamin D_2 see 10018
Oleovitamin D_3 see 10019
Oleptan [Bender] see 4228
Olestra see 8883
Oleth see 7577
Oleum see 8974
Oleum Abietis see 6793
Oleum Andropogonis Muricati see 6816

Oleum Rusci see 1238
Oleum Vitis Viniferae see 3835
Oleuropein, 6830
Oleyl Alcohol, 6831
Olibanum, 6832
Olicard [Solvay] see 5225
Oligomycin A see 6833
Oligomycin B see 6833
Oligomycin C see 6833
Oligomycin D see 6833
Oligomycins, 6833
Olimplex [Vaillant-Defresne] see 3168
Oliprevin [BMS] see 7714
Olivacine, 6834
Olivanic Acids, 6835
Olive Oil, 6836
Oliver [Sanzen] see 6886
Olive Spurge see 6170
Olivil, 6837
Olivin see 6838
Olivomycin A see 6838
Olivomycins, 6838
Olivoretin D see 9118
Olizumab see 6842
Olmelin see 4391
Olmesartan, 6839
Olmesartan Medoxomil see 6839
Olmetec [Sankyo] see 6839
Olmifon [Lafon] see 170
Ololiuqui see 5072
Olopatadine, 6840
Olprinone see 5575
Olsalazine, 6841
Olux [Connetics] see 2363
Olymp [DuPont] see 4206
Olympus [Bayer CropSci.] see 7838
Olynth [Pfizer] see 10086
OM-518 see 5851
OM-805 see 779
OM-853 see 9985
Omacor [Pronova] see 6844
Omadine [Olin] see 7994
Omadine Disulfide [Olin] see 7994
Omal see 9644
Omalizumab, 6842
Omapatrilat, 6843
Omca [BMS] see 4189
Omcilon [BMS] see 9595
OMD see 6056
OM-dopa see 6056
OMDS see 7994
Omebeta [Betapharm] see 6845
Omega-3 Acid Ethyl Esters, 6844
Omega-3 Polyunsaturated Fatty Acids
  Ethyl Esters see 6844
OmeLich [Winthrop] see 6845
Omelind [Lindopharm] see 6845
Omep [Hexal] see 6845
Omepral [AstraZeneca] see 6845
Omeprazen [Malesci] see 6845
Omeprazole, 6845
Ome-Puren [Alpharma] see 6845
Omeral [Simes] see 6264
Omeril [Bayer] see 5770
Omite [Uniroyal] see 7808
Omnes [Fumouze] see 6532
Omnibex [Bago] see 7262
Omnic [Astellas] see 9049
Omnicain [Daiichi] see 7757
Omnicef [Abbott] see 1920
Omniflox [Abbott] see 9132
Omnipaque [GE Healthcare] see 5052
Omnipen [Wyeth] see 586
Omniscan [GE Healthcare] see 4324
Omnopon [Roche] see 7018

Omoconazole, 6846
OMPA see 8395
Omperan [Taiho] see 8989
OMS-29 see 1787
OMS-45 see 3976
OMS-75 see 6358
OMS-115 see 3392
OMS-658 see 1431
OMS-659 see 1431
OMS-968 see 4246
OMS-1696 see 4805
OMS-1804 see 3142
OMS-2004 see 7770
OMS-3002 see 3876
OMS-3023 see 4010
OMS-3048 see 9565
Omtan see 5127
Onaka [Max Pharma] see 7419
Onapristone, 6847
ONB see 6592
Oncaspar [RPR] see 836
Onclast [Merck & Co.] see 229
Oncol [Otsuka] see 1042
Onconase [Alfacell] see 8112
OncoScint [Cytogen] see 8385
1-25-Oncostatin M (Human Precursor) Fusion Protein with CTLA-4 (Antigen)(human) Fusion Protein with Immunoglobulin G1 (Human Heavy Chain Fragment) see 4
Oncovin [Lilly] see 9986
Ondansetron, 6848
Ondena [Bayer] see 2832
Ondogyne [Roussel Diamant] see 2720
One-Alpha [Leo Pharm] see 4819
Onicit [Helsinn] see 6997
Onion Oil, 6849
Oniria [Lifepharma] see 8029
Onkotrone [Baxter] see 6217
ONO-802 see 4387
ONO-1078 see 7710
ONO-1101 see 5355
ONO-1206 see 5490
ONO-1308 see 6875
ONO-2235 see 3605
ONO-4128 see 737
ONO-5046 see 8558
ONO-RS-411 see 7710
Onoact [Ono] see 5355
Onokrein P [Ono] see 5279
Onon [Ono] see 7710
Ononin see 4244
Onsenal [Pfizer] see 1956
Onsukil [Otsuka] see 7759
Ontak [Ligand] see 2893
Ontosein [Diagnostic Data] see 9002
Onychomal [Hermal] see 9867
Onyxide see 3790
Oöcyan see 1219
Oolong Tea see 9088
Ooporphyrin see 7897
Oosporein, 6850
OP-1 see 1331
OP-1206 see 5490
Opacin see 5038
Opacist E.R. [Bracco] see 5011
Opacoron [Cilag] see 79
Opal see 8490
Opalène [Théraplix] see 9720
Opalgyne [Innothéra] see 1122
Opalmon [Ono] see 5490
Opalwax see 1899
Oparenol see 5040
Opatanol [Alcon] see 6840
OPC-31 see 785

OPC-1085 see 1866
OPC-2009 see 7759
OPC-7251 see 6345
OPC-8212 see 9970
OPC-12759 see 8124
OPC-13013 see 2277
OPC-14597 see 785
OPC-17116 see 4545
OPC-41061 see 9540
Opcon [Bausch & Lomb] see 6368
Opebacan see 938
Opegan [Santen] see 4757
Operidine [Janssen] see 7250
Ophiobolin D see 1977
Ophtacalm [Chauvin] see 2590
Ophtagram [Chauvin] see 4392
Ophthaine [BMS] see 7807
Ophthalamin (obsolete) see 10013
Ophthalgan [Wyeth-Ayerst] see 4484
Ophthalmadine [SAS] see 4891
Ophthetic [Allergan] see 7807
Ophtorenin [Winzer] see 1496
Ophtosol [Winzer] see 1391
Opian see 6718
Opianic Acid, 6851
Opianine see 6718
Opianyl see 5783
Opilon [Hansam] see 6292
Opiniazide, 6852
Opino [Bayropharma] see 6732
Opipramol, 6853
Opiran [Cassenne] see 7435
Opium, 6854
Opobalsam see 950
Opocarbyl see 1808
Oposim [Richet] see 7840
Oprelvekin see 5000
Opridan [Locatelli] see 1432
Opromazine, 6855
Opsins, 6856
α_2-Opsonins see 4075
Optaflexx [Elanco] see 8092
Optal see 7842
Optanox [Byk Gulden] see 9993
Optenyl [Stroschein] see 7019
Op-Thal-Zin [Alcon] see 10159
Opticrom [Sanofi-Aventis] see 2590
Optidase [Sanofi Winthrop] see 1900
Optiflex [Lilly] see 8716
Optilast [Viatris] see 906
OptiMARK [Mallinckrodt] see 4329
Optimax [Merck KGaA] see 9797
Optimine [Schering] see 901
Optimmune [Schering-Plough] see 2752
Optimycin [Novartis] see 5943
Optinate [Procter & Gamble] see 8232
Option [Bayer CropSci.] see 4234
Optipect [Thiemann] see 2913
Optipranolol [Bausch & Lomb] see 6140
Optiray [Mallinckrodt] see 5066
Optison [GE Healthcare] see 7158
Optocain [Bayer] see 5859
Optovit [Hermes] see 9495
Optovit-A [Hermes] see 10013
Optrin [Pharmacyclics] see 6282
Opturem [Kade] see 4881
Opus [BASF] see 3629
Opyrin [Taisho] see 4132
OR-611 see 3594
OR-1259 see 5471
Orabet [Berlin-Chemie] see 9507
Orabilex [Fougera] see 1486
Orabilix [Guerbet] see 1486
Orabolin [Organon] see 3805
Oracef [Lilly] see 1974

Oracéfal [BMS] see 1913
Oracilline [Schwarz] see 7100
Oracocin [Tobishi] see 1974
Oracon (obsolete) [Mead Johnson] see 3219
Oradexon [Organon] see 2943
Oradian [Chinoin] see 2186
Oradol [Novartis] see 3415
Ora-Gallin Purum [Nycomed] see 914
Oragest [Pharmagyn] see 5793
Orageston [Organon] see 291
Oragrafin Calcium [BMS] see 5071
Oragrafin Sodium [BMS] see 5071
Oraldene [Pfizer] see 4703
Oramorph [Boehringer, Ing.] see 6276
Oranabol [Farmitalia] see 6965
Orange I, 6857
Orange II, 6858
Orange III see 6105
Orange IV see 9776
Orange B, 6859
Orange Crush [Cyanamid] see 1244
Orange GS see 9776
Orange N see 9776
Orange Peel, 6860
Orange Root see 4769
Oranixon [Organon] see 5850
Orap [Janssen] see 7435
Orapem [Replidyne] see 3938
Orapred [BioMarin] see 7721
Oraprim [A.T.I.] see 8918
Orarsan [Boots] see 52
Oraseptic [Warner-Lambert] see 4703
Orasone [Solvay] see 7722
Oraspor [Novartis] see 1944
Orasthin [Aventis] see 6979
Oratane [Douglas] see 5228
Orathecin [SuperGen] see 8288
Oratrast [RPR] see 994
Oratrol [Alcon] see 3077
Oravir [SKB] see 3929
Oravue [BMS] see 5063
Oraxim [Menarini] see 1954
Orazamide, 6861
Orbax [Schering-Plough] see 6862
Orbenin [GSK] see 2419
Orbicin [Pfizer/Mack, Illert.] see 3005
Orbifloxacin, 6862
Orbinamon [Pfizer] see 9365
Orbit [BASF] see 2293
Orbit [Syngenta] see 7818
Orcanette see 256
Orcein, 6863
Orchil see 2615
Orchisterone [Negroni] see 9180
Orcin see 6864
Orcinol, 6864
Orcinolcarboxylic Acid see 6881
Orciprenaline see 5931
Orcl [Nippon Shinyaku] see 133
Ordeal Bark see 8382
Ordeal Bean see 7383
Ordiflazine see 5484
Ordimel [Lilly] see 62
Ordinary Lactic Acid see 5336
Ordinary Tartaric Acid see 9070
Ordinator [Dausse] see 3988
Oregon Grape Root see 1155
Oregovomab, 6865
Orelox [Sanofi-Aventis] see 1941
Orencia [BMS] see 4
Oreoselone Methyl Ether see 7191
Orestralyn [McNeil] see 3734
Oretic [Abbott] see 4781
Oreton [Schering-Plough] see 9180

Oreton Methyl [Schering] *see* 6125
Orexins, 6866
ORF-10131 *see* 6703
ORF-11676 *see* 6360
ORF-15244 *see* 9403
ORF-15817 *see* 3514
ORF-15927 *see* 8231
ORF-17070 *see* 4722
ORF-20485 *see* 9151
ORF-22164 *see* 865
Orfadin [Swedish Orphan] *see* 6570
Orfiril [Desitin] *see* 9913
Org-2969 *see* 2926
Org-3236 *see* 3884
Org-3770 *see* 6208
Org-5222 *see* 832
Org-6216 *see* 8226
Org-9426 *see* 8246
Org-9487 *see* 8113
Org-10172 *see* 2811
Org-31540 *see* 4232
Org-32489 *see* 4223
Org-34006 *see* 4892
Org-37462 *see* 4365
Org-GB-94 *see* 6172
Org-NA-97 *see* 7007
Org-NC-45 *see* 9941
Org-OD-14 *see* 9427
Orgabolin (obsolete) [Organon] *see* 3805
Orgaboral *see* 3805
Orgadrone [Han Wha] *see* 2943
Orgafol [Organon] *see* 4223
Orgalutran [Organon] *see* 4365
Orgametil *see* 5629
Orgametril [Organon] *see* 5629
Organoderm *see* 5700
Orgaran [Organon] *see* 2811
Orgasteron [Organon] *see* 6710
Orgastyptin [Organon] *see* 3707
Orgasuline [Organon] *see* 4980
Orgatrax [Organon] *see* 4849
Orgotein *see* 9002
Oricillin [Grünenthal] *see* 7817
Oriconazole *see* 5245
Oricur *see* 2105
Oriental Berry *see* 2456
Orientomycin *see* 2751
Orifungal M [Janssen] *see* 5302
Orimeten [Novartis] *see* 440
Orimon *see* 7252
Orinase [Pharmacia & Upjohn] *see* 9507
Oriodide [Abbott] *see* 8632
Oripavine, 6867
Oritavancin, 6868
Orix [Biomedica] *see* 6528
Orizaba Jalap Root *see* 5072
γ-Orizanol *see* 6886
Orkanet *see* 256
ORLAAM [BioDevelopment] *see* 5466
Orlipastat *see* 6869
Orlistat, 6869
Orlon [DuPont], 6870
Ormeloxifene *see* 1971
Ormetein (Rescinded) *see* 9002
Ormosanine *see* 6871
21-Ormosanin-20-yl Panamine *see* 6871
Ormosinine, 6871
Ornicetil [Logeais; Nordmark] *see* 5303
Ornidal [Selvi] *see* 6872
Ornidazole, 6872
Ornidyl [Aventis] *see* 3522
Ornipressin, 6873
L-Ornithine *see* 6874
Ornithine, 6874
L-Ornithine-L-aspartate *see* 6874

L(+)-Ornithine α-Ketoglutarate *see* 5303
8-L-Ornithinevasopressin *see* 6873
Ornitrol [Avitrol] *see* 892
Ornoprostil, 6875
Orn(8)-vasopressin *see* 6873
Orobronze [Applipharm] *see* 1753
Orofungin [SK & F] *see* 5847
Oroken [Bellon] *see* 1924
Oropur *see* 6876
Orospray [Vétoquinol] *see* 2192
Orotic Acid, 6876
Orotic Acid Compd with 5(or 4)-Amino-
  imidazole-4(or 5)-carboxamide (1:1)
  see 6861
Orotidine, 6877
Orotric [SAT] *see* 8871
Oroturic *see* 6876
Orotyl *see* 6876
Oroxine [GSK] *see* 9415
Oroxylin *see* 6878
Oroxylin A, 6878
Orphanin FQ *see* 6667
Orphanin FQ (Swine) *see* 6667
Orphenadrine, 6879
Orphol [Sanofi] *see* 3653
Orpiment *see* 806
Orris, 6880
Orris Root Oil *see* 6880
Orsanil [Orion] *see* 9359
Orseilles *see* 2615
o-Orsellinic Acid, 6881
Orsellinic Acid Methyl Ester 4-Methyl
  Ether *see* 8734
Orsin *see* 7285
Orstanorm [Novartis] *see* 3174
Ortacrone [Sanofi Winthrop] *see* 482
Ortazol *see* 4300
Ortensan [Cimex] *see* 47
Orthanilic Acid, 6882
Orthene [Valent] *see* 31
Ortho 9006 *see* 5947
Ortho 12420 *see* 31
Ortho Cyclen [Ortho] *see* 6703
Ortho Evra [Ortho] *see* 6694
Ortho Spotless [Ortho] *see* 3268
Ortho Tri-Cyclen [Ortho] *see* 6703
Orthoarsenic Acid *see* 795
[Orthoborato(3−)-*O*]phenylmer-
  curate(2−) Dihydrogen *see* 7303
Orthoboric Acid *see* 1336
Orthocaine, 6883
Ortho-Cept [Ortho] *see* 2926
Orthocide-406 *see* 1772
Orthoclase *see* 7604
Orthoclone OKT3 [J & J] *see* 6308
Orthocoll *see* 7634
Ortho-Creme [Ortho] *see* 6677
Orthodiazine *see* 7969
Orthodichlorobenzene *see* 3056
Orthoform [Winthrop] *see* 6883
Orthoformic Acid, 6884
Orthoform New *see* 6883
Ortho-Gynest [Cilag] *see* 3707
Ortho-Klor *see* 2082
Ortho-Novin 1/50 [Ortho-Cilag] *see* 6697
Ortho-Novum [Ortho] *see* 6697
Ortho-Novum 1/50 [Ortho] *see* 6697
Orthophosphoric Acid *see* 7344
Orthophthalic Acid Didiethylamide *see*
  9203
Orthotelluric Acid *see* 9120
Orthotitanic Acid *see* 9469
Orthoxenol *see* 7304
Orthoxine [Roberts] *see* 5998
Orthoxycol *see* 4785

Ortisporina [Turro] *see* 1974
Ortizon (obsolete) [Bayer AG] *see* 1782
Ortrel [Ortho] *see* 6703
Orudis [RPR] *see* 5305
Oruvail [RPR] *see* 5305
Orvagil [Galenika] *see* 6157
Oryvita [Ijaku] *see* 6886
Oryzaal [Sankei] *see* 6886
Oryzalin, 6885
γ-Oryzanol, 6886
Oryzanol A *see* 6886
Oryzanol C *see* 6886
OS-1897 *see* 3020
OS-2046 *see* 6165
Osalmid, 6887
Osaterone, 6888
Os-Cal [GSK] *see* 1657
Oscine *see* 8410
Oseltamivir, 6889
OSI-774 *see* 3672
O-sialic Acid *see* 8484
Osiren [Probiomed] *see* 6845
Osmarins *see* 6891
Osmaron B, 6890
Osmic Acid *see* 6893
Osmitrol [Baxter] *see* 5745
Osmium, 6891
Osmium Ammonium Chloride *see* 536
Osmium Hexafluoride, 6892
Osmium Octafluoride *see* 6892
Osmium Potassium Chloride *see* 7635
Osmium Tetroxide, 6893
Osmosal *see* 5745
Osnervan [Glaxo Wellcome] *see* 7763
Ospamox [Novartis] *see* 577
Ospen [Biochemie] *see* 7100
Ospolot [Bayer] *see* 8993
Osprey [Bayer CropSci.] *see* 5911
Ossalin [Chemipharm] *see* 8618
Ossein *see* 2480
Osseor [Servier] *see* 8106
Ossin [Sulzbach-Neuweiler] *see* 8618
Ossiten [Boehringer, Mann.] *see* 2371
Ossopan *see* 3467
Ostac [Boehringer, Mann.] *see* 2371
Ostelin *see* 10018
Osten [Takeda] *see* 5074
Osteocalcin [Tosi] *see* 1643
Osteocalcin, 6894
Osteo-F [Colgate-Hoyt] *see* 8618
Osteofix [Chiesi] *see* 5074
Osteofluor [Merck-Clévenot] *see* 8618
Osteogenic Protein-1 *see* 1331
Osteol [Yamanouchi] *see* 4378
Osteolite [DuPont] *see* 5792
Osteoscan-HDP [Mallinckrodt] *see* 6940
Osthole, 6895
Ostreogrycin A *see* 10004
Ostreogrycin B *see* 7753
Ostruthin, 6896
Ostruthol, 6897
Osvan [Takeda] *see* 1059
Osyritin *see* 8304
Osyritrin *see* 8304
Osyrol [Aventis] *see* 8760
Otavite *see* 1616
OTC *see* 6950
OTCA *see* 6950
Oterben [Chinoin] *see* 9507
Otifuril *see* 4294
Otilonium Bromide, 6898
Otobain, 6899
Otobite *see* 6899
Otokalixin *see* 5281
Otrasel [Cephalon] *see* 8428

Otreon [Sankyo] *see* 1941
Otrinol [Novartis] *see* 7916
Otrivine [Novartis] *see* 10086
Otto of Rose 6811
OU-1308 *see* 6875
Ouabagenin, 6900
Ouabain, 6901
Ourari *see* 2671
Oust [DuPont] *see* 8957
Outlook [BASF] *see* 3214
O-V Statin [BMS] *see* 6736
Ovaban [Schering] *see* 5805
Ovahormon [Teikoku Zoki] *see* 3703
Ovahormon Depot [Teikoku] *see* 3703
Ovalbumin, 6902
Ovalyse [Pharmacia & Upjohn] *see* 4061
Ovanon [Nourypharma] *see* 5629
Ovaras [Serono] *see* 3860
OvaRex [AltaRex] *see* 6865
Ovastol *see* 5917
Ovazyme *see* 4460
Ovcon [Warner-Chilcott] *see* 6697
Overal [Lusofarmaco] *see* 8276
Ovesterin *see* 3707
Ovestin [Organon] *see* 3707
Ovidrel [Serono] *see* 2216
Ovifollin *see* 3708
Oviol [Nourypharma] *see* 2926
Ovisot *see* 87
Ovitelmin [Cilag-Chemie] *see* 5768
Ovitrelle [Serono] *see* 2216
Ovoester *see* 855
Ovoresta [Organon] *see* 5629
Ovotransferrin *see* 9571
Ovo-Vinces [Wolff] *see* 3707
Ovral [Wyeth] *see* 6704
Ovran [Wyeth] *see* 6704
Ovranette [Wyeth] *see* 6704
Ovrette [Wyeth] *see* 6704
Ovulen *see* 3860
Ovysmen [Janssen-Cilag] *see* 6697
OX-373 *see* 2308
7-Oxabicyclo[2.2.1]heptane-2,3-dicar-
   boxylic Acid *see* 3575
22-Oxacalcitriol *see* 5760
Oxacarbazepine *see* 6929
Oxaceprol, 6903
2-Oxachlormadinone Acetate *see* 6888
Oxacillin, 6904
Oxacyclohexadecan-2-one *see* 3910
Oxacyclotetradecane Erythromycin
   Deriv *see* 8276
Oxadiargyl, 6905
1,3,4-Oxadiazole, 6906
Oxadiazon, 6907
22-Oxa-1α,25-dihydroxyvitamin D₃ *see*
   5760
Oxadixyl, 6908
6-Oxa-1,1,2,3,3,8-hexamethyl-2,3,5,6,-
   7,8-hexahydro-1*H*-benz[*f*]-indene *see*
   4715
Oxaine M [Wyeth] *see* 6933
Oxalacetic Acid, 6909
Oxalaldehyde *see* 4509
Oxalamide *see* 6918
Oxalato (1*R*,2*R*-Cyclohexanediamine)-
   platinum(II) *see* 6912
Oxalato (*trans-l*-1,2-Diaminocyclohex-
   ane)platinum (II) *see* 6912
Oxalatoplatin *see* 6912
Oxalatoplatinum *see* 6912
Oxalenediuramidoxime, 6910
Oxalic Acid, 6911
Oxalic Acid Bismuth Salt *see* 1272
Oxalic Acid Diamide *see* 6918

Oxalic Acid Diethyl Ester *see* 3125
Oxalic Acid Dinitrile *see* 2691
Oxalid [USV] *see* 6972
Oxaliplatin, 6912
Oxaloacetic Ester *see* 3836
Oxalodiacetic Acid *see* 5300
Oxalomolybdic Acid, 6913
[Oxalylbis(iminoethylene)]bis[(*o*-chloro-
   benzyl)diethylammonium Chloride]
   see 379
Oxalyl Chloride, 6914
Oxalylurea *see* 7022
Oxamarin, 6915
Oxametacine, 6916
Oxamic Acid, 6917
Oxamic Acid Hydrazide *see* 8445
Oxamide, 6918
Oxamidic Acid *see* 6917
Oxaminozoline *see* 8222
Oxammonium Hydrochloride *see* 4828
Oxammonium Sulfate *see* 4828
Oxamniquine, 6919
Oxamycin [Merck & Co.] *see* 2751
Oxamyl, 6920
Oxandrolone, 6921
Oxantel, 6922
Oxantel Embonate *see* 6922
22-Oxa-1,25(OH)₂D₃ *see* 5760
Oxaphenamide *see* 6887
Oxaphor *see* 4817
Oxapium Iodide *see* 2737
Oxapropanium Iodide, 6923
Oxaprozin, 6924
Oxarmin *see* 6944
Oxarol [Chugai] *see* 5760
Oxatomide, 6925
Oxatone [Baxter] *see* 3182
Oxazacort *see* 2862
Oxazepam, 6926
Oxazocilline *see* 6904
Oxazolam, 6927
Oxazolazepam *see* 6927
Ox Bile Extract, 6928
Oxcarbazepine, 6929
Oxedix [Labaz] *see* 6934
Oxedrine *see* 9012
Oxeladin, 6930
Oxendolone, 6931
Oxenin, 6932
Oxepinac *see* 5237
Oxetacaine *see* 6933
Oxetane *see* 9715
2-Oxetanone *see* 7820
Oxethazaine, 6933
Oxethazine *see* 6933
Oxetorone, 6934
Oxeze [AstraZeneca] *see* 4245
Oxfendazole, 6935
Oxiamine [Made] *see* 4975
Oxiarsolan *see* 57
Oxibendazole, 6936
Oxibuprokain *see* 1047
Oxibutinina *see* 6955
Oxichlorochine *see* 4818
Oxiconazole Nitrate, 6937
Oxidimethiin, 6938
Oxidized Cellulose, 6939
Oxidized Glutathione *see* 4475
Oxidronate Sodium *see* 6940
Oxidronic Acid, 6940
Oxilan [Cook Imaging] *see* 5068
Oxilapine *see* 5587
Oxilin [Allergan] *see* 6966
2-[4-(3-Oximinocyclohexyl)phenyl]-
   propionic Acid *see* 10078

Oxine *see* 4843
Oxiniacic Acid, 6941
Oxinofen *see* 6957
Oxinorm [Zambeletti] *see* 9002
Oxipendyl *see* 6970
Oxipethidine *see* 4836
Oxiracetam, 6942
Oxirane *see* 3802
Oxiranemethanol *see* 4490
Oxistat [GSK] *see* 6937
Oxitol *see* 3750
Oxitriptan *see* 4847
Oxitropium Bromide, 6943
Oxivent [Boehringer, Ing.] *see* 6943
Oxoacetic Acid *see* 4511
3-(3-Oxo-7α-acetylthio-17β-hydroxy-4-
   androsten-17α-yl)propionic Acid γ-
   Lactone *see* 8760
2-Oxo-acid Carboxylase *see* 8020
1-(2-Oxo-4-amino-1,2-dihydropyrimi-
   din-1-yl)-2-deoxy-2,2-difluororibose
   see 4386
α-Oxobenzeneacetaldehyde Aldoxime *see*
   5191
β-Oxobenzenepropanoic Acid Ethyl Ester *see* 3767
2-Oxo-2*H*-1-benzopyran-3-carboxylic
   Acid *see* 2563
4-Oxo-4*H*-1-benzopyran-2-carboxylic
   Acid *see* 2237
γ-Oxo-[1,1′-biphenyl]-4-butanoic Acid
   see 3963
2-Oxo-3,3-bis[*p*-aminophenyl]butane *see*
   581
d-2-Oxo-3-bornanecarboxylic Acid *see*
   1731
2-Oxo-10-bornanesulfonic Acid *see* 1734
2-Oxobutane *see* 6072
Oxobutanedioic Acid *see* 6909
Oxobutanedioic Acid Diethyl Ester *see*
   3836
3-Oxobutanoic Acid *see* 59
3-Oxobutanoic Acid Ethyl Ester *see* 3758
3-Oxobutanoic Acid Methyl Ester *see*
   6009
3-Oxobutanoic Acid 1-Methylethyl Ester
   see 5206
N-(1-Oxobutyl)adenosine Cyclic 3′,5′-
   (Hydrogen Phosphate) 2′-Butanoate
   see 1463
4-(3-Oxobutyl)-1,2-diphenyl-3,5-pyra-
   zolidinedione *see* 5288
δ-Oxo-α-butylene *see* 6134
d-2-Oxo-3-camphanecarboxylic Acid *see*
   1731
4-Oxo-β-carotene *see* 3495
4-Oxo-4*H*-chromene-2-carboxylic Acid
   see 2237
N-(4-Oxo-2,5-cyclohexadien-1-ylidene)-
   acetamide *see* 57
p-(3-Oxocyclohexyl)hydratropic Acid
   Oxime *see* 10078
(±)-*p*-[(2-Oxocyclopentyl)methyl]hydra-
   tropic Acid *see* 5589
(*E*)-9-Oxo-2-decenoic Acid *see* 8032
3-Oxodesogestrel *see* 3884
9-Oxo-11α,15α-dihydroxy-17*S*,20-di-
   methylprosta-*trans*-2,*trans*-13-dienoic
   Acid *see* 5104
6-Oxo-17*S*,20-dimethyl-PGE₁ Methyl
   Ester *see* 6875
1-Oxo-2-(2,6-dioxopiperidin-3-yl)-4-
   aminoisoindoline *see* 5436
Oxodiperoxymolybdenum(pyridine)(hexamethylphosphoric Triamide) *see* 9943

5,5′-Oxybis[3,4-dichloro-2(5*H*)-furan-one] *see* 6298
1,1′-Oxybisethane *see* 3806
N,*N*′-[Oxybis(2,1-ethanediyloxy-4,1-phenylene)]bisacetamide *see* 2974
2,2′-Oxybisethanol *see* 3119
1,1′-Oxybisethene *see* 9995
1,1′-Oxybis(2-ethoxy)ethane *see* 3118
Oxybismethane *see* 6071
1,1′-Oxybis[2-methoxyethane] *see* 3165
1,1′-Oxybis[3-methylbutane] *see* 5118
1,1′-[Oxybis(methylene)]bis[benzene] *see* 1132
1,1′-[Oxybis(methylene)]bis[4-(hydroxyimino)methyl]pyridinium Dichloride *see* 6738
3,3′-[Oxybis'(methylenecarbonylimino)]bis[2,4,6-triiodobenzoic Acid] *see* 5051
1,1′-Oxybis[2-methylpropane] *see* 5142
2,2′-Oxybis[2-methylpropane] *see* 3033
3,3′-[Oxybis[(1-oxo-2,1-ethanediyl)imino]]bis[2,4,6-triiodobenzoic Acid] *see* 5051
1,1′-Oxybispentane *see* 608
10,10′-Oxybis-10*H*-phenoxarsine *see* 6961
1,1′-Oxybispropane *see* 7857
2,2′-Oxybispropane *see* 5212
3,3′-Oxybis-1-propene *see* 292
1,1′-Oxybis[2,2,2-trifluoroethane] *see* 4201
Oxybuprocaine *see* 1047
Oxybutynin, 6955
Oxybutynin Chloride *see* 6955
Oxycamphor *see* 4817
Oxycel [Parke-Davis] *see* 6939
Oxychelidonic Acid *see* 5782
Oxychinolin *see* 4843
Oxychloroquine *see* 4818
Oxychlorosene, 6956
5-Oxychlorpromazine *see* 6855
Oxycinchophen, 6957
Oxyclozanide, 6958
Oxycodone, 6959
OxyContin [Purdue] *see* 6959
Oxydapatit *see* 1694
N,*N*-(Oxydiacetyl)bis[3-amino-2,4,6-triiodobenzoic Acid] *see* 5051
Oxydiazepam *see* 9133
4,4′-Oxydibenzamidine *see* 7208
4,4′-Oxydi-2-butanol, 6960
2,2′-Oxydiethanol *see* 3119
Oxydiformic Acid Diethyl Ester *see* 7998
1,1′-(Oxydimethylene)bis[4-formylpyridinium]dichloride Dioxime *see* 6738
Oxydimethylquinizine *see* 716
10,10′-Oxydiphenoxarsine, 6961
2,4:2′,4′-*O*-(Oxydistibylidyne)bis[D-gluconic Acid] *Sb*,*Sb*′-Dioxide Trisodium Salt Nonahydrate *see* 701
Oxydol *see* 4798
Oxyephedrin *see* 4824
Oxyethylated Tertiary Octylphenol Formaldehyde Polymer *see* 9833
8-(β-Oxyethyl)methylaminocaffeine *see* 1633
Oxyethyltheophylline *see* 3878
Oxyfan [Coli] *see* 4847
Oxyfedrine, 6962
Oxyflavil *see* 3523
Oxyfluorfen, 6963
Oxygen, 6964
Oxygen Fluoride *see* 4164
Oxygen Fluoride ((O₂)F₂) *see* 4163

Oxygent [Alliance] *see* 7156
3-Oxygermylpropionic Acid Polymer *see* 7795
Oxygeron [Will-Pharma] *see* 9983
Oxygesic [Mundipharma] *see* 6959
Oxyhemerythrin *see* 4641
Oxyhemocyanin *see* 4647
Oxyhemoglobin *see* 4648
Oxyjavanicin *see* 4315
Oxylidine *see* 8082
Oxylupanine *see* 4829
Oxymesterone, 6965
Oxymestrone *see* 6965
Oxymetazoline, 6966
Oxymethebanol *see* 3456
Oxymetholone, 6967
Oxymethurea, 6968
Oxymethylene *see* 4235
Oxymorphone, 6969
Oxy-Mycin [AgriPharm] *see* 6976
Oxyneurine *see* 1179
Oxynorm [Mundipharma] *see* 6959
Oxypaat [Katwijk] *see* 7465
Oxypangam [Sanorania] *see* 3197
Oxypendyl, 6970
Oxypertine, 6971
Oxypetidin *see* 4836
Oxyphedrine *see* 6962
Oxyphenbutazone, 6972
Oxyphencyclimine, 6973
(+)-Oxyphene *see* 2062
Oxyphenisatin Acetate, 6974
Oxyphenonium Bromide, 6975
Oxypropylated Cellulose *see* 4841
Oxyquinoline *see* 4843
Oxysept [Allergan] *see* 4798
Oxytetracycline, 6976
Oxytetrin [Schering-Plough] *see* 6976
Oxytheonyl *see* 3878
Oxythiamine, 6977
Oxythioquinox, 6978
Oxytocin, 6979
Oxytrimethylline *see* 2210
Oxyzin (Tabl.) *see* 7465
OYE *see* 6824
OZ *see* 6886
γ-OZ *see* 6886
Ozagrel, 6980
Ozex [Toyama] *see* 9555
Ozidia [Pfizer] *see* 4442
Ozolinone *see* 3891
Ozone, 6981
P₄₅₀ *see* 2792
P-4 *see* 7832
P-7 *see* 5386
p28ˢⁱˢ *see* 7525
P-30 Protein *see* 8112
P-50 *see* 586
P53 *see* 9247
P57 *see* 4743
P57AS3 *see* 4743
P-071 *see* 2022
P-71-0129 *see* 3971
P-113 *see* 8372
P-165 *see* 899
P-170 *see* 7195
P-253 *see* 3331
P-280 *see* 9098
P-286 *see* 5067
P-350 *see* 2265
P-607 *see* 2186
P-638 *see* 7943
P-652 *see* 4230
P-725 *see* 7151
P829 *see* 2911

P-1011 *see* 3084
P-1134 *see* 7438
P-1202 *see* 6016
P-1206 *see* 4693
P-1496 *see* 10121
P-1742 *see* 4188
P-1779 *see* 318
P-2647 *see* 1119
P-3693A *see* 3435
P-4000 *see* 6630
P-4599 *see* 3435
P-5604 *see* 5584
P-7138 *see* 6537
P-720549 *see* 5237
PA-93 *see* 6722
PA-94 *see* 2751
PA-105 *see* 6825
PA-155A *see* 4966
PA-248 *see* 7817
PA2024 *see* 8547
3PAA *see* 7971
PABA *see* 423
Pabanol [Valeant] *see* 423
Pabenol [Gentili] *see* 2843
PABG *see* 426
Pacerone [Upsher-Smith] *see* 482
Paceum [Orion] *see* 2994
Pacilan [Daltan] *see* 1655
Pacinol [Schering] *see* 4189
Pacitane [Wyeth] *see* 9695
Pacitron [Rorer] *see* 9797
Paclitaxel, 6982
Paclitaxel Poliglumex, 6983
Paclobutrazol, 6984
Pactamycin, 6985
Padan [Takeda] *see* 1865
PADGEM *see* 8426
Padimate A *see* 3232
Padimate O *see* 3232
Padisal [Bayer] *see* 9306
Padreatin *see* 5279
Padrin [Fujisawa] *see* 7742
Padukrein [Bayropharm] *see* 5279
Padutin [Winthrop] *see* 5279
Paederine *see* 7065
ψ-Paederine *see* 7065
Paediathrocin [Abbott] *see* 3681
PAF *see* 7524
PAF-acether *see* 7524
Pafnol [Yoshitomi] *see* 5241
Pagano-Cor [Helopharm] *see* 3710
Paginol [Jugoremedija] *see* 7082
PAH *see* 442
Paidomal [Malesci] *see* 9285
Paindor [Novartis Agro] *see* 2771
Paint White *see* 1284
Paka Oil *see* 5643
Palafer [GSK] *see* 4046
Palaprin [Nicholas] *see* 309
Palatinol A [Advanced Solvents] *see* 7371
Palatinol M *see* 3255
Palatinose [Süddeutsche Zucker; Shin Mitsui Sugar] *see* 5182
Palatone *see* 5713
Palavale [Otsuka] *see* 3502
Pale Catechu *see* 4359
Pale Gentian *see* 4393
Palfium [Purdue Frederick] *see* 2955
Palifermin, 6986
Palinum *see* 2711
Palisade [Syngenta] *see* 9725
Palitantin, 6987
Paliuroside *see* 8304
Palivizumab, 6988
Palladium, 6989

Palladium(II) Acetate *see* 6991
Palladium Chloride, 6990
Palladium Diacetate, 6991
Palladium Hydroxide On Carbon *see* 7060
Palladium Hydroxide (Pd(OH)$_2$) *see* 7060
Palladium Monoxide *see* 6993
Palladium Nitrate, 6992
Palladium Oxide, 6993
Palladone [Napp] *see* 4803
Palladous Chloride *see* 6990
Palladous Nitrate *see* 6992
Palladous Oxide *see* 6993
Pallidin [Merck KGaA] *see* 8934
Palmarosa Oil *see* 6796
Palmatine, 6994
Palmidrol, 6995
Palmitic Acid, 6996
Palmitic Acid Aluminum Salt *see* 357
Palmitic Acid Ammonium Salt *see* 538
Palmitic Acid Calcium Salt *see* 1687
Palmitic Acid Hexadecyl Ester *see* 2031
Palmitin *see* 9736
Palmityl Alcohol *see* 2028
Palm Kernel Oil *see* 6818
Palmofen [Zambon] *see* 4254
Palm Oil *see* 6818
Palm Olein *see* 6818
Palm Stearin *see* 6818
Palohex *see* 4979
Palonosetron, 6997
Palosein [Diagnostic Data] *see* 9002
Palphium *see* 2955
Paludrine [AstraZeneca] *see* 2090
Palustric Acid, 6998
Paluther [RPR] *see* 815
Palux [Taisho] *see* 7876
Palytoxin, 6999
Palytoxin (C51-55 Hemiacetal) *see* 6999
L-PAM *see* 5828
2-PAM *see* 7703
2-PAM Chloride *see* 7703
Pamabrom, 7000
Pamaquine, 7001
Pamaquine Embonate *see* 7001
Pamaquine Naphthoate *see* 7001
Pamedon(e) *see* 3337
Pameion [Simes] *see* 7019
Pamelor [Novartis] *see* 6715
Pamicogrel, 7002
Pamidronate Disodium *see* 7003
Pamidronic Acid, 7003
Pamine [Bradley] *see* 6003
Pamisyl Sodium [Parke-Davis] *see* 477
Pamiteplase, 7004
Pamoic Acid, 7005
Panacef [Lilly] *see* 1912
Panacid [Dainippon] *see* 7505
Panacur [Intervet] *see* 3960
Panadol [GSK] *see* 47
Panaldine [Daiichi] *see* 9429
Panaleve [Pinewood] *see* 47
Panama Bark *see* 8040
Panamicin [Gramon] *see* 3005
Panamine *see* 6871
Panaquilins *see* 4427
Panatus [Krka] *see* 1513
Panax *see* 4427
Panaxosides *see* 4427
Panazon [Toyama] *see* 6654
Panclar [Lematte et Boinot] *see* 2884
Pancoral [Eisai] *see* 3975
Pancrease *see* 7006
Pancreas Powder *see* 7006
Pancreatic Basic Trypsin Inhibitor *see* 757

Pancreatic Desoxyribonuclease *see* 2906
Pancreatic Dornase *see* 2906
Pancreatic Extract, 7006
Pancreatic Trypsin Inhibitor (Kunitz) *see* 757
Pancreatin *see* 7006
Pancreozymin *see* 2198
Pancreozymin C-Terminal Octapeptide *see* 8543
Pancrex-Vet [Pfizer] *see* 7006
Pancuronium Bromide, 7007
Pandermite *see* 1652
Panectyl [RPR] *see* 9704
Panergon [Mack, Illert.] *see* 7019
Panflavin [Chinosolfabrik] *see* 123
Panformin [Shionogi] *see* 1476
Panfungol [Esteve] *see* 5302
Pangamic Acid, 7008
Pangram [Virbac] *see* 4392
Panheprin [Abbott] *see* 4653
Panimit [Nattermann] *see* 1496
Panimycin [Meiji] *see* 3005
Panipenem, 7009
Panitumumab, 7010
Panmycin [Pharmacia & Upjohn] *see* 9196
Panodil [GSK] *see* 47
Panoral [Lilly] *see* 1912
Panorex [Centocor] *see* 3515
Panoxolin *see* 6928
PanOxyl [Stiefel] *see* 1116
Panpurol [Nippon Shinyaku] *see* 7471
Panretin [Ligand] *see* 249
Panrone [Panray] *see* 9290
Pansporin [Takeda] *see* 1935
Pansporin T [Takeda] *see* 1935
Pansporine [Cassenne-Takeda] *see* 1935
Pantecta [Pfizer] *see* 7014
Pantelmin [J & J] *see* 5768
Pantenyl [Kay] *see* 2947
Pantestone [Organon] *see* 9180
Pantetheine, 7011
Panthetine, 7012
Pantetina [Maggioni] *see* 7012
Panthecin [Sawai] *see* 7012
Pantheline [CP Protea] *see* 7805
Panthenol *see* 2947
Pantherine *see* 6312
Panthoderm [USV] *see* 2947
Pantholin [Lilly] *see* 7015
Pantocaine [Hoechst] *see* 9188
Pantocid [Abbott] *see* 4590
Pantogam *see* 4744
Pantoic Acid γ-Lactone *see* 7013
Pantoic Lactone *see* 7013
Pantolactone, 7013
Pantomicina [Abbott] *see* 3687
Pantomin [Daiichi] *see* 7012
Pantopan [Pharmacia] *see* 7014
Pantopaque [Lafayette] *see* 5060
Pantopon [Roche] *see* 7018
Pantoprazole, 7014
Pantorc [Altana] *see* 7014
Pantosin [Daiichi] *see* 7012
Pantostrep *see* 3179
Pantothenic Acid, 7015
Pantothenol *see* 2947
Pantothenyl Alcohol *see* 2947
N-(Pantothenyl)-β-aminoethanethiol *see* 7011
Pantothenylol *see* 2947
Pantovernil [BMS] *see* 2077
Pantoyl Lactone *see* 7013
N-Pantoyl-3-propanolamine *see* 2947
Pantozol [Altana] *see* 7014
Panurin *see* 4781

Panzid [Duncan] *see* 1946
Panzytrat [Axcan] *see* 7006
Papain, 7016
Papaveraldine, 7017
Papaveretum, 7018
Papaverine, 7019
Papaw *see* 7020
Papaya, 7020
Papayotin *see* 7016
Paper Red 4B [Crompton & Knowles] *see* 1101
Papital T.R. [Zemmer] *see* 7019
Papoose Root *see* 1320
PAPP *see* 470
Papra *see* 7547
Papuamine, 7021
Papulex [Euroderma] *see* 6523
Parabanic Acid, 7022
Parabis [Dow] *see* 3071
Parabolan *see* 9583
Parabromdylamine *see* 1443
(+)-Parabromdylamine *see* 1443
Paracarbinoxamine *see* 1799
Paracetaldehyde *see* 7027
Paracetamol *see* 47
Parachloramine *see* 5777
Parachlorometacresol *see* 2133
Parachlorometaxylenol *see* 2176
Paracide *see* 3057
Paracodin [Knoll] *see* 3171
Paradiazine *see* 7957
Paradichlorobenzene *see* 3057
Paradione [Abbott] *see* 7028
Paradise Plant *see* 6170
Paradisone [Firmenich] *see* 6052
Paradormalene *see* 5959
Paraffin, 7023
Paraffin Chlorinated, 7024
Paraffin Jelly *see* 7185
Paraffin Oil *see* 7186
Paraffin Wax *see* 7023
Paraflex [McNeil] *see* 2194
Paraflu [Dainippon] *see* 4132
Paraform *see* 7025
Paraformaldehyde, 7025
Paraguay Tea *see* 5756
Paraherquamide, 7026
(−)-Paraherquamide *see* 7026
Parahexyl *see* 9013
Paral [Forest] *see* 7027
Paralactic Acid *see* 5337
Paralaudin *see* 2967
Paraldehyde, 7027
Paralergin [Vita] *see* 856
Paralest [Parachemie] *see* 9695
Paralgin *see* 3350
Paralytic Shellfish Poison *see* 8389
Paramandelic Acid *see* 5717
Paramenyl *see* 5649
Paramethadione, 7028
Paramethasone, 7029
Paramezone [Recordati] *see* 7029
Paramicina [Raglionieri] *see* 7041
Paramidin [Takeda] *see* 1466
Paraminyl [Cooper] *see* 7984
Paramisan Sodium [Smith & Nephew] *see* 477
Paramorfan *see* 3177
Paramorphan *see* 3177
Paramorphine *see* 9276
Paramoth [Esquire] *see* 3057
Paraoxon, 7030
Paraoxypropiophenone *see* 7044
Paraplatin [BMS] *see* 1822
Paraquat, 7031

Paraquat I *see* 7031
Parasan *see* 1029
Parasepiolite *see* 5687
Parasitex [Virbac] *see* 2995
Parasiticol *see* 180
Parasorbic Acid, 7032
Paraspen [Pfizer] *see* 47
Parasympatol *see* 9012
Paratartaric Acid *see* 9069
Paratect [Pfizer] *see* 6266
Paratensiol [Yoshitomi] *see* 8144
Parathar [Rorer] *see* 9166
Parathiazan *see* 9300
Parathion, 7033
Parathion-methyl *see* 6108
Parathorm [Hormone-Chemie] *see* 7034
Parathormone *see* 7034
Para-thor-mone [Lilly] *see* 7034
Parathyroid Hormone, 7034
Paravermin *see* 7464
Parawollastonite *see* 1702
Paraxenol *see* 7305
Paraxin [Roche] *see* 2077
Para-zene [Reliable Chem.] *see* 3057
Parazine *see* 7464
Parbendazole, 7035
Parda [Parke-Davis] *see* 5464
Pardisol *see* 3747
Pardroyd [Parke-Davis] *see* 6967
Parecoxib, 7036
Paredrine [SK & F] *see* 4810
Paredrinex [SK & F] *see* 4810
Paredrinol [SK & F] *see* 7330
Pareira, 7037
Pareira Brava *see* 7037
Parenabol *see* 1324
Parenogen [Miles] *see* 4071
Parentamin [Pharmacia] *see* 7885
Parenzymol [Horner] *see* 9795
Parest *see* 5960
Parfenac [Lederle] *see* 1474
Parfenal [Cyanamid] *see* 1474
Parfuran [Parke-Davis] *see* 6599
Pargin [Gibipharma] *see* 3502
Pargitan [Abigo] *see* 9695
Pargluva [BMS] *see* 6303
Pargonyl *see* 7041
Pargyline, 7038
Paricalcitol, 7039
Paricina [Archifar] *see* 7041
Parid [Cooper] *see* 7464
Pariet [Eisai] *see* 8089
Parietic Acid *see* 8176
Parietin *see* 3561
Parietrope [Marcofina] *see* 8034
Parigenin *see* 8380
Pariprazole *see* 8089
Paris Blue *see* 7910
Paris Green *see* 2625
Paris Red *see* 5425
Paris White *see* 1657
Paris Yellow *see* 5405
Paritane [Berk] *see* 6952
Parizac [Lacer] *see* 6845
Parkazin *see* 3108
Parkemed [Parke-Davis] *see* 5798
Parkin [Yoshitomi] *see* 3747
Parkinane [Wyeth] *see* 9695
Parkinsan [Byk Gulden] *see* 1469
Park Lily *see* 2511
Park Nucleotide, 7040
Parkopan [Hexal] *see* 9695
Parks 12 [Novartis] *see* 7741
Parlay [Zeneca Ag Prod] *see* 6984
Parlef [Parke-Davis] *see* 4132

Parlodel [Novartis] *see* 1416
Parlodion [Mallinckrodt] *see* 8011
Parmal [Central] *see* 7984
Parmid [Lagap] *see* 6143
Parnate [GSK] *see* 9573
Parocin [Almirall] *see* 5826
Parodyne *see* 716
Paroidin [Parke-Davis] *see* 7034
Paroleine *see* 7186
Paromomycin, 7041
Paromomycin I *see* 7041
Parotin, 7042
Paroven [Zyma] *see* 9789
Paroxetine, 7043
Paroxon *see* 7044
Paroxypropione, 7044
Parphezein *see* 3747
Parphezin *see* 3747
Parrot Green *see* 2625
Parsal [Midy] *see* 7045
Parsalmide, 7045
Parsidol [Warner-Chilcott; Specia] *see* 3747
Parsitan *see* 3747
Parsley, 7046
Parsley Apiole *see* 734
Parsley Camphor *see* 734
Parsley Seed Oil *see* 7046
Parsol 1789 [DSM] *see* 888
Parsol HMS [DSM] *see* 4738
Parsol HS [DSM] *see* 3593
Parsol MCX [DSM] *see* 6769
Parsotil *see* 3747
Partel [Lilly] *see* 3369
Parterol *see* 3180
Parthenicin *see* 7047
Parthenin, 7047
Parthenolide, 7048
Partocon [Ferring] *see* 6979
Partricin, 7049
Partricin A *see* 7049
Partricin B *see* 7049
Partricin Methyl Ester *see* 5847
Partusisten [Boehringer, Ing.] *see* 3981
Parvaquone, 7050
Parvolex [Evans] *see* 88
Parzate *see* 6341
Parzone [Mallinckrodt] *see* 3171
PAS *see* 477
Pasalin [Takeda] *see* 3134
Pasalon [Bayer] *see* 477
PASER [Jacobus] *see* 477
Pasetocin [Kyowa] *see* 577
Pasiniazide *see* 5186
Paskalium [Glenwood] *see* 477
Pasminox [Beta] *see* 6898
Pasmus [Daiichi] *see* 4106
Pasolind N [Stada] *see* 47
Paspaline-P *see* 2790
Paspertin [Kali-Chemie] *see* 6143
Pasque Flower *see* 7938
Passiflora, 7051
Passiflorin *see* 4615
Passion Flower *see* 7051
Passion Vine *see* 7051
Pastaron [Sato] *see* 9867
Patanol [Alcon] *see* 6840
Patchouli Alcohol, 7052
Patchouli Camphor *see* 7052
Patchouli Oil *see* 6808
Patent Alum *see* 366
Paternoite *see* 5658
Pathfinder [Dow AgroSci.] *see* 9656
Pathilon [Lederle] *see* 9661
Pathocidin *see* 896

Pathocil [Wyeth] *see* 3084
Pathozone [Pfizer] *see* 1930
Patoran [Syngenta] *see* 6142
Patricin [Kaken] *see* 4096
Patronite *see* 9918
Pattonex [Makhteshim-Agan] *see* 6142
Patulin, 7053
Patupilone *see* 3628
Paucimycin *see* 7041
Pauly's Reagent *see* 2999
Pavabid [HMR] *see* 7019
Pavacen [Central Pharm.] *see* 7019
Pavadel [Canright] *see* 7019
Pavagen [Darby] *see* 7019
Pavakey [Key] *see* 7019
Pavased [Mallard] *see* 7019
Pavecef [IBP] *see* 1914
Paviin *see* 4266
Pavoninins, 7054
Pavulon [Organon] *see* 7007
Paxate [BMS] *see* 2994
Paxeladine [Beaufour] *see* 6930
Paxene [Ivax] *see* 6982
Paxil [GSK] *see* 7043
Paxipam [Schering] *see* 4589
Paxistil *see* 4849
Paylean [Elanco] *see* 8092
Payoff *see* 4124
Payzone [Am. Cyanamid] *see* 6654
Pazufloxacin, 7055
Pazufloxacin Mesylate *see* 7055
PB-89 *see* 4228
PB-94 *see* 8474
PB-868Cl *see* 5642
PBB *see* 4081
PBBs *see* 7563
PBN, 7056
PB-NOX [Roussel-Bio] *see* 7476
PBP *see* 4081
PBU *see* 7230
PBZ [Novartis] *see* 9738
PC *see* 7340
PC 1 *see* 3975
PC-904 *see* 724
PC-1421 *see* 7462
PCBs *see* 7564
PCBTF *see* 2126
PCC *see* 7974
PCDP *see* 7282
PCE [Abbott] *see* 3681
PCI-0120 *see* 6282
PCI-0123 *see* 6282
PCNB *see* 8080
PCP *see* 7109, 7219
PCPP-SA *see* 7559
PCV *see* 7083
PD-93 *see* 7505
PD-107779 *see* 3587
PD-109452-2 *see* 8051
PD-114720 *see* 5444
PD-127391 *see* 2355
PD-131501 *see* 8735
PD-144723 *see* 7725
PD-148515 *see* 884
PDB *see* 3057
3-PDC *see* 7110
PDDB *see* 3415
PDGA *see* 3291
PDGF *see* 7525
P-DHP *see* 240
P-DMEA *see* 2884
PDP *see* 6203
PDX Chloride *see* 7557
PEA *see* 7225
Peach Oil, Expressed, 7057

Peak [Syngenta] *see* 7881
Peanut, 7058
Peanut Oil, 7059
Pearl Ash *see* 7619
Pearlman's Catalyst, 7060
Pearl White *see* 1263
Pear Oil *see* 5111
Pearson's Creolin *see* 2570
Peau d'Espagne *see* 3766
PEBC *see* 7061
β-PEBG *see* 7231
Pebulate, 7061
PECA *see* 3787
Pecilocin, 7062
Pecitrol Veinogène *see* 1228
Pecnon [Sanken] *see* 5288
Pecram [Novartis] *see* 465
Pect [Rentschler] *see* 386
Pectamol [BDH] *see* 6930
Pectamon *see* 6930
Pectenine *see* 1847
Pectin, 7063
Pectin Sugar *see* 761
Pectobloc [Kytta-Siegfried] *see* 7443
Pectolin [Faulding] *see* 7329
Pectolinarigenin, 7064
Pectolinarin *see* 7064
Pectolitan [3M Pharma] *see* 2066
Pectox [Italfarmaco] *see* 1802
Pedameth [Forest] *see* 5975
Pederin, 7065
Pederine *see* 7065
ψ-Pederine *see* 7065
Pedestal [Uniroyal] *see* 6720
PEDG *see* 7231
Pediamycin [Abbott] *see* 3681
Pedisafe [Sagitta] *see* 2417
Peflacine [Bellon] *see* 7066
Peflox [Formenti] *see* 7066
Pefloxacin, 7066
Pefloxacine *see* 7066
Pefloxacin Mesylate *see* 7066
Pefurazoate, 7067
PEG *see* 7568
Peganine *see* 9937
Peganone [Abbott] *see* 3749
Pegaptanib Sodium, 7068
PEG-asparaginase *see* 836
Pegaspargase *see* 836
Pegasus [Novartis Agro] *see* 2969
Pegasyl [SweVet] *see* 4798
PEG Fatty Acid Esters *see* 7578
PEG-400 Monostearate *see* 7578
Pegorgotein *see* 9002
Pegosperse [Lonza] *see* 7578
Pegosperse 400-MS [Lonza] *see* 7578
Pegosperse 1750-MS [Lonza] *see* 7578
PEG-SOD *see* 9002
PEG-t44-OMe *see* 7068
Pegu Catechu *see* 1903
Pegvisomant, 7069
Pegylated Anti-(human Tumor Necrosis Factor α) Fab′ Fragment (Human-mouse Monoclonal CDP870 Heavy Chain) Immunoglobulin Disulfide with Human-mouse Monoclonal CDP870 Light Chain *see* 2003
Pegylated Somatotropin [18-Aspartic Acid, 21-Asparagine, 120-Lysine, 167-Asparagine, 168-Alanine, 171-Serine, 172-Arginine, 174-Serine, 179-Threonine] (Human) *see* 7069
Peimine *see* 9969
Peiminoside *see* 9969
PEITC *see* 7226

Pelanin Depot [Mochida] *see* 3703
Pelargidanon 1602 *see* 6424
Pelargidenolon 1497 *see* 5274
Pelargidenon 1449 *see* 730
Pelargonic Acid, 7070
Pelargonidin, 7071
Pelargonin *see* 7071
Pelentan *see* 3770
Peligal *see* 5918
Pellagra Preventive Factor *see* 6525
Pelletierine, 7072
(±)-Pelletierine *see* 7072
Pellitorine, 7073
Pellotine, 7074
Pelosine *see* 1016
PELS *see* 3683
α-Peltatin, 7075
β-Peltatin, 7076
β-Peltatin A *see* 7076
Peluces [Isei] *see* 4598
Pemal [Benzon] *see* 3748
Pemetrexed, 7077
Pemetrexed Disodium *see* 7077
Pemilaston [BMS] *see* 7078
Pemine [Lilly] *see* 7088
Pemirolast, 7078
Pemix [Prodes] *see* 7507
Pemoline, 7079
Pempidil [Farmigea] *see* 7080
Pempidine, 7080
Pempiten [I.G.I.] *see* 7080
Penamecillin, 7081
Penbristol [BMS] *see* 586
Penbritin [GSK] *see* 586
Penbutolol, 7082
Pencal [Tatsumi] *see* 1794
Penchlorol *see* 7109
Penciclovir, 7083
Pendimax [Dow AgroSci.] *see* 7084
Pendimethalin, 7084
Pendletonite *see* 2536
Penecort [Allergan] *see* 4787
Penetek *see* 7111
Penethamate Hydriodide, 7085
Penethecillin *see* 7085
Penetratin, 7086
Penetratin-1 *see* 7086
Penfluridol, 7087
Pengitoxin *see* 4434
Penglobe [AstraZeneca] *see* 931
Penicidin *see* 7053
Penicillamine, 7088
D-Penicillamine *see* 7088
Penicillamine Cysteine Disulfide, 7089
Penicillamine Disulfide, 7090
Penicillanic Acid, 7091
Penicillanic Acid 1,1-Dioxide *see* 8889
Penicillanic Acid Sulfone *see* 8889
Penicillic Acid, 7092
Penicillin II *see* 7094
Penicillin-152 *see* 7223
Penicillin-152 Potassium *see* 7223
Penicillin 356 *see* 2385
Penicillinase, 7093
Penicillin AT *see* 7099
Penicillin DF *see* 616
Penicillin G, 7094
Penicillin G Benethamine, 7095
Penicillin G Benzathine, 7096
Penicillin G Compd with 2-(Diethylamino)ethyl *p*-Aminobenzoate Monohydrate *see* 7097
Penicillin G *N*,*N*′-Dibenzylethylenediamine Salt *see* 7096
Penicillin G 2-Diethylaminoethyl Ester Hydriodide *see* 7085

Penicillin G Hydroxymethyl Ester Acetate *see* 7081
Penicillin G Procaine, 7097
Penicillin MV *see* 7223
Penicillin N, 7098
Penicillin O, 7099
Penicillin O 2-Chloroprocaine *see* 7099
Penicillin O Potassium *see* 7099
Penicillin P-12 *see* 6904
Penicillin Phenoxymethyl *see* 7100
Penicillin V, 7100
Penicillin V Benzathine *see* 7100
Penicillin V DBED *see* 7100
Penicilloyl Polylysine, 7101
Penicin *see* 458
Pénicline [Sanofi-Aventis] *see* 586
Penidural [Am. Home] *see* 7096
Penilevel [ERN] *see* 7094
Penimox [IBSA] *see* 577
Penin *see* 458
Penistaph *see* 5969
Penitardon [Woelm] *see* 6732
Penncap M [Cerexagri] *see* 6108
Penncozeb [Cerexagri] *see* 5716
Pennyroyal, 7102
Pennyroyal Oil *see* 7102
Penoxalin *see* 7084
Penoxsulam, 7103
Pensanate [Morishita] *see* 7471
Pen-Sint [Cophar] *see* 3084
Penspek (formerly) *see* 3961
Penstapho [BMS] *see* 6904
Penta *see* 7109
Penta-*O*-acetylgitoxin *see* 4434
Penta-*O*-benzylquercetin *see* 8034
Pentaborane(9), 7104
Pentaborane(11), 7105
Pentaboron Nonahydride *see* 7104
Pentaboron Undecahydride *see* 7105
Pentabromoacetone, 7106
1,1,1,3,3-Pentabromo-2-propanone *see* 7106
Pentac [Zoecon] *see* 3105
Pentacarbonyliron *see* 5099
Pentacarboxymethyl Diethylenetriamine *see* 7125
Pentacard [Cedona] *see* 5225
Pentacarinat [Sanofi-Aventis] *see* 7115
Pentacene, 7107
Pentachlorin *see* 2841
3,3′,5,5′,6-Pentachloro-2,2′-dihydroxybenzanilide *see* 6958
Pentachloroethane, 7108
3,3′,5,5′,6-Pentachloro-2′-hydroxysalicylanilide *see* 6958
Pentachloronitrobenzene *see* 8080
Pentachlorophenol, 7109
Pentacin *see* 7124
Pentacyclo[4.2.0.0²,⁵.0³,⁸.0⁴,⁷]octane *see* 2611
Pentacyclo[7.3.1.1⁴,¹².0²,⁷.0⁶,¹¹]tetradecane *see* 2499
6-(8-Pentadecenyl)-2-hydroxybenzoic Acid *see* 621
3-Pentadecyl-1,2-benzenediol *see* 7110
3-Pentadecylcatechol, 7110
6-Pentadecyl-2-hydroxybenzoic Acid *see* 621
3-Pentadecylpyrocatechol *see* 7110
6-Pentadecylsalicylic Acid *see* 621
Pentadoll [Showa Shinyaku] *see* 2408
Pentadorm *see* 5846
Pentaerythritol, 7111
Pentaerythritol Tetranicotinate *see* 6497
Pentaerythritol Tetranitrate, 7112

Pepo *see* 7941
Pepperidge Bush *see* 961
Peppermint, 7145
Peppermint Camphor *see* 5837
Pepsamar [Sanofi Winthrop] *see* 342
Pepsin, 7146
Pepstatin, 7147
Pepstatin A *see* 7147
Pepstatin B *see* 7147
Pepstatin C *see* 7147
Peptan [Merck & Co.] *see* 3930
Peptard [3M Pharma] *see* 4858
Peptarom [Fresenius] *see* 9889
Peptavlon [Ayerst] *see* 7113
Peptazol [Recordati] *see* 7014
Pepticum [Grünenthal] *see* 6845
Peptide T, 7148
Peptide Tyrosine-tyrosine *see* 7149
Peptide YY, 7149
Peptidoglycan *see* 6304
Peptilate [Dojin] *see* 223
Peptinimid [Iromedica] *see* 3748
Pepto-Bismol [Procter & Gamble] *see* 1285
Peptol [Horner] *see* 2279
Per-Abrodil *see* 5040
Peracef [Pfizer] *see* 1930
Peracetic Acid, 7150
Peracon [Kali-Chemie] *see* 5110
Peragit [AFI] *see* 9695
Peraprin [Taiyo] *see* 6143
Perazil [Burroughs Wellcome] *see* 2081
Perazine, 7151
Perazolin [Zenyaku Kogyo] *see* 8568
Perazyl *see* 2081
Perbenzoic Acid, 7152
Percapyl *see* 2105
Perchloracap [Mallinckrodt] *see* 7653
Perchloric Acid, 7153
Perchloric Anhydride *see* 2097
Perchlorobenzene *see* 4677
Perchlorobutadiene *see* 4678
Perchloroethane *see* 4679
Perchloroethylene *see* 9190
Perchloromethane *see* 1816
Perchloron *see* 1674
Perchloropentacyclo[5.2.1.0^{2,6}.0^{3,9}.0^{5,8}]-
    decane *see* 6207
Perchloryl Fluoride, 7154
Perclene *see* 9190
Percoccide [A.C.F.] *see* 8913
Percocet [Endo] *see* 6959
Percodan [Endo] *see* 6959
Percorten [Novartis] *see* 2901
Percutol [Pliva] *see* 6607
Perderm [Schering] *see* 220
Perdiem Fiber [RPR] *see* 7517
Perdilatal [Smith & Nephew] *see* 6732
Perdipina [Novartis] *see* 6495
Perdipine [Syntex] *see* 6495
Perdix [Schwarz] *see* 6229
Perdorm [Lagap] *see* 9133
Perduren *see* 9339
Perebral [Beytout] *see* 2704
Perebron [Angelini] *see* 6944
Pereirine *see* 4380
Peremesin [BMS] *see* 5777
Pérénan [Sanofi Winthrop] *see* 3653
Perenum [Delalande] *see* 9521
Perequil [Lepetit] *see* 5862
Perezone, 7155
Perfan [HMR] *see* 3589
Perfane [HMR] *see* 3589
Perfekthion [BASF] *see* 3220
Perflan [Dow AgroSci.] *see* 9095
Perfluamine *see* 4183

Perflubron, 7156
Perflunafene *see* 4183
Perfluoroacetic Acid *see* 9681
Perfluorobenzene *see* 4686
Perfluoroctyl Bromide *see* 7156
Perfluorocyclobutane *see* 6745
Perfluorodecalin *see* 4183
Perfluoroethene *see* 9205
Perfluorohexane, 7157
Perfluoro-*n*-hexane *see* 7157
Perfluoropropane, 7158
Perfluorotripropylamine *see* 4183
Perflutren *see* 7158
Perforin, 7159
Performic Acid, 7160
Perfosfamide, 7161
Perfusamine [Medi-Physics] *see* 5049
Pergamid [Scios-Nova] *see* 7161
Pergitral *see* 7112
Pergolide, 7162
Pergonal [Serono] *see* 4223
Pergotime [Serono] *see* 2386
Perhexilene *see* 7163
Perhexiline, 7163
N-(2-Perhydroazocin-1-ylethyl)guanidine
    see 4560
Perhydronaphthalene *see* 2846
Perhydrosqualene *see* 8767
Peri Acid *see* 6405
Periactin [Merck & Co.] *see* 2773
Periactinol [Merck & Co.] *see* 2773
Perichthol *see* 4885
Periciazine *see* 7164
Periciclina *see* 2886
Periclase *see* 5677
Peri-Colace *see* 1878
Peri-Colace [Roberts] *see* 3401
Pericyazine, 7164
Peridamol [Boehringer, Ing.] *see* 3346
Peridex [Procter & Gamble] *see* 2091
Peridon [Italchimici] *see* 3418
Peridys [Robapharm] *see* 3418
Perifadil [Sterling Winthrop] *see* 8948
Perifosine, 7165
Perifunal [Aristegui] *see* 7516
Perigen [Bayer CropSci.] *see* 7180
Perilax [Ferring] *see* 1242
Perilla Ketone, 7166
Perillaldehyde, 7167
l-Perillaldehyde α-*anti*-Oxime *see* 7167
l-Perillaldehyde α-*syn*-Oxime *see* 7167
Perillartine *see* 7167
"Perilla Sugar" *see* 7167
Perimetazine *see* 7168
Perimethazine, 7168
Perimycin, 7169
Perimycin A *see* 7169
Perin [Endo] *see* 7464
Perindopril, 7170
Perindoprilat *see* 7170
Perindopril Erbumine *see* 7170
Periodic Acid, 7171
Periodyl, 7172
Periograf *see* 3467
Periplanone A *see* 7173
Periplanone B *see* 7173
(−)-Periplanone B *see* 7173
Periplanones, 7173
Periplocin, 7174
Periplocoside *see* 7174
Periplocymarin, 7175
Periplogenin, 7176
Periplum [Italfarmaco] *see* 6551
Peripress [Pfizer] *see* 7717
Perisalol [Chugai] *see* 6521

Perisoxal, 7177
Peristim [Mead Johnson] *see* 1878
Periston [Bayer] *see* 7697
Peritol [EGYT] *see* 2773
Peritrate [Warner-Chilcott] *see* 7112
Perityl *see* 7112
Perivine, 7178
Perketan [Inverni] *see* 5296
Perlacton [Chassot] *see* 6979
Perlapine, 7179
Perlatan *see* 3708
Perlinganit [Schwarz] *see* 6607
Perlon *see* 6734
Perlopal *see* 5846
Perlutex [Leo Pharm] *see* 5793
Permanent Yellow *see* 972
Permanganic Acid Potassium Salt *see*
    7655
Permapen [Roerig] *see* 7096
Permasect [Mitchell Cotts] *see* 7180
Permastril [Cassenne] *see* 3448
Permax [Lilly] *see* 7162
Permeability Glycoprotein *see* 7195
Permease *see* 4758
Permethanoic Acid *see* 7160
Permethrin, 7180
Permiran [Laphal] *see* 10003
Permit [Nissan] *see* 4602
Permitil [Schering] *see* 4189
Permixon [Pierre Fabre] *see* 8388
Permonid [Roche] *see* 2927
Pernambuco, 7181
Pernazene [Synthelabo] *see* 9834
Pernovin [Chinoin] *see* 7233
Perocan [Toyo Jozo] *see* 5110
Perocef [Pulitzer] *see* 1930
Peroidin *see* 7653
Perolysen [M & B] *see* 7080
Peronine *see* 1141
Peronine Myristate *see* 6337
Perospirone, 7182
Perovskite *see* 9472
1,4-Peroxido-*p*-menthene-2 *see* 827
Peroxinorm [Grünenthal] *see* 9002
Peroxyacetic Acid *see* 7150
Peroxybenzoic Acid *see* 7152
Peroxyderm [Chassot] *see* 1116
Peroxyformic Acid *see* 7160
Peroxymonosulfuric Acid *see* 1851
Perparin [Chemopuro] *see* 3728
Perperine *see* 3728
Perphenan *see* 7183
Perphenazine, 7183
Perphenazine 3,4,5-Trimethoxybenzo-
    ate *see* 6145
Perprazole *see* 6845
Per-Radiographol *see* 5040
Persa-gel [J & J] *see* 1116
Persantine [Boehringer, Ing.] *see* 3346
Persedon [Roche] *see* 7995
Persephin *see* 4377
Persian Bark *see* 1880
Persian Berries *see* 4263
Persian Insect Powder *see* 7966
Persian Red *see* 5406
Persic Oil *see* 7057
Persio *see* 2615
Persistol [Chevron] *see* 9671
Persolv [Lepetit] *see* 9887
Perspex *see* 5941
Persulfuric Acid *see* 1851
Pertestis [Orma] *see* 9180
Pertofran [Novartis] *see* 2920
Pertofrane [Novartis] *see* 2920
Pertranquil [HMR] *see* 5862

Pertrombon see 3812
Pertscan [Abbott] see 8657
Peruvian Balsam see 949
Peruvian Bark see 2284
Peruviol see 6476
Pervetral [Viatris] see 6970
Pervincamine [Sanofi-Aventis] see 9983
Pervitin [Temmler] see 5948
Perviton see 7216
Perycit [Bofors] see 6497
Perylene, 7184
PES see 5617
Peson [Hoechst] see 5617
Pesos [Valeas] see 3973
Pestox III [FBC] see 8395
Pestox XIV see 3205
PET see 7569
Petalite see 5520
Peteha [Fatol] see 7891
Pethidine see 5849
Petidiol see 3718
Petidion [Gerot] see 3718
Petidon see 9706
Petimin see 5687
Petinimid see 3748
Petinutin [Parke-Davis] see 6004
Petisan [Gerot] see 3718
Petit Muguet see 10049
PETN see 7112
Petnidan [Desitin] see 3748
Petrin [Parke-Davis] see 7138
Petrohol see 5208
Petrolatum, 7185
Petrolatum, Liquid, 7186
Petrol (British) see 4372
Petroleum, 7187
Petroleum Benzin, 7188
Petroleum Jelly see 7185
Petroleum Naphtha see 7188
Petroleum Spirits see 6201
Petroselic Acid see 7189
Petroselinic Acid, 7189
Petrosulpho see 4885
Petty-morrel see 766
Petunidin, 7190
Petunidol see 7190
Petunin see 7190
Petylyl [Temmler] see 2920
Petzite see 4514
Peucedanin, 7191
Pevaryl [Cilag] see 3502
Pexelizumab, 7192
Pexid [Sigma] see 7163
Pexiganan, 7193
Peyocactine see 4746
Peyote see 5905
Peyrone's Chloride see 2317
Peyrone's Salt see 2317
Pezetamid [Hefa-Frenon] see 7956
PF-1593 see 1484
PF-804950 see 3512
PF-1022-221 see 3560
P-FAD see 4460
PFC-218 see 7158
Pfeiffer's Substance, 7194
Pfizer-E [Pfizer] see 3687
Pfizerpen [Roerig] see 7094
Pfizerpen-AS [Roerig] see 7097
PFOB see 7156
PFP see 7159
PFT Roche [Roche] see 1054
PFT-α see 7421
PG see 7859
PG490 see 9747
PG490-88 see 9747

PGA see 4221
PGE$_1$ see 7876
PGE$_2$ see 7877
PGF$_{2\alpha}$ see 7878
PGG$_2$ see 7875, 9388
PGH$_2$ see 7875
PGI$_2$ see 7875
P-Glycoprotein, 7195
[P(GMA-co-EA)] see 2514
P-gp see 7195
PGT/1A see 7419
PG-TXL see 6983
PGX see 7875
PH-60-40 see 3142
PH-70-23 see 4123
PH-1882 see 1419
PH-5776 see 6567
PHA-782615 see 3512
Phacetoperane see 5467
Phacetur see 7203
Phaenthine see 9231
Phaeomelanins see 5812
Phaeva [Schering AG] see 4413
Phalloidin, 7196
Phalloidine see 7196
Phaltan see 4224
Phanchinone see 7197
Phanodorm [Winthrop] see 2711
Phanodorn [Winthrop] see 2711
Phanquinone, 7197
Phanquone see 7197
Phanurane [Specia] see 1750
Phardol [Kreussler] see 4499
Pharmatex [Innothéra] see 1059
Pharorid [Wellmark] see 5983
Phaseolin, 7198
Phaseollin see 7198
Phaseolunatin see 5497
Phaseomannite see 4978
Phasil [Reed & Carnrick] see 3215
Phasin, 7199
Phasins see 5429
Phazyme [Reed & Carnrick] see 3215
Ph BC see 3975
PHD see 9388
Phe see 7271
Pheasant's Eye see 167
α-Phellandrene, 7200
β-Phellandrene, 7201
Phe^3-Lys^8-oxytocin see 5630
Phe^2-Lys^8-vasopressin see 3954
Phemeride [Parke-Davis] see 1074
Phe-Mer-Nite see 7302
Phemerol Chloride [Parke-Davis] see 1074
Phemiton [Pliva] see 5854
Phenacaine Hydrochloride, 7202
Phenacemide, 7203
Phenacetin, 7204
Phenacetolin, 7205
Phenacetylurea see 7203
Phenacide see 9557
Phenacite see 1161
Phenacylamine, 7206
Phenacyl Bromide see 1402
Phenacyl Chloride see 2115
Phenadoxone, 7207
Phenalzine see 7221
Phenamidine, 7208
Phenamin [Nycomed] see 2180
Phenamine see 7239
Phenamiphos see 3957
Phenamizole see 483
Phenampromid(e), 7209
9,10-Phenanthraquinone see 7213
Phenanthrene, 7212

9,10-Phenanthrenedione see 7213
Phenanthrenequinone, 7213
o-Phenanthroline, 7214
1,10-Phenanthroline see 7214
4,5-Phenanthroline see 7214
4,7-Phenanthroline-5,6-dione see 7197
4,7-Phenanthroline-5,6-quinone see 7197
Phenantoin see 5853
Phenarsazine Chloride, 7215
Phenatine, 7216
Phenatox see 9557
Phenazacillin see 4672
Phenazarsine Chloride see 7215
Phenazine, 7217
Phenazine [Jenkins] see 7220
2,3-Phenazinediamine see 2982
1,6-Phenazinediol 5,10-Dioxide see 5021
Phenazine Methosulfate see 6109
1-Phenazinol see 4645
Phenazocine, 7218
Phenazoline see 680
Phenazone see 716
Phenazone Salicylate see 717
Phenazopyridine, 7210
Phenazoxine see 7253
Phenbenicillin see 3961
Phenbutrazate see 3965
Phencamine see 3967
Phencyclidine, 7219
Phendimetrazine, 7220
Phénégic see 7252
Phenelzine, 7221
ν-Phenenyltris(oxyethylene)]tris[triethylammonium Triiodide] see 4343
Phenergan [Sanofi-Aventis] see 7786
Phenesin see 1522
Phenetharbital, 7222
Phenethicillin Potassium, 7223
Phenethyl Alcohol, 7224
Phenethylamine, 7225
4-[2-[[6-(Phenethylamino)hexyl]amino]-ethyl]pyrocatechol see 3424
N-Phenethyl Anthranilic Acid see 3580
Phenethylazocine see 7218
1-Phenethylbiguanide see 7231
Phenethyldiguanide see 7231
N'-β-Phenethylformamidinyliminourea see 7231
(2-Phenethyl)hydrazine see 7221
Phenethyl Isothiocyanate, 7226
N-(1-Phenethyl-4-piperidinyl)-N-phenyl-propionamide see 4001
N-(1-Phenethyl-4-piperidyl)propionani-lide see 4001
o-Phenetidine, 7227
p-Phenetidine, 7228
Phenetin [Alpinapharm] see 1522
p-Phenetolcarbamide see 3464
Phenetole, 7229
Phenetsal see 48
Pheneturide, 7230
p-Phenetylurea see 3464
Phenformin, 7231
Phenhydan [Desitin] see 7322
Phenibut see 464
Phenic Acid see 7241
Phenicin, 7232
Phenicol see 3768
Phenidiemal see 7222
Phenidone see 7309
Phenigamma see 464
Phenindamine, 7233
Phenindione, 7234

3-Phenyl-2-propenoic Acid *see* 2299

3-Phenyl-2-propenoic Acid Phenylmethyl Ester *see* 1130

3-Phenyl-2-propenoic Acid 3-Phenyl-2-propenyl Ester *see* 2304

3-Phenyl-2-propen-1-ol *see* 2302

3-Phenyl-2-propenoyl Chloride *see* 2301

3-Phenyl-2-propenyl Anthranilate *see* 2303

β-Phenylpropionic Acid *see* 4784

3-Phenylpropionic Acid *see* 4784

4-Phenyl-4-propionoxy-1,3-dimethyl-azacycloheptane *see* 7776

α-Phenyl-α-propoxybenzeneacetic Acid 1-Methyl-4-piperidinyl Ester *see* 7832

1-Phenylpropyl Alcohol *see* 3768

7-(3-Phenyl-2-propylaminoethyl)theophylline *see* 3972

γ-Phenylpropyl Carbamate *see* 7258

d-N-(1-Phenyl-2-propyl)-2-chlorobenzylamine *see* 2362

N-(3'-Phenyl-2'-propyl)-1,1-diphenyl-3-propylamine *see* 7737

3-(1-Phenylpropyl)-4-hydroxycoumarin *see* 7259

Phenylpropylmethylamine, 7308

Phenylpseudohydantoin *see* 7079

6-Phenyl-2,4,7-pteridinetriamine *see* 9599

1-Phenyl-3-pyrazolidinone, 7309

1-Phenyl-3-pyrazolidone *see* 7309

N'-(1-Phenylpyrazol-5-yl)sulfanilamide *see* 8935

1-Phenyl-1-(2-pyridyl)-3-dimethylaminopropane *see* 7235

(±)-1-Phenyl-1-(2-pyridyl)-4-(*cis*-2,6-dimethyl-1-piperidyl)butanol *see* 7501

3-Phenyl-3-(2-pyridyl)-N,N-dimethylpropylamine *see* 7235

1-[2-[Phenyl(2-pyridylmethyl)amino]-ethyl]piperidine *see* 7404

Phenyl-2-pyridylmethyl-β-N,N-dimethylaminoethyl Ether *see* 3441

N-Phenyl-N-(2-pyridylmethyl)-2-piperidinoethylamine *see* 7404

1-Phenyl-1H-pyrrole-2,5-dione *see* 7299

1-Phenyl-2,5-pyrrolidinedione *see* 8867

Phenylpyrrolidinopentane *see* 7781

1-Phenyl-2-pyrrolidylpentane *see* 7781

2-Phenyl-4-quinolinecarboxylic Acid *see* 2288

N-Phenylsalicylamide *see* 8330

Phenyl Salicylate, 7310

3-Phenylsalicylic Acid 2-Diethylaminoethyl Ester *see* 1234

Phenylselenotrimethylsilane, 7311

4-Phenylsemicarbazide, 7312

Phenyl Sodium *see* 1066

4-Phenylspiro[furan-2(3H),1'(3'H)-isobenzofuran]-3,3'-dione *see* 4158

4-Phenylspiro[furan-2(3H),1'-phthalan]-3,3'-dione *see* 4158

Phenylstibinic Acid *see* 1069

Phenylstibonic Acid *see* 1069

Phenyl Styryl Ketone *see* 2037

N-Phenylsuccinamic Acid *see* 8868

N-Phenylsuccinimide *see* 8867

1-Phenyl-3-p-sulfamoylanilino-1,3-propanedisulfonic Acid Disodium Salt *see* 6684

N¹-Phenylsulfanilamide *see* 8896

1-Phenyl-5-sulfanilamidopyrazole *see* 8935

N-Phenylsulfanilic Acid, 7313

Phenyl Sulfide, 7314

[5-(Phenylsulfinyl)-1H-benzimidazol-2-yl]carbamic Acid Methyl Ester *see* 6935

5-Phenylsulfinyl-2-carbomethoxyamino-benzimidazole *see* 6935

Phenylsulfohydrazide *see* 7598

Phenyl Sulfone *see* 3332

(5Z)-7-[(1R,2S,3S,4S)-3-[(Phenylsulfonyl)amino]bicyclo[2.2.1]hept-2-yl]-5-heptenoic Acid *see* 3416

(+)-(5Z)-7-[3-*endo*-[(Phenylsulfonyl)amino]bicyclo[2.2.1]hept-2-*exo*-yl]-5-heptenoic Acid *see* 3416

N-(Phenylsulfonyl)hydroxylamine *see* 7426

4-(Phenylsulfoxyethyl)-1,2-diphenyl-3,5-pyrazolidinedione *see* 8949

2-(6'-Phenyltetracyclo[5,4,2,0³,¹³,0¹⁰,¹²]-trideca-4',8'-dien-11'-yl)acetic Acid *see* 3571

(E)-4-(6'-Phenyltetracyclo[5,4,2,0³,¹³,-0¹⁰,¹²]trideca-4',8'-dien-11'-yl)but-2-enoic Acid *see* 3571

4-Phenyl-1-[2-[(tetrahydro-2-furanyl)methoxy]ethyl]-4-piperidinecarboxylic Acid Ethyl Ester *see* 4303

4-Phenyl-1-[2-(tetrahydrofurfuryloxy)-ethyl]isonipecotic Acid Ethyl Ester *see* 4303

1-Phenyl-1,2,3,4-tetrahydro-4-hydroxy-pyrrolo[2,3-b]-7-methylquinolin-4-one *see* 1317

(−)-6-Phenyl-2,3,5,6-tetrahydroimid-azo[2,1-b]thiazole *see* 5459

N-Phenyl-N'-1,2,3-thiadiazol-5-ylurea *see* 9313

5-Phenyl-2,4-thiazolediamine *see* 483

5-(Phenylthio)-2-benzimidazolecarbamic Acid Methyl Ester *see* 3960

[5-(Phenylthio)-1H-benzimidazol-2-yl]-carbamic Acid Methyl Ester *see* 3960

Phenylthiocarbamide *see* 7315

Phenylthiourea, 7315

Phenyltoloxamine, 7316

Phenyl Tolyl Ketone, 7317

2-(Phenyl-o-tolylmethoxy)ethyldimethylamine *see* 6879

Phenyl-o-tolylmethyl Dimethylaminoethyl Ether *see* 6879

6-Phenyl-2,4,7-triaminopteridine *see* 9599

6-Phenyl-1,3,5-triazine-2,4-diamine *see* 1089

1-Phenyltridecane *see* 9659

(+)-(1R)-1-Phenyl-1-[(3,4,5-trimethoxy)-benzyloxymethyl]-N,N-dimethyl-n-propylamine *see* 3949

Phenyltrimethylammonium Iodide, 7318

17-Phenyl-18,19,20-trinorprostaglandin F₂α Ethylamide *see* 1221

Phenylurea, 7319

Phenylurethan(e), 7320

Pheny-PAS-Tebamin [Purdue Frederick] *see* 7272

Phenyramidol, 7321

Phenytoin, 7322

Phenytoin Soluble *see* 7322

Phenyzene [C-Vet] *see* 7277

Phenzidole *see* 7274

Pheophytin *see* 2519

Phe²-Phe²-Lys⁸-oxytocin *see* 3954

Phetylureum [Katwijk] *see* 7203

PHGA *see* 7935

PhGABA *see* 464

Phillyrin, 7323

Phillyroside *see* 7323

Philodorm *see* 2711

Philosopher's Wool *see* 10147

PhIO *see* 5044

PhIP, 7324

pHisohex [Winthrop] *see* 4680

pHiso-Med *see* 2091

Phlogase [Adenylchemie] *see* 6972

Phlogistol [Spitzner] *see* 6972

Phlogont [Azupharma] *see* 4499, 6972

Phloguron [Steiner] *see* 5288

Phloionic Acid, 7325

Phloracetophenone 4,6-Dimethyl Ether *see* 10067

Phloretin, 7326

Phloretin-2'-β-glucoside *see* 7327

Phlorhizin, 7327

Phloridzin, 7327

Phlorizin, 7327

Phloroglucin *see* 7328

Phloroglucinol, 7328

Phlorol *see* 3839

Phloropropiophenone *see* 4106

Phlorrhizen *see* 7327

PHMB *see* 7560

Phoenicin *see* 7232

Phoenicochroite *see* 5405

Pholcodine, 7329

Pholedrine, 7330

Phomin *see* 2790

Phorate, 7331

Phorbol, 7332

Phorone, 7333

Phorwite RN *see* 1315

Phos *see* 4813

Phosalone, 7334

Phosdrin *see* 6165

Phoselit [Kytta-Siegfried] *see* 4813

Phosethyl Al *see* 4252

Phos-ex [Vitaline] *see* 1646

Phosgene, 7335

Phosgeniminium Chloride *see* 9977

Phosilite *see* 4813

Phoskill [United Phosphorus] *see* 6251

PhosLo [Nabi] *see* 1646

Phosmet, 7336

Phosote *see* 2573

Phosphacol *see* 7030

Phosphagen *see* 7340

Phosphaljel [Am. Home] *see* 358

Phosphalugel [Yamanouchi] *see* 358

Phosphamidon, 7337

Phosphate of Soda *see* 8659

"Phosphatidal Choline" *see* 7519

"Phosphatidal Ethanolamine" *see* 7519

Phosphatidic Acids *see* 4486

Phosphatidylcholine *see* 5428

Phosphatidylethanolamine *see* 1975

Phosphatidylglycerol *see* 7939

Phosphine, 7338

Phosphinic Acid, Sodium Salt *see* 8629

3,3',3''-Phosphinidynetrispropanoic Acid *see* 9085

1,1',1''-Phosphinothioylidynetrisaziri-dine *see* 9673

Phosphinothricin, 7339

1,1',1''-Phosphinylidynetrisaziridine *see* 9672

1,1',1''-Phosphinylidynetris[2-methyl-aziridine] *see* 5936

Phosphocol [Mallinckrodt] *see* 2227

Phosphocozymase *see* 6348

Phosphocreatine, 7340

Phosphocysteamine, 7341

3-Phosphoglyceraldehyde *see* 4482

Phosphorous Acid, 7346
Phosphorous Bromide see 7357
Phosphorous Chloride see 7358
Phosphorous Oxide (P_2O_5) see 7355
Phosphor-roesslerite see 5681
Phosphorus, 7347
Phosphorus Chloride see 7349
Phosphorus Oxybromide, 7348
Phosphorus Oxychloride, 7349
Phosphorus Pentabromide, 7350
Phosphorus Pentachloride, 7351
Phosphorus Pentafluoride, 7352
Phosphorus Pentaselenide, 7353
Phosphorus Pentasulfide, 7354
Phosphorus Pentoxide, 7355
Phosphorus Perbromide see 7350
Phosphorus Perchloride see 7351
Phosphorus Persulfide see 7354
Phosphorus Sesquisulfide see 9238
Phosphorus Sulfochloride, 7356
Phosphorus Tribromide, 7357
Phosphorus Trichloride, 7358
Phosphorus Trifluoride, 7359
Phosphorus Trioxide, 7360
Phosphorus Triselenide, 7361
Phosphoryl Bromide see 7348
Phosphoryl Chloride see 7349
Phosphorylcholine, 7362
Phosphorylcholine Chloride see 7362
Phosphoryldimethylaminoethanol see 2884
Phosphoryldimethylcolamine see 2884
Phosphoryldimethylethanolamine see 2884
O-Phosphoryl-4-hydroxy-N,N-dimethyl-tryptamine see 7926
(3-Phosphoryloxymethyl)phenytoin see 4258
Phosphoryl Tribromide see 7348
Phosphoserine, 7363
O-Phospho-DL-serine see 7363
Phosphosiderite see 4029
Phosphothion see 5700
Phosphotope [BMS] see 8661
Phosphotungstic Acid, 7364
Phostoxin [Degesch] see 359
Phosvel [Velsicol] see 5445
Phosvitin, 7365
Photine R see 1315
Photobiline see 5038
Photodyn see 4636
Photofrin [Axcan] see 7596
Photoglycine see 4837
Photol [Merck & Co.] see 6017
Photophor see 1695
Photopsins see 6856
Photo-Rex see 6017
Photosensitizer 101 see 7530
Photrex [Miravant] see 8269
Phoxim, 7366
Phrenazol see 7141
Phrenosin, 7367
Phrilon [Phrixwerke] see 6734
o-Phthalaldehyde, 7368
Phthalamide, 7369
Phthalamodine see 2193
Phthalamudine see 2193
Phthalazine, 7370
1(2H)-Phthalazinone (1,3-Dimethyl-2-butenylidene)hydrazone see 1470
1(2H)-Phthalazinone Hydrazone see 4763
3-(1-Phthalazinyl)carbazic Acid Ethyl Ester see 9502
2-(1-Phthalazinyl)hydrazinecarboxylic Acid Ethyl Ester see 9502

o-Phthaldialdehyde see 7368
Phthalic Acid, 7371
m-Phthalic Acid see 5197
p-Phthalic Acid see 9162
o-Phthalic Acid Bis[diethylamide] see 9203
Phthalic Acid Diamide see 7369
Phthalic Acid Dibutyl Ester see 3035
Phthalic Acid Dimethyl Ester see 3255
Phthalic Acid 1-Ethyl-1-methyl-2-pro-pynyl Ester see 7374
Phthalic Acid Potassium Acid Salt see 7612
Phthalic Anhydride, 7372
Phthalidyl D-α-Aminobenzylpenicil-lanate see 9033
Phthalidyl 2-(3-Trifluoromethylanilino)-nicotinate see 9044
Phthalidyl 2-(α,α,α-Trifluoro-m-toluidi-no)nicotinate see 9044
Phthalimide, 7373
α-Phthalimidoglutarimide see 9255
3-Phthalimidoglutarimide see 9255
Phthalin see 7244
(SP-4-1)-[29H,31H-Phthalocyaninato-(2−)-$N^{29},N^{30},N^{31},N^{32}$]copper see 2520
Phthalofyne, 7374
Phthalophos see 6354
Phthalophos (USSR) see 7336
Phthaloyl Chloride, 7375
N-Phthaloylglutamimide see 9255
Phthaloylsulfacetamide see 7376
Phthalthrin see 9223
2-(N^4-Phthalylaminobenzenesulfonami-do)thiazole see 7377
N-Phthalylglutamic Acid Imide see 9255
Phthalylsulfacetamide, 7376
Phthalylsulfacetimide see 7376
2-(N^4-Phthalylsulfanilamido)thiazole see 7377
Phthalylsulfathiazole, 7377
Phthalylsulfonazole see 7377
Phthiocol, 7378
Phtorazisin [Medexport] see 4113
PhXA-41 see 5376
Phycite see 3675
Phycobilin see 7379
Phycobiliproteins, 7379
Phycobilisomes see 7379
Phycocyanins see 7379
Phycoerythrins see 7379
Phygon see 3045
Phygon Paste see 3045
Phygon XL see 3045
Phylletten [Arznei Müller-Rorer] see 2913
Phyllocontin [Purdue Frederick] see 465
Phyllocormin N see 3878
α-Phyllohydroquinone see 7380
Phylloquinone, 7380
Phyllotemp [Mundipharma] see 465
Phyllyrin see 7323
Phyone see 8716
Physalaemin, 7381
Physalemin see 7381
Physalien see 10118
Physalin see 10118
Physcione see 3561
Physeptone [Glaxo Wellcome] see 5944
Physex [Leo Pharm] see 2216
Physiomycine see 5943
Physiotens [Giulini] see 6293
Physodalin see 7382
Physodic Acid, 7382
Physostigma, 7383
Physostigmine, 7384

Physostigmine Aminoxide see 3699
Physovenine, 7385
Phytane-1,2,3-triol see 7386
Phytantriol, 7386
Phytar [Monterey] see 1604
Phytat D. B. [Daniel-Brunet] see 7387
Phytic Acid, 7387
Phytin see 7387
Phytoagglutinins see 5429
Phytoalexins see 7928
Phytochlorin, 7388
Phytochlorin e see 7388
Phytochrome see 7379
Phytocor [Pharma Dynamics] see 7555
Phytoecdysteroids see 3491
Phytofluene, 7389
all-trans-Phytofluene see 7389
Phytohemagglutinin see 5429
Phytol, 7390
Phytolacca, 7391
Phytomelin see 8304
Phytomenadione see 7380
Phytomonic Acid see 5341
Phytonadiol see 7380
Phytonadiol Sodium Diphosphate see 7380
Phytonadione see 7380
α-Phytosterol see 8556
3-Phytylmenadione see 7380
Piazofolina see 6273
Piazolin see 6273
PIBCA see 5140
Piberaline, 7392
Piboserod, 7393
Picaridin, 7394
Piceid see 8158
Picein, 7395
Picene, 7396
Piceol see 7395
Piceoside see 7395
Picfume [Dow] see 2156
Picloram, 7397
Picloxydine, 7398
Pico [BASF] see 7399
Pi-Coli [Ist. Vitamine] see 7460
Picolinafen, 7399
α-Picoline, 7400
β-Picoline, 7401
γ-Picoline, 7402
4-Picoline see 7402
Picolinic Acid, 7403
γ-Picolinic Acid see 5187
Picolinic Acid N-Methylbetaine see 4729
7-(β-3′-Picolylaminoethyl)theophylline see 7430
2-Picolylidenebis(p-phenyl Sodium Sul-fate) see 7406
4,4′-(2-Picolylidene)bis(phenylsulfuric Acid) Disodium Salt see 7406
N-(2-Picolyl)-N-phenyl-N-(2-piperidino-ethyl)amine see 7404
Picoperidamine see 7404
Picoperine, 7404
Picoplatin, 7405
Pico-Salax [Ferring] see 7406
Picosulfate Sodium, 7406
Picosulfol see 7406
Picotamide, 7407
Picoxystrobin, 7408
Picragol [Wyeth] see 8526
Picramic Acid, 7409
Picrasmin see 5220
Picric Acid, 7410
Picric Acid Ammonium Salt see 547
Picric Acid Silver Derivative see 8526

Picrocine *see* 2929
Picrocrocin, 7411
Picrolonic Acid, 7412
Picromycin, 7413
Picronitric Acid *see* 7410
Picropodophyllic Acid *see* 7545
Picropodophyllinic Acid Lactone *see* 7546
Picrotin, 7414
Picrotol *see* 8526
Picrotoxin, 7415
Picrotoxinin, 7416
Picryl Chloride, 7417
Picrylmethylnitramine *see* 6573
Picrylnitromethylamine *see* 6573
Pictol [Mallinckrodt] *see* 6017
Picumast, 7418
PID *see* 7234
Pidilat [Solvay] *see* 6528
Pidorubicin *see* 3623
Pidotimod, 7419
Pierami [Fournier] *see* 405
PIFA *see* 7295
Pifarnine, 7420
Pifatidine *see* 8274
Pifazin [Pierrel] *see* 7420
Pifithrin-α, 7421
Pigitil [Fidia] *see* 7419
Piglet Pro-Gen V *see* 8578
Pigmentation Hormone *see* 6295
Pigmex *see* 6248
Pigweed *see* 376
Piketoprofen, 7422
Pikromycin *see* 7413
Pilagan [Allergan] *see* 7424
Pildralazine, 7423
Piliophen *see* 5038
Pill-bearing Spurge *see* 3903
Pilo [Novopharma] *see* 7424
Pilocarpine, 7424
β-Pilocarpine *see* 7424
Pilocarpus, 7425
Pilofrin [Allergan] *see* 7424
Pilogel [Alcon] *see* 7424
Pilopine HS [Alcon] *see* 7424
Piloral [Nippon Kayaku] *see* 2345
Pilosine, 5199
Pilostat [Bausch & Lomb] *see* 7424
Pilot [Schering] *see* 8086
Piloty's Acid, 7426
Pilsicainide, 7427
Pilzcin [Shionogi] *see* 2368
Pimadin *see* 7433
Pimafucin [Basotherm] *see* 6427
Pimagedine *see* 441
Pimaric Acid, 7428
α-Pimaric Acid *see* 7428
β-Pimaric Acid *see* 5468
d-Pimaric Acid *see* 7428
l-Pimaric Acid *see* 5468
Pimaricin *see* 6427
Pimavecort [Mycofarm] *see* 6454
Pimecrolimus, 7429
Pimefylline, 7430
Pimelic Acid, 7431
Pimelic Ketone *see* 2726
Pimenta, 7432
Pimenta Berry Oil *see* 7432
Pimenta Leaf Oil *see* 7432
Pimento Oil *see* 7432
Pimephylline *see* 7430
Pimexone [Formenti] *see* 5860
Piminodine, 7433
Pimobendan, 7434
Pimozide, 7435

Pimpernel *see* 7436
Pimpinella, 7436
Pimpinellin, 7437
Pinacidil, 7438
Pinacol, 7439
Pinacol Diborane *see* 1300
Pinacolin *see* 7440
Pinacolone, 7440
Pinacoloxymethylphosphoryl Fluoride *see* 8713
Pinacolyl Methylphosphonofluoridate *see* 8713
Pinacone *see* 7439
Pinacyanol Chloride *see* 8048
Pinakon *see* 4710
Pinang *see* 776
Pinaverium Bromide, 7441
Pinazepam, 7442
Pinbetol [Dolorgiet] *see* 7443
Pindac [Leo Pharm] *see* 7438
Pindione [Lipha] *see* 7234
Pindolol, 7443
Pindone, 7444
Pindoptan [Kanoldt] *see* 7443
"Pineapple Oil" *see* 3775
Pinene *see* 7445
Pinene [Diachem] *see* 7397
α-Pinene, 7445
β-Pinene, 7446
2-Pinene *see* 7445
Pinene Hydrochloride *see* 1340
(1R,5R)-(+)-2-Pinen-4-one *see* 9960
2-Pinen-7-one *see* 2252
Pine Oil, 7447
Pine Resin *see* 9826
Pineroro [Maruko] *see* 3311
Pine Tar, 7448
Pine Tar Oil *see* 9066
Pine Tulip *see* 2057
Pinguinain, 7449
Pinkroot *see* 8748
Pinnacle [DuPont] *see* 9316
Pinnoite *see* 5658
Pinolenic Acid, 7450
Pinol Hydrate *see* 8567
Pinorubin [Nippon Kayaku] *see* 7488
Pinosylvin, 7451
Pinozan *see* 7464
Pinrou [Century] *see* 7464
Pinus Montana Oil *see* 6791
Pinus Pumilio Oil *see* 6791
PIO *see* 7079
Pioglitazone, 7452
Pipacycline, 7453
Pipadone [Burroughs Wellcome] *see* 3337
Pipadox [Dagra] *see* 7465
Pipamazine, 7454
Pipamperone, 7455
Pipanol [Winthrop] *see* 9695
Pipazethate, 7456
Pipeacid [SIT] *see* 7460
Pipebuzone, 7457
Pipecolic Acid, 7458
Pipecolinic Acid *see* 7458
Pipecurium Bromide, 7459
Pipecuronium Bromide *see* 7459
Pipedac [Teofarma] *see* 7460
Pipemid [Gentili] *see* 7460
Pipemidic Acid, 7460
Pipenale [Fuso] *see* 7471
Pipenzolate Bromide, 7461
Pipenzolate Methylbromide *see* 7461
Pipenzolone Bromide *see* 7461
Piperacetazine, 7462
Piperacillin, 7463

Piperamic Acid *see* 7460
Piperate *see* 7464
Piperazate [Leeming] *see* 7464
Piperazidine *see* 7464
Piperazine, 7464
Piperazine Adipate, 7465
Piperazine-1,4-bis(N,N'-diethylenephos-phonediamide) *see* 3336
1,4-Piperazinebis(ethanesulfonic Acid) *see* 7479
Piperazine-N,N'-bis(2-ethanesulfonic Acid) *see* 7479
Piperazine Calcium Edathamil *see* 7464
1,4-Piperazinediethanesulfonic Acid *see* 7479
2,5-Piperazinedione, 7466
1,4-Piperazinediylbis[bis(1-aziridinyl)-phosphine Oxide] *see* 3336
1,1'-[1,4-Piperazinediylbis(imidocar-bonyl)]bis[3-(p-chlorophenyl)guani-dine] *see* 7398
N,N'-[1,4-Piperazinediylbis(2,2,2-tri-chloroethylidene)]bisformamide *see* 9691
Piperazine Estrone Sulfate *see* 3708
Piperazine Sultosylate *see* 8995
N-(1-Piperazinylacetyl)cyclohexylamine *see* 3695
1-Piperazinyl-4-methylenecarbonylcyclo-hexylamine *see* 3695
Piperic Acid, 7467
Piperidic Acid *see* 430
Piperidine, 7468
2-Piperidinecarboxylic Acid *see* 7458
3-Piperidinecarboxylic Acid *see* 6561
4-Piperidinecarboxylic Acid *see* 5189
2-Piperidineethanol 2-Aminobenzoate (Ester) *see* 7494
2-Piperidineethanol Anthranilate *see* 7494
1-Piperidineethanol Benzilate *see* 7471
3-Piperidino-4'-butoxypropiophenone *see* 3473
5-[3-(4-Piperidino-4-carbamoylpiperidi-no)propyl]-10,11-dihydro-5H-dibenz-[b,f]azepine *see* 1861
6-Piperidino-2,4-diaminopyrimidine 3-Oxide *see* 6203
2-(1-Piperidino)-4,4-diphenyl-5-hepta-none *see* 3337
6-Piperidino-4,4-diphenylheptan-3-one *see* 3337
3-Piperidino-1,1-diphenyl-1-propanol *see* 7741
2-(2-Piperidinoethoxy)ethyl 10H-Pyrido-[3,2-b][1,4]benzothiadiazine-10-car-boxylate *see* 7456
2-(2-Piperidinoethoxy)ethyl 10-Thia-1,9-diazaanthracene-10-carboxylate *see* 7456
2-(1-Piperidino)ethyl Benzilate *see* 7471
β-Piperidinoethyl-4-butoxyphenyl Ke-tone *see* 3473
2-Piperidinoethyl 3-Methylflavone-8-car-boxylate *see* 4096
2-Piperidinoethyl 3-Methyl-4-oxo-2-phenyl-4H-1-benzopyran-8-carboxy-late *see* 4096
N-(2-Piperidinoethyl)-N-(2-pyridylmeth-yl)aniline *see* 7404
3-(2-Piperidino-1-hydroxyethyl)-5-phen-ylisoxazole *see* 7177
2-Piperidinomethyl-1,4-benzodioxan *see* 7478
1-Piperidino-2-methyl-3-(p-tolyl)-3-pro-panone *see* 9522

3-Piperidino-1-phenyl-(Δ⁵-bicyclo[2.2.1]-hepten-2-yl)-1-propanol *see* 1233

3-Piperidino-1-phenyl-1-bicycloheptenyl-1-propanol *see* 1233
3-Piperidino-1-phenyl-(Δ^5-bicyclo[2.2.1]-hepten-2-yl)-1-propanol *see* 1233
1-Piperidino-2-(*N*-propionylanilino)propane *see* 7209
(*αS*)-*rel*-*α*-(2*R*)-2-Piperidinyl-2,8-bis(trifluoromethyl)-4-quinolinemethanol *see* 5801
N-(Piperidin-1-yl)-5-(4-chlorophenyl)-1-(2,4-dichlorophenyl)-4-methyl-1*H*-pyrazole-3-carboxamide *see* 8229
3-[2-(4-Piperidinyl)ethyl]-1*H*-indole *see* 4930
N-(2-Piperidinylmethyl)-2,5-bis(2,2,2-trifluoroethoxy)benzamide *see* 4098
1-(2-Piperidinyl)-2-propanone *see* 7072
3-(2-Piperidinyl)pyridine *see* 619
6-(1-Piperidinyl)-2,4-pyrimidinediamine 3-Oxide *see* 6203
Piperidione, 7469
Piperidolate, 7470
Piperidyl Amidone *see* 3337
α-(2-Piperidyl)benzhydrol *see* 7484
DL-*erythro*-*α*-2-Piperidyl-2,8-bis(trifluoromethyl)-4-quinolinemethanol *see* 5801
3-(1-Piperidyl)-1-cyclohexyl-1-phenyl-1-propanol Hydrochloride *see* 9695
3-(*N*-Piperidyl)-1,1-diphenyl-1-propanol *see* 7741
β-(2-Piperidyl)ethyl *o*-Aminobenzoate *see* 7494
β-Piperidylethyl Benzilate *see* 7471
2-(1-Piperidyl)ethyl *p*-Butoxyphenyl Ketone *see* 3473
2-(*β*-*N*-Piperidylethyl)-4,4-diphenyl-1,3-dioxolan-5-one Hydrochloride *see* 7483
2-(1-Piperidylmethyl)-1,4-benzodioxan *see* 7478
Piperilate, 7471
Piperine, 7472
Piperinic Acid *see* 7467
Piperinsäure (German) *see* 7467
Piperitone, 7473
Piperocaine, 7474
Piperonal, 7475
Piperonil [Lusofarmaco] *see* 7455
Piperonylaldehyde *see* 7475
Piperonyl Butoxide, 7476
Piperonylic Acid, 7477
10-[(4-Piperonyl-1-piperazinyl)acetyl]-phenothiazine *see* 3982
2-(4-Piperonyl-1-piperazinyl)pyrimidine *see* 7493
1-Piperonyl-4-(3,7,11-trimethyl-2,6,10-dodecatrienyl)piperazine *see* 7420
Piperoxan, 7478
(*E,E*)-1-Piperoylpiperidine *see* 7472
(*Z,Z*)-1-Piperoylpiperidine *see* 2049
Piperverm [Wild] *see* 7464
PIPES, 7479
Pipethanate *see* 7471
Pipitzahoic Acid *see* 7155
Pipizan Citrate [Merck & Co.] *see* 7464
Pipobroman, 7480
Piportil [Specia] *see* 7482
Piportil L4 [Specia] *see* 7482
Piportil M2 [Specia] *see* 7482
Piposulfan, 7481
Pipothiazine *see* 7482
Pipotiazine, 7482
Pipotiazine Palmitate *see* 7482
Pipotiazine Undecylenate *see* 7482

Pipoxolan Hydrochloride, 7483
Piperacid (syrup) [Universal Drug] *see* 7464
Pipracil [Wyeth] *see* 7463
Pipradol *see* 7484
Pipradrol, 7484
Pipram [RPR] *see* 7460
Pipril [Wyeth] *see* 7463
Piprinhydrinate *see* 3331
Piproxen *see* 6417
Piprozolin, 7485
Pipsissewa *see* 2057
Pipsyl Chloride, 7486
Piptal [Boehringer, Mann.] *see* 7461
Pipurin [Brocchieri] *see* 7460
Piracebral [Hexal] *see* 7487
Piracetam, 7487
Piracetrop [Holsten] *see* 7487
Piraldina [Bracco] *see* 7956
Pirarubicin, 7488
Pirate [BASF] *see* 2088
Pirbuterol, 7489
Pirecin [Yoshitomi] *see* 7903
Pirem [Gödecke] *see* 1833
Pirenoxine, 7490
Pirenzepine, 7491
Piretanide, 7492
Pirevan *see* 3353
Pirexyl [Pfizer] *see* 1049
Pirfenoxone *see* 7490
Piria's Acid *see* 6403
Piribedil, 7493
Piribenzil Methyl Sulfate *see* 1193
Piricef [CT] *see* 1984
Piridocaine, 7494
Piridolan [Janssen] *see* 7498
Pirifibrate, 7495
Pirilène [Cassenne] *see* 7956
Pirimicarb, 7496
Pirimiphos-ethyl, 7497
Pirimiphos-methyl *see* 7497
Pirimor [Syngenta] *see* 7496
Pirinitramide *see* 7498
Pirisudanol *see* 7991
Piritetrate *see* 5515
Piriton [GSK] *see* 2180
Piritramide, 7498
Piritrexim, 7499
Pirkam [DAK] *see* 7506
Pirlimycin, 7500
Pirmenol, 7501
Piroan [Towa Yakuhin] *see* 3346
Piroctone, 7502
Pirodal [SIT] *see* 7505
Piroflex [Lagap] *see* 7506
Piroheptine, 7503
Piromen, 7504
Piromidic Acid, 7505
Piroxicam, 7506
Piroxicam Cinnamate *see* 7506
Pirozadil, 7507
Pirsue [Pfizer] *see* 7500
Piscarol *see* 4885
Pisciol *see* 4885
Pistachia Galls *see* 5755
Pitavastatin, 7508
Pitayine *see* 8060
Pitchblende *see* 9855
Piteranometozine *see* 9970
Pithecolobine, 7509
Pitocin [Monarch] *see* 6979
Pitressin [Warner-Lambert] *see* 9938
Pituamin *see* 7510
Pituitary Growth Hormone *see* 8716
Pituitary Lactogenic Hormone *see* 7779

Pituitary Lipotropic Hormone *see* 5513
Pituitary, Posterior, 7510
Pituitrin [Parke-Davis] *see* 7510
Pivacef [Firma] *see* 7513
Pivadorm [Specia] *see* 1397
Pival [Kilgore] *see* 7444
Pivaldione *see* 7444
Pivalephrine [Santen] *see* 3338
Pivalic Acid, 7511
Pivalone [Jouveinal] *see* 9484
2-Pivaloyl-1,3-indandione *see* 7444
N-[*o*-(*p*-Pivaloyloxybenzene)sulfonylaminobenzoyl]glycine *see* 8558
Pivaloyloxymethyl D-*α*-Aminobenzylpenicillinate *see* 7512
Pivaloyloxymethyl Ampicillinate *see* 7512
Pivaloyloxymethyl 6-[(Hexahydro-1*H*-azepin-1-yl)methyleneamino]penicillanate *see* 390
Pivalyl Valone [Kilgore] *see* 7444
Pivalyl Indandione *see* 7444
2-Pivalyl-1,3-indandione *see* 7444
Pivalyn [Kilgore] *see* 7444
Pivamdinocillin *see* 390
Pivampicillin, 7512
Pivcefalexin, 7513
Pivcephalexin *see* 7513
Pivmecillinam *see* 390
Pivot [BASF] *see* 4907
Pix [BASF] *see* 5857
Pixalbol *see* 2426
Pixantrone, 7514
PIXY321 *see* 4995
Pizotifan *see* 7515
Pizotifen *see* 7515
Pizotyline, 7515
PJ-185 *see* 5571
PK-10169 *see* 3588
PK-26124 *see* 8223
PKC-412 *see* 6185
PKhNB *see* 8080
PK-Merz [Merz] *see* 374
PLA *see* 5338
Plac Out [Bernabo] *see* 2091
Placidyl [Abbott] *see* 3729
Plactamin [Morishita] *see* 7737
Plactidil [Novartis] *see* 7407
Plafibride, 7516
Planadalin *see* 1831
Planate [Mallinckrodt] *see* 2399
Plancol [Chugai] *see* 4787
Plandom [Nihon Nohyaku] *see* 3135
Planete [Zeneca] *see* 4681
Planetol *see* 6017
Planocaine [M & B] *see* 7757
Planochrome *see* 5867
Planofix [Hortichem] *see* 6371
Planoform *see* 1512
Planomycin *see* 4066
Planovin [Novo] *see* 5805
Planphylline [Viatris] *see* 465
Plantago Seed, 7517
Plantain Seed *see* 7517
Plant Amine Oxidase *see* 6247
Plantisul, 7518
Planum [Farmitalia] *see* 9133
Plaquenil Sulfate [Winthrop] *see* 4818
Plasdone [ISP] *see* 7697
Plasil [Lepetit] *see* 6143
Plasmalogens, 7519
Plasmasteril [Fresenius] *see* 4673
Plasma Thromboplastin Antecedent *see* 3924
Plasma Thromboplastin Component *see* 3922

Plasma Trypsinogen *see* 7521
Plasmin, 7520
Plasminogen, 7521
Plasminogen Activator (Desmodus Rotundus Isoform α1 Protein Moiety Reduced) *see* 3459
Plasminokinase *see* 8825
Plasmochin *see* 7001
Plasmocid, 7522
Plasmoquine *see* 7001
Plastenan [Isopharm] *see* 45
Plaster of Paris *see* 1706
Plastoquinone 9 *see* 7523
Plastoquinone 45 *see* 7523
Plastoquinone A *see* 7523
Plastoquinones, 7523
Platamine [Montedison] *see* 2317
Platelet Activating Factor, 7524
Platelet Activation-Dependent Granule-External Membrane Protein *see* 8426
Platelet-Derived Growth Factor, 7525
Platelet Glycoprotein IIb/IIIa *see* 4988
Plath-Lyse [Génévrier] *see* 3071
Platiblastin [Farmitalia] *see* 2317
Platifillin *see* 7531
Platilon [Toyo] *see* 7567
Platinex [BMS] *see* 2317
Platinic Ammonium Chloride *see* 548
Platinic Chloride, 7526
Platinic Oxide, 7527
Platinic Potassium Chloride *see* 7636
Platinol [BMS] *see* 2317
Platinous Ammonium Chloride *see* 549
Platinous Barium Cyanide *see* 991
Platinous Chloride, 7528
Platinous Lithium Cyanide *see* 5542
Platinous Potassium Chloride *see* 7682
Platinous Potassium Cyanide *see* 7685
Platinous Thorium Cyanide *see* 9378
Platinoxan [Degussa] *see* 2317
Platinum, 7529
Platinum Dioxide *see* 7527
cis-Platinum II *see* 2317
Platistin [Farmitalia] *see* 2317
Platonin, 7530
Platonin J *see* 7530
Platosin [Pharmachemie] *see* 2317
Plattnerite *see* 5407
Platyphylline, 7531
Plaunotol, 7532
Plavix [Sanofi] *see* 2396
Plazolite *see* 1648
Ple-1053 *see* 922
Plebilin *see* 6928
Pleconaril, 7533
Plegicil [Sanofi] *see* 32
Plegine [Ayerst] *see* 7220
Plegomazin [Servier] *see* 2185
Plemocil [Farmitalia] *see* 2766
Plenastril [Protochemie] *see* 6967
Plenaxis [Praecis] *see* 3
Plendil [AstraZeneca] *see* 3953
Plenum [Syngenta] *see* 7950
Plenur [Ipsen] *see* 5527
Plesium [Chiesi] *see* 1432
Plesmet [Link] *see* 4039
Plessy's Green *see* 2227
Pletal [Otsuka] *see* 2277
Pleurisy Root *see* 828
Pleuromutilin, 7534
Pleurotin(e), 7535
Plexamine [Biodica] *see* 4720
Plexiglas *see* 5941
Plexol 201 *see* 1251
Plicamycin, 7536

Plicatic Acid, 7537
Plictran [Dow] *see* 2760
Plitican [Synthelabo] *see* 250
PLS *see* 7595
Pluchine *see* 1179
Plumbagin, 7538
Plumbago *see* 4539
Plumbic Fluoride *see* 5424
Plumbous Fluoride *see* 5408
Plumbous Oxide *see* 5413
Plumbous Plumbate *see* 5417
Plumericin, 7539
Plumieride, 7540
Pluracol E [BASF] *see* 7568
Plurimen [Viatris] *see* 8428
Pluripoietin *see* 4537
Pluronic F68 [BASF] *see* 7562
Pluronic L62 *see* 7562
Pluronic L101 [BASF] *see* 7562
Pluropon [Boehringer, Ing.] *see* 8532
Plutonium, 7541
PLV-2 *see* 3954
PM-150 *see* 9942
PM-92102 *see* 5275
PM-185184 *see* 8419
PMA *see* 7300
PMAC *see* 7300
PMAS *see* 7300
PMEA *see* 151
PMP *see* 5233
*i*PMPA *see* 4924
(*R*)-PMPA *see* 9146
PMSF, 7542
PMSG *see* 2216
PN *see* 8018
PN-200-110 *see* 5240
PN-205-033 *see* 5240
PN-205-034 *see* 5240
PNB *see* 6593
Pneumorel [Stroder] *see* 3999
PNU-100766 *see* 5504
PNU-140690 *see* 9459
PNU-151774E *see* 8315
PNU-166196 *see* 1449
PNU-180638E *see* 304
PNU-200583E *see* 9525
P.O. 12 [Biothérax] *see* 3590
Poast [BASF] *see* 8473
Pocan *see* 7391
Podocarpic Acid, 7543
Pododacric Acid, 7544
Podofilox *see* 7546
Podophyllic Acids, 7545
Podophyllin *see* 7547
Podophyllinic Acid *see* 7545
Podophyllinic Acid 2-Ethylhydrazide *see* 7545
Podophyllinic Acid Hydrazide *see* 7545
Podophyllinic Acid Lactone *see* 7546
Podophyllotoxin, 7546
Podophyllum, 7547
Podophyllum Resin *see* 7547
POE Alcohol Ethers *see* 7577
POE Fatty Acid Esters *see* 7578
POE (40) Monostearate *see* 7578
POE Sorbitan Esters *see* 7582
POE (20) Sorbitan Monooleate *see* 7582
POE (8) Stearate *see* 7578
Pogy Oil *see* 5836
Poi, 7548
Poison Black Cherry *see* 1025
Poison Elder *see* 7551
Poison Hemlock *see* 2506
Poison Ivy, 7549
Poison Nut *see* 6730

Poison Oak, 7550
Poison Parsley *see* 2506
Poison Sumac, 7551
Poison Tobacco *see* 4859
Poison Vine *see* 7549
Poke Root *see* 7391
L-Polamidon [HMR] *see* 5944
Polamin [Schering-Plough] *see* 2180
Polaprezinc, 7552
Polaramine [Schering-Plough] *see* 2180
Polaronil [Schering-Plough] *see* 2180
Polar Yellow [Ciba], 7553
Poldine Methylsulfate, 7554
Poleon [Sumitomo] *see* 6359
Polibutin [Juste] *see* 9699
Policosanol, 7555
Policresulen, 7556
Policydal [Eisai] *see* 8910
Polidexide, 7557
Polidocanol, 7558
Polifeprosan, 7559
Polifeprosan 20 *see* 7559
Polihexanide, 7560
Polimod [Poli] *see* 7419
Polishing Powder *see* 8778
Polistin T-Caps [Trommsdorff] *see* 1799
Pollakisu [Kodama] *see* 6955
Pollucite *see* 2008
Polmiror [Poli] *see* 6532
Polo [Novartis Agro] *see* 2969
Polonium, 7561
Poloxamer 182 *see* 7562
Poloxamer 188 *see* 7562
Poloxamer 331 *see* 7562
Poloxamers, 7562
Poly *see* 8697
Polyacrylonitrile *see* 6870
Poly(allylamin-co-*N,N'*-diallyl-1,3-di-amino-2-hydroxypropane) *see* 8474
Polyamide *see* 6733
Polyaminopropylbiguanide *see* 7560
Polyanetholesulfonic Acid Sodium Salt *see* 8666
Polyanhydroglucuronic Acid *see* 6939
Poly[1,3-bis(*p*-carboxyphenoxy)propane-sebacic Acid] *see* 7559
Polybrene *see* 4682
Polybrominated Biphenyls, 7563
Polybromobiphenyls *see* 7563
Poly(butyl 2-Cyanoacrylate) *see* 1565
Poly(carbon monofluoride) *see* 4540
Poly-*trans*-[(2-carboxyethyl)germasesquioxane] *see* 7795
Polycell *see* 1829
Polychlorinated Biphenyls, 7564
Poly(2-chloro-1,3-butadiene) *see* 6461
Polychlorocamphene *see* 9557
Polychloroprene *see* 6461
Polychol [Croda] *see* 7577
Polychrome *see* 3698
Polycidine *see* 2913
Polycillin [BMS] *see* 586
Polycillin-N [BMS] *see* 586
Polyclar [ISP] *see* 7697
Polydatin *see* 8158
Polydextrose, 7565
Poly(dicarbon monofluoride) *see* 4540
Poly[2-(diethylamino)ethyl] Polyglycerylene Dextran Hydrochloride *see* 7557
Polydimethylsiloxane *see* 3215
Polyestradiol Phosphate, 7566
Polyetherin A *see* 6541
Poly(ethyl 2-Cyanoacrylate) *see* 3787
Polyethylene, 7567
Polyethylene Glycol, 7568

Polyethylene Glycol 200 *see* 7568
Polyethylene Glycol 400 *see* 7568
Polyethylene Glycol 600 *see* 7568
Polyethylene Glycol 1500 *see* 7568
Polyethylene Glycol 4000 *see* 7568
Polyethylene Glycol 6000 *see* 7568
Polyethylene Glycol Esters of Fatty Acids *see* 7578
Polyethylene Glycol Fatty Alcohol Ethers *see* 7577
Polyethylene Glycol *p*-Isooctylphenyl Ether *see* 6761
Polyethylene Glycol (9) Monododecyl Ether *see* 7558
Polyethylene Glycol 400 Monostearate *see* 7578
Polyethylene Glycol-polypropylene Glycol Block Copolymer *see* 7562
Polyethyleneglycols Mono(nonylphenyl) Ether *see* 6677
Polyethylene Sodium Sulfonate *see* 5617
Polyethylene Terephthalates, 7569
Polyferon [Biogen] *see* 4992
Poly-G [Olin] *see* 7568
L-Polyglutamic Paclitaxel *see* 6983
Poly(Glycidyl Methacrylate-co-Ethyl Acrylate) *see* 2514
Polyglycol E [Dow] *see* 7568
Polygodial, 7570
Polygris [Essex] *see* 4549
PolyHeme [Northfield] *see* 7572
Polyhexamethylene Biguanide Hydrochloride *see* 7560
Polyhexanide *see* 7560
Poly[imino-1,4-butanediylimino(1,6-dioxo-1,6-hexanediyl)] *see* 6735
Poly(iminocarbonimidoyliminocarbonimidoylimino-1,6-hexanediyl) Hydrochloride *see* 7560
Poly(iminocarbonylpentamethylene) *see* 6734
Poly[imino(1-oxo-1,6-hexanediyl)] *see* 6734
Poly I . Poly (C₁₂U) *see* 588
Poly(isobutyl 2-Cyanoacrylate) *see* 5140
Poly(lactic Acid) *see* 5338
Polylysine, 7571
Polymannuronic Acid *see* 242
Polymeric Sodium Metaphosphate *see* 5647
Polymerized Pyridoxylated Hemoglobin, 7572
Polymer of *N,N,N',N'*-Tetramethylhexamethylenediamine and Trimethylene Bromide *see* 4682
Polymetatelluric Acid *see* 9120
Poly(methyl 2-Cyanoacrylate) *see* 6046
Polymore [Unicrop] *see* 3078
Polymorphonuclear Elastase *see* 3535
Polymox [BMS] *see* 577
Polymyxin, 7573
Polymyxin B *see* 7573
Polymyxin B₁ *see* 7573
Polymyxin B₂ *see* 7573
Polymyxin D *see* 7573
Polymyxin D₁ *see* 7573
Polymyxin D₂ *see* 7573
Polymyxin E *see* 2479
Polymyxin E₁ *see* 2479
Polymyxin E₂ *see* 2479
Polymyxin F *see* 7573
Polymyxin K *see* 7573
Polymyxin M *see* 7573
Polymyxin P *see* 7573
Polymyxin S₁ *see* 7573

Polymyxin T₁ *see* 7573
Polynoxylin, 7574
Poly(octyl Cyanoacrylate) *see* 6766
Polyoxidonium, 7575
Polyoxin A *see* 7576
Polyoxin AL *see* 7576
Polyoxin B *see* 7576
Polyoxins, 7576
Poly[1-(2-oxo-1-pyrrolidinyl)ethylene] *see* 7697
Polyoxyaluminum Acetylsalicylate *see* 309
Polyoxyethylene Alcohols, 7577
Polyoxyethylene (20) Cetyl Ether *see* 7577
Polyoxyethylene Fatty Acid Esters, 7578
Polyoxyethylene Lauryl Ether *see* 7558
Polyoxyethylene(*n*)nonylphenyl Ether *see* 6677
Polyoxyethylene Sorbitan Esters *see* 7582
Polyoxyethylene (20) Sorbitan Monooleate *see* 7582
Polyoxyethylene (40) Stearate *see* 7578
Polyoxyl 8 Stearate *see* 7578
Polyoxyl 40 Stearate *see* 7578
Polyoxymethylene *see* 7025
Poly[oxy(1-methyl-2-oxo-1,2-ethanediyl)] *see* 5338
Polypeptide β₁ *see* 9405
Polyphase P-100 [Kop-Coat] *see* 5069
Polyphenolase *see* 9838
Polyphenoloxidase *see* 9838
Polyphlogin *see* 2288
Polyphosphazenes, 7579
Polyphosphoric Acid, 7580
Polyplasdone XL [ISP] *see* 7697
Polypodine A *see* 3491
Polypropylene, 7581
Poly(rI) . Poly[r(C₁₂U)ₙ] *see* 588
Polysaccharide B-1459 *see* 10057
Polysaccharide S-60 *see* 4383
Poly SFH-P *see* 7572
Poly-Solv DPM [Olin] *see* 3344
Polysorbate 80 *see* 7582
Polysorbates, 7582
Polystichalbin *see* 209
Polystichin *see* 846
Polystichocitrin *see* 4090
Polystictine *see* 2296
Polystyrene *see* 8860
Polysulfide Rubber *see* 9339
Polytef *see* 7583
Polytergent B [Olin] *see* 6677
Polytergent G [Union Carbide] *see* 6761
Polytetrafluoroethylene, 7583
Polytetrafluoroethylene Resin *see* 7583
Poly(tetramethyleneadipamide) *see* 6735
Poly(*N,N,N',N'*-tetramethyl-*N*-trimethylenehexamethylenediammonium Dibromide) *see* 4682
Polythene [DuPont] *see* 7567
Polythiazide, 7584
Polytrim [Wellcome] *see* 7573
Polyvidone *see* 7697
Polyvinyl Alcohol, 7585
Polyvinyl Chloride, 7586
Polyvinylpolypyrrolidone *see* 7697
Poly(4-vinylpyridine-*N*-oxide) *see* 7948
Polyvinylpyrrolidone *see* 7697
Polyvinylpyrrolidone-iodine Complex *see* 7698
Polyviol [Wacker] *see* 7585
Pomarsol [Bayer] *see* 9371
Pomarsol Z [Bayer] *see* 10172
POMC *see* 7791

Pomegranate, 7587
Ponalar [Parke-Davis] *see* 5798
Ponalide [Novartis] *see* 3756
Ponasterone A, 7588
Ponasterones *see* 7588
Ponazuril, 7589
Ponceau 3R, 7590
Ponceau SX, 7591
Poncho [Bayer CropSci.] *see* 2414
Poncuronium Bromide (rescinded USAN) *see* 7007
Poncyl-FP [Takeda] *see* 4549
Ponderal [Servier] *see* 3973
Ponderax [Selpharm] *see* 3973
Ponderex [Robins] *see* 3973
Pondimin [Robins] *see* 3973
Pondinil [Roche] *see* 5799
Pondinol [Roche] *see* 5799
Pondocil [Leo Pharm] *see* 7512
Pondocillin [Leo Pharm] *see* 7512
Pondocillina [Sigma-Tau] *see* 7512
Ponoxylan [Berk] *see* 7574
Ponsinomycin *see* 6204
Ponstan [Pfizer] *see* 5798
Ponstel [Warner-Lambert] *see* 5798
Ponstyl [Parke-Davis] *see* 5798
Pontal [Parke-Davis] *see* 5798
Pontamine White BR *see* 1315
Ponticin *see* 918
Pontocaine Hydrochloride [Sanofi Winthrop] *see* 9188
P.O.P. *see* 7044
POP *see* 4650
Popotillo *see* 3607
Poppy Capsules, 7592
Poppy Heads *see* 7592
Poppy Oil, 7593
Poppy-seed Oil *see* 7593
Populin, 7594
Populnetin *see* 5274
Populoside *see* 7594
POR-8 *see* 6873
Poractant Alfa, 7595
Porcelain Clay *see* 5282
Porcilene [Syntex] *see* 3995
Porcine Motilin *see* 6283
Porcine Somatotropin *see* 8716
Pore-forming Protein *see* 7159
Porfimer Sodium, 7596
Porfiromycin, 7597
Porofor-57 *see* 918
Porofor BSH [Bayer], 7598
Porphin *see* 7599
Porphine, 7599
21*H*,23*H*-Porphine *see* 7599
Porphobilinogen, 7600
Porphyrins *see* 7599
Porphyropsin, 7601
Portolac [Zyma] *see* 5340
Posaconazole, 7602
Posatirelin, 7603
Posedrine [Merck KGaA] *see* 1018
Posicor [Roche] *see* 6173
Posicycline [Alcon] *see* 6976
Posifenicol [Ursapharm] *see* 909
Posiformin [Ursapharm] *see* 1199
Posorutin [Ursapharm] *see* 9789
Posse [FMC] *see* 1826
Possipione [Recordati] *see* 7044
Postacton *see* 5630
Postafen [UCB] *see* 1464, 5777
Post-γ-globulin *see* 2778
Potaba [Glenwood] *see* 7606
Potasan *see* 4855
Potasoral [Bago] *see* 4456

Powder of Algaroth *see* 693
Powmil [Sumitomo] *see* 3109
PP-009 *see* 4116
PP-062 *see* 7496
PP-148 *see* 7031
PP-149 *see* 3740
PP-192 *see* 4117
PP-211 *see* 7497
PP-321 *see* 2758
PP-333 *see* 6984
PP-383 *see* 2767
PP-450 *see* 4214
PP-511 *see* 7497
PP-523 *see* 4681
PP-557 *see* 7180
PP-581 *see* 1379
PP-588 *see* 1494
PP-604 *see* 9564
PP-618 *see* 1498
PP-675 *see* 3217
PP-910 *see* 7031
PP-993 *see* 9111
PPACK, 7699
PPD *see* 9805
PPDA *see* 5108
P. P. Factor *see* 6525
PPG [Bago] *see* 7555
PPHF *see* 6821
PPI-149 *see* 3
PPL *see* 7101
PPN1011 *see* 9247
L-PPT *see* 7339
PQ-9 *see* 7523
PQs *see* 7523
PR-82/3 *see* 22
PR-934-423A *see* 8130
Practolol, 7700
Practon [Pfizer] *see* 8760
Pradif [Boehringer, Ing.] *see* 9049
Pradofloxacin, 7701
Praecicalm [Molimin] *see* 7130
Praeciglucon [Pfleger] *see* 4478
Praequine *see* 7001
Pragman Gelee [Milanfarma] *see* 9523
Pragmazone [UPSA] *see* 9579
Pragmoline [Specia] *see* 86
Praiden [Italchemie] *see* 1432
Prajmaline, 7702
Prajmaline Bitartrate *see* 7702
Prajmalium *see* 7702
Pralidoxime Chloride, 7703
Pralidoxime Iodide *see* 7703
Pralidoxime Mesylate *see* 7703
Prallethrin, 7704
Prälumin *see* 2711
Pramace [AstraZeneca] *see* 8103
Pramidex [Hospira] *see* 9507
Pramiel [Teikoku Kagaku] *see* 6143
Pramil [Hässle] *see* 8420
Pramindole (obsolete) *see* 5075
Pramipexole, 7705
Pramiracetam, 7706
Pramitol [Makhteshim-Agan] *see* 7788
Pramiverin, 7707
Pramiverine *see* 7707
Pramlintide, 7708
Pramocaine *see* 7709
Pramoxine, 7709
Prandase [Bayer] *see* 18
Prandin [Novo Nordisk] *see* 8136
Prandiol [Bottu] *see* 3346
Pranlukast, 7710
Pranoprofen, 7711
Pranosina [Newport] *see* 4976
Pranosine [Newport] *see* 4976

Pranoxen [Napp] *see* 6417
Prantal [Schering] *see* 3306
Präparat 5968 *see* 4763
Praseodymium, 7712
Prasterone *see* 2871
Pratensein, 7713
Praticef [Zambon] *see* 1929
Pravachol [BMS] *see* 7714
Pravacilin [Recordati] *see* 5925
Pravaselect [Menarini] *see* 7714
Pravasin [BMS] *see* 7714
Pravastatin Sodium, 7714
Pravidel [Novartis] *see* 1416
Praxadium [Bottu] *see* 6691
Praxilene [Lipha] *see* 6353
Praxiten [Teofarma] *see* 6926
Praxiten SP [Wyeth] *see* 387
Prazene [Pfizer] *see* 7715
Prazepam, 7715
Prazine [Wyeth] *see* 7783
Prazinil [Specia] *see* 1861
Praziquantel, 7716
Prazol [Corvi] *see* 3695
Prazosin, 7717
Prean [Chemil] *see* 5773
Prebediolone Acetate *see* 77
Precedex [Abbott] *see* 2946
Precef [BMS] *see* 1931
Preceptin [Ortho] *see* 6761
Precipitated Bismuth *see* 1257
Precipitated Calcium Carbonate *see* 1657
Precipitated Calcium Sulfate *see* 1706
Precipitated Chalk *see* 1657
Precipitated Silica *see* 8490
Precipitated Sulfur *see* 8977
Precipité Blanc *see* 5894
Precocene I *see* 7718
Precocene II *see* 7718
Precocenes, 7718
Precor [Wellmark] *see* 5983
Precortisyl [Aventis] *see* 7721
Precose [Bayer] *see* 18
Precursor to ACTH-LPH-β-endorphin
    see 7791
Pred Forte [Allergan] *see* 7721
Pred Mild [Allergan] *see* 7721
Predalon [Organon] *see* 2216
Predef [Pfizer] *see* 5174
Predenema [Forest] *see* 7721
Predfoam [Pharmax] *see* 7721
Prednacinolone *see* 2928
Prednicarbate, 7719
Prednicen [Central Pharm.] *see* 7721
Prednimustine, 7720
Prednisolone, 7721
Prednisolone 21-[4-[*p*-[Bis(2-chloroeth-yl)amino]phenyl]butyrate] *see* 7720
Prednisolone 17-Ethylcarbonate 21-Pro-pionate *see* 7719
Prednisolone 21-Pivalate *see* 7721
Prednisolone Sodium Metasulfobenzoate
    see 7721
Prednisolone Sodium Phosphate *see* 7721
Prednisolone Sodium Succinate *see* 7721
Prednisolone Steaglate *see* 7721
Prednisolone Tebutate *see* 7721
Prednisolone 17-Valerate *see* 7723
Prednisone, 7722
Prednitop [BASF] *see* 7719
Prednival, 7723
Prednylidene, 7724
Predonine [Shionogi] *see* 7721
Predsol [UCB] *see* 7721
Prefamone [Dexo] *see* 3127
Preferid [Yamanouchi] *see* 1468

Prefrin [Allergan] *see* 7286
Pregabalin, 7725
Preglandin [Ono] *see* 4387
Pregna-1,4-diene-11β,21-diol-3,20-di-one[17α,16α-*d*]-2′-methyloxazoline 21-Acetate *see* 2862
1,4-Pregnadiene-17α,21-diol-3,11,20-trione *see* 7722
Pregna-4,17(20)-diene-3,16-dione *see* 4573
(9β,10α)-Pregna-4,6-diene-3,20-dione *see* 3474
10α-Pregna-4,6-diene-3,20-dione *see* 3474
1,4-Pregnadiene-3,20-dione-11β,17α,-21-triol *see* 7721
Δ^{1,4}-Pregnadiene-16-methylene-11β,-17α,21-triol-3,20-dione *see* 7724
1,4-Pregnadiene-11β,17α,21-triol-3,20-dione *see* 7721
(17α)-Pregna-2,4-dien-20-yno[2,3-*d*]-isoxazol-17-ol *see* 2812
Pregnancy Urine Extract *see* 2216
Pregnane, 7726
(5α)-Pregnane *see* 266
5β-Pregnane *see* 7726
Pregnanediol, 7727
(3α,5α,20*R*)-Pregnane-3,20-diol *see* 268
(3β,5α,20*R*)-Pregnane-3,20-diol *see* 270
(3α,5β,20*S*)-Pregnane-3,20-diol *see* 267
(3α,5α,20*S*)-Pregnane-3,20-diol *see* 7727
(3β,5α,20*S*)-Pregnane-3,20-diol *see* 269
5α-Pregnane-3α,20α-diol *see* 267
5α-Pregnane-3β,20α-diol *see* 269
3,20-Pregnanedione, 7728
(5α)-Pregnane-3,20-dione *see* 272
(5β)-Pregnane-3,20-dione *see* 7728
11,20-Pregnanedione-3α,17α,21-triol
    see 9210
(3α,5β,11β,20*S*)-Pregnane-3,11,17,20,-21-pentol *see* 2541
5β-Pregnane-3α,11β,17,20α,21-pentol
    see 2541
5β-Pregnane-3α,11β,17,20β,21-pentol
    see 2541
3α,17α,20α,21-Pregnanetetrol-11-one
    see 2542
3α,17α,21-Pregnanetriol-11,20-dione
    see 9210
Pregnanolone *see* 7729
Pregnan-3α-ol-20-one, 7729
5α-Pregnan-3α-ol-20-one *see* 275
Pregnant Mare Serum Gonadotropin *see* 2216
4-Pregnene-11β,21-diol-3,20-dione *see* 2538
4-Pregnene-16α,17α-diol-3,20-dione *see* 239
4-Pregnene-17α,21-diol-3,20-dione *see* 2932
5-Pregnene-3β,21-diol-20-one 21-Ace-tate *see* 77
Δ^{4}-Pregnene-17α,21-diol-3,11,20-trione
    see 2539
Δ^{4}-Pregnene-3,20-dione *see* 7773
Pregn-4-ene-3,20-dione *see* 7773
4-Pregnene-11β,17α,20β,21-tetrol-3-one, 7730
4-Pregnene-11β,17α,21-triol-3,20-dione
    see 4787
4-Pregnene-17α,20β,21-triol-3,11-dione, 7731
4-Pregnene-17α,20β,21-triol-3-one, 7732
17α-Pregnenetriolone *see* 7732

Pregneninolone *see* 3741
4-Pregnen-17α-ol-3,20-dione *see* 4839
4-Pregnen-21-ol-3,20-dione *see* 2900
Pregnenolone, 7733
Δ⁵-Pregnen-3β-ol-20-one *see* 7733
Δ⁴-Pregnen-21-ol-3,11,20-trione *see* 2869
Pregnesin [Serono] *see* 2216
Pregnyl [Organon] *see* 2216
Prehemataminic Acid *see* 6483
Prelay [Sankyo] *see* 9769
Prelis [Novartis] *see* 6151
Prelital *see* 1506
Prelog-Djerassi Lactone, 7734
(+)-Prelog-Djerassi Lactonic Acid *see* 7734
Preludin [Boehringer, Ing.] *see* 7237
Premarin [Wyeth] *see* 2508
Premarrubiin *see* 5754
Premerge [Dow] *see* 3287
Premier [Bayer CropSci.] *see* 4910
Prempar [Duphar] *see* 8237
Premsyn PMS [Chattem] *see* 7000
Prenalex [Itherapia] *see* 9173
Prenalterol, 7735
Prenazone *see* 4012
Prenormine [AstraZeneca] *see* 859
Prenoxdiazine Hydrochloride, 7736
Prent [Bayer] *see* 19
Prentox [Prentiss] *see* 7476
Prenylamine, 7737
4-Prenyl-1,2-diphenyl-3,5-dioxopyrazo-lidine *see* 4012
4-Prenyl-1,2-diphenyl-3,5-pyrazoli-dinedione *see* 4012
Prep [Bayer CropSci.] *see* 3732
Pre-Par [Duphar] *see* 8237
Preparation K *see* 3384
Prepared Calcium Carbonate *see* 1657
Prepared Chalk *see* 1657
Pre-Pen [Kremers-Urban] *see* 7101
Prephenic Acid, 7738
Prepidil [Pharmacia & Upjohn] *see* 7877
Prepulsid [Janssen-Cilag] *see* 2316
Pres [Boehringer, Ing.] *see* 3567
Presamine [USV] *see* 4920
Pre-Sate [Warner-Lambert] *see* 2182
Prescal [Novartis] *see* 5240
Presdate [Alfa] *see* 5329
Presenilin 1 *see* 7739
Presenilin 2 *see* 7739
Presenilins, 7739
Preservex [BMS] *see* 22
Presfersul *see* 4057
Presidon *see* 7995
Presinex [Pliva] *see* 2924
Presinol [Bayer] *see* 6055
Presmode [Sankyo] *see* 1631
Pressalolo [Locatelli] *see* 5329
Pressamina [Zambeletti] *see* 3264
Pressionorm [HMR] *see* 4401
Pressunic [Unipharm] *see* 3169
Pressural [Polifarma] *see* 4935
Pressyn [Ferring] *see* 9938
Presuren *see* 4823
Prethcamide *see* 2591
Pretilachlor, 7740
Pretor [Aventis] *see* 1933
Pretyrosine *see* 790
Prevacid [TAP] *see* 5362
Prevangor *see* 7112
Preventol G-D *see* 3071
Preveon [Gilead] *see* 151
Prevex [Schering] *see* 3953
Previcox [Merial] *see* 4087

Previcur [Bayer CropSci.] *see* 7798
Previscan [Procter & Gamble] *see* 4134
Prexan [Lafare] *see* 6417
Prexidil [Bioindustria] *see* 6203
Prexige [Novartis] *see* 5601
Prezios [Chugai] *see* 5760
Priadel [Sanofi-Aventis] *see* 5527
Prialt [Elan] *see* 10122
Priamide [Janssen] *see* 5202
Priaxim [Ravizza] *see* 4148
Priceite *see* 1652
Pridinol, 7741
Pridinol Mesylate *see* 7741
Prifinium Bromide, 7742
Priftin [Aventis] *see* 8219
Prilagin [Gambar] *see* 6178
Prilan [IPESA] *see* 7806
Prilocaine, 7743
Prilon [Cassenne] *see* 6944
Prilosec [AstraZeneca] *see* 6845
Primacor [Sanofi-Synthelabo] *see* 6197
Primalan [Inava] *see* 5864
Primamycin *see* 4609
Primaquine, 7744
Primary Ammonium Phosphate *see* 543
Primary Calcium Phosphate *see* 1693
Primary Isoamyl Alcohol *see* 5195
Primary Magnesium Phosphate *see* 5682
Primary Sodium Phosphate *see* 8660
Primatene Mist [Wyeth] *see* 3619
Primaverine *see* 7707
Primaxin [Merck & Co.] *see* 4919
Primbactam [Menarini] *see* 925
Primcillin [AstraZeneca] *see* 7100
Primeral [Master] *see* 6417
Primeverose, 7745
Primexin [Wander] *see* 4218
Primicid [Zeneca] *see* 7497
Primidone, 7746
Primisulfuron-methyl, 7747
Primobolan-Depot [Schering AG] *see* 5967
Primobolan Tablets [Schering AG] *see* 5967
Primocarcin, 7748
Primofax [Rhône-Poulenc] *see* 6719
Primofenac [Streuli] *see* 3081
Primogonyl [Schering] *see* 2216
Primogyn C [Schering AG] *see* 3734
Primolut N [Schering AG] *see* 6697
Primolut-Nor [Schering AG] *see* 6697
Primonabol *see* 5967
Primonabol Depot *see* 5967
Primosiston [Schering AG] *see* 6697
Primoteston [Schering AG] *see* 9180
Primperan [Delagrange] *see* 6143
Primulaverin, 7749
Primulidin *see* 5715
Primulin *see* 5715
Primus [Dow AgroSci.] *see* 4108
Primycin, 7750
Prinadol [SK & F] *see* 7218
Princep [Syngenta] *see* 8533
Prince's Feather *see* 376
Prince's Pine *see* 2057
Principen [BMS] *see* 586
Prinil [Merck & Co.] *see* 5516
Prinivil [Merck & Co.] *see* 5516
Prinodolol *see* 7443
Prinomastat, 7751
Prinzide [Merck & Co.] *see* 5516
Priodax [Schering] *see* 5026
Prioderm *see* 5700
Priomicina [San Carlo] *see* 4254
Priscol [Novartis] *see* 9506

Priscoline [Novartis] *see* 9506
Prism [Valent] *see* 2349
Pristacin *see* 2032
Pristane, 7752
Pristinamycin, 7753
Pristinamycin IA *see* 7753
Pristinamycin II_A *see* 10004
Pritor [GSK] *see* 9129
Privaprol [Lepetit] *see* 5585
Privenal *see* 4704
Privine [Novartis] *see* 6368
PRN *see* 7316
Pro *see* 7780
Pro Dorm [Synthelabo] *see* 5579
Proaccelerin *see* 3919
Pro-Actidil [Wellcome] *see* 9746
ProAmatine [Roberts] *see* 6184
Proamipide *see* 8124
Proazamine *see* 7786
Probamyl [Continental Pharma] *see* 5862
Proban *see* 2785
Pro-Banthine [Roberts] *see* 7805
Probecid [Astra] *see* 7754
Proben [SCS] *see* 7754
Probenecid, 7754
Probilin [Gödecke; Warner-Lambert] *see* 7485
Probolin [Tennessee Pharm.] *see* 5950
Probon [Chinoin] *see* 8225
Probonal [Medipolar] *see* 8225
Probucol, 7755
Pro-Bumin [Probitas] *see* 8468
Probutylin [Rorer] *see* 7757
Procadil [Recordati] *see* 7759
Procainamide Hydrochloride, 7756
Procaine, 7757
Procaine Amide Hydrochloride *see* 7756
Procaine Benzylpenicillinate *see* 7097
Procaine Penicillin G *see* 7097
Procalmadiol *see* 5862
Procalmidol *see* 5862
Procamide [Sintesa] *see* 7756
Procanbid [Parke-Davis] *see* 7756
Procan-SR [Parke-Davis] *see* 7756
Procapan [Panray] *see* 7756
Procaptan [Stroder] *see* 7170
Procarbazine, 7758
Procardia [Pfizer] *see* 6528
Procaspase-1 *see* 1884
Procaspase-3 *see* 1885
Procaspase-8 *see* 1886
Procaspase-9 *see* 1887
Procaterol, 7759
Procef [BMS] *see* 1942
Processine [Sanko] *see* 2305
Procetofen *see* 3978
Procetofene *see* 3978
Procetoken [Bernabo] *see* 3978
Prochloraz, 7760
Prochlorpemazine *see* 7761
Prochlorperazine, 7761
Prochlorperazine Mesylate *see* 7761
Procholon [Squibb] *see* 2868
Prociclide [Crinos] *see* 2861
Proclaim [Syngenta] *see* 3554
Proclival [Houdé] *see* 1472
Proclorperazine *see* 7761
Procodazole, 7762
Procollagen *see* 2480
Proconazole *see* 7818
Proconvertin *see* 3920
Procoralan [Servier] *see* 5247
Procorum [Knoll] *see* 4356
Procrit [Ortho Biotech] *see* 3688
Proctocort [Solvay] *see* 4787

Proctofoam-NS [Schwarz] *see* 7709
Procyanidins *see* 1902
Procyclidine, 7763
Procylin [Kaken] *see* 1152
Procymate, 7764
Procymidone, 7765
Procysteine [Baxter] *see* 6950
Procytox [Baxter] *see* 2747
Pro-Dafalgan [UPSA] *see* 7792
Prodectin [Gedeon Richter] *see* 7975
Prodel *see* 3474
Pro-Diaban [Bayer; Schering AG] *see* 4444
Prodiamine, 7766
Prodif [Pfizer] *see* 4122
Prodigiosin, 7767
Prodigiosine *see* 7767
Prodigy [Dow AgroSci.] *see* 5993
(±)-α-Prodine *see* 310
(±)-β-Prodine Hydrochloride *see* 310
Prodipine, 7768
Prodium [Breckenridge] *see* 7210
Prodlure, 7769
Producil [Merck & Co.] *see* 3525
Proendotel [Fidia] *see* 2405
Pro-Entra [Wellcome-Sumitomo] *see* 9746
Pro-Epanutin [Pfizer] *see* 4258
Profasi [Serono] *see* 2216
Profemin [Yamanouchi] *see* 4309
Profenamine *see* 3747
Profender [Bayer] *see* 3560
Profenid [RPR] *see* 5305
Profenofos, 7770
Profenon [Morishita] *see* 4106
Profenone *see* 7044
Profibrinolysin *see* 7521
Profilate [Alpha Ther.] *see* 3921
Profilnine [Alpha Ther.] *see* 3922
Proflavine, 7771
Proflavine Hemisulfate *see* 7771
Proflax [Merck & Co.] *see* 9444
Proflex [Novartis] *see* 4881
Proflox [Esteve] *see* 6291
Proformiphen *see* 7258
Profume [Dow AgroSci.] *see* 8981
Progabide, 7772
Progallin P [Nipa] *see* 7859
Proge [Mochida] *see* 4839
Progeril [Midy] *see* 3653
Progesic [Lilly] *see* 3980
Progestasert [Alza] *see* 7773
Progesterone, 7773
Progestogel [Besins-Iscovesco] *see* 7773
Progeston [Fuji] *see* 7773
Proglicem [Essex] *see* 3004
Proglumetacin, 7774
Proglumide, 7775
Proglycem [Schering] *see* 3004
Prograf [Fujisawa] *see* 9025
Program [Novartis] *see* 5595
Proguanil *see* 2090
Progynon B [Schering AG] *see* 3703
Progynon C [Schering AG] *see* 3734
Progynon Depot [Schering AG] *see* 3703
Progynova [Schering AG] *see* 3703
ProHance [BMS] *see* 4328
Proheart 6 [Fort Dodge] *see* 6290
Proheptatriene *see* 2713
Proheptazine, 7776
Prohexadione, 7777
Prohormo [Pharmar] *see* 5915
Proin [PRN] *see* 7307
Proinsulin, 7778
Prokarbol *see* 3279
Prokayvit Oral [BDH] *see* 5830

Proketazine [Wyeth] *see* 1860
Prokine [Hoechst-Roussel] *see* 4538
Prokrein [Tobishi] *see* 5279
Prolactin, 7779
Proladone [Abbott] *see* 6959
Prolastin [Bayer] *see* 719
Prolate [Stauffer] *see* 7336
Prolax *see* 5850
Prolene [Industrial Rayon] *see* 7581
Proleukin [Chiron] *see* 4994
Prolift [Pfizer] *see* 8125
Proline, 7780
Proline [Bayer CropSci.] *see* 7887
L-Proline *see* 7780
25-L-Proline-28-L-proline-29-L-proline-amylin (Human) *see* 7708
Prolintane, 7781
Prolixan [Siegfried] *see* 726
Prolixin [Apothecon] *see* 4189
Prolonium Iodide, 7782
Prolopa [Roche] *see* 1050
Proloprim [Wellcome] *see* 9709
Proluton [Schering AG] *see* 7773
Proluton Depot [Schering AG] *see* 4839
L-Prolyl-L-leucylglycinamide *see* 5813
Promac [Zeria] *see* 7552
PromAce [Fort Dodge] *see* 32
Promacid *see* 2185
Promactil [Combiphar] *see* 2185
Promanide *see* 4463
Promaquid [Rhône-Poulenc] *see* 4231
Promassolax *see* 6974
Promaxol [Otsuka] *see* 7759
Promazine, 7783
Promecon [Searle] *see* 1119
Promedol, 7784
α-Promedol *see* 7784
γ-Promedol *see* 7784
Promegestone, 7785
ProMem [Bayer] *see* 9623
Promensil [Novogen] *see* 9690
Promethazine, 7786
Promethazine Teoclate *see* 7786
Promethestrol *see* 5968
γ-Promethestrol *see* 5968
Promethium, 7787
Prometon *see* 7788
Prometone *see* 7788
Prometryn, 7789
Promid [Kaken] *see* 7775
Promidione *see* 5077
Promin [Parke-Davis] *see* 4463
Prominal *see* 5854
Promintic [Ayerst] *see* 6160
Promit [Pharmacia] *see* 2948
Promixin [Profile] *see* 2479
Promizole [Parke-Davis] *see* 9309
Promotil [Boehringer, Ing.] *see* 7781
Promotin [Nippon Chemiphar] *see* 5279
Promwill [Will-Pharma] *see* 7783
Pronamid *see* 7872
Prondol [Wyeth] *see* 5075
Pronestyl [BMS] *see* 7756
Pronethalol, 7790
Pronon [Yamanouchi] *see* 7794
Pronox [Reiss] *see* 2711
Prontamid [SIT] *see* 8899
Prontobario [Bracco] *see* 994
Prontocalcin [Dompé] *see* 1643
Prontosil, 8923
Prontosil Album *see* 8925
Prontosil Flavum *see* 8923
Prontosil Rubrum *see* 8923
Prontylin *see* 8925
Proopiocortin *see* 7791

Pro-opiomelanocortin, 7791
Propabloc [Azupharma] *see* 7840
Propacetamol, 7792
Propachlor, 7793
Propacil [Chugai] *see* 7869
Propaderm [GSK] *see* 1019
1,2-Propadiene-1,3-dione *see* 1815
Propafenone, 7794
Propagermanium, 7795
Propal *see* 5217
Propalin [Vétoquinol] *see* 7307
Propallylonal, 7796
Propamidine, 7797
Propaminodiphen *see* 7707
Propamocarb, 7798
Propanal *see* 7823
Propanamide *see* 7824
1-Propanamine *see* 7843
2-Propanamine *see* 5209
Propane, 7799
1-Propanearsonic Acid, 7800
Propanedial *see* 5709
1,2-Propanediamine *see* 7852
1,3-Propanedicarboxylic Acid *see* 4473
Propane-diethyl Sulfone *see* 8960
Propanedinitrile *see* 5711
Propanedioic Acid *see* 5710
Propanedioic Acid Bis(1,1-dimethyl-ethyl) Ester *see* 3034
Propanedioic Acid Diethyl Ester *see* 3823
Propanedioic Acid Dimethyl Ester *see* 6096
1,2-Propanediol *see* 7855
1,3-Propanediol *see* 9714
1,3-Propanediol Bis[α-(p-chlorophen-oxy)isobutyrate] *see* 8537
1,3-Propanediol Bis[2-(4-chlorophen-oxy)-2-methylpropionate] *see* 8537
1,2-Propanediol-3-(p-chlorophenoxy)-1-carbamate *see* 2179
1,3-Propanedithiol, 7801
1,1'-[1,3-Propanediylbis[(dimethylim-ino)-3,1-propanediyl]]bis[4-(3-meth-yl-2(3H)-benzothiazolylidene)methyl]Quinolinium Tetraiodide *see* 9308
4,4'-[1,3-Propanediylbis(oxy)]bisben-zenecarboximidamide *see* 7797
4,4'-[1,3-Propanediylbis(oxy)]bis(3-bromobenzenecarboximidamide) *see* 3024
Propanenitrile *see* 7827
Propanethial S-Oxide, 7802
1,2,3-Propanetricarboxylic Acid *see* 9622
1,2,3-Propanetricarboxylic Acid 1,1'-[1-(12-Amino-4,9,11-trihydroxy-2-methyltridecyl)-2-(1-methylpentyl)-1,2-ethanediyl] Ester *see* 4289
1,2,3-Propanetriol *see* 4484
1,2,3-Propanetriol 1-(4-Aminoben-zoate) *see* 4487
1,2,3-Propanetriol Diacetate *see* 2961
1,2,3-Propanetriol Monoacetate *see* 6242
1,2,3-Propanetriol, Mono(dihydrogen Phosphate) Calcium Salt (1:1) *see* 1670
1,2,3-Propanetriol Mono(dihydrogen Phosphate) Disodium Salt *see* 8622
1,2,3-Propanetriol Triacetate *see* 9589
1,2,3-Propanetriol Trinitrate *see* 6607
Propanidid, 7803
Propanil, 7804
Propanoic Acid *see* 7825
Propanoic Acid Anhydride *see* 7826

(±)-4,4'-Propylenedi-2,6-piperazine-
dione *see* 8123
Propylene Glycol, 7855
Propylene Oxide, 7856
Propylene Polymer *see* 7581
Propyl Ether, 7857
Propyl Ethyl-*n*-butylthiolcarbamate *see*
7061
Propylethylene *see* 7122
Propyl Formate, 7858
Propyl Gallate, 7859
n-Propyl Gallate *see* 7859
3-(4-Propylheptyl)-4-morpholineethanol
see 2879
Propylhexedrine, 7860
Propyl Hydride *see* 7799
Propyl *p*-Hydroxybenzoate *see* 7866
Propylic Alcohol *see* 7842
Propylidene Chloride, 7861
Propyl Iodide, 7862
Propyliodone, 7863
D-6-*n*-Propyl-8β-methylmercaptometh-
ylergoline *see* 7162
n-Propyl Nitrate, 7864
n-Propyl Nitrite, 7865
19-Propylorvinol *see* 3888
Propylparaben, 7866
Propyl Parasept [Tenneco] *see* 7866
2-Propylpentamide *see* 9914
2-Propylpentanamide *see* 9914
2-Propylpentanoic Acid *see* 9913
1-(α-Propylphenethyl)pyrrolidine *see*
7781
l-*N*-*n*-Propylpipecolic Acid-2,6-xylidide
see 8258
(*S*)-(−)-1-Propyl-2',6'-pipecoloxylidide
see 8258
2-*n*-Propyl-Δ¹-piperidine *see* 2502
(2*S*)-2-Propylpiperidine *see* 2505
(3*S*-*trans*)-6-Propyl-3-piperidinol *see*
7914
6-Propylpiperonyl Butyl Diethylene Glycol Ether *see* 7476
N-Propyl-1-propanamine *see* 3343
Propyl Propionate, 7867
2-Propyl-4-pyridinecarbothioamide *see*
7891
N-Propyl-*N*-4-pyridinyl-1*H*-indol-1-
amine *see* 1176
1-(Propyl-4-pyridylamino)indole *see*
1176
Propyl Sulfide, 7868
2-*n*-Propyl-3,4,5,6-tetrahydropyridine
see 2502
[5-(Propylthio)-1*H*-benzimidazol-2-yl]-
carbamic Acid Methyl Ester *see* 210
2-Propyl-4-thiocarbamoylpyridine *see*
7891
5-(Propylthio)-2-carbomethoxyamino-
benzimidazole *see* 210
2-Propylthioisonicotinamide *see* 7891
Propylthiouracil, 7869
6-Propyl-2-thiouracil *see* 7869
Propyl-Thyracil [Frosst] *see* 7869
1-[*N*-Propyl-*N*-[2-(2,4,6-trichlorophen-
oxy)ethyl]carbamoyl]imidazole *see*
7760
N-Propyl-*N*-[2-(2,4,6-trichlorophen-
oxy)ethyl]-1*H*-imidazole-1-carbox-
amide *see* 7760
(*E*)-10-Propyl-5,9-tridecadien-1-ol Acetate *see* 7870
10-Propyl-*trans*-5,9-tridecadienyl Acetate *see* 7870
Propylure, 7870

2-Propylvaleramide *see* 9914
2-Propylvaleric Acid *see* 9913
2-Propynoic Acid *see* 7821
2-Propynoic Acid Ethyl Ester *see* 3846
2-Propyn-1-ol *see* 7809
2-Propynyl (*R*)-2-[4-(5-Chloro-3-fluoro-
2-pyridyloxy)phenoxy]propionate *see*
2370
1-(2-Propynyl)cyclohexanol Carbamate
see 4698
1-(2-Propynyl)cyclohexyl Carbamate *see*
4698
(*R*)-*N*-2-Propynyl-1-indanamine *see* 8116
Propyon [Makhteshim-Agan] *see* 7836
Propyphenazone, 7871
Propyzamide, 7872
Proquamezine *see* 467
Proquazone, 7873
Prorenal [Dainippon] *see* 5490
Prorennin *see* 8134
Prosaponin B *see* 3696
Proscar [Merck & Co.] *see* 4082
Proscillan [Streuli] *see* 7874
Proscillaridin, 7874
Proscillaridin A *see* 7874
Proscillaridin-4-methyl Ether *see* 7874
Prosedar [Schering-Plough] *see* 8029
Proserine *see* 6464
Proserout [Funai] *see* 5780
Proseryl [Funai] *see* 5780
Prosolvin [Intervet] *see* 5610
ProSom [Abbott] *see* 3702
Pro-Sonil *see* 2711
Prosopis *see* 5914
Prostacyclin, 7875
Prostaglandin E₁, 7876
Prostaglandin E₂, 7877
Prostaglandin F₂ₐ, 7878
Prostaglandin I₂ *see* 7875
Prostaglandin(s), 7879
Prostaglandin X *see* 7875
Prostaherb [Cesra] *see* 6482
Prostal [Teikoku Zoki] *see* 2102
Prostalene, 7880
Prostandin [Ono] *see* 7876
Prostanoic Acid *see* 7879
Prostap [Wyeth] *see* 5457
Prostaphlin [Apothecon] *see* 6904
Prostar [AgrEvo] *see* 4212
Prostarex [Biorex] *see* 1212
Prostarmon F [Ono] *see* 7878
Prostasal [TAD] *see* 8556
ProstaScint *see* 1762
Prostavet [Gifavet] *see* 3871
Prostenoglycine *see* 8809
Prostetin [Takeda] *see* 6931
Prostianol *see* 5610
Prostide [Sigma-Tau] *see* 4082
Prostigmin [Roche] *see* 6464
Prostigmin (Amp.) [Roche] *see* 6464
Prostin/15M [Pfizer] *see* 1823
Prostin E₂ [Pharmacia & Upjohn] *see* 7877
Prostin VR [Pharmacia & Upjohn] *see*
7876
Prostivas [Pharmacia & Upjohn] *see* 7876
Prostrumyl *see* 6128
Prosulfuron, 7881
Prosultiamine, 7882
Prosynap [Janssen] *see* 5590
Protacine *see* 7774
Protactinium, 7883
Protactyl [Wyeth] *see* 7783
Protagent [Alcon-Thilo] *see* 7697
Protalba *see* 7899
Protamine Zinc Insulin *see* 4980

Protamone-D [Agri-Tech] *see* 9413
Protanabol *see* 6967
Protangix [Lefrancq] *see* 3346
Protara [Gensia] *see* 16
Protargin *see* 8527
Protargol [Winthrop] *see* 8527
Protaxon [Opfermann] *see* 7774
α₁-Protease Inhibitor *see* 719
ProTec [Cell Therapeutics] *see* 5517
Protecadin [Taiho] *see* 5347
Protectins *see* 5429
Protecton [Yoshitomi] *see* 4927
α₁-Proteinase Inhibitor *see* 719
Protein C, 7884
Protein Hydrolysates, 7885
Protein P5 *see* 876
Protein P9 *see* 1910
Protein S *see* 7884
Protelos [Servier] *see* 8106
Protenolon [Showa] *see* 5915
Proterciclina [Proter] *see* 8252
Proternol *see* 5217
Prothazin [Rodleben] *see* 7786
Protheobromine, 7886
Prothiaden [Knoll] *see* 3429
Prothil [Kali-Chemie] *see* 5791
Prothioconazole, 7887
Prothionamide *see* 7891
Prothipendyl, 7888
Prothrombase *see* 7889
Prothrombin, 7889
Protiofate, 7890
Protionamide, 7891
Protirelin *see* 9588
Protium *see* 4792
Protium [Altana] *see* 7014
Protoactinium *see* 7883
Protoanemonin, 7892
Protocatechualdehyde, 7893
Protocatechualdehyde Dimethyl Ether
see 9951
Protocatechuic Acid, 7894
Protocatechuic Acid Methylene Ether *see*
7477
Protocatechuic Aldehyde *see* 7893
Protoenstatite *see* 5687
Protoescigenin *see* 3696
Protogen A *see* 9326
Protoheme *see* 4639
Protoheme IX *see* 4639
Protokylol, 7895
Protolipan [Millet] *see* 3978
Protomin *see* 4463
Protonix [Wyeth] *see* 7014
Proton Sponge *see* 3388
Protopam [Wyeth-Ayerst] *see* 7703
Protopic [Fujisawa] *see* 9025
Protopine, 7896
Protoporphyrin IX, 7897
Protopyrin *see* 3731
(+)-Protoquercitol *see* 8036
Protos [Servier] *see* 8106
Protosol *see* 3182
Protostephanine, 7898
Protostib *see* 6078
Protoveratrine A *see* 7899
Protoveratrine B *see* 7899
Protoveratrines, 7899
Protoverine, 7900
Protoxyl *see* 8578
Protriptyline, 7901
Protropin [Genentech] *see* 8716
Protugan [Makhteshim-Agan] *see* 5218
Pro-UK *see* 7902
Pro U-PA *see* 7902

Pro-Urokinase, 7902
Prourokinase (Enzyme-activating) *see* 7902
Prourokinase (Enzyme-activating) (Human Clone pUK4/pUK18 Protein Moiety Reduced) *see* 7902
Proustite *see* 8504
Provado [Bayer CropSci.] *see* 4910
Provas [Sanol Schwarz] *see* 1475
Provatene [Microbio] *see* 1853
Provell [Lilly] *see* 7899
Provenal [Pulitzer] *see* 8986
Provenge [Dendreon] *see* 8547
Proventil [Schering-Plough] *see* 216
Provera [Pharmacia & Upjohn] *see* 5793
Provigil [Cephalon] *see* 6228
Proviodine [Rougier] *see* 7698
Proviron [Schering AG] *see* 5916
Provisc [Alcon] *see* 4757
Provitamin D₃ *see* 2867
Provitar [Clin-Comar-Byla] *see* 6921
Provitina [Promonta] *see* 10019
Provocholine [Roche] *see* 5940
Prower Factor *see* 3923
Prowl [BASF] *see* 7084
Proxazocain *see* 7709
Proxazole, 7903
Proxen [Syntex] *see* 6417
Proxibarbal, 7904
Proxibarbital *see* 7904
Proxigermanium *see* 7795
Proxil [Rottapharm] *see* 7774
Proxine [Del Saz & Filippini] *see* 6417
Proxitane [Solvay Interox] *see* 7150
Proxol [AgrEvo] *see* 9623
Proxymetacaine *see* 7807
Proxyphylline, 7905
Prozac [Lilly] *see* 4185
Prozapine, 7906
Prozei [Kissei] *see* 589
Prozin [Lusofarmaco] *see* 2185
Prozinex [Makhteshim-Agan] *see* 7812
Prucalopride, 7907
Prulaurasin *see* 5720
Prulet [Mission Pharmacal] *see* 6974
Prulifloxacin, 7908
Prunasin *see* 5720
Prunetin, 7909
Prunetol *see* 4391
Prunitrin *see* 7909
Prunol *see* 9890
Prunusetin *see* 7909
Prussian Blue, 7910
Prussic Acid *see* 4795
Pryleugan [Temmler] *see* 4920
PS1 *see* 7739
PS2 *see* 7739
PS-60 *see* 4383
PS-207 *see* 9104
PS-341 *see* 1351
PSC-833 *see* 9917
P-Selectin *see* 8426
Pseudobaptigenin, 7911
Pseudobaptisin *see* 7911
Pseudobatrachotoxin *see* 1009
Pseudobutylbenzene *see* 1551
Pseudo-butylene *see* 1520
Pseudocef [Grünenthal] *see* 1945
Pseudochelerythrine *see* 8356
Pseudocholestane *see* 2523
Pseudocinchonine *see* 4783
Pseudococaine, 7912
Pseudocodeine, 7913
Pseudoconhydrine, 7914
Pseudocubebin *see* 8470

Pseudocumene, 7915
Pseudocumol *see* 7915
Pseudodigitoxin *see* 4434
Pseudoephedrine, 7916
Pseudofructose *see* 7924
Pseudohecogenin *see* 4622
Pseudoionone, 7917
Pseudolibethenite *see* 2648
Pseudomalachite *see* 2648
trans-Pseudomonic Acid *see* 6302
Pseudomonic Acid A *see* 6302
Pseudomonic Acid B *see* 7918
Pseudomonic Acid C *see* 7918
Pseudomonic Acid D *see* 7918
Pseudomonic Acid I *see* 7918
Pseudomonic Acids, 7918
Pseudomorphine, 7919
Pseudomorphine (C34 Alkaloid) *see* 7919
Pseudopaederine *see* 7065
Pseudopederin *see* 7065
Pseudopelletierine, 7920
Pseudopunicine *see* 7920
3-Pseudotropanol *see* 7921
Pseudotropine, 7921
Pseudotropine Benzoate *see* 9774
Pseudo-wollastonite *see* 1702
Pseudoyohimbine, 7922
Psicaine *see* 7912
Psicaine N *see* 7912
Psichial [Lang] *see* 2084
Psicofuranine, 7923
9β-D-Psicofuranosyladenine *see* 7923
9-β-D-Psicofuranosyl-9*H*-purin-6-amine *see* 7923
Psicopax [Schering] *see* 5579
Psicoperidol [Lusofarmaco] *see* 9684
D-Psicose, 7924
Psicosoma [Ferrer] *see* 4469
Psicoterina [Francia] *see* 2084
Psicronizer [Albert-Pharma] *see* 6673
Psilocin, 7925
Psilocybin, 7926
Psilocyn *see* 7925
Psiquium [Sintofarma] *see* 5786
PSK [Kureha], 7927
Psoil [Basotherm] *see* 9456
Psoraderm-5 [Sunlife] *see* 1157
Psoradrate [Procter & Gamble] *see* 684
Psoralen, 7928
Psorcon [Dermik] *see* 3140
Psorcutan [Schering AG] *see* 1641
Psorex [GSK] *see* 2363
Psoriderm [Istoria] *see* 684
Psorigel [Alcon] *see* 2426
P.S.P. *see* 7247
PSTMS *see* 7311
Psychoperidol [Ethnor] *see* 9684
Psychostyl *see* 6715
Psychotrine, 7929
Psychoverlan [Verla] *see* 4469
Psyllium Husk *see* 7517
Psyllium Hydrocolloid *see* 7517
Psyllium Hydrophylic Mucilloid *see* 7517
Psyllium Seed *see* 7517
Psyllium Seed Gum *see* 7517
Psymion [TAD] *see* 5748
Psyquil [Sanofi-Synthelabo] *see* 9685
PT *see* 7930
PT-14 *see* 7494
PTA *see* 3924
Ptaquiloside, 7930
PTC *see* 3922
Pteridine, 7931
2,4(1*H*,3*H*)-Pteridinedione *see* 5596
Pterin HB₂ *see* 1229

Pterocarpin, 7932
Pterofen *see* 9599
Pteroic Acid, 7933
Pterolyl-γ-glutamyl-γ-glutamylglutamic Acid *see* 7934
Pterophene *see* 9599
Pteropterin, 7934
Pteroyldiglutamic Acid *see* 3291
Pteroyldi-γ-glutamylglutamic Acid *see* 7934
Pteroylglutamic Acid *see* 4221
Pteroyl-α-glutamylglutamic Acid *see* 3291
N-[*N*-(*N*-Pteroyl-γ-glutamyl)-γ-glutamyl]glutamic Acid *see* 7934
Pteroylheptaglutamic Acid *see* 7935
Pteroylhexaglutamylglutamic Acid, 7935
Pteroyltriglutamic Acid *see* 7934
PTFE *see* 7583
PTGA *see* 7934
PTH *see* 7034
Ptimal [Egis] *see* 9706
PTK-787 *see* 9939
PTO *see* 7994
Pt(oxalato)(*trans*-*l*-dach) *see* 6912
PTX *see* 6999
Ptychotis Oil *see* 196
Puccoon Root *see* 8355
Pudding Pipe *see* 1894
Pudding-stick *see* 1894
Puerzym [Firma] *see* 7146
PUK *see* 7902
Pukateine, 7936
Pularin *see* 4653
Pulegone, 7937
Pulmadil [3M Pharma] *see* 8227
Pulmicort [AstraZeneca] *see* 1468
PulmiDur [Pharma-Stern] *see* 9285
Pulmoclase [UCB] *see* 1802
Pulmotil [Elanco] *see* 9439
Pulmo-Timelets [Temmler] *see* 9285
Pulmovet [Solvay] *see* 1465
Pulmozyme [Genentech] *see* 2906
Pulsan [Yamanouchi] *see* 4940
Pulsar [Medosan] *see* 2936
Pulsatilla, 7938
Pulsatilla Camphor *see* 642
Pulsoton *see* 4810
Pulsotyl [Chinoin] *see* 7330
Puma *see* 3984
Pumactant, 7939
Pumice, 7940
Pumpellyite *see* 1648
Pumpkin Seed, 7941
Punch [DuPont] *see* 4206
Punicin *see* 7071
Punicine *see* 7072
Punktyl [Krewel] *see* 5579
Purantix [Wander] *see* 2369
Purapuridine *see* 8709
Purapurine *see* 8710
Purecal [Wyandotte] *see* 1657
Puregon [Organon] *see* 4223
Purgaceen *see* 6974
Purging Agaric *see* 185
Purging Cassia *see* 1894
P¹-(uridine 5′)-P⁴-(2′-deoxycytidine 5′)-Tetraphosphate 2896
Purified Araroba *see* 2253
Purified Goa Powder *see* 2253
Purified Oxgall *see* 6928
Purified Ozokerite *see* 1987
Purified Poloxamer 188 *see* 7562
Purified Protein Derivative *see* 9805
Purified Rayon *see* 8122

Purim [Laphal] *see* 7505
1*H*-Purin-6-amine *see* 152
1*H*-Purine, 7942
1*H*-Purine-2,6-diamine *see* 2985
2,6(1*H*,3*H*)-Purinedione *see* 10059
Purine-6-thiol *see* 5871
Purinethol [GSK] *see* 5871
Puri-Nethol [GSK] *see* 5871
Purine-2,6,8-triol *see* 9875
Purine-2,6,8(1*H*,3*H*,9*H*)-trione *see* 9875
Purin-6(1*H*)-one *see* 4869
Purlytin [Pharmacia & Upjohn] *see* 8269
Purochin [Sclavo] *see* 9887
Purodigin [Wyeth] *see* 3163
Puromycin, 7943
Purosin-TC [Tatsumi] *see* 7874
Purostrophan [Kali-Chemie] *see* 6901
Purothionin, 7944
α_1-Purothionin *see* 7944
α_2-Purothionin *see* 7944
β-Purothionin *see* 7944
Purothionin A I *see* 7944
Purothionin A II *see* 7944
Purple Clover *see* 9690
Purple Coneflower *see* 3494
Purple Foxglove *see* 3159
Purple of Cassius *see* 4520
Purpurid [Promonta] *see* 3163
Purpurin, 7945
Purpurogallin, 7946
Purpurosamine *see* 4392
Pursennid [Novartis] *see* 8455
Purshiana Bark *see* 1880
Pursuit [BASF] *see* 4907
Putrescine, 7947
Putty Powder *see* 8778
PVA *see* 7585
PVC *see* 7586
PVNO, 7948
PVP *see* 7697
PVP-I *see* 7698
PVPNO *see* 7948
PVPP *see* 7697
PX-917 *see* 9763
Pycaril *see* 6526
Pydrin [Shell] *see* 4010
Pyelectan *see* 8633
Pyelokon-R [Mallinckrodt] *see* 79
Pyelosil *see* 5040
Pygeum Africanum Extract, 7949
Pykaryl *see* 6526
Pyknolepsinum [Rhein-Pharma] *see* 3748
Pyladox [Gedeon Richter] *see* 7603
Pylen [Toyo] *see* 7567
Pylorid [GSK] *see* 8110
Pylumbrin *see* 5040
Pymetrozine, 7950
Pynamin [Sumitomo] *see* 260
Pyocefal [Cassenne-Takeda] *see* 1945
Pyocianil [Farmitalia] *see* 1792
Pyocyanine, 7951
Pyoktanin [Merck KGaA] *see* 4395
Pyopen [SKB] *see* 1792
Pyoredol [Aventis] *see* 7322
Pyostacine [RPR] *see* 7753
Pyoxanthose *see* 4645
Py-Phe, 7952
β-Pyracine *see* 7981
Pyraclostrobin, 7953
Pyrafat [Fatol] *see* 7956
Pyrahexyl *see* 9013
Pyralene [Prodelec] *see* 7564
Pyralgin [Savage] *see* 3350
Pyralin *see* 1964
Pyramal [Roxane] *see* 7984

Pyramidon *see* 474
Pyramin *see* 9561
Pyramine *see* 9561
Pyranica [Mitsubishi Kasei] *see* 9094
Pyranine, 7954
Pyranisamine *see* 7984
Pyrantel, 7955
Pyrantel Embonate *see* 7955
Pyranton *see* 2964
Pyrargyrite *see* 8504
Pyrasanone *see* 7277
Pyrathyn [Flint] *see* 5959
Pyrazinamide, 7956
Pyrazine, 7957
N-(2-Pyrazine)carbonyl-L-phenylalanine-L-leucine Boronic Acid *see* 1351
Pyrazinecarboxamide *see* 7956
Pyrazine Carboxylamide *see* 7956
Pyrazinecarboxylic Acid *see* 7959
2,3-Pyrazinedicarboxylic Acid, 7958
Pyrazinemonocarboxylic Acid *see* 7959
Pyrazinobutazone *see* 7277
Pyrazinoic Acid, 7959
Pyrazinoic Acid Amide *see* 7956
Pyrazino[2,3-*d*]pyrimidine *see* 7931
N^1-2-Pyrazinylsulfanilamide *see* 8937
Pyrazole, 7960
1*H*-Pyrazole-3-ethanamine *see* 1183
2-Pyrazoline, 7961
1*H*-Pyrazolo[3,4-*d*]pyrimidin-4-ol *see* 279
Pyrazophos, 7962
Pyrcon [Meuselbach] *see* 8022
Pyrene, 7963
Pyrethrin I *see* 7964
Pyrethrin II *see* 7964
Pyrethrins, 7964
Pyrethrosin, 7965
Pyrethrum Flowers, 7966
Pyribenzamine [Novartis] *see* 9738
Pyricarbate *see* 7975
Pyricardyl *see* 6543
Pyrictal *see* 7222
Pyridaben, 7967
Pyridacil [Cilag] *see* 7210
Pyridate, 7968
Pyridazine, 7969
Pyridin [DuPont] *see* 4010
2-Pyridinamine *see* 473
3-Pyridinamine *see* 473
4-Pyridinamine *see* 3933
2*H*-Pyrid[4,3-*b*]indole *see* 1805
Pyridine, 7970
3-Pyridineacetic Acid, 7971
2-Pyridine Aldoxime Methiodide *see* 7703
2-Pyridine Aldoxime Methyl Chloride *see* 7703
3-Pyridinecarboxamide *see* 6523
Pyridine-β-carboxylic Acid *see* 6525
γ-Pyridinecarboxylic Acid *see* 5187
o-Pyridinecarboxylic Acid *see* 7403
2-Pyridinecarboxylic Acid *see* 7403
3-Pyridinecarboxylic Acid *see* 6525
4-Pyridinecarboxylic Acid *see* 5187
Pyridine-β-carboxylic Acid Benzyl Ester *see* 6526
3-Pyridinecarboxylic Acid 2,2-Bis[[(3-pyridinylcarbonyl)oxy]methyl]-1,3-propanediyl Ester *see* 6497
4-Pyridinecarboxylic Acid [(2-Carboxy-3,4-dimethoxyphenyl)methylene]hydrazide *see* 6852
3-Pyridinecarboxylic Acid 2-[2-(4-Chlorophenoxy)-2-methyl-1-oxopropoxy]-ethyl Ester *see* 3877

3-Pyridinecarboxylic Acid 2-[2-(4-Chlorophenoxy)-2-methyl-1-oxopropoxy]-1,3-propanediyl Ester *see* 1224
3-Pyridinecarboxylic Acid 3-[2-(4-Chlorophenoxy)-2-methyl-1-oxopropoxy]-propyl Ester *see* 8255
3-Pyridinecarboxylic Acid Compd with 3,7-Dihydro-7-[2-hydroxy-3-[(2-hydroxyethyl)methylamino]propyl]-1,3-dimethyl-1*H*-purine-2,6-dione (1:1) *see* 10060
Pyridine-3-carboxylic Acid Diethylamide *see* 6543
Pyridine-4-carboxylic Acid Diethylamide *see* 5188
4-Pyridinecarboxylic Acid [1-(2-Furanyl)ethylidene]hydrazide *see* 4308
4-Pyridinecarboxylic Acid Hydrazide *see* 5186
3-Pyridinecarboxylic Acid Hydroxymethylamide *see* 4833
3-Pyridinecarboxylic Acid Methyl Ester *see* 6100
4-Pyridinecarboxylic Acid 2-(1-Methylethyl)hydrazide *see* 5078
Pyridine-3-carboxylic Acid *N*-Methylolamide *see* 4833
3-Pyridinecarboxylic Acid 1-Oxide *see* 6941
4-Pyridinecarboxylic Acid 2-[3-Oxo-3-[(phenylmethyl)amino]propyl]hydrazide *see* 6491
3-Pyridinecarboxylic Acid Phenylmethyl Ester *see* 6526
4-Pyridinecarboxylic Acid 2-(Sulfomethyl)hydrazide *see* 5186
4-Pyridinecarboxylic Acid [(3-Sulfophenyl)methylene]hydrazide *see* 8959
3-Pyridinecarboxylic Acid 2-(1,2,3,6-Tetrahydro-1,3-dimethyl-2,6-dioxo-7*H*-purin-7-yl)ethyl Ester *see* 3879
3-Pyridinecarboxylic Acid 3,3,5-Trimethylcyclohexyl Ester *see* 2265
3,4-Pyridinediamine *see* 2986
2,3-Pyridinedicarboxylic Acid *see* 8073
2,5-Pyridinedicarboxylic Acid *see* 5159
3,4-Pyridinedicarboxylic Acid *see* 2283
2,6-Pyridinedimethanol Bis(methylcarbamate) (Ester) *see* 7975
2,6-Pyridinedimethanol Bis(3,4,5-trimethoxybenzoate) *see* 7507
2,6-Pyridinedimethanol Mono-*p*-chlorophenoxyisobutyrate *see* 7495
3-Pyridinemethanol *see* 6527
Pyridine *N*-Oxide *see* 7972
Pyridine 1-Oxide, 7972
2-Pyridinethiol 1-Oxide *see* 7994
Pyridinium Bromide Perbromide, 7973
Pyridinium Chlorochromate, 7974
Pyridinium Poly(hydrogen Fluoride) *see* 6821
2,3-Pyridino-(5′,6′)-5,6-benzo-4-(3″-dimethylaminopropyl)-1,4-thiazine *see* 7888
Pyridinol Carbamate, 7975
α-[(2-Pyridinylamino)methyl]benzenemethanol *see* 7321
N-2-Pyridinyl-[1,1′-biphenyl]-4-acetamide *see* 3137
2,6-Pyridinylenebis[methyl-*N*-methylcarbamate] *see* 7975
1-(3-Pyridinyl)ethanone *see* 6116
2-(3-Pyridinyl)-1-hydroxyethane Diphosphonic Acid *see* 8232

α-Pyrrolidone *see* 8016
2-Pyrrolidone, 8016
2-Pyrrolidoneacetamide *see* 7487
2-Pyrrolidone-5-carboxylic Acid *see* 8001
3-Pyrroline, 8017
Pyrrolnitrin, 8018
Pyrrolylene *see* 1509
Pyrrolysine, 8019
L-Pyrrolysine *see* 8019
Pyrro[*b*]monazole *see* 4912
Pyruvaldehyde *see* 6081
Pyruvaldehyde Bis(amidinohydrazone) *see* 6213
Pyruvaldoxime *see* 5190
Pyruvate Decarboxylase, 8020
Pyruvate Oxidation Factor *see* 9326
Pyruvic Acid, 8021
Pyruvic Carboxylase *see* 8020
Pyruvic Decarboxylase *see* 8020
Pyrvinium Chloride *see* 8022
Pyrvinium Embonate *see* 8022
Pyrvinium Pamoate, 8022
Pytetrahydroserpentine *see* 8119
Python [Dow AgroSci.] *see* 4141
PYY$_{1-36}$ *see* 7149
PYY$_{3-36}$ *see* 7149
PZ-51 *see* 3486
PZC *see* 7183
PZI Insulin *see* 4980
Q-35 *see* 944
Q-254 *see* 7523
Q-275 *see* 9843
Qari [Mediolanum] *see* 8294
QCD-84924 *see* 9209
QD-10733 *see* 4189
Q-Enzyme, 8023
Q-Gas *see* 4630
QHS *see* 817
Qinghao *see* 817
Qinghaosu *see* 817
Qing Hau Sau *see* 817
QNB *see* 8082
Q.T. (Quick Tan) *see* 3182
Quaalude *see* 5960
Quadrafos *see* 8667
Quadramet [Cytogen] *see* 8350
Quadris [Syngenta] *see* 924
Quadrisol [Intervet] *see* 9942
Quadrol [Wyandotte] *see* 3599
Quait [SIT] *see* 5579
Quaker Buttons *see* 6730
Quamonium *see* 2025
Quaname [Wyeth] *see* 5862
Quanil [Wyeth] *see* 5862
Quantalan [BMS] *see* 2202
Quantril [Roerig] *see* 1119
Quantum Dye, 8024
Quark [Polifarma] *see* 8103
Quartz *see* 8493
Quarzan [Roche] *see* 2354
Quasar [Abbott] *see* 9950
Quassia, 8025
Quassin, 8026
Quat *see* 5308
Quaternium-7 *see* 5370
Quaternium-15, 8027
Quaternium-18 *see* 1056
Quaternium 18-Bentonite *see* 1056
Quatrimycin, 8028
Quazepam, 8029
Quazium [Schering] *see* 8029
Quebrachamine, 8030
Quebrachine *see* 10102
Quebracho *see* 849
Quebracho Colorado, 8031

Quebrachol *see* 8556
Queen Bee Jelly *see* 8277
Queensland Asthma Weed *see* 3903
Queen's Root *see* 8818
Queen Substance, 8032
Queletox *see* 4002
Quelicin [Abbott] *see* 8875
Quellada [Block] *see* 5501
Quemicetina [Pharmacia] *see* 2077
Quensyl *see* 4818
Quentan [Boehringer, Ing.] *see* 1391
Quercetagetin, 8033
Quercetagitrin *see* 8033
Quercetin, 8034
Quercetin-3-glucoside *see* 5221
Quercetin-7-D-glucoside *see* 8035
Quercetin-3-L-rhamnoside *see* 8037
Quercetin-3-rutinoside *see* 8304
Quercimelin *see* 8037
Quercimeritrin, 8035
d-Quercitol, 8036
Quercitrin, 8037
Quercitroside *see* 8037
Quercus, 8038
Querto [Byk Gulden] *see* 1873
Querton 210CL [Kemanord] *see* 3099
Quest [Fort Dodge] *see* 6290
Quest [Am. Cyanamid] *see* 8716
Questran [BMS] *see* 2202
Quetiapine, 8039
Quick [Rhône-Poulenc] *see* 2152
Quick Grass *see* 9761
Quicklime *see* 1686
Quickphos [United Phosphorus] *see* 359
Quicksilver *see* 5898
Quide [HMR] *see* 7462
Quiess [Forest] *see* 4849
Quilan [Dow AgroSci.] *see* 1040
Quillaja, 8040
Quillaja Saponin, 8041
Quillay Bark *see* 8040
Quilonorm *see* 5521
Quilonum [GSK] *see* 5521
Quilonum-retard [GSK] *see* 5527
Quimoral *see* 2260
Quimotrase [Farmila] *see* 2260
Quin2, 8042
Quin-2 *see* 8042
Quin-2AM *see* 8042
Quinacillin, 8043
Quinacrine, 8044
Quinaglute [Berlex] *see* 8060
Quinagolide, 8045
Quinalbarbitone Sodium *see* 8420
Quinaldic Acid, 8046
Quinaldine, 8047
Quinaldine Blue, 8048
Quinaldine Red, 8049
Quinaldinic Acid *see* 8046
Quinaldofur *see* 6534
Quinalizarin, 8050
Quinalspan [Pharmax] *see* 8420
Quinambicide *see* 5031
Quinamm [Aventis] *see* 8061
Quinapril, 8051
Quinaprilat, 8051
Quinapyramine, 8052
Quinate [Aventis] *see* 8061
Quinazil [Malesci] *see* 8051
Quinazoline, 8053
Quince Seed, 8054
Quinestrol, 8055
Quinethazone, 8056
Quinfamide, 8057
Quinhydrone, 8058

Quinic Acid, 8059
Quinic Acid 1,5-Dicaffeic Ester *see* 2766
Quinicardine [Procter & Gamble] *see* 8060
Quinicine *see* 10003
Quinidex Extentabs [Robins] *see* 8060
Quinidine, 8060
α-Quinidine *see* 2286
Quinidine Bisulfate *see* 8060
Quiniduran [Teva] *see* 8060
Quinine, 8061
β-Quinine *see* 8060
Quinine Bimuriate *see* 8061
Quinine Dichloride *see* 8061
Quininic Acid, 8062
Quininone, 8063
Quiniofon *see* 4826
Quinisocaine *see* 3218
Quinizarin, 8064
Quinizarin Green SS, 8065
Quinmerac, 8066
Quinocide, 8067
Quinodis [Roche] *see* 4099
Quinofen *see* 2288
Quinofop-ethyl *see* 8086
Quinol *see* 4808
Quinoline, 8068
8-Quinolineboronic Acid, 8069
2-Quinolinecarboxylic Acid *see* 8046
8-Quinolinecarboxylic Acid, 8070
Quinoline Yellow, 8071
Quinoline Yellow A *see* 8072
Quinoline Yellow Base *see* 8072
Quinoline Yellow Spirit Soluble, 8072
Quinolinic Acid, 8073
2-Quinolinol *see* 1825
8-Quinolinol *see* 4843
2(1*H*)-Quinolinone *see* 1825
2-(2-Quinolinyl)-1*H*-indene-1,3-(2*H*)-dione *see* 8072
2(1*H*)-Quinolone *see* 1825
Quinomethionate *see* 6978
Quinomycin A *see* 3497
Quinone, 8074
p-Quinone *see* 8074
Quinone Monoxime *see* 6642
Quinone Oxime *see* 6642
Quinophan *see* 2288
Quinophthalone *see* 8072
Quinora [Key] *see* 8060
Quinotoxine *see* 10003
Quinotoxol *see* 10003
Quinova-bitter *see* 8076
Quinovaic Acid *see* 8075
Quinovatine *see* 784
Quinovic Acid, 8075
Quinovic Acid β-D-Glucoside *see* 8076
Quinovic Acid β-D-Quinovoside *see* 8076
Quinovin, 8076
Quinovose, 8077
Quinoxaline, 8078
"Quinoxaline Antibiotic" *see* 3497
"Quinoxaline Antibiotic Complex" *see* 9733
3-(2-Quinoxalinylmethylene)carbazic Acid Methyl Ester *N,N'*-Dioxide *see* 1780
(2-Quinoxalinylmethylene)hydrazinecarboxylic Acid Methyl Ester *N,N'*-Dioxide *see* 1780
N^1-(2-Quinoxalinyl)sulfanilamide *see* 8939
N^1-(2-Quinoxalyl)sulfanilamide *see* 8939
Quinoxyfen, 8078
Quinoxyl [Burroughs Wellcome] *see* 4826
Quintec [Dow AgroSci.] *see* 8079

Quintozene, 8080
Quintrate *see* 7112
Quinuclidine, 8081
3-Quinuclidinol, 8082
3-Quinuclidinyl Acetate *see* 8082
3-Quinuclidinyl Benzilate *see* 8082
3-Quinuclidinyl Benzoate *see* 8082
10-(3-Quinuclidinylmethyl)phenothiazine *see* 5864
(1*S*,3′*R*)-3′-Quinuclidinyl-1-phenyl-1,2,3,-4-tetrahydro-2-isoquinolinecarboxylate *see* 8712
5δ-[(3*S*)-3-Quinuclidinyl]thiomethylpristinamycin IA *see* 8084
Quinupramine, 8083
Quinupristin, 8084
Quinuronium Sulfate *see* 3353
Quinvet [Neopharmed] *see* 5637
Quisnon [Nippon Shinyaku] *see* 7908
Quisqualic Acid, 8085
L-Quisqualic Acid *see* 8085
Quitaxon [Boehringer, Mann.] *see* 3435
Quival [Schering] *see* 1697
Quixin [Santen] *see* 6771
Quizalofop-ethyl, 8086
Quorn [Marlow], 8087
Qvar [3M] *see* 1019
QZ-2 *see* 5960
R-3-ZON *see* 7277
R-11, 8088
R-32 *see* 3151
R-48 *see* 2108
R-75 *see* 5446
R-79 *see* 5202
R-100 *see* 387
R134a *see* 4714
R-148 *see* 5960
R-218 *see* 7158
R-242 *see* 8988
R-381 *see* 3965
R-400 *see* 7041
R-445 *see* 6267
R-658 *see* 1599
R-738 *see* 6440
R-773 *see* 8219
R-798 *see* 8227
R-802 *see* 4137
R-805 *see* 6548
R-818 *see* 4098
R-835 *see* 4872
R-837 *see* 4922
R-848 *see* 8151
R-875 *see* 2955
R-1132 *see* 3313
R-1504 *see* 7336
R-1513 *see* 913
R-1569 *see* 9493
R-1582 *see* 913
R-1608 *see* 3640
R-1625 *see* 4598
R-1658 *see* 6263
R-1881 *see* 6129
R-1910 *see* 1546
R-1929 *see* 898
R-2028 *see* 4114
R-2113 *see* 2930
R-2323 *see* 4415
R-2453 *see* 2888
R-2498 *see* 9684
R-2858 *see* 6289
R-3248 *see* 30
R-3345 *see* 7455
R-3365 *see* 7498
R-3746 *see* 1941
R-3763 *see* 1941

R-3959 *see* 2383
R-4263 *see* 4001
R-4318 *see* 4103
R-4584 *see* 1048
R-4749 *see* 3450
R-4845 *see* 1196
R-4929 *see* 1075
R-5020 *see* 7785
R-6128 *see* 4207
R-6238 *see* 7435
R-6700 *see* 5127
R-7315 *see* 6148
R-7465 *see* 6416
R-7904 *see* 5484
R-8299 *see* 5459
R-11333 *see* 1442
R-12563 *see* 5459
R-12564 *see* 5459
R-14827 *see* 3502
R-14889 *see* 6178
R-15403 *see* 3136
R-15454 *see* 5160
R-15889 *see* 5580
R-16341 *see* 7087
R-16470 *see* 2945
R-16659 *see* 3881
R-17147 *see* 2712
R-17635 *see* 5768
R-17889 *see* 4118
R-18553 *see* 5571
R-23979 *see* 3583
R-25061 *see* 9005
R-25788 *see* 3049
R-25831 *see* 1848
R-28644 *see* 641
R-30730 *see* 8887
R-31520 *see* 2411
R-33800 *see* 8887
R-33812 *see* 3418
R-34995 *see* 5556
R-35443 *see* 6925
R-39209 *see* 236
R-41400 *see* 5302
R-41468 *see* 5296
R-42470 *see* 9160
R-43512 *see* 856
R-49945 *see* 5296
R-50547 *see* 5463
R-51211 *see* 5245
R-51619 *see* 2316
R-55667 *see* 8235
R-58735 *see* 8310
R-64433 *see* 3080
R-64766 *see* 8233
R-65824 *see* 6432
R-66905 *see* 8362
R-67555 *see* 6432
R-68070 *see* 8212
R-75251 *see* 5475
R-76713 *see* 10035
R-83842 *see* 10035
R-85246 *see* 5475
R-87926 *see* 5590
R-93877 *see* 7907
R-115777 *see* 9458
R-151993 *see* 9111
R-152450 *see* 4214
RA-8 *see* 3346
Rabalan *see* 7376
Rabeprazole, 8089
Rabon [Shell] *see* 9192
Rabond [Shell] *see* 9192
Race-acetylmethadol *see* 5945
Racecadotril, 8090
Racemethionine *see* 5975

Racemethorphan, 8091
Racemic Acid *see* 9069
Racemic Ephedrine *see* 3608
Racemic Lactic Acid *see* 5336
Racemic Mandelic Acid *see* 5717
Racemic Propoxyphene *see* 7839
Racemic Tartaric Acid *see* 9069
Racemomycin A *see* 8829
Racemomycins *see* 8829
Racemorphan *see* 5470
Raceophenidol *see* 9301
Racephedrine *see* 3608
Racephedrine Hydrochloride *see* 3608
Racephenicol *see* 9301
Racepinephrine *see* 3619
Rachromate-51 [Abbott] *see* 8601
R Acid *see* 6387
Racobalamin-60 [Abbott] *see* 10015
Ractopamine, 8092
RAD-001 *see* 3907
Radanil [Roche] *see* 1084
Radapon *see* 2802
Raddeamine *see* 4926
Rad-e-cate [Vineland] *see* 8595
Radecol *see* 6527
Radedorm [AWD] *see* 6575
Radibud [Takeda] *see* 1452
Radical Weed *see* 8708
Radicicol *see* 6253
Radicinin, 8093
Radinyl [Roberts] *see* 3713
Radioactive Colloidal Gold *see* 4517
Radioactive Cyanocobalamin *see* 10015
Radioactive Sodium Phosphate *see* 8661
Radiocaps-131 [Abbott] *see* 8632
Radiocyanocobalamin *see* 10015
Radiogardase [Heyl] *see* 7910
Radio-gold (^{198}Au) Colloid *see* 4517
Radiographol *see* 5973
Radio-iodinated Insulin *see* 4980
Radiopaque [Schering AG] *see* 994
Radiostol *see* 10018
Radiotetrane *see* 5038
Radium, 8094
Radium Emanation *see* 8095
Radium F *see* 7561
Radon, 8095
Radsterin *see* 10018
Rafamebin *see* 5042
Raffinose, 8096
Rafoxanide, 8097
Raft [Rhone-Poulenc] *see* 6905
Ragadan [Hoechst] *see* 4664
Ralabol [Mallinckrodt Vet.] *see* 10121
Ralgro [Mallinckrodt Vet.] *see* 10121
Rally [Dow AgroSci.] *see* 6321
Ralone [Mallinckrodt Vet.] *see* 10121
Raloxifene, 8098
Raltitrexed, 8099
Ramace [AstraZeneca] *see* 8103
Ramatroban, 8100
Ramelteon, 8101
Rametin [Bayer] *see* 6354
Ramifenazone, 8102
Ramik [Hacco] *see* 3305
Ramipril, 8103
Ramiprilat *see* 8103
Ramoplanin, 8104
Ramosetron, 8105
R/AMP *see* 8216
Rampart [Platte Chemical] *see* 7331
Ramrod [Monsanto] *see* 7793
Ramycin *see* 4317
Rancho [Bayer] *see* 5797
Rancinamycin IV *see* 7893

Randa [Nippon Kayaku] *see* 2317
Randolectil [Bayer] *see* 1516
Ranelic Acid, 8106
Ranestol [Parke-Davis] *see* 1192
Ranexa [CV Therapeutics] *see* 8111
Raney Nickel [W. R. Grace], 8107
Raney Nickel Catalyst *see* 8107
Raniben [Firma] *see* 8110
Ranibizumab, 8108
Ranide [Merck & Co.] *see* 8097
Ranidil [Menarini] *see* 8110
Ranimustine, 8109
Raniplex [Fournier] *see* 8110
Ranitidine, 8110
Ranitidine Bismutrex *see* 8110
Ranman [Ishihara Sangyo] *see* 2700
Ranolazine, 8111
Ranomustine *see* 8109
Ranpirnase, 8112
Rantudil [Bayer] *see* 27
Ranunculin *see* 7892
Ranvil [Gentili] *see* 6495
RAPA *see* 8114
Rapacodin [Knoll] *see* 3171
Rapacuronium Bromide, 8113
Rapamune [Wyeth] *see* 8114
Rapamycin, 8114
Rapamycin 42-Ester with 2,2-Bis-(hy-
droxymethyl)propionic Acid *see* 9142
Rapamycin 42-[3-Hydroxy-2-(hydroxy-
methyl)-2-methylpropanoate] *see* 9142
Rapeseed Oil, 8115
Raphanus Rusticanus *see* 4749
Rapicidin *see* 9836
Rapifen [Janssen-Cilag] *see* 236
Rapilysin [Roche] *see* 8161
Rapinovet [Schering-Plough Vet.] *see* 7834
Rapitil [Aventis] *see* 6436
Rapitux [De Angeli] *see* 3452
Raplon [Organon] *see* 8113
Rapostan [Mepha] *see* 6972
Raptiva [Genentech] *see* 3519
Raptor [BASF] *see* 4904
Rapynogen [Maruko] *see* 7840
Rasagiline, 8116
Rasagiline Mesylate *see* 8116
Rasapen *see* 4749
Rasburicase, 8117
Rasilez [Novartis] *see* 247
Raspberry, 8118
Rastinon [Aventis] *see* 9507
Ratak [Sorex] *see* 3133
Ratanhine *see* 9007
Rat Antispectacled Eye Factor *see* 4978
Rathimed [Pfleger] *see* 6157
Raticate *see* 6687
Rattlesnake Root *see* 8453
Rattle Weed *see* 1312
Rattrack *see* 722
Raubasine, 8119
Raubixin [BMS] *see* 8120
Rauhimbine *see* 2548
Raunormine [Penick] *see* 2918
Raunova [Zambeletti] *see* 9017
Raupine *see* 8378
Rauserpol [Rhewie Pharma] *see* 8120
Rautensin [Sandoz] *see* 8120
Rauverid [OJ & F] *see* 8120
Rauwiloid [3M Pharma] *see* 8120
Rauwoldin [OJ & F] *see* 8120
Rauwolfemms [Truxton] *see* 8120
Rauwolfia Serpentina, 8120
Rauwolfine *see* 194
Rauwolscine *see* 10104
Ra-Valeas [Valeas] *see* 8120

Ravenil [Caber] *see* 7975
Ravenol [Caber] *see* 8986
Raviac [Lipha] *see* 2152
Ravocaine Hydrochloride [Cook-Waite]
see 7837
Ravuconazole, 8121
Ravyon [Bayer CropSci.] *see* 1787
Raxar [Glaxo Wellcome] *see* 4545
Raxil [Bayer CropSci.] *see* 9092
Rayon, 8122
Razadyne [J & J] *see* 4340
Razoxane, 8123
RB-1509 *see* 5564
RBPI$_{21}$ *see* 938
RC-61-91 *see* 4895
RC-160 *see* 9934
RC-172 *see* 223
RC-27109 *see* 6535
RCL I *see* 8209
RCL II *see* 8209
RCL III *see* 8209
RCL IV *see* 8209
RD-1572 *see* 4731
RD-4593 *see* 5784
RD-13621 *see* 4881
rDSPA alpha 1 *see* 3459
RDX *see* 2736
Re-1-0185 *see* 3523
RE-4355 *see* 6358
RE-40885 *see* 4205
RE-45601 *see* 2349
Reacid *see* 2680
Reactine [Pfizer] *see* 2022
Reactivan [Cascan] *see* 3966
Realgar *see* 799
Reasec [Janssen] *see* 3313
Reason [Bayer CropSci.] *see* 3956
Reazide *see* 2680
Rebamipide, 8124
Rebetol [Schering-Plough] *see* 8198
Rebif [Serono] *see* 4991
Reboxetine, 8125
Reboxetine Mesylate *see* 8125
Rec-7-0040 *see* 4096
Rec-7-0267 *see* 3204
Rec-15-0691 *see* 9426
Rec-15-1476 *see* 4005
Rec-15-2375 *see* 5446
Recanescine *see* 2918
Receptal [Intervet] *see* 1503
Recheton *see* 5288
Reclaim [Dow AgroSci.] *see* 2400
Recognan [Asahi] *see* 2319
Recolip [Benzon] *see* 2377
Recombinant Human Activated Protein
C *see* 7884
Recombinant Human Soluble Interleu-
kin-4 Receptor *see* 5002
Recombinant Methionyl Human G-CSF
see 4537
Recombinate [Baxter] *see* 3921
Reconin [Toyama] *see* 2345
Reconox *see* 7252
Recordil [Recordati] *see* 3523
Recormon [Roche] *see* 4808
Recruit [Dow AgroSci.] *see* 4683
Recruit II [Dow AgroSci.] *see* 4683
Recruit III [Dow AgroSci.] *see* 6721
Recruit IV [Dow AgroSci.] *see* 6721
Rectadione *see* 7234
Rectalad [Carter-Wallace] *see* 3401
Rectodelt [Trommsdorff] *see* 7722
Rectogesic [Strakan] *see* 6607
Rectovalone [Jouveinal] *see* 9484
Red-Al [Aldrich] *see* 8564

Red Arrow *see* 4374
Red Arsenic Glass *see* 799
Red Arsenic Sulfide *see* 799
Red Bole *see* 1327
Red Clover *see* 9690
Red Copper Oxide *see* 2664
Redeema [Merz] *see* 10159
Redeptin [SK & F] *see* 4207
Redergin [Lek] *see* 3653
Red Fluorescent Protein, 8126
Redigo [Bayer CropSci.] *see* 7887
Redisol [Merck & Co.] *see* 10014
Redisol H [Merck & Co.] *see* 4809
Red Lead *see* 5425
Red Lead Chromate *see* 5406
Red Liquor *see* 344
Red Mustard *see* 6315
Red No. 2 *see* 375
Red Oil *see* 9823
Redomex [Lundbeck] *see* 487
Red Orpiment *see* 799
Redoxon [Roche] *see* 830
Red Phosphorus *see* 7347
Red Precipitate *see* 5882
Red Prussiate of Potash *see* 7630
Red Puccoon *see* 8355
Red Quebracho *see* 8031
Red Raspberry *see* 8118
Redroot *see* 376
Red Root *see* 8355
Red Sandalwood *see* 8386
Red Tetrazolium *see* 9744
Reduced Hematin *see* 4639
Reduced Nicotinamide Adenine Di-
nucleotide Phosphate Dehydrogenase
see 6824
Reduced Ninhydrin *see* 4775
Reductic Acid, 8127
Reductil [Knoll] *see* 8485
Reductol [Wyeth-Ayerst] *see* 110
Reducymol [SePRO] *see* 631
Redul [Schering] *see* 4507
Red Uranium Oxide *see* 9860
Redux [Wyeth-Ayerst] *see* 3973
Red-water Tree Bark *see* 8382
Redwood *see* 7181
Reelon [Sanwa] *see* 7505
Reevon [Reeves] *see* 7567
Refacto [Wyeth] *see* 6271
Refined Solvent Naphtha *see* 5489
Refkas [Maruko] *see* 3681
Reflex [Syngenta] *see* 4227
Refludan [Aventis] *see* 4718
Refobacin [Merck KGaA] *see* 4392
Refosporin [Merck KGaA] *see* 1916
Refrigerant 134a *see* 4714
Refugal [Bayer] *see* 2066
Refungine [A.C.F.] *see* 8892
Regacholyl *see* 4835
Regaine [Pfizer] *see* 6203
Regelan [Zeneca] *see* 2377
Regenit [Hoechst] *see* 7719
Regenon [Temmler] *see* 3127
Regianin *see* 5269
Regitine [Novartis] *see* 7264
Reglan [Wyeth] *see* 6143
Regletin [Teikoku Zoki] *see* 313
Reglone [Syngenta] *see* 3352
Regolax [Corvi] *see* 7245
Regonol [Organon] *see* 7977
Regramostim *see* 4538
Regranex [Chiron] *see* 7525
Regulan [Procter & Gamble] *see* 7517
Regulin [Young] *see* 5816
Regulipid [Heilit] *see* 2378

Regulox see 5705
Regulton [Knoll] see 394
Regulus of Antimony see 692
Regu-Mate [Intervet] see 319
Regurin [Galen] see 9786
Regutol [Schering-Plough] see 3401
Rehibin [Thames] see 2720
Reicaf [San Carlo] see 8252
Reichstein's Substance C see 273
Reichstein's Substance Dehydro-C see 281
Reichstein's Substance E see 7730
Reichstein's Substance Fa see 2539
Reichstein's Substance G see 176
Reichstein's Substance H see 2538
Reichstein's Substance L see 271
Reichstein's Substance M see 4787
Reichstein's Substance Q see 2900
Reichstein's Substance R see 274
Reichstein's Substance S see 2932
Reichstein's Substance U see 7731
Reinecke Salt, 8128
Rela [Schering] see 1842
Relafen [GSK] see 6343
Relane [Cutter] see 3299
Relanium [Polfa] see 2994
Relaspium [Isei] see 9786
Relaxan [Hexal] see 4343
Relaxar see 5850
Relaxil see 5850
Relaxil G [Pannon] see 4555
Relaxin, 8129
Reldan [Dow AgroSci.] see 2189
Releasin (formerly) [Warner-Chilcott] see 8129
Relefact LH-RH [HMR] see 5474
Relenza [GSK] see 10113
Relestat [Allergan] see 3618
Relestrid see 5980
Reliberan [Geymonat] see 2084
Relicor see 3710
Relifen [GSK] see 6343
Relifex [GSK] see 6343
Reliveran [Finadiet] see 6143
Relpax [Pfizer] see 3544
Relvene [Pharmascience] see 9789
Rely [Bayer CropSci.] see 7339
Remacemide, 8130
Remantadin(e) see 8224
Remark [Nippon Zoki] see 1178
Remedy [Dow AgroSci.] see 9656
Remeflin [Recordati] see 3204
Remeron [Organon] see 6208
Remestan [Wyeth] see 9133
Remicade [Centocor] see 4972
Remid [TAD] see 279
Remifemin [Schaper & Brümmer] see 1312
Remifentanil, 8131
Remifentanyl see 8131
Reminyl [J & J] see 4340
Remivox [Janssen] see 5580
Remnos [DDSA] see 6575
Remodulin [United Ther.] see 9586
Remoxipride, 8132
Renacor [Merck & Co.] see 3567
Renagel [Genzyme] see 8474
Renal Natriuretic Peptide see 9886
Renarcol see 5850
Rencal [BMS] see 7387
Rendix [Boehringer, Ing.] see 2797
Renese [Pfizer] see 7584
Reneuron [Juste] see 4185
Renex 20 [ICI] see 7578
Renex 600'S [Atlas] see 6677
Renilan [Mochida] see 1938

Renin, 8133
Renin Substrate see 651
Renitec [Merck & Co.] see 3567
Reniten [Merck & Co.] see 3567
Renivace [Merck & Co.] see 3567
Rennase see 8134
Rennet see 8134
Rennin, 8134
Reno M [BMS] see 5807
Renografin [BMS] see 5807
Renoquid [Glenwood] see 8902
Renormax [Schering-Plough] see 8753
Ren-o-sal [Salsbury] see 8273
Renounce [Bayer CropSci.] see 2756
Renova [Ortho] see 8165
Renovist [BMS] see 5807
Renovue-65 [BMS] see 5011
Renovue-DIP [BMS] see 5011
Renpress [Sandoz] see 8753
Rentylin [Rentschler] see 7136
Renzapride, 8135
Renzepin [Bergamon] see 7491
Reocorin [Farmochimica] see 7737
Reomax [Bioindustria] see 3717
Reomucil [DOC] see 1802
ReoPro [Lilly] see 5
Reoxyl [Byk Gulden] see 4705
Repagermanium see 7795
Repaglinide, 8136
Repanidal [Leciva] see 9778
Reparil [Madaus] see 3696
Repel [WPC] see 2856
Repeltin [Fabre-Medikosma] see 9704
Repinotan, 8137
Repirinast, 8138
Replagal [Transkaryotic] see 4336
Repocal [Desitin] see 7130
Repodral [Winthrop] see 8813
Repoise [Robins] see 1516
Reprodin [Bayer] see 5610
Repronex [Ferring] see 4223
Reproterol, 8139
Reptilase [Knoll] see 1010
Repulson [Mochida] see 757
Requip [GSK] see 8257
Resacetophenone, 8140
Resantin see 3990
Resazoin see 8141
Resazurin, 8141
Resbenzophenone see 1106
Resbuthrin [Wellcome] see 1230
Rescinnamine, 8142
Rescriptor [Pharmacia & Upjohn] see 2877
Rescufolin [Nordic] see 4222
Rescula [Novartis] see 9849
Rescuvolin [Medac] see 4222
Resectisol [McGaw] see 5745
Reserpic Acid, 8143
Reserpilic Acid Dimethylaminoethyl Ester Dihydrochloride see 8144
Reserpiline, 8144
Reserpine, 8145
Reserpinine see 8142
Reserpinolic Acid see 8143
Resibufogenin, 8146
Resilin, 8147
Resimatil [Sanofi-Synthelabo] see 7746
Resin Benjamin see 4580
Resin Benzoin see 4580
Resin Copal see 2517
Resin Damar see 2807
Resin Guaiac see 4552
Resin Ipomea, 8148
Resin Jalap, 8149
Resin Kino see 5313

Resin of Mexican Scammony see 8148
Resin Scammony, 8150
Resin Tolu see 950
Resiquimod, 8151
Resistomycin [Bayer] see 5281
Resistomycin, 8152
Resitan [Takeda] see 9906
Resitox [Bayer] see 2558
Résivit [Oberlin] see 5452
Resloom M 75 [Monsanto] see 4691
Resmethrin, 8153
(+)-trans-Resmethrin see 1230
Resmit [Shionogi] see 5786
Resochin [Bayer] see 2163
Resolor [J & J] see 7907
Resolvable Tartaric Acid see 9069
Resonium A [Winthrop] see 8668
Resorantel, 8154
Resorcin see 8155
Resorcin Blue see 5332
Resorcinol, 8155
Resorcinolphthalein see 4159
Resorcinol Phthalein Sodium see 4159
Resorcinolphthalin see 4160
Resorcinol Yellow see 9775
β-Resorcylaldehyde, 8156
Resorcylam see 8154
β-Resorcylic Acid, 8157
Resorcylic Acid Lactones see 10116
Resotren [Bayer] see 4826
Resource [Valent] see 4142
Respacal [Bios-Coutelier] see 9811
Respbid [Boehringer, Ing.] see 9285
Respicort [Ivax] see 3870
Respicort [Mundipharma] see 9596
Respifral see 5217
Respigon [Taisho] see 8146
Respirase [Gibipharma] see 10170
Respiride [Schiapparelli] see 3999
Respirot [Novartis] see 2591
Respontin [GSK] see 5073
Resporisan [Kowa] see 8144
Restandol [Organon] see 9180
Restanolon [Isei] see 2408
Restar [Sumitomo] see 4213
Restas [Kanebo] see 4213
Restasis [Allergan] see 2752
Restenacht [Kabi] see 3558
Restenil [Recip] see 5862
Restetal [Kabi] see 3566
Rest-On see 5959
Restoril [Novartis] see 9133
Restrol [Central Pharm.] see 3104
Restryl see 5959
Resulax [AstraZeneca] see 8725
Resulfon [Nordmark] see 8908
Resveratrol, 8158
cis-Resveratrol see 8158
trans-Resveratrol see 8158
Resyl [Novartis] see 4555
Retabolil [Richter Gedeon] see 6365
Retalon see 3104
Retalon-Lingual see 4701
Retalon Oleosum see 4701
Retalon-Oral see 3104
Retamine, 8159
Retarcyl [Delagrange] see 6277
Retardon [Chassot] see 8934
Retavase [Centocor] see 8161
Retcin [DDSA] see 3681
Retene, 8160
Retens [Chiesi] see 3440
Reteplase, 8161
Reticulin, 8162
Reticuline, 8163

Riabal [Fujisawa] *see* 7742
Riacen [Chiesi] *see* 7506
Riamet [Novartis] *see* 5597
Riball [Schering AG] *see* 279
Ribamidine *see* 9063
Ribavirin, 8198
α-Ribazole, 8199
Ribena [GSK] *see* 830
Ribex [Formenti] *see* 3452
Ribitol *see* 168
Ribo [Tennessee Pharm.] *see* 8201
D-2-Ribodesose *see* 2908
Riboflavin, 8200
Riboflavin 5′-(Dihydrogen Phosphate) *see* 8201
Riboflavine 5′-Adenosine Diphosphate *see* 4091
Riboflavine 5′-(Trihydrogen Diphosphate) 5′ → 5′-Ester with Adenosine *see* 4091
Riboflavin Monophosphate, 8201
D-Ribofuranose-5-phosphoric Acid *see* 8205
9-β-D-Ribofuranosidoadenine *see* 153
1-β-D-Ribofuranosylcytosine *see* 2786
9-β-D-Ribofuranosylhypoxanthine *see* 4975
2-β-D-Ribofuranosylmaleimide *see* 8482
3-β-D-Ribofuranosylorotic Acid *see* 6877
9-β-D-Ribofuranosyl-9*H*-purin-6-amine *see* 153
9-β-D-Ribofuranosyl-9*H*-purine *see* 6433
9-β-D-Ribofuranosyl-9*H*-purine-2,6-diol *see* 10065
9-β-D-Ribofuranosyl-9*H*-purine-2,6-(1*H*,3*H*)-dione *see* 10065
N-(9-β-D-Ribofuranosyl-9*H*-purin-6-yl)-butyramide Cyclic 3′,5′-(Hydrogen Phosphate) 2′-Butyrate *see* 1463
3-β-D-Ribofuranosyl-1*H*-pyrrole-2,5-dione *see* 8482
7-β-D-Ribofuranosyl-7*H*-pyrrolo[2,3-*d*]-pyrimidin-4-amine *see* 9804
2β-D-Ribofuranosyl-4-thiazolecarboxamide *see* 9425
2-β-D-Ribofuranosyl-1,2,4-triazine-3,-5(2*H*,4*H*)-dione *see* 904
1-β-D-Ribofuranosyl-1*H*-1,2,4-triazole-3-carboxamide *see* 8198
1-β-D-Ribofuranosyl-1,2,4-triazole-3-carboxamidine *see* 9063
1-β-D-Ribofuranosyl-1*H*-1,2,4-triazole-3-carboximidamide *see* 9063
1-β-D-Ribofuranosyluracil *see* 9877
9-β-D-Ribofuranosyl Xanthine *see* 10065
D-Ribohexulose *see* 7924
Ribolact [Taiho] *see* 8200
Ribomustin [Ribosepharm] *see* 1034
Ribomycine [Delalande] *see* 8206
Ribonosine [Toyo Jozo] *see* 4975
Ribonuclease, 8202
Ribonuclease (*Rana pipiens* Reduced) *see* 8112
Ribonucleic Acid, 8203
D-Ribose, 8204
D-Ribose-5-phosphate *see* 8205
D-Ribose-5-phosphoric Acid, 8205
Ribosomal RNA *see* 8203
Ribostamin [Delalande] *see* 8206
Ribostamycin, 8206
Ribotrex [Fabre] *see* 915
Riboxamide *see* 9425
Ribrain [Yamanouchi] *see* 1178
D-Ribulose, 8207
Ricainide *see* 4937

Ricamycin [Toyo Jozo] *see* 8250
Rice Bran Oil, 8208
Rice Oil *see* 8208
Ricestar [Bayer CropSci.] *see* 3984
Richweed *see* 2483
Ricidine *see* 8210
Ricin, 8209
Ricin D *see* 8209
Ricinine, 8210
Ricinoleic Acid, 8211
Ricinolsulfuric Acid *see* 8211
Ricinstearolic Acid Diiodide *see* 7172
Ricinus Oil *see* 1898
Rickamicin *see* 8550
Ricketon *see* 10019
Ricobendazole *see* 210
Ricridene [Lipha] *see* 6540
Rid *see* 2839
Ridaura [Prometheus] *see* 878
Ridauran [Robapharm] *see* 878
Ridazin [Taro] *see* 9359
Ridect [Pfizer] *see* 7180
Ridene [Syntex] *see* 6495
Ridinol *see* 7741
Ridogrel, 8212
Ridomil [Syngenta] *see* 5922
Ridomil Gold [Syngenta] *see* 5922
Ridzol [Merck & Co.] *see* 8254
Riegel's Paper *see* 2498
Rifa [Grünenthal] *see* 8216
Rifabutin, 8213
Rifacol [Formenti] *see* 8220
Rifadin(e) [Aventis] *see* 8216
Rifalazil, 8214
Rifaldazine *see* 8216
Rifaldin [Aventis] *see* 8216
Rifamastene [Uce] *see* 8218
Rifamicine SV *see* 8218
Rifamide, 8215
Rifampicin *see* 8216
Rifampin, 8216
Rifamycin AG *see* 8217
Rifamycin AMP *see* 8216
Rifamycin B *see* 8217
Rifamycin B Diethylamide *see* 8215
Rifamycin L 105 *see* 8220
Rifamycin O *see* 8217
Rifamycins, 8217
Rifamycin S *see* 8217
Rifamycin SV, 8218
Rifamycin X *see* 8217
Rifapentine, 8219
Rifapiam [Piam] *see* 8216
Rifaprodin [Almirall] *see* 8216
Rifaxidin *see* 8220
Rifaximin, 8220
Rifit [Syngenta] *see* 7740
Rifloc [Avensa] *see* 5225
Rifocin [Lepetit] *see* 8218
Rifocin M [Lepetit] *see* 8215
Rifoldin [Aventis] *see* 8216
Rifomycins *see* 8217
Rifomycin SV *see* 8218
Rigelon [Dojin] *see* 9301
Rikamycin *see* 8250
Riker 52G *see* 757
Rilansyl *see* 2106
Rilaquil *see* 2106
Rilassol *see* 2106
Rilaten [Guidotti] *see* 8245
Rilmazafone, 8221
Rilmenidine, 8222
Rilutek [Aventis] *see* 8223
Riluzole, 8223
Rimactan(e) [Novartis] *see* 8216

Rimadyl [Pfizer] *see* 1862
Rimagina [Medipolar] *see* 8225
Rimantadine, 8224
Rimaon *see* 3716
Rimatil [Santen] *see* 1460
Rimazole [Cheil Sugar] *see* 2417
Rimazolium Metilsulfate, 8225
Rimexel [Organon] *see* 8226
Rimexolone, 8226
Rimifon [Pharmion] *see* 5186
Rimiterol, 8227
Rimitsid *see* 5186
Rimocidin, 8228
Rimon [Makhteshim-Agan] *see* 6720
Rimonabant, 8229
Rimostil [Novogen] *see* 9690
Rimso-50 [Britannia] *see* 3259
Rimsulfuron, 8230
Rinatec [Boehringer, Ing.] *see* 5073
Rinderon-DP [Shionogi] *see* 1180
Rinder-vasopressin *see* 9938
Rindex [Sidus] *see* 5943
Rinesal [Kissei] *see* 1974
Rineton [Sanwa] *see* 9596
Ringworm Powder *see* 768
Rinlaxer [Taisho] *see* 2179
Rino-Clenil [Chiesi] *see* 1019
Rinogutt [Boehringer, Ing.] *see* 9567
Rintal [Bayer] *see* 3944
Riol [Toa Eiyo] *see* 9112
Riomitsin *see* 6976
Riopan [Ayerst] *see* 5651
Rioprostil, 8231
Ripcord [BASF] *see* 2767
Ripercol [Am. Cyanamid] *see* 5459
Ripirin [Kabi] *see* 3558
Ripon *see* 5651
Riposon *see* 5846
Ripresil [Erba] *see* 2451
Riquent [La Jolla Pharmaceuticals] *see* 6
Riran [Yamanouchi] *see* 4928
rI$_n$ · r(C$_{12}$U)$_n$ *see* 588
Riripen [Daiichi] *see* 1122
Risamol [Yoshitomi] *see* 2316
Risatarun [Ravensberg] *see* 2843
Rischiaril [Piam] *see* 2843
Rise [Yoshitomi] *see* 2416
Risedronate Sodium *see* 8232
Risedronic Acid, 8232
Risolid [Dumex] *see* 2084
Risordan [Aventis] *see* 5225
Risperdal [J & J] *see* 8233
Risperidone, 8233
Ristocetin, 8234
Ristogen [Kowa Yakuhin] *see* 4132
Ristomycin *see* 8234
Ristomycin A *see* 8234
Ristomycin B *see* 8234
Riston *see* 8234
Ristosamine *see* 132
Risumic [Dainippon] *see* 394
Ritacetyl [R.I.T.A.] *see* 5358
Ritalan [R.I.T.A.] *see* 5358
Ritalin [Novartis] *see* 6110
Ritalmex [Alkaloida] *see* 6169
Ritanserin, 8235
Ritawax [R.I.T.A.] *see* 5359
Ritipenem, 8236
Ritipenem Acoxil *see* 8236
Ritmodan [Aventis] *see* 3360
Ritmos [Sanofi-Synthelabo] *see* 194
Ritmos Elle [Inverni] *see* 5577
Ritmusin [Gebro] *see* 754
Ritodrine, 8237
Ritonavir, 8238

Rituxan [Genentech] see 8239
Rituximab, 8239
RIV-2093 see 311
Rivadescin [Schaper & Brümmer] see 8120
Rivanol [Winthrop] see 3716
Rivasin [Solvay] see 8145
Rivastatin see 1993
Rivastigmine, 8240
Riversideite see 1702
Rivistel [Delagrange] see 311
Rivizor [J & J] see 10035
Rivoltan [Lichtwer] see 2942
Rivotril [Roche] see 2389
Rixapen [RIT] see 2385
Rizaben [Kissei] see 9570
Rizatriptan, 8241
Rize [Yoshitomi] see 2416
Rizen [Formenti] see 2416
Rizinsan K2 A2 see 4505
Rizolex [Sumitomo] see 9510
RJR-1734 see 5239
RL-50 see 6254
r-metHuG-CSF see 4537
RMI-17043 see 3589
RMI-71754 see 9978
RMI-71782 see 3522
RNA see 8203
RNase see 8202
Ro-1-5130 see 7977
Ro-1-5431 see 5470
Ro-1-5431/7 see 5470
Ro-1-5470 see 8091
Ro-1-5470/5 see 8091
Ro-1-5470/6 see 8091
Ro-1-6794 see 5470
Ro-1-7788 see 8091
Ro-1-7977 see 8865
Ro-1-9569 see 9182
Ro-2-2985 see 5373
Ro-2-3198 see 3516
Ro-2-3308 see 8082
Ro-2-3773 see 2354
Ro-2-7113 see 296
Ro-2-9578 see 9708
Ro-2-9757 see 4181
Ro-2-9915 see 4125
Ro-2-9945 see 4176
Ro-3-4787 see 1480
Ro-3-7008 see 202
Ro-4-1544/6 see 8812
Ro-4-1575 see 487
Ro-4-1577 see 2713
Ro-4-3780 see 5228
Ro-4-3816 see 221
Ro-4-4393 see 8906
Ro-4-4602 see 1050
Ro-4-5282 see 5799
Ro-4-5360 see 6575
Ro-4-6467 see 7758
Ro-4-8347 see 9584
Ro-5-0810/1 see 9653
Ro-5-0831 see 5157
Ro-5-2180 see 6691
Ro-5-2807 see 2994
Ro-5-3307/1 see 2844
Ro-5-3350 see 1385
Ro-5-3438 see 4128
Ro-5-4023 see 2389
Ro-5-4200 see 4146
Ro-5-5345 see 9133
Ro-5-6901 see 4198
Ro-6-4563 see 4438
Ro-7-0207 see 6872
Ro-7-1051 see 1084
Ro-7-1554 see 5079

Ro-7-4488/1 see 6340
Ro-7-6102 see 4209
Ro-7-6145 see 3199
Ro-8-6837 see 6141
Ro-9-1978 see 1754
Ro-10-1670 see 112
Ro-10-5970 see 1380
Ro-10-6338 see 1484
Ro-10-9070 see 389
Ro-10-9359 see 3892
Ro-11-780 see 8225
Ro-11-1163 see 6226
Ro-11-1430 see 6284
Ro-12-0068 see 9148
Ro-13-1042 see 5580
Ro-13-5057 see 662
Ro-13-5223 see 3987
Ro-13-8996 see 6937
Ro-13-9297 see 5582
Ro-13-9904/001 see 1953
Ro-14-3169/000 see 3993
Ro-14-4767/000 see 573
Ro-14-4767/002 see 573
Ro-15-1297 see 7983
Ro-15-1788 see 4135
Ro-15-8074 see 1923
Ro-15-8075 see 1923
Ro-17-2301 see 1871
Ro-17-3664 see 7806
Ro-18-0647 see 6869
Ro-19-5247 see 1947
Ro-19-6327 see 5394
Ro-20-5720/000 see 1862
Ro-20-7234 see 4158
Ro-21-3981/001 see 6182
Ro-21-3981/003 see 6182
Ro-21-5535 see 1644
Ro-21-5998 see 5801
Ro-21-6937 see 9723
Ro-21-8837 see 3706
Ro-21-9738 see 3437
Ro-22-7796 see 2269
Ro-22-8181 see 4990
Ro-22-9000 see 234
Ro-23-6019 see 4994
Ro-23-6240 see 4099
Ro-24-7375 see 2799
Ro-31-2848 see 2273
Ro-31-3113 see 2273
Ro-31-8959 see 8369
Ro-31-8959/003 see 8369
Ro-40-5967 see 6173
Ro-40-7592 see 9508
Ro 40-8757 see 6230
Ro-42-1611 see 814
Ro-44-9883 see 5349
Ro-47-0203 see 1353
Ro-61-0612 see 9252
Ro-61-1790 see 2342
Ro-63-9141 see 1952
Ro-65-5788 see 1952
Ro-107-9070/194 see 9907
Roaccutane [Roche] see 5228
Robac 22 [Robinson Bros.] see 3803
Robalate [Robins] see 3183
Robamol [Cenci] see 5980
Robamox [Wyeth] see 577
Robane [Robeco] see 8767
Robanul see 4501
Robaxin [Robins] see 5980
Robecote [Robeco] see 8477
Robenidine, 8242
Robenogatope I-131 [BMS] see 8262
Robenz [Am. Cyanamid] see 8242
Robenzidene see 8242

Robigenin see 5274
Robinin, 8243
Robinul [Robins] see 4501
Robison Ester see 4462
Robitet [Wyeth] see 9196
Robitussin [Wyeth] see 4555
Robizone-V [Robins] see 7277
Robnin [Nikken] see 10170
Robuoy [Robeco] see 7752
Rocain [Fuso] see 7757
Rocaltrol [Roche] see 1644
Roccal [Sanofi-Synthelabo] see 1059
Roccellic Acid, 8244
Rocefin [Roche] see 1953
Rocephin(e) [Roche] see 1953
Rochelle Salt see 7670
Rociverine, 8245
Rock Oil see 7187
Rock Salt see 8599
Rocornal [Rodleben] see 9574
Rocuronium, 8246
Rodeo [Dow AgroSci.] see 4512
Rodewod see 641
Rodex [Hacco] see 10038
Rodinal see 462
Rodipal see 3747
Rodiuran see 4789
Rody [Sumitomo] see 3991
(+)-Roemerine see 748
Roentgenium, 8247
Roeridorm [Roerig] see 3729
Rofecoxib, 8248
Roferon-A [Roche] see 4990
Roflual [Roche] see 8224
Roflumilast, 8249
Rogaine [Pfizer] see 6203
Rogitine [Novartis] see 7264
Rogojski's Salt see 2668
Rogor [Isagro] see 3220
Rohrbach's Soln see 982
Rohypnol [Roche] see 4146
Roinin [Mohan] see 7737
Roipnol [Roche] see 4146
Rökan [Intersan] see 4425
Rokital [Formenti] see 8250
Rokitamycin, 8250
Rolipram, 8251
Rolitetracycline, 8252
Roman Chamomile see 2041
Roman Chamomile Oil see 2041
Roman Laurel see 5382
Roman Vitriol see 2653
Romazicon [Roche] see 4135
Romensin [Elanco] see 6246
Romet [Mitsubishi] see 8138
Rometin see 5031
Romglizone see 9769
Romicil see 6825
Rompun [Bayer] see 10080
Romurtide, 8253
RonaCare [Merck KGaA] see 6820
RonaCare Ectoin [Merck KGaA] see 3505
Ronaxan [Merial] see 3440
Rondase see 4758
Rondomycin [Wallace] see 5943
Rongalite see 8620
Rongalite C see 8620
Roniacol [Roche] see 6527
Roniacol Tartrate [Roche] see 6527
Ronicol see 6527
Ronidase see 4758
Ronidazole, 8254
Ronifibrate, 8255
Ronilan [BASF] see 9984
Ronnel, 8256

Ruberythric Acid, 8280
Ruberythrinic Acid *see* 8280
Rubesol *see* 10014
Rubiadin, 8281
Rubian *see* 8280
Rubianic Acid *see* 8280
Rubiazol [Hoechst] *see* 8901
Rubiazol I *see* 8923
Rubichloric Acid *see* 844
Rubidazone [Bellon] *see* 10195
Rubidium, 8282
Rubidium Bromide, 8283
Rubidium Carnallite *see* 8282
Rubidium Chloride, 8284
Rubidium Hydroxide, 8285
Rubidium Iodide, 8286
Rubidomycin *see* 2832
Rubigan [Gowan] *see* 3958
Rubigervine *see* 8287
Rubijervine, 8287
Rubimycin [Nikken] *see* 6183
Rubinorm [IFI] *see* 8284
Rubitecan, 8288
Rubixanthin, 8289
Ruboxistaurin, 8290
Ruboxistaurin Mesylate Monohydrate
see 8290
Rubozinc [Labcatal] *see* 4456
Rubramin PC [BMS] *see* 10014
Rubratope-57 [BMS] *see* 10015
Rubratope-60 [BMS] *see* 10015
Rubriment [Nordmark] *see* 6526
α-Rubromycin *see* 2482
Rubus, 8291
Ruby [Spencer] *see* 6519
Ruby Arsenic *see* 799
Ruby Wood *see* 8386
Rudilin [Darby] *see* 6732
Rudotel [OPW] *see* 5786
Ruelene [Dow] *see* 2604
Rufast [AgrEvo] *see* 125
Rufigallic Acid *see* 8292
Rufigallol, 8292
Rufinamide, 8293
Rufloxacin, 8294
Rufol [Fournier] *see* 8916
Rugby [FMC] *see* 1632
Rugulovasine A *see* 8295
Rugulovasine B *see* 8295
Rugulovasines, 8295
Rulicalcin [HMR] *see* 1643
Rulid [Hoechst] *see* 8276
Rumatral [Nicholas] *see* 309
Rumensin [Elanco] *see* 6246
Rumex, 8296
Runner [Bayer CropSci.] *see* 5993
Rupafin [Uriach] *see* 8297
Rupatadine, 8297
Ruppert's Reagent *see* 9683
Rusa Oil *see* 6796
Rusat *see* 1156
Ruswut *see* 1156
Rusyde [CP] *see* 4309
Rutaecarpine *see* 8298
Rutamycin *see* 6833
Rutecarpine, 8298
Ruthenium, 8299
Ruthenium(VIII) Oxide *see* 8301
Ruthenium Oxychloride Ammoniated *see*
8300
Ruthenium Red, 8300
Ruthenium Tetroxide, 8301
Ruthenium Trichloride, 8302
Ruthenium Violet *see* 8300
Rutherfordium, 8303

Ruticina [Bernabo] *see* 5925
Rutile *see* 9472
Rutin, 8304
Rutinose, 8305
Rutoside *see* 8304
Ruven [Mepha] *see* 9789
RV-144 *see* 3647
RV-12424 *see* 4148
r-VIII SQ *see* 6271
RWJ-10553 *see* 6694
RWJ-17021-000 *see* 9547
RWJ-17070 *see* 4722
RWJ-20485 *see* 9151
RWJ-22164 *see* 865
RWJ-60235 *see* 7525
RX-5050M *see* 3340
RX-6029-M *see* 1497
RX-781094 *see* 4887
Ryanex *see* 8306
Ryania, 8306
Ryanicide [Penick] *see* 8306
Ryanodine, 8307
Ryanodol 3-(1*H*-Pyrrole-2-carboxylate)
see 8307
Rycarden [Syntex] *see* 6495
Rycoben [Novartis] *see* 210
Rycobendazole *see* 210
Rydar [Cutter] *see* 3299
Rydene [Syntex] *see* 6495
Rydrin [Kodama] *see* 6732
Ryegonovin [Aventis] *see* 6070
Rynacrom [Sanofi-Aventis] *see* 2590
Rythmatine [Burroughs Wellcome] *see*
5843
Rythmodan [Aventis] *see* 3360
Rythmodul [Aventis] *see* 3360
Rythmol [Abbott] *see* 7794
Rytmonorm [Abbott] *see* 7794
S-2-676 *see* 9234
S-7 *see* 4004
S-23/46 *see* 672
S-041 *see* 4324
S-73-4118 *see* 7492
S-77-0777 *see* 7719
S-94 *see* 4189
S-095 *see* 5722
S-145 *see* 3416
(+)-S-145 *see* 3416
S-165 *see* 3109
S-203 *see* 9700
S-222 *see* 3367
S-314 *see* 4313
S-596 *see* 791
S-640P *see* 1915
S-658 *see* 4295
S-768 *see* 3973
S-780 *see* 1039
S-805 *see* 5587
S-940 *see* 6354
S-992 *see* 1039
S-1006 *see* 1919
S-1108 *see* 1919
S-1153 *see* 1755
S-1320 *see* 1468
S-1452 *see* 3416
S-1520 *see* 4935
S-1530 *see* 6549
S-1574 *see* 9420
S-1605 *see* 3109
S-1694 *see* 409
S-1702 *see* 4439
S-1752 *see* 4002
S-1844 *see* 4010
S-1942 *see* 1431
S-2225 *see* 1431

S-2395 *see* 9173
S-2539 *see* 7211
S-2620 *see* 301
S-2703 *see* 2768
S-2703 Forte *see* 2768
S-3151 *see* 7180
S-3206 *see* 3991
S-3308-10 *see* 3268
S-3308L *see* 3268
S-3341 *see* 8222
S-3341-3 *see* 8222
S-3349 *see* 9510
S-3500 *see* 1525
S-4068 *see* 7704
S-4068SF *see* 7704
S-4084 *see* 2261
S-4522 *see* 8270
S-5602 *see* 4010
S-5602α *see* 4010
S-6059 *see* 6286
S-6810 *see* 4992
S-7131 *see* 7765
S-8527 *see* 2357
S-9318 *see* 7990
S-9490 *see* 7170
S-9490-3 *see* 7170
S-9780 *see* 7170
S-10036 *see* 4261
S-12911 *see* 8106
S-16257 *see* 5247
S-16257-2 *see* 5247
S-20098 *see* 190
S-21403 *see* 6211
S-23031 *see* 4142
S-25930 *see* 4872
S-26308 *see* 4922
S-28463 *see* 8151
S-31183 *see* 7990
S-31252 *see* 7177
S-32165 *see* 3109
S-50022 *see* 4428
S-53482 *see* 4143
SA *see* 9843
SA-79 *see* 7794
SA-96 *see* 1460
SA-97 *see* 4733
SA-504 *see* 9442
sab simplex [Pfizer] *see* 3215
Sabadilla, 8308
Sabalamin [Santen] *see* 2451
Sabcomeline, 8309
Sabeluzole, 8310
Sabidal [Zyma] *see* 2210
Sabiden [Szabo] *see* 7271
Sabril [HMR] *see* 9978
Sabromin [Sandoz] *see* 1451
Saccharase *see* 5005
Saccharated Ferric Oxide *see* 5101
Saccharic Acid *see* 4450
Saccharin, 8311
Saccharin Ammonium *see* 8311
Saccharin Insoluble *see* 8311
Saccharinol *see* 8311
Saccharinose *see* 8311
Saccharin Sodium *see* 8311
Saccharol *see* 8311
Saccharolactic Acid *see* 4331
Saccharolactone *see* 4450
L-Saccharopine, 8312
Saccharose *see* 8881
Saccharosonic Acid *see* 5126
Sacerno [EGYT] *see* 5853
Sacox [Intervet] *see* 8336
Sacred Bark *see* 1880
Sacysyl-cysteine *see* 2783

Sadopan *see* 4367
Safari [DuPont] *see* 9689
Safetray *see* 641
Saffan [Mallinckrodt] *see* 235
Safflor Carmine *see* 1867
Safflor Red *see* 1867
Safflower *see* 1868
Safflower Oil, 8313
Saffron, 8314
Saffron-bitter *see* 7411
Saffron Indian *see* 9824
Safinamide, 8315
Safinamide Mesylate *see* 8315
Safranal, 8316
Safranin B Extra *see* 7251
Safrole, 8317
Saga [Roussel-Uclaf] *see* 9565
Sagamicin [Kyowa] *see* 6181
Sagamicin (formerly) *see* 6181
Sage *see* 8343
Sagrotan [Schülke & Mayr] *see* 1059
SaH-42548 *see* 5762
SAHA *see* 10034
Saheli [Hindustan Latex] *see* 1971
SAICAR, 8318
Saigon Cinnamon *see* 2300
Saizen [Serono] *see* 8716
Sakarat X [Killgerm] *see* 10038
Sakuranetin, 8319
Sakuranin *see* 8319
Sal Acetosella *see* 7611, 7689
Saladjidi *see* 4885
Salagen [MGI] *see* 7424
Salamid [Hamilton] *see* 8328
Sal Ammoniac *see* 509
Salanil [Sato Yakuhin] *see* 4378
Salatrim, 8320
Salazolon *see* 717
Salazopyrin [Pfizer] *see* 8942
Salazosulfadimidine, 8321
Salazosulfapyridine *see* 8942
Salbulin [3M Pharma] *see* 216
Salbumol [GSK] *see* 216
Salbutamol *see* 216
Salbutard [Lusofarmaco] *see* 216
Salbuvent [Nycomed] *see* 216
Salcatonin *see* 1643
Salco *see* 2374
Salcyl *see* 8334
Salcylix *see* 8334
Saldox *see* 8327
Salen, 8322
Sal Enixum *see* 7613
Salep, 8323
Sal Ethyl *see* 3850
Salflex [Carnrick] *see* 8339
Salicain [Hoechst] *see* 4846
Salicin, 8324
Salicin Benzoate *see* 7594
Salicinerein *see* 7395
Salicoside *see* 8324
N-Salicoylaminophenol *see* 6887
Salicylacetylsalicylic Acid *see* 100
Salicyl Alcohol, 8325
Salicyl Alcohol Glucoside *see* 8324
Salicylaldehyde, 8326
Salicylaldehyde β-D-Glucoside *see* 4628
Salicylaldoxime, 8327
Salicylamide, 8328
Salicylamide *O*-Acetic Acid, 8329
Salicylamide *o*-Ethyl Ether *see* 3731
Salicylanilide, 8330
Salicylazosulfadimidine *see* 8321
Salicylazosulfamethazine *see* 8321
Salicylazosulfapyridine *see* 8942

Salicylhydroxamic Acid, 8331
Salicylic Acid, 8332
Salicylic Acid Acetate *see* 851
Salicylic Acid Acetate Calcium Salt *see* 1647
Salicylic Acid Acetate, Ester with 4-Hydroxyacetanilide *see* 1045
Salicylic Acid, Acid Sulfate *see* 8334
Salicylic Acid Benzyl Ester *see* 1144
Salicylic Acid Bimolecular Ester *see* 8339
Salicylic Acid Bornyl Ester *see* 1341
Salicylic Acid *p-tert*-Butylphenyl Ester *see* 1586
Salicylic Acid Choline Salt *see* 2209
Salicylic Acid Dihydrogen Phosphate *see* 4255
Salicylic Acid Ethyl Ester *see* 3850
Salicylic Acid Isopropyl Ester *O*-Ester with *O*-Ethyl Isopropylphosphoramidothioate *see* 5172
Salicylic Acid Monoammonium Salt *see* 550
Salicylic Acid Sulfuric Acid Ester *see* 8334
Salicylic Acid 3,3,5-Trimethylcyclohexyl Ester *see* 4738
Salicylic Aldehyde *see* 8326
Salicylic Ether *see* 3850
Salicyl Morpholide *see* 8333
Salicyloxysalicylic Acid *see* 8339
4-Salicyloylmorpholine, 8333
Salicyl Phosphate *see* 4255
Salicylsalicylic Acid *see* 8339
Salicylsulfonic Acid *see* 8964
Salicylsulfuric Acid, 8334
Salicyl-Vasogen *see* 550
Salicyl Yellow *see* 5919
Saligenin *see* 8325
Saligenin-β-D-glucopyranoside *see* 8324
Saligenol *see* 8325
Saliglutin [Streuli] *see* 8332
Salimid *see* 2745
Salinaphthol *see* 6415
Salinazid, 8335
Saliniazid *see* 8335
Salinidol [Doak] *see* 8330
Salinigrin *see* 7395
Salinomycin, 8336
Saliphenazon *see* 717
Salipran [Evans] *see* 1045
Salipurpol *see* 6424
Salipyrazolon *see* 717
Salipyrine *see* 717
Salit [Tenneco] *see* 1341
Saliuzid *see* 6852
Salizell [Byk Gulden] *see* 8328
Salizell (Amp.) [Byk Gulden] *see* 8329
Salizolo *see* 4913
Salmetedur [Menarini] *see* 8337
Salmeterol, 8337
Salmeterol Xinafoate *see* 8337
Salmiac *see* 509
Salmine Sulfate, 8338
Salmotonin [Yamanouchi] *see* 1643
Salocin [Intervet] *see* 8336
Salocoll *see* 7239
Salofalk [Falk] *see* 5904
Salol *see* 7310
Saloop *see* 8381
Salophen [Bayer] *see* 48
Salpetersäure (German) *see* 6577
Sal Polychrestum *see* 7674
Salsalate, 8339
Sal Soda *see* 8596
Salsoline, 8340

(+)-Salsoline *see* 8340
Salt *see* 8599
Salt Cake *see* 8680
Salt of Lemon *see* 7611
Salt of Saturn *see* 5397
Salt of Sorrel *see* 7611, 7689
Salt of Tartar *see* 7619
Saltpeter *see* 7648
Saltron *see* 2374
Saltucin [Boehringer, Mann.] *see* 1525
Salufer *see* 8624
Salures [Pfizer] *see* 1037
Saluric [Merck & Co.] *see* 2168
Salurin [Syntex] *see* 9624
Saluron [Apothecon] *see* 4789
Saluside *see* 6852
Salutaridine, 8341
Saluzid *see* 6852
Saluzide *see* 6852
Salvacard *see* 6543
Salvarsan *see* 811
Salverine, 8342
Salvia, 8343
Salvinin *see* 7071
Salvinorins, 8344
Salvizol *see* 1248
Salymid [Biochemie] *see* 8328
Salyrgan [Sterling Winthrop] *see* 5901
Salyzoron [Hishiyama] *see* 1122
Salzburg Vitriol *see* 2653
Samaderin A *see* 8345
Samaderin B *see* 8345
Samaderin C *see* 8345
Samaderins, 8345
Samaderoside A *see* 8345
Samandarine, 8346
Samandarone *see* 8346
Samarium, 8347
Samarium Cobalt, 8348
Samarium Diiodide *see* 8349
Samarium 153 Ethylenediaminetetramethylenephosphonic Acid *see* 8350
Samarium Iodide, 8349
Samarium(II) Iodide *see* 8349
Samarium Pentacobalt *see* 8348
Samarium [153]Sm Lexidronam, 8350
Sambucin *see* 2687
Sambucus, 8351
Sambunigrin *see* 5720
SAMe *see* 156
S-Amet [Europharma] *see* 156
Samid [Knoll] *see* 8328
Samli *see* 4417
Samorin [M & B] *see* 5183
Samorin, 8352
Samyr [Boehringer, Ing.] *see* 156
SAN-197 *see* 3893
SAN-322I *see* 7815
SAN-371F *see* 6908
SAN-582H *see* 3214
SAN-619F *see* 2771
SAN-835H *see* 3145
SAN-1269H *see* 3145
SAN-9789 *see* 6701
Sanamycin [FBA Pharm] *see* 1606
Sanapert *see* 6974
Sanasthmax [GSK] *see* 1019
Sanceller 22 [Sanshin] *see* 3803
Sanctura [Indevus] *see* 9786
Sand *see* 8493
Sandalwood, 8353
Sandalwood Oil *see* 8353
Sandarac, 8354
Sand-brier *see* 8708
Sandimmun(e) [Novartis] *see* 2752

Sandofan [Syngenta] *see* 6908
Sandolanid [Sandoz] *see* 3167
Sandolase [Sandoz] *see* 7902
Sandomigran [Novartis] *see* 7515
Sandonorm [Novartis] *see* 1333
Sandopart [Novartis] *see* 2842
Sandopril [Sandoz] *see* 8753
Sandoptal [Sandoz] *see* 1511
Sandostatin [Novartis] *see* 6762
Sandostene [Sandoz] *see* 9278
Sandoz 43-715 *see* 7873
Sanecta [Holland Sweetener] *see* 839
Sanger's Reagent *see* 4172
Sangrel *see* 8463
Sanguicillin [Zdravlje] *see* 7512
Sanguinaria, 8355
Sanguinarine, 8356
Sanifer [Esseti] *see* 4036, 8615
Saniflor [Esseti] *see* 1122
Sanlit [Sankyo] *see* 8534
Sanmigran [Novartis] *see* 7515
Sanmite [Nissan] *see* 7967
Sanocrisin [Ferrosan] *see* 2720
Sanocrysin *see* 4519
Sanodin *see* 1793
Sanofos [Sanonda] *see* 7770
Sanoma [Heilit] *see* 1842
Sanomigran [Novartis] *see* 7515
Sanorex [Novartis] *see* 5762
SANORG-34006 *see* 4892
Sanorin *see* 6368
Sanorin-Spofa *see* 6368
Sanotensin [Egis] *see* 4560
Sanoxit [Galderma] *see* 1116
Sansdolor *see* 5850
Sansert [Novartis] *see* 6137
α-Santalol, 8357
β-Santalol, 8358
Santavy's Substance F *see* 2887
Santemycin [Santen] *see* 6181
Santenol [Coop. Farm.] *see* 5431
Santobrite [Monsanto] *see* 7109
Santoflex *see* 3753
Santonica, 8359
Santonic Acid, 8360
α-Santonin, 8361
l-Santonin *see* 8361
Santophen 1 [Monsanto] *see* 2407
Santophen 20 [Monsanto] *see* 7109
Santoquin [Novus] *see* 3753
Santovar A *see* 3304
Santyl [Knoll] *see* 2481
Sanzyme [Sankyo] *see* 9031
SAPEP *see* 404
Saperconazole, 8362
Sapidan *see* 4367
l-Sapietic Acid *see* 5468
Sapilent [EGYT] *see* 9722
Sapoderm [Reckitt & Colman] *see* 9657
Saponaretin *see* 8364
Saponaria, 8363
Saponarin, 8364
Saponins, 8365
Saponite *see* 350
Saporin-6 *see* 8366
Saporins, 8366
Sapphire, 8367
Sapphirine *see* 350
Sapresta [Taiho] *see* 767
Saprol [Shell Agrar] *see* 9691
Sapropterin, 8368
Saquinavir, 8369
Saquinavir Mesylate *see* 8369
Sar *see* 8373
Sarafem [Lilly] *see* 4185

Sarafloxacin, 8370
Sarafotoxins, 8371
Sarafotoxins S6 *see* 3576
1-Sar-8-ala-angiotensin II *see* 8372
Saralasin, 8372
Saralasin Acetate *see* 8372
Saran [Dow] *see* 9996
Sarasar [Schering-Plough] *see* 5565
Sarcine *see* 4869
Sarcoclorin [Simes] *see* 5828
Sarcolactic Acid *see* 5337
Sarcolysine *see* 5828
D-Sarcolysine *see* 5828
L-Sarcolysine *see* 5828
Sarcomycin *see* 8376
Sarcosine, 8373
Sarelon *see* 7058
Sarenin [Procter & Gamble] *see* 8372
Sargenor [Viatris] *see* 840
Sargramostim *see* 4538
Sarin, 8374
Sarisol [Halsey] *see* 1506
Sarizotan, 8375
Sarkin *see* 4869
Sarkomycin, 8376
Sarkomycin A *see* 8376
Sarmentose, 8377
Sarolex *see* 2995
Saroten [Bayer] *see* 487
Sarotex [Lundbeck] *see* 487
Sarpagan-17-al *see* 9944
Sarpagan-10,17-diol *see* 8378
Sarpagine, 8378
Sarpul [Roche] *see* 662
Sarsaparilla, 8379
Sarsasapogenin, 8380
Sartosona [Sastre] *see* 1974
Saruplase *see* 7902
Sarvinal *see* 718
Saryuurin [Nippon Shoji] *see* 6887
SAS-643 *see* 3434
Sassafras, 8381
Sassolite *see* 1336
Sassy Bark, 8382
Sastridex [Lindopharm] *see* 4132
Sasulen [Andreu] *see* 7506
Satanolon [Tatsumi] *see* 3311
Satigrel, 8383
Satinite *see* 1706
Satin Spar *see* 1706
Satisfar [Sandoz] *see* 3893
Sativex [GW Pharma] *see* 1749
Satraplatin, 8384
Satumomab, 8385
Saturn Red *see* 5425
Saucy Bark *see* 8382
Saunders, Red, 8386
Saurol *see* 4885
Savac [Am. Cyanamid] *see* 5040
Saventrine [Pharmax] *see* 5217
Savey [Gowan] *see* 4713
Savin, 8387
Savinin *see* 8387
Saw Palmetto, 8388
Saxifrax *see* 8381
Saxin [Burroughs Wellcome] *see* 8311
Saxitoxin, 8389
Saxizon [Nikken] *see* 4787
Saxol *see* 7186
Saxoline *see* 7185
Saxon Bark *see* 8382
Sazio [Zyma] *see* 242
SB-58 *see* 8812
SB-75 *see* 2026
SB-5833 *see* 1725

SB-7505 *see* 4876
SB-202026 *see* 8309
SB-207266 *see* 7393
SB-207266A *see* 7393
SB-207499 *see* 2276
SB-209509 *see* 4272
SB-209509AX *see* 4272
SB-265805 *see* 4389
SB-393229 *see* 9554
SBA *see* 5429
SBB *see* 8885
SBB-I *see* 8885
SBB-II *see* 8885
α₂-SB Glycoproteins *see* 4075
SBP-1382 *see* 8153
SBP-1390 *see* 1230
SBP-1513 *see* 7180
SBR Rubber, 8390
SC-046 *see* 2914
SC-0051 *see* 8894
SC-0224 *see* 4512
SC-2910 *see* 5958
SC-7031 *see* 3360
SC-7525 *see* 1322
SC-9387 *see* 7454
SC-9420 *see* 8760
SC-9880 *see* 4200
SC-11800 *see* 3860
SC-12937 *see* 892
SC-13957 *see* 3360
SC-18862 *see* 839
SC-29333 *see* 6210
SC-40230 *see* 1204
SC-47111 *see* 5562
SC-48334 *see* 6188
SC-54684A *see* 10070
SC-54701A *see* 10070
SC-58635 *see* 1956
SC-59046 *see* 2914
SC-59735 *see* 9467
SC-65872 *see* 9900
SC-66110 *see* 3625
SC-69124A *see* 7036
SC-326421 *see* 6157
Scabecid [Stiefel] *see* 5501
Scabwort *see* 5003
Scala [Bayer CropSci.] *see* 7986
Scalibor [Intervet] *see* 2883
Scammony Root, 8391
Scandia *see* 8392
Scandicain [Bofors] *see* 5859
Scandine [Zambon] *see* 4876
Scandium, 8392
Scarlet Berry *see* 3463
Scarlet Red, 8393
scCO₂ *see* 1809
SCE-129 *see* 1945
SCE-963 *see* 1935
SCE-1365 *see* 1925
SCE-2174 *see* 1935
SCE-2787 *see* 1937
Scepter [BASF] *see* 4906
SCF *see* 8807
Sch-1000 *see* 5073
Sch-3132 *see* 5978
Sch-3940 *see* 7183
Sch-4831 *see* 1180
Sch-7056 *see* 126
Sch-10144 *see* 9519
Sch-10159 *see* 9655
Sch-10304 *see* 2392
Sch-10649 *see* 901
Sch-11460 *see* 1180
Sch-12041 *see* 4589
Sch-13475 *see* 8550

Name Index

Sch-13521 *see* 4208
Sch-14714 *see* 4147
Sch-14947 *see* 8261
Sch-15719W *see* 5329
Sch-16134 *see* 8029
Sch-18020W *see* 1019
Sch-19927 *see* 5329
Sch-20569 *see* 6479
Sch-21420 *see* 5106
Sch-21480 *see* 9455
Sch-22219 *see* 220
Sch-25298 *see* 4109
Sch-28316Z *see* 4940
Sch-29851 *see* 5578
Sch-30500 *see* 4990
Sch-32088 *see* 6241
Sch-32481 *see* 6480
Sch-33844 *see* 8753
Sch-33861 *see* 8753
Sch-34117 *see* 2922
Sch-39300 *see* 4538
Sch-39720 *see* 1949
Sch-52000 *see* 4999
Sch-56592 *see* 7602
Sch-58235 *see* 3918
Sch-66336 *see* 5565
Sch-209579 *see* 5760
Schaeffer's α-Acid *see* 6390
Schaeffer's β-Acid *see* 6392
Schaeffer's Salt *see* 6392
Schardinger Dextrins *see* 2718
Scheele's Green *see* 2626
Scheelite *see* 1712
Schering 36268 *see* 2085
Schering 38584 *see* 7236
Scherisolon [Schering] *see* 7721
Scheroson F [Schering AG] *see* 4787
Schiff Bases, 8394
Schizophyllan *see* 8559
Schleimsäure (German) *see* 4331
Schmiedeberg's Digitalin *see* 3158
Schöllkopf's Acid *see* 6386
Schradan, 8395
Schultenite *see* 5399
Schwartz's Reagent, 8396
Schwefelstickstoff *see* 9241
Schweine-Vasopressin *see* 5630
Schweinfurt Green *see* 2625
Schweizer's Reagent, 8397
Schwesinger P₄ Base, 8398
Scifluorfen *see* 109
Scillaren, 8399
Scillaren A *see* 8399
Scillaren B *see* 8399
Scillarenin, 8400
Scillarenin 3β-Rhamnoside *see* 7874
Scilliroside, 8401
Scobro [Ono] *see* 1588
Scobron [Mohan] *see* 1588
Scobutil [Rumanian] *see* 1588
Scoke *see* 7391
Scolecite *see* 1648
Scoline [Duncan Flockhart] *see* 8875
Scoparin, 8402
Scoparius, 8403
Scoparone, 8404
Scoparoside *see* 8402
Scopine Tropate *see* 8406
Scopoderm TTS [Novartis] *see* 8406
Scopola, 8405
Scopolamine, 8406
l-Scopolamine *see* 8406
Scopolamine Aminoxide *see* 8407
Scopolamine Bromobutylate *see* 1588
Scopolamine-*N*-butyl Bromide *see* 1588

Scopolamine Methobromide *see* 6003
Scopolamine Methyl Bromide *see* 6003
Scopolamine *N*-Oxide, 8407
Scopolammonium Bromide *see* 8406
Scopoletin, 8408
Scopolin, 8409
Scopoline, 8410
Score [Syngenta] *see* 3135
Scorprin [Fort Dodge] *see* 8903
Scotch Broom *see* 8403
Scotine [Unimed] *see* 2553
Scotophobin, 8411
Scotopsins *see* 6856
Scourge [Roussel Uclaf] *see* 7476
Scout [Roussel-Uclaf/AgrEvo] *see* 9565
SCP *see* 8597
S.C.T.Z. *see* 2384
Scu-PA *see* 7902
Scuroforme *see* 1512
Scutellarein, 8412
Scutellaria, 8413
Scutellarin *see* 8412
SD-271-12 *see* 2362
SD-709 *see* 3212
SD-1601 *see* 6264
SD-1750 *see* 3079
SD-3211 *see* 8446
SD-3562 *see* 3087
SD-4294 *see* 2600
SD-4402 *see* 5127
SD-7859 *see* 2089
SD-8447 *see* 9192
SD-9129 *see* 6251
SD-14114 *see* 3964
SD-15418 *see* 2685
SD-41706 *see* 3991
SD-43775 *see* 4010
SD-95481 *see* 2295
SD-208304 *see* 2087
S-Dimidine [Protea] *see* 8915
SDMH *see* 3248
SDS *see* 8636
Sdt-91 *see* 8813
SDX-105 *see* 1034
SDZ-205-502 *see* 8045
SDZ-212-713 *see* 8240
SDZ-215-811 *see* 7126
SDZ-ASM-981 *see* 7429
SDZ-CHI-621 *see* 1006
SDZ-DJN-608 *see* 6428
SDZ-ENA-713 *see* 8240
SDZ-HTF-919 *see* 9113
SDZ-ILE-964 *see* 4995
SDZ-PSC-833 *see* 9917
SDZ RAD *see* 3907
SE-780 *see* 1039
SE-1520 *see* 4935
SE-2395 *see* 9173
Seaborgium, 8414
Sea-Nine [Rohm & Haas] *see* 3070
Sea-oak *see* 4282
Sea Onion *see* 8770
Searlequin *see* 5042
Sea Salt *see* 8599
Sea-wrack *see* 4282
Sebacic Acid, 8415
Sebacil [Bayer] *see* 7366
Sebacil, 8416
Sebaclen [Carter-Wallace] *see* 1234
Sebacoin, 8417
Sebaklen [Fumouze] *see* 1234
Sebercim [ISF-Italseber] *see* 6700
Sebizon [Schering] *see* 8899
Secaclavine *see* 2042
Secalan [Zyma] *see* 2091

Secale Cornutum *see* 3660
Secalip [Fournier] *see* 3978
Secalonic Acid A *see* 8418
Secalonic Acid B *see* 8418
Secalonic Acid C *see* 8418
Secalonic Acid D *see* 8418
Secalonic Acid E *see* 8418
Secalonic Acid F *see* 8418
Secalonic Acid G *see* 8418
Secalonic Acids, 8418
Secalysat [Ysatfabrik] *see* 2552
Secbutobarbitone Sodium *see* 1506
Seccidin [Nippon Kayaku] *see* 7737
Secholex *see* 7557
Sechvitan *see* 7979
Seclar [Andromaco] *see* 1018
Secletan [Ipsen] *see* 2264
Seclin [Panthox & Burck] *see* 3168
Secnidazole, 8419
Secobarbital Sodium, 8420
(1α,3β,5Z,7E)-9,10-Secocholesta-5,7,-
   10(19)-triene-1,3-diol *see* 4819
(3β,5Z,7E)-9,10-Secocholesta-5,7,-
   10(19)-triene-3,25-diol *see* 1638
(1α,3β,5Z,7E)-9,10-Secocholesta-5,7,-
   10(19)-triene-1,3,25-triol *see* 1644
(1α,3β,5Z,7E,24R)-9,10-Secocholesta-
   5,7,10(19)-triene-1,3,24-triol *see* 9022
(3β,5Z,7E)-9,10-Secocholesta-5,7,-
   10(19)-trien-3-ol *see* 10019
(1S,1′E,3R,5Z,7E,20R)-9,10-Seco-20-
   (3′-cyclopropyl-3′-hydroxyprop-1′-
   enyl)-1,3-dihydroxypregna-5,7,-
   10(19)-triene *see* 1641
(1α,3β,5Z,7E,22E)-9,10-Secoergosta-5,-
   7,10(19),22-tetraene-1,3-diol *see* 3436
(3β,5Z,7E,22E)-9,10-Secoergosta-5,7,-
   10(19),22-tetraen-3-ol *see* 10018
(3β,6E,22E)-9,10-Secoergosta-5(10),6,-
   8,22-tetraen-3-ol *see* 9023
(3β,5Z,7E)-9,10-Secoergosta-5,7,-
   10(19)-trien-3-ol *see* 10020
(3β,5E,7E,10α,22E)-9,10-Secoergosta-
   5,7,22-trien-3-ol *see* 3180
Secoiridoid *see* 6830
Seconal Sodium [Lilly] *see* 8420
Secondary Ammonium Phosphate *see*
   542
Secondary Barium Phosphate *see* 990
Secondary Calcium Phosphate *see* 1692
Secondary Caprylic Alcohol *see* 6752
Secondary Magnesium Phosphate *see*
   5681
Secondary Propyl Alcohol *see* 5208
Secondary Sodium Phosphate *see* 8659
Secotil *see* 6855
Secrebil [Isnardi] *see* 7485
Secreflo [Repligen] *see* 8421
Secresolv [Refarmed] *see* 3647
γ-Secretase *see* 7739
Secretases *see* 615
Secretin, 8421
Secretin (Pig) *see* 8421
Secretin (Swine) *see* 8421
Secrosteron (obsolete) *see* 3219
Sectral [RPR] *see* 19
Securinan-11-one *see* 8422
Securinine, 8422
Securon [Abbott] *see* 9950
Securopen [Bayer] *see* 916
Securpres [Poli] *see* 4940
Sedaform *see* 2129
Sedagul [Wild] *see* 5482
Sedalande [J & J] *see* 4114
Sedalin [Chassot] *see* 32

tor (Human Tissue-type Reduced) Fusion Protein with Urokinase (Human Urine β-Chain Reduced) *see* 391
Sermaka [Lilly] *see* 4197
Sermion [Farmitalia] *see* 6496
Sermorelin, 8461
Sernevin [Toho Yakuhin] *see* 8989
Sernyl *see* 7219
Sernylan *see* 7219
Serocion *see* 7795
Seroden [Allen & Hanburys] *see* 9290
Serofene [Serono] *see* 2386
Seromycin [Lilly] *see* 2751
Serophene [Serono] *see* 2386
Seropram [Lundbeck] *see* 2318
Seroquel [AstraZeneca] *see* 8039
Serotinex *see* 2377
Serotone [Yoshitomi; Japan Tobacco] *see* 900
Serotonin, 8462
Serotropin [Teikoku] *see* 2216
Seroxat [GSK] *see* 7043
Serozyme *see* 7889
Serpasil [Novartis] *see* 8145
Serpax [Wyeth] *see* 6926
Serpentaria, 8463
Serpentine *see* 826
Serpentine (Alkaloid), 8464
Serpentine (Mineral) *see* 5687
Serpina [Himalaya] *see* 8120
Sertaconazole, 8465
Sertan [Valeant] *see* 7746
Sertindole, 8466
Sertraline, 8467
Serum Albumin, 8468
Serum Gonadotropin *see* 2216
Serum Lactic Dehydrogenase *see* 5334
Serum Prothrombin Conversion Accelerator *see* 3920
Serum Spreading Factor *see* 10026
Serum Transferrin *see* 9571
Serum Tryptase *see* 7520
Serutan [Menley & James] *see* 7517
Servispor [Servipharm] *see* 1974
Servizepam [Novartis] *see* 2994
L-**Seryl-**L-**aspartyl-**L-**asparaginyl-**L-**asparaginyl-**L-**glutaminyl-**L-**glutaminylglycyl-**L-**lysyl-**L-**seryl-**L-**alanyl-**L-**glutaminyl-**L-**glutaminylglycylglycyl-**L-**tyrosinamide** *see* 8411
N-(DL-**Seryl)-**N′-(2,3,4-**trihydroxybenzyl) Hydrazine** *see* 1050
Serzone [BMS] *see* 6438
Sesame Oil, 8469
Sesamin, 8470
Sesamodil *see* 8446
Sesamolin, 8471
Sesden [Tanabe] *see* 9442
Setastine, 8472
Sethotope [BMS] *see* 8441
Sethoxydim, 8473
Sethyl *see* 4730
Setous [Shionogi] *see* 10197
Setrol [Baxter] *see* 6973
Sevelamer, 8474
Seven Barks *see* 4766
Sevin [Bayer CropSci.] *see* 1787
Sevoflurane, 8475
Sevofrane [Maruishi] *see* 8475
Sevorane [Abbott] *see* 8475
Sevredol [Mundipharma] *see* 6276
Sexovid [Ferrosan] *see* 2720
Seyferth-Gilbert Reagent, 8476
SF-86-327 *see* 9156
SF-277 *see* 2960

SF-733 Antibiotic *see* 8206
SF-837 *see* 6183
SFAE *see* 8724
SG-75 *see* 6521
Sgd-301-76 *see* 6937
Sgd-12878 *see* 6846
S-GI *see* 2905
SH-100 *see* 2737
SH-261 *see* 3768
SH-406 *see* 9164
SH-437 *see* 5065
SH-582 *see* 4414
SH-617L *see* 5071
SH-714 *see* 2774
SH-717 *see* 4507
SH-770 *see* 4153
SH-818 *see* 2369
SH-863 *see* 2369
SH-881 *see* 2774
SH-926 *see* 5011
SH-80881 *see* 2774
SH B 331 *see* 4413
SH E 222 *see* 5856
SH K 203 *see* 4152
SH U 454 *see* 4335
SH U 508A *see* 4335
SHA-486300 *see* 4805
Shadocol *see* 5038
Shark Liver Oil, 8477
SHB-286 *see* 8991
SHCH-58 *see* 2621
Sheep Berry *see* 9974
Shekanin *see* 9107
Shellac, 8478
Shellolic Acid, 8479
Sheridanite *see* 350
Sherman [Calliope S.A.] *see* 2103
Shibagen [Ishihara] *see* 4097
Shigatox [Fawns & McAllan] *see* 8908
Shikalkin *see* 257
Shikimic Acid, 8480
Shikonin *see* 257
Shinbit [Nihon Schering] *see* 6529
Shiomarin [Shionogi] *see* 6286
Shionone, 8481
Shiosol [Shionogi] *see* 4518
Shirlan [Syngenta] *see* 4117
Shisonin A *see* 2687
SHL-451A *see* 4327
SHL-569B *see* 4330
Shock-Ferol *see* 10018
Showdomycin, 8482
Showersan *see* 5037
Shoxin *see* 6687
Shvo Catalyst, 8483
Siagoside *see* 4364
Sialic Acids, 8484
Sialor [Solvay] *see* 644
Sibelium [Janssen] *see* 4144
Siberian Pine Needle Oil *see* 6793
SIB-S1 *see* 5461
Sibutol *see* 1305
Sibutramine, 8485
Siccanin, 8486
Sicoclor [Gramon] *see* 3967
Sicorten [Novartis] *see* 4597
Sideramines *see* 2860
Siderin Yellow *see* 4020
Siderite *see* 5093
Sideromycins *see* 2860
Siderophilin *see* 9571
Siderophores *see* 6324
Sideros [Sanofi-Synthelabo] *see* 4036
Siderotil *see* 4057
Siduron, 8487

Sieromicin [Sierochimica] *see* 7453
Sifrol [Boehringer, Ing.] *see* 7705
Sigamopen [Alpharma] *see* 577
Sigaperidol [Dumex] *see* 4598
Sigaprim [Dumex] *see* 8918
Sigapurol [Siegfried] *see* 279
Sigmacef [Sigma Tau] *see* 7513
Sigmacort [Sigma] *see* 4787
Sigmafon [Fontana] *see* 5773
Sigmaform *see* 1291
Sigmart [Chugai] *see* 6521
SIL-4R *see* 5002
Silain [Wyeth] *see* 3215
Silane, 8488
Silarine [Vir] *see* 8532
Silbephylline [Berk] *see* 3479
Sildenafil, 8489
Silene *see* 1702
Silepar [Ibirn] *see* 8532
Silibinin *see* 8532
Silibrin [Silesia] *see* 2084
Silica *see* 8493
Silica Gel *see* 8490
Silicane *see* 8488
Siliceous Earth *see* 4973
Silicic Acid, 8490
Silicic Acid Tetraethyl Ester *see* 3851
Silicic Anhydride *see* 8493
Silicobromoform *see* 9615
Silicobutane *see* 9239
Silicochloroform *see* 9646
Silicoethane *see* 3356
Silicofluoric Acid *see* 4182
Silicon, 8491
Silicon Bromide *see* 8499
Silicon Carbide, 8492
Silicon Chloride *see* 8500
Silicon Dioxide, 8493
Silicon Disulfide, 8494
Silicone Glycol Copolymers *see* 8495
Silicone Glycols *see* 8495
Silicone Polyethers *see* 8495
Silicones, 8495
Silicon Fluoride *see* 8501
Silicon Monoxide, 8496
Silicon Nitride, 8497
Silicon Tetraacetate, 8498
Silicon Tetrabromide, 8499
Silicon Tetrachloride, 8500
Silicon Tetrafluoride, 8501
Silicon Tetrahydride *see* 8488
Silicon Tetramethyl *see* 9229
Silicopropane *see* 9754
Silicotungstic Acid, 8502
Silicristin *see* 8532
Silidianin *see* 8532
Silirex [Lampugnani] *see* 8532
Silkis [Galderma] *see* 1644
Silkweed *see* 829
Sillimanite *see* 362
Silliver [Abbott] *see* 8532
Silmar [Von Boch] *see* 8532
Silodosin, 8503
Silomat [Thomae] *see* 2365
Silosan [Zeneca] *see* 7497
Silubin *see* 1476
Silvadene [King] *see* 8903
Silver, 8504
Silver Acetate, 8505
Silverado [Bayer CropSci.] *see* 5911
Silver Balsam *see* 5271
Silver Benzoate *see* 1091
Silver Bromide, 8506
Silver Carbonate, 8507
Silver Chlorate, 8508

Silver Chloride, 8509
Silver Chromate(VI), 8510
Silver Citrate, 8511
Silver Cyanide, 8512
Silver Difluoride, 8513
Silver Drops *see* 5271
Silver Fluoride, 8514
Silver Iodate, 8515
Silver Iodide, 8516
Silver Lactate, 8517
Silver Leaf *see* 8818
Silver Manganate (VII) *see* 8524
Silver Monofluoride *see* 8514
Silver Nitrate, 8518
Silver Nitrite, 8519
Silver Nucleate *see* 8527
Silver Nucleinate *see* 8527
Silver Orthophosphate *see* 8525
Silver Oxalate, 8520
Silver Oxide, 8521
Silver(II) Oxide, 8522
Silver Perchlorate, 8523
Silver Permanganate, 8524
Silver Peroxide *see* 8522
Silver Phosphate, 8525
Silver Picrate, 8526
Silver Protein, 8527
Silver Proteinate *see* 8527
Silver Selenide, 8528
Silver Suboxide *see* 8522
Silver Sulfate, 8529
Silver Sulfide, 8530
Silver Tetraiodomercurate(II), 8531
Silver Trinitrophenolate *see* 8526
Silvisar 8595
Silvol [Parke-Davis] *see* 8527
Silybin *see* 8532
Silybum Substance E₆ *see* 8532
Silymarin, 8532
Silymarin I *see* 8532
Simactil [Rorer] *see* 3653
Simanex [Makhteshim-Agan] *see* 8533
Simatin [Geistlich] *see* 3748
Simazine, 8533
Simdax [Orion] *see* 5471
Simeconazole, 8534
(*R*)-Simendan *see* 5471
Simethicone *see* 3215
Simetride, 8535
Simetryn, 8536
Simfibrate, 8537
Simovil [Merck & Co.] *see* 8539
Simpadren *see* 9012
Simpalon *see* 9012
Simpatoblock *see* 4688
Simplesse [CP Kelco], 8538
Simplotan [Pfizer] *see* 9447
Simulect [Novartis] *see* 1006
Simvastatin, 8539
SIN-10 *see* 6234
Sinalbin, 8540
Sinan *see* 5850
Sinanomycin *see* 6481
Sinapic Acid Choline Ester *see* 8541
Sinapine, 8541
Sinapine Glucosinalbate *see* 8540
Sinapsan [Rodleben] *see* 7487
Sinapultide, 8542
Sinartrol [SPA] *see* 7506
Sinbar [DuPont] *see* 9155
Sincalide, 8543
Sincaline *see* 2204
Sincodix [Beta] *see* 1513
Sincomen [Schering AG] *see* 8760
Sindiatil *see* 1476

Sinecod [Zyma] *see* 1513
Sinefungin, 8544
Sinemet [Merck & Co.] *see* 1797
Sineptina [Antibioticos] *see* 5453
Sinequan [Pfizer] *see* 3435
Sinerem [Guerbet] *see* 4065
Sinerol *see* 6966
Sinesalin [MIT Gesundheit] *see* 1037
Sinetens [Erba] *see* 7717
Sinex [LaChartre] *see* 6966
Sinfibrate *see* 8537
Single-chain Pro-urokinase *see* 7902
Single-chain Urokinase-type Plasmino-
  gen Activator *see* 7902
Singulair [Merck & Co.] *see* 6258
Sinigrin, 8545
Sinigroside *see* 8545
Sinlestal [Daiichi Seiyaku] *see* 7755
Sinoaculine *see* 8341
Sinoflurol [Kaken] *see* 9112
Sinogan-Debil *see* 5986
Sinomenine, 8546
Sinomin [Shionogi] *see* 8918
Sinorphan *see* 8090
Sinorytmal [Giulini] *see* 9516
Sinos *see* 2740
Sinosid [SIF] *see* 7041
Sinovial [Irbi] *see* 7045
Sinox *see* 3279
Sinox W [FMC] *see* 3287
Sinthrome [Novartis] *see* 29
Sintisone [Pharmacia] *see* 7721
Sintoclar [Pulitzer] *see* 2319
Sintolexyn [ISF-Italseber] *see* 1974
Sintomicetina [Lepetit] *see* 2077
Sintomodulina [Italfarmaco] *see* 9403
Sintonal [Europharma] *see* 1450
Sintosulfa [Afi] *see* 8934
Sintotrat [Edmond] *see* 4787
Sintrom [Novartis] *see* 29
Sinvacor [Merck & Co.] *see* 8539
Sipeimine *see* 4926
Sipiri Bark *see* 1017
Siplarol [Erba] *see* 4187
Siptazin [Isei] *see* 2305
Sipuleucel-T, 8547
Siqualone [BMS] *see* 4189
SIR-8514 *see* 9678
Sirdalud [Novartis] *see* 9485
Siringina [Toyo Jozo] *see* 9017
Sirius Red, 8548
Sirius Red F3B *see* 8548
Sirolimus *see* 8114
Siroxyl [Aventis] *see* 1802
Sirtal [Dura] *see* 1781
Sisal, 8549
Siscard [Boehringer, Ing.] *see* 2275
Siseptin [Schering] *see* 8550
Sisobiotic [Von Boch] *see* 8550
Sisolline [Schering-Plough] *see* 8550
Sisomicin, 8550
Sisomin [Max] *see* 8550
Sisosamine *see* 8550
Sistalgin [Merck KGaA] *see* 7707
Sistan [DuPont] *see* 5949
Sisuril *see* 4789
Sitafloxacin, 8551
Sitagliptin, 8552
Sitagliptin Phosphate *see* 8552
Sitamaquine, 8553
Sitaxsentan, 8554
Sito-Lande [Delalande] *see* 8556
β-Sitostanol *see* 8814
Sitosterin *see* 8556
α₁-Sitosterol, 8555

β-Sitosterol, 8556
γ-Sitosterol, 8557
Sivastin [Sigma-Tau] *see* 8539
Sivelestat, 8558
Sivlor [Sidus] *see* 5586
Sizofiran, 8559
SJO 0498 *see* 4119
SK-7 *see* 7127
SK-331-A *see* 10060
SK-818 *see* 7795
Skanitrol [Schering] *see* 6633
Skatole, 8560
Skeetal *see* 932
Skelid [Sanofi] *see* 9441
SKF-51 *see* 6757
SKF-385 *see* 9573
SKF-478 *see* 3311
SKF-478-A *see* 3311
SKF-1700-A *see* 6732
SKF-2601-A *see* 2185
SKF-4657 *see* 7761
SKF-5137 *see* 2955
SKF-5883 *see* 9357
SKF-6574 *see* 7218
SKF-7988 *see* 10004
SKF-8542 *see* 9599
SKF-16214-A2 *see* 121
SKF-18667 *see* 7562
SKF-29044 *see* 7035
SKF-30310 *see* 6936
SKF-38095 *see* 6820
SKF-39162 *see* 878
SKF-40383 *see* 1833
SKF-41558 *see* 1917
SKF-60771 *see* 1915
SKF-62698 *see* 9430
SKF-62979 *see* 210
SKF-75073 *see* 1929
SKF-82526 *see* 3979
SKF-82526-J *see* 3979
SKF-83088 *see* 1926
SKF-88373 *see* 1951
SKF-92334 *see* 2279
SKF-96022 *see* 7014
SKF-96148 *see* 2806
SKF-101468 *see* 8257
SKF-101468A *see* 8257
SKF-102362 *see* 6545
SKF-102886 *see* 4594
SKF-104864 *see* 9548
SKF-104864A *see* 9548
SKF-105657 *see* 3634
SKF-108566 *see* 3635
SKF-108566J *see* 3635
Skimmetin *see* 9847
Skimmianine, 8561
Skimmin, 8562
Skimmiol *see* 9062
Skinoren [Schering AG] *see* 905
Skiodan [Winthrop] *see* 5973
Sklerolip [Mepha] *see* 2377
Skleromexe [L. Merckle] *see* 2377
Skleronorm [Grünenthal] *see* 3872
Sklero-Tablinen [Sanorania] *see* 2377
SK-Lygen [SKB] *see* 2084
Skullcap *see* 8413
SL-75.212 *see* 1182
SL-76.002 *see* 7772
SL-77.499 *see* 238
SL-77.499-10 *see* 238
SL-80.0750 *see* 10190
SL-80.0750-23N *see* 10190
SL-85.0324 *see* 6221
SL-160 *see* 4097
SL-950 *see* 6522

Sodium Prussiate Yellow *see* 8616
Sodium Pteroylglutamate *see* 8619
Sodium 7-(Pyrid-4-ylthioacetamido)-cephalosporanate *see* 1984
Sodium Pyroborate *see* 8590
Sodium Pyrocatechol-2,4-disulfonate *see* 9465
Sodium Pyrophosphate *see* 9240
Sodium Pyrosulfate *see* 8586
Sodium Pyrosulfite *see* 8638
Sodium Radio-chromate(^{51}Cr) *see* 8601
Sodium Radio-iodide (^{131}I) *see* 8632
Sodium Radiophosphate (^{32}P) *see* 8661
Sodium Rhodanide *see* 9327
Sodium Rhodizonate, 8670
Sodium Rose Bengal I 131 *see* 8262
Sodium Salicylate *see* 8332
Sodium Salicylsulfate *see* 8334
Sodium Salt of Metanilylazodiphenyl-amine *see* 5928
Sodium Salt of 1-Nitroso-2-hydroxy-naphthalene-3,6-disulfonic Acid *see* 6644
Sodium Selenate, 8671
Sodium Selenide, 8672
Sodium Selenite, 8673
Sodium Sesquicarbonate, 8674
Sodium Silicate, 8675
Sodium Silicate Solution, 8676
Sodium Silicofluoride *see* 8624
Sodium Stannate(IV), 8677
Sodium Stearate, 8678
Sodium Stibogluconate *see* 701
Sodium Succinate, 8679
Sodium Sulamyd [Schering] *see* 8899
Sodium Sulfate, 8680
Sodium Sulfhydrate *see* 8587
Sodium Sulfide, 8681
Sodium Sulfinylbismethane Ion(1−) *see* 8644
Sodium Sulfite, 8682
Sodium Sulfocarbolate *see* 8658
Sodium Sulfocarbonate *see* 8691
Sodium Sulfocyanate *see* 9327
Sodium β-Sulfopropionitrile, 8683
Sodium Sulfovinate *see* 8614
Sodium Sulfoxylate *see* 8626
Sodium Sulfuret *see* 8681
Sodium Superoxide *see* 8655
Sodium Tartrate, 8684
Sodium Taurocholate *see* 9075
Sodium Tellurate(IV), 8685
Sodium Tellurate(VI), 8686
Sodium Tellurite *see* 8685
Sodium L-Tenuazonate *see* 9149
Sodium Tetraborate *see* 8590
Sodium Tetrachloroaluminate, 8687
Sodium Tetrachloroaurate(III), 8688
Sodium Tetradecyl Sulfate, 8689
Sodium Tetrafluoroberyllate *see* 1174
Sodium Tetrafluoroborate *see* 8617
Sodium Tetrahydroborate *see* 8592
Sodium Tetraphenylborate, 8690
Sodium 2-Thenoate *see* 9354
Sodium Theobromine Acetate *see* 9283
Sodium Thiocarbonate, 8691
Sodium Thiocyanate *see* 9327
Sodium Thioglycolate, 8692
Sodium 2-Thiophenecarboxylate *see* 9354
Sodium Thiophosphate, 8693
Sodium Thiosulfate, 8694
Sodium Tin Oxide *see* 8677
Sodium *p*-Toluenesulfonchloramide *see* 2075
Sodium Triacetoxyborohydride, 8695

Sodium Trichloroacetate *see* 9627
Sodium L-Triiodothyronine *see* 5510
Sodium Trimetaphosphate, 8696
Sodium Trioxodinitrate *see* 648
Sodium Triphenyl-*p*-rosanilinetrisulfate *see* 6028
Sodium Triphosphate *see* 8697
Sodium Tripolyphosphate, 8697
Sodium (*T*-4)-Tris(acetato-*κO*)hydro-borate(1−) *see* 8695
Sodium Tungstate(VI), 8698
Sodium Tungstophosphate *see* 8665
Sodium Tyropanoate *see* 9837
Sodium Uranate(VI), 8699
Sodium Valproate *see* 9913
Sodium Vanadate(V), 8700
Sodium Xylan Polysulfate *see* 7134
Sodothiol *see* 8694
Sofalcone, 8701
Sofmin [Dainippon] *see* 5986
Soframycin [HMR] *see* 6454
Softenon *see* 9255
Soja Bean *see* 8730
Solacen [Wallace Labs.] *see* 9829
Solan, 8702
Solancarpidine *see* 8709
Solanesol, 8703
(3β,12α)-Solanid-5-ene-3,12-diol *see* 8287
(3β)-Solanid-5-en-3-ol *see* 8704
Solanidine, 8704
Solanidine-S *see* 8709
Solanine, 8705
Solanine-S *see* 8710
Solanocapsin *see* 8706
Solanocapsine, 8706
Solanone, 8707
Solantal [Fujisawa] *see* 9424
Solanum, 8708
Solapsone *see* 8711
Solar [BASF] *see* 2293
Solar NP [Swift] *see* 6677
Solart [Bioindustria] *see* 27
Solaskil [RPR] *see* 5459
Solasod-5-en-3β-ol *see* 8709
Solasodine, 8709
Solasonine, 8710
Solaspin [Indian Health] *see* 1647
Solasulfone, 8711
Solatene [Roche] *see* 1853
Solatubine *see* 8704
Solatunine *see* 8705
Solaxin *see* 2194
Solbrol A *see* 3837
Solbrol P [Bayer] *see* 7866
Solclot [Sumitomo] *see* 9468
Soldactone [Searle] *see* 1750
Soldesam [Farmacologico] *see* 2943
Solevar *see* 6696
Solfa [Takeda] *see* 490
Solganal [Schering] *see* 883
Solgol [BMS] *see* 6346
Solian [Synthelabo] *see* 485
Solicam [Syngenta] *see* 6701
Solid Crotonic Acid *see* 2597
Solid Green *see* 1374
Solid Green O *see* 5699
Solifenacin, 8712
Solimidin [Selvi] *see* 10188
Solinase [Yamanouchi] *see* 7004
Soliphylline *see* 2210
Solketal *see* 5213
Sol-Mycin [Roxane] *see* 3179
Solnhofen Stone *see* 5491

Solocalm [Microsules] *see* 7506
Solodelf [Cyanamid] *see* 9596
Solon [Taisho] *see* 8701
Solone [Abbott] *see* 7721
Solosin [Sanofi-Aventis] *see* 9285
Soloxine [Virbac] *see* 9415
Solozone *see* 8655
Sol Phenobarbital *see* 7238
Sol Phenobarbitone *see* 7238
Solprene [Phillips Petr.] *see* 8390
Solprin [Reckitt Benckiser] *see* 851
Solubacter [Pharmethic] *see* 9654
Solu-Biloptin [Schering AG] *see* 5071
Soluble Anhydrite *see* 1706
Soluble Aspirin *see* 1647
Soluble Barbital *see* 962
Soluble Fluorescein *see* 4159
Soluble Glass *see* 8675
Soluble Gun Cotton *see* 8011
Soluble Indigo Blue *see* 4944
Soluble Iodophthalein *see* 5038
Soluble Pentobarbital *see* 7130
Soluble Potash Glass *see* 7668
Soluble Potash Water Glass *see* 7668
Soluble Prussian Blue *see* 7910
Soluble RNA *see* 8203
Soluble Saccharin *see* 8311
Soluble Sulfacetamide *see* 8899
Soluble Sulfadiazine *see* 8903
Soluble Sulfamerazine *see* 8913
Soluble Sulfapyridine *see* 8938
Soluble Sulfathiazole *see* 8943
Soluble Tartar *see* 7677
Solucin *see* 6684
Solucort [Merck & Co.] *see* 7721
Solu-Cortef [Pfizer] *see* 4787
SoluDecadron [Merck & Co.] *see* 2943
Solu-Decortin-H [Merck KGaA] *see* 7721
Soludillar [Syntex] *see* 7029
Solufen [SMB] *see* 4881
Solufilin *see* 3479
Solufilina [Merck KGaA] *see* 3711
Solufontamide *see* 8944
Solufyllin *see* 3479
Soluglaucit *see* 7030
Solu-Glyc [Erco] *see* 4787
Solumédine [Specia] *see* 8913
Solu-Medrol [Pharmacia & Upjohn] *see* 6111
Solu-Medrone [Pharmacia] *see* 6111
Solupemid [Recordati] *see* 7460
Solupen N [Winzer] *see* 2943
Solupred [Aventis] *see* 7721
Solupsan [UPSA] *see* 1647
Soluran *see* 2374
Solurol [Delalande] *see* 9009
Soluseptasine *see* 6684
Soluseptazine *see* 6684
Solusetazine *see* 6684
Solustibosan [Bayer] *see* 701
Solutedarol [Specia] *see* 9596
Solu-Tracin [Alpharma] *see* 935
Solutrast [Bracco] *see* 5057
Solutrat [Labinca] *see* 9889
Solvay Soda *see* 8596
Solvazinc [Thames] *see* 10159
Solvazine [Solvay] *see* 10080
Solvent Naphtha *see* 5489
Solvezink [Tika] *see* 10159
Solvolan [Krka] *see* 386
Solvolip [Knoll] *see* 3994
Soma [Wallace Labs.] *see* 1842
Somac [Pfizer] *see* 7014
Somacton [Ferring] *see* 8716
Somadril [Dumex] *see* 1842

Somagard [Roberts] see 2923
Somagerol [Brenner-Efeka] see 5579
Somagrebove see 8716
Somalapor see 8716
Somalgen [Bago] see 9044
Somalgit [Inibsa] see 1842
Soman, 8713
Somason [Fujisawa] see 4986
Somatocrinin see 8714
Somatofalk [Falk] see 8715
Somatoliberin, 8714
Somatomedin see 4986
Somatomedin 1 see 4986
Somatomedin C see 4986
Somatonorm [Pfizer] see 8716
Somatostatin, 8715
Somatotropic Hormone see 8716
Somatotropin, 8716
Somatotropin Release Inhibiting Factor
    see 8715
Somatrem see 8716
Somatropin see 8716
Somatuline LP [Ipsen] see 5361
Somatyl [Teofarma] see 1179
Somavert [Pharmacia & Upjohn] see 7069
Somavubove see 8716
Somazina [Ferrer] see 2319
Sombrevin [Gedeon Richter] see 7803
Sombucaps see 4704
Sombulex [3M Pharma] see 4704
Somelin [Sankyo] see 4604
Somenopor see 8716
Sometribove see 8716
Sometripor see 8716
Somfasepor see 8716
Somidobove see 8716
Sominex [GSK] see 3309
Somio see 2072
Somlan [Sintyal] see 4198
Somnafac see 5960
Somnalert [Warren-Teed] see 4704
Somnased [GSK] see 6575
Somnatrol [Takeda] see 3702
Somnesin [Central Pharm.] see 5846
Somnibel [UCB] see 6575
Somnite [Norgine] see 6575
Somnos [Merck & Co.] see 2071
Somnovit [Hosbon] see 5574
Somnurol [Synochem] see 1397
Somon [Atlas] see 2112
Somsanit [Köhler] see 4815
Sonacide [Wyeth-Ayerst] see 4472
Sonaform see 2711
Sonalan [Dow AgroSci.] see 3719
Sonalen [Dow AgroSci.] see 3719
Sonata [Wyeth] see 10111
Sonate see 8578
Sone [Fawns & McAllan] see 7722
Soneryl [M & B] see 1521
Songar [Valeas] see 9604
Songorine, 8717
Sonicated Human Serum Albumin see
    8468
Sonifilan [Kaken] see 8559
Sonilyn [Carter-Wallace] see 8900
Sonin [Lipha] see 5574
Sonora see 5914
Soothe-N-Seal [Colgate-Palmolive] see
    6766
Sopental [Continental] see 7130
Sophocarpidine see 5759
Sophorabioside, 8718
Sophoretin see 8034
Sophoricoside see 4391
Sophorin see 8304

Sophorine see 2789
Sophorose, 8719
Sopivan [Aventis] see 10193
Soprol [Lederle] see 1295
Sorafenib, 8720
Sorbangil [Pharmacia] see 5225
Sorbic Acid, 8721
Sorbic Acid Potassium Salt see 7671
Sorbic Alcohol, 8722
Sorbichew [AstraZeneca] see 5225
Sorbic Oil see 7032
Sorbid SA [AstraZeneca] see 5225
Sorbidilat [AstraZeneca] see 5225
Sorbilande [Sanofi-Aventis] see 8725
Sorbilax [Vétoquinol] see 8725
Sorbin see 8726
Sorbinil, 8723
Sorbinose see 8726
Sorbistat [Ono] see 3605
Sorbit see 8725
Sorbitol, 8725
D-Sorbitol see 8725
Sorbitrate [AstraZeneca] see 5225
Sorbo [SPI] see 8725
Sorboquel [Schering] see 1697
Sorbose, 8726
L-Sorbose see 8726
Sorbostyl [Sanofi-Aventis] see 8725
Sorbsan [Maersk] see 242
Sordenac [Lundbeck] see 2394
Sordinol [Ayerst] see 2394
Sorensen's Phosphate see 8659
Sörensen's Potassium Phosphate see 7659
Sörensen's Sodium Phosphate see 8659
Soreton [Nippon Chemiphar] see 10112
Soriatane [Roche] see 112
Soricin see 8211
Soridermal [Rhône-Poulenc] see 6139
Soriflor [Nycomed] see 3140
Soripal [Specia] see 6139
Sorivudine, 8727
Sorlate [Abbott] see 7582
Sormetal see 3517
Sorot [Ravensberg] see 2913
Sortis [Pfizer] see 864
Sosegon see 7121
Sospitan [Kali-Chemie] see 7975
Sostril [Cascan] see 8110
Sotacor [BMS] see 8728
Sotal [Gramon] see 9457
Sotalex [BMS] see 8728
Sotalol, 8728
Soterenol, 8729
Sotradecol [Elkins-Sinn] see 8689
Soudan Coffee see 5318
Souframine see 7252
Sour-spine see 961
Soventol [Knoll] see 956
Sovran [BASF] see 5324
Sowberry see 961
Soxysympamine [Ferndale] see 5948
Soya Bean see 8730
Soybean, 8730
Soybean Agglutinin see 5429
Soybean Oil, 8731
Soy Sauce, 8732
SP see 8763, 8863

SP-54 [Bene-Chemie] see 7134
SP-63 see 6898
SP-281 see 9972
SP-732 see 7781
SP-1103 see 9223
SPA [Santen] see 5431
Spabucol [Lagap] see 9699
Spaderizine [Kotobuki] see 2305
Spametrin-M [Yamanouchi Seiyaku] see
    6070
Spamorin [Tanabe Seiyaku] see 4106
Span 20 [ICI] see 8724
Span 60 [ICI] see 8724
Span 80 [ICI] see 8724
Spandex, 8733
Spanidin [Nippon Kayaku] see 4582
Spanish Fly see 1751
"Spanish Fly" see 1752
Spanish Grass Wax see 3701
Spanish Saffron see 8314
Spanish Tea see 6785
Spanish White see 1284
Span-K [Aspen] see 7621
Spanon see 2085
Spanor [Bailleul] see 3440
Spantol [Nippon Chemiphar] see 7258
Spara [Dainippon] see 8735
Sparassol, 8734
Sparfloxacin, 8735
Sparicon [Yamanouchi] see 1588
Sparine [Wyeth] see 7783
Sparsamycin A see 9804
Sparsomycin, 8736
(+)-Sparsomycin see 8736
Spartakon [Janssen] see 5459
Sparteine, 8737
l-Sparteine see 8737
Spartrix [Janssen] see 1848
SPA-S-132 see 7049
SPA-S-160 see 5847
SPA-S-222 see 5847
SPA-S-510 see 7506
Spasen [Menarini] see 6898
Spasfon-Lyoc [Cephalon] see 7328
Spasmalex see 3168
Spasmaverine [Bellon] see 371
Spasmentral [Janssen] see 1075
Spasmex [Pfleger] see 9786
Spasmium [Donau] see 1857
Spasmoctyl [Menarini] see 6898
Spasmocyclon [3M] see 2704
Spasmodex [Crinex] see 3168
Spasmol see 5718
Spasmolyn see 5850
Spasmolysin [Kade] see 7905
Spasmolyt [Madaus] see 9786
Spasmolytin see 161
Spasmomen [Menarini] see 6898
Spasmonal [Norgine] see 371
Spasmo-Nit [Stroschein] see 7019
Spasmophen see 6975
Spasmopriv [Paillusseau] see 3982
Spasmoril see 4106
Spasmostenyl see 5718
Spassirex [Sanofi-Aventis] see 7328
Spasuret [Asche] see 4096
Spatomac see 1029
Spatonin see 3116
SP-B see 8542
SPC-97D see 910
SPCA see 3920
SPE see 8883
SPE-2792 see 668
Spearmint, 8738
Specifin [Bergamon] see 6359

Spectacillin [Sandoz] *see* 3614
Spectam [Abbott] *see* 8739
Spectamine [Medi-Physics] *see* 5049
Spectazole [Ortho] *see* 3502
Spectinomycin, 8739
Spectracide *see* 2995
Spectra-Sorb UV 24 [Am. Cyanamid] *see* 3303
Spectra-Sorb UV 284 [Am. Cyanamid] *see* 8983
Spectra-Sorb UV 531 [Am. Cyanamid] *see* 6742
Spectrazole [Mallinckrodt] *see* 1954
Spectrin, 8740
Spectro [Novartis Agro] *see* 3135
Spectrum [Sigma-Tau] *see* 1946
Speda [Byk Gulden] *see* 9993
"Speed" *see* 5948
Spergon *see* 2078
Spergualin *see* 4582
Spermaceti, 8741
Spermidine, 8742
Spermine, 8743
Spermine Oxidase *see* 6247
Spermine Phosphate *see* 8743
Sperm Oil, 8744
Spermwax [Robeco] *see* 8741
SPG *see* 8559
Sphaerocobaltite *see* 2436
Sphalerite *see* 10160
Sphene *see* 9470
Spheroidine *see* 9246
4-Sphingenine *see* 8747
Sphingofungin C *see* 8745
Sphingofungins, 8745
Sphingomyelins, 8746
Sphingosine, 8747
SP-I *see* 7545
Spice Berry *see* 766
Spiclomazine *see* 2412
Spigelia, 8748
Spignet *see* 766
Spike [Dow AgroSci.] *see* 9095
Spike Lavender *see* 5390
Spike Lavender Oil *see* 5390
Spikenard *see* 766
Spilanthol *see* 179
Spinacane *see* 8767
Spinacene *see* 8768
α-Spinasterin *see* 8749
α-Spinasterol, 8749
Spindle Tree *see* 3899
Spinnaker [Shell] *see* 9593
Spinosad *see* 8750
Spinosyn A *see* 8750
Spinosyn D *see* 8750
Spinosyns, 8750
SpinTor [Dow AgroSci.] *see* 8750
Spiperone, 8751
Spira 200 [RMB] *see* 8752
Spiramin [Mitsui] *see* 9569
Spiramycin, 8752
Spiramycin Adipate *see* 8752
Spiramycin I *see* 8752
Spiramycin II *see* 8752
Spiramycin III *see* 8752
Spirapril, 8753
Spiraprilat *see* 8753
Spiraprilic Acid *see* 8753
Spirein *see* 4628
Spirilloxanthin *see* 8194
Spirit of Ammonia, Aromatic, 8754
Spirit of Ants *see* 4241
Spirit of Ether, 8755
Spirit of Ether Compound, 8756

Spirit of Glonoin *see* 6607
Spirit of Hartshorn *see* 494
Spirit of Hartshorn, Aromatic *see* 8754
Spirit of Mindererus *see* 495
Spirit of Nitroglycerin *see* 6607
Spirit of Nitrous Ether *see* 3831
Spirit of Turpentine *see* 9826
Spiriva [Boehringer, Ing.] *see* 9454
Spiro-32 [Unimed] *see* 8758
Spirobeta [Betapharm] *see* 8760
Spirocid [Hoechst] *see* 52
Spirocort [AstraZeneca] *see* 1468
Spiroctan [Ferlux] *see* 8760
Spirodiclofen, 8757
Spirodon *see* 9234
Spiroform *see* 7270
Spirofulvin *see* 4549
Spirogermanium, 8758
Spirolair [3M Pharma] *see* 7489
Spirolone [APS] *see* 8760
Spiromesifen, 8759
Spironolactone, 8760
Spironone [Dexo] *see* 8760
Spiropent [Thomae; Boehringer, Ing.] *see* 2347
Spiropitan [Janssen] *see* 8751
(3β,5α,22β,25S)-Spirosolan-3-ol *see* 9544
(3β,5α,22β,25S)-Spirosolan-3-yl *O*-β-D-Glucopyranosyl-(1 → 2)-*O*-[β-D-xylopyranosyl-(1 → 3)]-*O*-β-D-glucopyranosyl-(1 → 4)-β-D-galactopyranoside *see* 9545
(3β,22α,25R)-Spirosol-5-en-3-ol *see* 8709
(3β,22α,25R)-Spirosol-5-en-3-yl *O*-6-Deoxy-α-L-mannopyranosyl-(1 → 2)-*O*-[β-D-glucopyranosyl-(1 → 3)]-β-D-galactopyranoside *see* 8710
(2α,3β,5α,25R)-Spirostan-2,3-diol *see* 4431
(3β,5α,6α,25R)-Spirostan-3,6-diol *see* 2143
(3β,5α,15β,25R)-Spirostan-3,15-diol *see* 3154
(3β,5α,25R)-Spirostan-3-ol *see* 9435
(3β,5β,25S)-Spirostan-3-ol *see* 8380
(25R)-Spirostan-3β-ol *see* 8565
(2α,3β,5α,15β,25R)-Spirostan-2,3,15-triol *see* 3160
(3β,25R)-Spirost-5-en-3-ol *see* 3295
(25R)-Spirost-5-en-3β-yl *O*-6-Deoxy-α-L-mannopyranosyl-(1 → 2)-*O*-[6-deoxy-α-L-mannopyranosyl-(1 → 4)]-β-D-glucopyranoside *see* 3292
Spiroxamine, 8761
Spizef [Grünenthal] *see* 1935
Splenda [McNeil Nutritionals] *see* 8880
Splendil [AstraZeneca] *see* 3953
Splendipherin, 8762
Splenin, 8763
Splenopentin *see* 8763
Split Nut *see* 7383
Splotin [Taiyo] *see* 8989
SPM-925 *see* 6229
SPM-927 *see* 5333
Spodumene *see* 5520
Spofa 325 *see* 6287
Spondyvit [Wyeth] *see* 9495
Spongoadenosine *see* 9976
Sponsin [Farmasan] *see* 3653
Spontin *see* 8234
Spoonwood *see* 5280
Sporamin [Hishiyama] *see* 1588
Sporanox [Janssen] *see* 5245
Sporeine *see* 932
Sporidesmin *see* 8764

Sporidesmin A *see* 8764
Sporidesmins, 8764
Sporidesmolide I *see* 8765
Sporidesmolide II *see* 8765
Sporidesmolide III *see* 8765
Sporidesmolide IV *see* 8765
Sporidesmolides, 8765
Sporidyn [Cyanamid] *see* 1935
Sporiline [Schering-Plough] *see* 9519
Sporostatin [Schering] *see* 4549
Sportak [Bayer CropSci.] *see* 7760
Sportak Delta [Aventis CropSci.] *see* 2771
Spotless [Sumitomo] *see* 3268
Spotlight [Dow AgroSci.] *see* 4203
Spotof [CCD] *see* 9569
Spotted Alder *see* 4606
Spotted Cowbane *see* 2506
Spotted Hemlock *see* 2506
SPP-100 *see* 247
Spreading Dogbane *see* 742
Spreading Factor *see* 4758
S-Protein *see* 10026
Sprout-Nip [PPG] *see* 2187
Spurge Flax *see* 6170
Spurred Rye *see* 3660
S.Q. [Merck & Co.] *see* 8939
SQ-1489 *see* 9371
SQ-4918 *see* 4189
SQ-9453 *see* 3259
SQ-9538 *see* 9179
SQ-10496 *see* 9305
SQ-10733 *see* 4189
SQ-11302 *see* 3614
SQ-11436 *see* 1986
SQ-11725 *see* 6346
SQ-13050 *see* 3502
SQ-13396 *see* 5057
SQ-14055 *see* 9419
SQ-14225 *see* 1774
SQ-15101 *see* 240
SQ-15860 *see* 4506
SQ-16144 *see* 4189
SQ-16150 *see* 3703
SQ-18566 *see* 4591
SQ-19844 *see* 8543
SQ-21983 *see* 5063
SQ-22022 *see* 1986
SQ-22947 *see* 9419
SQ-26776 *see* 925
SQ-26991 *see* 10186
SQ-27519 *see* 4256
SQ-28555 *see* 4256
SQ-29852 *see* 1994
SQ-30217 *see* 9103
SQ-31000 *see* 7714
SQ-32692 *see* 4328
SQ-32756 *see* 8727
SQ-200475 *see* 3595
Squalamine, 8766
Squalane, 8767
Squalene, 8768
Squalestatin 1 *see* 10114
Squalestatins *see* 10114
Squalestatin S1 *see* 10114
Squalidine *see* 8451
Square-stem Rose-gentian *see* 1970
Squaric Acid, 8769
Squaw Bush *see* 9973
Squaw Root *see* 1320
Squaw Weed *see* 8450
Squill, 8770
Squirrel Corn *see* 2545
SR-406 *see* 1772
SR-720-22 *see* 6147
SR-2508 *see* 3713

SR-4233 *see* 9461
SR-11247 *see* 1194
SR-25990 *see* 2396
SR-25990C *see* 2396
SR-29142 *see* 8117
SR-33557 *see* 3934
SR-33589 *see* 3449
SR-33589B *see* 3449
SR-34006 *see* 4892
SR-41319B *see* 9441
SR-47436 *see* 5083
SR-57746A *see* 10054
SR-90107A *see* 4232
SR-141716 *see* 8229
SR-141716A *see* 8229
SRA-3886 *see* 3957
SRA-5172 *see* 5947
SRA-12869 *see* 5172
Srendam [Kayaku] *see* 9005
SRG-95213 *see* 3004
SRIF *see* 8715
SRIF-14 *see* 8715
SRIF-25 *see* 8715
SRIF-28 *see* 8715
SRIF-A *see* 8715
Srilane [Medicia] *see* 4893
sRNA *see* 8203
SRS *see* 5455
SRS-A *see* 5455
SRTx *see* 8371
SS-578 *see* 5042
SS-717 *see* 6478
SSB *see* 8885
SSB-I *see* 8885
SSB-II *see* 8885
ST-21 *see* 7513
ST-37 *see* 4712
ST-52 [Baxter] *see* 4253
ST-155 *see* 2390
ST-200 *see* 84
ST-374 *see* 3967
ST-567 *see* 246
ST-679 *see* 596
ST-1085 *see* 6184
ST-1191 *see* 3885
ST-1396 *see* 1960
ST-1435 *see* 3538
ST-1512 *see* 4707
ST-2121 *see* 3639
ST-4331 *see* 4851
ST-7090 *see* 4705
ST-9067 *see* 914
Stabilene [Auclair] *see* 3770
Stabinol [Horner] *see* 2186
Stable Bixin *see* 1311
Stablon [Ardix] *see* 9420
Stachydrine, 8771
Stadacain [Stada] *see* 1531
Stadadorm [Stada] *see* 570
Stadalax [Stada] *see* 1242
Stadol [BMS] *see* 1530
Stafac [SKB] *see* 10004
Staff [Sigma-Tau] *see* 3885
Stafoxil [Yamanouchi] *see* 4111
Stag Bush *see* 9974
Staggerweed *see* 5372
Stagid [Merck KGaA] *see* 5938
Stagural [Stada-Chemie] *see* 6699
Stalcin [Locatelli] *see* 1643
Stalker *see* 2088
Stalleril [Pharmacal] *see* 9359
Stallimycin, 8772
Stam [Dow AgroSci.] *see* 7804
Stamine [Tutag] *see* 7984
Stampede [Dow AgroSci.] *see* 7804

STAN *see* 8796
Stanazol *see* 8794
Stangen [Phys. Drug] *see* 7984
Stangyl (amp) [Rhone-Poulenc] *see* 9722
Stangyl (tabl) [Rhone-Poulenc] *see* 9722
Stanilo [Pharmacia] *see* 8739
Stannic Anhydride *see* 8778
Stannic Bromide, 8773
Stannic Chloride, 8774
Stannic Chromate(VI), 8775
Stannic Fluoride, 8776
Stannic Iodide, 8777
Stannic Oxide, 8778
Stannic Selenide, 8779
Stannic Sulfide, 8780
Stannochlor *see* 8783
Stannous Acetate, 8781
Stannous Bromide, 8782
Stannous Chloride, 8783
Stannous Fluoride, 8784
Stannous Iodide, 8785
Stannous Oxalate, 8786
Stannous Oxide, 8787
Stannous Pyrophosphate, 8788
Stannous Selenide, 8789
Stannous Sulfate, 8790
Stannous Sulfide, 8791
Stannous Tartrate, 8792
Stanolene [Amoco] *see* 7185
Stanolone, 8793
Stanquinate *see* 5042
Stanyl [DSM] *see* 6735
Stapenor [Bayer] *see* 6904
Staphcillin [BMS] *see* 5969
Staphisagria, 8795
Staphlipen [Wyeth] *see* 4111
Staphylex [GSK] *see* 4111
Staphylokinase, 8796
Staphylomycin *see* 10004
Staphylomycine [SKB] *see* 10004
Staphylomycin M₁ *see* 10004
Staphylomycin S *see* 10004
Staple [DuPont] *see* 7993
Staporos [Cassenne] *see* 1643
STAR *see* 8796
Starane [Dow AgroSci.] *see* 4203
Star Anise, 8797
Starcef [Firma] *see* 1946
Starch, 8798
Starch Gum *see* 2953
Starch 2-Hydroxyethyl Ether *see* 4673
Starch Polymer with 2-Propenenitrile *see* 2587
Starch, Soluble, 8799
Star Grass *see* 230
Staril [BMS] *see* 4256
Starkle [Mitsui] *see* 3289
Starlix [Novartis] *see* 6428
Starsis [Yamanouchi] *see* 6428
Starwort *see* 230, 4631
Starycide [Bayer] *see* 9678
Stas-Hustenlöser [Stada] *see* 386
Staticin [Westwood] *see* 3681
Statine, 8800
Statobex [Lemmon] *see* 7220
Statocin [Yoshitomi] *see* 1839
Statolon, 8801
Statran [Delagrange] *see* 3566
Statyl [Ayerst] *see* 6472
Stauffer 2061 *see* 7061
Stauroderm *see* 4198
Staurosporine, 8802
Stavesacre *see* 8795
Stavudine, 8803

Stayban [Boots] *see* 4199
Staycept [Syntex] *see* 6677
Stazepine [Polfa] *see* 1781
St. Bartholomew's Tea *see* 5756
Steapyrium Chloride *see* 5370
Steareth 7577
Stearic Acid, 8804
Stearic Acid Aluminum Salt *see* 364
Stearic Acid Ammonium Salt *see* 553
Stearic Acid Calcium Salt *see* 1703
Stearic Acid Ester with Lactate of Lactic
   Acid Calcium Salt *see* 1704
Stearic Acid Lead Salt *see* 5418
Stearic Acid Potassium Salt *see* 7673
Stearic Acid Sodium Salt *see* 8678
Stearin *see* 9756
Stearyl Alcohol, 8805
Steatite *see* 9037
Steclin [BMS] *see* 9196
Stedicor [Procter & Gamble] *see* 911
Stédiril [Wyeth] *see* 6704
Steel Factor *see* 8807
Stefin A *see* 2778
Stefin B *see* 2778
Stefins *see* 2778
Steinbühl Yellow *see* 972
Stelabid [SK & F] *see* 5202
Steladone [Syngenta] *see* 2089
Stelazine [GSK] *see* 9680
Stellamicina *see* 3683
Stellar [Staley], 8806
Stellarid [GSK] *see* 7874
Stellerite *see* 1648
Stem Cell Factor, 8807
Stemetil [Aventis] *see* 7761
Stemex [Syntex] *see* 7029
Stemgen [Amgen] *see* 8807
Stem Peptide *see* 7040
Stemphylone *see* 8093
Stenbolone, 8808
Stenediol [Organon] *see* 5950
Stenobolone (rescinded USAN) *see* 8808
Stenol *see* 8805
Stenolon *see* 5951
Stenorol [Intervet] *see* 4596
Stephanine *see* 5929
Stepin [Basotherm] *see* 9456
Stepronin, 8809
Steranabol [Farmitalia] *see* 2413
Sterane [Pfizer] *see* 7721
Sterathal [Ward, Blenkinsop] *see* 7376
Sterax [Alcon] *see* 2928
Stercobilin *see* 9883
Stercorin *see* 2524
Sterculia *see* 5284
Sterecyt [Pharmaleo] *see* 7720
Stereocyt [Bellon] *see* 7720
Stereomycine [Toraude; Ayerst] *see* 5453
Stereon [Firestone] *see* 8390
Sterilon [Roter] *see* 2091
Sterinor [Heumann] *see* 9250
Sterisil [Warner-Lambert] *see* 4703
Steri/Sol [Warner-Lambert] *see* 4703
Steroderm [De Angeli] *see* 2928
Sterogyl [Roussel Diamant] *see* 10018
Sterosan [Novartis] *see* 2190
Sterox [Monsanto] *see* 6677
Steroxin [Novartis] *see* 2190
Sterretite *see* 358
Sterwin 904 *see* 232
Ster-Zac [Hough, Hoseason] *see* 9657
Stesolid [Alpharma] *see* 2994
Steviol *see* 8810
Stevioside, 8810
Steviosin *see* 8810

Steward [DuPont] *see* 4971
STH *see* 8716
STI-571 *see* 4902
"Stibic" Anhydride *see* 698
Stibine, 8811
Stibium *see* 692
Stibnal [Banyu] *see* 702
Stibnite *see* 713
Stibocaptate, 8812
Stibophen, 8813
Stibosamine *see* 3852
Stibron [Iwaki] *see* 1588
Stickstofflost *see* 5775
Stickstoffwasserstoffsäure (German) *see* 4774
Stiedex LP [Stiefel] *see* 2930
Stiemycin [Stiefel] *see* 3681
Stiglyn [Mallinckrodt Vet.] *see* 6464
(3β)-Stigmasta-5,7-dien-3-ol *see* 2875
(3β,5α,22E)-Stigmasta-7,22-dien-3-ol *see* 8749
(3β,5α,22E,24R)-Stigmasta-7,22-dien-3-ol *see* 2211
(3β,22E)-Stigmasta-5,22-dien-3-ol *see* 8815
(3β,24E)-Stigmasta-5,24(28)-dien-3-ol *see* 4280
Stigmastanol, 8814
(3β,5α)-Stigmastan-3-ol *see* 8814
Δ⁵-Stigmasten-3β-ol *see* 8556
(3β)-Stigmast-5-en-3-ol *see* 8556
(3β,24S)-Stigmast-5-en-3-ol *see* 8557
Stigmasterol, 8815
St. Ignatius' Bean *see* 4897
Stilalgin *see* 5850
Stilamin [Serono] *see* 8715
Stilbamidine, 8816
Stilbene, 8817
[Stilbene-(4,4′)]bis[ω-phenylurea]-2,2′-disulfonic Acid Disodium Salt *see* 1315
Stilbene-α-carboxylic Acid *see* 7281
4,4′-Stilbenedicarboxamidine *see* 8816
E-3,5-Stilbenediol *see* 7451
3,4′,5-Stilbenetriol *see* 8158
Stilbestrol *see* 3129
Stilbestrol Dimethyl Ether *see* 3211
Stilbestrol Diphosphate *see* 4253
Stilbetin [BMS] *see* 3129
Stilboestrol *see* 3129
Stilbostatin [Taro] *see* 4253
Stillacor [Wolff] *see* 3167
Stillingia, 8818
Stilnoct [Sanofi-Aventis] *see* 10190
Stilnox [Sanofi-Synthelabo] *see* 10190
Stilny [Will-Pharma] *see* 6691
Stilphostrol [Bayer] *see* 4253
Stilwet L [Union Carbide] *see* 8495
Stimate [ZLB Behring] *see* 2924
Stimol [Biocodex] *see* 2331
Stimolag [Lagap] *see* 7484
Stimsen [Lederle] *see* 9379
Stimulexin [Robins] *see* 3432
Stimulin *see* 6543
Stimulina *see* 4471
Stimu-TSH [HMR] *see* 9588
Stinger [Dow AgroSci.] *see* 2400
Stinging Nettle *see* 6482
Stinkweed *see* 8820
Stipolac [Burroughs Wellcome] *see* 5038
Stiptanon [Organon] *see* 3707
Stirofos *see* 9192
Stivane [Beaufour] *see* 7991
St. John's Wort *see* 4864
StL-1106 *see* 4191

Stock Guard *see* 4124
Stocrin [Merck & Co.] *see* 3521
Stoddard Solvent *see* 6201
Stogar [Fujirebio] *see* 5347
Stomamycin [Chassot] *see* 8752
Stomédine [GSK] *see* 2279
Stomp [BASF] *see* 7084
Stone Oil *see* 4885
Stone-root *see* 2483
Storax, 8819
Storinal *see* 1322
Storksbill *see* 4404
Storm [BASF] *see* 4102
Storocain [Eisai] *see* 6933
Stovaine *see* 614
Stovarsol [Abbott] *see* 52
Stoxil [SK & F] *see* 4891
Stozzon-Chlorophyll *see* 2155
STP *see* 3412
STPP *see* 8697
Straderm [ITA] *see* 4151
Stramonium, 8820
Stratene [Innothera; Sigma-Tau] *see* 2021
Strattera [Lilly] *see* 863
Strawberry Tree *see* 3899
Strengite *see* 4029
Strepogenin, 8821
Streptase [ZLB Behring] *see* 8825
Streptidine, 8822
Streptobrettin [Norbrook] *see* 8826
Streptocide [Frosst] *see* 8925
Streptococcal Deoxyribonuclease *see* 8823
Streptococcal Fibrinolysin *see* 8825
Streptodornase, 8823
Streptogramin A *see* 10004
Streptogramin B *see* 7753
Streptogramins, 8824
Streptokinase, 8825
Streptolin *see* 8829
Streptomagma [Wyeth] *see* 3179
Streptomycin, 8826
Streptomycin A *see* 8826
Streptomycin Hydrochloride *see* 8826
Streptomycin Hydrochloride-calcium Chloride Complex *see* 8826
Streptomycin Sulfate *see* 8826
Streptonigrin, 8827
Streptonivicin *see* 6722
L-Streptose, 8828
Streptothenat [Grünenthal] *see* 8826
Streptothricin VI *see* 8829
Streptothricin F *see* 8829
Streptothricins, 8829
Streptovaricin, 8830
Streptovaricin A *see* 8830
Streptovaricin B *see* 8830
Streptovaricin C *see* 8830
Streptovaricin D *see* 8830
Streptovaricin E *see* 8830
Streptovaricin F *see* 8830
Streptovaricin G *see* 8830
Streptovaricin J *see* 8830
Streptovarycin *see* 8830
Streptovirudin, 8831
Streptozocin, 8832
Streptozon *see* 8923
Streptozotocin *see* 8832
Stresam [Beaufour] *see* 3864
Strese & Hofmann's Hectorite *see* 4623
Stresnil [Janssen] *see* 898
Stresson [Boehringer, Ing.] *see* 1489
Striadyne [Am. Home] *see* 155
Striatran [Merck & Co.] *see* 3566
Strictylon *see* 6368

Strigol, 8833
Striped Alder *see* 4606
Strobane-T [Tenneco] *see* 9557
Strobilurin A *see* 8834
Strobilurins, 8834
Stroby [BASF] *see* 5324
Strodival [Herbert] *see* 6901
Stromba [Winthrop] *see* 8794
Strombaject [Winthrop] *see* 8794
Stromectol [Merck & Co.] *see* 5248
Strongarm [Dow AgroSci.] *see* 3083
Strongid [Pfizer] *see* 7955
Strong Silver Protein *see* 8527
Strontia *see* 8846
Strontianite *see* 8835, 8838
Strontium, 8835
Strontium Acetate, 8836
Strontium Bromide, 8837
Strontium Carbonate, 8838
Strontium Chlorate, 8839
Strontium Chloride, 8840
Strontium Chromate(VI), 8841
Strontium Fluoride, 8842
Strontium Hydrate *see* 8843
Strontium Hydride *see* 8835
Strontium Hydroxide, 8843
Strontium Iodide, 8844
Strontium Monoxide *see* 8846
Strontium Nitrate, 8845
Strontium Nitride *see* 8835
Strontium Oxide, 8846
Strontium Peroxide, 8847
Strontium Ranelate *see* 8106
Strontium Sulfate, 8848
Strontium Sulfide, 8849
Strontium Titanate, 8850
Strontium Titanium Oxide (SrTiO₃) *see* 8850
Strophadogenin *see* 8851
Strophanthidin, 8851
Strophanthidin α-L-Rhamnoside *see* 2512
Strophanthin, 8852
Strophanthus, 8853
Strophoperm [Sertürner] *see* 6901
Strotan [Strathmann] *see* 189
Structum [SKB] *see* 2214
Strumacil *see* 6128
Strumazol *see* 5971
Struvite, 8854
Strychnidin-10-one *see* 8855
Strychnidin-10-one 19-Oxide *see* 8856
Strychnine, 8855
Strychnine N⁶-Oxide *see* 8856
C-Strychnotoxine *see* 9558
Stryker's Reagent, 8857
Stryphnasal [Sertürner] *see* 171
Stryphnon [Salus-Braumapharm] *see* 171
STS-557 *see* 3106
Stuart Factor *see* 3923
Stuart-Prower Factor *see* 3923
Stugeron [Janssen] *see* 2305
Stutgeron [Janssen] *see* 2305
Stutgin *see* 2305
STX *see* 8389
Stylomycin *see* 7943
Stylophorin *see* 2053
Stylopine, 8858
Styphnic Acid, 8859
Styptic Collodion *see* 2484
Stypticin [Merck & Co.] *see* 2552
Styptol *see* 2552
Styquin *see* 1514
Styracin *see* 2304
Styrax *see* 8819

Name Index

6-Sulfanilamido-2,4-dimethylpyrimidine *see* 8951
2-Sulfanilamido-3-methoxypyrazine *see* 8910
2-Sulfanilamido-5-methoxypyrimidine *see* 8914
3-Sulfanilamido-5-methylisoxazole *see* 8918
4-Sulfanilamido-2-methyl-6-methoxypyrimidine *see* 8917
2-Sulfanilamido-4-methylpyrimidine *see* 8913
2-Sulfanilamido-5-methylpyrimidine *see* 8934
2-Sulfanilamido-5-methyl-1,3,4-thiadiazole *see* 8916
2-Sulfanilamidopyrazine *see* 8937
2-Sulfanilamidopyridine *see* 8938
2-Sulfanilamidopyrimidine *see* 8903
2-Sulfanilamidoquinoxaline *see* 8939
2-Sulfanilamidothiazole *see* 8943
Sulfanilanilide *see* 8896
m-Sulfanilic Acid *see* 5927
o-Sulfanilic Acid *see* 6882
Sulfanilic Acid Diazonium Salt *see* 2999
p-Sulfanilidobenzylamine *see* 8928
N-Sulfanilylacetamide *see* 8899
2-Sulfanilylaminopyrimidine *see* 8903
2-(Sulfanilylamino)thiazole *see* 8943
2-*p*-Sulfanilylanilinoethanol, 8927
N-Sulfanilylbenzamide *see* 8897
p-Sulfanilylbenzylamine, 8928
*N*¹-Sulfanilyl-*N*²-butylcarbamide *see* 1832
*N*¹-Sulfanilyl-*N*²-butylurea *see* 1832
Sulfanilylcarbamic Acid Methyl Ester *see* 857
N-Sulfanilylcarbamide *see* 8931
N-Sulfanilyl-β,β-dimethylacrylamide *see* 8904
N-Sulfanilyl-1-ethylcytosine *see* 8902
Sulfanilyl Fluoride, 8929
Sulfanilylguanidine *see* 8908
N-*p*-Sulfanilylphenylglycine *see* 23
N-Sulfanilylseneciamide *see* 8904
4′-Sulfanilylsuccinanilic Acid *see* 8878
*N*⁴-Sulfanilylsulfanilamide *see* 8930
1-Sulfanilyl-2-thiourea *see* 8944
Sulfanilylurea, 8931
N-Sulfanilyl-3,4-xylamide, 8932
Sulfanitran, 8933
Sulfaperine, 8934
Sulfaphenazole, 8935
Sulfaproxyline, 8936
Sulfapyrazine, 8937
Sulfapyrazinemethoxyine *see* 8910
Sulfapyrazole *see* 8945
Sulfapyridine, 8938
Sulfapyrimidine *see* 8903
Sulfaquinoxaline, 8939
Sulfarlem [Solvay] *see* 644
Sulfarsenobenzene *see* 8941
Sulfarside, 8940
Sulfarsphenamine, 8941
Sulfasalazine, 8942
Sulfasuxidine [Merck & Co.] *see* 8877
Sulfatase B *see* 819
Sulfated Castor Oil *see* 9823
Sulfated Potato Amylopectin Sodium Salt *see* 8577
Sulfatertiobutylthiadiazole *see* 4479
Sulfathiazole, 8943
Sulfathiocarbamide *see* 8944
Sulfathiourea, 8944

Sulfatreis [Ecobi] *see* 8934
Sulfaurea *see* 8931
Sulfavitina [CT] *see* 8943
Sulfazamet, 8945
Sulfazecin, 8946
Sulfenone *see* 8988
Sulfentrazone, 8947
Sulferrous [Conal] *see* 4057
Sulfethylic Acid *see* 3853
o-Sulfhydrylbenzoic Acid *see* 9360
Sulfinalol, 8948
Sulfinpyrazone, 8949
Sulfinylbismethane *see* 3259
Sulfiram, 8950
Sulfisomezole *see* 8918
Sulfisomidine, 8951
Sulfisoxazole, 8952
Sulfisoxazole Diolamine *see* 8952
Sulfitocobalamin *see* 4809
Sulfmidil [Tika] *see* 8924
Sulfoacetic Acid, 8953
3-Sulfoalanine *see* 2780
4-Sulfobenzenediazonium Inner Salt *see* 2999
Sulfobenzide *see* 3332
o-Sulfobenzimide *see* 8311
o-Sulfobenzoic Acid Imide *see* 8311
α-Sulfobenzylpenicillin *see* 8890
4,4′-[(3-Sulfo[1,1′-biphenyl]-4,4′-diyl)-bis(azo)]bis[3-amino-2,7-naphthalenedisulfonic Acid] Pentasodium Salt *see* 9793
4,4′-[(3-Sulfo-4,4′-biphenylene)bis-(azo)]bis(3-amino-2,7-naphthalenedisulfonic Acid) Pentasodium Salt *see* 9793
Sulfobromophthalein Sodium, 8954
Sulfobutanedioic Acid 1,4-Bis(2-ethylhexyl)ester Calcium Salt *see* 3400
Sulfobutanedioic Acid 1,4-Bis(2-ethylhexyl) Ester Sodium Salt *see* 3401
Sulfobutanedioic Acid 1,4-Bis(1-methylpentyl) Ester Sodium Salt *see* 1255
Sulfobutanedioic Acid 1,4-Dipentyl Ester Sodium Salt *see* 2989
Sulfocarbanilide *see* 3333
Sulfocarbolic Acid *see* 7246
12-Sulfodehydroabietic Acid *see* 3489
Sulfoethanoic Acid *see* 8953
Sulfogaiacol *see* 7634
Sulfogenol *see* 4885
Sulfolane, 8955
3-Sulfolene, 8956
Sulfometuron-methyl, 8957
Sulfomonoperacid *see* 1851
Sulfomyl *see* 5649
Sulfonal *see* 8960
Sulfona-Mae *see* 2822
p-Sulfonamidobenzoic Acid *see* 1876
1-(4-Sulfo-1-naphthylazo)-2-naphthol-3,-6-disulfonic Acid Trisodium Salt *see* 375
Sulfon-Cilag *see* 23
p-Sulfondichloramidobenzoic Acid *see* 4590
Sulfone Acid Blue R *see* 628
Sulfonediacetic Acid *see* 8961
Sulfonethylmethane, 8958
Sulfoniazide, 8959
Sulfonmethane, 8960
Sulfon-Niazone [Foscama] *see* 8959
Sulfonphthal *see* 7247
1,1′-Sulfonylbisbenzene *see* 3332
4,4′-Sulfonylbisbenzeneamine *see* 2822

2,2′-Sulfonylbis(ethanethiol) *see* 1254
Sulfonylbismethane *see* 3258
1,1′-[Sulfonylbis(4,1-phenyleneimino)]-bis[1-deoxy-1-sulfo-D-glucitol] Disodium Salt *see* 4463
1,1′-[Sulfonylbis(4,1-phenyleneimino)]-bis[3-phenyl-1,3-propanedisulfonic Acid] Tetrasodium Salt *see* 8711
Sulfonyldiacetic Acid, 8961
4,4′-Sulfonyldianiline *see* 2822
p,*p*′-Sulfonyldianiline-*N*,*N*′-di-D-glucose Sodium Bisulfite Compd *see* 4463
p,*p*′-Sulfonyldianiline *N*,*N*′-Diglucoside Disodium Disulfonate *see* 4463
N-(Sulfonyl-*p*-methylbenzene)-*N*′-*n*-butylurea *see* 9507
2-(Sulfooxy)benzoic Acid *see* 8334
1-*p*-Sulfophenylazo-2-naphthol-6-sulfonic Acid Disodium Salt *see* 9001
1-(4-Sulfophenyl)-3-ethylcarboxyl-4-(4-sulfonaphthylazo)-5-hydroxypyrazole Disodium Salt *see* 6859
p-Sulfophenylhydrazine *see* 4773
N-(3-Sulfopropyl)morpholine *see* 6265
Sulforal [Med-Pharmex] *see* 8905
Sulforaphane, 8962
Sulforidazine, 8963
Sulforthomidine *see* 8906
Sulfosalicylic Acid, 8964
5-Sulfosalicylic Acid *see* 8964
Sulfosate *see* 4512
Sulfosuccinic Acid 1,4-Bis(2-ethylhexyl) Ester *S*-Sodium Salt *see* 3401
Sulfosuccinic Acid Diisobutyl Ester *S*-Sodium Salt *see* 3194
Sulfosuccinic Acid Dipentyl Ester Sodium Salt *see* 2989
Sulfosulfuron, 8965
Sulfotep, 8966
Sulfotepp *see* 8966
Sulfothiorine *see* 8694
Sulfotrim [Nattermann] *see* 8918
Sulfovinic Acid *see* 3853
Sulfox-Cide [Penick] *see* 8967
Sulfoxide, 8967
Sulfoxine 33 [Univet] *see* 8915
Sulfoxine LA [Univet] *see* 8919
Sulfoxone Sodium, 8968
Sulfoxylic Acid Mono[[[5-[(3-amino-4-hydroxyphenyl)diarsenyl]-2-hydroxyphenyl]amino]methyl] Ester Monosodium Salt *see* 6447
Sulfoxyphenylpyrazolidine *see* 8949
Sulfuno [Nordmark] *see* 8924
Sulfur, 8969
Sulfurated Lime *see* 1707, 8977
Sulfurated Potash *see* 8977
Sulfur Chloride, 8970
Sulfur Dioxide, 8971
Sulfur Dioxide Soln *see* 8976
Sulfureted Hydrogen *see* 4800
Sulfuretin, 8972
Sulfur Hexafluoride, 8973
Sulfuric Acid, 8974
Sulfuric Acid Aluminum Salt Compd with Guanidine (2:1:1) Hexahydrate *see* 4563
Sulfuric Acid Ammonium Nickel(2+) Salt (2:2:1) *see* 6501
Sulfuric Acid Chromium(3+) Salt (3:2) *see* 2230
Sulfuric Acid Copper(2+) Salt (1:1) *see* 2653
Sulfuric Acid Diammonium Salt *see* 555
Sulfuric Acid Diethyl Ester *see* 3130

Sulfuric Acid Dimethyl Ester *see* 3256
Sulfuric Acid Monoanhydride with Nitrous Acid *see* 6648
Sulfuric Acid Monododecyl Ester Sodium Salt *see* 8636
Sulfuric Acid Monoethyl Ester *see* 3853
Sulfuric Acid Monomethyl Ester *see* 6122
Sulfuric Acid Nickel(2+) Salt (1:1) *see* 6517
Sulfuric Anhydride *see* 8979
Sulfuric Chlorohydrin *see* 2165
Sulfuric Ether *see* 3806
Sulfur Iodide, 8975
Sulfur Monochloride *see* 8970
Sulfur Mustard *see* 6316
Sulfurous Acid, 8976
Sulfurous Acid 2-(*p-tert*-Butylphenoxy)cyclohexyl 2-Propynyl Ester *see* 7808
Sulfurous Acid 2-[4-(1,1-Dimethylethyl)phenoxy]cyclohexyl 2-Propynyl Ester *see* 7808
Sulfurous Anhydride *see* 8971
Sulfurous Oxide *see* 8971
Sulfurous Oxychloride *see* 9348
Sulfur, Pharmaceutical, 8977
Sulfur Subchloride *see* 8970
Sulfur Tetrafluoride, 8978
Sulfur Trioxide, 8979
Sulfur Yellow S *see* 6393
Sulfuryl Amide *see* 8922
Sulfuryl Chloride, 8980
Sulfuryl Fluoride, 8981
Sulindac, 8982
Sulindac Sulfone *see* 3916
Sulinol [ICT] *see* 8982
Sulisobenzone, 8983
Sulla [Robins] *see* 8914
Sulmarin, 8984
Sulmazole, 8985
Sulmet [Am. Cyanamid] *see* 8915
Sulmetozine (rescinded INN) *see* 9760
Sulmycin [Essex] *see* 4392
Sulodexide, 8986
Sulpelin [Senju] *see* 8890
Sulperazone [Pfizer] *see* 8889
Sulphadione *see* 2822
Sulphafurazole *see* 8952
Sulphaloxic Acid *see* 8912
Sulphan Blue, 8987
Sulphaproxyline *see* 8936
Sulphasalazine *see* 8942
Sulphasolucin *see* 6684
Sulphasolutin *see* 6684
Sulphasomidine *see* 8951
Sulphation Factors *see* 4986
Sulphenone, 8988
Sulphetrone [Burroughs Wellcome] *see* 8711
7-(α-Sulphophenylacetamido)-3-(4′-carbamoylpyridinium)methyl-3-cephem-4-carboxylic Acid *see* 1945
Sulphormethoxine *see* 8906
Sulphur *see* 8969
Sulpiride, 8989
S(−)-Sulpiride *see* 8989
Sulpitil [Tillotts] *see* 8989
Sulpor [Rosemont] *see* 8989
Sulprim [Polfa] *see* 8918
Sulprofos, 8990
Sulprostone, 8991
Sulprotin [Taiyo] *see* 9005
Sulpyrin *see* 3350
Sulquin [Salsbury] *see* 8939
Sulreuma [Von Boch] *see* 8982
Sul-Spantab [SK & F] *see* 8907

Sultamicillin, 8992
Sultan Red 4B *see* 1101
Sultanol [GSK] *see* 216
Sulten-10 [Bausch & Lomb] *see* 8899
Sulthiame, 8993
Sultopride, 8994
Sultosilic Acid, 8995
Sulzol [Yoshitomi] *see* 8943
SUM-3170 *see* 5587
Sumach, 8996
Sumach Wax *see* 5256
Sumatra Camphor *see* 1338
Sumatriptan, 8997
Sumbul, 8998
Sumetrolim [EGYT] *see* 8918
Sumi-8 [Sumitomo] *see* 3268
Sumial [AstraZeneca] *see* 7840
Sumi-alpha [Sumitomo] *see* 4010
Sumicidin [Sumitomo] *see* 4010
Sumiferon [Sumitomo] *see* 4990
Sumilarv [Sumitomo] *see* 7990
Sumilex [Sumitomo] *see* 7765
Sumisclex [Sumitomo] *see* 7765
Sumisoya [Sumitomo] *see* 4143
Sumithion [Sumitomo] *see* 3976
Sumithrin [Sumitomo] *see* 7211
Sumitomo S-4084 *see* 2261
Summetrin *see* 7016
Summit [Mobay] *see* 9593
Sumycin [BMS] *see* 9196
SUN-208 *see* 3938
SUN-0588 *see* 8368
SUN-1165 *see* 7427
SUN-4936 *see* 872
SUN-5555 *see* 3938
Suncefal [Yamanouchi] *see* 1939
Suncide [Bayer] *see* 7836
Sundance [Monsanto] *see* 8965
SunDare [Texas Pharmacal] *see* 2310
Sundown *see* 3232
Sundralen [Delalande] *see* 9418
Sunette [Hoechst] *see* 37
Sunflower Seed Oil, 8999
Sunfural [Asahi Kasei] *see* 9112
Sungard [Miles] *see* 8983
Sunitinib, 9000
Sunrabin [Asahi] *see* 3586
Sunril [Emko] *see* 7000
Sunrythm [Suntory] *see* 7427
Sunset Yellow FCF, 9001
Supacal [Lederle] *see* 9585
Supanate [Nippon Shinyaku] *see* 4106
Supazlun [Kowa] *see* 4106
Superanabolon [Spofa] *see* 6365
Super-Caid [Lipha] *see* 1382
Super-Cel *see* 4973
Super Glue *see* 3787
Super-Hydride [Aldrich] *see* 5544
Superinone [Sanofi Winthrop] *see* 9833
Superoxide Dismutase, 9002
Super-Rozol [Lipha] *see* 1382
Super-Slurper *see* 2587
Supeudol [Sabex] *see* 6959
Supirdyl *see* 7038
Suplatast Tosylate, 9003
Suplexedil [Hépatrol] *see* 3986
Supona [BASF] *see* 2089
Supotran [Winthrop] *see* 2106
Supprelin [Roberts] *see* 4722
Suprachol *see* 2868
Supracid(e) [Syngenta] *see* 5970
Supracombin [Grünenthal] *see* 8918
Supracyclin [Grünenthal] *see* 3440
Supraene [Robeco] *see* 8768

Supral [Basotherm] *see* 7062
Supralgin *see* 7207
Supramox [Grünenthal] *see* 577
Supramycin [Grünenthal] *see* 9196
Suprane [Ohmeda] *see* 2919
Supranol [Cilag] *see* 9005
Suprarenin [Aventis] *see* 3619
Suprasec [J & J] *see* 5571
Suprasterol II, 9004
Supratonin [Grünenthal] *see* 394
Suprax [Wyeth] *see* 1924
Suprecur [Sanofi-Aventis] *see* 1503
Suprefact [Sanofi-Aventis] *see* 1503
Suprifen *see* 4824
Suprilent [Duphar] *see* 5238
Suprim [Valeas] *see* 8918
Supristol [Gallier] *see* 8924
Suprocil [Cilag] *see* 9005
Suprofen, 9005
Suprol [Cilag] *see* 9005
Suprotan *see* 2106
Sural [Chinoin] *see* 3720
Suralgan [Poli] *see* 9422
Suramin Sodium, 9006
Surbronc [Boehringer, Ing.] *see* 386
Surem [Novartis] *see* 1510
Surem [Galen] *see* 6575
Surestryl [Roussel Diamant] *see* 6289
Surexin [McNeil] *see* 7989
Surfacaine [Lilly] *see* 2735
Surfactal [Boehringer, Ing.] *see* 386
Surfactant Protein-B *see* 8542
Surfactant TA *see* 1151
Surfacten [Tokyo Tanabe] *see* 1151
Surfak [HMR] *see* 3400
Surfathesin *see* 2735
Surfaxin [Discovery Labs] *see* 8542
Surfen [Hoechst] *see* 475
Surfexo [Glaxo Wellcome] *see* 3917
Surflan [Dow AgroSci.] *see* 6885
Surfonic N [Jefferson] *see* 6677
Surgam [HMR] *see* 9422
Surgestone [Cassenne] *see* 7785
Surgi-Cen *see* 8989
Surheme [Merck KGaA] *see* 1510
Surika [Thiemann] *see* 4132
Surinam Balsam *see* 949
Surinamine, 9007
Surital [Warner-Lambert] *see* 9302
Surlid [HMR] *see* 8276
Surmax [Elanco] *see* 887
Surmontil (amp) [Rhone-Poulenc] *see* 9722
Surmontil (tabl) [Rhone-Poulenc] *see* 9722
Surofene *see* 4680
Surpass [Dow AgroSci.] *see* 61, 3049
Sursumid [Labif] *see* 8989
Survanta [Ross] *see* 1151
Survector [Eutherapie] *see* 409
Survivin, 9008
Suscard [Forest] *see* 6607
Suscardia [Pharmax] *see* 5217
Suspendol [Merckle] *see* 279
Sus-phrine [Forest] *see* 3619
Sustac [Forest] *see* 6607
Sustamycin [Boehringer, Mann.] *see* 9196
Sustane [UOP] *see* 1548
Sustane 1-F [UOP] *see* 1547
Sustiva [BMS] *see* 3521
Sutan Plus [Zeneca] *see* 1546
Sutent [Pfizer] *see* 9000
Sutoprofen *see* 9005
Suvipen [Midy] *see* 5925
Suvren [Ayerst] *see* 1773

Suxamethonium Bromide *see* 8874
Suxamethonium Chloride *see* 8875
Suxamethonium Iodide *see* 8876
Suxibuzone, 9009
Suxil [Eddé] *see* 8872
Suxilep *see* 3748
Suximal *see* 3748
Suxinutin [Parke-Davis] *see* 3748
Suzutolon [Tatsumi] *see* 1178
Swartziol *see* 5274
Swat [Allied Chemical] *see* 1330
Sweet Bay *see* 5382
Sweet Birch Oil *see* 6120
Sweet Bugle *see* 5624
Sweet Cane *see* 1637
Sweet Clover *see* 5821
Sweet Elder *see* 8351
Sweet Fennel *see* 3977
Sweet Flag *see* 1637
Sweet Grass *see* 1637
Sweet Orange Peel *see* 6860
Sweet Oriental Gum *see* 8819
Sweet Root *see* 4504
Sweet Spirit of Niter *see* 3831
Sweet Viburnum *see* 9974
Sweet-wood Bark *see* 1881
Sweroside-2′-(3″,5″,3‴-trihydroxydi-
    phenyl)-2″-carboxylic Acid Ester *see*
    377
Swertiamarin, 9010
Swiss Blue *see* 6060
Sword [Meiji] *see* 7908
SY-5555 *see* 3938
Sybron [Parke-Davis] *see* 4031
Sydnones, 9011
Sygen [Fidia] *see* 4364
Sykose *see* 8311
Sylvanite *see* 4514
Sylvic Acid *see* 7
Sylvine *see* 7621
Sylvite *see* 7621
Symclosene *see* 9641
Symetra [Forest] *see* 7220
Symlin [Amylin] *see* 7708
Symmetrel [Endo] *see* 374
Sympatektoman *see* 9199
Sympathol *see* 9012
Sympectothion *see* 3663
Symptom 3 [Parke-Davis] *see* 1443
Synacid [Sterivet] *see* 4757
Synaclyn [Syntex] *see* 4145
Synacort [Syntex] *see* 4787
Synacthen [Novartis] *see* 2551
Synadenylic Acid *see* 157
Synadrin [Hoechst] *see* 7737
Synagis [MedImmune] *see* 6988
Synalar [Syntex] *see* 4150
Synalate (rescinded) [Syntex] *see* 4151
Synamol [Syntex] *see* 4150
Synandone [Syntex] *see* 4150
Synandrol [Pfizer] *see* 9180
Synanthic [Fort Dodge] *see* 6935
Synapause [Organon] *see* 3707
Synaptic Laminin *see* 5351
SynaptoGreen [Biotium] *see* 4220
Synapton [Forest] *see* 7384
Synarel [Syntex] *see* 6351
Synasteron *see* 6967
Synatan [Ferring] *see* 2954
Synchrocept [Syntex] *see* 7880
Synchrocept B [Syntex] *see* 3995
Synchrodyn [Hoechst] *see* 314
Synchronate *see* 4200
Syncillin [Bayer] *see* 910, 7223
Syncl [Toyo Jozo] *see* 1974

Synclotin [Toyo Jozo] *see* 1982
Syncortyl [Roussel Diamant] *see* 2901
Syncro-Mate [Searle] *see* 4200
Syncuma [Philips Roxane] *see* 9492
Syncurine [Burroughs Wellcome] *see* 2847
Syndeins *see* 8740
Syndrox [McNeil] *see* 5948
Synédil [Beytout] *see* 8989
Synemol [Syntex] *see* 4150
Synephrin [Neukonigsforder] *see* 9012
Synephrine, 9012
Syneptine [Toraude] *see* 5453
Synercid [Rhône-Poulenc] *see* 2804
Synestrol [Schering] *see* 3104
Synexin *see* 676
Synflex [Recordati] *see* 6417
Syngacillin [Wyeth] *see* 2702
Synhexyl, 9013
Synkamin [Parke-Davis] *see* 10023
Synkavit [Roche] *see* 5830
Synkayvite [Roche] *see* 5830
Synklor *see* 2082
Synkonin *see* 4785
Synnematin B *see* 7098
Synogil [Basotherm] *see* 6427
Synopen [Novartis] *see* 2162
Synotic [Syntex] *see* 4150
Synpen [Novartis] *see* 2162
Synpenin [Sankyo] *see* 586
Synperonic PE/F68 [ICI] *see* 7562
Synpitan [Werfft] *see* 6979
Synpol *see* 7575
Synrelina [Syntex] *see* 6351
Synsac [Syntex] *see* 4150
Synsorb 90 *see* 9014
Synsorb CD [Synsorb Biotech] *see* 9014
Synsorb Pk [Synsorb Biotech] *see* 9014
Synsorbs, 9014
Synstigmin *see* 6464
Syntaris [Syntex] *see* 4145
Syntarpen [Polfa] *see* 3084
Syntecort [Medicamenta] *see* 7029
Syntes 12a *see* 3517
Syntestan [Syntex] *see* 2398
Syntetrin [BMS] *see* 8252
Synthenate *see* 9012
Synthovo *see* 4701
Synthroid [Knoll] *see* 9415
Syntocain [Sintetica] *see* 7757
Syntocinon [Novartis] *see* 6979
Syntometrine *see* 3655
Syntons *see* 7879
Syntopressin [Sandoz] *see* 5630
Syntrogène *see* 4701
Synulox [Pfizer] *see* 2341
Synvinolin *see* 8539
Syprine [Merck & Co.] *see* 9663
Syraprim [Wellcome] *see* 9709
Syringaldehyde, 9015
Syringic Acid δ-Guanidinobutyl Ester *see*
    5440
Syringic Aldehyde *see* 9015
Syringidin *see* 5715
Syringin, 9016
Syringopine *see* 9017
Syringoside *see* 9016
Syrosingopine, 9017
Syscor [Bayer] *see* 6565
Systamex [Schering-Plough] *see* 6935
Systemin, 9018
Systen [Janssen-Cilag] *see* 3703
Systhane [Dow AgroSci.] *see* 6321
Systox *see* 2889
Systral [Viatris] *see* 2181
Sytam [Murphy] *see* 8395

Sytasol [Murphy] *see* 3285
Szaibelyite *see* 5658
Szomolnikite *see* 4057
SZX-722 *see* 5080
T₃ *see* 5510
T₄ *see* 2736, 9415
2,4,5-T, 9019
T-20 *see* 3582
T 23P *see* 9751
T-34 *see* 1372
T-47 *see* 1372
T-113 *see* 9623
T-1220 *see* 7463
T-1258 *see* 9132
T-1384 *see* 6481
T-1551 *see* 1930
T-1824 *see* 3905
T-1982 *see* 1918
T-2525 *see* 1947
T-2588 *see* 1947
T-3033 *see* 7764
T-3262 *see* 9555
T-3761 *see* 7055
T-3762 *see* 7055
T-3811 *see* 4369
T-3811ME *see* 4369
TA-1 *see* 6274
TA-058 *see* 852
TA-064 *see* 2894
TA-870 *see* 3396
TA-903 *see* 1038
TA-0910 *see* 9045
TA-2711 *see* 3489
TA-3090 *see* 2348
TA-6366 *see* 4911
Tabalon [Teofarma] *see* 4881
Tabasco Pepper *see* 1770
Tabazur [Théraplix] *see* 6524
Tabe [Bernabo] *see* 7491
Taberdog [Nipa] *see* 2995
Tabergat [Nipa] *see* 2995
Tabernanthine, 9020
Table Salt *see* 8599
Table Spate *see* 1702
Tabloid [GSK] *see* 9337
Tabun, 9021
Tacalcitol, 9022
Tacaryl [Westwood] *see* 5964
Tace [HMR] *see* 2174
Tacef [Grünenthal] *see* 1925
Tachicol [Radiumfarma] *see* 2715
Tachigaren [Sankyo] *see* 4856
Tachionin [Sana] *see* 9624
Tachmalin [AWD] *see* 194
Tachostyptan [Consolidated Chem.] *see*
    9385
Tachydaron [AWD] *see* 482
Tachyrol [Duphar] *see* 3180
Tachysterol, 9023
Tacitin [Novartis] *see* 1087
Tackle [Sankyo] *see* 8486
Tacosal [Stada] *see* 7322
Tacrine, 9024
Tacrolimus, 9025
Tacryl, 9026
Tadalafil, 9027
Tadenan [Debat] *see* 7949
t-Adenylic Acid *see* 158
Tadeonal *see* 7570
TAED, 9028
TAED 4303 *see* 9028
Tafenoquine, 9029
Tafethion [Rallis] *see* 3736
Tafil [Pharmacia] *see* 312
TAG-72 *see* 8385

Tagamet [GSK] *see* 2279
Tagathen [Lederle] *see* 2167
D-Tagatose, 9030
Tagilite *see* 2648
Taicelexin [Taiyo] *see* 1974
Taidecanone [Taiyo] *see* 9843
Taiguic Acid *see* 5366
Tailed Pepper *see* 2612
TAK-375 *see* 8101
Takacillin [Torii] *see* 5437
Taka-Diastase, 9031
Takanarumin [Takata] *see* 279
Takaton *see* 3260
Takeoff [Takeda] *see* 4908
Takepron [Takeda] *see* 5362
Takesulin [Takeda] *see* 1945
Taketiam [Takeda] *see* 1935
Takizolite *see* 362
Taktic [Intervet] *see* 486
Takus [Montedison] *see* 2005
Taladren [Malesci] *see* 3717
Talampanel, 9032
Talampicillin, 9033
Talaporfin, 9034
Talaporfin Sodium *see* 9034
Talastine, 9035
Talat [Polifarma] *see* 9033
Talbutal, 9036
Talc, 9037
Talcid [Bayer] *see* 5660
Talcum *see* 9037
Talecid [Schering] *see* 7376
Talerc [Boehringer, Ing.] *see* 3618
Talin [Tate & Lyle] *see* 9273
Talinolol, 9038
Talion [Tanabe] *see* 1149
Talipexole, 9039
Talis [Kali-Chemie] *see* 5920
Talisomycin *see* 9043
Talisomycin B *see* 9043
Talleol *see* 9040
Tall Oil, 9040
Tallol *see* 9040
Tallow, 9041
Tallow Alcohol, 9042
Tallow Shrub *see* 1012
Tallysomycin, 9043
Tallysomycin A *see* 9043
Tallysomycin B *see* 9043
Talniflumate, 9044
Talodex *see* 4002
Talofen [Fournier] *see* 7783
Talon [Zeneca Ag Prod] *see* 1379
Taloxa [Schering-Plough] *see* 3950
Talpen [SKB] *see* 9033
Talsis [Wyeth] *see* 1296
Talstar [FMC] *see* 1209
Taltirelin, 9045
Talusin [Abbott] *see* 7874
Talwin [Sanofi-Synthelabo] *see* 7121
Tamarind, 9046
Tamaron [Bayer CropSci.] *see* 5947
Tamas [Schering] *see* 1122
Tambocor [3M Pharma] *see* 4098
TAME *see* 612
Tamed Iodine [West] *see* 5037
Tametin [ISF] *see* 2279
Tamex [CFPI] *see* 1532
Tamibaro [Toko] *see* 9047
Tamibarotene, 9047
Tamiflu [Roche] *see* 6889
Tamofène [Aventis] *see* 9048
Tamoxifen, 9048
Tamsulosin, 9049
Tamyl [Italchimici] *see* 1915

Tanacetin, 9050
Tanaclone [Amsa] *see* 3473
Tanadopa [Tanabe Seiyaku] *see* 3396
Tanafol *see* 2106
Tanakan [Ipsen] *see* 4425
Tanatril [Tanabe] *see* 4911
Tanbismuth *see* 1288
Tandearil [Novartis] *see* 6972
Tandix [Biofarma] *see* 4935
Tandospirone, 9051
Tanganil [Specia] *see* 95
Tangantangan Oil *see* 1898
Tannic Acid, 9052
Tannic Acid Bismuth Derivative *see* 1288
Tannigen *see* 104
Tannin *see* 9052
Tannyl Acetate *see* 104
Tanorama *see* 3182
Tanphetamin *see* 2954
Tantalic Acid Anhydride *see* 9056
Tantalite *see* 6556, 9053
Tantalum, 9053
Tantalum Chloride (TaCl₅) *see* 9054
Tantalum Oxide (Ta₂O₅) *see* 9056
Tantalum Pentachloride, 9054
Tantalum Pentafluoride, 9055
Tantalum Pentoxide, 9056
Tantarone [Mohan] *see* 5915
Tan Tone *see* 3182
Tantum [Angelini] *see* 1122
TAO [Roerig] *see* 9770
TAP-031 *see* 4061
TAP-144 *see* 5457
Tapazole [Lilly] *see* 5971
Taprostene, 9057
TAPS, 9058
TAPSO *see* 9058
Taquidil [Roemmers] *see* 9491
Taractan [Roche] *see* 2188
Tarasan [Roche] *see* 2188
Tarasyn [Syntex] *see* 5306
Taraxacum, 9059
Taraxast-20(30)-en-3β-ol *see* 9060
Taraxasterin *see* 9060
Taraxasterol, 9060
Taraxein, 9061
Taraxerol, 9062
Tar Camphor *see* 6370
Tarceva [OSI] *see* 3672
Tardamide [Grünenthal] *see* 8924
Tardastrex [Gruntex] *see* 2878
Tarden [Veterinaria] *see* 2878
Tardigal [Beiersdorf] *see* 3163
Tardisal [Sigma-Tau] *see* 8333
Tardocillin [Bayer] *see* 7096
Taredan [FMC] *see* 1632
Tareg [Novartis] *see* 9916
Targa [Nissan] *see* 8086
Targinine *see* 6022
Targocid [Aventis] *see* 9115
Targosid [Aventis] *see* 9115
Targretin [Ligand] *see* 1194
Taribavirin, 9063
Tarichatoxin *see* 9246
Tariquidar, 9064
Tarivid [Aventis] *see* 6771
Tarka [Abbott] *see* 9950
Taroctyl [Taro] *see* 2185
Tarodyl *see* 4501
Tarodyn *see* 4501
Tar Oil, 9065
Tar Oil, Rectified, 9066
Tarragon, 9067
Tarragon Oil *see* 3705
Tartar Emetic *see* 700

(+)-Tartaric Acid *see* 9070
(−)-Tartaric Acid *see* 9068
d-Tartaric Acid *see* 9070
dl-Tartaric Acid *see* 9069
D-Tartaric Acid, 9068
DL-Tartaric Acid, 9069
l-Tartaric Acid *see* 9068
L-Tartaric Acid, 9070
meso-Tartaric Acid, 9071
Tartaric Acid Bismuth Complex Potassium Salt *see* 1277
Tartaric Acid Bismuth Complex Sodium Salt *see* 1279
L-Tartaric Acid Monoammonium Salt *see* 503
Tartarized Antimony *see* 700
Tartarus Vitriolatus *see* 7674
Tartrated Antimony *see* 700
Tartrazine, 9072
Tartrol *see* 1279
Tartronic Acid, 9073
Tarugan [Ravensberg] *see* 6267
Taselin [Eisai] *see* 6750
Taseron [Janssen] *see* 5296
Tasis [Wyeth] *see* 1296
Task [Boehringer, Ing.] *see* 3079
Tasmaderm [Roche] *see* 6284
Tasmar [Valeant] *see* 9508
Tasnon (Elixir) [Tropon] *see* 7464
Tasnon (Tabl.) [Tropon] *see* 7464
Taste-modifying Protein *see* 6206
TAT-3 [Takeda] *see* 7404
TATBA *see* 9598
TATD *see* 6760
Tathiclon [Ohta] *see* 4475
Tathion [Yamanouchi] *see* 4475
Tationil [Boehringer Biochemia] *see* 4475
TATP *see* 9590
TAU-284 *see* 1149
Tauliz [HMR] *see* 7492
Taural [Roemmers] *see* 8110
Tauredon [Byk Gulden] *see* 4518
Taurine, 9074
Tauriscite *see* 4057
Taurocholic Acid, 9075
Tauroflex [Geistlich] *see* 9076
Taurolidine, 9076
Taurolin [HMR] *see* 9076
Tausonite *see* 8850
Tavanic [Aventis] *see* 6771
Tavegil [Novartis] *see* 2345
Tavegyl [Novartis] *see* 2345
Ta-Verm *see* 7464
Tavist [Novartis] *see* 2345
Tavor [Wyeth] *see* 5579
Taxicin-I *see* 9077
Taxicin-II *see* 9077
Taxicins, 9077
Taxilan [Schwarz] *see* 7151
Taxine, 9078
Taxine A *see* 9078
Taxine B *see* 9078
Taxine-I *see* 9078
Taxine-II *see* 9078
Taxinine *see* 9077
Taxodione, 9079
Taxol [BMS] *see* 6982
Taxol A *see* 6982
Taxotere [Aventis] *see* 3397
Taxusin *see* 6982
Tazalest [Wakamoto] *see* 9080
Tazanol [Wakamoto] *see* 9080
Tazanolast, 9080
Tazarotene, 9081
Tazarotenic Acid *see* 9081

Tazettine, 9082
Tazicef [GSK] see 1946
Tazidime [Lilly] see 1946
Tazin [Grelan] see 1789
Tazobactam, 9083
Tazocilline [Wyeth] see 9083
Tazocin [Wyeth] see 9083
Tazorac [Allergan] see 9081
TB-1 see 9820
TBAF see 9187
TBC-1269 see 1222
TBC-1269z see 1222
TBC-11251 see 8554
TBG-MINO see 9432
TBI see 9597
Tb I-698 see 9290
TBP see 1306
TBS see 1586, 9616
TBX see 7078
^{99m}Tc-Anti-SSEA-1 see 9100
^{99m}Tc Diisopropyl IDA see 3358
^{99m}Tc-DISIDA see 3358
^{99m}Tc-L,L-ECD see 9099
^{99M}Tc Hexakis(2-methoxyisobutyliso-nitrile) see 9102
^{99m}Tc-HEXAMIBI see 9102
^{99m}Tc-HIDA see 5483
^{99m}Tc-MAG$_3$ see 9101
^{99m}Tc-MDP see 5792
^{99m}Tc Mercaptoacetyltriglycine see 9101
^{99m}Tc-MIBI see 9102
^{99m}Tc-P246 see 9098
^{99m}Tc-P829 see 2911
^{99m}Tc-PPi see 8788
^{99m}Tc-PYP see 8788
^{99m}Tc-RP-30A see 9102
^{99m}Tc Tetrofosmin see 9247
$[^{99m}$Tc(Tetrofosmin)$_2$O$_2]^+$ see 9247
3TC see 5352
TC-80 see 5074
TC-109 see 9147
TC-1734 see 5239
Tc-924 (DPD) see 1517
TCA see 1643, 9627
TCAR see 9425
TCC see 9654
TCCA see 9641
TCDBD see 9084
TCDD, 9084
T-Cell Growth Factor see 4994
T-Cell Replacing Factor see 4993
T Cell Replacing Factor see 4997
TCEP, 9085
TCGF see 4994
TCl see 2721
TCMn see 6223
TCMTB, 9086
TCNE see 9195
TCP see 9763
TCT see 1643
TCTH see 2760
TCV-116 see 1739
TD-6424 see 9116
TDCPP see 9087
cis-9,trans-11-TDDA see 7769
TDE see 3061, 3880
p,p'-TDE see 3061
T-DET-N [Thompson-Hayward] see 6677
TDHL see 9164
TDI see 9530
TDP see 9296
TDZ see 9313
TE-031 see 2339
Tea, 9088
TEAB see 9199

Teaberry Oil see 6120
TEA Chloride see 9200
Teamsters' Tea see 3607
Tearisol [Novartis] see 6040
Tea Tree (Melaleuca alternafolia) Oil see 9089
Tea Tree Oil, 9089
Tebamin see 7272
Tebanicline, 9090
Tebanyl see 7272
Tebbe Reagent, 9091
Tebe [Simes] see 7886
Tebesium [Pharma Wernigerode] see 5186
Tebethion see 9290
Tebloc [Dukron] see 5571
Tebonin [Schwabe] see 4425
Tebraxin [Bracco] see 8294
Tebrazid [Searle] see 7956
Tebuconazole, 9092
Tebufenozide, 9093
Tebufenpyrad, 9094
Tebuthiuron, 9095
Tecadenoson, 9096
Tecaf [Farmochim. Ital.] see 8252
Técarine see 9283
Teceleukin see 4994
Teceos [Hoechst Roussel] see 1517
TechneScan Gluceptate [Mallinckrodt] see 4455
TechneScan HDP [Mallinckrodt] see 6940
TechneScan HIDA [Mallinckrodt] see 5483
TechneScan MAG3 [Mallinckrodt] see 9101
TechneScan MDP [Mallinckrodt] see 5792
TechneScan PYP [Mallinckrodt] see 8788
Technetium, 9097
Technetium ^{99m}Tc Apcitide, 9098
Technetium ^{99m}Tc Bicisate, 9099
Technetium ^{99m}Tc Ethyl Cysteinate Dimer see 9099
Technetium ^{99m}Tc Fanolesomab, 9100
Technetium ^{99m}Tc Gluceptate see 4455
Technetium ^{99m}Tc Gluheptonate see 4455
Technetium ^{99m}Tc Mertiatide, 9101
Technetium ^{99m}Tc Oxidronate see 6940
Technetium ^{99m}Tc Sestamibi, 9102
Technetium ^{99m}Tc Teboroxime, 9103
Teclosan see 9105
Teclosine see 9105
Teclothiazide, 9104
Teclozan, 9105
Teclozine see 9105
Tecomanine, 9106
Tecomin see 5366
Tecomine see 9106
Tecquinol see 4808
Tecramine see 4132
Tecto [Syngenta] see 9289
Tectochrysin see 2256
Tectoridin see 9107
Tectorigenin, 9107
Tectorigenin-7-glucoside see 9107
TECZA see 9663
Tedegliparin see 6349
Tedelparin see 2805
Tedion see 9198
Tedion-V18 [Solvay Duphar] see 9198
Tedisamil, 9108
Tedolan [Leo Pharm] see 3874
TEDP see 8966
Teel Oil see 8469
Teepol see 4367
Tefamin [Recordati] see 465
Tefilin [Hermal] see 9196

Teflon [DuPont] see 7583
Teflox [Abbott] see 9132
Teflubenzuron, 9109
Teflurane, 9110
Tefluthrin, 9111
Tefsiel C [Towa Yakuhin] see 9112
Tegafur, 9112
Tega-Pyrone [Ortega] see 3350
Tegaserod, 9113
Tegencia [Elmu] see 3999
Tegens [Inverni] see 1217
Tegison [Roche] see 3892
Tegopen [BMS] see 2419
Tegosept B see 1584
Tegosept M see 6107
Tegotin see 10025
Tegretol [Novartis] see 1781
TEI-6720 see 3948
TEI-7165 see 2358
TEI-9090 see 2358
Teichmann's Crystals see 4644
Teichoic Acids, 9114
Teichomycin A$_2$ see 9115
Teicoplanin, 9115
Teicoplanin A$_2$ see 9115
Teicoplanin A$_2$-1 see 9115
Teicoplanin A$_2$-2 see 9115
Teicoplanin A$_2$-3 see 9115
Teicoplanin A$_2$-4 see 9115
Teicoplanin A$_2$-5 see 9115
Teknar [Certis] see 932
Tektamer 38 [Lanxess] see 3021
Tektin A see 8740
TEL see 9202
Telar [DuPont] see 2191
Telavancin, 9116
Telbivudine, 9117
Telcyta [Telik] see 1745
Teldane [Aventis] see 9163
Teldanex [AstraZeneca] see 9163
Teldrin [SKB] see 2180
Telebar [Guerbet] see 994
Télémid [Procter & Gamble] see 8917
Teleocidin A see 9118
Teleocidin B see 9118
Teleocidin B$_4$ see 9118
Teleocidins, 9118
Telepaque [Winthrop] see 5058
Telepathine see 4616
Teleprim [Procter & Gamble] see 8918
Telesmin [Yoshitomi] see 1781
Telesol [Lasa] see 4847
Teletrast [Astra] see 5058
Telfast [Aventis] see 4068
Telgin-G [Takeda] see 2345
Teli see 8382
Telithromycin, 9119
Tell [Syngenta] see 7747
Telluric(IV) Acid see 9128
Telluric(VI) Acid, 9120
Telluric Bromide see 9125
Telluric Chloride see 9126
Tellurite see 9123
Tellurium, 9121
Tellurium Dichloride, 9122
Tellurium Dioxide, 9123
Tellurium Hexafluoride, 9124
Tellurium Oxide (TeO$_2$) see 9123
Tellurium Tetrabromide, 9125
Tellurium Tetrachloride, 9126
Tellurium Tetraiodide, 9127
Tellurobismuthite see 1289
Tellurous Acid, 9128
Tellurous Chloride see 9122
Telmicid [Lilly] see 3369

Telmid [Lilly] *see* 3369
Telmin [Janssen] *see* 5768
Telmisartan, 9129
Telodrin *see* 5127
Telomerase, 9130
Telomere Terminal Transferase *see* 9130
Telomycin, 9131
Telone II [Dow AgroSci.] *see* 3075
Telopar [Pfizer] *see* 6922
Telvar [DuPont] *see* 6261
Telzir [GSK] *see* 4250
TEM *see* 9671
Temac [Abbott] *see* 9132
Temafloxacin, 9132
Temaril [Allergan] *see* 9704
Temasept IV [Hexcel] *see* 9616
Temazepam, 9133
TEMED, 9134
Tementil [Aventis] *see* 7761
Temephos, 9135
Temesta [Wyeth] *see* 5579
Temetex [Sauter] *see* 3143
Temgesic [Schering-Plough] *see* 1497
Temik [Bayer CropSci.] *see* 222
Temina *see* 10025
Temocapril, 9136
Temocaprilat *see* 9136
Temocillin, 9137
Temodal [Schering-Plough] *see* 9139
Temodar [Schering-Plough] *see* 9139
Temopen [SKB] *see* 9137
Temoporfin, 9138
Temovate [GSK] *see* 2363
Temozolomide, 9139
TEMPO, 9140
Tempo [Bayer] *see* 2756
TEMPOL, 9141
Temposil [Lederle] *see* 1663
Tempra [BMS] *see* 47
Temserin [Merck & Co.] *see* 9444
Temsirolimus, 9142
Temur *see* 9230
Tenacid [Sigma-Tau] *see* 4919
Tenathan [Robins] *see* 1186
Tendor [Chinoin] *see* 2844
Tenecteplase, 9143
Tenelid [Helsinn] *see* 4558
Tenesdol [Hishiyama] *see* 3311
Tenex [ESP] *see* 4561
Tenicid *see* 5026
Tenidap, 9144
Teniposide, 9145
Tennecetin *see* 6427
Tenoblock [Leiras] *see* 859
Tenofovir, 9146
Tenofovir DF *see* 9146
Tenofovir Disoproxil *see* 9146
Tenonitrozole, 9147
Tenopt [Sigma] *see* 9444
Tenorite *see* 2646
Tenormal [Zeneca] *see* 7080
Tenormin [AstraZeneca] *see* 859
Tenovil [Schering-Plough] *see* 4999
Tenox BHA [Eastman Kodak] *see* 1547
Tenox BHT [Eastman Kodak] *see* 1548
Tenox PG [Eastman] *see* 7859
Tenoxicam, 9148
Tensatrin [Gedeon Richter] *see* 7899
Tensilon [Valeant] *see* 3516
Tensinol [Farmaroma] *see* 7080
Tensipine [Genus] *see* 6528
Tensobon [Schwarz] *see* 1774
Tensofin [BMS] *see* 4189
Tensoprel [Rubio] *see* 1774
Tensoral [Diana] *see* 7080

Tenso-Timelets *see* 2390
Tensozide [Mead Johnson] *see* 4256
Tenstaten [Ipsen] *see* 2264
Tenuate [Aventis] *see* 3127
Tenuazonic Acid, 9149
Tenyl [Nippon Kayaku] *see* 1178
Teofilcolina *see* 2210
Teokolin *see* 2210
Teonicon [Neopharmed] *see* 7430
Teoptic [Novartis] *see* 1866
Teorema [Panchemie] *see* 4448
Teoremac [Farmades] *see* 4448
Teosona [Phoenix] *see* 9285
TEPA *see* 9672
Tepanil [3M Pharma] *see* 3127
Tephroite *see* 5738
Tephrosin, 9150
Tephthol *see* 9162
Tepilta [Wyeth] *see* 6933
Tepirubicin *see* 7488
Tepoxalin, 9151
TEPP *see* 9204
Tepraloxydim, 9152
Teprenone, 9153
Tequin [BMS] *see* 4376
TER-286 *see* 1745
Téralithe [Aventis] *see* 5527
Teramine [Darby] *see* 2182
Terazol [Cilag] *see* 9160
Terazosin, 9154
Terbacil, 9155
Terbasmin [Farmitalia] *see* 9159
Terbia *see* 9157
Terbinafine, 9156
Terbium, 9157
Terbuconazole *see* 9092
Terbufos, 9158
Terbul [Hexal] *see* 9159
Terbutaline, 9159
Terbutaline Bisdimethylcarbamate *see* 953
Terbutrazole *see* 9092
Tercian [Théraplix] *see* 2683
Terconazole, 9160
Tercospor [Cilag] *see* 9160
Terebic Acid, 9161
Terebinic Acid *see* 9161
Terenol [Hoechst] *see* 8154
Terephthalic Acid, 9162
Terephthalylidene-3,3′-dicamphor-10,10′-disulfonic Acid *see* 3490
Terfenadine, 9163
Terfenadine Carboxylate *see* 4068
Terfex [Leiras] *see* 9163
Terflurane *see* 9110
Terfluzine [Aventis] *see* 9680
Tergal [Rhône-Poulenc] *see* 7569
Tergavon *see* 4367
Tergitol [Union Carbide] *see* 7577
Tergitol 4 *see* 8689
Tergitol NP [Union Carbide] *see* 6677
Tergitol TP-9 [Union Carbide] *see* 6677
Terguride, 9164
Teriam [Roussel Diamant] *see* 9599
Teridax [Schering] *see* 5061
Teriflunomide, 9165
Terion [Lusofarmaco] *see* 4228
Teriparatide Acetate, 9166
Terital [Montecatini] *see* 7569
Terlenka [Kunstzijde] *see* 7569
Terlipressin, 9167
Termidor [BASF] *see* 4085
Termierite *see* 362
Termitin *see* 10025
Tern [Syngenta] *see* 3992

Ternadin [Cantabria] *see* 9163
Ternelin [Novartis] *see* 9485
Terofenamate, 9168
Teronac [Novartis] *see* 5762
Teropterin *see* 7934
Terpate [Geneva] *see* 7112
"Terpene" Hydrochloride *see* 1340
Terpin, 9169
Terpinene, 9170
α-Terpineol, 9171
Terpin Hydrate *see* 9169
Terpinol *see* 9169
Terpinyl Thiocyanoacetate *see* 5129
Terposen [Vir] *see* 8110
Terra Alba *see* 1706
Terrachlor *see* 8080
Terraclor [Uniroyal] *see* 8080
Terracur P [Bayer] *see* 4000
Terra Japonica *see* 4359
Terralon [Virbac] *see* 6976
Terramycin [Pfizer] *see* 6976
Terranas [Nippon Organon] *see* 5563
Terratrex [Volpino] *see* 4557
Terreic Acid, 9172
Tersan [DuPont] *see* 9371
Tersigat [Boehringer, Ing.] *see* 6943
Tertatolol, 9173
α-Terthienyl, 9174
2,2′:5′2″-Terthiophene *see* 9174
Tertiapin, 9175
Tertiary Calcium Phosphate *see* 1694
Tertiary Magnesium Phosphate *see* 5683
Tertran [Wyeth] *see* 5075
Tertroxin [GSK] *see* 5510
Terylene [ICI] *see* 7569
TES, 9176
Tesaglitazar, 9177
Teslac [BMS] *see* 9179
Teslascan [Nycomed] *see* 5722
Tesmilifene, 9178
Tesnol [Kowa] *see* 7840
Tesoprel [Organon] *see* 1442
Tespamin [Sumitomo] *see* 9673
Tessalon [Forest] *see* 1096
Testarpen [Polfa] *see* 7101
Testex [Pasadena] *see* 9180
Testinon [Mochida] *see* 9180
Testoderm [Alza] *see* 9180
Testo-Enant [Geymonat] *see* 9180
Testogel [Schering AG] *see* 9180
Testolactone, 9179
Δ¹-Testolactone *see* 9179
Testolin [Pasadena] *see* 9180
Testosterone, 9180
trans-Testosterone *see* 9180
Testosterone 17-Chloral Hemiacetal *see* 2421
Testosterone Cypionate *see* 9180
Testosterone 17β-Undecylate *see* 9180
Testoviron [Schering AG] *see* 9180
Testred [Valeant] *see* 6125
Testriol *see* 2060
Testro AQ [Truxton] *see* 9180
TETA *see* 9663
Tetaine *see* 933
Tetiothalein Sodium *see* 5038
Tetmosol [Care] *see* 8950
N,N,N′,N′-Tetraacetylethylenediamine *see* 9028
2,3,4,6-Tetraacetyl-α-D-glucopyranosyl Bromide *see* 60
Tetra-*O*-acetylpentaerythritol *see* 7111
(2,3,4,6-Tetra-*O*-acetyl-1-thio-β-D-glucopyranosato-*S*)(triethylphosphine)-gold *see* 878

Tetrex [BMS] *see* 9196
Tetridin *see* 7995
Tetrin, 9245
Tetrin A *see* 9245
Tetrin B *see* 9245
Tetrodontoxin *see* 9246
Tetrodotoxin, 9246
Tetrofosmin, 9247
Tetrole *see* 4296
Tetron *see* 9204
Tetronasin, 9248
Tetropil *see* 9190
Tetroquinone, 9249
Tetroxoprim, 9250
L-*glycero*-Tetrulose *see* 3694
Tetryl *see* 6573
Tetryl Formate *see* 5143
Tetryzoline *see* 9219
Tetsol [Novartis] *see* 9196
Tetterwort *see* 8355
Tetucur [Teikoku Zoki] *see* 4057
Teturamin *see* 3364
Tevcodyne [Tevcon] *see* 7277
Teveten [Solvay] *see* 3635
Tevilon [Teikoku Rayon] *see* 7586
Texacort [Genderm] *see* 4787
Texanol Isobutyrate, 9251
Texmeten [Roche] *see* 3143
Texodil [Cassenne] *see* 1935
Texsolve S [Texaco] *see* 6201
Texsolve S-2 [Texaco] *see* 6201
Tezosentan, 9252
TF-1169 *see* 4116
TFE *see* 9205, 9682
TFM, 9253
TFMSA *see* 9676
TFPI *see* 9467
TFT Thilo [Alcon-Thilo] *see* 9687
Tg *see* 9072
TGB *see* 9417
T/Gel [Farillon] *see* 2426
TGF-*β* *see* 9572
TGS *see* 8880
TH-152 *see* 5931
TH-913 *see* 4908
TH-1165 *see* 3981
TH-1165a *see* 3981
TH-1395 *see* 4480
TH-2602 *see* 2683
TH-6040 *see* 3142
THA [Woods] *see* 9024
Thacapzol *see* 5971
Thalamonal *see* 3450
Thalamyd [Schering] *see* 7376
Thalazole [M & B] *see* 7377
Thalicarpine, 9254
Thalictrine *see* 5696
Thalidomide, 9255
Thalitone [Boehringer, Ing.] *see* 2193
Thallic Oxide *see* 9268
Thallium, 9256
Thallium Acetate, 9257
Thallium Bromide, 9258
Thallium Carbonate, 9259
Thallium Chloride, 9260
Thallium Cyanide, 9261
Thallium Fluoride, 9262
Thallium Hydroxide, 9263
Thallium Iodide, 9264
Thallium Mononitrate, 9265
Thallium(I) Nitrate *see* 9265
Thallium(III) Nitrate *see* 9271
Thallium Oxide, 9266
Thallium Peroxide *see* 9268
Thallium Selenide, 9267

Thallium Sesquioxide, 9268
Thallium Sulfate, 9269
Thallium Sulfide, 9270
Thallium Trinitrate, 9271
Thallous Acetate *see* 9257
Thallous Bromide *see* 9258
Thallous Carbonate *see* 9259
Thallous Chloride *see* 9260
Thallous Cyanide *see* 9261
Thallous Fluoride *see* 9262
Thallous Hydroxide *see* 9263
Thallous Iodide *see* 9264
Thallous Nitrate *see* 9265
Thallous Oxide *see* 9266
Thallous Selenide *see* 9267
Thallous Sulfate *see* 9269
Thallous Sulfide *see* 9270
Thalomid [Celgene] *see* 9255
THAM [Fisher Sci.] *see* 9772
Thanite [Hercules] *see* 5129
Thapsigargin, 9272
Thapsigargine *see* 9272
Thaumatin, 9273
R-THBP *see* 8368
Δ¹-THC *see* 9209
Δ⁶-THC *see* 9209
Δ⁸-THC *see* 9209
Δ⁹-THC *see* 9209
(3*R*,4*R*)-Δ⁶-THC-DMH-7-oic Acid *see*
198
THE *see* 9210
Theaflavine, 9274
Theal Ampules [Boehringer, Mann.] *see*
3479
Thearubigins, 9275
Thebacon *see* 3172
Thebaine, 9276
Thebainone, 9277
Thebainone-A *see* 9277
Theelin [Parke-Davis] *see* 3708
Theelol [Parke-Davis] *see* 3707
Thefylan *see* 3479
Thein *see* 1636
Theiomycetin *see* 1160
Thelestrin [Carnrick] *see* 3708
Thelin [Encysive] *see* 8554
Thelmesan *see* 3475
Thelykinin *see* 3708
Themalon [Burroughs Wellcome] *see* 9293
Thenaldine, 9278
Thenalidine *see* 9278
Thenardite *see* 8680
Thenclor *see* 2167
Thenfadil [Winthrop] *see* 9280
Thenitrazole *see* 9147
2-Thenoic Acid *see* 9354
3-Thenoic Acid, 9279
Thenophenopiperidine *see* 9278
2-(*α*-Thenoylamino)-5-nitrothiazole *see*
9147
p-(2-Thenoyl)hydratropic Acid *see* 9005
2-(*α*-Thenoylthio)propionylglycine *see*
8809
Thenyldiamine, 9280
Thenylene [Abbott] *see* 5959
Thenylpyramine *see* 5959
Theobid [Cipla] *see* 9285
Theobroma Oil, 9281
Theobromine, 9282
1-Theobromineacetic Acid, 9283
Theocalcin [Knoll] *see* 9282
Theochron [Forest] *see* 9285
Theofibrate, 9284
Theograd [Abbott] *see* 9285
Theolair [3M] *see* 9285

Theon [Bock] *see* 7905
Theon [Klinge] *see* 9285
Theophyllamine *see* 465
Theophylline, 9285
7-Theophyllineacetic Acid *see* 24
Theophylline Cholinate *see* 2210
Theophylline Compd with Ethylenedi-
amine *see* 465
Theophyllineethylamphetamine *see* 3972
Theophylline Ethylenediamine *see* 465
2-(7′-Theophyllinemethyl)-1,3-dioxolane
see 3438
Theophylline Salt of Choline *see* 2210
1-(Theophyllin-7-yl)ethyl 2-(*p*-Chloro-
phenoxy)isobutyrate *see* 9284
Theostat [Fabre] *see* 9285
Theoxylline *see* 2210
Thephorin [Sinclair] *see* 7233
Theprubicin [Aventis] *see* 7488
Therabloat [Pfizer] *see* 7562
Theraderm [BMS] *see* 1116
Therafectin [BLS] *see* 484
Theralene [Rhône-Poulenc] *see* 9704
Theranabol *see* 6965
Therapas [Smith & Nephew] *see* 1115
Therapav [Berlex] *see* 7019
Therarubicin [Meiji Seika] *see* 7488
Theratuss [Squibb] *see* 7456
Theriodide-131 [Abbott] *see* 8632
Thermolysin, 9286
Thermonatrite *see* 8596
Thermorubin, 9287
Thermorubin A *see* 9287
Thermovyl [Rhovyl] *see* 7586
Thesodate *see* 9282
Thevetigenin *see* 3162
Thevetin A, 9288
THFA *see* 9213
THF Glycol *see* 9212
THG *see* 9214
Thiabendazole, 9289
Thiabenzazonium Iodide *see* 9426
Thiabutazide *see* 1525
Thiacetarsamide *see* 793
Thiacetazone, 9290
Thiacetic Acid *see* 9320
Thiacloprid, 9291
Thiactin *see* 9364
Thiacyclopentane *see* 9218
1-Thia-3-cyclopentene 1,1-Dioxide *see*
8956
Thiadiazuron *see* 9313
3′-Thia-2′,3′-dideoxycytidine *see* 5352
Thialbarbital, 9292
Thialbarbitone *see* 9292
Thialbutone Sodium *see* 1524
Thialisobumalnatrium *see* 1524
Thiamazole *see* 5971
Thiambutene, 9293
Thiamcol [Morishita] *see* 9301
Thiamenidine *see* 9418
Thiamethoxam, 9294
Thiameturon-methyl *see* 9316
Thiamine, 9295
Thiamine Chloride Hydrochloride *see*
9295
Thiamine Dichloride *see* 9295
Thiamine Diphosphate, 9296
Thiamine Diphosphate Ester Chloride
see 9296
Thiamine Disulfide, 9297
Thiamine 8-(Methyl 6-Acetyldihydro-
thioctate) Disulfide *see* 6760
Thiamine Monochloride *see* 9295
Thiamine Monophosphate *see* 9296

Thioimidodicarbonic Diamide *see* 3371
2-Thio-4-ketothiazolidine *see* 8184
Thiokol [Thiokol], 9339
Thiokol A *see* 9339
Thiokol FA *see* 9339
Thiola [Coop. Farm.] *see* 9453
Thiolacetic Acid *see* 9320
Thiolactic Acid, 9340
Thiole *see* 9353
2-Thiolhistidine, 9341
Thiolhistidine-betaine *see* 3663
Thiolin *see* 4885
2-Thiolpropionic Acid *see* 9340
Thiolutin, 9342
Thiomalic Acid, 9343
Thiomebumal Sodium *see* 9350
Thiomerin Sodium [Wyeth] *see* 5870
Thiomersalate *see* 9317
Thiomethyl Alcohol *see* 5956
Thiomorpholine *see* 9300
Thiomucase [Sanofi Winthrop] *see* 4758
Thionalide, 9344
α-Thionaphthol *see* 6378
β-Thionaphthol *see* 6379
1-Thionaphthol *see* 6378
2-Thionaphthol *see* 6379
Thioneine *see* 3663
Thionembutal *see* 9350
Thionex [Makhteshim-Agan] *see* 3574
Thionic [UCB] *see* 10172
Thionicol [Mohan] *see* 9301
Thionine, 9346
5-Thio-2-nitrobenzoate Anion *see* 3551
Thiontan *see* 3108
Thionylan *see* 5959
Thionyl Bromide, 9347
Thionyl Chloride, 9348
Thionyl Difluoride *see* 9349
Thionyl Fluoride, 9349
2-Thio-4-oxo-6-propyl-1,3-pyrimidine
  see 7869
Thioparamizone [Smith & Nephew] *see*
  9290
Thiopental Sodium, 9350
Thiopentone Sodium *see* 9350
Thiopeptin, 9351
Thioperazine *see* 9357
Thioperoxydicarbonic Acid Diethyl Ester
  see 3384
Thiophanate, 9352
Thiophanate-methyl *see* 9352
Thiophan Sulfone *see* 8955
Thiophene, 9353
7-(Thiophene-2-acetamido)cephalospor-
  anic Acid *see* 1982
(2-Thiophenecarboxylato-κO², κS¹)-
  copper *see* 2521
2-Thiophenecarboxylic Acid, 9354
3-Thiophenecarboxylic Acid *see* 9279
2,2'-(2,5-Thiophenediyl)bis[5-(1,1-di-
  methylethyl)benzoxazole] *see* 1014
β-Thiophenic Acid *see* 9279
Thiophenicol [Clin Comar] *see* 9301
Thiophenol, 9355
Thiophenylpyridylamino-10-carboxylic
  Acid Piperidinoethoxyethyl Ester *see*
  7456
Thiophos *see* 7033
Thiophosphoric Acid 2-Isopropyl-4-
  methyl-6-pyrimidyl Diethyl Ester *see*
  2995
Thiophosphoric Anhydride *see* 7354
Thiophosphoryl Chloride *see* 7356
Thioproline *see* 9445

Thiopropanal *S*-Oxide *see* 7802
Thiopropazate, 9356
Thio-2-propene-1-sulfinic Acid *S*-Allyl
  Ester *see* 261
Thioproperazine, 9357
Thioproperazine Mesylate *see* 9357
Thiopropionaldehyde *S*-Oxide *see* 7802
2-Thio-6-propyl-1,3-pyrimidin-4-one
  see 7869
Thiopyrophosphoric Acid Tetraethyl
  Ester *see* 8966
Thioredoxin, 9358
Thioridazine, 9359
Thioridazine-2-sulfone *see* 8963
Thioridazine-2-sulfoxide *see* 5910
Thiorubber *see* 9339
Thiosalicylic Acid, 9360
Thiosarmine *see* 8941
Thioseconal *see* 9302
Thiosemicarbazide, 9361
Thioserine *see* 2781
Thiosinamine, 9362
Thiosol [Coop. Farm.] *see* 9453
1-Thiosorbitol, 9363
Thiostrepton, 9364
Thiotax *see* 5868
Thiotepa *see* 9673
Thiotepp *see* 8966
Thiotetrole *see* 9353
Thiothixene, 9365
2-Thiouracil, 9366
Thiourea, 9367
β-Thiovaline *see* 7088
Thioxamyl *see* 6920
Thioxanthene, 9368
Thioxanthen-9-one *see* 9369
Thioxanthone, 9369
2-Thioxo-3,5-dibenzyltetrahydro-1,3,5-
  thiadiazine *see* 8892
Thioxolone *see* 9456
2-Thioxo-4-thiazolidinone *see* 8184
4-[Thioxo(3,4,5-trimethoxyphenyl)-
  methyl]morpholine *see* 9760
Thiozin *see* 4885
THIP *see* 4321
Thiphenamil *see* 9370
Thiram, 9371
Thistle Saffron *see* 1868
Thiurad [Flexsys] *see* 9371
Thiuretic [Parke-Davis] *see* 4781
Thixokon [Mallinckrodt] *see* 79
Thomas Balsam *see* 950
Thomas Flour *see* 9372
Thomasin [Apogepha] *see* 3865
Thomas Phosphate, 9372
Thombolyse [Green Cross] *see* 7902
Thombran [Thomae] *see* 9579
Thonzylamine Hydrochloride, 9373
Thorazine [GSK] *see* 2185
Thoria *see* 9377
Thorium, 9374
Thorium Chloride, 9375
Thorium Dioxide *see* 9377
Thorium Nitrate, 9376
Thorium Oxide, 9377
Thorium Platinocyanide *see* 9378
Thorium Tetrachloride *see* 9375
Thorium Tetracyanoplatinate(II), 9378
Thorium(4+) Tetrakis(cyano-*C*)plati-
  nate(2−) (1:2) *see* 9378
Thorium X *see* 8094
Thorn Apple *see* 8820
Thoron *see* 8095
Thorotrast *see* 9377
Thoroughwort *see* 3902

Thousand-leaf *see* 105
Thoxan [Cutter] *see* 3889
Thoxidil *see* 5850
Thozalinone, 9379
THP *see* 7488, 9216
THP-ADM *see* 7488
THP-adriamycin *see* 7488
m-THPC *see* 9138
THQ *see* 9249
Thr *see* 9380
THR-221 *see* 1928
Thr²-cyclosporine *see* 2752
Threonine, 9380
L-Threonine *see* 9380
L-Threonyl-L-lysyl-L-prolyl-L-arginine
  see 9809
*N*²-[1-(*N*²-L-Threonyl-L-lysyl)-L-
  prolyl]-L-arginine *see* 9809
D-Threose, 9381
L-Threose, 9382
Thrombasal *see* 7234
Thrombin, 9383
Thrombinar [King] *see* 9383
Thrombin-sensitive Protein *see* 9387
Thrombocid [Bene-Chemie] *see* 7134
Thrombocytin *see* 8462
Thrombocytopoiesis-stimulating Factor
  see 9386
Thrombogen *see* 7889
Thrombogen [J & J] *see* 9383
Thrombokinase *see* 9385
Thrombokinin *see* 9385
Thromboliquine *see* 4653
Thrombolysin [Merck & Co.] *see* 7520
Thrombomodulin, 9384
Thrombophob [Nordmark] *see* 4653
Thromboplastin, 9385
Thrombopoietin, 9386
Thromboreductin [AOP Orphan Pharm.]
  see 622
Thrombospondin, 9387
Thrombostat [Pfizer] *see* 9383
Thrombotonin *see* 8462
Thromboxane A₂ *see* 9388
Thromboxane B₂ *see* 9388
Thromboxanes, 9388
THS-101 *see* 2943
THT *see* 9218
THTP *see* 9218
Thuja, 9389
(1*S*,4*R*,5*R*)-(−)-3-Thujanone *see* 9392
(1*S*,4*S*,5*R*)-(+)-3-Thujanone *see* 9392
3-Thujanone *see* 9392
β-Thujaplicin, 9390
Thujic Acid, 9391
Thujin *see* 8037
Thujone, 9392
α-Thujone *see* 9392
Thujopsene, 9393
Thulia *see* 9394
Thulium, 9394
Thurfyl Nicotinate, 9395
Thuricide [Certis] *see* 932
Thybon [Henning] *see* 5510
Thycapsol *see* 5971
Thylate [DuPont] *see* 9371
Thylogen [Rorer] *see* 7984
Thyloquinone [BMS] *see* 5831
Thymalfasin *see* 9405
Thyme, 9396
Thyme Camphor *see* 9399
Thymergix [Joulli] *see* 8010
Thymerin [Tokyo Tanabe] *see* 8109
Thymidine, 9397
L-Thymidine *see* 9117

p-Toluenesulfonylmethyl Isocyanide *see* 9556

Toluenethiol *see* 9325

α-Toluenethiol *see* 9322

Toluene Trichloride *see* 1109

Toluic Acid, 9535

α-Toluic Acid *see* 7268

m-Toluic Acid *see* 9535

o-Toluic Acid *see* 9535

p-Toluic Acid *see* 9535

p-Toluic Acid 4-[2-(*t*-Butylamino)-1-hy-droxethyl]-*o*-phenylene Ester *see* 1307

α-Toluic Acid Ethyl Ester *see* 3840

α-Toluic Aldehyde *see* 7265

Toluidine, 9536

m-Toluidine *see* 9536

o-Toluidine *see* 9536

p-Toluidine *see* 9536

Toluidine Blue O *see* 9520

Tolulexin *see* 5850

Tolulox *see* 5850

α-Tolunitrile *see* 1131

o-Tolunitrile, 9537

p-Tolunitrile, 9538

Toluol *see* 9529

p-Toluoylmethylcarbinolmono-*d*-cam-phoric Acid Ester Diethanolamine Salt *see* 9492

5-(*p*-Toluoyl)-1-methylpyrrole-2-acetic Acid *see* 9518

Tolurex [Makhteshim-Agan] *see* 2172

o-Toluylaldehyde *see* 9527

p-Toluyl-*o*-benzoic Acid *see* 9539

2-(*p*-Toluyl)benzoic Acid, 9539

Toluylene Blue, 9822

Toluylene Red *see* 6488

Tolvaptan, 9540

Tolvin [Organon] *see* 6172

Tolvon [Organon] *see* 6172

Tolycaine, 9541

Tolycar [Jugoremedija] *see* 1933

m-Tolylacetamide *see* 74

m-Tolyl Acetate *see* 2583

o-Tolyl Acetate *see* 2584

5-(*o*-Tolylazo)-2-aminotoluene *see* 420

1-*o*-Tolylazo-2-naphthylamine *see* 10096

4-(*o*-Tolylazo)-*o*-toluidine *see* 420

o-Tolylazo-*o*-tolylazo-β-naphthol *see* 8393

1-(4-*o*-Tolylazo-*o*-tolylazo)-2-naphthol *see* 8393

m-Tolylbromide *see* 1439

2,4-Tolylene Diisocyanate *see* 9530

1-*p*-Tolyl-1-ethanol *see* 3237

α-(*o*-Tolyl)glyceryl Ether *see* 5850

Tolylhydrazine, 9542

m-Tolylhydrazine *see* 9542

o-Tolylhydrazine *see* 9542

p-Tolylhydrazine *see* 9542

2-(*N'*-*p*-Tolyl-*N'*-*m*-hydroxyphenylamino-methyl)-2-imidazoline *see* 7264

p-Tolyliododifluoride *see* 3150

Tolylmercaptan *see* 9325

p-Tolylmethylcarbinol *see* 3237

p-Tolylmethylcarbinol Camphoric Acid Ester Diethanolamine Salt *see* 9492

1-(*p*-Tolyl)-1-oxo-2-pyrrolidino-*n*-pen-tane *see* 8010

3-(*o*-Tolyloxy)-1,2-propanediol *see* 5850

p-Tolyl Phenylacetate *see* 2585

1-(*p*-Tolyl)-2-pyrrolidino-1-pentanone *see* 8010

Tolylsulfonylbutylurea *see* 9507

3-(*p*-Tolyl-4-sulfonyl)-1-butylurea *see* 9507

1-(*p*-Tolylsulfonyl)-3-(2-*endo*-hydroxy-3-*endo*-D-bornyl)urea *see* 4438

p-Tolylsulfonylmethylnitrosamide, 9543

2-*p*-Tolyl-5,6,7,8-tetrahydrobenzo[*d*]-imidazo[2,1-*b*]thiazole *see* 7421

Tolyprin [DuPont] *see* 726

Tolyspaz [Conal] *see* 5850

Tomabef [Aandersen] *see* 1930

Tomanol [Byk Gulden] *see* 8102

5α-Tomatidan-3β-ol 9544

Tomatidine, 9544

Tomatine, 9545

Tombran [Boehringer, Ing.] *see* 9579

Tomieze [Yoshitomi] *see* 7902

Tomiporan [Toyama] *see* 1918

Tomiron [Toyama] *see* 1947

Tomoxetine *see* 863

Tomudex [AstraZeneca] *see* 8099

Ton *see* 362

Tonamil [Ecobi] *see* 9373

Tonedron [Grimault] *see* 5948

Toness [Angelini] *see* 7903

Tonexol [Pharmaton] *see* 9188

Tonibral [Bouchara] *see* 2843

Tonin, 9546

Tonka Bean Camphor *see* 2562

Tonocalcin [Searle] *see* 1643

Tonocard [Astra] *see* 9491

Tonocholin B *see* 86

Tonofolin [Zyma] *see* 4222

Tonofosan [Hoechst] *see* 9512

Tonoftal [Essex] *see* 9519

Tonolift [Teisan] *see* 6699

γ-Tonoplast Intrinsic Protein *see* 760

Tonopres [Boehringer, Ing.] *see* 3174

Tonsillosan (Lösung) [Spitzner] *see* 5336

Tony Red *see* 8884

Topalgic [Nippon Shoji] *see* 9005

Topamax [J & J] *see* 9547

Topaz *see* 340

Topazone *see* 4300

Tophol *see* 2288

Tophosan *see* 2288

Topicain [Chugai] *see* 6933

Topical Thrombin *see* 9383

Topicort [HMR] *see* 2930

Topicycline [Roberts] *see* 9196

Topifug [Wolff] *see* 2928

Topik [Syngenta] *see* 2370

Topilan [Syntex] *see* 2157

Topilar [Syntex] *see* 4121

Topinambur *see* 5263

Topiramate, 9547

Topisolon [HMR] *see* 2930

Topline [Intervet] *see* 486

TopNotch [Dow AgroSci.] *see* 61, 3049

Topocaine [Lilly] *see* 2735

Topotecan, 9548

Toprec [RPR] *see* 5305

Toprek [RPR] *see* 5305

Toprol-XL [AstraZeneca] *see* 6151

Topsin [Nippon Soda] *see* 9352

Topsin-M [Nippon Soda] *see* 9352

Topstar [Rhone-Poulenc] *see* 6905

Topsym [Grünenthal] *see* 4151

Topsymin [Grünenthal] *see* 4151

Topsyn [Syntex] *see* 4151

Topsyne [Cassenne] *see* 4151

Toracizin *see* 4113

Toradiur [Roche] *see* 9552

Toradol [Syntex] *see* 5306

Torasemide *see* 9552

Toratex [Syntex] *see* 5306

Torbugesic [Fort Dodge] *see* 1530

Torbutrol [BMS] *see* 1530

Torcetrapib, 9549

Torch [Sanwa] *see* 10085

Tordon [Dow AgroSci.] *see* 7397

Torecan [Novartis] *see* 9315

Torem [Roche] *see* 9552

Toremifene, 9550

Torental [Aventis] *see* 7136

Toresten [Sankyo] *see* 9315

Toricelocin [Torii] *see* 1982

Toril Oil, 9551

Toripamide *see* 9737

Tormosyl *see* 4193

Tornalate [Sterling Winthrop] *see* 1307

Torque [BASF] *see* 3964

Torrefaction Dextrin *see* 2953

Torsemide, 9552

Torularhodin, 9553

Torutilin *see* 10025

Torvast [Pfizer] *see* 864

Tosic Acid *see* 9533

Tositumomab, 9554

TosMIC *see* 9556

Tosmilen [Chemie Linz] *see* 2885

Tosnone [Nippon Shoji] *see* 1794

Tostram *see* 5246

Tosufloxacin, 9555

Tosufloxacin Tosylate *see* 9555

Tosuxacin [Dainabot] *see* 9555

Tosylchloramide Sodium *see* 2075

Tosyl Chloride *see* 9534

Tosylmethyl Isocyanide, 9556

D-3-*endo*-*p*-Tosylureidoborneol *see* 4438

Totabin *see* 6480

Totacef [BMS] *see* 1917

Totacillin N [GSK] *see* 586

Totalip [Guidotti] *see* 864

Totalon [Mallinckrodt] *see* 5459

Totapen [BMS] *see* 586

Totifen [Chiesi] *see* 5307

TOTO *see* 9308

Totocortin [Winzer] *see* 2943

Touchdown [Syngenta] *see* 4512

Touch Wood *see* 185

Tournesol *see* 5547

Tovene [Kali-Chemie] *see* 3297

Towk [Tanabe] *see* 9567

Toxakil *see* 9557

Toxalbumin *see* 9

Toxaphene, 9557

Toxicarol *see* 9150

Toxichlor *see* 2082

Toxiferine I, 9558

C-Toxiferine I *see* 9558

C-Toxiferine II *see* 9558

Toxiferine V *see* 9558

Toxiferine XI *see* 9558

Toxifren *see* 4090

Toxilic Acid *see* 5703

Toxilic Anhydride *see* 5704

Toxinal [Pharma-Selz] *see* 6976

Toxin HIL13-PE38QQR (Plasmid PhuIL13-Tx) *see* 2312

Toxoflavin, 9559

Toxogonin [Merck KGaA] *see* 6738

Toxohormone, 9560

Toxopyrimidine, 9561

Toyocamycin, 9562

Toyolysom-DS [Maruko] *see* 5640

Toyomycin *see* 2238

Tozalinone *see* 9379

TP *see* 6466, 9404

TP-1 *see* 9407

TP-5 *see* 9403

TP-21 *see* 9359

TPA *see* 7332, 9468

t-PA *see* 9468
TPD *see* 7882
TPMPA, 9563
TPN *see* 6348, 9175
TPN-12 *see* 8963
TPN$_Q$ *see* 9175
TPNH *see* 6348
TPO *see* 9386
TPP *see* 9296
TPP$^+$ *see* 9237
TPS-23 *see* 5910
TPTZ *see* 9744, 9750
TR-495 *see* 5960
TR-4698 *see* 8231
Trabectedin *see* 3503
Trabest [Hoei] *see* 2345
γ-Trace *see* 2778
Tracer [Dow AgroSci.] *see* 8750
Trachyl *see* 3830
Tracilon [Savage] *see* 9595
Tracker [DuPont] *see* 9565
Tracleer [Actelion] *see* 1353
Tracrium [GSK] *see* 868
Tractocile [Ferring] *see* 865
Tractur [Damor] *see* 7460
Tradon [Lilly] *see* 7079
Tradonal [Viatris] *see* 9566
Trafuril [Novartis] *see* 9395
Tragacanth *see* 4581
Tragacanthin *see* 4581
Tral [Abbott] *see* 4706
Tralate [DuPont] *see* 9565
Tralin *see* 4706
Tralkoxydim, 9564
Tralomethrin, 9565
Tralox [Roussel-Uclaf AH] *see* 9565
Tramacin [J & J] *see* 9596
Tramadol, 9566
Tramal [Grünenthal] *see* 9566
Tramat [Bayer CropSci.] *see* 3742
Tramazoline, 9567
Tramisol [Am. Cyanamid] *see* 5459
Trancalgyl *see* 3731
Trancolon [Fujisawa] *see* 5848
Trancopal [Winthrop] *see* 2106
Trancot [Truxton] *see* 5862
Trancote [Sawai] *see* 2106
Trandate [Allen & Hanburys] *see* 5329
Trandolapril, 9568
Trandolaprilat *see* 9568
Tranex *see* 9569
Tranexamic Acid, 9569
Tranexamic Acid *p*-(2-Carboxyethyl)-
    phenyl Ester *see* 2024
Trangorex [Sanofi Winthrop] *see* 482
Tranilast, 9570
Trankimazin [Pharmacia] *see* 312
Tran-Q [Pfizer] *see* 4849
Tranquilan [Bonin] *see* 5862
Tranquilax [Hokuriku] *see* 5786
Tranquinal [Bago] *see* 312
Tranquit [Promonta] *see* 6927
Tranquizine *see* 4849
Transacalm [Norgine] *see* 9699
Transamin [Daiichi] *see* 9569
Transanate [Teikoku Zoki] *see* 2106
Transbilix [Guerbet] *see* 5022
Transbronchin [Viatris] *see* 1802
Trans-citral *see* 2322
Transcobalamins *see* 10014
Transcop [Recordati] *see* 8406
Transcortin *see* 4787
Transcycline [HMR] *see* 8252
Transderm Scop [Novartis] *see* 8406
Transderm-Nitro [Novartis] *see* 6607

9,10-Transdihydrolisuride *see* 9164
Transducin *see* 4530
Transene [Clin-Comar-Byla] *see* 2403
Transferrins, 9571
Transfer RNA *see* 8203
Transforming Growth Factor-β, 9572
Transiderm-Nitro [Novartis] *see* 6607
Transithal [M & B] *see* 1524
Transline [Dow AgroSci.] *see* 2400
Translon [Daiichi] *see* 6439
Transthyretin *see* 9415
Transvaalin *see* 8399
Trantoin [McKesson] *see* 6599
Tranvet [Syntex] *see* 7829
Tranxene [Abbott] *see* 2403
Tranxilène [Clin-Comar-Byla] *see* 2403
Tranxilium [Mack, Illert.] *see* 2403
Tranylcypromine, 9573
Trapanal [Byk Gulden] *see* 9350
Trapex *see* 6092
Trapidil, 9574
Trapymin *see* 9574
Trasacor [Novartis] *see* 6952
Trasentine [Ciba-Geigy] *see* 161
Trasicor [Novartis] *see* 6952
Traslan [Gramon] *see* 2102
Trastuzumab, 9575
Trasulphane *see* 4885
Trasylol [Bayer] *see* 757
Tratul [Gador] *see* 2279
Traubensäure (German) *see* 9069
Traumacut [Brenner-Efeka] *see* 5980
Traumanase [Rorer] *see* 1388
Traumasept [Wolff] *see* 7698
Traumatic Acid, 9576
Traumatociclina [Biomed. Foscama] *see*
    5778
Traumon Gel [Troponwerke] *see* 3875
Trausabun [Promonta] *see* 5823
Travamin [Baxter] *see* 7885
Travatan [Alcon] *see* 9577
Travel-Gum [Chemofux] *see* 3207
Travelin *see* 3207
Travelmin *see* 3207
Travert [Baxter] *see* 5006
Travis *see* 2828
Travogen [Schering AG] *see* 5160
Travogyn [Keymer] *see* 5160
Travoprost, 9577
Traxam [Lederle] *see* 3951
Traxanox, 9578
Trazinin [Tobishi] *see* 757
Trazodone, 9579
Trazolan [Continental Pharma] *see* 9579
Trazyl [Angelini] *see* 4876
Treanda [Cephalon] *see* 1034
Trebiace [Mitsubishi] *see* 4933
Trecalmo [Bayer] *see* 2416
Trédémine [RPR] *see* 6519
Tree of Life *see* 9389
Treflan [Dow AgroSci.] *see* 9686
Trehalose, 9580
α,α-Trehalose *see* 9580
Trehalose 6,6′-Dimycolate *see* 2528
Tre-Hold [Amvac] *see* 6371
Trelibet [EGYT] *see* 7392
Trelstar [Watson] *see* 9748
Tremaril [Wander] *see* 5979
Tremarit [Wander] *see* 5979
Tremblex [Janssen] *see* 2945
Tremetone, 9581
Tremin [Schering-Plough] *see* 9695
Tremolite *see* 826
Tremonil [Wander] *see* 5979
Tremoquil *see* 5979

Tremorine, 9582
Trenbolone, 9583
Trenbolone Hexahydrobenzylcarbonate
    see 9583
Trengestone, 9584
Trenimon *see* 9603
Trentadil [Evans] *see* 955
Trental [Aventis] *see* 7136
Trepibutone, 9585
Trepidan [Max Farma] *see* 7715
Treprostinil, 9586
Tresanil [ISF] *see* 9760
Trescatyl [M & B] *see* 3737
Trescillin *see* 7817
Tresortil *see* 5980
Trest [Dorsey] *see* 5979
Tretamine *see* 9671
Trethylene *see* 9639
Tretinoin *see* 8165
Tretinoin Tocoferil *see* 9499
Tretoquinol, 9587
Trevintix [Théraplix] *see* 7891
Trevira [Hoechst] *see* 7569
TRF *see* 4993, 4997, 9588
TRH, 9588
Tri-4 [BASF] *see* 9686
Triac [Aché] *see* 9462
Triacana [Marcofina] *see* 9462
Triacetin, 9589
Triacetone Triperoxide, 9590
Triacetoxyperiodinane *see* 2933
1,3,4-Tri-*O*-acetyl-*N*-acetyl-6-deoxy-β-
    D-glucosamine *see* 2931
Triacetyl Glycerine *see* 9589
Triacetyloleandomycin *see* 9770
2-(2,3,5-Tri-*O*-acetyl-β-D-ribofurano-
    syl)-*as*-triazine-3,5(2*H*,4*H*)-dione *see*
    904
Triaconazole *see* 9160
1-Triacontanol, 9591
Triact [Misemer] *see* 5685
Triacylglycerol Lipase *see* 5511
Triadenyl [Henning] *see* 155
Triadimefon, 9592
Triadimenol, 9593
Trialkylaluminum *see* 326
Triallate, 9594
Triam [Lichtenstein] *see* 9596
Triamcinolone, 9595
Triamcinolone Acetonide, 9596
Triamcinolone 16α,17-Acetonide *see*
    9596
Triamcinolone Acetonide β-Benzoyl-
    aminoisobutyrate *see* 9597
Triamcinolone Acetonide *tert*-Butyl Ace-
    tate *see* 9598
Triamcinolone Benetonide, 9597
Triamcinolone Hexacetonide, 9598
Triamelin *see* 9671
2,4,7-Triamino-6-phenylpteridine *see*
    9599
2,4,6-Triamino-*s*-triazine *see* 5811
Triammonium Hexafluoroaluminate-
    (3−) *see* 524
Triammonium Hexafluorogallate(3−)
    see 525
Triammonium Hexakis(cyano-*C*)ferrate-
    (3−) *see* 519
Triammonium Hexakis(cyano-*C*)ferrate-
    (4−) *see* 520
Triammonium Pentafluorodioxouranate
    see 567
Triammonium Tris[ethanedioato(2−)-
    *O,O′*ferrate(3−) *see* 517
Triamterene, 9599

(*T*-4)-Trifluoro[2-methoxy-*N*-(2-meth-oxyethyl)ethanaminato-κ*N*]sulfur *see* 2897

2′,6′,8-Trifluoro-5-methoxy-*s*-triazolo-[1,5-*c*]pyrimidine-2-sulfonanilide *see* 4108

2-[3-(Trifluoromethyl)anilino]nicotinic Acid *see* 6531

(Trifluoromethyl)benzene *see* 1110

6-(Trifluoromethyl)-2*H*-1,2,4-benzothia-diazine-7-sulfonamide 1,1-Dioxide *see* 4139

5-(Trifluoromethyl)-2′-deoxyuridine *see* 9687

8-Trifluoromethyl-7-deschloroglafenine *see* 4103

5-Trifluoromethyl-*N*-[3(*R*)-[1-[5,6-dihy-dro-4-hydroxy-2-oxo-6(*R*)-(2-phen-ethyl)-6(*R*)-*n*-propyl-2*H*-pyran-3-yl]-propyl]phenyl]-2-pyridinesulfonamide *see* 9459

6-Trifluoromethyl-3,4-dihydro-7-sulfa-moyl-2*H*-1,2,4-benzothiadiazine 1,1-Dioxide *see* 4789

2-Trifluoromethyl-10-(γ-dimethylamino-propyl)phenothiazine *see* 9685

3′-Trifluoromethyldiphenylamine-2-car-boxylic Acid *see* 4132

Trifluoromethylhydrothiazide *see* 4789

2-Trifluoromethyl-9-[3-[4-(β-hydroxy-ethyl)-1-piperazinyl]propylidene]thio-xanthene *see* 4187

2-(Trifluoromethyl)-10-[3-[1-(β-hydroxy-ethyl)-4-piperazinyl]propyl]phenothia-zine *see* 4189

o-Trifluoromethyl-*m*′-isopropoxybenzoic Anilide *see* 4212

α,α,α-Trifluoro-5-methyl-4-isoxazole-carboxy-*p*-toluidide *see* 5432

2-Trifluoromethyl-10-[3′-(1-methyl-4-piperazinyl)propyl]phenothiazine *see* 9680

3-Trifluoromethyl-4-nitrophenol *see* 9253

1-(3′-Trifluoromethyl-4′-nitrophenyl)-4,4-dimethylimidazoline-2,5-dione *see* 6544

α,α,α-Trifluoro-2-methyl-4′-nitro-*m*-propionotoluidide *see* 4208

4-[3-[2-(Trifluoromethyl)-10*H*-phenothiazin-10-yl]propyl]-1-piperazine-ethanol *see* 4189

(+)-16-[3-(Trifluoromethyl)phenoxy]-17,-18,19,20-tetranorprostaglandin F$_{2α}$ Isopropyl Ester *see* 9577

2-[[3-(Trifluoromethyl)phenyl]amino]-benzoic Acid *see* 4132

2-[[3-(Trifluoromethyl)phenyl]amino]-benzoic Acid 2-(2-Hydroxyethoxy)-ethyl Ester *see* 3875

2-[[3-(Trifluoromethyl)phenyl]amino]-3-pyridinecarboxylic Acid *see* 6531

2-[[3-(Trifluoromethyl)phenyl]amino]-3-pyridinecarboxylic Acid 1,3-Dihydro-3-oxo-1-isobenzofuranyl Ester *see* 9044

1-(*m*-Trifluoromethylphenyl)-2-(β-ben-zoyloxyethyl)aminopropane *see* 1039

N-(3-Trifluoromethylphenyl)-*N*′,*N*′-di-methylurea *see* 4154

1-(3-Trifluoromethylphenyl)-4-methyl-amino-5-chloropyridazone *see* 6701

(*R*)-*N*-(3-(3-(Trifluoromethyl)phenyl)-propyl)-1-(1-napthyl)ethylamine *see* 2282

2-[4-[[5-(Trifluoromethyl)-2-pyridinyl]-oxy]phenoxy]propanoic Acid Butyl Ester *see* 4116

2-[[8-(Trifluoromethyl)-4-quinolinyl]-amino]benzoic Acid 2,3-Dihydroxy-propyl Ester *see* 4103

N-[8-(Trifluoromethyl)-4-quinolyl]an-thranilic Acid 2,3-Dihydroxypropyl Ester *see* 4103

6-Trifluoromethyl-7-sulfamoyl-4*H*-1,2,4-benzothiadiazine 1,1-Dioxide *see* 4139

6-Trifluoromethyl-7-sulfamyl-1,2,4-ben-zothiadiazine 1,1-Dioxide *see* 4139

Trifluoromethylthiazide *see* 4139

4-[3-[2-(Trifluoromethyl)-9*H*-thio-xanthen-9-ylidene]propyl]-1-pipera-zineethanol *see* 4187

Trifluoromethyltrimethylsilane, 9683

α,α,α-Trifluoro-4-nitro-*m*-cresol *see* 9253

1-[2-(3,3,3-Trifluoropropyl)phenylsul-fonyl]-3-(4-methoxy-6-methyl-1,3,5-triazin-2-yl)urea *see* 7881

α,α,α-Trifluorothymidine *see* 9687

α,α,α-Trifluorotoluene *see* 1110

2-(α,α,α-Trifluoro-*m*-toluidino)nicotinic Acid *see* 6531

N-(α,α,α-Trifluoro-*m*-tolyl)anthranilic Acid *see* 4132

N-(α,α,α-Trifluoro-*m*-tolyl)anthranilic Acid 2-(2-Hydroxyethoxy)ethyl Ester *see* 3875

2-(α³,α³,α³-Trifluoro-2,3-xylidino)nico-tinic Acid *see* 4147

Trifluperidol, 9684

Triflupromazine, 9685

Trifluralin, 9686

Triflurex [Makhteshim-Agan] *see* 9686

Trifluridine, 9687

Trifluron *see* 9678

Triflusal, 9688

Triflusulfuron-methyl, 9689

Trifoliin *see* 5221

Trifolitin *see* 5274

Trifolium, 9690

Triforine, 9691

Triformol *see* 7025

Triftazin *see* 9680

Trigard [Syngenta] *see* 2775

Trigenolline *see* 9694

Trigger [Polifarma] *see* 8110

Triglobe [AstraZeneca] *see* 8903

Triglycine *see* 6579

Triglycine Sulfate *see* 4492

Triglycollamic Acid *see* 6579

1-Triglycyl-8-lysinevasopressin *see* 9167

Triglyme, 9692

Trigonellamide Chloride, 9693

Trigonelline, 9694

Trigonyl [Hoyer] *see* 8918

Trigot [BMS] *see* 3653

3,3′,3″-Triheptyl-4,4′,4″-trimethyl-7-(2″-methylthiazolyl-2,2′-trimethine)-thiazolcyanine 3,3″-Diiodide *see* 7530

Trihexyphenidyl Hydrochloride, 9695

Trihistan 2081

(5*Z*,7*E*,22*E*,24*E*)-24a,26a,27a-Trihomo-9,10-secocholesta-5,7,10(19),22,24-pentaene-1α,3β,25-triol *see* 8456

2′,3′,4′-Trihydroxyacetophenone *see* 4342

11β,17α,21-Trihydroxyallopregnane-3,20-dione *see* 4764

1,2,3-Trihydroxy-9,10-anthracene-dione *see* 683

1,2,4-Trihydroxy-9,10-anthracene-dione *see* 7945

1,2,3-Trihydroxyanthraquinone *see* 683

1,2,4-Trihydroxyanthraquinone *see* 7945

3′,4′,6-Trihydroxyaurone *see* 8972

3′,4′,6-Trihydroxybenzalcoumaranone *see* 8972

1,2,3-Trihydroxybenzene *see* 8000

1,3,5-Trihydroxybenzene *see* 7328

3,4,5-Trihydroxy-1,2-benzenedicar-boxaldehyde *see* 4225

3,4,5-Trihydroxybenzoic Acid *see* 4345

3,4,5-Trihydroxybenzoic Acid, (2*R*,-3*R*)-3,4-Dihydro-5,7-dihydroxy-2-(3,4,5-trihydroxyphenyl)-2*H*-1-ben-zopyran-3-yl Ester *see* 3526

3,4,5-Trihydroxybenzoic Acid Propyl Ester *see* 7859

2-*C*-[[(3,4,5-Trihydroxybenzoyl)oxy]-methyl]-D-ribofuranose 5-(3,4,5-Tri-hydroxybenzoate) *see* 4607

[4a*S*-(4aα,5β,6α)]-3,3′,5-Trihydroxy-[1,1′-biphenyl]-2-carboxylic Acid 2-Ester with 5-Ethenyl-6-(β-D-gluco-pyranosyloxy)-4,4a,5,6-tetrahydro-1*H*,3*H*-pyrano[3,4-*c*]pyran-1-one *see* 377

(6*R*)-3,5,6-Trihydroxy-4,6-bis(3-meth-yl-2-butenyl)-2-(3-methyl-1-oxobu-tyl)-2,4-cyclohexadien-1-one *see* 4754

(3β,5β,11α)-3,11,14-Trihydroxybufa-20,22-dienolide *see* 4358

3β,14,16β-Trihydroxy-5β-bufa-20,22-dienolide 16-Acetate *see* 1477

(2*R*,3*R*)-2,3,4-Trihydroxybutanal *see* 3690

(2*R*,3*S*)-2,3,4-Trihydroxybutanal *see* 9382

(2*S*,3*R*)-2,3,4-Trihydroxybutanal *see* 9381

(2*S*,3*S*)-2,3,4-Trihydroxybutanal *see* 3691

(3*S*)-1,3,4-Trihydroxy-2-butanone *see* 3694

3β,22,23-Trihydroxy-24-(carboxy-methylene)cholest-5-en-7-one 23,24-Lactone *see* 681

(3β,5β)-3,5,14-Trihydroxycard-20(22)-enolide *see* 7176

(3β,5β,12β)-3,12,14-Trihydroxycard-20(22)-enolide *see* 3166

(3β,5β,16β)-3,14,16-Trihydroxycard-20(22)-enolide *see* 4433

3β,12β,14β-Trihydroxy-5β-card-20(22)-enolide-3-(4‴-*O*-methyltri-digitoxoside) *see* 3167

9α,11α,15-Trihydroxy-16-*m*-chloro-phenoxy-13-thia-17,18,19,20-tetra-nor-5-prostenoic Acid *see* 5610

(3α,5β,7α,12α)-3,7,12-Trihydroxycho-lan-24-oic Acid *see* 2203

Trihydroxycyanidine *see* 2698

[3*R*-(3α,4α,5β)]-3,4,5-Trihydroxy-1-cy-clohexene-1-carboxylic Acid *see* 8480

3,4,5-Trihydroxy-2,2-dimethyl-6-chro-manacrylic Acid δ-Lactone 4-Ace-tate 3-(2-Methylbutyrate) *see* 10010

2-(4,5-*cis*)-Trihydroxy-4,6-dimethyl-tetrahydropyran *see* 6318

3,16α,17β-Trihydroxy-Δ^{1,3,5}-estra-triene *see* 3707

Trihydroxyestrin *see* 3707

Tri(hydroxyethyl)rutoside *see* 9789

Trilafon [Schering] *see* 7183
Trilan [Esseti] *see* 8989
Trilene [Zeneca] *see* 9639
Trileptal [Novartis] *see* 6929
Tri-Levlen [Berlex] *see* 6704
Trilifan *see* 7183
Triline *see* 9639
Trilit *see* 9730
Trillekamin [Crookes] *see* 9625
Trillium, 9696
Trilobamine *see* 2819
Trilobine, 9697
Trilon A *see* 6579
Trilon B [BASF] *see* 3517
Trilophosphamide *see* 9768
Trilostane, 9698
Triludan [Aventis] *see* 9163
Trimagnesium Dicitrate *see* 5663
Trimagnesium Phosphate *see* 5683
Trimangol [Cerexagri] *see* 5721
Trimanyl [Tosse] *see* 9709
Trimar *see* 9639
Trimaton *see* 5949
Trimax [Bayer CropSci.] *see* 4910
Trimebutine, 9699
Trimecaine, 9700
Trimedlure, 9701
Trimellitic Acid, 9702
Trimellitic Acid 1,2-Anhydride *see* 9703
Trimellitic Anhydride, 9703
Trimeperidine *see* 7784
Trimepranol *see* 6140
Trimeprazine, 9704
Trimeprimine *see* 9722
Trimeproprimine *see* 9722
Trimeric Acetone Peroxide *see* 9590
Trimesulf [LPB] *see* 8918
Trimetaphan Camphorsulfonate *see* 9707
Trimetazidine, 9705
Trimethadione, 9706
Trimethaphan Camphorsulfonate *see* 9707
Trimethaphan Camsylate, 9707
Trimethaphen Camphorsulfonate *see* 9707
Trimethobenzamide, 9708
Trimethoprim, 9709
Trimethoquinol *see* 9587
1,2,10-Trimethoxy-6aα-aporphin-11-ol *see* 5162
2,10,11-Trimethoxy-6aα-aporphin-1-ol *see* 2546
3-(3,4,5-Trimethoxybenzamido)piperidine *see* 9790
3,4,5-Trimethoxybenzeneethanamine *see* 5905
3,4,5-Trimethoxybenzoic Acid 2-[4-[3-(2-Chloro-10H-phenothiazin-10-yl)-propyl]-1-piperazinyl]ethyl Ester *see* 6145
3,4,5-Trimethoxybenzoic Acid Diester with 3,3'-[Ethylenebis(methylimino)]di-1-propanol *see* 4705
3,4,5-Trimethoxybenzoic Acid Diester with Tetrahydro-1H-1,4-diazepine-1,4(5H)-dipropanol *see* 3200
3,4,5-Trimethoxybenzoic Acid 2-(Dimethylamino)-2-phenylbutyl Ester *see* 9699
3,4,5-Trimethoxybenzoic Acid 1,2-Ethanediylbis[(methylimino)-3,1-propanediyl] Ester *see* 4705
3,4,5-Trimethoxybenzoic Acid 2,6-Pyridinediylbis(methylene)ester *see* 7507

3,4,5-Trimethoxybenzoic Acid (Tetrahydro-1H-1,4-diazepine-1,4(5H)-diyl)di-3,1-propanediyl Ester *see* 3200
3,4,5-Trimethoxybenzoyl Methyl Reserpate *see* 8145
4-(3,4,5-Trimethoxybenzoyl)morpholine *see* 9720
N-β-(3,4,5-Trimethoxybenzoyloxy)-ethyl]-N'-γ-(3-chloro-10-phenothiazinyl)propyl]piperazine *see* 6145
N-(3,4,5-Trimethoxybenzoyl)tetrahydro-1,4-oxazine *see* 9720
1-(2,3,4-Trimethoxybenzyl)-4-[bis(4-fluorophenyl)methyl]piperazine *see* 5563
1-(3',4',5'-Trimethoxybenzyl)-6,7-dihydroxy-1,2,3,4-tetrahydroisoquinoline *see* 9587
2,9,10-Trimethoxyberbin-3-ol *see* 2549
3,9,10-Trimethoxy-13aα-berbin-2-ol *see* 5163
3,4,5-Trimethoxycinnamic Acid Ester of Methyl Reserpate *see* 8142
4-(3',4',5'-Trimethoxycinnamoyl)-1-(ethoxycarbonylmethyl)piperazine *see* 2290
4-(3,4,5-Trimethoxycinnamoyl)-1-piperazineacetic Acid Ethyl Ester *see* 2290
1-[4-[(3',4',5'-Trimethoxycinnamoyl)-1-piperazinyl]acetyl]pyrrolidine *see* 2291
6,7,8-Trimethoxycoumarin *see* 4265
6,6',7-Trimethoxy-2,2'-dimethylberbaman-12-ol *see* 1153
6,6',7-Trimethoxy-2,2'-dimethyloxyacanthan-12'-ol *see* 6953
(1β)-6,6',7'-Trimethoxy-2,2'-dimethyltubocuraran-12'-ol *see* 2213
7',10,11-Trimethoxyemetan-6'-ol *see* 1973
4,7,8-Trimethoxyfuro[2,3-b]quinoline *see* 8561
3,4,5-Trimethoxy-3'-hydroxy-4'-methoxy-(Z)-stilbene *see* 2494
Trimethoxymethane *see* 6884
(1α,6α,14α,16β)-1,6,16-Trimethoxy-4-(methoxymethyl)-20-methylaconitane-8,13,14-triol 8-Acetate 14-Benzoate *see* 2881
3,9,10-Trimethoxy-13aα-methyl-13aβ-berbin-2-ol *see* 5161
6,6',12'-Trimethoxy-2-methyloxyacanthan-7-ol *see* 2819
1,2,10-Trimethoxy-6aα-noraporphin-9-ol *see* 5388
1,1,1-Trimethoxypentane *see* 9717
3,4,5-Trimethoxyphenethylamine *see* 5905
1-[(2,3,4-Trimethoxyphenyl)methyl]-piperazine *see* 9705
5-[(3,4,5-Trimethoxyphenyl)methyl]-2,4-pyrimidinediamine *see* 9709
(2,4,6-Trimethoxyphenyl)-(3-pyrrolidinopropyl) Ketone *see* 1475
3,4,5-Trimethoxy-N-3-piperidinylbenzamide *see* 9790
1,2,4-Trimethoxy-5-(1-propenyl)benzene *see* 824
2,4,5-Trimethoxy-1-propenylbenzene *see* 824
2',4',6'-Trimethoxy-4-(1-pyrrolidinyl)-butyrophenone *see* 1475
4-(3,4,5-Trimethoxythiobenzoyl)morpholine *see* 9760

Trimethylacetic Acid *see* 7511
Trimethyl-β-acetoxypropylammonium Chloride *see* 5940
2-Trimethylacetyl-1,3-indandione *see* 7444
Trimethylamine, 9710
Trimethylamine N-Oxide, 9711
α,α',α''-Trimethylaminetricarboxylic Acid *see* 6579
1-Trimethylammonio-3-(3-indolyl)propionate *see* 4861
Trimethylammonium Chloride *see* 9710
N,N,N-Trimethylbenzaminium Iodide *see* 7318
sym-Trimethylbenzene *see* 5907
1,2,4-Trimethylbenzene *see* 7915
1,3,5-Trimethylbenzene *see* 5907
α,α,β-Trimethylbenzeneethanamine *see* 7133
N,α,α-Trimethylbenzeneethanamine *see* 5852
7,8,10-Trimethylbenzo[g]pteridine-2,4(3H,10H)-dione *see* 5599
(±)-7-(3,5,6-Trimethyl-1,4-benzoquinon-2-yl)-7-phenylheptanoic Acid *see* 8459
(±)-4-(α,2,3-Trimethylbenzyl)imidazole *see* 5787
endo-1,7,7-Trimethylbicyclo[2.2.1]heptan-2-ol *see* 1338
exo-1,7,7-Trimethylbicyclo[2.2.1]heptan-2-ol *see* 5128
1,7,7-Trimethylbicyclo[2.2.1]heptan-2-ol Acetate *see* 1339
(1S)-1,3,3-Trimethylbicyclo[2.2.1]heptan-2-one *see* 3968
1,7,7-Trimethylbicyclo[2.2.1]heptan-2-one *see* 1732
2,7,7-Trimethylbicyclo[3.1.1]heptan-6-one *see* 2252
2,6,6-Trimethylbicyclo[3.1.1]hept-2-ene *see* 7445
3,7,7-Trimethylbicyclo[4.1.0]hept-3-ene *see* 1836
(1R)-4,6,6-Trimethylbicyclo[3.1.1]hept-3-en-2-one *see* 9960
Trimethyl Borate, 9712
Trimethylbromo-IDA *see* 5772
Trimethylbromomethane *see* 1555
Trimethyl Carbinol *see* 1542
Trimethylchloromethane *see* 1562
trans-2,6,6-Trimethyl-1-crotonylcyclohexa-1,3-diene *see* 2809
2,2,6-Trimethyl-4,6-cyclohexadien-1-aldehyde *see* 8316
2,6,6-Trimethyl-1,3-cyclohexadiene-1-carboxaldehyde *see* 8316
(2E)-1-(2,6,6-Trimethyl-1,3-cyclohexadien-1-yl)-2-buten-1-one *see* 2809
3,3,5-Trimethylcyclohexanol α-Phenyl-α-hydroxyacetate *see* 2704
α,α,4-Trimethyl-3-cyclohexene-1-methanol *see* 9171
1,3,3-Trimethylcyclohexen-5-one *see* 5196
3,5,5-Trimethyl-2-cyclohexen-1-one *see* 5196
(E)-4-(2,6,6-Trimethyl-1-cyclohexen-1-yl)-3-buten-2-one *see* 5056
(E)-4-(2,6,6-Trimethyl-2-cyclohexen-1-yl)-3-buten-2-one *see* 5056
3,5,5-Trimethylcyclohexyl Amygdalate *see* 2704
3,3,5-Trimethylcyclohexyl Mandelate *see* 2704

1,3,7-Trimethylxanthine *see* 1636
Trimeton [Schering] *see* 7235
Trimetozine, 9720
Trimetrexate, 9721
Trimexolone *see* 8226
Tri-Minulet [Wyeth] *see* 4413
Trimipramine, 9722
Trimmit [Zeneca Ag Prod] *see* 6984
Trimogal [Lagap] *see* 9709
Trimol [Fujisawa] *see* 7503
Trimonase [Mipharm] *see* 9447
Trimopan [Berk] *see* 9709
Trimoprostil, 9723
Trimox [BMS] *see* 577
Trimpex [Roche] *see* 9709
Trimstat [Laser] *see* 7220
Trimtabs [Mayrand] *see* 7220
Trimustine *see* 9625
Trimyristin, 9724
Trimysten *see* 2417
Trinactin *see* 6675
Triniol [Syntex] *see* 7029
Trinitrin *see* 6607
1,3,3-Trinitroazetidine *see* 9487
sym-Trinitrobenzene, 9726
1,3,5-Trinitrobenzene *see* 9726
2,4,6-Trinitro-1,3-benzenediol *see* 8859
sym-Trinitrobenzoic Acid *see* 9727
2,4,6-Trinitrobenzoic Acid, 9727
2,4,7-Trinitrofluorenone, 9728
2,4,7-Trinitro-9*H*-fluoren-9-one *see* 9728
(2,4,7-Trinitro-9*H*-fluoren-9-ylidene)-propanedinitrile *see* 3094
Trinitroglycerol *see* 6607
1,3,5-Trinitrohexahydro-*s*-triazine *see* 2736
Trinitromethane, 9729
2,4,6-Trinitrophenol *see* 7410
2,4,6,-Trinitrophenol Ammonium Salt *see* 547
2,4,6-Trinitrophenol Silver Salt *see* 8526
sym-Trinitrophenylnitroaminoethyl Nitrate *see* 7139
2,4,6-Trinitroresorcinol *see* 8859
Trinitrosan [Merck KGaA] *see* 6607
sym-Trinitrotoluene *see* 9730
2,4,6-Trinitrotoluene, 9730
α-Trinitrotoluol *see* 9730
Trinitrotriazidobenzene, 9731
2,4,6-Trinitro-*N*-(2,4,6-trinitrophenyl)-benzenamine *see* 3335
18,19,20-Trinor-17-cyclohexyl-13,14-didehydro-PGF$_{2α}$ Methyl Ester *see* 234
Trinordiol [Wyeth] *see* 6704
[(5*Z*,13*E*,9α,11α,15*S*)-2,3,4-Trinor-1,5-inter-*m*-phenylene-6,9-epoxy-11,15-dihydroxy-15-cyclohexyl-16,17,18,-19,20-pentanor]prosta-5,13-dienoic Acid *see* 9057
Tri-Norinyl [Watson] *see* 6697
Trinosin [Toa Eiyo] *see* 155
Trinovum [Janssen-Cilag] *see* 6697
Trinoxol [Crystal Chem.] *see* 2796
Triocetin [OFF] *see* 9770
Triognost [Teva] *see* 2992
Triolein, 9732
Trional *see* 8958
Triosil *see* 6156
Triostin A *see* 9733
Triostin C *see* 9733
Triostins, 9733

Triovex *see* 3707
1,3,5-Trioxacyclohexane *see* 9734
s-Trioxane, 9734
1,3,5-Trioxane *see* 9734
1,3,5-Trioxane-2,4,6-triimine *see* 2682
Trioxazine [Labatec] *see* 9720
(5β)-3,7,12-Trioxocholan-24-oic Acid *see* 2868
2,4,6-Trioxohexahydropyrimidine *see* 963
Trioxone [Zeneca] *see* 9019
N,N',N''-(2,6,10-Trioxo-1,5,9-trioxa-cyclododecane-3,7,11-triyl)tris[2,3-dihydroxy]benzamide *see* 3596
N,N',N''-(2,6,10-Trioxo-1,5,9-trioxa-cyclododecane-3,7,11-triyl)tris-*o*-pyrocatechuamide *see* 3596
Trioxsalen, 9735
Trioxyethylrutin *see* 9789
"Trioxymethylene" *see* 7025
Trioxymethylene *see* 9734
2,6,8-Trioxypurine *see* 9875
Tripalmitin, 9736
Tripamide, 9737
Tripelennamine, 9738
Triperidol [Janssen] *see* 9684
Tripetroselin *see* 7189
Triphasil [Wyeth] *see* 6704
Triphedinon [Toho] *see* 9695
Triphenidyl [Leciva] *see* 9695
Triphenylcarbinol, 9739
Triphenylene, 9740
Triphenylmethane, 9741
Triphenylmethanol *see* 9739
Triphenyl Phosphate, 9742
Triphenylphosphine, 9743
Triphenylphosphine Copper(I) Hydride Hexamer *see* 8857
Triphenylphosphonium Anhydride Tri-fluoromethanesulfonate *see* 4650
3,5,6-Triphenyl-2,3,5,6-tetraazabicy-clo[2.1.1]hex-1-ene *see* 6613
Triphenyltetrazolium Chloride, 9744
2,3,5-Triphenyl-2H-tetrazolium Chlo-ride *see* 9744
Triphenyltin Acetate *see* 9745
Triphenyltin Hydroxide, 9745
Triphosphopyridine Nucleotide *see* 6348
Triphosphoric Acid Pentasodium Salt *see* 8697
Triphthasine *see* 9680
Triphylite *see* 5520
Tripiperazine Dicitrate *see* 7464
Tripolyphosphate *see* 8697
Tripotassium Citrate *see* 7623
Tripotassium Dicitrato Bismuthate *see* 2485
Tripotassium Hexakis(cyano-*C*)cobal-tate(3−) *see* 7637
Tripotassium Hexakis(cyano-*C*)ferrate-(3−) *see* 7630
Tripotassium Phosphate *see* 7660
Tripotassium Tris(ethanedioato)chro-mate(3−) *see* 2228
Tripotassium Tris(oxalato)antimonate-(3−) *see* 699
Tripotassium Tris(oxalato)chromate(3−) *see* 2228
Tripro-amylin *see* 7708
Triprolidine, 9746
Triptide *see* 4475
Triptil [Merck & Co.] *see* 7901
Triptizol [SIT] *see* 487
Tript-Oh [Sigma-Tau] *see* 4847
Triptolide, 9747

Triptorelin, 9748
Triptycene, 9749
Tripyridyltriazine *see* 9750
2,4,6-Tripyridyl-*s*-triazine, 9750
2,4,6-Tripyridyl-1,3,5-triazine *see* 9750
2,4,6-Tri-2-pyridyl-*s*-triazine *see* 9750
TRIS *see* 9772
1,1,1-Tris(acetyloxy)-1,1-dihydro-1,2-benziodoxol-3(1*H*)-one *see* 2933
Trisamine *see* 9772
2,3,5-Tris(aziridino)-1,4-benzoquinone *see* 9603
2,3,5-Tris(1-aziridinyl)-*p*-benzoquinone *see* 9603
2,3,5-Tris(1-aziridinyl)-2,5-cyclohexa-diene-1,4-dione *see* 9603
Tris(1-aziridinyl)phosphine Oxide *see* 9672
Tris(1-aziridinyl)phosphine Sulfide *see* 9673
2,4,6-Tris(1-aziridinyl)-1,3,5-triazine *see* 9671
Tris-BP, 9751
Tris Buffer *see* 9772
Triscabol [Elf Atochem] *see* 10172
Tris(2-carboxyethyl)phosphine *see* 9085
N-[[4,7,10-Tris(carboxymethyl)-1,4,7,-10-tetraazacyclododec-1-yl]acetyl]-D-phenylalanyl-L-cysteinyl-L-tyrosyl-D-tryptophyl-L-lysyl-L-threonyl-*N*-[(1*R*,2*R*)-2-hydroxy-1-(hydroxymeth-yl)propyl]-L-cysteinamide Cyclic-(2 → 7)-disulfide *see* 3513
Tris[2-chloro-1-(chloromethyl)ethyl]-phosphate *see* 9087
Tris(β-chloroethyl)amine *see* 9625
N,N,N'-Tris(2-chloroethyl)-*N'*,O-propyl-ene Phosphoric Acid Ester Diamide *see* 9768
N,N,3-Tris(2-chloroethyl)tetrahydro-2*H*-1,3,2-oxazaphosphorin-2-amine 2-Oxide *see* 9768
Tris(2,3-dibromopropyl) Phosphate *see* 9751
Tris(1,3-dichloroisopropyl)phosphate *see* 9087
1,2,3-Tris(2-diethylaminoethoxy)ben-zene Tris(ethyl Iodide) *see* 4343
Tris[7-[4-(dimethylamino)phenyl]-*N*-hy-droxy-4,6-dimethyl-7-oxo-2,4-hepta-dienamidato-*O*^{N}*O*^{1}]iron *see* 9649
2,4,6-Tris(dimethylamino)-*s*-triazine *see* 320
Tris(dimethylcarbamodithioato-*S,S'*)iron *see* 4013
Tris(dimethyldithiocarbamato)iron *see* 4013
Trisenox [Cell Therapeutics] *see* 804
Tris(ethylenediamine)cadmium Dihydr-oxide, 9752
Tris(ethylenediamine)cadmium Hydrox-ide *see* 9752
2,3,5-Tris(ethyleneimino)benzoqui-none *see* 9603
2,4,6-Tris(ethylenimino)-*s*-triazine *see* 9671
Tris(hydroxyethyl)amine *see* 9665
N,N,N'-Tris(2-hydroxyethyl)-*N'*-octa-decyl-1,3-diaminopropane Dihydro-fluoride *see* 6820
7,3',4'-Tris[*O*-(2-hydroxyethyl)]rutin *see* 9789
Tris(hydroxymethyl)aminomethane *see* 9772
N-Tris(hydroxymethyl)methyl-2-amino-ethanesulfonic Acid *see* 9176

N-Tris[(hydroxymethyl)methyl]-3-aminopropanesulfonic Acid *see* 9058
N-[Tris(hydroxymethyl)methyl]glycine *see* 9651
Tris(hydroxymethyl)nitromethane, 9753
Tris[2-(hydroxy-*κO*)propanoato-*κO*]aluminum *see* 348
Tris(8-hydroxyquinoline)aluminium *see* 370
Trisilane, 9754
Trisilicane *see* 9754
Trisilicon Octahydride *see* 9754
Trisilicon Tetranitride *see* 8497
Trisilicopropane *see* 9754
Tris(*p*-methoxyphenyl)chloroethylene *see* 2174
Tris[2-methyl-1-aziridinyl]phosphine Oxide *see* 5936
Tris[1-methylethylene]phosphoric Triamide *see* 5936
[[2,4,6-Tris(1-methylethyl)phenyl]acetyl]sulfamic Acid 2,6-Bis(1-methylethyl)phenyl Ester *see* 884
1,1,1-Tris(nitratomethyl)propane *see* 7811
Trisodium 4'-Anilino-8-hydroxy-1,1'-azonaphthalene-3,6,5'-trisulfonate *see* 628
Trisodium (*T*-4)-Bis[monothiosulfato-(2−)-*κO*,*κS*]-aurate(3−) *see* 4519
Trisodium Calcium Diethylenetriaminepentaacetate *see* 7124
Trisodium Carboxyphosphate *see* 4251
Trisodium Citrate *see* 8602
Trisodium Hexakis(nitrato-*N*)cobaltate-(3−) *see* 8603
Trisodium *N*-Hydroxyethylethylenediaminetriacetate *see* 9966
Trisodium Orthophosphate *see* 8662
Trisodium Phosphate *see* 8662
Trisodium Phosphonoformate *see* 4251
Trisomin [Lilly] *see* 5687
Trisoralen [Valeant] *see* 9735
Trisorcin [Merckle] *see* 7088
Tris(pentafluorophenyl)borane *see* 9755
Tris(pentafluorophenyl)boron, 9755
Tris(2-pyridinecarboxylato-*N*¹,*O*²)-chromium *see* 2236
Tris(8-quinolinolato-*κN*¹,*κO*⁸)aluminum *see* 370
Tristat [Salsbury] *see* 6612
Tri-Stat IU [Tri-K] *see* 4916
Tristearin, 9756
Tris(2,4,6-tribromophenoxy)bismuthine *see* 1291
1,2,3-Tris(2-triethylammonium Ethoxy)benzene Triiodide *see* 4343
Tris(trimethylsilyl)silane, 9757
Tristriphenylphosphine Rhodium Carbonyl Hydride, 9758
Trisulfurated Phosphorus *see* 9238
Tritace [Aventis] *see* 8103
Tritan *see* 9741
Tritanol *see* 9739
Tritec [GSK] *see* 8110
Triteren [Sumitomo] *see* 9599
Triterium *see* 9762
Tritheon [Ortho] *see* 410
4,5,9-Trithiadodeca-1,6,11-triene 9-Oxide *see* 195
Trithioacetaldehyde *see* 9318
Trithioanethole *see* 644
Trithiocarbonic Acid, 9759
Trithio-*p*-methoxyphenylpropene *see* 644
Trithiozine, 9760

Triticum, 9761
Tritiozine *see* 9760
Tritium, 9762
Tritocaline *see* 9765
Tritoftorol [Cerexagri] *see* 10165
Tritolyl Phosphate, 9763
Tri-*o*-tolyl Phosphate, 9764
Triton A-20 [Rohm & Haas] *see* 9833
Triton N [Rohm & Haas] *see* 6677
Triton WR-1339 [Rohm & Haas] *see* 9833
Triton X [Rohm & Haas] *see* 6761
Triton X-100 [Rohm & Haas] *see* 6761
Tritopine *see* 5379
Tritoqualine, 9765
Tritox *see* 9628
Trittico [Angelini] *see* 9579
Triuret, 9766
Trivastal [Itherapia] *see* 7493
Trivitan *see* 10019
Trizma [Sigma-Aldrich] *see* 9772
TRK-100 *see* 1152
tRNA *see* 8203
Trobicin [Pharmacia & Upjohn] *see* 8739
Trochol *see* 1189
Trocinate [Poythress] *see* 9370
Troclosene Potassium, 9767
Trodax *see* 6656
Trofan [Upsher-Smith] *see* 9797
Trofosfamide, 9768
Trofurit [Chinoin] *see* 4309
Troglitazone, 9769
Troillite *see* 4058
Trolamine *see* 9665
Trolamine Salicylate *see* 9665
Troleandomycin, 9770
Trolene [Dow] *see* 8256
Trolone [3M Pharma] *see* 8993
Trolovol [Dexo] *see* 7088
Tromantadine, 9771
Tromaril [Unichem] *see* 3580
Tromasin *see* 7016
Trombavar *see* 8689
Trombostop *see* 9385
Trombovar *see* 8689
Trometamol *see* 9772
Tromethamine, 9772
Tromethane *see* 9772
Tromexan [Novartis] *see* 3770
Trommsdorff's Starch *see* 10141
Trona *see* 8674
Tronolane [Abbott] *see* 7709
Tronothane [Abbott] *see* 7709
Tropacaine *see* 9774
Tropacine, 9773
Tropacocaine, 9774
Tropaeolin D *see* 6105
Tropaeolin G *see* 5928
Tropaeolin O, 9775
Tropaeolin OO, 9776
Tropaeolin OOO No. 1 *see* 6857
Tropaeolin OOO No. 2 *see* 6858
Tropaeolin R *see* 9775
Tropaic Acid *see* 9779
Tropane, 9777
1*αH*,5*αH*-Tropane *see* 9777
(*E*)-1*αH*,5*αH*-Tropane-3*α*,6*β*,7*β*-triol 3-(2-Methylcrotonate) *see* 5935
3-(3,6,7-Tropanetriol) Tiglate *see* 5935
1*αH*,5*αH*-Tropan-3*α*-ol *see* 9781
1*αH*,5*αH*-Tropan-3*β*-ol *see* 7921
3*β*-Tropanol *see* 7921
1*αH*,5*αH*-Tropan-3*α*-ol Atropate *see* 739
1*αH*,5*αH*-Tropan-3*α*-ol Benzilate *see* 9782
1*αH*,5*αH*-Tropan-3*β*-ol Benzoate *see* 9774

1*αH*,5*αH*-Tropan-3*α*-ol Diphenylacetate *see* 9773
1*αH*,5*αH*-Tropan-3*α*-ol Mandelate *see* 4730
(*E*)-1*αH*,5*αH*-Tropan-3*β*-ol 2-Methylcrotonate *see* 9434
1*αH*,5*αH*-Tropan-3*α*-ol (±)-Tropate (Ester) *see* 875
1*αH*,5*αH*-Tropan-3*α*-ol(−)-tropate (Ester) *see* 4858
3*α*-Tropanyl Diphenylacetate *see* 9773
1*αH*,5*αH*-Tropan-3*α*-yl Indole-3-carboxylate *see* 9783
3*α*-Tropanyl-1*H*-indole-3-carboxylic Acid Ester *see* 9783
3*α*-Tropanyl *S*-(−)-Tropate *see* 4858
Tropax [BMS] *see* 6955
Tropeic Acid *see* 9779
Tropeines *see* 9781
Tropene [Degussa] *see* 3885
Tropeolin O *see* 9775
Tropesin, 9778
Tropethydrylin *see* 3756
Trophicardyl *see* 4975
Trophicreme [Sanofi Winthrop] *see* 3707
Trophires *see* 9354
Trophosphamide *see* 9768
Trophy [Dow AgroSci.] *see* 61
Tropic Acid, 9779
Tropic Acid Ester with Scopine *see* 8406
Tropic Acid Ester with Tropine *see* 875
l-Tropic Acid Ester with Tropine *see* 4858
Tropicamide, 9780
2-Tropidinecarboxylic Acid *see* 3492
Tropin [Takeda] *see* 875
Tropine, 9781
ψ-Tropine *see* 7921
ψ-Tropine Benzoate *see* 9774
Tropine Benzohydryl Ether Methanesulfonate *see* 1121
Tropine Benzylate, 9782
Tropine Diphenylacetate *see* 9773
Tropine Mandelate *see* 4730
Tropine Tropate *see* 875
l-Tropine Tropate *see* 4858
Tropisetron, 9783
Tropium [DDSA] *see* 2084
Tropomyosins, 9784
Troponin, 9784
Tropylium Bromide, 9785
dl-Tropyl Tropate *see* 875
Trospium Chloride, 9786
Trosyd [Pfizer] *see* 9452
Trosyl [Pfizer] *see* 9452
Trotyl *see* 9730
Trovafloxacin, 9787
Trovafloxacin Mesylate *see* 9787
Trovan *see* 9787
Troxacitabine, 9788
Troxatyl [Shire Biochem] *see* 9788
Troxerutin, 9789
Troxidone *see* 9706
Troximin [Galenica] *see* 9250
Troxipide, 9790
Trozocina [Sigma-Tau] *see* 915
Trp *see* 9797
[D-Trp⁶,des-Gly¹⁰]-LH-RH Ethylamide *see* 2923
D-Trp⁶-gonadorelin *see* 9748
D-Trp⁶-LHRH *see* 9748
D-Trp⁶LRH *see* 9748
True Ammonium Sulfide *see* 556
True Lavender *see* 5390
True Unicorn Root *see* 230
Trusono *see* 5846

Trusopt [Merck & Co.] see 3426
Truxal [Lundbeck] see 2188
Truxaletten [Lundbeck] see 2188
Truxillic Acid, 9791
η-Truxillic Acid see 9791
Trycite [Dow] see 8860
Trycol [Henkel] see 7577
Trypaflavine see 123
Trypan Blue, 9792
Trypan Red, 9793
Tryparsamide, 9794
Tryparsone see 9794
Tryponarsyl see 9794
Trypothane see 9794
Trypoxyl see 8578
Trypsin, 9795
α₁-Trypsin Inhibitor see 719
Tryptamine, 9796
Tryptan [Valeant] see 9797
Tryptanol [Merck & Co.] see 487
Tryptizol [Merck & Co.] see 487
Tryptophan, 9797
L-Tryptophan see 9797
6-D-Tryptophan-9-(N-ethyl-L-prolin-amide)-10-deglycinamideluteinizing Hormone-Releasing Factor (Pig) see 2923
6-D-Tryptophan-LH-RH see 9748
6-D-Tryptophanluteinizing Hormone-Releasing Factor (Pig) see 9748
Tryptophol, 9798
Trypure [Novo] see 9795
TS-110 see 5582
TSAA-291 see 6931
TSE-424 see 1013
TSF see 9386
TSH see 9414
TSH-Releasing Factor see 9588
Tsiklamid see 62
Tsiklodol see 9695
Tsiklometiazid see 2745
Tsiklomitsin see 9196
TSP see 8662, 9387
TSPP see 9240
TSQ, 9799
Tsuduranine, 9800
TTC see 9744
TTC-909 see 2358
TTD see 3364
TTF see 9242
TTFD see 4311
TTMS see 8950
T-2 Toxin, 9801
TTP see 9298
TTPG see 8809
TTX see 9246
Tuads [Vanderbilt] see 9371
Tuamine [Lilly] see 9802
Tuaminoheptane, 9802
Tubarine [GlaxoWellcome] see 9807
Tuba Root see 2916
Tubazid see 5186
Tube Cucare see 2671
Tuberactin [Toyo Jozo] see 3600
Tuberactinomycin, 9803
Tuberactinomycin A see 9803
Tuberactinomycin B see 10001
Tuberactinomycin N see 3600
Tuberactinomycin O see 9803
Tubercidin, 9804
Tuberculin, 9805
Tuberin, 9806
Tubersol [Sanofi Pasteur] see 9805
Tubocurarine Chloride, 9807

Tubocurarine Dimethyl Ether Iodide see 6144
d-Tubocurarine Iodide Dimethyl Ether see 6144
d-Tubocurine see 2212
Tubulin, 9808
α-Tubulin see 9808
β-Tubulin see 9808
Tuclase [Pfizer] see 1794
Tuduranine see 9800
Tuff-Lite [Indust. Plastic] see 7581
Tuftsin, 9809
Tugon [Bayer] see 9623
Tulathromycin, 9810
Tulisan [Chiesi] see 6718
Tulobuterol, 9811
Tumenol see 4885
Tumeric see 9824
Tumil-K [Virbac] see 4456
Tumor Necrosis Factor, 9812
1-235-Tumor Necrosis Factor Receptor (Human) Fusion Protein with 236-467-Immunoglobulin G1 (Human γ1-Chain Fc Fragment) see 3712
Tums Smooth Dissolve [GSK] see 1657
Tung Oil, 9813
Tungsten, 9814
Tungsten Carbide, 9815
Tungsten Carbides see 9814
Tungsten Hexafluoride, 9816
Tungsten Oxide (WO₃) see 9817
Tungsten Trioxide, 9817
Tungstic(VI) Acid, 9818
Tungstic Anhydride see 9817
5-Tungsto-2-antimonate see 4750
21-Tungsto-9-antimonate see 4750
Tungstophosphoric Acid see 7364
Tungstosilicic Acid see 8502
Tunicamine see 9819
Tunicamycin, 9819
Tunichrome B-1, 9820
Tunichromes see 9820
Tunol see 2465
Tupersan [DuPont] see 8487
Turanose, 9821
Turbocalcin [SKB] see 3537
Turexan Crème [Turimed] see 9848
Turflon [Dow AgroSci.] see 9656
Turimycin P3 see 6183
Turinal [Gedeon Richter] see 291
Turixin [GSK] see 6302
Turkey Corn see 2545
Turkey-galls see 6728
Turkey-Red Oil, 9823
Turkish Geranium Oil see 6796
Turkish Laurel see 5382
Turlington's Balsam see 951
Turmeric, 9824
Turmeric Yellow see 2673
ar-Turmerone, 9825
Turnsole see 5547
Turoptin [Dispersa] see 6140
Turpentine, 9826
"Turpentine Camphor" see 1340
Turpentine Oil see 9826
Turpentine Substitutes see 6201
Tussafug [Robugen] see 1049
Tusseval [Marco Viti] see 7469
Tussirama [Serpero] see 4228
Tussistop see 2066
Tuss-Ornade [SKB] see 1776
Tutane see 1544
Tutin, 9827
Tuttomycin see 6454
TV-02 see 9022

TV-485 see 3875
TV-1322 see 27
TVP-1012 see 8116
TVX Q 7821 see 5081
TW 260/240 see 8740
Tween 80 [ICI] see 7582
Twist [Bayer CropSci.] see 9677
Twistane, 9828
Twiston [McNeil] see 1799
TWSb see 8812
Tx 60 see 10036
TXA₂ see 9388
TXB₂ see 9388
TXIB [Eastman Chemical] see 9251
Tybamate, 9829
Tybatran [Robins] see 9829
Tybraine [Nicholas] see 6068
Tydantil [Polichimica Sap] see 6532
Tygacil [Wyeth] see 9432
Tykerb [GSK] see 5367
Tylan [Elanco] see 9832
Tylcalsin see 1647
Tylciprine [Théraplix] see 9573
Tylenol [McNeil] see 47
Tylocrebrine, 9830
Tylonolide see 9832
Tylophorine, 9831
Tylose M [Clariant] see 6040
Tylose MGA see 1829
Tylosin, 9832
Tyloxapol, 9833
Tyloxypal see 9833
Tymazoline, 9834
Tymelyt [Lundbeck] see 5557
Tymium [Sapos] see 3945
Tympanol see 6121
Tymtran [Adria] see 2005
Tyr see 9839
Tyraminase see 6247
Tyramine, 9835
Tyrene see 9629
Tyri 10 [Lindopharm] see 9841
Tyrimide see 5202
Tyrocidine, 9836
Tyrocidine A see 9836
Tyrocidine B see 9836
Tyrocidine C see 9836
Tyropanoate Sodium, 9837
Tyropaque [Torii] see 9837
Tyrosamine see 9835
Tyrosinase, 9838
Tyrosine, 9839
L-Tyrosine see 9839
m-Tyrosine, 9840
[29-Tyrosine,104-glutamic Acid] CTLA-4 (Antigen) (Human Extracellular Domain-containing Fragment) Fusion Protein with Immunoglobulin G1 (Human Monoclonal Fc Domain-containing Fragment), Bimol. (120 → 120')-Disulfide see 1024
Tyrosur [Engelhard KG] see 9841
L-Tyrosylglycylglycyl-L-phenylalanyl-L-leucine see 3572
L-Tyrosylglycylglycyl-L-phenylalanyl-L-methionine see 3572
Tyrothricin, 9841
Tyrylen see 1516
Tysabri [Elan] see 6426
Tyzine [Pfizer] see 9219
TZB see 7277
TZP-4238 see 6888
TZU-0460 see 8274
U-27 see 7420
U-1363 see 3305

U-2032 see 5299
U-2043 see 9507
U-4527 see 2728
U-5956 see 4080
U-6013 see 5174
U-6591 see 6722
U-6987 see 1832
U-7800 see 4192
U-8344 see 9851
U-8471 see 5794
U-9586 see 7923
U-9889 see 8832
U-10071 see 9804
U-10136 see 7876
U-10149 see 5500
U-10858 see 6203
U-10997 see 6174
U-12062 see 7877
U-14583 see 7878
U-14743 see 7597
U-15167 see 6671
U-15800 see 6985
U-17835 see 9505
U-18496 see 890
U-19183 see 8736
U-19920 see 2354
U-21251 see 2356
U-22550 see 1722
U-24973A see 5823
U-26225A see 9566
U-26452 see 4478
U-26597A see 2475
U-27182 see 4199
U-28288D see 4559
U-28508 see 2354
U-28774 see 5297
U-31889 see 312
U-32070E see 1638
U-32921 see 1823
U-32921E see 1823
U-33030 see 9604
U-34865 see 3140
U-36059 see 486
U-36384 see 1823
U-41123 see 160
U-42585E see 5555
U-42718 see 5555
U-42842 see 769
U-53217 see 7875
U-53217A see 7875
U-57903E see 7500
U-62840 see 9586
U-63196 see 1938
U-63196E see 1938
U-64279E see 1950
U-67279A see 1950
U-69689E see 4061
U-70226E see 4883
U-72107A see 7452
U-74006F see 9463
U-76252 see 1941
U-76253 see 1941
U-76253A see 1941
U-90152 see 2877
U-90152S see 2877
U-100766 see 5504
Ub see 9844
Ubenimex, 9842
UBI-A1335 see 4123
Ubicardio [Tosi] see 9843
Ubichromenol 50 see 9843
Ubicor [Magis] see 9843
Ubidecarenone see 9843
Ubidenone [Esseti] see 9843
Ubifactor [San Carlo] see 9843

Ubimaior [Chiesi] see 9843
UBI-N252 see 6938
UBIP see 9844
Ubiquinone 10 see 9843
Ubiquinone 50 see 9843
Ubiquinones, 9843
Ubiquitin, 9844
Ubiquitous Immunopoietic Polypeptide
    see 9844
Ubisan [Leben's] see 9843
Ubiten-50 see 9843
Ubivis [AGIPS] see 9843
Ubretid [Nycomed] see 3362
Ubrocef [Novartis] see 1972
UC-7744 see 1787
UC-21149 see 222
UC-51762 see 9329
Ucarcide [Union Carbide] see 4472
UCB-1474 see 2080
UCB-1967 see 3452
UCB-2543 see 1794
UCB-3412 see 3385
UCB-3983 see 5909
UCB-4445 see 1464
UCB-4492 see 4849
UCB-5062 see 5777
UCB-6215 see 7487
UCB-22073 see 6220
UCB-28556 see 2022
UCB-34714 see 1377
UCB-L059 see 5461
UCC 974 see 2834
UD-CG 115 see 7434
UD-CG 115 BS see 7434
Udekinon [Tobishi] see 9843
Udicil [Pharmacia & Upjohn] see 2784
UDMH see 3247
Udolac [Mallinckrodt] see 2822
UDP see 9878
UDPG see 9879
UDP-Glucose see 9879
UDP-MurNAc-L-Ala-γ-D-Glu-X-D-Ala-
    D-Ala see 7040
Ue-5908 see 7998
U4Euh see 6018
UF-021 see 9849
Ugurol [Rottapharm] see 9569
UHF-8615 see 7067
UIC-94017 see 2827
Uintahite see 4422
Uintaite see 4422
Ujothion see 1051
UK-4271 see 6919
UK-14304 see 1375
UK-14304-18 see 1375
UK-20349 see 9452
UK-33274 see 3433
UK-33274-27 see 3433
UK-48340 see 491
UK-48340-11 see 491
UK-48340-26 see 491
UK-49858 see 4122
UK-61689 see 8443
UK-61689-2 see 8443
UK-67994 see 3425
UK-68798 see 3409
UK-73967 see 1742
UK-79300 see 1742
UK-81252 see 8352
UK-88525 see 2825
UK-92480 see 8489
UK-109496 see 10033
UK-116044 see 3544
UK-427857 see 5749
Ukidan [Serono] see 9887

Ularitide see 9886
Ulbreval see 1524
Ulcar [Houdé] see 8879
Ulcedin [AGIPS] see 2279
Ulcedine [Sanofi-Pharma] see 2279
Ulcerfen [Finadiet] see 2279
Ulcerlmin [Chugai] see 8879
Ulcerone [Yamanouchi] see 2485
Ulcesium [Zambon] see 4006
Ulcex [Guidotti] see 8110
Ulcimet [Temis Lostalo] see 2279
Ulcofalk [Interfalk Italia] see 2279
Ulcogant [Merck KGaA] see 8879
Ulcomedina [Pharmaland] see 2279
Ulcomet [Italfarmaco] see 2279
Ulcort see 4786
Ulcosan [Dompé] see 7491
Ulcuforton [Plantorgan] see 7491
Ulcus-Tablinen [Sanorania] see 1793
Uldumont see 5958
Ulexine see 2789
Ulfamid [Krka] see 3930
Ulfaret [Takeda] see 1945
UL-FS-49 see 10115
Ulgut [Shionogi] see 1038
Ulhys [Lafare] see 2279
Ulifloxacin see 7908
Uliginosin A see 9845
Uliginosin B see 9845
Uliginosins, 9845
Ulinastatin see 9882
Uliron C see 8930
ULO [3M Pharma] see 2066
Ulobetasol Propionate see 4593
Ulone [3M Pharma] see 2066
Ulsanic [Ferrer] see 3485
Ulstar [Roche] see 9723
Ulstron [ICI] see 7581
Ultidine [GSK] see 8110
Ultiva [Glaxo Wellcome] see 8131
Ultracain [HMR] see 1869
Ultracarbon see 1808
Ultracef [BMS] see 1913
Ultracid(e) [Syngenta] see 5970
Ultracillin [Grünenthal] see 2702
Ultracorten [Novartis] see 7722
Ultracortenol [Novartis] see 7721
Ultradol [Procter & Gamble] see 3874
Ultrafur see 4294
Ultralan Oral [Schering AG] see 4153
Ultralanum [Schering AG] see 4153
Ultram [Ortho] see 9566
Ultramarine, 9846
Ultramarine Green see 2234
Ultramarine Yellow see 972
Ultra-Mg [Melisana] see 4456
Ultramicina [Lisapharma] see 4254
Ultrapen see 7817
Ultraquinine see 2623
Ultrase [Axcan] see 7006
Ultrasulfon [Streuli] see 8905
Ultrasüss see 6630
Ultra-Technekow [Mallinckrodt] see 8657
Ultravate [BMS] see 4593
Ultravist [Schering AG] see 5062
Ultrax [Chemie Linz] see 8914
Ultroxim [Duncan Flockhart] see 1954
UM-792 see 6363
UM-952 see 1497
Umatrope [Lilly] see 8716
Umbellatine see 1154
Umbelliferone, 9847
Umbelliferone Glucoside see 8562
Umbradil see 5040
UML-491 see 6137

UMP *see* 9881
Unacid PD Oral [Pfizer] *see* 8992
Unacil [Firma] *see* 3440
Unacim [Pfizer] *see* 8889, 8992
Unagen *see* 3350
Unakalm [Pharmacia & Upjohn] *see* 5297
Unal *see* 462
Unasyn [Pfizer] *see* 8992
Unasyn (Inj.) [Pfizer] *see* 8889
Unat [Roche] *see* 9552
2-Undecanone *see* 6104
10-Undecenoic Acid *see* 9848
Undecylenic Acid, 9848
9-Undecylenic Acid *see* 9848
Unden [Bayer] *see* 7836
Unergol [Poli] *see* 3653
Ungernine *see* 9082
Unicide U-13 [Induchem] *see* 4916
Unicordium [Riom] *see* 1150
Unidasa *see* 4758
Unidone [Schering] *see* 668
Unidrox [Angelini] *see* 7908
Unifer [Tosi] *see* 4036
Uniflox [Bayer] *see* 2314
Unifur *see* 4294
Unifyl [Mundipharma] *see* 9285
Unihep [Leo Pharm] *see* 4653
Uniloc [Nycomed] *see* 859
Unipen [Wyeth-Ayerst] *see* 6352
Uniphyl [Purdue Frederick] *see* 9285
Uniphyllin [Mundipharma] *see* 9285
Unipril [Zambon] *see* 8103
Unipyranamide [Unichem] *see* 7956
Unisan [United Phosphorus] *see* 7300
Unisedil [Merck KGaA] *see* 2994
Unisept [Schering] *see* 2091
Unisom [Pfizer] *see* 3441
Unisom Sleepgels [Pfizer] *see* 3309
Unisomnia [Alliance] *see* 6575
Unispiran *see* 9203
Unistat *see* 6612
Unistat [Salsbury] *see* 8933
Unistat-3 [Salsbury] *see* 6612
Unitane *see* 9472
Unitiol *see* 3210
UNITOP [Roche] *see* 6340
Univasc [Schwarz] *see* 6229
Univer [Zeneus] *see* 9950
Unix [Syngenta] *see* 2772
Unixime [Firma] *see* 1924
Unizole *see* 3265
Unnatural Tartaric Acid *see* 9068
Unnilennium *see* 5809
Unnilhexium *see* 8414
Unniloctium *see* 4618
Unnilpentium *see* 3462
Unnilquadium *see* 8303
Unnilseptium *see* 1321
Unoprostone, 9849
Unresolvable Tartaric Acid *see* 9071
Ununbium *see* 3540
Ununhexium *see* 3542
Ununnilium *see* 2826
Ununquadium *see* 3541
Ununnium *see* 8247
Unusual Tartaric Acid *see* 9068
UP-33-901 *see* 2269
UP-83 *see* 6531
UP-106 *see* 7833
UP-34101 *see* 7792
Upbeet [DuPont] *see* 9689
UP₄dC *see* 2896
Upixon [Bayer] *see* 7464
Uprima [TAP] *see* 746
Upstene [Pharmuka] *see* 4930

UP₄U *see* 3351
UR-0003 *see* 7067
UR-112 *see* 2378
UR-1501 *see* 9688
UR-1521 *see* 4255
UR-4056 *see* 4215
UR-12592 *see* 8297
Urab [Hopkins] *see* 4009
Uracid [Hässle] *see* 342
Uracil, 9850
Uracil-6-carboxylic Acid *see* 6876
Uracil Deoxyriboside *see* 2910
Uracil Mustard, 9851
Uracil Riboside *see* 9877
Uractyl *see* 8931
Uradal *see* 1831
Uragon [Makhteshim-Agan] *see* 1381
Uralenic Acid *see* 3590
Uralgin [Ceccarelli] *see* 6359
Uramid [Spofa] *see* 8931
l-Uramidoglutaric Acid *see* 1838
Uramil, 9852
Uramite [DuPont] *see* 9868
Uramustine *see* 9851
Uramycin B *see* 9562
Uranediol, 9853
Uranic Oxide *see* 9860
Uranin(e) *see* 4159
Uranine Yellow *see* 4159
Uraninite *see* 9855
Uranium, 9854
Uranium Ammonium Carbonate *see* 566
Uranium Ammonium Fluoride *see* 567
Uranium Barium Oxide *see* 1001
Uranium Benzoate *see* 1091
Uranium Dioxide, 9855
Uranium Dioxydichloride *see* 9862
Uranium Hexafluoride, 9856
Uranium Oxide Orange *see* 7695
Uranium Oxide Yellow *see* 8699
Uranium Tetrachloride, 9857
Uranium Tetrafluoride, 9858
Uranium Trichloride, 9859
Uranium Trioxide, 9860
Uranium X₂ *see* 7883
"Uranium Yellow" *see* 565
Uranium Yellow *see* 8699
Uranium Z *see* 7883
Uranous Oxide *see* 9855
Urantoin [DDSA] *see* 6599
Uranyl Acetate, 9861
Uranyl Ammonium Carbonate *see* 566
Uranyl Ammonium Fluoride *see* 567
Uranyl Benzoate *see* 1091
Uranyl Chloride, 9862
Uranyl Nitrate, 9863
Uranyl Sulfate, 9864
Urao *see* 8674
Urapidil, 9865
Uraprene [IBI] *see* 9865
Urara [ISK] *see* 4105
Urari *see* 2671
Urate Oxidase *see* 9876
Urate Oxidase (*Aspergillus flavus* Clone
    9C/9A Reduced) *see* 8117
Urazole, 9866
Urbac [Merck-Clévenot] *see* 6533
Urbadan [HMR] *see* 2359
Urbanyl [HMR] *see* 2359
Urbilat [Hor-Fer-Vit] *see* 5862
Urdes [Errekappa] *see* 9889
Urea, 9867
Urea Amidohydrolase *see* 9870
Urea Calcium Acetylsalicylate *see* 1647
Urea Compd with Hydrogen Peroxide
    (1:1) *see* 1782

Ureaform, 9868
Urea Hydrogen Peroxide *see* 1782
Urea Nitrate, 9869
Ureaphil [Abbott] *see* 9867
Urease, 9870
Urea Stibamine, 9871
Urecholine [Merck & Co.] *see* 1185
Uredepa, 9872
Uregit [EGYT] *see* 3717
p-Ureidobenzenearsonic Acid *see* 1786
Ureidoglutaric Acid *see* 1838
5-Ureidohydantoin *see* 258
δ-Ureidonorvaline *see* 2331
4-Ureido-1-phenylarsonic Acid *see* 1786
Urem [Kade] *see* 4881
Urena, 9873
Urenil *see* 8931
Urepearl [Otsuka] *see* 9867
Urethan, 9874
Urethane *see* 9874
Urethimine *see* 9872
Urethylane *see* 6036
Uretrim [Bastian] *see* 9709
Urex [Mochida] *see* 4309
Urex [3M Pharma] *see* 5966
6,6′-Ureylenebis[1,1′-dimethylquino-
    linium] Sulfate *see* 3353
6,6′-Ureylenebis(1-methylquinolin-
    ium)bis(methosulfate) *see* 3353
Urfadyn [Zambon] *see* 6539
Urfamycine [Inpharzam] *see* 9301
Uriben [Rosemont] *see* 6359
Uric Acid, 9875
Uricase, 9876
Uricemil [Molteni] *see* 279
Uriclar [Crosara] *see* 6359
UriCon [ProLabs] *see* 7307
Urico-oxidase *see* 9876
Uricovac [Sanofi Winthrop] *see* 1065
Uric Oxidase *see* 9876
Uridine, 9877
Uridine 5′-Diphosphate, 9878
Uridine Diphosphate Glucose, 9879
Uridine-5′-diphosphoglucose *see* 9879
Uridine 5′-Monophosphate *see* 9881
Uridine 5′-(Pentahydrogen Tetraphos-
    phate) P‴ → 5′-Ester with 2′-Deoxycyti-
    dine *see* 2896
Uridine 5′-(Pentahydrogen Tetraphos-
    phate) P‴ → 5′-Ester with Uridine *see*
    3351
Uridine 5′-Phosphoric Acid *see* 9881
Uridine 5′-Pyrophosphate *see* 9878
Uridine 5′-Pyrophosphate Glucose Ester
    see 9879
Uridine-5-pyrophosphoric Acid *see* 9878
Uridine 5′-(Tetrahydrogen Triphosphate)
    see 9880
Uridine 5′-(Trihydrogen Diphosphate)
    see 9878
Uridine 5′-(Trihydrogen Diphosphate)
    P′-α-D-Glucopyranosyl Ester *see* 9879
Uridine 5′-Triphosphate, 9880
5′-Uridylic Acid, 9881
UriKoxidase *see* 9876
Urimeth [North Am. Pharm.] *see* 5975
Urinary HCG *see* 2216
Urinary Indican *see* 4941
Urinary Trypsin Inhibitor *see* 9882
Urinastatin, 9882
Urinorm [Torii] *see* 1065
Uriodone *see* 5040
Urion [Zambon] *see* 238
Uripurinol [Azupharma] *see* 279
Urisal [Sanofi-Synthelabo] *see* 8602

Ventavis [Schering AG] see 4901
Ventax [Robert] see 3438
Ventilastin [Viatris] see 216
Ventilat [Thomae] see 6943
Ventipulmin [Boehringer, Ing.] see 2347
Ventodisks [GSK] see 216
Ventolin [GSK] see 216
Ventox see 131
Ventramine see 6543
Ventrazol see 7141
Venturicidin A see 9947
Venturicidin B see 9947
Venturicidin B 3'-Carbamate see 9947
Venturicidins, 9947
Venzar [DuPont] see 5435
Venzoquimpe [Quimpe] see 5925
Vepesid [BMS] see 3886
Vepicombin [Nycomed] see 7100
VER-002 see 656
Veracillin [Ayerst] see 3084
Veracim [Cimex] see 9950
Veractil see 5986
Veracur [Typharm] see 4235
Veradol [Schering AG] see 6417
Veralcamine see 9949
Veralipride, 9948
Veralipril [Midy] see 9948
Veralkamine, 9949
Veramex [Sanofi-Synthelabo] see 9950
Veramix [Pharmacia] see 5793
Verapamil, 9950
Veraptin [Lagap] see 9950
Veratetrine see 7899
Veratraldehyde, 9951
Veratramine, 9952
Veratran [Latema] see 2416
Veratric Acid, 9953
Veratric Acid 4-[Ethyl(p-methoxy-α-
  methylphenethyl)amino]butyl Ester see
  5769
Veratric Aldehyde see 9951
Veratridine, 9954
Veratrine see 2033
Veratrine (Mixture), 9955
Veratrole, 9956
3-Veratroylveracevine see 9954
Veratrum Viride, 9957
Verax [Tosi] see 1122
Verbascose, 9958
Verbenalin, 9959
Verbenalol see 9959
d-Verbenone, 9960
Vercyte [Abbott] see 7480
Verel [Eastman Kodak] see 6227
Verelan [Elan] see 9950
Vergentan [Synthelabo] see 250
Vergonil see 4789
Veriloid [3M Pharma] see 9957
Veritol [Knoll] see 7330
Verladyn [Verla] see 3174
Vermicidin [Rivopharm] see 5768
Vermicompren (Tabl.) [Merck KGaA] see
  7465
Vermiculite, 9961
Vermilion see 5889
Verminum [Squibb] see 7035
Vermiparin see 5718
Vermirax [Biosintetica] see 5768
Vermitin see 7252
Vermizym see 7016
Vermouth see 10052
Vermox [Janssen] see 5768
Vernamycin A see 10004
Vernamycin B_α see 7753
Vernine see 4566

Vernitest Reagent see 8048
Vernolepin, 9962
Vernolic Acid, 9963
Verol see 6017
Veronal see 962
Veronal Sodium see 962
Verospiron [Richter Gedeon] see 8760
Veroxil [Baldacci] see 4935
Verrucarin A see 9964
Verrucarin B see 9964
Verrucarin J see 9964
Verrucarin K see 9964
Verrucarins, 9964
Verrucarol see 9964
Verrugon [Pickles] see 8332
Versalide [Givaudan-Delawanna], 9965
Versapen [BMS] see 4672
Versatrex [BMS] see 4672
Versed [Roche] see 6182
Versene 100 [Dow] see 3517
Versene Acid [Dow] see 3517
Versene Na₂ [Dow] see 3517
Versene-9 [Dow] see 3517
Versenol [Dow], 9966
Versus [Angelini] see 1035
Vertab [Chiesi] see 9950
Verteporfin, 9967
Verticillin A see 9968
Verticillin B see 9968
Verticillin C see 9968
Verticillins, 9968
Verticine, 9969
Vertigon [GSK] see 7761
Verucasep [Galen] see 4472
Verutal [Stiefel] see 4472
Verv-Ca see 1704
Verxite see 9961
Very Fast Death Factor see 627
Very Late Activation Antigens see 4988
Vesadin [Rhône-Mérieux] see 8915
Vésadol [Janssen] see 1599
Vesanoid [Roche] see 8165
Vesdil [AstraZeneca] see 8103
Vesicare [Yamanouchi] see 8712
Vesipyrin see 7270
Vesistol [Inverni] see 592
Vesnarinone, 9970
Vesperone [UCB] see 1361
Vesprin [BMS] see 9685
Vessel [Alfa] see 8986
Vestalin see 6702
Vestra [Pharmacia & Upjohn] see 8125
Vesulong [Novartis] see 8945
Vesuprim see 8903
Vesuvianite see 1648
Vesuvine see 1252
Vetacortyl [Vétoquinol] see 6111
Veta-K₁ [Sanofi] see 7380
Vetalar [Bioniche] see 5295
Vetalgina [ICC] see 5637
Vetalog [Solvay] see 9596
Vetalpha [A.T.I.] see 4819
Vetamox [Am. Cyanamid] see 53
Vetarsenobillon see 6447
Vetbond [3M] see 1565
Vetdectin [Fort Dodge] see 6290
Veteusan [Veterinaria] see 2594
Vetibenzamina [Novartis] see 9738
Vetimast [Novartis] see 1972
Vetiprost [Virbac] see 3871
Vetisulid [Fort Dodge] see 8900
Vetiver Oil see 6816
Vetiver Oil Haiti see 6816
Vetiver Oil Java see 6816
Vetiver Oil Reunion (Bourbon) see 6816

Vetivert Oil see 6816
α-Vetivone see 9971
β-Vetivone see 9971
Vetivones, 9971
Vetkelfizina [Centralvet] see 8910
Vetrabutine, 9972
Vetranquil [Sanofi] see 32
Vetrazin [Novartis] see 2775
Vetstrep [Merck & Co.] see 8826
Vetyver Oil see 6816
Vexol [Alcon] see 8226
Vfend [Pfizer] see 10033
Viaben [Schrholz] see 1432
Viacutan [Boehringer, Ing.] see 5507
Viadent [Vipont] see 8356
Viadil [Pharma Investi] see 1432
Viadril see 4823
Viadur [Alza] see 5457
Viagra [Pfizer] see 8489
Vianol see 1548
Viansin [Farmacosmici] see 2084
Viarespan [Servier] see 3999
Viarex [Schering-Plough] see 1019
Viarox [Byk Gulden] see 1019
Vibeline [Bellon] see 10010
Vibramycin [Pfizer] see 3440
Vibra-Tabs [Pfizer] see 3440
Vibraveineuse [Pfizer] see 3440
Vibravenös [Pfizer] see 3440
Vibriomycin see 3179
Viburnum Opulus, 9973
Viburnum Prunifolium, 9974
Vi-Cad [Vineland] see 1617
Vicard [Abbott] see 9154
Viccillin [Meiji] see 586
Viceton [Bimeda] see 2077
Vicilan [Zeneca] see 9980
Vicin see 9975
Vicine, 9975
Vicioside see 9975
Victan [Sanofi Winthrop] see 3821
Victoria Green B see 5699
Victoria Green W see 5699
Vidarabine, 9976
Vidaza [Pharmion] see 890
Vi-De-3 [Novartis] see 10019
Videobil [Bracco] see 5063
Videophel see 5038
Viderpen [Sintex] see 5925
Videx [BMS] see 3098
Vidine see 2204
Vidopen [APS] see 586
Vidora [Wyeth] see 4969
Viehe's Salt, 9977
Vienna Green see 2625
Vigabatrin, 9978
Vigamox [Alcon] see 6291
Vigantol [Merck KGaA] see 10019
Vigazoo [Am. Cyanamid] see 8891
Vigilor [Bouchard] see 4084
Vigorsan [Albert-Roussel] see 10019
Vikane [Dow AgroSci.] see 8981
Vilan [Lannacher] see 6520
Vildagliptin, 9979
Villiaumite see 8618
Viloxazine, 9980
Vimicon [Frosst] see 2773
Viminalol see 617
Viminol, 9981
Vinarol [Gen. Dyes] see 7585
Vinblastine, 9982
Vincafor [Pharmafarm] see 9983
Vincagil [Sanofi-Aventis] see 9983
Vincaleukoblastine see 9982
Vincamine, 9983

Name Index

Vincaminine *see* 9983
Vincamone *see* 3487
Vincanorine *see* 3487
Vincimax [Sanofi-Aventis] *see* 9983
Vincine *see* 9983
Vincinine *see* 9983
Vinclozolin, 9984
Vinconate, 9985
Vincrex [BMS] *see* 9986
Vincristine, 9986
Vindesine, 9987
Vindolidine *see* 9988
Vindoline, 9988
Vindorosine *see* 9988
Vinegar Naphtha *see* 3757
Vinesthene *see* 9995
Vinethene *see* 9995
Vinetine *see* 6953
Vinflunine, 9989
Vingsal [Stroschein] *see* 6699
Vinol [Air Prods. Chem.] *see* 7585
Vinorelbine, 9990
Vinpocetine, 9991
Vinyl Acetate, 9992
Vinylacetonitrile *see* 290
γ-Vinyl-γ-aminobutyric Acid *see* 9978
Vinylbenzene *see* 8860
Vinylbital, 9993
Vinyl Carbinol *see* 286
Vinyl Chloride, 9994
Vinyl Cyanide *see* 131
α-Vinyldiacetonalkamine Benzoate *see* 3894
Vinylestrenolone *see* 6702
17α-Vinyl-5(10)-estren-17β-ol-3-one *see* 6702
Vinyl Ether, 9995
Vinylethylene *see* 1509
Vinylformic Acid *see* 130
γ-Vinyl GABA *see* 9978
Vinylidene Chloride, 9996
Vinylidene Cyanide-vinyl Acetate Copolymer *see* 2828
5-Vinyl-5-(1-methylbutyl)barbituric Acid *see* 9993
17α-Vinyl-19-nortestosterone *see* 6717
(−)-5-Vinyl-2-oxazolidinethione *see* 4513
β-Vinylpyridine *see* 3730
N-Vinyl-2-pyrrolidinone *see* 7697
1-Vinyl-2-pyrrolidinone Polymers *see* 7697
1-Vinyl-2-pyrrolidinone Polymers, Iodine Complex *see* 7698
5-Vinyl-2-thiooxazolidone *see* 4513
Vinyl Trichloride *see* 9637
Vinyzene *see* 6961
Viocin [Pfizer] *see* 10001
Vio-D [Rowell] *see* 10018
Vioform [Novartis] *see* 5031
Viokase [Axcan] *see* 7006
Violacein, 9997
Violanin *see* 2880
Violaquercitrin *see* 8304
Violaxanthin, 9998
Viologen, 9999
Violuric Acid, 10000
Viomycin, 10001
Viophan *see* 2288
Viosterol *see* 10018
Vio-Thene [Rowell] *see* 6973
Vioxx [Merck & Co.] *see* 8248
Viozene *see* 8256
VIP, 10002
Viper [Dow AgroSci.] *see* 7103
Vipicil [Wyeth] *see* 2702

Viprinex [Knoll] *see* 630
Viprynium Chloride *see* 8022
Viprynium Embonate *see* 8022
Viquidil, 10003
Vira-A [Warner-Lambert] *see* 9976
Viracept [Agouron] *see* 6443
Viraferon [Schering-Plough] *see* 4990
Viramid [Alfa] *see* 8198
Viramidine [Valeant] *see* 9063
Viramune [Roxane] *see* 6490
Viras [Mect] *see* 8200
Virazide [Valeant] *see* 8198
Virazole [Valeant] *see* 8198
Viread [Gilead] *see* 9146
Virgimycin *see* 10004
Virginiamycin, 10004
Virginiamycin M₁ *see* 10004
Virginiamycin S₁ *see* 10004
Viridicatin, 10005
Viridin, 10006
Virilon [Star] *see* 9180
Virlix [Sanofi-Synthelabo] *see* 2022
Virmen [Menarini] *see* 146
Virofral [Novo] *see* 374
Virophta [Dulcis] *see* 9687
Viroptic [Burroughs Wellcome] *see* 9687
Virormone [Ferring] *see* 9180
Virosterone [Endo] *see* 9180
Virudermin [Robugen] *see* 10159
Virudox [Bioglan] *see* 4891
Virulizin [Lorus], 10007
Virulizin-2γ *see* 10007
Viru-Merz [Merz] *see* 9771
Viruseen [Hommel] *see* 146
Viruserol [Zyma] *see* 9771
Virusmin [Sumitomo] *see* 6272
Virustat [Delagrange] *see* 6272
Viruxan [Newport] *see* 4976
Viruzona *see* 5977
Visammin *see* 5309
Visano [Kade] *see* 5862
Visceralgina [SIT] *see* 9431
Visclair [Ranbaxy] *see* 5785
β-Viscol *see* 5608
Viscoleo [Lundbeck] *see* 4187
Viscose, 10008
Viscosin, 10009
Viscotiol [Erba] *see* 5449
Visha *see* 120
Visine [Pfizer] *see* 9219
Visipaque [GE Healthcare] *see* 5023
Viskaldix [Novartis] *see* 2393
Visken [Novartis] *see* 7443
Visnadine, 10010
Visnagin, 10011
Visnamine [Chinoin] *see* 10010
Visor [Dow AgroSci.] *see* 9311
Vista [AgrEvo] *see* 4196
Vista [Dow AgroSci.] *see* 4203
Vistagan [Allergan] *see* 5462
Vista-Methasone [Richard Daniel] *see* 1180
Vistamycin [Meiji] *see* 8206
Vistar [3M] *see* 5802
Vistaril Pamoate [Pfizer] *see* 4849
Vistaril Parenteral [Pfizer] *see* 4849
Vistide [Gilead] *see* 2268
Visual Purple *see* 8192
Visubeta *see* 1180
Visubutina *see* 6972
Visudyne [Novartis] *see* 9967
Vitabact [Faure] *see* 7398
Vitaberin [Taisho] *see* 9297
Vitacimin [Takeda] *see* 830
Vitacin [Towa Yakuhin] *see* 830

Vital Red, 10012
Vital Red Evans *see* 10012
Vitamin A, 10013
2-*cis*-Vitamin A *see* 6468
Vitamin A Acid *see* 8165
2-*cis*-Vitamin A Acid *see* 5228
Vitamin A Alcohol *see* 10013
Vitamin A Aldehyde *see* 8164
Vitamin A₁ *see* 10013
Vitamin A₂ *see* 2874
Vitamin A₂ Aldehyde *see* 2873
Vitamin B₁ *see* 9295
Vitamin B₁ O,S-Diacetate *see* 54
Vitamin B₁ Disulfide *see* 9297
Vitamin B₁ Propyl Disulfide *see* 7882
Vitamin B₂ *see* 8200
Vitamin B₂ Phosphate *see* 8201
Vitamin B₃ *see* 6523
Vitamin B₄ *see* 152
Vitamin B₅ *see* 7015
Vitamin B₆ Hydrochloride *see* 7982
Vitamin B₁₂, 10014
Vitamin B₁₂-Co(II) *see* 10016
Vitamin B₁₂ Coenzyme *see* 2451
Vitamin B₁₂, Radioactive, 10015
Vitamin B₁₂ₐ *see* 4809
Vitamin B₁₂ᵦ *see* 4809
Vitamin B₁₂ᵧ *see* 4809
Vitamin B₁₂ᵤ *see* 10159
Vitamin B₁₂ₚ *see* 3868
Vitamin B₁₂ᵣ, 10016
Vitamin B₁₂ₛ *see* 10016
Vitamin B₁₃ *see* 6876
Vitamin B₁₅ *see* 7008
Vitamin B₁₇ *see* 597
Vitamin Bᴛ *see* 1849
Vitamin Bₓ *see* 423
Vitamin Bc *see* 4221
Vitamin Bc Conjugate *see* 7935
Vitamin C *see* 830
Vitamin D₁, 10017
Vitamin D₂, 10018
Vitamin D₃, 10019
Vitamin D₄, 10020
Vitamin E, 10021
Vitamin G *see* 8200
Vitamin H *see* 1231
Vitamin K, 10022
Vitamin K₁ *see* 7380
Vitamin K₁ Epoxide *see* 7380
Vitamin K₁ Oxide *see* 7380
Vitamin K₂ *see* 5833
Vitamin K₂(₀) *see* 5831
Vitamin K₂(₂₀) *see* 5833
Vitamin K₂(₃₀) *see* 5833
Vitamin K₂(₃₅) *see* 5833
Vitamin K₃ *see* 5831
Vitamin K₄ *see* 5830
Vitamin K₅, 10023
Vitamin(s) L, 10024
Vitamin L₁ *see* 422
Vitamin M *see* 4221
Vitamin P Complex *see* 1228
Vitamin PP *see* 6523
Vitamin T, 10025
Vitamin T Goetsch *see* 10025
Vitamin U *see* 6098
Vitamogen [Tanabe] *see* 9297
Vitaneurin [Mepha] *see* 9295
Vitanevril [Sanofi Winthrop] *see* 1041
Vitarubin [Streuli] *see* 10014
Vitascorbol [Aventis] *see* 830
Vitaseptol [Faure] *see* 9317
Vitasprint B₁₂ [Brenner-Efeka] *see* 7363
VitaStain [Arapahoe] *see* 9744

Vitas-U [Kaken] *see* 6098
Vitavax [Uniroyal] *see* 1827
Vitavel K [Vitamins Ltd] *see* 5830
Vitazechs *see* 7979
Vitellin *see* 5428
Vitrasert [Chiron] *see* 4363
Vitravene [Novartis] *see* 4229
Vitride [Zeeland] *see* 8564
Vitronectin, 10026
Vivactil [Merck & Co.] *see* 7901
Vival [Alpharma] *see* 2994
Vivalan [Zeneca] *see* 9980
Vivarint [Zeneca] *see* 9980
Vivatec [Merck & Co.] *see* 5516
Vivelle [Novartis] *see* 3703
Vivelle-Dot [Novartis] *see* 3703
Vividrin [Mann] *see* 2590
Vividyl [Lilly] *see* 6715
Viviful [Kumiai] *see* 7777
VK-55 *see* 8907
VLA Antigens *see* 4988
VLA Integrins *see* 4988
VLB *see* 9982
Vleminckx's Lotion *see* 8977
VM-26 *see* 9145
VMA *see* 9933
VML-251 *see* 4272
VML-588 *see* 2342
V.M.&P. Naphtha *see* 5489
Voacamine, 10027
Voacangine *see* 10027
Voacanginine *see* 10027
Vodka, 10028
Vodol [Andromaco] *see* 6178
Voelicherite *see* 1694
Vogalene [Thraplix] *see* 6149
Vogan [Merck KGaA] *see* 10013
Vogesensäure (German) *see* 9069
Voglibose, 10029
Volatile Oil of Laurel *see* 5382
Volatile Oil of Mustard *see* 295
Volaton [Bayer] *see* 7366
Voldal [Novartis] *see* 3081
Volicitin, 10030
Volidan [BDH; Searle] *see* 5805
Volmax [GSK] *see* 216
Volon [BMS] *see* 9595
Volon A [BMS] *see* 9596
Volonimat [BMS] *see* 9596
Volpo [Croda] *see* 7577
Voltaren [Novartis] *see* 3081
Voltarol [Novartis] *see* 3081
Vomex A [Yamanouchi] *see* 3207
Vomicine, 10031
Vomit Nut *see* 6730
Vomitoxin, 10032
Vomit Wort *see* 5550
Vonamycin Powder V *see* 6454
Vondozeb [Cerexagri] *see* 5716
Vonedrine *see* 7308
Vontil [SKB] *see* 9357
Vontrol [SK & F] *see* 3311
Vonum [Sanofi-Synthelabo] *see* 4968
Voranil [USV] *see* 2410
Voriconazole, 10033
Vorinostat, 10034
Vorlan [Mallinckrodt] *see* 9984
Vorozole, 10035
VP-16-213 *see* 3886
VP-63843 *see* 7533
v-PA *see* 3459
V-Pen [Orion] *see* 7100
VPM *see* 5949
Vraap [Inverni] *see* 9983
V-Tablopen [Viatris] *see* 7100

Vucine *see* 3716
VUFB-6453 *see* 6140
VUFB-6638 *see* 9164
Vulgarobufotoxin *see* 1479
Vulkacit NPV/C [Mobay] *see* 3803
Vulkazit *see* 3324
Vulklor *see* 2078
Vumide [Burroughs Wellcome] *see* 2311
Vumon [BMS] *see* 9145
VX, 10036
VX-175 *see* 4250
VX-478 *see* 589
VX-497 *see* 5899
VX-710 *see* 1240
Vydate [DuPont] *see* 6920
Vyrene [U.S. Rubber] *see* 8733
W-37 *see* 1476
W-45 *see* 466
W-483 *see* 3747
W-554 *see* 3950
W-583 *see* 5773
W-1544a *see* 7221
W-2197 *see* 7138
W-2900A *see* 3891
W-2946M *see* 8139
W-2979M *see* 906
W-3566 *see* 8055
W-3699 *see* 7485
W-4020 *see* 7715
W-4565 *see* 6945
W-4869 *see* 7723
W-5219 *see* 7775
W-5759A *see* 9437
W-5975 *see* 1180
W-6309 *see* 3152
W-6421A *see* 5462
W-7000A *see* 5462
W-7320 *see* 219
W-19053 *see* 3862
W-36095 *see* 9491
WAC-104 *see* 1224
Wahoo *see* 3899
Wakaflavin L [Wakamoto] *see* 8200
Wakoboku *see* 5697
WAL-801 *see* 3618
WAL-801CL *see* 3618
Walconesin *see* 5850
Waldmeister (German) *see* 10049
Wandonorm [Novartis] *see* 1333
Wansar [Hoei] *see* 3311
Warbex *see* 3932
Warburganal, 10037
Warfarin, 10038
WARF Compound 42 *see* 10038
Warfilone [Merck & Co.] *see* 10038
Warfotox [Aimco] *see* 10038
Warrior [Syngenta] *see* 2758
Wartec [Kabi] *see* 7546
Warticon [Perstorp] *see* 7546
Waruzol [Farmanic] *see* 856
Washed Sulfur *see* 8977
Washing Soda *see* 8596
Water, 10039
Water-*d₂* *see* 2940
Water Bugle *see* 5624
Water Channel of Collecting Duct *see* 760
Water Elder *see* 9973
Water Glass *see* 8675
Water Hemp *see* 376
Watermelon, 10040
Water Shamrock *see* 5842
Wavellite *see* 358
Wax-O-Sol [Life Sci.] *see* 8767
Waxsol [Norgine] *see* 3401
WAY-140424 *see* 1013

WAY-TSE-424 *see* 1013
WBA-8119 *see* 1379
WCH-CD *see* 760
WE-941-BS *see* 1450
WEB-2086 *see* 723
Weedazol [CFPI] *see* 489
Weed Hoe [Vineland] *see* 5953
Weedone [Nufarm] *see* 2796
Weifacodine [Weifa] *see* 7329
Weinsäure (German) *see* 9070
dl-Weinsäure (German) *see* 9069
Weinstein *see* 782
Weinsteinsäure (German) *see* 9070
Weiselfuttersaft (German) *see* 8277
Weisspiessglanz *see* 711
Welchol [Sankyo] *see* 2473
Welfurin [GAP] *see* 6599
Wellbutrin [GSK] *see* 1499
Wellcome 33-A-74 *see* 868
Wellcome 248U *see* 146
Wellcome Prepn 47-83 *see* 2710
Wellcoprim [Wellcome] *see* 9709
Wellcovorin [Burroughs Wellcome] *see* 4222
Welldorm [Smith & Nephew] *see* 3046
Wellferon [Glaxo Wellcome] *see* 4990
Wellvone [GSK] *see* 866
Welvic [European Vinyls] *see* 7586
Wemid [Bernabo] *see* 3687
Weradys [Weimer] *see* 5805
Wescodyne [West Chemical] *see* 5037
Wespuril [Spitzner] *see* 3071
Westamine X *see* 5037
Westcort [Westwood] *see* 4787
Western Poison Oak *see* 7550
Westrosol *see* 9639
Weymouth Pine *see* 10043
WF-1360 *see* 8181
WG-253 *see* 8227
WG-696 *see* 9647
WGA *see* 5429
Wh-7286 *see* 10080
Wheat Germ Agglutinin *see* 5429
Wheat Germ Oil, 10041
Whey Factor *see* 6876
Whip *see* 3984
Whipcide *see* 7374
Whiskey *see* 10042
Whisky, 10042
White Agaric *see* 185
White Arsenic *see* 804
White Beeswax *see* 1020
White Bole *see* 5282
White Cedar *see* 9389
White Cinnamon *see* 1743
White Dextrin *see* 2953
White Flag *see* 6880
White Lead *see* 1005
White Mineral Oil *see* 7186
White Mustard *see* 6315
White Oak *see* 8038
White Oil of Camphor *see* 6780
White Phenolphthalein *see* 7243
White Phosphorus *see* 7347
White Pine, 10043
White Saunders *see* 8353
White Spirits *see* 6201
White Tin Oxide *see* 8778
White Vitriol *see* 10159
White Walnut *see* 5268
White Wax *see* 1020
Whiting *see* 1657
Whitlockite *see* 1694
Whorehouse Tea *see* 3607
Whortleberry *see* 1217

WHR-1142A *see* 5481
Widdrene *see* 9393
Widecillin [Meiji] *see* 577
WideMatch S [Dow AgroSci.] *see* 4203
Wieland-Gumlich Aldehyde, 10044
Wijs' Chloride *see* 5017
Wild Bergamot *see* 6243
Wild Black Cherry Bark *see* 10045
Wild Canilla *see* 1743
Wild Chamomile *see* 2041
Wild Cherry, 10045
Wild Cinnamon *see* 1743
Wild Cotton *see* 829
Wildfire Toxin, 10046
Wild Ginger *see* 825
Wild Indigo *see* 959
Wild Ipecac *see* 742
Wild Pepper *see* 6170
Wild Saffron *see* 2472
Wild Tobacco *see* 5550
Wild Woodbine *see* 4385
Wild Yam *see* 3293
Wilkinite *see* 1055
Wilkinson's Catalyst, 10047
Willemite *see* 10157
Wilpo [Dorsey] *see* 7262
Wilprafen [Mack, Illert.] *see* 5267
Wilzin [Orphan Europe] *see* 10128
Win [Bayer] *see* 1863
Win-771 *see* 4836
Win-1539 *see* 5301
Win-2848 *see* 9280
Win-3046 *see* 5170
Win-5063-2 *see* 9301
Win-8077 *see* 379
Win-8851-2 *see* 9837
Win-9317 *see* 7811
Win-11450 *see* 1045
Win-11831 *see* 5577
Win-13146 *see* 9105
Win-14098 *see* 7433
Win-14833 *see* 8794
Win-17757 *see* 2812
Win-18320 *see* 6359
Win-18446 *see* 4060
Win-18501-2 *see* 6971
Win-20228 *see* 7121
Win-20740 *see* 2705
Win-21904 *see* 232
Win-22005 *see* 9887
Win-22118 *see* 9002
Win-24540 *see* 9698
Win-32729 *see* 3627
Win-32784 *see* 1307
Win-35213 *see* 8268
Win-35833 *see* 2313
Win-39103 *see* 6155
Win-39424 *see* 5052
Win-40014 *see* 8057
Win-40680 *see* 592
Win-40808-7 *see* 8948
Win-41464 *see* 6754
Win-41464-2 *see* 6754
Win-41464-6 *see* 6754
Win-47203 *see* 6197
Win-59010 *see* 5722
Win-59075 *see* 9461
Win-63843 *see* 7533
Win-AM-13146 *see* 9105
Wincef [Fujisawa] *see* 1932
Wincoram [Sanofi Winthrop] *see* 592
Windaus-Grundmann Ketone *see* 4551
Wind Flower *see* 7938
Wine Ether *see* 3838
Wine Lees *see* 782

Win-Kinase [Winthrop] *see* 9887
Winobanin [Sanofi-Synthelabo] *see* 2812
Winstrol [Zambon] *see* 8794
Winter Bloom *see* 4606
Wintergreen Oil *see* 6120
Wintermin [Shionogi] *see* 2185
Wintersteiner's Compound D *see* 273
Wintersteiner's Compound F *see* 2539
Wintersteiner's Compound G *see* 271
Wintomylon [Daiichi] *see* 6359
Wintonin [Sanofi Winthrop] *see* 4401
Winuron [Sanofi Winthrop] *see* 8268
Wisdom [Amvac] *see* 1209
Witch Hazel *see* 4606
Withaferin A, 10048
Witherite *see* 969
WL-140 *see* 1697
WL-19805 *see* 2685
WL-41706 *see* 3991
WL-43775 *see* 4010
WL-108366 *see* 4102
WL-115110 *see* 4133
WL-136184 *see* 5934
WL-145158 *see* 9601
Wolfina [OJ & F] *see* 8120
Wolfram *see* 9814
Wolframite *see* 9814
Wolf's Bane *see* 116, 789
Wollastonite *see* 1702
Wometin *see* 4248
Wood Alcohol *see* 5957
Wood Creosote *see* 2573
Wood Oil *see* 947
Woodruff, 10049
Woodsour *see* 961
Wood Spirit *see* 5957
Wood Sugar *see* 10087
Wood Vinegar *see* 8003
Woodward Herb *see* 10049
Woodward's Reagent K, 10050
Woody Nightshade *see* 3463
Wool Alcohols *see* 5359
Wool Fat *see* 5358
Woollins' Reagent, 10051
Woorali *see* 2671
Woorari *see* 2671
Worm Away [Robins] *see* 7464
Worm Guard [SK & F] *see* 7035
Worm-Agen [Merz] *see* 4712
Wormgrass *see* 8748
Wormwood, 10052
Wortmannin, 10053
Wourara *see* 2671
WP-833 *see* 9080
WR-638 *see* 7341
WR-2721 *see* 404
WR-6026 *see* 8553
WR-142490 *see* 5801
WR-152520 *see* 4176
WR-171669 *see* 4594
WR-238605 *see* 9029
WRC-0470 *see* 1225
Wrightine *see* 2497
WS3 *see* 3825
WS23 *see* 9716
WS-4545 Antibiotic *see* 1202
WSM-5008 *see* 2386
WSX-8365 *see* 3287
Wulfenite *see* 5412
Wurster's Blue *see* 9228
Wurster's Reagent *see* 9228
Wurtzite *see* 10160
WV-569 *see* 6759
WX-2412 *see* 7169

Wy-401 *see* 3743
Wy-757 *see* 7776
Wy-806 *see* 6933
Wy-1094 *see* 7783
Wy-1359 *see* 7822
Wy-3263 *see* 5075
Wy-3277 *see* 6352
Wy-3467 *see* 2994
Wy-3475 *see* 6686
Wy-3478 *see* 4815
Wy-3498 *see* 6926
Wy-3707 *see* 6704
Wy-3917 *see* 9133
Wy-4036 *see* 5579
Wy-4082 *see* 5581
Wy-4508 *see* 2702
Wy-8138 *see* 1296
Wy-8678 *see* 4558
Wy-16225 *see* 2956
Wy-20788 *see* 7081
Wy-21743 *see* 6924
Wy-21901 *see* 4969
Wy-22811 *see* 5863
Wy-42422 *see* 9748
Wy-42462 *see* 9748
Wy-44635 *see* 1939
Wy-45030 *see* 9946
Wy-45651 *see* 9946
Wy-45655 *see* 9946
Wy-47663 *see* 872
WY-49605 *see* 3938
WY-90493-RD *see* 775
Wyamine [Wyeth] *see* 5852
Wycillin [Wyeth] *see* 7097
Wydase [Wyeth] *see* 4758
Wydora [Wyeth] *see* 4969
Wymox [Wyeth] *see* 577
Wynestron [Wyeth] *see* 3708
Wyovin [Wyeth] *see* 3097
Wypax [Yamanouchi] *see* 5579
Wypresin [Wyeth] *see* 4969
Wytensin [Wyeth] *see* 4558
Wytrion [Wyeth] *see* 9770
Wyvital [Wyeth] *see* 2702
X-340 *see* 8152
X-537A *see* 5373
X-1497 *see* 5969
X-5108 *see* 882
X-550007 *see* 6721
Xagrid [Shire] *see* 622
Xahl [SS Pharm.] *see* 1974
Xalatan [Pharmacia & Upjohn] *see* 5376
Xaliproden, 10054
Xamamina *see* 3207
Xametina [Zambeletti] *see* 9708
Xamoterol, 10055
Xanax [Pharmacia & Upjohn] *see* 312
Xanbon [Kissei] *see* 6980
Xanef [Merck & Co.] *see* 3567
Xanelim [Genentech] *see* 3519
Xanomeline, 10056
Xanomeline Tartrate *see* 10056
Xanteline *see* 5958
Xanthaline *see* 7017
Xanthan Gum, 10057
Xanthatin, 10058
9*H*-Xanthen-9-one *see* 10062
Xanthine, 10059
Xanthine Riboside *see* 10065
Xanthinol Niacinate, 10060
Xanthinol Nicotinate *see* 10060
Xanthium [Galephar] *see* 9285
Xanthocillin, 10061
Xanthocillin X *see* 10061
Xanthocillin Y$_1$ *see* 10061

Xanthocillin Y₂ see 10061
Xanthokermesic Acid see 5330
"Xanthomycin" see 4557
Xanthone, 10062
Xanthophyll, 10063
Xanthopterin, 10064
Xanthopuccine see 1736
Xanthosine, 10065
Xanthothricin see 9559
Xanthotoxin see 5988
Xanthoxime see 10062
Xanthoxyletin, 10066
Xanthoxylin, 10067
Xanthoxylin N see 10066
Xanthoxylin S see 823
Xanthoxyloin see 10066
Xanthurenic Acid, 10068
Xanthyletin, 10069
Xantium [Cyanamid] see 9588
Xantociclina [SPA] see 4557
Xantocillin see 10061
Xantomicina see 4557
Xantural [CP Kelco] see 10057
Xatral [Sanofi-Synthelabo] see 238
Xavin [Chinoin] see 10060
Xcytrin [Pharmacyclics] see 6281
XDE-007 see 6721
XDE-105 see 8750
XDE-564 see 3083
XE-779L see 3268
Xefo [Nycomed] see 5582
Xeloda [Roche] see 1754
Xemilofiban, 10070
Xenagol [Desbergers] see 7218
Xenalon [Mepha] see 8760
Xenar [Alfa] see 6417
Xenbucin, 10071
Xeneisol Xe 133 [Mallinckrodt] see 10072
Xenetix [Guerbet] see 5008
"Xenic Acid" see 10072
Xenical [Hoffmann-La Roche] see 6869
Xenid [RPG] see 3081
Xenon, 10072
Xenon Difluoride see 10072
Xenon Hexafluoride see 10072
Xenon Platinum Hexafluoride see 10072
Xenon Tetrafluoride see 10072
Xenon Trioxide see 10072
Xenylamine see 1235
α-(p-Xenyl)butyric Acid see 10071
p-Xenylcarbimide, 10073
Xenysalate see 1234
Xerac [Person & Covey] see 337
Xerac BP [Person & Covey] see 1116
Xerene [Martinet] see 5851
Xeroform [Warner-Chilcott] see 1291
X-gal, 10074
Xibenolol, 10075
Xibornol, 10076
Xibrom [ISTA] see 1390
XIFAM see 10078
Xifaxan [Salix] see 8220
Xigris [Lilly] see 7884
Xilopar [Cephalon] see 8428
Ximelagatran, 10077
Ximoprofen, 10078
Ximovan [Aventis] see 10193
Xinlay [Abbott] see 870
Xipamide, 10079
Xitix [Woelm] see 830
XK-62-2 see 6181
XL-7 see 1306
XL-90 see 4555
Xobaline [Albert-Roussel] see 2451
Xolair [Novartis] see 6842

Xolamin [Sanko] see 2345
Xonaltite see 1702
Xonotlite see 1702
Xopenex [Sepracor] see 216
X-Otag [Tutag] see 6879
XR-9576 see 9064
XRD-473 see 4683
"XTC" see 5767
XU 62-320 see 4218
Xumbradil [Astra Pharm.] see 5040
Xuret [Galen] see 6147
Xusal [UCB] see 2022
Xyduril [Dorsch] see 2377
Xylamide see 7775
Xylan Hydrogen Sulfate see 7134
Xylan Polysulfate see 7134
Xylans see 4642
Xylapan [Chassot] see 10080
Xylasol [Graeub] see 10080
Xylazine, 10080
Xylene, 10081
m-Xylene see 10081
o-Xylene see 10081
p-Xylene see 10081
Xylenol, 10082
as-m-Xylenol see 10082
as-o-Xylenol see 10082
p-Xylenol see 10082
sym-Xylenol see 10082
vic-m-Xylenol see 10082
vic-o-Xylenol see 10082
Xylenol Blue, 10083
p-Xylenolsulfonephthalein see 10083
Xylidine, 10084
Xylite see 10085
Xylitol, 10085
Xyliton [Morishita] see 10085
Xylocaine [AstraZeneca] see 5482
Xylocard [AstraZeneca] see 5482
Xylocitin [Jenapharm] see 5482
Xyloidin see 8011
Xylol see 10081
Xylomed [Bio-Medical] see 10087
Xylometazoline, 10086
Xylo-Mucine see 1829
Xylonest [AstraZeneca] see 7743
Xyloneural [Strathmann] see 5482
Xylo-Pfan [Savage] see 10087
6-O-β-D-Xylopyranosyl-D-glucose see 7745
Xylose, 10087
D-Xylose see 10087
Xylosecarboxylic Acid see 4577
6-(β-D-Xylosido)-D-glucose see 7745
Xylotocan [Astra] see 9491
o-Xylotocopherol see 9497
p-Xylotocopherol see 9496
Xylulose, 10088
N-(2,3-Xylyl)anthranilic Acid see 5798
1-Xylylazo-2-naphthol, 10089
1-(2,4-Xylylazo)-2-naphthol see 10089
Xylyl Bromide, 10090
m-Xylyl Bromide see 10090
o-Xylyl Bromide see 10090
p-Xylyl Bromide see 10090
[[(2,6-Xylylcarbamoyl)methyl]imino]-
    diacetic Acid see 5483
Xylyl Chloride, 10091
m-Xylyl Chloride see 10091
o-Xylyl Chloride see 10091
p-Xylyl Chloride see 10091
1-(2,6-Xylyloxy)-2-propylamine see 6169
Xymelin [Nycomed] see 10086
Xymiazole see 2764

Xynertec [Merck & Co.] see 3567
Xyotax [Cell Therapeutics] see 6983
Xyrem [Orphan Med.] see 4815
Xyzal [UCB] see 2022
XZ-450 see 915
Y-516 see 6278
Y-3642 see 9448
Y-4153 see 2366
Y-5350 see 1839
Y-6047 see 2416
Y-6124 see 1473
Y-7131 see 3873
Y-8004 see 7711
Y-9179 see 6661
Y-12141 see 9578
Y-24180 see 5241
Y-25130 see 900
Yageine see 4616
Yal [Ritter] see 3401
Yamacillin [Yamanouchi] see 9033
Yamaful [Yamanouchi] see 1844
Yambolap [Chinoin] see 5074
Yam, Mexican, 10092
Yangonin, 10093
Yara Yara see 5997
Yarmor [Hercules] see 7447
Yarrow see 105
Yasmin [Schering AG] see 3454
Yatren [Bayer] see 4826
Yaw Root see 8818
Yaxci see 8549
Yazumycin A see 8829
Yazumycins see 8829
Y2B8-MX-DTPA see 4878
YB-2 see 4940
YC-93 see 6495
YCs see 1727
⁹⁰Y-DOTA-hLL2 see 3631
Yeast, 10094
Yeast Adenylic Acid see 157
Yeast Nucleic Acid see 8203
Yellow AB, 10095
Yellow Arsenic Sulfide see 806
Yellow Beeswax see 1020
Yellow Cameleons see 1727
Yellow Copper see 2038
Yellow Cross Liquid see 6316
Yellow Cuprocide see 2664
Yellow Dextrin see 2953
Yellow Dock see 8296
Yellow Gentian see 4393
Yellow Indigo see 959
Yellow Jasmine see 4385
Yellow Jessamine see 4385
Yellow Melilot see 5821
Yellow Mercury Iodide see 5895
Yellow Moccasin Flower see 2770
Yellow Mustard see 6315
Yellow OB, 10096
Yellow Phenolphthalein see 7243
Yellow Precipitate see 5883
Yellow Prussiate of Potash see 7631
Yellow Prussiate of Soda see 8616
Yellow Puccoon see 4769
Yellow Resin see 8266
Yellow Root see 4769
Yellow Saunders see 8353
Yellow Sweet Clover see 5821
Yellow T see 9775
Yellow Ultramarine see 1660
Yentreve [Lilly] see 3465
Yerba Maté see 5756
Yerba Santa see 3669
Yermonil [Novartis] see 5629
YH-1 see 7079

YH-1885 *see* 8168
YI-5301 *see* 3890
Yig, 10097
Yingzhao *see* 10098
Yingzhaosu, 10098
Yingzhaosu A *see* 10098
Yingzhaosu C *see* 10098
(+)-Yingzhosu A *see* 10098
Yinyanghuo *see* 3617
YL-704B1 *see* 6183
Ylangene, 10099
α-Ylangene *see* 10099
Ylang-Ylang Oil, 10100
YM-026 *see* 6428
YM-060 *see* 8105
YM-087 *see* 2507
YM-175 *see* 4929
YM-177 *see* 1956
YM-617 *see* 9049
YM-866 *see* 7004
YM-905 *see* 8712
YM-08054-1 *see* 4938
YM-08310 *see* 404
YM-09151-2 *see* 6446
YM-09330 *see* 1934
YM-09538 *see* 575
YM-09730-5 *see* 1002
YM-11170 *see* 3930
YM-12617-1 *see* 9049
YM-14090 *see* 4990
YM-19020 *see* 3355
YM-35087 *see* 2507
YN-72 *see* 8727
Yobine [Lloyd] *see* 10102
Yobir [Maruko] *see* 313
Yochinol *see* 4826
Yocon [Palisades] *see* 10102
Yodoxin [Searle] *see* 5042
Yoghurt *see* 10101
Yogurt, 10101
Yohimbine, 10102
allo-Yohimbine, 10103
α-Yohimbine, 10104
δ-Yohimbine *see* 8119
Yohimex [Kramer] *see* 10102
Yohydrol [Riedel-Zabinka] *see* 10102
Yomesan [Bayer] *see* 6519
Yondelis [PharmaMar] *see* 3503
Yoristen [Kodama] *see* 4231
Yoshi 864 *see* 4927
Yoshicol [Yoshitomi] *see* 6887
Yoshimilon [Kowa Yakuhin] *see* 9705
Youthwort *see* 3453
Yovital [Kenwood] *see* 10102
Yperite *see* 6316
YRC-2388 *see* 4007
⁹⁰Y-SMT-487 *see* 3513
YTR-830 *see* 9083
YTR-830H *see* 9083
Ytterbia *see* 10105
Ytterbium, 10105
Ytterbium Triflate, 10106
Ytterbium(III) Trifluoromethanesulfonate *see* 10106
Yttria *see* 10107
Yttrium, 10107
Yttrium Iron Garnet *see* 10097
Yutopar [Astra] *see* 8237
Yxin [Pfizer] *see* 9219
Z-103 *see* 7552
Z-326 *see* 4006
Z-424 *see* 9981
Z-876 *see* 3137
Z-905 *see* 7442
Z-4828 *see* 9768

Z-4942 *see* 4896
ZA-1296 *see* 5912
ZA-1963 *see* 7408
Zabromin [Sandoz] *see* 1451
Zacin [Bioglan] *see* 1768
Zackal [SS Pharm.] *see* 4378
Zactane [Wyeth] *see* 3743
Zacutex [Brit. Biotech] *see* 5473
Zadaxin [SciClone] *see* 9405
Zadine [Schering] *see* 901
Zadipina [Zambeletti] *see* 6565
Zaditen [Novartis] *see* 5307
Zaditor [Novartis] *see* 5307
Zadorin [Mepha] *see* 3440
Zadstat [Wyeth] *see* 6157
Zafirlukast, 10108
Zagam [Specia] *see* 8735
Zalain [Robert] *see* 8465
Zalcitabine, 10109
Zaldaride, 10110
Zaleplon, 10111
Zaltoprofen, 10112
Zamadol [Viatris] *see* 9566
Zamanil *see* 6973
Zamocilline [Inpharzam] *see* 577
Zanaflex [Athena] *see* 9485
Zanamivir, 10113
Zanchol [Searle] *see* 4107
Zanidip [Napp] *see* 5446
Zanil *see* 6958
Zanosar [Pharmacia & Upjohn] *see* 8832
Zantac [GSK] *see* 8110
Zantic [GSK] *see* 8110
Zantrène [Lederle] *see* 1244
Zaragozic Acids, 10114
Zaratite *see* 6503
Zarnestra [Janssen] *see* 9458
Zarontin [Parke-Davis] *see* 3748
Zaroxolyn [Teofarma] *see* 6147
Zasten [Novartis] *see* 5307
Zavedos [Pharmacia & Upjohn] *see* 4886
Zavesca [Actelion] *see* 6188
ZD-443 *see* 3673
ZD-473 *see* 7405
ZD-1033 *see* 625
ZD-1694 *see* 8099
ZD-1839 *see* 4379
ZD-4522 *see* 8270
Z-DNA *see* 2907
ZE-101 *see* 6660
Zeal [Valent] *see* 3890
α-Zearalanol *see* 10121
Zearalenone, 10116
Zeatin, 10117
trans-Zeatin *see* 10117
Zeaxanthin, 10118
Zeaxanthin Diepoxide *see* 9998
Zeaxanthol *see* 10118
Zebedassite *see* 350
Zebeta [Lederle] *see* 1295
Zecovir [Guidotti] *see* 1378
Zeefra [Bouchara-Recordati] *see* 1986
Zefazone [Pharmacia & Upjohn] *see* 1926
Zeffix [GSK] *see* 5352
Zefnart [Tosoh] *see* 5515
Zegerid [Santarus] *see* 6845
Zein, 10119
Zelapar [Valeant] *see* 8428
Zeldox [Zeneca] *see* 4713
Zeldox [Pfizer] *see* 10171
Zelis [Proter] *see* 7506
Zelmac [Novartis] *see* 9113
Zelmid [Astra] *see* 10126

Zelnorm [Novartis] *see* 9113
Zemaira [ZLB Behring] *see* 719
Zemide [Alpharma] *see* 9048
Zemplar [Abbott] *see* 7039
Zemuron [Akzo] *see* 8246
Zen [Prophin] *see* 7506
Zenadrex [Veterinaria] *see* 2878
Zenapax [Roche] *see* 2799
Zeniquin [Pfizer] *see* 5750
Zenoxone [Biorex] *see* 4787
Zentel [GSK] *see* 210
Zentonil [Vétoquinol] *see* 156
Zentropil [Novartis] *see* 7322
Zenusin [Mepha] *see* 6528
Zeolites, 10120
Zepelin [De Angeli] *see* 4012
Zepharovicht *see* 358
Zephiran [Sanofi-Synthelabo] *see* 1059
Zephirol [Bayer] *see* 1059
Zephyr [Syngenta] *see* 2
Zepolas [Mikasa] *see* 4199
Zeranol, 10121
Zerit [BMS] *see* 8803
Zestoretic [AstraZeneca] *see* 5516
Zestril [AstraZeneca] *see* 5516
Zesulan [Toyo Jozo] *see* 5864
Zetamicin [Menarini] *see* 6479
Zeta Protein *see* 4075
Zetia [Merck/Schering-Plough] *see* 3918
Zettyn *see* 2017
Zevalin [IDEC] *see* 4878
Ziac [Am. Cyanamid] *see* 1295
Ziagen [GSK] *see* 1
Ziavetine *see* 1476
Zibeth *see* 2334
Zibren [Sigma-Tau] *see* 84
Ziconotide, 10122
Zidoval [3M Pharma] *see* 6157
Zidovudine, 10123
Zienam [Merck & Co.] *see* 4919
Zildasac [Chugai] *see* 1035
Zilden [Pharmacia] *see* 3202
Zileuton, 10124
Zilmax [Intervet] *see* 10125
Zilpaterol, 10125
Zimeldine, 10126
Zimelidine *see* 10126
Zimovane [Aventis] *see* 10193
Zimox [Pfizer] *see* 577
Zinacef [GSK] *see* 1954
Zinamide [Merck & Co.] *see* 7956
Zinat [GSK] *see* 1954
Zinc, 10127
Zinc Acetate, 10128
Zinc Acexamate *see* 45
Zinc Ammonium Chloride *see* 539
Zincaps [RPR] *see* 10159
Zincate [Paddock] *see* 10159
"Zincates" *see* 10127
Zinc Bacitracin *see* 936
Zinc Bis(dimethylthiocarbamoyl) Disulfide *see* 10172
Zinc Blende *see* 10160
Zinc Bromide, 10129
Zinc Caprylate, 10130
Zinc Carbonate, 10131
Zinc Carbonate Hydroxide *see* 10131
Zinc L-Carnosine *see* 7552
Zinc Chloride, 10132
Zinc Chromate(VI) Hydroxide, 10133
Zinc Citrate, 10134
Zinc Cyanide, 10135
Zinc Diethyl *see* 3131
Zinc Dimethyl *see* 3263
Zinc Dimethyldithiocarbamate *see* 10172

Zinc Ethylenebis(dithiocarbamate) *see* 10165
Zinc Fluoride, 10136
Zinc Fluosilicate *see* 10138
Zinc Formate, 10137
Zinc Gluconate *see* 4456
Zinc Hexafluorosilicate, 10138
Zinc *p*-Hydroxybenzenesulfonate *see* 10150
Zinc Insulin *see* 4980
Zinc Iodate, 10139
Zinc Iodide, 10140
Zinc Iodide-Starch, 10141
Zincite *see* 10147
Zinc Lactate, 10142
Zinc Manganese Ethylenebisdithiocar-bamate *see* 5716
Zinc Meta-arsenite, 10143
Zinc Nitrate, 10144
Zinc Oleate, 10145
Zincomed [Schwarz] *see* 10159
Zinc Orthosilicate *see* 10157
Zinc Oxalate, 10146
Zinc Oxide, 10147
Zinc Perchlorate, 10148
Zinc Peroxide, 10149
Zinc *p*-Phenolsulfonate, 10150
Zinc Phosphate, 10151
Zinc Phosphide, 10152
Zinc Propionate, 10153
Zinc 1,2-Propylene Bisdithiocarbamate *see* 7819
Zinc Pyridinethione *see* 7994
Zinc Pyrithione *see* 7994
Zinc Pyrophosphate, 10154
Zinc Salicylate, 10155
Zinc Selenide, 10156
Zinc Silicate, 10157
Zinc Silicofluoride *see* 10138
Zincspar *see* 10131
Zinc Stearate, 10158
Zinc Subcarbonate *see* 10131
Zinc Sulfanilate Tetrahydrate *see* 8926
Zinc Sulfate, 10159
Zinc Sulfide, 10160
Zinc Sulfocarbolate *see* 10150
Zinc Sulfocyanate *see* 10163
Zinc Sulfophenate *see* 10150
Zinc Superoxide *see* 10149
Zinc Tartrate, 10161
Zinc Telluride, 10162
Zinc Thiocyanate, 10163
Zinc Undecylenate *see* 9848
Zinc Valerate, 10164
Zinc Vitriol *see* 10159
Zinc White *see* 10147
Zinc Yellow *see* 10133
Zindaclin [Epitan] *see* 2356
Zineb, 10165
Zinecard [Pfizer] *see* 8123
Zingerone, 10166
Zingherone *see* 10166
Zingiberone *see* 10166
Zinnat [GSK] *see* 1954
Zinostatin, 10167
Zinpyr, 10168
Zinpyr-1 *see* 10168
Zinpyr-2 *see* 10168
Zinquin, 10169
Zinquin A *see* 10169
Zinquin E *see* 10169
Zinviroxime *see* 3601
Zipeprol, 10170

Ziprasidone, 10171
Ziram, 10172
Zircon *see* 10181
Zirconia *see* 10180
Zirconic Anhydride *see* 10180
Zirconium, 10173
Zirconium Chloride, 10174
Zirconium Dioxide *see* 10180
Zirconium Fluoride, 10175
Zirconium Hydride, 10176
Zirconium Hydroxide, 10177
Zirconium Iodide, 10178
Zirconium Nitrate, 10179
Zirconium Orthosilicate *see* 10181
Zirconium Oxide, 10180
Zirconium Oxychloride *see* 10184
Zirconium Potassium Fluoride *see* 7639
Zirconium Silicate, 10181
Zirconium Sulfate, 10182
Zirconium Tetrachloride *see* 10174
Zirconium Tetrafluoride *see* 10175
Zirconium Tetraiodide *see* 10178
Zirconyl Acetate, 10183
Zirconyl Chloride, 10184
Zirtek [UCB] *see* 2022
Zispin [Organon] *see* 6208
Zitazonium [Servier] *see* 9048
Zithromax [Pfizer] *see* 915
Zitoxil [Lifepharma] *see* 10170
Zitrix [Metapharma] *see* 1915
Zitromax [Pfizer] *see* 915
Zixoryn [Gedeon Richter] *see* 4136
Zizanal *see* 6816
ZK-30595 *see* 3454
ZK-31224 *see* 9164
ZK-36374 *see* 4901
ZK-39482 *see* 5065
ZK-57671 *see* 8991
ZK-62711 *see* 8251
ZK-93035 *see* 4327
ZK-98299 *see* 6847
ZK-222584 *see* 9939
ZL-101 *see* 6660
ZMA *see* 10143
ZN-6 *see* 4317
Zoalene [Dow] *see* 3269
Zoamix [Dow] *see* 3269
Zoapatanol, 10185
Zoaquin *see* 5042
Zocor [Merck & Co.] *see* 8539
Zocord [Merck & Co.] *see* 8539
Zofac [AirPharma] *see* 7939
Zofenil [Menarini] *see* 10186
Zofenopril, 10186
Zofenoprilat *see* 10186
Zofran [GSK] *see* 6848
Zoisite *see* 1648
Zoladex [AstraZeneca] *see* 4526
Zoledronate Disodium *see* 10187
Zoledronate Trisodium *see* 10187
Zoledronic Acid, 10187
Zoleptil [Abbott] *see* 10197
Zolicef [BMS] *see* 1917
Zolim [Schwarz] *see* 6221
Zolimidine, 10188
Zoliparin [Mann] *see* 146
Zoliridine *see* 10188
Zolmitriptan, 10189
Zoloft [Pfizer] *see* 8467
Zolone [Rhône-Poulenc] *see* 7334
Zolpidem, 10190
Zoltum [AstraZeneca] *see* 6845
Zolvera [Rosemont] *see* 9950

Zolyse [Alcon] *see* 2260
Zomacton [Ferring] *see* 8716
Zomaril [Novartis] *see* 4900
Zomax [McNeil] *see* 10191
Zomaxin [Cilag] *see* 10191
Zomepirac, 10191
Zometa [Novartis] *see* 10187
Zomig [AstraZeneca] *see* 10189
Zondel [Grelan] *see* 10192
Zonegran [Dainippon] *see* 10192
Zongorine *see* 8717
Zoniden [Irbi] *see* 9452
Zonisamide, 10192
Zooecdysteroids *see* 3491
"Zoomelanoidic" Acids *see* 4885
Zophren [GSK] *see* 6848
Zopiclone, 10193
Zopirac [Sintyal] *see* 10191
Zopolrestat, 10194
Zorac [Allergan] *see* 9081
Zorial [Syngenta] *see* 6701
Zoroxin [Merck & Co.] *see* 6700
Zorubicin, 10195
Zostex [Berlin-Chemie] *see* 1378
Zostrix [GenDerm] *see* 1768
Zosuquidar, 10196
Zosyn [Wyeth] *see* 9083
Zotepine, 10197
Zothelone *see* 3353
Zoton [Wyeth] *see* 5362
Zovant [Lilly] *see* 7884
Zovir [GSK] *see* 146
Zovirax [GSK] *see* 146
Zoxamide, 10198
Zoxan [Pfizer] *see* 3433
Zoxazolamine, 10199
Zoxium [Dow AgroSci.] *see* 10198
ZP-1 *see* 10168
ZP-2 *see* 10168
ZPO *see* 10149
ZR-512 *see* 4805
ZR-515 *see* 5983
ZR-2458 *see* 5983
ZR-3210 *see* 4217
Z Span [Goldshield] *see* 10159
Zubrin [Schering-Plough] *see* 9151
Zuclomiphene *see* 2386
Zuclopenthixol *see* 2394
Zumenon [Solvay] *see* 3703
Zunden [Luitpold] *see* 7506
ZY-15021 *see* 1111
ZY-15028 *see* 2361
ZY-17617B *see* 10110
Zyban [GSK] *see* 1499
Zydol [Searle] *see* 9566
Zyflo [Abbott] *see* 10124
Zygomycin A *see* 7041
Zyklolat [Mann] *see* 2746
Zylonite *see* 1964
Zyloprim [GSK] *see* 279
Zyloric [GSK] *see* 279
Zymafluor [Zyma] *see* 8618
Zymar [Allergan] *see* 4376
Zymofren [Specia] *see* 757
Zymoplastic Substance *see* 9385
Zymosan, 10200
Zyprexa [Lilly] *see* 6822
Zyrlex [UCB] *see* 2022
Zyrtec [Pfizer] *see* 2022
Zytrim [Isis Puren] *see* 902
Zytron [Dow] *see* 3392
Zyvox [Pharmacia & Upjohn] *see* 5504
Zyvoxid [Pharmacia & Upjohn] *see* 5504
Zyxorin [Gedeon Richter] *see* 4136

NOTES

NOTES

NOTES

NOTES